D1294127

HEMATOLOGY

BASIC PRINCIPLES AND PRACTICE

HEMATOLOGY

BASIC PRINCIPLES AND PRACTICE

SIXTH EDITION

Ronald Hoffman MD

Albert A. and Vera G. List Professor of Medicine, Tisch Cancer Institute, Department of Medicine, Mount Sinai School of Medicine, New York, New York

Edward J. Benz, Jr. MD

President and Chief Executive Officer, Dana-Farber Cancer Institute, Director and Principal Investigator, Harvard Cancer Center; Richard and Susan Smith Professor of Medicine, Professor of Pediatrics and Genetics, Harvard Medical School, Boston, Massachusetts

Leslie E. Silberstein MD

Director, Joint Program in Transfusion Medicine, Children's Hospital Boston; Director, Center for Human Cell Therapy, Boston, Massachusetts

Helen E. Heslop MD

Dan L. Duncan Chair, Professor of Medicine and Pediatrics; Director, Adult Stem Cell Transplant Program, Center for Cell and Gene Therapy, Baylor College of Medicine, The Methodist Hospital, Texas Children's Hospital, Houston, Texas

Jeffrey I. Weitz MD

Professor of Medicine and Biochemistry, McMaster University; HSFO/J.F. Mustard Chair in Cardiovascular Research; Canada Research Chair (Tier 1) in Thrombosis; Executive Director, Thrombosis & Atherosclerosis Research Institute, Hamilton, Ontario, Canada

John Anastasi MD

Associate Professor, Department of Pathology, University of Chicago, Chicago, Illinois

SAUNDERS

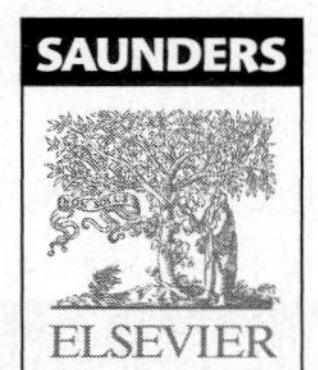

ELSEVIER

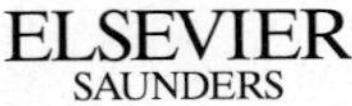

SAUNDERS

1600 John F. Kennedy Blvd.
Ste 1800
Philadelphia, PA 19103-2899

HEMATOLOGY: Basic Principles and Practice ISBN: 978-1-4377-2928-3

Notices

Knowledge and best practice in this field are constantly changing. As new research and experience broaden our understanding, changes in research methods, professional practices, or medical treatment may become necessary.

Practitioners and researchers must always rely on their own experience and knowledge in evaluating and using any information, methods, compounds, or experiments described herein. In using such information or methods they should be mindful of their own safety and the safety of others, including parties for whom they have a professional responsibility.

With respect to any drug or pharmaceutical products identified, readers are advised to check the most current information provided (i) on procedures featured or (ii) by the manufacturer of each product to be administered, to verify the recommended dose or formula, the method and duration of administration, and contraindications. It is the responsibility of practitioners, relying on their own experience and knowledge of their patients, to make diagnoses, to determine dosages and the best treatment for each individual patient, and to take all appropriate safety precautions.

To the fullest extent of the law, neither the Publisher nor the authors, contributors, or editors assume any liability for any injury and/or damage to persons or property as a matter of products liability, negligence, or otherwise, or from any use or operation of any methods, products, instructions, or ideas contained in the material herein.

Library of Congress Cataloging-in-Publication Data

Hematology : basic principles and practice / [edited by] Ronald Hoffman ...
[et al.]. – 6th ed.
p. ; cm.
Includes bibliographical references and index.
ISBN 978-1-4377-2928-3 (hardcover : alk. paper)
I. Hoffman, Ronald, 1945-
[DNLM: 1. Hematologic Diseases–diagnosis. 2. Hematologic Diseases–therapy. 3. Blood Physiological Phenomena. WH 120]
616.1′5–dc23

2012037059

Global Content Development Director: Judith Fletcher
Senior Content Strategist: Kate Dimock
Content Development Manager: Lucia Gunzel
Publishing Services Manager: Anne Altepeter
Project Manager: Jessica L. Becher
Design Direction: Lou Forgione

Printed in Canada
Last digit is the print number: 9 8 7 6 5 4 3 2

To the numerous authors who have toiled to create the timely and outstanding chapters that comprise this book. Their energy and perseverance is emblematic of their personal character and continued commitment to the value of scholarship and education in medicine. The work of each of these authors enhances the knowledge of practicing and research hematologists, which results in better care for patients with blood disorders. I would also like to recognize the continued support of my wife, Nan, and my children, Michael and Judith, who have encouraged me to continue this pursuit. This edition would not have happened without the continued support of the staff at Elsevier, especially Lucia Gunzel, who has made this book a reality. I would also like to acknowledge my colleagues at Mount Sinai School of Medicine who continue to value the contribution that this book represents. Last, but not least, our loyal readers, who have made this book a success for more than 20 years and continue to value and use it in a manner that enhances their professional pursuits.

Ronald Hoffman, MD

To my wife, Peggy, for your support, inspiration, and partnership; to our children, Tim, Jenny, Julie, and Rob, for your understanding; to my mentors, for your support and guidance; to Sharon Olsen, for your incredible skill, patience, and good humor throughout this project; and to the many patients and volunteers whose willingness to participate in clinical research made much of the knowledge conveyed by this book possible.

Edward J. Benz, Jr., MD

To my friends and family for their love and support; to my mentors, Eugene M. Berkman and Robert S. Schwartz, who have provided me with invaluable guidance; to my colleagues at the University of Pennsylvania and Harvard, who have helped me develop academic transfusion medicine programs; and to the trainees who make this endeavor enjoyable and worthwhile.

Leslie E. Silberstein, MD

To my family, friends, and all of my present and former colleagues and trainees for their support and encouragement; to all my mentors in hematology who have provided guidance, in particular, Michael Beard and Malcolm Brenner.

Helen E. Heslop, MD

To my wife, Julia, for her love and unwavering support: I would be lost without her; to my children, Daniel and Caileen, for their understanding and encouragement; to Gwen, for extending our family; to my colleagues for providing me with an environment for learning and growth; and to my trainees, for making this all worthwhile.

Jeffrey I. Weitz, MD

To my respected clinical colleagues with appreciation for trusting me with the diagnostic material from their patients; to my esteemed teachers, Jim Vardiman, Diana Variakojis, and from long ago, C. Robert Valeri, for your many lessons focused on things at both ends of the microscope; and to my awesome trainees; it is always a great pleasure to watch you grow to appreciate the serious, yet amazing, nature of our work.

John Anastasi, MD

CONTRIBUTORS

Janet L. Abrahm MD
Division Chief, Adult Palliative Care, Department of Psychosocial Oncology and Palliative Care, Dana-Farber Cancer Institute; Professor of Medicine, Harvard Medical School, Boston, Massachusetts
Indwelling Access Devices
Pain Management and Antiemetic Therapy in Hematologic Disorders
Palliative Care

Charles S. Abrams MD
Professor of Medicine, Division of Hematology and Oncology, University of Pennsylvania, Philadelphia, Pennsylvania
Molecular Basis for Platelet Function

Donald I. Abrams MD
Chief, Hematology and Oncology, San Francisco General Hospital, Integrative Oncology, University of California San Francisco Osher Center for Integrative Medicine, San Francisco, California
Integrative Therapies in Patients With Hematologic Diseases

Steven J. Ackerman PhD
Professor of Biochemistry and Molecular Genetics, and Medicine, Department of Biochemistry and Molecular Genetics, College of Medicine, University of Illinois at Chicago, Chicago, Illinois
Eosinophilia, Eosinophil-Associated Diseases, Chronic Eosinophil Leukemia, and the Hypereosinophilic Syndromes

Sharon Adams MT, CHS (ABHI)
National Institutes of Health, Clinical Center, Department of Transfusion Medicine, Human Leukocyte Antigen Laboratory Supervisor, Bethesda, Maryland
Human Leukocyte Antigen and Human Neutrophil Antigen Systems

Adeboye H. Adewoye MD
Assistant Professor of Medicine, Boston University School of Medicine; Attending Physician, Boston Medical Center, Boston, Massachusetts
Pathobiology of the Human Erythrocyte and Its Hemoglobins

Carl Allen MD, PhD
Assistant Professor, Department of Pediatrics, Texas Children's Cancer Center, Texas Children's Hospital, Baylor College of Medicine, Houston, Texas
Infectious Mononucleosis and Other Epstein-Barr Virus–Associated Diseases

Richard F. Ambinder MD, PHD
Murphy Professor of Oncology; Professor, Departments of Oncology, Medicine, Pathology, and Pharmacology; Director, Division of Hematologic Malignancies, Department of Oncology, Johns Hopkins School of Medicine, Baltimore, Maryland
Virus-Associated Lymphoma

Claudio Anasetti MD
Chair, Department of Blood and Marrow Transplantation, Moffitt Cancer Center, Tampa, Florida
Unrelated Donor Hematopoietic Cell Transplantation

John Anastasi MD
Associate Professor, Department of Pathology, University of Chicago, Chicago, Illinois
Progress in the Classification of Myeloid Neoplasms: Clinical Implications
Pathologic Basis for the Classification of Non-Hodgkin and Hodgkin Lymphomas

Julia A. Anderson MD
Department of Clinical and Laboratory Hematology, Royal Infirmary of Edinburgh, Edinburgh, United Kingdom; Associate Clinical Professor, Department of Medicine, McMaster University, Hamilton, Ontario, Canada
Hypercoagulable States

Michael Andreeff MD, PhD
Professor of Medicine, Haas Chair in Genetics, Departments of Leukemia and Stem Cell Transplantation and Cellular Therapy, The University of Texas MD Anderson Cancer Center, Houston, Texas
Pathobiology of Acute Myeloid Leukemia

Joseph H. Antin MD
Professor of Medicine, Chief, Stem Cell Transplantation Program, Dana-Farber Cancer Institute, Harvard Medical School, Boston, Massachusetts
Allogeneic Hematopoietic Stem Cell Transplantation for Acute Myeloid Leukemia and Myelodysplastic Syndrome in Adults

Aśok C. Antony MD
Professor of Medicine, Indiana University School of Medicine, Staff Physician, Roudebush Veterans Affairs Medical Center, Indianapolis, Indiana
Megaloblastic Anemias

Stavros Apostolakis MD, PhD
Lecturer in Cardiovascular Medicine, University of Birmingham Center for Cardiovascular Sciences, City Hospital, Birmingham, United Kingdom
Atrial Fibrillation

Scott A. Armstrong MD, PhD
Associate Professor, Division of Hematology and Oncology, Children's Hospital Boston, Dana-Farber Cancer Institute, Harvard Medical School, Boston, Massachusetts
Pathobiology of Acute Lymphoblastic Leukemia

Donald M. Arnold MDCM, MSc
Assistant Professor, Department of Medicine, McMaster University; Associate Medical Director, Canadian Blood Services, Hamilton, Ontario, Canada
Diseases of Platelet Number: Immune Thrombocytopenia, Neonatal Alloimmune Thrombocytopenia, and Posttransfusion Purpura

Andrew S. Artz MD, MS
Assistant Professor, Department of Medicine, Section of Hematology and Oncology, University of Chicago, Chicago, Illinois
Hematology in Aging

Farrukh T. Awan MD
Assistant Professor of Medicine Medical College of Georgia Augusta, Georgia
Chronic Lymphocytic Leukemia

Jacques Banchereau PhD
Chief Scientific Officer, Hoffman-La Roche, Inc., Nutley, New Jersey
Dendritic Cell Therapies

Juliet N. Barker MBBS (Hons), FRACP
Director of Cord Blood Transplantation Program, Associate Member, Department of Medicine, Adult Bone Marrow Transplant Service, Memorial Sloan-Kettering Cancer Center, New York, New York
Unrelated Donor Cord Blood Transplantation for Hematologic Malignancies

Linda G. Baum MD, PhD
Professor, Department of Pathology and Laboratory Medicine, David Geffen School of Medicine, University of California, Los Angeles, Los Angeles, California
Overview and Compartmentalization of the Immune System

Don M. Benson, Jr. MD
Department of Internal Medicine, Division of Hematology, Ohio State University Comprehensive Cancer Center, Columbus, Ohio
Natural Killer Cell Immunity

Edward J. Benz, Jr. MD
President and Chief Executive Officer, Dana-Farber Cancer Institute, Director and Principal Investigator, Harvard Cancer Center; Richard and Susan Smith Professor of Medicine, Professor of Pediatrics and Genetics, Harvard Medical School, Boston, Massachusetts
Anatomy and Physiology of the Gene
Pathobiology of the Human Erythrocyte and Its Hemoglobins
Anemia of Chronic Diseases
Hemoglobin Variants Associated With Hemolytic Anemia, Altered Oxygen Affinity, and Methemoglobinemias
Hematologic Manifestations of Systemic Disease: Renal Disease

Nancy Berliner MD
Chief, Division of Hematology, Brigham and Women's Hospital; Professor of Medicine, Harvard Medical School, Boston, Massachusetts
Anatomy and Physiology of the Gene
Granulocytopoiesis and Monocytopoiesis

Govind Bhagat MD
Professor of Clinical Pathology and Cell Biology in Medicine; Director, Division of Hematopathology, Department of Pathology and Cell Biology, Columbia University Medical Center, New York Presbyterian Hospital, Vanderbilt Clinic, New York, New York
T-Cell Lymphomas

Kapil N. Bhalla MD
University of Kansas Cancer Center, Kansas City, Kansas
Pharmacology and Molecular Mechanisms of Antineoplastic Agents for Hematologic Malignancies

Nina Bhardwaj MD, PhD
Professor, Departments of Medicine, Dermatology, and Pathology; Director, Tumor Vaccine Program, New York University School of Medicine, Langone Medical Center, New York, New York
Dendritic Cell Biology

Ravi Bhatia MBBS, MD
Professor, Department of Hematology and Hematopoietic Cell Transplantation; Director, Division of Hematopoietic Stem Cell and Leukemia Cell and Leukemia Research, City of Hope National Medical Center, Duarte, California
Chronic Myeloid Leukemia

Smita Bhatia MD, MPH
Professor and Ruth Ziegler Chair, Population Research; Associate Director, Population Sciences; Program Co-Leader, Cancer Control and Population Sciences, City of Hope Comprehensive Cancer Center, Duarte, California
Late Complications of Hematologic Diseases and Their Therapies

Craig D. Blinderman MD, MA
Assistant Professor of Palliative Care, Departments of Anesthesiology and Medicine, Columbia University College of Physicians and Surgeons; Division Chief, Adult Palliative Medicine, Department of Anesthesiology, New York Presbyterian Hospital, Columbia University Medical Center, New York, New York
Pain Management and Antiemetic Therapy in Hematologic Disorders

Catherine M. Bollard MBChB, MD
Associate Professor, Department of Pediatric Hematology Oncology, Baylor College of Medicine, Houston, Texas
Malignant Lymphomas in Childhood

Malcolm K. Brenner MB, BChir, PhD
Distinguished Service Professor and Fayez Sarofim Chair, Center for Cell and Gene Therapy, Baylor College of Medicine, Texas Children's Hospital, The Methodist Hospital, Houston, Texas
T-Cell Therapy of Hematologic Diseases

Gary M. Brittenham MD
James A. Wolff Professor of Pediatrics and Professor of Medicine, Department of Pediatrics, Columbia University College of Physicians and Surgeons; Attending Pediatrician, Department of Pediatrics, Children's Hospital of New York, New York, New York
Pathophysiology of Iron Homeostasis
Disorders of Iron Homeostasis: Iron Deficiency and Overload

Robert A. Brodsky MD
Professor of Medicine and Oncology; Director, Division of Hematology, Department of Medicine, Johns Hopkins University School of Medicine, Baltimore, Maryland
Paroxysmal Nocturnal Hemoglobinuria

Hal E. Broxmeyer PhD
Distinguished Professor; Mary Margaret Walther Professor Emeritus; Professor of Microbiology and Immunology; Program Leader, NCI-Designated Indiana University Simon Cancer Center Program on Hematopoiesis, Heme Malignancies, and Immunology, Department of Microbiology and Immunology, Indiana University School of Medicine, Indianapolis, Indiana
Principles of Cytokine Signaling

Kathleen Brummel-Ziedins PhD
Associate Professor, Department of Biochemistry, University of Vermont, Burlington, Vermont
Molecular Basis of Blood Coagulation

Francis K. Buadi MD
Assistant Professor of Medicine, College of Medicine, Cons-Hematology, Mayo Clinic, Rochester, Minnesota
Immunoglobulin Light-Chain Amyloidosis (Primary Amyloidosis)

Joseph H. Butterfield MD
Co-Chair Mast Cell and Eosinophil Disorders Program, Division of Allergy, Mayo Clinic, Rochester, Minnesota
Eosinophilia, Eosinophil-Associated Diseases, Chronic Eosinophil Leukemia, and the Hypereosinophilic Syndromes

John C. Byrd MD
Director, Division of Hematology, Ohio State University, Columbus, Ohio
Chronic Lymphocytic Leukemia

Paolo F. Caimi MD
Seidman Cancer Center, Division of Hematology and Oncology, Case Comprehensive Cancer Center, University Hospitals Case Medical Center, Cleveland, Ohio
Pharmacology and Molecular Mechanisms of Antineoplastic Agents for Hematologic Malignancies

Michael A. Caligiuri MD
Department of Internal Medicine, Division of Hematology, Ohio State University Comprehensive Cancer Center, Columbus, Ohio
Natural Killer Cell Immunity

Erica Campagnaro MD
Seidman Cancer Center, Division of Hematology and Oncology, Case Comprehensive Cancer Center, University Hospitals Case Medical Center, Cleveland, Ohio
Pharmacology and Molecular Mechanisms of Antineoplastic Agents for Hematologic Malignancies

Jonathan Canaani MD
Associate Scientist, Department of Immunology, Weizmann Institute of Science, Rehovot, Israel; Physician, Sourasky Medical Center, Tel Aviv, Israel
Dynamic Interactions Between Hematopoietic Stem and Progenitor Cells and the Bone Marrow: Current Biology of Stem Cell Homing and Mobilization

Michelle Canavan MD
Health Research Board Clinical Research Facility, National University of Ireland, Galway, Ireland
Stroke

Alan B. Cantor MD, PhD
Assistant Professor of Pediatrics, Division of Pediatric Hematology and Oncology, Children's Hospital Boston, Dana-Farber Cancer Institute, Harvard Medical School, Boston, Massachusetts
Thrombocytopoiesis

Manuel Carcao MD
Associate Professor, Division of Haematology and Oncology, Department of Pediatrics, Hospital for Sick Children, University of Toronto, Toronto, Canada
Hemophilia A and B

Michael C. Carroll PhD
Professor of Pediatrics, Harvard Medical School; Senior Investigator, Immune Disease Institute and Program in Cellular and Molecular Medicine, Children's Hospital Boston, Boston, Massachusetts
Complement and Immunoglobulin Biology

Shannon A. Carty MD
Division of Hematology and Oncology, Department of Medicine, Abramson Family Cancer Research Institute, University of Pennsylvania, Philadelphia, Pennsylvania
T-Cell Immunity

Richard E. Champlin MD
Professor and Chair, Department of Stem Cell Transplantation, The University of Texas MD Anderson Cancer Center, Houston, Texas
Mantle Cell Lymphoma

Anthony K.C. Chan MBBS, FRCPC, FRCPath
Professor, Department of Pediatrics, Chair in Pediatric Thrombosis and Hemostasis, McMaster Children's Hospital, Hamilton Health Sciences Foundation, McMaster University, Hamilton, Ontario, Canada
Disorders of Coagulation in the Neonate

Jacquelyn D. Choate MD
Blood Bank and Transfusion Medicine Fellow, Department of Laboratory Medicine, Yale University School of Medicine, New Haven, Connecticut
Transfusion Reactions to Blood and Cell Therapy Products

Peter Chung MD
Assistant Professor of Medicine, Department of Medicine, Olive View, University of California Los Angeles Medical Center, Sylmar, California; Health Sciences Assistant Clinical Professor of Medicine, David Geffen School of Medicine, University of California, Los Angeles, Los Angeles, California
Overview and Compartmentalization of the Immune System

John P. Chute MD
Professor of Medicine, Pharmacology and Cancer Biology, Division of Cellular Therapy and Stem Cell Transplantation, Duke University Medical Center, Durham, North Carolina
Hematopoietic Stem Cell Biology

Douglas B. Cines MD
Professor, Departments of Pathology and Laboratory Medicine; Director, Coagulation Laboratory, University of Pennsylvania Perelman School of Medicine, Philadelphia, Pennsylvania
Thrombotic Thrombocytopenic Purpura and the Hemolytic Uremic Syndrome

David B. Clark PhD
President, Platte Canyon Consulting, Inc., Shawnee, Colorado
Preparation of Plasma-Derived and Recombinant Human Plasma Proteins

Thomas D. Coates MD
Division Head, Hematology, Children's Center for Cancer and Blood Diseases; Professor of Pediatrics and Pathology, University of Southern California Keck School of Medicine, Children's Hospital Los Angeles, Los Angeles, California
Disorders of Phagocyte Function

Christopher R. Cogle MD
Associate Professor, Department of Medicine, Division of Hematology and Oncology, University of Florida College of Medicine, Gainesville, Florida
Regulation of Gene Expression, Transcription, Splicing, and RNA Metabolism

Nathan T. Connell MD
Teaching Fellow in Hematology and Medical Oncology, Department of Medicine, Warren Alpert Medical School of Brown University, Providence, Rhode Island
The Spleen and Its Disorders

Elizabeth Cooke RN, MS
Senior Research Specialist, Department of Nursing Research and Education, City of Hope Medical Center, Duarte, California
Psychosocial Aspects of Hematologic Disorders

Sarah Cooley MD
Assistant Professor of Medicine, Department of Medicine, Division of Hematology, Oncology, and Transplantation, University of Minnesota; Associate Director, Cancer Experimental Therapeutics Initiative, Masonic Cancer Center, Minneapolis, Minnesota
Natural Killer Cell-Based Therapies

Paolo Corradini MD
National Tumor Institute, Chair of Hematology, Milano, Italy
T-Cell Lymphomas

Mark A. Creager MD
Director, Vascular Center, Brigham and Women's Hospital, Simon C. Fireman Scholar in Cardiovascular Medicine, Cardiovascular Division; Professor of Medicine, Harvard Medical School, Boston, Massachusetts
Peripheral Artery Disease

Richard J. Creger MD
Seidman Cancer Center, Division of Hematology and Oncology, Case Comprehensive Cancer Center, University Hospitals Case Medical Center, Cleveland, Ohio
Pharmacology and Molecular Mechanisms of Antineoplastic Agents for Hematologic Malignancies

Caroline Cromwell MD
Assistant Professor of Medicine, Tisch Cancer Institute, Department of Medicine, Mount Sinai School of Medicine, New York, New York
Hematologic Changes in Pregnancy

Regina S. Cunningham PhD, RN
Associate Chief Nursing Officer for Cancer Services, Abramson Cancer Center, University of Pennsylvania Health System, Philadelphia, Pennsylvania
Nutritional Issues in Patients With Hematologic Malignancies

Melissa M. Cushing MD
Assistant Professor, Department of Pathology, Weill Cornell Medical College, New York, New York
Principles of Red Blood Cell Transfusion

Corey Cutler MD, MPH
Associate Professor, Department of Medical Oncology, Dana-Farber Cancer Institute, Harvard Medical School, Boston, Massachusetts
Allogeneic Hematopoietic Stem Cell Transplantation for Acute Myeloid Leukemia and Myelodysplastic Syndrome in Adults

Gary V. Dahl MD
Professor, Department of Pediatrics; Section Chief, Pediatric Oncology, Stanford University School of Medicine, Palo Alto, California
Acute Myeloid Leukemia in Children

Chi V. Dang MD, PhD
Professor of Medicine, Department of Medicine, Division of Hematology and Oncology; Director, Abramson Cancer Center, University of Pennsylvania Perelman School of Medicine, Philadelphia, Pennsylvania
Control of Cell Division

Nika N. Danial PhD
Assistant Professor, Cancer Biology, Dana-Farber Cancer Institute; Assistant Professor, Cell Biology, Harvard Medical School, Boston, Massachusetts
Cell Death

Sandeep S. Dave MD, MS
Assistant Professor, Department of Medicine, Division of Oncology, Duke Institute for Genome Sciences and Policy, Durham, North Carolina
Origin of Non-Hodgkin Lymphoma

Daniel J. DeAngelo MD, PhD
Clinical Director, Adult Leukemia; Associate Professor of Medicine, Harvard Medical School, Dana-Farber Cancer Institute, Boston, Massachusetts
Myelodysplastic Syndromes: Biology and Treatment

Madhav V. Desai MD
Student, Department of Lymphoma and Myeloma, The University of Texas MD Anderson Cancer Center, Houston, Texas
Mantle Cell Lymphoma

Bimalangshu R. Dey MD, PhD
Bone Marrow Transplant Program, Massachusetts General Hospital; Assistant Professor of Medicine, Harvard Medical School, Boston, Massachusetts
Haploidentical Hematopoietic Cell Transplantation

Volker Diehl MD, PhD
Professor Emeritus; Former Director, First Department of Internal Medicine, University Hospital of Cologne, Cologne, Germany
Hodgkin Lymphoma: Clinical Manifestations, Staging, and Therapy

Mary C. Dinauer MD, PhD
Fred M. Saigh Distinguished Chair of Pediatric Research, Departments of Pediatrics and of Pathology and Immunology, Washington University School of Medicine, St. Louis, Missouri
Disorders of Phagocyte Function

Reyhan Diz-Küçükkaya MD
Professor of Medicine and Hematology, Department of Internal Medicine, Division of Hematology, Istanbul Bilim University Faculty of Medicine, Istanbul, Turkey
Acquired Disorders of Platelet Function

Michele L. Donato MD
Collection Facility Medical Director, Blood and Marrow Transplantation Program, John Theurer Cancer Center, Hackensack University Medical Center, Hackensack, New Jersey
Practical Aspects of Hematologic Stem Cell Harvesting and Mobilization

Kenneth Dorshkind PhD
Vice-Chair of Research, Department of Pathology and Laboratory Medicine, David Geffen School of Medicine, University of California Los Angeles, Los Angeles, California
B-Cell Development

Gianpietro Dotti MD
Associate Professor, Center for Cell and Gene Therapy, Baylor College of Medicine, The Methodist Hospital, Houston, Texas
T-Cell Therapy of Hematologic Diseases

Yigal Dror MD
Associate Professor, Division of Hematology and Oncology; Scientist, Cell Biology Program, Research Institute, Hospital for Sick Children, Institute of Medical Sciences, University of Toronto, Toronto, Ontario, Canada
Inherited Forms of Bone Marrow Failure

Kieron Dunleavy MD
Attending Physician and Investigator, Center for Cancer Research, National Cancer Institute, Bethesda, Maryland
Diagnosis and Treatment of Diffuse Large B-Cell Lymphoma and Burkitt Lymphoma

Benjamin L. Ebert MD, PhD
Assistant Professor of Medicine, Division of Hematology, Brigham and Women's Hospital, Harvard Medical School, Boston, Massachusetts
Pathobiology of the Human Erythrocyte and Its Hemoglobins
Hemoglobin Variants Associated With Hemolytic Anemia, Altered Oxygen Affinity, and Methemoglobinemias

Michael J. Eck MD, PhD
Professor of Biological Chemistry and Molecular Pharmacology, Department of Cancer Biology, Dana-Farber Cancer Institute, Harvard Medical School, Boston, Massachusetts
Protein Architecture: Relationship of Form and Function

Dennis A. Eichenauer MD
Resident, First Department of Internal Medicine, University Hospital of Cologne, Cologne, Germany
Hodgkin Lymphoma: Clinical Manifestations, Staging, and Therapy

John W. Eikelboom MBBS, MSc
Department of Medicine, McMaster University, Hamilton, Ontario, Canada
Acute Coronary Syndromes

Andreas Engert MD
Professor, First Department of Internal Medicine, University Hospital of Cologne, Cologne, Germany
Hodgkin Lymphoma: Clinical Manifestations, Staging, and Therapy

William B. Ershler MD
Scientific Director, Institute for Advanced Studies in Aging and Geriatric Medicine, Washington, DC
Hematology in Aging

Charles T. Esmon PhD
Investigator, Howard Hughes Medical Institute; Member and Head, Coagulation Biology Laboratory, Oklahoma Medical Research Foundation; Professor, Departments of Pathology and Biochemistry and Molecular Biology, University of Oklahoma Health Sciences Center, Oklahoma City, Oklahoma
Regulatory Mechanisms in Hemostasis

Naomi L. Esmon PhD
Research Associate Member, Coagulation Biology Laboratory, Oklahoma Medical Research Foundation; Associate Professor, Department of Pathology, University of Oklahoma Health Sciences Center, Oklahoma City, Oklahoma
Regulatory Mechanisms in Hemostasis

William E. Evans PharmD
Director and CEO, St. Jude Children's Research Hospital; Professor, Pediatrics and Clinical Pharmacy, University of Tennessee, Colleges of Medicine and Pharmacy; Member and Professor, Pharmaceutical Sciences, St. Jude Children's Research Hospital, Memphis, Tennessee
Pharmacogenomics and Hematologic Diseases

Stefan Faderl MD
Professor, Department of Leukemia, The University of Texas MD Anderson Cancer Center, Houston, Texas
Clinical Manifestations and Treatment of Acute Myeloid Leukemia

James L.M. Ferrara MD, DSc
American Cancer Society Professor; Doris Duke Distinguished Clinical Scientist; Director, Blood and Marrow Transplant Program, University of Michigan, Ann Arbor, Michigan
Graft-Versus-Host Disease and Graft-Versus-Leukemia Responses

Alexandra Hult Filipovich MD
Division of Bone Marrow Transplantation and Immunodeficiency, Cincinnati Children's Hospital Medical Center, Cincinnati, Ohio
Histiocytic Disorders

Melvin H. Freedman MD
Professor Emeritus, Department of Pediatrics, University of Toronto Faculty of Medicine; Honorary Consultant, Department of Hematology and Oncology, Hospital for Sick Children, Toronto, Ontario, Canada
Inherited Forms of Bone Marrow Failure

Stephen J. Fuller MBBS, PhD
Senior Lecturer, Department of Medicine, Sydney Medical School Neapean, University of Sydney; Head of Academic Hematology, Neapean Hospital, Penrith, New South Wales, Australia
Heme Biosynthesis and Its Disorders: Porphyrias and Sideroblastic Anemias

David Gailani MD
Professor of Medicine, Pathology, Microbiology, and Immunology; Medical Director, Clinical Coagulation Laboratory, Vanderbilt University Medical Center, Nashville, Tennessee
Rare Coagulation Factor Deficiencies

Patrick G. Gallagher MD
Professor, Department of Pediatrics and Genetics, Yale University School of Medicine, New Haven, Connecticut
Red Blood Cell Membrane Disorders

Lawrence B. Gardner MD
Associate Professor, Departments of Medicine, Biochemistry, and Molecular Pharmacology, New York University School of Medicine, New York, New York
Anemia of Chronic Diseases Hematologic Manifestations of Cancer

Adrian P. Gee PhD
Professor of Pediatrics and Medicine, Center for Cell and Gene Therapy, Baylor College of Medicine, Houston, Texas
Graft Engineering and Cell Processing

Stanton L. Gerson MD
Professor of Medicine, Division of Hematology and Oncology, Case Western Reserve University, Cleveland, Ohio
Pharmacology and Molecular Mechanisms of Antineoplastic Agents for Hematologic Malignancies

Morie A. Gertz MD, MACP
Chair and Roland Seidler Jr. Professor, Mayo Distinguished Clinician, Department of Medicine, Mayo Clinic, Rochester, Minnesota
Immunoglobulin Light-Chain Amyloidosis (Primary Amyloidosis)

Patricia J. Giardina MD
Professor of Clinical Pediatrics, Weill Cornell Medical College, Department of Pediatrics, Division of Pediatric Hematology and Oncology, New York, New York
Thalassemia Syndromes

Karin Golan MsC
PhD student, Department of Immunology, Weizmann Institute of Science, Rehovot, Israel
Dynamic Interactions Between Hematopoietic Stem and Progenitor Cells and the Bone Marrow: Current Biology of Stem Cell Homing and Mobilization

Todd R. Golub MD
Chief Scientific Officer, Broad Institute of MIT and Harvard; Charles A. Dana Investigator, Dana-Farber Cancer Institute; Professor of Pediatrics, Harvard Medical School, Boston, Massachusetts
Genomic Approaches to Hematology

Stephen Gottschalk MD
Associate Professor, Departments of Pediatrics and Pathology and Immunology, Center for Cell and Gene Therapy, Texas Children's Cancer Center, Texas Children's Hospital, The Methodist Hospital, Baylor College of Medicine, Houston, Texas
Infectious Mononucleosis and Other Epstein-Barr Virus–Associated Diseases

Steven Grant MD
Virginia Commonwealth University, Massey Cancer Center, Richmond, Virginia
Pharmacology and Molecular Mechanisms of Antineoplastic Agents for Hematologic Malignancies

David L. Green MD, PhD
Department of Medicine, Division of Hematology, New York University School of Medicine, New York, New York
Hematologic Manifestations of Cancer

John G. Gribben MD
Hamilton Fairley Professor of Medical Oncology, Barts Cancer Institute, St. Bartholomew's Hospital, Queen Mary University of London, London, United Kingdom
Clinical Manifestations, Staging, and Treatment of Follicular Lymphoma

Joan Guitart MD
Associate Professor, Department of Dermatology, Northwestern University Medical School; Northwestern Memorial Hospital, Chicago, Illinois
T-Cell Lymphomas

Shiri Gur-Cohen MsC
PhD Student, Department of Immunology, Weizmann Institute of Science, Rehovot, Israel
Dynamic Interactions Between Hematopoietic Stem and Progenitor Cells and the Bone Marrow: Current Biology of Stem Cell Homing and Mobilization

Sandeep Gurbuxani MD
Department of Pathology, University of Chicago, Chicago, Illinois
Acute Lymphoblastic Leukemia in Adults

Alejandro Gutierrez MD
Instructor in Pediatrics, Division of Hematology and Oncology, Children's Hospital Boston, Dana-Farber Cancer Institute, Harvard Medical School, Boston, Massachusetts
Pathobiology of Acute Lymphoblastic Leukemia

Parameswaran Hari MD, MRCP, MS
Associate Professor of Medicine, Section Head, Blood and Marrow Transplantation, Division of Hematology Oncology, Department of Medicine, Medical College of Wisconsin, Milwaukee, Wisconsin
Indications and Outcome of Allogeneic Hematopoietic Cell Transplantation for Hematologic Malignancies in Adults

John M. Harlan
Professor, Department of Medicine, University of Washington; Chief, Section of Hematology and Oncology, Harborview Medical Center, Seattle, Washington
The Blood Vessel Wall

John H. Hartwig MD
Professor, Department of Medicine, Brigham and Women's Hospital, Harvard Medical School, Boston, Massachusetts
Megakaryocyte and Platelet Structure

Suzanne R. Hayman MD
Assistant Professor of Medicine, College of Medicine, Cons-Hematology, Mayo Clinic, Rochester, Minnesota
Immunoglobulin Light-Chain Amyloidosis (Primary Amyloidosis)

Catherine P.M. Hayward MD, PhD
Professor, Departments of Medicine and Pathology and Molecular Medicine, McMaster University; Hematologist, Division of Hematology and Thromboembolism, Hamilton Health Sciences and St. Joseph's Healthcare; Head, Coagulation, Hamilton Regional Laboratory Medicine Program, Hamilton, Ontario, Canada
Clinical Approach to the Patient With Bleeding or Bruising

Robert P. Hebbel MD
Regents Professor and Clark Professor, Department of Medicine; Director, Vascular Biology Center, University of Minnesota Medical School, Minneapolis, Minnesota
Pathobiology of Sickle Cell Disease

Helen E. Heslop MD
Dan L. Duncan Chair, Professor of Medicine and Pediatrics; Director, Adult Stem Cell Transplant Program, Center for Cell and Gene Therapy, Baylor College of Medicine, The Methodist Hospital, Texas Children's Hospital, Houston, Texas
Overview and Historical Perspective of Current Cell-Based Therapies
Overview of Hematopoietic Stem Cell Transplantation

Christopher D. Hillyer MD
Professor, Department of Medicine, Weill Cornell Medical College; President and Chief Executive Officer, New York Blood Center, New York, New York
Principles of Plasma Transfusion: Plasma, Cryoprecipitate, Albumin, and Immunoglobulins

David M. Hockenbery MD
Fred Hutchinson Cancer Research Center, Seattle, Washington
Cell Death

Ronald Hoffman MD
Albert A. and Vera G. List Professor of Medicine, Tisch Cancer Institute, Department of Medicine, Mount Sinai School of Medicine, New York, New York
Progress in the Classification of Myeloid Neoplasms: Clinical Implications
The Polycythemias
Essential Thrombocythemia
Primary Myelofibrosis
Eosinophilia, Eosinophil-Associated Diseases, Chronic Eosinophil Leukemia, and the Hypereosinophilic Syndromes
Mast Cells and Systemic Mastocytosis

Mary Horowitz MD
Robert A. Uihlein Professor of Hematologic Research; Chief, Division of Hematology and Oncology, Department of Medicine, Medical College of Wisconsin; Chief Scientific Director, Center for International Blood and Marrow Transplant Research, Medical College of Wisconsin, Milwaukee, Wisconsin
Indications and Outcome of Allogeneic Hematopoietic Cell Transplantation for Hematologic Malignancies in Adults

Edwin M. Horwitz MD, PhD
Associate Professor of Pediatrics, Department of Pediatrics and Oncology, University of Pennsylvania Perelman School of Medicine, Children's Hospital of Philadelphia, Philadelphia, Pennsylvania
Mesenchymal Stromal Cells

Robert A. Hromas MD
Professor and Chair, Department of Medicine, University of Florida College of Medicine, Gainesville, Florida
Regulation of Gene Expression, Transcription, Splicing, and RNA Metabolism

Franklin W. Huang MD, PhD
Clinical Fellow, Department of Hematology and Medical Oncology, Dana-Farber Cancer Institute, Brigham and Women's Hospital, Massachusetts General Hospital, Boston, Massachusetts
Indwelling Access Devices

David E. Isenman PhD
Professor Emeritus, Departments of Biochemistry and Immunology, University of Toronto, Toronto, Ontario, Canada*Complement and Immunoglobulin Biology*

Joseph E. Italiano, Jr. PhD
Associate Professor, Department of Medicine, Brigham and Women's Hospital; Associate Professor, Harvard Medical School; Assistant Professor, Department of Surgery, Vascular Biology Program, Children's Hospital Boston, Boston, Massachusetts
Megakaryocyte and Platelet Structure

Elaine S. Jaffe MD
Head, Hematopathology Section, Laboratory of Pathology, Center for Cancer Research, National Cancer Institute, Bethesda, Maryland
Pathologic Basis for the Classification of Non-Hodgkin and Hodgkin Lymphomas

Sundar Jagannath MD
Director, Multiple Myeloma Program, Mount Sinai Medical Center; Professor, Department of Hematology and Medical Oncology, Tisch Cancer Institute, Mount Sinai School of Medicine, New York, New York
Plasma Cell Neoplasms

Ulrich Jäger MD
Professor of Hematology; Head, Division of Hematology and Hemostaseology, Department of Medicine, Medical University of Vienna, Comprehensive Cancer Center, Vienna, Austria*Autoimmune Hemolytic Anemia*

Nitin Jain MD
Department of Leukemia, The University of Texas MD Anderson Cancer Center, Houston, Texas
Acute Lymphoblastic Leukemia in Adults

Paula James MD
Associate Professor, Department of Medicine, Queen's University, Kingston, Ontario, Canada
Structure, Biology, and Genetics of von Willebrand Factor

Sima Jeha MD
Director, Leukemia and Lymphoma Developmental Therapeutics, Department of Oncology, St. Jude Children's Research Hospital, Memphis, Tennessee
Clinical Manifestations and Treatment of Acute Lymphoblastic Leukemia in Children

Michael B. Jordan MD
Associate Professor of Pediatrics, Divisions of Immunobiology and Bone Marrow Transplant and Immunodeficiency, Department of Pediatrics, Cincinnati Children's Hospital, University of Cincinnati, Cincinnati, Ohio
Histiocytic Disorders

Cassandra Josephson MD
Associate Professor, Department Pathology and Pediatrics, Emory University School of Medicine; Director, Clinical Research, Center for Transfusion and Cellular Therapies; Program Director, Transfusion Medicine Fellowship; Medical Director, Children's Healthcare of Atlanta Blood and Tissue Services, Atlanta, Georgia
Pediatric Transfusion Medicine

Moonjung Jung MD
Fellow, Hematology Branch, National Heart, Lung, and Blood Institute, National Institutes of Health, Bethesda, Maryland
Neutrophilic Leukocytosis, Neutropenia, Monocytosis, and Monocytopenia

Leo Kager MD
Associate Professor of Pediatrics, Department of Hematology and Oncology, St. Anna Children's Hospital, Department of Pediatrics, Medical University of Vienna, Children's Cancer Research Institute, Vienna, Austria
Pharmacogenomics and Hematologic Diseases

Kala Y. Kamdar MD
Section of Hematology and Oncology, Department of Pediatrics, Baylor College of Medicine, Houston, Texas
Malignant Lymphomas in Childhood

Jennifer A. Kanakry MD
Hematology Fellow, Department of Hematology, Johns Hopkins Hospital, Baltimore, Maryland
Virus-Associated Lymphomas

Hagop M. Kantarjian MD
Professor, Department of Leukemia, Division of Cancer Medicine, Associate Vice President for Global Academic Programs, Department Chair, Kelcie Margaret Kana Research Chair, Department of Leukemia, Division of Cancer Medicine, The University of Texas MD Anderson Cancer Center, Houston, Texas
Clinical Manifestations and Treatment of Acute Myeloid Leukemia

Matthew S. Karafin MD
Transfusion Medicine Fellow, Department of Pathology, Johns Hopkins Hospital, Baltimore, Maryland
Principles of Plasma Transfusion: Plasma, Cryoprecipitate, Albumin, and Immunoglobulins

Aly Karsan MD
Professor, Pathology and Laboratory Medicine, University of British Columbia; Hematopathologist/Senior Scientist, British Columbia Cancer Agency, Vancouver, British Columbia, Canada
The Blood Vessel Wall

Louis M. Katz MD
Executive Vice President, Mississippi Valley Regional Blood Center, Davenport, Iowa; Adjunct Clinical Professor, Department of Internal Medicine, Division of Infectious Diseases, Carver College of Medicine, University of Iowa, Iowa City, Iowa
Transfusion-Transmitted Diseases

Randal J. Kaufman PhD
Director, Del E. Webb Neuroscience, Aging, and Stem Cell Research Center, Sanford Burnham Medical Research Institute, La Jolla, California
Protein Synthesis, Processing, and Trafficking

Richard M. Kaufman MD
Medical Director, Adult Transfusion Service, Brigham and Women's Hospital; Assistant Professor of Pathology, Harvard Medical School, Boston, Massachusetts
Principles of Platelet Transfusion Therapy
Transfusion Medicine in Hematopoietic Stem Cell and Solid Organ Transplantation

Frank G. Keller MD
Associate Professor of Pediatrics, Emory University School of Medicine, Aflac Cancer Center and Blood Disorders Service, Atlanta, Georgia
Hematologic Manifestations of Childhood Illness

Kara M. Kelly MD
Professor of Clinical Pediatrics, Division of Pediatric Oncology, Columbia University Medical Center, New York, New York
Integrative Therapies in Patients With Hematologic Diseases

John Kelton MD
Professor of Medicine and Pathology and Molecular Medicine, McMaster University, Michael G. DeGroote School of Medicine, Hamilton, Ontario, Canada
Diseases of Platelet Number: Immune Thrombocytopenia, Neonatal Alloimmune Thrombocytopenia, and Posttransfusion Purpura

Craig M. Kessler MD
Professor of Medicine and Pathology; Director, Division of Coagulation, Hemophilia and Thrombosis Comprehensive Care Center, Georgetown University Medical Center, Washington, DC
Inhibitors in Hemophilia A and B

Nigel S. Key MB, ChB
Harold R. Roberts Distinguished Professor, Department of Medicine and Pathology and Laboratory Medicine; Chief, Section of Hematology, Division of Hematology and Oncology; Director, Hemophilia and Thrombosis Center, University of North Carolina, Chapel Hill, North Carolina
Hematologic Problems in the Surgical Patient: Bleeding and Thrombosis

Alexander G. Khandoga MD
Department of Cardiology, German Heart Center Munich, Munich, Germany
Hematopoietic Cell Trafficking and Chemokines

Arati Khanna-Gupta MSc, PhD
Assistant Professor, Division of Adult Hematology, Brigham and Women's Hospital, Harvard Medical School, Boston, Massachusetts
Granulocytopoiesis and Monocytopoiesis

Harvey G. Klein MD
Chief, Department of Transfusion Medicine, W.G. Magnuson Clinical Center, National Institutes of Health, Bethesda, Maryland
Hemapheresis

Orit Kollet PhD
Associate Scientist, Department of Immunology, Weizmann Institute of Science, Rehovot, Israel
Dynamic Interactions Between Hematopoietic Stem and Progenitor Cells and the Bone Marrow: Current Biology of Stem Cell Homing and Mobilization

Barbara A. Konkle MD
Director, Translational Research; Medical Director, Hemostasis Reference Laboratory, Puget Sound Blood Center; Professor of Medicine and Hematology, University of Washington, Seattle, Washington
Inhibitors in Hemophilia A and B

Dimitrios P. Kontoyiannis MD
Frances King Black Endowed Professor, Infectious Diseases, Deputy Head, Division of Internal Medicine, The University of Texas MD Anderson Cancer Center, Houston, Texas
Clinical Approach to Infections in the Compromised Host

John Koreth MBBS, DPhil
Assistant Professor, Department of Medical Oncology, Dana-Farber Cancer Institute, Harvard Medical School, Boston, Massachusetts
Allogeneic Hematopoietic Stem Cell Transplantation for Acute Myeloid Leukemia and Myelodysplastic Syndrome in Adults

Gary A. Koretzky MD, PhD
Francis C. Wood Professor of Medicine, Department of Medicine, Division of Rheumatology, Abramson Family Cancer Research Institute, University of Pennsylvania, Philadelphia, Pennsylvania
T-Cell Immunity

Marina Kremyanskaya MD, PhD
Assistant Professor of Medicine, Tisch Cancer Institute, Department of Medicine, Mount Sinai School of Medicine, New York, New York
The Polycythemias
Essential Thrombocythemia
Primary Myelofibrosis
Eosinophilia, Eosinophil-Associated Diseases, Chronic Eosinophil Leukemia, and the Hypereosinophilic Syndromes
Mast Cells and Systemic Mastocytosis

Ralf Küppers PhD
Professor, Institute of Cell Biology and Cancer Research, University of Duisburg-Essen Medical School, Essen, Germany
Origin of Hodgkin Lymphoma

Timothy M. Kuzel MD, RACP
Professor, Division of Hematology and Oncology, Department of Medicine, Northwestern University Feinberg School of Medicine, Chicago, Illinois
T-Cell Lymphomas

Larry W. Kwak MD
Professor and Chair, Department of Lymphoma and Myeloma, The University of Texas MD Anderson Cancer Center, Houston, Texas
Mantle Cell Lymphoma

Viswanathan Lakshmanan PhD
Postdoctoral Scientist, Department of Microbiology and Immunology, Columbia University Medical Center, New York, New York
Dendritic Cell Biology

Wendy Landier PhD, RN
Clinical Director, Center for Cancer Survivorship, Department of Population Sciences, City of Hope Comprehensive Cancer Center, Duarte, California*Late Complications of Hematologic Diseases and Their Therapies*

Kfir Lapid PhD
Associate Scientist, Department of Immunology, Weizmann Institute of Science, Rehovot, Israel
Dynamic Interactions Between Hematopoietic Stem and Progenitor Cells and the Bone Marrow: Current Biology of Stem Cell Homing and Mobilization

Tsvee Lapidot PhD
Professor, Department of Immunology, Weizmann Institute of Science, Rehovot, Israel
Dynamic Interactions Between Hematopoietic Stem and Progenitor Cells and the Bone Marrow: Current Biology of Stem Cell Homing and Mobilization

Peter J. Larson
Director, Global Clinical Strategy, Biological Products, Research Triangle Park, North Carolina
Transfusion Therapy for Coagulation Factor Deficiencies

Klaus Lechner MD
Professor Emeritus of Medicine and Hematology, Department of Medicine, Division of Hematology and Hemostaseology, Medical University of Vienna, Vienna, Austria
Autoimmune Hemolytic Anemia

Andrea Lee MD
Associate Staff, Department of Medicine, Division of Hematology, Oakville-Trafalgar Memorial Hospital, Oakville, Ontario, Canada
Hematologic Manifestations of Liver Disease

William M.F. Lee MD, PhD
Associate Professor of Medicine, Department of Medicine, Division of Hematology and Oncology; Co-Program Leader, Tumor Biology, Abramson Cancer Center, University of Pennsylvania Perelman School of Medicine, Philadelphia, Pennsylvania
Control of Cell Division

Marcel Levi MD, PhD
Professor of Medicine, Academic Medical Center, University of Amsterdam, Amsterdam, The Netherlands
Disseminated Intravascular Coagulation

Russell E. Lewis PharmD
Professor, University of Houston College of Pharmacy, The University of Texas MD Anderson Cancer Center, Houston, Texas
Clinical Approach to Infections in the Compromised Host

Howard A. Liebman MA, MD
Professor of Medicine and Pathology, Jane Anne Nohl Division of Hematology and Center for the Study of Blood Diseases, University of Southern California Keck School of Medicine, Los Angeles, California
Hematologic Manifestations of HIV/AIDS

David Lillicrap MD
Professor, Department of Pathology and Molecular Medicine, Queen's University, Kingston, Ontario, Canada
Hemophilia A and B

Wendy Lim MD
Associate Professor, Department of Medicine, McMaster University, Hamilton, Ontario, Canada
Venous Thromboembolism
Hematologic Manifestations of Liver Disease

Thomas S. Lin MD
Associate Professor of Medicine, Ohio State University, Columbus, Ohio
Chronic Lymphocytic Leukemia

Robert Lindblad MD
Chief Medical Officer, The EMMES Corporation, Rockville, Maryland
Preclinical Process of Cell-Based Therapies

Gregory Y.H. Lip MD
Professor of Cardiovascular Medicine, University of Birmingham, Center for Cardiovascular Sciences, City Hospital, Birmingham, United Kingdom
Atrial Fibrillation

Jane A. Little MD
Associate Professor, Department of Medicine, University Hospitals Seidman Cancer Center, Case Western Reserve University, Cleveland, Ohio
Anemia of Chronic Diseases

Mignon L. Loh MD
Professor of Clinical Pediatrics, University of California San Francisco, Benioff Children's Hospital, Helen Diller Family Comprehensive Cancer Center, San Francisco, California
Myelodysplastic and Myeloproliferative Neoplasms in Children

A. Thomas Look MD
Professor of Pediatrics, Harvard Medical School, Vice-Chair for Research, Department of Pediatric Oncology, Division of Hematology and Oncology, Dana-Farber Cancer Institute, Children's Hospital Boston, Boston, Massachusetts
Pathobiology of Acute Lymphoblastic Leukemia

José A. López MD
Executive Vice-President for Research, Research Institute, Puget Sound Blood Center; Professor, Departments of Medicine and Biochemistry, University of Washington, Seattle, Washington
Acquired Disorders of Platelet Function

Francis W. Luscinskas PhD
Professor, Department of Pathology; Associate Director, Vascular Research Division, Brigham and Women's Hospital, Harvard Medical School, Boston, Massachusetts
Cell Adhesion

Christine A. Macartney MB, DCH, MRCP
Department of Pediatric Hematology, Royal Belfast Hospital for Sick Children, Belfast, Northern Ireland, United Kingdom
Disorders of Coagulation in the Neonate

Jaroslaw P. Maciejewski MD, PhD
Chairman and Professor of Medicine, Department of Translational Hematology and Oncology Research, Taussig Cancer Center, Cleveland Clinic, Cleveland, Ohio
Aplastic Anemia
Acquired Disorders of Red Cell, White Cell, and Platelet Production

Robert W. Maitta MD, PhD
Assistant Director of Transfusion Medicine, Blood Bank and Donor Apheresis Center; Assistant Professor, Department of Pathology, Case Western Reserve University, University Hospitals, Case Medical Center, Cleveland, Ohio
Transfusion Reactions to Blood and Cell Therapy Products

Navneet S. Majhail MD, MS
Medical Director, National Marrow Donor Program, Adjunct Associate Professor of Medicine, University of Minnesota, Minneapolis, Minnesota
Complications After Hematopoietic Stem Cell Transplantation

Olivier Manches PhD
Research Assistant, New York University School of Medicine, Langone Medical Center, New York, New York
Dendritic Cell Biology

Robert Mandle PhD
President, BioSciences Research Associates, Inc., Cambridge, Massachusetts
Complement and Immunoglobulin Biology

Kenneth G. Mann PhD
Departments of Biochemistry and Medicine, University of Vermont College of Medicine, Burlington, Vermont
Molecular Basis of Blood Coagulation

Catherine S. Manno MD
Pat and John Rosenwald Professor and Chair, Department of Pediatrics, New York University School of Medicine, New York, New York
Transfusion Therapy for Coagulation Factor Deficiencies

Enrica Marchi MD
Postdoctoral Fellow, New York University Cancer Institute, New York, New York
T-Cell Lymphomas

Guglielmo Mariani MD
Department of Internal Medicine, Section of Hematology, University of L'Aquila, Italy
Inhibitors in Hemophilia A and B

Francesco M. Marincola MD
Department of Transfusion Medicine, Clinical Center for Human Immunology, National Institutes of Health, Bethesda, Maryland
Human Leukocyte Antigen and Human Neutrophil Antigen Systems

Peter W. Marks MD, PhD
Associate Professor of Medicine, Department of Internal Medicine, Yale University School of Medicine, New Haven, Connecticut
Approach to Anemia in the Adult and Child
Hematologic Manifestations of Systemic Disease: Renal Disease

John Mascarenhas MD
Assistant Professor of Medicine, Tisch Cancer Institute, Department of Medicine, Mount Sinai School of Medicine, New York, New York
The Polycythemias
Essential Thrombocythemia
Primary Myelofibrosis
Eosinophilia, Eosinophil-Associated Diseases, Chronic Eosinophil Leukemia, and the Hypereosinophilic Syndromes
Mast Cells and Systemic Mastocytosis

Steffen Massberg MD
Professor of Cardiology, German Heart Center Munich, Technical University of Munich, Munich, Germany
Hematopoietic Cell Trafficking and Chemokines

Peter M. Mauch MD
Professor of Radiation Oncology, Dana-Farber Cancer Institute, Harvard Medical School, Boston, Massachusetts
Radiation Therapy in the Treatment of Hematologic Malignancies

Ruth McCorkle PhD, RN, FAAN
Florence Wald Professor of Nursing, Yale University School of Nursing, New Haven, Connecticut
Psychosocial Aspects of Hematologic Disorders

Keith R. McCrae MD
Professor of Molecular Medicine, Cleveland Clinic Lerner College of Medicine, Taussig Cancer Institute, Cleveland Clinic, Cleveland, Ohio
Thrombotic Thrombocytopenic Purpura and the Hemolytic Uremic Syndrome

Rodger P. McEver MD
Cardiovascular Biology Research Program, Oklahoma Medical Research Foundation, Department of Biochemistry and Molecular Biology, University of Oklahoma Health Sciences Center, Oklahoma City, Oklahoma
Cell Adhesion

Emer McGrath
Health Research Board Clinical Research Facility, National University of Ireland, Galway, Ireland
Stroke

Matthew S. McKinney MD
Fellow, Hematology and Oncology, Departments of Medicine and Cellular Therapy, Division of Oncology, Duke University, Durham, North Carolina
Origin of Non-Hodgkin Lymphoma

Amy Meacham MS
Senior Biological Scientist, Department of Medicine, Division of Hematology and Oncology, University of Florida College of Medicine, Gainesville, Florida
Regulation of Gene Expression, Transcription, Splicing, and RNA Metabolism

Jay E. Menitove MD
Clinical Professor of Pathology and Laboratory Medicine, University of Kansas School of Medicine, Kansas City, Kansas; Clinical Professor of Internal Medicine, University of Missouri-Kansas City School of Medicine; President, Chief Executive Officer, and Medical Director, Community Blood Center of Greater Kansas City, Kansas City, Missouri
Transfusion-Transmitted Diseases

Giampaolo Merlini MD
Director, Amyloidosis Research and Treatment Center, Foundation IRCCS Policlinico San Matteo, Department of Molecular Medicine, University of Pavia, Pavia, Italy
Waldenström Macroglobulinemia and Lymphoplasmacytic Lymphoma

Anna Rita Migliaccio MD
Professor of Medicine, Tisch Cancer Center, Mount Sinai School of Medicine, New York, New York
Biology of Erythropoiesis, Erythroid Differentiation, and Maturation

Jeffrey S. Miller MD
Professor of Medicine, Department of Medicine, Division of Hematology, Oncology, and Transplantation, University of Minnesota, Minneapolis, Minnesota
Natural Killer Cell-Based Therapies

Martha P. Mims MD, PhD
Associate Professor of Medicine; Chief, Department of Internal Medicine, Section of Hematology and Oncology, Baylor College of Medicine, Houston, Texas
Lymphocytosis, Lymphocytopenia, Hypergammaglobulinemia, and Hypogammaglobulinemia

Traci Heath Mondoro PhD
Deputy Branch Chief, Transfusion Medicine and Cellular Therapeutics, Division of Blood Diseases and Resources, National Heart, Lung, and Blood Institute, National Institutes of Health, Bethesda, Maryland
Preclinical Process of Cell-Based Therapies

Paul Moorehead MD
Pathology and Molecular Medicine, Queen's University, Kingston, Ontario, Canada
Hemophilia A and B

Nikhil C. Munshi MD
Associate Professor of Medicine, Harvard Medical School, Dana-Farber Cancer Institute, Boston, Massachusetts
Plasma Cell Neoplasms

Vesna Najfeld PhD
Professor of Pathology and Medicine, Departments of Pathology and Medicine; Director, Tumor Cytogenetics and Oncology, Molecular and Cellular Tumor Markers, Tisch Cancer Institute, Mount Sinai School of Medicine, New York, New York
Conventional and Molecular Cytogenetic Basis of Hematologic Malignancies
The Polycythemias
Essential Thrombocythemia
Primary Myelofibrosis

Ishac Nazi PhD
Assistant Professor, Biochemistry and Biomedical Sciences, McMaster University, Platelet Immunology, Hamilton, Ontario, Canada
Diseases of Platelet Number: Immune Thrombocytopenia, Neonatal Alloimmune Thrombocytopenia, and Posttransfusion Purpura

Anne T. Neff MD
Associate Professor of Medicine and Pathology, Microbiology, and Immunology; Director, Hemostasis and Thrombosis Clinic, Vanderbilt University Medical Center, Nashville, Tennessee
Rare Coagulation Factor Deficiencies

Paul M. Ness MD
Director, Transfusion Medicine, Department of Pathology, Johns Hopkins Hospital; Professor of Pathology, Medicine, and Oncology, Johns Hopkins University School of Medicine, Baltimore, Maryland
Principles of Red Blood Cell Transfusion

Andrea K. Ng MD, MPH
Associate Professor of Radiation Oncology, Dana-Farber Cancer Institute, Brigham and Women's Hospital, Harvard Medical School, Boston, Massachusetts
Radiation Therapy in the Treatment of Hematologic Malignancies

Luigi D. Notarangelo MD
Professor of Pediatrics and Pathology, Department of Medicine, Division of Immunology, Children's Hospital Boston, Harvard Medical School, Boston, Massachusetts
Congenital Disorders of Lymphocyte Function

Sarah H. O'Brien MD, MSc
Assistant Professor of Pediatrics, Division of Pediatric Hematology and Oncology, Nationwide Children's Hospital, Ohio State University, Columbus, Ohio
Hematologic Manifestations of Childhood Illness

Owen A. O'Connor MD, PhD
Associate Professor of Medicine, Director, Lymphoid Development and Malignancy Program, Herbert Irving Comprehensive Cancer Center, Columbia University; Chief, Lymphoma Service, College of Physicians and Surgeons, Presbyterian Hospital, Columbia University Medical Center, New York, New York
T-Cell Lymphomas

Diarmaid Ó Donghaile MD
Clinical Fellow, Department of Transfusion Medicine, W.G. Magnuson Clinical Center, National Institutes of Health, Bethesda, Maryland
Hemapheresis

Martin O'Donnell MD
Population Health Research Institute, Hamilton General Hospital, McMaster University, Hamilton, Ontario, Canada
Stroke

Stavroula Otis MD
Clinical Instructor, Department of Medicine and Hematology, Stanford University School of Medicine, Palo Alto, California
Red Blood Cell Enzymopathies

Zhishuo Ou MD
Instructor, Department of Lymphoma and Myeloma, The University of Texas MD Anderson Cancer Center, Houston, Texas
Mantle Cell Lymphoma

Sung-Yun Pai MD
Assistant Professor, Division of Hematology and Oncology, Children's Hospital Boston, Dana-Farber Cancer Institute, Harvard Medical School, Boston, Massachusetts
Congenital Disorders of Lymphocyte Function

Karolina Palucka MD, PhD
Investigator, Baylor Institute for Immunology Research, Dallas, Texas; Professor, Department of Oncological Sciences, Mount Sinai School of Medicine, New York, New York
Dendritic Cell Therapies

Reena L. Pande MD
Brigham and Women's Hospital, Cardiovascular Division, Instructor in Medicine, Harvard Medical School, Boston, Massachusetts
Peripheral Artery Disease

Thalia Papayannopoulou MD
Professor of Medicine, Division of Hematology, Department of Medicine, University of Washington, Seattle, Washington
Biology of Erythropoiesis, Erythroid Differentiation, and Maturation

Animesh Pardanani MBBS, PhD
Department of Hematology, Mayo Clinic, Rochester, Minnesota
Mast Cells and Systemic Mastocytosis

Nethnapha Paredes
Department of Pediatrics, McMaster University, Hamilton, Ontario, Canada
Disorders of Coagulation in the Neonate

Christopher Patriquin BHSc, MD
Hematology Fellow, Department of Medicine, Division of Hematology and Thromboembolism, McMaster University, Hamilton, Ontario, Canada
Diseases of Platelet Number: Immune Thrombocytopenia, Neonatal Alloimmune Thrombocytopenia, and Posttransfusion Purpura

Effie W. Petersdorf MD
Professor of Medicine, University of Washington; Member, Division of Clinical Research, Fred Hutchinson Cancer Research Center, Seattle, Washington
Unrelated Donor Hematopoietic Cell Transplantation

Stefania Pittaluga MD, PhD
Staff Clinician, Hematopathology Section, Laboratory of Pathology, Center for Cancer Research, National Cancer Institute, Bethesda, Maryland
Pathologic Basis for the Classification of Non-Hodgkin and Hodgkin Lymphomas

Edward F. Plow PhD
Professor of Molecular Medicine, Cleveland Clinic Lerner College of Medicine; Chairman, Robert C. Tarazi, MD Endowed Chair in Heart and Hypertension Research, Department of Molecular Cardiology, Joseph J. Jacobs Center for Thrombosis and Vascular Biology, Lerner Research Institute, Cleveland Clinic, Cleveland, Ohio
Molecular Basis for Platelet Function

Doris M. Ponce MD
Assistant Professor, Medicine, Adult Bone Marrow Transplantation, Memorial Sloan-Kettering Cancer Center, New York, New York
Unrelated Donor Cord Blood Transplantation for Hematologic Malignancies

Laura Popolo PhD
Associate Professor of Molecular Biology, Department of Biomolecular Sciences and Biotechnology, University of Milan, Milan, Italy
Protein Synthesis, Processing, and Trafficking

Leland D. Powell MD, PhD
Professor of Medicine, Department of Medicine, Olive View University of California Los Angeles Medical Center, Sylmar, California; Health Sciences Clinical Professor of Medicine, David Geffen School of Medicine, University of California Los Angeles, Los Angeles, California
Overview and Compartmentalization of the Immune System

Elizabeth A. Price MD, MPH
Assistant Professor, Department of Medicine, Division of Hematology, Stanford University School of Medicine, Palo Alto, California
Red Blood Cell Enzymopathies
Extrinsic Nonimmune Hemolytic Anemias

Ching-Hon Pui MD
Member; Chair, Department of Oncology; Co-Leader, Hematological Malignancies Program; Fahad Nassar Al-Rashid Chair of Leukemia Research; American Cancer Society Professor, St. Jude Children's Research Hospital, Memphis, Tennessee
Clinical Manifestations and Treatment of Acute Lymphoblastic Leukemia in Children

Pere Puigserver PhD
Associate Professor, Departments of Cancer Biology and Cell Biology, Dana-Farber Cancer Institute, Harvard Medical School, Boston, Massachusetts
Signaling Transduction and Regulation of Cell Metabolism

Alfonso Quintás-Cardama MD
Assistant Professor, Division of Cancer Medicine, Department of Leukemia, The University of Texas MD Anderson Cancer Center, Houston, Texas
Pathobiology of Acute Myeloid Leukemia

Janusz Rak MD, PhD
Professor, Department of Pediatrics; Jack Cole Chair in Pediatric Hematology and Oncology, McGill University, Research Institute of the McGill University Health Center, Montreal Children's Hospital, Montreal, Quebec, Canada
Vascular Growth in Health and Disease

Carlos A. Ramos MD
Assistant Professor, Center for Cell and Gene Therapy, Department of Medicine, Hematology and Oncology Section, Baylor College of Medicine, Houston, Texas
Clinical Manifestations and Treatment of Marginal Zone Lymphomas (Extranodal/MALT, Splenic, and Nodal)

Jacob H. Rand MD
Professor of Pathology and Medicine, Albert Einstein College of Medicine, Montefiore Medical Center, Bronx, New York
Antiphospholipid Syndrome

Farhad Ravandi MD
Professor of Medicine, Department of Leukemia, The University of Texas MD Anderson Cancer Center, Houston, Texas
Hairy Cell Leukemia

David J. Rawlings MD
Children's Guild Association Endowed Chair in Pediatric Immunology; Director, Center for immunity and Immunotherapies, Seattle Children's Research Institute; Chief, Division of Immunology, Seattle Children's Hospital; Professor of Pediatrics and Immunology, University of Washington School of Medicine, Seattle, Washington
B-Cell Development

Pavan Reddy MD
Associate Division Chief, Hematology and Oncology; Co-Director, Hematologic Malignancies and Bone Marrow Transplant Program, University of Michigan Cancer Center, Ann Arbor, Michigan
Graft-Versus-Host Disease and Graft-Versus-Leukemia Responses

Mark T. Reding MD
Associate Professor of Medicine, Division of Hematology, Oncology, and Transplantation; Director, Center for Bleeding and Clotting Disorders, University of Minnesota Medical Center, Minneapolis, Minnesota
Hematologic Problems in the Surgical Patient: Bleeding and Thrombosis

Charles Rhee MD
Department of Medicine, University of Chicago, Chicago, Illinois
Acute Lymphoblastic Leukemia in Adults

Lawrence Rice MD
Professor of Medicine, Weill Cornell Medical College; Chief of Hematology, Department of Medicine, Methodist Hospital; Adjunct Professor of Medicine, Baylor College of Medicine, Houston, Texas
Neutrophilic Leukocytosis, Neutropenia, Monocytosis, and Monocytopenia

Matthew J. Riese MD
Division of Hematology and Oncology, Department of Medicine, Abramson Family Cancer Research Institute, University of Pennsylvania, Philadelphia, Pennsylvania
T-Cell Immunity

Arthur Kim Ritchey MD
Chief, Division of Pediatric Hematology and Oncology, Children's Hospital, University of Pittsburgh Medical Center; Professor of Pediatrics, Vice-Chair for Clinical Affairs, Department of Pediatrics, University of Pittsburgh School of Medicine, Pittsburgh, Pennsylvania
Hematologic Manifestations of Childhood Illness

Stefano Rivella PhD
Associate Professor of Genetic Medicine, Departments of Pediatrics and Cell and Developmental Biology, Division of Hematology and Oncology, Weill Cornell Medical College, New York, New York
Thalassemia Syndromes

David J. Roberts MBChB, DPhil
Consultant Hematologist, National Health Service Blood and Transplant; Professor of Hematology, University of Oxford, Oxford, United Kingdom
Hematologic Aspects of Parasitic Diseases

Jorge E. Romaguera MD
Professor, Department of Lymphoma and Myeloma, The University of Texas MD Anderson Cancer Center, Houston, Texas
Mantle Cell Lymphoma

Elizabeth Roman MD
Assistant Professor of Pediatrics, Division of Pediatric Hematology and Oncology, New York University School of Medicine, New York, New York
Transfusion Therapy for Coagulation Factor Deficiencies

Cliona M. Rooney PhD
Professor, Departments of Pediatrics, Molecular Virology and Microbiology, and Pathology and Immunology, Center for Cell and Gene Therapy, Texas Children's Cancer Center, Texas Children's Hospital, The Methodist Hospital, Baylor College of Medicine, Houston, Texas
Infectious Mononucleosis and Other Epstein-Barr Virus–Associated Diseases

Steven T. Rosen MD
Professor of Medicine, Northwestern University Feinberg School of Medicine; Director, Robert H. Lurie Comprehensive Cancer Center, Northwestern Memorial Hospital, Chicago, Illinois
T-Cell Lymphomas

David S. Rosenthal MD
Professor of Medicine, Harvard Medical School; Co-Director, Leonard P. Zakim Center for Integrative Therapies, Dana-Farber Cancer Institute, Boston, Massachusetts; Director and Henry K. Oliver Professor of Hygiene, Harvard University, Cambridge, Massachusetts
Integrative Therapies in Patients With Hematologic Diseases

Rachel Rosovsky MD, MPH
Department of Medical Oncology, Massachusetts General Hospital, Boston, Massachusetts
Hematologic Manifestations of Systemic Disease: Renal Disease

Scott D. Rowley MD
Chief, Adult Blood and Marrow Transplantation Program, John Theurer Cancer Center, Hackensack University Medical Center, Hackensack, New Jersey
Practical Aspects of Hematologic Stem Cell Harvesting and Mobilization

Natalia Rydz MD
Hemostasis Fellow, Department of Pathology and Molecular Medicine, Queen's University, Kingston, Ontario, Canada
Structure, Biology, and Genetics of von Willebrand Factor

J. Evan Sadler MD, PhD
Professor and Director, Division of Hematology, Department of Medicine, Washington University School of Medicine, St. Louis, Missouri
Thrombotic Thrombocytopenic Purpura and the Hemolytic Uremic Syndrome

John T. Sandlund, Jr. MD
Department of Oncology, St. Jude Children's Research Hospital, University of Tennessee, Memphis, Tennessee
Malignant Lymphomas in Childhood

Steven Sauk MD, MS
Radiology Chief Resident, Mallinckrodt Institute of Radiology, Washington University School of Medicine, St. Louis, Missouri
Mechanical Interventions in Arterial and Venous Thrombosis

Yogen Saunthararajah MB, BCh
Staff, Cleveland Clinic, Taussig Cancer Institute, Cleveland, Ohio; Associate Professor, University of Illinois at Chicago, Chicago, Illinois
Sickle Cell Disease: Clinical Features and Management

David Scadden MD
Gerald and Darlene Jordan Professor of Medicine; Co-Director, Harvard Stem Cell Institute; Co-Chair, Department of Stem Cell and Regenerative Biology, Harvard Medical School; Director, Center for Regenerative Medicine, Massachusetts General Hospital, Boston, Massachusetts
Hematopoietic Microenvironment

Kristen G. Schaefer MD
Instructor, Director of Medical Student and Resident Education, Adult Palliative Care Division, Department of Psychosocial Oncology and Palliative Care, Dana-Farber Cancer Institute, Brigham and Women's Hospital, Harvard Medical School, Boston, Massachusetts
Palliative Care

Fred J. Schiffman MD
Sigal Family Professor of Humanistic Medicine; Vice-Chair, Department of Medicine, Warren Alpert Medical School, Brown University, Providence, Rhode Island
The Spleen and Its Disorders

Alvin H. Schmaier MD
Robert W. Kellermeyer Professor of Hematology and Oncology, Departments of Medicine and Pathology, Case Western Reserve University, University Hospital Case Medical Center, Cleveland, Ohio
Laboratory Evaluation of Hemostatic and Thrombotic Disorders

Stanley L. Schrier MD
Professor of Medicine, Division of Hematology; Active Emeritus, Stanford University School of Medicine, Palo Alto, California
Red Blood Cell Enzymopathies
Extrinsic Nonimmune Hemolytic Anemias

Edward H. Schuchman PhD
Genetic Disease Foundation, Francis Crick Professor, Vice-Chairman for Research, Genetics and Genomic Sciences, Mount Sinai School of Medicine, New York, New York
Lysosomal Storage Diseases: Perspectives and Principles

Bridget Fowler Scullion PharmD, BCOP
Clinical Pharmacy Manager, Department of Pharmacy, Clinical Pharmacy Specialist, Palliative Care, Division of Adult Palliative Care, Department of Psychosocial Oncology and Palliative Care, Dana-Farber Cancer Institute, Boston, Massachusetts
Pain Management and Antiemetic Therapy in Hematologic Disorders

Kathy J. Selvaggi MD, MS
Director of Intensive Palliative Care Unit, Psychosocial Oncology and Palliative Care, Dana-Farber Cancer Institute; Assistant Professor of Medicine, Harvard Medical School, Boston, Massachusetts
Pain Management and Antiemetic Therapy in Hematologic Disorders

Montaser Shaheen MD
Assistant Professor, Department of Internal Medicine, Division of Hematology and Oncology, University of New Mexico School of Medicine, Albuquerque, New Mexico
Principles of Cytokine Signaling

Beth H. Shaz MD
Chief Medical Officer, New York Blood Center, New York, New York; Clinical Associate Professor, Department of Pathology and Laboratory Medicine, Emory University School of Medicine, Atlanta, Georgia
Human Blood Group Antigens and Antibodies
Principles of Plasma Transfusion: Plasma, Cryoprecipitate, Albumin, and Immunoglobulins

Andrea M. Sheehan MD
Assistant Professor, Department of Pathology and Immunology, Department of Pediatrics, Section of Hematology Oncology, Baylor College of Medicine, Houston, Texas
Resources for the Hematologist: Interpretive Comments and Selected Reference Values for Neonatal, Pediatric, and Adult Populations

Samuel A. Shelburne MD, PhD
Assistant Professor, Department of Infectious Diseases Infection Control and Employee Health, The University of Texas MD Anderson Cancer Center, Houston, Texas
Clinical Approach to Infections in the Compromised Host

Mark J. Shlomchik MD, PhD
Professor, Laboratory Medicine and Immunobiology, Yale University School of Medicine, New Haven, Connecticut
Tolerance and Autoimmunity

Susan B. Shurin MD
Acting Director, National Heart, Lung, and Blood Institute, Bethesda Maryland
The Spleen and Its Disorders

Leslie E. Silberstein MD
Director, Joint Program in Transfusion Medicine, Children's Hospital Boston; Director, Center for Human Cell Therapy, Boston, Massachusetts
Overview and Historical Perspective of Current Cell-Based Therapies
Preclinical Process of Cell-Based Therapies

Lev Silberstein MD, PhD
Instructor, Harvard Medical School, Center for Regenerative Medicine, Massachusetts General Hospital, Boston, Massachusetts
Hematopoietic Microenvironment

Roy L. Silverstein MD
John and Linda Mellowes Professor and Chair, Department of Medicine, Medical College of Wisconsin; Senior Scientist, Blood Research Institute of Blood Center of Wisconsin, Milwaukee, Wisconsin
Atherothrombosis

Steven R. Sloan MD, PhD
Director, Pediatric Transfusion Medicine, Joint Program in Transfusion Medicine, Department of Laboratory Medicine, Children's Hospital Boston, Boston, Massachusetts
Pediatric Transfusion Medicine

Franklin O. Smith MD
Marjory J. Johnson Endowed Chair and Professor of Pediatrics and Medicine, University of Cincinnati College of Medicine, Cincinnati Children's Hospital Medical Center, Cincinnati, Ohio
Myelodysplastic and Myeloproliferative Neoplasms in Children

James Smith BSc
McMaster University, Hamilton, Ontario, Canada
Diseases of Platelet Number: Immune Thrombocytopenia, Neonatal Alloimmune Thrombocytopenia, and Posttransfusion Purpura

Edward L. Snyder MD
Professor, Department of Laboratory Medicine, Yale University School of Medicine, New Haven, Connecticut
Transfusion Reactions to Blood and Cell Therapy Products

Gerald A. Soff MD
Director, Benign Hematology Program, Memorial Sloan-Kettering Cancer Center, New York, New York
Hematologic Manifestations of Cancer

Thomas R. Spitzer MD
Department of Medicine, Massachusetts General Hospital; Professor of Medicine, Harvard Medical School, Boston, Massachusetts
Haploidentical Hematopoietic Cell Transplantation

Martin H. Steinberg MD
Professor, Department of Medicine, Pediatrics, Pathology and Laboratory Medicine, Boston University School of Medicine; Director, Center of Excellence in Sickle Cell Disease, Boston Medical Center, Boston, Massachusetts
Pathobiology of the Human Erythrocyte and Its Hemoglobins

Wendy Stock MD
Professor of Medicine, Section of Hematology and Oncology, Department of Medicine, University of Chicago Comprehensive Cancer Center, Chicago, Illinois
Acute Lymphoblastic Leukemia in Adults

Richard M. Stone MD
Associate Professor of Medicine, Harvard Medical School; Director of Clinical Research, Adult Leukemia Program, Dana-Farber Cancer Institute, Boston, Massachusetts
Myelodysplastic Syndromes: Biology and Treatment

Jill R. Storry PhD
Associate Professor, Clinical Immunology and Transfusion Medicine, University and Regional Laboratories, Lund, Sweden
Human Blood Group Antigens and Antibodies

Ronald G. Strauss MD
Professor Emeritus, Department of Pathology and Pediatrics, University of Iowa College of Medicine, Iowa City, Iowa; Associate Medical Director, LifeSource, Institute for Transfusion Medicine, Chicago, Illinois
Principles of Neutrophil (Granulocyte) Transfusions

David F. Stroncek MD
Chief, Cell Processing Section, Department of Transfusion Medicine, Clinical Center, National Institutes of Health, Bethesda, Maryland
Human Leukocyte Antigen and Human Neutrophil Antigen Systems

Zbigniew M. Szczepiorkowski MD
Section Chief, Clinical Pathology; Director, Transfusion Medicine Service, Cellular Therapy Center, Dartmouth-Hitchcock Medical Center, Lebanon, New Hampshire
Dendritic Cell Biology

Ramon V. Tiu MD
Assistant Professor of Molecular Medicine, Department of Translational Hematology and Oncology Research, Taussig Cancer Institute, Cleveland Clinic, Cleveland, Ohio
Acquired Disorders of Red Cell, White Cell, and Platelet Production

Lisa J. Toltl BSc, PhD
Department of Medicine, McMaster University, Hamilton, Ontario, Canada
Diseases of Platelet Number: Immune Thrombocytopenia, Neonatal Alloimmune Thrombocytopenia, and Posttransfusion Purpura

Angela Toms PhD
Director of X-ray Core Facility, Department of Cancer Biology; Research Fellow, Department of Biological Chemistry and Molecular Pharmacology, Dana-Farber Cancer Institute, Harvard Medical School, Boston, Massachusetts
Protein Architecture: Relationship of Form and Function

Christopher A. Tormey MD
Assistant Professor, Department of Laboratory Medicine, Yale University School of Medicine, New Haven, Connecticut
Transfusion Reactions to Blood and Cell Therapy Products

Steven P. Treon MD, MA, PhD
Associate Professor, Department of Medicine, Harvard Medical School; Director, Bing Center for Waldenström's Macroglobulinemia, Dana-Farber Cancer Institute, Boston, Massachusetts
Waldenström Macroglobulinemia and Lymphoplasmacytic Lymphoma

Anil Tulpule MD
Associate Professor of Medicine, University of Southern California Keck School of Medicine, Los Angeles, California
Hematologic Manifestations of HIV/AIDS

Suresh Vedantham MD
Professor of Radiology and Surgery, Mallinckrodt Institute of Radiology, Washington University School of Medicine, St. Louis, Missouri
Mechanical Interventions in Arterial and Venous Thrombosis

Michael R. Verneris MD
Associate Professor of Pediatrics, Department of Pediatrics, Division of Pediatric Hematology, Oncology, and Transplantation, University of Minnesota, Minneapolis, Minnesota
Natural Killer Cell-Based Therapies

Elliott P. Vichinsky MD
Hematology and Oncology Programs, Children's Hospital, Oakland Research Institute, Oakland, California
Sickle Cell Disease: Clinical Features and Management

Ulrich H. von Andrian MD, PhD
Mallinckrodt Professor of Immunopathology, Department of Microbiology and Immunobiology, Immune Disease Institute and Division of Immunology, Harvard Medical School, Boston, Massachusetts
Hematopoietic Cell Trafficking and Chemokines

Andrew J. Wagner MD, PhD
Medical Oncologist, Department of Medical Oncology, Center for Sarcoma and Bone Oncology, Dana-Farber Cancer Institute; Assistant Professor, Department of Medicine, Harvard Medical School, Boston, Massachusetts
Anatomy and Physiology of the Gene

Ena Wang MD
Staff Scientist, Immunogenetics Laboratory, Director of Molecular Science, Department of Transfusion Medicine, Clinical Center; Associate Director of Center for Human Immunology, National Institutes of Health, Bethesda, Maryland
Human Leukocyte Antigen and Human Neutrophil Antigen Systems

Jia-huai Wang PhD
Associate Professor of Pediatrics, Departments of Medical Oncology and Cancer Biology, Dana-Farber Cancer Institute, Harvard Medical School, Boston, Massachusetts
Protein Architecture: Relationship of Form and Function

Michael Wang MD
Associate Professor, Department of Lymphoma and Myeloma, Department of Stem Cell Transplantation and Cellular Therapy, The University of Texas MD Anderson Cancer Center, Houston, Texas
Mantle Cell Lymphoma

Theodore E. Warkentin MD
Professor, Departments of Pathology and Molecular Medicine and Medicine, Michael G. DeGroote School of Medicine, McMaster University; Regional Director, Transfusion Medicine, Hamilton Regional Laboratory Medicine Program; Hematologist, Service of Clinical Hematology, Hamilton Health Sciences, Hamilton General Hospital, Hamilton, Ontario, Canada
Thrombocytopenia Caused by Platelet Destruction, Hypersplenism, or Hemodilution
Heparin-Induced Thrombocytopenia

Melissa P. Wasserstein MD
Director, Program for Inherited Metabolic Diseases; Medical Director, International Center for Types A and B Niemann Pick Disease; Associate Professor, Departments of Genetics and Genomic Sciences and Pediatrics, Mount Sinai School of Medicine, New York, New York
Lysosomal Storage Diseases: Perspectives and Principles

Michael C. Wei MD, PhD
Instructor, Division of Pediatrics, Stanford University School of Medicine, Lucile Packard Children's Hospital, Palo Alto, California
Acute Myeloid Leukemia in Children

Howard J. Weinstein MD
R. Alan Ezekowitz Professor of Pediatrics, Department of Pediatrics, Harvard Medical School; Chief, Pediatric Hematology and Oncology, Massachusetts General Hospital, Boston, Massachusetts
Acute Myeloid Leukemia in Children

Daniel J. Weisdorf MD
Professor of Medicine; Director, Adult Blood and Marrow Transplant Program, University of Minnesota, Minneapolis, Minnesota
Complications After Hematopoietic Stem Cell Transplantation

Jeffrey I. Weitz MD
Professor of Medicine and Biochemistry, McMaster University; HSFO/J.F. Mustard Chair in Cardiovascular Research; Canada Research Chair (Tier 1) in Thrombosis; Executive Director, Thrombosis & Atherosclerosis Research Institute, Hamilton, Ontario, Canada
Overview of Hemostasis and Thrombosis
Hypercoagulable States
Acute Coronary Syndromes
Antithrombotic Drugs

Connie M. Westhoff PhD, SBB
Department of Immunohematology and Genomics, New York Blood Center, New York, New York; Adjunct Associate Professor, Division of Transfusion Medicine, University of Pennsylvania, Philadelphia, Pennsylvania
Human Blood Group Antigens and Antibodies

James S. Wiley MD
Principal Research Fellow, Florey Neuroscience Institutes, University of Melbourne, Victoria, Australia
Heme Biosynthesis and Its Disorders: Porphyrias and Sideroblastic Anemias

David A. Williams MD
Chief, Department of Hematology and Oncology, Children's Hospital Boston; Leland Fikes Professor of Pediatrics, Harvard Medical School, Boston, Massachusetts
Principles of Cell-Based Genetic Therapies

Wyndham H. Wilson MD, PhD
Senior Investigator, Center for Cancer Research, National Cancer Institute, National Institutes of Health, Bethesda, Maryland
Diagnosis and Treatment of Diffuse Large B-Cell Lymphoma and Burkitt Lymphoma

Joanne Wolfe MD
Division Chief, Pediatric Palliative Care, Department of Psychosocial Oncology and Palliative Care, Dana-Farber Cancer Institute; Director, Pediatric Palliative Care, Department of Medicine, Children's Hospital Boston; Associate Professor of Pediatrics, Harvard Medical School, Boston, Massachusetts
Palliative Care

Lucia R. Wolgast MD
Assistant Professor, Department of Pathology, Albert Einstein College of Medicine, Montefiore Medical Center, Bronx, New York
Antiphospholipid Syndrome

Deborah Wood BSMT (ASCP)
Project Manager, Production Assistance for Cellular Therapies Coordinating Center, The EMMES Corporation, Rockville, Maryland
Preclinical Process of Cell-Based Therapies

YanYun Wu MD, PhD
Associate Professor, Department of Laboratory Medicine, Yale School of Medicine, New Haven, Connecticut
Transfusion Reactions to Blood and Cell Therapy Products

Donald L. Yee MD
Associate Professor, Department of Pediatrics, Baylor College of Medicine, Houston, Texas
Resources for the Hematologist: Interpretive Comments and Selected Reference Values for Neonatal, Pediatric, and Adult Populations

Ken H. Young MD
Associate Professor, Department of Hematopathology, The University of Texas MD Anderson Cancer Center, Houston, Texas
Mantle Cell Lymphoma

Neal S. Young MD
Chief, Hematology Branch, National Heart, Lung, and Blood Institute; Director, Center for Human Immunology, Autoimmunity, and Inflammation, National Institutes of Health, Bethesda, Maryland
Aplastic Anemia

Steven R. Zeldenrust MD, PhD
Assistant Professor of Medicine, College of Medicine, Cons-Hematology, Mayo Clinic, Rochester, Minnesota
Immunoglobulin Light-Chain Amyloidosis (Primary Amyloidosis)

Liang Zhang MD
Instructor, Department of Lymphoma and Myeloma, The University of Texas MD Anderson Cancer Center, Houston, Texas
Mantle Cell Lymphoma

Ming-Ming Zhou PhD
Dr. Harold and Golden Lamport Professor and Chairman, Department of Structural and Chemical Biology; Co-Director, Experimental Therapeutics Institute, Mount Sinai School of Medicine, New York, New York
Protein Architecture: Relationship of Form and Function

PREFACE

Welcome to the sixth edition of *Hematology: Basic Principles and Practice*. This book has evolved over the past 2.5 decades and represents the collective efforts of the editorial team, which has focused on this book being informative, user friendly, and scholarly. The central hypothesis driving each edition remains unchanged—our belief that up-to-date knowledge of the ever-evolving science of hematology is essential to provide superior care to patients with blood disorders and that high-quality bench research into the pathogenesis of these disorders depends on an intimate understanding of the clinical manifestations of these diseases.

To meet these lofty ambitions, the educational team has continued to evolve. Three editors from the previous edition, Drs. Bruce Furie, Sanford J. Shattil, and Phillip G. McGlave, elected not to participate in this edition. The Editorial Board owes each of these individuals a debt of gratitude. Bruce and Sandy served as editors of the sections dealing with thrombosis and hemostasis for each of the previous five editions. Phil created the section on stem cell transplantation. The efforts and vision of each of these individuals have clearly been an important source of strength for this book. Dr. Jeffrey I. Weitz is the new editor for the sections dealing with thrombosis and hemostasis. Jeff is a professor of medicine and biochemistry at McMaster University and executive director of the Thrombosis and Atherosclerosis Research Institute in Hamilton, Ontario. He also holds the Canada Research Chair (Tier 1) in thrombosis as well as the Heart and Stroke Foundation of Ontario-Fraser Mustard Chair in Cardiovascular Research. He has modified the sections on thrombosis and hemostasis to meet the challenges encountered by clinicians and research scientists in 2013 while maintaining the high standards set by Drs. Shattil and Furie.

Dr. Helen Heslop from the Baylor College of Medicine has expanded her efforts in this edition. She has refocused and edited the section dealing with stem cell transplantation. Helen is intimately involved in efforts in both clinical and experimental stem cell transplantation and is uniquely suited to enhance the platform created by Dr. McGlave.

Dr. John Anastasi from the University of Chicago is now a full member of our editorial team. During development of the previous edition, he assisted in selecting images for many of the chapters, but he now plays a much larger role, enhancing the hematopathology sections of the numerous chapters dealing with cellular aspects of hematology.

During the past decades, medical publishing has undergone revolutionary changes, which have become possible with the increased availability and access to the Internet. In the sixth edition, *Hematology: Basic Principles and Practice* has capitalized on this new format. Although a print edition of the book will continue to be available, we expect that a growing number of readers will use the electronic version. We hope that the availability of these two formats will meet the needs of every reader and provide them with the desired information in a fashion with which they are most comfortable. To keep the edition updated, supplemental information will be provided through Internet access so that readers can remain informed.

Each one of us continues to enjoy the challenges that we have encountered in preparing this comprehensive textbook for our readership. We hope that this new edition continues to meet the expectations and growing needs of our readership.

Ronald Hoffman, MD
Edward J. Benz, Jr., MD
Leslie E. Silberstein, MD
Helen E. Heslop, MD
Jeffrey I. Weitz, MD
John Anastasi, MD

CONTENTS

HEMATOLOGY

BASIC PRINCIPLES AND PRACTICE

PART I

Molecular and Cellular Basis of Hematology

CHAPTER 1

ANATOMY AND PHYSIOLOGY OF THE GENE

Andrew J. Wagner, Nancy Berliner, and Edward J. Benz, Jr.

Normal blood cells have limited life spans; they must be replenished in precise numbers by a continuously renewing population of progenitor cells. Homeostasis of the blood requires that proliferation of these cells be efficient yet strictly constrained. Many distinctive types of mature blood cells must arise from these progenitors by a controlled process of commitment to, and execution of, complex programs of differentiation. Thus, developing red blood cells must produce large quantities of hemoglobin but not the myeloperoxidase characteristic of granulocytes, the immunoglobulins characteristic of lymphocytes, or the fibrinogen receptors characteristic of platelets. Similarly, the maintenance of normal amounts of coagulant and anticoagulant proteins in the circulation requires exquisitely regulated production, destruction, and interaction of the components. Understanding the basic biologic principles underlying cell growth, differentiation, and protein biosynthesis requires a thorough knowledge of the structure and regulated expression of genes because the gene is now known to be the fundamental unit by which biologic information is stored, transmitted, and expressed in a regulated fashion.

Genes were originally characterized as mathematical units of inheritance. They are now known to consist of molecules of deoxyribonucleic acid (DNA). By virtue of their ability to store information in the form of nucleotide sequences, to transmit it by means of semiconservative replication to daughter cells during mitosis and meiosis, and to express it by directing the incorporation of amino acids into proteins, DNA molecules are the chemical transducers of genetic information flow. Efforts to understand the biochemical means by which this transduction is accomplished have given rise to the discipline of molecular genetics.

THE GENETIC VIEW OF THE BIOSPHERE: THE CENTRAL DOGMA OF MOLECULAR BIOLOGY

The fundamental premise of the molecular biologist is that the magnificent diversity encountered in nature is ultimately governed by genes. The capacity of genes to exert this control is in turn determined by relatively simple stereochemical rules, first appreciated by Watson and Crick in the 1950s. These rules constrain the types of interactions that can occur between two molecules of DNA or ribonucleic acid (RNA).

DNA and RNA are linear polymers consisting of four types of nucleotide subunits. Proteins are linear unbranched polymers consisting of 21 types of amino acid subunits. Each amino acid is distinguished from the others by the chemical nature of its side chain, the moiety not involved in forming the peptide bond links of the chain. The properties of cells, tissues, and organisms depend largely on the aggregate structures and properties of their proteins. The central dogma of molecular biology states that genes control these properties by controlling the structures of proteins, the timing and amount of their production, and the coordination of their synthesis with that of other proteins. The information needed to achieve these ends is transmitted by a class of nucleic acid molecules called RNA. Genetic information thus flows in the direction DNA → RNA → protein. This central dogma provides, in principle, a universal approach for investigating the biologic properties and behavior of any given cell, tissue, or organism by study of the controlling genes. Methods permitting direct manipulation of DNA sequences should then be universally applicable to the study of all living entities. Indeed, the power of the molecular genetic approach lies in the universality of its utility.

One exception to the central dogma of molecular biology that is especially relevant to hematologists is the storage of genetic information in RNA molecules in certain viruses, notably the retroviruses associated with T-cell leukemia and lymphoma and the human immunodeficiency virus. When retroviruses enter the cell, the RNA genome is copied into a DNA replica by an enzyme called *reverse transcriptase*. This DNA representation of the viral genome is then expressed according to the rules of the central dogma. Retroviruses thus represent a variation on the theme rather than a true exception to or violation of the rules.

ANATOMY AND PHYSIOLOGY OF GENES

DNA Structure

DNA molecules are extremely long, unbranched polymers of nucleotide subunits. Each nucleotide contains a sugar moiety called deoxyribose, a phosphate group attached to the 5′ carbon position, and a purine or pyrimidine base attached to the 1′ position (Fig. 1-1). The linkages in the chain are formed by phosphodiester bonds between the 5′ position of each sugar residue and the 3′ position of the adjacent residue in the chain (see Fig. 1-1). The sugar phosphate links form the backbone of the polymer, from which the purine or pyrimidine bases project perpendicularly.

The haploid human genome consists of 23 long, double-stranded DNA molecules tightly complexed with histones and other nuclear proteins to form compact linear structures called *chromosomes*. The genome contains 3 billion nucleotides; each chromosome is thus 50 to 200 million bases in length. The individual genes are aligned along each chromosome. The human genome contains about 30,000 genes. Blood cells, similar to most somatic cells, are diploid. That is, each chromosome is present in two copies, so there are 46 chromosomes consisting of approximately 6 billion base pairs (bp) of DNA.

The four nucleotide bases in DNA are the purines (adenosine and guanosine) and the pyrimidines (thymine and cytosine). The basic chemical configuration of the other nucleic acid found in cells, RNA, is quite similar except that the sugar is ribose (having a hydroxyl group attached to the 2′ carbon rather than the hydrogen found in deoxyribose) and the pyrimidine base uracil is used in place of thymine. The bases are commonly referred to by a shorthand notation: the letters A, C, T, G, and U are used to refer to adenosine, cytosine, thymine, guanosine, and uracil, respectively.

The ends of DNA and RNA strands are chemically distinct because of the 3′ → 5′ phosphodiester bond linkage that ties adjacent bases together (see Fig. 1-1). One end of the strand (the 3′ end) has an unlinked (free at the 3′ carbon) sugar position and the other (the 5′ end) has a free 5′ position. There is thus a polarity to the sequence of bases in a DNA strand: the same sequence of bases read in a 3′ → 5′ direction carries a different meaning than if read in a 5′ → 3′ direction. Cellular enzymes can thus distinguish one end of a

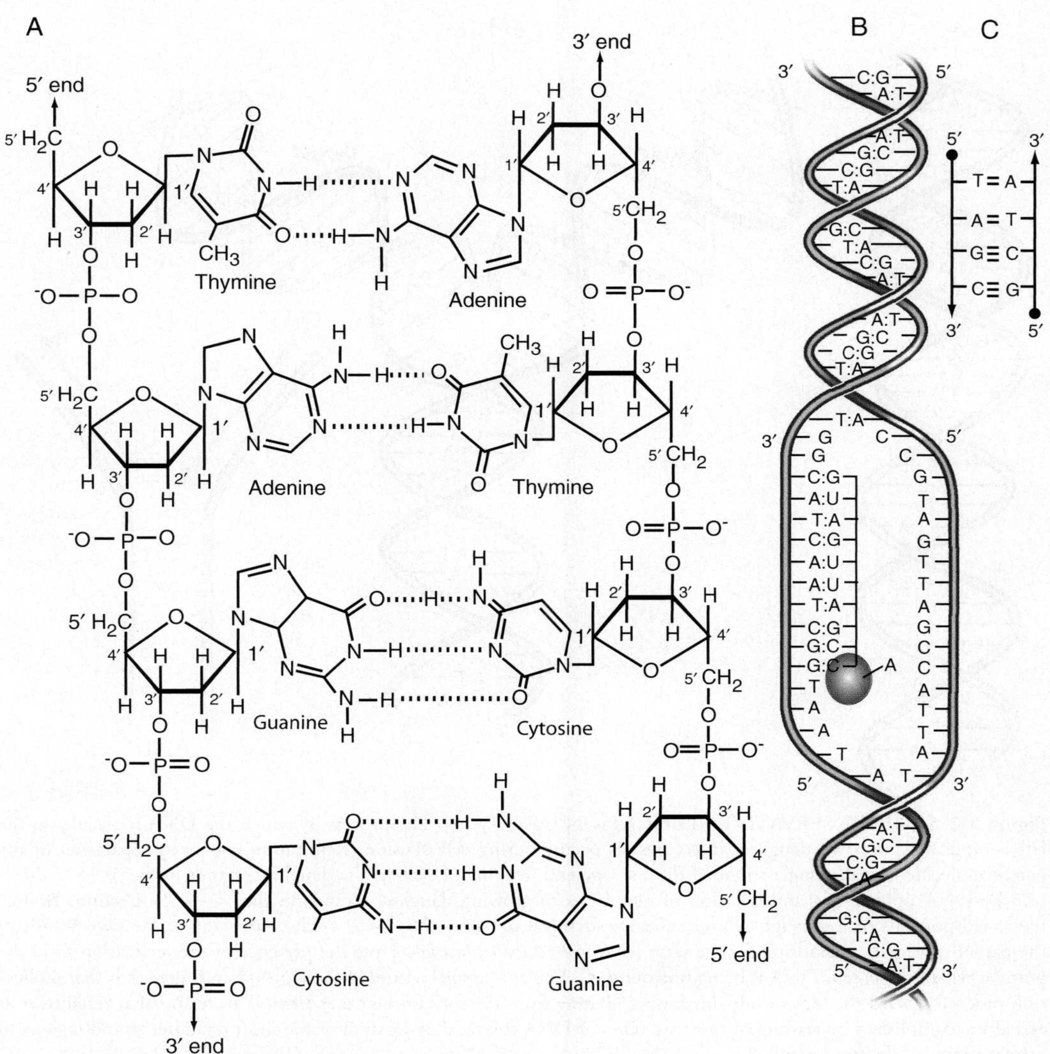

Figure 1-1 STRUCTURE, BASE PAIRING, POLARITY, AND TEMPLATE PROPERTIES OF DNA. **A,** Structures of the four nitrogenous bases projecting from sugar phosphate backbones. The hydrogen bonds between them form base pairs holding complementary strands of DNA together. Note that whereas A–T and T–A base pairs have only two hydrogen bonds, C–G and G–C pairs have three. **B,** The double helical structure of DNA results from base pairing of strands to form a double-stranded molecule with the backbones on the outside and the hydrogen-bonded bases stacked in the middle. Also shown schematically is the separation (unwinding) of a region of the helix by mRNA polymerase, which is shown using one of the strands as a template for the synthesis of an mRNA precursor molecule. Note that new bases added to the growing RNA strand obey the rules of Watson-Crick base pairing (see text). Uracil (U) in RNA replaces T in DNA and, like T, forms base pairs with A. **C,** Diagram of the antiparallel nature of the strands, based on the stereochemical 3′ → 5′ polarity of the strands. The chemical differences between reading along the backbone in the 5′ → 3′ and 3′ → 5′ directions can be appreciated by reference to part **A.** *A,* Adenosine; *C,* cytosine; *G,* guanosine; *T,* thymine.

nucleic acid from the other; most enzymes that "read" the DNA sequence tend to do so only in one direction (3′ → 5′ or 5′ → 3′ but not both). Most nucleic acid–synthesizing enzymes, for instance, add new bases to the strand in a 5′ → 3′ direction.

The ability of DNA molecules to store information resides in the sequence of nucleotide bases arrayed along the polymer chain. Under the physiologic conditions in living cells, DNA is thermodynamically most stable when two strands coil around each other to form a double-stranded helix. The strands are aligned in an "antiparallel" direction, having opposite 3′ → 5′ polarity (see Fig. 1-1). The DNA strands are held together by hydrogen bonds between the bases on one strand and the bases on the opposite (complementary) strand. The stereochemistry of these interactions allows bonds to form between the two strands only when adenine on one strand pairs with thymine at the same position of the opposite strand, or guanine with cytosine—the Watson-Crick rules of base pairing. Two strands joined together in compliance with these rules are said to have "complementary" base sequences.

These thermodynamic rules imply that the sequence of bases along one DNA strand immediately dictates the sequence of bases that must be present along the complementary strand in the double helix. For example, whenever an A occurs along one strand, a T must be present at that exact position on the opposite strand; a G must always be paired with a C, a T with an A, and a C with a G. In RNA–RNA or RNA–DNA double-stranded molecules, U–A base pairs replace T–A pairs.

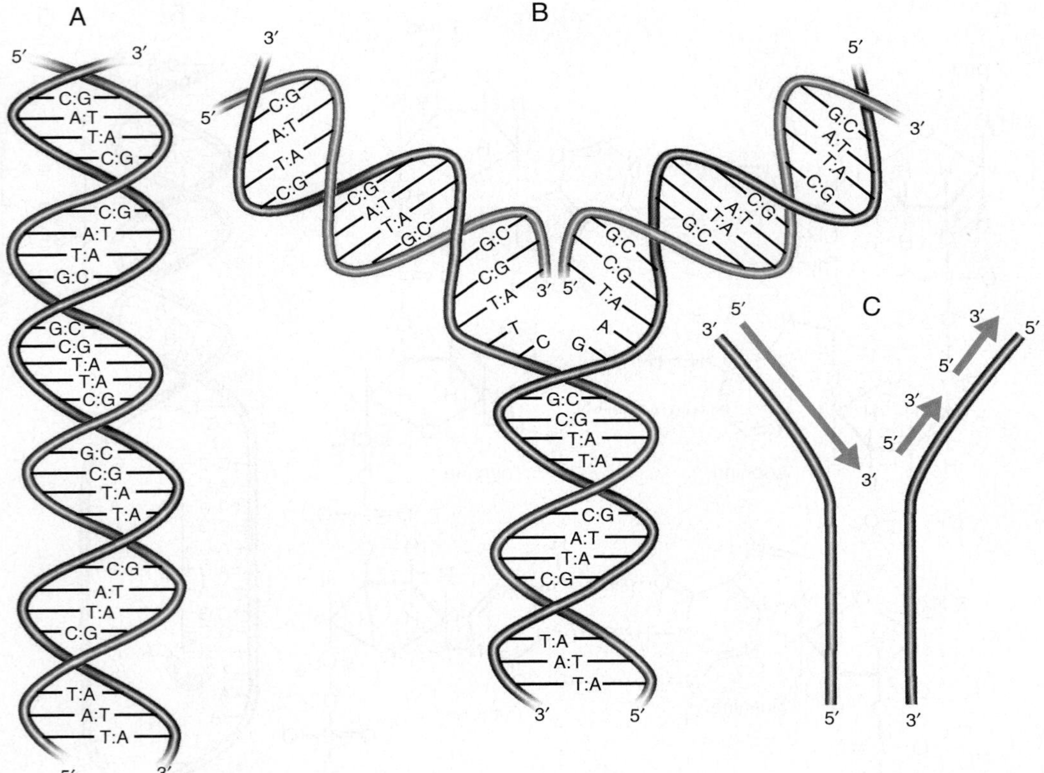

Figure 1-2 SEMICONSERVATIVE REPLICATION OF DNA. **A,** The process by which the DNA molecule on the left is replicated into two daughter molecules, as occurs during cell division. Replication occurs by separation of the parent molecule into the single-stranded form at one end, reading of each of the daughter strands in the 3′ → 5′ direction by DNA polymerase, and addition of new bases to growing daughter strands in the 5′ → 3′ direction. **B,** The replicated portions of the daughter molecules are identical to each other *(red)*. Each carries one of the two strands of the parent molecule, accounting for the term *semiconservative replication.* Note the presence of the replication fork, the point at which the parent DNA is being unwound. **C,** The antiparallel nature of the DNA strands demands that replication proceed toward the fork in one direction and away from the fork in the other *(red)*. This means that replication is actually accomplished by reading of short stretches of DNA followed by ligation of the short daughter strand regions to form an intact daughter strand.

STORAGE AND TRANSMISSION OF GENETIC INFORMATION

The rules of Watson-Crick base pairing apply to DNA–RNA, RNA–RNA, and DNA–DNA double-stranded molecules. Enzymes that replicate or polymerize DNA and RNA molecules obey the base-pairing rules. By using an existing strand of DNA or RNA as the template, a new (daughter) strand is copied (transcribed) by reading processively along the base sequence of the template strand, adding to the growing strand at each position only that base that is complementary to the corresponding base in the template according to the Watson-Crick rules. Thus, a DNA strand having the base sequence 5′-GCTATG-3′ could be copied by DNA polymerase only into a daughter strand having the sequence 3′-CGATAC-5′. Note that the sequence of the template strand provides all the information needed to predict the nucleotide sequence of the complementary daughter strand. Genetic information is thus stored in the form of base-paired nucleotide sequences.

If a double-stranded DNA molecule is separated into its two component strands and each strand is then used as a template to synthesize a new daughter strand, the product will be two double-stranded daughter DNA molecules, each identical to the original parent molecule. This semiconservative replication process is exactly what occurs during mitosis and meiosis as cell division proceeds (Fig. 1-2). The rules of Watson-Crick base pairing thus provide for the faithful transmission of exact copies of the cellular genome to subsequent generations.

EXPRESSION OF GENETIC INFORMATION THROUGH THE GENETIC CODE AND PROTEIN SYNTHESIS

The information stored in the DNA base sequence achieves its impact on the structure, function, and behavior of organisms by governing the structures, timing, and amounts of protein synthesized in the cells. The primary structure (i.e., the amino acid sequence) of each protein determines its three-dimensional conformation and therefore properties (e.g., shape, enzymatic activity, ability to interact with other molecules, stability). In the aggregate, these proteins control cell structure and metabolism. The process by which DNA achieves its control of cells through protein synthesis is called *gene expression.*

An outline of the basic pathway of gene expression in eukaryotic cells is shown in Fig. 1-3. The DNA base sequence is first copied into an RNA molecule, called *premessenger RNA,* by messenger RNA (mRNA) polymerase. Premessenger RNA has a base sequence identical to the DNA coding strand. Genes in eukaryotic species consist of tandem arrays of sequences encoding mRNA (exons); these sequences alternate with sequences (introns) present in the initial mRNA

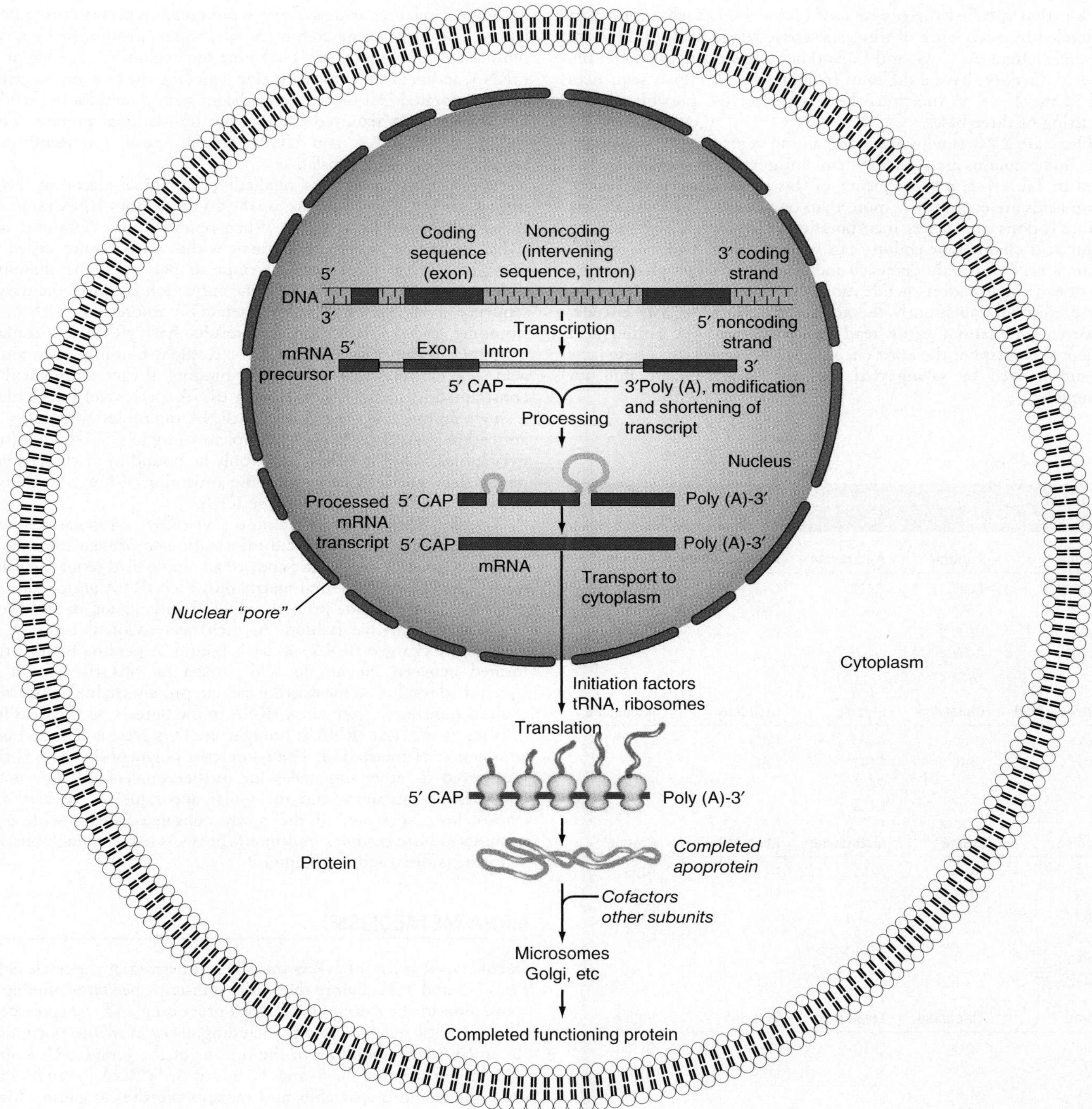

Figure 1-3 SYNTHESIS OF mRNA AND PROTEIN—THE PATHWAY OF GENE EXPRESSION. The diagram of the DNA gene shows the alternating array of exons *(red)* and introns *(shaded color)* typical of most eukaryotic genes. Transcription of the mRNA precursor, addition of the 5′-CAP and 3′-poly (A) tail, splicing and excision of introns, transport to the cytoplasm through the nuclear pores, translation into the amino acid sequence of the apoprotein, and posttranslational processing of the protein are described in the text. Translation proceeds from the initiator methionine codon near the 5′ end of the mRNA, with incorporation of the amino terminal end of the protein. As the mRNA is read in a 5′ → 3′ direction, the nascent polypeptide is assembled in an amino → carboxyl terminal direction.

transcript (premessenger RNA) but absent from the mature mRNA. The entire gene is transcribed into the large precursor, which is then further processed (spliced) in the nucleus. The introns are excised from the final mature mRNA molecule, which is then exported to the cytoplasm to be decoded (translated) into the amino acid sequence of the protein by association with a biochemically complex group of ribonucleoprotein structures called *ribosomes*. Ribosomes contain two subunits: the 60S subunit contains a single, large (28S) ribosomal RNA molecule complexed with multiple proteins, and the RNA component of the 40S subunit is a smaller (18S) ribosomal RNA molecule.

Ribosomes read mRNA sequence in a ticker tape fashion three bases at a time, inserting the appropriate amino acid encoded by each three-base code word or codon into the appropriate position of the growing protein chain. This process is called *mRNA translation*. The glossary used by cells to know which amino acids are encoded by each

DNA codon is called the *genetic code* (Table 1-1). Each amino acid is encoded by a sequence of three successive bases. Because there are four code letters (A, C, G, and U) and because sequences read in the $5' \rightarrow 3'$ direction have a different biologic meaning than sequences read in the $3' \rightarrow 5'$ direction, there are 4^3, or 64, possible codons consisting of three bases.

There are 21 naturally occurring amino acids found in proteins. Thus, more codons are available than amino acids to be encoded. As noted in Table 1-1, a consequence of this redundancy is that some amino acids are encoded by more than one codon. For example, six distinct codons can specify incorporation of arginine into a growing amino acid chain, four codons can specify valine, two can specify glutamic acid, and only one each methionine or tryptophan. In no case does a single codon encode more than one amino acid. Codons thus predict unambiguously the amino acid sequence they encode. However, one cannot easily read backward from the amino acid sequence to decipher the *exact* encoding DNA sequence. These facts are summarized by saying that the code is degenerate but not ambiguous.

Table 1-1 The Genetic Code* Messenger RNA Codons for the Amino Acids

Alanine	Arginine	Asparagine	Aspartic Acid	Cysteine
5′-GCU-3′	CGU	AAU	GAU	UGU
GCC	CGC	AAC	GAC	UGC
GCA	CGA			
GCG	AGA			
	AGG			
Glutamic Acid	**Glutamine**	**Glycine**	**Histidine**	**Isoleucine**
GAA	CAA	GGU	CAU	AUU
GAG	CAG	GGC	CAC	AUC
		GGA		AUA
		GGG		
Leucine	**Lysine**	**Methionine**	**Phenylalanine**	**Proline**‡
UUA	AAA	AUG†	UUU	CCU
UUG	AAG		UUC	CCC
CUU				CCA
CUC				CCG
CUA				
CUG				
Serine	**Threonine**	**Tryptophan**	**Tyrosine**	**Valine**
UCU	ACU	UGG	UAU	GUU
UCC	ACC		UAC	GUC
UCA	ACA			GUA
UCG	ACG			GUG
AGU				
AGC				
Chain Termination§				
UAA				
UAG				
UGA				

*Note that most of the degeneracy in the code is in the third base position (e.g., lysine, AA[G or C]; asparagine, AA[C or U]; valine GUN [where N is any base]).
†AUG is also used as the chain-initiation codon when surrounded by the Kozak consensus sequence.
‡Hydroxyproline, the 21st amino acid, is generated by posttranslational modification of proline. It is almost exclusively confined to collagen subunits.
§The codons that signal the end of translation, also called nonsense or termination codons, are described by their nicknames *amber* (UAG), *ochre* (UAA), and *opal* (UGA).

Some specialized codons serve as punctuation points during translation. The methionine codon (AUG), when surrounded by a consensus sequence (the Kozak box) near the beginning (5′ end) of the mRNA, serves as the initiator codon signaling the first amino acid to be incorporated. All proteins thus begin with a methionine residue, but this is often removed later in the translational process. Three codons, UAG, UAA, and UGA, serve as translation terminators, signaling the end of translation.

The adaptor molecules mediating individual decoding events during mRNA translation are small (40 bases long) RNA molecules called *transfer RNAs* (tRNAs). When bound into a ribosome, each tRNA exposes a three-base segment within its sequence called the *anticodon*. These three bases attempt to pair with the three-base codon exposed on the mRNA. If the anticodon is complementary in sequence to the codon, a stable interaction among the mRNA, the ribosome, and the tRNA molecule results. Each tRNA also contains a separate region that is adapted for covalent binding to an amino acid. The enzymes that catalyze the binding of each amino acid are constrained in such a way that each tRNA species can bind only to a single amino acid. For example, tRNA molecules containing the anticodon 3′-AAA-5′, which is complementary to a 5′-UUU-3′ (phenylalanine) codon in mRNA, can only be bound to or charged with phenylalanine; tRNA containing the anticodon 3′-UAG-5′ can only be charged with isoleucine, and so forth.

Transfer RNAs and their amino acyl tRNA synthetases provide for the coupling of nucleic acid information to protein information needed to convert the genetic code to an amino acid sequence. Ribosomes provide the structural matrix on which tRNA anticodons and mRNA codons become properly exposed and aligned in an orderly, linear, and sequential fashion. As each new codon is exposed, the appropriate charged tRNA species is bound. A peptide bond is then formed between the amino acid carried by this tRNA and the C-terminal residue on the existing nascent protein chain. The growing chain is transferred to the new tRNA in the process, so that it is held in place as the next tRNA is brought in. This cycle is repeated until completion of translation. The completed polypeptide chain is then transferred to other organelles for further processing (e.g., to the endoplasmic reticulum and the Golgi apparatus) or released into cytosol for association of the newly completed chain with other subunits to form complex multimeric proteins (e.g., hemoglobin) and so forth, as discussed in Chapter 3.

mRNA METABOLISM

In eukaryotic cells, mRNA is initially synthesized in the nucleus (see Figs. 1-3 and 1-4). Before the initial transcript becomes suitable for translation in the cytoplasm, mRNA processing and transport occur by a complex series of events including excision of the portions of the mRNA corresponding to the introns of the gene (mRNA splicing), modification of the 5′ and 3′ ends of the mRNA to render them more stable and translatable, and transport to the cytoplasm. Moreover, the amount of any particular mRNA moiety in both prokaryotic and eukaryotic cells is governed not only by the composite rate of mRNA synthesis (transcription, processing, and transport) but also by its degradation by cytoplasmic ribonucleases (RNA degradation). Many mRNA species of special importance in hematology (e.g., mRNAs for growth factors and their receptors, proto-oncogene mRNAs, acute-phase reactants) are exquisitely regulated by control of their stability (half-life) in the cytoplasm.

Posttranscriptional mRNA metabolism is complex. Only a few relevant details are considered in this section.

mRNA Splicing

The initial transcript of eukaryotic genes contains several subregions (see Fig. 1-4). Most striking is the tandem alignment of exons and introns. Precise excision of intron sequences and ligation of exons is critical for production of mature mRNA. This process is called

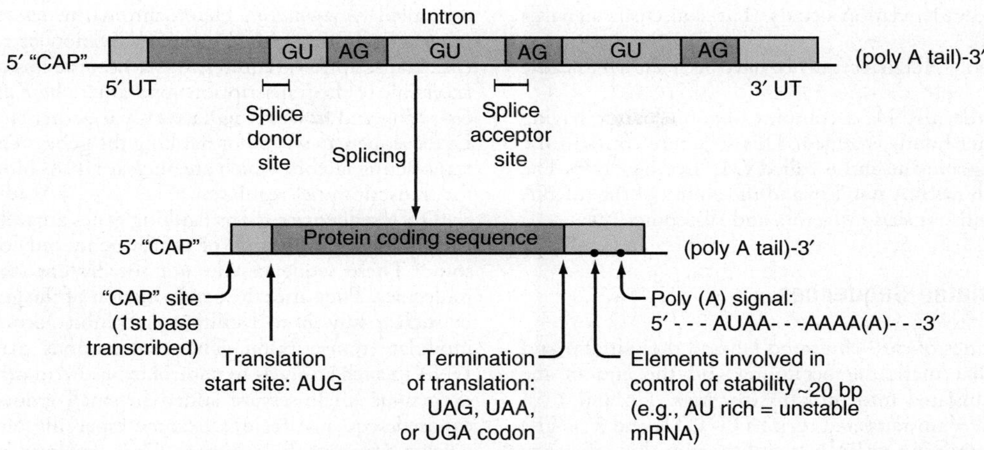

Figure 1-4 ANATOMY OF THE PRODUCTS OF THE STRUCTURAL GENE (mRNA PRECURSOR AND mRNA). This schematic shows the configuration of the critical anatomic elements of an mRNA precursor, which represents the primary copy of the structural portion of the gene. The sequences GU and AG indicate, respectively, the invariant dinucleotides present in the donor and acceptor sites at which introns are spliced out of the precursor. Not shown are the less stringently conserved consensus sequences that must precede and succeed each of these sites for a short distance.

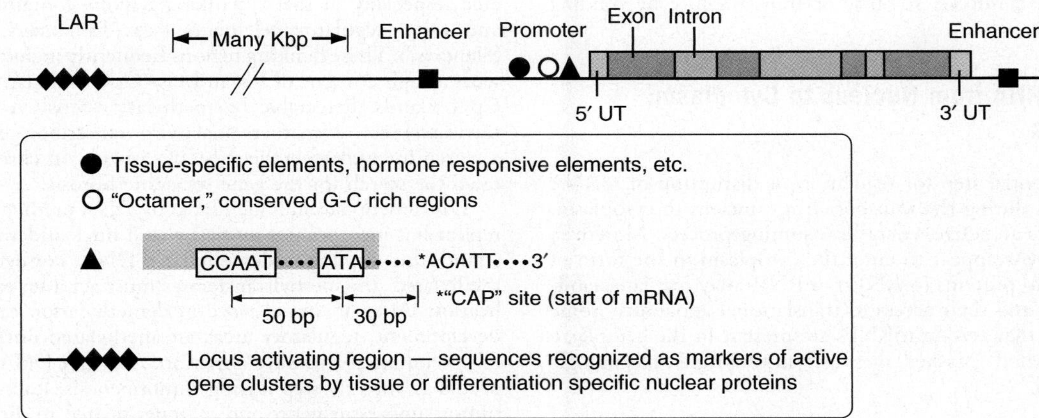

Figure 1-5 Regulatory elements flanking the structural gene.

mRNA splicing, and it occurs on complexes of small nuclear RNAs and proteins called snRNPs; the term *spliceosome* is also used to describe the intranuclear organelle that mediates mRNA splicing reactions. The biochemical mechanism for splicing is complex. A consensus sequence, which includes the dinucleotide GU, is recognized as the donor site at the 5′ end of the intron (5′ end refers to the polarity of the mRNA strand coding for protein); a second consensus sequence ending in the dinucleotide AG is recognized as the acceptor site, which marks the distal end of the intron (see Figs. 1-4 and 1-5). The spliceosome recognizes the donor and acceptor and forms an intermediate lariat structure that provides for both excision of the intron and proper alignment of the cut ends of the two exons for ligation in precise register.

Messenger RNA splicing has proved to be an important mechanism for greatly increasing the versatility and diversity of expression of a single gene. For example, some genes contain an array of more exons than are actually found in any mature mRNA species encoded by that gene. Several different mRNA and protein products can arise from a single gene by selective inclusion or exclusion of individual exons from the mature mRNA products. This phenomenon is called *alternative mRNA splicing*. It permits a single gene to code for multiple mRNA and protein products with related but distinct structures and functions. The mechanisms by which individual exons are selected or rejected remain obscure. For present purposes, it is sufficient to note that important physiologic changes in cells can be regulated by altering the patterns of mRNA splicing products arising from single genes.

Many inherited hematologic diseases arise from mutations that derange mRNA splicing. For example, some of the most common forms of the thalassemia syndromes and hemophilia arise by mutations that alter normal splicing signals or create splicing signals where they normally do not exist (activation of cryptic splice sites).

Modification of the Ends of the mRNA Molecule

Most eukaryotic mRNA species are polyadenylated at their 3′ ends. mRNA precursors are initially synthesized as large molecules that extend farther downstream from the 3′ end of the mature mRNA molecule. Polyadenylation results in the addition of stretches of 100 to 150 A residues at the 3′ end. Such an addition is often called the *poly-A tail* and is of variable length. Polyadenylation facilitates rapid early cleavage of the unwanted 3′ sequences from the transcript and is also important for stability or transport of the mRNA out of the nucleus. Signals near the 3′ extremity of the mature mRNA mark positions at which polyadenylation occurs. The consensus signal is AUAAA (see Fig. 1-4).

Mutations in the poly-A signal sequence have been shown to cause thalassemia.

At the 5′ end of the mRNA, a complex oligonucleotide having unusual phosphodiester bonds is added. This structure contains the nucleotide 7-methyl-guanosine and is called *CAP* (see Fig. 1-4). The 5′-CAP enhances both mRNA stability and the ability of the mRNA to interact with protein translation factors and ribosomes.

5′ and 3′ Untranslated Sequences

The 5′ and 3′ extremities of mRNA extend beyond the initiator and terminator codons that mark the beginning and the end of the sequences actually translated into proteins (see Figs. 1-4 and 1-5). These so-called 5′ and 3′ untranslated regions (5′ UTR and 3′ UTR) are involved in determining mRNA stability and the efficiency with which mRNA species can be translated. For example, if the 3′ UTR of a very stable mRNA (e.g., globin mRNA) is swapped with the 3′ UTR of a highly unstable mRNA (e.g., the c-myc proto-oncogene), the c-myc mRNA becomes more stable. Conversely, attachment of the 3′ UTR of c-myc to a globin molecule renders it unstable. Instability is often associated with repeated sequences rich in A and U in the 3′ UTR (see Fig. 1-4). Similarly, the UTRs in mRNAs coding for proteins involved in iron metabolism mediate altered mRNA stability or translatability by binding iron-laden proteins.

Transport of mRNA from Nucleus to Cytoplasm: mRNP Particles

An additional potential step for regulation or disruption of mRNA metabolism occurs during the transport from nucleus to cytoplasm. mRNA transport is an active, energy-consuming process. Moreover, at least some mRNAs appear to enter the cytoplasm in the form of complexes bound to proteins (mRNPs). mRNPs may regulate stability of the mRNAs and their access to translational apparatus. Some evidence indicates that certain mRNPs are present in the cytoplasm but are not translated (masked message) until proper physiologic signals are received.

GENE REGULATION

Virtually all cells of an organism receive a complete copy of the DNA genome inherited at the time of conception. The panoply of distinct cell types and tissues found in any complex organism is possible only because different portions of the genome are selectively expressed or repressed in each cell type. Each cell must "know" which genes to express, how actively to express them, and when to express them. This biologic necessity has come to be known as *gene regulation* or *regulated gene expression*. Understanding gene regulation provides insight into how pluripotent stem cells determine that they will express the proper sets of genes in daughter progenitor cells that differentiate along each lineage. Major hematologic disorders (e.g., the leukemias and lymphomas), immunodeficiency states, and myeloproliferative syndromes result from derangements in the system of gene regulation. An understanding of the ways that genes are selected for expression thus remains one of the major frontiers of biology and medicine.

EPIGENETIC REGULATION OF GENE EXPRESSION

Most of the DNA in living cells is inactivated by formation of a nucleoprotein complex called *chromatin*. The histone and nonhistone proteins in chromatin effectively sequester genes from enzymes needed for expression. The most tightly compacted chromatin regions are called *euchromatin*. Heterochromatin, less tightly packed, contains actively transcribed genes. Activation of a gene for expression (i.e., transcription) requires that it become less compacted and more accessible to the transcription apparatus. These processes involve both cis-acting and trans-acting factors. Cis-acting elements are regulatory DNA sequences within or flanking the genes. They are recognized by trans-acting factors, which are nuclear DNA–binding proteins needed for transcriptional regulation.

DNA sequence regions flanking genes are called *cis*-acting because they influence expression of nearby genes only on the same chromosome. These sequences do not usually encode mRNA or protein molecules. They alter the conformation of the gene within chromatin in such a way as to facilitate or inhibit access to the factors that modulate transcription. These interactions may twist or kink the DNA in such a way as to control exposure to other molecules. When exogenous nucleases are added in small amounts to nuclei, these exposed sequence regions become especially sensitive to the DNA-cutting action of the nucleases. Thus, nuclease-hypersensitive sites in DNA have come to be appreciated as markers for regions in or near genes that are interacting with regulatory nuclear proteins.

Methylation is another structural feature that can be used to recognize differences between actively transcribed and inactive genes. Most eukaryotic DNA is heavily methylated, that is, the DNA is modified by the addition of a methyl group to the 5 position of the cytosine pyrimidine ring (5-methyl-C). In general, whereas heavily methylated genes are inactive, active genes are relatively hypomethylated, especially in the 5′ flanking regions containing the promoter and other regulatory elements (see "Enhancers, Promoters, and Silencers"). These flanking regions frequently include DNA sequences with a high content of Cs and Gs (CpG islands). Hypomethylated CpG islands (detectable by methylation-sensitive restriction endonucleases) serve as markers of actively transcribed genes. For example, a search for undermethylated CpG islands on chromosome 7 facilitated the search for the gene for cystic fibrosis.

DNA methylation is facilitated by DNA methyltransferases. DNA replication incorporates unmethylated nucleotides into each nascent strand, thus leading to demethylated DNA. For cytosines to become methylated, the methyltransferases must act after each round of replication. After an initial wave of demethylation early in embryonic development, regulatory areas are methylated during various stages of development and differentiation. Aberrant DNA methylation also occurs as an early step during tumorigenesis, leading to silencing of tumor suppressor genes and of genes related to differentiation. This finding has led to induction of DNA demethylation as a target in cancer therapy. Indeed, 5-azacytidine, a cytidine analog unable to be methylated, and the related compound decitabine, are approved by the United States Food and Drug Administration for use in myelodysplastic syndromes, and their use in cases of other malignancies is being investigated.

Although it is poorly understood how particular regions of DNA are targeted for methylation, it is becoming increasingly apparent that this modification targets further alterations in chromatin proteins that in turn influence gene expression. Histone acetylation, phosphorylation, and methylation of the *N*-terminal tail are currently the focus of intense study. Acetylation of lysine residues (catalyzed by histone acetyltransferases), for example, is associated with transcriptional activation. Conversely, histone deacetylation (catalyzed by histone deacetylase) leads to gene silencing. Histone deacetylases are recruited to areas of DNA methylation by DNA methyltransferases and by methyl–DNA-binding proteins, thus linking DNA methylation to histone deacetylation. Drugs inhibiting these enzymes are being studied as anticancer agents.

The regulation of histone acetylation and deacetylation appears to be linked to gene expression, but the roles of histone phosphorylation and methylation are less well understood. Current research suggests that in addition to gene regulation, histone modifications contribute to the "epigenetic code" and are thus a means by which information regarding chromatin structure is passed to daughter cells after DNA replication occurs.

ENHANCERS, PROMOTERS, AND SILENCERS

Several types of cis-active DNA sequence elements have been defined according to the presumed consequences of their interaction with nuclear proteins (see Fig. 1-5). Promoters are found just upstream (to the 5′ side) of the start of mRNA transcription (the CAP). mRNA polymerases appear to bind first to the promoter region and thereby gain access to the structural gene sequences downstream. Promoters thus serve a dual function of being binding sites for mRNA polymerase and marking for the polymerase the downstream point at which transcription should start.

Enhancers are more complicated DNA sequence elements. Enhancers can lie on either side of a gene or even within the gene. Enhancers bind transcription factors and thereby stimulate expression of genes nearby. The domain of influence of enhancers (i.e., the number of genes to either side whose expression is stimulated) varies. Some enhancers influence only the adjacent gene; others seem to mark the boundaries of large multigene clusters (gene domains) whose coordinated expression is appropriate to a particular tissue type or a particular time. For example, the very high levels of globin gene expression in erythroid cells depend on the function of an enhancer that seems to activate the entire gene cluster and is thus called a *locus-activating region* (see Fig. 1-5). The nuclear factors interacting with enhancers are probably induced into synthesis or activation as part of the process of differentiation. Chromosomal rearrangements that place a gene that is usually tightly regulated under the control of a highly active enhancer can lead to overexpression of that gene. This commonly occurs in Burkitt lymphoma, for example, in which the MYC proto-oncogene is juxtaposed and dysregulated by an immunoglobulin enhancer.

Silencer sequences serve a function that is the obverse of enhancers. When bound by the appropriate nuclear proteins, silencer sequences cause repression of gene expression. Some evidence indicates that the same sequence elements can act as enhancers or silencers under different conditions, presumably by being bound by different sets of proteins having opposite effects on transcription. *Insulators* are sequence domains that mark the "boundaries" of multigene clusters, thereby preventing activation of one set of genes from "leaking" into nearby genes.

TRANSCRIPTION FACTORS

Transcription factors are nuclear proteins that exhibit gene-specific DNA binding. Considerable information is now available about these nuclear proteins and their biochemical properties, but their physiologic behavior remains incompletely understood. Common structural features have become apparent. Most transcription factors have DNA-binding domains sharing homologous structural motifs (cytosine-rich regions called zinc fingers, leucine-rich regions called leucine zippers, and so on), but other regions appear to be unique. Many factors implicated in the regulation of growth, differentiation, and development (e.g., homeobox genes, proto-oncogenes, antioncogenes) appear to be DNA-binding proteins and may be involved in the steps needed for activation of a gene within chromatin. Others bind to or modify DNA-binding proteins. These factors are discussed in more detail in several other chapters.

REGULATION OF mRNA SPLICING, STABILITY, AND TRANSLATION (POSTTRANSCRIPTIONAL REGULATION)

It has become increasingly apparent that posttranscriptional and translational mechanisms are important strategies used by cells to govern the amounts of mRNA and protein accumulating when a particular gene is expressed. The major modes of posttranscriptional regulation at the mRNA level are regulated alternative mRNA splicing, control of mRNA stability, and control of translational efficiency. As discussed elsewhere (see Chapter 3), additional regulation at the protein level occurs by mechanisms modulating localization, stability, activation, or export of the protein.

A cell can regulate the relative amounts of different protein isoforms arising from a given gene by altering the relative amounts of an mRNA precursor that are spliced along one pathway or another (alternative mRNA splicing). Many striking examples of this type of regulation are known—for example, the ability of B lymphocytes to make both IgM and IgD at the same developmental stage, changes in the particular isoforms of cytoskeletal proteins produced during red blood cell differentiation, and a switch from one isoform of the *c-myb* proto-oncogene product to another during red blood cell differentiation. Abnormalities in mRNA splicing due to mutations at the splice sites can lead to defective protein synthesis, as can occur in B-globin leading to a form of B-thalassemia. The effect of controlling the pathway of mRNA processing used in a cell is to include or exclude portions of the mRNA sequence. These portions encode peptide sequences that influence the ultimate physiologic behavior of the protein, or the RNA sequences that alter stability or translatability.

The importance of the control of mRNA stability for gene regulation is being increasingly appreciated. The steady-state level of any given mRNA species ultimately depends on the balance between the rate of its production (transcription and mRNA processing) and its destruction. One means by which stability is regulated is the inherent structure of the mRNA sequence, especially the 3′ and 5′ UTRs. As already noted, these sequences appear to affect mRNA secondary structure, recognition by nucleases, or both. Different mRNAs thus have inherently longer or shorter half-lives, almost regardless of the cell type in which they are expressed. Some mRNAs tend to be highly unstable. In response to appropriate physiologic needs, they can thus be produced quickly and removed from the cell quickly when a need for them no longer exists. Globin mRNA, on the other hand, is inherently quite stable, with a half-life measured in the range of 15 to 50 hours. This is appropriate for the need of reticulocytes to continue to synthesize globin for 24 to 48 hours after the ability to synthesize new mRNA has been lost by the terminally mature erythroblasts.

The stability of mRNA can also be altered in response to changes in the intracellular milieu. This phenomenon usually involves nucleases capable of destroying one or more broad classes of mRNA defined on the basis of their 3′ or 5′ UTR sequences. Thus, for example, histone mRNAs are destabilized after the S phase of the cell cycle is complete. Presumably this occurs because histone synthesis is no longer needed. Induction of cell activation, mitogenesis, or terminal differentiation events often results in the induction of nucleases that destabilize specific subsets of mRNAs. Selective stabilization of mRNAs probably also occurs, but specific examples are less well documented.

The amount of a given protein accumulating in a cell depends on the amount of the mRNA present, the rate at which it is translated into the protein, and the stability of the protein. Translational efficiency depends on a number of variables, including polyadenylation and presence of the 5′ cap. The amounts and state of activation of protein factors needed for translation are also crucial. The secondary structure of the mRNA, particularly in the 5′ UTR, greatly influences the intrinsic translatability of an mRNA molecule by constraining the access of translation factors and ribosomes to the translation initiation signal in the mRNA. Secondary structures along the coding sequence of the mRNA may also have some impact on the rate of elongation of the peptide.

Changes in capping, polyadenylation, and translation factor efficiency affect the overall rate of protein synthesis within each cell. These effects tend to be global rather than specific to a particular gene product. However, these effects influence the relative amounts of different proteins made. mRNAs whose structures inherently lend themselves to more efficient translation tend to compete better for rate-limiting components of the translational apparatus, but mRNAs that are inherently less translatable tend to be translated less efficiently in the face of limited access to other translational components. For example, the translation factor eIF-4 tends to be produced in higher amounts when cells encounter transforming or mitogenic events. This causes an increase in overall rates of protein synthesis but also leads to a selective increase in the synthesis of some proteins that were underproduced before mitogenesis.

Translational regulation of individual mRNA species is critical for some events important to blood cell homeostasis. For example, as discussed in Chapter 33, the amount of iron entering a cell is an exquisite regulator of the rate of ferritin mRNA translation. An mRNA sequence called the *iron response element* is recognized by a specific mRNA-binding protein but only when the protein lacks iron. mRNA bound to the protein is translationally inactive. As iron accumulates in the cell, the protein becomes iron bound and loses its affinity for the mRNA, resulting in translation into apoferritin molecules that bind the iron.

Tubulin synthesis involves coordinated regulation of translation and mRNA stability. Tubulin regulates the stability of its own mRNA by a feedback loop. As tubulin concentrations rise in the cell, it interacts with its own mRNA through the intermediary of an mRNA-binding protein. This results in the formation of an mRNA–protein complex and nucleolytic cleavage of the mRNA. The mRNA is destroyed, and further tubulin production is halted.

These few examples of posttranscriptional regulation emphasize that cells tend to use every step in the complex pathway of gene expression as points at which exquisite control over the amounts of a particular protein can be regulated. In other chapters, additional levels of regulation are described (e.g., regulation of the stability, activity, localization, and access to other cellular components of the proteins that are present in a cell).

SMALL INTERFERING RNA AND MICRO RNA

Recently, posttranscriptional mechanisms of gene silencing involving small RNAs were discovered. One process is carried out by small interfering RNAs (siRNAs): short, double-stranded fragments of RNA containing 21 to 23 bp (Fig. 1-6). The process is triggered by perfectly complementary double-stranded RNA, which is cleaved by Dicer, a member of the RNase III family, into siRNA fragments. These small fragments of double-stranded RNA are unwound by a helicase in the RNA-induced silencing complex. The antisense strand anneals to mRNA transcripts in a sequence-specific manner and in doing so brings the endonuclease activity within the RNA-induced silencing complex to the targeted transcript. An RNA-dependent RNA polymerase in the RNA-induced silencing complex may then create new siRNAs to processively degrade the mRNA, ultimately leading to complete degradation of the mRNA transcript and abrogation of protein expression.

Although this endogenous process likely evolved to destroy invading viral RNA, the use of siRNA has become a commonly used tool for evaluation of gene function. Sequence-specific synthetic siRNA may be directly introduced into cells or introduced via gene transfertion methods and targeted to an mRNA of a gene of interest. The siRNA will lead to degradation of the mRNA transcript, and accordingly prevent new protein translation. This technique is a relatively simple, efficient, and inexpensive means to investigate cellular phenotypes after directed elimination of expression of a single gene. The 2006 Nobel Prize in Physiology or Medicine was awarded to two discoverers of RNA interference, Andrew Fire and Craig Mello.

Micro RNAs (miRNAs) are 22-nt small RNAs encoded by the cellular genome that alter mRNA stability and protein translation. These genes are transcribed by RNA polymerase II and capped and polyadenylated similar to other RNA polymerase II transcripts. The precursor transcript of approximately 70 nucleotides is cleaved into mature miRNA by the enzymes Drosha and Dicer. One strand of the resulting duplex forms a complex with the RNA-induced silencing complex that together binds the target mRNA with imperfect complementarity. Through mechanisms that are still incompletely understood, miRNA suppresses gene expression, likely either through

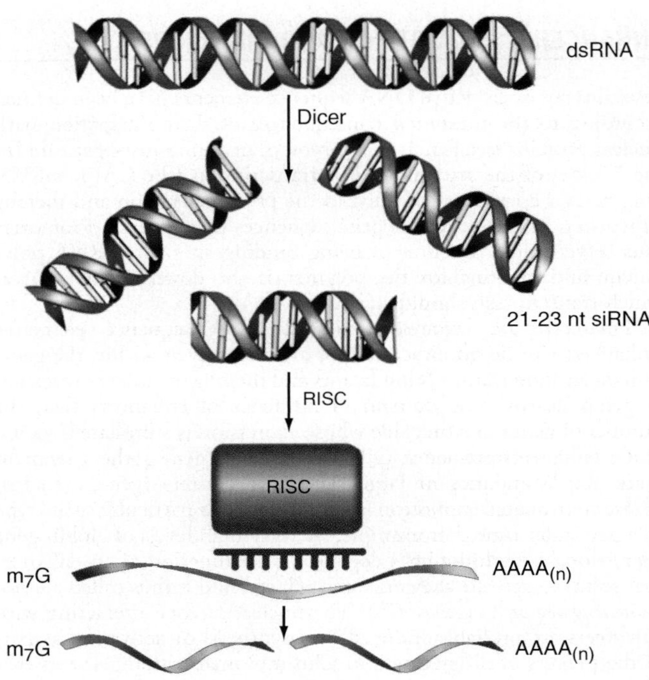

Figure 1-6 mRNA DEGRADATION BY siRNA. Double-stranded RNA is digested into 21- to 23-bp small interfering RNAs (siRNAs) by the Dicer RNase. These RNA fragments are unwound by RISC and bring the endonucleolytic activity of RNA-induced silencing complex (RISC) to messenger RNA (mRNA) transcripts in a sequence-specific manner, leading to degradation of the mRNA.

inhibition of protein translation or through destabilization of mRNA. miRNAs appear to have essential roles in development and differentiation and may be aberrantly regulated in cancer cells. The identification of miRNA sequences, their regulation, and their target genes are areas of intense study.

ADDITIONAL STRUCTURAL FEATURES OF GENOMIC DNA

Most DNA does not code for RNA or protein molecules. The vast majority of nucleotides present in the human genome reside outside structural genes. Structural genes are separated from one another by as few as 1 to 5 kilobases or as many as several thousand kilobases of DNA. Almost nothing is known about the reason for the erratic clustering and spacing of genes along chromosomes. It is clear that intergenic DNA contains a variegated landscape of structural features that provide useful tools to localize genes, identify individual human beings as unique from every other human being (DNA fingerprinting), and diagnose human diseases by linkage. Only a brief introduction is provided here.

The rate of mutation in DNA under normal circumstances is approximately $1/10^6$. In other words, one of 1 million bases of DNA will be mutated during each round of DNA replication. A set of enzymes called *DNA proofreading enzymes* corrects many but not all of these mutations. When these enzymes are themselves altered by mutation, the rate of mutation (and therefore the odds of neoplastic transformation) increases considerably. If these mutations occur in bases critical to the structure or function of a protein or gene, altered function, disease, or a lethal condition can result. Most pathologic mutations tend not to be preserved throughout many generations because of their unfavorable phenotypes. Exceptions, such as the hemoglobinopathies, occur when the heterozygous state for these mutations confers selective advantage in the face of unusual environmental conditions, such as malaria epidemics. These "adaptive" mutations drive the dynamic change in the genome with time (evolution).

Most of the mutations that accumulate in the DNA of *Homo sapiens* occur in either intergenic DNA or the "silent" bases of DNA, such as the degenerate third bases of codons. They do not pathologically alter the function of the gene or its products. These clinically harmless mutations are called *DNA polymorphisms*. DNA polymorphisms can be regarded in exactly the same way as other types of polymorphisms that have been widely recognized for years (e.g., eye and hair color, blood groups). They are variations in the population that occur without apparent clinical impact. Each of us differs from other humans in the precise number and type of DNA polymorphisms that we possess.

Similar to other types of polymorphisms, DNA polymorphisms breed true. In other words, if an individual's DNA contains a G 1200 bases upstream from the α-globin gene, instead of the C most commonly found in the population, that G will be transmitted to that individual's offspring. Note that if one had a means for distinguishing the G at that position from a C, one would have a linked marker for that individual's α-globin gene.

Occasionally, a DNA polymorphism falls within a restriction endonuclease site. (Restriction enzymes cut DNA molecules into smaller pieces but only at limited sites, defined by short base sequences recognized by each enzyme.) The change could abolish the site or create a site where one did not exist before. These polymorphisms change the array of fragments generated when the genome is digested by that restriction endonuclease. This permits detection of the polymorphism by use of the appropriate restriction enzyme. This specific class of polymorphisms is thus called *restriction fragment length polymorphisms* (RFLPs).

Restriction fragment length polymorphisms are useful because the length of a restriction endonuclease fragment on which a gene of interest resides provides a linked marker for that gene. The exploitation of this fact for diagnosis of genetic diseases and detection of specific genes is discussed in Chapter 137; Fig. 1-7 shows a simple example.

Restriction fragment length polymorphisms have proved to be extraordinarily useful for the diagnosis of genetic diseases, especially when the precise mutation is not known. Recall that DNA polymorphisms breed true in the population. For example, as discussed in Chapter 137, a mutation that causes hemophilia will, when it occurs on the X chromosome, be transmitted to subsequent generations attached to the pattern (often called a framework or haplotype) of RFLPs that was present on that same X chromosome. If the pattern of RFLPs in the parents is known, the presence of the abnormal chromosome can be detected in the offspring.

An important feature of the DNA landscape is the high degree of repeated DNA sequence. A DNA sequence is said to be repeated if it or a sequence very similar (homologous) to it occurs more than once in a genome. Some multicopy genes, such as the histone genes and the ribosomal RNA genes, are repeated DNA sequences. Most repeated DNA occurs outside genes, or within introns. Indeed, 30% to 45% of the human genome appears to consist of repeated DNA sequences.

The function of repeated sequences remains unknown, but their presence has inspired useful strategies for detecting and characterizing individual genomes. For example, a pattern of short repeated DNA sequences, characterized by the presence of flanking sites recognized by the restriction endonuclease Alu-1 (called Alu-repeats), occurs approximately 300,000 times in a human genome. These sequences are not present in the mouse genome. If one wishes to infect mouse cells with human DNA and then identify the human DNA sequences in the infected mouse cells, one simply probes for the presence of Alu-repeats. The Alu-repeat thus serves as a signature of human DNA.

Classes of highly repeated DNA sequences (tandem repeats) have proved to be useful for distinguishing genomes of each human individual. These short DNA sequences, usually less than a few hundred bases long, tend to occur in clusters, with the number of repeats varying among individuals (see Fig. 1-6). Alleles of a given gene can therefore be associated with a variable number of tandem repeats (VNTR) in different individuals or populations. For example, there is a VNTR near the insulin gene. In some individuals or populations, it is present in only a few tandem copies, but in others, it is present in many more. When the population as a whole is examined, there is a wide degree of variability from individual to individual as to the number of these repeats residing near the insulin gene. It can readily be imagined that if probes were available to detect a dozen or so distinct VNTR regions, each human individual would differ from virtually all others with respect to the aggregate pattern of these VNTRs. Indeed, it can be shown mathematically that the probability of any two human beings' sharing exactly the same pattern of VNTRs is exceedingly small if approximately 10 to 12 different VNTR elements are mapped for each person. A technique called *DNA fingerprinting* that is based on VNTR analysis has become widely publicized because of its forensic applications.

Variable-number tandem repeats can be regarded as normal sequence variations in DNA that are similar to, but far more useful than, single-base-change RFLPs. Note that the odds of a single base change altering a convenient restriction endonuclease site are relatively small, so that RFLPs occur relatively infrequently in a useful region of the genome. Moreover, there is only one state or variable that can be examined—that is, the presence or absence of the restriction site. By contrast, many VNTRs are scattered throughout the human genome. Most of these can be distinguished from one another quite readily by standard methods. Most important, the amount of variability from individual to individual at each site of a VNTR is considerably greater than for RFLPs. Rather than the mere presence or absence of a site, a whole array of banding patterns is possible, depending on how many individual repeats are present at that site (see Fig. 1-6). This reasoning can readily be extended to

A

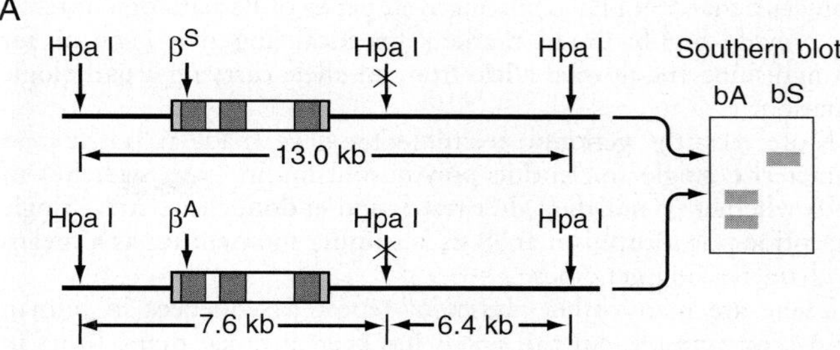

B

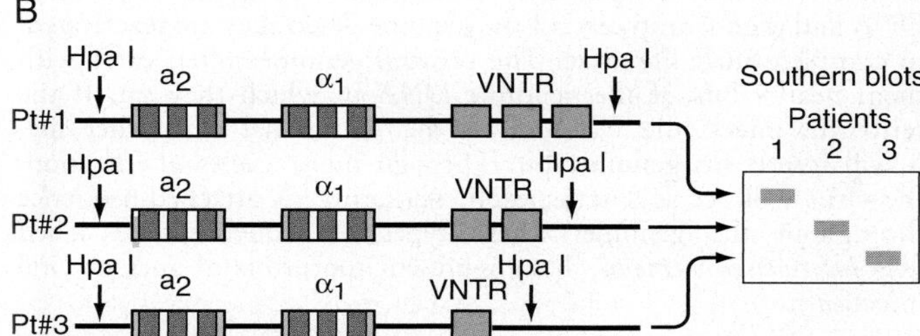

Figure 1-7 TWO USEFUL FORMS OF SEQUENCE VARIATION AMONG THE GENOMES OF NORMAL INDIVIDUALS. **A,** Presence of a DNA sequence polymorphism that falls within a restriction endonuclease site, thus altering the pattern of restriction endonuclease digests obtained from this region of DNA on Southern blot analysis. (Readers not familiar with Southern blot analysis should return to examine this figure after reading later sections of this chapter.) **B,** A variable-number tandem repeat (VNTR) region (defined and discussed in the text). Note that individuals can vary from one to another in many ways according to how many repeated units of the VNTR are located on their genomes, but restriction fragment length polymorphism differences are in effect all-or-none differences, allowing for only two variables (restriction site presence or absence).

appreciate that VNTRs occurring near genes of hematologic interest can provide highly useful markers for localizing that gene or for distinguishing the normal allele from an allele carrying a pathologic mutation.

More recently, genomic technologies have made it possible to characterize single nucleotide polymorphisms in large stretches of DNA whether or not they alter restriction endonuclease sites. Single nucleotide polymorphism analysis is gaining momentum as a means for characterizing genomes.

There are many other classes of repeated sequences in human DNA. For example, human DNA has been invaded many times in its history by retroviruses. Retroviruses tend to integrate into human DNA and then "jump out" of the genome when they are reactivated, to complete their life cycle. The proviral genomes often carry with them nearby bits of the genomic DNA in which they sat. If the retrovirus infects the DNA of another individual at another site, it will insert this genomic bit. Through many cycles of infection, the virus will act as a transposon, scattering its attached sequence throughout the genome. These types of sequences are called *long interspersed elements*. They represent footprints of ancient viral infections.

KEY METHODS FOR GENE ANALYSIS

The foundation for the molecular understanding of gene structure and expression is based on fundamental molecular biologic techniques that were developed in the 1970s and 1980s. These techniques allow for the reduction of the multibillion nucleotide genome into smaller fragments that are more easily analyzed. Several key methods are outlined here.

Restriction Endonucleases

Naturally occurring bacterial enzymes called *restriction endonucleases* catalyze sequence-specific hydrolysis of phosphodiester bonds in the DNA backbone. For example, EcoRI, a restriction endonuclease isolated from *Escherichia coli,* cleaves DNA only at the sequence 5′-GAATTC-3′. Thus, each DNA sample will be reproducibly reduced to an array of fragments whose size ranges depend on the distribution with which that sequence exists within the DNA. A specific six-nucleotide sequence would be statistically expected to appear once every 4^6 (or 4096) nucleotides, but in reality, the distance between specific sequences varies greatly. Using combinations of restriction endonucleases, DNA several hundred million base pairs in length can be reproducibly reduced to fragments ranging from a few dozen to tens of thousands of base pairs long. These smaller products of enzymatic digestion are much more manageable experimentally. Genetic "fingerprinting," or restriction enzyme maps of genomes, can be constructed by analyzing the DNA fragments resulting from digestion. Many enzymes cleave DNA so as to leave short, single-stranded overhanging regions that can be enzymatically linked to other similar fragments, generating artificially recombined, or recombinant, DNA molecules. These ligated gene fragments can then be inserted into bacteria to produce more copies of the recombinant molecules or to express the cloned genes.

DNA, RNA, and Protein Blotting

There are many ways that a cloned DNA sequence can be exploited to characterize the behavior of normal or pathologic genes. Blotting methods deserve special mention because of their widespread use in clinical and experimental hematology. A cloned DNA fragment can be easily purified and tagged with a radioactive or nonradioactive label. The fragment provides a pure and highly specific molecular hybridization probe for the detection of complementary DNA or RNA molecules in any specimen of DNA or RNA. One set of assays that has proved particularly useful involves Southern blotting, named after Dr E. Southern, who invented the method (Fig. 1-8). Southern blotting allows detection of a specific gene, or region in or near a gene, in a DNA preparation. The DNA is isolated and digested with one or more restriction endonucleases, and the resulting fragments are denatured and separated according to their molecular size by electrophoresis through agarose gels. By means of capillary action in a high salt buffer, the DNA fragments are passively transferred to a nitrocellulose or nylon membrane. Single-stranded DNA and RNA molecules attach noncovalently but tightly to the membrane. In this fashion, the membrane becomes a replica, or blot, of the gel. After the blotting procedure is complete, the membrane is incubated in a hybridization buffer containing the radioactively labeled probe. The probe hybridizes only to the gene of interest and renders radioactive only one or a few bands containing complementary sequences. After appropriate washing and drying, the bands can be visualized by autoradiography.

Digestion of a DNA preparation with several different restriction enzymes allows a restriction endonuclease map of a gene in the

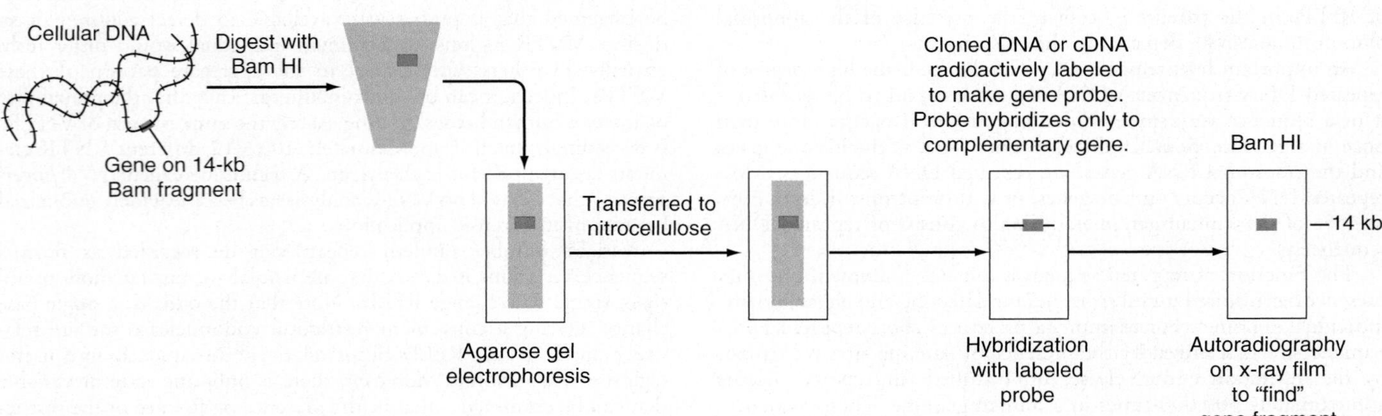

Figure 1-8 SOUTHERN GENE BLOTTING. Detection of a genomic gene *(red)* that resides on a 14-kb Bam HI fragment. To identify the presence of a gene in the genome and the size of the restriction fragment on which it resides, genomic DNA is digested with a restriction enzyme, and the fragments are separated by agarose gel electrophoresis. Human genomes contain from several hundred thousand to 1 million sites for any particular restriction enzyme, which results in a vast array of fragments and creates a blur or streak on the gel; one fragment cannot be distinguished from another readily. If the DNA in the gel is transferred to nitrocellulose by capillary blotting, however, it can be further analyzed by molecular hybridization to a radioactive cDNA probe for the gene. Only the band containing the gene yields a positive autoradiography signal, as shown. If a disease state were to result in loss of the gene, alteration of its structure, or mutation (altering recognition sites for one or more restriction enzymes), the banding pattern would be changed.

human genome to be constructed. Southern blotting has thus become a standard way of characterizing the configuration of genes in the genome.

Northern blotting represents an analogous blotting procedure used to detect RNA. RNA cannot be digested with restriction enzymes (which cut only DNA); rather, the intact RNA molecules can be separated according to molecular size by electrophoresis through the gel (mRNAs are 0.5-12 kilobases in length), transferred onto membranes, and probed with a DNA probe. In this fashion, the presence, absence, molecular size, and number of individual species of a particular mRNA species can be detected.

Western blotting is a similar method that can be used to examine protein expression. Cellular lysates (or another source of proteins) can be electrophoresed through a polyacrylamide gel so as to separate proteins on the basis of their apparent molecular sizes. The resolved proteins can then be electrically transferred to nitrocellulose membranes and probed with specific antibodies directed against the protein of interest. As with RNA analysis, the relative expression levels and molecular sizes of proteins can be assessed with this method.

Polymerase Chain Reaction

The development of the polymerase chain reaction (PCR) was a major breakthrough that has revolutionized the utility of a DNA-based strategy for diagnosis and treatment. It permits the detection, synthesis, and isolation of specific genes and allows differentiation of alleles of a gene differing by as little as one base. It does not require sophisticated equipment or unusual technical skills. A clinical specimen consisting of only minute amounts of tissue will suffice; in most circumstances, no special preparation of the tissue is necessary. PCR thus makes recombinant DNA techniques accessible to clinical laboratories. This single advance has produced a quantum increase in the use of direct gene analysis for diagnosis of human diseases.

The PCR is based on the prerequisites for copying an existing DNA strand by DNA polymerase: an existing denatured strand of DNA to be used as the template and a primer. Primers are short oligonucleotides, 12 to 100 bases in length, having a base sequence complementary to the desired region of the existing DNA strand. The enzyme requires the primer to "know" where to begin copying. If the base sequence of the DNA of the gene under study is known, two synthetic oligonucleotides complementary to sequences flanking the region of interest can be prepared. If these are the only oligonucleotides present in the reaction mixture, then the DNA polymerase can only copy daughter strands of DNA downstream from those oligonucleotides. Recall that DNA is double stranded, that the strands are held together by the rules of Watson-Crick base pairing, and that they are aligned in antiparallel fashion. This implies that the effect of incorporation of both oligonucleotides into the reaction mix will be to synthesize two daughter strands of DNA, one originating upstream of the gene and the other originating downstream. The net effect is synthesis of only the DNA between the two primers, thus doubling only the DNA containing the region of interest. If the DNA is now heat denatured, allowing hybridization of the daughter strands to the primers, and the polymerization is repeated, then the region of DNA through the gene of interest is doubled again. Thus, two cycles of denaturation, annealing, and elongation result in a selective quadrupling of the gene of interest. The cycle can be repeated 30 to 50 times, resulting in a selective and geometric amplification of the sequence of interest to the order of 2^{30} to 2^{50} times. The result is a millionfold or higher selective amplification of the gene of interest, yielding microgram quantities of that DNA sequence.

The PCR achieved practical utility when DNA polymerases from thermophilic bacteria were discovered; when synthetic oligonucleotides of any desired sequence could be produced efficiently, reproducibly, and cheaply by automated instrumentation; and when DNA thermocycling machines were developed. Thermophilic bacteria live in hot springs and other exceedingly warm environments, and their DNA polymerases can tolerate 100° C (212° F) incubations without substantial loss of activity. The advantage of these thermostable polymerases is that they retain activity in a reaction mix that is repeatedly heated to the high temperature needed to denature the DNA strands into the single-stranded form. Microprocessor-driven DNA thermocycler machines can be programmed to increase temperatures to 95° C to 100° C (203° F to 212° F) (denaturation), to cool the mix to 50° C (101° F) rapidly (a temperature that favors oligonucleotide annealing), and then to raise the temperature to 70° C to 75° C (141.4° F to 151.5° F) (the temperature for optimal activity of the thermophilic DNA polymerases). In a reaction containing the test specimen, the thermophilic polymerase, the primers, and the chemical components (e.g., nucleotide subunits), the thermocycler can conduct many cycles of denaturation, annealing, and polymerization in a completely automated fashion. The gene of interest can thus be amplified more than a millionfold in a matter of a few hours. The DNA product is readily identified and isolated by routine agarose gel electrophoresis. The DNA can then be analyzed by restriction endonuclease, digestion, hybridization to specific probes, sequencing, further amplification by cloning, and so forth.

USE OF TRANSGENIC AND KNOCKOUT MICE TO DEFINE GENE FUNCTION

Recombinant DNA technology has resulted in the identification of many disease-related genes. To advance the understanding of the disease related to a previously unknown gene, the function of the protein encoded by that gene must be verified or identified, and the way changes in the gene's expression influence the disease phenotype must be characterized. Analysis of the role of these genes and their encoded proteins has been made possible by the development of recombinant DNA technology that allows the production of mice that are genetically altered at the cloned locus. Mice can be produced that express an exogenous gene and thereby provide an in vivo model of its function. Linearized DNA is injected into a fertilized mouse oocyte pronucleus and reimplanted in a pseudopregnant mouse. The resultant transgenic mice can then be analyzed for the phenotype induced by the injected transgene. Placing the gene under the control of a strong promoter that stimulates expression of the exogenous gene in all tissues allows the assessment of the effect of widespread overexpression of the gene. Alternatively, placing the gene under the control of a promoter that can function only in certain tissues (a tissue-specific promoter) elucidates the function of that gene in a particular tissue or cell type. A third approach is to study control elements of the gene by testing their capacity to drive expression of a "marker" gene that can be detected by chemical, immunologic, or functional means. For example, the promoter region of a gene of interest can be joined to the cDNA encoding green jellyfish protein and activity of the gene assessed in various tissues of the resultant transgenic mouse by fluorescence microscopy. Use of such a reporter gene demonstrates the normal distribution and timing of expression of the gene from which the promoter elements are derived. Transgenic mice contain exogenous genes that insert randomly into the genome of the recipient. Expression can thus depend as much on the location of the insertion as it does on the properties of the injected DNA.

In contrast, any defined genetic locus can be specifically altered by targeted recombination between the locus and a plasmid carrying an altered version of that gene (Fig. 1-9). If a plasmid contains that altered gene with enough flanking DNA identical to that of the normal gene locus, homologous recombination can occur, and the altered gene in the plasmid will replace the gene in the recipient cell. Using a mutation that inactivates the gene allows the production of a null mutation, in which the function of that gene is completely lost. To induce such a mutation, the plasmid is introduced into an embryonic stem cell, and the rare cells that undergo homologous recombination are selected. The "knockout" embryonic stem cell is then introduced into the blastocyst of a developing embryo. The resultant animals are chimeric; only a fraction of the cells in the animal contain the targeted gene. If the new gene is introduced into some of the germline cells of the chimeric mouse, then some of the offspring of that mouse will carry the mutation as a gene in all of

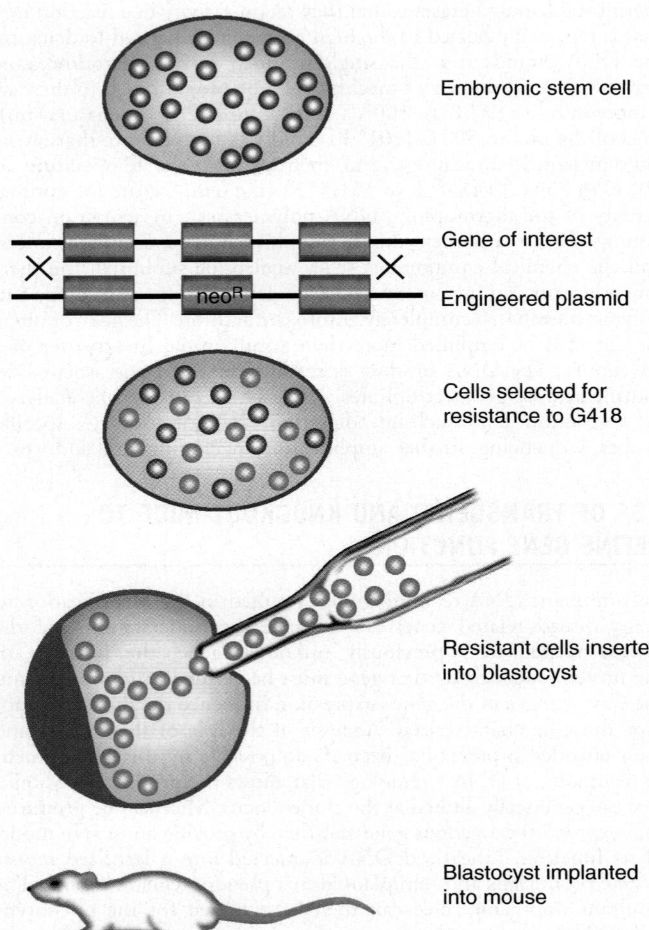

Figure 1-9 GENE "KNOCKOUT" BY HOMOLOGOUS RECOMBINATION. A plasmid containing genomic DNA homologous to the gene of interest is engineered to contain a selectable marker positioned so as to disrupt expression of the native gene. The DNA is introduced into embryonic stem cells, and cells resistant to the selectable marker are isolated and injected into a mouse blastocyst, which is then implanted into a mouse. Offspring mice that contain the knockout construct in their germ cells are then propagated, yielding mice with heterozygous or homozygous inactivation of the gene of interest.

their cells. These heterozygous mice can be further bred to produce mice homozygous for the null allele. Such knockout mice reveal the function of the targeted gene by the phenotype induced by its absence. Genetically altered mice have been essential for discerning the biologic and pathologic roles of large numbers of genes implicated in the pathogenesis of human disease.

DNA-BASED THERAPIES

Gene Therapy

The application of gene therapy to genetic hematologic disorders is an appealing idea. In most cases, this would involve isolating hematopoietic stem cells from patients with diseases with defined genetic lesions, inserting normal genes into those cells, and reintroducing the genetically engineered stem cells back into the patient. A few candidate diseases for such therapy include sickle cell disease, thalassemia, hemophilia, and adenosine deaminase–deficient severe combined immunodeficiency. The technology for separating hematopoietic stem cells and for performing gene transfer into those cells has advanced rapidly, and clinical trials have begun to test the applicability of these techniques. However, despite the fact that gene therapy has progressed to the enrollment of patients in clinical protocols, major technical problems still need to be solved, and there are no proven therapeutic successes from gene therapy. However, progress in this field continues rapidly. The scientific basis for gene therapy and the clinical issues surrounding this approach are discussed in Chapter 99.

Antisense Therapy

The recognition that abnormal expression of oncogenes plays a role in malignancy has stimulated attempts to suppress oncogene expression to reverse the neoplastic phenotype. One way of blocking mRNA expression is with antisense oligonucleotides. These are single-stranded DNA sequences, 17 to 20 bases long, having a sequence complementary to the transcription or translation start of the mRNA. These relatively small molecules freely enter the cell and complex to the mRNA by their complementary DNA sequence. This often results in a decrease in gene expression. The binding of the oligonucleotide may directly block translation and clearly enhances the rate of mRNA degradation. This technique has been shown to be promising in suppressing expression of bcr-abl and to suppress cell growth in chronic myelogenous leukemia. The technique is being tried as a therapeutic modality for the purging of tumor cells before autologous transplantation in patients with chronic myelogenous leukemia.

FUTURE DIRECTIONS

The elegance of recombinant DNA technology resides in the capacity it confers on investigators to examine each gene as a discrete physical entity that can be purified, reduced to its basic building blocks for decoding of its primary structure, analyzed for its patterns of expression, and perturbed by alterations in sequence or molecular environment so that the effects of changes in each region of the gene can be assessed. Purified genes can be deliberately modified or mutated to create novel genes not available in nature. These provide the potential to generate useful new biologic entities, such as modified live virus or purified peptide vaccines, modified proteins customized for specific therapeutic purposes, and altered combinations of regulatory and structural genes that allow for the assumption of new functions by specific gene systems.

Purified genes facilitate the study of gene regulation in many ways. First, a cloned gene provides characterized DNA probes for molecular hybridization assays. Second, cloned genes provide the homogeneous DNA moieties needed to determine the exact nucleotide sequence. Sequencing techniques have become so reliable and efficient that it is often easier to clone the gene encoding a protein of interest and determine its DNA sequence than it is to purify the protein and determine its amino acid sequence. The DNA sequence predicts exactly the amino acid sequence of its protein product. By comparing normal sequences with the sequences of alleles cloned from patients known to be abnormal, such as the globin genes in the thalassemia or sickle cell syndromes, the normal and pathologic anatomy of genes critical to major hematologic diseases can be established. In this manner, it has been possible to identify many mutations responsible for various forms of thalassemia, hemophilia, thrombasthenia, red blood cell enzymopathies, porphyrias, and so forth. Similarly, single base changes have been shown to be the difference between many normally functioning proto-oncogenes and their cancer-promoting oncogene derivatives.

Third, cloned genes can be manipulated for studies of gene expression. Many vectors allowing efficient transfer of genes into eukaryotic cells have been perfected. Gene transfer technologies allow the gene to be placed into the desired cellular environment and the expression of that gene or the behavior of its products to be analyzed. These surrogate or reverse genetics systems allow analysis of the normal physiology of expression of a particular gene, as well as the pathophysiology of abnormal gene expression resulting from mutations.

Fourth, cloned genes enhance study of their protein products. By expressing fragments of the gene in microorganisms or eukaryotic cells, customized regions of a protein can be produced for use as an immunogen, thereby allowing preparation of a variety of useful and powerful antibody probes. Alternatively, synthetic peptides deduced from the DNA sequence can be prepared as the immunogen. Controlled production of large amounts of the protein also allows direct analysis of specific functions attributable to regions in that protein.

Finally, all of the aforementioned techniques can be extended by mutating the gene and examining the effects of those mutations on the expression of or the properties of the encoded mRNAs and proteins. By combining portions of one gene with another (chimeric genes) or abutting structural regions of one gene with regulatory sequences of another, the researcher can investigate in previously inconceivable ways the complexities of gene regulation. These activist approaches to modifying gene structure or expression create the opportunity to generate new RNA and protein products whose applications are limited only by the collective imagination of the investigators.

The most important impact of the genetic approach to the analysis of biologic phenomena is the most indirect. Diligent and repeated application of the methods outlined in this chapter to the study of many genes from diverse groups of organisms is beginning to reveal the basic strategies used by nature for the regulation of cell and tissue behavior. As our knowledge of these rules of regulation grows, our ability to understand, detect, and correct pathologic phenomena will increase substantially.

SUGGESTED READINGS

Bentley D: The mRNA assembly line: Transcription and processing machines in the same factory. *Curr Opin Cell Biol* 14:336, 2002.

Dykxhoorn DM, Novina CD, Sharp PA: Killing the messenger: Short RNAs that silence gene expression. *Nat Rev Mol Cell Biol* 4:457, 2003.

Fischle W, Wang Y, Allis CD: Histone and chromatin cross-talk. *Curr Opin Cell Biol* 15:172, 2003.

Grewal SI, Moazed D: Heterochromatin and epigenetic control of gene expression. *Science* 301:798, 2003.

Kloosterman WP, Plasterk RHA: The diverse functions of microRNAs in animal development and disease. *Dev Cell* 11:441, 2006.

Klose RJ, Bird AP: Genomic DNA methylation: The mark and its mediators. *Trends Biochem Sci* 31:89, 2006.

Lee TI, Young RA: Transcription of eukaryotic protein-coding genes. *Annu Rev Genet* 34:77, 2000.

Tefferi A, Wieben ED, Dewald GW, et al: Primer on medical genomics, part II: Background principles and methods in molecular genetics. *Mayo Clinic Proc* 77:785, 2002.

Wilusz CJ, Wormington M, Peltz SW: The cap-to-tail guide to mRNA turnover. *Nat Rev Mol Cell Biol* 2:237, 2001.

CHAPTER 2

GENOMIC APPROACHES TO HEMATOLOGY

Todd R. Golub

The publication of the initial draft sequence of the human genome in 2001 heralded a new era of biomedical research. Just as molecular biology changed the face of research in the 1970s and 1980s, genomics promises a novel perspective into the biologic basis of human disease. Genomics involves the systematic study of biologic systems, typically focusing on aspects of the genome (e.g., DNA and its derivatives RNA and protein). However, a major tenet of genomics research involves *hypothesis-generating* data collection as opposed to *hypothesis-testing* experimentation. The latter has formed the basis of biomedical research, whereby existing knowledge and insight guide the testing of a particular hypothesis. In contrast, genome-based research tends to make few prior assumptions, favoring unbiased data generation and analysis as a path to discovery. Clearly, both approaches are powerful and essential, and both should continue full force in the future.

As attractive as unbiased, comprehensive genomic analysis may be, there have until recently been severe limitations to the approach. Most importantly, systematic approaches (e.g., to genome sequencing) have been cost prohibitive. However, sequencing costs have fallen dramatically over the past decade (by more than 10,000-fold), making it now possible to routinely characterize the genome at the level of DNA and RNA variation. Although less dramatic technical advances have been made in the area of protein analysis, proteomics is also undergoing technologic change that makes future prospects of systematic interrogation of entire proteomes conceivable in the near future.

With the ability to generate data of unprecedented scale comes the challenge of data analysis. This has driven an entirely new generation of computer scientists to focus on new approaches to genomic data analysis, leading to new methods of pattern recognition in voluminous, often noisy data. The challenge going forward will be that of translating these data into useful knowledge that provides biologic insight and clinical utility.

This chapter describes the principles underlying common genomic approaches in the study of hematologic and other diseases, focusing more on concepts than on technical detail. Although genomic approaches are just beginning to be introduced into clinical practice, it is likely that there will be an enormous acceleration of the pace of utilization of genomic approaches in clinical research and clinical care in the years ahead.

PRINCIPLES OF GENOMIC APPROACHES

Hypothesis-Generating Versus Hypothesis-Testing

Genomic approaches to hematology, similar to genomic approaches to other aspects of biomedical research, differ fundamentally from traditional, hypothesis-based investigation. The backbone of the entire biomedical research enterprise is the formulation of specific hypotheses based on an accumulation of knowledge in the field coupled to rigorous experimental strategies to test those hypotheses in physiologically relevant systems. This approach has been highly successful and should continue as a pillar of modern hematology research. However, such hypothesis-based approaches may not be sufficient for a complete elucidation of the molecular basis of hematologic disease. To complement hypothesis-driven research, genomics-based, hypothesis-generating approaches have proven powerful.

Genomics approaches can in the narrowest sense be seen as studies of DNA. However, a more liberal definition may be useful—namely, a systematic, unbiased approach that is not necessarily dependent on preexisting hypotheses. In this manner, one uses advanced technologies (focused on DNA, RNA, protein, or other measurements) to simply observe rather than to attempt to validate or invalidate a particular prior hypothesis. This approach can be particularly powerful when studying the biology of diseases without a known basis.

For example, the biology of polycythemia vera had been obscure despite decades of research until an unbiased search for mutations in the disease uncovered recurrent mutations in the gene encoding the tyrosine kinase Janus-activated kinase 2 (JAK2).[1,2] Nearly overnight, this finding established new directions for basic biologic research into the disease as well as mechanism-based drug development. Similarly, the molecular basis of certain myelodysplastic syndromes (MDS) has been entirely unknown, but recent unbiased genome sequencing approaches yielded common mutations in *SF3B1,* the gene encoding an RNA splicing factor in the majority of patients with refractory anemia with ringed sideroblasts.[3] Before this discovery, there was no reason to suspect defects in splicing machinery as the basis MDS.

Thus, although genomic approaches have been characterized by some as "fishing expeditions," it is clear that such strategies have the potential to dramatically accelerate understanding of disease, particularly in areas where the biologic basis is largely unknown.

Systematic and Comprehensive Measurements and Perturbations

A common feature of many genomic approaches is the systematic nature of the study (e.g., interrogating *all* kinases for their potential role in a particular biologic system). A more traditional approach would be to first determine (based on prior knowledge) the kinase (or kinases) most likely to be important and then develop highly validated assays for that particular kinase. A strength of the traditional approach is that the quality of the final assay is often high given the attention paid to the one (or a couple of) kinase(s) of interest. On the other hand, such an approach is limited by the quality of the initial hypothesis. In contrast, a genomic approach would be more systematic and comprehensive, attempting to screen all kinases for the phenotype of interest. Although this is compelling, it also comes with an important limitation—the quality of the assay for each kinase's activity may not be uniformly high. For example, a screen for kinase phosphorylation as surrogate for kinase activity has been reported.[4] Such an approach is limited by the sensitivity and specificity of kinase-directed antibodies, which can be enormously variable across kinase family members.

Although genomics is most commonly associated with systematic *observational* studies, the same principles can also be applied to *perturbational* studies (i.e., systematic modulation of proteins followed by a phenotypic read-out). A particularly powerful approach has been the systematic knock-down of mRNA transcripts using RNA interference (RNAi). In this manner, all genes within a particular class (e.g., kinases) can be knocked down and the phenotypic consequence of each assessed. Most recently, genome-wide RNAi studies have been reported using lentivirus-delivered short hairpin RNAs (shRNAs) (see the Functional Genomics section later). Although large-scale perturbational profiling studies are performed primarily in specialized research centers today, it is highly likely that such approaches will become increasingly common in the years ahead.

IMPORTANCE OF SAMPLE ACQUISITION

Acquisition of the appropriate samples for a genomic experiment is arguably the most crucial step for the production of a dataset that will be rich with biologic information. This is particularly true for gene expression analysis in which a number of processes may affect the data. Because gene expression is a dynamic process that can be affected by any type of cellular manipulation, RNA abundance measurements are potentially complicated by changes that occur between the time that the biopsy is taken and the time that the RNA is isolated from the specimen. In general, the highest quality RNA is obtained if, as soon as possible after harvesting a sample, cells are dissolved in a solution such as Trizol that inactivates RNAse enzymes, and the sample is stored at −80° Celsius until RNA can be extracted. A number of amplification procedures have been developed, including those that use two rounds of in vitro transcription and those that take advantage of the polymerase chain reaction (PCR); these manipulations make for the ability to analyze increasingly tiny samples (containing as few as 1000 cells or less). In addition, recent technical advances have made it possible to measure mRNA expression from formalin-fixed paraffin-embedded (FFPE) samples in which the mRNA is typically degraded to approximately 80 nucleotides in length.[5] These newer methods may make it feasible to analyze large archives of FFPE tissues with long-term clinical follow-up (which is often lacking from more recently collected, frozen samples) and may represent a suitable platform for routine clinical implementation when the collection of frozen specimens is often impractical.

Another extremely important but complicated issue is the complexity of the mixture of cells present in the sample. If one's goal is to assess genomic changes that represent somatic rather than germline differences, then the sample needs to be enriched (often to >75%) in the cell of interest. This may not be an issue for bone marrow samples from patients with newly diagnosed leukemia in whom the number of blasts often approaches 90% or greater. But it may become an issue if one's desire is to analyze leukemia at the time of relapse. In this scenario, the relapse is often detected long before the bone marrow is completely replaced with leukemia, and thus the blasts may represent less than 50% of the mononuclear cells. Multiple methods are available for enrichment and selection of cells of interest from a biopsy sample; these methods include flow cytometry, immunomagnetic bead sorting, and laser-capture microdissection.[6] All have the benefit of enrichment of the cell of interest but also increase the amount of processing time and sample manipulation. Alternatively, "contaminating," nonmalignant cells may be included in gene expression signatures because these cells may reflect the tumor environment and may therefore carry important information.[7] This is most obvious for solid tumors in which the tumor stroma and infiltrating inflammatory cells likely influence the neoplastic cells, but all diseased cells exist in a complex environment and are thus no doubt influenced by their interactions. Thus dismissing these cells as contamination must be done with caution.

As discussed in subsequent sections on next-generation sequencing technologies, the admixture of nonmalignant cells within a tumor may not obscure the presence of mutations in the tumor cells even if those cells represent a minority population. However, the detection of mutations in a subset of cells within a sample requires extra depth of sequencing beyond what would be required to sequence, for example, a normal diploid genome. Thus it becomes critical to have a rough estimate of the purity of a given sample so that the appropriate genomic approach can be taken subsequently.

ANALYTICAL CONSIDERATIONS

Unsupervised Learning Approaches

Unsupervised learning approaches (often referred to as *clustering*) have become an important part of the discovery process in genomic analysis. This type of analysis involves grouping samples based solely on the data obtained without regard to any prior knowledge of the samples or the disease. Thus, one can obtain the predominant "structure" of the dataset without imposing any prior bias. For example, unsupervised learning approaches have been used to cluster leukemia or lymphoma samples based on their gene expression profiles with the goal of uncovering the most robust classification schemes.[8-11] Clustering algorithms can also cluster genes that have a similar expression profile in a gene expression data set. There are a number of methods for clustering genes and samples, all of which have computational strengths and weaknesses. Comparing the clustering methods is beyond the scope of this chapter, but suffice it to say that all identify major associations within a given data set if the signature is strong and robust. Great care must be taken in the interpretation of clustering results because clusters with distinct gene expression profiles may be caused not only by biologically important distinctions but also by artifacts of sample processing. Unsupervised learning methods that have been used include hierarchical clustering, principle component analysis, non-negative matrix factorization, and *k*-means clustering.

Supervised Learning Approaches

Supervised learning approaches are best suited for comparing data among two or more classes of samples that can be distinguished by some known property (or class distinction) such as biologic subtype or clinical outcome. For example, to determine the gene expression differences between different leukemia subtypes with distinct genetic abnormalities, one would use a supervised approach (Fig. 2-1). The same genes might be clustered together based on the unsupervised approaches already described, but they might also be obscured by a more dominant gene expression signature that had nothing to do with the distinction of interest. For example, if there was another major signature within the data (i.e., a stage of differentiation signature), the differences that the investigator was searching for might be lost. A number of metrics can be used to identify genes that are differentially expressed between two groups of samples, all of which are best suited to identify genes that are uniformly highly expressed in one group. Although the different metrics may generate slightly different lists of gene expression differences, if the gene expression difference is robust, all should give comparable results.

Challenges of High-Dimensional Data

With the ability to generate large-scale genomic datasets comes a number of analytical issues that are unique to what is known as "big data." In particular, when the number of features analyzed in an experiment (e.g., the expression of each of 22,000 mRNA transcripts) exceeds the number of samples (e.g., 50 patients with a particular type of lymphoma), there is potential for finding patterns in the data simply by chance. The more features analyzed and the fewer the number of samples, the more likely such a phenomenon is to be encountered. For this reason, the use of nominal P values to estimate statistical significance of an observed observation is generally discouraged. Rather, some approach to correcting for multiple hypothesis testing is in order (in the present example, 22,000 hypotheses are effectively being tested). In the absence of such

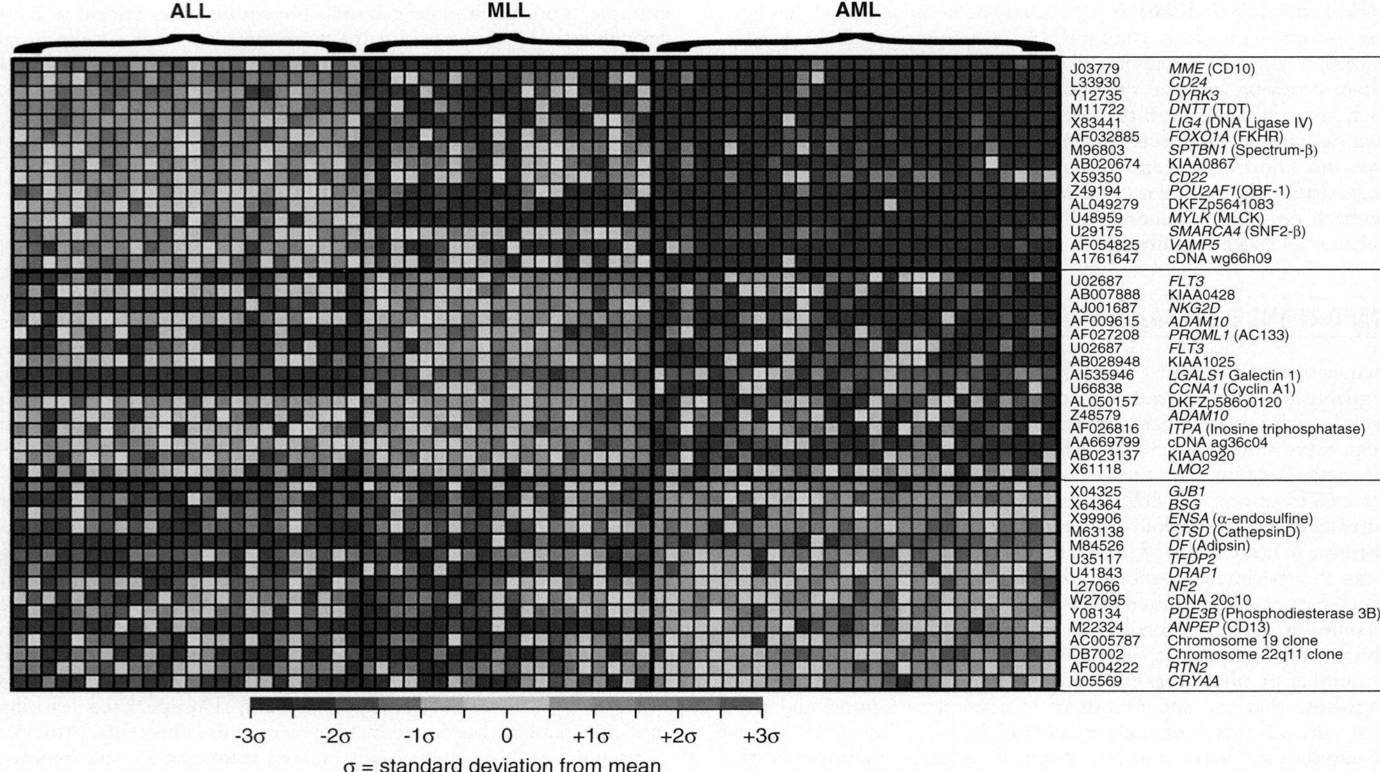

Figure 2-1 Comparison of gene expression in acute lymphocytic leukemia (ALL), *MLL*-rearranged ALL (designated MLL), and acute myelogenous leukemia (AML) samples using a supervised learning approach. Gene expression in leukemia samples was analyzed using Affymetrix microarrays containing 12,600 unique probe sets. Genes that are highly expressed in one type of leukemia relative to the other two are shown. Each column represents a patient sample, and each row represents a gene. *Red* represents relative high-level expression and relative low-level expression. *(From Armstrong SA, Staunton JE, Silverman LB, et al: MLL translocations specify a distinct gene expression profile that distinguishes a unique leukemia.* Nat Genet *30:41, 2002.)*

penalization, the significance of observations is likely to be grossly overestimated. Indeed, such misinterpretations of data were at the root of many of the early uses of gene expression profiling data in biomedical research.

Robustness of Pattern Recognition Algorithms

Related to the challenges with high-dimensional data described, special considerations of pattern-matching algorithms must be made. With the availability of high-dimensional gene expression profiling data in the late 1990s came a flood of computational innovation from computer scientists looking to find biologically meaningful patterns amid biologic data. With that early wave of computational analysis came the realization that with often limited numbers of samples (compared with the number of features analyzed) comes the possibility of "overfitting" a computational model to a particular dataset—that is, defining a pattern (e.g., a spectrum of genes that are differentially expressed) that is correlated with a phenotype of interest (e.g., survival) in an initial dataset but then does not predict accurately when applied to an independent dataset. This failure to reproduce initial findings was variously attributed to technical defects in the genomic data itself, insufficiently complex algorithms, and the possibility that perhaps the most important features were not being analyzed in the first place (e.g., noncoding RNAs). But, in fact, nearly all of the early failures of pattern recognition algorithms to validate when applied to new datasets were attributable to overfitting of the models to an initial, small dataset. The solution to this problem is to ensure that discovery datasets are sufficiently large to avoid overfitting and to insist that before any clinical or biologic claims are made the model is tested on completely independent samples.

NEXT-GENERATION SEQUENCING TECHNOLOGY

Distinguishing Features Compared With Sanger Sequencing

Beginning around 2006, a number of new approaches to DNA sequencing burst onto the scene. These technical advances have transformed the field of genomics and will likely equally transform the diagnostics field in the years to come. A number of novel sequencing approaches have been commercialized, and their details are beyond the scope of this chapter. However, they differ fundamentally from traditional Sanger sequencing that has been the mainstay for the past several decades. First, and most well-recognized, is the dramatically lower cost of current sequencing methods compared with Sanger sequencing. Costs have dropped by at least 10,000-fold over the past decade. This drop in cost has transformed genome sequencing from the work of an entire community over a decade (the initial sequencing of the human genome took 15 years and ~$3 billion) to a routine experiment done in a matter of weeks at a cost that is projected to drop to as low as $1000 by the end of 2012. These exponential cost reductions have come about not through dramatic drops in reagent costs but rather through dramatic increases in data output. A single lane on a modern sequencer generates vastly more data than a lane of conventional sequencing. This is relevant because to realize the lower costs of contemporary sequencing, large-scale projects must be undertaken. That is, devoting a single lane of sequencing to the sequencing of a plasmid, for example, is *more* expensive with current technologies than with traditional Sanger sequencing; the cost savings are only realized when large data outputs are required (e.g., the sequencing of entire genomes or of isolated genes across large numbers of patients).

Error Rates and Coverage

When executed and analyzed properly, next-generation sequencing technologies can yield nearly perfect fidelity of sequence. At the same time, the error rates for any given sequencing read can be as high as 1%, depending on the sequencing platform. How can these two statements both be correct? Although a 1% error rate (99% accurate) may seem low, when taken in the context of sequencing all 3 billion bases of the human genome, that would in principle result in 30 million errors! Thankfully, this is not the case because most sequencing errors are idiosyncratic—that is, they are not a function of a particular DNA sequence. The consequence of this is that by simply resequencing the same region multiple times and taking the consensus read, such idiosyncratic errors are lost; it is highly unlikely for them to occur over and over again at the same spot.

For normal, diploid genomes, sequencing is typically done 30-fold over (referred to as *30X coverage*). The consensus obtained by observing a given nucleotide 30 times is generally sufficient for rendering the correct read of that nucleotide. However, things get more complicated when dealing with (1) tumors containing gene copy number alterations (e.g., aneuploidy or regions or gene deletion or amplification) or (2) admixture of normal cells within the tumor sample. To compensate for copy number variation and normal cell contamination seen in most samples, typical cancer genome sequencing projects aim for a depth of coverage of at least 100X. Sequencing for diagnostic purposes may require even greater depth of coverage. And the analysis of samples containing only rare tumor cells (e.g., 10%) would require ultra-deep sequencing or any tumor-specific mutations would likely become false-negatives. Importantly, the frequency of cancer-associated mutations in studies performed using traditional Sanger sequencing methods may have been underestimated because of the lack of power to detect mutations in tumors with significant normal cell contamination. Whereas Sanger sequencing delivers the *average* allele observed in a sample, next-generation sequencing methods deliver a *distribution* of observed alleles, allowing for mutant alleles to be identified even if they represent a minority population.

Future of Sequencing Technologies

No one could have predicted the dramatic advances that have come to DNA sequencing technologies over the past several years. Costs have dropped dramatically, and it is predicted that costs will continue to drop, although less precipitously. It is likely that the cost of whole-genome sequencing will drop to $1000 by 2013, and some projections anticipate even further cost reductions. The details are unimportant, but the implications are clear: the cost of genome sequencing will soon shift from sequence *generation* to sequence *analysis*. Although future technologies may allow for the rapid sequencing of entire genomes for hundreds of dollars on a benchtop instrument, the interpretation of the observed sequence variants (whether germline or somatic) will be less obvious. The cost of storage of genome sequence may soon exceed the cost of generating the data in the first place, and a detailed analysis is far from straightforward. Nevertheless, it is likely that over the decade ahead, genome sequencing will become a routine component of both clinical research and routine clinical care.

DNA-LEVEL CHARACTERIZATION

Somatic Versus Germline Events

It is important to recognize the fundamental difference between *germline* variants and *somatic* variants in genome sequence. Germline variants are present in all cells of the body (with the exception of rare mosaicism), and these variants can contribute to the risk of future disease. Germline variants can be common (i.e., seen in ≥5% of the human population), or they can be rare (in principle, unique to a single individual). Each individual also carries 10s of de novo variants that are present in neither of the individual's parents' genome. It remains to be determined to what extent hematologic diseases (whether malignant or otherwise) are caused by germline genetic variation. Although it is clear that certain disorders (e.g., hemophilia) have a highly penetrant, Mendelian basis, it is less certain whether genetic variation explains a significant amount of disease that has been historically considered "sporadic."

In contrast, mutations present in tumors but absent in the normal cells from that individual are referred to as *somatic*. Somatic mutations are thought to be the major drivers of cancer behavior. However, all somatic mutations are not causal *drivers* of cancer. Indeed, the majority of somatic mutations observed in any individual tumor are likely to passenger mutations—that is, they play no functional role in the pathogenesis of the tumor but rather were present in a cell that subsequently acquired a driver mutation that resulted in the cell's clonal outgrowth. The proportion of passengers to drivers likely differs from tumor type to tumor type. For example, tumors associated with tobacco (e.g., lung cancer) or sunlight exposure (e.g., melanoma) have very high mutation frequencies with the majority of the observed mutations being "passengers." In contrast, many hematologic malignancies (e.g., acute myeloid leukemia) have relatively low mutation rates, and some cancers such as infant leukemias have extraordinarily low rates, with only a handful of protein-coding somatic mutations seen per patient.

Distinguishing passenger mutations from driver mutations is a major focus of cancer genome research. It is likely that the complete delineation of the biologically important mutations in cancer will require both large-scale sequencing studies (enabling the identification of recurrent mutations) and the functional characterization of observed mutations.

Point Mutations

The most common type of genetic variants (both germline and somatic) are single nucleotide variants, also known as point mutations. As more individuals are sequenced and deposited into databases, it is becoming possible to catalog all common variations in the human population. Still, it is estimated that every individual will harbor 50 to 100 coding mutations not present in any database. For these reasons, it is particularly important to compare the somatic genome of a tumor with its matched normal germline sequence or else "private" germline variants may be mistaken for somatic mutations.

Certain patterns of point mutation are characteristic of particular environmental exposures. For example, G>T/C>A transversions are characteristic of tobacco-associated lung cancer, and C>T/G>A transitions are characteristic of ultraviolet-associated skin cancers. Most hematologic malignancies lack a particular pattern of mutation, although B-cell lymphomas demonstrate a characteristic pattern of hotspots of mutations caused by activation-induced adenosine deaminase–mediated somatic hypermutation.[12,13]

Although not as common as point mutations, small somatic insertions or deletions (referred to collectively as *indels*) are also observed in tumors. These generally consist of the loss or gain of one or a few nucleotides that, when they occur within protein-coding regions, result in translation frame shifts that generally yield loss-of-function alleles.

Copy Number

Gains (amplifications) or losses (deletions) of genetic material at specific loci are recognized as playing an important role in the pathophysiology of disease. Germline copy number variants have recently been reported, although these are only rarely associated with hematologic disease. Trisomy 21, for example, predisposes to transient myeloproliferative disorders and acute megakaryoblastic leukemia.

Deletions at the RB1 locus encoding the retinoblastoma gene or deletions of the *TP53* gene encoding the p53 tumor suppressor predispose to the development of solid cancers, although only rarely hematologic malignancies. In a landmark set of studies, it was shown that tumors from patients who inherit a mutant copy of the retinoblastoma tumor suppressor gene often contain deletions of the remaining allele.[14] This process has been termed *loss of heterozygosity,* and the search for genetic loci showing loss of heterozygosity in tumor samples has identified a number of genes that are involved in critical cellular processes and are important for cancer progression. Similarly, amplification of genomic loci can play an important role in oncogenesis and cancer biology. For example, amplification of the ERBB2 (HER2) oncogene in human breast cancer predicts a poor prognosis, and ERBB2 has been shown to be an important therapeutic target in this disease.[15]

The search for gains and losses of genetic material can be done using a number of techniques that require various levels of expertise and allow assessment of genomic integrity at various resolutions. The first method developed to assess genomic integrity, *cytogenetic analysis,* is still used today, but it allows identification only of abnormalities that encompass large regions of the genome. Nevertheless, cytogenetic analysis has provided tremendous insight into the pathophysiology of disease, particularly for leukemogenesis.[16] Cytogenetic analysis remains a key part of the diagnostic workup for new cases of leukemia.

More recently developed methods for assessing copy number include *comparative genomic hybridization* (CGH) and high-density single nucleotide polymorphism (SNP) arrays. Although CGH is no longer extensively used, SNP arrays represent a powerful tool for assessing copy number variation. Commonly used SNP arrays contain nearly two million probes, allowing for small copy number aberrations (in some cases reflecting only certain exons of a single gene) to be routinely detected. Lastly, massively parallel genome sequencing can be used for copy number variant detection. The degree to which sequencing can yield as reproducible an assessment of copy number as SNP arrays has yet to be established.

Special note should be made of the analysis of copy number data. At the level of the individual sample (e.g., a tumor), one can easily visualize regions of aberration using tools such as the integrative genomics viewer (IGV) (Fig. 2-2).[17] Although this type of analysis highlights those aberrations in a *particular* sample, it does not reflect copy number abnormalities that are commonly observed across a *collection* of samples. Such recurrent copy number gains or losses tend to indicate biologically important events, as opposed to copy number aberrations that simply reflect genomic instability, but do not contribute to cancer pathogenesis (and therefore are nonrecurrent). To identify statistically significant regions of copy number abnormalities, algorithms such as the GISTIC (genomic identification of significant targets in cancer) method[18] can be applied, yielding a plot of regions of amplification and deletion that are commonly observed in a set of samples (as shown in Fig. 2-3 for 24 patients with multiple myeloma).

Rearrangements

Chromosomal rearrangements (including balanced and unbalanced translocations, inversions, and more complex aberrations) are particularly important in the hematologic malignancies. Translocations were among the very first genomic defects to be discovered in cancer because cytogenetic analysis of metaphase chromosome spreads was feasible for the acute leukemias long before more technically advanced methods become available. Two basic types of translocations are common: those that result in fusion proteins involving two distinct genes and those that result in overexpression of an otherwise structurally normal gene. Translocations resulting in fusion transcripts (e.g., *ETV6/RUNX1* in acute lymphoblastic leukemia)

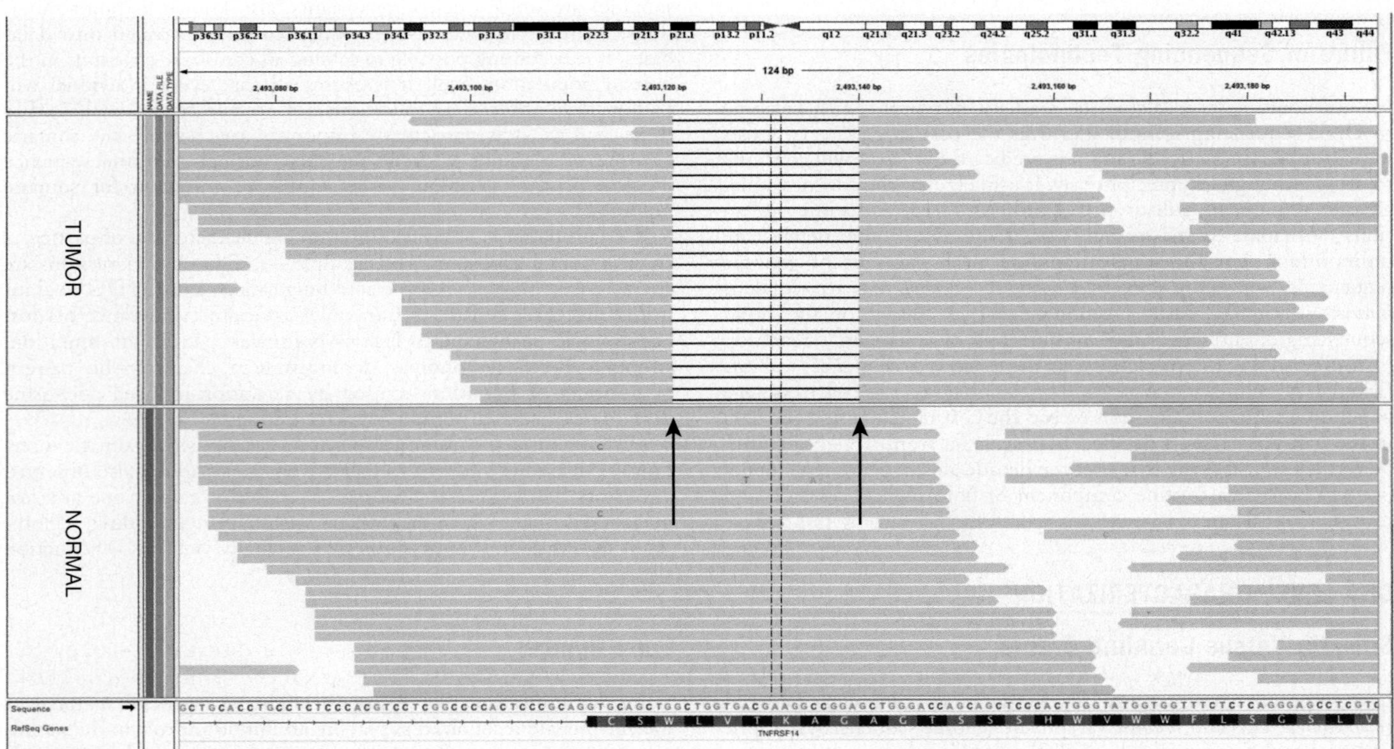

Figure 2-2 GENOME DELETION IN A PATIENT WITH DIFFUSE LARGE B-CELL LYMPHOMA (DLBCL). Genome sequencing of a patient with DLBCL revealed a clear region of genome deletion within the *TNFRS14* gene, as visualized in the integrative genomics viewer (IGV). The *grey bars* indicate the extent of the sequence read, with this region being interrogated multiple times. The *white block* in the middle (bracketed by *red arrows*) indicates the region of genome deletion captured by all of the reads in the tumor but in none of the reads from the matched normal DNA sample (*bottom portion* of figure).

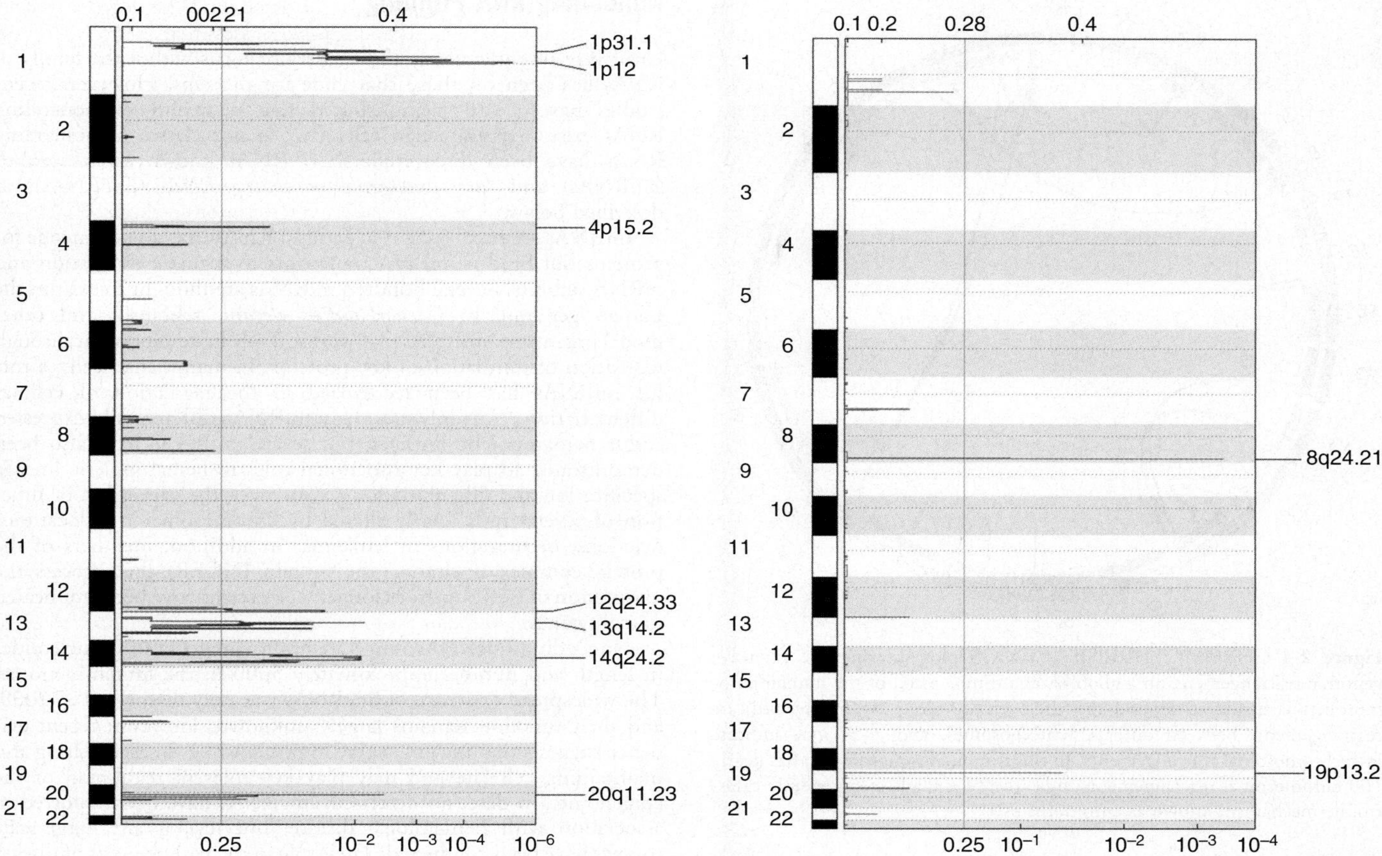

Figure 2-3 RECURRENT COPY NUMBER ABERRATIONS IN MULTIPLE MYELOMA. Output of the GISTIC (genomic identification of significant targets in cancer) algorithm indicates recurrent regions of gene copy number gain and loss. Recurrent gains are shown in *red* (including the *MYC* gene at 8q24), and recurrent losses are shown in *blue* (including the *RB* gene at 13q14). The height of each peak indicates the statistical significance of the event (a function of frequency and the rate expected by chance).

generally involve chromosomal breakage within intronic regions of the two genes, with in-frame fusion a result of the normal process of RNA splicing. In contrast, translocations resulting in overexpression typically involve the juxtaposition of a coding region next to a highly active promoter or enhancer region such as an immunoglobulin region in B cells. For example, in follicular lymphoma, translocations frequently involve juxtaposition of the antiapoptotic gene *BCL2* to the immunoglobulin heavy chain enhancer region, leading to massive overexpression of *BCL2* RNA and protein.

Translocations are best detected by either whole-genome sequencing or RNA sequencing ("RNAseq"), although their detection requires advanced computational analysis to distinguish them from artifactual errors in aligning sequence reads to a reference genome. For reasons that remain unclear, some tumors contain few, if any, translocations, but others contain hundreds, often involving multiple complex rearrangements. A particularly interesting phenomenon, recently termed *chromothripsis,* involves extensive complex genome rearrangements thought to occur via a single "big bang" genomic catastrophe (Fig. 2-4).[19] It has been speculated that chromothripsis may represent a mechanism by which a cell can acquire multiple oncogenic events required for cellular transformation in a single event rather than in a stepwise manner.

Methylation

Although the majority of information encoded in the genome is thought to emanate from its primary DNA sequence, it is clear that additional modifications of DNA play important regulatory roles. For example, DNA methylation can occur, particularly in CpG-rich regions of the genome, and such methylation can lead to the silencing of gene expression at that locus. Although methylation in normal tissues is relatively uncommon, widespread methylation appears frequently in cancer and may serve as an important mechanism of silencing tumor suppressor genes. Until recently, it has not been possible to systematically assess DNA methylation across the genome, but massively parallel sequencing instruments, coupled with bisulfite sequencing approaches, are now paving the way for the first genome-wide assessments of DNA methylation in development and disease. The extent to which aberrant methylation is an important driver of disease (as opposed to simply a reflection of it) remains to be determined.

RNA-LEVEL CHARACTERIZATION

mRNA Profiling

The most well developed and widely used genomic technology is genome-wide expression profiling of protein-coding RNAs (mRNAs). Most such profiling is done using an array format in which sequence-specific probes are immobilized onto a solid surface (or are synthesized in situ); mRNA is isolated from a sample of interest (e.g., a tumor biopsy or a cell line); the mRNA is labeled in some fashion, often with a fluorescent tag; and the extent of hybridization of the mRNA to the array is captured by a laser scanning device. In the early days of arrays, investigators made their own arrays, but at present

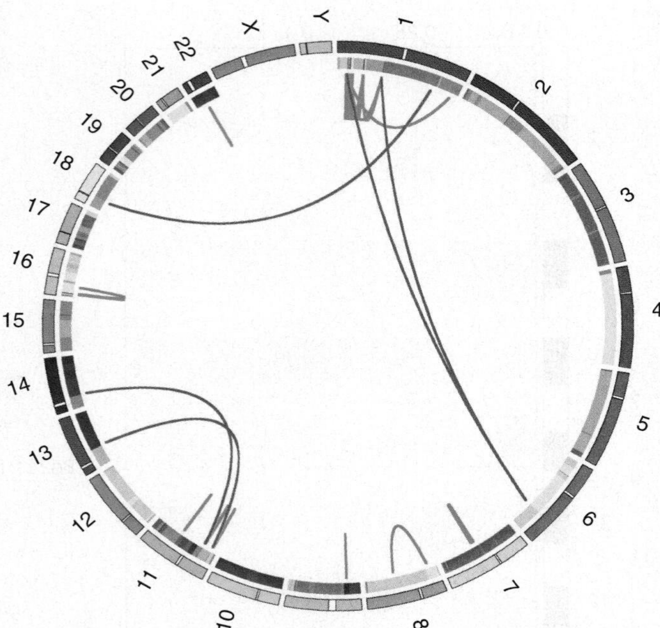

Figure 2-4 CHROMOTHRIPSIS. CIRCOS plot showing the extensive genomic rearrangements in a glioblastoma tumor. Each of the human chromosomes is displayed around the circle of the plot. *Purple lines* indicate rearrangements between different chromosomes, and *green lines* indicate intrachromosomal rearrangements. In this tumor, chromosome 1p has nearly 100 chromosomal rearrangements indicative of a single-step genomic catastrophe mechanism known as chromothripsis.

they are routinely available from a number of sources at high quality and relatively low cost, enabling the interrogation of all 22,000 or so mRNAs in the human and mouse transcriptomes.

Expression-profiling of FFPE tissues deserves special mention. Formalin fixation causes the degradation of mRNAs to fragments of only about 80 nucleotides in length. Conventional array-based profiling approaches therefore do not work well, particularly those that involve labeling of the mRNAs by priming of the 3′ polyadenylation tail. Two promising approaches have been recently developed, however, allowing for the profiling of FFPE-derived tissues. The first is a minor modification of standard arrays involving the use of 3′-biased probes for each mRNA transcript, such that even degraded mRNAs can be profiled. The other approach, known as the c**D**NA-mediated **a**nnealing, **s**election, extension, and **l**igation Method (DASL) method, involves highly multiplexed locus-specific, short PCR reactions.[5] Although it is likely that any method applied to FFPE samples will yield noisier data compared with frozen samples, the ability to analyze archived material, particularly those samples with long-term clinical outcome data, will prove invaluable.

Array-based approaches do not give absolute quantitation, but often this is not required. Rather, researchers wish to compare the expression level of a gene (or genes) in one sample with another (or one group of samples to another). Most gene expression profiling thus requires the *relative* assessment of expression across a set of samples, and absolute quantitation (e.g., number of mRNA copies per cell) is neither possible nor in most cases necessary. More recent sequencing-based approaches to expression profiling ("RNAseq"), however, provide the opportunity to provide a count of the number of transcripts in a given sample. In addition, RNA sequencing allows for the profiling of previously unknown genes (i.e., those not previously recognized to encode a transcript) as well as alternative splice forms of known mRNAs. The extent to which aberrant splicing underlies disease is at this time unknown. Until the advent of RNAseq, there was no way to systematically assess splicing patterns across the genome. The years ahead will likely bring significant new insights into this phenomenon.

Noncoding RNA Profiling

Until very recently, nearly the entirety of focus within the family of RNAs has been on those that code for proteins. However, recent studies have clearly demonstrated that a wealth of noncoding RNAs exist in mammalian cells. Two major classes of noncoding RNAs have been discovered: short RNAs known as *microRNAs* (miRNAs) and *large intergenic noncoding RNAs* (lincRNAs), as described below.

miRNAs are small (≈22 nucleotides) RNAs that do not encode for proteins but bind to mRNA transcripts to regulate translation and mRNA stability. Several hundred miRNAs are thought to exist in the human genome. In *Caenorhabditis elegans,* zebrafish, and other model organisms, miRNAs play a critical role in development through regulation of translation of key proteins. In mammalian cells, a role for miRNAs has been recognized in the regulation of cellular differentiation. Not only are many miRNAs differentially expressed across hematopoietic lineages, but several miRNAs have also been demonstrated to play key functional roles in hematopoietic lineage specification and differentiation.[20] Moreover, the expression or function of several miRNAs is altered by chromosomal translocations, deletions, or mutations in leukemia. In addition, members of the protein complex (including the protein DICER) that process the maturation of miRNAs from longer RNA forms have been implicated in malignancy.

Noncoding lincRNAs range are approximately 1000 nucleotides in length and number approximately 5000 in the human genome. The widespread existence of lincRNAs was only discovered in 2009, and their function remains largely unknown. However, recent evidence suggests that they may play important roles in establishing and maintaining cell fate and may play key roles in regulation of the epigenome. To date, no defects in lincRNAs have been reported in association with hematologic disease, but few, if any, large-scale surveys have been conducted. Their role in the pathogenesis of disease therefore remains unknown. Interestingly, lincRNAs appear to have exquisite tissue-specific patterns of expression, suggesting that they may have future diagnostic potential.

The expression of noncoding RNAs can be performed using hybridization-based arrays similar to those used for standard mRNA profiling. It is likely, however, that as the cost of sequencing continues to fall, comprehensive RNA sequencing will become the platform of choice, yielding in a single experiment the expression of all coding and noncoding RNAs.

PROTEIN-LEVEL CHARACTERIZATION

Unlike the characterization of DNA and RNA, which have become routine, the systematic, genome-wide characterization of proteins remains extremely technically challenging. Not long ago, comparative proteomic experiments largely consisted of the comparison of single proteins across various conditions or samples. However, a number of new advances in technology have made for a dramatic acceleration of the pace at which the abundance of proteins can be measured and their posttranslational modification (e.g., phosphorylation) assessed.

Mass Spectrometry

The workhorse of proteomics remains mass spectrometry. The fundamental principles of mass spectrometry have not changed over the years, but technical advances (the details of which are beyond the scope of this chapter) have led to increased ability to detect proteins in complex mixtures. Previously, extensive biochemical fractionation of the proteome was required to render mixtures of proteins sufficiently limited in number and with sufficient abundance so as to be reliably detected and identified. Such fractionation required extensive time, expertise, instrumentation, and a large amount of starting material, all of which tended to make systematic proteomic experiments difficult to perform routinely. However, newer instruments and methods allow for the analysis of significantly more complex mixtures. Today it is possible to quantitatively measure proteins and their modification with roughly 20-fold greater sensitivity and fivefold greater speed than just 5 years ago. Sequence assignment confidence, especially for modified peptides, has also been markedly improved owing to the more than 100-fold increase in both resolution and mass accuracy. For example, in mammalian cells, it is now possible to confidently detect more than 8000 unique proteins and more than 15,000 phosphopeptides in a few days on a single instrument. Experts believe that the coming years will bring the ability to perform proteome-wide analysis of complex samples such as entire cells and tissues without extensive fractionation. If this comes to pass, the interrogation of the proteome is likely to become a routine part of biomedical research.

Reverse Phase Lysates

An attractive alternate to mass spectrometry involves the use of *reverse phase lysate arrays* (RPPAs). RPPAs involve the robotic spotting of minute amounts of total cell protein lysates onto glass slides (thus creating an array of lysates from different samples) (Fig. 2-5). The slides can then be probed with antibodies against particular proteins of interest, including phosphorylation-specific antibodies.[21] The advantage of RPPAs is that only a tiny amount of cellular material is required, and hundreds of samples can be tested on a single array. The downside is that the method requires the availability of high-quality antibodies that are both sensitive and specific for the protein of interest. Unfortunately, such high-quality antibodies are available for only a minority of human proteins. In addition, RPPAs are not suitable for the analysis of large numbers of proteins because each protein to be interrogated requires a separate slide. Nevertheless, RPPA remains a powerful new tool in the armamentarium of proteomic research and may prove particularly useful for the comparison of proteins of interest across a large panel of samples (e.g., across a collection of patient samples or cell lines).

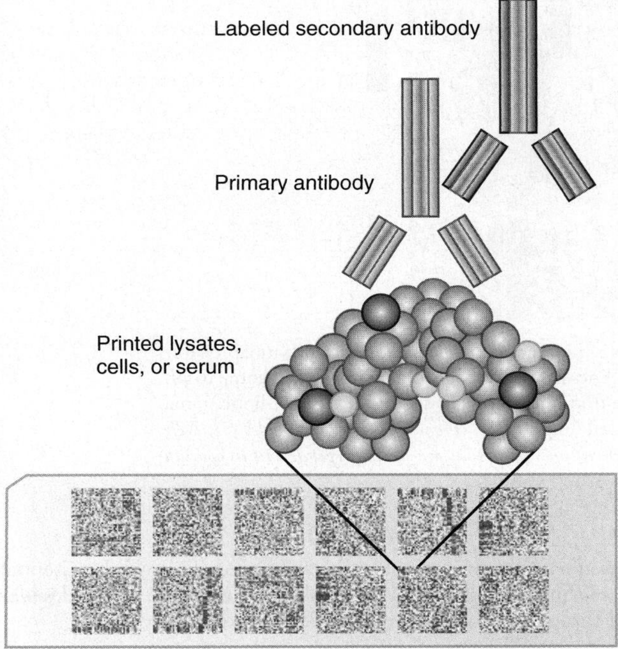

Figure 2-5 REVERSE PHASE PROTEIN ARRAYS (RPPAs). Schematic illustrating the concept of RPPA. Cellular lysates from patient samples or cell lines are robotically spotted onto a glass slide. Next, a primary antibody specific for a protein of interest is added to the slide, with the antibody sticking to the array in proportion to the abundance of the protein in question. To visualize the antibody-binding event, a secondary antibody that recognizes the primary antibody (generally fluorescently labeled) is added, and the slide examined by microscopy or a laser scanning instrument.

Bead-Based Profiling

Another new proteomic method involves the multiplexed analysis of protein abundance or phosphorylation. Phosphorylation involves the use of Luminex microspheres (beads). In this approach, a different protein-specific antibody is coupled to beads of distinct color. A mixture of antibody-coupled beads is then mixed with protein lysate and then binding events are detected with a labeled secondary antibody (e.g., anti-phosphotyrosine antibody). Multiple analytes are thereby simultaneously profiled in a single sample. This approach was successfully used to profile the tyrosine phosphorylation status of nearly all protein tyrosine kinases across a panel of cell lines.[4] The advantage of this approach is that multiple proteins (as many as 100 or more) can be simultaneously assessed in a single sample. But, similar to RPPA, the method depends on the availability of high-quality antibodies, and this limitation makes the approach difficult to generalize broadly. Nevertheless, the method may prove useful for interrogating particular classes of proteins such as kinases, for which suitable antibodies exist.

METABOLITE-LEVEL CHARACTERIZATION

Beyond nucleic acid and protein characterization, systematic profiling of small-molecule metabolites has also recently become possible. Such unbiased approaches to the assessment of metabolite levels have yielded new insights into the pathogenesis of metabolic diseases such as diabetes.[22] In addition, the recent discovery of mutations in metabolic enzymes in acute myeloid leukemia has spurred interest in the metabolic consequences of these mutations on the "metabolome."[23] Metabolite profiling is at present not routinely used in biomedical research, but it is likely that the years ahead will see a significant surge in its use.

FUNCTIONAL GENOMICS

Although the bulk of genomics research takes the form of observational studies (i.e., determining the spectrum of mutations in a tumor), increasingly, functional approaches to genomic research are becoming feasible. For example, the discovery of RNAi technology has now made it possible to knock down the expression of all genes in a given cell line and measure the consequence. This approach has been taken most extensively in the area of cancer, where the complete set of genes that are essential for the survival of a cancer cell line can be identified via genome-wide RNAi screens conduct genome-wide screens (Fig. 2-6). For example, a recent report elucidated the genes required for survival of each of approximately 100 cancer cell lines.[24] Similar approaches have been reported for hematologic malignancies, such as in multiple myeloma, in which new therapeutic targets were suggested.[25] In addition to pointing to new potential therapeutic targets for cancer, large-scale RNAi screens hold the promise of identifying genetic predictors of gene dependency. Such predictors will be key for the translation of these in vitro approaches to the clinic.

In addition to loss-of-function RNAi screens, it is also becoming possible to perform systematic gain-of-function screens by overexpressing a library of cDNAs and then selecting for a phenotype of interest. This approach was recently piloted in the study of drug resistance in melanoma, leading to the discovery of the kinase COT that appears to confer resistance to BRAF inhibitors by providing an alternate path to activating the mitogen-activated protein (MAP) kinase pathway.[26]

Other approaches to functional genomics include various strategies aimed at insertional mutagenesis, whereby endogenous genes in the genome are either activated or inactivated via the ectopic insertion

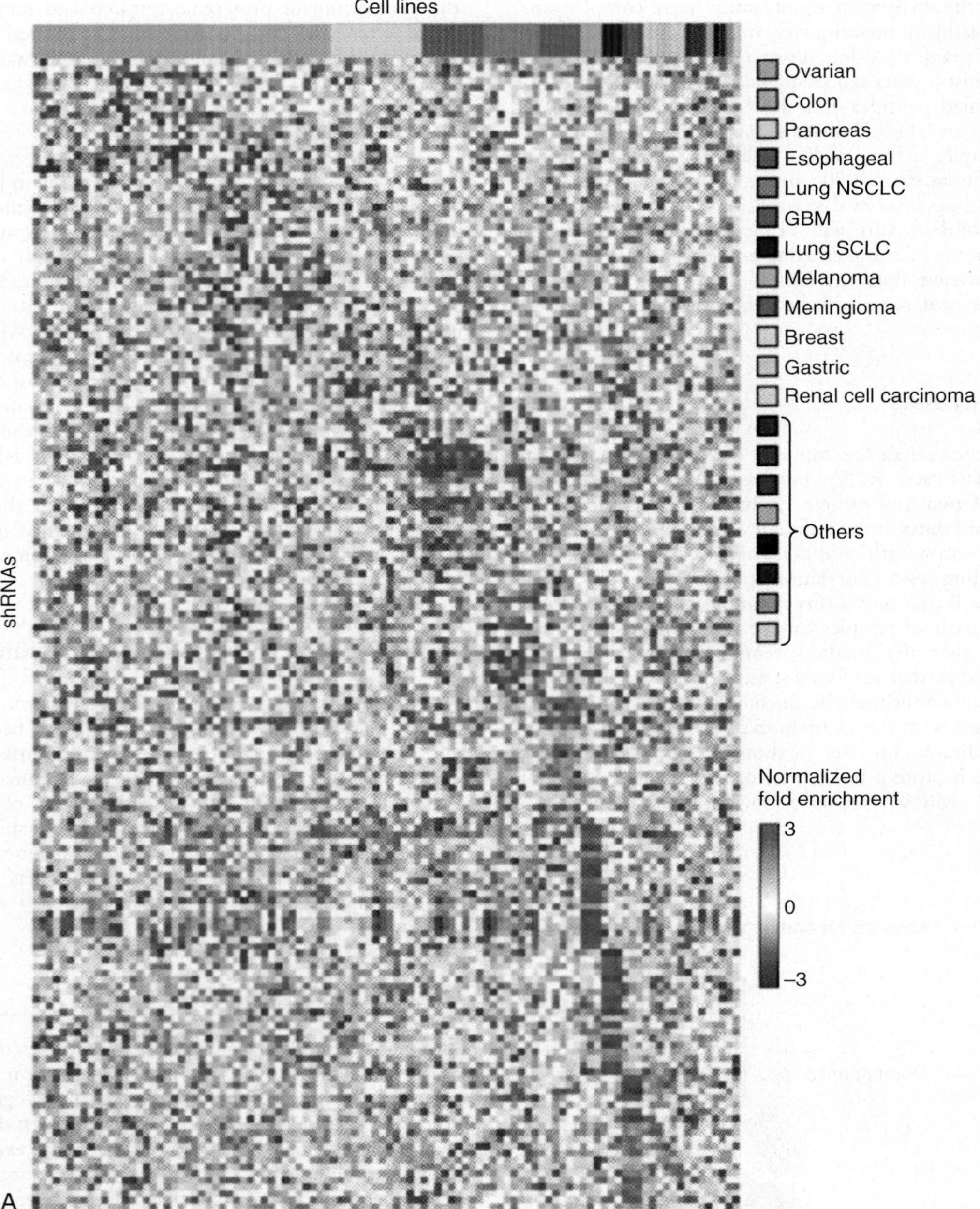

Figure 2-6 SYSTEMATIC RNA INTERFERENCE SCREENS. Lineage-specific dependencies. Heatmap of differentially antiproliferative short hairpin RNAs (shRNAs) in cell lines from individual cancer lineages in comparison with all others. The top 20 shRNAs that distinguish each lineage from the others are displayed. *GBM,* Glioblastoma multiforme; *NSCLC,* non–small cell lung cancer; *SCLC,* small cell lung cancer. *(From Cheung HW, Cowley GS, Weir BA, et al: Systematic investigation of genetic vulnerabilities across cancer cell lines reveals lineage-specific dependencies in ovarian cancer.* Proc Natl Acad Sci U S A *108:12372, 2011.)*

of foreign genetic material such as a transposon. These approaches can be powerful methods of mutagenizing the genome to find functionally important elements. Similarly, random mutagenesis can be performed chemically with agents such as *N*-ethyl N-nitrosourea (ENU).

Last, new and potentially powerful methods for genome engineering have been recently described, whereby transcription activator-like effectors (TALEs) have been used to either modulate transcription or edit the genome sequence at any locus of interest within the genome.[27] This approach may prove particularly useful in the functional testing of disease-associated genetic variants; the ability to experimentally revert a variant allele to its wild-type version should allow for the consequence of the variant to be monitored. This will be essential in establishing the functional role of disease-associated risk alleles identified through genome-wide association studies.

PHARMACOGENOMICS

The use of the genome to study drug response deserves special mention and is the subject of an entire chapter of this book (see Chapter 7). As the cost of genome sequencing continues to fall, it will become increasingly feasible to perform population-scale genetic studies to identify genetic determinants of drug toxicity and response.

Although some examples of such pharmacogenomic markers have been discovered (e.g., genetic predictors of antimetabolite chemotherapy), the field is still in its infancy and awaits truly large-scale, systematic studies of large numbers of patients with known drug response data.

CLINICAL USE OF GENOMICS

Expression-Based Diagnostics

It has been over a decade since the first proof-of-principle studies were published demonstrating the possibility of using gene expression profiling to classify diseases such as cancer. Those studies raised the possibility that such promising gene expression signatures might be further validated and then implemented in the routine clinical setting as powerful diagnostic tests. The reality is that few such transitions to clinical practice have been made. The notable exception to this is the OncoType Dx test, which consists of a tumor gene expression signature of 21 genes capable of determining the requirement for chemotherapy in women with early stage breast cancer. This test has now become part of the standard of care at many cancer centers nationwide.

One should ask, however, why, despite thousands of papers being published on potential diagnostic applications of gene expression profiling, so few have progressed to routine clinical implementation. There are likely several reasons to explain the slow pace of advancement. First, to develop truly valid diagnostic tests, the test must be applied to large numbers of patients with known clinical outcome, and in many cases, such cohorts of patients simply do not exist, making validation challenging. Second, because gene expression signatures are based on relative transcript abundance (as opposed to, for example, genome sequencing), it is subject to technical variation such as stromal admixture of tumors that can distort a diagnostic signature. Third, although the academic publishing system tends to reward *initial* discoveries (which are often published in high-profile journals), the essential follow-up *validation* studies tend to be valued less, and therefore investigators are not incentivized to follow up initial observations. And finally, the economics of molecular diagnostics have in general not been favorable, thereby discouraging companies from making major investments in the validation and commercialization of promising diagnostic tests. It is likely that diagnostic tests will command more of a premium in the future as a mechanism to use expensive therapeutics only in patients likely to benefit, but the time required for this to evolve is uncertain.

Sequencing-Based Diagnostics

With the recent dramatic fall in the cost of genome sequencing has come the prospect of introducing comprehensive sequencing into the clinical setting. Compared with RNA-based analysis, DNA-based diagnostics have the advantage of being more definitive in that one is looking, for example, for the presence of a mutation (an A, G, C, or T) as opposed to a relative abundance of a particular transcript or transcripts. Also, because modern sequencing approaches allow for allele separation, the admixture of tumors with normal cells can be overcome simply by increasing depth of sequencing coverage, as described in the preceding sections. Therefore, it is likely that in the years ahead, we will see an explosion of sequencing-based diagnostic applications for cancers, including hematologic malignancies, whereby clinically actionable mutations will be assessed by sequencing a panel of genes (hundreds of candidate genes). As the cost of sequencing continues to drop, this will likely give way to more systematic approaches that include whole-exome sequencing and whole-genome sequencing. It is likely, however, that the pace of technology advancement will outstrip our understanding of clinical utility and financial reimbursement by health insurance payers, so the rate at which sequencing-based diagnostics will become mainstream remains to be established.

Sequencing-based diagnostics will also likely have an increasingly important role in nonmalignant conditions, such as blood clotting disorders, in which it will become possible to systematically resequence all genes in the coagulation cascade, thereby identifying either common or highly rare sequence variants that might explain or predict disease. The widespread use of germline sequencing to predict disease also raises a large set of ethical questions that must be addressed in the years ahead, particularly those relating to children and family members of individuals undergoing sequence analysis. Whether whole-genome sequencing will become a routine part of routine health care in the future remains to be determined, but it is almost certain that much of our current diagnostic approach to medicine will eventually be supplanted by DNA-level analysis.

FUTURE DIRECTIONS

The field of genomics has matured greatly over the past decade. Major analytical advances have made it possible to analyze and interpret complex datasets beyond what was previously possible. And dropping costs have made it possible to generate data at a scale that was never before imaginable. For example, it is likely that by the year 2015, there will be more than 100,000 tumor genomes available for analysis to the research community (the first such genome sequence became available only in 2008). We will also witness an explosion of functional genomic studies involving, for example, the genome-wide interrogation of gene dependencies across as many as 1000 cancer cell lines. Each of these approaches, although powerful, has its own limitations, and it is likely that most progress will be made by integrating across many disparate experimental strategies and datasets. The implication of this is that researchers will increasingly need strong quantitative analytical skills to be successful in modern biomedical research. Last, as costs drop and our knowledge base increases, so too will diagnostic opportunities increase. The integration of such genomic approaches into clinical research and routine clinical care is likely to be one of the greatest challenges and opportunities in medicine in the decade ahead.

REFERENCES

1. James C, Ugo V, Le Couédic JP, et al: A unique clonal JAK2 mutation leading to constitutive signalling causes polycythaemia vera. *Nature* 434:1144, 2005.
2. Levine RL, Wadleigh M, Cools J, et al: Activating mutation in the tyrosine kinase JAK2 in polycythemia vera, essential thrombocythemia, and myeloid metaplasia with myelofibrosis. *Cancer Cell* 7:387, 2005.
3. Papaemmanuil E, Cazzola M, Boultwood J, et al: Chronic Myeloid Disorders Working Group of the International Cancer Genome Consortium: Somatic SF3B1 mutation in myelodysplasia with ring sideroblasts. *N Engl J Med* 365:1384, 2011.
4. Du J, Bernasconi P, Clauser KR, et al: Bead-based profiling of tyrosine kinase phosphorylation identifies SRC as a potential target for glioblastoma therapy. *Nat Biotechnol* 27:77, 2009.
5. Hoshida Y, Villanueva A, Kobayashi M, et al: Gene expression in fixed tissues and outcome in hepatocellular carcinoma. *N Engl J Med* 359:1995, 2008.
6. Emmert-Buck MR, Bonner RF, Smith PD, et al: Laser capture microdissection. *Science* 274:998, 1996.
7. Hanahan D, Weinberg RA: Hallmarks of cancer: The next generation. *Cell* 144:646, 2011.
8. Alizadeh AA, Eisen MB, Davis RE, et al: Distinct types of diffuse large B-cell lymphoma identified by gene expression profiling. *Nature* 403:503, 2000.
9. Armstrong SA, Staunton JE, Silverman LB, et al: MLL translocations specify a distinct gene expression profile that distinguishes a unique leukemia. *Nat Genet* 30:41, 2002.
10. Shipp MA, Ross KN, Tamayo P, et al: Diffuse large B-cell lymphoma outcome prediction by gene-expression profiling and supervised machine learning. *Nat Med* 8:68, 2002.

11. Yeoh EJ, Ross ME, Shurtleff SA, et al: Classification, subtype discovery, and prediction of outcome in pediatric acute lymphoblastic leukemia by gene expression profiling. *Cancer Cell* 1:133, 2002.
12. Auclair D, Chapuy B, Sougnez C, et al: Discovery and prioritization of somatic mutations in diffuse large B-cell lymphoma (DLBCL) by whole-exome sequencing. *Proc Natl Acad Sci U S A* 109:3879, 2012.
13. Morin RD, Mendez-Lago M, Mungall AJ, et al: Frequent mutation of histone-modifying genes in non-Hodgkin lymphoma. *Nature* 476:298, 2011.
14. Dryja TP, Rapaport JM, Epstein J, et al: Homozygosity of chromosome 13 in retinoblastoma. *N Engl J Med* 310:550, 1984.
15. Slamon DJ, Leyland-Jones B, Shak S, et al: Use of chemotherapy plus a monoclonal antibody against HER2 for metastatic breast cancer that overexpresses HER2. *N Engl J Med* 344:783, 2001.
16. Rowley JD: The critical role of chromosome translocations in human leukemias. *Annu Rev Genet* 32:495, 1998.
17. Robinson JT, Thorvaldsdóttir H, Winckler W, et al: Integrative genomics viewer. *Nat Biotechnol* 29:24, 2011.
18. Beroukhim R, Getz G, Nghiemphu L, et al: Assessing the significance of chromosomal aberrations in cancer: Methodology and application to glioma. *Proc Natl Acad Sci U S A* 104:20007, 2007.
19. Stephens PJ, Greenman CD, Fu B, et al: Massive genomic rearrangement acquired in a single catastrophic event during cancer development. *Cell* 144:27, 2011.
20. Shivdasani RA: MicroRNAs: Regulators of gene expression and cell differentiation. *Blood* 108:3646, 2006.
21. Paweletz CP, Charboneau L, Bichsel VE, et al: Reverse phase protein microarrays which capture disease progression show activation of pro-survival pathways at the cancer invasion front. *Oncogene* 20:1981, 2001.
22. Wang TJ, Larson MG, Vasan RS, et al: Metabolite profiles and the risk of developing diabetes. *Nat Med* 17:448, 2011.
23. Mardis ER, Ding L, Dooling DJ, et al: Recurring mutations found by sequencing an acute myeloid leukemia genome. *N Engl J Med* 361:1058, 2009.
24. Cheung HW, Cowley GS, Weir BA, et al: Systematic investigation of genetic vulnerabilities across cancer cell lines reveals lineage-specific dependencies in ovarian cancer. *Proc Natl Acad Sci U S A* 108:12372, 2011.
25. Shaffer AL, Emre NC, Lamy L, et al: IRF4 addiction in multiple myeloma. *Nature* 454:226, 2008.
26. Johannessen CM, Boehm JS, Kim SY, et al: COT drives resistance to RAF inhibition through MAP kinase pathway reactivation. *Nature* 468:968, 2010.
27. Sanjana NE, Cong L, Zhou Y, et al: A transcription activator-like effector toolbox for genome engineering. *Nat Protoc* 7:171, 2012.

CHAPTER 3

REGULATION OF GENE EXPRESSION, TRANSCRIPTION, SPLICING, AND RNA METABOLISM

Christopher R. Cogle, Amy Meacham, and Robert A. Hromas

The function of a cell is governed by the sum of the specific proteins expressed. Protein expression is most commonly regulated at the level of gene transcription into ribonucleic acid (RNA), which is then processed and translated. The life of a cell is the life of its RNA. Therefore, to understand how a cell behaves, one must understand the expression of a gene through RNA.

Transcription of deoxyribonucleic acid (DNA) into RNA controls cellular differentiation, proliferation, and apoptosis in all differentiating cell systems, but especially in hematopoiesis. For example, through regulation of transcription, hematopoietic stem cells maintain a balance between quiescence and differentiation to mature blood cell types. Regulation of transcription is also necessary for erythroid progenitors to produce vast quantities of hemoglobin, for myeloid cells to generate granules of immune responses, for lymphocytes to control immunoglobulin levels, and for platelets to regulate levels of thrombotic receptors.

Aberrant gene expression can result in hematologic disorders such as lymphomas, leukemias, and myelodysplastic and myeloproliferative syndromes, as will be discussed later. Understanding the process behind RNA synthesis is also crucial for the diagnosis and treatment of hematologic disorders. Converting genetic information contained in the DNA sequence of a gene into a finished protein product is a complex process consisting of several steps, with each step involving distinct regulatory mechanisms. Beginning with the basics of gene structure, this chapter will present the foundation necessary to understand the process of gene expression through RNA synthesis and processing, including transcription, splicing, posttranscriptional modification, and nuclear export. Subsequent chapters will present regulation of protein translation and posttranslational modifications.

The first step of gene expression is transcription, where RNA polymerases decode the DNA using specific start and stop signals to synthesize RNA. In the subsequent step, splicing removes portions of the RNA that do not code for protein. Next, the spliced RNA is modified for export out of the nucleus and into the cytoplasm, where ribosomes translate RNA into protein products.

HOW GENES ARE ORGANIZED IN DNA

The gene is the fundamental unit for storage and expression of genetic information. Genes are made up of nucleotide sequences of DNA and are transferred to daughter cells during mitosis (and meiosis in gametes) via semiconservative replication. Each cell in the human body contains about 25,000 genes, which are distributed unevenly across the 46 individual chromosomes found within the nucleus. Chromosomes are dense DNA-protein complexes that are made up of individual linear DNA helices packed tightly together by specific protein repeats. Unwound completely and stretched out, the largest chromosome is about one meter in length, demonstrating that the cell, even to exist, must be an expert at packaging.

Only 1% to 2% of human DNA actually serves as genes, which are the templates for protein production. Most genes are broken down into separated coding sections known as *exons* (Fig. 3-1). These exons are separated from each other by intervening, noncoding sequences known as *introns*. Genes also have other noncoding DNA, typically short sequences near or within genes that function as regulatory sequences critical for controlling gene expression. Together, these regulatory sequences determine in which cell, at what time, and in what amount the gene is converted into the corresponding protein.

In order for transcription to begin, RNA polymerase must attach to a specific DNA region at the beginning of a gene. These regions, known as *promoters*, contain specific nucleotide sequences and response elements. These provide a secure initial binding site on the gene for RNA polymerase. RNA polymerase often requires other proteins called *transcription factors* for proper recruitment to a given gene. Not all transcription factors are activating; some may inhibit RNA polymerase and repress gene expression by attaching to specific promoters and blocking binding of RNA polymerase. Promoters can additionally function together with other more distant regulatory DNA regions (termed *enhancers, silencers, boundary elements,* or *insulators*) to direct the level of transcription of a given gene. Unlike RNA polymerase, transcription factors are not limited to the promoter region but can be directed by these other regulatory DNA sequences to either promote or repress transcription. The minimum essential transcription factors needed for transcription to occur are termed *basal transcription factors,* and they include transcription factor IIA (TFIIA), as well as TFIIB, TFIID, TFIIE, TFIIF, and TFIIH. These ubiquitous proteins bind to the recognition sequence in the promoter, forming a transcription initiation complex that recruits the RNA polymerase. Basal transcription factors cannot by themselves increase or decrease the rate of transcription but may be linked to activators by coactivator proteins that can.

The promoter is a regulatory sequence located near the start of the gene, to provide the exact start site recognized by the transcription machinery where conversion of the DNA template into intermediary molecules begins. The promoter contains the consensus sequence to bind the transcription factors and then RNA polymerase needed to initiate transcription. The best-known example of this sequence is the TATA box sequence, TATAAA, which binds RNA polymerase and associated transcription factors. However, more than 80% of mammalian protein-coding genes are driven by TATA-less promoters, which contain different recognition sequences—often GC boxes. The GC promoters are repeats of guanine and cytosine nucleotides, frequently have multiple transcriptional start sites, and require alternative transcription factors, such as specificity protein 1 (Sp1).

Genes can have more than one promoter. This results in different sized mRNAs, depending on how far the promoter is from the 5′ end of the gene. The binding strength between a promoter and the transcription factors determines the avidity of RNA polymerase binding and, subsequently, of transcription. Some genetic diseases are associated with mutations in promoters, such as β-thalassemia, which can involve single nucleotide substitutions, small deletions, or insertions, in the β-globin promoter sequence. The promoter mutations in β-thalassemias result in decreased RNA polymerase binding to the transcriptional start site and thereby reduce β-globin gene expression.

Globin gene expression in erythroid cells is also dependent on another regulatory unit: the enhancer. Unlike promoters, which are

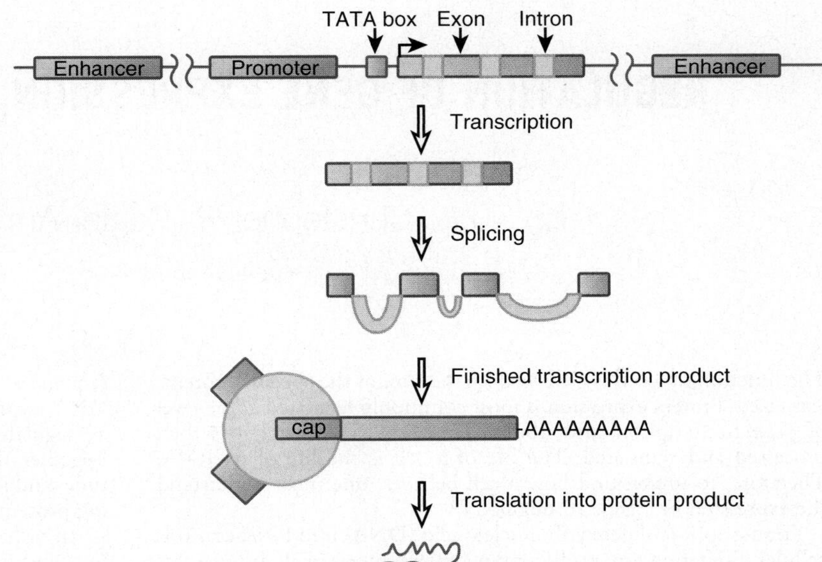

Figure 3-1 OVERVIEW OF GENE TRANSCRIPTION FROM DNA TO RNA AND THEN TRANSLATION FROM RNA TO PROTEIN. Protein synthesis requires multiple processes and regulatory steps including transcript of DNA into RNA, splicing and post-transcription modification of RNA, translation of RNA into protein, and post-translational protein modification.

situated close to the start site of the gene, enhancers can be positioned far to either side of the gene, or even within it. This means that there may be several signals determining whether a certain gene can be transcribed. In fact, multiple enhancer sites may be linked to one gene, and each enhancer may be bound by more than one transcription factor. The determining factor in whether or not such a gene is transcribed is the sum of the activity of these transcription factors bound to the different enhancers. Enhancers can compensate for a weak promoter by binding activator transcription factors. For instance, regulation of gene expression during T-lymphocyte differentiation requires multiple activating transcription factors, such as lymphocyte enhancer factor (LEF1), GATA3, and ETS1, binding to the T-cell receptor alpha (TCRA) gene enhancer.

Transcription factors can also influence multiple genes in coordination, like the globin family. Enhancers are often the major determinant of transcription of developmental genes in the differing lineages and stages of hematopoiesis. They can also inhibit transcription of specific genes in one cell type while, at the same time, activating it in another cell type. When gene sequences routinely negatively regulate gene transcription, they are termed *silencers*. Insulators, another type of DNA regulatory sequence, define borders of multigene clusters to prevent activation of one set of genes from affecting a nearby set of genes in another cluster.

TRANSCRIPTION OF GENES

The first phase of gene expression occurs when the RNA polymerase synthesizes RNA from a DNA gene template. As described in the previous section, this is called *transcription*. The encoded material on the transcribed gene determines the kind of RNA synthesized. For example, proteins are coded for by messenger RNA (mRNA), which will later undergo the process of translation. Alternatively, the transcribed gene may encode transfer RNA (tRNA), which carries specific amino acids to the ribosome for incorporation into the growing protein chain during translation. Another type of RNA synthesized from genes in DNA is ribosomal RNA (rRNA), which serves as the backbone of ribosomes and interacts with tRNA during translation. Ribosomes catalyze the formation of proteins, using the mRNA as the code and the tRNA to obtain the amino acids to build the proteins. Each amino acid is attached to the previous one by hydrolysis and aminotransferase activity residing within the ribosome. Transcription of the different classes of RNAs in eukaryotes is carried out by three different RNA polymerase enzymes. RNA polymerase I (i.e., Pol I) synthesizes the rRNAs, except for the 5S species. RNA polymerase II (i.e., Pol II) synthesizes the mRNAs and some small nuclear RNAs (snRNAs) involved in RNA splicing. RNA polymerase III (i.e., Pol III) synthesizes the 5S rRNA and the tRNAs.

The most intricate controls of eukaryotic genes are those that govern the expression of RNA Pol II-transcribed genes, the genes that encode mRNA. Most eukaryotic mRNA genes contain a basic structure consisting of alternating coding exons and noncoding introns and have one of two major types of basal promoters as defined earlier. These protein-coding genes also can have a variety of transcriptional regulatory domains, such as the enhancers or silencers mentioned earlier. In addition to management of gene expression by the RNA polymerase binding strength of the promoters at the beginning of a given gene, the interaction between activator and inhibitor transcription factor proteins binding to the given promoter also exerts regulatory action on transcription.

To initiate transcription, the RNA polymerase must bind to the promoter sequence. However, as mentioned earlier, this can only happen with help from gene-specific transcription factors that mediate RNA polymerase binding to the promoter. These transcription factors are sequence-specific DNA binding proteins that can be modified by cell signals. Many transcription factors, such as STAT proteins, require phosphorylation in order to bind DNA. Because transcription factors can be targeted by kinases and phosphatases, phosphorylation can effectively integrate information carried by multiple signal transduction pathways, thus providing versatility and flexibility in gene regulation. For example, the Janus kinase (JAK) signal transducer and activator of transcription (STAT) pathway is widely used by members of the cytokine receptor superfamily, including those for granulocyte colony-stimulating factor (G-CSF), erythropoietin, thrombopoietin, interferons, and interleukins. Normally, ligand-bound growth factor receptors lead to JAK2 phosphorylation, which then activates STAT, also by phosphorylation. Activated STAT then dimerizes, translocates to the hematopoietic cell nucleus, binds DNA, and promotes transcription of genes for hematopoiesis. Alteration of JAK2, such as a V617F mutation, results in a constitutively active kinase capable of driving STAT activation. This leads to constitutive transcription of STAT target genes and results in myeloproliferative disorders such as polycythemia vera.

Mutations in promoter sequences that result in decreased transcription factor binding, and therefore less RNA polymerase binding, result in decreased gene expression. One of the best examples of a mutation in a transcription factor binding site associated with a human disease is in the factor IX gene. The transcription factor HNF4α is required to bind to the factor IX promoter before this gene can be transcribed. Patients with a mutation in the HNF4α

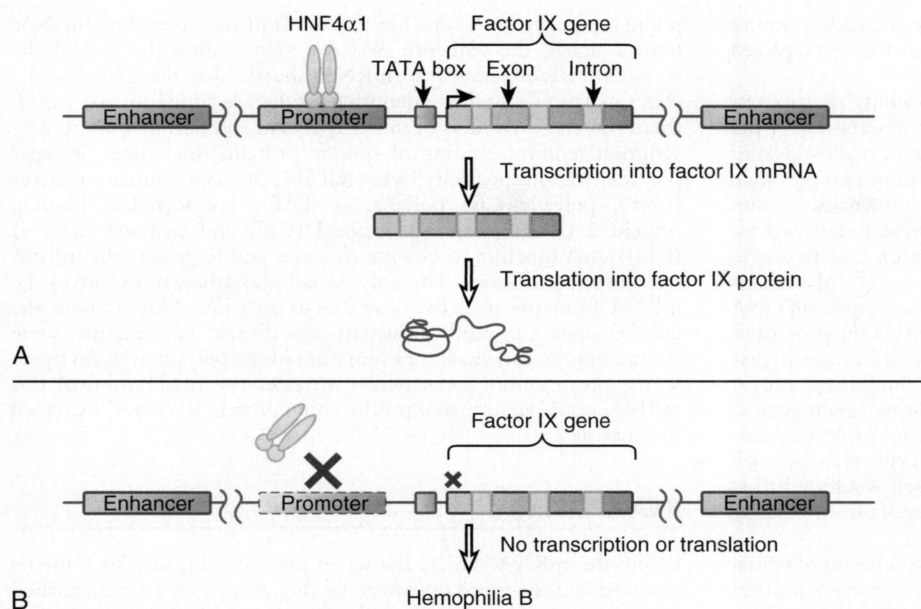

Figure 3-2 ROLE OF TRANSCRIPTION FACTOR BINDING SITES IN THE REGULATION OF EUKARYOTIC GENE EXPRESSION. **A,** Schematic diagram of a eukaryotic promoter showing transcription factor binding sites in promoter region before the factor IX gene, the TATA box, and the start site of transcription *(red X)*. Not shown are histones, co-regulators, mediator or chromatin remodeling complexes. **B,** Effect of a mutation in the HNF4α1 binding site on expression of the blood coagulation gene factor IX.

binding site can develop hemophilia B, an X-linked recessive bleeding disorder primarily affecting males (Fig. 3-2).

The ability of transcription factors and RNA polymerases to access specific promoters and transcribe genes is also regulated by the packaging of DNA into discrete packets by proteins generically termed *chromatin*. Chromatin can package DNA tightly or loosely, and this regulates the availability of a gene for transcription. Several factors affect the openness of chromatin and therefore regulate availability of the DNA to transcription factors and RNA polymerases. There are two types of chromatin: euchromatin and heterochromatin. *Euchromatin* refers to loosely packaged DNA, where RNA polymerases can freely bind to DNA and genes are actively transcribed. *Heterochromatin* refers to tightly packaged DNA that is protected from transcription machinery, sequestering genes away from transcription. The basic unit of chromatin is the nucleosome, which contains eight histone proteins packaging 146 base pairs of DNA wound 1.7 times around the histone complex (Fig. 3-3).

These histones can be extensively modified to regulate the accessibility of the DNA to the transcriptional apparatus. Histones can be chemically modified by acetylation, methylation, or phosphorylation. In general, acetylation opens the nucleosome to increase transcription, whereas phosphorylation marks damaged DNA. Histone methylation can either open chromatin to increase transcription or close it to repress transcription, depending on where the histone is methylated. Transcription factors can themselves recruit histone-modifying enzymes that can regulate transcription. In hematopoiesis, transcription factors, including GATA1, ELKF, NF-E2, and PU.1, recruit histone acetyltransferases (HATs) and histone deacetylases (HDACs) to promoters of target genes, leading to addition or subtraction of acetyl groups from histones, thereby affecting chromatin structure and the openness of DNA to transcription. A gene essential to erythroid maturation and survival—GATA1, for instance—directly recruits HAT complexes to the β-globin locus to stimulate transcription activation.

Chromatin usually tightly packages DNA, which is essential for the cell to have a functional size and shape. Therefore, for transcription to take place, the DNA must be unwound from the chromatin. This process of unpackaging, called *chromatin remodeling*, is mediated by a family of proteins with switch/sucrose nonfermentable (SWI/SNF) domains. These proteins use ATP hydrolysis to shift the nucleosome core along the length of the DNA, a process also known as *nucleosome sliding*. By sliding nucleosomes away from a gene sequence, SWI/SNF complexes can activate gene transcription.

SWI/SNF proteins also contain helicase enzyme activity, which unwinds the DNA by breaking hydrogen bonds between the complementary nucleotides on opposite strands. By unwinding the DNA into two single strands, the DNA can then be read by RNA polymerases in the direction 3′ to 5′. A new antiparallel RNA strand, 5′

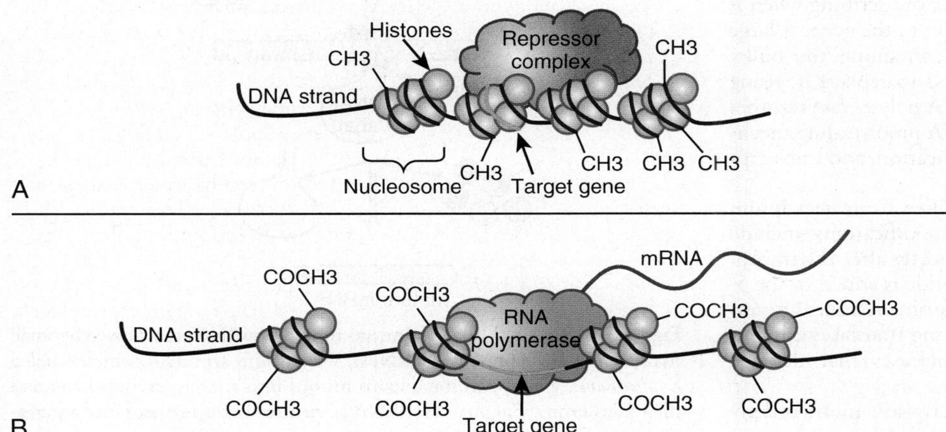

Figure 3-3 CHROMATIN STRUCTURE. **A,** The nucleosome is the fundamental unit of chromatin and is made up of DNA coiled around histone proteins. In a condensed state, the DNA is tightly wrapped around histone complexes and target genes are inaccessible to transcription machinery. **B,** Histones and DNA can be epigenetically modified by acetylation and methylation, rendering the target genes more accessible to transcription machinery.

to 3′, is produced by RNA polymerases to mirror the coding strand of the DNA, with the exception of all thymine nucleotides replaced by uracil nucleotides.

DNA itself can be chemically modified to amplify or suppress transcription. Stretches of cytosine and guanine repeats (i.e., CpG sites because of the single phosphate linking these to nucleotides) in promoters can be chemically modified by methylation enzymes such as DNA methyltransferases (DNMTs), which subsequently alter binding of RNA polymerase and associated transcription factors. Hypermethylation, which blocks DNA transcription and results in gene silencing, has been observed in bone marrow cells of patients with myelodysplastic syndromes (MDS), with the degree of DNA hypermethylation correlating to disease stage. In MDS the promoters of genes that are important for myeloid differentiation are hypermethylated, repressing their transcription and inhibiting proper maturation of the myeloid lineages. Hypomethylating agents such as azacitidine and decitabine can induce remission and prolonged survival in MDS patients. The regulation of gene expression by such chemical modifications of chromatin or DNA itself is referred to as *epigenetic*, since the alteration of cell function results from changes outside of the DNA sequence.

Such epigenetic modifications are crucial to the behavior of hematologic diseases. Mutation of the DNMT3 genes may have indirect effects on gene expression without altered DNA methylation, as have been observed in 20% of acute myeloid leukemia (AML) cases and correlated with poor clinical outcome. The Ten-Eleven-Translocation oncogene member TET2, which plays a role in DNA methylation, and therefore epigenetic stability, is mutated in AML, MDS, chronic myelomonocytic leukemia (CMML), and other myeloproliferative neoplasms (MPNs). Another recurring observation in hematologic malignancies is aberrant histone methylation, for example, at H3K27, seen in myelodysplasia. This is associated with altered gene expression affecting cell cycle, cell death, and cell adhesion pathways.

Before a final mRNA product is made, several proofreading regulatory steps must take place. The RNA polymerase may not even clear the promoter, in which case it will slip off, producing truncated transcripts. Once the transcript reaches approximately 23 nucleotides, the RNA polymerase no longer slips off, and full transcript elongation can occur. RNA polymerase then continues to traverse the template DNA strand, using ATP while complementarily pairing bases and forming the phosphodiester-ribose backbone. Many RNA transcripts may be rapidly produced from a single copy of a gene, as multiple RNA polymerases may transcribe the gene simultaneously, spaced out from one another. An important proofreading mechanism during elongation allows the substitution of incorrectly incorporated bases, usually by permitting short pauses during which the appropriate RNA editing factors can bind. RNA editing mechanisms in mRNAs include nucleoside modifications of cytidine to uridine (C-U) and adenosine to inosine (A-I) by deamination, as well as nucleotide insertions and additions without a DNA template by proteins called *editosomes*.

Another repair mechanism is transcription-coupled nucleotide excision repair, in which RNA polymerase stops transcribing when it comes to a bulky lesion in one of the nucleotides in the gene. A large protein complex excises the DNA segment containing the bulky lesion, and a new DNA segment is synthesized to replace it, using the opposite strand as a template. Then the RNA polymerase resumes transcribing the gene. However, in general, RNA proofreading mechanisms are not as effective as those in DNA replication, and transcription fidelity is lower.

After a gene is transcribed, mRNA is modified to protect it and target it for translation to protein. These modifications include *capping* and *polyadenylation*. Capping occurs shortly after the start of transcription, when a modified guanine nucleotide is added to the 5′ end of the mRNA. This terminal 7-methylguanosine residue is necessary for proper attachment to the ribosome during translation. It also protects the RNA from endogenous ribonucleases that degrade uncapped RNA, which is often viral in origin.

RNA polymerases do not terminate transcription in an orderly manner. They tend to be processive; yet the cell cannot tolerate a population of mRNAs that are enormous in size. Therefore mRNAs have a signal, the sequence AAUAA, that defines the end of the transcript. Ribonucleases cut mRNAs shortly after that signal, and a chain of several hundred adenosine residues is added to that free 3′ transcript end. Synthesis of this poly(A) tail and termination of transcription requires binding of specific proteins, including cleavage/polyadenylation specificity factor (CPSF), cleavage stimulation factor (CstF), polyadenylate polymerase (PAP), polyadenylate binding protein 2 (PAB2), cleavage factor I (CFI) and cleavage factor II (CFII), that function to catalyze cleavage, and to protect the mRNA from exoribonucleases. The poly(A) tail also assists in export of the mRNA from the nucleus, as well as translation. Mutations in the poly(A) signal can result in hematologic disease. For example, some thrombophilic patients have a mutation in the polyadenylation signal in the prothrombin gene, which increases the stabilization of this mRNA, resulting in higher prothrombin protein levels and increased thrombosis.

RNA SPLICING

Before the mRNA can be translated into protein, introns must be removed and the exons re-connected (Fig. 3-4). This process, termed *splicing*, requires a series of reactions mediated by the spliceosome, a complex of small nuclear ribonucleoproteins (snRNPs). The types of snRNPs in the spliceosome determine the mechanism of splicing. Canonical splicing, also called the *lariat pathway*, utilizes the major spliceosome and accounts for more than 99% of splicing. The major spliceosome is composed of the nuclear active snRNPs U1, U2, U4, U5, and U6, along with specific accessory proteins, U2AF and SF1. This complex recognizes the dinucleotide GU at the 5′ end of an intron and an AG at the 3′ end. Intermediately, a lariat structure forms, connecting these ends, providing for both excision of the intron and proper alignment of the ends of the two bordering exons to allow precise ligation. When the intronic flanking sequences do not follow the GU-AG rule, noncanonical splicing removes these rare introns with different splice site sequences using the minor spliceosome. The same U5 snRNP is found in the minor spliceosome, in addition to the unique yet functionally similar U11, U12, U4atac, and U6atac. Furthermore, there are splicing mechanisms, including tRNA splicing and self-splicing, that function without any spliceosome.

Splicing is central to proper gene expression and is therefore required for appropriate hematopoietic development. One of the best

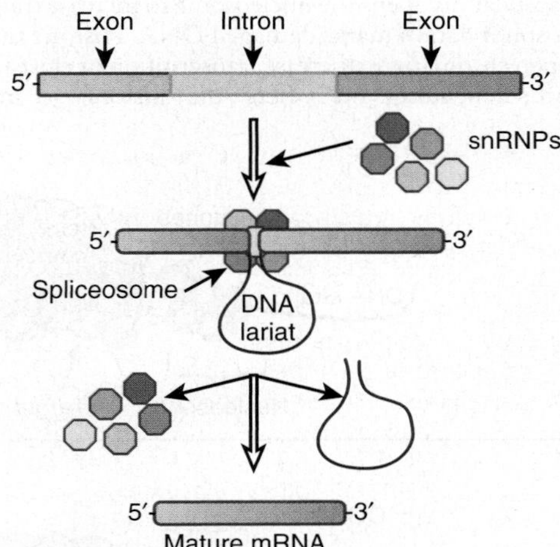

Figure 3-4 RNA SPLICING. Introns from pre-mRNA are removed by small nuclear ribonucleoproteins (snRNPs), which form a protein complex called a *spliceosome*. The spliceosome loops introns into a lariat, excises them, and then joins exons. The mature mRNA is then ready for further posttranscription processing.

examples of inappropriate splicing leading to hematologic disease is β-thalassemia, in which there are a number of different mutations that occur in the GU-AG splicing signals, resulting in aberrant β-globin mRNAs. Abnormal splicing can also lead to AML. The translocation liposarcoma (TLS) protein recruits splicing complexes to mRNAs, and it is involved in the TLS-ERG fusion oncogene in t(16;21) in AML. This fusion of TLS with the transcription factor ERG alters the splicing profile of immature myeloid cells, blocking the expression of genes required for proper differentiation and resulting in accumulation of immature myeloid cell precursor cells. Recently, whole exome sequencing of MDS specimens led to the discovery of frequently occurring mutations in RNA splicing machinery, including U2AF35, ZRSR2, SRSF2 and SF3B1. These results suggest the possibility of aberrant splicing in the pathogenesis of MDS and highlight new targets for treatment.

Trans-splicing is a form of splicing that joins two exons that are not within the same mRNA transcript. Some trans-splicing events occur when the intron splice donor sites are not filled by spliceosomes. They can lead to mRNAs displaying exon repetitions or chimeric fusion RNAs, which can mimic the presence of a chromosomal translocation in normal cells. For example, specific chimeric fusion mRNAs seen in acute leukemias (such as MLL-AF4, BCR-ABL, TEL-AML1, AML1-ETO, PML-RAR, NPM-ALK, and ATIC-ALK) have been found in blood cells from healthy individuals with normal chromosome karyotype. Of interest, these individuals do not develop leukemia, indicating that these fusion oncoproteins must be heritable (in DNA) and that they must occur in the appropriate hematopoietic precursor cell for leukemogenesis.

Alternative splicing can enhance the versatility and diversity of a single gene. By alternatively excising different introns along with the intervening exons, a wide range of unique proteins of differing sizes can be generated. These alternative proteins, termed *isoforms*, come from one gene that generates a variety of mRNA with varying exon composition. Alternative splicing is common and is essential for the proper function of almost all hematopoietic cells. For example, B cells are able to produce both immunoglobulin M (IgM) and immunoglobulin D (IgD) at the same developmental stage using alternative splicing. Additionally, erythrocytes use alternative splicing to produce differing isoforms of cytoskeletal proteins. However, alternative splicing does not always give beneficial results. The mutations in the splicing signals in β-globin gene, mentioned earlier for β-thalassemia, result in abnormal alternative splicing. In addition, in patients with chronic myeloid leukemia (CML), resistance to tyrosine kinase inhibitor therapy has been linked to alternative splicing of the BCR-ABL transcript.

NUCLEAR EXPORT OF RNA

The nuclear envelope serves as a major regulator of gene expression by controlling the flow of RNA to the cytoplasm for translation. Nuclear pore complexes (NPCs) inserted within the nuclear envelope regulate the transport of molecules in and out of the nucleus. Ions, small metabolites, and proteins under 40 kilodaltons (kDa) passively diffuse across NPC channels. However, larger proteins and mRNA are transported through NPCs via energy-dependent (as with guanosine triphosphate [GTP]) and signal-mediated processes that require chaperoning transport proteins.

NPCs are composed of three major parts: (1) a central core containing a 10-nm channel, (2) a nuclear basket that can dilate in response to large cargoes, and (3) flexible fibrils that extend from the central core into the cytoplasm (Fig. 3-5). These large NPCs are composed of nucleoporins, or Nups. Demonstrating how crucial nuclear export of mRNA is for correct hematopoietic development, mutations or deletions in Nups can result in MDS and leukemia. For example, point mutations of Nup98 in hematopoietic precursors results in myelodysplasia and eventual AML. Furthermore, multiple translocations involving Nup98 (up to 29 recognized partners) have been found in patients with MDS and AML as the sole cytogenetic abnormality.

Naked RNA cannot be exported through NPC channels. Rather, RNA export from the nucleus requires that newly synthesized RNAs undergo the previously described processing steps, 5′ capping, splicing, and 3′ polyadenylation. In addition, RNA binding proteins are required to fold and shuttle the modified RNA through NPCs. Several of these RNA-binding proteins have been identified as important in hematopoiesis. For example, the eukaryotic translation initiation factor 4E (eIF4E) enhances nuclear export of specific RNA transcripts and is critical for proper granulocyte differentiation. Overexpression of eIF4E impedes myeloid maturation and can result in AML. Inhibiting eIF4E with ribavirin has shown activity in early-phase clinical trials of AML and may represent a promising novel class of leukemia therapy.

RNA METABOLISM

RNA does not live forever, and that is a good thing. In mammalian cells, mRNA lifetimes range from several minutes to days. The limited lifetime of mRNA enables a cell to alter protein synthesis in response to its changing needs. The stability of mRNA is regulated by the untranslated regions (UTRs) of mRNA. UTRs are sections of the mRNA before the start codon (5′) and after the stop codon (3′) that are not translated. These regions govern mRNA half-life, localization, and translational efficiency. Translational efficiency, both enhancement and inhibition, can be controlled by UTRs. Both proteins and small RNA species can bind to either the 5′ or 3′ UTRs, and these can either regulate translation or influence survival of the transcript. There are several fascinating mechanisms by which this occurs, and these will be described later. UTR sequence regulation of mRNA survival is essential for proper hematopoietic differentiation. The best example of this is globin synthesis, in which its mRNA is quite stable because of UTR sequences. This long half-life meets the needs of reticulocytes to synthesize globin for up to 2 days after terminally mature erythroblasts lose the ability to make new mRNA.

Some of the elements contained in UTRs form a characteristic secondary structure that alters the survival of the mRNA transcript. Riboswitches, one class of these mRNA elements, can sense the concentration of what the mRNA codes for and can alter mRNA survival. For example, the mRNA for several enzymes in the cobalamine pathway have riboswitches that bind adenosylcobalamine, and this regulates the survival of these mRNAs. Thus in states of high cobalamine, riboswitches sense the high cobalamine concentration and decrease survival of the mRNA for enzymes used in this synthetic pathway.

Another class of UTR secondary structures that regulate stability is exemplified by the prothrombin 3′ UTR. This mRNA is constitutively polyadenylated at seven or more positions, and the 3′ UTR is folded into at least two distinct stem-loop conformations. These alternate structures expose a consensus binding site for trans-acting factors—such as heterogeneous nuclear ribonucleoproteins (hnRNPs), polypyrimidine tract-binding protein 1 (PTB1), and nucleolinin—with translational regulatory properties. Another type of 3′ UTR regulatory sequence involves selenocysteine insertion sequence (SECIS) elements. These represent another stem-loop RNA structure found in mRNA transcripts that serve as protein-binding sites on UTR segments and direct the ribosome to translate the codon UGA as selenocysteines rather than as a stop codon. An example of this regulation can be found in selenoprotein P in plasma.

Another class of UTR binding site that affects the stability of mRNA is represented by the adenine- and uracil-rich (AU-rich) elements (AREs). AREs are lengths of mRNA consisting mostly of adenine and uracil nucleotides. These sequences destabilize mRNA transcripts through the action of riboendonucleases that stimulate poly(A) tail removal. Loss of the poly(A) tail is thought to promote mRNA degradation by facilitating attack by both the exosome complex and the decapping complex. Rapid mRNA degradation via AREs is a critical mechanism for preventing the overproduction of potent cytokines such as tumor necrosis factor (TNF) and granulocyte-macrophage colony-stimulating factor (GM-CSF). AREs also

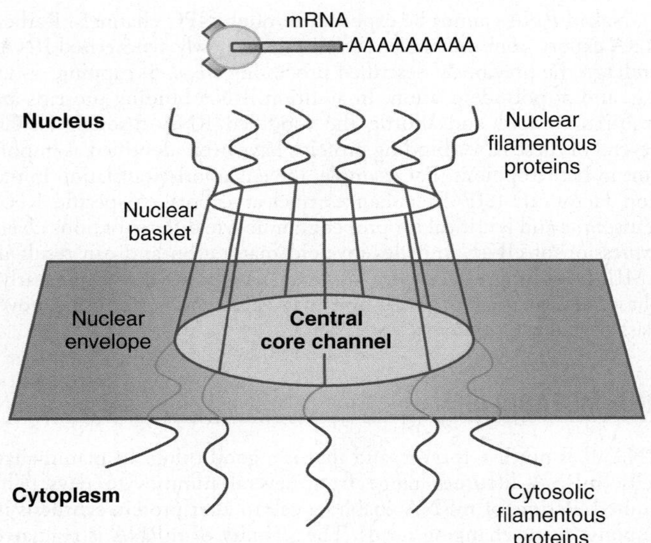

Figure 3-5 NUCLEAR EXPORT OF RNA THROUGH NUCLEAR PORE COMPLEXES. The central core of the nuclear pore complex consists of ring structure embedded in the nuclear envelope. Radiating in toward the nucleus is a nuclear basket that extends filamentous proteins in surveillance for mRNA. The central ring structure also radiates cytosolic protein filaments, which act to facilitate release of cargo into the cytoplasm.

regulate the synthesis of mRNA for proto-oncogenic transcription factors such as c-Jun and c-Fos. The AREs in these genes' mRNA target destruction of their mRNA transcripts in quiescent cells, preventing inappropriate cell proliferation that would occur if c-Jun and c-Fos were still active.

Eukaryotic mRNA messages are also subject to surveillance for accuracy by a mechanism termed *nonsense mediated decay (NMD)*. The NMD complex surveys the transcript for the presence of premature stop codons (nonsense codons) in the message. These premature stop codons can arise via either incomplete splicing mutations in DNA, transcription errors, or leaky scanning by the ribosome causing frame shifts. Detection of a premature stop codon by NMD triggers mRNA degradation by 5′ decapping, 3′ poly(A) tail removal, or endonucleolytic cleavage.

Translational efficiency can be regulated by cellular factors that bind mRNA in a sequence-specific manner. Iron metabolism is an excellent example of how cells coordinate uptake and sequestration of an essential metabolite in response to availability. Transferrin is a plasma protein that carries iron. Receptors for transferrin are expressed on cells requiring iron for maturation, such as erythroid progenitor cells. They mediate internalization of transferrin loaded with iron into the cytoplasm through receptor-mediated endocytosis. When a cell becomes iron deficient, a Krebs cycle enzyme, aconitase, is structurally altered, becoming an iron-responsive protein (IRP) so that it can bind to iron-responsive elements (IREs) in the UTR of transferrin receptor (TfR) mRNA (Fig. 3-6). UTR binding leads to stabilization of the TfR mRNA transcript and thus to greater availability for translation, which results in increased protein expression. However, when a cell has sufficient iron, aconitase is not altered, and TfR mRNA becomes unstable and prone to degradation. In that situation TfR receptor expression is low, and the fewer receptors import less iron.

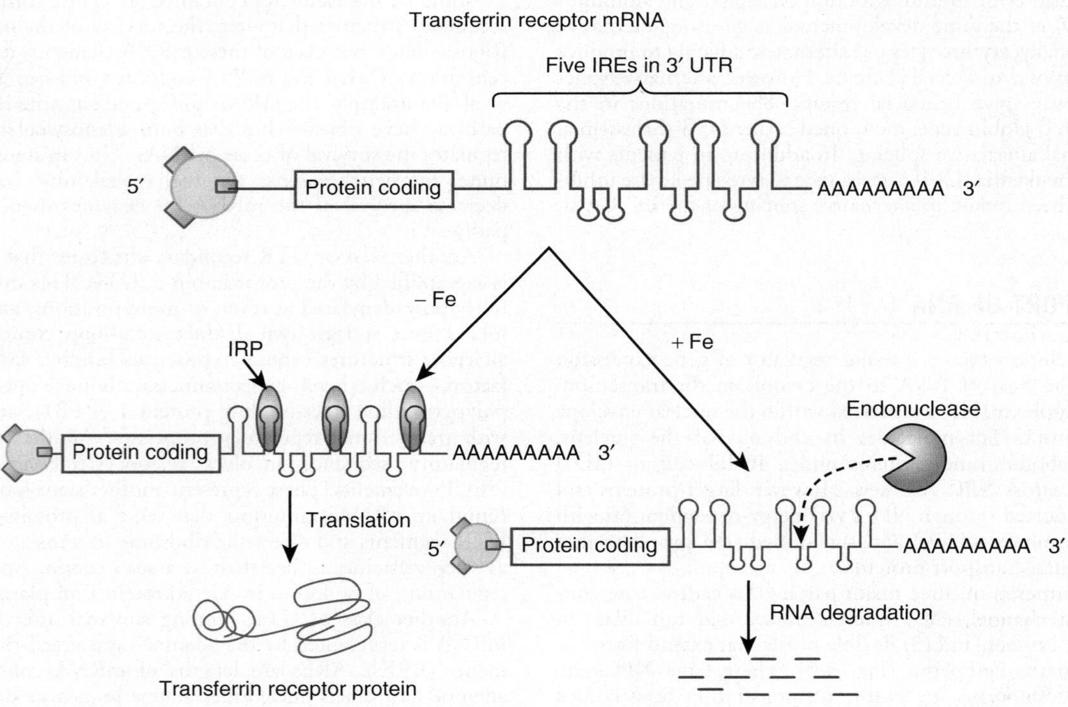

Figure 3-6 CONTROL OF TRANSFERRIN RECEPTOR GENE EXPRESSION. The transferrin receptor mRNA has five iron-responsive elements (IREs) in the 3′ end of its untranslated region (UTR). In an iron-deficient state (–Fe), iron-responsive proteins (IRPs) bind to IREs and stabilize the mRNA transcript for translation into protein product. In an iron-replete state (+Fe), IRPs are downregulated and the transferrin receptor mRNA is susceptible to endonucleases. Endonuclease cleavage of mRNA leads to RNA degradation and reduced availability of transcript for protein production.

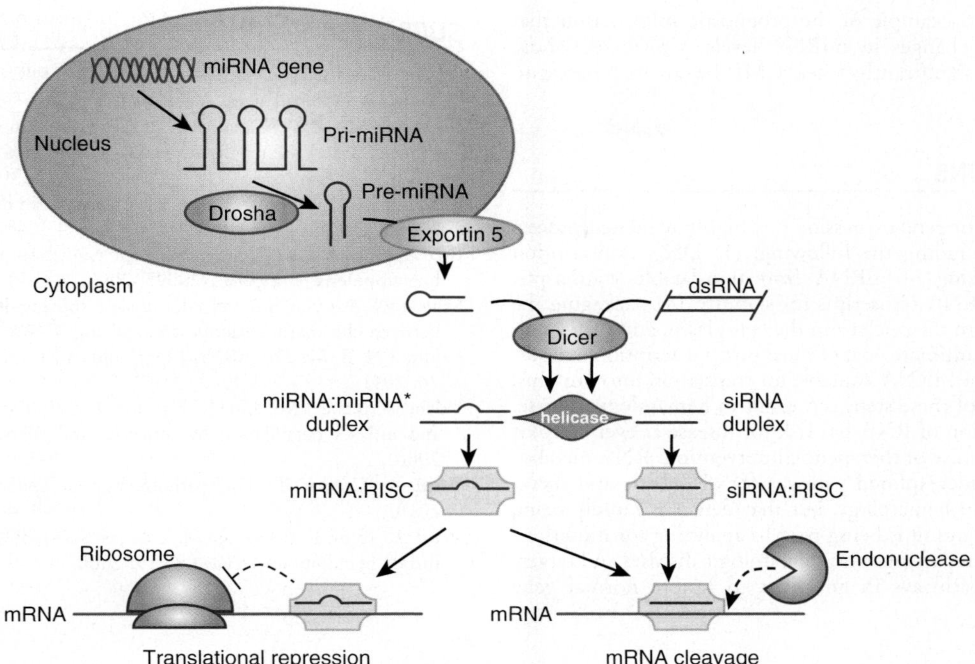

Figure 3-7 RNA INTERFERENCE AND CONTROL OF GENE EXPRESSION. The stem-loop of the primary miRNA (pri-miRNA) gene transcript is first cleaved through the action of the RNase III–related activity called Drosha, which takes place in the nucleus and generates the precursor miRNA (pre-miRNA). In the siRNA pathway the duplex RNAs are cleaved into 22 to 25 nucleotide pieces through the action of the enzyme Dicer in the cytosol. Processed miRNA stem-loop structures are transported from the nucleus to the cytosol via the activity of exportin 5. In the cytosol the processed miRNA stem-loop is targeted by Dicer, which removes the loop portion. The nomenclature of the mature miRNA duplex is miRNA:miRNA*, where the miRNA* strand is the nonfunctional half of the duplex. Ultimately, fully processed miRNAs and siRNAs are engaged by the RNA-induced silencing complex (RISC), which separates the two RNA strands. The active strand of RNA derived either from the miRNA or siRNA pathway is complementary or anti-sense to a region of the target mRNA. RNA interference results in blockade of translation by ribosomes and/or degradation of mRNA.

MICRO-RNA

Another powerful mechanism of regulating of gene expression at the RNA level involves small RNA molecules, termed *micro-RNA (miRNA),* bind to complementary (i.e., anti-sense) sequences on target mRNA transcripts. This binding results in either degradation or inhibition of translation and consequent silencing of gene expression. There are roughly 1000 miRNA molecules coded in the human genome, indicating how robust this regulatory mechanism is. miRNA usually contain 18 to 25 nucleotides, and each miRNA has the potential to target about 500 genes. Conversely, an estimated 60% of all mRNAs have one or more sequences that are predicted to interact with miRNAs. This biology, termed *RNA interference (RNAi)*, has also been exploited in the laboratory, where investigators design small interfering RNA (siRNA) to specifically repress expression of target genes to study artificially induced phenotypes. In these studies siRNAs are synthetically created to bind to complementary sequences within specific mRNAs. siRNAs are then transfected into cells, where they mediate destruction of their target mRNA through endogenous ribonucleases. Repression of gene expression in this manner has become known as "gene knockdown," a phrase widely used to describe the function of genes by assessing what function the cell lacks in the absence of the target gene's expression.

Naturally occurring miRNAs are produced from transcripts that form stem-loop structures, whereas laboratory-created siRNAs are produced from long, double-stranded RNA (dsRNA) precursors (Fig. 3-7). Similarly, both miRNAs and siRNAs are processed in the nucleus by a multiprotein complex called the RNA-induced silencing complex (RISC), which contains the ribonuclease III (RNase III) enzyme Dicer, DGCR8, and Argonaute. The specificity of miRNA and siRNA interactions with their target mRNAs mediates how they regulate gene expression. For example, the specificity of miRNA targeting is ruled by Watson-Crick complementarities between positions 2 to 8 from the 5′ end of the miRNA, with the 3′ UTR of their target mRNAs.

Two models have been proposed to explain how miRNAs and siRNAs interfere with the expression of target genes. The mechanisms involve both directed degradation and interference with translation of the target mRNA. In the case of directed mRNA degradation, the proposed model involves miRNA-mRNA binding and recruitment of RISC, which ultimately leads to degradation of the target mRNA. In the interference model it is believed that the interaction of miRNA, RISC, and mRNA blocks the ribosomal machinery along the mRNA transcript, preventing translation, yet sparing the mRNA from degradation. This latter model was hypothesized based on work with the *Caenorhabditis elegans* gene lin-14. In this example the amount of lin-14 mRNA does not decrease, but the protein product of the lin-14 mRNA is reduced. In the degradation model, the paired miRNA-mRNA becomes a target for double-stranded ribonucleases, which are thought to be part of the innate immune system as a defense against dsRNA viruses, such as rotavirus.

Various disease states have aberrant expression of miRNA. One example in chronic lymphocytic leukemia (CLL) is the *miR-15a/miR-16-1* cluster (located on chromosome 13q). When this cluster is deleted in B lymphocytes, there are higher levels of antiapoptotic proteins such as BCL2 and MCL1, but also higher levels of the tumor suppressor protein 53 (TP53). High levels of antiapoptosis yet with an intact TP53 tumor suppressor pathway could explain why 13q deletions in CLL are associated with an indolent form of the disease. Patterns of miRNA expression are correlated with disease progression in CML, although it is not clear whether these changes are causative or epiphenomena. An example of the prognostic information that can be provided by changes in miRNA levels is *miR328,* whose expression levels fall significantly when CML begins to progress to blast crisis.

FUTURE DIRECTIONS

In summary, control of gene expression is a highly regulated process with several steps including the following: (1) DNA transcription into RNA, (2) splicing of mRNA into translatable transcripts, (3) modifying the mRNA transcripts for stability, (4) packaging the mRNA for export from the nucleus to the cytoplasm, and (5) regulation by miRNA. The ultimate goal of most posttranscriptional modifications is to make the mRNA available for translation into proteins. Perturbations in any of these steps can result in hematologic disease. Although the regulation of RNA has risk for disease at every step, it also possesses the promise of therapeutic intervention. RNA metabolism is a relatively underexplored pathway for diagnostic and therapeutic development in hematology, but that deficit is rapidly being overcome as more attention is being paid to analyzing for mutations of RNA metabolism in patients with hematologic diseases and targeting aberrant RNA pathways in an effort to restore normal gene expression.

SUGGESTED READINGS

Garzon R, Marucci G, Croce C: Targeting microRNAs in cancer: Rationale, strategies and challenges. *Nat Rev Drug Disc* 9:775, 2010.

Kowarz E, Merkens J, Karas M, et al: Premature transcript termination, trans-splicing and DNA repair: A vicious path to cancer. *Am J Blood Res* 1:1, 2011.

Li B, Carey M, Workman J: The role of chromatin during transcription. *Cell* 128:707, 2007.

Rice K, Hormaeche I, Licht J: Epigeneic regulation of normal and malignant hematopoiesis. *Oncogene* 26:6697, 2007.

Schwartz S, Ast G: Chromatin density and splicing destiny: On the cross-talk between chromatin structure and splicing. *EMBO* 29:1629, 2010.

Siddiqui N, Borden K: mRNA export and cancer. *Wiley Interdiscip Rev RNA 10,* 2011.

Valencia-Sanchez M, Liu J, Hannon G, et al: Control of translation and mRNA degradation by miRNAs and siRNAs. *Genes Dev* 20:515, 2006.

Ward A, Cooper T: The pathobiology of splicing. *J Pathol* 220:152, 2010.

Ward A, Touw I, Yoshimura A: The Jak-Stat pathway in normal and perturbed hematopoiesis. *Blood* 95:19, 2000.

CHAPTER 4

PROTEIN SYNTHESIS, PROCESSING, AND TRAFFICKING

Randal J. Kaufman and Laura Popolo

The final step in the transfer of the genetic information stored in deoxyribonucleic acid (DNA) into proteins is the translation of the intermediary messenger molecules, mRNAs (see Chapter 3). Protein synthesis occurs in the cytoplasm and generates a great variety of products endowed with a wide spectrum of functions. The complete set of proteins produced by a cell is called a *proteome* and is responsible for the remarkable diversity in cell specialization that is typical of metazoan organisms. In order to be functional, proteins need to be properly folded, assembled, and transported to the final destination if required. The cell has in its interior several membrane-bound compartments, termed *organelles,* such as the mitochondria, the peroxisomes, the nucleus, and the endoplasmic reticulum, to which the proteins may be targeted. Since each compartment serves a particular purpose, protein transport is crucial to maintain the identity and functions of each organelle. The intracellular physiology depends on the proper functioning of the organelles. In many cases, protein folding and processing are coupled with protein trafficking so that the targeting process is unidirectional and irreversible.

This chapter briefly describes how proteins are synthesized and then focuses on their processing and delivery to their appropriate destinations within the cell. An understanding of the machines that catalyze protein folding, assembly, and targeting is relevant to the study of hematology, providing a basis for an explanation of how malfunctions in these processes can cause blood disorders.

PROTEIN SYNTHESIS

Among the biosynthesis of macromolecules occurring in a cell, protein synthesis is the most important in quantitative terms. It is a highly energy-consuming process and proceeds through a mechanism that has been conserved during evolution. Proteins are synthesized by the joining of amino acids, each of which has characteristic physical-chemical properties (see Table 4-1 for single-letter designations). Peptide bonds are created by the condensation of the carboxyl group (COOH) of one amino acid with the amino group (NH_2) of the next. The free NH_2 and COOH groups of the terminal amino acids define the amino- or N-terminal end and the carboxyl- or C-terminal end of the resulting polypeptide chain. In many cases, multiple polypeptide chains assemble into a functional protein. For example, hemoglobin is formed by four polypeptide chains, two α-globin chains and two β-globin chains that assemble with heme, an iron-containing prosthetic group, to yield the functional protein designed to deliver molecular oxygen to all cells and tissues.

The whole process of protein synthesis is orchestrated by a large ribonucleoprotein complex, called the *ribosome.* The ribosome 80S (S stands for Svedberg unit and refers to the rate of sedimentation) is typical of mammalian cells and is constituted by a large subunit of 60S and a small one of 40S. Additional components are mRNAs, tRNAs, amino acids, soluble factors, ATP, and GTP. Preliminarily to protein synthesis is the activation of amino acids and their coupling to the cognate tRNAs. This crucial function is carried out by the aminoacyl-tRNA synthetases, which generate aminoacyl-tRNAs at the expenses of ATP and operate a quality control on the coupling reaction. Eukaryotic mRNA molecules typically contain a 5′-untranslated region (5′-UTR), a protein coding sequence that begins with the start codon AUG and ends with one of three stop codons (UAA, UAG, UGA), and a 3′-untranslated segment (3′UTR). The 5′ end carries a 7-methylguanosine forming a structure called a "cap" (m^7GpppN mRNA), whereas the 3′ end is polyadenylated. These modifications are required to protect the mRNA from degradation, for export out of the nucleus and for efficient recruitment of ribosomes for translation. Once in the cytoplasm, the 40S ribosomal subunit binds to the cap and then scans the mRNA toward the 3′ end until the translation start codon is encountered, usually the first AUG (underlined) located in a nucleotide context optimal for translation initiation called the Kozak sequence (A/GNNAUGG). The assembly of the 60S subunit with the 40S produces an 80S ribosome. A special tRNA specific for methionine, called the initiator ($tRNA_i^{Met}$) is required for the initiation of protein synthesis at the start codon. Aminoacyl-tRNAs ferry amino acids to the ribosome being joined together in sequence as the ribosome moves toward the 3′ end of the mRNA. The codons in the mRNA interact by base-pairing with the anticodon of the tRNAs so that amino acids are incorporated into the nascent polypeptide chain in the right order. Translation is terminated on encounter of a stop codon where the polypeptide is released. Typically, multiple ribosomes are engaged in the translation of a single mRNA molecule in a complex termed a *polyribosome* or *polysome.*

Protein synthesis is divided into three phases: initiation, elongation, and termination. Each phase requires soluble proteins (or factors) that transiently associate with the ribosomes and are called initiation, elongation, and termination (or release) factors; these factors are in turn termed *eIFs*, *eEFs*, and *eRFs*, respectively, where the prefix *e* indicates their eukaryotic origin. Many soluble factors required for protein synthesis belong to the G protein (guanine nucleotide-binding proteins) superfamily, which comprehends regulatory molecules of important cellular processes such as hormone or growth factors signaling pathways, membrane trafficking, or neurotransmission. Dysfunctions of G proteins are involved in human diseases such as cancer.

REGULATION OF mRNA TRANSLATION

There are two major general regulatory steps in mRNA translation that are mediated by the initiation factors eIF2 and eIF4. All cells regulate the rate of protein synthesis through reversible covalent modification of eIF2, a soluble factor required for the binding and recruitment of the Met-$tRNA_i^{Met}$ to the 40S ribosomal subunit.

eIF2 is a heterotrimeric G protein that can exist in an inactive form bound to GDP or an active form bound to GTP. The eIF2-GTP/Met-$tRNA_i^{Met}$ ternary complex binds to the 40S subunit. Joining of the 60S subunit triggers hydrolysis of GTP to GDP and thus converts eIF2 to the inactive form whereas the opposite reaction is catalyzed by a guanine nucleotide exchange factor (GEF) called *eIF2B.* Phosphorylation regulates eIF2 function. In reticulocytes, which synthesize hemoglobin almost as a sole protein, heme starvation blocks the synthesis of α- and β-globins by activating a protein kinase, called *hemin-regulated inhibitor (HRI),* that specifically phosphorylates the α-subunit of eIF2. The phosphorylated form of eIF2 binds more tightly than usual to eIF2B, so that eIF2B is sequestered and not available for the exchange reaction. Thus eIF2 molecules remain in the GDP-bound form and translation of globin mRNA comes to a halt. This mechanism of translational inhibition is of more general significance because eIF2 is a target of phosphorylation by additional protein kinases that cause translational arrest in response to different conditions of cell stress, such as amino acid starvation, glucose starvation, and viral infection. Overall, phosphorylation by different stress-activated protein kinases converges on eIF2, which is thus a central key element of the so-called integrated stress response.

A second major control point of general protein synthesis is mediated by the eIF4 complex, which binds the cap and uses an ATP-dependent RNA helicase (eIF4A) activity and its stimulatory subunit (eIF4B) to unwind structural elements in the 5′ end of mRNA to make it accessible for 40S ribosome subunit binding. The subunit that binds the cap, eIF4E, is the least abundant factor regulating translation in mammalian cells. Increased levels of eIF4E stimulate protein synthesis and can contribute to oncogenesis. The cap-binding activity of eIF4E is inhibited by eIF4E-binding protein (eIF4EBP), which is regulated by phosphorylation mediated by the protein kinases AKT (also named *PKB*) and TOR. Since phosphorylated eIF4BP cannot bind eIF4E, eIF4EBP phosphorylation stimulates translation initiation. Extracellular factors, such as insulin, activate signaling pathways that stimulate protein synthesis through this mechanism. Insulin also activates eIF2B exchange activity and in the long term also increases the cellular ribosome content.

The efficiency of translation can also be modulated by cellular factors that bind mRNA in a sequence-specific manner. An example of this mode of regulation is the control of iron metabolism in animal cells. Key players of this system are (1) the iron-responsive element (IRE), a hairpin structure that is formed in the untranslated regions of the mRNAs, and (2) iron regulatory proteins (IRPs) that bind IRE. In the transferrin receptor (Tfr) mRNA and ferritin mRNA, IREs are located in the 3′-UTR and 5′-UTR, respectively. In iron-starved cells, the binding of IRPs to IREs results in the stabilization of Tfr mRNA and inhibition of translation initiation of ferritin mRNA. Conversely, when iron is abundant IRPs have a lower affinity to IREs and as a result Tfr mRNA is degraded whereas ferritin mRNA translation is stimulated. In this manner, cells can coordinately regulate iron uptake and iron sequestration in response to the changes in iron availability.

PROTEIN FOLDING

As the polypeptide emerges from the ribosome, it must fold in order to become a mature functional protein. The conformation of a protein is dictated chiefly by the primary structure. Some proteins can spontaneously acquire their mature three-dimensional conformation as they are synthesized in the cell and can even fold in a test tube by a self-assembly process. However, most polypeptides require assistance by other proteins in order to fold. These proteins are *molecular chaperones* that either directly assist protein folding or act to prevent aberrant interactions, such as aggregation that can occur in a densely packed environment like that of the cytosol of eukaryotic cells (protein concentrations of 200 to 300 mg/mL). Most molecular chaperones are heat-shock proteins (Hsps) and, in particular, are members of the Hsp70 family. Chaperones bind to short-sequence protein motifs, in many cases containing hydrophobic amino acids. By undergoing cycles of binding and release (linked to ATP hydrolysis), chaperones help the nascent polypeptide to find its native conformation, one aspect of which is hiding hydrophobic sequence motifs in the protein interior so that they no longer contact the hydrophilic environment of the cytosol. Some properly folded protein monomers are assembled with other proteins to form multi-subunit complexes. The population of chaperones that assist folding and assembly in the cytosol is distinct from those that operate within the endoplasmic reticulum (ER) or mitochondria.

PROTEIN DEGRADATION

Proteins can contain mutations that prevent them from folding properly. Such misfolded proteins are marked for destruction and then degraded. The breakdown of these molecules is achieved in two major phases. First, the molecules are tagged with a polypeptide called ubiquitin, which is 76 residues long and covalently linked to the substrate protein. Second, the tagged molecules are ferried to an ATP-dependent protease complex called the *26S proteasome*, a multi-subunit molecular machinery specialized in protein destruction.

Since its first discovery in carrying out the disposal of damaged and misfolded proteins, protein ubiquitylation was found in association with an increasing number of specific regulatory events involving a selective degradation of key regulatory proteins. Thus ubiquitylation is responsible for regulating a wide array of cellular processes, including differentiation, tissue development, induction of inflammatory responses, antigen presentation, cell cycle progression, and programmed cell death, also called *apoptosis* (see Chapter 16 for a review of cell death). In addition, ubiquitylation of surface receptors is involved in endocytosis, whereas ubiquitylation of histones activates DNA repair.

SORTING FROM THE CYTOSOL INTO OTHER COMPARTMENTS

Most of the proteins synthesized on free polysomes remain in the cytosol as cytosolic or soluble proteins. These include enzymes involved in many metabolic and signal transduction pathways, proteins required for mRNA translation or assembly of cytoskeleton. Other proteins are imported from the cytosol into the organelles, including the nucleus, the mitochondrion, and the peroxisome (Fig. 4-1).

In general, there are two types of protein trafficking. In one type, the protein crosses a lipid bilayer. The polypeptide crosses the membrane in an unfolded state through an aqueous channel composed of proteins. In the second type, the protein does not traffic across a lipid bilayer and is exemplified by trafficking into the nucleus or from the ER to the Golgi compartment. In these cases, proteins and protein complexes are transported in their folded/assembled state.

The sorting events are governed by sorting signals (i.e., short linear sequences or three-dimensional patches of particular amino acids) and by their cognate receptors (see some examples in Table 4-1). The first sorting decision occurs after approximately 30 amino acids of the nascent polypeptide have been extruded from the ribosome. If the nascent polypeptide lacks a "signal sequence," most often found near the amino-terminal end, the translation of the polypeptide is completed in the cytosol. Then the protein can either stay in the cytosol or be posttranslationally incorporated into one of the indicated organelles (see Fig. 4-1). If the protein does contain an amino-terminal signal, sequence is imported cotranslationally into the ER from where it can be targeted to the other compartments of the secretory pathway (see Fig. 4-1).

Targeting of Nuclear Proteins

One of the distinctive features of the eukaryotic cells is that the genome is contained in an intracellular compartment called a *nucleus.* This organelle is bounded by a double membrane that forms the nuclear envelope (NE) (see Fig. 4-1). The outer nuclear membrane is continuous with the ER and has a polypeptide composition distinct from that of the inner membrane. About 3000 nuclear pore complexes (NPCs) perforate the NE in animal cells. Although NPCs allow unrestricted, bidirectional movement of molecules smaller than 40,000 daltons, traversal of NPCs by larger molecules is tightly regulated. NPCs are approximately 120 nm in external diameter and comprise approximately 50 different proteins (nucleoporins), arranged in a complex cylindrical structure with an octagonal symmetry. Nucleoporins constitute the scaffold of the NPC and are

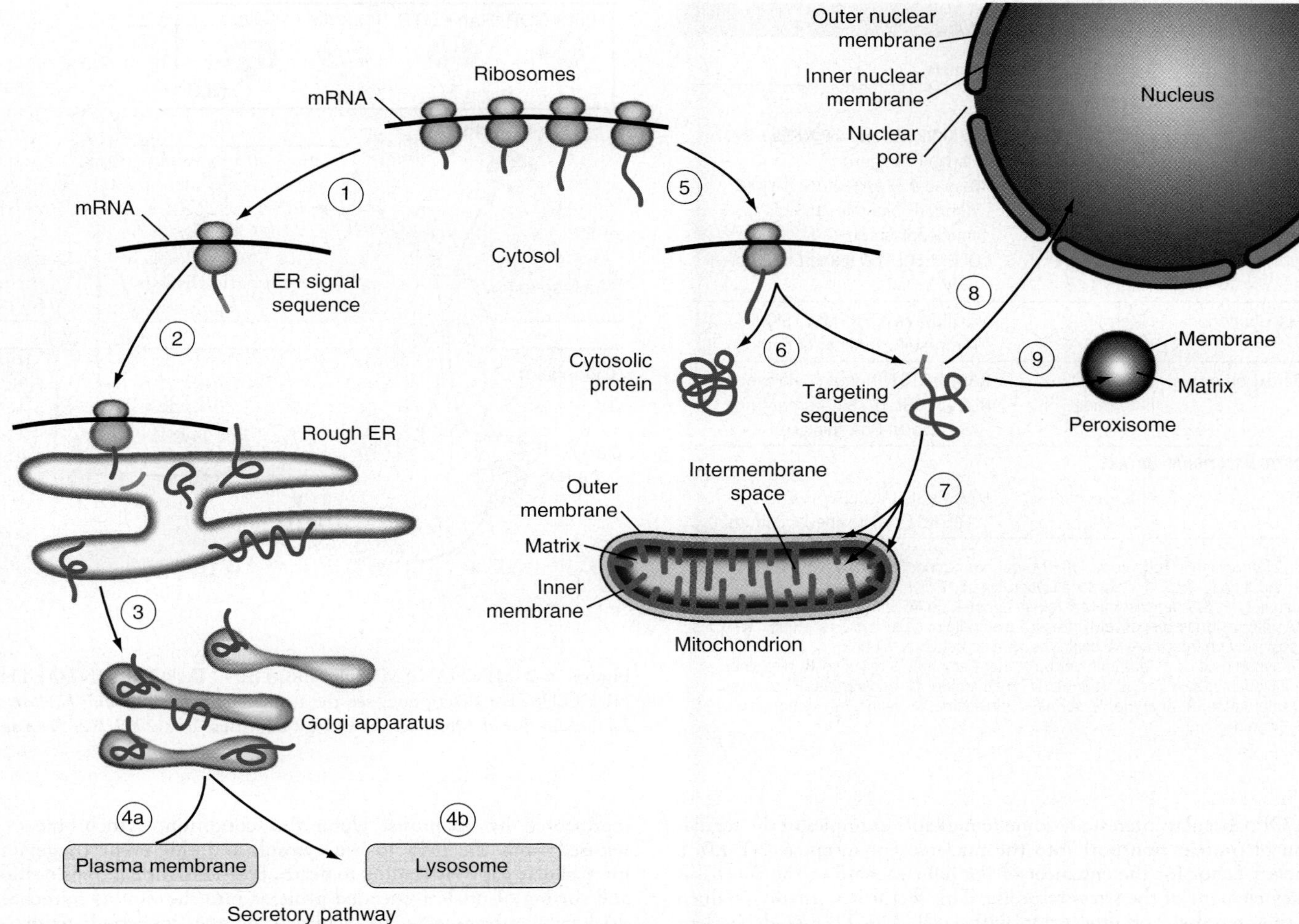

Figure 4-1 SORTING OF PROTEINS FROM THE CYTOSOL TO DIFFERENT DESTINATIONS. *Left,* Steps 1 to 4a and 4b: Sorting of proteins destined to organelles of the secretory pathway, ER, Golgi, plasma membrane, lysosome, or extracellular space. *Right,* Steps 5 and 6: Synthesis of a cytosolic protein. Steps 7, 8, and 9: Sorting of proteins to mitochondrion, nucleus, and peroxisome.

arranged in rings. In the inner ring, nucleoporins containing repeats of the hydrophobic amino acids phenylalanine and glycine (FG-repeats) seem to be essential for the movement of the cargo-carrier complexes and for creating a selectivity barrier against the diffusion of nonnuclear proteins. The FG-nucleoporin filaments protrude toward the inner core of the NPC, and the weak hydrophobic interactions between the FG-repeats and the cargo-carrier complexes mediate the passage of molecules.

NPCs are capable of importing and exporting molecules or complexes, provided that the molecules have an exposed nuclear localization signal (NLS) or nuclear export signal (NES). These signals are not always easy to predict. Some of the best-known signals are listed in Table 4-1. The function of these signals in importing or exporting a protein was analyzed by critically testing both the effects of amino acid substitutions on transport and the capability of the signal to target an attached reporter protein in or out of the nucleus. The nuclear localization signals are not cleaved off as occurs for other signals (see later discussion) and thus can function repetitively. Candidates exposing signals for nuclear import (e.g., transcription factors, coactivators or corepressors, DNA repair enzymes, ribosomal proteins, mRNA processing factors) or export (ribosomal subunits, mRNA-containing particles, tRNAs, etc.) are transported through the NPC in association with soluble carrier proteins, called *karyopherins* (also called *importins, exportins,* or *transportins*), which function as shuttling receptors of different protein cargos. According to the direction of transport, these carrier proteins are divided into two groups: (1) importins, if they bind their cargo on the cytoplasmic side of the NPC and release it on the other; and (2) exportins, if they bind their cargo in the nucleus and release it in the cytoplasm.

A small Ras-like GTPase, belonging to the G protein superfamily and called *Ran*, controls both the docking of carrier proteins with their cargo and the directionality of transport through cycles of GTP binding and hydrolysis. Fig. 4-2 exemplifies a cycle of import in the nucleus. An importin binds the cargo in the cytosol and then moves to the nucleus, where its association with Ran-GTP triggers the release of the cargo. The importin bound to Ran-GTP is transported back to the cytoplasm, where the conversion of GTP to GDP stimulated by a Ran-GAP protein (GTPase-activating protein) causes dissociation of Ran from the importin, which can initiate a new cycle. Ran-GDP is transported to the nucleus, where a Ran-GEF (guanine-nucleotide exchange factor) regenerates Ran-GTP. The movement from the nucleus to the cytoplasm occurs by formation of a Ran-GTP-exportin-cargo complex that is transported to the cytoplasm, where Ran-GAP triggers the hydrolysis of GTP. The conformational change of the exportin releases the cargo in the cytoplasm. The different localization of Ran-GEF and Ran-GAP and the continuous transport of Ran-GDP in the nucleus create an asymmetry that is important for the directionality of the process. In conclusion, karyopherins possess a cargo-binding domain but also binding domains for nucleoporins and Ran-GTPase.

The lack of NLS/NES removal during transport through the NPC enables multiple cycles of nuclear entry and exit, which is a particularly important mechanism for regulating the activity of proteins involved in DNA and RNA metabolism.

Table 4-1 Examples of Sorting Signals

Organelle	Signal Location*	Example
POSTTRANSLATIONAL UPTAKE		
Nucleus	Internal	SP**KKKRK**V*E* (import; NLS of SV40 large T antigen)
		KR-spacer (PAATKKAGQ)-**KKKK** (import; bipartite NLS of nucleoplasmin)
		LQLPPL*E***R**LTL*D* (export; NES of HIV-1 rev)
Mitochondrion	N-terminal	MLGI**R**SSV**K**TCF**K**PMSLTS**KR**L (iron-sulfur protein of complex III)
Peroxisomes	C-terminal	**K**ANL (PTS1, human catalase)
	N-terminal	**R**LQVVLG**H**L (PTS2, human 3-ketoacyl-CoA thiolase)
COTRANSLATIONAL UPTAKE		
ER	N-terminal	MMSFVSLLLVGILFWAT*E*A*E* QLT**K**C*E*VFQ (ovine lactalbumin)

ER, Endoplasmic reticulum; *HIV,* human immunodeficiency virus; *NES,* nuclear export signal; *NLS,* nuclear localization signal; *PTS1,* peroxisomal targeting signal-1; *PTS2,* peroxisomal targeting signal-2; *SV40,* simian virus 40.
*Acidic residues (negatively charged) are in italic type; basic residues (positively charged) are in bold type. Amino acids: A, alanine; C, cysteine; *D,* aspartic acid; *E,* glutamic acid; F, phenylalanine; G, glycine; **H**, histidine; I, isoleucine; **K**, lysine; L, leucine; M, methionine; N, asparagine; P, proline; Q, glutamine; **R**, arginine; S, serine; T, threonine; V, valine; W, tryptophan; Y, tyrosine.

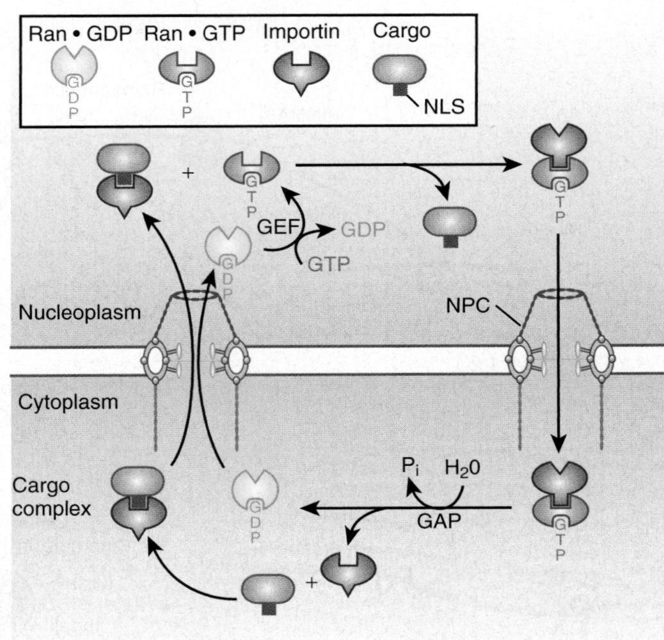

Figure 4-2 MECHANISM OF PROTEIN IMPORT INTO THE NUCLEUS. For description, see the text. *(Modified from Lodish H, Berk A, Matsudaira P, et al:* Molecular cell biology, *ed 5, New York, 2003, WH Freeman.)*

Of particular interest are some remarkable examples of the regulation of protein transport into the nucleus. For instance, NF-κB, a nuclear factor for the enhancer of the light κ chain in the B cells, is a key element of the stress response. This factor is normally retained in the cytoplasm by interaction with I-κB. The TNF-α–dependent phosphorylation of I-κB releases NF-κB, which exposes an NLS and migrates into the nucleus, where it activates transcription of several target genes. For the glucocorticoid receptor (GR), which is localized in the cytoplasm, the binding to the lipophilic ligand exposes an NLS, which is recognized by an importin and allows the translocation into the nucleus, where GR activates genes by binding to GR-responsive elements in their promoter.

Targeting of Mitochondrial Proteins

The mitochondrion is an essential cellular compartment in eukaryotes. Although it contains a genome organized in a circular DNA molecule and independent transcriptional/translational machinery, 98% of the approximately 1500 proteins that constitute mitochondrion proteome are encoded by nuclear DNA and are imported from the cytosol after their synthesis. A small number of highly hydrophobic proteins is encoded by mitochondrial DNA and is synthesized inside the organelle by a translational machinery of bacterial derivation using organelle-transcribed mRNAs.

Like nuclei, mitochondria have two membranes: the outer membrane (MOM) contacts the cytosol, whereas the inner one (MIM) forms numerous infoldings named *cristae,* in which reside the enzymes that synthesize ATP through reactions of the electron transport chain and oxidative phosphorylation. Whereas the MOM is permeable to small molecules (less than 5 kDa) and ions, the inner membrane is highly impermeable, a property essential to create an electrochemical gradient necessary to drive the synthesis of ATP. The space enclosed by the two membranes is the intermembrane space (IMS) and the space enclosed in the inner membrane is the *matrix.* The transport in the mitochondria seems to be unidirectional, and no known proteins are exported from these organelles. A remarkable exception is represented by apoptosis. Upon this condition, cytochrome c is released from the IMS to the cytosol, and this event triggers an intracellular pathway leading to death. Posttranslational translocation and sorting of nuclear-encoded proteins into the various mitochondrial subcompartments are achieved by the concerted action of translocases.

Precursor proteins usually have one of two targeting signals: (1) an amino-terminal presequence that is generally between 10 and 80 amino acid residues long and forms an amphipathic α-helix, which is rich in positively charged, hydrophobic, and hydroxylated amino acids (see Table 4-1); or (2) a less well-defined, hydrophobic targeting sequence distributed throughout the protein. The TOM (translocase of the outer membrane) complex functions as a single entry point into the mitochondria and is crucial for the biogenesis of the organelle and for the viability of eukaryotic cells. Preproteins translocate through it in an unfolded state in an N-to-C direction. TOM translocase is a heteromolecular protein complex whose central component is TOM40, an essential protein that forms the protein-conducting channel. After crossing the outer membrane, proteins segregate according to their signals and recognize two distinct translocases of the inner membrane, or TIMs (TIM23 and TIM22). Presequence-containing proteins are directed to the TIM23 complex, which mediates transport across the inner membrane, a process that requires the electrochemical membrane potential and the ATP-driven action of the matrix heat shock protein 70 (mtHsp70). Once in the matrix, the presequence is often cleaved by a mitochondrial processing peptidase. Proteins with internal targeting signals are guided to the TIM22 complex. Membrane insertion at the TIM22 is also dependent on the membrane potential.

In the context of cell biology, mitochondria play relevant roles in apoptosis, in the communication with the ER, and in oxidative stress. Among the proteins associated with the cytosolic side of MOM, those of the BCL2 family have both pro- and antiapoptotic functions. In addition, recent studies unveiled an ER-mitochondria linkage that is important in Ca^{++} homeostasis and phospholipids biogenesis, whereas oxidative stress generated in the mitochondria is connected to cell aging and senescence.

Targeting of Peroxisomal Proteins

Peroxisomes are membrane-bound compartments in which oxidative reactions that generate hydrogen peroxide, such as β-oxidation of fatty acids, occur. In this organelle, hydrogen peroxide is rapidly degraded by catalase to prevent oxidative reactions that have potential damaging effects on cellular structures. A single membrane surrounds the peroxisome, which encloses an interior matrix. This organelle lacks a genetic system and a transcriptional/translational machinery. Therefore all peroxisomal proteins are imported posttranslationally from the cytosol by proteins called *peroxins.*

The targeting of matrix proteins is directed by two types of peroxisomal targeting signals (PTSs). Type 1 (PTS1) is a carboxyl-terminal tri- or tetrapeptide, whereas type 2 (PTS2) is an amino-terminal peptide of nine amino acids (see Table 4-1). Two cytosolic peroxins, PEX5 and PEX7, recognize PTS1 and PTS2, respectively. These proteins function as cargo receptors. They bind cargo proteins in the cytosol, release them into the matrix, and cycle back to the cytosol. Other peroxins are involved in the import of membrane proteins. Although the mechanism of translocation is still elusive, soluble cargo proteins appear to cross the membrane in a folded state, or even as oligomers. At the peroxisomal membrane, the cargo-receptor complex associates with the docking complex, consisting of the peroxisomal membrane proteins PEX13 and PEX14. Ubiquitylation has been proposed to function in concert with ATPases associated to diverse activities (AAA^+ ATPases) to move proteins across the membrane using an ATP-dependent mechanism that resembles the retrotranslocation of misfolded proteins from ER lumen to the cytosol (see later discussion on ERAD).

One consequence of the existence of two different mechanisms for protein import is that when the import of matrix proteins is defective, membrane ghosts of peroxisomes persist in the cells. In contrast, when the import of membrane proteins is impaired, neither normal peroxisomes nor membrane ghosts are present. Defects in PEX3 underlie Zellweger syndrome, which is characterized by the presence of empty peroxisomes and abnormalities of the brain, liver, and kidney that cause death shortly after birth.

COTRANSLATIONAL PROTEIN TRANSLOCATION IN THE ENDOPLASMIC RETICULUM

The ER is an extensive membranous network that is continuous with the outer nuclear membrane and is responsible for the synthesis of the massive amounts of lipid and protein used to build the membranes of most cellular organelles. The ER comprises three interconnected domains: rough ER, smooth ER, and ER exit sites. The rough ER is so called because it is studded with bound ribosomes that are actively synthesizing proteins. Cells specialized in protein secretion, such as cells of the exocrine glands and plasma cells, are rich in rough ER. Smooth ER lacks ribosomes, is not very abundant in most cells (except hepatocytes), and is thought to be the site of lipid biosynthesis and of cytochrome P450-mediated detoxification reactions. Finally, ER exit sites are specialized areas of the ER membrane where transport cargo is packaged into transport vesicles en route to the Golgi apparatus.

Nascent secretory proteins are marked for import in the ER by the presence of an amino-terminal signal sequence (see Table 4-1). This sequence has a length of about 15 to 30 amino acids and displays no conservation of amino acid sequence, although it contains a hydrophobic core flanked by polar residues that preferentially have short side chains in proximity to the cleavage site. As the signal sequence emerges from the ribosome, it is recognized by the signal recognition particle (SRP), a ribonucleoprotein, and this binding induces a temporary arrest in translational elongation (Fig. 4-3). The docking of ribosomes to the ER occurs by interaction of the SRP with the SRP receptor. Upon binding of GTP to both the SRP and its receptor, the ribosome and the nascent chain are transferred to the Sec61 complex, allowing translation to resume. Preproteins translocate through the Sec61 complex in an N-to-C direction. As the nascent polypeptide emerges from the luminal side of the translocon, its signal sequence is cleaved by a signal peptidase.

In the absence of specific targeting sequences, proteins that completely translocate into the ER lumen traffic through bulk flow to the cell surface. In contrast, proteins that have specific targeting signals may be localized to the lumen of the ER, the Golgi compartment,

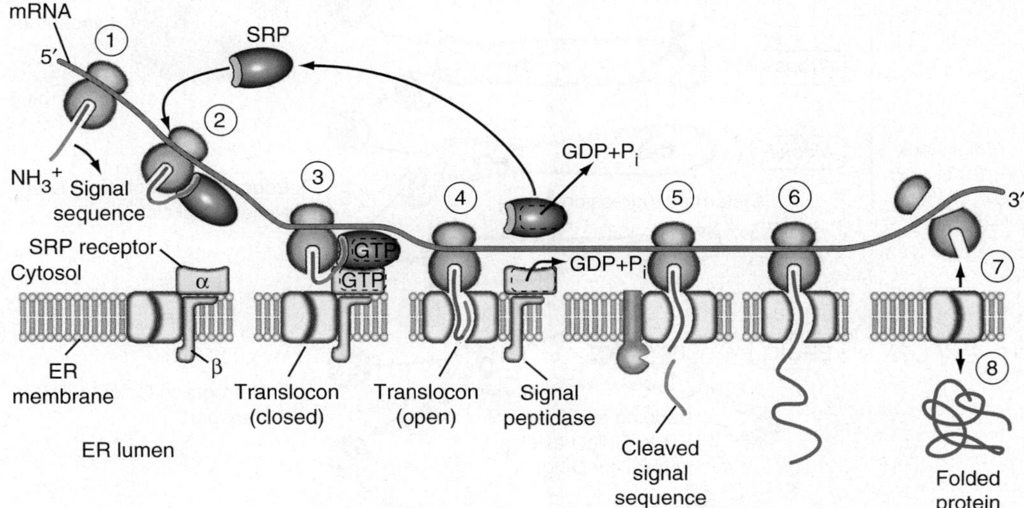

Figure 4-3 SYNTHESIS OF PROTEINS SORTED FOR IMPORT IN THE ER. The figure depicts the main steps of the cotranslational translocation of a secretory protein in the ER. *Steps 1 and 2:* The signal sequence of the emerging polypeptide is recognized by the SRP and binding induces a translation arrest. *Steps 3 and 4:* The binding of the SRP-nascent polypeptide-ribosome complex to the SRP-receptor triggers GTP hydrolysis of both SRP and SRP-receptor. The translocon channel (Sec61) opens and translation resumes. SRP is recycled. *Step 5:* The polypeptide chain elongates and emerges on the luminal side of the ER, where a signal peptidase removes the signal sequence. *Steps 6, 7, and 8:* The synthesis of the polypeptide proceeds until the end of translation and the protein assumes its native conformation (concurrent glycosylation is not shown). Ribosome dissociates and the single subunits are released.

or lysosomes. Other proteins that reside in membranes of the cell contain topologic sequences called *transmembrane (TM) domains* that consist of ≈20 largely apolar amino acids. When a transmembrane domain enters the translocon, the polypeptide is released laterally from the Sec61 channel into the lipid bilayer. Membrane proteins can assume different topologies according to the number and type of TM domains.

PROTEIN TRAFFICKING WITHIN THE SECRETORY PATHWAY

Proteins that enter the ER are transported toward the plasma membrane through a route that is called the *secretory pathway* (Fig. 4-4). Specific signals cause resident proteins to be retained in the ER, Golgi, or plasma membrane. Proteins may also be targeted from the Golgi compartment to lysosomes or from the plasma membrane to endosomes (see Fig. 4-4, pathways 8 and 9). Initially, the study of this complex protein trafficking took advantage of the use of yeast genetics to isolate temperature-sensitive mutants *(sec)*, which were defective at different stages of the secretory pathway. The subsequent characterization of *SEC* genes, thanks to the advent of DNA recombinant techniques, made possible the isolation of the counterparts in mammalian cells and the beginning of molecular and biochemical investigation of secretion. Many genes encoding products involved in secretion were found to be strikingly conserved from yeast to mammals, indicating the importance of this pathway for the life of a eukaryotic cell.

Transport through the secretory pathway is mediated by vesicles. Different sets of structural and regulatory proteins control the fusion of the appropriate vesicles with the target membrane. Sorting motifs dictate the selective incorporation of cargo proteins into those vesicles and their delivery to the intended destination. A major question in cell biology today is how the identity of the compartments of the secretory pathway is maintained while allowing unimpeded transit of other nonresident proteins.

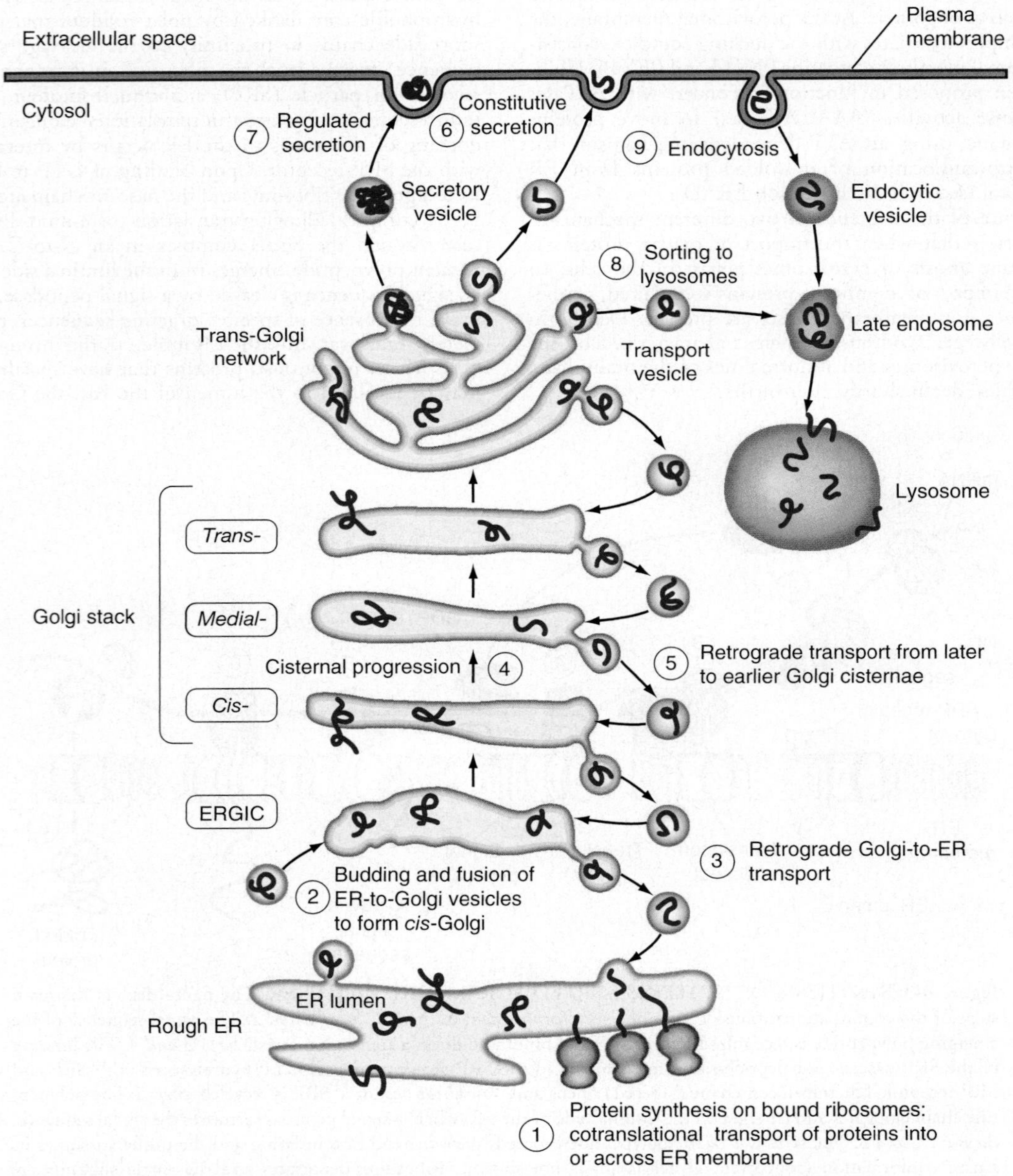

Figure 4-4 PROTEIN TRAFFICKING THROUGH THE SECRETORY PATHWAY. For details, see the text.

Processing of Proteins in the Endoplasmic Reticulum

Protein Folding in the Lumen of the ER

Protein chaperones facilitate protein folding in the ER, but amino acid posttranslational modifications such as asparagine(N)-linked glycosylation and disulfide bond formation are also involved. Proteins start to fold cotranslationally by interaction with a host of chaperones, among which is the Hsp70 family member BiP. In addition, there are folding catalysts that increase the rate of protein folding. For example, the proper pairing and formation of disulfide bonds is catalyzed by oxidoreductases, such as protein disulfide isomerase (PDI), which also shuffles nonnative disulfide bonds. In the current model the oxidation of two thiols produces a disulfide bond (S-S) in the substrate protein and concomitantly reduces two thiols of PDI, which return to the oxidized state by another thiol-disulfide exchange catalyzed by ERO1, a membrane-associated oxidoreductase. ERO1, a flavoprotein that was first discovered in yeast, returns to the oxidized state by transfer of electrons to molecular oxygen via its cofactor FAD. In contrast to the highly reducing environment of the cytosol, where disulfide bonds do not typically form, the lumen of the ER is very oxidizing so that disulfide bonds formation is favored.

Protein Modifications in the ER

Most proteins that enter the secretory pathway are modified by N-glycosylation (Fig. 4-5). This process starts with the transfer of a core oligosaccharide from a lipid-linked donor to an asparagine residue within the consensus sequence N-X-S/T of a nascent polypeptide (X can be any amino acid except proline). The N-linked oligosaccharide is composed of a glucose$_3$-mannose$_9$-N-acetylglucosamine$_2$ unit ($Glc_3Man_9GlcNac_2$). Further processing of the terminal sugars occurs in the ER and after the polypeptide transits the Golgi compartment (see Fig. 4-5).

Many blood proteins (e.g., immunoglobulins, antiproteases, coagulation factors) and many membrane proteins of the cell are glycosylated. Although glycan chains are often not required for the enzymatic activity of glycoproteins, they are important for the physical properties they confer and for many physiologic functions. Glycans protect proteins from protease digestion and heat denaturation, confer hydrophilicity and adhesive properties to the proteins, and mediate interaction with other proteins or receptors. A remarkable example is the hormone erythropoietin that requires a particular complex type of N-glycan chains for its biologic function to stimulate erythropoiesis.

In the recent years, several studies have revealed the importance of protein N-glycosylation in promoting folding. The addition of glycan chains may prevent aggregation or provide steric influences that affect polypeptide folding and disulphide bond formation and also mediate interaction with specific chaperones. In mammalian cells, N-linked oligosaccharides are also used as signal for monitoring protein folding. They are substrates for a complex chaperone system composed of the lectin chaperones calnexin (CNX) and calreticulin (CRT), Erp57 (an oxidoreductase), two glucosidases (GI and GII) and one folding sensor (UGT1) endowed with reglucosylation activity (UDP-glucose: glycoprotein glucosyltransferase). GI and GII remove the two terminal glucose residues to form a monoglucosylated N-linked chain (see Fig. 4-5) that is a ligand for CNX and CRT. Then another glucose residue is removed. UGT1 recognizes and reglucosylates N-linked oligosaccharides on proteins that have not completed the folding process. The addition of glucose residues allows reassociation with the CNX/CRT chaperone system for another attempt for the polypeptide to attain its proper conformation. Beside N-core glycosylation and oxidative folding, the ER is also the site of other kinds of protein modifications. A remarkable one is γ-carboxylation of glutamic acid residues. Although this is a

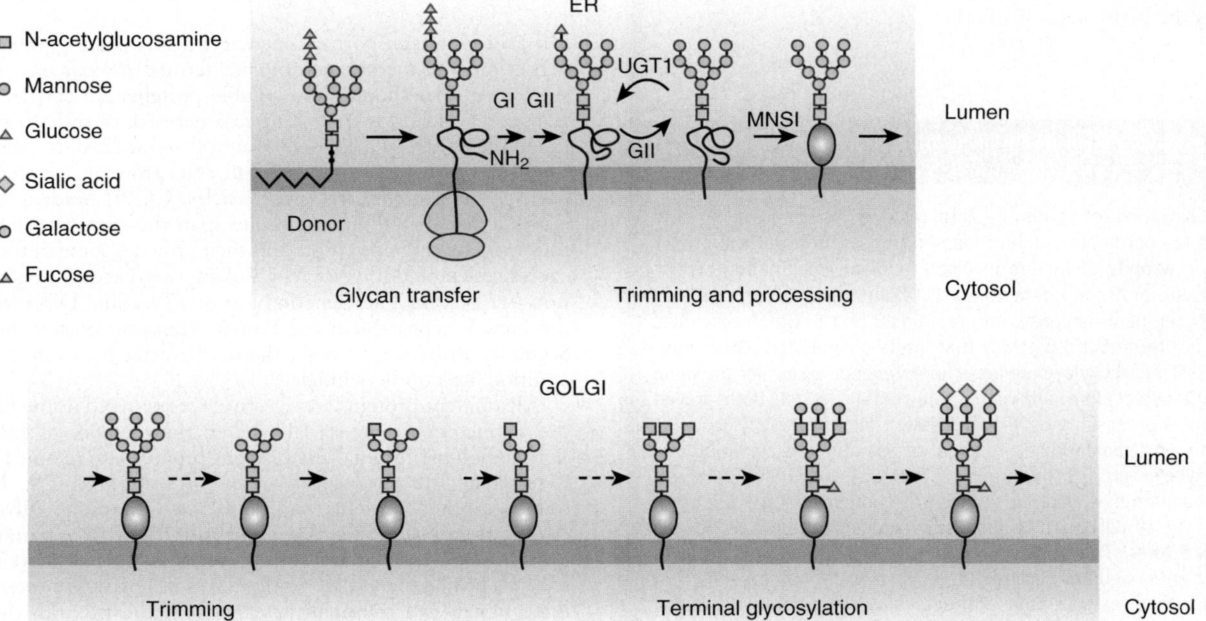

Figure 4-5 N-GLYCOSYLATION OF PROTEINS. In the lumen of the ER, a core oligosaccharide, $Glc_3Man_9GlcNac_2$, is transferred from a lipid-linked precursor (donor) to the asparagine residue of an N-X-S/T motif in a nascent polypeptide chain. The terminal glucoses are removed by GI and GII, and cycles of reglucosylation by UGT1 can occur *(curved arrows)*. When the protein is folded, one mannose is trimmed by ER-mannosidase I and the protein is transported to the Golgi. Core oligosaccharides are further trimmed by mannosidases to produce a $Man_5GlcNac_2$ unit. Further elaboration is catalyzed by glycosyltransferases that add various sugars and create branches. Bi-, tri-, and tetraantennary chains are generated. In the figure, only one pathway of terminal glycosylation is shown. *(Modified from Helenius A, Aebi M: Intracellular function of N-linked glycans.* Science *291:2364, 2001.)*

rather rare modification, it is crucial for the functionality of specific proteins and is essential for life (see box on Protein γ–Carboxylation: A Rare ER Posttranslational Modification Crucial for Life).

Destruction of Misfolded or Misassembled Proteins: ER-Associated Degradation

In the ER, proteins undergo a so-called quality control, which ensures that only correctly folded proteins exit the ER. Consequently, misfolded proteins are extracted from the ER folding environment for disposal. This mode of degradation is referred to as *endoplasmic reticulum-associated degradation* (ERAD). The destruction of proteins that undergo ERAD occurs in three major steps: (1) detection by the ER quality control machinery and targeting for ERAD, (2) transport across the ER membrane into the cytosol, and (3) ubiquitylation and release in the cytosol for degradation by the proteasome. One model for misfolded protein recognition is that hydrophobic patches or sugar moieties, which remain exposed on the protein for an extended period of time, are recognized by chaperone proteins such as PDI or by the CNX/CRT chaperone system. In a number of cases, retrotranslocation appears to require reduction of disulfide bridges by PDI. Similarly, BiP association with substrates (e.g., unassembled immunoglobulin light chains) can direct them to ERAD. If a protein remains in its unfolded state for an extended period of time, trimming of the $Man_8GlcNac_2$ also occurs. This processing is catalyzed by ER-degradation enhancer mannosidase α-like proteins EDEM1, EDEM2, EDEM3 (Htm1p in yeast). The current model postulates that the N-glycan structure generated by extensive de-mannosylation is the signal for glycoprotein degradation. ER-resident lectins (OS-9 and XTP3-B) bind to the remaining mannose residues and assist the retrotranslocation.

Proteins retrotranslocate to the cytosol through a protein-conducting channel, possibly formed by Derlin-1 and/or the complex. On their emergence at the cytosolic face of the ER membrane, substrates targeted for degradation start undergoing ubiquitylation. Tagged peptides are released into the cytosol in an ATP-dependent fashion, where they are degraded by the 26S proteasome. Fig. 4-6 illustrates the main steps of ERAD.

Protein γ–Carboxylation: A Rare ER Posttranslational Modification Crucial for Life

γ-Carboxylation of glutamic acid residues in the Gla domain serves to coordinate calcium ions and is essential for the proper biologic activity of factors involved in blood coagulation. These factors are prothrombin factors VII, IX, and X, which are involved in the coagulant response, and proteins C and S, which play roles in an antithrombotic pathway that limits coagulation. Other substrates of γ-carboxylase are less characterized, excect for the bone proteins osteocalcin and matrix Gla protein, which both proved to require processing by γ-carboxylation for full activity.

This posttranslational modification is catalyzed by γ-glutamyl carboxylase, an ER membrane protein. Its obligate cofactor, reduced vitamin K, is produced by the action of vitamin K–epoxide reductase (VKOR), which converts oxidized vitamin K to the reduced form. The activity of VKOR is inhibited by warfarin, a potent anticoagulant compound. γ-Carboxylase homozygous null mutants manifested dramatic effects on development with partial midembryonic loss and postnatal hemorrhage. Similar effects were observed in prothrombin or factor V–deficient mice. Thus the results of these studies have suggested that the functionally critical substrates for γ-carboxylation are primarily restricted to components of the blood coagulation cascade. These results highlight the importance of a rare protein modification for blood coagulation.

The Unfolded Protein Response

The ER monitors the amount of unfolded protein in its lumen. When that number exceeds a certain threshold, ER sensors activate a signal transduction pathway. The set of responses activated by this pathway is called the unfolded protein response (UPR). A number of cellular insults disrupt protein folding and cause unfolded protein accumulation in the ER lumen. The UPR is an adaptive response signaled through three ER-localized transmembrane proteins: PERK, IRE1, and ATF6. These proteins function as sensors through the properties of their ER-lumenal domains and trigger a concerted response through the function of their cytosolic domains. The activation of the sensors result in a complex response aimed to (1) limit accumulation of unfolded protein through reducing protein synthesis, (2) increasing the degradation of unfolded protein, and (3) increasing the ER protein-folding capacity.

IRE1 is conserved in all eukaryotic cells and has protein kinase and endoribonuclease activities that, upon activation, mediate unconventional splicing of a 26-base intron from the XBP1 mRNA to produce a potent basic leucine zipper (bZIP) transcription factor. ATF6, upon accumulation of unfolded protein in the ER lumen, is transported to the Golgi compartment, where it is cleaved by two proteases, S1P and S2P. These enzymes release a cytosolic fragment of ATF6 containing a bZIP-transcription factor that migrates to the nucleus to activate gene transcription. S1P and S2P are two important Golgi proteases because they are also involved in the regulation of cholesterol metabolism. Finally, PERK-mediated phosphorylation of eIF2α attenuates general mRNA translation but, paradoxically, increases translation of the transcription factor ATF4 mRNA to also induce transcription of UPR genes. If the UPR adaptive response is not sufficient to correct the protein-folding defect, the cells enter apoptotic death. Activation of the UPR and defects in UPR are now known to be important factors that contribute to a wide range of disease processes, including metabolic disease, neurologic disease, infectious disease, and cancer.

Control of Exit From the Endoplasmic Reticulum

On achieving transport competence, proteins are granted access to higher-ordered membrane domains termed *ER exit sites.* At ER exit sites, membrane-bound and soluble proteins are concentrated into transport vesicles for trafficking to a network of smooth membranes called the *ER-Golgi intermediate compartment* (ERGIC, see Fig. 4-4). COPII complexes, composed of *co*at *p*roteins, concentrate and package the protein cargo into vesicles. COPII binds to cargo molecules either directly (if molecules span the membrane) or through intermediate cargo receptors and then provides some of the force that causes vesicle budding, thereby linking cargo acquisition to vesiculation (see box on The Genetic Basis of a Bleeding Disorder Revealed the First Receptor-Mediated Protein Transport System in the Early Secretory Pathway). Overall, the mechanisms involved in cargo recognition are poorly defined.

ER resident proteins are selectively sequestered in the ER both for the absence of export signals and to the presence of ER retention signals. Soluble luminal ER resident proteins are retained through a C-terminal ER tetrapeptide retention motif KDEL. Frequently, transmembrane proteins have either a C-terminal dilysine motif KKXX or an N-terminal diarginine motif XXRR, or variants thereof for transmembrane proteins. However, it is more accurate to indicate ER localization signals as "retrieval motifs" because proteins bearing these signals can transiently escape from the ER into the ERGIC, from which they are returned to the ER through the retrograde vesicular transport (see Fig. 4-4).

For the KDEL motif of luminal ER proteins, a specific retrieval receptor has been identified, first in yeast and then in mammals. The KKXX motif has been shown to interact directly with the COPI coat protein complex that is involved in retrograde transport from the ER to the Golgi. Retrograde transport also serves to replenish the vesicle components lost as a result of anterograde (forward) transport. In

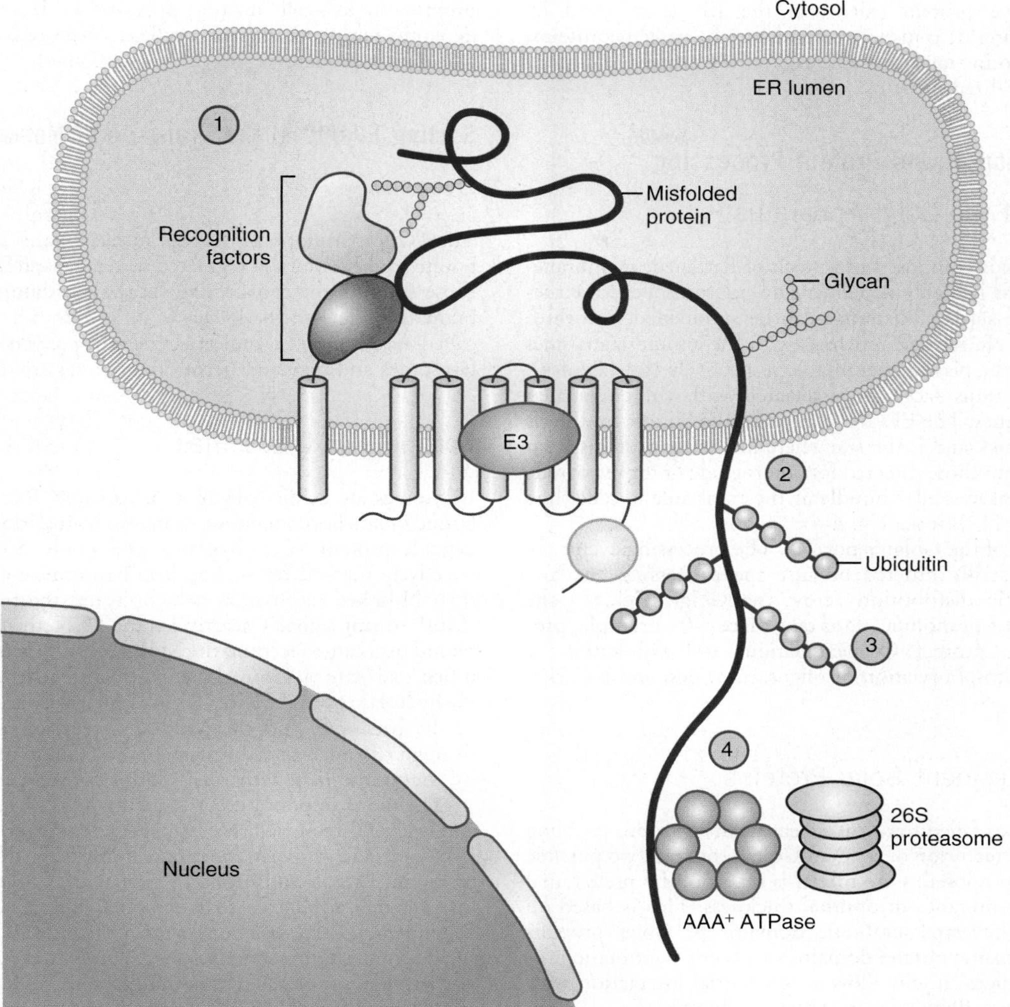

Figure 4-6 ER-ASSOCIATED PROTEIN DEGRADATION (ERAD). The figure depicts the steps in the degradation process of misfolded proteins in the ER. *Step 1:* Recognition factors (some of which are lectins), and ubiquitin ligases of the ER membrane cooperate in recognizing substrate proteins. *Step 2:* Proteins are exported into the cytosol via a so-far unidentified channel. *Step 3:* On the cytosolic face of the ER, the protein is ubiquitylated by an ER ligase. *Step 4:* The substrate is removed from the membrane by the AAA$^+$ ATPase Cdc48 and directed to the 26S proteasome. *(From Hirsch C, Gauss R, Horn SC, et al: The ubiquitylation machinery of the endoplasmic reticulum.* Nature *458:453, 2209.)*

The Genetic Basis of a Bleeding Disorder Revealed the First Receptor-Mediated Protein Transport System in the Early Secretory Pathway

In 2003 a form of bleeding disorder (hemophilia A) was found to be caused by defective secretion of coagulation factors V and VIII, two glycoproteins secreted into blood by specialized cells. Studies of human genetics combined with molecular biology led to the identification of two genes, *LMAN1* and *MCFD2*. LMAN1, or lectin mannose-binding protein1 (also referred to as ERGIC-53), is a transmembrane protein with a C-terminal cytoplasmic tail containing an ER-exit-motif (two phenylalanine residues, FF). This motif allows the interaction of LMAN1 with the COPII-coat proteins. The luminal domain of LMAN1 recognizes mannose residues and binds MCFD2 (multiple coagulation factor deficiency 2), a luminal protein, in a Ca^{++}-dependent manner. Both LMAN1 and MCFD2 are required in a complex for the recruitment of coagulation factors V and VIII into specific cargo vesicles. Of interest, loss of function mutations in either *LMAN1* or in *MCFD2* causes a bleeding disorder as a result of the combined deficiency of factors V and VIII. It has been shown that mutant forms of both LMAN1 and/or MCFD2 fail to recruit factor VIII into the vesicles. Thus the clotting factor deficiency is caused by a block in their export from the ER. Intriguingly, the LMAN1-MCFD2 complex appears to be required only for the secretion of factors V and VIII, as there are no significant reductions in any other plasma proteins. To date, the LMAN1-MCFD2 complex is the only well-defined cargo receptor in mammalian cells.

conclusion, selective protein exit from the ER is achieved by monitoring/regulating (l) transport competence of nascent proteins, (2) capture of cargo in transport vesicles, and (3) protein retention/retrieval for ER-localized proteins.

Intra-Golgi Transport and Protein Processing

Organization of the Golgi Apparatus

The Golgi complex is composed of a stack of flattened, membrane-bound cisternae that is highly dependent on microtubules for structural integrity. The stack of cisternae can be subdivided into three parts referred to as *cis, medial,* and *trans* with the cis and trans sides facing the ER and the plasma membrane, respectively (see Fig. 4-4). Both the cis and trans faces are associated with tubulovesicular bundles of membranes. The ERGIC comprises the bundle on the cis side of the Golgi stack and is the site where incoming proteins from the ER are sorted into those directed for anterograde or for retrograde transport. The tubulovesicular bundle at the trans side is called the *trans-Golgi network* (TGN; see Fig. 4-4).

A major feature of the Golgi is polarity. The processing events are temporally and spatially ordered because the processing enzymes have a characteristic distribution across the Golgi stack. In the Golgi, different types of modifications take place—for example, proteolytic processing, protein O-glycosylation, and elaboration of N-linked chains, phosphorylation of oligosaccharides, and sulfation of tyrosines.

Retention of Resident Golgi Proteins

Extensive analysis has failed to reveal a clear retention motif enabling subdomain-specific retention of resident Golgi proteins. Two possible models have been proposed. One model is retention by preferential interaction with membranes of optimal thickness. This is based on the finding that the transmembrane domains of Golgi proteins are shorter than transmembrane domains of plasma membrane proteins. These differences should allow a preferential interaction with the Golgi membrane lipid bilayer, which is thinner than that of plasma membrane. The other model is kin-recognition/oligomerization. This model postulates that proteins of a given subdomain of the Golgi membrane can aggregate into large detergent-insoluble oligomers as a way of minimizing lipid-protein contact. This would prevent the entry of proteins into the vesicles and thus their traffic to more distal cisternae. There is evidence in support of both models.

Protein Trafficking to and Through the Golgi Apparatus

Cargo proteins exit the ER in COPII-coated vesicles that enter the ERGIC and are ultimately delivered to the cis-Golgi either in vesicles or along extended tubules. However, the means whereby cargo proteins move across the Golgi complex from cis to trans remain controversial. Two models have been proposed. The vesicular transport model contends that anterograde transport occurs in vesicles or tubules and vesicles convey cargo in an anterograde direction. The second model suggests that there is a cisternal progression and maturation. This alternative model proposes that Golgi cisternae are not fixed structures but move forward from the cis side to the trans side, generating an anterograde movement. As cisternae mature, resident Golgi proteins that belong to more cis-like cisternae must be selectively pinched off in vesicles and trafficked back to the cis side of the Golgi stack. This would occur by COPI-mediated retrograde vesicular transport (see Fig. 4-4). Although which of these models is correct is currently unclear, most of the experimental data support the cisternal maturation model. In particular, technical progress in live-cell imaging provided evidence supporting a very dynamic nature of this organelle as expected by the progression/maturation model.

Sorting Events at the Trans-Golgi Network

Overview

The TGN is an important site of intracellular sorting, where proteins bound for lysosomes or regulated secretory vesicles are separated from those entering the constitutive pathway leading to the plasma membrane (see Fig. 4-4, pathways 6, 7, and 8). The secretion process is called *exocytosis.* The molecular basis for diversion of proteins into lysosomes and regulated secretory granules are described later.

Sorting Into Lysosomes

Lysosomes are acidic (pH of approximately 5.0 to 5.5), membrane-bound organelles containing numerous hydrolytic enzymes designed to degrade proteins, carbohydrates, and lipids. Soluble hydrolases are selectively marked for sorting into lysosomes by phosphorylation of their N-linked saccharides, which creates the mannose-6-phosphate (M6P) sorting signal. On arrival at the TGN, the modified hydrolase is bound by a cargo receptor, the M6P-receptor (M6P-R), which delivers it first to a "late endosomal compartment," where the low pH releases the hydrolase from the M6P-R. Subsequently, the hydrolase is delivered to the lysosome, and the M6P-R is recycled from the endosomes through retromer-coated vesicles to the TGN to be reused (for simplicity, the endosome to Golgi transport is not represented in Fig. 4-4).

The motif responsible for targeting M6P-R to lysosomes is YSKV and is recognized by all three distinct adaptor protein (AP) complexes (AP-l, -2, and -3) that contribute to delivery of cargo to lysosomes by linking cargo acquisition to vesiculation. Cargo recruitment occurs in a manner similar to that described for the COPI- and COPII-dependent vesicles, except that the cytosolic coat complex is clathrin. In addition to luminal hydrolases, lysosomes also contain a wide array of membrane proteins that are targeted to lysosomes via one of two consensus motifs: (1) YXXe, where X is any amino acid and e is any amino acid with a bulky hydrophobic side chain; and (2) a leucine-based motif (LL or LI). Trafficking of these membrane-bound proteins to lysosomes is indirect, proceeding first to late endosomes or the plasma membrane before their retrieval to lysosomes. Failure to accurately target lysosomal hydrolases underlies two well-known human diseases, Hurler syndrome and I-cell disease. Hurler syndrome is caused by a mutation in a hydrolase responsible for breakdown of glycosaminoglycans that prevents the hydrolase from acquiring the M6P modification, consequently preventing targeting to lysosomes. Similarly, in I-cell diseases undigested material accumulates in lysosomes because a mutation in the enzymes that create the M6P modification causes missorting of lysosomal hydrolases. Chapter 51 provides an overview of the lysosome storage diseases.

Autophagy: A Lysosomal Degradation Pathway

Autophagy, the most common name for *macroautophagy,* consists of the capture and degradation of cellular components and organelles. Cellular material is sequestered inside double-membrane vesicles, called *autophagosomes,* and degraded upon fusion with lysosomal compartments (Fig. 4-7). Raw precursors are then recycled for new biosyntheses. Constitutive autophagy serves to demolish damaged organelles or cytosolic components and contributes to the maintenance of cell homeostasis.

Autophagy is also stress responsive. It accelerates the catabolism of cellular components to sustain the demand of energy in adverse conditions and promotes cell survival. From yeast to human cells, starvation typically activates autophagy. Yeast has been a useful model microorganism to identify the first autophagy genes *(ATG),* which

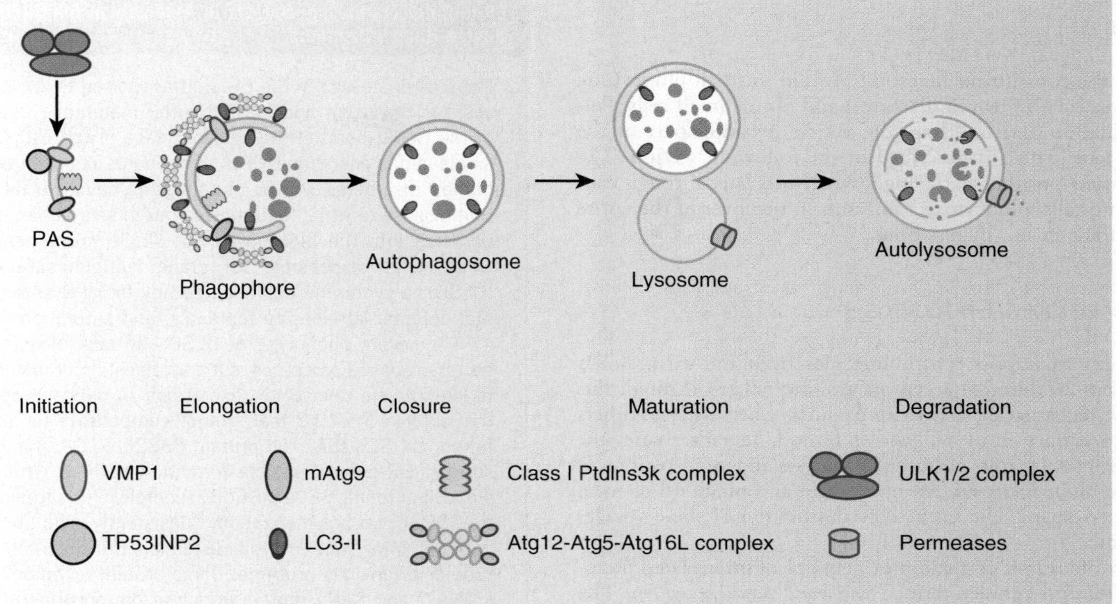

Figure 4-7 STEPS IN THE AUTOPHAGY PATHWAY. The scheme depicts different steps in mammalian autophagy. Shown on the left are the initiation at the PAS (phagophore assembly site); elongation and expansion of the phagophore; closure and completion of the autophagosome; autophagosome maturation via docking and fusion with an endosome and/or lysosome; breakdown and degradation of the autophagosome inner membrane and cargo; and recycling of the resulting molecules. In the lower part, some components of the molecular machinery are shown. The ULK complex is under the regulation of the protein kinase mTOR. *(Modified from Yang Z, Klionsky DJ: Mammalian autophagy: Core molecular machinery and signaling regulation.* Curr Opin Cell Biol *22:124, 2010.)*

allowed the subsequent isolation of the mammalian counterparts. ATG proteins are involved in the basic mechanism of autophagy, on which a complex regulation has been superimposed in mammals to respond to a wider variety of hormonal, environmental, and intracellular signals. An increasing body of evidence suggests that autophagy plays an important role in development and cell differentiation by facilitating cell and tissue remodeling. Remarkably, reticulocyte maturation in erythrocytes, which involves a mitochondria loss whose basis remained mysterious for decades, is partly dependent on autophagy (mitophagy).

Defects in constitutive autophagy compromise cell fitness. As a consequence, cells become more susceptible to tumorigenesis, neurodegenerative disorders, liver disease, aging, inflammatory diseases, and host defense against pathogens. However, recent evidence suggests that in established tumor cells, autophagy may represent an advantage for survival in hostile environments of the human body. Thus the autophagy may be regarded both as a target for tumor prevention or for cancer therapy.

Sorting Into Regulated Secretory Granules

In regulated secretion, proteins are condensed into stored secretory granules that are released to the plasma membrane after the cell has received an appropriate stimulus (see Fig. 4-4, pathway 7). After budding from TGN, the granule proteins are concentrated (up to 200-fold in some cases) by selective removal of extraneous contents from clathrin-coated vesicles. Mature secretory granules are thought to be stored in association with microtubules until the stimulation of a surface receptor triggers their exocytosis. One example of stimulus-induced exocytosis is the binding of a ligand to the T-cell antigen receptor (TCR) complex on a cytotoxic T lymphocyte. Conjugation of a cytotoxic T cell with its target causes its microtubules and associated secretory granules to reorient toward the target cell. Subsequently, the granules are delivered along microtubules until they fuse with the plasma membrane, releasing their contents for lysis of the target cell. Following release of the granule contents, the granule membrane components are internalized and transported back to the TGN, where the granule can be refilled with cargo proteins.

Endocytic Traffic

Overview

Substances are imported from the cell exterior by a process termed *endocytosis* (see Fig. 4-4, pathway 9). Endocytosis also serves to recover the plasma membrane lipids and proteins that are lost by ongoing secretory activity. There are three types of endocytosis: (1) phagocytosis (cell eating), (2) pinocytosis (cell drinking), and (3) receptor-mediated endocytosis. Defects in endocytosis can underlie human diseases. For example, patients with familial hypercholesterolemia (FH) have elevated serum cholesterol because of mutations in the low-density lipoprotein (LDL) receptor that prevent the endocytic uptake of LDL and its catabolism in lysosomes.

Phagocytosis

During phagocytosis cells are able to ingest large particles (greater than 0.5 μm in diameter). Phagocytosis serves not only to engulf and destroy invading bacteria and fungi but also to clear cellular debris at wound sites and to dispose of aged erythrocytes. Primarily, specialized cells such as macrophages, neutrophils, and dendritic cells execute phagocytosis. Phagocytosis is triggered when specific receptors contact structural triggers on the particle, including bound antibodies, complement components as well as certain oligosaccharides. Then the polymerization of actin is stimulated, driving the extension of pseudopods, which surround the particle and engulf it in a vacuole called *phagosome*. The engulfed material is destroyed when the phagosome fuses with a lysosome, exposing the content to hydrolytic enzymes. In addition, phagocytosis is a means of "presenting" the pathogen's components to lymphocytes, thus eliciting an immune response.

Pinocytosis

Pinocytosis is the constitutive ingestion of fluid in small pinocytotic (endocytic) vesicles (0.2 μm in diameter) and occurs in all cells. Following invagination and budding, the vesicle becomes part of the endosome system, which is described in the following section. The plasma membrane portion that is ingested returns later through exocytosis. In some cells, pinocytosis can result in turnover of the entire plasma membrane in less than 1 hour.

Receptor-Mediated Endocytosis

This is a means to import macromolecules from the extracellular fluid. More than 20 different receptors are internalized through this pathway. Some receptors are internalized continuously whereas others remain on the surface until a ligand is bound. In either case, the receptors slide laterally into coated pits that are indented regions of the plasma membrane surrounded by clathrin and pinch off to form clathrin-coated vesicles. The immediate destination of these vesicles is the endosome.

The endosome is part of a complex network of interrelated membranous vesicles and tubules termed the *endolysosomal system.* The endolysosomal system comprises four types of membrane-bound structures: early endosomes (EEs), late endosomes (LEs), recycling vesicles, and lysosomes. It is still a matter of debate whether these structures represent independent stable compartments or whether one structure matures into the next. The interior of the endosomes is acidic (pH about 6). Endocytosed material is ultimately delivered to the lysosome, presumably by fusion with LE. Lysosomes are also used for digestion of obsolete parts of the cell in the process of autophagy (described in more detail earlier).

During the formation of clathrin-coated vesicles, clathrin molecules do not recognize cargo receptors directly but rather through the adaptor proteins, which form an inner coat. The AP-2 components bind both clathrin and sorting signals present in the cytoplasmic tails of cargo receptors close to the plasma membrane. These internalization motifs are YXXϕ (where ϕ is a hydrophobic amino acid), the most common motif, and the NPXY signal that was first identified in the LDL receptor. For receptors that are internalized in response to ligand binding, the internalization signal may also be generated by a conformational change induced by the binding of the ligand. Through the specificity of the AP-2 complex, the capture of a unique set of cargo receptors is linked to vesiculation, resulting in concentration of the cargo. The coated pit pinches off from the plasma membrane by the action of a GTP binding protein, dynamin, which forms a ring around the neck of each bud and contributes to the vesicle formation. After release and shedding of the clathrin coat, the vesicle fuses with the EE compartment.

SPECIFICITY OF VESICULAR TARGETING

As described earlier, COPI- and COPII-vesicles transport material early in the secretory pathway, whereas clathrin-coated vesicles transport material from the plasma membrane and Golgi. Coating proteins assemble at specific areas of the membrane in a process controlled by the coat-recruitment GTPases: ARF1 is responsible for the assembly of COPI coats and clathrin coats at Golgi membranes, whereas SAR1 is responsible for COPII coat assembly at the ER membrane. In yeast the process of vesiculation in the transport from the ER to Golgi has been dissected at a molecular level. On the cytosolic face of the ER membrane, Sar1p is activated by the ER-localized GEF Sec12p. Sar1-GTP assembles with the Sec23-Sec24 complex whose Sec24 subunit binds directly or through a membrane receptor to specific signals displayed by the cargo. This prebudding cargo complex recruits the outer layer Sec13-Sec31 complex leading to coat polymerization, membrane deformation, and COPII-vesicle formation. Mutations in gene encoding the human homolog of Sec24 or Sar1 are responsible for severe human diseases (see box on ER-to-Golgi Trafficking: Defects in Assembly of the COPII Coat Cause Severe Human Disorders).

Clathrin-coat assembly at the plasma membrane is also thought to involve a GTPase, but its identity is unknown. These regulatory proteins also ensure that membrane traffic to and from an organelle are balanced.

After budding, vesicles are transported to their final destination by diffusion or motor-mediated transport along the cytoskeletal network (microtubules or actin). The molecular motors kinesin, dynein, and myosin have been implicated in this process. The vesicles undergo an uncoating process before fusion with the correct target membrane. Both transport vesicles and target membranes display surface markers that selectively recognize each other.

Three classes of proteins guide the selectivity of transport vesicle docking and fusion: (1) complementary sets of vesicle SNAREs (v-SNAREs; *SNARE* derived from SNAP receptor, or *soluble NSF association protein receptor*) and target membrane SNAREs (t-SNAREs), which are crucial for the fusion; (2) a class of GTPases, called *Rabs*; and (3) protein complexes called *tethers,* which, together with Rabs, facilitate the initial docking of the vesicles to the target membrane.

Although Rab GTPases function as the master regulators of membrane traffic, they are themselves regulated by factors that control their activation by GEFs or their inactivation by GAP, proteins that stimulate the intrinsic GTPase activity.

ER-to-Golgi Trafficking: Defects in Assembly of the COPII Coat Cause Severe Human Disorders

Proteins processed in the ER are transported to the Golgi through vesicles that form and bud from the membrane upon assembly of the COPII coat on the cytosolic face of the ER. Mutations in single genes encoding COPII components result in two inherited human disorders. *SAR1B* mutant gene causes a fat malabsorption disease in which enterocytes fail to secrete large lipoprotein particles into the bloodstream. A single missense mutation in *SEC23A* is responsible for cranio-lenticulo-sutural dysplasia (CLSD), a syndrome characterized by facial dysmorphism, skeletal defects, late-closing fontanels, and sutural cataracts.

The severe phenotype of CLSD and lack of defects in other secretion-based processes, such as digestion or insulin signaling, is likely to be due to low expression in calvarial osteoblasts of the isoform *SEC23B* that cannot compensate for the lack of a functional SEC23A. The mutant F382L-*SEC23A* is incapable to support ER-derived vesicle formation both *in vitro* and *in vivo* since it impairs SEC13-SEC31 complex recruitment necessary for COP II coat polymerization. Consistently, skin fibroblasts from patients with CLSD exhibit distended ER cisternae from which tubular extensions protrude. Cargo protein receptors (ERGIC-53/LMNA1) and SAR1 protein enrich at the presumed ER exit sites of the tubular protrusions.

FUTURE DIRECTIONS

The mechanisms regulating protein synthesis, processing, degradation, and transport are under intense investigation. Protein motifs and their cognate receptors have been identified for many intracellular sorting and processing reactions. Studies are now directed to elucidate these processes at a molecular level by resolution of the three-dimensional structures of the proteins involved in protein processing and trafficking. The future challenge will be to find ways of exploiting this knowledge to intervene in the numerous disease states that result from errors in these processes.

SUGGESTED READINGS

Aebi M, Bernasconi R, Clerc S, et al: N-Glycan structures: Recognition and processing in the ER. *Trends Biochem Sci* 35:74, 2009.

Bagola K, Mehnert M, Jarosch E, et al: Protein dislocation from the ER. *Biochim Biophys Acta* 1808:925, 2010.

Baines AC, Zhang B: Receptor-mediated protein transport in the early secretory pathway. *TIBS* 32:381, 2007.

Bernasconi R, Molinari M: ERAD and ERAD tuning: Disposal of cargo and of ERAD regulators from the mammalian ER. *Curr Opin Cell Biol* 23: 176, 2011.

Brocker C, Engerlbrecht-Vandrè S, Ungermann C: Multisubunit tethering complexes and their role in membrane fusion. *Curr Biol* 20:R943, 2010.

Cal H, Reinisch K, Ferro-Novick S: Coats, Tethers, Rabs and SNAREs work together to mediate the intracellular destination of a transport vesicle. *Dev Cell* 12:671, 2007.

Dancourt J, Barlowe C: Protein sorting receptors in the early secretory pathway. *Ann Rev Biochem* 79:777, 2010.

Fromme JC, Ravazzola M, Hamamoto S, et al: The genetic basis of a craniofacial disease provides insight into the COPII coat assembly. *Dev Cell* 13:623, 2007.

Helenius A, Aebi M: Roles of N-linked glycans in the endoplasmic reticulum. *Annu Rev Biochem* 73:1019, 2004.

Hirsch C, Gauss R, Horn SC, et al: The ubiquitylation machinery of the endoplasmic reticulum. *Nature* 458:453, 2009.

Jones B, Jones EL, Bonney SA, et al: Mutations in a Sar1 GTPase of COPII vesicles are associated with lipid absorption disorders. *Nat Genet* 34:29, 2003.

Kroemer G, Mariño G, Levine B: Autophagy and the integrated stress response. *Mol Cell* 40:280, 2010.

Kundu M, Lindsten T, Yang C, et al: Ulk1 plays a critical role in the autophagic clearance of mitochondria and ribosomes during reticulocyte maturation. *Blood* 112:1493, 2008.

Malhi H, Kaufman RJ: Endoplasmic reticulum stress in liver disease. *J Hepatol* 54:795, 2011.

Malhotra JD, Kaufman RJ: The endoplasmic reticulum and the unfolded protein response. *Semin Cell Dev Biol* 18:716, 2007.

Margittai E, Sitia R: Oxidative protein folding in the secretory pathway and redox signaling across compartments and cells. *Traffic* 12:1, 2011.

Mizushima N, Levine B: Autophagy in mammalian development and differentiation. *Nat Cell Biol* 12:823, 2010.

Nakano A, Luini A: Passage through Golgi. *Curr Opin Cell Biol* 22:471, 2010.

Pfeffer S, Novick P: Membrane traffic. *Curr Opin Cell Biol* 22:419, 2010.

Proud CG: Regulation of protein synthesis by insulin. *Biochem Soc Trans* 34:213, 2006.

Rouault TA: The role of iron regulatory proteins in mammalian homeostasis and disease. *Nat Chem Biol* 2:406, 2006.

Schliebs W, Girzalsky W, Erdmann R: Peroxysomal protein import and ERAD: Variations on a common theme. *Nat Rev Mol Cell Biol* 11:885, 2010.

Schmidt O, Pfanner N, Meisinger C: Mirochondrial protein import: From proteomics to functional mechanisms. *Nat Rev Mol Cell Biol* 11:655, 2010.

Schroder M, Kaufman RJ: The mammalian unfolded protein response. *Annu Rev Biochem* 74:739, 2005.

Tabas I, Ron D: Integrating the mechanisms of apoptosis induced by endoplasmic reticulum stress. *Nat Cell Biol* 13:184, 2011.

Vucic D, Dixit V, Wertz IE: Ubiquitylation in apoptosis: A post-translational modification at the edge of life and death. *Nat Rev Mol Cell Biol* 12:439, 2011.

Wente S, Rout MP: The nuclear pore complex and nuclear transport. *Cold Spring Harb Perspec Biol* 2:a000562, 2010.

Zhang B: Recent developments in the understanding of the combined deficiency of FV and FVIII. *Br J Haematol* 145:15, 2009.

CHAPTER 5

PROTEIN ARCHITECTURE: RELATIONSHIP OF FORM AND FUNCTION

Jia-huai Wang, Angela Toms, Ming-Ming Zhou, and Michael J. Eck

Previous chapters have outlined the central dogma of molecular biology: the storage of genetic information in DNA and its regulated transcription into messenger RNA and eventual translation into proteins. In this chapter, we briefly outline the chemical structure of proteins and their posttranslational modifications. We explain how the properties of the 20 amino acids of which proteins are composed allow these polymers to fold into compact, functional domains and how particular domains and motifs have been assembled, modified, and reused in the course of evolution. Finally, we describe a sampling of proteins and domains of relevance to the hematologist and explore briefly how point mutations, chromosomal translocations, and other genetic alterations may modify protein structure and function to cause disease.

AMINO ACIDS AND THE PEPTIDE BOND

Proteins are linear polymers of the 20 naturally occurring amino acids, linked together by the peptide bond. All of the amino acids share a common core or backbone structure and differ only in the side chain emanating from the central α-carbon of this core. The common backbone elements include an amino group, the central α-carbon, and a carboxylic acid group. Peptide bonds are formed by reaction of the carboxylic acid of one amino acid with the amino group of the next amino acid in the chain. This reaction is templated and catalyzed by the ribosome and leads to the release of water formed by the loss of an –OH group from the carboxylic acid of one amino acid residue and a hydrogen atom from the amino group of the next residue in the chain. Coupling of multiple amino acids together via the peptide bond produces the repeating main-chain structure of the polypeptide chain, composed of the amide (NH) nitrogen, alpha carbon (Cα), and carbonyl carbon (CO), followed by the amide nitrogen of the next amino acid in the chain (Fig. 5-1, *A*). The resonant, partial double-bond character of the peptide bond prevents rotation about this bond; thus the five main-chain carbon, nitrogen, and oxygen atoms of each peptide unit lie in a plane. The conformational flexibility in the polypeptide chain is conferred by rotation about the bonds on either side of the α-carbon atom; these bond angles are referred to as *phi* and *psi angles*. The angle of the N–Cα bond is known as the *phi angle* (Φ), and the angle of the Cα–CO bond is known as the *psi angle* (ψ).

The primary structure or primary sequence of a protein is the order in which various residues of the 20 amino acids are assembled into the polypeptide chain, and this sequence is critically important for determining the three-dimensional fold and thus function of the protein. It is the diverse chemical structure and physicochemical properties of the 20 amino acid side chains that guide the three-dimensional fold of proteins and also provide for the enormous repertoire of protein function—from catalysis of myriad chemical reactions to immune recognition to establishment of muscle and skeletal structure.

The amino acids can be divided into general classes based on the properties of their side chains and, in particular, their propensity to interact with water. Hydrophobic amino acids have aliphatic or aromatic side chains and include alanine, valine, leucine, isoleucine, proline, methionine, and phenylalanine. The hydrophobic amino acids predominate in the interior of proteins, where they are sequestered from water. They tend to pack against each other via van der Waals interactions, which contribute to the overall stability of folded protein domains. Charged amino acids include those with acidic side chains (aspartic acid and glutamic acid) and those with basic side chains (lysine, arginine, and histidine). Histidine merits special mention, because it is the only amino acid whose side chain can be protonated or unprotonated, and therefore charged or uncharged, in physiologic ranges of pH. For this reason, histidine is part of many enzyme-active sites. For example, in the serine proteases of the coagulation cascade, an active-site histidine acts as a general base, accepting and then releasing a proton in sequential steps of the enzymatic reaction. Polar amino acids include serine, threonine, tyrosine, asparagine, glutamine, cysteine, and tryptophan. Both polar and charged residues can form hydrogen bonds with each other, with the protein main chain, and with water or ligand molecules. Hydrogen bonds refer to the attractive interaction of a proton covalently bonded to one electronegative atom (usually a nitrogen or oxygen in proteins) with another electronegative atom. Hydrogen bonds are an important contributor to the stability of proteins and to the specificity of protein-protein and protein-ligand interactions. Some polar amino acids (e.g., threonine, lysine, tyrosine, and tryptophan) are amphipathic—that is, they have both polar and hydrophobic traits. This dual nature makes them well suited for participating in protein-protein interactions, where they may be alternately exposed to solvent or buried upon formation of a complex.

Protein Secondary Structure

The alternating pattern of hydrogen bond donating amide groups and hydrogen bond accepting carbonyl groups gives rise to repeating elements of protein structure that are stabilized by hydrogen bonds between these main-chain groups. These secondary structure elements include α-helices and β-sheets. In an α-helix, the main chain adopts a right-handed helical conformation in which the carbonyl oxygen of the ith residue in the polypeptide chain accepts a hydrogen bond from the amide nitrogen of the $(i + 4)^{th}$ residue (see Fig. 5-1, *B*). The pattern may repeat for only a few residues, forming a single turn of α-helix, or for more than 100 residues, forming dozens of turns of helix. There are 3.6 residues per turn of helix, and the pitch or rise of the helix is 1.5 Å per residue or 5.4 Å per turn. The side chains of residues in an α-helix project outward, away from the central axis of the helix. Often a polar side chain will "cap" the end of a helix by forming a hydrogen bond with the otherwise unpartnered amide or carbonyl group at the N- or C-terminal end of the helix.

In β-sheet secondary structure, the protein backbone adopts an extended conformation and two or more strands are arranged side by side, with hydrogen bonds between the strands. The strands can run in the same direction (parallel β-sheet) or antiparallel to one another. Mixed sheets with both parallel and antiparallel strands are also possible (see Fig. 5-1, *C*). In β-sheets, the side chains of a given strand extend alternately above and below the plane defined by the hydrogen-bonded main chains. Other common types of secondary structure include a variant of the helix with an $i + 3$ hydrogen bonding pattern

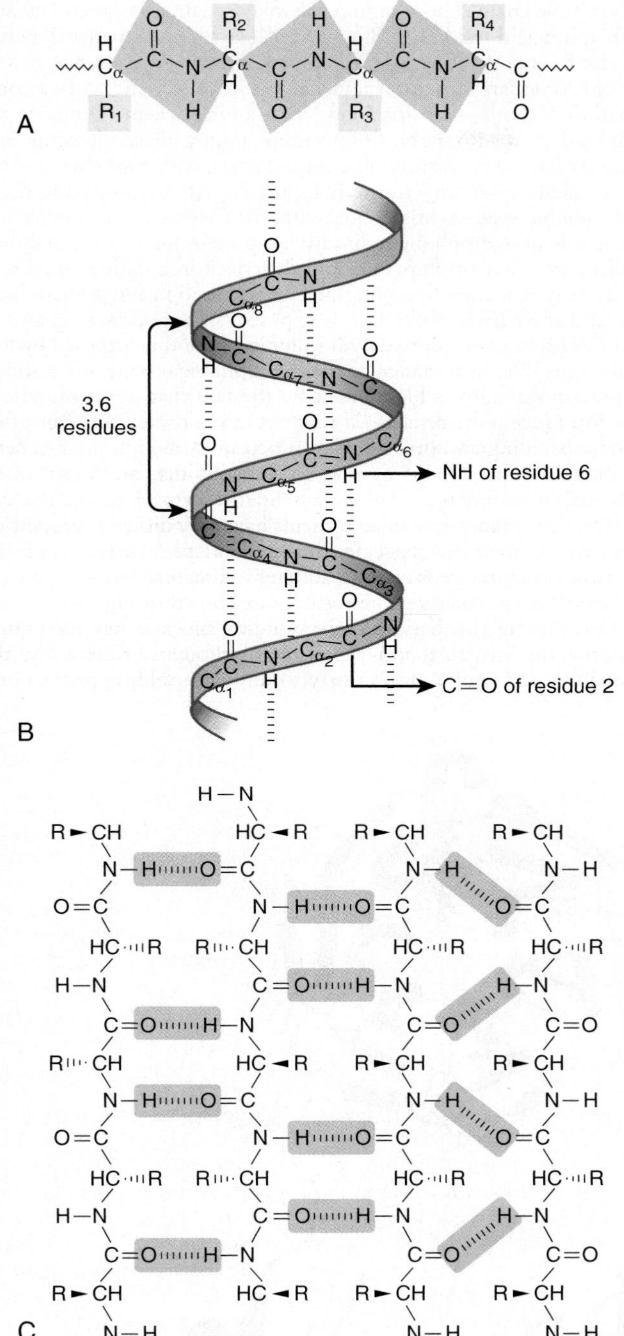

Figure 5-1 **A,** Diagram showing a polypeptide chain where the main-chain atoms are represented as peptide units, linked through the Cα atoms. Each peptide unit is a planar, rigid group *(shaded in pink)* and has two degrees of freedom; it can rotate around the Cα-CO bond and the N-Cα bond. The peptide bonds are depicted in the trans conformation; adjacent Cα carbons and their side chains *(highlighted in blue)* on opposite sides of the N- Cα bond. This is the preferred configuration for most amino acids, because it minimizes steric hindrance. **B,** The α-helix. The hydrogen bonds between residue *n* and residue *n* + 4, which stabilizes the helix, are shown as dashed lines. **C,** Schematic drawing of a mixed β-sheet. The first three β-strands are antiparallel to one another, whereas the last two β-strands are parallel. The hydrogen bonds that stabilize these structures are highlighted.

(the 3_{10} helix) and specific types of β-turns, short segments connecting other elements of secondary structure that are stabilized by β-sheet–like hydrogen bonds. Although any of the amino acids can be found within α-helices or β-sheets, the special characteristics of proline and glycine merit mention. The cyclic structure of proline means that it lacks an amide proton; thus it introduces an irregularity in hydrogen bonding, for example, leading to a "kink" in an α-helix. Glycine lacks a side chain—it has only a second hydrogen atom on its α-carbon—and therefore has less steric restriction and can adopt a wider range of backbone phi and psi angles. This added flexibility means that glycine tends to disfavor regular secondary structure.

Because proteins are large and complicated structures, they are typically illustrated with "ribbon" diagrams that trace the path of the polypeptide backbone. In such representations, helices are drawn as helical coils or cylinders, and β-strands appear as elongated rectangles with an arrow as a guide to the direction of the protein chain from its amino- to carboxy-terminal end. Specific side chains of amino acids of functional interest can then be added to illustrate a particular feature.

Disulfide Bonds and Posttranslational Modifications

The covalent structure of proteins is commonly modified in structurally and functionally important ways beyond the linear coupling of amino acids via the peptide bond. Regulated proteolysis can be considered a posttranslational modification and can serve an important regulatory role, as in the cleavage of prothrombin in the blood-clotting cascade. The structure of cell-surface and extracellular proteins is often stabilized by disulfide bonds, which are covalent bonds formed between the thiol groups of juxtaposed cysteine residues. In general, disulfide bonds are not found in intracellular proteins, where the reducing environment disfavors their formation. Disulfide bonds can form between cysteines within the same polypeptide chain, stabilizing the fold of the polypeptide backbone, or they may covalently join two different polypeptide chains, for example, the heavy and light chains of immunoglobulins. In addition to their role in disulfide bond formation, cysteine residues often contribute to protein stability via their participation in metal ion coordination, in particular zinc, which is often bound by conserved sets of cysteine and histidine residues in small protein domains.

A number of functional groups are appended to proteins to regulate their function, localization, protein interactions, and degradation. Examples of these posttranslational modifications (PTMs) include phosphorylation, glycosylation, ubiquitylation, methylation, acetylation, and lipidation. PTMs occur at distinct amino acid side chains or peptide linkages and are most often mediated by enzymatic activity and can occur at any step in the "life cycle" of a protein. As discussed later, a number of protein domains have evolved to recognize and bind specifically to proteins labeled by a particular PTM. Protein phosphorylation on serine, threonine, or tyrosine residues is one of the most important and well-studied posttranslational modifications. Phosphorylation is mediated by protein kinases and can activate or deactivate many enzymes through conformational changes and thus plays a critical role in the regulation of many cellular processes, including cell cycle, growth, apoptosis, and signal transduction pathways. Protein glycosylation encompasses a diverse selection of sugar-moiety additions to proteins that ranges from simple monosaccharide modifications to highly complex branched polysaccharides. Glycosylation has significant effects on protein folding, conformation, distribution, stability, and activity. Carbohydrates in the form of asparagine-linked (N-linked) or serine/threonine–linked (O-linked) oligosaccharides are major structural components of many cell-surface and secreted proteins. Protein methylation on arginine or lysine residues is carried out by methyltransferases with S-adenosyl methionine (SAM) as the primary methyl group donor.[1] Methylation is an important mechanism of epigenetic regulation—histone methylation and demethylation influence the availability of DNA for transcription. N-acetylation, the transfer of an acetyl group to the amine nitrogen at the N-terminus of the polypeptide chain, occurs in a majority of eukaryotic proteins.

Lysine acetylation and deacetylation is an important regulatory mechanism in a number of proteins. It is best characterized in histones, where histone acetyltransferases (HATs) and histone deacetylases (HDACs) regulate gene expression via modification of histone tails. Many cytoplasmic proteins are also acetylated, and therefore acetylation seems to play a greater role in cell biology than simply transcriptional regulation.[2] Lipidation is a modification that targets proteins to membranes in organelles, vesicles, and the plasma membrane. Examples of lipidation include myristoylation, palmitoylation, and prenylation. Each type of modification gives proteins distinct membrane affinities, although all types of lipidation increase the hydrophobicity of a protein and thus its affinity for membranes. In N-myristoylation, the myristoyl group (14-carbon saturated fatty acid) is transferred to a N-terminal glycine by N-myristoyltransferase. The myristoyl group does not always permanently anchor the protein in the membrane; in a number of proteins the N-terminal myristoyl group has been observed to pack into the protein core. N-myristoylation can therefore act as a conformational localization switch, in which protein conformational changes influence the availability of the handle for membrane attachment.

The Domain Structure of Proteins

In general, the minimal biologically functional unit of three-dimensional protein structure is the protein domain. Domains are locally compact and semi-independent units of usually contiguous polypeptide chain. The common size of a domain is between 100 and 200 amino acid residues, although much larger and smaller domains are also frequently observed. Protein domains are composed of closely packed secondary structure elements—α-helices, β-sheets, or a combination of both—and the loops that connect them. Domains are stabilized by hydrophobic interactions among these elements and typically have very hydrophobic central cores, with more hydrophilic amino acids extending from their surface. Alternating patterns of hydrophobic residues in secondary structure elements are a reflection of the role of hydrophobicity in driving protein folding and stability. Helices are often amphipathic, and they pack in a folded domain in such a way that their hydrophobic face is buried in the domain interior and their hydrophilic face is exposed on the surface. Likewise, β-sheets often have a buried hydrophobic face and an exposed hydrophilic face. The importance of the hydrophobic core to the stability of protein domains is highlighted by the fact that point mutations that introduce polar or charged residues into a protein interior often cause misfolding and thus a loss of function. Although these general characteristics are shared by protein domains that are found in an aqueous environment, such as that on the cytosol or on the cell surface, membrane-embedded proteins have very different properties, reflective of their residence in the lipid bilayer. Several common domain structures representing different categories with regard to their secondary structure composition are shown in Fig. 5-2.

Deciphering this basic protein building block is key for understanding the structure and evolution of proteins. Kinetically, the domain structure of a protein may simplify the folding process into

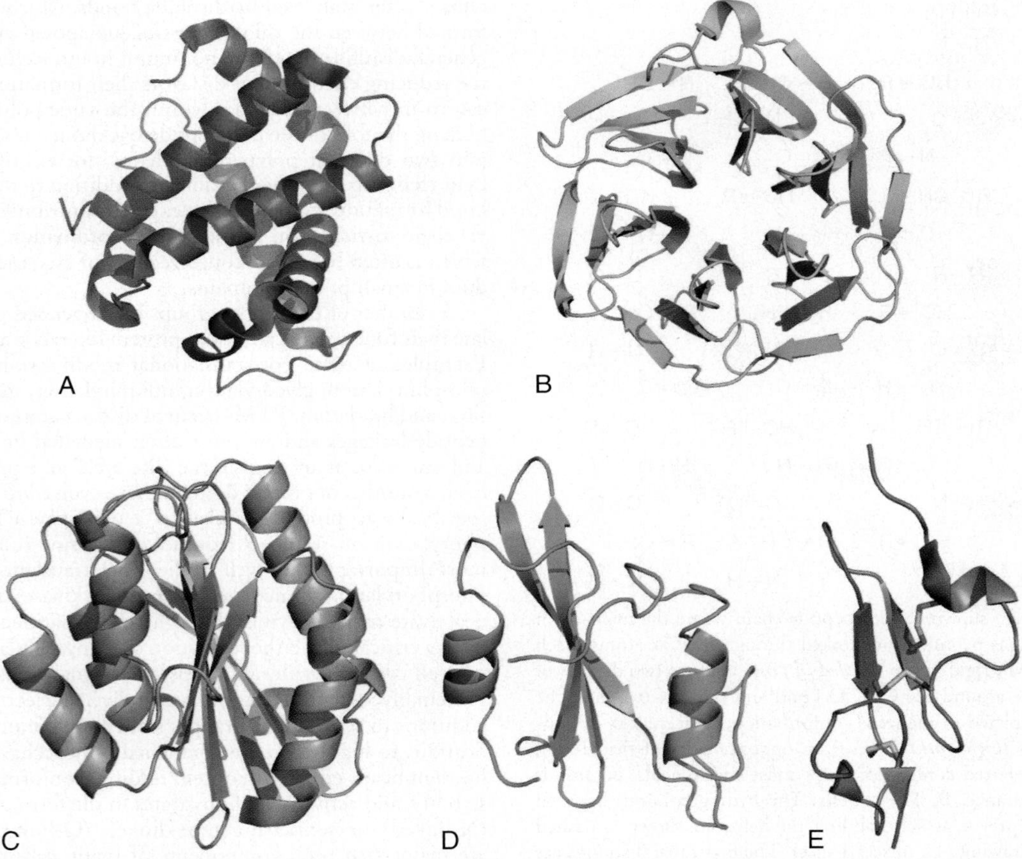

Figure 5-2 SEVERAL COMMON DOMAIN STRUCTURES. **A,** The α-globin domain of hemoglobin, made up by all α-helices (PDB entry 2MHB). **B,** The β-propeller domain, composed of all β-strands, existed in many extracellular matrix and cell surface proteins (PDB entry 1NPE). **C,** The I domain, comprising alternate β-strand and α-helix, from integrin (PDB entry 1ID0). **D,** SH2 (Src homologue 2) domain, consisting of sequentially separate β-strands and α-helices, typically found in tyrosine kinases (PDB entry 1FMK). **E,** The EGF (epidermal growth factor) domain, mainly maintained by 3-4 disulfide bonds, found in many extracellular matrix proteins and cell adhesion molecules (PDB entry 1UZJ).

a stepwise course.[3] Thus a long amino acid sequence may fold into multiple domains rapidly and correctly. For many proteins, individual domains fold in a cotranslational manner; from the N-terminal region, a growing nascent polypeptide chain immediately begins to fold domain-by-domain during translation from the ribosome in a very efficient manner.[4] Genetically, it was long suspected that the exon structure of genes was correlated with the domains structure of proteins.[5] Recent multigenome analysis does find a strong correlation between domain organization and exon-intron arrangement in genomic DNA. The exon-domain correlation facilitates extensive exon shuffling events during evolution,[6] although it is not necessarily always one-exon/one-domain. This mechanism ensures that a stable and functionally efficient domain can be repeatedly used as a module assembled into many proteins with shared functions. A well-known early example is the nucleotide-binding domain identified in various dehydrogenases; its robust alternate β-strand–α-helix–β-strand fold provides a common structural unit for these enzymes.[7]

Recent computational approaches demonstrate that almost all of a growing number of known sequences come from new combinations of individual protein domains, and as a consequence more than 70% of all sequences can be partially modeled from known structures with homologous domains.[8] This has been reflected in the human genome sequence.[9] Impressive progress has already been made in computational protein prediction and design, principally based on the known structural elements.[10]

Many proteins are composed of multiple domains, which may confer multiple functions, couple a targeting function to a catalytic function, or provide for allosteric regulation. The following sections will highlight the structure of a few proteins and domains that are of central and recurring importance in hematology in order to illustrate the relationship between domain architecture and function. Representative examples have been chosen from the extracellular space (the immunoglobulin domain), intracellular signaling (protein kinase domain), and nuclear gene regulation (transcription factors and domains involved in epigenetic regulation).

The Immunoglobulin Domain and Variations

As implied by its name, the immunoglobulin (Ig) domain was first recognized in antibodies.[11] A detailed discussion on antibody biology can be found in Chapter 22. The human genome project has identified the Ig superfamily (IgSF) as the largest superfamily in the human genome, owing to its extensive usage in more recently developed immune system in vertebrates.[9] In fact, the Ig domain is an evolutionarily ancient structural unit that can be found in *Caenorhabditis elegans*.[12] Although Ig-like domains also exist in a few intracellular proteins, they are found predominately in the extracellular space and are the most abundant structural unit found in cell surface receptors, serving key recognition functions in both the immune and nervous systems. Along with a handful of other modular domains such as fibronectin type III domains and EGF domains, they form modular structures of most receptor molecules on the cell surface.[13]

An Ig domain is composed of roughly 100 residues, folding into two β-sheets packing face-to-face, forming a β-barrel. This distinctively folded structure is commonly known as the Ig fold. Since an antibody consists of a variable domain and one (in light chain) or three (in heavy chain) constant domains, Ig domains have correspondingly been classified into V-set and C-set. A V-set Ig domain has β-strands A, B, E, and D on one sheet and A′, G, F, C, C′, and C″ strands on the other (Fig. 5-3, *A*), whereas a C-set Ig domain lacks A′, C′, and C″ strands on either edges (see Fig. 5-3, *B*). The two sheets are linked together by a conserved disulfide bond between B strand and F strand (reviewed in Williams et al[14]). The V-set Ig domains of heavy chain and light chain combine to make up the antigen-binding site, where hypovariable sequences cluster into three CDR (complementarity-determining region) loops that connect β-strands (see Fig. 5-3, *A*). Fig. 5-4, *A*, depicts how a broadly neutralizing antibody 2F5's CDR loops form an antigen-binding pocket, grabbing the antigenic peptide from the HIV surface protein.[15] In the figure, only the antibody's two variable domains are shown. A similar structural platform is used in cellular immunity by T-cell receptors (TCR), which, distinct from antibodies, recognize an antigenic peptide along with the MHC (major histocompatibility complex) molecule that presents the peptide on the infected cell surface. In this case, CDR3 loops of TCR's variable domains play a key role in antigen recognition, whereas germline-encoded CDR1 and CDR2 loops are responsible for contacting the polymorphic region of the MHC molecule, with CDR1 also taking part in peptide binding.[16,17] Fig. 5-4, *B*, illustrates a typical structure of a TCR in complex with an antigenic peptide bound to the MHC molecule. An extensive discussion on the role of these proteins in cellular immunity can be found in Chapter 19.

A number of variations on the Ig fold are found in other cell surface receptors. These Ig-like domains include the topologically similar fibronectin type III domains[18] and the domains of cadherins, which also assumes the same strand topology.[19] The fibronectin domains and cadherins lack the disulfide bridge found in the Ig domain, which demonstrates the thermodynamic robustness of the immunoglobulin fold.

Further variations are found in modular cell surface receptors, which often have a V-set Ig-like domain as their most N-terminal

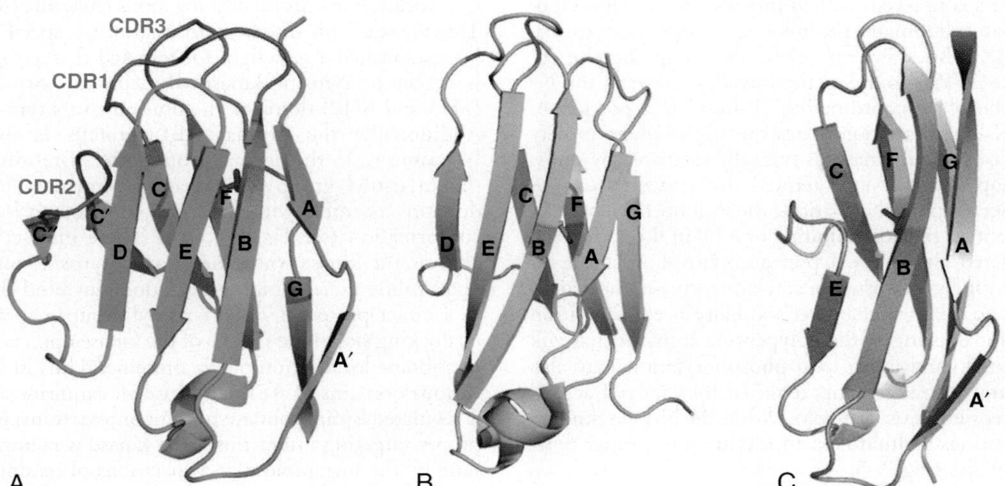

Figure 5-3 Ig DOMAIN TYPES. **A,** V-set Ig domain (PDB entry 3IDG). **B,** C-set Ig domain (3IDG). **C,** I-set Ig domain, which can be described as a truncated V-set (PDB entry 2V5M). Highlighted in orange are the disulfide bonds.

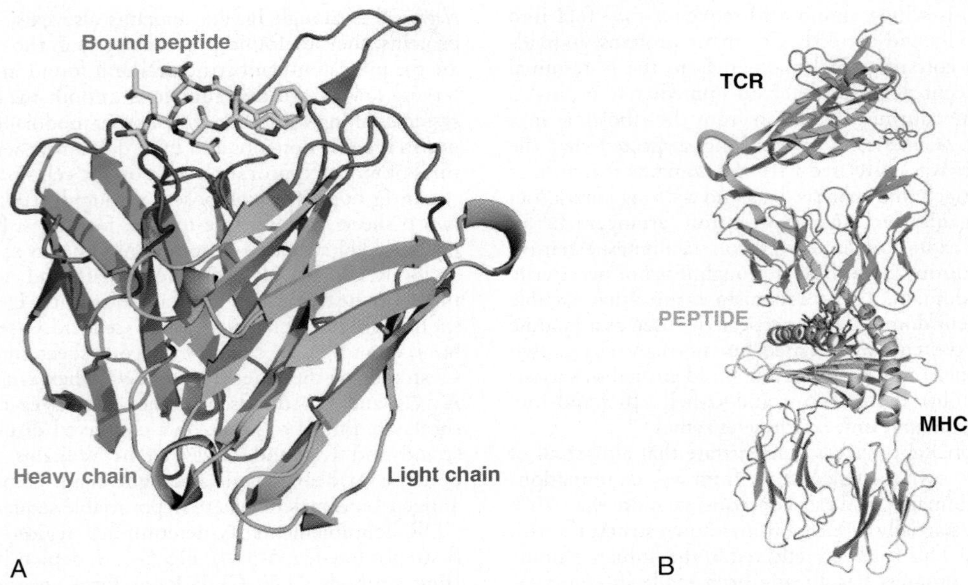

Figure 5-4 A, Complex structure of an antigenic peptide with a neutralizing antibody (3IDG). **B,** Structure of an antigenic peptide bound to the MHC molecule in complex with TCR (2CKB).

element, positioned to extend from the plasma membrane for ligand binding, serving a role analogous to antigen recognition. By contrast, I-set Ig-like domains (see Fig. 5-3, *C*) usually function as one of the building blocks lined up in tandem to present the ligand-binding V-set domain on the cell surface. This can be seen in many immune receptors such as CD2[20] and CD4.[21] There is also a large pool of receptors that are exclusively composed of I-set domains, including immune receptor ICAM1 (intercellular adhesion molecule 1),[22] neural cell adhesion molecule (NCAM),[23] and Down syndrome cell adhesion molecule (Dscam).[24,25] Thus the I-set variant is the most abundant Ig-like domain and plays a critical biologic role in cell surface receptors.

The Protein Kinase Domain

Protein kinases catalyze the transfer of a phosphate group from ATP to specific sites on target proteins. More than 500 protein kinases have been identified in the human genome. Approximately 90 of these are tyrosine kinases; the remaining protein kinases are specifically phosphorylate serine or threonine residues. Both ser/thr and tyrosine kinases share a conserved bilobed protein fold, composed of a smaller N-terminal subdomain (N-lobe) and larger C-terminal subdomain (C-lobe).[26] The active site cleft, including the site for binding the substrate ATP, is found at the interface between the N- and C-lobes. The phosphate-coordinating "P-loop" is a portion of the β sheet in the N-lobe that coordinates the triphosphate moiety of ATP. The activity of protein kinases is typically regulated by phosphorylation on a loop in the C-lobe termed the *activation loop* or *A-loop*. In the absence of phosphorylation, the A-loop may play an inhibitory role, sometimes blocking binding of ATP in the active site, or it may be disordered altogether. Upon autophosphorylation, or phosphorylation in *trans* by an upstream activating kinase, the activation loop rearranges to adopt a characteristic hairpin conformation that creates the site for docking of the polypeptide segment that will become phosphorylated. Activation loop phosphorylation may also induce other structural rearrangements required for catalytic activation, in particular a reorientation of a helix within the N-lobe (known as the C-helix) that brings a glutamic acid residue into proper position within the active site (Fig. 5-5, *A*).

Deregulated tyrosine kinases are the cause of a number of hematologic malignancies. Two general classes of tyrosine kinases can be defined: receptor and nonreceptor tyrosine kinases. Receptor tyrosine kinases are transmembrane proteins with an extracellular ligand-binding domain—often composed of Ig-like domains as described earlier, a single transmembrane domain and the cytoplasmic tyrosine kinase domain. They are generally activated by dimerization upon binding of ligands to their extracellular region, which induces autophosphorylation and activation of their catalytic domains inside the cell.[27] Chromosomal translocations that underlie a number of human leukemias fuse a tyrosine kinase domain to an oligomerization domain from an otherwise unrelated protein, often the dimerization domain of a transcription factor, to generate a constitutively dimeric, and therefore constitutively active, kinase. Examples of such oncogenic translocations include (1) the fusion of the dimerization domain of an ETS-family transcription factor to a JAK-family tyrosine kinase in the leukemogenic TEL-JAK2 fusion[28] and (2) the fusion of the oligomerization domain of nucleophosmin with the tyrosine kinase domain of ALK in the NPM-ALK fusion in anaplastic large-cell lymphoma.[29] These translocations are further described in Chapters 54 and 72, respectively.

Perhaps the best-characterized kinase translocation is the BCR-ABL fusion protein produced by the (9 : 22) chromosomal translocation in chronic myelogenous leukemia (see also Chapter 66). Treatment of this disease with imatinib, a specific inhibitor of ABL, has established a paradigm for targeted therapy in cancer.[30] ABL is a nonreceptor tyrosine kinase that contains Src homology 3 and 2 (SH3 and SH2) domains in addition to its tyrosine kinase domain. Additionally, the normal ABL protein is myristoylated at its N-terminus. In the normal protein, the N-terminal region including the myristoyl group and adjacent sequences, the SH3 and SH2 domains assemble with the kinase domain to lock it in an inactive conformation (see Fig. 5-5, *B*).[31] These interactions are released to activate the kinase when the phosphotyrosine-binding SH2 domain and proline motif–binding SH3 domains bind their cognate ligands in a target protein.[32] The myristoyl group may also be release from its docking site in the C-lobe of the kinase upon activation to promote membrane localization of the protein.[33] Thus in its normal state, the various domains of ABL comprise an exquisite signaling switch that is regulated by appropriate binding interactions; in the absence of the proper targeting interactions, the kinase is maintained in an inactive state by the intramolecular associations of its domains. In the oncogenic BCR-ABL fusion protein, this regulatory control is lost because the N-terminal regulatory region is truncated and replaced with unrelated sequences from the BCR protein.

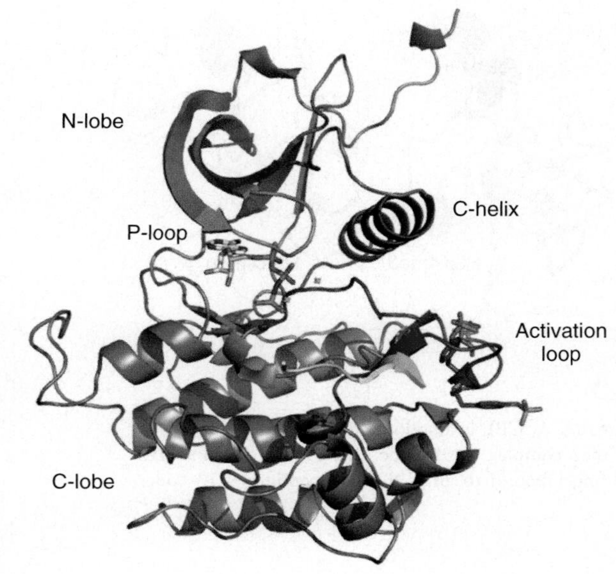

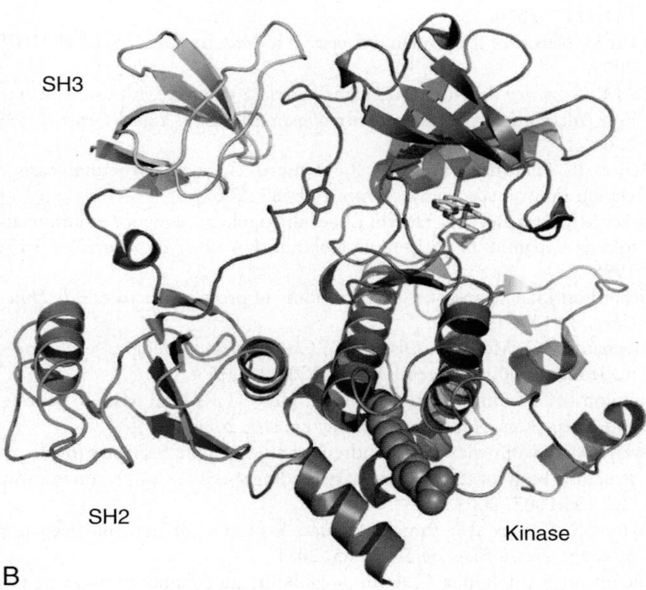

Figure 5-5 **A,** A kinase domain in complex with an ATP analog and peptide substrate (PDB entry 1IR3). The phosphate-binding loop is highlighted in *purple,* the activation loop is red, the substrate peptide is *yellow,* and the ATP analog is shown in *grey.* **B,** The autoinhibited structure of Abelson tyrosine kinase (c-ABL) in complex with the kinase inhibitor PD166326 (PDB entry 1OPK). The Src homology 3 (SH3), SH2, and kinase domains are shown in *yellow, green,* and *blue,* respectively. The SH2–kinase-domain linker and the SH3-SH2 connector are shown in *red.* The myristate is shown in *orange* spheres in the C-lobe of the kinase.

Molecular Interactions and Regulation of Gene Expression

Genomic DNA is packaged into chromatin, an ordered structure composed of the building block called the *nucleosome*. In each nucleosome, DNA of 147-bp wraps in two superhelical turns around a histone octamer formed by an H3-H4 tetramer and two H2A-H2B dimers. Nucleosome core particles are linked by short stretches of DNA bound to "linker" histones H1 and H5 to form a nucleosomal filament that is folded into higher-order structure of chromatin fiber. Epigenetic regulation of gene expression involves a host of protein complexes, conserved structural modules and molecular interactions mediated by DNA (i.e., methylation of cytosine) and histone modifications (i.e., acetylation, methylation, phosphorylation, SUMOylation, and ubiquitylation), which work together to compose a balanced and heritable system.[34] The addition, removal, and interpretation of these covalent chemical modifications to chromatin allow for an additional level of complex control of gene transcription beyond the genetic code. Early processes such as cell differentiation and embryonic development, as well as aging and environmental effects on mature organisms are all controlled by epigenetic processes.[35] Dysregulation of these mechanisms has been shown to lead to cancer and other diseases. Manipulating the occurrence of these modifications has therefore inspired new clinical therapies. Toward this goal, many studies have focused on examining functional mechanisms of the proteins that are involved in chromatin remodeling and epigenetic control of gene transcription at a molecular and structural level.

Notably, many chromatin-associated proteins contain one or more structurally conserved domains that are, for the large part, exclusive to chromatin remodeling and may recognize DNA, RNA, or covalent histone modifications. Few of these domains occur or behave alone; many are found in multiple copies or in tandem with other chromatin-associated domains in a single protein. Contrary to the earlier "histone code hypothesis," which postulated that different combinations of modifications, either in combinatorial or sequential manner, can elicit different transcriptional outcomes by recruiting proteins that recognize these modifications,[36,37] mounting evidence from recent studies show that these histone modifications work in combination and exert context-dependent functions in control of gene transcription in chromatin, thus allowing for a far more nuanced functional response.[38]

Of all the known histone modifications, lysine acetylation and methylation are best characterized thus far for their role in control of gene transcription through modification-dependent interactions with the modular domains present in chromatin and transcription-associated proteins. Lysine acetylation by HATs, such as Gcn5, PCAF, TAFII250, and CBP/p300, serves as a means to facilitate protein complex assembly through binding to the bromodomain (BrD), which until very recently (see later) was the only known acetyl-lysine binding domain.[39] Originally identified in the *Drosophila* protein brahma (hence the name),[40] the bromodomain is a conserved module found in many chromatin-associated proteins and HATs.[41] Structural analysis of the bromodomain from PCAF reveals that the bromodomain structure consists of a left-handed 4-helix bundle in which loops connecting the helices form the acetyl-lysine binding pocket (Fig. 5-6, *A*). The functions of bromodomains in gene transcription include directing remodeling complexes (such as the SWI/SNF, RSC, or PBAF complexes) to open chromatin for gene activation; recruitment of the bromodomain-containing HATs such as CBP/p300 for acetylation on histones and transcription-associating proteins; and facilitating the assembly of active transcription machinery complexes by transcription factors such as p53, NF-κB, and STAT3.

Chromodomains bind specifically to methyl-lysine sites on histones.[43,44] Various families of chromodomain have been defined (e.g., the "Royal Family" domains, which include the Tudor, PWWP, MBT [malignant brain tumor], and Agenet domains), but all contain a three-strand β-sheet capped on one side by an α-helix (see Fig. 5-6, *B*).[45] The chromodomain of heterochromatin protein 1 (HP1) binds to H3K9me3 to form transcriptionally silent heterochromatin. The importance of chromodomain/methyl-lysine binding is epitomized by polycomb repressive complexes (PRC1 and PRC2) in transcriptional gene silencing.[46]

An additional methyl-lysine targeting domain is the PHD finger, a small zinc-binding motif (50-80 amino acids) that appears in chromatin-associated proteins.[47] The conserved PHD fold consists of a two-stand antiparallel β-sheet and a C-terminal α-helix that is

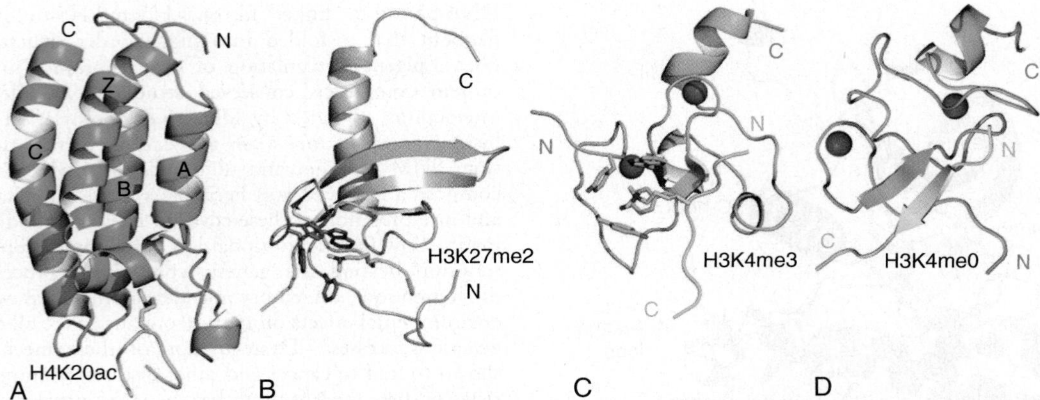

Figure 5-6 Three-dimensional structures of histone binding domains. **A,** CBP bromodomain bound to an H4K20ac peptide (PDB code: 2RNY). **B,** CBX7 chromodomain/H3K27me2 complex (PDB code: 2KMV). **C,** BPTF PHD finger/H3K4me3 complex (PDB code: 2F6J). **D,** AIRE PHD finger bound to an H3K4me0 peptide (PDB code: 2KFT).

stabilized by two zinc atoms anchored by the Cys4-His-Cys3 motif. Functional versatility of the PHD fold is underscored by the extraordinary ability of some PHD fingers to recognize histone H3 in an H3K4 methylation sensitive manner (positively or negatively), typifying it as an epigenetic "reader" module. One type of PHD finger is the human BPTF or ING2, which binds the trimethylated H3K4me3 (a mark for gene activation) in an "aromatic cage" (see Fig. 5-6, *C*).[48] Another type of PHD finger lacks this aromatic cage (e.g., AIRE or BHC80) and specifically recognizes the nonmethylated H3K4 site (a mark for gene repression) using an N-terminal aspartic acid (see Fig. 5-6, *D*).

SUGGESTED READINGS

Barreca A, Lasorsa E, Riera L, et al: Anaplastic lymphoma kinase in human cancer. *J Mol Endocrinol* 47:R11, 2011.

Bork P, Holm L, Sander C: The immunoglobulin fold. Structural classification, sequence patterns and common core. *J Mol Biol* 242:309, 1994.

Boggon TJ, Murray J, Chappuis-Flament S, et al: C-cadherin ectodomain structure and implications for cell adhesion mechanisms. *Science* 296:1308, 2002.

Chothia C, Jones EY: The molecular structure of cell adhesion molecules. *Annu Rev Biochem* 66:823, 1997.

Cunningham BA, Hemperly JJ, Murray BA, et al: Neural cell adhesion molecule: Structure, immunoglobulin-like domains, cell surface modulation, and alternative RNA splicing. *Science* 236:799, 1987.

Das R, Baker D: Macromolecular modeling with rosetta. *Annu Rev Biochem* 77:363, 2008.

Druker, BJ: Translation of the Philadelphia chromosome into therapy for CML. *Blood* 112:4808, 2008.

Gilbert W: Why genes in pieces? *Nature* 271:501, 1978.

Glozak MA, Sengupta N, Zhang X, Seto E: Acetylation and deacetylation of non-histone proteins. *Gene* 363:15, 2005, doi:10.1016/j.gene.2005.09.010.

Golub TR, McLean T, Stegmaier K, et al: The TEL gene and human leukemia. *Biochim Biophys Acta* 1288:M7, 1996.

Jones EY, Davis SJ, Williams AF, et al: Crystal structure at 2.8: A resolution of a soluble form of the cell adhesion molecule CD2. *Nature* 360:232, 1992.

Kolb VA, Makeyev EV, Spirin AS: Co-translational folding of an eukaryotic multidomain protein in a prokaryotic translation system. *J Biol Chem* 275:16597, 2000.

Lander ES, et al: Initial sequencing and analysis of the human genome. *Nature* 409:860, 2001, doi:10.1038/35057062.

Lemmon MA, Schlessinger J: Cell signaling by receptor tyrosine kinases. *Cell* 141:1117, 2010.

Levitt M: Nature of the protein universe. *Proc Natl Acad Sci U S A* 106:11079, 2009.

Liu M, Grigoriev A: Protein domains correlate strongly with exons in multiple eukaryotic genomes–evidence of exon shuffling? *Trends Genet* 20:399, 2004.

Meijers R, Puettmann-Holgado R, Skiniotis G, et al: Structural basis of Dscam isoform specificity. *Nature* 449:487, 2007.

Parker MJ, Dempsey CE, Hosszu LL, et al: Topology, sequence evolution and folding dynamics of an immunoglobulin domain. *Nat Struct Biol* 5:194, 1998.

Richardson JS: The anatomy and taxonomy of protein structure. *Adv Protein Chem* 34:167, 1981.

Rossmann MG, Moras D, Olsen KW: Chemical and biological evolution of nucleotide-binding protein. *Nature* 250:194, 1974.

Rudolph MG, Stanfield RL, Wilson IA: How TCRs bind MHCs, peptides, and coreceptors. *Annu Rev Immunol* 24:419, 2006.

Sawaya MR, Wojtowicz WM, Andre I, et al: A double S shape provides the structural basis for the extraordinary binding specificity of Dscam isoforms. *Cell* 134:1007, 2008.

Taylor SS, Kornev AP: Protein kinases: Evolution of dynamic regulatory proteins. *Trends Biochem Sci* 36:65, 2011.

Teichmann SA, Chothia C: Immunoglobulin superfamily proteins in *Caenorhabditis elegans. J Mol Biol* 296:1367, 2000.

Walsh C: *Posttranslational modification of proteins: Expanding nature's inventory.* Englewood, Colo, 2006, Roberts and Co. Publishers.

Wang JH, Reinherz EL: Structural basis of T cell recognition of peptides bound to MHC molecules. *Mol Immunol* 38:1039, 2002.

Williams AF, Davis SJ, He Q, Barclay AN: Structural diversity in domains of the immunoglobulin superfamily. *Cold Spring Harb Symp Quant Biol* 54:Pt 2, 637, 1989.

Wu H, Kwong PD, Hendrickson WA: Dimeric association and segmental variability in the structure of human CD4. *Nature* 387:527, 1997.

Yang Y, Jun CD, Liu JH, et al: Structural basis for dimerization of ICAM-1 on the cell surface. *Molecular Cell* 14:269, 2004.

Zwick MB, Delgado K, Binley FM, et al: The long third complementarity-determining region of the heavy chain is important in the activity of the broadly neutralizing anti-human immunodeficiency virus type 1 antibody 2F5. *J Virol* 78:3155, 2004.

For complete list of references log on to www.expertconsult.com.

CHAPTER 6

SIGNALING TRANSDUCTION AND REGULATION OF CELL METABOLISM

Pere Puigserver

Hematopoiesis is a cellular process in which self-renewing stem progenitor cells differentiate into mature blood cells, which carry out specific biologic functions. These functions include oxygen delivery, clot formation, and defense of the host from infection. Homeostasis of the whole hematopoietic system in vivo requires a tight control of systems and networks governing proliferation, cell fate, cell death, differentiation, cell–cell interaction, and migration. An imbalance in or dysregulation of these processes results in pathologic alterations. For example, uncontrolled cell proliferation is a signature of leukemias, and defective lymphocyte differentiation can lead to immunodeficiency. A better understanding at the molecular level of these biologic events will help to identify new therapeutic targets for the design of better drugs to treat hematologic diseases.

Because of the diversity in cellular types and their respective, specific biologic functions, hematopoietic cells respond to a broad array of extrinsic and intrinsic signals transduced through molecular (signaling and metabolic) pathways. It is therefore important to recognize that these molecular pathways serve to ultimately define a specific functional response in a given cell type. These regulatory signals (Table 6-1) can be general, such as growth factors (e.g., insulin growth factor [IGF], fibroblast growth factor [FGF]) or amino acids that control proliferation, or highly specific, such as the antigen signaling response in immune cells or 2,3-diphosphoglycerate in erythrocytes. Importantly, the action of these signals—as well as their integration inside the cell—is needed to accomplish a specific cellular task (either a physiologic or cellular fate decision). Moreover, as discussed later in this chapter, these signals also serve to tightly control metabolic pathways in hematopoietic cells, such as anaerobic glycolysis for energy generation in red blood cells (RBCs).

Extrinsic cellular signals, often polypeptides, are recognized by plasma membrane receptors that trigger a phosphorylation cascade (using tyrosine or serine or threonine residues) that propagates through the cytoplasm and cellular organelles, including the nucleus. Thus, the sequential activation of this cascade occurs in a temporal and spatial manner to define the specific biologic response. In general, there are two types of signals (Fig. 6-1): (1) signals that transduce immediate or short-term biologic outputs without changes in gene expression and (2) signals that transduce medium- and long-term biologic outputs with changes in gene expression. In the first case, for example, chemoattractants induce the PI3K and Cdc42 pathways to rapidly establish neutrophil polarity. One example in the second case is the signaling transduced through frizzled receptors and the transcription factor T-cell specific transcription factor (TCF-1) necessary for T-cell development. In both cases, the signals transduced are amplified through a series of physical interactions and chemical modifications on proteins, the most common being phosphorylation, but others such as ubiquitination, acetylation, sumoylation also play important roles.

This chapter provides a general survey of the different key signaling and metabolic pathways that operate in hematopoietic cells. The goal is to provide the molecular basis by which signals are transduced and control fundamental cellular processes that define the different lineages of the hematopoietic system.

SIGNALING TRANSDUCTION

Hematopoietic cells use general signaling transduction pathways that are common to most cell types. The specificity in these signaling transduction pathways is often established at the beginning of the pathway's activation (e.g., by specific antigen-binding or ligand-membrane receptor complexes) (Table 6-2), and at downstream targets, including transcription of the specific genes that will serve to define a particular biologic response (see Fig. 6-1). Here, we will review these general signaling transduction pathways, illustrating some of the specific components of hematopoietic cells.

Receptor Tyrosine Kinases, Phosphoinosite-3-Kinase, and Mitogen-Activated Protein Kinase Pathways

Receptor Tyrosine Kinases

Receptor tyrosine kinases (RTKs) are enzyme-linked receptors localized at the plasma membrane containing an extracellular ligand-binding domain, a transmembrane domain, and an intracellular protein-tyrosine kinase domain. In general, the ligands for RTKs are proteins such as IGF, epidermal growth factor (EGF), platelet-derived growth factor (PDGF), and FGF. Ephrins that bind to Eph receptors also form a large subset of RTK ligands. The colony stimulating-factor 1 (CSF-1), which is important for macrophage function, is another example of RTK ligand. RTKs can function as monomers or multimeric subunits assembled at the plasma membrane that, upon ligand binding, cause oligomerization or conformational changes followed by tyrosine (trans)-phosphorylation in the kinase activation loop. Activation of RTKs results in phosphorylation of additional sites in the cytoplasmic part of the receptor, leading to docking of protein substrates, which initiate the intracellular signaling cascade. These substrates bind to RTKs phosphorylated tyrosines through SH2 (Src homology domain-2) or PTB (phosphotyrosine-binding) domains. Examples of these types of proteins are insulin receptor substrates and the p85 regulatory subunit of the phosphoinosite-3 kinase (PI3K). RTKs recruit, assemble, and phosphorylate different proteins, including adaptors and enzymes.

There are mechanisms to terminate the ligand-induced RTK activity through cellular processes, including receptor-mediated endocytosis or through a family of regulated protein–tyrosine phosphatases (PTPs), some of which are transmembrane and have extracellular domains, suggesting the possibility of ligand-mediated regulation. Interestingly, there is also intracellular regulation of PTPs through negative feedback loops to attenuate the signal or direct control through reactive oxygen species (ROS) (see later discussion).

Phosphatidylinositol-3-Kinase Pathway

One of the key signaling components associated with RTKs is the phosphatidylinositol-3-kinase (PI3K) signaling transduction pathway.

This pathway is also activated by cytokine receptors and G protein–coupled receptors. Among many functions of this pathway in hematopoietic cells, the interleukin-3 (IL-3)–dependent survival of these cells largely depends on the activation of the PI3K pathway. PI3K is a heterodimeric complex formed by a regulatory and a catalytic subunit. The regulatory protein subunits are encoded by isoforms (which include p85α and p85β) that contain SH3 binding domains that mediate binding to activated RTKs. This binding allows additional recruitment and activation of the PI3K catalytic subunits (p110α, p110β, and p110*). At the plasma membrane, activated PI3K phosphorylates PIP2 (phosphoinosite-2) at position 3 of the inositol to produce PIP3. In addition, Ras, a small guanosine triphosphate (GTP)–binding protein and potent oncogene, also activates PI3K. An important lipid phosphatase and tumor suppressor, phosphatase and tensin homologue (PTEN), dephosphorylates PIP3, counteracting PI3K and decreasing the intensity of the pathway. Accumulation of PIP3 at the plasma membrane recruits several pleckstrin homology domain (PHD) containing proteins, among them PDK and AKT serine/threonine kinases, which are key components in transducing the PI3K signaling. Activated AKTs target different protein substrates for initiation of a biologic response. For example, the Bad protein, phospho-Bad does not bind Bcl-2 and functions as an anti-apoptotic mechanism and promoting cell survival. Another key target of AKTs are the forkhead transcription factors FoxOs (Fig. 6-2). When phosphorylated by AKT, phospho-FoxOs are sequestered and inactive in the cytoplasm through direct binding to 14-3-3 proteins. Dephosphorylated FoxOs, on the other hand, activate gene expression associated with stress resistance and cell growth arrest. Another major component downstream of AKT is mTOR (mammalian target of rapamycin, a kinase that belongs to the phosphoinositide 3-kinase related protein kinases family), which is involved in metabolism, growth and proliferation. Akt phosphorylates TSC2 that forms a complex with TSC1 decreasing its GTPase activating protein (GAP) activity for small GTPase Rheb, as a consequence increases in GTP-Rheb activate mTORC1 (one of the mTOR complexes). Among the key downstream targets of mTOR are S6K and 4EBP1, which control

Table 6-1 Signals in the Hematopoietic System

Types of Ligands	Examples
Peptide or Protein	
Soluble	Growth factors or cytokine
ECM	Fibronectin, collagen
Cell surface bound	ICAM, Kit ligand
Small organics	Thyroid hormone
Nucleotides	
Soluble	ADP
DNA	Double-strand breaks
Lipids	Eicosanoids, LPA
Gases	H_2O_2, nitric oxide*

ADP, Adenosine diphosphate; *ECM,* extracellular matrix; *ICAM,* intercellular adhesion molecule; *LPA,* lipopolysaccharide.
*Function in hematopoietic system not well-defined.

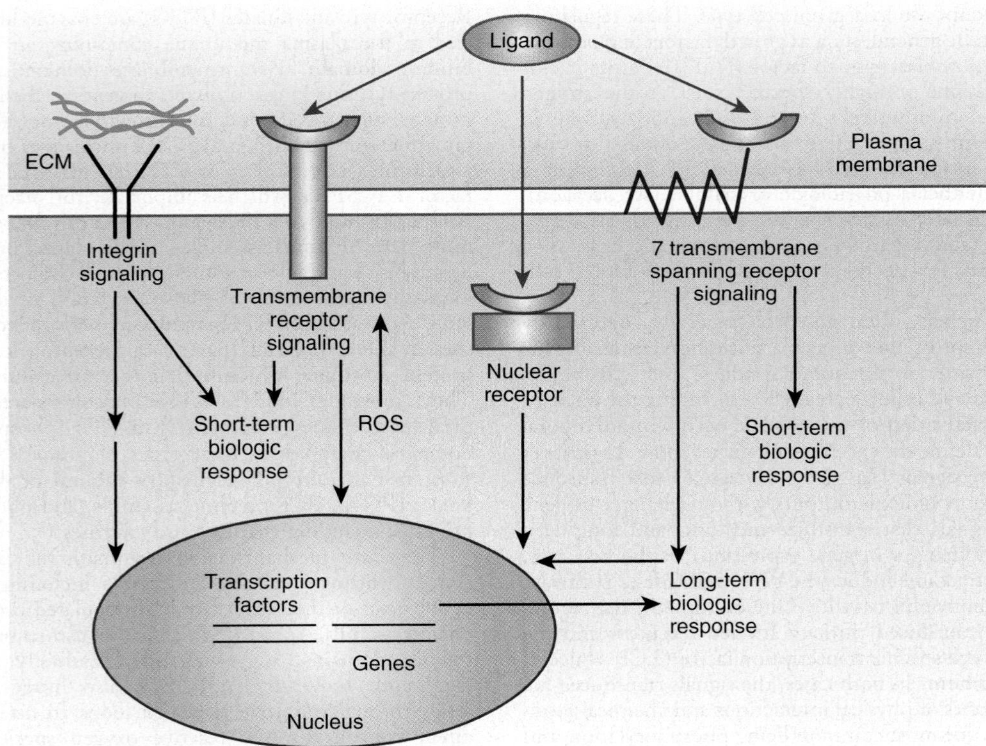

Figure 6-1 EXAMPLES OF LIGANDS AND RECEPTORS THAT TRANSDUCE BIOLOGIC RESPONSES. Signals can originate from fixed ligands (e.g., extracellular matrix [ECM]) or soluble ligands that are not membrane permeable bind to extracellular regions of transmembrane receptors. Membrane-permeable ligands bind to intracellular receptors, such as the nuclear receptor family. Signals can also originate from within the cell, such as increases in reactive oxygen species (ROS) levels. These signals cause short short-term biologic outputs without changes in gene expression or transduce medium- and long-term biologic outputs with changes in gene expression.

Table 6-2 Receptors in the Hematopoietic System

Types of Receptors	Examples	Types of Ligands
RTK	Insulin, Kit, Fms	Kit ligand, M-CSF
RSK	TGFβ receptors	Activin, BMPs, TGF-β
GPCR	Thrombin receptor, CXC, CC receptors	Thrombin chemokines
PTK-associated MIRR	Cytokine receptors BCR/TCR/FcR	Epo, interleukins, IFN peptide/MHC, Fc domains
TNF family	Fas, TNFR, CD40	Fas, TNF, CD40L
Notch	Notch	Delta-serrate-LAG-2
Frizzled family	Wnt receptors	Wnts
Toll receptors	TLR1-10	Bacterial DNA, LPS
RPTP	CD45	Unknown
Nuclear receptors	AR, RAR	Testosterone, retinoids
Adhesion receptors	Integrins	Fibronectin, collagen

AR, Androgen receptor; *BCR,* B-cell antigen receptor; *BMP,* bone morphogenetic protein; *CC,* CXC, types of chemokine receptors; *CD40L,* ligand for CD40; *Epo,* erythropoietin; *FcR,* receptors for Fc portion of antibodies; *GPCR,* G protein–coupled receptor; *LPA,* lipopolysaccharide; *M-CSF,* macrophage colony-stimulating factor; *MIRR,* multichain immune recognition receptor; *RAR,* retinoic acid receptor; *RPTP,* receptor protein-tyrosine phosphatase; *RSK,* receptor serine kinase; *RTK,* receptor tyrosine kinase; *TCR,* T-cell antigen receptor; *TGFβ,* transforming growth factor β; *TNF,* tumor necrosis factor.

protein translation. mTOR can also be activated independently of RTKs through nutrients, including branched chain amino acids. Interestingly, mTORC1 inhibitors such as rapamycin are used as immunosupressors in organ transplantation.

MAPK/ERK Pathway

Activated RTKs recruit docking proteins, such as Grb2 and SOS, that allow binding of GTP to Ras to become active and trigger a kinase cascade signaling. Ras activates RAF kinase, which in turn triggers a series of MEK kinases, which finally activate mitogen-activated protein kinase (MAPK) or extracellular signal-related kinase (ERK) . ERK phosphorylates many proteins involved in cell growth, including ribosomal S6K, which is involved in protein translation and AP-1 and c-myc transcription factors, which increase many different cell cycle and antiapoptotic related genes (see Fig. 6-2). Other MAPKs include the stress-activated kinases c-Jun-terminal kinase (JNK) and p38. Constitutive MAP kinase in hematopoietic stem cells is known to induce myeloproliferative disorders.

Transforming Growth Factor-β Pathway

The transforming growth factor-β (TGFβ) family of cytokines contains two subfamilies, the TGFβ/activin/nodal and the BMP (bone morphogenetic protein)/GDF (growth and differentiation factor)/ MIS (Müellerian inhibiting substance) subfamilies. At the plasma membrane, TGFβ ligands bind with high affinity to the ectodomain of type II receptors, which then recruit type I receptors. This forms a large ligand–receptor complex involving a ligand dimer and four receptor subunits. Upon ligand binding, the type II receptor phosphorylates multiple serine and threonine residues in the cytoplasmic GS-rich region of the type I receptor, leading to its activation. The phosphorylated TGFβ type I receptor binds to and phosphorylates Smad2 and Smad3 transcription factors, which are critical mediators of TGFβ signaling and function. Upon phosphorylation, Smad proteins translocate to the nucleus to activate gene expression through

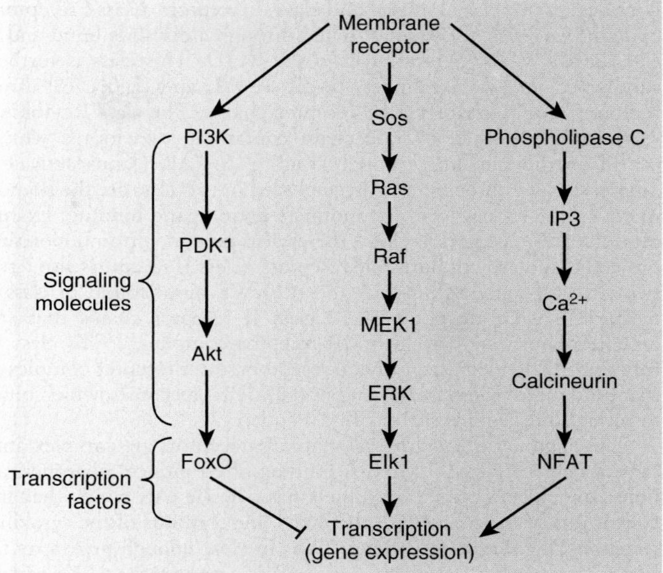

Figure 6-2 EXAMPLES OF SIGNALING AND TRANSCRIPTIONAL PATHWAYS PROGRAMMING GENE EXPRESSION. Proteins involved in gene expression are a common target of many signaling pathways, and receptors often stimulate multiple pathways that can regulate common and distinct transcription factors. In the examples shown here, production of PtdIns-3,4,5-P3 by phosphoinositide 3-kinase (PI3K) leads to the activation of the serine/threonine kinase Akt. Akt phosphorylates and inactivate FoxO transcription factors. Ras is activated by the guanine nucleotide exchange factor son of sevenless (Sos). Ras activation initiates a cascade of serine/threonine kinase activity: Ras activates Raf, Raf phosphorylates and activates MEK1, and MEK1 phosphorylates and activates extracellular signal-related kinase (ERK). Phosphorylation of the transcription factor Elk1 by ERK activates gene expression. Increased intracellular calcium is also a common signaling event. Activation of phospholipase C leads to hydrolysis of PtdIns-4,5-P2 and production of IP3. IP3 binds to its receptor, leading to intracellular calcium release and then extracellular calcium influx. Calcium activates the serine phosphatase calcineurin, which dephosphorylates nuclear factor of activated T cells (NFAT proteins), allowing them to enter the nucleus and stimulate transcription.

binding to specific DNA-binding sites. There are several mechanisms to terminate Smad activation that include proteasomal degradation and dephosphorylation. TGFβ-1 has been shown to be associated with active centers of hematopoiesis and lymphopoiesis in developing fetuses.

Signaling Through Receptors Associated With Protein-Tyrosine Kinases

Three different types of receptors and their signaling are discussed here: (1) cytokine receptors, (2) multi-chain immune recognition receptors, and (3) Integrin receptors.

Cytokine Receptors and JAK Signaling

The cytokine receptor superfamily mediates many of the central specific responses in hematopoietic cells. Ligands for these receptors include interleukins, thrombopoietin, erythropoietin, and so on. Cytokine receptors possess a conserved extracellular region (cytokine receptor homology domain [CDH]) and several structural modules, including extracellular immunoglobulin or fibronectin type III-like domains, transmembrane domain, and intracellular homology regions. Based on the divergence of the CHD, cytokine receptors are classified in two classes, class I and class II receptors. Class I receptors contain two pairs of cysteines linked through a disulfide bond and a C-terminal WSXWS motif within the CHD. This class is further subdivided into three families, IL-2R, IL-3R, and IL-6R. All three receptor families share similar receptor chains. The class I cytokine receptors are formed by one chain containing two motifs which transduce the signaling through binding to JAK (Janus activated kinase; see later discussion). Also included in this class are the homomeric receptors that form homodimers upon ligand binding. Examples of these receptors include the erythropoietin, thrombopoietin, prolactin, and growth hormone receptors. Class II receptors also have two pairs of cysteines but lack the WSXWS motif found in class I receptors. There are pools of 12 class II receptor chains that are capable of forming a total of 10 receptor complexes. This class is functionally divided into antiviral receptors (three receptor complexes that bind interferons [INFs]) and non-antiviral receptors, which bind to several interleukins such as IL-10 and IL-20.

The oligomeric structures of cytokine receptors are complex and cannot be generalized. Cytokine binding often induces oligomerization that activates protein tyrosine kinases in the JAK family that are constitutively associated with the Box 1 and 2 motifs of the cytokine receptor. Oligomerization brings JAKs in close enough proximity to transphosphorylate on Tyr residues. This activates the JAK, which results in the phosphorylation of other cytokine receptors as well as other substrate proteins. Among these substrates, the STAT (signal transducers and activators of transcription) family of transcription factors is pivotal to JAK-mediated cytokine signaling. STATs are phosphorylated on Tyr residues by JAKs upon cytokine binding to the receptor. Phospho-STATs homo- or heterodimerize and translocate to the nucleus to activate gene expression. STATs are also phosphorylated on a serine residue via MAPK, which serves to strengthen the intensity of the signal. As part of the cytokine signaling attenuation, STATs induce genes encoding for SOCS (suppressors of cytokine signaling) proteins that bind to phosphotyrosine residues of the cytokine receptor and JAK through SH2 binding domains.

Multichain Immune Recognition Receptors

This family of receptors include antigen receptors in B and T lymphocytes, activating receptors in natural killer (NK) cells, and immunoglobulin E (IgE) and Fc receptors. This class of receptors contains different integral membrane subunits that bind the ligand at the cell surface and transduce the signal. Ligand-binding induces oligomerization of receptor subunits that contain immunoreceptor tyrosine-based activation motifs (ITAMs) within their cytoplasmic domains. These domains become phosphorylated on tyrosine residues upon receptor activation. These phosphotyrosines are involved in activation of a series of protein tyrosine kinases containing SH2 domains that include Src (SFK), Syk (Syk or ZAP-70), and Tec (Btk, Itk, Rlk) that mediate immune signaling through downstream pathways that include MAPK, calcium signaling and nuclear factor kappa-B (NF-κB), among others. The precise mechanism of this activation is not completely understood, and in some cases, such as T-cell receptors, a protein tyrosine phosphatase (-CD45, which counteracts the action of SFKs) is regulated upon ligand binding. In the case of Tec kinases, additional downstream targets include enzymes such as phospholipase C γ (PLCγ).

Integrin Signaling

Integrin receptors are involved in cell adhesion, migration, survival, and growth. This signaling is central in hematopoietic cell function, such as at places of inflammation or infection, wherein integrins trigger a cascade that by which leukocytes exit the vasculature. Interestingly, these receptors signal bidirectionally through the plasma membrane in pathways referred to as *inside-out* and *outside-in signaling*. Integrins are a class of receptors that are heterodimeric type I transmembrane proteins consisting of α and β subunits. These subunits contain a large extracellular domain, a single transmembrane domain, and a short cytoplasmic tail. There are 18 α and 8 β subunits that are associated and form 24 different integrins with different affinities for ligands. Most of the ligands are extracellular membrane (ECM) proteins containing one of the two motifs, arginine–glycine–aspartate (RGD) or leucine–aspartate–valine (LDV). Examples of integrin ligands are intercellular adhesion molecule 1 (ICAM-1), which is present at the plasma membrane of antigen-presenting cells and binds to the integrin receptor LFA-1 to promote cell–cell adhesion.

Ligand binding to the extracellular domain induces clustering of integrins, allowing separation of the different subunits cytoplasmic portions forming interactions with cytoskeleton proteins involved in actin polymerization (outside-in signaling). Signals arising from the cellular interior, including phosphorylation, can also separate these cytoplasmic domains and can affect ligand binding (inside-out). Ligand binding to integrin receptors also signals to protein tyrosine kinases such as the Src family kinases (SFK) and focal adhesion kinase (Fak). This part of the signaling is not completely understood but appears to involve a domain in the β-integrin tail (NPXY motif) that binds talin, which in turn recruits paxillin that binds Fak, which once activate phosphorylates SFKs to mediate integrin response.

Tumor Necrosis Factor Receptors and Signaling

Tumor necrosis factor receptors (TNFRs) influence inflammation, innate immunity, lymphoid organization, and T-cell responses. There are approximately 19 different ligands for TNFR that mediate cellular responses through 29 TNFRs. TNFRs are a family of single membrane-spanning proteins that contain an extracellular TNF binding region and a cytoplasmic tail. As in the case of other cytokine receptors, ligand binding causes oligomerization and the formation of a mature receptor complex that is required to transduce the signal. TNFRs fall into three classes: (1) death domain (DD) containing receptors (FAS, TNFR,1 and DR3), which activate the caspase cascade via the DD-initiating extrinsic apoptotic pathway; (2) decoy receptors, which lack the cytoplasmic tail and therefore cannot transmit the signal, making these receptors ligand sequesters; and (3) TNFR-associated factor (TRAF) receptors such as TNFR2, which lack the DD recruiting TRAF proteins. In general, TRAFs are associated with either proapoptotic or survival pathways through activation of the NF-κB family of transcription factors and MAPK signaling (ERK, JNK, and p38). TRAFs activate NF-κB through ubiquitin-mediated degradation of its inhibitor IκBα, which retains NF-κB inactive in the cytoplasm. This process is initiated by phosphorylation of IκBα by IκBα kinase (IKK) complex, mainly by the IKKb catalytic subunit, and requires a regulatory subunit (also known as NEMO [NF-κB essential modulator]). Upstream of IKKs are other kinases, including NF-κB–inducing kinase (NIK) that binds to TRAFs. Nuclear activated NF-κB modulates gene expression that mediates TNF biologic responses.

Toll-like Receptors and Signaling

Toll-like receptors (TLR) play essential roles in the innate immune response. Ten TLRs have been identified and can be grouped into two classes based on their extracellular domain: (1) TLRs with leucine-reach repeats and (2) TLRs with immunoglobulin domains. The ligands for TLRs are diverse and include the different constituent components of microorganism, such as lipopolysaccharide, and heat shock proteins (which bind to TLR2 and TLR4). The host defense against organisms mainly relies on signals originated from the TIR (Toll/IL-1) intracellular domain (domain present in TLR and IL-1R). The TLR signaling pathway is similar to the one triggered by the IL-1R. Ligand-binding induces TLR multimeric receptor complexes, recruiting adaptor proteins such as MyD88, which contains a TIR domain and a DD that in turn binds to the IRAK (IL-1R-associated kinase). IRAK is activated by phosphorylation and then associates with TRAF6, leading to activation of mainly two different pathways, JNK and NF-κB, to activate the innate immune response, including release of inflammatory cytokines.

Wnt Signaling

Wnt proteins are lipid-modified, secreted proteins of approximately 400 amino acids that bind to Wnt cell surface transmembrane receptors, called frizzled (Fz), to initiate the canonical Wnt signaling transduction pathway. At the plasma membrane, binding of Wnt ligands to Fz receptors connect through direct binding to several intracellular proteins, including disheveled (Dsh), glycogen synthase kinase-3β (GSK3β), axin, and adenomatous polyposis coli (APC) inhibiting proteasomal-mediated degradation of the transcriptional protein β-catenin. This degradation is regulated through a GSK3β-mediated phosphorylation of β-catenin. As a consequence, β-catenin accumulates in the cytoplasm and translocates to the nucleus, where it interacts with transcription factors such as lymphoid enhancer-binding factor 1 (LEF-1)/TCFTCF to modulate gene expression.

Notch Signaling

Notch ligands are plasma single-pass transmembrane proteins named delta-like and jagged. Thus, cells expressing the ligands are adjacent to cells expressing the Notch receptors, which are also transmembrane proteins. Notch receptor interacts with a Notch ligand on a contacting cell; this interaction produces a Notch receptor cleavage that releases the Notch intracellular domain (NICD). NICD translocates to the nucleus, where it binds to several DNA binding proteins, including CBF1/suppressor of hairless/LAG-1 (CSL). As a result of this interaction between NICD and CSL, changes in Notch target genes occur. In contrast to the other signaling pathways discussed in this chapter that mainly function through phosphorylation, there is no amplification from the initial Notch ligand binding to the receptor. Moreover, this core pathway is modulated through auxiliary proteins that influence the response to the Notch ligand. Among these proteins are acute myeloid leukemia 1 (AML1), discoidin domain receptor family (DDR1), NECD, Notch extracellular domain, and CBF1 interacting protein.

Nuclear Hormone Receptor Superfamily

Nuclear hormones include steroid hormones (sex hormones, glucocorticoids, and mineralocorticoids), sterol hormones (vitamin D and its derivatives), thyroid hormones, and retinoids. These hormones are lipophilic and need carrier proteins to be transported in the blood. Because of this hydrophobicity, they can diffuse across the plasma membrane to reach the receptor proteins inside the cells, either in the cytoplasm or in the nucleus. These receptors are called the nuclear hormone receptor (NHR) superfamily. What distinguishes this receptor family from those discussed previously is their ability to directly bind to DNA and coordinate gene expression, which effectively makes them a form of transcription factor. NHRs contain a central DNA-binding domain, which targets the receptor to DNA sequences known as hormone response elements. In addition, the C-terminal part of the receptor contains a ligand-binding domain where the ligand or hormone binds. Upon ligand binding, nuclear hormone receptors control expression of diverse sets of genes related to the hormonal response. Based on the types of ligands that they can bind, NHRs can be grouped into four classes: (1) steroid receptors, which include receptors for glucocorticoids (GRs), mineralocorticoids (MRs), progesterone (PR), androgen (AR), and estrogen (ER); (2) RXR (retinoid X receptor) heterodimers, such as thyroid receptor (TR), retinoic acid receptor (RAR), vitamin D receptor (VDR), and peroxisome proliferator activated receptors (PPARs); (3) dimeric orphan receptors, such as COUPTF and HNF4; and (4) monomeric orphan receptors, such as NGFI. The cognate ligands for orphan receptors have yet to be identified.

G Protein–Coupled Receptor and Chemokine Signaling

GPCR Signaling

The G protein–coupled receptor (GPCR) superfamily comprises a large collection of proteins, with approximately 2000 annotated genes in the human genome (≈10% of the entire genome). GPCRs are involved in a large array of physiologic functions, including platelet aggregation and leukocyte chemotaxis. GPCRs are single polypeptides with seven-pass transmembrane domains containing both cytoplasmic and extracellular regions. Ligands for GPCRs are very diverse and include proteins or peptides, amino acids, lipids, and nucleotides that bind at the cell surface where GPCRs are localized. Despite its vast size and variety of activational ligands, the GPCR superfamily relies on three main intracellular signaling cascades for communicating receptor activation: the cAMP (cyclic adenosine monophosphate)–protein kinase A (PKA), the phosphatidylinositol–phospholipase C, and the Rho GTPase-based cascades.

G protein–coupled receptors are coupled to a heterotrimeric G protein formed from three unique subunits (α, β, and γ), which are membrane bound. The G-α subunit contains a GTPase domain, which is capable of hydrolyzing guanosine triphosphate (GTP) to guanosine diphosphate (GDP). When bound to GDP, the complex is functionally inactive, with the G-α subunit remaining tightly associated with the other subunits of the GPCR complex. Upon ligand binding to the GPCR, structural conformational changes produce release of GDP from the heterotrimeric complex, allowing GTP to bind to the G-α subunit. In this GTP-bound form, G-α subunit dissociates from G-β and G-γ subunits with which it interacts. The G-α subunit then proceeds to interact with its downstream cognate targets to affect a particular signal response, depending on the GPCR and the specific G-αsubunit isoform. Among these second-messenger effectors are the cAMP–PKA pathway, ion channels, Rho GTPase, MAPK, PI3K, and InsP3–DAG (inositol 3-phosphate–diacylglycerol) pathways. In the case of the cAMP pathway, adenylate cyclase is downstream of different GPCRs (e.g., adrenergic receptors) and is activated by GTP-bound G-α. Adenylate cyclase converts adenosine triphosphate (ATP) to cAMP, a freely diffusible second messenger molecule. A key effector of intracellular cAMP is PKA, an inactive tetrameric protein complex consisting of two regulatory and two catalytic subunits. Binding of cAMP to the regulatory subunits causes release and activation of the catalytic subunits that phosphorylate different cellular targets. Among them are the transcription factor cAMP-responsive element (CREB) and several ion channels. In addition to adenylate cyclase, there are other common effectors downstream of GPCRs, such as phospholipase C, a plasma membrane bound enzyme that cleaves phosphatidyl inositol, PIP2, in two products and messengers; inositol triphosphate (IP3); and DAG. IP3 can diffuse through the cytoplasm and bind receptors in the endoplasmic reticulum, resulting in calcium release to the cytoplasm. Importantly, calcium propagates the signaling cascade through different proteins such as calcineurin and nuclear factor of activated T cells (NFAT) transcription factors (see Fig. 6-2), which are involved in, for example, IL-2 gene expression. DAG at the plasma membrane binds and activates, in conjunction with calcium, protein kinase C (PKC), which phosphorylates other downstream targets. Rho guanine nucleotide exchange factor (RhoGEF) is also a target for some G-α subunits. Binding of the G-α subunit to Rho allosterically activates its, causing GTP to be preferentially bound. This in turn allows RhoGEFs to activate Rho kinase, which is involved in the cytoskeletal reorganization necessary for changes in cell shape and motility.

Chemokine Signaling

Chemokines mediate cell migration in immune surveillance, inflammation, and development. There are nearly 50 human chemokines divided into four families (CXC, CC, C, and CX3C) on the basis of the pattern of internal cysteine residues; thus, C stands for cysteine and X/X3 stands for one or three noncysteine amino acids. Expression of some of these chemokines is induced by inflammatory signals such as TNF-α, INF-γ, trauma, or microbial infection. There are approximately 20 signaling chemokine receptors, and they are all GPCR receptors; thus, the chemokine acts as a ligand and activation of the chemokine receptor follows the principles described above. The major downstream effectors are cAMP and calcium messengers. Interestingly, some of the chemokine receptors also bind HIV viral proteins.

REGULATION OF CELL METABOLISM

There are three important general pathways by which metabolism impact cellular function (Fig. 6-3): (1) activity of catabolic pathways that supply energy in the form of ATP, such as glycolysis or oxidative phosphorylation; (2) activity of anabolic pathways that synthesize molecules that are used for cellular growth or an specific function; and (3) generation of metabolites that control cellular intrinsic and extrinsic activities. This regulation is intimately connected to signaling transduction because most of the pathways described in the previous section directly control cellular metabolism. Here, this part of the review covers the main metabolic pathways, taking into consideration their implications in hematopoietic cells.

Glucose Metabolism

Glucose is the one of the three basic macronutrients and certain cells such RBCs, because they are devoid of mitochondria, entirely depend on glucose or other monosaccharides as an energy source. Hematopoietic cells have different types of glucose transporters (e.g., activation of T cells) that cause dramatic increases in Glut1 expression to maintain immune homeostasis. After transport into the cell, glucose is metabolized through different biochemical pathways to provide energy and building blocks for macromolecules that constitute the cell or regulatory metabolites. Glucose can be stored in cells in form of glycogen, which constitutes a rapid source of energy through its breakdown to free glucose (glycogenolysis), although this pathway is limited to certain number of hematopoietic cells. Chemotaxins (FMLP, C5ades arg, arachidonic acid) activate granulocytes to catabolize significant amounts of endogenous glycogen.

Glycolysis

Glycolysis is a series of reactions by which six-carbon glucose is converted into two three-carbon ketoacids (pyruvate). Importantly, these oxidative reactions generate energetic molecules such as ATP and NADH (nicotinamide adenine dinucleotide) and can occur in the absence of oxygen and mitochondria. In some cells such as erythrocytes, anaerobic glycolysis produces lactate, but in most cell types, pyruvate is completely oxidized to acetyl coenzyme-A and carbon dioxide by the mitochondrial pyruvate dehydrogenase complex and the tricarboxylic acid (TCA) cycle coupled to oxidative phosphorylation. In general, whereas hematopoietic stem cells are thought to largely depend on glycolysis, more differentiated cells, except for erythrocytes, use mitochondrial oxidative metabolism. Glycolytic fluxes are under intrinsically tight control through intermediate metabolites in the pathway. The most powerful control is exerted by

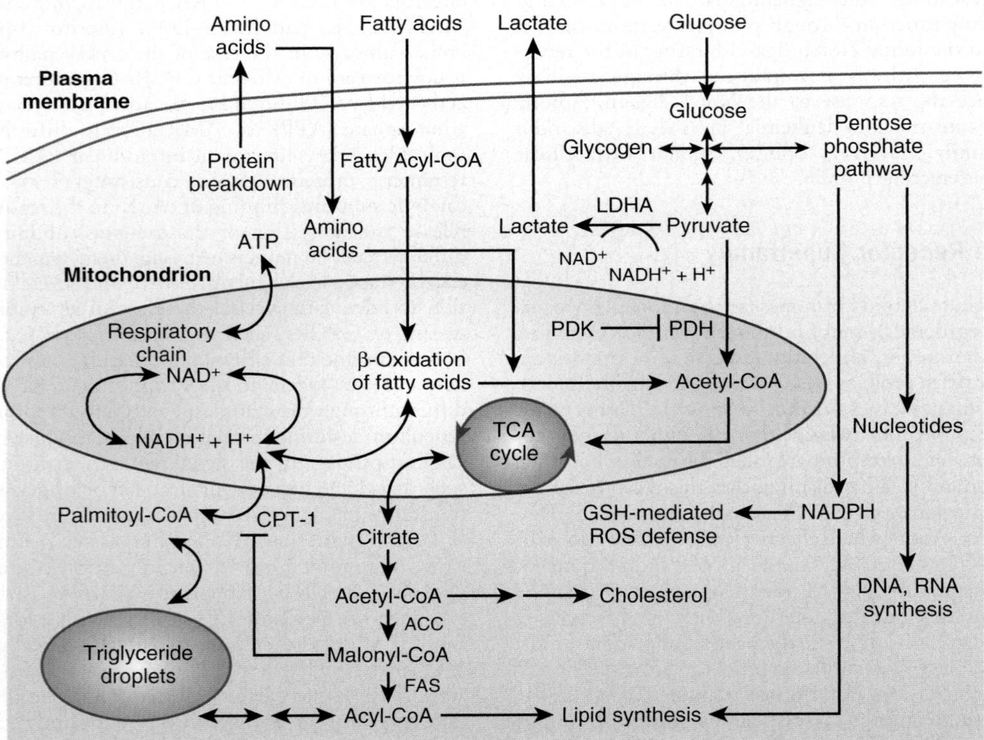

Figure 6-3 INTEGRATION OF CENTRAL METABOLIC PATHWAYS. The metabolic fluxes within anabolic and catabolic routes are controlled by different signals, including metabolite concentrations. These metabolic pathways are localized in different cellular compartments to adequately provide cellular energetic and nutrient homeostasis necessary for growth and survival. See text for further details. *ACC,* Acetyl-CoA carboxylase; *ATP,* adenosine triphosphate; *CPT-1,* carnitine palmitoyltransferase I; *FAS,* fatty acid synthase; *NAD,* nicotinamide adenine dinucleotide; *NADH,* nicotinamide adenine dinucleotide, reduced form; *PDH,* pyruvate dehydrogenase; *PDK,* pyruvate dehydrogenase kinase; *TCA,* tricarboxylic acid.

fructose 2,6-bisphosphate (F-2,6-BP), which is generated by phosphofructokinase 2. F-2,6-BP allosterically activates phosphofructokinase, providing a "feedforward" mechanism of stimulation. Activation of growth factor signaling pathways potently stimulate glycolysis at different points, including phosphorylation of phosphofructokinase 2 and pyruvate kinase. The PI3K pathway is a major signaling pathway that controls glycolysis.

Interestingly, in erythrocytes, 1,3-diphosphoglycerate can be diverted from glycolysis to synthesize 2,3-diphosphoglycerate (2,3-DPG) via the enzyme diphosphoglycerate (Rapoport-Laubering shunt). 2,3-DPG is an important metabolite that regulates oxygen binding to hemoglobin; thus, increased levels of 2,3 DPG—for example, under hypoxic conditions—allow hemoglobin to release oxygen under low partial oxygen tensions.

Pentose Phosphate Pathway

The pentose phosphate pathway (PPP) derives from glycolysis in the cytoplasm. The first enzyme in this pathway is glucose-6-phosphate dehydrogenase (G6PDH) and produces NADPH (nicotinamide adenine dinucleotide phosphate), a substrate used for lipogenesis and glutathione regeneration by glutathione reductase. The regulation of NADPH production through G6PDH is through NADPH-mediated product inhibition. The PPP is also important in generating ribose-5 phosphate, which is a precursor for nucleotide synthesis in proliferating cells. Interestingly, G6PDH deficiency leads to low levels of NADPH, which is essential for controlling reactive oxygen species through glutathione reductase. It is one of the most common erythrocyte enzymopathies, and these cells cannot prevent oxidative damage in critical molecules such as heme, causing overall irreparable damage to the cell at a much higher rate than normal, particularly in response to certain environmental triggers such as drugs and stress. The damaged erythrocytes are removed from circulation in the spleen and destroyed by macrophages at an elevated rate, leading to anemia. This enzymopathy occurs in areas with high malarial burden, partly because the mutated recessive allele confers malarial resistance. This resistance is because RBCs with low G6PDH activity, when infected with the parasite, are continuously removed from the circulation.

Tricarboxylic Acid or Krebs Cycle

A major route for pyruvate oxidation is conversion to acetyl-CoA, a reaction catalyzed by the mitochondrial pyruvate dehydrogenase enzymatic complex. Acetyl-CoA is a high-energy intermediate that can be further oxidized by the TCA cycle or used for fatty acid synthesis. The TCA cycle is initiated by the condensation of oxaloacetic acid with acetyl-CoA, forming citrate. In reactions involving decarboxylation and oxidation, CO_2 is produced, and NADH and FADH (flavin adenine dinucleotide) are produced for use in the mitochondrial respiratory chain. The flux of the TCA cycle is regulated by the levels of acetyl-CoA and oxaloacetic acid, which are entry points in the cycle, and by the availability of NAD^+ and FAD^+ substrates. The rate of oxidation through the TCA cycle depends on mitochondrial electron transport activity, which is governed in part by NADH levels. The TCA cycle also produces metabolites for biosynthetic processes (anaplerotic reactions). For example, citrate is converted to fatty acids and sterols, and succinyl CoA is an intermediate in heme and porphyrin synthesis. Aside from the bioenergetic and anaplerotic aspect of this cycle, several reactions have important clinical implications. Recently, for instance, gain-of-function mutations of isocitrate dehydrogenase 1 and 2 (IDH1 is cytoplasmic and is unrelated to the TCA cycle; IDH2 is the TCA mitochondrial form) have been found in 20% of patients with acute leukemia. In three identified mutations, the enzyme undergoes a change in its normal physiologic catalytic reaction (i.e., oxidative decarboxylation of isocitrate to produce α-ketoglutarate and CO_2 while converting NAD[P] to NAD[P]H) and instead produces 2-hydroxyglutarate, which is now considered to be an a pro-oncometabolite.

Oxidative Phosphorylation

In most cell types, oxidative phosphorylation is dominant on ATP generation. Exceptions include RBCs that lack mitochondria. Oxidative phosphorylation complexes are located at the inner mitochondrial membrane and receive high-energy electrons from NADH (produced from the oxidation of acetyl-CoA). These electrons are passed through the different oxidative phosphorylation complexes (which contain heme, copper iron-sulfur groups, and flavins as electron carriers) until they reach the final electron acceptor, molecular oxygen. As a consequence of electron transfer, protons are pumped into the mitochondrial intermembrane space, generating an electrochemical gradient used to synthesize ATP. There are five oxidative phosphorylation complexes: complex I (NADH-CoQ reductase complex), complex II (succinate–CoQ reductase complex), complex III (CoQH2–cytochrome C reductase complex), complex IV (cytochrome C oxidase complex), and complex V (ATP synthase complex). In general, hematopoietic stem cells are located in low-oxygen niches and largely depend on glycolysis instead of oxidative phosphorylation to maintain ATP levels. The differentiation process is associated with increases in mitochondria, which allow for the generation of ATP through the respiratory chain. For example, this occurs in quiescent T cells that are in a catabolic phase producing ATP mainly through oxidative phosphorylation. Upon stimulation, activated T cells shift toward an anabolic phase, relying on a high rate of glycolysis for ATP generation. Mitochondrial DNA encodes for several oxidative phosphorylation subunits and mutations in this DNA produces mitochondrial diseases. Interestingly, anemia is a symptom associated with patients having Pearson syndrome and is caused by accumulation of mutated mitochondrial DNA in sideroblasts. This suggests that hematopoietic cell–specific respiration defects can be responsible for anemia by inducing abnormalities in erythropoiesis during development.

Reactive Oxygen Species Metabolism

Reactive oxygen species (ROS) are chemically reactive small molecules with oxygen in different oxidation states, such as partially reduced oxygen ions and peroxides. The three major species are superoxide, hydrogen peroxide, and hydroxyl radicals. The major cellular sites for ROS production are the mitochondria and NADPH oxidase, a plasma membrane or phagosome-bound enzyme. Approximately 85% of cellular ROS is a subproduct of normal oxidative phosphorylation. Superoxide is the initial ROS produced in the electron transport chain and is transformed to hydrogen peroxide by the enzyme superoxide dismutase. Hydrogen peroxide is the substrate of catalase or glutathione peroxidase, which reduces it to water. Hydrogen peroxide, however, is also converted to hydroxyl radicals, the most reactive oxygen species, in a Fenton reaction with ferrous iron. NADPH oxidase catalyzes the NADPH-dependent reduction of oxygen into the superoxide anion.

Reactive oxygen species cause cellular damage through oxidation and chemical modifications of proteins, lipids, and DNA. Nuclear and mitochondrial DNA can be oxidized, producing strand breaks. Intracellular levels of ROS are regulated through different signaling transduction pathways. Growth factor–mediated signaling increases ROS levels, for instance. Conversely, ROS also affect this signaling through modulation of protein tyrosine phosphatases that contain cysteine-sensitive residues that modulate their enzymatic activity and regulate the biological responses associated with this signaling.

Reactive oxygen species are particularly deleterious to hematopoietic stem cells because of their effect on genomic stability and survival. In phagocytic cells (neutrophils, macrophages, or eosinophils), NADPH oxidase is responsible for the oxidative burst that is triggered upon phagocytosis of pathogens. Superoxide generated by NADPH oxidase is rapidly converted to other ROS, which, in cooperation with pH-sensitive proteases, are responsible for killing the microorganisms in the phagosome vacuole.

Lipid Metabolism

Fatty acids and triglycerides (storage form of fatty acids) constitute an energetic reserve in the body. Most of the cells are able to synthesize fatty acids, but essential fatty acids such as linoleic acid, α-linoleic, and arachidonic acid cannot be synthesized. Arachidonic acid is made from linoleic acid and is the precursor for prostaglandins, thromboxanes, and leukotrienes which participate in different pathways such as the inflammatory response. Drugs that block the enzyme cyclooxygenase and prostaglandin synthesis such as acetaminophen, ibuprofen, and acetylsalicylate provide pain relief. Fatty acids can directly mediate transcriptional responses acting as ligands for PPARs, a family of nuclear hormone receptors.

Fatty Acid Synthesis

In the mitochondrial matrix, acetyl-CoA is generated from pyruvate and is the precursor for fatty acid synthesis. Acetyl-CoA cannot cross the mitochondrial membrane; thus, acetyl-CoA condenses with oxaloacetate (first reaction in the TCA cycle) to form citrate and is exchanged into the cytoplasm through TCA translocases. In the cytoplasm, citrate is converted to acetyl-CoA by ATP citrate lyase. The rate-limiting reaction of fatty acid synthesis is the carboxylation of acetyl-CoA to form malonyl CoA, which is catalyzed by acetyl-CoA carboxylase (ACC). Malonyl CoA is a potent inhibitor of fatty acid oxidation. ACC is allosterically regulated by citrate to form active enzyme polymers, which are depolymerized by the end product of fatty acid synthesis: long chain fatty acids. Growth factors positively control ACC dephosphorylation. Catecholamines, on the other hand, result in the phosphorylation and inhibition of ACC via PKA. Fatty acids are synthesized in the cytoplasm by a multifunctional enzyme, fatty acid synthase (FAS). Two of these functional domains are the acyl carrier protein (ACP) and the condensing enzyme (CE). After completion of the different rounds of synthesis, the palmityl group is transferred to CoASH. In macrophages, LPS activates lipogenesis through activation of SREBP (sterol regulatory element-binding protein), a key transcriptional mediator of cholesterol and fatty acid synthesis.

Fatty Acid Oxidation

Fatty acids are "charged" before oxidation to form acyl-SCoA, a cytoplasmic reaction catalyzed by the enzyme fatty acyl-CoA synthetase. Fatty acid β-oxidation, however, occurs in the mitochondrial matrix, and charged fatty acids must first be conjugated to carnitine to cross the mitochondrial membranes. This transport is carried out by the carnitine acyltransferases I and II. These enzymes constitute a rate-limiting step for β-oxidation of fatty acids and are allosterically regulated by malonyl CoA, allowing the cell to avoid a futile cycle of fatty acid synthesis and breakdown. Inside the mitochondria, acyl-CoA undergoes a cycle of reactions removing acetyl-CoA from the main chain. This acetyl-CoA is then processed through the TCA cycle.

Cholesterol

Cholesterol is an important component of cellular membranes and is a substrate for the production of steroid hormones. Free cholesterol is tightly control in cells through synthesis, storage, and transport. Excess cholesterol in cells is secreted through reverse cholesterol transport or stored in the cytoplasm as cholesterol ester, produced by acyl-CoA: cholesterol acyltransferase located in the endoplasmic reticulum. Cholesterol is transported in plasma by lipoproteins, including chylomicrons and very low-density lipoprotein (VLDL). The main sources of cellular cholesterol for hematopoietic cells are the cholesterol-rich lipoprotein, low-density lipoprotein (LDL), and de novo synthesis from acetyl-CoA. The rate-limiting step for cholesterol synthesis is catalyzed by HMG-CoA reductase, the direct target of the cholesterol-lowering statin drugs, and converts hydroxymethylglutaryl CoA to mevalonic acid. Cellular cholesterol levels are sensed in the endoplasmic reticulum through the SREBP transcription factor, which directly controls most the enzymes in cholesterol synthesis as well as LDL transport. Excess of LDL becomes oxidized and taken by macrophages, a main cause of atherosclerosis. The SREBP pathway is also important for T-cell activation under antigenic challenge because its activation favors cholesterol synthesis and transport, which is used for membrane biogenesis and cell proliferation in the activated T cell.

Amino Acid Metabolism

The major sources of amino acids are from the diet or protein breakdown. Non-essential amino acids are synthesized from carbon skeletons using different metabolic pathways. Amino acids conjugated to tRNA are used in protein synthesis; however, in excess, they can be used for energy production. In addition, amino acids are necessary for the synthesis of other compounds. For example, tryptophan catabolism constitutes a route for de novo NAD^+ synthesis in a pathway that is important in leukocytes for the replenishment of NAD^+ levels after oxidative stress. Interestingly, different metabolites derived from tryptophan catabolism via kynurenine pathway play a role in immune tolerance. Plasma amino acids are transported in cells against a concentration gradient. Amino acid transporters are specific for neutral (small and larger), basic, and acidic amino acids. Depending on the cell type and specific state—growth, hypoxia, or fasting—intracellular amino acids are used in anabolic or catabolic pathways.

Most of the regulation of amino acid metabolism is achieved through substrate fluxes affecting specific enzyme kinetics. However, two major regulatory pathways involve amino acid–sensing mechanisms and metabolic control: (1) GCN2 (general control nonrepressed 2) is a protein kinase that senses amino acid deficiency through direct binding to uncharged tRNA. GCN2 controls the transcription factor ATF4 affecting different enzymes of amino acid metabolism. (2) mTOR (mammalian target of rapamycin) is a protein kinase activated in response to increased amino acid concentrations (particularly, branch chain amino acids). mTOR controls many aspects involved in protein synthesis, inhibition of protein degradation, and amino acid biosynthetic enzymes. The high asparagine requirement of certain acute lymphoblastic leukemias has resulted in the use of asparaginase to deplete circulating levels of asparagine. Limited amounts of asparagine result in activation of GCN2 in the leukemic cells and reduce their proliferation and viability rates.

Biosynthesis of the Non-Essential Amino Acids

Non-essential amino acids are synthesized by most of the cells, including hematopoietic lineages. Non-essential amino acids are mainly synthesized from glucose (alanine, arginine [from the urea cycle in hepatic cells], asparagine, aspartate, cysteine (from methionine) glutamate, glutamine, glycine, proline, and serine), except tyrosine, which is synthesized from phenylalanine. The rest of the nine amino acids are essential, and the body needs to obtain them from the diet. Serine, glycine, and cysteine are synthesized from glycolytic intermediates. Serine synthesis has recently been found to be increased and necessary in stem cells. For some hematopoietic cells, the synthesis of cysteine and glycine is of elevated importance because of their use in the synthesis of the tripeptide glutathione. Aspartate and asparagines are synthesized by transamination of oxalacetate by glutamate and amide transfer from glutamine respectively. Glutamate, glutamine, proline, and arginine are formed from the TCA cycle intermediate α-ketoglutarate.

Amino Acid Catabolism

Two central reactions in amino acid catabolism are the generation of ammonia through transamination (catalyzed by amino transferases) and oxidative deamination (catalyzed by glutamate dehydrogenase) in which the α-amino group of the different amino acids is transferred to α-ketoglutarate to form glutamate, which undergoes the release of free NH_3. Free ammonium is added to glutamate to generate glutamine that is then exported into circulation to the liver and enter the urea cycle. The urea cycle only occurs in the liver and has two purposes: (1) to get rid of free ammonium and (2) to supply arginine. Interestingly, one of the enzymes of the urea cycle, arginase (which converts arginine to ornithine), is expressed in immune cells. Myeloid cell arginase depletes arginine and suppresses T-cell immune response and is an important mechanism of inflammation-associated with immunosuppression. Arginase is viewed as a promising strategy in the treatment of cancer and autoimmunity. Arginine is also essential for the differentiation and proliferation of erythrocytes.

Nucleotide Metabolism

Nucleotides are involved in a diverse array of cellular functions, including (1) energy metabolism (ATP, NAD^+, $NADP^+$, and FAD^+ and their corresponding reduced forms); (2) units of nucleic acids (NTPs are substrates for RNA and DNA polymerases); (3) physiologic mediators such as adenosine, ADP (which is critical in platelet aggregation), cAMP and cGMP (second messenger molecules), and GTP (which participates in signal transduction via GTP binding proteins).

Most of the regulatory pathways that are associated with nucleotide synthesis and degradation are strictly controlled by regulatory components of the cell cycle machinery. The amount of intracellular nucleotides has to reach certain levels for the cell to proceed through the S phase checkpoint. In addition, several of the key cell cycle regulators, including the c-myc oncogene (which is translocated in certain myelomas), directly increase the expression of most of the key enzymes associated with nucleotide synthesis.

Nucleotide Synthesis

There are two pathways for the synthesis of nucleotides, salvage and de novo. The salvage pathway uses free bases by a reaction with phosphoribosyl pyrophosphate (PRPP) and generation of nucleotides. De novo pathways synthesize pyrimidines and purine nucleotides from amino acids, carbon dioxide, folate derivatives, and PRPP. Importantly, both salvage and de novo pathways depend on PRPP, which is produced from ATP and ribose-5-phosphate (generated in the pentose phosphate pathway) by PRPP synthetase, an enzyme that is inhibited by metabolic markers of low energy AMP, ADP, and GDP to avoid nucleotide synthesis in these conditions. In general, PRPP levels are low in postmitotic cells but high in proliferating cells. Folate is essential in nucleotide biosynthesis, and lack of folate in the diet can lead to anemias caused by inhibition of proliferation of RBC precursors.

Nucleotide Degradation

Nucleotidases and nucleosidases initially participate in purine nucleotide degradation. For example, adenosine is deaminated to produce inosine that, after ribose is removed, generates hypoxanthine, which is used by xanthine oxidase to form uric acid. Immune cells have potent nucleotide salvage pathways, and a lack of adenosine deaminase causes a severe combined immune deficiency (SCID) syndrome. SCID is associated with a large accumulation of dATP in immune cells, which, through a negative feedback mechanism on ribonucleotide reductase, blocks production of dNTPs and results in a failure to replicate DNA.

FUTURE DIRECTIONS

This short review summarizes the central signaling and metabolic pathways that play a pivotal role in all the processes executed by hematopoietic cellular systems. In normal physiologic conditions, these pathways are regulated and operating to achieve homeostatic cellular functions in healthy individuals. In pathologic conditions, however, dysregulation or failure of these pathways leads to diseases of lymphohematopoietic tissues. To a large extent, the main components and regulatory circuitries of these pathways have been elucidated, but the challenge for the future is to fully integrate them and identify therapeutic targets that will enable the development of effective treatments for these diseases.

SUGGESTED READINGS

Abram CL, Lowell CA: The ins and outs of leukocyte integrin signaling. *Annu Rev Immunol* 27:339, 2009.

Aggarwal BB: Signaling pathways of the TNF superfamily: A double-edged sword. *Nat Rev Immunol* 3:745, 2003.

Bolanos JP, Almeida A, Moncada S: Glycolysis: A bioenergetic or a survival pathway? *Trends Biochem Sci* 35:145, 2010.

Brown MS, Goldstein JL: The SREBP pathway: Regulation of cholesterol metabolism by proteolysis of a membrane-bound transcription factor. *Cell* 89:331, 1997.

Chan DI, Vogel HJ: Current understanding of fatty acid biosynthesis and the acyl carrier protein. *Biochem J* 430:1, 2010.

Engelman JA, Luo J, Cantley LC: The evolution of phosphatidylinositol 3-kinases as regulators of growth and metabolism. *Nat Rev Genet* 7:606, 2006.

Evans DR, Guy HI: Mammalian pyrimidine biosynthesis: Fresh insights biosynthesis: Fresh insights into an ancient pathway. *J Biol Chem* 279:33035, 2004.

Fritsche K: Fatty acids as modulators of the immune response. *Ann Rev Nutr* 26:45, 2006.

Gordon MD, Nusse R: Wnt signaling: Multiple pathways, multiple receptors, and multiple transcription factors. *J Biol Chem* 281:22429, 2006.

Hamanaka RB, Chandel NS: Mitochondrial reactive oxygen species regulate cellular signaling and dictate biological outcomes. *Trends Biochem Sci* 35:505, 2010.

Hurlbut GD, Kankel MW, Lake RJ, et al: Crossing paths with Notch in the hyper-network. *Curr Opin Cell Biol* 19:166, 2007.

Kim C, Ye F, Ginsberg MH: Regulation of Integrin activation. *Annu Rev Cell Dev Biol* 27:321, 2011.

Kolch W: Coordinating ERK/MAPK signaling through scaffolds and inhibitors. *Nat Rev Mol Cell Biol* 6:827, 2005.

Lemmon MA, Schlessinger J: Cell signaling by receptor tyrosine kinases. *Cell* 141:1117, 2010.

Levine AJ, Puzio-Kuter AM: The control of the metabolic switch in cancer by oncogenes and tumor suppressor genes. *Science* 330:1340, 2010.

Lunt SY, Vander-Heiden MG: Aerobic glycolysis: Meeting the metabolic requirements of cell proliferation. *Annu Rev Cell Dev Biol* 27:441, 2011.

Mangelsdorf DJ, Thummel C, Beato M, et al: The nuclear receptor superfamily: The second decade. *Cell* 83:835, 1995.

Mitin N, Rossman KL, Der CJ: Signaling interplay in Ras superfamily function. *Curr Biol* 15:R563, 2005.

Munder M: Arginase: An emerging player in the mammalian immune system. *Br J Pharmacol* 15:638, 2009.

Norlund P, Reichard P: Ribonucleotide reductases. *Ann Rev Biochem* 75:681, 2006.

Owen OE, Kalhan SC, Hanson RW: The key role of anaplerosis and cataplerosis for citric acid cycle function. *J Biol Chem* 277:30409, 2002.

Saggerson D: Malonyl-CoA, a key signaling molecule in mammalian cells. *Annu Rev Nutr* 28:253, 2008.

Shi Y, Massague J: Mechanisms of TGF-beta signaling from cell membrane to the nucleus. *Cell* 113:685, 2003.

Sigalov A: Multi-chain immune recognition receptors: Spatial organization and signal transduction. *Semin Immunol* 17:51, 2005.

Takeda K, Kaisho T, Akira S: Toll-like receptors. *Annu Rev Immunol* 21:335, 2003.

Wallace DC, Fan W, Procaccio V: Mitochondrial energetics and therapeutics. *Annu Rev Pathol* 5:297, 2010.

Waters C, Pyne S, Pyne NJ: The role of G-protein coupled receptors and associated proteins in receptor tyrosine kinase signal transduction. *Semin Cell Dev Biol* 15:309, 2004.

Watowich SS, Wu H, Socolovsky M, et al: Cytokine receptor signal transduction and the control of hematopoietic cell development. *Annu Rev Cell Dev Biol* 12:91, 1996.

Watts TH: TNF/TNFR family members in costimulation of T cell responses. *Annu Rev Immunol* 23:23, 2005.

Zoncu R, Efeyan A, Sabatini DM: mTOR: From growth signal integration to cancer, diabetes and ageing. *Nat Rev Mol Cell Biol* 12:21, 2011.

CHAPTER 7

PHARMACOGENOMICS AND HEMATOLOGIC DISEASES

Leo Kager and William E. Evans

The fundamental hypothesis pursued in genetics is that heritable genetic variation (i.e., genotypes or haplotypes) translates into inherited phenotypes (e.g., disease risk, drug response). On the basis of this hypothesis, the aim of medical genetics and pharmacogenomics is to understand the myriad associations between individual genotypes and specific phenotypes of disease or drug response, with the ultimate goal of better defining the risk for, or outcome of, diseases and the response to specific medications. Many seminal discoveries in medical genetics were made in the course of investigating hematologic disorders, as exemplified by the fact that the most prevalent monogenic disorders, the hemoglobinopathies, affect approximately 7% of the world's population. Pharmacogenomics also has a long tradition in hematology; one of the first documented clinical observations of inherited differences in drug effects was the relationship between hemolysis after antimalarial therapy and the inherited glucose-6-phosphate dehydrogenase activity in erythrocytes.[1]

In the pregenomic era, efforts concentrated on mapping highly penetrant monogenic (Mendelian) loci, for both specific diseases and drug-metabolizing pathways that influence the effects of medications. Since the completion of the first draft of the human genome sequence, genome-wide approaches are being increasingly used to define markers for polygenic loci in complex diseases, identify genetic factors that modify the phenotype of a monogenic disease, and elucidate the interplay of genes encoding proteins involved in multiple pathways of drug metabolism, disposition, and effects.[2] This chapter provides a brief overview of pharmacogenomics, using selected examples to illustrate its impact on the treatment of hematologic diseases.

VARIATION IN THE HUMAN GENOME

The genome-wide systematic identification of heritable (i.e., germline) and acquired (i.e., somatic) variants and the functional analysis of genes, their variants, and related products (i.e., proteins) are revolutionizing the study of disease, the development of new medications, and the optimization of drug therapy. Genomics increasingly enable clinicians to make reliable assessments of a person's risk for acquiring a particular disease, to identify drug targets, and to explain interindividual differences in the effectiveness and toxicity of medications.[3]

The Human Genome Project and subsequent projects such as the International HapMap Project and the 1000 Genomes Project have unveiled many types of variations within the 3 billion base pairs of the human haploid genome (Table 7-1); the spectrum ranges from single–base-pair differences to large chromosome events. Variations encompass single-nucleotide polymorphisms (SNPs) and structural variants (SVs, or genomic rearrangements that affect >50 bp of sequence). Comparisons among human genomes showed that they differ more as a consequence of structural variation than as a result of single nucleotide variation. For practical purposes, the term *sequence variation* is mainly used herein. *Polymorphisms* are defined as common variations in the DNA sequence, that is, typically, although somewhat arbitrarily, as the least common allele having a frequency of 1% or more in the population.

SINGLE-NUCLEOTIDE POLYMORPHISMS

The most common and important inherited sequence variations are SNPs, positions in the genome where individuals have inherited a different nucleotide, and it is now estimated that several million SNPs exist in humans. Many efforts are under way to catalog these variants, because a comprehensive SNP catalog offers the possibility to pinpoint important variants in which nucleotide changes alter the function or expression of a gene that influences diseases or response to pharmacologic treatment. The main public database is dbSNP, and the increase in the number of SNPs (currently about 20 million) is driven largely by the International HapMap Project and the 1000 Genomes Project (see Table 7-1).[3]

SINGLE-NUCLEOTIDE POLYMORPHISMS AND PHENOTYPES

SNPs are present in exons, introns, promoters, enhancers, and intergenic regions. To elucidate the relationship between SNPs and phenotypes of interest, initial efforts have concentrated mainly on SNPs that are likely to alter the function or expression of a gene. However, only a small portion of the identified SNPs lie within coding regions, and only about half of those SNPs cause amino acid changes in expressed proteins. SNPs that cause amino acid changes are referred to as *nonsynonymous SNPs* (nsSNPs). nsSNPs are the main sequence variants underlying most of the highly penetrant inherited monogenic diseases currently known, such as hemoglobinopathies. The likelihood that an nsSNP will result in disease or functional change in drug metabolism depends on the localization and nature of the amino acid change within the encoded protein; software algorithms have been developed to "predict" whether a certain amino acid change is likely to have a major or minor effect on protein function.

Although it is intuitively obvious that amino acid substitutions have the potential to change the function of a protein, gene expression also can be affected by SNPs positioned in regulatory sequences or intronic regions. For example, a "silent" or synonymous SNP has been identified that affects protein folding and function of an important drug transporter, namely ATP-binding cassette transporter ABCB1 (or P-glycoprotein), and this variant has the potential to influence the pharmacology of drugs that are substrates for P-glycoprotein.[4]

As the knowledge of the topology of the genome has evolved, a new class of noncoding RNAs has emerged called micro-RNAs (miRNAs). miRNAs are small (19- to 22-nucleotide-long), single-stranded RNA molecules that can influence cellular mRNA levels or impair translation after binding to miRNA binding sites at the target gene's 3′ untranslated region. SNPs in miRNA binding sites have the potential to alter binding and function of miRNAs. Indeed, a so-called miRSNP, which is defined as a functional SNP that can interfere with micro-RNA (miRNA) function, had been identified to affect the expression of the antifolate target dihydrofolate reductase (DHFR), thereby influencing antifolate pharmacodynamics.[5]

Collectively, these examples demonstrate that SNPs in functionally different genomic regions can influence drug disposition and response.

HAPLOTYPES, LINKAGE DISEQUILIBRIUM, AND HAPMAP

Combinations of SNPs are commonly inherited together in the same region of DNA, forming haplotypes. Genome-wide haplotypes can be constructed by linkage disequilibrium (LD) analysis. LD analysis is a statistical measure of the extent to which particular alleles or SNPs at two loci are associated with each other in the population, and LD occurs when haplotype combinations of alleles or SNPs at different loci occur more frequently than would be expected from random association. SNPs and alleles of interest are presumably inherited together if they are physically close to each other (usually <50 kilobases [kb]), producing strong LD. Therefore SNPs that are in LD with a disease phenotype or response-to-drug phenotype can *mark* the position on the chromosome where a susceptibility gene is located, even though the SNP itself may not be the cause of the phenotype.

By studying millions of SNPs in hundreds of individuals from geographically diverse populations, the international HapMap consortium created genome-wide maps of haplotypes. The HapMap project has revealed a block-like structure of LD, as well as the existence of areas of low or high recombination rate, and this has helped to identify so-called tagging (tag) SNPs. Such tag SNPs can be used to predict with high probability the alleles at other co-segregating "tagged" SNPs, and the number of identified tag SNPs considerably varies among ethnic groups. Of note, recent investigations have demonstrated that common SNPs are also in LD with other common variants in the human genome (i.e., structural variants).[3]

STRUCTURAL GENOMIC VARIANTS

Along with point mutations, SVs have been identified to be the primary sources of variation in the human genome; SVs include insertions, deletions, inversions, mobile element transpositions, duplications, and translocations of DNA segments that are >50 bp or larger. Unbalanced SVs that change the number of base pairs in comparison with a reference genome are defined as copy number variants (CNVs).[6] Many efforts focus on the identification, validation, and mapping of these variants, and the Database of Genomic Variants (dbVAR) currently contains data on more than 66,000 CNVs, 950 inversions, and 34,000 InDels (insertions and deletions; 100 bp to 1 kb) (see Table 7-1). CNVs are found in a wide spectrum of genomic regions; therefore many pharmacologically relevant genes can be affected by these variants. Indeed, CNVs have been described to influence activity of some of the most important drug-metabolizing enzymes, such as cytochrome P450 enzymes and glutathione S-transferases.

SOMATIC GENOMIC VARIANTS

Genomic instability is a "hallmark of cancer cells." Nonrandom genetic abnormalities, including aneuploidy (gains and losses of whole chromosomes) and structural rearrangements that often result in the expression of chimeric fusion genes (e.g., ETV6-RUNX1, BCR-ABL), can be found in the majority of hematologic malignancies. These acquired (somatic) genomic variations can differ significantly from inherited (germline) genomic variations and can, for example, create allele-specific copy number differences between normal host cells and cancer cells. Such differences can have pharmacologically relevant consequences. Indeed, it was shown that the cellular acquisition of additional chromosomes in leukemia cells—for example, the gain of additional chromosomes 21 in hyperdiploid acute lymphoblastic leukemia (ALL) (ALL blast cells with more than 50 chromosomes)—can cause discordance between germline genotypes and leukemia cell phenotypes, which are important when these discordant genotypes/phenotypes influence the disposition of antileukemic agents.[7] Moreover, somatic deletions of genes encoding proteins that regulate the stability of the DNA mismatch repair enzyme MSH2 have been identified in approximately 11% of children with newly diagnosed ALL. These deletions in ALL cells have been shown to cause DNA mismatch repair deficiency and increased resistance to thiopurines, representing a novel genomic mechanism by which leukemia cells can acquire MSH2 deficiency with numerous downstream consequences.[8]

Table 7-1 Relevant Web Sites in the Context of Pharmacogenomics and Hematology

Topic	Web site Address
GENOMIC VARIANTS	
Human Genome Project	http://www.genome.gov/
International HapMap Project	http://www.hapmap.org/
The 1000 Genomes Project	http://www.1000genomes.org/
dbSNP Database	http://www.ncbi.nlm.nih.gov/SNP/
Database of Genomic Variants	http://projects.tcag.ca
The Encyclopedia of DNA Elements (ENCODE)	http://www.genome.gov/encode
PHARMACOGENOMICS	
Pharmacogenomics Knowledge Base	http://pharmgkb.org
U.S. Food and Drug Administration—Pharmacogenomic Biomarkers	http://www.fda.gov/drugs/scienceresearch/researchareas/pharmacogenetics/ucm083378.htm
Connectivity map	http://www.broad.mit.edu/cmap/
Cytochrome P450 Homepage	http://drnelson.uthsc.edu/CytochromeP450.html
Human CYP Allele Nomenclature Committee	http://www.cypalleles.ki.se/
Warfarin Dosing	http://www.warfarindosing.org
Therapeutically Applicable Research to Generate Effective Treatments	http://target.cancer.gov/
Pediatric Cancer Genome Project	http://www.pediatriccancergenomeproject.org/site/

CATALOGUES OF GENOMIC VARIANTS, GENOTYPING PLATFORMS, AND GENOME-WIDE ASSOCIATION STUDIES

Cataloguing the pattern of genome variation in diverse populations is fundamental in understanding areas of human phenotypic diversity such as interindividual and interethnic differences in drug responses; increasingly detailed maps of human genomic variation are provided in public databases (see Table 7-1). Information from these maps has been used to design high-throughput genotyping platforms (e.g., SNP chips that can now assay up to 2 million variants simultaneously), thereby providing tools to interrogate the relationship between genetic variation across the human genome and important phenotypes such as disease or response to medications in a relatively unbiased (agnostic) fashion.[3] Current SNP catalogues encompass roughly up to 95% of variants that are found in at least 10% of humans, and these catalogues have been used in genome-wide association studies to pinpoint genes important to diseases and drug responses.

GENETIC VARIATIONS INFLUENCING DRUG RESPONSE: PHARMACOGENETICS–PHARMACOGENOMICS

Until relatively recently, genetics has played little or no role in finding the right drug and the optimal dosage for individual patients. Mostly empiric approaches are used to select drug therapy, despite the fact that there is great heterogeneity in the way people respond to medications, in terms of both host toxicity and treatment efficacy. Unfortunately, for almost all medications, interindividual differences are the rule, not the exception, and these differences result from the interplay of many variables, including genetics and environment. Variables influencing drug response include pathogenesis and severity of the underlying disease being treated; drug interactions; the patient's age (i.e., developmental pharmacology), sex, nutritional status, and renal and liver function; presence of concomitant illnesses; and other medications. In addition to these clinical variables, increasing evidence points to a substantial inherited component of interindividual differences in drug response. Clinical observations of inherited differences in drug effects (based on family studies and twin studies) were first documented in the 1950s, and the concept of pharmacogenetics was defined initially in 1959 by Friedrich Vogel as "the study of the role of genetics in drug response." The number of recognized clinically important pharmacogenetic traits grew steadily in the 1970s; the elucidation of the molecular genetics underlying these traits began in the late 1980s and 1990s, and their translation to molecular diagnostics is well under way in the 2000s. Of interest, during the last 2 decades, the field of pharmacogenetics was rediscovered by the pharmaceutical industry and by a broader spectrum of researchers in academia. This rediscovery has been driven in large part by the Human Genome Project, and by the recognition that inheritance can play a major role in determining drug effects. The study of pharmacogenetics began with the analysis of genetic variations in drug-metabolizing enzymes and how those variations translate into inherited differences in drug effects. More recently, the field has incorporated genome-wide approaches to identify networks of genes that govern the clinical response to drug therapy (i.e., pharmacogenomics). The terms *pharmacogenetics* and *pharmacogenomics*, however, are synonymous for all practical purposes.

Overall, pharmacogenomics can be viewed as a broad strategy to establish pharmacologic models by integrating information from functional genomics, high-throughput molecular analyses, and pharmacodynamics. Approaches to establish pharmacogenomic models include candidate gene analyses (which focus on the analysis of single genes or sets of functionally related genes in pathways) and genome-wide analyses. Pharmacogenomic models can be used to maximize efficacy and reduce toxicity of existing medications, as well as to identify novel therapeutic targets.

Recent comprehensive reviews on pharmacogenomics are available elsewhere.[1,2,7,9-12] Herein, clinically relevant examples are provided to illustrate how pharmacogenomics can be used to improve current drug therapy for hematologic disorders, to prevent hematologic toxicity, and to identify novel targets for developing new therapeutic approaches in hematology.

OPTIMIZATION OF DRUG THERAPY

Most drug effects are determined by the interplay of several gene products that influence the pharmacokinetics and pharmacodynamics of medications. Pharmacokinetics is the study of the absorption, distribution, metabolism, and excretion (ADME) of drugs. Pharmacodynamics is the relationship between the pharmacokinetic properties of drugs and their pharmacologic effects, either desired or adverse. The ultimate goal of pharmacogenomics in this context is to elucidate the inherited determinants for drug disposition and response to select medications and dosages on the basis of each patient's inherited ability to metabolize, eliminate, and respond to specific drugs. A model of how polygenic variables can determine drug response is illustrated in Fig. 7-1.

GENETIC VARIATIONS THAT INFLUENCE DRUG DISPOSITION

Drug Metabolism

Metabolism often involves reactions that make lipophilic drugs more water soluble and thus more easily excreted. Pathways of drug metabolism are classified as either phase I reactions (which catalyze changes of functional moieties by oxidation, reduction, or hydrolysis) or phase II conjugation reactions (which conjugate functional moieties by acetylation, glucuronidation, sulfation, or methylation). The process of metabolic reactions that inactivate drugs or prodrugs is referred to as *catabolism*. Drug metabolism also includes reactions that convert prodrugs into therapeutically active compounds; these processes are referred to as *anabolism*. Additionally, metabolic reactions can form toxic metabolites.

Essentially all genes encoding drug-metabolizing enzymes (there are more than 30 families of enzymes in humans) exhibit genetic variations, many of which translate into functional changes in the proteins encoded. Inheritance of genes containing sequence variations that alter the function of enzymes encoded or CNVs that alter the expression of functionally relevant genes can influence drug disposition and ultimately determine drug effects (either desired or adverse), if those enzymes are involved in crucial pathways of elimination or activation of the administered medication. Numerous variant enzymes have been characterized; the focus here is on two extensively investigated examples: thiopurine S-methyltransferase (TPMT) and cytochrome P450 (CYP) enzymes.

Thiopurine S-Methyltransferase and Thiopurines

The genetic sequence variation of TPMT provides one of the best and most thoroughly studied examples of a clinically important pharmacogenetic trait. Studies have established that variations within the TPMT gene locus are a major determinant of the effects of thiopurines, which are widely prescribed structural analogs of purines. The prodrugs mercaptopurine (MP) and thioguanine are among the agents that constitute the "backbone" of treatment for childhood ALL.

The hydrophilic thiopurines are transported into target cells, where they undergo extensive metabolism. Metabolic reactions include anabolism (via a series of enzymes, the first of which is hypoxanthine phosphoribosyltransferase) to form active cytotoxic thioguanine nucleotides (TGNs) and catabolism, including phase I (oxidation via xanthine oxidase) and phase II (S-methylation via TPMT) reactions. In hematopoietic cells such as leukemic blasts, xanthine oxidase is low or absent; therefore degradation via TPMT is essentially the only path by which thiopurines can be inactivated. TPMT activity determines how much of these intracellular prodrugs are inactivated to methylated metabolites and how much remains available for activation to TGNs. TGNs are responsible for the efficacy in leukemic blasts and toxicity in normal hematopoietic tissues.[13]

TPMT activity is inherited as an autosomal codominant trait. Approximately 90% to 95% of persons are homozygous for the wild-type (wt) allele (TPMT*1) and have "normal" enzyme activity; approximately 5% to 10% are heterozygous for the polymorphism and have intermediate levels of enzyme activity; 1 in 300 persons inherit two variant (nonfunctional) TPMT alleles that cause TPMT deficiency. TPMT activity typically is measured in erythrocytes, because this measure correlates with the activity in other normal and neoplastic tissues.[13]

Three nsSNPs account for more than 95% of the clinically relevant TPMT variant alleles, namely, TPMT*2 (238G>C, rs1800462), TPMT*3C (719A>G, rs1800460), and TPMT*3A (contains two nsSNPs: 460G>A, rs1142345; and 719A>G, rs1800460). Other TPMT variants are very rare. These sequence variants of TPMT do not affect its messenger RNA (mRNA) expression; rather, they render the variant protein more susceptible to

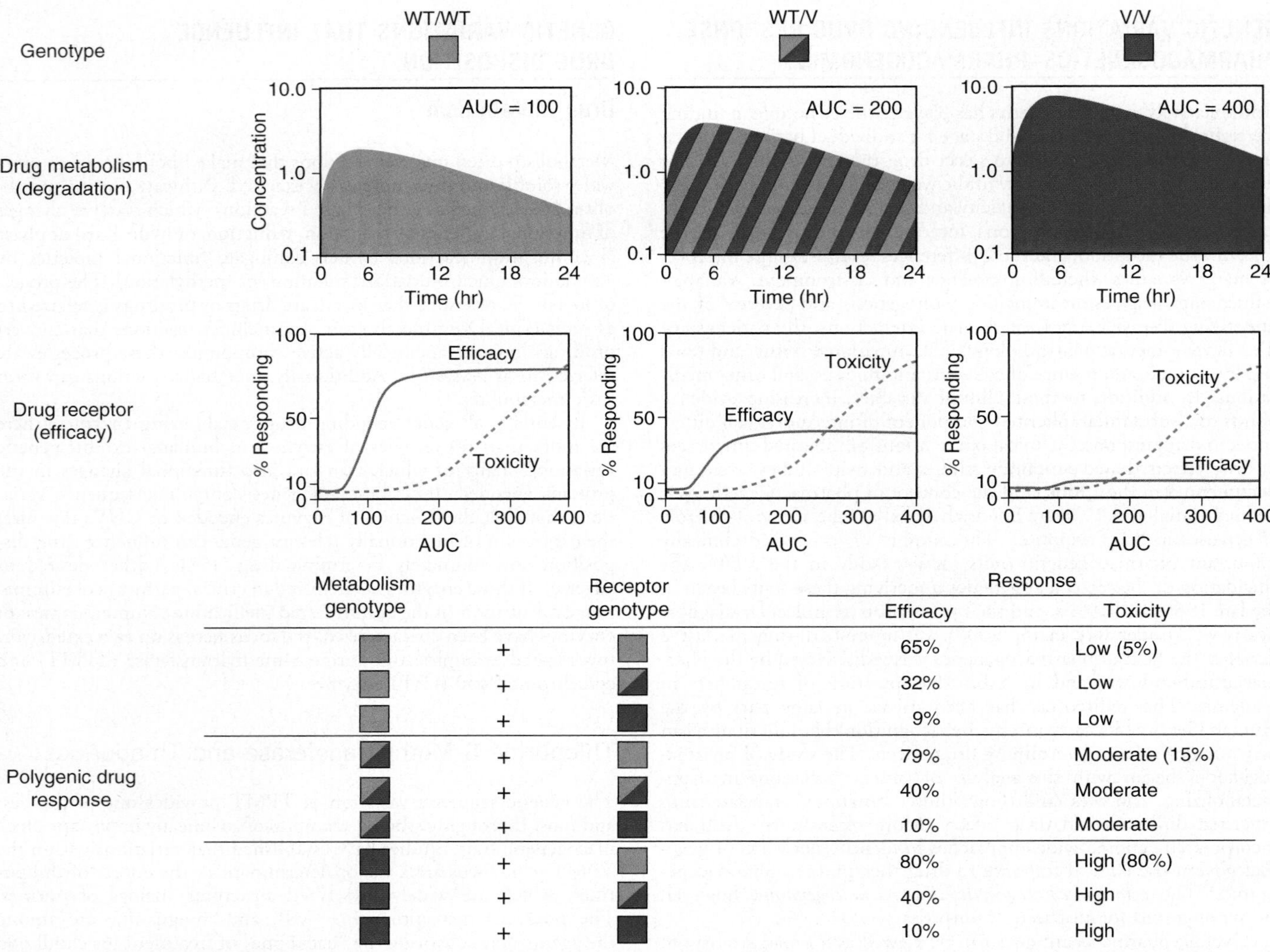

Figure 7-1 POLYGENIC DETERMINANTS OF DRUG RESPONSE. The potential effects of two genetic variants are illustrated. One genetic variant involves a drug-metabolizing enzyme *(top)*, and the second involves a drug receptor *(middle)*. Differences in drug clearance (or the area under the plasma concentration–time curve [AUC]) and receptor sensitivity are depicted in patients who are either homozygous for the wild-type allele *(WT/WT)* or heterozygous for one wild-type and one variant *(V)* allele *(WT/V)*, or have two variant alleles *(V/V)* for the two genetic variants. At the *bottom* are shown the nine potential combinations of drug metabolism, drug-receptor genotypes, and the corresponding drug-response phenotypes, which were calculated with data from the top. The therapeutic indexes (efficacy-to-toxicity ratios) ranged from 13 (65%:5%) to 0.125 (10%:80%). *(Modified with permission from Evans WE, McLeod HL: Pharmacogenomics: Drug disposition, drug targets, and side effects.* N Engl J Med *348:538, 2003. Copyright 2003 Massachusetts Medical Society. All rights reserved.)*

proteasome-mediated degradation, and persons inheriting these alleles have a low (in heterozygotes) or undetectable (in the *variant/variant* genotype) level of TPMT activity. Subsequent studies demonstrated that the TPMT*3A variant disrupts the structure of the encoded enzyme, resulting in misfolding, protein aggregation (so-called aggresome formation) and rapid degradation of TPMT monomers and aggregates. The prevalence of TPMT allelic variants differs among ethnic populations. TPMT*3A is the most common variant in Caucasians, and TPMT*3C is the predominant variant in Asians and Africans.[13]

Childhood ALL studies have shown that essentially all homozygous TPMT-deficient patients experience dose-limiting hematotoxicity, and some experience life-threatening hematotoxicity if given conventional doses of thiopurines. Patients with only one nonfunctional TPMT allele have intermediate tolerance to thioguanine therapy. Although many patients with only one nonfunctional TPMT allele can tolerate thiopurine therapy at essentially full doses, they are at higher risk for dose-limiting hematotoxicity than are those patients who have a wild-type TPMT genotype (e.g., 35% cumulative risk versus 7% cumulative risk in a study of ALL patients).[7]

In TPMT-deficient patients, the thiopurine dose must be reduced to 10% to 15% of the conventional doses (i.e., an 85% to 90% dose reduction of the conventional 75 mg/m^2/day MP dose) to avoid severe hematopoietic toxicity. At these very low thiopurine doses, TPMT-deficient patients have erythrocyte TGN levels that are comparable to (or greater than) those of "wild-type patients" given full doses. Although many patients with one nonfunctional TPMT allele can tolerate essentially full doses of thiopurines (dependent on starting dose and other therapy), thiopurine-intolerant heterozygous patients typically require a 50% dose reduction. Multivariate analyses have demonstrated that children who have ALL and at least one *TPMT*-variant allele tend to respond well to MP therapy (i.e., 75 mg/m^2/day) and may experience better leukemia control than is obtained in those who have two wild-type TPMT alleles. However, it was observed in the same patient group (St. Jude Children's Research Hospital Total protocols) that those who are treated with thiopurines and have deficient TPMT activity (i.e., all patients except those with a *1/*1 genotype) are at an increased risk for epipodophyllotoxin-related acute myeloid leukemia (therapy-related AML, or t-AML) or irradiation-induced brain tumors.[7] Similar results (with similar MP doses) have been reported from the Scandinavian Nordic Society of Pediatric Haematology and Oncology (NOPHO) ALL-92 trial, with a significantly higher risk for t-AML or myelodysplastic syndrome in patients with lower TPMT activity compared with control patients. Of note, in children treated on Berlin–Frankfurt–Muenster (BFM) protocols with lower starting doses of MP in continuation therapy (i.e., 50 mg/m^2/day versus 75 mg/m^2/day) and lower doses of MP in combination with high-dose methotrexate infusions (i.e., 25 mg/m^2/day versus 75 mg/m^2/day), TPMT genotype was not associated with a higher risk for secondary malignant disease.

On the other hand, another study from the BFM ALL group raised the question whether dose escalation in patients with wild-type TPMT would yield greater efficacy in protocols that routinely use lower MP doses (i.e., 50 to 60 mg/m^2/day). In this investigation, the TPMT genotype was linked to early ALL treatment response, which was determined by measuring minimal residual disease after induction and consolidation treatment that included a 4-week cycle of MP 60 mg/m^2/day. Children with the *1/*1 genotype were found to have a 2.9-fold higher risk for positive minimal residual disease than did TPMT-heterozygous patients. In contrast to TPMT-heterozygous patients treated at St. Jude Children's Research Hospital (who received more prolonged MP treatment with modestly higher MP doses of 75 mg/m^2/day), for whom the risk for dose-limiting hematopoietic toxicity is increased, TPMT-heterozygous patients treated with lower MP doses according to BFM protocols did not have higher toxicity compared with TPMT wild-type patients. Furthermore, in the St. Jude Total protocols, prospective MP dose adjustments (i.e., reduced doses in heterozygotes) were associated with less toxicity without compromise in treatment efficacy.[7]

Of note, in children treated with combination chemotherapy for ALL in whom MP dose was adjusted according to TPMT genotypes, a sequence variant in inosine triphosphate pyrophosphatase (ITPA, another enzyme involved in purine metabolism) was identified as a significant determinant of MP metabolism and of severe febrile neutropenia, illustrating that when treatment is adjusted for the most penetrant (strongest) genetic polymorphism, less penetrant polymorphisms can emerge as clinically important.[14]

More than 98% concordance exists between TPMT genotype and phenotype, and genotyping is very reliable (90% sensitivity, 99% specificity) in identifying patients who have inherited one or two nonfunctional alleles. In 2004 the U.S. Food and Drug Administration (FDA) prompted additions to the label for MP providing TPMT testing and dosage recommendations for TPMT-deficient patients. Evidence suggests that TPMT genotyping before initiation of MP treatment can be cost effective in children with ALL. By using the TPMT genotype to individualize thiopurine therapy, clinicians can now diagnose inherited differences in drug response, thereby preventing serious toxicities. Guidelines for TPMT genotype and thiopurine dosing are available from the Clinical Pharmacogenetics Implementation Consortium (CPIC); these guidelines are periodically updated at the Pharmacogenomics Knowledge Base (PharmGKB)[15] (also see Table 7-1, box on Relevance to Clinical Hematology, and Fig. 7-2).

Relevance to Clinical Hematology

Mercaptopurine Dosage Adjustment Based on TPMT Genotypes in Acute Lymphoblastic Leukemia

Mercaptopurine (MP) is a mainstay of treatment of childhood acute lymphoblastic leukemia (ALL). However, conventional doses of this prodrug can induce severe hematotoxicity in patients who have impaired thiopurine metabolism in hematopoietic tissues owing to less-stable thiopurine S-methyltransferase (TPMT) enzyme variants. The three major variant alleles (TPMT*2, TPMT*3C, and TPMT*3A) encoding the variant proteins can quickly be determined by commercially available Clinical Laboratories Improvement Act–certified molecular diagnostics or in special laboratories (e.g., Prometheus Labs, San Diego, Calif) using samples obtained from peripheral blood before MP therapy. In patients with two nonfunctional alleles (1 out of 300), MP dosage must be reduced to 10% to 15% of conventional 75 mg/m^2/day dosages. Patients with one variant allele (5% to 10% of the population) can tolerate MP at full dosage; however, in intolerant patients, a dose reduction of 50% often is required.[15] For more details, refer to this chapter's text discussion.

Cytochrome P450 Enzymes

The cytochrome P450 (CYP) superfamily is a system of phase I enzymes involved in the metabolism of endogenous substances (e.g., steroids, arachidonic acid, vitamin D_3) and exogenous compounds (e.g., drugs, environmental chemicals, pollutants). In humans, the CYP enzymes are encoded by more than 57 genes, and the majority of genes are polymorphic. Updated information regarding the nomenclature and properties of the variant alleles with links to the dbSNP database is available at the human CYP allele Web site (see Table 7-1). On the basis of the composition of CYP variant alleles, individuals have been categorized into four major phenotypes: poor metabolizers (PM, having two loss-of-function alleles), intermediate metabolizers (IM, being deficient in one allele), extensive metabolizers (EM, having two copies of functional alleles), and ultrarapid metabolizers (UM, having three or more functional gene copies, or two increased-activity alleles, or one functional allele plus one increased activity allele).

Different populations of metabolizers have been linked to variants in the coding region of CYP genes, SNPs in intronic regions, which alter CYP gene mRNA expression, CNVs (e.g., gene deletions, gene duplications) of CYP genes, or differences in the methylation at CpG islands in promoter and 5′ regions, which alter expression of CYP genes.[16]

Many pharmacologically relevant variants in CYP genes have been identified. The focus here is on the variants in CYP2C9 and CYP2C19. These CYP enzymes strongly influence the metabolism of two extensively prescribed medications: warfarin and clopidogrel.

CYP2C19 and Clopidogrel

Platelets play a crucial role in thrombosis and the development of acute coronary syndromes (ACS) because a platelet-rich thrombus forms at the site of the ruptured atherosclerotic plaque. Thus inhibition of platelet function is an effective strategy in the treatment and prevention of thrombosis of arteriosclerotic origin, especially after percutaneous coronary interventions (PCI). Main classes of antiplatelet agents for clinical use include aspirin, the thienopyridines (clopidogrel and prasugrel), the nonthienopyridine $P2Y_{12}$ receptor antagonists (ticagrelor), and intravenous GPIIb/IIIa antagonists.

Clopidogrel is an orally administered antiplatelet prodrug, and dual antiplatelet treatment with aspirin and clopidogrel is currently (2011) the guideline-approved standard of care in patients with ACS and PCI with stenting. According to the American Heart Association, approximately 470,000 persons in the United States will have a recurrent heart attack annually; therefore it is not surprising that clopidogrel was reported to be amongst the best-selling drugs in the world in 2009. However, about 20% of patients have been reported to be "resistant" to clopidogrel treatment.

Intestinal absorption of clopidogrel is diminished via the P-glycoprotein transporter (encoded by the polymorphic ABCB1 gene); once absorbed, 85% of clopidogrel is inactivated via esterases, and only about 15% of the prodrug is available for the two-step activation via hepatic CYP enzymes. The active drug selectively and irreversibly binds to the ADP-dependent $P2Y_{12}$ receptor on thrombocytes and thereby inhibits platelet activation and aggregation for the platelets' life span, which is about 10 days.

Candidate gene investigations identified a "high-risk" pharmacokinetic profile for clopidogrel, and functional variants in the drug

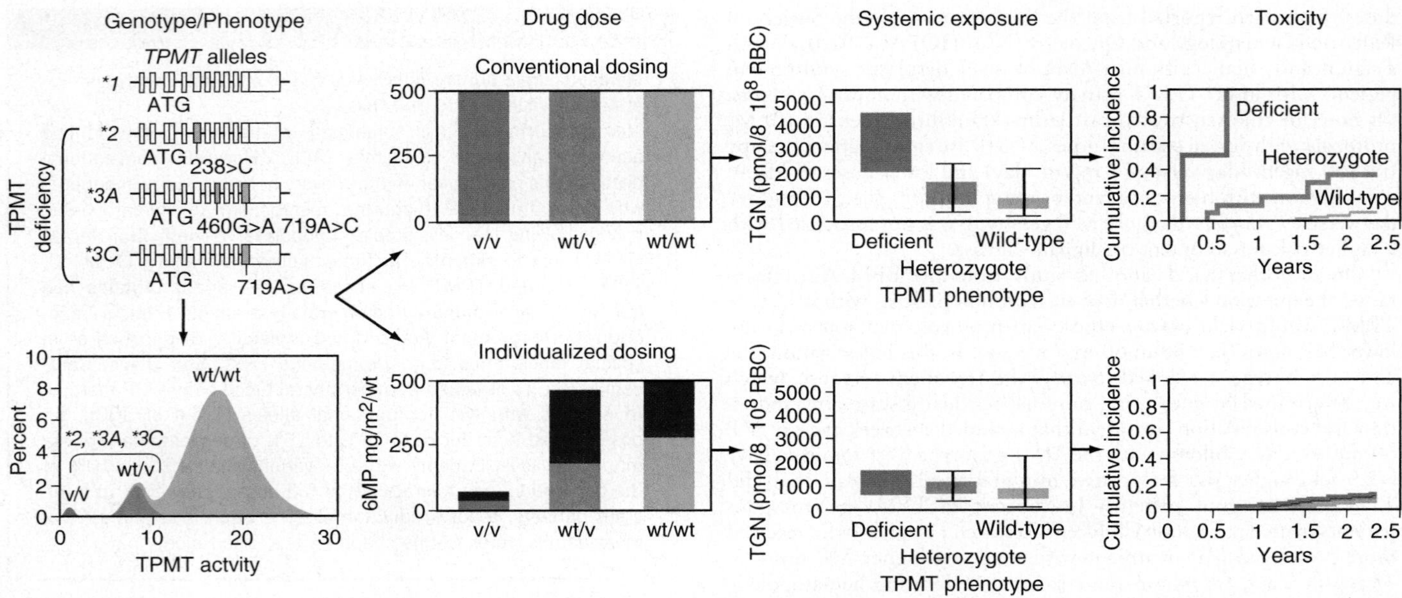

Figure 7-2 Genetic polymorphism of thiopurine methyltransferase (TMPT) and its role in determining toxicity to thiopurine medications. Under "Genotype/Phenotype" *(far left)* are depicted the predominant *TPMT* mutant alleles that cause autosomal codominant inheritance of TPMT activity in humans. As shown in the graphs under "Drug Dose," "Systemic Exposure," and "Toxicity," when uniform (conventional) dosages of thiopurine medications (e.g., azathioprine, mercaptopurine [6MP], thioguanine) are administered to all patients, TPMT-deficient patients accumulate markedly higher (10-fold) cellular concentrations of the active thioguanine nucleotides (TGN), and TPMT-heterozygous patients accumulate approximately twofold higher TGN concentrations, which translate into a significantly higher frequency of toxicity *(far right)*. As depicted in the bottom row of graphs, when genotype-specific dosages of thiopurines are administered, comparable cellular TGN concentrations are achieved, and all three TPMT phenotypes can be treated without acute toxicity. In the two graphs under "Drug Dose," the *solid* or *striped* portion of each bar depicts the mean 6MP doses that were tolerated in patients who presented with hematopoietic toxicity; the *stippled* portion depicts the mean dosage tolerated by all patients in each genotype group, not just those patients presenting with toxicity. *v,* Variant; *wt,* wild-type. *(Reproduced with permission from Evans WE: Thiopurine S-methyltransferase: A genetic polymorphism that affects a small number of drugs in a big way.* Pharmacogenetics *12:421, 2002.)*

activating cytochrome P450 enzyme CYP2C19 were shown to significantly affect drug response.[12] In a recent metaanalysis that included almost 10,000 patients, a significantly higher risk for adverse cardiovascular events was found in individuals who had reduced-function variants of CYP2C19, because these patients cannot activate the parent drug to its active metabolites, as well as patients with the wild-type CYP2C19 genotype.[17] The most important poor metabolizer alleles in CYP2C19 are *2 (681G>A, rs 4244285, ≈15% in Caucasians and Africans, ≈30% in Asians) and the less frequent *3 (636G>A, rs 4986893, 2% to 9% in Asians, less than1% in Caucasians and Africans). Other CYP2C12 variant alleles (*4 to *8) that encode enzymes with low or absent activity are very rare, with allele frequencies of less than 1%.[18]

On the other hand, the CYP2C19*17 gain-of-function allele (806C>T, rs12248560, multiethnic allele frequencies from 3% to 21%) results in enhanced CYP2C19 enzyme activity and can place these ultra-metabolizing individuals at a higher risk for bleeding because of increased drug activation.[18]

In a small study including 40 patients, increased doses of clopidogrel in PM patients resulted in better antiplatelet response. However, the first large randomized controlled trial addressing this important issue was not able to confirm this, and a metaanalysis and systematic review in 2011 did not find a consistent influence of CYP2C19 genotypes on clinical efficacy of clopidogrel.[9,12,19] Potential reasons for these negative trials have been reviewed, including differences among patient groups (e.g., differences in the percentage of patients who had undergone PCIs) and differences in study designs.[9,10,12,18]

The FDA has issued a "black box" warning for clopidogrel in regard to reduced effectiveness in PM individuals carrying two defective CYP2C19 alleles, and genotyping for the important variants is widely available in the United States. Further prospective trials are underway to clarify whether clopidogrel dosing based on genetic biomarkers is clinically useful. The CPIC has recently published guidelines for CYP2C19 genotype-directed antiplatelet therapy; these guidelines are periodically updated at the Web site of the PharmGKB (see Table 7-1).[18]

Other strategies to overcome the drug resistance mechanism of clopidogrel (i.e., low functional variants of CYP2C19) focus on bypassing of the "high-risk" pharmacokinetic pathway. The third-generation thienopyridine prasugel, for example, is mainly metabolized by the less polymorphic CYP3A4 enzyme. The pharmacokinetics of the nonthienopyridine $P2Y_{12}$ inhibitor ticagrelor are not affected by CYP2C19 variants.[9,12]

CYP2C9, VKORC1, and Warfarin

In the United States, the oral vitamin K antagonist warfarin is widely used to prevent thromboembolic events in patients with chronic conditions such as atrial fibrillation, and the drug is prescribed to more than 1 million persons annually. A narrow therapeutic index with a risk for serious hemorrhage and interindividual variability in response to warfarin necessitate individualization of treatment, which has been based primarily on monitoring prothrombin time via the international normalized ratio (INR) testing.

Several candidate gene studies have demonstrated that CYP2C9 genotype influences warfarin anticoagulant dose requirements and bleeding risks. CYP2C9 is the principal CYP2C isoenzyme in the human liver, and it is involved in the oxidative metabolism of several clinically important drugs, including oral anticoagulants, phenytoin, and various nonsteroidal antiinflammatory drugs.[16]

To date, numerous polymorphic alleles (CYP2C9*1 to *35) have been identified for the known CYP2C9 gene, at least half of which are associated with diminished enzyme activity in vitro. The two most common CYP2C9 variants are CYP2C9*2 (430C>T; rs1799853, Arg144Cys) and CYP2C9*3 (1075A>C; rs1057910, Ile359Leu).

Approximately 35% of Caucasians have one or two of these variant alleles; the overall allelic frequency of CYP2C9*2 is approximately 10%, and that of CYP2C9*3 is 8%. The *2 and *3 variants are virtually nonexistent in Africans and Asians; 95% of these persons express the wild-type genotype (i.e., extensive metabolizers).

Both CYP2C9*2 and CYP2C9*3 are important in the metabolism of the anticoagulants warfarin, acenocoumarol, and phenprocoumon. The required dose of warfarin is lowest if CYP2C9*3 is present, as predicted by in vitro studies that compared the functional effects of the two variant alleles. In addition, heterozygosity for CYP2C9*2 significantly affects overall CYP2C9 activity. Warfarin is a racemic mixture of R- and S-enantiomers that differ in their patterns of metabolism and in their potency of pharmacodynamic effect. Although S-warfarin exhibits a three- to fivefold higher inhibitory effect on the target enzyme vitamin K epoxide reductase, differences in metabolism result in an approximately twofold higher plasma concentration of R-warfarin. It has therefore been suggested that S-warfarin accounts for 60% to 70% of the overall anticoagulation response and R-warfarin accounts for 30% to 40%.[20]

A number of CYP isoforms contribute to warfarin metabolism; however, 6- and 7-hydroxylation by CYP2C9 is the most important inactivation pathway of S-warfarin. Compared with the amount of S-warfarin metabolized by wild-type enzyme (encoded by the CYP2C9*1 allele), metabolism by the enzyme encoded by the CYP2C9*2 variant is reduced by approximately 30% to 50%, and the amount metabolized by the enzyme encoded by the CYP2C9*3 variant is reduced by 90%. The substantial reduction in turnover seen with the CYP2C9*3 variant may be caused by the amino acid substitution Ile359Leu within the substrate-binding site of the enzyme.

It was well established that *CYP2C9* genotype is correlated with warfarin, acenocoumarol, and phenprocoumon metabolism and dose requirement. However, because interindividual variability in the dose requirement occurred within the various CYP2C9 groups, genotyping for additional polymorphic genes that encode clotting factors, transporters, and warfarin targets was performed.

An important pharmacogenomic finding was the identification of a novel pharmacodynamic mechanism underlying warfarin resistance—the discovery of sequence variants in the warfarin target gene VKORC1, which encodes the vitamin K epoxide reductase complex 1.[20] This complex regenerates reduced vitamin K for another cycle of catalysis, which is essential for the posttranslational γ-carboxylation of vitamin K–dependent clotting factors II (prothrombin), VII, IX, and X (Fig. 7-3). The identification of common variants in VKORC1 has quickly emerged as one of the most important genetic factors determining coumarin dose requirements.

Main VKORC haplotypes include the putative ancestral haplotype VKORC1*1, the haplotype VKORC1*2 (which is more sensitive to warfarin), and the haplotypes VKORC1*3 and *4 (which are more resistant to warfarin). There are major differences in the distribution of VKOCR1 haplotypes among ethnic groups, and this may explain interethnic differences in coumarin requirement. For example, the significantly higher average warfarin requirement in Africans is in line with significantly lower occurrence of the VKORC1*2 haplotype in Africans.

Genome-wide association (GWA) studies in patients treated with warfarin and acenocoumarol showed two major signals in and around VKORC1 and CYP2C9 and identified a much weaker additional association with CYP4F2. These GWA studies indicated that any other genetic factors are of much less importance in determining warfarin dose. CYP2F4 was subsequently identified to catalyze vitamin K oxidation. Overall, the hereditary pharmacodynamic factor VKORC1 explains approximately 25% of the variance in coumarin dose requirement, the hereditary pharmacokinetic factor CYP2C9 explains about 15%, and CYP4F2 explains about 3%.[20]

The FDA has updated the label on warfarin, providing VKORC1 and CYP2C9 genotype-specific ranges of doses and suggesting that VKORC1 and CYP2C9 genotypes be taken into consideration when the drug is prescribed. Additionally, dosing algorithms are available online, including genetic and nongenetic information that can help to optimize warfarin starting dose (see Table 7-1). In comparison with a matched historic control group that started on warfarin treatment without genotyping, 900 patients who were treated with warfarin and for whom CYP2C9 and VKORC1 genotypes were available had a 28% lower risk for being hospitalized for hemorrhage.[9,10,12,20] Before this can become the standard of care, findings of trials currently underway will be important to further confirm the benefit of including safety, cost-effectiveness, and feasibility of individualized dosing regimens that include genomic biomarkers. Alternative anticoagulants are being developed; for example, the dosing of dabigatran, which acts as a direct thrombin inhibitor, is not influenced by these genetic polymorphisms, which makes this drug a potential alternative for patients in whom heredity is associated with extreme variations in warfarin effects.

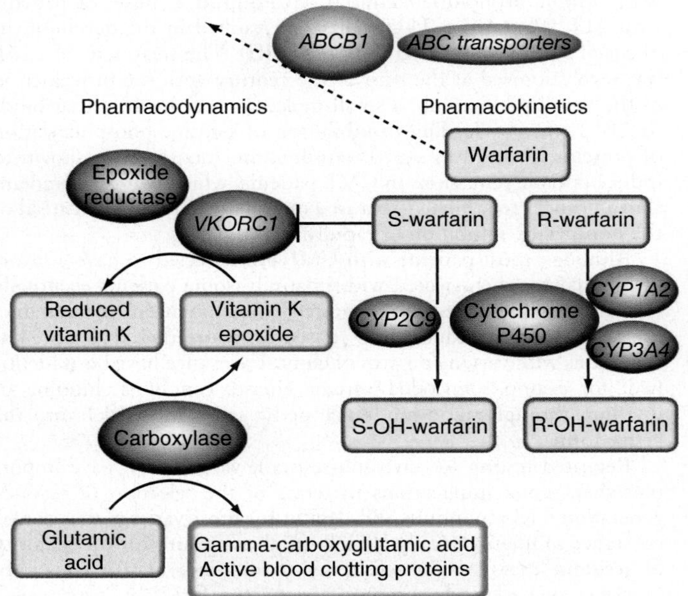

Figure 7-3 The cytochrome P450 isoenzymes CYP2C9 (to a much lesser extent CYP3A4 and CYP1A2) and vitamin K epoxide reductase complex 1 VKORC1 genotypes influence warfarin dose requirement. The racemic mixture of R- and S-warfarin (higher pharmacodynamic effect of S-warfarin) inhibits the reductase in the vitamin K cycle, impairing the synthesis of active vitamin K-dependent clotting factors in liver cells and causes bleeding. R- and S-warfarin are metabolized via hepatic CYP isoenzymes and there is evidence that warfarin is transported out of the liver into the bile via the ATP-dependent transporter (ABC transporter) ABCB1 (or P-glycoprotein).

DRUG TRANSPORTERS

Although passive diffusion accounts for tissue distribution of some drugs and metabolites, an increased emphasis is being placed on the role of membrane transporters. Membrane transporters move drugs and metabolites across the gastrointestinal tract into systemic circulation and across hepatic and renal tissue into the bile and urine for excretion. They also distribute drugs into "therapeutic sanctuaries," such as the brain and testes, and transport them into and out of sites of action, such as leukemic blast cells, cardiovascular tissue, and infectious microorganisms.

Adenosine Triphosphate-Binding Cassette Transporters

The most extensively studied transmembrane transporters are the adenosine triphosphate (ATP)-binding cassette (ABC) family of membrane transporters, which utilize ATP to move substrates across membranes. There are seven subfamilies of ABC transporters, including the P-glycoprotein MDR1, which is encoded by the multidrug-resistance gene 1 (MDR1; i.e., ABCB1), the nine multidrug-resistance proteins (MRP1 to MRP9; i.e., ABCC1 to ABCC9), and other proteins such as breast cancer-resistance protein (BCRP; i.e., ABCG2) and bile salt export protein (BSEP; i.e., ABCB11). The function, substrate specificity, and organ distribution among different transporters vary. For example, a principal function of the P-glycoprotein (MDR1) is the energy-dependent cellular efflux of numerous substrates (e.g., anticancer drugs, immunosuppressive agents, glucocorticoids, antiplatelet drugs, and bilirubin). The expression of MDR1 in many tissues, including the kidney, liver, intestinal tract, and choroid plexus, suggests that this membrane transporter plays an important role in the absorption and distribution of xenobiotics. MDR1 excretes xenobiotics and their metabolites into urine, bile, and the intestinal lumen and transports substances across the blood-brain barrier. Genetic polymorphisms of the ABC transporters are being increasingly investigated in the field of hematology.

For example, individuals who are homozygous for an ABCB1 (putative gain-of-function) coding region variant allele (3435C>T, rs1045642) have been identified as more likely to display failure of efficacy during antiplatelet therapy with clopidogrel, because in these individuals the prodrug may be stronger effluxed into the intestine. Moreover, an SNP in the ABCC4 gene (2269G>A, rs3765534) that strongly reduces the function of the encoded MRP4 protein has been identified, and this ABCC4 variant may be a locus accounting for enhanced thiopurine sensitivity among susceptible populations.

Although transporters such as MDR1 transport various substrates and thus have rather low substrate specificity, other transporters (e.g., the reduced folate carrier SLC19A1) transport only a few specific molecules and their analogs and thus have much higher substrate specificity. Functionally important polymorphisms in transporters with high substrate specificity might be of even greater interest in pharmacogenomics than those with low specificity, because the former can affect the distribution of specific drugs.

Organic Anion-Transporting Polypeptide 1B1 (OAT1B1) and Methotrexate

The solute carrier organic anion-transporter family member 1B1 gene (SLCO1B1), which is localized on chromosome 12, encodes a transporter molecule (OATP1B1) that is located primarily on the sinusoidal face of human hepatocytes. OATP1B1 mediates the hepatic uptake of many endogenous compounds (e.g., bilirubin, bile acids) and xenobiotics such as HMG-CoA reductase inhibitors (e.g., simvastatin), antibiotics (e.g., benzylpenicillin) and cytostatic drugs (e.g., irinotecan) from sinusoidal blood, resulting in their net excretion from blood (likely via biliary excretion).[21]

A common sequence variant in the coding region of SLCO1B1 (521T>C, rs4149056, protein V174A) decreases the transport activity of the encoded protein and results in markedly increased plasma concentrations of drugs that are eliminated from the blood via hepatic uptake. Using genome-wide pharmacogenomic association studies, correlations have been established between variants in SLCO1B1 and myopathy after treatment with the HMG-CoA reductase inhibitor simvastin.[21]

In the field of hematology, a GWA study (interrogating 500,568 germline SNPs) was performed in a discovery cohort of 434 children with ALL in order to identify determinants for MTX clearance, which is important for MTX clinical antileukemic effects and toxicity. Of interest, two SNPs in the SLCO1B1 gene—namely, rs11045879 and rs4149081—were identified to be associated with MTX clearance and gastrointestinal (GI) toxicity. These associations were confirmed in a validation cohort of 206 children. Of note, the rs11045879 and the rs4149081 SNPs were in complete linkage disequilibrium ($r^2 = 1$) with each other and also showed a significant correlation with the 521T>C SNP (rs4149056) ($r^2 > 0.84$), which was not included in the genome-wide genotyping. The rs4149056 was genotyped in a subset of the patients, and the 521C allele was found to be associated with a reduced clearance of MTX at the genome-wide significance level. Of note, no inherited variants in other genes were associated with MTX clearance.[22]

Whereas the mechanisms behind the observed effects remain to be determined, this investigation illustrates how GWA studies can help to identify pharmacologically relevant candidate genes.

GENETIC VARIATIONS INFLUENCING DRUG TARGETS

To exert their pharmacologic effects, most drugs interact with specific target proteins, such as receptors, enzymes, or proteins involved in signal transduction, cell cycle control, or other cellular events. Molecular studies have revealed that many of the genes encoding these drug targets exhibit genetic variations, which can alter the sensitivity of these targets to specific medications (e.g., *VKORC1* and warfarin effects). The following section illustrates this, focusing on somatic genetic variants in hematologic malignancies that alter the targets of tyrosine kinase inhibitors.

BCR-ABL and Tyrosine Kinase Inhibitors

The increased tyrosine kinase activity of the BCR-ABL1 protein—a reciprocal translocation t(9;22)(q34;q11) causes the fusion of the tyrosine kinase ABL1 to BCR, leading to constitutive activation of ABL1—is the driving oncogenic event in the majority of patients with chronic myeloid leukemia (CML) and in a subset of patients with ALL (Ph+ ALL). This realization resulted in the development of specific tyrosine kinase inhibitors (TKI). The treatment of CML was revolutionized at the turn of the century with the introduction of the first TKI imatinib, a small molecular-weight drug that binds to ABL1, thereby leading to inhibition of tyrosine phosphorylation of proteins involved in signal transduction. Imatinib was shown to induce durable remissions in CML patients, which led to a paradigm shift in cancer treatment—that is, a more targeted therapy instead of the nonspecific inhibition of rapidly dividing cells.

Although most patients with CML are expected to have a favorable outcome when treated with imatinib, some patients eventually fail on therapy as a result of acquired point mutations in the target kinase ABL1 that induce drug resistance. More than 100 different mutations with varying degrees of clinical relevance have been identified; for example, encoded variant kinases can block binding of imatinib through steric hindrance or by switching ABL1 into the active form.

Repeated testing for imatinib-resistant variants can have important therapeutic implications in terms of the selection of second-generation TKIs (nilotinib and dasatinib); most variants that confer resistance to imatinib (only a small number account for the majority of resistant cases) retain sensitivity to nilotinib and/or dasatinib. However, one relatively common variant, the T315I or "gatekeeper" variant, confers resistance to all three drugs by stabilizing the active form of ABL1 to block imatinib and nilotinib binding and introducing a steric clash with dasatinib in the ATP pocket. To overcome these resistance mechanisms of the T315I variant, a "switch-control inhibitor" (DCC-2036) was recently designed that is able to stabilize the BCR-ABL1 T315I variant in the inactive confirmation; phase I clinical trials with this promising drug are underway.[23] In addition, novel TKIs such as ponatinib (which specifically target the T315I gatekeeper mutation) are already entering advanced clinical development stages.

Upfront and repeated monitoring of the mutational status in patients with BCR-ABL1–positive leukemias can help select appropriate TKIs and tailor TKI treatment and also has the potential to provide valuable information on mechanisms underlying selection of resistant clones during TKI therapy.

C-KIT and Tyrosine Kinase Inhibitors

Imatinib and other TKIs do not just target the ATP-folding site of BCR-ABL1; they also inhibit kinases, including C-KIT, platelet-derived growth factor receptor (PDGFR), and others. The C-KIT proto-oncogene encodes the type III transmembrane receptor tyrosine kinase (RTK), which plays an important role in the development of stem cells in the bone marrow and other tissues. C-KIT is expressed in hematopoietic progenitor cells, mast cells, interstitial cells in the gastrointestinal tract, melanocytes, germ cells, and in a subset of cerebellar neurons. Upon binding the dimeric C-KIT ligand, stem cell factor (SCF), C-KIT undergoes dimerization and autophosphorylation, resulting in consecutive activation of the intrinsic C-KIT tyrosine kinase. C-KIT activates multiple downstream signal transduction pathways (e.g., phosphatidylinositol-3-kinase/AKT and Janus-activated kinase [JAK]/signal transducer and activator of transcription [STAT] pathways) and thus has an important role in cell proliferation, self-renewal, differentiation, and other processes.

Gain-of-function mutations in c-KIT can be found in numerous human cancers. For example, up to 70% of gastrointestinal stromal tumors (GISTs) harbor a mutation in the juxtamembrane domain (exon 11) of c-KIT, and this variant is more responsive to imatinib treatment. In aggressive systemic mastocytosis (ASM), a disease with clonal neoplastic proliferation of mast cells that infiltrate hematopoietic (and other) tissues, about 90% of affected individuals have the activating c-KIT 2447A>T, resulting in the C-KIT D816V variant. The activation c-KIT mutation D816V seems to lead to conformational changes in the KIT molecule, which block binding of imatinib and result in resistance to imatinib.[24]

The examples of TKIs and variants in their targets (e.g., BCR-ABL, c-KIT, PDGFR) provide clear evidence that the use of genetic biomarkers can help select drugs and tailor therapy. This has also been recognized by regulatory authorities; for example, the FDA approved imatinib only for adults with ASM without D816V c-KIT mutations or with unknown c-KIT mutational status.

ADVERSE DRUG EFFECTS PRESENTING AS HEMATOLOGIC DISORDERS

Adverse drug reactions (ADRs) constitute a major clinical problem, and strong evidence indicates that ADRs account for approximately 5% of all hospital admissions and increase the length of hospitalization by 2 days. Although the factors that determine susceptibility to ADRs are unclear in most cases, there is increasing interest in the role of genetics; therefore the availability of a genetic test that identifies patients at risk for rare but serious adverse effects has particular appeal. Based on the clinical relevance of ADRs, the FDA has provided advice on the use of certain biomarkers (e.g., variants in TPMT, UGT1A1, CYP2C19) to avoid serious adverse drug effects; a full list of these biomarkers is available at the FDA Web site (see Table 7-1). This list includes, for example, a dosage and administration warning label for irinotecan to prevent severe hematotoxicity based on the assessment of sequence variants in the uridine diphosphate glucuronosyltransferase (UGT) 1A1 gene (i.e., a reduction in the starting dose is recommended for patients homozygous for UGT1A1*28 allele).[10,11] Several medications whose adverse effects have been associated with variability in candidate genes and manifest predominantly as hematologic abnormalities are listed in Table 7-2.

DRUG DEVELOPMENT

Optimizing the selection and dosage of medications is a principal goal of pharmacogenomics. Another important application is in drug development, which is evolving in parallel with improved insights into the mechanisms by which medications exert their pharmacologic effects. Such improved insights into the mechanism(s) of drug action in target cells can help elucidate mechanisms that confer drug resistance, and they will facilitate the development of strategies to further enhance efficacy. This knowledge can be used as a basis to engineer drugs that amplify treatment effects or bypass resistance mechanisms, or both.

Here we focus on examples to show how insights from pharmacogenomic investigations have helped to develop novel strategies to further improve outcome in subgroups of children with ALL who still have a poor outcome despite intensive treatment with current multiagent risk-adapted therapies (so-called high-risk ALL, or HR-ALL). Although excellent outcomes with 5-year event-free survival of higher than 80% can be achieved in childhood ALL in industrial countries, ALL is still a leading cause of death from disease in children older than 1 year of age, and treatment of children with HR-ALL remains one of the greatest challenges in pediatric oncology. HR-ALL features include the resistance of leukemia cells to steroids (i.e., poor steroid responders in BFM-based treatment trials) and multidrug therapy (clearance of leukemia blasts in the peripheral blood, bone marrow, and sanctuary sites), and the presence of certain genetic alterations in leukemia cells—for instance, mixed-lineage leukemia (MLL)–rearrangements (especially in infants), the BCR-ABL1 fusion gene (Ph+ ALL), and (recently identified) alterations in the IKZF1 gene, which is encoding the early lymphoid transcription factor IKAROS.[7,25]

The introduction of TKIs in the treatment of Ph+ ALL has led to a dramatic improvement in outcome, as demonstrated by results from the Children's Oncology Group (COG) AALL0031 trial.[25] The following sections focus on further examples of the development of novel approaches to treat children with HR-ALL; these approaches have in part been the result of the collaborative TARGET (Therapeutically Applicable Research to Generate Effective Treatments) initiative (see Table 7-1).

Connectivity Map and Steroid Resistance

Genome-wide analyses of gene expression profiles by means of high-density microarrays provide powerful tools to study mechanisms of drug action. This approach offers the opportunity to identify previously unknown drug targets. The feasibility of this method has been demonstrated in studies of several hematologic diseases. For example, pharmacogenomic studies have shed light on the biologic basis of treatment failure in childhood ALL, by investigating gene expression signatures that were associated with in vitro sensitivity of diagnostic ALL cells to prednisolone, vincristine, L-asparaginase, and daunorubicin. Of note, only a few of the identified intrinsic drug resistance genes had been previously linked to drug resistance, and the identified gene expression signatures discriminated patients who were at higher risk for relapse.[7]

A novel approach was used to computationally connect disease-associated gene expression signatures (e.g., ALL blast cells that are intrinsically sensitive or resistant to glucocorticoid [GC]-induced apoptosis in vitro) to drug-associated gene expression profiles (i.e., the so-called Connectivity Map) in order to identify molecules that reverse a drug-resistance signature.[26] This strategy builds on prior

Table 7-2 Selected Pharmacogenetic Defects That Lead to Adverse Drug Reactions Manifesting as Hematologic Disorders

Adverse Drug Reaction	Drug(s) That Cause ADR	Altered Protein	Important Genetic Variant(s)	Hypotheses on Pathophysiology
Myelosuppression	6-Mercaptopurine 6-Thioguanine azathioprine	Thiopurine-6-methyltransferase (TPMT)	TPMT*2: 238G>C; TPMT*3A: 460G>A; 719A>G; and TPMT*3C: 719A>G	In hematopoietic cells, TPMT inactivates cytotoxic thioguanine nucleotides (TGNs) by methylation. Accumulation of TGNs due to the functionally defective TPMT variants causes hematotoxicity (see text for details).
Myelosuppression (diarrhea)	Irinotecan (CPT-11) Active metabolite: 7-ethyl-10-hydroxycamptothecine (SN-38)	UDP-Glucuronosyltransferase (UGT) isoenzyme 1A1 (UGT1A1)	UGT1A1*28: promotor polymorphism; dinucleotide insertion in the TATA box [wild-type: $(TA)_6TAA$] resulting in $(TA)_7TAA$	The cytotoxic metabolite of CPT-11, SN-38, is mainly inactivated by UGT1A1. Accumulation of cytotoxic SN-38 in hematopoietic and intestinal cells is due to decreased inactivation (glucuronidation) by the variant enzyme.
Myelosuppression (mucositis, neurotoxicity)	5-flourouracil (5-FU)	Dihydropyrimidine Dehydrogenase (DPD)	DPYD*2A: G to A mutation in the invariant GT splice donor site flanking exon 14 (IVS14+1G>A), leading to skipping of exon 14 during splicing	DPD is the rate-limiting enzyme in 5-FU catabolism. Skipping exon 14 during splicing renders the enzyme inactive and can, therefore, be one cause of severe 5-FU toxicity due to prolonged 5-FU exposure.
Venous thrombosis	Oral contraceptives	Prothrombin (FII, F2)	Factor II 20210G>A; SNP in the 3 untranslated region (UTR) at position 20210	Factor II 20210G>A causes elevated prothrombin level, which a risk factor for thrombosis. Oral contraceptives are an additional independent risk factor, and both (FVL) raise the risk for thrombosis
Venous thrombosis	Oral contraceptives	Factor V (FV, F5)	FVL: 1691G>A (in exon 10 of the FV gene) leads to Arg506Gln change lies within the activated protein C cleavage site	FVL causes activated protein C resistance, which is a thrombotic risk factor. Oral contraceptives are an additional independent risk factor, and both (+ factor II 20210G>A) raise the risk for thrombosis.
Bleeding risk	Warfarin and other coumarin derivatives	Cytochrome P450 isoenzyme 2C9 (CYP2C9)	CYP2C9*2: 430C>T in exon 3 leads to an Arg144Cys change. CYP2C9*3: 1075A>C in exon 7 leads to an Ile359Leu change.	CYP2C9 is the most important enzyme in the catabolism of S-warfarin. The CYP2C9*3 allele leads to an amino acid change in the substrate binding site, a decrease in enzyme activity (additionally seen in CYP2C9*2 allele), and an accumulation of S-warfarin, which enhances the risk for bleeding.
Bleeding risk	Clopidogrel	CYP2C19	CYP2C19*17: -806C>T	The prodrug clopidogrel is activated via CYP2C19. CYP2C19*17 results in enhanced transcription and higher enzyme activity, leading to enhanced drug activation and platelet inhibition (ultrarapid metabolizers).

Ig, Immunoglobulin; *SNP*, single-nucleotide polymorphism; *UDP*, uridine diphosphate.
*Nucleotide bases: *A*, adenine; *C*, cytosine; *G*, guanine; *T*, thymine.

findings that small molecules can induce treatment-specific changes in gene expression in leukemia cells in vivo. Indeed, the profile induced by the mTOR inhibitor rapamycin was found to match the signature of GC sensitivity in ALL cells.[7] Moreover, it was shown that rapamycin sensitized a resistant leukemia cell line to GC-induced apoptosis via a modulation of antiapoptotic protein MCL1. This is consistent with earlier work revealing MCL1 overexpression in steroid-resistant ALL. This work suggests that GC in combination with rapamycin could be an effective approach to overcome intrinsic GC resistance in ALL and provides evidence that such a chemical genomic approach based on gene expression might be useful to identify molecules with the potential to overcome intrinsic drug resistance in leukemia.[7]

FMS-Like Tyrosine Kinase-3 (FLT3) and FLT3 Inhibitors

The FMS-like tyrosine kinase-3 (FLT3) is a class III receptor tyrosine kinase (RTK) and is primarily expressed in early myeloid and lymphoid progenitors, where it plays an important role in their proliferation and differentiation. Activating mutations and overexpression of TKIs are well known to be involved in the pathogenesis of many hematologic malignancies. For example, internal-tandem duplications (ITDs) in the FLT3 gene, which led to constitutive activation of FLT3, are found in up to 30% of patients with AML, and FLT3-ITD–positive AML is associated with a poor response to chemotherapy and a poor prognosis.[25]

Using genome-wide gene expression analyses, the FLT3 wild-type gene was identified as being overexpressed in MLL-rearranged and hyperdiploid childhood ALL. FLT3 inhibitors have been shown to inhibit growth in cells that overexpress FLT3, and infants with MLL-rearranged ALL and high FLT3 expressions have been identified to have a very poor prognosis when treated with standard ALL medications. Thus the inclusion of FLT3 inhibitors seems worthy of being investigated in the treatment of children with the poor-prognostic ALL subtype with MLL rearrangements and perhaps those with hyperdiploid ALL, which also overexpresses FLT3. Indeed, the COG trial AALL0631 already investigates the combination of the FLT3 inhibitor lestaurtinib in combination with an intensive chemotherapy backbone in children with MLL-rearranged infant ALL, and this approach may help to improve outcome in this poor-prognostic ALL subtype.[25]

Janus Kinases (JAKs) and JAK Inhibitors

Janus kinases (JAKs) are a family of tyrosine kinases (JAK1, JAK2, JAK3, and nonreceptor protein-tyrosine kinase 2 [TYK2]) that associate with the intracellular tail of cytokine receptors and activate downstream signaling via the STAT family of transcription factors, which bind specific promoters that regulate proliferation and differentiation.

It has long been recognized that the JAK-STAT pathway is essential in hematopoiesis, and its deregulation may play an important role in hematologic malignancies. Indeed, in 2005, a recurrent somatic gain-of-function mutation in the JAK2 gene (1849G>T, rs77375493, V617F) was discovered in a significant proportion of patients with myeloproliferative neoplasms (MPNs)—polycythemia vera (PV), more than 95%; essential thrombocytosis (ET), approximately 50%; and primary myelofibrosis (PM), approximately 40%; this led to the development of JAK2 inhibitors. It is important to note that the JAK-STAT pathway is essential for normal hematopoiesis, and blocking wt-JAK can lead to potentially severe hematologic and/or immunologic side effects; thus inhibitors that selectively target mutant JAK would be an attractive alternative. Early trials with the JAK inhibitor ruxolitinib have already shown clinical benefits in MPN, with manageable toxicity (primarily decreased erythropoiesis and thrombopoiesis); JAK inhibitors, however, have not thus far shown disease-modifying activity, and results of future trials and research will clarify their role in the treatment of MPN.[27] Whereas variants in the JAK genes are often found in myeloid neoplasms, their occurrence seems to be rare in lymphoid neoplasms.

In childhood ALL, however, JAK mutations have recently been identified in a subcohort of children with HR-ALL. This exciting discovery began with genome-wide gene expression analyses that identified a subtype of HR-ALL, which has a gene expression profile similar to that of BCR-ABL1 positive (Ph+) ALL. In contrast to Ph+ ALL, leukemia cells in the identified subtype do not harbor the BCR-ABL1 fusion gene; therefore this HR-ALL subtype has been named BCR-ABL1–like ALL.[25] It was speculated that genetic alterations that can influence tyrosine kinase signaling pathways similar to those downstream of BCR-ABL1 might be involved in the pathogenesis of BCR-ABL1-like ALL; indeed, alterations in the lymphoid transcription factor gene IKZF1 (encoding IKAROS), the lymphoid signaling receptor gene CRLF2 (encoding cytokine receptor like factor 2), and the JAK family of tyrosine kinases, have been identified. Activating mutations in JAK2 (rare in JAK1 and JAK3) have been identified in approximately 10% of children with HR-ALL, and these mutations have been shown to result in increased sensitivity to JAK inhibitors in vitro.[28] Therefore the combination of JAK inhibitors with an intensive chemotherapy backbone seems to be an attractive strategy to improve outcomes in a subgroup of children (those who have activating JAK mutations) with HR-ALL.

FUTURE DIRECTIONS

Pharmacogenomics has already proven to be an important approach to improve drug therapy, and as of August 2011, the FDA has included information on pharmacogenomic biomarkers in the labels of more than 70 drugs. A full list of these medications and further details are available at the FDA's Web site (see Table 7-1). There is, however, a relatively slow pace of translating pharmacogenomics into clinical practice. Laboratory tests (e.g., liver and kidney function tests) are widely used to adjust drug dosages, but even though technology for testing relevant pharmacogenomic biomarkers is widely available, simple, robust, and inexpensive genotyping tests are rarely used to adjust drug dosage.[29] A major difference among these tests is the time lag from the blood sampling to the result. As genotyping becomes faster and cheaper, this issue may no longer be an obstacle. In addition, educative and legislative initiatives and the implementation of user-friendly decision support systems will help to make pharmacogenomic biomarkers a routine part of clinical care. A major advantage to the use of biomarkers is that a patient's genotype, unlike a renal function test, needs to be performed only once in a patient's lifetime.

The recent unprecedented gain of insights into the human genome and genomic variations among individuals has already changed the practice of medicine. High-throughput technologies, such as hybridization-based microarray approaches and next-generation sequencing (NGS) technologies,[6] are available for genome-wide analyses of genomic variants, gene expression patterns, epigenetic patterns, and proteomic and metabonomic profiles. The recent application of these genome-wide tools has already yielded novel insights into drug actions and led to important drug discoveries.

Moreover, these tools are being used to elucidate differences between genomes of normal cells and cancer cells (e.g., the Pediatric Cancer Genome Project; see Table 7-1), and this knowledge has the potential to illuminate paths toward novel prognostic markers (those that can be used for risk stratification in clinical trials) and/or novel therapeutic targets (those that can be used to discover new medications).

Once novel candidate genes have been identified via GWA studies, functional investigations such as systematic mutagenesis, RNA interference, use of overexpression systems (cDNA, open reading frame [ORF] and miRNA expression libraries), and chemistry-based approaches are necessary to establish valid pharmacogenomic mechanisms.[30] The outputs of such studies will advance understanding of the pharmacology of existing medications and will help to identify genes and pathways involved in drug resistance and novel therapeutic targets.

One important consideration in modern medicine is that clinically useful approaches must also be cost-effective. About a decade ago, the cost for the first full human genome sequence was approximately $3 billion; within the next decade, this cost is expected to be about $1000. The markedly lower cost for robust genotyping points to an exciting future for pharmacogenomics research and translation, suggesting that the current approach to selecting medications (often "trial and error") will continue to evolve into more scientific methods for selecting the optimal medications and doses for individual patients—with genomics playing an increasing role in such therapeutic decisions.

REFERENCES

1. Evans WE, Relling MV: Moving towards individualized medicine with pharmacogenomics. *Nature* 429:464, 2004.
2. Ma Q, Lu AY: Pharmacogenetics, pharmacogenomics, and individualized medicine. *Pharmacol Rev* 63:437, 2011.
3. Lander ES: Initial impact of the sequencing of the human genome. *Nature* 470:187, 2011.
4. Kimchi-Sarfaty C, Oh JM, Kim IW, et al: A "silent" polymorphism in the MDR1 gene changes substrate specificity. *Science* 315:525, 2007.
5. Rukov JL, Shomron N: MicroRNA pharmacogenomics: Post-transcriptional regulation of drug response. *Trends Mol Med* 17:412, 2011.
6. Alkan C, Coe BP, Eichler EE: Genome structural variation discovery and genotyping. *Nat Rev Genet* 12:363, 2011.
7. Cheok MH, Pottier N, Kager L, et al: Pharmacogenetics in acute lymphoblastic leukemia. *Semin Hematol* 46:39, 2009.
8. Diouf B, Cheng Q, Krynetskaia N, et al: Somatic deletions of genes regulating MSH2 protein stability cause DNA mismatch repair deficiency and drug resistance in human leukemia cells. *Nature Medicine* 17:1298, 2011.
9. Wang L, McLeod HL, Weinshilboum RM: Genomics and drug response. *N Engl J Med* 364:1144, 2011.

10. Sim SC, Ingelman-Sundberg M: Pharmacogenomic biomarkers: New tools in current and future drug therapy. *Trends Pharmacol Sci* 32:72, 2011.
11. Paugh SW, Stocco G, McCorkle JR, et al: Cancer pharmacogenomics. *Clin Pharmacol Ther* 90:461, 2011.
12. Roden DM, Wilke RA, Kroemer HK, et al: Pharmacogenomics: The genetics of variable drug responses. *Circulation* 123:1661, 2011.
13. Wang L, Weinshilboum R: Thiopurine S-methyltransferase pharmacogenetics: Insights, challenges and future directions. *Oncogene* 25:1629, 2006.
14. Stocco G, Cheok MH, Crews KR, et al: Genetic polymorphism of inosine triphosphate pyrophosphatase is a determinant of mercaptopurine metabolism and toxicity during treatment for acute lymphoblastic leukemia. *Clin Pharmacol Ther* 85:164, 2009.
15. Relling MV, Gardner EE, Sandborn WJ, et al: Clinical Pharmacogenetics Implementation Consortium guidelines for thiopurine methyltransferase genotype and thiopurine dosing. *Clin Pharmacol Ther* 89:387, 2011.
16. Ingelman-Sundberg M, Sim SC, Gomez A, et al: Influence of cytochrome P450 polymorphisms on drug therapies: Pharmacogenetic, pharmacoepigenetic and clinical aspects. *Pharmacol Ther* 116:496, 2007.
17. Mega JL, Tabassome S, Collet JP, et al: Reduced function CYP2C19 genotype and risk of adverse clinical outcomes among patients treated with clopidogrel predominantly for PCI: A meta-analysis. *JAMA* 204:1821, 2010.
18. Scott SA, Sangkuhl K, Gardner EE, et al: Clinical Pharmacogenetics Implementation Consortium Guidelines for Cytochrome P450-2C19 (CYP2C19) Genotype and Clopidogrel Therapy. *Clin Pharmacol Ther* 90:328, 2011.
19. Bauer T, Bouman HJ, van Werkum JW, et al: Impact of CYP2C19 variant genotypes on clinical efficacy of antiplatelet treatment with clopidogrel: Systematic review and meta-analysis. *BMJ* 343:d4588, 2011.
20. Kamali F, Wynne H: Pharmacogenetics of warfarin. *Annu Rev Med* 61:63, 2010.
21. Niemi M, Pasanen MK, Neuvonen PJ: Organic anion transporting polypeptide 1B1: A genetically polymorphic transporter of major importance for hepatic drug uptake. *Pharmacol Rev* 63:157, 2011.
22. Trevino LR, Shimasaki N, Yang W, et al: Germline genetic variation in an organic anion transporter polypeptide associated with methotrexate pharmacokinetics and clinical effects. *J Clin Oncol* 27:5972, 2009.
23. Chan WW, Wise SC, Kaufman MD, et al: Conformational control inhibition of the BCR-ABL1 tyrosine kinase, including the gatekeeper T315I mutant, by the switch-control inhibitor DCC-2036. *Cancer Cell* 19:556, 2011.
24. Quintas-Cardama A, Jain N, Verstovsek S: Advances and controversies in the diagnosis, pathogenesis, and treatment of systemic mastocytosis. *Cancer* 117:5439, 2011.
25. Pui CH, Carroll WL, Meshinchi S, et al: Biology, risk stratification, and therapy of pediatric acute leukemias: An update. *J Clin Oncol* 29:551, 2011.
26. Lamb J, Crawford ED, Peck D, et al: The connectivity map: Using gene-expression signatures to connect small molecules, genes, and disease. *Science* 313:1929, 2006.
27. Quintas-Cardama A, Kantarjian H, Cortes J, et al: Janus kinase inhibitors for the treatment of myeloproliferative neoplasias and beyond. *Nat Rev Drug Discov* 10:127, 2011.
28. Mullighan CG, Zhang J, Harvey RC, et al: JAK mutations in high-risk childhood acute lymphoblastic leukemia. *Proc Natl Acad Sci U S A* 106:9414, 2009.
29. Relling MV, Altman RB, Goetz MP, et al: Clinical implementation of pharmacogenomics: Overcoming genetic exceptionalism. *Lancet Oncol* 11:507, 2010.
30. Boehm JS, Hahn WC: Towards systematic functional characterization of cancer genomes. *Nat Rev Genet* 12:487, 2011.

PART

II

Cellular Basis of Hematology

CHAPTER 8

HEMATOPOIETIC STEM CELL BIOLOGY

John P. Chute

Hematopoietic stem cells (HSCs) are characterized by their unique ability to self-renew and give rise to the entirety of the blood and immune system throughout the lifetime of an individual.[1-3] HSCs are very rare cells, representing approximately one in 100,000 bone marrow (BM) cells in the adult.[4] The concept of the existence of an HSC that is capable of reconstituting hematopoiesis in vivo was first introduced more than 60 years ago, when Jacobsen et al[5] demonstrated that lead shielding of the spleen protected mice from otherwise lethal γ irradiation.[5] Subsequently, Jacobsen and colleagues[6] demonstrated that similar radioprotection of mice could be achieved via shielding of one femur. Shortly thereafter, it was demonstrated that intravenous injection of BM cells also provided radioprotection of lethally irradiated mice.[7] Interestingly, investigators initially hypothesized that the radioprotected spleen or BM provided soluble factors that mediated radiation protection.[8,9] However, subsequent experiments by Nowell et al[10] and Ford et al[11] critically demonstrated that transplanted BM cells provided radioprotection directly via cellular reconstitution of the blood system. The historical significance of these studies cannot be overestimated because they provided the basis for not only the ultimate isolation and characterization of HSCs but also for the field of hematopoietic cell transplantation.

Subsequent landmark studies by Till and McCulloch[12] demonstrated that transplantation of limiting doses of BM cells gave rise to myeloid and erythroid colonies in the spleens of irradiated recipient mice. Importantly, Till and McCulloch showed that the numbers of colonies detected in recipient mice was proportional to the numbers of BM cells injected into the irradiated mice, suggesting that a particular population of hematopoietic cells was capable of reconstituting hematopoiesis in vivo.[12-14] The clonogenic nature of a subset of BM cells was definitively shown when these investigators irradiated BM cells and then transplanted the cells into lethally irradiated mice. Persistent chromosomal aberrations were demonstrated in spleen colonies in recipient mice.[15] It was subsequently shown that cells within the spleen colonies were radioprotective of lethally irradiated mice and contained myeloid, erythroid, and lymphoid cells.[12,16] Taken together, these data strongly suggested the presence of hematopoietic stem or progenitor cells that were capable of in vivo engraftment and provision of multilineage progeny from a small number of parent cells.[17]

EMBRYONIC ORIGIN OF HEMATOPOIETIC STEM CELLS

During embryogenesis, cells from the ventral mesoderm migrate to the extraembryonic yolk sac, wherein primitive hematopoiesis occurs at **E7.5.**[4] Primitive hematopoiesis in mammals is transient and encompasses the generation of primarily erythroid cells and macrophages.[4,18] Careful anatomic analysis has demonstrated erythroid cells and vascular endothelium in close proximity during primitive hematopoiesis, suggesting perhaps a common cell of origin or hemangioblast.[4] Early studies by Shalaby et al[19,20] showed that mice lacking Flk1, a tyrosine kinase expressed on endothelial progenitor cells (EPCs), failed to develop both vascular endothelium and blood islands during embryogenesis. Choi et al[21] subsequently demonstrated via gene tracing studies in vitro that vascular endothelial and hematopoietic cells arose from a common precursor cell, the hemangioblast. More recently, studies of human embryonic stem cells (ESCs) revealed that cytokine stimulation of human ESCs can induce the development of cells with both hematopoietic and vascular features.[4,22] Taken together, these studies suggest that a cell consistent with a hemangioblast provides the origin of primitive hematopoiesis in mammals.

In contrast to the extra-embryonic origin of primitive hematopoiesis, definitive hematopoiesis originates in the intraembryonic aorto–gonado–mesonephros (AGM) region.[4,19,21,23,24] The onset of definitive hematopoiesis was shown by several different investigators to occur at the site of the dorsal aorta at **E10.5-11.5** within the AGM region.[23,24] Several complementary studies using lineage tracing experiments in both mice and zebrafish have subsequently demonstrated that HSCs arise from hemogenic endothelium within the ventral aspect of the dorsal aorta.[25-27] Runx1 is required for this process to occur in mice,[28] and HSCs that arise from hemogenic endothelium migrate properly to the fetal liver and to the BM and are capable of self-renewal and multilineage differentiation.[25]

DEFINITION OF HEMATOPOIETIC STEM CELLS

Phenotype

Murine Hematopoietic Stem Cells

The HSC is the most well-defined somatic, multipotent cell in the body. With the emergence of antibody technology and flow cytometry[17,29,30] and coupled with *in* vitro and in vivo functional assays,[31-36] biologists have developed reproducible methods to analyze and isolate murine and human HSCs with a high level of enrichment. In mice, Weissman and colleagues were able to show that antibody-based depletion of BM cells expressing myeloid, B cell, T cell, and erythroid cells along with positive selection for cells expressing c-kit, sca-1, and Thy1.1^{lo} ("KTLS" cells), allowed for enrichment for HSCs to approximately 1 of 10 to 30 cells as measured by the capacity to provide long-term, multilineage hematopoietic reconstitution in a competitively transplanted, lethally irradiated congenic mouse.[32,37-40] Because Thy 1.1 is not expressed on many strains of mice,[38] additional markers were developed, including Flk2 (Flt-3), the absence of which was shown to substantially enrich for murine LT-HSCs.[41,42] Similarly, it has been demonstrated that the isolation of murine BM KSL cells based upon the lack of expression of CD34 (34^-KSL) enriches for HSCs with long-term reconstituting capability at the level of one of 5 to 10 cells (Fig. 8-1).[43]

An alternative and effective method for isolating BM HSCs involves the use of intravital dyes, Hoescht 33342 and Rhodamine 123.[44-48] HSCs, unlike more committed progenitor cells, efficiently efflux these dyes such that HSCs display low-intensity staining for these dyes.[48,49] Li and Johnson[47] demonstrated that HSCs capable of long-term, multilineage repopulation in lethally irradiated mice were significantly enriched in the Rhodamine 123 lo Sca-1+Lin- cells, but Rho hi Sca-1+Lin- cells possessed little repopulating activity. Similarly, McAlister et al[46] showed that isolation of Hoescht lo BM mononuclear cells significantly enriched for both CFU-S14 and cells capable of radioprotection and multilineage reconstitution in lethally irradiated mice. A subsequent and important refinement in the use of Hoescht 33342 (Ho 33342) to isolate HSCs was made by Goodell

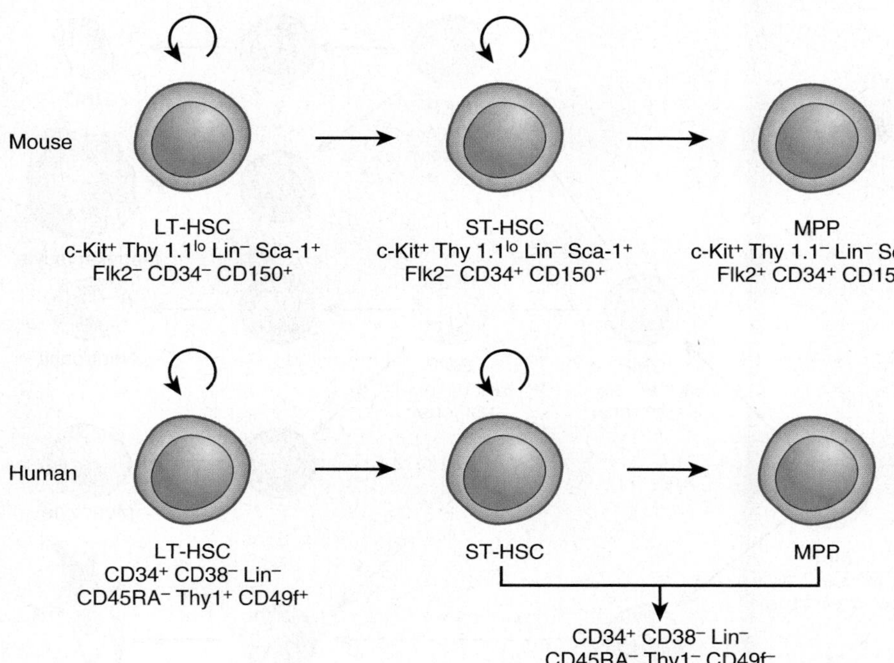

Figure 8-1 PHENOTYPE OF MURINE AND HUMAN HEMATOPOIETIC STEM CELLS (HSCs). Long-term HSCs (LT-HSCs), short-term HSCs (ST-HSCs), and multipotent progenitor cells (MPPs) have precise cell surface markers that discriminate them from more committed progenitor cells. *(Adapted from Prohaska S, Weissman I: Chapter 5. Biology of hematopoietic stem and progenitor cells. In Appelbaum FR, Forman SJ, Negrin RS, et al, editors:* Thomas' Hematopoietic Cell Transplantation, *ed 4, 2009, John Wiley and Sons.)*

et al,[48] who showed that a Ho 33342 side population (SP) can be identified via the emission of Ho 33342 at 2 wavelengths, which yields a tail profile on flow cytometric analysis. Importantly, isolation of Ho 33342 SP cells has been shown to yield variable enrichment for HSCs compared with 34^-Flt3^-KSL cells, and this may be caused by the sensitivity of the assay to variations in staining techniques and batch-to-batch differences in Hoescht 33342 dye.[50-52] However, Matsuzaki et al[53] demonstrated that transplantation of single Ho 33342 SP 34^-KSL cells into lethally irradiated C57Bl6 mice yielded donor cell multilineage engraftment greater than 1% in more than 95% of transplanted mice. Therefore, the combination of Ho 33342 SP cells with 34^-KSL markers provides a basis for isolation of highly enriched LT-HSCs from mice.[29,50,52]

A major advance in this field involved the discovery by Kiel et al[54] that the surface expression of CD150, a member of the signaling lymphocyte activation molecules (SLAM) family, significantly enriched for murine BM HSCs. It was also shown that the absence of CD41 and CD48 on $CD150^+$ cell enriches further for the HSC population and that $CD150^+CD41^-CD48^-$KSL cells reconstitute approximately half of all mice competitively transplanted with limiting numbers of cells.[54] Taken together, isolation of $SLAM^+$KSL BM cells has become a reproducible and efficient strategy to isolate murine LT-HSCs with maximal enrichment (see Fig. 8-1).[55]

Although this chapter focuses on the phenotypic and functional characterization of HSCs, it is worth noting that some controversy exists regarding whether adult T-cell progenitors possess myeloid potential.[56-58] It was independently suggested by Bell et al[57] and Wada et al[56] that adult T-cell thymic progenitors possessed myeloid differentiation potential. However, whereas these studies primarily involved in vitro culture of T cells on stromal cells, subsequent in vivo transplantation studies failed to demonstrate the myeloid potential of adult T cells.[58] Taken together, these data suggest that although common lymphoid progenitors may possess myeloid differentiation potential, it may not be physiologically relevant but rather may be an artifact of specialized co-culture conditions.[58] Recent studies have also clarified the nature of common lymphoid progenitor cells (CLPs) and has dissected this population further into an all-lymphoid progenitor (ALP) cell, which retains full lymphoid potential and thymic seeding capability, and B lymphoid progenitor cells (BLPs), which is restricted to the B-cell lineage.[59] Whereas ALPs are characterized by the lack of surface expression of Lyd6, BLPs demonstrate expression of Lyd6 and upregulate the B-cell–specific factors, Ebf1 and Pax5.[59] The phenotypic markers of the hematopoietic hierarchy through myeloid and lymphoid differentiation are shown in Fig. 8-2.

Human Hematopoietic Stem Cells

Significant progress has also been made in the phenotypic characterization of human HSCs via flow cytometric analysis combined with in vivo transplantation assays in immune-deficient mice.[60,61] Of particular note, although murine HSCs can be characterized by the absence of CD34 expression on the cell surface, human HSCs are primarily enriched using CD34 surface expression, and this provides the basis for confirming sufficient HSC content to allow for successful hematopoietic cell transplantation in patients.[17,62,63] There is also some controversy in this area because some investigations have suggested that LT-HSCs can be isolated from $CD34^-$ human hematopoietic cells.[64-67] Of note, only a small percentage (<0.1%) of $CD34^+$ human hematopoietic cells possess the capacity to engraft following intravenous injection into nonobese diabetic/severe combined immune deficient (NOD/SCID) mice.[4,61] Further enrichment of human HSCs has been demonstrated via negative selection for surface expression of CD38 and depletion of lineage surface markers.[61,68,69] Thy 1.1 (CD90) surface expression also enriches for multilineage colony-forming ability and in vivo reconstituting capacity of human hematopoietic cells.[17,70] Majeti et al showed that the $CD34^+$ $CD38^-Thy1.1^+CD45RA^-lin^-$ population in human cord blood (CB) was enriched at the level of 1 in 10 cells for LT-HSCs.[70] The authors also showed that candidate multipotent progenitor cells (MPPs) were demarcated by the $CD34^+CD38^-Thy1.1^-CD45RA^-lin^-$ population, suggesting that the loss of Thy1.1 reflects the transition of LT-HSCs to ST-HSCs/MPPs.[17,70]

$CD49f^+$ Human Hematopoietic Stem Cells

Although it is possible to enrich murine BM HSCs to the level of nearly single-cell purity using various combinations of cell surface

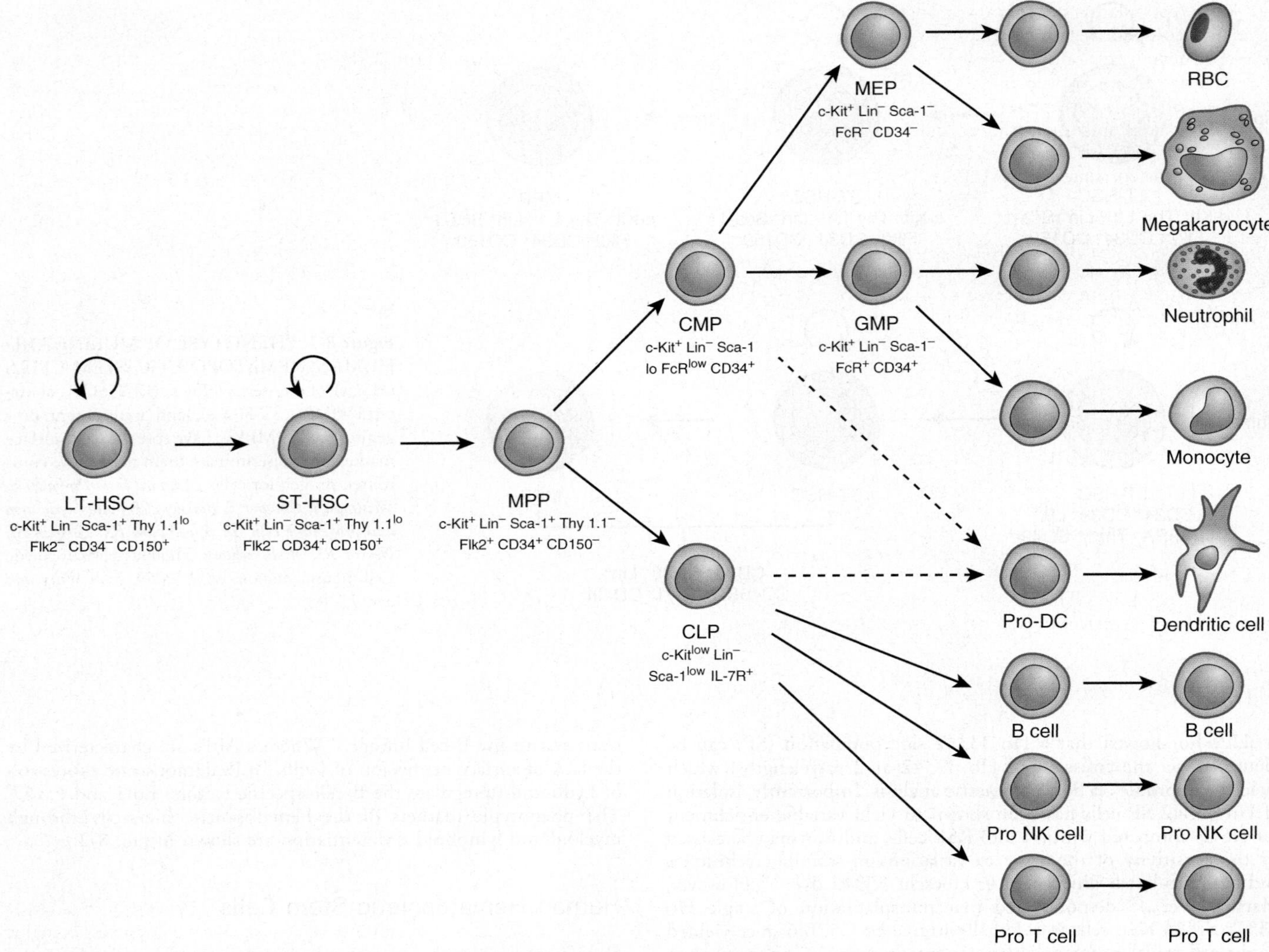

Figure 8-2 HEMATOPOIETIC CELLULAR HIERARCHY. The phenotypes of murine hematopoietic stem cells (HSCs) and committed progenitor cells are shown. *CLP,* Common lymphoid progenitor cell; *CMP,* common myeloid progenitor cell; *DC,* dendritic cell; *GMP,* granulocyte-macrophage progenitor cell; *MEP,* megakaryocytic-erythroid progenitor cell; *NK,* natural killer; *RBC,* red blood cell. *(Adapted from Prohaska S, Weissman I: Chapter 5. Biology of hematopoietic stem and progenitor cells. In Appelbaum FR, Forman SJ, Negrin RS, et al, editors:* Thomas' Hematopoietic Cell Transplantation, *ed 4, 2009, John Wiley and Sons.)*

markers, isolation of human BM HSCs to the same level of purity has not been achieved.[48,54,71] However, a recent study indicates that intrafemoral injection of a FACS-purified population of human CB $CD34^+CD38^-CD45RA^-Thy1^+$ cells that were additionally purified based on surface expression of the integrin α6 (CD49f$^+$) yielded 6.7-fold increased human donor chimerism at 20 weeks in NOD-SCID IL2R-γ-/- (NSG) mice compared with injection with the identical dose of $CD34^+CD38^-CD45RA^-Thy1^+CD49f^-$ cells.[72] Only the $Thy1^+CD49f^+$ cells could be serially transplanted in this study, and the enrichment for LT-HSCs via limiting dilution analysis was estimated to be approximately 1 in 11 $CD34^+CD38^-CD45RA^-Thy1^+CD49f^+$ cells.[72] Further purification of this population of cells using Rhodamine dye demonstrated that single-cell transplantation of $Thy1^+Rho^{lo}$ CD49f$^+$ cells yielded long-term, multilineage engraftment in 5 of 18 transplanted recipients. Serial transplantation was also successful in two of four secondary mice, suggesting that at least some of the $Thy1^+Rho^{lo}CD49f^+$ cells undergo self-renewal.[72] Of note, because mice were transplanted via intrafemoral injection in these studies, it remains unknown whether this panel of markers equally identifies human HSCs capable of homing properly to the BM after intravenous injection. Nonetheless, these studies reveal that the addition of CD49f$^+$ to the panel of human LT-HSC markers provides an improved capability to isolate human HSCs at a level of purity that is comparable to that applied to murine HSC isolation.

FUNCTIONAL ASSAYS

In Vitro Assays

The colony-forming cell (CFC) assay does not measure HSC content but rather committed myeloid progenitor cell content via a 14-day assay for colonies within methylcellulose media that is supplemented with specific growth factors.[52] The CFC assay measures CFU–granulocyte monocyte (CFU-GM), burst forming unit-erythroid (BFU-E) and CFU–granulocyte, erythroid, macrophage, megakaryocyte (CFU-GEMM). The CFU-GEMM, or CFU-mix colonies, represent a more immature progenitor cell population. B- and T-cell progenitor cell content can also be measured via in vitro assay but requires specialized co-culture conditions, which are described elsewhere.[52,73,74]

The long-term culture-initiating cell (LTC-IC) assay is a 6-week in vitro assay in which BM cells are co-cultured with murine stromal cells for 4 weeks followed by replating of the entire culture system into methylcellulose and additional 2-week assay for colony formation.[52,75] The LTC-IC, unlike the CFC, measures a more immature stem/progenitor cell population, although the results of the LTC-IC are inherently dependent and limited by technical variabilities in stromal co-culture experiments.[52] Importantly, the LTC-ICs lack long-term repopulating cells because transplantation of LTC-ICs into mice in a competitive transplantation assay does not result in any long-term reconstitution.[52,60]

The cobblestone area–forming cell (CAFC) assay also involves co-culture of HSCs with preestablished stromal cell monolayers and relies on microscopic quantification of cobblestone-forming cells embedded underneath the stromal layer.[75,76] It has been shown that CAFC content correlates well with CFU-S-12 content and marrow repopulating capacity.[52,75] However, similar to the LTC-IC, the CAFC assay does not measure LT-HSCs. An advantage of the CAFC and LTC-IC assays is that the estimate of stem/progenitor cell content is not confounded by the homing capacity of the cell population being tested. However, competitive transplantation assays provide a more physiologically relevant measure of functional HSC content and allow quantification of LT-HSC content as well as homing efficiency.[38,52,77]

In Vivo Assays

Colony-Forming Unit–Spleen Assay

The first reproducible in vivo assay for hematopoietic progenitor cells was the CFU–spleen assay (CFU-S), which was developed by Till and McCullough.[12,62] In this assay, BM cells are injected into lethally irradiated mice, and macroscopic spleen colonies are measured from 1 to 3 weeks after injection.[52] These colonies represent short-term repopulating cell and MPP activity but do not measure long-term HSC content.[4,52]

Competitive Repopulation Assay

A significant advance in the study of hematopoiesis was the development of the competitive repopulating assay.[52,78] In this assay, an unknown population of hematopoietic cells is transplanted via intravenous injection into lethally irradiated syngeneic mice along with a competing dose of host-derived BM cells.[52,79,80] This assay has been refined over time such that it is typically performed using a limiting dilution method in which several cell doses (typically >–three to five doses; n = 10 mice/dose level) of BM cells or purified HSCs (e.g., 34^-KSL cells) are injected into lethally irradiated mice along with a fixed dose of host competitor BM cells, such that a fraction of the recipient mice can be predicted to have non-engraftment.[52,81,82] This approach allows the application of Poisson statistical analysis to provide an estimate of competitive repopulating units (CRUs) within the donor hematopoietic cell population.[52,81-83] An important feature of the CRU assay is the potential to estimate the frequency of LT-HSCs in a given hematopoietic cell population. Donor cell engraftment that is detected within the first 8 to 12 weeks after transplantation, reflects the contribution of ST-HSCs, which extinguish at or beyond 12 weeks posttransplant. Therefore, measurement of LT-HSC cannot be convincingly estimated until more than 12 to 20 weeks posttransplantation.[52,84] Dykstra et al.[85] showed that competitive transplantation of single, phenotypic HSCs results in stable donor cell engraftment in lethally irradiated mice beyond 16 weeks, and retroviral marking of HSCs revealed that stable donor-derived hematopoiesis was not observed in recipient mice until 6 months posttransplant.

A commonly used and rigorous approach to estimate the presence of LT-HSCs is the performance of secondary, tertiary, and quaternary HSC transplants.[52] This approach is based on the principle that a singular feature of primitive LT-HSCs is the capacity to serially reconstitute multilineage hematopoiesis in vivo without exhaustion.[52,86-88] In this method, whole BM is typically collected from primary recipient mice and then injected, along with host competitor BM cells, into lethally irradiated syngeneic mice. Donor cell repopulation is then measured at 12 to 20 weeks posttransplantation. Serial transplantation assays have the limitation of being potentially confounded by variables such as homing efficiency of the donor cells.[52,89,90] Therefore, as pointed out by Purton and Scaddon[52] in an excellent review of this subject, serial transplantation assays may be better suited to studies of wild type hematopoietic cell populations as opposed to mutant mice-derived hematopoietic cells, which may have alterations in homing or engraftment mechanisms independent of HSC content.[52] Utilization of whole BM avoids issues regarding the fidelity of phenotypic markers of HSCs in mutant mice and is perhaps more broadly feasible than FACS-isolated HSC populations at some centers.[52,91-94] However, the use of purified HSCs avoids the potential confounding effects of accessory cells contained within the BM graft on donor cell repopulation and allows for precise determination of effects of growth factors on HSC content in vitro compared with unmanipulated BM.[77,95] Lastly, Poisson statistical analysis and estimation of CRU frequency is based on particular criteria for "positive" donor engraftment in recipient mice, typically 0.1 to 1.0% multilineage donor engraftment.[77,96] Therefore, the estimation of CRU frequency can be substantially altered depending on what criteria for engraftment is established. Given the limitations of flow cytometric analysis for accurate multilineage engraftment of hematopoietic cells, it is recommended that a criteria of greater than 1% multilineage engraftment be used for evidence of donor cell repopulation using the competitive repopulating assay.[52]

REGULATION OF HEMATOPOIETIC STEM CELL FATE

Intrinsic Pathways

Transcription Factors

The HSC pool must be maintained throughout the lifetime of an individual to replenish the blood and immune system over time. Sustainment of the HSC pool over time is regulated by both intrinsic and extrinsic mechanisms. Remarkably, numerous transcription factors have been shown to be necessary for HSC self-renewal as measured by competitive transplantation assay.[1] For example, GATA2, GFI1, JunB, PU.1, Myb, CREB-binding protein, Smad4, and ZFX have each been shown to be necessary for maintenance of adult HSCs in vivo.[1,97-104] Zon[1] and others[105] have articulated that a competitive balance exists between transcription factors, thereby providing fine control of HSC self-renewal and differentiation processes. Whether such a balance occurs via direct binding or competition for target genes or modulation of activator–repressor complexes remains unknown.[1] However, the interaction of PU.1, which drives myeloid differentiation,[105] and GATA1, which drives erythroid differentiation, provides an example as to how transcription factors can govern progenitor cell fate.[1,106,107] PU.1 and GATA1 can bind each other as a means of preventing binding of lineage-specific target genes, and lineage differentiation has been shown to be directly related to the levels of PU.1 and GATA1 in the cell.[1]

Recent studies have implicated numerous intracellular proteins as regulators of HSC content in vivo. For example, genetic deletion of the cyclin-dependent kinase inhibitor, p21, resulted in an expansion of the HSC pool in vivo, but BM cells from $p21^{-/-}$ mice demonstrated impaired capacity for serial transplantation. Therefore, p21 appears to be essential for maintenance of LT-HSCs in vivo.[108] Similarly, genetic deletion of PTEN, a negative regulator of the PI3K-Akt pathway, resulted in expansion of ST-HSCs in mice but depletion of LT-HSCs with serial repopulating capacity.[109] Interestingly, Akala et al showed that deletion of the cyclin dependent kinase inhibitors, p16lnk4a and p19Arf, along with p53 in mice yields a 10-fold increase in BM cells capable of long term hematopoietic repopulation.[110,111] These results suggest that p16, p19, and p53 have an important function in controlling the expansion potential of BM stem/progenitor cells.[110] Taken together, these results indicate that targeting of intracellular proteins that regulate HSC proliferation has therapeutic potential as a means to expand the HSC pool.[111,112]

HOX PROTEINS

HOX proteins have been shown to be necessary for normal development in *Drosophila* and mice.[1] Several proteins within the HOX family, including HOXB4, HOXA9, and HOXA10, have been shown to have an important role in the induction of HSC self-renewal.[113-115] Virally-mediated overexpression of HOXB4 in mouse HSCs causes a pronounced (>40-fold) expansion of HSCs in vitro and in vivo.[116,117] Nonviral culture with a TAT-HOXB4 protein also induces a four- to sixfold amplification compared with input HSC numbers after 4-day culture, suggesting the translational potential of expanding HSCs using this approach.[116] An important aspect of *HOXB4* overexpression is the apparent lack of development of leukemia in mice transplanted with *HOXB4*-overexpressing hematopoietic cells followed long term.[116,117] Enforced expression of *HOXA9* also promotes the expansion of adult HSCs.[114] However, mice transplanted with BM cells that overexpress *HOXA9* develop leukemia over time.[1,118] Overexpression of other *HOX* genes, including *HOXA10 and HOXA7,* have also been shown to induce HSC expansion[1,119]; however, overexpression of *HOXA10* blocks myeloid and lymphoid differentiation and leads to acute myeloid leukemia.[120] Recently, Ohta et al[121] reported that retroviral-mediated overexpression of NUP98/HOXA10 fusion protein in murine BM ckit$^+$sca-1$^+$lin$^-$ (KSL) cells caused more than 1000-fold expansion of HSCs in 10-day cultures. Interestingly, mice that are deficient in HOXB4 or HOXB3 display only a mild proliferative defect in HSCs,[122,123] and HOXA9-deficient mice demonstrate moderate decreases in leukocyte counts but no effects on HSC content.[124] However, compound deletion of *HOXA9, HOXB4,* and *HOXB3* in mice causes severe hematopoietic defects.[125] These results suggest that although overexpression of *HOX* genes can induce HSC self-renewal and, in some cases, leukemogenesis,[1,118,119,126] these genes are not necessary for HSC self-renewal and can be compensated for by other mechanisms.

Importantly, *HOX* gene expression is regulated by members of the caudal-type homeobox (CDX) proteins, which can bind to and activate *HOX* gene expression.[1,127] The homeobox protein, MEIS 1, and the homeodomain protein, PBX, also regulate *HOX* gene expression.[1,118] Davidson et al[127] demonstrated that zebrafish lacking CDX4 failed to generate HSCs during development, and these mutants could be rescued from this phenotype by delivery of *HOXA9* mRNA.[1] Similarly, Schnabel et al[118] showed that HOXA9-mediated expansion of hematopoietic progenitor cells required expression of PBX and MEIS1 motifs.[1] Taken together, these results demonstrate the important role of CDX, PBX, and MEIS1 in regulating HOX-protein activity in the hematopoietic system.

Epigenetic Regulation of Hematopoietic Stem Cells Self-Renewal

In the steady state, most DNA in a cell is inaccessible to the transcriptional machinery, coiled in tightly packed chromatin, but certain active genes are highly accessible.[1,128,129] The accessibility of genes to transcriptional activity is regulated by several factors, including methylation status, histone modification, and nucleosome activity. During development, cells undergo processes in which they progressively lose pluripotency and become committed to various lineages.[128,129] It has now been demonstrated that this process is regulated substantially via epigenetic mechanisms. For example, it has been shown that the enforced expression of OCT4, SOX2, c-Myc, and KLF4 in mouse or human somatic cells can induce the generation of pluripotent stem cells (iPS).[130-137] Kim et al[130] subsequently showed that ectopic expression of an unmethylated copy of OCT4 was sufficient to generate induced pluripotent stem (iPS) cells from human neural stem cells.

Epigenetic regulation has also been shown to be important in the differentiation and the lineage commitment of HSCs.[129] For example, Lck, which encodes a SRC kinase responsible for initiating T-cell receptor signaling, is methylated in HSCs but demethylated in CLPs.[129,138,139] Similarly, myeloperoxidase (Mpo), a microbicidal enzyme important in neutrophils, is methylated in HSCs and demethylated in granulocyte monocyte progenitor cells (GMPs).[129] More importantly, from a functional standpoint, Bröske et al[140] and Trowbridge et al[141] have demonstrated directly that DNA methylation regulates the HSC self-renewal process. Mice with deficient DNA methyltransferase 1 (DNMT1) activity demonstrated severe depletion of BM HSC and progenitor cell content over time and skewed myeloid differentiation in vivo.[140] Similarly, conditional deletion of DNMT1 in the hematopoietic system was shown to block HSC self-renewal and niche retention as measured in a competitive transplantation assays.[141] Interestingly, targeted deletion of DNMT3A or DNMT3B does not affect HSC self-renewal, but deletion of both DNMT3A and DNMT3B causes a repopulating defect in HSCs.[1,142] Therefore, the combination of DNMT3A and DNMT3B is also necessary for normal HSC self-renewal.

Another example of epigenetic modulation of HSC self-renewal is the BMI protein.[1,143-145] BMI1 is a chromatin-associated factor that is a component of the polycomb repressive complex.[1] Mice that are deficient in BMI1 demonstrate exhaustion of HSCs, but overexpression of BMI1 increases HSC self-renewal.[1,143-145] It was also shown that BMI1-deficient mice have markedly increased levels of INK4 (p16), a cell cycle regulator, suggesting that BMI1 represses the expression of this gene.[1,146,147] Therefore, BMI1 may promote HSC self-renewal via repression of cell cycle regulatory genes.[1] Several additional examples of chromatin-associated factors that regulate HSC homeostasis have been described, and this topic is well summarized in the comprehensive review by Cedar and Bergman.[129]

MicroRNA Regulation

An additional and important level of regulation of gene transcription is mediated by microRNAs.[148,149] MicroRNAs are small, noncoding RNAs that regulate gene expression by binding with target mRNAs, yielding transcriptional repression or mRNA destabilization.[148,150-152] MicroRNAs can target hundreds of different mRNAs, and mRNAs have multiple microRNA binding sites, allowing for highly complex regulation of gene expression.[148,153] Array analysis has revealed numerous miRNAs to be enriched in HSCs, including miR-155, miR-125b, miR-126, and miR-130a.[154-157] Several miRNAs have been implicated in regulating hematopoietic progenitor cell differentiation, including miR-155 (lymphoid and myeloid development),[154,158,159] miR-223 (myeloid development),[160,161] and the miR-181/miR-150/miR-17-92 cluster (lymphoid development).[162-165] Recently, Gerrits et al[148] demonstrated that overexpression of the miR cluster of miR-99b/let-7e/125a or miR-125a alone in hematopoietic progenitor cells caused a significant increase in CAFC content in vitro and accelerated myeloid differentiation after transplantation into lethally irradiated mice. In a parallel study, Guo et al[149] reported that this same miRNA cluster was enriched in CD34$^-$Flt-3$^-$KSL cells and that overexpression of miR-125a alone was capable of expanding the HSC pool. Importantly, these authors also showed that miR-125a modulated this expansion of HSCs, at least in part, via inhibition of the pro-apoptotic gene, Bak1.[149] Although numerous additional miRNAs, including miR-125b, miR-29a, and miR-146a, have been implicated in regulating HSC fate,[156,166,167] the critical objective going forward will be to identify and validate the miRNA gene targets in HSCs.[148] This will allow a comprehensive map of miRNA regulation of HSC fate to be developed.

EXTRINSIC REGULATION

The past 3 decades have yielded substantial progress in the discovery and characterization of mechanisms that regulate HSC self-renewal and differentiation. Despite this, the translation of these discoveries into the development of translatable methods to expand human HSCs ex vivo or therapeutics to induce HSC expansion in vivo has proven to be difficult. Therefore, dissection of both intrinsic signaling pathways and extrinsic mechanisms that regulate HSC self-renewal, differentiation, and regeneration continues to be a high priority. The following pathways are extrinsically controlled and reflect unique mechanistic targets for the development of therapeutics to amplify the human HSC pool.

Notch Signaling

The Notch signaling pathway has been shown to have an important role in regulating the development of the central nervous system, eye, mesoderm, and ovaries.[111,168,169] To date, four Notch receptors have been identified (Notch 1-4) as well as five ligands for Notch receptors (Jagged 1 and 2 and Delta 1, 3, and 4).[111,170] Notch ligands bind Notch receptors on HSCs, causing cleavage of the Notch-intracellular domain (NICD), which then translocates to the nucleus and binds with the transcription factor CSL (CBF1/RBPJκ).[111,171] RBPJκ then activates target transcription factors, such as HES1 and HES5,[1,111,172,173] which can inhibit both myeloid and B-cell differentiation. Notch 1 and 2 are expressed on murine and human hematopoietic progenitor cells and BM microenvironmental cells express Jagged 1 and Delta 1, providing the basis for extrinsic regulation of Notch signaling in HSCs in the physiologic niche.[111,174,175] Retroviral-mediated expression of the constitutively active form of the NICD in murine HSCs causes the generation of an immortal, cytokine-dependent cell line capable of multilineage in vivo repopulating capacity,[176] thereby demonstrating that activation of Notch signaling is sufficient to induce HSC expansion.[111] Culture of murine HSCs with immobilized Delta 1 promotes a several-fold expansion of HSCs ex vivo.[177] Similarly, MSCV-mediated or Jagged 2–mediated activation of Notch signaling inhibits the differentiation of human CB CD34+ cells,[178] and culture of human CB HSCs with soluble human Jagged 1 induces HSC expansion ex vivo.[175] Notch signaling also appears to have a role in regulating the physiologic maintenance of the HSC pool in vivo.[179] BM osteoblasts express Jagged 1 and administration of γ-secretase inhibitor significantly decreases murine HSC expansion in BM osteoblast co-cultures.[179] Conversely, deletion of Jagged 1 was shown to have no effect on HSC content in mice, and Notch 1–deficient HSCs displayed normal reconstituting capacity in vivo.[180] Deletion of RBPJ, which is required for canonical Notch signaling, also caused no defect in defect in HSC repopulating capacity.[181] Therefore, although activation of Notch signaling clearly induces HSC expansion, Notch signaling may not be necessary for maintenance of the functional HSC pool.[111,180,181] A schematic overview of Notch 1 and 2 regulation of HSC self-renewal and differentiation is shown in Fig. 8-3.

In keeping with the evidence in mice that activation of Notch signaling can induce HSC expansion, Delaney et al[182] showed that serum-free culture of human CB progenitor cells with immobilized Delta 1 plus cytokines for 3 weeks yielded a 5.3-fold increase in human hematopoietic cell engraftment in transplanted non-obese diabetic/severe combined immunodeficient (NOD/SCID) mice. This group subsequently completed a phase I clinical trial showing that transplantation of CB cells expanded with immobilized Delta 1 along with an unmanipulated CB unit was associated with earlier time to neutrophil recovery (median, 16 days) compared with a cohort that received 2 unmanipulated CB units (median, 26 days).[183] Of note, in this phase I study, the unmanipulated CB cells demonstrated dominant engraftment by day +80 and in seven of eight reported recipients, and ex vivo expanded CB cells were not detectable in recipients by day +40 posttransplant.[183] The extinction of the Delta 1–expanded grafts may have been explained by T-cell depletion of the ex vivo expanded products because donor CB CD8+ T cells have been shown to mediate the rejection of second CB units in the setting of double CB transplantation.[184]

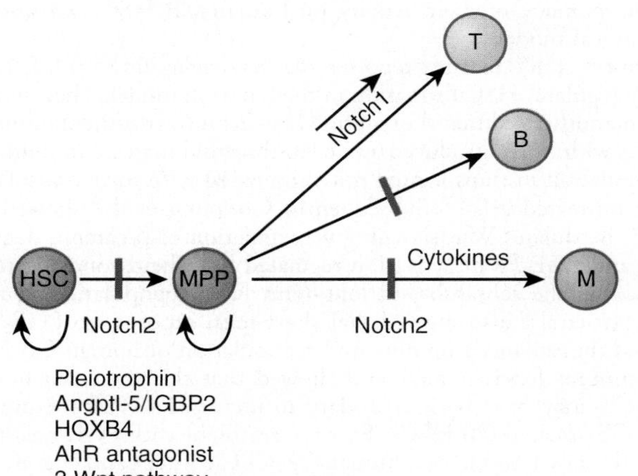

Figure 8-3 MODEL OF NOTCH REGULATION OF HEMATOPOIETIC STEM CELL (HSC) SELF-RENEWAL. Notch2 promotes HSC self-renewal by blocking differentiation into multipotent progenitor cells (MPPs) and the myeloid lineage (M). Notch1 promotes T-cell differentiation and inhibits B-cell differentiation. Molecules and growth factors with proposed roles in regulating HSC self-renewal are also shown. Angptl2, Angiopoietin-like 2; IGBP, insulin-like growth factor binding protein . *(Figure used with permission from American Society of Hematology, Dahlberg A, Delaney C, Bernstein ID: Ex vivo expansion of human hematopoietic stem and progenitor cells.* Blood *117:6083, 2011.)*

Wnt Signaling

Several lines of evidence implicate Wnt signaling in the regulation of HSC self-renewal and differentiation. First, Wnt proteins have been shown to be expressed at sites of fetal hematopoiesis, and the Wnt-responsive transcription factors, LEF/TCF, are expressed by adult HSCs.[185-187] Using BM from bcl2 transgenic mice,[188] Willert et al[189] showed that treatment of BM c-kit+Thy1.1losca-1+lin− (KTLS) cells with purified Wnt3a protein differentially maintained cells in culture capable of providing multilineage reconstitution in competitively transplanted recipient mice. Reya et al[187] showed that retroviral-mediated overexpression of the active form of β-catenin, a transcriptional co-regulator which mediates Wnt signaling, in BM KTLS cells from bcl2 transgenic mice resulted in expansion of HSCs capable of multilineage reconstitution in competitively transplanted mice. Furthermore, these investigators showed that overexpression of β-catenin caused upregulation of HoxB4 and Notch 1 in HSCs, suggesting cross-talk between these pathways in regulating HSC self-renewal.[187] In vivo activation activation of Wnt signaling via systemic administration of Wnt5a was also shown to induce a greater than threefold increase in human hematopoietic progenitor cell repopulation in NOD/SCID mice.[190] Of note, no effect of Wnt5a was observed on the ex vivo expansion of human HSCs.[190] Nemeth et al[191] reported that treatment of murine HSCs with Wnt5a inhibited canonical Wnt signaling and maintained HSC repopulating activity in culture via inhibition of HSC cycling. In a related study, culture of human CB cells with an inhibitor of glycogen synthase kinase–3b (GSK-3B), which antagonizes Wnt signaling, failed to expand CB HSCs in culture but did improve CB engraftment in immune-deficient mice when delivered in vivo.[192] Interestingly, although activation of Wnt signaling can induce HSC expansion, it is uncertain whether Wnt signaling is indispensable for normal hematopoiesis to occur. Cobas et al[193] demonstrated that conditional deletion of β-catenin had no significant effect on hematopoiesis in an MxCre-loxP mouse model. Conversely, Zhao et al[194] reported that conditional deletion of β-catenin in VavCre mice caused a deficiency in both HSC growth and maintenance in vivo. The differences observed in these studies may have reflected the different mouse models because administration of polyI-polyC, as required in the MxCre model, can cause HSC toxicity.[195] However, Kirstetter et al[196] also reported that activation of the canonical Wnt pathway under control of the ROSA26 locus led to exhaustion of the HSC pool in vivo. These results raise the possibility that the prior report of HSC expansion in response to retroviral-mediated overexpression of β-catenin may have been affected by the use of bcl-2 transgenic mice.[187] Nonetheless, the abundance of evidence suggests that activation of Wnt signaling is capable of promoting HSC expansion *in* vitro and perhaps in vivo.[185,187,189-191] Importantly, Duncan et al[197] demonstrated that Wnt-mediated maintenance of the HSC pool depended on intact Notch signaling, suggesting a deterministic role for the Notch pathway in controlling the effects of Wnt signaling on the undifferentiated HSC pool.[185]

Smad Signaling Pathway

The Smad pathway represents a signaling mechanism that can be activated by members of the transforming growth factor-β (TGF-β) superfamily and bone morphogenetic proteins.[1,185] TGF-β has strong antiproliferative effects on HSCs, and deletion of TGF-β releases HSCs from quiescence.[198-201] It has been suggested that TGF-β mediates cell cycle inhibition of HSCs via upregulation of cyclin dependent kinase inhibitors, p21 and p57, and downregulation of cytokine receptors.[185,202-209] The role of TGF-β as a negative regulator of hematopoiesis is further supported by the observation that deletion of TGF-β1 causes augmented myelopoiesis in mice.[185,210] Conversely, TGF-β type 1 receptor null mice display normal HSC self-renewal and regeneration in vivo.[185,211,212] These differences between the in vitro activity of TGF-β and in vivo phenotype may reflect activities of other ligands (e.g., activin), which can also signal through the Smad pathway.[185]

The bone morphogenetic protein 4 (BMP4), which also signals through the Smad pathway, has been shown to have an essential role in regulating hematopoietic development across different species.[185,213-215] BMP4 has been shown to modulate adult human HSC maintenance and proliferation in culture in a concentration-dependent manner[216] but does not induce significant proliferation of murine HSCs in vitro.[217] Studies by Bhardwaj et al[218] suggest an intersection between BMP4 and hedgehog signaling in the hematopoietic system. Hedgehog proteins, similar to BMPs, regulate the formation of the early mesoderm and specify several nonhematopoietic tissues during development.[219-222] In humans, there are three hedgehog proteins: Sonic hedgehog, Indian hedgehog, and Desert hedgehog.[218,223,224] Bhardwaj et al[218] reported that culture of human CB progenitor cells with Sonic hedgehog promoted the expansion of cells capable of multilineage repopulation in NOD/SCID mice. The addition of Noggin, a natural inhibitor of BMP4, blocked the effect of Sonic hedgehog on CB stem cell proliferation in culture, suggesting that BMP4 acts downstream of Sonic hedgehog in regulating human HSC growth.[218] Although these results suggest that hedgehog signaling regulates human HSC growth, it has also been shown that deletion of Smoothened, the downstream effector of Sonic hedgehog signaling, had no effect on HSC content or hematopoiesis in adult mice.[225-227] Similarly, pharmacologic inhibition of hedgehog signaling in adult mice had no effect on hematopoiesis.[227] Last, Gao et al[226] demonstrated that mice with MxCre-driven Smoothened activation displayed no expansion of the HSC pool in vivo. Taken together, these results provide conflicting results as to the role of hedgehog signaling and BMP4 in regulating HSC fate.

Although the role of BMP4 and hedgehog signaling in regulating adult hematopoiesis is not clear, the importance of Smad proteins in regulating HSC self-renewal has been unambiguously demonstrated.[103,185] Using an MxCre model, Smad4, the essential mediator of Smad pathway signaling, was shown to be essential for HSC self-renewal in vivo.[103] Interestingly, retroviral-mediated overexpression of Smad7, an inhibitor of the Smad pathway, also promoted HSC self-renewal in vivo.[228] Taken together, these results have been interpreted to indicate that Smad4 positively regulates HSC self-renewal independently from its role as a mediator of Smad pathway signaling.[185,229] This hypothesis is supported by evidence demonstrating that Smad proteins can activate Wnt signaling, which has been shown to promote HSC expansion.[185,187,229]

NOVEL GROWTH FACTORS FOR HEMATOPOIETIC STEM CELLS

Recently, several novel proteins and small molecules have been reported to promote potent expansion of murine or human HSCs in culture (Table 8-1).[87,230,231] Zhang et al[232] reported the discovery of the proteins, angiopoietin-like 2 (Angptl2) and Angptl3, in a fetal liver stromal cell line and demonstrated that the addition of Angptl2 or Angptl3 to cytokine cultures supported a 24- to 30-fold expansion of human BM cells capable of long-term repopulation in NOD/SCID mice. Subsequently, Zhang et al[233] demonstrated that the addition of Angptl5 and IGFBP2 to the combination of SCF, TPO, and FGF1 supported up to a 20-fold increase in human CB cells capable of 8-week engraftment in NOD/SCID mice. Of note, the receptor for Angptl proteins has not yet been cloned, so the mechanism through which Angptl proteins facilitate HSC expansion remains unknown.[232] Also, because the addition of Angptl 5 and IGFBP2 did not substantially increase total cell expansion compared with SCF, TPO, and FGF1 alone, it remains possible that treatment with Angptl proteins or IGFBP2 may enhance the homing of HSCs in immune-deficient transplant models.[233] Nonetheless, Angptl proteins represent attractive targets for translation into the clinic on the basis of the potency of their activity on human CB HSC expansion in preclinical models.

Table 8-1 Soluble Proteins and Small Molecules that Regulate Hematopoietic Stem Cell Self-Renewal

Growth Factor	Function in HSC Self-Renewal	Reference(s)*
Notch ligands	Sufficient, not necessary	176,177,181-183
Wnt proteins	Sufficient, ? necessary	187,189,193,194
BMPs	? Sufficient, Smad4 necessary	103
SCF	Necessary, not sufficient	230
TPO	Necessary, not sufficient	231
RAR-γ	Necessary	87
Ang-PTL	Sufficient	232,233
PGE_2	Sufficient	234,237
PTN	Sufficient, ? necessary	77,242
AhR antagonist	Sufficient	244

Adapted from Zon L: Intrinsic and extrinsic control of haematopoietic stem cell self-renewal. *Nature* 453:306, 2008, with permission.
AhR, Aryl hydrocarbon receptor; *Ang-PTL*, angiopoietin-like protein; *BMP*, bone morphogenetic protein; *HSC*, hematopoietic stem cell; *PGE_2*, prostaglandin E_2; *PTN*, pleiotrophin; *RAR-γ*, retinoic acid receptor γ; *SCF*, stem cell factor; *TPO*, thrombopoietin.
*References are representative, not all-inclusive.

North et al[234] recently reported that prostaglandin E_2 (PGE_2) positively regulates HSC formation in the zebrafish model. These authors also demonstrated that short-term (1- to 2-hour) treatment of murine HSCs with PGE_2 produced a two- to threefold increase in donor cell repopulation in transplanted mice compared with mice transplanted with untreated cells.[234] Subsequently, Goessling et al[235] showed that PGE_2 modulates Wnt signaling via regulation of β-catenin degradation and PGE_2/Wnt activation regulated both hematopoietic regeneration in the zebrafish and long-term HSC repopulation in mice. Hoggatt et al[236] also showed that short-term exposure to PGE_2 promoted the enhanced homing and repopulation of human CB HSCs in immune-deficient mice and showed that this increased homing capacity may have been secondary to increased CXCR4 expression on PGE_2-treated CB HSCs. Ex vivo treatment with $PGE_2$was subsequently shown to increase human CB CFC content and engraftment capacity after transplant into immune-deficient mice, and PGE_2-treated BM cells were also found to provide more than 1 year of multilineage reconstitution in a non-human primate model.[237] Based on these encouraging results, a phase I clinical trial has been initiated in which 1 unmanipulated CB unit and the progeny of a second CB unit cultured with PGE_2 will be transplanted into adult patients after nonmyeloablative conditioning.[111]

Recently, screening strategies have been successfully used to identify novel growth factors for HSCs. Himburg et al identified pleiotrophin (PTN), a heparin binding growth factor, from a gene expression analysis of human brain-derived endothelial cells (ECs) that support human HSC expansion in vitro.[238-241] Treatment of murine BM HSCs with PTN produced a 1-log expansion of long-term repopulating HSCs in culture, and systemic administration of PTN to irradiated mice caused a 20-fold increase in the recovery of BM LTC-ICs in vivo.[77] Mechanistically, PTN signaling caused the upregulation of PI3k/Akt signaling and Hes1 expression in HSCs, suggesting that activation of these signaling cascades may contribute to PTN-mediated HSC expansion.[77] Recently, these authors reported that mice lacking PTN ($PTN^{-/-}$ mice) had 11-fold less BM HSC content than $PTN^{+/+}$ mice.[242] Subsequently, it was reported that chimeric mice that had deletion of PTN in the BM microenvironment (WT;$PTN^{-/-}$ mice) contained increased LT-HSC content compared with WT;$PTN^{+/+}$ mice, as measured in tertiary and quaternary transplants.[243] Taken together, these results suggest that PTN is a potent mediator of BM HSC expansion and regeneration, but persistent PTN signaling may result in exhaustion of the most primitive HSC pool in vivo.[77,243] Further studies will be necessary to resolve these questions and define the potential therapeutic efficacy of PTN. Boitano et al[244] described a screening approach of more than 100,000 heterocyclic compounds for capacity to maintain human $CD34^+$ cells in 5-day culture. This yielded the discovery of a purine derivative (StemRegenin 1), which was shown to promote the expansion of human CB repopulating cells in vitro.[244] Three-week cultures of human CB $CD34^+$ cells with thrombopoietin, SCF, Flt-3 ligand, interleukin-6 (IL-6), and StemRegenin 1 promoted a 17-fold increase in SCID-repopulating cells compared with the progeny of cultures containing thrombopoietin, SCF, Flt-3 ligand, and IL-6 alone.[244] This purine derivative appears to mediate its effects via inhibition of the aryl hydrocarbon receptor. Aryl hydrocarbon receptors are expressed by HSCs, but the downstream signaling mechanism through which StemRegenin 1 mediates HSC expansion remains unknown.[244]

Methods for Hematopoietic Stem Cell Expansion in Clinical Testing

In addition to the novel preclinical methods to amplify HSCs described earlier, several different approaches to expand human CB HSCs have been tested in early clinical trials. Jaroscak et al[245] tested the combination of flt-3 ligand, a GM-CSF/IL-3 fusion protein, and erythropoietin in a continuous perfusion culture system as a means to expand human CB cells before transplant. Similarly, Shpall et al[246] tested the capacity of stem cell factor, granulocyte colony-stimulating factor (GCSF), and megakaryocyte growth and differentiation factor to expand human CB cells that were then transplanted in adult CB transplant recipients. An alternative approach to cytokine-based expansion of human CB cells was suggested by Peled et al,[247-249] who demonstrated a 159-fold increase in human $CD34^+$ cells in 7-week culture with a copper chelator, tetraethylenepentamine (TEPA), and cytokines. Subsequently, de Lima et al[250] reported the safety and feasibility of culturing human CB cells with TEPA and SCF, flt-3 ligand, IL-6, and thrombopoietin followed by transplantation into patients in a phase I/II clinical trial. Although each of these clinical trials has shown the feasibility of transplanting ex vivo–cultured CB cells, none demonstrated substantial acceleration in hematopoietic cell engraftment in CB transplant recipients compared to historical controls. However, the TEPA plus cytokine strategy is being tested further in a phase II/III study in several countries, including the United States.[111] In addition, de Lima et al recently described a dual CB transplant study in which patients were transplanted with 1 unmanipulated CB unit and the progeny of a second CB unit co-cultured for 14 days with either related donor mesenchymal stromal cells (MSCs) or third-party MSCs supplemented with SCF, Flt-3 ligand, GCSF, and thrombopoietin.[251] The authors reported a 40-fold expansion of $CD34^+$ progenitor cells and a median time to neutrophil engraftment of 15 days.[251] These results compare favorably with historical data regarding the engraftment kinetics of dual CB transplantation in adults and suggest the potential for ex vivo expansion methods to facilitate CB engraftment in adult patients.

HEMATOPOIETIC STEM CELL REGENERATION

Although much is now known about the intrinsic and extrinsic mechanisms that regulate adult HSC self-renewal and differentiation,[1,111,185] the process through which HSCs regenerate after injury (e.g., chemotherapy or radiation) remains less well understood. Successful delineation of the mechanisms that control HSC regeneration has significant therapeutic potential because a large proportion of patients with cancer receive myelosuppressive or myeloablative therapy during the course of their disease. Signaling through the BMP and Wnt signaling pathways has been shown to be necessary for hematopoietic regeneration to occur in zebrafish after sublethal irradiation.[252] These authors further demonstrated that Smad and TCF, the downstream effectors of BMP and Wnt signaling, respectively, couple with master regulators of myeloid and erythroid differentiation (C/EBPα and GATA1) to drive lineage-specific regeneration.[252] In a murine model of hematopoietic injury, Congdon et al[253] showed that Wnt10b expression is increased in BM stromal cells in response to irradiation, and Wnt signaling is activated in BM HSCs after irradiation. Interestingly, in a zebrafish model, activation of Wnt signaling during hematopoietic regeneration is modulated by PGE_2.[235] Wnt reporter activity was responsive to PGE_2 treatment, and the effect of Wnt8 toward enhancing hematopoietic recovery after sublethal irradiation was inhibited by administration of indomethacin, a PGE_2 antagonist.[235] Notch signaling has also been implicated in the regulation of hematopoietic regeneration after stem cell transplantation.[254] Deletion of Notch 2, but not Notch 1, was shown to delay myeloid reconstitution in mice after stem cell transplantation.[254] These data suggest that the BMP, Wnt, and Notch pathways are attractive mechanistic targets for strategies to augment hematopoietic regeneration after myelosuppressive therapy.

Additional signaling pathways have been implicated in regulating hematopoietic regeneration. Deletion of plasminogen (Plg), a fibrinolytic factor, was shown to prevent hematopoietic progenitor cell proliferation and recovery after fluorouracil (5FU)-induced myelosuppression in mice.[255] Conversely, administration of tissue plasminogen activator promoted hematopoietic progenitor cell proliferation and differentiation after myelosuppression, and this effect was dependent on matrix metallopeptidase 9–mediated release of c-kit ligand.[255] Similarly, Trowbridge et al[256] reported that mice that were heterozygous for Patched 1 ($Ptc1^{+/-}$), the receptor for hedgehog, displayed earlier recovery of hematopoiesis after 5FU-induced myelosuppression compared with littermate $Ptc1^{+/+}$ mice. Hedgehog binding blocks Patched 1–mediated inhibition of Smoothened, thereby promoting downstream hedgehog signaling. Therefore, $Ptc1^{+/-}$ mice have enhanced hedgehog signaling, and these results implicate hedgehog signaling as positively regulating short-term hematopoietic regeneration after injury. However, this acceleration in hematopoietic recovery in $Ptc1^{+/-}$ mice occurred at the expense of LT-HSCs, which were exhausted in these mice.[256] Genetic studies have similarly demonstrated that deletion of SHIP (SH2-containing inositol phosphatase, $SHIP^{-/-}$ mice) is associated with increased loss of HSCs in mice after 5FU exposure compared with $SHIP^{+/+}$ mice.[257] In a similar model of 5FU-mediated myelosuppression, Nemeth et al[258] reported that mice deficient in the high-mobility group 3 (HMGB3) DNA binding protein exhibited more rapid recovery of phenotypic HSCs compared with wild-type mice. The enhanced recovery of the stem/progenitor pool in HMGB3-deficient mice was associated with activation of Wnt signaling, suggesting that activation of the Wnt pathway may accelerate HSC recovery after myelosuppression. Of note, overexpression of the signal transducer and activator of transcription 3 (STAT3) in HSCs increases their regenerative capacity after transplant into lethally irradiated mice.[259] In this study, it was not determined whether alteration in STAT3 expression affected HSC regeneration after myelosuppression (e.g., 5FU or irradiation).[259]

At the cellular level, increasing evidence suggests an important role for BM ECs in promoting hematopoietic regeneration after myelotoxic stress.[260-263] Genetic deletion or antibody-based inhibition of vascular endothelial growth factor receptor 2 (VEGFR2), which is expressed by sinusoidal BM ECs, was shown to delay both BM vascular and hematopoietic recovery after total-body irradiation (TBI).[260] Systemic infusion of syngeneic or allogeneic ECs has also been shown to significantly accelerate the recovery of both the HSC pool and overall hematopoiesis in mice after high-dose TBI.[261,264] Salter et al[261] and Butler et al[265] further demonstrated that hematopoietic regeneration after irradiation is dependent on vascular endothelial (VE)-cadherin–mediated vascular reorganization because administration of a neutralizing anti VE-cadherin antibody caused significant delay in hematologic recovery in mice after TBI. The mechanisms through which BM ECs regulate HSC regeneration in vivo remain unclear, but it was recently shown that systemic administration of PTN, a heparin binding protein that is secreted by both BM and brain ECs, causes a rapid increase in recovery of the HSC pool in mice after high-dose TBI.[77] Taken together, these studies suggest that the BM vascular niche may be an important reservoir for the discovery of growth factors and membrane-bound proteins that mediate HSC regeneration.

Lastly, the effect of age on the capacity for HSCs to regenerate after myelosuppressive challenge remains an important question.[266] Not surprisingly, older mice with defects in DNA damage repair mechanisms (nucleotide excision repair, nonhomologous end-joining) and telomere maintenance displayed severe defects in their capacity to reconstitute hematopoiesis after transplantation into lethally irradiated recipient mice compared with age-matched control subjects that retained the DNA repair and telomerase genes.[267] Therefore, therapeutic targeting to accentuate these DNA repair mechanisms may facilitate the recovery of the functional HSC pool after myelosuppression and may lessen the oncogenic risk incurred via repeated exposure to DNA-damaging therapies (e.g., alkylators and irradiation).[267]

GENERATING HEMATOPOIETIC STEM CELLS FROM EMBRYONIC STEM CELLS AND INDUCED PLURIPOTENT STEM CELLS

After the successful isolation of ESCs from both mice and humans, it has been shown that ESCs can be induced to differentiate into tissues representative of all three germ layers, raising the potential for regenerative therapy.[268,269] There has been particular optimism that human HSCs could be generated from ESCs or iPS cells.[268] Indeed, initial studies demonstrated that murine hematopoietic progenitor cells could be generated from murine ESCs in vitro.[46] However, subsequent studies indicated that without further genetic manipulation, hematopoietic progenitor cells generated from murine ESCs lacked complete in vivo multilineage repopulating potential.[268,270,271] To overcome this obstacle, investigators leveraged knowledge from studies of hematopoietic development in the zebrafish and in mice to demonstrate the feasibility of generating HSCs with in vivo repopulating capacity from ESCs and iPS cells.[127,268,272] Cdx and Hox genes were shown to be essential for embryonic blood formation in the zebrafish,[127,268,272] and Cdx gene–deficient murine ESCs displayed impaired hematopoietic potential that could be rescued via ectopic expression of Cdx4.[273] In a complementary study, it was shown that the ectopic expression of Cdx4 in murine ESCs promotes hematopoietic specification and, coupled with HoxB4 expression, increases the multilineage hematopoietic repopulating potential of ESC-derived HSCs as measured in lethally irradiated recipient mice.[274] Subsequently, Lengerke et al[275] demonstrated that hematopoietic specification of murine ESCs is directed by BMP4, which activates Wnt3a and upregulates both Cdx and Hox genes.

With the successful generation of iPS cells from somatic cells via the retroviral introduction of OCT4, SOX2, c-Myc, and KLF4 transcription factors[131-133,135] and the subsequent demonstration that human iPS cells can be generated via coupling of the histone deacetylase inhibitor, valproic acid, with retroviral expression of OCT4 and SOX2,[276] scientists are now poised to generate human HSCs with long-term repopulating capacity from iPS cells.[268,274] Lengerke et al[268] reported that fibroblast-derived human iPS cells can be induced to generate hematopoietic progenitor cells via culture with BMP4 and hematopoietic cytokines. In this study, iPS-derived hematopoietic cells were confirmed via cell surface expression of CD34 and CD45, colony-forming cell content, and expression of hematopoietic-specific genes *(SCL, GATA2)*.[268] However, the authors did not describe whether these human iPS-derived hematopoietic progenitors retained multilineage in vivo repopulating capacity.[268] Tolar et al[277] subsequently demonstrated that human iPS cells could be generated from both keratinocytes and mesenchymal stromal cells from patients with mucopolysaccharidosis type I (Hurler syndrome), and these cells could be induced to develop a hematopoietic phenotype and gene expression profile after culture with BMP4 and hematopoietic cytokines. Taken together, these studies suggest that the generation of HSCs from human iPS cells is at least feasible and provide a conceptual framework for how iPS-derived hematopoietic cells could be used for the autologous correction of hematopoietic disorders.

SUGGESTED READINGS

Antonchuk J, Sauvageau G, Humphries RK: HOXB4-induced expansion of adult hematopoietic stem cells ex vivo. *Cell* 109:39, 2002.

Bertrand JY, Chi NC, Santoso B, et al: Haematopoietic stem cells derive directly from aortic endothelium during development. *Nature* 464:108, 2010.

Bhatia M, Wang JC, Kapp U, et al: Purification of primitive human hematopoietic cells capable of repopulating immune-deficient mice. *Proc Natl Acad Sci U S A* 94:5320, 1997.

Blank U, Karlsson G, Karlsson S: Signaling pathways governing stem-cell fate. *Blood* 111:492, 2008.

Boitano AE, Wang J, Romeo R, et al: Aryl hydrocarbon receptor antagonists promote the expansion of human hematopoietic stem cells. *Science* 329:1345, 2010.

Calvi LM, Adams GB, Weibrecht KW, et al: Osteoblastic cells regulate the haematopoietic stem cell niche. *Nature* 425:841, 2003.

Cedar H, Bergman Y: Epigenetics of haematopoietic cell development. *Nat Rev Immunol* 11:478, 2011.

Dahlberg A, Delaney C, Bernstein ID: Ex vivo expansion of human hematopoietic stem and progenitor cells. *Blood* 117:6083, 2011.

Delaney C, Heimfeld S, Brashem-Stein C, et al: Notch-mediated expansion of human cord blood progenitor cells capable of rapid myeloid reconstitution. *Nat Med* 16:232, 2010.

Gerrits A, Walasek MA, Olthof S, et al: Genetic screen identifies microRNA cluster 99b/let-7e/125a as a regulator of primitive hematopoietic cells. *Blood* 2011.

Guo S, Lu J, Schlanger R, et al: MicroRNA miR-125a controls hematopoietic stem cell number. *Proc Natl Acad Sci U S A* 107:14229, 2010.

Himburg HA, Muramoto GG, Daher P, et al: Pleiotrophin regulates the expansion and regeneration of hematopoietic stem cells. *Nat Med* 16:475, 2010.

Hooper AT, Butler JM, Nolan DJ, et al: Engraftment and reconstitution of hematopoiesis is dependent on VEGFR2-mediated regeneration of sinusoidal endothelial cells. *Cell Stem Cell* 4:263, 2009.

Kiel MJ, Yilmaz OH, Iwashita T, et al: SLAM family receptors distinguish hematopoietic stem and progenitor cells and reveal endothelial niches for stem cells. *Cell* 121:1109, 2005.

Morrison SJ, Weissman IL: The long-term repopulating subset of hematopoietic stem cells is deterministic and isolatable by phenotype. *Immunity* 1:661, 1994.

North TE, Goessling W, Walkley CR, et al: Prostaglandin E2 regulates vertebrate haematopoietic stem cell homeostasis. *Nature* 447:1007, 2007.

Notta F, Doulatov S, Laurenti E, et al: Isolation of single human hematopoietic stem cells capable of long-term multilineage engraftment. *Science* 333:218, 2011.

Osawa M, Hanada K, Hamada H, et al: Long-term lymphohematopoietic reconstitution by a single CD34-low/negative hematopoietic stem cell. *Science* 273:242, 1996.

Park IH, Zhao R, West JA, et al: Reprogramming of human somatic cells to pluripotency with defined factors. *Nature* 451:141, 2008.

Prohaska SS, Weissman I: Biology of hematopoietic stem and progenitor cells. In Appelbaum F, Forman S, Negrin R, et al, editors: *Thomas' Hematopoietic Cell Transplantation,* United Kingdom, 2008, Wiley-Blackwell, p 36.

Purton LE, Scadden DT: Limiting factors in murine hematopoietic stem cell assays. *Cell Stem Cell* 1:263, 2007.

Reya T, Duncan AW, Ailles L, et al: A role for Wnt signalling in self-renewal of haematopoietic stem cells. *Nature* 423:409, 2003.

Salter AB, Meadows SK, Muramoto GG, et al: Endothelial progenitor cell infusion induces hematopoietic stem cell reconstitution in vivo. *Blood* 113:2104, 2009.

Takahashi K, Yamanaka S: Induction of pluripotent stem cells from mouse embryonic and adult fibroblast cultures by defined factors. *Cell* 126:663, 2006.

Till JE, McCulloch EA: A direct measurement of the radiation sensitivity of normal mouse bone marrow cells. *Radiat Res* 14:213, 1961.

Trowbridge JJ, Snow JW, Kim J, et al: DNA methyltransferase 1 is essential for and uniquely regulates hematopoietic stem and progenitor cells. *Cell Stem Cell* 5:442, 2009.

Varnum-Finney B, Brashem-Stein C, Bernstein ID: Combined effects of Notch signaling and cytokines induce a multiple log increase in precursors with lymphoid and myeloid reconstituting ability. *Blood* 101:1784, 2003.

Wang Y, Yates F, Naveiras O, et al: Embryonic stem cell-derived hematopoietic stem cells. *Proc Natl Acad Sci U S A* 102:19081, 2005.

Zhang CC, Kaba M, Ge G, et al: Angiopoietin-like proteins stimulate ex vivo expansion of hematopoietic stem cells. *Nat Med* 12:240, 2006.

Zon LI: Intrinsic and extrinsic control of haematopoietic stem-cell self-renewal. *Nature* 453:306, 2008.

For complete list of references log on to www.expertconsult.com.

CHAPTER 9

HEMATOPOIETIC MICROENVIRONMENT

Lev Silberstein and David Scadden

EVOLUTION OF THE NICHE CONCEPT

In 1868, Ernest Neumann first suggested that blood cells are being replenished throughout postnatal life, and this proposal led to the attempts to localize the place of hematopoiesis.[1] His proposal that blood cell production takes place in the bone marrow (BM) was experimentally validated by selective lead shielding of limbs in irradiated animals almost a century later.[2] Notably, these and other studies showed that differentiation pathways of immature blood cells are determined by their location and are different between the spleen and the BM.[3] Based on this difference between BM and spleen, Schofield first proposed that there is a specialized place or niche where stem cells reside and are governed. He succinctly proposed in 1978 that "stem cell is seen in association with other cells which determine its behavior."[4] Stem cells reside in a defined microanatomic site and respond to local and systemic signals.

Trentin further clarified how different sites affected hematopoietic stem cell (HSC) differentiation.[5] Although both spleen and marrow support multiple cell lineages (erythropoietic and granulocytopoietic, for example), the ratios of differentiating cells were different—spleen favored erythropoiesis, but BM predominantly supported granulopoiesis. This controlling influence of the "stroma" was further illustrated by implanting BM stroma into the spleen and showing that hematopoietic cells abruptly changed showed that abrupt change from erythropoiesis to granulopoiesis at the spleen–BM demarcation. These observations suggest that immature differentiating progenitors require interactions with specific other cell types in a defined *micro*environment.

Niches are not static, however. Although HSCs migrate in early development and throughout adult life, so do the niches that support their dynamic ability change in function and in number. For example, the niche has to have the ability to respond to stress signals from the sympathetic nervous system or granulocyte colony-stimulating factor (G-CSF) and control the exit of hematopoietic cells from the bone marrow to the peripheral blood.[6] Moreover, the niches can be created anew in the context of disease and development. Therefore, a proper functioning of the hematopoietic system can be achieved through the ability of the niche not only to maintain the resident pools of functional cells but also respond to physiologic need.

This chapter reviews the current knowledge of the hematopoietic microenvironment during development and in postnatal life, with a particular focus on recent in vivo data. The chapter also reviews the evidence for the contribution of the microenvironment toward development and maintenance of leukemia and myelodysplasia and the opportunities for therapeutic manipulation of the niche in the treatment of these disorders. For the related topics on stem cell mobilization, hematopoietic cytokines and the role of microenvironment in lymphoid malignancies, plasma cell disorders, and myeloproliferative conditions, readers are referred to other chapters of this book.

HEMATOPOIEITIC MICROENVIRONMENT DURING DEVELOPMENT

In mammals, hematopoiesis during development takes place in distinct extra-embryonic and embryonic sites. Sequentially, it moves from the yolk sac to the aorta-gonad-mesonephros (AGM) region, fetal liver, placenta, and bone marrow (for details, see Chapter 8).

The first definitive adult HSCs emerge from the floor of the dorsal aorta, more precisely from AGM region in midgestation mouse embryo, and the HSC clusters appear in close association with the aortic endothelium.[7] Recent reports indicate that phenotypically defined HSCs (Sca1+ c-kit + CD41+) arise directly from ventral aortic endothelial cells and that fluid shear stress may be important for this process.[8,9] Although direct cellular interactions during hematopoietic stem cells (HSCs) emergence in the embryo remain to be dissected, bone morphogenetic protein 4 (BMP4), fibroblast growth factor (FGF), transforming growth factor (TGF), and vascular endothelial growth factor (VEGF)-Flk1 signaling pathways are involved in early mouse hematopoiesis.[10,11]

Recently, placenta has been identified as a hematopoietic organ during development.[12] Placenta is known to produce hormones that influence vascularization and therefore may affect blood cell production because hematopoiesis and vasculogenesis are tightly coupled.[13] The hematopoiesis-promoting factors may be either produced by the placental trophoblast cells or enter via maternal circulation. Hematopoietic progenitors appear in the placenta at E9, but their number declines by E13. The cells and local factors providing placental hematopoietic support are currently unknown, but mesenchymal/stromal cells have been suggested as candidates. Placental microenvironment is thought to be geared toward supporting the expansion or maturation of HSCs without their concomitant differentiation.

In the fetal liver, the HSCs are first detected on day 9 of mouse embryonic development, and large expansion of the HSCs occurs between days 12 and 15 before migration to the bone on day 18. Stromal cell lines obtained from the fetal liver are able to support primitive hematopoietic cells in ex vivo cultures.[14,15] Some of these cells (termed *myelosupportive stroma*) are able to differentiate in vitro into mesenchymal components (osteoblasts, chondrocytes, and adipocytes).[10] Although the nature of fetal liver cells participating in the HSC niche remains enigmatic, recent studies point to a nonhematopoietic hepatic population that express Dlk-1, a member of delta-like family of cell surface transmembrane proteins, and stem cell factor, and can be prospectively isolated based on the expression of these molecules.[16] These cells express angiopoietin ligand 3 and CXCL12, and in combination with stem cell factor, thrombopoietin, FGF1 and FGF2, and either angiopoietin ligand 2 or 3 are able to produce more than 30 expansion of the murine HSCs in culture.

Despite the differences in the hematopoietic microenvironment between the sites of fetal and adult hematopoiesis, the key components of the molecular milieu are likely to be shared, as evidenced by successful (although limited) engraftment of HSCs across developmental barriers. For example, AGM- or fetal liver–derived HSCs are able to engraft in the adult BM. Notably, they have a competitive advantage over their BM-derived counterparts, with the long-term repopulating ability exceeding that of the BM by five-fold.[17] Vice versa, BM HSCs engraft in fetal liver when transplanted in utero, although at low efficiency (<5% for the whole BM and 0.43% for highly enriched HSCs), which may be partly attributable to the absence of pretransplant conditioning.[18]

Multilineage hematopoiesis during development occurs largely by the virtue of sequential HSC migration from the AGM region to the fetal liver and the BM, as opposed to de novo HSC generation.[19,20] Failure of migration to the "next niche," as exemplified by the targeted disruption of the guanine-nucleotide–binding protein stimulatory α-subunit (GS-α), calcium-sensing receptor, or CXCL12/CXCR4 axis (discussed in detail in Chapter 11 on HSC migration) leads to severe impairment in hematopoiesis.[21-23] This suggests even in the absence of cell-intrinsic HSC defects, proper progression of blood cell production throughout developmental critically depends on the ability of the HSC to sequentially move to the appropriate microenvironmental compartments.

ADULT BONE MARROW MICROENVIRONMENT

Hematopoietic Stem Cell Niches

In mammals, BM is a major site of hematopoiesis throughout life. Over the recent years, animal studies revealed tremendous complexity in cellular and molecular organization of the HSC BM niche (Fig. 9-1). In evaluating the results of these studies, it is important to be aware of formidable experimental challenges in the field, as outlined below. These account for inherent limitations to our knowledge and often generate considerable controversies.

First, the HSC niche is a dynamic entity. However, the majority of current experimental approaches are not suitable for adequately capturing cell interactions within the niche in real time. This problem is being gradually circumvented by in vivo imaging studies (see below), although they are limited to providing a largely descriptive picture of the niche.

Second, current studies are mainly focused on the "conditioned" niches, usually by total-body irradiation (TBI), in a transplant model. The HSC niches can be identified in vivo only spatially (i.e., on the basis of co-localization between a nonhematopoietic "niche cell" and an HSC). However, endogenous HSCs are extremely rare (1 : 10,[5]

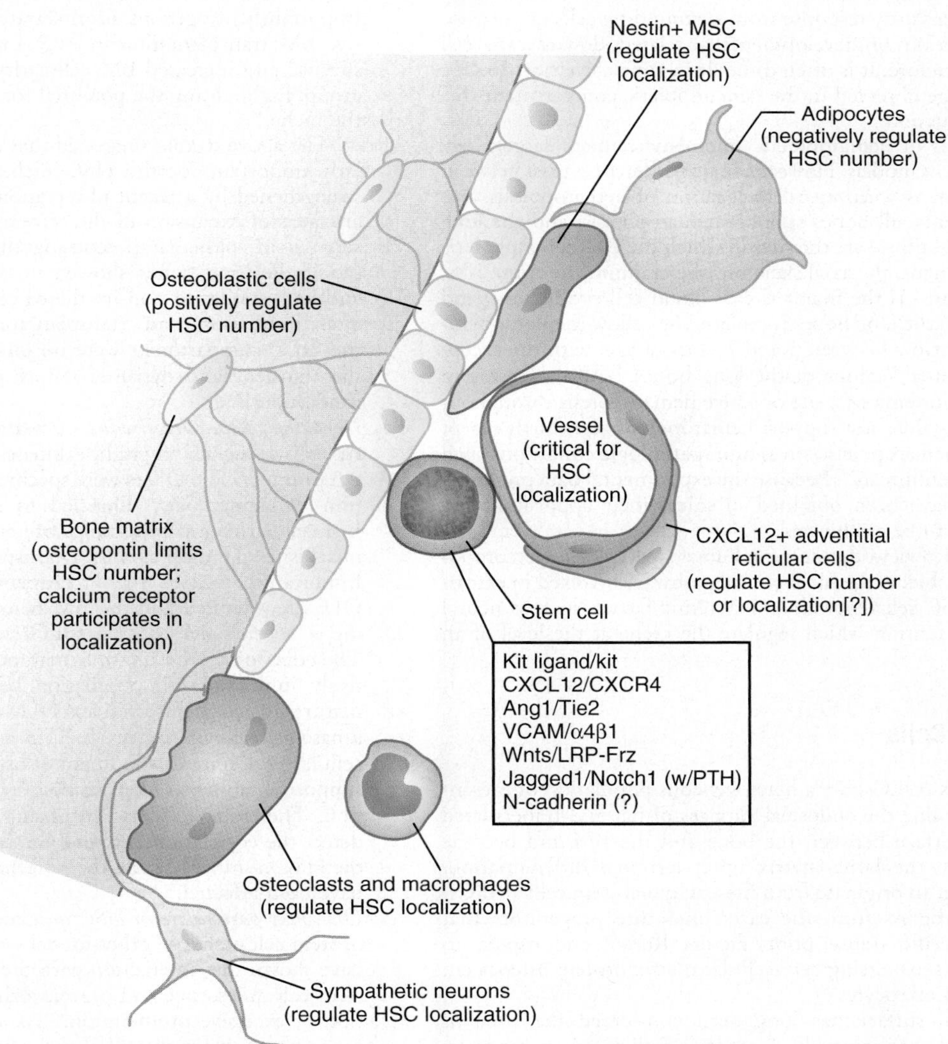

Figure 9-1 BONE MARROW HEMATOPOIETIC NICHE COMPONENTS TO DATE. *Ang1,* Angiopoietin-like 1; *HSC,* hematopoietic stem cell; *MSC,* mesenchymal stem cell.

nucleated cells)[24] and lack reliable markers for visualization in normal tissues with the same specificity as they can be isolated from the BM by fluorescence-activated cell sorting (FACS). Therefore, the vast majority of studies that focused on the HSC niche do so by injecting highly purified FACS-sorted HSCs into an animal recipient. This approach has the advantage of standardized and homogeneous input HSC and progenitor population but involves conditioning of the recipient niche, usually by TBI. Irradiation has a profound effect on the BM microenvironment.

For example, irradiation largely destroys the vascular compartment[25] and is also able to make the niche more "receptive" to HSCs; post-irradiation increase of CXCL12, a major HSC chemoattractant, is well documented.[26] In addition, irradiation increases the number of available niches, which is limited under physiologic conditions; transplantation of the BM into nonconditioned recipient in both neonatal[27] and adult mice results in a very low level of chimerism (0.1.%), suggesting that "empty" niches that are made vacant by circulating HSCs can be saturated. Interestingly, these niches can be "emptied" by using a cytotoxic antibody against HSC surface molecule c-kit, and the level of engraftment increases proportionally to the number of transplanted HSCs.[28] Thus, "conditioned" niches are likely to be different from those that exist under physiologic conditions, both in quality and number, and the effect of these factors on experimental readout is unknown.

Third, an important caveat inherent to those experimental systems, which use genetic tools to either increase or delete a target cell population within the niche, is that these manipulations often produce a compensatory response from surrounding cells or are associated with deletion of developmentally related downstream cell populations. Therefore, it is often difficult to conclusively attribute a phenotypic change observed in the hematopoietic compartment to a specific cell population.

Finally, studies of hematopoietic microenvironment largely rely on the use of rodent models. However, major differences exist between rodents and humans with regard to location of hematopoiesis. For example, in rodents, all bones support hematopoiesis, and the long bones (femurs and tibias) are the sites in which the BM hematopoiesis is studied. In humans, the axial skeleton (the cranium, sternum, ribs, vertebra, and ilium) is the major site of blood cell production, and the red marrow in the long bones is replaced by yellow (hematopoietically inactive) marrow between 5 and 7 years of age, with the exception of the proximal regions of the long bones.[29] Also, whereas in rodents, the spleen remains a site of active hematopoiesis throughout life, in humans, it does not support hematopoiesis after birth except for the times of hematopoietic stress or in pathologic conditions such as idiopathic myelofibrosis.[30] Because the experimental data presented in this section have been obtained in mice, their applicability to humans remains to be established.

Here, we will review the current knowledge of cellular components of the HSC niche, the biochemical pathways involved in extrinsic control of HSC self-renewal, and systemic factors such as neural input or oxygen tension which regulate the niche at the level of an organism.

Osteolineage Cells

Osteolineage cells (OLCs) are a heterogeneous population of mesenchymal cells that line the endosteal surfaces of flat and trabeculated bones at the interface between the bone and the BM and become embedded within the bone matrix upon terminal differentiation. OLCs are thought to originate from mesenchymal stem cells (MSCs) and gradually progress from the early immature progenitors that express OLC-specific transcription factors Runx2 and osterix to mature osteoblasts expressing extracellular matrix protein osteocalcin and eventually to osteocytes.[31]

The endosteal surface has long been considered the zone in which HSCs are preferentially located.[32] Failure to engage the endosteal niche, as seen in animals with homozygous deletion of Ca-sensing receptor, leads to a marked reduction of the HSC pool,[23] and augmented lodgement at the endosteal surface because of pharmacologic stimulation of the same receptor leads to enhanced HSC engraftment.[33] It therefore seems intuitive that OLCs influence hematopoiesis. Indeed, both mouse and human OLCs have been shown to produce hematopoietic growth factors (GCSF, granulocyte-macrophage colony-stimulating factor [GM-CSF], and others) and stimulate proliferation of hematopoietic cells in vitro.[34,35] Several lines of recent in vivo evidence also argue in favor of a functional role of the OLCs in the HSC niche.

1. *Activation of OLCs increases HSC pool size.* Two simultaneously published studies used genetically modified OLCs to show that increase in number of activated OLCs leads to a corresponding increase in the number of long-term HSCs. In one, the OLCs and other cells in the microenvironment harbored a deletion in the bone morphogenic protein receptor 1A, which resulted in ectopic formation of trabecular bone area and correlated with a twofold increase in the number of HSCs, both by immunophenotypic and functional assays.[36] In the other study, the OLCs specifically expressed a constitutively activated form of the parathyroid hormone–related peptide receptor (PPR).[37] Similar to the other model, these animals had an increased trabecular bone area and an elevated number of trabecular osteoblasts that expressed the Notch ligand Jagged 1 and displayed a twofold increase in HSCs. This effect was abolished in the absence of osteopontin, an extracellular matrix protein produced by the OLCs, thus shown to negatively control the HSC pool size.[38] Importantly, exogenous administration of PTH after myeloablative BM transplantation in PPR animals significantly improved survival and increased BM cellularity compared with the control group, highlighting the potential for therapeutic manipulation of the niche.[39]

   The above studies suggested that trabecular OLCs are particularly important for the HSC niche function. This notion was strengthened by a recent observation that after irradiation, there are areas of expansion of the trabecular OLC population, which serve as sites of hematopoietic engraftment.[40] OLCs in the epiphyses of the long bones showed no visible proliferative response and look similar to non-irradiated controls. Remarkably, 10 days after irradiation and transplantation, the above changes in the OLC compartment were no longer detectable, underscoring the transient and dynamic nature of the OLC niche in post-irradiation BM.
2. *Depletion of the OLCs reduces hematopoiesis.* Using a suicide gene strategy in which thymidine kinase was driven by the collagen 2.3 promoter, the OLCs were specifically deleted after administration of gancyclovir.[41] This led to a marked reduction in the BM cellularity and appearance of hematopoiesis in the extramedullary sites, arguing against a nonspecific toxicity of ganciclovir. Importantly, after the treatment was discontinued, the OLCs regenerated and the BM hematopoiesis returned, suggesting a specific role of the OLCs within hematopoietic niche. The effect of the OLCs on hematopoiesis was restricted to a relatively immature cell population because depletion of a more mature (osteocalcin-positive) OLC using the same thymidine kinase/ganciclovir strategy had no appreciable effect on the BM cellularity despite development of osteoporosis.[42] Thus, the HSC-supporting ability is likely to be restricted to a specific OLC fraction. Therefore, it is not surprising that some studies failed to detect the correlation between OLC deletion and expansion and the HSC number because the "effector" OLC population may not have been affected.[43,44]
3. *OLC may participate in HSC quiescence and mobilization.* Studies of stem cell niches in other model systems (e.g., *Drosophila* testis) have shown that interaction with the niche is necessary to induce stem cell quiescence and prevent exhaustion through differentiation or excessive proliferation.[45] As already mentioned, a similar niche function for the HSC niche was proposed by Schofield in his original conception of the niche and found experimental support in several in vivo studies aimed at identifying the

molecular mediators of HSC-OLC cross-talk. In the experiments using OLC-specific expression of the paninhibitor of canonical Wnt signaling Dickkopf1 (Dkk1), HSCs were found to have increased cycling and progressive loss of regenerative function.[46] These results contradict the work with pharmacologic doses of Wnt3a in vitro,[47] suggesting the importance of dose and cell context for the Wnt effects. Another OLC-derived inhibitor of HSC proliferation is angiopoietin 1, which interacts with receptor thyrosine kinase Tie-2 to induce HSC quiescence, and this interaction protects HSCs from myelosuppressive stress.[48] Similarly, OLC-secreted thrombopoietin increases the number of quiescent HSCs by acting through its receptor c-mpl, although when administered exogenously, its effect is transient.[49a] Given that both angiopoietin 1 and thrombopoietin can be produced by other cell types, these studies provide only indirect evidence for the OLC involvement in the HSC niche.

OLCs also participate in regulating OSC localization. HSCs egress into blood and return to the BM, a process that forms the basis for clinical peripheral blood stem cell collection for transplantation. After administration of GCSF, the OLCs in the trabecular bone adapt a flattened morphology with short projections, associated with HSC egress from the niche.[6] Also, in studies in which mature OLCs were deleted from bone, GCSF was not able to induce HSC mobilization into the blood.[49b] OLCs therefore have a role in regulation of HSC traffic.

4. *In vivo imaging shows that transplanted HSCs are located adjacent to osteolineage and perivascular cells.* Until recently, our knowledge of HSC microenvironment came from studies that used immunostaining to visualize engrafting HSCs and surrounding cells. However, histologic sections are unable to represent the three-dimensional structure of the BM, making it difficult to capture the spatial relationship between HSCs and other niche components. Moreover, they only provide a static assessment of cell interactions and do not account for the changes that occur within the HSC niche over time.

The advent of two-photon confocal microscopy enables examination of intact tissue at the depth of multiple cell layers (150-μm), and application of this technology to live animal imaging allowed microanatomic analysis of the HSC–OLC interaction in real time[25] (Fig. 9-2). Currently, in vivo imaging is limited to calvarial BM, an area in the mouse skull where the bone is very thin, thus permitting penetration of the laser beam into the BM cavity. Using this technique and simultaneous multicolor fluorescent labeling of OLCs, HSCs, and the vasculature, studies showed that in irradiated recipients, transplanted HSCs home closest to the endosteal surface and individual OLCs compared with more differentiated progenitors, and are "anchored" to their niches at least through 72 hours. Importantly, the endosteal location of transplanted HSCs was observed in animals in which no preconditioning with radiation or chemotherapy was required. Similar results were observed in studies that used comparable techniques to visualize HSC–OLC interactions in the long bones, although performing these experiments in live animals remains a challenge.[50] Although descriptive in nature, imaging studies complement the results of molecular and genetic experiments by bridging the functional role of the OLCs in the niche and their intimate microanatomic relationship with HSCs.

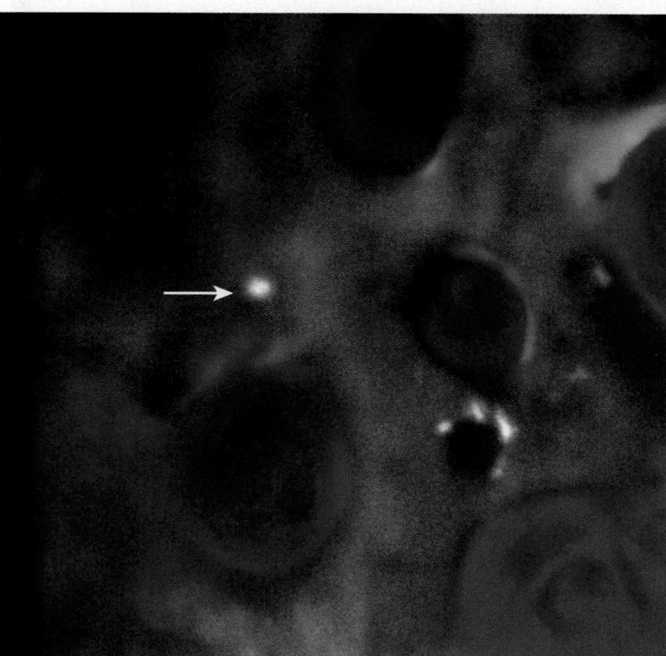

Figure 9-2 IN VIVO IMAGING OF THE HEMATOPOIETIC STEM CELL (HSC) NICHE. Engraftment of single fluorescently labeled HSC *(arrow)* in calvarial bone marrow 1 day after injection into irradiated recipient. *Blue,* bone matrix; *red,* vasculature; *green,* osteolineage cells; *white,* HSC progeny. *(Adapted from Lo Celso C, Fleming HE, Wu JW, et al: Live-animal tracking of individual haematopoietic stem/progenitor cells in their niche.* Nature *457:92, 2009.)*

Endothelial Cells

Endothelial cells are known to secrete hematopoietic cytokines and express several adhesion molecules such as E-selectin, P-selectin, vascular cell adhesion molecule 1 (VCAM-1), and intercellular adhesion molecule 1 (ICAM-1),[51,52] raising the possibility of their involvement in the HSC niche. The existence of vascular niche for the HSCs has been suggested by in vivo imaging studies showing early homing of transplanted BM progenitors to specific subdomains of the vascular tree,[53] as well as by histologic assessment of the BM using CD150 antibody when HSCs were found to be in a close proximity to the BM sinusoids.[24] In vivo evidence delineating the role of vascular endothelium in HSC homeostasis is sparse, and it is therefore possible that close association of HSCs with blood vessels simply reflects their "transit" to and from the marrow as opposed to being indicative of functional interaction. However, observations that selected activation of Akt 1 in endothelial cells promotes expansion of long-term HSC number in vivo suggests that endothelial cells may be involved in modulating the balance between HSC quiescence, self-renewal, and differentiation.[54] Given that OLCs are perivascular,[55] any microanatomic distinction between the vascular and "osteoblastic" niche seems artificial, although it is possible that both cell types make functionally distinct contributions toward HSC homeostasis.

Adipocytes

An observation that adipocyte-rich vertebrae in mice contained significantly fewer cycling HSCs compared with adipocyte-poor thoracic vertebrae led to discovery of their role in HSC regulation.[56] In a genetic mouse model of lipoatrophy (i.e., a condition with reduced adipocyte number), posttransplant hematopoietic recovery was accelerated, although a concomitant increase in trabecular bone could have contributed to this result.

Osteoclasts

Osteoclasts are BM-derived cells that are located in close proximity to stem cell–rich endosteum and play a critical role in bone remodeling. During stress and GCSF-induced mobilization, the activity of the osteoclasts increases and is accompanied by secretion of proteolytic enzymes and reduction in the endosteal niche components, as evidenced by downregulation of the osteopontin expression by the OLCs.[57] Conversely, inhibition of the osteoclasts leads to reduced HSC and progenitor egress.

Nestin-Positive Cells

The BM has long been known as a home for two stem cells—skeletal and hematopoietic. Skeletal stem cells—more commonly known as MSCs—are located in the perisinusoidal space. They are bona fide stem cells because they possess self-renewal capacity and an ability to differentiate into multiple skeletal or stromal tissues—bone, cartilage, and fat.[58] In mice, these cells can be identified through the expression of green fluorescent protein (GFP) under control of the regulatory elements of the intermediate filament protein nestin.[59] Nestin-positive cells receive innervation from sympathetic nervous system and are located in close proximity to endogenous and transplanted HSCs. Nestin-positive cells express the genes associated with HSC retention in the niche (Cxcl12, kit-ligand, and angiopoietin 1), which are downregulated upon GCSF mobilization. Selective deletion of Nestin-positive cells in mice resulted in 50% reduction in the number of long-term HSCs and their relocation to the spleen, although it is not clear whether this effect was mediated directly by Nestin-positive cells or through their more differentiated downstream progeny.

CXCL12-Abundant Reticular Cells

CXCL12 (also known as stromal-derived factor 1) is a major chemokine responsible for HSC trafficking to the BM. CXCL12-abundant reticular cells were identified in a mouse model in which GFP was driven by CXCL12 promoter.[60] Similar to the other components of the niche, CXCL12-abundant reticular (CAR) cells are found in a close proximity to HSCs. It is likely that they are genetically and phenotypically related to Nestin-positive cells because their ablation also severely impaired adipogenic and osteogenic differentiation of nonhematopoietic BM cells in addition to reducing the number of HSCs and increasing HSC quiescence. The effect of deletion was not limited to HSCs but also affected mature lineages, such as lymphoid cells (see below).

Bone Marrow Macrophages

During experiments investigating the mechanisms of GCSF-induced HSC mobilization, it was noted that in addition to previously reported reduction in the endosteal OLCs, BM macrophages were also decreased in number. In vivo depletion of this cell population by clodronate administration produced the same result. It therefore appears that macrophages play a critical role in supporting the OLC niche compartment. A similar role for the macrophages, but with regard to supporting Nestin-positive MSCs, has been suggested by another study that used clodronate-mediated macrophage ablation.[61,62] Again, this resulted in HSC egress from the BM, perhaps through the effect on Nestin-positive cells, which showed a marked downregulation of genes responsible for HSC retention in the niche (see earlier discussion). Thus, macrophages appear to function at a level of regulation upstream of OLCs and Nestin-positive cells.

EXTRINSIC REGULATION OF THE HEMATOPOIETIC STEM CELL NICHE

Innervation

Sensory and autonomic innervation of the BM is critical for its ability to respond to hematopoietic stress. As mentioned above, increase in sympathetic tone promotes HSC mobilization and down-regulates the components of the endosteal niche, mainly through the activation of β_2-adrenergic receptor.[6] Nestin-positive cells express both β_2 and β_3 receptors and act as another mediator between sympathetic signaling and HSCs, again facilitating egress from the BM.[59] In a mouse model of streptozocin-induced diabetes, diabetic autonomic dysfunction was shown to disrupt this regulatory circuit, alter the function of Nestin-positive cells, and lead to impaired GCSF-induced HSC mobilization, providing a biologic explanation for a higher frequency of peripheral blood stem cell mobilization failure in diabetic patients.[49b] The sympathetic nervous system is also involved in regulation of HSC egress from the BM as governed by circadian rhythms, a remarkable discovery based on a chance observation that continuous exposure to light (because of a broken light switch in the animal house) significantly altered the number of HSCs mobilized after GCSF administration.[63] Thus, niche innervation is essential for relaying and integrating extrinsic signals, and acts as a responsive and finely tuned tool, which regulates HSC traffic between peripheral blood and the BM.

Hypoxia

Several studies using the intracellular hypoxic marker pimonidazole have provided indirect evidence that the HSC niche is hypoxic.[64,65] Hypoxia is associated with upregulation of stromal cell–derived factor 1 (SDF-1) expression in the endosteal region and HSC traffic to the BM; in contrast, hyperbaric oxygen (exposure to 100% oxygen under increased atmospheric pressure) mobilizes HSC and progenitors away from the BM.[66,67]

Hypoxic responses in the HSCs are mediated through a family of hypoxia-inducible factors (HIFs). The best studied species of HIFs is HIF1-α, which induces SDF-1 expression and directs metabolic circuits within HSCs toward anaerobic metabolism.[68] HIF1-α also stimulates secretion of VEGF, thereby promoting bone formation and angiogenesis.[69]

What is a physiologic role of hypoxia? Firstly, hypoxia is believed to protect HSCs in the niche from oxidative stress.[70] Indeed, HSCs within the niche contain a lower level of reactive oxygen species. Moreover, it appears that hypoxic conditions are indeed beneficial for the HSC function because culturing human BM HSCs under lower oxygen tension leads to increase in their ability to engraft and repopulate nonobese diabetic/severe combined immune deficient (NOD/SCI) mice.[71] Finally, hypoxia may also protect the HSC pool from exhaustion by promoting cell cycle quiescence.[65] Therefore, manipulating hypoxia within the niche may serve as a powerful strategy to increase the number of self-renewing HSCs or shield them from cytotoxic stress by inducing quiescence.

These observations are in an apparent contradiction with the data suggesting that the HSC niche at the endosteal surface is perivascular and should in theory be highly oxygenated. Whether capillary flow is particularly slow in the sinusoidal networks of the BM vessels, the niche endothelium is highly specialized and allows oxygen diffusion at a very low rate, or BM vasculature has a low baseline level of oxygen is a subject of ongoing investigation.

LYMPHOID NICHES

Bone marrow is the site of *B-cell lymphopoiesis.* Several cell types involved in the HSC niche also participate in formation of the lymphoid niches. Interestingly, B-cell niche counterparts are determined by the maturation stage—whereas OLCs, osteoclasts, and CAR cells are necessary for the less mature stages of development, interleukin-7 (IL-7) secreting cells and sinusoidal endothelial cells are important for more differentiated cells.[72-74] These observations come from targeted deletion of each supporting cell population using genetic means and analyzing the effect on B-cell homeostasis. For example, deletion of the OLCs leads to a considerable decrease in pre-pro and pro-B cells. This process appears to be mediated by the heterotrimeric G protein α subunit because its deletion in the OLCs leads to 60% decrease in the percentage of B-cell precursors in the BM.[75] A similar phenotype is seen upon deletion of CAR cells.[74]

Naïve recirculating B and T cells are located in the perisinusoidal space and co-localize with dendritic cells, which are thought to deliver supportive signals, because as their deletion leads to significant decrease in B-cell number and reduction in IgM production after immunization.[76,77]

Plasma cells are the product of terminal differentiation of B cells after antigen exposure. In vitro and in vivo studies showed that plasma cells receive multiple extrinsic survival signals, including CXCL12, IL-6, BAFF (B-cell activating factor of the TNF family), and APRIL (a proliferation-inducing ligand), which may account for their longevity.[78] Mice deficient in CXCR4 displayed impaired homing of plasmablasts, illustrating the involvement of CXCL12–CXCR4 axis in plasma cell trafficking.[79] Eosinophil- and megakaryocyte-derived APRIL and BAFF appear to regulate the number of plasma cells, which is greatly reduced upon eosinophil or megakaryocyte deletion.[80]

The majority of long-lived *memory T cells* reside in the BM and appear to require a close contact with IL-7 secreting stromal cells to ensure that they remain quiescent in the absence of antigen stimulation.[74] The BM also contains a large proportion of *regulatory T cells,* which have recently been found to exclusively protect HSCs and early progenitors from rejection after allogeneic transplantation, arguing that the endosteal surface act as an immune privileged site.[81]

ERYTHROID NICHES

Erythroblastic islands were first described by a French hematologist Marcel Bessis more than 50 years ago and consist of developing erythroblasts surrounding a central macrophage.[82] They are present in the BM, fetal liver, and the spleen and in in vitro long-term BM cultures. The number of erythroblasts per island ranges from 10 cells observed in sections of rat femur to 5 to 30 erythroblasts seen in human BM. Some islands are located adjacent to the BM sinusoids, and the others are scattered throughout the BM cavity. Within erythroid islands, the macrophage functions as a "nurse cell" providing iron to the developing erythroblasts and phagocytosing the extruded nuclei at the end of erythroid differentiation.

Adhesion between maturing erythroblasts and central macrophage is mediated by several molecules, including erythroblast macrophage protein (Emp via homophilic binding),[83] $\alpha4\beta1$ integrin (VCAM-1),[84] and αv integrin (ICAM-4)[85]; antibody-mediated blockade each of these molecule results in disruption of the islands. The most striking effect is seen with the blockade of Emp, which causes significant increase in proliferation, maturation, and apoptosis of maturing erythroblasts in vitro. Of note, Emp-null fetuses die in utero from severe anemia.[83]

In addition to interaction within macrophages, maturing erythroblasts adhere to extracellular matrix proteins, fibronectin, and laminin for the maturation to proceed. Fibronectin protects erythroblasts from apoptosis, partly through anti-apoptotic bcl-xL, and laminin is thought to localize reticulocytes to sinusoids as the initial step before their release into circulation.[86,87]

MEGAKARYOCYTIC NICHES

Megakaryocytes localize to BM endothelial cells in vivo and release platelets into the marrow intravascular–sinusoidal space or the lung capillaries. Although CXCL12 induces platelet production by megakaryocytes if preceded by migration through endothelial cells, this is not observed in the absence of endothelial cells, suggesting that megakaryocyte interaction with specific molecules present on the endothelial cells is necessary for thrombopoiesis.[88] FGF4 and CXCL12 enhance the interaction of megakaryocytes with endothelial cells and restore thrombopoiesis in mice deficient in thrombopoietin or its receptor c-mpl. Thus, chemokine-mediated localization of megakaryocytes within a specific vascular microenvironment is necessary for their maturation and platelet production.

HUMAN BONE MARROW MICROENVIRONMENT

Because direct mechanistic studies of human BM microenvironment cannot be undertaken, the bulk of our knowledge comes from experiments in xenotransplantation models.[89] These initially involved fetal sheep and heavily irradiated or nude mice as recipients, but only very low level of human hematopoietic engraftment was observed. The discovery of SCID mice led to development of two powerful models. The first, known as SCID-hu mouse, was generated by engrafting human thymus and fetal liver. This model was most informative for the study of human lymphoid development and is still used for testing novel HIV drugs.[90] The second model, hu-SRC (for SCID-repopulating cell), through the pioneering work of John Dick and colleagues,[91] enabled investigation of human HSC engraftment and differentiation. Further modifications of the SCID model led to generation of NOD/SCID–IL2 receptor γ chain knock-out (NSG) strain, which supports robust normal human multilineage (myeloid and lymphoid) hematopoietic engraftment, as well as engraftment of acute myeloid leukemia (AML) and acute lymphoblastic leukemia (ALL) cells from patients.[92] The sensitivity of the transplant assay is further increased by direct intrafemoral injection into the BM cavity[93]; remarkably, in NSG recipients, human hematopoietic engraftment can be detected after intrafemoral transplantation of a single highly purified human HSC.[94] Just as the case in the study of murine microenvironment, the xenotransplantation model has an inherent limitation of requiring conditioning by sublethal irradiation to enable human hematopoietic engraftment.

Similar to mouse HSCs, human HSCs transplanted into mouse recipients also preferentially traffic to the trabecular bone and home next to the endosteal surface.[95] They are guided to their niches by the CXCL12–CXCR4 pathway and cell adhesion molecules such as very late antigen-4 (VLA-4), very late antigen-5 (VLA-5), and lymphocyte function-associated antigen-1 LFA-1; of note, CXCL12 is expressed by human OLCs, mesenchymal stromal, Nestin-positive, and endothelial cells. CD44 and hyaluronic acid cooperate with CXCL12 in human HSC homing.[96] Recent experiments identified $\alpha6$ integrin CD49f as a novel marker for human HSCs, alluding to functional importance of HSC anchorage within BM microenvironment.[94]

The cellular components of the human HSC niche are yet to be identified. One potential candidate is a population of mesenchymal subendothelial cells expressing CD146, which can be prospectively isolated from human BM.[58] These perivascular cells were able to establish both bone and hematopoietic microenvironment upon subcutaneous transplantation; had a documented self-renewal capacity; and produced angiopoietin 1, a cytokine known to induce HSC quiescence. CD271 has been suggested as another marker for human hematopoiesis-supporting mesenchymal population[97]; in addition to CD146+ perivascular cells, it labels CD146-endosteal population, which co-localizes with hematopoietic CD34+ cells in human BM.

The limitations of our knowledge of human hematopoietic microenvironment led to current difficulties in achieving in vitro stem cell expansion using noncell autonomous means despite the potential benefits of doing so, especially in the context of cord blood transplantation when the number of donor cells is small. Although some of the cytokines involved in the maintenance of stem cell pool are known, very few factors that lead to a net increase in the HSC number have been discovered. One of them Sonic hedgehog protein, which has been shown to induce proliferation of primitive human hematopoietic cells when added to highly purified CD34+ CD38- lineage human cells[98]; this effect translated into increased level of progenitor expansion in NOD/SCID mice. The other two molecules are an engineered Notch ligand Delta 1[99] and prostaglandin E_2.[100] The latter molecule was identified in a high-throughput screen in zebrafish and found to enhance murine HSC localization in the BM after brief in vitro exposure to the compound. This resulted in a two- to threefold increase in the number of HSCs compared with control (vehicle-exposed) cells. Current phase 1 studies are in progress to test the efficacy of these molecules for in vitro HSC expansion before cord blood transplantation.

HEMATOPOIEITIC MICROENVIRONMENT IN ACUTE LEUKEMIA AND MYELODYSPLASIA

Given a critical role of hematopoietic microenvironment in safeguarding cellular homeostasis in the BM, it is not surprising that alterations within it—either primary or induced by the presence of malignant cell population—have been proposed to be a contributing factor toward tumor initiation, maintenance, and resistance to treatment. Here, we will summarize recent experimental data, which reveal the role of specific cellular and molecular alterations within microenvironment in the pathogenesis of acute leukemia and myelodysplasia. For the review of this topic in other hematologic neoplasms, readers are referred to disease-specific chapters of this book.

Early in vitro studies alluded to significant contribution of nonhematopoietic BM cells (collectively termed *stroma*) to the pathogenesis of acute leukemia. For example, fibroblastic stromal cells from patients with AML were unable to support normal granulocytic-macrophage colony formation in contrast to those obtained from normal individuals. However, when the stromal cells were tested from patients in remission, they maintained growth of GM colonies similar to normal stroma.[101] Strikingly, when the patients relapsed, this GM colony-supporting ability was lost. In another series of observations, when nonadherent cells from continuous marrow cultures or GM-CSF–dependent progenitor cell lines were co-cultured with mouse stromal cells that had been previously irradiated, they developed factor-independence and multiple distinct karyotypic abnormalities[102]; upon subcutaneous injection, these newly transformed cell lines produced granulocytic monomyeloid tumors that spread to spleen, lymph nodes, and BM. Although by no means definitive, these studies suggested that either the altered stromal cells may contribute to the emergence of leukemia, or leukemia itself may affect the nonhematopoietic compartment. Both of these hypotheses found confirmation in the later studies reviewed below.

The idea of "niche-induced oncogenesis," or contribution of the microenvironment to the emergence of malignant disease, is supported by the clinical observation of donor-induced leukemia.[103] In this condition, which has a reported incidence between 0.12% and 5%, the leukemic clone arises from an apparently normal donor hematopoietic cells after allogeneic BM transplantation. Although the etiology is clearly multifactorial, damage to the BM microenvironment, either because of previous chemotherapy or pretransplant conditioning, may be an important contributing factor. In keeping with this idea, several experimental mouse models illustrate that microenviromental damage, either alone or in conjunction with corresponding molecular lesions in the hematopoietic compartment, can play a critical role in the initiation of malignant disease. The mice with deficiency of phosphatase and tensin homologue (PTEN) both in the microenvironment and HSC developed a myeloproliferative disorder, but PTEN deficiency in HSCs alone did not result in the disease.[104] Similarly, widespread deletion of retinoblastoma protein or retinoic acid receptor led to the development of myeloproliferative disorder, in the latter case purely because of gene deletion in the microenvironment deletion.[105,106] In the most recent study addressing this question, targeted deletion of the micro-RNA processing enzyme Dicer 1 in immature OLCs resulted in development of myelodysplasia and acute leukemia associated with independent complex genetic changes.[107] The effect of Dicer-1 deletion was entirely attributable to the microenvironment because transplantation of Dicer 1-deleted BM into normal microenvironment resulted in reversal of the myelodysplastic phenotype. Remarkably, hematopoietic abnormalities were observed when Dicer-1 was deleted in very immature OLCs (osterix+) but not in those at a more mature differentiation stage (osteocalcin+). Deletion of Scwachman-Diamond-Bodian syndrome gene in immature OLCs recapitulated the key features of the Dicer-1 deletion phenotype and implicated their role of OLCS in its pathogenesis. Taken together, the above data suggest that microenvironment is capable of contributing to dysplasia and possibly leukemogenesis by selecting for abnormal hematopoietic cells. Microenvironment-induced signals are therefore potential therapeutic targets in the setting of myelodysplasia.

In addition to the microenvironment contributing to disordered hematopoiesis, it may be affected by it. It has been shown that primary ALL and AML blasts are able to downregulate CXCL12 expression in the BM, causing the egress of normal CD34+ HSCs from the BM.[108] This process was mediated by the stem cell factor (CSF) secreted by leukemic blasts because neutralization of this cytokine with an antibody reversed the above changes. The "niche-modifying" ability of the leukemic cells in vivo is an area of ongoing investigation because it suggests that the leukemic niche can be molecularly distinct from the normal and therefore therapeutically targeted.

CXCR4 is expressed by LSCs, and the CXCR4–CXCL12 pathway is critical for homing and subsequent adhesion of LCSs to the BM microenvironment.[109,110] Of note, the level of CXCR4 is elevated in patients with AML and is associated with a poor outcome.[111] The presence of Flt3 internal tandem duplication (a poor prognostic factor in AML) is in turn associated with increased CXCR4 expression.[112] Experimentally, treatment of NOD/SCID mice transplanted with primary human AML cells using a neutralizing antibody against CXCR4 reduced the leukemic burden.[110] Follow-up studies confirmed the antileukemic effect of blocking CXCL12–CXCR4 axis using competitive antagonists of CXCR4 (AMD3100 and AMD3254) in mouse models of AML.[113,114] These findings formed the basis for ongoing clinical trials of CXCR4 antagonist AMD3100 (Plerixafor) as a chemosensitizing agent in AML.

Another example of LSC niche dependence is a cell adhesion molecule CD44, which is present on the surface of leukemic cells and interacts with hyaluronan on the endosteal surface. Blocking the interaction between CD44 and hyaluronan using activating CD4 antibody had significant effect on LSC eradication and even cured some mice.[115] The therapeutic effect of the antibody was more marked when it was administered soon after injection of human leukemic cells compared with the animals with established disease, suggesting that it acts predominantly at the stage when LCSs engage their respective niches. It is also possible that some of the effect of the CD44 antibody was attributable to differentiation induction in the LSCs. Nevertheless, this study provided a proof-of-principle demonstration that LSCs interaction with the niche is required for their survival and leukemia progression and thereby raised the potential for targeting therapy.

Other molecular mediators of LSC–microenvironment interaction have also been identified. B4 integrin (also known as very late antigen 4) mediates lodgment of leukemic cells in the BM and interacts with fibronectin to confer resistance to cytosine arabinoside-induced apoptosis.[116] Integrin ligation triggers prosurvival pathways, and the blocking antibody leads to reduction in the level of leukemic burden and a modest prolongation of the lifespan in human AML-transplanted animals. Similar protective role for AML blasts has been observed for β1 and β2 integrins. IL-3 receptor α chain (CD123) also contributes to LSC survival, at least partly through being involved in controlling LSC homing to the BM[117]; CD123 blocking antibody demonstrated considerable antileukemic activity, which was also attributable to promoting immune-mediating destruction of leukemic cells—the idea that has been explored further in the studies of blocking a macrophage-associated molecule CD47 (see below).

Little is known about the cells that make up the leukemic niche and the mechanisms by which they control LSC behavior. Most experiments addressing this question are based on co-localization of transplanted leukemic cells with one of the "niche" cells, which are either fluorescently labeled or morphologically defined. However, to date, no cell ablation experiments have been performed to show a nonredundant role of a particular cell type within a leukemic niche, and given a microanatomic proximity between "niche" cells as discussed above, it is likely that several of them participate in formation of leukemic microenvironment. Currently, there is circumstantial evidence for the role of endothelial cells, OLCs, and macrophages in the leukemic microenvironment.

Endothelial Cells

Increased vascularization is seen in AML, ALL and preleukemic conditions such as myelodysplastic syndrome and myeloproliferative neoplasms. Leukemic blasts and BM microenvironment secrete several angiogenic growth factors such as VEGF, basic FGF, and angiopoietins.[118] Abnormal expression of matrix metalloproteinases, which are involved in regulation of angiogenesis, has also been documented. In vivo imaging studies examining early homing pattern of Nalm-6 ALL cells point to specific vascular subdomains within CD31-positive endothelium, which express CXCR4 and E-selectin and favor the lodgment of leukemic cells.[53] Importantly, these subdomains are shared by normal hematopoietic progenitors, suggesting that leukemic cells outcompete their normal counterparts for the vascular niches during disease progression. Several phase II studies are currently underway to assess the clinical efficacy of inhibition of VGEF–VEGF receptor axis in refractory and resistant AML.[119] It is becoming clear that antiangiogenic agents in leukemia are insufficient as monotherapy, but larger studies and longer follow-up are needed to assess their benefit as a part of multiagent chemotherapy.

Osteolineage Cells

Osteolineage cells are thought to participate in formation of protective leukemic niche and confer cell cycle quiescence and chemoresistance.[120] This would be consistent with the role of OLCs in normal HSC niche, such as induction of quiescence and negative regulation of HSC self-renewal (see earlier discussion). Transplanted human AML LSCs home next to the endosteal surface, and the majority of them remain in the G0 phase of the cell cycle.[121] The endosteal surface serves as the main site of residual disease after administration of cytosine arabinoside. The proportion of cycling LSCs increases after GCSF-induced mobilization, and this has a chemosensitizing effect on the LSCs, resulting in prolongation of survival in AML-engrafted animals treated with a combination of GCSF and cytosine arabinoside compared with cytosine arabinoside alone. However, it is unclear whether this effect is because of a specific LSC-OLC interaction or simply the result of LSC "moving away" from the niche after G-CSF treatment. Further studies are therefore required to more definitively address the role of OLC in microenvironment-influenced sensitivity to chemotherapy.

Macrophages

Bone marrow macrophages are emerging as another key functional component of the leukemic niche because the interaction of signal regulatory protein α (SIRPα) on the macrophages and CD47 on LSCs appears to protect the LSCs from phagocytosis.[122,123] CD47 is more highly expressed on LSCs, is associated with Flt3-ITD mutation, and independently predicts worse prognosis. Mechanistically, CD47 acts as a "do not eat me" signal for the macrophages. Blocking CD47 antibody produces depletion of AML in xenotransplantation models and specific eradication of LSCs. Strikingly, CD47 antibody also demonstrated potent antitumor effect in xenotransplantation models of ALL and non-Hodgkin lymphoma.[124,125]

Hypoxia

Emerging experimental evidence (using the chemical marker of hypoxia pimidazole) suggests that leukemic BM niches are hypoxic and that leukemic cells adapt to hypoxic conditions.[126] Although low oxygen tension within the leukemic niche remains to be directly demonstrated, the findings of overexpression of the key hypoxia-response factor HIF1α in clusters of ALL cells, together with increased angiogenesis and production of VEGF by the ALL blasts support this hypothesis.[127] In several xenograft models, hypoxia-activated dinitrobenzamide mustard, PR-104, prolonged survival of NSG mice engrafted with ALL cell line Nalm-6.[126] Although very preliminary, these important results identify hypoxia as another potential avenue of niche-based antileukemic therapy.

FUTURE DIRECTIONS

Although the concept of specific microenvironment for different hematopoietic compartments was first proposed more than 100 years ago, it was not until recently that the existence of the "niches" has been experimentally proven and the molecular factors involved in cellular interactions have been discovered.

Our current knowledge of the hematopoietic microenvironment has been evolving in parallel and often leading that in other stem cell systems. It appears that fundamental components and molecular pathways are highly conserved among evolutionary diverse species, although their role in specific niches may vary. These include supporting stromal cells secreting soluble molecules regulating stem cell self-renewal (bone morphogenic protein and Wnt signaling), extracellular matrix proteins that serve as stem cell anchors (integrins), blood vessels that are responsible for nutritional support and transit of stem cells in and away from the niche, and neural inputs for integrating signals from different systems. It is therefore likely that future studies in spatial and molecular organization of other stem cell niches will inform the knowledge of hematopoietic niches and vice versa.

With a rapidly increasing number of cell types known to be involved in hematopoietic niches (and the number of different cytokines they produce, which will inevitably follow), it will be important to use a "network" approach—similar to the one used for analysis of transcriptional networks—to understand how these multiple factors act in concert to control location, proliferation, and trafficking of HSCs and more mature cells in the BM. It is possible that these factors work in combinatorial manner, ultimately creating a "niche code" that is designed to suit a specific physiologic situation.[128]

A particularly notable development over the recent years has been our improvement in understanding of the role of microenvironment in initiation and maintenance of malignant disease, although many questions remain. We still know very little about the molecular mediators of "niche-induced oncogenesis" and those involved in microenvironment-induced chemoresistance. Recent advances in xenotransplantation assay using highly immunocompromised mouse strains for the study of normal and leukemic hematopoiesis, together with further molecular insights into biology of leukemic stem cells, will provide an opportunity to address these issues.

Therapeutic manipulation of the hematopoietic microenvironment remains an ultimate goal of ongoing research. Clearly, the effort of the next several years will be focused on translating the wealth of data obtained from the animal models into human biology and the clinic. This work has already started with the clinical trials of ex vivo HSC expansion before cord blood transplantation. A number of clinical trials are also underway to examine the efficacy of niche-directed therapies in hematologic malignancies. Although the animal data suggest that targeting the niche alone is often insufficient to achieve cure, especially in established disease, this approach has been successful in regaining leukemia chemosensitivity to commonly used agents and may become a valuable component of future treatment protocols. Gaining a deeper insight into the molecular distinctions between normal and malignant niches will enable better understanding of "niche competition" between normal and leukemic populations and lead to development of novel approaches based on eradication of leukemic cells and fostering normal hematopoiesis through manipulation of niche-derived signals.

SUGGESTED READINGS

Adams GB, Alley IR, Chung UI, et al: Haematopoietic stem cells depend on Galpha(s)-mediated signalling to engraft bone marrow. *Nature* 459:103, 2009.

Adams GB, Chabner KT, Alley IR, et al: Stem cell engraftment at the endosteal niche is specified by the calcium-sensing receptor. *Nature* 2005.

Arai F, Hirao A, Ohmura M, et al: Tie2/angiopoietin-1 signaling regulates hematopoietic stem cell quiescence in the bone marrow niche. *Cell* 118:149, 2004.

Calvi LM, Adams GB, Weibrecht KW, et al: Osteoblastic cells regulate the haematopoietic stem cell niche. *Nature* 425:841, 2003.

Chasis JA, Mohandas N: Erythroblastic islands: Niches for erythropoiesis. *Blood* 112:470, 2008.

Colmone A, Amorim M, Pontier AL, et al: Leukemic cells create bone marrow niches that disrupt the behavior of normal hematopoietic progenitor cells. *Science* 322:1861, 2008.

Cumano A, Godin I: Ontogeny of the hematopoietic system. *Annu Rev Immunol* 25:745, 2007.

Dominici M, Rasini V, Bussolari R, et al: Restoration and reversible expansion of the osteoblastic hematopoietic stem cell niche after marrow radioablation. *Blood* 114:2333, 2009.

Dzierzak E, Speck NA: Of lineage and legacy: The development of mammalian hematopoietic stem cells. *Nat Immunol* 9:129, 2008.

Ferraro F, Celso CL, Scadden D: Adult stem cells and their niches. *Adv Exp Med Biol* 695:155, 2010.

Fujisaki J, Wu J, Carlson AL, et al: In vivo imaging of Treg cells providing immune privilege to the haematopoietic stem-cell niche. *Nature* 474:216, 2011.

Jaiswal S, Jamieson CH, Pang WW, et al: CD47 is upregulated on circulating hematopoietic stem cells and leukemia cells to avoid phagocytosis. *Cell* 138:271, 2009.

Jin L, Hope KJ, Zhai Q, et al: Targeting of CD44 eradicates human acute myeloid leukemic stem cells. *Nat Med* 12:1167, 2006.

Katayama Y, Battista M, Kao WM, et al: Signals from the sympathetic nervous system regulate hematopoietic stem cell egress from bone marrow. *Cell* 124:407, 2006.

Keith B, Simon MC: Hypoxia-inducible factors, stem cells, and cancer. *Cell* 129:465, 2007.

Kobayashi H, Butler JM, O'Donnell R, et al: Angiocrine factors from Akt-activated endothelial cells balance self-renewal and differentiation of haematopoietic stem cells. *Nat Cell Biol* 12:1046, 2010.

Konopleva MY, Jordan CT: Leukemia stem cells and microenvironment: Biology and therapeutic targeting. *Journal of Clinical Oncology* 5:591, 2011.

Lapidot T, Dar A, Kollet O: How do stem cells find their way home? *Blood* 106:1901, 2005.

Lo Celso C, Fleming HE, Wu JW, et al: Live-animal tracking of individual haematopoietic stem/progenitor cells in their niche. *Nature* 457:92, 2009.

Mazurier F, Doedens M, Gan OI, et al: Rapid myeloerythroid repopulation after intrafemoral transplantation of NOD-SCID mice reveals a new class of human stem cells. *Nat Med* 9:959, 2003.

Mendez-Ferrer S, Lucas D, Battista M, et al: Haematopoietic stem cell release is regulated by circadian oscillations. *Nature* 452:442, 2008.

Mikkola HK, Orkin SH: The journey of developing hematopoietic stem cells. *Development* 133:3733, 2006.

Naveiras O, Nardi V, Wenzel PL, et al: Bone-marrow adipocytes as negative regulators of the haematopoietic microenvironment. *Nature* 460:259, 2009.

North TE, Goessling W, Walkley CR, et al: Prostaglandin E2 regulates vertebrate haematopoietic stem cell homeostasis. *Nature* 447:1007, 2007.

Notta F, Doulatov S, Laurenti E, et al: Isolation of single human hematopoietic stem cells capable of long-term multilineage engraftment. *Science* 333:218, 2011.

Ottersbach K, Dzierzak E: The placenta as a haematopoietic organ. *Int J Dev Biol* 54:1099, 2010.

Raaijmakers MH, Mukherjee S, Guo S, et al: Bone progenitor dysfunction induces myelodysplasia and secondary leukaemia. *Nature* 464:852, 2010.

Sacchetti B, Funari A, Michienzi S, et al: Self-renewing osteoprogenitors in bone marrow sinusoids can organize a hematopoietic microenvironment. *Cell* 131:324, 2007.

Sipkins DA, Wei X, Wu JW, et al: In vivo imaging of specialized bone marrow endothelial microdomains for tumour engraftment. *Nature* 435:969, 2005.

Suda T, Takubo K, Semenza GL: Metabolic regulation of hematopoietic stem cells in the hypoxi niche. *Cell Stem Cell* 9:298, 2011.

Visnjic D, Kalajzic Z, Rowe DW, et al: Hematopoiesis is severely altered in mice with an induced osteoblast deficiency. *Blood* 103:3258, 2004.

For complete list of references log on to www.expertconsult.com.

CHAPTER 10

CELL ADHESION

Rodger P. McEver and Francis W. Luscinskas

Cell adhesion is essential for the development and maintenance of multicellular organisms. Cell-to-cell and cell-to-matrix adhesion provide a mechanism for intercellular communication and to define the architecture of organs. The regulated nature of cell adhesion is particularly evident in the hematopoietic system, where blood cells routinely make transitions between nonadherent and adherent phenotypes during differentiation and in response to stimuli in the circulation or extravascular tissues.

In the bone marrow (BM), hematopoietic stem cells reside in a specialized microenvironment called the *stem cell niche,* and their proliferation and differentiation are controlled not only by soluble growth factors but also by adhesion to stromal cells and matrix molecules. Weakening of these adhesive interactions is required for mature blood cells to enter the circulation. Circulating erythrocytes normally remain nonadhesive until they are finally cleared by the reticuloendothelial system. Other circulating blood cells often participate in regulated adhesive events during their lifespan. For example, prothymocytes adhere to components of the thymus, where they undergo further maturation before reentering the circulation. T cells regularly stick to the specialized high endothelial venules of lymphoid tissues, migrate into these tissues for sampling of processed antigens, and then exit via the lymphatics. During inflammation, specific classes of leukocytes roll at very low velocity on the endothelium that line all blood vessels, then adhere more tightly, and finally emigrate between endothelial cells into the tissues. There, neutrophils and monocytes phagocytose invading pathogens, and lymphocytes adhere to antigen-presenting cells such as dendritic cells, B cells, and macrophages. During hemorrhage, platelets stick to exposed subendothelial matrix components, spread, and recruit additional platelets into large aggregates that serve as an efficient surface for thrombin and fibrin generation. Leukocytes also adhere to activated platelets and to other leukocytes, and platelets roll on the endothelium. When activated, endothelial cells increase expression of molecules that affect the adhesiveness of platelets or leukocytes. Tight contacts between adjacent endothelial cells also regulate access of blood cells to the underlying tissues.

ADHESION MOLECULES

Cells adhere through noncovalent bond formation between macromolecules on cell surfaces with macromolecules on other cell surfaces or in extracellular matrix (ECM). These interactions involve either protein–protein or protein–carbohydrate recognition. Although some adhesion molecules are expressed only by blood or endothelial cells, most also are synthesized by other cells. Many adhesion molecules can be grouped into families according to related structural and functional features.

EXTRACELLULAR MATRIX PROTEINS

The ECM provides structural and mechanical support for many tissues and spatial cues that enable cell–cell communication and signaling. The principal constituents of the ECM are adhesive proteins and proteoglycans. The major proteins are collagens, von Willebrand factor (vWF), thrombospondin, elastin, fibronectin, laminin, and vitronectin. These proteins are large and often highly extended and consist of multiple domains with different binding functions. In some proteins such as fibronectin, alternative splicing can increase diversity by producing molecules with variable numbers of domains. In addition, stretching of fibronectin can expose cryptic binding sites. The many binding domains allow adhesive proteins to interact with each other as well as with cell-surface receptors, resulting in multipoint contacts that stabilize matrix structure. One adhesive protein, fibrinogen, is found predominantly in plasma but also may be deposited in exposed subendothelial matrix after vascular injury. Fibronectin, vitronectin, thrombospondin, and vWF are located predominantly in the ECM but also are found in plasma. Several adhesive proteins also are stored in α-granules of platelets, where they are secreted after platelet activation at sites of vascular injury. Similarly, the endothelium stores adhesive proteins in storage granules, called *Weibel-Palade bodies,* that are released upon injury or activation.

Proteoglycans contain protein cores to which are covalently attached many glycosaminoglycans-long linear polymers of repeating disaccharides. Most proteoglycans are in the ECM, but some are anchored on cell surfaces through a core protein that contains a membrane-spanning domain. Hyaluronan is a unique glycosaminoglycan that forms polymers with molecular masses up to several million daltons that are not covalently attached to a protein. Hyaluronan forms noncovalent interactions with globular domains on the protein core of proteoglycans and with a small molecule called *link protein*. The resultant hyaluronan–proteoglycan complexes can become very large, contributing to the structural stability of matrix and function as space fillers during embryonic development. Hyaluronan can also bind to cell-surface receptors and is also abundantly produced during wound healing.

INTEGRINS

Integrins are a broadly distributed group of cell-surface adhesion receptors that consist of noncovalently associated α- and β-subunits (Fig. 10-1 and Table 10-1). There are 18 α chains and eight β chains that pair in many, but not all, of the possible combinations. All blood cells have several different integrins. The four β2 integrins, each paired with a unique α subunit, are expressed only by leukocytes, and the αIIbβ3 integrin (glycoprotein IIb–IIIa [GPIIb–IIIa]) is expressed only by megakaryocytes and platelets. Multidomain adhesive proteins of the ECM are ligands for many integrins. Integrins are unusual adhesion molecules because they usually reside in an inactive state on the cell surface until they receive an activating signal. Some integrins bind to specific domains of several different proteins, and some adhesive proteins bind to several different integrins. These interactions generally mediate cell–matrix adhesion. A unique feature of integrins is transmission of signals in both directions across the cell plasma membrane. Integrin binding to matrix informs the interior of the cell (outside-in) and intracellular signals or conditions inside cells transmit signals outward (inside-out) that regulate binding to matrix or to adhesion receptors on the surface of adjacent cells. Force can also regulate integrin adhesive function. The application of tension to integrins can increase ligand binding, and a reduction in

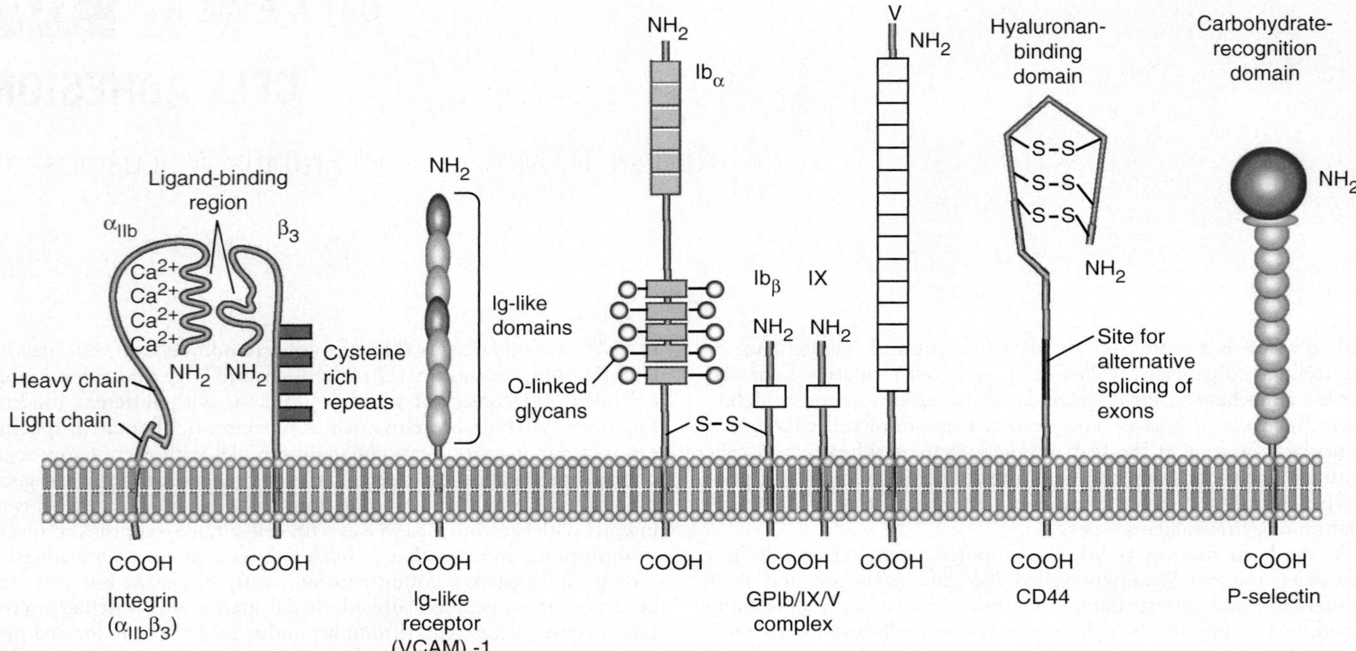

Figure 10-1 SCHEMATIC DIAGRAMS OF SEVERAL TYPES OF CELL-SURFACE ADHESION RECEPTORS. Integrins consist of noncovalently linked α and β subunits, both of which contribute to ligand binding. The platelet αIIbβ3 integrin is illustrated at *far left*. Immunoglobulin (Ig)-like receptors contain a variable number of Ig homology domains, of which some bind ligands and others extend the ligand-binding domains from the membrane. Shown *second from left* is vascular cell adhesion molecule-1 (VCAM-1), which contains seven Ig domains; the two domains that bind to integrins are *shaded*. The platelet glycoprotein Ib–IX–V (GPIb–IX–V) complex, depicted in the *middle diagram*, consists of several leucine-rich protein subunits. CD44, illustrated next, contains an amino-terminal (*N*-terminal) domain that binds to hyaluronan. Each of the selectins contains an *N*-terminal carbohydrate recognition domain that binds sialylated and fucosylated oligosaccharides on specific cell-surface GP ligands. Illustrated at *far right* is P-selectin, the largest of the three selectins.

tension lessens integrin adhesiveness. Cell–cell interactions result from integrin recognition of cell-surface members of the immunoglobulin superfamily. Binding of fibrinogen to αIIbβ3 integrins on adjacent platelets creates a molecular bridge that promotes platelet aggregation. Furthermore, fibrinogen simultaneously binds to the αMβ2 integrin on leukocytes and to an immunoglobulin-like receptor on endothelial cells, promoting leukocyte adhesion to the endothelium.

IMMUNOGLOBULIN-LIKE RECEPTORS

Immunoglobulin superfamily members contain a variable number of disulfide-stabilized motifs similar to those in antibodies, which are linked to transmembrane and cytoplasmic domains (Table 10-2; see also Fig. 10-1). The immunoglobulin-like motif provides a framework on which specific recognition structures for other proteins can be added. Some of these motifs also recognize glycoconjugates. The immunoglobulin-like molecules, intercellular adhesion molecule 1 and 2 (ICAM-1 and ICAM-2), and vascular cell adhesion molecule 1 (VCAM-1), expressed on endothelial cells, as well as ICAM-3, expressed on leukocytes, mediate cell–cell contact through recognition of specific integrins on leukocytes. ICAM-4, expressed on erythroid precursors, binds to integrins on stromal cells of BM, which may regulate erythropoiesis. ICAM-5 is restricted to neural tissues. The immunoglobulin-like GPVI on platelets promotes cell activation by binding to collagen exposed on damaged blood vessels. Interactions between immunoglobulin-like molecules help to mediate adhesion between T cells and antigen-presenting cells. Thus, whereas the immunoglobulin-like molecules CD8 and CD4 on T cells bind to the conserved membrane-proximal domains of class I and class II major histocompatibility complex (MHC) proteins, respectively, the T-cell receptor (CD3) binds to the polymorphic antigen-presenting domain. In addition, the immunoglobulin-like proteins CD2 and CD28 on T cells bind to the immunoglobulin-like protein leukocyte function-associated antigen-3 (LFA-3) and B7-1, respectively, on antigen-presenting cells. The immunoglobulin-like receptor platelet and endothelial cell adhesion molecule-1 (PECAM-1) (CD31) uses homotypical interactions to promote contacts between adjacent endothelial cells and to mediate adhesion of leukocytes to platelets and endothelium. The immunoglobulin-like junctional adhesion molecules (JAMs), expressed on endothelial and epithelial cells and leukocytes, regulate endothelial and epithelial cell junctions, paracellular permeability, and leukocyte trafficking between endothelial and epithelial cells by homotypical interactions or by heterotypical interactions with integrins. JAM-A, the founding member of this family, functions as a homodimer and transmits intracellular signals critical for its function in regulation of endothelial and epithelial permeability.

OTHER ADHESION RECEPTORS THAT MEDIATE PROTEIN–PROTEIN INTERACTIONS

Cadherins are cytoskeletally linked membrane proteins that mediate cell–cell contact in many organs through homotypical binding to cadherins on adjacent cells (Table 10-3). Cadherins have not been described on blood cells but are found on endothelial cells, where, similar to PECAM-1 and JAMs, they help form cell junctions and participate in the process of leukocyte migration across endothelial cell-to-cell borders, termed *diapedesis* or *transendothelial migration*.

The GPIb–IX–V complex on platelets consists of leucine-rich protein subunits (see Fig. 10-1). Under conditions of high shear stress such as those found in arterial circulation, this complex promotes the initial platelet adhesion to injured vessels by binding to vWF exposed in the subendothelium. It also may assist interactions with other

Table 10-1 Integrins on Blood Cells

Integrin Designation	Other Name(s)	Expressed by	Ligand(s)	Function(s)
$\alpha_1\beta_1$	VLA-1	Leukocytes, other cells	Collagens, LM	Adhesion to ECM
$\alpha_2\beta_1$	VLA-2 GPIa/IIa	Leukocytes, platelets, other cells	Collagens, LM	Adhesion to ECM
$\alpha_3\beta_1$	VLA-3	Leukocytes, other cells	Collagens, LM, FN	Adhesion to ECM
$\alpha_4\beta_1$	VLA-4	Monocytes, lymphocytes, eosinophils	VCAM-1, FN	Adhesion to cells, ECM
$\alpha_5\beta_1$	VLA-5 GPIc/IIa	Leukocytes, platelets, other cells	FN	Adhesion to ECM
$\alpha_6\beta_1$	VLA-6 GPIc/IIa	Leukocytes, platelets, other cells	LM	Adhesion to ECM
$\alpha_9\beta_1$		Neutrophils	VCAM-1	Adhesion to ECs
$\alpha_L\beta_2$	LFA-1 CD11a/CD18	Leukocytes	ICAM-1, -2, -3	Leukocyte aggregation and adhesion
$\alpha_M\beta_2$	MAC-1 CR3 CD11b/CD18	Neutrophils, monocytes	ICAM-1, FIB, CR for iC3b	Neutrophil aggregation and adhesion to ECs
$\alpha_X\beta_2$	P150,95 CD11c/CD18	Neutrophils, monocytes	CR for iC3b	Adhesion to ECs
$\alpha_D\beta_2$	CD11d/CD18	Eosinophils, monocytes, lymphocytes	VCAM-1, ICAM-3	Adhesion to leukocytes and to ECs
$\alpha_{IIb}\beta_3$	GPIIb/IIIa	Platelets	FIB, FN, vWF, VN, TSP	Platelet adhesion and aggregation
$\alpha_V\beta_3$	VN receptor	Platelets, ECs	FIB, FN, vWF, VN, TSP, collagens	Platelet adhesion, angiogenesis
$\alpha_4\beta_7$	LPAM-1	Lymphocytes	VCAM-1, MAdCAM-1, FN	Lymphocyte adhesion to ECs and ECM

CR, Complement receptor; *EC*, endothelial cell; *ECM*, extracellular matrix; *FIB*, fibrinogen; *FN*, fibronectin; *GP*, glycoprotein; *LFA-1*, leukocyte function-associates antigen; *LM*, laminin; *LPAM-1*, lymphocyte Peyer patch adhesion molecule; *MAdCAM-1*, mucosal addressin cell adhesion molecule-1; *TSP*, thrombospondin; *VCAM-1*, vascular cell adhesion molecule-1; *VLA*, very late-appearing antigen; *VN*, vitronectin; *vWF*, von Willebrand factor.

Table 10-2 Immunoglobulin-Like Receptors

Name	Other Name	Expressed by	Ligand	Function(s)
ICAM-1		Macrophages, EC, other cells	$\alpha_M\beta_2$, $\alpha_L\beta_2$, FIB	T-cell responses, leukocyte adhesion to EC
ICAM-2		EC	$\alpha_L\beta_2$	Leukocyte adhesion to EC
ICAM-3		Leukocytes	$\alpha_L\beta_2$	T-cell responses, leukocyte aggregation
ICAM-4		Erythroid precursors	$\alpha_4\beta_1$, $\alpha_V\beta_3$, $\alpha_{IIb}\beta_3$	Regulate erythropoiesis
GPVI		Platelets	Collagen	Platelet adhesion and activation
PECAM-1	CD31	Leukocytes, platelets, EC	PECAM-1	EC junctions, leukocyte transmigration, cell signaling
VCAM-1		Activated EC, smooth muscle cells	$\alpha_4\beta_1$, $\alpha_4\beta_7$	Mononuclear cell adhesion to EC
MAdCAM-1		EC of Peyer patches	$\alpha_4\beta_7$	Lymphocytes homing
Siglecs		Leukocyte subsets	Sialylated glycans	Regulate B-cell activation, innate immunity?, hematopoiesis?
JAMs		EC	JAMs, $\alpha_L\beta_2$, $\alpha_4\beta_1$	EC junctions, leukocyte transmigration
CD2		T cells	LFA-3*	T-cell responses
CD4		T cells	Class II MHC*	T-cell responses
CD8		T cells	Class I MHC*	T-cell responses
CD3	T-cell receptor	T cells	Antigen on MHC*	T-cell responses
CD28	Costimulatory molecule	T cells	B7-1 (CD80)	T-cell responses

ICAM-1, -2, -3, -4, Intercellular adhesion molecules; *JAM*, junctional adhesion molecule; *MHC*, major histocompatibility complex; *PECAM-1*, platelet and endothelial cell adhesion molecules-1. For other abbreviations, see Table 10-1 footnotes.
*LFA-3 and classes I and II MHC molecules are also immunoglobulin-like receptors.

Table 10-3 Other Adhesion Receptors

Name	Other Name	Expressed by	Ligand	Function(s)
Cadherins		EC, many other cells	Homotypic binding	Formation of EC junctions
GPIb/IX/V		Platelets	vWF	Platelet adhesion to ECM under shear
CD36	GPIV	Platelets, many other cells	Collagens, TSP	Platelet adhesion to ECM
CD44		Leukocytes, other cells	Hyaluronan, serglycin	Lymphopoiesis, lymphocyte activation
DC-SIGN		Dendritic cells	Mannosylated glycans, other glycans	Regulate T-cell–dendritic cell interactions, recognize pathogens
NK cell receptors		NK cells	MHC molecules	Recognition of virus-infected or other foreign cells

DC-SIGN, Dendritic cell-specific ICAM-3 grabbing nonintegrin; *MHC,* major histocompatibility complex; *NK,* natural killer. For other abbreviations, see Table 10-1 footnotes.

Table 10-4 Selectins

Name	Other Name	Expressed by	Ligand	Ligands Expressed by	Function(s)
P-selectin	CD62P GMP-140 PADGEM	Thrombin-activated platelets and EC, cytokine-activated EC	PSGL-1, GPIbα	Leukocytes, platelets	Leukocyte adhesion to activated EC and platelets
E-selectin	CD62E ELAM-1	Cytokine-activated EC	PSGL-1, other sialylated and fucosylated GPs	Leukocytes	Leukocyte adhesion to activated EC
L-selectin	CD62L LECAM-1 LAM-1	Leukocytes	PSGL-1, also GlyCAM-1, CD34, and other mucins on EC of lymph nodes	Leukocytes, EC or lymph nodes	Leukocyte adhesion to other leukocytes; lymphocyte homing to lymph nodes

EC, Endothelial cell; *ELAM-1,* endothelial leukocyte adhesion molecule-1; *Gly-CAM-1,* glycosylation-dependent cell adhesion molecule-1; *GMP-140,* granule membrane protein-140; *LAM-1,* leukocyte adhesion molecule-1; *LECAM-1,* leukocyte endothelial cell adhesion molecule-1; *PADGEM,* platelet activation-dependent granule external membrane protein; *PSGL-1,* P-selectin glycoprotein ligand-1.
The selectins bind to sialylated, fucosylated, and (in some cases) sulfated oligosaccharides on specific glycoproteins, of which only some have been identified.

platelets or with endothelial cells by binding to P-selectin, which normally binds to glycoconjugates, and it may assist platelet adhesion to leukocytes by binding to the integrin $\alpha_m\beta_2$.

CD36 is a receptor with at least two membrane-spanning domains that is expressed on many cell types. On platelets, it has been implicated as a receptor for collagen and perhaps for thrombospondin; both interactions could facilitate adhesion to the subendothelial matrix at sites of hemorrhage.

LECTIN ADHESION RECEPTORS

CD44 is an unusual transmembrane GP expressed to variable degrees on many subsets of leukocytes (see Fig. 10–1). It has a membrane-distal domain that is structurally related to link protein of ECM, and similar to link protein, can bind to hyaluronan. CD44 also binds to the serglycin, a proteoglycan secreted by hematopoietic cells. The hyaluronan-binding function of CD44 may modulate a number of leukocyte responses. The most clearly demonstrated function is in lymphopoiesis, where maturation of lymphocyte precursors requires contacts with BM stromal cells bearing surface hyaluronan. CD44–hyaluronate interactions also may promote lymphocyte entry to and transit through organized lymphoid tissues. The membrane-proximal regions of CD44 are structurally diverse because of the insertion of variable numbers of domains through alternative splicing. These insertions may regulate the ability of CD44 to bind hyaluronan and may mediate postbinding events that affect cell signaling.

The selectins are a group of three receptors that terminate in a membrane-distal carbohydrate-recognition domain related to those in Ca^{2+}-dependent (C-type) animal lectins such as the hepatic asialoglycoprotein receptor (see Fig. 10-1). L-selectin is expressed on leukocytes, E-selectin on cytokine-activated endothelium, and P-selectin on macrophages, platelets, and endothelial cells exposed to secretagogues such as thrombin or histamine (Table 10-4). The selectins mediate leukocyte adhesion to platelets, endothelium, or other leukocytes through Ca^{2+}-dependent interactions of the carbohydrate-recognition domains with cell-surface carbohydrates on apposing cells. High-affinity binding appears to require specific carbohydrate structures displayed on a limited number of membrane GPs. The best-characterized GP ligands for selectins are mucins that have large numbers of clustered, sialylated *O*-linked oligosaccharides. Site-specific construction of *O*-glycans with specific sialylated, fucosylated, and (in some cases) sulfated moieties is required for these mucins to bind optimally to selectins. In the case of one mucin, P-selectin GP ligand-1 (PSGL-1), sulfation of tyrosine residues near a specific *O*-glycan is required for binding to P- and L-selectin.

Dendritic cells and related macrophages express a novel group of C-type lectins, of which the best-characterized is dendritic cell-specific ICAM-3–grabbing nonintegrin (DC-SIGN). DC-SIGN binds to particular oligosaccharides on ICAMs, thereby regulating T-cell and dendritic cell function during antigen presentation. It also binds to glycans on a variety of pathogens, which may have critical roles in innate immunity. Natural killer cells express a different group of proteins with some containing membrane-distal C-type lectin-like domains. Although these receptors are important for interactions of natural killer cells with target cells, they may bind to proteins rather than to glycoconjugates.

Siglecs are a subgroup of membrane proteins of the immunoglobulin superfamily that bind to carbohydrates instead of to proteins (see Table 10-2). The first two amino-terminal (*N*-terminal) domains appear to be necessary and sufficient for carbohydrate recognition. The *N*-terminal domain is a V-type structure that includes an unusual disulfide bond that is not found in the more common C-type immunoglobulin domains. Siglecs bind well to sialylated glycans on some but not all GPs. Different siglecs preferentially recognize sialic acid that is linked α2,6-, α2,8-, or α2,3- to an underlying galactose residue. Most siglecs have immune receptor tyrosine-based inhibitory motifs and transmit inhibitory signals. Siglecs can form *cis* interactions with other GPs on the same cell or *trans* interactions with GPs on another cell. The best-characterized example is CD22, which negatively regulates B-cell activation when it engages sialylated GPs. Sialoadhesin, expressed on BM macrophages, may regulate hematopoietic cell differentiation.

LIGAND BINDING VERSUS CELL ADHESION

As with all noncovalent macromolecular interactions, adhesion molecules bind to each other with equilibrium affinities that are defined by their association and dissociation rates. However, the efficiency of cell adhesion is not simply a function of the solution-phase equilibrium affinities of adhesion molecules for one another. Adhesion molecules in cell membranes and matrix are limited primarily to two dimensions, and even low-affinity molecular interactions may stabilize adhesion if there is time for sufficient bonds to form along the plane of cell contact. The efficiency of cell attachment and the ensuing strength of adhesion reflect multiple factors that dictate the probability of formation of bonds between adhesion molecules on cell or matrix surfaces. The kinetics of bond formation and dissociation are especially important for certain kinds of cell adhesion. Furthermore, interactions between cell adhesion molecules are subjected to force, which affects the lifetimes of adhesive bonds. This is particularly true in the circulation, where platelets and leukocytes must rapidly adhere to the blood vessel wall and withstand forces applied by the wall shear stresses of flowing blood. Other factors that affect bond formation include the number of adhesion molecules on a cell or matrix surface, the distance the binding domain of an adhesion receptor protrudes from the cell membrane, the lateral mobility of receptors, receptor dimerization, and the clustering of receptors on microvilli or other membrane domains. Cell adhesion can be further stabilized by events that occur after the initial interactions of adhesion molecules. For example, the cytoplasmic domains of many adhesion molecules bind to cytoskeletal components, allowing clustering of receptors into surface patches that strengthen adhesion, thereby promoting cell spreading or migration.

REGULATION OF ADHESION RECEPTORS

To prevent inappropriate interactions of cells with each other or with ECM, the expression and function of adhesion receptors must be tightly controlled. Three primary control mechanisms are used: (1) the rate of synthesis of the receptor, (2) the time during which the receptor is displayed on the cell surface, and (3) the binding affinity or avidity of the receptor for ligands (Table 10-5). All of these mechanisms are used to control interactions of blood and vascular cells.

Table 10-5 Regulation of Adhesion Receptors

Mechanism	Example
Synthesis	Erythroid precursor synthesis of $\alpha_5\beta_1$ Lymphocyte synthesis of CD44 Cytokine-induced synthesis of E-selectin, P-selectin, ICAM-1, and VCAM-1 by endothelial cells
Surface expression	Proteolytic cleavage of L-selectin from leukocytes Redistribution of P-selectin from granule membranes to plasma membrane of platelets and endothelial cells Endocytosis of P- and E-selectin on endothelial cells
Ligand affinity	Activation-induced increased affinity of many integrins for their ligands Activation-induced increased affinity of CD44 for hyaluronan

For abbreviations, see Table 10-1 footnotes.

REGULATION OF SYNTHESIS

The synthesis of many adhesion receptors is regulated. Erythroid precursors synthesize integrins that mediate their interactions with stromal cells and with ECM in the BM. As the precursors mature, synthesis ceases, resulting in loss of expression of cell-surface integrins by the time a mature erythrocyte enters the circulation. Lymphocyte precursors synthesize CD44 during differentiation in the BM, stop synthesis before release, and resume synthesis during maturation in the thymus. On exposure to antigens, immunologically naive lymphocytes synthesize increased amounts of several adhesion receptors and chemokine receptors during their conversion to the effector phenotypes; this process presumably allows these cells to become more adhesive in response to a subsequent antigenic challenge. Endothelial cells in postcapillary venules of the peripheral vasculature express very low, if any, levels of adhesion molecules that bind leukocytes. When exposed to inflammatory cytokines such as tumor necrosis factor-α and interleukin-1 (IL-1) or bacterial endotoxin, endothelial cells transiently increase synthesis of E- and P-selectin, ICAM-1, and VCAM-1, resulting in an adhesive surface for leukocytes.

REGULATION OF SURFACE EXPRESSION

The surface expression of some adhesion receptors is tightly controlled. L-selectin is present on the plasma membrane of leukocytes, where it is available to bind to ligands on the endothelial cell surface. Stimulation of the leukocyte causes L-selectin to be shed into the plasma by proteolytic cleavage. P-selectin is constitutively synthesized by megakaryocytes (where it is incorporated into platelets) and by endothelial cells. Rather than being directly delivered to the plasma membrane, it is sorted into secretory storage granules: the α granules of platelets and the Weibel–Palade bodies of endothelial cells. On stimulation of these cells by agonists such as thrombin, P-selectin is rapidly transported to the cell surface during fusion of granule membranes with the plasma membrane. When they are on the surface of the endothelium, both E-selectin and P-selectin are internalized and delivered to lysosomes for degradation. The cytoplasmic domain of P-selectin contains signals that direct sorting into secretory granules, internalization through coated pits of the plasma membrane, and movement from endosomes to lysosomes; the latter two signals probably also are present in the cytoplasmic domain of E-selectin. The net result of these events is to control the duration of exposure of E- and P-selectin on the endothelium, where they can mediate adhesion of leukocytes. Activation of leukocytes also mobilizes a pool of β_2 integrins from storage compartments to the plasma membrane, although some of these molecules also are constitutively expressed on the cell surface. Finally, platelet activation redistributes a portion of the GPIb–IX–V complexes from ligand-accessible positions on the plasma membrane to sequestered, invaginated membrane domains known as the *surface-connected canalicular system*. This process, which requires interactions of the cytoplasmic domain of GPIb–IX–V with the cytoskeleton, may serve to downregulate GPIb-mediated adhesion of platelets to immobilized vWF.

REGULATION OF BINDING AFFINITY

Regulation of binding affinity is an important control mechanism for other adhesion receptors. Many integrins are constitutively present on the cell surface but interact poorly with their ligands. Cell activation by a number of agonists induces conformational changes in integrins so that they effectively recognize their ligands. An example is the $\alpha_{IIb}\beta_3$ integrin, which requires platelet stimulation to bind fibrinogen; if this binding affinity were not regulated, circulating platelets would indiscriminately aggregate in the fibrinogen-rich plasma milieu. The cytoplasmic domains of integrins can exert both positive and negative influences on binding affinity. Binding of specific cytoplasmic proteins to these domains may propagate structural changes to the extracellular ligand-binding regions of the integrins. Three-dimensional structures of integrins suggest that the integrin "headpiece" that contains the ligand-binding site faces down toward the membrane in the inactive conformation and rapidly extends upward in a "switchblade"-like opening motion on activation. Low-affinity ligand binding may stabilize some active conformations of integrins, perhaps explaining why integrins on unactivated cells will sometimes bind to immobilized, multivalent adhesive proteins but not to the same proteins in solution. Cellular activation also may regulate the binding avidities of CD44, L-selectin, P-selectin, and some integrins through changes in membrane distribution engineered by interactions of their cytoplasmic domains with the cytoskeleton or with clathrin-coated pits.

CELL SIGNALING THROUGH ADHESION MOLECULES

In addition to their roles in cell–cell and cell–matrix contacts, adhesion molecules may cause cell signaling through indirect or direct mechanisms. Proteoglycans in the ECM can sequester growth factors that can be released to bind to surface receptors on nearby cells. Some chemoattractants bind to proteoglycans on the surface of endothelial cells, where they can activate adherent leukocytes. Binding of adhesive ligands to cell-surface integrins, GPIb–IX–V, CD44, cadherins, CD36, PECAM-1, selectins, and perhaps other receptors can directly trigger intracellular events. The consequences of such signaling include changes in affinity or avidity of other adhesion receptors for their ligands, shape change, secretion, proliferation, synthesis of cytokines and other molecules, and migration. In some cases, binding of a monovalent adhesive ligand to a receptor may induce a signal. More commonly, signaling requires cross-linking of several receptors through interactions with multivalent ligands in matrix or on apposing cells.

Many studies of adhesion receptor signaling have focused on integrins. Binding of the same ligand to different integrins can mediate different responses in the same cell. Furthermore, ligand binding to the same integrin expressed in different cells can result in different signals. These data suggest that very specific interactions occur between ligand-occupied integrins and intracellular components. The cytoplasmic domains of integrins are essential for initiating signaling. Tyrosine kinases have been localized at the interaction zones between integrins, the cytoskeleton and several adaptor and effector molecules, and tyrosine phosphorylation of a number of proteins accompanies integrin-mediated cell signaling. Tyrosine phosphorylation initiates a cascade of signaling events, including the activation of serine/threonine kinases, which cause a variety of cellular responses. Ligand binding to integrins also results in generation of lipid second messengers, alkalization of the cytoplasm, and influxes of Ca^{2+}.

COOPERATIVE INTERACTIONS BETWEEN SIGNALING AND ADHESION MOLECULES

Signaling and adhesion molecules frequently function cooperatively in sequential cascades to enhance the specificity of cell adhesion. Three examples of how these cooperative interactions facilitate blood cell responses are described next.

Platelet Adhesion and Aggregation

At sites of blood vessel injury in the arterial circuit, platelets rapidly tether to and then translocate or roll along the damaged vessel through reversible interactions of GPIb–IX–V receptors with immobilized vWF exposed in the subendothelial matrix of injured vessels (Fig. 10-2). These interactions are facilitated by arterial flow, perhaps because of complex effects of high wall shear stresses on the lifetimes of bonds between GPIb and vWF. An important feature of this initial reversible adhesive event is that prior activation of the platelets is not required. After adhesion, however, the interaction of immobilized vWF with GPIb receptors triggers intracellular signals that lead to platelet activation. These signals synergize with those produced by engagement of the collagen receptor GPVI. Platelet activation, in turn, increases the affinity of platelet integrins for collagen and fibronectin, which stabilizes adhesion. Binding of these ligands transduces signals that propagate further activation responses such as spreading, secretion of granule contents, and recruitment of additional platelets through cell–cell contact mediated by binding of fibrinogen to activated $\alpha_{IIb}\beta_3$ integrins. This adhesion cascade allows unstimulated platelets to home to the site of vascular injury and then be activated by locally generated mediators.

Neutrophil Rolling, Spreading, and Migration

Near sites of extravascular bacterial infections, neutrophils first tether to and roll on the endothelial surface of venules through the interactions of selectins with cell-surface carbohydrate ligands (Fig. 10-3). Little, if any, leukocyte adhesion occurs in nearby arterioles. Neutrophil rolling on the endothelium occurs under shear forces, just as platelets adhere to subendothelial matrix under shear forces, although the shear flow in postcapillary venules is lower than that in arterioles. Rolling requires a balance between the formation of selectin–ligand bonds at the leading edge of the cell and the dissociation of bonds at the trailing edge of the cell. Whereas shear forces affect the lifetimes of selectin–ligand bonds; lower forces prolong lifetimes (catch bonds), higher forces shorten lifetimes (slip bonds). Catch bonds help explain why a minimum shear force is required to support leukocyte rolling, particularly through L-selectin. Just as the initial adhesion to vWF does not require prior activation of platelets, selectin-mediated rolling does not require prior activation of neutrophils. Instead, locally generated inflammatory mediators induce expression of E- or P-selectin

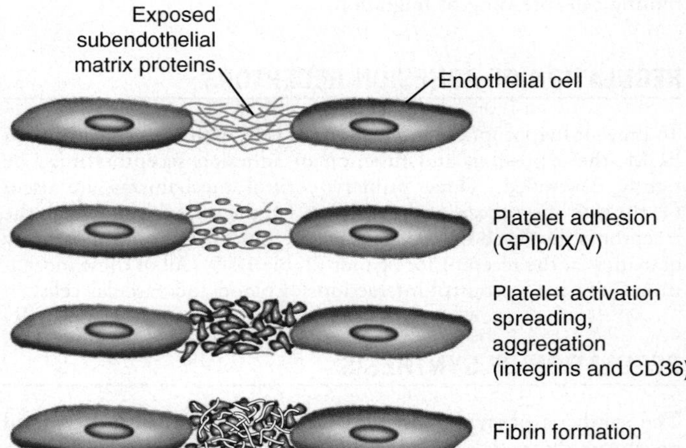

Figure 10-2 PLATELET ADHESION AND AGGREGATION. In response to arterial injury under high shear forces, platelets rapidly adhere to the subendothelial matrix of injured vessels. The initial contacts are made between glycoprotein Ib–IX–V (GPIb–IX–V) on platelets and von Willebrand factor (vWF) in the matrix. These molecular interactions help activate platelets, thereby increasing the affinity of several platelet integrins for other adhesive matrix proteins such as fibronectin, laminin, and collagen. GPVI further activates platelets by binding to collagen. CD36 also interacts with both collagen and thrombospondin. Fibrinogen cross-links activated platelets into aggregates by binding to $\alpha_{IIb}\beta_3$ integrins. The platelet plug then serves as an efficient surface for generation of thrombin and fibrin.

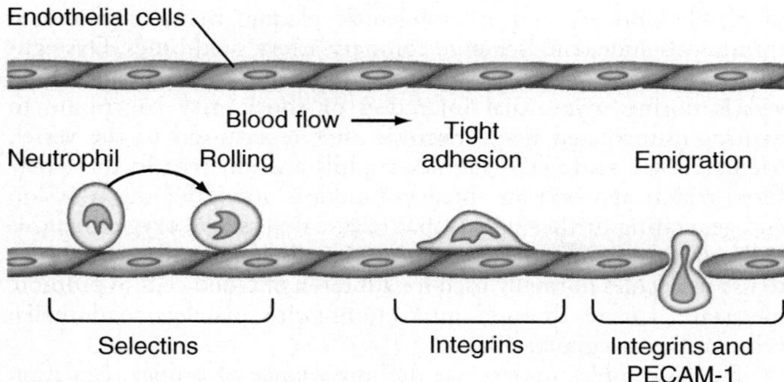

Figure 10-3 NEUTROPHIL ROLLING, SPREADING, AND EMIGRATION. At sites of tissue injury or infection, neutrophils first roll on the endothelial cells in postcapillary venules. These transient adhesive interactions are mediated by activation-induced transcription-dependent expression of E- or P-selectin on the endothelial cell surface. E- and P-selectin bind to carbohydrate ligands on the neutrophil. These molecular bonds can form under the shear forces in the venular circulation. The rolling neutrophils are then activated by locally generated inflammatory mediators that increase the affinity of β_2 integrins for immunoglobulin-like receptors such as intercellular adhesion molecule-1 (ICAM-1) on the endothelium. These bonds slow rolling and then promote firm adhesion to the endothelium. Neutrophil migration between endothelial cells into tissues at the site of infection requires disengagement of old adhesive bonds and formation of new bonds among integrins, platelet and endothelial cell adhesion molecule-1 (PECAM-1), and their respective ligands.

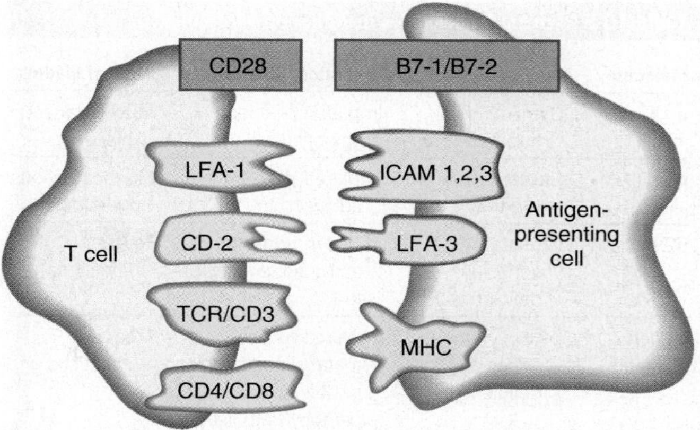

Figure 10-4 ADHESION BETWEEN T LYMPHOCYTES AND ANTIGEN-PRESENTING CELLS (APCs). The initial contact is mediated by the T-cell receptor (TCR), or CD3, which binds with low affinity but high specificity to a specific antigen presented by a major histocompatibility complex (MHC) molecule. Additional contacts, also of low affinity, are between CD4 (on helper cells) or CD8 (on cytotoxic cells) and MHC and between costimulatory molecules CD2 and leukocyte function-associated antigen-3 (LFA-3) and CD28 and CD80 (B7-1) and CD86 (B7-2). These interactions signal the T cell to increase transiently the affinity of the β_2 integrin LFA-1 for the immunoglobulin-like molecules intercellular adhesion molecule ICAM-1 on the APC. These bonds strengthen adhesion, and the costimulatory molecules transduce further signals to the T cell that cause increased gene transcription, proliferation, and cytokine secretion. Not shown is the redistribution of these adhesion molecules into different regions of the contact zone as adhesion strengthens. Additional signals result from binding of β_1 integrins on the T cell to adhesive proteins in the extracellular matrix.

on the endothelial cell surface. The requirement for activation of endothelial cells rather than leukocytes allows the latter to adhere to vessels only at the site of vessel inflammation. After being situated on the vessel wall through selectin-mediated contacts, however, the neutrophils become exposed to activators such as platelet-activating factor, a phospholipid signaling molecule, activated complement proteins, and IL-8, a potent chemoattractant cytokine or chemokine, both of which are presented on the surface of activated endothelial cells. These signals cooperate with others directed by engagement of selectin ligands and promote very slow rolling of neutrophils on the surface of activated endothelium. Neutrophil activation increases the affinity of β_2 integrins for immunoglobulin counterreceptors on the endothelial cell surface such as ICAM-1. Although flowing cells cannot form these bonds, neutrophils rolling on selectins can do so because of their slower velocities. The integrin–ICAM interactions further slow rolling and then arrest the cells on the endothelium. The leukocytes then migrate, presumably because of disengagement of integrin–ICAM bonds and redistribution of integrins to the leading edge of the cell, where new bonds form. Interactions of leukocytes with JAMs and PECAM-1 and other molecules at interendothelial cell junctions facilitate transendothelial migration of the neutrophils into the underlying tissues. Adhesion of leukocytes to the endothelium disrupts cytoskeletal tethers to the endothelial cadherins; this disruption leads to dissociation of homotypical cadherin interactions that normally prevent passage of leukocytes. Both the integrin- and the PECAM-1–mediated adhesive events may signal cytoskeletal redistributions in leukocytes that enhance migration toward chemotactic molecules released in the vicinity of the infection. When leukocytes enter in the tissues, integrin recognition of ECM protein ligands may trigger secretion of proteolytic enzymes and production of superoxide anions, both required for optimal bactericidal function.

Adhesion of T Cells to Antigen-Presenting Cells

The initial engagement of T cells with antigen-presenting cells requires that the T-cell receptor (CD3) recognize antigen presented by the polymorphic domain of MHC molecules (Fig. 10-4). Subsequent interactions include the binding of CD8 or CD4 to MHC class I or II molecules, respectively, plus the binding of CD2 to LFA-3 and CD28 binding to B7 molecules. These molecular contacts are all of low affinity but are highly specific because they first require specific antigen presentation to the appropriate T cell. The combination of these binding events triggers inside-out signals that increase the affinity of LFA-1 ($\alpha_L\beta_2$), a β_2 integrin on T cells, for its ligand, ICAM-1 on antigen-presenting cells, strengthening and prolonging the length of time cells stably adhere. During this time, the T cell is further activated by a second or costimulatory signal delivered by T cell CD28 binding to B7 molecules expressed by antigen-presenting cells. Together these interactions drive TCR-induced gene activation (IL-2 production) and cell proliferation and differentiation into different effector T cells that exit the secondary lymph node and migrate to immune reactions (see Chapter 19 for detailed discussion of T cell–antigen-presenting cell activation).

The first principle of these three responses is that the initial adhesive event, although relatively limited, is highly specific. Thus, platelets bind to exposed subendothelial matrix in injured vessels, neutrophils bind to hyperadhesive endothelium near the site of infection, and T cells bind to cells presenting specific antigen in secondary lymph nodes. The second principle is that subsequent activation events strengthen cell adhesion and lead to further responses such as secretion, fibrin formation, cellular migration, and release of cytotoxic mediators or cell activation and proliferation. Activation often results from cooperative signaling by soluble agonists and by binding of ligands to adhesion receptors. Costimulation by multiple signals can amplify and provide specificity to cellular responses by mechanisms not always feasible for individual mediators. Thus, adhesion and cell signaling are highly interrelated processes.

The process of reversing cell adhesion, although less well understood, is equally important for the control of cell behavior. Some molecules such as the selectins can be proteolytically cleaved or internalized. The activation-induced increases in affinity of integrins and CD44 for their ligands are generally transient, but the mechanisms for return to the inactive conformation are obscure.

Table 10-6 Genetic Deficiencies in Adhesion Molecules

Molecule	Disease	Laboratory Finding(s)	Clinical Finding
$\alpha_{IIb}\beta_3$	Glanzmann thrombasthenia	Impaired platelet aggregation	Mucocutaneous bleeding
GPIb/IX/V	Bernard–Soulier syndrome	Impaired platelet adhesion to vWF	Mucocutaneous bleeding
β2 integrins	Leukocyte adhesion deficiency-1	Impaired adhesion of activated leukocytes to EC	Frequent infections
Selectin ligands	Leukocyte adhesion deficiency-2	Impaired fucose metabolism resulting in defective carbohydrate ligands for selectins, impaired rolling of leukocytes on venules	Frequent infections
β1, β2, β3 integrins	Leukocyte adhesion deficiency-3	Impaired platelet adhesion and aggregation and impaired adhesion of activated leukocytes to EC	Mucocutaneous bleeding and frequent infections

For abbreviations, see Table 10-1 footnotes.

ALTERED EXPRESSION OF ADHESION MOLECULES

The highly regulated nature of adhesive events by hematopoietic cells suggests that defects in or excessive expression of adhesion molecules may contribute to the pathogenesis of disease. A variety of clinical observations support this hypothesis.

Genetic Deficiencies in Adhesion Molecules

Genetic deficiencies in platelet adhesion receptors such as the GPIb complex (as in Bernard-Soulier syndrome) and the $\alpha_{IIb}\beta_3$ integrin (as in Glanzmann thrombasthenia) result in hemorrhagic symptoms similar to those in patients with thrombocytopenia (Table 10-6). Genetic deficiencies in the leukocyte β_2 integrins (as in leukocyte adhesion deficiency-1) are associated with frequent severe bacterial infections and a failure of neutrophils to enter the infected tissues. Similar symptoms are seen in patients with a congenital defect in fucose metabolism that prevents synthesis of the carbohydrate ligands for selectins (leukocyte adhesion deficiency-2). A recently identified set of patients has both hemorrhagic symptoms and life-threatening infections (leukocyte adhesion deficiency-3). The molecular mechanism is attributable to mutations in an intracellular protein kindlin-3, which binds to β1, β2, and β3 integrin cytoplasmic tails upon cell activation. These patients have normal levels of integrin surface expression (see Table 10-6).

Dysregulated Expression of Adhesion Molecules

Inappropriate expression of adhesion molecules has been implicated in thrombotic and inflammatory disorders and in tumor metastasis. For example, erythrocytes from patients with sickle cell anemia adhere to each other, to leukocytes, and to the endothelium, contributing to vasoocclusive crises. These adhesive events may reflect, in part, the expression of integrins and selectin ligands not normally found on mature erythrocytes. Inappropriate adhesion and activation of platelets on exposed atherosclerotic plaques may contribute to thrombosis and acute ischemic coronary artery syndromes. Dysregulated expression of selectins on the endothelium of ischemic blood vessels during myocardial infarction or shock may contribute to neutrophil-mediated tissue necrosis after reperfusion of the vessel. Mediators released while the neutrophils are adherent in the reperfused vessels may activate integrin function, strengthening adhesion and generating further signals that release destructive oxygen radicals and proteases within the vasculature. Finally, malignant cells appear to use molecules normally used for adhesion of blood cells to promote metastatic spread through interactions with platelets, endothelial cells, and extravascular matrix.

These examples underscore the importance of proper regulation of adhesion molecule expression in the physiology of blood cells.

SUGGESTED READINGS

Alcaide P, Auerbach S, Luscinskas FW: Neutrophil recruitment under shear flow: It's all about endothelial cell rings and gaps. *Microcirculation* 16:43, 2009. *Erratum in: Microcirculation* 16:782, 2009.

Berndt MC, Shen Y, Dopheide SM, et al: The vascular biology of the glycoprotein Ib-IX-V complex. *Thromb Haemost* 86:178, 2001.

Bunting M, Harris ES, McIntyre TM, et al: Leukocyte adhesion deficiency syndromes: Adhesion and tethering defects involving β2 integrins and selectin ligands. *Curr Opin Hematol* 9:30, 2002.

Cambi A, Koopman M, Figdor CG: How C-type lectins detect pathogens. *Cell Microbiol* 7:481, 2005.

Cao H, Crocker PR: Evolution of CC33-related siglecs: Regulating host immune functions and escaping pathogen exploitation? *Immunology* 132:18, 2010.

Chen J, Lopez JA: Interactions of platelets with subendothelium and endothelium. *Microcirculation* 12:235, 2005.

Fooksman DR, Vardhana S, Vasiliver-Shamis G, et al: Functional anatomy of T cell activation and synapse formation. *Annu Rev Immunol* 28:79, 2010.

Hickey MJ, Kubes P: Intravascular immunity: The host-pathogen encounter in blood vessels. *Nat Rev Immunol* 9:364, 2009.

Hogg N, Patzak I, Willenbrock F: The insider's guide to leukocyte integrin signalling and function. *Nat Rev Immunol* 11:416, 2011.

Hynes RO: Integrins: Bidirectional, allosteric signaling machines. *Cell* 110:673, 2002.

Koppel EA, van Gisbergen KP, Geijtenbeek TB, et al: Distinct functions of DC-SIGN and its homologues L-SIGN (DC-SIGNR) and mSIGNR1 in pathogen recognition and immune regulation. *Cell Microbiol* 7:157, 2005.

McEver RP: Adhesive interactions of leukocytes, platelets, and the vessel wall during hemostasis and inflammation. *Thromb Haemost* 86:746, 2001.

McEver RP, Zhu C: Rolling cell adhesion. *Annu Rev Cell Dev Biol* 26:363, 2010.

Muller WA: Mechanisms of leukocyte transendothelial migration. *Annu Rev Pathol* 28:323, 2011.

Ponta H, Sherman L, Herrlich PA: CD44: From adhesion molecules to signalling regulators. *Nat Rev Mol Cell Biol* 4:33, 2003.

Ruggeri ZM: Platelet adhesion under flow. *Microcirculation* 16:58, 2009.

Shattil SJ, Kim C, Ginsberg MH: The final steps of integrin activation: The end game. *Nat Rev Mol Cell Biol* 11:288 2010.

Sperandio M, Gleissner CA, Ley K: Glycosylation in immune cell trafficking. *Immunol Rev* 230:97, 2009.

Springer TA, Wang JH: The three-dimensional structure of integrins and their ligands, and conformational regulation of cell adhesion. *Adv Protein Chem* 68:29, 2004.

Tailor A, Cooper D, Granger DN: Platelet-vessel wall interactions in the microcirculation. *Microcirculation* 12:275, 2005.

Vestweber D, Winderlich M, Cagna G, et al: Cell adhesion dynamics at endothelial junctions: VE-cadherin as a major player. *Trends Cell Biol* 19:8, 2009.

Wang H, Lim D, Rudd CE: Immunopathologies linked to integrin signalling. *Semin Immunopathol* 32:173, 2010.

CHAPTER 11

HEMATOPOIETIC CELL TRAFFICKING AND CHEMOKINES

Steffen Massberg, Alexander G. Khandoga, and Ulrich H. von Andrian

The mammalian immune system has evolved to prevent infection while preserving self-tolerance and restraining immune-mediated pathology. Accomplishing these tasks requires billions of motile cells that continually travel throughout the body. The migration profiles vary substantially among individual types of leukocytes. However, their distinct traffic patterns are not random but follow a precisely organized process that is essential for proper immune surveillance and serves to maximize the likelihood that leukocytes will encounter and eliminate or contain pathogens.

During differentiation in the bone marrow (BM) (innate immune cells and B cells) or thymus (naive T cells), leukocytes are equipped with characteristic repertoires of traffic molecules that enable and restrict their migration to certain microenvironments and tissues. For example, whereas naive lymphocytes are poorly responsive to inflammatory signals, but they migrate efficiently to lymphoid organs, innate immune cells and antigen-experienced lymphocytes can respond to inflammation-induced traffic cues, although at least some subsets also travel to noninflamed (lymphoid and nonlymphoid) target tissues.[1-4] Notably, not only mature leukocytes migrate from one tissue to another via the circulation or lymphatic systems; some hematopoietic stem cells (HSCs) and progenitor cells also travel continuously throughout the body.[5-13] The characteristic trafficking of each leukocyte subset is coordinated by adhesion molecules expressed on leukocytes and endothelial cells (see Chapter 10) and through chemoattractants and their receptors. Chemoattractants are generated in a target tissue and can be sensed by passing leukocytes that express the appropriate receptor. Leukocyte chemoattractants include a number of lipid mediators; microbial factors; and a variety of peptides, such as activated complement 5 (C5a) and members of the chemokine family. This chapter will discuss chemokines as master navigation signals for leukocyte trafficking and then focuses on specific trafficking pathways that direct discrete leukocyte subsets to distinct target tissues.

CHEMOKINES IN CONTROL OF LEUKOCYTE TRAFFICKING

Nomenclature and Structure of Chemokines

Chemokines (short for *chemo*tactic cyto*kines*) are critical messengers in the complex cellular communication network used by the immune system. At least 47 chemokines have been identified to date (Table 11-1).[14-20] The two major subclasses of chemokines are distinguished as CC- or CXC-chemokines, depending on the arrangement of two canonical cysteine residues within the conserved chemokine motif, which are either adjacent (CC) or separated by a single amino acid (CXC). The XC (XCL1 and XCL2) and CX3C chemokines (CX3CL1) constitute two additional structural subfamilies of chemokines. Most chemokines are secreted proteins of 67 to 127 amino acids, only CXCL16 and CX3CL1 possess a transmembrane domain, but also exist in a cleaved, soluble form. Traditionally, chemokines were grouped into functional subfamilies termed "inflammatory" chemokines, that are induced by inflammatory signals and control the recruitment of effector leukocytes in infection, inflammation, tissue injury and malignancies, and "homeostatic" chemokines that navigate leukocytes during hematopoiesis in the BM and thymus during initiation of adaptive immune responses in secondary lymphoid organs and in immune surveillance of healthy peripheral tissues (e.g., CCL19, CCL21, or CXCL12). However, many chemokines cannot be assigned unambiguously to one of these two categories and are therefore referred to as *dual-function chemokines* (e.g., CXCL16, CXCL9).

Chemokine Signaling Through G-Protein–Coupled Receptors

Chemokine messages are decoded through specific cell-surface G protein–coupled receptors (GPCRs) with seven transmembrane domains.[21-25] The human chemokine receptor repertoire identified at present consists of 20 different GPCRs (Table 11-2).[26] The tremendous specificity and plasticity observed in leukocyte migration and anatomic distribution is largely owed to this system because each leukocyte subset expresses a distinct repertoire of chemokine receptors and each chemokine receptor can bind different sets of chemokines with various binding affinities.[27,28] Chemokine receptors function as allosteric molecular relays where chemokine binding to the extracellular portion modifies the tertiary structure of the receptor. This allows the intracellular domain of the engaged receptor to bind to and activate heterotrimeric G proteins. In response, the activated G proteins exchange guanosine 5′-diphosphate (GDP) for guanosine 5′-triphosphate (GTP) and in the process dissociate into Gα and Gβγ subunits. The dissociated Gβγ subunits mediate most chemokine-induced signals by activating different phosphoinositide-3-kinase (PI3K) isoforms, which in turn lead to the formation of phosphatidyl-3,4,5-triphosphate (PIP_3). PI3K and its product PIP_3 then translocate to the pseudopod at the leading edge of migrating leukocytes, where they colocalize with the small GTPase Rac.[29-32] PIP_3 activates Rac through specific guanine nucleotide exchange factors (GEFs).[33,34] Rac in turn acts through the downstream effectors p21-activated kinase (PAK) and the Wiskott-Aldrich syndrome protein (WASP) homologue WAVE, that stimulate actin-related protein (Arp) 2/3. Together, this process induces focal cytoskeleton polymerization, which is required for the development and forward extension of the pseudopod, a critical step in leukocyte chemotaxis.[35] The importance of PI3K-dependent signaling for leukocyte chemotaxis is evidenced by the lack of migration of myeloid leukocytes to chemokines in mice lacking PI3Kγ.[36-41] Notably, though, distinct signaling pathways or at least other PI3K isoforms appear to be involved in the trafficking of different subsets of immune cells. For example, whereas neutrophil and B-cell migration requires PI3Kδ, T-cell chemotaxis is not impaired in PI3K-deficient mice but depends on the Rac guanine exchange factor DOCK2.[42-48]

Termination of Chemokine Signaling

Different pathways have been identified that can terminate chemokine signaling through their GPCRs. The Gα subunit possesses an intrinsic GTPase activity to hydrolyze GTP. In a negative feedback loop, this GTPase activity allows the Gα subunits to reassociate with the Gβγ subunits, thereby restoring the heterotrimeric G protein to its inactive state. In addition, another class of molecules, known as

Table 11-1 Chemokines and Chemokine Receptors

Chemokine	Chemokine Receptor	Physiologic Function	Tissue Expression	Disease Connection[‖]
		CC FAMILY		
CCL1 (I309)	CCR8*	Attracts monocytes, NK cells, and immature B cells as well as DCs	Lung, skin, synovial fluid, brain	Asthma, COPD, atopic dermatitis, juvenile arthritis, cancer, MS
CCL2 (MCP-1)	CCR2* DARC/Duffy[§] D6[§]	Recruits monocytes, memory T cells, and DCs	Lung, kidney, joint, large arteries, intestinum, skin, brain, lymphatic endothelium	Asthma, glomerulonephritis, rheumatoid arthritis, osteoarthritis, atherosclerosis, inflammatory bowel disease, psoriasis, bacterial and viral meningitis, diabetes, HIV infection, pulmonary tuberculosis, cardiomyopathy in human Chagas disease, HBV clearance, HCV severity
CCL3 (MIP-1α)	CCR1* CCR5* D6[§]	Attracts eosinophil, basophil, monocyte, and T cell	Lung, joint, intestinum, brain, lymphatic endothelium	Asthma, rheumatoid arthritis, osteoarthritis, inflammatory bowel disease, bacterial meningitis, MS
CCL3L1 (MIP-1αP)	CCR1* CCR3* CCR5* D6[§]	Attracts lymphocytes to sites of infection or tissue damage	Lymphatic endothelium	Co-receptor for HIV, various infectious diseases, including chronic hepatitis and Kawasaki disease
CCL4 (MIP-1β)	CCR5* D6[§]	Attracts NK cells, monocytes, and a variety of other immune cells	Joint, brain, lymphatic endothelium, tear fluid, vessels, skin	Major HIV-suppressive factor produced by $CD8^+$ T cells; involved in rheumatoid arthritis, osteoarthritis, bacterial meningitis, dry eye syndrome, dermatomyositis, psoriasis
CCL4L1 (MIP-1β2)	CCR5* D6[§]	Similar to CCL4	Lymphatic endothelium, skin	HIV infection, psoriasis
CCL5 (RANTES)	CCR1* CCR3* CCR5* DARC/Duffy[§] D6[§]	Chemotactic for T cells, eosinophils, and basophils; recruits leukocytes into inflammatory sites; induces the proliferation and activation of NK cells	Lung, kidney, lymphatic endothelium, skin, joint, large arteries	Asthma, glomerulonephritis, allergic rhinitis, atopic dermatitis, SLE, rheumatoid arthritis, MS, HIV infection, hepatitis C infection, sarcoidosis, atherosclerosis, diabetes
CCL7 (MCP-3)	CCR1* CCR2* CCR3* CCR5[†] D6[§]	Attracts monocytes Regulates macrophage function	Lymphatic endothelium, macrophages, some tumor cell lines	HIV infection, MS
CCL8 (MCP-3)	CCR1* CCR2* CCR3* CCR5[†] D6[§]	Chemotaxis and activation of mast cells, eosinophils, and basophils; recruits monocytes, T cells, and NK cells; potent inhibitor of HIV-1 by virtue of its high-affinity binding to the receptor CCR5	Lymphatic endothelium, skin, stromal cells	HIV infection, MS, atopic dermatitis
CCL11 (eotaxin)	CCR2[†] CCR3* CCR5* CXCR3A[‡] CXCR3B[‡] DARC/Duffy[§] D6[§]	Recruits eosinophils, basophils, monocytes, and T cells	Lung, intestinum, lymphatic endothelium, skin, large arteries	Asthma, inflammatory bowel disease, atopic dermatitis, myocardial infarction, MS
CCL13 (MCP-4)	CCR1* CCR2* CCR3* DARC/Duffy[§] D6[§]	Induces chemotaxis of monocytes, eosinophils, T lymphocytes, and basophils	Lung, large arteries, brain, kidney, placenta, lymph nodes, spleen	Asthma, atherosclerosis, MS
CCL14 (HCC1)	CCR1* CCR5* DARC/Duffy[§] D6[§]	Activates monocytes	Kidney, heart, liver	Chronic renal failure, herpes simplex infection, HIV infection, hepatitis, amyloidosis, dilated cardiomyopathy
CCL15 (HCC2, MIP-1δ)	CCR1* CCR3*	Activates monocytes	Liver, small intestine, colon	MS, sarcoidosis, renal insufficiency, psoriasis, cirrhosis, hepatitis

Table 11-1 Chemokines and Chemokine Receptors—cont'd

Chemokine	Chemokine Receptor	Physiologic Function	Tissue Expression	Disease Connection[‖]
CCL16 (HCC4)	CCR1* CCR2* CCR5*	Chemoattractive for monocytes and lymphocytes	Liver, thymus, spleen	Drug-induced liver damage, angiogenesis
CCL17 (TARC)	CCR4* DARC/Duffy[§] D6[§]	Chemoattractive for lymphocytes	Thymus, DCs, endothelial cells, keratinocytes, fibroblasts, skin	Autoimmune diseases, SLE, allergy, asthma, pulmonary fibrosis, allergic dermatitis, atopic dermatitis, bullous pemphigoid, atherosclerosis, allergic rhinitis
CCL18 (PARC)	CCR3[†]	Chemoattractive for lymphocytes	Lung, lymphoid tissues	HIV infection
CCL19 (ELC)	CCR7* CCX-CKR[§]	Homeostatic chemokine controlling lymphocyte recirculation and homing, trafficking of T cells into thymus, T- and B-cell migration to secondary lymphoid organs	Spleen, lymph nodes, placenta, kidney, brain, lung	Asthma, atherosclerosis, allergic rhinitis, HIV infection, rheumatoid arthritis, pulmonary sarcoidosis, inflammatory bowel disease, renal disease
CCL20 (MIP-3 β, LARC)	CCR6*	Strongly chemotactic for lymphocytes, DCs, weakly attracts neutrophils	Mucosal lymphoid tissues, lymphocytes, lymph nodes, liver, appendix, fetal lung	Inflammatory bowel disease, pulmonary sarcoidosis, asthma, COPD, colitis, psoriasis
CCL21 (SLC)	CCR7* CCX-CKR[§]	Homeostatic chemokine, controls trafficking of lymphocytes in(to) secondary lymphoid-tissues	Spleen, lymph nodes, placenta, kidney, brain, leukocytes, liver	Cancer metastasis, melanoma, lymphoma, renal fibrosis, chronic hepatitis, cardiomyopathy
CCL22 (MDC)	CCR4* D6[§]	Recruits regulatory T cells, macrophages	DCs, macrophages	Autoimmune diabetes, pleural effusion, autoimmune encephalomyelitis
CCL23 (MPIF-1, SCYA23)	CCR1*	Highly chemotactic for naive T cells and monocytes; weakly chemotactic for neutrophils	Lung, liver, bone marrow, myeloid cells	Rheumatoid arthritis, *Bordetella* pertussis, fibrosarcoma, atherosclerosis, systemic sclerosis
CCL24 (Eotaxin-2)	CCR3*	Inhibits the proliferation of HPCs; recruitment of eosinophils	Thymus, spleen, intestine, activated monocytes and T cells	Asthma, ulcerative colitis, dermatitis, fibrosis, leukemia, certain types of neoplasia
CCL25 (TECK)	CCR9* CCX-CKR[§]	Chemotactic for thymocytes, macrophages, and DCs; controls T cell development	Thymus, liver, intestine	Inflammatory bowel disease, prostate cancer, primary sclerotic cholangitis
CCL26 (Eotaxin-3)	CCR3* CCR2[†]	Chemotactic for eosinophils and basophils	Lung, ovary, endothelial cells, heart	Allergic dermatitis, asthma, rheumatoid arthritis, allergic rhinitis, bullous pemphigoid
CCL27 (CTACK)	CCR10*	Homing of memory T lymphocytes to the skin	Gonads, thymus, skin	Dermatitis, psoriasis, mycosis fungoides
CCL28 (MEC)	CCR3* CCR10*	Drives mucosal homing of T and B lymphocytes; induces migration of eosinophils	Columnar epithelial cells in the gut, lung, breast, and salivary glands; colon	Atopic dermatitis, antimicrobial activity against *Candida albicans*, psoriasis, bullous pemphigoid, Hodgkin disease
		CXC FAMILY		
CXCL1 (GROα)	CXCR2* DARC/Duffy[§]	Recruitment of neutrophils; melanoma growth stimulating activity	Lung, skin, brain	ARDS, psoriasis, bacterial meningitis, MS, wound healing, melanoma, tumor genesis, angiogenesis, hemolytic transfusion reactions
CXCL2 (GROβ)	CXCR2* DARC/Duffy[§]	Chemotactic for neutrophils	Lung, blood, bone, bone marrow, brain, cervix, connective tissue, eye, intestine, kidney	ARDS, severe sepsis, septic peritonitis, autoimmune diseases, rheumatoid arthritis
CXCL3 (GROγ)	CXCR2* DARC/Duffy[§]	Controls adhesion and migration of monocytes	Lung, blood, adipose tissue	ARDS, Influenza, *Escherichia coli* infection
CXCL4 (PF4)	CXCR3B*	Chemotactic for neutrophils, fibroblasts, and monocytes; regulates T cell trafficking and B lymphopoiesis	Lung, liver, kidney, bone marrow, ovary	Putative antigen in HIT, thrombosis, wound healing, ARDS, liver fibrosis, arthritis, atherosclerosis, arterial hypertension, allergic dermatitis, HIV infection, cancer, metastasis

Continued

Table 11-1 Chemokines and Chemokine Receptors—cont'd

Chemokine	Chemokine Receptor	Physiologic Function	Tissue Expression	Disease Connection[‖]
CXCL5 (ENA-78)	CXCR2*	Neutrophil chemotaxis; modulates connective tissue remodelling	Lung, joint, blood	Bacterial pneumonia, rheumatoid arthritis, osteoarthritis
CXCL6 (GCP2)	CXCR1* CXCR2*	Chemoattractant for neutrophils	Adipose tissue, bladder, bone, connective tissue, eye, intestine, kidney, liver, lung, pancreas, placenta, prostate, spleen, uterus	Several types of malignancies (chondrosarcoma, leukemia, liver tumor, non-neoplasia, pancreatic tumor, uterine tumors, small cell lung cancer), tonsillitis, inflammatory bowel disease
CXCL7 (NAP-2)	CXCR2* DARC/Duffy[§]	Stimulates mitogenesis, synthesis of ECM, regulates glucose metabolism and synthesis of plasminogen activator	Platelets, monocytes, DCs, bronchial mucosa, brain	COPD, bronchial dysplasia, cancer, metastasis
CXCL8 (IL-8)	CXCR1* CXCR2* DARC/Duffy[§]	Chemoattractant for neutrophils; potent angiogenic factor	Lung, joint, intestinum, skin, brain, kidney, pancreas	ARDS, bacterial pneumonia, diffuse parabronchiolitis, rheumatoid arthritis, osteoarthritis, inflammatory bowel disease, psoriasis, bacterial meningitis, SLE, nephritis, acute pancreatitis, acute pyelonephritis, cancer, AIDS-related Kaposi sarcoma
CXCL9 (MIG)	CXCR3A* CXCR3B* CCR3[†]	Chemoattractant for T cells and NK cells	Skin, thyroid glands, synovia, lymphoid tissue, joint	Psoriasis, kidney disease, rheumatoid arthritis, inflammatory bowel disease, Sjögren syndrome, Hashimoto thyroiditis, Graves disease, ocular sarcoidosis, arterial hypertension, allograft rejection, cancer, cerebral malaria, inflammatory bowel disease
CXCL10 (IP-10)	CXCR3A* CXCR3B* CCR3[†]	Chemoattracts monocytes, macrophages, T cells, NK cells, and DCs	T cells, monocytes, neutrophils, kidney, larges arteries, intestinum, skin, brain	Hepatitis C, sarcoidosis, glomerulonephritis, atherosclerosis, inflammatory bowel disease, psoriasis, viral meningitis, MS, rheumatoid arthritis
CXCL11 (I-TAC)	CXCR3A* CXCR3B* CXCR7 CCR3[†]	Chemotactic for activated T cells	Liver, lung, kidney, brain, thyroid glands, intestine	COPD, pulmonary fibrosis, hepatitis C virus infection, nephritis, Sjögren syndrome, autoimmune encephalomyelitis, autoimmune thyroiditis, arthritis, inflammatory bowel disease, atherosclerosis
CXCL12 (SDF-1)	CXCR4* CXCR7*	Activates different leukocyte subsets; strongly chemotactic for lymphocytes; homeostatic chemokine directing the migration of hematopoietic cells from fetal liver to bone marrow and the formation of large blood vessels	Pancreas, spleen, ovary, small intestine, joint, tumor tissue, endothelium, hematopoietic tissue	Angiogenesis, carcinogenesis, metastasis, HIV-1 infection, atherosclerosis, acute myeloid leukemia, lymphoma, chronic myeloproliferative disease, type 1 diabetes, rheumatoid arthritis
CXCL13 (BCA-1)	CXCR5* CCX-CKR[§]	Selectively chemotactic for B cells	Liver, spleen, lymph nodes, gut	Lyme disease, SLE, rheumatoid arthritis, neurosyphilis, MS, myasthenia gravis, Sjögren syndrome, prostatic disease
CXCL14 (BRAK)	Unknown	Chemotactic for monocytes; potent chemoattractant and activator of DCs; can stimulate the migration of activated NK cells; inhibits angiogenesis	Many normal tissues, where its cellular source is thought to be the fibroblast	Cancer, liver failure, Alzheimer disease, Charcot-Marie-Tooth disease type 1A, angiogenesis, obesity
CXCL16 (SR-PSOX)	CXCR6*	Migration of T cells and NK cells	DCs, T cells, lymph nodes, spleen	Atherosclerosis, inflammatory bowel disease, chronic kidney failure
		CX$_3$C FAMILY		
CX3CL1 (fractalkine)	CX3CR1*	Chemoattractant for T cells and monocytes; patrolling of resident monocytes in the steady state	Endothelial cells	Inflammatory bowel disease, myocardial infarction, acute renal failure, end-stage renal disease, periodontal tissue, cirrhosis, Parkinson disease, atherosclerosis, cancer metastasis

Table 11-1 Chemokines and Chemokine Receptors—cont'd

Chemokine	Chemokine Receptor	Physiologic Function	Tissue Expression	Disease Connection‖
		XC FAMILY		
XCL1 (lymphotactin, SCM-1α)	XCR1*	Attracts T cells	Spleen, thymus, intestine, peripheral blood leukocytes, lung, ovary, prostata	Wegener granulomatosis, baculovirus, acute lymphoblastic leukemia, HIV
XCL2 (SCM-1β)	XCR1*	Leukocyte chemotaxis	Activated T cells	Atherosclerosis, chlamydial infection, atopic dermatitis, scleroderma, sarcoidosis, meningitis, biliary tract disease, Alzheimer disease

ARDS, Acute respiratory distress syndrome; *CCL,* chemokine ligand; *COPD,* chronic obstructive pulmonary disease; *DARC,* Duffy antigen receptor for chemokines; *DC,* dendritic cell; *ECM,* extracellular matrix; *HBV,* hepatitis B virus; *HCV,* hepatitis C virus; *HIT,* heparin-induced thrombocytopenia; *HIV,* human immunodeficiency virus; *HPC,* hematopoietic progenitor cell; *IL,* interleukin; *MIG,* monokine induced by interferon-γ; *MIP,* macrophage inflammatory protein; *MS,* multiple sclerosis; *NAP,* neutrophil-activating protein; *NK,* natural killer; *RANTES,* regulated upon activation, normal T-cell expressed, and secreted; *SLE,* systemic lupus erythematosus.
*Agonistic.
†Antagonistic interaction.
‡Nonagonist–nonantagonistic interaction.
§"Atypical" interaction, signal transduction as yet undefined.
‖Connection can be supportive or preventive.

regulators of G protein signaling (RGS), also modulates signaling through chemokine GPCRs. RGS are a large and diverse protein family initially identified as GTPase-activating proteins (GAPs) of heterotrimeric G-protein Gα-subunits.[49,50] At least some RGS can also influence Gα activity through either effector antagonism by competing with effector molecules for GTP-bound Gα-subunits or by acting as guanine nucleotide dissociation inhibitors (GDIs).[49] To date, more than three dozen genes have been identified within the human genome that encode proteins containing an RGS or RGS-like domain.

Fine Tuning of Chemokine Signaling by Chemokine Cleavage and Inactivation

In addition to termination of GPCR signaling, fine tuning of chemokine communication is also achieved by proteolytic cleavage and inactivation of chemokines, chemokine receptors, or both, further adding to the plasticity of the chemokine system. Proteases, such as dipeptidyl peptidase CD26, elastase, and the a disintegrin and metalloproteinase (ADAM) family, as well as matrix metalloproteinases (MMPs), have been implicated in the control of chemokine-mediated navigation of leukocyte trafficking.[51-54] The MMPs are a family of more than 20 enzymes with important functions in matrix degradation. They also act on chemokines to regulate varied aspects of inflammation and immunity.[55] The ADAM family of disintegrins and MMPs, which has been implicated in the shedding of adhesion receptors, including L-selectin, vascular cell adhesion molecule (VCAM), and junctional adhesion molecule A (JAM-A) (see Chapter 10), also modulates trafficking by cleavage of the chemokine CX3CL1. Other chemokines, such as CCL2 (MCP-1), CXCL10 (IP-10), and CXCL12 (stromal cell–derived factor-1 α [SDF-1α]), are cleaved and inactivated by MMP-2 and -9.[56-58] Apart from MMPs, proteases stored in neutrophil granules, particularly cathepsin G and elastase, inactivate chemokines, such as SDF-1α and its receptor CXCR4, that regulate not only the migration of mature leukocytes but also the mobilization and homing of immature HSCs.[59,60] Hence, proteases by means of their chemokine-modifying properties must be regarded as integral components in the control of trafficking of mature leukocytes and their precursors.

The expression of chemokines and their GPCRs, but also the termination of chemokine signaling (including chemokine and GPCR cleavage) within the local micromilieu, act together to tailor the trafficking of specific leukocyte subsets under steady-state conditions and during inflammatory diseases.

The remainder of this chapter gives an overview on trafficking for different leukocytes. In general, leukocyte trafficking can be classified into three distinct patterns of migration (1) **entry into tissues** from the circulation, (2) **migration within tissues,** and (3) **exit from tissues.** Each of these steps in leukocyte trafficking is discussed in the following sections.

LEUKOCYTE ENTRY INTO TISSUES

The emigration of leukocytes from the circulation is governed by (1) cell surface receptors that mediate the process of adhesion to the vascular endothelium (see Chapter 10) and (2) signaling molecules particularly chemokines, (see section above), which fine tune adhesion and control subsequent leukocyte migration.[29,61-66] The initial phase of leukocyte entry into tissues involves five distinct steps: (1) **leukocyte tethering and rolling** mediated by selectins (a family with three members, P-, E-, and L-selectin) that interact with specialized carbohydrate ligands on opposing cells (also see Chapter 10); (2) **firm leukocyte adhesion** mediated by the concerted action of chemokines and a group of leukocyte adhesion receptors, the integrins (e.g., β-2 integrins LFA-1 [CD11a/CD18], Mac-1 [CD11b/CD18], and α4 β1 integrin VLA-4) interacting with their endothelial ligands belonging to the Ig-superfamily (e.g., intercellular adhesion molecule 1 [ICAM-1], ICAM-2, and VCAM-1); (3) subsequent Mac-1– and ICAM-1–dependent **postadhesion strengthening and crawling;** (4) **transendothelial migration** mediated predominantly through adhesion receptors expressed on the endothelial cell contacts; and (5) subsequent **interstitial leukocyte migration** to their target site within the tissue. The adhesion receptors involved in leukocyte–endothelium interactions are discussed in greater detail in Chapter 10. The following sections therefore only give a brief overview of the molecular events relevant to each of the five steps involved in leukocyte accumulation.

Tethering and Rolling of Leukocytes

Initially, tethers are formed between leukocytes and endothelial cells through adhesion receptors that are characterized by the ability to rapidly bind their ligands with high tensile strength. The most important initiators of leukocyte tethering are selectins, expressed on leukocytes (L-selectin), endothelial cells (E- and P-selectin), and platelets (P-selectin). The most relevant selectin ligands are sialomucins that

Table 11-2 Chemokine Receptors

Receptor	Chemokine Ligands	Cell Types
	CC FAMILY	
CCR1	CCL3 (MIP-1α), CCL5 (RANTES), CCL7 (MCP-3), CCL14 (HCC1)	T cells, monocytes, eosinophiles, basophiles
CCR2	CCL2 (MCP-1), CCL8 (MCP-2), CCL7 (MCP-3), CCL13 (MCP-4), CCL16 (HCC4)	Monocytes, dendritic cells (immature), memory T cells
CCR3	CCL11 (eotaxin), CCL13 (eotaxin-2), CCL7 (MCP-3), CCL5 (RANTES), CCL8 (MCP-2), CCL13 (MCP-4)	Eosinophiles, basophiles, mast cells, Th2, platelets
CCR4	CCL17 (TARC), CCL22 (MDC)	T cells (Th2), dendritic cells (mature), basophiles, macrophages, platelets
CCR5	CCL3 (MIP-1α), CCL4 (MIP-1β), CCL5 (RANTES), CCL11 (eotaxin), CCL14 (HCC1), CCL16 (HCC4)	T cells, monocytes
CCR6	CCL20 (MIP-3 β, LARC)	T cells (T regulatory and memory), B cells, dendritic cells
CCR7	CCL19 (ELC), CCL21 (SLC)	T cells, dendritic cells (mature), antigen-experienced B cells
CCR8	CCL1 (I309)	T cells (Th2), dendritic cells
CCR9	CCL25 (TECK)	T cells, IgA$^+$ plasma cells
CCR10	CCL27 (CTACK), CCL28 (MEC)	T cells
	CXC FAMILY	
CXCR1	CXCL8 (interleukin-8), CXCL6 (GCP2)	Neutrophils, monocytes
CXCR2	CXCL8, CXCL1 (GROα), CXCL2 (GROβ), CXCL3 (GROγ), CXCL5 (ENA-78), CXCL6	Neutrophils, monocytes, microvascular endothelial cells
CXCR3-A	CXCL9 (MIG), CXCL10 (IP-10), CXCL11 (I-TAC)	Th1 helper cells, mast cells, mesangial cells
CXCR3-B	CXCL4 (PF4), CXCL9 (MIG), CXCL10 (IP-10), CXCL11 (I-TAC)	Microvascular endothelial cells, neoplastic cells
CXCR4	CXCL12 (SDF-1)	Widely expressed
CXCR5	CXCL13 (BCA-1)	B cells, follicular helper T cells (T_{FH})
CXCR6	CXCL16 (SR-PSOX)	CD8$^+$ T cells, SK cells, memory CD4$^+$ T cells
CXCR7	CXCL12 (SDF-1), CXCL11 (I-TAC)	Tumor cell lines, activated endothelial cells, murine fetal liver cells
	CX$_3$C FAMILY	
CX$_3$CR1	CX3CL1 (fractalkine)	Macrophages, endothelial cells, smooth-muscle cells
	XC FAMILY	
XCR1	XCL1 (lymphotactin), XCL2	T cells, NK cells

BCA-1, B-cell chemoattractant 1; *CTACK,* cutaneous T cell–attracting chemokine; *ELC,* Epstein Barr virus–induced molecule 1 ligand chemokine; *ENA,* epithelial-cell-derived neutrophil-activating peptide; *GCP,* granulocyte chemotactic protein; *GRO,* growth-regulated oncogene; *HCC,* hemofiltrate chemokine; *IP-10,* interferon-inducible protein 10; *I-TAC,* interferon-inducible T cell alpha chemoattractant; *LARC,* liver and activation-regulated chemokine; *MCP,* monocyte chemoattractant protein; *MDC,* macrophage-derived chemokine; *MEC,* mammary-enriched chemokine; *MIG,* monokine induced by interferon-γ; *MIP,* macrophage inflammatory protein; *NK,* natural killer; *SDF-1,* stromal cell-derived factor-1; *SLC,* secondary lymphoid-tissue chemokine; *SR-PSOX,* scavenger receptor for phosphatidylserine-containing oxidized lipids; *TARC,* thymus and activation-regulated chemokine; *TECK,* thymus-expressed chemokine.

are decorated with oligosaccharides related to sialyl-Lewis^x, including P-selectin glycoprotein ligand (PSGL)-1 and the peripheral node addressin (PNAd). Selectin-mediated adhesive adhesion bonds that are formed in the bloodstream are transient and do not allow prolonged leukocyte arrest. As the bonds continuously dissociate at the cell's upstream end, new bonds form downstream, resulting in a characteristic slow rolling motion of the tethered leukocyte.

Firm Adhesion of Leukocytes

To undergo firm adhesion, the rolling cell must engage additional adhesion receptors belonging to the integrin family, particularly CD11a/CD18 (LFA-1) and the α4 integrins, α4β1 (VLA-4) and α4β7. However, whereas selectins are constitutively active, integrins first need to be activated to assume a high-affinity state that promotes efficient adhesion to endothelial ligands. Integrin activation is induced on leukocytes by chemoattractant signals that trigger a reversible change in integrin conformation (leading to enhanced ligand binding affinity) or in integrin clustering (enhancing avidity) or both.[22] Some (but not all) chemokines presented on the luminal surface of microvascular endothelial cells can trigger rapid integrin activation and efficiently induce leukocyte arrest. The retention and presentation of chemokines on the vessel endothelium is mediated through binding to glycosaminoglycans (GAGs) in the luminal glycocalix. Chemokines that are produced in the abluminal space can be transported across the endothelial monolayer to the luminal surface with the help of the Duffy antigen receptor for chemokines (DARC).[67]

Chemokines signal through the Gα_i subfamily of large heterotrimeric G proteins to promote integrin activation. Gα_i can be inhibited by pertussis toxin (PTX); consequently, intravital microscopy studies have shown that lymphocytes treated with PTX undergo normal tethering and rolling interactions in high endothelial venules in lymph nodes (LNs) and Peyer patches (PPs), but unlike control cells, the PTX-treated cells are unable to engage in integrin-dependent firm arrest. Chemokine receptor activation precipitates a cascade of intracellular signaling events, which (among other effects) trigger integrin activation. This integrin activation involves proteins that impinge upon the cytoplasmic tail of integrins, including kindlins and talin. Binding of these adapter molecules to the cytoplasmic tails of the integrin α and β chains is critical to regulate leukocyte adhesion to integrin ligands, such as the binding and spreading of neutrophils on ICAM-1 and the complement C3 activation product iC3b.[68]

Postadhesional Leukocyte Crawling

Once arrested, the adherent leukocytes rapidly polarize and slowly migrate within the vessel in random directions.[69-71] This process is called *intraluminal crawling* and is thought to be essential for enabling leukocytes to find exit points within the vessel through which they can leave the vasculature.[29] Whereas neutrophils crawl only in inflammatory settings, a subset of monocytes crawl constitutively within noninflamed microvessels under steady-state conditions.[63,72,73] These "patrolling monocytes" are poised to provide immune surveillance via rapid tissue invasion into the extravascular space in case of damage and infection. After emigration, these cells can differentiate into macrophages or dendritic cells (DCs).[73,74] Interactions among ß2-integrins, LFA-1, and Mac-1 with endothelial ICAMs are required for intravascular crawling.[69,73,75]

Leukocyte Transendothelial Migration

The transendothelial migration or diapedesis is a critical event allowing leukocytes to cross the vascular wall and enter their target tissue. Two routes of leukocyte diapedesis have been described so far: a paracellular route that dominates most extravasation processes and a transcellular route reported for neutrophils and some T cells.[76-82] Both routes involve the action of apical and junctional endothelial ICAM-1 and, at least in some settings, VCAM-1. In inflammatory conditions, additional junctional endothelial ligands, such as ICAM-2, platelet endothelial cell adhesion molecule 1 (PECAM-1), vascular endothelial (VE)-cadherin, endothelial cell-selective adhesion molecule (ESAM), CD99, CD99L2, and JAM, can contribute to leukocyte diapedesis.[77,83-89]

Interstitial Leukocyte Migration

After penetration of the endothelial barrier, leukocytes move in the interstitium to their target sites within the tissue. This interstitial migration occurs along gradients of chemotactic agents, guiding them toward their destination.[90,91] This process is called *leukocyte chemotaxis* and depends on the ability of migrating cells to sense gradients of chemoattractants.[92-94] The spatiotemporal formation of chemokine gradients in the interstitial tissue is mediated by glycosaminoglycans, which bind chemokines using low-affinity interaction and control the site and durability of the soluble chemokine gradients.[95,96] The exact mechanisms involved in interstitial migration of distinct leukocyte subsets remain controversial.[97] Only recently, it has been reported that interstitial leukocyte migration involves integrin-independent flowing and squeezing.[98] Proteolytic enzymes (proteases) such as heparase, elastase, and MMPs (MMP-2 and MMP-9) seem to play a critical role in leukocyte interstitial migration because they are required for the degradation of the components of the basement membrane as well as of the extracellular matrix during leukocyte locomotion.[53,99]

All of these consecutive steps—(1) leukocyte tethering and rolling, (2) exposure to a chemotactic stimulus and firm arrest, (3) postadhesive strengthening and intraluminal crawling, (4) diapedesis, and (5) interstitial migration—are essential for leukocytes to enter lymphoid and nonlymphoid tissues and to migrate to sites of inflammation. Correspondingly, in patients with leukocyte adhesion deficiency syndrome, a genetic defect either in ß2 integrins (type 1) or in fucosylated selectin ligands (type 2), neutrophils cannot stop or roll, respectively; this syndrome is characterized by marked leukocytosis and frequent and severe soft tissue infections.[100-102]

The following sections discuss the mechanisms that control the entry of different subsets of leukocytes into their specific target tissues.

CHEMOKINE CONTROL OF LYMPHOCYTE HOMING TO SECONDARY LYMPHOID ORGANS

Migration of bloodborne lymphocytes to secondary lymphoid organs is the best-characterized example of leukocyte trafficking from the circulation into distinct target tissues.[2,4,103-108] Lymphocytes constantly survey secondary lymphoid organs, which include the spleen, tonsils, the appendix, PPs and LNs, to determine whether an antigen is present that poses a threat to the body. This information is provided to T cells by DCs, which collect and trap antigen and then present it to T cells together with costimulatory molecules and cytokines. Mature DCs that have captured antigen in peripheral tissues and some memory cells reach the LNs through afferent lymph vessels.[109-111] In contrast, circulating T and B lymphocytes gain access to LN and PP through specialized postcapillary microvessels lined with cuboid endothelial cells that are known as *high endothelial venules* (HEVs).[112-115] HEVs in different secondary lymphoid organs express distinct patterns of trafficking molecules to serve as tethering platforms for defined subsets of lymphocytes. For example, whereas HEVs in LN express PNAd, HEV in PP express mucosal addressin-cell adhesion molecule (MAdCAM-1). Other mucosa-associated lymphoid organs, such as mesenteric LN, express both MAdCAM-1 and PNAd. Although T and B lymphocytes are recruited by similar multistep cascades to home to secondary lymphoid organs, the role of individual traffic molecules is not necessarily identical even when both subsets interact with the same microvessel.[2]

Specific mechanisms control homing to different secondary lymphoid organs. To illustrate this, the following section gives an overview on two prominent examples of lymphocyte homing: (1) lymphocyte homing to LNs and (2) lymphocyte homing to the PPs patches of the gut.

Homing of T and B Lymphocytes in High Endothelial Venules of Lymph Nodes

The first step in the homing cascade in LNs is mediated by L-selectin/CD62L expressed on all lymphocytes, except effector/memory cells. PNAd, an O-linked sulfated core 1 carbohydrate moiety that is exclusively found in HEV, is the major endothelial L-selectin ligand.[116-120] Binding of L-selectin to PNAd initiates lymphocyte rolling in HEV and slows down and marginates the free-flowing lymphocytes.[2,66,119] Although the L-selectin-PNAd interaction is required, it is not by itself sufficient to promote firm leukocyte adhesion. The subsequent firm arrest of rolling T and B lymphocytes is mediated by the α4ß1 integrin, ß2-integrin CD11a/CD18 (LFA-1), CD11b/CD18 (Mac-1), and ß7-integrin, which bind ICAMs, particularly ICAM-1 and ICAM-2; VCAM-1; or MAdCAM-1 on high endothelial cells.[119-124]

Chemokines that are presented in the lumen of HEV function as triggers of integrin activation.[125,126] On naive T cells, integrin activation is primarily mediated by CCL21 (also called SLC, TCA4, exodus 2, or 6-C-kine), which is constitutively expressed and secreted by HEV. The secreted chemokine is noncovalently bound to glycosaminoglycans on the surface of HEV, where it activates rolling lymphocytes through binding to CCR7, which is expressed on naive B and T cells. Another CCR7 ligand, CCL19 (also termed ELC or macrophage inflammatory protein [MIP] 3β), also supports T-cell homing to LN.[126] CCL19 is not expressed by high endothelial cells themselves; however, CCL19 and other chemokines are released by extravascular cells in LN or in tissues that discharge lymph to a local LN. Lymphborne chemokines can be transported to the luminal aspect of HEV. Correspondingly, chemokines, including CCL2, CCL19, and CCL21, injected under the skin of mice accumulate on the luminal surface of the HEV in draining LN, where they promote integrin activation on rolling leukocytes bearing the cognate receptors.[127-129]

Endothelial heparan sulfate has been shown to be essential in controlling chemokine presentation on the endothelium, contributing to the recruitment of lymphocytes to LN.[130]

B cells use largely the same trafficking molecules as naive T cells to home to LN. However, B cell–HEV interactions are only moderately affected by the absence of CCR7 or its ligands.[131] Correspondingly, LNs of mice lacking CCR7 contain few T cells, but the B-cell compartment (and the memory T-cell compartment) is less affected.[132,133] Similar observations were made in *plt/plt* mice, which have a spontaneous genetic defect resulting in deletion of CCL19 and the HEV-expressed form of CCL21 (mice, unlike humans, have a second *ccl21* gene that is only expressed in lymph vessels), demonstrating that B cells are not absolutely dependent on CCR7 to adhere to HEV.[131] In fact, rolling B cells can be induced to arrest in HEVs by either CCR7 agonists or by CXCL12 (also called SDF-1α), the ligand for CXCR4.[134] An additional chemokine pathway involving CXCL13 (also called BLC) and its receptor CXCR5 has also been implicated in B-cell homing to secondary lymphoid tissues.[135] Of note, although B cells encounter several distinct integrin-activation signals in HEV, B-cell homing to LN is nonetheless less efficient than that of T cells. A likely reason is that the B cells express only approximately half the number of L-selectin molecules expressed on T cells, which greatly affects their ability to initiate the adhesion cascade in HEV.[115,136]

Homing in the High Endothelial Venules of the Peyer Patches

In HEVs of PP, similar homing mechanisms are encountered as described above for LNs. However, the levels of L-selectin ligands (which are immunologically distinct from PNAd) expressed by HEV in PP are considerably lower compared with LN.[137,138] As a result, L-selectin itself is not sufficient to initiate a successful homing cascade for most lymphocytes in PP.[137] Indeed, HEV in PP (and in mucosa-associated LN) additionally express MAdCAM-1, a ligand for the α4β7 integrin.[138-140] The α4β7 heterodimer, which comprises an α4 integrin chain (CD49d) linked to the β7 integrin chain, is expressed at low levels by naive T and B cells and is required for the successful homing of these cells in PP HEV.[137,140] After formation of an initial L-selectin-dependent tether, the α4β7-MAdCAM-1 pathway stabilizes and slows the rolling lymphocytes without requiring chemokine activation. After a chemokine signal has been transmitted, both α4β7 and LFA-1 become activated and jointly mediate firm arrest.[137]

Of note, α4β7 is strongly upregulated on gut-homing effector/memory lymphocytes but completely absent on skin-homing memory T and B cells; these differential levels of α4β7 integrin expression allow certain antigen-experienced lymphocyte subsets to acquire tissue selectivity.[141] The mechanisms underlying this specificity and plasticity of lymphocyte homing are addressed later. Similar to the case in LNs, chemokines are essentially involved in promoting integrin activation and allowing firm lymphocyte arrest in HEV of PP. Thus, CXCR4, CXCR5, and CCR7 have been implicated in B-cell homing, and CCR7 seems exclusively responsible for T-cell homing. Interestingly, although T and B cells are recruited across the same HEV in LNs, there is segmental segregation of T- and B-cell recruitment in PP. HEV supporting B-cell accumulation in PP are concentrated in or near B follicles and present CXCL13, but not CCL21, but T cells preferentially accumulate in interfollicular HEV (i.e., within the T-cell area), which express high levels of CCL21, but not CXCL13.

The above examples clearly show that each leukocyte must undergo a specific sequence of distinct molecular steps to arrest within microvessels. Notably, this sequence differs among different lymphoid and nonlymphoid tissues and between steady-state and inflammatory conditions. This explains why only certain leukocyte subsets gain access to lymphoid tissues and others are excluded. Granulocytes, for example, express LFA-1 and L-selectin but not CCR7. Consequently, although granulocytes can roll in HEV (via L-selectin), these leukocytes do not perceive an integrin-activating stimulus and therefore fail to accumulate in noninflamed LNs or PPs. Likewise, mature DCs express CCR7 and CD11a/CD18 but not L-selectin. Because these cells are thus incapable of rolling in HEV, they fail to home to noninflamed LN from the blood (although mature DCs readily access LN via afferent lymph). Hence, the GPCR-mediated integration activation step is critical for imparting specificity to the process of lymphocyte homing to LNs.

TRAFFICKING OF LEUKOCYTES FROM BLOOD INTO NONLYMPHOID TISSUES

General Principles of Leukocyte Trafficking to Nonlymphoid Tissues

As already outlined, naive lymphocytes migrate most efficiently to secondary lymphoid organs from which innate immune cells are excluded. However, both innate immune cells and subsets of lymphocytes can respond to inflammatory or activation signals by modulating the expression or activity of traffic molecules in a way that allows them to migrate to nonlymphoid tissues but also to inflamed lymphoid tissues. For example, in response to an inflammatory stimulus, granulocytes, including neutrophils, eosinophils, and basophils, are rapidly recruited to the affected site and provide the first line of defense. Thereafter, additional immune cells, including monocytes, DCs, and effector cells as well as memory lymphocytes, may be recruited. Essentially, all of these different recruitment events depend on distinct multistep adhesion cascades.

Many of the inflammation-seeking traffic molecules required for access to nonlymphoid tissues are shared by the different leukocyte subsets. The key receptors that initiate capture of neutrophils, monocytes, natural killer cells, eosinophils, and effector T and B cells at peripheral sites of injury and inflammation are the three selectins, the leukocyte-expressed L-selectin as well as P- and E-selectin, which are induced on both acutely and (in some settings) chronically stimulated endothelial cells.[142-146] In addition, leukocyte–leukocyte-interactions, mediated through PSGL-1 and L-selectin can also support accumulation of immune cells in inflamed tissues.[147-150] Subsequent firm arrest of leukocytes in nonlymphoid tissues involves integrins, including CD11a/CD18 (and its ligand ICAM-1 and possibly also ICAM-2), VLA-4 (and its ligand VCAM-1), as well as Mac-1 (and its ligand ICAM-1).[1,29,151] As discussed earlier for lymphoid tissues, chemoattractants, including chemokines and other GPCR agonists, such as formyl peptides, activated complement fragments (particularly C5a), and lipid mediators (e.g., PAF and LTB4), contribute essential integrin-activation signals for leukocytes at sites of inflammation. The molecular diversity and selective action of these different chemoattractants on distinct leukocyte subsets as well as their restricted temporal and spatial expression patterns provide a crucial mechanism for the fine tuning of cellular immune responses.[66,152,153]

Mechanisms of Tissue-Tropic Lymphocyte Trafficking

In most innate immune cells, the changes that are induced by activation signals are relatively uniform. In contrast, the migratory properties acquired by T and B lymphocytes in response to activation are diverse depending on the strength, the quality, and the context of the antigenic stimulus.[141] Specifically, antigen stimulation of naive lymphocytes results in the generation of effector and memory cells that express specific repertoires of trafficking molecules that guide them back to tissues containing the stimulatory antigen.[154-156] Thus, whereas a cutaneous challenge generates preferentially a skin-tropic memory response, oral stimulation induces preferentially gut-homing effector and memory cells.

Recent studies have shown that DCs play a critical role in fine tuning the tropism of lymphocytes. In addition to presenting antigen, DCs in different lymphoid organs are endowed with information indicating the tissue from which the antigen was obtained. DCs in mucosa-associated lymphoid tissues (unlike those in other lymphoid organs) possess the enzymatic machinery to synthesize retinoic acid (RA) from vitamin A.[157] Exposure of activated T cells to RA induces the expression of gut-homing receptors (i.e., α4β7 and CCR9) and suppresses skin-homing molecules.[155,158] In the absence of RA, T-cell stimulation induces few or no gut-homing molecules but instead promotes the expression of P- and E-selectin ligands as well as CCR4, which are needed for homing to the skin. Additionally, when activated T cells are exposed to interleukin-2 (IL-12) and high levels of vitamin D3, which is physiologically induced by sunlight in the skin, they upregulate CCR10, the receptor for the epidermal chemokine CCL27.[159] This organ-specific information can reprogram and "imprint" the tissue-tropic memory cells as they differentiate from naive lymphocytes.[156]

Similar to T cells, B-cell subsets also express homing receptors that permit their selective trafficking to specific tissues. For example, distinct B-cell subsets produce the immunoglobulin isotype IgA that is present in secreted body fluids, including tears, breast milk, and mucus. IgA$^+$ B cells are characterized by their expression of CCR10.[160,161] The ligand for CCR10, MEC/CCL28, is expressed predominantly in mucosal tissues that secrete IgA.[162] Hence, CCR10 may function as a homing receptor that allows IgA-secreting B cells to migrate to tissues where IgA is required. A large subset among the IgA secreting B cells are those in the small intestine, which in addition to CCR10 express the gut-homing receptors, α4β7 and CCR9. When naive B cells are activated in the presence of intestinal DCs, they upregulate not only these two traffic receptors but also undergo class switching to IgA. This imprinting effect is dependent on RA, which is sufficient to induce gut-homing receptors, but must be combined with DC-derived IL-5 or IL-6 to promote IgA class switching.[158] At least 50 additional subtypes of lymphocytes have been characterized in human blood, and it is likely that multiple similar associations among homing receptors, immunologic effector function, and tissue specificity will be revealed in future.

MIGRATION OF HEMATOPOIETIC STEM CELLS TO THE BONE MARROW

Role of Adhesion Molecules for Hematopoietic Stem Cell Trafficking

The BM is the principal site of hematopoiesis in the adult body. Correspondingly, most HSCs are lodged in the BM cavity. Within the BM, maintenance of HSCs and regulation of their self-renewal and differentiation is thought to depend on the specific microenvironment, which has historically been termed the *stem cell niche* (see Chapter 12).[6,8,163-165] The central role of stem cell niches for HSC function has been recognized with the discovery that *Sl/Sl^d* (steel-Dickie) mice bearing a mutation in the gene encoding membrane-bound stem cell factor (SCF, also known as KIT ligand) show failure of BM HSC maintenance.[166] However, the exact localization as well as the composition of BM HSC niches and the molecular crosstalk that controls the retention of HSC within the niches are subject of intense ongoing research.[167-170]

Notably though, not all HSCs reside within the BM. In fact, it has been known for almost 4 decades that a small amount of hematopoietic precursors are also present in peripheral blood.[10-13] Bloodborne HSCs continuously migrate back to the BM cavity, presumably to fill any vacant stem cell niches.[13] Although the exact physiologic relevance of bloodborne HSCs remains to be determined, the intrinsic capacity of HSCs to home to the BM compartment is the prerequisite for successful clinical BM and stem cell transplantation. Homing of HSCs to the BM is a rapid process because murine and human progenitors injected intravenously are quickly cleared from the recipient circulation.[13,171,172] Similar to mature lymphocytes, HSCs and hematopoietic progenitor cells (HPCs) interact through a multistep adhesion cascade with BM microvessels.[7,172-177] Initially, HPCs tether and roll along BM microvessels.[178,179] This process involves α4β7 integrin on HSC/HPC, which binds VCAM-1, as well as E- and P-selectin on BM sinusoidal endothelial cells, which bind α (1-3)-fucosylated ligands, including CD44 and PSGL-1 on the surface of HPCs.[172] The subsequent firm arrest is mediated by activated α4β1 and VCAM-1, which is constitutively expressed in BM sinusoids. In addition to α4β1 integrin, the integrins α4β7, α5β1, and α6β1, CD44 as well as JAM-B have recently been implicated in HSC homing to the BM.[177,180-183] β1 integrin-mediated adhesion is important for HSC and HPC movement not only in adulthood but also during embryogenesis. Correspondingly, it has been shown that fetal HSCs/HPCs lacking β1 integrins form normally and differentiate, but they cannot colonize the FL, suggesting an essential role of β1 integrins in fetal HSC/HPC trafficking. In contrast to β1 integrins, the role of the β2-integrins LFA-1 (CD11a/CD18) and Mac-1 (CD11b/CD18) for HSC and HPC trafficking is controversially discussed. Although some studies have reported their involvement in HSC and HPC retention, others have indicated that the effect of β2 integrins becomes apparent only in synergy with α4β1.[184-186]

Role of Chemokines for Homing and Retention of Hematopoietic Stem Cells and Hematopoietic Progenitor Cells in the Bone Marrow

The chemokine CXCL12, the ligand for CXCR4 expressed by most hematopoietic cells, including HSCs, is thought to play a pivotal role in BM homing of HSC. BM endothelial cells (in addition to immature osteoblasts and other stromal cells) constitutively express and secrete CXCL12.[173,187-190] However, alternate pathways appear to exist because fetal liver–derived mouse HSCs home to the BM of adult recipients independent of CXCR4, and adult HSCs treated with a CXCR4 antagonist are still able to home sufficiently to the BM.[191,192] This indicates that HSCs may use different receptors or respond to distinct integrin-activation signals. In this context, the recent description of CXCR7, an alternate receptor for CXCL12, may explain some of the seemingly contradictory findings.[193]

Of note, the CXCL12/CXCR4 axis is not only involved in the homing process of HSCs to the BM but (among others) has also been linked to the retention of HSCs within stem cell niches and to the regulation of the maturation of more committed HPCs (particularly B-cell progenitor cells).[60,194-198] Correspondingly, disruption of the CXCL12/CXCR4 pathway leads to premature release of HPCs into the peripheral blood.[199,200] HPCs lacking CXCR4 accumulate in the circulation and fail to undergo normal lymphopoiesis and myelopoiesis, most likely because the cells do not receive the required maturation signals. Interestingly, upregulation of MMPs (see earlier discussion), which cleave and inactivate CXCR4 and CXCL12, has recently been implicated in HSC mobilization.[201-204] Mechanisms that modulate the CXCR4/CXCL12 axis are also thought to play a role in the coordinated mobilization of HPCs in response to cytokines that are used for this purpose in clinical practice.[59]

Regulation of Hematopoietic Stem Cell and Hematopoietic Progenitor Cell Homing in the Bone Marrow by the Nervous System

The nervous system has recently been shown to play a critical role in the regulation of the migration of HSCs and HPCs to and from the BM.[205-207] Signals from the sympathetic nervous system control the function of BM stromal cells, particularly osteoblasts, and regulate the attraction of stem cells to the BM niche by modulating stromal CXCL12 expression. Notably, trafficking of HSCs into and from the BM is not static but rather follows a physiologically regulated circadian rhythm. This circadian HSC migration is orchestrated in the nervous system through the rhythmic secretion of noradrenaline from nerve terminals in the BM, which leads to activation of the β_3-adrenergic receptor and downregulation of Cxcl12, the major BM chemoattractant for HSCs and HPCs. From a clinical point of view, the timing of stem cell harvest or infusion may influence the yield or engraftment, respectively, and could affect the therapeutic outcomes.[206]

LEUKOCYTE MIGRATION WITHIN TISSUES

Trafficking Patterns of Lymphocytes

After a leukocyte has accessed a tissue, it must migrate to specific interstitial positions. As already discussed, homing typically requires that the bloodborne leukocyte completes a complex tissue- and subset-specific multistep adhesion cascade. One exception to this rule is the spleen, where most bloodborne lymphocytes can leave the circulation even when multiple traffic molecules are inhibited. However, chemokines are essential in all lymphoid organs, including the spleen, to guide the newly arrived lymphocytes to their proper position within the organ.

Multiphoton intravital microscopy was recently used as a tool to decipher the mechanisms that control the extravascular traffic patterns of homed lymphocytes within lymphoid and nonlymphoid tissues.[208-216] For example, imaging experiments have shown that T cells that have entered an LN move incessantly within the paracortex (T-cell area), where they query the resident DCs for the presence of antigens that activate their T-cell receptor. B cells that home to LN migrate to the more superficial B-cell–rich follicles, where they may detect antigens presented by follicular DCs. Activated B cells that encounter antigens then move to the margins of the B- and T-cell zones,[211] where they can receive help from antigen-specific CD4 T cells. Analogous specific microenvironments for T and B cells exist also in the other lymphoid tissues.

Migration of T Cells to T Zones within Secondary Lymphoid Organs

After homing to secondary lymphoid organs, T cells migrate within the T zones. They engage in highly motile ameboid movement (average speed, ~12 μm/min) and undergo multiple brief encounters with resident DCs.[217-219] A network of fibroblastic reticular cells guides T cells to the T zone and defines the limits of T-cell movement within this domain.[220,221] As a consequence of high T-cell motility, it has been estimated that every DC in an LN touches as many as 5000 naive T cells within 1 hour. When T cells encounter a specific antigen, they progressively decrease their motility, become activated, and form long-lasting stable conjugates with DCs. Finally, antigen-experienced T cells start to proliferate and resume their rapid migration while contacting DC only briefly.[219,222]

The positioning and high motility of T cells in the T-cell area is dependent on CCR7 and its ligands CCL19 and CCL21.[104,132,133,208,223,224] Both ligands are abundantly expressed in T zones by radiation-resistant stromal cells. Notably, ectopic expression of CCL21 induces the formation of LN-like structures in the pancreas of mice.[225] The expression of CCL19 and CCL21 but also of CXCL13, which attracts B cells to B cell follicles (see later discussion), by lymphoid stromal cells is strongly dependent on the cytokine lymphotoxin-$\alpha 1\beta 2$ heterotrimers signaling via lymphotoxin β receptor.[226-228] Correspondingly, mice deficient in lymphotoxin have no morphologically detectable LNs or PPs.[229] CCL21 and CXCL13 have been shown to be transiently downregulated in activated or inflamed lymphoid tissues in a process controlled by the cytokine interferon-γ, alternating the positioning of T cells.[230,231]

POSITIONING OF B CELLS WITHIN SECONDARY LYMPHOID ORGANS

Similar to T cells, B cells enter secondary lymphoid organs from the blood to search for their specific antigens.[232] As previously outlined, the homing and entry of B cells into secondary lymphoid organs such as the LNs and PPs depends on chemokine–receptor interactions that finally result in firm adhesion of integrins on the surface of HEV. This adherence is followed by movement into lymphoid tissue.[134,230,233,234] After entering secondary lymphoid organs, the naive B cells migrate to B-cell–rich areas, termed B cell follicles. This migration depends on the presence of CXCR5 on the surfaces of B cells and the localized expression of CXCL13 by follicular stromal cells.[103,228,234] Follicular B cells are also highly motile migrating on a network of follicular DCs (FDCs), a process that is thought to be necessary to ensure optimal surveillance of the FDC for surface-displayed antigen. After a period of random migration within follicles, B cells that have not encountered a cognate antigen return to the circulation via the lymph or, in case of the spleen (also see later discussion), via the blood. In contrast, B cells that become stimulated by antigen relocate to the B-cell–T-cell boundary area to solicit help from T cells, which is necessary for further differentiation. To achieve this repositioning, activated B cells rapidly upregulate CCR7. This permits their chemotaxis toward CCR7 ligands expressed in the T-cell–rich zones of the secondary lymphoid organs.[211] Real-time imaging has been performed to further characterize the timing of this relocalization process. Antigen-engaged follicular B cells initially reduce their migration velocity upon antigen exposure. About 6 hours later, the activated B cells move toward the follicle border with the T-cell–rich zone and undergo highly dynamic interactions with helper T cells during the following several days.[211]

In the spleen, a subpopulation of B cells is lodged in the marginal zone (MZ) immediately adjacent to the marginal sinus that surrounds the white pulp cords. The exact extent to which chemokine-induced attraction and adhesion affect the positioning of MZ B cells is still unclear. However, recent studies indicate that the lodgment of B cells in the MZ is dependent upon interactions of $\alpha L\beta 2$ and $\alpha 4\beta 1$ on MZ B cells with their ligands (ICAM-1 and VCAM-1, respectively).[235,236] As with follicular B cells in LN, antigen encounter of MZ B cells causes their rapid repositioning to the B-cell–T-cell boundary area. The retention of naive B cells in the MZ and their relocalization to the B-cell–T-cell boundary area upon antigen encounter is thought to involve signaling through the phospholipid sphingosine-1 phosphate (S1P) and its receptor $S1P_1$.[237]

LEUKOCYTE EXIT FROM TISSUES

Although the coordinated role of adhesion molecules and chemokines governing lymphocyte entry into tissues has been examined in great detail, less is known about the exit of these cells from tissues. The final sections of this chapter discuss examples of emerging research on the diverse mechanisms that regulate exit of distinct leukocyte subsets from tissues.

Reprogramming Dendritic Cells to Exit Tissues Toward Secondary Lymphoid Organs

Lymphocyte homing remains without consequence unless lymphocytes encounter DCs that present their cognate antigen. DCs capture and present antigen to T cells more efficiently than any other antigen-presenting cell. In general, two routes of antigen delivery to LNs have been described to date: (1) antigenic material becomes lymph borne and is taken up by DCs that reside in the LN a priori and (2) antigen is acquired by DCs that reside in peripheral tissues and then transport the material to the draining LN. DCs constitutively patrol all tissues and engulf microorganisms, dead cells, and cellular debris. In the absence of inflammatory stimuli, the cells remain in an immature state that is only weakly immunogenic and often stimulates T-cell tolerance rather than activation. However, multiple signals associated with infection or tissue damage can induce DC maturation. Immature DCs express a variety of chemokine receptors, including as CCR1, CCR5, and CCR6, which are believed to result in the constitutive homing of immature DCs into tissues, particularly sites of inflammation, where ligands for these receptors are abundant.[4,109,238-240] After exposure to a maturation stimulus, such as Toll-like receptor

(TLR) agonists (e.g., LPS, bacterial lipoproteins, peptidoglycans, or CpG dinucleotides), which often originate from infectious pathogens,[241,242] whereas DCs lose CCR1, CCR5, and CCR6, expression of GPCRs for lymphoid chemokines, particularly CCR7 and CXCR4, is upregulated.[243] Lymphatic endothelial cells in peripheral tissues express CCL21, the ligand for CCR7.[244] The loss of chemokine receptors that keep the DCs within the tissue together with the increased expression of CCR7 results in the exit of the mature DCs via the lymphatic drainage system.[132,245] Recently it was shown that CCL21 is a more potent directional cue for DC migration than CCL19.[246] DC migration into the draining lymphatics requires also β2 integrin binding to ICAM-1 expressed by lymphatic endothelial cells. The JAM-A, which is expressed by DCs and the lymphatic endothelium, represses DC migration to LNs because the absence of JAM-A expression by DCs facilitates their migration to LNs.[111,247] Likewise, ß1-integrins, which mediate the interaction of DCs with extracellular matrix components, favor retention of DCs in the periphery.[111] While traveling to the draining LN, DCs upregulate the expression of molecules for efficient antigen presentation and T-cell stimulation and begin to generate chemokines and other cytokines that allow them to attract and stimulate T cells.[245,248,249]

Egress of Lymphocytes from Secondary Lymphoid Organs

When naive lymphocytes do not encounter antigen on antigen-presenting DCs after a period of random walk, they exit secondary lymphoid organs through efferent lymph vessels or, in case of the spleen, by directly returning to the blood. Several adhesion receptors have been implicated in the egress of lymphocytes into lymphoid sinusoids, including PECAM-1 (CD31), the mannose receptor, which interacts with L-selectin, and common lymphatic endothelial and vascular endothelial receptor 1 (CLEVER-1).[250]

We still have very limited information about the signals that determine the dwell time of lymphocytes in secondary lymphoid organs (≈12 to 24 hr for T cells). However, the recent observation that the egress of both T and B cells from LNs can be prevented by the immunosuppressant molecule FTY720 has revealed some of the principal mechanisms underlying lymphocyte egress. FTY720 is a synthetic derivative of myricin, a metabolite of the fungus *Isaria sinclairii,* which has been used in Chinese traditional medicine. FTY720 induces lymphocyte sequestration in LNs and causes profound lymphopenia. In animal models of transplantation and autoimmunity, FTY720 causes immunosuppression, and it has been shown to exert significant therapeutic effects in a placebo-controlled clinical trial of relapsing multiple sclerosis.[251-253] Although lymphocyte sequestration in LN and lymphopenia in response to FTY720 have been reported some time ago, the underlying molecular mechanisms were uncovered only recently.[108] Upon in vivo administration, FTY720 becomes rapidly phosphorylated and then binds to four of the five known S1P receptors, $S1P_1$and $S1P_{3-5}$.[103,254-256] Naive B and T cells express substantial levels of $S1P_1$, and it appears to be this receptor that plays a predominant role in lymphocytes egresses from lymphoid tissues into the efferent lymph vessels. Studies using gene-targeted mice have shown that T lymphocytes deficient in $S1P_1$ cannot exit secondary lymphoid organs (and in case of T cells, also the thymus).[257,258] Reports using FTY720 and $S1P_1$-selective agonists also supported a role for S1P–$S1P_1$ signaling in the regulation of lymphocyte egress from secondary lymphoid organs. Notably, $S1P_1$ receptors not only regulate lymphocyte exit from tissues but also modulate lymphocyte homing capacity.[114]

Whereas the sphingolipid S1P is abundant in blood and lymph, low levels of S1P are maintained within lymphoid tissues. This S1P gradient is established by the action of the S1P degrading enzyme S1P lyase.[259-261] Based on these findings, it has been proposed that S1P gradients between blood, lymphoid tissue, and lymph fluid together with cyclical ligand-induced modulation of $S1P_1$ on recirculating lymphocytes regulates lymphocyte egress and determines the lymphoid organ transit time of lymphocytes.[6,262] Indeed, recent observations support that concept by showing that $S1P_1$ on lymphocytes is downregulated in the blood, upregulated in lymphoid organs, and downregulated again in the lymph.[263] Notably, CD69, which is rapidly induced when T cells become activated, negatively regulates $S1P_1$ and thus promotes lymphocyte retention in lymphoid organs.[264,265]

Egress of Hematopoietic Stem Cells and Hematopoietic Progenitor Cells from Non-Marrow Tissues

Although the mechanisms that control HSC and HPC homing and egress from the BM are well investigated (see earlier discussion), little is known about the signals regulating the exit of HSCs and HPCs out of tissues other than the BM. HSCs and HPCs arrive in peripheral organs via blood but leave them predominantly via the draining lymphatics.[6,266] Interestingly, it has been shown that S1P and S1P receptors not only mediate egress of lymphocytes from LN but also control the egress of HSPCs from peripheral tissues.[6-8] Correspondingly, inhibition of S1P–S1P receptor signaling decreases the number of HSCs and HPCs in tissue-draining lymph because of impaired egress from the tissue. Stress signals that mimic an infection (induced by administration of a TLR4 agonist) reduce $S1P_1$ expression on HPCs, leading to the prolonged retention in peripheral organs. This prolonged tissue dwell time is necessary for HSC and HPCs to allow them to differentiate into immune cells on the spot. Tuning of HSC and HPC retention in peripheral tissues through the S1P– $S1P_1$ axis could support innate immune responses by fostering a local and versatile supply of effector cells.

FUTURE DIRECTIONS

This chapter has outlined three distinct modes of leukocyte trafficking, (1) **leukocyte entry into tissues** from the circulation, (2) **migration within tissues,** and (3) **exit from tissues.** The constitutive and inducible migration of leukocytes throughout the body is essential for lymphocyte development and warrants proper immune surveillance. The processes involved in leukocyte migration are tightly regulated by chemoattractants and adhesion molecules. Leukocyte migration is characterized by a tremendous level of plasticity and specificity because different leukocyte subsets express unique patterns of traffic molecules that enable their navigation to target tissues. Our expanding knowledge of the mechanisms that control leukocyte trafficking will likely influence the development of multiple therapeutic strategies, including stem cell mobilization; immunotherapy of cancer; and the treatment of tissue-specific autoimmune, inflammatory, and infectious diseases.

SUGGESTED READINGS

Bonasio R, von Andrian UH: Generation, migration and function of circulating dendritic cells. *Curr Opin Immunol* 18:503, 2006.

Butcher EC, Picker LJ: Lymphocyte homing and homeostasis. *Science* 272:60, 1996.

Campbell DJ, Kim CH, Butcher EC: Chemokines in the systemic organization of immunity. *Immunol Rev* 195:58, 2003.

Charo IF, Ransohoff RM: The many roles of chemokines and chemokine receptors in inflammation. *N Engl J Med* 354:610, 2006.

Cyster JG: Chemokines, sphingosine-1-phosphate, and cell migration in secondary lymphoid organs. *Annu Rev Immunol* 23:127, 2005.

Glodek AM, Honczarenko M, Le Y, et al: Sustained activation of cell adhesion is a differentially regulated process in B lymphopoiesis. *J Exp Med* 197:461, 2003.

Lapidot T, Petit I: Current understanding of stem cell mobilization: The roles of chemokines, proteolytic enzymes, adhesion molecules, cytokines, and stromal cells. *Exp Hematol* 30:973, 2002.

Luster AD, Alon R, von Andrian UH: Immune cell migration in inflammation: Present and future therapeutic targets. *Nat Immunol* 6:1182, 2005.

Massberg S, von Andrian UH: Fingolimod and sphingosine-1-phosphate—modifiers of lymphocyte migration. *N Engl J Med* 355:1088, 2006.

Parks WC, Wilson CL, Lopez-Boado YS: Matrix metalloproteinases as modulators of inflammation and innate immunity. *Nat Rev Immunol* 4:617, 2004.

Rosen SD: Ligands for L-selectin: Homing, inflammation, and beyond. *Annu Rev Immunol* 22:129, 2004.

Scadden DT: The stem-cell niche as an entity of action. *Nature* 441:1075, 2006.

Spiegel S, Milstien S: Sphingosine-1-phosphate: An enigmatic signalling lipid. *Nat Rev Mol Cell Biol* 4:397, 2003.

Sumen C, Mempel TR, Mazo IB, et al: Intravital microscopy: Visualizing immunity in context. *Immunity* 21:315, 2004.

von Andrian UH, Mackay CR: T-cell function and migration: Two sides of the same coin. *N Engl J Med* 343:1020, 2000.

von Andrian UH, Mempel TR: Homing and cellular traffic in lymph nodes. *Nat Rev Immunol* 3:867, 2003.

Zou Y-R, Kottmann AH, Kuroda M, et al: Function of the chemokine receptor CXCR4 in haematopoiesis and in cerebellar development. *Nature* 393:595, 1998.

For complete list of references log on to www.expertconsult.com.

CHAPTER 12

DYNAMIC INTERACTIONS BETWEEN HEMATOPOIETIC STEM AND PROGENITOR CELLS AND THE BONE MARROW: CURRENT BIOLOGY OF STEM CELL HOMING AND MOBILIZATION

Shiri Gur-Cohen, Karin Golan, Kfir Lapid, Jonathan Canaani, Orit Kollet, and Tsvee Lapidot

The hallmark of hematopoietic stem cells (HSCs) is their motility and developmental program. The initial migration route of murine HSCs occurs during ontogeny in the embryo's yolk sac and the aorta–gonad–mesonephros (AGM) region[1] in which the first set of hematopoietic precursors develops. The initial wave of hematopoiesis is followed by the migration of HSC precursors to the fetal liver, where they undergo proliferation and differentiation to fetal blood cell lineages.[1,2] During the final stages of embryonic development, HSCs migrate from the fetal liver to the bone marrow (BM), guided by signals coming from the newly constructed bones. HSCs migrate via the blood circulation across the physical blood–BM endothelial cell barrier and extracellular matrices and finally home to their niches, supported by BM stromal cells. The murine BM stromal microenvironment, revealed as a negative regulator of hematopoietic stem and progenitor cells' (HSPCs) proliferation and differentiation via adhesion interactions, is believed to be part of the mechanism to preserve the quiescent HSPC pool in the BM while maintaining their migration and developmental potential.[3] Importantly, murine embryos that lack the chemokine stromal cell–derived factor-1 (SDF-1, also termed CXCL12),[4] which is highly expressed by many BM stromal cell types, or its major receptor CXCR4,[5] which is highly expressed by HSPCs, have multiple lethal defects, including lack of BM seeding and repopulation by fetal liver HSPCs. This abnormal phenotype reveals the essential role of the SDF-1–CXCR4 axis in HSC homing and repopulation during embryonic development. The adult BM is the major hematopoietic organ, where hematopoietic progenitor cells continuously replenish the blood with new maturing myeloid and lymphoid cells with a finite lifespan.[6] Bidirectional trafficking between the BM and the periphery, referred to as *homing, steady-state egress, stress-induced recruitment,* and *clinical mobilization,* is a hallmark of HSPC physiology.

This chapter discusses recent findings concerning the biology of HSPC homing and mobilization, emphasizing the major roles of the SDF-1/CXCR4 signaling cascade and the brain–bone–blood triad, which dynamically regulate stem cell migration and development.

HEMATOPOIETIC STEM AND PROGENITOR CELL HOMING

The prerequisite critical first step leading to successful clinical engraftment is homing of HSPCs to ablated BM of transplanted recipients, which is their predominant physiologic site of hematopoiesis.[7,8] Intravenously infused into the peripheral blood, HSPCs find their way to the BM and lodge there to initiate hematopoiesis and BM reconstitution.[8] This process requires the tropic SDF-1/CXCR4 guiding signal and firm adhesion and docking to the vascular sinusoidal wall followed by movement across the physical BM–blood endothelial cell boundary and extracellular matrix barrier toward the marrow cavity.[6,9] During the early stages of the homing process to the BM, murine HSPCs are directed preferentially to the trabecular-rich metaphysis of the femurs in nonablated mice at all time points from 15 minutes to 15 hours after transplant.[10] The homing process ends with selective access and anchorage of HSPCs to their specialized stromal niches within the BM. The choice of the BM microenvironment as the HSPCs' preferred residence is not casual. The BM is highly organized in a complex architectural and cellular structure, whereby HSPCs are localized and anchored in special stromal niches via adhesion interactions, providing signals that prevent their motility, proliferation, and uncontrolled differentiation. The murine HSPCs supporting stromal reticular niche cells express the highest levels of SDF-1, which is essential for stem cell quiescence and maintenance.[11,12] Dynamic signals produced by the brain–bone–blood triad via circadian rhythms and bone turnover, generate stress signals which coordinately turn the BM into the preferred environment for adult HSPCs.[8,13]

Studying Human Hematopoietic Stem and Progenitor Cell Homing: Use of Preclinical Immunodeficient Mice Models

To understand the complex mechanisms regulating human HSPC homing, functional preclinical animal models have been developed to study human stem cell engraftment. Human and murine SDF-1 are cross reactive and differ in only one amino acid, enabling engraftment of human HSPCs in transplanted immune deficient mice.[8] The severe combined immunodeficiency (SCID) mouse was one of the first immune-deficient models.[14,15] Additional murine models were developed throughout the years based on the initial SCID model, including the immunodeficient nonobese diabetes/SCID (NOD/SCID) mouse, which exhibits additional reduced immunity and was used to identify primitive human $CD34^+/CD38^-$ and $CD34^-/CD38^-$ SCID repopulating cells (SRC),[16,17] and the NOD/SCID/interleukin (IL)-$2R\gamma^{null}$ mouse, with further reduced innate immunity because of the lack of natural killer cell activity.[18] The homing of immature human $CD34^+$ cells to the recipient BM requires host preconditioning with sublethal total-body irradiation (TBI) or chemotherapy. These myeloablative regimens have been shown to induce a dramatic elevation of SDF-1 production and secretion by BM stromal cells,[19] disruption of the physical BM endothelium barrier,[20-22] and attraction of transplanted human $CD34^+/CXCR4^+$ cells to the BM microenvironment. Functional, preclinical immune-deficient murine models, which tolerate human HSPC xenografts, are important for understanding the mechanisms involved as well as identification of molecules participating in the biologic regulation of HSPC trafficking to and from the BM with clinical relevance.

Homing: Essential Role of the SDF-1–CXCR4 Axis

A major role in the regulation of HSPC homing is attributed to interactions between SDF-1 and its receptor CXCR4. Both human and murine BM stromal cells, including endothelial cells and endosteal bone lining osteoblasts, express high levels of SDF-1. In parallel, circulating HSPCs express CXCR4 which allows them to be preferentially chemoattracted toward high levels of SDF-1 found in the BM, thus facilitating the homing process.[9] CXCR4-dependent homing is also observed in aging neutrophils, which express high levels of CXCR4 and migrate back to the BM across the mechanical barrier for their eventual apoptotic cell death.[23] Blocking of CXCR4 by neutralizing antibodies impaired homing of immature adult human CD34$^+$ progenitor cells to the BM of transplanted immuno-deficient mice,[24,25] but genetic overexpression of CXCR4[26] or cytokine-induced increased surface expression of CXCR4[24,27] enhanced the homing capacity of transplanted human HSPCs. Given the important clinical challenge of improving HSPC engraftment and repopulation, upregulation of CXCR4 expression is a promising approach.[28]

Of interest, immature human CD34$^-$/CD38$^-$ SRC express low levels of CXCR4, have poor SDF-1 induced migration and cannot home when transplanted into the veins of immune deficient mice, hence requiring direct intra-bone transplantation.[29] Pre-incubation of CD34$^-$/CD38$^-$ cells on a murine stromal cell line induces CD34$^+$ expression on these cells and as a result improves their repopulation potential.[29]

The murine stem cell niche contains a rare population of reticular Nestin-positive mesenchymal stem cells (MSCs), which express the highest levels of SDF-1 in the BM microenvironment and form a niche for most HSCs.[11] Depletion of Nestin-positive stromal supporting niche cells results in defective hematopoiesis and reduced homing of transplanted HSPCs to the BM, demonstrating the crucial role of SDF-1 in homing of HSPCs.[11] Homing of human CD34$^+$ progenitors is largely regulated by the bioavailability of the SDF-1 guiding signal in the BM cavity. Functional, noncleaved SDF-1 is translocated from the blood circulation to the BM tissue through endothelial cells, which also express CXCR4[30] (as well as CXCR7, another SDF-1 receptor[31]). Once SDF-1 is bound to its receptor on the surface of the endothelial cell, it is internalized and transcytosed via clathrin-coated pit vesicles. The increase in SDF-1 levels in the BM functionally enhances the homing capacity of transplanted human CD34$^+$ progenitors to the BM of NOD/SCID mice.[30]

Dynamic changes in BM SDF-1 and CXCR4 levels affect HSPC homing. BM progenitor cells from mobilized individuals home better compared with nonmobilized BM progenitor cells because of elevated levels of CXCR4.[32] Prostaglandin E_2 (PGE_2), known to act through cAMP-mediated regulation of the Wnt signaling pathway to control HSC self-renewal and proliferation in-vivo,[33,34] is also capable of improving the homing efficiency of human and murine progenitor cells because of upregulation of surface CXCR4 expression,[28,35] resulting in consequently improved engraftment.[28] Enhanced CXCR4 expression as well as inhibition of SDF-1 degradation is important to enable a stable chemotactic response, directing the homing of HSPCs to the BM. Indeed, inhibition of the dipeptidyl peptidase CD26, a membrane-bound extracellular serine-protease with SDF-1 cleavage activity, improves homing to the BM and the engraftment potential of murine HSPC[36] and human CD34$^+$ SRC in transplanted immune-deficient recipients.[37,38] SDF-1 bound to CXCR4 was also found to enhance the expression of CD9, a member of the tetraspanin family of proteins expressed on primitive human CD34$^+$/CD38$^{-/low}$ and the more mature CD34$^+$/CD38$^+$ progenitor cells. Blockage of CD9 activity in immature human cord blood CD34$^+$ progenitors inhibits SDF-1–mediated migration, as well as conferring enhanced adhesion to fibronectin and endothelial cells. Moreover, CD9 blockage also impaired CD34$^+$ progenitor cell homing to the BM and spleens of transplanted NOD/SCID mice.[39]

Another important cytokine regulating progenitor cell homing is stem cell factor (SCF, c-Kit ligand), which plays an important role in hematopoiesis.[40] In contrast to immature cord blood CD34$^+$/CD38$^-$ cells, which home successfully to the murine BM and spleen, mature cord blood CD34$^+$/CD38$^+$ cells home poorly unless prestimulated with cytokines, such as SCF in vitro, for 1 to 2 days.[29] Prestimulation of human or murine HSPCs with SCF improved their in vivo homing abilities through increased migration and adhesion via very late antigen 4 (VLA-4) and VLA-5 integrins.[24,40,41] Moreover, the homing of murine progenitor cells to the BM of mice deficient in P- and E-selectin is impaired,[42] demonstrating the pivotal role of adhesion interactions for proper homing, allowing HSPCs rolling on BM endothelium and attachment to their stromal supportive niches.

Interestingly, SDF-1 is not the only chemoattractant factor in HSPC homing. The chemoattractant lipid sphingosine-1-phosphate (S1P) and ceramide 1-phosphate (C1P) were shown recently to have a role in inducing murine HSPCs homing to the BM by increasing progenitor adhesion to stromal cells.[43] The adhesion molecule CD44, expressed by murine and human HSPCs, is required for cell spreading and adhesion to hyaluronan and osteopontin, both of which are expressed by blood vessel walls and along the endosteum.[10] Blocking of CD44 prevents homing of immature human CD34$^+$ cells to the BM and spleen of NOD/SCID mice.[9,44] The importance of CD44–hyaluronan interaction in enhancing HSPC homing is further supported in physiologic conditions, showing that murine HSPCs home preferentially to the metaphysis of nonirradiated recipients, a process mediated by hyaluronan expression on endothelial cells in this area.[10] Changing the glycosylation of CD44 on MSC allows their interaction with selectins and navigation of human MSC to the murine BM.[45] Homing of murine and human HSPCs to the endosteal surface of the BM followed by their lodgment and engraftment also requires active sensing of calcium levels,[46,47] demonstrating the interplay between bone turnover and HSPC trafficking.

Taken together, manipulation of SDF-1 levels in the target organ and CXCR4 on the transplanted stem cells can be used to navigate stem cells in vivo to their target organs. Enhanced SDF-1 production by BM stromal cells after host preconditioning, crossing the blood–BM barrier and activation of the adhesion machinery are required for HSPC attraction and attachment to the BM supporting niches, allowing their subsequent self-renewal and differentiation.

RETENTION OF HEMATOPOIETIC STEM AND PROGENITOR CELLS IN THE BONE MARROW

After HSPCs home to the BM, they lodge at specialized niches, where they subsequently reside and contribute to ongoing hematopoiesis. The BM is highly organized in a complex architectural and cellular structure, where HSPCs are localized and anchored in stromal niches that prevent their motility, proliferation, and differentiation. Primitive murine HSPCs preferentially localize to endosteal regions rather than the central marrow along the bone shaft[48,49] and predominantly in the trabecular-rich metaphysis, which is also rich in blood vessels.[10] Retention at those BM niches is important for the support and maintenance of HSPCs,[50] and various cell types have been demonstrated to fulfill this supportive function in mice, including osteoblasts,[51,52] CXCL12-abundant reticular (CAR) progenitors adjacent to vascular cells,[12] reticular sinusoidal endothelial cells,[53,54] and Nestin-positive pluripotent MSC.[11] CAR and Nestin reticular progenitor cells have been shown to highly express various genes that are essential for HSC retention, such as SDF-1, SCF, vascular cell adhesion molecule 1 (VCAM-1), osteopontin, and angiopoietin-1.[11,12] In humans, reticular CD146$^+$ mesenchymal progenitors were identified as HSPC supporting cells,[55] and with similarity to mouse MSC, have been shown to express Nestin.[56] Whereas depletion of murine BM niche cells results in loss of HSPCs,[11,54,57,58] their increase is accompanied by higher HSPC numbers.[11,51] For example, increased numbers of osteoblasts caused by parathyroid hormone (PTH) administration or osteoblast-specific constitutively-active parathyroid hormone-related protein (PTHrP) receptors expand murine HSCs via Notch signaling.[51] Interestingly, preliminary results indicate that basic fibroblast growth factor (FGF2), a downstream mediator of PTH, expands HSCs by upregulating membrane bound SCF on stromal cells and c-Kit expression on HSPCs and downregulating SDF-1 expression by stromal cells.[59]

Apart from the current concept of HSC-supporting niche cells, another less established concept is the metabolic niche.[60] HSCs are predominantly located in hypoxic regions in the BM[61,62] and preferentially use glycolysis over mitochondrial oxidative phosphorylation to meet their energy demands.[63] Thus, it is not surprising that balanced levels of the hypoxia-induced transcription factor hypoxia-inducible factor 1α (HIF-1α) are crucial for HSC function.[64] It was long hypothesized that mutual interactions among HSCs and their stromal supporting cells exert inhibitory feedback on proliferation and differentiation, keeping HSCs dormant in a nonmotile mode.[3,65] One such important interaction is mediated via angiopoietin-1 expression by BM osteoblasts and Tie-2 expression by HSCs, triggering cell cycle arrest as well as tight adhesion required for retention.[66] Thus, interference with the adhesion interactions may lead to their loss of function and mobilization. For example, conditional deletion of CXCR4[12,67] or SDF-1[68] leads to increased cycling and exhaustion of the stem cell pool, as well as loss of retention and protection from DNA-damaging agents. Deficiency in the cell cycle regulator CDC42 also results in increased cycling, impaired homing and retention, and massive mobilization.[69] Robo4 is predominantly expressed by murine HSCs, and mice that lack Robo4 expression exhibit reduced retention of HSCs, correlating with poor repopulation capacity.[70] Annexin2, which is expressed by murine HSPCs, assists in localizing to the endosteum by binding to SDF-1; therefore, transplantation of Annexin2-deficient HSPCs results in impaired engraftment.[71] It should be noted that homing and retention may be regulated by different mechanisms. In other words, a stem cell may home and reach the BM, but as long as it is not retained, successful engraftment is not achieved. For example, HSPCs that lack the G protein Rac1, calcium-sensing receptor or the guanine nucleotide exchange factor Vav-1 home normally but demonstrate impaired localization to the endosteum or to Nestin-positive MSCs, resulting in poor repopulation.[46,72,73] Inhibition of Rac1 also causes mobilization of HSPCs because of loss of retention.[72] Because adhesion interactions are crucial for retention of HSPCs in their BM niches, targeting these molecules is expected to induce mobilization. Indeed, administration of neutralizing antibodies to the integrin VLA-4,[74] which is expressed by HSPCs, or to its receptor VCAM-1,[75] which is expressed by the BM stroma, induces HSPC mobilization. Mice deficient in each of these adhesion molecules have higher numbers of circulating HSPCs.[76,77] The major adhesion molecule CD44 is an important player in homing and engraftment of HSPCs, assisting in localizing to hyaluronan-rich regions in the BM.[44] Thus, whereas CD44 blockage leads to HSPC mobilization,[78] mice that are devoid in one of the hyaluronan synthases show reduced lodgment of transplanted HSPCs to the endosteum.[10] It is therefore not surprising that breakdown of adhesion interactions is an integral part of mobilization mechanisms, induced by granulocyte colony-stimulating factor (G-CSF) or AMD3100 administration. SDF-1, which is essential for quiescent HSC retention and function is downregulated in the BM following repetitive G-CSF stimulations[79,80] or rapid AMD3100 treatment[81] as discussed later in this chapter. Of note, genes that are necessary for retention are downregulated in Nestin-positive MSCs after administration of G-CSF or agonists to β-adrenergic receptors, leading to detachment of HSPCs and allowing their enhanced egress.[11] Intriguingly, apart from adherence to osteopontin, which participates in murine HSPC lodgment at the endosteum region,[82] HSC proliferation is also negatively regulated by ostepontin,[82,83] demonstrating an inhibitory feedback role for retention in the niche. Retention of HSPCs in the BM is monitored by the endothelial BM–blood barrier. Although the levels of HSPCs in the circulation and spleen are similarly distributed in murine parabiotic partners (pairs of mice with connected blood vessels and a shared circulation), the BM HSPCs are mostly of host origin because of the presence of the aforementioned BM–endothelial barrier.[84] The low levels of partner derived HSPCs are dramatically increased after G-CSF mobilization, indicative of increased permissiveness of the barrier, enabling enhanced egress, which is followed by enhanced HSPC homing. Indeed, upon irradiation, chemotherapy, or G-CSF administration, the permeability of BM vasculature increases, thus disrupting the BM–endothelial barrier.[20,22,85] Altogether, proper retention of HSPCs at their BM niches is required for ongoing hematopoiesis and repopulation capacity, and the loss of retention is an integral part of mobilization physiology.

HEMATOPOIETIC STEM AND PROGENITOR CELL MOBILIZATION

Stress Signals and Extensive Hematopoietic Stem and Progenitor Cell Recruitment

Hematopoietic stem cells are maintained primarily in a homeostatic quiescent nonmotile state, mostly because of a complex tight regulation by the BM niche microenvironment.[3,12,86] Although most of the adult HSC compartment is located and preserved within the BM during homeostatic conditions, a small and rare population of HSPCs is constitutively released and circulates in the peripheral blood.[8] In the early 1960s, circulating HSPCs were described for the first time to have repopulation potential.[87] Psychologic stress such as anxiety,[88] as well as physiologic stress caused by bleeding, injury, inflammation, and DNA damage induced by radiation or chemotherapy, prompt dramatic changes that have a significant impact on HSPC fate.[8] These systemic and direct changes include the detachment of immature leukocytes from their anchored BM lodgment and initiation of cell cycle entry and progression followed by increased motility and massive recruitment of HSPCs to the circulation as part of host defense and repair.

The host immune response is associated with increased production of the myeloid cytokines granulocyte macrophage colony-stimulating factor (GM-CSF) and G-CSF, which trigger HSPC proliferation, differentiation, recruitment, and clinical HSPC mobilization.[89] Clinical mobilization protocols take advantage of the motile nature of HSPCs. Repetitive, once-daily G-CSF stimulations mimic stress conditions and provide proinflammatory signals. This cytokine induces HSPC detachment from their stromal niches and triggers massive accelerated progenitor proliferation and differentiation, involving a rapid increase in neutrophil counts and a gradual increase in HSPC numbers in the circulation, peaking between days 4 and 5 of G-CSF administration. Recruitment of HSPCs to the peripheral blood is not a passive release of proliferating HSPCs but rather an active process in which the impetus toward gaining motility is triggered by tightly regulated guiding signals, repressing the BM stromal inhibitory attachment machinery, which in turn allows mobilization of HSPCs to the circulation. HSPC mobilization is a complex multistep process involving the secretion of various cytokines and chemokines and the activity of proteolytic enzymes, which inhibit BM retention-inducing signals and increase the cells' trafficking capacity. The chemokine SDF-1 and its major receptor CXCR4 are essential components in the tightly regulated process of HSPC recruitment and mobilization. SDF-1 is produced by many BM resident cell types, including osteoclasts,[90] osteoblasts, endothelial cells,[30,81] reticular Nestin-positive MSCs,[11] and CAR stromal progenitor cells.[12] SDF-1 is a known powerful chemotactic factor for primitive human $CD34^+/CD38^-$ and murine $Sca\text{-}1^+/c\text{-}Kit^+/$ (SKL) cells enriched with repopulating HSCs.[91,92] An increase in SDF-1 levels in injured peripheral organs recruits $CXCR4^+$ progenitor cells from the BM reservoir and directs them to the site of injury.[93] Modulation in SDF-1 concentration also contributes to the delicate balance between hematopoiesis and directed motility: whereas low levels of SDF-1 induce proteolytic enzymes secretion by human $CD34^+$ progenitors (including matrix metalloproteinase-2 and 9; MMP2/9), directional migration, and proliferation, high levels induce internalization and desensitization of CXCR4,[94,95] progenitor cell quiescence,[96] and inhibition of cell motility. Thus, basal levels of SDF-1 in the BM are required for HSPC homeostatic maintenance, acting via CXCR4 to ensure cell quiescence and retention. Perturbation of the fundamental balanced SDF-1/CXCR4 signaling axis in the BM during mobilization is associated with a transient increase of SDF-1 levels because of its secretion by BM stromal cells followed by its release to the circulation. Local expression of SDF-1 in the BM is further reduced in response to active proteolytic cleavage by many enzymes that are activated by the secreted SDF-1, and BM HSPC gain increased CXCR4 expression and thereafter are guided into the periphery.[79,81,97] G-CSF–induced mobilization of murine HSPCs from their BM niches inhibits SDF-1 transcription and production by BM stromal cells, including osteoblasts[97] and reticular Nestin-positive MSCs.[11] Dynamic perturbation in the guiding signal SDF-1 in the surrounding BM niche supporting cells is also accompanied by increased CXCR4 expression on the surface of immature human BM CD34+ cells[79,98] and primitive CD34+CD38− cells.[79] This direct HSPC regulation as well as indirect inhibitory effect of BM stromal cell function demonstrates the importance of interactions between SDF-1 and CXCR4 in retaining HSPCs; disruption of this fine-tuned axis leads to HSPC mobilization.

Rapid HSPC mobilization is a fast process that does not involve proliferation, typically peaking within minutes to hours after administration. One such agent is the rapid mobilizer AMD3100 (also known as Plerixafor and Mozobil), which was first characterized as a CXCR4 antagonist according to its ability to inhibit migration toward SDF-1 in vitro[99,100] because it reversibly blocks SDF-1 binding to CXCR4. Upon its administration in vivo, AMD3100 disrupts the SDF-1–CXCR4 axis, thus facilitating both human CD34+ and murine HSPC mobilization in the time frame of a few hours.[101] AMD3100 is approved for clinical HSPC mobilization protocols in combination with G-CSF in patients with non-Hodgkin lymphoma and multiple myeloma undergoing autologous transplantation.[102] Prolonged G-CSF-induced HSPC mobilization shares some similarities with rapid mobilization protocols but also reveals mechanistic differences. AMD3100 and G-CSF act in synergy to facilitate enhanced HSPC egress from the BM.[103] In addition to the kinetic differences, the gene expression profile signatures of immature human CD34+ cells following G-CSF, AMD3100 or the combined treatment is largely different, demonstrating unique mechanisms of activity driving these two powerful mobilizers.[104] Disrupting the SDF-1–CXCR4 axis by the antagonistic effect of AMD3100 cannot fully explain the mechanism leading to rapid HSPC mobilization because neutralizing antibodies against CXCR4, which also inhibit SDF-1–induced migration in vitro, are incapable of inducing in vivo HSPC mobilization.[79,81,105] Current understanding suggests that HSPC mobilization by AMD3100 is an active process, consistent with the notion that stem cell detachment from their nursing microenvironment and recruitment to the circulation is a highly regulated process. Recent findings suggest that AMD3100 has also an agonistic effect by mediating rapid SDF-1 secretion from murine BM CXCR4+ stromal cells followed by its rapid release to the circulation.[81] Mobilized human CD34+ progenitor cells following AMD3100 and G-CSF treatment have increased SDF-1 chemotaxis in vitro,[101] suggesting that AMD3100 inhibition in vivo is transient and short lived. SDF-1 secretion from BM stromal cells could induce the removal of AMD3100 from CXCR4+ HSPCs, allowing their enhanced SDF-1–mediated migration and rapid mobilization in vivo. These dynamic fluctuations, enabling transient and local SDF-1 gradients toward the blood, emerge as an essential mechanism for egress and rapid mobilization of immature progenitor cells and are less important for mature leukocytes egress.[81] SDF-1 secretion by human and murine BM stromal cells, driven by either pharmacologic manipulation or homeostatic condition, is a cell-contact–dependent event mediated by connexin 43/45 gap junctions.[56] Enhanced SDF-1 release from BM stromal cells and its translocation to the circulation, together with the short transient inhibitory effect of AMD3100, actively promotes HSPC recruitment from the BM in the course of rapid mobilization. Of note, murine Sca-1+/c-Kit+/Lin− progenitor cells recruitment to sites of injury is also associated with rapid SDF-1 secretion from thrombin-activated platelets, thereby supporting host defense and repair mechanisms.[106] Thrombin and its receptor protease-activated receptor-1 (PAR-1) play an important role in coagulation after injury and bleeding. Interestingly, thrombin stimulation results in rapid SDF-1 secretion from murine BM stromal cells, including from rare Nestin-positive MSCs, which functionally express PAR-1.[107] Accordingly, PAR-1 activation in vivo induces rapid murine HSPC mobilization within 1 hour via CXCR4 upregulation and a dramatic decrease of SDF-1 in the BM.[107] Indeed, PAR-1 was found to be significantly increased on mobilized human CD34+, suggesting the involvement of PAR-1 signaling in human HSPC trafficking to the circulation as part of G-CSF mobilization.[108]

Collectively, the SDF-1–CXCR4 axis plays a pivotal role in directing steady-state egress and enhanced recruitment of HSPCs. Altering SDF-1 levels in the BM and the blood thereby dynamically affects circulating HSPC numbers and may be exploited for future clinical protocols.

Stem Cell Trafficking is Coordinated by the Brain–Bone–Blood Triad

The sympathetic nervous system (SNS) interacts with the immune system and exerts direct and indirect influences on stem and progenitor cells function. Human and murine BM are highly innervated.[109-111] The mammalian nervous system regulates the immune system in many acute physiologic conditions, especially during mental stress, as part of the "fight-or-flight" response of the adrenergic SNS.[112] Acute and chronic psychologic stresses, mediated by neuronal signals, can affect HSPC function and recruitment to the periphery as a front line of defense.[88,113] Neuronal receptors are dynamically expressed on primitive human CD34+/CD38− HSPCs, with a gradual decrease as the cells progressively differentiate. G-CSF–mobilized human CD34+ show higher catecholaminergic receptor expression compared with nonstimulated human cord blood or BM-derived CD34+ progenitor cells,[114] suggesting a role for the SNS in regulating HSPC recruitment and clinical mobilization. The involvement of the SNS in the regulation of HSPC trafficking was further supported by murine models showing that mice lacking norepinephrine synthesis and mice that were subjected to pharmacologic catecholaminergic ablation exhibited inability to induce mobilization in response to G-CSF.[115] Neurotransmitters that have a chemotactic activity for both resting and G-CSF–stimulated human CD34+ HSPCs induce HSPC motility and BM repopulation of immune deficient NOD/SCID mice via activation of the canonical Wnt signaling pathway.[114] Human HSPC mobilization is also regulated in a paracrine fashion by the endocannabinoid system, representing a pivotal neuroprotective mechanism whereby BM stromal cells express endocannabinoids and HSPCs express the cannabinoid receptor CB2. Indeed, cannabinoid receptor activation reduced CXCR4 expression, rapidly mobilized murine HSPCs, and enhanced mobilization by G-CSF.[116]

Bone marrow SDF-1 levels oscillate in a circadian manner, a process orchestrated by rhythmic β_3 adrenergic signals delivered by the nervous system,[117] verifying the notion that HSPC egress from the murine BM is not a random event but is rather triggered and synchronized by functional BM SDF-1 expression. Accordingly, expression of CXCR4 by murine BM HSPCs also demonstrates circadian oscillations.[118] Enforced mobilization by G-CSF or AMD3100 is also controlled by the molecular clock, such that synchronized CXCR4 and SDF-1 levels can influence the yield of collected HSPCs.[118] Studies in humans have revealed circadian fluctuations of human CD34+/CD38− stem cells in peripheral blood, suggesting the importance of circadian rhythms in pharmacologic mobilization protocols to increase the success of HSPC transplantation.[118] Circadian rhythms of HSPC egress during low SDF-1 levels in the BM are coupled to environmental dark–light cycles, demonstrating how signals initiated in the eyes and brain can synchronize bone remodeling and HSCs egress via the SNS.[119] The molecular clock in the nervous system is only one arm by which it controls HSPC egress. The essential course of SDF-1 secretion from BM stromal cells to the circulation, in order to induce HSPC mobilization, was also found to be regulated by neurotransmitter signaling. Catecholaminergic stimulation with norepinephrine induces rapid SDF-1 release to the periphery from BM stromal cells expressing the β_2-adrenergic receptor, thus enabling murine HSPC mobilization within 1 hour.[81] The SNS also affects murine HSPC steady-state egress and promotes G-CSF–induced mobilization indirectly by suppression of endosteal osteoblasts function, hence resulting in downregulation of SDF-1 expression in the BM.[97,115]

Adrenergic stimulation reduces bone formation via leptin dependent neuronal regulation, indicating that bone formation and osteoblast function are regulated by the SNS as well.[120] Accordingly, repetitive

G-CSF treatments in mice inhibit the transcription of genes that regulate HSPC maintenance and retention in the BM in the supportive Nestin-positive niche cells, such as SDF-1 and Kit ligand.[11] By contrast, in vivo PTH administration primes Nestin-positive MSCs to differentiate more rapidly into osteoblasts[11] and doubles the HSPC pool.[51] PTH stimulates osteoblasts to produce the cytokines receptor activator of nuclear factor κ-B ligand (RANKL) and macrophage colony-stimulating factor (M-CSF), therefore facilitating marrow monocyte differentiation into mature osteoclasts that initiate remodeling by enhanced bone resorption.[121] The bone is a highly dynamic tissue through the process of bone remodeling. Changes within the BM microenvironment after administration of RANKL, the osteoclast differentiation cytokine, were associated with preferential mobilization of immature murine progenitors.[90] Bone resorption by HSC-originated osteoclasts and bone formation by osteoblasts, originated from mesenchymal progenitors, are two coupled processes whereby bone resorption is normally followed by new bone formation.[122] This balanced process is tightly regulated by complex signals of hormones, cytokines, chemokines, and inflammatory factors.[123] Inhibition of osteoblast function by the powerful mobilizing agent G-CSF dictates osteoclasts recruitment and increased activity. It should be noted, however, that after G-CSF administration, osteoblasts first proliferate before their suppression, thus enabling HSPC expansion before the subsequent mobilization.[124] The endosteal stem cell niche is dynamic, producing hematopoietic cells on demand, and is dramatically accelerated in response to alarm signals because of injury.[123] Concomitantly, bone-degrading osteoclasts are directly involved in mobilization of progenitor cells from the BM to the circulation, both in homeostatic and stress conditions.[90] Robust activation of bone resorbing tartrate-resistant acid phosphatase (TRAP)-positive active osteoclasts along the bone-interface endosteum regions in various physiologic stress conditions, such as bleeding and bacterial infection, induces preferential HSPC mobilization.[123] The involvement of osteoclast activation in mediating HSPC egress and mobilization is also evident in CD45-deficient mice, possessing defective osteoclast activity and altered metaphysial trabecules, which exhibit impaired HSPC release to the circulation during G-CSF mobilization.[125] One of the driving forces behind HSPC mobilization after osteoclast activation may be an alteration in intercellular communication among the stromal supporting cells in the BM microenvironment. SDF-1 secretion is cell contact dependent mediated via connexin 43/45 gap junctions,[56] suggesting that osteoclast activation transiently breaks the tight BM stromal cell syncytium, which results in SDF-1 downregulation, reduced retention, and HSPC mobilization.

Myeloid BM macrophages are emerging as additional key participants in the systemic response to G-CSF stimulation. The endosteal-specific murine macrophages, osteomacs, which support bone-forming osteoblast function, are dramatically depleted after repetitive G-CSF stimulations followed by suppression of osteoblasts and their adhesion interactions with HSPCs, leading to HSPC release into the blood.[126,127] Depletion of another BM-derived macrophage subpopulation, defined as CD169$^+$ macrophages, known to support the function of Nestin-positive MSC, induced marked HSPC egress and mobilization.[127] BM macrophages might also serve as a connecting link between signals of the SNS and osteoblast suppression.[80,128] Taken together, complex hierarchical differentiation of monocytic precursors, including CD169$^+$ macrophages, osteomas, and bone-degrading osteoclasts, dictate HSPCs' fate via a wide variety of signals.

Proteolytic Enzymes and Hematopoietic Stem and Progenitor Cell Mobilization

The BM microenvironment is highly vascularized, containing large blood vessels and sinusoids. This endothelial gatekeeper function is essential to preserve HSPCs confined to the BM. Mobilization upon clinical G-CSF administration or chemotherapy is associated with disrupted endothelial integrity and increased permeability of BM sinusoids, the site at which active transition of HSPCs from the BM to the circulation takes place.[9,129] Bordering endothelial gaps, as part of the complex mechanism to enhance HSPC mobilization, are believed to be under the regulation of proteolytic enzymes including MMP-9. This enzyme is highly produced in the BM after G-CSF treatment[130] and is capable of degrading components that comprise the endothelial tight junctions and are responsible for endothelial integrity.[131] Functional osteoclasts secrete several proteolytic enzymes, including MMP-9 and the major bone-resorbing enzyme cathepsin K during homeostasis, and more intensively under stressed conditions, such as after G-CSF administration. These events are followed by proteolytic deactivation of factors providing stem cell retention signals in the endosteum region such as SDF-1, osteopontin, and SCF, eventually leading to HSPC mobilization.[90,123] Release of membrane-bound SCF, an important lodgment factor for murine stem cells[132] from the BM to the peripheral blood because of SDF-1–induced proteolytic activity of MMP-9 further demonstrates the involvement of MMP-9 in the mobilization process.[130] The transient increase of SDF-1 levels in the marrow cavity followed by its rapid secretion to the circulation during AMD3100 administration[81] or secretion and degradation after repetitive G-CSF stimulation,[79] emerges as a pivotal event in the mechanism of HSPC mobilization. In response to the G-CSF regimen, the adult BM becomes a highly proteolytic microenvironment caused by neutrophil proliferation and activation, resulting in the release of large amounts of neutrophil proteases such as neutrophil elastase, cathepsin G, and MMP-9 directly into the BM cavity.[133] The chemotactic potential of SDF-1 is reduced after cleavage of its N-terminal domain as a consequence of proteolytic activity by several degrading enzymes, including CD26/dipeptidylpeptidase IV,[134] neutrophil proteases,[135] and cathepsin K.[90] Secretion of functional MMP-9 is also associated with AMD3100 administration, suggesting the involvement of the proteolytic enzyme MMP-9 in rapid HSPC mobilization.[136,137] Another important enzyme, the cell surface protease membrane type 1 MMP (MT1-MMP), which is expressed by immature human CD34$^+$ cells and by mature myeloid cells, can inactivate SDF-1 and CD44 by proteolytic cleavage.[138] Upon G-CSF treatment, MT1-MMP expression is increased on human CD34$^+$ progenitor cells followed by downregulation of its endogenous inhibitor RECK and CD44, facilitating loss of progenitor cell retention and allowing their egress and mobilization.[139] Importantly, MT1-MMP expression positively correlates with egress and G-CSF mobilization of human CD34$^+$ progenitors[139]; thus, MT1-MMP may predict clinical mobilization outcome. The thrombolytic agent plasminogen, which is activated by tissue-type and urokinase-type plasminogen activator (tPA and uPA) to plasmin, was found to be a critical regulator of murine HPSC mobilization,[81,140-142] mediating MMP-9 secretion in a CXCR4-dependent manner.[98] Current understanding strongly suggests that proteases and MMPs are part of the major stem cell migration and mobilization regulatory machinery, inactivating BM-derived growth factors and chemokines, which are responsible for immature and maturing leukocyte adhesion and retention, thus facilitating enhanced movement across the physical barrier of the marrow extracellular matrix in response to AMD3100 or G-CSF stimulations.

Additional Control of Hematopoietic Stem and Progenitor Cell Mobilization

One of the major pathways by which HSPCs directly and indirectly gain motility is the generation of reactive oxygen species (ROS). Repetitive G-CSF–induced mobilization involves ROS generation directly in primitive hematopoietic progenitors, correlating with their enhanced egress and motility, involving hepatocyte growth factor (HGF) and its cognate receptor c-Met signaling.[105] Concomitantly, inhibition of ROS by the antioxidant NAC (*N*-acetyl cysteine) led to a preferential inhibition of AMD3100-induced and G-CSF–induced murine HSPC mobilization.[81,105] HSPC recruitment to the peripheral blood is also regulated by the chemoattractant lipid S1P as part of steady state egress as well as stress-induced mobilization.[143,144] In humans, S1P induces chemotaxis of immature CD34$^+$ cells that express the S1P receptor sphingosine-1-phosphate receptor-1

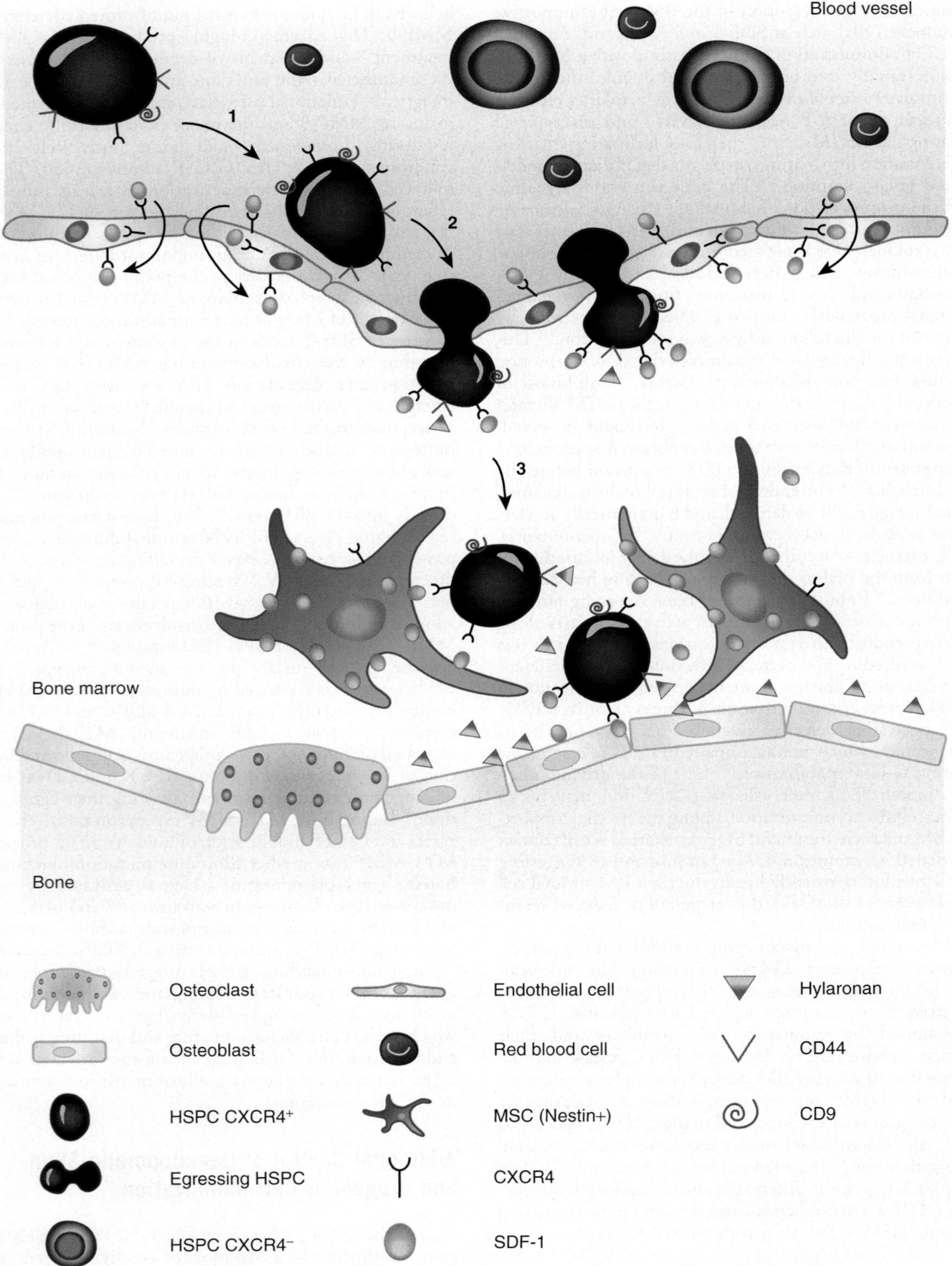

Figure 12-1 HOMING OF TRANSPLANTED HEMATOPOIETIC STEM AND PROGENITOR CELLS (HSPCs) TO THE BONE MARROW (BM). Rolling and firm adhesion *(1)* of navigating HSPC from the blood circulation via the BM sinusoid after their transplantation is followed by transendothelial migration across the physical blood–BM barrier *(2)*. Stromal cell–derived factor-1 (SDF-1)–CXCR4 interaction, including translocation of SDF-1 to the abdominal side of the endothelium and its sequential secretion to the BM, as well as CD44–hyaluronan interaction and CD9, are key regulators of human stem cell homing to BM stromal supportive niches *(3)*.

($S1P_1$).[145,146] Accordingly, murine HSPC egress from extramedullary tissues depends on S1P receptor upregulation and migration toward higher S1P concentrations in the lymph and blood circulations.[147] During G-CSF–induced mobilization, S1P concentration is augmented in the peripheral blood[143,144] and concomitantly decreases in BM fluids,[143] suggesting a potential chemotaxis induced mobilization mechanism via the formation of a S1P gradient toward the blood.[143,144] The S1P–$S1P_1$ axis is also an important regulator of rapid mobilization by AMD3100 because inhibition of this axis reduced the level of progenitor cell recruitment to the blood in mice.[144]

Altogether, immunosurveillance by hematopoietic progenitor cell trafficking, as part of the host defense and repair mechanism, is enabled via a dynamic complex interplay of mediators, governed by SDF-1–CXCR4 signaling, proteolytic enzymes, bone remodeling, and signals from the nervous system, regulating HSPC egress and mobilization under stress conditions.

FUTURE DIRECTIONS

*"In order to keep your **balance,** you must keep **moving.**"*
—*Albert Einstein*

*"I find the great thing in this world is not so much where we stand, as in **what direction we are moving.**"*
—*Oliver Wendell Holmes*

This chapter discusses mechanisms and pathways involved in the regulation of HSPC homing and retention, as well as HSC egress, recruitment, and mobilization, emphasizing the major role that the SDF-1–CXCR4 axis plays in the regulation of these complex processes. The brain–bone–blood triad dynamically regulates both HSCs and BM stromal stem cells via bone turnover, circadian rhythms, and stress signals, producing leukocytes on demand as part of host defense and repair mechanism. Successful BM reconstitution requires directed stem cell movement from the circulation, across the blood–marrow barrier into their specialized niches in the BM wherein stem cells proliferate and differentiate to give rise to multilineage hematopoietic cells, while maintaining a small pool of primitive stem cells (Fig. 12-1). Most HSPCs reside in the BM, anchored to the endosteal region and perivascular sites. However, a rare population of circulating progenitors continuously egresses to the blood as part of homeostasis. Although these low circulating levels are dramatically increased together with maturing leukocytes as part of host defense and repair mechanisms, it is yet unknown what is the biologic advantage of an active directional migration of immature stem cells from the safe shore of the BM cavity to the turbulent blood circulation during homeostasis. Clinical protocols such as repeated G-CSF and rapid AMD3100 stimulation induce massive recruitment of stem and progenitor cells to the circulation (Fig. 12-2). This process is used clinically to harvest HSPCs for transplantation.

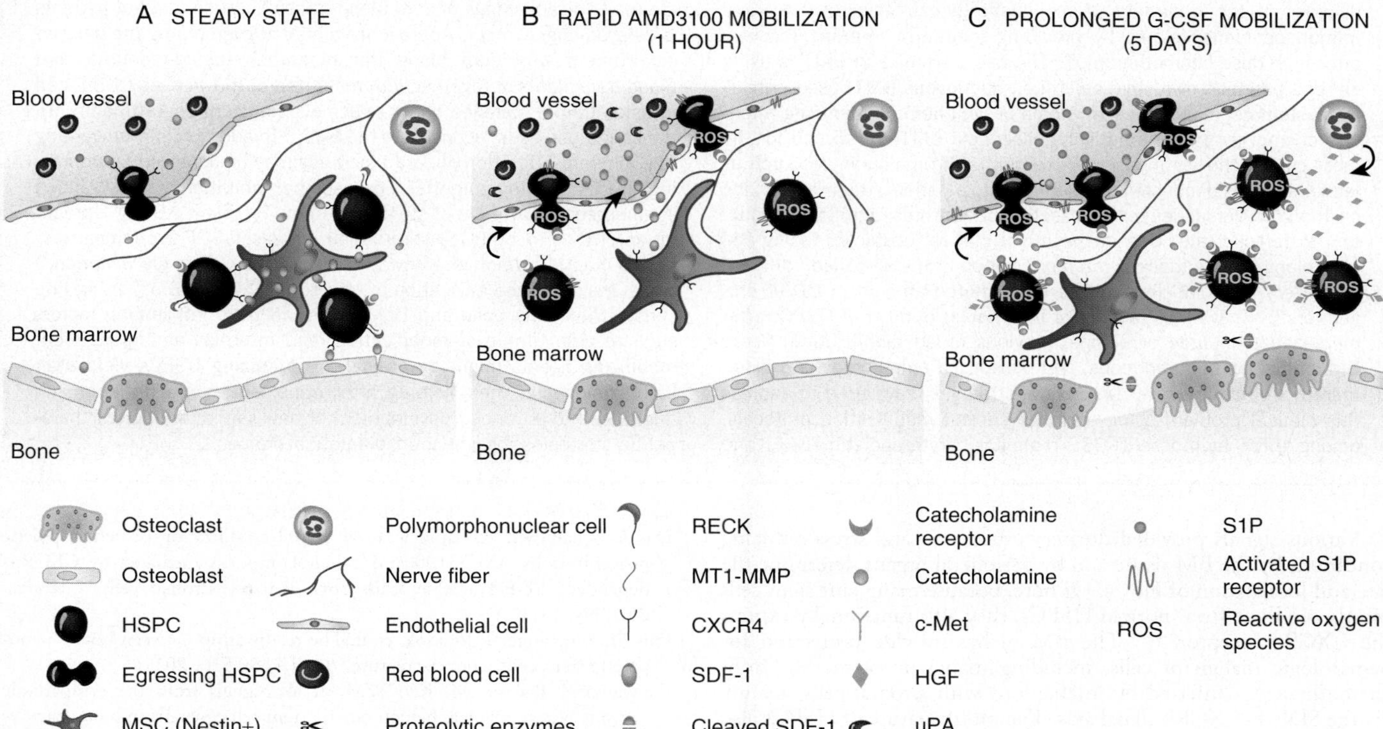

Figure 12-2 HEMATOPOIETIC STEM AND PROGENITOR CELL (HSPC) EGRESS AND MOBILIZATION. **A,** During steady state, HSPCs are localized and anchored in special stromal niches, closely associated with bone marrow (BM)–supporting cells, including osteoblasts and Nestin-positive mesenchymal stem cells (MSCs) that prevent their uncontrolled differentiation. The quiescent state of HSPCs is maintained via signaling of the stromal–cell derived factor-1 (SDF-1)–CXCR4 axis and inhibition of membrane type 1 metalloprotease (MT1-MMP) by RECK. **B,** Rapid HSPC mobilization after AMD3100 stimulation temporarily disrupts SDF-1–CXCR4 interactions and induces rapid SDF-1 secretion from BM $CXCR4^+$ stromal cells, including SDF-1–enriched Nestin-positive MSCs, resulting in local increase in SDF-1 levels in the BM followed by its release to the circulation. Secretion and rapid release of SDF-1 to the circulation enhance urokinase-type plasminogen activator (uPA) activation and increase expression of sphingosine-1-phosphate (S1P) receptors on HSPCs' surfaces. Consequently, an increase in intracellular reactive oxygen species (ROS) levels mediates HSPC recruitment and rapid mobilization within 1 hour. **C,** Repetitive granulocyte colony-stimulating factor (G-CSF) stimulation induces HSPC mobilization via osteoclast activation, alternation of sympathetic nervous system (SNS) signaling, and attenuation of osteoblast and MSC function followed by reduction of SDF-1 in the BM, CXCR4 upregulation, and proteolytic enzyme activation (including upregulation of surface MT1-MMP), leading to HSPC proliferation, differentiation, and increased mobilization to the circulation. During G-CSF–induced mobilization, S1P levels in the circulation are increased, thus intensifying the gradient between the blood and the BM. Increased production of hepatocyte growth factor (HGF) from polymorphonuclear cells in the BM results in HGF–c-Met axis activation, which in turn augment intracellular ROS generation and facilitating HSPC mobilization.

Relevance to Clinical Hematology

Optimal HSC migration from the BM to the circulation (mobilization) for donor cell transplant harvest and from the recipient blood into the BM (homing) for stem cell lodgment is an essential prerequisite for successful BM reconstitution in clinical transplantation. Discussed in this chapter, experimental systems involving human and murine HSPCs enable dissecting these migration processes to identify regulatory mechanisms to improve clinical settings. Current understanding of HSPC biology reveals that these cells home to the BM homeland, where they proliferate and differentiate, giving rise to multilineage hematopoietic cells while maintaining a small pool of primitive stem cells. The majority of HSPCs remain confined to the BM cavity in a nonmotile mode, adjacent to niche supportive cells that preserve them in a quiescent, nonproliferative mode, but a very low level of primitive progenitors and stem cells also continuously egress to the circulation as part of homeostasis. The levels of these rare migrating HSPCs are dramatically enhanced during alarm situations caused by injury and inflammation as part of host defense and repair mechanism. The physiologic process of enhanced HSPC recruitment from the BM has been used clinically to accelerate stem and progenitor cell migration to the circulation. Thus, collection of HSPCs from the donor's peripheral blood, rather than from their BM became the most common clinical protocol for BM transplantation (BMT).

Clinical BMT has gained immense success within the past 4 decades in the treatment of malignant hematologic diseases and immunodeficiency states by providing long-term immune recovery after high-dose chemotherapy.[152] The basic premise in BMT is using either a patient's own stem cells (i.e., autologous BMT) used primarily as stem cell support for myeloma or lymphoma undergoing intensive chemotherapy. Alternatively, allogeneic BMT, performed for the most part in the setting of marrow-infiltrating malignancies such as leukemia, uses donor stem cells infused to a patient, thus capitalizing on the graft-versus-leukemia effect, which affords significant reduction in relapse rate. One of the major clinical obstacles facing BM transplant experts today is the mobilization of the so-called "difficult mobilizers" who fail to mobilize the required amount of CD34 progenitors.[153] Known risk factors for insufficient number of HSPCs after mobilization include older age, previous failed mobilization, heavy BM infiltration by tumor cells, and previous chemotherapy and radiotherapy, to name just a few. Several strategies have tried to address this clinical problem using optimize current mobilization protocols, among them high-dose G-CSF regimens, erythropoietin, SCF, and chemomobilization achieved by chemotherapy treatment combined with G-CSF. Despite the wide gamut of therapeutic strategies used, most of them have either failed to show a clear advantage to standard mobilization regimens or were associated with substantial adverse effects (chemomobilization). With the recent introduction of the CXCR4 antagonist AMD3100 (also termed Mozobil and Plorexifor), there is renewed optimism in the management of difficult to mobilize patients. AMD3100 mediates rapid secretion of SDF-1 from BM stromal cells and its release to the circulation,[81] resulting in $CD34^+$ progenitor mobilization.[101] Treatment with AMD3100 exhibits marked synergism with G-CSF, suggesting their different and complementary mechanisms of action to induce HSPC mobilization. Several studies have shown its success in mobilization of previously failed myeloma in non-Hodgkin lymphoma and Hodgkin lymphoma patients.[154]

Clearly, because BMT is used increasingly in elderly adults and patients previously exposed to intense chemotherapy, novel approaches for optimizing mobilization are warranted. Several promising approaches are looming over the clinical horizon, among them are novel mobilization agents such as AMD3465,[155] SB-251353,[156] T140,[157] and PTH[158] acting in its capacity as a pivotal regulator of the hematopoietic niches. Additional avenues to be explored in this area include the use of cord blood, which at present is limited to pediatric patients and adults of low body weight because of the low number of $CD34^+$ progenitors contained in each cord blood unit. For this reason, the major disadvantage of cord blood transplantation in adult patients is delayed engraftment. Approaches aimed at overcoming the delayed engraftment with cord blood transplantation include double cord blood transplants or together with mobilized or BM-derived $CD34^+$ cell infusion from a matched donor to achieve transient engraftment until the cord blood cells reconstitute the BM.[159] In addition, circumventing this inherent limitation of cord blood use may be achieved by improving HSPCs' homing potential. For instance, inhibition of CD26 allows augmented engraftment of stem cells to the recipient's BM.[38] Upregulation of CXCR4 by PGE_2 stimulation increases SDF-1 chemoattraction to the BM.[28] Another pathway is activated by CD44 glycozilation,[45] which may enhance navigation of treated MSC to the BM. Taking into consideration the bone and BM niches integrity, influencing factors such as age, timing of mobilization, and interplay among different mobilizing agents might be crucial in optimizing HSPCs yield after mobilization and their homing after transplantation. This approach might lead to advanced development of new safe and efficient therapeutic strategies for HSC transplantation protocols.

Various signals provided during homeostasis and stress-inducing conditions by the BM tissue and by peripheral organs determine the fate and localization of HSCs. Of note, because malignant stem cells mostly originate from normal HSPCs, they also functionally express the CXCR4 receptor.[148,149] The BM niches provide protection for hematologic malignant cells, including malignant stem cells from chemotherapy, conferred by interactions with stromal cells, mainly via the SDF-1–CXCR4 signal axis. The motile nature of HSPCs also holds true for hematologic malignant cells. Priming of patients with mobilizing agents, such as G-CSF and AMD3100, might break the protective machinery provided by BM stromal cells, induce cell chemosensitization, and subsequently will provide eradication of the malignant disease.[150,151]

SUGGESTED READINGS

Broxmeyer HE, Orschell CM, Clapp DW, et al: Rapid mobilization of murine and human hematopoietic stem and progenitor cells with AMD3100, a CXCR4 antagonist. *J Exp Med* 201:1307, 2005.

Christopher MJ, Liu F, Hilton MJ, et al: Suppression of CXCL12 production by bone marrow osteoblasts is a common and critical pathway for cytokine-induced mobilization. *Blood* 114:1331, 2009.

Dar A, Schajnovitz A, Lapid K, et al: Rapid mobilization of hematopoietic progenitors by AMD3100 and catecholamines is mediated by CXCR4-dependent SDF-1 release from bone marrow stromal cells. *Leukemia* 25:1286, 2011.

Ellis SL, Grassinger J, Jones A, et al: The relationship between bone, hemopoietic stem cells, and vasculature. *Blood* 118:1516, 2011.

Katayama Y, Battista M, Kao WM, et al: Signals from the sympathetic nervous system regulate hematopoietic stem cell egress from bone marrow. *Cell* 124:407, 2006.

Kollet O, Dar A, Lapidot T: The multiple roles of osteoclasts in host defense: Bone remodeling and hematopoietic stem cell mobilization. *Annu Rev Immunol* 25:51, 2007.

Kollet O, Dar A, Shivtiel S, et al: Osteoclasts degrade endosteal components and promote mobilization of hematopoietic progenitor cells. *Nat Med* 12:657, 2006.

Lapid K, Vagima Y, Kollet O, et al: *Egress and mobilization of hematopoietic stem and progenitor cells.* StemBook [Internet] Cambridge MA, 2008, Harvard Stem Cell Institute.

Lapidot T, Dar A, Kollet O: How do stem cells find their way home? *Blood* 106:1901, 2005.

Lapidot T, Kollet O: The brain-bone-blood triad: Traffic lights for stem-cell homing and mobilization. *Hematology Am Soc Hematol Educ Program* 2010:1, 2010.

Mendez-Ferrer S, Lucas D, Battista M, et al: Haematopoietic stem cell release is regulated by circadian oscillations. *Nature* 452:442, 2008.

Mendez-Ferrer S, Michurina TV, Ferraro F, et al: Mesenchymal and haematopoietic stem cells form a unique bone marrow niche. *Nature* 466:829, 2010.

Papayannopoulou T, Scadden DT: Stem-cell ecology and stem cells in motion. *Blood* 111:3923, 2008.

Petit I, Szyper-Kravitz M, Nagler A, et al: G-CSF induces stem cell mobilization by decreasing bone marrow SDF-1 and up-regulating CXCR4. *Nat Immunol* 3:687, 2002.

Ratajczak MZ, Lee H, Wysoczynski M, et al: Novel insight into stem cell mobilization-plasma sphingosine-1-phosphate is a major chemoattractant that directs the egress of hematopoietic stem progenitor cells from the bone marrow and its level in peripheral blood increases during mobilization due to activation of complement cascade/membrane attack complex. *Leukemia* 24:976, 2010.

Sackstein R, Merzaban JS, Cain DW, et al: Ex vivo glycan engineering of CD44 programs human multipotent mesenchymal stromal cell trafficking to bone. *Nat Med* 14:181, 2008.

Schajnovitz A, Itkin T, D'Uva G, et al: CXCL12 secretion by bone marrow stromal cells is dependent on cell contact and mediated by connexin-43 and connexin-45 gap junctions. *Nat Immunol* 12:391, 2011.

Spiegel A, Kalinkovich A, Shivtiel S, et al: Stem cell regulation via dynamic interactions of the nervous and immune systems with the microenvironment. *Cell Stem Cell* 3:484, 2008.

Sugiyama T, Kohara H, Noda M, et al: Maintenance of the hematopoietic stem cell pool by CXCL12-CXCR4 chemokine signaling in bone marrow stromal cell niches. *Immunity* 25:977, 2006.

Vagima Y, Avigdor A, Goichberg P, et al: MT1-MMP and RECK are involved in human CD34+ progenitor cell retention, egress, and mobilization. *J Clin Invest* 119:492, 2009.

Zipori D, Sasson T: Adherent cells from mouse bone marrow inhibit the formation of colony stimulating factor (CSF) induced myeloid colonies. *Exp Hematol* 8:816, 1980.

For complete list of references log on to www.expertconsult.com.

CHAPTER 13

VASCULAR GROWTH IN HEALTH AND DISEASE

Janusz Rak

HEMOSTATIC, HEMATOPOIETIC, AND VASCULAR SYSTEMS AS A FUNCTIONAL CONTINUUM

Although specific demands of practice, concepts, and methodologies may have defined the unique scope of current hematology, the underlying biologic processes do not occur in isolation. Thus it is increasingly obvious that diseases affecting bone marrow and peripheral blood are closely intertwined with the state of the vascular system,[1] which acts as a niche, conduit, and regulator of many of these events.[2] This is exemplified by the anatomic proximity and interactions among several related cellular populations, including hematopoietic progenitors, their derivatives, endothelial cells and their precursors, platelets, and other components involved in blood vessel formation, repair, homeostasis, and patency.[2,3] The remarkable recent progress in understanding the molecular mechanisms involved in communication between these cells increasingly informs medical considerations and drug discovery efforts.[2,4,5] For instance, agents that block vascular growth (antiangiogenics), which are currently used to treat solid tumors, elicit hematologic perturbations[6] and are being considered for treatment of hematopoietic malignancies.[7] Indeed, hematopoietic, hemostatic, and vascular compartments can be viewed as a functional continuum, both in health and in disease.

CONSTITUENTS OF THE VASCULAR SYSTEM

The hematopoietic and vascular systems emerge from a common progenitor cell (hemangioblast) early during embryogenesis. Subsequently the vascular lineage evolves to form a network of channels that integrate, control, and reflect the structure and function of the tissues (parenchyma) and organs that they supply.[8] Local characteristics of the vascular system are superimposed on a more general, hierarchical branching pattern (arborization) and arteriovenous directionality of the circulation. Structurally, distinct lymphatics emerge from the venous system to return extravascular (interstitial) fluid and extravasated cells to the venous circulation.[2]

Blood vessels are not only the essential supply routes of nutrients and oxygen to tissues (parenchyma), but also conduits of long-range regulatory signals (hormonal/endocrine) and an important source of paracrine cues that act on surrounding cells in a perfusion-independent (angiocrine) manner.[2,9] Postnatal tissue maturation imposes a quiescent phenotype throughout the vascular system, a state that is interrupted by only a small number of transient growth events, such as posttraumatic tissue regeneration, wound healing, vascular repair, or cyclic changes in reproductive organs. This quiescent state may be chronically compromised in certain pathologic conditions (inflammation, hyperplasia, or cancer), which can lead to unscheduled or abnormal vascular growth.[2] Out of several forms of such growth, vasculogenesis and angiogenesis stand out as fundamentally important and distinct. In vasculogenesis, endothelial progenitor cell self-assembly results in the formation of new vascular channels (e.g., during embryogenesis). In contrast, angiogenesis is a process whereby preexisting vascular channels are extended to form additional capillary loops (e.g., during tissue remodeling and in cancer).[2]

Cells Involved in Vascular Growth

Specialized endothelial cells (ECs) constitute the crucial structural and functional element of the adult vasculature. ECs create antithrombotic luminal surfaces within all blood vessels, produce an active interface between the blood and the surrounding tissues, control the flux of fluids and macromolecules (permeability), and are the key component of vascular growth processes. Such growth not only involves cessation of the quiescent state in subsets of resident ECs, but is also associated with multiple systemic events, such as emission of cytokines into the circulation and mobilization of cells from the bone marrow, including putative endothelial progenitor cells (EPCs), hematopoietic stem cells, and myeloid cells (bone marrow–derived cells [BMDCs]).[10] These cells serve as surveillance and regulatory mechanisms that control and coordinate the responses of the peripheral vasculature (Fig. 13-1).[11,12] In established blood vessels the functionality of the endothelial tube is dependent on the support of abluminal basement membrane (BM), which is shared between these cells and one or more layers of contractile mesenchymal cells of the blood vessel wall (mural cells). Sparse networks of these cells (here called pericytes) are associated with capillary endothelium, whereas continuous sheets of mural smooth muscle cells cover the precapillary/postcapillary vascular segments (arterial and venous, respectively).[2] The thickness and complexity of the vessel wall differs between veins and arteries and increase with vascular hierarchy. So much so, that the multilayered walls of large arteries contain their own capillary networks *(vasa vasorum),* the growth of which can contribute to the formation of atherosclerotic plaques.[13] Blood vessel integrity and growth are also dependent on platelets and the hemostatic system (tissue factor, thrombin, thrombin receptor/protease-activated receptor 1 [PAR1]), other PARs the fibrinolytic system, and other effectors), all of which play important parts in the regulation of vascular continuity, patency, and permeability.[2] Coagulation proteases not only regulate clot formation upon injury but also elicit signals within the surrounding vascular, inflammatory, and parenchymal cells, thereby modulating these processes.[9]

Molecular Regulators of Vascular Responses

The state of the vascular networks is controlled by a web of intercellular communications, which are executed by soluble growth factors, adhesion molecules, extracellular matrix (ECM) molecules, cell-cell contacts, the hemostatic system, various proteases, and the intercellular exchange of molecules (proteins, messenger ribonucleic acid [mRNA] and micro-RNA [miRNA]) by membrane microvesicles.[12] This array of mediators includes those essential for vascular homeostasis and ones that are more pleiotropic in nature, serving to stimulate or inhibit vascular growth (Table 13-1).[1,2]

Vascular Endothelial Growth Factors

Vascular endothelial growth factor-A (VEGF-A), is also known as VEGF or vascular permeability factor.[3] VEGF is the key member of a larger family of related polypeptides, which includes VEGF-B,

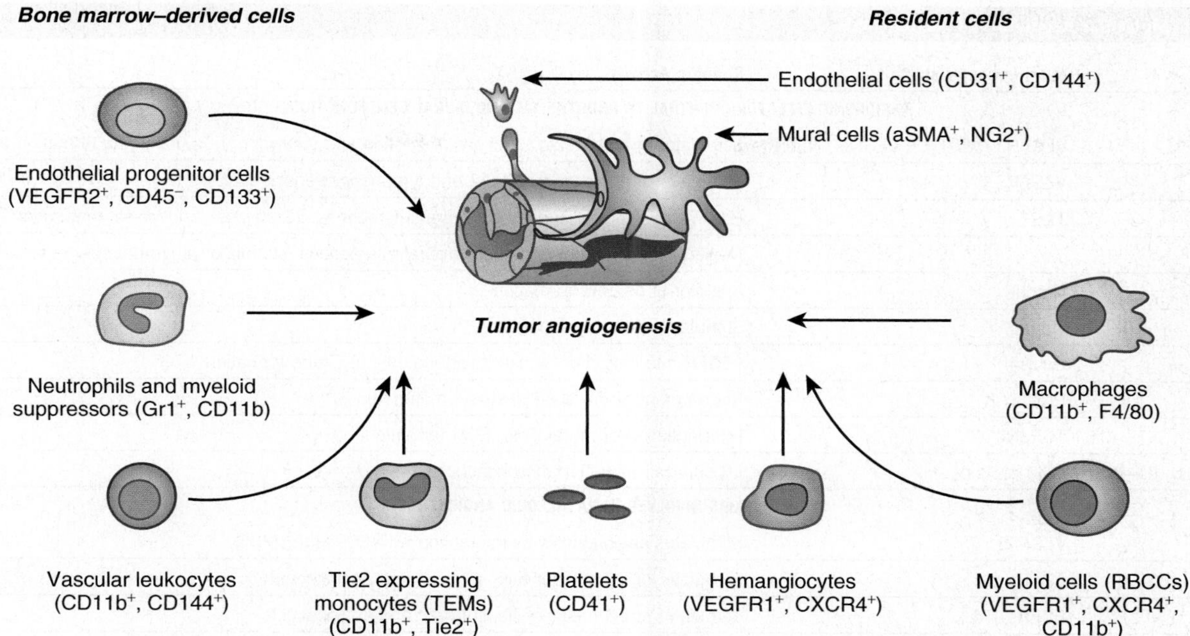

Figure 13-1 CELL POPULATIONS INVOLVED IN TUMOR ANGIOGENESIS. Cells involved in blood vessel formation include endothelial cells, their progenitor cells, mural cells (pericytes), and several population of bone marrow–derived cells, as well as angiogenic fibroblasts, cancer cells, and immune effectors not included in this diagram. *VEGFR,* Vascular endothelial growth factor receptor. *(Modified from Kerbel RS: Tumor angiogenesis.* N Engl J Med *358:2039, 2008.)*

VEGF-C, VEGF-D, VEGF-E, VEGFR-F, and placenta growth factor (PlGF).[5] Upon dimerization these factors bind to their tyrosine kinase receptors (RTKs/VEGFRs), including VEGFR1/Flt-1, VEGFR2/KDR/Flk-1, and VEGFR3/Flt-4, often acting in conjunction with their neuropilin coreceptors (NRP1, NRP2).[2] The specificity of these interactions is relatively restricted, as indicated in Fig. 13-2. For instance, VEGF-A interacts with VEGFR2, VEGFR1, and VEGFR3, whereas PlGF is selective for VEGFR1. The distribution of different VEGFRs on vascular (VEC) and lymphatic (LEC) endothelial cell subsets, as well as among EPCs, hematopoietic, myeloid, and certain tumor cells defines the known biologic activities of various VEGF ligands. The effects of VEGF include stimulation of VEC mitogenesis, migration, survival, morphogenesis, and vascular permeability (e.g., through formation of intercellular gaps or transcellular structures know as *fenestrae*). The signaling activity of VEGFR2 is crucial for these processes, whereas VEGFR1 is often expressed as a soluble splice variant (sFlt-1) that neutralizes VEGF (acts as VEGF "sink"), thereby inhibiting angiogenesis.[2]

VEGF activity is also regulated by splicing of the corresponding mRNA, which results in the generation of several protein isoforms, including VEGF121, VEGF145, VEGF165, VEGF189, and VEGF206 (designations based on the number of amino acids).[5] These variants differ in their cell association, solubility, the ability to bind heparinoids, or interact with neuropilins, all of which define the formation of extracellular gradients and determine their biologic activity. In this regard, VEGF165 is an especially potent inducer of angiogenesis. VEGF-C and VEGF-D stimulate growth of lymphatics (lymphangiogenesis), via activation of VEGFR3, whereas VEGF-B and PlGF interact with VEGFR1 and are involved in vascular pathologic conditions and inflammation.[2]

Platelet-Derived Growth Factors

The platelet-derived growth factor (PDGF) family of VEGF-related growth factors consists of four members: PDGF-A, PDGF-B, PDGF-C, and PDGF-D, the homodimers or heterodimers of which interact preferentially with one of the three known cellular RTKs, namely PDGFR-α, PDGFR-β, and PDGFR-γ, each endowed with different cellular functions. For example, PDGF-BB is expressed by endothelial cells and mediates their capacity to attract mural cells harboring PDGFR-β.[2]

Prokineticins

This group of factors consists of the endocrine gland–derived vascular endothelial growth factor/prokineticin 1 (EG-VEGF/PK1) and *Bombina variegata*–secreted protein 8/prokineticin 2 (Bv8/PK2), both of which interact with their respective G protein–coupled receptors on endothelial cells (PKR1 and PKR2). These mediators induce VEGF-like effects in endothelial cells and may render tumors resistant to VEGF inhibition.[5]

Angiopoietins and Tie Receptors

Angiopoietins (Ang1, Ang2, and Ang4) interact with the Tie2/TEK receptor (RTK) that is preferentially expressed by endothelial cells and some myeloid cells (see Fig. 13-1). A related orphan receptor, known as Tie1, remains poorly characterized and likely acts by modulating Tie2 activity.[2] Ang1 emanates from perivascular tissues and serves as the main Tie2 agonist to stabilize endothelial-mural cell interactions and to promote endothelial cell survival, vascular quiescence, and the nonpermeable state. Ang2, which is produced by VEGF-stimulated endothelium, exerts the opposite effects and stimulates pericyte detachment, permeability, vascular growth or regression, and lymphangiogenesis.[2]

Notch Pathway

Delta-like (Dll1, 3, and 4) and Jagged (1 and 2) are membrane-bound ligands that activate Notch receptors on adjacent cells. During vascular development and growth Dll4 and Jagged1 are expressed by subsets of endothelial and mural cells, respectively, and regulate their

Table 13-1 Molecular Regulators of Angiogenesis

Regulator	Main Receptor(s)	Biologic Activity
		ANGIOGENIC EFFECTORS CENTRAL TO ENDOTHELIAL AND MURAL CELL FUNCTION
VEGF-A/VEGF	VEGFR2 (VEGFR3, VEGF1), NRP1	Stimulator of angiogenic functions, migration and survival of ECs, including formation of tip cells
VEGF-C	VEGFR3 (VEGFR2)	Stimulator of angiogenesis (ECs) and lymphangiogenesis (LECs)
Ang1	Tie2	Positive regulator of endothelial-mural interactions, EC survival, and vessel maturation
Ang2	Tie2	Negative regulation of endothelial-mural interactions, stimulator of lymphangiogenesis
Dll4	Notch	Inhibitor of tip cells formation
Jagged1	Notch	Stimulator of tip cell formation
ephrinB2	EphB4	VEGFR internalization/signaling, arterial identity, tube formation
PDGF-B	PDGFR-β	Recruitment of mural cells, vessel maturation
TGFβ1	TGFβRII	Differentiation of mural cells, ECM formation
Integrins (αv, β1, β5)	ECM proteins	EC survival, migration morphogenesis
		STIMULATORS INVOLVED IN PATHOLOGIC ANGIOGENESIS
PIGF	VEGFR1	Stimulates angiogenesis by interaction with ECs and BMDCs
Acidic FGF (FGF1)	FGFRs 1-4	Stimulator of EC mitogenesis, survival, and angiogenesis
Basic FGF (FGF2)	FGFRs 1-4	Stimulator of EC mitogenesis, survival, and angiogenesis
FGF3	FGFRs 1-4	Stimulator of EC mitogenesis, survival, and angiogenesis
FGF4	FGFRs 1-4	Stimulator of EC mitogenesis, survival, and angiogenesis
IL-8	CXCR1	Stimulator of ECs and inflammatory cells
IL-6	IL-6R	Stimulator of inflammatory angiogenesis
TNF-α	TNFR1 (55)	EC stimulator and VEGF inducer
Bv8	GPCR	Stimulator of endocrine and tumor ECs
PD-ECGF/TP	Unclear	Stimulator of angiogenesis
Angiogenin	170-kDa receptor	Stimulator of angiogenesis and RNase
MMP-9	ECM proteins	Matrix metalloproteinase that breaks down ECM and releases angiogenic growth factors
		ENDOGENOUS ANGIOGENESIS INHIBITORS
Inhibitor	**Biologic Activity**	
TSP1	Interacts with CD36 receptor, integrins, and other proteins causing growth inhibition and apoptosis of angiogenic ECs	
Endostatin	Proteolytic fragment of collagen XVIII with antiangiogenic activity	
Angiostatin	Proteolytic fragment of plasminogen with antiangiogenic activity	
Tumstatin	Proteolytic fragment of collagen IV alpha 3 chain	
sFlt-1/sVEGFR1	Soluble splice variant of VEGFR1 neutralizing VEGF and blocking VEGFR2 signaling	
VEGF165b	Splice variant of VEGF with antiangiogenic activity	
PEX	Inhibitor of EC invasion and MMP activity	
IFN-α (β)	Inhibits release of angiogenic growth factors	

Ang, Angiopoietin; *BMDC,* bone marrow–derived cell; *Bv8, Bombina variegata*–secreted protein 8; *Dll4,* delta-like ligand 4; *EC,* endothelial cell; *FGF,* fibroblast growth factor; *FGFR,* fibroblast growth factor receptor; *GPCR,* G protein–coupled receptor; *IFN,* interferon; *IL,* interleukin; *LEC,* lymphatic endothelial cell; *MMP-9,* matrix metalloproteinase 9; *NRP,* neuropilin; *PD-ECGF/TP,* platelet-derived endothelial cell growth factor/thymidine phosphorylase; *PDGF,* platelet-derived growth factor; *PDGFR,* platelet-derived growth factor receptor; *PIGF,* placenta growth factor; *TGF,* transforming growth factor; *TNF-α,* tumor necrosis factor-α; *TNFR,* tumor necrosis factor receptor; *TSP1,* thrombospondin 1; *VEGF,* vascular endothelial growth factor; *VEGFR,* vascular endothelial growth factor receptor; see text and references for details.[2]

distinct functions within the capillary outgrowths (sprouts), as depicted in Figs. 13-2 and 13-3.[14] Dll1 is also involved in circumferential vascular enlargement (arteriogenesis).[2]

Ephrins and Eph Receptors

The arterial or venous identity of endothelial cells in the evolving microcirculation is preprogrammed by the expression of transmembrane guidance molecules, especially ephrinB2 and its EphB4 receptor. Bidirectional signals emanating from these molecules, together with mechanosensory cues, govern the arteriovenous vascular arborization that is essential for, and maintained by, proper blood flow. Other ephrins are implicated in endothelial-pericyte interactions, communication between blood vessels and tumor cells. They may also cooperate in VEGFR2 endocytosis and signaling.[2]

Vascular Integrins, Cadherins, and Cell Adhesion Molecules

Quiescent endothelial cells are anchored to the BM, a structured layer of ECM composed mainly of laminin and collagen type IV. In

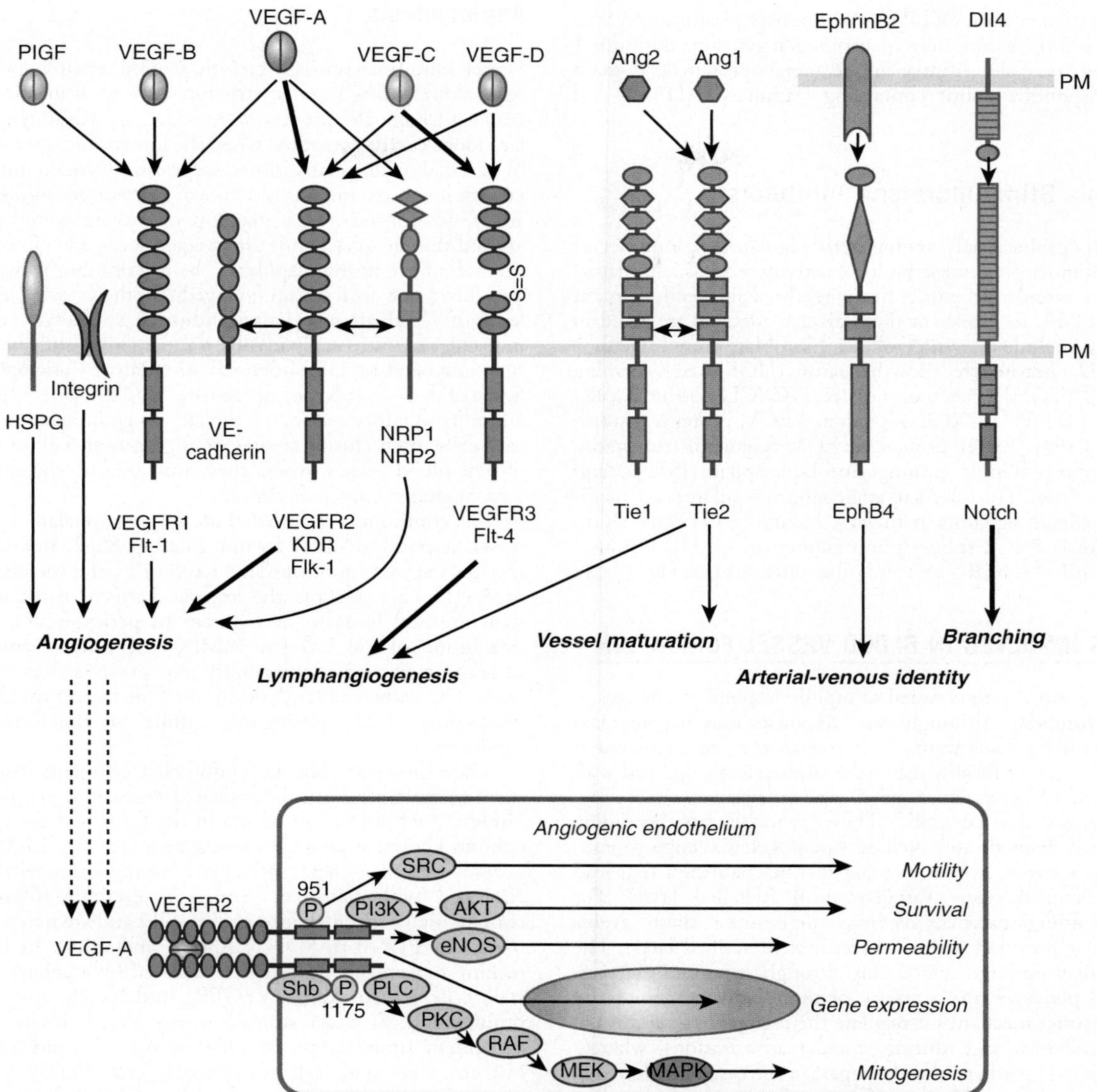

Figure 13-2 Some of the key elements of the signaling circuitry involved in blood vessel formation and tumor angiogenesis. Receptors and coreceptors involved in angiogenic, lymphangiogenic, and regulatory signaling. *Bottom panel:* outline of signaling pathways and their effector mechanisms downstream of VEGF-A/VEGF. *Ang,* Angiopoietin; *Dll,* Delta-like ligand; *eNOS,* endothelial nitric oxide synthase; *HSPG,* heparan sulfate proteoglycan; *NRP,* neuropilin; *PLC,* phospholipase C; *PlGF,* placenta growth factor; *PM,* plasma membrane; *VE-cadherin,* vascular endothelial cadherin; *VEGF,* vascular endothelial growth factor; *VEGFR,* vascular endothelial growth factor receptor.

contrast, growing (angiogenic) endothelial cells are surrounded by provisional ECM containing fibrin, vitronectin, fibronectin, and partially degraded collagens. Growth factors upregulate the expression of dimeric integrin receptors ($\alpha v\beta 3$, $\alpha v\beta 5$, $\alpha 1\beta 1$, $\alpha 2\beta 1$, $\alpha 4\beta 1$, $\alpha 5\beta 1$), which recognize specific motifs in ECM molecules (often, the RGD sequence). The angiogenesis-related integrin, $\alpha v\beta 3$, is the target of blood vessel–directed therapies.

Vascular endothelial cadherin (VE-cadherin/CD144) is selectively expressed by endothelial cells and contributes to their barrier function, homotypic adhesion, and growth regulatory signals. Other cadherins, as well as claudins (e.g., endothelial claudin 5) and connexins, contribute to homotypic and heterotypic endothelial cell interactions, and the formation of gap and tight junctions and transmission of long-range signals that propagate within the vascular wall upstream of the blood flow.[2] On the other hand, interactions between endothelium and circulating immune, myeloid, inflammatory, and progenitor cells, as well as platelets, are mediated by selectins (e.g., P-selectin, L-selectin, and E-selectin), integrins ($\alpha 4\beta 1$/very late antigen 4 [VLA4]), and members of the immunoglobulin family of cell adhesion molecules (intercellular adhesion molecule 1 [ICAM1]/ICAM2 and vascular cell adhesion molecule 1 [VCAM1]), all of which play distinct roles in angiogenesis.[2,15]

Proteases

Proteases regulate remodeling, growth and invasion of new blood vessels, liberation of ECM-bound angiogenic growth factors, generation of regulatory peptides (e.g., angiogenesis inhibitors), clotting and fibrinolysis, intracellular signaling, and numerous other steps involved in vascular maintenance and remodeling. For example, matrix metalloproteinases (MMPs) and their tissue inhibitors (TIMPs 1 to 4) participate in the controlled ECM/BM breakdown, which is required for invasiveness of the angiogenic endothelium.[15] The key enzymes in this group include MMP-1, MMP-2, MMP-9, and MMP-14, coagulation factors (VIIa and thrombin) and their receptors (tissue factor and PAR1), urokinase plasminogen activators (uPAs) and their inhibitors (plasminogen activator inhibitor 1 [PAI-1]), members of the disintegrin and metalloproteinase domain and thrombospondin motif–containing families (ADAM and ADAMTS).

Angiogenesis Stimulators and Inhibitors

In addition to "professional" angiogenesis regulators, a number of molecules with more pleiotropic biologic activity serve as stimulators or inhibitors of vascular growth, either directly or indirectly (e.g., as inducers of VEGF). Examples of these diverse effectors are listed in Table 13-1 and include certain cytokines (fibroblast growth factor 1 [FGF1], FGF2, hepatocyte growth factor [HGF], transforming growth factorβ [TGFβ]), chemokines (IL-8/CXCL8, stromal cell–derived factor 1 [SDF-1]/CXCL12), secreted ECM proteins (thrombospondin 1 [TSP1], TSP2), proteolytic ECM fragments (tumstatin, angiostatin), phospholipids (sphingosine-1-phosphate [S1P]), and several other entities.[1] The effects of angiogenesis regulators are mediated by intracellular signaling pathways, including GTPases (Ras), kinases (src, AKT, PKC), transcription factors (ERG, HIF), microRNA species (miR-17, miR-155), and other effectors (see Fig. 13-2).[2]

PROCESSES INVOLVED IN BLOOD VESSEL FORMATION

The vascular system is programmed to rapidly respond to changes in the microenvironment. Although these responses may be provoked by local factors (e.g., tissue injury or hypoxia), they are regulated at several levels, including locally, regionally, and systemically, and with the involvement of perivascular, vessel wall–associated, circulating, and bone marrow–derived cells.[2] These processes are becoming increasingly well defined, and include vasculogenesis, angiogenesis, and lymphangiogenesis, as well as other distinct pathways that lead to increased/changed tissue vascularization (detailed later). For example, expanding parenchyma may orchestrate these events through vascular cooption or intussusception (described later). The vascular wall may undergo remodeling through structural changes, recruitment of pericytes (maturation), or lumen enlargement (arteriogenesis). Distinct mechanisms regulate the regression (pruning) of superfluous capillaries (e.g., during vascular arborization), whereas progenitor cells may mediate vascular repair in the case of endothelial damage (i.e., denudation). New vessel segments may also form when transdifferentiation of nonendothelial stem cells results in the formation of endothelial-like luminal layers (vasculogenic mimicry). Each of these processes is driven by specialized cellular and molecular circuitry and plays a unique role in vascular growth, homeostasis, and pathology, as outlined briefly later.[1,2,5,14]

Vasculogenesis and Vascular Repair

Processes involving the recruitment of endothelial precursors, such as angioblasts or EPCs, and their self-assembly, differentiation, and/or structural integration within the endothelial lining are referred to as vasculogenesis. These events are central to the origin of the vascular system (primary capillary plexus formation) during embryogenesis.[8] Although EPC-like cells can be detected during postnatal life, especially in the bone marrow, walls of large vessels, and in the circulating blood (circulating endothelial progenitors [CEPs]), they have a more restricted role, which is mainly regulatory and reparative in nature. For instance, EPCs may accumulate at sites of angiogenesis, but they rarely form complete vascular segments. However, EPCs may contribute to the endothelialization of denuded luminal surfaces, vascular grafts, or damaged larger vessels (vascular repair) or to the recanalization of occlusive thrombi.[16] Several molecular mechanisms control the recruitment of EPCs and their retention at sites of vascular growth, including high levels of circulating VEGF, SDF-1, expression of certain integrins, and other factors.[4,10]

Angiogenesis

Under conditions of tissue growth, wound repair, hypoxia, or disease (e.g., cancer), new vascular structures emerge from preexisting blood vessels through the process of angiogenesis. Although smaller capillary loops can be generated when the lumens of larger vessels are split by external tissue pillars (intussusception), the main mode of capillary growth involves a mechanism known as *sprouting angiogenesis* (see Fig. 13-3). In this process, a gradient of proangiogenic activity forms around the site of ischemia and triggers a cascade of responses within the wall of the nearest capillary. The reaction begins with local capillary distension to form an enlarged "mother vessel." Although high levels of VEGF are sufficient to induce these changes,[3] the underlying molecular events usually involve a more global shift in levels of multiple angiogenesis inhibitors and stimulators ("angiogenic switch").[1] Some of these factors may upregulate VEGF in parenchymal, stromal, and inflammatory cells or act directly on endothelial cells. Inflammatory cells often cluster at sites of angiogenesis before the formation of new blood vessels, where they contribute to the consolidation of a proangiogenic microenvironment.[2]

The continuous endothelial monolayers (phalanx cells) of mother vessels respond to VEGF by upregulating Ang2, an event that blocks the tonic activation of the Tie2 receptor by the constitutive presence of Ang1. This disrupts the key mechanism maintaining capillary structure and leads to detachment of pericytes, followed by local dissolution of the BM (by MMPs) and other events, such as an increase in vascular permeability and extravasation of plasma proteins. The extravascular deposition of fibrin and the formation of a provisional ECM provide the scaffold for the formation of new capillaries.[2]

These processes liberate endothelial cells and instruct some of them to emigrate from the activated vascular segment in an orderly fashion. Such migration occurs in the form of a directional cellular column known as an angiogenic sprout (see Fig. 13-3). Each sprout is composed of a single, specialized leading endothelial cell (tip cell) equipped with hair-like, sensing projections (filopodia), which contain high concentrations of VEGFR2 and are rich in other regulators (e.g., PDGF-B, SDF-1, Apelin, and Dll4). In their gradient-seeking movement, tip cells are followed by a cohort of endothelial stalk cells, which express VEGFR1 and Notch, and are capable of proliferation. Stronger stimulation by VEGF results in VEGFR2-dependent upregulation of Dll4 in tip cells and allows them to instruct their stalk cell counterparts (via Notch) to retain their phenotype, refrain from independent branching, and maintain VEGF signaling at lower levels. The latter is mediated, at least in part, by upregulation of soluble VEGFR1 (the "VEGF sink" molecule). Consequently, the exogenous blockade of the Dll4/Notch pathway leads to excessive generation of tip cells and sprouts (from stalk cells), resulting in the formation of overly branched, hyperdense, nonperfused, and dysfunctional capillary network ("non-productive angiogenesis").[14] Stimulation of Notch by Jagged1 ligand modulates the effects of Dll4 on stalk cells and fine-tunes the branching pattern. The neighboring sprouts eventually connect (anastomose) to form new capillary loops. This process is mediated by interaction with tissue macrophages expressing Tie2 and NRP1.[17] Subsequent generation of the vascular lumen and resumption of blood flow occur through formation of intercellular spaces between endothelial stalk cells.[2]

Vascular Maturation

Maturation of vessels involves a buildup of a mural cell layer around the newly formed endothelial tube and is driven by several molecular mechanisms.[2] Thus endothelial tip cells secrete PDGF-B, which attracts regional pericytes, which provide structural support and vessel-stabilizing Ang1 activity.[18] S1P regulates N-cadherin, which further links endothelial cells and pericytes. Upon their attachment to the endothelial tube, pericytes assume a more mature phenotype

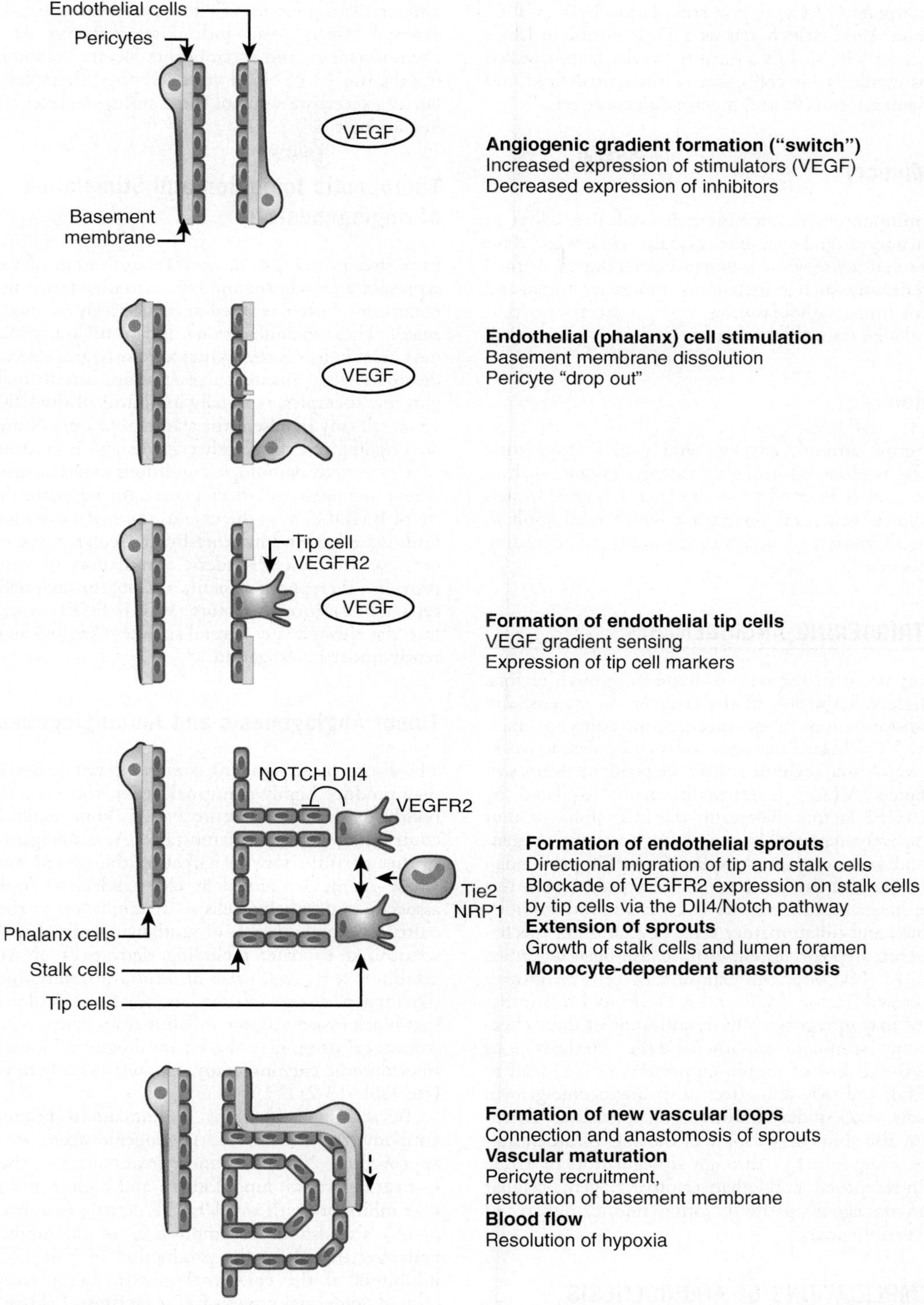

Figure 13-3 SPROUTING ANGIOGENESIS. The change in balance between angiogenesis stimulators and inhibitors (angiogenic switch) and especially gradient of vascular endothelial growth factor (VEGF) leads to sprouting angiogenesis. This causes changes in the vessel wall (endothelial phalanx cells) resulting in formation of mother vessels, endothelial tip cells, stalk cells, capillary loops, and eventually anastomoses, as depicted (details are in the text and in Carmeliet and Jain[2]). *Dll,* Delta-like ligand; *NRP,* neuropilin; *VEGFR,* vascular endothelial growth factor receptor.

under the influence of TGFβ1.[18] Endothelial prolyl hydroxylase 2 (PHD2), an oxygen-sensing enzyme, also regulates pericyte recruitment. These mechanisms ensure vascular integrity, mechanical resistance, endothelial cell survival, diminished dependence on VEGF, and restricted permeability.[2]

Lymphangiogenesis

As mentioned earlier, sprouting of new lymphatics is described as lymphangiogenesis. LECs express distinct markers (VEGFR3, Prox-1, LYVE-1) but otherwise exhibit up to 98% molecular similarity to their vascular counterparts (VECs). Upon stimulation by VEGF-C, VEGF-D, VEGF, and Ang2 (which acts as a Tie2 agonist in LECs and a Tie2 antagonist in VECs), LECs form networks of thin-walled vessels that serve as conduits for collection of interstitial fluid and cells, including inflammatory cells and metastatic cancer cells.[19]

Vasculogenic Mimicry

In some instances, multipotential, nonendothelial cells may adopt an endothelial-like phenotype and can line vascular channels.[20] This process, which is termed *vasculogenic mimicry,* occurs during normal placentation and in tumors, such as melanoma, mouse teratoma, and in certain regions of human glioblastoma, where cancer stem cells undergo such endothelial transdifferentiation.[20]

Vascular Cooption

Cancer cells may grow around, envelop, and exploit preexisting vessels.[21] This process is observed in highly vascular organs, such as the lung and brain, and is referred to as *cooption.* Coopted vessels may undergo additional structural alterations, which may result in remodeling and the formation of occlusive thrombi and regression that can lead to ischemia.[22]

MECHANISMS TRIGGERING ANGIOGENESIS

Vascular growth may occur in response to hypoxia, growth factors, inflammatory mediators, activation of the coagulation system, and after malignant transformation. These mechanisms converge upon the regulation of the VEGF gene[5] but also involve complex networks of other effectors, which may exhibit context-dependent degrees of functional redundancy.[2] VEGF is transcriptionally regulated by dimeric HIF1 and HIF2 factors. Normally, the HIF alpha subunit (HIF-1α) is constitutively degraded by a pathway involving oxygen-dependent prolyl and asparaginyl hydroxylases, von Hippel-Lindau (VHL) ubiquitin ligase, and the proteasome.[23] Hypoxia blocks this process, resulting in increased HIF activity and VEGF production by parenchymal, stromal, and inflammatory cells. Several other mechanisms of proangiogenic, hypoxic responses have also been described (e.g., NFκB, EGR1).[24] Likewise, the exposure of cells to growth factors (epidermal growth factor [EGF], FGF, HGF) and inflammatory cytokines (IL-6) may upregulate VEGF, and some of these effectors may also directly stimulate endothelial cells.[2] Activation of oncogenes (e.g., Ras) and loss of tumor suppressors (VHL) lead to upregulation of VEGF and may also affect other angiogenic growth factors in cancer cells, even under conditions of normoxia.[9] Oncogenic transformation also shuts down some of the angiogenic inhibitors, contributes to coagulopathy (through upregulation of tissue factor and thrombin receptors), and enhances proangiogenic cellular vesiculation. Indeed oncogenic pathways often mimic, distort, or exacerbate the effects of hypoxia.[9]

THERAPEUTIC IMPLICATIONS OF ANGIOGENESIS IN HEMATOLOGY

Vascular events associated with cancer, hemangioma, or vascular malformation have the potential to trigger hematologic consequences, either spontaneously or during therapeutic angiogenesis or antiangiogenesis. These linkages are poorly understood but often include one or more of the following factors: (1) endothelial cell activation associated with intravascular upregulation of tissue factor, adhesion molecules, and other factors; (2) disruption of the vascular wall; (3) recruitment of inflammatory cells and BMDCs (e.g., by cytokines); (4) enhanced vascular permeability, resulting in the extravasation and activation of coagulation factors; (5) platelet activation; (6) contact between procoagulant cells (e.g., metastatic cancer cells) and circulating blood; (7) flow perturbations and stasis; (8) indirect external effects (e.g., indwelling catheters or administration of chemotherapy); and several other factors.[9] Nonetheless, understanding the impact of blood vessel–directed therapies, which can modulate or exacerbate some of these events, represents a new direction in hematology.

Therapeutic Inhibition and Stimulation of Angiogenesis

Excessive, protracted, or aberrant activation of vascular growth may represent a correlative and/or a causative factor in several pathologic conditions (often referred to collectively as *angiogenesis-related diseases*).[1] These include chronic inflammation, certain forms of blindness, metabolic diseases, atherosclerosis, and cancer.[1] In some of these disorders (e.g., macular degeneration, certain malignancies) antiangiogenic therapies, especially inhibitors of the VEGF pathway (Table 13-2), already represent the standard of care. Numerous clinical trials are ongoing to explore other agents and indications.[2]

Conversely, pathologic conditions may also arise because of insufficient angiogenesis, arteriogenesis, or regulatory/repopulating activity of BMDCs, as is the case in the myocardium after infarction, in limb ischemia, and in other hypovascular states, especially in elderly persons. In these disorders, stimulation of vascular growth may provide a therapeutic benefit, notably through delivery of angiogenic cells (EPCs), growth factors (VEGF, FGF), or gene therapy vectors into the affected site. Several such (proangiogenic) strategies are currently under investigation.[2]

Tumor Angiogenesis and Antiangiogenesis

The disorganized signaling cues that occur during tumor angiogenesis may produce highly abnormal, leaky, tortuous, prothrombotic, and poorly perfused vasculature (vessel "abnormalization"), which may contribute to aberrant hemostasis.[2] Antiangiogenic agents may cause further perturbations by targeting the related molecular anomalies. These agents are aimed at either selective destruction of tumor-associated endothelial cells or at inhibition of their stimulatory circuitry.[1] Several classes of antiangiogenic compounds have been scrutinized to date, including derivatives of natural angiogenesis inhibitors (e.g., endostatin or tumstatin), inhibitors of proangiogenic signaling pathways (antibodies, small molecule agents), and agents that block proangiogenic inflammatory pathways (e.g., thalidomide). Anticancer drugs may also be administered in low but frequent doses (metronomic chemotherapy) to preferentially target endothelial cells (see Table 13-2).[1,4,25]

Bevacizumab (Avastin), a humanized monoclonal anti-VEGF antibody was the first antiangiogenic agent to be developed and approved (in 2004) for cancer treatment, and the drug is now used to treat colorectal, lung, kidney, and brain tumors.[2] Several multikinase inhibitors with anti-VEGFR activity (sunitinib, sorafenib, pazopanib) are also in common use, as are inhibitors of oncogenic pathways that drive the production of VEGF.[9] The latter include inhibitors of the epidermal growth factor receptor (EGFR) and human epidermal growth factor receptor 2 (HER2) (cetuximab and trastuzumab, respectively), and other oncogene inhibitors.[9] These VEGF/VEGFR antagonists are mostly used in combination with chemotherapy, which suggests that they serve as chemosensitizers.[4] Studies are under way to develop drugs that specifically target pathologic angiogenesis (e.g., blockers of PlGF), or established tumor blood vessels (e.g., vascular disrupting agents [VDAs]).[4]

The overall objective of antiangiogenic therapy in cancer is to induce tumor hypovascularity, thereby causing hypoxic damage to tumor cells. Of note, blockade of Dll4 may result in hypoxia through a process that involves "nonproductive" angiogenesis and tumor hypervascularity.[14] Alternatively, antiangiogenic agents may also induce "vessel normalization" and improved tumor perfusion, which can lead to increased sensitivity to chemotherapy and radiation.[2]

Table 13-2 Blood Vessel–Targeting Agents: Antiangiogenic Agents

Drug	Type	Target	Stage of Development
TARGETED AGENTS DESIGNED TO OBLITERATE DEFINED ANGIOGENIC PATHWAYS			
Bevacizumab (Avastin)	Neutralizing huMoAb	VEGF	Approved for human use
Sunitinib (Sutent)	TKI	VEGFR1-3, PDGFR-α/β, KIT, Flt-3, RET, CSF1R	Approved for human use
Sorafenib (Nexavar)	TKI	VEGFR2-3, C-Raf, B-Raf, VEGF-C, Flt-3, FGFR1, PDGFR-β, KIT, p38	Approved for human use
Pazopanib (Votrient)	TKI	VEGFR1-3; PDGFR-α/β; KIT; FGFR1, 3, 4; FMS	Approved for human use
Vandetanib (Caprelsa) ZD6474	TKI	VEGFR2, EGFR, RET	Approved for human use
Axitinib (AG-013736)	TKI	VEGFR1-3, PDGFR, KIT	Approved for human use
XL184	TKI	VEGFR2, MET, RET, KIT, Flt-3, Tie2	In clinical development
VEGF Trap (Aflibercept)	Soluble VEGF "receptor-body"	VEGF-A, -B, PIGF	Approved for human use
Cilengitide	Cyclic peptide	αvβ3/β5 Integrin	In advanced clinical trials
AGENTS WITH DIRECT ANTIANGIOGENIC ACTIVITY			
Endostar	Protein fragment	Unclear	In human use (China)
ABT-510	Peptide	Endothelial CD36	In clinical development
2ME2	Sterol	HIF-1α, tubulin	Investigational agent
TNP-470 (Lodamin)	Small molecule (slow release)	Complex activity	Investigational agent
INDIRECT-ACTING AGENTS DESIGNED TO BLOCK ONCOGENIC PATHWAYS DRIVING ANGIOGENESIS			
Trastuzumab (Herceptin)	Neutralizing huMoAb	HER2	Approved for human use
Cetuximab (Erbitux)	Neutralizing huMoAb	EGFR	Approved for human use
Gefitinib (Iressa)	TKI	EGFR	Approved for human use
Erlotinib (Tarceva)	TKI	EGFR	Approved for human use
Lapatinib (Tykerb)	TKI	EGFR, HER2	Approved for human use
Imatinib (Gleevec)	TKI	ABL, PDGFR-β, KIT	Approved for human use
PF-00299804	TKI	Irreversible pan-ErbB inhibitor	In development
Tipifarnib	FTI	Ras, farnesylated proteins	In clinical development
AGENTS WITH ANTIANGIOGENIC AND NONANTIANGIOGENIC ACTIVITIES			
Chemotherapy (metronomic)	Various agents (CTX, VBL, TMZ, TAX)	Stress response pathways, DNA, cytoskeleton	Under clinical exploration
Celecoxib (Celebrex)	Small molecule	COX-2	Under clinical exploration
Thalidomide and analogues (lenalidomide)	Small molecule	Inflammatory pathways	Approved in multiple myeloma, under investigation
ANTIVASCULAR AGENTS/VASCULAR DISRUPTING AGENTS			
ASA404	Flavonoid	EC survival	Advanced clinical trials
CA4P	Tubulin binding	Tubulin assembly	Advanced clinical trials
AVE8062	Tubulin binding	Tubulin assembly	Advanced clinical trials
ABT-751	Tubulin binding	Tubulin assembly	Advanced clinical trials
OXi4503	Tubulin binding	Tubulin assembly	In clinical trials

COX-2, Cyclooxygenase-2; *CSF1R,* colony-stimulating factor 1 receptor; *CTX,* cyclophosphamide; *DNA,* deoxyribonucleic acid; *EGFR,* epidermal growth factor receptor; *FGFR,* fibroblast growth factor receptor; *FTI,* farnesyltransferase inhibitor; *HER2,* human epidermal growth factor receptor 2; *HIF-1α,* hypoxia-inducible factor-1α; *huMoAb,* humanized monoclonal antibody; *2ME2,* 2-methoxyestradiol; *PDGFR,* platelet-derived growth factor receptor; *PIGF,* placenta growth factor; *TAX,* paclitaxel; *TKI,* tyrosine kinase inhibitor; *TMZ,* temozolomide; *VBL,* vinblastine; *VEGF,* vascular endothelial growth factor; *VEGFR,* vascular endothelial growth factor receptor; see text and references for more details.[2]

Angiogenesis and Antiangiogenesis in Hematopoietic Malignancies

The vascular bone marrow stroma plays a pivotal role in leukemogenesis. Indeed, angiogenesis, increased vascular density, and increased levels of angiogenic growth factors have all been observed in the bone marrow of patients with hematopoietic malignancies.[26] VEGF may play multiple roles in this context, including as a (1) vascular growth stimulator, (2) paracrine growth factor for leukemic stem cells,[7] and (3) inducer of angiocrine interactions between these cells and the endothelium.[27] Consequently, a wide spectrum of antiangiogenic agents, including VEGF antagonists (bevacizumab, sorafenib, sunitinib, cediranib) are now being investigated for the treatment of hematologic disorders such as acute myeloid leukemia, chronic myeloid leukemia, acute lymphoblastic leukemia, myelodysplastic syndrome, non-Hodgkin lymphoma, multiple myeloma, and others.[7] Additional agents with antiangiogenic activity have also been explored (bortezomib), but the antiinflammatory antiangiogenics (thalidomide and lenalidomide) are the only drugs to be licensed thus far (in multiple myeloma and myelodysplastic syndrome, see Medinger and Mross[7] for review).

Hematologic Complications Associated With Blood Vessel–Directed Agents

Manipulation of endothelial and mural cells in the course of proangiogenic and antiangiogenic therapy creates the potential for side effects.[28] The most extensive clinical experience is in the area of cancer, where some toxicities (e.g., hypertension, proteinuria, fatigue, hypothyroidism), have been observed, along with hematologic side effects, mainly thrombosis and/or bleeding. Although cancer patients are prone to thrombosis,[29] additional risk for venous and arterial thromboembolism may also be associated with antiangiogenic therapy.[6] A considerable variability in this regard has been reported with different agents, and their effects found to be exacerbated by the accompanying chemotherapy or hormonal therapy.[29] This is of particular concern in patients with multiple myeloma who receive thalidomide derivatives in combination with anthracyclines and dexamethasone. In this case the reported risk for thrombosis could be as high as 75%.[29] Bevacizumab may also provoke an up to twofold increase in arterial thrombosis in patients with solid tumors, especially in the presence of additional risk factors and old age. These estimates are variable, however (0.9% to 19.4% according to different studies), and drug specific, because small-molecule kinase inhibitors acting on VEGFR are less likely to trigger venous thromboembolism (0% to 3%).[29]

Bleeding episodes were also recorded with several of these agents, ranging from minor to life threatening.[30] In general, however, antiangiogenic agents are relatively well tolerated, and their side effects are usually manageable with careful monitoring and standard supportive care[6] (see box on Advantages, Disadvantages, and Resistance to Antiangiogenic Therapy in Cancer).

Advantages, Disadvantages, and Resistance to Antiangiogenic Therapy in Cancer

Advantages of Antiangiogenesis

- Is directed against unique molecular targets
- Interferes with unusual deregulation of vascular cells and has moderate toxicity
- Targets the "angiocrine" niche for cancer and leukemic stem cells
- The target (blood vessels) is readily accessible to therapeutics
- Targets a rate-limiting process for tumor growth and dissemination
- Circumvents certain forms of drug resistance in cancer
- In some cases resistance to antiangiogenics is reversible
- Improves the efficacy of chemotherapy and radiation (vessel "normalization")

Disadvantages of Antiangiogenesis

- May facilitate hypoxic selection of more aggressive cancer cells
- May provoke cytokine emission and reactive bone marrow mobilization
- Bone marrow activation and pericyte damage may stimulate invasion and metastasis
- May cause toxicity related to housekeeping effects of angiogenic factors (e.g., vascular endothelial growth factor)
- Causes vessel regression and may activate coagulation
- May compromise wound healing
- May cause some unspecific toxicities

Mechanisms of Resistance to Antiangiogenic Agents

- Oncogenic mutations in cancer cells rendering them refractory to ischemia
- Redundancy of proangiogenic pathways in cancer cells ("evasive" resistance)
- Influx of proangiogenic host cells (fibroblasts, myeloid cells)
- Formation of more mature (pericyte-rich) vessels
- Onset of alternative modes of neovascularization (cooption, vasculogenic mimicry)
- Rapid vascular regrowth
- Genetic alterations in tumor endothelial cells
- Rebound effects involving angiogenesis, lymphangiogenesis, invasion, and metastasis

FUTURE DIRECTIONS

The functional integration of the vascular system, bone marrow, and circulating blood results in a high degree of biologic interdependence. Although this may not always be clinically obvious, the existence of these subtle links necessitates a greater inclusion of blood vessel–regulating processes into pathogenetic analysis and therapy of hematologic disorders.

REFERENCES

1. Folkman J: Angiogenesis: An organizing principle for drug discovery? *Nat Rev Drug Discov* 6:273, 2007.
2. Carmeliet P, Jain RK: Molecular mechanisms and clinical applications of angiogenesis. *Nature* 473:298, 2011.
3. Dvorak FH, Rickles FR: Malignancy and hemostasis. In Coleman RB, Marder VJ, Clowes AW, et al, editors: *Hemostasis and thrombosis: Basic principles and clinical practice*, Philadelphia, 2006, Lippincott Williams & Wilkins, p 851.
4. Kerbel RS: Tumor angiogenesis. *N Engl J Med* 358:2039, 2008.
5. Ferrara N, Kerbel RS: Angiogenesis as a therapeutic target. *Nature* 438:967, 2005.
6. Hurwitz HI, Saltz LB, Van CE, et al: Venous thromboembolic events with chemotherapy plus bevacizumab: A pooled analysis of patients in randomized phase II and III studies. *J Clin Oncol* 29:1757, 2011.
7. Medinger M, Mross K: Clinical trials with anti-angiogenic agents in hematological malignancies. *J Angiogenes Res* 2:10, 2010.
8. Ema M, Rossant J: Cell fate decisions in early blood vessel formation. *Trends Cardiovasc Med* 13:254, 2003.
9. Rak J: Ras oncogenes and tumour vascular interface. In Thomas-Tikhonenko A, editor: *Cancer genome and tumor microenvironment,* New York, 2009, Springer, p 133.
10. Rafii S, Lyden D, Benezra R, et al: Vascular and haematopoietic stem cells: Novel targets for anti-angiogenesis therapy? *Nat Rev Cancer* 2:826, 2002.
11. De Palma M, Naldini L: Role of haematopoietic cells and endothelial progenitors in tumour angiogenesis. *Biochim Biophys Acta* 1766:159, 2006.
12. Rak J: Microparticles in cancer. *Semin Thromb Hemost* 36:888, 2010.
13. Lusis AJ: Atherosclerosis. *Nature* 407:233, 2000.
14. Thurston G, Noguera-Troise I, Yancopoulos GD: The Delta paradox: DLL4 blockade leads to more tumour vessels but less tumour growth. *Nat Rev Cancer* 7:327, 2007.
15. Kessenbrock K, Plaks V, Werb Z: Matrix metalloproteinases: Regulators of the tumor microenvironment. *Cell* 141:52, 2010.
16. Xu Q: The impact of progenitor cells in atherosclerosis. *Nat Clin Pract Cardiovasc Med* 3:94, 2006.

17. Fantin A, Vieira JM, Gestri G, et al: Tissue macrophages act as cellular chaperones for vascular anastomosis downstream of VEGF-mediated endothelial tip cell induction. *Blood* 116:829, 2010.
18. Gaengel K, Genove G, Armulik A, et al: Endothelial-mural cell signaling in vascular development and angiogenesis. *Arterioscler Thromb Vasc Biol* 29:630, 2009.
19. Tammela T, Alitalo K: Lymphangiogenesis: Molecular mechanisms and future promise. *Cell* 140:460, 2010.
20. Ricci-Vitiani L, Pallini R, Biffoni M, et al: Tumour vascularization via endothelial differentiation of glioblastoma stem-like cells. *Nature* 468:824, 2010.
21. Holash J, Maisonpierre PC, Compton D, et al: Vessel cooption, regression, and growth in tumors mediated by angiopoietins and VEGF. *Science* 284:1994, 1999.
22. Brat DJ, Van Meir EG: Vaso-occlusive and prothrombotic mechanisms associated with tumor hypoxia, necrosis, and accelerated growth in glioblastoma. *Lab Invest* 84:397, 2004.
23. Rey S, Semenza GL: Hypoxia-inducible factor-1-dependent mechanisms of vascularization and vascular remodelling. *Cardiovasc Res* 86:236, 2010.
24. Majmundar AJ, Wong WJ, Simon MC: Hypoxia-inducible factors and the response to hypoxic stress. *Mol Cell* 40:294, 2010.
25. Cook KM, Figg WD: Angiogenesis inhibitors: Current strategies and future prospects. *CA Cancer J Clin* 60:222, 2010.
26. Perez-Atayde AR, Sallan SE, Tedrow U, et al: Spectrum of tumor angiogenesis in the bone marrow of children with acute lymphoblastic leukemia. *Am J Pathol* 150:815, 1997.
27. Butler JM, Kobayashi H, Rafii S: Instructive role of the vascular niche in promoting tumour growth and tissue repair by angiocrine factors. *Nat Rev Cancer* 10:138, 2010.
28. Verheul HM, Pinedo HM: Possible molecular mechanisms involved in the toxicity of angiogenesis inhibition. *Nat Rev Cancer* 7:475, 2007.
29. Zangari M, Fink LM, Elice F, et al: Thrombotic events in patients with cancer receiving antiangiogenesis agents. *J Clin Oncol* 27:4865, 2009.
30. Elice F, Rodeghiero F: Bleeding complications of antiangiogenic therapy: Pathogenetic mechanisms and clinical impact. *Thromb Res* 125:S55, 2010.

CHAPTER 14

PRINCIPLES OF CYTOKINE SIGNALING

Monteaser Shaheen and Hal E. Broxmeyer

CYTOKINE AND RECEPTOR FAMILIES AND SIGNAL TRANSDUCTION

Cytokines are secreted molecules that regulate cellular interactions through binding to defined receptors and inducing intracellular signaling. Cytokines are classified based on the primary structural features of the extracellular domains of their receptors.[1] Class or type I cytokines (often referred to as *hematopoietins*) regulate development, differentiation, and activation of hematopoietic and immune cells. Type I cytokine receptors include those for colony-stimulating factors (CSFs), interleukins (ILs), erythropoietin (EPO), thrombopoietin (TPO), and some hormones such as growth hormone and leptin. Class II cytokines consists of type I interferons (IFNs), including IFN-α, IFN-β, IFN-ω, IFN-ε, IFN-κ, IFN-τ, IFN-ς/lumitin, IFN-δ and IFN-ν, type II IFN consisting of the single IFN-γ, and the IL-10 family of cytokines (which includes several cytokines, including IL-19, IL-20, IL-22, IL-24, IL-26) and type III IFNs, including IFN-λ1 (IL-29), IFN-λ2 (IL-28A), and IFN-λ3 (IL-28).

The structural similarities of type I cytokines were not initially recognized. However, cloning of their receptors revealed significant homology in that the extracellular regions contain a common domain with four conserved cysteines (C4) in the N-terminal segment and a tryptophan-serine doublet near the C-terminal end.[2] This 200–amino acid region, which is derived from a tandem of two fibronectin-like domains, has been named the *hematopoietin receptor domain*. Two conserved Box1/Box2 regions are located in the proximal intracytoplasmic segment. Fig. 14-1 depicts the general structure of a type 1 cytokine receptor. By contrast, type II cytokine receptors contain two cysteine doublets (C2-C2) located in the C-terminal end of both fibronectin-derived domains. They retain Box1/2 regions but lack the tryptophan(Trp)-serine(ser)-x(any amino acid)-serine(ser)-tryptophan(Trp) motif. Both types of receptors bind ligands that display common spatial four α-helix bundle organization and utilize intracellular signaling mediators of the Janus kinase (JAK) and signal transducer and activator of transcription (STAT) families. Because of these shared features, type I and II cytokine receptors represent a homogeneous structural group of proteins. However, sequence homology is observed in a limited number of cases, such as for the growth hormone (GH)/prolactin (PRL) family and for the IL-6 family. Nonetheless, evidence of common ancestry of cytokines can be observed in the similar four-helix bundle structure[3] in addition to the similar intron–exon relationship and the clustering observed for certain cytokine genes such as genes of the IL-4 family.[4]

The receptors can be composed of dimers of a single chain (granulocyte-colony stimulating factor receptor [G-CSFR], EPO receptor [EPOR], TPO receptor [TPOR or c-mpl]) or can be heterodimeric with a common signaling subunit and a unique ligand-binding chain. These heterodimeric receptors can be grouped into families based on whether they share the common β-chain (granulocyte macrophage [GM]-CSFRα, IL-3Rα, IL-5Rα) or those that share the gp130 receptor (IL-6Rα, leukemia inhibitory factor receptor β, ciliary neurotrophic factor receptor α, IL-11Rα, oncostatin M receptor α, cardiotrophin-like cytokine factor 1) and those that share the common γ-chain (IL-2Rα, IL-2R β, IL-4Rα, IL-7Rα, IL-9Rα, IL-13Rα, IL-15Rα, and IL-21Rα). Fig. 14-2 demonstrates the shared receptors' units among type 1 cytokine receptor families. Cytokines bind their cognate receptors with high affinity. This binding triggers receptor homodimerization (e.g., G-CSFR), heterodimerization or oligomerization of receptor subunits (e.g., granulocyte macrophage colony-stimulating factor receptor [GM-CSFR]), or it induces a conformational change in preformed receptor dimers (EPOR), resulting in the activation of the JAKs. Unlike other receptors with intrinsic enzyme activity (e.g., receptor tyrosine kinases [RTKs] such as Flt3 and c-Kit), most cytokine receptors are constitutively associated with kinases. These cytoplasmic kinases comprise the four members of the JAK family: JAK1, JAK2, and tyrosine kinase 2 (Tyk2), which bind to a wide range of receptors, and JAK3, which binds to only one receptor, the common gamma chain, or γc. This binding is mediated by interactions between the 4.1, ezrin, radixin, moesin (FERM) domain of JAK and the Box1 membrane proximal intracytoplasmic region of the receptor. Upon ligand binding, JAKs come into juxtaposition and phosphorylate themselves and their associated receptors. Mutagenesis studies have shown that there are distinct regions of individual phosphorylated receptors that transmit signals for cell survival, proliferation, differentiation, or activation via interaction with adaptor molecules. Phosphorylation of certain residues generates docking sites for the Src homology (SH2) domains of the STATs. After bound to the receptor–JAK complex, STATs are themselves phosphorylated, which induces a conformational change that generates active STAT dimers via reciprocal phosphotyrosine and SH2 domain interaction. The dimers translocate to the nucleus, where they bind to DNA sequences in the promoters of target genes to activate transcription.

Multiple mechanisms exist to attenuate cytokine signaling, which ensures controlled cellular responses to cytokines and prevents pathologic hyperactivation. Because the signaling is mediated by extensive phosphorylation, phosphatases have emerged as important negative regulators. Examples of these include the Src-homology 2 containing phosphatase (SHP) proteins. Other regulators have been identified including protein inhibitors of activated STAT (PIAS), suppressor of cytokine signaling (SOCS) proteins, and cytokine-inducible SH2-domain-containing proteins (CIS). Fig. 14-3 simplifies the intracellular events that are triggered by cytokine-receptor engagement. This chapter discusses in some details the proposed mechanisms of inhibition of these proteins. Expression of receptors is also regulated at the level of gene transcription, protein translation, internalization, and degradation.

MODELS OF LIGAND-RECEPTOR BINDING AND ACTIVATION

Cytokines bind with high affinity to their cognate receptors. The presence and the density of the receptors may determine the biologic response in a hematopoietic progenitor or lymphocytic cell population.[5] The crystal structures of cytokines bound to the receptors have been illustrated for multiple cytokine families. It can be concluded, for most cytokine–receptor couples, that more than one cytokine molecule engages more than one receptor unit at one time to form a complex. For example, two IL-6 molecules aggregate with four receptor chains to form a hexameric and interlocking assembly

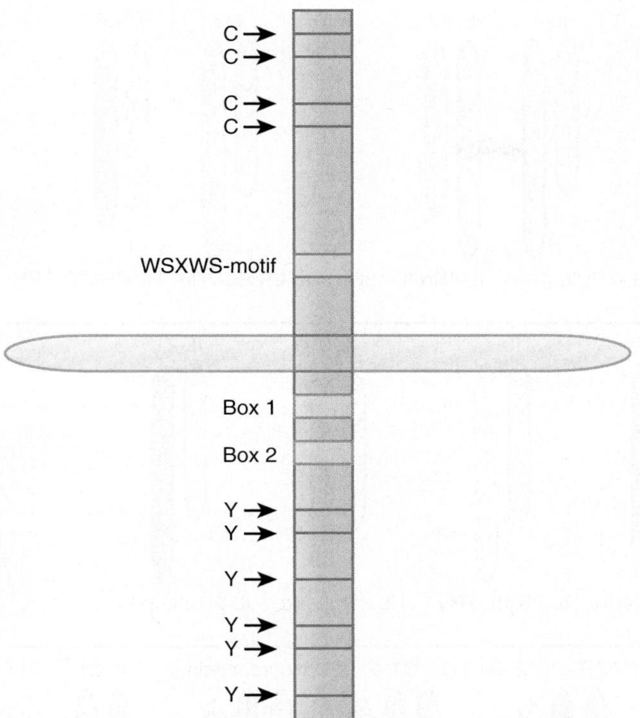

Figure 14-1 CYTOKINE RECEPTOR SUPERFAMILY. The general structure of cytokine receptor superfamily. In the extracellular cytokine receptor module (CRM) 4 conserved cysteine residues exist and are involved in disulfide bonds. A WSXWS (Trp, Ser, any, Trp, Ser) motif that is essential for receptor processing, ligand binding, and activation of the receptor is also located in the extracellular domain. In the intracellular portion, two short domains termed *box 1* and *box 2* are important for Janus kinase (JAK) binding. Tyrosine residues are present on the intracellular part to be phosphorylated upon receptor activation.

mediated by a total of 10 symmetry-related, thermodynamically coupled interfaces.[6] The assembly of this hexameric complex occurs sequentially: IL-6 is first engaged by IL-6Rα and then is presented to gp130 in the proper geometry to facilitate a cooperative transition into the high-affinity, signaling-competent hexamer (Fig. 14-4). This structure also reveals that gp130 is bent such that the membrane-proximal domains of gp130 are close together at the cell surface, enabling activation of intracellular signaling. Variation in the receptor bend angles suggests a possible conformational transition from open to closed states upon ligand binding. Reconstruction of full-length JAK1 in conjunction with gp130/IL–6/IL–6Rα complex reveals a three-lobed structure of JAK1 possessing extensive intersegmental flexibility that likely facilitates allosteric activation[7] (Fig. 14-5). Single-particle imaging of the gp130/IL–6/IL–6Rα/JAK1 holocomplex shows JAK1 associated with the membrane proximal intracellular regions of gp130, abutting the would-be inner leaflet of the cell membrane. JAK1 association with gp130 appears to be enhanced by the presence of a membrane environment.

It has been debated how the 16 human type I IFN molecules signal through the same receptors, IFNAR1 and IFNAR2, yet they can evoke different physiologic effects. Recently, structural analysis of this family in complex with this single receptor complex indicates that the receptor–ligand cross-reactivity is enabled by conserved receptor-ligand "anchor points" interspersed among ligand-specific interactions that "tune" the relative IFN-binding affinities in an apparent extracellular "ligand proofreading" mechanism that modulates biologic activity.[8] This differential binding leads to variable conformational changes in the receptor complex, resulting in different STAT phosphorylation profiles, receptor internalization rates, and downstream gene expression patterns.

Signaling networks are typically measured in either their basal (minimum) or hyperstimulated (maximum) states. Recent investigations[9] indicate that the cytokine signal "dynamic range," defined as the responsiveness of cell outcomes to incremental changes in signal activation is more important for biologic outcome than signal strength per se.

The following describes information on JAK and STAT proteins. Table 14-1 summarizes the abnormalities in mice associated with deletion of specific JAK and STAT genes.

Janus Kinases

Janus kinase proteins are Tyks of approximately 1000 amino acids. They have clear nonredundant in vivo functions defined by the analysis of gene deletion in mice and mutations of JAK3 or Tyk2 in humans that lead to primary immunodeficiency syndromes of severe combined immunodeficiency (SCID) type and autosomal recessive hyperimmunoglobulin E syndrome (AR-HIES), respectively.[10] In addition, somatic mutations of JAKs are seen in human neoplastic conditions. Below is a brief description of functions of the JAKs in cytokine signaling. Fig. 14-6 depicts the general structure of JAK proteins.

Janus Kinase 1

Janus kinase 1 is widely expressed and associates with the IFN receptors and receptors that use gp130 or γ chain (γc). $JAK1^{-/-}$ mice have grossly normal nonlymphoid organogenesis[10,11]; however, the neonates fail to nurse and die perinatally of a poorly characterized defect that may be neurologic. It is believed that this morbid phenotype is attributable to the failure of signaling via cytokines that promote neuronal cell survival via gp130. Defective cytokine signaling is observed with class II cytokine receptors (IFNs) and IL-2, IL-6, and IL-7 families. There is a severe lymphocyte defect in the newborn mice consistent with the fact that JAK1 binds to the ligand-specific receptor subunit of γc. Somatic JAK1 activating mutations have been described in occasional cases of acute leukemia and solid tumors.

Janus Kinase 2

Janus kinase 2 is widely expressed and is involved in signaling by single-chain hormone receptors, the common β chain family, and certain members of the class II receptor cytokine family. JAK2 deficiency is lethal at day 12.5 because of failure of erythropoiesis,[12] and this explains lack of reports on individuals with germline loss-of-function JAK2 mutations. Receptor stimulation by EPO induces tyrosine phosphorylation of JAK2, which is required for EPO function.[13] Defective responses of cells from $JAK2^{-/-}$ mice also reveal its essential role in the signaling of IL-3, GM-CSF, IL-5, TPO, and IFN-γ but not IL-6 and IFN-α/β.[14] Transfer of $JAK2^{-/-}$ fetal liver cells into irradiated $JAK3^{-/-}$ recipients resulted in normal thymic subsets, arguing that JAK2 is not essential for T-cell development. In 2005, multiple groups identified activating mutations in JAK2 as the etiology for virtually all cases of polycythemia vera, and significant percentages of cases of essential thrombocythemia and idiopathic myelofibrosis. JAK2 mutations have also been described in other hematopoietic neoplasms. JAK2 inhibitors have shown efficacy at least in decreasing spleen size and constitutional symptoms in patients with JAK2 mutation–positive myeloproliferative disorders.

Janus Kinase 3

In contrast to the ubiquitous expression of the other JAKs, JAK3 is predominantly expressed in hematopoietic tissues. JAK3 selectively associates exclusively with the γc, which is a component of multiple

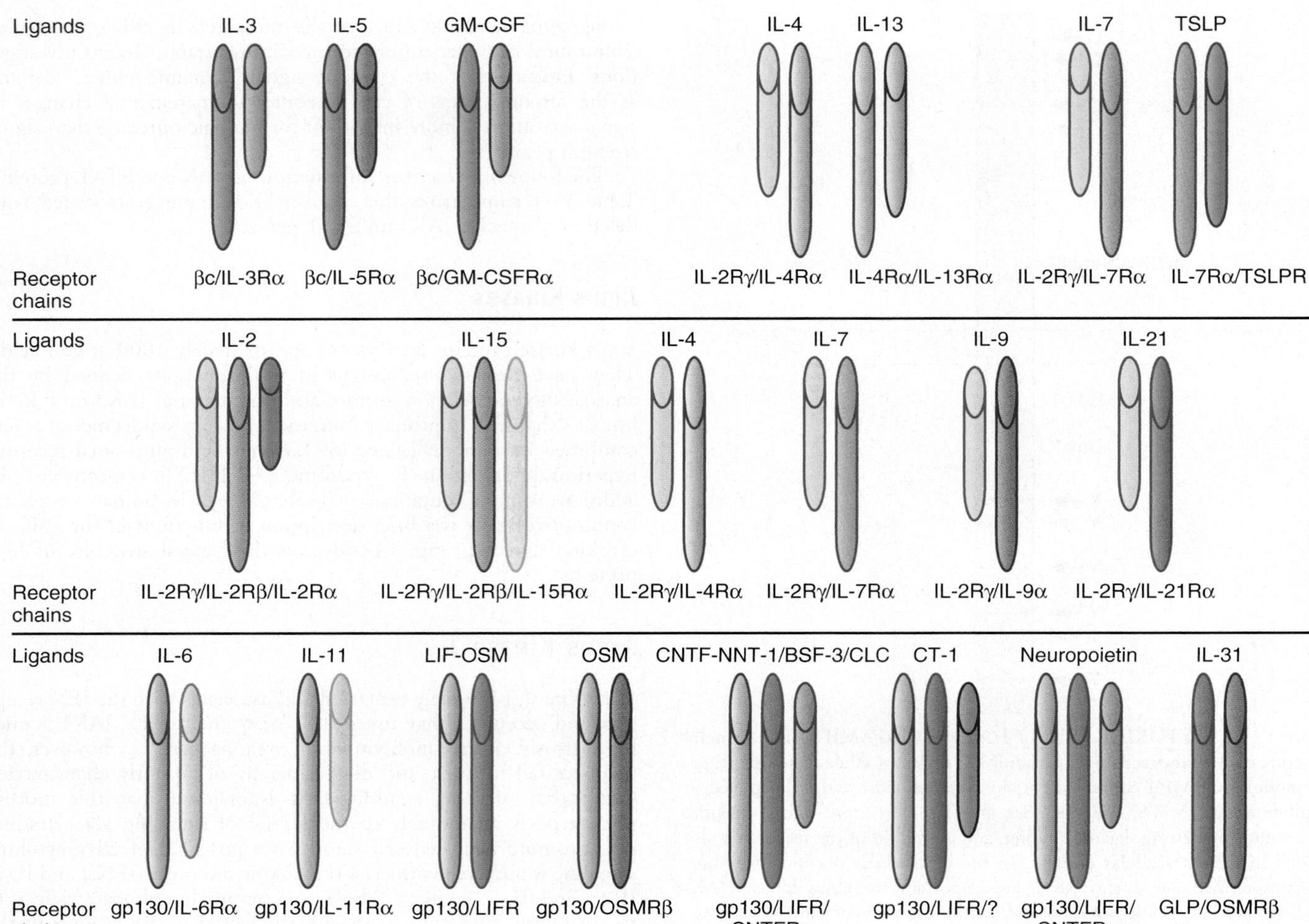

Figure 14-2 SIMPLE DEPICTION OF TYPE 1 CYTOKINE RECEPTOR SUBFAMILIES THAT SHARE RECEPTOR UNITS. Interleukin-3R (IL-3R), IL-5R, and granulocyte macrophage colony-stimulating factor receptor (GM-CSFR) share a common βc chain that place them in one group. Multiple cytokines (IL-2, IL-4, IL-7, IL-9, IL-15, and IL-21) share the IL-2Rγ chain, which is mutated in a subset of patients with severe combined immunodeficiency. IL-4R shares a subunit with IL-13R. Both IL-4 and IL-13 drive Th2 response. IL-7R shares one subunit with the thymic stromal lymphopoietin (TSLP). This sharing of receptor subunit may explain why deletion of the gene encoding IL-7R affects the lymphoid system more severely than deleting the IL-7 gene. Finally, the IL-6 family includes multiple cytokines that all share the common signal transducer gp130. Deleting gp130 results in embryonic lethality. Some IL-6 family members activate more than one receptor. Oncostatin M (OSM) can work through a heterodimer receptor consisting of gp130 with OSMRβ or gp130 with leukemia inhibitory factor receptor (LIF-R). Ciliary neurotrophic factor (CNTF) shares its receptor with novel neurotrophic-1/B cell–stimulating factor-3/cardiotrophin-like cytokine (NNT/BSF-3/CLC). Cardiotrophin-1 (CT-1) uses a receptor composed of gp130, LIF-R, and another yet to be identified subunit. Neuropoietin shares the same receptor as CNTF. IL-31 receptor is composed of gp130-like receptor (GLR) and OSMRβ.

cytokine receptors. Accordingly, a mutation of γc or JAK3 results in SCID in humans, characterized by the lack of T and natural killer (NK) cells, but B-cell numbers are preserved; thus, this abnormality is designated T^-B^+ NK^- SCID.[15] Mice homozygous for JAK3 null mutation have severe defects in lymphoid cells. B-cell precursors in bone marrow, thymocytes, and both T and B cells are drastically decreased,[10] although these defects can improve as aging occurs.[16] Peripheral lymph nodes, NK cells, dendritic cells (DCs), epidermal T cells, and intestinal intraepithelial γ δ T cells are absent in these mice. Normal numbers of bone marrow HPCs and a similar capability of these marrow cells to generate myeloid and erythroid colonies as wild-type mice indicates that specific defects in lymphoid progenitor cells exist. Thymic progenitors are severely deficient. This phenotype is attributable to failure of IL-7 and IL-2 signaling, which explains the T-cell deficiency; the absence of NK cell development has been attributed to an impairment in IL-15 signaling. There is a high apoptotic rate in the lymphocytes generated in these mice, and this is consistent with the identified function of JAK3 in regulating Bcl-2 and Bax.

Activation of JAK3 caused by gain-of-function mutations is found in several human hematologic malignancies, including acute megakaryoblastic leukemia and cutaneous T-cell lymphoma.

Given the essential role of JAK3 in cytokine signaling through γc and given its limited tissue expression, inhibition of JAK3 activity has emerged as a promising strategy for immunosuppression for autoimmune disorders and immune rejection.

Tyrosine Kinase 2

Tyrosine kinase 2 was the first JAK family member identified in cytokine signaling. Tyk2 was discovered as an essential component in a screen for mutants in IFN-α signaling. Type I IFN receptors require Tyk2 and JAK1, but IFN-γ signaling depends on the combination of Tyk2 and JAK2.[17] The combination of Tyk2 with JAK2 is not only required for IFN-γ signaling but also for the differentiation of IFN-γ–producing Th1 cells from naive Th cells. Lymphocyte development and proliferation are not affected in Tyk2-deficient mice, but

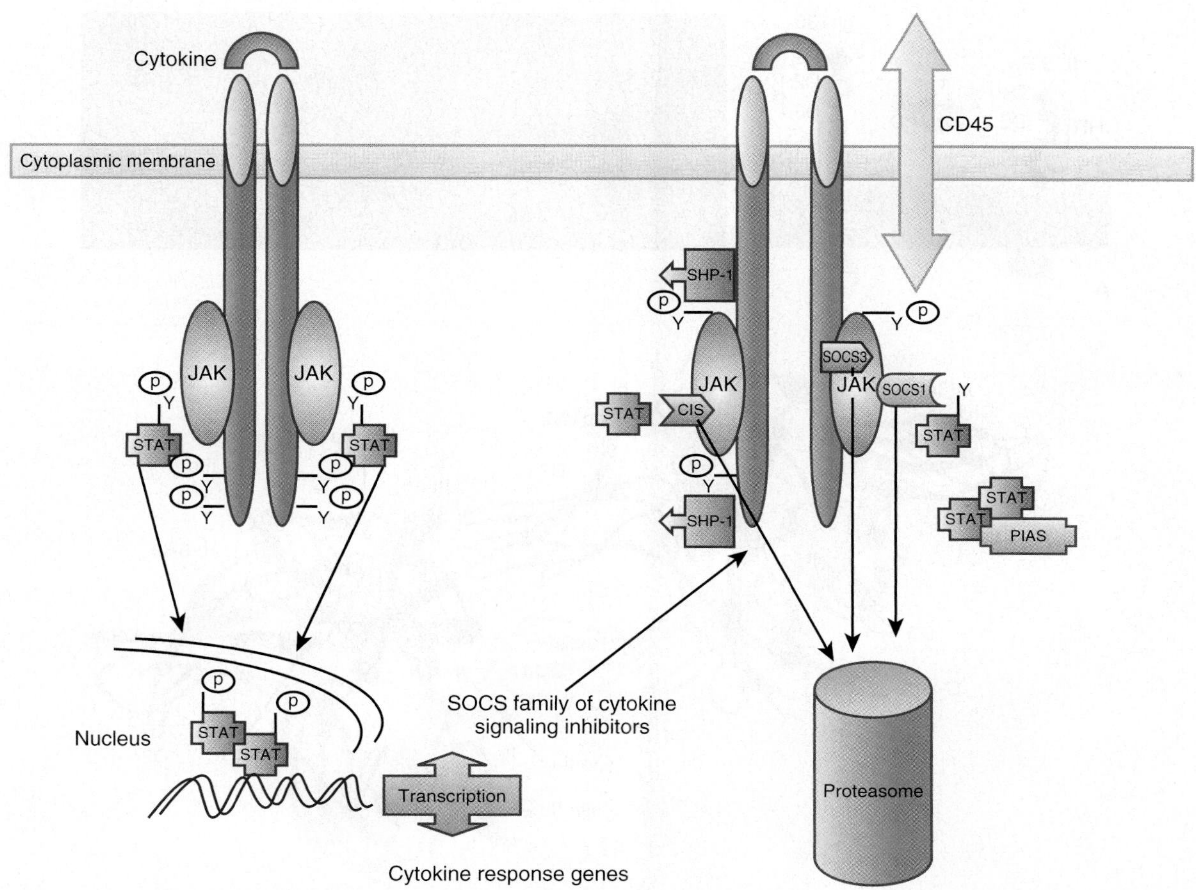

Figure 14-3 CYTOKINE–RECEPTOR INTERACTIONS. A general depiction of signal transduction by cytokine receptor superfamily. Ligand binding leads to dimerization or oligomerization of the receptor, which brings into proximity the associated Janus kinases (JAKs). The Latter phosphorylate tyrosine residues on the receptor and JAKs. This phosphorylation creates docking sites for proteins containing Src homology (SH2) domains such as signal transducers and activators of transcription (STATs). These hetero- or homodimerize and translocate to the nucleus, where they affect transcription of target genes. Several mechanisms exist to reverse this cytokine-activated state. STATs trigger a negative feedback loop by inducing transcription of suppressors of cytokine (SOCSs). There are eight SOCS members. SOCS1 interacts directly with JAK1 and inhibits its catalytic activity. Cytokine-inducible SH2-domain-containing proteins (CIS), another SOCS, binds the receptor and blocks binding and phosphorylation of STATs. SOCS3 binds the receptor before inhibiting JAK. SOCS proteins contain a SOCS box that leads to proteosomal degradation of the SOCS-associated molecules. Src-homology 2 containing phosphatase 1 (SHP1) is a tyrosine phosphatase that negatively regulates the cytokine transduction process by dephosphorylating JAKs and the cytokine receptors. CD45 is a transmembrane phosphatase that inactivates JAKSs. Protein inhibitors of activated STAT (PIAS) family members interact with STAT dimers and inhibit their functions as described in the main text.

signaling by cytokines that are important for host defense is impaired.[18] The IL-12 receptor (IL-12R) is associated with Tyk2 and JAK2 and activates mainly the transcription factor STAT4. IL-12 signaling is strongly impaired in the absence of Tyk2, and downstream activation of STAT3 and STAT4 is clearly reduced, resulting in the inability of IFN-γ production by T cells. Both STAT3 and STAT1 activation by type I and type II IFNs is reduced in Tyk2-deficient mice, although at high concentration, IFN-α can fully transduce its signal in the absence of Tyk2. IL-10 signaling is essentially normal. Because of all of the above, Tyk2-deficient mice are susceptible to viral and bacterial infections. This susceptibility can be explained by impaired Th1 lineage development, but Th17 differentiation also seems to be affected in the absence of Tyk2. Because IL-4 is essential in generating Th2 cells and because its signaling is independent of Tyk2, there is no disruption of Th2 in Tyk2-deficient mice. Th2 cell differentiation can also be inhibited by Tyk2-mediated signals derived from IL-12 or IFNs. As expected, Th2-induced diseases such as allergic bronchitis are enhanced in the background of Tyk2 deficiency. One example is a mouse asthma model in which pronounced lung inflammation is noted because of an enhanced Th2 response with an increase of IL-4 production, increased IgE levels, and recruitment of eosinophils.[19]

Signal Transducers and Activators of Transcription

There are seven STAT family members that share a similar structure, but mediate distinct biologic functions.[20] Fig. 14-6 shows the general structure of a STAT. STAT1, for example, harbors an *N*-terminal domain followed by an α-helical coiled-coil and a DNA-binding domain and a linker that connects to the C terminus. The C terminus contains an SH2 domain followed by a short region containing a tyrosine residue, which is critical for the activation by JAK-mediated phosphorylation, and a transactivation domain, which is the most divergent part within the STAT family. STAT proteins can be tyrosine phosphorylated by receptor-associated JKs, by growth factor receptor Tyks, or by nonreceptor Tyks. Latent STATs diffuse freely in the cytoplasm. Upon STAT phosphorylation and

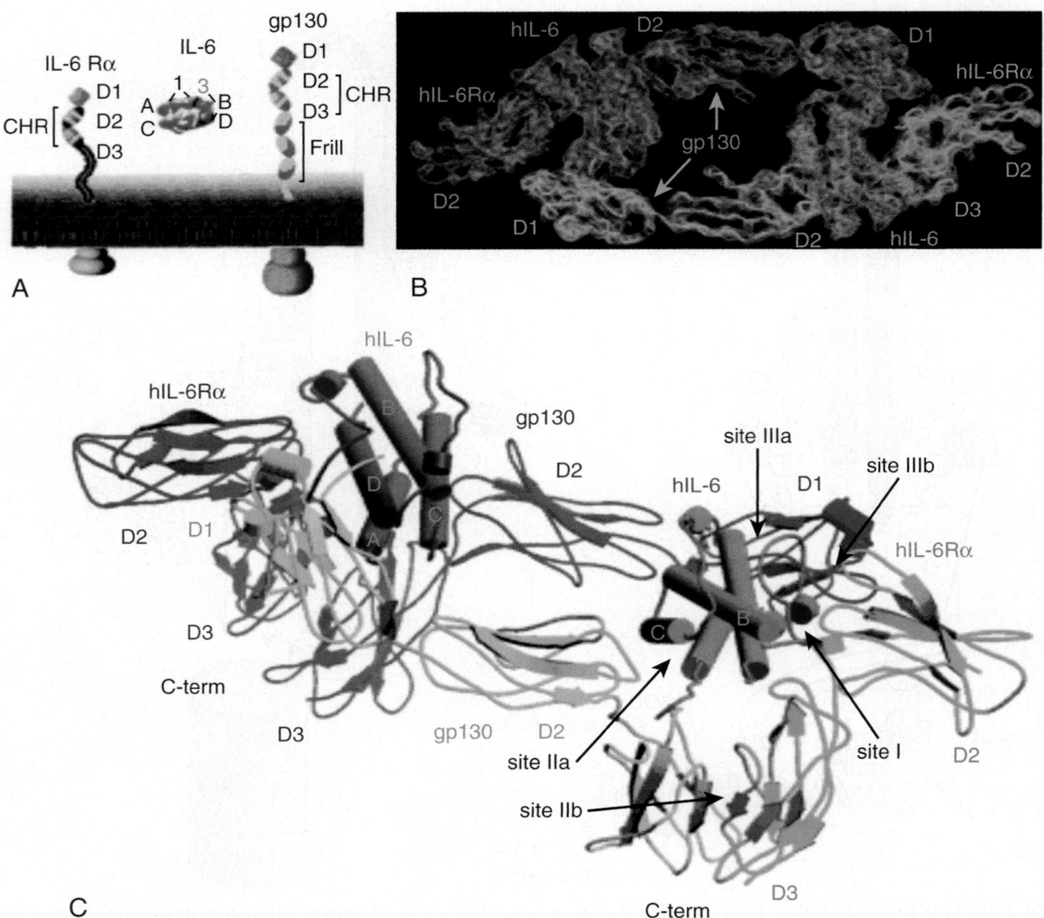

Figure 14-4 INTERLEUKIN-6 (IL-6) COMPLEX STRUCTURE. **A,** The complex is a hexamer consisting of interleukin-6 (IL-6), the IL-6 α-receptor (IL-6Rα), and the shared signaling receptor gp130. **B,** The 3.65 angstrom–resolution shows a hexameric, interlocking assembly mediated by a total of 10 symmetry-related, thermodynamically coupled interfaces. Assembly of the hexameric complex occurs sequentially: IL-6 is first engaged by IL-6Rα and then presented to gp130 to activate the downstream signaling. **C,** The domain structure of IL-6 engaging its receptor complex. *(Adapted from Boulanger MJ, Chow DC, Brevnova EE, et al: Hexameric structure and assembly of the interleukin-6/IL-6 alpha-receptor/gp130 complex.* Science *300:2101, 2003.)*

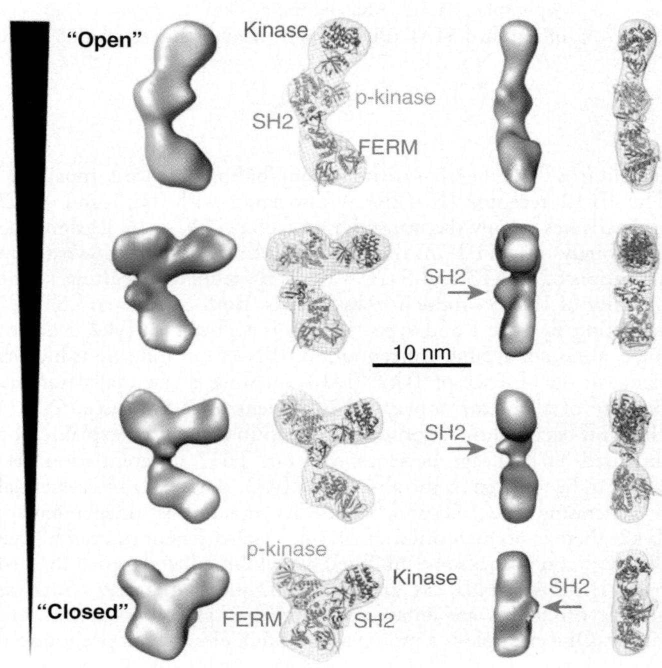

Figure 14-5 3D REPRESENTATION OF JAK1 SHOWING IT FORMING THREE LOBES. It switched *in vitro* from an open to a closed conformation. The orientations of the reconstructions in the left column represent the particles face-on, while the orientations to the right are rotated 90°, reflecting the flatness of the surface on which Jak1 is lying. It is uncertain whether the open or the closed conformation represents the active state. *FERM,* 4.1, ezrin, radixin, moesin; *SH2,* Src homology. *(Adapted from Lupardus PJ, Skiniotis G, Rice AJ, et al: Structural snapshots of full-length Jak1, a ransmembrane gp130/IL-6/IL-6Rα cytokine receptor complex, and the receptor-Jak1 holocomplex.* Structure *19:45, 2011.)*

dimerization with a partner, the dimer quickly translocates to the nucleus (Fig. 14-7). This is done through an active process mediated by the nuclear transport machinery. For example, phosphorylated STAT1 transport is facilitated by the importin-α5/importin-β1 heterodimer. This nuclear movement culminates in DNA binding and transcriptional activity. For example, IFN-γ binding to its receptor leads to tyrosine phosphorylation of STAT1. The STAT1 dimer was originally called the *IFN-γ activated factor* (GAF). It recognizes a DNA sequence termed the *IFN-γ activated sequence* (GAS), which contains an inverted repeat of GAAA residues spaced by two to four nucleotides. Below we will briefly discuss the biologic activities of STAT proteins largely inferred from gene targeting experiments.

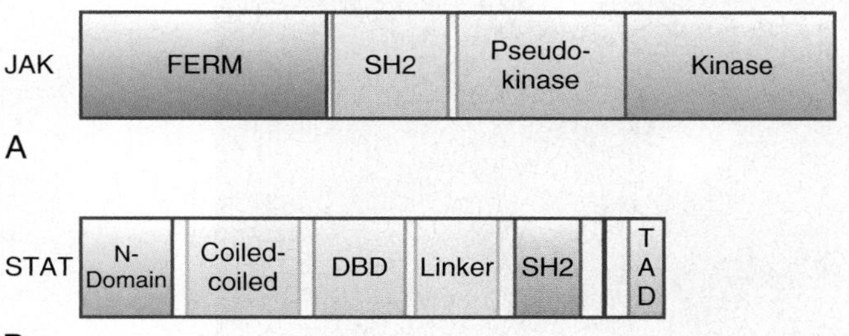

Figure 14-6 GENERAL STRUCTURE OF JANKUS KINASE (JAK) AND STAT PROTEINS. **A,** JAK protein consists of the 4.1, ezrin, radixin, moesin (FERM) domain (which modulates the kinase activity), Src homology (SH2) domain for phospho-tyrosine binding, pseudokinase (which can exert inhibitory function), and kinase domain. **B,** STAT protein consists of an N-terminus domain, coiled-coiled domain for protein interaction, DNA binding domain (DBD), linker domain, SH2 domain, conserved tyrosine, and transactivation domain (TAD), which binds transcription regulators.

Signal Transducer and Activator of Transcription 1

STAT1 mediates signaling from IFNs. STAT1-deficient mice show no significant developmental abnormalities, but they display a complete lack of responsiveness to either IFN-α or IFN-γ and are highly sensitive to infection by microbial pathogens and viruses.[21] The induction of IFN-inducible genes is disrupted. A missense mutation of STAT1 was initially identified in a patient with atypical mycobacterial infections, similar to individuals with mutations of IFNγR subunits. However, this STAT1 mutation was not associated with susceptibility to viral infections.[22] Since then, other families have been described with mutations in STAT1 that lead to viral and mycobacterial infections. Recently, families with mucocutaneous candidiasis have been reported with STAT1 mutations.[23] These families have defective Th1 and Th17 responses. Not all IFN-dependent signaling is regulated by STAT1 because there is a large number of STAT1-independent genes that are induced by IFN-γ, and this may explain the observations that STAT1$^{-/-}$ mice are less susceptible to infection

Table 14-1 Consequence of Deficiencies in Genes Encoding Intracellular Signaling Molecules*

Signal Transduction Molecule	Phenotype of Deficient Mice
JAK1	Perinatal mortality, defects in IL-6, IL-2, and cytokine receptor type II families
JAK2	Embryonic lethality caused by defective definitive hematopoiesis; defects in EPO, TPO, IL-2 family, IL-3, and IFN-γ signaling
JAK3	Immunodeficiency caused by absent common γ chain signaling; JAK3 expression is restricted to the hematopoietic system
TYK2	Reduced responses to IFN-α/β, IL-12, and IFNγ
STAT1	Complete lack of responsiveness to either IFN-α/β or IFN-γ and high sensitivity to infections by viruses and other microbial pathogens; normal response to other cytokines such as GH and IL-10
STAT2	Lack of responsiveness to IFN-α/β; susceptibility to viral infections
STAT3	Early embryonic lethality before gastrulation
	STAT3 $^{-}$/+ mice demonstrate decreased HSC/HPCs
STAT4	Defective Th1 and Th17 responses caused by defective IL-12, IL23 signaling
STAT5a	Defective mammary gland development and lactogenesis; GM-CSF and FL signaling is impaired but no gross hematopoietic abnormalities
STAT5b	Disrupted sexual dimorphism of body growth rates; defective GH signaling
STAT5a/b	Anemic embryos of the double knock-outs with apoptotic erythroid progenitors caused by impaired EPO signaling; adult mouse erythrocyte RBC number is normal; loss of GH and prolactin signaling; infertile females; severe impairment of IL-2–induced T-cell responses
STAT6	Defective Th2 response with defective IL-4 signaling
SHP-1	Natural mutation in *moth-eaten* mice results in hair loss, immunodeficiency, autoimmune disorders, enhanced SDF-1 chemotactic activities, and enhanced hematopoietic progenitor proliferation in response to cytokines such as GM-CSF
CD45	Enhanced cytokine and IFN-receptor–mediated activation of JAKs and STATs
SOCS1	Neonatal lethality probably caused by excessive IFN-γ responses, with hematopoietic infiltration of multiple organs, lymphopenia, and fatty liver degeneration
SOCS2	Gigantism caused by GH or IGF-1 excessive signaling
SOCS3	Embryonic lethality with placental defect; erythrocytosis in embryos

EGF, Epidermal growth factor; *EPO,* erythropoietin; *FL,* Flt-Ligand; *GH,* growth hormone; *GM-CSF,* granulocyte macrophage colony-stimulating factor; *HPC,* hematopoietic progenitor cell; *HSC,* hematopoietic stem cell; *IFN,* interferon; *IGF-1,* insulin-like growth factor-1; *IL,* interleukin; *JAK,* Janus kinase; *RBC,* red blood cell; *SDF-1,* stromal derived factor-1; *SHP,* Src homology 2 containing phosphatase; *SOC,* suppressor of cytokine signaling; *STAT,* signal transducer and activator of transcription.
*This table outlines the phenotypes of mice deficient in the major signaling molecules that directly interact with the cytokine receptors. The phenotypes range from significant embryonic lethality caused by hematopoietic impairment to less remarkable defects in other organ systems. Please refer to the main text for more details on the functions of these molecules.

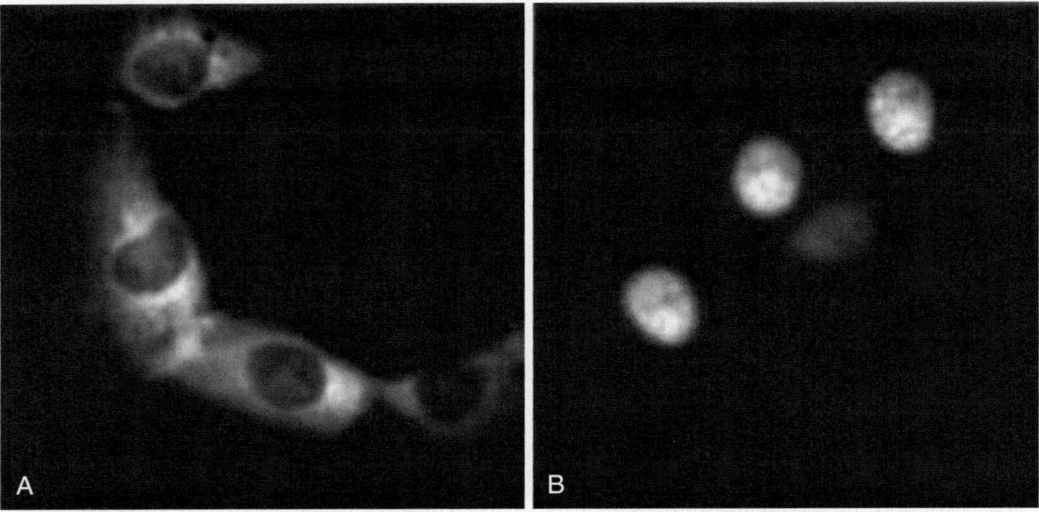

Figure 14-7 DEMONSTRATION OF STAT PROTEIN LOCATION RESPONSE TO CYTOKINE SIGNALING. U3A cells expressing STAT-Green Fluorescent Protein (STAT-GFP) were untreated **(A)** or treated **(B)** with interferon-γ for 30 min. One can observe the migration of STAT1 from the cytoplasm to the nucleus. *(Adapted from McBride KM, McDonald C, Reich NC: Nuclear export signal located within the DNA-binding domain of the STAT1 transcription factor.* EMBO J *19:6196, 2000.)*

than mice lacking both IFN-γ and IFN-α/β receptors. Other less pronounced defects have been described in STAT1-deficient mice such as a subtle decrease in bone marrow erythroid progenitors. STAT1 regulates other cytokine/growth factor signaling. One example is its role in the inhibitory activity of fibroblast growth factor on chondrocytes mediated by transcriptional activation of cell cycle inhibitors. Another example of IFN-independent activity of STAT1 is the regulation of NK cells whose function is more severely impaired by STAT1 deficiency than by deficiencies of both IFN-γ and IFN-α/β receptors.

Because IFNs have antineoplastic activities, a role for STAT1 in tumor suppression was suspected, and indeed, STAT1-deficient mice have higher incidence of tumor formation in response to chemical carcinogens and also on a background of P53 deletion. However, given the involvement of STAT1 in other cellular pathways such as myc regulation and apoptosis, it cannot be concluded with certainty that this tumor-promoting phenotype is completely caused by a lack of immune surveillance.

Signal Transducer and Activator of Transcription 2

The main function of STAT2 is to mediate IFN-α/β signaling. STAT2 is constitutively associated with a non-STAT protein, IFN regulatory factor 9 (IRF-9). Tyrosine phosphorylated STAT1–STAT2–IRF-9 multimeric complex is called the IFN-stimulated gene factor 3 (ISGF3). This complex binds to a specific DNA sequence in type I IFN-induced genes called the IFN-stimulated response element (ISRE). Because of the impaired IFN-α/β responsiveness, STAT2 knockout mice are susceptible to viral infections.[24] As is the case with STAT1-deficient mice, STAT2-deficient mice are viable and develop normally. The absence of STAT2 results in reduced tyrosine phosphorylation and activation of STAT1 because STAT2 facilitates recruitment and activation of STAT1 by the IFN-α/β receptor complex.

Signal Transducer and Activator of Transcription 3

STAT3 mediates signaling from multiple cytokines. It was originally cloned as an acute-phase response factor activated by IL-6. Murine embryos deficient in STAT3 die at postcoital day 7.5. One potential explanation for this early embryonic death is failure of extraembryonic trophoblast caused by impaired leukemia inhibitory factor signaling. Cell line–specific conditional STAT3 deletions have been reported for multiple lineages with no major developmental abnormalities.[25] STAT3-deficient T cells and hepatocytes have poor responses to IL-6. Deletion of STAT3 in macrophages results in constitutively activated cells and increased sensitivity to lipopolysaccharide. This is attributed to the role for STAT3 in the antiinflammatory responses induced by IL-10. CD4+ T cells can differentiate into the Th17 cells whose development and function are critically dependent on STAT3. These cells produce the inflammatory cytokine IL-17 and are responsible for recruitment and activation of neutrophils and other inflammatory cells. Th17 cells can be generated from naive CD4+ T cells by IL-6 and TGF-β but can also produce another cytokine IL-21, which promotes IL-17 production in an autocrine–paracrine manner. Another cytokine, IL-23, also acts to expand and maintain Th17 cells. The importance of IL-23 signaling in inflammation is exemplified by recent discoveries that polymorphisms in *IL23R* are associated with an increased risk of developing inflammatory bowel disease, ankylosing spondylitis, and psoriasis. IL-6, IL-21, and IL-23 all activate STAT3 by binding to their cognate receptors. The importance of STAT3 in Th17 cell development and function is appreciated in patients with Job syndrome, an autosomal dominant disorder caused by STAT3 mutations, which is associated with a failure to make Th17 cells.

STAT3 deficiency in multiple types of T cells results in decreased IL-21 production, which is required for hematopoietic progenitor proliferation. STAT3 promotes optimal Th2 cell differentiation and cytokine production in the presence of activated STAT6.

Selective targeting of the STAT3b isoform has been reported, and these mice exhibit diminished recovery from endotoxic shock. STAT3 deletions in other cell lineages have been described. For example, STAT3 deletion in mammary glands result in a delay in involution after weaning because of a decrease in apoptosis. STAT3-deficient epidermal cells show defective wound healing and in vitro migration of epidermal cells.

STAT3 is activated in multiple tumor types. This activation enhances tumor cell survival mediated by multiple mechanisms, including enhanced levels of prosurvival genes (e.g., Bcl-2 and Bcl-X_L). STAT3 is also frequently activated in cells that are transformed by a variety of oncogenes (e.g., v-src and BCR-abl). The enforced expression of a constitutively active STAT3 homodimer is sufficient to transform immortalized fibroblasts. STAT3 inhibitors are in early clinical trials for advanced malignancies.

Signal Transducer and Activator of Transcription 4

STAT4 is predominantly activated in response to IL-12, which drives T-helper cell differentiation into the Th1 and Th17 pathways. The phenotype of STAT4 deficient mice is very similar to that of mice lacking IL-12. IL-12 promotes differentiation of naive CD4$^+$ T cells to Th1 cells, which produce IFN-γ and augment cell-mediated immune responses. Th1 cells are critical in host defense against intracellular pathogens and tumors and in the pathogenesis of autoimmune diseases. Thus, the phenotype of STAT4-deficient mice includes impaired Th1 differentiation, IFN-γ production, and cell-mediated immunity.[26] IL-12–, IL-12 receptor–, and STAT4-deficient mice have increased susceptibility to infection with intracellular organisms. STAT4-deficient mice are resistant to autoimmune diseases characterized by a Th1 response. A common single nucleotide polymorphism of the STAT4 gene has been shown to be associated with susceptibility to rheumatoid arthritis, systemic lupus erythematosus, and primary Sjögren syndrome.[27] In acute sepsis, whereas STAT4 deficiency is associated with improved survival, STAT4$^{-/-}$ mice had *increased* lethality in a noninfectious sepsis model. It appears that STAT4 may have either pro- or antiinflammatory effects, depending on the context.

STAT4 is also activated by IL-23. Additionally, in humans but not in mice, IFN-α/β induces STAT4 phosphorylation. This is notable because IFN-α/β can promote Th1 differentiation in humans and not in mice. This has been explained by the finding that the STAT4/STAT2 dimer is recruited to the human type I IFN receptor via the carboxy terminus of STAT2. STAT4 also mediates IFN-γ production by DCs and macrophages induced by IL-12, and this may explain the mechanisms by which DCs promote Th1 differentiation.

Signal Transducer and Activator of Transcription 6

STAT6 is primarily activated by IL-4 and IL-13. STAT6-deficient mice lack most of the physiologic functions associated with IL-4. In particular, the ability of IL-4 to induce the in vitro differentiation of Th2 cells is lost.[26] STAT6 is critically involved in several distinct aspects of allergic inflammatory disease, such as airway hyperresponsiveness, eosinophilic infiltration, and responses of mast cells. B cells of STAT6-deficient mice cannot undergo class switching to produce IgE against helminthes and allergens. As expected, STAT6$^{-/-}$ mice have impaired expulsion of helminthic parasites and reduced pathology in models of asthma. STAT6$^{-/-}$ mice have increased lethality, inflammation, and cytokine production in a noninfectious model of endotoxemia but reduced lethality and enhanced clearance of bacteria in an infectious model.

STAT6 induces expression of GATA3, which is considered a Th2 cell master regulator. Transgenic mice expressing IL-4 or constitutively active STAT6 are characterized by the development of spontaneous allergic inflammation. Certain chemokines such as CCL11, CCL17, CCL22, and CCL26 have been reported to be regulated in a STAT6-dependent manner and are involved in allergic disorders. Although a number of pathways, including the mitogen-activated protein kinase (MAPK) and the phosphoinositide-3-kinase (PI-3-K), are involved in the signal transduction of IL-4, IL-4-induced T-cell differentiation appears to occur almost exclusively via STAT6. IL-4 also antagonizes Th1 responses through STAT6. In fact, residual STAT4-independent Th1 differentiation becomes apparent in doubly deficient STAT4/STAT6 knockout mice. A study on murine mast cells demonstrated IL-15-inducible STAT6 phosphorylation, involving Tyk2, although IL-15 was less potent than IL-4.

Signal Transducer and Activator of Transcription 5

The genes encoding STAT5A and STAT5B are juxtaposed, and the transcriptional start sites are within 10 kb of each other. Although the *STAT5a* and *STAT5b* gene promoters might share certain regulatory elements, lineage-specific expression has been reported. The highly related STAT5 proteins (a and b) are activated in response to a variety of cytokines and Tyk receptors. Mice lacking STAT5a, STATb, and STAT5a/b display distinct phenotypes, suggesting discrete functions for these proteins. STAT5a deficiency results in the loss of prolactin-dependent mammary gland development, which is necessary for lactation. STAT5b-deficient mice are sexually dimorphic with growth retardation. In contrast, a good portion of STAT5a/b double knockout mice die within a few weeks of birth, and these mice are infertile with defective corpus luteum development, and have defective mammary gland development. Both male and female STAT5a/b-deficient mice are small with small fat pads and reduced levels of insulinlike growth factor-1 (IGF-1). STAT5a/b double knockout mice have hypocellular bone marrows, lymphopenia, neutrophilia, and modest anemia and thrombocytopenia.[28] Moreover, the hematopoietic progenitors of STAT5a/b-deficient have defective bone marrow repopulating capacity. Myeloid development is grossly normal in STAT5a/b knockout mice, but in vitro cytokine-dependent proliferation, survival, and migration of myeloid cells are impaired. With respect to T- and B-cell development, complete deletion of the STAT5a/b locus results in severely impaired lymphoid development and differentiation with abrogated T-cell receptor γ rearrangement and survival of peripheral CD8$^+$ T. In other words, complete STAT5 deficiency results in SCID, similar in lymphoid phenotype to deficiencies of IL-7R, γc, and JAK3. Whereas deficiency of both STAT5a and STAT5b results in loss of CD4$^+$ regulatory T (Treg) cells, which express the transcription factor Foxp3, constitutive activation of STAT5b enforces Foxp3-positive Treg-cell development, bypassing the requirements for upstream cytokine or costimulatory signals to activate foxp3 transcription. STAT5 deficiency abrogates transformation by Tel-JAK but not by v-Abl or BCR-abl. Mutations in the *STAT5B* gene in a few patients with severe growth retardation have been described. Loss of functional STAT5B is associated with severe IGF-1 deficiency, indicating that this pathway is responsible for most of the GH-induced IGF-1 production.

NEGATIVE REGULATORS OF CYTOKINE SIGNALING

Src-Homology 2 Containing Phosphatase 1

SHP1 is a cytoplasmic phosphotyrosine phosphatase whose expression is limited to the hematopoietic system. SHP1 was identified as the protein encoded by the mutated locus *(Hcph)* in *moth-eaten (me)* mice.[29] These mice display severe immunologic dysfunction, particularly enhanced proliferation of macrophages and neutrophils in the lungs, which leads to pneumonitis, and in the skin, which causes patchy dermatitis that results in the "moth-eaten" phenotype. SHP1 associates with cytokine receptors and dephosphorylates JAK kinases. For example, it downregulates EPO-induced signaling by binding to the EPOR and dephosphorylating JAK2 associated with the EPOR. SHP1 also dephosphorylates JAK1 because IFN-α–induced phosphorylation of JAK1 is enhanced in SHP1 deficient macrophages. SHP1 also interacts with JAK3. This interaction may explain the activation of JAK3/STAT3 pathway in some cases of ALK (+) anaplastic large cell lymphoma in which SHP1 appears to be suppressed by promoter methylation. The expression of an inactive SHP1 in the cytokine-dependent cell line Ba/F3 increased the proliferative response to IL-3, STAT5 phosphorylation, and cell survival after IL-3 withdrawal.

Consistent with a negative role of SHP1 in the JAK–STAT pathway, silencing of SHP1 by promoter methylation is often associated with various kinds of leukemias, lymphomas, and myeloma, and the effect caused by SHP1 silencing is at least partially attributed to increased activities in the JAK–STAT pathway. On the other hand, in a limited number of cases, SHP1 was described to have a positive role in promoting JAK/STAT signaling. For example, the epidermal growth factor, and IFN-γ–induced STAT activation was suppressed by expressing a catalytically inactive form of SHP1 in HeLa cells, but this pathway was essentially unaffected by the expression of WT SHP1. There is no molecular explanation described for this observation.

Src-Homology 2 Containing Phosphatase 2

SHP2 is a protein–tyrosine phosphatase that is widely expressed, with high level expression in hematopoietic cells. It contains 2 tandem Src homology 2 (SH2) domains (N-SH2 and C-SH2), a protein tyrosine phosphatase (PTP) domain, and a C-terminal tail. SHP2 has low basal enzymatic activity because of autoinhibition of the PTP domain by the N-SH2 domain. SHP2 directly or indirectly (via adaptor proteins) associates with activated receptor protein Tyks or cytokine receptors via its two SH2 domains. Binding of SH2 domains to phosphotyrosine sites of these receptors alters the conformation of the N-SH2 domain, releasing its binding to PTP domain and causing catalytic activation. Despite being a phosphatase, SHP2 promotes activation of the Ras and ERK pathway by cytokines. Its catalytic activity is required for cytokine activation of the phosphatidylinositol 3–kinase pathway. SHP2 plays an essential role in hematopoietic cell development. Embryonic lethality is observed at day 8.5 in mice with a truncated version of SHP2 because of severe defects in gastrulation and mesodermal patterning.[30] Complete loss of SHP2 causes embryonic death in the peri-implantation period, and SHP2 is required for trophoblast stem cell survival. Hematopoietic stem cells (HSCs) from SHP2 haploinsufficient mice display a competitive repopulating defect. Embryonic stem (ES) cells lacking SHP2 exhibit severely decreased differentiation to erythroid and myeloid progenitors in vitro and fail to contribute to erythroid and myeloid lineages in chimeric mice derived from SHP2$^{-/-}$ ES cells and wild-type embryos. SHP2 loss of function causes an early block of lymphocyte development before pro-T and pro-B stages. The exact mechanisms through which SHP2 regulates cytokine signaling and hematopoiesis are uncertain. SHP2 both enhances and inhibits signaling in the JAK–STAT pathway depending on the context. It was shown, for example, to dephosphorylate STAT1 and STAT5. At the same time, SHP1 is required for optimal JAK2 activation.

Activating germline mutations of *PTPN11* (the gene encoding for SHP2 protein) are seen in persons with Noonan syndrome, and loss-of-function mutations are seen in LEOPARD (lentigines, electrocardiographic conduction abnormalities, ocular hypertelorism, pulmonary stenosis, abnormal genitalia, retarded growth, and deafness: sensorineural) syndrome. Both are congenital disorders associated with abnormal hematopoiesis. Somatic activating mutations are seen in approximately 35% of juvenile patients with myelomonocytic leukemia. PTPN11 mutations are also seen in patients with myelodysplastic syndrome, acute lymphoblastic leukemia, and acute myelogenous leukemia. These gain-of-function mutations induce hyperactivation of the Ras pathway, which results in growth factor– and cytokine-independent proliferation and survival of hematopoietic progenitor cells (HPCs). Increased SHP2 expression has also been observed in acute leukemia specimens, suggesting a potential role in leukemogenesis.

CD45, PTP1B, TC-PTP, PTPRT, and PTP-BL

CD45 is a receptor-like tyrosine phosphatase highly expressed by hematopoietic cells. CD45 was identified as a JAK family phosphatase.[31] CD45 is able to dephosphorylate all JAKs in murine cells and dephosphorylate JAK1 and JAK3 in human cells.[32] Targeted disruption of the CD45 gene leads to enhanced cytokine and IFN receptor–mediated activation of JAK and STAT proteins. The removal of CD45 also increased erythroid colony formation and antiviral activity, which is consistent with the fact that CD45 negatively regulates EPO and IFN signaling. The Src family kinase members Lck and Lyn are key substrates for CD45 in T and B lymphocytes, respectively. CD45 lowers the threshold of antigen receptor signaling, which impacts T- and B-cell activation and development.

Protein tyrosine phosphatase 1B (PTP1B) and T-cell PTP (TC-PTP) are closely related PTPs, sharing 74% homology in their catalytic domain.[33] Although PTP1B is expressed in many tissues, TC-PTP (gene name, *PTPN2*) is ubiquitously expressed with particularly high expression in hematopoietic tissues. PTP1B is involved in multiple signaling pathways by downregulating several Tyks. For example, PTP1B-deficient mice display attenuated insulin signaling. Increased phosphorylation of JAK2, Tyk2, STAT3, and STAT5 has been observed in PTP1B-deficient embryonic fibroblasts. TC-PTP targets multiple STAT and JAK proteins in addition to growth factor receptors for dephosphorylation. TC-PTP–deficient mice develop anemia, lymphadenopathy, and splenomegaly and die at an early age. These mice display excessive inflammation but demonstrate increased number of BM HSCs and HPCs. Other phosphatases, such as PTP-receptor type T (PTPRT) and PTP-basophil like (PTP-BL), have also been implicated in cytokine signaling but will not be discussed here further.

Protein Inhibitor of Activated STAT

Protein inhibitor of activated STAT3 (PIAS3) was the first family member to be identified as a repressor of STAT3 activity. Three additional family members PIAS1, PIASy (or PIAS4), and PIASx (or PIAS2) were later identified with high-sequence homology. Other proteins with weak homology (hZIMP7 and hZIMP10) have been reported. PIAS1 was identified as a STAT1-interacting protein and subsequently found to inhibit STAT1-mediated transcriptional activation. The PIAS family members PIASx and PIASy were identified based on sequence similarity to PIAS1 and have been shown to inhibit STAT1 and STAT4, respectively. PIAS proteins have been shown to impact on the function of many different proteins, with particular involvement in gene transcription.

PIAS proteins contain a domain known as Siz/PIAS-RING (SP-RING) with structural similarity to ubiquitin E3 ligase RING fingers (Fig. 14-8). It was shown that PIAS binds the protein modifier small ubiquitin-like modifier (SUMO)[34] and recruits the E2 SUMO ligase UBC9, which transfers SUMO to target proteins, particularly to transcription factors such as STATs. PIAS1, PIAS3, and PIASx all sumoylate STAT1 at Lys-703 close to the site at which it is phosphorylated by JAKs (Tyr-701), and mutation of Lys-703 results in an increased response to IFN-γ (IFN-γ).

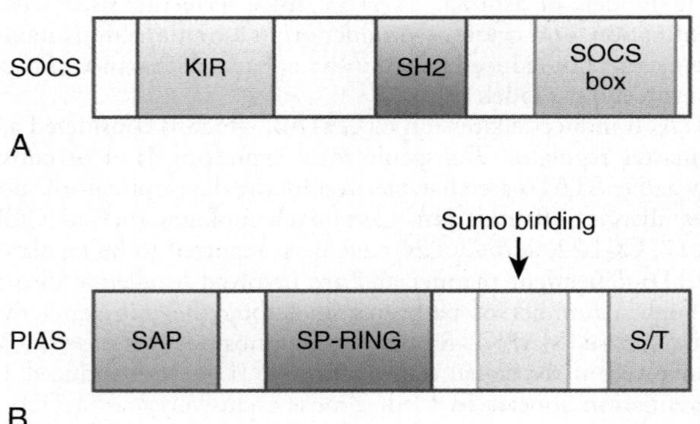

Figure 14-8 THE GENERAL STRUCTURE OF A SUPPRESSOR OF CYTOKINE SIGNALING (SOCS) AND A PROTEIN INHIBITORS OF ACTIVATED STAT (PIAS) PROTEIN. **A,** SOCS protein has a central Src homology (SH2) domain; an amino-terminal domain of variable length; and divergent sequence, which contains a kinase inhibitory region (KIR) and a carboxy-terminal 40-amino-acid SOCS box. **B,** PIAS protein contains a SAP (SAFA/B, ACINUS, PIAS) domain that is present in other chromatin-associated proteins. PIAS proteins which are Small Ubiquitin-like MOdifier (SUMO) E3 ligases contain a conserved SP-RING domain that shares sequence similarity to RING domains of ubiquitin E3 ligases. This domain recruits the SUMO E2 ligase (UBC9).

Thus, the binding of PIAS to STAT results in the inhibition of STAT-mediated gene activation. PIAS1 and PIAS3 inhibit STAT DNA binding activity, and PIASy and PIASx repress STAT1 and STAT4-mediated gene activation without affecting DNA binding. PIAS proteins also act by recruiting other corepressor molecules. One example is the inhibition of natural regulatory T-cell differentiation by PIAS1 through chromatin–based epigenetic repression.[35] Sumoylation may impact nuclear localization of proteins because it is the case for the transcriptional factor LEF1, where LEF1 sumoylation by PIASy results in its sequestration into nuclear bodies hindering its transcriptional activity. Given its impact on STAT1 and by that on IFN signaling, PIAS1 has a tangible role in innate immunity. The antiviral activity of IFNs is significantly increased in PIAS1-/- cells.[36] In addition, PIAS1-/- mice show increased protection against bacterial and viral infection.

Suppressor of Cytokine Signaling

The suppressor of cytokine signaling (SOCS) family consists of eight proteins that antagonize the signaling of STAT proteins. STATs activate the transcription of genes encoding the SOCS family as a negative feedback regulation.[37] For example, expression of SOCS3 is activated by several transcription factors, including STAT1, STAT3, and MAPK p38, but expression of SOCS1 is dependent on the production of IRF-1, a STAT1-inducible transcription factor. Each SOCS has two major domains, an SH2 domain and a Socs box, which mediates a complex formation with elongins B and C, a cullin, and Rbx2, to form E3 ubiquitin ligase (see Fig. 14-8). SOCS proteins function in a negative feedback loop to inhibit cytokine signaling by binding to either phospho-JAK or phospho-receptor through SH2 domain, and this inhibits JAK activity directly or by targeting the receptor complex for ubiquitylation and subsequent proteasome-mediated degradation. Gene-targeting studies have delineated the distinct in vivo functions of SOCS proteins. For example, SOCS1 -/- mice die as neonates from an inflammatory disease caused by dysregulated IFN signaling and which presents as lymphopenia, infiltration of macrophages and T cells into the liver and other organs, and fatty degeneration of the liver.[22] A SOCS3 deletion results in embryonic lethality at 12 to 16 days associated with marked erythrocytosis.[38] In addition, the in vitro proliferative capacity of high-proliferative potential progenitor cells is greatly increased.

FUTURE DIRECTIONS

A short review of cytokine signaling from a historical perspective has been published.[39] The past 4 decades have witnessed significant progress in our understanding of cytokines and their diverse functions, starting with cloning cytokines, identifying their receptors, cloning the receptors, and elucidating the complex signaling pathways triggered by ligand–receptor engagement. This has reflected positively on human health, particularly in the field of hematology and immunology, where the pathogenesis of multiple disorders has been uncovered and connected to defective cytokine signaling. We are witnessing, as a result, a plethora of targeted therapies that aim at abnormal cytokine signaling as a strategy to reverse morbid phenotypes.

REFERENCES

1. Boulay J, O'Shea J, Paul W: Molecular phylogeny within type I cytokines and their cognate receptors. *Immunity* 19:159, 2003.
2. Bazan J: Structural design and molecular evolution of a cytokine receptor superfamily. *Proc Natl Acad Sci U S A* 87:6934, 1990.
3. Rozwarski D, Gronenborn A, Clore GM, et al: Structural comparisons among the short-chain helical cytokines. *Structure* 2:159, 1994.
4. Boulay JL, Paul WE: The interleukin-4 family of lymphokines. *Curr Opin Immunol* 4:294, 1992.
5. McKinstry WJ, Li CL, Rasko JE, et al: Cytokine receptor expression on hematopoietic stem and progenitor cells. *Blood* 89:65, 1997.
6. Boulanger MJ, Chow DC, Brevnova EE, et al: Hexameric structure and assembly of the interleukin-6/IL-6 alpha-receptor/gp130 complex. *Science* 300:2101, 2003.
7. Lupardus PJ, Skiniotis G, Rice AJ, et al: Structural snapshots of full-length Jak1, a ransmembrane gp130/IL-6/IL-6Rα cytokine receptor complex, and the receptor-Jak1 holocomplex. *Structure* 19:45, 2011.
8. Thomas C, Moraga I, Levin D, et al: Structural linkage between ligand discrimination and receptor activation by type I interferons. *Cell* 146:621, 2011.
9. Janes KA, Reinhardt HC, Yaffe MB: Cytokine-induced signaling networks prioritize dynamic range over signal strength. *Cell* 135:343, 2008.
10. Ghoreschi K, Laurence A, O'Shea JJ: Janus kinases in immune cell signaling. *Immunol Rev* 228:273, 2009 Mar.
11. Rodig SJ, Meraz MA, White JM, et al: Disruption of the Jak1 gene demonstrates obligatory and nonredundant roles of the Jaks in cytokine-induced biologic responses. *Cell* 93:373, 1998.
12. Neubauer H, Cumano A, Müller M, et al: Jak2 deficiency defines an essential developmental checkpoint in definitive hematopoiesis. *Cell* 93:397, 1998.
13. Witthuhn BA, Quelle FW, Silvennoinen O, et al: JAK2 associates with the erythropoietin receptor and is tyrosine phosphorylated and activated following stimulation with erythropoietin. *Cell* 74:227, 1993.
14. Parganas E, Wang D, Stravopodis D, et al: Jak2 is essential for signaling through a variety of cytokine receptors. *Cell* 93:385, 1998.
15. Roberts JL, Lengi A, Brown SM, et al: Janus kinase 3 (JAK3) deficiency: Clinical, immunologic, and molecular analyses of 10 patients and outcomes of stem cell transplantation. *Blood* 103:2009, 2004.
16. Park SY, Saijo K, Takahashi T, et al: Developmental defects of lymphoid cells in Jak3 kinase-deficient mice. *Immunity* 3:771, 1995.
17. Bacon CM, McVicar DW, Ortaldo JR, et al: Interleukin 12 (IL-12) induces tyrosine phosphorylation of JAK2 and TYK2: Differential use of Janus family tyrosine kinases by IL-2 and IL-12. *J Exp Med* 181:399, 1995 Jan 1.
18. Karaghiosoff M, Neubauer H, Lassnig C, et al: Partial impairment of cytokine responses in Tyk2-deficient mice. *Immunity* 13:549, 2000.
19. Seto Y, Nakajima H, Suto A, et al: Enhanced Th2 cell-mediated allergic inflammation in Tyk2-deficient mice. *J Immunol* 170:1077, 2003.
20. Cytokine signaling in 2002: New surprises in the Jak/Stat pathway. *Cell* 109:S121, 2002.
21. Meraz MA, White JM, Sheehan KC, et al: Targeted disruption of the Stat1 gene in mice reveals unexpected physiologic specificity in the JAK-STAT signaling pathway. *Cell* 84:431, 1996.
22. Marine JC, Topham DJ, McKay C, et al: SOCS1 deficiency causes a lymphocyte-dependent perinatal lethality. *Cell* 98:609, 1999.
23. van de Veerdonk FL, Plantinga TS, Hoischen A, et al: STAT1 mutations in autosomal dominant chronic mucocutaneous candidiasis. *N Engl J Med* 365:54, 2011.
24. Park C, Li S, Cha E, Schindler C: Immune response in Stat2 knockout mice. *Immunity* 13:795, 2000.
25. Akira S: Roles of STAT3 defined by tissue-specific gene targeting. *Oncogene* 19:2607, 2000 May 15.
26. Wurster AL, Tanaka T, Grusby MJ: The biology of Stat4 and Stat6. *Oncogene* 19:2577, 2000.
27. Remmers EF, Plenge RM, Lee AT, et al: STAT4 and the risk of rheumatoid arthritis and systemic lupus erythematosus. *N Engl J Med* 357:977, 2007.
28. Teglund S, McKay C, Schuetz E, et al: Stat5a and Stat5b proteins have essential and nonessential, or redundant, roles in cytokine responses. *Cell* 93:841, 1998.
29. Shultz LD, Schweitzer PA, Rajan TV, et al: Mutations at the murine motheaten locus are within the hematopoietic cell protein-tyrosine phosphatase (Hcph) gene. *Cell* 73:1445, 1993.
30. Saxton TM, Henkemeyer M, Gasca S, et al: Abnormal mesoderm patterning in mouse embryos mutant for the SH2 tyrosine phosphatase Shp-2. *EMBO J* 16:2352, 1997.
31. Irie-Sasaki J, Sasaki T, Matsumoto W, et al: CD45 is a JAK phosphatase and negatively regulates cytokine receptor signaling. *Nature* 409:349, 2001.

32. Xu D, Qu CK: Protein tyrosine phosphatases in the JAK/STAT pathway. *Front Biosci* 13:4925, 2008.
33. Bourdeau A, Dubé N, Tremblay ML: Cytoplasmic protein tyrosine phosphatases, regulation and function: The roles of PTP1B and TC-PTP. *Curr Opin Cell Biol* 17:203, 2005.
34. Johnson ES, Gupta AA: An E3-like factor that promotes SUMO conjugation to the yeast septins. *Cell* 106:735, 2001.
35. Liu B, Tahk S, Yee KM, Fan G, Shuai K: The ligase PIAS1 restricts natural regulatory T cell differentiation by epigenetic repression. *Science* 330:521, 2010.
36. Liu B, Mink S, Wong KA, et al: PIAS1 selectively inhibits interferon-inducible genes and is important in innate immunity. *Nat Immunol* 5:891, 2004.
37. Wormald S, Hilton DJ: The negative regulatory roles of suppressor of cytokine signaling proteins in myeloid signaling pathways. *Curr Opin Hematol* 14:9, 2007.
38. Marine JC, McKay C, Wang D, et al: SOCS3 is essential in the regulation of fetal liver erythropoiesis. *Cell* 98:617, 1999.
39. O'Shea JJ, Gadina M, Kanno Y: Cytokine signaling: Birth of a pathway. *J Immunol* 187:5475, 2011.

CHAPTER 15

CONTROL OF CELL DIVISION

William M.F. Lee and Chi V. Dang

Somatic cells undergo one of several general fates: They proliferate by mitotic cell division, differentiate and acquire specialized functions, and senesce or die and are eliminated. Cell proliferation is necessary for growth of the organism and ensures repletion of cells lost to terminal differentiation, cell death, or cell shedding. In the case of lymphocytes, it serves the additional function of amplifying immune responses to specific antigens. Differentiation provides the organism with a supply of cells to execute specific and specialized functions. In some cell types, such as muscle and nerve cells, differentiation and proliferation are mutually exclusive fates, and cells undergo "terminal differentiation." In other cell types, such as those of the hematopoietic lineage, proliferation may continue after cells acquire differentiated characteristics. For example, erythroblasts, myeloblasts, and megakaryoblasts are committed to particular differentiation pathways and possess lineage-specific markers yet continue to proliferate. T and B lymphocytes are fully differentiated and express antigen-specific receptors but can be induced to proliferate when appropriately stimulated. Cell death is an active process when it is initiated by the cell itself in the process known as apoptosis and can be as important as cell proliferation and differentiation for maintaining the integrity of the organism. It allows tissue renewal and changes in cellular composition without undesirable cell accumulation.

When the regulation of any of these three cellular processes—proliferation, death, and differentiation—goes awry and their balance becomes abnormal, the consequences to the organism are usually dire and result in either functional insufficiency or neoplasia. The relevance of these events to normal tissue function and neoplasia has led to investigations of their mechanisms and regulation at a molecular level. This chapter focuses on cell proliferation and its regulation. Cell death is discussed in Chapter 16, and differentiation of specific hematopoietic cell types is discussed in chapters focused on these cell types.

SIGNAL TRANSDUCTION AND CELL PROLIFERATION

Cells normally proliferate and differentiate and sometimes senesce or die in response to signals from their environment. Of these, cell proliferation or mitogenic signals and signaling mechanisms are the best studied and provide a paradigm for how cells respond to environmental signals in general. Cell proliferation normally is stimulated by extracellular growth factors interacting with specific receptors located at the cell surface providing that there are sufficient nutrients to support the proliferative cellular bioenergetic needs. Signal transduction is the process by which information about growth factors at the cell surface is transmitted to the nucleus, where ultimate control of most cellular events resides. Signal transduction pathways leading to cell differentiation operate on similar principles and use similar mechanisms but produce different outcomes. A brief overview of some of the biochemical events involved in mitogenic signal transduction is provided as introduction and context for the following discussion of cell cycle regulation. A detailed discussion of signal transduction is found in Chapter 6.

Much of what is known about signal transduction is based on studies of the cellular biochemical response to mitogens such as platelet-derived growth factor (PDGF) and epidermal growth factor (EGF).[1,2] When these ligands bind to their cognate cell-surface receptors (PDGF-R and EGF-R, respectively), the receptors dimerize, activate their intrinsic tyrosine kinase activity, and catalyze the transfer of phosphate groups from adenosine triphosphate (ATP) to tyrosine residues of specific cellular proteins, including the receptors themselves (Fig. 15-1).[3] Some other types of receptors, such as the T-cell antigen receptor and CD4 and CD8 coreceptors, are not tyrosine kinases, and the tyrosine phosphorylation that they induce on ligand binding is mediated by associated nonreceptor tyrosine kinases-ZAP-70 in the case of T-cell antigen receptors and Lck in the case of CD4 and CD8.[4]

The presence of phosphotyrosines in target proteins enables them to form noncovalent complexes with proteins containing SH2 domains (Src homology region 2; defined by homology to a region in the Src retroviral oncoprotein), which are peptide domains that bind phosphotyrosine-containing peptides.[5] Thus, phosphorylation of the EGF-R and PDGF-R enables them to interact with SH2-containing proteins near or at the plasma membrane, which initiates downstream signaling events. Certain enzymes with SH2 domains, such as the γ1 isoform of phospholipase C (PLCγ1), directly associate with phosphorylated EGF-R and PDGF-R and become tyrosine phosphorylated by them, which, in the case of PLCγ1, results in enhancement of enzymatic activity. Activation of PLCγ1 catalyzes the hydrolysis of phosphatidylinositol (PIP3) into diacylglycerol (DAG) and inositol 1,4,5-triphosphate (IP3), both of which act as "second messengers" that launch additional actions inside cells: DAG activates protein kinase C (PKC), a kinase that phosphorylates serine–threonine residues in substrate proteins, and IP3 induces Ca^{2+} release from intracellular stores, which in turn activates Ca^{2+}/calmodulin-dependent serine–threonine protein kinases and other Ca^{2+}-dependent events.[6]

Another signaling pathway activated when mitogen receptors bind ligand and become phosphorylated stems from activation of Ras proteins. These are low-molecular-weight guanosine triphosphate (GTP)-binding proteins that are active in their GTP-bound state but inactive in their guanosine diphosphate (GDP)-bound state. The intrinsic GTPase activity of Ras, enhanced by the presence of GTPase-activating proteins (GAPs), hydrolyzes bound GTP to GDP and maintains Ras in its inactive state.[7,8] After EGF binding by EGF-R, two cytoplasmic proteins, Grb2 and SOS, that exist as heterodimers in unstimulated cells physically link EGF-R with Ras in a quaternary complex through binding of phosphorylated EGF-R with the SH2 domain of Grb2 and the binding of SOS to Ras. Formation of this complex activates the function of SOS as a guanine nucleotide exchange factor (GEF), resulting in the conversion of Ras-GDP to Ras-GTP and Ras activation. Activation of Ras initiates a cascade of serine–threonine kinase activation involving a trio of kinases.[9] Beginning with the association of GTP-Ras with Raf-1 (a mitogen-activated protein kinase [MAPK]), which activates the latter's serine–threonine kinase function, Raf-1 phosphorylates and activates MEK (MAPK kinase). MEK is a kinase that phosphorylates and activates MAPK, which is also known as ERK (extracellular signal-regulated kinase). Modules composed of three sequentially activated serine–threonine kinases are a recurring motif in signaling from the plasma membrane, where Ras and Ras-like molecules reside, to the nucleus, which phosphorylated MAPK or ERK can enter.

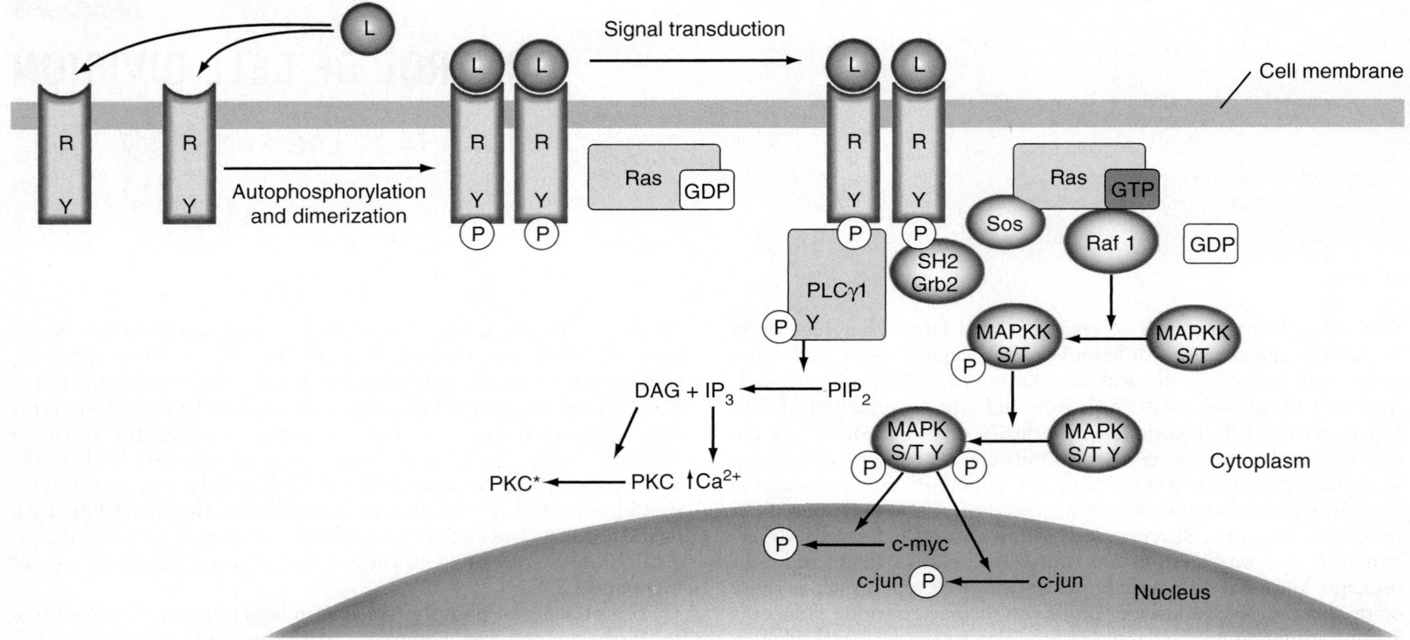

Figure 15-1 MITOGENIC SIGNAL TRANSDUCTION. Shown are signal transduction pathways activated by the binding of mitogenic ligands (L), to their cognate receptors (R) at the cell surface. Binding results in dimerization and autophosphorylation (P) of the receptors on tyrosine residues (Y). This enables them to associate with and activate specific SH2 domain-containing downstream components of the signaling pathway. In the case of phospholipase Cγ1 (PLCγ1), association leads to tyrosine phosphorylation by the receptor kinase and an enhanced ability to hydrolyze phosphoinositol bisphosphate (PIP_2) to diacylglycerol (DAG) and inositol trisphosphate (IP_3); in turn, DAG activates protein kinase C (PKC) and IP_3 mobilizes Ca^{2+} from intracellular stores. In the case of Grb2-SOS, association with phosphorylated receptors stimulates its ability to facilitate Ras GTP-GDP exchange; GTP-Ras activates the MAP kinase (MAPK) cascade, which eventually induces serine (S)–threonine (T) phosphorylation of nuclear proteins that modulate gene transcription. Note that MAPK is activated by serine–threonine and tyrosine phosphorylation and that both result from the activity of a single dual-function kinase, MAPK kinase. *EGF,* Epidermal growth factor; *MAP,* mitogen-activated protein; *PDGF,* platelet-derived growth factor.

Serine–threonine kinases activated after mitogen exposure phosphorylate diverse cellular proteins and modulate their activities.[10] Prominent among these targets are transcription factors.[11] Phosphorylation may directly alter the ability of these factors to bind DNA or activate transcription. Alternatively, phosphorylation may indirectly activate transcription factors by inactivating an antagonist of these factors. Mitogen stimulation may result in activation of protein phosphatases that dephosphorylate specific phosphorylated residues in certain transcription factors to alter function.[12] The end result of these rapid posttranslational protein modifications is the first wave of change in cell transcription, which can occur independent of new protein synthesis. "Immediate early" is the description collectively applied to genes whose messenger RNA (mRNA) is rapidly induced by growth factor stimulation in the absence of de novo protein synthesis. Included in their number are genes encoding transcription factors. These initial changes lead to changes in expression of other transcription factor genes (which do require de novo protein synthesis) and culminate in the transcriptional reprogramming of the cell that eventually enables them to undergo DNA synthesis and cell cycling. It should not be surprising that many of the components of the mitogenic signaling pathway are oncogenic when they are inappropriately activated.[1]

Ligands other than EGF and PDGF may use different schemes for signal transduction. Neuroactive and vasoactive peptides (e.g., epinephrine and thrombin) activate responsive cells through specific receptors that have seven membrane-spanning domains. These receptors are typically coupled to heterotrimeric G proteins that resemble Ras in being regulated by GTP and GDP.[7,13] These receptor-coupled G proteins are linked to effector enzymes (e.g., adenylyl cyclases) that generate molecular signaling intermediates (e.g., cyclic adenine monophosphate [cAMP]) on ligand binding. Steroid and thyroid hormones and retinoids can enter cells by virtue of their lipophilic nature. Their receptors are intracellularly located and able to bind sequence-specific DNA and directly modulate the transcription of responsive genes. Thus, the receptors are transcription factors whose activities are influenced by binding of the cognate hormone.[14]

Interferon signaling uses a different signal transduction paradigm. Tyrosine kinases of the Janus kinase (Jak) family associate with interferon receptor subunits. On ligand binding, association of the receptor subunits allows these Jaks to phosphorylate and activate each other and to phosphorylate the associated receptors. Specific members of the STAT (signal transducers and activators of transcription) family of latent cytoplasmic transcription factors, which have SH2 domains, dock to the receptor phosphotyrosines and become phosphorylated by Jak. Tyrosine phosphorylation allows STATs to dimerize and translocate to the nucleus, where they bind sequence-specific DNA and modulate transcription of interferon-responsive genes.[15] Signal transduction using Jak-STAT protein is used by many peptide ligands and cytokines of hematologic interest (e.g., erythropoietin; interleukins IL-2, IL-3, IL-4, IL-6, and IL-12).

The signal transduction schemes outlined permit a single event, ligand-receptor interaction, to have several downstream consequences. Its multiplex, frequently cascading nature allows signal amplification and diversification but also permits their modulation and fine regulation. Signaling pathways can intersect and interact at different levels, allowing one ligand to modify the signals generated by another ligand. For example, STATs can be phosphorylated by receptor tyrosine kinases, such as PDGF-R and EGF-R, as well as by Jak, and can undergo serine–threonine phosphorylation, which modulates their transcriptional activity.[15] This allows PDGF and EGF to initiate some events usually initiated by cytokines and interferons, and the phenotypic changes brought about by cytokines and interferons may be altered in the presence of PDGF and EGF.

Transcription factors are final participants in afferent signal transduction pathways and initiators of cellular responses to these signals.[11] In general, they are sequence-specific DNA-binding proteins that modulate the expression of genes to which they bind. When these factors bind their cognate DNA sequence, they interact with the basal transcription machinery either directly or via intermediary proteins ("coactivators" and "corepressors") to initiate, enhance, or inhibit transcription. Transcription factors have peptide domains with characteristic secondary structures that are responsible for their ability to bind DNA. Many bind DNA only as dimers, making the peptide domain responsible for dimerization essential for DNA binding.

Transcription factors use one of a number of peptide motifs to dimerize and bind DNA, among them the zinc finger, the basic region-leucine zipper (bZip), the basic region–helix–loop–helix (bHLH), and the helix–turn–helix motifs.[16] Factors that activate gene transcription generally do so because they have a distinct transcriptional activation domain that is frequently acidic in nature, glutamine rich or proline rich. Transcriptional gene regulation is highly complex, not only because of the multitude of transcription factors present in cells but also because of the ability of many factors to heterodimerize and form combinatorial pairs that have DNA-binding, transactivation, or regulatory properties that differ from those of the parental homodimers. A striking example is provided by heterodimers containing the Id protein, which is an HLH protein that can dimerize with selected bHLH proteins, such as the myogenic transcription factor MyoD, but that does not possess a DNA-binding basic region. Id-containing heterodimers are incapable of binding DNA, making Id a negative transcriptional regulator that inhibits the function of positive factors.

Negative gene regulation also occurs by active repression of transcription, and certain transcriptional repressors have been shown to recruit factors that bind histone deacetylases. Histones are a family of nuclear proteins that interact with DNA and organize it into higher order structures consisting of DNA wrapped around a histone core (nucleosomes). Acetylation of histones masks their basic residues, destabilizes their interaction with DNA, "loosens" nucleosome DNA, and facilitates transcription. Deacetylation of histones, in contrast, stabilizes their interaction with DNA, which "tightens" nucleosome DNA and inhibits transcription. Reversible, regional histone acetylation, through recruitment of coactivators with acetyltransferase activity or recruitment of corepressors with deacetylase activity, is a general mechanism by which transcription factors facilitate or repress expression of specific genes.[17]

THE CELL DIVISION CYCLE

A cell stimulated to divide passes through a series of states, defined by biochemical and morphologic criteria, collectively termed the *cell cycle* (Fig. 15-2). Passage through the cell cycle provides an ordered sequence to the complex series of events necessary for the production of two identical progeny cells. The normal cell cycle is divided into discrete and sequential phases: S, G_2, M, and G_1.

S Phase

S phase is the period of wholesale DNA synthesis during which the cell replicates its genetic content; a normal diploid somatic cell with a 2N complement of DNA at the beginning of S phase acquires a 4N complement of DNA at its end. (Recall that N = 1 copy of each chromosome per cell [haploid]; 2N = 2 copies [diploid].) The duration of S phase may vary from only a few minutes in rapidly dividing, early embryo cells to a few hours in most somatic cells. Early embryo cells generally "live off" the accumulated stores of maternal RNA and proteins present in the egg and are transcriptionally silent, but cells in later development and mature organisms must actively transcribe subsets of their genes to survive and maintain specialized functions. The longer time required for the latter to complete S phase probably allows these cells to coordinate DNA replication with transcription and to preserve higher order gene and chromatin structural information that influences gene expression for transmission to progeny cells.

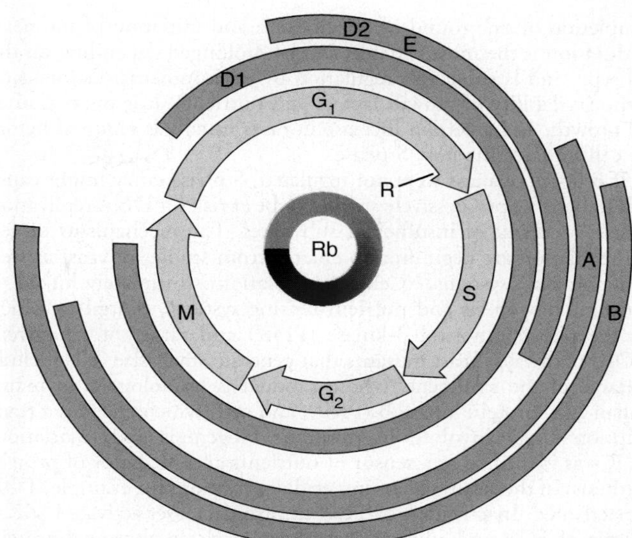

Figure 15-2 THE CELL CYCLE. The somatic cell cycle is divided into phases of DNA replication (S), mitosis (M), and the "gaps" in between (G_1 between M and S; G_2 between S and M). G_0 is not shown for the sake of simplicity but would be a side loop exiting and entering G_1. The point in late G_1 at which cells become committed to DNA replication is called the restriction point (R). The *inner circle* shows the pattern of Rb phosphorylation through the cell cycle, with the density of stippling indicating the degree of Rb phosphorylation. Places in the cell cycle where individual cyclins (A, B, D1, D2, E) appear are shown by the outer arcs.

M Phase

Mitosis, or M phase, is the period of actual nuclear and cell division during which the duplicated chromosomes are divided equally between two progeny cells. It is obvious microscopically as the period of chromosome condensation and segregation, nuclear division (karyokinesis), and physical separation of the two daughter cells (cytokinesis). A cell entering M phase has a 4N DNA content and finishes as two cells, each with an identical 2N complement of DNA. The complex sequence of changes that take place allows M to be subdivided into prophase, prometaphase, metaphase, anaphase, and telophase. Prophase is the period of chromatin and chromosome condensation, centrosome separation and migration to opposite poles, and nuclear membrane breakdown. The centrosomes are microtubule organization centers that eventually give rise to the bipole mitotic spindle apparatus that will separate the sister chromatids of each duplicated chromosome. During prometaphase, chromosomes attach to microtubules of the mitotic spindle, so that sister chromatids become attached to opposite poles. In metaphase, the condensed chromosomes align at the equatorial plate. The cohesive "bond" between sister chromatids of duplicated chromosomes is dissolved, allowing anaphase, the period of sister chromatid separation, to proceed. On reaching their poles, nuclear membranes form to envelop each of the two separated sets of chromosomes, which also begin to decondense, marking telophase and karyokinesis. This is soon followed by cytokinesis and exit from M.

G_1 and G_2 Phases

$G_1$and G_2 phases were originally conceived of as "gaps" between the distinctive M and S phases of the cell cycle. G_1, which occupies the period or gap between M and S, is the interval between the completion of one round of cell division and initiation of the next. Its duration is the most variable, can be prolonged depending on the cell type, and is subject to regulation by environmental factors such as the availability of growth factors and nutrients. It is the period of cell growth, and a certain increase in mass usually is required before the cell initiates the next S phase.

If cell size or mass were not regulated, S phase entry might cause cells to become progressively smaller or be at risk for DNA replication errors as a result of insufficient substrates. The mechanisms of cell size regulation are beginning to emerge from studies of yeast as well as mammalian systems.[18] Cell size regulation is intimately linked to ribosome biogenesis and nutrient-sensing systems, central to which are the phosphoinositol 3-kinase (PI3K) and target of rapamycin (TOR) pathways. Yeast mutants that generate small-size cells include mutants of the *sch9* gene, whose product is homologous to mammalian Akt–protein kinase B (PKB), and *sfp1,* which encodes a transcription factor involved in ribosome biogenesis and translation. TOR was identified as a sensor of nutrients and mediator of protein synthesis. In the setting of amino acid deprivation, for example, TOR is inactivated. Inactivation of TOR in turn decreases activated S6K1, a target of TOR and a kinase that phosphorylates ribosomal protein S6 in response to proliferative signals. A decrease in TOR function also activates 4EBP, which binds to and inhibits the translational initiator eIF4E. In an intriguing line of evidence, a class of *Drosophila* small-body-size mutants, termed *Minutes,* also has been shown to be defective in ribosomal protein genes as well as in signal transduction pathways. Specifically, whereas mutations in the *Drosophila* insulin receptor, PI3K, TOR, S6K and Akt–PKB result in the *Minute* phenotype, mutation of Pten (phosphatase and tensin homolog deleted on chromosome 10), which negatively regulates the PI3K and Akt–PKB pathways, produces large flies with large cells.

Remarkably, mutations in the *Drosophila Myc* gene also resulted in fewer, smaller cells and small body size, suggesting that protooncogenic *Myc* regulates size as well as cell proliferation. Because *Myc* pleiotropically affects gene expression, it has emerged as an integrator of cell size regulation and cell proliferation. In particular, mammalian c-Myc regulates both cyclins and CDK genes as well as ribosomal protein genes and genes involved in translation. Overexpression of c-Myc in lymphocytes results in both cell size increase and a detectable increase in cell proliferation. However, germline mutation of myc in the mouse results in small mice that have fewer but normal-sized cells. An interpretation of these observations is that mammalian cells may be less tolerant of cell size depletion than lower metazoans. In aggregate, studies from a variety of organisms indicate that cell size regulation is linked to cell proliferation except in specialized cells that undergo endoreplication (see Specialized Cell Cycle).

As a first approximation, the amount of time a cell spends in G_1 is inversely related to its rate of proliferation. When conditions are unsuitable for proliferation (e.g., because of insufficient nutrients or absence of mitogens), cells arrest in G_1, and those that are already in S, G_2, or M usually complete the round to which they have been committed and arrest only when they reach G_1again. On the other hand, when rapid cell proliferation is mandated, as in embryos shortly after fertilization, $G_1$is virtually undetectable, and there is no cell enlargement. As a result, the original mass of egg cytoplasm is partitioned among thousands of cells within a few hours without a noticeable increase in size. G_1has been subdivided into segments and regulatory points based largely on the study of the proliferative response of cells to sequential application of different growth factors, nutrients, and metabolic inhibitors. From the standpoint of cell cycle regulation, a particularly important point in $G_1$is the restriction point, or R, which occurs near the G_1–S boundary. This is the point at which cells become committed to entering S phase, regardless of subsequent availability of growth factors or essential nutrients, and is analogous to the commitment point in the yeast cell cycle called Start.

G_2 is the period or gap between S and M when cells have finished replicating their DNA, are preparing to divide, and have a 4N DNA content. For most cells entering S phase, passage through G_2 is "automatic," and the duration of G_2 is fixed except under unusual circumstances. For example, G_2 duration can be extremely short and is essentially undetectable in rapidly proliferating, early embryonic cells.

G_0 Phase

G_0 is a nonproliferative phase in which viable cells may remain for prolonged periods. Cells in G_0 have 2N DNA content and have exited the cell cycle. They may be difficult to distinguish morphologically from cells in a prolonged G_1 phase but in some cases can be distinguished biochemically because they differ in protein and RNA metabolism. Terminally differentiated cells, such as neutrophilic granulocytes, muscle cells, and neurons, have irreversibly exited the cell cycle during the process of differentiation and are examples of cells that have irreversibly entered G_0. Other cells reversibly enter G_0 and may be induced to return to G_1 and begin cycling with appropriate stimuli. For example, hepatocytes usually are in G_0 unless partial hepatectomy induces them to proliferate to reconstitute the functional mass of the liver. Resting, antigen-specific lymphocytes are in G_0 until antigen and cytokine stimulation induces them to proliferate.

The enforced sequence G_1–S–G_2–M during normal progression through the cell cycle means that a cell must duplicate its DNA before dividing and that it must divide before duplicating its DNA again. This sequence ensures euploidy, and its enforcement maintains genetic stability. The dependence of later events in the cell cycle on successful completion of earlier events is ensured by checkpoint control mechanisms that prevent a cell that has not successfully completed one phase of the cycle from entering the next.[19,20] Certain cell types, such as megakaryocytes, become polyploid as part of their normal development and differentiation. In these cases, the normal cell division cycle script obviously is not followed: M fails to follow S, and DNA replication is allowed to repeat despite this lack of follow-through.

RB AND TRANSCRIPTIONAL REGULATION OF THE CELL DIVISION CYCLE

Progression through the different phases of the cell cycle requires successful execution of a complex series of events. Although each of these is indispensable for a cell to give rise to two identical progeny, the pivotal event during cell proliferation is the replication of its genes. Not surprisingly, therefore, entry into S phase and initiation of DNA replication constitute a highly regulated decision. Without trivializing the other processes involved in cell cycling, those preceding DNA synthesis may be viewed as ensuring that conditions warrant genome replication and preparing for it, and those following genome replication may be viewed as making sure that the products are apportioned correctly to progeny cells. The actual process of DNA replication requires the coordinate presence and activity of substrates for DNA synthesis (deoxynucleotide triphosphates), DNA-synthetic enzymes, mechanisms for copying template DNA, mechanisms for checking the integrity of the results and correcting defects if present, and mechanisms for deconstructing and reconstructing chromatin composition and chromosome structure. The task of replicating cellular DNA is complex, as are the enzymatic and regulatory mechanisms that carry them out. Cells entering S phase must possess the proteins and substrates necessary for DNA synthesis (acquiring substrates essentially means acquiring the relevant biosynthetic enzymes), so S phase entry can happen only in cells that have activated expression of genes encoding the needed proteins.

Studies of the Rb protein have revealed fundamental principles underlying transcriptional regulation of cell entry into S phase and DNA replication.[21] Rb is the product of the Rb gene, which when defective is responsible for childhood susceptibility to retinoblastoma tumors.[22] Only one functional copy of Rb is present in the germline of patients with familial susceptibility to retinoblastomas. Retinoblasts become transformed and proliferate uncontrollably when there

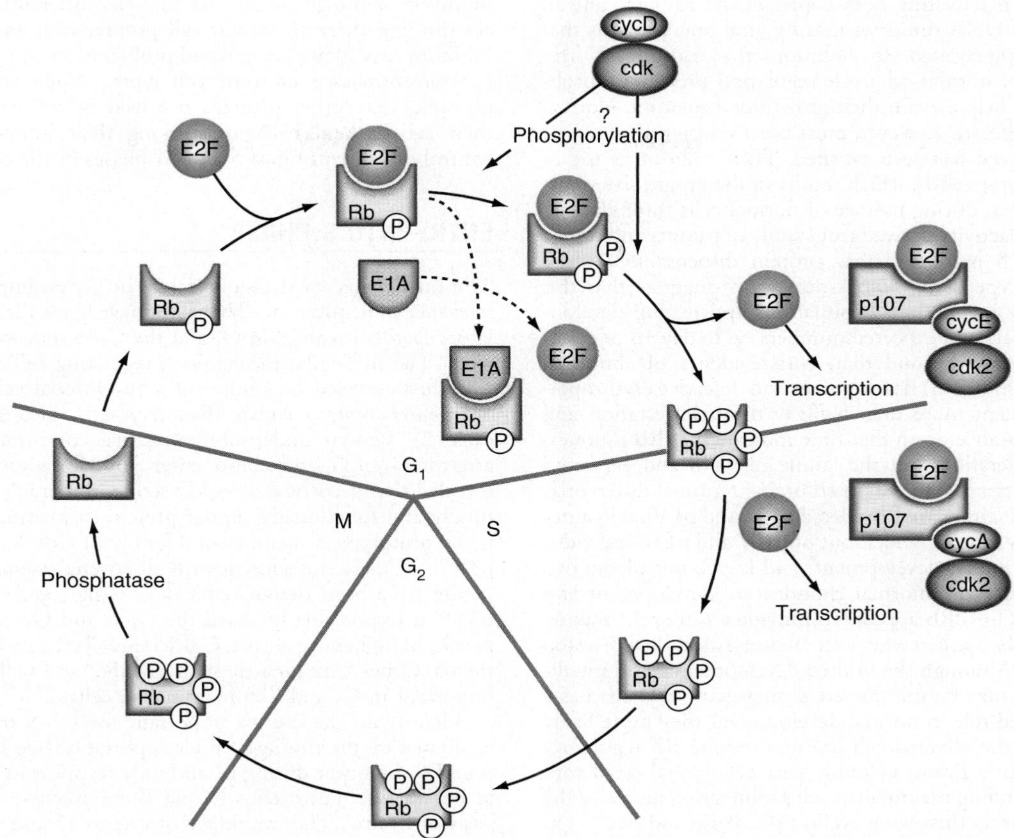

Figure 15-3 REGULATION OF THE RETINOBLASTOMA SUSCEPTIBILITY GENE PRODUCT (Rb) THROUGH THE CELL CYCLE. Rb is regulated by serine–threonine phosphorylation (P) through the cell cycle. Non- or hypophosphorylated Rb present in early and mid-G_1 can bind transcription factor E2F and thereby alter or sequester its activity. In late G_1, Rb becomes hyperphosphorylated (perhaps caused by Cdk–cyclin D kinase activity), releasing E2F for transcriptional duties or formation of other complexes. Removal of phosphate groups in M restores Rb to its hypophosphorylated form. In cells transformed by adenovirus E1A, SV40 large T, or HPV E7, these oncoproteins can bind hypophosphorylated RB and displace E2F *(dashed lines)*. The Rb-like p107 protein also binds E2F and is found in quaternary complexes with cyclin E–Cdk2 in G_1 or with cyclin A–Cdk2 in S phase.

is no functional Rb after the remaining good copy of Rb is lost or rendered nonfunctional in retinoblastoma tumor cells from these patients. This mechanism is supported by the observation that introduction of wild-type but not mutant Rb into cells without Rb causes them to arrest in G_1.[23] Thus, Rb can prevent cell entry into S phase, and retinoblastomas arise when retinoblast proliferation is no longer restrained by Rb.

Rb is widely expressed in normal cells and present at similar levels throughout the cell cycle, indicating that cell proliferation is not regulated primarily by levels of Rb protein. On the other hand, Rb phosphorylation changes markedly in different phases of the cell cycle. It is hypophosphorylated in early G_1, becomes progressively more phosphorylated on serine and threonine residues as cells progress through G_1 and approach S, and maintains this hyperphosphorylated state until M, at which time it is dephosphorylated and returned to its hypophosphorylated, early G_1 state.[24-26]

How Rb phosphorylation controls cell proliferation is understood in terms of Rb binding to transcription factors of the E2F family (Fig. 15-3).[27,28] Originally described as a cellular factor necessary for adenovirus E2 gene transcription, E2F proteins heterodimerize with members of the DP family of proteins to activate gene transcription. E2F-responsive genes include many that encode proteins necessary for DNA synthesis, such as dihydrofolate reductase, thymidine kinase, and others. Hypophosphorylated Rb binds E2F, rendering it transcriptionally inactive or an active repressor of E2F-mediated transcription.[29] Phosphorylation of serine–threonine residues in Rb near or at the site of E2F binding abrogates this interaction and Rb inhibition of E2F transcriptional activity. Thus, E2F activation of gene expression needed for S phase is inhibited by hypophosphorylated Rb in early G_1 and is reinstated as Rb becomes increasingly phosphorylated as cells progress through G_1. The importance of E2F activity for S phase transition is shown by the fact that its gratuitous expression can induce cells to enter S phase. In addition to p105 Rb (molecular mass of 105 kD), two related cellular proteins, p107 and p130, possess similar functional properties, such as the ability to bind E2F.[30] These two Rb-related proteins undoubtedly participate in cell cycle regulation, but their precise roles are still being defined.

The importance of hypophosphorylated Rb in control of cell cycling is underscored by the mechanisms tumorigenic DNA viruses use to deregulate proliferation of infected cells.[31] These viruses possess oncogenes that encode proteins responsible for transforming the infected cells. The E1A oncoprotein of adenovirus, E7 oncoprotein of human papillomavirus, and large T antigen of SV40 virus preferentially bind Rb in its hypophosphorylated state. These oncoproteins interact with Rb in the same molecular pocket as that of E2F, preventing Rb from binding E2F and permitting E2F to carry out its function unimpeded. Thus, transformation by these DNA tumor viruses is associated with cell cycle deregulation caused by viral oncoprotein inactivation of hypophosphorylated Rb function.

In the widely accepted model just described, the key to cell proliferation is release of E2F and other proteins important for S phase from Rb inhibition. This is solved in retinoblastoma and some other tumor cell types by inactivating both copies of the Rb gene and in cells transformed by DNA tumor viruses by viral oncoproteins that inactivate hypophosphorylated Rb. Solutions that cause total, irreversible disruption of normal cell cycle regulation present no problems for tumors and help explain their growth deregulation. Normal cells needing to proliferate, however, must use a solution that can be reversed when the need has been satisfied. Their solution is use of kinases that phosphorylate Rb, which results in the progressive phosphorylation of Rb seen during passage of normal cells through G_1.

The model of Rb activity derived from study of tumors and tumor cells implies that Rb is a regulatory protein dispensable for cell cycling. The phenotype of Rb knock-out mice[32] suggests that this view also may apply in physiologic situations and during development. $Rb^{-/-}$ embryos arise in expected numbers up to day 14 of gestation but fail to develop beyond that, with evidence of abnormal central nervous system (CNS) development and defective erythropoiesis. Their development more than halfway through gestation and grossly normal appearance up to that time indicate that Rb is nonessential for cell proliferation, but the failure of CNS and erythroid development supports a role for Rb in enforcing terminal differentiation in these tissues. Neither are Rb-related p107 and p130 obligatory components of the cell cycle: Knock-out of p107 and p130 individually permits normal mouse development, and knock-out of the two in combination results in abnormal chondrocyte development and neonatal lethality.[30] Thus, Rb appears to provide a cell cycle braking mechanism that can be applied whenever circumstances dictate a stop to cell proliferation. Although the limited developmental abnormalities in *Rb*$^{-/-}$ embryos may be interpreted as suggesting that Rb has a rather tissue-restricted role in normal development, they more likely reflect the fact that the affected cell lineages require Rb regulatory intervention first. Rb is almost certainly part of a global regulatory mechanism for controlling mammalian cell proliferation based on the fact that the Rb pathway (involving cyclin D–Cdk4,6 and $p16^{INK4a}$ in addition to Rb, discussed next) is corrupted in many types of cancers originating in diverse tissues.

CYCLINS, CYCLIN-DEPENDENT KINASES, AND CELL CYCLE REGULATION

Discovery of the mechanisms responsible for Rb phosphorylation and mammalian cell cycle regulation had origins in studies in yeast and invertebrate and frog embryos and was aided by the phylogenetic conservation of the molecular mechanisms involved. Many of the molecules found to be important in yeast and nonmammalian cells, which can be experimentally manipulated and studied far more easily, have close counterparts and functional equivalents in mammalian cells.

Identification and subsequent functional analysis of the factors and cofactors involved in mammalian cell cycle regulation have led to the current view that progression through the cell division cycle is driven and regulated by the activity of serine–threonine kinases of the Cdk (cyclin-dependent kinase) family. As their name implies, the activity of these kinases is under the stringent control of associated regulatory proteins called *cyclins*. These were so named because levels of the first to be described, cyclins A and B, were seen to fluctuate periodically with the cell cycle. Binding to cyclins alters Cdk structure and activates their catalytic function.[33] Numerous Cdk kinases and cyclins exist in the cell, forming combinatorial pairs with distinct activities.

Control of cyclin–Cdk activity occurs at many levels. First is the appearance and disappearance of different cyclins at specific phases of the cell cycle, which dictates the cyclin–Cdk complexes that can form in each phase. Regulation at this level is a result of highly regulated synthesis and degradation of cyclin mRNA and protein at different points in the cell cycle. A second level of regulation is afforded by posttranslational modification of Cdk kinases, which is often necessary to activate their function. A third level of regulation is provided by proteins that inhibit the activity of Cdk kinases or cyclin–Cdk complexes. The importance of regulation by Cdk inhibitors is shown by the fact that cell differentiation signals often act through them to inhibit cell proliferation and by the fact that inhibitor loss allows deregulated proliferation and promotes neoplastic transformation of some cell types. When active, Cdk kinases phosphorylate other proteins involved in cell cycling, modulating their activity and behavior. Among their important functions is control of cell entry into S and M phases of the cell cycle.

ENTRY INTO S PHASE

The importance of decisions made in G_1 leading into S and their relevance to neoplastic cell behavior have made identification of regulatory factors involved in G_1 and the G_1–S transition a prime objective.[34] The molecular mechanisms regulating cell entry into S phase were first revealed by studies of a conditional cell cycle mutant of *Schizosaccharomyces pombe* (fission yeast) called *cdc2* (cell division cycle 2). Grown under nonpermissive conditions, these mutants arrest in G_1 or G_2 and cannot enter S or M. Cloning of the *cdc2* gene revealed that it encodes a 34-kD serine–threonine kinase. The structurally and functionally similar protein in mammalian cells, $p34^{cdc2}$, is the prototypical member of a family of Cdk kinases. The protein $p34^{cdc2}$ is Cdk1, and subsequently discovered members of this kinase family have been designated Cdk2, Cdk3, and so forth. Whereas $p34^{cdc2}$ is responsible for both the G_1–S and G_2–M transitions in *S. pombe,* in higher organisms, Cdk1 is involved only in G_2 and M phase events. Other Cdk kinases, such as Cdk2 and Cdk4, are the kinases important in G_1 and S in mammalian cells.

Identifying the cyclins important for G_1–S transition has been facilitated by the timing of their appearance (see Fig. 15-2). Cyclins A and B disappear during M and only reappear in S and are unlikely to have a role, but cyclins D and E are excellent candidates on the basis of timing. The candidacy of cyclins D and E is supported by their ability to functionally complement *Saccharomyces cerevisiae* (budding yeast) mutants deficient in G_1 cyclin genes *(CLN)*.[35,36] D-type cyclins were independently suspected as being important when their genes turned up during the search for an oncogene involved in parathyroid adenomas[37] and for genes induced during mitogenic stimulation of macrophages.[38] Studies indicate that D-type cyclins, of which there are three (D1, D2, and D3), associate predominantly with Cdk4 and Cdk6. Cyclin E associates with Cdk2, which also can associate with cyclin A, once it appears in S phase.

Cyclin D–Cdk4,6 and cyclin E–Cdk2 are considered the kinases primarily responsible for phosphorylating Rb and allowing cells to progress through G_1, past R in late G_1, and into S phase. Several lines of evidence support cyclin D–Cdk4,6 as regulators of G_1 progression and entry into S phase: D-type cyclins appear in early G_1 and are induced by mitogenic signals; they can phosphorylate Rb; neutralization of D-type cyclins prevents cell entry into S; and overexpression of D-type cyclins can accelerate entry into S.[39,40] D-type cyclins appear to be mitogen sensors for the cell cycle, with many steps in their accumulation being sensitive to the presence of extrinsic growth factors and mitogenic signaling. The generally accepted view is that cyclin D–Cdk4,6 complexes initiate Rb phosphorylation in mid-G_1, which leads up to the subsequent complete inactivation of Rb that is needed for the G_1–S transition. Other studies, however, have raised questions about the absolute requirement for cyclin D–Cdk4,6 in the G_1–S transition.[41,42] In mitogen-stimulated cells, cyclin E appears later in G_1, peaks near the G_1–S boundary, and declines in S (see Fig. 15-2). Cyclin E–Cdk2 associates with Rb in G_1 and can phosphorylate Rb, and inhibition of Cdk2 activity blocks cell entry into S. If all of these observations are taken into account, cyclin E–Cdk2 is probably responsible for phosphorylating Rb at additional sites in late G_1, producing a hyperphosphorylated Rb that can no longer bind E2F.

Cyclin E associates primarily with Cdk2, and the two can be found in complex with transcription factor E2F and members of the Rb family of proteins in cells in G_1. Of interest, this complex disappears as cells enter S, just as a similar complex containing cyclin A instead of E makes its appearance. Thus, cyclin A–Cdk complexes may maintain Rb in its hyperphosphorylated state past this point in the cell cycle. Cyclin A first appears at the beginning of S and declines in G_2 and M and has an expression pattern that parallels but precedes that of cyclin B (see Fig. 15-2). These data and the results of cyclin A inhibition and addition experiments 43 have led to the view that cyclin A–Cdk2 plays a major role in driving events when cells enter S phase. Later in S and G_2, cyclin A in complex with p32cdc2 may help trigger the G_2–M transition by phosphorylating Cdc25 and initiating activation of cyclin B–p32cdc2.

ENTRY INTO M PHASE

Studies initiated in *S. pombe cdc2* mutants, which arrest in G_1 or G_2 and do not enter S or M, led to the cloning of the evolutionarily conserved $p34^{cdc2}$ (Cdk1) serine–threonine kinase.[44] An independent line of study examining the effect of cytoplasmic extracts from mature *Xenopus* frog eggs microinjected into immature frog oocytes showed that these extracts contain a material that induces oocytes to mature and undergo M phase changes such as nuclear membrane breakdown. After purification, the maturation-promoting factor (MPF) in these extracts was found to contain two proteins: One is $p34^{cdc2}$, and the other is a B-type cyclin. Cyclin B has a regulatory role in the MPF complex, shown by the fact that $p34^{cdc2}$ exhibits kinase–MPF activity only in association with cyclin B.

Cyclin B levels increase during S and G_2 (see Fig. 15-2), and levels of cyclin B–$p34^{cdc2}$ complex sufficient for the G_2-M transition are reached well before the onset of M. Mitosis is not prematurely triggered because the complex accumulates in an inactive form (Fig. 15-4). During S and G_2, the $p34^{cdc2}$ complexed with cyclin B accumulates as a multiply phosphorylated protein. In mammalian cells, phosphorylation of $p34^{cdc2}$ threonine (Thr) 161 stabilizes its association with cyclin B and is essential for activity. The kinase responsible for Thr 161 phosphorylation, CAK (Cdk-activating kinase), is itself a Cdk (designated Cdk7) that associates with a novel cyclin, cyclin H. On the other hand, phosphorylation of $p34^{cdc2}$ Thr 14 and tyrosine (Tyr) 15 suppresses its kinase activity and keeps the cyclin B–$p34^{cdc2}$ complex inactive. The kinase responsible for Tyr 15 phosphorylation is the homolog of the product of the *S. pombe wee1* gene.[45]

Activation of the cyclin B–$p34^{cdc2}$ complex is the key to cell entry into M and occurs just before M through the action of the dual-specificity phosphatase, Cdc25, causing dephosphorylation of both Thr 14 and Tyr 15. The activities of wee1 kinase and Cdc25 phosphatase are themselves regulated with phosphorylation, inhibiting

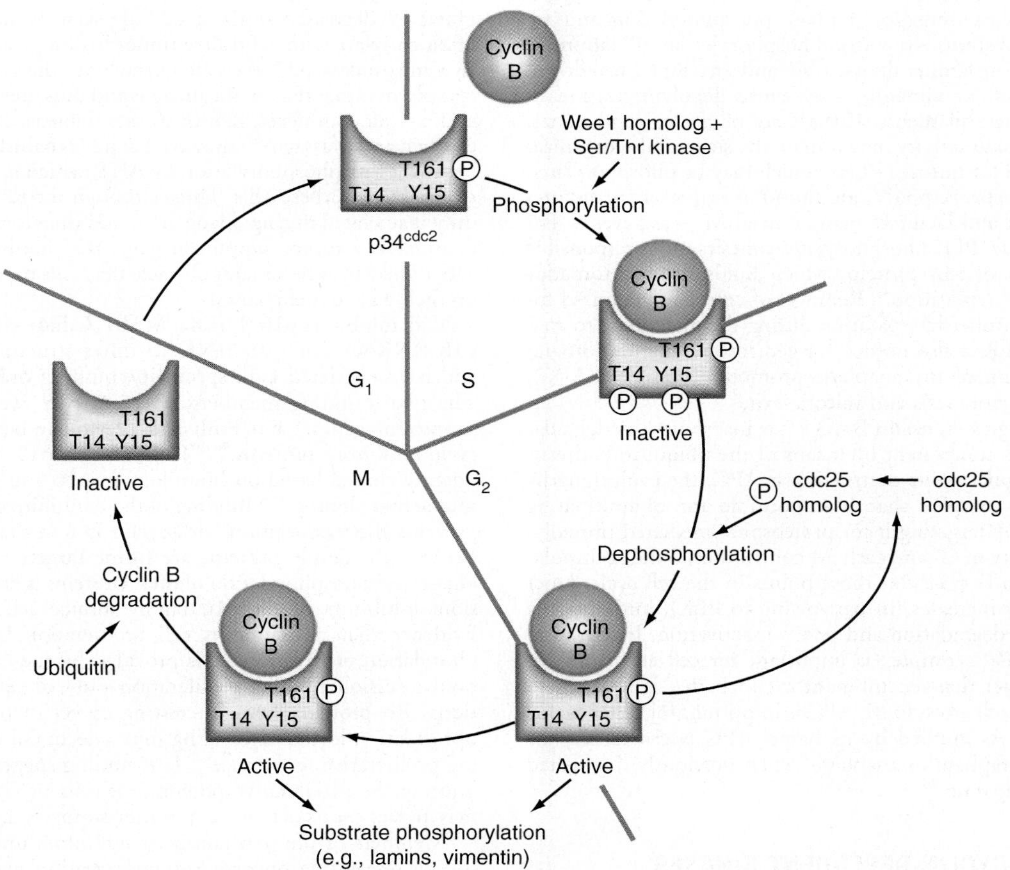

Figure 15-4 Regulation of cell entry into M by cyclin B–$p34^{cdc2}$ or Cdk1 (maturation-promoting factor [MPF]). $p34^{cdc2}$ kinase activity controls cell entry into M and is regulated during the cell cycle. Association with cyclin B, which first appears during S phase, is necessary for its kinase activity, and formation of the cyclin B–$p34^{cdc2}$ or Cdk1 complex (MPF) is stabilized by phosphorylation of Thr(T)161. Accumulating MPF is maintained in an inactive state by phosphorylation of Thr14 and Tyr(Y)15, which is catalyzed by the homolog of the *Schizosaccharomyces pombe wee1* gene product and another kinase. At the G_2–M transition, MPF is activated by dephosphorylation of Thr14 and Tyr15 by the homolog of the *S. pombe cdc25* gene product. This may be a self-amplifying reaction because activated MPF can phosphorylate and activate more Cdc25. Activated MPF phosphorylates cellular substrates and brings about the biochemical changes needed for M phase. During progression through M, degradation of cyclin B generates inactive $p34^{cdc2}$ and permits cell exit from M.

wee1 kinase function and enhancing Cdc25 phosphatase function. After a little cyclin B–p34^{cdc2} is activated, it can phosphorylate Cdc25 and create a self-amplifying feedback loop that generates more active cyclin B–p34^{cdc2} from the large preexisting stock of inactive complex.

What starts this sequence of events by initially phosphorylating and activating Cdc25 is unclear. Cyclin A–Cdk complexes have been suggested as candidates because they are active before cyclin B–p34^{cdc2} activation and have MPF activity and because inhibition of cyclin A during S prevents entry into M.[43] However, it is unclear how cyclin A–Cdk complexes, which are abundant and active throughout S, would suddenly initiate the cascade of cyclin B–p34^{cdc2} activation that marks cell entry into M phase. Polo-like kinases (PLKs), named after polo kinase, the prototypical member of this evolutionarily conserved serine–threonine kinase family,[46] are reasonable candidates because they, too, can phosphorylate and activate Cdc25 and because amplification of cyclin B–p34^{cdc2} activity does not occur until PLK becomes activated. Additionally, PLK phosphorylation of cyclin B and Cdc25 promotes nuclear localization of these proteins, enhancing nuclear accumulation of active cyclin B–p34^{cdc2} complex.[47]

Cyclin B–p34^{cdc2} can phosphorylate serine–threonine residues in many cellular proteins. Discerning its direct physiologic substrates is not simple, however, because many other kinases and cyclin–Cdk kinases are concurrently active. Candidate substrates include the lamins and vimentin, which are, respectively, nuclear and cytoplasmic proteins important for the structural organization of their compartments. These proteins undergo M phase phosphorylation and are cyclin B–p34^{cdc2} substrates in vitro. Phosphorylation of lamins is important for nuclear lamina disassembly and envelope breakdown, and phosphorylation of vimentin may cause depolymerization of vimentin intermediate filaments. If these are physiologic substrates, p34^{cdc2}–cyclin B kinase activity may initiate the structural reorganization that is essential for mitosis. PLKs, which may be phosphorylated and activated by cyclin B–p34^{cdc2}, are found at important structures and sites during M and facilitate many crucial M phase events. For example, in prophase, PLK phosphorylates cohesin and is responsible for removing most of this protein, which holds sister chromatids together after DNA replication.[48] Removal of cohesin is required for subsequent sister chromatid separation during the metaphase to anaphase transition. PLK is also needed for centrosome maturation and separation, activation of the anaphase promoting complex (APC), and regulation of cytokinesis and mitotic exit.[49]

As M phase progresses, cyclin B–p34^{cdc2} is inactivated by degradation of the cyclin B component by means of the ubiquitin pathway. A critical factor regulating its destruction is APC, the evolutionarily conserved protein complex that is responsible for ubiquitinating cyclin B and thereby targeting it for proteosome-mediated proteolysis. Low APC activity in G_2 and early M contributes to the accumulation of active cyclin B–p34^{cdc2} at those points in the cell cycle. Later in M, APC activity increases (in part owing to PLK), initiating the process of cyclin B degradation and p34^{cdc2} inactivation. Inactivation of the cyclin B–p34^{cdc2} complex is important for cell exit from M, evidenced by the fact that recombinant cyclin B that is resistant to proteolysis induces cell arrest in M. APC is important for other events during M as well. As implied by its name, APC is critical for the transition from metaphase to anaphase, when previously duplicated sister chromatids separate.[50]

INHIBITORS OF CYCLIN-DEPENDENT KINASES

Inhibitors of Cdk and cyclin–Cdk activity impose an additional layer of complexity on cell cycle regulation.[51] These inhibitors fall into two major categories. So-called "universal" inhibitors, which include p21, p27, and p57, inhibit by binding cyclin–Cdk complexes. The second group of inhibitors, which include p16, p15, p18, and p19, are more restricted in their activity and inhibit by complexing with Cdk kinases that associate with D-type cyclins (i.e., Cdk4 and Cdk6). The latter group of inhibitors are also known as INK4 because of their role as inhibitors of Cdk4.

The first inhibitor to be identified and cloned in mammalian cells was p21 (Waf1, Cip1, Sdi1), which binds several different cyclin–Cdk complexes and is the prototypical "universal" inhibitor.[52,53] The proteins p27 (Kip1) and p57 (Kip2) were subsequently identified as Cdk inhibitors with structural and functional similarities to those of p21.[54-56] The regulation of p21 expression sheds light on its function. Expression is transcriptionally induced by p53, the tumor suppressor protein activated by DNA damage (see following), and induction of p21 expression provides a mechanism for halting cell proliferation after DNA damage to allow time for damage assessment and repair.[57] The p21 protein also can be expressed in cells lacking functional p53, indicating that p53-independent pathways of expression exist. These other pathways may account for increased p21 expression in other circumstances associated with cell cycle arrest, such as senescence and terminal differentiation.

The p27 protein was originally cloned as the Cdk inhibitor associated with G_1 arrest in cells treated with transforming growth factor-β (TGFβ) or experiencing contact inhibition of growth,[54] but levels also increase in cells induced to differentiate.[58] These observations indicate that p27 often mediates the cell cycle arrest induced by extrinsic inhibitors of cell proliferation. In marked contrast with the transcriptional regulation of p21, regulation of p27 occurs posttranscriptionally, such that mRNA levels remain constant while levels of the protein change. In accordance with the ability of p21 and p27 to inhibit cyclin–Cdk activity and cell cycling, p21 and p27 are candidate tumor suppressor genes, but silencing or loss of these genes is very uncommon in cancers. However, decreased levels of p27 are seen in many carcinomas and often correlate with aggressive tumor histology and poor prognosis.[58] In some cancers, p27 levels are normal, but the protein is found in the cytoplasm rather than in the nucleus and thus unable to inhibit nuclear cyclin–Cdk complexes. Recent studies in breast cancer cells (reviewed by Blain and Massague[59]) showed that p27 is banished from the nucleus because of its phosphorylation by AKT, which is frequently constitutively active in these cells. Thus, although the *p27* gene is not genetically inactivated during oncogenesis and therefore cannot be formally counted as a tumor suppressor gene, p27 inhibition of cyclin–Cdk activity seems to be a major obstacle that cells may have to circumvent on their way to malignancy.

Cdk inhibitors p16 (INK4a, MTS1, Cdk4), p15 (INK4b, MTS2), p18 (INK4c), and p19 (INK4d) differ structurally from p21–p27 and have restricted Cdk specificity, binding only Cdk4 and Cdk6. The two founding members, p16 and p15, were cloned as tumor suppressor genes,[60] but both had previously been identified as cell cycle inhibitory proteins.[61,62] The p18 and p19 proteins were subsequently cloned based on homology to p16 and p15 and by protein interaction cloning.[63,64] Binding of these inhibitors to Cdk4 and Cdk6 prevents their association with cyclin D and their kinase activation. Because Rb family proteins are prime targets of cyclin D–Cdk4,6 kinase and phosphorylation of these proteins is crucial for G_1 progression, inhibitors of the p16 family induce cell cycle arrest in G_1. Evidence that p16 inhibits cell proliferation by preventing phosphorylation of Rb proteins is provided by the observation that p16 overexpression inhibits proliferation only of cells containing functional Rb proteins.[65] An interesting aspect of p16 expression is its upregulation in tissues of aging mice and in cultured cells approaching proliferative senescence.[66] This finding suggests a role for p16 in limiting the proliferative potential of cells in vivo and in vitro and may reflect on its activity as a tumor suppressor.

Members of the p16 family of inhibitors unquestionably have a role in preventing oncogenic transformation in vivo. This role was originally established by the cloning of the *p16* and *p15* genes from the region of chromosome 9p21 mutated in the germline of patients with familial melanoma and in the genome of many human tumor cell lines. Their importance during oncogenesis was reinforced when it was observed that *p16* knock-out mice are cancer prone[67] and by the finding that the normal *p16* and *p15* genes found in many human tumors are silenced by the epigenetic mechanism of promoter hypermethylation (reviewed by Ruas and Peters[68]). A lingering issue concerning these genes in oncogenesis stems from the fact that the 9p21 locus containing p16 also contains the *p14ARF* (in humans) or *p19ARF* (in mice) genes.[69] Because these genes overlap, *p14–p19ARF* mRNA shares sequence with p16 mRNA but produces a totally different protein because of translation in an alternative reading frame (i.e., ARF). This overlap also means that many inactivating mutations of *p16* (including engineered mutations in mice) also inactivate *p14–p19ARF*. Because *p14–p19ARF* is a positive regulator of p53 expression and a tumor suppressor protein in its own right, attribution of tumor suppressor effect to each of these two genes is difficult. The more recent results of individual knock-out of each these two genes in mice indicate that loss of either *p14–p19ARF* or *p16INK4a* predisposes mice to tumors and results in abnormal regulation of cell proliferation.[70,71]

The idea that Cdk inhibitors act simply as negative regulators of kinase activity and cell cycling and that *p16–p15INK4* arrests cell cycling solely through inhibition of Cdk4,6 activity has been revised (reviewed in 1999 by Sherr and Roberts[51]). It was observed that complexes such as cyclin E–Cdk2 bound to p21–p27 were inactive but that cyclin D–Cdk4,6 complexes containing these inhibitors remained active. This suggested that the latter might sequester inhibitors while maintaining activity and prevent inactivation of Cdk2-containing complexes. Keeping cyclin E–Cdk2 active by preventing its inhibition by p21–p27 is a noncatalytic function of cyclin D–Cdk4,6 that complements and augments its catalytic function of promoting Rb hyperphosphorylation and cell cycling. In addition, p21–p27 was found to promote assembly and nuclear accumulation of active cyclin D–Cdk complexes, suggesting that the presence of these inhibitors in cyclin D–Cdk complexes may actually be facilitatory or obligatory rather than merely optional. If cyclin D–Cdk complexes are positively regulated by p21–p27 and prevent p21–p27 from inactivating cyclin E–Cdk2, the effect of p16–p15 extends beyond inhibition of Cdk4,6 complexes. In binding Cdk4,6 and preventing assembly of cyclin D–Cdk complexes, p16–p15 causes redistribution of p21–p27 onto cyclin E–Cdk2 complexes, resulting in their inactivation and an inability to hyperphosphorylate Rb. Thus, G_1 cell cycle arrest induced by p16–p15INK4 may require and be mediated by p21–p27 proteins.

CELL CYCLE CHECKPOINTS

The welfare of an organism depends on production, by its constituent cells, of normal copies of themselves during mitotic replication. If errors arise, one or both of the progeny cells develop defects in their genome that will be transmitted to successive cell generations in subsequent rounds of mitotic proliferation. Perpetuation and amplification of genetic flaws are fundamentally detrimental, and cell cycle checkpoints, which are control mechanisms that monitor and enforce proper execution of the cell division cycle, defend against development of genomic error and instability.[19]

Cell cycle checkpoints are positioned before entry into S (G_1 checkpoint), in S (S phase checkpoint), and before entry into M (G_2 checkpoint). They enforce the orderly progression of cell cycle events, such that cells must fully duplicate their DNA before they divide and divide before they duplicate their DNA again. They also check for damage sustained by genomic DNA. When problems are detected, checkpoint mechanisms interrupt cell cycling to allow correction of the problem or elimination of the defective cell. Where the mechanisms are known, cell cycling is stopped through inhibition of the cyclins and Cdk kinases that drive normal cell cycle progression. Checkpoints also exist within M, but mitotic checkpoints may exist mostly to prevent chromosome missegregation by enforcing the sequence of M phase events that distribute duplicated genetic material equally between progeny cells. The operation of checkpoints and the consequences of their failure are illustrated by yeast mutants defective in the *RAD9* gene. Although yeasts normally cannot enter M phase until their DNA is fully replicated, defects in the *RAD9* gene allow yeasts to enter M phase even if they are prevented from completing DNA replication. Affected yeasts die more rapidly because progeny inherit incomplete or damaged genetic material.

The activity of checkpoints in mammalian cells usually is observable after they have been exposed to DNA-damaging agents, such as ionizing radiation, ultraviolet (UV) light, or certain chemotherapy agents. Checkpoint activation by these genotoxic insults results in cell division cycle arrest in G_1, S, or G_2 phase, allowing cells time to repair the fault before resuming the cycle or, if the damage is irreparable, to execute a program of programmed cell death or apoptosis. Mechanisms that detect and signal the presence of damaged cellular DNA are incompletely understood, but the ATM (ataxia-telangiectasia–mutated) and ATR (AT and RAD3-related) protein kinases are clearly important components (Fig. 15-5). ATM kinase is activated by ionizing radiation and the double-strand DNA breaks it causes.[72] Defects in ATM result in cell sensitivity to ionizing radiation, defects in all DNA damage-induced cell cycle checkpoints and susceptibility of

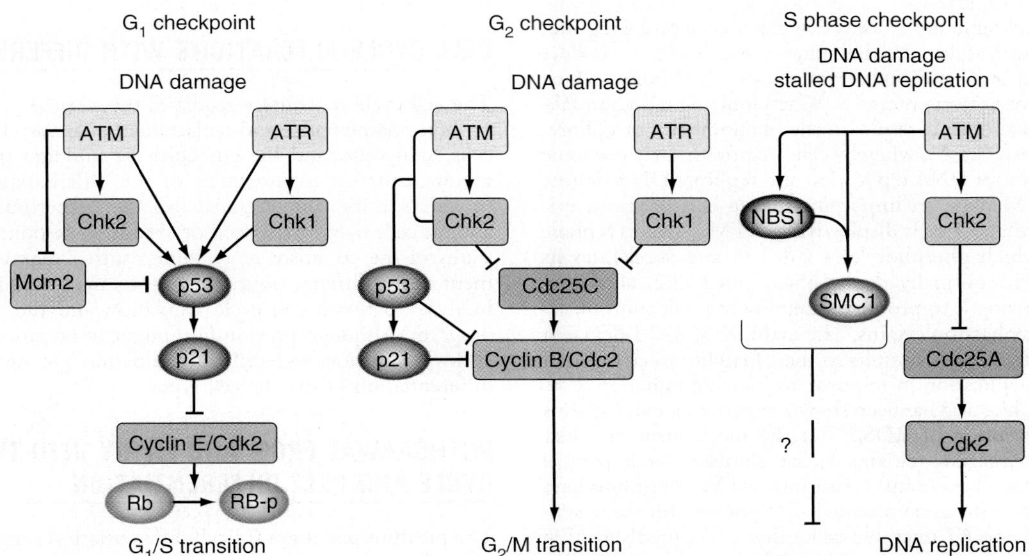

Figure 15-5 CELL CYCLE CHECKPOINTS. Pathways for activating G_1, G_2, and S phase checkpoints are shown. Arrows (Ø) designate activating interactions, and (→) designate inhibitory or inactivating interactions.

patients with ataxia-telangiectasia (AT) to cancer. The ATR kinase responds to UV-induced DNA damage, to stalled intermediates of DNA replication, and to damage from ionizing radiation.

ATM and ATR, both of which bind DNA, plus other proteins with homology to proteins involved in DNA replication, are responsible for sensing damaged DNA or failed DNA replication and initiating checkpoint signaling. As ATM and ATR kinase function is activated in the process, they also transduce the signals by phosphorylating downstream effectors of the checkpoint response (reviewed by Abraham[73]). Among the recipients of ATM–ATR signaling are Chk1 and Chk2. These two structurally distinct serine–threonine kinases are phosphorylated and activated by ATM–ATR. Whereas Chk1 is regulated primarily by ATR,[74] Chk 2 is regulated primarily by ATM,[75] but other factors, such as BRCA1, clearly influence their activation in response to DNA damage.[76] When active, Chk1–Chk2 join ATM–ATR to phosphorylate and activate effectors of the checkpoint response.

Prominent among the effectors activated by these kinases is p53, the tumor suppressor protein missing or inactivated in more than 50% of human cancers and an essential component of the G_1 DNA damage checkpoint. ATM–ATR directly phosphorylate p53 and indirectly promote its phosphorylation through Chk1–Chk2 phosphorylation of p53 at additional sites. The effect of this p53 phosphorylation is protein stabilization, a result that is augmented by ATM phosphorylation of the Mdm2 protein and inhibition of its ability to direct rapid p53 turnover.[77] Through this combination of mechanisms, p53 is rapidly induced following DNA damage. A transcription factor, p53 engenders cell cycle arrest by activating transcription of p21(Waf1–Cip1–Sdi1) and inhibiting cyclin–Cdk2 activity. The pathway leading from ATM–ATR to Cdk2 inhibition activates the G_1 DNA damage checkpoint by preventing Rb hyperphosphorylation.

Enforcement of the G_2 DNA-damage checkpoint involves Chk1 and Chk2 phosphorylation of Cdc25C, allowing this phosphatase to bind the 14–3-3σ protein and be sequestered in the cytoplasm. Excluded from the nucleus, Cdc25C cannot dephosphorylate Cdc2 and activate the cyclin B–Cdc2 complex needed for M phase entry.[78] Although signaling from ATM–ATR to Chk1–Chk2 to Cdc25C is one G_2 checkpoint mechanism, p53 also plays a role. The p53 protein induces p21 and represses cyclin B and Cdc2 gene expression, reducing levels and activity of cyclin B–Cdc2 complex.[79,80] These effects, plus effects on expression of other genes, result in p53-dependent G_2 arrest after DNA damage. Because p53 induction stems from ATM–ATR activation, this pathway complements Cdc25C sequestration to provide multiple ways by which ATM–ATR activation can enact G_2 arrest.

The S phase checkpoint arrests cells that experience problems after beginning DNA replication (i.e., cells that are in S phase). It does not depend on p53 and is distinct from the G_1 checkpoint, which affects cells that have not yet entered S. When ionizing radiation fails to activate this checkpoint, it results in the phenomenon of radioresistant DNA synthesis (RDS), whereby cells inappropriately continue to initiate new origins of DNA replication and replicate DNA despite DNA damage. ATM plays an important role in this pathway, evidenced by the fact that AT cells display RDS. ATM activates S phase arrest via Chk2, which phosphorylates Cdc25A and accelerates its degradation. Cdc25A normally dephosphorylates Cdk2, activating this kinase and allowing it to promote assembly of replication initiation complexes at replication origins. The inability of ATM-deficient cells to downregulate Cdc25A results in their inability to curb Cdk2 activity and DNA replication in response to ionizing radiation.[81]

More recently, Chk1 also has been shown to participate in Cdc25A regulation and prevention of RDS,[82] but the mechanism of Chk1 activation in this situation remains to be clarified. In a parallel pathway of S phase checkpoint activation, ATM phosphorylates NBS1, the product of the gene mutated in Nijmegen breakage syndrome (NBS). NBS and AT resemble each other in the predisposition of patients to cancer and of their cells to chromosome instability, radiation sensitivity, and RDS. NBS1 is part of a protein complex that binds to and helps repair double-strand DNA breaks,[83,84] and its phosphorylation by ATM is important for inducing S phase arrest after DNA damage and preventing RDS. Recently, the SMC1 (structure maintenance of chromosomes-1) protein, which has a role in chromosome structure and DNA repair, was found to be phosphorylated by ATM after ionizing radiation exposure. Phosphorylation depended on NBS1 and was important for S phase checkpoint activation.[85,86] Although many details are still unclear, ATM–NBS1–SMC1 and ATM–Chk2–Cdc25A appear to provide parallel and cooperative pathways for S phase checkpoint activation.[87]

The importance of checkpoint mechanisms is shown by the fact that mutant yeasts defective in checkpoint genes and proteins exhibit difficulties with mitotic replication, genomic instability, and death. In mammals, the consequences of failed checkpoint mechanisms can be just as devastating. *ATR* knock-out in mice is lethal at a very early stage (7.5 days) of embryonic development, with cells cultured from the embryos exhibiting loss of genomic integrity and widespread death by apoptosis.[88] Defective checkpoint mechanisms compatible with survival beyond birth, such as loss of *ATM* or *NBS1,* must have less catastrophic consequences but nevertheless produce growth retardation and developmental abnormalities.[89-91] Because organisms deficient in ATM or NBS1 survive, the impact of these proteins on neoplasia can be seen. Deficient mice and humans are predisposed to neoplasia, especially the development of thymic lymphomas. Some humans and mice heterozygous for *ATM* mutations (carriers) also are prone to developing cancers.[92,93] This occurs when the mutant *ATM* allele produces nonfunctional protein that inhibits the function of normal ATM present in the cells (i.e., exerts a dominant-negative effect).

Mutation of *p53* is the single most common genetic abnormality leading to cancer and may best illustrate the importance of checkpoint effector mechanisms as safeguards against neoplasia. p53 knock-out mice and humans heterozygous for mutated *p53* (Li-Fraumeni syndrome) have no developmental abnormalities but are predisposed to the development of a variety of malignancies. This predisposition may not be solely caused by defective p53-dependent checkpoint mechanisms, however, because p53 also has apoptosis-activating functions, and defective p53-dependent apoptotic mechanisms are known to contribute to neoplasia. The fact that p53 is important for both cell cycle arrest and apoptosis makes it almost certain that p53 plays a critical role in the cell's decision whether or not to die following genotoxic damage. In view of the fact that radiation therapy and many types of cancer chemotherapy act by damaging cellular DNA, the death or repair response of cells after genotoxic insults has impact beyond tumor development and also may influence tumor response to cancer therapy.

CELL CYCLE ALTERATIONS WITH DIFFERENTIATION

The cell cycle machinery regulates the normal proliferation of cells for both maintenance and replacement purposes. For example, blood cells, skin cells, and the gut epithelia undergo rapid turnover and require constant maintenance of the differentiated cell pools that provide specific differentiated functions. In contrast, liver, muscle, and fat cells may be replaced or expand in response to the metabolic status of the organism or to injury. Either maintenance or replacement of the differentiated cell compartment requires an orchestrated interplay between cell cycle regulation and the cell differentiation program. Although previously thought to be mutually exclusive, cell cycle progression and cell differentiation are tightly linked in the differentiation of specific cell types.

WITHDRAWAL FROM AND ENTRY INTO THE CELL CYCLE AND CELL DIFFERENTIATION

The previous paradigm for cell differentiation suggested, on the basis of studies performed with cell lines, that cell cycle progression and cell differentiation are mutually exclusive. It has become more evident, however, that cell cycle progression is inherently necessary for the differentiation of specific cell types. For example, the hematopoietic stem cell (HSC) compartment is quiescent until these cells are called on by certain stresses to activate the hematopoietic differentiation program. The cell cycle inhibitors p21 and p27 participate in the regulation of HSC cycle. Using mice null for either p21 or p27, transplantation experiments have revealed distinct roles for these two cell cycle inhibitors. HSCs depleted of p21 proliferated, and the absolute number of stem cells doubled.[94] This unrestricted proliferation caused diminished self-renewal potential, resulting in hematopoietic failure in animals that received serially transplanted p21-null bone marrow. In contrast with the findings for p21, depletion of p27 does not affect stem cell numbers, but its absence increases progenitor cell proliferation and pool size.[95] The absence of p27, however, does not affect self-renewal potential. These findings indicate that HSCs differentiate through an orderly progression through the cell cycle for the generation of progenitor cells and the ensuing more differentiated lineage-specific cells.

COUPLING OF MANDATORY CELL CYCLE PROGRESSION AND CELL DIFFERENTIATION

Cell cycle progression required for cell differentiation is illustrated by a number of different systems, including lymphopoiesis, myeloerythropoiesis, and adipocyte and keratinocyte differentiation. In the case of lymphopoiesis, upstream regulators of the cell cycle such as the Myc–Max and Mad–Max transcriptional regulators permit cell cycle progression of pre-B lymphocytes for their sequential differentiation down the B-lymphocyte lineage. For example, overexpression of Mad, which blocks cell cycle progression, results in the paucity of mature B lymphocytes.[96] The fact that myeloid and erythroid hematopoiesis requires several generations of differentiating cells to proliferate further supports the requirement of concurrent cell expansion and differentiation.

Perhaps one of the best-studied models of cell differentiation is the adipocyte model. In this model, specific fibroblasts are triggered to initiate the adipogenesis program through a series of cell culture manipulations, including exposure of confluent fibroblasts to specific factors such as insulin, dexamethasone, and methylisobutylxanthine. An intriguing observation is that after exposure to these differentiation-inducing agents, there is a "mitotic clonal expansion" phase that is mandatory for adipogenesis of 3T3L1 fibroblasts.[97] During this phase, preadipocytes traverse through the G_1–S checkpoint with the concurrent activation of Cdk2 activity and turnover of p27. After several rounds of synchronous cell divisions, these cells cease to proliferate and start to express markers of adipocytes.

SPECIALIZED CELL CYCLE: ENDOREPLICATION AND DIFFERENTIATION

A special type of cell cycle progression is featured in the differentiation of cells that have high metabolic profiles required for synthesis of specific proteins, such as plasma proteins produced by hepatocytes, or for the production of platelets by megakaryocytes. Both cell types display endoreplication, or the repeated phases of DNA replication without cell division, resulting in cells that are gigantic and could have large nuclei with DNA content well over 128N.[98] Endoreplication also features prominently in specific plant and insect tissues, indicating that this mechanism is well used through evolution.

It stands to reason that endoreplicating cells permit G_1–S transition but have mechanisms to prevent entry into or completion of mitosis. Studies of many types of endoreplicating cells in fact support this notion. In particular, megakaryocytes endoreplicate in response to thrombopoietin with upregulation of cyclin D3. Overexpression of cyclin D3 results in increased megakaryocyte ploidy.[99] As suspected, megakaryocyte endoreplication occurs at levels of the mitotic cyclin B–Cdk1 significantly below levels in cells that undergo cytokinesis. Similarly, mammalian trophoblasts, which also undergo endoreplication, display increased cyclins D1, E, and A, but the levels of cyclin B are diminished. These observations indicate that depending on the specific cell types, cell cycle progression may be critically required for differentiation of specialized cells.

SUGGESTED READINGS

Blain SW, Massague J: Breast cancer banishes p27 from nucleus. *Nat Med* 8:1076, 2002.

Falck J, Petrini JH, Williams BR, et al: The DNA damage-dependent intra-S phase checkpoint is regulated by parallel pathways. *Nat Genet* 30:290, 2002.

Helt AM, Galloway DA: Mechanisms by which DNA tumor virus oncoproteins target the Rb family of pocket proteins. *Carcinogenesis* 24:159, 2003.

Iritani BM, Delrow J, Grandori C, et al: Modulation of T-lymphocyte development, growth and cell size by the Myc antagonist and transcriptional repressor Mad1. *EMBO J* 21:4820, 2002.

Kang J, Bronson RT, Xu Y: Targeted disruption of NBS1 reveals its roles in mouse development and DNA repair. *EMBO J* 21:1447, 2002.

Kim ST, Xu B, Kastan MB: Involvement of the cohesin protein, Smc1, in Atm-dependent and independent responses to DNA damage. *Genes Dev* 16:560, 2002.

Narlikar GJ, Fan HY, Kingston RE: Cooperation between complexes that regulate chromatin structure to transcription. *Cell* 108:475, 2002.

Saucedo LJ, Edgar BA: Why size matters: Altering cell size. *Curr Opin Genet Dev* 12:565, 2002.

Shiloh Y: ATM and related protein kinases: Safeguarding genome integrity. *Nat Rev Cancer* 3:155, 2003.

Sorensen CS, Syljuasen RG, Falck J, et al: Chk1 regulates the S phase checkpoint by coupling the physiological turnover and ionizing radiation-induced accelerated proteolysis of Cdc25A. *Cancer Cell* 3:247, 2003.

Spring K, Ahangari F, Scott SP, et al: Mice heterozygous for mutation in *Atm*, the gene involved in ataxia-telangiectasia, have heightened susceptibility to cancer. *Nat Genet* 32:185, 2002.

Sumara I, Vorlaufer E, Stukenberg PT, et al: The dissociation of cohesin from chromosomes in prophase is regulated by Polo-like kinase. *Mol Cell* 9:515, 2002.

Tang QQ, Otto TC, Lane MD: Mitotic clonal expansion: A synchronous process required for adipogenesis. *Proc Natl Acad Sci U S A* 100:44, 2003.

Toyoshima-Morimoto F, Taniguchi E, Nishida E: Plk1 promotes nuclear translocation of human Cdc25C during prophase. *EMBO Rep* 3:341, 2002.

Yarden RI, Pardo-Reoyo S, Sgagias M, et al: *BRCA1* regulates the G2/M checkpoint by activating Chk1 kinase upon DNA damage. *Nat Genet* 30:285, 2002.

Yazdi PT, Wang Y, Zhao S, et al: SMC1 is a downstream effector in the ATM/NBS1 branch of the human S-phase checkpoint. *Genes Dev* 16:571, 2002.

For complete list of references log on to www.expertconsult.com.

CHAPTER 16

CELL DEATH

Nika N. Danial and David M. Hockenbery

Cell death is a highly organized fundamental activity that is equally complex in regulation as cell division and differentiation. In the physiologic contexts of embryonic development and tissue renewal, or as a pathologic response to cell injury and infectious pathogens, cell deaths are orchestrated for multiple purposes that benefit the organism. These include maintenance of epithelial barrier function, destruction of microbes, adaptive immune responses, recycling of biologic macromolecules, intracellular signaling, and preservation of genomic integrity. The majority of mammalian cell deaths have morphologic and biochemical features of apoptosis (Fig. 16-1), a self-inflicted death program encoded in the genetic material of all cells (Fig. 16-2). Necrosis, an alternative mechanism of cell death, occurs in the aftermath of extreme cellular insults and could be viewed as a failure of cellular homeostasis. Recently, a programmed pathway of necrosis, referred to as *necroptosis,* has been identified. Although cells contain their own death apparatus, cell death in multicellular organisms is exquisitely sensitive to the advice and consent of neighboring cells. As might be expected, the internal cell death machinery is tightly interwoven with other essential cell pathways. Investigations of cell death have also informed our understanding of living cells (e.g., the recognition that cellular remodeling shares some pathways with apoptotic cell death).

PHYSIOLOGIC CELL TURNOVER

An adult human loses approximately 10^{11} cells/day, with skin, intestine, and hematopoietic tissues accounting for the majority. Physiologic cell death in adults occurs in the context of continuously (skin, intestine) or cyclically renewing (endometrium, breast) tissues. In most instances, homeostatic mechanisms balance generation of new cells with loss of terminally differentiated cells. In the intestinal epithelium, as an example, one stem cell per epithelial crypt asymmetrically divides to produce a daughter cell that rapidly divides, terminally differentiates (and exits from cell cycle), migrates onto the epithelium surface, and undergoes a specialized form of apoptosis that leaves behind cytoplasmic bridges that preserve epithelial barrier function, all within 2 to 3 days.

Neutrophils recruited to sites of inflammation undergo apoptosis upon removal of the inflammatory stimulus. Apoptotic neutrophils are unable to degranulate and reprogram macrophages to an antiinflammatory phenotype when phagocytosed. This clearance mechanism is specialized to apoptotic neutrophils, as necrotic neutrophils and opsonized cells trigger macrophages to secrete inflammatory cytokines.

Reversible physiologic cell deaths also provide a reserve production capacity for functionally mature cells. The glycoprotein hormone erythropoietin (EPO) is produced by kidney mesangial cells and stimulates excess red blood cell (RBC) production in proportion to the demand for blood oxygen-carrying capacity. The EPO receptor is expressed on committed erythrocyte precursors (erythroid colony-forming unit [CFU-E] and proerythroblasts). Growth factors, in general, also generate survival signals. The primary in vivo effect of EPO is to rescue erythroid precursors from physiologic death. The EPO-responsive erythroid compartment in the bone marrow is maintained at a constant size and rate of cell proliferation under various demands (hypoxia, hypertransfusion) despite widely differing production rates of mature erythroid cells. The raison d'être appears to be to overproduce CFU-Es and proerythroblasts at low altitudes with excess cells removed before the erythroblast stage; this scheme provides a rapidly accessible reserve under conditions of higher demand. Similar arrangements of excessive production with apoptosis of maturing cells are found in small intestinal crypts and spermatogenesis.

A final physiologic application for apoptosis is as a mechanism for selection of specific cell phenotypes. A well-known example occurs in the immune system after clonal diversification of T- and B-lymphocyte antigen receptors by gene recombination and error-prone DNA replication. Positive and negative clonal selection to match T-cell receptors to cognate class I and class II histocompatibility antigens on accessory cells and eliminate receptors reacting with self-antigens takes place in the thymus. Affinity maturation of immunoglobulin-bearing B cells takes place in germinal centers of lymphoid organs. In each case, cells run through a gauntlet of near-death experiences, with death and survival signals directly linked to the binding properties of the antigen receptor on individual cells.

EMBRYOGENESIS AND SCULPTING

During development, apoptosis is extensively used to sculpt the final shape of the embryo. Regression of vestigial tails, interdigital webs, and the pro- and mesonephros are all accomplished by an autophagic type of cell death with biochemical hallmarks of classical apoptosis. Certain anatomic structures, such as hollow viscus organs, are formed by apoptotic excavation of interior cell masses; the final forms of other structures, such as the forebrain, are shaped by patterns of apoptotic death within neural precursor cells. A more refined example is the matching of numbers of projecting neurons to the size of a target field, which is accomplished by apoptosis of surplus neurons. Excess or misdirected neurons fail to find the trophic factors produced by their designated targets. Localized activity of caspases may even selectively prune neural processes, leaving the neuron intact.

EXECUTIONERS OF APOPTOSIS

Caspases

The central effectors of apoptosis are a family of cysteine proteases known as caspases (cysteinyl aspartate-specific protease).[1] All caspases are aspartases with a four-residue recognition sequence P4-P1 (Fig. 16-3). A serine protease that also recognizes aspartic acid motifs, granzyme B, is similarly involved in cytolytic T-cell killing. Often only one or two caspase cleavage sites are found in a variety of cellular proteins, in many cases members of the same complex or biochemical pathway, leading to limited digestion of substrate proteins. Proteins truncated by caspase cleavage frequently exhibit altered functions, demonstrating that caspases can act as signaling proteases. The number of identified caspase substrates is approaching 1000.[2] These can be grouped in several categories (Fig. 16-4).

Although no single caspase substrate has been identified that is obligate for cell death, some progress has been made in attributing biochemical and morphologic features of apoptotic death to proteolysis of specific substrates. Caspase-mediated cleavage and activation of Rho-associated kinase-1 (ROCK1) stimulates actin–myosin contractility, leading to membrane blebbing and fragmentation of the nucleus weakened by cleavage of nuclear lamins. DNA fragmentation is mediated by an endonuclease, DNA fragmentation factor 40 (DFF40) or caspase-activated DNase (CAD), that is activated after caspase-mediated degradation of an inhibitory binding partner, ICAD/DFF45.

In the intracellular battle between survival and proapoptotic factors, caspases can also swing the advantage toward death by altering the balance of forces. The mitochondrial survival proteins BCL-2 and BCL-X_L are subject to N-terminal cleavage by caspases. Not only does N-terminal truncation eliminate a survival function, but the cleaved versions also behave as proapoptotic factors. Activation of a proapoptotic BCL-2-family member, BH3 interacting domain death agonist (BID), also features caspase-mediated processing to a truncated factor, tBID, which then traffics to its mitochondrial site of action.

ACTIVATION OF PROCASPASES

Caspases are expressed in healthy cells as zymogens with low to absent protease activity, with association as homodimers and proteolytic processing into large and small subunits required for strong activation (Fig. 16-5). Downstream or executioner caspases (caspase-3, -6, and -7) exist as preformed dimmers.[1] Cleavage of a flexible interchain connector between subunits facilitates the movement of surface loops to form an open active site. Processing of procaspases occurs immediately after aspartate residues within caspase recognition motifs. Subsite specificities are distributed among caspases so that many caspase zymogens must be processed in trans by a different caspase, creating a hierarchy of proteolytic activation. Apical caspases (caspase-2, -8, -9, -10) have proteolytic (including autocatalytic) activity at

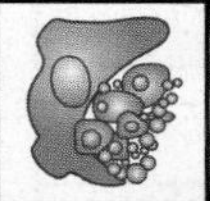 Apoptosis	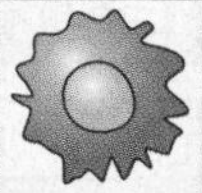 Necrosis
Cell shrinkage and fragmentation	Cell swelling and lysis
Nuclear condensation	Karyolysis
Internucleosomal DNA fragmentation	Random DNA breaks
Loss of asymmetry of phospholipids in plasma membrane bilayer	Loss of plasma membrane integrity
Detachment and engulfment by phagocytes	Recruitment of inflammatory cells

Figure 16-1 MORPHOLOGIC FEATURES ASSOCIATED WITH APOPTOSIS AND NECROSIS.

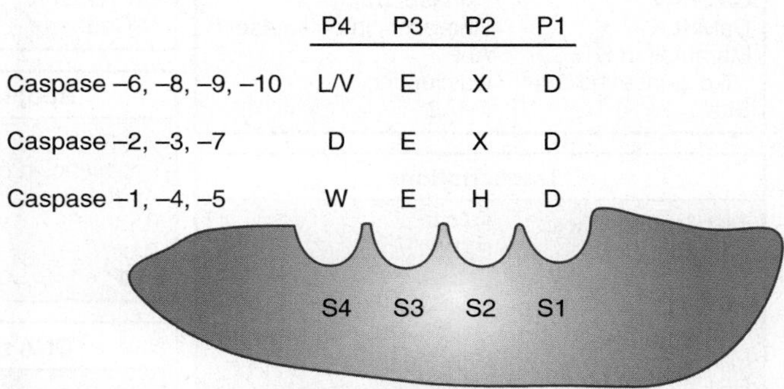

Figure 16-3 SUBSTRATE SPECIFICITY OF CAPASES. Substrate specificity of caspases is determined by geometry of specificity binding pockets S4 to S1, recognizing peptide side chains numbered P1 to P4 on acyl side of scissile peptide bond. All caspases require Asp in S1 pocket.

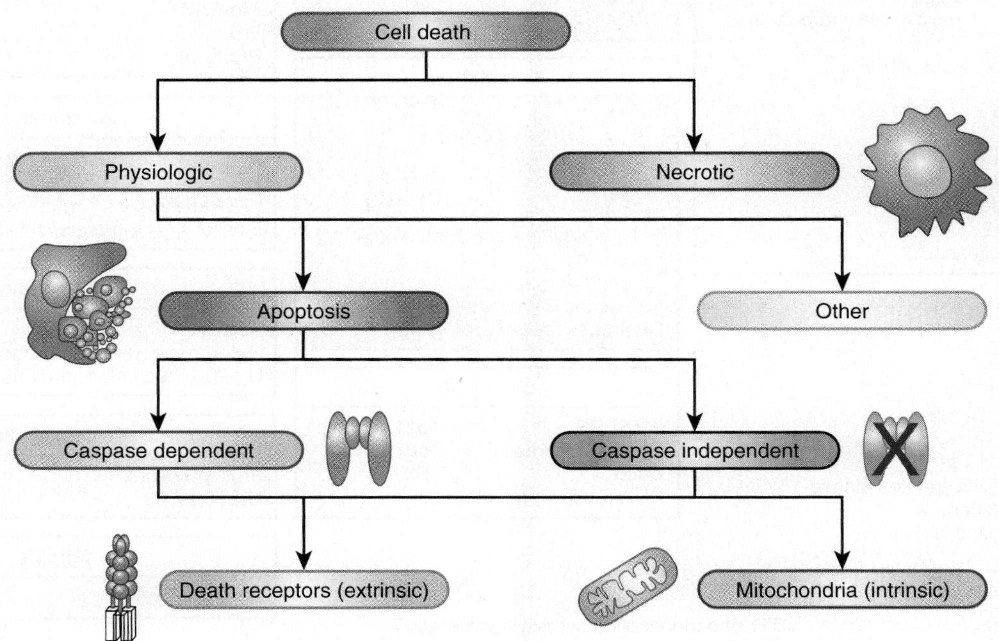

Figure 16-2 CLASSIFICATION OF CELL DEATH PATHWAYS.

Cytoskeletal proteins

Paxillin-γ, α/β-Actin, α-Adducin, Vimentin, Tau, Gas2, Myosin light chain, Tensin 4, Plectin-1, α-Actinin, Cytoplasmic dynein 1 intermediate chain 1, Cortacin, Filamin, α, β-II-Fodrin, HIP-55, HS1, Plectin, β-I-Spectrin, Troponin T, Gelsolin, Keratins (14, 17, 18, 19)

Protein kinases/phosphatases

Protein kinase C-related kinase 2, Fyn, Lyn, PIP5K1-α, MAP4K1, ETK/BMX, CaMK IV, CaMKLK, Mammalian STE20-like kinase-1/2/3/4, SLK, SPAK, AKT, MEKK-1, PKC-δ, ε, η, μ, θ, ζ, PKR, p21-activated kinase-2, Receptor-interacting kinase-1/2, Rho-associated kinase-1, Abl, Calcineurin, PPA2

Transcription

Transcription factor AP-2α, Sp1, SRF, MEF2A, C, D, Max, CREB, c-Rel, IκB-α, NRF2, STAT1, BTF3, KHSRP, NONO/p54nrb, RNA helicase A, Splicing factors, arginine/serine-rich-1, 9, GATA-1, NF-κB p65, TAF(II)80-δ

Protein and membrane sorting

Clathrin assembly protein (CALM), POM121, Nup153, TPR, GRASP65, Kinectin, Signal recognition particle 72 kD, Farnesyltransferase, Geranylgeranyltransferase I, Calcium-independent phospholipase A2, Cytosolic phospholipase A2, SET-β, BAP31, Golgin-160, Vesicle-docking protein p115, Rabaptin-5

Receptor signaling

TRAF 1/3, Netrin receptor UNC5B, TNFR1, EGF-R, ErbB-2, GluR1, TCR ζ, GrpL/Gads, Vav-1, Phosphodiesterase 4A5, 6, 10A2, Phospholipase C-γ1, Androgen receptor, Deleted in colon cancer, RET

Cell adhesion

p130cas, α, γ-Catenin, Desmoglein-3, Desmocollin 3, Desmoplakin, E-Cadherin, N-Cadherin, P-Cadherin, HEF1, Connexin 45.6, Plakophilin-1, APC, Focal adhesion kinase

Apoptosis regulators

Bcl-2, Prothymosin α, Apaf-1, Bad, Bax, FLIP, IAP-1, Bid, Bcl-xL, ICAD/DFF45, Procaspases (2, 3, 6, 7, 9)

DNA repair/topology

Topoisomerase 1, Bloom syndrome BLM, ATM, Helicard, PolyADP ribose glycohydrolase, PolyADP ribose polymerase-1/2, DNA-dependent protein kinase catalytic subunit RAD51, Lens epithelium-derived growth factor p75, BRCA1

Translation

eIF2-α, eIF3, eIF4B, eIF4E-BP, eIF4GI/II, Polypyrimidine tract binding protein 1, Nucleolin, SS-B/La-autoantigen, 60S acidic ribosomal protein P0, Death-associated protein 5

Cell cycle

PITSLRE, DNA polymerase ε, Cdc6, DNA replication factor C, p21waf1/cip1, p27kip1, Rb

Protein degradation

HDM2, MDMX, Proteasome activator 28γ, UBE4B, UFD2, Calpastatin

Neurodegenerative disorders

Amyloid-like protein 1, Ataxin-3, Atrophin-1, Huntingtin, β-Amyloid precursor protein, Presenilin-1/2

G-Protein signaling

Rho GDIβ, Rac, D4-GDI, Ras-Gap, TIAM1, CDC42

Intermediary metabolism

CAD, SREBP-1/2, CTP: phosphocholine cytidylyltransferase α, Carbamoyl-phosphate synthetase II, Glutamate-L-cysteine ligase catalytic subunit, Pyruvate dehydrogenase complex-E2

Nuclear organization

Special AT-rich sequence binding protein 1, Lamina-associated polypeptide 2-α, NuMA, Lamins A, B1, C, Scaffold attachment factor-A

Cytokines

Pro-IL-1b, Pro-IL16, Pro-IL-18, Pro-IL-33

Ion transport

Kv channel interacting protein 3, Plasma membrane calcium-transporting ATPase 2/4, Inositol 1, 4, 5-triphosphate receptor-1/2

RNA splicing

Acinus, Heterogeneous nuclear ribonucleoproteins, U1-70 kDa small nuclear ribonucleoproteins

Protein folding

Prothymosin-α, Hsp90-α/β

Mitosis

RAD21 homolog

*The following caspase substrates are activated

Bid, Procaspases, Pro-IL 1-β, 16, 18, 33, FLIP, MEKK-1, Mammalian STE20-related kinase-1/2/3/4, p21-activated kinase-2, Rho-activated kinase-1, MAP4K1, Ras-GAP, PITSLRE, ETK/BMX, Protein kinase C-δ, ε, η, θ, ζ, Calcineurin, PP2A, CTP: phosphocholine cytidylyltransferase α, SREBP-1/2

Figure 16-4 DIVERSITY OF CASPASE SUBSTRATES.

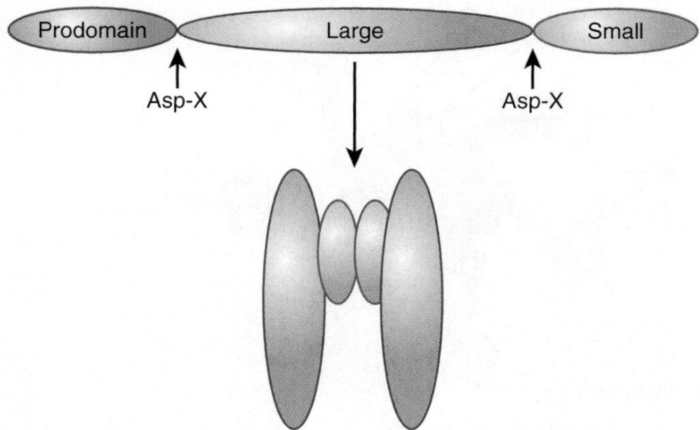

Figure 16-5 MATURE CASPASES ARE FORMED BY PROTEOLYTIC PROCESSING OF PROCASPASES TO DIVIDE LARGE AND SMALL SUBUNITS AND REMOVE N-TERMINAL PEPTIDES. Caspase substrate motifs at cleavage sites enable sequential caspase activation or, in the case of initiator caspases, autoactivation. Caspase dimers are assembled from two large and two small subunits. *Asp,* Aspartate.

high concentrations without a requirement for processing. Interactions at a dimer interface (induced proximity model) reorient and stabilize the binding pocket conformation of these caspases. Normally monomeric, these zymogens are distinguished by the presence of a long prodomain that serves as a docking site for recruitment into a self-activating complex. Protein associations within these complexes are built around homomeric interactions between three binding cassettes, the death domain (DD), death effector domain (DED), and caspase activation and recruitment domain (CARD).

DISCS, APOPTOSOMES, INFLAMMASOMES, AND PIDDOSOMES

Four distinct caspase-activating assemblies are known (Fig. 16-6). Caspase-8 and -10 are engaged by a family of cell surface receptors known as death receptors, including tumor necrosis factor receptor I (TNFR1), Fas/CD95, death receptor 4 (DR-4), and death receptor 5 (DR-5).[3,4] Ligand binding to trimerized death receptors induces conformational changes that promote binding of adaptor proteins, Fas-associated death domain protein (FADD) and TNFR1-associated death domain protein (TRADD), to the cytoplasmic tail of the death receptor by dimerization of homologous DDs from each molecule. A second interaction domain in FADD, a DED, binds to a similar DED in the prodomain of caspase-8/10, leading to caspase dimerization and localized autocatalysis. The prodomain of caspase-8/10 is severed during processing, dispersing active caspases to cellular substrates. Analysis of unprocessed caspase-8 dimers demonstrated that active sites can be formed in the absence of processing, stabilized by hydrophobic interactions at the dimer interface. The death receptor, FADD, and caspase complex is known as the death-inducing signaling complex (DISC) (see Fig. 16-6, *A*).

The second assembly, the apoptosome, is specialized for activating caspase-9, which has a CARD-type prodomain. Formation of the cytoplasmic apoptosome is initiated by release of the soluble electron carrier, cytochrome *c,* from mitochondria. Cytochrome *c* binds to an adaptor protein, apoptosis protease activating factor-1 (APAF-1), enabling adenosine triphosphate (ATP)/dATP-dependent oligomerization of APAF-1 in a heptameric wheel and exposure of its own CARD domain (see Fig. 16-6, *B*). Docking of caspase-9 to the apoptosome through CARD–CARD interactions is both necessary and sufficient for proteolytic activity. Unprocessed caspase-9 dimers contain one active site; thus, induced dimerization of caspase-9 initiates autocatalytic processing and eventual dissociation from the apoptosome with loss of proteolytic activity. Both pathways converge with proteolytic activation of caspase-3 by caspase-8, -9, or -10.

Inflammasomes are multiprotein complexes dedicated to activating caspase-1 in response to molecular cues from infectious pathogens (pathogen-associated molecular patterns [PAMPs]) or endogenous signals (danger-associated molecular patterns [DAMPs]).[5] A family of Nod (nucleotide-binding oligomerization domain)-like receptors (NLRs) detect PAMPs and DAMPs through leucine-rich repeats (LRRs), triggering oligomerization of Nod domains. A third, N-terminal region contains one of several protein interaction motifs, including CARD and pyrin domains, for direct interaction with caspase-1 or via an adaptor protein, apoptosis-associated speck-like protein containing a CARD (ASC) (see Fig. 16-6, *C*). The three inflammasomes best characterized to date are named after the NLR protein involved. Whereas NLRP1 and NLRC4 recognize bacterial muramyl dipeptide and flagellins, respectively, NLRP3 recognizes multiple stimuli, including lipopolysaccharide, bacterial RNA, and urate crystals. The inflammasome scaffold is postulated to trigger caspase-1 activity according to the induced proximity model.

Caspase-2 is activated after genotoxic damage via PIDD in a complex known as the PIDDosome. Similar to death receptors, death domains in PIDD bind to an adaptor protein, RAIDD, which in turn recruits caspase-2 through DED interactions, generating a large (>670 kD) multiprotein complex (see Fig. 16-6, *D*). PIDD also activates nuclear factor kappa-B (NF-κB) downstream of DNA damage responses through competing interactions with the receptor-interacting protein-1 (RIP1) serine/threonine kinase and I-kappa-B kinase (IKK) scaffold, NF-κB essential modulator (NEMO).

NON-APOPTOTIC ROLES FOR CASPASES

Although justifiably known for their apoptotic functions, accumulating evidence indicates that caspases also function in healthy cells.[6] Caspase-1 was originally identified as the processing enzyme for interleukin-1β (IL-1β) and recently shown to process another proinflammatory cytokine, IL-18. Caspases can also be involved in negative feedback control of erythroblast differentiation by mature erythroblasts through degradation of GATA-1. Several dramatic structural alterations associated with cell differentiation also appear to require transient caspase activation. Cleavage of a limited number of caspase substrates precede nuclear and chromatin changes during terminal erythroid differentiation, and caspase inhibitors block proplatelet formation from megakaryocytes. The more limited caspase activation in these instances may involve some degree of compartmentalization. Because the activity of unprocessed apical caspases requires persistent binding to adaptor proteins, this constraint may allow for localized, limited caspase activity under some circumstances consistent with a nonapoptotic role.

INHIBITOR OF APOPTOSIS PROTEINS

The only known endogenous caspase inhibitors are members of the inhibitor of apoptosis proteins (IAP) family. IAPs were originally described in insect viruses as viral proteins produced during cellular infection to block host cell apoptosis.[7] In mammalian cells, X-linked inhibitor of apoptosis (XIAP) is the only direct caspase inhibitor. XIAP binds to the active sites of specific caspases[3,7] to block catalytic activity or interferes with dimerization (caspase-9). IAP proteins contain one to three baculovirus IAP repeat (BIR) domains that coordinate zinc, and one or more additional protein-interaction domains. IAP-binding motifs (IBM) consist of a short peptide sequence with an amino-terminal alanine and bind to a surface groove on certain BIR domains. Initial processing of caspase-3, -7, and -9 generates an IBM at the amino-terminal end of the short subunit, providing an anchor point for additional physical interactions with IAP proteins. XIAP uses different BIR domains to bind IBMs of specific caspases.

IAPs also function as ubiquitin E3 ligases. In most cases, this function is linked to a RING domain, mediating interactions with an E2 ubiquitin conjugating enzyme. Although protein

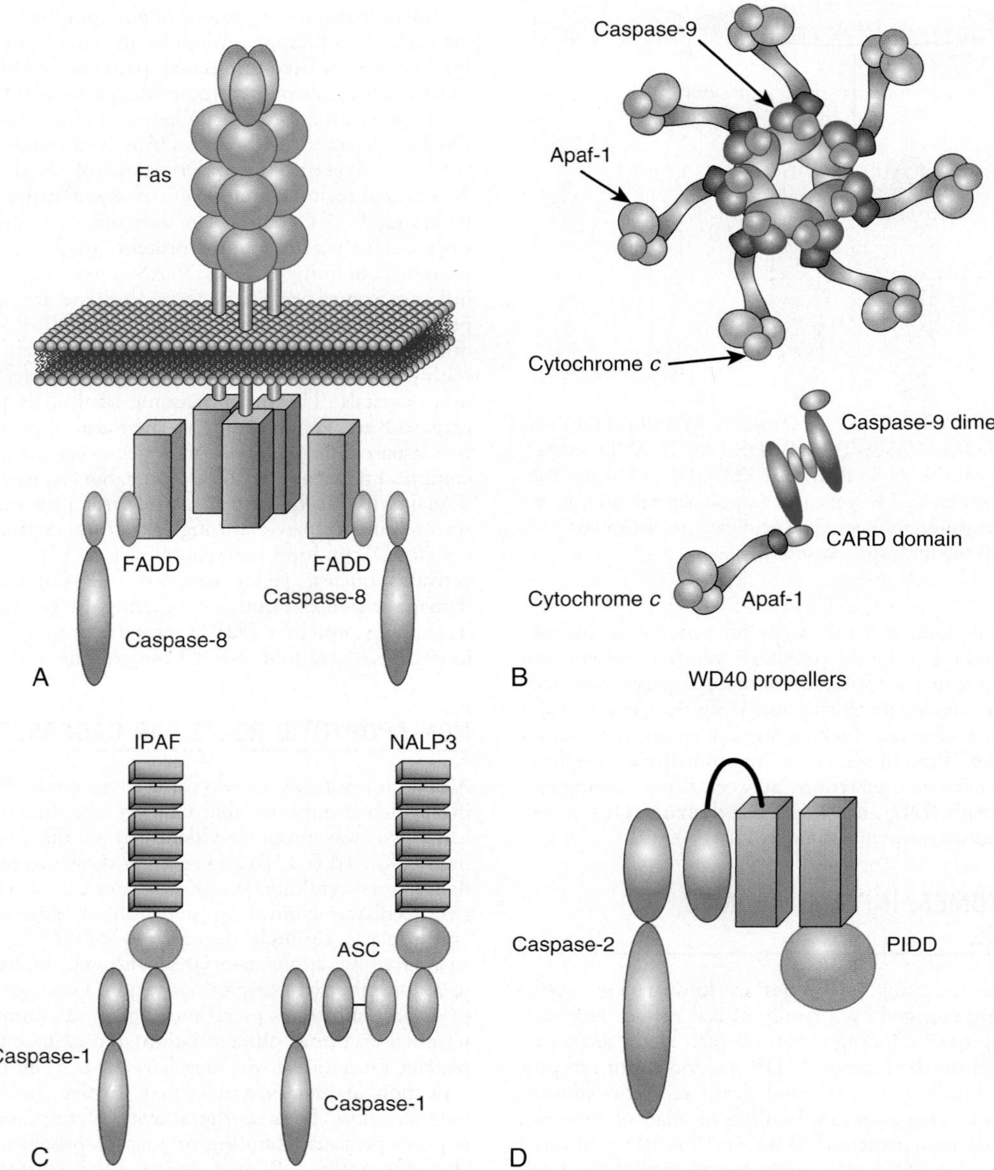

Figure 16-6 CASPASE ACTIVATION PLATFORMS. **A,** DISC (death-inducing signaling complex) is assembled after binding of ligand (Fas) to death receptor (CD95) at cell surface. Protein interaction domains (death domain [DD] and death effector domain [DED]) mediate associations between death receptor, initiator caspase (caspase-8), and adaptor protein (FADD). **B,** Apoptosome resembles a seven-spoked disc, with procaspase-9 molecules bound at the hub extending above one surface and apoptosis protease activating factor-1 (APAF-1) adaptors aligned as spokes, presenting caspase activation and recruitment domain (CARD) interaction domains at hub and WD40 propellers bound to cytochrome *c* at rim. **C,** Inflammasomes are multiprotein complexes containing either IPAF or NALPs as adaptor proteins that recruit caspase-1 and contain oligomerization domains. IPAF binds procaspase-1 through its CARD domain, and NALP-based inflammasomes recruit procaspase-1 indirectly through apoptosis-associated speck-like protein containing a CARD-1 (ASC-1), which possesses pyrin domain for NALP binding and CARD domain for caspase-1 recruitment. **D,** PIDDosome is a molecular platform consisting of the DD-containing p53-inducible protein PIDD, which binds another DD containing protein RAIDD (RIP-associated Ich-1/CED homologous protein with death domain). RAIDD recruits procaspase-2 through DD-based interactions.

degradation of polyubiquitylated caspase substrates may be involved in the apoptotic effects of XIAP, a clearer role for the ubiquitin ligase activity of IAPs has been established in NF-κB signaling.[7] TNF binding promotes assembly of a multiprotein signaling complex at the TNF-R1 receptor, including TRAF2; TRAF5; RIP1 kinase; and two IAPs, cIAP1 and cIAP2. Lysine-63 linked ubiquitylation of RIP1 by cIAP1/cIAP2 recruits two kinase complexes, IKKγ/IKKα/IKKβ and the mitogen-activated protein kinase (MAPK) TAK1/TAB2/TAB3. TAK1 phosphorylates IKKβ, which in turn phosphorylates IkB proteins, allowing NF-κB to enter the nucleus. The noncanonical pathway of NF-κB activation is also negatively regulated by cIAP1/cIAP2-mediated attachment of K48-linked polyubiquitin chains to the NF-κB–inducing kinase (NIK), leading to its degradation.

INHIBITOR OF APOPTOSIS PROTEIN ANTAGONISTS

Two proteins normally localized in the mitochondrial intermembrane space, SMAC (second mitochondria-derived activator of caspase)/Diablo and Omi/HtrA2, can bind IAPs via an NH2-terminal IBM sequence and competitively displace bound caspases. Whereas the NH2-terminus of active SMAC/Diablo is generated by removal of a presequence during mitochondrial import, Omi/HtrA2 is a stress-activated serine protease that is cleaved by autoprocessing. Cytoplasmic translocation of SMAC/Diablo and Omi/HtrA2 during apoptosis provides an additional mechanism for caspase activation. The reaper, grim, hid, and sickle proteins in *Drosophila* function similarly with fly IAPs and have NH2-terminal sequence homology to SMAC/Diablo and Omi/HtrA2.

CORE APOPTOSIS PATHWAYS

In mammals, the execution of apoptosis downstream of death signals is governed by two molecular programs that terminate in caspase activation, which may be linked in certain cell types. The extrinsic pathway operates downstream of death receptors, such as Fas and other members of the TNF receptor family, which recruit DISC upon ligand binding. This complex in turn recruits and activates caspase-8 and -10, leading to activation of other downstream caspases. The second program, also known as the *intrinsic pathway,* is marked by the involvement of mitochondria.[8-10] Besides providing most of the cellular ATP, mitochondria participate in apoptosis by releasing factors such as cytochrome *c,* a component of the mitochondrial electron transport chain. The permeabilization of the outer mitochondrial membrane (MOMP) marks the "point of no return" in the intrinsic pathway of apoptosis. After being released, cytochrome *c* is assembled with APAF-1 and caspase-9 to form the "apoptosome," which in turn triggers downstream effector caspases (see Fig. 16-6, *B*). Other apoptogenic factors released from mitochondria, including apoptosis-inducing factor (AIF), SMAC/Diablo, Omi/HtrA2, and endonuclease G, augment apoptosis.

BCL-2 FAMILY PROTEINS AND THE INTRINSIC PATHWAY OF APOPTOSIS

The BCL-2 family of proteins constitutes a critical control point in apoptosis residing immediately upstream to irreversible cellular damage, where the members control the release of apoptogenic factors from mitochondria.[8-10] Several Bcl-2 proteins reside at subcellular membranes, including the mitochondrial outer membrane, endoplasmic reticulum (ER), and nuclear membranes. The different anti- and proapoptotic members of this family form a highly selective network of functional interactions that ultimately governs the permeabilization of the mitochondrial outer membrane and subsequent release of apoptogenic factors such as cytochrome *c.* The founding member of this family, *BCL2,* was discovered as the defining oncogene in follicular lymphomas, located at one reciprocal breakpoint of the t(14;18) (q32;q21) chromosomal translocation. Cells transduced with *BCL2* remained viable for extended periods in the absence of growth factors. Transgenic mice bearing a *BCL-2-Ig* mini-gene recapitulating the t(14:18) chromosomal translocation displayed B-cell follicular hyperplasia and progressed over time to diffuse large B-cell lymphomas. BCL-2 expression specifically blocked the morphologic features of apoptosis, including the plasma membrane blebbing, nuclear condensation, and DNA cleavage. Importantly, unlike other oncogenes known at that time, BCL-2 did not promote proliferation, defining a new category of oncogenes, namely regulators of cell death. The first proapoptotic BCL2 homologous protein to be identified, BAX, co-immunoprecipitated in stoichoimetric amounts with BCL-2. *BAX*-transfected cells died rapidly in the absence of growth factor and BAX was subsequently shown to be capable of directly triggering apoptosis. Since the discovery of BCL-2 and BAX, the BCL-2 family in mammals has expanded with several acting principally as prosurvival proteins and others hastening cell death in various experimental systems (Fig. 16-7). Homologues of BCL-2 proteins exist in all metazoans studied to date as well as several animal DNA viruses.

The BCL-2 family is marked by the conserved homology domains, BH1-4 (see Fig. 16-7).[8-10] BH (BCL-2 homology) domains correspond to α-helical and connecting segments that dictate structure and function. All antiapoptotic members, such as BCL-2 and BCL-X_L, and a subset of proapoptotic family members, such as BAX and BAK, are "multidomain" proteins sharing sequence homology within 3-4 BH domains. The "BH3-only" subset of proapoptotic molecules, including BAD (BCL2 antagonist of cell death), BID, BIM (BCL2 interacting mediator of cell death), NOXA, and PUMA (p53 upregulated modulator of apoptosis), show sequence homology only within a single α-helical segment, the BH3 domain, which is also known as the critical death domain required for binding to "multidomain" BCL-2 family members. The ability of BCL-2 family proteins to selectively bind each other is integral to their function in apoptosis. The BH1, -2, and -3 domains of the antiapoptotic proteins form a hydrophobic groove that binds to the hydrophobic face of the amphipathic α-helical BH3 domain from a proapoptotic binding partner.

BAX AND BAK AND THE MITOCHONDRIAL GATEWAY TO APOPTOSIS

A combination of genetic approaches, biochemical experiments, and pharmacologic studies has begun to unravel the molecular mechanisms underlying the function of BCL-2 family proteins (Fig. 16-8). The combination of two multidomain proapoptotic members, BAX and BAK, that are absolutely required to execute death by all apoptotic signals that activate the intrinsic pathway, nominating these molecules as the requisite gateway to the mitochondrial apoptotic machinery.

Mitochondrial intramembranous homo-oligomerization of BAX and BAK is a prime candidate mechanism of MOMP that would release cytochrome *c* and involves conformational changes that result in exposure of specific epitopes. Conversely, antiapoptotic BCL-2 family members prevent the mitochondrial release of cytochrome *c.* Conformational changes during BAX and BAK activation are ultimately linked to their mitochondrial intramembranous homo-oligomerization. However, the mechanisms underlying these changes are distinct for each of these proteins. Whereas BAX is a soluble monomeric protein in the cytosol or peripherally attached to mitochondrial membrane that inserts into the mitochondrial outer membrane (MOM) upon receipt of a death stimulus, BAK is a mitochondria-resident protein (Fig. 16-9). The three-dimensional structure of inactive BAX revealed that its C-terminal tail, which is required for its insertion into the MOM, is folded back into the BAX hydrophobic cleft formed by the BH1, -2, and -3 domains. Soon after induction of apoptosis, cytosolic BAX undergoes a conformational change that releases the COOH-terminal tail, allowing BAX docking to mitochondria and exposing an NH2-terminal epitope. Membrane integrated monomers subsequently oligomerize to form pores in a manner that is dependent on the exposed NH2 terminal epitope. This is distinct from other pore-forming proteins that oligomerize before membrane insertion. Multiple conformer-specific binding partners of BAX have been identified and proposed to regulate BAX translocation, insertion, or oligomerization.[11] Among these, roles for both antiapoptotic BCL-2 proteins and BH3-only proapoptotic molecules have been proposed (see below). A growing body of evidence also shows that, in addition to protein–protein interactions, protein–lipid interactions influence BAX conformation and its ability to permeabilize the MOM.

Unlike BAX, BAK monomers are integrated into the MOM before induction of apoptosis. Select BH3-only proteins can conformational changes necessary for BAK activation. Upon activation, the

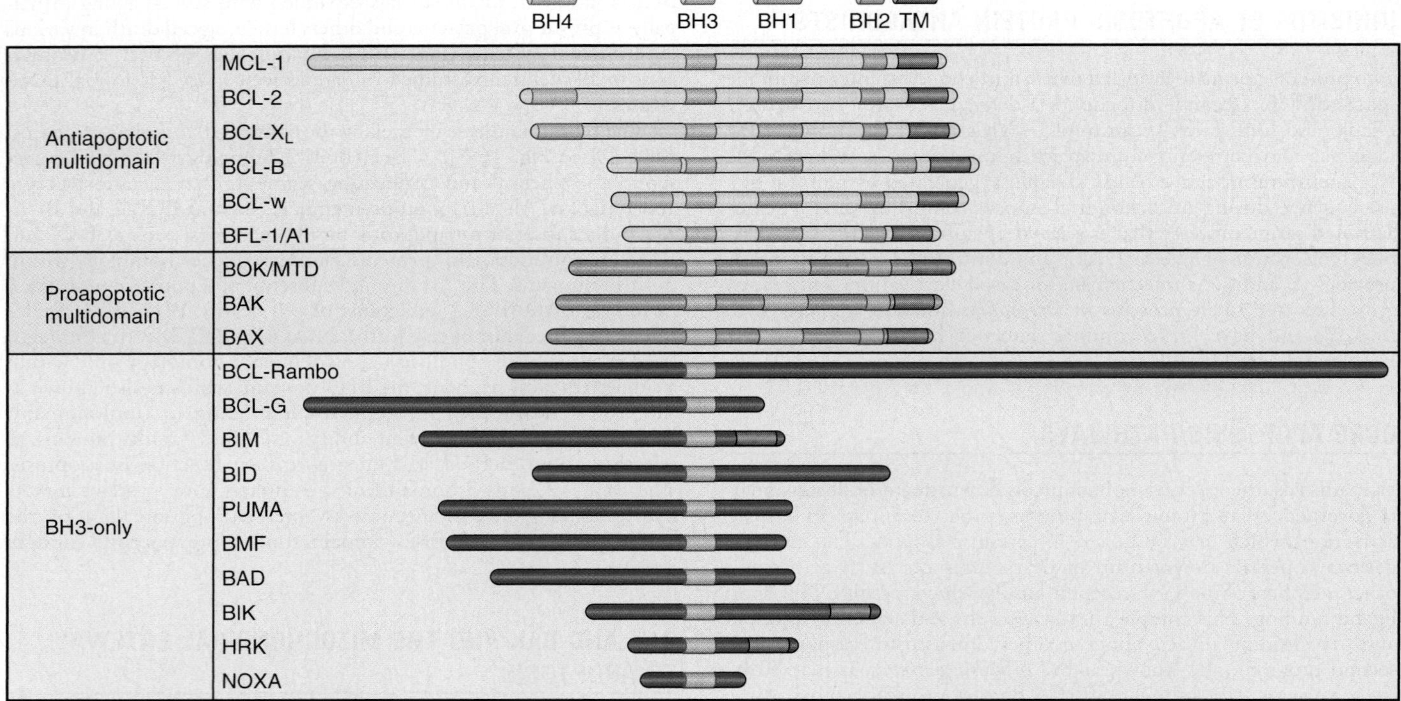

Figure 16-7 CLASSIFICATION OF BCL-2 FAMILY ACCORDING TO CONSERVED DOMAINS. BH1-3 domains form a surface hydrophobic groove capable of binding BH3 domains of other family members. C-terminal hydrophobic sequences function to target or anchor Bcl-2 family proteins to intracellular lipid membranes. *BAD,* BCL2 antagonist of cell death; *BAK,* BCL2 antagonist/killer; *BAX,* BCL2-associated x protein; *BCL,* B-cell lymphoma; *BID,* BH3 interacting domain death agonist; *BIK,* BCL2-interacting killer; *BIM,* BCL2 interacting mediator of cell death; *BMF,* BCL2 modifying factor; *BOK,* BCL2-related ovarian killer; *HRK,* harakiri; *MCL-1,* myeloid cell leukemia sequence 1; *PUMA,* p53 upregulated modulator of apoptosis; *TM,* transmembrane domain.

BH3 domain of BAK is exposed and binds to a hydrophobic binding pocket in an adjacent BAK molecule to form a symmetric dimer. Interaction between BAK dimers may lead to higher order oligomers. Several studies suggest that membrane-activated conformers of BAX or BAK can subsequently activate other latent BAX or BAK molecules through an autoactivation mechanism, serving to amplify the signal leading to MOMP.[11]

BH3-ONLY PROTEINS

BAX and BAK oligomerization is directly or indirectly triggered by BH3-only subgroup of proapoptotic BCL-2 family members[8-10] (see Fig. 16-8). BH3-only molecules are upstream sentinels that selectively respond to proximal death and survival signals and require BAX/BAK to induce death.[12] Genetic loss of function models together with biochemical studies point to an emerging paradigm for BH3-only proteins, which consists of latent lethality requiring transcription or posttranslational modifications for activation in a tissue-restricted and signal-specific manner. Proapoptotic activity of any given BH3-only protein is associated with exposure of the hydrophobic face of its BH3 helix, enabling it to interact with the hydrophobic groove of multidomain dimerization partners. For example, cytosolic BID is activated upon cleavage by caspase-8, leading to mitochondrial translocation, BAX/BAK activation, and cytochrome *c*. On the other hand, the ability of the BH3-only molecule BAD to engage antiapoptotic BCL-2 partners is regulated though phosphorylation on three serine residues. Among the three serine sites, the phosphorylation status of serine at position 155 within the BAD BH3 domain is a critical determinant of its availability for binding to BCL-2/BCL-X_L.[13] Other BH3 proteins interact with distinct extramitochondrial targets. For example, BIM is localized to the microtubule dynein motor complex by binding to the dynein light chain, DLC1, and BMF associates with dynein light chain 2 (DLC2) in the myosin V actin motor complex. Lastly, the activation of NOXA and PUMA is under direct transcriptional regulation by p53, a finding that is consistent with their roles as specialized death sentinels during DNA damage. Thus, the large number of "BH3-only" members is indicative of specialization rather than redundancy. The unique localizations, protein associations, and mechanisms of activation for the individual proapoptotic BH3-only members BAD, BID, BIM, NOXA, and PUMA suggest that each acts as a sentinel for distinct damage signals, thereby increasing the range of inputs for endogenous death pathways.

Proapoptotic activity of BH3-only proteins is associated with exposure of the hydrophobic face of their BH3 helix, enabling it to interact with the hydrophobic groove of multidomain dimerization partners. Extensive binding studies using peptides derived from the BH3 domain of BH3-only molecules have assessed the affinities and selectivity of their interactions with multidomain BCL-2 proteins.[12] Experimental evidence based on mutational analysis, loss-of-function models and in vitro studies with isolated mitochondria has given rise to several models of how upstream BH3-only molecules directly or indirectly trigger activation of BAX and BAK to induce MOMP.[12] The complex and selective molecular interactions between the multidomain anti- and proapoptotic molecules also involve both cytosolic and membrane conformers of select family members, each of which is subjected to distinct regulatory mechanisms, including binding affinities, on/off rates, and association with membrane lipids and other binding proteins.[11]

These findings suggest that compounds capable of occupying the hydrophobic pocket of antiapoptotic BCL-2 molecules may mimic the function of sensitizer BH3-only molecules to lower the threshold for apoptosis. It has been suggested that cancer cells, which normally violate many intracellular checkpoints, already possess a significant amount of activator BH3-only molecules, "priming" these cells for death. However, antiapoptotic BCL-2 proteins are also upregulated in many cancers, sequestering the activator BH3-only molecules and

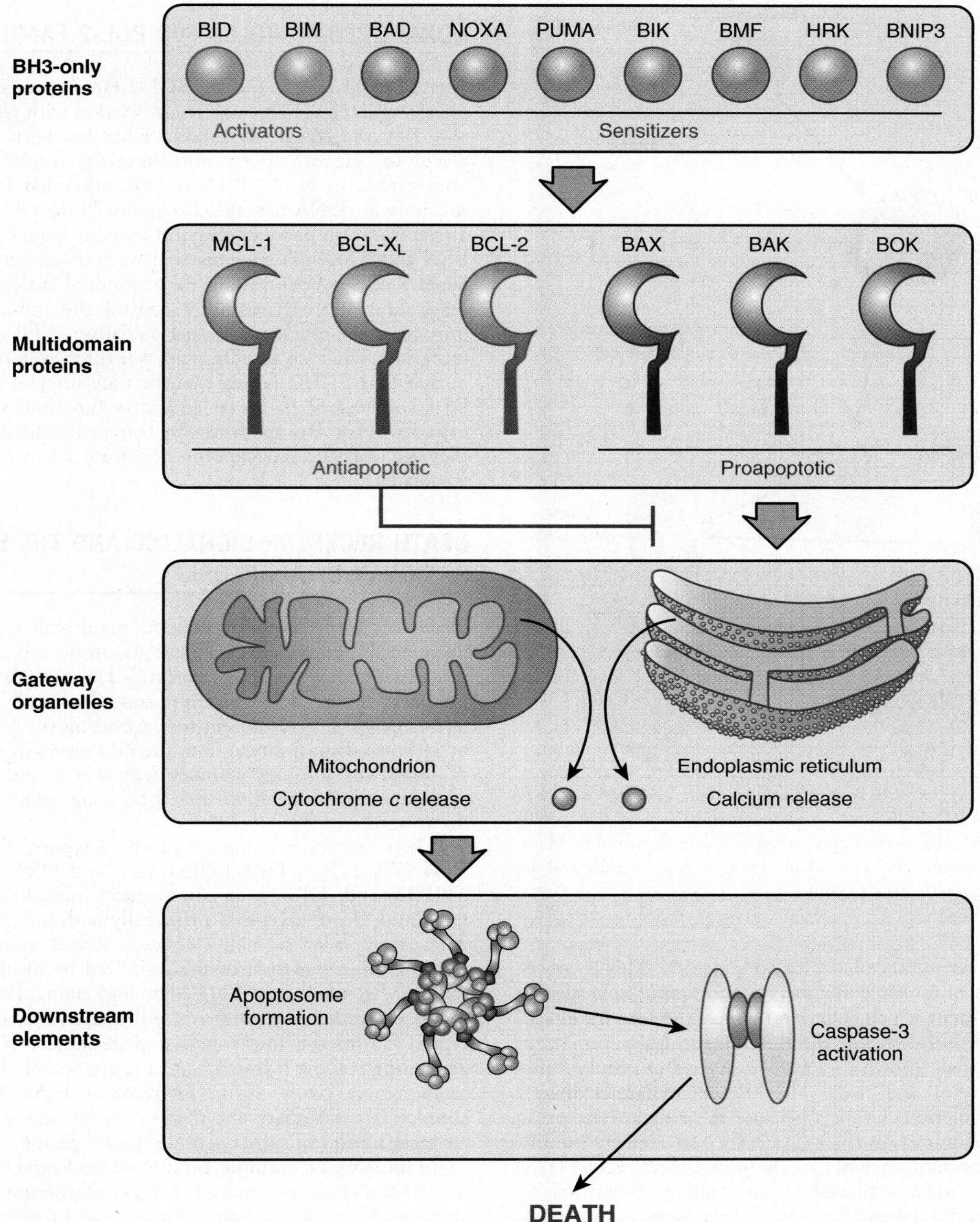

Figure 16-8 SCHEMATIC REPRESENTATION OF THE INTRINSIC APOPTOTIC PATHWAY IN WHICH A BH3-ONLY MOLECULE SERVE AS UPSTREAM SENTINELS THAT SELECTIVELY RESPOND TO SPECIFIC DEATH SIGNALS. BH3-only molecules ultimately regulate BAX and BAK (BCL2 antagonist/killer) activation directly or indirectly. This process is in turn inhibited by antiapoptotic BCL-2 family members. BAX and BAK serve as gateways to apoptosis, regulating both cytochrome *c* release from mitochondria and Ca^{2+} release from the endoplasmic reticulum (ER). See Fig. 16-7 for definitions of abbreviations.

preventing them from inducing the oligomerization of BAX/BAK. Indeed a class of small molecule inhibitors of BCL-X_L and BCL-2 mimic the sensitizer function of BAD BH3 domain and have shown efficacy in several tumor models.[14] Other approaches to manipulate the function of BCL-2 family members include peptidic compounds based on the BH3 domains of BH3-only molecules. These compounds, referred to as stabilized α-helices of BCL-2 domains (SAHBs) are generated using a synthetic strategy known as hydrocarbon stapling that allows retention of the α-helical structure and binding specificity to dimerization partners and additionally imparts membrane permeability and protease resistant properties.[15] In addition to BH3 mimetics, other approaches for manipulation of this pathway are being actively pursued.

BCL-2 FAMILY PROTEIN AND THE ENDOPLASMIC RETICULUM GATEWAY TO APOPTOSIS

Apart from cytochrome *c* release, the control of Ca^{2+} dynamics at the ER by BCL-2 family proteins has recently emerged as an important

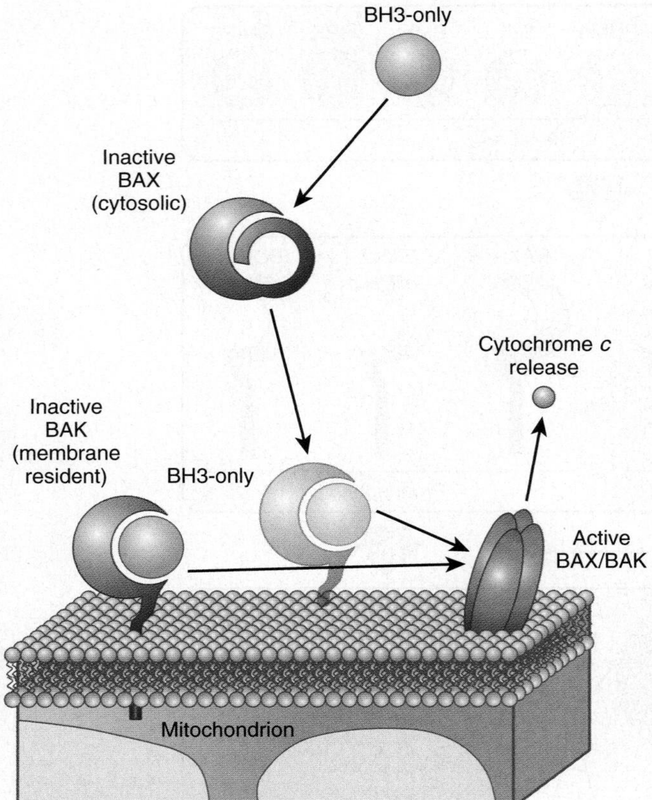

Figure 16-9 REGULATION OF BAX AND BAK (BCL2 ANTAGONIST/KILLER) OLIGOMERIZATION. BAX is a cytosolic protein that inserts into mitochondria and oligomerizes upon receipt of a death stimulus. Membrane resident BAK monomers are held in check in healthy cells and are activated to form oligomers during apoptosis.

parameter in affecting the threshold for apoptosis.[16,17] This is consistent with the ability of multiple members of this family to localize to the ER. ER Ca^{2+} content is a chief determinant of the amount of Ca^{2+} that can be released in the cytosol and thus constitutes an important regulator of Ca^{2+} signals known to control a myriad of cellular functions, including survival and death. The ER Ca^{2+} dynamics directly affect the function of mitochondria because these organelles are in close proximity, and mitochondria take up Ca^{2+} released by the ER. Ca^{2+} stimulates important enzymes in the tricarboxylic acid (TCA) cycle and influences oxidative phosphorylation and ATP synthesis by mitochondria. Supraphysiologic levels of Ca^{2+}, however, can prompt the opening of a mitochondrial innermembrane large conductance channel known as the permeability transition (PT) pore, which can eventually cause the swelling and rupture of mitochondria.

Cells overexpressing BCL-2 or deficient for both BAX and BAK show lower levels of ER Ca^{2+} and consequently lower Ca^{2+} entry into the mitochondrion. Lower ER Ca^{2+} content in these cells is associated with higher rate of ER Ca^{2+} leak. Consequently, Ca^{2+} mobilizing death stimuli specifically require the function of BAX and BAK at the ER. Genetic and pharmacologic approaches demonstrated that reduced ER Ca^{2+} content and inhibition of IP3R-mediated Ca^{2+} release is an important component of the prosurvival effect of antiapoptotic BCL-2 proteins, which is reversed by the proapoptotic members of the family. Evidence suggests that the effect of multidomain anti- and proapoptotic BCL-2 proteins on ER Ca^{2+} is likely independent of their pore-forming properties observed in synthetic membranes. Rather, modulation of ER Ca^{2+} content by BCL-2 proteins is mediated, at least in part, by their direct or indirect modulation of IP3R and SERCA.[16] The functional consequence of these interactions in regulation of ER Ca^{2+} handling and the underlying molecular mechanisms are under active investigation.

NONAPOPTOTIC ROLES FOR BCL-2 FAMILY PROTEINS

Beyond regulating apoptosis, BCL-2 family proteins may have other physiologic roles.[18] Through its association with glucokinase (hexokinase IV), the BH3-only protein BAD has been shown to regulate glycolysis, glucose-driven mitochondrial respiration, and glucose homeostasis in vivo.[13] BID, on the other hand, is a downstream substrate for DNA damage checkpoint kinases ATM/ATR and plays a role in intra-S phase checkpoint separate from its role in apoptosis. BAX and BAK influence the dynamics of mitochondrial tubules in healthy cells by controlling mitochondrial fusion and fission, processes known to dynamically control the mitochondrial network impacting the efficiency of fuel oxidation, ATP synthesis, and Ca^{2+} buffering. The above findings are but three examples of an emerging notion that BCL-2 family members are integral component of cellular homeostatic pathways and carry functions separate from their capacity to regulate apoptosis. By being embedded in these processes, they act as critical checkpoints for death when cellular homeostasis is violated.

DEATH RECEPTOR SIGNALING AND THE EXTRINSIC PATHWAY OF APOPTOSIS

Death receptors are expressed on many cell types, especially the immune system, where they have apoptotic and nonapoptotic functions, depending on cell context.[19] The cytoplasmic sequences of members of the death receptor superfamily all contain the death domain (DD 80 aa) protein-interaction motif. After being clustered by receptor–ligand interaction, the DD serves to nucleate formation of DISC for initiator caspases (caspases 8 and 10) with distinct protein interaction motifs in their long prodomains (see earlier discussion).

There are six mammalian death receptors, TNFR1, Fas, DR3, DR4 (TRAILR1), DR5 (TRAILR2), and DR6. Signaling through TNFR1 and DR3 is predominantly proinflammatory, but the remaining death receptors principally activate cell death pathways. The extracellular segments contain several cysteine-rich domains forming an extended structure stabilized by disulfide bonds. Death receptor ligands share a TNF homology domain and bind as trimers to the corresponding receptors. All known ligands are expressed as type II transmembrane proteins and are subject to limited proteolysis generating soluble forms. In most cases, soluble ligands are inferior to membrane-bound forms for receptor activation. Thus, cell–cell contacts are necessary for death-receptor signaling, justifying the characterization of subsequent apoptotic deaths as "fratricides."

In the simplest example, binding of Fas ligand to CD95/Fas receptor triggers clustering and allosteric conformational activation of an apparently trimeric receptor. An adaptor protein, FADD, binds at the Fas cytoplasmic domain using homotypic DD associations. Similarly, procaspase-8 (or procaspase-10) is bound to FADD by homotypic DED interactions. The induced proteolytic activity of procaspase-8 associated with the DISC appears to be sufficient for auto-processing in trans of neighboring procaspase molecules. A NH2-proximal cleavage separates the caspase-8 prodomain from the catalytic subunits, allowing untethering of active caspase-8 from the DISC and initiation of a cascade of effector caspase processing. Certain cells (e.g., thymocytes) can bypass Bcl-2 interdiction at the mitochondria and activate sufficient effector caspases downstream of death receptor signaling to kill cells (type I cells). Others (e.g., hepatocytes) rely on an amplification loop in which BID cleavage triggers mitochondrial apoptosis (type II cells).

Superimposed on this three-component model are additional factors that can substitute for one of the core components. FLIP (FLICE/caspase-8 inhibitory protein) is homologous to caspase-8 but devoid of protease activity (the active site cysteine is replaced). Different splice forms of FLIP retain the DED motif and compete with caspase-8 for binding to FADD. The long splice variant of FLIP, $FLIP_L$, forms heterodimers with caspase-8. Caspase-8 bound to $FLIP_L$

has catalytic activity but is processed inefficiently and remains associated with the DISC. Importantly, the caspase-8-FLIP$_L$ heterodimer is unable to cleave caspase-3 or BID. Thus, FLIP can either suppress caspase-8 activation or allow local, nonapoptotic activity. Moreover, FLIP$_L$ is also a substrate for caspase-mediated cleavage in the DISC. The cleaved product may assist with the recruitment of RIP1 kinase to the DISC, promoting activation of NF-κB and MAPKs (see above). Rapid turnover of FLIP explains the sensitization of death receptor–induced apoptosis by protein synthesis inhibition.

Recent evidence indicates that the signaling output of TNFR1 and other death receptors arises from distinct complexes.[19] The TNFR1-bound complex triggers apoptosis or NF-κB/MAPK signaling depending on the level and splice form of FLIP expressed. Notably, NF-κB upregulates expression of FLIP in a positive feedback pathway. Alternatively, a cytosolic complex lacking the TNFR1 is established after d-ubiquitination of RIP1 kinase by the CYLD deubiquitinase. This complex, designated the ripoptosome, is also capable of apoptosis signaling via caspase-8 but in the absence of caspase-8 (or presence of caspase inhibitors) triggers necroptosis, a programmed necrosis pathway characterized by cell swelling and rupture.[20] This requires association with another RIP kinase family member, RIP3. Curiously, deletion of both caspase-8 and RIP1/RIP3 is synthetically viable in mice, indicating that the embryonic lethality associated with caspase-8 is attributable to RIP1/RIP3-dependent necroptosis.[19] The downstream targets of RIP1/RIP3 in necroptosis are unknown at present. Similarly, the mechanism of caspase-8 suppression of necroptosis is unknown, although FLIP is required. Necrostatin 1, a RIP1 kinase inhibitor, is a potent inhibitor of necroptosis.[20]

Two arenas where death receptors have physiologic roles involve lymphocytes. Activation-induced cell death upon antigen restimulation involves Fas receptor signaling. Fas ligand (FasL) and Fas are induced during T-cell activation downstream of lck and NF-κB. Engagement of Fas on one cell by Fas ligand on a second cell triggers apoptosis. Autocrine suicide from FasL and Fas on the same cell has also been reported. Thus, the Fas–FasL system provides an upper limit on the density of activated T cells at sites of inflammation. Lymphocyte cell death is also directed by FasL expression on dissimilar cells. Fas expression in germinal center B lymphocytes appears to play a role in eliminating cells bearing self-reactive surface immunoglobulin because mice expressing Fas only on T lymphocytes acquire high levels of autoantibodies. In this case, FasL expression on T cells may deliver the fatal blow. T lymphocytes can also be eliminated by FasL expressed on nonlymphoid cell types.

SPECIFIC APOPTOTIC PATHWAYS

Unfolded Protein Response

Protein stress responses have been recently recognized to link into apoptotic pathways. These highly conserved mechanisms provide feedback fidelity control of protein folding, glycosylation, and secretory pathways in the ER and other subcellular compartments. Multiple inputs (amino acid deficiency, glucose deprivation, calcium dysregulation, proteasomal activity) trigger this pathway via their effects on ER protein folding. Protein stress responses are a recent addition to apoptotic pathways. These highly conserved mechanisms provide feedback fidelity control of protein folding, glycosylation, and secretory pathways in the ER.

Three protein sensors—PERK (protein kinase-like ER kinase), ATF-6 (activating transcription factor 6), and IRE1 (inositol requiring transmembrane kinase/endonuclease 1)—are triggered in response to unfolded proteins and activate a homeostatic process that reduces production of new client proteins for the ER folding machinery, helps refold misfolded proteins, and degrades protein aggregates.[21] The activity of these sensors is normally held dormant because of association with the ER chaperone BiP. During UPR, BiP is bound and sequestered by unfolded proteins, leading to derepression of each UPR sensor. PERK is activated by dimerization and autophosphorylation to subsequently phosphorylate the translation initiation factor eIF2α, leading to inhibition of general protein translation and selective increase in ATF-4 translation. The transcription factor ATF-4 in turn increases expression of select chaperones and antioxidant defense genes. ATF-6 is activated upon translocation to the Golgi and subsequent proteolytic cleavage to a fragment that translocates to the nucleus and binds the UPR response element found in the promoters of target genes. Another UPR sensor, the bifunctional protein kinase IRE1, is activated by dimerization and transphosphorylation, leading to stimulation of its inherent endoribonuclease activity and processing of mRNA encoding the basic leucine zipper transcription factor XBP-1 (X-box binding protein-1). XBP-1 together with ATF-6 regulates transcription of additional genes required for UPR, including chaperones, folding enzymes, protein disulfide isomerase (PDI), ER-associated degradation (ERAD) components, and autophagy genes. Increased ERAD components and autophagy help clear unfolded protein, protein aggregates, and damaged organelles. Remarkably, increased ER biogenesis is also part of the UPR transcriptional program to ensure sufficient ER mass matches this protein quality control response. If the integrated outcome of these signaling pathways does not salvage the ER load of unfolded and aggregated proteins, these same UPR sensors can engage the intrinsic pathway of apoptosis.[16] P53 and CHOP/GADD153, a transcription factor induced by ATF-4, initiate an ER stress-associated transcription program that is marked by changes in expression levels of several BCL-2 family members, death receptors such as FAS and DR5, and attenuation of AKT survival pathway. In addition, recruitment of the adaptor protein TRAF-2 to IRE1 may further sensitize cells to ER-stress mediated apoptosis through activation of ER-linked caspases or c-Jun-terminal kinase (JNK). JNK-1 phosphorylation of BCL-2 inhibits its survival function.

Emerging evidence from multiple experimental systems indicates that select protein modulators of UPR can be both prosurvival or prodeath depending on the extent of ER damage or the duration of UPR. The discovery of BAX and BAK association with IRE1 and modulation of its downstream effectors, such as XBP-1, suggest cross talk between BCL-2 family proteins and UPR.[22] Importantly, genetic reconstitution of DKO cells with an ER-targeted BAK restored signaling to XBP-1, suggesting that the role of BAX and BAK in UPR is distinct from their function at mitochondria. How BAX and BAK modulate IRE1 activity and signaling and whether they execute a direct role or an accessory function during each of the adaptive and protective or apoptotic phases of UPR and ER stress remain to be determined.

Oncogene-Induced Apoptosis

Hyperactivity of mitogenic oncogenes such as Myc, adenovirus E1A, and Ras triggers a common pathway of p53 accumulation via induction of the ARF tumor suppressor gene. p14ARF (or p19ARF in mice) is encoded by an alternative reading frame in the p16INK4a locus. ARF inhibits Mdm2, the p53 E3 ubiquitin ligase, and exhibits p53-independent functions, including binding to Myc and E2F transcription factors, inhibiting transactivation of target genes. The nature of the oncogenic stress leading to induction of ARF is still poorly understood but may involve DNA replication stress.

Autophagy

The main function of survival factor signaling is to support growth and proliferation through activation of metabolism, including regulation of glucose uptake, glycolysis, and mitochondrial membrane potential.[23] PI3 kinase activation downstream of growth factor receptors, including activation of the serine/threonine kinase AKT, is essential in mediating the metabolic effect of growth factors. Consequently, growth factor withdrawal is associated with a decline in metabolism, including a drop in cellular ATP levels, blunted glycolytic rates, decrease in O_2 consumption, inhibition of protein synthesis, and induction of apoptosis.

In response to such metabolic stress and nutrient starvation, the cell activates a homeostatic pathway known as autophagy (from Greek meaning to eat ["phagy"] oneself ["auto"]). Autophagy is primarily a housekeeping mechanism that normally serves to degrade long-lived proteins and damaged organelles. It involves the formation of a double membrane vesicle termed the *autophagosome*, which engulfs cytoplasmic cargo followed by fusion with the lysosome and subsequent degradation of internal contents. Autophagy is best known as a response to starvation, in which the recycling of proteins and organelles supplies required nutrients to the cell.[24,25] This process is regulated by an evolutionarily conserved set of proteins that ultimately orchestrate the recruitment of protein and organelle cargo to vesicles that will deliver their contents to lysosomes. Autophagy serves multiple functions, including tissue remodeling during development in addition to survival in face of nutrient starvation or other environmental stress.[24,25]

The survival signaling pathway and autophagy are hardwired to preserve the cellular bioenergetic balance. Survival signaling inhibits autophagy. Downstream of AKT, the mTOR (mammalian target of rapamycin kinase) serves as a nutrient sensor that is activated by high levels of ATP, glucose, or amino acids and in turn stimulates protein synthesis and inhibits autophagy. In the presence of growth factors and extracellular nutrients, mTOR inhibits autophagy through inactivation of ATG1, an autophagy-related serine/threonine kinase that is important for autophagy induction. During nutrient starvation the activity of mTOR is inhibited by AMPK (adenosine monophosphate–activated protein kinase), another nutrient sensor kinase that is activated when the ratio of ATP to AMP decreases during metabolic stress. Through inactivation of mTOR, AMPK releases the brake on autophagy. Upon cellular metabolic decline and nutrient starvation, breakdown of organelles and proteins in autophagosomes produces amino acids and metabolites that can then feed into the mitochondrial TCA cycle, sustaining the production of $FADH_2$ and NADH, ensuring that the flow of electrons through the mitochondrial respiratory chain complexes remain uninterrupted. The bioenergetic benefits of autophagy are temporary until the metabolic stress is eliminated (e.g., growth factor or oxygen availability). Inactivation of autophagy during metabolic decline and nutrient stress leads to apoptosis unless apoptosis is inactivated (e.g., BAX/BAK deficiency), in which case cell death occurs through necrosis. Whether autophagy is primarily a form of cell death or a means of cellular survival is the subject of intense investigation. Current findings support the notion that autophagy is primarily a self-limiting survival pathway and a temporary adaptive response during metabolic stress. Current findings support the notion that autophagy is primarily a self-limiting survival pathway, which can promote cell death if not terminated.

The interrelationship between apoptosis, autophagy, and necrosis carries significant relevance in tumor settings, where defects in the apoptotic pathway (e.g., overexpression of BCL-2 or BAX/BAK deficiency) and abnormal upregulation of proliferation (e.g., constitutive activation of PI3 kinase/AKT pathway) are common.[24] Before vascularization, malignant cells in the center of tumors are exposed to hypoxia and metabolic stress, where autophagy meets the bioenergetic demands of tumor cells until vascularization supplies oxygen and nutrients. When exposed to hypoxia and nutrient limitation, such apoptosis-resistant tumor cells cannot undergo autophagy because of constitutive activation of AKT. They revert instead to necrosis, which through inflammation and stimulation of cytokine and chemokine production has been proposed to initiate a cellular repair program analogous to wound healing, further promoting proliferation and angiogenesis. Indeed, necrotic tumors are known to have a poor prognosis. These findings also explain, in part, why defects in autophagy are tumorigenic despite the notion that autophagy is primarily a survival pathway during metabolic stress.

CLINICAL APPLICATIONS

Abnormal regulation of cell death pathways is believed to contribute significantly to several diseases associated with excess cell number or function (e.g., neoplasia, autoimmune disorders) or accelerated cell loss (bone marrow failure syndromes, neurodegenerative diseases). The clearest supporting evidence is linkage to an altered gene sequence or epigenetic alteration followed by mechanism testing in cellular and animal models. As previously discussed, *Bcl-2* gene rearrangement is associated with t(14;18) in follicular B-cell lymphomas, leading to transcriptional activation and high expression levels. Mutations in the BAX coding region are found in approximately 50% of colorectal and gastric cancers associated with mismatch repair defects, representing frame-shift mutations at a poly(G)8 tract in the coding region.

One of the anticipated benefits of basic research on cell death pathways is the ability to selectively manipulate cell survival or cell death through rational drug design. Members of the Bcl-2 protein family, p53, and caspases have been targets of intensive efforts at drug discovery and design. Two small molecule inhibitors of Bcl-2 and related antiapoptotic proteins (BCL-X_L and MCL-1) have advanced to phase I to II clinical trials for chronic lymphocytic leukemia, Hodgkin and non-Hodgkin lymphoma, and myelofibrosis.[26,27] These and several other inhibitors in late preclinical development bind to the hydrophobic groove in similar manner to proapoptotic BH3 peptides and are understood to act by preventing antiapoptotic proteins from sequestering proapoptotic BH3-only proteins. In addition, a broad-spectrum oxamyl dipeptide caspase inhibitor has completed phase II trials in treatment-resistant hepatitis C and orthotopic liver transplantation.[28]

FUTURE DIRECTIONS

Apoptosis is an evolutionarily conserved, highly regulated mechanism for maintaining homeostasis in multicellular organisms. Numerous signals are capable of modulating cell death. After a death stimulus, the signal is propagated and amplified through the activation of caspases, culminating in the ordered disassembly of the cell. The process may transpire through an intrinsic, mitochondria-dependent pathway, or an extrinsic pathway depending on the death signal and cell type involved. The BCL-2 family of proteins is situated upstream of irreversible cell damage in the apoptotic pathway, providing a pivotal checkpoint in the fate of a cell after a death stimulus. The proapoptotic molecules BAX and BAK undergo an allosteric conformational activation to permeabilize mitochondria upon receipt of a death stimulus. BH3 only members connect distinct upstream signal transduction pathways with the common, core apoptotic pathway. The distribution and responsiveness of the BH3-only members suggests that they function as sentinels for recognizing cellular damage. For example, BID amplifies minimal caspase-8 activation, and BAD patrols for metabolic stress after loss of critical survival factors or glucose. This model explains how seemingly diverse cellular injuries converge on a final common pathway of cell death.

REFERENCES

1. Pop C, Salvesen GS: Human caspases: Activation, specificity, and regulation. *J Biol Chem* 284:21777, 2009.
2. Crawford ED, Wells JA: Caspase substrates and cellular remodeling. *Annu Rev Biochem* 80:1055, 2011.
3. Mace PD, Riedl SJ: Molecular cell death platforms and assemblies. *Curr Opin Cell Biol* 22:828, 2010.
4. Wilson NS, Dixit V, Ashkenazi A: Death receptor signal transducers: Nodes of coordination in immune signaling networks. *Nat Immunol* 10:348, 2009.
5. Schroder K, Tschopp J: The inflammasomes. *Cell* 140:821, 2010.
6. Algeciras-Schimnich A, Barnhart BC, Peter ME: Apoptosis-independent functions of killer caspases. *Curr Opin Cell Biol* 14:721, 2002.
7. Gyrd-Hansen M, Meier P: IAPs: From caspase inhibitors to modulators of NF-kappaB, inflammation and cancer. *Nat Rev Cancer* 10:561, 2010.
8. Chipuk JE, Moldoveanu T, Llambi F, et al: The BCL-2 family reunion. *Mol Cell* 37:299, 2010.

9. Danial NN, Korsmeyer SJ: Cell death: Critical control points. *Cell* 116:205, 2004.
10. Youle RJ, Strasser A: The BCL-2 protein family: Opposing activities that mediate cell death. *Nat Rev Mol Cell Biol* 9:47, 2008.
11. Leber B, Lin J, Andrews DW: Still embedded together binding to membranes regulates Bcl-2 protein interactions. *Oncogene* 29:5221, 2010.
12. Shamas-Din A, Brahmbhatt H, Leber B, et al: BH3-only proteins: Orchestrators of apoptosis. *Biochim Biophys Acta* 1813:508, 2011.
13. Danial NN: BAD: Undertaker by night, candyman by day. *Oncogene* 27:S53, 2008.
14. Oltersdorf T, Elmore SW, Shoemaker AR, et al: An inhibitor of Bcl-2 family proteins induces regression of solid tumours. *Nature* 435:677, 2005.
15. Walensky LD, Kung AL, Escher I, et al: Activation of apoptosis in vivo by a hydrocarbon-stapled BH3 helix. *Science* 305:1466, 2004.
16. Heath-Engel HM, Chang NC, Shore GC: The endoplasmic reticulum in apoptosis and autophagy: Role of the BCL-2 protein family. *Oncogene* 27:6419, 2008.
17. Orrenius S, Zhivotovsky B, Nicotera P: Regulation of cell death: The calcium-apoptosis link. *Nat Rev Mol Cell Biol* 4:552, 2003.
18. Danial NN, Gimenez-Cassina A, Tondera D: Homeostatic functions of BCL-2 proteins beyond apoptosis. *Adv Exp Med Biol* 687:1, 2010.
19. Oberst A, Green DR: It cuts both ways: Reconciling the dual roles of caspase 8 in cell death and survival. *Nat Rev Mol Cell Biol* 12:757, 2011.
20. Yuan J, Kroemer G: Alternative cell death mechanisms in development and beyond. *Genes Dev* 24:2592, 2010.
21. Ron D, Walter P: Signal integration in the endoplasmic reticulum unfolded protein response. *Nat Rev Mol Cell Biol* 8:519, 2007.
22. Hetz C, Martinon F, Rodriguez D, et al: The unfolded protein response: Integrating stress signals through the stress sensor IRE1α. *Physiol Rev* 91:1219, 2011.
23. DeBerardinis RJ, Lum JJ, Hatzivassiliou G, et al: The biology of cancer: Metabolic reprogramming fuels cell growth and proliferation. *Cell metabolism* 7:11, 2008.
24. Karantza-Wadsworth V, Patel S, Kravchuk O, et al: Autophagy mitigates metabolic stress and genome damage in mammary tumorigenesis. *Genes Dev* 21:1621, 2007.
25. Levine B, Kroemer G: Autophagy in the pathogenesis of disease. *Cell* 132:27, 2008.
26. Manion MK, Fry J, Schwartz PS, et al: Small-molecule inhibitors of Bcl-2. *Curr Opin Investig Drugs* 7:1077, 2006.
27. Shore GC, Viallet J: Modulating the bcl-2 family of apoptosis suppressors for potential therapeutic benefit in cancer. *Hematology Am Soc Hematol Educ Program* 226, 2005.
28. Linton SD, Aja T, Armstrong RA, et al: First-in-class pan caspase inhibitor developed for the treatment of liver disease. *J Med Chem* 48:6779, 2005.

PART III

Immunologic Basis of Hematology

CHAPTER 17

OVERVIEW AND COMPARTMENTALIZATION OF THE IMMUNE SYSTEM

Leland D. Powell, Peter Chung, and Linda G. Baum

The human immune system is assigned the seemingly impossible role of keeping at bay the universe of pathogens seeking to invade and take advantage of the permissive conditions found in mammals for growth. It also plays a less celebrated but equally important role in the clearance of dead cells and tissues, promoting wound healing, and recognition of transformed cells. It is a complex, multilayered system that has evolved over millions of years, and early vestiges of our current immune system can be found in simple invertebrate species. The tasks assigned to it are to recognize and rapidly neutralize invading pathogens and their toxins, with minimal damage to host tissues in the process; to recognize new pathogens, including those with a high degree of likeness to the host; to discriminate between trace amounts of virulent organisms or toxins and more abundant amounts of foreign yet benign dietary or environmental structures; and to distinguish between healthy viable cells and apoptotic or necrotic cells. Disorders that are the consequence of immune under- or over-reactivity are found in all medical specialties. Methods of manipulating the immune system in the areas of infectious disease, transplantation biology, autoimmunity, and tumor immunology are active frontiers of medical research and drug development.

Conceptually, the immune response may be divided into innate and adaptive systems (Table 17-1). The innate system is evolutionarily the oldest, with many components found in invertebrate species. It is a system of cells and constitutively expressed membrane-bound or soluble receptors on those cells that recognize specific pathogens without the requirement of prior exposure. Pathogen–receptor binding results in the immediate activation of specific protective humoral and cellular responses. In contrast, cells of the adaptive system do not mount an effective response on first encounter with a pathogen because of the limited numbers of antigen-specific T and B cells present in a naive host. However, recurrent infections or infections by pathogens that escape the innate immune system result in the expansion of populations of pathogen-specific lymphocytes (i.e., formation of immunologic memory). Although superficially separate, there is extensive cross-talk between the innate and humoral systems, so that pathogens that activate one lead to the recruitment and activation of the other.

The innate and adaptive immune systems have been characterized in depth at the cellular and molecular levels. The principal goal of these systems is defense against pathogens seeking entry through one of four anatomic sites: the respiratory, gastrointestinal, and genitourinary tracts and the skin. Consequently, immune function can be fully understood only by examining the anatomy of these four entry points and their relation to lymphatics, blood vessels, and lymphoid organs. This chapter provides an introduction to the molecular and cellular components of innate and adaptive immunity with an overview of their anatomic relationships.

THE INNATE IMMUNE SYSTEM

Pathogen Recognition Receptors and Pathogen-Associated Molecular Patterns

Pathogen recognition molecules or receptors (PRRs) are proteins that recognize and bind to pathogen-associated molecular patterns (PAMPs); they are the cornerstones of the innate immune response.[1,2] PAMPs are molecular motifs common to bacteria, fungi, and some viruses but not viable mammalian cells. They frequently are characterized by a repeating pattern of hydrophobic or charged molecules. Common PAMPS include lipopolysaccharide (LPS or endotoxin of gram-negative bacteria), peptidoglycans and teichoic acids (gram-positive and negative bacteria), mannans (fungi), single- or double-stranded RNA (viruses), and dsDNA (viruses or necrotic/apoptotic cells). An important feature of PAMPs is that they are derived from structures essential for the viability of the particular pathogen, properties that make them ideal targets for immune recognition by a host organism, which is accomplished by the PRRs (Table 17-2). PRRs are germ-line encoded and constitutively expressed, key features that distinguish them from the adaptive immune system. PRRs may be soluble proteins found in the serum, lymphatic fluid, or cell cytosol or as type I transmembrane proteins expressed on the surface of bone marrow (BM)–derived effector cells. They are also produced by epithelial cells in the gut,[3] bronchial airways,[4] renal tubules,[5] uterus,[6] skin,[7] and endothelial cells in the liver.[8] As such, they are poised at the four major portals of pathogen entry.

Pathogen recognition molecules or receptors encompass several different structural families (see Table 17-2). Two PRR families—peptidoglycan receptor proteins (PGRPs) and the Toll-like receptors (TLRs)—were first identified in *Drosophila* and only later demonstrated in vertebrate organisms.[9] In humans, four PGRPs have been identified and are secreted by neutrophils, hepatocytes, and epithelial cells on mucous membranes and defend against gram-positive and -negative organisms. Ten TLRs have been identified; their ligands include bacterial lipopeptides (TLR1, TLR2, TLR6), peptidoglycans (TLR2), LPS (TLR2, TLR4), fungal saccharides (TLR2, TLR6), ds- and ssRNA (TLR3, TLR7, TLR8), flagellin (TLR5), and dsDNA and CpG DNA fragments (TLR9).[10,11] Other PRR families include the C-type lectins (including the mannose-binding lectin [MBL] and pulmonary surfactant proteins),[12,13] dectin-1,[14] macrophage scavenger receptors, NOD-like receptors (NLRs),[15] and RNA helicases.[16] Many of these receptors are transmembrane proteins and function as cellular receptors and activation molecules, but others are soluble serum proteins and function by neutralizing or inducing the opsonization of pathogens. Other PRRs are found as soluble proteins within the cytoplasm of cells, where they recognize intracellular bacterial components resulting from lysosomal degradation or the products of replicating viruses (NLRs and RNA helicases).

Consequences of PRR–PAMP Ligation: Phagocytosis, the Cytokine Response, and Priming the Adaptive Immune Response

PRR–PAMP ligation triggers immune and inflammatory responses in three stages. In the first, ligation induces clearance of pathogens or foreign molecules by monocytes, macrophages, and neutrophils. This process is initiated by pathogen binding directly to PRRs on the surfaces of these cells or the opsonization of pathogens bound by a soluble PRR. Internalized pathogens are destroyed by a combination of hydrolytic and oxidation reactions within vacuoles inside the phagocytic cells. Phagocytosis also triggers degranulation and the

Table 17-1 Human Innate Versus Adaptive Immune System

Feature	Innate	Adaptive
Response time	Hours to days	>5 days
Expression	Constitutive	Induced by pathogen exposure
Shaped by pathogen exposure	No	Yes
Approximate number of gene products involved in direct pathogen recognition	10^2 to 10^3	10^{10} to 10^{14}
Clonal response	No	Yes
Found in invertebrate species	Yes	No

release into tissues of bactericidal or bacteriostatic molecules such as lysozyme, lactoferrin, myeloperoxidase, antimicrobial peptides, nitrous oxide, and superoxide radicals. These products are toxic to pathogens and induce a local inflammatory response that can lead to tissue injury. Other molecules released, including elastase and collagenase, participate in tissue injury and wound healing.[17-20]

The second stage is cytokine production. Despite the diversity of the PRRs, intracellularly they share common pathways, leading to the synthesis and secretion of proinflammatory cytokines, chemokines, and type I interferons (IFNs), molecules that are essential for the initiation, amplification, and maintenance of innate and adaptive immune responses. Many PRRs function by activating NF-κB (nuclear factor κ-light-chain-enhancer of activated B cells), but others signal through the caspases, IRF3/5/7, MyD88, and other kinase cascade pathways. Cytokines may be categorized according to similarities in cell source, receptor structure, or biologic consequences. In general, interleukins are produced by monocytes or macrophages, lymphocytes, or specialized or inflamed epithelial cells. They act on these and other cells to amplify the innate and initiate the adaptive immune responses. The INFs are produced by virtually all cells. Acting on T and natural killer (NK) cells, they propagate antiviral and antitumor responses. Chemokines are produced primarily by cells of the innate immune system and function dually as chemoattractants (i.e., recruiting cells) and cytokines (i.e., activating cells). Members of the tissue necrosis factor family mediate the sepsis response and cell death and participate in the development of lymphoid organs. A simplified organization of some of the better-characterized cytokines by biologic effects is presented in Table 17-3, and a more detailed discussion of some cytokines can be found in Chapter 14.

The final stage is activation of the adaptive immune response. Both by the production of cytokines, which activate lymphocytes, and by the processing, transport, and presentation of antigens directly to T cells (primarily done by dendritic cells [DCs]), PRRs and cells of the innate immune system are essential for the development of adaptive immune responses. The biology of T cells, B cells, and DCs is discussed in detail in Chapters 18 to 21.

IMMUNE DEFICIENCY CONDITIONS CAUSED BY MUTATIONS IN THE INNATE IMMUNE SYSTEM

Although studies in mice have been instrumental in characterizing the roles of many PRRs listed in Table 17-2, their significance to humans is established by diseases linked to naturally occurring mutations or polymorphisms in either the PRRs or their intracellular signaling molecules. For instance, 10 different MBL haplotypes have been identified with serum levels varying by up to 1000-fold. Low levels can be associated with increased severity of infections with encapsulated organisms in immunocompromised or chronically infected hosts.[21] Mutations or polymorphisms in TLRs are associated with sepsis response, asthma, and the rare immunodeficiency syndrome ectodermal dysplasia with immunodeficiency. Although the absolute absence of a molecule or a critical mutation (e.g., stop codon mutation) can certainly be viewed as a mutation, other polymorphisms are common and thus could be more accurately viewed in the continuum of phenotypic variation of the species.[22]

INNATE IMMUNITY AND TISSUE HOMEOSTASIS

Pathogen recognition molecules or receptors and cells of the innate immune system also play roles in normal tissue homeostasis. Specific PRRs are involved in the clearance of serum clotting factors, hormones, lysosomal hydrolases, senescent cells, and proteins and in wound healing.[23,24] The class A scavenger receptor on macrophages is involved in the internalization of oxidized low-density lipoprotein, the development of atherosclerosis, and the clearance of apoptotic T cells in the thymus.[12] Another aspect of tissue homeostasis is the surveillance against transformed or malignant cells, which involves IFN-γ, γδ T cells, NK cells, and cytotoxic T lymphocytes (CTLs).

ADAPTIVE IMMUNE RESPONSE

The adaptive immune response deals primarily with the generation of T-cell receptor (TCR) and B-cell receptor ([BCR] or immunoglobulin [Ig]) diversity. The adaptive system achieves two goals not met by the innate system: generation of a receptor repertoire far more diverse than that represented by PRRs and the amplification of specific populations of pathogen-specific cells as a consequence of pathogen exposure (i.e., generation of specific immunologic memory). Whereas innate immune function depends on germ line–encoded molecules, the adaptive immune response arises from somatic mutations in TCR and BCR/Ig genes that occur during T- and B-cell development. This process results in a remarkable diversification and amplification of the repertoire of pathogen-specific recognition molecules (see Table 17-1).

The complex steps involved in TCR and BCR/Ig generation require a close interplay between the innate and adaptive immune systems. A particular pathogen gaining entry through a specific anatomic site first encounters the innate defense. The initial response, which depends on PRRs, triggers the production of cytokines that activate resident DCs. DCs phagocytize and process the antigens by cleaving them into small peptides. These peptides are then presented on the DCs' surfaces bound to MHC molecules. T and B cells that recognize the processed antigens become activated and begin to divide. This antigen presentation step may occur at the site of pathogen exposure, or it may require the migration of antigen-containing DC from the point of pathogen entry through lymphatic channels to lymphoid tissues. Other consequences of the inflammatory response induced by the innate response include changes in vascular permeability, chemotaxis, and lymphocyte adhesion. These steps result in local inflammation and the recruitment of additional lymphocytes to the site of pathogen entry. DCs, B cells, and T cells are discussed in depth in Chapters 18 to 21.

CELLS OF THE INNATE AND ADAPTIVE IMMUNE SYSTEMS

Lymphocytes

The major lymphocyte subsets are B and T cells, and NK cells are an important but less common, a specialized lymphoid population. Lymphocytes initially arise in the BM and subsequently undergo maturation in peripheral lymphoid organs (i.e., thymus for T cells and lymph nodes [LNs], spleen, or other lymphoid tissues for B cells). Subsets of T and B cells can be identified by unique surface phenotypes, a characteristic that has been useful in understanding normal biology and in the diagnosis of inflammatory or malignant conditions.

Table 17-2 Human Pathogen Recognition Receptors

Receptor	Location	Ligands or PAMPs	Features
TLRs (leucine-rich protein)	Leukocytes and some epithelial cells in bronchial airways, urogenital tract, and gut	Cell wall components of gram-positive and -negative bacteria (peptidoglycans and lipopeptides), viral dsDNAs, ds- and ssRNAs, bacterial flagellin, and other pathogen-derived molecules	A family of 10 different proteins (TLR1–TLR10) found as transmembrane proteins on the surface of cells or internal endosomes or as free cytosolic proteins; trigger cell activation and cytokine response
CD14 (leucine-rich protein)	Soluble and membrane-bound forms found on monocytes, macrophages, and endothelial cells	LPS from gram-negative bacteria	Binding of LPS on the cell surface forms a complex, including TLR4, which results in cytokine production and the sepsis response
Serum MBL (C-type lectin)	Soluble protein found in serum and lymphatic fluid	Pathogen-derived carbohydrate structures containing mannose, fucose, or *N*-acetylglucosamine	Secreted by hepatocytes; binding to pathogen triggers complement activation and assembly of the membrane attack complex
Pulmonary surfactant proteins (C-type lectin)	Soluble proteins found extracellularly on pulmonary mucosal surfaces	Carbohydrate structures or lipid motifs on viral, bacterial, or fungal pathogens and inhaled irritants, including pollens	Secreted by alveolar type II cells and nonciliated bonchiolar epithelial cells; binding to pathogen induces opsonization and leukocyte activation (including alveolar macrophages)
Macrophage mannose receptor (C-type lectin)	Surface of monocytes and macrophages	Pathogen-derived carbohydrate structures similar to MBP	Ligand binding results in phagocytosis and monocyte or macrophage activation
NKG2 (C-type lectin)	Surface of NK cells	Carbohydrates on HLA molecules or other host molecules	Involved in recognition and destruction of virally infected or transformed host cells
Dectin-1 (C-type lectin)	Surface of macrophages, neutrophils, and DCs	β-Glucan structures on fungi and plants	Binding results in cell activation, cytokine production, and internalization of pathogen
Class A scavenger receptors (SR-A I/II/III) (Scavenger receptor family)	Monocytes, macrophages, and epithelial cells	Modified, cell wall components of gram-positive and -negative organisms	Phagocytosis of nonopsinized particles and macromolecules triggers macrophage activation and cytokine release; plays a role in the generation of atherosclerotic plaques and diabetic nephropathy
MARCO (scavenger receptor family)	More restricted macrophage populations than SR-A, including alveolar, peritoneal, and thymic macrophage populations	Similar to SR-A, including silica particles	Phagocytosis of nonopsinized particles and macromolecules triggers macrophage activation and cytokine release
RNA helicases (RIG-I, Mda-5)	Cell cytoplasm	dsRNA	Bind to dsRNA produced during intracellular replication of certain classes of viruses
CRPs and serum amyloid P (Pentraxins)	Serum proteins	Bind to and affect clearance or activation of host proteins (C1q and DNA fragments) as well as constituents of some pathogenic organisms	Secreted by the liver during early acute-phase response and influence clearance and complement activation of recognized macromolecules
Peptidoglycan recognition proteins	Soluble proteins found intracellularly in leukocyte granules or synthesized by the liver and secreted into the serum	Peptidoglycan structures	Direct bacteriocidal or bacteriostatic activity by interfering with bacterial peptidoglycan wall biosynthesis
NOD-LRR receptor family (NLR) (includes NOD, NALP, CIITA, IPAF, and NAIP proteins)	Soluble intracellular proteins	NOD1 and NOD2 bind bacterial peptidoglycan; PAMPs for other proteins not identified	Survey intracellular compartment for intracellular pathogens, binding to bacterial wall fragments produced either during bacteria proliferation or lysozomal degradation; ligand binding triggers activation of NF-κB inflammation pathway
$\alpha_v\beta_3$ (integrin)	Epithelial cells	*Trypanosome cruzi*	Binding induces opsonization and cell activation
CD11b/CD18 (also CR3) (integrin)	Monocytes, macrophages, and epithelial cells	LPS, constituents of *Mycobacterium tuberculosis,* yeast saccharides (including zymosan)	Binding induces opsonization and cell activation
Sialic acid–binding immunoglobulin-like lectins (Siglecs)	Surface receptors on onocytes, macrophages, NK cells, and myeloid cells	Sialylated complex carbohydrates (found on endogenous proteins and some pathogenic organisms)	Role for binding and phagocytosis of pathogenic organisms proposed

CIITA, Class II transcription activator; *CRP,* C-reactive protein; *DC,* dendritic cell; *HLA,* human leukocyte antigen; *IPAF,* ICE-protease activating factor; *LDL,* low-density lipoprotein; *LPS,* lipopolysaccharide; *MARCO,* macrophage receptor with collagenous domain; *MBL,* mannose-binding lectin; *MBP,* mannose binding protein; *NAIP,* neuronal apoptosis inhibitory protein; *NALP,* NACHT, LRR, and PYD containing proteins; *NF-κkB,* nuclear factor κ-light-chain-enhancer of activated B cells; *NK,* natural killer; *NLR,* NOD-like receptor; *NOD-LRR,* nucleotide-binding oligomerization domain leucine rich repeats; *PAMPs,* pathogen-associated molecular patterns; *SR-A,* scavenger receptor type A; *TLR,* Toll-like receptor.

Table 17-3 The Cytokines

Cytokines and Cellular Targets	Examples	Biologic Consequences
	Interleukins	
Monocyte and macrophages, endothelial cells	IL-1, IL-2, IL-6, IL-10, IL-13, IL-16, TNF-α	Local inflammation, cell recruitment, hepatic acute phase reaction, sepsis response
B cells	IL-2, IL-4, IL-6, IL-7, IL-9, IL-14	Recruitment, activation, differentiation of B cells
T cells (type 1 cytokines)	IFN-α/β/γ, IL-2, IL-12, IL-15	T helper(T_H)1 response: defense against intracellular pathogens
T cells (type 2 cytokines)	IL-4, IL-5, IL-6, IL-10, IL-13	T_H2 response: defense against parasitic infections
Neutrophils, epithelial cells	IL-17, IL-22	T_H17 response: defense against extracellular pathogens; mucosal inflammation and release of anti-microbial peptides, neutrophil recruitment, and autoimmunity
	Interferons	
T cells and NK cells	IFN-α, IFN-β, IFN-γ	Upregulate activity of T cells and NK cells against virally infected cells and malignant cells
	Tissue Necrosis Factors	
All cells except erythrocytes	TNF-α, TNF-β	Pyrexia, tissue hyperemia, capillary leak, sepsis/shock syndrome, enhancement of target cell effector functions, expansion of lymphoid compartments
	Chemokines	
Monocytes and macrophages, granulocytes, dendritic cells, lymphocytes	MCPs, eotaxin, TARC, MDC, MIPs, RANTES, PF4	Recruit and activate cells of innate and adaptive immune system to specific sites of pathogen exposure, inflammation, or tissue damage
	Hematopoietic Growth Factors	
Hematopoietic cells in marrow and peripheral compartments	G-CSF, GM-CSF, M-CSF, SCF	Maintenance, growth, and differentiation of hematopoietic cells

G-CSF, Granulocyte colony-stimulating factor; *GM-CSF,* granulocyte-macrophage colony-stimulating factor; *IFN,* interferon; *IL,* interleukin; *MCP,* macrophage/monocyte chemotactic protein; *M-CSF,* macrophage colony-stimulating factor; *MDC,* macrophage-derived chemokine; *MIP,* macrophage inflammatory protein; *PF4,* platelet factor 4; *RANTES,* regulated on activation, normally T-cell expressed and segregated chemokine; *SCF,* stem cell factor; *TARC,* thymus and activation–regulated chemokine; *TNF,* tumor necrosis factor.

Mature B cells express CD19 and CD20. Most B cells, called *B2 cells,* have a $CD5^-$ phenotype and require T-cell cooperation for function. A minority population of B cells, called *B1 cells,* expresses CD5, does not require T-cell help, and appears to function in pleural and peritoneal immunity. Given their $CD20^+CD5^+$ phenotype, B1 lymphocytes may be the population from which chronic lymphocytic leukemia arises. B cells represent approximately 10% of the lymphocytes in the BM or in circulation but account for up to 50% of the population in spleen and LNs.

After emerging from the BM compartment, T cells develop further into αβ T-cell or γδ T-cell populations. The αβ T cells are the most abundant subset and include $CD3^+CD8^+$ and $CD3^+CD4^+$ T-cell populations. $CD3^+CD8^+$ T cells, which develop into CTLs, are involved in defense against virally infected or transformed cells. $CD3^+CD4^+$ T cells can be further subdivided into T helper (TH)1 cells (stimulate development of CTLs), TH2 cells (stimulate isotype switching and antibody production in B cells), TH17 cells (induce or enhance tissue damage secondary to autoimmune or infectious processes), or T-regulatory (Treg) cells (control or limit autoimmune responses).[25-27] The γδ T cells are $CD3^+CD4^+CD8^-$ T cells that can develop in the thymus and the gut.[28] Because the γδ antigen receptor on this T-cell subset is rearranged embryonically before antigen exposure, these cells may function in innate immunity. The γδ T cells represent only 1% to 5% of circulating T cells but up to 50% of the T cells in certain epithelial sites (e.g., skin and intestinal tract), where their activity is influenced by local inflammation. Stimulatory and suppressive roles of γδ T cells' response to bacterial and viral infections and possibly malignant transformation have been demonstrated in experimental systems.

Natural killer cells are a distinct lymphocyte subset and comprise approximately 10% of the circulating lymphocyte population. NK cells are identifiable by their $CD3^-CD56^+$ phenotype. They function in defense against virally infected cells and transformed cells through the generation of cytotoxic cytokines, direct cytolytic activity, and antibody-dependent cellular cytotoxicity. Pathogen recognition is accomplished through three classes of receptors, including killer cell Ig receptors (KIRs), C-type lectins (CD94/NKG2s), and natural cytotoxicity receptors (NCRs).[29]

Monocytes, Macrophages, and Dendritic Cells

Monocytes develop in the BM and then circulate through the blood and lymphatics with an average half-life of 1 to 3 days before migrating into tissues and maturing into macrophages.[30,31] Macrophages can be found in all tissues, particularly at points of entry for pathogens such as the skin, respiratory tract, gastrointestinal tract, and genitourinary tract. Tissue-specific macrophage populations include Kupffer cells (liver), alveolar macrophages (lung), osteoclasts (bone), microglia (central nervous system), and type A lining cells (synovia), which can be identified morphologically and by surface immunophenotype.

Dendritic cells are specialized antigen-presenting cells (APCs). Similar to macrophages, DCs are found at points of pathogen entry, including the skin and mucosal surfaces, and locations of lymphocyte proliferation, such as germinal centers (GCs). DC biology is described further in Chapter 21.

Granulocytes

Granulocytes can be further subclassified into neutrophils, basophils, and eosinophils by the types of cytoplasmic granules that they contain. Neutrophils mature in the BM, where 80% to 90% of the body's store of mature neutrophils resides. The recruitment of neutrophils from the BM into the circulation and inflamed tissues can occur within hours of exposure to bacterial endotoxin. Neutrophil effector functions include phagocytosis and cytokine production, both of which are activated through PRR-, FcR-, or CR3-dependent triggering. Neutrophils have multiple functions, including the direct killing of foreign organisms via phagocytosis or release of hydroxylases and oxidative enzymes from primary and secondary granules, release of PRRs, and the formation of neutrophil extracellular nets (webs of degraded nucleic acids and histones), which trap organisms.[32] Neutrophils (via chemokines and cytokines) also recruit and activate the cells of the adaptive immune system (lymphocytes and DCs).

The basophilic leukocytes—mast cells and basophils—have several structural and functional similarities. They are key mediators of immediate allergic and inflammatory responses, with mast cells being more predominant in tissues and basophils in circulation. Both cell types express FcεR, which induces rapid degranulation when triggered by aggregated IgE, and have granules containing histamine, platelet-activating factor, and bioactive proteoglycans. Degranulation can be rapid, producing anaphylaxis, or sustained, inducing a more sustained inflammatory response. Differences between basophils and mast cells include the expression of receptors on basophils for IgG, C3a, and C5a and receptors on mast cells for stem cell factor, interleukin-2 (IL-2), and IL-3 and in the spectrum of cytokines produced by each cell type. Basophils and diseases related to basophils are discussed in Chapter 71.

Eosinophils are found predominantly in tissues, with a smaller fraction found in circulation. The eosinophilic granules of this subset contain hydrolytic enzymes that may be damaging to invading pathogens and host tissues. Eosinophil activation also triggers leukotriene production and the release of an array of cytokines. A role in allergic responses and defense against helminth pathogens has long been presumed according to the eosinophilia characteristic of these conditions; however, the true physiologic necessity of eosinophils has yet to be demonstrated. Eosinophils may be viewed as effector cells of the adaptive immune system because they are acutely triggered by a B-cell product (IgE) and their development in part depends on T cells. Disorders of eosinophils are discussed in Chapter 70.

Non–Bone Marrow–Derived Cells Involved in Immune Function

Populations of non–BM-derived cells function in innate immunity. Renal tubular cells and epithelial cells in the gut, bronchial airways, reproductive organs, and dermis express different PRRs. In these cells, the receptors function in pathogen clearance or by triggering pathogen-dependent inflammatory responses. Bronchial airway cells secrete pulmonary surfactants and antimicrobial peptides, creating a very localized antimicrobial barrier. Liver endothelial cells use several PRRs, including the Fcγ, scavenger, and mannose receptors, to clear senescent serum proteins and pathogens. The functions of these cells dovetail with those of the leukocytes in pathogen defense and tissue homeostasis.[5,6,8,33-35]

ANATOMY OF THE IMMUNE SYSTEM

An array of soluble mediators and a repertoire of immune cells mediate the host response to microbial pathogens, to tumors, to self-antigens in autoimmunity, and to foreign antigens in graft rejections. Where do these cells and mediators come from, and where do these interactions take place?

Immune Cell Development: Primary and Secondary Lymphoid Organs

The organs and tissues of the immune system are divided into the primary *(or generative) lymphoid organs* and *secondary (or peripheral) lymphoid organs*. The *primary lymphoid organs* consist of the BM and thymus and are the sites where cells of the innate and adaptive immune system are generated and produced. The *secondary lymphoid organs* include the spleen, LNs, and epithelial and mucosa associated lymphoid tissues such as Peyer patches in the small intestine and are the sites where the adaptive immune response is generated.

Most immune cells arise in the BM. Anatomy of the BM and hematopoiesis is discussed in detail in Chapter 8. The cellular components of the innate immune response—neutrophils, eosinophils, basophils, and monocytes—leave the BM as mature, functional cells. In contrast, the cellular components of the adaptive immune response leave the BM as immature precursors that undergo further development in the thymus or secondary lymphoid organs.

T-Cell Maturation

T-cell precursors mature into functional T cells in the thymus (Fig. 17-1).[26,36,37] The thymus is composed of lymphocytes, DCs, epithelial cells, and stromal components. The thymic stroma arises primarily

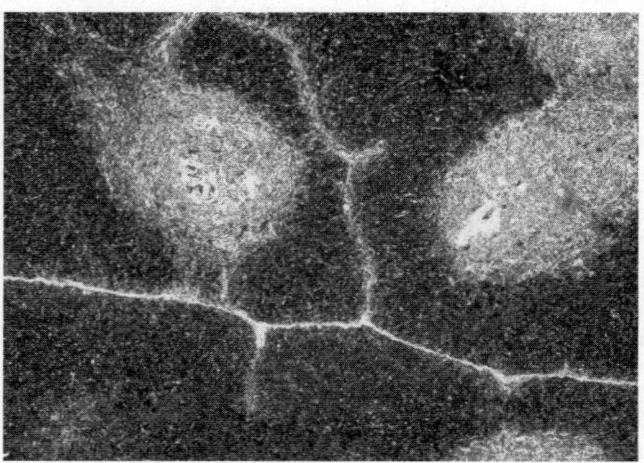

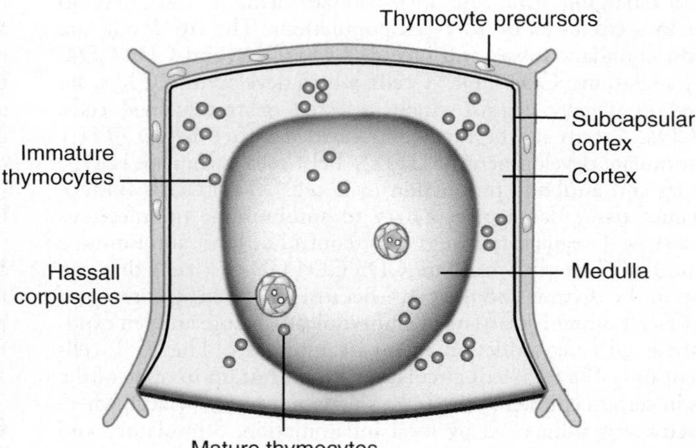

Figure 17-1 ANATOMY OF THE THYMUS. The human thymus *(left)* is composed of lobules, each separated by a thin capsule. Immediately under the capsule is a narrow zone called the *subcapsular cortex* that surrounds the larger zone of the cortex, the darkly staining region. In the center of each lobule is the medulla, the lighter staining region. In the medulla, nests of epithelial cells called *Hassall corpuscles* are visible. T-cell precursors *(right)* arising in the bone marrow migrate through the blood and enter the thymus as immature cells. During maturation in the cortex, most of the immature thymocytes fail to produce functional T-cell receptors (TCRs) and die. Cells that produce functional TCRs are positively selected to survive and migrate to the thymic medulla. Mature, naive T cells exit the medulla to the peripheral circulation.

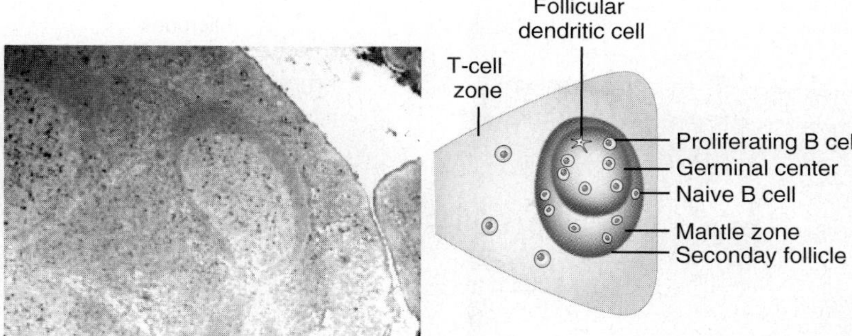

Figure 17-2 B-CELL PROLIFERATION IN LYMPH NODES. B cells primarily populate the lymphoid follicles. A section of tonsil *(left)* demonstrates a secondary follicle with a pale germinal center filled with proliferating B cells, scattered T cells, and specialized antigen-presenting cells called *follicular dendritic cells (dark staining).* The germinal center is surrounded by a darker mantle zone populated by nonproliferating B cells. Adjacent to the follicle is the T cell–rich zone of the cortex. The schematic of a section of lymph node *(right)* demonstrates a secondary follicle with a germinal center and a mantle zone. The T cells reside primarily adjacent to the follicles. However, scattered T cells can be found in the germinal center and are typically helper-T cells stimulating B-cell proliferation.

from the third and fourth pharyngeal pouches during fetal development, and the stroma is then populated with lymphocyte precursors emigrating from the BM. The stromal meshwork of the thymus, including various types of epithelial cells, is essential for thymic development. The requirement for thymic stroma in T-cell development is demonstrated in patients with DiGeorge syndrome, otherwise known as 22q11 deletion (del22q11) syndrome. These patients have deletions of one or more genes critical for fetal development, resulting in failure of involution of the third and fourth pharyngeal pouches and consequent absence of thymic stroma. Although patients with DiGeorge syndrome have T-cell precursors in the BM, they have no thymus organ and have markedly reduced numbers of mature T cells in the peripheral circulation and in tissues. As discussed in "Secondary Lymphoid Tissue," the observation that most patients with DiGeorge syndrome do have small numbers of circulating mature T cells suggests that extrathymic sites in these patients may partially substitute for the thymus in promoting T-cell maturation.

The thymus is divided histologically into two general zones, the cortex and the medulla, although these zones have microdomains thymocytes are phenotypically and functionally distinct.[37-39] Thymic precursors leave the BM, circulate in the blood, and selectively home to the thymus, entering to populate the subcapsular cortex. At this site, TCR rearrangement begins, and maturing thymocytes move to the cortex and continue to proliferate. Interactions among TCRs expressed by developing T cells and self-peptide/MHC-I complexes presented by resident thymic cortical and medullary epithelial cells (cTECs and mTECs) mediate the process known as selection.[40,41] A large fraction of thymocytes, however, fail to express a functional TCR and are never able to interact with cTECs; as a result, these cells do not receive critical survival signals from cTECs and thus die of nonselection (i.e., programmed cell death). T cells that do express a functional TCR undergo one of two fates—positive selection or negative selection. In positive selection, thymocytes that have successfully assembled a TCR with low to intermediate affinity for self-peptide–MHC complexes expressed by cTECs are selected to survive and mature. In negative selection, thymocytes bearing TCRs with a high affinity to self-peptide–MHC complexes of cTECs undergo apoptosis, resulting in the deletion of dangerous autoreactive T cells, which is proposed to reduce self-reactivity and autoimmune disease.

T cells that survive the selection process in the cortex proceed to the medulla, where they commit to a particular T-cell lineage (CD4 or CD8) and undergo further negative selection by interactions with mTECs that express tissue specific antigens promiscuously.[41-43] Negative selection by the mTECs is partially regulated by the transcription factor termed *autoimmune regulator* (AIRE). AIRE deficiency results in inadequate deletion of self reactive T lymphocytes and manifests clinically as autoimmune polyendocrinopathy–candidiasis–ectodermal dystrophy in humans (APECED).[44,45]

Only 1% to 3% of the initial thymic progenitor cells succeed in surviving the selection process and thus emigrate from the thymus as non–self-reactive, functional CD4 or CD8 cells.[41,46] T-cell development is elaborated on in Chapter 19.

B-Cell Maturation

Naive B cells leave the BM and traffic to *secondary lymphoid tissues,* where the mature cells of the adaptive immune system encounter non–self-antigens and become activated. Briefly, naive cells enter primary follicles in the cortex of the secondary lymphoid tissue, such as the LN shown in Fig. 17-2.[47] When B cells in primary follicles encounter non–self-antigens that are recognized by their surface BCR/Ig, the B cells begin to proliferate and undergo somatic hypermutation (SHM) of immunoglobulin genes in an attempt to express a higher affinity BCR. B cells bearing a high-affinity BCR are positively selected to proliferate. When B-cell proliferation begins, the primary follicle becomes a secondary follicle.[48] The secondary follicle has two general regions: (1) a GC filled with the proliferating B cells, some T cells, macrophages, and DC and a (2) surrounding mantle zone of nonproliferating B cells that have not encountered an antigen they recognize. The GC can be further divided into dark and light zones, depending on the stage of proliferation, as discussed later in "Systemwide Surveillance." Chapter 18 discusses B-cell development in depth.

ENCOUNTERS WITH ANTIGEN: THE INFLAMMATORY RESPONSE

A primary function of the immune system is to protect against microbial pathogens. The most common sites for microbes to breach the protective barriers of epithelium are the skin and the respiratory, gastrointestinal, and genitourinary tracts. These tissues directly encounter the outside world and possess complex, multifaceted mechanisms for dealing with antigens.[49,50]

The local defense system is immediately activated when pathogens disrupt the epithelial barriers in these sites. These tissues are rich in components of the innate immune system, including macrophages and DCs, which perform a surveillance function in tissues. Some tissues have specialized or unique populations of macrophages and

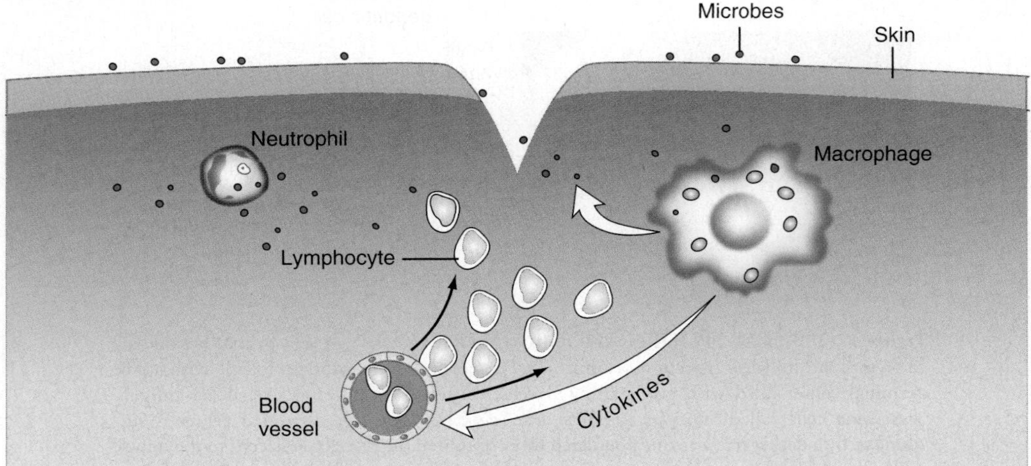

Figure 17-3 ENCOUNTERS WITH ANTIGEN. The immune system evolved primarily to protect against invading microorganisms that penetrate the epithelial coverings of the body. In this schematic, microbes entering through a break in the skin epithelium are phagocytosed by resident macrophages as the first line of defense in innate immunity. The macrophages can secrete products that are directly microbicidal as well as cytokines and other mediators that cause vasodilatation and endothelial cell separation to allow influx of soluble mediators and inflammatory cells such as neutrophils and lymphocytes into the skin. Neutrophils, as a component of innate immunity, can also directly kill microorganisms, typically by releasing granular contents. Lymphocytes responding to microbial antigens proliferate and contribute to the adaptive immune response against microbes.

DCs (see Chapter 21), although these cells have many common features in different tissues. Macrophages provide a critical first line of defense against pathogens by directly phagocytizing the microorganisms. Macrophages also send the first signals that recruit granulocytes from the circulation into the tissues (Fig. 17-3). These signals include cytokines, nitrous oxide, and leukotrienes that cause vasodilatation, endothelial cell activation, leukocyte adhesion to endothelial cells at the inflammatory site, and diapedesis of leukocytes into the tissues (see Chapter 11). The resulting exudate fluid at the site of vasodilatation is also rich in plasma proteins that participate in innate immunity, such as complement and soluble PRRs. The soluble mediators may be directly toxic to microbes or may opsonize microbes to facilitate phagocytosis and killing by granulocytes. The soluble and cellular components of the innate immune system provide the first line of defense at the tissues where pathogens invade.

The epithelial barriers also contain resident lymphocytes and plasma cells. The lymphoid cells can also respond to cytokines secreted by resident macrophages, such as IL-2, which stimulates T-cell proliferation. The ability of macrophages to secrete mediators that cause vasodilatation and recruitment of granulocytes, as well as initiate T-cell activation, illustrates the interplay between innate and adaptive immunity in tissues where antigens are encountered and underscores the point that the innate and adaptive immune systems work in concert in host defense. Resident T cells and plasma cells in the tissue can respond to antigen, with local activation of antigen-specific effector T cells and increased antibody secretion, respectively, so that the adaptive immune response is stimulated locally after pathogens are sensed by the innate immune system.

SYSTEMWIDE SURVEILLANCE: THE ROLE OF LYMPHATIC CIRCULATION

Lymphatics are an essential component of the vascular system (Fig. 17-4). Even in the absence of inflammation, a fraction of the fluid component of blood continually leaves the capillary bed during circulation because of the pressure drop between the arterial and venous sides. This fluid bathes the tissues of the body picking up antigens and cells and then drains into lymphatic channels that interdigitate in every capillary bed.

At sites of inflammation, the amount of fluid and cells draining into the local lymphatics increases because of changes in the vascular tone and permeability mediated by macrophage and neutrophil-derived chemokines, lipid mediators, and oxygen radicals. During the local inflammatory response, the exuded fluid, along with antigen-loaded DCs, T cells, and cytokines, drains from the tissues back through the lymphatic channels.

Lymphatic fluid eventually returns to blood circulation via the thoracic duct, which drains into the vena cava. However, before returning to the venous circulation, lymphatic fluid travels through the secondary lymphoid tissues and undergoes sampling for foreign antigens, thus providing a mechanism of systemic immune surveillance. The complex organization and structure of these secondary lymphoid tissues create a close interface among antigens, APCs, and lymphocytes to optimize cellular interactions to produce an efficient and robust adaptive immune response. Signals from cells within the LNs can also expand the lymphatic vessel network, again resulting in increased drainage of DCs and antigens into the LNs.[51] The movement of lymphatic fluid through secondary lymphoid tissue is an essential component of the adaptive immune system.

Lymph node anatomy is shown schematically in Fig. 17-5; the anatomy of LNs and the spleen is also discussed in Chapter 18. Fluid and cells enter the lymphatics in body tissues and gain entry to the convex surface of the LN via afferent lymphatic vessels that drain into the subcapsular sinus. Lymphatic fluid in the subcapsular sinus then courses into the trabecular sinus network that runs perpendicular to the capsule through an area called the cortex. The cortex region is composed mainly of B and T cells arranged into follicles and interfollicular zones. Follicles consist mainly of B cells, some T cells, and APCs, and interfollicular zones consist mainly of T cells and additional APCs. These zones are separate but contiguous compartments where initial B-cell and T-cell antigen encounters occur within the LN. The movement of antigen-rich fluid into these B- and T-cell zones in the cortex stimulates the proliferation of antigen-specific lymphocytes. Local B-cell proliferation in the LN further stimulates lymphatic drainage to the node.[51] In the follicles, additional processing of antigens may be carried out by local APCs, such as follicular DCs.

Follicles are functionally characterized as either primary or secondary follicles. Primary follicles are composed of nonproliferating

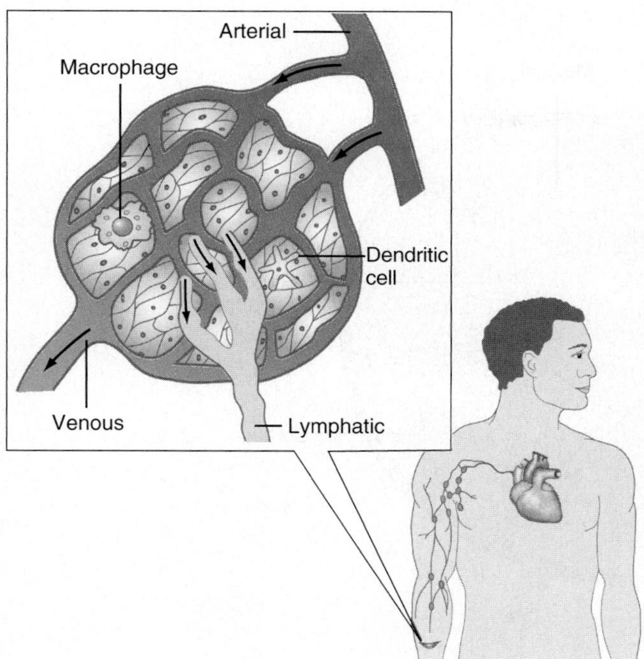

Figure 17-4 LYMPHATIC DRAINAGE IS A CRITICAL PART OF IMMUNE SURVEILLANCE. As shown in Fig. 17-3, fluid and cells leave the vasculature at sites of inflammation. Hydrostatic pressure across the capillary bed continually drives transudation of fluid from the blood into tissues. The extravasated fluid, along with antigen-presenting cells (APCs) such as macrophages and dendritic cells, collects in lymphatics *(inset)*. Lymphatics drain past series of lymph nodes *(dark ovals),* affording the APCs the opportunity to migrate to lymph nodes and stimulate lymphocytes in the nodes. Fluid in lymphatics passing through chains of lymph nodes eventually collects in the thoracic duct, which returns the fluid to the vascular circulation by draining into the vena cava.

naive B cells that have yet to encounter antigen recognized by their surface BCR/Ig complex. B-cell recognition of an antigen displayed by a Th cell or other APC results in activation and clonal expansion. A fraction of these activated proliferating B cells form GCs, which are surrounded by a mantle zone of naive B cells, which together comprise a secondary follicle.

Germinal centers are classically divided into two compartments, denoted as the dark and light zone based on their appearance under light microscopy.[52,53] Dark zones contain a high density of proliferating B cells termed *centroblasts,* which do not express surface immunoglobulin (sIg) and are located adjacent to T-cell areas.[53] The light zone are termed such, as they appear less opaque because of the reduction in cellular density secondary to the presence of an extensive loose network of follicular DCs (FDCs).[54,55] B cells in the light zone are termed *centrocytes,* which in contrast to the centroblasts, are small, nondividing B cells expressing sIg. Some of these cell types, such as centrocytes and centroblasts, are discussed in Chapter 72 in the context of lymphoid malignancies.

The GC reactions, colloquially known as the B-cell selection process, are viewed as a series of sequential events within the dark and light zone where B cells undergo cyclic shuttling and reentry to and from these two zones. The cyclic reentry model proposes that centroblasts in the dark zone undergo cell division and SHM of variable light chain genes mediated by the enzyme activation-induced cytosine deaminase (AID).[56] Next they reexpress BCR/sIg and exit the cell cycle, migrating into the light zone to interact with antigen-presenting FDCs. In light zones, B cells with increased affinity for antigen are preferentially selected for survival receiving vital signals from T follicular helper cells; in contrast, B cells with impaired or absent antigen binding undergo apoptosis and clearance by resident macrophages.[53,57] Selected centrocytes in the light zone are thought to return to the dark zone to undergo further rounds of proliferation, affinity maturation, and selection to improve the affinity of B-cell repertoire.[54] Positively selected GC B cells eventually leave the GC, differentiating into memory B cells or plasma cells possessing somatically mutated immunoglobulin genes that encode for a high-affinity BCR/Ig.[53] The genetically modified capability of B cells to generate a fast, highly specific humoral immune response upon a second encounter with the same pathogen forms the mechanistic basis of humoral memory.[52,53,55,57,58] Memory B cells may circulate through secondary lymphoid organs and colonize the splenic marginal zone. Plasma cells take residence in the BM and spleen for a long period of time.[59]

The lymphatic fluid within the cortical trabecular sinus network continues to drain toward the medullary sinus, which lies deep to the cortex, forming the central part of the LN, known as the *hilum*. The medullary sinus contains additional APCs, some T cells, and numerous plasma cells that have migrated from the cortex to the medulla. There, plasma cells may leave the LN in the lymphatic fluid via the efferent lymphatic vessel at the hilum, to traffic to peripheral tissue such as the BM. Lymphatic fluid travels through additional LNs on the way to the thoracic duct; thus, antigens and cells draining from sites of inflammation travel through chains of LNs. In the lymphatic system, trace amounts of microbial proteins or toxins, together with activated monocytes, macrophages, DCs, lymphocytes, and the cytokines produced (the direct consequence of PAMP–PRR ligation), are kept in anatomic proximity, providing numerous opportunities for the antigens to encounter antigen-specific lymphocytes and stimulate the adaptive immune response.

In addition to lymphatic fluid, blood must also travel through LNs to provide oxygen and nutrients and to deliver new B and T cells to the tissue. Although lymphatic fluid contains lymphocytes from tissues that have already encountered antigens, lymphocytes in blood are predominantly naive T cells that have emigrated from the thymus but have not yet encountered antigens. Arterial blood enters the LN at the hilum, where arterioles arborize toward each follicle. Naive T cells leave the blood to enter LNs through specialized vessels called *postcapillary venules,* which arise from follicular capillary beds, and travel through the T-cell–rich interfollicular zones.[55] Naive T cells exit from postcapillary venules into the T-cell zone, and if the naive T cells encounter antigens they recognize, the cells remain in the node to proliferate and differentiate. If the naive T cells do not encounter antigens they recognize, the cells drain by means of lymphatic fluid back to the blood and continue the circular route from the blood through LNs to lymphatics and back to blood (refer to Chapter 18 for further information on T-cell immunity).

Egress of lymphocytes from LNs and from the thymus is regulated by a specialized lipid produced in lymphoid tissue known as sphingosine-1-phosphate (S1P). Lymphocytes express S1P receptor-1 ($S1P_1$) receptors that facilitate their egress from tissues into blood. Novel immunosuppressive therapeutics are being developed that are S1P antagonists; these S1P antagonists reduce release of lymphocytes from lymphoid tissues into blood.

SECONDARY LYMPHOID TISSUE: COMMON AND UNIQUE ANATOMY AND FUNCTIONS

The spleen is an important site for B-cell development and for antigen presentation and stimulation of the adaptive immune system.[60-62] Lacking afferent lymphatics, the spleen serves to sample blood for foreign antigens (rather than lymphatic fluid), which gains access via the splenic artery. The spleen is divided into two functionally and morphologically distinct compartments, the white pulp and the red pulp. The white pulp is composed mainly of lymphoid cells and is the site of antigen detection and presentation to splenic B and T cells. The red pulp consists mainly of myeloid cells, including macrophages that ingest opsonized antigens and damaged erythrocytes from the systemic circulation. The red pulp functions also as a site of extramedullary hematopoiesis early in fetal life and is a storage

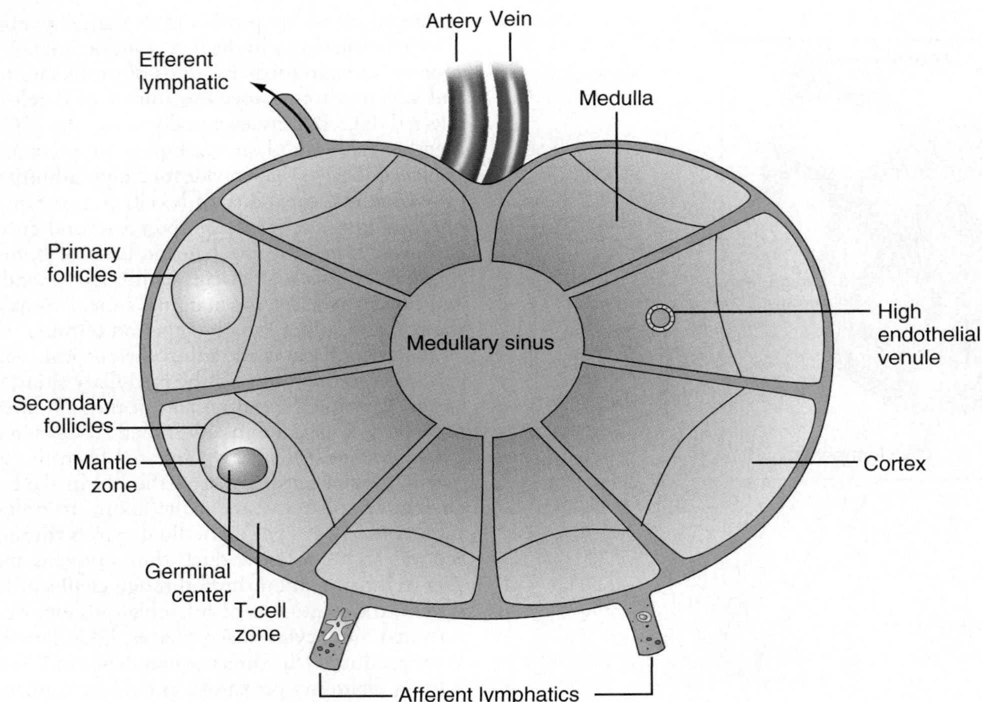

Figure 17-5 LYMPH NODE ANATOMY. The lymph node is surrounded by a capsule. Afferent lymphatics draining tissues enter the node on the convex side into the capsule. Fluid and cells drain through the node and collect in the medullary sinus, where the fluid leaves the node through efferent lymphatics to rejoin the lymphatic circulation. The outer rim of the node is called the *cortex* and contains primary follicles composed of naive, nonproliferating B cells that have not encountered antigens and secondary follicles with proliferating B cells in the germinal center. The germinal center can be subdivided into dark and light zones. Each lymph node is supplied with blood by the arterial circulation. Arterioles expand into a meshwork of capillaries within each follicle, and venous blood drains back out of the node. Naive T cells in the peripheral circulation can exit the blood and enter the lymph node through the high endothelial venules.

site for iron, erythrocytes, and platelets. Extramedullary hematopoiesis in the spleen may also occur postnatally in patients with diseases in which the BM is not competent to support hematopoietic cell development.

In many mammalian species, including humans, splenic blood flows through a unique vascular circulation that ensures the interposing of blood (and therefore bloodborne antigens) with the lymphoid areas of the white pulp. This has been best characterized in the murine model.[61,62] In this model, the splenic white pulp consists of three compartments—the periarteriolar lymphoid sheath (PALS), follicles, and the marginal zone—that interact with blood through an open sinusoidal arterial network.[61,63] The PALS is the spleen's T-cell zone and is found surrounding the central artery. Follicles in the spleen are found adjacent to the PALS and are capable of generating primary and secondary follicles with GCs as in LNs. The marginal zone, composed of subsets of B cells and macrophages, surrounds the follicles in the spleen and serves as the major route of entry of bloodborne antigens and lymphocytes from the blood into the white pulp. Unlike other organs that have a closed vascular circulation in which blood travels from arterial to venous circulation through capillary beds, branches of the splenic artery penetrate the white pulp, forming an open sinusoidal network termed the *marginal sinuses*.[63,64] From the marginal sinuses, blood filters through the white pulp regions of the spleen to be sampled by resident B and T lymphocytes. The spleen does have efferent lymphatics, and fluid and cells that do not exit through the splenic vein collect by means of lymphatics that originate in the white pulp and drain into the lymphatic circulation. Beyond the white pulp, the splenic artery sends additional branches into the red pulp for further blood antigen surveillance and filtration that is accomplished by macrophages.

In addition to LNs and the spleen, there are numerous other sites of secondary lymphoid tissue.[65] A critical part of the secondary lymphoid system is the mucosa-associated lymphatic tissue (MALT). As the name implies, the MALT is in physical proximity with the mucosa (i.e., the epithelium and associated connective tissue that line the surfaces of the body). MALT is found at sites where antigens most commonly breach these epithelial barriers: the gastrointestinal, respiratory, and genitourinary tracts. In some tissues, the MALT forms relatively large structures that can be clearly distinguished histologically, such as the Peyer patches in the ileum and in the lymphoid tissue under the epithelium of the appendix. In these sites, perhaps because of the constant stimulation by microbial pathogens in the intestine, the MALT resembles lymphatic tissue in the spleen and LNs, with well-demarcated primary and secondary follicles that contain primarily B cells and intervening T-cell rich zones.

In other tissues, such as the genitourinary tract and the salivary glands, the microscopic anatomy of the MALT may not be as well defined as seen in Peyer patches; but the stromal tissue underlying the epithelium contains numerous lymphocytes and APCs. These sites provide an additional compartment of secondary lymphoid tissue where antigens can accumulate, be processed, and be presented to lymphocytes to stimulate an adaptive immune response.

In addition to serving as part of the secondary lymphoid tissue, the MALT may also provide an alternative site of primary lymphoid tissue for T-cell development.[66] In support of this theory, it has been observed that children with DiGeorge syndrome, in whom the thymus does not develop, do have some circulating mature T cells, although the number of T cells is greatly reduced. This suggests that the T-cell precursors emigrating from the BM can mature in other sites, such as the intestine, if the thymus is absent.

Whereas the MALT constitutes a lymphoid population beneath the surface epithelium, a separate population of lymphocytes, primarily T cells, traffics directly through the epithelium in certain tissues, such as the gastrointestinal tract, on surveillance for pathogens. These intraepithelial lymphocytes (IELs) include $\alpha\beta$ T-cells and $\gamma\delta$ T-cells, and comprise 1 in every 5 to 10 cells in the intestinal epithelium. Because the lining of the intestine is the largest organ surface area of the body, IELs are one of the largest T-cell populations. These IEL T-cells are composed of different subpopulations, some of which are conventional T cells that recognize foreign antigens; others are regulatory T cells that limit the extent of an immune response and maintain immune homeostasis, a critical function in the antigen-rich milieu of the gut.[34,50]

SUGGESTED READINGS

Akira S, Uematsu S, Takeuchi O: Pathogen recognition and innate immunity. *Cell* 124:783, 2006.

Belardelli F, Ferrantini M: Cytokines as a link between innate and adaptive antitumor immunity. *Trends Immunol* 23:201, 2002.

Borregaard N: Neutrophils, from marrow to microbes. *Immunity* 33:657, 2010.

Cheroutre H: IELs: Enforcing law and order in the court of the intestinal epithelium. *Immunol Rev* 206:114, 2005.

Gowthaman U, Chodisetti SB, Agrewala JN: T cell help to B cells in germinal centers: Putting the jigsaw together. *Int Rev Immunol* 29:403, 2010.

Greaves DR, Gordon S: The macrophage scavenger receptor at 30 years of age: Current knowledge and future challenges. *J Lipid Res* 50:S282, 2009.

Kumar H, Kawai T, Akira S: Pathogen recognition by the innate immune system. *Int Rev Immunol* 30:16, 2011.

Mantovani A, Cassatella MA, Costantini C, et al: Neutrophils in the activation and regulation of innate and adaptive immunity. *Nat Rev Immunol* 11:519, 2011.

Misch EA, Hawn TR: Toll-like receptor polymorphisms and susceptibility to human disease. *Clin Sci (Lond)* 114:347, 2008.

Papayannopoulos V, Zychlinsky A: NETs: A new strategy for using old weapons. *Trends Immunol* 30:513, 2009.

Sansonetti PJ: To be or not to be a pathogen: That is the mucosally relevant question. *Mucosal Immunol* 4:8, 2011.

Steinman L: A brief history of T(H)17, the first major revision in the T(H)1/T(H)2 hypothesis of T cell-mediated tissue damage. *Nat Med* 13:139, 2007.

Trinchieri G, Sher A: Cooperation of Toll-like receptor signals in innate immune defence. *Nat Rev Immunol* 7:179, 2007.

Turvey SE, Hawn TR: Towards subtlety: Understanding the role of Toll-like receptor signaling in susceptibility to human infections. *Clin Immunol* 120:1, 2006.

Villasenor J, Benoist C, Mathis D: AIRE and APECED: Molecular insights into an autoimmune disease. *Immunol Rev* 204:156, 2005.

For complete list of references log on to www.expertconsult.com.

CHAPTER 18

B-CELL DEVELOPMENT

Kenneth Dorshkind and David J. Rawlings

B cells are the subset of lymphocytes specialized to synthesize and secrete immunoglobulin (Ig). Their name derives from the finding, made in the mid-1950s, that removal of the avian *b*ursa of Fabricius severely compromises antibody production. In contrast to birds, B-cell production in mammals occurs in the bone marrow (BM) during postnatal life. The generation of B cells in that tissue is referred to as *primary* B-cell production.

B lymphocytes, similar to all blood cells, are derived from hematopoietic stem cells (HSCs). HSCs generate B–cell–specified progenitors that mature through a series of defined stages into surface Ig–expressing B lymphocytes. These newly generated B lymphocytes then migrate into *secondary* lymphoid organs, the spleen in particular, where they undergo final maturation. At this point, the mature B cells may remain in the spleen or relocate via the circulation to additional tissues such as lymph nodes, where they are poised to respond to antigenic challenge.

The aim of this chapter is to summarize B-cell development in primary and secondary lymphoid tissues. The discussion focuses initially on primary B-cell development in the BM and the regulation of that process by local and systemic signals. The final sections of the chapter outline B-cell maturation in secondary lymphoid tissues. The information presented provides a basis for understanding abnormalities of B-cell development, such as leukemia, lymphoma, and immunodeficiency states that are discussed in other chapters. Studies in mice have contributed much to what is known about B-cell development and have served as a basis for understanding human B lymphopoiesis. Thus, although we emphasize the human literature as much as possible, frequent reference to findings in mice are made.

THE HEMATOPOIETIC HIERARCHY AND STAGES OF B-CELL DEVELOPMENT

B lymphocytes, similar to all hematopoietic cells, are derived from HSCs that can sustain long-term, multilineage blood cell production for the lifetime of the organism.[1] HSCs are able to function in this capacity because they can self-renew, thereby producing additional stem cells, as well as generate lineage committed progenitors from which mature myeloid and lymphoid cells derive (Fig. 18-1).

Advances in the development of monoclonal antibodies to leukocyte cell surface antigens and in flow cytometry have made it possible to isolate murine and human B lineage progenitors at various stages of development. For example, a cell termed the *common lymphoid progenitor* (CLP) is one of the earliest B-cell progenitors. Murine CLPs can be resolved by their lineage–negative (Lin^-) c-kit^{low} Sca-1^{low} interleukin-7 (IL-7) receptor-positive ($IL\text{-}7R^+$) phenotype while human CLPs are $CD34^+$, $CD45RA^+$, $CD7^+$, $CD10^+$ $IL\text{-}7R^+$ cells.[2,3] Lin^- indicates that the cells lack expression of determinants present on mature myeloid, erythroid, and lymphoid lineage cells. Many schemes of hematopoiesis indicate that the CLP is the precursor from which all T and B cells arise. However, an emerging view based on murine studies is that CLPs are primarily destined to generate B lymphocytes.[2]

The stages of B-cell development between the CLP and IgM^+ B cells are well defined in both mice and humans. The earliest B-lineage progenitor in both species is termed the *pro-B cell.* Ig heavy chain gene rearrangements have initiated in these cells, and if the rearrangement is successful, an Ig heavy chain of the μ class is expressed in the cytoplasm. At this stage, the cells are defined as *pre-B cells*. Finally, after light chain gene rearrangements have occurred and light chain protein is expressed, pre-B cells mature into B lymphocytes that express the assembled Ig molecule on their surface. The designation of a cell as a B lymphocyte should be restricted to cells that express surface Ig.

The phenotypic subdivision of cells within the pro-, pre- and B-cell compartments based on the differential expression of cell surface antigens is possible as shown in Fig. 18-1.[2] For example, human pro-B cells can be resolved based on their expression of CD10, CD34, and CD19. After an Ig heavy chain gene has undergone productive rearrangement and is expressed, μ heavy chain protein is detected in the cytoplasm of pre-B cells that no longer express CD34. Finally, productive rearrangement and expression of an Ig light chain gene result in maturation of pre-B cells into surface IgM expressing B-cells.[3] Developing and mature B-lineage cells also express additional cell surface determinants, which include CD20, CD21, CD22, CD24, CD38, and CD40, several of which are linked to critical intracellular signaling pathways. Antibodies against the CD20 determinant (Rituximab) are in widespread clinical use for the treatment of lymphoma and, increasingly, autoimmune diseases.

TRANSCRIPTIONAL REGULATION OF B-CELL DEVELOPMENT

The ability to resolve specific stages of B-cell differentiation has made it possible to determine when the expression of transcription factors critical for B-cell development occurs. These observations, combined with the analysis of genetically engineered strains of mice in which the genes encoding specific transcription factors have been deleted, have made it possible to obtain a sophisticated understanding of the transcriptional regulation of B-cell development.[4]

Early blood cell development is dependent on PU.1, an Ets family member. Mice in which PU.1 is not expressed produce erythroid and megakaryocytic but not monocytic, granulocytic, and lymphoid cells. As a result of this severe defect, *PU.1* knock-out mice die during embryonic development. The developmental potential of hematopoietic cells is specified toward a lymphoid fate by products of the *Ikaros* gene. Ikaros is an interesting transcription factor because rather than activating gene expression, it acts as a repressor by associating with transcriptionally silent genes in foci containing heterochromatin.

Further specification toward the B-cell lineage is dependent on expression of additional transcription factors that include early B-cell factor (EBF) and the *E2A*-encoded splice variants E12 and E47. Each of these DNA-binding proteins regulates the expression of a variety of B-lineage target genes and induces expression of additional transcription factors that play a role in B-cell development. That EBF and E2A expression play a critical role in B lymphopoiesis has been demonstrated by the fact that mice in which they are not expressed exhibit an almost complete block in B-cell development at the pro-B-cell stage.

Early B-cell factor– and E2A-expressing progenitors can still exhibit some non-B lineage potential, indicating that the expression

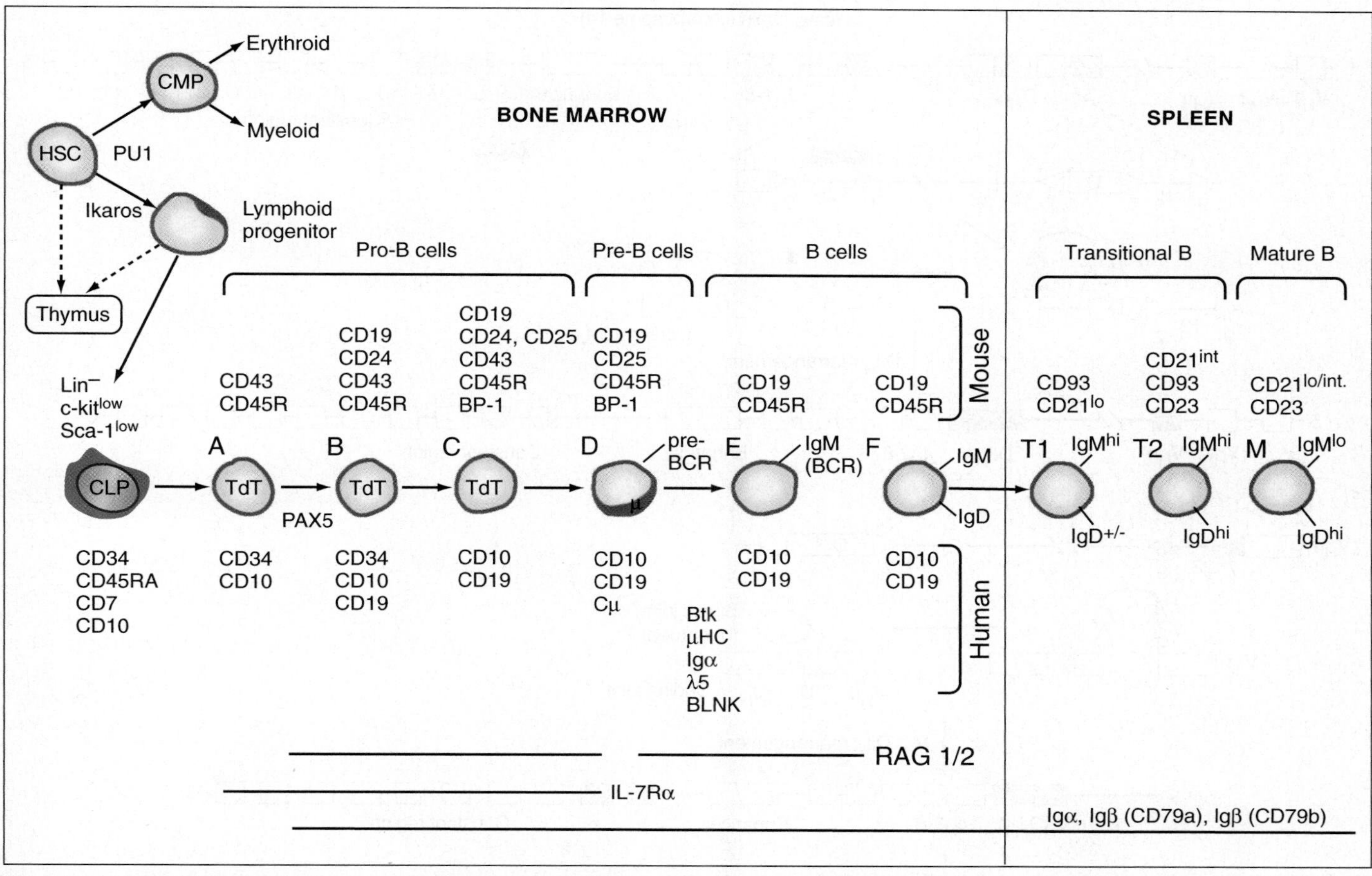

Figure 18-1 HEMATOPOIESIS WITH AN EMPHASIS ON B-CELL DEVELOPMENT. Stages of human and murine B-cell development and selected cell surface, cytoplasmic, and nuclear determinants expressed at various stages of differentiation are shown. The *dashed lines* leading to the thymus indicate that the precise identity of the bone marrow (BM)–derived, thymus-seeding cells is unclear. After leaving the BM, newly produced B cells migrate to the spleen and mature through transitional cell stages into marginal zone or follicular B cells. The phenotype of mature B cells refers to the latter population. *CLP,* common lymphoid progenitor; *CMP,* common myeloid progenitor; *HSC,* hematopoietic stem cell; *Ig,* immunoglobulin; *M,* mature, naïve B cells; *RAG,* recombinase-activating gene; *T1,* transitional 1 B cells; *T2,* transitional 2 B cells.

of these DNA binding proteins does not result in absolute commitment of cells to the B lineage. Instead, this is dependent on expression of the Pax5 transcription factor. Phenotypically identifiable B-cell precursors are present in *Pax5* knock-out mice, and when placed under appropriate conditions, they can differentiate into myeloid, T, and natural killer (NK) cells. However, if the gene encoding Pax5 is introduced into Pax5-deficient precursors, this developmental promiscuity is no longer observed. Thus, a critical function of Pax5 is to suppress non–B lineage potential.[5] One way in which this is accomplished is by extinguishing expression of myeloid growth factor receptors, such as those for macrophage colony-stimulating factor. Pax5 also may inhibit the T-cell potential of lymphoid-restricted progenitors by antagonizing expression of Notch1, a cell-surface receptor whose stimulation activates signaling pathways required for commitment to the T-cell lineage. In addition to regulating commitment to the B-cell lineage, continued Pax5 expression is necessary to maintain lineage fidelity even in relatively mature B cells.

DEVELOPMENTAL CHECKPOINTS DURING B-CELL DIFFERENTIATION

As cells mature from pro-B cells into B lymphocytes, they pass through two critical checkpoints. The first occurs at the pro-B to pre-B-cell transition and is dependent on successful recombination of the Ig heavy chain gene and expression of Ig heavy chain protein. The second occurs at the pre-B to B-cell transition, where signaling through the pre-B-cell receptor (pre-BCR [B-cell receptor]) leads to expression of light chain protein and surface expression of the mature BCR.[6] The events that must occur at each of these checkpoints for a B-cell progenitor to survive and mature are discussed in the following sections.

THE PRO-B TO PRE-B CELL TRANSITION

The expression of Ig heavy chain protein is dependent on the functional rearrangement of an Ig heavy chain gene.[7] If this occurs successfully, Ig heavy chain protein of the μ class is expressed in the cytoplasm of pre-B cells.

The genes that encode Ig heavy chain protein are located on human chromosome 14 (Fig. 18-2). The heavy chain gene consists of distinct variable (V), diversity (D), joining (J), and constant (C) regions. The V region genes are located at the 5′ end of the Ig heavy chain locus, and each consists of approximately 300 base pairs. These genes, which are separated by short intron sequences, are organized into seven families based on sequence homology. There are about 25 human D region genes located 3′ to the V region. These also are grouped into families, and at least 10 have been described. Downstream of the D region are six human J region genes. Finally, 10 C region genes representing alternative Ig isotypes are arranged in tandem.

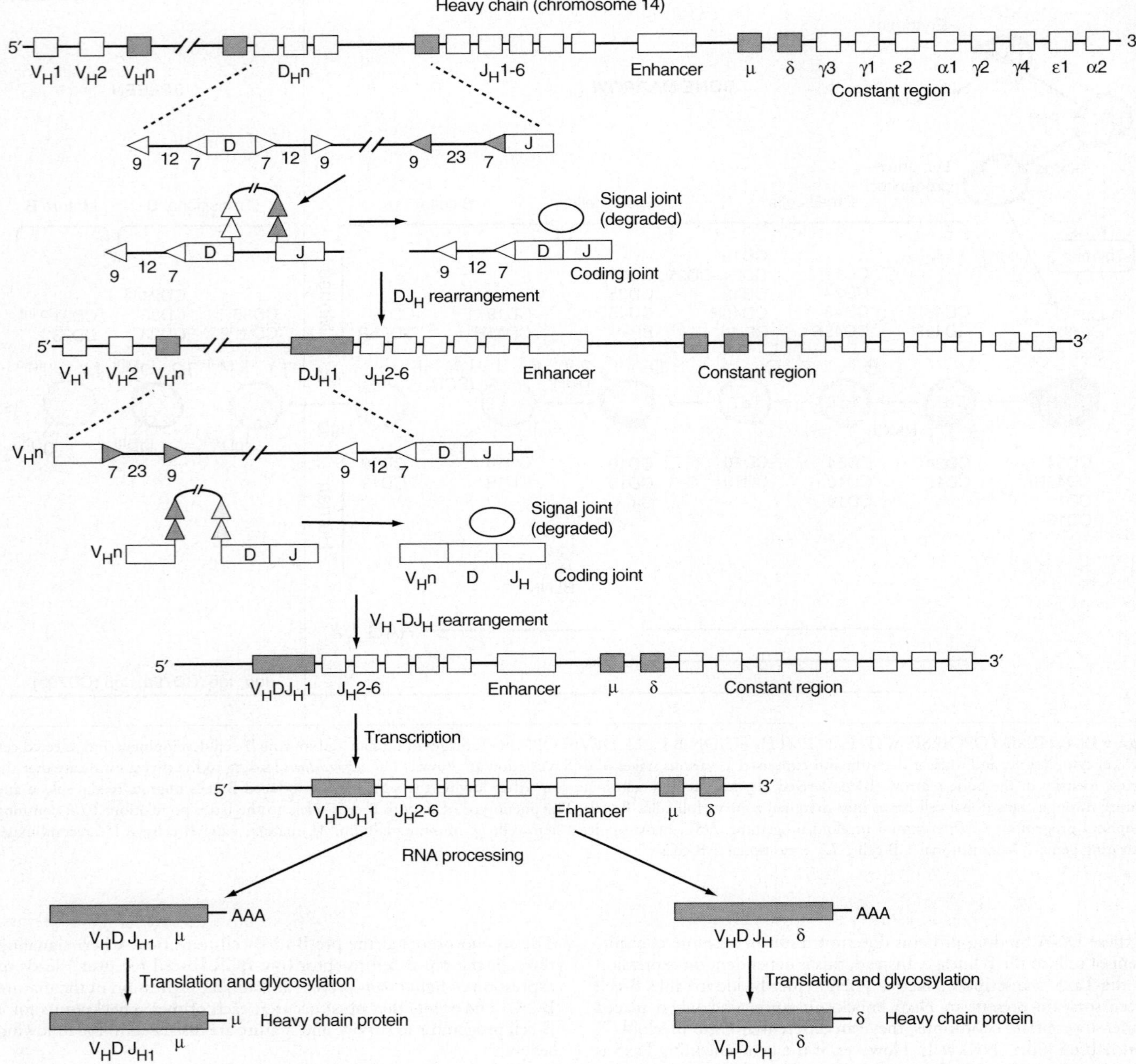

Figure 18-2 REARRANGEMENT AND EXPRESSION OF THE HUMAN IMMUNOGLOBULIN HEAVY CHAIN GENE. The figure shows the Ig heavy chain gene and the signal sequences 3′ of each V region locus, 5′ and 3′ of each D region locus, and 5′ of each J region locus. These consist of heptamer and nonamer sequences separated by either 12 or 23 base pairs. During immunoglobulin (Ig) recombination, a signal sequence of 12 base pairs can only join to another of 23 base pairs (the so-called 12-23 rule). As shown in the figure, initial heavy chain gene rearrangements form coding joints between D and J regions as well as signal joints that are ultimately degraded. Subsequently, the joining of the V region gene to the DJ complex occurs. After a successful rearrangement, the VDJ complex, the μ intron, and portions of the constant regions are transcribed. RNA processing and differential splicing results in formation of an mRNA molecule that is then translated. In the example shown, the rearranged VDJ complex and the constant region, with the μ and δ C region genes, is transcribed. After RNA processing and translation, a particular B cell could then express μ protein, δ protein, or both.

Sterile Transcripts

Ig heavy chain gene rearrangement is preceded by transcription of the unrearranged heavy chain locus. This results in the production of developmentally regulated transcripts of unrearranged Ig genes, referred to as *germline* or *sterile transcripts*. Multiple species of sterile transcripts have been described, and some could conceivably encode proteins. A mechanistic link between transcription and Ig gene rearrangement has been hypothesized. For example, transcription might make unrearranged Ig genes accessible to both RNA polymerase and V(D)J recombinase, the germline transcripts could function in the rearrangement reaction, or transcription could alter structural characteristics of DNA, making the recombination signal sequences (see later) better targets for recombination.

Immunoglobulin Heavy Chain Gene Rearrangement and Expression

Subsequent to the appearance of sterile transcripts, Ig heavy chain gene rearrangements occur. Because the coding regions of the V, D, and J region segments are separated from one another, their juxtaposition with deletion of the intervening intron must occur. The initial event during heavy chain gene rearrangement juxtaposes a D region segment to a JH segment. Although in theory any D region gene can join with equal frequency to any one JH region gene, there may be preferential utilization of selected D and JH region genes at various times during fetal and adult B-cell development. After successful D–JH recombination, a VH region gene rearranges to the D–JH complex. Evidence suggests that biased usage of JH proximal VH genes occurs in the newly generated repertoire of neonatal mice and humans. The heavy chain C region remains separated from the rearranged VHDJH complex by an intron, and this entire sequence is transcribed. RNA processing subsequently leads to deletion of the intron between the VHDJH complex and the most proximal C region genes. After translation, μ heavy chain protein is expressed in the cytoplasm of pre-B cells.

The process just described is dependent on an enzymatic machinery that deletes intronic sequences and joins coding segments of DNA. The enzymes that mediate these functions act through recognition of recombination signal sequences that are located 3′ of each heavy chain V region exon, 5′ of each heavy chain J segment, and 5′ and 3′ of each heavy chain D region gene. Fig. 18-2 shows the association of these recognition sequences with the various heavy chain exons. Each recombination signal sequence consists of conserved heptamer and nonamer sequences separated by nonconserved DNA segments of 12 or 23 base pairs. During Ig gene recombination, these recognition sequences form loops of DNA, which in turn bring the coding exons in apposition to one another. These noncoding loops are subsequently deleted and degraded.

The expression of two highly conserved proteins, referred to as recombinase-activating genes-1 (RAG-1) and RAG-2, is required for heavy and light chain gene recombination.[8] Mice and humans in whom RAG genes are not expressed do not generate B or T cells. Results from cell-free systems that measure V(D)J recombination indicate that RAG proteins are involved in cleavage of DNA at recombination signal sequences and the subsequent joining of coding sequences to one another. In addition to the RAG proteins, general DNA repair enzymes, those encoded by the Ku complex of genes in particular, also play a critical role in Ig heavy chain gene recombination.

After the productive rearrangement of at least one heavy chain gene, transcription of the rearranged locus occurs. Transcription is dependent on the binding of various transcription factors to specific promoter sequences located 5′ of each heavy chain V region and one or more heavy chain enhancer regions located 3′ of the J region genes and downstream from the CH region genes (see Fig. 18-2). Many of the transcription factors that bind within these sites have been identified. These include the previously described E12 and E47 proteins encoded by the *E2A* gene. Before Ig gene rearrangement, E12 and E47 proteins may be in an inactive state owing to their heterodimeric association with another protein known as Id. In this configuration, DNA binding by E12 and E47 does not occur. Thus, successful transition from the pro-B to pre-B-cell stage is dependent on cessation of Id expression. This conclusion is consistent with the fact that mice expressing an Id transgene have a complete block in B-cell differentiation.

Allelic Exclusion

Each pro-B cell has two Ig heavy chain genes, but only one of these encodes μ protein in any given cell. This phenomenon is known as *allelic exclusion*. One theory for how this occurs is that functional Ig rearrangements are rare, so the chance that two functional rearrangements will occur in an individual cell is extremely low. An increasingly accepted, second model of allelic exclusion is that the expression of μ protein from a successfully rearranged allele inhibits rearrangements at the other heavy chain allele. As discussed subsequently, these signals may be mediated through the pre-BCR complex. However, if rearrangements are unsuccessful at one heavy chain locus during B-cell development, recombination will initiate at the second one. If productive, these cells will then mature into pre-B cells. If this rearrangement is also defective, cells will undergo apoptosis.

Expression of the Pre-B Cell Receptor

When μ heavy chain protein is first synthesized, it associates with a chaperone protein known as binding immunoglobulin protein (Bip) in the endoplasmic reticulum. However, it subsequently appears on the cell surface with the *surrogate light chains,* encoded by genes located on chromosome 16 in mice and on chromosome 22 in humans, that together function in a manner analogous to that identified for conventional light chains. The surrogate light chain proteins, referred to as Vpre-B and λ5, are noncovalently linked to one another.[9] λ5 in turn is covalently linked to the CH1 domain of the μ heavy chain via a carboxyl-terminal (C-terminal) cysteine. This μ heavy chain–surrogate light chain complex is associated with two additional transmembrane proteins, Igα and Igβ, and the entire complex is referred to as the pre-BCR. The intracellular tails of both Igα and Igβ contain immunoreceptor tyrosine activation motifs (ITAMs) critical to the signaling function of the pre-BCR (Fig. 18-3, *upper panel*).

One role of the surrogate light chains is to select heavy chains that will ultimately be capable of pairing with conventional light chains. In fact, pre-B cells that pair with surrogate light chains to form the pre-BCR have a significant proliferative advantage, thus ensuring that their numbers will increase and they will generate progeny that will contribute to the B-cell repertoire. Another function, as described previously, may be to mediate allelic exclusion. As soon as the pre-BCR is expressed, the genes encoding RAG-1 and RAG-2 are turned off, and the previously synthesized proteins are degraded. This effectively halts further Ig heavy chain gene rearrangements.

Lipid rafts that contain mediators of intracellular signaling such as Lyn are constitutively associated with the pre-BCR in human pre-B cells.[10] Cross-linking of the pre-BCR leads to an increase in Lyn kinase activity; phosphorylation of the Igβ chain; and recruitment and activation within the pre-BCR complex of additional signaling intermediates, including spleen tyrosine kinase (Syk), B cell linker protein (BLNK), phosphoinositide-3 kinase (PI3K), Bruton's tyrosine kinase (Btk), VAV, and phospholipase C-γ (PLCγ2). These events lead to calcium flux and activation of signaling cascades within the pre-B cell. Pre-B cells in which signaling through the pre-BCR occurs have a marked growth advantage over pre-B cells that do not express a pre-BCR. A logical assumption is that these events are initiated by binding of the extracellular portion of the pre-BCR to an environmental ligand, but no definitive pre-BCR ligand has been identified to date. Thus, precisely how these signaling events are initiated in the absence of external cross-linking ligand remains unclear, although it appears likely that constitutive signaling after pre-BCR surface expression may be sufficient. Recent structural studies suggest that the pre-BCR constitutively assembles as an oligomer providing a potential mechanism for this behavior.[11]

These signaling pathways are crucial in developing pre-B cells. One of the best examples of this requirement is the prototypical humoral immunodeficiency, X-linked agammaglobulinemia (XLA), first described in 1952 by Bruton. XLA results from mutations within the gene segments that encode the nonreceptor tyrosine kinase, Btk. In males who express a defective Btk protein, pre-B-cell clonal expansion is markedly depressed, and there is an almost complete loss of immature B cells in the BM and in secondary lymphoid organs. As a result, affected males develop recurrent bacterial infections early in life because of a profound decrease in circulating Ig. A nearly identical clinical phenotype also has been observed in persons with mutations

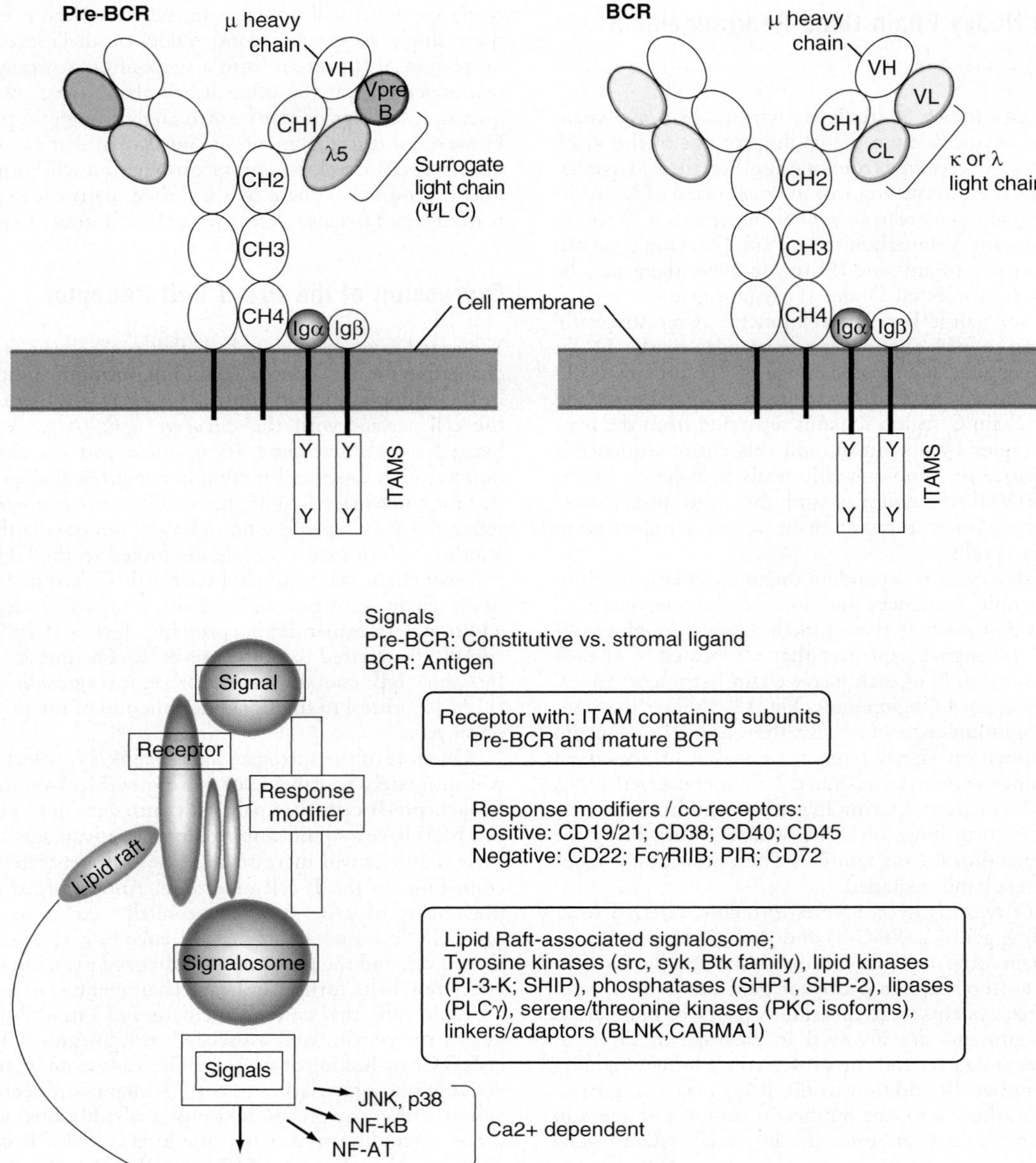

Figure 18-3 THE PRE-B-CELL RECEPTOR (PRE-BCR) AND B-CELL RECEPTOR (BCR) AND ASSOCIATED SIGNALING INTERMEDIATES. *Top,* μ heavy chain protein in pre-B cells is associated with the surrogate light chains v-pre-B and λ5 *(left).* In newly produced B lymphocytes, μ heavy chain is associated with conventional light chain *(right).* Associated with heavy chain in both pre-B and B cells are two additional transmembrane proteins, Ig–α and Ig–β, that contain immunoreceptor tyrosine activation motifs (ITAMs) critical to the signaling function. *Bottom,* Expression of the pre-BCR (or possibly its binding to a stromal ligand) or binding of antigen to the mature BCR, respectively, initiates the assembly of a lipid raft, BCR-associated "signalosome" composed of multiple signaling molecules, ultimately leading to transcriptional events that promote cell proliferation, survival, and differentiation. *ERK,* Extracellular-signal-regulated kinase; *Ig,* immunoglobulin; *JNK,* Janus kinase; *NF-κB,* nuclear factor kappa-light-chain enhancer of activated B cells; *NFAT,* nuclear factor of activated T cells; *SHIP,* src homology 2 containing inositol phosphatase. *SHP,* src homology 2-containing protein tyrosine phosphatase;

in additional components of the pre-BCR signaling complex, including the μ–heavy chain, λ5, Igα, and the key B-cell adaptor protein BLNK (see Fig. 18-1).

THE PRE-B TO B-CELL TRANSITION

At some point, pre-BCR–expressing cells cease to proliferate and enter a resting phase. This change occurs coordinately with a cessation of surrogate light chain expression, reactivation of the recombinatorial machinery, and initiation of conventional light chain gene rearrangement. These events culminate in the expression of light chain protein.

Ig light chain protein can be encoded by the kappa (κ) or lambda (λ) genes (Fig. 18-4). Greater than 90% of murine B cells express κ protein. However, the proportions of human κ and λ proteins are more equivalent, with approximately 60% of human B cells expressing κ light chain protein. The human κ gene is located on

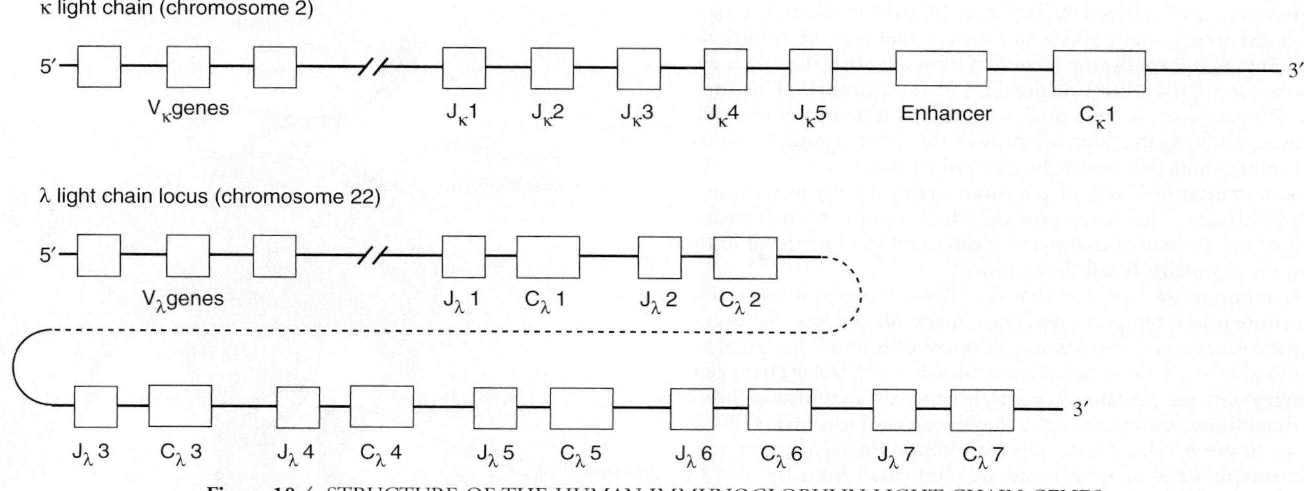

Figure 18-4 STRUCTURE OF THE HUMAN IMMUNOGLOBULIN LIGHT CHAIN GENES.

chromosome 2 and includes around 40 Vκ region genes, clustered in up to seven families, five functional Jκ region genes, and one C κ region gene. The human λ locus is located on human chromosome 22. Approximately 30 human Vλ genes exist and are grouped into 10 families. There are seven human Cλ genes, four of which are functional and three of which are pseudogenes. Each Cλ gene is located 3′ of a respective J λ gene. Light chain genes do not include D region loci.

Although B cells can express κ or λ light chain protein, rearrangements initiate at the κ locus, where the initial event is the joining of a V κ segment to a J κ segment. The VκJκ complex remains separated from the light chain C region by an intron, the entire complex is transcribed, and further splicing of the intron between the κ and C κ segment results in formation of a mature Vκ– Jκ–cκ transcript. If rearrangements at the first κ allele are unsuccessful, attempts are made to rearrange the second κ gene. If this fails, the λ locus is used. The regulation of light chain gene rearrangement is similar to that for heavy chain gene recombination. For example, the same enzymatic machinery involving the RAG proteins is necessary.

IMMUNOGLOBULIN CLASS SWITCHING

At the terminal stage of primary B-cell development, newly produced B cells can express both IgM and IgD. This coexpression occurs by means of alternative processing of a primary RNA transcript. As noted previously, the rearranged VHDJH heavy chain, part of the C region, and the intron separating these exons is transcribed after productive rearrangements in a cell. If the intron is spliced, resulting in association of the Cμ region with the VDJ complex, the B cell expresses IgM. Alternatively, if the Cμ exon is deleted along with the heavy chain intron, the VDJ complex and the Cδ exon become contiguous and the B cell expresses IgD. The differential processing of heavy chain transcripts within a single cell explains why some newly produced B cells coexpress both IgM and IgD (see Fig. 18-2).

These primary developmental events are distinguished from Ig class switching that allows the newly produced B cell to express the same VDJ complex associated with additional heavy chain C regions other than IgM and IgD. Deletions of germline DNA resulting in religation of the VDJ complex to these downstream heavy chain C region genes, such as γ3, γ1 γ2b, γ2a, ε and α are the mechanism by which this takes place. These DNA deletions are believed to occur at or near nucleotide sequences called *switch regions* that are located in the intron 5′ to each CH exon. As discussed subsequently, these class-switching events are highly regulated, secondary-differentiation events that occur in spleen and lymph nodes and are potentiated by helper T cells and their secreted products.[12]

THE B-CELL RECEPTOR

The structure of the BCR is similar to that described for the pre-BCR, except that κ or λ, rather than surrogate light chain proteins are associated with the Ig heavy chain. As shown in Fig. 18-3, the BCR consists of the Ig molecule and the associated Igα and Igβ proteins that are required for initiation of the intracellular signaling cascade after binding of antigen. This requirement exists because even though Ig heavy chains span the cell membrane, their cytoplasmic carboxyl tails are relatively short. For example, the intracellular C terminus of IgM and IgD consists of only three amino acids.

Antigen engagement of the BCR initiates assembly of a lipid raft, BCR-associated "signalosome," composed of multiple signaling molecules that include tyrosine kinases, serine/threonine kinases, lipid kinases, lipases, phosphatases, and linkers and adaptors.[13] This signalosome mediates a cascade of intracellular signals that includes the initiation of calcium influx. Additional calcium-dependent and -independent downstream signals that include the mitogen-activated protein (MAP) kinase cascade (c-jun N-terminal kinase [JNK], p38, extracellular-signal-regulated kinase [ERK]) and activation of key transcription factors that include JUN, c-fos, nuclear factor of activated T cells (NFAT), and nuclear factor kappa-light-chain enhancer of activated B cells (NF-κB) in turn mediate transcriptional events leading to cell proliferation, survival, and differentiation. The level and duration of receptor activation and hence transcriptional output are further modified by a series of cell surface coreceptors or "response modifiers" that bind to complement or to receptors on the surface of stromal cells, activated T cells, or other populations present in secondary lymphoid organs.

GENERATION AND SELECTION OF THE PRIMARY B-CELL REPERTOIRE

For the organism to mount an effective humoral immune response, an array of Igs with unique antigen-binding specificities, together referred to as the *Ig repertoire,* must be generated. Several mechanisms have evolved to ensure that this occurs.[14]

First, heavy and light chain proteins can be encoded by multiple germline V, J, and, in the case of the heavy chain, D region genes, and the combinatorial diversity among them is enormous. Second, nucleotides not encoded in the germline can be added to D-JH and VH-DJH junctions by a nuclear enzyme known as terminal deoxynucleotidyl transferase (TdT). Two splice variants of TdT, encoded by a single gene, have been identified, and it is the short (509-amino-acid) variant that catalyzes the addition of nontemplated nucleotides at coding joints. The long (529-amino-acid) form is a 3′-5′ exonuclease that catalyzes the deletion of nucleotides at coding joints. Thus,

N region diversity catalyzed by TdT may be attributable to the coordinated activities of short and long forms of that enzyme. Third, the DNA joints that form during recombination are often imprecise and can occur at any of several nucleotides in the germline. This junctional diversity has the potential to generate different amino acid sequences, resulting in added diversity of the Ig repertoire. However, out-of-frame joints that cannot be transcribed also may result. Finally, somatic mutation of V region genes can occur, usually in secondary lymphoid tissues. This latter process, which results in an increased affinity of the antibody for antigen, is discussed in more detail in the section on secondary B-cell development.

It is important to recognize that not all B-cell progenitors successfully mature into B lymphocytes. The remarkable cell loss that occurs during the process of differentiation of pro-B cells into B lymphocytes is attributable to a series of selection events. First, Ig heavy chain gene rearrangements are productive in approximately one-third of pro-B cells. In addition, functional light chain gene rearrangements do not occur in all pre-B cells. Those cells with nonproductive Ig gene rearrangements undergo apoptosis and are eliminated from the BM by resident macrophages and stromal cells.

Selection events also are operative on cells that have matured to the surface IgM stage of development. As a result, although approximately 2×10^7 IgM^+ immature B cells are produced daily in murine BM, only 10% to 20% of these cells survive to exit the BM and enter the spleen as transitional B cells. Some of these surface IgM^+ cells are eliminated because they are potentially self-reactive. Such self-reactive B cells may be generated because the process of Ig gene recombination is random.

Several mechanisms have been proposed to account for the fate of such self-reactive cells.[15] In some cases, the presence of self-antigen may not activate self-reactive B cells. This scenario may result from weak B-cell affinity for the antigen, or the autoantigen may be present at an extremely low concentration. In other instances, interaction of antigen with the autoreactive B cell may result in anergy. The level of membrane Ig on such anergic B cells may be reduced up to 20-fold, the cell's ability to proliferate may be impaired, and differentiation into Ig-secreting cells may be blocked. Finally, self-reactive B cells may be clonally deleted. Clonal deletion may result from cytolysis by other cells, such as BM macrophages, or autoreactive B cells may undergo a physiologic change resulting in cell death after receptor engagement.

The recognition of self-antigen by a B cell may not necessarily result in anergy or deletion but instead may lead to *receptor editing*. In this process, rearranged κ light chain alleles can be replaced by secondary rearrangements of upstream Vκ genes to downstream, unrearranged Jκ segments. These secondary rearrangements, which may delete the primary VκJκ complex or separate it from Cκ by inversion, are possible because of the continual presence of unrearranged Vκ regions upstream of the joined VκJκ coding segments. Receptor editing also can occur in peripheral B cells in response to antigen stimulation, as discussed subsequently.

REGULATION OF PRIMARY B-CELL DEVELOPMENT

Hematopoiesis occurs in the intersinusoidal spaces of the medullary cavity in association with a fixed population of stromal cells.[16] Stromal cells are largely sessile and form a three-dimensional hematopoietic microenvironment with which developing blood cells associate (Fig. 18-5). Before 1980, little was known about how stromal cells and their secreted products regulate B-cell development. However, advances in molecular biology, the isolation of BM stromal cells, and the development of long-term culture methods for growing B-lineage cells have converged in the past 3 decades. As a result, considerable insights into the regulation of B-cell development by extracellular signals have been obtained.

Cell–Cell Interactions

Direct contact between developing B-lineage and stromal cells can be observed on analysis of intact BM or of B lymphopoiesis in long-term

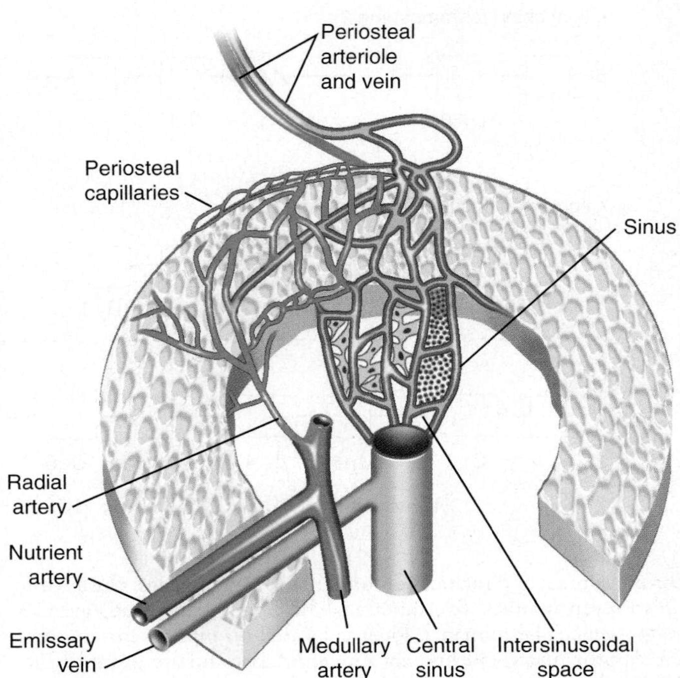

Figure 18-5 CROSS-SECTION OF BONE SHOWING ELEMENTS OF THE MEDULLARY CIRCULATION, THE MARROW SINUSOIDS, AND THE LOCATION OF STROMAL CELLS. *(From Dorshkind K: Regulation of hematopoiesis by bone marrow stromal cells and their products.* Annu Rev Immunol *8:111, 1990. Reprinted by permission from the Annual Review of Immunology.)*

BM cultures, and the molecular basis for these associations is being defined in both humans and mice. For example, both murine and human pre-B cells express the very late antigen 4 (VLA-4) integrin that interacts with a stromal cell ligand identified as vascular cell adhesion molecule-1 (VCAM-1). VLA-4 also promotes binding to fibronectin, an extracellular matrix protein. CD44 on developing B-lineage cells also has been implicated in mediating stromal cell–lymphocyte interactions in the mouse through binding to stromal cell–derived hyaluronate. These intercellular interactions presumably would allow B cells to receive proliferative or developmental signals (or both) from stromal cells. It is important to appreciate that the stromal cells may not be passive populations that constitutively provide these signals. Instead, the binding of the B-lineage cell may stimulate the stromal cell in turn to produce such differentiation or growth-potentiating activities.

Cytokines

An additional means by which BM stromal cells regulate the growth and differentiation of B-lineage cells is via the secretion of soluble mediators. The literature describing the effects of cytokines on B-cell development is extensive, and a discussion of each one is beyond the scope of this chapter. However, the focus can be narrowed considerably when only those factors with obligate effects on B-cell development are considered.

The critical B lymphopoietic cytokine in mice is IL-7, which binds to a cell-surface receptor formed by the IL-7 receptor α chain and the common cytokine γ chain. That IL-7 is required for murine B-cell development was demonstrated by studies showing that mice administered antibodies to IL-7 exhibit severe lymphopenia. Subsequent analysis of IL-7 and IL-7 receptor knock-out mice corroborated these studies. These animals also exhibit a severe T-cell depletion because IL-7 is required for thymopoiesis. Cells that have initiated Ig heavy chain D-JH rearrangements are particularly responsive to the growth-stimulating effects of IL-7. However, by the time they have

Table 18-1 Characteristics of B Cell Subpopulations in Mice and Humans

Cells	Function	Phenotype	Properties	Localization
B-1a (mouse)	Innate immunity	$IgM^{high}IgD^{low}CD11b^{+}CD5^{+}$ (in serous cavities)	Secretion of IgM natural antibodies	Serous cavities, spleen, gut
B-1b (mouse)	Innate immunity	$IgM^{high}IgD^{low}CD11b^{+}CD5^{-}$ (in serous cavities)	Antibody production is induced	Serous cavities, spleen, gut
MZ (mouse and human)	Innate immunity	$IgM^{+}IgD^{low}$ (human MZ B cells also include $CD27^{+}$ IgM^{+} unswitched memory cells)	Strong response to T-independent antigens	Splenic MZ
Follicular (mouse and human)	Adaptive immunity	$IgM^{low}IgD^{high}$	Strong response to T-dependent antigens	Spleen and lymph nodes; recirculate

IgD, Immunoglobulin D; *IgM*, immunoglobulin M; *MZ*, marginal zone.

matured to the late pre-B-cell stage of development, responsiveness to IL-7 attenuated. Subsequent murine studies revealed that in addition to its growth-promoting effects, IL-7 acts as a differentiation factor that potentiates the recombination of a VH region gene segment to an already rearranged DJH complex.

The precise role of IL-7 during human B-cell development remains to be determined. Human B-cell progenitors are IL-7 responsive, as shown in studies in which $CD34^{+}CD19^{+}$ pro-B cells proliferate in response to IL-7. The issue is whether IL-7 is an obligate human B-lymphopoietic factor as in mice. This question arises because B-cell development is normal in patients with X-linked severe combined immunodeficiency. These individuals have mutations in the gene encoding the cytokine common γ chain, which is part of the receptor for IL-2, IL-4, IL-9, and IL-15, in addition to IL-7. Further suggesting that IL-7 is not an obligate B lymphopoietic factor is that B-cell development also is normal in patients whose B-lineage cells express a mutated IL-7Rα chain. Additional studies to identify factors required for human B-cell development are needed.

Systemic Factors

In addition to regulation by microenvironmental factors, there is a growing appreciation that systemic factors, and those of endocrine origin in particular, also regulate B-cell development. For example, B-cell development in mice is dependent on the integrity of the pituitary–thyroid axis because mice deficient in the production of thyroid hormone or expression of the thyroid hormone receptor exhibit suppressed BM B lymphopoiesis. Whether or not these events also occur in human B lymphopoiesis has not been established. It also has been demonstrated that hormones can negatively affect B-cell development. In particular, increased levels of estrogens occurring during pregnancy inhibit lymphopoiesis.

B-1 B CELLS

The B cells that are produced in adult BM and that constitute the majority of B cells in the peripheral lymphoid tissues such as the spleen and lymph node are often referred to as B-2 B cells. This nomenclature serves to contrast them with another functionally distinct population of mature B cells that are referred to as B-1 B cells. B-1 B cells have been extensively studied in mice.[17,18] B-1 B cells constitute around 5% of total B lymphocytes in that species and are found in multiple tissues that include the spleen and serous cavities. Approximately half of the B cells present in the latter sites, including the pleural and peritoneal cavities, in most strains are B-1 B cells. B-1 B cells in serous cavities can be distinguished by their unusual phenotype. For example, peritoneal cavity B-1 B cells can be defined by their expression of high levels of sIgM; low levels of sIgD; and CD11b, a determinant expressed on myeloid cells. B-1 B cells can be further subdivided based on the differential expression of cell surface CD5 into $sIgM^{high}$ $sIgD^{low}$ $CD11b^{+}$ $CD5^{+}$ B-1a B cells, and $sIgM^{high}$ $sIgD^{low}$ $CD11b^{+}$ $CD5^{-}$ B-1b B cells. Both B-1 subpopulations are generally considered to be part of the innate immune system, although each mediates distinct functions. B-1a B cells are distinguished by their spontaneous secretion of IgM, which are often referred to as *natural antibodies,* and antibody production by B-1b B cells is induced after exposure to antigen (Table 18-1). Antibodies from both subpopulations of B-1 B cells have been shown to be required for protection against pathogens such as *Streptococcus pneumoniae.*

Classic studies demonstrating that the transplantation of neonatal liver cells into irradiated murine recipients most efficiently generated B-1 B cells but adult BM most efficiently repopulated B-2 B cells suggested that B-1 cells were a distinct B-cell lineage derived from progenitors that preferentially arose during fetal life.[18] The description of a phenotypically identifiable B-1 B cell–specified progenitor that is preferentially generated in fetuses has provided strong support that a significant number of B-1 cells are derived from distinct progenitors. In addition to this "lineage model," the "selection model" proposes that B-1 cells are conventional B-2 B cells that develop the distinguishing B-1 characteristics because of selective pressures after antigen exposure. That some B-1 cells are generated in this manner cannot be excluded.

Based on the expression of CD5 by murine B-1a cells, many studies have claimed to have identified human B-1 cells based on simultaneous expression of CD5 and sIgM. These reports must be viewed with caution because CD5 is not a B-1–restricted determinant. Thus, the existence of human B-1 cells has remained controversial. However, a $CD20^{+}$ $CD27^{+}$ $CD43^{+}$ $CD70^{-}$ population of cord blood B cells that has properties consistent with their being classified as human B-1 cells was recently described.[19]

FETAL B-CELL DEVELOPMENT

Murine blood cell formation initiates during embryogenesis, with the extraembryonic yolk sac and intraembryonic paraaortic splanchnopleura region being two of the earliest sites of hematopoiesis.[20] The potential of cells from both of those tissues to generate B lymphocytes has been demonstrated. Subsequently, cells that express B-lineage antigens that include cytoplasmic Ig can be detected in fetal liver and BM, and by late gestation, surface IgM^{+} B cells are present in multiple fetal tissues that include the spleen.

The analysis of human fetal B-cell development is more limited, but what is known generally parallels the murine data. For example, hematopoiesis initiates in the human yolk sac at 3 weeks of gestation, although whether or not B-cell potential is present at that time is unclear. Pre-B cells are present in human fetal liver by week 8 of gestation, and surface IgM^{+} cells are present at week 9. IgM expressing cells have also been observed in additional human fetal tissues that include the omentum, the peritoneal cavity, and the spleen.

Evidence from mouse studies suggests that the first B-cell potential to arise in fetuses is associated with the B-1 lineage.[21] For example, the B-cell precursors in day 9.5 yolk sac and paraaortic splanchnopleura primarily generate B-1 cells. Also, the first B lineage cells to arise in fetal liver have a phenotype consistent with B-1 progenitors.[22] Only later during gestation and subsequent to the emergence of HSCs on day 10.5 are B-2 progenitors detected in appreciable numbers. The sequential emergence of B-1 and B-2 cells is consistent with the layered immune system hypothesis, which proposes that distinct waves of lymphopoiesis that generate B cells with increasingly sophisticated functions emerge.[23] Evidence indicates that selected T cells, γδ T cells in particular, also develop in a layered manner. It has been suggested that B-cell development occurs in distinct waves in the human fetus as well.[24]

SECONDARY LYMPHOID COMPARTMENTS

After newly produced B cells exit the BM, they migrate to the spleen, where they undergo further maturation into follicular (FO) B cells or marginal zone (MZ) B cells. In general, FO B cells are poised to respond to T-dependent antigens, which, as their name implies, require help from T cells. The T cells in the spleen that provide this help are located in the periarterial lymphoid sheath (PALS) (see Fig. 18-6).

The spleen (but not lymph nodes) contains additional B cells located at the outer limit of the splenic white pulp (see Fig. 18-6). This area, known as the MZ, is where the MZ B cells localize, and the region also contains macrophages and dendritic cells. MZ B cells present in this region play a critical role in the response to T-independent antigens (see later discussion). Human MZ B cells are clearly heterogeneous and include a large proportion of $CD27^+$ IgM^+ unswitched memory B cells with somatically mutated Ig heavy chains. The origin of this cell population is unclear but is presumed to be antigen driven yet may not require T-cell help. Although MZ B cells in rodents appear to be a static, nonrecirculating population, cells with a $CD27^+$ IgM^+ phenotype are clearly present in human peripheral blood as well as other lymphatic tissues. This circulating population becomes detectable in parallel with seeding of the splenic MZ (typically after 2 years of age), increases in number after exposure to polysaccharide antigens, and appears to play an essential role in the rapid response to infection with encapsulated bacteria.[25]

Marginal zone and FO B cells are the progeny of $sIgM^+$ B cells produced in the BM. However, the latter cells are functionally immature and migrate to the spleen, where they undergo maturation through various transitional B-cell stages that results in the generation of MZ and FO B cells. The most immature transitional cells are referred to as *transitional 1 (T1) B cells,* which localize at the outer edge of the PALS (see Fig. 18-6). The PALS in mice is occupied by a considerable number of T cells but in humans few T cells are present in this region. T1 B cells give rise to a more mature population of splenic B cells, referred to as *transitional 2 (T2) cells.*[26]

The T1 and T2 populations respond differentially to developmental stimuli, and a considerable degree of selection occurs during the T1 to T2 transition. For example, T1 cells with BCR specificities for bloodborne self-antigens are deleted by negative selection. Positive selection via BCR signaling must occur, and if it does not, the T2 cells will die by neglect. The survival of T2 cells, but not T1 cells, is also dependent on the B-cell growth factor BAFF (BLyS, TALL-1, THANK, zTNF4), which is produced by the splenic microenvironment. A fraction of T2 cells are no longer in G_0 phase of the cell cycle, suggesting they are in a more activated state than is the case for T1 cells.

Various signals determine whether T2 cells mature into MZ or FO B cells. Weak signaling through the BCR along with engagement of the Notch2 receptor promotes entry into the MZ B-cell compartment. There is a marked depletion of MZ B cells when the Notch2 pathway is blocked. Self-reactive B cells are enriched within the MZ population, suggesting that weak self-antigens may play an important role in their generation. This feature may permit them to respond rapidly to cross-reactive epitopes on pathogens as discussed later. BCR signals, along with activation of the alternative NF-κB pathway, are required for T2 cells to mature into an FO B cell. It is estimated based on murine studies that only 1% to 3% of splenic transitional B cells develop into mature, naïve B cells. When mature, naïve B cells are generated, they recirculate and take up residence in various lymphoid tissues that include lymph nodes, intestinal Peyer patches, and the spleen itself. Within these tissues, mature naïve cells localize in clusters of B lymphocytes, and each such cluster is termed a *primary follicle* (see Fig. 18-6). Within these regions, the FO B cells are poised to respond to antigen and undergo the germinal center reaction described below.

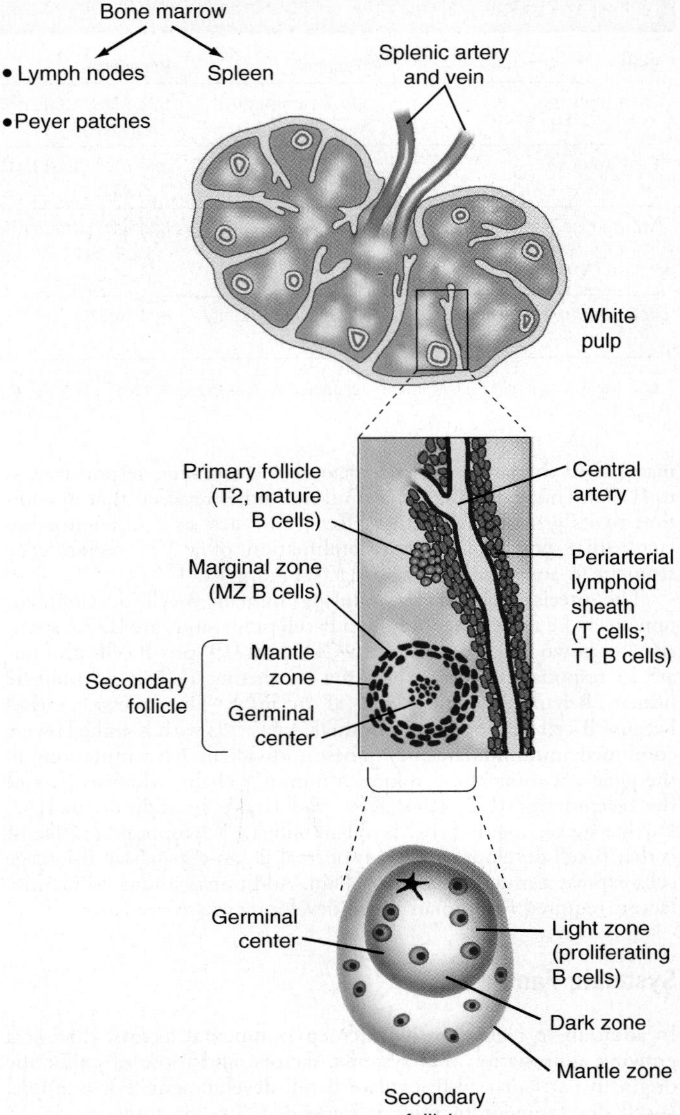

Figure 18-6 ORGANIZATION OF B CELLS IN SECONDARY LYMPHOID ORGANS WITH EMPHASIS ON THE SPLEEN.

The molecular signals responsible for the intraorgan localization of specific B-cell populations and their migration patterns after antigenic challenge are being identified.[27] Proper segregation of splenic B cells in follicles and the MZ is dependent on expression of tumor necrosis factor (TNF) and lymphotoxins α and β (LTα and LTβ). Signaling through lymphocyte function-associated antigen (LFA-1) and α4β1 integrins also has been implicated in localization and retention of MZ B cells. These molecules and their receptors may also transmit signals required for the development of stromal cells that produce chemokines required for movement of cells among different anatomic locations within secondary lymphoid organs. A role for chemokines in B-1 B-cell localization to the peritoneal cavity has also been demonstrated.

T-INDEPENDENT B-CELL RESPONSES

T-independent responses are elicited by polymeric antigens, such as polysaccharides, that are composed of repetitive antigenic epitopes. MZ B cells play a critical role in these responses. On antigen binding, MZ B cells undergo rapid proliferation and maturation into plasma cells that secrete low-affinity IgM.

The rapid response of MZ B cells to antigen has led to the idea that this effector population, similar to B-1 B cells, constitutes a key element of the innate immune response to bacterial and other selected pathogens. Because they have a low activation threshold, MZ B cells rapidly differentiate into antibody-forming cells in response to antigen. These cells secrete primarily low-affinity IgM and IgG3 antibodies that provide a first line of defense. This response may be reinforced by B-1 B cells, whose Ig repertoire is designed for responsiveness to the polymeric antigens that characterize the T-independent response. In view of this, it is not surprising that many of the properties of MZ B cells overlap with those of B-1 B cells (see Table 18-1). The poor response of infants to some types of T-independent antigens correlates with the fact that the MZ is not fully formed until the age of 1 to 2 years. In addition, splenectomized individuals are more susceptible to infection with some bacteria, owing to the deficient antibody response to capsular polysaccharides.

T-DEPENDENT RESPONSES

Although some B cells in the MZ can respond to T-dependent antigens, most B cells that do so are the mature, naive FO B cells located in primary follicles. As described previously, these cells are derived from T2 B cells and have subsequently migrated into the primary follicle. After their binding of a T-dependent antigen (as soluble antigen, indirectly via presentation by a local antigen presenting cell, or as an immune complex) mature, naïve B cells in primary follicles undergo a blastogenic response. Some of these cells will immediately mature into plasma cells that secrete low-affinity IgM to provide a rapid initial response to infection. In response to T-cell help, however, other B cells undergo further proliferation and differentiation. The histologic appearance of the follicle changes as these events evolve. The nonresponsive B cells form an outer *mantle zone* surrounding the proliferating, antigen-responsive B cells in a central germinal center.[28]

Germinal center B cells are shielded from soluble antigens and are exposed only to a unique set of antigens presented by follicular dendritic cells. Two regions can be distinguished within the germinal center of the secondary follicle. At one pole, the cycling B-cell blasts are referred to as *centroblasts* and form the *dark zone*. The other pole, referred to as the *light zone,* consists of nonproliferating cells referred to as *centrocytes*. Some of these centrocytes go on to become plasma cells, but others become memory B cells (see Fig. 18-6). The end result of the germinal center reaction is the formation of plasma cells that secrete high-affinity Ig. Other germinal center B cells convert to memory B cells, which constitute about 40% of all B cells and are responsible for the relatively rapid response observed on secondary exposure to the same antigen.

AFFINITY MATURATION AND LYMPHOMAGENESIS

After the initial low-affinity IgM response that helps to keep a developing infection in check, the response of B cells in the germinal centers to T-dependent antigens involves Ig class switching and selection of B-cell clones of higher affinity antigen-binding potential. This process is known as *affinity maturation.*

Affinity maturation results in the selection of B cells estimated to have a 10-fold or even greater, increase in antigen-binding potential. Analysis of Ig gene sequences of pre– and post–germinal center B cells indicates that this increased affinity is secondary to changes in the genes that encode the antigen-binding domain of the Ig molecule. These genomic changes result from three types of modifications. First, as described previously, B cells may undergo receptor editing. Receptor editing usually involves modifications of the existing light chain in which an upstream V region segment joins to a downstream J region gene. As a result, the genetic region encoding the originally expressed light chain is deleted. For this process to occur, RAG-1 and RAG-2 expression are required. It has been proposed that B cells in germinal centers might reactivate *RAG* gene expression to mediate events such as receptor editing. However, that this occurs has been questioned. Instead, receptor editing in splenic B cells may be limited to a small subset of recent immature BM immigrants that enter germinal centers before their *RAG* gene expression has been extinguished.

Somatic hypermutation provides a second means to increase antibody affinity. During this process, single-nucleotide exchanges, deletions, and mutations are introduced into the genes encoding the antibody-binding regions of the Ig receptor. Finally, Ig class switching (see earlier) can occur. Class switching results in the replacement of the existing heavy chain constant region by a downstream constant region gene. Recently, a B cell–specific gene that encodes activation-induced cytidine deaminase (AID), which is expressed in germinal center B cells, has been identified. AID is a putative RNA-editing enzyme that acts as a cytidine deaminase and has been shown to be indispensable for somatic hypermutation and class switch recombination.[29]

Affinity maturation is dependent on signals delivered to the antigen-responsive B cells by antigen-specific T lymphocytes that migrate into the germinal center from the PALS. T cells mediate their effects on B cells through the secretion of cytokines as well as through direct intercellular contacts, and these stimuli result in B-cell growth, differentiation, and Ig class switching. For example, CD40 is a T cell–surface glycoprotein encoded by a member of the tumor necrosis gene family, and its ligand is expressed on B cells. CD40 ligand knock-out mice do not form germinal centers, and humans who do not express CD40 ligand have X-linked hyper IgM immunodeficiency. Another key T-cell costimulatory signal includes the cytokine IL-10, which is secreted by T cells in response to their activation via the "inducible costimulator" ICOS. Humans lacking expression of ICOS on T cells have adult-onset common variable immune deficiency, leading to a severe deficit in generation of class-switched and memory B cells.

There are two unintended consequences of affinity maturation. One is that autoreactive clones may be inadvertently generated. The other is the development of B-cell lymphoma. Lymphomagenesis results in part from the fact that vigorous B-cell proliferation combined with the changes at the DNA level that lead to molecular alterations promoting or support malignant transformation. Numerous studies have assigned B-cell lymphomas to each of the normal B-cell counterparts (as described). Events that limit differentiation of immature or activated mature B cells can also promote malignant transformation.

AGING AND B-CELL DEVELOPMENT

Studies of both rodents and humans have demonstrated that the quality of the immune response is diminished with age. Such declines are not incompatible with life, but they may become a factor when the individual is required to mount an immune response to a novel pathogen, respond to vaccination or when considering the use of BM-derived from older donors. Consequently, defining how aging affects the immune system is critical in order to develop strategies to augment immunity in the elderly.

Studies of mice have established that the production of B cells from HSCs is severely attenuated with age. For example, the frequency and total number of CLP, pro-B cells, and pre-B cells is significantly reduced in the BM of old mice. This also seems to be the case for human B-cell development as well. B-cell progenitors from young and old mice have been compared in order to identify patterns of gene expression that underlie the decline in B-cell production with age. This has led to the identification of multiple genes that include E2A as well as p16^{Ink4a} and Arf. The latter two genes are part of the Cdkn2a locus, and the proteins they encode function as potent tumor suppressors. Levels of p16^{Ink4a} and Arf expression increase in pro-B cells with age, and this in turn results in diminished proliferation and increased apoptosis of B-cell progenitors.

Why these changes in primary B-cell development occur is under intense study. One possibility is that HSCs and lymphoid progenitors are genetically programmed to age. An alternative hypothesis is that aging in HSCs and lymphoid progenitors is secondary to changes in the local and systemic environments. Further studies to distinguish between these possibilities are needed.

Regardless of why B-cell production declines, the end result is a lower number of newly produced, naïve B cells that enter secondary lymphoid tissues such as the spleen. Senescence also affects mature B cells resident in peripheral lymphoid tissues. For example, in addition to an accumulation of memory B cells in the spleen of old mice, the Igs they produce are less protective because of low titer and affinity. Some of these defects may be intrinsic to the B cells but others may be secondary to age-related defects in T cells.[30]

REFERENCES

1. Notta F, Doulatov S, Laurenti E, et al: Isolation of single human hematopoietic stem cells capable of long-term multilineage engraftment. *Science* 333:218, 2011.
2. Hardy RR, Kincade PW, Dorshkind K: The protean nature of cells in the B lymphocyte lineage. *Immunity* 26:703, 2007.
3. Blom B, Spits H: Development of human lymphoid cells. *Annu Rev Immunol* 24:287, 2006.
4. Nutt SL, Kee BL: The transcriptional regulation of B cell lineage commitment. *Immunity* 26:715, 2007.
5. Cobaleda C, Schebesta A, Delogu A, et al: Pax5: The guardian of B cell identity and function. *Nat Immunol* 5:463, 2007.
6. Mårtensson IL, Keenan RA, Licence S: The pre-B-Cell receptor. *Curr Opin Immunol* 19:137, 2007.
7. Subrahmanyam R, Sen R: RAGs' eye view of the immunoglobulin heavy chain gene locus. *Sem Immunol* 22:337, 2010.
8. Schatz D, Ji Y: Recombination centres and the orchestration of V(D)J recombination. *Nat Rev Immunol* 11:251, 2011.
9. Melchers F: The pre-B-cell receptor: Selector of fitting immunoglobulin heavy chains for the B-cell repertoire. *Nat Rev Immunol* 5:578, 2005.
10. Hendriks R, Middendorp S: The pre-BCR checkpoint as a cell-autonomous proliferation switch. *Trend Immunol* 25:249, 2004.
11. Bankovich AJ, Raunser S, Juo ZS, et al: Structural insight into pre-B cell receptor function. *Science* 316:291, 2007.
12. Stavnezer J, Guikema J, Schrader C: Mechanism and regulation of class switch recombination. *Annu Rev Immunol* 26:261, 2008.
13. Moreno-Garcia M, Sommer K, Bandaranayake A, et al: Proximal signals controlling B-cell antigen receptor (BCR) mediated NF-kappaB activation. *Adv Exp Med Biol* 584:89, 2006.
14. Ganesh K, Neuberger M: The relationship between hypothesis and experiment in unveiling the mechanisms of antibody gene diversification. *FASEB J* 25:1123, 2011.
15. Yarkoni Y, Getahun A, Cambier J: Molecular underpinning of B-cell anergy. *Immunol Rev* 237:249, 2010.
16. Kiel M, Morrison SJ: Uncertainty in the niches that maintain haematopoietic stem cells. *Nat Rev Immunol* 8:290, 2008.
17. Montecino-Rodriguez E, Dorshkind K: New perspectives in B-1 B cell development and function. *Trends Immunol* 27:428, 2006.
18. Kantor AB, Herzenberg LA: Origin of murine B cell lineages. *Annu Rev Immunol* 11:501, 1993.
19. Griffin DO, Holodick NE, Rothstein TL: Human B1 cells in umbilical cord and adult peripheral blood express the novel phenotype CD20$^+$ CD27$^+$ CD43$^+$ CD70$^-$. *J Exp Med* 208:67, 2011.
20. Medvinsky A, Rybstov S, Taoudi S: Embryonic origin of the adult hematopoietic system: Advances and questions. *Development* 138:1017, 2011.
21. Yoshimoto M, Montecino-Rodriguez E, Prashanth P, et al: B-1 and marginal zone B progenitor cells emerge from yolk sac hemogenic endothelium. *Proc Natl Acad Sci U S A* 108:1468, 2011.
22. Montecino-Rodriguez E, Leathers H, Dorshkind K: Identification of a B-1 B cell-specified progenitor. *Nat Immunol* 7:293, 2006.
23. Herzenberg LA, Herzenberg L: Toward a layered immune system. *Cell* 59:953, 1989.
24. Sanz E, Munoz-A N, Monserrat J, et al: Ordering human CD34$^+$CD10$^-$CD19$^+$ pre/pro-B-cell and CD19$^-$ common lymphoid progenitor stages in two pro-B-cell development pathways. *Proc Natl Acad Sci U S A* 107:5925, 2010.
25. Carsetti R, Rosado MM, Wardmann H: Peripheral development of B cells in mouse and man. *Immunol Rev* 197:179, 2004.
26. Allman D, Pillai S: Peripheral B cell subsets. *Curr Opin Immunol* 20:149, 2008.
27. Pereira J, Kelly L, Cyster J: Finding the right niche: B-cell migration in the early phases of T-dependent antibody responses. *Int Immunol* 22:413, 2010.
28. Klein U, Dalla-Favera R: Germinal centres: Role in B-cell physiology and malignancy. *Nat Rev Immunol* 8:22, 2008.
29. Maul R, Gearhart P: AID and somatic hypermutation. *Adv Immunol* 105:159, 2010.
30. Cancro M, Hao Y, Scholz J, et al: B cells and aging: Molecules and mechanisms. *Trends Immunol* 30:313, 2009.

CHAPTER 19

T-CELL IMMUNITY

Shannon A. Carty, Matthew J. Riese, and Gary A. Koretzky

Thymus-derived (T) lymphocytes play an essential role in the immune response to pathogens and against host cells that have undergone malignant transformation. T cells are critical regulators of other arms of the immune system via soluble mediators they produce and through direct interactions between ligands on the T-cell surface and receptors on other immune cells. This chapter first reviews T-cell activation after engagement by specific antigen and how signals delivered by the antigen receptors shape the repertoire of mature T cells in secondary lymphoid organs. The chapter then discusses how different populations of mature T cells exert their effector functions. Because homeostasis of the immune system requires not only that T cells become activated under appropriate conditions but also that their activity be curtailed when the pathogenic challenge has been met, the chapter describes several means by which T-cell activation is terminated. Finally, the chapter reviews advances in drug development that make use of our understanding of the molecular basis for T-cell activation.

T-CELL ACTIVATION

T-cell activation begins when a T cell encounters a specific antigen that engages and then initiates signal transduction through the T-cell antigen receptor (TCR). Unlike B cells that respond to soluble antigens, T cells are stimulated by small peptides presented on the surface of other cells. These peptides are incorporated into the binding groove of proteins of the major histocompatibility complex (MHC, known in humans as human leukocyte antigen [HLA] complexes) through a process called *antigen presentation*. Thus, the ligand for the TCR is a peptide surface that is generated by both amino acids from the antigenic peptide and residues found in the MHC molecules themselves. Engagement of peptide–MHC complexes by the TCR induces a series of intracellular biochemical events that culminate in T-cell activation. Although T cells make use of many of the same biochemical pathways used by other cells for activation, a number of molecules are unique to immune cells that are critical for T-cell activation. This section discusses TCR signal transduction, focusing on immune cell specific molecular events.

Antigen Presentation: Creating the Ligand for the T-Cell Receptor

Invading pathogenic bacteria and viruses use different strategies to survive within infected hosts. Many bacteria, such as the pathogens staphylococci, streptococci, and various enteric Gram-negative bacilli, survive in the extracellular milieu, but viruses and other bacteria, such as *Listeria* spp., survive inside host cells. Successful elimination of pathogens in each of these locations requires distinct responses from the host. T cells play a central role in the control of extracellular and intracellular pathogens; however, the subset of T cells differs for each type of pathogen, with T cells expressing the cell surface marker CD4 most important for the response against extracellular pathogens and those expressing the CD8 marker essential for control of intracellular organisms. Whereas stimulated $CD4^+$ T cells act on other cells of the immune system by producing cytokines, soluble mediators that elicit a variety of cellular responses important for clearance of extracellular pathogens, $CD8^+$ T cells function largely by directly lysing host cells that have become infected with an intracellular organism. It is therefore critical for antigens derived from extracellular sources to stimulate $CD4^+$ T cells and for antigens derived from within the cell to stimulate $CD8^+$ T cells. Whether a particular antigenic peptide stimulates a $CD4^+$ versus a $CD8^+$ T cell is determined by which MHC proteins present the peptide to the TCR.

Class II MHC proteins are found on cells of the innate immune system known as "professional" antigen-presenting cells (APCs) as well as B cells and the thymic epithelium. Professional APCs include dendritic cells (DCs) and various tissue macrophages, which engulf extracellular organisms (often after these are coated with host antibodies), host cells that have undergone apoptosis (programmed cell death), and cellular debris through an endocytic pathway that brings the ingested material into contact with degradative enzymes. The peptides that are formed in these reactions are bound to the MHC class II proteins for presentation to $CD4^+$ T cells. The MHC class II complex is a dimer consisting of a single α chain and a single β chain. Both α and β contribute to peptide binding and interaction with the TCR. As they are being synthesized within the cell, MHC class II complexes bind invariant chain (Ii), a protein that directs the newly formed MHC proteins into an acidic vesicle. During this trafficking event, a portion of the Ii occupies the peptide binding site. When the MHC class II protein reaches the acidic vesicle, Ii is proteolyzed by cathepsin S, leaving behind a small fragment that remains lodged within the peptide-binding cleft of the MHC class II complex. This fragment is termed the *class II–associated invariant chain peptide (CLIP)*. The MHC class II containing vesicles then fuse with other vesicles containing the peptide fragments from the endocytosed particles. There, CLIP is replaced with a peptide, thus stabilizing the MHC class II complex and allowing it to be transported to the cell surface, where it interacts with $CD4^+$ T cells (Fig. 19-1).

All cells of the body are at risk of being infected with intracellular pathogens or becoming transformed. Because protection against such challenges requires a $CD8^+$ T-cell response, all nucleated cells in the body express class I MHC, the protein complex that presents antigen to $CD8^+$ T cells. Similar to class II MHC, class I MHC is a protein dimer. However, in contrast to class II, only the α chain of class I is variable. This α chain is associated with $\beta 2$ microglobulin, which stabilizes the complex but plays no direct role in antigen presentation. During its assembly in the endoplasmic reticulum (ER), the MHC class I complex comes into contact with peptides derived from proteins being translated in the cell. During protein synthesis, small amounts of protein are modified by ubiquitinylation. This serves as a targeting sequence, directing the modified protein to the proteosome, where it is degraded into small peptide fragments. These fragments are transported back into the ER by the transporters associated with antigen processing (TAP-1 and TAP-2), where they become available for binding to the newly synthesized MHC class I complexes. Peptide association completes the folding and assembly of MHC class I, which is then transported to the cell surface, where it can be recognized by $CD8^+$ T cells.

T cells can only respond to antigenic peptides if these peptides fit into the binding pocket of either MHC class I or II. Although a large number of peptides are able to bind to a specific MHC complex, the

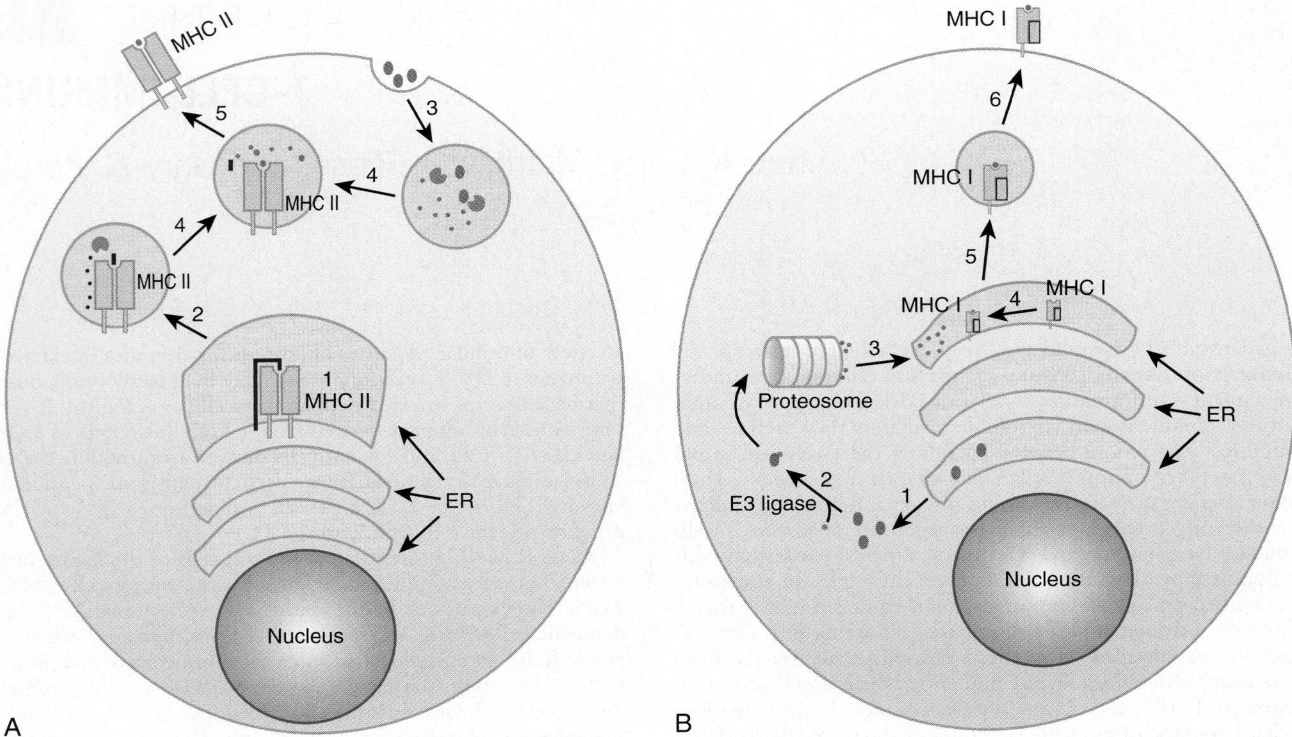

Figure 19-1 ANTIGEN PRESENTATION. Presentation of peptides by major histocompatibility complex (MHC) class I and class II molecules occurs by different mechanisms. **A,** Processing and presentation of class II peptides is limited to specialized antigen-presenting cells (APCs). *(1)* MHC class II molecules are synthesized in the APC endoplasmic reticulum (ER) in conjunction with a stabilizing protein known as invariant chain (Ii) *(purple)*. *(2)* After transport into intracellular vesicles, proteases degrade Ii chain, leaving only the peptide class II–associated invariant chain peptide (CLIP) in the antigen presentation cleft of the class II molecule. *(3)* Peptides for MHC class II molecules are generated from extracellular proteins that are endocytosed from the surrounding milieu and degraded by proteases in intracellular vesicles after vesicle acidification. *(4)* Class II peptides are exposed to MHC molecules after fusion of peptide-containing vesicles and vesicles containing CLIP-loaded MHC class II complexes. After exposure to peptide, CLIP is replaced with a peptide derived from the ingested materials, and the vesicle moves to the plasma membrane, depositing the peptide-loaded class II molecule at the cell surface *(5)*. **B,** All nucleated cells are capable of processing and presenting MHC class I peptides. Peptides for MHC class I molecules are generated from intracellular proteins that are synthesized in the ER *(1)* and transported into the cytosol. *(2)* A fraction of these cytosolic proteins become ubiquitinated by E3 ubiquitin ligases that target their proteolysis by the proteosome. Resultant peptides are subsequently transported back into the ER *(3)* and loaded onto MHC class I molecules *(4)*. Peptide-loaded MHC class I molecules bud into vesicles *(5)* that fuse with the plasma membrane *(6)*, resulting in cell surface expression.

diversity of antigen presentation is enhanced through expression of three different MHC class I alleles (in humans, HLA A, B, and C) and class II alleles (in humans, HLA DR, DP, and DQ). To increase the spectrum of peptides any particular cell may present even further, MHC alleles are always co-dominantly expressed. Thus, any individual expresses a large number of different class II dimers on its APCs and class I dimers on all nucleated cells, providing excellent protection against potential pathogenic organisms. It is possible, however, that even with this degree of potential for antigen presentation, pathogens may evolve that do not possess unique proteins with sequences to fit into the MHC grooves. To circumvent this problem, the MHC locus evolved to be highly polymorphic, thus providing enormous diversity within the population for antigen presentation, ensuring that some individuals will express MHC dimers that can present antigen from virtually any pathogen. Interestingly, predominant MHC alleles exist in different parts of the world, suggesting that there is local pressure, perhaps based on prevailing microorganisms, that shapes selection of MHC expression.

Neither MHC class I nor class II complexes distinguish foreign from host peptides as they fill their peptide binding grooves. Because MHC class II samples all ingested antigens and class I is stabilized by a sampling of all proteins produced by the cell, the majority of the MHC complexes are filled with self peptides. The T cell must distinguish self from nonself to ensure that a response is only directed against that which is foreign. Control over what antigens elicit a T-cell response is accomplished through selection of a population of T cells expressing appropriate TCRs, as discussed later (see T-Cell Development).

The T-Cell Receptor Complex

The TCR is a multimolecular complex with separate components able to bind ligand or to transduce an activating signal to the cell. The peptide–MHC binding regions of the TCR consist of an α/β heterodimer in the majority of T cells and the related γ/δ heterodimer in a smaller subset of T cells. Both α and β and γ and δ consist of variable and constant regions. Similar to antibodies (see Chapters 18 and 22), the variable regions of the TCR antigen-binding proteins arise from rearranging gene segments that are imprecisely joined during T-cell development. This process allows for an extraordinarily diverse repertoire of potential antigen reactivity, although there are in total only several hundred genes that make up the α, β, γ, and δ loci. The germline configuration of the α and β loci are different, such that the α-chain locus comprises about 70 variable (V) segments, 60 joining (J) segments, and one (C) constant segment, but the β-chain locus comprises 50 V regions, 2 diversity (D) segments, 13 J segments, and 2 C regions. Greater diversity is generated by the addition of nucleotides between the V and J gene segments on α chains and the V, D, and J segments in β chains during the formation of the mature TCR. In total, it has been calculated that approximately 10^{18} different TCRs can be created from these segments, although the functional population is much smaller because of the requirements for selection during maturation in the thymus (see T-Cell Development). Thus, after it has completed its developmental program, an individual T cell expresses a unique TCR encoded by a combination of gene segments that have been altered and rearranged (Fig. 19-2). The T cells circulating through the lymphatics, lymph nodes (LNs), and spleen possess sufficient diversity so that nearly all pathogens encountered express an antigenic sequence recognized by a circulating T cell, which then expands in number to combat that pathogen.

Soon after identification of the genes encoding TCR α and β, gene transfer studies in cell lines provided definitive proof that the α/β heterodimer itself contains all of the information necessary for peptide–MHC binding and is the protein complex that confers specific antigen reactivity on a particular T-cell clone. It also became apparent that although sufficient to bind peptide–MHC, the α/β heterodimer is not capable of transmitting an intracellular signal after ligand is bound. A series of studies, first in cell lines and then in mouse models, demonstrated that the signal transduction function of the TCR complex resides in a protein complex that associates noncovalently with the α/β dimer. This complex, CD3, is required

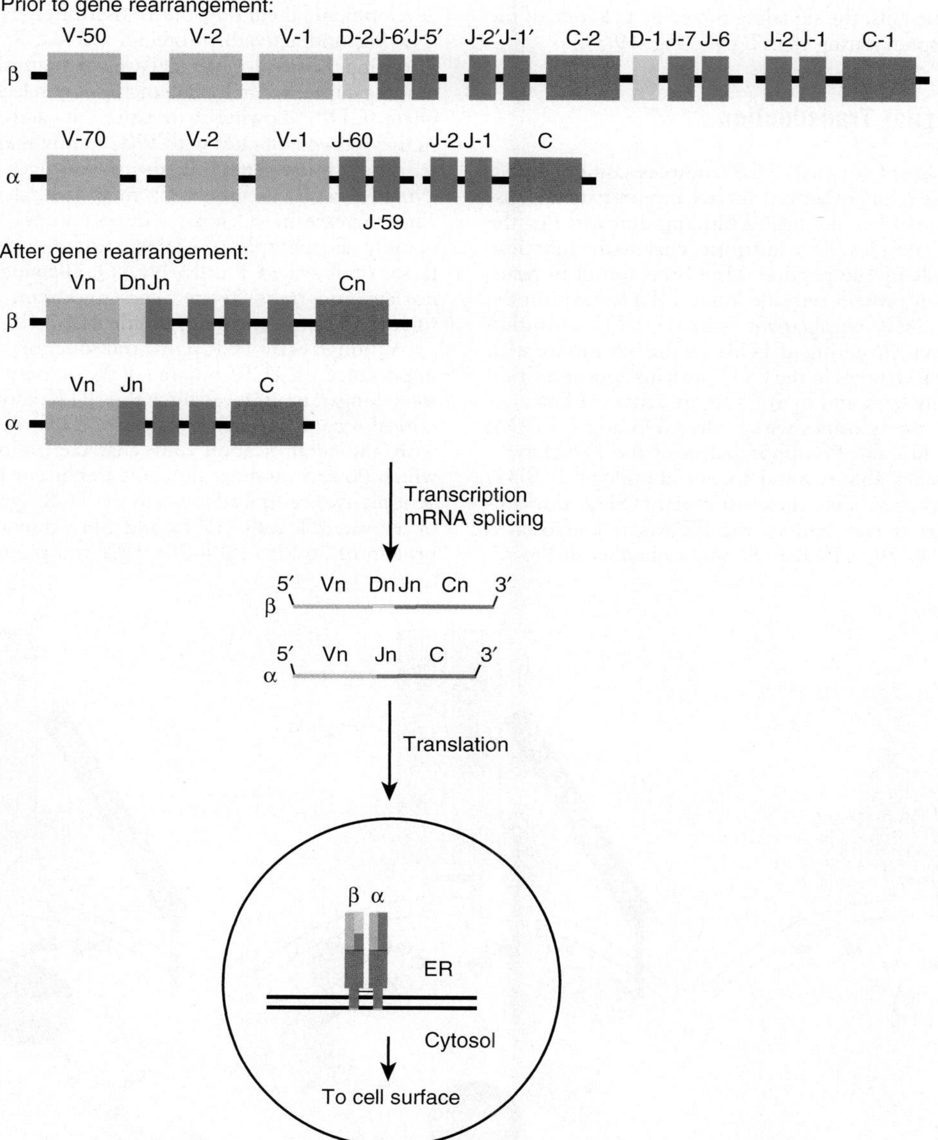

Figure 19-2 GENERATION OF DIVERSITY OF THE T-CELL ANTIGEN RECEPTOR. To generate the diverse repertoire of antigen receptors needed for protective T-cell immunity, the genetic loci encoding the two proteins of the T-cell receptor (TCR) undergo multiple rearrangements to form the mature α and β chains. For the β chain, DNA recombination occurs between a variable (V) segment, a diversity (D) segment, and a joining (J) segment to create, along with remaining joining segments and a constant region, an mRNA transcript. This transcript is spliced to remove intervening joining regions, creating the final mature β chain mRNA. For the α chain, recombination takes place between a V segment and a J segment, with the insertion of additional nucleotides between the recombined segments. As with the β chain, mRNA processing removes intervening J segments to permit translation of the mature α chain. After translation, β chains and α chains pair to form the TCR heterodimer that is transported to the cell surface. Note that peptide-binding regions of the TCR are generated from the recombined V(D)J segments of the TCR gene.

both for stable expression of the ligand-binding components of the TCR and for signal transduction. CD3 is composed of three subunits, δ, ε, and γ, expressed as heterodimers (γ/ε and δ/ε) along with the ζ subunit, which is present as a homodimer. Each subunit contains immunoreceptor tyrosine-based activation motifs (ITAMs), a stretch of amino acids with discretely placed tyrosine residues: one ITAM in δ, ε, and γ and three ITAMS in ζ. The ITAM tyrosines are key for the CD3 and ζ chains to transduce signals and are inducibly phosphorylated upon engagement of the α/β TCR chains by peptide–MHC. Upon their phosphorylation, the ITAMs become docking sites for other proteins that initiate the signaling cascade for T-cell activation. Notably, the CD4 or CD8 protein also plays a role in mediating signal transduction. These coreceptors bind both the appropriate MHC complex (MHC I for CD8, MHC II for CD4), and via their cytoplasmic tails, the signaling molecule Lck, one of the kinases capable of phosphorylating the ITAMs (Fig. 19-3).

T-Cell Receptor Signal Transduction

After the genes were cloned for each TCR complex component, it became clear that unlike many other cell surface receptors that transduce activating signals, neither the ligand-binding domains nor the CD3 proteins of the complex have intrinsic enzymatic function. Engagement of the TCR by the peptide–MHC was found to result in the rapid activation of protein tyrosine kinases (PTKs) within the T cells. Exactly how TCR engagement initiates PTK activation remains unclear; however, clustering of TCRs on the cell surface with resultant conformational changes in the CD3 proteins appears critical in the process. Src family (Lck and Fyn) PTKs are activated first after TCR stimulation, and the tyrosines within the CD3 and ζ ITAMs are substrates of these kinases. Phosphorylation of the ITAM tyrosines makes these residues able to bind to Src homology 2 (SH2) domains of other proteins. The most important SH2 domain-containing protein that is recruited to the ITAMs is ζ-associated protein of 70 kDa (ZAP-70), a PTK itself and a member of the syk family of proteins. Thus, binding of the TCR by ligand converts an enzymatically inactive receptor complex into an active PTK through recruitment and activation of cytosolic proteins.

Activation of ZAP-70 leads to tyrosine phosphorylation of a number of substrates, including enzymes that catalyze reactions generating second messengers important for T-cell activation. Phospholipase Cγ1 (PLCγ1) is activated by its tyrosine phosphorylation to cleave phosphatidylinositol-(4,5)-bisphosphate (PIP_2) into the second messengers diacylglycerol (DAG) and inositol-(1,4,5)-triphosphate (IP_3). DAG is a lipid second messenger that binds to and activates downstream signaling components, including protein kinase Cθ(PKCθ) and the Ras guanine exchange factor RasGRP. PKCθ, a member of the PKC family of serine/threonine kinases, regulates numerous effectors of gene transcription and T-cell effector function development, including the transcription factors nuclear factor κB (NF-κB) and activator protein-1 (AP-1). RasGRP is responsible for activating the small-molecular-weight guanosine triphosphate (GTP)-binding protein Ras by enhancing Ras release of guanosine diphosphate (GDP) allowing it to assume its activated GTP-bound form. Active Ras collaborates with PKC family members to stimulate transcription of new genes by activating mitogen-activated protein kinase (MAPK) family members. IP_3 mobilizes calcium stores from the ER. This increase in calcium is important for enzyme function, most notably the phosphatase calcineurin that dephosphorylates nuclear factor of activated T cells (NFAT), allowing it to translocate to the nucleus and transactivate genes important for T-cell proliferation, such as the gene encoding interleukin-2 (IL-2).

Although early TCR signal transduction studies demonstrated the importance of TCR-initiated PTK activity for T-cell activation, it took longer to unravel how this PTK activation drives the many critical second messenger cascades. This mechanism was elucidated with the identification and characterization of adapter proteins, which possess modular domains important for intermolecular interactions. Two central adapters in the TCR signaling pathway are linker of activated T cells (LAT) and SH2 domain-containing leukocyte protein of 76 kDa (SLP-76). LAT is a transmembrane protein with

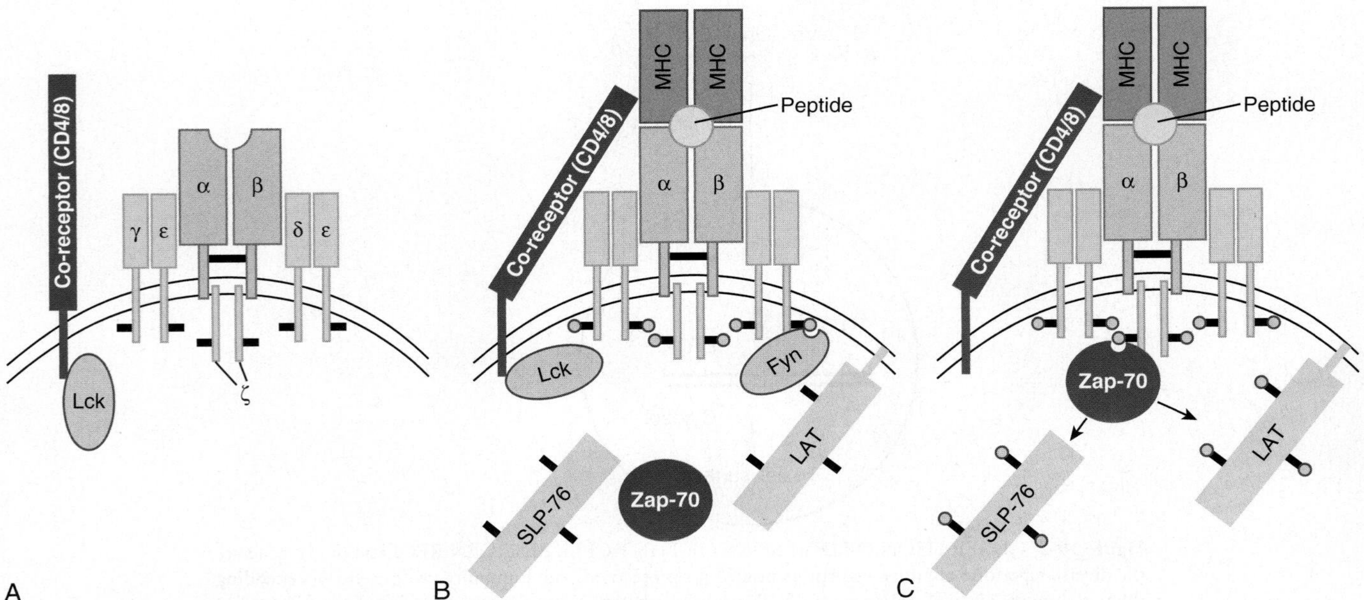

Figure 19-3 PROXIMAL T-CELL RECEPTOR (TCR) SIGNAL TRANSDUCTION. Binding of major histocompatibility complex (MHC) and peptide to the TCR and corresponding coreceptor (CD4 for MHC class II complexes and CD8 for MHC class I complexes) results in a series of molecular events that culminate in T-cell activation. **A,** At rest, the TCR exists in a complex with CD3, which consists of heterodimers between δ, ε, or γ (δ/ε, γ/ε) chains (*olive, left* or *right* of the TCR) and homodimers of ζ chains (*olive,* between TCR chains). **B,** Initially after ligand binding, the src-family kinases Lck (associated with CD4 and CD8) and Fyn (cytoplasmic) phosphorylate immunoreceptor tyrosine-based activation motifs (ITAMs) of CD3 and ζ *(black lines)*. **C,** These phosphorylated ITAMs in turn serve as docking sites for the kinase Zap-70 that subsequently phosphorylates the adapter proteins linker of activated T cells (LAT) and (SH2) domain-containing leukocyte protein of 76 kDa (SLP-76), which serve to nucleate the complex containing signaling proteins.

cytoplasmic tyrosines that are phosphorylated by the PTKs activated by the TCR. SLP-76 is a cytosolic adapter protein that is also phosphorylated by these PTKs. Because these tyrosine phosphorylation events create docking sites for other proteins with SH2 domains, when the TCR is engaged, SLP-76 and LAT nucleate a large complex of signaling molecules at the membrane in the vicinity of the activated TCR. This cluster of molecules initiates the signaling cascades that are integrated to result in T-cell activation. Key proteins in this complex are Vav1, a guanine nucleotide exchange factor important for cytoskeletal reorganization; inducible T-cell kinase (ITK), a member of the Tec family of PTKs (a third family of PTKs essential for T-cell activation); adhesion and degranulation-promoting adapter protein (ADAP), an adapter that is a key regulator of integrins to promote T-cell interactions with other cells; PLCγ, the enzyme described earlier that initiates both the calcium and Ras/MAPK pathway in T cells; and growth factor receptor-bound protein 2 (Grb2) and son of sevenless (SOS), two proteins important for activating Ras through a RasGRP independent pathway (Fig. 19-4).

For T-cell immunity to be effective, T cells must possess TCRs that are exquisitely sensitive to specific antigen. Because the TCR is generated through random reassortment of and alteration of gene segments, it is impossible to prevent generation of TCRs that have the potential to respond to self antigens. Although the developmental program of T cells in the thymus provides a mechanism to eliminate most potentially self reactive T cells (see T-Cell Development section later), this process is not 100% effective. Hence, mechanisms exist to prevent mature T cells from responding against normal host tissues. One such mechanism is the requirement for T cells to receive two signals to become activated, one mediated by the TCR and the second through a costimulatory receptor. Although several different T-cell molecules can provide this costimulatory function, the best studied is the surface protein CD28. This additional requirement for T-cell activation helps to prevent autoimmunity because the ligands for CD28, CD80, and CD86 are upregulated on APCs only in the presence of "danger signals" generated largely by bacterial and viral components or in the setting of cellular stress. (The mechanism of how bacterial and viral components signal through Toll-like receptors to activate APCs is described in Chapter 21.)

For CD28 engagement to provide the second signal for T-cell activation, it must also initiate signal transduction pathways (Fig. 19-5). CD28 augments many of the TCR-stimulated pathways described earlier and in particular activates phosphatidylinositol 3-kinase (PI3K), a protein that phosphorylates PIP_2 to form phosphatidylinositol-(3,4,5)-trisphosphate (PIP_3). Although the formation of PIP_3 induces broad changes within cells, the PIP_3 effector molecule that has been studied most intensively is Akt, a serine/threonine kinase responsible for maintaining cell survival and proliferation in a variety of cell types, including T cells, and for altering the metabolism of those cells to favor cell division. The importance of CD28 costimulation of T cells goes beyond its requirement for T-cell activation because engagement of the TCR in the absence of CD28 signaling induces an impaired functional state within T cells termed *anergy* (see Anergy section later in this chapter).

Spatial Coordination of T-Cell Receptor Signal Transduction: The Immunologic Synapse

As the biochemical signaling events that occur after TCR engagement by peptide–MHC became known, investigators sought to define the

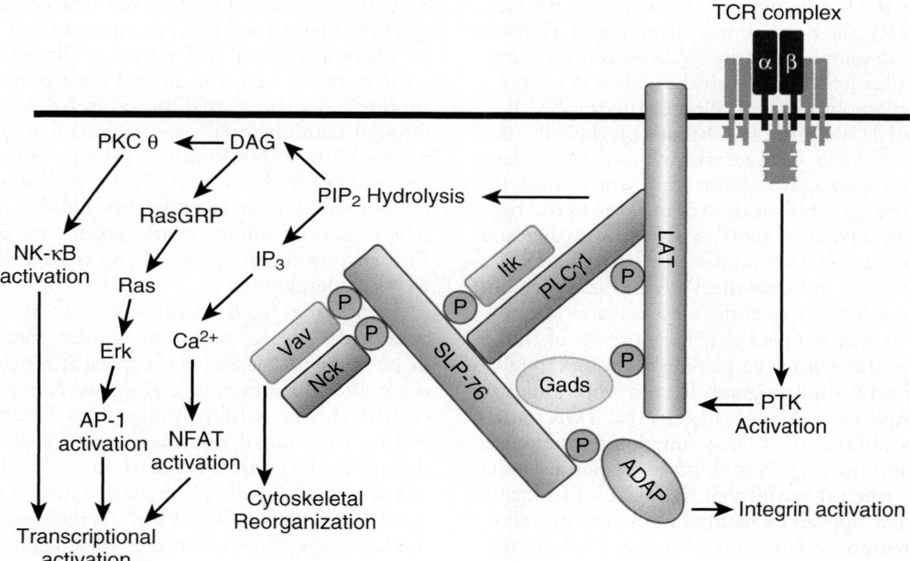

Figure 19-4 INTEGRATION OF T-CELL RECEPTOR (TCR) SIGNALS BY ADAPTER PROTEINS. After engagement of the TCR and activation of protein tyrosine kinases, several hematopoietic specific adapter proteins are phosphorylated, enabling the formation of a multimolecular signaling complex. The transmembrane adapter protein linker of activated T cells (LAT) recruits SH2 domain-containing leukocyte protein of 76 kDa (SLP-76) through the Grb2 family member Gads. This SLP-76 nucleated complex associates with PLCγ1, Itk, Vav1, and adhesion and degranulation-promoting adapter protein (ADAP). After phosphorylation by Itk, PLCγ1 catalyzes the cleavage of PIP_2 into inositol-(1,4,5)-triphosphate (IP_3) and diacylglycerol (DAG). IP_3 induces calcium flux from the endoplasmic reticulum, leading to activation of the transcription factor nuclear factor of activated T cells (NFAT). DAG binds and activates proteins important in signaling such as PKCθ, a kinase whose substrates initiate the activation of the transcription factor nuclear factor κB (NF-κB), and RasGRP, a Ras activating protein that induces activation of Erk and formation of the transcription factor AP-1. Apart from transcriptional changes, T cells also undergo cytoskeletal changes after TCR stimulation mediated in part by Vav1, an activating protein for the actin-modulating protein Rac1, and activation of cell surface integrins, mediated in part by the adapter protein ADAP.

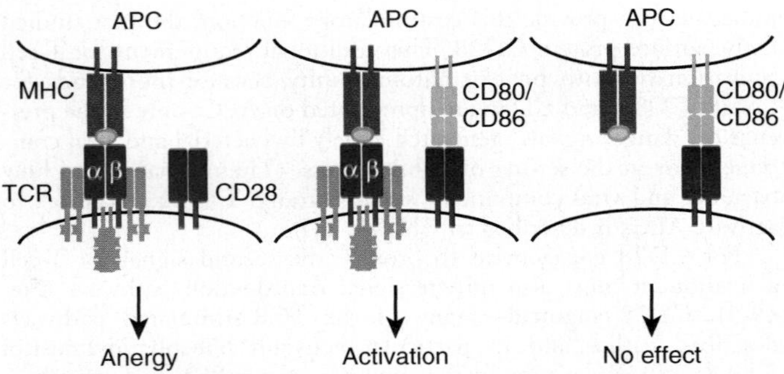

Figure 19-5 TWO SIGNALS ARE REQUIRED TO ACTIVATE T CELLS. T-cell activation requires two signals, one through the T-cell receptor (TCR) and one mediated by a costimulatory molecule, such as CD28. An APC will activate a T cell if it presents appropriate peptide : major histocompatibility complex (MHC) to the T cell and expresses a ligand to engage CD28. If CD28 is engaged without a concomitant TCR signal, the T cell is neither activated nor inactivated. However, if a T cell is stimulated through the TCR in the absence of costimulation through CD28, then it becomes anergic, unresponsive to the initial as well as subsequent stimulations.

topography of the activation events. Sophisticated imaging technologies were applied to visualize the contact site between the APC and the T cell, and this interaction was modeled by visualizing the contact between key receptors on T cells and ligands fixed to a solid support. These studies revealed a stepwise reorganization of the T-cell membrane at the contact site called the immunologic synapse (IS). The first step in IS formation is an interaction between integrins on the surface of the T cell and their ligands on the APC that brings the T cell and APC into close proximity. If a productive interaction occurs between the TCR and peptide–MHC, the next event is clustering of TCRs in the central portion of the developing IS (the so-called central supramolecular activation complex [cSMAC]) with the activated integrins forming the peripheral supramolecular activation complex (pSMAC), a ring around the clustered TCRs. Although ligands on the APC initially direct the formation of the IS, changes within the T cell, including reorganization of the actin cytoskeleton, are also critical for stabilization of this structure. As sophistication of imaging in real time has advanced and with the advent of tools to visualize smaller and smaller numbers of molecules, it has become clear that the IS is a dynamic structure that includes not only the TCR and integrins but also many of the signaling molecules essential for T-cell activation.

When first described, it was assumed that the purpose of the IS was to cluster the TCR together with key signaling molecules to initiate and sustain the T-cell activation program. Recent work indicates that this notion is too simplistic. Evidence suggests that TCR signaling precedes IS formation and that the IS may function to internalize activated receptors, thus terminating their ability to respond. Under other conditions, perhaps when the avidity of the TCR for its ligand is not as great, the IS does appear to maintain contact and allow signaling to occur. Moreover, recent work suggests that another important function of the IS is to focus the release of cytokines from T cells toward other cells of the immune system or materials from the lytic granules of cytotoxic T cells toward their targets, thus enhancing the ability of T cells to exert their appropriate effector functions.

T-Cell Proliferation

The number of naive T cells potentially responsive to any particular peptide antigen (the precursor frequency of the responding population) is quite small, yet a large number of antigen-specific T cells are required to combat pathogens. Accordingly, a consequence of TCR plus costimulatory receptor engagement is the clonal expansion of an activated T cell. One outcome of the second messenger cascades stimulated by the TCR and CD28 is the production of IL-2, an essential cytokine for T-cell proliferation. Another outcome of TCR signaling is upregulation of the high affinity receptor for IL-2, hence making the activated T cell able to respond to local concentrations of this cytokine. Signaling through the IL-2 receptor is necessary for the proliferative response. Similar to the TCR, the IL-2 receptor makes use of cytoplasmic PTKs (in this case members of the Janus kinase [JAK] family) to initiate a cascade of second messengers that lead ultimately to T-cell proliferation.

T-CELL DEVELOPMENT

Protective T-cell immunity requires populating the secondary lymphoid organs with a large number of mature T cells. This population collectively must possess a diverse TCR repertoire capable of recognizing the enormous universe of foreign antigens that will be encountered over life. Because the TCR binds antigenic peptide plus amino acid residues of self MHC molecules, it is essential that only cells with a TCR able to recognize self MHC, albeit with limited affinity, be exported from the thymus to the periphery. It is also critical, however, that the population of peripheral T cells be restricted to those that respond to foreign antigens, and cells possessing TCRs recognizing self peptides plus MHC must not be allowed to complete their developmental program. Ensuring that only those cells with an appropriate TCR mature in the thymus relies heavily on many of the same TCR signal transduction events described earlier.

Unlike most hematopoietic cells that complete the transition from progenitors to mature cells in the bone marrow, T cells develop primarily in the thymus. Experiments in mice demonstrated 50 years ago that neonatal thymectomy results in fatal viral infection, thereby revealing a key role of the thymus in the immune system and paving the way for the identification of the thymus as the site of T-cell development. In the ensuing decades, much has been learned about how progenitor cells enter the thymus and develop into mature T cells.

There are several T lymphocyte lineages. αβ T cells (discussed earlier) are the best studied and most numerous lineage. γδ T cells, another population that possesses an antigen receptor generated through combinatorial rearrangement of gene segments, as well as natural killer T (NKT) cells, a subtype of lymphocytes that has characteristics of both NK and T cells, are also generated in the thymus. It has become clear recently that additional small populations of T cells possessing unique characteristics are produced in the thymus. This chapter focuses primarily on αβ T cells and touches briefly on γδ T-cell development.

Identifying T-cell progenitors is an area of intense investigation because developing tools to manipulate these cells has great therapeutic potential for increasing the speed at which T-cell repopulation may occur after bone marrow transplant. A population of bone marrow-derived thymic settling progenitors (TSPs) that can give rise to mature T-cell populations has been identified. As these cells enter the thymus at the corticomedullary junction, they develop into double-negative (DN) T cells, characterized by lack of expression of the CD4 or CD8 coreceptors (Fig. 19-6). As these early T cells progress though the DN stage, they are further classified as DN1, DN2, DN3, and DN4 stages based on the cell surface receptors they express. During DN1, TSPs lose the ability to differentiate into non-T lineages and begin to proliferate in the deep cortex of the thymus. As the early thymocytes progress to the DN2 phase, they begin to express certain T-cell specific markers, such as Thy-1 (CD90), CD24, and CD25 and initiate TCR gene rearrangement at the TCRγ, TCRδ, and TCRβ loci. Throughout the DN1 to DN3 stages, as the cells migrate from the cortex to the subcapsular zone, interactions between Notch receptors on the developing T cells and specific Notch ligands collaborate with signaling through the IL-7 receptor to regulate differentiation and progression.

During the DN3 stage, rearrangement of TCRγ, TCRδ, and TCRβ loci occurs with maximal efficiency, and initial expression of the TCR proteins these genes encode occurs. From this time onward in T-cell development, the proliferation and survival of the developing thymocytes depend on TCR signals. Two key checkpoints must

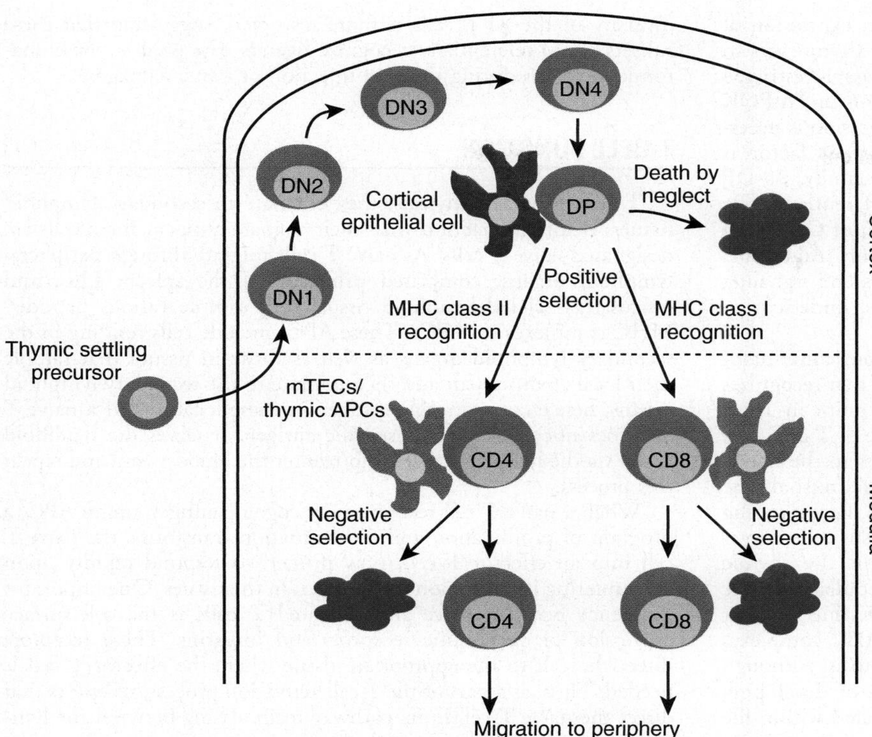

Figure 19-6 T-CELL DEVELOPMENT IN THE THYMUS. Thymic settling precursors (TSPs) from the bone marrow enter the thymus at the corticomedullary junction. These hematopoietic precursors develop into double-negative (DN) thymocytes, at which time they lose the ability to differentiate into non-T lineages, express T-cell markers, and begin TCR gene rearrangement. Developing αβ thymocytes pass through the β-selection checkpoint before progression to the double-positive (DP) stage to ensure that the rearranged TCR proteins are able to transduce signals. DP thymocytes undergo positive selection if their TCR is able to recognize self major histocompatibility complex (MHC) molecules; otherwise, they undergo "death by neglect." Negative selection occurs in the thymic medulla when cells bearing TCRs that bind with strong avidity to self-MHC with self-peptide undergo apoptosis, thereby promoting central tolerance. Mature CD4 SP and CD8 single-positive (SP) cells then emigrate to the periphery.

be passed for full T-cell development to occur. First, upon productive rearrangement of the TCR β locus, the TCRβ protein forms a "pre-TCR" complex with an invariant cytosolic protein designated pre-Tα. This complex engages the TCR signaling machinery, including the PTKs Lck, Fyn, and Syk (a ZAP-70 related PTK) and the adapters SLP-76 and LAT, to initiate the TCR signaling cascade. The resultant biochemical second messengers suppress rearrangement of the other β allele, resulting in "allelic exclusion" or silencing of the nonrearranged allele to ensure each T cell expresses only one TCR specificity. These signals also induce continued T-cell development by promoting rearrangements at the α locus, maintaining cellular survival, initiating a proliferative burst, and inducing expression of CD4 and CD8. For effective signaling to occur, the rearranged β locus must encode a protein that folds correctly and pairs with pre-Tα. Because the rearrangement of the genes that eventually makes up the β chain is a random process, it is often the case that the rearranged allele encodes a dysfunctional protein. In this circumstance, signaling does not occur, and the cell initiates rearrangement at the other β chain allele. Again, if this does not result in a functional protein, no signaling occurs, and the cell undergoes apoptosis. In other cells, a similar rearrangement process occurs in the γ and δ loci. Productive rearrangements of these gene families create a functional, mature γδ TCR that also associates with the TCR signaling complex to propagate signals to trigger further cellular development.

Although the determining factors that result in either γδ or αβ T-cell development have not been fully elucidated, several molecular processes are thought to contribute. The expression of a TCR gene rearrangement product likely plays a role in lineage determination because evidence suggests that developing thymocytes with a functional γδ TCR are often excluded from the αβ cell fate. However, TCR expression is not the only factor in determining lineage fate; cytokine signals and TCR signal strength may also play a role. Experiments have shown that DN2 thymocytes distinguished according to IL-7 receptor expression differentiate into αβ or γδ T cells, with DN2 cells expressing high IL-7 receptor levels preferentially developing into γδ T lymphocytes and those with lower expression more likely to differentiate into the αβ lineage. Other studies have suggested that the strong signals propagated by the γδ TCR compared with those of the pre-TCR complex may promote γδ lineage commitment.

Developing αβ T cells that have passed the first checkpoint demonstrating functional β chain rearrangement transition into the double-positive (DP; $CD4^+CD8^+$) stage and complete TCRα rearrangement to produce a mature αβ TCR heterodimer. The stochastic nature of TCR gene rearrangements guarantees that a significant proportion of cells expressing TCRαβ complexes will not be able to interact with self-MHC proteins and hence would not be stimulated by peptide–MHC complexes in the periphery. DP thymocytes therefore undergo a series of tests, collectively known as *positive and negative selection*, to determine TCR fitness. If the TCR is not stimulated via peptide–MHC complexes presented by thymic APCs, the developing cell undergoes "death by neglect" through apoptosis. Approximately 90% of developing αβ DP thymocytes express a TCR that cannot recognize self peptide–MHC and die by neglect. In contrast, DP thymocytes that interact with self peptide–MHC complexes on thymic cortical epithelial cells with sufficient strength pass this "positive selection" test and are protected from apoptosis.

The MHC specificity of the TCR on a positively selected DP thymocyte influences lineage fate. Cells signaled through a MHC class I–restricted TCR develop into CD8 single-positive (SP; $CD4^-CD8^+$) cells, and those that receive signals via MHC class II–restricted TCRs develop into CD4 SP T cells. The underlying molecular mechanisms governing CD4/CD8 lineage choice is much debated. Predicated on the thought that TCR signals during positive selection result in the termination of either CD4 or CD8 gene transcription, the two classical models of lineage fate are the stochastic selection and instructive models. In the stochastic selection model, TCR signals in a positively selected DP thymocyte randomly terminate either CD4 or CD8 expression. In the instructive model, certain TCR signal qualities, such as strength of signal, direct termination of mismatching coreceptor expression. More recently, a kinetic signaling model has emerged, which proposes that CD4 or CD8 lineage fate is determined by TCR signal duration. Experimental models continue to be tested to fully elucidate the mechanisms underlying lineage fate.

Among the many proteins that are involved in CD4 or CD8 lineage choice are key transcription factors. One such example is Th-POK, a zinc finger protein that is expressed exclusively in $CD4^+$

T cells and not in $CD8^+$ T cells. In transgenic mice, expression of this protein forces the majority of positively selected thymocytes to adopt $CD4^+$ T-cell fate, even those with MHC class I–restricted TCRs. In addition, mice with a spontaneous mutation in Th-POK lack virtually all $CD4^+$ T cells, indicating that its expression is necessary for $CD4^+$ T-cell development. Another important factor is Runx3, a member of the Runx transcription factor family. As DP thymocytes differentiate, Runx3 regulates CD8 differentiation by silencing CD4 transcription, promoting the initiation of CD8 gene transcription, and downregulating Th-POK expression. Additional studies have identified other key transcription factors and signaling proteins important for lineage choice in the thymus, underscoring the complexity of this stage of T-cell development.

Although positive selection ensures that the random combinatorial rearrangement of gene segments results in a TCR that recognizes antigen presented by self MHC proteins, until this point in T-cell development, there is no guard against the emergence of T cells that possess TCRs with high reactivity against self peptides in the MHC binding pockets. Thus, to prevent autoimmunity, there must also be a mechanism to eliminate developing T cells with TCRs expressing these potentially autoreactive specificities. This process is called *negative selection*. Negative selection occurs primarily in the thymic medulla, where thymocytes serially interact with medullary thymic epithelial cells (mTECs) and other thymic APCs, including DCs. At this stage, if thymocytes with TCRs engage peptide–MHC complexes with high affinity, a strong TCR signal initiates apoptosis. Although it is easy to see how this model allows for deletion of developing thymocytes with reactivity against self antigens generated within the thymus itself, it was difficult to imagine how cells with reactivity against antigens known to be expressed outside of the thymus would also be deleted. An explanation for how this occurs came from the discovery of the autoimmune regulator (AIRE) protein. Initially identified as the gene mutated in a rare human autoimmune disorder, autoimmune polyendocrinopathy–candidiasis–ectoderm dystrophy syndrome (APECED), AIRE was later found to be essential for the expression of peripheral tissue specific antigens by mTECs. Although AIRE does not regulate thymic expression of all peripheral antigens, its contribution to the elimination of autoreactive cells is highlighted by the widespread, multiorgan autoimmunity seen in individuals with APECED. Identifying additional mechanisms responsible for thymic expression of tissue-specific genes is an area of active investigation.

Negative selection is one mechanism for development of "tolerance" or immune unresponsiveness to self antigens; however, negative selection is not 100% effective. Hence, other means exist to promote self-tolerance after T cells leave the thymus. One such mechanism relies on development of regulatory T cells (Tregs), which actively interfere with effector T-cell function. Similar to conventional αβ T cells, a subset of Tregs (known as *natural* or *nTregs*) also develops in the thymus. Tregs are characterized by the surface expression of CD4 and CD25 (the α chain of the IL-2 receptor) and depend on the transcription factor forkhead box protein 3 (FoxP3) for their lineage commitment. The gene encoding FoxP3 was originally identified as the causal mutation in a rare human autoimmune disease, immunodysregulation polydendocrinopathy and enteropathy, X-linked (IPEX) syndrome. A mutation in the mouse gene for FoxP3 causes a similar disease (scurfy mice). These naturally occurring loss-of-function mutations demonstrate the necessity for Tregs in maintaining self-tolerance. In the thymus, development into a Treg is enhanced in cells that have high-affinity TCR–peptide–MHC interactions, suggesting that these cells develop specifically to counter autoreactive responses. The exact mechanism that drives these cells to adopt a Treg fate and avoid negative selection during development is being investigated.

The path of developing γδ thymocytes contrasts with that of αβ T-cell development, which is likely related to the function of mature γδ T cells. In the periphery, γδ T cells reside in secondary lymphoid organs with conventional αβ T cells but also are enriched in epithelial tissues of various organs, such as the skin, intestinal epithelium, reproductive tract, and lung. In these distinct settings, the TCR diversity of the γδ T cells is more restricted, suggesting that these subsets may preferentially recognize ligands expressed at these anatomic locations during times of infection or tissue damage.

T-CELL FUNCTION

As T cells leave the thymus, they circulate to secondary lymphoid tissues. Before interaction with their cognate antigen, these cells are designated naïve T cells. As naïve T cells migrate through peripheral lymphoid organs, comprised primarily of the spleen, LNs, and mucosal associated lymphoid tissue, they sample various peptide–MHC complexes on APCs. These APCs include cells residing in the secondary lymphoid organs as well as those in tissues that sample their local environment and then migrate to the secondary lymphoid organs, hence concentrating antigen in these locations. If a naïve T cell does not encounter its specific antigen, it leaves the lymphoid tissue via the lymphatic system to reenter the bloodstream and repeat this process.

When a naïve T cell recognizes its cognate antigen on an APC, a program of proliferation and differentiation transforms the naïve T cell into an effector T cell, now primed to respond rapidly upon encountering its corresponding antigen in the tissues. One important difference between naïve and activated T cells is the cell surface expression of chemokine receptors and integrins. These receptors direct the cell to the appropriate tissue where the effector T cell is needed. Thus, as a part of the T-cell activation process, receptors that direct the naïve T cell in its pathway recirculating between the lymphatic organs and blood vessels are altered for those that direct the activated cell to the tissues, so that the effector T cell reaches the site of pathogen challenge.

$CD4^+$ and $CD8^+$ T cells undergo analogous differentiation processes to acquire functional maturity but play distinct roles in the adaptive immune response to infection. Naïve cells of both lineages are activated through peptide–MHC interaction with their TCRs, and their differentiation is influenced by a combination of signals, including TCR signal strength, costimulation by ligands that interact with other T-cell surface receptors, and the local cytokine environment during antigen encounter. Integration of these signals promotes expression of signature transcription factors and key effector molecules, which allow the mature cell to perform its individualized function. Activated $CD8^+$ T cells possess the machinery to induce death in host cells that express the appropriate peptide within the binding groove of MHC class I, and $CD4^+$ T cells exert their functions through the production of cytokines or through interacting with other immune cell types through direct cell–cell contact after restimulation of their TCR by peptide presented by class II MHC. These so-called "helper" functions marshal and activate other cells of the immune system (Fig. 19-7). Until they encounter peptide–MHC, naïve $CD4^+$ T cells have the potential to develop into one of several effector subsets, including Th1, Th2, Th17, and T follicular helper (Tfh) cells. Additional subsets have been defined recently, but these remain less well characterized and are not discussed in this chapter.

Th1 Cells

Th1 cells activate macrophages, NK cells, and $CD8^+$ T cells to combat intracellular pathogens. Th1 cells also stimulate immunoglobulin (Ig) class switching in B cells for the production of IgG2a antibodies that optimize clearance of viruses and extracellular bacteria. During priming of naïve $CD4^+$ T cells, several factors combine to promote differentiation along the Th1 pathway, including characteristics of the antigen, costimulatory signals from the presenting APC, and the cytokine microenvironment. Several cytokines are implicated in Th1 differentiation, but the two most critical are interferon-γ (IFN-γ) and IL-12. IFN-γ produced by innate immune cells promotes Th1 differentiation, by activating signal transducer and activator of transcription 1 (STAT1), a key signaling molecule that regulates T-bet, one of

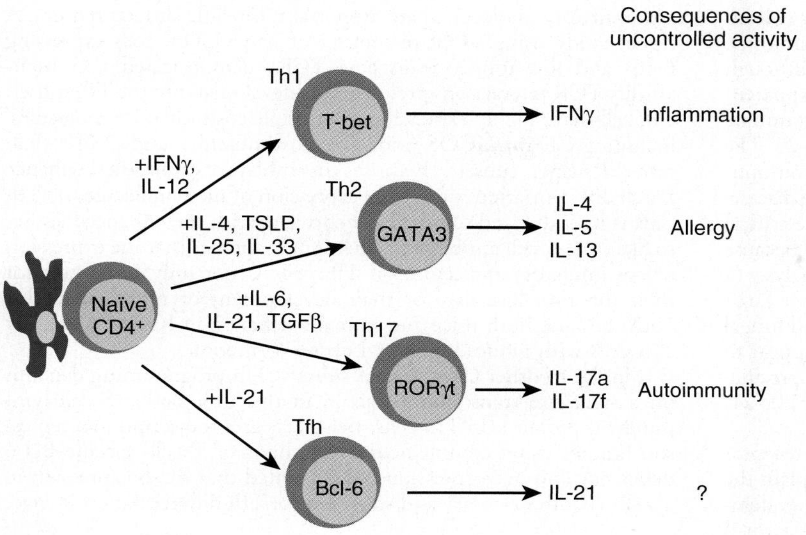

Figure 19-7 DIFFERENTIATION OF CD4$^+$ T HELPER SUBSETS. When activated, CD4$^+$ T cells differentiate into distinct, functionally mature effector subsets. Various factors, including the cytokine milieu, promote the expression of signature transcription factors and effector molecules. CD4$^+$ helper subsets are defined largely by their cytokine production driven by these key transcription factors. Th1 cells are induced by interferon-γ (IFN-γ) and interleukin-12 (IL-12), express the transcription factor T-bet and produce IFN-γ. IL-4 is the primary cytokine that promotes Th2 differentiation. Th2 cells are characterized by expression of GATA-3 and production of IL-4, IL-5, and IL-13. Naive CD4$^+$ cells that are activated in the presence of IL-6 and IL-21 differentiate into Th17 cells, typified by the expression of ROR-γt and production of the IL-17 family of cytokines. T follicular helper (Tfh) cell differentiation is mediated by IL-21. These cells are characterized by the transcription factor Bcl-6 and production of IL-21. If CD4$^+$ helper differentiation and activity are not adequately controlled, imbalanced responses can lead to pathologic conditions.

the signature transcription factors associated with Th1 cells. IL-12, produced by activated APCs and other innate immune cells, acts through a separate STAT4-dependent pathway to promote IFN-γ production. IL-12 also signals to upregulate its own receptor and the IL-18 receptor, thereby allowing IL-18 to act in concert with IL-12 to promote IFN-γ production, thus creating a "feedforward" cycle to amplify the Th1 response.

T-bet, a T-box family member, is the key transcription factor associated with Th1 differentiation and function. T-bet–deficient T cells are defective in their ability to differentiate into Th1 cells either in vitro or in vivo, and T-bet–deficient mice are unable to control *Leishmania major* infection, a well-characterized intracellular pathogen model that depends on the characteristic Th1 cytokines for its clearance. Although T-bet is considered the "essential" factor that directs Th1 lineage determination, other transcription factors, such as Runx3 and Hlx, are important for optimal Th1 function.

After differentiation, Th1 effector cells are characterized by production of proinflammatory cytokines such as IFN-γ and tumor necrosis factor α (TNF-α) that stimulate macrophages, NK cells, and CD8$^+$ T cells to promote pathogen clearance. It is clear, however, that Th1 function must be balanced. Evidence from both animal models and human patients indicates that overexuberant Th1 responses drive inflammatory conditions and may lead to tissue destruction.

Th2 Cells

Th2 cells are critical for the immune response against extracellular parasites, such as helminths, through production of IL-4, IL-5, and IL-13. At initial sites of parasitic infection, epithelial cells of the target organs, including the skin, lungs, and intestines, and resident cells of the innate immune system sense parasite-derived products and produce Th2-inducing cytokines, including thymic stromal lymphopoietin (TSLP), IL-4, IL-25, and IL-33. These cytokines then act on innate immune cells, including basophils and DCs, as well as directly on naïve CD4$^+$ cells to promote Th2 differentiation.

Recent work has provided insight into how cytokine signaling, particularly IL-4 signaling, promotes Th2 differentiation. Through interaction with its receptor, IL-4 activates STAT6. STAT6 plays a vital role in Th2 differentiation, as evidenced by the profound reduction in development of this lineage in *Stat6*-deficient mice. STAT6 activation leads to its nuclear translocation and subsequent induction of the transcription factor GATA-3, which, similar to T-bet for Th1 cells, is considered the master regulator of Th2 differentiation. GATA3 regulates Th2 cytokine production by binding and activating the "Th2 locus," which includes the genes encoding IL-4, IL-5, and IL-13. When GATA3 function is abrogated, Th2 differentiation is virtually absent both in vitro and in vivo. In mature differentiated Th2 cells, GATA3 deficiency results in loss of IL-5 and IL-13 production. GATA3 is both necessary and sufficient for Th2 differentiation because forced expression either by retroviral constructs or transgenic expression promotes Th2 differentiation and represses Th1 differentiation. Repression of Th1 development is as least partially through GATA3-dependent inhibition of STAT4, thus interfering with *Ifng* gene transcription.

TCR signal strength also is involved in determining if a naïve T cell will differentiate into a Th1 or Th2 cell. Studies in mice using altered peptide ligands that have decreased affinity for particular TCRs and experiments using limiting dose of antigen have demonstrated that diminished TCR stimulation promotes Th2 cell differentiation. Differences in costimulation also affect Th2 pathway differentiation. Mice deficient in CD28 or CD80/CD86 have a more pronounced defect in Th2 responses, suggesting that these molecules may play a greater role in promoting Th2 differentiation than Th1 differentiation.

IL-4 produced by mature Th2 cells acts in a positive feedback loop to promote further Th2 cell differentiation in naïve T cells as they encounter antigen. Th2-derived IL-4 also mediates IgE class switching in B cells. Soluble IgE binds to and crosslinks its high-affinity receptor FcεRI on basophils and mast cells, promoting production of histamine and serotonin as well as several cytokines, including IL-4, IL-13, and TNF-α. IL-5 produced from Th2 cells recruits eosinophils, and Th2-derived IL-13 promotes both the expulsion of helminths during parasitic infection and the induction of airway hypersensitivity.

Th2 responses are critical for immunity against extracellular parasites, but excessive Th2 responses are associated with the pathologic conditions of allergy and airway hypersensitivity. The recent increase in asthma in the developed world has been linked to an imbalance of Th subsets with skewing towards "Th2-ness" in the population. Additional work is necessary to more firmly establish a molecular immunologic link to the epidemiology of these diseases.

Th17 Cells

The original description of Th1 and Th2 cells, indicating that not all mature CD4$^+$ T cells were alike, led to the search for other CD4$^+$ subsets. One such cell type was identified after unexpected results were observed in experimental autoimmune disease models. For many years, mouse models of multiple sclerosis and rheumatoid arthritis were thought to be dependent on excessive Th1-driven inflammation. Because IL-12 is a key factor in Th1-mediated responses, blocking IL-12 signaling was predicted to ameliorate experimental autoimmunity. IL-12 is a heterodimeric protein that includes a larger (p40) and smaller (p35) subunit. Experiments in mice in which p40 was deleted revealed the expected result with marked resistance to autoimmunity. Surprisingly, however, mice lacking p35 still exhibited disease, although IL-12 function was abrogated. An explanation for this apparent paradox emerged as it was learned that the p40 subunit was not unique to IL-12 but also dimerized with p19 to form the cytokine IL-23. The hypothesis then arose that IL-23 was the critical driver of autoimmunity in the mice, and IL-23–deficient animals were resistant to disease. These findings led to further studies that revealed IL-23 to be critical for the generation of another Th subset, later designated Th17 because of the production of its signature cytokine IL-17. Extensive analyses of IL-17 and the cells that produce this cytokine demonstrate that Th17 cells are important for the control of extracellular bacterial and fungal infections. With excessive activity, however, these cells also appear to play an important role in autoimmune diseases through the production of proinflammatory cytokines, including IL-17A, IL-17F, IL-21, and IL-22.

Although IL-23 is a key regulator of Th17 cells, the IL-23 receptor is not expressed on naïve $CD4^+$ cells and hence could not explain the differentiation of cells into the Th17 subset. Subsequent studies demonstrated that the combination of transforming growth factor-β (TGF-β) with either IL-16 or IL-21 induces Th17 differentiation in mice; however, in human cells, IL-6, IL-1 and IL-23 are sufficient to induce Th17 differentiation. Studies are ongoing to clarify the differential cytokine requirements for Th17 differentiation in mice and humans. The cytokines that are key mediators of Th17 differentiation and survival, including IL-6, IL-21, and IL-23, all activate STAT3. The critical role of this STAT family member was demonstrated in murine studies, when its deletion abrogated the ability of T cells to undergo Th17 differentiation. In humans, the importance of STAT3 was highlighted when it was identified as the genetic mutation present in many patients with hyper-IgE syndrome (HIES, or Job syndrome). HIES is a rare immunodeficiency syndrome characterized by recurrent staphylococcal skin abscesses, elevated serum IgE, and pneumatocele-forming pneumonias. HIES patients with STAT3 mutations have an impaired ability to form Th17 cells, which may explain part of their immunodeficiency. STAT3 regulates expression of many cytokine and cytokine receptor genes involved in Th17 generation or function, including IL-17A, IL-17F, IL-21, IL-21R, and IL-23R.

STAT3 is also important for induction of the signature Th17 transcription factor ROR-γt, which is a member of the retinoic acid–related orphan receptor family. In naïve $CD4^+$ cells, ROR-γt induces IL-17 gene transcription and promotes expression of the IL-23 receptor. Overexpression of ROR-γt induces Th17 differentiation, but deficiency of ROR-γt only partially affects Th17 cells in vivo because of expression of the related transcription factor RORα, which is also expressed in T cells and is induced by IL-6/TGF-β in a STAT3-dependent manner. Cells deficient in both ROR-γt and RORα lose the ability to undergo Th17 differentiation, both in vitro and in vivo.

Th17 cells are induced during the response to extracellular bacteria and fungi, including *Klebsiella pneumoniae, Bacteroides* spp., and *Candida albicans*. Indeed, some patients with chronic mucocutaneous candidiasis have been shown to have mutations in IL-17F and the IL-17 receptor genes. Excessive Th17 cell function also plays a role in autoimmune disease, such as rheumatoid arthritis, psoriasis, and Crohn disease.

Tfh Cells

In addition to Th1, Th2, and Th17 subsets, naïve $CD4^+$ cells develop other functions dependent on the cytokines produced. Examples include newly described Th9, Th22, and Tfh cells. This latter subset enhances the humoral immune response by providing help to B cells during germinal center reactions. Tfh cells express high levels of CXCR5, the receptor for the chemokine CXCL13. The expression of CXCR5 allows differentiating Tfh cells to migrate from the T-cell zone to the CXCL13-rich B-cell follicle, thereby allowing Tfh cells to interact with B cells and exert their function. In addition to CXCR5 expression, other signals, such as TCR signal strength and costimulatory molecules, are important for Tfh differentiation. A recent study using adoptive transfer of naïve $CD4^+$ cells expressing high- and low-affinity transgenic TCRs demonstrated that high-affinity TCR interactions preferentially developed into the Tfh subset. Tfh cells have higher expression of multiple costimulatory molecules, including CD40L, ICOS (inducible costimulator), and OX40, than other T-helper subsets. Because costimulatory molecules enhance B-cell differentiation, the higher expression of these molecules on Tfh cells is hypothesized to positively correlate with the enhanced ability to facilitate B-cell antibody production. It appears that the expression of costimulatory molecules on Tfh cells is not only important for their function but also for their development or maintenance (or both) because both mice and humans deficient in ICOS have fewer Tfh cells with reduced germinal center formation.

Similar to other $CD4^+$ helper subsets, Tfh programming depends on a signature transcription factor, in this case Bcl-6 (B-cell lymphoma 6 protein). In Tfh cells, Bcl-6 acts as a transcriptional repressor. Studies using complementary methods of T cell–specific Bcl-6 deficiency and overexpression demonstrated that Bcl-6 expression in T cells is both necessary and sufficient for Tfh differentiation in vivo.

$CD8^+$ Cytotoxic T Cells

The principal function of $CD8^+$ cytotoxic T cells (CTLs) is to kill host cells that have been infected with pathogens or that have undergone deleterious changes, such as malignant transformation. Similar to $CD4^+$ cells, naïve $CD8^+$ cells initially encounter peptide antigen and MHC on the surface of APCs in the secondary lymphoid organs. However, unlike $CD4^+$ cells, which are stimulated by class II MHC alleles on the APCs, $CD8^+$ cells are engaged by class I MHC plus peptide. For many years, it remained unclear how APCs, which acquire peptide antigens largely by engulfing materials generated outside of the cell, are able to present MHC class I–restricted peptides, which typically are generated within the cell (see earlier discussion). This mystery was solved with the description of "cross presentation," a mechanism by which APCs present engulfed antigens on both class I and class II alleles. Thus, tissue-resident phagocytic cells ingest virally infected or malignantly transformed host cells, degrade the ingested material, and present the peptide antigens in the binding grooves of both class I and class II MHC alleles. These activated phagocytic cells then migrate to the LNs, where they encounter recirculating naïve $CD8^+$ cells. TCR engagement of foreign peptide–MHC class I complexes triggers activation of the $CD8^+$ T cells and initiates CTL differentiation. As part of its activation program, the CTL changes its expression of integrins and chemokine receptors so that it can leave the circulation and enter the tissues, looking for host cells displaying the same antigen that induced CTL activation by the APC in the LN.

After an appropriate target cell has been identified in the tissues, the CTL is again stimulated through its TCR, this time by the peptide–MHC class I combination on the target cells. A structure similar to the IS forms between the CTL and the target cell. The CTL contains specialized granules that are transported to the contact site between the CTL and target. These granules are modified lysosomes that contain effector proteins, including perforin, granzymes, and granulysin. Perforin facilitates the entry of the granzymes into the cytosol of the target cell. The granzyme family, consisting of granzymes A, B, H, K, and M, are proteases that degrade host cell proteins. Granzyme B is the most well-studied family member and is known to cleave caspase 3, activating a proteolytic cascade leading to DNA degradation and apoptosis of the target cell (Fig. 19-8). Granzyme B also promotes cell death in a caspase-independent manner through cleavage of the proapoptotic protein Bid, promoting its migration to and disruption of the outer mitochondrial membrane, resulting in the release of cytochrome c. CTLs also produce cytokines, including IFN-γ, TNF-α, and IL-2. IFN-γ acts to inhibit viral replication in the affected tissues and induces increased class I MHC expression, hence improving the ability of cells to stimulate the TCR on CTLs. IFN-γ synergizes with TNF-α for macrophage activation.

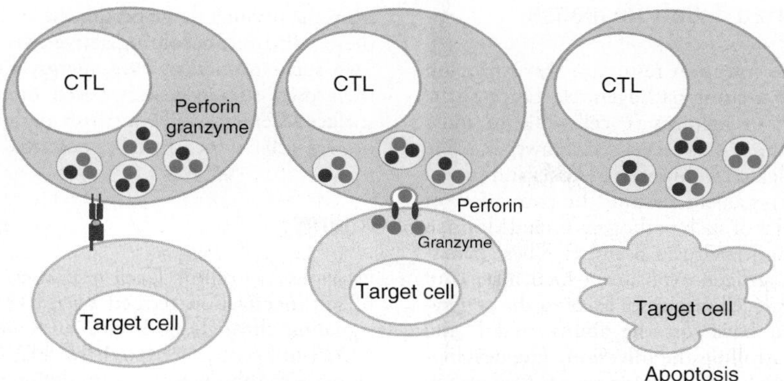

Figure 19-8 CD8⁺ CYTOLYTIC FUNCTION. Cytotoxic CD8⁺ T cells function primarily to kill host cells that have been infected by intracellular pathogens or that have undergone malignant transformation. After naïve CD8⁺ cells encounter peptide-major histocompatibility complex (MHC) class I plus costimulation in secondary lymphoid organs, these activated cytotoxic T cells (CTLs) leave the circulation and enter the tissues. There, upon interaction with a target expressing that same peptide-MHC class I, a CTL forms a lytic synapse, similar to the immunologic synapse (IS), with the target. Cytoplasmic granules containing perforin and granzymes congregate at the synapse, and granule contents are exocytosed into the cleft between the CTL and its target cell. Perforin molecules facilitate entry of the cytolytic molecules into the target cells and granzymes act to promote apoptosis of the target cell.

The transcription factors important for CD8⁺ T-cell effector differentiation include two members of the T-box family, T-bet and Eomesodermin (Eomes). Initially identified as the master Th1 determining transcription factor in CD4⁺ cells, T-bet also plays an essential role in CD8⁺ effector cell differentiation. Recent work has shown that T-bet expression is highest in short-lived effector cells and lower in CD8⁺ T cells destined to become memory cells (see later discussion), suggesting that a gradient of T-bet expression controls the balance between different CD8⁺ effector fates. Eomes cooperates with T-bet in CTL function, and cells deficient in both factors are unable to generate CTLs in response to viral infection.

MATURATION OF T CELL–MEDIATED IMMUNITY

T-Cell Memory

The activation of naïve T cells does not complete their maturation process; instead, it is the starting point for the changes that result in T cell–mediated immunity. At the initiation of an infection, individual antigen-specific T cells become activated and expand robustly to combat the pathogen. As the pathogen is eradicated, the large population of activated T cells must contract dramatically to ensure homeostasis of the immune system. However, a discrete but relatively small population of antigen-specific T cells persists. These long-lived T cells have properties distinct from naïve or activated T cells, including self-renewal through homeostatic proliferation and the ability to rapidly proliferate and regain effector function upon reexposure to antigen. These are the cardinal features of cell-mediated immunologic memory.

Immunologic memory refers to the observation that after an initial exposure and mounting of an effective immune response to a pathogen, subsequent interactions with that pathogen elicit rapid and robust T-cell activation with more efficient clearance of the pathogen. Memory is the foundation of vaccination because immunization with pathogen-specific antigens induces a memory response so that the first exposure of the host to the pathogen itself results in a rapid, effective response, thus abrogating signs and symptoms of the infection.

Within days of infection, subsets of activated effector T cells can be identified with different cell fates: those that are terminally differentiated and those that have the potential to develop into memory cells. How memory cells develop from naïve T cells is a subject of ongoing debate, and several models have been proposed. In one model, memory T cells are thought to develop from a broad pool of activated effector T cells with most effector cells undergoing apoptosis and others surviving to provide memory. A second model suggests that when activated, naïve T cells randomly differentiate into either effectors or memory cells. Most recently, it was postulated that memory cells develop from naïve cells at the first contact with peptide–MHC complexes but not in a random fashion. Instead, asymmetric partitioning of various proteins into the daughter cells during the first cell division determines effector versus memory lineage formation.

Similar to effector T cells, there are different subsets of memory cells. The two main classes are effector memory and central memory T cells. Effector memory T cells, characterized by loss of expression of LN homing molecules CD62L and CCR7, rapidly produce cytokines in response to restimulation with previously encountered antigen, thereby allowing for rapid responses to invading pathogens. These cells preferentially reside in nonlymphoid tissues, such as lung and intestinal mucosa, which are frequently sites of pathogen entry. In contrast, central memory cells express high levels of CD62L and CCR7, are more prevalent in lymphoid tissues, and mount a robust proliferative response after reencountering antigen.

As with differentiation of naïve T cells into efficient effectors, cytokines play an important role in memory T-cell development and maintenance. IL-2 is essential for initial memory cell differentiation, and IL-7 and IL-15 are crucial for memory cell persistence. Other signals, such as the strength of antigenic and inflammatory signals during T-cell activation, also influence memory cell development and maintenance. An important consideration for memory development is cell–cell interactions because CD4⁺ T cells are required during initial priming of CD8⁺ cells for development of fully functional CD8⁺ memory cells. A number of infectious disease models have demonstrated that in the absence of CD4⁺ T-cell help, fewer CD8⁺ memory T cells are maintained, and those that do persist are of the central memory phenotype. Although great progress has been made elucidating the molecular underpinnings of immunologic memory, much remains to be learned. As additional discoveries are made, it is anticipated that new approaches will develop to improve vaccines against infectious agents and to harness host T-cell responses to combat tumors.

T-Cell Exhaustion: An Aborted T-Cell Response

Under most circumstances, acute infection results in the expansion of T lymphocytes specific for the inciting pathogen, clearance of the pathogen, and the development of memory T cells able to more effectively clear that pathogen if the host is reexposed. However, some pathogens cannot be efficiently cleared from infected hosts and persist throughout the lifetime of the organism despite the formation of pathogen-specific T cells. Examples of such pathogens include human immunodeficiency virus and hepatitis viruses B and C. These persistent infections result in chronic antigen exposure, which instead of continuing to induce productive T-cell responses leads to the generation of "exhausted" T cells that have lost the ability to kill and produce cytokines capable of controlling the infection. The development of T-cell memory and the exhaustion response are initiated in similar ways, with the formation of cells that are capable of responding to antigen challenge through proliferation and the secretion of cytokines. However, during exhaustion, the persistence of pathogen causes T cells to become increasingly ineffective in response to stimulation. At early time points in this process, exhausted $CD8^+$ T cells lose the ability to secrete IL-2 or TNF-α and cannot induce cytolysis of infected host cells. At later time points, $CD8^+$ T cells become completely unresponsive and ultimately undergo apoptosis.

Concurrent with the loss of functional responses, exhausted cells upregulate inhibitory cell surface receptors. The best-studied of these inhibitory receptors is programmed death 1 (PD-1), which binds its ligand, PD-L1, expressed on activated macrophages and other APCs. Engagement of PD-1 dampens the T-cell response, likely by recruiting phosphatases that oppose the PTKs necessary for T-cell activation. PD-1 is normally expressed on T cells after initial activation, likely to prevent excessive responses, and is then downregulated as T cells acquire a memory phenotype after the pathogen clearance. Exhausted T cells, however, continue to express this inhibitory receptor. Early during exhaustion, PD-1 blockade reversed T-cell exhaustion in experimental models; however, other inhibitory receptors are expressed on these cells. Blockade of PD-1 with these other receptors has been shown to improve T-cell responsiveness even at later stages of exhaustion. Better understanding of the biology of PD-1 and other key inhibitory receptors and how these molecules interfere with T-cell responses will guide the development of new therapies to combat pathogens that are difficult to eradicate.

INHIBITION OF T CELL–MEDIATED IMMUNITY

Efficient signaling through the TCR and other cell surface molecules is required for initial T-cell activation. Similarly, appropriate maturation of the T-cell response to generate effectors and memory cells is critical for adequate responses to pathogens. Because of the potential for activated T cells to damage host tissues, an integral aspect of the immune system is to negatively regulate T-cell activities. The mechanisms for inhibiting T-cell responses are critical for the prevention of inappropriate activation of naïve T cells at the initiation of an immune response, for limiting the robustness of an appropriate T-cell response as effector cell functions are developed, and for terminating the T-cell response when an antigenic challenge has been met. This section discusses examples of how T-cell activation is modulated at each of these three critical steps of T-cell immunity.

Prevention of Inappropriate Initiation of T-Cell Responses

Given the enormous power of immune effector cells to damage tissues, it is essential that the immune system be nonreactive (tolerant) to self. As already described, T-cell tolerance is achieved centrally through the requirement to pass selection checkpoints during thymic development. However, negative selection in the thymus is not sufficient to eliminate all cells with potential autoreactivity, and some T cells bearing TCRs that may respond to self antigens are exported from the thymus to the periphery. Mechanisms are in place to prevent these cells from becoming active effectors as they encounter antigen. Two such mechanisms are anergy, a process by which T cells limit their own responsiveness based on engagement of particular cell surface receptors (a cell intrinsic path to inactivation), and the action of Treg cells, which instruct potential effectors to remain quiescent.

Anergy

One means to limit T-cell responses against host tissues is a process of self-inactivation termed *anergy*. As noted earlier, T cells require signaling through both the TCR and the costimulatory receptor CD28 to become activated (see Fig. 19-5). Stimulation of the TCR alone in the absence of costimulation through CD28 produces T cells that fail to secrete IL-2 or upregulate high-affinity receptors for this cytokine and hence fail to clonally expand. Cells that have been rendered anergic fail to respond to subsequent stimulation even if ligands for both the TCR and CD28 are available. This two signal requirement ensures that only APCs activated by pathogens or other "danger signals" can initiate an immune response because CD80 and CD86, the ligands for CD28, are upregulated only in activated APCs. Thus, under circumstances of pathogen invasion, APCs present peptide antigens to T cells in addition to CD28 ligands. In the absence of an immune challenge, APCs express only low levels of CD80 or CD86. If a T cell encounters an APC that presents a stimulatory peptide–MHC complex but lacks sufficient expression of CD28 ligands, the T cell does not become activated. In this situation, the absence of ligands for CD28 implies that there is no "danger" and that the antigen being recognized is derived from a self protein. The result of such an encounter leaves the T cell in an anergic state, refractory to activation even in the face of subsequent TCR stimulation by an activated APC.

The role of anergy in human immunology remains unclear because investigators have largely utilized in vitro models systems and animal models. However, several lines of evidence indicate that there are self antigen–reactive T cells that remain quiescent in normal human hosts. The biochemical basis of anergy also remains incompletely understood, but intriguing models suggest that an imbalance between the strength of Ras versus calcium signaling may be crucial. In this paradigm, it is the activation of calcium-dependent transcription factors, such as NFAT, in the absence of transcription factors activated by Ras signaling, such as AP-1, that confers an anergic state. Although anergy is classically thought to persist indefinitely, under some circumstances, there is apparent plasticity because exposure of T cells to high concentrations of IL-2 can improve functional responses in previously anergic cells. Thus, the physiologic importance of anergy in limiting endogenous T-cell activation and preventing autoimmunity and whether there are times when anergy must be reversed for appropriate immune responses are areas of active investigation.

Regulatory T Cells

Tregs are a subset of $CD4^+$ T cells that suppress the proliferation and cytokine production of activated T cells whose TCRs have been engaged by peptide–MHC, even in the presence of costimulation. Hence, as opposed to anergy, which operates in a cell intrinsic fashion, Tregs block responsiveness in *trans* by modulating responses of other cells. Tregs arise in two ways: "natural" Tregs (nTregs) that acquire function during development in the thymus (described earlier), and "inducible" Tregs (iTregs) that are generated through the differentiation of naïve $CD4^+$ T cells in the periphery. Both natural and inducible Tregs are characterized by expression of the key transcription factor FoxP3 and by surface expression of CD25, a subunit of the receptor for IL-2.

As noted, multiple steps and checkpoints occur during the development of T cells in the thymus. After reaching the DP stage, T cells test their TCR for reactivity against peptide–MHC complexes presented by thymic APCs and epithelial cells. Cells bearing TCRs with no reactivity undergo apoptosis (failed positive selection) as do cells with very strong TCR reactivity (through negative selection). Only cells whose TCRs have moderate affinity for peptide–MHC continue to mature. Within this continuum of permitted reactivity, cells with TCRs exhibiting the highest affinity for peptide–MHC are induced to express FoxP3 and develop into Tregs. In the periphery, these cells respond to TCR stimulation by diminishing the response of "conventional" T effector cells, thus downregulating immune responses.

iTregs act similarly to nTregs, but these cells do not leave the thymus poised to have suppressive function. Instead, these cells arise from naïve T cells that encounter antigen in the secondary lymphoid structures. Similar to other $CD4^+$ subsets, iTregs are induced based on the prevailing cytokine conditions and what receptor–ligand interactions predominate during this initial antigen encounter. Regardless of whether they arise in the thymus or are induced in the periphery, Tregs exert their immunosuppressive functions on a variety of immune cells, including $CD4^+$ and $CD8^+$ T cells, DCs, B cells, macrophages, and NK cells, within their microenvironment. Tregs mediate these immunosuppressive effects through the secretion of suppressor cytokines such as IL-10 and TGF-β, the consumption of local concentrations of IL-2, and the induction of apoptosis or cell cycle arrest through direct cell-to-cell contact (Fig. 19-9).

Limiting T-Cell Responses After Stimulation by Foreign Antigen

Even when stimulated appropriately to combat an invading pathogen, it is essential to limit T-cell activation. Unchecked T-cell effector functions present a danger to the host through production of proinflammatory cytokines that recruit other cells of the immune system and through direct damage of self tissues. T-cell effector functions are limited by modulating the T-cell activation pathways through activation of signaling molecules that counter the second messengers stimulated by TCR engagement; through inducible expression of cell surface receptors that compete with activating receptors on the T cell; or by targeting key activating proteins for destruction, thus limiting their ability to promote T-cell effector function. Additionally, the local environment in which the T cell exists may change, with cell extrinsic factors (e.g., inhibitory cytokines) becoming available to dampen T-cell responses (Fig. 19-10).

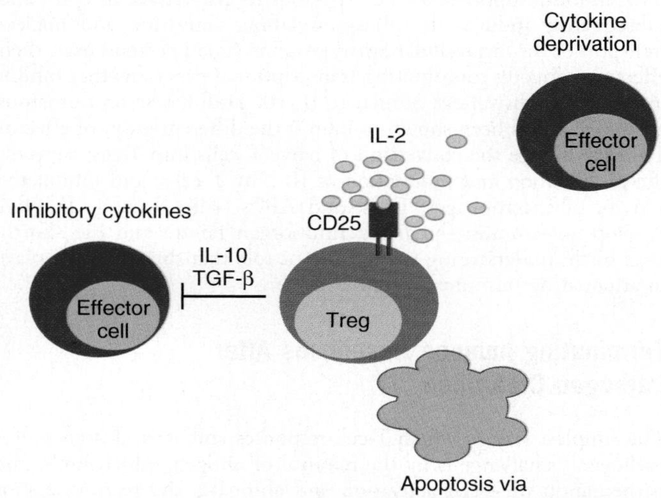

Figure 19-9 T-REGULATORY CELL (Treg) ACTIONS. Tregs act to suppress other T cells through a multitude of mechanisms, including the secretion of suppressor cytokines interleukin-10 (IL-10) and transforming growth factor β (TGF-β), consumption of local concentrations of IL-2 and induction of cell cycle arrest or apoptosis.

Limitation of T-Cell Activity From Cell-Intrinsic Components

Protein Tyrosine Phosphatases

As already noted, the most proximal known biochemical event to occur after engagement of the TCR by peptide–MHC results is activation of PTKs, including Lck and Zap-70, enzymes central to the T-cell activation program. Thus, one means to limit TCR signaling is to oppose the activating PTKs with deactivating protein tyrosine phosphatases, reversing the phosphorylation events that drive T-cell activation. Several such phosphatases have now been identified, including SH2 domain-containing phosphatase-1 (SHP-1) and protein tyrosine phosphatase, nonreceptor type 1 (PTPN1). Although the direct targets of these phosphatases have yet to be demonstrated conclusively, there is increasing evidence in murine systems that they are important for control of T-cell activation as well as for regulating function of other cells of the immune system. Experiments show that SHP-1–deficient T cells demonstrate enhanced proliferation and cytokine production after stimulation compared with wild-type cells. These cells also show prolonged phosphorylation of TCR signaling molecules, consistent with a role for SHP-1 in reversing these events. Overexpression of SHP-1 within T-cell lines inhibits TCR-mediated signaling events. Furthermore, SHP-1 is recruited into the IS after

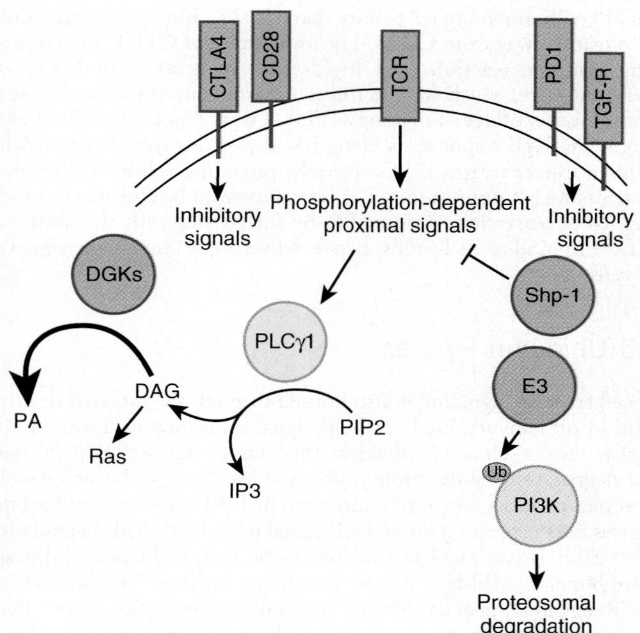

Figure 19-10 INHIBITORY PATHWAYS IN T CELLS. Negative influences on T cells and T-cell receptor (TCR) signaling take place at multiple levels within T cells and are crucial for the prevention of autoimmunity. Examples (indicated in *red*) include the protein tyrosine phosphatase 2 domain-containing phosphatase-1 (SHP-1) that opposes early phosphorylation events mediated by kinases after TCR activation; E3 ubiquitin ligases such as cbl-b that ubiquitinate key signaling mediators, such as PI3K, resulting in proteosome-mediated degradation; and diacylglycerol kinases (DGKs), which terminate TCR signaling by metabolizing signaling intermediates such as diacylglycerol (DAG). Cytotoxic T lymphocyte antigen-4 (CTLA-4), a T-cell surface receptor upregulated after activation, also induces T-cell inhibition, both by sequestering B7 away from the activating costimulatory molecule CD28 and by transducing its own inhibitory signals after B7 binding. Other well-established inhibitory T-cell surface receptors are PD-1, which is expressed under prolonged antigenic stimulation or "exhaustion", and the transforming growth factor β receptor (TGFβ-R), a receptor for one a cytokine key for Treg-mediated suppression.

engagement of the TCR, thus providing an appropriate physical localization for SHP-1 to directly engage targets of the TCR-stimulated PTKs. SHP-1 inhibitory activity appears to be crucial in vivo because mice that lack functional SHP-1 develop fatal autoimmunity, likely because of alterations of function of both innate and adaptive immune cells. Accumulating evidence indicates that other phosphatases are also critical for interfering with T-cell activation, both in animal models and more recently in studies of human patients. Polymorphisms in the genes encoding several protein tyrosine phosphatases, including CD45 and *PTPN22*, align with susceptibility to human immune-mediated disorders. These intriguing findings are being pursued actively by a number of laboratories to uncover the molecular basis of how these phosphatases exert their control on immune cell function.

CTLA-4

A second strategy to limit T-cell activity is through the induced expression and activation of inhibitory cell surface receptors (e.g., cytotoxic T lymphocyte antigen-4 [CTLA-4]). As already discussed, activation of T cells requires two independent signals, one through the TCR and a second through a costimulatory receptor such as CD28. Several days after initial T-cell activation, however, another member of the CD28 superfamily, CTLA-4, becomes upregulated on T cells. CTLA-4 differs from CD28 in that instead of serving as an essential costimulatory receptor, engaged CTLA-4 actively interferes with T-cell activation. Moreover, CTLA-4 binds CD80 and CD86 with much higher affinity than CD28, thus sequestering these key ligands away from CD28. The importance of CTLA-4 in controlling immune reactions was highlighted in a study of CTLA-4–deficient mice, which were found to die from autoimmune disease at 3 to 4 weeks of age. Targeting CTLA-4 with blocking antibodies to augment T-cell responses is being tested as a therapeutic strategy for human cancer treatment. Conversely, providing soluble CTLA-4 to patients with autoimmunity has been shown to be effective at blocking T-cell activation, presumably by interfering with the ability of CD28 to bind to its ligands, hence delivering an anergizing signal to T cells.

E3 Ubiquitin Ligases

T-cell receptor signaling is also limited through the targeted destruction of proteins required for TCR signal transduction. E3 ubiquitin ligases are a class of proteins that target intracellular proteins for degradation by the proteosome, the large multisubunit cytosolic complex essential for protein turnover. In T cells, several E3 ubiquitin ligases target components of TCR signal transduction for degradation after TCR activation. These include c-cbl, Itch, and Casitas b-lineage lymphoma-b (cbl-b). As with other negative modulators of TCR signaling, genetic deletion of E3 ubiquitin ligases, either alone or in combination, results in dysregulation of immune function or the development of frank autoimmune disease in mice. The targeted degradation of crucial signaling modulators after T-cell activation thus serves as an additional physiologic mechanism to limit T-cell responses.

Diacylglycerol Kinases

Intrinsic cellular components limit T-cell activity through degradation of second messengers of T-cell signal transduction, such as metabolism of diacylglycerol (DAG) by diacylglycerol kinases (DGKs). As described earlier, engagement of the TCR results in the activation and recruitment of PLCγ1 that cleaves PIP_2 into the second messengers DAG and IP_3. DAG levels are regulated in T cells through the activity of DGKs that metabolize DAG to terminate its ability to transduce signals. Two DGK isoforms, DGKα and DGKζ, are important for limiting TCR signaling because deletion of either in mice results in enhanced proliferation and cytokine production after TCR stimulation. Moreover, deletion of DGKα leads to impaired induction of T-cell anergy. Mice deficient in either isoform of DGK do not develop overt autoimmune disease, likely because of the functional overlap of these two isoforms. However, enhanced functional responses to viral infection and tumors have been reported in DGK-deficient T cells, defining an important role for DGKs in limiting immune responses.

Limitation of T-Cell Activity From Cell-Extrinsic Components

Extrinsic factors also help limit the function and activation state of T cells. The predominant influences of T cells in this respect are inhibitory cytokines that bind cell surface receptors and influence transcriptional changes that favor decreased activation. Two cytokines that serve as a paradigm for understanding cytokine-mediated inhibition of T cells are IL-10 and TGF-β.

Interleukin-10 is a major negative regulator of immune effector function. Its central role is underscored by the fact that pathogenic viruses, such as cytomegalovirus and Epstein-Barr virus, use homologs of IL-10 to subvert immunologic activity and create environments more favorable for viral spread and replication. IL-10 is produced by both innate and adaptive immune cells in response to activation. As with other cytokines, binding of IL-10 to the IL-10 receptor induces signaling through JAKs, resulting in the nuclear translocation of STAT proteins and the implementation of a transcriptional program that results in decreased expression of inflammatory cytokines and in antagonism of crucial signaling molecules.

Interleukin-10 exerts broad changes within the immune system. In monocytes, IL-10 decreases the production of inflammatory mediators and antigen presentation. In T cells, the effects of IL-10 are generally inhibitory, resulting in decreased capacity for proliferation and a decreased capacity to secrete cytokines. These effects vary by T-cell subtype, however, because IL-17 secretion by Th17 cells is not impaired in the presence of IL-10. As in other proteins important in the negative regulation of T cells, *il10* germline deletion often results in fatal autoimmunity, in this case a gastrointestinal disease resulting from the inability to control inflammation caused by commensal bacteria.

TGF-β is important for upregulating the transcription factor FoxP3 in Tregs. This cytokine also elicits more global changes that favor immunosuppression. TGF-β binds its cell surface receptor and subsequently induces the phosphorylation, activation and nuclear transport of the intracellular Smad proteins. Smad proteins exert their effects by directly coordinating transcriptional programs that inhibit immune responsiveness. Similar to IL-10, TGF-β acts on numerous cell types. It has been shown to inhibit the differentiation of effector Th cells; induce the conversion of naïve T cells into Tregs; suppress the proliferation and production of IL-2 by T cells; and inhibit the activity of macrophages, DCs, and APCs. Mice lacking TGFβ-1 develop autoimmune-mediated multiorgan failure and die shortly after birth, underscoring the important role that this molecule plays in attenuating immune reactions.

Terminating Immune Responses After Pathogen Clearance

The simplest way in which T-cell responses end after clearance of a pathogenic challenge is by the removal of antigen, which limits the perpetuation of T-cell activation and abrogates the recruitment of new effector cells. Effector functions of T cells that were stimulated to respond to the pathogen challenge also diminish as the inhibitory mechanisms already described exert their effects. However, homeostasis of the immune system also requires that the majority of the T cells that emerged from the clonal expansion of antigen stimulated cells (at its peak representing several percent of the hosts' T-cell pool) be eliminated, retaining only the small population of memory T cells responsive to the inciting antigens. Elimination of the expanded population occurs through activation-induced cell death (AICD).

Activation-induced cell death is initiated when CD95 (also called Fas), a T-cell surface receptor present on the activated effector cells, is engaged by its ligand, CD95 ligand, expressed on multiple immune cells, including the activated cells themselves. CD95 is a member of the TNF family of receptors and, when stimulated, recruits the adapter molecule Fas-activating via death domain (FADD). FADD creates a multimolecular complex that triggers the activation of several intracellular caspases that induce DNA damage and apoptosis of the effector T cell. During T-cell activation, both CD95 and CD95 ligand are upregulated on the surface of the cell, and all of the machinery is present to initiate AICD. Hence, the default pathway for activated T cells is apoptosis, an event that is blocked when T cells are appropriately stimulated to respond to antigen. After antigen is cleared and the stimulatory events cease, AICD takes over, reducing the expanded population of cells (Fig. 19-11).

Experiments of nature have taught us much about the biology and importance of both CD95 and CD95 ligand. Loss of these proteins as well as components of their signaling machinery results in autoimmune lymphoproliferative syndrome (ALPS). ALPS is characterized by massive enlargement of lymphoid organs, autoimmune cytopenias, and an increased risk of hematologic malignancy.

THERAPEUTIC MANIPULATION OF T CELL–MEDIATED IMMUNITY

A comprehensive description of the myriad ways in which the manipulation of T cells has led to important clinical advances is beyond the scope of this chapter. However, it is worth appreciating some of the ways in which an enhanced understanding of T cell–mediated immunity has resulted in changes in clinical practice. Many human diseases are related to T-cell dysfunction, both in cases of overexuberant immune responses, as in autoimmune diseases and rejection of transplanted organs, and in insufficient immune responses, as in the case of some chronic infections and in uncontrolled malignancy. Here, we briefly address T-cell responses in graft rejection and in malignancy as paradigms for how T-cell immunity has been modulated therapeutically.

The success of solid organ transplantation depends greatly on the ability to control the immune response of the recipient against the donor organ. Donor tissues express foreign MHC alleles and other proteins to which endogenous T cells have not been exposed (and tolerized against) during thymic development, and thus these tissues serve as potential targets for T cell–mediated immunity. Initially, the only medications capable of permitting graft survival were high-dose steroids, medications with potent effects in essentially all organ systems and with severe side effects not limited to the immune system. Subsequently, however, several classes of medications were identified that act more specifically on T cells, first cyclosporine and subsequently tacrolimus and sirolimus. These medications target the IL-2 axis: cyclosporine and tacrolimus inhibit IL-2 transcription, and sirolimus inhibits mammalian target of rapamycin (mTOR), a group of proteins crucial in facilitating IL-2 signal transduction. Because T cells, depending on the treatment agent, are either unable to produce IL-2 or respond to IL-2, they fail to proliferate despite conditions favorable for stimulation, leading to impaired T cell–mediated immunity and improved survival of transplanted organs.

Other agents currently in use in the clinic were also designed precisely because of insights that emerged from studies probing the molecular basis of immune cell function. For example, antibodies directed against CD3 are potent T-cell inhibitors and are now used in the setting of acute solid organ transplant rejection. Similarly, blocking the IL-2 receptor with monoclonal antibodies prevents IL-2 receptor signaling and thus abrogates division of stimulated T cells, thereby quelling T cell–mediated immune destruction.

Given the importance of costimulation for T-cell activation and the success in interfering with CD28 signaling in various autoimmune disorders, recent studies have demonstrated efficacy in transplant with blockade of the CD28–CD80/CD86 interaction using soluble CTLA-4 as a competitive inhibitor of the interaction between CD28 and CD80/CD86. A soluble CTLA-4 fusion protein has recently been approved in the setting of transplant rejection. Additional studies are in progress to examine ways in which modulation of other costimulatory receptors, alone or in combination with soluble CTLA-4, may be used to preserve allografts. As our understanding of how different T-cell subsets are induced is becoming more precise, new therapeutics on the horizon are designed to redirect immune responses by changing the balance of the various effector subsets that emerge as the recipient responses to the transplanted organ. Additional agents directed against receptors and signaling molecules discovered to be key for T-cell activation are currently being tested for clinical efficacy and safety and likely will soon be available to block T-cell responses in the setting of solid organ transplant.

In contrast to the need to impede immune responses in organ transplant, in the setting of malignancy, the desire is to intervene to enhance T-cell activity. T cells face several hurdles in their response to spontaneous malignancy. First, they must recognize peptides and proteins that are unique to tumor tissue. These include oncogenic mutant proteins, fusion proteins that may have formed during the course of tumor development, or aberrantly expressed embryonic proteins that result from altered transcription often found in malignant tissue. Second, T cells must overcome the lack of costimulation provided by tumor cells. Because tumor cells originate from normal host tissue, they fail to generate the bacterial or viral products crucial for activating APCs. Third, T cells must overcome the generally immunosuppressive microenvironment within tumor tissue, which may include an abundance of TGF-β, Tregs, immunosuppressive macrophages, the induction of an anergic-like state, and persistent antigen-induced exhaustion.

One approach to enhance T cell–mediated responses to tumors also makes use of the biology of CTLA-4. In this case, however, instead of using soluble CTLA-4 as an agent to inhibit T-cell responses by interfering with costimulation, antibodies against CTLA-4 are being tested as a means to block the ability of CTLA-4 expressed on activated T cells to inhibit T-cell function. Preliminary studies have shown that CTLA-4 blocking antibodies may prolong T-cell activation in response to malignancy, and their use has resulted in long-term disease remission in a small percentage of patients with metastatic melanoma, an otherwise uniformly fatal disease. Whether CTLA-4 antibodies mediate their effect by inducing the expansion of newly activated tumor-specific cells or by reversing the immunosuppressive microenvironment on existing cells remains to be determined. In addition to targeting CTLA-4 to abrogate its ability to inhibit T-cell responses, preliminary approaches are underway to block other inhibitory receptors or ligands to enhance T-cell immunity. One promising example is targeting of PD-1, the inhibitory receptor present on activated and exhausted T cells, with the hope of boosting T-cell responses against cancers and promoting clearance of pathogenic viruses that now typically persist in the host.

In addition to targeting inhibitory receptors on T cells to augment antitumor responses, studies are underway to engineer APCs to more effectively stimulate effector T-cell responses (e.g., through enhanced expression of ligands for activating costimulatory receptors). Such APCs are being tested in clinical trials for effectiveness as tumor vaccines. Investigators are making use of our understanding of the most proximal events important for T-cell activation to develop chimeric antigen receptors (CARs). These engineered molecules include a binding site for an antigen thought to be expressed selectively (or relatively so) by tumor cells coupled to the transmembrane and cytoplasmic signaling components of the ζ chain of the TCR complex and other key activating receptors. T cells are removed from patients and then transfected with cDNA encoding these "engineered" receptors ex vivo. The modified T cells are then administered back into the patients with the anticipation that these T cells will engage the tumor through the CAR, which will also transduce a signal to activate the T

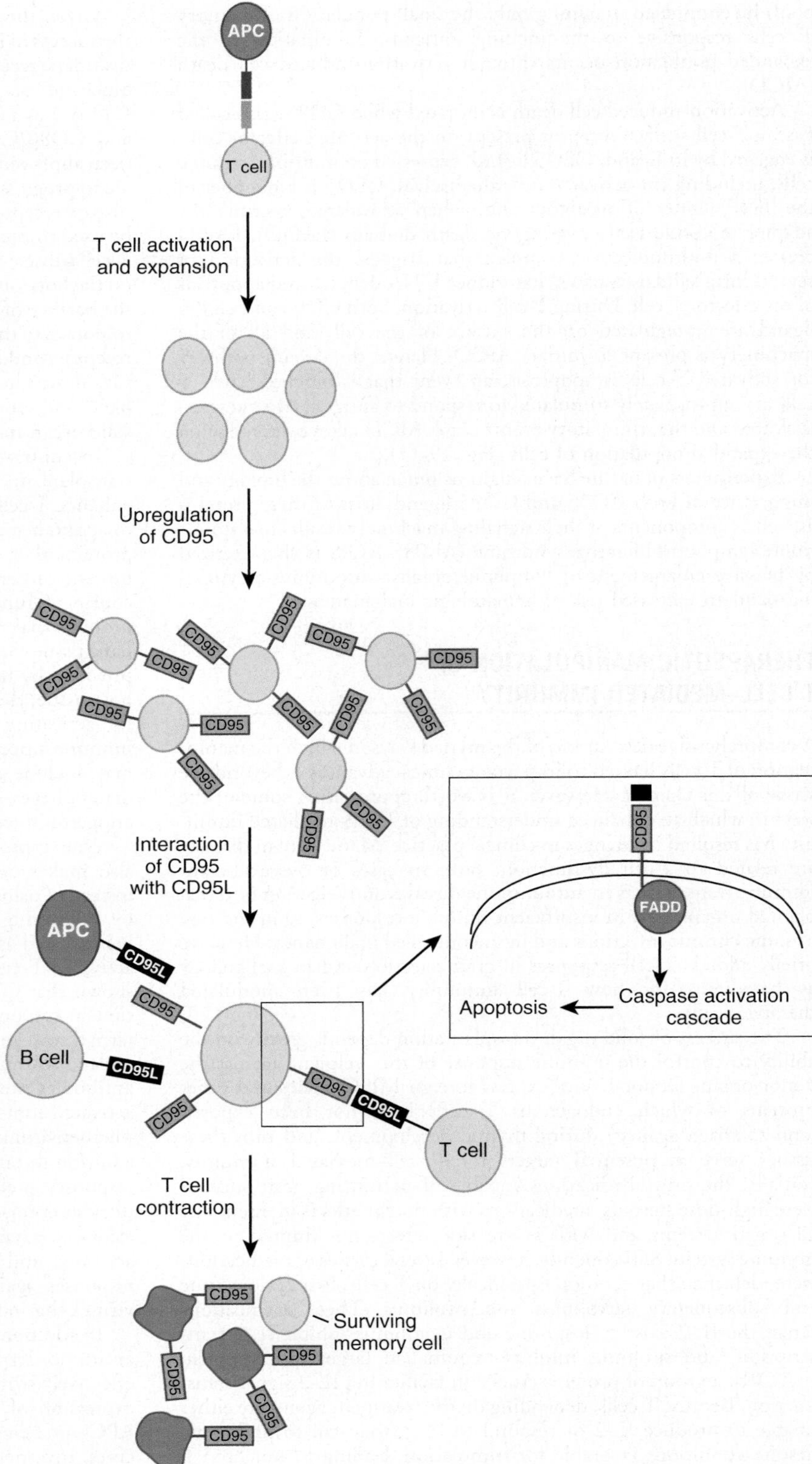

Figure 19-11 CD95-DEPENDENT ACTIVATION-INDUCED CELL DEATH. After T-cell activation and resultant expansion, T cells begin to upregulate the cell death receptor CD95. The ligand for CD95, CD95L, is expressed on many cell types, including APCs, B cells, and the activated T cells themselves. Binding of CD95 to CD95L triggers recruitment of the adapter protein Fas-activating via death domain (FADD), resulting in activation of caspases and the induction of cell death through apoptosis. The process of CD95 upregulation and apoptosis leads to contraction of activated T-cell populations.

cell. These activated T cells with reactivity against the tumor are designed to mount a robust antitumor response, bolstering antitumor immunity sufficiently to eliminate the cancer. Although studies using such agents are only beginning, early results are promising.

The examples presented here are only a small subset of novel approaches in use or being tested to modulate immune cell function based on our understanding of the molecular basis of T-cell activation. It is anticipated that as more is learned about the molecules and pathways critical for control of T cell–mediated immunity, additional new agents with greater efficacy and improved safety profiles will become available for clinical use. The advent of these new therapeutics and their potential to improve treatments for serious human diseases underscore the importance of continued efforts to understand the mechanisms of T-cell development and function.

SUGGESTED READINGS

Anderson MS, Venanzi ES, Klein L, et al: Projection of an immunological self shadow within the thymus by the aire protein. *Science* 298:1395, 2002.

Chan AC, Iwashima M, Turck CW, et al: ZAP-70: A 70 kd protein-tyrosine kinase that associates with the TCR zeta chain. *Cell* 71:649, 1992.

Chang JT, Palanivel VR, Kinjyo I, et al: Asymmetric T lymphocyte division in the initiation of adaptive immune responses. *Science* 315:1687, 2007.

Clements JL, Yang B, Ross-Barta SE, et al: Requirement for the leukocyte-specific adapter protein SLP-76 for normal T cell development. *Science* 281:416, 1998.

Crotty S: Follicular helper CD4 T cells (TFH). *Annu Rev Immunol* 29:621, 2011.

Day CL, Kaufmann DE, Kiepiela P, et al: PD-1 expression on HIV-specific T cells is associated with T-cell exhaustion and disease progression. *Nature* 443:350, 2006.

Dembi Z, Haas W, Weiss S, et al: Transfer of specificity by murine alpha and beta T-cell receptor genes. *Nature* 320:232, 1986.

Dustin ML, Depoil D: New insights into the T cell synapse from single molecule techniques. *Nat Rev Immunol* 11:672, 2011.

Huang F, Gu H: Negative regulation of lymphocyte development and function by the Cbl family of proteins. *Immunol Rev* 224:229, 2008.

Irving BA, Weiss A: The cytoplasmic domain of the T cell receptor zeta chain is sufficient to couple to receptor-associated signal transduction pathways. *Cell* 64:891, 1991.

Jin HT, Ahmed R, Okazaki T: Role of PD-1 in regulating T-cell immunity. *Curr Top Microbiol Immunol* 350:17, 2011.

Kremer JM, Westhovens R, Leon M, et al: Treatment of rheumatoid arthritis by selective inhibition of T-cell activation with fusion protein CTLA4Ig. *N Engl J Med* 349:1907, 2003.

Love PE, Bhandoola A: Signal integration and crosstalk during thymocyte migration and emigration. *Nat Rev Immunol* 11:469, 2011.

Monks CR, Freiberg BA, Kupfer H, et al: Three-dimensional segregation of supramolecular activation clusters in T cells. *Nature* 395:82, 1998.

Porter DL, Levine BL, Kalos M, et al: Chimeric antigen receptor-modified T cells in chronic lymphoid leukemia. *N Engl J Med* 365:725, 2011 Aug 25.

Rieux-Laucat F, Le Deist F, Fischer A: Autoimmune lymphoproliferative syndromes: Genetic defects of apoptosis pathways. *Cell Death Differ* 10:124, 2003.

Rudd CE, Taylor A, Schneider H: CD28 and CTLA-4 coreceptor expression and signal transduction. *Immunol Rev* 229:12, 2009.

Sakaguchi S, Ono M, Setoguchi R, et al: Foxp3+ CD25+ CD4+ natural regulatory T cells in dominant self-tolerance and autoimmune disease. *Immunol Rev* 212:8, 2006.

Sallusto F, Lanzavecchia A, Araki K, et al: From vaccines to memory and back. *Immunity* 33:451, 2010.

Singer A, Adoro S, Park JH: Lineage fate and intense debate: Myths, models and mechanisms of CD4- versus CD8-lineage choice. *Nat Rev Immunol* 8:788, 2008.

Smith-Garvin JE, Koretzky GA, Jordan MS: T cell activation. *Annu Rev Immunol* 27:591, 2009.

Vang T, Miletic AV, Arimura Y, et al: Protein tyrosine phosphatases in autoimmunity. *Annu Rev Immunol* 26:29, 2008.

Vyas JM, Van der Veen AG, Ploegh HL: The known unknowns of antigen processing and presentation. *Nature Rev Immunol* 8:607, 2008.

Waterhouse P, Penninger JM, Timms E, et al: Lymphoproliferative disorders with early lethality in mice deficient in Ctla-4. *Science* 270:985, 1995.

Webber A, Hirose R, Vincenti F: Novel strategies in immunosuppression: Issues in perspective. *Transplantation* 91:1057, 2011.

Williams MA, Bevan MJ: Effector and memory CTL differentiation. *Annu Rev Immunol* 25:171, 2007.

Zhang W, Sommers CL, Burshtyn DN, et al: Essential role of LAT in T cell development. *Immunity* 10:323, 1999.

Zhu J, Paul WE: Peripheral CD4+ T-cell differentiation regulated by networks of cytokines and transcription factors. *Immunol Rev* 238:247, 2010.

CHAPTER 20

NATURAL KILLER CELL IMMUNITY

Don M. Benson, Jr., and Michael A. Caligiuri

Natural killer (NK) cells are large granular lymphocytes comprising about 10% to 15% of the peripheral circulation.[1,2] First characterized by their ability to lyse targets independent of activating or initiating stimuli,[3] NK cells are a critical cellular component of the innate immune system. In addition, NK cells secrete cytokines that help to marshal and shape the innate and adaptive immune response to infection and malignant transformation. There has been a recent surge of interest in NK cells as new discoveries in both the laboratory and the clinic have characterized the crucial contributions of NK cells in shaping the early immune response.[4] NK cells play a key role in maintaining host defense as exemplified in human NK cell deficiency syndromes (which carry increased susceptibility to overwhelming viral, intracellular, and atypical mycobacterial infections),[5] and animal models of NK cell deficiency (e.g., such mice are particularly susceptible to developing cancer).[6,7] This chapter reviews current understanding of NK cell biology, the role of NK cells in human diseases, and the recent clinical applications of NK cells in cancer therapy.

FUNDAMENTAL BIOLOGY

Natural Killer Subsets

Natural killer cells are phenotypically recognized by surface expression of CD56 (also called neural cell adhesion molecule [NCAM]) and the absence of the T-cell–specific surface antigen CD3 as well as the T-cell receptor(TCR).[8,9] Based on the intensity of CD56 surface expression, two functional subsets (so-called $CD56^{bright}$ and $CD56^{dim}$) of NK cells may be discriminated from one another. $CD56^{dim}$ NK cells comprise 85% to 90% of the NK cells in peripheral circulation and are potent mediators of cytotoxicity. About 10% to 15% of NK cells in the circulation are $CD56^{bright}$, and upon activation, this subset is capable of robust cytokine and chemokine production.[2] Fig. 20-1 graphically represents the NK subsets described below, and Table 20-1 summarizes major surface antigens associated with each NK cell subset.

$CD56^{dim}$ Natural Killer Cells

$CD56^{dim}$ NK have exquisite cytolytic properties, able to kill infected as well as tumor cell targets without prior sensitization.[10] They constitutively express the interleukin-2/15 (IL-2/15) receptor (R) β and common γ-receptor chains, which together form a receptor complex through which cells may respond to stimulation by either IL-2 or IL-15.[11,12] $CD56^{dim}$ NK cells can lyse tumor cell targets through at least three distinct mechanisms. First, they can execute cytotoxicity through granule exocytosis of perforin and granzyme.[13,14] Second, cytotoxicity can be mediated through FasL and TRAIL associated with production of cytokines, including interferon-γ (IFN-γ), tumor necrosis factor α (TNF-α), and granulocyte macrophage colony-stimulating factor (GM-CSF).[15] Third, $CD56^{dim}$ NK cells can mediate antibody-dependent cytotoxicity (ADCC) via the high-density surface expression of CD16 (the FcγRIII receptor).[2,16] Freshly isolated, unstimulated $CD56^{dim}$ NK cells have intrinsically greater cytotoxicity against NK-sensitive targets such as the K562 cell line in vitro compared with the $CD56^{bright}$ NK cells.[17]

Other antigens are differentially expressed by $CD56^{dim}$ NK cells and provide insight into their functional role in the immune response. For example, $CD56^{dim}$ NK cells also exhibit relatively high surface density expression of killer immunoglobulin-like receptors (KIRs). NK cell KIR expression appears important in preventing autoimmunity and in surveying against malignant transformation.[16,18]

Both $CD56^{dim}$ and $CD56^{bright}$ NK cells express modest levels of the chemokine receptor CXCR3. However, in contrast to $CD56^{bright}$ NK cells, $CD56^{dim}$ NK cells display relatively abundant surface expression levels of CXCR1, CXCR4, and CX3CR1.[19] CXCR1 binds IL-8, and CXCR4 binds SDF-1 (stromal cell-derived factor). These cytokines are associated with local inflammatory response; for example, IL-8 levels are increased in the setting of acute viral infections,[20] and IL-8 and SDF-1 levels are increased with solid[21,22] and hematopoietic malignancies.[23,24] Thus, expression of these chemokine receptors allows NK cells to traffic to local areas of inflammatory response to mediate antiviral and antitumor activity.

$CD56^{bright}$ Natural Killer Cells

$CD56^{bright}$ NK cells play more of an immunoregulatory role. $CD56^{bright}$ NK produce a multitude of cytokines and chemokines, have a relatively high proliferative capacity, reside primarily in the parafollicular T cell–rich region of secondary lymphoid tissue (SLT), and have modest cytolytic granules, KIR, and FcγRIII expression (see Table 20-1).[10] $CD56^{bright}$ NK cells are unique among cytotoxic effector cells in constitutive expression of the high-affinity IL–2Rαβγ complex, making them responsive to picomolar concentrations of IL-2 released by activated T cells in the parafollicular T cell–rich region of SLT.[25] As noted, $CD56^{bright}$ NK cells comprise only about 10% of the circulating NK population but predominate almost to the exclusion of the $CD56^{dim}$ NK subset in SLT.[2,26] This likely results from their selective expression of a number of receptors that assist in homing cells to and retaining cells in SLT (e.g., CCR7 and CD62L).[10]

The ability of $CD56^{bright}$ NK cells to produce an abundant variety of cytokines and chemokines compared with the $CD56^{dim}$ subset likely relates more to the differential expression of both negative and positive regulators of cytokine/chemokine production and less to constitutive expression of cytokine-activating receptors. For example, $CD56^{bright}$ NK cells have little or no expression of two negative regulators of cytokine/chemokine production, namely SHIP-1 (Src homology-2 domain-containing inositol 5-phosphatase 1) and HLX (H2.0-like homeobox 1),[27,28] but $CD56^{dim}$ NK lack constitutive expression of a positive regulator of cytokines called SET.[29]

NATURAL KILLER CELL DEVELOPMENT

Interleukin-15 is required for NK cell development in mouse and humans,[30,31] and as with B cells and T cells, human NK cells are derived from $CD34^{(+)}$ hematopoietic stem cells in bone marrow (BM). However, NK cell precursors in human BM have not been

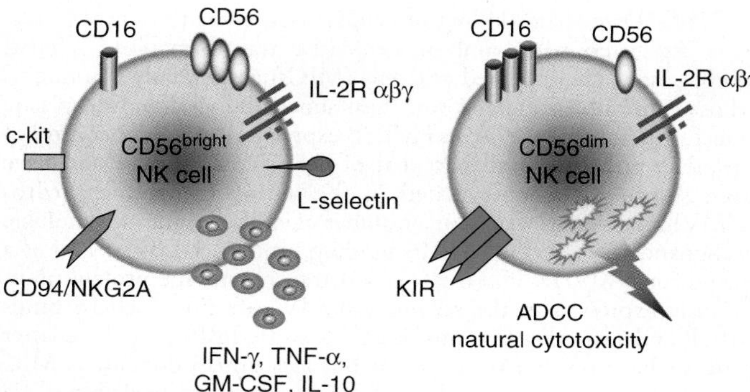

Figure 20-1 SIMPLIFIED REPRESENTATION OF NATURAL KILLER CELL SUBSETS. CD56^{bright} cells have immunoregulatory function whereas CD56^{dim} cells have cytolytic function. *ADCC,* Antibody-dependent cellular cytotoxicity; *GM-CSF,* granulocyte macrophage-colony stimulating factor; *IFN,* interferon; *IL,* interleukin; *KIR,* killer immunoglobulin-like receptor; *R,* receptor; *TNF,* tumor necrosis factor. *(Adapted from Cooper MA, Fehniger TA, Caligiuri MA: The biology of human natural killer cell subsets.* Trends Immunol *22:633, 2001.)*

Table 20-1 Human Natural Killer Cell Subsets Display Different Repertoires of Surface Antigens

Antigen	CD56^{dim}	CD56^{bright}
CD16 (FcγRIIIa)	+++	–/+
KIR	+++	–/+
CXCR1	+	–
CXCR3	++	–
CX3CR3	+	–
CXCR4	++	–
CD94	–	++
NKG2A	–/+	+
NKG2D	+	+
c-kit	–	+
CCR7	–	++
CD2	++	+++
CD62L (L-selectin)	+	++
CD44	+	++

Adapted from Cooper MA, Fehniger TA, Caligiuri MA: The biology of human natural killer cell subsets. *Trends Immunol* 22:633, 2001.
KIR, Killer immunoglobulin-like receptor.

identified, suggesting that maturation may occur elsewhere.[2,32] Freud et al identified a CD34^{dim}CD45RA(+)α4β7^{bright} cell to be the only CD34(+) subset in SLT.[26] Found within the parafollicular T cell–rich region of SLT in the same region as the CD56^{bright} NK cell, this CD34^{dim}CD45RA(+)α4β7^{bright} cell can differentiate into a CD56^{bright} NK cell in the presence of IL-15.[22] With evidence for a CD34(+) NK precursor and CD56^{bright} NK cell in the same region within SLT, five novel, discrete stages of NK cell development were characterized in situ within the same parafollicular region of SLT, each by their differential expression of CD34, CD117, and CD94.[33,34] As development proceeds along this continuum, cells acquire the ability to secrete cytokines (e.g., INF-γ); display natural cytotoxicity; and lose the ability to differentiate into dendritic cells (DCs), T cells, or both. This orderly development in SLT from a CD34(+) subset to CD56^{bright} NK cells suggests that CD56^{dim} NK cells represent a terminally differentiated NK stage that follows CD56^{bright} NK development and exit into the periphery. Interestingly, the expression of CD94 may mark

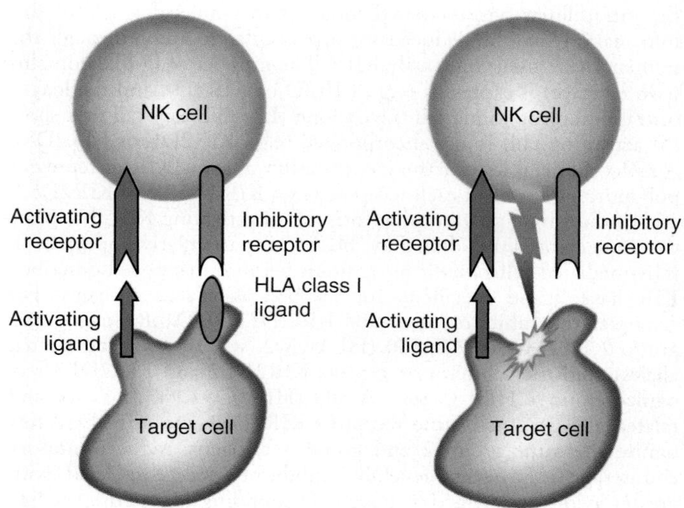

Figure 20-2 SIMPLIFIED REPRESENTATION OF NATURAL KILLER (NK) CELL CYTOTOXICITY MEDIATED THROUGH THE BALANCE OF ACTIVATING AND INHIBITORY SIGNALING IN RESPONSE TO LIGANDS ON POTENTIAL TARGETS. The target cell on the left is spared, but the target cell on the right is lysed. *(Adapted from Farag SS, Fehniger TA, Ruggeri L, et al: Natural killer cell receptors: new biology and insights into the graft-versus-leukemia effect.* Blood *100:1935, 2002.)*

a functional intermediary step between C56^{bright} and CD56^{dim} human NK cells.[35] The abundance of CD56^{dim} NK cells in blood versus SLT and their loss of both CD117 (c-kit) expression and proliferative capacity along with their acquisition of KIR, FcRγRIII, and cytolytic granules are all consistent with this notion.[2] More recently, CD57 has been identified as a surface marker of terminally differentiated NK cells.[36]

NATURAL KILLER CELL RECEPTORS

Natural killer cells, as opposed to B and T lymphocytes, do not undergo clonotypic gene rearrangement in order to express antigen receptors; however, through the expression of a complex repertoire of surface molecules, NK cells may efficiently determine nonself from self and rapidly initiate an appropriate response.[37] NK cell receptors may be activating or inhibitory—in other words, binding of the receptor to its ligand expressed on a target cell either activates or suppresses a functional NK response. Such receptors fall into three general categories: those which are members of the immunoglobulin-like superfamily (KIR), one type that belongs to the C-type lectin receptor (CLR) superfamily,[38] and finally NK cell–specific receptors (NKRs). The complex function of these receptor subsets is still a matter of intense research; however, a model by which NK cell receptors KIR may recognize particular features of major histocompatibility complex (MHC) class I alleles (e.g., human leukocyte antigen A [HLA-A],[39] HLA-B,[40] HLA-C[41]) or recognize other surface antigens on target cells has been developed.[42,43] Fig. 20-2 is a simplified, schematic representation of what we currently understand regarding the ability of NK cells and their receptors to survey the immune system.

Killer Immunoglobulin-Like Receptors

KIRs provide one method by which NK cells recognize self from nonself to mediate the appropriate cytotoxic response. There are at least 15 KIRs identified on chromosome 19q13.4.[18,42,43] Structurally, KIRs contain two or three extracellular immunoglobulinlike domains and recognize MHC class I proteins.[18,39,40] KIRs may be either inhibitory or activating, a functional feature associated with the intracellular tyrosine-based motif of the molecule.[18] All of this information may be deduced for a particular receptor through the nomenclature used to identify KIRs. The number of Ig-like domains (two or three) is expressed (e.g., KIR2D or KIR3D), and the length of the intracytoplasmic tail (i.e., a long [L] inhibitory tail or a short [S] activating tail) is also incorporated (e.g., KIR2DL or KIR2DS). A suffix numeral follows the identification of some KIR to represent polymorphic forms of each receptor (e.g., KIR2DS2 and KIR2DS3, each indicating a polymorphic form of an activating KIR that bears the same extracellular domains). HLA-C is particularly important in KIR-mediated self/nonself recognition because many well-described KIR have ligand specificity for HLA-C associated antigens. For example, the inhibitory receptor KIR2DL1 (CD158a) recognizes group 2 HLA-C Asn77Lys80 (HLA-Cw2, w4, w5, w6 and related alleles), and the inhibitory receptors KIR2DL2 and KIR2DL3 recognize group 1 HLA-C Ser77Asn80 (HLA-Cw1, w3, w7, w8 and related alleles).[43] Activating receptors KIR2DS1 and KIR2DS2 recognize the same group 2 and group 1 antigens as the inhibitory counterparts; however, generally, inhibitory receptors bind with greater avidity or attraction for a corresponding HLA antigen than activating receptors.[44] Complementary activating and inhibitory KIRs recognize the same cognate extracellular domains on target cells; thus if an NK cell expresses both activating and inhibitory KIR for an identical ligand, the cell will generally be inhibited from killing.

The KIR family is likely not all inclusive for human classical type I HLA allotypes; for instance, only one inhibitory KIR directed against HLA-A (KIR3KL2) and none toward HLA-B alleles have been found.[43] Additionally, specific KIRs may have particular roles in maintaining host immunity in unique settings. For example, KIR2DL4 recognizes the nonclassical HLA-G molecule that is only expressed on fetal extravillous trophoblasts that invade the maternal decidua during pregnancy.[45] Controversy surrounds the exact nature of this KIR; however, KIR2DL4 is likely not clonally distributed as other KIRs but is present on the surfaces of most mature NK cells.[46] Interestingly, despite having an inhibitory intracellular signaling moiety, KIR2DL4 serves to promote IFN-γ secretion but not cytolytic activity.[46] It is possible that this KIR functions to facilitate immune tolerance to developing fetuses.[47]

C-Type Lectin Receptors

C-type lectin receptors (CTLRs), located on human chromosome 12p.12.3, share a common subunit (CD94) covalently bonded to one of four closely related gene products of the NKG2 family.[48,49] CTLR represent a second type of NK cell receptor–mediating killing and include NKG2A (and splice variant B), NKG2C, NKG2E (and splice variant H), and NKG2F.[49] NKG2D, which does not bind CD94 and shares little sequence homology to other NKG2 proteins, is discussed later. All but one of the CTLRs are activating and expressed on NK cells and cytotoxic T lymphocytes. CD94/NKG2A is inhibitory and is expressed on NK cells as well as cytotoxic T lymphocytes where they serve to regulate CD8(+) T-cell antiviral responses.[50] CD94/NKG2A specifically recognizes the nonclassical HLA-E Class I molecule.[51] Interestingly, HLA-E specifically presents leader peptides from other HLA receptor antigens; thus, sensitivity to HLA-E provides a mechanism for NK cells to sense functional overexpression of class I MHC molecules on cell surfaces. As with KIR, binding between CD94/NKG2A and HLA-E is more avid than binding of activating CTLRs to other epitopes, however, unlike KIR, the target antigens for activating and inhibitory CTLR are not the same.[52]

NKG2D is a CTLR, however, it has only modest sequence homology with other members of the NKG2 family and does not associate with CD94.[51] NKG2D exists as a homodimer and does not have inherent signaling capability but rather signals via the PI3K pathway as recruited through DAP10Wu or KAP10.[53] This unique signal transduction arrangement renders NKG2D signaling privileged from inhibitory, intracellular intermediaries that modulate signal transduction of other CTLR systems. NKG2D is constitutively expressed on all NK cells, γδ T cells, and CD8(+) T cells.[54]

NKG2D mediates killing of cellular targets expressing two antigens associated with viral or neoplastic transformation.[43,55] First, MHC class I chain-related antigens (MICs) are a family of proteins whose expression correlates with heat shock and viral and neoplastic transformation.[54,56] MICA and MICB expression are under control of promoter elements similar to that of heat shock proteins and have been shown to be upregulated in the setting of cytomegalovirus (CMV) infection as well as in a number of epithelial and hematologic malignancies.[56,57] Second, UL16 binding protein (ULBP) serves as a ligand for NKG2D. UL16 is a type I transmembrane protein ubiquitously expressed in the setting of CMV infection.[58] UL16 binds MICB and two other proteins, ULBP-1 and ULBP-2.[59] (These latter proteins have α1 and α2 domains but lack an α3 domain as MIC and MHC class I molecules have; furthermore, they are expressed via a glycosylphosphatidyl inositol [GPI] anchor and thus have no requirement for β2 microglobulin.) In binding MICB, ULBP-1, and ULBP-2, CMV-produced UL16 counteracts cell surface expression of these NKG2D ligands, thus providing a mechanism of immune evasion from NK cell surveillance and cytotoxicity.[60] In a similar fashion, some human tumors downregulate expression of NKG2D ligands or release soluble forms of such (e.g., MICA or ULBPs) as a mechanism of immune escape from NK cells.[61-63] Although ULBPs are expressed more ubiquitously than MIC proteins, some tissues with high mRNA levels express no protein, implying important post-transcriptional control of these antigens.[59] IL-15 stimulation enhances the NK cell NKG2D-mediated response to tumors expressing ULBP.[64]

Other Activating Natural Killer Receptors

A third family of NK receptors that mediate cell killing are called natural cytotoxicity receptors (NCRs).[57,65] In addition to NKG2D, NCRs comprise an important family of activating NK cell receptors involved in the process of target recognition and elimination. NCRs include three receptors called NKp46 and NKp30, which are exclusively and constitutively expressed on NK cells, and NKp44, which is expressed after IL-2 stimulation on NK and some γδ T cells.[57,65,66] Infectious, pathogen-specific ligands for NCR have been identified (e.g., NKp46 and NKp44) that recognize and engage virus specific hemagglutinin and hemagglutinin-neuraminidase.[67] This provides a mechanistic understanding of how NK cells can target and eliminate cells infected with influenza and parainfluenza virus (e.g., although such target cells have not downregulated MHC class I expression).[67] Recently, B7-H6 has been identified as a ligand for NKp30; however, endogenous ligands for other NCR remain to be identified.[68-70]

ADAPTIVE IMMUNE PROPERTIES OF NATURAL KILLER CELLS

Recent findings regarding NK cell biology have blurred the functional borders between the innate and adaptive arms of the immune system. Although NK cells have traditionally been dichotomized into the innate immune system, emerging data suggest that NK cells demonstrate sophisticated adaptive properties and do not interact in an invariant manner in the microenvironment.[71]

Natural Killer Cell Education

The potential for NK cell autoreactivity exists because some NK cells may lack inhibitory receptors, but others may express activating receptors for self ligands. This can occur because the receptor array that individual NK cells express occurs largely at random and ligands to these receptors are inherited independently.[72] Potentially autoreactive NK cells are not clonally deleted but rather rendered hyporesponsive. For example, NK cells lacking inhibitory receptors for self MHC are unresponsive to self cells.[73] And in a complementary manner, humans who lack MHC class I expression do not experience NK cell–mediated autoimmunity. By comparison, through an

MHC-dependent processing termed *licensing,* NK cells that express receptors for self MHC exhibit greater responsiveness to stimulation; however, their effector function against normal cells is blocked by engagement of inhibitory receptors for self MHC.[74] Whether responsiveness is determined by interaction with cells expressing ligands for NK cell receptors (so-called "arming") or hyporesponsiveness is induced via encounters with normal cells lacking MHC ligands ("disarming" or "anergy") is unclear; however, experimental data suggest that persistent stimulation results in hyporesponsiveness but persistent stimulation with concomitant inhibition leads to NK cell responsiveness.[75,76] Studies such as these and others suggest that NK cells may be sensitive to changes in the microenvironment and may modulate responsiveness to stimuli.

Natural Killer Cell Memory

Immunologic memory has long been reserved as a process of the adaptive immune system; however, recent data suggest that NK cells possess a form of memory as well. This idea was first demonstrated in a recombinase-activating genes-1 (RAG-1) deficient mouse lacking T and B cells. Hapten-induced hypersensitivity was mediated by NK cells in this model, and "memory" NK cells were described as residing in the liver and bearing Thy1 and CXCR6 on their surfaces.[77]

This concept has also been demonstrated in the setting of viral infection in mice with vesicular stomatitis virus, HIV-1, influenza, and murine CMV (MCMV).[77,78] In regards to MCMV, for instance, Ly49H(+) NK cells recognize MCMV m157 glycoprotein, resulting in NK-cell mediated control of the disease. These Ly49H$^+$ NK cells preferentially expand in the setting of infection and contract after infection is controlled. However, "memory" NK cells could be detected months after infection, and upon restimulation, these NK cells exhibited augmented cytotoxicity and cytokine production against MCMV.[78] Although a unique marker of memory is unclear, these NK cells stably express KLRG1, a cadherin-recognizing inhibitory receptor, and could be detected 2 months after infection control even in adoptive transfer models.[78]

THE ROLE OF NATURAL KILLER CELLS IN HUMAN DISEASE

Natural killer cell deficiencies are rare; however, such conditions provide insight into the role NK cells play in response to infectious pathogens, autoimmune disorders, and the development of malignancy. Selective NK cell deficiency has not been associated with a particular Mendelian disorder[79]; however, studies have shed new light on the genetic mechanisms responsible for proper NK development and function. Many syndromes have been linked to increased susceptibility to infection, and others may predispose to autoimmune disease.

Natural Killer Deficiency Syndromes Linked to Increased Infectious Risks

The first gene directly implicated in NK deficiency was FCGR3A, which codes for FcγRIIIa (CD16) expressed on NK cells. A "T ◇ A" substitution at position 230 leads to coding of a lysine residue at position 48, normally a histidine. Although the protein expressed appears phenotypically normal, patients present with increased susceptibility to severe and disseminated herpes simplex virus (HSV) infections.[80] Other patients present with progressive Epstein-Barr virus and varicella infections.[81] Patients have variable deficits in NK cytotoxicity and responsiveness to cytokine stimulation. Population studies have subsequently suggested that the H48 allele may be necessary but not sufficient to produce clinical disease.[82]

Clinical examples of patients entirely lacking any CD56$^+$ lymphocyte subsets have been reported. The first report was a young patient who presented with life-threatening varicella infection. She subsequently developed CMV pneumonia and cutaneous HSV infection. Analysis of her lymphocyte subsets demonstrated a striking and selective absolute absence of CD56$^+$ or CD16$^+$ cells.[5] The patient went on to develop aplastic anemia and expired from complications of stem cell transplantation.[82] A second patient presented with disseminated *Mycobacterium avium* went on to die of disseminated varicella.[83] Other patients have been described with an isolated deficiency of CD56$^+$/CD3$^-$ lymphocytes but with normal or even increased populations of CD56$^+$/CD3$^+$ cells. One such patient presented with severe, recurrent human papilloma virus–related condylomatous disease.[84] Although the genetic mechanisms of these diseases remain unknown, they highlight the functional role of NK cells in providing immunity toward infectious pathogens.

Natural killer cell deficiencies have been described as a component of other disease processes affecting multiple hematopoietic and immune lineages. The genetic deficiencies responsible for many of these disorders have been described and can be found in Table 20-2.

The Role of Natural Killer Cells in Autoimmunity

Interestingly, NK cells have been implicated in both the regulation and pathogenesis of autoimmune disorders. For example, in a murine experimental autoimmune encephalomyelitis (EAE) model of multiple sclerosis in which disease is induced with myelin oligodendrocyte glycoprotein (MOG), NK depletion leads to enhanced T-cell response to MOG. Similarly, in human multiple sclerosis, NK cells have been implicated in the maintenance of disease remission.[85] NK cells have also been shown to control inflammation in an experimental model of autoimmune colitis.[86] NK cells may exert this effect through recognition and elimination of T cells activated against autoantigens.[87]

There are also examples of NK cells promoting autoimmune disorders. For instance, experimental evidence supports the idea that NK cells may promote development of type 1 diabetes mellitus through targeted elimination of pancreatic islet β cells after viral infection.[88] Other studies suggest that NK cells can promote humorally mediated autoimmune diseases such as myasthenia gravis through potentiation of autoreactive B cells.[89] Synoviocytes of patients with rheumatoid arthritis (RA) have been shown to express abnormally high levels of MICA, the previously described ligand for NKG2D.[90,91] In fact, NK cells present in acute RA joint effusions may perpetuate this autoimmune inflammatory response.[92]

Finally, NK cell receptor polymorphisms have been implicated in the pathogenesis and progression of autoimmune disease. For example, a T ◇ G substitution at position 559 in the FcγRIIIA (CD16) gene leads to a phenylalanine to valine substitution at residue 176 of the FcγRIIIA protein.[93] Although the receptors are expressed similarly on the cell membrane, the V/V homozygous state is associated with a higher affinity for IgG binding than the F/F state. The low binding state (F/F) is associated with lupus nephritis.[94] Others have confirmed this observation by genetic linkage studies in patients with systemic lupus erythematosis.[95] Another polymorphism in the FcγRIIIA receptor (158V/F) has been associated with RA in certain ethnic groups.[96] This mutation may also be associated with development of subcutaneous rheumatoid nodules in patients with established RA.[96] As CD16 expressed on a number of immune cells, the specific role of NK cells contributing to pathology is unclear; however, as discussed later, these polymorphisms have also been linked to response to enhanced response to monoclonal antibody therapy of cancer.

THE THERAPEUTIC POTENTIAL OF NATURAL KILLER CELLS

T lymphocytes depend on recognition of tumor-specific antigens to effect antitumor immune response, an approach limited by our inability to identify such targets for the vast majority of nonviral neoplasms. NK cells, on the other hand, have long been recognized

Table 20-2 Human Disorders Characterized in Part by Natural Killer Cell Deficiency

Disease	Gene	Protein	Cell Count	Cytotoxicity	ADCC	Cytokine Response
X-linked SCID	*1.1.1.1.1.1.1.1 IL2Rg*	Common g chain	Low/absent	Low/absent	N/A	Reduced
Autosomal recessive severe combined immunodeficiency	*1.1.1.1.1.1.1.2 JAK3*	Janus kinase 3	Low/absent	Low/absent	N/A	N/A
Bloom syndrome	*1.1.1.1.1.1.1.3 BLM*	Bloom helicase	Normal	Low	N/A	Normal
Chediak-Higashi syndrome	*1.1.1.1.1.1.1.4 LYST*	Lysosome trafficking regulator	Normal	Absent	Absent	Reduced
Xeroderma pigmentosum	*1.1.1.1.1.1.1.5 XPAG*	DNA repair enzymes	Normal	Low	N/A	Normal
Familial erythrophagocytic lymphohistiocytosis	*1.1.1.1.1.1.1.6 PFP1*	Perforin	Normal	Absent	Absent	Reduced/absent
X-linked lymphoproliferative syndrome	*1.1.1.1.1.1.1.7 SH2-DIA*	SLAM-associated protein	Normal	Absent	Normal	Normal
Paroxysmal nocturnal hemoglobinuria	*1.1.1.1.1.1.1.8 PIG-A*	Phosphatidylinositol glycan class A	Low	Absent	Normal	Reduced/absent
von Hippel-Lindau syndrome	*1.1.1.1.1.1.1.9 NKTR*	Tumor recognition molecule	Normal	Absent	Normal	Reduced
Wiskott-Aldrich syndrome	*1.1.1.1.1.1.1.10 WASP*	WAS protein	High	Low	Low/normal	N/A
X-linked agammaglobulinemia	*1.1.1.1.1.1.1.11 BTK*	Bruton tyrosine kinase	Normal	Low	Low	N/A
Ectodermal dysplasia with immunodeficiency	*1.1.1.1.1.1.1.12 IKBKG*	NEMO	Normal	Low	Low/normal	Reduced
Common variable immunodeficiency	*TACI*	TNF receptor family member	Low	Low/normal	Low/normal	Normal

Adapted from Orange J: Human natural killer cell deficiencies and susceptibility to infection. *Microbes Infect* 4:1545, 2002.
ADCC, Antibody-dependent cytotoxicity; *N/A*, not applicable; *NEMO*, nuclear factor-κB essential modulator; *SCID*, severe combined immunodeficiency; *SLAM*, signaling lymphocyte-activation molecule; *TNF*, tumor necrosis factor.

as being capable of antitumor rejection independent of such tumor antigens. As the understanding of how NK cells identify and eliminate targets has advanced, novel roles for the application of NK in clinical anticancer therapy have been defined. Three general approaches have been developed.

First, direct infusion of NK cells into patients with therapeutic intent has been performed.[97] This strategy has developed based on observations such as that in the allogeneic peripheral blood stem cell transplant (PBSCT) setting, where higher doses of transplanted NK cells have been associated with better outcomes as evidenced by reductions in posttransplant infections as well as reduction in nonrelapse mortality.[98] Several studies have shown this approach to be safe and associated with at least a modicum of effectiveness in the autologous setting.[99,100] At least one trial evaluating direct NK cell infusion has been reported in the allogeneic setting, correlating successful transfer and expansion of haploidentical NK cells with hematologic remission of leukemia.[101]

Second, NK cells have been successfully expanded in vivo in patients with cancer through the exogenous administration of recombinant human cytokines, such as low-, intermediate-, or high-dose IL-2.[102-106] The tumor nonspecificity of these strategies is being explored by concomitantly administering a tumor-specific monoclonal antibody whose Fc portion can bind to CD16 expressed on the cytokine-expanded NK cells, thus initiating a process called *antibody-dependent cellular cytotoxicity*.[105,107,108]

A third methodology under development to enhance the antitumor response of NK cells is based on the emerging understanding of KIR biology.[109] More than 20 years ago, an inverse relationship was reported between expression of MHC class I molecules on target cells and the ability of NK cells to kill such targets successfully.[37] As this "missing self" model was further characterized, three principal, common HLA class I allele specificities were identified that serve as ligands for three specific NK cell inhibitory KIR receptors. These have been termed "group 1" HLA-C alleles expressing Asn80 (e.g., HLA-Cw1, w3, w7, w8, and related alleles), "group 2" HLA-C alleles expressing Lys80 (e.g., HLA-Cw2, w4, w5, w6, and related alleles), and HLA-Bw4 alleles (e.g., HLA-B27). As one's NK receptor repertoire, including inhibitory KIRs, is dictated during development by the HLA class I genotype, ultimately every NK cell expresses at least one inhibitory KIR specific to self HLA class I molecules.[18] Moreover, allogeneic targets sensitive to NK cytotoxicity are identified by their lack of self MHC class I inhibitory KIR ligands.

These principles have been applied in a number of therapeutic settings. Perhaps most dramatically, Aversa and colleagues[110] have demonstrated an impressive improvement in survival after allogeneic stem cell transplantation–based therapy for patients with acute myeloid leukemia. Donor-versus-recipient NK cell alloreactivity has been shown to contribute to enhanced survival in this setting, as well as improved engraftment, and protection against graft-versus-host-disease.[111,112] In a series of patients receiving haploidentical grafts, 68% of patients without NK alloreactivity had relapsed disease, but only 15% of patients with NK alloreactivity relapsed with a median follow-up of 4 years.[111] Similarly, KIR-mismatch has been shown to improve outcome after reduced-intensity chemotherapy followed by allogeneic stem cell transplantation in multiple myeloma patients.[102,113] Fig. 20-3 shows how mismatching KIR epitopes facilitates NK-mediated tumor cytotoxicity in a haploidentical setting.

Others have extended on these transplantation-based findings by manipulating the relationship between NK receptors and MHC class I receptors through the means of monoclonal antibodies. For example, a murine model lends support to the notion that tumor expression of MHC class I molecules become engaged by inhibitory NK cell receptors and thus mediate NK tolerance.[114] When antibody fragments were introduced to disrupt this ligand–receptor interaction, increased NK cytotoxicity and decreased tumor growth were observed. Furthermore, adoptive transfer of murine NK cells pretreated with an antibody to block inhibitory NK receptor expression into leukemia-bearing mice led to enhanced survival as compared with transfer of untreated NK cells. These findings support the notion that blocking inhibitory NK receptors may be beneficial in increasing the

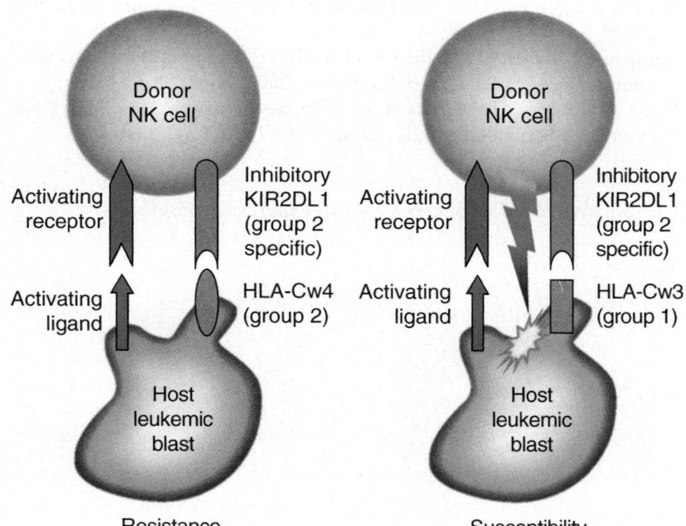

Figure 20-3 SIMPLIFIED REPRESENTATION OF HAPLOTYPE MISMATCHED ALLOGENEIC STEM CELL TRANSPLANT FOR ACUTE MYELOID LEUKEMIA: PROPER MAJOR HISTOCOMPATIBILITY COMPLEX (MHC) CLASS I MISMATCH CAN LEAD TO DONOR NATURAL KILLER (NK) CELL KILLING HOST LEUKEMIC BLASTS. As the human leukocyte antigen C (HLA-C) ligand binds to the NK cell inhibitory killer immunoglobulin-like receptor (KIR) on the left, the inhibitory signal interrupts the activation signal, and no killing occurs. However, when the HLA-C ligand does not bind the NK inhibitor KIR on the right, no inhibitory signal is sent, and tumor killing occurs. *(Adapted from Farag SS, Fehniger TA, Ruggeri L, et al: Natural killer cell receptors: new biology and insights into the graft-versus-leukemia effect.* Blood *100:1935, 2002.)*

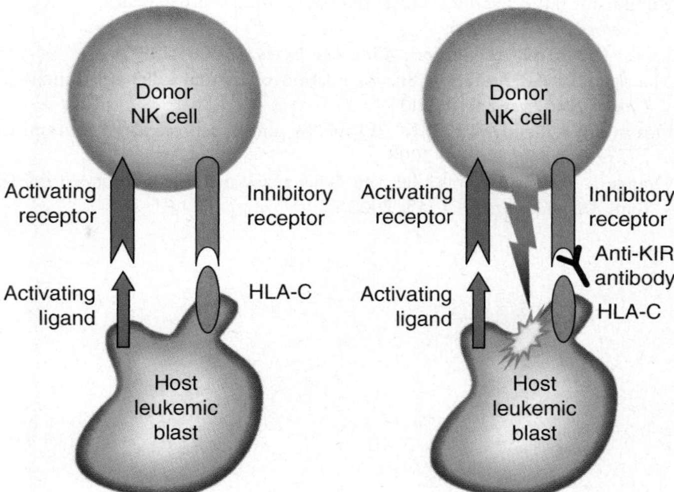

Figure 20-4 SIMPLIFIED REPRESENTATION SHOWING THE GENERAL EQUILIBRIUM BETWEEN ACTIVATING AND INHIBITORY SIGNALING THAT FAVORS NO KILLING AS SHOWN ON THE LEFT. However, the introduction of an antibody to the inhibitory receptor tips this balance towards activation and elimination of the target cell, as shown on the right. *HLA-C,* Human leukocyte antigen C; *NK,* natural killer. *(Adapted from Farag SS, Fehniger TA, Ruggeri L, et al: Natural killer cell receptors: New biology and insights into the graft-versus-leukemia effect.* Blood *100:1935, 2002.)*

efficacy of cancer immunotherapy.[114,115] In fact, phase 1 clinical trials of anti-KIR antibodies are underway in humans. Fig. 20-4 demonstrates this principle.

In complementary fashion, other approaches have sought to enhance activating NK receptors, such as NKG2D. One group has created a novel bivalent protein (ULBP2-BB4) which recognizes NKG2D and CD138, a protein overexpressed in a number of malignancies, including multiple myeloma. Although such an approach is limited by knowledge of particular tumor antigens, the concept of enhancing NK function was demonstrated in this model through increases in NK cytokine secretion as well as abrogation of tumor cell growth in the presence of the molecule.[116]

Finally, the use of monoclonal antibodies directed against tumor cell antigens has significantly advanced treatment of some malignancies. For example, treatment with the monoclonal, immunoglobulin G (IgG), chimeric anti-CD20 antibody rituximab has been shown to improve survival of patients with non-Hodgkin lymphoma. As discussed, genotypic, single nucleotide polymorphisms in the FcγRIIIA (CD16) receptor expressed on NK cells and other immune cells may convey functional differences in the receptor that have clinical consequences. Patients with the V/V homozygous state at residue 176 have a higher affinity for the Fc portion of the rituximab, and these patients show enhanced clinical response to the antibody.[117] Such a finding supports the notion that enhanced ADCC function in CD16-bearing cells, including NK cells, is one key mechanism of action of rituximab and suggests that antibody-mediated cancer therapies could be advanced by enhancing NK cell numbers and cytotoxic potential in vivo.

FUTURE DIRECTIONS

Natural killer cells are a critical cellular component of innate immunity. Rapid secretion of powerful immunomodulatory cytokines and chemokines support the role of NK cells as "first responders" to immune insults, facilitating mobilization and tailoring of the innate and adaptive immune response. Potent natural cytotoxicity, unrestricted by classical antigen presentation, and costimulation required for adaptive immune cells, suggest that NK cells have an important, complementary role to that of cytotoxic T lymphocytes, which provide antigen-specific cytotoxicity and lasting memory. Further understanding of the functional differences between $CD56^{dim}$ and $CD56^{bright}$ subsets, their cytotoxicity and cytokine receptor expression, and their developmental biology will certainly shed more light on the therapeutic potential for NK cells in the pathogenesis, prevention, and treatment of human disease.

SUGGESTED READINGS

Becknell B, Caligiuri MA: Interleukin-2, interleukin-15, and their roles in human natural killer cells. *Adv Immunol* 86:209, 2005.

Borrego F, Masilamani M, Marusina AT: The CD94/NKG2 family of receptors: From molecules and cells to clinical relevance. *Immunol Res* 35:263, 2006.

Caligiuri MA: Human natural killer cells. *Blood* 112:461, 2008.

Colucci F, Caligiuri MA, Di Santo JP: What does it take to make a natural killer? *Nat Rev Immunol* 3:413, 2003.

Cooper MA, Fehniger TA, Caligiuri MA: The biology of human natural killer cell subsets. *Trends Immunol* 22:633, 2001.

Cooper MA, Fehniger TA, Turner SC: Human natural killer cells: A unique innate immunoregulatory role for the CD56(bright) subset. *Blood* 97:3146, 2001.

Djeu JY, Jiang K, Wei S: A view to a kill: Signals triggering cytotoxicity. *Clin Cancer Res* 8:636, 2002.

Farag SS, Fehniger TA, Ruggeri L, et al: Natural killer cell receptors: New biology and insights into the graft-versus-leukemia effect. *Blood* 100:1935, 2002.

Freud AH, Yokohama A, Becknell B, et al: Evidence for discrete stages of human natural killer cell differentiation in vivo. *J Exp Med* 203:1033, 2006.

Jie HB, Sarvetnick N: The role of NK cells and NK cell receptors in autoimmune disease. *Autoimmunity* 37:147, 2004.

Klingmann HG: Natural killer cell-based immunotherapeutic strategies. *Cytotherapy* 7:16, 2005.

Lanier L: NK cell recognition. *Annu Rev Immunol* 2005;23:225.

Makrigiannis AP, Anderson SK: Regulation of natural killer cell function. *Cancer Biol Ther* 2:610, 2003.

Ogasawara K, Lanier LL: NKG2D in NK and T cell-mediated immunity. *J Clin Immunol* 25:534, 2005.

Orange J: Human natural killer cell deficiencies and susceptibility to infection. *Microbes Infect* 4:1545, 2002.

Paust S, von Andrian UH: Natural killer cell memory. *Nat Immunol* 12:500, 2011.

Sentman CL, Barber MA, Barber A, et al: NK cell receptors as tools in cancer immunotherapy. *Adv Cancer Res* 95:249, 2006.

Vivier E, Raulet DH, Moretta A, et al: Innate or adaptive immunity? The example of natural killer cells. *Science* 331:44, 2011.

For complete list of references log on to www.expertconsult.com

CHAPTER 21

DENDRITIC CELL BIOLOGY

Olivier Manches, Viswanathan Lakshmanan, Zbigniew M. Szczepiorkowski, and Nina Bhardwaj

Dendritic cells (DCs) are a sparsely distributed population of bone marrow (BM)–derived mononuclear cells that exist in an "immature" form in virtually all tissues in the body.[1] DC serve as professional antigen-presenting cells (APCs) with an extraordinary capacity to stimulate naïve T lymphocytes (as well as B, natural killer [NK], and NK T cells) and initiate primary immune responses. In their immature state, DCs detect and capture "danger signals" originating from microorganisms or their macromolecular constituents in their resident tissues. Upon encountering such danger signals, DCs undergo a complex series of events leading to their "maturation."[1] Maturation of DCs is characterized by migration of DCs to draining lymph nodes and processing and presentation of antigens in the context of antigen presenting molecules such as major histocompatibility complex (MHC) and CD1 to naïve T, B, and NK cells. This chapter provides a snapshot of our current understanding of DC function as well as DCs' potential clinical applications as immunotherapeutic agents in diseases such as cancer, HIV and autoimmunity.[2]

DENDRITIC CELL SUBSETS AND DEVELOPMENT

Extensive research has demonstrated that DCs exist in many "flavors."[3,4] However, our understanding of DC differentiation and the different DC subsets is complicated by the heterogeneity of data obtained from in vitro human and mouse studies and in vivo animal studies and limited in vivo human studies. The generation of functionally distinct DC subtypes follows two generally accepted models: (1) the functional plasticity model postulating the existence of a single DC lineage possessing functional plasticity and (2) the specialized lineage model postulating the existence of multiple DC lineages displaying functional diversity.[5] Both models assume four stages of DC development, namely hematopoietic precursors, DC precursors (pre-DC), immature DCs (imDCs), and mature DCs (mDCs) (Fig. 21-1). It is likely, however, that elements of both models are involved in DC subset development. In this chapter, we concentrate on human DCs with little reference to murine models. Readers are encouraged to seek additional information in several comprehensive reviews.[5-14]

Most studies on the developmental origin of human DC subsets have used in vitro culture systems. DC precursors and imDCs, similar to other cell types in the immune system, are continuously produced in a steady rate and pathogen-independent manner from $CD34^+$ hematopoietic stem cells (HSCs) within the BM. Fms-like tyrosine kinase-3 ligand (Flt-3-L) and granulocyte colony-stimulating factor (G-CSF) represent the key DC growth and differentiation factors.[15] The $CD34^+$ HSC differentiate into hypothetical common lymphoid progenitors (CLPs) and common myeloid progenitors (CMPs) in the BM. Subsequently, CMPs differentiate into $CD34^+CLA^+$ and $CD34^+CLA^+$ populations (CLA, skin homing receptor cutaneous lymphocyte-associated antigen), which give rise to phenotypically distinguishable $CD11c^+CD1a^+$ and $CD11c^+CD1a^+$ immature DCs, respectively.[16] The former migrate into the skin epidermis and differentiate into Langerhans cells, and the latter localize to skin dermis and other tissues and become interstitial imDCs.[17] The human Langerhans cell DC subset has distinct markers, including the presence of Birbeck granules; the expression of CD1a; and langerin, a member of the C-type lectin family of receptors involved in the uptake of pathogens.[18]

The $CD34^+$ hematopoietic progenitor cells (HPCs) and blood monocytes are commonly used as precursor cells for generating DC in culture in vitro for both research and immunotherapeutic purposes. HPCs are treated with c-kit ligand and tumor necrosis factor-α (TNF-α) that yield subsets of myeloid DCs, including Langerhans cells. Monocytes, obtained by simple adherence of HPCs to plastic, when exposed to a combination of GM-CSF and interleukin-4 (IL-4), yield imDCs that are comparable to some degree to tissue interstitial DCs. Maturation of these different DCs can be induced by the addition of various stimuli.

The pre-DC subset expresses several myeloid markers, including CD11b, CD11c, CD13, CD14, and CD33, indicating that they may derive from a CMP. In contrast to the blood "myeloid DCs" derived from CMP, which we will refer to here as conventional DCs (cDCs), the "plasmacytoid DCs" contain "lymphoid" mRNA transcripts for pre-T α chains, germline IgK, and Spi-B and are also called interferon (IFN) type I producing cells (IPCs). These latter cells display distinct plasma cell morphology, contain abundant endoplasmic reticulum (ER), and express CD4 and high levels of the IL-3αR but lack myeloid antigens, including CD11c and most lineage markers. Plasmacytoid DCs (pDC) are found in peripheral blood, thymus, and many lymphoid tissues. The production of extraordinarily high levels of IFN type 1 by pDC is unique to this cell type and may be important for initiating a strong antiviral innate response and promote maturation of bystander $CD11c^+$ cDC to protect them from the cytopathic effect of viruses.[18-21] It is hypothesized that human cDCs and pDCs have evolved to recognize and respond to different pathogens in unique ways owing to their complementary expression of receptors for "pathogen-associated molecular patterns" (see Antigen Acquisition section), capacity to secrete either IFN type I or IL-12, antigen presentation, and migration into secondary lymphoid organs. As mentioned, pDCs secrete high amounts of IFN-α upon viral infection but no IL-12 and display poor antigen capture and presentation capacity. Upon activation, pDCs differentiate into cells bearing similar characteristics to activated cDCs (i.e., with a dendritic morphology, high expression of MHC class II molecules, and the capacity to prime naïve T cells)[22,23] but express low levels of CD11c and lack typical myeloid markers. The functional properties of these latter pDC-derived DC is still to be investigated thoroughly,[24] although they may differ from cDCs, especially in their cross-presentation[25] or T-cell skewing capacities. Thus, whereas DCs derived from pDCs upon culture with IL-3 and activation by CD40-L preferentially prime naïve $CD4^+$ T cells toward a Th2 profile, DCs derived from pDCs by viral/Toll-like receptor (TLR) stimulation prime toward a Th1 profile in an IFN-α–dependent and IL-12–independent pathway.[20] Upon activation, immature cDCs migrate through afferent lymph from nonlymphoid tissues to the T cell–rich areas of lymph nodes. Plasmacytoid DCs, which also migrate into T-cell areas of secondary lymphoid tissues, do so through high endothelial venules (HEVs) of lymph nodes and marginal zone of the spleen, likely using CCR7 and CD62-L.[26] Both activated blood cDCs and pDCs can migrate in response to lymph node homing chemokines (CCL19 and

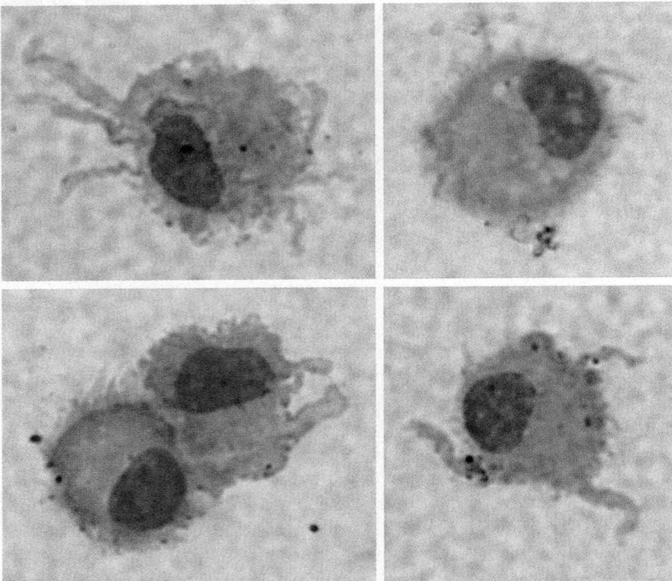

Figure 21-1 EXAMPLES OF MONOCYTE-DERIVED MATURE DENDRITIC CELLS. The mononuclear cells were enriched by adherence, cultured with interleukin-4 (IL-4) and granulocyte colony-stimulating factor (G-CSF) for 6 days and underwent maturation with IL-1, IL-6, tumor necrosis factor-α (TNF-α), and prostaglandin E_2 (PGE_2) for 24 hours.

CCL21) through expression of CCR7. Although cDCs can be found in virtually every peripheral tissue as well as in lymphoid organs, pDCs seem to display a more restricted distribution. They can be found mostly in the T-cell area of lymphoid organs (lymph node, tonsils, spleen, thymus, BM, and Peyer patches), blood, and some peripheral tissues (liver, nasal mucosa). Although cDCs and pDCs express a similar array of chemotactic receptors (e.g., CCR2, CCR5, CXCR2, CXCR4), pDCs do not respond to a number of inflammatory chemokines. However, they accumulate in inflamed tissues, such as in systemic lupus erythematosus (SLE) and contact dermatitis, probably through their expression of ChemR23 and CXCR4.

This division of DCs into cDC and pDC subsets is likely to be an oversimplified view of DC heterogeneity. For example splenic DCs are heterogenous with regard to expression of CD4, CD11b, and CD11c, but most of the thymic DCs are CD11c$^+$ but lack other myeloid markers, thereby not fitting into either of the classical categories of cDCs and pDCs in blood.[27]

An important role for CD103$^+$ (αE integrin) has recently been uncovered. CD103$^+$ DC reside in the intestinal mucosa and play a crucial role in tolerance to commensal bacteria and food antigens. These cells originate in the lamina propria (LP) and migrate to the mesenteric lymph nodes (MLNs), where they drive the differentiation of gut-homing FoxP3+ regulatory T cells by producing retinoic acid from dietary vitamin A.

In addition, the BDCA3$^+$ (CD141) DC subset has been found to be the equivalent of murine CD8α$^+$ DCs, which are most potent at cross-presenting antigens to CD8$^+$ T cells. They express the chemokine receptor XCR1 and the DC NK lectin group receptor-1 (DNGR1) C type lectin, a sensor for necrotic cells, and mediate the phagocytosis of dead cells. They also express basic leucine zipper transcriptional factor ATF-like-3 and INF regulatory factor-8, which may be essential for their development. BDCA3$^+$ DCs express high levels of TLR3 and TLR8, and upon stimulation by TLR3 agonists (e.g., poly I:C), they secrete high amounts of IL-12 and IFN-β, both Th1-skewing cytokines. These combined characteristics make them attractive targets for DC-based vaccines in cancer and chronic immune diseases.

Although Langerhans cells and microglia seem to be capable of self renewal in ectodermal tissues, epidermis and brain, other DC arise from bloodborne precursors from BM. DC arise from a macrophage and DC precursor (MDC), giving rise to monocytes and DCs, and a common DC precursor (CDP).[28] Recent studies of human immunodeficiencies have highlighted the transcription factors directing the development of DCs and emphasized their role in defense against microbial pathogens. Thus, in DC, monocyte, B, and NK lymphoid deficiency (DCML), blood and interstitial DCs are absent along with monocytes and pDCs. The DCML is attributable to GATA-binding factor 2 (GATA2) mutations, a transcription factor involved in the homeostasis of HSCs. Patients with DCML deficiency have increased susceptibility to *Mycobacteria* spp., fungi, and viruses. Another DC deficiency syndrome is caused by INF regulatory factor 8 (IRF8) mutations. The autosomal recessive K108E mutations leads to defects in peripheral cDCs, pDCs, and monocytes, with increased susceptibility to *Mycobacteria* spp., other intracellular bacteria, and viruses and is accompanied by a myeloproliferative syndrome. The dominant sporadic mutation T80A induces a specific loss of CD1c$^+$ DC, with increased susceptibility to mycobacterial infection but otherwise a normal life expectancy.

The developmental origin of pDCs versus cDCs is still debated because pDCs and cDCs can be derived from both CLP and CMP, suggesting that pDCs and cDCs may arise during hematopoiesis from progenitors with already distinct and restricted lineage potential.[29] It seems that whereas cDC differentiation is dependent on the transcription factor Ikaros, pDC development is dependent on the Ets family transcription factor SpiB and probably PU.1. A recent study also described an important role for the upregulation of basic helix–loop–helix transcription factor (E-protein) E2-2 in developing pDCs, and E2-2–deficient hematopoietic progenitors do not produce pDC.[30] Studies in mice described the conversion of BM pDCs into cDCs upon viral infection, again highlighting the complexity and plasticity of DC development.[31]

The migration of myeloid DC and plasmacytoid DC precursors from the BM can be increased by administration of Flt-3-L up to 50-fold for pre-DCs and 15-fold for pDCs.[32,33] G-CSF is also known to increase the number of pDCs in the circulation. With the advent of newer technologies, it has also become feasible to generate large numbers of DC subsets in vitro.

THE CONCEPT OF MATURATION

In their resting state, imDCs are primed to acquire antigens in situ through a variety of receptors and mechanisms. Upon encountering pathogens or other "activating stimuli," DCs undergo a complicated series of phenotypic and functional changes referred here to as "activation" and "maturation," respectively.[1] The process of DC activation is an intricate differentiation process under tight control that is closely associated with antigen acquisition. It is induced by various stimuli (Table 21-1) or danger signals (e.g., signs of pathogenic infection or cell injury), including cytokines (e.g., IFN type I, TNF-α, and IL-1), microbial products (e.g., lipopolysaccharide [LPS], flagellin), intracellular products (e.g., heat shock proteins), growth factors (e.g., thymic stromal lymphopoietin [TSLP]), immune complexes and T-cell molecules (e.g., CD40). The process of activation is characterized by upregulation of adhesion and costimulatory molecules such as CD54, CD80, CD86, MHC class I and II molecules, cytokines (e.g., TNF-α, IL-12, IL-18) and chemokines (e.g., RANTES, MIP-1 α, IP-10). The latter enable the recruitment of T cells, monocytes, and other DCs into the local environment. In their mature state, DC express markers, which distinguish them from imDCs such as CD83 (a molecule involved in thymic T-cell selection and DC–DC interactions) and DC-LAMP, a lysosomal protein. Maturation also changes the migratory properties of DCs. They express CCR7 and acquire responsiveness to the chemokines CCL19 and CCL21 that are expressed in the T-cell areas of lymph nodes where mature DCs generate immune responses. Concomitantly, DCs downregulate their receptors for CCL3, CCL4, and CCL5, which are secreted at sites of inflammation, reduce their capacity for phagocytosis, macropinocytosis, antigen uptake, and processing but acquire potent immunostimulatory ability through enhanced T-cell–DC immune synapse

Table 21-1 Agents That Cause Dendritic Cell Maturation*

Agent Property	Molecules
Stimulatory agents	TNF family members (TNF-α, CD40L, FasL, TRANCE) TLR ligands (dsRNA, LPS, imiquimod, CpG ODNs) Growth factors (TSLP) Interferons (IFN-α) Adhesion molecules (CECAM-1 (CD66a) Costimulatory molecules (LIGHT, B7-DC) Receptors (FcR via Ag-Igs; TREM-2 via Dap-12) Viruses or microbes (influenza, bacteria, bacterial products) Chemokines (MCP, MIP1α, RANTES, IP10, IL-8, MDC, TARC) Chemokine receptors (CCR7 and loss of CCR2 and CCR5)
Inhibitory agents	Drugs (rapamycin, FK506, cyclosporin A, dexamethasone, IVIg) Chemokines (IL-10) Viruses (EBV, vaccinia, canarypox, HSV) Others (β2 microglobulin)
Survival signals	CD40 L, TRANCE, B7-DC, Bcl-2
Cell–cell interaction	Activated cells (CD4 and CD8 cells [via CD40L]) NK cells, NK T cells Vδ1+, γδ T cells

Ag-Igs, Antigen-immunoglobulin immune complexes; *Bcl-2,* B-cell lymphoma 2; *CCR,* chemokine (C-C motif) receptor; *CECAM-1,* carcinoembryonic antigen-related cell adhesion molecule-1; *CpG ODNs,* CpG oligodeoxynucleotides; *dsRNA,* double-stranded DNA; *EBV,* Epstein-Barr virus; *FcR,* Fc receptor; *HSV,* herpesvirus; *IFN,* interferon; *IL,* interleukin; *IP10,* interferon gamma-induced protein 10; *IVIg,* intravenous immunoglobulin; *LIGHT,* homologous to lymphotoxins, exhibits inducible expression, and competes with HSV glycoprotein D for herpesvirus entry mediator, a receptor expressed by T lymphocytes; *LPS,* lipopolysaccharide; *MCP,* macrophage/monocyte chemotactic protein; *MDC,* macrophage and dendritic cell precursor; *MIP1α,* macrophage inflammatory protein 1 alpha; *NK,* natural killer; *RANTES, regulated* on activation, normal T expressed and secreted; *TARC,* thymus and activation-regulated chemokine; *TNF,* tumor necrosis factor; *TRANCE,* TNF-related activation-induced cytokine; *TREM-2,* triggering receptor expressed on myeloid cells 2; *TSLP,* thymic stromal lymphopoietin.
*Maturation is a complex process tightly linked to antigen acquisition and the surrounding microenvironment. See text for more details.

Table 21-2 Antigen Recognition and Uptake Receptors Expressed by Dendritic Cells*

Receptor	Antigenic Ligand
C-type lectins (DC-SIGN, MMR, DEC-205)	Mannosylated molecules, viruses, bacteria, fungi
FcγR (CD32, CD64)	Immune complexes, antibody-coated tumor cells
CD1 a, b, c, d	Biphosphonate moieties in *Mycobacterium tuberculosis,* BCG, and *Listeria monocytogenes;* lipid and glycolipid foreign and self-antigens
Integrins (αVβ5, CR3, CR4)	Opsonized antigens, apoptotic cells
Scavenger receptors (CD36, LOX-1)	Opsonized antigens, apoptotic cells, heat shock proteins
TLRs and other PRRs	TLR 2–8 (myeloid DC) peptoglycans, endotoxin, flagellin TLR 7 (plasmacytoid DC) bacterial DNA; RIG-I, MDA5, STING, DAI, AIM2, PKR, NOD proteins
HSP-R (CD91)	Heat shock proteins
Aquaporins	Fluids

AIM2, Absent in melanoma 2; *BCG,* Bacillus Calmette-Guérin; *DAI,* DNA-dependent activator of IFN-regulatory factors; *DC,* dendritic cell; *DC-SIGN,* dendritic cell-specific intercellular adhesion molecule-3-Grabbing non-integrin; *HSP-R,* heat shock protein receptor; *MDA5,* melanoma differentiation-associated protein 5; *NOD,* nucleotide oligomerization domain; *PKR,* protein kinase R; *PPR,* pattern recognition receptor; *RIG-1,* retinoid-inducible gene I; *STING,* stimulator of interferon genes; *TLR,* Toll-like receptor.
*The table lists some of the receptors expressed by DCs that are involved in antigen acquisition. The antigen receptor repertoire dictates that range of antigens captured by the DC. Ligation of some of these receptors induces DC maturation.

formation, production of immunoproteosomes, and upregulation of unique DC-specific costimulatory molecules such as B7-DC.[34] However, although increased expression of costimulatory molecules and migration to secondary lymphoid organs often correlates with their capacity to prime CD4 and CD8 immunity, activated DCs may also induce tolerization of T cells, as when $CD4^+$ T cell help is missing[35,36] or on activation by inflammatory cytokines in the absence of TLR engagement,[37] and can potentially induce the generation of regulatory T cells (Tregs). Some stimuli, such as thymic stromal lymphopoietin (TSLP), can induce phenotypic maturation of DCs without concomitant secretion of proinflammatory cytokines such as IL-12, IL-6, TNF-α, or IL-1.[38] Therefore, DC maturation is more appropriately used in a functional sense, with mature DCs being defined as able to prime naïve T-cell responses. What makes a phenotypically activated DC capable of priming instead of tolerizing a T cell appears multifactorial and dependent on such factors as the state of the microenvironment and the DC subset in question, although this remains to be clearly defined.

ANTIGEN ACQUISITION AND DENDRITIC CELL ACTIVATION

Immature DCs sample their environment through several mechanisms, including micropinocytosis, macropinocytosis, receptor-mediated endocytosis, and phagocytosis. They display an array of surface receptors, which facilitate acquisition of antigens and pathogens and at the same time induce differentiation into activated DCs. An important class of receptors is the pattern recognition receptors (PRRs), which recognize pathogen-associated molecular patterns (PAMPs) expressed by many microorganisms. PRRs serve as an important link between innate and adaptive immunity because they directly mature DCs while also inducing the production of a variety of cytokines and chemokines. PRRs consist of several groups of receptors, including secreted (e.g., MBL, CRP, SAP, LBP), cell-surface (e.g., CD14, MMR, MSR, MARCO),[39] and intracellular molecules (e.g., RIG-I and MDA5, which are RNA helicases involved in the recognition of nucleic acids upon viral infection; STING, DAI, AIM2 [absent in melanoma 2], which recognize intracellular DNA[40]; NOD receptors, which recognize peptidoglycan subcomponents or other bacterial molecules; inflammatory caspases, such as caspase-1 and caspase-5, which form an intracellular complex with NALP1 or NALP2 and NALP3 called the inflammasome that recognize bacterial RNA and other danger signals and induce the production of the proinflammatory cytokines IL1β and IL-18) (Table 21-2). TLRs, which constitute another group of PRRs, are expressed by imDCs and mediate activation by microbial components such as peptidoglycan, LPS, flagellin, and unmethylated CpG DNA motifs. Ligation of the TLRs results in the activation of Rel family members, particularly the transcription factor nuclear factor kappa-B (NF-κB), c-Jun-terminal kinase (JNK), and p38 MAP kinase, leading to the initiation of the maturation process.[41,42] TLRs are unevenly distributed among DCs, with myeloid DCs expressing TLR 2, 3, 4, 5, 8 and plasmacytoid DC strongly expressing TLR 7 and 9 (Table 21-3). Another important feature of some TLRs is their capacity to induce secretion of IFN type I for antiviral defense and immune regulation. cDCs express TLR3 and 4, mediating recognition of viral double-stranded

Table 21-3 Toll-Like Receptors Expressed by Dendritic Cells*

mDC	pDC	Ligand(s)
TLR1	TLR1	?
TLR2		Peptidoglycan *(Staphylococcus aureus)* Lipoproteins and lipopeptides from several bacteria Glycophopshotidylinositol anchors from *Trypanosoma cruzi* Lipoaminomannan from *Mycobacterium tuberculosis* Zymosan (yeast)
TLR3		Double-stranded RNA (e.g., poly I:C)
TLR4		LPS + MD-2, taxol, hsp 60 (?), heparan sulfate (?), RSV, fibronectin
TLR5		flagellin (*Salmonella typhimurium, Listeria* spp.)
TLR6	TLR6	? or undergoes dimerization with TLR2
	TLR7	Imiquimod (Aldara), R-848 (resiquimod), single-stranded RNA
TLR8	TLR8	Imiquimod (Aldara), R-848 (resiquimod), single-stranded RNA
	TLR9	CpG ODNs, DNA from bacteria and viruses, chromatin-IgG complexes
	TLR10	?

CpG ODNs, CpG oligodeoxynucleotides; *RSV,* respiratory syncytial virus.
*Toll-like receptors (TLRs) can form heterodimeric receptor complexes consisting of two different TLRs or homodimers (as in the case of TLR4). The TLR4 receptor complex requires supportive molecules (MD-2) for optimal response to its ligand lipopolysaccharide (LPS). A common feature of the TLR receptors is the cytoplasmic TIR domain that serves as a scaffold for a series of protein–protein interactions that result in the activation of a unique signaling module consisting of MyD88; interleukin-1 receptor associated kinase (IRAK) family members; and Tollip, which is used exclusively by TIR family members. Subsequently, several central signaling pathways are activated in parallel, the activation of nuclear factor kappa-B (NF-κB) being the most prominent event of the inflammatory response. Recent developments indicate that in addition to the common signaling module MyD88/IRAK/Tollip, other molecules can modulate signaling by TLRs, especially of TLR4, resulting in differential biologic responses to distinct pathogenic structures. TLR2 is also involved in cross-presentation.

RNA and LPS, respectively, and on triggering secrete low amounts of IFN-β through a signaling pathway using the adaptor TRIF and the transcription factor IRF3. Although cDCs can also induce IFN type I through RIG-I and MDA-5 upon viral infection, pDCs seem to rely mostly on a specialized MyD88-dependent signaling pathway, allowing them to secrete very high amounts of IFN-α upon triggering of TLR7 and 9. This is because of their constitutive high expression of IRF7, a crucial IFN-α gene transcription factor, and because of a specialized spatiotemporal regulation of TLR7 and 9 signaling, allowing IRF7 to interact with MyD88 docked onto TLR in the endosomal membrane.[43]

The inflammasome consists of a family of PRRs that induce IL-1 and IL-18 secretion. IL-1β secretion can be triggered through the NLRP3, NLRC4, and NLRP1 inflammasomes, as well as by the DNA sensor AIM2. Activation of the inflammasome occurs through activation of the nucleotide-binding domain, leucine-rich repeat-containing proteins (NLRs). NLRs are composed of three domains: at the N-terminus a pyrin domain, a caspase recruitment domain, or a baculovirus inhibitory repeat domain; the central domain is the nucleotide binding domain (NBD) responsible for dNTPase activity and oligomerization; and the leucine-rich repeat domain at the C-terminus. IL-1 and IL-18 secretion is dependent on synthesis of pro-IL-1 and pro-IL-18, which can be induced in response to TLR-NF-κB signaling. Activation of the inflammasome leads to caspase-1–mediated processing of pro-IL-1 and pro-IL-18 for IL-1β or IL-18 secretion and inflammatory cell death (pyropoptosis and pyronecrosis). The inflammasome can be activated by sterile (nonmicrobial) activators, including host (adenosine triphosphate [ATP], uric acid crystals, amyloid β) and microenvironment derived molecules (alum, silica, asbestos). It can also be activated by pathogen-derived products, including PAMPs. Microbial activators include pore-forming toxins, RNA and DNA, flagellin, β-glucans, and zymosan. The best studied inflammasome is the NLRP3 inflammasome, and the mechanisms of activation are being deciphered. It is believed that inflammasome activation can occur through three main mechanisms: generation of reactive oxygen species (ROS), possibly by the phagosomal NADH (nicotinamide adenine dinucleotide) oxidase, release of cathepsin B upon phagolysosomal destabilization, and pore formation at the plasma membrane through the P2X7 receptor, allowing K+ efflux.

C-type lectins are calcium-dependent carbohydrate-binding proteins with a broad range of biologic functions, many of which are involved in immune responses. They are well represented on DCs and include the following: DC-SIGN, responsible for binding of HIV-1, HIV-2, simian immunodeficiency virus, Ebola viruses, dengue virus, *Candida* spp., *Leishmania* spp.; blood dendritic cell antigen 2 (BDCA-2), potentially responsible for delivering tolerogenic signals; BDCA-4/neuropilin-1, capable of binding vascular endothelial growth factor (VEGF); langerin, responsible for uptake and processing of antigens in Langerhans cells; DEC-205 (CD205) involved in the uptake and processing of antigens in MIIV (vesicles enriched for MHC class II molecules and proteases such as the cathepsins that mediate antigen processing and MHC class II peptide complex formation), and generation of tolerogenic signals; and macrophage mannose receptor (MMR), which is involved in the processing of microbial organisms.

Other receptors expressed by DCs include FcR, which is involved in cross-presentation of immune complexes and antibody opsonized dead cells; integrins such as αVβ5, scavenger receptors CD36, and Mer-family tyrosine kinases for phagocytosis of apoptotic cells and lipoxygenase-1 (LOX-1) or CD91 for uptake of heat shock proteins (HSPs); complement receptors that play a role in uptake of opsonized microbes and apoptotic cells; receptors for viruses (e.g., CD4, CCR5, and CXCR4 for HIV and CD46 for measles virus); and the CD1 family of receptors that activate CD4, CD8, γδT cells, and NK T cells through binding and processing of antigens such as sphingolipids, sulfatides, glycosphingolipids glycosylphosphatidylinositol (GPI)-anchored mucin-like glycoproteins (GPI mucins), glycoinositolphospholipids (GIPLs), and their phosphatidylinositol moieties. Altogether, these various receptors provide substantial avenues for DCs to efficiently capture multitudes of antigens in their environment.

Antigen capture is tightly coupled to DC activation and antigen presentation, and triggering of TLR or exposure to inflammatory cytokines first induces a transient increase in the macropinocytic uptake followed by a near complete downregulation of the uptake process. Furthermore, it has been suggested that TLR engagement also enhances microbe-loaded phagosome maturation, potentially discriminating between nonimmunogenic antigens (apoptotic cells) and microbial antigens at the antigen processing level.[44]

ANTIGEN PROCESSING

Dendritic cells have a remarkable ability to process and present antigens restricted by major histocompatibility complex (MHC) and CD1 molecules. The processing is tightly associated with DC activation.

Major Histocompatibility Complex Class I Antigen Presentation (Endogenous Route)

The process of antigen processing and presentation to $CD8^+$ T cells begins with degradation of proteins synthesized within the cytoplasm, either as mature proteins or as neosynthesized defective proteins (defective ribosomal products [DRiPS]), into oligopeptides by the ubiquitin–proteasome pathway. Misfolded proteins are also a source of antigenic peptides after retrotranslocation from the ER to the cytosol through the ER-associated degradation (ERAD) pathway. Subsequently, aminopeptidases cleave N-terminal precursors into peptides of appropriate length for presentation on MHC class I molecules. Antigen processing via this route is regulated through activation of the catalytically active subunits of the proteasome, the PA28 proteasome activator, and leucine aminopeptidase, which are upregulated by IFN.[45] Mature DCs, in particular, express immunoproteosomes containing the active site subunits latent membrane protein 2 (LMP2), LMP7, and MECL-1, which can enhance antigen processing.[46] After transport into the ER through the transporter associated with antigen processing (TAP) (Fig. 21-2), long peptides are further trimmed by ER aminopeptidase-1 (ERAP-1) to 8-mer or 9-mer peptides for loading onto MHC class I molecules.

Dendritic cells also have the capacity to acquire antigens exogenously and process them for presentation on MHC class I molecules. This phenomenon, referred to as *cross-presentation,* allows the immune system to recognize antigens that are not otherwise presented or that may not access DCs directly (e.g., tumor cells, viruses). DCs can acquire such antigens in the form of apoptotic cells, necrotic cells, antibody opsonized cells, immune complexes, and heat shock proteins (intracellular chaperones for antigenic peptides, which are released by necrotic cells).[47] DCs even acquire antigens via phagocytosis of particles released from intracellular vesicles (referred to as *exosomes*).[48] Finally, DCs may even nibble bits of live cells to acquire antigens.[49] Mechanistically, cross-presentation may involve cathepsin-S dependent processing of antigenic peptides within the endocytic/phagocytic vacuole and subsequent binding to recycling MHC class I molecules within the same organelle (vacuolar pathway) (see Fig. 21-2).[50] Alternatively, the antigens may be transferred from the endocytic vacuole to the cytoplasm followed by processing by the proteasome and loading onto newly formed MHC class I molecules (phagosome-to-cytosol pathway), with a possible recruitment of the ER machinery for antigen processing and MHC class I loading (see Fig. 21-2).[51-54] Activation of DCs through TLR triggering or exposure to fever-like temperatures induces transient formation of large polyubiquitinated protein aggregates called DC aggregosome-like induced structures (DALIS), the role of which might be to temporarily concentrate and store endogenous antigens to reduce self-antigen presentation.[55,56] This phenomenon of cross-presentation is especially efficient in, if not unique to, DCs compared with other APCs.

Major Histocompatibility Class II Antigen Presentation (Exogenous Route)

Assembly of MHC class II molecules, which present antigen in the form of short peptides to $CD4^+$ T lymphocytes, occurs in the ER of DC. After being assembled, these MHC class II molecules are transported to specialized compartments in the lysosomal system involved in the processing of exogenous antigens. These include MIIVs, which are protease rich compartments containing newly synthesized MHC class II molecules. Epidermal DCs or Langerhans cells contain cytoplasmic tubules with internal striations called *Birbeck granules.* Birbeck granules are rich in langerin (CD205), a C-type lectin necessary for granule formation and possibly for capture of pathogens.[57] After being endocytosed by imDCs, antigens are partially retained within lysosomes. Upon receiving a maturation signal, the pH of lysosomes decreases to less than 5 (owing to the activation of a vacuolar H^+ ATPase). Concomitantly there is antigen degradation caused by activation of proteases such as cathepsins. Cystatin C, a protein that blocks the activity of cathepsin S, is also degraded, thereby allowing the degradation of invariant chain peptide (Ii chain), which

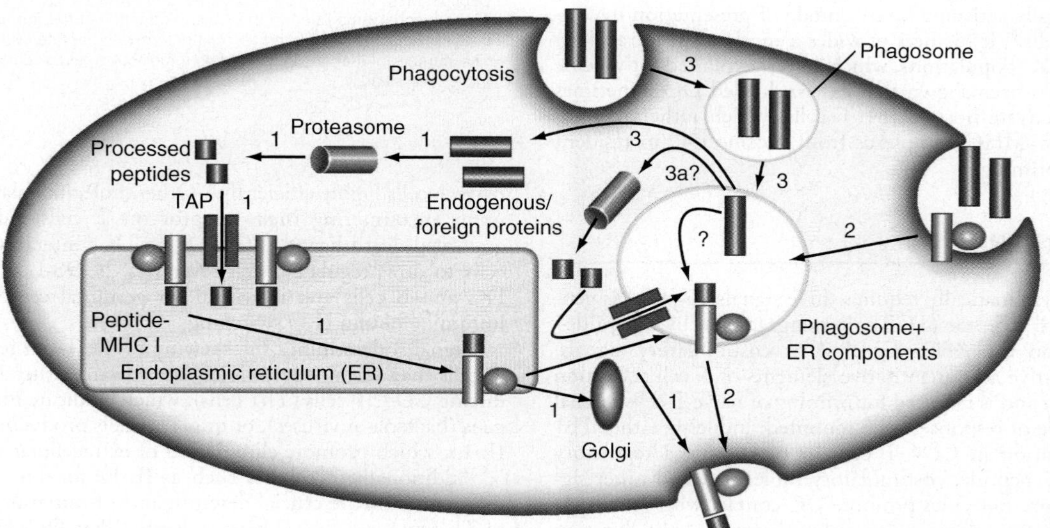

Figure 21-2 PATHWAYS FOR MAJOR HISTOCOMPATIBILITY COMPLEX (MHC) CLASS I PRESENTATION. The classical pathway for MHC class I presentation *(1)* involves degradation of endogenous or viral antigens into peptides by the proteasome followed by transport into the endoplasmic reticulum (ER). After further trimming in the ER, the peptides are loaded onto newly synthesized MHC class I molecules, and the peptide–MHC class I complexes are transported to the plasma membrane. Two main pathways of cross-presentation *(2, 3)* have been described that allow presentation of exogenous antigens in association with MHC class I molecules. Antigens endocytosed or phagocytosed can be cleaved into peptides by proteases and loaded onto recycling MHC class I molecules within the same phagosome or on the cell surface (vacuolar pathway) *(2)*. Alternatively, antigens may escape from the phagosome and enter the cytosol (phagosome-to-cytosol pathway) *(3)* to be processed via the classical MHC class I pathway. It has been suggested recently that elements of ER can be associated with phagosomes, allowing transfer of antigens into the cytosol by the ER-associated degradation (ERAD) pathway and degradation by the phagosome-associated proteasome *(3a)*. The importance of each pathway *(2, 3)* for cross-presentation in vivo and the precise mechanisms and the locations of antigen processing in each model are under investigation. *TAP,* Transporter associated with antigen processing.

normally blocks access of antigenic peptides to MHC class II molecules. These changes occur in late endosomes and lysosomes (the MIIV compartment). After antigenic peptide is bound to MHC class II molecules, they exit the lysosomes through the formation of long tubular structures, which simultaneously deliver costimulatory molecules such as CD86 to the cell surface.[58,59]

Dendritic cells handle internalized antigens in a specialized way unlike other phagocytic cells such as macrophages, which degrade most of the internalized material, leaving only limited amounts of antigenic peptides for presentation onto MHC molecules. On the contrary, internalized antigens in cDCs are preserved for longer times, thereby allowing their transport by maturing DC to secondary lymphoid organs, where actual presentation occurs. Mature DCs display higher levels of proteolysis than imDCs, allowing appropriate degradation of the antigens for loading onto MHC molecules. These differences are accounted for by several features unique to DCs, such as low levels of lysosomal proteases in immature stages compared with macrophages, expression of protease inhibitors (cystatin C), regulation of lysosomal pH (and hence activity of proteases) by regulation of the acidifying V-type H+ ATPase activity, and consumption of H^+ upon reaction with superoxide radicals generated by NADPH (nicotinamide adenine dinucleotide phosphate) oxidase NOX2 in maturing DCs.[60] During maturation, trafficking of MHC class II molecules to the surface is dramatically increased, probably because of degradation of Ii chain (containing endosome-lysosome targeting signal) in acidic compartments, leading to transport of MHC class II via the constitutive secretory pathway to the cell membrane.

In addition to direct presentation of intracellular antigens and cross-presentation of internalized material, DCs can acquire preformed MHC class I molecules in complex with antigens from other cells by the process of trogocytosis (transfer of cell-membrane patches or individual proteins between cells) or through gap junctions, in a process termed *cross-dressing;* this allows rapid presentation without processing of antigens. It has been suggested that memory CD8 T cells are preferentially activated by this mode of presentation in contrast to naïve T cells.[61] It furthers provides a mechanism for antigen transfer between DC populations, which can be exploited for vaccine design. Thus, it has been shown that ex vivo loaded DC sometimes do not directly activate host CD8+ T cells, which rather requires transfer of peptide–MHC complexes from vaccine DC to resident DC for efficient priming.[62]

Table 21-4 Costimulatory Molecules Involved in the Interaction Between Dendritic Cells and T Cells (Signal 2)*

Dendritic Cell	T Cell	Signal
	B7 FAMILY	
B7-1(CD80)/B7-2(CD86)	CD28	Activating
B7-1(CD80)/B7-2(CD86)	CTLA4	Inhibitory
B7-H1(PDL1)/B7-DC(PDL2)	?	Activating
B7-H1(PDL1)/B7-DC(PDL2)	PD1	Inhibitory
B7-H2 (B7h; B7PR1; ICOSL)	ICOS	Activating
B7H3	?	Activating
B7H4 (B7S1; B7x)	?	Inhibitory
	TNF RECEPTOR FAMILY	
4–1BBL	4–1BB	Activating
CD27L	CD27	Activating
OX40L	OX40	Activating
LIGHT	LIGHT-R	Activating
	CYTOKINES	
IL-2	IL-2R	T-cell proliferation
IL-12	IL-12R	T-cell proliferation
IL-18		

From Moretta A: Natural killer cells and dendritic cells: Rendezvous in abused tissues. *Nat Rev Immunol* 2:957, 2002.
CTLA, Cytotoxic T-lymphocyte antigen 4; *IL,* Interleukin; *LIGHT,* homologous to lymphotoxins, exhibits inducible expression, and competes with HSV glycoprotein D for herpesvirus entry mediator, a receptor expressed by T lymphocytes; *PD1,* programmed death 1; *TNF,* tumor necrosis factor.
*T-cell activation requires two signals. The T-cell receptor interaction with a peptide–MHC complex (signal 1) is accompanied by signal 2 delivered by one of the mechanisms listed in this table. Formation of the immunologic synapse between a dendritic cell and a T cell determines the fate of the lymphocyte. The number of identified costimulatory molecules responsible for signal 2 is increasing steadily.

T-CELL ACTIVATION

T-cell activation systematically requires three signals. Signal 1 is generated by the T-cell receptor (TCR) after engagement by a peptide–MHC complex on the APC. Signal 2 or costimulatory signals, determines qualitative and quantitative elements of T cell activation and differentiation and is required for priming of naïve T cells. Signal 3 specifies the type of response to be mounted, inducing either Th1 or Th2 differentiation in CD4 T cells or promoting a regulatory phenotype. MHC–peptide, costimulatory molecules, and other signaling and adhesion molecules promote DC contact with T cells via formation of an immunologic synapse that determines the duration and strength of signals transduced to T cells, leading to their subsequent activation. The minimum time for productive interaction between naïve T cells and DCs is 6 to 30 hours, with lesser time periods required for memory T-cell activation.[63,64] Although only a few peptide–MHC complexes (<10) are sufficient to trigger calcium fluxes in T cells,[65] only mature DC can prime naïve CD4 and CD8 T cells.[66] Remarkably, relatively few peptide–MHC complexes (<200) are necessary on mature DCs to activate T cells. Compared with other APCs such as B cells and monocytes, DCs are up to 1000-fold more efficient at activating T cells.[67]

Costimulatory molecules include the CD80 and CD86 members of the B7 family, which ligate to CD28 on T cells and members of the TNF family, such as CD40 (Table 21-4).[12] Notably, one new member of the B7 family, B7-DC, is unique to DC and stimulates naïve T cells highly efficiently.[68] Other molecules play inhibitory roles upon encountering their receptor on T cells. For example, programmed death ligand 1 (PDL1) on DCs interacts with PD1 on T cells to downregulate T-cell responses. ICOS-L is present on both DC and B cells and is critical for germinal center formation and immunoglobulin class switching.

Signal 3 determines the skewing of the T-cell response such that T cells may terminally differentiate toward either IFN-gamma producing $CD4^+$ T cells (Th1 cells), which eradicate intracellular pathogens (bacteria or viruses), or into Th2 cells producing IL-4, IL-5, and IL-13, which promote elimination of extracellular infections.

Additionally, cytokines such as IL-12 for Th1 or IL-4 for Th2 differentiation are crucial determinants of initiation or amplification of Th responses. It has been suggested that DCs express the Notch ligands delta or jagged under Th1 or Th2 conditions, respectively, and that these ligands promote differentiation of naïve T cells toward one or the other Th profile.[69] Thus, whereas factors and pathogens, which stimulate DC maturation and IL-12 production, promote Th1 responses (e.g., *Escherichia coli*), inducers of IL-4 production prime Th2 responses (e.g., *Porphyromonas gingivalis*).

Furthermore, the Th1 polarizing capacity of DCs depends on a number of variables that include the expression of certain transcription factors, the microenvironment, exposure to various maturation stimuli, the kinetics of maturation, and the antigen dose. For example, expression by DCs of the transcription factor T-bet, which controls IFN-γ expression in $CD4^+$ T cells, appears to be required for optimal development of Th1 responses.[70] Epithelial DCs in the respiratory tract may by default induce Th2 responses upon production of factors such as TSLP by epithelial cells.[38] The duration of DC activation and antigen dose also determines the direction of T-cell skewing. Prolonged activation causes IL-12 depletion and results in "exhausted DCs."[34] DCs presenting low amounts of antigen skew towards Th2 whereas high doses skew toward Th1, which in turn depends on the maturation state of the DCs and consequences of environmental exposure.[71,72]

Recently, a new lineage of effector CD4 T cell was discovered.[73] Named Th17 because of their characteristic secretion of IL-17, this lineage of cells is implicated in several chronic inflammatory disorders. The IL-12 family member IL-23 and transforming growth factor β (TGFβ) have been implicated in the generation of Th17 cells, but the precise role of DCs in the formation of these cells remains to be determined.[73] LPS-stimulated DCs secrete inflammatory cytokines, notably IL-6, and in combination with TGFβ seem to divert differentiation of Tregs into Th17 cells.[74,75] TGFβ upregulates the expression of the pivotal transcription factor RORγt in a concentration-dependent manner, but high TGFβ concentration favors Treg development over Th17 differentiation, partly through Foxp3 inhibitory interaction with RORγt.[76] The pathogenic role of Th17 may depend on the cytokine milieu in which they are differentiated or expand, and DC-derived IL-23 or IL-1β could contribute to enhanced pathogenicity of TH17 cells. On the other hand, Th17 cells display heightened levels IL-10 receptor and are more susceptible to IL-10–mediated regulation, a cytokine secreted by DC upon ligation of some TLRs (e.g., TLR2, TLR4). Therefore, the flexibility of DC activation and cytokine secretion profile may impact on the pathogenic potential of developing Th17 cells.

It is important to note that T-cell priming depends on mDCs because imDCs may induce immunosuppressive or Tregs.[77,78] In fact, antigen presentation by imDCs in vivo is an important pathway by which tolerance is maintained at both the CD4 and CD8 T-cell level, either through the induction of Tregs or through the deletion of autoreactive T cells.[79] Nevertheless, recent data suggest that in some conditions, mDCs can also induce the generation of $CD4^+$ $CD25^+$ Tregs.[80,81]

$CD8^+$ T cells[78] and generation of effective CD8 memory cells in turn requires CD4 T-cell help.[82-84] This help is provided through activation of DC via CD40L–CD40 interactions and the production of cytokines such as IL-2, although some studies have suggested that when cytotoxic T-lymphocyte precursor frequencies are high, priming of CD8 T cell responses may be CD4 T cell independent. In these cases though, memory generation is likely to be hampered because of the absence of IL-2 during priming,[85] and primed T cells may commit fratricide through expression of TRAIL,[86] or become functionally tolerant upon receiving signals through the inhibitory receptor PD-1.[87]

Evidence is accumulating that pDCs, which were believed to play a role only in the innate immune response because of their ability to produce high levels of IFN type I, can present viral and tumor antigens to initiate both $CD4^+$ and $CD8^+$ T-cell responses.[88,89] Plasmacytoid DCs mature in response to certain viral infections (e.g., influenza and HIV), thereby providing an important link between innate and adaptive arms of the immune response. Similar to their myeloid counterparts, however, pDCs display plasticity, even inducing immunosuppressive responses depending on their microenvironment or the stimuli to which they are exposed.[90] Genetic depletion of pDCs, using transgenic mice expressing diphtheria toxin receptor under the control of BDCA-2 promoter, has allowed dissecting precisely the role of pDC in antiviral responses. In the case of vesicular stomatitis virus infection, depletion of pDCs resulted in decreased specific $CD8^+$ T-cell responses, but depletion of pDCs during lymphocytic choriomeningitis virus (LCMV) did not affect the magnitude of LCMV-specific $CD8^+$ T-cell response. This suggests that pDC may be required to enhance weak cytotoxic T-cell responses.[91] A recent study targeting Siglec-H by conditional genetic ablation specifically induced specific pDC depletion and demonstrated a complex role of pDC. Siglec-H and pDC depleted pDC suppressed antigen-specific $CD4^+$ T-cell responses in vivo, but they were required to enhance $CD8^+$ T-cell response to soluble and microbial antigens.[92]

B-CELL ACTIVATION

In addition to affecting T-cell function, DCs can also influence B-cell proliferation, isotype switching, and plasma cell differentiation.[93] DC produce factors that activate and induce B-cell proliferation (B-Lys and APRIL).[94] Furthermore, DCs stimulate antibody responses in a T–cell–independent manner against polysaccharide antigens. The initial interactions between B cells and DCs occur in the T-cell area of lymph nodes and in the germinal centers of lymph nodes or splenic red pulp (or both). Importantly, antigen-exposed cDCs possess a specialized nondegradative pathway, which allows them to present internalized antigens in their native state for the engagement of B-cell receptors (BCRs) on B cells. This is mediated by endocytosis of antigenic immune complexes through the inhibitory Fc receptor FcγRIIB and recycling of the endocytic vesicle to the surface without antigen degradation.[95] The follicular DCs, which are present in germinal centers of lymph nodes and which constitute a different class of DCs, participate in the maintenance of B-cell memory by formation of multiple antigen–antibody complexes and continuous stimulation of B cells. The antigen–antibody complexes may remain in the lymph node for an extended period of time (up to months or years).

NATURAL KILLER CELL ACTIVATION

The interactions between DCs and NK cells are complex and further underscore a role of DCs as a link between innate and adaptive immunity.[8] Direct interactions between NK cells and mature DCs can result in NK cell activation as well as the potentiation of their cytolytic activity, and conversely, NK cells can induce further DC maturation. NK cells and DCs can form an immune synapse, probably helping directional and confined secretion of cytokines as well as facilitating receptor–ligand interactions on one another. Activated NK cells induce DCs through both cell contact (involving NKp30) and TNF-α and IFN-γ secretion. In turn, activated DCs secrete IL-12/IL-18, IL-15, and IFN-α/β, which enhance IFN-γ secretion, proliferation, and cytotoxicity of NK cells. In some conditions, NK cells can lyse DCs through NKp30, although mature DCs are protected from cytolysis. This might represent a form of "cellular editing" whereby immature and tolerogenic DCs are cleared by NK cells in the course of an ongoing immune response.[96]

It is thus possible that DC and NK cells play complementary roles in sensing pathogens such that DCs could be the first to detect microbes through their expression of PRR (TLR, NOD proteins), whereas NK may get activated in the absence of overt inflammation but in the presence of ligands for activating NK-cell receptors, such as in the settings of tumors (which frequently lose MHC class I expression or express NKG2D ligands, such as MIC-A/B). In both situations, either DCs or NK cells could create an inflammatory environment and induce the integrated activation of other cell types. Thus, in mice, infection by murine cytomegalovirus (CMV) induces pDCs to secrete high levels of IFN-α/β, bit $CD8\alpha^+$ DC are the major producers of IL-12, and resistance to the virus is associated with expansion of $Ly49H^+$ NK cells, driven by IL-12/IL-18.

The interaction between NK cells and DC is likely to take place early during the course of an immune response. This allows DC to exploit the ability of NK cells to kill tumor or virus- or parasite-infected cells and to cross-present this material to T cells.[97]

ACTIVATION OF OTHER ELEMENTS OF THE IMMUNE SYSTEM

Dendritic cells have proven to be quite versatile in their ability to interact with many constituents of the immune system. For example, they can activate NK T cells by presentation of the synthetic ligand α-galactosyl ceramide on CD1, inducing the production of cytokines such as IFN-γ and resistance to tumors.[98] CD1 restricted γ δ T cells, which respond to microbial antigens from *Mycobacterium tuberculosis*

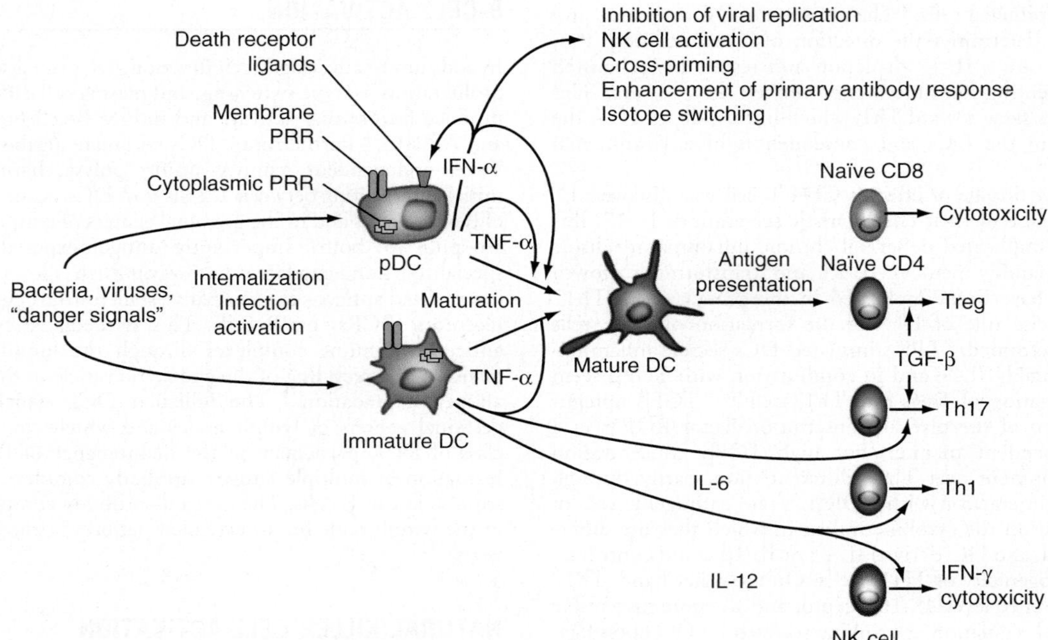

Figure 21-3 DENDRITIC CELLS (DCs) LINK INNATE AND ADAPTIVE IMMUNITY. Through the expression of pattern-recognition receptors (PRRs), such as Toll-like receptors, DCs act as sensors of pathogen intrusion. Upon signaling by PRRs, DCs secrete cytokines and express receptors allowing stimulation of the innate immune system. Interferon-α (IFN-α) or interleukin-12 (IL-12) stimulate natural killer (NK) cell activation while also inducing the expression of death-receptor ligands (TRAIL) on DCs, harnessing them for direct killing of infected cells. They take up antigens through direct infection or phagocytosis, undergo a complex program of maturation by upregulating the expression of costimulatory and major histocompatibility complex (MHC) molecules, migrate to the secondary lymphoid organs, and stimulate naïve T cells. They secrete cytokines, skewing the type of response induced toward Th1, Th2, regulatory T cell (Treg), or Th17 differentiation, inducing the generation of cytotoxic CD8 T cells, or participating in the generation of antibody responses. *pDC,* Plasmacytoid dendritic cell; *TGF,* transforming growth factor.

and other organisms, induce maturation of resting DC, and induce IL-12 production. This pathway and the IFN-γ secretion by activated γδ T cells, provide the immune system with a source of activated APCs, which can polarize Th1 responses.[99]

In summary, the influence of DCs on other cell types of the immune system is broad and integrative (Fig. 21-3). Future studies will ascertain the interplay between the myriad of host cells and the innate and adaptive immune response.

TOLERANCE AND AUTOIMMUNITY

Dendritic cells play a pivotal role in the balance between immunity and tolerance. DCs are important in the induction of both central and peripheral tolerance. In the former, DCs play a role in deletion of autoreactive T cells in the thymus. In the latter, imDCs in their steady state induce T-cell deletion, anergy, or generation of regulatory T cells, which interfere with IL-2 production and proliferation of effector T cells against self.[100] Regulatory T cells are $CD4^+$ or $CD8^+$ in nature and express CD25, CTLA-4, and the transcription factor Foxp3 (a member of the forkhead transcription factor family). These cells exert their tolerogenic effects either via cell contact or through release of immunosuppressive cytokines such as IL-10[101] or TGF-β, preventing proliferation and cytotoxicity of activated CD4 or CD8 T cells, and can also inhibit TLR-mediated maturation of cDCs but not pDCs.[102] It was recently suggested that a subset of human thymic DCs, upon activation by TSLP from epithelial cells of Hassall corpuscles, positively selects $CD4^+$ Tregs in the thymic medulla, thereby playing a central role in the generation of naturally occurring Tregs.[103] How might DC in peripheral tissues induce tolerance is an open question. One report suggests that uptake of antigens via receptors such as DEC-205, a member of the C-type lectin family, can induce T-cell deletion or generation of antigen-specific Tregs.[104]

Dendritic cells may also be actively rendered tolerogenic via a number of mechanisms. Resting imDCs acquire self-antigens through phagocytosis of apoptotic bodies formed as a consequence of physiologic cell turnover. In the absence of a maturation signal, these DCs induce tolerance to such self-antigens.[105] Some studies have suggested that ligation of specific receptors on DCs such as complement receptors CR3 and CR4[106] by apoptotic cells inhibit their maturation,[106] thereby ensuring the delivery of a tolerogenic rather than stimulatory signal. Others include MER, CD91/calreticulin, and CD36/αvβ5. External factors such as steroids, IL-10, and TGF-β may also compromise DC immunostimulatory function by inhibiting their full maturation.[107] For example, DCs isolated from tumor environments are poorly immunostimulatory because of the presence of immunosuppressive cytokines or the induction of costimulatory molecules such as PDL-1, which deliver negative signals.[108] Moreover, there may exist distinct tolerogenic DC subsets. A particular DC subset was identified in normal mice that were CD11c-low/CD45RB high), secreted IL-10 after activation, and induced tolerance through induction of Tregs.[109] Recently in mice, pDCs have been shown to induce tolerance against a vascularized cardiac allograft upon administration of a tolerizing regimen.[110] After capturing pDC alloantigens from the graft, they migrated to peripheral lymph nodes and induced specific Tregs.[110] Human DC deficiencies are associated with a loss of Tregs, and it seems that DC and Treg reciprocally control each other's expansion, where DCs control Treg expansion and Tregs control DC numbers through a Flt3-dependent feedback loop.

Recently, production of indoleamine 2,3-dioxygenase (IDO) has been proposed to account for some of the tolerogenic potential of DC.[111] IDO is an enzyme that degrades the indole moiety of tryptophan and other molecules and induces the production of immunoregulatory metabolites known as kynurenines. Local depletion of tryptophan and increase in proapoptotic kynurenines affects T-cell proliferation and survival. Induction of IDO in DCs has been postulated as one means by which deletional tolerance occurs. This is compounded by the observation that Tregs may directly act on DCs via CTLA-4-B7 interactions to promote IDO production.[111] Also, pDCs activated through TLR7 or TLR9 upregulate the expression of IDO and can induce the generation of Tregs from naïve $CD4^+$ T cells. Moreover, expression of death-inducing ligands such as FasL may render DCs capable of killing activated T cells.[104,112] Altogether, these properties of DCs make them attractive candidates for inducing tolerance in the setting of transplantation or autoimmunity. Indeed, injection of antigen pulsed immature DCs in vivo induces antigen specific IL-10–producing $CD8^+$ Tregs, which supplant their IFN-γ–producing effector cell counterparts.[78,113]

Dendritic cells are also believed to be important for the induction of the chronic phase of autoimmune diseases. IFN-α produced by pDCs is thought to contribute to the autoimmune response in SLE.[114,115] Plasmacytoid DC can be activated through TLR7 and 9 by immune complexes containing RNA and DNA, respectively, from dead cells and induced to secrete high amounts of IFN-α. This can further promote the differentiation of monocytes into activated cDCs, thus enhancing presentation of self-antigens, increasing the cytotoxicity of CD8 and NK cells, and promoting plasma cell differentiation and subsequent generation of pathogenic autoantibodies. Several host factors can convert self DNA into triggers of pDC activation. For example, the antimicrobial peptide LL-37 forms large aggregates with self-DNA released from dying cells, protecting it from extracellular nuclease digestion, and is taken in pDCs for induction of type I INF. LL-37 has been found to be overexpressed in psoriatic skin, and the gene encoding LL-37 is the most upregulated in the blood of lupus patients.[116]

A role of cDCs during disease onset is also strongly suggested in arthritis, multiple sclerosis, diabetes, and atherosclerosis.[117-119] The similarity between outcomes of microbial infection and autoimmunity suggests that TLRs or PRRs triggered by microbial molecules on DCs induce their maturation and secretion of cytokines and chemokines. This may cause DCs to upregulate presentation of self-antigens in such instances as apoptosis or necrosis induced directly by pathogens or antimicrobial immune response. Endogenous ligands such as extracellular matrix breakdown products (heparan sulfate and hyaluronate), molecules released from necrotic cells (high-mobility group box 1 protein [HMGB1], uric acid, or even endogenous nucleic acids), fibronectin and heat-shock proteins, which can activate TLRs on cDCs, may also contribute to the generation of autoimmune responses.[120]

SUBVERSION OF DENDRITIC CELL FUNCTION BY PATHOGENS AND TUMORS

Several pathogens have evolved different mechanisms to inhibit DC functions, allowing them to downregulate specific immune responses and hence persist in the host. Numerous viruses, such as measles, vaccinia, herpes simplex, smallpox, and lymphocytic choriomeningitis virus, can impair antigen presentation by infected cells through different mechanisms. Thus, human CMV induces downmodulation of MHC class I or class II molecules and can inhibit activated T cells through secretion of a virally encoded IL-10 homolog. Directly targeting DCs allows viruses to impair the generation and quality of the antiviral immune responses. In mice, murine CMV has been shown to trigger paralysis of infected DCs, preventing them from secreting IL-12 or IL-2 upon TLR4 triggering, impairing their capacity to mature, eventually rendering them unable to prime an effective T cell response.[121] Some viral products interfere with IFN-α secretion pathways, such as the E6 oncoprotein of human papillomavirus, inhibiting transactivation of IRF3 or IRF7, or NS3/4A inhibiting RIG-I and MDA5-mediated activation of IRF3.

It is now well documented that in HIV-infected patients that not only the number of pDCs and cDCs in blood is reduced, but cDCs are also less efficient at stimulating primary T-cell responses and may generate IL-10–secreting T cells with a potential regulatory role. DCs may be the first cells to encounter HIV in mucosal tissues and may mediate the spread of virus to $CD4^+$ T cells in lymphoid organs. Formation of virions and release from the cell surface is counteracted by tetherin, an interferon-regulated restriction factor, that retains virions at the cell surface. The Vpu accessory protein antagonizes tetherin activity to allow virion release. cDCs can mediate transinfection of $CD4^+$ T cells through the formation of an infectious synapse, carrying the virus with or without infection of the DCs themselves. DCs express the coreceptors CD4, CCR5, CXCR4, and the C-type lectin DC-SIGN necessary for binding or entry of HIV, albeit at lower levels than CD4+ T cells, although the expression of DC-SIGN remains to be firmly demonstrated. HIV can infect DCs, but its replication is not as efficient as in $CD4^+$ T cells because of expression of the viral restriction factor SAMHD1, a deoxynucleoside triphosphate triphosphohydrolase. The viral envelope protein gp120 can bind to CD4 and C-type lectins such as DC-SIGN and mannose receptor, but the contribution of each receptor to binding and internalization may vary depending on the particular type of DC encountered by HIV. Thus, although DCs are not the main reservoir of HIV, the virus can "highjack" DCs to mediate its spread to $CD4^+$ T cells from mucosal tissues to lymphoid organs. Nevertheless, although cDCs only get minimally activated by HIV, pDCs can get infected and be strongly activated by HIV, causing them to secrete high amounts of IFN-α and other antiviral molecules. This can inhibit the replication of HIV in $CD4^+$ T cells, suggesting that the two subsets play different and opposing roles during HIV infection. However, pDCs may also function to downregulate the response by secreting TRAIL.[122,123] Furthermore, the continuous secretion of IFN-α by pDCs stimulated by HIV may be detrimental to the host by participating to chronic immune activation and $CD4^+$ T-cell depletion.

Tumors also evolve mechanisms to negate the functionality of DCs. For example, the number of cDCs (but not pDCs) is reduced in blood of cancer patients, and these numbers of DCs are restored upon surgical removal of the tumor, indicating a systemic defect orchestrated by the tumor cells. Moreover, increased numbers of imDCs are found in blood and tumor tissue, also displaying an impaired response to activation stimuli. A subset of immature myeloid cells, composed of immature macrophages, DCs, granulocytes, and myeloid cells at early stages of differentiation, accumulate in the secondary lymphoid organs and tumors of tumor-bearing mice and presumably humans. These myeloid suppressor cells are endowed with suppressive activity toward antitumor T cells through various mechanisms such as regulation of arginine metabolism and release of ROS. In some tumors, IDO-expressing pDCs are found in significant numbers, thereby decreasing availability of tryptophan and generating tryptophan catabolites. IDO expressing pDCs can activate intratumor Tregs. It seems that tumors impair early myeloid, and in particular DC, differentiation at a systemic level by secreting soluble factors such as VEGF, M-CSF (macrophage colony-stimulating factor), IL-6, IL-10. Many tumors constitutively express activated STAT3, a transcription factor partially implicated in the production of these cytokines, the constitutive activation of which also impairs the secretion of proinflammatory cytokines. STAT3 (signal transducer and activator of transcription 3) is also responsible for abnormal differentiation of hematopoietic precursor cells, suggesting that inhibition of its activity may be a promising route toward restoring DC function in cancer. The tumor microenvironment thus profoundly impact on the function of infiltrating DCs and T cells, and it has recently been shown that overexpression of matrix metalloproteinase-2 (MMP-2) conditions DCs to produce low levels of IL-12 and to express OX40-L, which biases anti-tumor CD4+ T cells toward a suboptimal Th2 differentiation.[124]

IMMUNOTHERAPEUTIC STRATEGIES AND CLINICAL TRIALS

The past decade has seen an increasing interest in clinical applications of DCs, harnessing the growing knowledge about DC biology. It is becoming apparent that any effective vaccine must activate and induce antigen presentation by DCs, the most potent cells at stimulating T-cell immunity. A number of clinical trials (mostly phase I and II) have been completed describing the use of DCs in cancer immunotherapy (e.g., non-Hodgkin lymphoma, malignant melanoma, multiple myeloma, prostate cancer, renal cell carcinoma, breast cancer) and in the immunotherapy of human pathogens such as HIV. Most of these studies have relied on monocyte-derived DCs, but a few have used DCs prepared from $CD34^+$ HPC. A critical issue is the antigen delivery to the DCs, with the nature of the antigen and the vehicle for delivery probably being decisive. DCs can be pulsed with defined antigens in the form of HLA-binding antigenic peptides or whole proteins or the whole assortment of tumor antigens upon phagocytosis of dying or opsonized autologous tumor cells. Artificial fusion of DCs with tumor cells allows the generation of hybrid cells with characteristic of DCs but expressing the whole set of tumor antigens as well. Because autologous tumor cells are not always available from patients with advanced disease, allogeneic tumor cells of the same histologic origin expressing shared tumor antigens are also used for loading DCs.

Dendritic cells themselves can also be genetically modified through transfection. However, DCs are terminally differentiated nondividing cells and difficult to transfect. Methods using RNA electroporation and infection by recombinant viruses (lentivirus, poxvirus, herpes virus, and adeno-associated virus) lead to foreign transgene expression in DC. Another strategy is to target DC in situ using antibodies recognizing DC-specific molecules, such as DEC-205, as demonstrated in mouse models.[125] Recently a phase II trial involved priming by a recombinant vaccinia virus encoding prostate-specific antigen and the "tricam" CD80, ICAM-1, and LFA-3, and boosting by a fowlpox virus. GM-CSF was injected at the same time to further amplify immune stimulation. This vaccine was designed to mimic antigen presentation by DCs, even in an incomplete way, and induce significant overall survival benefit.[126]

Because the activation state of antigen-presenting DCs is a determining factor in shaping the ensuing immune response, genetic engineering of DCs or triggering activating receptors also allows enhancing their secretion, migration, and antigen presentation capacity. Thus, DCs can be activated by artificial TLR ligands (e.g., R848, which is a ligand for TLR7; unmethylated CpG oligonucleotides, which are ligands for TLR9; or inflammatory cytokines, such as IL-1β, IL-6, or TNF-α) that can be used in a clinical setting to activate DCs before injection or even in vivo.[127] DCs can also be transfected for immunostimulatory molecules, such as cytokine genes (e.g., IL-2, IL-12), or inhibitory siRNA for molecules dampening DC activation (e.g., SOCS1).

Anticancer vaccination can be used in synergy with chemotherapy and radiotherapy. The rationale is that chemotherapy and radiotherapy triggers tumor cell death, which provides a source of tumor antigens to DCs while at the same time inducing exposure of immunogenic molecules on tumor cells. Thus, anthracycline-treated tumor cells expose the ER chaperones calreticulin (CRT) and ERp57 because of induction of an ER stress response and potentiate dying tumor cells phagocytosis. Death of tumor cells is also accompanied by release of non histone chromatin binding nuclear protein HMGB1, which can trigger TLR4, and ATP, which upon binding to P2RX7 potentiates inflammasome activation and IL-1β release. Increased uptake of tumor antigen in the context of maturion signals strongly enhances cross-presentation and cross-priming of tumor antigens by DCs.

Recent successes in DC vaccination trials have been witnessed using intratumoral injection of the CpG oligonucleotide (PF-3512676) in low-grade B-cell lymphoma, thus targeting TLR9 on pDCs and B cells. Complete and partial clinical responses were observed in several patients with induction of tumor-specific CD8 T cells responses.[128,129] Tumor regressions were observed in injected and distant tumor sites. Another phase III clinical trial in metastatic prostate cancer, consisting of enriched blood APCs pulsed with a fusion of prostatic acid phosphatase with GM-CSF, led to about 4 months of prolonged median survival. This vaccine (sipuleucel-T [APC8015]) has recently been approved by the Food and Drug Administration for treatment of metastatic prostate cancer. A phase III trial in metastatic melanoma using peptide vaccination with high-dose IL-2 showed a significantly increased overall response rate and progression-free survival. Another phase III trial in patients with follicular lymphoma using idiotype vaccination increased the duration of chemotherapy-induced remission. Although the target APCs in these vaccines has not been defined yet, they most likely involved DCs to induce or expand antitumor immune responses.

It is likely that to achieve significant clinical responses upon vaccination for cancer, combining DC vaccination with other strategies will improve the therapeutic outcome. For example, some strategies aim at depleting or inactivating Tregs (using a toxin targeting CD25, a molecule expressed by Tregs, or cyclophosphamide), alleviating T-cell anergy (using antagonistic CTLA-4 or PD-1), differentiating myeloid suppressor cells into nonimmunosuppressive cells (by injection of retinoic acid derivative ATRA [all-trans-retinoic acid]), common γ chain cytokines such as IL-7, which have potent effects on T-cell survival and function, or adoptive immunotherapy of in vitro activated T cells.[130,131] Finally, it seems that irradiation of the tumor tissue conditions it for enhanced migration of APCs and T cells, augments MHC class I expression on tumor cells, and induces apoptotic cells death, thus augmenting delivery of tumor antigens to DCs.[132-134] The identification of specific surface receptors regulating DC–T-cell interaction and T-cell activation and differentiation allowed using targeting antibodies functioning as immune modulators. Thus, agonistic antibodies targeting GITR, OX40, CD137, or CD40 or cytokines potently enhancing cytotoxic T-cell responses, such as IL-15, can be harnessed to enhance vaccine-induced antitumor immune responses.

Thus far, DC vaccines have not met the desired endpoints in clinical studies (i.e., tumor regression) in the majority of patients despite clear evidence that DC vaccination can induce measurable cellular or humoral immune responses in cancer patients.[135-138] In a recent phase III trial, vaccination of stage IV melanoma patients by DCs loaded with multiple peptides could not be demonstrated to be more effective than the standard chemotherapy treatment.[139] However, the optimal DC type, optimal maturation signal(s), mechanism of antigen delivery, nature of antigen, frequency of immunization, and route of administration still remain to be determined. Furthermore, it may be that only a subset of patients may be able to respond to DC vaccination, or in the case of advanced stage cancer patients, to any vaccination. In the authors' opinion, DC immunotherapy will be most efficacious when coadministered with an adjuvant and when the tumor burden is low. The timing of vaccination is probably also crucial, and frequent immunizations may dramatically improve the clinical efficacy.[140] In the setting of HIV infection, a recent study in a small group of chronically infected individuals showed that vaccination with DCs loaded with chemically inactivated virus allows stabilization and even suppression of viral load for an extended period of time without any other treatment.[141] Vaccination with DCs holds great promise in cancer and infectious diseases, but its potential is likely to be best exploited in combination with other strategies manipulating other arms of the immune system.

Although DCs are considered the most potent cells in inducing T-cell responses, they can also function as tolerizing cells, a function that can be harnessed against autoimmune diseases and in a transplantation setting. Thus, it is possible to differentiate in vitro maturation-resistant imDCs or differentially activated DCs using biologic agents such as IL-10, TGF-β, or the fusion protein CTLA-4-Ig, and pharmacologic agents such as corticosteroids, cyclosporine, rapamycin, mycophenolate mofetil, vitamin D3, or prostaglandin E_2. The clinical relevance of some of these strategies is being evaluated. Another way to dampen pathologic immune responses is to use antagonists for TLRs or other innate immune sensor participating in amplifying damaging responses. Thus, because the role of DNA-immune complexes has been established as important in the etiology of SLE, synthetic inhibitory oligodeoxyribonucleotides have been developed that can prevent or inhibit activation through TLR9 on pDCs and B cells and block SLE in animal models. Finally, significant challenges remain with respect to DCs based immunotherapy ranging from applicability of preclinical models to humans to regulatory and funding hurdles.

FUTURE DIRECTIONS

Dendritic cells are a sparsely distributed population of BM derived mononuclear cells that exist in an immature form in virtually all tissues in the body. DCs serve as professional APCs with extraordinary capacity to stimulate naïve T lymphocytes (as well as B cells, NK cells, and NK T cells) and initiate primary immune response. They link innate and adaptive immunity and are responsible for activation and inhibition of effector cells. Their clinical applications in cancer, transplantation, and chronic virus infections are under investigation.

SUGGESTED READINGS

Ackerman AL, Giodini A, Cresswell P: A role for the endoplasmic reticulum protein retrotranslocation machinery during crosspresentation by dendritic cells. *Immunity* 25:607, 2006.

Akira S, Takeda K, Kaisho T: Toll-like receptors: Critical proteins linking innate and acquired immunity. *Nat Immunol* 2:675, 2001.

Barber DL, Wherry EJ, Masopust D, et al: Restoring function in exhausted CD8 T cells during chronic viral infection. *Nature* 439:682, 2006.

Cella M, Facchetti F, Lanzavecchia A, et al: Plasmacytoid dendritic cells activated by influenza virus and CD40L drive a potent TH1 polarization. *Nat Immunol* 1:305, 2000.

Hawiger D, Inaba K, Dorsett Y, et al: Dendritic cells induce peripheral T cell unresponsiveness under steady state conditions in vivo. *J Exp Med* 194:769, 2001.

Kadowaki N, Antonenko S, Lau JY, et al: Natural interferon alpha/beta-producing cells link innate and adaptive immunity. *J Exp Med* 192:219, 2000.

Kapsenberg ML: Dendritic-cell control of pathogen-driven T-cell polarization. *Nat Rev Immunol* 3:984, 2003.

Lu W, Arraes LC, Ferreira WT, et al: Therapeutic dendritic-cell vaccine for chronic HIV-1 infection. *Nat Med* 10:1359, 2004.

Medzhitov R: Toll-like receptors and innate immunity. *Nat Rev Immunol* 1:135, 2001.

Moretta A: The dialogue between human natural killer cells and dendritic cells. *Curr Opin Immunol* 17:306, 2005.

Rapoport AP, Stadtmauer EA, Aqui N, et al: Restoration of immunity in lymphopenic individuals with cancer by vaccination and adoptive T-cell transfer. *Nat Med* 11:1230, 2005.

Shortman K, Liu YJ: Mouse and human dendritic cell subtypes. *Nat Rev Immunol* 2:151, 2002.

Skoberne M, Beignon AS, Larsson M, et al: Apoptotic cells at the crossroads of tolerance and immunity. *Curr Top Microbiol Immunol* 289:259, 2005.

For complete list of references log on to www.expertconsult.com.

CHAPTER 22

COMPLEMENT AND IMMUNOGLOBULIN BIOLOGY

David E. Isenman, Robert Mandle, and Michael C. Carroll

This chapter is divided into two parts. The first part details the current understanding of the activation and biology of the complement system and how it links innate and adaptive immunity. The second part focuses on immunoglobulins and their importance in protecting against disease. The goal of this chapter is to impart to the reader the underlying role of the complement system and antibody in protecting the host from microbial insult and disease.

THE COMPLEMENT SYSTEM: AN OVERVIEW

Complement refers to a family of distinct proteins that play a pivotal role in host defense against infection. In the 1880s, the serum factors involved in host response to pathogens were placed into two categories based on sensitivity to heat. Whereas the heat-stable component, antibody, was recognized as being specific for the invading pathogen and arose after immunization, the heat-labile (>56° C [133° F]) fraction displayed nonspecific killing activity. The heat-labile fraction acted to complement the antibody-mediated lytic killing of targeted organisms.[1-3]

In addition to its lytic role in the effector arm of the antibody response, the complement system serves several other functions. First, components of the complement system are involved in clearance of targeted microorganisms by the process of opsonization. *Opsonization* is the coating of a particle with proteins that facilitate phagocytosis of the particle by tissue macrophages and activated follicular dendritic cells (FDCs) as well as binding by receptors on peripheral blood cells.[4,5] Second, complement promotes inflammation by releasing small peptide fragments from complement proteins. These peptides cause mast cell degranulation, smooth muscle contraction, and directed migration (chemotaxis) of motile cells to sites of inflammation.[6,7]

Complement can be activated via three distinct pathways: classical, lectin, and alternative. Although all depend on different molecules for their initiation, eventually they converge to generate the same set of effector molecules. Each of these pathways is described here (Fig. 22-1).

Classical Pathway

The classical pathway (CP), so called because it was the earliest studied arm of the complement system, directly links the innate and acquired immune systems. There are nine proteins in the CP. As a matter of terminology, each CP component protein is designated with an uppercase C followed by a number. Fragments of these proteins generated by cleavage during the complement cascade are designated with a lower case letter suffix (e.g., C3a, C3b). In general, the smaller product arising from a proteolytic activation step is given the fragment designation "a," and the larger product is designated "b." The sole exception to this rule is for the naming of the C2 proteolytic activation fragments, where, for historical reasons, the larger fragment is C2a and the smaller one is C2b.

C1, the first component of the CP, binds and is activated by the Fc portion of the antibody molecule. C1q is a macromolecule complex composed of three individual protein subunits: C1q, C1r, and C1s.[8-12] The largest of these subunits, C1q, is an 18-chain molecule with six copies each of three chains: A, B, and C. Structurally, C1q consists of a central core with six radiating arms. Each arm possesses a triple helical structure similar to collagen that is capped at the end with a head region consisting of a quaternary assembly of the globular domains from each of chains A, B, and C. C1q, largely through ionic interactions, links the C1 complex to the antibody molecule. In addition to its capacity for binding to antibody molecules, C1q possesses the capability to bind directly to the surfaces of some microorganisms and apoptotic cells, not unlike mannan-binding lectin (MBL; see lectin pathway discussion, later).

Associated with C1q are two molecules each of C1r and C1s. In unactivated C1, C1r and C1s are proenzyme serine esterases. Upon binding of C1q with an array of target-associated immunoglobulin G (IgG) Fc regions, or directly to surface molecules of the pathogen, a conformational change occurs that leads to reciprocal autoactivation of the associated C1r molecules. The active form of C1r then cleaves its associated C1s to generate an active serine protease.

Activated C1s is responsible for cleaving C4 and C2, the next two proteins in the complement pathway. Cleavage of C4 yields two fragments: C4a and C4b. C4b possesses a highly reactive thioester group that allows it to bind covalently to molecules in the immediate vicinity of its active site. Only a small proportion of the C4b produced binds to proteins or carbohydrates on the targeted surface; the rest is inactivated by reaction with water in the surrounding milieu. This helps to prevent inadvertent C4b binding to surrounding host cells.

C2, the next substrate in the CP cascade, is susceptible to cleavage by C1s. Upon association with C4b, C2 is cleaved by activated C1s into two fragments: C2a and C2b. C2a, which is now an active serine protease, remains bound to C4b, thereby confining it to the targeted surface. C4b2a is termed the *C3 convertase,* an enzymatic complex that is responsible for binding and cleaving C3, the next component in the cascade. The function of the C3 convertase is to cleave large numbers of C3 molecules to produce C3b and C3a. Nascently activated C3b, similar to C4b, also possesses a highly reactive thioester bond, allowing a portion of the nascent C3b to covalently bind to the targeted surface (opsonization of the target) and thereby mark it for phagocytosis. The activated thioester in the bulk of the nascent C3b becomes water hydrolysed and can no longer bind to a target. By contrast, all of the C3a fragment remains in solution, where it initiates a local inflammatory response.

An Ig-independent mechanism for activation of C1q has been identified.[13] The lectin protein Sign R1, which is expressed on a subset of macrophages within the outer marginal zone sinus of the spleen, is capable of capturing to the surface of the marginal zone macrophage both C-polysaccharide–containing bacteria and C1q. The recruited C1 becomes activated and propagates the CP to deposit C3b on the captured bacterium. Recently, Sign R1 was identified on the surface of resident dendritic cells (DC) in draining lymph nodes and shown to be important in capture and transport of inactivated influenza virus.[14] This novel pathway provides an alternative innate recognition of pathogens leading to activation of the CP of complement.

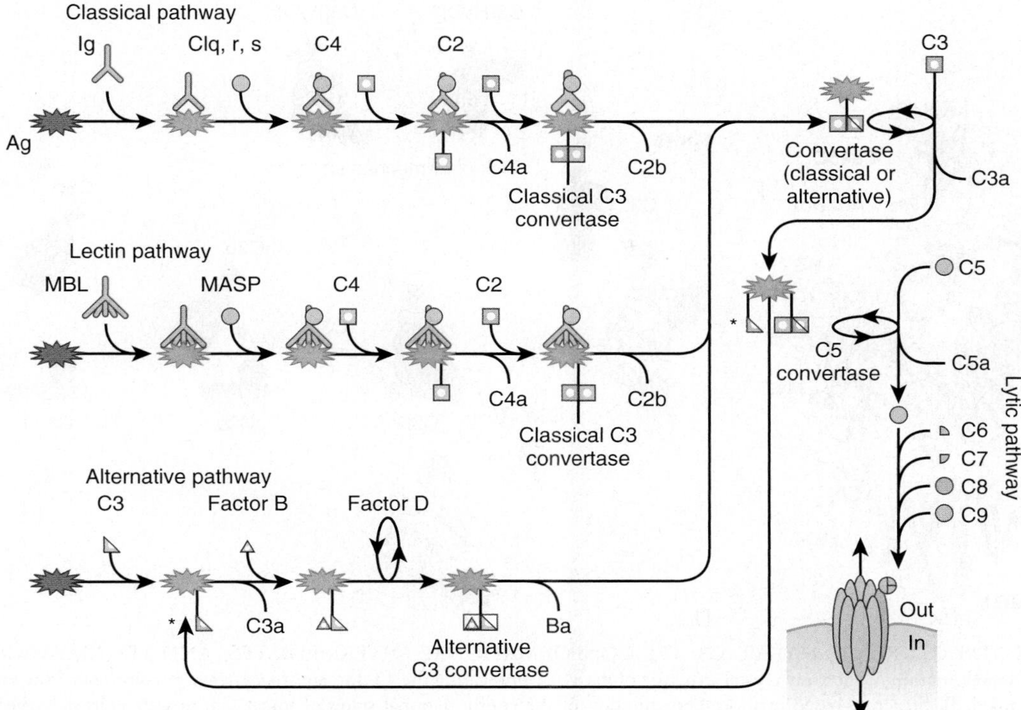

Figure 22-1 SCHEMATIC OVERVIEW OF THE COMPLEMENT CASCADE. Classical, lectin, and alternative pathways commence from the left side of the figure, leading to the converging point of C3 activation *(top right).* In every subsequent proteolytic step, the position of the new addition to the antigen complex is shown in *black* for clarity. From the central C3 activation step downward, the C3 amplification loop through the alternative pathway is indicated by *asterisks.* The lytic pathway is initiated with the formation of C5 convertase and leads to the assembly of the C5–C6–C7–C8–C9 membrane attack complex, which interferes with the target's structural integrity by penetrating the cellular membrane *(bottom right). MASP,* mannan-binding lectin–associated serine protease; *MBL,* mannan-binding lectin.

Lectin Pathway

Before continuing with the discussion of the complement cascade at the point of C3 cleavage by convertase, we turn our attention to the other two complement-activating pathways: the lectin pathway (LP) and the alternative pathway (AP). What will become evident is that all of these pathways converge at C3.

The lectin pathway is a relatively recently described pathway for complement activation.[15,16] Mannan-binding lectin (MBL), similar to C1q, is a triple helical structure with collagen-like arms (most commonly four) coupled to globular domains, which form carbohydrate recognition domains that bind repeating polysaccharides present on the surfaces of many microorganisms. MBL attaches to the terminus of polymeric carbohydrate chains in the following order: mannose > GlcNAc > fucose > glucose. The greatest avidity appears to be for repeating mannose-based structural patterns typical of microbial surfaces. On vertebrate cells, these sugars are not as dense as on microbial surfaces, thus decreasing the avidity of the MBL-binding interaction, and furthermore, they often are covered by sialic acid residues, thus limiting recognition by MBL. Upon binding to polysaccharides on a pathogen surface, MBL activates the serine proteases MBL-associated serine protease (MASP)-1 and MASP-2. MASP-2 acts similar to C1s, cleaving C4 and C2 and thereby forming a C3 convertase, C4b2a, as found in the CP.[17] The role of MASP-1 in the LP is less well defined. Because it cleaves C2, but not C4, its role may be more augmentory than essential. Along similar lines, although complexes consisting of MBL and only MASP-2 are activatable, the availability of MASP-1, in a yet to be clarified manner, augments the activation process.[14]

Mannan-binding lectin serum concentration can differ by up to 1000-fold among individuals, with those having low circulating MBL apparently more vulnerable to infections. MBL insufficiency appears to be a particular risk factor for infections in infants and individuals undergoing chemotherapy or immunosuppression treatment.[18]

Given the relatively recent discovery of the MBL pathway in the 1990s, progress into fully understanding this pathway is now just beginning. Gene-targeted knock-out mouse models deficient in MBL components have been described. Generally, in pathogenic microbe infection models, such as *Candida albicans* or *Staphylococcus aureus,* MBL knock-out mice showed increased susceptibility to systemic infection and relatively much higher mortality compared to wild type.[19,20]

Alternative Pathway

The AP may represent one of the earliest forms of innate immunity. Unlike the CP or LP pathway, the AP can be fully activated in the absence of specific pathogen binding by a "recognition" equivalent to C1q or MBL.[21] In fact, the AP is always "on" at a low level. In addition, the AP forms and uses the distinct C3 convertase C3bBb.[22]

Complement C3 is a two-chain protein with an apparent molecular weight of approximately 200 kDa. The crystal structure of native C3, shown as a domain-colored ribbon model in Fig. 22-2, *A,* identified 13 distinct domains, including the thioester domain (TED), which contained the covalent binding site.[23] In the native molecule, the intramolecular thioester bond, formed between the side chains of cysteine and glutamine residues within the sequence CGEQ, is buried within a hydrophobic interface formed between the TED and MG8 domains, which is nevertheless close to the protein's

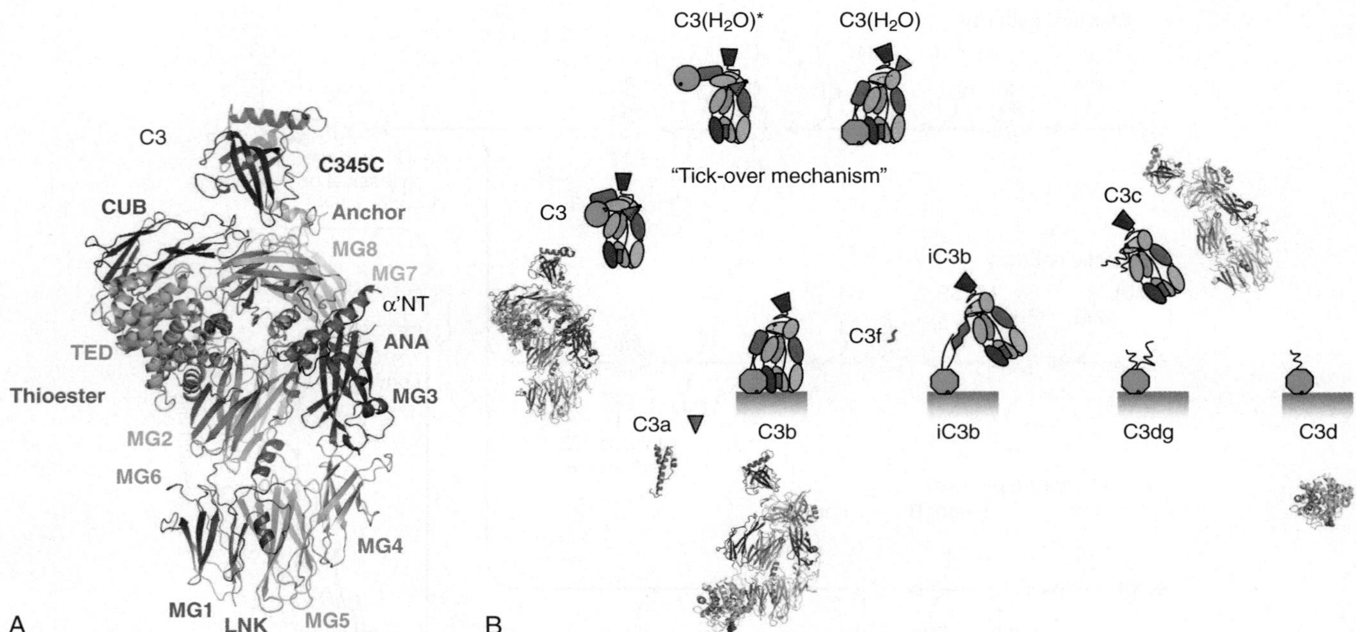

Figure 22-2 THE STRUCTURE OF NATIVE C3, ITS CONFORMATIONAL INTERMEDIATES, AND ITS CLEAVAGE FRAGMENTS. **A,** Ribbon diagram representation of the x-ray crystal structure of native C3 indicating the 13 domains (*bold lettering,* color-coded the same as the domain) of which it is composed. **B,** Structure-based cartoon representation of the conformational states of intact C3, as well as its cleavage fragments. Where these cartoons are derived from x-ray structures, those structures are depicted as ribbon diagrams adjacent to the cartoon. The remaining cartoons are based on electron micrograph images,[199] as well as established biochemical data. In all cases, the domain colors in the cartoons correspond to those in the ribbon diagrams. Proteolytic activation of C3 to C3b results in an approximate 90-Å downward movement of the thioester domain (TED), a significant repositioning of the CUB (complement C1r/C1s, urchin EGF, bone morphogenic protein 1), and a flipping of the positions macroglobulin 7 (MG7) and MG8 domains. The reorientation of these domains creates binding sites for ligands of C3b that were not present in the native molecule. The reactive thioester produced during this conformational transition is capable of binding a portion of the C3b molecules covalently to a target surface *(grey-shaded boxes).* Subsequent cleavage of C3b by factor I releases a small C3f fragment and results in a reorientaction of the C3c portion of the molecule relative to C3d/TED within iC3b, a molecule that remains bound to the target. This reorientation relative to C3b relieves the steric blockage by MG1 of a portion of the binding site for CR2/CD21, as iC3b is an equivalent ligand to C3dg and C3d with respect to CR2 binding. C3dg and C3c are the products of an additional cleavage by factor I within the CUB domain. A noncomplement protease removes an N-terminal segment from C3dg, yielding the still target-associated C3d fragment. The remaining "squiggle" on C3d represents 16 residues at its C-terminus that are sufficiently flexible that they were not visible in the x-ray crystal structure of C3d. Although the thioester in native C3 is protected from the solvent, native C3 is in conformational equilibrium with a stable conformational intermediate, C3(H_2O)*, in which the thioester become susceptible to hydrolysis. Although the equilibrium strongly favors the native state, if hydrolysis of the thioester in C3(H_2O)* occurs, it cannot reform, and the molecule undergoes a unidirectional conformational change to the C3(H_2O) stage, which adopts both a C3b-like conformation and functional profile. This conformational transition of intact C3 is the basis of the "tick-over mechanism" for alternative pathway initiation. *(Modified from P. Gros, Utrecht University; contains elements previously published in Gros P, Milder FJ, Janssen BJ: Complement driven by conformational changes.* Nat Rev Immunol *8:48, 2008.)*

surface. The subsequent determination of the atomic structure of the activated form of C3 (i.e., C3b) demonstrated a dramatic shift in the location of the TED.[24,25] Proteolytic cleavage releases the C3a anaphylatoxin peptide, and the TED becomes fully exposed to engage potential targets (see structure-based cartoon depiction of C3b in Fig. 22-2, *B*). Thus, the dramatic shift in structure also exposes potential binding sites for factor B of the AP and competing sites for regulators of C3b, such as factor H (FH), membrane cofactor protein (MCP), complement receptor type 1 (CR1), and decay accelerating factor (DAF; all described later in this section). At a low so-called "tickover" level, the thioester bond undergoes spontaneous hydrolysis, forming C3(H_2O). This conformationally altered C3b-like form of C3 (see Fig. 22-2, *B*) allows for binding to factor B, a plasma protein. Factor B is a serine protease that is approximately 30% identical to C2. The binding of factor B by C3(H_2O) allows factor D, another protease, to cleave factor B to form Ba and Bb. Bb remains associated with C3(H_2O) to form the C3(H_2O)Bb complex. Factor D appears to function as a serine protease in its native state but can cleave factor B only when bound to C3. Recently, there has been an interesting connection found between factor D and MASP-1, a component of the LP. It was found that a *MASP-1/MASP-3* knockout mouse (the proteins MASP-1 and MASP-3 are alternative splice products of the same gene) completely lacked AP functionality. Upon further investigation, it was determined that the secreted factor D in this mouse possessed a five residue propeptide at its amino terminus. Removal of this propeptide from factor D by the addition of MASP-1 resulted in restoration of AP functionality.[26]

C3(H_2O)Bb is an enzymatic complex capable of cleaving native C3. This complex is a fluid-phase C3 convertase. Although it is formed only in small amounts, it can cleave many molecules of C3. Much of the C3b produced in this process is inactivated by hydrolysis, but some attaches covalently to the surface of host cells or pathogens. C3b bound in this way is able to bind factor B, allowing its cleavage by factor D to yield Ba and Bb. The result is the formation of C3bBb, a C3 convertase akin to C4b2a found in the classical and MBL pathways, with the capability of initiating an amplification cascade.

In light of the nonspecific nature of C3b binding in the AP, it is not surprising that a number of complement regulators exist both in the plasma and on host cell membranes to prevent complement activation on self tissues. Some of these regulatory components are mentioned now for the sake of clarity; more detailed attention is provided later in this chapter (Table 22-1). CR1 and DAF (CD55) compete with factor B for binding to C3b on the cell surface and can

Table 22-1 Control Proteins of the Classical and Alternative Pathways

Name	Role in the Regulation of Complement Activation
C1 inhibitor (C1INH)	Binds to activated C1r, C1s, removing it from C1q
C4-binding protein (C4BP)	Binds C4b, displacing C2a; cofactor for C4b cleavage by factor I
Complement receptor 1 (CR1)	Binds C4b, displacing C2a, or C3b displacing Bb; cofactor for FI
Factor H (FH)	Binds C3b, displacing Bb; cofactor for factor I
Factor I (FI)	Serine protease that cleaves C3b and C4b: aided by factor H, MCP, C4BP, or CR1
Decay-accelerating factor	Membrane protein that displaces Bb from C3b and C2a from C4b
Membrane cofactor protein	Membrane protein that promotes C3b and C4b inactivation by factor I
CD59 widely	Prevents formation of membrane attack complex on autologous cells expressed on membranes

displace Bb from a convertase that has already formed.[27] Factor I (FI), a serum protease, in concert with CR1 or MCP (CD46) can prevent convertase formation by converting C3b into its inactive derivative, iC3b.[28] CR1 is unique among the FI cofactors in facilitating an additional proteolytic cleavage of iC3b to yield C3c and C3dg (see Fig. 22-2, *B*). Trimming of the latter by noncomplement proteases yields the proteolytic limit fragment C3d, which structurally corresponds to the TED domain (see Fig. 22-2, *B*). Another complement regulatory protein found in the plasma is FH. FH binds C3b and is able to compete with factor B and displace Bb from the convertase. In addition, FH acts as a cofactor for FI to convert C3b to iC3b. In addition to interaction sites for C3b, FH possesses two distinct binding sites for polyanionic molecules, particularly various sulphated glycosaminoglycans (e.g., heparan sulphate) or arrays of sialic acid (e.g., from membrane surface glycoproteins) found on host surfaces in contact with blood plasma. Although these polyanion binding sites are not required for FH to regulate fluid phase AP C3 convertase, they are required for its activity on surface-bound C3bBb. In fact, this is the basis for FH being able to discriminate between AP C3 convertase adventitiously deposited on host tissue versus that deposited on a microbial surface because the latter do not possess either the sulphated glycosaminoglycans or the sialic acid arrays.[29,30]

Pathogen surfaces normally are not afforded the protection offered by these regulators. Persistence of the C3bBb convertase on microbial surfaces may additionally be favored by the positive regulator properdin (factor P). This positive modulation of the AP by properdin has traditionally been thought to be attributable to its ability to prolong the lifetime of the AP C3 convertase by forming a C3bBbP complex. This mechanism is still valid, but recently, evidence has been presented that properdin, which circulates predominantly as a homotrimer, may also be able to recognize AP targets directly. Specifically, it has been shown to bind to microbial surfaces, such as to *Neisseria gonorrhoeae* or yeast cell walls, that are known AP activators, but not to strains of *Escherichia coli* that are known to be nonactivators of the AP of complement. Because it is a homotrimer, even if factor P uses two of its subunits to bind to the microbial surface, one is still left that can recruit C3b, or C3(H_2O), from the fluid phase to the microbial surface. The properdin-bound C3b/C3(H2O) can then act as a platform for recruiting factors B and D, thereby forming a surface-bound AP C3 convertase.[31] Consistent with this target recognition model for properdin functionality, individuals with deficiencies in factor P have a heightened susceptibility to infection with *Neisseria* spp.[32]

After forming, the C3bBb convertase rapidly cleaves more C3 to C3b, which can participate in the formation of more molecules of C3bBb convertase. The AP thereby activates an amplification loop that can proceed on the surface of a pathogen but not on a host cell. An additional point regarding amplification by the AP is that C3b deposited on a target as a result of activation of either the CP or the LP can act as a nidus for the formation of an AP C3 convertase.

Although specific antibody is not required for AP activation, many classes of immunoglobulin can facilitate AP activation.[33] The mechanism by which this occurs remains elusive, although some evidence indicates that C3b covalently bound to IgG displays a reduced rate of inactivation to iC3b by factors H and I.[34] However, in contrast to CP activation, which requires Fc, AP activation can occur with $F(ab)'_2$ fragments.

An instructive demonstration for the role of antibody in continuing the AP cascade, with possible ramifications for human disease, comes from a murine model of rheumatoid arthritis. Mice do not spontaneously develop rheumatoid arthritis.[35] However, a murine model has been developed in which expression of antibodies specific for the ubiquitously expressed cytoplasmic protein glucose-6-phosphate can cause joint destruction reminiscent of human rheumatoid arthritis. Interestingly, the disease state, through complement-mediated joint destruction, can occur even if the specific antibodies are of isotypes incapable of fixing complement through the CP. The response may be localized to the joints because of the absence of complement cascade regulators on cartilage.

C3, C5, and the Membrane Attack Complex

The formation of the C3 convertase, C4b2a (CP and LP) and C3bBb (AP), is the point at which the three pathways converge (see Fig. 22-1). The function of these complexes is to convert C3 to C3a and C3b. C3 is the most abundant complement protein in plasma, occurring at a concentration of 1.2 mg/mL, and up to 1000 molecules of C3b can bind in the vicinity of a single C3 convertase.[36]

The covalent attachment of C3b to either C4b2a or C3bBb converts this enzyme into a trimeric complex (C5 convertase) capable of binding and cleaving C5 into C5a and C5b. Mechanistically, the "adduct" C3b molecule increases the binding affinity of the C5 convertase for its substrate C5 such that its K_M is now well below the physiologic concentration of C5 in plasma.[37] C5b is the initiating component of the membrane attack complex (MAC). The MAC is a multiprotein complex whose components are C5b, C6, C7, C8, and multiple C9s.[38,39] The constituent components of the MAC associate in the numerical order C5b–C6–C7–C8–C9.

The MAC, when viewed by electron microscopy, resembles a cylinder that possesses a hydrophobic outer face and a hydrophilic central core. If assembled near a lipid bilayer, such as a cell or the bacterial membrane of a gram-negative strain, the MAC can associate with and insert into the lipid bilayer. Such insertion can be thought as "punching holes" into the membrane, allowing for passage of water and small ions into the cell. Osmotic equilibrium is thereby lost, leading to eventual lysis of the targeted cell or bacterium. C5b678 are sufficient to form small pores in the target membrane. The role of C9 appears to be to enlarge the channel through multiple C9 polymerization, thereby causing more rapid loss of membrane function and lysis. Deficiencies in complement components C5 to C9 have only been associated with increased susceptibility to *Neisseria* spp.–based infections, such as gonorrhea and bacterial meningitis. Also, the extended cell wall peptidoglycan layer of gram-positive strains of bacteria make them resistant to the lytic arm of complement. It can be concluded from these observations that the requirement for MAC is limited in host protection.

Complement Receptors and Their Role in Immune Complex Clearance and Activation

As described in the previous section, complement can act by the direct lysis of targeted cells. Another important function of complement in host protection is facilitating the uptake and destruction of pathogens by phagocytic cells. This occurs by the specific recognition of C3b/C4b–coated (opsonized) particles by complement receptors.[40,41]

The best characterized complement receptor for the uptake of C4-coated immune complexes is CR1 (CD35). CR1 binds C4b/C3b–bearing immune complexes. CR1, similar to most proteins that bind activation products of C4 and C3 molecules, shares a structural motif known as the short consensus repeat (SCR). Each short consensus repeat consists of approximately 60 amino acids. CR1 in humans is composed of 30 linked short consensus repeats. CR1 possesses three binding sites for C4b and two for C3b.

CR1 is expressed on a wide variety of cell types in humans, including erythrocytes, macrophages, polymorphonuclear leukocytes, B cells, monocytes, and FDCs. The role of CR1 expression on B cells and FDCs in activating and maintaining the adaptive immune response is detailed subsequently. For now, the focus is on the other cell types that express CR1.

Because CR1 is not directly associated on its cytoplasmic side with any intracellular signaling molecules, binding of C3b by CR1 expressed on phagocytic cells is not in itself capable of inducing endocytosis of the C3b-opsonized target. A secondary signal is required to induce phagocytosis. This second signal can be provided by IgG binding to the phagocyte's Fc receptor, by carbohydrates commonly found on bacterial surfaces, or by exposure of the phagocytic cell to the appropriate cytokines. In addition, some phagocytic cells, such as macrophages, are activated by binding of C5a through C5a receptor (C5aR, [CD84]) (see Biologic Activity of C3a and C5a, later). What these secondary ligands have in common is that they all bind to receptor domains that are the ligand recognition units of a cell signaling molecule or complex.

The largest pool of CR1-expressing cells is erythrocytes.[42] Erythrocytes bearing opsonized material are removed from the circulation presumably to prevent deposition in tissue sites such as the renal glomerulus. Erythrocytes bearing opsonized material traverse the sinusoids of the liver and spleen, where they come into close contact with fixed phagocytic cells. These phagocytic cells effect the transfer of opsonized material from the erythrocyte onto their own membranes. The transfer of complexes is enhanced by cleavage of C3b to iC3b by FI, as iC3b is a poor ligand for CR1, but is a good ligand for CRIg, a complement receptor of the Ig superfamily present on tissue-resident phagocytic cells (see later for further discussion of CRIg).

Given its central position in the complement cascade, the presence of C3b is tightly regulated. This regulation is brought about by cleaving C3b into inactive derivatives that cannot participate in forming an active convertase. One of the conformationally altered inactive derivatives of C3b, iC3b (see Fig. 22-2, *B*), can act as an opsonin in its own right for complement receptors CR2 (CD21), CR3 (CD11b/CD18) and CR4 (CD11c/CD18). CR3 binds iC3b and plays a major role in inducing phagocytosis but probably not activation in the absence of a second signal (e.g., Fc receptor or pattern recognition receptor). CR4 also binds iC3b-opsonized particles, resulting in direct endocytosis. Although its role as a phagocytic receptor is not well characterized, CD11c is the major marker for DCs. It is important to understand the functional importance of this complement receptor on DC and how it participates in uptake of antigen for presentation to T lymphocytes.

CR2 expressed on B cells augments cognate antibody receptor signaling (see later section). This receptor recognizes targets that are coated with iC3b, as well as the subsequent degradation products C3dg and C3d, all of which remain covalently bound to the target (see Fig. 22-2, *B*). CR2 is the only complement receptor that recognizes C3d/TED as its ligand. However, the CR2 binding site on TED only becomes accessible after degradation of C3 to at least the iC3b stage. Activation of complement plays a contributing role in producing a strong antibody response. An interesting aside is that CR2 is the cell surface receptor on human B cells that is recognized by the Epstein-Barr virus.[43]

CRIg is a recently described complement receptor that plays an important role in the clearance of C3b opsonized complexes by phagocytic cells of the liver.[44] It is also expressed on subsets of macrophages, but less is known about this role. The recent cocrystallization of C3b and CRIg revealed binding to the C3b β chain, which is in contrast to all other known C3-interacting partners, in which binding to the activated C3 occurs via the α chain.

Biologic Activity of C3a and C5a

The role of the complement fragments C3a and C5a in the immune response is to produce localized inflammation.[45] C3a and C5a are anaphylatoxins and are structurally similar to chemokines. When produced in large amounts or injected systemically, they induce a generalized circulatory collapse and shocklike syndrome similar to that seen in a systemic allergic reaction involving IgE antibodies.[46]

Of the two fragments, C5a is the most stable and possesses the best characterized and possibly highest specific biologic activity. Both C3a and C5a induce smooth muscle contraction and increased vascular permeability. C5a and C3a also act on endothelial cells lining blood vessels to induce adhesion molecule expression.[47,48] Additionally, C3a and C5a can activate the mast cells that populate submucosal tissues and line vessels throughout the body to release histamine, tumor necrosis factor α (TNF-α), and protease.[6] The changes induced by C3a and C5a recruit antibody, complement, and phagocytic cells to the site of infection, thereby hastening the adaptive immune response. C5a also induces the upregulation of CR1 and CR3 on the surfaces of these cells. C5a is the only complement chemotactic agent for neutrophils, macrophages, and basophils. By contrast, both C3a and C5a possess chemotactic activity for mast cells.[49] Although a similar fragment, C4a, is produced in the course of C4 activation, its physiologic relevance as an anaphylatoxin is highly questionable. First, human C4a binds to neither C3aR nor C5aR, the two well characterized complement anaphylatoxin receptors, and a specific C4a binding entity has not been identified. Second, anaphylatoxin activity for human C4a has only been reported on guinea pig targets, but even there, it is two to three orders of magnitude less potent than human C3a.[49]

Regulation of Complement Activation

Activation of the complement system must be tightly regulated to prevent autologous tissue damage (see Table 22-1).[50] Some of the proteins involved in regulating complement action have been described (see Alternative Pathway earlier). In addition to these regulators, a number of other checkpoints limit the scope and target of complement activation.

As a result of binding to antibody or pathogen, conformational changes to C1q induce the enzymatic activity of C1r and C1s. Both of these enzymes are regulated by the C1 inhibitor (C1-INH). C1-INH is a member of a family of *ser*ine *p*rotease *in*hibitors termed *serpins*.[51] Serpins provide a bait sequence that mimics the active site of the substrate. When C1r or C1s proteolytically attacks this sequence, the net result is that their respective active site serine hydroxyls become permanently covalently bound to the C1-INH bait site, thereby destroying their proteolytic activity. C1-INH works in a similar fashion in regulating the activated MASP proteases of the LP. Finally, C1-INH is also responsible for preventing spontaneous fluid-phase activation of C1 in plasma, but this activity can be overridden by immune complexes.

Although C1 is capable of cleaving multiple C4 molecules, only approximately 10% of the produced C4b clusters about the targeted antigen.[52] The rest is released into the fluid phase. C4b in the fluid phase is rapidly bound by C4 binding protein (C4BP), which is a cofactor for FI. Factor I cleaves C4b into two fragments, C4c and C4d, which are quickly cleared from the circulation.

In addition to their FI cofactor activities, the soluble regulators C4BP and FH, respectively, promote the dissociation of the CP (C4b2a) and AP (C3bBb) C3 convertases into their constituent components. This decay-dissociation is unidirectional because neither C2a nor Bb can reassociate on its own with their respective C3 convertase subunits. The membrane-bound regulators CR1 and DAF similarly possess decay-accelerating functionality toward both the CP and AP C3 convertases. The importance of CR1 or CR1-like molecules in curbing the complement response can be witnessed in a rather unexpected condition. Complement receptor 1–related gene (*Crry*) is a murine homologue of the human *CR1* gene, although its near-ubiquitous tissue distribution more closely resembles that of MCP (a somewhat more distant homologue).[53,54] Mice lacking Crry are unable to properly regulate C3. Crry-deficient mice spontaneously abort because of C3-dependent injury to the fetus. This presumably is the result of uncontrolled C3 deposition on the placenta. This observation in mice sheds light on the possibility that MCP (or perhaps CR1) plays a role in recurrent fetal loss manifest in patients with antiphospholipid syndrome.

Biologic Consequences of Complement Cascade Deficiencies

The important role of the complement system in preventing disease is witnessed in cases in which components of the system are absent either because of random mutation in the human population or by design in gene-targeted "knock-out" mice. Some complement cascade deficiencies have been described. This section focuses on the biologic consequences of deficiencies in complement cascade activation that have profound biologic consequences followed by a discussion on deficiencies in complement regulatory proteins.

Homozygous deficiencies in C1q, the most common form of C1 deficiency in humans, is a powerful susceptibility factor for the development of systemic lupus erythematosus (SLE).[55,56] Patients lacking C1q nearly always present with SLE. They have increased susceptibility to viral and bacterial infections, but it is not nearly as pronounced as in C3 deficiency (see later discussion). C1q knock-out mice show increased mortality, with up to 25% of mice having histologic evidence of glomerulonephritis.

C4 in humans is encoded by two separate loci giving rise to two distinct protein products, C4A and C4B.[57] Complete C4 deficiency correlates with a 75% prevalence of SLE in humans. However, at least in certain human populations, the absence, or even haploinsufficiency, of C4A, but not C4B, is associated with elevated risk for development of autoimmune diseases such as SLE and other lupus-like autoimmune disease. The reason for the protective effect of C4A is not settled, but it is worth noting that the one indisputable functional difference between C4A and C4B is in the nature of the covalent bond formed upon target deposition. Whereas C4A transacylates onto amino group nucleophiles, forming amide bonds, C4B shows a strong preference for forming ester linkages to hydroxyl group nucleophiles. The approximately threefold greater propensity of C4A, relative to C4B, to bind to amino-group-rich C1-bearing IgG aggregates,[58] as would be present in immune complexes in need of complement-dependent clearance, is one possible reason for the association of C4A null states with SLE. Finally, as with C1q, mice deficient in C4 are predisposed to SLE-like disease.

C2 deficiency appears to be relatively benign.[59] Humans lacking C2 appear to have a normally functioning immune system, although autoimmune disorders and, less commonly, infections are observed with increased frequency.

In light of the central role of C3 in the complement cascade, it is not surprising that C3 deficiency has dire consequences for the host organism. Of all known cases of C3 deficiency among humans, no patients have been reported as disease free. Infectious complications, predominately pyogenic in nature, occur frequently and recurrently. *Streptococcus pneumoniae* and *Neisseria meningitidis* are the major pathogens reported. In addition, SLE, vasculitic syndromes, and glomerulonephritis have been documented in up to 21% of C3-deficient patients. Mice deficient in C3 show, similar to humans, greatly increased susceptibility to streptococcal infection and death.[60] The 50% lethal dose (LD_{50}) is 50-fold less for C3-deficient mice than for C3-sufficient control subjects. This may be attributable in large part to the inability of mice deficient in C3 to effectively opsonize the bacteria. Moreover, the deficient mice have an impaired humoral response (see later section).

Biologic Consequences of Complement Regulatory Protein Deficiencies

Deficiencies in C1-INH have been observed in the human population.[61] C1-INH deficiency can be inherited as an autosomal dominant trait or can result from autoantibodies that recognize C1-INH, blocking its function.[51] The inherited form of this deficiency is the cause of hereditary angioedema. Patients with hereditary angioedema experience chronic spontaneous complement activation leading to the production of excess cleaved fragments of C4 and C2. The biochemical cause of angioedema in these patients is not definitively elucidated. One line of reasoning points to excess production of C2 kinin and bradykinin. The peptide C2 kinin is a breakdown product of C2a after cleavage of C2. This peptide causes extensive swelling; the most dangerous is local swelling in the trachea, which can lead to suffocation. Bradykinin, which has similar actions to C2 kinin, also is produced in an uncontrolled fashion in this disease as a result of the lack of inhibition of another plasma protease, kallikrein, which is activated by tissue damage and is regulated by C1-INH. Although C1 is unregulated in patients with hereditary angioedema, large-scale cleavage of C3 is prevented by C4 and C2 control mechanisms and by regulation of C3 convertase formation on host cells. An increased risk of infection is not associated with C1-INH deficiency. This disease can be fully corrected by infusion of purified C1-INH.

Acquired C1-INH deficiency may be associated with lymphoproliferative disorders and in most cases represents development of an autoantibody that binds to and neutralizes C1-INH. In two examined cases, autoantibodies abrogate C1-INH activity by preventing formation of the C1s–C1-INH complex. However, after the complex formed, the autoreactive antibodies had no effect on C1-INH function. To date, there is no uniform, fully effective therapy for these patients.

The role of FI in complement cascade regulation can be witnessed in patients with FI deficiency.[62] In the presence of a cofactor protein, FI cleaves C3b, producing iC3b, the inactive form of C3b. iC3b is incapable of reacting with factor B to form the AP C3 convertase, thereby preventing uncontrolled AP activation. In the absence of FI, unrestrained C3 consumption occurs secondary to accelerated spontaneous AP turnover. Patients with FI deficiency have recurrent infections caused by pyogenic organisms, including meningococcal meningitis.

Likewise, mice deficient in the central protein FH exhibit unrestrained C3 activation via the AP, leading to near depletion of serum C3. An important outcome of the failure to regulate C3 activation is glomerulonephritis. Strikingly, mice deficient in FH develop a disease resembling the human disorder membrane glomerulonephritis. The phenotype of the mice confirms the general notion that the AP is always "on" and that failure to regulate activated C3 results in consumption of circulating C3 and tissue injury.

Another example of the importance of FH regulation are reports of genetic association between variant alleles of FH and the human diseases age-related macular degeneration (AMD) and atypical hemolytic uremic syndrome (aHUS). Whereas AMD is a fairly common condition—indeed, it is the leading cause of blindness in the Western world—it has been the elucidation of the etiology of the much rarer aHUS condition (two cases per million) that has led to a fuller appreciation of the diverse ways through which dysregulation of the AP of complement can give rise to severe pathology. Classically, HUS is a clinical triad of microangiopathic hemolytic anemia, thrombocytopenia, and acute renal failure. The disease is characterized by a precipitating injury of endothelial cells. In contrast to the fairly common classical form of HUS, which is diarrhea associated and is usually caused by a Shiga toxin–secreting pathogen, the atypical form of HUS is nondiarrheal and is caused by genetic predisposition. Even haploinsufficency of variants of FH, MCP, and FI resulting from either loss of expression—or more commonly, loss of regulatory function—results in disease pathology. Additionally, gain-of-function variants of factor B have been described that either form the AP C3 convertase more efficiently than wild-type factor B or are more resistant to decay-dissociation by FH or DAF. Finally, several C3 variants have been described in aHUS patients that are gain of function in the sense that as C3b there is decreased binding affinity for MCP and FH and thus AP C3 convertases formed with this C3b as subunit would have a prolonged lifetime relative to wild type C3b.[63,64]

Because FH mutations account for at least 30% of reported aHUS cases and approximately 70% of these are caused by missense mutations in SCR domains 19 and 20, the molecular basis of this disease association has been intensively investigated, and the findings of these studies are best understood in the context of a structure-based domain model[65] of FH bound to C3b on a nonactivator (i.e., host) surface (Fig. 22-3). FH consists of 20 SCR domains, where some domains in the middle of the molecule appear to play mainly a structural role, likely allowing the molecule to bend back on itself, but domain clusters near the ends mediate specific functions. SCRs 1 to 4 bind to C3b and mediate both decay-accelerating and FI-cofactor functionalities. Indeed, FH(SCR1-4) on its own is able to regulate a fluid-phase AP C3 convertase, but it cannot do so for surface-bound AP C3 convertases. For regulation of the latter, there are three additional binding interactions that become relevant. Two of these are located within SCRs 19 to 20, specifically, a site localized mainly to SCR19 binds to the C3d/TED domain of the surface-bound C3b molecule, and a site within SCR20 binds to surface-associated polyanions such as sulphated glycosaminoglycans or sialic acid arrays. The aHUS-associated missense mutations found within SCRs 19 to 20 affect one or other of these two binding functions and lead to dysregulation of the AP C3 convertase at the surface of host tissue. In particular, complement-mediated damage to the kidney basement membrane is often a hallmark of aHUS. As a tissue devoid of the membrane-associated complement regulators MCP, DAF, or CR1, but rich in sulphated glycosaminoglycans, the functionality of the soluble AP regulator FH becomes even more crucial for host protection and likely explains the high incidence of missense mutations within SCRs 19 to 20 in aHUS patients. Interestingly, missense mutations in FH SCRs 19 to 20 do not result in systemic C3 consumption, as would be the case for complete deficiencies of FH. This is because SCRs 1 to 4 of the mutant molecule are still capable of regulating spontaneously formed AP C3 convertases in the fluid phase.

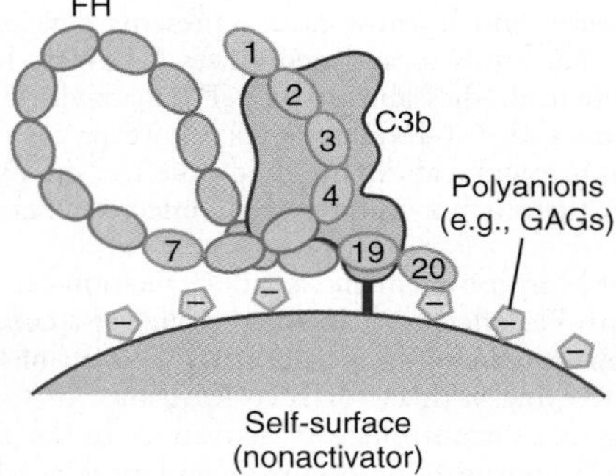

Figure 22-3 A STRUCTURE-BASED MODEL OF THE FACTOR H (FH)–MEDIATED REGULATION OF THE ALTERNATIVE PATHWAY ON HOST CELLS BEARING ADVENTITIOUSLY DEPOSITED C3b. Whereas the depicted interaction of FH domains SCR(1-4) with C3b is sufficient to prevent C3b in solution from becoming a subunit of an AP C3 convertase, for surface-bound C3b, at least two additional interactions are necessary. The first is the interaction indicated between FH SCR19 and the thioester domain (TED)/C3d domain of the C3b molecule. The second is between FH SCR20 and cell surface–associated sulphated glycosaminoglycans (GAGs) or arrays of sialic acid containing glycans, in both cases denoted by *pentagons with an internal minus sign.* Mutations affecting either the C3d binding site or the polyanion binding site within FH SCR(19-20) lead to alternative pathway dysregulation and the disease atypical hemolytic uremic syndrome (aHUS). There is an additional polyanion binding site in SCR7, which appears to be important for regulating the AP on some host surfaces, most particularly Bruch's membrane in the eye because the SCR7 Y402H polymorphism is a risk factor for AMD. *(Adapted from Kajander T, Lehtinen MJ, Hyvärinen S, et al: Dual interaction of factor H with C3d and glycosaminoglycans in host-nonhost discrimination by complement.* Proc Nat Acad Sci U S A *108:2897, 2011; reproduced with permission of the National Academy of Science.)*

In addition to the polyanion binding site in FH SCR 20, there is also one in SCR 7. This SCR is the site of an amino acid polymorphism in FH (tyrosine to histidine at residue 402, Y402H) that is a significant risk factor for AMD but interestingly does not correlate with disease susceptibility for aHUS. Heterozygotes and homozygotes for H402 are respectively 2.7-fold and 7.4-fold more at risk for AMD than homozygous Y402 individuals, and this single polymorphism can account for up to 50% of the risk of AMD.[66,67] Two significant functional differences have been observed for the Y402 and H402 variants of FH. First, the affinity and specificity for a spectrum of sulphated glycosaminoglycans is different for the two variants of FH. Secondly, the affinity of the H402 variant of FH for C-reactive protein (CRP), an acute-phase protein that binds to damaged tissue, is substantially lower than that of the Y402 variant. It is notable that Bruch membrane of the macula, similar to the kidney basement membrane, is devoid of membrane-associated complement regulators and so is highly dependent of FH for local AP regulation. Indeed, the spectrum of sulphated glycosaminoglycans found on Bruch membrane appear to be more dependent on the polyanionic binding site in SCR 7 for the interaction than that in SCRs 19 to 20 because even with non-AMD eye tissue, there is preferential binding of the Y402 variant to Bruch membrane.[68] Thus, the lower binding affinity of the H402 FH variant, coupled with a possible age-related change in the bisynthesized spectrum of sulphated glycosaminoglycans on Bruch membrane, could account for the dysregulation of the AP in the macula with the ensuing inflammation of the macula seen in AMD patients. There may also be a contribution from the differential binding of the FH variants to CRP present on the particulate debris (drusen) residing in between the retinal pigment epithelium and Bruch membrane.

The MAC is one mechanism used by the host to rid itself of certain microorganisms. Host cells are protected from MAC-mediated lysis by CD59 (protectin), a membrane-bound protein. CD59 performs its function by inhibiting the binding of C9 to the C5b–C6–C7–C8–C9 complex. CD59 and DAF are linked to the cell surface by a phosphoinositol glycolipid (PIG) tail. One of the enzymes involved in the synthesis of PIG tails is encoded on chromosome X. Mutation of this gene leads to a failure to synthesize PIG tails and with it an inability to express CD59 or DAF on the cell surface.[60-71] Lack of CD59 and DAF expression on host cell surfaces is the cause of paroxysmal nocturnal hemoglobinuria. This disease is characterized by episodes of chronic intravascular hemolysis and propensity to thrombosis.

Autoimmunity and Complement Deficiencies

There exists a strong correlative relationship between the lack of certain components of the complement system (i.e., C1 and C4) and autoimmune disease, particularly SLE. Two general nonmutually exclusive hypotheses have been put forward to explain the increased incidence of SLE among complement deficient individuals—the clearance hypothesis and the tolerance hypothesis.[56,72,73] The clearance hypothesis is based on the known role of the CP of complement in binding to foreign antigens and transporting them to the liver and spleen for degradation and removal from the circulation. Thus, defects in clearance of apoptotic cells or debris would lead to inappropriate accumulation of self-antigen and overstimulation of self-reactive lymphocytes.

The tolerance model proposes that innate immunity protects against SLE by delivering lupus autoantigens to sites where immature B lymphocytes are tolerized, thereby eliminating a source of autoreactive antibody molecules. SLE is characterized by high-affinity antibodies specific for autoantigens such as double-stranded DNA (dsDNA), ribonuclear proteins, and histones. Validation of the model comes in part from studies with human B cells demonstrating that self-reactive B cells are eliminated or anergized at two major checkpoints, bone marrow (BM) and spleen. Thus, counterselection of potentially pathogenic B cells is an active process and most likely involves components of innate immunity.

Recent studies in a mouse model (strain 564 Igi) in which the B cells express an Ig receptor specific for the lupus antigen SSB/LA suggests a third possible explanation for why C4 is critical for protection against SLE. Accordingly, this hypothesis suggests that C4-dependent defects in clearance of immune complexes leads to a loss of tolerance of certain autoreactive B cells. Thus, accumulation of immune complexes composed of lupus antigens that bear DNA or RNP ligands that trigger Toll-like receptors (TLRs) TLR 7 and TLR 9 may induce myeloid cells to release excess type I interferon (IFN-α). In a feed forward loop, IFN-α release induces increased sensitivity of TLR 7 and 9 receptors, in particular on B cells, such that the combined effects of engagement of DNA or RNP self-antigen and increased TLR 7 and 9 leads to escape of B-cell tolerance (MCC, unpublished).

The first part of this section familiarized the reader with the general aspects of the complement system. The remainder of this section focuses on the role of the complement system in the initiation and propagation of the adaptive immune response and begins with a description of natural antibody.

Natural Antibody

Natural antibody, in contrast to antibody secreted in response to active immunization, is continuously released, mostly by the B1 subpopulation of lymphocytes. Predominantly IgM but also IgA and IgG3 (in mice), natural antibodies tend to be polyreactive, with low-affinity binding for antigens such as nuclear proteins, DNA, and phosphatidylcholine, which are common structures among both pathogens and host tissue. These antibodies rarely show evidence of somatic mutation. It has been speculated that the variable region genes that predominate among natural antibodies have been selected evolutionarily for their ability to recognize pathogens and act as a rapid response to infection, thereby acting as a stop gap to provide sufficient time for the adaptive immune response to form. Natural antibody mediates its protective effects via the CP of complement.

IgM natural antibody is important in initiating the CP, leading to enhanced humoral immunity. In addition to its role in protecting against pathogens, natural antibody protects against lupuslike disease based on studies in mice. Thus, similar to C1q and C4, deficiency in IgM predisposes to an SLE-like phenotype.

Complement Links Innate and Adaptive Immune Responses

One of the critical functions of CP complement is providing a bridge between innate and acquired immune systems. The process is achieved through attachment of complement products to the antigen or pathogen, either directly to the surface or via antibody (see earlier section). This complement "tag" consists of breakdown products of C3 (i.e., C3b, C3dg, and C3d) that facilitate recognition of pathogens by the immune system. The recognition phase is mediated principally through complement receptors CD21 (CR2) and CD35 (CR1). This section details complement-dependent mechanisms of immune detection and humoral responses to thymus (T)-dependent antigens.

Soluble Complement Mediators of Antibody Responses

The first clue that complement is important in regulating B-lymphocyte responses came from the observation that B lymphocytes bind activated C3 fragments.[74] Soon thereafter, it was noted that mice depleted of serum C3 by treatment with cobra venom factor had diminished responses to T-dependent antigens.[75] The discovery of naturally occurring genetic deficiencies in C3, C4, and C2 in species as diverse as guinea pigs,[76,77] dogs[78] and humans[79,80] allowed description of impaired antibody responses as well. Because the impaired responsiveness is comparable among animals deficient in CP activators (C4, C2) and C3-deficient or C3-depleted animals, a model emerged suggesting that the effect is mediated through the CP of the complement system. That the impaired responsiveness is comparable among diverse animal species indicated the importance of CP complement in regulating antibody responses to T-dependent antigens.

The advance of gene-targeting technology in the murine system led to development of engineered strains devoid of various components of CP complement. C1q-, C4-, and C3-deficient mouse strains generate reduced antibody responses to T-dependent antigens.[81-84] Furthermore, these strains fail to switch Ig isotypes normally, suggesting that germinal center responses are impaired.[83] Germinal centers are microanatomic structures whose purpose is to provide for increasing affinity of serum antibody for antigens (affinity maturation), isotype switching, and development and differentiation of memory B lymphocytes and plasma cells.[85] Consistent with this theory, immunized complement-deficient mice produce fewer and smaller germinal centers compared with immunized wild-type mice.[83] Importantly, humoral responses in each of the C1q-, C4-, and C3-deficient strains can be rescued by transplantation of wild-type BM.[55,86,87] Therefore, BM-derived cells can produce sufficient complement to reconstitute antibody responses to T-dependent antigens administered intravenously.

It is suggested that the CP potentiates antibody responses through involvement of immune complex formation. The implication is that natural antibodies or specific IgM released early in the response by B cells responding to antigen recognize and bind pathogens, thereby activating the CP. In support of this model, genetically engineered mice producing only membrane IgM (i.e., with gene-targeted deletion of secretory signals) produce significantly reduced antibody responses to T-dependent antigens.[88] A second mechanism for initial CP activation on the antigen, which may be relevant to a subset of antigens bearing a repeating epitope, involves binding of the antigen by B cells through the surface IgM of two or more B-cell receptors (BCRs). The cross-linking and distortion that is imparted to the Fc_{μ} regions of adjacent BCRs is sufficient to activate the CP at the B-cell surface. Indeed, this mechanism does not work if the BCR μ-chain contains a mutation that abolishes C1q binding.[89] Finally, a third permutation of these mechanisms may apply to monovalent soluble T-dependent antigens. The antigen is first captured by the BCR, creating an antigen array on the B-cell surface, to which low-affinity natural repertoire IgM can bind by virtue of avidity effects and initiate the CP.[90] As illustrated by these examples, immune complex formation is only important for initiating the CP, leading to the deposition of C3 activation products on the antigen or immune complex. Indeed, antigens directly conjugated to C3b or C3d fragments are more potent immunogens compared to unconjugated antigen.[91,92] Furthermore, the magnitude of the immune response is directly influenced by the number of C3d fragments conjugated to the antigen.[91] Therefore, activated products of complement component C3 act as a natural adjuvant in driving efficient antibody responses.

Complement Receptors and Antibody Responses

B-Lymphocyte Coreceptors

The effects of complement-coated antigens on antibody responses are mediated primarily through complement receptors CD21 and CD35. CD21 and CD35 are expressed predominantly on B lymphocytes and FDCs.[93,94] CD35 is also found on polymorphonuclear cells, macrophages, mast cells, and DCs.[93] CD21 and CD35 are encoded for by separate yet closely linked genes in humans.[95] In mice, CD21 and CD35 originate from the same locus (Cr2) and are generated by alternative splicing events at the RNA level.[96,97]

Two novel sets of experiments demonstrated that CD21 and CD35 are important in regulating B-lymphocyte responses to T-dependent antigens. In the first set of experiments, antibodies specific for both CD21 and CD35 or CD35 alone were administered to immunized mice.[98-101] In the second set of experiments, a soluble form of CD21 was administered to immunized mice, thereby competing for C3d-coupled antigen interactions.[102] In both sets of experiments, treatment impaired antibody responses. In the first approach, the antibody that specifically blocked the interaction of C3d with CD21 was much more effective at blocking antibody responses compared with anti-CD35 antibody treatment, which blocked only the binding of C3b to CD35. This suggested that although both receptors contribute, CD21 is more important in regulating antibody responses.[99]

Because CD21 and CD35 are found on B lymphocytes and FDCs, two important cell types for humoral responses, two nonmutually exclusive models are proposed for their function. In the first model, CD21 augments antibody responses through activity as a coreceptor on B lymphocytes[103] (Fig. 22-4, *A*). The second model proposes that CD21/CD35 on FDCs trap and focus antigen such that B lymphocytes can efficiently cross-link their antigen receptor to become activated[104] (see Fig. 22-4, *B*).

As is apparent from the schematics in Fig. 22-4, *A* and *B* and as will be elaborated upon further in the ensuing discussion, the key ligand receptor–receptor interaction mediating the linkage between complement and the adaptive humoral immune system is that between the C3d fragment that is covalently coupled to antigen and CD21 (CR2) present on B cells and FDC. The extracellular region of CD21 is composed of 15 or 16 SCR domains (because of the usage of alternative splice sites for exon 11), but the C3d binding site is confined to the two *N*-terminal–most SCR domains.[105] In what is an instructive lesson on the need to have concordance between x-ray crystallographic structures and biochemical data, the nature of this important interface had been hotly debated for the past decade because of discrepancies between a structure of the CR2(SCR1-2):C3d complex published[106] in 2001 with both preexisting and subsequent biochemical data in the literature. A recent de novo structure of this complex[107] depicted in Fig. 22-4, *C* appears to have resolved the issue because the interactions seen in the new structure are fully supported by the biochemical data in the literature. For example, the biochemical data suggesting that there should be multiple ionic bonds mediating the binding is fully rationalized in terms of the five such bonds seen in the structure between a very negatively charged interface on a concave face of C3d that is remote from the covalent attachment site and positively charged lysine and arginine side chains from CR2 sticking down and interacting with oppositely charged residues on the C3d interface, as can be appreciated in Fig. 22-4, *C*.

As a coreceptor, engagement of CD21 by complement-coupled antigen on the surface of a B lymphocyte, in combination with membrane Ig (BCR) cross-linking, would lower the strength of signal through the BCR to activate the cell.[103] Accordingly, naïve B lymphocytes bear low-affinity receptors for antigen; therefore, especially under conditions of limiting antigen, as would be the case during initial encounter with a microbial pathogen, additional signaling by the CD21 coreceptor is required for efficient activation. This was demonstrated in vitro by culturing B lymphocytes with cognate antigen, either uncoupled or coupled to C3d. By measuring intracellular Ca^{2+} levels as a measure of cell activation, it was estimated that 100- to 1000-fold less C3d-conjugated antigen was required to activate B lymphocytes compared with unconjugated antigen.[91]

The opportunity to test the importance of CD21 and CD35 as B-lymphocyte coreceptors in vivo came from studies using mice with targeted disruption in the *Cr2* locus. Importantly, *Cr2*-deficient mice have impaired humoral responses similar to C1q-, C4- and C3-deficient mice (Fig. 22-5).[108-110] Using embryonic stem cells with a disrupted *Cr2* locus, Croix et al[111] used blastocyst complementation of $Rag2^{-/-}$ mice, such that chimeric mice expressed CD21/CD35 on FDCs but not on B lymphocytes. These chimeric mice displayed impaired antibody responses to the T-dependent antigen NP-KLH compared with control subjects. Therefore, CD21/CD35 on B lymphocytes is important for normal antibody responses. Although CD21/CD35 on FDC is on its own insufficient for normal antibody responses, as discussed in the next section, CD21/CD35 on FDC does have a specific role in the memory response of B cell–mediated immunity.

Complement's covalent attachment to antigen engages CD21 as a complex with CD19/CD81 and BCR on the cell surface (see Fig. 22-4, *A*).[103,112,113] Dual binding of CD21/CD19/CD81 with BCR generates a stronger signal compared with BCR engagement alone.[103] If the combined signal is sufficient, the B lymphocyte is activated. If insufficient, then the B lymphocyte likely is eliminated by apoptosis.[86,114-118] The major ligand-binding receptor within the CD21/CD19/CD81 complex is CD21. CD19's major role is in initiating a signaling cascade within the cell.[119] CD81 is a tetra-spanning molecule that stabilizes the complex within the membrane. After co-ligation of the BCR with the CD21/CD19/CD81 complex, CD81 gets S-palmitoylated on a cysteine side chain, and this in turn mobilizes the co-ligated complexes to a special compartment of the plasma membrane known as a lipid raft. Localization to this compartment facilitates prolonged intracellular signaling because the compartment is rich in signal-propagating phosphokinases but is relatively devoid of the regulatory phosphatases.[120] Absence of any of the CD21/CD19/CD81 components adversely affects antibody responses to T-dependent antigens, although the degree of impairment varies.[108,121-123]

Focusing Antigen on Follicular Dendritic Cells

The second role of complement receptors CD21 and CD35 in regulating humoral responses is that they permit FDCs to trap antigen (Fig. 22-6).[104,124] FDCs concentrate in regions of ongoing immune responses, such as germinal centers, and they appear necessary for antibody responses. Germinal centers (see earlier section) promote somatic hypermutation within Ig heavy- and light-chain genes along with isotype switching and production of memory B lymphocytes and plasma cells. They can be divided into two regions, dark zone and light zone. To gain entry into the dark zone, B lymphocytes are activated by receiving above threshold signals from the CD21/CD19/CD81 and BCR in combination with costimulation from helper T lymphocytes.[125-127] Within the dark zone, activated B lymphocytes divide and mutate their Ig receptor genes.[126-129] After several rounds of proliferation in the dark zone, B lymphocytes enter the light zone, where they are subjected to selection on antigen deposited on FDCs (i.e., clonal selection).[130,131] The selection of high-affinity B lymphocyte clones into memory B-lymphocyte and plasma cell pools ensures future protection against repeat antigen exposure.

How antigen is retained on FDCs, both for primary B-lymphocyte responses and for long-term memory responses, is subject to intense research. However, supporting evidence indicates that complement receptors on FDCs are important in both short- and long-term B-lymphocyte responses. Papamichail et al[104] demonstrated that retention of antigen–IgG immune complexes on FDCs was reduced upon depletion of C3 using cobra venom factor. Therefore, it appears that immune complex deposition on FDCs is complement dependent. In addition, antibody production in vitro using FDCs demonstrates that antibody production is dependent on CD21/CD35.[132]

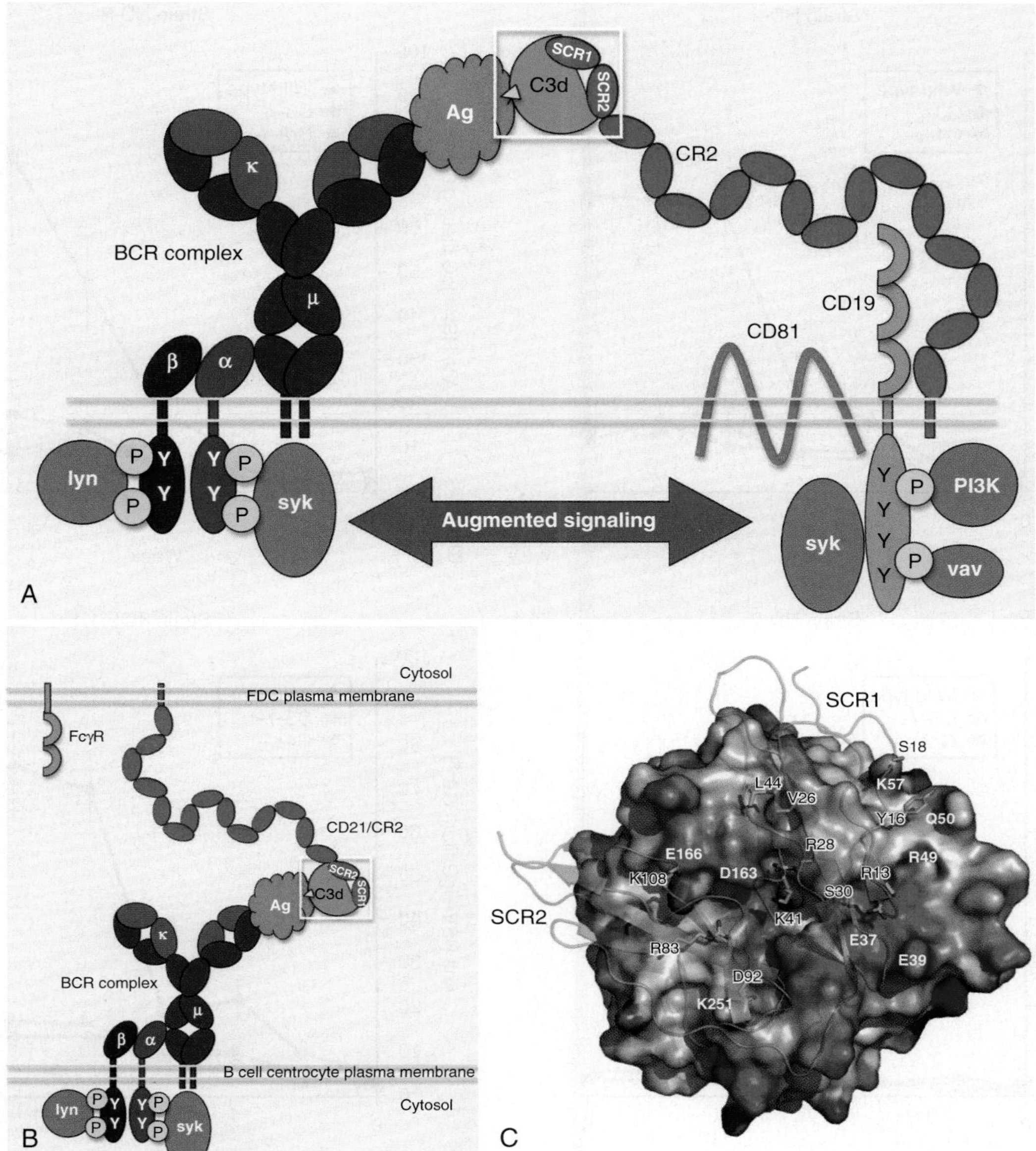

Figure 22-4 COUPLING OF C3D TO ANTIGEN ALTERS ITS FATE IN B-CELL RESPONSE. **A,** Coligation of the B-cell receptor (BCR) with the CD19/CD21/CD81 complex by antigen coated with C3d regulates essential functions for naïve B-cell activation. The *boxed area* indicates the key binding interaction between CD21/CR2(SCR1-2), and the C3d fragment that is covalently bound *(yellow triangle)* to the antigen recognized by this B cell's BCR. **B,** C3d-coated antigens are also captured on the surface of the follicular dendritic cells (FDCs) by CD21, allowing for efficient stimulation of previously antigen-engaged B-cell centrocytes in the germinal centers during the process of affinity maturation and the generation of memory B cells. **C,** The structure of the CR2(SCR1-2):C3d complex as a surface representation of C3d colored for electrostatic potential (*red,* negative; *blue,* positive) and an overlayed, semi-transparent, ribbon diagram of CR2(SCR1-2) showing stick models of the side chains of some of the interacting residues. Note the charge complementarity for many of the interacting amino acids. *(**C** reproduced with permission from van den Elsen JM, Isenman DE: A crystal structure of the complex between human complement receptor 2 and its ligand C3d.* Science *332:608, 2011.)*

Availability of *Cr2*-deficient mice has shed light on the importance of FDC-derived CD21/CD35 on humoral responses. Because FDCs are radioresistant, it was possible to generate chimeric mice that restricted CD21/CD35 expression to B lymphocytes by BM transplantation. Ahearn et al[108] made chimeric mice with *Cr2*-deficient FDCs by transplanting wild-type BM (B-lymphocyte $Cr2^{+/+}$) into lethally irradiated *Cr2*-deficient recipient mice (FDC-$Cr2^{-/-}$). After secondary challenge with antigen, the chimeric mice failed to sustain high-level antibody production, suggesting that CD21/CD35 on FDCs is important for recall or memory responses. Fang et al[133] came to a similar conclusion regarding the importance of CD21/35 expression on FDC for a strong immune response.

CD21/CD35 do appear important for persistence of antibody titers, normal frequencies of memory B lymphocytes and plasma cells, and affinity maturation. Adoptively transferring memory B lymphocytes into recipient mice lacking FDC-derived CD21/CD35 demonstrated that complement receptors on recipient mice stroma were required for each of these elements of memory.[114] Importantly,

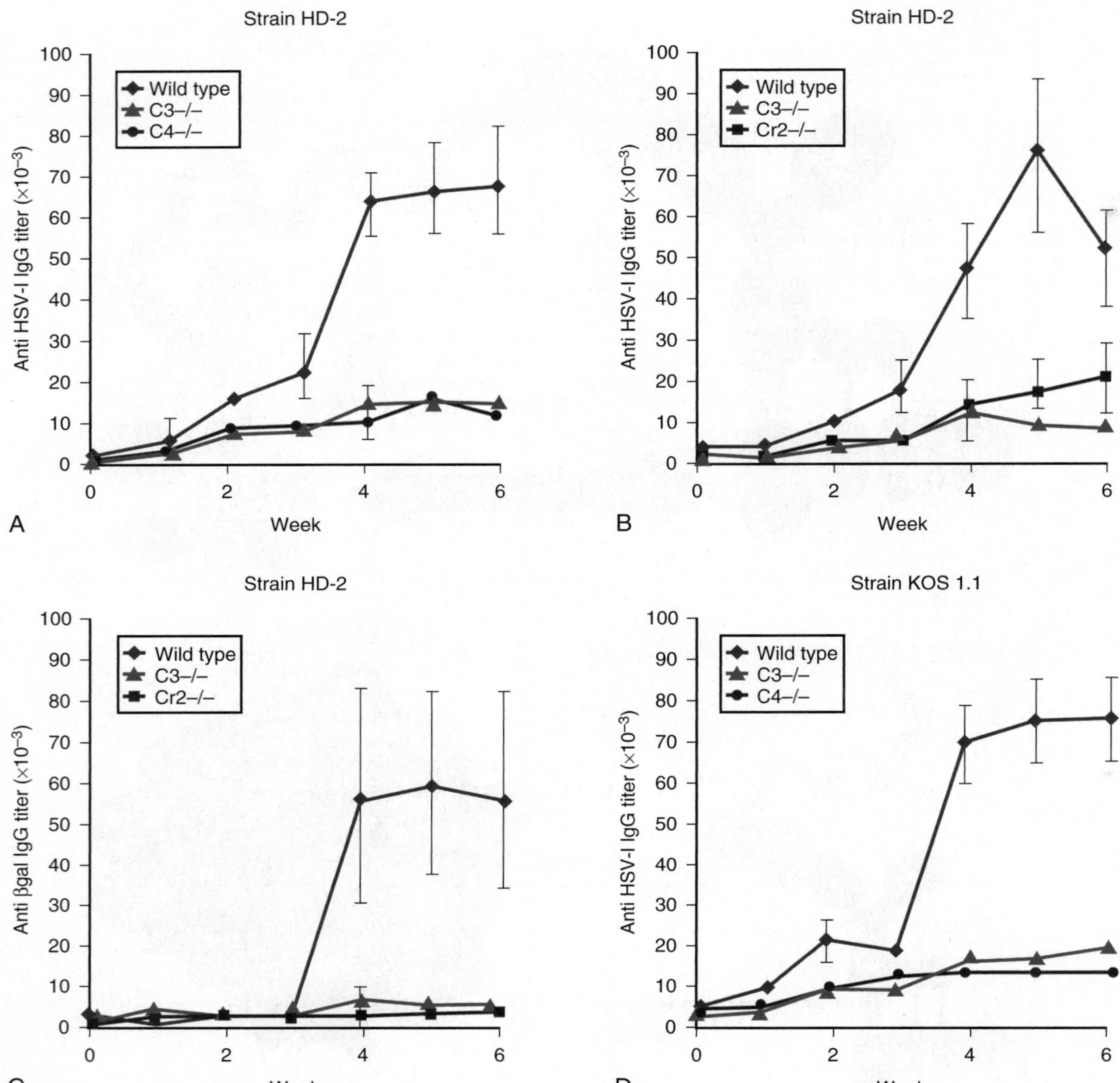

Figure 22-5 Classical pathway complement and complement receptors CD21/CD35 are required for the humoral response to replication-defective HD-2 virus or replication-sufficient KOS1.1 wild-type (WT) virus. Mice were injected at days 0 and 21 with 2×10^6 plaque forming units of replication-defective (**A** to **C**) or replication-sufficient (**D**) virus, HD-2, and KOS1.1, respectively. Antibody titers were determined by enzyme-linked immunosorbent assay. Mean titer ± SD represents at least five mice analyzed in two separate experiments. **A,** Deficiency in either C3 or C4 results in an impaired secondary humoral response to infectious herpes simplex virus (HSV). **B,** Cr2–/– mice have an impaired secondary response similar to mice deficient in C3. **C,** Humoral response to recombinant virus-expressed heterologous protein (β-galactosidase) is also impaired in mice deficient in C3 or CD21/CD35. **D,** Secondary humoral response to replication-sufficient HSV-1 (strain KOS1.1) depends on complement C3 and C4. *(From Da Costa XJ, Brockman MA, Alicot E, et al: Humoral response to herpes simplex virus is complement-dependent.* Proc Nat Acad Sci U S A *96:12708, 1999; reproduced with permission of the National Academy of Science.)*

chimeric mice lacking CD21/CD35-bearing FDCs had severely impaired recall responses several months after transfer of memory B lymphocytes compared with wild-type recipients.[114] These studies suggest that CD21/CD35 on FDCs have an important role in long-term storage of antigen, thereby facilitating B-lymphocyte memory.

Complement and T-Cell Immunity

The complement system is important not only in humoral immunity; it also enhances responses by both CD4 and CD8 T cells.[134] Studies with influenza in C3-deficient mice first identified an important role for C3 in both the CD8 and CD4 response to infectious virus.[135] Although the mechanism is not clear, given the importance of DC in uptake and presentation of antigen, one likely role is C3 opsonization of virus. Moreover, the anaphylatoxins C3a and C5a released during complement activation stimulate cytokine releases by mast cells via their respective complement receptors. Studies of mice deficient in C3a receptor identified reduced responsiveness of a subset on CD4 T cells.[136] Likewise, C5a receptor appears to play an important role in the lung in T cell–dependent allergic responses.

T-cell responses are also "tuned down" via complement receptor. Interestingly, cross-linking of the CD46 complement receptor via C3b on activated CD4 T cells induces differentiation to a T-regulatory

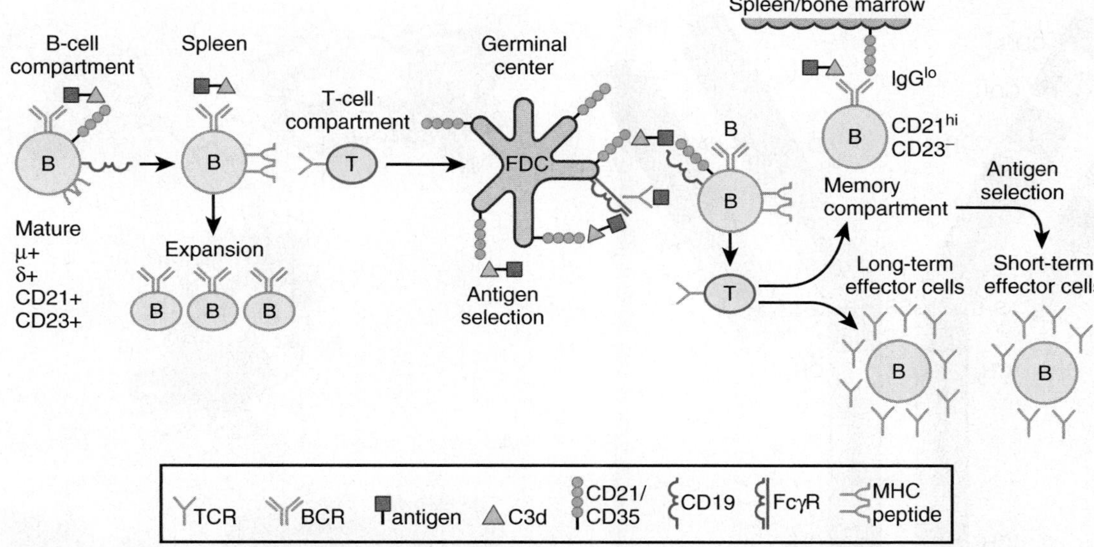

Figure 22-6 ROLE OF COMPLEMENT-TAGGED ANTIGEN IN DIRECTING B-LYMPHOCYTE ACTIVATION AND FORMATION OF MEMORY B LYMPHOCYTES. Mature B lymphocytes survey secondary lymphoid tissues in search of antigen. Survival of mature B lymphocytes after antigen contact and T-cell help within splenic follicles depends on coreceptor signals through CD21/CD35. Lymphocytes receiving requisite signals expand and continue to differentiate within germinal centers, where CD21/CD35 is again important. B lymphocytes not receiving complement–ligand interactions in germinal centers die. In addition, complement-mediated deposition may localize antigen to follicular dendritic cells (FDCs), thereby providing the substrate for B-lymphocyte selection. Selection and differentiation in germinal centers lead to production of long-lived memory B lymphocytes and effector cells. The lifespan of memory B lymphocytes may also depend on continued interaction of antigen deposited on FDCs with CD21/CD35 in the spleen and in bone marrow. *IgG*, Immunoglobulin G.

phenotype.[137] Further investigation on this topic will reveal additional examples whereby the complement system participates in activation and regulation of T cells.

Conclusion

Over the past 15 years, a new appreciation for the complement system has come to light. Not only is the complement system required for host protection and innate immunity, but it also plays a critical role in "directing" the humoral response to thymus-dependent and -independent antigens. Covalent attachment of split products of C3 (i.e., C3d) alters the fate of antigen and targets it to FDC within the lymphoid compartment. Other studies are uncovering additional roles for complement in the regulation of self-reactive B cells. The next decade likely will witness a similar revolution on our understanding of how complement participates in protection against autoimmune diseases such as SLE.

IMMUNOGLOBULINS

Properties and Structure

The mammalian immune system responds to the almost unlimited array of antigens by producing antibodies that react specifically with the molecules that induced their production. During the immune response, the structure of the inducing antigen is imprinted on the immune system, and subsequent challenges with the same or structurally related molecule(s) causes a more rapid rise in antibody levels to much greater concentrations than were achieved after the primary antigenic challenge. Thus, the hallmarks of the humoral immune system include induction, specific protein interaction, and memory.

Antibodies belong to the family of proteins called the *immunoglobulins*. The basic structure of all immunoglobulins consists of a monomer that contains four polypeptide chains: two identical heavy (H) chains and two identical light (L) chains covalently linked by disulfide bonds (Fig. 22-7).[138] The x-ray crystallographic structure of a monomeric immunoglobulin, specifically a mouse IgG2a monoclonal antibody (mAb), is shown depicted in both ribbon and space-filling models in Fig. 22-8.[139] Depending on the angle between the constituent Fab (fragment antigen-binding) monomers, an immunoglobulin monomer consists of a Y- or T-like structure. The size of the Fab arms is 80 × 50 × 40 Å, and the size of base, called the Fc (fragment crystallizable) region, is approximately 70 × 45 × 40 Å according to the x-ray structure models. The Ig molecule exhibits considerable flexibility. In electron microscopic, low-angle x-ray scattering, transient electric birefringence, and resonance energy transfer studies, the angle between the Fab domains has been observed to vary from 0 to 180 degrees. All antibodies have two identical combining sites for each antigen located at the ends of the Fab domains.

Fab and Fc represent functional domains in immunoglobulins. They were discovered by performing limited proteolytic digestion of the molecule. Both the H and L chains contribute amino acids that constitute the antigen-binding site in Fab. The monovalent Fab fragment will bind to, but will not precipitate, multivalent antigens, in contrast to native IgG. A fragment can be prepared, called $F(ab')_2$, that is devoid of Fc but still precipitates antigen. This form of immunoglobulin consists of two Fabs disulfide bonded at a part of the molecule called the *hinge region*. The hinge region is the part of the Ig molecule that is responsible for the molecular flexibility exhibited by all immunoglobulins. The other major function of immunoglobulins, binding to specific receptors on cells and certain effector proteins such as C1q, is associated with binding site(s) also found in Fc. The Fc region of IgG, one of the classes of immunoglobulin, also interacts with protein A, an immune evasion molecule on the cell walls of *S. aureus*. When bound to protein A, the binding of IgG to host effector molecules such as C1q is sterically interfered with.

The chain structure of immunoglobulins explains neither antibody structural diversity nor antibody binding to antigen. The discovery of variable and constant regions of amino acid sequence formed the basis for understanding both phenomena. Thus, in the L

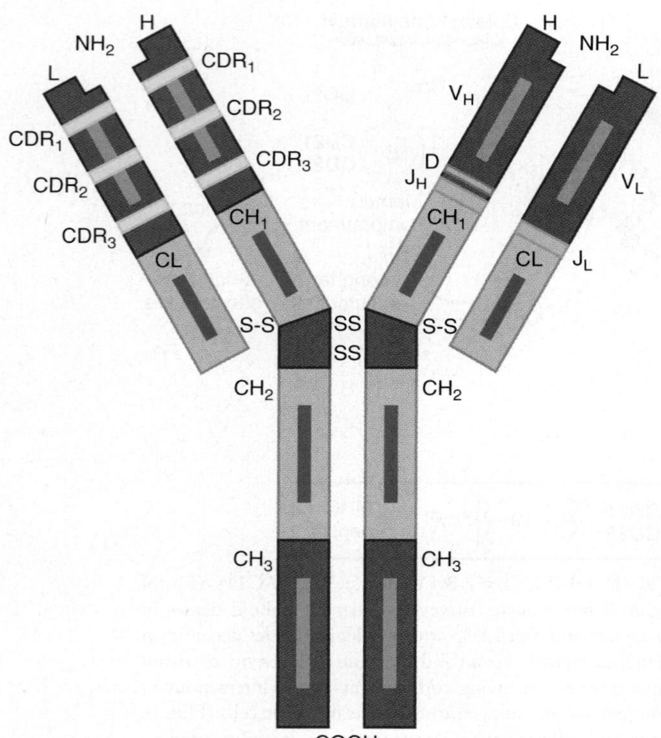

Figure 22-7 DIAGRAMMATIC REPRESENTATION OF THE STRUCTURAL FEATURES OF AN IMMUNOGLOBULIN G (IgG) MOLECULE. NH_2 indicates the NH_2-terminus and COOH the C-terminus. V_H, C_{H1}, V_L, and C_L homology domains are shown as *boxes*. Only the disulfide linkages that join H and L chains are shown. *Left,* Approximate boundaries of the complementarity-determining region (CDR) regions in the V_L and V_H regions. *Right,* Sequences encoded by V_H, D, J_H, V_L, and J_L segments in the V_H and V_L regions.

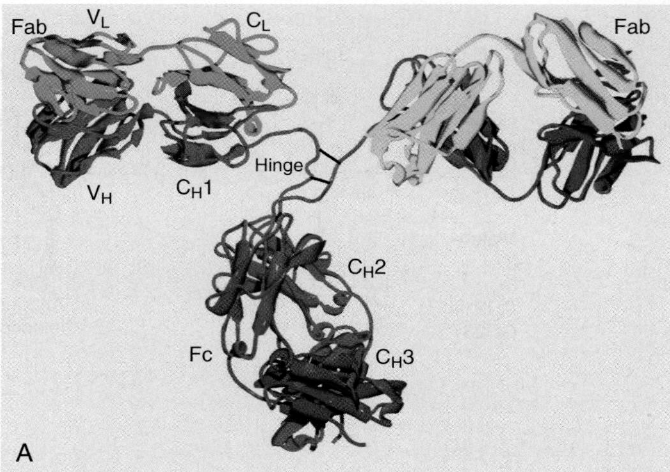

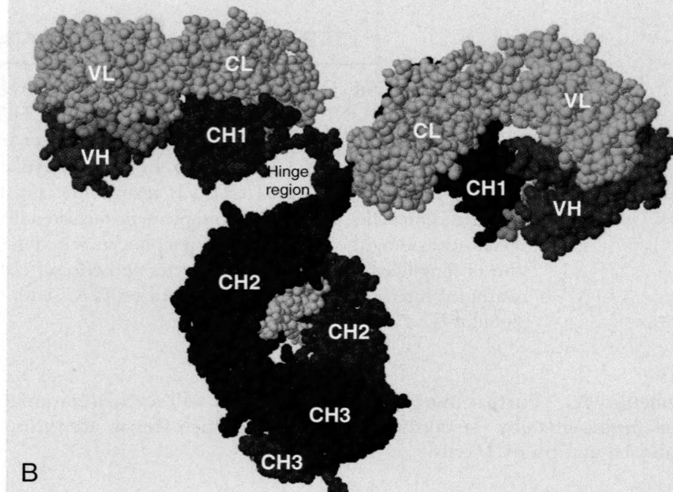

Figure 22-8 X-RAY CRYSTALLOGRAPHIC STRUCTURE OF AN INTACT IgG MOLECULE shown as a ribbon diagram **(A),** or a space-filling model **(B).** The structure is that of a mouse immunoglobulin G2a (IgG2a) monoclonal antibody (protein data base (PDB) file 1IGT) and it was the first intact IgG to have its structure determined. **A,** The two-layer β-sandwich characteristic of the "immunoglobulin fold" is clearly visible within each of the constituent domains of the γ-heavy chains *(blue and red)* and κ-light chains *(green and yellow)*, respectively. *Black lines* indicate the positions of inter-heavy chain disulfide bonds in the hinge region. **B,** The constant domains of the heavy chains and light chains are in various shades of *blue,* and the glycan chain lining a region between apposing C_H2 domains is in *white*. The variable regions are colored according to the genetic segment encoding them. *Dark green* denotes the polypeptide region encoded by the V segment of V_H and *orange* the DJ segment of V_H. *Light green* denotes the polypeptide encoded by the V segment of V_L and *yellow* that encoded by the J segment of V_L. *(**A** modified from http://www.proteopedia.com/wiki/images/4/4a/Opening_1igt.png; **B** from http://www.imgt.org/IMGTeducation/Tutorials/IGandBcells/_UK/3Dstructure/Figure2.html.)*

chain, the 100 or so amino acids in the amino-terminal half of the protein (variable region [V_L]) vary among antibody molecules, but in the second half (constant region [C_L]), there is virtual complete correspondence in amino acids, position for position, to the carboxy-terminus. The H chains exhibit a similar pattern and can be divided likewise into V_H and C_H1, C_H2, and C_H3. Comparison of the amino acid sequence of many V_Ls has revealed that whereas certain parts of the variable region exhibit excess variability, others are less variable. The former regions are called *hypervariable* or *complementarity-determining regions* (CDRs). The latter framework regions function as a structural scaffold to support the CDRs. Antigen binding is mediated by six CDRs, three in each of the V_H and V_L domains. The combining site for antigen is a trough, cavity, or even flat surface composed of parts of the hypervariable regions of both the H and L chains. It is a small region, representing only 25% of the antibody V region. The region that interacts directly with the epitope on the antigen is even smaller and is formed by the association of the CDR regions, each of which consists of approximately 20 amino acids. Thus, the variation in a few amino acids accounts for the specificity and diversity of antibodies with respect to antigen binding.[140]

Immunoglobulins exhibit additional physical heterogeneity, which imparts to each immunoglobulin a special effector function that is reflected in unique biologic properties independent of antigen-binding activity. In the pre-genome era of immunochemical research, heterologous and autologous antisera raised against immunoglobulins were used to classify three types of physical heterogeneity. The first kind is based on the antigenic heterogeneity exhibited by immunoglobulin when it is used as an immunogen in other species. This is called *class* or *isotypic variation*. In humans, five isotypes can be distinguished based on unique antigenic (isotypic) determinants found on the H chain. These are designated by capital Roman letters as IgG, IgM, IgA, IgD, and IgE. The H chain of each class is designated by the lower case Greek letter corresponding to the Roman letter of the class. Thus, the H chain for IgG is γ, for IgM is μ, for IgA is α, for IgD is δ, and for IgE is ε. Some of the immunoglobulin classes are composed of polymers of the basic monomer. In humans, the two antigenic varieties of the L chain are kappa (κ) and lambda (λ). Each Ig has two identical L chains; the κ and λ are shared by all classes. The monomeric form of any immunoglobulin is described by its chain structure. The molecular mass of the immunoglobulins can vary from 150 to 1000 kDa. This variation is attributable to polymerization of the basic monomer form. None of the immunoglobulins are polymeric forms of another class. IgG is the most prevalent, constituting 75% of the total Ig in blood. It is present in normal adults at concentrations of 600 to 1500 mg/dL. IgG is designated $\gamma2\kappa2$ or $\gamma2\lambda2$. It is the only class of Ig that crosses the placenta (Table 22-2).[141]

The isotype IgM is predominantly a pentamer consisting of five monomeric units disulfide linked at the C-terminus of the H chain. Each monomer of IgM is 180 kDa because of the presence of an additional C_H domain, specifically the $C\mu2$ domain, which replaces the hinge segment. The complete protein has a sedimentation coefficient of 19 S, which corresponds to a molecular mass of 850 kDa. IgM is designated $(\mu2\kappa2)_5$ or $(\mu2\lambda2)_5$. IgM also contains a 15-kDa protein called the *J chain*. In the current structural model of IgM, the J chain forms a disulfide-bonded clasp at the C-terminus of two H chains (Fig. 22-9).[138]

The structure of the other isotypes of immunoglobulins are summarized as follows. The isotype IgA has a variable number of monomeric units and is designated $(\alpha2\kappa2)_n$ or $(\alpha2\lambda2)_n$, where n = 2 to 5. Serum IgA constitutes 20% of the total serum immunoglobulin, and 80% of this is monomeric. The remainder exists as polymers, where n = 2 to 5. The other form of IgA is found in external secretions such as saliva, tracheobronchial secretions, colostrum, milk, and genitourinary secretions. Secretory IgA consists of four components: a dimer of two monomeric molecules, a 70-kDa secretory component that binds noncovalently to the IgA dimer, and the 15-kDa J chain that is believed to form a disulfide-bonded clasp at the C-terminus of the H chains (see Fig. 22-9). The isotype IgD has a molecular mass of 180 kDa. Its serum concentration is very low, approximately 3 mg/dL. IgD apparently functions as a membrane molecule, being associated on mature but unstimulated B cells in association with IgM. IgE is the homocytotropic or reaginic Ig and mediates immediate hypersensitivity. It has a molecular mass of 180 kDa and, similar to IgM, has four C domains. The Fc portion of IgE binds strongly to a receptor on mast cells, FcεR, and this is how this immunoglobulin exerts its particular activity. The overall properties of the immunoglobulins are summarized in Table 22-2.

Subclasses of isotypes IgG, IgA, and IgM have been identified. The structural basis for this antigenic heterogeneity is variation in amino acid sequence in the Fc portion of the H chain of a given class. The subclasses of human IgG, called IgG1, IgG2, IgG3, and IgG4, are the best characterized. Each has a slightly different structure, with the most notable differences being in the length of the hinge and in the number of interchain disulfide bonds (see Fig. 22-9 and Table 22-2). IgG1 constitutes 70% of the total IgG and IgG2 20%. IgG3 and IgG4 constitute 8% and 2%, respectively, of the total IgG. The subclasses of IgG exhibit different catabolic rates and bind differentially to cell-associated Fc receptors (FcγR) and to C1q. Specifically, IgG2 does not bind to the FcγRs and IgG4 binds about 10-fold less well than do IgG1 and IgG3. For C1q binding, the rank order of affinities is IgG3 > IgG1 > IgG2 » IgG4. Despite the most obvious sequence differences among the human IgG isotypes being in their hinge regions, studies using engineered domain-swapped chimeric molecules have demonstrated that it is the more subtle amino acid sequence differences within the respective $C\gamma2$ domains that account for the differences in binding to C1q and to the FcγRs. Transport across the placenta is mediated by the Fc-neonatal receptor (FcRn) and for this functional activity IgG2 crosses the placenta slightly more slowly than the other three subclasses. The other known subclasses of Ig isotypes are associated with IgM (IgM1 and IgM2) and IgA (IgA1 and IgA2). The properties and function of these subclasses are less well known.

The second type of variation is called *allotypic variation*. It is attributable to genetically controlled antigenic determinants found on both the H and L chains. Although each human has all immunoglobulin isotypes, an individual has only one form of each allotype on his or her immunoglobulin molecules. Allotypes are codominantly expressed, but an individual B lymphocyte secretes only one of the parental forms. This phenomenon is called *allelic exclusion*.

The third type of variation is attributable to antigenic determinants that are unique to each particular antibody molecule produced by an individual. These markers are called *idiotypic determinants,* and they are associated with a single species of antibody. The antiidiotypic antibodies that recognize a particular idiotype will not react with any

Table 22-2 Human Immunoglobulins: Properties and Functions

	IgG1	IgG2	IgG3	IgG4	IgM	IgA1	IgA2	IgD	IgE
H chain	$\gamma1$	$\gamma2$	$\gamma3$	$\gamma4$	μ	$\alpha1$	$\alpha2$	δ	ε
Molecular weight (kDa)	146	146	170	146	970	160	160	194	199
Molecular weight of H chain (kDa)	51	51	60	51	65	56	52	70	73
Number of H chain domains	4	4	4	4	5	4	4	6	5
Carbohydrate (%)	2-3	2-3	2-3	2-3	12	7-11	7-11	9-14	12
Hinge inter-heavy chain disulfides	2	5	11	2	NA	2	1	1	NA
Serum concentration (mg/dL)	900	300	100	50	150	300	50	3	0.005
Classical pathway complement fixation	++	+	+++	+	+++	–	–	–	
Alternative pathway complement activity			–			+	+		–
Placental transfer	+	+	+	+	+				–
Binding to mononuclear cells	+	–	+					–	–
Binding to mast cells and to basophils	–	–	–	–	–			–	+++
Reaction with protein A from *Staphylococcus aureus*	+	+	–	+	–			–	–
Half-life (days)	21	20	7	21	10	6	6	3	2
Distribution (% intravascular)	45	45	45	45	80	42	42	75	50
Fractional catabolic rate (% Intravascular pool catabolized/day)	7	7	17	7	9	25	25	37	71
Synthetic rate (mg/kg/day)	33	33	33	33	33	24	24	0.4	0.002

Data from Golub, ES: *Immunology: A synthesis.* Sunderland, Mass, 1987, Sinaur.

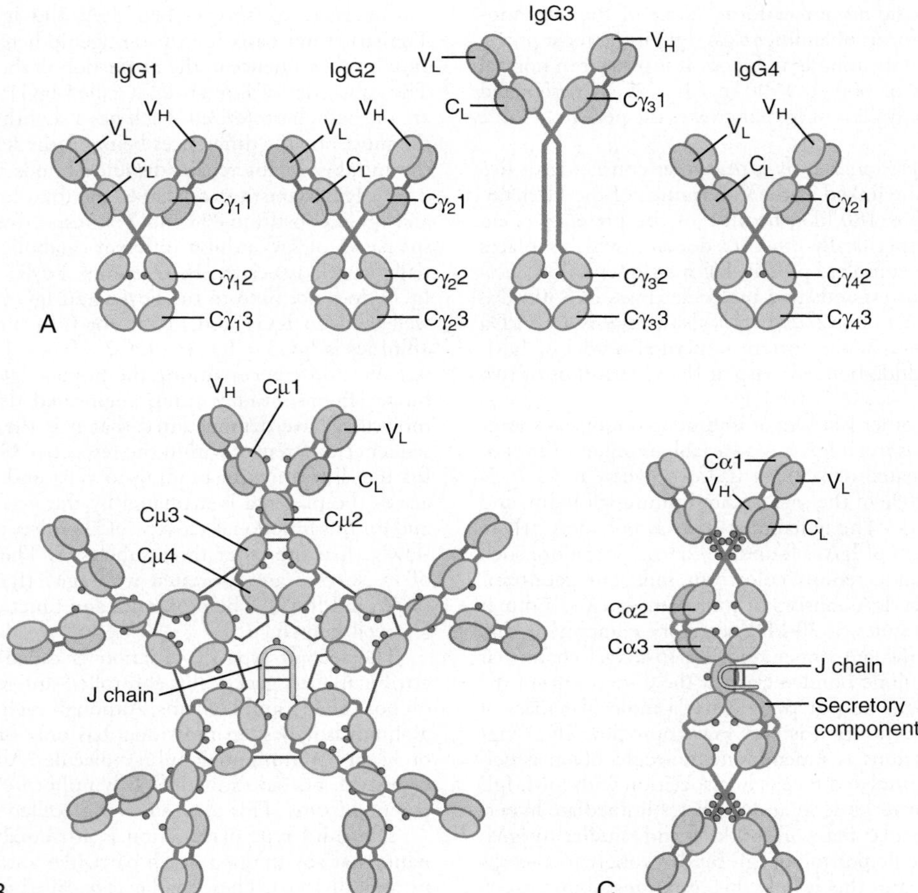

Figure 22-9 A, Structure of the four subclasses of human immunoglobulin G (IgG). Constant region domains are indicated by C_nN, where n is the subclass and N is the domain. **B,** Structure of human IgM. The J chain is shown in the model as disulfide linked to two μ-chains. Other models have been proposed. *Filled circles* indicate carbohydrate. **C,** Structure of human secretory IgA. This model shows the possible arrangement of the two IgA monomers in relation to the secretory component and J chain. As the IgA molecule passes through the epithelial cells, the secretory components are synthesized and attached covalently to the Fc domain of the α-chains that have previously been joined to the J chain with disulfide links. Light chains are shown in *blue,* heavy chains in *purple,* disulfide bonds as *gray lines,* and carbohydrates as *red circles. (From Turner M:* Molecules which recognize antigens. *In Roitt DK, editors:* Immunology, *London, 1989, Gower, p 51.)*

other immunoglobulins in the donor other than the purified antibody that was used to raise the antiidiotype antibody. In most cases, the immune response to an antigen results in a mixture of several antibodies, each of which has identical binding specificity but distinct idiotypic determinants. Thus, there can be many idiotypes for a given antigenic specificity, which has been interpreted as being a reflection of physical heterogeneity in or near the antibody combining site, for example, in the variable region domains. In some species (notably certain strains of mice), the response to antigen results in a predominant idiotype on all antibodies of a given specificity. Because this quality is inherited, the idiotypes are called major, cross-reactive, or public. Some public idiotypes have been found in certain species (again, most notably mice) to be genetically linked to allotypes. Three kinds of antiidiotype antibodies have been described, those that function as an internal image of the original antigen by mimicking the antigen structure, those that recognize antibody combining site-associated idiotypes, and those that are specific for framework-associated determinants. The internal image antiidiotypic antibodies are of clinical interest.

Every immunoglobulin is a glycoprotein, and the critical glycan is attached to the H chain in the Fc domain at the conserved asparagine at position 297 (Asn297). This single, N-linked glycan is essential for maintaining an open conformation of the two H chains as it lines the opposing faces of the pair of C_H2 subdomains of Fc (see Fig. 22-8, *B*). The core structure of the N-linked glycan is a biantennary heptapolysaccharide containing *N*-acetylglucosamine plus additional sugars (fucose, galactose), with bisecting *N*-acetylglucosamine and sialic acid variably present. Effector functions depend on the Asn297-linked glycan and are influenced by its structure.[142] Deglycosylated IgG does not interact effectively with Fcγ receptors (FcγRs) and cannot support in vivo effector responses, including antibody-dependent cell-mediated cytotoxicity or complement-dependent cytotoxicity.[143] Individual glycoforms contribute to modulating inflammatory responses and have disease association. For example, glycosylation differs in patients with rheumatoid arthritis[144] or vasculitis[145] compared with the normal population. Addition of sialic acid to the N-linked glycan reduces binding of IgG to FcγRs and reduces in vivo cytotoxicity. Regulation of sialylation of IgG contributes to the antiinflammatory homeostasis of serum IgG. Upon antigen challenge, reduced sialic acid–IgG can mediate immune clearance and protective immunity through interaction with subclass-specific FcγRs. Kaneko et al[146] have proposed that the protective effect of intravenous immunoglobulin (IVIg) therapy is attributable to the minor fraction of sialylated IgG species in the total IVIg preparation and that the high doses required (1-3 g/kg body weight) for antiinflammatory activity could be significantly reduced by increasing the percentage of sialylated IgG.

Therapeutic Use

Immunoglobulin G was one of the first plasma proteins prepared in a purified state as a therapeutic drug for treatment of clinical disorders. It remains, along with albumin and α-proteinase inhibitor, the most widely used therapeutic plasma derivative and is currently the major plasma product on the global market. Polyvalent human immunoglobulin preparations have been used to reconstitute humoral immunity in agammaglobulinemic patients for more than 3 decades. Until 25 years ago, intramuscular treatment was the mode of administration. Intramuscular preparations caused severe adverse reactions when injected intravenously.[147-149] The most serious were anaphylactoid reactions and were probably complement mediated. Efforts to reduce anticomplementary activity and the prekallikrein activator activity were initiated in the early 1980s and safer IVIg preparations became available.

Intravenous immunoglobulin is prepared from pooled human plasma pools of 3000 to 50,000 L. The World Health Organization requires more than 1000 donors per lot. The majority of IVIg is produced by cold ethanol fractionation procedures,[150,151] with filtration and polishing chromatography steps added to increase yield and decrease pathogen transmission.[152,153] Gamunex (Talecris Biotherapeutics) is produced from cold ethanol fractionation followed by caprylate precipitation and chromatograpy.[152,154] This is the first significant change in commercial IVIg production in 20 years. IVIg contains concentrated IgG with normal plasma ratios of IgG1 and IgG2, lower percentages of IgG3 and IgG4, and only trace amounts of IgA and IgM. It retains the antibody repertoire, reflecting the combined immunologic experience of the donors.[155,156] Hyperimmune IVIg is purified from donor plasma selected for high titer toward a specific pathogen. Prophylaxis for cytomegalovirus and respiratory syncytial virus are two approved clinical applications.[156,157]

The availability of safe IVIg preparations and the fortuitous observation that IgG treatment of a patient with thrombocytopenia and IgG deficiency increased the patient's platelet count began an intense period of clinical use of IVIg for indications other than primary immune deficiency. In 1990, the National Institutes of Health sponsored a Consensus Development Conference, which produced the first consensus statement on IVIg clinical indications.[158] As a result, six disease indications—primary immunodeficiency, Kawasaki syndrome, chronic lymphocytic leukemia, human immunodeficiency virus (HIV) infections during childhood to prevent infections, BM transplantation to prevent graft-versus-host disease or bacterial infections in adults, and idiopathic purpura—were approved by the Food and Drug Administration (FDA) for labeling and marketing. The licensed indications remain unchanged, but off-label uses include more than 100 conditions (for further discussion, see Chapter 117).[159,160]

The experience with IVIg clinical development has been largely empirical and anecdotal. The mechanisms for patient benefit or harm are poorly understood, especially for high-dose immune modulation therapy. Various known and some yet undiscovered functions of immunoglobulins in immune homeostasis may contribute, including modulation of the function and expression of Fc receptors, interaction with complement and cytokine systems, antiidiotypic antibodies, and regulation of T-cell and B-cell function.[161-163]

Many effects of IVIg are explained by mechanisms beyond antigenic recognition of pathogens. IVIg preparations contain up to 30% dimers composed of idiotype–antiidiotype antibody pairs. These dimers appear to be very effective as a sink for activated complement and can inhibit complement activation.[164] Benefit for treatment of immune thrombocytopenia purpura seems to be mediated by Fc-receptor blockade of the reticuloendothelial cell salvage receptor, also known as FcRn, combined with an antiidiotypic neutralization of antiplatelet antibody that together eliminates antiplatelet antibody from the blood. Other indications of antibody neutralization can be seen in IVIg treatment of myasthenia gravis. The dramatic success of IVIg in treating Kawasaki syndrome may be attributable to several mechanisms, including antiidiotypic neutralization of antiendothelial antibodies, inhibition of cytokine production and function, and elimination of causative superantigens.[165,166] IVIg inhibits B-cell activation and autoantibody production by enhancing $CD8^+$ suppressor T-cell function. Cell-mediated immunity also is affected.[161] As mentioned earlier, Kaneko et al[146] ascribe much of the effect of IVIg to a small fraction of it which is sialylated. A 2011 report from this group suggests a mechanism for the way which sialylated IgG in IVIg downmodulates the inflammatory response of the immune system.[167] They suggest that the sialylated IgG Fc region binds to DC-SIGN, a molecule on the surface of "regulatory" myeloid cells, including DCs. In response to DC-SIGN ligation by sialylated IgG, these cells secrete the cytokine IL-33, which in turn stimulates IL-4 production by basophils. IL-4 upregulates the synthesis of the "inhibitory" class of FcγR on effector macrophages, namely FcγRIIB. Because ligation of this class of FcγR by immune complexes actually results in the recruitment of regulatory phosphatases, which shut down intracellular signaling cascades, the net effect is to increase the activation threshold required to initiate inflammation by these effector cells.

Adverse Events Related to Intravenous Immunoglobulin Infusion

Adverse events associated with IVIg can be characterized as (1) early systemic events, (2) infectious disease transfer, and (3) high-dose treatment-related adverse effects.[148]

Early Systemic Events

Common transfusion-related early events are listed in Table 22-3. Most early events are self-limiting and infusion rate dependent. Premedication with steroids, aspirin, or other nonsteroidal antiinflammatory drugs often decreases symptoms. Prophylaxis with propranolol can be effective for induced migraine. Aseptic meningitis is a rare early event, is observed 1 to 2 days postinfusion, is unrelated to infusion rate, and can be treated with intravenous steroids and analgesics.[148,168]

The frequency of reported adverse events varies considerably, ranging from 10% to 85%.[148,158,169-171] There are many reasons for this

Table 22-3 Early Systemic Adverse Events Associated With Intravenous Immunoglobulin Infusion

Fever	Rash or urticaria
Chills	Chest tightness
Sore throat	Dyspnea
Face flush	Wheezing
Tachycardia	Low or high blood pressure
Palpitations	Shock
Lumbar pain	Anxiety
Abdominal pain	Nervousness
Nausea	Headache
Vomiting	Migraine
Shaking	Anaphylaxis
Fatigue	Malaise
Myalgia	Leukopenia

high variability in reporting, including (1) differences in product,[153,169,172] (2) infusion rate, (3) dose and frequency of dosing, (4) patient population, and (5) relative experience of patient and physician. Both patients and physicians become steeled to the adverse events, and because incidents are not life threatening and often respond to prophylaxis medication, they are ignored as "normal." Nonetheless, these events are common and affect health and quality of life of patients.[159,169]

Infectious Disease Transfer

A few early preparations of IVIg transmitted hepatitis C virus. Manufacturers have added viral inactivation and partitioning steps, and current licensed products are safe with respect to HIV, hepatitis C virus, hepatitis B virus, and other bloodborne pathogens (see Chapter 117).[173] The industry has responded to the threat of prions with process validation,[170,174] donor screening, donor testing, inventory management (look back), and plasma pool testing.

High-Dose Treatment-Related Adverse Events

Intravenous immunoglobulin treatment for immune modulation of neurologic diseases requires doses of 1 to 2 kg/kg body weight or two to five times the dose recommended for replacement therapy. Adverse events with high-dose administration include those listed in Table 22-3 and occasionally thromboembolic events, renal complications, and anemia.[148,171,175-178] Thromboembolic events include deep venous thrombosis, pulmonary embolism, myocardial infarction, and stroke. Thromboembolic events and renal failure seem to be independent of infusion rate. The cause of thromboembolic events is not known. Dalakas[179] has suggested that increased serum viscosity plays a role. Factor XIa has also been identified in IVIg preparations.[172] Factor XIa could directly lead to shortening of coagulation time and risk of thrombosis. Renal complications are rare but result in high morbidity and mortality. Whether IgG, contaminants, or excipients are responsible is not clear. Of the 88 renal adverse events reported to the FDA, 90% were stabilized with sucrose.[148,168] Whether the adverse events observed with IVIg treatment of neurologic diseases are related to a preexisting medical condition or the high doses required for treatment is not clear.

Monoclonal Antibody Therapy

Monoclonal antibody technology as described in 1975 by Kohler and Milstein[180] is now well established for the production of diagnostic and therapeutic mAb. Despite early enthusiasm and much research and development effort, the development of clinical mAb was frustrated for 20 years by reports of severe toxicity and poor clinical efficacy. Only one mAb, OKT3, an anti-CD3, was licensed for clinical use before 1994. Over the past 15 years, the situation has changed. mAb products constitute as much as 25% of new biologicals in clinical development, with a first in humans to regulatory approval success rate of 27%, which compares very favorably with the 11% rate for small-molecule drugs.[181,182] Table 22-4 lists the more than 22 mAbs that have received FDA approval as of early 2009.

The list includes antibodies for diverse clinical conditions, including oncology, chronic inflammatory conditions, solid organ transplantation, infectious disease, and cardiovascular medicine. Approved antibody therapy includes unmodified mAb, radioimmunoconjugates, immunodrug conjugates, and antibody fragments. More than 150 mAbs are in clinical development, with at least 33 in clinical trials for conditions, including colorectal cancer, melanoma, postmenopausal osteoporosis, cutaneous T-cell lymphoma, rheumatoid arthritis, and respiratory syncytial virus infection.[182] Part of the progress is attributable to the advent of genetic engineering, which has allowed the production of "humanized" mAbs. Human–mouse chimerized Ab with limited mouse determinants or fully human mAb now are produced by DNA technology or with transgenic mice. The humanization of mAbs provides some protection from the patient's immune system, prolonging the circulation half-life from less than 24 hours for murine mAbs in humans and approaching the 21-day half-life of native IgG. Increased circulation time is partly attributable to the reduction in immune reactivity and subsequent opsonization of mAbs but also because human but not murine IgG is recycled by FcRn on human epithelial cells.[183,184]

ReoPro (abciximab) is a chimeric Fab fragment directed to glycoprotein IIb/IIIa and is one of the early successful clinical mAbs (approved for marketing in 1994). ReoPro prevents thrombus formation in patients undergoing procedures such as percutaneous coronary intervention.[185] Another example of a chimeric mAb (IgG1) is Remicade (infliximab), which is an anti–TNF-α. Remicade was approved in 1998 for treatment of Crohn disease and in 1999 for treatment of rheumatoid arthritis.[186,187]

Monoclonal antibodies for cancer therapy are divided into two stratagems. "Naked" mAbs target specific tumor-related antigens or cell receptors to recruit the immune system or to modify the growth of tumor cells. Examples of approved naked mAbs are Rituxan (rituximab),[188] an anti-CD20 approved for non-Hodgkin lymphoma, and Herceptin (trastuzumab),[189] an anti-HER2 approved for advanced breast cancer. To date, most naked mAb candidates have been disappointing, and the most efficacious are used as adjuvant therapy. The most promising naked mAbs may not directly affect the tumor cell but instead may modify the patient's immune response to the tumor. An example of immune-modulating mAbs in development is anti-CD152,[190] which may modulate the way T cells respond to cancer cells.

The second strategy is to attach or conjugate an antitumor agent to an antitumor mAb. The mAbs deliver the toxic agent to the tumor or tumor cells in an attempt to obliterate the cancer cells. Both radioactive and chemical toxins have been conjugated to a variety of tumor-specific mAbs. Two mAbs that deliver radioactivity directly to the tumor are Zevalin (ibritumomab tiuxetan) and Bexxar (tositumomab), which were approved in 2002 and 2003, respectively, for B-cell non-Hodgkin lymphoma.[191,192] Many immunotoxins have been developed but without much clinical success. Mylotarg (gemtuzumab ozogamicin), an anti-CD33 mAb, is approved for myelogenous leukemia when chemotherapy is not effective or appropriate.[193]

A listing of approved mAb therapy for cancer can be found online on the American Cancer Society's web page (at www.cancer.org) under Monoclonal Antibody Therapy (Passive Immunotherapy). For a review of therapeutic MAbs, see Carter.[194]

Finally, the humanized anti-C5 mAb Soliris (eculizumab) provides an interesting tie-together between the complement section of this chapter and the present section on therapeutic monoclonal antibodies. Soliris binds to C5 in a way that prevents its cleavage by C5 convertases of either the classical or APs. As such, it not only blocks the generation of C5a, the most powerful of the complement inflammatory agents, but also prevents formation of the MAC. At the same time, its activity does not grossly impair the opsonic function of complement against most pathogenic microorganisms, the exception being *N. meningitidis,* whose clearance depends on the activity of the lytic complement pathway. Fortunately, there is a vaccine for this microorganism that can be administered prophylactically before commencement of treatment with Soliris. In 2007, Soliris received FDA approval for treatment of paroxysmal nocturnal hemoglobinuria (PNH), a very rare complement-mediated hemolytic disease resulting from the absence of the MAC regulator CD59 on all host cells, particularly on erythrocytes, which, unlike nucleated host cells, have no way of repairing a MAC-generated membrane lesion. Biweekly administered Soliris has proven to be extremely effective in keeping PNH patients symptom free.[195] In addition to treatment of PNH, beginning in 2009, there have been an ever-increasing number of case reports in the literature in which Soliris is being used off-label for the effective management of aHUS, which as discussed earlier, is a disease caused by dysregulation of the alternative complement pathway.[196] The problem, however, is cost, being approximately $400,000 per year because of the very high development and manufacturing costs, contrasted with a very small market owing to the rarity of both PNH and aHUS. AMD is another AP dysregulation disease that in a mouse model of the wet form of human AMD, has been shown to be C5-,

Table 22-4 Monoclonal Antibodies Approved by the Food and Drug Administration for Therapeutic Use*

Trade Name	Company	Target	Source	Year	Indication
Orthoclone	Ortho Biotech, Inc. (subsidiary of J&J)	CD3	All rodent	1986	Transplantation rejection
ReoPro	Centocor, Inc. (subsidiary of Johnson & Johnson) and Eli Lilly	GPIIb/IIIa	Chimeric	1994	High risk angioplasty
Rituxan	Biogen Idec and Genentech, Inc.	CD20	Chimeric	1994	Non-Hodgkin lymphoma, rheumatoid arthritis
REMICADE	Centocor, Inc. (subsidiary of Johnson & Johnson)	TNF-α	Chimeric	1998	Crohn disease
Simulect	Novartis	CD25	Chimeric	1998	Transplantation rejection
Synagis	Medimmune	RSV F protein	Humanized	1998	RSV infection
Zenapax	Hoffmann-La Roche Inc., Protein Design Labs	CD25	Humanized	1997	Transplantation rejection
Herceptin	Genentech	HER-2	Humanized	1998	Breast cancer
Mylotarg	UCB and Wyeth	CD33	Humanized	2000	Acute myeloid leukemia
Campath	Millenium Pharmaceuticals, Inc. and Berlex Laboratories, Inc.	CD52	Humanized	2001	Chronic lymphotic leukemia, T-cell lymphoma
Zevalin	Idec Pharmaceuticals Corporation	CD20	Murine with yttrium90 or indium-111	2002	Non-Hodgkin lymphoma
HUMIRA	Abbott Laboratories/Cambridge Antibody Technology	TNF-α	Human	2002	Inflammatory diseases—mostly autoimmune disorders such as rheumatoid arthritis, psoriadic arthritis, Crohn disease
Bexxar	Corixa Corp. and GlaxoSmithKline	CD20	Murine covalently bound to iodine-131	2003	Non-Hodgkin lymphoma
Xolair	Genentech, Tanox, Inc., Novartis Pharmaceuticals	IgE	Humanized	2003	Severe (allergic) asthma
Avastin	Genentech	VEGF	Humanized	2004	Metastatic colorectal cancer, non–small cell lung cancer, metastatic breast cancer
TYSABRI	Biogen Idec and Elan Corp.	α4 subunit of α4β1	Humanized	2004	Multiple sclerosis, Chron disease
Erbitux	Merck KG aA/Bristol-Myers Squibb/ImClone Systems	EGFR	Chimeric	2004	Colorectal cancer, head and neck cancer
Vectibix	Amgen	EGFR	Human	2006	Metastatic colorectal carcinoma
LUCENTIS	Genentech	VEGFA	Humanized Fab	2006	Wet macular degeneration
Soliris	Alexion Pharmaceuticals, Inc.	C5	Humanized	2007	Paroxysmal nocturnal hemoglobinuria
CIMZIA	UCB	TNF-α	Humanized (Fab)	2008	Crohn disease, rheumatoid arthritis
Simponi	Centocor (subsidiary of Johnson & Johnson)	TNF-α	Human	2009	Rheumatoid and psoriatic arthritis, active ankylosing spondylitis

From http://www.actip.org/pages/library/Table_Monoclonal_Antibodies.pdf.
EGFR, Epidermal growth factor receptor; *GP*, glycoprotein; *HER-2*, human epidermal growth factor receptor 2; *RSV*, respiratory syncytial virus; *TNF*, tumor necrosis factor; *VEGF*, vascular endothelial growth factor.
*In total, 22 monoclonal antibodies were approved by the U.S. Food and Drug Administration for therapeutic use as of early 2009. The table gives a chronologic listing.

and indeed MAC-dependent.[197] Unlike PNH and aHUS, AMD is not a rare disease, and thus if Soliris were to be an effective therapeutic, the cost of the treatment would likely drop to the range of other monoclonal antibodies needed for continuous therapy (~$40,000-$100,000 per year). Very recently, a patient enrolled in a clinical trial of Soliris use for a neurologic condition, who also happened to have symptoms of the wet form of AMD (i.e., macular edema and widespread exudates), was found to have a significant improvement in his vision, as well as resolution of his exudates, shortly after the commencement of the treatment with Soliris.[198] This observation is encouraging but of course needs to be confirmed in a proper clinical trial.

SUGGESTED READINGS

Ahearn JM, Fischer MB, Croix D, et al: Disruption of the Cr2 locus results in a reduction in B-1a cells and in an impaired B cell response to T-dependent antigen. *Immunity* 4:251, 1996.

Bayary J, Dasgupta S, Misra N, et al: Intravenous immunoglobulin in autoimmune disorders: An insight into the immunoregulatory mechanisms. *Int Immunopharm* 6:528, 2006.

Carroll MC: The complement system in regulation of adaptive immunity. *Nat Immunol* 5:981, 2004.

Carter RH, Fearon DT: CD19: Lowering the threshold for antigen receptor stimulation of B lymphocytes. *Science* 256:105, 1992.

Dalakas MC: Mechanisms of action of IVIG and therapeutic considerations in the treatment of acute and chronic demyelinating neuropathies. *Neurology* 59:S13, 2002.

Fischer MB, Goerg S, Shen L, et al: Dependence of germinal center B cells on expression of CD21/CD35 for survival. *Science* 280:582, 1998.

Gros P, Milder FJ, Janssen BJ: Complement driven by conformational changes. *Nat Rev Immunol* 8:48, 2008.

Helmy KY, Gorgani NN, Kljavin NM, et al: CRIg: A macrophage complement receptor required for phagocytosis of circulating pathogens. *Cell* 124:915, 2006.

Hopken UE, Lu B, Gerard NP, et al: The C5a chemoattractant receptor mediates mucosal defence to infection. *Nature* 383:86, 1996.

Jordan SC, Vo AA, Peng A, et al: Intravenous gammaglobulin (IVIG): A novel approach to improve transplant rates and outcomes in highly HLA-sensitized patients. *Am J Transplant* 6:459, 2006.

Kang YS, Do Y, Lee HK, et al: A dominant complement fixation pathway for pneumococcal polysaccharides initiated by SIGN-R1 interacting with C1q. *Cell* 125:47, 2006.

Kelsoe G: Life and death in germinal centers (redux). *Immunity* 4:107, 1996.

Kemper C, Chan AC, Green JM, et al: Activation of human CD4+ cells with CD3 and CD46 induces a T-regulatory cell 1 phenotype. *Nature* 421:388, 2003.

Kopf M, Abel B, Gallimore A, et al: Complement component C3 promotes T-cell priming and lung migration to control acute influenza virus infection. *Nat Med* 8:373, 2002.

Minard S, Papa SM, Campiglio M, et al: Biologic and therapeutic role of HER2 in cancer. *Oncogene* 29:6570, 2003.

Thiel S, Vorup-Jensen T, Stover CM: A second serine protease associated with mannan-binding lectin that activates complement. *Nature* 386:506, 1997.

van den Elsen JM, Isenman DE: A crystal structure of the complex between human complement receptor 2 and its ligand C3d. *Science* 332:608, 2011.

For complete list of references log on to www.expertconsult.com.

CHAPTER 23

TOLERANCE AND AUTOIMMUNITY

Mark J. Shlomchik

The immune system must balance the capacity to respond to foreign antigens and the need not to respond to self-antigens. A complex and multilayered approach has evolved to successfully handle this problem. However, autoimmune diseases, in which this balance is upset, are remarkably common in the population. The diversity and variable severity of such diseases most likely reflects the various approaches the immune system takes to regulate antiself responses and thereby the various points at which this multilayered system can break down. The normal functions that may prevent autoimmune disease are collectively known as *self-tolerance mechanisms*.

Autoimmune diseases are relevant to hematology at several levels. Autoimmune hemolytic anemia (AIHA) and idiopathic thrombocytopenic purpura are syndromes in which spontaneous autoimmunity to formed blood components may require transfusion support that is rendered difficult because of the presence of autoantibodies. Some cases of aplastic anemia may also fall into this category. Autoantibodies to red blood cells (RBCs), whether pathogenic or not, are often problematic in terms of typing and screening. Another class of diseases are those induced by transfusion but that are nonetheless autoimmune in nature: these include posttransfusion purpura (PTP)[1-3] and possibly AIHA associated with transfused thallasemia.[4-6] Finally, graft-versus-host disease (GVHD), a common complication of allogeneic stem cell transplantation, although not a classical autoimmune disease, shares many features of autoimmune syndromes.[7,8]

An important principle in understanding the etiology of autoimmune diseases is that no special mechanisms, cells, antibody types, or reactions are specific to autoimmune diseases. Rather, the pathogenesis involves the inappropriate or dysregulated triggering of the normal mechanisms of immunity. Therefore, an understanding of autoimmune disease induction and pathogenesis requires a grounding in the basic immune cell functions and interactions, which can be found in the preceding chapters.

SELF-REACTIVE LYMPHOCYTES: ORIGIN AND CONTROL

Origins

Inevitably, autoreactive lymphocytes are generated as a consequence of the fact that B-cell receptor (BCR) and T-cell receptor (TCR) genes are encoded in pieces that rearrange in the DNA of precursor lymphocytes to ultimately form a complete gene. This process allows for many possible gene segment combinations (e.g., 4000 different ones for the human Ig heavy chain alone), and in addition, small deletions and random additions at the sites where the pieces are joined together create additional diversity. There are two implications of this process for self-tolerance. First, it is impossible to prevent the assembly of a self-reactive receptor by filtering these out of the germline gene repertoire. Second, a developing lymphocyte cannot be considered autoreactive until the assembly process is complete and the BCR or TCR is expressed. Thus, autoreactive lymphocytes are produced every day, and it is at this key developmental stage—when the BCR or TCR is first expressed by the cell—that the immune system can first eliminate these potentially harmful cells. For B cells, this occurs in the bone marrow (BM), the primary central lymphoid organ (Fig. 23-1); for T cells, it occurs in the thymus. The process is thus termed *central tolerance*.

Regulation: Central Tolerance

Clonal Deletion

The classical experiments of Pike and Nossal were the first to demonstrate that developing autoreactive B cells can be eliminated in the BM.[9-11] The details of this process remained murky until the Goodnow and Nemazee groups each developed a BCR transgenic mouse system for the study of self-tolerance.[12-14] These mice have been genetically altered to carry the preformed immunoglobulin (Ig) variable (V) genes that encode a specific autoantibody. Mice that have undergone this genetic transfer are termed *transgenic,* and the gene that is transferred is termed the *transgene* (Fig. 23-2). The presence of this preformed transgene short circuits and prevents the normal rearrangement process at the natural Ig gene loci. Thus, each B cell in the animal expresses only the transgene and has the same specificity. By choosing a target antigen that is carried by only some strains of mice (e.g., the polymorphic major histocompatibility complex class I genes used by Nemazee), it is possible to render the transgenic B cells autoreactive when crossed onto one strain (Fig. 23-3) but not autoreactive in a different strain. The results of such systems were dramatic. A complete loss or deletion of the B cells was demonstrated in the strain of mice that had the autoantigen, but perfectly good expression of the B cells was observed when the autoantigen was absent. This provided clear proof of B-cell clonal deletion. Furthermore, it was shown that this deletion occurred at the immature B-cell stage, just when the cells first express their BCR.[15-17] It has been since discovered that deletion is just the final step in controlling autoreactive B cells.[15,17-19] B cells that have completed H- and L-chain rearrangement and then recognize self-antigen while still immature in the BM may actually undergo a second round of V gene rearrangement. This most likely occurs at the L-chain loci, which are particularly suited to secondary V to J rearrangements. This process has been termed *receptor editing.* Evidently, a cell has a certain period of time in which to produce a second L-chain rearrangement that will inactivate the cell's self-reactivity. If this does not occur, the cell fails to mature and is eventually eliminated. The physiologic role of the editing process is still unclear, but it could represent a way to maximize the efficiency of B-cell generation while still maintaining an effective filter against strongly self-reactive B cells.

More recently, evidence has been accumulating that autoreactive B cells are similarly filtered out of the human repertoire. Polyreactive and antinuclear B cells are progressively eliminated during the progression of B-cell development; however, even in healthy individuals, some B cells with detectable autoreactivity remain among mature B cells.[20]

Clonal Anergy

Another type of self-tolerance mechanism was also revealed by similar experiments in mice. This form, clonal anergy, involves inactivation of the self-reactive cell but not its elimination.[10,14] Such B cells remain in the peripheral lymphoid circulation, albeit with a shorter lifespan than normal B cells. In addition, these cells have a lower amount of

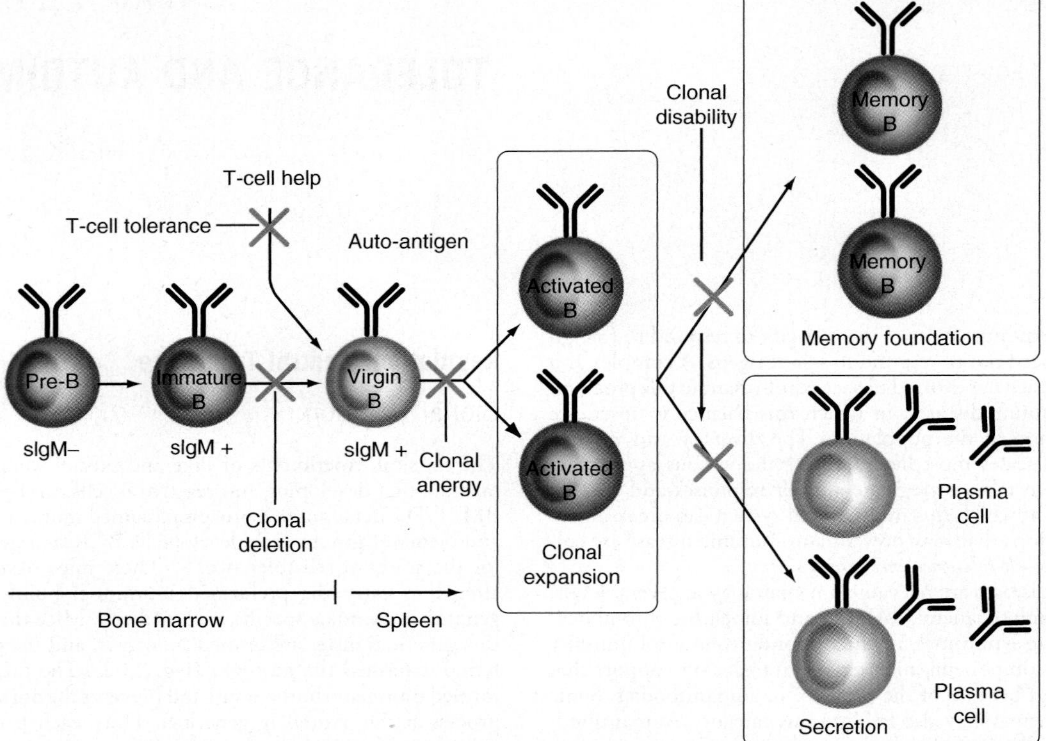

Figure 23-1 STAGES AT WHICH SELF-TOLERANCE CAN BLOCK B-CELL DEVELOPMENT. *Arrows* indicate the normal pathway of development. *X* indicates where these differentiation steps can be interrupted for self-reactive B cells as a consequence of encountering self-antigen. Each X is labeled with the type of self-tolerance it represents. The clonal disability steps are somewhat more hypothetical than the earlier steps. See text for details. *sIgM*, Surface immunoglobulin M.

surface Ig (sIg) and, moreover, are much less capable of sensing the presence of antigen when the sIg receptor is triggered. This second form of B-cell tolerance, demonstrated dramatically through the use of Ig transgenic mice, was also anticipated in the experiments of Pike and Nossal.[10] The physiologic advantage of maintaining these anergic cells is unclear. They can be activated by strong stimulation under certain conditions; thus, it has been suggested that they are maintained as a secondary repertoire to maintain greater B-cell diversity and thus better protect against a broader spectrum of pathogens. However, the presence of these cells also raises a danger that they may be activated by self-antigens as well, which could represent a source of autoantibodies. Indeed, it has been suggested that autoantibody-secreting B cells can arise by the activation of anergic B cells.

Clonal deletion, receptor editing, and clonal anergy are often referred to as "central" self-tolerance because they can occur in the central lymphopoietic organs and act on immature lymphocytes that have just expressed their antigen receptors. Central tolerance is probably most important in purging or controlling very high-affinity antiself lymphocytes.

Tolerance of Memory B Cells

Fig. 23-1 indicates that there are yet other stages of B-cell development at which one could imagine that self-tolerance should occur. The most important of these is development of memory B cells, the long-lasting cells that harbor the ability of the immune system to respond better and faster to antigens that have already been encountered once. An important and unique process occurs during memory cell development—the genes that encode the antibody receptor molecule undergo a process of random mutation.[21-23] This process is thought to provide mutants with an increased affinity for the immunizing antigen, and in fact, the secondary immune response is known to be of higher affinity. However, a side effect of any random process, just as in the receptor rearrangement itself, is the potential to create novel antiself specificities.[24,25] Thus, many have postulated that there should be a screening of cells for self-reactivity during memory B-cell development.[26-28] In fact, some evidence suggests this process exists, but it is much more elusive than clonal deletion or clonal anergy. Moreover, some new evidence indicates that the normal human IgG memory B-cell compartment does contain autoreactive B cells that nonetheless do not normally cause disease.[29]

T Cells

In many respects, self-tolerance for T cells is similar to that for B cells; both deletion and anergy exist.[30-34] The principle differences reflect the basic differences in B- and T-cell development. Deletion for T cells occurs in the thymus (where TCR gene rearrangement occurs), not in the BM. In addition, the self-antigens for T cells consist of self-peptides, just as the foreign antigens for T cells are foreign peptides. One key implication of these differences is that it may be difficult to tolerize developing T cells to peptides derived from proteins that are not expressed in the thymus. Over the past 10 years, data have emerged supporting the concept that many peripheral tissue proteins are "ectopically" expressed in the thymus, presumably to promote self-tolerance. These self-proteins are expressed in specialized thymic epithelial cells concentrated in the thymic medulla. Strikingly, a gene known as Aire (autoimmune regulator) was found to be required for the expression of a large number of these peripheral tissue proteins. This gene is nonfunctional in humans with the autoimmune polyglandular syndrome-type I (APS-1, also known as APECED); people with the condition have autoimmune-based failure of multiple endocrine organs as well as autoimmunity in a variety of target tissues

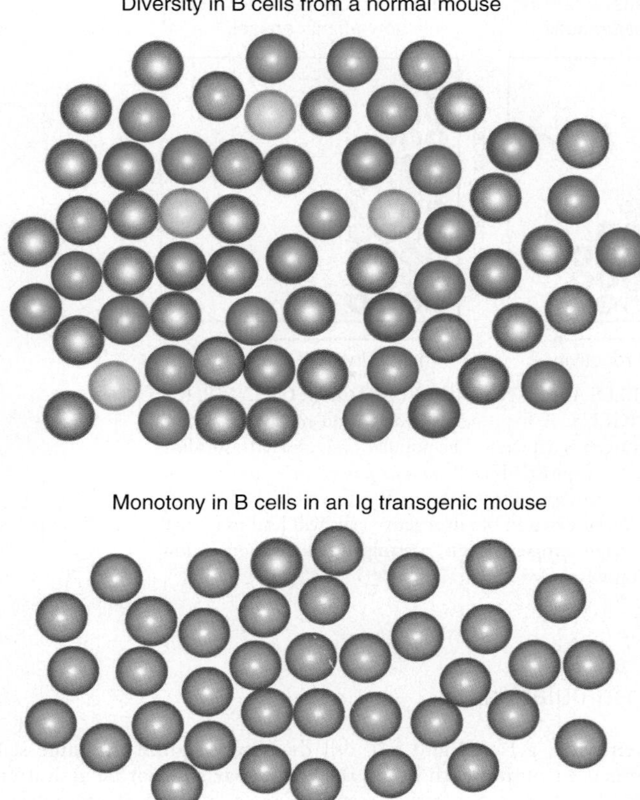

Figure 23-2 CLONAL DIVERSITY IN A NORMAL VERSUS TRANSGENIC MOUSE. The great diversity of B-cell specificities found in a normal mouse is indicated by the different patterns in each type of B cell. In contrast, in a transgenic mouse, each B cell expresses the same specificity because each carries the genes for a preformed heavy- and light-chain immunoglobulin (Ig) gene (the transgenes). This is indicated by the same pattern in each B cell. The one B cell with a different pattern signifies that occasional cells will express a unique specificity even in a transgenic because the system is imperfect.

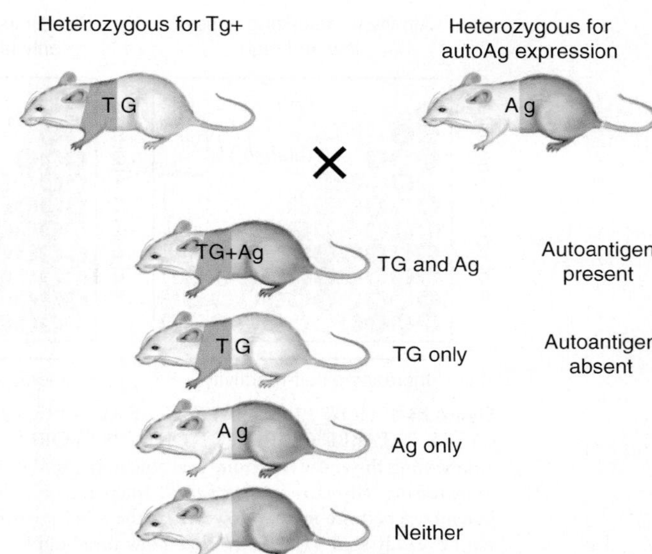

Figure 23-3 MATING STRATEGY TO GENERATE TRANSGENIC (TG) MICE WITH AND WITHOUT A POLYMORPHIC AUTOANTIGEN (Ag). Two mice are crossed, each of which is heterozygous, one for the transgene and the other for a polymorphic autoantigen (much as people can be heterozygous for blood group antigens). Shown are the possible resulting progeny of such a cross, each of which would occur at one-fourth frequency. The first two types of mice, one with TG and Ag and the other control with TG and not the Ag, are compared in experiments to determine how autoantigen affects the development of the autoreactive B cells.

such as the stomach. Mice with an induced mutation on Aire have a similar phenotype. Hence, specific mechanisms enhance thymic T-cell tolerance to otherwise sequestered peripheral antigens.[35]

Limitations of Central Tolerance

Although these mechanisms to eliminate or inactivate self-reactive B cells as they first emerge are clearly critical for the viability of an animal, they only account for part of the overall system that protects against autoimmunity. There are many reasons to believe that central tolerance cannot and should not be perfectly efficient. One is that the ability to tolerate self must be balanced against the ability to efficiently respond to a wide variety of foreign antigens. Each cell that is eliminated in the interests of self-tolerance is one that cannot respond to a potential foreign antigen. This concept is illustrated metaphorically in Fig. 23-4. Thus, one must suppose that it might be advantageous to allow some (weakly) antiself cells to escape these purging mechanisms. This is indeed the case. A second way to view this same problem is that even if it were desirable to have complete elimination of antiself lymphocytes, it would be impossible. It is unlikely that during development, each cell will be exposed to a sufficient quantity of each and every self-antigen in the body to be functionally tested for self-reactivity. Furthermore, some antigens are tissue specific, such as thyroglobulin, and are unlikely to be found in the circulation at appreciable quantities.

Persistence of Self-Reactive Lymphocytes

Thus, despite central tolerance, self-reactive cells nonetheless exist in peripheral lymphoid organs of normal animals. It has been observed for some time that many immune responses are accompanied by transient antiself antibody responses.[36-40] For example, rheumatoid factors with specificity for self-IgG often accompany strong secondary immune responses to foreign proteins or viruses.[36-38] The simplest explanation for such phenomena is that the B cells that make these autoantibodies already exist in the peripheral lymphoid compartment but are quiescent until they receive the proper stimulus. (How such cells get activated and why in normal animals this does not pose a threat are discussed following.)

Transgenic mouse models similar to those described above have provided the most convincing evidence of the existence of such B cells. One of particular relevance to hematology was generated by Honjo et al[41] These workers isolated the V genes that came from an actual anti-RBC autoantibody originally obtained from an NZB mouse with AIHA. Similar to Goodnow and Nemazee, they used the transgenic approach to express the anti-RBC antibody in a normal nonautoimmune mouse. Although central deletion was seen in most of the transgenic mice studied, many also had some residual autoreactive B cells in the spleen and lymph nodes, and some otherwise normal mice even developed frank AIHA. These results were interpreted as follows: central tolerance is not completely efficient even in a nonautoimmune mouse, and some autoreactive B cells can be stimulated to cause disease. Shlomchik et al, also using a transgenic approach, demonstrated that a rheumatoid factor autoantibody that was isolated from a diseased mouse was not subject to self-tolerance when expressed in a normal BALB/c mouse.[42] These B cells generally remained quiescent in a normal animal, suggesting that B cells that are not usually regulated by self-tolerance (perhaps because they recognize the self-antigen only weakly) may be the precursors of pathogenic autoantibodies in disease.

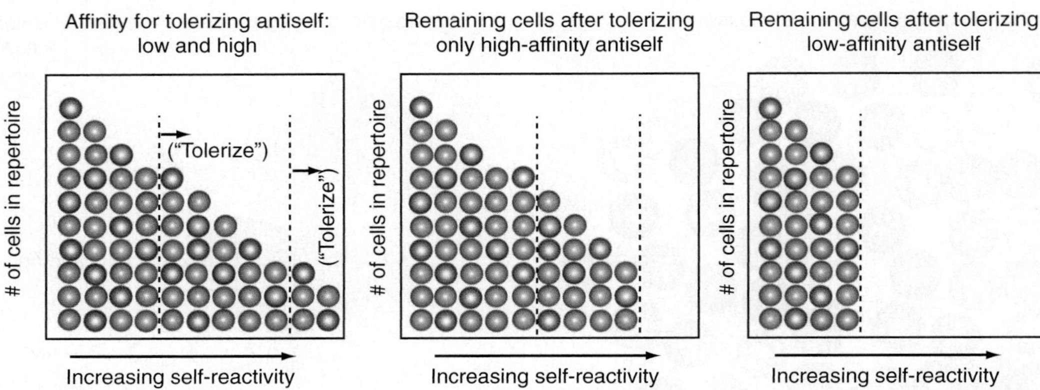

Figure 23-4 HOW ELIMINATION OF AUTOREACTIVE CELLS AFFECTS THE REPERTOIRE OF LYMPHOCYTES CAPABLE OF RESPONDING TO FOREIGN ANTIGENS. A hypothetical population of diverse B cells representing the entire repertoire available to respond to foreign antigen is depicted. The population is arrayed according to increasing self-reactivity *(left panel)*. Tolerizing only the high-affinity antiself B cells *(middle panel)* leaves most of the potential repertoire intact. However, as the affinity cutoff for self-reactivity increases, fewer B cells will be included. It can be readily seen *(right panel)* that a low threshold for inactivation or deletion of self-reactive cells will lead to a small number of competent residual cells available for responses to foreign antigens. Thus, a stringent tolerization of low affinity antiself cells will compromise the ability to respond to nonself.

Control of Self-Reactive Lymphocytes: Preventing Activation

The recognition that potentially self-reactive lymphocytes exist in the peripheral lymphoid repertoire of normal individuals,[43] despite central tolerance, raises the question of why they do not usually cause disease. One reason is the second layer of immune tolerance that prevents activation of self-reactive lymphocytes that exist in the periphery. This layer consists of several facets, which are described in the following sections.

Absence of Self-Antigen

The simplest explanation for why a self-specific lymphocyte is not spontaneously activated in the peripheral lymphoid compartment is the absence of self-antigen. This may be the reason why it was not eliminated in the first place. This situation has been termed clonal ignorance. It is related to the scenario described for rheumatoid factor B cells above in that the cell does not seem to care about the concentration of its autoantigen. In the case of rheumatoid factor, though, this is because the cell has relatively low affinity for self-IgG; in the case of thyroglobulin, for example, this is because the antigen concentration is vanishingly small. However, a change in antigen concentration, such as after thyroid damage from a viral infection, might then precipitate activation of these heretofore ignorant cells, leading to autoimmunity.

This antigen sequestration concept only applies to a limited set of autoantigens. A more general reason that self-specific lymphocytes remain quiescent, despite the ubiquity of self-antigens, is that for the vast majority of self-antigens, T and B cells are dependent on each other for activation (see Chapter 18).[44-47] It is evident that for this to occur, B and T cells specific for the same self-antigen must be in the same place at the same time. If such cells are rare, then the requisite coexistence of two such cells will happen very infrequently, minimizing the chance of starting an autoimmune reaction. A second consequence of T–B interdependence is that specific inefficiencies of central tolerance in one limb can be compensated for in the other. For example, T cells are probably very efficiently purged of cells that react with thymus-specific antigens, but B cells are probably not. However, antithymus B-cell responses are unlikely even though many thymus-specific B cells probably circulate; the cognate T cell with specificity for the same self-antigen simply does not exist.

Costimulation

Even when a B cell and a T cell that do recognize the same self-antigen encounter each other, the result may still not be activation. This is because a positive response by a lymphocyte to antigen encounter also requires a second signal aside from the stimulus of antigen recognition itself. These signals are transmitted through a series of ligand–receptor molecular pairs known as costimulatory molecules (see Chapter 19). The most important of these are: CD80 and CD86[48-53]1 (expressed on B cells, macrophages, and dendritic cells) and CD28[52,53] (expressed on T cells). Another important pair is CD40[54,55] (expressed on B cells, macrophages, and dendritic cells) and CD40 ligand[56-61] (CD40L, expressed on T cells and missing in patients with X-linked immunodeficiency/hyper-IgM syndrome[63-65]). CD40 stimulation is especially important for B cells, as it is for other antigen-presenting cells (APCs) as well. Other significant costimulatory molecules in T–B interactions include ICOS and ICOS-L (not shown in the figure), which are critical for germinal center responses and isotype switching.[66] Also in this category are lymphokine signals. For B cells, interleukin-4 (IL-4) signaling is important, but other cytokines such as IL-2, IL-5, IL-6, IL-21 also play roles in growth and differentiation. As shown in Fig. 23-5, some of these molecules are constitutively expressed, but others are induced in activated cells. This pattern of expression and induction leads to a cascade of events that occur during immune activation.

In general, for proper transmission of this second signal, one or the other of the lymphocytes must have been previously activated. This concept generates a paradox in that if one lymphocyte must already be activated, how is it possible to start an immune response at all? This is resolved in several ways. First, it is indeed difficult to start immune responses, and this is one of the mechanisms by which nonresponsiveness to self is maintained. However, a strong or prolonged first signal to a T or B cell may be sufficient for it to induce its costimulatory molecules.[48,67] Second, inflammation of any type is a powerful nonspecific inducer of these same costimulatory molecules.[68-70] Thus, in the presence of ongoing inflammation, such as would occur with infection or trauma, immune responses are much easier to start. Indeed, recent evidence suggests an important role in systemic autoimmunity for Toll-like receptors (TLRs), which recognize molecules specific to pathogens and induce costimulatory molecules and immune system activation. Ligands for TLRs include lipopolysaccharide (TLR4), bacterial DNA enriched for CpG dinucleotides (TLR9), and ss and dsRNA (TLR7 and TLR3). TLRs can

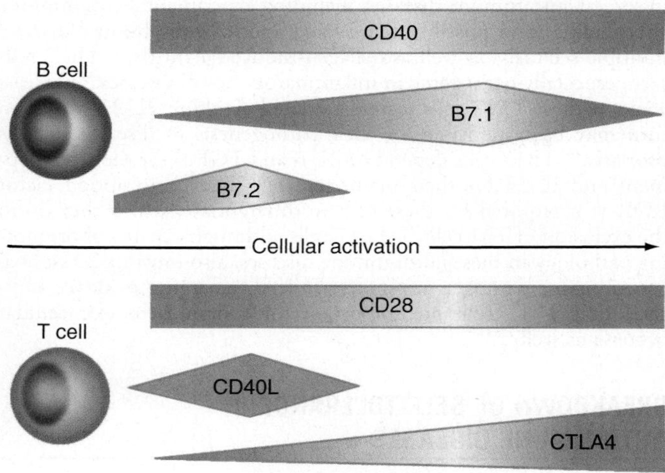

Figure 23-5 TIMING OF EXPRESSION OF COSTIMULATORY MOLECULES. The schematic shows the regulated expression of the CD40–CD40 L family *(light red)* and the B7-CD28–CTLA4 family *(dark red)* of molecules. From left to right is depicted increasing cellular activation as time elapses after initial encounter with antigen. The expression level of each molecule over time is indicated by a *polygonal shape*. The vertical width of the shape at any time reflects the degree of expression at that time. For example, CTLA4 is expressed little at the start and the expression increases continuously over time. The shapes depicting expression of molecules that are thought to deliver signals are outlined in ***bold,*** and those of molecules thought to receive signals are in *fine line*. The top three molecules are chiefly expressed on B cells and the lower three on T cells.

be activated by infection and may provide a mechanism by which some infections can trigger autoimmunity. However, in the right context some self (as opposed to pathogen) molecules, such as DNA found in chromatin, a target for systemic lupus erythematosus (SLE) autoantibodies, can also activate TLRs (TLR9 in the case of DNA).[71] Third, certain "professional" APCs, such as dendritic cells, may constitutively express these costimulatory molecules at moderate levels and can start the cascade, for example, by activating T cells, which is then amplified by T–B interactions.[70] In summary, there are two main functions of costimulatory requirements: (1) they focus the interactions between two antigen-specific T and B cells and limit nonspecific interactions, and (2) they restrict immune responses in the absence of inflammation. Both of these features of costimulation tend to prevent the activation of self-reactive lymphocytes that exist in peripheral lymphoid organs. For B cells, this means that tolerance in the T-cell compartment alone will prevent many self-reactive B cells from being activated.

Even with antigen sequestration and costimulatory regulation, mechanisms that prevent the activation of self-reactive lymphocytes are incomplete at best. For example, it seems likely during infection or trauma that antiself responses could initiate because costimulatory molecules will be nonspecifically induced. Indeed, this is the case. Furthermore, during infection and tissue damage, self-proteins that ordinarily are sequestered can be released. This leads to activation of the ignorant cells circulating in the body.[72-77] In fact, (usually) self-limited autoimmune responses after infection are well known, such as poststreptococcal glomerulonephritis or postmycoplasmal cold agglutinins. Although these syndromes can cause serious clinical problems, they are self-limited, unlike autoimmune diseases such as SLE.

Control of Self-Reactive Lymphocytes: Downregulation

The difference between transient autoimmune responses and chronic severe autoimmunity may lie in the third layer of protection against autoimmunity: downregulation of ongoing responses. Again, this layer is a normal part of the immune system, functioning to regulate both normal and autoimmune responses. Initially, in a normal response to a viral pathogen, there is great proliferation of lymphocytes specific for viral antigens. This process leads ultimately to the elimination of the pathogen, which was traditionally thought of as the signal to stop an immune response. However, when the pathogen is eliminated, in the absence of any other regulatory mechanism, there would be many residual cells that had been responding to the pathogen. Although a few such cells could be retained to provide immunologic memory, most of these are no longer useful in the short term. In addition to unnecessarily filling the lymphoid compartment, these cells may be a risk for causing autoimmunity. This is because of the possibility of the generation of newly autoreactive B cells by virtue of random somatic mutation.[25] B cells responding to foreign antigens begin to mutate their antibody V region genes. Mutation is a random process, and thus a mutation could occur that converts a nonautoimmune B cell into a self-reactive B cell.[25] No clear mechanism exists by which the body can discriminate and specifically eliminate these newly self-reactive mutant B cells. However, at a minimum, elimination of most of the reactive B cells regardless of specificity would mitigate this problem.

Over the past several years, several pathways for the removal of such postexpansion cells have been elucidated. One seems to be an inborn program that causes cells to apoptose after undergoing a certain amount of proliferation.[78-80] Particularly important in this program in lymphocytes are the Bcl2-inhibitable pathways that are activated in large part by Bim.[81,82] In B cells, CD40 signaling in concert with BCR and IL-4 signaling may rescue some cells from this self-destructive fate, and it is believed that these cells become long-lived memory cells.[83-86] There are also active mechanisms that signal cells to apoptose. One receptor–ligand pair called Fas and FasL is central in this process. Generally, when Fas is ligated by FasL, the cell expressing Fas is triggered to die by apoptosis.[87-90] Fas and FasL are not expressed at high levels on unstimulated resting lymphocytes. On activation, whereas T cells express both Fas and FasL, B cells express Fas.[90,91] Sensitivity to the Fas signal may be regulated in the Fas-expressing cell as well. Thus, after a certain degree of activation and proliferation, a T cell (expressing FasL) encountering an activated B cell (expressing Fas) may actually kill that B cell. There are likely other ligand pairs, particularly those in the tumor necrosis factor (TNF) family, that may serve similar functions, both for B and T cells.

A particularly interesting and instructive receptor ligand pair that downregulates ongoing responses has been elucidated. The receptor, CTLA4, is expressed on activated T cells, and when ligated, causes inactivation or death of the receptive T cell; it is said to therefore transduce a "negative" signal.[92-95] The other ligands in this pair are CD80 and to a lesser extent CD86, the same ligands that gives a positive signal to naïve T cells by ligating CD28. Thus, the same molecule can promote activation early on in the immune response while, through a change in the receptive T cell, it can inhibit activation at a later time. An analogous receptor pair of the B7 family are PD-1, an inhibitory receptor similar to CTLA-4, and its ligands PD-L1 and PD-L2. PD-1 is expressed on a number of activated lymphocytes and its ligands are constitutively and inducibly expressed on a variety of parenchymal cells (PD-L1) and dendritic cells (PD-L2).[96] Absence of these molecules leads to exaggerated immune responses and autoimmunity.[97-99] Most recently, data are emerging that PD-L1 and CD80 also interact strongly, with negative regulatory consequences that could be important for organ transplant rejection and autoimmunity in vivo.[100] These examples underscore the careful means by which the immune system regulates and dampens activation presumably to prevent autoimmunity.

Suppressor, or more commonly termed, *regulatory* T cells play critical roles in restraining many aspects of immune and autoimmune responses. The best-studied regulatory cell expresses CD25, the receptor for IL-2,[101,102] and its development and function is dependent on the expression of a key transcription factor, FoxP3.[103-105] These cells can prevent autoimmune syndromes such as inflammatory bowel disease, diabetes, and autoimmune encephalomyelitis in murine models and can even be used to treat active disease.[106,107] They are also active in preventing transplantation rejection and GVHD. These cells may function by secreting suppressive cytokines, such as IL-10 and TGF-β, and also by cell–cell contact. Their critical role of regulatory T cells in humans is underscored by a rare and fatal inherited autoimmune disorder, IPEX (immune dysregulation, polyendocrinopathy, enteropathy, and X-linked inheritance), that results from a lack of FoxP3, which is needed for the development of CD25+ regulatory cells.[108,109]

How does regulation of ongoing immune responses prevent autoimmunity? In the first place, these normal forms of downregulation undoubtedly prevent common transient autoimmune responses from becoming chronic. More subtly, elimination or control of cells after immune responses will prevent the accumulation of a large number of self-specific memory cells. As long as such cells are rare, it is unlikely for autoreactive T cells and B cells, each specific for the same self-antigen, to wind up in the same place at the same time. Thus, downregulation and elimination of responding cells prevents a critical mass of self-reactive cells from ever forming.

Control of Self-Reactive Lymphocytes: Channeling the Type of Effector Response

A final layer of protection against self-inflicted immune damage involves channeling of responses so they are not harmful. Depending on the context, only certain effector functions will effectively eliminate certain pathogens. For example, antibodies will not be effective against intracellular pathogens. By analogy, only certain effector functions may cause autoimmune disease, depending on the circumstances. It is clear that there are two major types of T-helper cell responses, Th1 and Th2, that in turn lead to very different effector functions.[110-112] The propensity to make these various types of responses depends on a number of ill-understood factors, but these include genetics, route of antigen exposure, and dose of antigen.[113,114] Intriguingly, in certain murine models of autoimmunity such as the nonobese diabetic (NOD) model, experimental manipulations that shift responses away from Th1 and toward Th2 are highly protective against disease.[115-117] This is also relevant to B-cell autoimmunity per se because, through the use of different isotypes of Ig, different effector functions can occur. The cytokines secreted by Th1 and Th2 cells have profound effects on the isotypes of immunoglobulins that are produced during a response. Thus, not only is the T-cell component of the response channeled in this way, but the humoral response is also influenced. Recently, a new subset of T cells that secrete IL-17, thus dubbed Th17, has been recognized as important pathogenic cells in several autoimmune diseases, including experimental autoimmune encephalitis (and possibly the related spontaneous human disease, multiple sclerosis) as well as collagen-induced arthritis.[118] Th17 cells seem especially pathogenic in inflammatory bowel diseases.[119] At least some of these Th17 cells secrete a related cytokine, IL-22, which in turn may be responsible for their pathogenesis in diseases such as psoriasis.[120] Th17 cells depend on IL-6 and TGF-β for their development and IL-23 for their maintenance.[118] The transcription factor ROR-γt is required for these cells to differentiate, which they do to the exclusion of Th1 cells.[121] Th17 cells, although capable of promoting pathology in these autoimmune diseases, also must have essential functions for pathogen resistance. Indeed, emerging evidence indicates that Th17 cells are important for responses to extracellular bacteria as well.[118,122]

BREAKDOWN OF SELF-TOLERANCE IN AUTOIMMUNE DISEASES

Presumably, for autoimmune diseases and autoantibody production to occur, one or more of the multilayered mechanisms to prevent autoimmunity must fail. Surprisingly, the precise nature of these failures is not well understood. The mechanism of failure are likely different for the various autoimmune diseases and perhaps even for different patients with similar syndromes. Moreover, it seems likely both from phenomenologic and genetic studies that failures at several levels are required to generate clinically significant autoimmunity. In the following section, some examples of the current state of knowledge are given.

This chapter is not meant to review the nature of autoimmune diseases; however, before considering the likely points at which self-tolerance mechanisms break down, it is useful to review some basic concepts about these diseases. Grossly, autoimmune diseases have often been divided into organ-specific and systemic autoimmune syndromes. This classification is useful, but as these diseases are becoming better understood, the dividing lines are blurring; pathogeneses of all these diseases are likely to have much in common. In particular, systemic autoimmune diseases are actually much more specific in their antigenic targets than is commonly realized. Table 23-1 shows the types of autoantibodies commonly found in several systemic autoimmune diseases. Certain autoantibodies are diagnostic for specific autoimmune diseases, such as anti-Sm in SLE. Thus, Sm is a specific target in SLE, but patients with autoimmune diseases, such as rheumatoid arthritis, do not respond to this autoantigen. In fact, only 30% of all patients with SLE make anti-Sm, meaning that the other 70% are tolerant of their own Sm despite having a systemic

Table 23-1 Patterns of Autoantibody Expression in Systemic Autoimmune Diseases

Autoantigen/Autoimmune Diseases (% of Patients with Autoantibody)	Systemic Lupus Erythematosus	Rheumatoid Arthritis	Scleroderma	Sjögren Syndrome
dsDNA	40			
ssDNA	70			
Histones	70			
Sm	30			
nRNP	30			
Ro (SS-A)	35			60
La (SS-B)	15			40
IgG (RF)	20	90		10-20
Scl-70 (Topo I)			70	
Centromere			70	

From Tan EM: Antinuclear antibodies: Diagnostic markers for autoimmune diseases and probes for cell biology. *Adv Immunol* 44:93, 1989.
dsDNA, Double-stranded DNA; *nRNP*, native ribonucleoprotein; *Scl-70*, scleroderma 70-kd antigen (topoisomerase I); *Sm*, Smith ribonucleoprotein; *ssDNA*, single-stranded DNA. *Blank space* indicates rarely or never detected.

autoimmune disease.[123] Another salient feature of most human autoimmune diseases is adult onset. Both the selective nature of disease and its late onset argue against gross defects in the basic central tolerance mechanisms as being the cause.

Instead, these considerations suggest that most clinical autoimmune diseases are likely to arise from defects in the later stages of self-tolerance, such as preventing the activation of autoreactive cells or downregulating them when they are activated. Because in no case is the primary cause of a polygenic autoimmune disease known, it cannot be excluded that subtle defects in the earlier stages, including central tolerance, may also play a role; in fact, for some diseases, recent data suggest that there is a role for more "leaky" central self-tolerance.[124,125] However, it does seem clear that a gross defect in central tolerance would lead to a severe syndrome of congenital autoimmunity.

Genetic and Environmental Factors

Genetic Factors

Both genetic and environmental factors help to explain why autoimmunity occurs in some individuals and not others.[126] The most well-known genetic factor is the major histocompatibility complex, known as human leukocyte antigen (HLA) in humans. Many different autoimmune diseases are more or less associated with specific genotypes at this polymorphic locus. Among these are ankylosing spondylitis (HLA-B27), insulin-dependent diabetes mellitus (HLA-DR3/4), rheumatoid arthritis (HLA-DR4), and to some degree SLE (HLA-DR2/3).[127] It should be emphasized that although individuals with these genotypes are relatively more prone, most will not develop the autoimmune disease. How certain HLA genes predispose to autoimmunity is not very clear. These genes could be involved in the efficiency or specificity of central tolerance in the thymus but could also be involved in the activation of autoreactive T cells in the periphery. They could even control the efficiency with which the regulatory compartment of T cells develops.

Inheritance patterns of all systemic autoimmune diseases suggest that multiple genes, in addition to the HLA locus, contribute to susceptibility. Such genes are beginning to be identified in human and in animal models. This work has used "gene chips" that detect common variant single-nucleotide polymorphisms to identify and map genes that are associated with autoimmune phenotypes across large numbers of patients and control participants. This is currently being supplemented with whole-exon and in some cases whole-genome sequencing, which promises to find more rare genetic variants that are also likely to contribute to disease risk. Interestingly, risk alleles have been identified for a number of the same genes in more than one autoimmune disease; these include CTLA-4, STAT-4, PTPN-22, TNFAIP3, and IRF-5, all of which are known to regulate inflammation.[128-130] Analogous work—this time using crosses between susceptible and resistant strains—has allowed a number of predisposing genetic loci to be identified in murine autoimmune disease and their phenotypes investigated in greater detail.[131-135] Interestingly, most of them seem to have direct effects on B-cell function or activity. Table 23-2 lists categories of genes that are likely involved in genetic predisposition to autoimmune disease, drawing from both human and murine studies. Note that these include genes involved in the processes of antigen sequestration, T–B collaboration, and immune response downregulation that were discussed earlier as key features of the self-tolerance mechanisms that normally prevent autoimmune disease. In ongoing work, of the precise nature of defects in these genes may be defined; these include noncoding polymorphisms that affect expression levels in addition to structural alleles. This will in turn permit screening for defects in human autoimmune disease patients with the ultimate goals of aiding diagnosis, providing insights into pathogenic mechanisms, and guiding patient-specific therapies.

Although human genetic studies and animal models suggest multigenic inheritance, there are certain instructive cases in which single-gene defects play a major role. A well-studied example of mutations

Table 23-2 Genes Involved in Regulation of Autoimmune Responses

Category	Types of Genes*	Known Examples†
Central and peripheral deletion and anergy	Receptor signaling, MHC genes, receptor V genes	CD45,[126] PTPN22,[127-129] HLA (certain types2),[102] CD3,[131] CD4, CD8, CD28/B7[35]
Initiation of response	Receptor signaling, co-stimulatory molecules, adhesion molecules	BLK, STAT-4, IRF5, ITGAM, PTPN22, FcγRII[128,130]
Downregulation of response	Apoptosis genes, interleukins, negative costimulatory molecules	Fas,[110,112] TNF,[132,133] CTLA4,[89] CD40, CD3,[134] TNFAIP3,[130] CD28/B7[52,135]
Channeling of response	Interleukins, interleukin receptors	STAT-4,[130] IL-4, IL-10, IL-12, IFN-γ[98,99]
Autoantigen metabolism and apoptosis	Complement components, apoptosis signaling	C1q, C2, C4, DNAse I, MER[145,146]

BLK, B lymphocyte kinase; *CTLA*, cytotoxic T lymphocyte activation; *IFN*, interferon; *IL*, interleukin; *IRF*, interferon response factor; *MER*, C-mer tyrosine kinase; *MHC*, major histocompatibility complex; *PTP*, posttransfusion purpura; *STAT*, signal transducers and activators of transcription.
*Indicates some of the categories of genes that may be involved in regulating autoimmunity at the indicated step.
†Some genes in the "Types of Genes" category that have been shown to play a role in the process indicated in the left column. Some have also been directly shown to play a role in autoimmunity.

in these genes is the lpr/lpr mouse, a natural variant originally discovered at the Jackson Laboratories, which carries an inactivated murine Fas.[87,147,148] The gld mutation (another natural variant discovered at Jackson), which inactivates murine Fas ligand (FasL),[90] has a very similar phenotype to the lpr. Both of these mutations lead to an age-dependent autoimmune syndrome with autoantibody profiles that remarkably resemble human SLE.[148] These mice die prematurely of renal failure. They also have an accumulation of lymphocytes that leads to marked lymphadenopathy.[149] Presumably, this is the result of failure to eliminate postactivation T and B cells by the Fas-based mechanism.[150-152] Exactly how defects in the apoptotic Fas pathway lead to autoimmunity has yet to be elucidated. Interestingly, a rare syndrome in humans with incomplete penetrance, called *autoimmune lymphoproliferation syndrome,* has been traced to mutations in human Fas.[153] Often these patients are misdiagnosed with leukemia or lymphoma, and some have even been treated for (and survived) these neoplasms. Clonality and chromosomal studies in autoimmune lymphoproliferation syndrome reveal polyclonal B- and T-cell proliferations with normal karyotypes, in distinction with true lymphoma or leukemia. The phenotypes of these mutants in the Fas pathway, although more fulminant than most human autoimmune syndromes, illustrate two important points. They demonstrate the critical nature of the late downregulatory controls in preventing autoimmune disease. They also point out pathways in which less severe mutations might be discovered that account for human disease.

A final category of genes regulate the clearance of self-antigens and dead cells, which is particularly important in systemic autoimmune diseases such as SLE. These include complement components C4, C3, and C2, C1q, and less-known genes such as *MER,* which plays a role in signaling for the uptake of apoptotic fragments by macrophages.[145,146] Evidently, when self-antigens are not cleared promptly after cell death, they can become targets of the immune system, leading to autoimmunity to intracellular components such as chromatin.

As noted, TLRs can recognize some of these molecules when they are present in high concentrations, thus providing proinflammatory signals. In murine models of lupus, it has been demonstrated in vivo that TLR9 is required to generate antichromatin autoantibodies[154] and that TLR7, which recognizes RNA, is required for the generation of autoantibodies to RNA-related antigens.[155] Indeed, a mutant mouse with a double dose of TLR7 develops spontaneous lupus with high levels of RNA antibodies.[156,157] Stimulation of these TLRs on specialized plasmacytoid dendritic cells leads to release of abundant type I interferon, which itself may be causally linked to lupus in mice and humans.[158] These findings highlight a genetic basis for recognizing self-molecules in autoimmune diseases and suggest new therapeutic targets that are currently being explored. Whether this theme extends to other autoimmune diseases beyond lupus remains to be determined.

Environmental Factors

Environment plays a role that is at least as important as genetics. This is illustrated by the fact that concordance rates among identical twins, even raised in the same household, are surprisingly low. Only 20% of twins of patients with rheumatoid arthritis also get rheumatoid arthritis.[127] There are many examples of environmental factors causing either chronic or transient autoimmune diseases. There are postinfectious syndromes such as postmycoplasmal cold agglutinin disease. The pattern of incidence of multiple sclerosis suggests a viral etiology, although no causative virus has ever been convincingly demonstrated. Another category of infectious associations includes postviral myocarditis, which follows certain coxsackievirus infections.[76] It is sometimes conceptually difficult to draw a line between viral damage and consequent immune system damage; however, if sensitization to self-antigens occurs as a consequence of viral infection and these later are pathogenic targets independent of viral antigens, it seems reasonable to consider the syndrome as autoimmune.

Infections are not the only source of environmental stimuli for autoimmunity. Toxins, such as mercury, cause autoimmunity in animal models.[159,160] Another form more familiar to those in hematology is drug-induced autoimmunity, as in AIHA. Drugs, such as procainamide, that cause lupus-like syndromes are particularly prominent examples.[161,162] Despite these specific examples, the environmental factors that play a role in promoting common autoimmune diseases such as rheumatoid arthritis or SLE are unknown.

Examples in Hematology: Epitope Spreading in Posttransfusion Purpura

One potential way to break self-tolerance may be particularly relevant to syndromes found in hematology and is worthy of elaboration. This is a form of environmental stimulation, albeit iatrogenic. In PTP, transfusion with allogeneic platelets that contain a platelet-specific antigen (e.g., HPA-1a) lacking in the recipient (which in this case would be HPA-1b) leads to rapid destruction of the transfused platelets and antibody formation to the foreign platelet antigen.[3,163] However, several days later, the recipient becomes severely thrombocytopenic owing to increased destruction of the recipient's own platelets. Although how such destruction of self-platelets occurs secondary to destruction of allogeneic platelets may still be controversial,[3,163,164] the best explanation is an autoimmune response.[1-3] How does this response get stimulated? The probable pathway bears significant parallels to one demonstrated in mice a number of years ago by Janeway and colleagues.[165,166] These workers immunized normal mice with human cytochrome c, which differed slightly from endogenous murine cytochrome c. The mice made both an antibody response and a T-cell response to the human cytochrome c; however, because the human and mouse cytochromes are so similar, the antibody response (but not the T-cell response) cross-reacted with murine cytochrome c. Presumably, this reflected activation of ignorant B cells with specificity for self-cytochrome c (and also human). However, several weeks later, if the mice were given a dose of self-cytochrome c, now both a vigorous B-cell and T-cell antiself response ensued. These authors suggested that priming with the cross-reactive antigen first induced self-reactive B cells, which in turn could then break tolerance in anergic or ignorant self-reactive T cells.

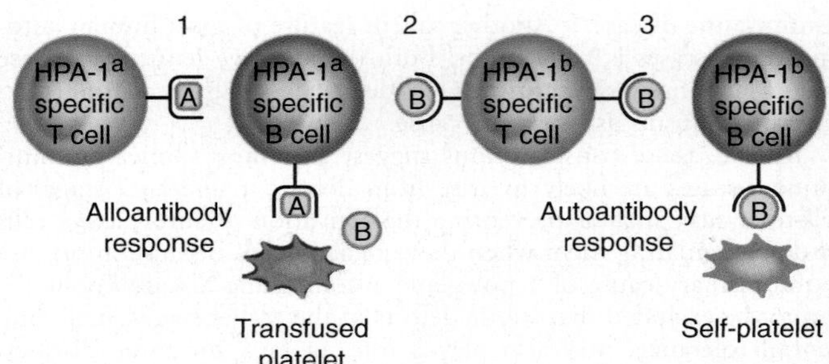

Figure 23-6 EPITOPE SPREADING AS A POSSIBLE AUTOIMMUNE MECHANISM FOR POSTTRANSFUSION PURPURA (PTP). Events are depicted as progressing from left to right. An HPA-1^b person is transfused with an HPA-$1^{a/b}$ platelet product. An alloantibody response ensues as an HPA-1^a-specific B cell recognizes the platelet, becomes activated to secrete antibody, and presents the HPA-1^a antigen to an anti-HPA-1^a T cell *(step 1)*. In addition, the activated B cell may now activate a previously ignorant anti-HPA-1^b-specific T cell to initiate an autoimmune response *(step 2)*. The activated B cell acquired the self-HPA-1^b antigen as a passenger on the HPA-$1^{a/b}$ allogeneic platelet. This autoreactive T cell can then activate an ignorant anti-HPA-1^b B cell to make an autoantibody response *(step 3)* in response to autologous platelets. Note that the sensitization involved in *steps 1 and 2* may take place in a primary response during the first transfusion or exposure and that *step 3* may take place in a clinically noticeable way only after a secondary exposure to homologous platelets.

How does this relate to PTP? Fig. 23-6 illustrates the author's hypothetic adaptation of this mechanism to the platelet transfusion situation. The foreign platelets actually share many common antigens with the host, as well as differ at the HPA-1a locus. The foreign antigenic difference allows ignorant self-specific B cells (as well as HPA-1a-specific B cells) to interact with helper T cells that are specific for the foreign HPA-1a antigen and become activated. Moreover, these activated B cells can then present self-platelet antigens along with costimulatory signals to self-reactive T cells. When this happens, the immune response can perpetuate even in the absence of the foreign platelets. This is exactly what is seen in PTP, in which a delayed response continues to eliminate self-platelets for many days after the disappearance of the transfused platelets. Thus, a foreign platelet is analogous to foreign cytochrome c in having a few different antigens along with many shared antigens. In the same way as shown experimentally with cytochrome c, it is hypothesized that the few foreign antigens existing on the same particle (in the case of cytochrome c, it is the same molecule) allow spreading of autoimmunity from a foreign antigen to self-antigens. The key events are the activation of ignorant B cells that cross-react with both self and foreign molecules and then the activation by these B cells or T cells that are specific for self.

It is reasonable to question how such antiself responses are ever stopped once started. PTP, for example, is a self-limited syndrome. In fact, the answer is not known; however, both downregulation of antigen as the platelet count falls to near zero, and the natural mechanisms that cause apoptosis of responding lymphocytes probably play a role. Regulatory T cells could also help bring the response under control. In the absence of an autoimmune-prone host who has mutations affecting the downregulation of immune responses, these autoimmune reactions will remain transient. It is speculated that when similar events—for example, a response to a viral DNA-binding protein that eventually spreads to allow for responses to self-DNA and chromatin, as in SLE—occur in people who do have genetically based problems in downregulating such responses, a chronic autoimmune syndrome can be induced.

IMPLICATIONS AND THERAPY

The significance of this issue to hematology ranges from syndromes such as AIHA and idiopathic thrombocytopenic purpura to iatrogenically induced autoimmunity as in PTP. In the latter case, a phenomenon known as *epitope spreading*, which is documented in murine models, but little discussed in terms of PTP, is speculated to be a relevant pathogenetic mechanism. A basic understanding of the mechanisms of self-tolerance and their breakdown in autoimmune disease raises the possibility of many types of specific therapeutic interventions. One of the clearest would be to identify initiating factors, such as infections, and to prevent or treat them. A second approach would be to reset tolerance. Some of the previous examples, such as in PTP, illustrate how an initiating event can be amplified, leading to broken tolerance. If the system can be set back to the state before that event, the disease could be cured. At present, it is unclear how to do this; however, an autologous or even allogeneic hematopoietic stem cell transplant may have the desired effect. In fact, this sort of radical therapy has been tried in selected cases of severe SLE and seems to have some efficacy.[167] Another promising area is in channeling the immune response, particularly as the steering mechanisms are becoming better understood at the molecular level. Work in this area is currently active. A third area is to design more specific modulators of inflammation, including interfering with costimulatory signals. These latter approaches have seemed promising in various animal models, although issues with unexpected effects on clotting have arisen in clinical trials of CD40L inhibition.

Current therapy is much more crude and typically involves general nonspecific immunosuppression either with steroids or cytotoxic drugs. Although these therapies can be effective, they have numerous undesirable side effects, not the least of which is increased susceptibility to infection caused by immunosuppression. More promising are drugs that inhibit the effects of TNF-α, which have proven successful in modifying progression of rheumatoid arthritis and also in inflammatory bowel disease, psoriasis, and GVHD.[168-170] Recently, additional proinflammatory cytokines, such as IL-6 and IL-12/23, have been targeted by monoclonal Ab as effective therapies in patients.[171,172] This approach, although a result of modern biotechnology and our understanding of immunopathogenesis, still targets effector function of the immune system and does not modify the root cause of disease. Therapies should ultimately be directed toward either prevention or else specific downregulation of ongoing responses. Recently, rituximab, an antibody to CD20 that depletes B cells and is effective in treating non-Hodgkin lymphoma, has been used to treat a variety of autoimmune syndromes. It is showing great promise[173,174] and it has been approved to treat some rheumatoid arthritis patients.[175] In a similar vein, BLyS (B-lymphocyte stimulator), which is a survival factor for B cells, has been successfully targeted via a monoclonal Ab that leads to B-cell depletion.[176,177] This compound, belimumab, was recently granted U.S. Food and Drug Administration approval for the treatment of SLE. It will be interesting to determine whether B-cell depletion leads to long-term remissions, perhaps by interrupting positive feedback loops such as illustrated in Fig. 23-6. Future work will include continuing to define how self-tolerance is imposed and how it is broken in disease, what the critical triggers and autoantigens are, and how to use immunomodulation to treat autoimmune diseases on the basis of a better understanding of the pathogenesis.

SUGGESTED READINGS

Allen RC, Armitage RJ, Conley ME, et al: CD40 ligand gene defects responsible for X-linked hyper-IgM syndrome. *Science* 259:990, 1993.

Anderson MS, Su MA: Aire and T cell development. *Curr Opin Immunol* 23:198, 2011.

Aster RH: Platelet-specific alloantigen systems: History, clinical significance and molecular biology. In Nance ST, editor: *Alloimmunity: 1993 and Beyond*, Bethesda, MD, 1993, American Association of Blood Banks, p 83.

Christensen SR, Kashgarian M, Alexopoulou L, et al: Toll-like receptor 9 controls anti-DNA autoantibody production in murine lupus. *J Exp Med* 202:321, 2005.

Christensen SR, Shupe J, Nickerson K, et al: TLR7 and TLR9 dictate autoantibody specificity and have opposing inflammatory and regulatory roles in a murine model of lupus. *Immunity* 25:417, 2006.

Coyle AJ, Lehar S, Lloyd C, et al: The CD28-related molecule ICOS is required for effective T cell-dependent immune responses. *Immunity* 13:95, 2000.

Flesher DL, Sun X, Behrens TW, et al: Recent advances in the genetics of systemic lupus erythematosus. *Expert review of clinical immunology* 6:461, 2010.

Fontenot JD, Gavin MA, Rudensky AY: Foxp3 programs the development and function of CD4(+)CD25(+) regulatory T cells. *Nat Immunol* 4:330, 2003.

Gay D, Saunders T, Camper S, et al: Receptor editing: An approach by autoreactive B cells to escape tolerance. *J Exp Med* 177:999, 1993.

Goodnow CC, Crosbie J, Adelstein S, et al: Altered immunoglobulin expression and functional silencing of self-reactive B lymphocytes in transgenic mice. *Nature* 334:676, 1988.

Ivanov II, McKenzie BS, Zhou L, et al: The orphan nuclear receptor RORgammat directs the differentiation program of proinflammatory IL-17+ T helper cells. *Cell* 126:1121, 2006.

Keir ME, Butte MJ, Freeman GJ, et al: PD-1 and its ligands in tolerance and immunity. *Ann Rev Immunol* 26:677, 2008.

Kisielow P, Swat W, Rocha B, et al: Induction of immunological unresponsiveness in vivo and in vitro by conventional and super-antigens in developing and mature T cells. *Immunol Rev* 122:69, 1991.

Leadbetter EA, Rifkin IR, Hohlbaum AM, et al: Chromatin-IgG complexes activate B cells by dual engagement of IgM and Toll-like receptors. *Nature* 416:603, 2002.

Liu Y-J, Joshua DE, Williams GT, et al: Mechanism of antigen-driven selection in germinal centres. *Nature* 342:929, 1989.

Mamula MJ, Lin R-H, Janeway Jr CA, et al: Breaking T cell tolerance with foreign and self co-immunogens: A study of autoimmune B and T cell epitopes of cytochrome c. *J Immunol* 149:789, 1992.

Nemazee DA, Burki K: Clonal deletion of B lymphocytes in a transgenic mouse bearing anti-MHC class-I antibody genes. *Nature* 337:562, 1989.

Nishimura H, Nose M, Hiai H, et al: Development of lupus-like autoimmune diseases by disruption of the PD-1 gene encoding an ITIM motif-carrying immunoreceptor. *Immunity* 11:141, 1999.

Tiegs SL, Russell DM, Nemazee D: Receptor editing in self-reactive bone marrow B cells. *J Exp Med* 177:1009, 1993.

Tivol EA, Borriello F, Schweitzer AN, et al: Loss of CTLA-4 leads to massive lymphoproliferation and fatal multiorgan tissue destruction, revealing a critical negative regulatory role of CTLA-4. *Immunity* 3:541, 1995.

Wallace DJ, Stohl W, Furie RA, et al. A phase II, randomized, double-blind, placebo-controlled, dose-ranging study of belimumab in patients with active systemic lupus erythematosus. *Arthritis Rheum* 61:1168, 2009.

Walport MJ: Lupus, DNase and defective disposal of cellular debris. *Nat Genet* 25:135, 2000.

Wardemann H, Nussenzweig MC. B-cell self-tolerance in humans. *Adv Immunol* 95:83, 2007.

Weaver CT, Harrington LE, Mangan PR, et al: Th17: An effector CD4 T cell lineage with regulatory T cell ties. *Immunity* 24:677, 2006.

Yurasov S, Wardemann H, Hammersen J, et al: Defective B cell tolerance checkpoints in systemic lupus erythematosus. *J Exp Med* 201:703, 2005.

For complete list of references log on to www.expertconsult.com.

PART IV

Disorders of Hematopoietic Cell Development

CHAPTER 24

BIOLOGY OF ERYTHROPOIESIS, ERYTHROID DIFFERENTIATION, AND MATURATION

Thalia Papayannopoulou and Anna Rita Migliaccio

The production of erythroid cells is a dynamic and exquisitely regulated process. The mature red cell is the final phase of a complex but orderly series of genetic events that initiates when a multipotent stem cell commits to the erythroid program. Expression of the erythroid program occurs several divisions later in a greatly amplified population of erythroid cells, which have a characteristic form and structure, maturation sequence, and function. These maturing cells are termed *erythroid precursor cells* and *reticulocytes*. Terminally differentiated cells have a finite life span, and they are constantly replenished by influx from earlier compartments of progenitor cells that are irreversibly committed to express the erythroid phenotype. During ontogeny, successive waves of erythropoiesis occur in distinct anatomic sites. Erythroid cells developing in these sites have distinguishable phenotypes and intrinsic programs that are dependent on gestational time and their microenvironment. At each site, erythroid cells are in intimate contact with other cells (e.g., stromal cells, hematopoietic accessory cells, and extracellular matrix) composing their microenvironment. Within this microenvironment, erythroid development is influenced by cytokines, which are either elaborated by microenvironmental cells or produced elsewhere and then entrapped in the extracellular matrix.

Knowledge of the properties of erythroid progenitor and precursor cells and their complex interactions with the microenvironment is essential for understanding the pathophysiology of erythropoiesis. Aberrations in the generation and/or amplification of fully mature and functional erythroid cells or in the regulatory influences of microenvironmental cells or their cytokines/chemokines form the basis for various clinical disorders, including aplasias, dysplasias, and neoplasias of the erythroid tissue.

ERYTHROID PROGENITOR CELL COMPARTMENT

The erythroid progenitor cell compartment, situated functionally between the multipotent stem cell and the morphologically distinguishable erythroid precursor cells, contains a spectrum of cells with a parent-to-progeny relationship, all committed to erythroid differentiation. A complete understanding of how erythroid commitment is achieved at the biochemical or molecular level is lacking, although some attempts at determining the molecular basis have been made.[1-4] Evidence from in vitro cultures of single multipotent progenitor cells allowed to differentiate in competent environments, as well as evidence obtained by studying the phenotype of leukemic cells, suggests that commitment to a specific hematopoietic lineage is accomplished not by acquisition of new genetic information but by restriction (probably on a stochastic basis) to specific programs from a wider repertoire available to pluripotent progenitor cells.[5,6] Molecular evidence supports this view.[6-8] Although all erythroid progenitor cells share the irreversible commitment to express the erythroid phenotype, the properties of these cells progressively diverge as the cells become separated by several divisions.

Erythroid progenitor cells are sparse (Table 24-1) and difficult to isolate in sufficient purity and numbers for study. For these reasons, the existence and characteristics of these cells were inferred from their ability to generate hemoglobinized progeny in vitro in clonal erythroid cultures (Fig. 24-1). Two classes of progenitors have been identified using this approach.[9] The first, more primitive class consists of the burst-forming unit–erythroid (BFU-E), named for the ability of BFU-E to give rise to multiclustered colonies (erythroid bursts) of hemoglobin-containing cells. BFU-E represent the earliest progenitors committed exclusively to erythroid differentiation and a quiescent reserve, with only 10% to 20% in cycle at any given time. However, once stimulated to proliferate in the presence of appropriate cytokines, BFU-Es demonstrate a significant proliferative capacity in vitro, giving rise to colonies of 30,000 to 40,000 cells, which become fully hemoglobinized after 2 to 4 weeks, with a peak incidence at 14 to 16 days. They have a limited self-renewal capacity; at least a subset of BFU-E is capable of generating secondary bursts upon replating. In contrast to this class of progenitor cells, a second, more differentiated class of progenitors consists of the colony-forming unit–erythroid (CFU-E). Most (60% to 80%) of these progenitors already are in cycle and thus proliferate immediately after initiation of culture, forming erythroid colonies within 7 days. Because CFU-E are more differentiated than BFU-E, they require fewer divisions to generate colonies of hemoglobinized cells, and the colonies are small (8 to 64 cells per colony).

Although the two classes of committed erythroid progenitors (BFU-E and CFU-E) appear distinct from each other, in reality progenitor cells constitute a continuum, with graded changes in their properties. Only progenitor cells at both ends of the differentiation spectrum have distinct properties. Perhaps the earliest cell with the potential to generate hemoglobinized progeny is an oligopotent progenitor, which is capable of giving rise to mature cells of at least one other lineage (granulocytic, macrophage, or megakaryocytic) in addition to the erythroid. This progenitor, a multilineage colony-forming unit (CFU) called a *colony-forming unit–granulocyte, erythrocyte, macrophage, megakaryocyte* (CFU-GEMM) or *common myeloid progenitor,* and the most primitive BFU-E have physical and functional properties that are shared by both pluripotent stem cells and progenitor cells committed to nonerythroid lineages. These properties include high proliferative potential, low cycling rate, response to a combination of cytokines, and presence of specific surface antigens or surface receptors (see Table 24-1). In contrast, the latest CFU-E have many similarities with erythroid precursor cells and little in common with primitive BFU-E. Their proliferative potential is limited, they cannot self-renew, they lack the cell surface antigens common to all early progenitors, and they are exquisitely sensitive to erythropoietin (EPO; see Table 24-1).

Although clonal erythroid cultures are indispensable for the study of erythroid progenitors, they do not faithfully reproduce the in vivo kinetics of red cell differentiation/maturation, and many maturing cells have a megaloblastic appearance and lyse before they reach the end stage of red cell development. In vivo, erythropoiesis probably occurs faster than predicted from culture data. For example, studies in dogs with cyclic hematopoiesis, a genetic stem cell defect leading to pulses of hematopoiesis, provide evidence that BFU-E mature to CFU-E over 2 to 3 days in vivo, although this process may require 5 to 6 days in canine marrow cultures.[10]

Erythroid progenitors can be cultured in serum-depleted media,[11,12] as well as in serum-containing media. The effects of recombinant growth factors can be studied in serum-depleted cultures without the complicating influences of multiple or unknown factors present in

Table 24-1 Changes in the General Properties During the Differentiation of Erythroid Progenitors

	CFU-GEMM (CMP)	BFU-E	CFU-E
GENERAL FEATURES			
Self-renewal	++	+	0
Differentiation potential	Multipotent	Erythroid committed	Erythroid committed
Cycling status % suicide with ^{3}H thymidine	15-20	30-40	60-80
Cell density (g/mL)	<1.077	<1.077	<1.077
Incidence/10^5 cells	2-5	40-120	200-600
Circulate in blood	+	+	0
GROWTH FACTOR RESPONSE			
EPO	+	+	++
TPO	+	+	+
KL	+	+	–
GM-CSF, IL-3	+	+	–
FL	+	0	0
G-CSF, IL-6, IL-1	+	0	0
Insulin, insulin-like growth factor, activin	0	0	+
TGFβ1	–	–	++
Hyper-IL-6	+	+	+
RECEPTOR/ANTIGEN			
CD34	++	++	–
CD33	+	+	0
C-KIT	++	++	–
HLA-DR (-DP, -DQ)	++	++	+

	CFU-GEMM (CMP)	BFU-E	CFU-E
EPO receptor	+	+	++
gp130	+	+	+
Tumor necrosis factor receptor	+	+	++
P67 laminin	–	+	–
EP-1[163]	+	+	++
23.6*	0	0	+
CD36	0	±	+
Glycophorin A	0	0	+
ABH, Ii†	0	+	+
ADHESION MOLECULES			
VLA4 (CD49d/CD29)	++	++	++
VLA5 (CD49e/CD29)	+	+	++
CD41	+	+	
CD11a/CD18	+	+	
CD44	+	+	
HCAM‡	+	+	
TRANSCRIPTION FACTORS			
GATA2	++	+	–
GATA1	+	++	+++
SCL	+	+	+
EKLF	+	+	++
Myb	++	+	–
Id1, Id2	++	+	–

BFU-E, Burst-forming unit–erythroid; *CFU-E,* colony-forming unit–erythroid; *CFU-GEMM (CMP),* colony-forming unit–granulocyte, erythrocyte, macrophage, megakaryocyte (common myeloid progenitor); *EKLF,* erythroid Krüppel-like factor; *EPO,* erythropoietin; *FL,* Flt-3 ligand; *G-CSF,* granulocyte colony-stimulating factor; *GM-CSF,* granulocyte-macrophage colony-stimulating factor; *HCAM,* homing-associated cytoadhesion molecule; *HLA,* human leukocyte antigen; *IL,* interleukin; *KL,* KIT ligand; *SCL,* stem cell leukemia; *TGF,* transforming growth factor; *TPO,* thrombopoietin.
*23.6 (SFL 23.6) is a monoclonal antibody reactive with CFU-E, erythroblasts, and erythrocytes.[577]
†ABH and Ii are blood group antigens.
‡Presence of other cytoadhesion molecules (i.e., CD31, L-selectin, P-selectin, E-cadherin) has been described in progenitors (see text). However, the extent of their presence in BFU-E as compared to other cells is not clear.

serum. Conditions that imitate lower oxygen pressures, found in bone marrow in vivo, favorably influence erythroid development in culture and may be advantageous.[13]

BFU-E are generated from multipotent or oligopotent progenitors within the marrow, and their survival and proliferation are dependent on the presence of cytokines, elaborated by either stromal cells or accessory cells within the microenvironment. A number of cytokines influence proliferation and/or survival of early progenitors. Among the cytokines, KIT ligand (KL, also known as *stem cell factor,* SCF), which is produced by stromal cells, and interleukin (IL)-3, which is produced by a subset of T cells, alone and in synergy, have a profound proliferative effect on BFU-E and its progeny. Other cytokines, such as granulocyte-macrophage colony-stimulating factor (GM-CSF), IL-11, and thrombopoietin (TPO), stimulate a subset of BFU-E.[14-16] Cytokines exert their effects through interaction with specific receptors present on the BFU-E surface. The presence of such receptors also has been documented in the leukemic counterparts of normal BFU-E and in leukemic cell lines.[17] BFU-E in culture cannot survive for more than a few days in the absence of cytokines. If they are deprived of cytokines for more than 6 days, more than 80% of BFU-E are lost.[18] In addition to positive regulators (IL-3, GM-CSF, TPO, KL, and IL-11), substances with negative influences on BFU-E proliferation have been identified. They include tumor necrosis factor-α (TNF-α), tumor necrosis factor–related apoptosis-inducing ligand (TRAIL), transforming growth factor-β (TGFβ), and interferon-γ.[19-21] These negative regulators are responsible, at least in part, for the anemia associated with chronic inflammatory states. The effects of TNF-α and TRAIL are mediated through induction of apoptosis at specific stages of erythroid maturation. In the case of TRAIL, a complex system of signaling and decoy receptor isoforms determines the precise cell window susceptible to TRAIL-induced apoptosis.[21] TRAIL probably induces apoptosis by competing with EPO for activation of Bruton tyrosine kinase. Its effects are counteracted by KL[22,23] and protein kinase Cε[24] signaling. TRAIL also is involved in the pathobiology of the anemia associated with multiple myeloma (TRAIL is overproduced by the malignant plasma cells of these patients[25]) and myelodysplastic syndrome (MDS) (myelodysplastic erythroid progenitors overexpress the adaptor Fas-associated death domain of the TRAIL receptor[26]). On the other hand, the negative effects of TGFβ[27] are mainly achieved by accelerating cell

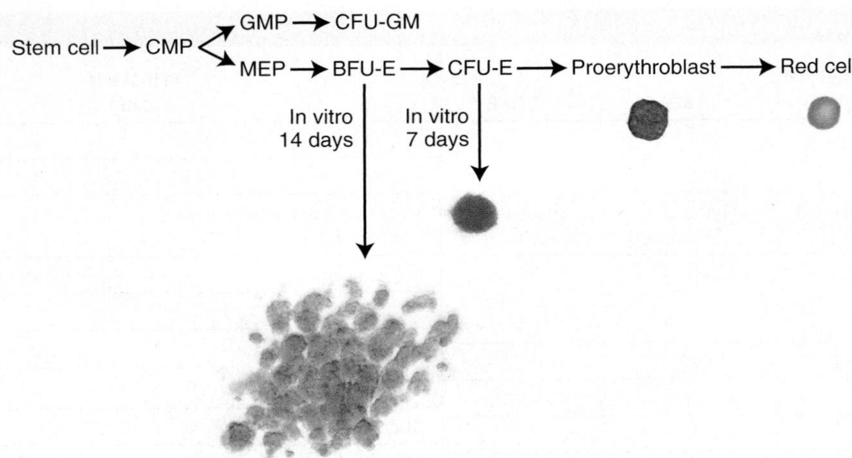

Figure 24-1 CELLULAR MODEL OF ERYTHROID DIFFERENTIATION. Multipotent stem cells generate cellular compartments defined on the basis of their antigenic profile and restricted toward the myeloid differentiation pathway–defined common myeloid progenitor (CMP).[68,69] CMP in turn give rise to granulocyte/macrophage progenitor (GMP) and megakaryocyte-erythroid progenitor (MEP), which probably correspond to the burst-forming unit–erythroid (BFU-E). Lastly, MEP generate cells capable of unilineage differentiation toward either the megakaryocytic (colony-forming unit-megakaryocyte [CFU-Mk], not shown) or the erythroid pathway (colony-forming unit–erythroid [CFU-E]). These cells occur infrequently in the marrow (approximately 0.3% of mononuclear cells) and are defined on the basis of clonogenic assays. If marrow is placed in semisolid medium (e.g., methylcellulose) to decrease cell motility, with appropriate nutrients and growth factors (e.g., transferrin, insulin, erythropoietin, and interleukin-3), CFU-E (after approximately 7 days) differentiate into small clusters of hemoglobinized or red cells termed *erythroid colonies*. Most BFU-E present in the inoculum differentiate to form multiclustered colonies of hemoglobinized cells, or erythroid bursts, by days 14 to 16. Each erythroid colony or burst derives from one BFU-E or CFU-E, respectively. *CFU-GM,* Colony-forming unit–granulocyte-macrophage.

differentiation, whereas data on mouse models of chronic exposure indicate that interferon-γ reduces the erythrocyte life span and inhibits erythropoiesis by promoting the expression of PU.1, a transcription factor that antagonizes GATA1, a master transcriptional regulator of erythropoiesis[28,29] (see Transcription Factors in Erythropoiesis).

In addition to the negative growth factors, overexpression of hepcidin, a key regulator of systemic iron homeostasis (see Chapter 33), is involved in determining the anemia associated with chronic inflammation.[30] The increased hepcidin synthesis that occurs during inflammation traps iron in macrophages, decreases plasma iron concentrations, and causes iron-restricted erythropoiesis characteristic of the anemia of inflammatory states. Hepcidin deficiency induces iron overload in transgenic mice, whereas hepcidin excess induces iron accumulation in macrophages similar to observations in patients with chronic inflammation.[31] Hepcidin might inhibit proliferation of erythroid progenitors at low EPO concentrations.[32]

BFU-E and immediate progeny (but not CFU-E) are motile cells found in significant numbers in peripheral blood. As with BFU-E, the ability of stem cells and progenitor cells to circulate is physiologically important for the redistribution of marrow cells in cases of local damage to the microenvironment and for reconstitution of hematopoiesis after transplantation. The spectrum of BFU-E in circulation probably is narrower (consisting mostly of early, quiescent BFU-E) than that of BFU-E in the bone marrow; otherwise, their properties are similar to those of marrow BFU-E. The number of circulating BFU-E (along with other progenitors and stem cells) can increase to significant levels after cytokine/chemokine treatments and after chemotherapy, a finding that has been exploited for transplantation purposes.[33] At present, mononuclear cells contained in the blood from subjects mobilized with granulocyte colony-stimulating factor (G-CSF) are routinely used as a source of stem/progenitor cells in autologous and allogeneic transplantation,[34] alone or in combination with AMD3100, a CXCR4 inhibitor.[35]

In addition to forming colonies in semisolid medium, hematopoietic progenitors from different sources can generate erythroid cells in liquid culture.[36] Liquid cultures do not allow progenitor cell enumeration but may generate more differentiated cells per progenitor cell than do semisolid cultures.[37,38] The number of erythroblasts generated in liquid cultures can be further increased by adding to the media glucocorticoid steroids,[37,39] which exert a reversible inhibition on proerythroblast maturation.[40,41] In theory this culture system may generate numbers of erythroid cells equivalent to 1 unit of blood from discarded stem cell sources (cord blood <50 mL and from buffy coats produced during the leukoreduction process of blood donations).[42,43] This recognition led to the belief that red blood cells generated ex vivo may one day be used for transfusion. Recently it has been demonstrated that red blood cells generated *in vitro* from mobilized CD34^{pos} cells collected by apheresis have normal survival when transfused into an autologous recipient.[44] Although production of red blood cells in numbers required for transfusion is currently a challenging proposition (approximately 2.5×10^{12}), this first-in-man proof-of-principle has fostered great interest in studies addressing the various aspects of the complex process of making red blood cells in vitro to ultimately translate this approach into clinical transfusion practice.

Surface antigens of human BFU-E have been defined through the use of monoclonal antibodies.[45,46] The antibodies tested include two broad categories: antibodies raised against leukemic cells or cell lines with progenitor cell properties, and antibodies raised against normal, terminally differentiated red cells. Enrichment in BFU-E (or CFU-E) after labeling with these antibodies, or their loss after complement-dependent lysis, is considered indicative of the presence of test antigens on the BFU-E surface. Reactivities of BFU-E with several antibodies directed against defined surface antigens are listed in Table 24-1. Like other hematopoietic progenitors, BFU-E display human leukocyte antigen (HLA) class I (A, B, C) and class II (DP, DQ, DR) antigens on their surface. Class II antigens (especially the products of the DR locus), in contrast to class I, are variably expressed among BFU-E. This may relate to variations in their cycling status, because myeloid progenitors in S phase have relatively higher expression of class II antigens.[47] The presence of HLA class II antigens (DR and, to a lesser extent, DP and DQ) most likely allows BFU-E to recognize and interact with the immunoregulatory cells (e.g., T cells, monocytes), which also express class II determinants.[48] In addition to HLA antigens, several other antigenic structures are found on cells within the BFU-E compartment (see Table 24-1). The best representative of these is the CD34 antigen, which has been successfully exploited for isolation of BFU-E and other progenitors. CD34 is a highly *O*-glycosylated cell surface glycoprotein. It is expressed in all hematopoietic progenitors and vascular endothelial cells.[49] The role of CD34 in human hematopoiesis is not clearly defined. The numbers of all hematopoietic progenitors were reduced in CD34 "null" murine embryos and adult animals, but no other abnormalities were identified.[50] Expression of CD34 was low or absent in a population of adult long-term repopulating cells in mouse[51] and in man.[52] However, the clinical significance of this finding is not clear because of the fluctuating expression of CD34[53] and the difference in regulatory mechanisms of CD34 gene expression in mouse and human stem cells.[54] Furthermore, use of antibodies or conjugated ligands determined that BFU-E present in enriched progenitor preparations display receptors for KL, EPO, TPO, GM-CSF, IL-3, IL-6, and IL-11. However, the majority of BFU-E, in contrast to myeloid progenitors (colony-forming unit–granulocyte-macrophage), do not express the restricted hematopoietic phosphatase CD45RA.[55,56] Furthermore, BFU-E appear to share with late colony-forming unit-megakaryocyte progenitors the expression of the TPO receptor (c-Mpl or TPO-R)[56,57] and glycoprotein IIb/IIIa (CD41), a marker of the divergence between definitive hematopoiesis and endothelial cells during development.[58]

As BFU-E mature to the CFU-E stage, they begin to express surface proteins characteristic of erythroblasts, the morphologically recognizable erythroid cells. For example, CFU-E express Rh antigens and the erythroid-specific sialoglycoprotein glycophorin A. Blood group antigens of the ABH Ii type are detectable in a subset of CFU-E. In contrast, CD34 molecules, class II antigens, and certain growth factor receptors (i.e., IL-3R, C-KIT) are greatly diminished or virtually absent at the CFU-E stage (see Table 24-1). The most important functional difference between BFU-E and CFU-E is the abundance of erythropoietin receptors (EPORs) on CFU-E and their dependence on EPO for cell survival. CFU-E, in contrast to BFU-E, cannot survive in vitro even for a few hours in the absence of EPO. Although greater than 80% of CFU-E have detectable EPORs,[59] only a small proportion of BFU-E have receptors[60,61] and can terminally differentiate in culture in the presence of EPO alone.[62] Direct binding studies show that the number of EPORs peaks at the CFU-E/proerythroblast level and progressively declines when cells mature further (see Table 24-1),[59] reflecting the declining influence of EPO. In addition to the abundance of EPORs, erythroid progenitors are distinguished from other marrow progenitors by the presence of high levels of transferrin receptors (TfRs).[60,63,64] Peak levels of TfRs are seen on CFU-E and erythroid precursors, and lower levels are present on reticulocytes.[57,63] (For a detailed review of iron metabolism and heme synthesis in erythroid cells, see references 65 to 67).

In addition to the functional definition, the hemopoietic compartments in the marrow of a normal adult mouse have been prospectively identified on the basis of expression of specific cell surface antigens and subsequent differentiation in vitro and in vivo.[68] The $Lin^{neg}IL\text{-}7R^{neg}Thy1^{neg}C\text{-}KIT^{pos}Sca1^{neg}$ fraction of the marrow of normal adult mice has been subdivided into three populations based on the expression of CD34 and CD16/CD32: $CD16/CD32^{low}CD34^{high}$ representing the common myeloid progenitor (CMP), $CD16/CD32^{low}CD34^{low}$ representing the megakaryocyte/erythroid progenitor (MEP), and $CD16/CD32^{high}CD34^{high}$ representing the granulocyte/macrophage progenitor (see Fig. 24-1).[68] Many laboratories have also prospectively identified the corresponding human compartments.[69-71] In humans, the transition from CMP to MEP is characterized by loss of aldehyde dehydrogenase activity[72] and acquisition of c-Mpl expression.[73]

The correlation between phenotype and function of cells isolated on the basis of these antigenic expression profiles is not maintained under conditions of perturbed or stressed erythropoiesis. Stress activates the bone morphologic protein 4 (BMP4)/hedgehog signaling, which induces the generation of erythroid progenitor cells with a unique phenotype, KIT^{pos}, $CD71^{pos}$ and $TER\text{-}119^{pos}$ (TER-119 recognizes the murine equivalent of glycophorin A).[74,75] The expression on these cells of "true" markers of terminal erythroid maturation suggests that stress-specific erythroid progenitors may be related to the proerythroblasts with extensive proliferative potential generated in mice after EPO treatment or anemia challenge,[76,77] thereby indicating that stress may uncouple proliferation and differentiation programs during terminal erythroid maturation. The proliferation and differentiation programs are also uncoupled during ontogenesis. The number of erythroblasts generated in vitro by embryonic/primitive (E7.5 yolk sac), embryonic/definitive (E8.5-9.5 yolk sac and E12.5 fetal liver), and adult/definitive murine erythroid progenitors in the presence of EPO, KL, and dexamethasone differ widely.[78] Embryonic/definitive proerythroblasts originating from a transient wave of early fetal erythropoiesis are capable of generating large numbers (10^{10}- to 10^{30}-fold expansion) of proerythroblasts that, because of their great expansion potential, were characterized as extensively self-renewing erythroblasts (ESREs). By contrast, under the same conditions, embryonic/primitive proerythroblasts failed to expand and adult/definitive proerythroblasts expanded only 10^2- to 10^5-fold. Interestingly, human erythroblasts generated in the presence of dexamethasone also express high levels of C-KIT and acquire self-renewal potential.[79] In addition to steroids, polymeric immunoglobulin A1 (IgA1) has also been shown to control erythroblast proliferation and to accelerate erythropoiesis recovery in anemia.[80] These observations challenge the notion that erythroblasts are capable of a limited (at most two to four) number of divisions.

More recently, erythroid cells have been derived in vitro from stem cell sources with unlimited proliferation potential such as human embryonic stem cells (hESCs) and induced pluripotent stem cells (iPSCs).[81] Seminal studies in 2008 from Hiroyama et al established that red blood cells generated from murine ESCs are functional in vivo because they protect mice from lethal hemolytic anemia.[82] Methods for generating red blood cells from human ESCs have also been published, and the biologic properties of these human ESC-derived red blood cells have been extensively characterized.[83,84] A number of groups have also published methods for generating red blood cells from iPSCs.[85,86] In general, independently of their origin, ES- or iPS-derived erythroid cells express mostly embryonic and fetal globins. In addition, several investigators are exploring the feasibility of reprogramming somatic cells directly into erythroid cells, bypassing the pluripotent state and/or generating stem cells with unlimited expansion potential by epigenetic or genetic in vitro treatments.[87,88] In both cases, the modified cells generated erythroblasts that mature into circulating red cells when injected into immunodeficient NOD/SCID/γc^{null} mice.

ERYTHROID MORPHOLOGICALLY RECOGNIZABLE PRECURSOR CELL COMPARTMENT

The erythroid precursor cell compartment, also termed the *erythron,* includes cells that, in contrast to the erythroid progenitor cells (BFU-E and CFU-E), are defined by morphologic criteria. The earliest recognizable erythroid cell is the *proerythroblast,* which after four to five mitotic divisions and serial morphologic changes gives rise to mature erythroid cells. Its progeny include basophilic erythroblasts, which are the earliest daughter cells, followed by polychromatophilic and orthochromatic erythroblasts. Their morphologic characteristics reflect the accumulation of erythroid-specific proteins (i.e., hemoglobin) and the decline in nuclear activity (Fig. 24-2). After the last mitotic division, the inactive dense nucleus of the orthochromatic erythroblast moves to one side of the cell and is extruded, encased by a thin cytoplasmic layer with differential partitioning of membrane/cytoplasmic proteins.[89] Expelled nuclei are ingested by marrow

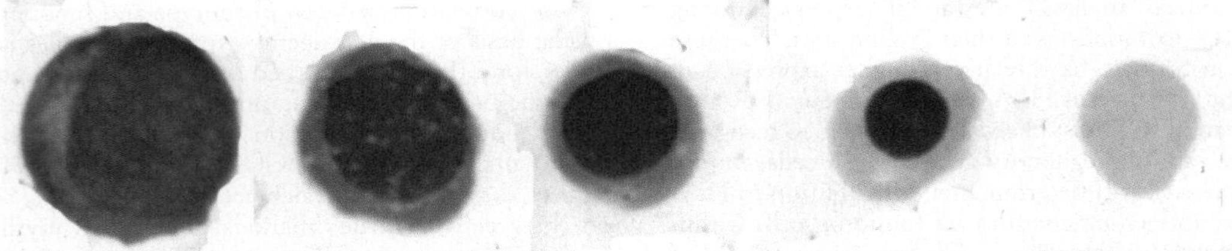

Figure 24-2 ERYTHROID MATURATION SEQUENCE. As proliferation parameters (i.e., rates of deoxyribonucleic acid [DNA] and ribonucleic acid [RNA] synthesis) and cell size decrease, accumulation of erythroid-specific proteins (i.e., heme and globin) increases, and the cells adapt their morphologic characteristics. *(Modified from Granick S, Levere R: Heme synthesis in erythroid cells. In Moore CV, Brown EB, editors:* Progress in hematology, *vol 4, Orlando, Fla, 1964, Grune & Stratton, p 1.)*

macrophages, and the resulting enucleated cell is a reticulocyte. Although all mammals have enucleated cells in their circulation, the evolutionary advantage of enucleation is not readily apparent. It may allow for more red cell deformability when traveling through the small vasculature, or it may minimize cardiac workload.

Maturation from proerythroblast to reticulocyte likely does not always adhere to a rigid sequence in which each division is associated with the production of two more differentiated and morphologically distinct daughter cells (i.e., basophilic erythroblast gives rise to two polychromatophilic ones). Rather, significant flexibility, both in the number and rate of divisions and in the rate of enucleation, may be allowed. Such deviations from the normal orderly maturation sequence may be dictated by the level of EPO or "stress" conditions. Thus in cases of acute demand for red cell production (because of blood loss or hemolysis), the kinetics of formation of new reticulocytes are significantly more rapid. Resulting red cells may be larger (i.e., with increased mean corpuscular volume). This has led to the concept of "skipped" divisions.[90] The orderly unilineage differentiation pathway shown in Fig. 24-1 likely is restricted to conditions of steady-state hematopoiesis. Similar to occurrences in the lymphoid system,[91] alternative routes are taken under conditions of "stress." Murine models have been developed to address phenotype-function cell relationships during recovery from acute and chronic erythroid stress. A model for acute stress is represented by the hemolytic anemia induced by phenylhydrazine treatment. Recovery from this acute anemia involves recruitment of the spleen as an additional erythropoietic site and is dependent on EPO. The amount of ^{3}H-thymidine incorporated by splenic erythroblasts produced in response to this stress initially represented the biologic assay for EPO.[92] Genetic evidence indicates that recovery from this hemolytic anemia is controlled by a receptor complex formed between the EPOR and a truncated version of the Stk receptor encoded by Fv2^{s}, a locus that also determines strain susceptibility to Friend virus infection.[93] An additional control on the response to acute erythroid stress in mice is exerted by the glucocorticoid receptor (GR), because mice in which this receptor is targeted recover poorly from phenylhydrazine treatment.[94] On the other hand, experimentally induced mutations in genes involved in the regulation of erythroid differentiation, such as signal transducer and activator of transcription 5 (STAT5^{null} [95]) and GATA1^{LOW}[96], or inability of response to reactive oxygen species (ROS) challenge (i.e., Foxo3 deficiency)[97] increase the rate of erythroblast apoptosis. The spleen is also recruited as a hemopoietic site in response to chronic erythroid stress.[95,96] Several studies in aggregate suggest that the erythron does not respond to stress only by amplifying the normal erythroid progenitor cell compartments (i.e., CMP, MEP, and CFU-E), but by generating alternative routes of differentiation, possibly through cooperation between EPOR and other receptors (e.g., Stk, GR, soluble KL, BMP4/hedgehog pathway) specifically recruited as part of the stress response.[76,77,98,99] Genetic heterogeneity in the control of gene expression of these receptors may add another layer of variability in recovery from anemia in humans.

The importance of GR in the control of stress erythropoiesis was established by studies in transgenic mice harboring a dimerization-defective GR (GR$^{dim/dim}$ mice).[100] These mice have normal steady-state erythropoiesis but were unable to increase red blood cell production in response to hypoxia. Gene deletion studies established that GR facilitates stress erythropoiesis in mice by blocking maturation of erythroid precursors and inducing a limited self-renewal state.[101] Although clinical observations indicating that the GR ligand such as dexamethasone stimulates erythropoiesis have been available since 1961,[102,103] the precise role of GR in human erythropoiesis is still unclear. Murine GR is not polymorphic, whereas human GR (GR/NR3C1 located in the 5q31-32 region of chromosome 5 and deleted in 5q- syndrome) contains several single-nucleotide polymorphisms (SNPs).[104-107] Because of this genetic diversity, human cells may express more than 260 isoforms with slightly or greatly different biologic activities. The most studied isoform is GRα, an isoform similar to the murine GR. Alternative splicing between exon 3-4 generates GRγ, an isoform containing an additional arginine in the deoxyribonucleic acid (DNA)-binding domain that reduces the transactivation potential by half. An alternative splicing of exon 9 generates messenger ribonucleic acid (mRNA) encoding the dominant-negative GRβ isoform.[107] It is debatable whether an isoform with dominant-negative action similar to GRβ exists in mice.[105,108] It is generally accepted that responses to GR ligands depend on the signal transduction potential of the GR isoforms expressed by different cells and tissues. Studies in human nonerythroid cell types have identified that GR isoform expression predicts the variegation of cellular response to dexamethasone in vitro.[109-111] Recently clinicians have established important correlations between GR haplotype and variability in patients' responses to glucocorticoids and in the development of glucocorticoid resistance in several disorders.[112] GR polymorphism and/or epigenetic changes are emerging as the leading cause for dexamethasone unresponsiveness or for development of dexamethasone resistance in patients with inflammatory and autoimmune diseases[113] (i.e., Crohn disease, systemic lupus) and in chronic depression.[112,114-116]

Similarly, several in vitro and in vivo studies suggest that variegation of GR isoform expression may also have biologic and clinical effects on terminal erythroid maturation. The numbers of erythroblasts generated by murine erythroid progenitors in response to dexamethasone is fairly consistent, whereas the number generated by human erythroid progenitors from different individuals may vary by 1 to 2 logs,[43,117] likely reflecting the genetic background of human GR. In addition, the frequency of the rs6198 SNP is greater than normal in patients with polycythemia vera (PV) (55%, $P = 0.0028$)[118] and with Diamond-Blackfan anemia (DBA) (43%, $P = 0.03$),[118] suggesting that genetic conditions favoring GRβ expression may represent host genetic modifiers in diseases with altered terminal erythroid differentiation.

The morphologic alterations that occur as erythroid precursor cells mature (see Fig. 24-2) are determined by complex biochemical changes, which accommodate the accumulation of erythroid-specific proteins and the progressive decline in proliferation.[119] Compared with erythroid progenitor cells, erythroid precursor cells have been more accessible to study, and considerable information is available about their maturation-related biochemical changes.

The shape and deformability of the red cells are determined by the appropriate assembly of their membrane proteins with the cytoplasmic cytoskeleton. Red cells survive shear forces in the microvasculature because transmembrane complexes embedded in the lipid bilayer attach to the cytoskeleton, ensuring its flexibility. These complexes contain clinically relevant blood group antigens determined by genetic polymorphisms in proteins of these complexes.[120-122] The similarity between the amino acid sequence of the blood group antigens and that of proteins present on the surface of bacteria and the increased frequency of certain blood group antigens in regions with high incidence of malaria suggest that blood group antigens, in addition to ensuring appropriate membrane structure, may facilitate development of appropriate immunoreactivity toward opportunistic infections.

Most membrane cytoskeletal proteins (spectrin, glycophorin, band 3, band 4.1, and ankyrin) accumulate after the CFU-E stage (i.e., within the precursor cell compartment). Specifically, expression of membrane glycoproteins such as band 3 and band 4.1 is greatly enhanced at the later stages of erythroid maturation.[119,123,124] Likewise, the quantity of polylactosaminoglycan, a specific carbohydrate chain that carries blood group ABH and Ii antigenic determinants, is much higher in mature erythrocytes than in erythroblasts.[125] Whereas a linear, virtually unbranched polylactosamine structure is present in fetal and newborn erythroid cells (reflected by i antigenic reactivity), a branched polylactosaminyl structure is present in adult erythroblasts (reflected by I antigenic reactivity), and branching increases further as maturation progresses.[125,126] A correctly assembled cytoskeleton is important for the deformability and dynamic plasticity of red blood cells in circulation. A recently recognized player required for actin assembly in red cells, Rac GTPase, has been identified.[127] Glycophorins, especially glycophorin A, are expressed fully at the CFU-E or proerythroblast level just before expression of globin, and few changes occur during maturation.[46] In contrast, the membrane glycoproteins p105 and p95 decline during the later stages of maturation,[125] and yet other membrane glycoproteins, such as vimentin (an intermediate filament protein), are totally lost.[119] Loss of vimentin expression at the late erythroblastic stages most likely facilitates enucleation.

The process of erythroblast enucleation involves membrane remodeling,[128] chromatin condensation to form pyknotic nuclei, and formation of spindle independent motors driving the separation of the reticulocyte from the pyrenocyte (the pyknotic nuclei surrounded by a cytoplasmic rim).[129] Partitioning of erythroblast plasma membrane components to reticulocytes is regulated by the degree of skeletal linkage,[130] whereas chromatin condensation is mediated by the histone deacetylase (HDAC) 2,[131] suggesting that impairment of HDAC2 activity may contribute to the development of anemia observed in HDAC-based cancer treatments. Nonmuscle myosin appears to represent the motor driving the separation between the reticulocyte and the pyrenocyte.[132] Reticulocytes are released in the blood, where they undergo extensive cytoplasmic remodeling to reduce the number of ribosomes and mitochondria and to become mature red cells. This process is mediated by autophagic machinery,[133] whereas engulfment of pyrenocytes, and subsequent degradation by macrophages, occurs only after pyrenocytes are totally disconnected from reticulocytes. Phosphatidylserine, the "eat me" flag for apoptotic cells, is also used for engulfment of pyrenocytes expelled from erythroblasts,[134] whereas expression of CD47, the "eat me not" signal, by interacting with SIRP1α expressed by the macrophages, prevents engulfment and destruction of erythroblasts and reticulocytes.[135] The enucleation process is caspase independent[136] but erythroblast macrophage protein dependent.[137] Erythroblast macrophage protein is expressed by both erythroblasts and macrophages, and it is necessary for proper enucleation to occur.[137] The fact that proper enucleation requires interaction with macrophages explains the old observation that erythroid differentiation in the marrow occurs in discrete sites, the "erythroblastic islands," which are composed of erythroblasts surrounding a central macrophage.

In addition to quantitative changes that occur during maturation, gradual switches in subunit composition of some cytoskeletal proteins occur. For example, exclusively erythroid subunits of α- and β-spectrin are displayed only in end-stage cells.[50] Likewise, multiple transcripts of ankyrin or protein 4.1 have been identified, and the ratios of these transcripts change during maturation.[138] Initial expression of many of these membrane components likely begins at the progenitor cell level. However, in these cells, final assembly may be discouraged because of the higher turnover of these proteins, which minimizes mutual interactions, or because of asynchrony in protein synthesis. Prevention of cytoskeletal assembly at these early stages may secure more membrane fluidity and cell motility needed during this proliferative phase of differentiation. Because molecular probes for many of the red cell cytoskeletal components have been developed, detailed information about the transcription and processing of most of these proteins is beginning to emerge.[124] For example, band 3, the major anion transport protein of human erythrocytes, is a key component of a multicomplex that also contains protein 4.2. Appropriate display of this protein complex on the cell membrane is dependent on critical interactions established between newly synthesized band 3 and protein 4.2 already at the proerythroblast stage.[139]

Expression of the majority of genes encoding cytoskeletal components is not restricted to red cells. Dissecting hemopoietic from nonhemopoietic consequences of abnormalities in these genes has been difficult, but the development of mouse models that mimic defects found in human diseases has been helpful in this respect.[140]

Gene activity during erythroid maturation is dominated by globin expression. Globin represents less than 0.1% of protein at the proerythroblast level but constitutes 95% of all protein at the reticulocyte level.[141] Globin expression has been extensively studied, and its gene regulation is well understood in molecular terms. Major steps in globin transcription and processing are known in considerable detail and are summarized elsewhere in this text (see Chapter 31). The globin type synthesized by adult precursors is hemoglobin A (HbA; $\alpha_2\beta_2$). In addition, two other minor globin components, HbA_2 ($\alpha_2\delta_2$) and HbF ($\alpha_2\gamma_2$), are present. Of significant biologic interest are the low amounts of HbF that continue to be synthesized throughout life.

The small amount of HbF, which is present in all normal individuals, has the following characteristics.[142] (1) It is confined to a small fraction of red cells, called *F cells*, which are detected by sensitive immunofluorescence assays or acid elution techniques and usually constitute 2% to 5% of all red cells. Within each F cell, HbF or γ-globin constitutes 14% to 25% of total globin. (2) The number of F cells is genetically determined, and the gene(s) linked or nonlinked to the β-locus is responsible for F-cell formation. (3) F cells do not display other features of "fetalness" because their membrane components and enzymes are characteristically adult. (4) Synthesis of HbF peaks earlier than that of HbA, so the proportion of HbF is higher in immature cells compared with mature, fully hemoglobinized cells. (5) F cells and cells that contain only HbA are not derived from distinct stem cell populations but from a common adult stem cell. Whether the latter will form F or non-F (i.e., A) cells is determined at the BFU-E level and throughout the CFU-E level.[143] In vitro the great majority of BFU-E have the potential to express HbF, whereas in vivo only a very small proportion of red cells contain HbF. This potential appears to be lost during normal cell differentiation and maturation in vivo. This concept links the potential for HbF expression to the pathway of erythroid differentiation and thus may have implications for interpreting the reactivation of HbF that occurs in adults under diverse circumstances (e.g., after chemotherapy or with acute bleeding).[142] Many of these circumstances seem to influence HbF levels by directly or indirectly modifying the kinetics of the normal differentiation/maturation process.[144,145] HbF levels in red cells can be increased by exposing the cells during maturation to chemical inhibitors of HDAC. This class of enzymes nonspecifically suppresses gene transcription by catalyzing histone deacetylation and consequently chromatin condensation.[146] Therefore they can directly activate transcription of γ-globin genes in vitro and in vivo[147-149] and in a number of patients with β-thalassemia.[150,151]

Synthesis of globin appears to be coordinated with synthesis of heme throughout erythroid maturation so that functional hemoglobin tetramers are formed rapidly and spontaneously after release of newly synthesized globins from polysomes. Information about the accumulation of heme and its synthetic intermediaries has been provided by crude biochemical approaches (see Fig. 24-2). However, now that the genes for several enzymes in the heme synthetic pathway (e.g., δ-5-aminolevulinic acid synthase, porphobilinogen deaminase, ferrochelatase) have been cloned, information about their regulation is rapidly emerging.[65,67]

An important role in coordinating heme and globin chain assembly during hemoglobin production is exerted by α-hemoglobin-stabilizing protein (AHSP). AHSP is a protein abundantly expressed in erythroid cells[152] whose function is to bind free α-chains, stabilizing their structure and limiting their ability to participate in chemical reactions that generate ROS.[153,154] In addition, AHSP binding increases the affinity of α-chains for β-chains, accelerating the formation of Hb tetramers. The essential role exerted by this gene in erythroid development has been demonstrated by the fact that its deletion in normal mice impairs red cell production. AHSP^{null} red cells have a decreased half-life, contain Hb precipitates, and exhibit signs of oxidative damage.[152] The observation that double AHSP^{null} β-thalassemic mutant mice have an exacerbated phenotype[155] suggests that AHSP is a gene modifier that, like the hereditary persistence of HbF mutations, ameliorates the phenotype of thalassemic patients. However, the search for AHSP polymorphisms that might correlate with milder clinical phenotypes in thalassemia has not provided consistent results. Gene mapping, direct genomic sequencing, and extended haplotype analysis did not reveal any mutation or specific association between haplotypes of AHSP in 120 β-thalassemic patients.[156] On the other hand, a polymorphism in the putative AHSP promoter leading to a threefold higher expression of the gene in reticulocytes has been observed in the normal population,[157] but the clinical consequences of this observation are unknown.

Crucial to the functional response of erythroid precursors is the expression of EPORs and TfRs. EPORs decrease progressively (from approximately 1000 to <300 receptors per cell) as proerythroblasts mature, and they are undetectable at the reticulocyte level.[59,158] Through these receptors, EPO exerts its proliferative influence on proerythroblasts and basophilic erythroblasts, but maturation beyond these stages can proceed in the absence of EPO.

TfRs are found in characteristic abundance in erythroid cells (300,000 to 800,000 TfRs per cell).[159] This composition reflects not only the proliferative needs of erythroid cells but also their extreme requirements for iron uptake for hemoglobin synthesis. For this reason, TfRs persist in maturing nondividing erythroblasts and in reticulocytes. TfRs belong to a large group of receptors that internalize their ligand through receptor-mediated endocytosis. This cycle allows for reuse both of the ligand (transferrin) for resaturation with iron and of the receptor for entering another route of endocytosis.[160] TfRs' density decreases with maturation. After the reticulocyte stage, receptors appear to be shed as small lipid vesicles.[161] An inverse relationship exists between receptor density and iron availability. Deprivation of iron results in receptor induction, and excess iron results in receptor suppression.[160] However, the mechanisms that regulate the number of TfRs throughout the maturation of precursors (even within progenitors) are largely unknown. Erythroid precursor cells differ from nonerythroid cells not only by requiring a higher number and higher occupancy of TfRs, but also by displaying immunologically distinct receptor isoforms.[64] A second gene for transferrin receptor (TfR2) has been identified,[162] and monoclonal antibodies recognizing distinct receptor isoforms are useful in isolating erythroid cells from bone marrow.[64,163] TfR1 and TfR2 are members of a family of genes encoding at least seven different homologous proteins in primates.[164] TfR1 is a type II membrane glycoprotein that, as a cell surface homodimer, binds iron-loaded transferrin as part of the process of iron transfer and uptake. TfR2 is expressed in two forms—membrane-bound (TfR2-α) and nonmembrane (TfR2-β)—both of which bind transferrin with low affinity. The specific role of TfR2 in hematopoietic cells is unclear. In cells from 67 patients with de novo acute myeloid leukemia (AML), high levels of TfR2-α expression were correlated with better prognosis, and higher levels of both TfR2-α and TfR2-β were associated with longer survival, suggesting that TfR-independent iron uptake plays a role in in vivo proliferation of AML cells.[165] TfR2 plays its most prominent role in the liver[166] as the key regulator of iron metabolism. Maintenance of stable extracellular iron concentrations requires the coordinate regulation of iron transport into plasma from dietary sources in the duodenum, recycled senescent red cells in macrophages, and storage in hepatocytes. Diferric transferrin is present in the liver due to complex machinery involving the product of the hereditary hemochromatosis (HFE) gene (a protein of the major histocompatibility complex class I), TfR2, and the product of the hemojuvelin (HJV) gene (also known as HFE2). Given that the levels of TfR2 expression are exclusively regulated by holotransferrin, TfR2 expressed by hepatocytes likely is the first element of the iron sensory pathway in the liver.[167] Hepatocytes respond to iron sensoring by modulating hepcidin expression and secretion. Hepcidin, a 25–amino acid disulfide-rich peptide, acts as a systemic iron regulatory hormone that regulates both dietary iron absorption by the enterocytes and iron recycling by the macrophages. Because ferroportin shuttles iron from the enterocytes to the macrophages and hepcidin is required for ferroportin internalization and degradation, decreased hepcidin expression blocks iron export in the two cell types.[168] Each gene involved in iron metabolism has a role in regulating the expression of the other genes. In particular, reduced expression of HEF, TfR2, and HJV reduces expression of hepcidin. It is not surprising then that mutations altering the function of all of these genes have been found to be associated with hereditary hemochromatosis. The most prevalent form of hereditary hemochromatosis (type 1; HFE1) involves mutations in HFE.[169] Most families with juvenile hemochromatosis (HFE2) have mutations in the HJV gene.[170] Homozygous nonsense[171] and single-point mutations causing methionine→lysine substitution at position 172 of the protein M172K[172] have been detected in the gene encoding TfR2 in patients with familial hemochromatosis HFE3. Autosomal dominant iron overload is associated with previously unrecognized ferroportin 1 mutations (p.R88T and p.I180T)[173] and with mutations in the divalent metal transporter 1 gene DMT1, which mediates apical iron uptake in duodenal enterocytes and iron transfer from the TfR endosomal cycle into the cytosol in erythroid cells.[174] The observation that targeted deletions of any of these genes (including TfR2) induce a hemochromatosis-like syndrome in mice provides proof of direct involvement of the mutations in disease development.[175-178] On the other hand, the finding that hepcidin is a gene modifier of the HEF^{null} mouse model of hemochromatosis suggests that heterogeneity at the hepcidin locus mediates the low penetrance of the genetic disease.[179] In addition to its role in determining the pathobiology of hereditary hemochromatosis, hepcidin plays an important role in determining the anemia of chronic diseases. Based on the central involvement of hepcidin in iron regulation and its pathologic conditions, a hepcidin assay has been proposed as a useful tool for diagnosing iron disorders and monitoring their treatment. On the other hand, development of hepcidin agonists and antagonists may provide useful therapeutics for treatment of iron disorders.[180]

The patterns of TfR and glycophorin A expression during erythroid maturation have been exploited to define flow cytometric criteria that distinguish the different populations of erythroid precursors in mice and men. By coupling size and forward scatter (both progressively reduced) with CD71 (TfR) and TER-119, murine erythroid precursors were divided into the classes TER-119^{med}CD71^{high}, TER-119^{high}CD71^{high}, TER-119^{high}CD71^{med}, and TER-119^{high}CD71^{low}, which correspond to proerythroblasts and basophilic, chromatophilic, and orthochromatophilic erythroblasts, respectively.[95] However, such distinction is not conserved in all mouse strains. For example, in C57Bl/6 mice, CD71 expression levels remain constant during maturation.[181] CD44/glycophorin A expression provides a better flow cytometric definition of the maturation stage of murine erythroblasts.[182] Unfortunately, maturation of human erythroblasts is not associated with significant changes of CD44 expression. Double CD71/glycophorin A staining is therefore still used as criteria to define human erythroblast precursors by flow cytometry. However, the pattern of CD71 expression during erythroid maturation presents a high level of donor variability. Given that downmodulation of CD36 expression during erythroid maturation is relatively independent of genetic variability, an alternative flow cytometric definition of erythroblast subclasses is proposed by the phenotype CD36^{high}/glycophorin A^{medium}, CD36^{high}/glycophorin A^{high}, and CD36^{low}/glycophorin A^{high}, corresponding to basophilic, polychromatic, and orthochromatic erythroblasts, respectively.[183] Flow cytometric criteria for reticulocytes and red cells are instead provided by size (reticulocytes and red cells are distinctively smaller than erythroblasts) and by lack of reactivity for DNA (both reticulocytes and red cells) and RNA (reticulocyte only) staining.

ERYTHROPOIETIN AND EPOR

EPO, a 35-kd glycoprotein,[184] is the physiologically obligatory growth factor for erythroid development. It is produced mainly in the kidney by peritubular cells.[185] A heme-containing protein senses oxygen need and then triggers the synthesis of EPO and its release into the bloodstream.[186,187] Through the interaction of EPO with receptor-bearing cells within the bone marrow, physiologic oxygen demands are translated into increased red cell production. Thus EPO is a true hormone, manufactured at one anatomic site and transported through the bloodstream to the site of activity.

According to the prevailing model of hematopoiesis, progenitor cells committed to erythroid differentiation (i.e., BFU-E) are generated in a stochastic fashion from pluripotent stem cells.[4,5] Neither EPO nor other lineage-restricted regulators play any role in determining lineage commitment. According to this model, EPO influences erythroid differentiation by rescuing (from apoptosis) cells that express EPOR and amplifying them further. Whether EPORs are present on all BFU-E (detectable only in a subset of BFU-E) is not clear.[61] Thus whether the presence of EPOR in BFU-E is synchronous with the initial commitment event or follows it is not known. In addition to the permissive role of EPO ascribed by the stochastic theory, experiments in vivo, in anemic states, or after pharmacologic doses of EPO suggest that high levels of EPO hasten the transition from BFU-E to hemoglobin-synthesizing cells by decreasing either the number of divisions required for this transition[90] or the resting periods between cell divisions.[188] Autoradiographic studies of purified BFU-E populations indicate that EPORs increase as BFU-E mature to CFU-E, with the highest level observed at the CFU-E/proerythroblast boundary.[61] That the transition from BFU-E to CFU-E occurs under the influence of EPO suggests ligand (EPO)-induced receptor upregulation. Whether the magnitude of such upregulation is dependent on EPO dose and whether it can modulate the rate of entry of these cells into the maturing compartment is unclear.

BFU-E and CFU-E can be generated in vitro[189] and in vivo,[190] in the absence of EPO or EPOR (in EPO or EPOR^{null} mice), but their survival and terminal maturation normally are dependent on EPO. For CFU-E, EPO seems to stimulate all the biochemical processes characterizing erythroid cells (i.e., heme synthesis, globin synthesis, and synthesis of cytoskeletal proteins). However, the necessity of EPO in these processes is not absolute. In vitro experiments showing complete maturation of BFU-E in the absence of EPO suggest that other factors or combinations of factors can influence red cell maturation. Activation of the gp130 signaling pathway by use of soluble IL-6 receptor and IL-6 leads to full terminal erythroid maturation (in the presence of stem cell factor and IL-3 but in the absence of EPO), suggesting some form of cross-circuiting in signaling pathways among hematopoietic growth factor receptors.[191,192] Furthermore, stimulation by TPO of erythroid colony formation from yolk sac cells in the absence of EPOR (in EPOR$^{-/-}$ embryos)[193] can be explained by the same reasoning and the finding of a very high proportion of bipotent erythroid/megakaryocytic progenitors in yolk sac carrying both EPO and TPO receptors (c-Mpl) compared to adult bone marrow.[56,194,195]

Whatever the precise mode of EPO action, it directly affects the number of CFU-E and the maturation of their progeny. This control is achieved by influencing CFU-E survival and not their cycling status.[196] CFU-E are irrevocably lost after one cycle of DNA synthesis if EPO is not present.[197]

With the availability of radiolabeled recombinant EPO and purified or enriched populations of progenitors and precursors has come information about the characteristics of EPORs in erythroid cells. Direct binding studies have shown that a progressive decrease in the number of EPORs occurs as CFU-E and proerythroblasts mature to reticulocytes.[60,61,158] Pure reticulocyte populations show no detectable binding to EPO. The maturation-associated decline in the number of EPORs parallels the declining influence of EPO on erythroid cells during the terminal phase of maturation. The exquisite role of EPO in determining red cell numbers in the circulation has been clearly established by direct correlations between hematocrit and EPO plasma concentrations in individuals exposed to hypoxia and in patients with compromised kidney functions.[198] However, the variabilities around the mean of hematocrit and EPO plasma levels found in normal individuals under steady-state conditions are not correlated, indicating that other factors (sex and age) cooperate with EPO in determining the fluctuations in red cell mass under steady-state hematopoiesis.[199]

Cloning and expression of EPOR has allowed for a better understanding of the role of EPO in the regulation of erythroid development. The EPOR polypeptide is a 66-kd membrane protein that is a member of the cytokine receptor superfamily.[200,201] Many of the structural features of the cell surface EPOR have been previously reviewed.[202] Like other members of the cytokine receptor superfamily, which includes the receptors for IL-3, GM-CSF, and IL-5, the EPOR polypeptide contains four conserved cysteine residues and a WSXWS motif in the extracellular region. Additional extracytoplasmic sequences of EPOR determine the specificity for EPO binding. The cytoplasmic region of EPOR does not contain a tyrosine kinase catalytic domain; instead it interacts with cytoplasmic tyrosine kinases. Cross-linking of radiolabeled EPO to cell surface EPOR results in formation of at least two major cross-linked protein complexes of 140 and 120 kd.[203] The molecular composition of these complexes remains unsolved but suggests that EPOR contains additional subunits or accessory proteins.[204] The extracytoplasmic region of the EPOR polypeptide contains the EPO binding activity of the receptor.[205-207] Therefore additional EPOR subunits may provide other structural and functional elements of the receptor but are not required for high-affinity EPO binding. The extracytoplasmic region of the EPOR polypeptide has been crystalized.[208-210] The crystal structure confirms the dimeric structure of the activated receptor. Interestingly, small synthetic peptides are capable of inducing EPOR dimerization, suggesting a profitable avenue for EPO-mimetic and EPO-antagonist drug design.[211] EPO-mimetic agents are represented by polypeptides restricted to the portion of the protein that binds the receptor, by forms of the protein molecularly engineered to increase its glycosylation state and therefore its stability in vivo, or by dimeric forms of proteins obtained by genetic introduction of bridging sites or chemical cross-linking.[212] It also is possible that nonpeptide chemicals sharing the same stereo and electric properties of the receptor-binding domain of the protein might be identified. As shown for carbamylated EPO, modified isoforms may have biologic activity that partially differs from, and is possibly more effective than, the native protein,[213] especially with regard to the activity of the growth factor in nonhematopoietic tissues.[214]

EPOR mRNA, originally isolated from murine erythroblast cell lines (MEL and HCD57)[184] and from a human erythroid cell line (OCIM1),[215] has been found in nonerythroid cells as well. EPO promotes the differentiation of megakaryocytes at physiologic concentrations of hormone, suggesting that megakaryocytes have functional cell surface EPORs. Rat and mouse placenta also have cell surface EPOR, detected by radiolabeled EPO cross-linking. EPO promotes a chemotactic effect on endothelial cells,[216,217] suggesting the presence of a cell surface receptor in these cells. Other studies suggest that EPOR is expressed in neural cells[218] and smooth muscle cells.[219] Adverse effects in cancer patients treated with EPO have been attributed to the effects of EPO on tumor cells.[220] The functional importance of EPOR expression in nonerythroid cells has been revealed by rescue experiments in EPOR^{null} mice.[221] Because EPOR^{null} mutant mice die of severe anemia between days 13 and 15 of embryonic development, the mutant embryos can be rescued by transgenic expression of EPOR under the control of the hemopoietic-specific

GATA1 regulatory domain. Under steady-state conditions, the rescued animals are normal, because the gene is expressed only in erythroid cells. However, in comparison with normal mice, the increase in plasma EPO concentration in response to induced anemia was delayed in the rescued animals, suggesting that one of the major functions of EPOR expression in nonerythroid cells is fine-tuning the regulation of the response to stress.[221]

The existence of naturally occurring splice variants of the EPOR gene encoding EPOR polypeptides of variable length and activity has been shown.[222-225] The soluble secreted form of EPOR[226] binds EPO and thereby competes with the cell surface receptor isoform. The biologic function of alternative forms of the cell surface EPOR, including a truncated form of EPOR found in early progenitors,[227] remains unknown but may be related either to differential EPO signaling and responses (survival, proliferation, differentiation) at different stages in erythroid development or to the establishment of erythroid-specific versus myeloid-specific niches in the marrow microenvironment.

SIGNAL TRANSDUCTION BY EPOR

Considerable progress has been made in our understanding of EPOR-mediated signal transduction. Early studies demonstrated that stimulation of EPOR on primary erythroid cells resulted in increased calcium ion flux and increased globin mRNA synthesis.[228] Since the cloning of the EPOR polypeptide and its stable expression in heterologous cell systems, such as the Ba/F3 cell system,[229] considerable molecular insight has been gained.[230] For instance, it now is clear that EPO induces homodimerization of the EPOR polypeptide.[231,232] Following receptor dimerization at the cell surface, a series of tyrosine phosphorylation events occurs, resulting in a mitogenic signal and a differentiative signal.[233,234] Initial studies of the EPOR signal transduction pathway made use of mutant forms of EPOR stably expressed in the indicator cell line Ba/F3. Ba/F3 cells are a murine IL-3–dependent pro–B lymphocyte cell line. These cells can be readily transfected with the complementary DNA (cDNA) for EPOR, resulting in stable expression of the receptor on the cell surface. Expression of the full-length, wild-type EPOR polypeptide in these cells resulted in EPO-dependent growth and partial EPO-induced erythroid differentiation.[233,234] Expression of truncated forms of the EPOR polypeptide in these cells resulted in variable growth responses. For instance, truncation of the membrane proximal region of EPOR demonstrated a critical positive regulatory domain of EPOR required for mitogenesis.[229] Furthermore, truncation of the carboxy-terminal 40 amino acids of EPOR resulted in increased EPO-dependent growth, suggesting that the carboxy-terminal region contained a negative regulatory domain normally required for downmodulating EPOR mitogenic signals.[229]

The biochemical basis for these positive and negative regulatory domains has been elucidated. The membrane proximal positive regulatory region of EPOR binds constitutively to Janus-activated kinase 2 (JAK2),[235] a cytoplasmic tyrosine kinase necessary for erythroid differentiation, as evidenced by mice lacking the corresponding gene dying at an early embryonic stage.[236] Upon EPO binding to the receptor, the receptor dimerizes, resulting in activation of prebound JAK2. The JAK2 next tyrosine phosphorylates multiple signaling proteins in the cell, leading to various mitogenic and differentiative responses. The negative regulatory domain of EPOR is required for recruiting the phosphatase SHP1 to EPOR.[237] SHP1 binds to an activated tyrosine phosphate on the EPOR polypeptide and rapidly downregulates JAK2 activity and dephosphorylates the EPOR polypeptide. Failure to recruit the SHP1 phosphatase can result in increased EPOR signaling and a polycythemic state (see Alterations in EPOR and Its Signaling in Disorders of Erythropoiesis).

JAK2 is required for appropriate Golgi processing and cell surface expression of EPOR.[238] Once activated by EPO/EPOR binding on the cell surface, JAK2 initiates several events in EPOR-mediated signal transduction. JAK2 initially activates tyrosine phosphorylation of several tyrosine residues of the cytoplasmic tail of EPOR. These phosphorylated tyrosine residues next serve as docking sites for binding of other cytoplasmic effector proteins containing Src homology 2 (SH2) domains, such as the p85 subunit of phosphatidylinositol 3-kinase,[239] the adaptor protein Shc,[240,241] and STAT5.[242,243] (Examples of signal transduction proteins expressed in primary human erythroblasts are given in Table 24-2). Once these proteins have docked on EPOR, they become tyrosine phosphorylated and engage other downstream signaling events. In addition, JAK2 activates the Ras/Raf/MAPK (mitogen-activated protein kinase) pathway, further contributing to the EPO-induced mitogenic signal.[244,245] The molecular mechanism of Ras activation by JAK2 remains unknown but may entail direct binding of the proteins and tyrosine phosphorylation.[245]

Activation of the JAK2/STAT5 signaling pathway has been studied in considerable detail. Upon EPOR tyrosine phosphorylation, STAT5 protein binds to a specific phosphorylated tyrosine residue of the EPOR.[242,246] Binding is mediated by the SH2 domain of STAT5. Following EPOR binding, STAT5 itself becomes tyrosine phosphorylated at amino acid Y694.[247] Activated STAT5 then disengages from EPOR, undergoes homodimerization, and translocates to the cell nucleus, where it activates transcription of EPO-inducible genes. Some EPO-inducible genes, such as MYC and FOS, are common to other hematopoietic growth factor signaling pathways. Other EPO-inducible genes are specifically expressed in erythroid cells and are not shared by other growth factor responses.[248]

Other signal transduction pathways downstream from cytokine receptors have been identified. For instance, EPO and IL-3 activate tyrosine phosphorylation of the signaling protein CBL and the subsequent binding and tyrosine phosphorylation of the signal protein CrkL.[249] The mechanism of activation of this pathway by EPOR is not known, and the relative role of this pathway in EPO-induced growth and erythroid differentiation remains largely unexplored. Inositide-specific phospholipases C (PLCs) and the protein kinase C (PKC) pathway also are involved in EPO signaling. PLCs catalyze hydrolysis of phosphatidylinositol 4,5-bisphosphate to generate diacylglycerol and inositol 3,4,5-bisphosphate, a well-known intracellular messenger for PKC activation and intracellular Ca^{2+} mobilization. PLCs are classified into four isoform families (α, β, γ, and δ), and each family has multiple isoforms.[250,251] The involvement of PLCs in erythroid differentiation was suggested by early studies demonstrating that stimulation of EPOR in primary erythroid cells results in increased calcium ion flux.[228] More recent studies demonstrated that primary erythroblasts express only some (i.e., PLC β_1, β_2, β_3, δ_1, γ_1, and γ_2) PLC isoforms. Among these, PLCβ_1 most likely is involved in EPO signaling, based on findings that its expression is induced within 6 hours of stimulation with the growth factor.[22,183,252] On the other hand, PKC represents a family of nine different serine-threonine kinases genes, encoding a total of 12 different isoforms, involved in the regulation of many cellular functions.[253] These enzymes exert their biologic functions as a cytoplasmic-nuclear shuttle of the transduction machinery and become phosphorylated, and hence activated, in response to a variety of stimuli. Human multipotent $CD34^+$ progenitor cells express all of the PKC isoforms.[254,255] Commitment of these cells along the erythroid lineage requires suppression of PKCε.[254,256] PKCε exerts a positive control on erythropoiesis, because its inhibitors specifically impair the ability of erythroid cells to respond to EPO[257] and to phosphorylate EPOR, STAT5, GAB1, ERK1/2, and AKT.[258] It also is possible that different PKC isoforms are active at different ontogenic stages, because PKCα and PKCδ are differentially phosphorylated, and hence activated, during differentiation of neonatal and adult erythroblasts.[259]

EPO signaling activates also Lyn, a tyrosine kinase member of the Src family[260] physically associated with EPOR.[261] Lyn acts upstream to both the STAT5[261] and the PLCγ_2/PI3K pathways.[262] Failure to activate Lyn prevents erythroid differentiation of the J2E cell line[260] and Lyn^{null} mice have a phenotype remarkably similar to that of $GATA1^{LOW}$ mice (normal hematocrit in spite of reduced levels of GATA1, erythroid Krüppel-like factor (EKLF), and STAT5 expression due to development of extramedullary hematopoiesis in spleen).[263] In addition to STAT5 and PLCγ2/PI3K signaling, Lyn activates Liar,

Table 24-2 Major Transcription Factors/Signaling Molecules Involved in the Control of Erythropoiesis

Transcription Factor	Binding Motif	Role in Hematopoiesis	Knock-Out Phenotype	Mutations/Human Disease
GATA1	(A/T)GATA(A/G)	↑ Erythroid differentiation	• No terminal erythropoiesis • Arrest in Mk development (with hyperproliferation)	• X-linked thalassemia/ thrombocytopenia • Leukemia (Down syndrome)
GATA2	(A/T)GATA(A/G)	↑Proliferation ↓Differentiation	↓ Proliferative expansion of primitive and definitive erythropoiesis Absence of mast cells	MonoMAC syndrome, MDS, AML
FOG-1	None	GATA1 cofactor	↓ Erythroid maturation Block in megakaryocyto poiesis	
EKLF	CACCC	Promotes terminal erythroid differentiation	Severe anemia β-globin deficiency	β-Thalassemia, Lu-negative blood phenotype, HPFH, Nan phenotype in mice
SCL	CANNTG (E-box)	Specification of hematopoiesis	Absence of prenatal hematopoiesis ↓ Erythro/Mk in adults	Translocation in T-cell ALL
LMO2	LIM domain		Absence of hematopoiesis	T-cell ALL
Myb	(T/C)AAC(G/T)G	↓ Definitive erythropoiesis	Block in definitive erythropoiesis	HPFH, Myb-GATA1 fusion gene in acute basophilic leukemia
Fli-1	Winged helix-turn-helix	Inhibition of GATA1 expression		
BKLF	CACC		Myeloproliferative disorder	
SHP1 (BKLF activated?)				Erythroleukemia Polycythemia vera
STAT5	GAS		Transient fetal anemia due to apoptosis of erythroid progenitors Mild anemia, exacerbated by stress in adult life	
PU.1	GGAA	↓ Erythropoiesis	Absence of myelomonocytic differentiation	
Id		Blocks terminal differentiation of all cell types		
IaPI-3 kinase (p85)		↓ Proliferation/differentiation	↓ Fetal erythropoiesis Perinatal death	
Gfi-1b	Zinc finger domain	↑ Proliferation (↑ GATA2)		
Sp3			↓ Fetal erythropoiesis Perinatal death	
NF-E2	TGAGTCA	Promotes terminal erythroid differentiation in vitro	Thrombocytopenia Absence of erythroid abnormalities (?)	

ALL, Acute lymphoblastic leukemia; *AML*, acute myeloid leukemia; *BKLF*, basic Krüppel-like factor; *EKLF*, erythroid Krüppel-like factor; *FOG-1*, Friend of GATA1; *HPFH*, hereditary persistence of fetal hemoglobin; *LMO2*, LIM domain only 2; *MDS*, myelodysplastic syndrome; *SCL*, stem cell leukemia; *↓ Erythro/Mk*, decrease in erythropoiesis/megakaryocytopoiesis.

a Lyn-binding nuclear/cytoplasmic shuttling protein[264] specifically responsible for downregulating KIT expression in response to EPO.[265] In humans, Lyn is responsible for the phosphorylation of several membrane proteins, and failure to activate Lyn results in the formation of acanthocytic red cells, a diagnostic marker of chorea-acanthocytosis, a rare autosomal recessive neurodegenerative disorder.[266]

Erythroblasts generated under conditions of stress retain C-KIT expression. Several studies have investigated the relationship between KIT signaling and erythroid cell fate. In human and murine erythroid progenitors, KL induces rapid, within 15 minutes, ERK activation, which lasts only 1 hour.[267,268] In human erythroleukemic K562 and myeloid MO7e cells, the rapid KL-dependent ERK activation is associated with proliferation, whereas the late sustained ERK activation is responsible for differentiation.[269,270] Whether KL activates the STAT5 pathway in erythroid cells is controversial. Although KL was found to be unable to activate STAT5 in prospectively isolated human erythroid progenitor cells,[267] more recent single-cells fluorescence-activated cell sorter (FACS) analyses indicate that KL activates STAT5 in bipotent erythroid/megakaryocytic but not in myelomonocytic progenitor cells.[271] KL has also been described to activate the PI3K/AKT pathway in murine erythroid progenitors[268] and in human MO7e cells.[270] Finally, coexpression of KIT and EPOR deletion mutants in 32D cells have identified that KIT intracellular tyrosines play an essential role in EPOR cosignaling,[272] providing a mechanism for the signaling synergy observed between KL and EPO.

A critical question in the field of EPOR signal transduction is the mechanism of EPO specificity. Most, if not all, of the signal transduction pathways activated by EPOR (i.e., Ras/Raf/MAPK and JAK/STAT) are shared by other hematopoietic cytokine receptors, such as the receptors for IL-3, GM-CSF, and IL-5. How EPOR triggers a specific growth factor response resulting in erythroid differentiation is unclear. Several models are possible. First, EPOR may activate unique but unknown signaling pathways specific to EPOR and distinct from other cytokine receptors. Alternatively, EPOR may activate identical pathways, activated by other cytokine receptors. In the latter model, the specificity of the EPO signal is derived not from EPOR itself but from interactions with other developmentally programmed events in the erythroid cell, such as expression of erythroid-specific transcription factors.

Activation of EPOR in the murine IL-3–dependent cell line Ba/F3 results in induction of both mitogenesis and globin accumulation.[158] In contrast, the murine IL-2–dependent cell line CTLL-2, when engineered to express the heterologous EPOR, grows in EPO but does not differentiate into globin-bearing cells. These data suggest that expression of EPOR is necessary for erythroid differentiation but not sufficient alone. Other erythroid-specific markers, such as GATA1 and NF-E2, or EKLF, likely are required for cells to differentiate down the erythroid pathway. Other cytokine receptors, such as IL-3R and IL-2R, do not drive β-globin synthesis in these cell lines. Taken together, these results suggest that EPOR generates a differentiation-specific signaling within the context of a proper transcriptional environment.

Regardless of the mechanism of cytokine specificity, each cytokine receptor activates a similar but not identical pattern of signaling events. For instance, EPOR shows a preferential activation of the JAK2/STAT5 pathway in cultured erythroid cells in vitro. In contrast, IL-2R shows preferential activation of the JAK1/JAK3/STAT6 pathway.[247,273,274] Interestingly, although EPO activates STAT5a and STAT5b in cultured cells, knockout of the STAT5a or STAT5b gene by homologous recombination results in a mouse phenotype with slightly impaired stem cell activity but apparently normal baseline erythroid development.[275,276] More extensive analysis of this phenotype has revealed that the mice experience increased apoptotic rates at erythroblast levels that are compensated by a cellular compensatory mechanism very similar to that described for GATA1^{LOW} mutants,[95] involving expansion of hemopoietic progenitors in the marrow and recruitment of the spleen as an additional hemopoietic site. These results suggest that, in vivo, other STAT proteins are at least partially capable of substituting for STAT5 and functioning downstream of the EPOR. These findings emphasize the importance of in vivo studies in confirming the phenotypic relevance of in vitro studies.

Studies have suggested that EPO functions synergistically with other multilineage growth factors, such as KL and IL-3. EPO and KL function together, resulting in increased erythroid colony cell growth in methylcellulose culture. Studies with the EPOR polypeptide suggest a molecular mechanism for such synergy.[277] Activation of the KIT receptor by KL results in transphosphorylation of EPOR at the cell surface. A direct interaction between EPOR and the KIT receptor has been demonstrated.[278] Physical interaction between EPOR and the β common chain of the IL-3 receptor in erythroid cells has been demonstrated.[279] This interaction might be involved in the neuroprotective action exerted by EPO.[280] In fact, a carbamylated derivative of EPO prevents motoneuron degeneration in vitro and in vivo[280] and ameliorates recovery in several in vivo models of brain and heart injuries, such as chronic autoimmunoencephalomyelitis in mice,[281] radiosurgery- or ischemia-induced brain injury,[282] and myocardium ischemia–reperfusion injury[283] in rats. (For a review of the nonhematopoietic activity of EPO, see reference 284) Taken together, these results suggest that receptor cross-talk at the cell surface may account, at least in part, for the physiologic interaction of some cytokines in controlling hematopoietic versus nonhematopoietic effects of EPO.

ALTERATIONS IN EPOR AND ITS SIGNALING IN DISORDERS OF ERYTHROPOIESIS

As discussed earlier, the normal role of EPO is to stimulate cell surface EPOR in developing erythroid cells. The latter cells respond to EPO via a proliferative and differentiation response. EPO-activated signal transduction of EPOR is quickly downregulated in the cell, and continuing presence of EPO is required for optimal differentiation.

In some cells, the EPOR may become constitutively activated. In these cases, erythroid progenitor cells are placed into a sustained proliferative state. Interestingly, these mechanisms underlie several murine and human examples of erythrocytosis (erythroid overproduction). Multiple mechanisms exist by which EPOR may become constitutively activated. First, the Friend spleen focus-forming virus of the Friend erythroleukemia complex encodes the glycoprotein F-gp55, which binds and activates murine EPOR.[285-287] F-gp55 appears to bind to EPOR via its transmembrane region. EPO and F-gp55 binding sites are discrete; tertiary complexes of EPOR, EPO, and F-gp55 have been detected on the surface of Friend virus-infected cells.[288] Second, EPOR can be constitutively activated by a point mutation (R129C) in the extracytoplasmic region of the polypeptide.[289] This mutation occurs in the "dimerization domain" of EPOR and results in constitutive homodimerization of the EPOR polypeptide, presumably through a disulfide bond. This mutation further underscores the importance of receptor dimerization in the initiation of a receptor signaling response. Third, EPOR can be constitutively activated in an autocrine manner. Murine erythroleukemia cell lines have been established that coexpress EPOR and EPO. A fourth mechanism of EPOR constitutive activation results from EPOR overexpression. For instance, some murine erythroleukemia cell lines have increased EPOR mRNA, resulting from spleen focus-forming virus proviral integration within the first intron of the murine EPOR gene.[290] Overexpression of the normal murine EPOR polypeptide may thereby contribute to oncogenesis.

Soon after the cDNA of mouse and human EPOR were cloned, the mouse and human genomic structures were identified. The gene for mouse EPOR was found to map to mouse chromosome 9,[291] whereas the human gene was found on human chromosome 19p.[292] Mapping of the EPOR genes led to their implication in various human disease states. For instance, studies demonstrated that a chromosomal breakpoint 3′ to the human EPOR gene results in increased EPOR expression.[293] The rearranged EPOR allele appears to encode a mutated EPOR polypeptide with increased activity, perhaps secondary to loss of the carboxy-terminal negative regulatory domain.

EPOR plays a role in the rare congenital disease familial erythrocytosis. Familial erythrocytosis is a heterogeneous group of hereditary conditions characterized by an increase in red blood cell mass in the setting of low serum EPO levels. A few families that demonstrate autosomal dominant inheritance have been identified.[294] The linkage between the EPOR gene and familial erythrocytosis was first established by the observation that a mutant EPOR allele segregates with the disease in one familial erythrocytosis kindred. This allele contains a nonsense mutation in the coding region of the gene that results in synthesis of a truncated EPOR that lacks the negative regulatory domain of its carboxy-terminal region.[295,296] Since that report, several other frameshift and deletion EPOR gene mutations, all encoding carboxy-terminal–truncated forms of the protein providing EPO hypersensitivity and resulting in familial erythrocytosis, have been reported.[297-301]

Congenital polycythemia may arise not only from gene mutations leading to abnormal EPOR signaling but also from gene mutations altering EPO production. The T598T mutation in one of the genes controlling oxygen sensoring (von Hippel-Lindau (VHL) gene), which leads to increased EPO production by the kidney, is associated with congenital erythrocytosis, the Chuvash polycythemia.[302,303] The C598T VHL mutation is endemic in Chuvashia, Russian Federation, and in the small island of Ischia, in southern Italy. The frequency of the mutation on this small island is higher than in Chuvashia (0.07% versus 0.02%), but the haplotype of Italian patients matches that identified in the Chuvash cluster, supporting a single-founder hypothesis.[304]

Acquired mutations in the EPOR signaling pathway have been identified in PV, essential thrombocythemia, and idiopathic myelofibrosis, a class of myeloproliferative neoplasm that lacks the

Philadelphia chromosome (Ph) abnormality and therefore cannot be cured with inhibitors, such as Gleevec, which are specific for the signaling pathway altered by the Ph abnormality. These diseases originate at the level of the pluripotent hematopoietic stem cell and are characterized by proliferation of one or more of the myeloid lineages but relatively normal hematopoietic cell maturation. Several investigators have reported a mutation in the JAK2 gene resulting in a valine→phenylalanine substitution at position 617 of the protein (JAK2V617F mutation) in patients with Ph-negative chronic proliferative disorders.[305-308] Since the early reports, the presence of JAK2V617F in patients with Ph-negative myeloproliferative disorders has been confirmed by numerous publications. Depending on the study, JAK2V617F has been reported in 60% to 90% of patients with PV, 30% to 50% of patients with essential thrombocythemia (ET), and 30% to 60% of patients with primary myelofibrosis (PMF). The mutation is harbored at either the heterozygous or, by somatic recombination, the homozygous stage. It is detectable in all myeloid cells up to the clonal hematopoietic stem cells.[309] The mutation affects the domain of the protein that is directly involved in signal transduction but is necessary to return the protein to its resting configuration after signaling. As a consequence, after its first engagement with EPO, EPOR signaling becomes constitutively activated. Because JAK2 is the earliest element of the EPOR pathway, it is conceivable that the high red cell numbers found in patients with PV carrying the JAK2V617F mutation is a direct consequence of constitutive EPO signaling in erythroid cells. The extent to which the downstream EPOR signaling pathway is altered as a consequence of this constitutive activation is a debatable issue. The observation that erythroblasts derived in vitro from patients with PV carrying the JAK2V617F mutation are highly resistant to TRAIL-induced apoptosis[310] suggests that the mutation exquisitely increases erythroblast survival. However, additional abnormalities induced by the presence of JAK2V617F are represented by hypersensitivity to insulin-like growth factor I[311] and increased EPOR recycling from the Golgi apparatus.[238] Therefore inhibitors directly targeting the JAK2V617F mutation might represent the best candidates for PV therapy. More difficult to understand is why the mutation is also present in some patients with ET and PMF. JAK2, in addition to EPOR, has an important role in transducing the signal from c-Mpl, the TPO receptor.[312] The protein has two opposing effects on the intracellular p rocessing of the two receptors after growth factor stimulation: it favors EPOR recycling from the Golgi apparatus,[238] but it determines retention and degradation of c-Mpl in the cytoplasm.[313] As such, the JAK2V617F mutation should increase the number of EPOR on the surface of erythroid cells while reducing that of c-Mpl on megakaryocytes. This hypothesis explains why the mutation is found preferentially in PV. However, megakaryocytes originating from JAK2V617F stem cells might express a reduced number but constitutively active c-Mpl, so it can be argued that the mutation manifests itself prevalently in the erythroid or the megakaryocytic lineage, depending on genetic polymorphisms outside the JAK2 locus present in the population. This hypothesis is supported by the observation that mice transplanted with JAK2V617F hematopoietic stem cells develop either a PV- or an ET–like syndrome, depending on their genetic background[314] and/or level of JAK2V617F expression.[315,316] One of the genetic factors that may determine the phenotype expressed by JAK2V617F-positive myeloproliferative neoplasms may be represented by the GR locus. The blood mononuclear cells from PV patients, but not those from ET or PMF, express increased levels of the dominant negative GRβ isoform. Increased levels of GRβ are also expressed by the erythroblasts expanded in vivo from PV patients. The observations that these erythroblasts lack nuclear STAT5 activity, in spite of constitutive STAT5 phosphorylation induced by the presence of JAK2V617F mutation, and do not mature in response to EPO[118] suggest that constitutive inhibition of the EPO maturation signal provided by GRβ expression may confer a self-renewal state to PV erythroblasts, contributing to erythrocytosis. Expression of GRβ may be favored by the increased frequency of the rs6198 SNP, which stabilize GRβ mRNA observed in these patients.[118]

Studies on the biology and biochemistry of the JAK2V617F mutation are actively being pursued by many investigators. Furthermore, in JAK2V617F-negative PV or idiopathic erythrocytosis patients, several other gain-of-function mutations affecting JAK2 exon 12 with a distinct phenotype (idiopathic erythrocytosis) have been identified.[317] The identification of specific mutations and the availability of the crystal structures of EPO, EPOR, and JAK2 should allow use of computer modeling to design targeted protein-signaling inhibitors for treatment of Ph-negative myeloproliferative neoplasms.[318]

HEMATOPOIETIC MICROENVIRONMENT

In invertebrates such as worms and sessile marine creatures, erythropoiesis occurs adjacent to peritoneal and endothelial cells. In premammalian species, the spleen is the primary site of erythropoiesis. With evolutionary advancement, the function gradually shifts to the liver and the sinusoidal cavities of bones.[9] These observations suggest that sufficient oxygen, a stagnated flow of blood to avoid dispersion of factors produced locally, and extensive and redundant surfaces for cell-cell interactions are essential to supporting red cell production. Similar sites support erythropoiesis during human development (see Ontogeny of Erythropoiesis). During both phylogeny and ontogeny, the liver and spleen are primarily erythropoietic organs; granulocytic cells dominate in the bone marrow.[9] Within the bone marrow, hematopoiesis is restricted to the extravascular space, where compact collections of cells are interspersed among venous sinuses. These sinuses originate adjacent to the endosteal bone surface and empty into a central longitudinal vein. Studies in mice demonstrate that BFU-E follow a bimodal distribution with peaks adjacent to the periosteum and midcavity, whereas CFU-E and later erythroid cells have a broad distribution with highest incidence toward the axis of the femur, adjacent to the central vein,[9,319] thus suggesting that the local anatomy (specialized niches?) influences the maturation of erythroid cells.

The bone marrow microenvironment consists of three broad components: stromal cells (e.g., fibroblasts, endothelial cells, mesenchymal stem cells and their diverse descendant progeny), accessory cells (monocytes, macrophages, megakaryocytes, T cells), and extracellular matrix (a protein-carbohydrate scaffold). In the bone marrow, although early studies described two distinct hematopoietic niches for hematopoietic stem cells /progenitor cells (i.e., the "endosteal" niche and the "endothelial or vascular niche" within the medulla), more recent studies suggest that this distinction may be artificial, because both cellular structures can be intimately associated in trabecular bone. Thus mesenchymal stem cell–derived osteoprogenitor cells and stromal reticular cells (nestin+ or leptinR+) are intimately associated with sinusoidal endothelium and seem to be pivotal organizers of the bone marrow niche.[320-322] Reciprocal communication of hematopoietic stem cells with cells/matrix in their bone marrow niche ensures both their quiescent state and self-renewal dynamics.

EPO, in addition to promoting erythropoiesis directly, enhances erythropoiesis indirectly by decreasing the interaction of hematopoietic stem cells with their niches, reducing the amount of trabecular bone[323] and downregulating CXCR4 expression, the receptor for CXCR12L/SDF1, on hematopoietic stem cells[324]).

Accessory cells are progeny of hematopoietic stem cells; hence after marrow transplantation these cells are of donor origin, whereas stromal cells remain mostly host derived.[325,326] Extracellular matrix molecules are synthesized and secreted by microenvironmental cells and include collagens (types I, III, IV, and V), glycoproteins (fibronectin, laminins, thrombospondins, hemonectin, and tenascin), and glycosaminoglycans (hyaluronic acid, chondroitin, dermatan, and heparan sulfate).[327,328] The production of extracellular matrix proteoglycans by mesenchymal stromal cells may be regulated by the Wnt pathway.[329]

Besides providing structure to the marrow space and a surface for cell adhesion, the microenvironment is important for hematopoietic cell homing, engraftment, migration, and the response to physiologic stress and homeostasis. Although the functional consequences of the microenvironment ultimately must be defined by in vivo studies in mice, dissection of the cellular components of the microenvironment, definition of the cytokines that are produced by individual cells, and the nature of cell-cell interactions have been aided by in vitro models. Long-term bone marrow cultures provide an experimental approach for such studies.[330,331] Under these in vitro conditions, murine hematopoiesis can be maintained for 8 to 10 months and human hematopoiesis for 2 to 3 months.[330] An adherent layer consisting of fibroblasts, adipocytes, and macrophages is a crucial component of the culture system. Progenitor cells adherent to stroma are generally quiescent (dormant), whereas those in the nonadherent cell compartment are in active cell cycle.[331,332]

In vitro studies have demonstrated that stromal cells, including endothelial cells and fibroblasts, elaborate cytokines such as GM-CSF, G-CSF, IL-1, IL-3, IL-6, IL-11, KL, Flt-3 ligand, activin A, and basic fibroblast growth factor, which influence, alone or in combination, the growth of adjacent marrow progenitors.[330-333] In addition to positive regulators of replication and differentiation, stromal cells elaborate factors such as TGFβ, TPO, CXCL12L, interferon-γ, and TNF-α, which exert a negative influence on proliferation and may help maintain a dormant (noncycling) state.[331,332,334-336] Because some regulators inhibit differentiation along certain lineages but not others, there is an intriguing possibility that lineage-specific regulation within the microenvironment can be achieved through negative, rather than positive, factors.[337] Several cytokines are expressed in a transmembrane, form as well as a soluble (secreted) product. Others bind extracellular matrix, a mechanism that not only allows for high concentrations of a factor within the microenvironment that metabolically stabilizes these factors but also keeps them adjacent to developing progenitors.

Among the factors elaborated by stromal cells, KL has the most profound effect on erythropoiesis. Mice unable to synthesize KL die in utero because of severe anemia. Steel-Dickie (Sl^d) mice that are unable to make the membrane-restricted form of KL are viable but severely anemic, whereas other lineages in these animals are marginally affected or not affected by this defect.[338] The fact that erythropoiesis is abnormal, despite high levels of circulating EPO and the presence of soluble KL, suggests that normal erythroid differentiation and maturation require both a functional membrane-restricted KL/KIT and an EPO signaling pathway. Cross-phosphorylation of EPOR by KL may provide a basis for the predominately erythroid effect.[278] Furthermore, data suggest that tyrosine cross-phosphorylation of EPOR is sustained longer when cells are cultured on steel stromal cells engineered to express the membrane-restricted form of KL than cells expressing the soluble form.[339]

The soluble form of KL is produced by proteolytic cleavage of membrane KL and is released in the circulation. Soluble KL effectively supports erythroid maturation in vitro[340] but is dispensable for steady-state erythropoiesis, because targeted mutant mice expressing exclusively the more stable membrane isoform of KL, KL2, lacking the major proteolytic cleavage site, have normal hematocrit values.[341] However, these mice recover poorly from radiation-induced anemia.[341] In wild-type mice, sublethal radiation induced a transient fourfold increase in KL in the serum (from <0.5 up to >2 ng/mL), reaching a peak after 7 days. In contrast, the proteolytic-cleavage mutant $KL^{KL2/KL2}$ mice did not release soluble KL into the serum after sublethal radiation, and survival was significantly diminished because of anemia. These observations suggest that soluble KL plays an important regulatory role under conditions of stress.

The pathway(s) that regulate erythropoiesis under conditions of acute or chronic anemia are starting to emerge.[342] In mice, stress induces the formation of an erythroid permissive microenvironment in the spleen and other extramedullary sites. In fact, recent evidence suggests that, in addition to increasing EPO production by the kidney, in order to raise the levels of soluble KL in the serum and to activate GR response, this pathway activates spleen-specific microenvironmental cues (BMP4/hedgehog), which generate stress-specific hematopoietic compartments.[76,343] The identity of the hematopoietic stem cell niche in the spleen and the human equivalent of this cell are yet to be determined.

Besides cell-cytokine interactions, (paracrine) cell-cell adhesion and adhesion of cells to the extracellular matrix are important functions of the microenvironment.[344,345] Perhaps most studied are the β_1 integrins VLA4 and VLA5, which mediate the adherence of hematopoietic cells to stromal cells, fibronectin, or other components of the extracellular matrix.[345,346] In mice lacking β_1 integrins, hematopoietic stem cells fail to colonize the fetal liver during embryonic development,[347] and cells lacking α_4 integrin fail to contribute to normal hematopoiesis postnatally.[348] Antibodies to VLA4 or to the vascular cellular adhesion molecule 1 (VCAM1, a VLA4 ligand on endothelial cells) impair homing and lead to mobilization of progenitor cells and stem cells in adult mice and primates.[349-352] In in vitro studies, hematopoietic progenitors bind to specific domains of fibronectin in a differentiation-dependent manner (long-term culture-initiating cell and day 12 colony-forming unit–spleen in mice adhere mainly through the heparin-binding domain and CS-1). BFU-E and other progenitor cells adhere to both the cell-binding (Arg-Gly-Asp-Ser [RGDS]) and heparin-binding domains, whereas CFU-E preferentially bind the RGDS sequence, and reticulocytes fail to adhere to fibronectin.[328,353-356] This differential binding could influence the proliferation and especially the maturation and survival of developing erythroid cells, particularly under stress,[357] as well as the migration of progenitor cells in and out of the bone marrow cavity.[348,349] Hematopoietic cytokines/chemokines present in the microenvironment also can modulate the affinity of β_1 integrins for ligand,[358,359] adding complexity to the regulation of erythropoiesis within the marrow microenvironment.

Many observations suggest that hematopoietic progenitor cells at one stage of fetal development may not be supported by a hematopoietic microenvironment of a different ontogenetic stage. For example, cells present in the murine yolk sac are not able to repopulate adult recipients,[360] although they can repopulate newborn recipients with active fetal liver hematopoiesis.[361] Targeted disruption of CXCL12/SDF1, a member of the CXC chemokine family that is constitutively expressed by bone marrow stromal cells (i.e., reticular/endothelial cells or osteoblasts), leads to inhibition of marrow hematopoiesis, although fetal liver hematopoiesis is unaffected,[362] suggesting that this chemokine is important in maintaining normal bone marrow hematopoiesis. Other factors with distinct function on fetal versus adult hematopoiesis have also been described: Sox17 for fetal hematopoiesis[363] or TEL (translocation-ETS [E26 transformation-specific]-leukemia)[364] and Bmi-1 for adult hematopoiesis.[365]

Accessory cells, such as stromal cells, in addition to secreting cytokines, express adhesion molecules, and they may influence marrow hematopoiesis by their nonrandom distribution in the marrow cavity. T cells (along with mast cells) are the only source of IL-3 and, through secretion of TNF-α and interferon-γ, may negatively impact erythropoiesis. In histologic sections of normal marrow, islands of maturing erythroblasts (erythroblastic islands) often surround a central macrophage, termed a *nurse cell*.[366] Adhesion may be mediated through the binding of VLA4 (on erythroid cells) to VCAM1 (on central macrophages),[367] or through several other molecules.[368] These molecular interactions have been identified as being critical for erythroblastic island integrity. Erythroblast macrophage protein expressed on erythroblasts and macrophages mediates cell-cell attachment through homophilic binding, and erythroblast intercellular adhesion molecule 4 (ICAM4) links erythroblasts to macrophages by interacting with α_v integrin expressed in macrophages.[369-371] Mice with targeted deletion of erythroblast macrophage protein are severely anemic and die at an embryonic stage,[137] and $ICAM4^{null}$ mice[370] have markedly reduced erythroblastic islands. Of interest, retinoblastoma (RB)-deficient macrophages do not bind RB^{null} erythroblasts,[372] and failure of this interaction may mediate the defect in fetal liver erythropoiesis observed in RB^{null} mice. RB normally stimulates macrophage differentiation by counteracting inhibition of Id2 (a helix-loop-helix protein) on PU.1, a transcription factor crucial in macrophage differentiation. In addition to the aforementioned pathways, macrophage CD163 can serve as an erythroblast adhesion receptor in erythroblastic islands, promoting erythroid proliferation and/or survival.[373] More studies addressing the specific interactions between macrophages and erythroid cells that promote erythroid differentiation are needed for definite conclusions regarding specialized "erythroid niches." Of note, tissue macrophages express RNA for EPO[374] and may also influence erythropoiesis through this mechanism.

The microenvironment is not only a passive surface for the adherence of progenitor cells; it exerts a crucial and interactive role in development and maturation. Some interactions are lineage (red cell) specific, whereas other interactions affect hematopoiesis more broadly. Stromal and accessory cells secrete cytokines and/or express them in a transmembrane form on their cell surface. Cytokines are retained via binding to components of the extracellular matrix. All components of the microenvironment are involved in adhesive interactions, some of which maintain quiescence (i.e., interactions of stem cells with endosteal surfaces[375,376]), whereas other cell-cell interactions or interactions of cells with matrix components induce proliferation and/or differentiation.[377-379] An individual progenitor cell, in an anatomic niche adjacent to certain stromal cells, accessory cells, and extracellular matrix molecules, likely responds to the sum of the signals that it uniquely receives. In this way, erythropoiesis, or the entire hematopoiesis, is influenced by the complexity of the interaction network.

ONTOGENY OF ERYTHROPOIESIS

During human development, distinct anatomic areas for production of erythroid cells are recruited sequentially, in a temporal succession that allows overlap (Fig. 24-3). In addition, parallel changes occur in the morphologic and functional properties of the erythroid cells themselves.

During the phase of embryonic erythropoiesis in the blood islands of yolk sac, aggregates of immature erythroid cells undergo maturation synchronously as a single cohort. Before their maturation is completed, they begin to circulate, and by gestational week 5 they are found in the vascular spaces of the rudimentary liver (Fig. 24-4). At about the same time, foci of immature erythroid cells emerge within the fetal liver as the fetal (or hepatic) phase of erythropoiesis commences.[380] From week 7 onward, the liver is progressively filled with erythroid precursors and becomes the dominant site of erythroid cell production until approximately gestational week 30. Although some red cell production can be found in the thymus, the spleen, or occasionally in the lymph nodes, these other sites are never dominant. However, recently placenta has been recognized as an important local erythropoietic site.[381] From month 6 onward, the cavities of long bones are invaded by vascular sprouts and become competent to support red cell development. Shortly after birth, all bone cavities are actively engaged in erythroid production, and the hepatic (fetal) phase of erythropoiesis comes to an end, as the final (adult) phase of erythropoiesis unfolds exclusively within the bone marrow.

In addition to the anatomic shifts in the sites of erythropoiesis are associated shifts in the phenotypic characteristics of erythroid cells. Embryonic erythroid cells (derived from the yolk sac) are large (approximately 200 μm), circulate as nucleated cells, and have a megaloblastic appearance (see Fig. 24-4). The fact that primitive erythroblasts of mammals, like erythroid cells of lower vertebrates, retain their nuclei at terminal stages of maturation may serve as an example of embryonic recapitulation of the phylogenetic evolution of the erythroid system. However, a study has identified the presence of enucleated megaloblasts in the blood of the mouse embryo at late stages of development, indicating that the enucleation process predominantly in the fetal liver is at least partially at work.[382] Other studies using genetic reporter models further suggest that embryonic (primitive) cells represent a stable cell population that persists through the end of gestation.[383] Fetal erythroid cells (produced in the fetal liver and later in fetal bone marrow spaces) are smaller than embryonic cells (approximately 125 μm) but have a macrocytic appearance compared with adult normocytic red cells (approximately 80 μm). However, like adult cells, fetal erythroid cells eject their nuclei during maturation.

Apart from variations in size and morphologic characteristics, embryonic and fetal erythroid cells differ from each other and from their adult counterparts in several other characteristics, including hormonal or growth factor requirements, proliferative status, and transplantation potential. For example, whereas fetal erythropoiesis is under the control of EPO,[384] the extent of EPO's influence on embryonic erythropoiesis is disputed. Most convincing are the results of EPO/EPOR knockouts[190] that showed only partial effects on embryonic erythropoiesis, in contrast to fetal erythropoiesis. Single-lineage transcriptosome analyses indicate that TGFβ may represent a primary regulator of embryonic erythropoiesis.[385] Evidence suggests that precursor cells from the extraembryonic mesoderm are dependent on EPO for proliferation and erythroid differentiation.[386] EPO levels increase between weeks 9 and 32 of gestation, and fetuses respond to hypoxia or anemia with increased EPO as early as 24 weeks. Fetal erythroid progenitors when studied in vitro appear more sensitive to EPO and KL than adult progenitors. In contrast, their in vitro response to lymphokines (e.g., IL-3 or GM-CSF) is minimal compared to that of adult erythroid progenitors.[387,388] Of note, in the early stages of fetal liver erythropoiesis, mainly erythroid differentiation/maturation is promoted.[241] Progenitors committed to other lineages are abundant in the fetal liver, but few mature cells (granulocytes, megakaryocytes) from other lineages are seen. In addition to their heightened sensitivity to EPO, fetal erythroid progenitors and precursors are characterized by high proliferative potential and shorter doubling times than adult cells when cultured in vitro.[387,389] The dependency of stem/progenitor cells on KL changes during ontogeny. Although generation of repopulating stem cells (C-KIT$^+$/Sca1$^+$/Thy1^{lo}/Lin$^-$) and colony-forming unit–spleen is minimally

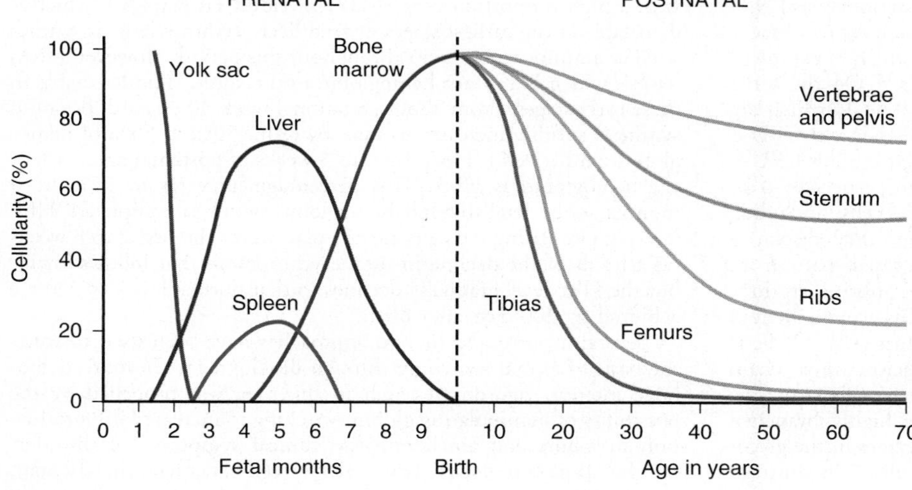

Figure 24-3 SITES OF HEMATOPOIESIS DURING FETAL DEVELOPMENT AND AFTER BIRTH. Only erythroid cells and possibly lymphocytes are generated by the yolk sac and early embryo. Significant megakaryocytopoiesis and granulopoiesis develop at 4 to 5 months. After birth, hematopoiesis occurs in the sinusoidal cavities of the tibias, femurs, and axial skeleton. *(Modified from Erslev A, Gabuzda T: Pathophysiology of blood, ed 2, Philadelphia, 1979, WB Saunders.)*

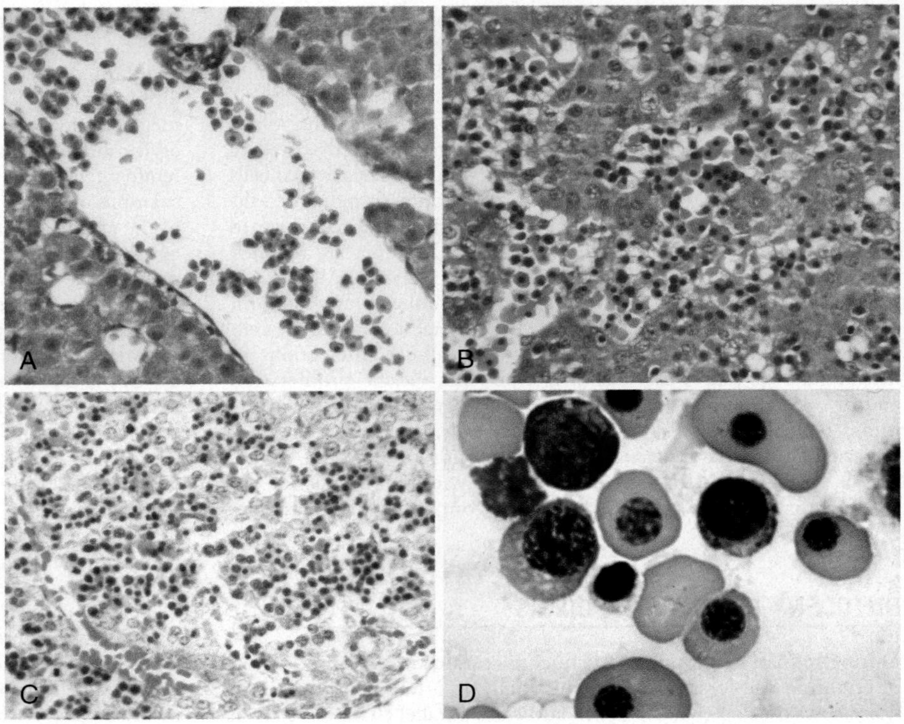

Figure 24-4 EMBRYONIC/FETAL ERYTHROPOIESIS. **A,** Section of an 8-mm embryo depicting a portion of hepatic parenchymal cells with embryonic erythroblasts present within primitive sinusoidal cavities. **B,** At 6 to 8 weeks, discrete aggregates of definitive erythroblasts appear within the liver parenchyma, whereas mature embryonic erythroblasts persist in well-developed sinusoids. **C,** Definitive erythroblasts are spread throughout the liver (100-day fetus). **D,** Cytologic spread from disaggregated fetal liver cells of a 55-day embryo. Characteristic form of embryonic erythroblasts and immature (basophilic) definitive erythroblasts is shown. (**A** to **C,** hematoxylin-eosin stain; **D,** Wright-Giemsa stain.)

affected during fetal life in mice that cannot produce KL, adult steel-Dickie (Sl/Sl^d) mutant mice (which produce only some soluble KL) display greatly impaired erythropoiesis and hematopoiesis, suggesting that the KL/C-KIT pathway plays a role in the recruitment and self-renewal behavior of adult stem cells in vivo.[390,391] The long-term transplantation potential is impaired in cells with mutations of C-KIT kinase activity.[391] Transplantable stem cells from the yolk sac, in contrast to fetal liver cells, cannot engraft adult recipients, because of altered homing behavior or inability of bone marrow to support their development,[361] as suggested by their engraftment in neonatal liver.[392] The homing properties of fetal stem cells transplanted into adult irradiated recipients were found to be inferior to those of their adult counterparts.[393] Whether this finding is related to their increased cycling or other reasons is unclear. However, fetal liver stem cells, despite their reduced homing potential,[393] have higher engraftment levels, likely because of their proliferative prowess compared to adult stem cells.[394]

The surface antigenic profiles of erythroid progenitors and precursors are distinct at each ontogenic stage. For example, HLA class I and class II antigens are not detected in embryonic erythroid progenitor cells but reach adult levels at approximately gestational week 9.[395] CD34$^+$ hematopoietic progenitors present in yolk sac express Mac-1 but are negative for stem cell antigen 1 (Sca-1), which is expressed in fetal and adult CD34$^+$ murine progenitor cells.[396] On the other hand, adult CD34$^+$ progenitors lack Mac-1 and AA4.1, which are expressed in fetal CD34$^+$ progenitor cells. Fetal BFU-E and CFU-E express similar levels of HLA class II antigens, whereas adult CFU-E are largely devoid of these antigens.[395,397] β_1 integrins, especially $\alpha_4\beta_1$ and α_5, are expressed widely in all hemopoietic cells, including nucleated erythroid cells. However, in the latter, they display a differentiation-dependent, developmentally segregated pattern of expression, because they are absent in embryonic murine erythroblasts,[398] and among adult cells, stem/progenitor cells express them in a constitutively active form in contrast to more mature cells.[399-401] Fetal red cells display a straight, unbranched polylactosaminyl chain (i antigen) on their surface, whereas in adult cells, this structure, which bears ABH blood group determinants, is highly branched (I antigen).[124] The enzymatic activity of several enzymes in the glycolytic pathway is greater in fetal than in adult red cells.[402] In contrast, carbonic anhydrase levels are very low during intrauterine and early neonatal life.[403] Distinct isozyme patterns for several enzymes (i.e., phosphoglycerate kinase, acetylcholinesterase) also distinguish fetal from adult red cells.[404,405]

The most widely studied changes during red cell ontogeny are the shifts or "switches" in globin types. Embryonic erythroblasts are characterized by their avid accumulation of iron, which is stored as ferritin[406] (0.3% to 1% of total protein) and by the synthesis of the unique hemoglobins Gower I ($\zeta_2\varepsilon_2$), Gower II ($\alpha_2\varepsilon_2$), and hemoglobin Portland ($\zeta_2\gamma_2$). The ζ- and ε-globin chains are embryonic α-like and β-like chains, respectively.[88] These three embryonic types of hemoglobin are most likely synthesized in succession, because the concentration of Gower I is highest in smaller embryos. Thus a switch from ζ- to α- and ε- to γ-globin gene production begins during the embryonic phase of erythropoiesis but is not complete until fetal erythropoiesis is well established. During the transition from yolk sac to fetal liver erythropoiesis (6 to 9 weeks), erythroid precursors within the fetal liver coexpress embryonic (ζ- or ε-) and fetal (α- or γ-) globin both in vivo and in vitro.[407,408] The predominant type of hemoglobin synthesized during fetal liver erythropoiesis is HbF ($\alpha_2\gamma_2$), with a high proportion of $^G\gamma$:$^A\gamma$ (7:3). Adult HbA ($\alpha_2\beta_2$), which is detectable at the earliest stages of fetal liver erythropoiesis, is synthesized as a minor component throughout this period. However, HbA_2 ($\alpha_2\delta_2$), which is a minor hemoglobin in the adult, is undetectable in these early stages. From about gestational week 30 onward, β-globin synthesis steadily increases so that, by term, 50% to 55% of hemoglobin synthesized is HbA. By 4 to 5 weeks of postnatal age, 75% of the hemoglobin is HbA. This percentage increases to 95% by 4 months as the fetal-to-adult hemoglobin switch is completed. HbF levels in circulating red cells are at a plateau for the first 2 to 3 weeks (as a result of the decline in total erythropoiesis that follows birth), but the HbF level gradually declines so that normal levels (<1%) are achieved by 200 days after birth.[409]

Several in vitro and in vivo approaches have been used to study the basis of globin switching through development. Beyond its biologic interest, rigorous research in this area was propelled by the possibility of manipulating globin switching to increase HbF production in adults and ameliorate the clinical symptoms of disorders of the β-globin locus (e.g., sickle cell anemia, thalassemia).

Transplantation experiments and ablative endocrine maneuvers in the sheep model have failed to provide convincing support for the effects of environmental or humoral factors on the switching process, although some modulation of the rate of switching was seen in these models.[410,411] Similar conclusions were reached with transplantation of human fetal liver cells to adult recipients.[412,413] The most important determinant of fetal-to-adult hemoglobin switching seems to be post-conceptual age, with the sharpest period for transition between 30 and 52 weeks. The fetal-to-adult switch appears to be unaffected by the time at which birth occurs or by changes in the kinetics of erythropoiesis induced by perinatal hemolysis.[414] A delay in switching usually is observed in cases of general developmental retardation, in patients with certain chromosomal abnormalities (e.g., trisomy 13), and in diabetic infants because of increased circulating levels of α-aminobutyric acid, which directly affects HbF synthesis.[415] Integration of data from studies using in vitro and in vivo approaches indicates that developmental control of globin switching is intrinsic to erythroid cells. Stage-specific transcriptional forces with negative or positive influences (or both) on specific globin genes may provide the molecular basis for differential transcriptional activity during development. This view is favored by experiments in transgenic mice[416] and in heterokaryons (produced by fusion of human with mouse cells),[417] as well as by isolation of stage-specific transcription factors in other erythroid systems (e.g., avian).[418] Furthermore, because α-like and β-like globin genes are activated sequentially in the order of their location in chromosome 11 or 16, respectively, it is possible that polarity of the transcriptional activity and globin promoter competition for the locus control region and developmental stage–specific transcription factors contribute to this regulation.[419]

Recently genetic linkage and genome-wide association studies in individuals with increased levels of HbF or hereditary persistence of fetal hemoglobin (HPFH) syndromes have provided new and important insights in the control of fetal to adult globin switching.[420,421] Of interest, besides cis control of switching (deletions in β-globin cluster or mutations in the γ-globin gene promoters), trans control was revealed through direct and indirect interactions of γ-globin with molecules (controlled by loci unlinked to the β-globin cluster) exerting repressive fetal globin activity. These molecules were BCL11A, a transcription factor involved in juvenile leukemia, and HBS1L-Myb. The full-length BCL11A is expressed in adult but not fetal erythroid cells, and adult individuals with high hemoglobin F/BCL11A genotype have reduced expression of full-length BCL11A. Suppression of its expression reactivates HbF expression in adult erythroid cells in vitro,[422] and deletion of BCL11A interferes with fetal hemoglobin silencing during development and rescues the phenotype of a mouse model of sickle cell disease.[423] Myb-HBS1L is downregulated in individuals with elevated HbF levels and overexpression of Myb inhibits γ-globin in human erythroleukemia cells. The levels of Myb were found to be controlled by micro-RNA 15a and 16-1 in patients with human trisomy 13 and high HbF levels.[424] In addition to the above molecules with γ-globin repressive activity, recent data support a role of KLF1, the major erythroid transcriptional regulator, in globin gene switching. Valuable insights were obtained from families with haploinsufficiency of KLF1 (missense mutations affecting DNA binding) and increased fetal hemoglobin levels.[425,426] However, this was not always the case, and a compound heterozygosity was required in other families for high HbF expression.[427] It appears that KLF1 targets genes such as BCL11A, EPB4.9, and CD44, which are very sensitive to KLF1 activity, whereas effects on other genes like γ-globin, or BCAM (carrying the Lutheran blood group antigens) are variable. Collectively, it turned out that KLF1 has a critical role in globin gene switching both by directly activating β-globin and indirectly by suppressing γ-globin through its control of BCL11A. Overall, genetic data account for approximately 70% of the HPFH phenotypes observed in human populations, suggesting that new factors are yet to be identified. In this context, it is of interest that three β^0-thalassemia major patients who failed to engraft after stem cell transplantation became transfusion independent because they expressed sustained levels of increased HbF in autologous red cells post transplantation without evidence of any known HPFH genotypes.[428] From all of these studies, it has become apparent that switching is very complex, involving many players, cis and trans, with distinct and variable roles. The many models of globin switching proposed previously (i.e., the competitive model, the chromosome looping, the gene silencing) are not mutually exclusive and may complement each other.

In summary, throughout human development, waves of hematopoiesis are initiated sequentially in newly recruited sites. The first wave of erythropoiesis is seen in yolk sac between days 15 and 18 (7.5 days after conception in mice). In addition to erythroid cells, uncommitted progenitors and progenitors for nonerythroid cells are present in the yolk sac and are thought to be the source of cells colonizing the fetal liver.[195,429-431] However, in addition to yolk sac, foci of hematopoietic activity have been detected within the embryo around the developing aorta (in para-aortic–splanchnopleura [P-Sp] and aorto-gonad-mesonephros [AGM] area).[432-434] In fact, the P-Sp/AGM site in mice was shown to harbor progenitor cells before circulation begins and 1 day before these cells are found in the yolk sac. Long-term repopulating cells after their transplantation in adult recipients were detected only in the AGM area, leading to speculation that this intraembryonic site is the main or only source of fetal liver colonization,[434] in contrast to earlier experiments implicating the yolk sac in that role.[429-431] Establishment of blood flow and the concentration of nitric oxide appear to play an important role in determining the number of definitive hematopoietic stem cells generated in the AGM region.[435] Presence of mesodermally derived hematopoietic cells in two distinct anatomic sites, one intraembryonic and the other extraembryonic, has been seen in explant studies of *Xenopus* and after analysis of chick-quail chimeras.[436] More recent experiments with human cells have led to similar conclusions.[437] Although the presence of progenitors for definitive hematopoiesis in two independent sites (extraembryonic and within the embryo proper) is indisputable, the extent to which these two sites contribute to fetal liver colonization has been a matter of dispute. The conclusion that only the AGM area contributes to fetal liver colonization was based on transplantation experiments in adult recipients and has been challenged.[361] Transplantation experiments using newborn mice with active fetal liver hematopoiesis as recipients showed that adult long-term repopulating cells are detectable in the yolk sac at day 9 post conception and are 37-fold greater in number than repopulating cells present in the P-Sp/AGM area at the same time. Therefore failure of yolk sac cells (or AGM cells before day 10 post conception) to engraft adult recipients may be caused by either compromised homing or impaired survival and proliferation within the adult bone marrow environment (because of positive regulators or inhibition by negative regulators). In light of this information, the 30-year-old theory that yolk sac colonizes the fetal liver has been revived.[429] A question that remains unanswered is whether stem cell activity 9 days post conception in yolk sac and P-Sp/AGM is generated autonomously and independently or is derived from a common precursor cell with migratory properties. Murine studies comparing newborn transplant outcomes before the onset of systemic circulation between the yolk sac site and the intraembryonic AGM site have emerged,[438] and these, together with the identification of placenta as an autonomous circulation-independent site with terminal erythroid maturation of primitive cells,[439] have added an additional layer of complexity.

A common precursor cell giving rise to erythroid cells with either yolk sac or fetal liver characteristics has been identified by culture of murine and human embryonic stem cells in vitro.[440,441] Environmental regulation of specification to the primitive or definitive lineage has been shown in *Xenopus*.[442] However, because BFU-E present in yolk sac, fetal liver, and fetal bone marrow have a definitive-like progeny and these progenitors were not present after ablation of core binding factor (CBF)-β[443] despite the presence of normal embryonic erythropoiesis, the derivation of embryonic erythroblasts from a distinct progenitor, not present in subsequent life, remains a viable hypothesis. Of further interest is the observation that deletion of Mdm2 and Mdm4, two critical negative regulators of p53, exerted distinct outcomes on primitive and definitive hematopoiesis. Whereas Mdm2 is required for primitive erythropoiesis, Mdm4 is required for massive expansion of definitive erythropoiesis in fetal liver and is dispensable for adult erythropoiesis. These data are also consistent with the distinct molecular control between fetal and adult cells[444] discussed earlier.

TRANSCRIPTION FACTORS IN ERYTHROPOIESIS

Lineage-specific transcription factors are widely believed to be responsible for regulating the expression of erythroid genes during both ontogeny and the course of erythroid differentiation. The majority of erythroid-specific transcription factors has been identified from cloning of breakpoints or translocations associated with human leukemias or from expression libraries obtained from erythroid cell lines. The precise role exerted by each of these factors in erythropoiesis was later clarified by painstaking experiments with somatic cell fusions and in transgenic mice.[417,445,446] Some of the major transcription factors implicated in the control of erythropoiesis are listed in Table 24-2.

Studies of mice with targeted gene disruption have provided key insights into the complex molecular pathways that regulate hematopoiesis in general and erythropoiesis in particular.[1,2] These studies, complemented by in vitro differentiation of mutated embryonic stem cells into different lineages, have provided clear evidence about distinct regulatory requirements of primitive (yolk sac) versus definitive (fetal liver and bone marrow) erythropoiesis, or of early versus late stages of erythroid differentiation. Because erythropoiesis is the first differentiated lineage in embryonic yolk sac hematopoiesis and the predominant lineage in fetal liver hematopoiesis, factors that affect hematopoiesis in general will disturb erythropoiesis during early stages of development and lead to lethality at different gestational days, depending on the defect. The time in development at which disruption of each specific gene manifests its phenotype is used to establish a hierarchical control among the different transcription factors. The earliest disruption of erythroid differentiation is observed in mice lacking the bHLH factor TAL1/SCL, which is encoded by a gene initially identified on the basis of its localization in a chromosomal breakpoint region frequently associated with T-cell acute leukemia.[447] SCL^{null} embryos are bloodless and die very early, with abrogation of both yolk sac and fetal liver erythropoiesis.[448] Because of the requirement for SCL in the formation of the transcription complex with the nuclear protein Rbtn2/LMO2 rhombotin 2/LIM domain only 2 (Rbtn2/LMO2) and GATA1 (detailed later), it is not surprising that targeted disruption of Rbtn2 and LMO2 also produces a bloodless phenotype.[449]

Mice lacking expression of GATA2, a member of the GATA family of transcription factors, exhibit an early and severe quantitative defect in hematopoiesis that influences all lineages.[450] Other regulatory factors seem to totally spare embryonic (yolk sac) hematopoiesis and have a specific effect only on fetal liver hematopoiesis, with death occurring at later days (12.5 days post conception). In this category are the proto-oncogene c-Myb and the core-binding factors CBF-α_2/AML1 and CBF-β.[451-453] Embryonic erythropoiesis is spared in mice with targeted ablation of these genes. Both c-Myb, the cellular homologue of v-Myb proto-oncogene, and the heterodimeric transcription factor CBF are abundantly expressed early in normal myelolymphoid cells, with decreasing expression as differentiation proceeds. Their expression pattern and their functional influence on growth factor receptor genes (i.e., IL-3, GM-CSF, CSF1, T-cell antigen receptor [TCR] α, β) may underlie their importance in the development of all definitive hematopoietic lineages.[1]

Of paramount importance for adult erythropoiesis is the transcription factor GATA1, the founder of the GATA family of factors.[1] The GATA1 protein controls erythroid differentiation at several levels by controlling (in cooperation with GATA2) the proliferative capacity of erythroid progenitor/precursor cells, the apoptotic rate of erythroblasts, and the expression of lineage-specific genes. These effects are mediated through activation of expression of target genes by binding to specific sequences (WGATAR) present in the regulatory domains of virtually any erythroid gene, including EPOR and GATA1 itself. However, WGATAR binding sites also are present in genes specific for megakaryocytic, eosinophilic, mast cell, and dendritic lineages, as well as in genes expressed in testicular Sertoli cells. Insights into the specificity of GATA1 in erythroid differentiation have been provided by studies on the organization of WGATAR sites in erythroid-specific regulatory sequences. A minimal erythroid transcription-activation sequence that consists of a core-binding motif flanked by two canonical GATA1 binding sites has been identified. The core-binding motif is composed of one SCL binding site and one GATA binding site separated by 10 bp.[2] Different domains of the GATA1 protein are responsible for binding to the core and the flanking sequences. At least three functional domains in the GATA1 protein have been identified: two zinc finger domains (amino-terminal finger [NF] and carboxyl-terminal finger [CF)]) and an active amino-terminal domain. The NF domain is required for association with Friend of GATA1 (FOG-1), a protein encoded by a gene identified using GATA1 as bait in the two-hybrid yeast assay.[454] FOG-1 contains 10 zinc finger domains, only the first of which is required for GATA1 binding. The function of its other 9 zinc finger domains is not clear because they appear to be dispensable in structure-function studies, but they are well conserved in evolution. The GATA1-FOG-1 heterodimeric complex binds to the two flanking sites of the minimal erythroid transcription activation domain. Experimentally induced genetic mutations, such as $GATA1^{V205M}$, impairing GATA1-FOG-1 interaction in mice lead to impaired megakaryocytopoiesis and absence of definitive erythropoiesis, whereas primitive erythropoiesis is normal.[455] Rescue experiments indicate that $GATA1^{V205M}$ newborns are severely anemic with anisocytosis and spherocytosis with striking reduction mainly in the expression of genes encoding membrane proteins, whereas expression of other erythroid-specific genes, such as Alas2, was not affected.[456] These results indicate that DNA binding of the GATA1-FOG-1 complex is necessary for activation of a subset of GATA1 target genes in definitive erythroid cells but is dispensable for their activation in primitive erythroblasts. It should be emphasized that GATA1-FOG-1 interaction, while activating the expression of erythroid genes, inhibits target gene activation in testicular Sertoli cells.[457] This result provides insight into how one factor regulates more than one differentiation program by suggesting that its function, but not its expression, is different depending on the cellular context. Whether GATA1-FOG-1 interaction inhibits erythroid gene expression in myelomonocytic cells has not been investigated.

The CF domain, on the other hand, recognizes and binds to the GATA site localized in the core of the minimal erythroid transcription sequence 10 bp downstream to the SCL binding site. SCL and GATA1 bind simultaneously to their respective sites of the core as multimeric complexes formed by SCL/E47/LMO2 on the one hand and by GATA1/LMO2 on the other. Binding of the two complexes to the core is stabilized by Lbd1, which forms a physical bridge between them. The paramount importance of the CF finger for GATA1 function is proved by the fact that GATA1 genes lacking the region encoding this domain are unable to rescue erythroid differentiation in $GATA1^{null}$ embryonic stem cells,[458] whereas minigenes containing only the CF of either GATA1 or GATA2 are sufficient to induce megakaryocytic differentiation of myeloid cell lines.[459] In addition to forming heterodimers with LMO2, CF can form complexes with Sp1 and PU.1, two factors essential for myelomonocytic differentiation. The GATA1-PU.1 complex is unable to bind DNA, so its function might be to establish either an erythroid- or a myeloid-permissive cellular environment depending on which factor is expressed at the highest concentration.[2] The presence of relatively higher concentrations of GATA1 would favor the formation of GATA1-LMO2 complexes leading to activation of erythroid-specific genes, whereas the presence of relatively higher concentrations of PU.1 would lead mainly to the formation of the transcriptionally inactive GATA1-PU.1 complexes.

Although early experiments on cell lines failed to identify any function for the amino-terminal domain of GATA1,[459,460] knock-in experiments in mice indicated that this domain, although dispensable for primitive erythropoiesis, is required for appropriate production of definitive red cells.[458] A truncated GATA1 gene lacking the amino-terminal domain is 10 times less efficient than the full-length gene in rescuing erythroid differentiation in GATA1^{null} mice.[458] This experiment suggests that interaction of the amino-terminal domain of GATA1 with a suitable partner(s) is required for optimal definitive erythropoiesis. Structure function studies have identified that interaction between the amino-terminal domain of GATA1 and the product of the retinoblastoma (RB) gene is essential for proper terminal erythroid maturation, providing a unifying mechanism for the similar phenotype of several Gata1 and RB mouse mutants and of human diseases associated with mutations in these two genes.[461]

In addition to all the evidence pointing to GATA1 as exerting a predominant but ontogenetic-specific role in the control of erythroid differentiation, other evidence indicates that this gene exerts exquisite control in the differentiation of other hemopoietic lineages, such as megakaryocytes,[1] mast cells,[462] eosinophils[463] and dendritic cells.[464] The mechanism used by one single factor in guiding differentiation along different lineages does not rely on specific domains in the GATA1 protein itself. In fact, the structure of all the GATA proteins is so well conserved among different family members and in evolution that GATA1^{null} embryonic stem cells are rescued not only by reintroduction of the GATA1 gene itself but also by introducing any other member of the GATA family, such as GATA3.[465] The lineage-specific action of GATA1 in regulating gene expression is achieved through the presence of lineage-specific regulatory sequences in the promoter regions of the target genes. Therefore the relative concentration of GATA1, as opposed to the levels of a few key regulatory partners, may establish a lineage-permissive microenvironment. Furthermore, the existence of lineage-specific regulatory sequences in the GATA1 gene itself ensures that such concentrations are achieved only in the right cell. Although GATA1 is expressed in erythroid, megakaryocytic, mast, dendritic, and eosinophilic cells, its level of expression differs greatly among the various cell types, with erythroid cells expressing the most. Three DNase hypersensitive sites (HS) have been recognized within the 8 Kb upstream and the first intron of the murine GATA1 gene, defined as HSI, HSII, and HSIII. Targeted deletion mutants in the mouse have shown that each of these sites functions as an enhancer in different cell types. HSI is required for GATA1 expression in megakaryocytes,[466] mast cells,[462] and also for upregulation of GATA1 expression during the process of antigen presentation in dendritic cells[467] and during the progression of erythroid maturation.[468] HSIII is capable of sustaining low levels of GATA1 expression in erythroid and dendritic cells. HSII, which is dispensable for erythroid and megakaryocyte expression, is absolutely required for gene expression in eosinophils.[463] All of the 317 bp of HSI are required for GATA1 expression in megakaryocytes, but only the first 5′ 62 bp are needed for erythroid-specific reporter activity.[469] The HSI region contains a canonical minimal erythroid activation sequence, and point mutations in the GATA site, but not in the E-box, abolish HSI function in both erythroid and megakaryocytic cells. Of note, GATA1 mRNA has an unusually long half-life (>9 hours). Two GATA1 bands, corresponding to the native and processed (acetylated and phosphorylated) forms of the protein, have been detected by Western blot analysis.[470] The processed form binds DNA with higher affinity than the native form. Furthermore, although the half-life of the native form is short (approximately 0.5 hour) and stabilized by EPO, the processed form is extremely stable (half-life >6 hours) and EPO independent.[470] Because the cell cycle of hemopoietic cells in vivo is as short as 6 hours, erythroid cells accumulate GATA1 mRNA and protein as they proliferate. Because maturation is dependent on the levels of GATA1 expressed by cells, the cellular GATA1 content might represent the biologic clock that, by controlling the number of precursors, determines the cellular output of the differentiation process. This hypothesis suggests that EPO-induced GATA1 processing through the ubiquitin-proteasome pathway is an important element in the regulation of erythroid differentiation. On the other hand, the TRAIL–Bruton kinase death pathway has as an end point caspase 3, the protein specifically responsible for GATA1 cleavage. However, caspase 3 is unable to cleave GATA1 if the protein is complexed in the nucleus with the chaperone protein heat shock protein 70 (Hsp70). EPO-receptor signaling counteracts the apoptotic pathway by favoring Hsp70-GATA1 colocalization in the nucleus.[471] The equilibrium between TRAIL and EPO-dependent control on Hsp70 localization may be perturbed under pathologic conditions. As an example, defective nuclear localization of Hsp70 and increased GATA1 cleavage is associated with dyserythropoiesis in myelodysplastic disorders.[472] These biochemical studies detailing the biochemical link between EPO and TRAIL from one side and GATA1 from the other are consistent with studies indicating that EPO signaling also induces GATA1 phosphorylation at Ser310 and that this phosphorylation plays an important role in regulating GATA1 function in erythroid cell lines.[473,474] Although GATA1 mutants expressing only the native form of GATA1 do not have a detectable erythroid phenotype under steady-state conditions,[475] more studies on the response of these mice to erythroid stress will clarify the role of GATA1 processing in stress erythropoiesis.

Another gene of the GATA family important for erythroid differentiation is GATA2. Both GATA1 and GATA2 are expressed early in multipotential progenitors; however, their expression ratios change as the cells differentiate (see Table 24-1),[476] suggesting that the ratio of these two factors may be important at specific stages of erythroid differentiation. Knock-out experiments with both of these genes have borne this out. Thus in contrast to GATA2, which is expressed at high levels in early cells and affects expansion of all hematopoietic lineages,[450] GATA1 expression increases as differentiation advances and seems to be the obligatory factor required for survival and terminal differentiation of erythroid cells. In mice with targeted disruption of GATA1, erythropoiesis proceeds only up to the stage of proerythroblasts; these mice die early and fail to mature further.[477,478] Furthermore, transgenic mice with partial loss of function (knockdown alleles, GATA1^{LOW}) of GATA1 show that erythroid differentiation is dose dependent with respect to GATA1.[468] High levels of GATA1 are necessary to form complexes with its cofactor FOG-1[454] and with the other proteins described earlier (LM02, SCL, or Hsp70) during terminal erythroid differentiation.

The realization that minute differences in transcription factor concentrations are required for lineage specification under physiologic conditions supports the idea that the differentiation system allows more flexibility in both the choice and the reversibility of pathway commitment toward a specific lineage. For example, a CFU-E was thought to have no other choice than to became an erythroid cell or to die.[6] More recently, experiments with forced expression of transcription factors in fully committed or even mature cells have demonstrated that the system has some degree of plasticity and that forced expression of FOG-1 into mast cells may turn them into erythroblasts,[479] whereas forced expression of GATA1 into common myeloid progenitor cells induces their transdifferentiation into MEP.[480] It is foreseen that future experiments will demonstrate that any cell type may be turned into an erythroblast by overexpression of an appropriate combination of transcription factors. All of these manipulations were performed in vitro. Of interest, experimentally decreased expression of GATA1 in progenitor cell compartments in vivo does not alter the frequency of individual compartments (i.e., does not decrease MEP by increasing the granulocyte/macrophage progenitor) but results in alternative differentiation pathways. Although the numbers of cells phenotypically recognizable as MEP in these animals are much higher than normal, MEP with reduced GATA1 expression, unlike normal cells, have the potential also to differentiate into mast cells.[481]

Another factor with special importance in the erythroid lineage is the CACCC binding protein designated EKLF (also known as KLF1), which is expressed at all stages of erythropoiesis but binds preferentially to CACCC sites in the β-globin promoter. EKLF is a zinc finger protein that binds not only DNA, but also, after appropriate posttranslational modifications, is a key regulatory protein that modulates chromatin structure of the β-globin locus.[482] Mice lacking EKLF (EKLF^{null}) die of a thalassemic-like defect due to severe deficiency of β-globin expression.[483] Microarray analysis of EKLF^{null} erythroid cells and promoter-specific expression of reported genes in EKLF^{null} cells have identified that the first GATA1-dependent molecular control of erythroid differentiation is followed by a second EKLF-dependent phase.[484,485] Primarily GATA1-dependent genes include, in addition to *EPOR* and those involved in the control of apoptosis, α- and δ-globin. EKLF-dependent genes, in addition to β-globin[486,487] and AHSP, are represented by those required for appropriate membrane assembly, such as β-spectrin, ankyrin, and band 3 (but not α-spectrin). These results are consistent with the notion that, in erythroid differentiation, activation of α-globin gene expression precedes that of β-globin[488] and that loss of GATA1 binding sites in the promoter of the gene is found in α-thalassemia,[489] in the Greek nondeletion HPFH (guanine to adenine at nucleotide position-–117 of γ-globin),[490] and in δ-thalassemia (point mutation leading to G→A substitution at position +69 of the δ-globin gene),[491] whereas loss of EKLF binding site is present in other forms of HPFH. In addition to regulating globin gene expression directly, EKLF inhibits γ-globin expression indirectly by activating BCL11A expression.[492]

Intrinsic control of erythroid differentiation also is exerted by genes that, until repressed, prevent terminal cell maturation. The most studied of these genes is ID1,[493] which as its name indicates, inhibits differentiation along almost all mesenchymal cell lineages, including the erythroid lineage.[494,495] ID1 appears to act between GATA1 and EKLF by preventing EKLF from executing its program.

Because common transcription factors are present in erythroid and megakaryocytic cells, and bipotent erythroid/megakaryocytic progenitors exist both in vitro (in the form of cell lines) and in vivo,[56] exciting insights regarding subtleties in the molecular control of these two lineages by the same transcription factors have surfaced. Modified gene–targeting strategy ("knockdown") of GATA1 uncovered a largely unanticipated role of this transcription factor in the control of proliferation and maturation of megakaryocytes.[468] In addition to GATA1, other important transcription factors essential for terminal megakaryocytic development are NF-E2[496] and its partner mafG.[497]

Nevertheless, the fact that several regulators are necessary for primitive (yolk sac), as opposed to definitive (fetal liver and bone marrow), erythropoiesis provides evidence that molecular control between these two hemopoietic sites is different and may include both ubiquitous and hematopoietic-specific factors. In fact, evidence suggests that GATA1 transcription is differentially regulated in yolk sac cells compared to fetal liver erythroid cells, with alternative promoter use and an additional intron element requirement for promoter activation in fetal liver cells.[498]

In addition to transcription factors/oncogenes influencing erythropoiesis, targeted ablation and naturally existing mutations of hematopoietic growth factor receptors, especially of the tyrosine kinase family, have disclosed important insights into the control of erythropoiesis. Whereas deletion of the vascular endothelial growth factor (VEGF)/flk-1 receptor affects both endothelial and hematopoietic development[499] through its presumed presence in the hemangioblast, the common endothelial/hematopoietic stem cell, mutations affecting the tyrosine kinase KIT receptor (present in hematopoietic cells) or of its ligand KL (present in stromal cells) seem to predominantly affect erythropoiesis in the fetal liver and the adult animal. Mice with KIT mutations (W mutations) leading to absence of or compromised kinase activity and steel mice with mutations of KL have disproportionate and severe reduction of the numbers of late erythroid progenitors, CFU-E, and differentiated erythroid precursors resulting in anemia.[500] Studies showing cross-phosphorylation of EPOR following activation of KIT/KL signaling may be relevant to the effect.[277] Mutations or targeted ablations of some downstream signaling substrates for KIT or other receptors (i.e., SHP2 phosphatase or gp130) seem to produce a hematopoietic picture not unlike the one produced by receptor mutations.[501,502]

Taken together, these studies have significantly expanded our understanding of the molecular basis of hematopoietic cell development in general and of erythropoiesis in particular. The emerging picture is that certain genes, such as SCL, are absolutely required for hematopoietic development, whereas other genes, such as GATA2, c-Myb, CBF, TEL, and some downstream signal transducing molecules, such as gp30 and SHP2, are responsible for expansion and maintenance of a normal pool of fetal liver and adult hematopoietic progenitors. The participation of many of these molecules in multicomponent molecular complexes with protein/protein and protein/DNA interactions (i.e., LM02/Lbd1/SCL/E2A/GATA), during the early proliferative stages of hematopoiesis[503] may underlie their role in the proliferation and maintenance of immature progenitor/precursor pools in erythropoiesis. Other genes such as GATA1, its partner FOG-1, and EKLF are necessary to direct high levels of function of erythroid-specific genes in cells already committed to terminal differentiation. Thus a hierarchical requirement in the expression of specific regulators during early versus late erythroid differentiation or during yolk sac versus fetal liver/adult erythropoiesis is demonstrated. However, this does not exclude the involvement of some factors (i.e., SCL, TEL) at both early and late stages of erythropoiesis. In fact, more recent studies on conditional knockouts have clarified that SCL exerts two different levels of control in the development of the hemopoietic system. First, SCL is required for the determination event that induces one (or few) mesenchymal cell(s) to become a hematopoietic stem cell(s) in the early embryos.[181] After this initial event has taken place, its presence becomes dispensable, as demonstrated by the fact that conditional SCL deletion in the adult animals impairs only erythropoiesis and megakaryocytopoiesis.[181,504]

With information from innovative applications of molecular approaches becoming available at a fast pace, the list of regulators with a biologic impact on hematopoiesis/erythropoiesis not only is continuously expanding but is starting to fill the gap between the individual transcription factors and the epigenetic control of erythroid cells. Actively expressed genes are localized in areas on the chromosome in an open configuration. The DNA switch from a closed to an open configuration is determined by the tightness of its binding to the histones by which it is surrounded.[505] A series of enzymes regulates the chromosome configuration state by modifying either the DNA (cytosine methylation mediated by specific methylases) or the histones (e.g., histone acetyltransferase [HAT] and deacetylase [HDAC], polycomb repressive complexes). HAT exerts a positive control (promoting the formation of an open configuration state), whereas methylases and HDAC exert a negative control (inducing a closed chromatin configuration state) on gene expression. Once the chromatin is in an open configuration state, appropriate enzymatic complexes (e.g., polymerases, spliceosomes) are recruited to the locus for appropriate expression to occur. Because of their ability to recognize specific DNA sequences, transcription factors play an important role in the recruitment of the epigenetic and/or transcriptional protein machinery to a specific locus. The link between epigenetic and transcriptional control of gene expression in erythroid cells is emerging. The first global methylation status of erythroid cells as they mature has been determined.[506] The relationship between chromatin architecture and transcription factor occupancy in the loci encoding key erythrocyte membrane proteins has been established.[507] In addition to binding GATA1, FOG-1 is also capable of binding NuRD, a complex that contains HDAC1.[508] The multicomplex GATA1/FOG-1/NuRD is responsible for appropriate activation/repression of several erythroid specific genes, including the GATA2-GATA1 switch occurring at early stages of erythroid development.[509]

TRANSCRIPTIONAL AND POSTTRANSCRIPTIONAL IMPAIRMENT IN DISORDERS OF ERYTHROPOIESIS

The transcription factor found most frequently altered in inherited and acquired human diseases of the erythroid and megakaryocytic lineage is GATA1. The mutations often involve the region of the gene encoding the NF domain. Mutations in the GATA1 NF domain interrupting its interaction with FOG-1, such as V205M and G208S, are responsible for familial dyserythropoietic anemia and X-linked thrombocytopenia, respectively.[510,511] A different mutation at position 208 leading to G→A substitution is associated with dyserythropoietic anemia and macrothrombocytopenia.[512] Mutations in the NF terminal domain of GATA1 responsible for DNA binding, such as A216G[513] and D218G,[514] instead have been found to be associated with X-linked thalassemia and/or thrombocytopenia. The phenotype of X-linked thrombocytopenia was mimicked in mice by knock-in experiments of the mutant V205G GATA1 gene.[515] However, the same A216G mutation has been found associated with X-linked gray platelet syndrome, a mild bleeding disorder characterized by thrombocytopenia and large agranular platelets.[516] Furthermore, a mutation at codon 216 changing arginine to tryptophan (R216W) was detected in a 3-year-old boy with congenital erythropoietic porphyria, an autosomal recessive disorder usually due to mutations of the uroporphyrinogen III synthase gene (UROS). The boy also presented with microcytic anemia and red cell morphologic characteristics and a globin chain pattern compatible with β -thalassemia and increased HbF levels (59.5%).[517] The different phenotype expressed by patients carrying mutations either in the FOG-1 or the DNA binding portion of NF supported the notion that the two domains influence erythroid versus megakaryocytic maturation.[518] However, the observation that, in certain cases, a mutation in the same codon or even the same mutation results in a different phenotype suggests that the phenotype induced by mutations in the GATA1 gene is extremely sensitive to genetic modifiers outside the GATA1 locus. This hypothesis has been demonstrated in mice in which the same mutation induces embryonic lethality, thrombocytopenia, or myelofibrosis, depending on the mouse background in which it is harbored.[519]

On the other hand, frameshift and splice mutations encoding GATA1s, a protein lacking the amino-terminal domain, not only are associated with impaired erythropoiesis[520] but also are found in patients with megakaryocytic leukemia in Down syndrome,[521,522] in newborns with transient myeloproliferative syndromes,[523] and in one adult patient with megakaryocytic leukemia.[524] A mutation equivalent to that found in patients with acute megakaryoblastic leukemia and Down syndrome was created in mice by *N*-ethyl-*N*-nitrosourea mutagenesis screening. The reduced expression of the full-length GATA1 was not compensated in mice by expression of GATA1s. The mutation was embryonic lethal in hemizygous males and induced thrombocytopenia in heterozygous females.[525] However, when introduced in mice the GATA1s mutation increased proliferation of a "unique" fetal stem/progenitor cell extinguished in adult life.[526] The association between a mutation of GATA1 and the development of leukemia supports the concept that GATA1 controls the proliferation of hematopoietic progenitors. Reduced GATA1 expression, by increasing progenitor cell proliferation, may predispose hematopoietic cells to leukemia by favoring accumulation of secondary mutations. These mutations may involve the GATA1 itself because transforming Myb-GATA1 fusion genes have been associated with reduced GATA1 levels in acute basophilic leukemia.[527,528] Alterations of hematopoietic proliferation appear to be achieved through quantitative, rather than structural, GATA1 alterations. The GATA1s protein is far less efficient than the full-length GATA1 in rescuing the phenotype of GATA1^{null} embryonic stem cells,[458] and hypomorphic mutations in mice induce either leukemia[529] or a phenotype similar to idiopathic myelofibrosis,[530] depending on the severity of the reduction of the expression. Interestingly, the reduced content of GATA1 in megakaryocytes, through an as yet unidentified molecular defect rather than the presence of JAK2V617F, distinguishes primary myelofibrosis from all the other myeloproliferative neoplasms in humans.[531] (For a more complete review on the role of GATA factors in hematologic diseases, see reference 532.)

Point mutations in the EKLF/KLF1 gene have been associated with human diseases of terminal erythroid maturation (see Table 24-2). E325K substitution in the conserved residue of the zinc finger domain 2 is associated with congenital dyserythropoietic anemia.[533,534] Premature stop codons (L127X, K292X), point mutations in conserved residues of the zinc finger 1 (H299Y) and 2 (R328L, R328H, R331G), frameshift (X47 and X34), and hypomorphic mutations (deletion of the GATA1 binding site in the promoter region) have been associated with lack of Lutheran group antigen (Lu negative phenotype),[535] whereas neutral substitution (M39L), premature stop codon (K288X), and premature stop codon plus point mutations in the conserved residue of zinc finger 2 (S270X plus K332Q) have been associated with the HPFH phenotype with or without elevated zinc protoporphyrin.[425,427] Hereditary spherocytosis has also been observed in mice carrying the spontaneous Nan mutation (E339D substitution in the conserved residue of zinc finger 2).[536]

Another disease associated with abnormalities in the molecular machinery of red cell differentiation is represented by DBA, a rare congenital red cell hypoplasia characterized by anemia, bone marrow erythroblastopenia (lack of late erythroid forms), and congenital anomalies. The disease is associated with heterozygous mutations in the ribosomal protein S19 gene (RPS19) in approximately 25% of probands.[537] In a large cohort of 172 new families with familial history of DBA, mutations affecting the coding sequence of RPS19 or splice sites were found in 34 cases (19.8%), whereas additional mutations in noncoding regions were found in 8 patients (4.6%). Mutations included nonsense, missense, splice site, and frameshift mutations. More recently, de novo nonsense and splice-site mutations in another ribosomal protein, RPS24 (encoded by RPS24 [10q22-q23]), was identified in approximately 2% of RPS19 mutation-negative probands.[538] The molecular defect of the other families is yet to be uncovered. No correlation between the nature of mutations and the different patterns of clinical expression, including age at presentation, presence of malformations, and therapeutic outcome, has been documented. The lack of a consistent relationship between the nature of the mutations and the clinical phenotype implies that as yet unidentified factors modulate the phenotypic expression of the primary genetic defect in families with RPS19 mutations.[539] Two not mutually exclusive hypotheses had been proposed to explain the pathobiologic role of RPS19 (and RPS24) in the pathogenesis of the disease: (1) loss of unknown functions not directly connected with RPS19's structural role in ribosomes and (2) altered protein synthesis because of poor ribosome organization. The first hypothesis was suggested by findings based on a proteomic approach that identified numerous proteins bound to RPS19. In addition to FGF2, complement component 5 receptor 1, a nucleolar protein called RPS19 binding protein, and Pim-1, the other RPS19-binding proteins fall in the following Gene Ontology categories: NTPases (ATPases and GTPases; 5 proteins), hydrolases/helicases (19 proteins), isomerases (2 proteins), kinases (3 proteins), splicing factors (5 proteins), structural constituents of ribosome (29 proteins), transcription factors (11 proteins), transferases (5 proteins), transporters (9 proteins), DNA/RNA-binding protein species (53 proteins), other (1 dehydrogenase protein, 1 ligase protein, 1 peptidase protein, 1 receptor protein, 1 translation elongation factor), and 13 proteins with unknown function.[540] However, more recent studies have identified that RPS19 plays an essential role in the biogenesis and maturation of the 40S small ribosomal subunit in human cells[541,542] because of reduced gene expression of clustered ribosomal proteins due to abnormal pre-mRNA processing.[543] Such a defective ribosomal gene expression results in alterations of the transcription, translation, apoptosis, and oncogenic pathways.[544] Expression of RPS19 mRNA and protein decreases during terminal erythroid differentiation.[545] A mouse model of the disease has been generated by disrupting the endogenous Rps19 gene.[546-548] Cellular models of the disease have been established by small interfering RNA (siRNA) technology against RPS19 protein.[549-551] These models are establishing that RPS19 deficiency is accompanied by an unanticipated activation of p53 and death of the erythroid cells. Treatment of RPS19^{null} cells with dexamethasone prevents p53 activation and restores terminal erythroid maturation,[552] providing a molecular mechanism for the therapeutic effects exerted by dexamethasone in these patients. Alternatively, it has been proposed that dexamethasone may rescue defective protein synthesis in ribosomal-deficient erythroid cells by increasing expression of a subset of GR target genes (such as Zfp36l2, which controls RNA stability and/or translation).[553] Only 40% to 50% of DBA patients respond to steroids.[554] The mechanism underlying this lack of response has been the subject of recent investigation. The increased frequency of rs6198 GR SNP observed in these patients suggests that the failure to respond to steroids may be influenced by genetic and/or epigenetic modifications of the GR locus.

RSP19 deficiency and p53 activation is also observed in the 5q− MDS syndrome,[552] and p53 activation associated with reduced ribosomal gene dosage has been reported in low-risk MDS.[555] Whole-exome sequencing of MDS has recently uncovered mutations in genes involved in RNA splicing.[556,557] Whether these mutations also activate p53 has yet to be determined. These results suggest that defective mRNA splicing/translation may represent a unifying mechanism for the etiology of MDS. Interestingly, MDS has also been associated with mutations in GATA2. In fact, in spite of its importance in the early phases of erythroid maturation, GATA2 mutations have not been detected in erythroid diseases so far. However, a gain-of-function GATA2 mutation has been reported in one patient with chronic myelomonocytic leukemia[558] and loss-of-function GATA2 mutations have been systematically detected in patients with a rare genetic immunodeficiency distinguished by reduced levels of all the immune cells produced in the marrow (monocytes, dendritic, NK and B cells, MonoMAC syndrome)[559,560] (see Table 24-2). The marrow of these patients is hypocellular, with absent/reduced levels of multilymphoid and myeloid progenitor cells and dysplasia of the myeloid as well as the erythroid and megakaryocytic lineage. These patients may eventually develop MDS and AML. Mutations in the coding region of GATA2 have also been found in four patients with MDS without immunodeficiency.[561] In addition, quantitative alterations (reduced levels) in GATA2 expression, possibly secondary to the primary lesions, have been described in the $CD34^+$ cells from patients with aplastic anemia[562] and in blasts from AML,[563] and although hypomorphic GATA2 mutations do not induce a strong phenotype in mice,[561] genome-wide analyses of transcriptional reprogramming of mouse models of AML have identified GATA2 as one of the few key transcription factors whose expression is reduced in leukemic blasts.[563]

CELLULAR DYNAMICS IN ERYTHROPOIESIS

The primary function of the mature red cell, which is the end product of erythropoiesis, is to transport oxygen efficiently through the circulation to the tissues. To achieve this goal, the adult marrow must release approximately 3×10^9 new red cells, or reticulocytes, per kilogram per day.[564] This number of reticulocytes represents (1%) of the total red cell mass and is derived from an estimated 5×10^9 erythroid precursors per kilogram.[564] In addition to maintaining homeostasis (i.e., a stable hematocrit), the erythron must be able to respond quickly and appropriately to increased oxygen demands, either acute (e.g., following red cell loss) or chronic (e.g., with hypoxia from pulmonary disease or a right-to-left cardiac shunt). It is well established that EPO is responsible both for maintaining normal erythropoiesis and for increasing red cell production in response to oxygen needs. However, the overall marrow response is complex and requires not only the participation of erythroid cells responsive to EPO but also a structurally intact microenvironment and an optimal iron supply within the marrow.

EPO stimulation elicits two types of measurable responses: changes in proliferative activity (including improved survival) and changes in maturation rates. The first detectable response to increased serum EPO is amplification of CFU-E and erythroid precursors, cells that are extremely sensitive to EPO. Because virtually all these cells are already in cycle, increases in their numbers cannot be achieved by increasing their fraction in cycle. Either additional divisions are involved, or new cells are recruited to the CFU-E pool (from a pre-CFU-E pool). Additional divisions of CFU-E or precursor cells would increase their transit time within the marrow and potentially delay the delivery of new red cells to the periphery. Because a shortened maturation time has been observed instead and the proliferative potentials of CFU-E and proerythroblasts are finite, high levels of amplification cannot be achieved through this mechanism. Therefore such needs are met by influx into the CFU-E and precursor pools of newly differentiating cells from earlier progenitor compartments.

Such a surge of newly produced cells has been observed in prior experiments.[188,565,566] A rapid influx of fresh cells was particularly notable in polycythemic mice that were experimentally depleted of CFU-E and erythroid precursors at the time the stimulus was applied.[160,188] Because of the rapidity of response (i.e., within 24 hours in the polycythemic animals), it appeared that the orderly progression from BFU-E to CFU-E to proerythroblast had been compressed. Such acceleration of differentiation is possible through shortened intermitotic intervals, fewer mitotic divisions, or differentiation without divisions. This short-circuiting in differentiation requires high serum levels of EPO and adequate numbers of BFU-E (i.e., these conditions are met in a previously hypertransfused, polycythemic animal stimulated by EPO or in marrow suddenly recovering from acquired pure erythroid aplasia). Once CFU-E and precursors are expanded through this mechanism, most persisting erythropoietic demands can be met through this pool without excess input from pre-CFU-E pools. Thus acute demand for erythropoiesis is met by influx from pre-CFU-E pools through an accelerated differentiation and maturation sequence. In contrast, chronic demands (i.e., demands due to a chronic hemolytic anemia) are mainly satisfied through a greatly amplified late erythroid pool and with a minimum distortion in the differentiation sequence.[142,567] The fact that the kinetics of erythroid differentiation/maturation are different in acute versus chronic marrow regeneration is supported by differing qualitative changes in the newly formed red cells. An increase in i antigen and HbF expression as well as an increase in cells with higher mean corpuscular volumes is seen with an acute response, whereas these alterations are minimal or less pronounced with chronic responses.[142,568] When severe anemia persists from birth onward, erythroid production can increase up to 10-fold above baseline.[567] This is possible not only because of maximally expanded erythropoietic pools but also because the sites of active erythropoiesis may extend to include those that support red cell differentiation during fetal life. Thus although the marrow space in axial bones (vertebrae, pelvis, ribs, sternum, clavicles) is sufficient for normal erythropoiesis or for response to moderate anemia, the femur, humerus, spleen and/or liver, and (rarely) thymus may support red cell production in children with congenital hemolytic anemia (e.g., thalassemia major). Expanded erythropoiesis may lead to skeletal deformities, hepatosplenomegaly, or erythropoiesis in the soft tissues adjacent to bone.

Quantitative assessments of changes in erythroid progenitor cell pools in response to EPO stimulation can be made through cultures of bone marrow cells. Despite sampling errors, erythroid cultures can provide rough estimates of relative progenitor abundance within an aspirated marrow specimen and have shown consistent increases in the frequency of CFU-E in proportion to the level of EPO stimulation.[569,570] Conversely, with increases in the hematocrit or in polycythemic animals, a decrease in CFU-E frequency has been observed.[571,572] In contrast to CFU-E, the incidence of BFU-E was found to fluctuate less with either acute or chronic expansion of erythropoiesis, probably because a few BFU-E can generate several thousand cells. Furthermore, BFU-E can increase their fraction in cycle and thus increase the number of differentiated progeny without a significant change in their total numbers. Most BFU-E detectable in marrow or blood erythroid cultures probably represent a reservoir of progenitors not normally participating in day-to-day erythropoiesis. The parameters needed to maintain a healthy or appropriate BFU-E pool in hematopoiesis are not defined. That hematopoietic expansion is curtailed in mice with steel mutations and anemia develops in mice treated with anti–C-KIT antibody[573] suggests that adequate levels of normal KL may be crucial for early erythropoietic expansion.[189]

The rate of red cell production also can be accurately evaluated by ferrokinetic studies (i.e., study of iron incorporation into developing red cells). In addition, a marrow scan, typically with technetium Tc 99m, can document the extent of active erythropoiesis. However, these approaches seldom are necessary in clinical practice because estimates of erythropoiesis can be obtained from the reticulocyte index.[567] First, the observed percentage of reticulocytes is normalized to the hematocrit to calculate the total marrow output of reticulocytes. Alternatively, the absolute number of reticulocytes per microliter can be counted directly using fluorescent RNA labeling. However, because younger reticulocytes are prematurely released into the circulation under conditions of acute need, the total number of reticulocytes overestimates the true level of red cell production as measured by iron kinetics.[567] Therefore a second correction is made to account for the maturation of early circulating reticulocytes, or "shift" cells (polychromatophilic red cells), when present in the blood smear. The resulting reticulocyte index gives excellent estimates of effective red cell production.

Although the presence, density, or both of EPORs on developing erythroid cells determines the responses to EPO, other properties (e.g., surface antigens on BFU-E versus CFU-E versus end-stage red cells) may provide the basis for selective suppression of CFU-E versus BFU-E or selective immune destruction of red cells versus erythroblasts. For example, suppression of CFU-E or erythroblasts can occur in acquired pure red cell aplasia[574] or B19 parvovirus infection,[575] respectively, whereas BFU-E in both these conditions remain largely unperturbed. Thus the boundary from BFU-E to CFU-E and erythroblast may be biologically important for the pathophysiology of these disease states. Furthermore, in acquired hemolytic anemia, selective destruction at a given stage of maturation (of red cells only or of both erythroblasts and red cells) can be observed depending on the type of antibody produced and the density of its antigen on maturing erythroid cells. Qualitative aberrations in the response of erythroid progenitors to cytokines or EPO may underlie the abnormalities of congenital erythroid hypoplasia (Diamond-Blackfan syndrome).[361] Analogous qualitative or functional defects can be observed in neoplastic erythropoiesis, because erythroid progenitors from patients with polycythemia vera and other myeloproliferative neoplasms have altered sensitivities to EPO.[576]

Detailed knowledge of the structural and functional properties of erythroid cells throughout their differentiation may provide significant insights into the pathogenesis of hematopoietic disorders affecting the red cell lineage.

SUGGESTED READINGS

Abdel-Wahab O, Levine R: The spliceosome as an indicted conspirator in myeloid malignancies. *Cancer Cell* 20:420, 2011.

Agarwal N, Gordeuk RV, Prchal JT: Genetic mechanisms underlying regulation of hemoglobin mass. *Adv Exp Med Biol* 618:195, 2007.

Andrews NC: Closing the iron gate. *N Engl J Med* 366:376, 2012.

Anstee DJ: The relationship between blood groups and disease. *Blood* 115:4635, 2010.

Baron MH, Isern J, Fraser ST: The embryonic origins of erythropoiesis in mammals. *Blood* 2012.

Bianco P: Bone and the hematopoietic niche: A tale of two stem cells. *Blood* 117:5281, 2011.

Bieker JJ: Putting a finger on the switch. *Nat Genet* 42:733, 2010.

Bissels U, Bosio A, Wagner W: MicroRNAs are shaping the hematopoietic landscape. *Haematologica* 97:160, 2012.

Bowie MB, Kent DG, Copley MR, et al: Steel factor responsiveness regulates the high self-renewal phenotype of fetal hematopoietic stem cells. *Blood* 109:5043, 2007.

Bowman TV, Trompouki E, Zon LI: Linking hematopoietic regeneration to developmental signaling pathways: A story of BMP and Wnt. *Cell Cycle* 11:424, 2012.

Bresnick EH, Lee HY, Fujiwara T, et al: GATA switches as developmental drivers. *J Biol Chem* 285:31087, 2010.

Bunn HF: New agents that stimulate erythropoiesis. *Blood* 109:868, 2007.

Byon JC, Papayannopoulou T, MicroRNAs: Allies or foes in erythropoiesis? *J Cell Physiol* 227:7, 2012.

Choesmel V, Bacqueville D, Rouquette J, et al: Impaired ribosome biogenesis in Diamond-Blackfan anemia. *Blood* 109:1275, 2007.

Di Baldassarre A, Di Rico M, Di Noia A, et al: Protein kinase Cα is differentially activated during neonatal and adult erythropoiesis and favors expression of a reporter gene under the control of the Aγ globin-promoter in cellular models of hemoglobin switching. *J Cell Biochem* 101:411, 2007.

Dore LC, Crispino JD: Transcription factor networks in erythroid cell and megakaryocyte development. *Blood* 118:231, 2011.

Fabriek BO, Polfliet MM, Vloet RP, et al: The macrophage CD163 surface glycoprotein is an erythroblast adhesion receptor. *Blood* 109:5223, 2007.

Flygare J, Aspesi A, Bailey JC, et al: Human RPS19, the gene mutated in Diamond-Blackfan anemia, encodes a ribosomal protein required for the maturation of 40S ribosomal subunits. *Blood* 109:980, 2007.

Fraser ST, Isern J, Baron MH: Maturation and enucleation of primitive erythroblasts during mouse embryogenesis is accompanied by changes in cell-surface antigen expression. *Blood* 109:343, 2007.

Ghinassi B, Sanchez M, Martelli F, et al: The hypomorphic Gata1low mutation alters the proliferation/differentiation potential of the common megakaryocytic-erythroid progenitor. *Blood* 109:1460, 2007.

Hattangadi SM, Wong P, Zhang L, et al: From stem cell to red cell: Regulation of erythropoiesis at multiple levels by multiple proteins, RNAs, and chromatin modifications. *Blood* 118:6258, 2011.

Higgs DR, Engel JD, Stamatoyannopoulos G: Thalassaemia. *Lancet* 379:373, 2012.

Kaneko H, Shimizu R, Yamamoto M: GATA factor switching during erythroid differentiation. *Curr Opin Hematol* 17:163, 2010.

Kerenyi MA, Orkin SH: Networking erythropoiesis. *J Exp Med* 207:2537, 2010.

Lambert LA, Mitchell SL: Molecular evolution of the transferrin receptor/glutamate carboxypeptidase II family. *J Mol Evol* 64:113, 2007.

Liu J, Mohandas N, An X: Membrane assembly during erythropoiesis. *Curr Opin Hematol* 18:133, 2011.

Maetens M, Doumont G, Clercq SD, et al: Distinct roles of Mdm2 and Mdm4 in red cell production. *Blood* 109:2630, 2007.

Migliaccio AR, Whitsett C, Papayannopoulou T, et al: The potential of stem cells as an in vitro source of red blood cells for transfusion. *Cell Stem Cell* 10:115, 2012.

Mohandas N, Gallagher PG: Red cell membrane: Past, present, and future. *Blood* 112:3939, 2008.

Narla A, Ebert BL: Translational medicine: Ribosomopathies. *Blood* 118:4300, 2011.

Orru S, Aspesi A, Armiraglio M, et al: Analysis of the ribosomal protein S19 interactome. *Mol Cell Proteomics* 6:382, 2007.

Palis J: Ontogeny of erythropoiesis. *Curr Opin Hematol* 15:155, 2008.

Phillips JD, Steensma DP, Pulsipher MA, et al: Congenital erythropoietic porphyria due to a mutation in GATA1: The first trans-acting mutation causative for a human porphyria. *Blood* 109:2618, 2007.

Ribeil JA, Zermati Y, Vandekerckhove J, et al: Hsp70 regulates erythropoiesis by preventing caspase-3-mediated cleavage of GATA-1. *Nature* 445:102, 2007.

Roy CN, Mak HH, Akpan I, et al: Hepcidin antimicrobial peptide transgenic mice exhibit features of the anemia of inflammation. *Blood* 109:4038, 2007.

Scott LM, Tong W, Levine RL, et al: JAK2 exon 12 mutations in polycythemia vera and idiopathic erythrocytosis. *N Engl J Med* 356:459, 2007.

Siatecka M, Bieker JJ: The multifunctional role of EKLF/KLF1 during erythropoiesis. *Blood* 118:2044, 2011.

Tober J, Koniski A, McGrath KE, et al: The megakaryocyte lineage originates from hemangioblast precursors and is an integral component both of primitive and of definitive hematopoiesis. *Blood* 109:1433, 2007.

Tubman VN, Levine JE, Campagna DR, et al: X-linked gray platelet syndrome due to a GATA1 Arg216Gln mutation. *Blood* 109:3297, 2007.

Wallace DF, Summerville L, Subramaniam VN: Targeted disruption of the hepatic transferrin receptor 2 gene in mice leads to iron overload. *Gastroenterology* 132:301, 2007.

Wilber A, Nienhuis AW, Persons DA: Transcriptional regulation of fetal to adult hemoglobin switching: New therapeutic opportunities. *Blood* 117:3945, 2011.

Zambidis ET, Sinka L, Tavian M, et al: Emergence of human angiohematopoietic cells in normal development and from cultured embryonic stem cells. *Ann N Y Acad Sci* 1106:223, 2007.

For complete list of references log on to www.expertconsult.com.

CHAPTER 25

GRANULOCYTOPOIESIS AND MONOCYTOPOIESIS

Arati Khanna-Gupta and Nancy Berliner

GRANULOCYTOPOIESIS

Granulocytes (neutrophils, eosinophils, and basophils) are short-lived cells that are critical to both antimicrobial and inflammatory responses. The bone marrow (BM) produces granulocytes, especially neutrophils, at a prodigious rate to supply the baseline needs of circulating cells that survive in the peripheral blood for only 3 to 6 hours. It also has the capacity to upregulate granulocyte production sharply in response to a wide range of stresses. The regulation of granulocyte production is controlled by a variety of cytokines that induce the myeloid differentiation program through the carefully orchestrated interaction of multiple general and myeloid-specific transcription factors. Understanding this intricate maturation sequence provides important insights into normal neutrophil responses to infectious, inflammatory, and allergic stresses, as well as into the dysregulation of differentiation contributing to the origins of myelodysplasia and leukemia.

Granulocyte Ontogeny

Stages of Neutrophil Differentiation

Granulocytes differentiate from early progenitor cells in the BM in a process that takes 7 to 10 days. The cells pass through several identifiable maturational stages, during which they acquire the morphologic appearance and granule contents that characterize the mature granulocyte.[1] The earliest identifiable granulocyte precursor is the myeloblast, a minimally granulated cell with scant cytoplasm and a prominent nucleolus (Fig. 25-1). Transition to the promyelocyte stage is associated with the acquisition of abundant primary granules. Primary granules are found in both granulocytes and monocytes and contain many of the proteins necessary for intracellular killing of microbes. The transition to the myelocyte stage is associated with the acquisition of secondary or "specific" granules, which give the characteristic staining that differentiates neutrophils from eosinophils and basophils.

Neutrophil precursors account for approximately half of the cells in the marrow of normal persons, with a majority at the metamyelocyte stage and more differentiated forms. Promyelocytes and myelocytes represent the primary proliferative pool of granulocyte precursors in the BM. Beyond the myelocyte stage, cells mature as nondividing cells. Bands and segmented neutrophils constitute greater than 50% of the total granulocyte mass, primarily as a mobilizable pool of cells in the BM. Only 5% of total neutrophils circulate in the periphery, where 60% are marginated in the spleen and on vessel walls. Mature neutrophils circulate in the peripheral blood for 3 to 12 hours and then migrate to the tissues, where they survive 2 to 3 days. Hence, the peripheral blood count reflects roughly 2% of the total neutrophil cell mass spanning approximately 1% of the neutrophil lifespan.

Biochemical events that accompany these physical changes include the sequential acquisition of primary granules and their content proteins (e.g., myeloperoxidase, lysozyme, neutrophil elastase [NE, also known as ELANE], defensins, myeloblastin), secondary granules and their content proteins (lactoferrin, neutrophil collagenase matrix metalloproteinase 8 or MMP-8), neutrophil gelatinase [MMP-9], neutrophil gelatinase-associated lipocalin [NGAL], transcobalamin 1), and tertiary granules containing neutrophil gelatinase (Table 25-1). The progressive gain of characteristics of differentiated cells is accompanied by a loss of proliferative potential. This carefully coordinated process is disrupted in acute myeloid leukemias (AMLs), in which a block in the myeloid maturation pathway usually results in the circulation of immature blasts in the peripheral blood.

Markers of Granulocytic Maturation

Stem cells have been characterized primarily by their marrow-repopulating potential, as outlined in Chapters 4. Early granulocytic progenitors form hematopoietic colonies in vitro and their more differentiated progeny express specific cell surface proteins that are critically important to myeloid differentiation and function. They mediate both the adhesion of precursors within the marrow and the vascular adhesion of mature neutrophils that is critical to normal neutrophil activation. Other proteins serve as receptors that recognize pathogens or as stimulatory peptides that facilitate activation of phagocytosis and killing of organisms. Appropriate expression of these surface proteins plays an important role in normal neutrophil function, and abnormalities of their expression are implicated in a wide range of diseases affecting the neutrophil compartment. For example, congenital abnormalities in the surface expression of integrin proteins are responsible for failure of neutrophil adhesion in leukocyte adhesion deficiency, and acquired abnormalities of expression of the same proteins are hypothesized to underlie the abnormal peripheral circulation of immature precursors in myeloproliferative disease.[2] These markers also serve to help distinguish among the stages of myeloid commitment and maturation.

The phenotype of the early hematopoietic stem cells is $CD34^+/CD33^-$, with absence of lineage-specific markers. The common myeloid progenitor, colony-forming unit granulocyte, erythrocyte, macrophage, megakaryocyte (CFU-GEMM), is characterized by the coexpression of CD33 and CD34. CD33 is expressed at high levels on committed myeloid progenitors and on early precursors of both the granulocytic and monocytic lineages. Expression of CD33 wanes with granulocytic maturation, and it is absent or nearly absent beyond the myelocyte stage. CD33 is a member of the sialic acid-binding immunoglobulin (Ig)-like lectins (siglecs), which generally mediate cell–cell interactions and cell signaling. The precise biologic function of CD33 remains unknown.

Characteristic granulocyte markers acquired as the early myeloid progenitor cells become committed to the neutrophil lineage include CD45RA, myeloperoxidase (MPO), and CD38, all of which are expressed on the myeloblast. Further differentiation beyond the myelocyte stage is associated with acquisition of increased expression of CD16, CD11b/CD18 (Mac-1), and leukocyte alkaline phosphatase (LAP), all of which are expressed at high levels in mature neutrophils.

Neutrophil Granules and Their Content Proteins

The acquisition of granules and their content proteins is a critical part of the developmental program of granulocytes.[3] Acquired at specific identifiable stages of neutrophil maturation, these

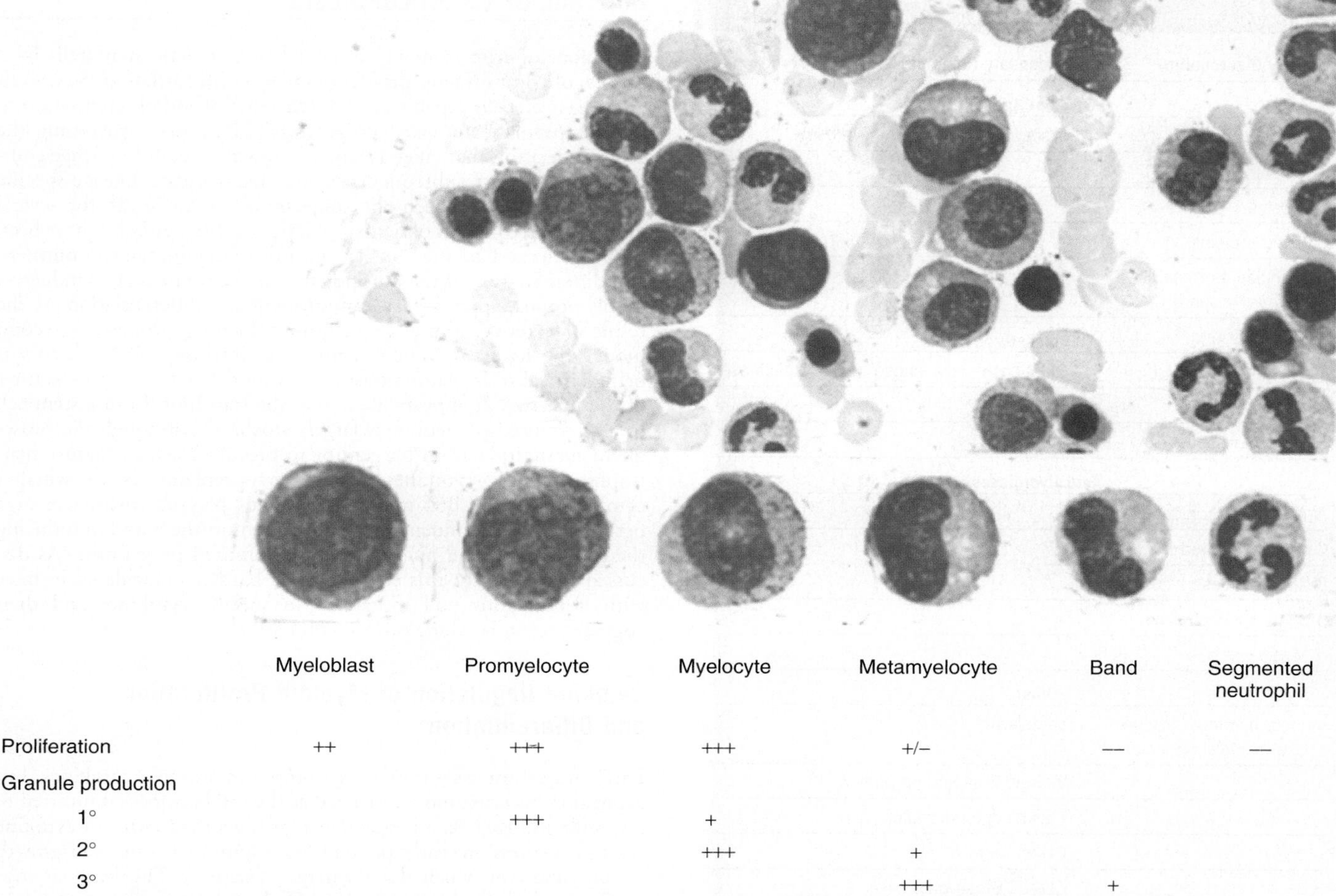

	Myeloblast	Promyelocyte	Myelocyte	Metamyelocyte	Band	Segmented neutrophil
Proliferation	++	+++	+++	+/–	—	—
Granule production						
1°		+++	+			
2°			+++	+		
3°				+++	+	

Figure 25-1 NEUTROPHIL MATURATION. Neutrophil maturation stages with associated acquisition of stage-specific granules.

intracellular and secretory organelles contain many of the requisite enzymes that mediate the oxidative and nonoxidative killing functions of neutrophils (see Table 25-1).

Primary (azurophilic) granules are acquired at the promyelocyte stage and contain a wide array of proteins, including myeloperoxidase, defensins, cathepsins, and ELANE. Secondary granules are secretory granules acquired at the transition to the myelocyte stage. Neutrophil secondary granules contain lactoferrin, the vitamin B_{12}–binding protein transcobalamin I, and the MMPs (neutrophil collagenase and gelatinase), as well as NGAL. With the exception of gelatinase, which is also expressed by monocytes, expression of the secondary granule proteins is restricted to neutrophils. Secondary granules and the synthesis of their contents therefore constitute a definitive marker of commitment to terminal neutrophil maturation. Furthermore, characteristic secondary granules are acquired at the same stage by eosinophils and basophils. Tertiary granules, containing primarily gelatinase, are formed during later stages of neutrophil maturation. Secretory vesicles are formed by endocytosis and contain plasma proteins.[4]

On stimulation, the neutrophil first mobilizes secretory vesicles, which contribute their membrane proteins, including abundant integrin receptors, to the plasma membrane. They may thus increase cellular adhesion by upregulating surface integrin expression in response to selectin stimulation or inflammatory mediators. Primary granules fuse with the phagosome and contribute to bacterial killing. Secondary and tertiary granules have a complex function. They are secretory granules, releasing the matrix-modifying MMPs collagenase (MMP-8) and gelatinase (MMP-9) into the extracellular milieu, enhancing neutrophil penetration into sites of inflammation. The function of lactoferrin and transcobalamin I remains poorly defined, but they are hypothesized to contribute to the antimicrobial response by sequestering iron and cobalamin, respectively, away from infecting organisms. Secretion also results in the contribution of membrane proteins to the plasma membrane and is the source of the prominent upregulation of surface integrin receptor Mac-1 (CD11b/CD18) expression that occurs on neutrophil activation. Finally, they also fuse intracellularly with the phagosome to help promote bactericidal activity.

The fusion of azurophilic and peroxidase-negative granules allows for cross-exposure to their contents within the phagosome. These proteins are carefully sequestered in separate organelles, preventing premature activation and damage to the resting neutrophil; on fusion, the contents of the two granule subtypes cooperate in generating the antimicrobial response. Hydrogen peroxide, a byproduct of nicotinamide adenine dinucleotide phosphate (NADPH) oxidase in the secondary granule, in combination with MPO from the primary granules, produces hypochlorous acid, a highly toxic microbicidal agent. Additionally, both neutrophil gelatinase (MMP-9) and neutrophil collagenase (MMP-8) (secondary granule proteins) are produced as zymogens and are converted to their active forms by the action of ELANE released from the primary granules.

Current evidence largely supports the hypothesis that the content of neutrophil granules is determined primarily by the timing of synthesis of their respective content proteins. Studies have demonstrated that each distinct granule population is generated not by a sophisticated protein sorting mechanism but rather by a highly regulated transcriptional process that results in sequential gene expression. For example, because myeloperoxidase and the other primary granule proteins are expressed between the promyelocyte and the myelocyte stages of neutrophil development, they are packaged into the primary granules. Secondary granule proteins such as lactoferrin, on the other hand, are expressed between the myelocyte and the metamyelocyte

Table 25-1 Neutrophil Granules: Major Classes and Contents

Primary (Azurophilic)	Secondary (Specific)	Tertiary
Microbial Agents		
Lysozyme	Lysozyme	
Myeloperoxidase		
Defensins		
Cationic proteins		
Bactericidal permeability–increasing agent		
Proteases		
Elastase	Gelatinase, collagenase	Gelatinase
Cathepsin G		
Other proteases		
Acid Hydrolases		
N-Acetylglucuronidase		
Cathepsins B and D		
β-Glucuronidase		
β-Glycerophosphatase		
α-Mannosidase		
Other		
Kinin-generating enzyme C5a-inactivating factor	Lactoferrin	
	Vitamin B_{12}–binding protein	
	Plasminogen activator	
	Cytochrome *b**	
	CD11/1B complex*	
	Formyl peptide receptor*	
	Histaminase*	
	NGAL	

Adapted from Boxer LA, Smolen JE: Neutrophil granule constituents and their release in health and disease. *Hematol Oncol Clin North Am* 2:101, 1988.
NGAL, Neutrophil gelatinase-associated lipocalin.
*These granule constituents are conventionally assigned to the secondary granule, but their exact compartment remains controversial. Some may be located in the tertiary granule or possibly in one of the other, heterogeneous small-granule populations.

stages and are hence packaged into the secondary granules. Overexpression of the secondary granule protein NGAL in HL60 cells, a leukemic cell line that is arrested at the myeloblast stage of differentiation, resulted in its incorporation into primary granules, lending empirical support to the concept that gene expression and protein sorting into granules are coordinate events. This hypothesis may, however, be a somewhat oversimplified view of granule protein sorting because there is some overlap of expression between certain primary and secondary granule protein genes. Whereas secondary granule protein gene transcription appears to be coordinately regulated, the sequence of primary granule protein gene expression is much less synchronous. The defensins are expressed later than the other primary granule proteins, and defensin transcription appears to be regulated by the same transcriptional regulatory pathway as the secondary granule proteins gelatinase (MMP-9) and lactoferrin.[5] Indeed, the defensins are the only primary granule proteins that are absent in patients with neutrophil-specific granule deficiency (SGD). This suggests that the presence of defensin would be targeted to the secondary granule.[6] Consequently, how defensins are directed exclusively to the primary granule remains unclear.

CONTROL OF GRANULOPOIESIS

Granulocytes arise from pluripotent hematopoietic stem cells by a process of commitment, proliferation, and differentiation. Stem cells are long-lived cells capable of both self-renewal and differentiation to lineage-specific–committed progenitors. The process governing the cell fate decision that takes a stem cell down the path to lineage commitment and the subsequent factors that regulate lineage-specific differentiation have been the subjects of intense study for several decades. Three models of hematopoietic cell differentiation have been proposed to address the mechanism underlying lineage commitment and differentiation of the pluripotent stem cell. The first or inductive model proposes that lineage commitment and differentiation are the result of external stimuli (e.g., growth factors, stroma). A second model, the stochastic model, emphasizes intrinsic cellular factors as being critical to hematopoiesis; a third model combines the features of the first two. It appears likely that the transition from a stem cell to a committed progenitor is largely stochastic, although the subsequent maturation from progenitor to precursor cell to mature neutrophil requires cytokines. Controversy remains as to whether cytokines and the BM microenvironment play an instructive or a permissive role in influencing stem cell commitment and in inducing the proliferation and maturation of committed progenitors. As discussed subsequently, this complex issue has been elucidated in mice with homologous null mutations in specific cytokines and their cognate receptors, alone or in combination.

Cytokine Regulation of Myeloid Proliferation and Differentiation

Early progenitor cells express receptors for multiple cytokines, but expression becomes more restricted as the cell becomes committed to a specific lineage.[7] As a consequence of this broad range of cytokine receptor expression, early progenitors respond to combined growth factors, many of which show synergy of activity. The “early-acting” cytokines include the interleukins IL-1 and IL-6; stem cell factor (SCF); FLT3 ligand; and several others, including granulocyte colony-stimulating factor (G-CSF). IL-3 is important in directing the pluripotent stem cell toward the myelomonocytic lineage, giving rise to the mixed myeloid progenitor (CFU-GEMM). Subsequent stages leading to commitment- and lineage-restricted differentiation are governed by more “late-acting” cytokines (Fig. 25-2).

The major cytokines mediating neutrophil maturation are G-CSF and granulocyte macrophage colony-stimulating factor (GM-CSF). G-CSF not only supports the survival and proliferation of developing myeloid cells at all stages of differentiation but also increases the functional activity of mature neutrophils. Although the major role of G-CSF is thought to be the induction of neutrophil proliferation and differentiation, the G-CSF receptor (G-CSFR) is expressed on a wide range of cell types. In addition to myeloid progenitors and precursors at all stages of neutrophil differentiation, G-CSFR is expressed on platelets; monocytes; lymphocytes; and several nonhematopoietic cells, including endothelial cells and placenta. The role of G-CSF as both an early- and late-acting cytokine is underscored by the successful use of G-CSF to mobilize early progenitors into the peripheral blood for stem cell collection and to speed neutrophil recovery after chemotherapy.

The G-CSFR is a member of the cytokine receptor superfamily that signals through activation of the JAK–STAT (Janus kinase signal transducer and activator of transcription) pathway and the Ras pathway. Ligand binding induces homodimerization of the receptor, leading to a cascade of downstream phosphorylation events. Dimerization leads to phosphorylation of associated JAK kinases that in turn phosphorylate STAT1 and STAT3. In addition, the activated G-CSFR also phosphorylates mediators of the Ras–mitogen-activated protein (MAP) kinase pathway by tyrosine phosphorylation of Shc.[8]

The importance of G-CSF in myeloid proliferation and differentiation has been studied in G-CSF–null and G-CSFR–null mice. Mice lacking G-CSF or G-CSFR had markedly decreased myeloid

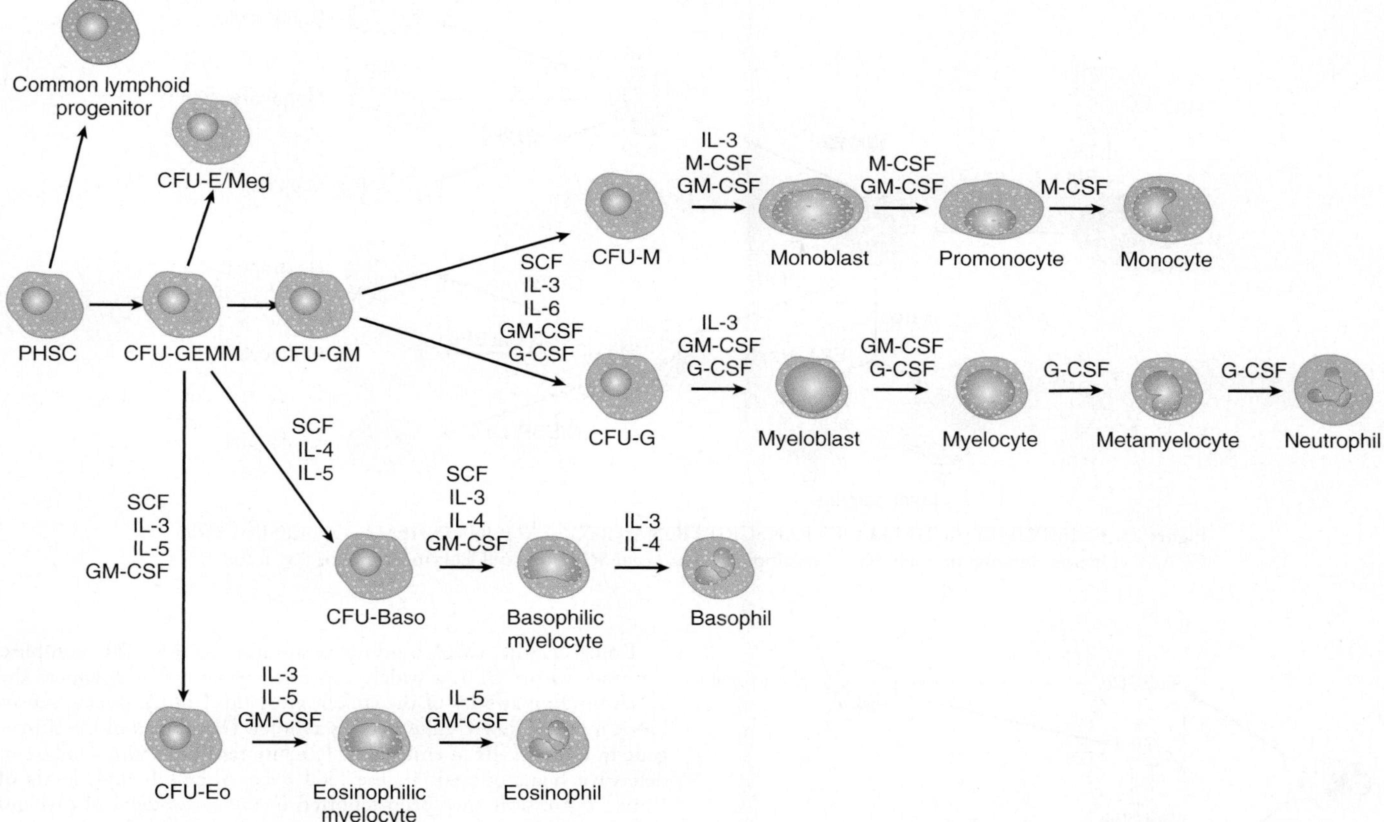

Figure 25-2 CYTOKINE REGULATION OF GRANULOCYTIC PROGENITORS. *CFU-Baso,* Colony-forming unit-basophil; *CFU-E/Meg,* colony-forming unit-erythrocyte/megakaryocyte; *CFU-Eo,* colony-forming unit-eosinophil; *CFU-G,* colony-forming unit-granulocyte; *CFU-GEMM,* colony-forming unit-granulocyte, erythrocyte, macrophage, megakaryocyte; *CFU-GM,* colony-forming unit-granulocyte macrophage; *CFU-M,* colony-forming unit-macrophage; *G-CSF,* granulocyte colony-stimulating factor; *GM-CSF,* granulocyte macrophage colony-stimulating factor; *IL,* interleukin; *M-CSF,* monocyte colony-stimulating factor; *PHSC,* pluripotent hematopoietic stem cell; *SCF,* stem cell factor.

progenitors and impaired neutrophil production, with low circulating neutrophil counts. In addition, G-CSF–null mice had impaired neutrophil mobilization, and mature neutrophils from G-CSFR–null mice had increased susceptibility to apoptosis, supporting the role of the G-CSF pathway in sustaining the mobilization, survival, and function of mature neutrophils as well. However, despite all of these profound abnormalities, G-CSF/G-CSFR knock-out mice continue to make some neutrophils, suggesting that alternative overlapping cytokine pathways support granulocyte development.

GM-CSF also induces proliferation and differentiation of myeloid precursors. The GM-CSFR is a heterodimeric protein composed of an α- and a β-subunit. The α-subunit binds GM-CSF. The β-subunit is shared by the GM-CSFR and the receptors for IL-3, IL-5, and IL-6. The β-subunit does not bind ligand but is necessary for the high-affinity ligand binding to the αβ-heterodimer of each receptor. Signaling through the GM-CSFR also depends on the JAK–STAT pathway, signaling through JAK2, and serves to activate the Ras–MAP kinase pathway. Of interest, however, the GM-CSF–null mouse lacks any defect in hematopoiesis. Mice with null mutations in both G-CSF and GM-CSF had more profound neutropenia in the perinatal period but the same levels of neutrophils in adulthood as those mice solely lacking G-CSF only.

Transcriptional Regulation of Myeloid Differentiation

Lineage-specific maturation of committed hematopoietic progenitor cells is ultimately driven by transcription factors, which have been hypothesized to be the final common pathway leading to commitment and differentiation of the pluripotent stem cell.[9] The role of transcription factors in cellular proliferation, differentiation, and survival of stem cells during hematopoiesis in the mammalian BM has been well established. Studies of the regulation of individual genes that show tissue- and stage-specific myeloid expression have implicated a small number of transcription factors that are responsible for directing both phenotypical myeloid maturation and the expression of functionally important myeloid genes. As described in detail subsequently, this role is underscored by the observations in AML, in which disruption of differentiation and defective myeloid-specific gene expression are linked to pathognomonic chromosomal translocations that result in the dysregulation of transcription factor expression.

Maturation of multipotent progenitor stem cells into specialized blood cells (lymphocytes, erythrocytes, neutrophils, monocytes, and eosinophils, among others) is regulated by a well-orchestrated interplay of transcription factors that are capable of instructing the expression of a specific set of genes within a specific lineage. Gene knock-out technology and overexpression studies, in conjunction with newer techniques that involve the use of multicolor fluorescence-activated cell sorting (FACS), have aided in delineating several transcription factors critical to the development of specific hematopoietic lineages. On the basis of these studies, critical transcription factors have been classified into two major categories. The first category includes factors such as stem cell leukemia transcription factor (SCL), GATA2, and AML factor-1 (AML-1) now known as Runx1, that influence differentiation to all of the hematopoietic lineages; the second category comprises the master regulators of lineage development, including GATA1, PU.1, and CCAAT enhancer–binding protein-α (C/EBPα).

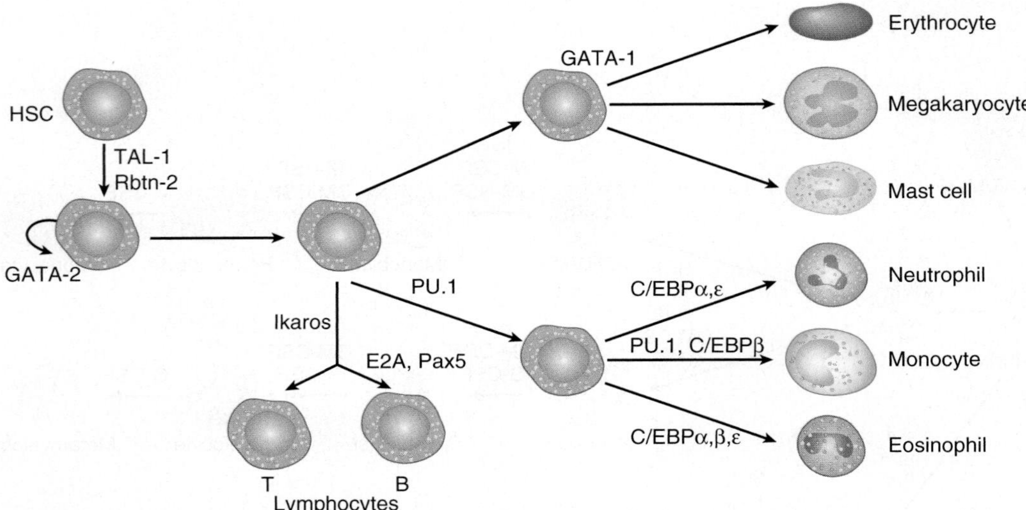

Figure 25-3 SIMPLIFIED SCHEMA OF TRANSCRIPTIONAL REGULATION OF HEMATOPOIESIS. *C/EBP,* CCAAT enhancer–binding protein; *HSC,* hematopoietic stem cell; *SCL,* stem cell leukemia transcription factor.

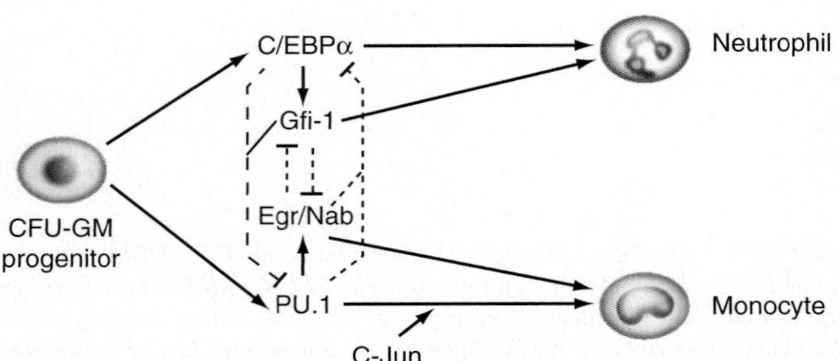

Figure 25-4 TRANSCRIPTION FACTOR CROSS-TALK AFFECTING NEUTROPHIL AND MONOCYTE DEVELOPMENT.

These factors not only promote lineage-specific gene expression but also suppress alternative lineage pathways. Fig. 25-3 summarizes the postulated role of several key transcription factors during hematopoietic development. Myeloid progenitors exhibit multilineage patterns of gene expression. Studies by Laslo et al[10] elegantly demonstrated that cell fate determination is dependent on subtle changes in expression levels of transcription factors, which regulate differential lineage maturation. For example, levels of PU.1 expression are increased by Egr-1/Nab-2 in developing macrophages; at the same time, Egr-1 represses the expression of the neutrophil specific Gfi-1 transcription factor, thereby simultaneously repressing the neutrophil development program (Fig. 25-4).

Transcription Factors Regulating Myeloid Differentiation and Myeloid-Specific Gene Expression

Runx1

Runx1 (AML-1) belongs to a family of highly conserved transcription factors that harbors a 128-amino-acid motif referred to as the *Runt domain.* The Runt domain functions in DNA binding, protein–protein interaction, and adenosine triphosphate binding and contributes to nuclear localization.[11] This family of transcription factors, also known as the core binding factor (CBF) family, has been implicated in specification of cell fate and has a role in myeloid differentiation and lineage-specific granulocytic function.

Runx1 is the DNA-binding α-subunit of the CBF complex. Together with CBFβ, a widely expressed protein that enhances the DNA-binding affinity of the α-subunit, Runx1 binds the consensus DNA motif 5′ Pu ACCPuCA 3′ as a dimer. Disruption of the Runx1 gene in mice results in embryonic lethality resulting from a failure of definitive hematopoiesis in the fetal liver. Although high levels of Runx1 expression have been reported in the early stages of myeloid differentiation, its expression levels decrease beyond the promyelocytic stage of differentiation. In concordance with its pattern of expression, Runx1 has been implicated in regulating a number of genes expressed early in the myeloid development pathway, including GM-CSF, macrophage colony-stimulating factor (M-CSF) receptor, myeloperoxidase, ELANE, and IL-3, among others. In addition to activating lineage-specific myeloid markers, Runx1 has been shown to stimulate the G1 to S transition in myeloid and lymphoid cell lines.

A significant percentage (10%-20%) of human leukemias have been found to be associated with mutations in the Runx1 gene. Most common of these is the t(8;21) translocation, which results in the Runx1-ETO (8, 21 oncoprotein) fusion protein. In Runx1-ETO, the Runt domain of Runx1 is fused in frame with the ETO transcriptional corepressor. The fusion protein has been hypothesized to function predominantly as a repressor that inhibits expression of genes that are normally activated by Runx1. For example, the tumor suppressor gene p14/p19(ARF), a critical Runx1 target gene that is necessary for the activation of p53 function, is normally activated by Runx1 but is repressed by Runx1-ETO. The mechanisms underlying Runx1 function through its target genes are not yet fully understood. Studies in sea urchins, however, have suggested that AML-1 regulates genes that contribute to chromatin architecture during cell proliferation. It has also been shown that Runx1 functions within a narrow window during development by assisting in the opening of chromatin associated with genes that are vital to hematopoietic development and for the formation of transcription factor complexes on these genes.[12]

Studies involving mouse knock-in models of Runx1-ETO expression have indicated that the fusion protein alone is not sufficient to cause leukemia. These animals are more susceptible to mutagen-induced AML, however, suggesting that Runx1-ETO is part of a multistep process that contributes to leukemogenesis. Although the fusion partner of Runx1 (e.g., ETO) may contribute to the role of the Runx1 fusion protein in leukemogenesis, the primary cause of the disease is thought to be the dysregulation of Runx1-specific target genes that are directly dependent on the Runt domain of Runx1.

CCAAT Enhancer–Binding Protein Family of Transcription Factors

CCAAT enhancer–binding proteins (C/EBPs) are a family of basic region-leucine zipper (b-ZIP) transcription factors that recognize the consensus DNA-binding sequence 5′TKN NGYAAK3′ (Y = C or T; K = T or G) within the regulatory regions of target genes. C/EBP family proteins have been shown to bind DNA as either homo- or heterodimers. This family of transcription factors, which plays a crucial role in hematopoiesis, includes C/EBPα,-β,-γ, -δ,-ε, and -ζ (CHOP-GADD 153), all of which contain highly homologous carboxyl-terminal (C-terminal) dimerization (leucine zipper) domains and DNA-binding (basic region) motifs but differ in their amino-terminal (N-terminal) transactivation domains, with the exception of CHOP-GADD 153, which lacks this domain altogether.[9] Of interest, CHOP-GADD 153 can dimerize with and inhibit transactivation by C/EBPα,-β, and -ε and is found at a breakpoint in liposarcomas resulting in the TLS-CHOP fusion protein.

With the exception of C/EBPε, which is expressed exclusively in the late stages of granulopoiesis and in T lymphocytes, the other C/EBP members are expressed in a wide variety of cells, including liver, adipose tissue, lung, intestine, adrenal gland, and peripheral blood mononuclear cells and placenta. Both C/EBPβ and C/EBPδ are expressed at high levels in late-stage granulocytes. The C/EBP family members are known to exert pleiotropic effects in the tissues in which they are expressed. This may be because of their tissue- and stage-specific expression, their ability to dimerize with members of their own family and of the Fos/Jun and ATF/CREB families of transcription factors, and their ability to interact with other transcription factors such as nuclear factor-κB (NF-κB) and specificity protein-1 (Sp-1).

The C/EBP factors have been implicated in regulating the differentiation of a variety of tissues. C/EBPα plays a role in adipocyte differentiation: Inhibition of C/EBPα blocks adipocyte differentiation, and overexpression of C/EBPα induces adipocyte differentiation. Regulation of constitutive hepatic genes as well as acute-phase response genes in the liver involves several C/EBP family members, particularly C/EBPα. Modulation of myelomonocytic differentiation is also attributed to the activity of C/EBP family members. The importance of this family of transcription factors in myeloid differentiation has been demonstrated by the study of hematopoietic abnormalities observed in mice with targeted disruption of C/EBPα, -β, and -ε.

C/EBPα

C/EBPα has been postulated to be a master regulator of the granulocytic developmental program. It is expressed at high levels throughout myeloid differentiation and has been shown to bind to the promoters of multiple myeloid-specific gene promoters regulating gene expression at many different stages of myeloid maturation. Although C/EBPα$^{-/-}$ mice die perinatally because of defects in gluconeogenesis that result in fatal hypoglycemia, they also have a selective early block in the differentiation of granulocytes without affecting either monocyte/macrophage maturation or the differentiation of other hematopoietic lineages. Myeloid cells from C/EBPα$^{-/-}$ mice lack the G-CSFR, and it has been postulated that lack of mature neutrophils in these mice may be caused by the lack of G-CSFR. However, the myeloid defect in C/EBPα$^{-/-}$ mice is more severe than that seen in G-CSFR$^{-/-}$ mice, suggesting that C/EBPα has additional functions vital to granulocytic maturation.

C/EBPα is a single exon gene, but it is expressed as two isoforms that arise from alternate translation start sites that give rise to a full-length C/EBPαp42 and a truncated dominant negative C/EBPαp30 isoform.[13] Translational control of C/EBPα isoform expression is orchestrated by a conserved upstream open reading frame (uORF) in the 5′ untranslated region (5′UTR). This region is thought to be responsive to the activities of the translation initiation factors eIF4E and eIF2[14] such that an increase of eIF2 or eIF4E activity results in an increase in expression of the shorter p30 isoform.[13]

Several groups have reported mutations in the C/EBPα gene in a subset of patients (~10%) with AML presenting with a normal karyotype.[15] These mutations can be broadly classified into two main categories. The first includes in-frame mutations clustered in the highly conserved C-terminus of the C/EBPα protein. The second category involves frame-shift mutations at the N-terminus of C/EBPα, resulting in the premature termination of the full length C/EBPαp42 isoform while keeping the truncated C/EBPα p30 protein intact.[16] The remaining C/EBPαp42 is thought to be rendered inactive by the dominant-negative activity of the p30 isoform by an unknown mechanism. Additionally, a recent study has shown that mice homozygously expressing p30 C/EBPα from the *C/EBPα* locus develop AML with complete penetrance.[17] Thus, changes in the expression ratio of the two C/EBPα isoforms play a role in cell fate.[15,18]

The expression of C/EBPα is associated with growth arrest and differentiation of granulocyte precursor cells. This block in proliferation is thought to occur via the interaction of C/EBPα with the cyclin-dependent protein kinases cdk2 and cdk4, resulting in a block in cell proliferation by inhibiting these cell cycle kinases. In addition, C/EBPα inhibits E2F-dependent transcription, which in turn contributes to inhibition of cell proliferation and induction of differentiation associated with C/EBPα-induced granulopoiesis.

C/EBPβ

Expression of C/EBPβ increases during myeloid maturation and has been shown to be important for monocyte/macrophage gene expression and development. Mice lacking the C/EBPβ gene demonstrate decreased B-cell levels and defects in macrophage activation and function and are more prone to microbial infections. The C/EBPβ knock-out studies reveal that this transcription factor is not essential for myeloid development per se, but knock-in of C/EBPβ into the C/EBPα locus of C/EBPα$^{-/-}$ mice rescues granulopoiesis. Several monocyte/macrophage-specific genes are activated by C/EBPβ, including the G-CSF receptor, lysozyme, CD11c, monocyte chemoattractant protein-1 (MCP-1), IL-6, IL-8, and nitric oxide synthase, among others. Similar to C/EBPα, multiple isoforms of C/EBPβ are generated from a single transcript through the use of three translation initiation sites and a leaky ribosome scanning mechanism. The shortest of these isoforms, initiated at the most 3′ AUG, results in the formation of liver-enriched inhibitory protein (LIP), which lacks the N-terminal activation domain present in full-length C/EBPβ and has been implicated as a negative regulator of C/EBPβ function. It has been suggested that the ratio of C/EBPβ to LIP may affect cellular proliferation and differentiation. The activity of C/EBPβ is regulated posttranscriptionally through protein–protein interactions and covalent modifications. For example, in early myeloid progenitor cells, C/EBPβ is found in an unphosphorylated state in the cytoplasm. However, on differentiation, C/EBPβ becomes phosphorylated and translocates to the nucleus.[19]

C/EBPγ

C/EBPγ is a ubiquitously expressed C/EBP family member that was first identified by its affinity for *cis*-regulatory sites in the Ig heavy chain promoter and enhancer. C/EBPγ contains a C/EBP-like b-Zip domain but lacks an N-terminal transactivation domain and can inhibit transcriptional activation of other C/EBP members in some cell types. Impairment of natural killer cytotoxic activity and of interferon-γ production has been reported in C/EBPγ$^{-/-}$ mice.

C/EBPδ

C/EBPδ is expressed at low or undetectable levels in several tissues of adult mice and humans. Expression has been shown to dramatically increase on induction with bacterial lipopolysaccharide (LPS) and inflammatory cytokines, suggesting a role for C/EBPδ in acute-phase and inflammatory response. Double-knock-out experiments using C/EBPβ and C/EBPδ suggest a synergistic role for these two

C/EBP family members in controlling terminal adipocyte differentiation. Of interest, both C/EBPβ and C/EBPδ are expressed during late neutrophil development and have been postulated to play roles in late neutrophil gene expression.

C/EBPε

CCAAT enhancer-binding protein ε (C/EBPε) is the most recently described C/EBP protein. The human C/EBPε gene resides on chromosome 14 and is transcribed by two alternative promoters, Pα (thought to function in mature neutrophils) and Pβ (thought to function in BM). A combination of differential splicing and alternate promoter usage results in four messenger RNA (mRNA) isoforms 2.6 kilobases and 1.3 to 1.5 kilobases in size, from which three proteins of 32.2 kd, 27.8 kd, and 14.3 kd have been described. C/EBPε$^{-/-}$ mice produce hyposegmented granulocytes that are functionally defective. Late in life, these mice develop myelodysplasia. Absence of C/EBPε is thought to block the later steps in terminal differentiation of mature segmented granulocytes. Mutant mice usually survive 2 to 5 months and eventually succumb to low-pathogenicity bacterial infections. C/EBPε thus plays a crucial role in terminal granulocytic differentiation.

C/EBPε$^{-/-}$ mice have wild-type levels of the G-CSF receptor, and the defects manifested in these mice are confined to late-stage gene expression associated with the function of the mature neutrophil. Recently, it has been demonstrated that the ability of G-CSF to regulate myeloid differentiation is dependent on the induction of C/EBPε. The mRNA of several genes, including p47 phox (a component of the neutrophil NADPH oxidase complex), as well as the secondary granule protein (SGP) genes, are either absent or abnormal in the BM of C/EBPε$^{-/-}$ mice. C/EBPε is suggested to play a critical role in the regulation of host antimicrobial defense.

Neutrophils from C/EBPε$^{-/-}$ mice have morphologic and biochemical features very similar to those observed in patients with neutrophil-specific SGD. SGD is an extremely rare congenital disorder that is characterized by frequent and severe bacterial infections. Patients with SGD have defects in neutrophil function, including atypical nuclear morphology, impaired bactericidal activity, and abnormalities in neutrophil migration; they also lack both neutrophil and eosinophil secondary granule proteins. Recent sequence analyses of genomic DNA from two patients with SGD revealed mutations within the C/EBPε gene, resulting in a mutant protein lacking the dimerization and DNA-binding domains and hence transcriptional activity. Lack of functional C/EBPε activity has been postulated to underlie the observed pathology in these patients.

C/EBPζ

C/EBPζ-C/EBP homologous protein (CHOP) is a C/EBP family member that was originally isolated as the product of a gene induced in response to DNA-damaging agents. It has subsequently been shown to be induced by various extracellular or endoplasmic reticulum stresses. The basic region of CHOP is less well conserved than that of the other C/EBP family members, and CHOP does not seem to bind to canonical C/EBP *cis* elements. CHOP has been shown to interfere with the transcriptional activity of C/EBPβ in a manner dependent on its leucine zipper.

PU.1

PU.1 is a member of the Ets family of transcription factors and is expressed abundantly in B cells and macrophages. Expression of PU.1 has also been reported in granulocytes and eosinophils as well as in CD34^{+} hematopoietic progenitor cells. Whereas high levels of PU.1 expression in fetal livers of mice preferentially direct macrophage development, low levels of PU.1 result in B-cell development. C-Jun, another member of the b-Zip family of transcription factors, serves as a coactivator of PU.1 during macrophage development. It has been demonstrated that overexpression of c-Jun in myeloid progenitor cells results in macrophage development. Recent studies have revealed that downregulation of c-Jun by C/EBPα is necessary for granulocytic maturation and appears to be the mechanism through which C/EBPα blocks macrophage development. C/EBPα not only binds to the promoter of the *c-jun* gene and decreases its expression but also binds PU.1, thereby inhibiting its activity.

PU.1-binding sites have been reported in almost all myeloid-specific promoters reported to date, including those for M-CSF, GM-CSF, and G-CSF receptors, all of which play critical roles in myeloid cell development. PU.1 activity is modulated both by covalent modifications and by protein–protein interactions. For example, phosphorylation of PU.1 by casein kinase II or by JNK kinase leads to increased transcriptional activity.

Abrogation of PU.1 expression in PU.1$^{-/-}$ mice results in perinatal lethality accompanied by the absence of mature monocytes/macrophages and B cells and delayed and reduced granulopoiesis. After in vitro differentiation, embryonic stem cells derived from PU.1$^{-/-}$ blastocysts fail to express mature myeloid cell markers, suggesting that PU.1 is not essential for the initial events associated with myeloid lineage commitment but is necessary for the later stages of development.

Growth Factor Independence-1

The growth factor independence-1 (Gfi-1) gene was first identified as a target of proviral insertion after infection with Moloney murine leukemia virus (MoMuLV) resulting in interleukin-2 factor independence of a rat lymphoma cell line.[20] Gfi-1 is a highly conserved gene that encodes a 55kD nuclear proto-oncogene that harbors six C_2H_2 type zinc finger domains at the carboxy terminus and a 20–amino acid stretch at the N-terminus known as the SNAG domain.[20] The SNAG domain, which appears to be conserved in the Snail/Slug family of proteins, has been shown to confer transcriptional repressor activity on Gfi-1. The human Gfi-1 gene is located on chromosome 1p22, and its closely related paralog Gfi1b maps to chromosome 9q34. Whereas Gfi-1 is expressed at high levels in the thymus and BM, Gfi1B expression is confined to the BM and spleen. Homozygous knockout of Gfi-1B results in embryonic lethality at day E15 even though myelopoiesis is normal. Death in these mice has been attributed to a failure of erythropoiesis and megakaryopoiesis.

The essential role of Gfi1 in neutrophil differentiation became apparent after two reports of gene disruption in mice. Gfi1-null mice are severely neutropenic and eventually succumb to bacterial infections. In addition, these mice lack mature neutrophils, and their granulocyte precursors are unable to differentiate into mature neutrophils upon induction with G-CSF. These cells also lacked SGP expression reminiscent of C/EBPε$^{-/-}$ granulocytes. Gfi-1$^{-/-}$ BM contained an atypical Gr1^{+}Mac1^{+} myeloid precursor cell that appears to share characteristics of both granulocyte and macrophage precursors. Ectopic expression of Gfi1 in ex vivo sorted Gfi1$^{-/-}$ progenitor cells restored G-CSF–mediated neutrophil maturation to these cells. These observations provide evidence for the critical role of Gfi1 in the neutrophil maturation program. Recent studies have further demonstrated that Gfi-1 together with C/EBPε synergize to transactivate the promoters of late myeloid genes. This synergy is lost in a patient with SGD, who has a heterozygous substitution mutation in the C/EBPε gene and decreased levels of Gfi-1 in the BM.

Recently, heterozygous dominant negative mutations in the Gfi1 gene have been described in two patients with severe congenital neutropenia (SCN), underscoring the role of Gfi1 in the neutrophil maturation pathway. It has been suggested that mutant Gfi1 in these patients alters the expression of ELANE mutations that are commonly associated with SCN (see below). This observation confirms the vital role Gfi1 plays in human granulopoiesis.

CCAAT Displacement Protein

CCAAT displacement protein/cut (CDP) is a ubiquitously expressed, highly conserved, homeodomain (HD) protein with extensive homology to the *Drosophila* cut protein. CDP has been shown to act as a repressor of developmentally regulated genes, including the phagocyte-specific cytochrome heavy chain gene (gp91 phox), which is expressed exclusively in differentiating granulocytes.[21] Overexpression of CDP in 32Dcl3 myeloid cells blocks G-CSF–induced expression of SGP genes without blocking phenotypical maturation. CDP therefore acts as a negative regulator of stage-specific expression of both early and late neutrophil-specific genes.

The CDP homeobox protein contains three highly conserved DNA-binding repeats referred to as *cut repeats* (CR1, CR2, CR3) and a HD, each of which is capable of recognizing and binding specific DNA motifs in target genes. This may explain why the CDP molecule as a whole does not have a well-defined consensus DNA-binding sequence. The cut repeats cannot bind DNA as monomers but in combination exhibit high DNA-binding affinity. It has further been suggested that CDP-binding activity is restricted to proliferating cells, in which CDP target genes are repressed. These targets are upregulated as cells undergo cell cycle arrest and terminal differentiation in association with a decrease in CDP binding. Target genes of CDP include c-myc, c-mos, and the thymidine kinase (TK), cdk inhibitor p21(WAF1/CIP1), cystic fibrosis transmembrane conductance regulator (CFTR), transforming growth factor-β (TGF-β) type II receptor, gp91 phox, major histocompatibility complex (MHC) class I locus, and neutrophil SGP genes.

During myeloid differentiation, CDP binding has been shown to regulate genes that are expressed at widely disparate stages of differentiation. For example, it represses the gp91 phox gene, which is expressed at a much earlier time in myelopoiesis than is the case for the lactoferrin gene. The mechanism by which CDP mediates repression and the means by which it modulates stage-specific gene expression at different stages of differentiation within a single lineage are not fully understood. CDP is reported to have repressive activity associated with its ability to be displaced by a positive transacting factor involving the CR1 and CR2 cut repeats. However, other modes of repressive activity involving the two active repression domains within the C terminus of CDP also have been reported. CDP has been shown to function as a repressor of transcription via chromatin modification through recruitment of histone deacetylases (HDACs), consistent with the notion that transcriptional silencing is associated with hypoacetylated histones. Both acetylation and phosphorylation of CDP are posttranscriptional modifications that have been postulated to regulate CDP function. Thus, differential modification, by phosphorylation or acetylation, of CDP-DNA complexes binding the promoters of target genes could result in the observed differential repression exerted by CDP during neutrophil development.

ROLE OF DEVELOPMENTALLY IMPORTANT NEUTROPHIL-SPECIFIC GENES IN DISEASE

Our understanding of the role of neutrophil-specific genes has been enhanced by the study of mice in which targeted disruption of a gene results in phenotypically important defects in neutrophil differentiation and function. Similarly, the importance of these genes has been underscored by the analysis of naturally occurring genetic events within these genes that result in human disease. The links between some genes and the diseases induced by their dysfunction may be anticipated by their important roles in neutrophil differentiation and function, but the pathophysiologic links between others and the diseases they induce remain elusive (Table 25-2).

Disruption of neutrophil transcriptional regulation is a recurring theme in the pathogenesis of leukemia. Nearly half of patients with AML have pathognomonic translocations resulting in the fusion of a transcription factor with a tissue-specific gene. These translocations have been shown to interfere with myeloid differentiation and emphasize the role of transcription factors in that process.

As discussed previously, the same transcription factors that are implicated in the induction of neutrophil differentiation also direct the expression of genes encoding neutrophil-specific functional proteins. The link between morphologic differentiation and synthesis of neutrophil functional proteins is illustrated by the demonstration that disruption of C/EBPε signaling results in SGD associated with both morphologic abnormalities and increased infections attributable to neutrophil functional defects. It is intriguing that C/EBPε$^{-/-}$ mice share these abnormalities while also demonstrating a predilection for the development of myelodysplasia (i.e., myelodysplastic syndrome [MDS]). Although the development of MDS or AML has not been reported in patients with SGD, the deficiency is a rare disease described in less than a dozen patients, so a tendency to develop MDS or AML might be difficult to document.

Table 25-2 Differentiation-Specific Genes Implicated in Neutrophil Disorders

TRANSCRIPTION FACTORS
C/EBPα, PU.1, RARα, AML1, and others in AML
C/EBPε and Gfi-1 in specific granule deficiency
Gfi-1 in neutropenia
GRANULE AND FUNCTIONAL PROTEINS
Neutrophil elastase in Kostmann syndrome and cyclic hematopoiesis
gp91 phox in chronic granulomatous disease
ADHESION MOLECULES, RECEPTORS
Common β-chain of integrin receptors in LAD
G-CSF receptor mutations in AML arising in patients with Kostmann syndrome

AML, Acute myeloid leukemia; *C/EBP,* CCAAT enhancer–binding protein; *G-CSF,* granulocyte colony-stimulating factor; *gp91 phox,* glycoprotein 91 phagocyte nicotinamide adenine dinucleotide phosphate oxidase; *LAD,* leukocyte adhesion deficiency.

Other diseases have been linked to defects in functionally important neutrophil proteins. Abnormalities in integrin expression, notably, loss of the common β-chain of the integrin receptors, result in leukocyte adhesion deficiency, and absence of any of the components of the reduced NADPH oxidase leads to chronic granulomatous disease.

Abnormalities in granule protein gene expression again underscore the complexity of the granulocyte functional program. Congenital absence of many individual granule proteins, including myeloperoxidase, lactoferrin, and transcobalamin, has been described. In the absence of the more global defects seen in SGD, which presumably reflect more complex abnormalities than simple protein deficiency, these defects tend to be incidental laboratory findings with minimal or no associated pathology.

One prominent exception to that observation is the association between point mutations in the gene encoding NE (ELA2; neutrophil elastase, ELANE) and SCN, or Kostmann syndrome. The pathogenesis of SCN originally was sought in studies of G-CSFR, supported by the observation of a truncation mutation in G-CSFR in select patients with Kostmann syndrome.[22] It was later demonstrated that these were acquired mutations that may predispose the patient to secondary AML but did not constitute the pathologic basis for the neutropenia itself. Subsequent studies have implicated ELANE in the pathogenesis of SCN. ELANE is a primary granule protein that digests elastin and has been implicated in the pathogenesis of emphysema. Linkage studies have linked heterozygous abnormalities in the NE gene to both SCN (Kostmann syndrome) and cyclic hematopoiesis. The link between elastase and the control of neutrophil cell mass remains a mystery.

Role of microRNAs in Controlling Gene Expression in Granulopoiesis

MicroRNAs (miRNAs) are 18 to 24 nucleotides long, noncoding RNAs that regulate eukaryotic gene expression in general by binding to specific sites in the 3′UTR of target genes and altering expression by destabilizing mRNA or blocking mRNA translation. miRNAs are encoded in the genome and are initially transcribed by RNA polymerase II as long primary transcripts referred to as primary miRNAs (pri-miRNAs). These transcripts are recognized and processed by a ribonuclease called Drosha into 60 to 80 nucleotide intermediates called *precursor miRNAs* (pre-miRNAs), which are then exported to the cytoplasm, where a second ribonuclease termed *Dicer* cleaves pre-miRNAs to generate double-stranded 18- to 24–nucleotide-long miRNAs. The miRNAs are then incorporated into the RNA-induced silencing complex (RISC), a large protein complex that also contains the Argonaute or mRNA cleaving proteins. The miRNA guides the RISC complex to target complementary regions in the 3′UTRs of mRNAs, leading to repression of translation or destabilization of the mRNA by deadenylation.[23]

An increasing body of evidence implicates miRNA activity in mediating both normal and abnormal myelopoiesis.[24] MiRNAs have been shown to activate or be activated by myeloid-specific transcription factors such as C/EBPα and Gfi-1. For example, mir-223 is thought to be a direct target of C/EBPα, and its expression increases during granulopoiesis. Ablating mir-223 in mice results in the expansion of granulocyte precursor cells resulting from a cell autonomous increase in the number of granulocytic progenitors.[25] Additionally, overexpression of mir-223 in acute promyelocytic leukemia cells results in an enhanced capacity for granulocytic differentiation.[26] Mir-223 is thus thought to be a positive regulator of granulopoietic differentiation. Additionally, it has been shown that mir-223 targets E2F1, a master cell cycle regulator, by inhibiting translation of its mRNA. Thus, granulopoiesis appears to be regulated by a C/EBPα–miR-223–E2F1 axis, wherein miR-223 functions as a key regulator of myeloid cell proliferation associated with E2F1 in a mutual negative feedback loop.[27]

Eiring et al[28] have demonstrated another role for miRNAs in granulopoiesis. They demonstrated that mir-328 is downregulated in CML patients in blast crisis. Restoration of mir-328 expression restores differentiation by interaction with both the C/EBPα translational inhibitor hnRNP-E2 and the mRNA for PIM1, a survival factor. The interaction with hnRNP-E2 leads to the release of C/EBPα mRNA from hnRNA-E2–mediated translational inhibition through an interaction that is independent of its seed sequence. Thus, mir-328 appears to control cell fate by its ability to base pair with the 3′UTR of target mRNAs (PIM1) as well as by acting as a decoy for hnRNP binding, thus interfering with cell fate by releasing C/EBPα from translational inhibition.[28]

A role for mir-27 in granulopoiesis has also been documented. This miR targets the myeloid transcription factor Runx1, whose expression decreases during granulocytic differentiation in a mir-27–dependent manner. Anti-mir-27 treatment of immature myeloid progenitors resulted in an increase in the expression of Runx1 and impaired granulocytic differentiation.[29] In a separate study, the transcription factor Gfi-1 was shown to bind to the promoter of miR-196b and repress its expression, thereby promoting granulocytic maturation while repressing monocytic lineage development. Overexpression of miR-196b blocked granulopoiesis in granulocyte monocyte precursor cells.[30]

Thus, a growing number of feedforward and feedback regulatory loops involving specific miRNAs and myeloid-specific transcription factors that determine lineage development and fate have been recognized in recent years, thereby underscoring a vital role of miRNAs in granulopoiesis.

EOSINOPHIL PRODUCTION

Eosinophil precursors constitute approximately 3% of marrow progenitors, of which about two-thirds are myelocyte precursors and the remainder mature eosinophils (Fig. 25-5). Eosinophilic myelocytes are large cells with a single-lobed nucleus. The characteristic specific granules of eosinophils contain major basic protein, eosinophil cationic protein, eosinophil peroxidase, and eosinophil-derived neurotoxin. Eosinophils also contain primary granules that contain Charcot-Leyden crystal protein. Mature eosinophils are released from the marrow, where they circulate up to 18 hours before migrating to the tissues.

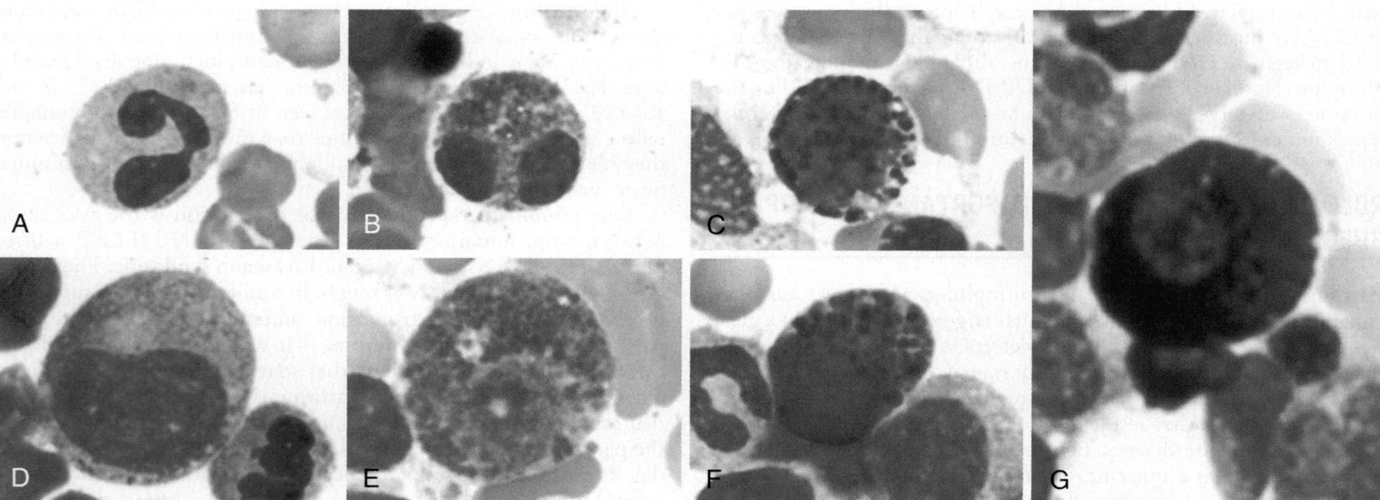

Figure 25-5 NEUTROPHILIC, EOSINOPHILIC, AND BASOPHILIC GRANULOCYTES; THEIR MYELOCYTE PRECURSORS; AND MAST CELLS. Eosinophilic and basophilic granulocytes are always best viewed compared with neutrophilic granulocytes because staining can vary from laboratory to laboratory and even from case to case. When compared with a neutrophil **(A),** the eosinophil **(B)** has larger and more red/orange-colored and almost refractile granules than the pink and barely perceivable granules in the neutrophil. Mature eosinophils are also frequently bilobed, but neutrophils tend to have three or four lobes. The basophil **(C)** has dense, dark blue granules that frequently overly the condensed and lobulated nucleus. The granules frequently obstruct the nucleus and are a much larger than the primary granules of promyelocytes. The myelocyte stage of maturation is when the secondary granules first appear **(D** to **F).** In the neutrophilic myelocyte **(D),** the secondary granules first appear in the Golgi region and have been describes as resembling the sunrise over the horizon, the "dawn of neutrophilia." The eosinophilic and basophilic myelocytes **(E** and **F)** are relatively infrequent in the bone marrow and are usually enumerated together with the mature forms. Mast cells **(G)** must be distinguished from basophils and basophilic myelocyte. Mast cells are larger and have quite numerous granules mostly in the cytoplasm. Mast cells have round nuclei, which are frequently obscured by the granules. A toluidine blue cytochemical reaction will be positive (metachromatic) in the granules of both basophils and mast cells. However, a mast cell tryptase immunostain used on a tissue section will be positive only in mast cells.

Eosinophils proliferate and mature under the influence of IL-3, IL-5, and GM-CSF. Evidence suggests that these cytokines are secreted by T cells as the stimulus to eosinophil production in many disorders associated with eosinophilia. Studies of idiopathic hypereosinophilic syndrome have described activating mutations in the platelet-derived growth factor receptor-α (PDGFR-α) that result in constitutive tyrosine kinase activation and eosinophil proliferation.

Transcriptional regulation of eosinophilic differentiation is mediated through PU.1 C/EBPα and -β. Because these same factors serve to induce myeloid differentiation, the modulation of the signals determining the choice between these two lineages is not well defined. It has been proposed that levels of GATA1 may be important in determining whether C/EBP expression induces the eosinophilic or the myeloid maturation program (see Chapter 70).

BASOPHIL AND MAST CELL PRODUCTION

Basophils and mast cells mediate allergic responses, where they are the central cells involved in IgE-induced immune responses to parasites and other allergens. Both cell types are derived from marrow precursors, but they have a very different ontogeny (see Fig. 25-5 and Chapter 71).

Basophils have a bilobed nucleus and characteristic intensely staining purple granules that may cover the nucleus. These granules contain glycosaminoglycans, predominantly heparin. Basophils differentiate from marrow progenitors and are released from the marrow as mature cells, where they circulate briefly, with a lifespan similar to that of neutrophils. Maturation occurs in response to IL-3, which serves both to induce basophilic differentiation and to mediate activation of mature basophils. Although IL-3 is the primary mediator of basophil development, studies of IL-3–null mice have demonstrated that it is not required for baseline production of basophils. It is, however, required for the induction of basophilia in response to parasitic infection. Other cytokines that influence basophil proliferation include GM-CSF, IL-5, and SCF.

Mast cells arise from marrow precursors but are released into the circulation as immature cells. They circulate only briefly in the peripheral blood before migrating to the tissues, where they complete their maturation. There remains some question about whether mast cells and basophils arise from a common precursor. In vitro studies showed that adding SCF and IL-3 to cultured $CD34^+$ cells results in an increased proliferation and maturation of both basophils and mast cells but did not establish a common progenitor cell for the two lineages. It is clear that SCF is especially effective in inducing mast cell proliferation; in fact, activating mutations in c-Kit, the SCF receptor, is the underlying molecular defect in cases of systemic mastocytosis.

MONOCYTOPOIESIS

Monocyte Ontogeny

Stages of Monocyte Differentiation

Monocytes originate in the BM from promonocytes, which constitute approximately 3% of the total cells in the normal marrow (Fig. 25-6). Promonocytes have round nuclei and basophilic cytoplasm. Differentiation occurs rapidly, with a maturation time of 50 to 60 hours, associated with two rounds of replication and morphologic maturation marked by progressive lobulation of the nucleus. Stress-induced release of monocytes occurs primarily through their premature release from the proliferating pool. Survival in the blood is short, approximately 8 to 72 hours. Monocytes then enter the tissues, where they develop into macrophages that may survive 2 to 3 months. Tissue-fixed macrophages are found in the lung (alveolar macrophages), the liver (Kupffer cells), the spleen, and the central nervous system (glial cells).

Monocytes also may serve as precursors to a subset of dendritic cells. Dendritic cells are professional antigen-presenting cells that arise from both myeloid and lymphoid precursor cells. The myeloid subset of dendritic cells arises from a precursor that can alternatively differentiate into macrophages. Similar cells have been generated for immunotherapy by exposing peripheral blood monocytes to GM-CSF and IL-4 in vitro.

Markers of Monocyte Maturation

Unique surface markers of monocyte maturation have been difficult to identify. In mice, the marker F4/80 was identified as a nearly universal marker of monocytes and macrophages; this antigen has been shown to be homologous to the human epidermal growth factor module containing mucin-like hormone receptor 1. The function of this receptor is unknown because knock-out mice have no phenotype.

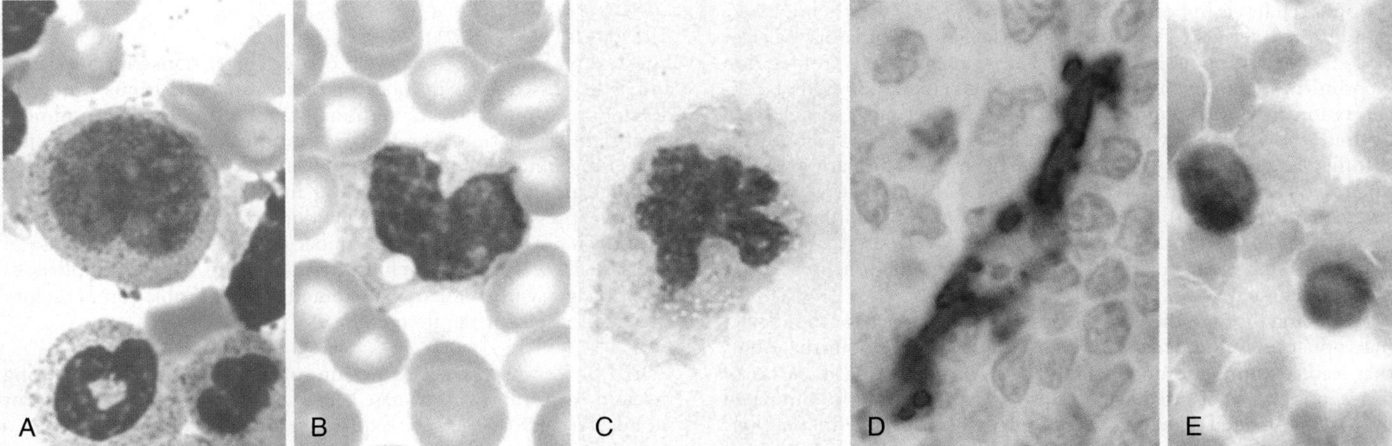

Figure 25-6 A PROMONOCYTE, MONOCYTE, MACROPHAGE, AND HISTIOCYTE. Promonocytes are rare in the bone marrow (BM) **(A)** and are more frequently seen during recovery or during marrow regeneration after chemotherapy or other insult. They are typically slightly folded and have nucleoli. The cytoplasm is moderately abundant and blue/grey with very faint granules. Monocytes seen in the blood **(B)** typically have more folded or horseshoe-shaped nuclei and more abundant grey cytoplasm frequently with vacuoles and rare granules. The macrophage **(C)** is seen in body fluid specimens such as peritoneal fluid or cerebrospinal fluid and resembles the blood monocyte. Tissue histiocytes are fixed in the tissues and are seen on tissue sections. The histocyte illustrated **(D)** is stained with CD68 and is from a lymph node. It likely represents a dendritic cell in a germinal center. Monocytes in the BM can be more easily enumerated with a nonspecific esterase cytochemical reaction such as alpha-naphthyl acetate esterase, which gives an orange/brown reaction product **(E)**.

Monocyte precursor cells express the M-CSF receptor, lysozyme, the Fcγ receptor (II/III), and the scavenger receptor. Mature monocytes, similar to neutrophils, show high-level expression of CD11b/CD18. After differentiation to macrophages, the cells acquire expression of macrosialin (CD68), a glycoprotein of unknown function that may play a role in lipoprotein metabolism. Macrophages also express sialoadhesin, a member of the sialic acid–binding receptor family. Although its precise function has not been proved, sialoadhesin mediates binding to sialic acid moieties on cell surfaces and probably plays a role in macrophage cell–cell interactions and cell–extracellular matrix interactions.

CD14 is a major functional surface protein of the monocyte/macrophage lineage. CD14 is the receptor for LPS, leading to monocyte/macrophage activation. More recent studies have suggested that CD14 also may have a role in apoptosis.

Monocytes contain both primary (peroxidase-positive) and secondary (peroxidase-negative) granules. The primary granules of monocytes, similar to those of neutrophils, contain myeloperoxidase. Secondary granule fusion with the membrane on stimulation of monocytes results in upregulation of Mac1 and p150 and is thought to play a role in adhesion and diapedesis of stimulated monocytes.

Control of Monocytopoiesis

Cytokine Regulation of Monocyte Proliferation and Differentiation

The effects of colony-stimulating factor 1 (CSF-1 also known as M-CSF), the primary regulator of mononuclear phagocyte production, are thought to be mediated by the high-affinity receptor tyrosine kinase CSF-1 receptor (CSF-1R), encoded by the c-fms proto-oncogene. A total of five human or mouse mRNAs result from alternative splicing, and the alternative use of the 3′ untranslated region results in three isoforms of the CSF-1 protein, a secreted proteoglycan, a secreted glycoprotein, and a membrane-spanning cell surface proteoglycan.

The phenotypes of Csf1-null mice and of mice harboring an inactivating mutation in the coding region of CSF-1 (Csfop/Csf1op) (osteopetrotic mice) are virtually identical; features include toothlessness, low body weight, low growth rate, and deficient tissue macrophages. Additionally, the mutant mice have defects in both male and female fertility. Compared with their wild-type littermates, splenic erythroid burst-forming unit and high-proliferative-potential colony-forming cell levels in both Csf1op/Csf1op and $Csf1^-/Csf1^-$ mice were significantly elevated, consistent with a negative regulatory role for CSF-1 on erythropoiesis and on the maintenance and proliferation of primitive hematopoietic progenitors. The circulating CSF-1 concentration in CSF receptor-null ($Csf1R^-/Csf1R^-$) mice was elevated 20-fold, in agreement with clearance of circulating CSF-1 by CSF-1R–mediated endocytosis. Despite their overall similarity, several phenotypical characteristics of the $Csf1R^-/Csf1R^-$ mice were more severe than those of the Csf1op/Csf1op mice. The results indicate that all of the effects of CSF-1 are mediated via the CSF-1R but that additional effects of the CSF-1R could result from its CSF-1-independent activation.

Signaling through the CSF-1R appears to be critical for monocyte/macrophage development. Although little is known about the events that lead to stimulation of a monocyte/macrophage specific array of genes, it is clear that several transcription factors, probably stimulated by M-CSF–related signaling events, play vital roles in the development of this lineage. It should be noted, however, that the ability of phorbol esters to induce monocytic differentiation of myeloid cell lines through activation of the protein kinases Cα and Cδ suggests a role for the protein kinase C pathway in monopoiesis.

IL-3, G-CSF, and tumor necrosis factor all have been shown to synergize with M-CSF in the proliferation of macrophages. G-CSF also has been shown to induce the increased release of monocytes; this is an indirect effect dependent on the presence of M-CSF. Monocytes also have been demonstrated to have functional G-CSF receptors, although G-CSF appears to function mainly to decrease monokine secretion rather than to increase monocyte proliferation.

Transcriptional Regulation of Monocyte Differentiation

Of the several transcription factors that regulate the development of the monocyte/macrophage lineage, the most well-established is PU.1 because abrogation of PU.1 expression in $PU.1^{-/-}$ mice results in perinatal lethality accompanied by the absence of mature monocytes/macrophages and B cells and delayed and reduced granulopoiesis. A number of factors, the most notable of which is c-Jun, cooperate with PU.1 to regulate monocyte-specific genes.

c-Jun

The c-*jun* proto-oncogene encodes the transcriptional activator protein AP-1. As a member of the early response genes, *c-jun* is rapidly and transiently activated in response to external proliferative signals. The expression of c-Jun as well as related family members JunB and JunD is upregulated during monocytic differentiation. In addition, overexpression of c-Jun in M1, U937, or WEHI-B D^+ myeloid cell lines, as well as in myeloid progenitor cells, was found to result in partial monocytic differentiation. However, $c\text{-}Jun^{-/-}$ fetal liver cells are capable of reconstituting hematopoiesis in syngeneic recipients, suggesting that c-Jun is not required for myeloid development. This finding may reflect a compensatory role played by other Jun family proteins.

As discussed, c-Jun serves as a coactivator of PU.1 during macrophage development. Recent studies have revealed that downregulation of c-jun by C/EBPα is necessary for granulocytic maturation and appears to be the mechanism through which C/EBPα blocks macrophage development (see Fig. 25-4). C/EBPα not only binds to the promoter of the c-jun gene and decreases its expression but also binds to PU.1, thereby inhibiting its activity. Such transcription factor cross-talk resulting in subtle changes in the levels of transcription factors within a given lineage appears to be an emerging paradigm through which master regulators of lineage specification, such as C/EBPα and PU.1, direct lineage-specific development by directly upregulating lineage-specific genes as well as by blocking the progression of alternate lineages.

Other Transcription Factors Modulating Monocyte Development

Egr-1. Egr-1 belongs to a family of zinc finger transcription factors and is expressed in a number of tissues and at various points in development, including the terminal stages of macrophage and neutrophil differentiation. Egr-1 is necessary for monocytic differentiation of myeloid cell lines U937 and M1 and prevents factor-induced granulocytic differentiation of HL60 and 32Dcl3 cells. Additionally, ectopic expression of Egr-1 in myeloid marrow progenitors was found to result in an increase in the number of CFU-M at the expense of CFU-G. However, mice lacking Egr-1 develop normal numbers of macrophages, a phenomenon attributed to the possible compensatory effects of other Egr family members.

C/EBPβ. As discussed, expression of C/EBPβ increases during myeloid maturation and has been shown to be important for monocyte/macrophage gene expression and development.

MafB and c-Maf. The transcription factors MafB and c-Maf belong to a family of basic-leucine zipper (b-Zip) factors that bind DNA as dimers. The Maf proteins can dimerize with members of other b-Zip family proteins, including c-Jun, fos, and NF-E2 in erythroid cells. Whereas ectopic expression of MafB in myeloblasts directed their expression to macrophages, overexpression of c-Maf in HL60 and U937 myeloid cells resulted in monocytic differentiation.

REFERENCES

1. Dao C, Metcalf D, Zittoun R, Bilski-Pasquier G: Normal human bone marrow cultures in vitro: Cellular composition and maturation of granulocytic colonies. *Br J Haematol* 37:127, 1977.
2. Verfaillie C: Adhesion receptors as regulators of the hematopoietic process. *Blood* 92:2609, 1998.
3. Borregaard N, Theilgaard-Monch K, Sorensen O, et al: Regulation of human neutrophil granule protein expression. *Curr Opin Hematol* 8:23, 2001.
4. Borregaard N, Kjeldsen L, Rygaard K, et al: Stimulus-dependent secretion of plasma proteins from human neutrophils. *J Clin Invest* 90:86, 1992.
5. Khanna-Gupta A, Zibello T, Sun H, et al: Chromatin immunoprecipitation (ChIP) studies indicate a role for CCAAT enhamcer binding proteins alpha and epsilon (C/EBPa and C/EBPe) and CDP/cut in myeloid maturation induced lactoferrin gene expression. *Blood* 101:3460, 2003.
6. Johnston JJ, Boxer LA, Berliner N: Correlation of messenger RNA levels with protein defects in specific granule deficiency. *Blood* 80:2088, 1992.
7. Metcalf D: Hematopoietic regulators: Redundancy or subtlety? *Blood* 82:3515, 1993.
8. Avalos B: Molecular analysis of the granulocyte-colony stimulating factor receptor. *Blood* 88:761, 1996.
9. Tenen D: Disruption of differentiation in human cancer: AML shows the way. *Nature Rev: Cancer* 3:89, 2003.
10. Laslo P, Spooner CJ, Warmflash A, et al: Multilineage transcriptional priming and determination of alternate hematopoietic cell fates. *Cell* 126, 2006.
11. Coffman J: Runx transcription factors and the developmental balance between cell proliferation and differentiation. *Cell Biol Int* 27:315, 2003.
12. Lichtinger M, Hoogenkamp M, Krysinska H, et al: Chromatin regulation by RUNX1. *Blood Cells Mol Dis* 44:287, 2010.
13. Calkhoven C, Müller CAL: Translational control of C/EBPalpha and C/EBPbeta isoform expression. *Gene Dev* 14:1920, 2000.
14. Khanna-Gupta A: Regulation and deregulation of mRNA translation during myeloid maturation. *Exp Hematol* 39:133, 2011.
15. Muller B, Pabst T: C/EBPa and the pathophysiology of acute myeloid leukemia. *Curr Opin Hematol* 13:7, 2006.
16. Pabst T, Muller B, Zhang P: Dominant negative mutations of CEBPA encodong CCAAT/enhancer binding protein-a (C/EBPa), in acute myeloid leukemia. *Nat Genet* 27:263, 2001.
17. Kirstetter P, Schuster MB, Bereshchenko O, et al: Modeling of C/EBPalpha mutant acute myeloid leukemia reveals a common expression signature of committed myeloid leukemia-initiating cells. *Cancer Cell* 13:299, 2008.
18. Koschmieder S, Halmos B, Levantini E, et al: Dysregulation of the C/EBPalpha differentiation pathway in human cancer. *J Clin Oncol* 27:619, 2009.
19. Ford AM, Bennett CA, Healy LE, et al: Regulation of the myeloperoxidase enhancer binding proteins PU.1, C-EBPa, -b and -d during granulocytic-lineage specification. *Proc Natl Acad Sci USA* 93:10838, 1996.
20. van der Meer L, Jansen JH, van der Reijden BA: Gfi1 and Gfi1b: Key regulators of hematopoiesis. *Leukemia* 24:1834, 2010.
21. Nepveu A: Role of the multifunctional CDP/cut/cux homeodomain transcription factor in regulating differentiation, cell growth and development. *Gene* 270:1, 2001.
22. Berliner N: Lessons from congenital neutropenia: 50 years of progress in understanding myelopoiesis. *Blood* 111:5427, 2008.
23. Manikandan J, Aarthi JJ, Kumar SD, et al: Oncomirs: The potential role of non-coding microRNAs in understanding cancer. *Bioinformation* 8:330, 2008.
24. Pelosi E, Labbaye C, Testa U: MicroRNAs in normal and malignant myelopoiesis. *Leukemia Res* 33:1584, 2009.
25. Johnnidis J, Harris MH, Wheeler RT, et al: Regulation of progenitor cell proliferation and granulocyte function by microRNA-223. *Nature* 451:1125, 2008.
26. Fazi F, Rosa A, Fatica A, et al: Aminicircuitry comprised of microRNA-223 and transcription factors NFI-A and C/EBPalpha regulates human granulopoiesis. *Cell* 123:819, 2005.
27. Pulikkan J, Dengler V, Peramangalam PS, et al: Cell-cycle regulator E2F1 and microRNA-223 comprise an autoregulatory negative feedback loop in acute myeloid leukemia. *Blood* 115:1768, 2010.
28. Eiring A, Harb JG, Neviani P, et al: miR-328 functions as an RNA decoy to modulate hnRNP E2 regulation of mRNA translation in leukemic blasts. *Cell* 140:652, 2010.
29. Feng J, Iwama A, Satake M, et al: MicroRNA-27 enhances differentiation of myeloblasts into granulocytes by post-transcriptionally downregulating Runx1. *Brit J Haematol* 145:412, 2009.
30. Velu C, Baktula AM, Grimes HL: Gfi1 regulates miR-21 and miR-196b to control myelopoiesis. *Blood* 113:4720, 2009.

CHAPTER 26

THROMBOCYTOPOIESIS

Alan B. Cantor

Platelets, once regarded simply as "blood dust," are now recognized to play essential roles in hemostasis. Not only do they form a hemostatic plug and initiate thrombus formation in the event of vascular injury, but they also repair minute vascular damage that occurs on a daily basis. Platelets are also thought to be involved in wound healing and angiogenesis via delivery of key growth factors, such as VEGF, PDGF, and TGF-β to sites of vascular injury. Disorders associated with platelet production carry significant morbidity and mortality in humans due to hemorrhage, thrombosis, bone marrow fibrosis, bone marrow failure, and/or hematologic malignancy. Platelets are generated from their precursor cells, megakaryocytes, via a complex process. For a long time, the extreme rarity of megakaryocytes significantly hampered studies aimed at understanding the molecular mechanisms underlying platelet biogenesis. However, the purification and cloning (in 1994) of thrombopoietin (TPO), the major megakaryocyte cytokine, has enabled considerable progress to be made. These new insights provide an important foundation for improved diagnosis and treatment of disorders of thrombocytopoiesis. This chapter reviews the current understanding of megakaryocyte biology and platelet production, highlighting connections with human disease.

MEGAKARYOCYTE BIOLOGY

Megakaryocyte Development

Although platelets were described as early as the 1840s, it was not until 1906, in a seminal study by James Homer Wright, that their origin from megakaryocytes was first recognized.[1] Megakaryocytes are large polyploid cells that reside predominantly within the bone marrow during postnatal life. They are rare cells, constituting only about 0.1% of nucleated cells under normal steady-state conditions. They develop from common bipotential megakaryocyte-erythroid progenitor (MEP) cells, which are themselves derived from common myeloid progenitor (CMP) cells, and ultimately from pluripotential hematopoietic stem cells (HSCs). Once committed to the megakaryocytic lineage, megakaryocyte progenitors undergo a series or dramatic maturational steps ultimately tailored to their final task of platelet production and release. These include changes in proliferative capacity, cell size, nuclear content, organelle biogenesis, membrane development, and cytoskeletal rearrangement. The large increase in cell size is linked to an unusual process termed *endomitosis,* in which cells replicate their DNA but fail to undergo cytokinesis. Mature megakaryocytes reach diameters of approximately 100 microns and contain DNA content as high as 128N. They contain a multilobulated nucleus enclosed by a single nuclear membrane. Their abundant cytoplasm is filled with ribosomes, platelet-specific granules, mitochondria, and complex intracellular membrane systems. Although megakaryocytes reside predominantly within the bone marrow, they are also found in peripheral blood, spleen, and lung under normal conditions. These extramedullary megakaryocytes release platelets, but their contribution to total thrombocytopoiesis is estimated to account for at most 7% to 15%.

Megakaryocyte Progenitors

Like other hematopoietic progenitor cells, megakaryocyte progenitors can be cultured in vitro using semisolid media. Animal studies using these colony assays have allowed delineation of hierarchal developmental pathways of megakaryocyte progenitor maturation based on proliferative potential, DNA content, morphologic criteria, and gene expression pattern (Fig. 26-1). This pathway can be conceptually divided into three broad stages: proliferating megakaryocytic progenitors, which contain normal DNA content (2N/4N), nonproliferating immature megakaryocytes (4N-8N DNA content), and nonproliferating mature megakaryocytes (DNA content 8N-128N). Within the proliferating megakaryocyte progenitor compartment, the earliest detectable cell is the megakaryocyte high-proliferative-potential colony-forming cell (Mk-HPP-CFC), which is capable of generating macroscopically visible colonies containing a few thousand megakaryocytes. This corresponds to a proliferative capacity of ≈8 to 10 replicative cycles. These cells require IL-3 and simultaneous activation of the protein kinase C and cyclic adenosine monophosphate (cAMP) signaling pathway.

The burst-forming unit-megakaryocyte (BFU-Mk), which is thought to be a direct progeny of Mk-HPP-CFC, is more mature than the Mk-HPP-CFC, but retains a high degree of proliferative potential, developing "bursts" of individual colony-forming cells. These colonies contain approximately 100 to 500 megakaryocytes, representing ≈5 to 7 replicative cycles. In humans, BFU-Mk cells require mitogenic stimulation with IL-3 or GM-CSF and synergistic signaling with SCF (stem cell factor; also called *kit-ligand*), IL-11, IL-1α, and TPO. They are also resistant to treatment in vitro with 5-fluorouracil (5-FU).

The most mature proliferating cell is the colony-forming cell-megakaryocyte (CFU-Mk), which has very limited proliferative potential, representing only 2 to 5 cell divisions (4 to 32 megakaryocytes per colony). This progenitor responds to a variety of single growth factors, such as IL-3 and GM-CSF, and co-regulators such as SCF, FLT3 ligand, and TPO. They express early markers of differentiation such as glycoprotein IIb (GPIIb) and platelet factor 4 (PF4) before initiating endomitotic cell cycles.

Immature Megakaryocytes: Promegakaryoblasts

Promegakaryoblasts are transitional cells intermediate between proliferating progenitor cells and postmitotic, mature megakaryocytes. These cells are not readily observed morphologically in vitro or in bone marrow specimens but may be identified by their expression of megakaryocyte- or platelet-specific markers, such as platelet peroxidase, platelet GPIIb/IIIa, and von Willebrand factor (vWF). They have DNA content levels intermediate between proliferating progenitors and mature megakaryocytes. Promegakaryoblasts respond to a variety of cytokines in vitro, including IL-3, SCF, IL-6 and TPO, to produce large polyploid megakaryocytes. At least three distinct

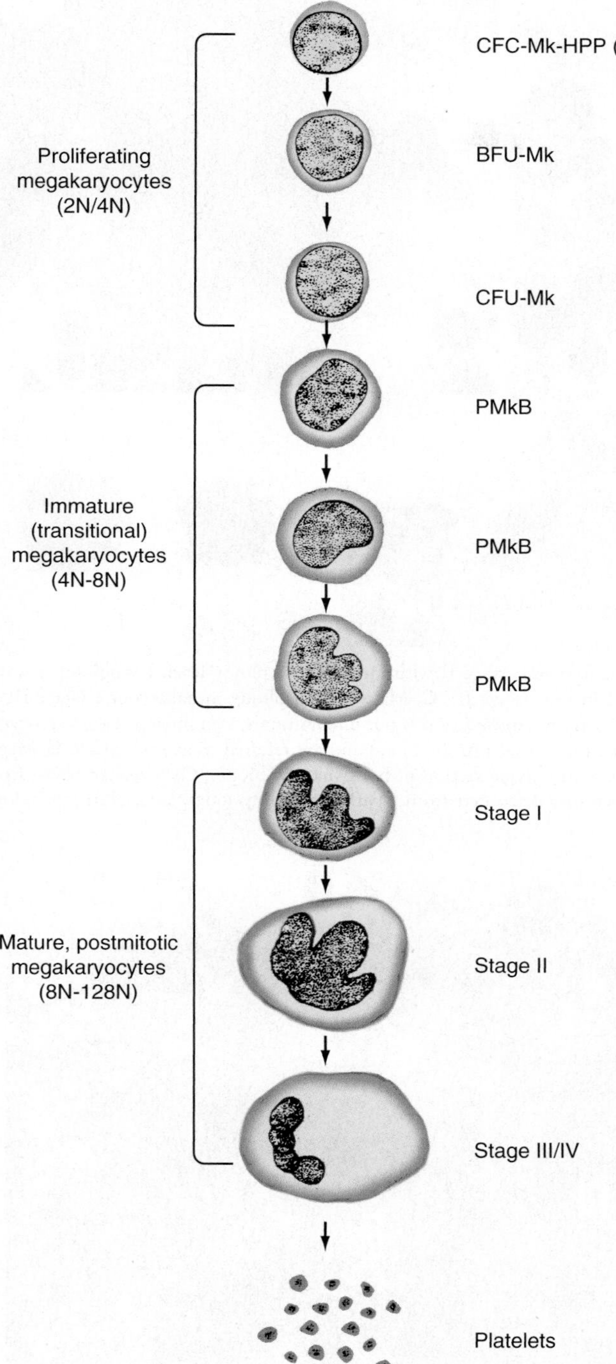

Figure 26-1 CELLULAR HIERARCHY OF MEGAKARYOCYTE DEVELOPMENT. Megakaryocyte development can be conceptually divided into three stages: The proliferating progenitor cells, which have the typical 2N/4N DNA content; the immature megakaryocytes, which have an intermediate DNA content and are transitional between the progenitor cells and the more mature cells; and the mature, postmitotic cells, which have an 8N to 128N DNA content. *BFU-Mk,* Burst-forming unit-megakaryocyte; *CFC-Mk-HPP,* colony-forming unit-megakaryocyte high-proliferative potential; *CFU-Mk,* colony-forming unit-megakaryocyte; *PMkB,* promegakaryoblast.

subpopulations of promegakaryoblasts have been identified based on different physiochemical characteristics, morphology, antigen expression, and enzyme content.

Mature Megakaryocytes

Morphologically recognizable megakaryocytes exist in at least four distinct maturation stages as defined morphologically (Fig. 26-2). The megakaryoblast (stage I) is characterized by a high nucleus-to-cytoplasm ratio and scanty basophilic cytoplasm, reflecting the large amount of protein synthesis occurring in these cells. The promegakaryocyte (stage II) is the cell in which the cytoplasmic volume and number of platelet-specific granules increase. The granular or "platelet shedding" megakaryocyte (stages III and IV) is the most mature cell. In reality, these stages likely represent a continuum.

Prospective Isolation of Megakaryocyte Progenitor Cells

Weissman and colleagues have reported the prospective isolation of clonogenic committed megakaryocyte progenitor cells from the bone marrow of adult C57BLKa-Thy1.1 mice based on selection of a unique cell surface immunophenotype: c-kit(+)Sca-1(-)IL7Ralpha(-)Thy1.1(-)Lin(-)CD9(+)CD41(+)FcgammaR(lo).[2] This fraction represents approximately 0.01% of the total nucleated bone marrow cells and gives rise to CFU-Mk and occasionally BFU-Mk in colony assays. The immunophenotype Lin(-)c-kit (+)Sca1(-)CD150 (+) CD41(+) has also been used to enrich for committed murine Mk progenitors. Identification of a comparable set of surface markers for human megakaryocyte progenitors has not been reported.

Structure of Mature Megakaryocytes

Mature megakaryocytes contain a large multilobulated polyploid nucleus often situated toward the periphery of the cell. They have abundant cytoplasm, which contains platelet-specific secretory granules, alpha (α-) granules and dense granules (Fig. 26-3).[3] The biogenesis of α-granules and dense granules begins in immature megakaryocytes, and both granule types develop concomitantly. α-Granules are 200 to 500 nm in diameter and have a dense center and fine granular matrix. Megakaryocytes synthesize many of the constituents of α-granules and target them to the granules. These include von Willebrand factor (vWF), fibronectin, P-selectin, fibrinogen receptors, platelet factor 4 (PF4), coagulation factor V, plasminogen activator inhibitor-1 (PAI-1), among others. In addition, some constituents, such as fibrinogen, are taken up by megakaryocytes via endocytosis and/or pinocytosis and stored in α-granules. It was once thought that α-granules were a homogeneous population of vesicles. However, it has become clear that there are distinct populations of α-granules containing different constituents, and these can be differentially released during platelet activation.[4] Dense granules are 200 to 300 nm in diameter and consist of a halo encircling an electron opaque core. They contain many soluble hemostatic factors such as serotonin, catecholamines, adenosine, adenosine 5′-diphosphate, adenosine 5′-triphosphate, and calcium. Their limiting membranes contain glycoproteins such as αIIbβ3, glycoprotein Ib (GPIb), and P-selectin, which are also present in α-granules, as well as unique membrane proteins such as granulophysin. Multivesicular bodies (MVBs) serve as intermediates in the biogenesis of both α-granules and dense granules. It has been proposed that they constitute a sorting compartment between α-granule and dense granule components.

The megakaryocyte cytoplasm contains at least two complex membranous systems: the demarcation membrane system (DMS) and the dense tubular network (DTS) (see Fig. 26-3). The DMS consists of an extensive network of tubular and flattened membranous structures that interconnect with one another and communicate

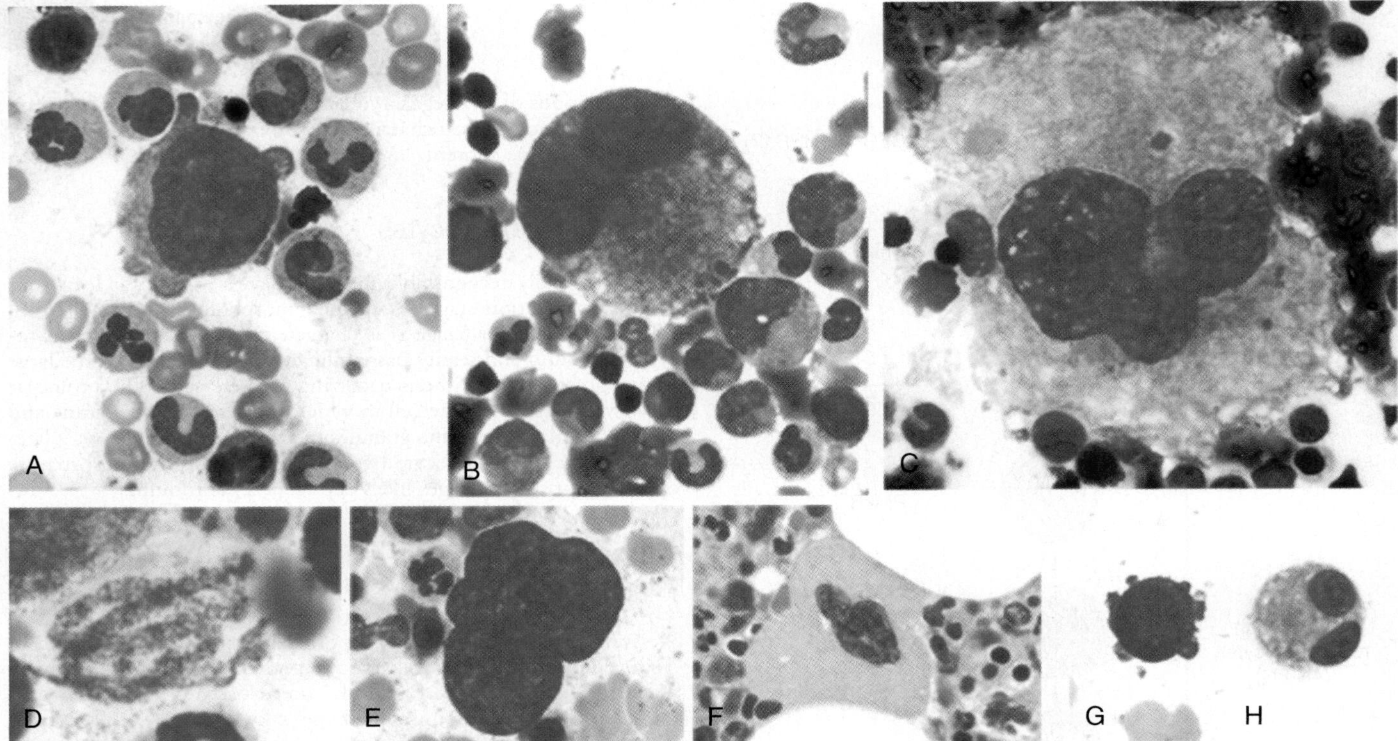

Figure 26-2 MEGAKARYOCYTOPOEISIS AND MEGAKARYOCYTES. **A,** Megakaryoblast (stage I) with intermediate ploidy level. Cytoplasm is scant. Note prominent cytoplasmic pseudopods. **B,** Promegakaryocyte with early platelet production (stage II). **C,** Mature, high-ploidy megakaryocyte (stage III or IV) with abundant cytoplasm. Note cells traveling through cytoplasm. This is referred to as *emperipolesis* and is not uncommonly seen in large megakaryocytes. **D,** Portion of megakaryocyte cytoplasm in a long strand. Fragments of these can sometimes be seen in the blood and are referred to as *proplatelets*. **E,** Megakaryocyte nucleus denuded of its platelets and cytoplasm. **F,** Mature megakaryocyte seen in a tissue section of bone marrow biopsy. **G,** Megakaryoblast from a patient with acute megakaryoblastic leukemia. Note cytoplasmic pseudopods. **H,** Micromegakaryocyte from a patient with myelodysplasia. Note small, low-ploidy (2-4N) nucleus, but mature cytoplasm.

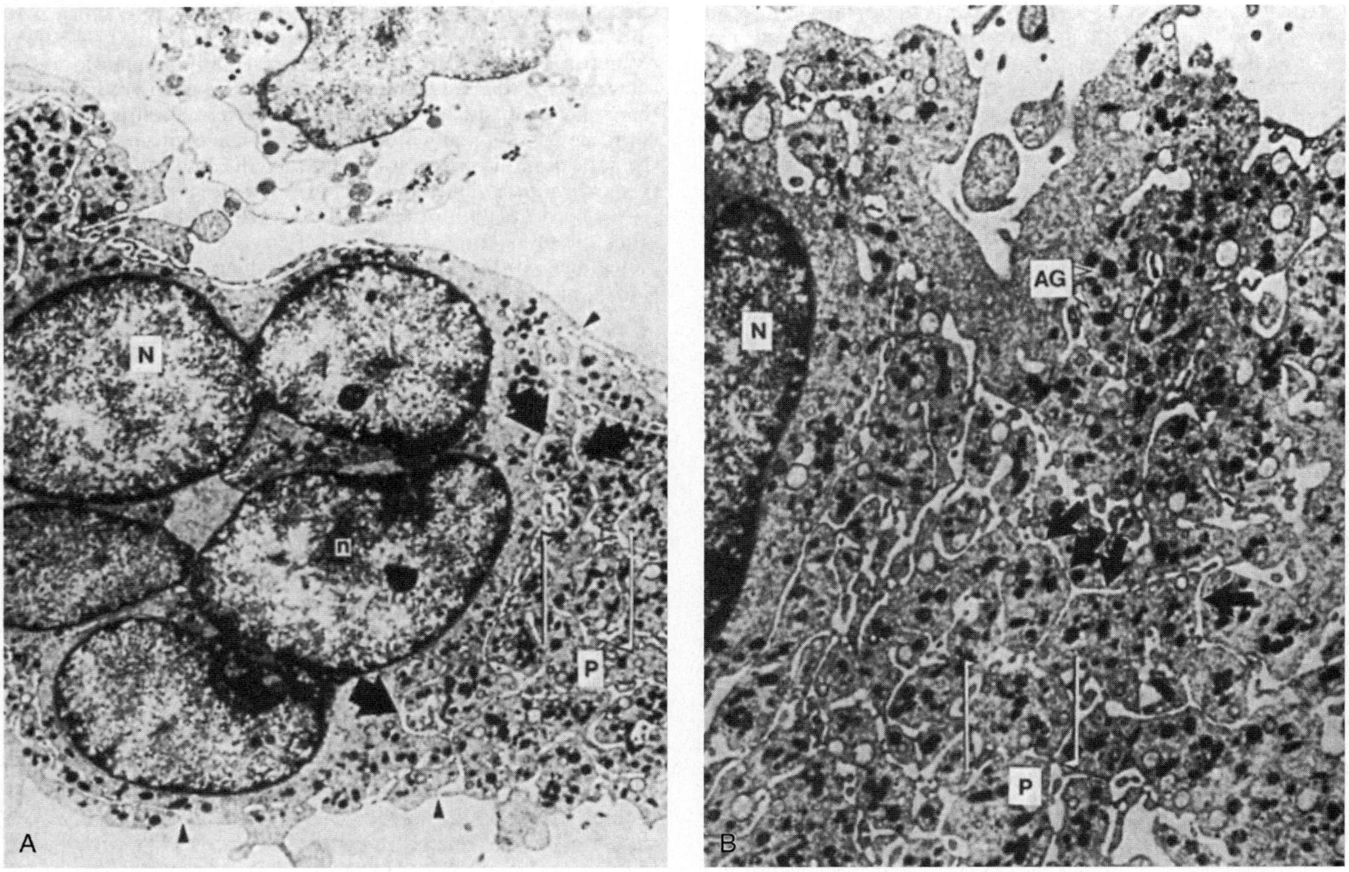

Figure 26-3 MATURE HUMAN MEGAKARYOCYTE ULTRASTRUCTURE. **A** and **B,** Transmission electron micrographs of two stage III and IV human megakaryocytes. *AG,* α-granules; *n,* nucleolus; *N,* nucleus; *P,* a platelet field within the megakaryocyte cytoplasm; *arrowheads,* openings of the demarcation membrane system (DMS). *(Courtesy Dr. Maryann Weller.)*

with the extracellular space. Whole cell patch-clamp studies in living rat megakaryocytes show that they are electrophysiologically contiguous with the plasma membrane. The open canalicular system (OCS) of platelets shares many features of the megakaryocyte DMS and may represent a remnant of this structure. The DMS serves as a vast membrane reservoir for proplatelet and platelet formation. The DTS of megakaryocytes is distinct from the DMS. Unlike the DMS, it fails to stain with surface membrane tracer dyes, indicating a lack of communication with the plasma membrane. The DTS is thought to be a site of platelet prostaglandin synthesis.

Ontogeny of Megakaryopoiesis

Hematopoiesis develops in distinct waves during embryonic development.[5] In mammals, the first hematopoietic progenitors are found in blood islands of the yolk sac. These give rise to a distinct population of large erythrocytes, termed *primitive erythrocytes,* which express unique globin genes and retain their nucleus longer than adult-type or "definitive" erythrocytes. "Definitive" hematopoiesis arises later during embryogenesis from hematopoietic stem cells that develop de novo from the ventral aspect of the dorsal aorta in the aorto-gonad-mesonephros (AGM) region. These then seed the fetal liver, which serves as a major site of hematopoiesis during gestation. Eventually, hematopoiesis shifts to the bone marrow (and spleen in mice), where it is sustained postnatally.

Megakaryocyte progenitors have been detected in yolk sac as early as embryonic day 7.5 (e7.5) of mouse development.[6] They are capable of generating proplatelets and platelets after in vitro culture. Circulating platelets have been detected in the mouse embryo as early as e10.5. Megakaryocytes cultured from early yolk sac have features somewhat distinct from those cultured from adult bone marrow, such as lower modal ploidy, smaller size, different cytokine requirements, and faster kinetics of platelet generation. These unique progenitors disappear by e13.5. In addition, mixed erythroid-megakaryocyte colonies derived from the early yolk sac give rise to primitive erythrocytes. It has therefore been suggested that a separate wave of "primitive megakaryocytes," akin to "primitive erythrocytes," exists during early yolk sac stages of hematopoiesis. These rapidly maturing megakaryocytes may prevent hemorrhage from the developing vasculature until definitive hematopoiesis is available to provide a steady supply of platelets.

Several pieces of evidence suggest that fetal liver megakaryocytes also have unique features compared with adult bone marrow–derived megakaryocytes.[7] This could be due to either intrinsic differences in the progenitors, or possibly their interactions with a distinct microenvironment. Megakaryocytes that develop from murine neonatal liver progenitors after transplantation into myeloablated mouse recipients are smaller and have lower ploidy levels than those derived from transplanted adult bone marrow. However, these differences are no longer apparent 1 month after transplant. In addition, several congenital disorders of megakaryopoiesis in humans, such as Down syndrome transient myeloproliferative disorder (DS-TMD) and thrombocytopenia with absent radii (TAR) resolve spontaneously after the newborn period, suggesting specific effects on fetal megakaryocytopoiesis (see additional discussion of GATA1 mutations in DS-TMD later). It is possible that these differences account for the delayed platelet engraftment often observed when umbilical cord blood is used as a graft for allogeneic stem cell transplantation for humans.

Platelet Biogenesis

It has been estimated that each megakaryocyte produces between a few hundred to several thousand platelets. The exact mechanism by which this occurs has been controversial, with several competing models proposed in the past. It was initially suggested that the DMS established platelet fields, which defined territories of prepackaged platelet contents. These fields would generate platelets directly upon breakdown of the megakaryocyte cytoplasm. However, prevailing evidence supports an alternate model in which platelets are released from dynamic megakaryocyte pseudopod extensions called *proplatelets.* This model was first proposed by Becker and DeBruyn in 1976 and supported by ultrastructural studies later in the 1980s. Italiano and associates extended these earlier studies on proplatelet formation and platelet biogenesis using videomicroscopy of cultured murine megakaryocytes[8] (see Chapter 126). These in vitro experiments demonstrate that platelet biogenesis begins with a reorganization of unique cortical microtubules within the megakaryocyte to produce large pseudopodia structures from one pole of the megakaryocyte. This spreads across the megakaryocyte generating extensions that elongate into complex branching tubular proplatelet processes. During this time, organelles travel along microtubules within the shafts of the proplatelets and are loaded into the proplatelet tips where they are captured.[9] It is only at the tips of the proplatelet processes that platelets are shed. During proplatelet formation, extensive remodeling and branching occurs, allowing for marked amplification of proplatelet ends. This phenomenon likely accounts for the ability of each megakaryocyte to generate such a large number of platelets. The DMS serves as an extensive membrane reservoir for these processes.[10] Proplatelet formation is regulated by a pathway involving Rho GTPase proteins, Rho-associated kinase (ROCK), and the *MYH9* gene product myosin IIA.[11]

Bone Marrow Spatial Cues and Megakaryocyte Maturation

There is mounting evidence that the proliferation and terminal maturation of megakaryocyte progenitors occur in distinct spatial compartments within the bone marrow (see Chapter 9). In a simplified model, the bone marrow space can be conceptually divided into distinct regions, a space adjacent to the cortical bone (an "osteoblastic niche"), an intermediate zone, and a "vascular niche" containing sinusoidal vessels lined with specialized bone marrow endothelial cells (BMECs). HSCs are thought to reside in a quiescent state adjacent to the bone. Under appropriate conditions, they are recruited to generate hematopoietic multipotent progenitor cells, which leave the osteoblastic niche, perhaps in part under the regulation of metalloproteinases such as MMP-9. The multipotent progenitors are then subject to expansion and lineage commitment under the influence of various cytokines and likely other signaling molecules. This is where TPO is postulated to affect megakaryocyte progenitor proliferation and survival. Rafii and coworkers have shown that the chemokines stromal derived factor-1 (SDF-1; also called CXCL12) and fibroblast growth factor-4 (FGF-4) promote migration and attachment of murine megakaryocyte progenitor cells (which express the receptor for SDF-1, CXCR4) to the vascular endothelium, where they physically attach, mature, and produce intercalating pseudopod structures.[12] In fact, exogenous SDF-1 and FGF-4 restores thrombopoiesis in $TPO^{-/-}$ or TPO receptor $(c\text{-}Mpl)^{-/-}$ mice to near wild-type levels. This occurs in the absence of enhanced megakaryocyte progenitor proliferation and requires direct physical interaction with BMECs. Based on these findings, Rafii and colleagues have proposed a model in which megakaryocyte progenitors proliferate in an immature developmental state (in response to TPO) in a nonvascular niche (Fig. 26-4). However, once the progenitors reach and adhere to the sinusoidal vessels in the vascular niche in response to chemokines (Fig. 26-5), proliferation ceases and terminal maturation and platelet release ensues. Work from other investigators supports this model. Multiple electron microscopic studies have captured megakaryocytes extending proplatelet processes through vascular endothelium and into bone marrow sinusoids, and a recent in vivo imaging study documented this process in living mice.[13] Isolated megakaryocytes can be induced to form proplatelets after adhering to bovine corneal endothelial cells-derived extracellular matrix or via binding of the megakaryocyte surface integrin $\alpha IIb\beta 3$ to fibrinogen, which is present in bone marrow vascular sinusoids. Conversely, culture of megakaryocytes with bone marrow stromal cells inhibits megakaryocyte differentiation.

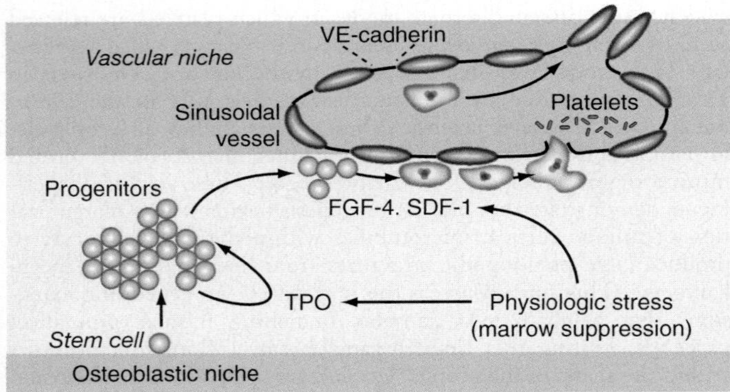

Figure 26-4 MODEL OF TERMINAL MATURATION OF MEGAKARYOCYTES AT THE BONE MARROW VASCULAR SINUSOID. Schematic diagram showing hematopoietic stem cells (HSCs) located predominantly adjacent to the cortical bone ("osteoblast niche"), megakaryocyte progenitors proliferating in the bone marrow space, and migration of progenitor cells to the vascular sinusoid ("vascular niche") under the influence of chemokines such as SDF-1 and fibroblast growth factor 4 (FGF-4). Once attached to the sinusoidal vascular endothelium, megakaryocyte progenitors cease proliferating, undergo terminal maturation and proplatelet formation, and shed platelets into the vascular sinusoidal space. *(From Avecilla ST, Hattori K, Heissig B, et al: Chemokine-mediated interaction of hematopoietic progenitors with the bone marrow vascular niche is required for thrombopoiesis,* Nat Med *10:64, 2004. Reproduced with permission.)*

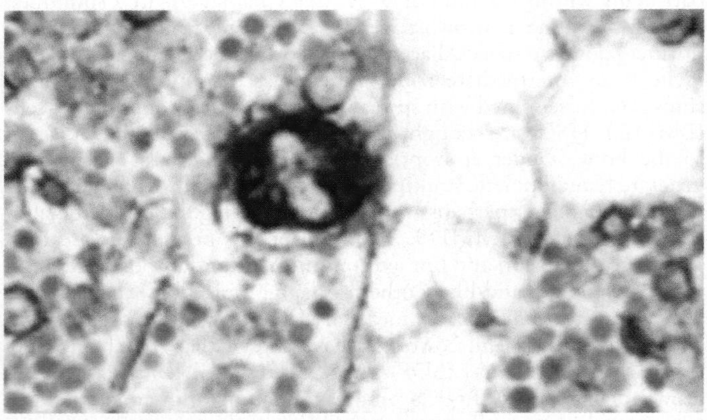

Figure 26-5 MEGAKARYOCYTE ATTACHED TO SINUSOIDAL VASCULAR ENDOTHELIUM. Bone core biopsy with megakaryocyte (stained with CD31) attached to the endothelium of a sinusoidal vessel *(right)*.

CYTOKINE REGULATION OF THROMBOCYTOPOIESIS

Thrombopoietin Signaling

Thrombopoietin

It has been estimated that an adult human produces nearly 2×10^{11} platelets per day, and this number can increase four- to eight-fold during times of increased demand.[14] The regulation of this process has been the subject of intense investigation. Kelemen first used the term *thrombopoietin* in 1958 to describe a humoral substance responsible for enhancing platelet production following the onset of thrombocytopenia. However, it was not until 1994 that five independent groups succeeded in purifying and cloning the responsible cytokine, now known as thrombopoietin (TPO) (previously referred to as *c-Mpl ligand, megakaryocyte growth and development factor [MGDF],* and *megapoietin*).[15] The gene for thrombopoietin is located on

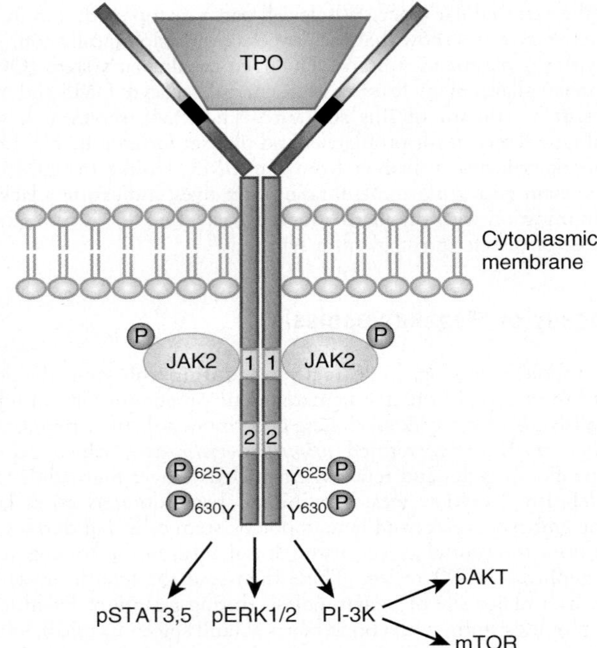

Figure 26-6 THE THROMBOPOIETIN RECEPTOR. Schematic diagram of the TPO receptor depicted as a homodimer with TPO bound. Binding of JAK2 at box 1 of the cytoplasmic tail is shown. Conformational changes in the TPO receptor upon TPO binding results in juxtaposition of the two cytoplasmic tails, as well as JAK2 autophosphorylation and JAK2-mediated phosphorylation of the c-Mpl cytoplasmic tail (Tyr^{625} and Tyr^{630}). Activation of STAT, ERK, phosphoinositol-3 kinase (PI-3K)-Akt, and PI3K- mTOR signaling pathways then occurs. *(Modified from Geddis AE: Megakaryopoiesis,* Semin Hematol *47:212, 2010.)*

chromosome 3q27. It encodes a 30 kDa glycoprotein of 353 amino acids that can be divided into two structural domains: an amino terminal region with homology to human erythropoietin, and a carboxyl terminal region that contains multiple N- and O-linked oligosaccharides. The amino terminal 155 residues of human thrombopoietin share 21% sequence identity and 46% overall sequence similarity to human erythropoietin. This region mediates binding to the TPO receptor (c-Mpl). The carboxyl region does not share sequence homology with any known protein. Thrombopoietin is reported to enhance multiple stages of megakaryocyte maturation, including cell size, cell ploidy, and platelet production. The predominant sites of TPO production are the liver and kidney, which secrete it constitutively. Inducible expression of TPO has been detected by more sensitive methods in bone marrow stroma and spleen in the setting of thrombocytopenia, although this likely accounts for only a minor fraction of total TPO production. Low-level expression has also been reported in the amygdala and hippocampus of the brain.

Thrombopoietin Receptor (c-Mpl)

The receptor for TPO (TPO receptor; c-Mpl) is the normal homologue of the oncogene v-Mpl, the transforming gene of murine myeloproliferative leukemia virus. It is a 635 amino acid protein that contains a number of distinct functional domains: a 25 amino acid signal peptide, a 465 amino acid extracellular domain, a 22 residue transmembrane domain, and an intracellular domain that contains two conserved motifs, termed *box 1* and *box 2* (Fig. 26-6). The extracellular domain contains of a distal region that negatively influences TPO signaling. It is a member of the type I cytokine receptor superfamily. Like the erythropoietin receptor, it is thought to function as a homodimer. The TPO receptor is expressed on megakaryocyte progenitors, as well as earlier multipotential progenitors, including MEPs, CMPs, and HSCs. TPO receptors are present on the surface of platelets at an estimated density of 20 to 200 receptors per platelet and bind TPO with an affinity of 200 to 560 pM. Binding of TPO to platelets plays an important role in the regulation of total body platelet mass by the TPO-TPO receptor system. Both TPO receptor$^{-/-}$ (c-Mpl$^{-/-}$) and TPO (TPO$^{-/-}$) knock-out mice contain ≈85% to 90% lower platelet and megakaryocyte numbers as compared with wild-type mice.[16,17] The structure of the megakaryocytes and platelets in these animals is normal, reinforcing the notion that TPO signaling plays an important role in expansion and development of megakaryocyte progenitors, but not in terminal maturation and proplatelet release. In addition, the residual platelet production in these mice suggests alternate cytokine, or possibly cytokine-independent, pathways for thrombocytopoiesis. Interbreeding experiments of TPO receptor$^{-/-}$ mice with knock-out mice for IL-3, IL-6, IL-11, or LIF or their receptors, show that these other cytokines are not responsible for the residual platelet production.

TPO Receptor Downstream Signaling Pathways

The TPO receptor lacks intrinsic tyrosine kinase activity. Instead, ligand binding is thought to induce a conformational change in the homodimeric receptor and stimulates the cytoplasmic tyrosine kinase JAK2 (Janus-kinase 2), which binds to box 1 of the cytoplasmic tail. This results in tyrosine phosphorylation of multiple targets, including STATs (signal transducers and activators of transcription), Shc adaptor protein, and the TPO receptor itself (Tyr^{625} and Tyr^{630}).[18] Additional signaling pathways activated upon TPO receptor engagement include the mitogen-activated protein kinase (MAPK) p38, p42/p44 extracellular signal-regulated kinase 1 (ERK1/ERK2), phosphoinositol-3-kinase-AKT (PI3K-AKT), and PI3K-Mammalian target of rapamycin (mTOR) signaling pathways.

Several of these downstream signaling pathways have been shown to be functionally important in TPO-mediated effects on megakaryocytopoiesis. Double STAT5a/STAT5b–deficient mice have impaired platelet production as well as defects in early multipotent progenitor cells. Moreover, megakaryocyte-selective overexpression of a dominant negative mutant STAT3 in transgenic mice reduces platelet recovery following 5-fluorouracil–induced myelosuppression. These findings suggest a functional role for STAT family members in thrombopoiesis.

Studies in primary megakaryocytes show a requirement for PI3-AKT signaling in TPO-induced cell cycling. This involves silencing of the Forkhead O (FOXO) family of transcription factors. Activation of the p42/p44-MAPK plays an important role in TPO-induced maturation and endomitosis. The mTOR signaling pathway is involved in TPO-mediated megakaryocytic progenitor proliferation and possibly terminal megakaryocyte size determination, ploidy, and cellular maturation.[19]

Negative Regulation of TPO Signaling

As with other receptor-mediated signaling processes, feedback mechanisms exist to limit or turn off the signal once initiated to avoid uncontrolled growth. Lnk, an adaptor protein implicated in immunoreceptor and cytokine receptor signaling negatively modulates TPO signaling in megakaryocytes. Overexpression of Lnk decreases TPO-dependent megakaryocyte growth and polyploidization in bone marrow (BM)–derived cultures. Conversely, loss of Lnk expression by gene targeting results in increased numbers of megakaryocytes, accentuated megakaryocyte polyploidization, and a myeloproliferative disorder in mice.[20] This correlates with enhanced and prolonged TPO-mediated induction of STAT3, STAT5, AKT, and MAPK signaling pathways.

Following TPO binding, the TPO receptor is internalized and subsequently degraded. This process depends on dileucine repeats, and Tyr^{591} and Tyr^{625} within the TPO receptor cytoplasmic tail, and involves ubiquitinylation via the E3 ubiquitin ligase c-Cbl.

TPO Signaling in Hematopoietic Stem Cells

It has recently been recognized that the TPO-TPO receptor signaling system is not only important for megakaryocyte proliferation and development, but also plays a role in hematopoietic stem cell survival, self-renewal, and expansion.[21] TPO receptor$^{-/-}$ HSCs compete poorly with wild-type HSCs, even at a ratio of 10:1, in murine bone marrow competitive repopulation studies. The role of TPO signaling in HSC expansion is in part due to its activation of the homeobox domain containing transcription factor HOXA9, via a mechanism involving phosphorylation and nuclear translocation of its partner protein MEIS1.

Congenital Amegakaryocytic Thrombocytopenia

Bi-allelic mutations in the TPO receptor gene cause congenital amegakaryocytic thrombocytopenia (CAMT) (see Chapter 27). In this disorder, megakaryocytes are absent or greatly diminished in number in the bone marrow. Patients typically present shortly after birth with petechiae, bruising, or bleeding. Patients with severe CAMT are at high risk for developing progressive bone marrow failure, typically within the first few years of life. This is consistent with a role of TPO signaling in maintaining hematopoietic stems cells and/or multipotential progenitor cells. Of interest, no mutations in the gene encoding TPO itself have been reported in patients with CAMT. It should also be noted that in contrast to the humans, TPO receptor$^{-/-}$ (as well as TPO$^{-/-}$) mice do not develop bone marrow failure states. The reason for this discrepancy is not known, but it highlights important differences between human and mouse hematopoiesis.

Essential Thrombocythemia

Essential thrombocythemia (ET) is a chronic myeloproliferative neoplasm associated with sustained excessive megakaryocyte hyperproliferation, thrombocytosis, and abnormal platelet function leading to either hemorrhage or thrombosis (see Chapter 68). In 2005, an acquired activating mutation in the JAK2 family (V617F JAK2) was identified by four independent groups in a large proportion (≈50%) of patients with ET. The identical mutation has also been identified in several other myeloproliferative neoplasms, including polycythemia vera (95% of patients) and primary myelofibrosis (50% of patients). How the identical mutation leads to distinct clinical entities is not well understood but may be related to the allelic dosage of the mutation. Mutations leading to constitutive activation of the TPO receptor or enhanced translation efficiency of the TPO gene have also been reported in rare cases of familial thrombocytosis. These two classes of disorders can be distinguished by measuring circulating TPO levels, which are elevated with mutations enhancing TPO mRNA translation efficiency, and decreased with mutations leading to constitutive TPO receptor activation (see Chapter 68).

Regulation of Platelet Mass by Thrombopoietin

Platelet counts are typically held at a relatively fixed level in humans, ranging from 150,000 to 400,000/mm^3. The maintenance of platelet number by the TPO-TPO receptor system involves an unusual homeostatic mechanism among hematopoietic cytokine-mediated regulation. This is sometimes referred to as the "sponge" model (Fig. 26-7). Unlike other cytokines, TPO is secreted predominantly in a constitutive manner, mostly from the liver and kidney. High affinity TPO receptors present on the platelet surface bind free TPO and internalize it, where it is degraded. Therefore, when platelet counts are low, less TPO is removed, and more is available to stimulate megakaryocytopoiesis in the bone marrow. Conversely, when platelet counts rise above a given set point, they act as a "sink" for TPO, binding and destroying it before it can stimulate megakaryocytopoiesis in the bone marrow. Thus total platelet mass is preserved,

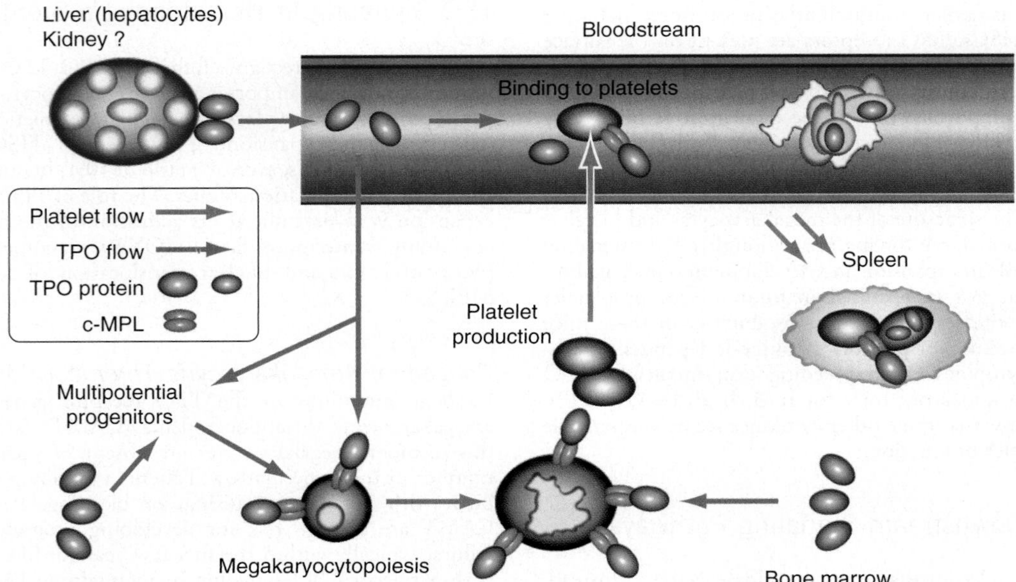

Figure 26-7 REGULATION OF PLATELET COUNT BY THROMBOPOIETIN: THE "SPONGE" MODEL. Thrombopoietin is secreted at a constitutive rate primarily from liver, and perhaps other sources such as the kidney, into the circulation. There it binds with high affinity to TPO receptors (c-Mpl) present on the surface of platelets. The TPO is then internalized by the platelets and degraded. Free TPO (i.e., TPO not bound to platelets) enters the bone marrow and stimulates megakaryocytopoiesis. Thus in the presence of high platelet counts, little free TPO is available to stimulate megakaryocytopoiesis. Conversely, low platelet numbers lead to increased free TPO and active megakaryocytopoiesis. The net result is preservation of total platelet mass.

rather than absolute platelet number. This may explain the mild-moderate thrombocytopenia seen in certain disorders associated with large platelets, such as Bernard-Soulier syndrome (BSS).

Several pieces of evidence support this model. First, it has been known for over 40 years that the peripheral blood platelet count varies inversely with plasma TPO activity. Second, TPO receptor deficient mice (c-Mpl$^{-/-}$) have elevated levels of circulating TPO, and this is reduced when the mice are transfused with washed platelets from normal mice. Third, in contrast to platelets from TPO receptor–deficient mice, platelets from normal mice bind purified radiolabeled TPO and degrade it. Fourth, TPO levels are low to intermediate in normal individuals and in those with idiopathic thrombocytopenic purpura (where the bound TPO is destroyed along with the platelets). However, following chemotherapy, or in individuals with aplastic anemia, levels are markedly elevated.

Although the model described above likely explains the predominant basal regulation of platelet number by the TPO-TPO receptor signaling system, overlying inducible mechanisms also probably exist. It has been shown that the TPO gene is transcriptionally activated in bone marrow stroma and spleen during times of thrombocytopenia, although the degree to which this may contribute to total TPO levels is uncertain. In addition, IL-6 mediates up regulation of hepatic TPO mRNA transcripts in inflammation-related thrombocytosis.

Additional Cytokines Involved in Megakaryocytopoiesis

Although TPO is the major cytokine regulating megakaryocytopoiesis, other cytokines have been shown to be active in vitro, particularly during earlier stages of megakaryocyte development. These include SCF, IL-3, IL-6, IL-11, leukemia inhibitory factor (LIF), G-CSF, and erythropoietin (EPO). None of these factors are megakaryocyte-specific, but act as synergistic co-regulators with TPO. Only SCF and TPO have been shown to affect megakaryocyte development and platelet production in vivo using genetic ablation experiments in mice. No effects were seen with knockout of IL-3, IL-6, IL-11 receptor, or LIF.

Therapeutic Cytokine Stimulation of Megakaryocytopoiesis

Since the identification of TPO as a major activator of megakaryocyte growth and maturation, there has been considerable interest in developing recombinant forms of TPO for clinical use in the treatment of chemotherapy-related thrombocytopenia and immune-mediated thrombocytopenia. Small pilot studies using a polyethyleneglycol (PEG)ylated, truncated form of human TPO (PEG-MGDF) showed activity in stimulating megakaryocyte growth and maturation, resulting in elevated platelet counts. However, some recipients subsequently developed thrombocytopenia as a result of the generation of a neutralizing anti-TPO antibody that cross-reacted with endogenous TPO. The agent was therefore withdrawn from further testing. Since then, several nonimmunogenic thrombopoietic peptides and small, nonpeptide molecules have been developed.[22] Romiplostim (formerly called *AMG 531*), a synthetic molecule consisting of an immunoglobulin Fc domain fragment linked to two identical peptide chains that activate the TPO receptor, stimulates platelet production and has been approved by the Food and Drug Administration (FDA) for the treatment of adults with chronic immune thrombocytopenia purpura (ITP). It is given intravenously or subcutaneously. Eltrombopag, an orally administered small molecule that binds to a portion of the TPO receptor distinct from the normal TPO binding site, also stimulates thrombopoiesis and is FDA approved for the treatment of chronic ITP. Additional agents that stimulate the TPO receptor are also under development.

IL-11 has multiple effects on in vivo and in vitro megakaryocytopoiesis. It affects IL-3–dependent megakaryocyte colony formation and has a potent effect on megakaryocyte maturation. Administration of recombinant IL-11 to mice results in increased numbers of megakaryocyte progenitors, increased megakaryocyte polyploidization, and increased peripheral platelet counts. Recombinant IL-11 has been approved for use in humans for the treatment of chemotherapy-induced thrombocytopenia.

ENDOMITOSIS

The Endomitotic Cell Cycle

Megakaryocytes derive their name from their large and complex nuclei. This arises from an atypical cell cycle, termed the *endomitotic* cell cycle (see comprehensive review by Ravid and colleagues[23]) (Fig. 26-8). Like normal diploid cells, the cycle begins with a G1 phase, followed by S phase (DNA replication), and a G2 phase. The cells then enter M phase, but unlike normal diploid mitotic cells, fail to complete anaphase B, telophase, or cytokinesis. A cleavage furrow initially develops but then regresses. The cells then proceed directly to the next G1 phase and subsequent rounds of DNA replication. As DNA ploidy increases, multiple spindle poles and centrosomes form, but chromosome segregation is incomplete and asymmetric. During each endomitotic cell cycle (Fig. 26-9), the nuclear envelope breaks down and later reforms as a single nuclear membrane around all of the sister chromatids. The end result is a polyploid cell with a multilobulated nuclei encapsulated by a single nuclear membrane. Mature human megakaryocytes have been observed to reach ploidy levels as high as 128N. The term *endoreduplication* has at times been used

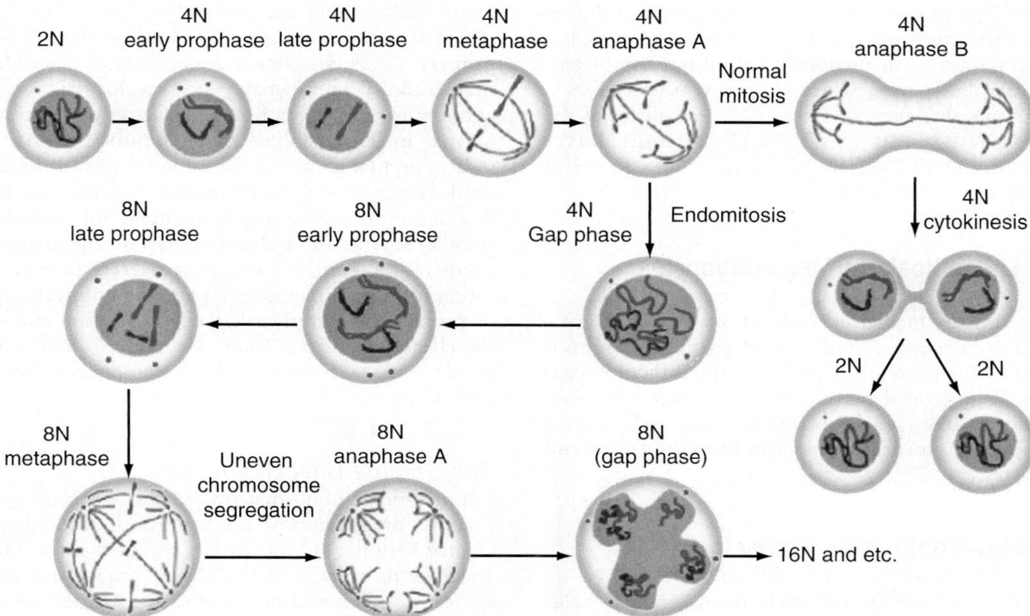

Figure 26-8 THE ENDOMITOTIC CYCLE IN MEGAKARYOCYTES. Schematic diagram depicting stages of the cell cycle in cells undergoing endomitosis *(bottom left)* versus normal mitosis *(right)*. Endomitotic and mitotic cells share all stages of the cell cycle until anaphase A. Normal mitotic cells proceed through anaphase B and complete cytokinesis, yielding two daughter cells, each with 2N DNA content. In contrast, endomitotic cells fail to undergo anaphase B or cytokinesis, and proceed to the next cycle following a gap phase. Subsequent rounds produce multicentric spindles with uneven chromosome segregation. A single nuclear membrane *(shown in pink)* reforms after each round of endomitosis. Centrosomes are shown as *blue dots. (From Ravid K, Lu J, Zimmet JM, et al: Roads to polyploidy: The megakaryocyte example,* J Cell Physiol *190:7, 2002. Reproduced by permission.)*

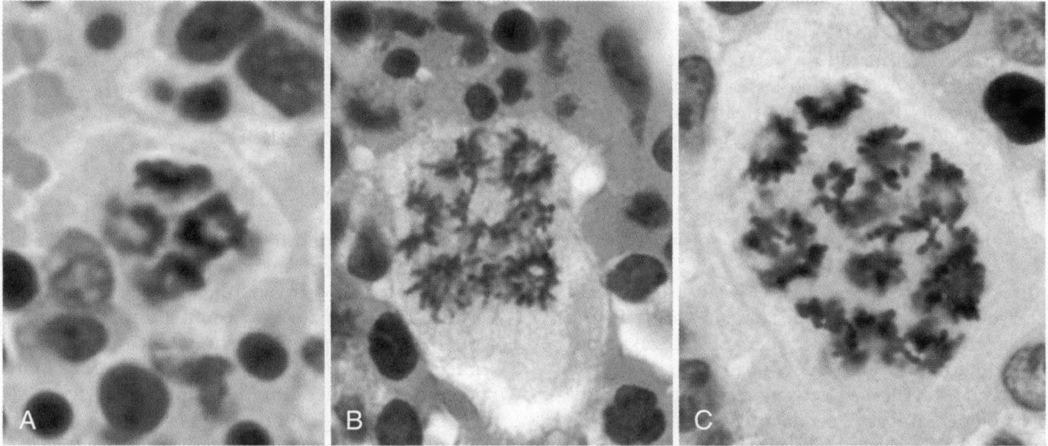

Figure 26-9 MEGAKARYOCYTES IN ENDOMITOSIS. Polyploid megakaryocytes in endomitosis at 8N stage **(A)**, 16N stage **(B)**, and probably 32N stage **(C)**.

erroneously to describe megakaryocyte polyploidization. *Endoreduplication* correctly refers to a cell cycle that involves DNA replication but no entry into M phase.

Role of Endomitosis in Thrombocytopoiesis

The reason that megakaryocytes undergo endomitosis is not known. It has been speculated that it provides a means for generating the abundant membrane, protein, biosynthetic cargo, and energy required for the dramatic final stages of proplatelet elaboration and platelet release. Several circumstantial pieces of evidence support this model. First, it is known that megakaryocyte DNA content correlates with megakaryocyte cell size, mRNA content, protein production, and eventual numbers of platelets released. Second, an increased DNA content of megakaryocytes precedes increases in platelet count during recovery from acute thrombocytopenia. Third, increases in cytoplasmic volume and maturation occur predominantly, if not completely, in stage II and III megakaryocytes, which do not synthesize DNA. Fourth, in polyploid megakaryocytes (4N to 32N), all alleles of the genes studied (i.e., ITGA2B [GPIIb], VWF, ACTB [β-actin], HSPA1 [HSP70], MPL, FLI1, and ZFPM1 [FOG-1]) have been found to be transcriptionally active.

Mechanisms of Endomitosis in Megakaryocytes

The molecular mechanisms mediating endomitosis in megakaryocytes are incompletely understood. Studies investigating endomitosis have been hampered by the rarity of megakaryocytes, difficulty separating direct effects from general perturbations of cell maturation, complications associated with synchronizing the cell cycle, use of transformed cell lines, and potential differences between rodent and human megakaryocytes.

Cyclins and Cyclin-Dependent Kinases

Two classes of proteins control the cell cycle in mammalian cells. These are the cyclins, so named for their cyclical synthesis and degradation during the cell cycle, and cell division kinases (Cdks, also known as *cyclin-dependent kinases*). Together, these two families of proteins form a protein-kinase complex in which the regulatory unit is the cyclin and the catalytic unit is the Cdk. The role of these kinase complexes in cell cycle control is complex. At least seven members of the cyclin gene family and seven distinct Cdk genes have been identified.

Given the importance of cyclins and Cdks in controlling cell cycle, they have been the focus of considerable attention in investigations of the mechanisms underlying megakaryocyte endomitosis. The most compelling evidence probably exists for a role of the D-type cyclins in megakaryocyte endomitosis. The D-type cyclins are unique in that their activity can be modulated by extracellular mitogens. Megakaryocytes express cyclin D3 and, to a lesser extent, cyclin D1. Levels of both of these factors increase after treatment with TPO. Overexpression of cyclin D3 results in increased megakaryocyte ploidy in transgenic mouse models. Complexes of cyclin D3 and its major kinase subunit, Cdk2, show high kinase activity in polyploid cells. Antisense knockdown of cyclin D3 levels suppresses endomitosis and abrogates normal development of primary mouse megakaryocytes.

Cyclin D1 is a direct target gene of GATA1, a transcription factor required for megakaryocyte polyploidization and maturation. Overexpression of cyclin D1 in transgenic mice increases megakaryocyte modal ploidy compared with nontransgenic littermates, and the combination of cyclin D1 and Cdk4 kinase activity restores polyploidization of GATA1-deficient murine megakaryocytes. Conversely, enforced expression of $p16^{ink4a}$, a cell cycle inhibitor of Cdk4/6, blocks polyploidization in murine megakaryocytes. $p16^{ink4a}$ is also potently repressed by GATA1.

Cyclin $E^{-/-}$ mice have impaired megakaryocytopoiesis with reduced modal ploidy. These mice also have defective trophoblast development, another tissue characterized by endomitosis. Cyclin B1/CDC2 is a mitotic cyclin complex. Yeast strains deficient in cyclin B1 or CDC2 undergo an additional round of DNA replication without cytokinesis. Several studies have shown that low levels of cyclin B1/CDC2 are required for progression of endomitosis in megakaryocytic cell lines. However, studies of primary megakaryocytes have shown normal cyclin B1 and CDC2 levels and functional mitotic activity during endomitosis.

Other Mitotic Kinases

Aurora-B kinase (also called *AIM-1 kinase*) is involved in late anaphase and cytokinesis, and mRNA transcript levels of Aurora-B kinase have been reported to decrease during polyploidization of primary megakaryocytes and megakaryocytic cell lines. This suggests that Aurora-B kinase may play a mechanistic role in megakaryocyte endomitosis. However, functional activity of Aurora-B kinase appears normal in late anaphase of endomitotic primary megakaryocytes, indicating that simple deficiency of Aurora-B kinase activation is an unlikely mechanism to explain endomitosis. Polo-like kinase (PLK-1) is a serine-threonine kinase required for assembly of the mitotic spindle, separation of chromosomes during anaphase, and exit from mitosis. PLK-1 mRNA and protein levels decrease during polyploidization of murine megakaryocytes, and enforced expression of PLK-1 in primary murine megakaryocytes impairs endomitosis. However, the effects of overexpression are modest, preferentially affect lower-ploidy megakaryocytes, and are complicated by alterations in cell cycle kinetics.

The Spindle Checkpoint

During mitosis of normal diploid cells, a spindle assembly checkpoint prevents progression of anaphase until all of the chromosomes are aligned with the mitotic spindle and each sister chromatid is properly attached to spindle microtubules originating from the opposing spindle pole. This ensures that each daughter cell receives the proper complement of chromosomes. The anaphase-promoting complex (APC) is a multisubunit protein complex with ubiquitin ligase activity that regulates chromosome segregation and anaphase progression by targeting key factors for degradation. Since some chromosomal missegregation occurs during megakaryocyte endomitosis, several groups have examined the expression levels and/or activity of certain APC components and associated factors. These studies have shown no significant difference in protein levels of the core APC protein CDC27 or the kinetochore-associated signaling protein hsMAD2 in primary murine megakaryocytes undergoing polyploidization compared with nonendomitotic precursors. Haploinsufficiency of BUBR1, a key component of the spindle checkpoint, perturbs megakaryocyte development and polyploidization in mice, but does not cause alterations in circulating platelet counts.

Microtubule Regulation

Microtubules play key roles in mitosis. Therefore factors that regulate their assembly have also been investigated as candidates involved in megakaryocyte endomitosis. PRC-1 is involved in mitotic spindle elongation and cytokinesis. However, no differences in PRC-1 levels were detected in primary murine megakaryocytes undergoing polyploidization compared with nonendomitotic precursors. Stathmin is a microtubule-depolymerizing factor that plays an important role in regulation of the mitotic spindle. Levels of stathmin are inversely related to the level of ploidy of megakaryocytic cell lines and primary megakaryocytes. Inhibition of stathmin in K562 cells increases their propensity to undergo endomitosis when induced to differentiate into megakaryocytes, and overexpression of stathmin prevents the transition from mitotic to endomitotic cell cycles. Together, these findings support a possible role of stathmin in modulating endomitosis.

Contractile Ring Activity

Cytokinesis requires the assembly and activity of a contractile ring. The failure to complete cytokinesis during endomitotic cell cycles in megakaryocytes may involve functional defects in the Rho/Rock pathway.[24] Further studies will be required to fully dissect the molecular pathways involved in megakaryocyte endomitosis.

TRANSCRIPTIONAL CONTROL OF MEGAKARYOCYTOPOIESIS

Since platelets do not contain nuclei, all transcriptional regulation of platelet-specific genes must occur at the level of the megakaryocyte. Significant strides have been made recently in identifying key transcription factors involved in megakaryocyte development and platelet-specific gene expression. Of note, mutations in several of these factors have been linked to various hematologic disorders providing significant new insights into the pathogenesis of these diseases (see Chapters 4 and 152; see also box on Inherited Causes of Thrombocytopenia.

GATA Family Transcription Factors

GATA1

GATA transcription factors comprise a family of zinc finger proteins that bind the consensus DNA sequence (T/A))GATA(A/G). There are six known members of the GATA family in vertebrates. GATA1, -2, -3 play roles predominantly, although not exclusively, within the hematopoietic system. GATA4, -5, and -6 are expressed in nonhematopoietic tissues and play diverse developmental roles within the cardiac, gastrointestinal, endocrine, and gonadal systems. Functionally important binding sites for GATA factors have been identified in cis-acting regulatory elements of essentially every megakaryocytic and erythroid gene that has been studied. GATA1, the founding member of this family, is highly expressed in erythroid and megakaryocytic cells and, to a lesser extent, in eosinophils and mast cells. GATA1 plays an essential role in erythroid development, with loss of function resulting in blocked erythroid maturation and apoptosis of erythroid progenitor cells. GATA1 is also required for megakaryocyte maturation and growth control. Lineage-selective loss of GATA1 in megakaryocytes results in marked thrombocytopenia in mice with platelet counts of only ≈15% of wild-type littermates. Megakaryocytes are present in the mutant animals but have a disorganized DMS, paucity of platelet-specific granules, reduced expression of multiple megakaryocyte-specific genes (including GPIbα, GPIbβ, PF4, c-Mpl, and p45 NF-E2), and marked hyperproliferation as compared with wild-type mice. Gene expression studies of GATA1-deficient versus wild-type murine megakaryocytes have revealed a large number of potential GATA1 target genes, although evidence for direct targets has only been established for a few. Mice containing reduced megakaryocyte-specific expression of GATA1 ($GATA1^{low}$) develop myelofibrosis as they age, a frequent finding with disorders of megakaryocyte progenitor hyperproliferation. A GATA binding site mutation in the GPIbβ promoter has been described in a patient with Bernard-Soulier syndrome, which is characterized by deficiency of the GPIb/IX/V complex and a bleeding diathesis. Taken together, these findings suggest that GATA1 acts as master regulator of megakaryocyte maturation and proliferative control.

> **Inherited Causes of Thrombocytopenia**
>
> Although the most common cause of thrombocytopenia is immune thrombocytopenic purpura (ITP), it is important to maintain a high index of clinical suspicion for inherited disorders of thrombocytopoiesis. This is a particular problem because ITP is essentially a diagnosis of exclusion, and many inherited disorders mimic the macrothrombocytopenia seen in ITP. Making the correct diagnosis early is paramount, since it may spare patients unnecessary treatment with corticosteroids, other immunosuppressants, and/or splenectomy. In addition, it may be important in guiding decisions about surveillance for myelodysplasia or leukemia, screening for additional associated clinical problems, and/or possible family planning. Obtaining a careful family history, and sometimes obtaining blood counts on first-degree relatives, is important in fully evaluating patients with chronic thrombocytopenia. Associated abnormalities may provide important clues to the presence of a nonimmune familial thrombocytopenia. For instance, associated erythroid abnormalities and/or an X-linked inheritance pattern (GATA1 mutations) (obligate female carriers may have dimorphic populations of platelets); leukocyte Döhle bodies, +/– nephritis and sensineural hearing loss (Myh9 mutations); family history of myelodysplasia or myeloid leukemia (RUNX1 mutations); developmental delay, congenital cardiac anomalies, hand/face dysmorphogenesis (Paris-Trousseau/Jacobsen syndrome; Fli-1 [ETS-1] mutations); bleeding diathesis out of proportion to degree of thrombocytopenia (Bernard-Soulier syndrome). Mutations in the 5-UTR of the ANKRD26 gene have been described in a large number of families with autosomal dominant macrothrombocytopenia. A superb review of inherited thrombocytopenias and an excellent diagnostic algorithm has been provided by Savoia and colleagues.[29]

Friend of GATA (FOG-1)

All vertebrate GATA factors contain two zinc fingers. The carboxyl zinc finger mediates high-affinity DNA binding, whereas the amino zinc finger stabilizes the DNA interaction at certain double GATA sites. Important to note, the amino zinc finger also interacts with Friend of GATA (FOG) proteins, a family of large multitype zinc finger transcriptional cofactors. This interaction occurs on the surface of the zinc finger opposite to its DNA binding surface. FOG-1 (also called zfpm1), the founding member, is expressed predominantly within erythroid and megakaryocytic cells. Knockout of FOG-1 in mice results in embryonic lethality caused by severe anemia from a block in erythroid maturation similar to that observed in $GATA1^{-}$ mice. In addition, $FOG\text{-}1^{-/-}$ mice have complete failure of megakaryocytopoiesis, establishing FOG-1 as the first identified transcription-associated factor selectively required to generate the entire megakaryocyte lineage. FOG-1's role in megakaryocyte and erythroid development requires direct physical interaction with GATA factors. The discrepancy between the relatively late block in megakaryocyte development seen in GATA1-deficient animals and the complete loss of megakaryocytopoiesis in $FOG\text{-}1^{-/-}$ mice is explained by overlapping FOG-dependent roles of GATA1 and GATA2 during early stages of megakaryocytopoiesis.

X-Linked Dyserythropoietic Anemia and Thrombocytopenia Due to GATA1 Mutations

Germline GATA1 mutations that impair binding to FOG-1 and/or DNA have been identified in several families with X-linked macrothrombocytopenia and/or anemia (GATA1 is located on the X chromosome in both humans and mice). The first case, reported by Weiss and colleagues, involved a woman with mild chronic thrombocytopenia who had two pregnancies with male offspring that were both complicated by severe fetal anemia and thrombocytopenia requiring in utero transfusions. Bone marrow examination after birth revealed marked dyserythropoiesis and an overabundance of immature-appearing, dysplastic megakaryocytes that share many of the features of GATA1^{low} murine megakaryocytes. Remarkably, sequencing of the GATA1 gene from affected family members identified substitution of valine by methionine at codon 205 within the amino zinc finger. This mutation (GATA1^{V205M}) significantly impairs FOG-1 binding, but retains normal DNA affinity based on electromobility shift assays using synthetic oligonucleotides. This is consistent with the location of this residue on the surface of the zinc finger opposite the DNA binding face.

Several other GATA1 mutations have been linked to cases of familial X-linked macrothrombocytopenia with or without anemia (Table 26-1). These substitutions all impair FOG-1 binding, although to different degrees. Substitution of glycine by serine at codon 208 (GATA1^{G208S}) results in moderate to severe thrombocytopenia and mild dyserythropoiesis, but no anemia. Substitution of the same residue by arginine (GATA1^{G208R}) results in thrombocytopenia with anemia and severe dyserythropoiesis. Similarly, substitution of aspartic acid by glycine at codon 218 (GATA1^{D218G}) leads only to thrombocytopenia, whereas substitution of this same codon by tyrosine (GATA1^{D218Y}) leads to severe thrombocytopenia, moderate anemia, and marked dyserythropoiesis. The severity of the phenotype appears to correlate with the degree of FOG-1 binding impairment, suggesting that megakaryocytic development is more sensitive to affinity changes in GATA1: FOG-1 interactions than is erythroid development.

X-Linked Thrombocytopenia and β-Thalassemia Due to GATA1 Mutations

Mutations mapping to the DNA binding surface of the amino zinc finger of GATA1 have also been described (GATA1^{R216Q}). As expected, this reduces DNA affinity to double (palindromic) GATA sites but not to single GATA sites. FOG-1 binding is not substantially altered. Affected family members exhibit an X-linked β-thalassemia syndrome characterized by imbalance of alpha and beta globin chain synthesis, reticulocytosis and hemolysis. They also have mild to moderate thrombocytopenia. In vitro platelet aggregation studies are normal, but there is a prolonged bleeding time. Substitution of the same residue by tryptophan (R216W) produces thrombocytopenia, β-thalassemia intermedia, and congenital erythropoietic porphyria (CEP). The CEP is likely due to dysregulation of the GATA1 target gene uroporphyrinogen III synthase.

X-Linked Gray Platelet-Like Syndrome

Gray platelet syndrome (GPS) refers to a disorder of large platelets with absent or markedly reduced α-granules and/or α-granule proteins. Platelets from individuals with GATA1^{Arg261Gln} share some features with classical GPS. Ultrastructural studies of platelets from a different family with GATA1-related X-linked macrothrombocytopenia (GATA1^{G208S}) also demonstrate hypogranular platelets that contain small vacuoles, likely representing membranes of empty α-granules. However, the GATA1 mutant platelets also possess unique features such as masses of dense tubular system channels, dense double membranes, and platelets within platelets, not seen in classical GPS, suggesting a more general disorder of platelet biogenesis.

GATA1 Mutations in Down Syndrome Transient Myeloproliferative Disorders and Acute Megakaryoblastic Leukemia

About 10% of children with Down syndrome (DS; trisomy 21) are born with a transient myeloproliferative disorder (TMD), which is

Table 26-1 Reported GATA1 Mutations in Hematologic Disease With Associated Clinical and Biochemical Features

Mutation	Thrombo-cytopenia	Platelet Features	Anemia	Erythroid Features	Other Features	FOG-1 Binding	DNA Binding
V205M	Severe	Large*	Severe; fetal hydrops	Dyserythropoiesis	Cryptorchidism	Markedly reduced	Normal
G208S	Moderate	Large; decreased platelet aggregation	None			Moderately reduced	Normal
G208R	Severe	Large*	Moderate	Dyserythropoiesis	Cryptorchidism†	Not studied	Not studied
D218G	Moderate	Large; decreased platelet aggregation	None	Dyserythropoiesis		Moderately reduced	Normal
D218Y	Severe	Large*	Severe		Platelets in carrier female expressed only WT allele	Markedly reduced	Normal
R216Q	Moderate	Large; normal platelet aggregation in vitro, but prolonged bleeding time; grey platelet syndrome	Mild	Mild β-thalassemia	Splenomegaly	Normal	Decreased
R216W	Moderate	*	Mild	Mild β-thalassemia	Congenital erythropoietic anemia	Not studied	Not studied
G332C‡	None	Decreased platelet aggregation; dysplastic megakaryocytes	Variable	Macrocytosis	Neutropenia	Not studied	Not studied

Adapted from GATA1-related X-linked cytopenia. Available at: http://www.genetests.org/profiles/gata1.
*Function not studied.
†Cryptorchidism also in two siblings with wild type GATA1.
‡Germline splice mutation results in exclusive production of the amino truncated GATA1s molecule.

characterized by an abundance of circulating erythromegakaryocytic precursor cells, pancytopenia, and in some cases, severe liver fibrosis. Remarkably, this myeloproliferation resolves spontaneously over the first few months of life. In about 20% to 30% of cases, Down syndrome–associated acute megakaryocytic leukemia (DS-AMKL) develops within a few years, sometimes preceded by a myelodysplastic phase. In 2002, Crispino and colleagues reported that DS-AMKL cells harbor acquired mutations in their GATA1 gene. Since then, several groups have reproduced these findings and identified similar mutations in DS-TMD cells.[25] Although a wide spectrum of mutations have been found, including missense, deletion, insertion, and splice-site mutations, they all involve exon 2 and result in the same outcome: generation of an amino terminal truncated protein (loss of amino acids 1-83) due to translation initiation from a downstream ATG codon (Fig. 26-10). This removes a region that functions as a transcriptional activation domain in transient transfection reporter assays. The mutations are detectable in bone marrow from DS-AMKL patients but disappear when patients enter remission, indicating a strong correlation between the mutated clone and the leukemic phenotype. Mutations involving exon 2 of GATA1 are highly specific for DS-AMKL and DS-TMD, or AMKL with acquired trisomy 21. There is only one reported case of such a mutation in AMKL without trisomy 21, and no mutations have been detected in DS-acute lymphoblastic leukemia or a large number of healthy individuals.

Analysis of stored neonatal blood spots shows the coexistence of several different GATA1 mutations (all resulting in the generation of GATA1s) in patients who subsequently developed DS-AMKL, suggesting an oligoclonal expansion. In a few cases in which material was available, identical GATA1 mutations have been found in both the DS-TMD and DS-AMKL cells from the same patient. DS-AMKL cells often harbor additional genetic abnormalities, such as trisomy 8 or tetrasomy 21, not observed in DS-TMD cells. Taken together, these findings support a clonal evolution model of DS-AMKL, with GATA1 mutations associated with an early initiating event.

Generation of knock-in mice that recapitulate the truncating GATA1 mutations show unexpected stage-specific effects on megakaryocytopoiesis. During fetal liver hematopoiesis, the mutant megakaryocytes markedly hyperproliferate, similar to what is observed for GATA1-deficient megakaryocytes. However, during adult-stage bone marrow hematopoiesis, megakaryocytopoiesis and thrombocytopoiesis appear normal. This suggests that the fetal liver and bone marrow cellular contexts interact differentially with the GATA1 truncated molecule. This may also explain the restriction of TMD to the neonatal period. A family has been described with members containing a germline GATA1 gene splice site mutation (G332C) that results in exclusive production of the GATA1s protein product. Affected individuals exhibit a unique phenotype characterized by trilineage bone marrow dysplasia, macrocytic anemia, and neutropenia. None of the family members has developed leukemia, suggesting that trisomy 21 plays a role in DS-TMD progression to DS-AMKL.

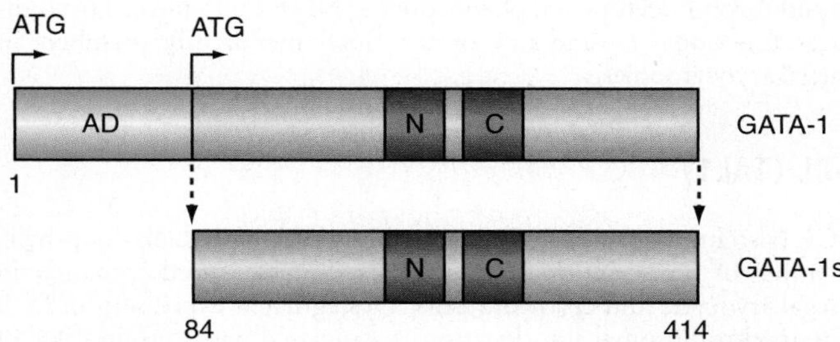

Figure 26-10 GENERATION OF AN AMINO TERMINAL TRUNCATED ISOFORM OF GATA1 BY MUTATIONS ASSOCIATED WITH DS-TMD AND DS-AMKL. Schematic representation of full-length GATA1 is shown on top; the truncated form (GATA1s), on bottom. The amino terminal transcriptional activation domain, as defined by reporter assays in transiently transfected cells, is indicated *(AD)*. The amino *(N)* and carboxyl *(C)* zinc fingers are shown as *gray boxes*. In DS-TMD and DS-AMKL, mutations involving exon 2 of GATA1 (point mutations, deletions, insertions, and/or splice site mutations) lead to exclusive translation from a downstream in-frame methionine at codon 84, producing the amino terminal truncated GATA1 protein (GATA1s).

Of note, Santoro and his colleagues previously reported that GATA1s is produced naturally at low levels in erythroid cells. They proposed that this might serve a regulatory role during normal hematopoiesis by acting as a dominant negative molecule at specific times/environmental stimuli. Endogenous GATA1s has also been detected in normal mouse fetal liver megakaryocytes and adult human bone marrow megakaryocytes. Thus it has been proposed that the ratio of GATA1 to GATA1s plays a role in developmental aspects of megakaryocytopoiesis and that acquired GATA1 mutations observed in DS-TMD and DS-AMKL, or germline mutations in the family described earlier, perturb hematopoiesis by altering this ratio.

ETS Family Transcription Factors

A common feature of megakaryocyte-specific genes is the presence of tandem binding sites for GATA and ETS transcription factors in their promoters and enhancers. The ETS transcription factor family is composed of a diverse group of proteins that share a common ETS DNA-binding domain, which recognizes a GGAA core sequence. Over 30 different ETS factors have been identified, at least nine of which (ELF1, ELF2, Fli-1, PU.1, TEL, GABPα, ETS1, ETS2, ELK4) are expressed in megakaryocytes. Functional studies have implicated several of these, including Fli-1, ETS1, TEL, and GABPα, in megakaryocytopoiesis.

Fli-1

The role of Fli-1 megakaryocytopoiesis is the best characterized of the ETS factors in terms of its functional role in megakaryocyte development. Fli-1$^{-/-}$ mice die during embryogenesis from hemorrhage, likely due to both vascular defects and dysmegakaryocytopoiesis. Colony assays show an increased number of megakaryocyte progenitors in Fli-1$^{-/-}$ embryos as compared with wild-type mice. However, the megakaryocytes from these colonies are small, contain a high nuclear/cytoplasm ratio, and have hypolobulated nuclei, disorganized platelet demarcation membranes, and reduced number of α-granules. Expression of the late megakaryocyte marker gene GPIX is markedly reduced, whereas expression of the early genes, TPO receptor, and αIIb are normal or mildly reduced, consistent with a role of Fli-1 in late megakaryocyte maturation. Fli-1 is involved in the synergistic transcriptional activation of several megakaryocyte-specific genes by GATA1 and FOG-1. Work by Poncz and colleagues shows that different ETS factors act in a stage-specific manner during megakaryocytopoiesis, with GABPα predominantly regulating genes active during early stages of megakaryocytopoiesis and Fli-1 during later stages.

Fli-1 has been implicated in the lineage commitment of bipotent erythroid-megakaryocyte progenitor cells to the megakaryocyte pathway. Fli-1 expression is downregulated as bipotent cells commit to the erythroid lineage, and its overexpression in the bipotent human erythroleukemia cell line K562 enhances the expression of several megakaryocyte-specific genes and induces a megakaryocyte phenotype. In addition, functional cross-antagonism occurs between Fli-1 and the erythroid-specific transcription factor EKLF.

Paris-Trousseau syndrome (OMIM 188925) and Jacobsen syndrome (OMIM 147791) are overlapping contiguous gene-deletion disorders in humans involving the long arm of chromosome 11 (11q23). The constellation of findings in these syndromes includes severe congenital cardiac abnormalities, trigonocephaly, mental retardation, dysmorphogenesis of the hands and face, and macrothrombocytopenia. The etiology of the thrombocytopenia in these patients appears to be related to impaired platelet production, since platelet survival time is normal. Examination of bone marrow reveals significant dysmegakaryocytopoiesis with an abundance of micromegakaryocytes and death of large numbers of megakaryocytes during terminal stages of maturation. Peripheral blood platelets contain giant α-granules, which are thought to arise from aberrant α-granule fusion during prolonged residence in the bone marrow. The minimal chromosome regions deleted in Paris-Trousseau and Jacobsen syndromes associated with thrombocytopenia includes the genes for the ETS factors Fli-1 and ETS-1. Lentiviral expression of Fli-1 in $CD34^+$ cells from patients with Paris-Trousseau thrombocytopenia rescues megakaryocyte differentiation in vitro, providing strong evidence that it is deficiency of Fli-1 that is the cause of impaired thrombopoiesis in these patients. Of interest, Favier and colleagues have shown that in normal individuals, expression of Fli-1 is mostly monoallelic in early megakaryocytic progenitors ($CD41^+$/$CD42^-$ cells) but predominantly biallelic in later stages. They propose that the different populations of megakaryocytes seen in patients with Paris-Trousseau disorder arise from expression of the normal allele in the normally differentiating megakaryocytes, and the deleted allele (leading to complete loss of Fli-1 expression) in the dying population of megakaryocytes.

TEL (ETV6)

Generation of a fusion protein between TEL (ETV6) and RUNX1 is the most frequent chromosome translocation in childhood pre–B cell acute lymphoblastic leukemia. Although TEL is required for the ontogeny of all definitive hematopoiesis, a recent conditional knockout study of the TEL gene in mice demonstrates its specific requirement for adult-stage megakaryocytopoiesis.

RUNX1

In 1999, Gilliland and colleagues used positional cloning to identify the genetic cause of a rare dominant disorder characterized by thrombocytopenia, an aspirin-like functional platelet defect, and increased risk for developing acute myelogenous leukemia (FPD/AML; OMIM 601399).[26] They identified nonsense mutations, intragenic deletions, or missense mutations on one allele of the gene for RUNX1 (formerly called *AML-1* and *CBFA2*) that co-segregated with the disease in six separate pedigrees. These mutations all resulted in loss of function, indicating that haploinsufficiency of RUNX1 plays a causal role in this disorder. Bone marrow or peripheral blood from these patients were characterized by reduced megakaryocyte colony formation, indicating that RUNX1 dosage affects megakaryocytopoiesis.

RUNX1 is a member of an evolutionarily conserved family of transcription factors that share a conserved 128 amino acid domain in their amino half with homology to Drosophila *runt* gene. This region mediates binding to DNA (consensus [C/T]G[C/T]GGT), as well as to its heterodimeric binding partner CBF-β via protein-protein interactions. RUNX1 is the most frequently mutated transcription factors in human leukemia. In addition, acquired mutations in RUNX1 have been identified in significant number of patients with myelodysplastic syndrome (MDS), particularly those that progress to AML. Homozygous knockout of either RUNX1 or CBF-β in mice is embryonic lethal due to a complete failure of definitive hematopoiesis. This is thought to arise from a defect in the ontogeny of hematopoietic stem cells in the AGM region. More recent studies using conditional knockout of RUNX1 in adult hematopoiesis demonstrate a specific role of RUNX1 in megakaryocytopoiesis. Bone marrow deletion of RUNX1 in adult mice results in up to ≈80% reduction in peripheral blood platelet numbers, although no bleeding diathesis. Bone marrow megakaryocytes are small, lack lobulated nuclei, have poorly developed demarcation membranes, and reduced polyploidization. These findings are reminiscent of the abnormal "micromegakaryocytes" seen in humans with myelodysplastic syndromes. Paradoxically, there is an increase in in vitro megakaryocyte colony plating efficiency, suggesting an expansion of early megakaryocyte progenitors. These effects are cell-autonomous. No defects are seen in the erythroid lineage. Reduced dosage of RUNX1's essential cofactor CBF-β also perturbs megakaryocytopoiesis in vivo. Taken together, these findings indicate a specific role of RUNX1/CBF-β in megakaryocyte terminal maturation.

NF-E2 p45

NF-E2 is a heterodimeric transcription factor composed of two basic region-leucine zipper (bZip) subunits: a hematopoietic-specific 45 kDa protein (p45) and a widely expressed 18 kDa subunit (p18). NF-E2 p45 is expressed in erythroid, megakaryocytic and mast cell lineages. In vitro studies implicated NF-E2 p45 as a critical factor for β-globin expression. Unexpectedly, NF-E2 $p45^{-/-}$ mice were found to have only mild perturbations of the erythroid lineage. However, these mice fail to produce platelets secondary to a maturational arrest in the megakaryocyte lineage, and succumb to hemorrhage in the neonatal period. Since the initial studies, NF-E2 p45 has been recognized as being a major regulator of terminal megakaryocyte maturation and platelet release. Notably, although NF-E2 $p45^{-/-}$ mice are severely thrombocytopenic, they have normal serum levels of TPO. In addition, megakaryocytes from these animals proliferate in vivo in response to TPO administration. These findings suggest that NF-E2 p45 regulates target genes independent of the action of TPO.

Several important target genes of NF-E2 p45 have been identified, including β-1 tubulin, 3β-hydroxysteroid dehydrogenase (3β-HSD), thromboxane synthase, caspase 12, and Rab27b. β-1 tubulin is a megakaryocyte-restricted isoform of β-tubulin that plays a key role in the marginal band structure of platelets and is essential for their discoid shape. Deficiency of β-1 tubulin leads to spherocytic platelets. Heterozygosity for a polymorphism (Q43P, due to the double nucleotide substitution AG>CC) in the human β1-tubulin gene is present in about 11% of individuals in a Caucasian northern European population and correlates with a reduced risk for cardiovascular disease in man. This may be due to alterations in platelet structure and function. 3β-HSD catalyzes autocrine biosynthesis of estradiol within megakaryocytes and plays an important role in proplatelet formation.

p18 (also called mafK) is a member of a family of small maf proteins (mafF, mafG, mafK) related to the chicken v-maf oncoprotein. Knockout of mafK, and the related mafF, in mice has no discernable phenotypes, whereas deficiency of mafG leads to mild thrombocytopenia. Compound mafK::mafG null mice have profound thrombocytopenia, phenocopying NF-E2 p45 mice. This indicates functional redundancy of the small maf family members in megakaryocytopoiesis.

SCL (TAL1)

SCL (also known as *TAL1*) is a member of the basic helix-loop-helix member of transcription factors and is expressed predominantly in megakaryocytic and erythroid cells. Dysregulated expression of SCL due to chromosomal translocation is associated with certain cases of T-cell acute lymphoblastic leukemia. SCL forms obligate heterodimers with ubiquitously expressed E proteins (such as E12 and E47), which bind to E-box motifs (sequence CANNTG). It participates in multiprotein complexes that include E2A, GATA1, LMO2, LDB1, and the repressor ETO-2. $SCL^{-/-}$ mice die during embryogenesis as a result of failure of all hematopoiesis and defective vasculogenesis. However, conditional SCL knock-out models show a specific role for SCL in late stages of megakaryopoiesis and stress thrombopoiesis during adult hematopoiesis. SCL-null megakaryocytes have disorganized demarcation membrane systems and a reduced number of platelet granules. SCL modulates thrombopoiesis, in part, by direct transcriptional activation of NF-E2 p45.

Other Transcription Factors

The transcription factors discussed thus far are those that have received the most in-depth study in terms of their roles in megakaryocytopoiesis. Additional factors involved in megakaryocytopoiesis and/or thrombopoiesis have been identified, although their roles are just beginning to be explored. Gfi-1b (*Gfi* standing for "growth factor independent") is a member of a family of hematopoietic expressed zinc finger transcription factor proto-oncogenes that contain a unique amino terminal transcriptional repressor SNAG domain. Knockout of Gfi-1b in mice results in embryonic lethality due to severe anemia. The fetal liver of mutant mice contains erythroid and megakaryocytic progenitors that are blocked in their maturation. Culture of these cells in the presence of thrombopoietin, in contrast to those from wild-type animals, generates only small colonies and the cells are acetylcholinesterase negative (a marker of maturing megakaryocytes in mice). They contain markedly reduced mRNA transcript levels of vWF, NF-E2 p45, c-Mpl, and GPIIb, compared with wild-type, suggesting a requirement for Gfi-1b in at least relatively early stages of megakaryocytopoiesis. Gfi-1 has been shown to repress target genes by recruitment of histone lysine methyltransferases.

Warren and colleagues performed an ENU mutagenesis screen in TPO receptor$^{-/-}$ mice in order to identify factors that might influence thrombocytopoiesis. They identified two independent loss-of-function alleles of the transcription factor c-Myb (substitution of valine for aspartic acid at residue 152 within the DNA binding domain and residue 384 within the leucine zipper domain). Both TPO receptor$^{-/-}$ and wild-type mice containing these mutations have supraphysiologic production of platelets as a result of excessive megakaryocytopoiesis, at the expense of erythroid and lymphocyte development. Megakaryocytes from these animals have a 200-fold increased sensitivity to GM-CSF, suggesting dysregulation of signaling pathways. Similar megakaryocytic hyperplasia and thrombocytosis occur in mice containing germline c-Myb mutations that disrupt binding the transcriptional coactivator p300. Thus c-Myb may play an important negative regulatory function in megakaryocytopoiesis and thrombocytopoiesis.

Megakaryocyte Enhancesome Complex

A number of biochemical and genome-wide chromatin occupancy studies have provided evidence for physical and functional interactions between a core set of megakaryocyte transcription factors that includes GATA1, GATA2, Fli-1, RUNX1, and SCL/TAL1.[27] This suggests that a specific "enhancesome complex" involving these factors drives megakaryocyte-specific gene expression.

MICRORNAS IN MEGAKARYOCYTOPOIESIS

MicroRNAs (miRNAs) are a recently discovered class of small (typically 19-25 nucleotide) noncoding RNAs that interact in a sequence-specific manner with mRNAs (typically in their 3′ untranslated region in mammals) and modulate gene expression through either enhanced mRNA decay or inhibiting translation. There is increasing evidence that they play significant roles in development and differentiation, likely by fine-tuning tissue-specific transcription factor expression. Each miRNA can have multiple target genes, and conversely, each mRNA can be subject to regulation by multiple miRNA species. In addition, transcription of miRNAs is itself mediated by RNA polymerase II and subject to control by transcription factors. Therefore complex regulatory networks can exist between miRNAs and transcription factors. A number of miRNAs have been shown to influence thrombopoiesis.[28] miR-150 enhances megakaryocytopoiesis at the expense of erythropoiesis, suggesting a critical role in the cell fate decision of bipotent megakaryocyte-erythroid progenitor cells. This is mediated, at least in part, via targeting the 3′-UTR of c-MYB mRNA transcripts. Thrombopoietin signaling increases miR-150 levels. miR-155 inhibits megakaryocytopoiesis by targeting ETS1 and Meis1 transcription factors. Other miRNAs have been implicated in controlling thrombopoiesis, but the evidence supporting a functional role is not as strong as for miR-150 and miR-155. miRNAs are also present in platelets. Further studies are needed to examine their potential role in platelet activation and function.

FUTURE DIRECTIONS

Although the molecular details regarding the regulation and generation of platelets remain to be fully elucidated, considerable progress has been made over the past few decades. This has been significantly facilitated by the isolation of TPO and its receptor. Important models of thrombocytopoiesis have now been tested rigorously in vivo, yielding new insights into the final stages of platelet formation and shedding. These studies highlight the efficient mechanisms that have developed to satisfy the demands for dynamic and high-output platelet production. Several important transcription factors have been identified that regulate different stages of megakaryocytopoiesis, and mutations in these, and other genes, have been linked to human disorders of thrombocytopoiesis. The role of miRNAs in controlling thrombopoiesis is beginning to be appreciated. Although mouse models have played important roles in the analysis of these genes, it is becoming clear that they do not always faithfully recapitulate human disease. In addition, several studies have documented important differences between rodent and human platelets, including differences in size, circulating numbers, and DMS ultrastructural features. Thus some caution must be exercised when extrapolating results of mouse studies to human thrombocytopoiesis. The advent of megakaryocyte in vitro differentiation systems using human embryonic stem (ES) cells and/or CD34^{+} cells should provide important tools for future studies geared toward understanding and treating human disorders of megakaryocytopoiesis and thrombocytopoiesis.

REFERENCES

1. Wright J: The origin and nature of the blood platelets. *Boston Med Surg J* 23:643, 1906.
2. Nakorn TN, Miyamoto T, Weissman IL: Characterization of mouse clonogenic megakaryocyte progenitors. *Proc Natl Acad Sci U S A* 100:205, 2003.
3. King SM, Reed GL: Development of platelet secretory granules. *Semin Cell Dev Biol* 13:293, 2002.
4. Italiano JE, Jr, Battinelli EM: Selective sorting of alpha-granule proteins. *J Thromb Haemost* 7:173, 2009.
5. Tavian M, Peault B: Embryonic development of the human hematopoietic system. *Int J Dev Biol* 49:243, 2005.
6. Tober JM, Koniski A, McGrath KE, et al: The megakaryocyte lineage originates from hemangioblast precursors and is an integral component both of primitive and of definitive hematopoiesis. *Blood* 109:1433, 2007.
7. Liu ZJ, Sola-Visner M: Neonatal and adult megakaryopoiesis. *Curr Opin Hematol* 18:330, 2011.
8. Italiano JE, Jr, Lecine P, Shivdasani RA, et al: Blood platelets are assembled principally at the ends of proplatelet processes produced by differentiated megakaryocytes. *J Cell Biol* 147:1299, 1999.
9. Richardson JL, Shivdasani RA, Boers C, et al: Mechanisms of organelle transport and capture along proplatelets during platelet production. *Blood* 106:4066, 2005.
10. Schulze H, Korpal M, Hurov J, et al: Characterization of the megakaryocyte demarcation membrane system and its role in thrombopoiesis. *Blood* 107:3868, 2006.
11. Chang Y, Aurade F, Larbret F, et al: Proplatelet formation is regulated by the Rho/ROCK pathway. *Blood* 109:4229, 2007.
12. Avecilla ST, Hattori K, Heissig B, et al: Chemokine-mediated interaction of hematopoietic progenitors with the bone marrow vascular niche is required for thrombopoiesis. *Nat Med* 10:64, 2004.
13. Junt T, Schulze H, Chen Z, et al: Dynamic visualization of thrombopoiesis within bone marrow. *Science* 317:1767, 2007,

14. Harker LA, Finch CA: Thrombokinetics in man. *J Clin Invest* 48:963, 1969.
15. Kaushansky K: The molecular mechanisms that control thrombopoiesis. *J Clin Invest* 115:3339, 2005.
16. Gurney AL, Carver-Moore K, de Sauvage FJ, et al: Thrombocytopenia in c-mpl-deficient mice. *Science* 265:1445, 1994.
17. Bunding S, Widmer R, Lipari, T, et al: Normal platelets and megakaryocytes are produced in vivo in the absence of thrombopoietin. *Blood* 90:3423, 1997.
18. Kirito K, Kaushansky K: Transcriptional regulation of megakaryopoiesis: Thrombopoietin signaling and nuclear factors. *Curr Opin Hematol* 13:151, 2006.
19. Raslova H, Baccini V, Loussaief L, et al: Mammalian target of rapamycin (mTOR) regulates both proliferation of megakaryocyte progenitors and late stages of megakaryocyte differentiation. *Blood* 107:2303, 2006.
20. Bersenev A, Wu C, Balcerek J, et al: Lnk constrains myeloproliferative diseases in mice. *J Clin Invest* 120:2058, 2010.
21. Kimura S, Roberts AW, Metcalf D, et al: Hematopoietic stem cell deficiencies in mice lacking c-Mpl, the receptor for thrombopoietin. *Proc Natl Acad Sci U S A* 95:1195, 1998.
22. Stasi R, Bosworth J, Rhodes E, et al: Thrombopoietic agents. *Blood Rev* 24:179, 2010.
23. Ravid K, Lu J, Zimmet JM, et al: Roads to polyploidy: The megakaryocyte example. *J Cell Physiol* 190:7, 2002.
24. Lordier L, Jalil A, Aurade F, et al: Megakaryocyte endomitosis is a failure of late cytokinesis related to defects in the contractile ring and Rho/Rock signaling. *Blood* 112:3164, 2008.
25. Muntean AG, Ge Y, Taub JW, et al: Transcription factor GATA-1 and Down syndrome leukemogenesis. *Leuk Lymphoma* 47:986, 2006.
26. Song WJ, Sullivan MG, Legare RD, et al: Haploinsufficiency of CBFA2 causes familial thrombocytopenia with propensity to develop acute myelogenous leukaemia. *Nat Genet* 23:166, 1999.
27. Tijssen MR, Cvejic A, Joshi A, et al: Genome-wide analysis of simultaneous GATA1/2, RUNX1, FLI1, and SCL binding in megakaryocytes identifies hematopoietic regulators. *Dev Cell* 20:597, 2011.
28. Edelstein LC, Bray PF: MicroRNAs in platelet production and activation. *Blood* 117:5289, 2011.
29. Balduini CL, Cattaneo M, Fabris F, et al: Inherited thrombocytopenias: A proposed diagnostic algorithm from the Italian Gruppo di Studio delle Piastrine. *Haematologica* 88:582, 2003.

CHAPTER 27

INHERITED FORMS OF BONE MARROW FAILURE

Yigal Dror and Melvin H. Freedman

Inherited bone marrow (BM) failure is defined herein as decreased production of one or more of the major hematopoietic lineages due to mutations that were derived from the parents or occurred de-novo (Table 27-1). Although outdated, the term "constitutional" has been used interchangeably with "inherited" and similarly implies that a genetic abnormality causes the BM dysfunction. The designation "congenital" has a looser connotation and refers to conditions that manifest early in life, often at birth, but does not imply a particular causation. Therefore, "congenital BM failure" is not necessarily inherited and may be caused by a de novo gene mutation during early embryogenesis or by acquired factors such as viruses, drugs, or environmental toxins.

Hematopoiesis is an orderly but complex interplay of stem and progenitor cells, growth factors, BM stromal elements, and positive and negative cellular and humoral regulators. Thus, BM failure can potentially occur at several critical points in the hematopoietic lineage pathways. With regard to inherited BM disorders, genetic mutations interfere with orderly hematopoiesis and cause the BM failure. The discovery of specific, high-penetrance mutant alleles associated with discrete inherited BM failure syndromes provides evidence for this. Many of these alleles are of genes that directly affect physiologic cell survival and function pathways that are essential for normal hematopoiesis (e.g., DNA repair, telomere maintenance, ribosome biogenesis, microtubule stabilization, chemotaxis, signaling from hematopoietic growth factors, signal transduction related to hematopoietic cell differentiation, and granulocytic enzymes). Modifying genes, epigenetic processes, acquired factors, and chance effects may also be operative and interact with the mutant genes to produce overt disease with varying clinical expression. Hence, the disorders listed in Table 27-1 can be transmitted in a simple Mendelian pattern determined primarily by mutant genes with inheritance patterns of autosomal dominant, autosomal recessive, or X-linked types. Alternatively, some or all of these can be multifactorial in origin caused by an interaction of multiple genes and a variety of exogenous or environmental determinants.

The incidence of the inherited BM failure syndromes (IBMFSs) can be approximated from experience at large centers. Data from Children's Hospital Boston show that the inherited syndromes comprise about 30% of cases of pediatric BM failure with Fanconi anemia (FA) cases leading the list. Data from the Canadian Inherited Marrow Failure Registry (CIMFR) suggest an incidence of about 65 cases diagnosed per million live births per year. Importantly, none of these syndromes is restricted to the pediatric age group. Patients with dyskeratosis congenita (DC) and FA may be detected for the first time in adulthood. Similarly, cases of Shwachman-Diamond syndrome (SDS), Diamond-Blackfan anemia (DBA), and Kostmann (KS) (congenital) neutropenia may first become evident in young adults.

BI-LINEAGE AND TRI-LINEAGE CYTOPENIAS

Fanconi Anemia

Background

Fanconi anemia is inherited in an autosomal recessive manner in 98% of cases. In about 2% of cases, it is transmitted in an X-linked recessive mode caused by a mutant *FA type B* gene.

Although the original report of FA in 1927 by Dr. Guido Fanconi described pancytopenia combined with physical anomalies in three brothers, a published summary in 2010 of more than 2000 FA cases has underscored the clinical variability of the condition. Basically, FA is a *genomic instability disorder* characterized by chromosomal fragility and breakage, a defect in DNA repair, progressive BM cellular underproduction, peripheral blood cytopenias, developmental anomalies, and a strong propensity for hematologic and solid tumor cancers.

There are four possible clinical presentations: FA patients may have (1) typical physical anomalies but normal hematology; (2) normal physical features but abnormal hematology; (3) normal physical features *and* normal hematology; or (4) physical anomalies and abnormal hematology, the so-called classic phenotype that fits the original description (Fig. 27-1). There can also be sibling heterogeneity in presentation with discordance in clinical and hematologic findings, even in affected monozygotic twins. FA patients show abnormal chromosome fragility that is readily seen in metaphase preparations of peripheral blood lymphocytes cultured with phytohemagglutinin (PHA) and enhanced by adding a DNA interstrand cross-linking agent, either mitomycin C (MMC) or diepoxybutane (DEB) (see Abnormal Chromosome Fragility section later). Using published information, the median age at diagnosis of FA is about 6.5 years with a reported range from birth to 49 years.

Epidemiology

The overall prevalence of FA is 1 to 5 cases per million with a carrier frequency of one in 200 to 300 in most populations. Data from the CIMFR showed a prevalence of 11.4 cases per million live births per year. It occurs in all racial and ethnic groups. Spanish Gypsies have the world's highest prevalence of FA with a carrier frequency of one in 64 to one in 70 for a common founder mutation. A founder effect has also been demonstrated in Afrikaners in South Africa in whom one specific mutation is common (frequency, one in 83), as well as in Ashkenazi Jews (one in 89), Moroccan Jews, Tunisians, sub-Saharan African blacks, Indian, Israeli Arabs, Brazilians, and Japanese.

Etiology and Genetics

Complementation Subtyping

A breakthrough in the search for FA genes evolved from the important observation that fusion of normal cells with FA cells (i.e., cell hybridization) resulted in correction of MMC hypersensitivity of the FA cells in a growth inhibition assay. Thus, the cell hybridization corrected the abnormal FA chromosome fragility, a process known as *complementation*. It was further demonstrated that cell hybridization in several unrelated FA patients could also produce the corrective effect on chromosomal fragility by complementation, which led directly to subtyping of patients into discrete complementation groups. A second method for complementation testing, which is currently used more often for research and clinical purposes, is retroviral transduction. The cDNA of each wild-type FA gene can be transfected into T cells from a newly diagnosed patient using retroviral

Table 27-1 Inherited Bone Marrow Failure Syndromes: Inheritance and Mutated Genes

Group	Disorder	Gene	Protein	Gene Locus	Inheritance
IBMFSs with pancytopenia	Fanconi anemia	*FANCA*	FANCA	16q24.3	AR
		FANCB	FANCB	Xp22.31	XL
		FANCC	FANCC	9q22.3	AR
		FANCD1/BRCA2	FANCD1/BRCA2	13q12.3	AR
		FANCD2	FANCD2	3p25.3	AR
		FANCE	FANCE	6p21.3	AR
		FANCF	FANCF	11p15	AR
		FANCG/XRCC9	FANCG	9p13	AR
		FANCI	FANCI	15q25-q26	AR
		FANCJ/ BRIP1	FANCJ/BRIP1	17q22	AR
		FANCL/ PHF9	FANCL/PHF9	2p16.1	AR
		FANCM	FANCM	14q21.3	AR
		FANCN/ PALB2	FANCN/PALB2	16p12	AR
		FANCP/ SLX4	FANCP/SLX4	16p13.3	AR
		FANCO/RAD51C	FANCO/RAD51C	17q22	AR
		Monosomy 21q22.11-q22.13	UK	UK	UK
	Shwachman-Diamond syndrome	*SBDS*	7q11.2	7q11	AR
	Dyskeratosis congenita	*DKC1*	Dyskerin	Xq28	XL
		TINF2	TIN2	14q12	AD
		TERC	TERC	3q21-q28	AD
		TERT	Telomerase	5p15.33	AD
		NOP10	NOP10	15q14-q15	AR
		NHP2	NHP2	5q35.3	AR
		TCAB1	*TCAB1*	17p13	AR
	Congenital amegakaryocytic thrombocytopenia	*MPL*	Thrombo-poietin receptor	1p34	AR
	Reticular dysgenesis	*AK2*	Adenylate kinase 2	1p34	AR
	Pearson syndrome	*mDNA*	Variable	Mitochondrial DNA	Maternal
	Lig4-associated aplastic anemia	*LIG4*	DNA Ligase IV	1q22-q34	UK
IBMFSs with predominantly anemia	Diamond-Blackfan anemia	*RPS19*	RPS19	19q13.3	AD
		RPL5	RPL5	1p22.1	AD
		RPS26	RPS26	12q	AD
		RPL11	RPL11	1p35-p36.1	AD
		RPS24	RPS24	10q22-q23	AD
		RPL35a	RPL35a	3q29	AD
		RPS7	RPS7	15q	AD
		RPS17	RPS17	15q	AD
		RPS10	RPS10	6p	AD
	Inherited sideroblastic anemia	*ALAS2*	ALAS	Xp11.21	XL
		ABC7	ATP-binding cassette transporter 7	Xq13.1-q13.3	XL
		SLC19A2	Thiamine transporter 2	1q23.3	AR
		PUS1	Pseudo-uridine synthase 1	2p16.1	AR
		SLC25A38	SLC25A38	3p22.1	AR
	Congenital dyserythropoietic anemia type I	*CDAN1*	Codanin-1	15q15	AR
	Congenital dyserythropoietic anemia type II	*SEC23B*	SEC23B	20p11.2	AR
	Congenital dyserythropoietic anemia type III	*CDAN3*	UK	15q21	AD
	Congenital dyserythropoietic anemia, unclassified	*KLF1*	KLF1	19p13.12-p13.13	UK
IBMFSs with predominantly neutropenia	Kostmann syndrome and severe congenital neutropenia	*ELA2*	Neutrophil Elastase	19p13.3	AD
		HAX1	HAX1	1q21.3	AR
		GLI1	GLI1	1p22	AD
		WASP	WASP	Xp11.23-p11.22	XL
	Dursun syndrome	*G6PC3*	Glucose-6-phosphatase catalytic unit 3	17q21	AR
	Cyclic neutropenia	*ELA2*	Neutrophil Elastase	19p13.3	AD
	WHIM syndrome	*CXCR4*	CXCR4	2q21	AD
	Glycogen storage diseases Ib	*G6PT*	G6PT	11q23	AR
	Barth syndrome	*TAZ*	Taffazin	Xq28	XL
	Poikiloderma with neutropenia	*C16orf57*	Not determined	16q13	AR

Table 27-1 Inherited Bone Marrow Failure Syndromes: Inheritance and Mutated Genes—cont'd

Group	Disorder	Gene	Protein	Gene Locus	Inheritance
IBMFSs with predominantly thrombocytopenia	Thrombocytopenia absent radii	*RBM8A*	Y14	1q21.1	AR
	Epstein, Fechtner, Sebastian, May-Hegglin, Alport syndrome	*MYH9*	Nonmuscle myosin heavy chain IIA	22q11-q13	AD
	Mediterranean platelet disorder	*GPIBA*	GPIb	17pter-p12	AD
	Familial AD nonsyndromic thrombocytopenia	*MASTL*	Microtubule-associated serine/threonine-like kinase	10p11-12	AD
		ACBD5	ACBD5	10p12.1	AD
		ANKRD26	ANKRD26	10q22.1	AD
	Thrombocytopenia with dyserythropoiesis	*GATA1*	GATA1	Xp11.23	XL
	Thrombocytopenia with associated myeloid malignancies	*CBFA2*	CBFA2	21q22.1-22.2	AD
	X-linked thrombocytopenia	*WASP*	WASP	Xp11.23	XL
	Thrombocytopenia with radio-ulnar synostosis	*HOXA11*	HOXA11	7p15-p14.2	AD

Modified from Dror Y: Inherited bone marrow failure syndromes: Genetic complexity of monogenic disorders. In Genetic Disorders. InTech Open Access Publisher. Available at http://www.intechweb.org.

AD, Autosomal dominant; *AR,* autosomal recessive; *IBMFSs, inherited* bone marrow failure syndromes; *UK,* unknown; *WHIM,* warts, hypogammaglobulinemia, infections, and myelokathexis; *X-L,* X-linked recessive.

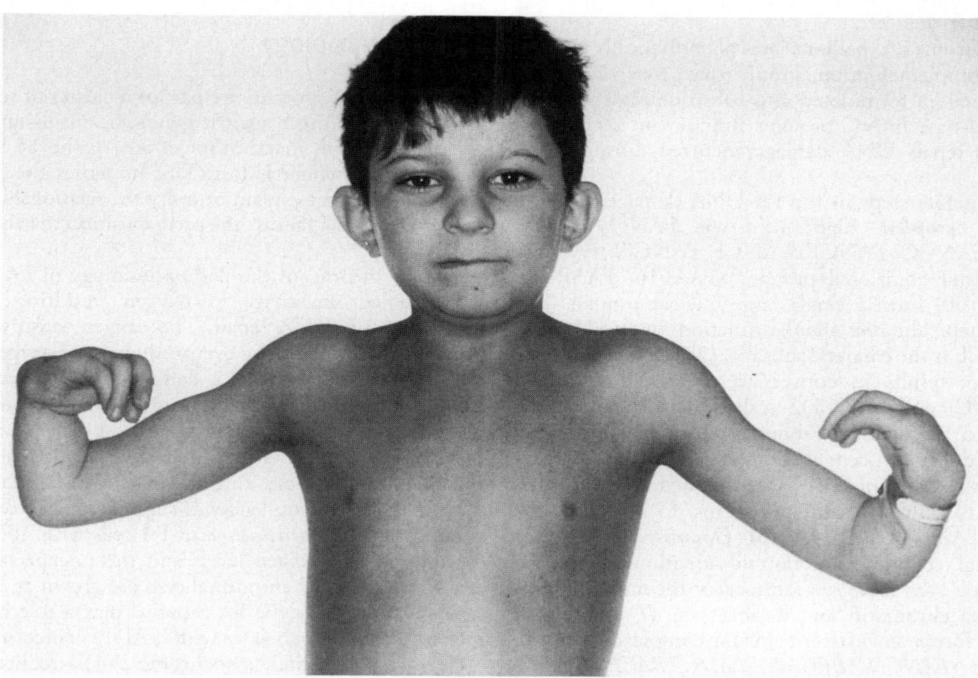

Figure 27-1 CLASSIC PHENOTYPE OF FANCONI ANEMIA. The patient has pigmentary changes around the neck, shoulders, and trunk; short stature; absent radii and absent thumbs bilaterally; microcephaly; and low-set ears.

vectors. If a specific wild-type FA gene corrects (complements) the abnormal chromosome breakage in the patient's T cells in culture on exposure to DEB, the mutant gene is identified. At least 15 complementation groups (termed types A, B, C, D1/BRCA2, D2, E, F, G, I, J, L, M, N, O, and P) have been distinguished on the basis of somatic cell hybridization or retroviral transduction experiments.

Fanconi Anemia Genes

The identification of the 15 subtypes facilitated the cloning of the 15 corresponding FA or *FANC* genes by 2011 (see Table 27-1). The first gene, *FANCC* on chromosome 9q22.3, was discovered in 1992 in Toronto, and then the other genes, corresponding to each of the other complementation groups, were subsequently cloned: *FANCA* on 16q24.3, *FANCB* on Xp22.31, *FANCD1/BRCA2* on 13q12.3, *FANCD2* on 3p25.3, *FANCE* on 6p21.3, *FANCF* on 11p15, *FANCG* on 9p13, *FANCI* on 15q26.1, *FANCJ/BACH1/BRIP1* on 17q22, *FANCL* on 2p16.1, *FANCM* on 14q21.3, *FANCN/PALB2* on 16p12, *FANCO/RAD51C* on 17q22, and *FANCP/SLX4* on 16p13.3.

Of patients tested, up to 70% have mutant *FANCA*, 14% *FANCC*, 10% *FANCG*, 3% *FANCD1*, 3% *FANCD2*, 3% *FANCE*, and 2% or less for the others. FA complementation groups can now be accurately determined clinically by identifying which cDNA of the 15 FA-related genes, when expressed in cells from a newly diagnosed FA patient, corrects the MMC hypersensitivity phenotype.

Murine Models

There are at least 7 FA mouse models, each resulting from targeted disruption of one of the following: FancA, FancC, FancG, FancN, FancD1, FancD2, and the Usp1 gene that encodes the enzyme that deubiquitinates FANCD2. With the exception of FancC and FancG mice, not all other knock-out mouse models recapitulate the hypocellularity and cytopenia that characterizes FA. However, these models provide insight into the various functions of the genes and the role of individual FA mutations. Consistent findings in some or all of the mice include impaired proliferation of BM hematopoietic progenitors, hypogonadism, impaired fertility, growth retardation, microphthalmia, development of cancers, hypersensitivity of BM progenitor cells to administered MMC, as well as to interferon-γ (INF-γ) or tumor necrosis factor-α (TNF-α) in vitro and in vivo. The phenotype of these mutant mice shows abnormal G_2/M progression of the cell cycle similar to FA patients.

Function of FANC Proteins

Cells and cell lines from FA patients are phenotypically similar regardless of the complementation group that they represent. A hypothesis was therefore formulated and subsequently substantiated that the 15 wild-type FANC proteins function in a common response pathway to repair DNA damage incurred during DNA replication.

There are three discrete steps in the FA DNA damage response pathway: (1) ***Core complex***. Eight wild-type FANC proteins (FANCA, FANCB, FANCC, FANCE, FANCF, FANCG, FANCL, and FANCM) and four additional proteins (FAAP16, FAAP 20, FAAP24, and FAAP100) form a single large nuclear protein *"core complex"* as the first step. The *core complex* functions as an ubiquitin ligase of which FANCL is the catalytic subunit. (2) ***ID complex***. The activated *core complex* results in conversion of two downstream protein targets, FANCI and FANCD2 (called the *"ID complex"*), from unubiquitinated isoforms to monoubiquitinated isoforms. Monoubiquitination does not occur if the *core complex* upstream of the *ID complex* is not intact or if FANCL is mutated, and therefore FA cells from patients with upstream mutations do not show the monoubiquitinated FANCI/FANCD2. (3) ***Downstream effector complexes***. In normal cells after monoubiquitination of the *ID complex*, the wild-type *core complex* translocates the monoubiquitinated *ID complex* to chromatin and localizes the *ID complex* to nuclear foci, where it forms downstream effector complexes with five other FANC genes *FANCD1/BRCA2, FANCJ/BACH1/BRIP1, FANCN/PALB2, FANCO/Rad51C,* and *FANCP/SLX4*), as well as with DNA-repair proteins such as BRCA1, RAD51, MRE11-RAD50-NBS1, replication protein A, PCNA, and *BLM* to complete the final step of the DNA repair response.

There are important protein–protein interactions between FA proteins and non-FA "binding partners" for cell survival. FANCC and FANCD2 form complexes with members of the signal transducer and activator of transcription (STAT) family of transcription factors in cytokine-mediated biologic responses. Secondly, heat shock proteins provide several cell survival functions, and FANCC protein specifically facilitates the anti-apoptotic role of Hsp 70. FANCC also interacts with cdc2, PKR, and p53, suggesting that FANCC has other roles that are independent of DNA damage recognition and repair. Finally, GSTP1 is an enzyme that detoxifies byproducts of redox stress and xenobiotics and *FANCC* protein enhances GSTP1 activity in cells exposed to apoptosis inducers.

Genotype–Phenotype Correlations

The clinical severity of FA is partly determined by the specific *FANC* gene involved and by the type of mutation. ***FANCA*** patients who are homozygous for null mutations and produce no protein tend to have an earlier onset of anemia and a higher propensity to leukemic transformation compared with hypomorphic *FANCA* patients who produce protein, albeit abnormal. Compared with other ***FANCC*** mutations, *FANCC* IVS4+4A>T, commonly found in Ashkenazi Jews, is particularly severe and linked with early-onset anemia; early BM failure; and severe physical anomalies, including some cases with physical features of VACTERL-H syndrome (a well-known malformation association, including vertebral, anal, tracheoesophageal, renal, and limb abnormalities). Of genetic-ethnic interest, the identical IVS4+4A>T mutation in Japanese FA patients manifests with a *milder* phenotype than in Ashkenazi Jews. ***FANCD1/BRCA2*** and ***FANCN/PALB2*** mutations are both associated with a significant predisposition to develop acute myeloid leukemia (AML) and with a severe physical anomaly phenotype. The VACTERL-H cluster of anomalies is closely linked with biallelic mutations of *FANCD1/BRCA2*. Null mutations of ***FANCG*** correlate with very severe manifestations compared with most other *FANC* mutations and correlate with early-onset anemia and BM failure, a higher incidence of AML, and severe physical anomalies. ***FANCD2*** and ***FANCI*** mutations also correlate with severe anomalies, and *FANCI* is associated with early-onset anemia.

Pathophysiology

Wild-type FA proteins are part of a cluster of survival signaling molecules that protect against genotoxic insult and suppress apoptosis signaling. With inactivation of any of the 15 known FA genes, the prosurvival benefit is lost. This underlies the phenotype of clinical FA but does not explain or unify the relationship between congenital anomalies, BM failure, the predisposition to cancer, and chromosome fragility.

Two theories of the pathophysiology of FA relate to either (1) a heightened sensitivity to oxygen, resulting in cell damage; or (2) defective DNA repair. The oxygen sensitivity phenotype of FA cells is characterized by overproduction of oxygen radicals, a deficient oxygen radical defense, a deficiency in superoxide dismutase, and poor cell growth at ambient oxygen, all producing shortened cell survival. A cardinal phenotype of FA cells is an abnormality in cell cycle distribution with an increased number of cells with 4N DNA content arising from a delay in the G_2/M or late S phase of the cell cycle. The strongest evidence supporting an oxygen metabolism deficiency in FA is a *reduction* of FA cells with 4N DNA content when grown at *low* oxygen levels and the unexpected appearance of 4N DNA content when normal cells are grown at *high* oxygen levels. Of note, some wild-type FA proteins play a role in redox-related functions. FANCC associates with NADPH (nicotinamide adenine dinucleotide phosphate), cytochrome P-450 reductase, and glutathione S-transferase, proteins with redox functions. FANCA and FANCG are redox-sensitive proteins that multimerize after H_2O_2 treatment, prompting the notion that the FA pathway may function in oxidative stress management.

The best evidence supporting the theory that the primary defect is in DNA repair relates to the critical role of wild-type FANC proteins in the DNA damage response pathway. Whereas clastogenic bifunctional cross-linker agents such as MMC and DEB induce chromosomal breakage in FA cells, monofunctional chemical agents do not, indicating that FA cells cannot repair interstrand cross-links. There were also experiments in the 1980s in which the frequency of mutations induced by 8-methoxypsoralen plus near-ultraviolet radiation at the *HPRT* locus was lower in FA cells than in control participants. These results indicated that FA cells cannot repair cross-links through the normal pathway involving mismatch repair, recombinational repair after bypass of the lesion, or both. Additional evidence for defective DNA repair in FA cells includes an accumulation of DNA adducts, a failure to arrest DNA synthesis in response to DNA damage, increased homologous recombination, defective nonhomologous end joining, abnormal induction of p53, and increased apoptosis.

The two theories for the pathophysiology of FA can be reconciled theoretically. We speculate that biallelic gene inactivation in autosomal recessive FA and monoallelic gene inactivation in X-linked recessive FA could either make the repair pathway sensitive to oxidative damage or cause a transient increase of oxidative damage to which the repair machinery is particularly sensitive.

Hematopoietic Dysfunction

Hematologic abnormalities in FA are evident at the hematopoietic progenitor cell level in BM and peripheral blood. The frequencies of CFU-E (colony-forming unit-erythroid), BFU-E (burst-forming unit-erythroid), and CFU-GM (colony-forming unit-granulocyte macrophage) colony-forming cells are reduced fairly consistently in almost all patients after aplastic anemia ensues as well as in a few patients before the onset of aplastic anemia. Although FA BM cells show normal transcripts for the α and β chains of the GM-CSF (granulocyte macrophage colony-stimulating factor)/interleukin-3 (IL-3) receptor and for c-kit protein, there is a deficient proliferative response of CFU-GEMM (colony-forming unit granulocyte, erythrocyte, macrophage, megakaryocyte), BFU-E, and CFU-GM progenitors in response to GM-CSF plus stem cell factor (SCF) (c-kit ligand) or to IL-3 plus SCF. Because all hematopoietic lineages are affected, the basic defect is presumed to be at the hematopoietic stem cell (HSC) level. Cure of FA BM failure by HSC transplantation (HSCT) supports this view. Confirmatory data for defective stem cells in FA using long-term BM cultures were reported by one group but not confirmed by another. Decreased colony numbers in these studies can be interpreted as the result of an absolute decrease in progenitors and/or progenitors that have faulty proliferative properties and cannot form colonies in vitro.

Additional factors are operative in FA BM failure. Telomeres, the non-encoding DNA at each end of chromosomes, shorten with each round of cell division in normal human somatic cells. Their length is a reflection of the mitotic history of the cell. Telomerase, a ribonucleoprotein reverse transcriptase that can restore telomere length, is variably present in hematopoietic progenitors. Leukocyte telomere length is significantly shortened in FA patients but there is increased telomerase activity, suggesting an abnormally high proliferative rate of progenitors which ultimately leads to their premature senescence. In parallel, increased BM cell apoptosis has been demonstrated in FA patients and in knock-out mouse models and is mediated by Fas, a membrane glycoprotein receptor containing an integral death domain. FA cells exposed to TNF-α, INF-γ, MIP-1α, Fas ligand, and double-stranded RNA undergo exaggerated apoptotic responses.

Studies of cytokines in FA patients have shown varied abnormalities. Although FA fibroblasts showed no deficiencies in SCF or M-CSF (macrophage colony-stimulating factor) production, variability ranging from diminished production to augmentation of production of IL-6, GM-CSF, and G-CSF (granulocyte colony-stimulating factor) has been observed in different patients. A consistent finding that may relate directly to pathogenesis is diminished IL-6 production in FA patients and markedly increased TNF-α generation.

Clinical Features

History and Physical Examination

Historically, the diagnosis of FA was based on signs and symptoms related to aplastic anemia and the presence of characteristic congenital physical anomalies. However, about 30% of FA patients may lack anomalies. The older historical terms *Estren-Dameshek aplastic anemia* and *constitutional aplastic anemia type II* referred to such patients. Confirmatory diagnostic chromosome testing data from the International Fanconi Anemia Registry (IFAR, Rockefeller University) showed that 39% of FA patients had aplastic anemia and anomalies, 30% had aplastic anemia but no anomalies, 24% had anomalies but not aplastic anemia, and 7% had neither. Hence, the Estren-Dameshek cases that lack anomalies should not be considered a separate entity but as part of the continuum of FA.

Table 27-2 lists the characteristic physical abnormalities and their approximate frequency based on more than 2000 published case reports. The two most common anomalies are *skin hyperpigmentation* and *short stature,* each with a frequency of 40% of cases. Characteristically, the hyperpigmentation is a generalized brown melanin-like splattering that is most prominent on the trunk, neck, and intertriginous areas and that becomes more obvious with age. Café-au-lait spots are common alone or in combination with the generalized hyperpigmentation and sometimes with vitiligo or hypopigmentation. The skin pigmentation should not be confused with hemosiderosis-induced bronzing in transfusion-dependent patients who have not been adequately iron chelated. In those with short stature (growth failure), most are less than the third percentile for height. In some patients, growth failure is associated with endocrine abnormalities. In one report, spontaneous overnight growth hormone secretion was abnormal in all patients tested, and 44% had a subnormal response to growth hormone stimulation. Approximately 40% of patients also have overt or compensated hypothyroidism, sometimes in combination with growth hormone deficiency.

Malformations involving the upper limbs are common, especially hypoplastic, supernumerary, bifid, or absent thumbs. Hypoplastic or absent radii are always associated with hypoplastic or absent thumbs in contrast to the thrombocytopenia with absent radii (TAR) syndrome in which thumbs are always present. Less often, anomalies of the feet are seen, including toe syndactyly, short toes, a supernumerary toe, clubfoot, and flat feet. Congenital hip dislocation and leg abnormalities are occasionally seen. Male patients often have gonadal and genital abnormalities, including an underdeveloped penis or micropenis, undescended, atrophic, or absent testes, hypospadias, phimosis, and an abnormal urethra. Female patients occasionally have malformations of the vagina, uterus, or ovary. Renal anomalies occur but require imaging for documentation. Ectopic, pelvic, or horseshoe kidneys are detected often, as are duplicated, hypoplastic, dysplastic, or absent organs. Occasionally, hydronephrosis or hydroureter is present.

Table 27-2 Characteristic Physical Anomalies in More Than 2000 Published Case Reports of Patients With Fanconi Anemia

Anomalies	Approximate Frequency (%)
Skin pigment changes or café-au-lait spots	40
Short stature	40
Upper limb anomalies (thumbs, hands, radii, ulnae)	35
Hypogonadal and genitalia changes (mostly male)	27
Other skeletal findings (head or face, neck, spine)	25
Eye, eyelid, or epicanthal fold anomalies	20
Renal malformations	20
Gastrointestinal or cardiopulmonary malformations	11
Ear anomalies (external and internal), deafness	10
Hips, legs, feet, toe abnormalities	5
CNS imaging anomalies	3

From Shimamura A, Alter BP: Pathophysiology and management of inherited bone marrow failure syndromes. *Blood Rev* 24:101, 2010.
CNS, Central nervous system.

Many patients have a *Fanconi facies,* and unrelated patients can resemble each other almost as closely as siblings. The head and facial changes vary but commonly consist of microcephaly; small eyes; epicanthal folds; and abnormal shape, size, or positioning of the ears (see Fig. 27-1). Anomalies in the tympanic membrane and middle ear ossicles are seen in almost 70% of patients, resulting in hearing loss in most affected patients. Approximately 10% of FA patients are cognitively impaired.

Laboratory Manifestations

Peripheral Blood and Bone Marrow Findings

A cardinal feature is the gradual onset of BM failure usually in the first decade of life, with declining values in one or more hematopoietic lineages. Of 754 FA patients followed prospectively by the IFAR, 80% had hematologic abnormalities other than acute leukemia or myelodysplastic syndrome (MDS). The cumulative incidence of BM failure by 40 years of age was 90%. Patients with *FANCC* mutations appeared to have the earliest onset of changes and the highest incidence (see Phenotype-Genotype Correlations section). Thrombocytopenia with red blood cell (RBC) macrocytosis usually develops initially, with subsequent onset of granulocytopenia and then anemia. Severe BM aplasia eventually ensues in most cases, but the degree of pancytopenia is variable and evolves over a period of months to years. The development of aplastic anemia can be accelerated by intercurrent infections or by drugs such as chloramphenicol. Within families, there is a tendency for the hematologic changes to occur at approximately the same age in affected siblings.

The RBCs are macrocytic with mean corpuscular volumes (MCVs) often above 100 fl even before the onset of significant anemia. Erythropoiesis is characterized by increased fetal hemoglobin (HbF) levels and increased expression of i antigen but not necessarily both features in individual cells. The increased HbF production is not clonal and has a heterogeneous distribution. Ferrokinetic studies indicate that most patients have an element of ineffective erythropoiesis. The RBC lifespan may be slightly shortened, but this is a minor contributory factor to the anemia.

In the early stages of the disease, the BM can show erythroid hyperplasia, sometimes with dyserythropoiesis, myelodysplastic changes, and even megaloblastic-appearing cells. Dysplastic changes may be very prominent with nuclear–cytoplasmic dyssynchrony, hypolobulated megakaryocytes, and binucleated erythroid cells; the findings are difficult to distinguish from MDS. As the disease progresses, the BM becomes hypocellular and fatty, sometimes in a patchy manner, and shows a relative increase in lymphocytes, plasma cells, reticulum cells, and mast cells. When full-blown BM failure occurs, the morphology of the BM biopsy is identical to severe acquired aplastic anemia.

Abnormal Chromosome Fragility. A major finding in FA is abnormal chromosome breakage seen in metaphase preparations of peripheral blood lymphocytes cultured with PHA. The karyotype is characterized by chromatid breaks, rearrangements, gaps, endoreduplications, and chromatid exchanges. Cultured skin fibroblasts also show the abnormal karyotype, underscoring the systemic nature of the disorder. The abnormal lymphocyte chromosome patterns and the number of breaks per cell have no direct correlation with the hematologic or clinical course of individual patients.

Although the breakage is increased in these baseline lymphocyte cultures, it is strikingly enhanced by adding a bifunctional DNA interstrand cross-linking agent, either DEB or MMC. This is the recommended diagnostic test for FA. Indeed, homozygous FA cells are hypersensitive to many oncogenic and mutagenic inducers such as ionizing radiation; SV40 viral transformation; and alkylating and chemical agents, including cyclophosphamide, nitrogen mustard, and platinum compounds, but DEB and MMC have supplanted them for diagnostic testing.

For a definitive diagnosis of FA, the IFAR has defined FA as being associated with increased numbers of chromosome breaks per cell occurring after exposure to DEB with a range of 1.06 to 23.9 compared with the normal control range of 0.00 to 0.10. Further supportive features are unusual chromosome abnormalities such as tri-radial and quadri-radial figures. This pattern of abnormal chromosome breakage can also be used to make a prenatal diagnosis of FA. Diagnostic testing can be performed on fetal amniotic fluid cells obtained at week 16 of gestation or on chorionic villus biopsy specimens at 9 to 12 weeks of gestation. A very high degree of prenatal diagnostic accuracy has been obtained by looking at both spontaneous and DEB-induced breaks in fetal tissue. DEB testing of heterozygote carriers is unreliable for diagnosis because there is overlap of results with normal individuals.

A scoring system was developed for the probability of an accurate diagnosis of FA using discriminating clinical and laboratory variables in patients enrolled in the IFAR whose diagnosis was confirmed by DEB-induced chromosomal breakage analysis. The scoring system was useful in proving that DEB-induced chromosomal breakage results could be correlated with common FA findings. DEB testing is considered by the IFAR to be the gold standard for diagnosis, but MMC testing is still used in many laboratories.

DEB and MMC also induce cell cycle arrest in G2/M in cultures of FA lymphocytes or fibroblasts leading to a resultant 4N DNA cellular content. This alteration can be detected by flow cytometry and has been used to diagnose FA. It requires sophisticated instrumentation and is not used as widely as the DEB or MMC chromosome breakage assay.

Somatic Mosaicism. About 10% to 15% of patients with clinical FA do not show increased chromosome breakage when tested with DEB or MMC. These patients usually have hematopoietic cell somatic mosaicism as a result of a molecular genetic correction in a stem cell, resulting in one normal allele. The mechanisms for this phenomenon include gene conversion events, back mutations, or compensatory deletions or insertions. The end result is mixed populations of somatic cells, some with two abnormal alleles and some with one. If FA is strongly suspected, a skin biopsy is performed to assess chromosomal breakage in cultured fibroblasts with DEB or MMC rather than in lymphocyte cultures.

Immunoblotting for FANCD2. An accurate diagnostic and subtyping assay for FA has been introduced in research laboratories. Primary lymphocytes or fibroblasts are assayed for FANCD2 after exposure to MMC or radiation by immunoblotting, which distinguishes the unubiquitinated and monoubiquitinated forms. The testing is useful in three situations for screening FA mutations: (1) in FA patients with diagnostic MMC-induced chromosomal breakage assays, FANCD2 null mutations are presumed if no full-length FANCD2 is detected by immunoblotting; (2) if FANCD2 is detected but is not monoubiquitinated, mutations of one of the upstream core complex genes are predicted; and (3) if FANCD2 is detected and is monoubiquitinated, a mutation of FANCD1/BRCA2, FANCJ/BACH1/BRIP1, FANCN/PALB2, FANCO/Rad51C, or FANCP/SLX4 is expected because all five localize downstream of FANCD2. Monoubiquitination of FANCD2 is normal in other BM failure syndromes and chromosomal breakage disorders.

Other Findings. Fanconi anemia cells exposed to alkylating agents arrest in the G_2/M phase of the cell cycle. The transfected wild-type FA gene that reduces G_2/M arrested cells as determined by cell cycle kinetics using flow cytometry pinpoints the mutant gene.

Apparently, the majority of FA patients have stable, elevated levels of serum α-fetoprotein expressed constitutively that are independent of liver complications and of androgen therapy. Levels are also unchanged after HSCT. The clinical utility of these findings is limited.

Ultrasonographic examination of the abdomen may reveal congenital anomalies of the kidneys and urogenital system. Echocardiography may reveal cardiac anomalies. Radiography and computed tomography (CT) can be informative in revealing bone, intestinal, or other anomalies. Imaging using radiation should be minimized as much as possible because of the carcinogenic risk.

Predisposition to Malignancy

A major feature of the FA phenotype is the propensity to develop cancer. The chromosome fragility, the defects in DNA repair, the genomic instability, and the cellular damage that occur in FA patients translate into a significant predisposition to develop a malignancy. Because there are at least 15 genetic mutations that lead to FA and alterations in the FA pathway are relevant to the pathogenesis of common types of cancers, the disorder is a critical human model of the genetic determinants of hematologic cancers and solid tumors.

Fanconi anemia is a member of two families of cancer predisposition syndromes. The first is composed of genetic disorders of DNA repair that include ataxia telangiectasia, xeroderma pigmentosum, and Bloom syndrome. The close relationship between FA and ataxia telangiectasia, for example, is underscored by data showing convergence of signaling pathways in both conditions. The second family of predisposition syndromes consists of other inherited BM failure disorders described herein, including SDS and DC that show a propensity for malignant myeloid transformation or solid tumors.

The magnitude of the risk of developing malignancy in FA has been defined in three comprehensive reports: a literature review of more than 2000 published cases, the IFAR prospective registry of 754 patients, and a retrospective North American cohort survey of 145 cases. The median patient age for the development of all cancers in the literature review was 16 years of age, which is strikingly different from the median age of 68 years for the same types of cancer in the general population. It was apparent from the three reports that the crude risk of cancer in FA patients is extraordinarily high: 5% to 10% for leukemia, about 5% for MDS, and 5% to 10% for solid tumors. The IFAR data indicate that by the age of 40 years, the cumulative incidence of leukemia and nonhematologic cancers is 33% and 28%, respectively.

The literature review identified 175 cases of leukemia, mostly AML, and 110 cases of MDS. Previous observations by the IFAR showed that the risk of developing MDS and AML was higher for patients in whom a prior clonal BM cytogenetic abnormality had been detected. Monosomy 7, rearrangement or partial loss of 7q, rearrangements of 1p36 and 1q24-34, and rearrangements of 11q22-25 are frequent recurring cytogenetic clonal changes. Additional data indicate a strong correlation in FA BM cells of chromosome 3q26q29 partial trisomies and tetrasomies and rapid progression to MDS or AML. When interpreting the significance of clonal cytogenetic abnormalities in FA patients, note that clonal variation is frequent, including appearances of new clones, inability to detect established clones on repeat examination, and clonal evolution. Similar to the literature review, the IFAR verified that the risk of developing hematologic and nonhematologic cancer in FA increased with advancing age, but the IFAR did not show an age-related plateau for the risks for MDS and AML, possibly because both diagnoses were analyzed together.

The literature review also identified 320 patients with other forms of cancer, 25 of whom had up to three separate types of solid tumors, and 14 additional cases of solid tumors who also had leukemia. None of these patients had received a BMT before developing cancer. The most frequent solid tumor reported was squamous cell carcinoma involving head and neck and upper and lower esophagus followed by the vulva or anus, cervix, and skin. There were additional cases of tongue and oral squamous cell carcinoma that occurred after HSCT. Liver tumors, benign and malignant, were second most frequent. Most of these hepatoma and adenoma patients had received prior androgen therapy for aplastic anemia. Androgen administration has therefore been implicated in liver tumor pathogenesis. In descending order of frequency, cancers were also reported in brain, kidney, breast, and adrenal gland. The IFAR 20-year prospective observational study and the North American cohort survey corroborated the literature review in terms of type of cancer, site, and risk.

Heterozygote Phenotype

Heterozygote carriers of FANC gene mutations do not develop peripheral blood cytopenias or aplastic anemia, and cell lines from heterozygote carriers do not show excessive chromosome fragility in culture when exposed to DEB or MMC. The mean chromosomal breakage level of lymphocytes from FA carriers tested in cultures with a clastogenic agent may be higher than controls, but individual carrier testing may show overlap with normal values and severely limits its diagnostic utility. Literature from the early 1980s describes congenital anomalies of the hand and the genitourinary system in relatives of patients with FA, and parents of children with FA may have short stature. FA carriers may have increased levels of HbF, decreased natural killer (NK) cell counts, and diminished reactivity to mitogen stimulation.

Monoallelic carriers for *FANCD1, FANCN,* and *FANCJ* are at increased risk of developing cancer. Female carriers of *FANCD1* have an increased risk of breast cancer ranging from 40% at age 80 years to a lifetime risk of about 80%. Carriers also are predisposed to develop ovarian cancer with a risk of up to 20% at age 70 years. Male carriers have a 7% risk of breast cancer and a 20% risk of prostate cancer before age 80 years. Mutant FANCN and FANCJ are low-penetrance breast cancer susceptibility alleles with about a twofold increased risk in carriers compared with the general population.

Differential Diagnosis

About 30% of FA patients do not have physical anomalies, and such individuals may not be recognized until they present with aplastic anemia, MDS, AML, unilineage cytopenias, or macrocytic RBCs. Thus, FA should be part of the differential diagnosis in children and adults with unexplained cytopenias, characteristic birth defects, a diagnosis of aplastic anemia, MDS or AML in patients up to the age of 40 years and possibly higher, unusual sensitivity to chemo- or radiotherapy, cancer typical of FA but at an atypical age such as cancer of the cervix when younger than 30 years, or squamous cell carcinoma of the head and neck when younger than 50 years of age. Any of these should prompt consideration of FA as the underlying problem. All patients with idiopathic aplastic anemia who are younger than 40 years should have chromosomal fragility testing. However, if the test was not performed at diagnosis, patients with "idiopathic" aplastic anemia who fail to respond to immunosuppressive therapy with ATG and cyclosporine should be tested.

Although neutropenia is a consistent feature of SDS, anemia or thrombocytopenia (or both) is seen in more than 50% of the patients and can be confused with FA. Because growth failure is also a manifestation of SDS, differentiating between the two disorders can initially be difficult. The major difference between them is that SDS is a disorder of exocrine pancreatic dysfunction that produces gut malabsorption. This can be confirmed by fecal fat analysis; by pancreatic stimulation studies using intravenous secretin or cholecystokinin that confirm markedly impaired enzyme secretion; and by showing reduced levels of serum trypsinogen, serum isoamylase, or fecal elastase. CT, ultrasonography, or magnetic resonance imaging (MRI) of the pancreas may also demonstrate fatty changes within the pancreatic body. Other skeletal distinguishing features found in some patients with SDS are short flared ribs, thoracic dystrophy at birth, delayed bone maturation, and metaphyseal dysostosis of the long bones. Chromosomes analyses do not show spontaneous breaks in SDS, and there is no increased breakage after clastogenic stress testing using DEB or MMC. Specific diagnostic confirmation is obtained by demonstrating the mutant *SBDS* gene.

Dyskeratosis congenita shares some features with FA, including development of pancytopenia, a predisposition to cancer and leukemia, and skin pigmentary changes. However, the pigmentation pattern is somewhat different in DC and manifests with a lacy reticulated pattern affecting the face, neck, chest, and arms, often with a telangiectatic component. At some point, usually in the first decade of life, DC patients also develop dystrophic nails of the hands and feet and, somewhat later, leukoplakia involving the oral mucosa, especially the tongue. Other findings seen only in DC and not in FA are teeth abnormalities with dental decay and early tooth loss, hair loss, and hyperhidrosis of the palms and soles. Chromosomal fragility with DEB testing is normal in DC patients, who contrast sharply with FA patients. In the X-linked form of DC, mutations can be identified in the *DKC1* gene. A *TERC, TERT,* or *TINF2* gene mutation confirms an autosomal dominant form of the disorder. A *NOP10* or *NHP2* mutation accounts for autosomal recessive DC.

Congenital amegakaryocytic thrombocytopenia (CAMT) and **TAR syndrome** both manifest in the neonatal period with thrombocytopenia. A neonatal hematologic presentation is atypical for FA; fewer than 5% of patients are diagnosed during the first year of life. Neither of the thrombocytopenic syndromes shows chromosome fragility, which separates them from FA, and a mutant *MPL* gene is diagnostic of CAMT. In the TAR syndrome, thumbs are always preserved and intact despite the absence of radii, but in FA, the thumbs are hypoplastic or absent when the radii are absent.

Seckel syndrome, or **"bird-headed dwarfism"** manifests with short stature; microcephaly; cognitive delay; sinopulmonary infections; and a predisposition to developing lymphomas, pancytopenia, and AML. Some patients may show increased chromosomal breakage in lymphocyte cultures with DEB or MMC and mimic FA. There are possibly four genes linked to Seckel syndrome: mutant *ATR* has been confirmed for Seckel 1 subtype, and mutant *CENPJ* has been postulated to account for Seckel 4 subtype. Genotyping will distinguish FA from Seckel syndrome.

Nijmegen breakage syndrome (NBS) is an autosomal recessive disorder caused by mutations in the *NBS1* gene and is characterized by stunted growth, microcephaly, a distinctive facies, café-au-lait spots, immunodeficiency, and a predisposition to lymphoid malignancy. Some patients resemble those with FA, have BM failure, and may show increased chromosome breakage in lymphocyte cultures with MMC. The genetic defect is a mutant *NBS1* gene whose wild-type protein product is involved in DNA repair. Because NBS can mimic and be confused with FA, genotyping is essential and diagnostic.

Cells from patients with **Bloom syndrome** show abnormal spontaneous breakage, but unlike FA cells, the breakage does not increase in vitro in response to DEB. **Ataxia telangiectasia** is characterized by sister chromatid exchange without hypersensitivity to DEB or BM failure.

Natural History and Prognosis

The most serious early consequence in most FA patients is BM failure. The exceptions are patients with biallelic FANCD1/*BRCA2* mutations who have a cumulative probability of 97% of developing a malignancy by age 6 years, including AML, Wilms tumor, and medulloblastoma. Judging from the literature, the overall risk for FA patients developing solid malignant tumors, liver tumors, acute leukemia, and MDS is at least 15%, but it is likely higher in older patients. Treatment for cancer imposes additional problems and probably increases the risk for additional cancers secondary to therapy. Thus, the major causes of death in FA are sepsis and bleeding from BM failure, complications of HSCT, and progressive cancer or consequences of its treatment.

Despite these serious issues, the prognosis for FA patients is improving. Based on a literature review of more than 2000 FA case reports, the median survival from 1927 to 1999 was 21 years. In contrast, the median survival from 2000 to 2009 was 29 years of age. FA patients are now predicted to reach adulthood because more than 80% of patients reach age 18 years or more. Earlier diagnosis, especially of mild cases, diagnosis of FA in young adults with AML or a solid tumor, comprehensive clinical and laboratory surveillance programs, timely therapeutic interventions, and HSCT are attributed to the improved outlook.

Therapy

Because of their clinical and psychosocial complexity, patients with FA should be supervised by a hematologist at a tertiary care center using a comprehensive and multidisciplinary approach (see www.fanconi.org for *Fanconi Anemia Guidelines for Diagnosis and Management,* 3rd edition, 2008). On the initial visit, the practitioner should take a detailed personal and family history, a careful physical examination with emphasis on physical anomalies, complete blood counts and chemistries, a BM biopsy for cellularity and morphology, and an aspirate for additional morphology, cytogenetics, and an iron stain for ringed sideroblasts. DEB or MMC chromosome fragility testing on peripheral blood lymphocytes on patients and siblings should be arranged. If FA is confirmed by DEB or MMC testing, the complementation group assignment and mutation analysis can be initiated. On a separate visit, imaging studies should be requested to search for internal anomalies. When all the results from the workup have been compiled, a follow-up visit with the patient and family is arranged to discuss the diagnosis, management options, and prognosis. A referral to a genetic counselor should ensue. High-resolution human leukocyte antigen (HLA) typing of the patient and immediate family members is recommended shortly after the diagnosis is established to determine potential matched-related donors in case HSCT becomes necessary.

If the patient is stable, has only minimal to moderate hematologic changes, and does not have transfusion requirements, a period of observation is indicated. During this time, subspecialty consultations (e.g., with orthopedic surgeons, urologists, gynecologists, and otolaryngologists) can be arranged during this interval. Blood counts should be monitored every 1 to 3 months to determine their stability. In a stable patient with mild cytopenias, blood counts can be monitored every 3 months, and BM evaluation should be performed annually. Falling counts, a clonal BM cytogenetic abnormality, or prominent multilineage dysplasia require more frequent clinic visits and blood and BM sampling to monitor for progression to severe aplastic anemia, AML, or MDS. Spectral karyotyping (SKY), fluorescent in situ hybridization (FISH), and comparative genomic hybridization of BM cells can enhance the diagnostic capability.

A surveillance program for solid cancers should be initiated at least annually. After the age of 10 years or after HSCT, the oral cavity should be examined every 6 months for signs of malignant change because the risk in untransplanted FA patients is 700-fold that of the general population. Oral cancers can occur within 1 year after HSCT. Dentists, oral surgeons, or head and neck surgeons should be recruited after the age of 10 years or after HSCT to screen for head and neck squamous cell carcinomas by rhinopharyngoscopy using a flexible endoscope. Beginning at age 13 years, all women with FA should undergo annual gynecologic screening because the relative risk of vulvar squamous cell carcinoma is 4000-fold higher and cervical cancer is 200-fold higher than that of the general population. Human papilloma virus (HPV) DNA can be detected in 84% of FA squamous cell carcinoma specimens from various anatomic sites. Although the role of HPV in FA carcinogenesis is controversial, quadrivalent HPV vaccine is still recommended for boys and girls with FA at 9 years of age as a possible preventive approach.

Growth should be serially documented, and when growth velocity or stature falls below expectations, endocrine evaluation is needed to identify growth hormone deficiency. Impaired glucose tolerance, hyperinsulinemia, and diabetes mellitus occur more commonly in FA, and patients should be screened annually or biannually depending on the degree of hyperglycemia found on initial testing. Screening for hypothyroidism also should be performed annually.

Hematopoietic Stem Cell Transplantation

Hematopoietic stem cell transplantation is the only curative therapy for the hematologic abnormalities of FA: aplastic anemia, AML, and MDS. The best donor source is an HLA-matched sibling in whom thorough history, physical examination, blood counts, HbF, chromosome breakage testing, and ideally genetic testing have excluded a diagnosis of FA. Initial efforts to transplant FA patients using standard preparative regimens and graft-versus-host disease (GVHD) prophylaxis were plagued by two serious and often lethal problems, severe cytotoxicity from chemotherapy and irradiation and exaggerated GVHD. Reduced-intensity HSCT protocols that remain myeloablative for FA patients were subsequently introduced and improved outcomes ensued. Research is constantly ongoing for the most effective strategies.

Absolute indications for a matched sibling donor HSCT are (1) severe underproductive cytopenias and transfusion dependency; (2) high-risk MDS with chromosomal clonal abnormalities like monosomy 7, or partial trisomies and tetrasomies of 3q26q29, or a BM blast count of greater than 5%; or (3) overt AML. Serious consideration for transplantation should also be considered for FA with high-risk mutations for AML such as biallelic *FANCD1/BRCA2*. Decision to transplant for milder, relative indications should be made on a case-by-case basis.

Three caveats about transfusional supportive care before HSCT are (1) more than 20 exposures to blood products is a risk factor that adversely affects engraftment and survival posttransplant; (2) use of directed donations from family members may cause alloimmunization to an antigen that can increase the risk of graft rejection after a matched sibling donor or haploidentical related HSCT; and (3) single-donor apheresis platelets should be requested when required and the product should be leukodepleted and irradiated.

Cytoreductive regimens for matched sibling donor HSCT have gradually excluded total-body irradiation (TBI). Most published studies have adopted one of the following protocols: (1) cyclophosphamide, ATG, and TBI; (2) fludarabine, cyclophosphamide, and ATG; or (3) cyclophosphamide alone. Fludarabine, a purine antimetabolite with potent immunosuppressive and myeloablative properties with minimal toxicity to other tissues, continues to gain favor as an effective adjunct to preparative regimens. Some centers currently prefer fludarabine, cyclophosphamide, and TBI because of improved rates of engraftment, reduction of T-cell mosaicism and its deleterious effects, and improved survival. All four regimens are successful and have their advocates. Transplant centers usually intensify the cytoreductive regimen when the patient has MDS or AML. Disease-free survival data for TBI-based protocols vary between 64% and 89%. Disease-free survivals for non-TBI protocols are as high as 93% using cyclophosphamide alone. The risk of primary or secondary graft failure is 5% to 10%, and the risk of acute GVHD ranges from 8% using cyclosporine and methotrexate prophylaxis to 55% using cyclosporine alone.

Hematopoietic stem cell transplantation using HLA-mismatched related donors, matched or one-antigen mismatched unrelated donors, or cord blood carries a higher risk of complications and a lower disease-free survival than matched sibling donor HSCT. The best outcome predictors are recipients younger than 10 years old, recipient seronegativity for CMV, history of fewer than 20 exposures to blood products, and use of fludarabine in the cytoreductive regimen. Risk factors adversely affecting survival are an HLA-mismatched donor, an FA phenotype with three or more congenital malformations, and prior administration of androgen therapy. The latter factor might be related to the delay in transplant rather than the therapy itself. Indications for an alternate donor HSCT are identical to those for a matched sibling donor HSCT.

Provided that no extended family members are suitable BM or peripheral blood stem cell donors, unrelated BM donors are sought and identified by searching donor and umbilical cord blood registries. An acceptable unrelated donor should be fully matched by high-resolution typing for all HLA-A, B, C, and DRB1 antigens, a so-called *8/8 match*. A second choice is a one-antigen mismatch in a BM donor. Matched or one-antigen mismatched banked umbilical cord blood is equally suitable to a one-antigen mismatched BM donor and is an option. The last choice is a two-antigen mismatched cord blood. Using cord blood cells from unrelated donors, engraftment and survival are comparable to related or unrelated BM, although engraftment is slower with cord blood. The incidence of acute and chronic GVHD is reduced with cord blood grafts even in 1 or 2 HLA antigen mismatched transplants. Three-year published survival rates after unrelated HSCT for FA range between 40% and 75%.

Molecular technology has led to preimplantation genetic diagnosis (PGD) coupled with in vitro fertilization. This is an option for parents who have a child with FA and a defined *FANC* mutation but without a matched sibling donor. If the mother is fertile, eggs are harvested and fertilized with the father's sperm in vitro, resulting in a number of blastomeres. Using single-cell polymerase chain reaction (PCR) technology, isolated cells from several blastomeres can be tested for an HLA match and for absence of the *FANC* mutation. The selected HLA-compatible normal blastomeres can then be transferred and implanted in utero, resulting in a successful pregnancy and subsequent birth of a matched unaffected sibling. Cord blood from the PGD-selected healthy infant sibling can be banked for a HSCT for the affected sibling. The notion of "designer babies" is still debated in ethical circles.

Despite the successes of HSCT in correcting the BM failure of FA patients, there is a subset of survivors who develop cancers, particularly squamous cell carcinoma of the head and neck. These malignancies reflect the ongoing genetic susceptibility of FA nonhematopoietic tissue to cancer despite successful transplantation for aplastic anemia, MDS, or AML. Published data comparing cancer risks in transplanted and nontransplanted FA patients show a 4.4-fold increase in age-specific hazard rate of squamous cell carcinoma in the transplanted cohort. The causes for the increased cancer risk are not proven, but GVHD, especially chronic, and the preparative regimens of chemotherapy and irradiation are highly suspect. T-cell depletion has been introduced in some protocols to reduce GVHD, and irradiation has been reduced or eliminated in others to address this issue.

G-CSF mobilization and collection of peripheral blood $CD34^+$ cells from FA patients before the onset of severe pancytopenia has not attained broad application. These cells in theory can be used as targets for gene therapy; however, their cryopreservation and infusion later when severe BM failure ensues or as an autologous rescue after chemotherapy in the event of leukemic transformation is unlikely to reconstitute the hematopoietic system or confer a survival benefit.

Hematopoietic Growth Factors

Both G-CSF and GM-CSF can induce a neutrophil response in neutropenic FA patients. G-CSF is indicated for a patient with recurrent or serious bacterial infection, especially if the neutrophil counts are less than $500/mm^3$. In a published clinical trial of G-CSF in 12 FA patients, all 12 had an increase in absolute neutrophil numbers, five had a significant increment in hemoglobin levels, and four had an increase in platelet counts. Concurrent with the impressive improvements in blood counts, 8 of 10 patients who finished 40 weeks of G-CSF treatment showed elevations in the percentage of BM and peripheral blood CD34+ cells. The starting dose for subcutaneous G-CSF is 5 μg/kg/day, and after a neutrophil response occurs, the dose can be decreased to every second day or 2 to 3 times a week. Long-acting pegylated G-CSF has not been studied in FA.

In another published clinical trial, combination cytokine therapy consisting of subcutaneous G-CSF 5 μg/kg once daily with erythropoietin 50 units/kg administered subcutaneously or intravenously three times a week was given to FA patients. Androgen therapy was added if the response was inadequate. Of 20 patients treated, 19 had improved neutrophil numbers, 6 had an increase in hemoglobin levels, and 4 achieved a sustained rise in platelets.

Because genomic instability and a marked predisposition to leukemia and cancer are features of FA, the wisdom of using granulopoietic growth-promoting cytokines on a long-term basis for FA is an issue. There may be a heightened risk of inducing or promoting expansion of a leukemic clone, especially one with monosomy 7. Therefore, before starting cytokine therapy, a baseline BM aspirate and biopsy is recommended and then repeated every 6 months to document changes in morphology and cytogenetics.

Androgens

Androgen therapy has been used to treat FA for decades. The overall response rate in the literature is about 50% heralded by reticulocytosis and a rise in hemoglobin within 1 to 2 months. If the other lineages respond to androgens, white blood cells increase next and then platelets, but it may take many months to achieve the maximum response. When the response is deemed maximal, the androgens should be slowly tapered but not stopped entirely. Accepted indications for treating with androgens are one or more of the following: hemoglobin level less than 8 g/dL or symptoms from anemia, platelet count less than 30,000/mm^3, and neutrophil count less than 500/mm^3. Oxymetholone, an oral 17-α alkylated androgen, is used most frequently at 1 to 5 mg/kg once a day. The authors' practice is to start with 0.5 mg/kg/day and increase it monthly if there are no major side effects and an insufficient response. Although unproven, some clinicians add corticosteroids to offset androgen-induced growth acceleration and to prevent thrombocytopenic bleeding by promoting vascular stability. For this purpose, 5 to 10 mg of prednisone is given orally every second day. If an injectable androgen is preferred to decrease the risk of liver toxicity and growth of hepatic tumors, nandrolone decanoate, 1 to 2 mg/kg/wk, is given intramuscularly followed by the application of local pressure and ice packs to prevent the development of hematomas. There are insufficient comparative data on the efficacy of the attenuated androgen, Danazol, compared with oxymetholone to make a recommendation, but a Danazol clinical trial for FA at Children's Hospital Boston is underway. Another androgen, oxandrolone, is also in clinical trial for FA at Cincinnati Children's Hospital. Claims of reduced masculinizing side effects in female FA patients treated with Danazol compared with those treated with oxymetholone have not been substantiated in clinical trials.

Almost all patients relapse when androgens are stopped. The few who successfully discontinue treatment are often in the puberty age range when temporary "spontaneous hematologic remissions" have been observed to occur. Most patients on long-term androgens eventually become refractory to therapy as BM failure progresses. Potential side effects include masculinization, which is especially troublesome in female patients, and elevated hepatic enzymes, cholestasis, *peliosis hepatis,* and liver tumors. Five complications of androgen therapy require consideration.

1. *Peliosis hepatis* is a cystic dilation of hepatic sinusoids that fill with blood and can be life threatening if they rupture. They may be clinically silent or produce right upper quadrant pain. Liver function test results are normal. Ultrasonographic examination is a safe way to diagnose the abnormality. The lesions may regress after stopping the androgens.
2. *Androgens also damage hepatocytes* nonspecifically. This may be manifest as cholestatic jaundice or elevated liver enzymes. Stopping androgen therapy usually leads to complete resolution. Hepatic cirrhosis may develop in patients on continued androgen therapy. If resolution of enzyme elevation does not occur after androgen withdrawal, a liver biopsy is indicated.
3. *Hepatocellular adenomas* are associated with androgen therapy. These are benign, noninvasive tumors. They can, however, rupture, leading to life-threatening bleeding. FA patients may develop these tumors rapidly, but they can be readily detected by imaging. The tumor may regress after stopping the androgens. If persistent, surgical resection or radiofrequency ablation may be necessary.
4. *Hepatocellular carcinoma* (HCC; hepatoma) occurs with androgen use, and some studies have suggested that FA patients on treatment may be at increased risk for HCC. The HCC associated with androgens characteristically does not produce α-fetoprotein in serum, distinguishing it from de novo HCC. Patients developing HCC should discontinue androgen therapy.
5. Androgen therapy for FA patients is recognized by HSCT physicians as an important *adverse prognostic factor* for those receiving a transplant. Several centers with experience in FA transplants firmly recommend that androgens *not* be given to FA patients unless a suitable donor cannot be identified. The cause of the association is unknown but may be related to delay in HSCT rather than the drug itself.

Those receiving androgens should be evaluated serially with liver enzyme profiles every 2 to 3 months and ultrasonography or CT scan of the liver every 6 to 12 months. If liver enzymes increase to above normal or if abnormalities appear on imaging, the androgen dose should be decreased or stopped. It is strongly recommended by many transplant centers that an FA patient not receive androgens if it is known that the patient has a matched donor available.

Future Directions

The premise for gene therapy in FA is based on the assumption that corrected hematopoietic cells would have a growth advantage. Strengthening this supposition are FA patients with hematopoietic somatic mosaicism who show spontaneous disappearance of cells with the FA phenotype. These *mosaic* patients may show spontaneous hematologic improvement, suggesting that hematopoiesis was derived from stem cells with a normal phenotype. In the context of gene therapy, evidence suggests that even one genetically corrected HSC may be able to repopulate the BM of an FA patient.

Despite encouraging preclinical studies more than a decade ago using retroviral vectors showing that wild-type *FANCC* and *FANCA* could be integrated into normal and FA CD34$^+$ cells, the ensuing clinical trials in *FANCC* and *FANCA* patients were disappointing, and gene therapy still remains at a developmental stage. A central problem is suboptimal wild-type gene integration into FA cells in culture. Because of the apoptotic phenotype and the sensitivity to oxidative stress, FA cells die rapidly in vitro before efficient gene transfer is accomplished. Changing the tissue culture conditions and introducing lentiviral vectors that can infect noncycling human cells were deemed the solutions, but obstacles persist. Ongoing research is directed at novel vector design, transduction methodology, and improved strategies for preparing HSCs. One caveat: a successful FA gene therapy protocol may correct BM failure and possibly the propensity for MDS and AML, but the predisposition for cancer in other tissues will continue unchecked.

Shwachman-Diamond Syndrome

Shwachman-Diamond syndrome is an autosomal recessive multisystem disorder characterized by varying degrees of BM failure, a high risk of leukemia, and exocrine pancreatic insufficiency. Additional features may include short stature and skeletal abnormalities. The mutant gene responsible for this complex pleiotropic phenotype, termed *Shwachman-Bodian-Diamond syndrome (SBDS),* has been identified and has been confirmed in 90% of patients with the classic presentation. *SBDS* seems to be multifunctional and promotes cell survival, ribosome biogenesis, mitotic spindle stability, and chemotaxis. To date, though, no unifying pathogenesis has been able to account for all of the multisystem features of SDS.

Epidemiology

Shwachman-Diamond syndrome has been reported among all ethnic groups. Older studies suggested a higher incidence in males. However, recent data suggest an equal distribution between genders as expected from an autosomal recessive disorder. Based on data from the CIMFR, SDS is the third most common inherited BM failure syndrome with an incidence of 8.5 cases per million live births.

Pathobiology

The identification of *SBDS* on chromosome 7q11 was the entry point for studies on the molecular basis for SDS. There is an adjoining pseudogene *(SBDSP)* with 97% homology in its coding regions to *SBDS*. The gene encodes a 250 amino acid protein product, which is a member of a highly conserved protein family of previously unknown function with putative orthologs in diverse species, including Archaea and eukaryocytes. Based on structural studies of the ortholog in Archae and the human protein, the SBDS protein has three main domains (N-terminal, middle, and C-terminal) with predicted protein–protein, protein–DNA, and protein–RNA binding motifs.

The common *SBDS* mutations are composed of sequences that are homologous to *SBDSP*. Hence, these mutations are believed to result from recombination events whereby segments of *SBDSP* become incorporated into wild-type *SBDS* and interfere with its function. These recombinational events result in three common gene conversion mutations in exon 2 that account for 75% of *SDS* alleles: (1) a nonsense mutation, 183_184TA>CT, introduces an in-frame stop codon (K62X); (2)) a splice-site mutation, 258+2T>C, which may either cause premature truncation of the SBDS protein by frameshift (C84fs3) or use an alternative splice site; and (3) an extended conversion mutation, 183_184TA>CT and 258+2T>C, encompasses both mutations. In the Toronto database of 210 SDS families, 89% of unrelated SDS individuals carry a gene conversion mutation on one allele, and 60% carry conversion mutations on both alleles. Thus, the vast majority of patients are compound heterozygotes with respect to K62X and C84fsx3. Additional rare mutations in the *SBDS* gene have been identified in SDS patients. These include dozens of insertion, deletion, and missense mutations that have not arisen from gene conversion events. Most *SBDS* mutations alter the N-terminal domain of the protein and lead to markedly reduced protein levels.

SBDS protein is essential for life because no patients with homozygous null mutations have been reported, and residual protein levels can usually be detected in SDS patients. Furthermore, a complete loss of the protein in mice causes developmental arrest before embryonic day 6.5 and early lethality. SBDS seems to be multifunctional and play a role in several cellular pathways, including ribosomal biogenesis, cell survival, chemotaxis, mitotic spindle formation, and protection from cellular stress.

The SBDS protein phylogeny is shared with proteins that are enriched for RNA metabolism and/or ribosome-associated functions. The SBDS protein can be detected in human cell nuclei and cytoplasm. It concentrates in the nucleolus during G1 and G2. Synthetic genetic arrays of YHR087W, a yeast homolog of the N-terminal domain of SBDS, suggested interactions with several genes involved in RNA and rRNA processing. Loss of the protein in humans and yeast results in failure to remove eukaryotic initiation factor 6, elf6 or its homologue in yeast, Tif6, from the ribosomal large subunit in the cytoplasm and impairs the assembly of the large and small ribosome subunits to form the mature ribosomes. SBDS directly interacts with the GTPase elongation factor-like 1 (EFL1). The interaction promotes eIF6 removal from the 60S subunit by a mechanism that requires guanosine triphosphate (GTP) binding and hydrolysis by EFL1. SBDS interacts with multiple proteins with diverse molecular functions; many of them are involved in ribosome biogenesis, such as RPL4, and DNA metabolism, such as RPA70.

SBDS is critical for cell survival. When *SBDS* is lost in SDS BM cells or in *SBDS*-knockdown K562 and HeLa cells, the cells undergo accelerated apoptosis. The accelerated apoptosis in BM cells and *SBDS*-knockdown cells seems to be through the Fas pathway and not through the Bax/Bcl-2/Bcl-XL pathway. SBDS deficiency in primary SDS cells and in *SBDS*-knockdown cells results in abnormal accumulation of functional Fas at the plasma membrane level.

Patients with SDS have a defect in leukocyte chemotaxis. Consistent with this observation, the *SBDS* homologue in amoeba was found to localize to the pseudopods during chemotaxis. These observations suggest that the *SBDS* protein deficiency in SDS causes a chemotaxis defect in patients.

Shwachman-Bodian-Diamond syndrome has been shown to colocalize to the mitotic spindle and bind microtubles and stabilize them. Its deficiency results in centrosomal amplification and multipolar spindles.

The pathophysiologic link between *SBDS* mutations and BM failure is still unclear. Initial studies in the 1970s and early 1980s showed reduced CFU-GM and BFU-E colony formation in most patients compatible with a defective stem cell origin of the BM failure. Recent investigations have characterized a much more extensive hematopoietic phenotype (Table 27-3). SDS BM has decreased numbers of $CD34^+$ cells as well as an impaired ability for $CD34^+$ cells to form multilineage hematopoietic colonies in vitro, confirming that they are intrinsically defective. Patients' BM cells overexpress Fas, the membrane receptor for Fas ligand, and show increased patterns of apoptosis after preincubation with activating anti-Fas antibody, pinpointing this as a central pathogenetic mechanism for the BM failure. Induction of differentiation (at least toward erythroid lineage) results in markedly accelerated apoptosis in SBDS-deficient cells, with only a minimal effect on proliferation. Importantly, oxidative stress is increased during differentiation of SBDS-deficient erythroid cells, and antioxidants enhance the expansion capability of both differentiating *SBDS*-knockdown K562 cells and colony production of SDS patient HSCs and progenitors. Erythroid differentiation also results in reduction of all ribosomal subunits and global translation. These studies indicate that when *SBDS* protein is deficient, several biologic pathways may be dysfunctional during hematopoietic cell development; this may be the cause of the high predilection for BM failure in patients with SDS.

Two other abnormalities have been identified in SDS. When the averages of telomere lengths adjusted to age are compared with those of control participants, a tendency toward shortening of telomeres is found in patient leukocytes, reflecting premature cellular aging. This may represent either an inherent defect in telomere maintenance or compensatory stem cell hyperproliferation. In addition to an inherent hematopoietic defect, it has also been shown that the BM stroma is markedly defective in terms of its ability to support and maintain normal hematopoiesis.

Clinical Features

The many clinical manifestations that occur in varying combinations are shown in Table 27-4. Most patients present in infancy with evidence of growth failure, feeding difficulties, diarrhea, and infections. Steatorrhea and abdominal discomfort are frequent. Approximately 50% of patients exhibit a modest improvement in pancreatic function and do not require further pancreatic enzyme replacement therapy. Hepatomegaly is a common physical finding in young children but typically resolves with age and does not have clinical significance.

Patients with SDS are particularly susceptible to bacterial and fungal infections, including otitis media, bronchopneumonia, osteomyelitis, septicemia, and recurrent furuncles. Overwhelming sepsis is a well-recognized fatal complication of this disorder, particularly early in life.

Short stature is fairly consistent feature of the syndrome. When treated with pancreatic enzyme replacement, most patients show a

Table 27-3 Hematopoietic Phenotype in Shwachman-Diamond Syndrome

Decreased BM $CD34^+$ cells
Decreased colonies from $CD34^+$ cells
Abnormal telomere shortening of leukocytes
Increased apoptosis of BM cells
Apoptosis is mediated by Fas pathway
Impaired BM stromal cell function
Abnormal lymphoid immune function
Increased BM microvessel density
BM cell upregulation of specific oncogenes
Increased levels of reactive oxygen species
Accentuation of the ribosome biogenesis defects with reduced ribosome subunits, ribosomes, and polysomes
Accentuation of the protein translation defect

BM, Bone marrow.

Table 27-4 Clinical and Hematologic Features of Shwachman–Diamond Syndrome

Major Features	Patients (%)
Pancreatic insufficiency (decreased digestive enzymes)	86-100
HEMATOLOGIC CYTOPENIAS	
Neutropenia	88-100
Thrombocytopenia	24-70
Anemia	42-66
Pancytopenia	10-44
MDS/AML	≈30
Other Features	
Short stature	50
Delayed bone maturation	100
Metaphyseal dysplasia	44-77
Rib cage anomalies	32-52
Hepatomegaly or elevated enzymes	<50
Poor oral health (caries, ulcers, tooth loss)	>50
Learning and behavioral problems	>50

AML, Acute myeloid leukemia; *MDS*, myelodysplastic syndrome.

normal growth velocity yet remain consistently below the third percentile for height and weight, indicating an intrinsic growth defect. The occasional adult achieves the 25th percentile for height. Although metaphyseal dysplasia is a common radiologic abnormality (44%-77% of patients), particularly in the femoral head and the proximal tibia, in most patients it fails to produce any symptoms. Occasional patients have clinical joint deformities, resulting in pain, functional impairment, or cosmetic problems, necessitating surgery. Some patients present at birth with respiratory distress caused by thoracic dystrophy. Others may have asymptomatic short and flared ribs.

The majority of the patients have deficits in cognitive abilities at varying levels of severity. These include delayed language development, low intellectual ability, impaired visual-motor integration, and failure to achieve higher order language functioning and problem solving. About one-fifth of the children have behavioral challenges such as attention deficit hyperactivity disorder, pervasive developmental disorder, or oppositional defiant disorder.

Some additional clinical features are seen very infrequently in SDS. Endocrine abnormalities include insulin-dependent diabetes, growth hormone deficiency, hypogonadotropic hypogonadism, hypothyroidism, and delayed puberty. Cardiomyopathies have been noted in some cases. Urinary tract anomalies, renal tubular acidosis, and cleft palate also occur.

Laboratory Findings

Peripheral Blood and Bone Marrow Findings. Published data accurately represent the spectrum of hematologic findings (see Table 27-4). Neutropenia is present in almost all patients on at least one occasion. The neutropenia can be chronic or intermittent. Neutropenia has been identified in some SDS patients in the neonatal period during an episode of sepsis. Anemia is recorded in about half of the patients. RBC MCV and fetal hemoglobin are elevated in 60% and 75% of the patients, respectively, after the age of 1 year. Whether this reflects stress hematopoiesis or ineffective erythropoiesis concomitant with chronic infections has not been clarified. The combination of isolated neutropenia and high MCV or high HbF after the first year of life is seen in up to 28% of SDS patients and almost never in other IBMFSs. Reticulocyte responses are inappropriately low for the levels of hemoglobin in 75% of patients. Thrombocytopenia can be seen in about 40% of the patients.

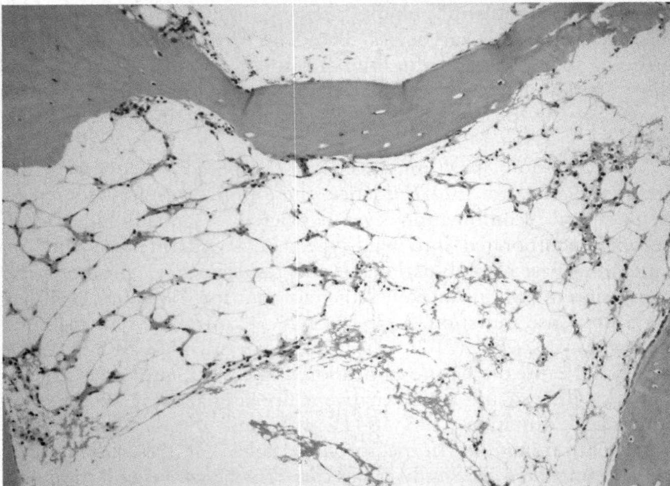

Figure 27-2 BONE MARROW BIOPSY IN SEVERE SHWACHMAN-DIAMOND SYNDROME SHOWING STRIKING HYPOCELLULARITY, FATTY CHANGES, AND TRILINEAGE APLASIA. *(Courtesy Dr. Mohamed Abdelhaleem, Toronto.)*

More than one lineage can be affected, and pancytopenia is observed in up to 65% of cases. The pancytopenia can be profound as a result of severe aplastic anemia (Fig. 27-2). However, BM biopsies and aspirates vary widely with respect to cellularity; varying degrees of BM hypoplasia and fat infiltration are the usual findings. BM with normal or even increased cellularity has also been observed, typically in young children. The severity of neutropenia does not always correlate with BM cellularity, nor is the severity of the pancreatic insufficiency concordant with the hematologic abnormalities.

Shwachman-Diamond syndrome neutrophils may have defects in mobility, migration, and chemotaxis. There appears to be a diminished ability of SDS neutrophils to orient toward a gradient of *N*-formyl-methionyl-leucyl-phenylalanine. An unusual surface distribution of concanavalin A has also been reported that reflects a cytoskeletal defect in SDS neutrophils. Whatever the magnitude of the chemotaxis abnormality is in vitro in SDS, neutrophil recruitment into abscesses or empyemas ensues robustly in vivo.

Immune Dysfunction. Impaired immune function can be significant in SDS and underlie recurrent infections even if adequate numbers of neutrophils are present. Patients have various B-cell abnormalities, including one or more of the following: low immunoglobulin G (IgG) or IgG subclasses, low percentage of circulating B lymphocytes, decreased in vitro B-cell proliferation, and lack of specific antibody production. Patients may also have T-cell abnormalities, including a low percentage of circulating T lymphocytes or subsets or NK cells, and decreased in vitro T-cell proliferation. Inverted CD4:CD8 ratios have also been described.

Exocrine Pancreatic Tests. The exocrine pancreatic pathology is caused by failure of pancreatic acinar development (Fig. 27-3). Pathologic studies reveal normal ductular architecture but extensive fatty replacement of pancreatic acinar tissue, which can be visualized by CT, ultrasonography, or MRI. Pancreatic function studies using intravenous secretin or cholecystokinin confirm the presence of markedly impaired enzyme secretion averaging 10% to 14% of normal but with preserved ductal function. Because of its invasive nature, this test has largely been replaced by measuring the levels of pancreatic enzymes in the serum.

During the first 3 years of life, serum trypsinogen is typically reduced and can be used for diagnostic purposes. Serum isoamylase

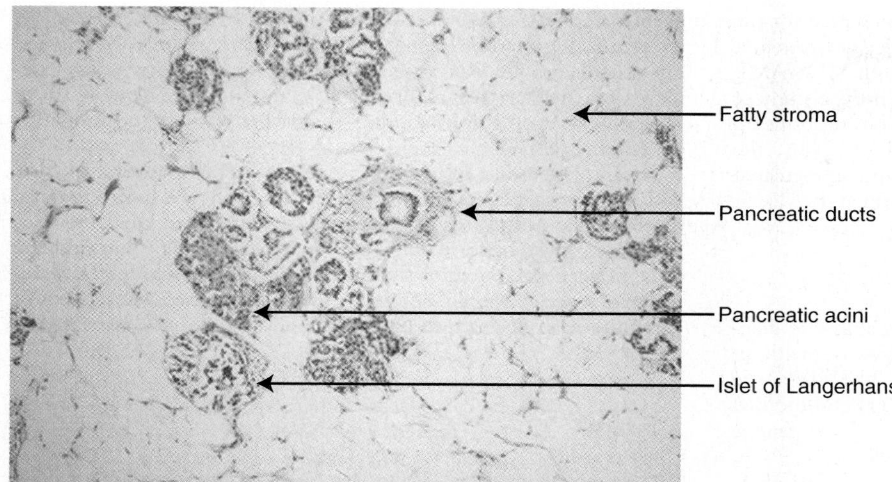

Figure 27-3 PANCREATIC TISSUE PATHOLOGY IN SEVERE SHWACHMAN-DIAMOND SYNDROME. The two classic features, deficiency of acinar tissue and fatty replacement, are shown. Islets of Langerhans are intact. *(Provided by Dr. Peter Durie, Toronto.)*

levels are low in SDS patients of all ages. However, normal children younger than 3 years have low isoamylase levels, so its measurement is not diagnostically useful at this age. Fecal elastase is another pancreatic enzyme that is reduced in SDS. Approximately 50% of patients exhibit a modest improvement in enzyme secretion with advancing age and normal fat absorption when assessed by 72-hour fecal fat balance studies. These patients do not require further pancreatic enzyme replacement therapy.

Skeletal Imaging. Radiographs of the bone are useful to establish a diagnosis. Osteopenia is seen in most patients but rarely results in clinical osteoporosis. Metaphyseal dysplasia has been reported in about 50% of the patients, particularly of the femoral heads, knees, humeral heads, wrists, ankles, and vertebrae. Rib-cage abnormalities can be found in 30% to 50% of patients. These include a narrow rib cage, short ribs, flared anterior rib ends, and costochondral thickening. Digital abnormalities such as clinodactyly, syndactyly, and supernumerary thumbs have been reported but are rare. Spinal deformities, including kyphosis and scoliosis, have been reported.

Imaging of the Brain. Patients with SDS do not have macroscopic brain malformations. However, they may have a decreased global brain volume (both gray matter and white matter) and a smaller posterior fossa, cerebellar vermis, corpus callosum, brainstem, and occipitofrontal head circumferences compared with control participants. These anomalies might be the basis for the neurocognitive and neurobehavioral difficulties.

Leukemia Predisposition. Shwachman-Diamond syndrome is characterized by a high propensity to develop MDS and leukemia, particularly AML. The published crude rate for MDS or AML (MDS/AML) in patients with SDS ranges from 8% to 33%. Of 55 SDS patients followed prospectively in the French Severe Chronic Neutropenia Registry, seven patients developed MDS or AML with an estimated risk of 19% at 20 years and 36% at 30 years. A literature search revealed 99 SDS cases with MDS/AML of whom 38 were reported as having leukemia either at first presentation with malignant transformation or after progressive MDS. Almost 90% of the patients had clonal BM cytogenetic abnormalities at transformation.

There is an increased frequency of BM clonal cytogenetic abnormalities as the sole evidence for a clonal disease in an otherwise hypocellular BM without excess blast counts or major prominent multilineage dysplasia. The incidence is roughly estimated to be 7% to 41% based on pooled published data. Isochromosome 7q [i(7q)], an extremely uncommon finding rarely described in MDS or AML in patients without SDS, was seen in 44% of SDS patients. This high occurrence suggests that it is a fairly specific marker for SDS and might be related to the mutant gene on 7q(11). Other chromosome 7 abnormalities are seen in 33% of SDS patients and include monosomy 7, i(7q) combined with monosomy 7 and deletions or translocations involving part of 7q. The prognostic significance of the cytogenetic changes requires prospective monitoring for clarification. Of the patients with i(7q), progression to MDS with excess blasts or to AML has rarely been reported. Similarly, SDS patients with del(20q) rarely evolve into MDS/AML. In a prospective 5-year follow-up Canadian study of SDS patients, progression to overt transformation was not seen in two patients with del(20q), one patient with i(7q), and one with combined del (20q) and i(7q). Similarly, no progression was seen in six additional patients with i(7q) from several hospitals in the United Kingdom. In contrast, approximately 40% of patients with the other chromosomal 7 abnormalities progress to either advanced MDS or to AML.

The pathophysiologic link between *SBDS* mutations and propensity to MDS and AML is unknown. It is possible that patients with SDS cells develop more frequent mutations caused by genomic instability possibly because of mitotic spindle dysregulation or telomere shortening. It is also possible that impaired ribosome biogenesis and accelerated apoptosis cause a growth disadvantage for SDS BM cells, allowing for a growth advantage and expansion of malignant clones. Although molecular and cellular parameters do not distinguish SDS patients with transformation from SDS patients without transformation, it is remarkable that all SDS BM demonstrates many characteristic features observed in MDS. These include impaired BM stromal support of normal hematopoiesis, increased BM cell apoptosis mediated by the Fas pathway, telomere shortening of leukocytes, increased BM neovascularization, high frequency of clonal cytogenetic abnormalities, and abnormal leukemia-related gene expression in BM progenitor cells.

The vast majority of the published cases of SDS-associated MDS/AML developed without previous G-CSF therapy. None of the six patients with SDS-associated MDS/AML from our institution were treated with G-CSF before transformation. However, it is still unclear whether G-CSF increases the risk of developing leukemia or promotes the expansion of existing malignant clones. Because G-CSF might increase neutrophil counts and prevent infections in SDS, a fraction of the reported patients with SDS-associated MDS/AML had been previously treated with G-CSF. For example, two of the 29 SDS patients on the Severe Chronic Neutropenic International Registry who received G-CSF therapy developed MDS/leukemia.

Shwachman-Bodian-Diamond syndrome must play a critical role in preventing leukemic myeloid transformation because up to one-third of SDS patients develop MDS/AML. To address whether an acquired mutant *SBS* gene is associated with leukemic transformation in de novo AML, 77 AML BM samples at diagnosis or relapse were analyzed for *SBS* mutations, and none were identified. To see if a subset of previously undiagnosed SDS patients presented for the first time with AML, 48 AML BM samples were studied at remission, but no *SBDS* mutations were found. SDS patients with MDS/AML have common *SBDS* mutations, and a genotype–phenotype study of 21 patients with SDS with MDS/AML showed no relationship (Linda Ellis, RN, Toronto, personal communication). Thus, the link between mutant SBDS; hematologic cancer; and upregulated oncogenes, including *LARG,* and *TAL1,* is undetermined.

Differential Diagnosis

The introduction of genetic testing has improved the ability to diagnose the disorder and particularly has helped identify cases with an atypical presentation (Y. Dror, unpublished data). The diagnostic criteria include having at least two of the following: (1) chronic BM failure, (2) exocrine pancreatic insufficiency, (3) positive genetic testing results, and (4) a first degree-relative with SDS.

The syndrome of refractory sideroblastic anemia with vacuolization of BM precursors, or **Pearson syndrome,** is clinically similar to SDS but characterized by very different BM morphology. Severe anemia requiring transfusions rather than neutropenia is often present at birth and by 1 year of age in all cases. In contrast to SDS, the major BM morphologic findings are ringed sideroblasts with decreased erythroblasts and prominent vacuolation of erythroid and myeloid precursors. The disorder shares clinical similarities with SDS because of exocrine pancreatic dysfunction. Malabsorption and severe failure to thrive occur in approximately half of cases within the first 12 months of life. Qualitative pancreatic function tests show depressed acinar function and reduced fluid and electrolyte secretion. Approximately 50% of reported patients die early in life from sepsis, acidosis, and liver failure; the others appear to improve spontaneously with reduced transfusion requirements. At autopsy, the pancreas shows acinar cell atrophy and fibrosis; fatty infiltration as seen in SDS is not a prominent feature. The need for long-term pancreatic enzyme replacement is unclear. These patients have a diagnostic deletion of mitochondrial deoxyribonucleic acid (mtDNA). mtDNA encodes enzymes in the mitochondrial respiratory chain that are relevant to oxidative phosphorylation, including the reduced form of nicotinamide adenine dinucleotide dehydrogenase (NADH), cytochrome oxidase, adenosine triphosphatase (ATPase), transfer ribonucleic acids (tRNAs), and ribosomal RNAs. The degree of heteroplasmy affects the disease expression. Transplantation of mouse BM cells carrying mitochondrial DNA with a large-scale deletion into normal mice leads to macrocytic anemia in mice with hematopoietic cells carrying a high proportion of abnormal mitochondria. The deletion impairs erythroid differentiation and erythropoietic response to stress.

Shwachman-Diamond syndrome shares some manifestations with **FA** such as BM dysfunction and growth failure, but patients with SDS can usually be distinguished because of malabsorption syndrome, fatty changes within the pancreatic body that can be visualized by imaging, and characteristic skeletal abnormalities not seen in patients with FA. In difficult cases with incomplete disease expression, the distinction relies on normal clastogenic stress-induced chromosome fragility testing and genetic testing. Mutational analysis for mutant *SBDS* is definitive, but 10% of classic clinical SDS do not have a mutant *SBDS.*

Atypical SDS cases with only little evidence of pancreatic changes can be difficult to distinguish from early-onset **dyskeratosis congenita** with no mucocutaneous manifestations. Establishing a diagnosis in such cases can be assisted by telomere length screening, which might show telomere shortening but typically not in the very severe range seen in dyskeratosis congenita.

Prognosis

Because of the broad pleiotropy in SDS, the number of undiagnosed patients with mild or asymptomatic disease is unknown. Hence, the overall prognosis may be better than previously thought. The majority of *SBDS* mutations represent hypomorphic alleles with reduced but variable protein expression. Also, there is phenotypic heterogeneity in patients carrying identical *SBDS* mutations. Therefore, until more information is forthcoming, the natural history and prognosis are not yet defined.

From a literature review, the projected median survival of SDS patients was calculated as 35 years. During infancy, morbidity and mortality are mostly related to malabsorption, infections, and thoracic dystrophy. Later in life, the major problems are hematologic or complications related to their treatment. Cytopenias tend to fluctuate in severity but do not fully resolve spontaneously. The most common cause of death in late childhood or adulthood is related to MDS/AML.

Therapy

Patient management is ideally shared by a multidisciplinary team consisting of a hematologist and a gastroenterologist as core members and other subspecialists such as a dentist and a psychologist as required. The malabsorption component of SDS responds to treatment with oral pancreatic enzyme replacement with meals and snacks using guidelines similar to those for cystic fibrosis. Supplemental fat-soluble vitamins are also usually required. When monitored over time, approximately 50% of patients convert from pancreatic insufficiency to sufficiency because of spontaneous improvement in pancreatic enzyme secretion. This improvement is particularly evident after 4 years of age. A long-term plan should be initiated for early detection of severe cytopenias that require corrective action or malignant myeloid transformation. There are currently no data about the cost effectiveness of a specific leukemia surveillance program in SDS. However, it is generally accepted that it should include periodic blood counts with differentials and blood smears every 3 to 4 months, a clinical evaluation by a hematologist every 6 months, and BM testing every 1 to 3 years. The latter includes aspirates for smears and cytogenetics analyses. Concomitant BM biopsies are recommended when the patient's clinical status changes.

G-CSF

G-CSF given for profound neutropenia has been very effective in inducing a clinically beneficial neutrophil response. Of 16 SDS patients in the Severe Chronic Neutropenia International Registry (SCNIR) treated with G-CSF, 14 had brisk neutrophil responses that were sustained in some cases for more than 11 years (Beate Schwinzer, Hannover, Germany, personal communication).

Steroids and Androgens

A small number of patients have been treated with corticosteroids with hematologic improvement in 50%. A smaller number received androgens plus steroids in the manner of treating FA, and improved BM function was also noted. Anecdotal cases treated with androgens alone, cyclosporine, or erythropoietin do not allow broad therapeutic conclusions.

Blood Products and Other Supportive Care

Anemia and thrombocytopenia are managed with transfusions of RBCs or platelets when symptoms appear or prophylactically for profound cytopenias. Antifibrinolytic therapy with tranexamic acid can also be given for mild mucosal bleeding. Broad-spectrum antibiotics are indicated for febrile episodes and severe neutropenia.

Hematopoietic Stem Cell Transplantation

At present, the only curative option for severe BM failure in SDS is allogeneic HSCT. The indications for HSCT include BM failure with severe or symptomatic cytopenia, MDS with excess blasts (5%-29%), or leukemia. Published data are limited and derived from case reports or small case series with a mix of sibling and matched unrelated donors. Two registries in Europe have provided additional information.

The European Group for Blood and Bone Marrow Transplantation (EBMT) Registry reported 26 transplanted SDS patients. The indications included aplastic anemia (n = 16), MDS/AML (n = 9), or other (n = 1). Patients were transplanted with myeloablative conditioning regimens that included either busulfan or total-body irradiation. The majority of the donors were unrelated (n = 19). Eighty-one percent engrafted. The incidence of grade III to IV GVHD was 24%; chronic GVHD was 29%. The overall survival was 65% at 1.1 years. Deaths were primarily caused by infections, GVHD, or major organ toxicities. Factors associated with adverse outcome included MDS/AML or usage of total-body irradiation.

The French Neutropenia Registry reported 10 transplanted SDS patients. The indications included severe BM failure (n = 5) or MDS/leukemia (n = 5). Patients were conditioned with myeloablative regimens incorporating busulfan or total-body irradiation. Six received grafts from unrelated donors and four from a sibling donor. BM engraftment occurred in eight patients. The 5-year overall survival was 60%. Causes of death included infections related to neutropenia, GVHD, relapse, and transplant-related toxicity. Factors associated with adverse outcome included MDS/AML.

A note of caution is sounded regarding HSCT for SDS. Left ventricular fibrosis and necrosis without coronary arterial lesions have been reported in 50% of SDS patients at autopsy, suggesting that there may be an increased risk of cardiotoxicity as well as other problems with the intensive preparatory chemotherapy used in HSCT. Indeed, published data emphasized that complications are more common in SDS patients who receive chemotherapy or undergo transplantation than in non-SDS patients with aplastic anemia. Complications include cardiotoxicity, neurologic and renal complications, venoocclusive disease, pulmonary disease, posttransplant graft failure, and severe GVHD. The heightened risk for patients with SDS after transplantation can be explained in three ways; (1) the presence of the SDS BM stromal defect that is not corrected by the allograft and might be aggravated by the conditioning regimen; (2) increased sensitivity to chemotherapy and radiation, resulting in massive apoptosis in various organs; or (3) performing HSCT relatively late and at an advanced disease stage.

Results of reduced intensity HSCT regimens have been published by two groups. In a study from Cincinnati published in 2008, six patients with severe cytopenia with or without clonal BM cytogenetic abnormalities and one patient with AML in remission were transplanted. The conditioning regimen included Campath-1H, fludarabine, and melphalan. Four patients received matched related MB, two received unrelated peripheral blood, and one had unrelated BM. All patients engrafted and were alive at a median follow-up of 548 (range, 93-920) days. In another study from Hannover, three patients received conditioning with fludarabine, treosulfan, and melphalan in addition to Campath-1H or rabbit ATG. Donor sources were matched sibling BM, matched unrelated BM, or 9/10 matched cord blood. The indications were severe BM failure (n = 2) and MDS (n = 1). The patients who received BM cells survived at 9 and 20 months posttransplant. The other patient died of idiopathic pneumonitis.

Future Directions

Mutant *SBDS* causes SDS in 90% of clinically diagnosed patients. The hunt for additional causative mutant genes in the other 10% is still underway. Identification of such gene(s) may expand our understanding of pathogenesis. Several other clinical and basic research questions in SDS must be addressed. First, the various biochemical functions of the *SBDS* gene require further study. How SBDS protein maintains normal hematopoiesis and protects from apoptosis as well as cancer is unclear. The complete clinical phenotype, natural history, and risk factors for the development of complications need to be determined. There is also a need to understand the mechanism for the heightened sensitivity of SDS patients to chemotherapy and irradiation and to develop low-intensity regimens for HSCT. Research should continue on the efficacy of innovative drugs such as antiapoptotic agents in increasing the growth potential of HSCs and relieving the severity of cytopenia. Determining risk factors and molecular events during malignant myeloid transformation might prompt strategies for prevention and screening for complications.

Dyskeratosis Congenita

Background

Dyskeratosis congenita is an inherited multisystem disorder of the mucocutaneous and hematopoietic systems in association with a wide variety of other somatic abnormalities. Originally, it was considered a dermatologic disease and was termed *Zinsser-Cole-Engman syndrome*. The traditional diagnostic ectodermal triad consists of reticulate skin pigmentation of the upper body, mucosal leukoplakia, and nail dystrophy. The skin and nail findings usually become apparent during the first 10 years of life, but the oral leukoplakia is observed later. These manifestations tend to progress as patients get older.

Hematologic manifestations were subsequently recognized to be a major component of the syndrome and are responsible for substantial morbidity and mortality. Indeed, the full diagnostic dermatologic triad is present only in about 46% of the patients, but BM failure of varying severity is reported in up to 90% of cases. With the recent advances in understanding the molecular basis of the disease, patients with hematologic abnormalities but without dermatologic findings have been identified that dramatically changed the historical definition of the disease. Dyskeratosis congenita patients also have a predisposition to develop cancer and MDS.

Epidemiology

About 550 cases have been reported in the literature. The incidence of dyskeratosis congenita in childhood is about 4 cases per million per year. In older literature, most DC patients were reported as males. However, with better understanding and broadening of the clinical spectrum of the disease and with more autosomal cases being identified, the proportion of males is much lower.

Pathobiology

Multiple genes have been associated with DC (see Table 27-1). All are components of the telomerase complex or the shelterin protein complex. The **X-linked recessive** disease is a common form of DC. It was originally estimated to comprise as many as 75% of DC cases, but with the identification of more DC genes and more patients with autosomal dominant inheritance, the true incidence is approximately 30%. The X-linked disease is caused by mutations in *DKC1* on chromosome Xq28. *DKC1* encodes for the protein dyskerin. Dyskerin associates with the H/ACA class of RNA. Dyskerin binds to the 3′ H/ACA small nucleolar RNA-like domain of the *TERC* component of telomerase. This stimulates telomerase to synthesize telomeric repeats during DNA replication. Dyskerin is also involved in maturation of nascent rRNA. It binds to small nucleolar RNA through the 3′ H/ACA domain and catalyzes the isomerization of uridine to pseudouridine through its peudouridine synthase homology domain. This might be the mechanism for impaired translation from internal ribosome entry sites seen in mice and human DC cells.

Several genes are mutated in families with **autosomal dominant** inheritance. *TINF2* is probably the most commonly mutated gene in this group and accounts for approximately 11% to 25% of the DC families. TINF2 protein is part of the shelterin protein complex that binds to and protects telomeres by allowing cells to distinguish between telomeres and regions of DNA damage. In the complex, TINF2 binds to TRF1, TRF2, POT1, TPP1, and RAP1.

Heterozygous mutations in *TERT* also results in autosomal dominant disease. *TERT* encodes for the enzyme component of telomerase. Telomerase is a ribonucleoprotein polymerase that maintains telomere ends by synthesis and addition of the telomere repeat TTAGGG at the 3′-hydroxy DNA terminus using the *TERC* RNA as a template.

Heterozygous mutations in the *TERC* gene are another cause of autosomal dominant DC. *TERC* encodes for the RNA component of telomerase and has a 3′ H/ACA small nucleolar RNA -like domain.

The **autosomal recessive** forms of DC are caused by biallelic mutations in *NOP10, NHP2, TERT,* or *TCAB1*. In the telomerase complex, the H/ACA domain of nascent human telomerase RNA forms a pre-ribonucleoprotein with NAF1, dyskerin, NOP10, and NHP2. Initially, the core trimer dyskerin-NOP10-NHP2 forms to enable incorporation of NAF1, and efficient reverse transcription of telomere repeats. NOP10 and NHP2 also play an essential role in the assembly and activity of the H/ACA class of small nucleolar ribonucleoproteins that catalyze the isomerization of uridine to pseudouridine in rRNAs.

TCAB1 facilitates trafficking of telomerase to Cajal bodies. Mutations in this gene impair this trafficking activity and lead to misdirection of telomerase RNA to nucleoli; thereby preventing elongation of telomeres by telomerase.

Dyskeratosis congenita cells are characterized by very short telomeres. In several acquired and inherited BM failure syndromes, telomeres are short compared with those from age-matched control participants. However, because the telomerase function is profoundly impaired in DC, the telomeres in this disease are very short (lower than the first percentile of the normal range). Shortening of telomeres results in cellular senescence, apoptosis ("cellular crisis"), or chromosome instability. However, some cells may survive the crisis by harboring compensatory genetic mutations that confer proliferative advantage and neoplastic potential.

Dyskeratosis congenita is a chromosome "instability" disorder of a different type than FA. Results of clastogenic stress studies of DC cells are normal. There is no significant difference in chromosomal breakage between patient and normal lymphocytes with or without exposure to bleomycin, DEB, MMC, or γ-radiation. This contrasts sharply with FA cells and distinguishes one disorder from the other. However, metaphases of cultured patient peripheral blood cells, BM cells, and fibroblasts show numerous spontaneous unbalanced chromosome rearrangements such as dicentrics, tricentrics, and translocations. These are probably caused by short telomeres.

Dyskeratosis congenita with mutations in the *DKC1* (X-linked recessive DC) or *TINF2* and biallelic *TERT* mutations (autosomal recessive DC) can result in a severe form of DC called **Hoyeraal Hreidarsson syndrome**. It is characterized by hematologic and dermatologic manifestations of DC in addition to cerebellar hypoplasia. Immune deficiency is common when this syndrome is caused by *DKC1* mutations. **Revez syndrome** is a combination of classical manifestations of DC and exudative retinopathy. It is caused by mutations in *TINF2* and is an autosomal dominant form of the disease. *TINF2* mutations have also been in children with severe **aplastic anemia** without physical anomalies. Biallelic mutations in *TERT* are also associated with a severe form of DC. However, heterozygosity for mutations in *TERT* is associated with a milder phenotype, late presentation, severe aplastic anemia without physical malformations, isolated pulmonary fibrosis, isolated hepatic fibrosis, or a combination of these clinical manifestations. Heterozygosity for mutations in *TERC* is associated with a milder phenotype, late presentation and severe aplastic anemia, or MDS without physical malformations.

Most studies of the pathogenesis of the aplastic anemia in DC have shown a marked reduction or absence of CFU-GEMM, BFU-E, CFU-E, and CFU-GM. Long-term DC BM cultures have shown that hematopoiesis is severely defective in all patients with a low frequency of colony-forming cells. The function of DC BM stromal cells is normal in their ability to support growth of hematopoietic progenitors from normal BM, but generation of progenitors from DC BM cells seeded over normal stroma is reduced, suggesting that the defect in DC is of stem cell origin. Telomerase is activated in HSCs; however, how mutations that impair telomere maintenance disrupt hematopoiesis is unclear. The BM failure in this disorder may be a result of a progressive attrition and depletion of HSCs. Alternatively, the BM dysfunction may represent a failure of replication, maturation, or both.

Induced pluripotent stem cells (iPSCs) from dyskeratosis congenita patients have been shown to have defects in telomere elongation during programming in a mechanism that is concordant with the mutated gene in the patients. In iPSCs from patients with heterozygous mutations in *TERT,* telomerase activity is directly affected. iPSCs from patients with mutant *DKC1* manifest reduced telomerase activity because of impaired telomerase assembly. iPSCs from a patient with *TCAB1* mutations are characterized mislocalization of telomerase from Cajal bodies to nucleoli. It was also shown that extended culture of *DKC1*-mutant iPSCs leads to progressive telomere shortening and eventual loss of self-renewal. In contrast, another group studied telomerase reactivation and *TERC* regulation during reprogramming and showed that reprogramming restores telomere elongation in dyskeratosis congenita cells despite genetic lesions affecting telomerase. This group showed that *TERC* upregulation is a feature of the pluripotent state and that several telomerase components are targeted by pluripotency associated transcription factors.

Clinical Features

Clinical manifestations in dyskeratosis congenita often appear during childhood. The skin pigmentation and nail changes typically appear first; mucosal leukoplakia and excessive ocular tearing appear later; and by the mid-teens, the serious complications of BM failure and malignancy begin to develop. In a portion of the patients, BM abnormalities appear before or without the skin manifestations.

The DC Registry data from England have detailed the prevalence of somatic abnormalities in families with classic DC. Cutaneous findings are a typical feature of the syndrome. Lacy reticulated skin pigmentation affecting the face, neck, chest, and arms is a common finding (89%). The degree of pigmentation increases with age and can involve the entire skin surface. There may also be a telangiectatic erythematous component. Nail dystrophy of the hands and feet is the next most common finding (88%) (Fig. 27-4). It usually starts with longitudinal ridging, splitting, or pterygium formation and may progress to complete nail loss. Leukoplakia usually involves the oral mucosa (78%), especially the tongue (Fig. 27-5), but may also be seen in the conjunctiva, anal, urethral, or genital mucosa. Hyperhidrosis of the palms and soles is common, and hair loss is sometimes seen. Eye abnormalities are observed in approximately 50% of cases. Excessive tearing (epiphora) secondary to nasolacrimal duct obstruction is common. Other ophthalmologic manifestations include conjunctivitis, blepharitis, loss of eyelashes, strabismus, and cataracts and optic atrophy. Abnormalities of the teeth, particularly an increased rate of dental decay and early loss of teeth, are common. Skeletal abnormalities such as osteoporosis with recurrent long bone fractures, avascular necrosis, abnormal bone trabeculation, scoliosis, and mandibular hypoplasia are seen in approximately 20% of cases. Genitourinary abnormalities include hypoplastic testes, hypospadias, phimosis, and urethral stenosis and horseshoe kidney. Gastrointestinal findings, such as esophageal strictures, hepatomegaly, or cirrhosis, are seen in 10% of cases. A subset of patients develops idiopathic pulmonary fibrosis with reduced diffusion capacity or a restrictive defect. In fatal cases, lung tissue shows pulmonary fibrosis and abnormalities of the pulmonary vasculature. Hepatic fibrosis may also occur. Vasculopathy of the gut, kidneys, liver, chest, or other organs is seen in severe cases and may cause massive bleeding.

Laboratory Findings

Peripheral Blood, Bone Marrow, and Immunologic Findings

The incidence of cytopenias caused by BM failure has been reported in up to 90% of the patients. Severe aplastic anemia occurs in about

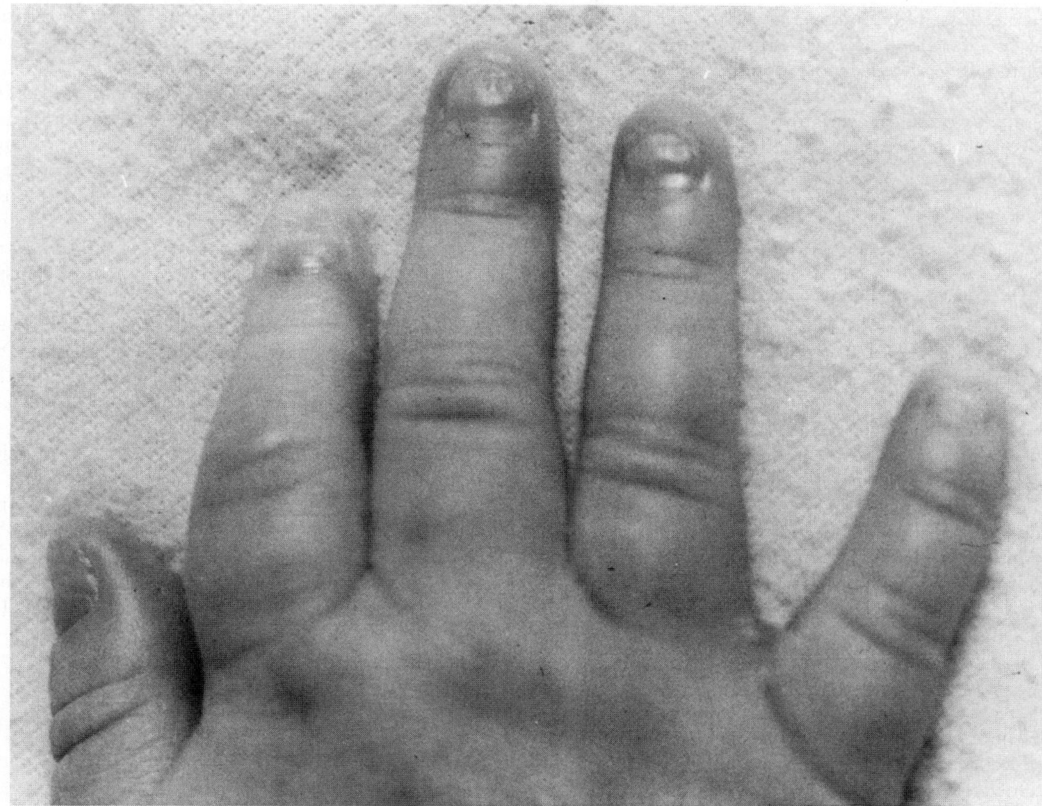

Figure 27-4 DYSTROPHIC NAILS IN DYSKERATOSIS CONGENITA.

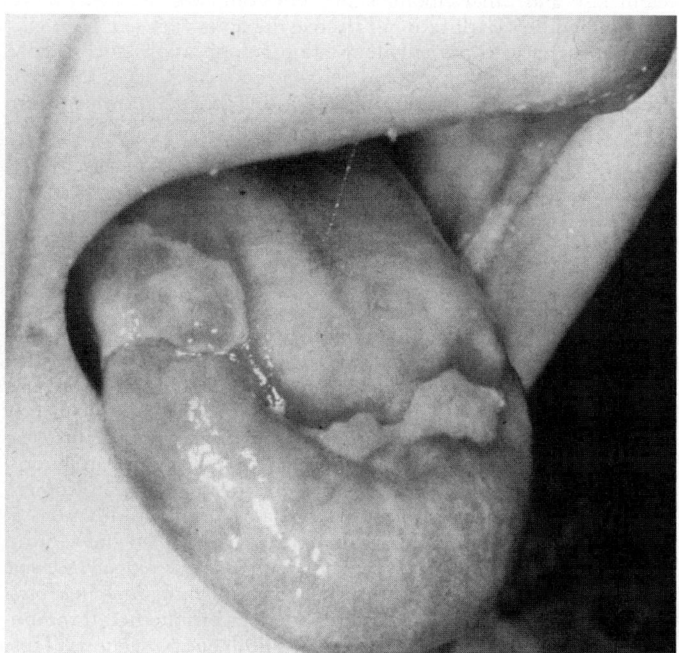

Figure 27-5 LEUKOPLAKIA OF THE TONGUE IN DYSKERATOSIS CONGENITA.

50% of the patients. When BM failure is evident, most patients already have physical manifestations of DC, but this is variable. The initial hematologic change is usually thrombocytopenia, anemia, or both followed by full-blown pancytopenia caused by aplastic anemia. The RBCs are often macrocytic, and the fetal hemoglobin can be elevated. In is noteworthy that early BM specimens and biopsies may be normocellular or hypercellular; however, with time, the cellular elements decline with a symmetrical decrease in all hematopoietic lineages. Ferrokinetic studies at this point are consistent with aplastic anemia. Some patients with DC, particularly those with *DKC1* mutations, have immunologic abnormalities, including reduced immunoglobulin levels, reduced B- or T-lymphocyte numbers, and reduced or absent proliferative responses to PHA. Severe immunodeficiency necessitating HSCT has also been described.

On imaging studies, a small-sized cerebellum may give a clue to the diagnosis in patients with atypical presentations. Imaging of the skeleton usually shows nonspecific osteopenia.

Telomere length is a useful screening testing for DC. In the vast majority of patients, the telomeres are very short (i.e., lower than the first percentile adjusted to age).

Cancer Predisposition

Cancer develops in about 10% to 15% of patients, usually in the third and fourth decades of life. Similar to FA, DC patients can develop solid tumors as well as MDS/AML. However, the incidence of MDS/AML in DC is much lower than in FA. At the age of 50 years, the cumulative risk of solid cancers and MDS/AML is estimated as 40% and 3%, respectively. Most of the cancers are squamous cell carcinomas or adenocarcinomas, and the oropharynx and gastrointestinal tract are involved most frequently. Some patients have multiple separate primaries in different sites involving the tongue and nasopharynx. Thus, the sites of most of the cancers involve areas known to be abnormal in DC, such as mucous membranes and the gastrointestinal tract.

Differential Diagnosis

Several physical findings can be used to distinguish **FA** from DC. The following abnormalities are seen only in DC and not FA: nail dystrophy, leukoplakia, abnormalities of the teeth, hyperhidrosis of the palms and soles, and hair loss. There are overlap syndromes that share some of the features of DC. The **Hoyeraal-Hreidarsson syndrome** variant of DC and the **Revesz syndrome** variant of DC are two examples. Mutant *TINF2* was identified in Revesz syndrome and hence is an autosomal dominant variant of DC. **The ataxia–pancytopenia syndrome** at least in some families is a variant of DC with mutations in *TINF2*.

Natural History and Prognosis

In classical DC, nail dystrophy and skin pigmentation present first, often in the first 10 years of life. BM failure usually follows in the teenage years and twenties. The primary causes of death are hemorrhage secondary to thrombocytopenia or intestinal vascular anomalies, sepsis from severe neutropenia, and complications after HSCT. In the patients who develop cancer or MDS, the disease or its treatment can prove fatal. Pulmonary fibrosis can develop in 20% of cases and is typically progressive and culminates in death caused by respiratory failure. Considerable clinical heterogeneity exists even within the same family, and some patients live into their forties with only moderate nail changes and mild cytopenias. The median survival in the cases reported in the past decade was estimated at 49 years.

Therapy

Androgens

Management of aplastic anemia is similar to treatment for FA. Androgens improve BM function in about 50% of patients. If a response is achieved and deemed to be maximal, the androgen dose can be slowly tapered but not stopped. As in FA, patients typically become refractory to androgens as aplastic anemia progresses. Immunosuppressive therapy is not effective for this disorder, and a portion of the patients with DC are only diagnosed after failure to respond to immunosuppressive therapy for severe aplastic anemia.

G-CSF

A small number of patients were reported who responded to G-CSF therapy with significant increases in absolute neutrophil counts (ANCs). Similarly, two other patients received GM-CSF therapy that resulted in improved neutrophil numbers. G-CSF with erythropoietin resulted in a trilineage hematologic response in one patient. G-CSF plus androgens has led to splenic peliosis and rupture in DC and is not recommended as a long-term treatment if a donor for HSCT is available. Although the reports are scanty, cytokine therapy appears to offer potential benefit, at least in the short term, especially for improving granulopoiesis.

Hematopoietic Stem Cell Transplantation

The outcomes of about 70 patients with DC who have undergone HSCT have been reported. However, the publications are mostly isolated case reports or a small series that limit one's ability to make meaningful correlations of the types of regimens, donors, and indications with outcome. The older literature consists of patients who received myeloablative regimens resulting in a median survival of approximately 3 years after HSCT. Causes of death include unusual complications related to DC that are not prevented by HSCT such as vascular lesions of the gut, kidneys, liver, and lung (≈50% of the patients) and fibrosis involving the lung and liver (≤40% of the patients). These striking complications after HSCT probably reflect the natural history of the disease. However, it is not known whether HSCT can accelerate their course. These unusual complications, uniquely seen in DC, have not been reported in other inherited BM failure syndromes such as FA.

Dyskeratosis congenita is a disorder with chromosomal instability caused by flawed telomere maintenance. This might explain the hypersensitivity to irradiation and chemotherapy. The increased hypersensitivity of DC patients to transplant conditioning can be related to the telomere shortening from DC combined with the accelerated telomere shortening that occurs after HSCT. Further, because of the high degree of mucocutaneous involvement, DC patients may be more susceptible to endothelial damage, which occurs after HSCT as a result of various factors, including the conditioning regimen, cyclosporine A, infectious diseases, GVHD, and cytokine storm. The increased predisposition to posttransplant complications and the tendency to develop tumors highlight the need to avoid certain conditioning agents such as busulfan and irradiation and possibly reduce the intensity of the transplant preparative regiments.

The strategy of using low-intensity fludarabine-based protocols for HSCT has produced encouraging results for DC patients. From 2002 to 2011, 14 patients were transplanted using fludarabine-based reduced intensity protocols. Overall, 11 of the 14 were reported alive at 10 to 72 months posttransplant. These regimens appear to be well tolerated and allow prompt engraftment without significant complications. However, the benefit in reducing the risk of disease-related complications, such as bleeding from vascular lesions and respiratory failure caused by pulmonary fibrosis, is not clear. A Toronto patient reported in 2003 did develop these two complications 7 years after transplant. Also, the role of these conditioning regimens in increasing the additive risk of cancer caused by HSCT is still to be determined.

Future Directions

Although six mutated genes for the three forms of DC have been identified, only 50% of the patients can now be genotyped. Clearly, there is a need to discover additional DC genes. Furthermore, the mechanism by which impaired activity, transport, and stability of telomerase and other ribonucleoprotein complexes influence HSC function requires clarification. Effective therapies with reduced toxicity are necessary to prevent devastating complications such as BM failure, pulmonary fibrosis, and vascular anomalies. Last, there is a need for studies focusing on translating this genetic knowledge into gene therapy.

Congenital Amegakaryocytic Thrombocytopenia

Background

Congenital amegakaryocytic thrombocytopenia (CAMT) is an autosomal recessive syndrome that typically presents in infancy with isolated thrombocytopenia caused by reduced or absent BM megakaryocytes with preservation initially of granulopoietic and erythroid lineages (see Chapters 26). Aplastic anemia subsequently ensues in the vast majority of the patients, usually in the first few years of life. Most patients do not have physical malformations; therefore, the diagnosis depends on the exclusion of other acquired and inherited causes of thrombocytopenia in early life. Mutations of the thrombopoietin receptor, MPL, have been identified and confirm that sporadic and familial cases are inherited in an autosomal recessive manner. *CAMT* is a distinct genetic entity, but mutations in several other genes have been described in a number of inherited thrombocytopenias that must be considered in the differential diagnosis (Table 27-5).

Epidemiology

More than 100 cases have been reported in the literature. However, with the recent identification of patients with *MPL* mutations and relatively late presentation, it is possible that the incidence is higher and includes a portion of the patients with aplastic anemia who do not respond to immunosuppressive therapy. The incidence of diagnosed cases is estimated at one case per million births per year.

Table 27-5 Miscellaneous Inherited Thrombocytopenia Disorders and Their Major Hematologic Features

Disorder	Genetics	Mutant Gene	Platelet Size*	Features
Amegakaryocytic thrombocytopenia	AR	*MPL*	Normal	± Physical anomalies
Thrombocytopenia absent radii	AR	Unknown	Normal	Physical anomalies
MYH9-related thrombocytopenia: May-Hegglin anomaly	AD	*MYH9*	Large	Neutrophil inclusions
Fechtner syndrome	AD	*MYH9*	Large	Neutrophil inclusions, hearing loss, nephritis
Epstein syndrome	AD	*MYH9*	Large	No inclusions, hearing loss, nephritis
Sebastian syndrome	AD	*MYH9*	Large	Neutrophil inclusions
X-linked macrothrombocytopenia	X-L	*GATA1*	Large	Anemia, dyserythropoiesis, thalassemia
Wiskott-Aldrich syndrome	X-L	*WAS*	Small	Immune deficiency, eczema
X-linked thrombocytopenia	X-L	*WAS*	Small	No associated features
Thrombocytopenia and radio-ulnar synostosis	AD	*HOXA11*	Normal	Fused radius, limited range of motion
Familial platelet disorder/AML	AD	*AML1 (RUNX1; CBFA2)*	Normal	MDS, AML
Familial dominant thrombocytopenia	AD	*FLJ14813*	Normal	No associated features
Paris-Trousseau thrombocytopenia	AD	*FLI1* (hemizygous deletion)	Large	Dysmegakaryocytopoiesis, Jacobsen syndrome
Bernard-Soulier syndrome	AR	*GP1BA*	Large	No associated features
Bernard-Soulier carrier/Mediterranean macrothrombocytopenia	AD	*GP1BA*	Large	No associated features

AD, Autosomal dominant; *AML*, acute myeloid leukemia; *AR*, autosomal recessive; *MDS*, myelodysplastic syndrome; *MPV*, mean platelet volume; *X-L*, X-linked recessive.
*Platelet size: small, MPV <7 fL; normal, MPV 7-11 fL; large or giant, MPV >11 fL.

Pathobiology

The defect in CAMT is directly related to mutations in *MPL*, the gene for the thrombopoietin receptor that maps to 1p34 in 94% of the patients. Heterozygote carriers of the mutant gene have normal blood cell counts. Affected individuals have mutations in both alleles in either homozygous or compound heterozygous state. Mutations have been found throughout the *MPL* gene, including nonsense, missense, frameshift, and splicing mutations. A genotype–phenotype correlation has been identified in CAMT patients and two prognostic groups established, types I and II.

Type 1

Frameshift and nonsense mutations produce a complete loss of function of and signaling from the thrombopoietin receptor in type I by deletion of all or most of the intracellular domain. This causes persistently low platelet counts and a rapid progression to pancytopenia. Thrombopoietin plays a critical role in the proliferation, survival, and differentiation of early and late megakaryocytes. This clearly explains the thrombocytopenia. However, *MPL* is also highly expressed in HSCs and promotes their quiescence and survival. Thus, MPL protein insufficiency may account for depletion of HSCs and pancytopenia. Evolution into severe aplastic anemia is particularly common in type I.

Type II

Congenital amegakaryocytic thrombocytopenia with missense and splicing mutations cause reduced expression of the protein, reduced localization to the plasma membrane (e.g., R102P in the extracellular domain), or an inability to bind thrombopoietin (e.g., F104S). Patients with these mutations have a milder course; a transient increase in platelet counts during the first years of life; and delayed onset, if any, of pancytopenia, indicating residual receptor function.

Serial studies of CAMT hematopoiesis using clonogenic assays have been informative. Initially, when the only hematologic abnormality is isolated thrombocytopenia, the numbers of hematopoietic progenitors are comparable to those of control participants, including the number of megakaryocyte precursors, CFU-MK (colony-forming unit megakaryocytes; CFU-Meg). As the disease evolves into aplastic anemia, the peripheral blood counts decline, and colony numbers from progenitors belonging to each myeloid lineage also decline in parallel. When added to the BM cultures, patient plasma is not inhibitory to control or to patient colony growth. Similarly, no cellular inhibition of hematopoiesis is observed when the patient BM is cultured after depleting the sample of T lymphocytes or after adding them back. Stromal cells established in short- and long-term cultures of patient BM show normal proliferative activity and yield a "fertile" BM microenvironment for patient and control BM colony growth. The findings are consistent with current knowledge about *MPL* mutations, namely, that the central problem in CAMT is an intrinsic HSC defect rather than an abnormality of the BM milieu.

Other data demonstrate measurable numbers of CFU-MK progenitors in vitro from patients with CAMT when studied early in the disease in response to IL-3, GM-CSF, or a combination of both but defective CFU-MK colony formation in response to recombinant human thrombopoietin that fits with *MPL* mutations. Plasma thrombopoietin levels in patients with CAMT are always elevated and are among the highest seen in any patient population.

The pathogenesis of the associated neurologic abnormalities (see Clinical Features) is less understood; however, MPL is expressed in the neuronal cells and might be important for their development.

Clinical Features

Almost all patients present with a petechial rash, bruising, or bleeding during the first year of life. Most cases are obvious at birth or within the first 2 months. Almost all of the patients with proven *MPL* mutations have normal physical and imaging features, but isolated cases with anomalies have been identified. A patient in the Canadian Registry with an *MPL* mutation had a cystic fourth ventricle and Dandy Walker malformation (unpublished data).

Before the availability of genotyping, physical anomalies were an important part of the clinical phenotype in published case reports and small series. The commonest anomalies in published phenotypic CAMT patients are neurologic, including varying degrees of cerebellar hypoplasia or agenesis, cerebral atrophy, cortical dysplasia and lissencephaly, and hypoplasia of the corpus callosum and brainstem. Facial malformations have also been described. Developmental delay is a prominent feature among those with physical malformations. Patients may also have microcephaly and an abnormal facies.

Congenital heart disease with a variety of malformations can be detected, including atrial septal defects, ventricular septal defects, patent ductus arteriosus, tetralogy of Fallot, and coarctation of the aorta. Some of these occur in combinations. Other anomalies include abnormal hips or feet, kidney malformations, eye anomalies, and cleft or high-arched palate. Some affected sibships manifested both normal and abnormal physical findings in the same family.

Laboratory Findings

Thrombocytopenia is the major laboratory finding with normal hemoglobin levels and white blood cell counts initially. Although there are usually measurable but reduced platelet numbers, peripheral blood platelets may be totally absent. Those that can be identified are of normal size and appearance. Similar to other inherited BM failure syndromes, RBCs may be macrocytic. HbF is increased in most but not all patients, and there may be increased expression of i antigen. BM aspirates and biopsies initially show normal cellularity with markedly reduced or absent megakaryocytes (Fig. 27-6). In patients who develop aplastic anemia, BM cellularity is decreased with fatty replacement, and the erythropoietic and granulopoietic lineages are symmetrically reduced.

Predisposition to Leukemia

Cases with CAMT have been reported with secondary clonal BM cytogenetic abnormalities such as monosomy 7 and trisomy 8, MDS, or AML. Several published cases clearly demonstrate a typical progression of thrombocytopenia, aplastic anemia, and clonal or malignant myeloid transformation. One boy with a normal physical appearance had amegakaryocytic thrombocytopenia from day 1 of life, developed aplastic anemia at 5 years of age, responded poorly to androgens and steroids, and then developed AML at age 16 years with death at age 17 years. A girl had thrombocytopenia at 2 months of age, pancytopenia at 5 months, and thereafter developed a preleukemic picture with clonal abnormalities involving chromosome 19. Another patient had thrombocytopenia at 6 months of age, developed progressive aplastic anemia over the next 2 years, acquired monosomy 7 in BM cells at 5 years of age, and then developed MDS with an activating *RAS* oncogene mutation in hematopoietic cells. Hence, the current evidence indicates that CAMT is another inherited BM failure disorder that is preleukemic. The risk or incidence of malignant conversion is difficult to determine because of the rarity of the disease and the paucity of published data, and because patients frequently require early HSCT.

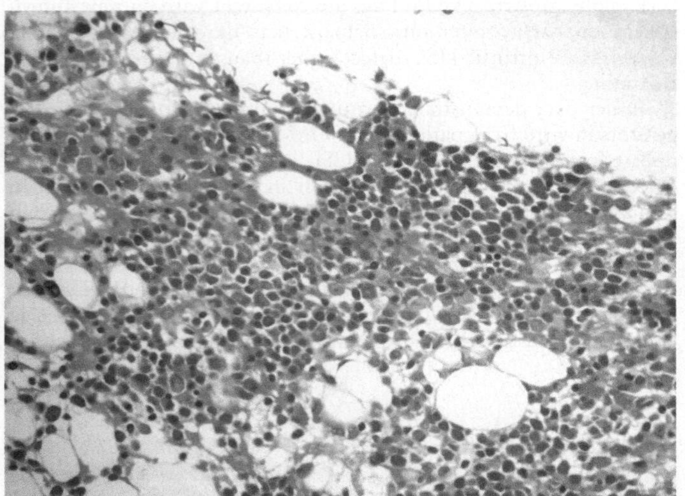

Figure 27-6 LOW-POWER VIEW OF A BONE MARROW ASPIRATE FROM A NEWLY DIAGNOSED PATIENT WITH CONGENITAL AMEGAKARYOCYTIC THROMBOCYTOPENIA. The three findings are normal cellularity, normal granulopoiesis and erythropoiesis, and absent megakaryocytes. *(Photomicrograph prepared by Dr. Mohamed Abdelhaleem, Toronto.)*

Differential Diagnosis

If CAMT presents at birth or shortly after, it must be distinguished from other causes of severe neonatal thrombocytopenia, which most commonly are caused by severe systemic congenital infections collectively designated as the **TORCH** (***To**xoplasma gondii,* **r**ubella, **c**ytomegalovirus, and **h**erpes simplex virus) **syndrome** or **other neonatal infections** caused by bacteria or viruses. Usually, these infectious etiologies are characterized by increased peripheral destruction of platelets or a combination of peripheral destruction and BM suppression.

Passive transplacental passage of IgG antiplatelet antibodies into fetal circulation can cause rapid destruction of fetal platelets. This occurs in two circumstances: a (1) **maternal autoimmune disease** such as idiopathic thrombocytopenic purpura or systemic lupus erythematosus and (2) in **neonatal alloimmune thrombocytopenia** by alloimmunization of the pregnant mother to fetal antigens inherited from father but absent in the mother. In the former situation, the mother has thrombocytopenia or a history of such; in the latter situation, the mother has a normal platelet count and serum antibodies to human platelet alloantigens.

Thrombocytopenia with absent radii syndrome is distinguished from CAMT because in TAR, the radii are absent. Peripheral blood chromosomes analysis is not associated with increased breakage with DEB or MMC clastogenic stress testing, which allows CAMT to be distinguished from **FA.** Increased platelet destruction also occurs in newborns with giant benign hemangiomas of skin, liver, or spleen, the so-called **Kasabach-Merritt syndrome.**

In an infant or young child with a CAMT clinical diagnosis but without mutant *MPL*, **other inherited forms of thrombocytopenia** should be addressed (see Table 27-5). These can generally be classified according to inheritance pattern (autosomal dominant, autosomal recessive, or X-linked recessive), size of the platelets (small, normal, or large or giant), and presence or absence of associated clinical features. Identification of the specific mutant gene for each disorder confirms the diagnosis.

If CAMT presents beyond the neonatal age period, it must be distinguished from causes of peripheral platelet destruction such as in chronic immune thrombocytopenia purpura, acquired amegakaryocytic thrombocytopenia or aplastic anemia, other inherited BM failure syndromes, MDS, and acute leukemias. The medical history of the patient and family, physical examination, and initial laboratory test results may help to exclude other disorders. However, a BM aspirate and biopsy will point to the diagnosis, and a *MPL* mutational analysis will confirm the diagnosis.

Therapy and Prognosis

Supportive treatment has been largely unsatisfactory to date, and the mortality rate from thrombocytopenic bleeding, complications of aplastic anemia, or malignant myeloid transformation has been very close to 100%. For that reason, HLA typing of family members should be performed as soon as the diagnosis is confirmed to determine if a matched related donor for HSCT exists. If not, a search for a matched unrelated donor or for a cord blood graft should ensue as soon as the severity of the clinical picture is appreciated. The need for transfusional support is a cogent indication.

Platelet transfusions should be used discretely. Platelet numbers should not be a sole indication; clinical bleeding is a more appropriate trigger for the use of platelets. Single-donor filtered platelets are preferred to multiple unfiltered random donor platelets to minimize sensitization, and if HSCT is a realistic possibility, all blood products should be free of cytomegalovirus and irradiated.

Corticosteroids have been used for thrombocytopenia with no apparent efficacy. Androgens with or without low-dose corticosteroid therapy may induce a partial response, but the effect is short-lived and does not after the long-term outcome.

Based on the in vitro augmentation of megakaryocyte progenitor colony growth in response to IL-3, a small phase I/II clinical trial was initiated for CAMT. IL-3 resulted in improved platelet counts in two of five patients and decreased bleeding and transfusion requirements in the other three. Prolonged IL-3 administration in two additional patients also resulted in platelet increments. This pilot study illustrates that IL-3 may have been an important adjunct to the medical management of CAMT, but it was not adopted broadly and is no longer commercially available. GM-CSF has a positive in vitro effect but not in vivo. Thrombopoietin has not been tried for the treatment of severe type I CAMT and would likely fail because endogenous thrombopoietin levels are markedly increased and the mutated thrombopoietin receptor is nonfunctional. Nevertheless, thrombopoietin agonists that bind to the transmembrane domain might prove efficacious, similar to the in vitro effect of LGD-4665 on cells carrying the F104S *MPL* mutation. LGD-4665 binds to the transmembrane domain of the MPL receptor. Initial application of such a strategy should be assessed as part of clinical trials because of a potential risk of developing hematologic malignancies.

Congenital amegakaryocytic thrombocytopenia can be cured by HSCT. Most of the recent published cases have had successful outcomes. Matched sibling donor sources are ideal even if the donor is a carrier with one mutant allele. Reduced-intensity conditioning regimens for CAMT have been successfully used even in a case with monosomy 7 and in the unrelated donor setting. HSCT using T cell–depleted BM with relatively high $CD34^+$ cell numbers and enhanced T cell–specific immunosuppression in the transplant cytoreductive regimens that have also been successful.

Future Directions

Novel therapy with thrombopoietin receptor agonists may be suitable for type I and type II CAMT patients who retain some MPL function. The cellular consequences of specific gene mutations need to be further studied because this might help to develop novel strategies in patients who do not respond to such therapies. CAMT is also a candidate disease for gene therapy because restoration of wild-type *MPL* would provide in vivo selection of corrected HSCs.

Other Inherited Syndromes With Associated Pancytopenia

Bone marrow failure and cancer predisposition can occur as part of several specific other inherited syndromes and in familial settings that do not exactly correspond with the entities already described.

Down Syndrome

Down syndrome, or constitutional trisomy 21 (+21), has a unique association with aberrant hematologic abnormalities. Three related events can occur. In the neonatal period, a myeloproliferative blood picture with large numbers of circulating blast cells has been observed in approximately 10% of these infants. The blasts show somatic *GATA1* mutations and apparently are clonal but, remarkably, disappear spontaneously over several weeks in most cases. The term *transient myeloproliferative disorder* is often used to describe this unusual clinical picture.

Second, in 20% to 30% of these transient cases, *true* acute megakaryoblastic leukemia (AMKL), also with *GATA1* mutations, appears later and requires treatment. Acute lymphoblastic and myeloblastic leukemias are also seen in Down syndrome, but AMKL is the most common form of myeloblastic leukemia and is estimated to be 500 times greater in children with trisomy 21 than in other children.

Third, the onset of AMKL is frequently preceded by an interval of MDS characterized by thrombocytopenia; abnormal megakaryocytopoiesis; megakaryoblasts in the BM; and an abnormal karyotype, commonly trisomy 8 or monosomy 7. In addition to the propensity for leukemia, a few patients have been reported with aplastic anemia. Of five trisomy 21 with aplastic anemia cases in the literature, three died of BM failure and two responded to androgen therapy.

Dubowitz Syndrome

This is an autosomal recessive disorder characterized by a peculiar facies, infantile eczema, small stature, and mild microcephaly. The face is small with a shallow supraorbital ridge, a nasal bridge at the same level as the forehead, short palpebral fissures, variable ptosis, and micrognathia. This is a rare disorder, and incidence rates for complications are difficult to establish; however, there appears to be a predilection to develop cancer as well as hematopoietic disorders in children with Dubowitz syndrome. Patients have developed acute leukemia, neuroblastoma, and lymphoma. Approximately 10% of patients also develop hematologic abnormalities varying from hypoplastic anemia, moderate pancytopenia, and full-blown aplastic anemia. The mutant gene has not been identified.

Seckel Syndrome

Sometimes called *bird-headed dwarfism,* patients with this autosomal recessive developmental disorder have marked intrauterine and postnatal growth failure, mental deficiency, severe microcephaly, a hypoplastic face with a receding forehead and chin, a prominent curved nose, and low-set or malformed ears. Some patients may show increased chromosomal breakage in lymphocyte cultures with DEB or MMC and mimic FA. About 25% of patients develop aplastic anemia or malignancies. There are possibly five genes linked to Seckel syndrome, all in different cytogenetic locations. Four have been identified: mutant *ATR* has been confirmed for the Seckel 1 subtype; *RBBP8* is responsible for Seckel 2; *CENPJ* for Seckel 4; and *CEP152* for Seckel 5. The abnormal gene for Seckel 3 has been mapped to 14q21-q22. Genotyping will distinguish FA from Seckel syndrome.

Reticular Dysgenesia (Dysgenesis)

This is an immunologic deficiency syndrome coupled with congenital agranulocytosis. The mode of inheritance is autosomal recessive caused by biallelic mutations in mitochondrial *AK2*. The disorder is a variant of severe combined immune deficiency in which cellular and humoral immunity are absent; patients also have severe lymphopenia and neutropenia. Because of profoundly compromised immunity, the syndrome presents early with severe infection at birth or shortly thereafter. A striking feature is absent lymph nodes and tonsils and an absent thymic shadow on radiographs. In addition to lymphopenia and neutropenia, anemia and thrombocytopenia may be present. BM specimens are hypocellular with markedly reduced myeloid and lymphoid elements. Clonogenic assays of hematopoietic progenitors consistently show reduced to absent colony growth, indicating that the disorder has its origins at the HSC level. The only curative therapy is HSCT.

Schimke Immunoosseous Dysplasia

Schimke immunoosseous dysplasia is an autosomal recessive disorder caused by mutations in the chromatin remodelling gene *SMARCAL1* in 50% to 60% of patients. Patients manifest spondyloepiphyseal dysplasia with exaggerated lumbar lordosis and a protruding abdomen. They have pigmentary skin changes and abnormally discolored and configured teeth. Renal dysfunction can be problematic with proteinuria and nephrotic syndrome. Approximately 50% of patients have hypothyroidism and 50% have cerebral ischemia; 50% have anemia, 50% have neutropenia, 30% have thrombocytopenia, and 10% have aplastic anemia. Lymphopenia and altered cellular immunity are present in 80% of patients. One patient has undergone a successful stem cell transplantation.

Noonan Syndrome

Noonan syndrome (NS) is a developmental disorder characterized by the *Noonan facies* (hypertelorism, ptosis, short neck, low-set ears), short stature, congenital heart disease, and multiple skeletal and hematologic abnormalities. The literature describes several NS patients who developed amegakaryocytic thrombocytopenia and another who developed pancytopenia and a hypocellular BM. NS is an autosomal dominant disorder with genetic heterogeneity. So far, heterozygous germline mutations in nine genes (*PTPN11, SOS1, KRAS, NRAS, RAF1, BRAF, SHOC2, MEK1,* and *CBL*) underlie the disorder in 75% of cases. These genes encode for proteins in the RAS-mitogen–activated protein kinases signal transduction pathway. A variant of neurofibromatosis type 1(NF1) caused by germline mutations in the *NF1* gene shares a phenotypic overlap disorder with NS, the so-called *neurofibromatosis–Noonan syndrome*. Remarkably, children with NF1 and with NS both have an increased risk of juvenile myelomonocytic leukemia (JMML), a rare, aggressive hematologic cancer with onset in the first few years of life. Of note, three of the mutated genes that cause NS (*PTPN11, KRAS,* and *NRAS*) are also found as somatic mutations in BM cells from children with JMML.

Cartilage-Hair Hypoplasia

Cartilage-hair hypoplasia (CHH) is an autosomal recessive syndrome characterized by metaphyseal dysostosis; short-limbed dwarfism; and fine, sparse hair. Additional skeletal findings include scoliosis, lordosis, chest deformity, and varus lower limbs. Aganglionic megacolon and other gastrointestinal abnormalities have been reported. Most cases in the literature are Finnish or Amish. Mutations in the noncoding RNA gene *RMRP* are seen in more than 80% of cases. Macrocytic anemia of varying severity is seen in the majority of patients. Most patients have mild and self-limited anemia, but some are severe and persistent resembling Diamond-Blackfan anemia and require RBC transfusions. Severe immunodeficiency can occur, often with the severe anemia. HSCT has been used successfully to reconstitute the immune system. Neutropenia has been reported in 25% of CHH cases and lymphopenia in 65%. Lymphomas and basal cell carcinoma also occur at an increased frequency.

Pearson Syndrome

Pearson syndrome is an inherited failure of BM and, in 30% of cases, impaired exocrine pancreatic function caused by acinar cell atrophy and fibrosis. Patients with Pearson syndrome have a maternally inherited diagnostic deletion of mtDNA that encodes enzymes that are critical to oxidative phosphorylation. The genetic deletion results in a syndrome of refractory anemia with ringed sideroblasts and prominent vacuolization of BM erythroid and myeloid precursors. Physical malformations are rarely observed. Severe anemia requiring transfusions is present within the first year of life, sometimes at birth. Pancytopenia may occur alone or in association with hepatic failure and a renal tubulopathy leading to lactic acidosis. The projected median survival time is 4 years. Anemia is managed with RBC and platelet transfusional support. Erythropoietin has been used for the anemia of renal failure. G-CSF is indicated for severe neutropenia. The need for pancreatic enzyme replacement is unclear.

Other Unclassified Inherited Forms of Bone Marrow Failure

Bone marrow failure can cluster in families, but many of these cases cannot be readily classified into discrete diagnostic entities such as FA, SDS, or DC. The phenotype of these familial conditions can be complex with varying combinations of cytopenias, macrocytosis, elevated levels of HbF, hypocellular BM, immunologic deficiency, physical malformations, and predisposition to leukemia. The BM failure appears to be the result of a complex interplay of mutant genes, modifying genes, epigenetic processes, acquired factors, and chance effects that may be specific to each affected family. Published examples of unclassified familial forms of BM failure have been reviewed and divided into inheritance patterns, and then subdivided into cases with and without physical anomalies.

Using the Canada-wide database of the CIMFR, a unique study was launched on IBMFs cases that were deemed unclassifiable at study entry. Of 162 enrolled patients, 39 were registered as having an unclassified disorder. Although the hematologic phenotypes were similar to the classified syndromes in the registry (single- or multilineage cytopenia, severe aplastic anemia, MDS, AML, and cancer), the patients presented at an older age (median, 9 months vs. median 1 month for classified), and the variation in clinical presentations was substantial. Grouping patients according to physical abnormalities and hematologic phenotype was not always sufficient to characterize or diagnose a condition because affected members from several families fit into different phenotypic groupings. It was difficult to formulate a sensible and cost-effective diagnostic workup based on the family histories and hematologic and physical findings. Compared with workups of classifiable syndromes, clastogenic chromosomal fragility testing and extensive genotyping efforts of the unclassified cases required use of several-fold higher specific diagnostic tests at a cost that was 4.5 times higher per evaluated patient. Despite these efforts and the huge, recent explosion of gene discovery, only 20% of unclassified patients were diagnosed with a specific syndrome, underscoring ongoing diagnostic limitations for these disorders.

Treatment of Unclassified Familial Forms of Bone Marrow Failure

Because these disorders are rare, broad conclusions about management are difficult to formulate. For full-blown aplastic anemia with a hypocellular, fatty BM or for MDS/AML, curative therapy with HSCT remains the first choice if a suitable donor is identified. In the familial cases, potential related stem cell donors must be thoroughly assessed clinically, hematologically, and by diagnostic laboratory testing to ensure that latent or masked BM dysfunction is not present. If a matched sibling donor is not available, an unrelated donor search should be initiated, and in the interim, principles of medical management used for FA and for acquired aplastic anemia should be used.

UNILINEAGE CYTOPENIAS

Diamond-Blackfan Anemia

Background

Diamond-Blackfan anemia, previously called *congenital hypoplastic anemia,* is an inherited form of pure RBC aplasia. The syndrome is heterogeneous with respect to genetic causes, clinical and laboratory findings, in vitro data, and therapeutic outcome. DBA is the first disease to be identified as a *ribosomopathy*. It is also the best example of the ribosomopathies because all currently known DBA genes are components of the small or large ribosome subunits. However, only about 55% of the patients can now be genotyped; thus, it is still possible that different pathways are affected by undiscovered DBA genes. All genetically proven cases show autosomal dominant inheritance with variable penetrance. Recessive inheritance was inferred in more than 30 families published in the literature that had affected siblings with normal parents, affected cousins, or consanguinity. However, these cases have not been confirmed as autosomal recessive. Some of these may be autosomal dominant with partial penetrance or arise from gonadal mosaicism.

Epidemiology

Based on data from a European registry of DBA patients, the estimated incidence of the disorder as assessed for France over a 13-year period was 7.3 cases per million live births. Data from the Canadian Registry show an incidence of 10.4 cases per million live births as assessed over a 9-year period. Although the majority of published patients are white, DBA has been recognized in several ethnic groups, including African blacks, Arabs, East Indians, and Japanese.

In terms of gender distribution, both sexes are equally affected. About 80% of DBA cases are sporadic.

Etiology, Genetics, and Pathophysiology

The discovery of nine DBA genes (see Table 27-1) demonstrates heterozygosity for mutations in the respective genes consistent with autosomal dominant inheritance in all currently known genetic groups. All known DBA proteins are structural components of either the small or large ribosomal subunits.

In most DBA cases peripheral blood karyotype is normal, although alterations of chromosomes 1 and 16 have been reported. Discovery of a balanced reciprocal translocation t(x;19) in a sporadic female case of DBA and the identification of microdeletions on chromosome 19 in some other DBA patients led to the identification of the first DBA gene mutation. Subsequent studies revealed mutations in one allele for the gene in 25% of patients, and it is currently the most common known mutant DBA gene.

RPS19 protein is a component of the ribosomal 40S subunit. Multiple other genes encoding either the 40S small ribosome subunit or 60S ribosome subunit have been subsequently identified in DBA. The second most commonly mutated gene in DBA is *RPL5*. It is mutated in 12% to 21% of the patients. Other mutated genes are *RPL11* (7%-9% of the patients), *RPS26* (10%), *RPS10* (4%), *RPS24* (2%), *RPL35a* (2%), *RPS17* (<1%), and *RPS7* (<1%). Alterations in *RPL30, RPS15,* and *RPS27a* have also been identified, but the etiologic significance of these alterations is still unclear. Despite the identification of many mutated genes in DBA, only about 55% of the patients with DBA can now be genotyped.

Recent studies have shed light on the function of the RPS19 protein in ribosome biogenesis. RPS19 associates with the ribosomal subunit 40S. It is critical for normal maturation of rRNA because its deficiency causes defective cleavage of the pre-rRNA at the ITS1 sequence and abnormal maturation of the 40S subunit. This leads to accumulation of faulty pre-40S ribosome subunits.

Other ribosomal proteins that are mutated in DBA are also critical for ribosome biogenesis, For example, it has been shown that the yeast RPL11 is positioned at the intersubunit cleft of the large ribosome subunit central protuberance, thereby forming an intersubunit bridge with the small subunit protein S18. Mutations in this region such as F96 and A66 lead to halfmer formation. Mutations in RPS24 also impair pre-rRNA processing of the 18S rRNA and decrease the production of the 40S ribosomal subunit. On the other hand, depletion of RPL35A reduces the amount of the 60S subunit and of the mature 80S ribosomes.

The mechanism by which RP gene mutations impairs RBC development remains unknown. In 25% of cases with mutant *RPS19,* the prevailing opinion is that the disorder results from protein haploinsufficiency. In support of this, two classes of *RPS19* mutations have been described: quantitative defects resulting in undetectable protein and hotspot mutations leading to loss of function. Additional links between *RPS19* and erythropoiesis have now been clearly established. Defective erythropoiesis ensues when *RPS19* is knocked down in cellular models. In addition, wild-type gene transfer corrects the defective erythropoiesis in *RPS19*-deficient DBA CD34+ cells resulting in a threefold increase in erythroid colony growth. In yeast, the introduction of *RPS19* mutations found in DBA results in a defect in the processing of pre-rRNA similar to that observed in DBA cells with decreased expression of *RPS19*.

A large body of evidence indicates that the erythroid progenitor compartment is intrinsically defective in DBA. Standard clonogenic assays for CFU-E and BFU-E progenitors consistently have shown reduced or absent colonies in most DBA patients and intermediate, normal, or occasionally increased numbers in the rest. The DBA erythroid progenitors are relatively insensitive to erythropoietin in vitro and to burst-promoting activity, but the hyporesponsiveness to erythropoietin can be corrected in some cases by the addition of glucocorticoids in vitro or by clinically administering prednisone.

The data underscore the fact that the intrinsic defect of DBA erythroid progenitors is an inability to respond normally to inducers of erythroid proliferation, differentiation, or both. Indeed, DBA $CD34^+$ HSCs/early progenitors differentiate normally along megakaryocytic and granulocytic pathways in short-term cultures but aberrantly along the erythroid lineage. Accelerated programmed cell death (apoptosis) plays a central role in this pathogenesis as it does in many, if not all, inherited BM failure disorders. A role for induction of apoptosis by the Fas–Fas ligand system in DBA was suggested because of elevated serum soluble Fas ligand in patients compared with control participants. Based on the various patterns of erythroid colony growth seen with DBA patients, a model for the aberrant erythropoiesis was developed that proposes maturational arrest at varying sites along the differentiation pathway.

The combination of recombinant IL-3 and Steel factor (SCF) increases the in vitro clonogenicity of DBA BM progenitors. The size and number of DBA BFU-E colonies are dramatically increased. The data on the effect of IL3, SCF, or GM-CSF as single agents is less conclusive. The human ligand for flt-3 apparently has no effect on DBA BM colony growth. However, addition of IL-9 to SCF, IL-3, and erythropoietin does potentiate DBA BFU-E growth.

There are significant age-related changes in erythroid and granulopoietic progenitors in DBA patients. Despite profound anemia, seven of 10 patients studied within 1 year of diagnosis had normal numbers of CFU-E and BFU-E that showed a normal response to cytokines. In contrast, 12 of 14 patients followed more than 3 years had decreased erythroid progenitors and, in seven cases, decreased CFU-GM. The data are consistent with the idea that the DBA defect involves other hematopoietic lineages and worsens with time.

Strong support for this conclusion comes from a detailed study that examined the interaction between DBA $CD34^+$ cells and the hematopoietic microenvironment using long-term BM cultures. Stromal adherent layers from DBA patients did not show evidence of any morphologic, phenotypic, or functional abnormality, and the stroma sustained the proliferation of normal $CD34^+$ cells. A major finding was an impaired capacity of DBA $CD34^+$ cells in the presence of normal stromal cells to proliferate and differentiate along not only the erythroid pathway but also along the granulocytic–macrophage pathway. These results indicate an intrinsic defect of a hematopoietic progenitor with at least bilineage potential that places it earlier than previously suspected and that was only unmasked by testing in long-term cultures. This observation, however, is in keeping with the clinical observation that in addition to anemia, patients may have neutropenia and thrombocytopenia. These findings were extended with evidence in long-term culture initiating assays for a trilineage defect in DBA refractory to treatment. The data broaden the definition of DBA and explain generalized BM dysfunction and hypoplasia in some cases of DBA that have puzzled investigators for years.

The molecular mechanism that links ribosome protein haploinsufficiency to the erythroid defect is unclear. One hypothesis is that it is related to translation insufficiency. It is well known that during early stages of erythropoiesis, translation is increased. It is possible that the need for protein synthesis is not met during this critical developmental stage. A second hypothesis is that *RP* gene mutations lead to accumulation of abnormal rRNA precursors as well as dysregulation of multiple ribosomal protein genes and protein expression as shown with *RPS19*. This leads to defective ribosome biogenesis, unassembled ribosome proteins, and possibly cellular stress.

A third hypothesis and the one considered most plausible is that defective ribosome biogenesis leads to activation of p53, thereby causing apoptosis and cell cycle arrest. A role of p53 is supported by a recent mouse model with mutations in *RPS19* that is characterized by RBC underproduction and small mouse size and by zebrafish models of *RPS19* inhibition that manifest impaired erythropoiesis and malformations. Activation of p53 may involve the interactions of MDM2 with specific ribosomal proteins such as RPL5, RPL11, and RPL23. These interactions may lead to dissociation of p53 from MDM2, impairment of p53 targeting to the proteosome, and prevention of proteosome degradation. However, these models do not explain how haploinsufficiency of RPL5 and RPL11 leads to p53 activation.

Extraribosomal functions have been ascribed to various RP genes that might mediate BM failure. For example, RPS19 has been shown to interact with a nucleolar protein S19-binding protein (S19BP), fibroblast growth factor 2, and the PIM-1 oncoprotein. PIM-1 is an ubiquitous serine-threonine kinase, the expression of which can be induced in erythropoietic cells by several growth factors, including erythropoietin. Thus, there may be a possible link between erythropoietic growth factor signaling and RPS19.

The erythroid lineage is predominantly impaired in DBA for unknown reasons. Studies have shown that the heme exporter FLVCR1 is critical for CFU-E development. Knocking out FLVCR1 in mice causes impaired CFU-E development. A partial block in human FLVCR1 in $CD34^+$ HSCs recapitulates the hematologic features of DBA, including $CD36^+/CD135a^+$ erythroid progenitor cell development but not myeloid cell development. Importantly, 55% to 95% of the *FLVCR1* transcript is alternatively spliced in DBA cells compared with 4% to 24% in normal immature erythroid cells. The spliced variants in DBA encode *FLVCR1* proteins that are defective in their cellular and surface expression and in their function. It is possible that expression of *FLVCR1* splicing variants leads to impaired export of intracellular iron and apoptosis because of accumulation of iron.

Patients with mutations in *RPL5* and *RPL11* are more likely to have multiple physical malformations. For example, thumb anomalies are seen in 56% and 39% of the patients with *RPL5* and *RPL11* mutations, respectively, compared with 7% in patients who have *RPS19* gene mutations. Interestingly, cleft lip or palate was reported in 42% of the patients with *RPL5* mutations compared with 6% and 0% of the patients with *RPL11* and *RPS19* gene mutations, respectively.

Clinical Features

Diamond-Blackfan anemia registries with longitudinal data and a summary of published cases provide comprehensive information about clinical aspects of the disorder. Aside from findings associated with anemia, about half of infants at presentation look healthy and are normal physically. Unless the baby develops cardiac failure as a result of anemia, hepatosplenomegaly and edema are absent.

Pregnancy, birth history, or both are often abnormal. In a survey from the French and German DBA registries of 64 pregnancies in 26 women with DBA, complications were seen in 42 pregnancies (66%) and included abortion, preeclampsia, in utero fetal death, in utero growth retardation, retroplacental hematoma, and preterm delivery. Thirteen of 34 children born alive had DBA. Fetal DBA with hydrops fetalis has been reported. More than 90% of cases present in the first 12 months of life.

About 30% to 47% of patients present with one or more congenital anomalies. Most of these phenotypic abnormalities belong to the following categories: (1) craniofacial dysmorphism, including hypertelorism, microcephaly, microphthalmos, congenital cataract or glaucoma, strabismus, microretrognathism, and a high-arched palate or cleft palate; (2) prenatal or postnatal growth failure independent of steroid therapy; (3) neck anomalies, which may consist of a pterygium coli or the fusion of cervical vertebrae with flaring of the trapezius muscle (Klippel-Feil syndrome), giving a Turner syndrome appearance or there may also be the Sprengel deformity (congenital elevation of the scapula) as an isolated anomaly or a combination of the two anomalies; and (4) thumb malformations, such as bifid thumb (Fig. 27-7), duplication, subluxation, hypoplasia, or absence of the thumb. There is a characteristic association of triphalangeal thumbs with DBA (Fig. 27-8) commonly referred to as "Aase syndrome II" or "Aase-Smith syndrome." In addition, some patients have a flat, hypoplastic thenar eminence, weak or absent radial pulses, or both, which probably represent variations of the thumb malformations.

Some patients have a characteristic facial appearance. The facies of individuals with DBA is said to consist of tow-colored hair, a snub nose, wide-set eyes, a thick upper lip, and an intelligent expression. Another facies observed in two unrelated girls of markedly different ancestries consists of small heads, almond-shaped eyes with a slight antimongoloid slant, a "fish-like" smile, and a pointed chin. These patients resemble each other more than they resemble their own

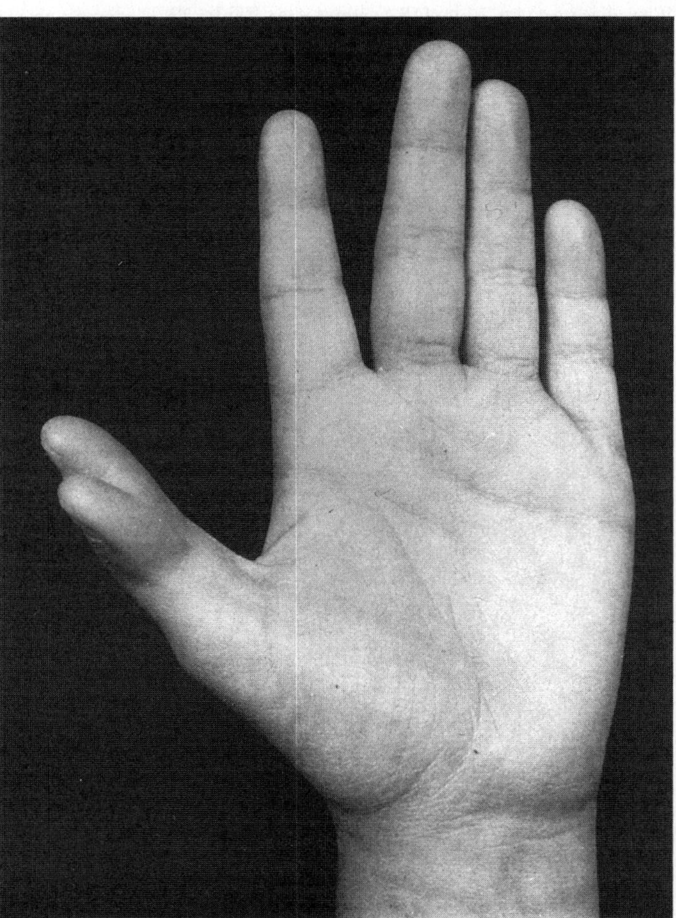

Figure 27-7 BIFID THUMB IN DIAMOND-BLACKFAN ANEMIA.

family members (Figs. 27-9, *A* and 27-9, *B*). Some patients with DBA have a phenotype indistinguishable from Treacher-Collins syndrome, a disorder of ribosome biogenesis caused by *TCOF1* mutations.

Various other anomalies are occasionally reported in association with DBA. There may be urogenital malformations, such as dysplastic or horseshoe kidneys, duplication of ureters, or renal tubular acidosis. There may also be congenital heart disease, mainly ventricular and atrial septal defects, or hypogonadism, ear malformations, mental retardation, congenital hip dislocation, or tracheoesophageal fistula.

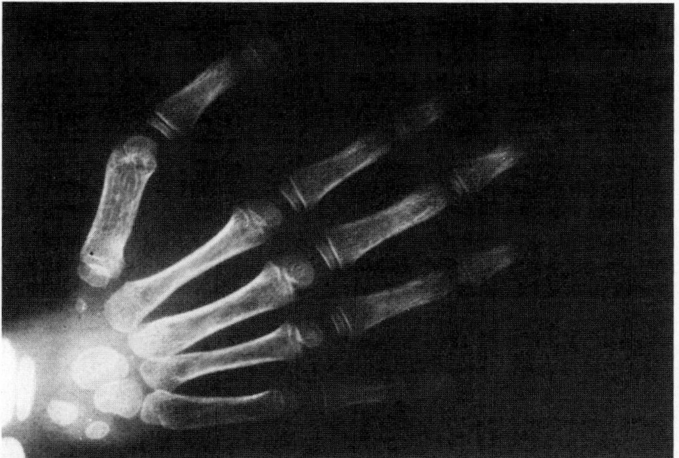

Figure 27-8 RADIOGRAPH OF A TRIPHALANGEAL THUMB IN DIAMOND-BLACKFAN ANEMIA.

Laboratory Findings

Peripheral Blood and Bone Marrow. The main hematologic findings in DBA are summarized in Table 27-6. The anemia is usually profound at the time of diagnosis. Hemoglobin levels average 6.5 g/dL in patients diagnosed in the first 2 months of life (range, 1.7-9.1 g/dL) and 4.0 g/dL (range, 1.8-7.4 g/dL) in those diagnosed later. In the vast majority of patients, the MCV is above the expected values for age. The peripheral blood smear may show, in addition to macrocytes, a mild degree of nonspecific anisocytosis and poikilocytosis. The aregenerative component of the anemia is reflected by the absence of both polychromasia and nucleated RBCs on the blood film. Decreased RBC production is confirmed by the absence of a reticulocyte response and by characteristic findings on BM examination.

In more than 90% of patients, the BM aspirate is normocellular, but erythroblasts are markedly decreased or absent. Proerythroblasts, if present, account for less than 3% of all nucleated elements, with a myeloid-to-erythroid ratio of 10 to 1 (Fig. 27-10). In 5% to 10% of cases, proerythroblasts may be present in normal numbers, with or without a maturation arrest. The other cell lines are normal. White blood cell counts and platelet counts are usually normal at diagnosis, but platelets may be decreased or increased and with normal function. Mild to moderate neutropenia, thrombocytopenia, or both may occur later in the course of the disease. Progression of the single-lineage erythroid deficiency of DBA into pancytopenia and severe aplastic anemia is rare but occurs. Of 36 deaths reported to the American Diamond-Blackfan Anemia Registry (DBAR), one died from severe aplastic anemia.

Erythrocyte Findings. Erythrocytes in DBA express a number of fetal characteristics. The level of HbF is increased persistently even during remission. It remains at a level of 5% to 10% after the age of

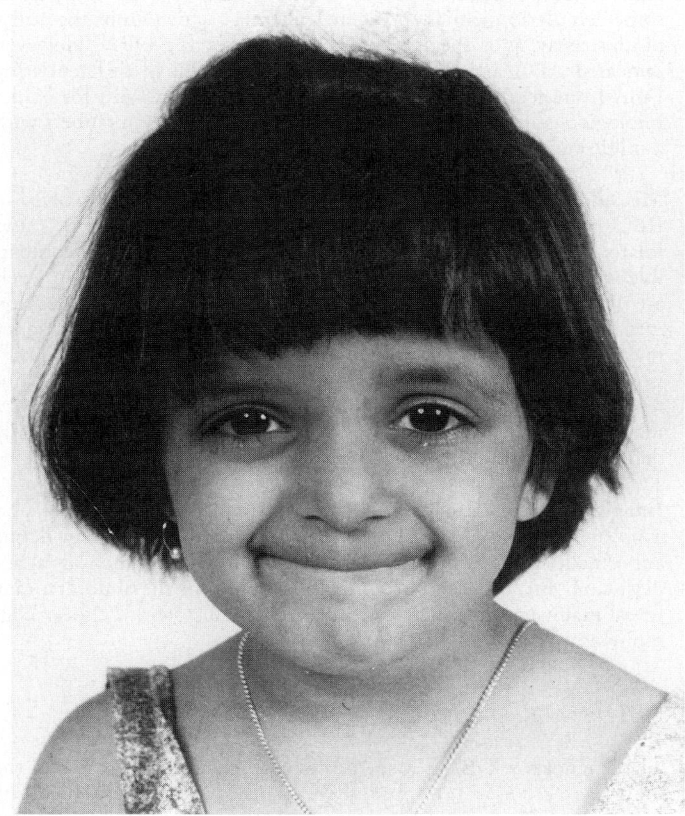

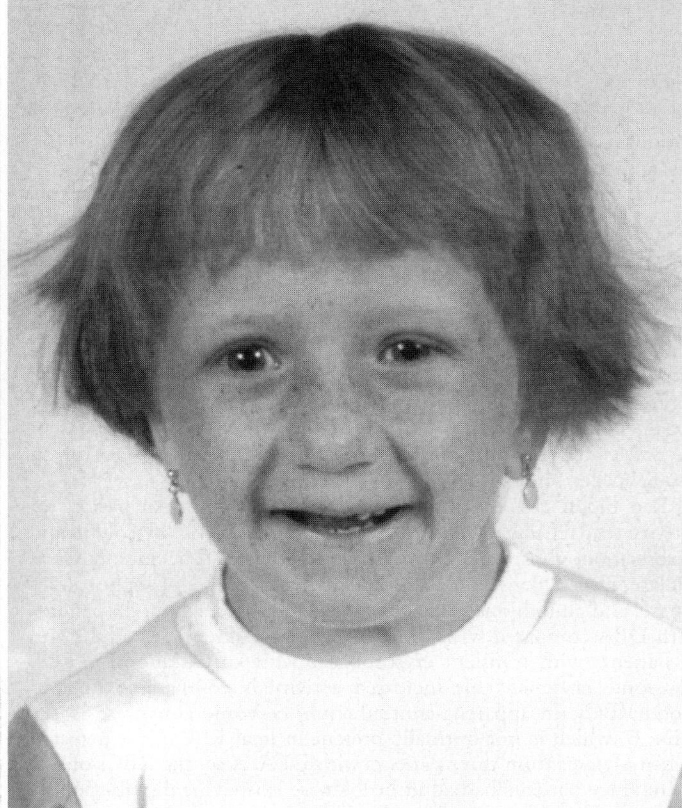

A B

Figure 27-9 SIMILAR DIAMOND-BLACKFAN FACIES IN TWO UNRELATED GIRLS OF DIFFERENT ANCESTRIES CONSSTING OF A SMALL HEAD, ALMOND-SHAPED EYES WITH A SLIGHT ANTIMONGOLOID SLANT, A "FISH-LIKE" SMILE, AND A POINTED CHIN.

Table 27-6 Hematologic Features in Diamond-Blackfan Anemia at Diagnosis Based on Data on 21 Toronto Cases and on 41 Cases From the Canadian Inherited Marrow Failure Registry

Hematologic Parameters	Laboratory Findings
Mean hemoglobin value (range) *Newborns* younger than 2 months of age *Children* 2 months of age or older	 6.5 g/dL (1.7-9.1 g/dL) 4.0 g/dL (1.8-7.4 g/dL)
High MCV for age after the age of 1 year	87%
Low reticulocyte for the degree of anemia	100% (usually markedly decreased to <1%)
Increased HbF for age after 1 year of age	100%
RBC adenosine deaminase activity	77%
RBC i antigen	Expression increased beyond first year of life
RBC enzymes	Fetal pattern
Neutropenia	31%
Thrombocytopenia	11%
BM cellularity	Normal or increased in 90%; mildly reduced in 10%
BM erythropoiesis	Markedly reduced/absent erythroid precursors in >90% of cases
BM myeloid and megakaryocytic lineages	Normal in 100% of the cases

BM, Bone marrow; *HbF,* fetal hemoglobin; *MCV,* mean corpuscular volume; *RBC,* red blood cell.

6 months and has a heterogeneous distribution in RBCs. The HbF has a specifically fetal amino-acid profile with a high glycine-to-alanine ratio (G-γ:A-γ). Similarly, the i antigen, which normally disappears from the erythrocyte surface by 1 year of age, is expressed at near fetal levels in older patients with DBA.

The precise cause of this fetal-like erythropoiesis is unclear. It is clearly distinct from the fetal erythropoiesis implicated in various types of leukemia, notably in juvenile myelomonocytic leukemia in which the fetal RBCs presumably arise from the leukemic clone. The situation in DBA may be analogous to that in other forms of BM failure and in the hematologic recovery phase after BMT. In all of these conditions, the fetal (or "stress") erythropoiesis may represent an accelerated recapitulation of RBC ontogeny in the face of an increased demand for new RBCs in peripheral blood.

Red blood cell enzymes often display an abnormal pattern of activity that reflects a fetal expression pattern of RBC glycolytic and hexose monophosphate shunt enzyme activities. Enzymes, such as enolase, glyceraldehyde-3-phosphate dehydrogenase, phosphofructokinase, and glutathione peroxidase, have increased activity in patients with DBA compared with those in normal children and adults and in patients with transient erythroblastopenia of childhood (TEC). For some enzymes, this increased activity is comparable to cord blood RBCs. In apparent contradiction, carbonic anhydrase isoenzyme B, which is not normally present in fetal RBCs, was detected in hemolysates from three patients with DBA. Also, the RBCs of two of the three patients had adult hexokinase isoenzyme distribution by isoelectric focusing.

Abnormalities in purine and pyrimidine metabolism are reflected by increased activity of RBC adenosine deaminase (ADA) in 60% to 90% of the patients with DBA. Also, increased orotidine decarboxylase (ODC) activity is seen in some patients. ADA activity is raised in DBA erythrocytes but not in cord blood RBCs from normal newborns or from patients with any of several hematologic conditions associated with "stress" erythropoiesis. Thus, this enzymatic abnormality cannot be simply attributable to a "reversion" to fetal erythropoiesis. Raised ADA activity may also be detected in some hemolytic anemias and acute leukemias, which limits the utility of this assay as a specific diagnostic marker for DBA. However, increased ADA activity does appear to be useful in differentiating DBA from acquired pure cell anemias such as TEC and for epidemiologic testing of DBA pedigrees to identify family members with a mild phenotype.

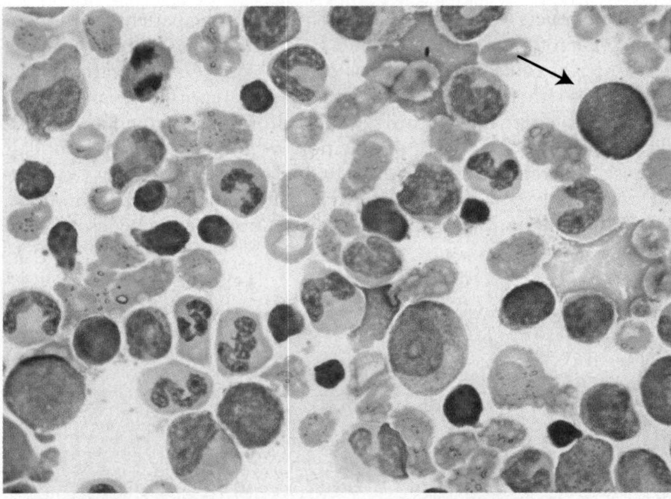

Figure 27-10 HIGH-POWER VIEW OF A BONE MARROW ASPIRATE FROM A NEWLY DIAGNOSED INFANT WITH DIAMOND-BLACKFAN ANEMIA. The findings are active granulopoiesis; normal lymphoid activity for age; and an isolated pronormoblast *(arrow)* with total absence of early-, intermediate-, and late-stage nucleated red blood cells. *(Photomicrograph prepared by Dr. Mohamed Abdelhaleem, Toronto.)*

Miscellaneous Findings. Serum levels of various factors involved in RBC production, such as erythropoietin, iron, vitamin B_{12}, and folate, are appropriately elevated in DBA. These findings are compatible with any form of chronic hypoplastic anemia. Riboflavin levels are normal in the serum but not in the erythrocytes. This observation initially aroused interest because experimental riboflavin deficiency may be corrected by corticosteroids similar to DBA. However, administration of large doses of riboflavin to several DBA patients did not result in a hematopoietic response. RBC serology is usually unremarkable at the time of diagnosis, but alloantibodies are frequently detected in chronically transfused patients.

Imaging Studies. Imaging studies are frequently informative and assist in establishing a diagnosis. Skeletal radiography may define abnormalities suspected from physical examination, such as hypoplastic, absent, or extra phalanges. Ultrasound of the abdomen may reveal malformations such as of the urogenital system. Echocardiography may reveal undiagnosed cardiac defects.

Differential Diagnosis

The diagnosis of DBA is made if the patients have at least two of the following criteria (1) pure RBC aplasia as documented by normochromic-macrocytic anemia, relative reticulocytopenia, and normocellular BM with a selective deficiency of RBC precursors; (2) classical constellation of physical malformations; (3) a first-degree relative with DBA; or (4) a mutation in a DBA gene.

Table 27-7 Distinguishing Features Between Diamond–Blackfan Anemia (DBA) and Transient Erythroblastopenia of Childhood (TEC)

	DBA	TEC
Etiology	Genetic	Acquired
Immune mediated	None	Common
Family history	≈10%	Occasional siblings with concurrent TEC
Antecedent history	None	Viral infection
Age at diagnosis	90% by 1 year	6 months-4 years
Physical anomalies	≈50%	None
Neurologic findings	None	Occasional
Transfusion dependence	Yes, if steroid refractory	None
Course	Chronic	Full recovery
Risk of cancer	Increased	Not increased
Risk of MDS or leukemia	Increased	Not increased
Laboratory findings at diagnosis:		
RBC size	Macrocytic	Normocytic
HbF	Increased	Normal*
i Antigen	Increased	Normal*
RBC enzyme activities	Fetal levels	Adult levels
RBC adenosine deaminase	Increased in 40%-90%	Normal

HbF, Fetal hemoglobin; *MDS,* myelodysplastic syndrome; *RBC,* red blood cell; *TEC,* transient erythroblastopenia of childhood.
*During spontaneous recovery, values may be increased.

In clinical practice, after excluding a viral etiology, particularly parvovirus B_{19}, **TEC** is usually the main diagnosis that is confused with DBA (Table 27-7). Both entities share the same morphologic findings in the BM. However, TEC is a self-limited disorder with an excellent prognosis and needs no specific therapy except for RBC transfusions in the most profoundly anemic patients. The definition of TEC includes the following features: (1) gradual onset of pallor in previously healthy children usually 1 to 4 years of age (85% of cases); (2) normochromic-normocytic anemia with varying reticulocytopenia unless recovery has already ensued; (3) BM erythroid hypoplasia (60% of cases) or aplasia (10% of cases) or a recovery picture (30% of cases); and (4) spontaneous recovery usually within 4 to 8 weeks without recurrence, with rare exceptions.

There are some additional important features of TEC. It can occur in siblings simultaneously and in seasonal "clusters" from June to October and from November to March. Of concern are the transient neurologic changes that can accompany TEC and that appear to be linked to the disorder. Affected children may have one or more of the following: hemiparesis, papilledema, abnormal extraocular movements, seizures, and unsteadiness of gait. The affected patients in the published reports recovered without sequelae, and the precise relationship of these neurologic changes to the pathogenesis of TEC has not been determined.

It was claimed initially that only the erythroid lineage was affected in TEC and all other hematopoietic lineages were normal. Nevertheless, significant neutropenia also occurs in many patients with TEC, being associated in some with hypocellular BM or with a granulopoietic maturational arrest. The neutropenia may be caused by a common pathogenetic mechanism that produces anemia. An unusual presentation of TEC as a leukoerythroblastic anemia has been recorded, possibly reflecting a recovery stage.

Although one case of TEC was caused by parvovirus B19, no data firmly incriminate other infectious agents in the etiology of TEC, although a history of a preceding viral-like illness can be obtained in more than half of the patients. The most plausible explanation proposed to date is that TEC is caused by transient immunosuppression of erythropoiesis and possibly of granulopoiesis in those with neutropenia. Increased numbers of $CD10^+$ lymphoid cells in BM of TEC patients might be an indication for such a mechanism. Most supportive evidence for this hypothesis comes from in vitro studies. Two reports described an inhibitory effect of TEC serum and fractionated IgG on erythroid colony growth that disappeared as TEC improved. An IgG inhibitor of erythropoiesis was discovered in one case and an IgM inhibitor in a second patient. A summary of other published studies suggests that more than 60% of TEC patients have autologous or allogeneic serum inhibitors of erythroid colony formation. Autologous or allogeneic cell-mediated immune suppression of erythropoiesis has also been identified in about 25% of cases. All of the in vitro studies have generated varying patterns of erythroid colony growth in TEC. Colony numbers can be normal, but reduced numbers of BFU-E and CFU-E progenitors have been recorded in 30% and 50% of cases, respectively.

Therefore, TEC has an autoimmune pathogenesis. TEC cases are not caused by DBA mutations. The transient nature of TEC is similar to other autoimmune hematologic disorders of childhood such as immune thrombocytopenia purpura and some cases of autoimmune hemolytic anemia. The decreased activities of virtually all RBC enzymes in TEC compared with control participants probably relate to the aged population of peripheral blood erythrocytes being tested.

Regarding **viral causes** of non-DBA RBC aplasia, Epstein-Barr virus, hepatitis virus, human T-cell leukemia virus-1, and human immunodeficiency virus-1 have all been implicated and should be excluded if the etiology of the anemia remains unclear. Parvovirus B_{19} stands out as a major causal agent of RBC aplasia in the context of an underlying chronic hemolytic anemia in infants and children with chronic congenital and acquired forms of immunosuppression. Fetuses are uniquely susceptible to parvovirus infection, and in utero transmission is a well-documented cause of nonimmune hydrops fetalis. Parvovirus infection should be ruled out in every case of childhood RBC aplasia by serial measurements of serum IgM and IgG and by BM examination for the characteristic giant pronormoblasts. Parvovirus may also be detected in BM by gene amplification using PCR and confirmed by direct in situ hybridization.

Rarely, the initial hematologic manifestation of several other inherited BM failure syndrome such as **FA** and **congenital hair hypoplasia** is isolated macrocytic anemia. Specific screening testing for these conditions might be necessary. Milder forms of **mitochondrial DNA deletion syndromes** can also present with macrocytic anemia.

Predisposition to Malignancy

Diamond-Blackfan anemia is associated with hematologic cancer and with solid tumors, albeit to a much lesser degree than FA, DC, SDS, and Kstmann/severe congenital neutropenia (K/SCN). The link between DBA and hematologic cancer is more understandable from the data described herein that implicate an early pluripotent BM progenitor in the pathobiology of DBA. From published data, 10 DBA patients developed AML, 2 developed MDS, 1 had acute lymphoblastic leukemia, 3 had Hodgkin lymphoma, and 1 had non-Hodgkin lymphoma. Regarding solid tumors, a predilection to osteosarcoma was reported in 6 of the 11 solid tumors. The other solid tumors included HCC, breast carcinoma, gastric carcinoma, vaginal melanoma, and malignant fibrous histiocytoma. Although the actuarial risk of cancer in DBA is unknown, the risk exists, and hence DBA is considered to be a cancer predisposition syndrome. The published cases implicate several possible operative factors, including genetic predisposition, transfusional iron overload, use of androgens, immunosuppression from corticosteroids, thymic and skeletal irradiation during childhood as "therapy" for DBA in one case, and cyclophosphamide "treatment" in another. It is noteworthy that inhibition of ribosome protein genes in zebrafish is associated with the development of cancer.

Natural History and Prognosis

Historically, the only treatment for DBA was blood transfusions. Without this, patients died of anemia. When corticosteroids were introduced as an effective therapy for DBA, all patients were assigned to one of the two therapeutic interventions, and the "natural history" of the disorder took on a different dimension.

A notable phenomenon is spontaneous remission that occurs in about 20% of cases that allows patients to discontinue whatever treatment they are receiving, either chronic transfusion therapy or corticosteroids. The DBAR has actuarial data showing that 75% of these patients remit before their 10th birthday, and in most cases, the remission is sustained. It appears that an equal number of patients remit from either corticosteroids or transfusions. A relapse of DBA requires reintroduction of treatment.

The overall actuarial survival for DBA patients greater than 40 years of age is 75% ± 4.8%. For those in sustained spontaneous remission, it is 100%; for corticosteroid responders, it is 57% ± 8.9%; and for transfusion-dependent patients, it is 8.9%. Causes of death mostly relate directly to the development of cancer or its treatment, complications from corticosteroid-induced immunosuppression, stem cell transplant–related complications, and transfusional hemosiderosis.

Therapy

In younger children and infants, it is important to determine whether the RBC aplasia is DBA or TEC (see Table 27-7). Until a firm diagnosis is established, the initial treatment in children is almost always transfusions. This allows the flexibility to complete the viral workup and other investigations and to await a spontaneous remission if the anemia is caused by TEC or another self-limited condition. Demonstration of a mutant ribosomal protein gene would clinch the diagnosis, but it occurs in only about 55% of patients.

If transfusions are used, it is recommended to aim for a moderate but not full correction of anemia so that erythropoiesis is not suppressed and recovery from TEC not delayed. Generally, the nadir should not be less than 6 g/dL and should not allow the development of significant symptoms. Most patients with TEC usually recover within a few weeks after receiving only one transfusion. Occasionally, recovery from TEC is slow and may mimic DBA in chronicity. If there is confusion about the proper diagnosis, it is appropriate to withhold corticosteroids in favor of a further transfusion to allow more observation time.

Transfusions for Patients With Diamond-Blackfan Anemia

Before the first transfusion, it is recommended that a full RBC phenotype be performed on the patient. This information is valuable for prevention and management of alloantibody formation caused by sensitization. For patients in whom corticosteroids are either ineffective or excessively toxic, a regular program of RBC transfusions is usually required. During the course of this program, a small number of steroid-resistant patients may show responsiveness to corticosteroids when retreated or even proceed to a spontaneous transient or prolonged remission. If not, leukocyte-depleted packed RBCs are given monthly to keep the hemoglobin concentration at a level compatible with normal activity; usually above 9 g/L. CMV-negative packed cells should be used if stem cell transplantation is contemplated. Several complications may arise from transfusions such as bloodborne infections and sensitization, but the major long-term threat is iron overload, which causes delayed puberty, growth retardation, diabetes mellitus, hypoparathyroidism, and eventually liver cirrhosis and cardiac failure. These complications can be delayed and possibly prevented by the early administration of an iron chelator.

Two iron chelators are available in North America. The first, deferoxamine (Desferal), is administered by a battery-powered pump as a daily 12-hour subcutaneous infusion. It has been the main chelator used for the past 4 decades. Deferasirox (Exjade) is an effective oral iron chelator in patients with iron overload and is approved for children older than 2 years of age. The initial dose is 20 to 30 mg/kg/ by mouth once daily. In a randomized trial of Desferal versus Exjade in patients with transfusional iron overload, the two chelators showed similar efficacy. In an international multicenter study in which the efficacy of Exjade was assessed in patients with anemia of various etiologies, 30 patients with DBA were included. Successful chelation was observed in 54% of the DBA patients as defined by reduction of liver iron concentration by biopsy to less than 7 mg/g dry weight within 1 year. Given its oral route of administration, it is predicted that Exjade will replace Desferal as the iron chelator of choice.

There are uncertainties about the optimal age at which to start patients younger than 2 years old with transfusion-dependent anemia with desferal therapy. There have been reports of abnormal linear growth and metaphyseal dysplasia in patients with thalassemia major treated with Desferal before the age of 3 years. This adverse event has prompted recommendations for starting Desferal later. However, a progressively rising serum ferritin level or, more accurately, excessive hepatic iron concentration obtained by biopsy after 1 year of regular transfusions would be an appropriate indication to commence chelation therapy. The daily starting subcutaneous infusion dose of Desferal should not exceed 50 mg/kg. Ascorbate supplementation should be considered if there is sustained loss of efficacy of deferoxamine, especially if tissue ascorbate concentrations are reduced.

Corticosteroids

Steroid responsiveness occurs in 50% to 75% of DBA patients. Upon administration of prednisone at a dose of 2 mg/kg/day in three divided doses, reticulocytosis is usually seen within 1 to 4 weeks and is followed by a rise in hemoglobin concentration. When the hemoglobin level reaches 9.0 to 10.0 g/dL, prednisone can be slowly tapered by reducing the number of daily doses. If a single daily dose of prednisone maintains the desired hemoglobin level, the dose can be doubled and given on alternate days, but this may not prevent significant steroid toxicity.

The dose of prednisone can be further reduced by small decrements on a weekly basis or more slowly until the minimal effective dose is determined. This dose is extremely variable. A few patients can be maintained on minute, nonpharmacologic doses, but other patients need large doses that preclude long-term therapy because of serious side effects such as Cushingoid features, pathologic fractures, cataracts, growth failure, diabetes, and avascular necrosis of the femoral or humeral heads. There is no known predictor of steroid responsiveness or any way to anticipate the type of individual responses. In general, a corticosteroid dose equivalent of prednisone, 0.5 mg/kg/day, is suggested as a maximum "maintenance" dose after the initial dose of 2 mg/kg/day. About one-third of patients can maintain a response at a low prednisone dose. The rest are usually managed with chronic RBC transfusions.

There are several patterns of response to corticosteroid therapy, some of which may occur at different times in the same patient. Most children who respond to steroids cannot be completely weaned off the medication and become steroid dependent. About one-third of these patients, however, enter steroid-free remission after a prolonged period of treatment. Between 1% and 5% of responders immediately enter a durable steroid-independent remission. However, late relapses, sometimes precipitated by an infectious illness or by hormonal changes such as in pregnancy or with the use of birth control pills, are common. In other cases, a progressive resistance to steroids occurs, requiring escalating doses of prednisone or alternative therapy. After a relapse, some patients are responsive to steroids again, but others are refractory to subsequent trials. Initial refractoriness to steroids is observed in 36% of cases. In more than 60% of patients, long-term steroid therapy is hampered by the development of resistance or by side effects of the treatment. In adolescent responders on long-term steroids, an option is to stop prednisone temporarily to allow a normal growth spurt. Infants with DBA on high doses of steroids are at risk for pneumocystis pneumonia and should be given prophylactic antibiotics.

High-Dose Methylprednisolone. Megadose steroid therapy for DBA patients who were refractory to conventional-dose prednisone has been reported to induce a sustained erythroid response leading to transfusion independence in 8 of 13 cases. Eleven had been treated with 100 mg/kg/day intravenously, and two additional patients had been treated with 30 mg/kg/day orally. Another report showed only a transient response in one of eight patients after intravenous treatment with 30 mg/kg/day and a sustained response after a higher dosage (100 mg/kg/day) in three of eight patients, but side effects were weight gain, oral moniliasis, increase in hepatic transaminases, transient hyperglycemia, and bacteremia related to a central venous catheter. A conclusive study of nine refractory DBA patients using megadose oral methylprednisolone showed no response in five cases and a partial or complete response in the other four during the initial 4 to 8 weeks of therapy, but all of these patients relapsed with a taper and became transfusion dependent. Thus, none of the cases exhibited a clinically significant or durable response.

Cytokine Therapy

Because of the "corrective" effect on erythropoiesis by IL-3 in vitro, clinical trials were introduced for steroid-refractory and steroid-dependent DBA patients and for those in whom HSCT was considered too risky. The early enthusiasm generated by sustained remissions in some patients was tempered by the realization that IL-3 is effective in only a very small number of cases of steroid-refractory, transfusion-dependent DBA. Of 49 patients treated with IL-3 in a European multicenter compassionate-need study, only three children had a significant response with sustained remissions off therapy. A comparison of individual patient characteristics confirmed that patients who had never achieved significant in vivo erythropoiesis in response to steroids or during a spontaneous remission were highly unlikely to respond to IL-3. Thus, the overall response rate in all published studies averaged 10% to 20%. Currently, there are no IL-3 or other growth factor clinical trials in North America for DBA. Serum erythropoietin levels are elevated in DBA, and attempts at treatment with high-dose erythropoietin have been ineffective.

Hematopoietic Stem Cell Transplantation

Hematopoietic stem cell transplantation is a therapeutic option for DBA, but the risks must be weighed against the benefits on a case-by-case basis. The fundamental issue centers on the defined mortality rate with HSCT when used for a nonlethal medical disorder, at least a disorder that is nonlethal in the short term. In steroid-responsive patients on low-dose maintenance and in properly transfused and adequately chelated patients, quality of life is not threatened by life-threatening complications. Thus, the decision for intervention with HSCT in this setting is difficult.

Nevertheless, experience has broadened since the first HSCT was performed for DBA in 1976. Preparative regimens, supportive measures, and GVHD management have progressively become more refined, thereby reducing the overall risks of the procedure. For consideration in the decision-making process, though, there are still lethal risks, including interstitial pneumonia, cardiac failure, fatal complications associated with chronic GVHD, graft failure, graft rejection, and sepsis. Results from the International Bone Marrow Transplant Registry show a 64% 3-year probability of overall survival of 61 transplanted DBA patients. The DBAR and the Aplastic Anemia Committee of the Japanese Society of Pediatric Hematology report an 87.5% and an 85% survival, respectively, but express caution that alternative donors pose a much higher risk than matched sibling donors. From the DBAR database, the survival rate for patients younger than the age of 10 years receiving matched related HSCT is greater than 90%. Related and unrelated umbilical cord blood as a stem cell source has been used for DBA HSCT with favorable results. Given the generally favorable results with related donors, this procedure can now be offered to patients approximately after the age of 5 years when no spontaneous remission is apparent. However, HSCT from an unrelated donor is not recommended unless the patient has severe aplastic anemia, MDS, or leukemia or as part of a clinical trial.

This success with related donors has sparked interest in PGD with in vitro fertilization to "create" HLA-matched sibling donors without a mutated DBA gene, and a number of patients worldwide have been successfully transplanted using umbilical cord–derived stem cells from donors produced in this way. The religious, ethical, and economic questions generated by PGD to find a healthy matched donor for DBA and other inherited BM failure transplantations is ongoing.

Other Therapeutic Options

Based on the role of the DBA genes in ribosome biogenesis and global protein translation and in vitro studies aimed to stimulate translation in BM cells, a trial was performed in which the branched amino acid leucine was administered to a patient with DBA patient. The patient had an impressive response. Based on this, two leucine trials are ongoing in the United States and Europe. Leucine stimulates translation by enhancing the activation of translation initiation factors that regulate mRNA binding to the ribosomal complex and by activation of the ribosomal protein S6 kinase and the mTOR (mammalian target of rapamycin) pathway.

A number of uncontrolled therapeutic trials have been performed in steroid-refractory patients using various medications and treatments with varying anecdotal successes in a few patients. The medications include cyclosporine, metoclopramide, lenalidomide, androgens, riboflavin, vitamin B_{12}, folate, iron and other "hematinic" agents, 6-mercaptopurine, cyclophosphamide with antilymphocyte globulin, and antithymocyte globulin alone. There is a case report claiming efficacy of valproic acid for DBA and another report of an 8-month transfusion-free remission after rituximab therapy. Plasmapheresis has also been tried. Splenectomy, used in the past, shows no effect on erythropoiesis but may be helpful in transfused patients with proven hypersplenism.

Future Directions

Registries and DBA patient databases will continue to broaden our understanding of the genetic origins and epidemiology of DBA. Specimen collection and distribution to qualified research laboratories globally will identify the remaining DBA genes. Genetically based DBA diagnosis and pedigree analysis will underscore the broad dimensions of the DBA phenotype, from clinically silent to life-threatening severe. Genotype–phenotype correlations will facilitate HSCT donor selection, allow counseling for reproductive options, and be predictive of cancer risk. Deciphering the pathogenesis of BM failure and other disease manifestations using animal models and iPSCs may allow the development of effective erythropoietic stimulators for use in this disease.

Kostmann Syndrome and Severe Congenital Neutropenia

Background

Kostmann syndrome and SCN refer to inherited types of neutropenia with onset in early childhood of profound neutropenia (ANC <200/μL), recurrent life-threatening infections, and a maturation arrest of myeloid precursors at the promyelocyte-myelocyte stage of differentiation. Some experts in the field refer to KS as the autosomal recessive type of severe inherited neutropenia and to SCN to all the other inherited neutropenia with similar phenotype. However, because many IBMFSs are inherited in different modes and because

SCN and KS are indistinguishable phenotypically in the majority of the patients, the option to "split" the two disorders is debatable. In this chapter, we will refer to them as K/SCN.

The initial description of syndrome made by Dr. Kostmann in 1956 included several neutropenic patients in a large intermarried Swedish kinship. An autosomal recessive mode of inheritance in 24 cases was deduced by inference because of hematologically normal parents with two or more neutropenic children in several families. Recently, homozygous germline *HAX1* mutations have been identified in patients with KS, including some from Kostmann's original pedigree, confirming an autosomal recessive inheritance in these families. Nevertheless, it is now clear that K/SCN are genetically heterogeneous despite a shared hematologic phenotype (see Table 27-1). The first identified K/SCN gene was the neutrophil elastase 2 gene *(ELA2),* which was found mutated one one allele in patients with K/SCN, indicating an autosomal dominant inheritance in many cases.

Epidemiology

K/SCNs are rare. The estimated incidence based on Canadian data from CIMFR from 2001 to 2010 was 4.7 cases per million live births per year. There is equal distribution of the disease between genders. There might be different frequency of specific genetic groups in different countries. For example, no *HAX1* mutations were found among cases from the United States or Canada.

Etiology, Genetics, and Pathophysiology

The discovery of heterozygous mutations in the *ELA2* gene encoding neutrophil elastase in 22 of 25 sporadic and dominantly inherited patients with K/SCN was the entry point for understanding the molecular basis of the disorder in many patients. As experience with genetic testing has broadened, it appears that 60% to 80% of cases have spontaneously occurring or inherited point mutations in *ELA2* and, less commonly, mutations in other genes. Mutant *ELA2* also occurs in all cases of classical cyclic neutropenia, but the mutations cluster in exon 4 or 5 on the gene on chromosome 19p13.3 or at the junction of exon 4 with intron 4. Patients with congenital neutropenia have mutations more widely distributed over exons 2, 3, 4, and 5.

Although typical K/SCN patients present early in life with severe neutropenia and life-threatening infections, rare cases with *ELA2* mutations in phenotypically healthy family members were reported. For example, two siblings with congenital neutropenia inherited the same heterozygous ELA2 mutation from their hematologically normal father. In another family, a healthy father of a congenital neutropenia patient was mosaic for his daughter's Cys42Arg mutation in peripheral blood hematopoietic cells. The mutation was found in about 50% of his T lymphocytes but only in 10% of his neutrophils. This is congruent with a lack of recurrent infection phenotype in the father. The mutation was evident in myeloid precursors but was selectively lost during myelopoiesis or failed to mature to neutrophils.

The exact mechanism whereby mutant *ELA2* causes neutropenia is under intense study. *ELA2* encodes neutrophil elastase; a glycoprotein synthesized in the promyelocyte/myelocyte stages and packed in the azurophilic cytoplasmic granules. It is released in response to infection and inflammation. The wild-type neutrophil elastase diffusely localizes throughout the cytoplasm, but the mutated protein in cases of congenital neutropenia abnormally concentrates in the nucleus and plasma membrane. There are several lines of evidence that mutant ELA2 protein triggers accelerated apoptosis of developing neutrophil precursors. Mutant protein leads to accumulation of nonfunctional protein in the endoplasmic reticulum, activation of unfolded protein response, and apoptosis of K/SCN neutrophils. In addition, decreased expression of Bcl-2 was observed in K/SCN myeloid progenitor cells along with constitutive mitochondrial release of cytochrome C and excessive cellular apoptosis. Of note, administration of G-CSF restored Bcl-2 expression and improved survival of myeloid progenitor cells. Another proposed mechanism is downregulation of lymphoid enhancer-binding factor 1 (*LEF-1*) in K/SCN. This leads to reduced transcription of *LEF1*-target genes such as *C/EBP-α* and impaired granulocytic differentiation.

HAX1 was reported to be mutated in 40% of patients with K/SCN in a European study but in none of the patients in the American studies and in none of the patients in the Canadian Inherited Marrow Failure Study. HAX1 localizes to the mitochondria. It contains two domains reminiscent of a BH1 and BH2 of the BCL-2 family. It promotes normal potential of the inner mitochondrial membrane and protects myeloid cells from apoptosis. The direct function of HAX1 in promoting survival may explain the accelerated apoptosis reported in K/SCN neutrophils. *HAX1-mutant* K/SCN cells are also characterized by reduced LEF1 levels as in *ELA2-mutant* K/SCN cells.

A constitutively activating mutation in the Wiskott-Aldrich syndrome protein encoded by the *WASP* gene was discovered in five males from a three-generation family. The phenotype of the resulting X-linked immunodeficiency syndrome was composed of severe neutropenia from birth, bacterial infections, monocytopenia, and shifts of lymphocyte subsets. BM morphology showed a selective maturation arrest at the promyelocyte/myelocyte stage similar to K/SCN. Mutant *WASP* leads to constitutive activation of the WASP protein because of disruption of an autoinhibitory domain in the wild-type protein. This increased WASP protein activity produces marked abnormalities of cytoskeletal structure and dynamics, disruption of mitosis, genomic instability, and apoptosis of neutrophils.

Mutations in the proto-oncogene *GFI1* also cause K/SCN with severe neutropenia and a maturation arrest at the promyelocyte–myelocyte stage. GFI1-deficient mice exhibit severe neutropenia with accumulation of abnormal arrested progenitors and increased HSC/P proliferation. GFI1 is a transcriptional repressor of several transcription programs. The first transcription program is active during the progenitor stage. During this stage, GFI1 downregulates the HoxA9-Pbx1-Meis1 transcription factor complex. Because HOXA9 drives progenitor proliferation, GFI1 deficiency leads to uncontrolled HOXA2 activation and accumulation of arrested-differentiation myeloid progenitors. The second transcription program is activated during terminal granulopoietic differentiation. During this stage, GFI1 represses genes that promote differentiation of nongranulocytic cells such as CSF1. Patient-related mutations also disable the GFI1 repressor activity on *ELA2* expression, which leads to accumulation of neutrophil elastase in all subcellular compartments and might underlie the mechanism for premature apoptosis. Another potential mechanism for neutropenia when GFI1 is deficient might be related to loss of GFI1-mediated regulation of the expression of the micoRNAs miR-21 and miR-196b, which regulate myeloid maturation.

A constitutive point mutation was discovered in the extracellular domain of the G-CSF receptor in a patient with K/SCN who also had a mutant *ELA2* gene. The receptor mutation affected ligand–receptor complex formation with severe consequences for intracellular signal transduction; the patient was totally unresponsive to G-CSF therapy. As demonstrated in vitro and then clinically, corticosteroids combined with G-CSF produced a corrective action through synergistic activation of STAT5, and the patient responded to G-CSF therapy. Three subsequent patients with cell-surface G-CSF receptor mutations were also refractory to G-CSF therapy and suggest that this may be a common finding in cases unresponsive to treatment.

Regarding the cellular pathology of K/SCN, many cell culture studies performed in the 1970s and 1980s provided clonogenic data that pointed to intrinsically defective granulocytic progenitors. Further reports confirmed this and excluded other possible pathogenetic factors. To summarize: (1) K/SCN BM myeloid colony growth is defective, (2) K/SCN serum contains normal or increased levels of G-CSF, (3) endogenous K/SCN G-CSF has normal biologic activity,

(4) G-CSF receptors are expressed in slightly increased numbers on myeloid cells from K/SCN patients, and (5) the binding constant for G-CSF to its receptor in K/SCN is normal.

Regarding correlation between the mutated gene and phenotype, *ELA2* mutations are associated with severe and early-onset neutropenia with differentiation arrest at the stage of promyelocyte-myelocyte. Typically, the patients do not have physical malformations. The patients have a high risk of MDS/AML but no known risk of solid tumors. Patients with mutations in *HAX1* typically have severe and early-onset neutropenia with differentiation arrest at the stage of promyelocyte–myelocyte. They also have a high risk of MDS/AML but no known risk of solid tumors. About 30% of the patients with *HAX1* mutations have neurologic abnormalities such as seizures, learning disabilities, and developmental delay. This is usually attributable to nonsense mutations (e.g., p.Gln155ProfsX14) that affect both *HAX1* transcripts. Mutations in *WAS* are associated with moderate to severe neutropenia, reduced phagocyte activity, monocytopenia, lymphopenia, reduced NK cells, reduced lymphocyte proliferation, and recurrent infections (but usually not as frequent as in the classical K/SCN). MDS/monosomy 7 has also been reported. *GFI* mutations are associated with severe to moderate neutropenia, and monocytosis, reduced B and T cells with normal lymphocytic function. There are no clear data about the BM findings in this type of neutropenia, and the risk of MDS/AML is unknown.

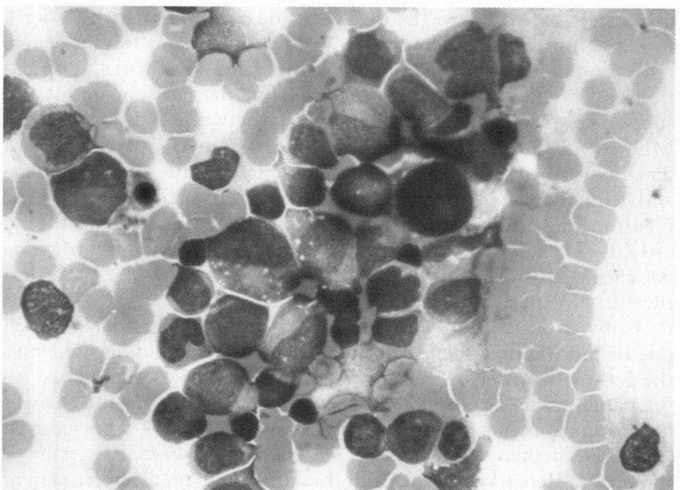

Figure 27-11 HIGH-POWER VIEW OF A BONE MARROW ASPIRATE FROM A PATIENT WITH KOSTMANN SYNDROME (CONGENITAL NEUTROPENIA) BEFORE GRANULOCYTE COLONY-STIMULATING FACTOR THERAPY. The findings are a "maturation arrest" with recognizable myeloblasts, promyelocytes, myelocytes, and occasional metamyelocytes but total absence of band forms and neutrophils. *(Photomicrograph prepared by Dr. Mohamed Abdelhaleem, Toronto.)*

Clinical Features

Approximately half of patients develop clinically significant infections within the first month of life and almost all others develop them by 6 months. Skin abscesses are common, but deep-seated tissue infections and septicemias also occur. Data from the SCNIR illustrate examples of every conceivable form of bacterial and fungal infection in the precytokine era. Especially troublesome in survivors were recurrent episodes of otitis media and pneumonia; advanced gingival stomatitis, sometimes with tooth loss; and in the extreme, gut bacterial flora overgrowth, leading to malabsorption requiring total parenteral nutritional therapy.

In contrast to some of the other IBMFSs, physical malformations are uncommon. Birth weights are generally unremarkable, and physical examination findings are usually normal. There are a small number of reports of short stature, cataracts, microcephaly, seizures, developmental delay, and mental retardation. As mentioned earlier, neurologic manifestations are part of a small group of patients with *HAX1* mutations. Data from the SCNIR indicate that some patients with K/SCN develop bone demineralization that may be an intrinsic component of the disorder; it has been observed before and during G-CSF therapy. The underlying pathogenesis is unclear, but patients can develop bone pain and unusual fractures. Osteopenia is a common theme with the IBMFSs.

Laboratory Findings

Peripheral Blood and Bone Marrow

Neutropenia is profound and persistent in K/SCN, usually less than 200/μL. A small number of patients have intermittent cycling patterns with regular periodicity that ranges in a low to severely low neutrophil count range. A compensatory two- to fourfold increase in monocytes is seen, sometimes accompanied by eosinophilia. At diagnosis, platelet numbers are normal or increased, and hemoglobin values are usually normal. In survivors in the precytokine era, anemia of chronic disease associated with recurrent infections and inflammation was common. Aside from neutropenia, humoral and cellular immunity is completely normal.

Bone marrow specimens are usually normocellular. The striking classical finding is a maturation arrest at the promyelocyte or myelocyte stage with a paucity of more mature elements. Promyelocytes are abundant and may have atypical nuclei and the cytoplasm may be vacuolated. Neutrophils and bands are usually absent (Fig. 27-11). BM eosinophilia and monocytosis is common. The other hematopoietic lineages are normal, active, and undisturbed.

Predisposition to Leukemia and Myelodysplastic Syndrome

Clearly, K/SCN carries a high risk of leukemia. There were three case reports of patients who developed AML before the use of hematopoietic growth factors and one more recent patient diagnosed with acute leukemia before starting G-CSF. As a rough estimate, in the literature, there were 128 cases of congenital neutropenia reported and three cases of AML up to 1989 (the first year that G-CSF was available for general use), leading to a crude estimated risk of leukemia of 2%. Nevertheless, because most patients with congenital neutropenia died at a young age from bacterial sepsis or pneumonia in the precytokine era, the true risk of patients with congenital neutropenia developing MDS/AML was not clearly defined.

G-CSF therapy completely changed clinical outcomes of K/SCN. Before G-CSF, the median duration of survival was about 3 years; the current median age is more than 40 years. The number of documented cases of MDS/AML has dramatically increased since 1989, which likely reflects the natural history of the disease that is now allowed to manifest by prolonging life. However, whether G-CSF increases this risk or hastens the appearance of leukemia is still debatable. From 1987 to year-end 2005, data at the SCNIR identified 50 of 422 patients with K/SCN who developed MDS/leukemia (crude rate of 11.8%).

To determine if the incidence of MDS/AML in the SCNIR patients is related to G-CSF dosage or duration of therapy or to other patient demographics, a detailed analysis was conducted on 374 patients who received G-CSF for at least 10 years. After 10 years on G-CSF, the annual risk of MDS/AML was stable at 2.3% per year. After 15 years on G-CSF, the cumulative incidence of MDS/AML was 22%.

The risk of MDS/AML is higher in patients requiring higher doses of G-CSF. According to SCNIR data, less responsive patients, defined as those having ANCs of less than 2.1×10^9/L on G-CSF doses greater than 8 μg/kg/d had a cumulative incidence of MDS/AML of 34% after 15 years; more responsive patients, defined as having ANCs of greater than 2.1 $\times 10^9$/L on G-CSF doses lower than 8 μg/kg/d had a cumulative incidence of 15%. The data were interpreted as indicating that a poor response to G-CSF defines an "at-risk" population and predicts an adverse outcome. The data do not necessarily support a cause-and-effect relationship between development of MDS/AML and G-CSF therapy. The results may only mean that patients requiring higher G-CSF therapy have a more severe clinical and hematologic phenotype. A report from the French Severe Chronic Neutropenia Study Group confirmed that increased exposure to G-CSF with respect to dose and duration in congenital neutropenia patients was associated with a heightened risk of MDS/AML, but they do not speculate on the mechanism.

Conversion to MDS/AML in K/SCN patients is associated with one or more cellular genetic abnormalities that provide insight into the pathobiology of the transformation and may be useful in identifying patients who are at high risk. Several cellular and genetic changes have been found in the BM of patients with K/SCN who received G-CSF. Whether these changes are coupled to G-CSF therapy is unknown. Remarkably, the abnormalities have predictable, similar characteristics in most patients and underscore a fairly specific multistep pathogenesis in the evolution into MDS/AML. At varying time points after starting G-CSF therapy, about half of the congenital neutropenia patients who transform acquire the same activating RAS oncogene mutation, namely a GGT (glycine) to GAT (aspartic acid) substitution at codon 12. More than 90% of patients who transform also show an acquired cytogenetic clonal alteration in BM cells, usually −7 or 7q- but also +21 or +8. Complex cytogenetics (e.g., −7 and +21) have also been identified. More than 80% of patients develop one or more G-CSF receptor point mutations. These G-CSF-R mutations are nonsense mutations that result in the truncation of the C-terminal cytoplasmic region, a subdomain that is crucial for G-CSF–induced maturation. The acquired mutation is directly operative in the conversion to MDS/AML. In murine models, the mutation results in impaired ligand internalization, defective receptor downmodulation, and enhanced growth signaling that produces an exaggerated hyperproliferative effect in response to G-CSF. This also confers resistance to apoptosis and enhances cell survival that favors clonal expansion in vivo. The detection of G-CSF-R mutations places patients at high risk for malignant conversion, but the time course from detection of mutations to overt MDS/AML varies considerably and may take years.

Although patients requiring higher doses of G-CSF to attain safe neutrophil levels are at a higher risk of developing MDS/AML, there is no definitive evidence that G-CSF directly causes malignant transformation. G-CSF may simply be an "innocent bystander" that corrects the neutropenia, prolongs patient survival, and allows time for the malignant predisposition to declare itself. Alternatively, G-CSF may accelerate the propensity for MDS/AML in the genetically altered stem and progenitor cells in congenital neutropenia. G-CSF may rescue malignant clones that would otherwise be destined for apoptosis. The clinical interplay between G-CSF and the receptor mutation was underscored in the report of a patient with congenital neutropenia on G-CSF who developed a receptor mutation and AML. When G-CSF was stopped, the blast count in blood and in BM fell to undetectable levels on two occasions without giving chemotherapy, although the mutant receptor was persistently detectable during the remissions. A similar patient has been observed in Toronto (Y. Dror, unpublished data).

An axiom of oncogenesis is that rapidly dividing cells are more susceptible to mutational events. Because therapeutic G-CSF provides a powerful proliferative signal for BM cells, it is a reasonable hypothesis that congenital neutropenia BM progenitors acquire new mutations. From the evidence cited herein, acquisition of a G-CSF receptor mutation in the face of therapeutic G-CSF in congenital neutropenia can provide the hyperresponsive replicative scenario that can relentlessly evolve into MDS/AML. Is recombinant human G-CSF a carcinogen? This would seem highly unlikely. As a physiologic regulator of hematopoiesis, it would be unexpected for G-CSF to break molecular bonds and cause DNA damage even when used in therapeutic dosages.

Differential Diagnosis

The commonest cause of isolated neutropenia in very young children is **viral-induced BM suppression.** An antecedent history of good health, the occurrence of a viral illness, and the transient nature of the neutropenia distinguish this disorder from K/SCN.

Autoimmune neutropenia of infancy is recognized as a fairly specific syndrome of early childhood. Low neutrophil numbers are often discovered during the course of routine investigation for a benign febrile illness. The illness abates, but the neutropenia persists, sometimes for months and occasionally for years. A BM biopsy is normocellular, and an aspirate shows active granulopoiesis up to the band stage; neutrophils may be normally represented, reduced or absent. The neutropenia is caused by increased peripheral destruction and the diagnosis can be supported by demonstrating specific antigranulocyte antibodies on neutrophils. The prognosis is good, the neutropenia is self-limited albeit protracted, and patients seldom develop serious bacterial infections as a result of it. Other infrequent acquired causes of severe, isolated neutropenia in this age group include BM suppression from a drug or toxin and neutrophil sequestration as part of a hypersplenism syndrome.

Of the IBMFSs, **SDS** can also manifest as isolated neutropenia but can be identified because of growth failure, the malabsorption component caused by pancreatic insufficiency, fatty changes in the pancreas seen on CT scanning or ultrasonography, and characteristic skeletal abnormalities. **Glycogen storage disease type 1b (GSD-1b)** and **Barth syndrome** are also in the differential diagnosis. Neutropenia can also be a prominent part of **antibody deficiency syndromes** and **cellular immunodeficiency disorders** (Table 27-8); investigation of chronic neutropenia of childhood should include an immunoglobulin electrophoresis, T-cell proliferative studies, and quantitation of T-cell subsets and NK cell activity. **Cyclic neutropenia** is distinguished by predictable symptomatology, especially mouth sores about every 3 weeks (19-23 days), often associated with chronic gingivitis. A complete blood count two or three times a week for 4 to 8 weeks demonstrates the diagnostic oscillation pattern with a cyclic nadir. Other **unclassified inherited neutropenia syndromes** with vertical transmission or in siblings have been described. The neutropenia in such cases are typically mild to moderate. When severe **neutropenia is diagnosed in the newborn period,** the cause may be passive transfer transplacentally of IgG antineutrophil antibodies from the mother. This can occur if the mother has an autoimmune disorder with neutropenia or by alloimmunization caused by fetomaternal incompatibility for a neutrophil-specific antigen.

Therapy and Prognosis

Before the introduction of G-CSF as a specific therapy of K/SCN, there was limited treatment. Antibiotics were the mainstay of management for active infection and for prophylaxis. Attempts to mobilize neutrophils with lithium had limited application.

Cytokine Therapy

G-CSF has supplanted all other forms of management because more than 90% of K/SCN patients respond. It is recommended to begin G-CSF therapy as front-line treatment when the diagnosis is established. GM-CSF in crossover trials with G-CSF for K/SCN is not as effective and does not induce a neutrophil response consistently. If the ANC remains below 1.0×10^9/L after initiation of G-CSF at 5 μg/kg/dose once a day subcutaneously, the dose may be escalated to 10 μg/kg/dose and then by increments of 10 μg/kg/dose at 14-day intervals until a response is seen. As soon as the ANC can be maintained at 1.0×10^9/L or above, the G-CSF dose does not have to be increased further because the occurrence of bacterial infection is reduced dramatically with an ANC at this level. Patients who are proven to be infection free with ANC of 0.75 to 1.0 may continue on the same G-CSF doses. The G-CSF dose can be reduced if the ANC increases to 5.0×10^9/L or above to find the lowest dose

Table 27-8 Miscellaneous Inherited Neutropenia Disorders

Diagnosis	Genetics	Mapping	Mutant Gene	Additional Features
Hyper IgM syndrome, type 1	X-L	Xq26	*CD40L*	↓IgG, IgA, IgE, autoimmune cytopenias
Hermansky-Pudlak syndrome, type 2	AR	5q14.1	*AP3B1*	↓IgG, partial albinism, platelet dysfunction
Griscelli syndrome, type 1	AR	15q21	*MYO5A*	Neurologic dysfunction, partial albinism
Griscelli syndrome, type 2	AR	15q21	*RAB27A*	Same as type 1 plus hemophagocytosis
Chediak-Higashi syndrome	AR	1q42.1-q42.2	*LYST (CHSI)*	Immunodeficiency, partial albinism
Poikiloderma with Neutropenia	AR	16q13	*C16ORF57*	Rash, short stature, dystrophic nails
P14 deficiency	AR	1q22	*MAPBPIP*	Immunodeficiency, hypopigmentation
Cohen syndrome	AR	8q22-q23	*VPS13B/COH1*	Retinopathy, retardation, skeletal anomalies
Charcot-Marie-Tooth syndrome, type 2	AD	19p13.2	*DMN2*	Axonal demyelinating neuropathy

Data compiled from Online Mendelian Inheritance in Man (http://ncbi.nlm.nih.gov/omim).
AD, Autosomal dominant; *AR,* autosomal recessive; *Ig,* immunoglobulin; *X-L,* X-linked recessive.

necessary for maintaining a neutrophil count at 1.0×10^9/L or greater. The SCNIR co-investigators defined nonresponders as patients who do not respond to G-CSF levels exceeding 120 μg/kg/day. Partial responders show an increase of their ANC to 0.5 to 1.0×10^9/L with the highest dose, but they still experience bacterial infections. In these patients, the dose of G-CSF cannot be increased because of the large volume and frequency of injections required. In some of these patients, a combination of G-CSF with SCF can induce a further increase in the ANC, but the potential allergic side effects of SCF have limited the use of this treatment combination to hospitalized patients with severe infections who also receive concomitant antihistamines. The only currently available treatment for patients who do not respond to G-CSF treatment alone or in combination with SCF is HSCT. In one published case of a G-CSF nonresponder, the addition of small dose of prednisone (5 mg/day) to a standard G-CSF dose of about 5 μg/kg resulted in a long-term complete response.

All patients on G-CSF therapy should be seen by a physician every 3 to 6 months. Patients requiring more than 8 μg/kg/day are at higher risk for MDS/AML and should be evaluated more often. Blood counts (white blood cells, hemoglobin, platelets, and differential blood counts) should be obtained and a physical examination performed at least every 3 months, including assessment for weight and height in pediatric patients and documentation of intercurrent infections. BM examination for morphology and cytogenetics is recommended once a year to search for acquired cytogenetic abnormalities such as monosomy 7 or trisomy 21.

From SCNIR data, a sustained hematologic response in patients treated with G-CSF for more than 15 years has been confirmed. With therapy, neutrophil counts rise in more than 90% of K/SCN patients and are maintained at a plateau for protracted periods, resulting in vast clinical benefits. In no instance has there been BM or hematopoietic lineage "exhaustion" or depletion with G-CSF therapy.

Hematopoietic Stem Cell Transplantation

The SCNIR transplant data was reported in 2000. Of 29 who were transplanted, 18 had transformed to MDS, AML, or both, and the dual goal was to cure the malignancy and the neutropenia. Only three of the 18 were successful. The causes for failure included mismatched transplants, progressive refractory AML, serious illness at the time of the procedure, and transplants performed in desperation. The other 11 patients underwent HSCT for reasons other than malignant transformation, mostly because of no response or only partial response to G-CSF. Eight patients received stem cells from an HLA-matched sibling after conditioning mainly with busulfan–cyclophosphamide alone or with additional immunosuppression. In sharp contrast to the MDS/AML group, nine of the 11 were cured with resolution of neutropenia.

A summary of 18 K/SCN cases transplanted between 1989 and 2005 in Japan for lack of or a partial response to treatment with G-CSF but without MDS/AML was published in 2010. Nine patients received stem cells from an HLA-identical sibling donor and nine from an alternative donor. Twelve received myeloablative regimens, and 6 patients received varying nonmyeloablative conditioning regimens. Sixteen of the patients were reported alive and in complete remission at a median follow-up of 6.5 years.

A multicenter retrospective analysis of umbilical cord transplants for IBMFs in Europe published in 2011 included 16 patients with K/SCN. The conditioning regimens were myeloablative in nature. One patient received a related cord blood graft, and the other 15 received unrelated grafts. Three patients were transplanted for leukemia or MDS using unrelated cord blood; two died. The other 13 patients were transplanted because of a lack of response to G-CSF. At a median follow-up of 41 months, 11 of the 13 were alive; one received an untreated graft, and 10 received unrelated grafts.

In the literature, seven patients received nonmyeloaplastive regimens. However, the small number of patients, the different regimens, and the different indications (refractoriness to G-CSF or MDS/AML) do not allow meaningful conclusions.

In general, the best scenario for a curative HSCT is when the procedure is performed before developing MDS/AML using a matched-related donor and when the patient is in good physical condition. In a small series of six transplanted patients for MDS or AML, two with MDS who underwent the procedure without being given induction chemotherapy survived, but four with AML given induction chemotherapy had significantly more morbidity and died posttransplant, raising questions about conditioning strategies for these patients.

The discovery of an isolated BM clonal cytogenetic abnormality without other evidence of MDS or AML in patients with congenital neutropenia raises management issues. One option is to perform HSCT if there is a matched donor as soon as feasible. This has generally been recommended for patients with −7, 7q-, or +21. The a priori argument is that the chance for cure is higher when the patient is well and has a low burden of malignant cells. The problem with this decision centers on not knowing the tempo of progression from cytogenetic evolution to clear-cut MDS or AML. Thus, there may not be a need to rush to transplant in all patients. Instead, one recommendation is to lower the G-CSF to the lowest dose that maintains neutrophil counts greater than 0.5×10^9/L and to monitor the patient regularly with blood counts and by serial BM testing.

Opinions also vary about the best way to manage patients with other genetic changes such as *G-CSF-R* or *RAS* mutations but without clonal BM cytogenetic abnormalities or morphologic evidence of transformation. In one patient with an isolated G-CSF receptor mutation, an HSCT was performed to eliminate the risk of leukemic conversion. Debate about this approach continues, and watchful waiting is an acceptable option.

Bisphosphonates for Osteoporosis

In 50% of K/SCN patients on G-CSF, bone density measurements show varying degrees of osteopenia and osteoporosis. Most of these are subclinical and asymptomatic, but some patients complain of bone pain and have fractures. Evidence shows that bisphosphonates are effective treatment for the majority of these cases.

Future Directions

The list of K/SCN genes is by no means complete, and further studies are necessary to discover novel genes. It is also not clear if there is an association between specific mutations and the risk of evolution to MDS and acute leukemia, but studies are ongoing to try to answer this clinical question. At present, diagnosis of cyclic and congenital neutropenia still depends primarily on observations of serial blood cell counts, but it is expected that mutational analysis of the *ELA-2* gene will become a routine part of making the diagnosis and the establishment of a prognosis for these patients in the years ahead. Because apoptosis is a central mechanism of neutropenia in these patients, future studies will determined whether the term *maturation arrest* should be replaced by *accelerated apoptosis* as a descriptive term for the BM findings. It appears that cellular models involving transfection of the mutant genes into human myeloid cell lines provide evidence of how neutropenia occurs. Potentially, these models can also be used to examine new approaches to preventing apoptosis and serve to provide clues to new and more effective therapies. Considerable data now confirm the effectiveness of G-CSF in the treatment of various forms of K/SCN. However, the inconvenient administration, potential long-term effects, and lack of response in 10% of the patients require the development of alternative therapies.

Other Inherited Neutropenia Syndromes

Barth Syndrome

Barth syndrome is a rare multisystem metabolic disorder inherited in an X-linked recessive mode. It is the first human disease in which the primary causative factor is an alteration of cardiolipin remodeling. Cardiolipin is a component of the inner mitochondrial membrane necessary for proper functioning of the electron transport chain. The findings in typical cases are mild to severe neutropenia, dilated or hypertrophic cardiomyopathy, underdeveloped skeletal musculature and muscle weakness, exercise intolerance, growth delay, cardiolipin abnormalities, and 3-methylglutaconic aciduria. ANCs are variable, but total agranulocytosis has been reported. BM morphology includes a maturation arrest at the myelocyte stage. On electron microscopy, mitochondria show concentric, tightly packed cristae and occasional inclusion bodies in various tissues, including granulocyte precursors. Clinically, the cardiomyopathy dominates the clinical picture, but gingivitis, oral problems, and bacterial sepsis from neutropenia can be problematic. Anecdotal reports and the authors' experience (Y. Dror, unpublished data) suggest that G-CSF is highly effective in correcting the neutropenia and preventing infections. The myriad of clinical problems requires a multidisciplinary approach. Female carriers are healthy and hematologically normal, likely because of extreme skewing of X-inactivation. The initial impression that Barth syndrome was a lethal infantile disease has been modified; age distribution in 54 living patients ranges from 0 to 49 years and peaks around puberty.

The Barth syndrome gene was mapped to Xq28, which led to the cloning of the *TAZ* gene and the various mutations that account for the phenotype. *TAZ* produces several different mRNAs with resultant proteins called tafazzins. Mutations in *TAZ* result in a decrease in tetralinoleoyl species of cardiolipin and an accumulation of monolysocardiolipin within cells. A murine model of Barth syndrome has been developed. Knocked-down cellular models and patient BM cells are characterized by accelerated apoptosis.

Kostmann/Severe Congenital Neutropenia: Granulocyte Colony-Stimulating Factor Versus Hematopoietic Stem Cell Transplantation as First-Line Therapy

Therapeutic options for newly diagnosed patients with K/SCN must be constantly reevaluated. It is largely accepted that G-CSF induces robust neutrophilic responses and eliminates infections almost completely in more than 90% of K/SCN patients. Therefore, it should be the first treatment choice. HSCT has been regarded as "salvage" therapy for patients who either acquire evidence of malignant myeloid transformation or fail to respond to G-CSF altogether. For KS patients transplanted with a fully matched donor before transforming to MDS/AML and in stable health, the chance for cure is at least 85%, possibly higher. The SCNIR data support this estimate. Not only is the neutropenia fully corrected by HSCT, but the risk of MDS/AML is also eliminated. The onerous burden of daily subcutaneous injections is removed, the financial expense is relieved, and the side effects of G-CSF are prevented. Clearly, an 85% cure rate stacks up favorably against the high cumulative incidence of incurable MDS/AML over time, particularly in patients who require large doses of G-CSF. HSCT is a reasonable option as front-line therapy for selected higher risk patients instead of G-CSF, and the option should be discussed fairly and sensibly with newly diagnosed patients and families.

Glycogen Storage Disease Type 1b

Glycogen storage disease type 1b is caused by a deficiency in glucose-6-phosphate translocase (transporter) because of mutant *G6PT1 (SLC37A4)*. GSD-1b patients experience disturbed glucose homeostasis and quantitative or qualitative neutrophil abnormalities. The translocase transports glucose-6-phosphate into the lumen of the endoplasmic reticulum, where it is hydrolyzed into glucose and inorganic phosphate. Absence of translocase results in an inability to liberate glucose from glucose-6-phosphate. Consequently, patients with GSD-1b are susceptible to fasting hypoglycemia, lactic acidosis, hepatomegaly, poor linear growth, delayed pubertal development, and other systemic complications.

Most patients have neutropenia, which ranges from mild to severe. A strict correlation between genotype and the degree of neutropenia has not been established. Some studies reported hypocellular BM; however, BM testing on nine patients from the City of Hope National Medical Center in 2001 before G-CSF therapy revealed normal to hypercellularity in all patients. Maturation arrest at the myelocyte stage or later is a feature. Neutrophil apoptosis appears to be a central mechanism leading to granulopoietic failure. Neutrophil dysfunction with defective chemotaxis and an impaired respiratory burst is an additional feature. Patients are consequently susceptible to recurrent infections and to inflammatory bowel disease. Infections most commonly involve the skin, perirectal area, ears, and urinary tract, but septicemia, pneumonia, and meningitis may also occur. The most frequently isolated organisms include *Staphylococcus aureus,* group A streptococci, *Streptococcus pneumoniae, Escherichia coli,* and *Pseudomonas.*

G-CSF therapy is extremely effective in almost all GSD-1b patients. BM cellularity increases, the ANCs increase exuberantly, and impaired oxygen radical formation is corrected. AML while on G-CSF is a rare event. Prospective data on GSD-1b patients receiving G-CSF therapy from the SCNIR identified 40% with splenomegaly before starting G-CSF, 81% with splenomegaly by the first year of treatment, and 100% with splenomegaly by 3 years. Hypersplenism can occur but can be overcome by reducing the G-CSF dosage or by splenectomy. Histology of the surgically excised spleens shows extramedullary hematopoiesis.

Cyclic Neutropenia

Cyclic neutropenia is an autosomal dominant disorder characterized by a regular, repetitive reduction in peripheral blood neutrophils for 3 to 4 days every 19 to 23 days. Between nadirs, the patients have normal or nearly normal neutrophil counts. Patients usually present in infancy or childhood and have a less severe infectious course compared with those with K/SCN. However, life-threatening infections have been reported. Daily treatment with G-CSF typically improves symptoms in most patients.

Cyclic neutropenia is caused by heterozygous mutations in the *ELA2 (ELANE)* gene that normally encodes neutrophil elastase. The mutations usually occur at the active site of neutrophil elastase without disrupting the enzymatic substrate cleavage by the active site. The mutations seem to disturb a predicted transmembrane domain, leading to excessive granular accumulation of elastase and defective membrane localization of the enzyme. The myeloid precursors are characterized by cyclic increases in apoptosis. However, the precise molecular mechanism for the cycling hematopoiesis has not been defined. It is also not clear why the same mutations in *ELA2* are associated with both cyclic and K/SCN phenotypes.

Myelokathexis and WHIM Syndrome

Myelokathexis is a rare autosomal dominant disorder with recurrent bacterial infections caused by a reduced number and function of neutrophils. Neutropenia is typically moderate to severe. Degenerative changes in the granulocytes are characteristic and include pyknotic nuclear lobes, fine chromatin filaments, and hypersegmentation. The BM is usually hypercellular with granulocytic hyperplasia. The pathophysiology of myelokathexis has been attributed to a defective release of BM cells into the peripheral blood. Neutrophil precursors are characterized by decreased expression of BCL-X and accelerated apoptosis. G-CSF ameliorates the neutropenia and leads to clinical improvement during episodes of bacterial infection.

WHIM syndrome refers to the association of myelokathexis with other features (**w**arts, **h**ypogammaglobulinemia, **i**nfections, and **m**yelokathexis). Most cases are caused by mutations in the chemokine receptor gene *CXCR4* but dysfunction of GRK3, a negative regulator of CXCR4, has also been implicated. The mutations result in enhanced chemotactic response of neutrophils in response to the CXCR4 ligand CXCL12 (stroma-derived factor 1) and pathologic retention of neutrophils in the BM. Patients with wild type *CXCR4* might have other genetic defects that lead to an enhanced interaction between CXCR4 and CXCL12 and an enhanced chemotactic response, such as reduced inhibition of CXCL12-promoted internalization, and desensitization of CXCR4 by G protein–coupled receptor (GPCR) kinase-3 caused by decreased transcription of the GPCR kinase-3. G-CSF induces a prompt increase in neutrophil numbers and gamma globulin levels may also increase.

Dursun Syndrome

Dursun syndrome is an autosomal recessive form of SCN caused by biallelic mutant *G6PC3*. Wild-type *G6PC3* encodes glucose-6-phosphatase catalytic subunit 3, which, when mutated, confers an increased susceptibility of neutrophils to apoptosis. BM samples show a marked decrease in mature neutrophils, rendering patients susceptible to severe bacterial infections. Lymphopenia and thrombocytopenia may occur. Structural heart defects, urogenital abnormalities, venous angiectasia on the trunk and extremities, and a broad range of other physical abnormalities are additional features.

Other Inherited Neutropenias

Other inherited neutropenia disorders are associated with specific mutant genes, but they do not necessarily have the K/SCN BM phenotype, nor is their pathophysiology necessarily similar (see Table 27-8). Immune deficiency appears to be an important component of these syndromes. These miscellaneous forms tend to have distinguishing physical abnormalities such as partial albinism and are not predisposed to MDS/AML.

Thrombocytopenia With Absent Radii Syndrome

Background

Thrombocytopenia absent radii syndrome (see Chapters 20) has two essential features, hypomegakaryocytic thrombocytopenia and bilateral radial aplasia with thumbs present. It is one of a group of inherited hematologic disorders that includes FA and DBA with radial ray anomalies. The manifestations of the phenotype vary widely, and patients can present with abnormalities involving skeletal, skin, gastrointestinal, brain, renal, and cardiac systems. The mode of inheritance is not known. Autosomal recessive and autosomal dominant modes with variable penetrance have both been suggested. From published information, families with normal parents have been observed with more than one affected sibling. Additionally, in reports of two sets of identical twins, each child had TAR, but one of a pair of fraternal twins had the syndrome. Almost always, parents of patients with TAR are phenotypically normal. Women with TAR syndrome can conceive and give birth to hematologically and phenotypically normal offspring. The disease is caused by biallelic mutations in *RBM8A*. Three cases of AML and one case of acute lymphoid *(lymphoidic)* leukemia in TAR syndrome patients have been reported. Using a denominator of about 300 published cases of TAR, four leukemic episodes (1%-2% crude rate) suggests a predisposition to the development of hematologic malignancies.

Etiology and Pathophysiology

Thrombocytopenia in TAR syndrome is the result of a defect in megakaryocytopoiesis and thrombocytopoiesis. It was previously shown that TAR patients have submicroscopic deletions at 1q21.1 in one allele in 100% of cases. However, since the deletion was found in about 25% of unaffected parents, the pathogenetic significance of the deletion was unclear. Recently, a group from Cambridge found that TAR syndrome is caused by compound inheritance of a null allele of the RBM8A gene at 1q21.1 and one of two low-frequency SNPs in the regulatory regions of RBM8A, encoding the Y14 subunit of exon-junction complex, which processes mRNA. The mutations caused reduced expression of the protein in platelets from affected individuals.

Thrombopoietin levels in plasma or serum are consistently elevated in TAR syndrome, thereby excluding a cytokine production defect as a cause for thrombocytopenia in this disorder. BM CFU-Meg (CFU-MK) progenitors are either absent or are present in low to normal frequencies but produce small colonies in vitro with abnormal morphology. CFU-GM and BFU-E colony growth is often increased.

In a detailed study of $CD34^+$ cells, the thrombocytopenia of TAR syndrome was associated with a dysmegakaryocytopoiesis characterized by cells remaining at an early stage of differentiation. Cells expressing CD41 without CD42 accumulated behind the block, and there was a decrease in c-mpl transcripts and mpl protein. The response of platelets to adenosine diphosphate or to the thrombin receptor agonist peptide SFLLRN (TRAP) is normal in TAR patients. However, in contrast to control participants, there is no in vitro platelet activation of platelets from TAR patients to recombinant thrombopoietin as measured by testing thrombopoietin synergism to adenosine diphosphate and TRAP in platelet activation. Thrombopoietin-induced tyrosine phosphorylation of platelet proteins in this setting is completely absent or markedly decreased. The results indicate that there is a lack of response to thrombopoietin downstream the c-mpl signal transduction pathway.

No recurrent chromosomal changes are seen in TAR syndrome. Some karyotypic abnormalities found in a few patients are of unclear significance. Clastogenic induced chromosomal breakage analysis in TAR syndrome is normal.

Clinical Features

History and Physical Examination

The diagnosis is made during the newborn period because of the absent radii, and about half of patients develop a petechial rash and overt hemorrhage such as bloody diarrhea. Patients have bilateral radial aplasia (Fig. 27-12) with preservation of the thumbs and fingers on both sides. Additional upper extremity deformities include radial club hands; hypoplastic carpals and phalanges; and hypoplastic ulnae, humeri, and shoulder girdles. Syndactyly and clinodactyly of the toes and fingers are also seen. Characteristic findings include a selective hypoplasia of the middle phalanx of the fifth finger and altered palmar contours. Upper extremity involvement ranges from isolated absent radii to true, often asymmetric, phocomelia. The lower extremities are involved in about half of cases. Malformations include hip dislocation, coxa valga, femoral torsion, tibial torsion, abnormal tibiofibular joints, small feet, and valgus and varus foot deformities. Abnormal toe placement is commonly seen, especially the fifth toe overlapping the fourth. Similar to upper limb involvement, lower extremity deformities range from minimal involvement to complete phocomelia. An asymmetric first rib, a cervical rib, cervical spina bifida, and a fused cervical spine can occur, but trunk involvement is usually minimal. Micrognathia has been associated with the TAR syndrome in up to 65% of cases.

Cardiac abnormalities occur in 15% of the patients, including atrial septal defect, tetralogy of Fallot, and ventricular septal defect. Capillary hemangiomas are common (24%) as well as redundant nuchal folds.

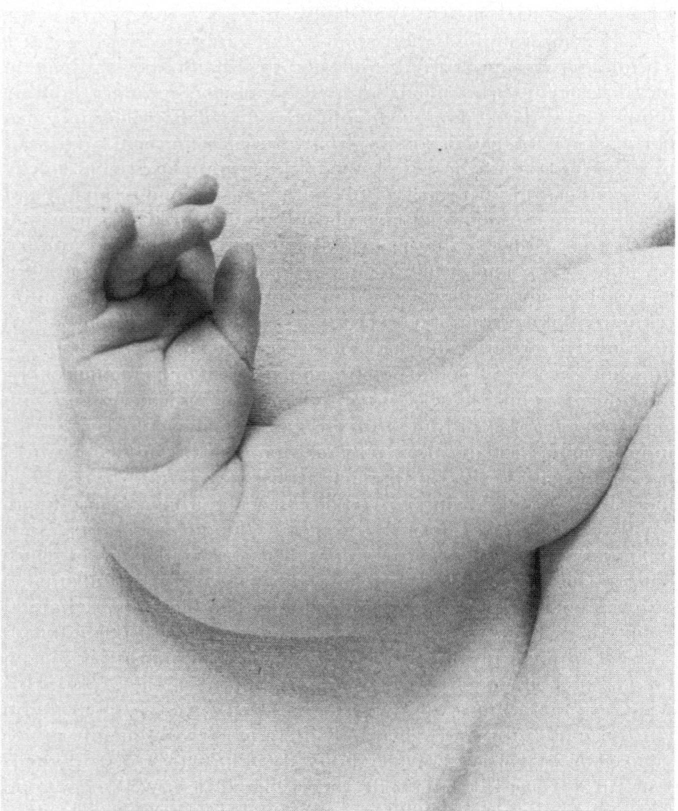

Figure 27-12 RADIAL APLASIA WITH PRESERVATION OF THE THUMB IN A NEWBORN WITH THROMBOCYTOPENIA WITH ABSENT RADII SYNDROME.

Genitourinary tract malformations are detected in 23% of cases. About 95% of patients have short stature, 76% have macrocephaly, and 53% show facial dysmorphism. Structural brain abnormalities may be present. Additional findings are dorsal pedal edema, hyperhidrosis, and gastrointestinal disturbances such as diarrhea and feeding intolerance; almost 50% of patients are intolerant of cow's milk.

Prenatal diagnosis can be made by ultrasound imaging of absent radii with thumbs present and by measuring platelet numbers obtained by fetoscopy or cordocentesis. A published case describes a prenatal diagnosis of TAR followed by an in utero platelet transfusion to facilitate safe delivery.

Laboratory Findings

Thrombocytopenia as a result of BM underproduction is a consistent finding. BM specimens show normal to increased cellularity with decreased to absent megakaryocytes. The erythroid and myeloid lineages are normally represented. When a few megakaryocytes can be identified in biopsies, they are small, contain few nuclear segments, and show immature nongranular cytoplasm. If platelet counts increase spontaneously in patients after the first year of life, megakaryocytes increase in parallel and appear more mature morphologically. At diagnosis, leukocytosis is seen in the majority of patients and is sometimes extreme to greater than 100,000/μL with a "left shift" to immature myeloid forms. The cause of this leukemoid reaction is unclear, but it is usually transient and subsides spontaneously. If anemia is present, it is likely attributable to blood loss caused by thrombocytopenia. When platelet numbers are adequate for study, their size is generally normal, and routine testing of function is unremarkable, although some patients may show abnormal platelet aggregation and storage pool defects. Compared with other inherited BM failure syndromes, RBC size and fetal hemoglobin levels are normal.

Differential Diagnosis

Important clinical differences distinguish TAR syndrome from **FA.** In FA, when radii are absent, the thumbs are hypoplastic or absent. FA patients do not have skin hemangiomas like some patients with TAR, but TAR patients do not show abnormal skin pigmentation like 40% of Fanconi patients. Confirmation of FA is made by the clastogenic chromosome stress test showing increased fragility and by mutational analysis. TAR patients do not have increased chromosomal breakage.

Some infants with **trisomy 18** (+18) have absence or hypoplasia of radii and thrombocytopenia. However, in +18, thumbs are absent if radii are absent, and the disorder can also be distinguished from TAR syndrome cytogenetically. There are several syndromes with radial abnormalities but with *normal* platelet counts that can be diagnosed by mutational gene analysis. These include **Roberts syndrome** (mutant *ESC02*); **Holt-Oram syndrome** (mutant *TBX5*); and the clinical spectrum of three disorders caused by mutant *RECQL4:* **Rothmund-Thomson syndrome, Baller-Gerold syndrome,** and **RAPADILINO syndrome.**

Therapy and Prognosis

The risk of hemorrhage is greatest in the first year of life. Deaths are usually caused by intracranial or gastrointestinal bleeding. If patients survive the first year, platelet counts spontaneously increase inexplicably to levels that are hemostatically safe and do not require platelet transfusional support. A minority of patients have sustained, profound thrombocytopenia that does not improve spontaneously. Published cases of TAR syndrome show an actuarial survival curve plateau of 80% by age 1 to 2 years. Many reports of TAR patients antedated the modern use of platelet transfusions so the survival is likely much better currently. TAR patients do not evolve into having BM failure with pancytopenia but may develop acute leukemia in 1% to 2% of cases.

Platelet Transfusions

As in other inherited BM failure disorders associated with thrombocytopenia, platelet transfusions should be used judiciously. Bleeding and prophylaxis for orthopedic surgical procedures are appropriate indications. Persistent platelet counts below 10,000/μL may require preventative platelet transfusions on a regular basis, especially in the first year of life when the expectation is that a spontaneous improvement in platelet number will ensue with time in most infants. Single-donor platelets are preferred to multiple random donor platelets to minimize the risk of alloimmunization. HLA-partially matched or fully matched donors for platelets may be required if patients become refractory to transfusions.

Other Therapies

Supportive management is the mainstay, but in exceptional situations, profound, persistent life-threatening thrombocytopenia can be successfully treated by HSCT. Thrombopoietin receptor agonists, such as romiplostim and eltrombopag, have not been studied in TAR syndrome. Elevated serum thrombopoietin levels at baseline in TAR patients may predict a poor response to these products. IL-11, another thrombopoietic cytokine, has not been studied in clinical trials either; however, endogenous IL-11 serum levels in TAR patients are also elevated. Androgens, corticosteroids, and splenectomy are ineffective therapies for TAR syndrome.

Congenital Dyserythropoietic Anemias

Background

The designation *congenital dyserythropoietic anemia* (CDA) refers to a family of inherited refractory anemias characterized by BM erythroid multinuclearity, ineffective erythropoiesis, and secondary hemosiderosis. The ineffective erythropoiesis is reflected by BM erythroid hyperplasia, inappropriately low reticulocyte counts for the degree of anemia, and intramedullary RBC destruction. Splenomegaly and chronic or intermittent jaundice are additional features. Granulopoiesis and thrombopoiesis are normal. Although these disorders are not classical BM failure syndromes per se, they are genetically transmitted and result in anemia with a blunted erythropoietic response. Some patients, especially with CDA type I, have congenital anomalies.

Three classical forms of CDA have been described as well as a number of variants. An arbitrary classification used in practice for these three is based on the inheritance pattern, the peripheral blood and BM morphology, and the serologic findings in each case. The distinguishing features of the three types of CDA are as follows:

- Type I: Autosomal recessive; macrocytosis; megaloblastic erythroid precursor cells; 2% to 5% binucleated erythroid precursor cells; internuclear chromatin bridges involving polychromatic erythroblasts; negative acidified serum lysis test result (neg Ham test)
- Type II: Autosomal recessive; normocytic RBCs; normoblastic erythroid precursor cells; 10% to 40% binucleated late normoblasts; positive acidified serum lysis test result (pos Ham test)
- Type III: Autosomal dominant (or sporadic); macrocytosis; megaloblastic erythroid maturation; giant multinucleated erythroid precursors with up to 12 nuclei per cell; negative acidified serum lysis test result (neg Ham test)

The designation "type IV" is defunct but was briefly used to classify cases of morphologic CDA type II with a *negative* Ham acidified serum test result. Because some of these were reclassified as CDA type II after retesting using a large panel of heterologous sera, "type IV"

Inherited Marrow Failure and Malignant Leukemic Transformation

Historically, the inherited marrow failure syndromes were classified as "benign" hematology to contrast sharply with hematologic cancer. Patients with KS/congenital neutropenia, SDS, FA, DC, CAMT, DBA, or TAR syndrome often died early in life from complications of cytopenias. However, in the current era of advanced supportive care and availability of recombinant cytokines and other effective therapeutics, patients with these conditions usually survive the early years of life and beyond. With the extended lifespan of patients, the natural history of these disorders has dramatically changed. One of the most sobering observations is that the seven disorders cited above confer an inordinately high predisposition to developing MDS and AML. Thus, the distinction between "benign" and "malignant" hematology in the context of the inherited BM failure disorders has become blurred, and a new clinical and hematologic continuum is evident.

Carcinogenesis occurs as a multistep sequence of events that is driven by genetic damage and by epigenetic factors. In the traditional view, the initiation of cancer starts in a normal cell through mutations from exposure to carcinogens. In the proliferative phase that follows, the genetically altered, initiated cell undergoes selective clonal expansion that enhances the probability of additional genetic damage from endogenous mutations or DNA-damaging agents. Activation of proto-oncogenes, inactivation of tumor-suppressor genes, or inactivation of genomic stability genes may be central in this process. Finally, during malignant conversion and cancer progression, malignant cells show phenotypic changes, gene amplification, chromosomal alterations, and altered gene expression.

With respect to the seven inherited BM failure syndromes that are predisposed to develop hematologic cancers, there is reason to believe that leukemogenesis is also a multistep process. The first genetic "hit" or leukemia-initiating step may be the syndrome-specific inherited genetic abnormality itself, which initially manifests as the single- or multiple-lineage marrow failure state. The "predisposed" progenitor, already initiated, could conceptually develop decreased responsiveness to the signals that regulate homeostatic growth, terminal cell differentiation, or programmed cell death. Leukemic promotion and progression with clonal expansion leading to MDS or AML could then ensue readily. Because many of the mutant genes that produce the inherited BM failure syndromes have been discovered, the nature of the leukemogenic-initiating events in these conditions should become evident.

Three of the syndromes illustrate the point. The best example is the multistep evolution of leukemic transformation over time in patients with congenital neutropenia while taking G-CSF. The acquisition of activating RAS oncogene mutations, cytogenetic abnormalities involving primarily +7, 7q- and +21, and G-CSF receptor mutation occurs in the majority of patients who transform.

Other than clonal cytogenetic changes, we know little about the timeline or sequence of events that characterize the malignant phenotype of SDS. It is striking, though, that the syndrome from early age already shares many of the findings of de novo adult MDS, including abnormal hematopoietic colony growth, abnormally short leukocyte telomeres, elevated apoptotic index mediated by FAS/FAS ligand, an abnormal immune system, an aberrant marrow microenvironment that shows impaired support of normal hematopoiesis, and increased microvessel density. Many, if not all, of these findings may evolve in utero.

Finally, FA has a "short cut" mechanism to leukemic conversion. Biallelic mutant genes from conception result in genomic instability, compromised DNA repair and chromosome breakage. The opportunities for blood cancers in this setting are infinite. Actuarial data from the IFAR showed that the risk of acquiring clonal cytogenetic abnormalities was 67% by 30 years of age in patients with BM failure. The actuarial risk of MDS or AML was 52% by 40 years of age. This steady tempo of leukemic evolution implies a stepwise acquisition over time of additional, critical genetic "hits" before overt MDS/AML.

is no longer used as a category. There are also several other forms of CDA that are distinct from CDA types I, II, and III. Some of these variants have been identified in three or more families and have been tentatively classified phenotypically into CDA *groups* (not types) IV, V, VI, and VII (see section below, Other CDAs). Additional CDA's are associated with specific gene mutations other than those seen in CDA I and II. The growing number of variants underscores the complex nature of CDA and the current direction to reclassify these disorders accurately by genotype rather than by morphology.

Etiology, Genetics, Pathophysiology, and Clinical Features

CDA Type I

Congenital dyserythropoietic anemia I is inherited in an autosomal recessive manner. The disorder is caused by biallelic mutant *CDAN1*. The gene was identified in highly inbred Israeli Bedouins. The gene product, codanin-1, may be involved in nuclear envelope integrity, but this is uncertain, and little is known about pathogenesis.

In several reported families, more than one sibling was affected, and the disorder has been seen in fraternal and identical twins. The onset of anemia, jaundice, and other symptoms may be noted at any age, especially in neonates. Eighty percent of infants in a recent large series required blood transfusions during the first month of life. One case was reported with anemia in utero requiring intrauterine exchange transfusions at 28 and 30 weeks' gestation. Affected patients often have some degree of icterus and splenomegaly.

Congenital dyserythropoietic anemia I can be associated with a variety of congenital anomalies. The following have been catalogued: patches of brown skin pigmentation, syndactyly in the feet, absence of phalanges and nails in the fingers and toes, an additional phalanx, duplication or hypoplasia of metatarsals, short stature, pigeon chest deformity, varus deformity of hips, flattened vertebral bodies, a hypoplastic rib, congenital ptosis, Madelung deformity of the wrist, and deafness. The pigmentation, syndactyly and absence of phalanges and nails are not common in CDA I patients but appear to be quite specific for this subtype. Dysmorphic features are seen in up to 65% of patients. Three siblings from a Bedouin family presented with neonatal pulmonary hypertension. In a French family, three siblings had sensorineural deafness and a lack of motile sperm cells.

Laboratory Abnormalities. The degree of anemia is usually mild to moderate (hemoglobin in the range of 6.6-11.6 g/dL), and RBCs appear macrocytic. Peripheral blood RBC morphology is characterized by anisocytosis and poikilocytosis, and occasionally Cabot rings are seen. Cabot rings appear to be unique to CDA I and are not seen in types II and III. White blood cells and platelets are normal. Examination of the BM reveals erythroid hyperplasia with some megaloblastic erythropoiesis and a small number of erythroblasts with dyserythropoietic features. The unique morphologic abnormality seen in CDA I is the presence of chromatin bridges between nuclei of two separate erythroblasts, a reflection of impaired cellular division (Fig. 27-13). This internuclear bridging of erythroblasts seen with light microscopy is also a common feature in MDS. Electron microscopy reveals additional abnormalities that include widening of the nuclear membrane pore space with cytoplasmic invagination into the nucleus, separation of nuclear chromatin, and chromatin condensation, all of which give the general appearance of a spongy nucleus (Fig. 27-14). Dyserythropoiesis seems limited mostly to more mature RBC precursors. In contrast to CDA II, there are no unique serologic features.

The defect in CDA I is at the stem cell level. The numbers of CFU-E and BFU-E colonies are normal but contain a mixture of normal and abnormal cells when examined by electron microscopy. This suggests that the abnormality is expressed variably in the mature progeny of each stem cell. Erythroid precursors also demonstrate S phase arrest and morphologic features of apoptosis. In some CDA I patients, hemoglobin A_2 levels are increased. Also, some cases show unbalanced globin chain synthesis. Patients do not have thalassemia, and the cause of these findings is not known.

CDA Type II (HEMPAS)

Congenital dyserythropoietic anemia II is commonly known as HEMPAS, an acronym for hereditary erythroblastic multinuclearity with a positive acidified serum test. It is inherited in an autosomal recessive manner. The disorder is caused by biallelic mutant *SEC23B*. The wild-type gene encodes the SEC23B component of the coat protein (COP) II complex. COP II vesicles transport secretory proteins from the endoplasmic reticulum to the Golgi complex. Mutations result in misglycosylation and an impaired clearance of endoplasmic reticulum cisternae past a given point during erythroid differentiation.

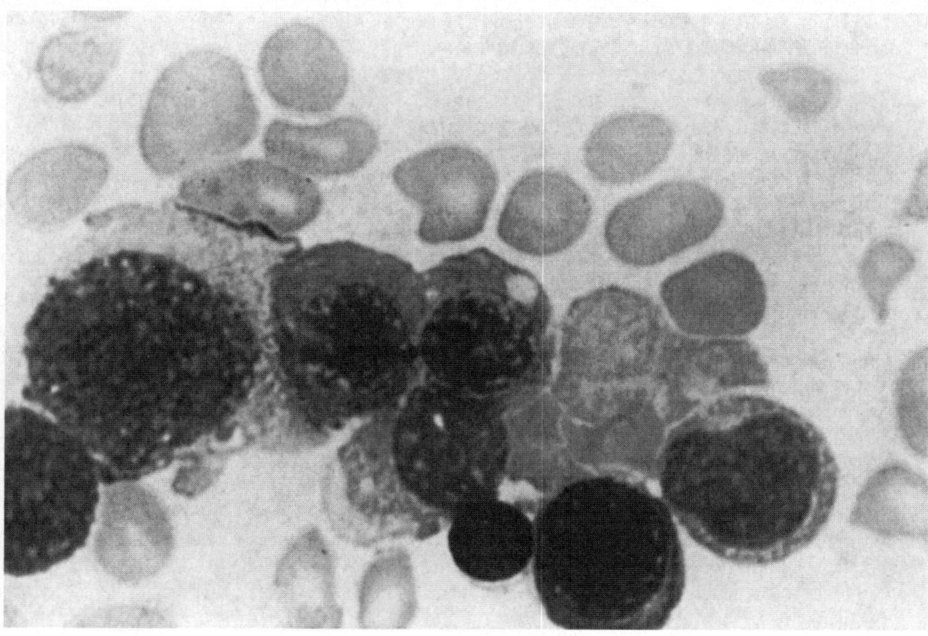

Figure 27-13 BONE MARROW FROM PATIENT WITH CONGENITAL DYSERYTHROPOIETIC ANEMIA TYPE I. Erythroblasts are connected by internuclear bridges between two cells. *(Provided by Dr. Jean Shafer, Rochester, NY.)*

Compared with the other CDAs, the pathogenesis of CDA II has been almost completely clarified. At the stem cell level, in vitro culture of CDA II erythroid progenitors produces CFU-E and BFU-E colonies with erythroblast multinuclearity. Initially, studies of peripheral blood CDA II RBCs identified a number of chemical abnormalities, including unbalanced globin chain synthesis, increased membrane glycolipids, and altered RBC membrane protein patterns demonstrated by two-dimensional electrophoresis. Furthermore, glycoproteins on CDA II RBCs were found to have an abnormal carbohydrate structure, leading to aberrant reactivity with anti-i sera. Additional data suggested that the IgM antibody responsible for hemolysis in the acidified-serum lysis test (Ham test) recognized an abnormal glycolipid structure sharing homology with i and I antigens. Thus, a variety of data predicted and confirmed that abnormalities in the glycosylation pathway were involved in the etiology of CDA II.

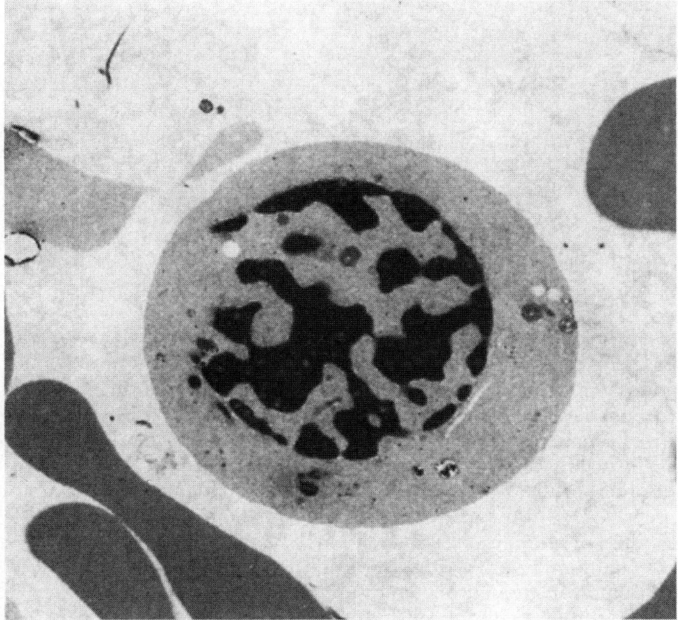

Figure 27-14 ELECTRON MICROSCOPY OF BONE MARROW FROM CONGENITAL DYSERYTHROPOIETIC ANEMIA TYPE I. Note the "spongy" appearance of the nucleus resulting from uneven chromatin with cytoplasmic invagination into the nucleus. *(Provided by Dr. Raoul Fresco, Maywood, Ill.)*

The two major defects in the CDA II glycosylation enzymatic pathway are a deficiency of α-mannosidase II and of *N*-acetylglucosaminyl transferase II. A third defect in a CDA II variant is deficient levels of the membrane-bound form of galactosyl transferase. All three of these enzymatic deficiencies lead to abnormal oligosaccharides on major erythrocyte proteins such as the anion transporter Band 3 that could cause disruption of the structural network of erythrocytes and their precursors, thereby leading to their premature demise. Defective glycosylation on the RBC surface may also affect the regulation of complement on the surface of erythrocytes. Enhanced functional activity of the alternative pathway C3 convertase and of the membrane attack complex may result from the improper glycosylation of glycophorin A, which has been proposed to serve as a complement regulatory protein. These abnormalities are not a consequence of quantitative or functional deficiencies of the complement regulatory proteins CD55 or CD59.

Laboratory Abnormalities. There is overlap of some clinical and laboratory manifestations between CDA I and CDA II, but there are three major differences. The first is that the magnitude of anemia is usually more severe, and patients, especially children, often require RBC transfusions. Peripheral blood RBCs are usually normocytic but show anisocytosis and poikilocytosis (Fig. 27-15). The second difference is that the BM in CDA II reveals greater numbers of abnormal erythroblasts with binuclearity in up to 35% late erythroblasts, as well as multinuclearity and abnormal lobulation (Fig. 27-16). These nuclear abnormalities are seen only in the late erythroblasts, not in basophilic erythroblasts. Karyorrhexis is commonly observed, and pseudo-Gaucher cells may be present, representing the ingestion of debris by histiocytic cells from ineffective erythropoiesis. Electron microscopy of late erythroblasts also reveals an excess of endoplasmic reticulum parallel to the cell membrane, giving the appearance of a double cell membrane (Fig. 27-17). A third difference, which is also a pathognomonic finding, is that CDA II RBCs are lysed by acidified (pH, 6.8) sera obtained from approximately 30% to 60% of fresh ABO-compatible sera from normal persons (i.e., a positive Ham test result), but there is no lysis when RBCs are incubated with the patient's own acidified serum. This lysis is a result of a naturally occurring IgM antibody that recognizes an antigen on CDA II cells and binds complement; this antibody can be removed by

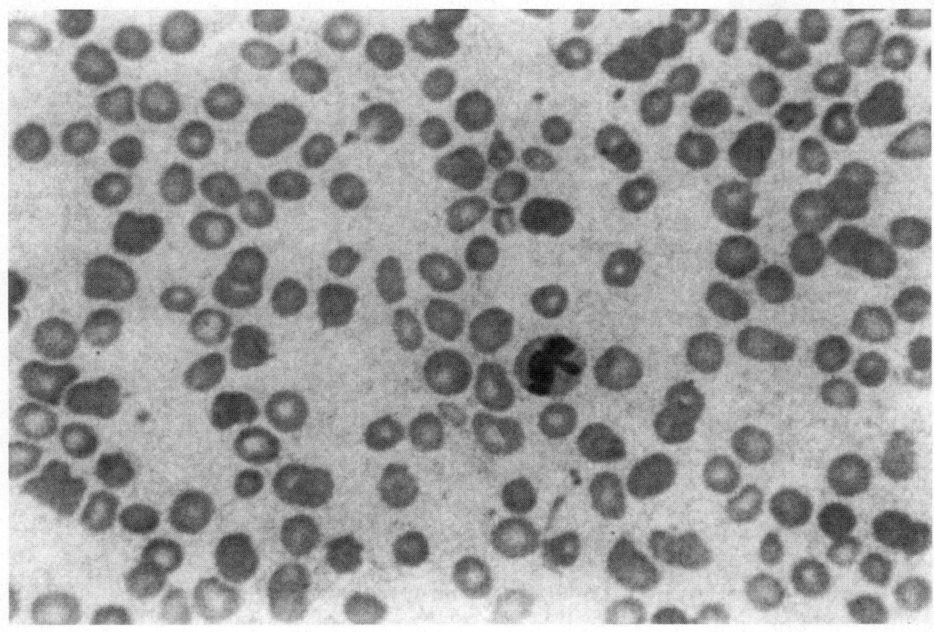

Figure 27-15 PERIPHERAL BLOOD SMEAR FROM A PATIENT WITH CONGENITAL DYSERYTHROPOIETIC ANEMIA TYPE II. Note the marked variation in red blood cell size and shape.

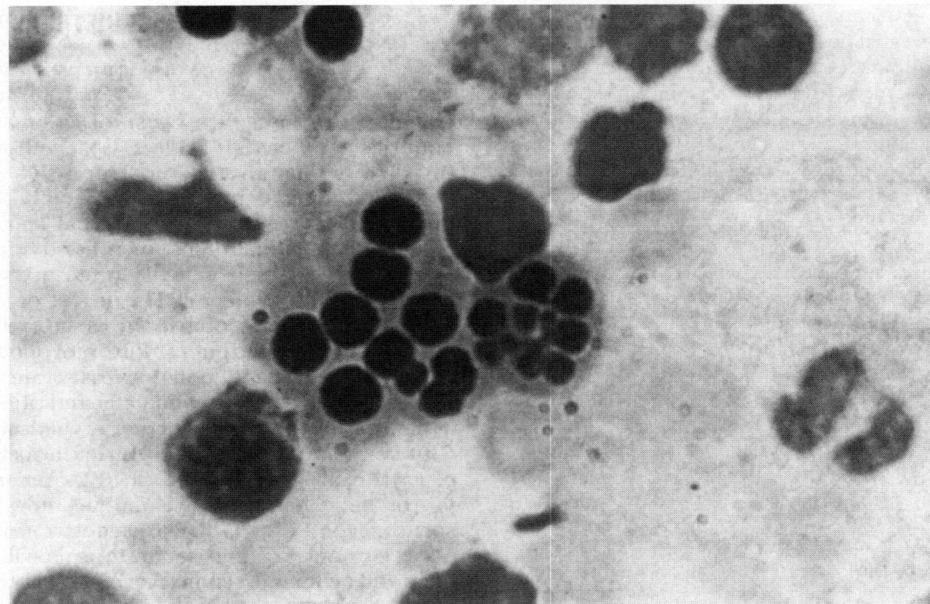

Figure 27-16 BONE MARROW ASPIRATE FROM A PATIENT WITH HEMPAS (CONGENITAL DYSERYTHROPOIETIC ANEMIA TYPE II) SHOWING ERYTHROID HYPERPLASIA AND MULTINUCLEATED ERYTHROBLASTS. *(Provided by Dr. Jean Shafer, Rochester, NY.)*

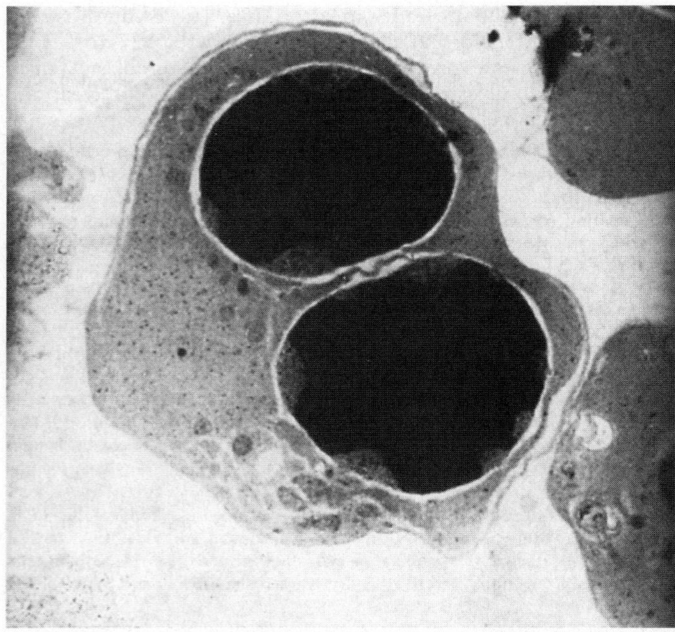

Figure 27-17 ELECTRON MICROSCOPY OF A BONE MARROW ERYTHROBLAST FROM A PATIENT WITH HEMPAS (CONGENITAL DYSERYTHROPOIETIC ANEMIA TYPE II). Note the appearance of a double cell membrane, reflecting an excess of endoplasmic reticulum. *(Provided by Dr. Raoul Fresco, Maywood, Ill.)*

preincubating normal sera with HEMPAS erythrocytes. However, the specific HEMPAS antigen recognized by this antibody is not known. In contrast to HEMPAS, the erythrocytes of patients with paroxysmal nocturnal hemoglobinuria (PNH) undergo lysis when the acidified serum is from the PNH patient or from normal donors. Another difference is that PNH erythrocytes undergo lysis in isotonic sucrose (sugar water test), but HEMPAS RBCs do not lyse in isotonic sucrose.

The erythrocytes from patients with CDA II also exhibit an increased agglutinability and lysis to anti-i and anti-I sera and manifest increased expression of both antigens. These surface antigens are complex carbohydrate structures found predominantly on fetal and adult RBCs, respectively. Increased expression of i antigen can be demonstrated on all RBCs in CDA II using fluorescent labels. Relatives of patients with CDA II who have normal BM but increased agglutinability to anti-i appear to be heterozygote carriers of this disorder. HEMPAS erythrocytes bind a normal amount of complement (C1), but more antibody and less C4 than normal. This causes binding of an excess of C3 and hemolysis.

The number of erythroid progenitors is probably normal in BM and blood. Although one study found only normal morphology of the erythroblasts produced in culture, subsequent studies reported multinuclearity similar to that seen in the BM. As in CDA I, the defect in CDA II is in the erythroid progenitor cell and is expressed variably in more mature erythroblasts.

Patients with CDA II may develop progressive, lifelong iron overload even in the absence of transfusions, and approximately 20% develop cirrhosis as a consequence. Splenomegaly occurs in the majority of patients with CDA II. A number of other clinical associations with CDA II have been reported such as mental retardation, Sweet syndrome, von Willebrand disease, and Dubin-Johnson syndrome, among others. Rather than true associations, it is likely that the majority represent coincidental occurrences. An adult patient was reported with an extramedullary hematopoietic mass in the posterior mediastinum that was a result of BM expansion associated with ineffective erythropoiesis. In a retrospective study of 41 patients, coinheritance of Gilbert syndrome was associated with a significantly increased risk of hyperbilirubinemia and early-onset gallstone formation.

CDA Type III

Based on reported CDA cases, type II is the most common CDA, type I is next, and CDA III is the rarest of the three major forms. In contrast to the other two forms, CDA III is inherited as an autosomal dominant disorder. The responsible gene maps to chromosome 15q21-q25, but little is known about CDA III pathophysiology. Sporadic cases have also been described. These latter cases with hematologically normal parents and relatives may represent autosomal recessive inheritance or may have been caused by spontaneous dominant mutations. In a Swedish family with 31 cases inherited in an autosomal dominant mode, an excess number of cases with a monoclonal gammopathy and myeloma have occurred. Also, an adult patient with CDA III was described with T-cell non-Hodgkin lymphoma. These cases, plus a case of Hodgkin disease occurring in an additional patient, may indicate an increased incidence of lymphoproliferative diseases in CDA III.

Laboratory Abnormalities. In CDA III, splenomegaly is usually minimal or absent. The anemia is usually mild to moderate, but transfusion-dependent patients have been observed. The circulating RBCs can be normal or mildly macrocytic. BM examination shows erythroid hyperplasia. Giant erythroblasts with up to 12 nuclei are the most distinctive feature of CDA III observed on light microscopic examination of the BM. These may appear similar to some of the large multinucleated cells seen in CDA II (see Fig. 27-16). Abnormally large lobulated nuclei and discordance in nuclear maturation are also found. Although they are hallmarks of CDA III, these findings are not pathognomonic and may be seen in erythroleukemia. Electron microscopy demonstrates nuclear clefts and blebs, autolytic areas within the cytoplasm, and iron-filled mitochondria. In some dominantly inherited and sporadic cases of CDA III, electron microscopy reveals that an occasional erythroblast section contains stellate or branching electron-dense intracytoplasmic inclusions. These are morphologically indistinguishable from those in HbH disease and consist of precipitated β-globin chains.

The acidified-serum lysis test result is negative in CDA III. Agglutination and lysis of erythrocytes to anti-i antibody has only been examined in a few cases of CDA III with conflicting findings. Serum thymidine kinase was measured in 20 CDA III patients and 10 healthy siblings. Elevated thymidine kinase was found in all 20 cases but was normal in the siblings. It is suggested that measuring thymidine kinase levels can allow clinicians to discriminate between affected individuals and healthy siblings without performing a BM aspirate.

Other CDAs: Classifiable and Nonclassifiable Variants

Dozens of cases of CDA have been reported that do not conform to the classification of types I, II, and III. Some of the earlier reports of variants may or may not have been CDAs. In an attempt to sort out some of the better-documented cases, a phenotype-based classification was proposed that assigns patients to one of four groups (not types), designated groups IV, V, VI, and VII. To qualify for inclusion in this classification, each group contains cases from three or more unrelated families. The features of each are as follows.

CDA Group IV. This group has severe anemia, transfusion dependence from birth, marked erythroid hyperplasia, normoblastic or mild to moderate megaloblastic changes, up to 8% BM erythroblasts with markedly irregular or karyorrhectic nuclei, and an absence of precipitated protein within erythroblasts by electron microscopy. An infant with group IV CDA presented with hydrops fetalis. The spleen is enlarged. The inheritance is not clear.

CDA Group V. Patients have normal or near-normal hemoglobin levels, a normal or slightly elevated MCV, and an increased serum unconjugated bilirubin. The BM shows marked erythroid hyperplasia and normoblastic or mild to moderate megaloblastic changes. The spleen may be palpable. The condition has been previously described as "primary shunt hyperbilirubinemia." Inheritance is variable and appears to be autosomal recessive in some cases but possibly autosomal dominant or X-linked in others. In CDA group V, the BM macrophages engulf morphologically normal but functionally abnormal erythroblasts.

CDA Group VI. This group is characterized by marked macrocytosis (MCV 119-125 fL) with little or no anemia and grossly megaloblastic erythropoiesis. There may be mild jaundice and an increased serum bilirubin. The differential diagnosis includes orotic aciduria and thiamine-responsive anemia. Vitamin B_{12} and RBC folate levels are normal.

CDA Group VII. These patients have severe transfusion-dependent anemia from birth, marked erythroid hyperplasia, normoblastic or nonspecific dysplastic changes, markedly abnormal nuclear shapes in many erythroblasts, and intraerythroblastic inclusions resembling precipitated α globin chains. The inclusions do not react with monoclonal antibodies against α and β globin chains. The diagnosis requires the exclusion of β-thalassemia trait in the parents.

Unclassifiable cases of CDA have been reported with lifelong anemia that was probably inherited. These cases were characterized by marked aniso- and poikilocytosis and occasional teardrop and fragmented erythrocytes in the peripheral blood. Hyperplastic BM showed megaloblastoid features without multinuclearity or ringed sideroblasts, but a case with prominent ringed sideroblasts was also described. Unlike classical CDA, neutropenia or thrombocytopenia has been observed in some of these patients. Cytogenetic studies of BM revealed no clonal chromosomal abnormalities. Reticulocyte response to anemia was absent or inappropriately low in all. Most studies of parents failed to reveal abnormalities, suggesting an autosomal recessive mode of transmission.

Variant CDAs Associated With Specific Gene Mutations

GATA1 is a transcription factor closely linked with erythropoiesis and megakaryopoiesis. The Val205Met mutation in the ***GATA1*** gene underlies a CDA with dyserythropoiesis and thrombocytopenia**.** The ***KLF1*** gene encodes an erythroid transcription factor. A specific mutation of *KLF1* produced a severe form of CDA with basophilic stippling of polychromatic erythroblasts and erythrocytes, marked abnormalities of nuclear shape, and increased expression of embryonic and fetal hemoglobin. A case of hereditary cryostomatocytosis and dyserythropoiesis was caused by a de novo erythroid anion exchanger **band 3 mutation.** The BM morphology showed dyserythropoiesis characteristic of CDA I and CDA II. Mutant ***MVK*** resulted in mevalonate kinase deficiency, dyserythropoietic anemia, and BM findings similar to those in CDA II. A syndrome of dyserythropoietic anemia, exocrine pancreatic insufficiency, and calvarial hyperostosis was caused by a mutation in ***COX412,*** a gene highly expressed in BM.

Differential Diagnosis

Marrow erythroblast multinuclearity is seen with other hematologic disorders, but these can be readily distinguished from CDA. The **megaloblastic anemias** have a different clinical presentation and are identified in the laboratory by the presence of hypersegmented neutrophils, decreased RBC folate values, or reduced serum levels of vitamin B_{12}. The **MDS** may manifest as an isolated refractory anemia, but they often present with bi- or trilineage cytopenias that contrast sharply with CDA. The MDS subsets may also show BM granulocytic and megakaryocytic morphologic abnormalities, the presence of myeloblasts, ringed sideroblasts, and clonal cytogenetic changes. **Erythroleukemia** (AML, M6) is another cause of marked dyserythropoiesis, but typically there is pancytopenia, the erythroblasts are avidly positive for the periodic acid-Schiff stain, and the BM cells may show a clonal cytogenetic marker. The **β-thalassemia syndromes** differ from CDA by the presence of marked microcytosis with elevated levels of hemoglobin A_2, fetal hemoglobin, or both.

Therapy and Prognosis

In general, the CDAs are associated with a favorable long-term prognosis. For example, CDA I can be diagnosed late in life. One reported case was associated with a relatively benign course over a 30-year follow-up. Clinical manifestations of the CDAs may include intermittent jaundice and dark urine caused by increased hemoglobin catabolism or signs and symptoms of anemia. Rarely, hyperbilirubinemia without anemia may be the initial presentation of CDA patients. Cholelithiasis may be present as a consequence of chronic hyperbilirubinemia.

Anemia is typically mild in most cases of CDA and requires no intervention, but in more severe presentations, especially those requiring transfusional support, splenectomy may be beneficial. Most of the experience showing an improvement in hemoglobin levels after splenectomy has been in CDA II; the benefit of splenectomy in CDA I is less clear. Splenectomy may cause a persistent thrombocytosis in CDA types I and II and contribute to the development of Budd-Chiari syndrome and portal vein thrombosis.

Treatment of all forms of CDA with androgens, corticosteroids, vitamin E, vitamin B_{12}, folic acid, pyridoxine, or iron is ineffective in ameliorating the anemia. Iron therapy is also contraindicated because of the underlying propensity for hemosiderosis secondary to ineffective erythropoiesis, transfusional iron overload, increased gut iron absorption, and downregulation of the primary regulator of iron absorption, hepcidin. Even if regular RBC transfusions are not initiated, patients should be routinely monitored for evidence of iron overload. Iron chelation with daily subcutaneous infusions of deferoxamine (Desferal) has been underused in CDA even though deaths have been recorded from hemochromatosis. The value of the oral iron chelator deferasirox (Exjade) has not been defined yet for the CDAs.

Phlebotomy has been carried out to remove iron in selected CDA patients, but this could result in a worsening of the anemia and theoretically enhance gut iron absorption. An additional concern is that CDA patients seem predisposed to hepatic cirrhosis irrespective of body iron burden. The pathogenesis of this is unclear.

Interferon-α-2a or INF-α-2b therapy given two or three times a week or peg-INF-α-2a once a week, increase hemoglobin levels and decrease iron overload in most CDA I patients who require repeated transfusions for moderately severe anemia. Erythrokinetic studies demonstrate a striking reduction of ineffective erythropoiesis in patients receiving INF, and electron microscopy shows a reduction in nuclear structural abnormalities. INF therapy should also be considered in moderately anemic CDA I patients before treatment of iron overload with phlebotomy. Patients with CDA II do not respond to INF-α.

Hematopoietic stem cell transplantation has been curative in a few severe cases of CDA, including transfusion-dependent CDA type I, CDA type II, Ham test–negative "CDA type II," and an unclassifiable CDA.

Asymptomatic extramedullary hematopoiesis may mimic tumors of the mediastinum, abdomen, and vertebral column. Because of the increased RBC production that occurs, the development of sites of extramedullary hematopoiesis may result in an amelioration of the degree of anemia. Technetium-99m sulfur colloid scintigraphy is useful in delineating the extent of these regions.

Future Directions

Identification of the various mutant genes for the CDA types will facilitate a more precise classification than the phenotype-based system used currently. The wild-type protein product of *CDAN1* requires further research to clarify its function in health and its role in producing CDA type I when mutated. Strategies are required for managing iron overload similar to those for Diamond-Blackfan anemia and thalassemia major. In this regard, the therapeutic benefit of oral iron chelators such as Exjade should be explored fully.

SUGGESTED READINGS

General

Shimamura A, Alter P: Pathophysiology and management of inherited bone marrow failure syndromes. *Blood Reviews* 24:101, 2010.

Tsangaris E, Klaassen R, Fernandez CV, et al: Genetic analysis of inherited bone marrow failure syndromes from one prospective, comprehensive and population-based cohort and identification of novel mutations. *J Med Genet* 48:618, 2011.

Fanconi Anemia

Auerbach AD: Fanconi anemia and its diagnosis. *Mutat Res* 668:4, 2009.

Kee Y, D'Andrea AD: Expanded roles of the Fanconi anemia pathway in preserving genomic stability. *Genes Dev* 15;24:1680, 2010.

Kutler DI, Singh B, Satagopan J, et al: A 20-year perspective on the International Fanconi Anemia Registry (IFAR). *Blood* 15;101:1249, 2003.

Shwachman-Diamond Syndrome

Finch AJ, Hilcenko C, Basse N, et al: Uncoupling of GTP hydrolysis from eIF6 release on the ribosome causes Shwachman-Diamond syndrome. *Genes Dev* 25:917, 2011

Hashmi SK, Allen C, Klaassen R, et al: Comparative analysis of Shwachman-Diamond Syndrome to other Inherited Marrow Failure Syndromes. *Clin Genet* 79:448, 2011.

Sen S, Wang H, Nghiem CL, et al: The ribosome-related protein, SBDS, is critical for normal erythropoiesis. Blood 118:6407, 2011.

Dyskeratosis Congenita

Alter BP, Giri N, Savage SA, et al: Cancer in dyskeratosis congenita. *Blood* 25;113:6549, 2009.

Walne AJ, Dokal I: Advances in the understanding of dyskeratosis congenita. *Br J Haematol* 145:164, 2009.

Congenital Amegakaryocytic Thrombocytopenia

Geddis AE: Congenital amegakaryocytic thrombocytopenia. *Pediatr Blood Cancer* 57:199, 2011

Germeshausen M, Ballmaier M, Welte K: MPL mutations in 23 patients suffering from congenital amegakaryocytic thrombocytopenia: The type of mutation predicts the course of the disease. *Hum Mutat* 27:296, 2006.

Diamond-Blackfan Anemia

Boria I, Garelli E, Gazda HT, et al: The ribosomal basis of Diamond-Blackfan Anemia: Mutation and database update. *Hum Mutat* 3:1269, 2010.

Clinton C, Gazda HT: Diamond-Blackfan anemia. In: Pagon RA, Bird TD, Dolan CR, Stephens K, editors: *GeneReviews [Internet],* Seattle (WA), 1993-2009 Jun 25 [updated 2011 Jan 27], University of Washington, Seattle, See:www.ncbi.nlm.nih.gov/books/NBK1116/.

Daniella Maria Arturi Foundation, Proceedings of the 9th Annual Diamond-Blackfan Anemia International concensus conference, 2008 (contact Foundation Director, Lauren Carroll: lcarroll@dmaf.org).

Ellis SR, Gleizes PE: Diamond Blackfan anemia: Ribosomal proteins going rogue. *Semin Hematol* 48:89, 2011.

Lipton JM, Atsidaftos E, Zyskind I, et al: Improving clinical care and elucidating the pathophysiology of Diamond-Blackfan anemia: An update from the Diamond-Blackfan Anemia Registry. *Pediatr Blood Cancer* 46:558, 2006.

Kostmann or Severe Congenital Neutropenia

Dale DC, Welte K: Cyclic and chronic neutropenia. *Cancer Treat Res* 157:97, 2011.

Grenda DS, Murakami M, Ghatak J, et al: Mutations of the ELA2 gene found in patients with severe congenital neutropenia induce the unfolded protein response and cellular apoptosis. *Blood* 110:4179, 2007.

Rosenberg PS, Zeidler C, Bolyard AA, et al: Stable long-term risk of leukaemia in patients with severe congenital neutropenia maintained on G-CSF therapy. *Br J Haematol* 150:196, 2010.

Skokowa J, Fobiwe JP, Dan L, et al: Neutrophil elastase is severely downregulated in severe congenital neutropenia independent of ELA2 or HAX1 mutations but dependent on LEF-1. *Blood* 114:3044, 2009.

Congenital Dyserythropoietic Anemias

Iolascon A, Russo R, Delaunay J: Congenital dyserythropoietic anemias. *Curr Opin Hematol* 18:146, 2011.

Wickramasinghe SN, Wood WG: Advances in the understanding of the congenital dyserythropoietic anaemias. *Br J Haematol* 131:431, 2005.

CHAPTER 28

APLASTIC ANEMIA

Neal S. Young and Jaroslaw P. Maciejewski

Aplastic anemia (AA), the paradigm of the bone marrow (BM) failure syndromes, is most simply defined as peripheral blood pancytopenia and a hypocellular BM (Fig. 28-1). From epidemiologic and clinical features, pathophysiologic studies, and response to therapy, AA is a distinctive disease. However, the diagnosis of AA requires excluding other causes of pancytopenia (Table 28-1). AA can occur as a primary hematologic disorder, most often idiopathic, or apparently result from various proximate causes, including obvious physical and chemical toxins but also drugs and viruses that can act indirectly. Although AA is usually characterized by a severe diminution in BM function that affects all the hematopoietic lineages, granulocyte, platelet, and red blood cell (RBC) levels may not be depressed uniformly, and less severe degrees of BM hypoplasia and odd combinations of bicytopenias and monocytopenias can occur. AA can be especially difficult to distinguish from hypocellular myelodysplasia, a diagnostic dilemma that can rest on real biologic similarities. Even typical AA can vary in its clinical presentation and course, from a fulminant illness marked by continuous or recurrent hemorrhage and major infections to an indolent process manageable by transfusion therapy alone. Readers are referred to previous editions of this textbook for references, as well as to the authors' recent reviews.[1,2]

HISTORY

The study of BM failure dates to 1888, when Paul Ehrlich described a young woman who died after an explosive short illness marked by severe anemia, bleeding, and high fever. As a pathologist, Ehrlich was struck by the absence of nucleated RBCs and the fatty quality of the femoral BM. Vaquez and Aubertin, in a 1904 case report of "pernicious anemia with yellow marrow," named the disease and emphasized a pathophysiology of "anhematopoiesis." The etymologic root of the term *aplastique* is the Greek verb *pl¿Jw,* to create and give shape to (*¿plaztká,* the adjective, unformed). Early inferences about the cause of the disease were made from the BM appearance at autopsy. Pathologically, the watery, yellow BM seen uniquely characterized the aplasia, but the limited and rather general clinical signs were less helpful in distinguishing this type of a regenerative BM failure from other anemias.

CLASSIFICATION

AA is a major sequela of irradiation and exposure to cytotoxic chemotherapy. It has been associated with the use of chemicals and drugs, viral infections, and other diseases (Table 28-2). Most patients have an idiopathic form of the disease. Too strict a division of cases into categories can obscure important pathophysiologic relationships. Historical associations of environmental exposures and causation are interesting but should be considered with some skepticism because of biases of observation and reporting and lack of direct evidence in most cases.

EPIDEMIOLOGY

Incidence and Geographic and Age Distribution

The largest and most comprehensive study of the epidemiology of BM failure was the International Aplastic Anemia and Agranulocytosis Study (IAAAS) conducted in Europe and Israel from 1980 to 1984.[3] IAAAS was performed prospectively and applied strict case definition to pathologically confirmed cases. Using stringent criteria, the overall annual incidence of AA was two cases per 1 million people. The incidence rates reported in the IAAAS are three- to fourfold lower than rates reported in many earlier, mainly retrospective, and far less well-designed surveys.

A remarkable feature of the epidemiology of AA is the unexplained geographic variation in its incidence. The incidence of AA in Bangkok and two rural regions of Thailand has been accurately determined using the same methods as those used by the IAAAS researchers in Europe and Israel; the annual incidence was 4.0 cases per 1 million people in the capital and 5.6 cases per 1 million people in the northeastern province of Khonkaen.[4] The incidence in China has been estimated to be 7.4 cases per 1 million people annually. From published, hospital-based series, personal communications, and firsthand observations, AA appears more prevalent in less developed regions of the world. There are no major sex or racial differences in the occurrence of AA.[3]

Aplastic anemia is a disease of the young (Fig. 28-2). Most patients present between 15 and 25 years of age or older than 60 years of age.

Epidemiologic Clues to Causality

Population-based studies have investigated possible causal associations. Drugs are implicated in only approximately 25% of cases of AA in the West; in Thailand, AA was attributed to drug exposure in only approximately 15% of cases.[4] There are associations with chemical exposures, exposures to viruses, hepatitis, and occupation. There is evidence that geographic variation in AA might result from environmental causes[4] and a genetic predisposition.

Genetic Aspects

In children and young adults, acquired AA should be distinguished from the main inherited forms of BM failure, Fanconi anemia (FA) and dyskeratosis congenita (DKC). Identification of constitutional AA has important therapeutic implications. Patients with FA and DKC can lack typical physical anomalies, and the pancytopenia can develop long after childhood (see Chapter 27), mimicking acquired disease. The distinction between inherited and acquired AA has been blurred with the identification of mutations in the telomerase genes that appear to be risk factors rather than determinants of clinical BM

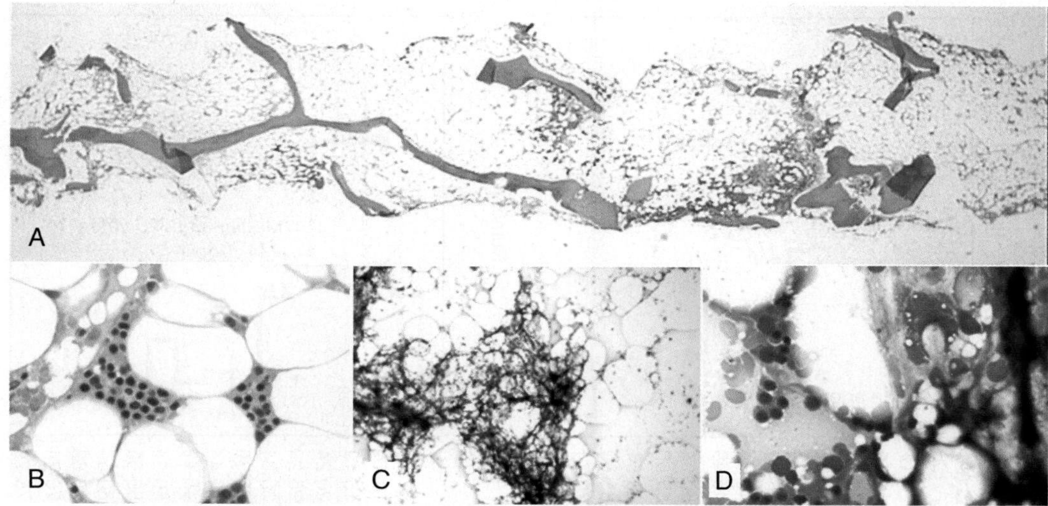

Figure 28-1 BONE MARROW MORPHOLOGY IN SEVERE APLASTIC ANEMIA. Bone marrow biopsy specimen of sufficient length **(A)** shows severe hypocellularity with a few "hot spots" of hematopoietic activity. These are sometimes predominantly erythroid **(B).** The corresponding aspirate (**C** and **D**) shows empty marrow spicules and residual stoma, including lymphoid cells, plasma cells, histiocytes, mast cells, and a few hematopoietic elements.

Table 28-1 Differential Diagnosis of Pancytopenia

Pancytopenia With Hypocellular Bone Marrow
Acquired aplastic anemia
Inherited aplastic anemia (Fanconi anemia and others)
Some myelodysplasia syndromes
Rare aleukemic leukemia (acute myeloid leukemia)
Some acute lymphoblastic leukemias
Rare lymphomas of bone marrow
Pancytopenia With Cellular Bone Marrow
Primary bone marrow diseases
Myelodysplasia syndromes
Paroxysmal nocturnal hemoglobinuria
Myelofibrosis
Some aleukemic leukemias
Myelophthisis
Bone marrow lymphoma
Hairy cell leukemia
Secondary to systemic diseases
Systemic lupus erythematosus, Sjögren syndrome
Hypersplenism
Vitamin B_{12}, folate deficiency (familial defect)
Overwhelming infection
Alcohol
Brucellosis
Ehrlichiosis
Sarcoidosis
Tuberculosis and atypical mycobacteria
Hypocellular Bone Marrow ± Cytopenia
Q fever
Legionnaires disease
Mycobacteria
Tuberculosis*
Anorexia nervosa, starvation
Hypothyroidism

*Pancytopenia in tuberculosis only rarely is associated with a hypocellular bone marrow at biopsy or autopsy. Marrow failure in the setting of tuberculosis is almost always fatal; exceptional patients probably had underlying myelodysplasia or acute leukemia.

Table 28-2 A Classification of Aplastic Anemia

Acquired Aplastic Anemia
Secondary aplastic anemia
Irradiation
Drugs and chemicals
Regular effects
Cytotoxic agents
Benzene
Idiosyncratic reactions
Chloramphenicol
Nonsteroidal antiinflammatory drugs
Antiepileptics
Gold
Other drugs and chemicals
Viruses
Epstein-Barr virus (infectious mononucleosis)
Hepatitis virus (non-A, non-B, non-C, non-G hepatitis)
Parvovirus (transient aplastic crisis, some pure red blood cell aplasia)
Human immunodeficiency virus (acquired immunodeficiency syndrome)
Immune diseases
Eosinophilic fasciitis
Hyperimmunoglobulinemia
Thymoma and thymic carcinoma
Graft-versus-host disease in immunodeficiency
Paroxysmal nocturnal hemoglobinuria
Pregnancy
Idiopathic aplastic anemia
Inherited Aplastic Anemia
Fanconi anemia
Dyskeratosis congenita
Shwachman-Diamond syndrome
Reticular dysgenesis
Amegakaryocytic thrombocytopenia
Familial aplastic anemias
Preleukemia (e.g., monosomy 7)
Nonhematologic syndromes (e.g., Down, Dubowitz, Seckel)

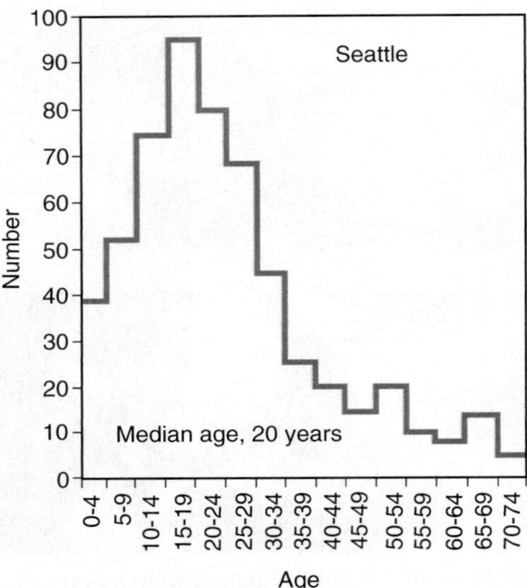

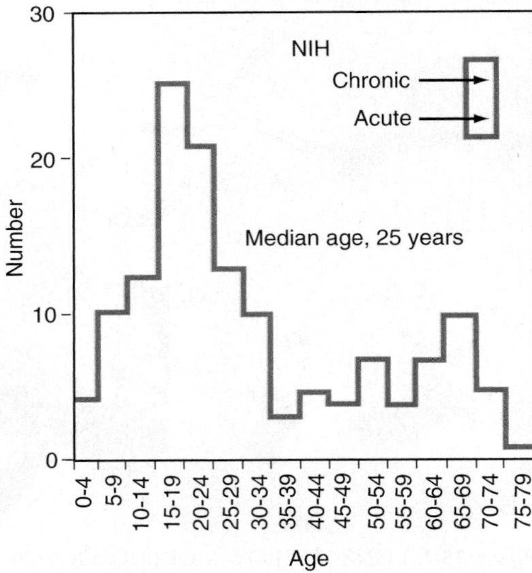

Figure 28-2 DISTRIBUTION OF APLASTIC ANEMIA BY AGE. For the patients at the University of Washington, a major transplantation center, the age given is at the time of first treatment. For the patients at the National Institutes of Health (NIH), where immunosuppressive therapy is offered, the age given is at the time of diagnostic bone marrow biopsy. Acute disease is defined as less than 3 months between diagnosis and presentation at NIH, and chronic disease is defined as more than 3 months. *(Seattle statistics courtesy Rainer Storb, University of Washington.)*

failure (see later discussion). Genomic approaches to the study of AA are likely to uncover other genetic contributions to susceptibility to BM failure.[5,6]

A few histocompatibility types have also been associated with AA, most consistently human leukocyte antigen (HLA)-DR2. HLA-DR subtypes have proved useful in predicting response to immunosuppressive therapy; in a large cohort of U.S. AA patients, HLA-DR15 was associated with the presence of the paroxysmal nocturnal hemoglobinuria (PNH) clone and responsiveness to immunosuppression. Genetic predisposition may be responsible for some idiosyncratic reactions to drugs and chemicals leading to the development of AA. Polymorphisms in cytokine genes, associated with an increased immune response, also are more prevalent in AA; examples include a nucleotide polymorphism in the tumor necrosis factor-α (TNF-α; *TNF2*) promoter at −308, homozygosity for a variable number of dinucleotide repeats in the gene encoding γ-interferon (IFN-γ), and polymorphisms in the interleukin 6 (IL-6) gene. Genome-wide transcriptional analysis of T and natural killer cells from AA patients has implicated pathologic expression of components of innate immunity, including Toll-like receptors.

ETIOLOGY AND PATHOGENESIS

Hematopoiesis in Bone Marrow Failure

Stem Cells

A consistent laboratory finding for patients with AA is a very low number of hematopoietic progenitor cells. Deficient colony formation by BM cells of AA patients remains unresponsive even to high levels of hematopoietic growth factors. The total number of progenitors in a BM sample is reduced, and the number of colony progenitor cells assayed from a purified CD34 population is low. Long-term culture-initiating cells (LTC-ICs), a stem cell surrogate assay, also are profoundly deficient in all patients with severe AA. At clinical presentation, the number of LTC-ICs is usually less than 10% of normal; combined with a reduction in total BM cellularity to 10% or less, the stem cell number is estimated to be reduced to 1% or less than normal in patients with AA (Fig. 28-3).

Telomeres and Bone Marrow Failure

One peculiar feature of white blood cells (WBCs) in AA is short telomeres. The discovery, first by linkage analysis in large pedigrees, that the X-linked form of DKC was caused by mutations in *DKC1* and subsequently purposeful identification of mutations in *TERC* in some autosomal dominant patients with this constitutional BM failure syndrome implicated a genetic basis for telomere deficiency. Central to the repair machinery is an RNA template, encoded by *TERC,* on which telomerase, a reverse transcriptase encoded by *TERT,* elongates the nucleotide repeat structure; other proteins, including the *DKC1* gene product dyskenin, are associated with the telomere repair complex. Systematic surveys of DNA disclosed first *TERC* and later *TERT* mutations in some patients with apparently acquired AA, including older adults.[5] Family members who share the mutation, despite normal or near normal blood counts, have hypocellular BMs, reduced CD34 cell counts and poor hematopoietic colony formation, increased hematopoietic growth factor levels, and of course short telomeres; however, their clinical presentation is much later than in typical DKC, and they lack typical physical anomalies. Chromosomes are also protected by several proteins that bind directly to telomeres. Mutations in the gene for shelterin, one such protein, produces very severe DKC, and polymorphisms in *TERF1* and *TERF2* are also more or less prevalent in AA compared with healthy control participants. A few patients with apparently acquired AA have heterozygous mutations in the Shwachman-Bodian-Diamond syndrome *(SBDS)* gene. Almost all children with this form of constitutional AA are compound heterozygotes for mutations in *SBDS,* and their WBCs have extremely short telomeres; however, the *SBDS* gene product has not been directly linked to the telomere repair complex or to telomere binding. A parsimonious inference from these data is that inherited mutations in genes that repair or protect telomeres are genetic risk factors in acquired AA, probably because they confer a quantitatively reduced hematopoietic stem cell compartment that may also be qualitatively inadequate to sustain immune-mediated damage. Accelerated telomere attrition in AA not currently explicable by mutations may be caused by more subtle genetic lesions or follow from the pathophysiology of BM stress and excessive stem cell turnover.

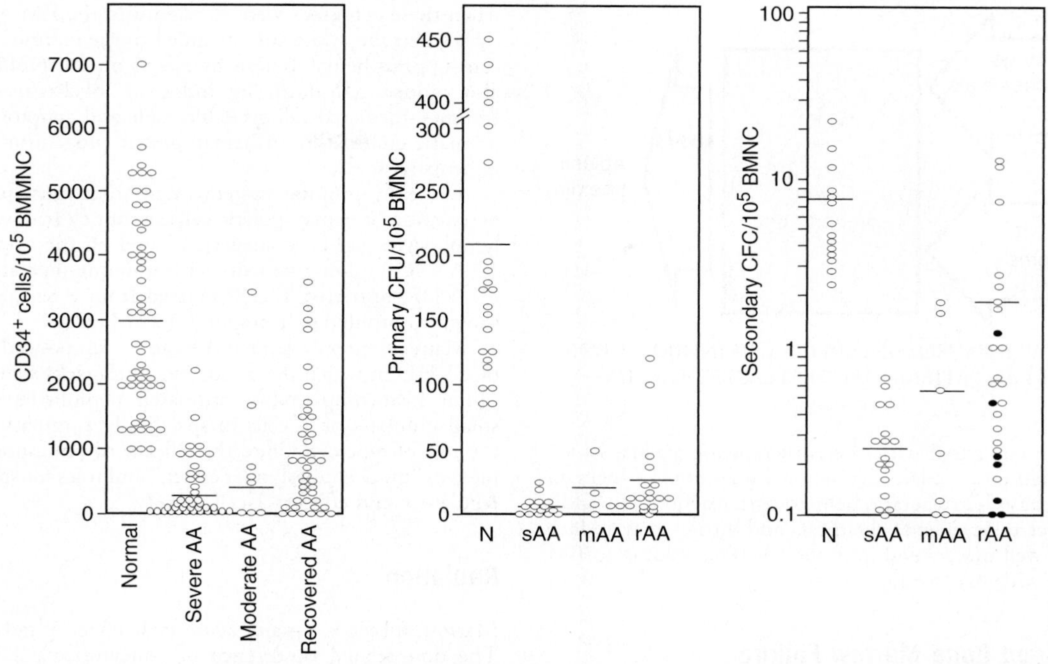

Figure 28-3 The numbers of CD34 cells, primary colony-forming cells (CFCs), and long-term culture-initiating cells (LTC-ICs) were measured in the bone marrow of patients with aplastic anemia. Each *dot* represents an individual patient's sample studied. Severe aplastic anemia (sAA) includes patients at presentation, cases refractory to immunosuppressive therapy, and patients who relapsed after a period of recovery. Primary CFCs were measured in short-term methylcellulose cultures. Secondary CFCs after long-term bone marrow cultures reflect LTC-IC numbers. *BMNC,* Blood mononuclear cell; *CFU,* colony-forming unit; *mAA,* moderate aplastic anemia; *N,* normal; *rAA,* recovered from aplastic anemia.

Stromal and Hematopoietic Growth Factors

Stromal cell function is usually not defective in cases of AA. Whereas adherent cells from patients support hematopoiesis by normal CD34 cells, no hematopoietic colonies develop when patients' CD34 cells are cultured in the presence of normal stroma (Fig. 28-4). Stromal cells cultured from patients' BM generally produce normal quantities of hematopoietic growth factors. Serum levels of erythropoietin, thrombopoietin, granulocyte colony-stimulating factor (G-CSF), and granulocyte-macrophage colony-stimulating factor (GM-CSF) are almost always normal or elevated. Cytokines that act at very early stages of hematopoiesis have been studied as possible etiologic factors in the pathobiology of AA. Blood levels of FLT3 ligand are highly elevated in AA, stem cell factor (SCF) levels are modestly decreased, and SCF stromal cell production is normal. Adequate stromal function is implicit in the success of BM transplantation (BMT) in AA because important stromal elements remain of host origin.

PATHOPHYSIOLOGIC PATHWAYS LEADING TO APLASTIC ANEMIA

Direct Hematopoietic Injury

The most common form of AA is iatrogenic; transient BM failure often follows treatment with cytotoxic chemotherapeutic drugs or irradiation (Fig. 28-5). Certain chemical or physical agents directly injure proliferating and quiescent hematopoietic cells. However, patients with community-acquired AA rarely have a history of exposure to such physicochemical agents. Even benzene, which can act as a particularly inefficient cytotoxic chemical, is an infrequent cause of AA in developed countries.[3] Medical drugs are associated with acquired AA, and in some instances, they can directly cause BM

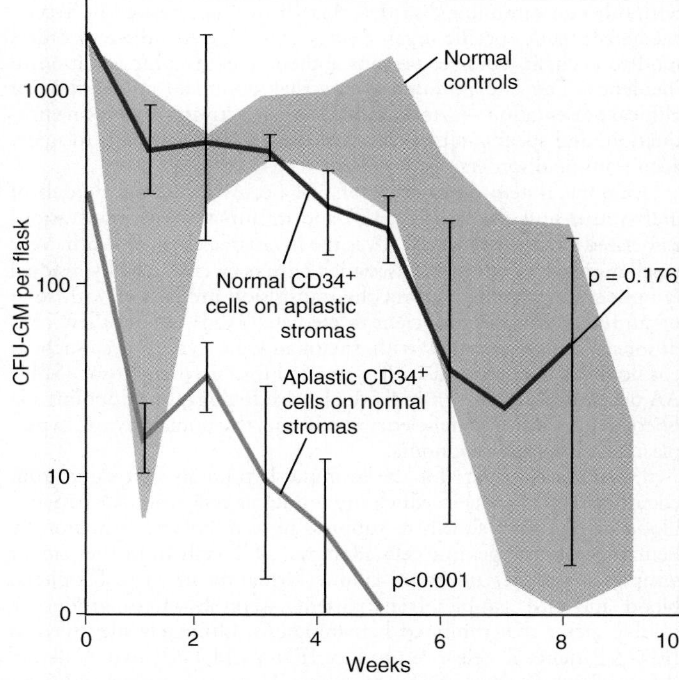

Figure 28-4 NORMAL STROMAL CELL FUNCTION IN LONG-TERM CULTURE OF APLASTIC ANEMIA BONE MARROW. *AML,* Acute myelogenous leukemia; *MDS,* myelodysplastic syndrome. *(Courtesy Dr. Judith Marsh, St. George's Hospital Medical School, London.)*

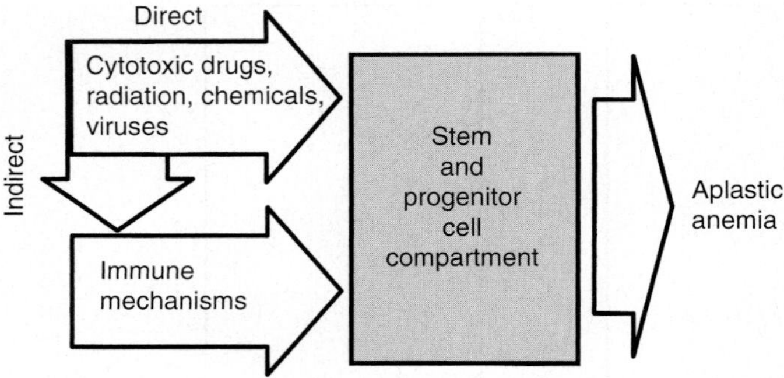

Figure 28-5 POSSIBLE CAUSES OF DIRECT AND INDIRECT BONE MARROW FAILURE IN PATIENTS WITH APLASTIC ANEMIA.

damage. However, compared with chemotherapeutic agents, which are delivered in high doses, relatively low total quantities of ingested drug apparently cause idiosyncratic hematologic reactions. In addition to their direct toxic effects, chemicals and viruses may induce complex and not well understood immune reactions leading to BM failure in persons with AA (see Fig. 28-5).

Immune-Mediated Bone Marrow Failure

In the 1970s, Mathé and colleagues observed unexpected improvement of pancytopenia after failed BMT. They speculated that the immunosuppressive conditioning regimen, intended to allow engraftment of the donor BM, might instead have promoted the recovery of host BM function. The effectiveness of diverse treatments that reduce lymphocyte number or block T-cell function and the superior results obtained when agents are combined strongly suggest that such therapeutic success is caused by the immunosuppressive effects of the drugs employed. AA shares clinical and pathophysiologic features with other autoimmune disorders that all are characterized by T-cell–mediated, tissue-specific organ destruction. Like AA, these disorders tend to occur in younger persons and show geographic variation in incidence. The late immune events that dominate at the time of clinical presentation—cytotoxic lymphocyte activation, cytokine production, and specific target cell elimination—are common to many autoimmune disorders.

Immune system destruction of BM occurs in animal models of graft-versus-host disease (GVHD) and in humans with transfusion-associated GVHD, in which AA is the invariable cause of death. Very small numbers of effector cells, which have been conveyed by residual lymphocytes contained within the transfusion product or with solid organ transplants, are sufficient to mediate GVHD under these conditions. AA is associated with rheumatologic syndromes, such as eosinophilic fasciitis, and with systemic lupus erythematosus (SLE). AA occasionally occurs in individuals with hypogammaglobulinemia or congenital immunodeficiency syndrome, thymoma, thymic hyperplasia, and thymic carcinoma.

Laboratory support for the immune hypothesis first came from coculture experiments in which mononuclear cells from AA patients' blood or BM were shown to suppress in vitro colony formation by hematopoietic progenitor cells. Removal of T cells from the patient samples sometimes improved colony formation in vitro. Peripheral blood and BM samples from patients were shown to produce a soluble factor that inhibited hematopoiesis, ultimately identified as IFN-γ. Patients' T cells overproduce IFN-γ and TNF, two cytokines that inhibit hematopoietic proliferation. Tbet, a transcriptional regulator that is critical to Th1 polarization, is constitutionally expressed in a majority of AA patients. AA blood and BM also contains elevated numbers of activated cytotoxic lymphocytes, and activity and levels of these cytotoxic cells decreased appropriately with antithymocyte globulin (ATG) therapy.

Interferon-γ and TNF negative effects on the proliferation of early and late hematopoietic progenitor and stem cells is far more potent when these cytokines were secreted into the BM microenvironment than when they were simply added to the cultures, IFN-γ and TNF can suppress hematopoiesis by effects on cell proliferation, but they also induce cell death by induction of Fas-mediated apoptosis. Immune-mediated cell cycle blockade and apoptosis can lead to the dramatic elimination of hematopoietic progenitor and stem cells in patients with AA.

The early immune system events that must precede the global destruction of hematopoietic cells are not clear. Involvement of CD4 lymphocytes has been suggested based on the overrepresentation of HLA-DR15 among patients with immune-mediated AA. Clones of HLA-DR–restricted T cells derived from a few patients have been shown to proliferate in response to BM cells.[7]

Many features of human AA can be reproduced in mouse models of GVHD in which the donor inoculum lacks stem cells. Major and minor histocompatibility mismatch demonstrates the efficacy of small numbers of T cells in specifically eliminating hematopoiesis, the role of type cytokines, the efficacy of immunosuppressive therapies, an "innocent bystander effect," and roles for specific lymphocyte regulatory and effector T-cell subsets.[8]

Radiation

Marrow aplasia is a major acute toxic effect of radiation (Fig. 28-6). The dose-related occurrence of pancytopenia 2 to 4 weeks after exposure to radiation is caused by injury of actively replicating progenitor cells. Mortality from hematologic toxicity is a function of the BM's ability to tolerate depletion of hematopoietic cells and damage to the stem cell. The capacity for recovery of hematopoietic function after even massive single irradiation exposures is considerable, reflecting the resistance of the quiescent stem cell to damage and the enormous BM repopulating potential of even a greatly reduced stem cell pool. At intermediate radiation doses around the median lethal dose (LD50), at which BM toxicity limits survival, supportive efforts can drastically alter outcome. Autopsies of atomic bomb victims in Japan showed acellular BMs in the first weeks of the explosion, but there frequently was regenerating BM in those who survived longer. The histologic picture of radiation-mediated aplasia includes necrosis, nuclear pyknosis and karyorrhexis, nuclear lysis, and ultimately cytolysis; the associated phagocytosis, marked congestion, and hemorrhage are rapidly followed by fatty replacement. BM hypoplasia occurs with radiation doses higher than 1.5 to 2 Gy to the whole body. Precise LD50 figures for humans do not exist, and estimates are based on the limited direct human data and extrapolation from animal experiments. The LD50 is highly dependent on the quality of medical care, and improved support may double the tolerated radiation dose. From assessment of the outcome of radiation accidents and high-dose therapeutic irradiation, the LD50 has been estimated at approximately 4.5 Gy (see Fig. 28-6).

Although the principles of management of pancytopenia after a single large dose of irradiation are similar to those for treating AA in general, some unique points should be made concerning immediate evaluation and long-term prognosis. The type and intensity of the source of radiation and the distance and shielding of the subject are the major determinants of radiation injury; because of the nature of the exposure, these factors are often difficult to assess. Early recognition of the nature of the accident provides the best opportunity for dosimetry by accident reconstruction and can allow employment of blocking, displacement, or chelation agents. Exposure correlates well with the degree of pancytopenia. Because lymphocytes are particularly sensitive to radiation, their rate of decline can be used to estimate the dose of total-body exposure to a level of approximately 3 Gy. At higher doses, the fall in granulocytes and the severity of thrombocytopenia and reticulocytopenia can be used as gauges. The survival of some patients who received doses higher than 9 Gy suggests in retrospect that autologous BM reconstitution may occur in most persons who survive the immediate consequences of radiation exposure.

Pancytopenia may be a late consequence of a single radiation dose, but AA is not well documented as a delayed event after radiation

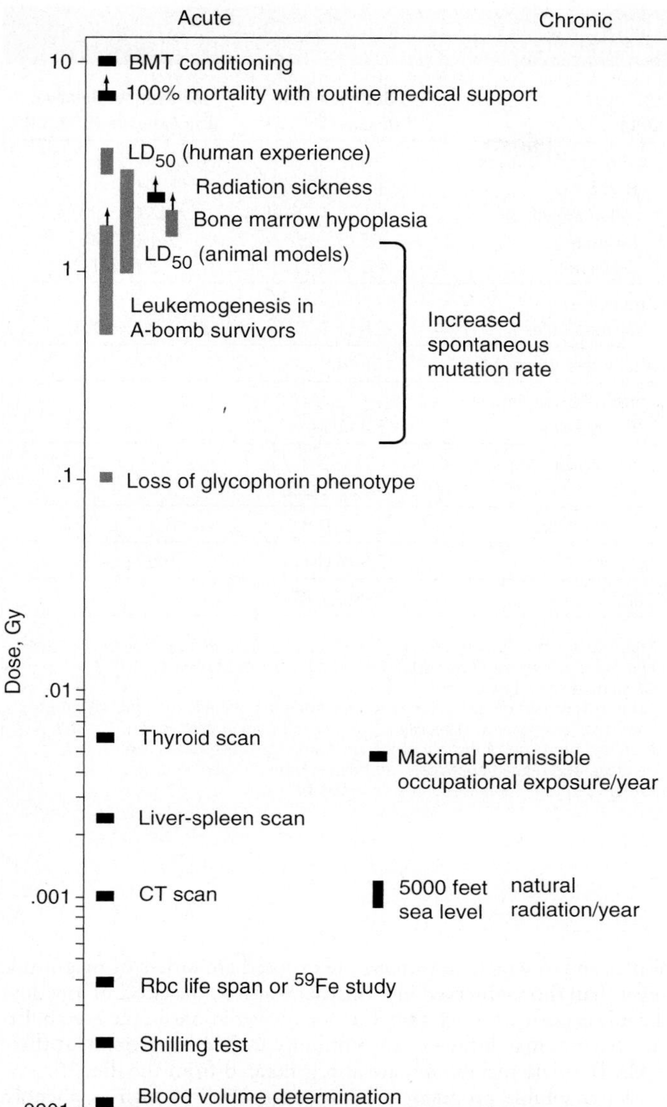

Figure 28-6 SCALE OF WHOLE-BODY RADIATION DOSES. A Gray (Gy) is a measure of absorbed dose equivalent to 1 J/kg unit mass, and 1 Gy equals 100 rads. Radiation represents radiant energy. When absorbed by biologic tissue, radiant energy causes release of electrons and molecular ionization, which result in further energy release. Radiant energy can directly break chemical bonds and indirectly damage macromolecules through generation of high-energy free radical forms. The relationship between increased mutation rate and radiation dose is very approximate *(hatched bars)*. Measurement of the phenotype of an autosomal recessive gene such as for glycophorin would be expected to be a very sensitive indicator. Because malignant transformation is almost certainly a two-step process, increased leukemogenesis is probably an underestimation of the effect of radiation on a single gene. Even the extensive data on the atomic bomb survivors of Hiroshima are subject to statistical errors because of the small number of cases; a linear or exponential curve fit gives various results, and very high doses of radiation may not be associated with as high a risk of leukemia because of stem cell death. Other data that can bear on mutation frequency lie outside the range shown. In a patient with ankylosing spondylitis who underwent irradiation of the spine, leukemogenesis was observed at relatively low doses (doubling of the leukemia rate can be extrapolated to approximately 7 Gy), but such individuals can be predisposed to leukemia. An increased risk of thyroid cancer after irradiation of the mediastinum in childhood occurred at approximately 4 Gy. *BMT,* Bone marrow transplantation; *CT,* computed tomography; LD_{50}, median lethal dose; *RBC,* red blood cell.

exposure. A variety of hematologic abnormalities are associated with chronic low-level radiation exposure, most commonly lymphocytosis, neutropenia, immature or dysmorphic WBCs, and giant platelets (see Fig. 28-6). Cytogenetic abnormalities accumulate with time after chronic exposure, but they may not be reliably related to dose. Repeated low doses of radiation can damage BM and have been associated with AA, but even in these circumstances, only a small proportion of exposed individuals develop hematologic disease. AA does not appear to be more frequent among nuclear power plant or thorium processing factory workers or among residents living close to the plants. Excessive numbers of deaths from AA were reported after therapeutic irradiation of the spine for ankylosing spondylitis, later analysis has suggested that the risk may have been overestimated. AA has not been found in unexpected numbers in a large population of cancer patients who had received therapeutic irradiation. BM failure has not been observed with abnormally high frequency among persons exposed to higher natural background radiation.

Drugs and Chemicals

Aplastic anemia is frequently associated with medical drug use (Table 28-3). At the end of the 19th century, chemicals were linked to BM function through observations of benzene effects on workers. Establishment of a relationship between the analgesic amidopyrine and agranulocytosis in the early 20th century, and an apparent epidemic of AA after the introduction of chloramphenicol in the 1960s also supported this concept. Initially suggested by the accumulation of case reports, drug associations have been established in formal case-control population-based epidemiologic studies. In the IAAAS, relative risks were estimated for individual drugs and large classes of pharmaceutical agents, including nonsteroidal antiinflammatory drugs (NSAIDs), drugs affecting thyroid function, certain cardiovascular agents, some psychotropics, and sulfa-based antibiotics (Table 28-4).[3] Approximately 25% of the cases of AA identified in the IAAAS could be attributed to drug use. Drug use as a risk factor was also assessed by similar methods in Thailand, where the incidence of AA is higher than in the West. Surprisingly, chloramphenicol was not shown to be a risk factor; the etiologic fraction for drugs in AA was only 15%.

Associations between drug exposure and AA can be divided into two classes. Drugs used in cancer chemotherapy are selected for their cytotoxicity, and their regular, dose-dependent induction of BM aplasia is an expected effect. Most AA associated with medical drug use in the community is described as idiosyncratic, meaning that its occurrences are unexpectedly rare. Many of the drugs implicated in AA also appear to cause other, milder forms of BM suppression such as neutropenia. Although difficult to prove, some dose relationship probably does exist even for idiosyncratic reactions. In most case reports, patients received normal or high doses of the agent, usually for a period of weeks to months. Drug-induced aplasia cannot be distinguished by history from idiopathic forms of the disease; the clinical course, including the favorable response to immunosuppressive therapy, of patients with histories of drug exposure is the same as in idiopathic disease.

The low probability of developing AA after a course of drugs may be a reflection of the gene frequency for metabolic enzymes (for direct chemical effects) or immune response genes (for immune-mediated BM failure) in the population.[9] The rarity of idiosyncratic drug reactions could then arise from the infrequent combination of unusual circumstances: exposure, genetic variations in drug metabolism, the physical properties of the agent, enzymatic pathways that chemically alter the drug, and the susceptibility of the host to the action of a toxic compound. Many drugs and chemicals, especially if they have limited water solubility, must be enzymatically degraded before conjugation and excretion. Degradative pathways for xenobiotics are complex, specific, redundant, and interrelated. Intermediate metabolites in complex degradation pathways can be toxic, highly reactive, and responsible for some adverse effects of the primary agents. Examples of detoxifying enzyme systems directly applicable

Table 28-3 Classification of Drugs and Chemicals Associated With Aplastic Anemia

I. Agents That Regularly Produce Bone Marrow Depression as a Major Toxic Effect When Used in Commonly Used Doses or Normal Exposures

Cytotoxic drugs used in cancer chemotherapy
Alkylating agents (busulfan, melphalan, cyclophosphamide)
Antimetabolites (antifolic compounds, nucleotide analogs) antimitotics (vincristine, vinblastine, colchicine)
Some antibiotics (daunorubicin, doxorubicin [Adriamycin])
Benzene (and less often benzene-containing chemicals: kerosene, carbon tetrachloride, Stoddard solvent, chlorophenols)

II. Agents Probably Associated With Aplastic Anemia But With a Relatively Low Probability Relative to Their Use

Chloramphenicol
Insecticides
Antiprotozoals (quinacrine and chloroquine)
Nonsteroidal antiinflammatory drugs (including phenylbutazone, indomethacin, ibuprofen, sulindac, diclofenac, naproxen, piroxicam, fenoprofen, fenbufen, aspirin)
Anticonvulsants (hydantoins, carbamazepine, phenacemide, ethosuximide)
Gold, arsenic, and other heavy metals such as bismuth and mercury
Sulfonamides as a class
Antithyroid medications (methimazole, methylthiouracil, propylthiouracil)
Antidiabetes drugs (tolbutamide, carbutamide, chlorpropamide)
Carbonic anhydrase inhibitors (acetazolamide, methazolamide, mesalazine)
D-Penicillamine
2-Chlorodeoxyadenosine

III. Agents More Rarely Associated With Aplastic Anemia

Antibiotics (streptomycin, tetracycline, methicillin, ampicillin, mebendazole and albendazole, sulfonamides, flucytosine, mefloquine, dapsone)
Antihistamines (cimetidine, ranitidine, chlorpheniramine)
Sedatives and tranquilizers (chlorpromazine, prochlorperazine, piperacetazine, chlordiazepoxide, meprobamate, methyprylon, remoxipride)
Antiarrhythmics (tocainide, amiodarone)
Allopurinol (can potentiate marrow suppression by cytotoxic drugs)
Ticlopidine
Methyldopa
Quinidine
Lithium
Guanidine
Canthaxanthin
Thiocyanate
Carbimazole
Cyanamide
Deferoxamine
Amphetamines

Table 28-4 Drugs Associated With Aplastic Anemia in the International Aplastic Anemia and Agranulocytosis Study*

Drug	Stratified Risk Estimate (95% CI)	Multivariate Relative Risk Estimate (95% CI)
Nonsteroidal Analgesics		
Butazones	3.7 (1.9-7.2)	5.1 (2.1-12)
Indomethacin	7.1 (3.4-15)	8.2 (3.3-20)
Piroxicam	9.8 (3.3-29)	7.4 (2.1-26)
Diclofenac	4.6 (2.0-11)	4.2 (1.6-11)
Antibiotics		
Sulfonamides†	2.8 (1.1-7.3)	2.2 (0.6-7.4)
Antithyroid drugs	16 (4.8-54)	11 (2.0-56)
Cardiovascular Drugs		
Furosemide	3.3 (1.6-7.0)	3.1 (1.2-8.0)
Psychotropic drugs		
Phenothiazines	3.0 (1.1-8.2)	1.6
Corticosteroids	5.0 (2.8-8.9)	3.5 (1.6-7.7)
Allopurinol	7.3 (3.0-17)	5.9 (1.8-19)
Gold	29 (9.7-89)	

From Kaufman DW, Kelly JP, Levy M, et al: *The drug etiology of agranulocytosis and aplastic anemia.* New York, 1991, Oxford University Press.
CI, Confidence interval.
*The multivariate model included the following factors: age, gender, geographic area, date of interview, reliability of the patient, person interviewed, transfer from another hospital, history of blood disorder or tuberculosis, exposure to benzene and related chemicals, and use of other suspected drugs.
†Other than trimethoprim–sulfonamide combination.

to BM failure and that also demonstrate genetic variability include arylhydrocarbon hydroxylase (e.g., benzene toxicity), epoxide hydrolases (e.g., phenytoin toxicity), *S*-methylation (e.g., 6-mercaptopurine, 6-thioguanine, azathioprine), and *N*-acetylation (e.g., sulfa drugs). Genomic approaches have revealed the complex role of genetic variation in metabolic pathways that process arylhydrocarbons and even links to the immune function.

Benzene

Benzene exposure is linked to AA. Benzene myelotoxicity can be placed between the predictable effects of chemotherapeutic agents and idiosyncratic drug reactions. Industrial emissions add greatly to the biologic sources of ambient benzene. Significant benzene exposure can also occur outside of industry. Although the concentrations of benzene to which consumers are exposed are orders of magnitude lower than those observed in industrial workers, the effect of low-dose chronic exposure is uncertain, but genetic variations in the metabolizing enzymes may influence susceptibility to BM suppression at these levels. Benzene metabolites are also generated from the diet.

Water-soluble products of benzene metabolism such as phenols, hydroquinones, and catechols mediate the toxicity to the BM. Benzene and its intermediate metabolites covalently and irreversibly bind to BM DNA, inhibit DNA synthesis, and introduce DNA strand breaks. Benzene acts as a "mitotic poison" and as a mutagen. Acutely, the more mature, actively cycling BM precursor cells are preferentially damaged over the more primitive progenitors. Intermittent exposure may be more damaging to the stem cell compartment than is continuous exposure. BM stroma can also be damaged by benzene.

The range of hematologic disease attributable to benzene is broad, from relatively frequent mild alterations in blood counts to AA or leukemia. Studies of exposed North American workers earlier in the 20th century suggested that the risk of AA was 3% to 4% in men exposed to concentrations higher than 300 ppm and that 50% of individuals exposed to 100 ppm developed some blood cell count depression. The prevalence of some form of BM suppression, manifest as leukopenia, for example, with heavy exposure can be high. Leukopenia, anemia, thrombocytopenia, and lymphocytopenia are common consequences of benzene; other manifestations include macrocytosis, acquired Pelger-Huet anomaly, eosinophilia, and basophilia and less often, polycythemia, leukocytosis, thrombocytosis, or splenomegaly. The BM is usually normocellular but can show hypocellularity or hypercellularity; a hypercellular phase can precede complete aplasia. In addition to hypocellularity, chronically exposed workers can have BM necrosis, fibrosis, edema, and hemorrhage. Conversely, pancytopenia can precede acute leukemia. BM failure and leukemia in benzene workers can manifest decades after exposure.

Aromatic Hydrocarbons

The common perception that other molecules resembling benzene or containing a benzene ring can also cause BM suppression is not well supported. Neither the closely related alkylbenzenes nor pure toluene or xylene is an established BM toxin. Often, an aromatic hydrocarbon has been implicated as causative by a clinician only for lack of another apparent etiology. For some substances, toxicity might result from the presence of benzene as a contaminant of the synthesis of the molecule or in the petroleum distillates used to dissolve the compound. However, the total number of AA cases reported with aromatic hydrocarbon exposures is small when the large populations exposed to this heterogeneous group of chemicals are considered. For example, the significance of a handful of case reports associated with insecticide exposure in the context of the vast use of these compounds is questionable. However, the very high prevalence of aromatic hydrocarbons in daily life would greatly amplify even a small individual risk. Pesticides and insecticides have been associated with AA for decades, with almost 300 medical case reports appearing in the medical literature. The most frequently cited insecticides are chlordane, lindane, and dichlorodiphenyltrichloroethane (DDT). For the miscellaneous aromatic hydrocarbons, case reports also greatly outnumber series of patients, and systematic epidemiologic surveys have shown mixed results.

Chloramphenicol

A structural similarity of chloramphenicol to amidopyrine, a drug known to cause agranulocytosis, led to early prediction of possible hematotoxicity. During the period of its unrestrained use, chloramphenicol was considered the most common cause of AA in the United States, accounting for 20% to 30% of total cases and 50% of drug-associated cases. Estimates of the risk of AA after a course of chloramphenicol ranged from one case per 20,000 to one case per 800,000 people. Based on these figures, a course of chloramphenicol was estimated to increase the risk of AA 13-fold. Although the introduction of chloramphenicol into the American market was perceived as having increased the total number of cases of AA, this assumption was only weakly supported by epidemiologic data, and the mortality rate from AA remained essentially constant during the period of chloramphenicol's introduction and extensive use and after the withdrawal of chloramphenicol from the market. Chloramphenicol has not been associated with AA in Thailand despite its high rate of use there. In Hong Kong, where the use of chloramphenicol is almost 100 times higher than in the West, drug-associated AA occurs infrequently. The early epidemiologic surveys stressed excessive dosage, high blood levels, repeated or intermittent courses, young age, and oral route of administration as particular risks for chloramphenicol BM toxicity.

At ordinary doses, a pattern of reversible alterations in erythropoiesis occurs in most patients treated with chloramphenicol. In vitro, chloramphenicol can decrease hematopoietic colony formation[3] or diminish colony size, although usually at doses greater than those achieved in patients. There is no consistent evidence of abnormal BM sensitivity to the drug in affected individuals.

Nonsteroidal Antiinflammatory Drugs

Compared with chloramphenicol, it took far longer to associate phenylbutazone with AA. Mortality estimates have ranged from one case per 100,000 to one case per 1 million treatment courses. The use of other NSAIDs is associated with case reports of AA. A large case-control led investigation in Europe confirmed the risk of AA with phenylbutazone use and identified even higher probabilities with other NSAIDs. There was a suggestion of increased risk with drugs taken regularly for a prolonged period at very high doses, and in some cases, hematologic reactions were reproduced on repeat exposure.

Neuroleptics and Psychotropic Drugs

A variety of drugs used to treat disorders of the central nervous system have been associated with AA: the hydantoins and carbamazepine, antidepressants, tranquilizers, and felbamate. The marketing of felbamate was severely affected by the occurrence of aplasia in more than 30 patients. Monitoring of drug blood levels and peripheral blood counts in patients receiving carbamazepine was recommended despite fewer than two dozen AA cases reported by 1982. Doubt about the validity of many cases reported in the literature, as well as several large series of patients who did not develop hematologic toxicity and an estimated AA case rate of approximately one in 200,000 treated patients, have led to questions concerning the relationship between carbamazepine and AA.

Gold and Heavy Metals

Gold salts have an extraordinarily high frequency of fatal adverse reactions, estimated at 1.6 cases per 10,000 prescriptions. Dose-dependent leukopenia is common, but several dozen cases of AA have been reported. In the IAAAS, exposure to gold salts was the most significant drug association for developing AA, with a relative risk of 29 and an excess risk of 23 cases per 1 million users in 1 week.[3] Spontaneous recovery rarely occurs. Patients have been successfully treated with stem cell transplantation or immunosuppressive therapy; chelation therapy usually has not been helpful. High concentrations of gold salts inhibit hematopoietic colony formation in vitro; there is some evidence for a dose relationship.

TYPICAL AND ATYPICAL PRESENTATIONS

Most patients with AA seek medical attention for symptoms that occur as a result of low blood counts (Table 28-5 and Fig. 28-7). Some patients can be diagnosed incidentally and show remarkable few symptoms despite severely depressed blood counts. All of the blood elements can be depressed or a single lineage cytopenia can dominate the clinical picture. The differential diagnosis of pancytopenia includes a variety of diseases (see Table 28-1). Most patients do not have systemic symptoms; weight loss, persistent fever, pain, and loss of appetite point to an alternative diagnosis.

Bleeding is the most alarming manifestation of pancytopenia and most frequently sends the patient to a doctor. Thrombocytopenia usually does not cause massive bleeding. Instead, the patient reports easy bruisability and the appearance of red spots, especially over dependent surfaces; gum bleeding with tooth brushing and episodic nose bleeds are common. Heavy menstrual flow or irregular vaginal bleeding can occur in younger women. In AA associated with PNH, red or dark urine may be reported that is caused by free hemoglobin, but visible bleeding from the genitourinary and gastrointestinal tracts

Table 28-5 Clinical Presentation of Aplastic Anemia

Symptoms	Patients (*n*)
Bleeding	41
Anemia	27
Bleeding and anemia	14
Bleeding and infection	6
Infection	5
Routine examination	8
Total	101

Adapted from Williams DM, Lynch RE, Cartwright GE: Drug induced aplastic anemia. *Semin Hematol* 10:195, 1973.

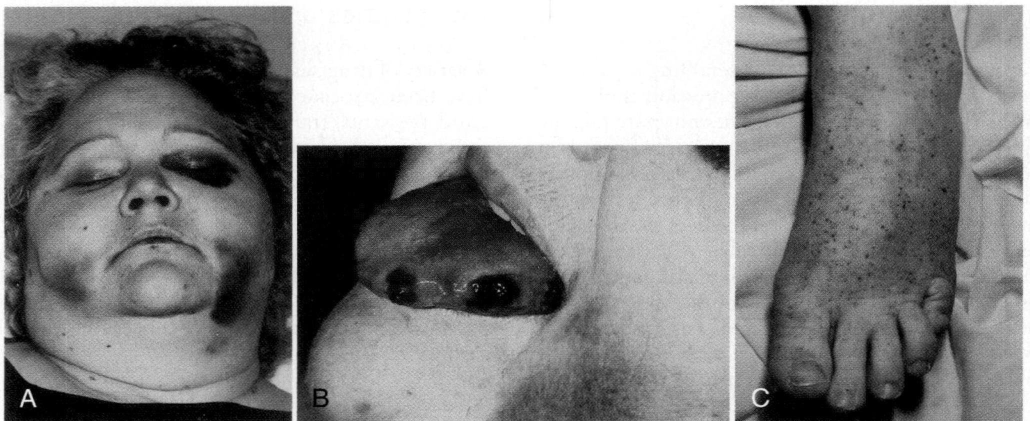

Figure 28-7 CLINICAL PRESENTATIONS OF APLASTIC ANEMIA. **A,** Ecchymosis in pancytopenic women. **B,** Submucosal hematomas. **C,** Petechial eruptions in a thrombocytopenic patient.

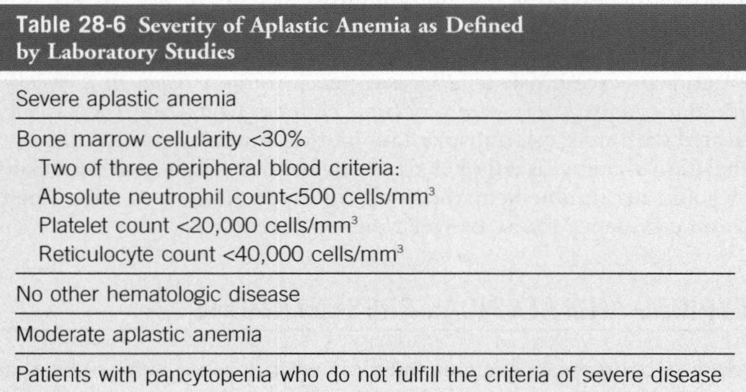

Table 28-6 Severity of Aplastic Anemia as Defined by Laboratory Studies

Severe aplastic anemia
Bone marrow cellularity <30%
Two of three peripheral blood criteria:
Absolute neutrophil count<500 cells/mm^3
Platelet count <20,000 cells/mm^3
Reticulocyte count <40,000 cells/mm^3
No other hematologic disease
Moderate aplastic anemia
Patients with pancytopenia who do not fulfill the criteria of severe disease

is rare on presentation in AA. Extensive hemorrhage from any organ can occur but usually late in the course of the disease and almost always associated with infections, drug therapy (e.g., corticosteroids), or invasive procedures.

The ability to adapt to a gradual reduction in hemoglobin concentration is remarkable. Patients with anemia might mention fatigue, lassitude, shortness of breath, or ringing in the ears, but some individuals can tolerate astonishingly low hemoglobin levels without complaint. Even abrupt cessation of erythropoiesis leads to only a slow decline in hemoglobin (≈1 g/dL each week).

Infection is an uncommon presentation in patients with AA. The sore throat of agranulocytosis is not often observed, presumably because other alarming symptoms appear earlier.

Retrospective studies of AA associated with drugs and viruses and the observation of the occasional patient with serially monitored blood counts suggest a latent period of 6 to 8 weeks between the inciting event and the onset of pancytopenia. The interval can be more prolonged when pancytopenia is well tolerated or moderate. For purposes of diagnosis and management, a history of blood diseases in other family members is very important and should trigger appropriate genetic tests for constitutional causes.

With identification of genetic risk factor, the family history has assumed great importance in the evaluation of pancytopenia. Leukemia and myelodysplastic syndrome (MDS) can occur in FA and DKC pedigrees. In the telomeropathies secondary to *TERT* and *TERC* mutations, hematologic findings in other family members may be mild, such as modest thrombocytopenia or macrocytosis with or without anemia. These mutations also are etiologic of cirrhosis and pulmonary fibrosis, which may be present as diagnoses in the pedigree. Early graying of the hair is a less reliable sign but is sometimes prominent in the telomere diseases.

Findings on physical examination usually reflect the severity of the pancytopenia (Table 28-6). However, patients with severe disease

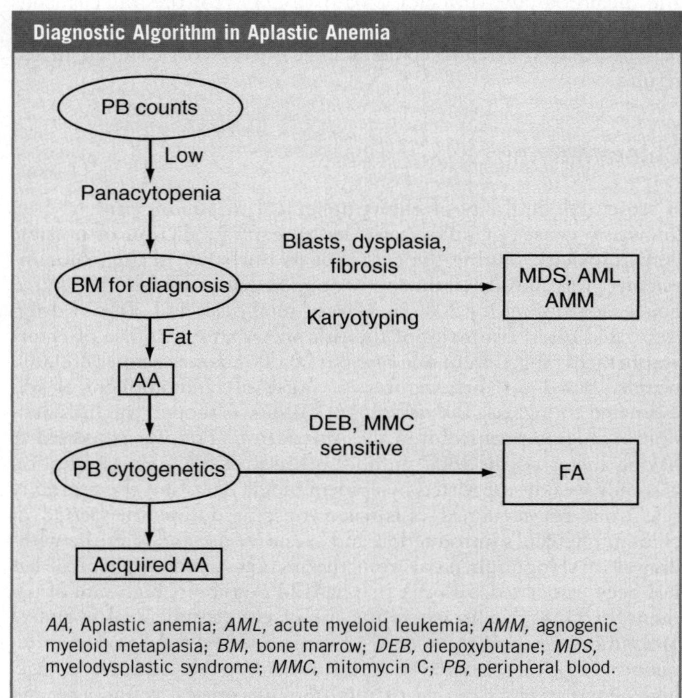

can look well. The patient may present with subtle variations from normal or with a dramatic, even toxic appearance. Petechiae are often present over the pretibial surface of the lower leg and the dorsal aspects of the forearm and wrist; a few petechiae can be seen in the oropharynx and on the palate. Scattered ecchymoses typically appear in areas exposed to minor trauma. With severe thrombocytopenia, retinal hemorrhages can be present on funduscopic examination, there can be gingival oozing or blood in the nares, and hemorrhage can be apparent at the uterine cervical os. The stool can contain traces of heme. Pallor is common and is best appreciated on the mucosal membranes and palmar surfaces. A new patient can be febrile, but specific or localizing signs of infection are uncommon on presentation. Cachexia, splenomegaly, and lymphadenopathy are not associated with AA, and these findings should strongly suggest another diagnosis. The examiner should look carefully for café au lait spots and other physical anomalies of FA and for typical nail changes, leukoplakia, hypopigmentation of the skin, and grey hair of telomere disease in children *and* adults.

Several atypical presentations of AA should be pointed out. A physician might encounter an elderly patient with pancytopenia in

Table 28-7 Bone Marrow Morphologic Findings that Discriminate Myelodysplasia From Aplastic Anemia

Characteristic*	Myelodysplasia	Aplastic Anemia
Cellularity	Usually normal to increased	Decreased
Erythropoiesis		
Megaloblastic	Very common	Common
Dyserythropoietic	Very common	Unusual
Maturation defects	Common	Not found
Ringed sideroblasts	Common	Not found
Myelopoiesis		
Monocyte prominence	Very common	Unusual
Midmyeloid predominance	Very common	Unusual
Increased blasts	Yes	Not found
Megakaryocytes		
Atypical morphology	Very common	Not found

Adapted from Bagby GC: The preleukemic syndrome (hematopoietic dysplasia). In Shahidi NT, editor: *Aplastic anemia and other bone marrow failure syndromes,* New York, 1990, Springer-Verlag, p 199. Provides percentages for myelodysplasia.
*Ringed sideroblasts and myeloblasts are observed by definition in some of the myelodysplastic syndromes. Dyserythropoietic red blood cell precursors show bizarre forms with multiple or irregular nuclei. Megakaryocytes can show defective nuclear polyploidization and increased internuclear spaces, or they can be small with only a few nuclei and peculiar granulation.

whom subsequent BM examination reveals dysplastic features (see box on Diagnostic Algorithm in Aplastic Anemia and Table 28-7). Although the history of the illness in a newly diagnosed patient is typically short—in the range of months—some patients may recall a long history of bruisability, anemia, and low blood cell counts reported to them by previous physicians during routine examinations. These patients can have a moderately severe, chronic disease that is stable for years, and pancytopenia from childhood should suggest a constitutional AA.

CLINICAL ASSOCIATIONS

A number of clinical syndromes, usually revealed through a careful history and physical examination, are associated with AA (see box on Diagnostic Algorithm in Aplastic Anemia and Tables 28-2 and 28-3).

Posttransfusion Graft-Versus-Host Disease

Almost uniformly fatal, AA is a constant feature of transfusion-associated GVHD produced by the transfusion of competent lymphocytes into immunodeficient hosts, including children with congenital syndromes, cancer patients receiving high-dose chemotherapy, and patients with adoptive cellular immunotherapy for leukemia. Rarely, posttransfusion GVHD occurs in an apparently immunocompetent recipient in the special circumstance in which the donor is homozygous for an HLA haplotype also shared by the recipient, as can occur among first-degree family members. Small numbers of lymphocytes are sufficient to produce the syndrome, which is surprisingly resistant to immunosuppressive therapy. Pancytopenia with BM hypoplasia is an almost constant feature of posttransfusion GVHD. Runt disease in animals is a model of this immune-mediated BM failure syndrome.

Pregnancy

Pregnancy is common in the age groups most susceptible to BM failure, and in many cases, its association is probably only coincidental. The true frequency of AA in pregnancy is unknown, but from the number of cases reported, it appears rare, although BM hypoplasia may be relatively common during pregnancy. A causal relationship is suggested by the temporal relationship between the onset of pancytopenia and that of pregnancy and by resolution after delivery and spontaneous or induced abortion; some patients have developed AA that remitted after each delivery. Survival rates for AA in pregnancy have been relatively high for the mother and baby, with most pregnancies being successful. Hemorrhage is the most common cause of death from AA during pregnancy. The published data are insufficient to guide the management of pregnant women with AA, especially because it is clear that AA in some cases is serendipitously diagnosed and can persist beyond parturition. A woman who desires a child can be maintained with transfusions with the understanding that any clinical deterioration is a criterion for interruption or termination of the pregnancy. The hazard of pregnancy to a woman who has recovered from idiopathic AA is unknown, but most hematologists, recognizing the risk of relapse, advise patients not to become pregnant, especially if thrombocytopenia and a PNH clone are present.[10]

Post-Hepatitis AA

Hepatitis-associated AA has several peculiar features. Typically, an uneventful episode of apparent viral hepatitis in a young man is followed in 1 to 2 months, during convalescence from the liver inflammation, by very severe pancytopenia. Depression of blood cell counts during the course of hepatitis is common; leukopenia, atypical lymphocytosis, erythroid macrocytosis, and thrombocytopenia mimic in milder forms the hematologic changes of AA. However, posthepatitis AA has a very poor prognosis, with early estimates of mortality of 90% at 1 year, and a history of hepatitis in AA has been considered an indication for early BMT. Patients with posthepatitis AA can successfully undergo BMT without an increased risk of veno-occlusive disease. Patients with hepatitis-associated aplasia have markers of immune system activation and respond well to intensive immunosuppressive therapy. Almost all cases have been seronegative, non-A, non-B, and non-C hepatitis. Posthepatitis AA is linked to fulminant hepatitis of childhood and acute seronegative hepatitis. Acute viral hepatitis that is seronegative differs clinically from hepatitis C disease; parenteral exposure is not a risk factor, liver functions abnormalities are more severe during the acute phase, and late complications are more common.

Postmononucleosis Aplastic Anemia

Acute infection with Epstein-Barr virus (EBV) causes infectious mononucleosis that is commonly associated with neutropenia and other hematologic abnormalities but, similar to acute hepatitis, is only rarely complicated by AA. However, EBV may be involved in the cause of AA more frequently than originally appreciated because a large number of primary EBV infections are unrecognized. Pancytopenia can be first observed during the acute mononucleosis syndrome or shortly after disappearance of symptoms. Some patients have recovered spontaneously, others after therapy with corticosteroids or immunosuppressive therapy. EBV can occasionally be demonstrated in the BM cells of patients with apparently idiopathic AA in association with serologic evidence of a primary or reactivated viral infection.

Hemophagocytic Syndrome

The BM is hypocellular in approximately one-third of cases with hemophagocytic syndrome. In this disorder, there can be progression from BM hypercellularity to aplasia; myelofibrosis is also common. Pancytopenia occurs in most of cases; anemia is a universal finding; thrombocytopenia and neutropenia are also common. In contrast to typical AA, these patients appear systemically ill, with fever and constitutional symptoms, and peripheral blood cell count depression is often associated with abnormalities of other organ systems, including hepatosplenomegaly, lymphadenopathy, cutaneous eruptions, and pulmonary infiltrates. The syndrome is associated with a large variety of diseases, including immunodeficiency, malignancy, and infections. In the infectious category, viral infections are most common and include EBV, cytomegalovirus, herpes simplex, herpes zoster, B19 parvovirus, and HIV-1; bacterial and parasitic infections also have been associated with hemophagocytosis. Hemophagocytosis is often observed on supravital or Wright-Giemsa staining of the BM of patients with idiopathic AA, and it is also a morphologic feature of graft rejection after BMT. In virus-associated hemophagocytosis, there is evidence of immune system activation. The sera of patients have been shown to contain high levels of IFN-γ, TNF-α, IL-6, soluble CD8, and soluble interleukin-2 (IL-2) receptor, and T cells overproduce IFN-γ in vitro. The clinical response to cyclosporine is consistent with a T cell–mediated pathophysiology of hematopoietic failure.

Paroxysmal Nocturnal Hemoglobinuria and Aplastic Anemia

There is a strong association between AA and PNH (see Chapter 29). These diseases frequently are diagnosed concurrently or sequentially in the same individual, and they share similar clinical and pathologic features (i.e., pancytopenia and BM hypocellularity). The presence of an expanded PNH clone is associated with HLA-DR15 and has been reported as a good prognostic factor for the responsiveness to immunosuppressive therapy. Clinical BM failure can be present at the onset of PNH or can develop after diagnosis. By flow cytometry of granulocytes for glycosylphosphoinositol-anchored proteins, there is expansion of a PNH clone in 50% or more of AA cases at presentation.[11]

Longitudinal studies of patients with de novo PNH or PNH developing from AA indicate a low probability of spontaneous remission; in most patients, the contribution of the PNH clones remains stable for years, but hemolytic disease can develop.

Collagen Vascular Diseases

Aplastic anemia is a component of the collagen vascular syndrome called eosinophilic fasciitis. This severe, scleroderma-like disease is characterized by fibrosis of subcutaneous and fascial tissue, localized skin induration, eosinophilia, hypergammaglobulinemia, and an elevated erythrocyte sedimentation rate. The rheumatologic symptoms of fasciitis respond to corticosteroids, but the associated AA has a very poor prognosis. A few patients have survived after BMT or immunosuppressive therapy. More rarely, AA has complicated SLE and rheumatoid arthritis, but in many cases, the role of concomitant drug therapy is confounding. Rarely, AA can accompany Sjögren syndrome, multiple sclerosis, and immune thyroid disease. AA occasionally occurs in individuals with hypogammaglobulinemia or congenital immunodeficiency syndrome, thymoma, or thymic hyperplasia.

LABORATORY EVALUATION

Peripheral Blood

In typical cases of AA, all of the blood cell counts are depressed. The blood smear usually shows obvious paucity of platelets and leukocytes but normal RBC morphology; toxic granulations can be present in neutrophils. Automated cell counting shows erythrocyte macrocytosis and a normal RBC distribution of width. Platelet size is normal and not increased as in immune peripheral destruction, but the low number can cause greater heterogeneity of size. Prior transfusions alter platelet numbers, relative reticulocyte counts, and hemoglobin values. Although relative lymphocytosis is very common, most patients also have decreased absolute numbers of monocytes and lymphocytes. The severity of AA can be graded based on the peripheral blood cell counts (see Table 28-6 and box on Diagnostic Algorithm in Aplastic Anemia).

DIAGNOSIS OF APLASTIC ANEMIA

Although the ultimate diagnosis of AA rests on the interpretation of an adequate BM biopsy specimen, important clues to the cause of pancytopenia can be obtained from the history, physical examination, and laboratory data. Pancytopenia that is not primarily hematologic in origin but secondary to other disease processes is usually an obvious diagnosis. Patients with severe liver disease and splenomegaly, SLE, or overwhelming sepsis can have low blood cell counts, but their clinical presentation is not subtle. Similarly, BM aplasia follows cytotoxic drug therapy for cancers and is an anticipated and transient toxic effect for a variety of nonmalignant diseases. In challenging cases, obvious medical causes of pancytopenia usually have already been excluded. Pancytopenia almost never results from peripheral blood cell destruction alone. In AA, the blood smear does not show reticulocytes, band forms, or the large platelets typical of increased compensatory BM efforts.

Acquired AA is a disease of the young, as is constitutional aplasia. Patients with FA often, but not always, have physical abnormalities. In the absence of a suggestive family history or the presence of physical anomalies, the distinction between acquired and constitutional disease depends on the results of a clastogenic-stress culture of peripheral lymphocytes (for FA) and telomere length of leukocytes (for DKC and the telomeropathies).

In older patients, the major differential diagnosis is between AA and myelodysplasia. There is a gray area between hypocellular myelodysplasia and moderate AA, and even competent hematologists might not agree on the final diagnosis. BM cytogenetics can help in establishing the proper diagnosis.

Myelofibrosis can also produce pancytopenia, but the BM is not aspirable, the spleen is often enlarged, and the peripheral blood smear shows characteristic abnormalities. Acute leukemia in children and elderly adults can manifest as BM hypocellularity, requiring a careful search for lymphoblasts or myeloblasts, including phenotypic analysis by flow cytometry. Peripheral blood flow cytometry for glycophosphoinositol-anchored proteins should be performed to diagnose PNH (see Chapter 29).

The patient's history can provide clues, such as benzene exposure for myelodysplasia and acute leukemia or a suspicious drug history for AA. Discontinuation of exposure to the incriminated drugs or chemicals is mandatory, and in some instances, patients may then recover. However, given the difficulty of assigning blame with absolute certainty to environmental agents, the authors treat all patients similarly and do not advocate protracted observation for possible spontaneous recovery. For patients with severe disease (see Table 28-6), suitable and early preparation for BMT should be undertaken or immunosuppression begun, but for those with moderate disease, the clinical status should be evaluated, and serial blood cell counts are required to assess progression of the disease.

BONE MARROW

The BM must be assessed quantitatively and qualitatively for cellularity and the morphology of residual cells (Fig. 28-8 and see Fig. 28-1). BM aspiration and biopsy should always be performed, and the core specimen should be at least 1 cm long. There should be no compromise in obtaining adequate specimens and no hesitation in performing a second procedure if required.

Bone marrow cellularity is estimated from the core biopsy. Point counting under microscopic cross hairs in many parts of a histologic section is the most accurate method of determining cellularity, but hematologists commonly rely on visual estimation only. A crude

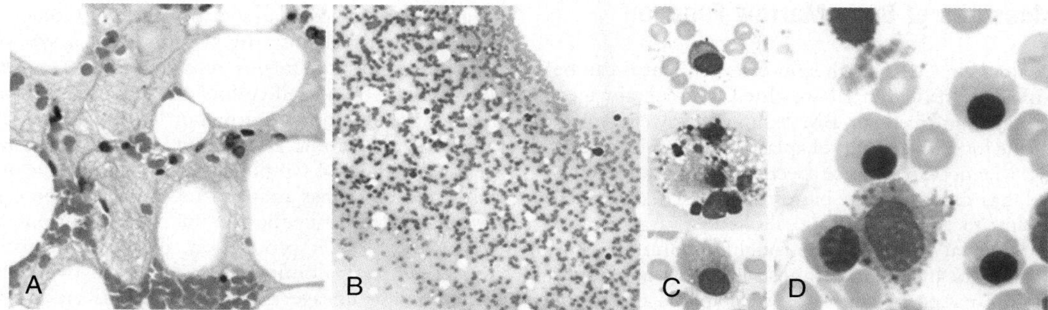

Figure 28-8 SOME MORPHOLOGIC FEATURES OCCASIONALLY OBSERVED IN PATIENTS WITH APLASTIC ANEMIA. Empty marrow with eosinophilic ground substance consistent with serous atrophy or stomal injury **(A),** possibly indicative of marrow damage. Scanty bone marrow aspirate in severe disease **(B)** showing only rare nucleated elements, many of which are from blood. The presence of plasma cells, histiocytes, and osteoblasts **(C)** confirms the bone marrow nature of the aspirate. Note: Sometimes the histiocytes can show hemophagocytosis. Megaloblastoid erythropoiesis **(D)** is sometimes seen in aplastic anemia and in recovery.

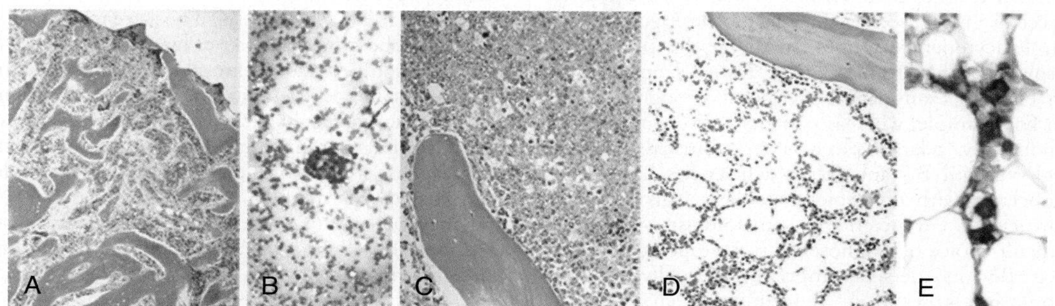

Figure 28-9 MORPHOLOGY OF OTHER DISEASES THAT MAY MANIFEST WITH PANCYTOPENIA. Bone marrow biopsy from patient with pancytopenia showing myelofibrosis and osteosclerosis associated with metastatic prostate cancer **(A).** The aspirate was hypocellular but did show occasional tumor clusters **(B).** Another case where the patient presented with pancytopenia and was found to have a bone marrow packed with lymphoma cells **(C).** Hairy cell leukemia can present with pancytopenia and with a hypocellular bone marrow **(D)** difficult to distinguish from aplastic anemia. The diagnosis rests on identifying a B-cell infiltrative process with immunohistochemical stains **(E,** CD20).

"eyeball" approximation is almost always adequate in severe aplasia because the hematopoietic content of the BM specimen is usually close to zero. Estimates of BM cellularity based on examination of the aspirate smear and biopsy specimen are correlated, but dilution of the aspirate by sinusoidal blood often occurs, and the aspirate can be hypocellular when the biopsy specimen is hypercellular or can show focal areas of active hematopoiesis. Normal BM cellularity decreases with age, a variation that is of some importance in assessing older patients with aplasia or myelodysplasia. In autopsy samples from normal young children, approximately 80% of the BM space of the iliac crest is cellular. BM cellularity gradually decreases from age 20 to 70 years and more precipitously in very elderly adults to approximately 30% in the eighth decade of life. For practical purposes, the lower limit of normal BM cellularity in adults is accepted at approximately 30%, but the differences at the extremes of life should be recalled when evaluating infants and elderly adults. In most patients with AA, total BM cellularity is extremely low, but there can be significant residual lymphocytosis. The increase in BM fat in aplasia is caused by increases in the size and number of individual fat cells. "Hot pockets" of hematopoiesis can be present. The BM tends to contract centripetally with age, and a similar process can be observed in pathologic states, so the sternal BM can be more cellular than iliac crest samples.

Examination of the BM (Fig. 28-9 and see Figs. 28-1 and 28-8) is basic for the diagnosis of most primary hematologic causes of pancytopenia (see Table 28-1 and box on Diagnostic Algorithm in Aplastic Anemia). Information can be gained by observing the BM aspirate itself. A fatty, even watery specimen can usually be aspirated without difficulty from an aplastic patient, but a truly dry tap is more typical of a hypercullular ("packed") or fibrotic BM. The morphology of individual cells is best seen in the Wright-Giemsa–stained aspirate smear, and the architecture of the BM is appreciated in a biopsy section. In acellular specimens, the only cells visible are usually lymphocytes, plasma cells, and stromal elements—fibroblastoid and histiocytic cells. Some degree of dyserythropoiesis is common, usually the megaloblastoid features of macrocytosis and some nuclear-cytoplasmic maturation asynchrony, but sometimes more complex degenerative changes in nuclei and cytoplasm can be observed by light and electron microscopy (see Fig. 28-8). These features are common to AA and myelodysplasia (see Table 28-7), which can be very difficult to distinguish. Hemophagocytosis of RBCs can also be seen in AA. Examination of the cells close to the spicules of a sparse aspirate smear can disclose a distinctive population of leukemic blasts; increased numbers of myeloblasts are not seen in AA and are evidence of aleukemic leukemia or herald the evolution of leukemia from pancytopenia. Histochemistry for CD34 cells should show staining only of vascular elements in AA, and increased CD34 is typical of MDS and AML. Lymphoid aggregates, nests of tumor cells, granulomas, and infectious particles can be apparent on examination of the fixed biopsy specimen.

Karyotyping of BM cells is diagnostically important. Unfortunately, the yield of cells from a hypocellular BM can be inadequate to perform cytogenetic analysis. Chromosome analysis is usually normal in AA but frequently reveals a clonal abnormality in myelodysplasia. Cytogenetic studies, including interphase fluorescent in situ hybridization (FISH) and single nucleotide polymorphisms array-based karyotyping may produce informative results, including detection of cryptic chromosomal abnormalities.[12]

Radiographic Measures of Bone Marrow Function

Magnetic resonance imaging (MRI) with spin-echo sequences can be useful in the study of BM disease. On T1-weighted spin-echo images, fatty BM appears bright, and cellular BM exhibits a lower density signal (Fig. 28-10). The high fat content of aplastic BM can be readily appreciated on MRI. Magnetic resonance spectroscopy, which detects the type of fat signal, has shown diverse patterns among AA patients. MRI is complementary to tissue sampling, allowing a large area of BM to be visualized and fat content to be roughly quantified. The technique appears to be worthwhile in diagnosis because the patterns of fat and cell distribution appear to differ between aplasia and hypocellular myelodysplasia, and in prognosis, to monitor improvements in hematopoiesis after treatment.

DIFFERENTIAL DIAGNOSIS OF PANCYTOPENIA

Aplastic anemia is not the most common cause of pancytopenia (see Table 28-1). A rational diagnostic algorithm can be very helpful in establishing a correct diagnosis (see box on Diagnostic Algorithm in Aplastic Anemia). Pancytopenia is unlikely to be the presenting feature of hypersplenism in cirrhosis or of Evans syndrome in SLE. Findings on physical examination can point strongly toward another diagnosis. For example, whereas patients with myelofibrosis usually have splenomegaly, a large spleen is very unusual in those with AA. Although vitamin B_{12} and folate deficiencies have been reported to be associated with erythroid hypoplasia, this must be an exceedingly rare event. For practicing hematologists, the most important and difficult choice of diagnoses in pancytopenic patients is among the primary BM disorders. An empty BM is usually obvious, but diagnostic confusion arises from the equivocal character of moderate AA; alterations in the BM appearance in patients with chronic disease; and real overlaps among AA, myelodysplasia, and leukemia.

In moderate AA, the modest depression of BM cellularity can muddle the single most reliable diagnostic criterion. BM cellularity is imprecisely quantitated at best, and further uncertainty is introduced by large sampling errors. "Hot spots" of hematopoietic activity in an otherwise acellular specimen reflect biologic heterogeneity in the pattern of cell loss. In patients with a syndrome of transient pancytopenia, spontaneous recovery occurs within a few months; although the blood cell counts can be severely depressed, the BM is much more commonly normal or hypercellular than hypoplastic. In patients with chronic BM failure, serial BM specimens may not be identical because of sampling error or because the original disease was misdiagnosed or has changed its character. Some patients with AA are not pancytopenic; they do not have uniform depressions of RBC, WBC, and platelet production, despite an empty BM, and their clinical course is dominated by failure in two cell lines or a single hematopoietic lineage. Related conditions such as pure RBC aplasia, amegakaryocytic thrombocytopenia, and agranulocytosis, although usually distinctive in their clinical presentation, can evolve into more generalized BM failure. In the absence of better markers, sometimes the only accurate diagnosis is a description of the clinical features and the specific BM morphology.

A hypocellular BM often precludes the proper morphologic diagnosis. This problem can be especially evident in the case of an MDS with hypoplastic BM (see Table 28-7).

Bone marrow cytogenetics, if positive for chromosome abnormalities, established the diagnosis of leukemia or MDS (see Chapter 27). However, some random chromosomal abnormalities may be transient, and some believe that typical AA is not incompatible with the abnormal karyotype, particularly when somatic mosaicism is present. Often, acellular specimen precludes successful culture and generation of metaphase smears. In such cases, single nucleotide polymorphisms arrays-based karyotyping can be performed on interphase cells and may be helpful in detection of clonal abnormalities.[13] Screen for monosomy-7, and trisomy-8 can also be performed using interphase FISH.

TREATMENT

Aplastic anemia should be considered a medical emergency. Lives are lost, mainly because the grave consequences of severe pancytopenia go unrecognized. The ultimate benefits of definitive therapies such as transplantation or immunosuppression will be unrealized if the

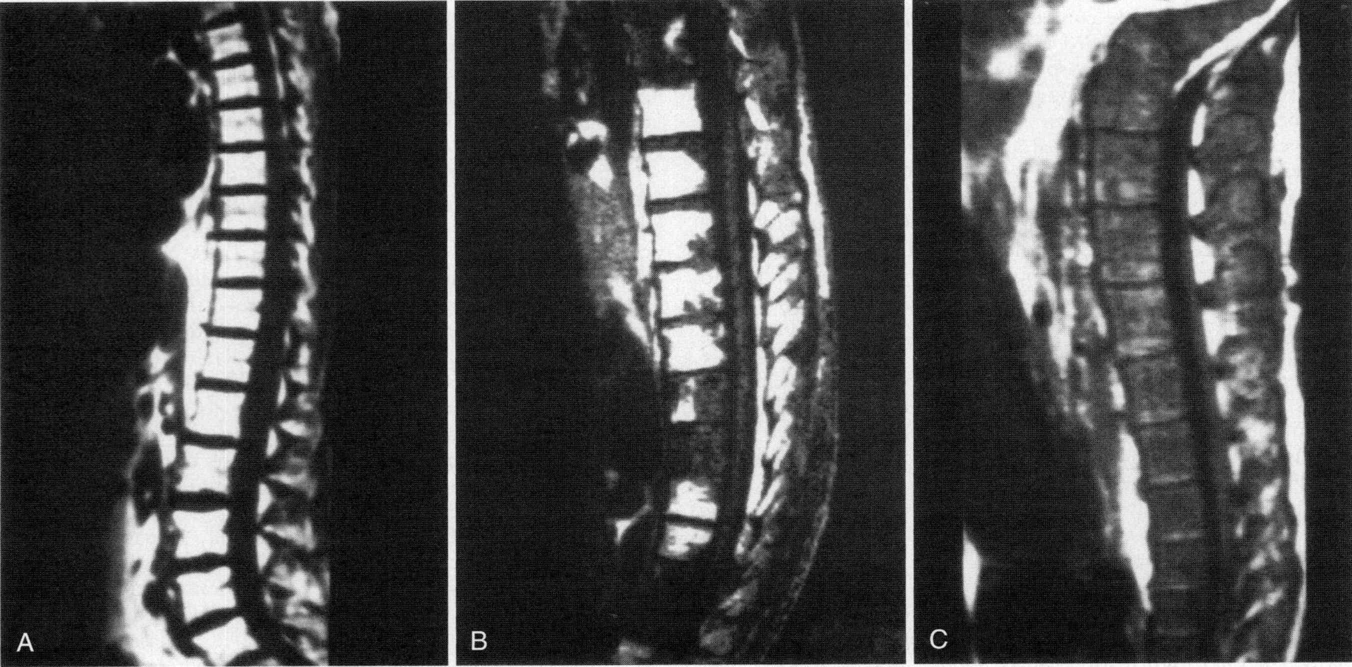

Figure 28-10 MAGNETIC RESONANCE IMAGING OF BONE MARROW. **A,** Bone marrow in a young man with severe aplastic anemia, a middle-aged woman with severe aplastic anemia (**B**), and a middle-aged woman with myelodysplasia (**C**).

patient succumbs to an early clinical catastrophe. A haphazard transfusion policy increases the risk of graft rejection after BMT, but an overly conservative approach to transfusion can jeopardize the patient's life and increase morbidity. Supportive management therefore requires meticulous attention to the daily problems that occur as a consequence of pancytopenia and appreciation of their impact on the ultimate possibilities for cure or amelioration of AA. AA can be cured by replacement of stem cells, by BMT, and by immunosuppressive therapy. Androgens and hematopoietic growth factors have secondary roles (see box on Treatment Algorithm in Aplastic Anemia).

Supportive Management

Bleeding

Bleeding was historically a common symptom in AA, and death from hemorrhage occurred frequently in the premodern era. Platelet transfusions have substantially improved survival in patients with this disease. Measurable correction of the platelet count by transfusion almost always alleviates the minor mucocutaneous bleeding common in thrombocytopenic patients. Major bleeding usually is not caused by thrombocytopenia alone, and ancillary explanations for massive hemorrhage should be sought. The bleeding time improves after erythrocyte transfusion in patients with anemia, and there is a strong inverse correlation between the hematocrit and bleeding. The treatment of serious hemorrhage should include correction of severe anemia and RBC transfusions.

Modern transfusion practice has made platelets readily available and safe to administer. Other than cost and convenience, the major problem related to platelet transfusions is the development of alloimmunization in the recipient. The life span of the transfused platelet in the circulation is dramatically shortened by host antibodies, almost always directed to HLA-A and HLA-B antigens. Alloimmunization is suggested by poor recovery of the 1-hour posttransfusion platelet count and confirmed by finding specific HLA antibodies in serum. Refractoriness can often be overcome by selection of HLA-matched donors, but perfectly HLA-matched transfusions can fail. Alloimmunization can be prevented or delayed by the use of single-donor platelets rather than pooled platelets and by physical leukocyte depletion by filtration or ultraviolet treatment of blood products. Avoidance of platelet transfusions except when there is active bleeding is another alternative to prevent alloimmunization, but the dose relationship between exposure to different donors' platelets and the probability of developing refractoriness is not clearly established, and only after more than about 40 units have been administered does the risk of alloimmunization clearly increase.

Prophylactic transfusion of platelets is not standard. The primary indication for platelet prophylaxis is to prevent intracranial hemorrhage, but the risk of this complication in chronically thrombocytopenic patients, although real, is low. Prophylactic platelet transfusions have not been shown to alter survival. Nevertheless, the beneficial effects of avoiding bleeding complications and improving the quality of life justifies their use. Although the 20,000 platelets/μL value has long been used to trigger transfusion, many reports have suggested little difference in the risk of bleeding over a wide range of platelet counts between 5000 and 100,000 platelets/μL. In a randomized trial

Treatment Algorithm in Aplastic Anemia

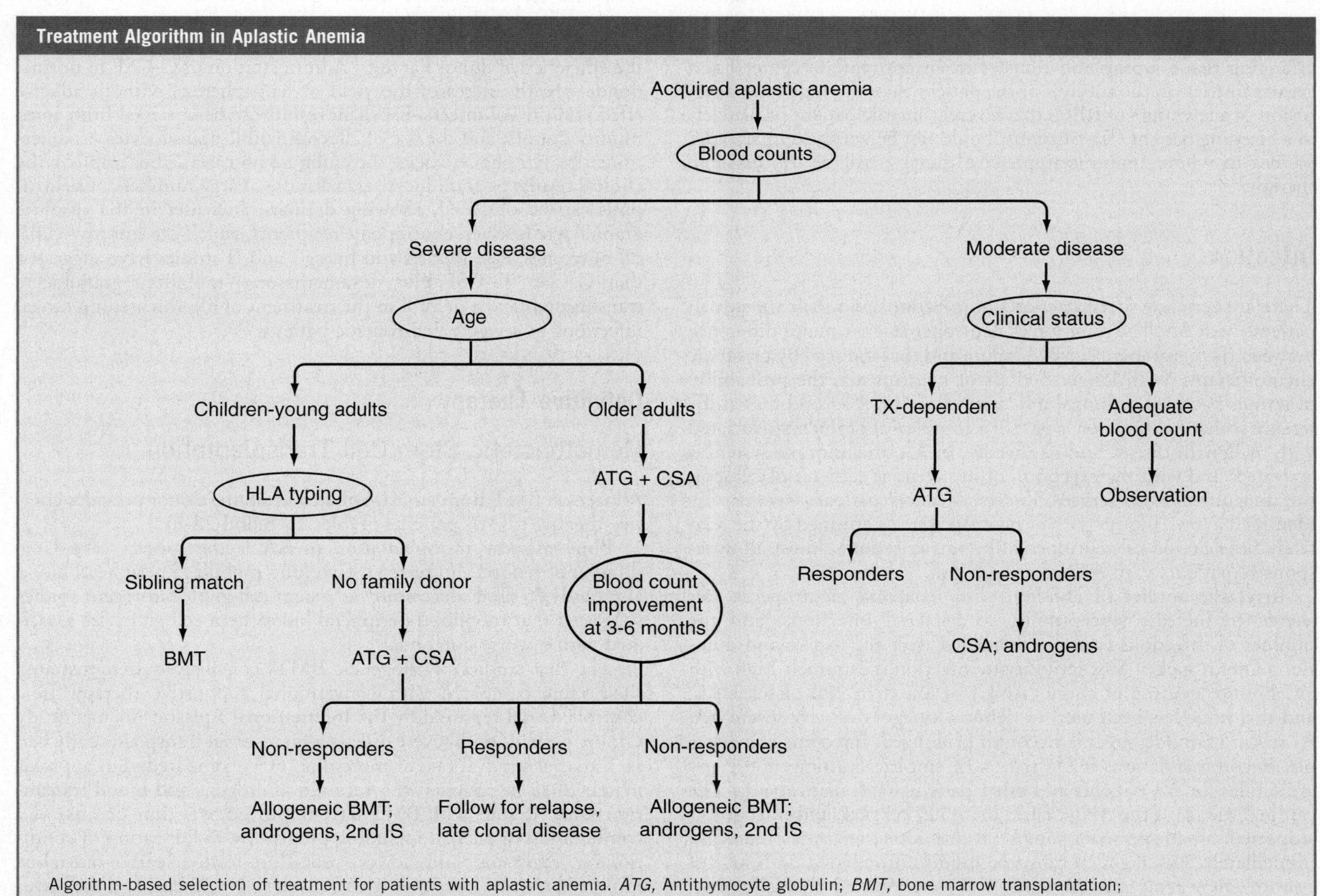

Algorithm-based selection of treatment for patients with aplastic anemia. *ATG,* Antithymocyte globulin; *BMT,* bone marrow transplantation; *CSA,* cyclosporine A; *HLA,* human leukocyte antigen; *IS,* immunosuppression; *TX,* treatment.

of patients with AML, the risk of major bleeding was no different when 10,000 or 20,000 platelets/μL was chosen as the threshold, but the lower value led to a 20% reduction in platelet use. Any prophylaxis program must be modified to address the individual patient, but a goal of maintaining platelet counts higher than 10,000 platelets/μL is reasonable.

Major surgery can be accomplished in the setting of thrombocytopenia. In one study, blood loss and morbidity rates were low even at platelet counts of less than 30,000 platelets/μL.

Anemia

Other than to reduce the risk of graft rejection after receiving an allogeneic transplant, there is no reason to allow a patient to suffer the symptoms of anemia. After equilibrium is achieved, a constant amount of blood will be required to maintain a given hemoglobin concentration. Physically fit individuals are usually not symptomatic at hemoglobin concentrations higher than 7 g/dL; patients with underlying cardiovascular disease should be maintained at a higher level (≥9 g/dL). Iron chelation should be used in patients with unresponsive chronic anemia who have a reasonable expectation of survival.

Alloimmunization as a result of blood product administration increases the probability of graft rejection and mortality after BMT. Blood products from a potential BM donor such as a sibling or a parent (who share histocompatibility antigens) should be avoided. Small numbers of transfusions do not have a major deleterious effect on survival. The 5% risk of graft rejection after transplantation in entirely untransfused patients was increased to 15% with receipt of 1 to 40 units and to higher than 25% only in more heavily transfused patients. Graft rejection would be anticipated to be lower with leucocyte-depletion methods of platelet preparations. Speed in arranging tissue typing and transfer to an appropriate center has a greater impact on the survival of the patient than the judicious transfusion of a few units of RBCs to a severely anemic patient or platelets to a bleeding patient. Transfusions should not be withheld in an older patient in whom immunosuppressive therapy will be the first-line therapy.

Infection

There are very few specific reports of infections and their therapy in patients with AA. The duration of neutropenia is the major difference between the neutropenia of BM failure and that induced by cytotoxic chemotherapy. With longer periods of neutropenia, the probability of serious bacterial or fungal infection increases. A second major difference is that neutropenia is part of a complex of problems associated with malignant disease and its therapy. In AA, the immune system is activated, and with the exception of intravenous catheter placement, the integument is preserved. Studies of cancer patients have usually identified a low-risk category of neutropenia, determined by the relatively brief period of neutropenia; by this criterion, almost all unresponsive patients with AA are at high risk.

In classic studies of children with leukemia, neutropenia was shown to increase susceptibility to bacterial infections, and the number of infectious episodes correlated with the degree and duration of neutropenia. Susceptibility to infection is extremely high with an absolute neutrophil count (ANC) of less than 200 platelets/μL, and this value has been used to define a category of very severe AA. As severe granulocytopenia becomes prolonged, infection is inevitable. Recommendations for initiation of empirical antibiotic therapy are similar for AA patients and other patients with neutropenia. The cardinal rule is, if the ANC is less than 500 cells/μL and infection is suspected, broad-spectrum parenteral antibiotic therapy should begin immediately. Any regimen can need modification based on results of cultures, new symptoms or signs, or a deteriorating clinical course. Bacteremia is present in only 20% of febrile neutropenic episodes, and in only approximately 40% of those can a microbiologic cause or localizing physical findings be identified. Early discontinuation of antibiotics when cultures are unrevealing in persistently neutropenic patients is dangerous.

Patients often remain febrile despite antibiotic therapy or fever reappears. In the absence of additional microbiologic data or clinical clues from the patient's complaints or physical examination, antifungal therapy should be instituted in patients who have remained febrile despite adequate antibacterial therapy. Earlier addition of anti-fungal drugs is advisable in AA patients, especially if there are findings on chest tomography and a positive test result for galactomannan protein. Fungemia during an initial febrile episode is rare, but fungal infection becomes more likely with repeated courses of antibiotics and ultimately is the major cause of death in AA patients in whom definitive therapy fails. *Candida* and *Aspergillus* spp. account for almost all fungal diseases in AA. Early aggressive treatment of neutropenic patients can reverse fungal disease. Large randomized trials have shown that newer antifungal agents such as voriconazole and caspofungin are less toxic and as effective or superior compared with amphotericin and liposomal amphotericin for the treatment of both persistent neutropenic fever and established *Candida* and *Aspergillus* infection. Improved survival in severe AA is caused in some part by better antifungal drug therapies.[14]

Polymorphonuclear cells have a relatively brief life span in the circulation, and their major activity is in infected tissue. There are no simple measures of the therapeutic efficacy of WBC transfusions. The ANC is not measurably increased by standard transfusions. Several controlled trials performed in the 1970s reported improved survival in patients who received granulocyte transfusions; negative studies may have used relatively low numbers of granulocytes transfused ($<10^{10}/m^2$/day). Granulocyte transfusions are expensive and associated with serious toxicity, including severe febrile reactions, pulmonary capillary leak syndrome, an increased risk of infection, and inevitable alloimmunization. Cytokines offer a strategy for increasing the efficiency of donor harvests. Administration of G-CSF to normal donors greatly increases the yield of leukapheresis without adverse effects on the volunteers. Excellent results can be obtained from community donors, and the use of allocompatible granulocytes (as determined by lymphocytoxicity screening assay) can further improve the clinical results of granulocyte transfusions. Large numbers of neutrophils can be obtained, allowing dramatic increases in the absolute granulocyte levels in neutropenic recipients, which can improve clinical outcomes; case reports and phase I and II studies have suggested that G-CSF (G-CSF plus dexamethasone)–mobilized granulocyte transfusions can be helpful in the treatment of life-threatening fungal infections in severely neutropenic patients.[15]

Definitive Therapy

Hematopoietic Stem Cell Transplantation

Allogeneic BMT from an HLA-matched sibling donor provides curative therapy for AA patients (Tables 28-8 and 28-9).[16]

Bone marrow transplantation in AA is the subject of a large number of reports and reviews. Cytokine-mobilized peripheral blood also has been used successfully as a stem cell graft, but recent studies suggested that mobilized peripheral blood stem cell grafts are associated with a worse outcome.[17]

The first studies of allogeneic BMTs conclusively demonstrated their value compared with conventional supportive therapy. In a controlled trial reported by the International Aplastic Anemia Study Group, patients with severe disease who received transplants early had an actuarial survival rate of more than 60% compared with approximately 20% in patients who received androgens and blood transfusions only. Results with BMT have improved over time because of a combination of factors, including progressive modification of conditioning regimens and lower procedure-related early mortality, improved transfusion support and antibiotic regimens, and the introduction of cyclosporine as prophylactic therapy for GVHD. Analysis of the International Bone Marrow Transplant Registry data showed

Table 28-8 Results of Matched Sibling Donor Allogeneic Marrow Transplantation for Aplastic Anemia

Institution/Study	Years of Study	Patients (*n*)	Age (Median in Years)	Graft Rejection or Failure (%)	Acute GVHD (%)	Chronic GVHD (%)	Actuarial Survival Rate
IBMTR	1988-1992	471	20 (1-51)	16	19	32	66% at 5 years
Vienna	1982-1996	20	25 (17-37)	0	26	53	95% at 15 years
EBMT	1991-1998	71	19 (4-46)	3	30	35	86% at 5 years
Seoul	1990-1999	22	22 (14-43)	5	10	33	95% at 5 years
Seoul	1990-2001	64	28 (14-43)	18	31	19	79% at 6 years
Hamburg	1990-2001	21	25 (7-43)	5	5	5	86% at 5 years
Paris	1994-2001	33	20 (8-42)	6	0	42	94% at 5 years
Sao Paulo	1993-2001	81	24 (3-53)	22	37	39	56% at 6 years
Taipei	1985-2001	79	22 (4-43)	8	7	35	74% at 5 years
Tunis	1998-2001	31	19 (4-39)	16	11	3	86% at 2 years
Seoul	1995-2001	113	28 (16-50)	15	11	12	89% at 6 years
London	1989-2003	33	17 (4-46)	24	14	4	81% at 5 years
Seattle	1988-2004	94	26 (2-59)	4	24	26	88% at 6 years
Mexico City	2000-2005	23	25 (4-65)	26	17	26	88% at 4 years

EBMT, European Group for Bone Marrow Transplant; *GVHD,* graft-versus-host disease; *IBMTR;* International Blood and Marrow Transplant Registry.
GVHD results are generally for grades II–IV and in patient at risk.
Only studies reporting ≥20 patients are tabulated.
In contrast to Table 28-1, response rates are not provided because, in surviving patients who do not experience primary graft rejection or secondary graft failure, full hematologic recovery with donor hematopoiesis is anticipated.

that 5-year survival rates climbed from 48% in the years 1976 to 1980 to 66% in 1988 to 1992. Some hospitals now report very high rates of survival: 89% in Seattle at 8 years, 79% in Baltimore, 89% and 95% at Viennese centers. Registry data indicate lower survival values as the general experience for the same period, with 64% of patients who received transplants during the period of 1985 to 1991 alive at 5 years after the procedure. Between 1990 and 1994, the European Group for Bone Marrow Transplantation (EGBMT) reported a 72% survival rate at 3.5 years. In the latest updates of the EGBMT, the long-term survival had further improved over the past 5 years to 80%.[18]

In the most favorable subgroup—untransfused or minimally transfused young, uninfected patients—survival rates of 80% to 90% should be routinely achieved (see Fig. 28-10). Overall, the survival rates reported from major centers are approximately 70%.

Therapy for Aplastic Anemia

After the diagnosis of acquired AA has been established, treatment options must be identified, considered carefully, and chosen with alacrity (see box on Treatment Algorithm in Aplastic Anemia). For patients with moderate disease (see Table 28-6), an expectant approach can be chosen based on a stable course and adequate blood counts, or for patients dependent on transfusion support, horse ATG (40 mg/kg/day for 4 days) can be given. Intradermal sensitivity testing with 50 ng/mL of ATG solution should be performed, and patients showing an immediate reaction should be desensitized. After assessment of the response, patients who improve should be monitored for hematologic signs of relapse and nonresponders can be offered alternative therapy, such as androgens or cyclosporine. In severe disease for which the prognosis with blood transfusion and antibiotic support alone is very poor, BMT from a histocompatible sibling or immunosuppression are accepted and effective therapies. Although large, retrospective analyses have shown that long-term survival rates from transplantation or immune therapy are equivalent, each has its own advantages and disadvantages. For children, BMT remains the treatment of choice if an appropriate family donor is available because these patients have a low rate of GVHD, and the BM disease is cured by stem cell replacement. The risk of therapy-related cancers can be increased, especially in children, after BMT. Adults with AA also successfully receive transplants, although the risk and severity of chronic GVHD and other treatment-related complications increase with age. BMT has been performed in patients older than 50 years of age, and it is a reasonable approach in a younger adult, especially with more severe degrees of neutropenia.

Most patients with AA do not have an HLA-matched sibling donor, and immunosuppression is the treatment of choice in these cases. Patients with severe disease should receive a combination of ATG and cyclosporine. The authors recommend a regimen consisting of 40 mg/kg/day of horse ATG on days 1 to 4 followed by cyclosporine for 6 months at a dose of 12 mg/kg. Corticosteroids are added in moderate doses (1 mg/kg of prednisone or methylprednisolone) during the first 2 weeks to ameliorate serum sickness. Improvement should be expected within 6 months. This regimen has produced hematologic responses in approximately 70% of treated patients, who then have an excellent 5-year survival rate.

Although immunosuppressive therapy is relatively nontoxic, patients frequently relapse and require further treatment; however, relapse is not associated with a poor prognosis. A more serious problem is the development of late-onset hematologic clonal diseases, PNH (which may not be clinically significant); MDS; and rarely, acute myeloid leukemia. Immunosuppression can be considered ameliorative therapy in which BM destruction may continue and abnormal stem cell clones develop.

For patients in whom immunosuppressive therapy fails, there are a number of options. For children, alternative donor BMT should be seriously considered; at the best centers, survival rates now are almost as good as with sibling donors. Adults do less well, primarily because of transplant-related mortality from the intensive conditioning regimen. Some patients respond to androgen therapy and others to combinations of growth factors. Repeated immunosuppression in a

Table 28-9 Alternative Donor Stem Cell Transplantation for Severe Aplastic Anemia

Study	Year of Publication	Patients (*n*)	Donor Source	Conditioning	Age (Median in Years)	Acute GVHD* (%)	Chronic GVHD (%)	Survival Rate
Nagoya	2001	15	MUD—11 MMUD—4	Cy/ATG/TBI	11 (3-19)	33	13	100% at 4 years
Great Britain	2001	8	MUD—7 MMUD—1	Cy/CP/TBI	7 (0-10)	25	0	100% at 3 years
Japan Marrow Donor Program	2002	154	MUD—79 MMUD—75	Cy ± TBI or LFI; Cy/ATG ± TBI or LFI	17 (1-46)	29	30	56% at 5 years
Memphis	2004	9	MUD—4 MMUD—5	High CD34+ cell dose, TCD, Cy/ATG/TLI or TBI ± thiotepa	11 (6-16)	0	0	89% at 4 years
Gyeonggi-do	2004	5	MUD	Cy/Flu/ATG	13 (7-18)	0	0	80% at 2 years
Guangzhou	2004	6	UCB	Cy/ATG	26 (22-37)	0	33	66% at 2 years
Genova	2005	38	MUD—33 MMRD—5	Cy/Flu/ATG	14 (3-37)	11	24	73% at 2 years
Philadelphia	2005	12	MUD—4 MMUD—8	Partial TCD, TBI + Cy/Ara-C or Cy/TT or ATG	9 (1-20)	33	25	75% at 4 years
Seoul	2005	13	MUD—12 MMUD—1	Cy/ATG	22 (15-34)	31	62	75% at 3 years
IBMTR	2006	318	MUD—181 MMRD—86 MMUD—51	Various	16 (1-55)	48 for MUD	29 for MUD	39% at 5 years for MUD
Seattle	2006	87	MUD—62 MMUD—25	Cy/ATG/TBI	19 (1-53)	70 for MUD	5% for MUD	61% at 5 years for MUD

ATG, Anti-thymocyte globulin; *CP,* Campath; *Cy,* cyclophosphamide; *Flu,* fludarabine; *GVHD,* graft-versus-host disease; *IBMTR,* International Blood and Marrow Transplant Registry; *LFI,* limited field irradiation; *MMRD,* mismatched related donor; *MMUD,* mismatched unrelated donor; *MUD,* matched unrelated donor; *TBI,* total-body irradiation; *TCD,* T-cell depletion; *TLI,* total lymphoid irradiation; *TT,* thiotepa; *UCB,* umbilical cord blood.
*GVHD results are generally for grades II-IV and in patient at risk.
Only studies reporting ≥5 patients are tabulated.

patient in whom a first course of ATG and cyclosporine has failed is successful in about 30% of cases. High-dose cyclophosphamide can also be effective therapy for AA at presentation and in patients who are refractory to ATG.

Patients with severe AA should not be subjected to useless early trials of corticosteroids or hematopoietic growth factors as the primary treatment. For the occasional patient who must decide between BMT and immunosuppression, the advice of experts familiar with this disease and careful counseling of the patient are advisable. Age and severity of neutropenia are decisive factors. A limited number of transfusions can be necessary to optimize the patient's condition before definitive therapy and are acceptable. Single-donor platelets should be given and can be obtained from HLA-compatible donors. In severely neutropenic patients, G-CSF therapy can decrease the risk of life-threatening infections.

Graft rejection and GVHD are the major complications of allogeneic transplantation in AA. Graft rejection is a major predictor of posttransplantation survival. The rate of graft rejection decreased with intensification of the immunosuppressive conditioning regimen from 15% to 4% in Europe and from 35% to between 10% and 15% in Seattle and has remained stable in the past decade. Graft rejection can be caused by the pathophysiology of AA, a finding supported by the unexpectedly high proportion of failures in unprepared patients receiving syngeneic transplants and even in adequately preconditioned patients receiving syngeneic transplants. In a group of untransfused patients who received allogeneic stem cells, the incidence of graft rejection was 10%, indicating that AA patients may be particularly sensitive to alloimmunization. Nevertheless, the influence of the number of transfusions on graft rejection is relative, and modest numbers of blood donations (40 units in the International Bone Marrow Transplant Registry experience and less than 10 units of erythrocytes or 40 units of platelets in Seattle) did not greatly increase the risk of graft rejection.[19]

Matched Sibling Donor (Hematopoietic Stem Cell Transplantation [see Table 28-8])

Intensification of immunosuppressive conditioning regimens with the use of total-body or lymphoid irradiation, cyclosporine, or ATG reduces the risk of graft rejection. Such measures, however, have not been shown to influence long-term survival.[16] The effect of the conditioning program on graft rejection probably is achieved through elimination of the recipient's lymphocytes and of subsequent mixed hematologic chimerism, which is associated with rejection. More rapid regeneration of BM grafts has been observed when cyclosporine was used, and second transplantations have been successful when ATG was added to the conditioning regimen. The effect of ATG or cyclosporine in the conditioning regimen on the rate of graft rejection has been tested in randomized studies. Conditioning regimens that do not include irradiation now regularly achieve engraftment and avoid many of irradiation's long-term complications, especially late cancers. In patients who were prepared by cyclophosphamide plus ATG, sustained engraftment can be achieved by more than 90%, and patients who reject the graft can still be successfully retransplanted. The combination of cyclophosphamide plus fludarabine, with or without ATG, has achieved high rates of graft acceptance and survival even in heavily transfused patients who are transplanted with mobilized peripheral blood stem cells, months after proving refractory to immunosuppressive drugs. The use of methotrexate and cyclosporine has not improved rates of GVHD compared with cyclosporine, but surprisingly, methotrexate was associated with a better survival rate for patients with AA transplanted from matched sibling donors.[20] Overall, the reported rejection rates range between 10% and 15%, account for 14% of deaths in the first 100 days after transplantation and 23% of deaths thereafter.

Rates of chronic GVHD vary and are related to patient selection and treatment regimens. Historically, age was the major risk factor for the development of chronic GVHD. The incidence of chronic GVHD ranged from 19% to 90% for patients between 0 and 10 years and older than 31 years in an older Seattle series. With improved treatment regimens, patients have fared better, but additional studies have confirmed a higher incidence and more serious consequences of GVHD in older patients. Children have a lower probability of suffering and dying from chronic GVHD. In an EGBMT analysis, a significant survival difference was observed between those younger than 20 years of age (65%) and those older than 20 years of age (56%), but there was no survival difference between patients 21 to 30 years old and those 31 to 55 years old. Young adults have fared better in other series, although morbidity from severe GVHD disease was far more prevalent in the young adults than in children (43% vs. 10%). Overall, the acute GVHD rate between 1991 and 1997 was approximately 20% for patients younger than 20 years of age and 40% for those older than 40 years of age. In general, similar numbers were cited for chronic GVHD.[16]

In summary, excellent survival rates and low morbidity in younger patients make allogeneic BMT the treatment of choice for children and adolescents. Older adults have a higher risk of transplant-related morbidity and mortality. Younger adults have a good opportunity for cure with transplantation but face more complications than children. In addition to age, a prolonged interval between diagnosis and transplantation, multiple transfusions, and serious infections before transplantation are poor risk factors.

Matched Unrelated and Nonhistocompatible Family Donors (see Table 28-9)

Until recently, the lack of an HLA genotypically identical sibling donor has precluded BMT, excluding approximately 70% of patients with AA from access to this therapeutic option. Alternative potential donors include relatives who are phenotypically matched or partially matched and HLA phenotypically matched but unrelated volunteers. Although phenotypically identical family donors are occasionally available, mismatched family members and matched but unrelated donors represent a much larger pool.

Haplotype sharing between parents occasionally has allowed identification and successful transplantation between phenotypically matched relatives. Long-term survival after even one-locus-mismatched family donation is inferior to genotypically matched transplants, mainly because of graft rejection and GVHD. In the large European experience, for phenotypically identical family matches, the actuarial survival rate was 45%; for patients with a single-locus mismatch, it was 25%; and for those with two to three loci mismatched, the survival rate was 11%. In a report from Seattle, although all patients who received fully HLA-matched transplants survived, those with mismatches at one or more loci had a much poorer outcome, and even with total-body irradiation added to the conditioning regimen, the survival rate was only 50%. Most large studies of unrelated donors have shown inferior long-term survival and higher rates of complications such as graft rejection, GVHD, and delayed immune system reconstitution. Even more than in standard sibling transplants, age is a crucial risk factor in unrelated transplants and probably more important than the level of match, conditioning regimen, or use of T-cell depletion. For patients with AA who received unrelated transplants and who were enrolled in the National Marrow Donor Program, the survival rate at 2 years was 29%. In the EGBMT's 1994 report, the survival rate for 110 recipients of BM grafts from other than a matched sibling was 34%, approximately half of the rate of standard transplantation. Superior results were obtained at Children's Hospital in Milwaukee, where T-cell depletion of the donor graft was combined with a rigorous conditioning program of cytosine arabinoside, cyclophosphamide, and TBI. For 28 transfused and previously treated children with severe AA, a survival of 54% was reported at a median follow-up of almost 3 years, with no incidence of chronic GVHD. Similar results have been reported in a series of 154 transplantations performed in patients between the ages of 1 and 46 years of age (median, 17 years of age), with delayed transplantation (>3 years after diagnosis), HLA-A or HLA-B mismatch, and age being poor risk factors. In a meta-analysis, for fully matched, unrelated recipients, the survival rate was 25% to 50%, with rates of graft failure and GVHD of 0% to 50% and 28% to 100%, respectively. The degree of match clearly impacts the outcome of the unrelated BMT. As shown in the recent study with mismatched related and unrelated transplantation, the survival was highly related upon degree of mismatch with survivals of 49%, 30%, 39%, and 36% for after 1-antigen mismatched related donor, more than 1-antigen mismatched related donor, matched unrelated donor and mismatched unrelated donor transplants, respectively.[21]

Retrospective analysis of 71 AA patients treated with umbilical cord transplantation showed the estimated probability of 3-year overall survival of 38% (median follow-up, 35 months); the cell dose appeared to be the most important factor impacting survival.[22]

Despite progress, matched but unrelated transplantation is associated with a high mortality rate, and perhaps refractory, high-risk patients are therefore often selected for this procedure. It is likely the poor results may be a consequence of this referral bias. However, alternative-donor transplantation is feasible; the rare phenotypic match from within the family may be equivalent to a sibling donor, but with other family members or unrelated donors, there is a high risk of transplantation-related mortality. Because unrelated-donor transplantation takes months to arrange, it should be considered early. At the best centers, alternative-donor transplantation represents an option, especially for the young patient with very severe pancytopenia in whom immunosuppressive therapy has failed. In Japan, an unrelated but matched transplant has been reported to produce better results in refractory pediatric cases when used early rather than after repeated courses of immunosuppression. In an analysis from Seattle, patients who failed one or more courses of immunosuppression had an overall survival rate of 36% at 3 years.

Late Complications of Bone Marrow Transplantation

Recent study analyzing outcomes of children with AA over the 4 decades indicates that the majority of long-term survivors after transplantation during childhood can have normal, productive lives, with a 30-year survival rate of 82%.[23]

Very late complications after transplantation include effects on growth and development, as well as on the function of endocrine, neurologic, and other organ systems. A high rate of secondary malignancies has been recorded after transplantation. In a National Cancer Institute retrospective analysis of almost 20,000 transplantations, the risk of late-onset cancer was eightfold higher at 10 years than in the general population and even higher for young patients, for whom the risk of malignancy was increased approximately 40-fold. Multivariate analysis suggested that high-dose radiation was a risk factor for the development of malignancies. For AA, among 320 patients who received transplants in Seattle, 4 developed cancer, leading to a calculated risk seven times higher than for normal control participants. In a recent update, 12% of patients who survived more than 2 years after transplantation developed solid tumors. In a French survey, 4 of 147 AA patients developed solid tumors, an 8-year cumulative incidence rate of 22%. In an analysis of 700 transplantation patients with AA and FA, the risk of developing a secondary malignancy was 14% at 20 years. The hazard of lymphoid malignancies decreased with the time after transplantation, but the risk of solid tumors progressively increased. Secondary solid cancers developed in the radiation fields of 5 of 147 AA patients whose conditioning regimens included irradiation of the thorax and abdomen. In general, the rates of secondary malignancies after BMT for AA and other diseases are similar. Immune events such as acute GVHD, treatment with ATG or monoclonal antibodies, and irradiation have been related to the development of secondary malignancies. Patients with these secondary cancers have a poor prognosis. The risk of cancer after BMT must be evaluated in the context of other therapeutic options, especially immunosuppression, because a significant risk of late malignancy exists in AA patients independent of transplantation therapy. The risk of malignancy in the large registry of the EGBMT was equivalent for patients who received immunosuppression and those who underwent transplantation. Compared with the general European population, the relative risk of malignancy was calculated at 5.15 for AA patients treated with immunosuppression (confidence interval [CI], 3.26-7.94) and at 6.67 (CI, 3.05-12.65) for patients receiving transplants. Overall, the rate of malignancy after BMT has been calculated to be 3.8-fold higher than in the age-matched population.

Immunosuppression

Antithymocyte Globulins

Immunosuppressive therapy is an effective alternative treatment for patients who are not candidates for BMT (Table 28-10 and see box on Treatment Algorithm in Aplastic Anemia).[2]

Immunoglobulin preparations made from the sera of horses immunized against human thymocytes are the mainstays of current regimens. Horse ATG is licensed for use in the United States as ATGAM (Pfizer) and SAA is an approved indication. Thymoglobulin (Genzyme), a rabbit ATG, is more available worldwide.

The efficacy of antilymphocyte globulin (ALG) in BM failure was discovered serendipitously in the late 1960s, when Mathé observed recovery of autologous hematopoietic function in patients who received antilymphocyte serum as conditioning for BMT. Observations and formal studies in Europe showed that 40% to 70% of patients responded with hematologic improvement and improved survival. Similar results were also obtained in American randomized and multicenter protocols in which about half of patients treated with ATG or ALG show hematologic improvement, broadly defined as an end to transfusion dependence and an improvement in a neutrophil number to a level protective against infection.

Table 28-10 Intensive Immunosuppression in Severe Aplastic Anemia

Study	Patients (*n*)	Median Age (Years)	Response (%)	Relapse (%)	Clonal Evolution (%)	Survival Rate
German	84	32	65	19	8	58% at 11 years
EGMBT	100	16	77	12	11	87% at 5 years
NIH	122	35	61	35	11	55% at 7 years
Japan*	119	9	68	22	6	88% at 3 years
NIH†	104	30	62	37	9	80% at 4 years

*With androgens and ± granulocyte colony-stimulating factor.
†With mycophenolate mofetil.
Only studies of more than 20 enrolled patients are tabulated. Responses to immunosuppressive therapy are usually partial; blood counts may not become normal, but transfusions are no longer required, and the neutrophil count is adequate to prevent infection. Relapse is usually responsive to further immunosuppressive therapies. Clonal evolution is to dysplastic bone marrow changes or cytogenetic abnormalities. For details, see accompanying text.

The putative cause of AA is not a factor that predicts response. Virus- and drug-induced aplasia and posthepatitis AA respond similarly compared with idiopathic disease. Cytogenetic abnormalities do not preclude a response because AA with chromosome abnormalities and some cases of frank myelodysplasia improve after ATG. The response rate to ATG or ALG is not improved by the addition of androgens or very high doses of corticosteroids.

A hematologic response to ATG is usually apparent within a few months of therapy; in some cases, all blood counts rise dramatically, but in others, increases in platelets or RBCs can be delayed (see box on Treatment Algorithm in Aplastic Anemia). The average time to improvement in neutrophil number is 1 to 2 months; transfusion independence occurs approximately 2 to 3 months after initiation of treatment. Continued improvement without further therapy commonly occurs after 3 months; nevertheless, clinical status by 3 months is strongly correlated with long-term survival. Blood cell counts above the critical values for severity and platelets and reticulocyte counts of more than 50,000 cells/μL are highly prognostic. Patient selection is important; in general, survival correlates with disease severity. However, in most recent series, reticulocyte count, perhaps reflecting the stem cell reserve, has been the best predictor of response and survival.[24] With new and better tolerated antifungal drugs, survival even of nonresponders has improved, and a very low neutrophil count may no longer have prognostic value.

Antithymocyte globulin has three major toxic effects: immediate allergic phenomena, serum sickness, and transient blood cell count depression (Fig. 28-11). Fever, rigors, and an urticarial cutaneous eruption are common on the first or second day of ATG therapy, and these symptoms respond to antihistamines and meperidine therapy. Anaphylaxis is rare but can be fatal. A positive immediate wheal-and-flare reaction to the cutaneous application of 50 mg/mL of stock solution of horse ATG can be predictive of massive histamine release on systemic infusion, and desensitization with gradually increasing doses of horse ATG administered intradermally, subcutaneously, and then intravenously has permitted use in allergic individuals. Corticosteroids are administered in moderate doses (1 mg/kg of prednisone or methylprednisolone) during the first 2 weeks to ameliorate the symptoms of serum sickness. Doses of ATG and ALG have varied from 5 to 50 mg/kg, and the duration of administration has varied from 4 to 28 days. It is more rational to administer equivalent doses of horse ATG by the schedule originally used in Europe (40 mg/kg/day for 4 days); antiserum will then have reached low levels in the circulation by the time host antibody appears. A short course of therapy is easier to administer, associated with less serum sickness, and equally effective as the same dose given over a more prolonged course. Thymoglobulin, rabbit ATG, has been approved for use in the United States. Although rabbit ATG is more potent by weight than horse ATG, a recent randomized trial showed it markedly inferior to horse ATG in achieving hematologic response, and survival was poorer as well.[25]

Antilymphocyte globulins are immunosuppressive. ATGs contain a heterogeneous mix of antibody specificities for lymphocytes, including reactivity to antigens such as CD2, CD3, CD4, CD8, CD25 (the receptor for IL-2), and HLA-DR. Horse sera fix human complement efficiently, and all preparations are T-cell cytotoxic in vitro, with little difference among ATGs or among lots for lymphocyte killing in vitro. In vitro, ALGs efficiently inhibit T-cell proliferation and block IL-2 and IFN-γ production, and IL-2 receptor expression ATG induces Fas-mediated apoptosis of T cells, especially after activation. In patients, the administration of ATG results in rapid reduction in the number of circulating lymphocytes, usually to less than 10% of starting values, and lymphocytopenia persists for several days after discontinuing therapy. Although lymphocyte numbers return to pretreatment values by 3 months, reductions in activated lymphocyte numbers in recovered patients persist. It seems likely that these inhibitory effects on T cells are responsible for the efficacy of ALGs in AA. Nevertheless, the ability of ATG to stimulate lymphocyte function by acting as a mitogen may also have a role in their therapeutic efficacy. Notably, rabbit ATG can stimulate regulatory T cell development in vitro and in patients, although this effect in AA is overwhelmed by rabbit ATG's more potent CD4 cell depletion compared with horse ATG.

Reliable methods to predict which patients will respond to ATG are lacking.

Cyclosporine

Several groups reported anecdotal success with cyclosporine therapy combined with androgens in individual patients with AA, in many of whom other therapies had failed. Some studies suggested efficacy of cyclosporine in patients refractory to ALG or ATG alone, with salvage rates of approximately 50%. The optimal regimen has not been determined. In the United States, cyclosporine has usually been used in high doses (12 mg/kg/day for adults and 15 mg/kg/day for children), with adjustment according to plasma drug concentrations and serum creatinine levels. In Europe, lower doses (3-7 mg/kg/day) have been reported to be equally efficacious. Hematologic improvement can occur in a few weeks or months. A 6-month trial is warranted. Remissions, when achieved, usually have been durable, but some patients relapse when cyclosporine is discontinued. Most patients who relapse will respond to the reinstitution of cyclosporine; the lowest possible dose should be sought by tapering, but some patients may require long-term maintenance treatment.

Cyclosporine has considerable toxicity. Hypertension and azotemia are the most common serious side effects; hirsutism and gingival hypertrophy are also frequent complaints. Increasing serum creatinine levels are an indication for dose reduction. Chronic cyclosporine nephropathy characterized by interstitial fibrosis and tubular atrophy can be irreversible. The risk of nephropathy is increased by high doses and longer durations of therapy and occurs more commonly in older than in younger patients. Cyclosporine, especially in combination with corticosteroids, converts patients with AA to a temporary immunodeficiency state and puts them at high risks for opportunistic infections. Monthly aerosolized pentamidine prophylaxis can prevent *Pneumocystis carinii* pneumonia in patients receiving cyclosporine. Convulsions, possibly related to hypomagnesemia, are another serious complication of cyclosporine therapy.

Combined or Intensive Immunosuppressive Therapy

The combination for the treatment of AA of an agent that lyses lymphocytes (ATG) with a drug that blocks lymphocyte function is

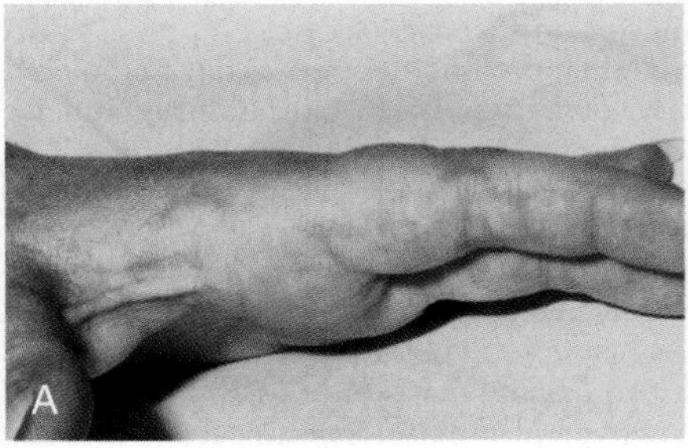

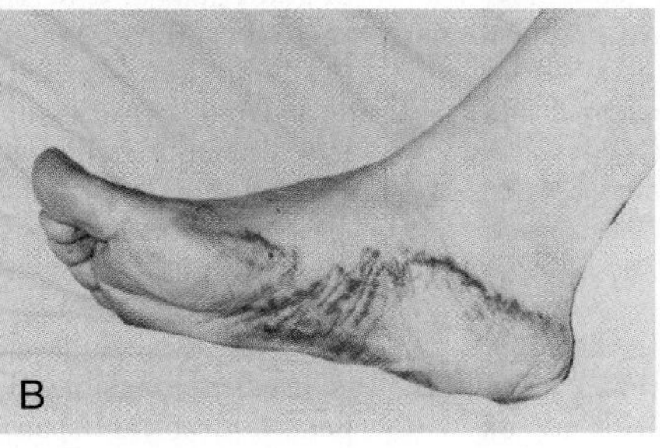

Figure 28-11 CUTANEOUS ERUPTIONS OF SERUM SICKNESS. On the hand **(A)** and on the foot **(B)**.

rational (see Table 28-10). The strategy has resulted in a striking increase in the response rate to immunosuppressive therapy in randomized and multicenter trials, to 60% to 80% at 1 year compared with about 40% with ATG alone; more complete response;, and better 5-year survival rates for responding patients at 80% to 90%. Children do especially well with combined therapy, elderly patients less so, partly because of more toxicity from therapy and poor tolerance of pancytopenia complications in the presence of comorbidities.

In disease refractory to initial therapy with ATG and cyclosporine, a repeat course is often administered as a salvage regimen and can rescue about one-third or more of patients.

Cyclophosphamide

High-dose cyclophosphamide (45-50 mg/kg/day for 4 days) without stem cell rescue can induce hematologic recovery in severe AA, with an overall response rate claimed similar to that achieved with ATG therapy but a higher proportion of complete responses and less relapse and clonal evolution. However, cyclophosphamide severely depresses the neutrophil count, resulting in prolonged hospitalization for suspected or actual infection and a higher risk of invasive fungal infections and death compared with ATG and cyclosporine.

Corticosteroids

Methylprednisolone in modest doses (1 mg/kg/day) is administered with ATG to ameliorate the symptoms of serum sickness. Very-high-dose corticosteroid regimens can be effective, especially in recently diagnosed patients. High-dose methylprednisolone also has been added to ATG therapy, with inconsistent results. However, ATG is associated with better response rates and many fewer associated toxic effects than high-dose steroid therapy, and ATG is generally preferable as initial therapy. Modest doses of corticosteroids do not have roles in the treatment of AA except in combination with ATG. There is little evidence of their effectiveness in reversing BM failure or improving hemostasis, and even limited courses of steroids can contribute to the development of aseptic vascular necrosis and the increase in the rate of fungal infections.

Late Complications of Immunosuppressive Therapy

Relapse after immunosuppressive therapy is common. About one-third or more of responding patients may be expected to require reinstitution of immunosuppressive drugs or another course of ATG. Relapse can manifest as a gradual decline in one blood count, need for transfusion after a period of transfusion independence, or abrupt recurrence of severe pancytopenia. Most relapse responds to retreatment, and there is no clear relationship with worse survival.

A much more serious complication is the development of late-onset clonal hematologic disorders, especially myelodysplasia and AML. Some of these events likely represent part of the natural history of AA. Before recent improvements in treatment, leukemia was considered an unusual complication, but late-onset clonal disorders do not appear to be the result of the introduction of immunosuppressive therapy. In European and National Institutes of Health trials, the overall rate of clonal evolution is 12% to 15% at about 1 decade. Children appear to be at similar risk for the development of clonal complication as adults, and evolution to MDS can occur in responders and in refractory patients. MDS that develops after AA can progress to AML but can also be surprisingly indolent. BM chromosomes are almost always abnormal in clonal evolution, and cytogenetics are predictive. Monosomy 7 is the most frequent finding and confers a poor prognosis; in contrast, patients with trisomy 8 patients often remain responsive to cyclosporine and have good prospects for survival. Trisomy 6 and 13q− also behave benignly in most cases.

A PNH clone can be detected in up to 50% of patients on their presentation. Usually the clone size remains stable, and it may decrease; over time, only a minority of patients develop a large clone and the hemolytic or thrombotic form of PNH.

Immunosuppression Versus Bone Marrow Transplantation

Immunosuppression and transplantation are both effective therapies for AA[2] (Figs. 28-12 and 28-13). Lack of a matched sibling donor; the expense and availability of transplantation; and risk factors such as active infections, advanced age, or a heavy transfusion burden lead most patients to treatment with ATG and cyclosporine. For a few patients with AA, a choice does exist between transplantation and immunosuppressive therapy. BMT offers a permanent cure. Its disadvantages are cost, procedure-related morbidity and mortality (especially GVHD in older patients), and an increased incidence of solid organ malignancies. Immunosuppressive therapy is easier and initially cheaper. However, many patients do not achieve normal blood cell counts and remain at high risk for relapse and the more serious complications of late-onset clonal hematologic disease, especially MDS.

Retrospective analyses of the large number of European patients reported to the EGBMT show consistently improved results with both therapies but have repeatedly failed to demonstrate a survival advantage for transplantation over immunosuppression. Single-center studies are similar. Certain categories of patients, defined by neutrophil number and age, probably benefit from one therapy or the other. In general, BMT yields superior results in children and immunosuppression in older adults.[16]

Remarkable improvements in results using unrelated donors have made this transplant available to many patients who lack a sibling donor. Increasingly, children who have failed a single course of immunosuppression and adults refractory to multiple courses of ATG are offered this procedure.

Androgens

Testosterone and synthetic anabolic steroids appeared to be major advances in the treatment of AA when they were introduced in the 1960s. The high response rates in some early series may be retrospectively attributed to the inclusion of patients with moderate acquired and constitutional AA. For severe AA, controlled trials in general have not demonstrated efficacy, as measured by survival rates or hematologic improvement. When added to immunosuppressive therapies, androgens failed to result in any increase in response rates.

Although BMT or immunosuppressive therapy is generally preferred, certain androgen regimens have their advocates. Androgens continue to be helpful in occasional patients when used as a second-line therapy. Most hematologists have observed patients who appeared to respond or even to develop hormone dependence. Androgen therapy remains popular in developing countries because it is inexpensive, well tolerated, and seemingly effective. Various preparations of androgens in different doses have resulted in similar response rates of 35% to 60% after 6 months of therapy.

Useful androgens include nandrolone decanoate, oxymetholone, and danazol; unfortunately, their popularity and abuse by athletes have led to restrictions of their availability and manufacture. The hemoglobin response frequently is more impressive than improvements in granulocyte or platelet levels. An adequate trial is considered to be a full dose given for at least 3 months. Complications occur infrequently, although some are serious and can limit effective therapy, especially in elderly patients. The associated liver cholestasis is usually reversible. Hepatotoxicity (e.g., bile duct proliferation, peliosis, atypical hepatocyte hyperplasia, tumors) can occur but is less

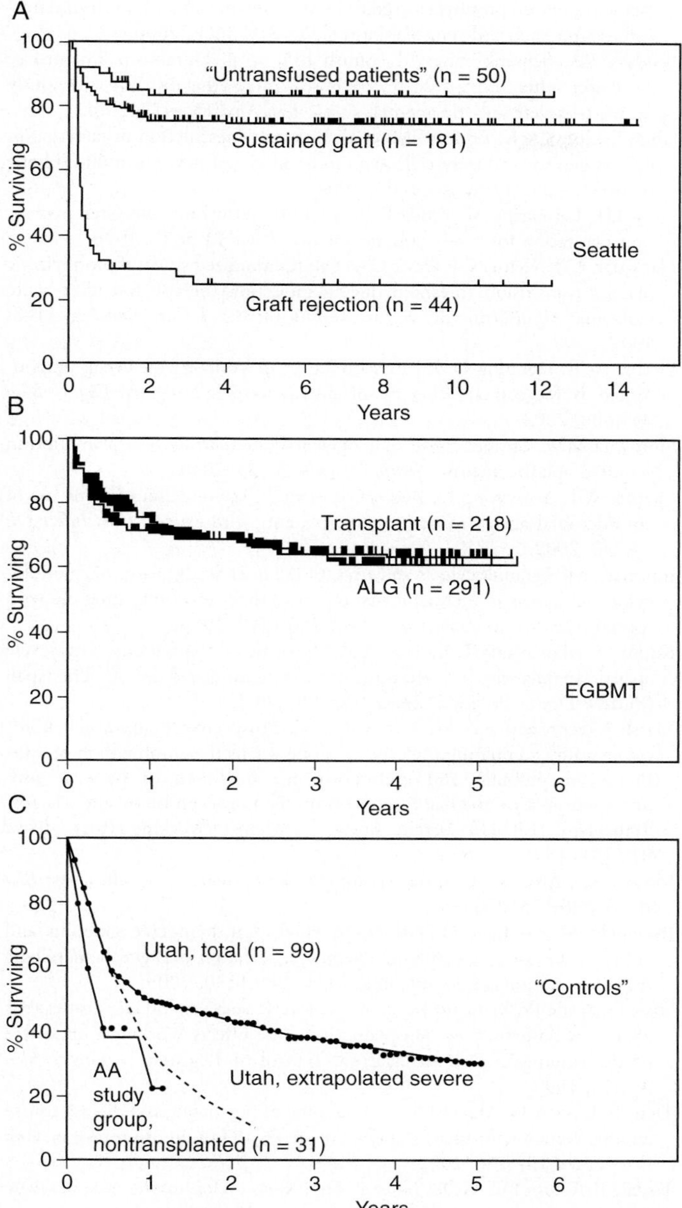

Figure 28-12 ACTUARIAL SURVIVAL RATES FOR PATIENTS WITH APLASTIC ANEMIA (AA). **A,** Data on bone marrow transplantation from the University of Washington. **B,** Data from the European Group for Bone Marrow Transplantation on bone marrow transplantation versus immunosuppression with antilymphocyte globulin (ALG). **C,** Natural history as indicated by survival with supportive and other treatments. Two groups are illustrated. Extrapolated survival curves for patients with severe disease are derived from retrospective reviews from the University of Utah of 101 records collected from the late 1940s to early 1970s. The patients received blood transfusions and, later in this period, also received platelets. Almost all were treated with corticosteroids, and one-half were also treated with androgens. Data for patients who did not receive transplants come from a multicenter study of the efficacy of bone marrow transplantation performed in the early 1970s; this control group was treated with androgens.

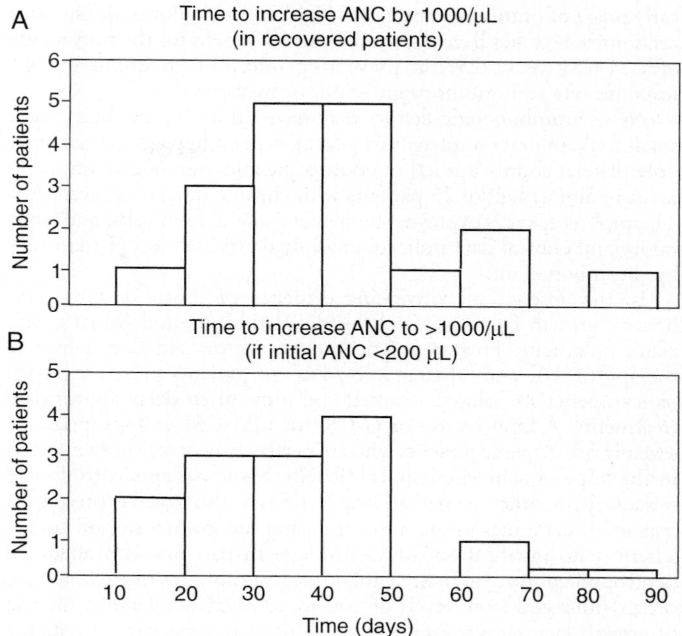

Figure 28-13 TIME TO RESPONSE AFTER TREATMENT WITH ANTILYMPHOCYTE GLOBULIN (ATG). **A,** Distribution of patients with severe aplastic anemia by time to achieve an increase in the absolute neutrophil count (ANC) of 1000 cells/mm^3. **B,** Distribution of patients with an initial ANC of less than 200 cells/mm^3 by time to achieve an ANC of 1000 cells/mm^3.

common with parenteral formulations. Children appear to tolerate high doses of androgens without lasting effects on growth or maturation.

Hematopoietic Growth Factors

Hematopoietic growth factor production is normal or increased in most patients with AA. Nevertheless, many patient are treated with pharmacologic high doses of cytokines, often with uncertain justification. G-CSF and GM-CSF in some cases can increase neutrophil numbers in patients with AA. In general, neutrophil responses to growth factors are transient, dependent on their continuous administration, and usually restricted to patients with less severe AA. Nevertheless, bilineage and trilineage responses have been observed. Children may be more sensitive to the effects of prolonged administration of G-CSF.

A concern has been the possibility that prolonged administration of G-CSF might increase the probability of late clonal disease, especially monosomy 7. In retrospective analyses of Japanese children and adults with severe AA, this syndrome appeared to occur most frequently among patients who had received growth factor; a modest increase in the risk of myelodysplasia and leukemia and monosomy 7 was also seen in European cases. The mechanism of G-CSF's relationship to monosomy may be selection of aneuploid cells bearing an isoform of G-CSF; these cells are less sensitive to G-CSF, but when triggered by the cytokine, they proliferate and do not differentiate.

Anemia and pancytopenia in rare patients have responded to prolonged administration of high doses of erythropoietin alone, GM-CSF and erythropoietin, and with IL-3 and G-CSF. In one randomized protocol, the combination of G-CSF and high doses of erythropoietin improved hemoglobin values, mainly in patients with moderate disease.

Growth factors have also been combined with definitive medical therapy for the purpose of improving neutrophil counts during the early phase of immunosuppression. Neither small pilot trials nor large randomized studies have shown substantial benefit for the routine use of GM-CSF or G-CSF, in preventing infection, in improving the response rate to immunosuppression, or in survival.

New thrombopoietic factors may have utility in AA. In a recent small trial, an oral c-mpl agonist peptide, eltrombopag, increased not only platelet counts but led to erythrocyte and granulocyte improvement in almost half of 25 patients with chronic refractory severe AA. The mpl receptor is expressed by hematopoietic stem cells, and laboratory and clinical data indicate physiologic stimulation of stem cells by thrombopoietin.

In the absence of convincing evidence of short- or long-term benefit, growth factor use in AA is dictated by the individual physician's judgment. Hematopoietic growth factors are not definitive therapy of AA, and "therapeutic trials" in patients presenting with pancytopenia are seldom justified and most often delay appropriate treatments. A brief course of G-CSF or GM-CSF is appropriate in severely neutropenic patients who are persistently or seriously infected in the hope of achieving clinical benefit. Some patients with disease refractory to other forms of treatment can also receive prolonged courses of cytokines in the hope of raising the low neutrophil count. There is no justification for G-CSF use in patients with adequate neutrophil counts, yet many patients inexplicably are treated increase the granulocytes from levels of 500 to 1000/μL. Preferably, the use of growth factors over long treatment periods, especially in patients who are not severely neutropenic, should be in the context of a formal study. Physicians and patients should be aware of possibly significant risks associated with such treatment.

PROGNOSIS

The initial blood cell counts of a patient with AA are important indicators of prognosis. The popular "Camitta" criteria used to define severe disease are the presence of two of the following three: neutrophil count of less than 500 cells/μL, platelet count of less than 20,000 cells/μL, and corrected reticulocyte level of less than 1% (<40,000 cells/μL). In the more modern era, absolute reticulocytes (>25,000/μL) and absolute lymphocytes predicted good response to immunosuppression and survival.[26] The robustness of the platelet and reticulocyte response after immunosuppression also correlates with long-term survival. Clonal evolution, especially monosomy 7, is a poor prognostic factor, and age-adjusted telomere length of leukocytes at diagnosis may predict this serious complication.[27]

The rate of spontaneous recovery is difficult to estimate, but most observers believe it to be low. Untreated severe disease is almost invariably fatal. In contrast, moderate AA has a good prognosis, and some patients with minimal blood cell count depression recover normal blood cell counts with limited or no therapy.

SUGGESTED READINGS

Adkins DR, Goodnough LT, Shenoy S, et al: Effect of leukocyte compatibility on neutrophil increment after transfusion of granulocyte colony-stimulating factor-mobilized prophylactic granulocyte transfusions and on clinical outcomes after stem cell transplantation. *Blood* 95:3605, 2000.

Brodsky RA, Sensenbrenner LL, Smith BD, et al: Durable treatment-free remission after high-dose cyclophosphamide therapy for previously untreated severe aplastic anemia. *Ann Intern Med* 135:477, 2001.

Chen J, Lipovsky K, Ellison FM, et al: Bystander destruction of hematopoietic progenitor and stem cells in a mouse model of infusion-induced bone marrow failure. *Blood* 104:1671, 2004.

Deeg HJ, Leisenring W, Storb R, et al: Long-term outcome after marrow transplantation for severe aplastic anemia. *Blood* 91:3637, 1998.

Heckman KD, Weiner GJ, Davis CS, et al: Randomized study of prophylactic platelet transfusion threshold during induction therapy for adult acute leukemia: 10,000/microL versus 20,000/microL. *J Clin Oncol* 15:1143, 1997.

Herbrecht R, Denning DW, Patterson TF, et al: Voriconazole versus amphotericin B for primary therapy of invasive aspergillosis. *N Engl J Med* 347:408, 2002.

Horowitz MM: Current status of allogeneic bone marrow transplantation in acquired aplastic anemia. *Semin Hematol* 37:30, 2000.

Hughes WT, Armstrong D, Bodey GP, et al: 2002 Guidelines for the use of antimicrobial agents in neutropenic patients with cancer. *Clin Infect Dis* 34:730, 2002.

International Agranulocytosis and Aplastic Anemia Study: Risks of agranulocytosis and aplastic anemia: A first report of their relation to drug use with special reference to analgesics. *JAMA* 256:1749, 1986.

Kojima S, Matsuyama T, Kato S, et al: Outcome of 154 patients with severe aplastic anemia who received transplants from unrelated donors: The Japan Marrow Donor Program. *Blood* 100:799, 2002.

Marsh J, Schrezenmeier H, Marin P, et al: Prospective randomized multicenter study comparing cyclosporin alone versus the combination of antithymocyte globulin and cyclosporin for treatment of patients with nonsevere aplastic anemia: A report from the European Blood and Marrow Transplant (EBMT) Severe Aplastic Anaemia Working Party. *Blood* 93:2191, 1999.

Morgan GJ, Alveres CL: Benzene and the hemopoietic stem cell. *Chem Biol Interact* 30:153, 2005.

Rosenfeld SJ, Follman D, Nunez O, et al: Antithymocyte globulin and cyclosporine for severe aplastic anemia. Association between hematologic response and long-term outcome. *JAMA* 289:1130, 2003.

Socie G, Stone JV, Wingard JR, et al: Long-term survival and late deaths after allogeneic bone marrow transplantation. Late Effects Working Committee of the International Bone Marrow Transplant Registry. *N Engl J Med* 341:14, 1999.

Tichelli A, Socie G, Marsh J, et al: Outcome of pregnancy and disease course among women with aplastic anemia treated with immunosuppression. *Ann Intern Med* 137:164, 2002.

Tisdale JF, Dunn DE, Geller N, et al: High-dose cyclophosphamide in severe aplastic anaemia: A randomised trial. *Lancet* 356:1554, 2000.

Walsh TJ, Teppler H, Donowitz GR, et al: Caspofungin versus liposomal amphotericin B for empirical antifungal therapy in patients with persistent fever and neutropenia. *N Engl J Med* 351:1391, 2004.

Young NS, Calado R, Scheinberg P: Current concepts in the pathophysiology and treatment of aplastic anemia. *Blood* 108:2511, 2006.

For complete list of references log on to www.expertconsult.com

CHAPTER 29

PAROXYSMAL NOCTURNAL HEMOGLOBINURIA

Robert A. Brodsky

Paroxysmal nocturnal hemoglobinuria (PNH) is a clonal hematopoietic stem cell disorder that has fascinated hematologists for more than a century because of its protean clinical manifestations and captivating pathophysiology. One of the earliest descriptions of PNH was by Dr. Paul Strübing, who in 1882 described a 29-year-old Cartwright who presented with fatigue, abdominal pain, and severe nocturnal paroxysms of hemoglobinuria that were exacerbated by excess alcohol, physical exertion, and iron salts.[1] Strübing deduced that the hemolysis was occurring intravascularly as the patient's plasma turned red after severe attacks of hemoglobinuria. Decades later, his prescient deduction was confirmed. Later reports by Marchiafava and Micheli led to the eponym Marchiafava-Micheli syndrome, but it was Enneking, in 1925, who introduced the term *paroxysmal nocturnal hemoglobinuria*.

In 1937, Thomas Ham found that PNH erythrocytes were hemolyzed when incubated with normal, acidified serum. This seminal discovery resulted in the first diagnostic test for PNH, the acidified serum or Ham test. The cell lysis after acidified serum appeared to be complement dependent because heat inactivation abrogated the reaction; however, it was not until 1954, with the discovery of the alternative pathway of complement activation, that complement was formally proven to cause the hemolysis of PNH red blood cells (RBCs). After the emergence of specific diagnostic tests, additional disease manifestations such as venous thrombosis, bone marrow (BM) failure, and development of myelodysplastic syndromes (MDS) and acute leukemia were associated with PNH. These nonerythroid manifestations of the disease foreshadowed the discovery that PNH results from the clonal expansion of a mutated hematopoietic stem cell (HSC).

In the 1980s, roughly 100 years after Strübing's initial description of the disease, it was discovered that PNH cells display a global deficiency in a group of proteins affixed to the cell surface by a glycosylphosphatidylinositol (GPI) anchor. Interestingly, several of the missing proteins (e.g., CD55 and CD59) are important complement regulatory proteins. A few years later, the genetic mutation *(PIGA)* responsible for the GPI-anchor protein deficiency was discovered,[1,2] and most recently, a humanized monoclonal antibody that inhibits terminal complement activation has been shown to ameliorate hemolysis and disease symptoms in PNH patients.[3] Although the pathophysiology of many of PNH's clinical manifestations are now understood, the mechanism of thrombosis, the mechanism of clonal dominance, and the close association with aplastic anemia continue to be subjects of intense investigation. PNH is an extremely rare condition; however, the risk for developing PNH in patients with acquired aplastic anemia is 20% to 30%. In addition, more than half of patients with acquired aplastic anemia harbor a small- to moderate-sized PNH population at diagnosis.

PATHOPHYSIOLOGY

The Glycosylphosphatidylinositol Anchor

Covalent linkage to GPI is an important means of anchoring many cell-surface glycoproteins to the cell membrane. Alkaline phosphatase was the first GPI-anchor protein recognized after it was discovered that cell surface alkaline phosphatase could be removed by a bacterial enzyme, phosphatidylinositol-specific phospholipase C (PIPLC). PIPLC cleaved the phosphate from phosphatidylinositol (PI) and left the enzyme with full activity after its release, suggesting that the protein structure was unperturbed. This fundamental observation led to the discovery of dozens of GPI-anchored proteins.

The GPI anchor consists of a highly conserved glycan core (ethanoloamine-*P*-6Manα1-2Manα1-6Manα1-4GlcN) linked to the 6-position of the D-*myo*-inositol ring of PI (Fig. 29-1). The anchor is synthesized in the endoplasmic reticulum membrane and involves at least 10 reactions and more than 20 different genes (Table 29-1). The first step in GPI anchor biosynthesis is the transfer of *N*-acetylglucosamine (GlcNAc) from uridine diphosphate (UDP)-GlcNAc to PI to yield GlcNAc-PI. This step is catalyzed by GlcNAc-PI α1-6 GlcNAc transferase, an enzyme whose subunits are encoded by seven different genes: *PIGA, PIGC, PIGH, GPI1, PIGY, PIGP,* and *DPM2.* In the second step, GlcNAc-PI is deacetylated by the gene product of *PIGL* to form glucosamine (GlcN)-PI. GPI anchor assembly continues in the endoplasmic reticulum with acylation of the inositol and stepwise addition of mannosyl and phosphoethanolamine residues. The preassembled GPI is linked to nascent proteins that contain a C-terminal GPI-attachment signal peptide, displacing it in a transamidase reaction. The GPI-anchored protein then transits the secretory pathway to reach its final destination at the plasma membrane in compartments known as *lipid rafts.* If the GPI anchor is not attached to the protein, it is degraded intracellularly, probably in lysosomes.

Given the numerous gene products involved in GPI anchor assembly, it seemed improbable that PNH would be the consequence of a single genetic mutation. However, after intense scrutiny of this pathway, it became apparent that in all PNH cases, the defect could be attributed to mutations in the *PIGA* gene, whose product is essential for the first step of GPI anchor biosynthesis. Later it was determined that the *PIGA* gene is on the X chromosome and that its product is part of a complex that transfers *N*-acetylglucosamine to PI to form GlcNAc-PI. Thus, a single "hit" will generate a PNH phenotype because males have only one X chromosome, and in females, one X chromosome is inactivated through lyonization. Conceivably, a mutation in any one of the genes in this pathway would cause the disease; however, other genes involved in GPI anchor biosynthesis are located on autosomes (see Table 29-1). Inactivating mutations in these genes would have to occur on both alleles to produce the PNH phenotype. Congenital *PIG-A* mutations resulting in an absence of GPI anchored proteins are embryonic lethal; however, germline mutations have been described in mannosyltransferases in the GPI pathway. A *PIGM* promoter mutation causing reduced GPI-linked protein expression was described in two consanguineous families. Individuals presented with portal and hepatic vein thrombosis and persistent seizures. Missense *PIGV* mutations cause hyperphosphatasia mental retardation syndrome (HPMR).

Acetylcholinesterase from erythrocytes and alkaline phosphatase from leukocytes were the first GPI-anchored proteins shown to be missing in PNH. Since then, more than a dozen GPI-anchored proteins with heterogeneous expression on hematopoietic cells have been found to be missing in PNH (Table 29-2). The functions of these cell surface GPI-anchored proteins are manifold; they can serve as

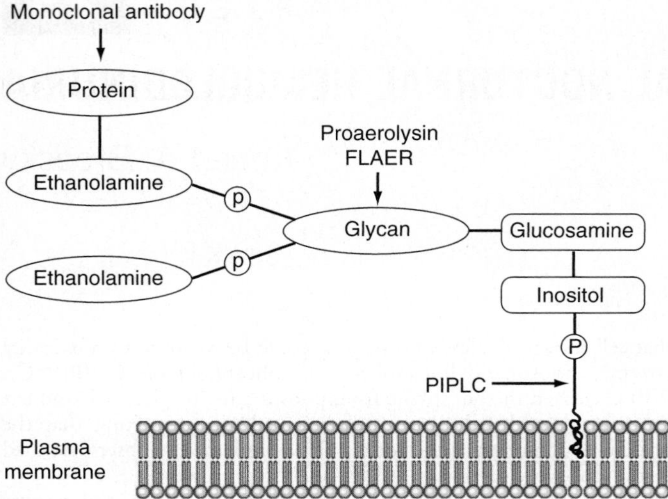

Figure 29-1 STRUCTURE OF THE GLYCOSYLPHOSPHATIDYLINOSITOL (GPI) ANCHOR. Phosphatidylinositol is inserted into the lipid bilayer of the plasma membrane. The glycan core, which serves as the binding site for aerolysin, proaerolysin, and FLAER, consists of a molecule of *N*-glucosamine, three molecules of mannose, and one molecule of ethanolamine. The representative protein (e.g., CD55, CD59, and so on) is covalently attached through an amide bond to an ethanolamine on the terminal mannose. Individual monoclonal antibodies used for the diagnosis of PNH (e.g., CD55, CD59, and so on) bind to the protein but not the GPI anchor. Phosphatidylinositol-specific phospholipase C (PIPLC) cleaves the phosphate from phosphatidylinositol and leaves the enzyme with full activity after its release *P,* Phosphate.

complement regulatory proteins, enzymes, blood group antigens, receptors, and adhesion molecules. Membrane inhibitor of reactive lysis (CD59) and decay accelerating factor (CD55)—both complement regulatory proteins—are the most widely expressed GPI-anchored proteins and can be found on all hematopoietic lineages, including $CD34^+CD38^-$ progenitor cells.[4] Certain proteins, CD58 (LFA3) and CD16 (FcγRIII), may exist in both GPI-linked and transmembrane forms.

Table 29-1 Genes Involved in Glycosylphosphatidylinositol Anchor Biosynthesis

Number	Gene	Location
1	*PIG-A**	Xp22.1
2	*PIG-C**	1q23.3
3	*PIG-H**	14q11-q24
4	*PIG-P**	21q22.2
5	*GPI1 (PIG-Q)**	16p13.3
6	*PIG-L*	17p12
7	*PIG-M*	1q22
8	*PIG-N*	18q21
9	*PIG-B*	15q21-q22
10	*PIG-F*	2q16-p21
11	*PIG-O*	9
12	*GPI8 (PIG-K)*†	1p22.2-p22.3
13	*GAA1 (GPAA1)*†	8q24.3
14	*PIG-S*†	17
15	*PIG-T*†	20q12-q13
16	*DPM1*	20q13.1
17	*DPM2*	9q33
18	*DPM3*	1q21.2
19	*SL15 (MPDU1)*	17p13.1
20	*PIG-U*†	20q11
21	*PIG-V*	1p36.11
22	*PIG-W*	17p12
23	*PIG-X*	3q29
24	*PIG-Y**	4q21

GPI, Glycosylphosphatidylinositol.
*Genes involved in the first step of GPI anchor biosynthesis.
†Genes involved in the transamidase reaction.

PIGA Gene

Investigators in Osaka, Japan, first identified the gene that was defective in PNH.[5] The gene was isolated by expression cloning and named *PIGA* (phosphatidylinositol–glycan complementation class A). *PIGA* was then cloned into an expression vector and transfected into GPI-deficient cell lines derived from PNH patients; cell surface expression of all the missing GPI-anchored proteins was restored, confirming that *PIGA* mutations are responsible for causing PNH. Since this seminal discovery, somatic mutations of the *PIGA* gene have been found in all PNH patients to date. Little to no GPI anchor is made when the *PIGA* gene is mutated. Consequently, the translated protein (e.g., CD59, CD55, and so on) residing in the cisterna of the endoplasmic reticulum cannot be attached to the GPI anchor and is degraded in situ.

The human *PIGA* gene contains 6 exons and 5 introns and extends over 17 kb (Fig. 29-2); it encodes for a protein that contains 484 amino acids (60 kd). In humans, a single copy of the gene is located on the short arm of the X chromosome (Xp22.1), although an intronless pseudogene has been found on chromosome 12q21. A wide range of somatic mutations interspersed throughout the entire coding region of the *PIGA* gene have been described in PNH patients. There are no true mutational "hot spots," although exon 2, which contains almost half of the coding region, is the exon where most mutations occur. Most *PIGA* mutations are small insertions or deletions, usually one or two base pairs, which result in a frameshift in the coding region and consequently a shortened, nonfunctional product. Although *PIGA* function is abolished by these frameshift mutations, missense mutations, where the product of the mutated *PIGA* gene has some residual activity, have also been described. In most patients studied, a single (monoclonal) *PIGA* mutation has been discovered. However, two different mutations (biclonal)—and in one case, four separate *PIGA* mutations—have been found in PNH patients.

Paroxysmal Nocturnal Hemoglobinuria Stem Cell

Paroxysmal nocturnal hemoglobinuria is a clonal hematopoietic disorder. The first evidence to support the notion that PNH arises through the mutation of an abnormal multipotent HSC was derived from glucose 6-phosphate dehydrogenase studies of the RBCs of women with PNH. Subsequently, flow cytometric analyses revealed that all hematopoietic lineages—myeloid, erythroid, and lymphoid—were involved. Furthermore, *PIGA* mutations found in granulocytes match those found in other lineages, and $CD34^+CD38^-$ progenitor cells have been shown to be missing GPI-anchored proteins in PNH patients. Thus, the "hit" in PNH clearly involves a multipotent HSC and appears to involve an earlier stem cell than diseases such as chronic myelogenous leukemia, MDS, or acute leukemia. In the latter disorders, B cells are sometimes derived from the leukemia clone, but T cells are seldom involved. In PNH, both B cells and T cells have been shown to be derived from the malignant clone.[6]

Table 29-2 Cell Surface Glycosylphosphatidylinositol-Anchored Protein Absent on Paroxysmal Nocturnal Hemoglobinuria Blood Cells

Antigen	Hematopoietic Lineage	Classification
CD55—decay accelerating factor	All blood cells	Complement regulator
CD59—membrane inhibitor of reactive lysis	All blood cells	Complement regulator
CD58—lymphocyte function associated antigen-3	All blood cells	Adhesion molecule
Acetylcholinesterase	RBCs	Enzyme
CD14—monocyte differentiation antigen	Granulocytes, monocytes, macrophages	Endotoxin-binding receptor
CD16—Fcγ receptor III	Granulocytes, NK cells	Receptor
CD66b	Granulocytes	Adhesion
Neutrophil alkaline phosphatase	Granulocytes	Enzyme
CD87—urokinase (plasminogen activator) receptor	Monocytes, granulocytes	Receptor
Leukocyte alkaline phosphatase	Granulocytes	Enzyme
CDw52—Campath-1 antigen	Lymphocytes, monocytes	Unknown
CD24	B lymphocytes, granulocytes	B-cell differentiation
CD48	All leukocytes	Adhesion molecule
CD73—ecto-5'-nucleotidase	Some B and T lymphocytes	Enzyme
Dombrock-Holley/Gregory-bearing protein	Red cells	Blood group antigen
Folate receptor	Myeloid and erythroid cells	Receptor

NK, Natural killer; *RBC,* red blood cell.

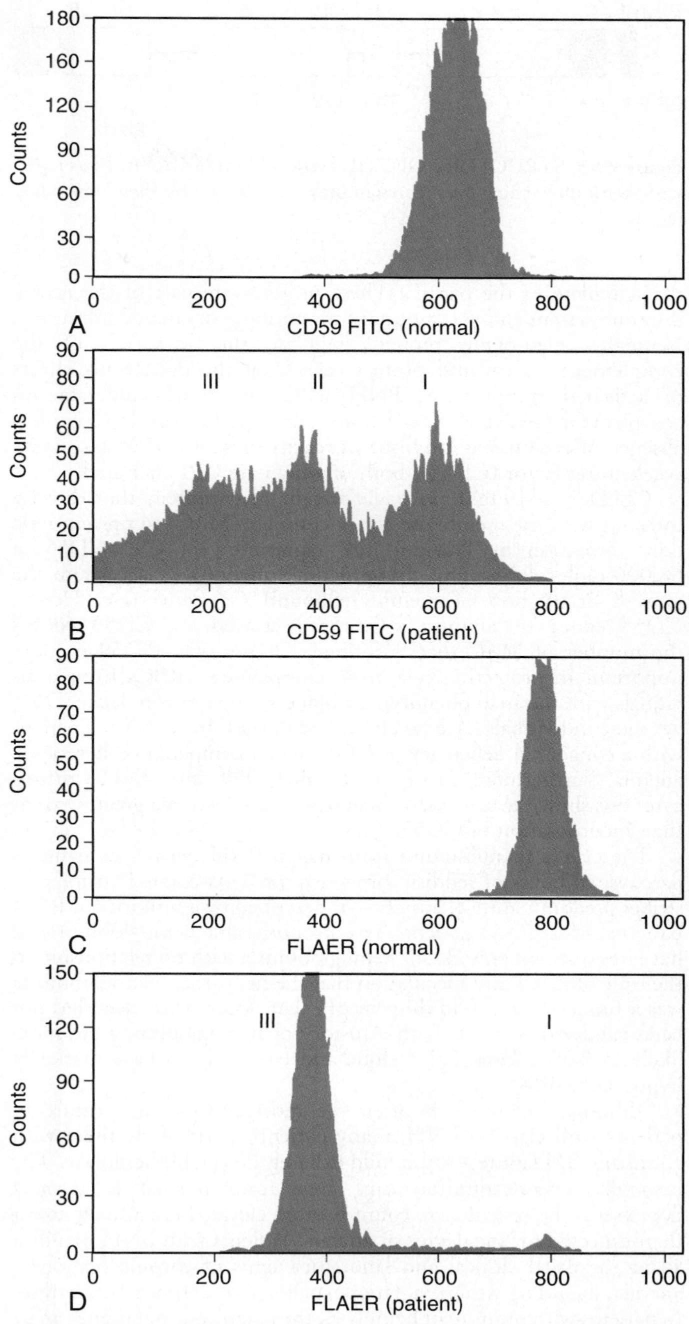

Figure 29-2 FLOW CYTOMETRIC ANALYSIS OR PERIPHERAL BLOOD CELLS FROM A PATIENT WITH PAROXYSMAL NOCTURNAL HEMOGLOBINURIA (PNH). **A,** Fluorescence intensity of erythrocytes from a healthy control participant after staining with anti-CD59. **B,** Fluorescence intensity of erythrocytes from an untransfused PNH patient after staining with anti-CD59. Type II cells are "blended" between the type I (normal) and type III cells. **C,** Fluorescence intensity of granulocytes from a healthy control participant stained with FLAER. **D,** Fluorescence intensity of granulocytes from the same PNH patient as in **B** after staining with FLAER. Note that the granulocytes are almost exclusively type III cells. A small population of type I granulocytes is present. *FITC,* Fluorescein isothiocyanate.

Paroxysmal Nocturnal Hemoglobinuria Red Blood Cells

Paroxysmal nocturnal hemoglobinuria cells can display one of three phenotypes (Fig. 29-3): cells with normal expression of GPI-anchored proteins (type I cells), cells with intermediate expression of GPI anchor proteins (type II cells), and cells with no expression of GPI anchor proteins (type III cells). These three populations are most easily seen in the erythrocyte and granulocyte populations. Patients with three discreet granulocyte populations (type I, type II, and type III cells) usually have more than one PNH clone. Whereas the type II cells are usually the consequence of a missense mutation, the type III cells commonly result from frameshift mutations caused by small base pair insertions or deletions. However, in many PNH patients, the type II cells are not a distinct population but represent a "spectrum" between the type III and type I cells (see Fig. 29-3).

CLINICAL FEATURES

Hemolytic Anemia and Hemoglobinuria

Hemolysis in PNH results from the increased susceptibility of PNH RBCs to complement. Complement consists of a battery of proteins

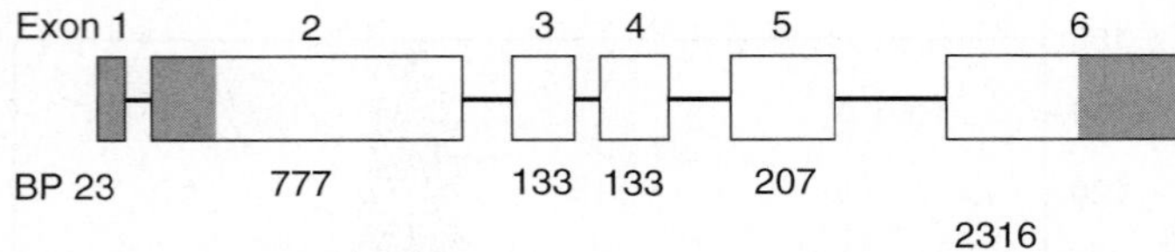

Figure 29-3 STRUCTURE OF THE HUMAN *PIGA* GENE. *Boxes* represent exons; intervening *lines* represent introns. *Shaded areas* show noncoding regions.

that circulate in the plasma. These proteins are part of the innate immune system and are important for antibody-mediated immunity. Normally, membrane proteins regulate the activation of the complement system and protect cells from the deleterious effects of activated complement. PNH RBCs are more vulnerable to complement-mediated lysis because of a reduction or complete absence of membrane inhibitor of reactive lysis (CD59) and decay accelerating factor (CD55), both of which are GPI anchored.

CD59 is a 19,000-molecular-weight glycoprotein that directly interacts with the membrane attack complex (MAC) to prevent lytic pore formation by blocking the aggregation of C9.[7] CD55, a 68,000-molecular-weight glycoprotein, functions to accelerate the rate of destruction of membrane-bound C3 convertase. Hence, CD55 reduces the amount of C3 that is cleaved, and CD59 reduces the number of MAC that is formed. Of the two, CD59 is more important in protecting cells from complement. RBCs from individuals with the Inab phenotype, a blood group antigen, lack CD55, yet these individuals have no clinical hemolysis. In contrast, a patient with a congenital deficiency of CD59 had a compensated hemolytic anemia. Furthermore, incorporation of CD59 onto PNH erythrocytes was shown to ameliorate acidified serum lysis to a greater extent than incorporation of CD55.

The classic manifestation from which PNH derives its name—paroxysmal bouts of reddish, brownish, or "cola-colored" urine that strikes predominantly overnight—is described by a minority of PNH patients. Most PNH patients have no noticeable hemoglobinuria or have intermittent episodes of hemoglobinuria with no relationship to the time of day. Early speculation that the nocturnal hemoglobinuria was a function of a mild drop in pH that occurs with sleep has not been validated. Patients with a history of hemoglobinuria are more likely to have a large PNH clone and less likely to have markedly hypocellular BM.

Although hemolysis is often the most conspicuous feature in patients with classical PNH, many patients, particularly those with coexisting BM failure, exhibit mild to barely detectable hemolysis. The hemoglobin concentration can range from normal to severely depressed. The reticulocyte count is often elevated but usually lower than expected for the degree of anemia. Patients with PNH manifest all of the usual clinical and laboratory signs of chronic hemolytic anemia, including weakness, fatigue, pallor, and dyspnea on exertion. In patients with prominent hemolysis, the magnitude of fatigue can be out of proportion to the degree of anemia. Morphologically, the RBCs appear normal, although some cases display mild to moderate poikilocytosis and anisocytosis. The haptoglobin levels are usually low, and the lactate dehydrogenase (LDH) level is frequently elevated, sometimes greater than 3000 IU/L, depending on the degree of hemolysis.

Multiple factors influence the degree of hemolysis in PNH, including the size and type of the PNH clone and the degree of complement activation. In general, the percentage of PNH erythrocytes correlates with the degree of hemolysis. However, the type of PNH erythrocytes may also influence the degree of hemolysis. Type III erythrocytes are more readily lysed than type II erythrocytes and almost always constitute a larger percentage of the PNH RBCs. Thus, patients with a large percentage of type III erythrocytes tend to have more hemolysis than patients with a large percentage of type I or type II cells. Finally, hemolysis is frequently exacerbated by infections (especially gastrointestinal infections), surgery, strenuous exercise, excessive alcohol intake, blood transfusions, and anything else that increases complement activation.

Smooth Muscle Dystonia and Nitric Oxide

Many clinical manifestations of PNH are readily explained by hemoglobin-mediated nitric oxide scavenging.[8] Failure of complement regulation on the PNH erythrocyte membrane leads to intravascular hemolysis, resulting in the release of large amounts of free hemoglobin into the plasma. Free plasma hemoglobin leads to increased consumption of nitric oxide, resulting in manifestations that include fatigue, abdominal pain, esophageal spasm, erectile dysfunction, and possibly thrombosis. Indeed, hemoglobinuria, thrombosis, erectile dysfunction, and esophageal spasm are more common in patients with large PNH populations (>60% of granulocytes) than in patients with relatively small PNH populations. In a study of 49 PNH patients diagnosed using flow cytometry, Moyo and colleagues[5] demonstrated that large PNH clones were associated with an increased risk for thrombosis, hemoglobinuria, abdominal pain, esophageal spasm, and male impotence. Thus, many of the clinical manifestations of PNH appear to be a direct consequence of intravascular hemolysis, leading to the release of free hemoglobin, scavenging of nitric oxide, and smooth muscle dystonias.

Renal Manifestations

Patients with PNH can experience renal manifestations that resemble those observed with sickle cell anemia. Perturbed tubular function and declining creatinine clearance are found in a high percentage of patients. Radiologically, patients may exhibit large kidneys, cortical infarcts, cortical thinning, and papillary necrosis. PNH patients display marked hemosiderin deposition in the proximal tubules; however, microvascular thrombosis can be responsible for many of the renal abnormalities in PNH.[9] Acute renal failure after massive hemolysis occurs infrequently and usually resolves in days to weeks.

Thrombosis and Paroxysmal Nocturnal Hemoglobinuria

Thrombosis is an ominous complication of PNH and was the leading cause of death before the availability of pharmacologic complement inhibition. Thrombosis occurs in approximately 40% of PNH patients and most commonly involves the venous system, but arterial clots may also occur. Patients with a large percentage of PNH cells and classical symptoms (hemolytic anemia and hemoglobinuria) have a greater propensity for thrombosis than patients with a small percentage of PNH cells. According to logistic regression modeling, for a 10% change in PNH clone size, the odds ratio for risk of thrombosis is estimated to be 1.64. Patients with PNH granulocyte clones of greater than 60% appear to be at greatest risk for thrombosis. The mechanism of thrombosis in PNH is not entirely understood and is probably multifactorial, but similar to other manifestations of the disease, it is probably related to the GPI anchor protein deficiency and activation of complement. Indeed, C5a is proinflammatory and may increase the risk for thrombosis. Furthermore, nitric oxide depletion (as a consequence of intravascular hemolysis and nitric oxide scavenging) has been associated with increased platelet aggregation, increased platelet adhesion, and accelerated clot formation. In an attempt to repair damage, PNH platelets undergo exocytosis of the complement attack complex. This results in the formation of microvesicles with phosphatidylserine externalization, a potent in vitro procoagulant. These prothrombotic microvesicles have been detected in the blood of PNH patients. Fibrinolysis can also be perturbed in PNH given that PNH blood cells lack the GPI-anchored urokinase receptor. Lastly, tissue factor pathway inhibitor (TFPI), a major inhibitor of tissue factor, has been shown to require a GPI-anchored chaperone protein for trafficking to the endothelial cell surface. Although the mechanism of thrombosis in PNH is not entirely clear, the sites of venous thrombosis in PNH are manifold with the abdominal veins and the cerebral veins being the most commonly involved regions.

Liver

Hepatic vein thrombosis (Budd-Chiari syndrome) is a common site of thrombosis in PNH and may be fatal without appropriate therapy. The clinical manifestations of hepatic vein thrombosis include abdominal pain, hepatomegaly, jaundice, ascites, and weight gain. The onset of symptoms can be abrupt or insidious. Hepatic vein thrombosis in PNH tends to inexorably progress with periodic exacerbations followed by intervals of relatively stable disease. Although some patients live many years with the condition, it frequently results in death unless complement inhibition or BM transplantation (BMT) is initiated. The best noninvasive tests to confirm the diagnosis include computed tomography scanning, magnetic resonance imaging (MRI), and ultrasonography. Thrombosis can involve the small hepatic veins, large-sized hepatic veins, or both. Thrombolytic therapy has been used successfully to restore venous patency and reverse the hepatic congestion; however, because of the potential danger of this approach, it should be used judiciously. Patients with acute-onset disease, preserved platelet counts (>50,000 cells/mm^3), and large vessel involvement are the best candidates for thrombolysis. For patients with massive ascites who are not suitable candidates for thrombolytic therapy, transjugular intrahepatic portal-systemic shunting or surgical shunting can successfully palliate some patients. Orthotopic liver transplantation was once considered contraindicated in PNH, but now that the thrombotic risk can be mitigated using complement inhibition, this is no longer true. Long-term survival after liver transplantation and eculizumab administration has been reported.[9]

Portal vein thrombosis is also common in PNH and can occur with or without hepatic vein thrombosis. Patients frequently present with nausea, vomiting, abdominal pain, and liver dysfunction. Management is similar to that of hepatic vein thrombosis.

Other Abdominal Veins

Venous thrombosis in PNH has been described in all abdominal and retroperitoneal venous systems, including the splenic veins, mesenteric veins, renal veins, and inferior vena cava. Thrombosis of minor veins can also occur and can be difficult to diagnose because of the protean manifestations and their relapsing and remitting nature. Often such patients present with recurrent, severe abdominal pain crises sometimes mimicking intestinal obstruction. The consequence of these microthromboses can sometimes be visualized with esophagogastroduodenal endoscopy or colonoscopy. Patients with intestinal thromboses can present with ischemic colitis and can be misdiagnosed as having Crohn disease. Upper gastrointestinal bleeding can be caused by esophageal or gastric varices that develop as a consequence of portal hypertension or splenic vein thrombosis.

Cerebral Veins

Cerebral veins, particularly the sagittal veins and sinuses, are also highly prone to thrombosis in PNH. Patients can present with severe headaches or focal neurologic deficits depending on the location of the thrombosis. Similar to hepatic vein thrombosis, cerebral vein thrombosis is an ominous complication that can result in substantial morbidity and mortality. MRI to carefully examine the cerebral blood flow is helpful in establishing the diagnosis.

Other Sites

Dermal venous thrombosis can occur virtually anywhere on the body. Patients usually complain of pain, discolorations, and swelling. The lesions can reach several centimeters in diameter and are firm and tender. Necrosis and the formation of a black eschar can occur. Anticoagulation and warm compresses can ameliorate the attacks. Pulmonary emboli and deep venous thrombosis have also been reported in PNH but are uncommon; arterial thrombosis is rare.

CLONALITY AND BONE MARROW FAILURE

PIGA Mutations in Aplastic Anemia and Myelodysplastic Syndrome

Small to moderate PNH clones are found in up to 70% of patients with acquired aplastic anemia, demonstrating a pathophysiologic link between these disorders.[10,11] Typically, less than 20% GPI anchor protein–deficient granulocytes are detected in aplastic anemia patients at diagnosis, but occasional patients can have larger clones. DNA sequencing of the GPI anchor protein–deficient cells from aplastic anemia patients reveals clonal *PIGA* gene mutations that arise from a multipotent HSC. Moreover, many of these patients exhibit expansion of the *PIGA* mutant clone and progress to clinical PNH. Although it was once thought that PNH evolving from aplastic anemia is more benign than classical PNH, this observation is probably a consequence of lead time bias because many of these patients eventually develop classical PNH symptoms.

GPI anchor protein–deficient cells have also been reported in patients with MDS, but sequencing of the *PIGA* gene to establish clonality has not been performed in most of these studies. MDS patients reported to have small PNH populations tend to be classified as refractory anemia and often have the following characteristics: a hypocellular marrow, human leukocyte antigen (HLA)-DR15 positivity, normal cytogenetics, moderate to severe thrombocytopenia, and a high likelihood of response to immunosuppressive therapy. Thus, it is possible that many of these patients have moderate aplastic anemia rather than MDS. Distinguishing hypoplastic MDS from aplastic anemia is often difficult; however, quantitative analysis of BM CD34 positive cells is useful for discriminating between these two entities.

PIGA Mutations in Healthy Controls

Paroxysmal nocturnal hemoglobinuria is an uncommon disease, with only two to five new cases per million U.S. inhabitants annually; however, *PIGA* mutations can be found in the blood from virtually all healthy control participants. Araten and coworkers[7] used flow cytometric analysis of blood from nine healthy control participants and found an average of 22 GPI anchor protein–deficient granulocytes per 10^6 cells, yet none of these subjects developed PNH. GPI anchor protein–deficient lymphocytes have also been detected in patients with lymphoid malignancies or rheumatoid arthritis after treatment with alemtuzumab (Campath-1H). Alemtuzimab is a monoclonal antibody that recognizes CD52, a GPI-anchored protein expressed on monocytes, B cells, and T cells. None of these patients developed PNH; furthermore, when alemtuzimab was discontinued, the GPI anchor protein–deficient cells regressed.

How can such a common mutation, *PIGA,* be so specific for PNH yet so rarely result in disease? One hypothesis to explain the close relationship between PNH and aplastic anemia, and the mechanisms whereby the PNH clone achieves dominance, involves a "two-step" model. This model proposes that HSCs randomly and spontaneously acquire *PIGA* mutations at a very low frequency (step one). Step two in this model proposes that the immunologic attack that targets HSCs in aplastic anemia spares PNH cells, ostensibly because they lack GPI-anchored proteins.[12] Indeed, *PIGA* mutant cells are found at low frequency in most healthy control participants. More recent data suggest that most, if not all, *PIGA* mutations in healthy control participants arise from colony-forming cells rather than HSCs.[6] Because colony-forming cells lack self-renewal capacity and only produce new blood cells for a few months, *PIGA* mutations arising in these cells do not result in PNH. Similarly, the *PIGA* mutations found in some MDS patients also arise in colony-forming cells, explaining why MDS patients with small populations of PNH-like cells seldom, if ever, progress to PNH. Furthermore, no direct evidence supports a GPI-anchored protein being the target of the immune attack in aplastic anemia. Importantly, this two-step model does not explain the similarly high incidence of MDS in patients with aplastic anemia.

An alternative hypothesis that could explain the predisposition of patients with aplastic anemia to develop both PNH and MDS has been proposed.[13] MDS and PNH evolving in the setting of aplastic anemia could be analogous to the *field cancerization effect* described in aerodigestive and other solid tumors to explain second primary tumors in the affected tissue. That is, a single insult to the BM, such as generalized toxic damage or a genetic predisposition, may be responsible for bringing about different forms of BM disorders; these disorders can occur alone, simultaneously, or sequentially. In aplastic anemia, the BM injury may primarily trigger an autoimmune attack on the hematopoietic stem progenitor compartment, perhaps by exposing cryptic epitopes through molecular mimicry or by sending a "danger" signal. In primary PNH or MDS, the injury may primarily produce a genetic mutation that leads to clonal dominance of the affected clone. In other patients, BM injury may induce both an autoimmune hematopoietic attack and a clonal genetic mutation that presents either simultaneously or sequentially. Examples of simultaneous presentation are the aplastic anemia–PNH overlap and hypoplastic MDS. A third hypothesis proposes that additional mutations occurring in *PIGA* mutant stem cells are required for clonal expansion PNH. These hypotheses may not be mutually exclusive; thus, further investigation is needed to fully understand the mechanism of clonal dominance in PNH.

Clinical observations also provide clues to understanding clonal dominance in PNH and the relationship between aplastic anemia and PNH. Up to 30% of patients with aplastic anemia treated with conventional immunosuppressive therapy (antithymocyte globulin [ATG] and cyclosporine) develop PNH or MDS, usually several years after therapy. In contrast, allogeneic BMT appears to eliminate the risk for developing PNH in patients with aplastic anemia. These data suggest that secondary clonal disorders (PNH and MDS) are part of the natural history of aplastic anemia. Although immunosuppressive therapy unequivocally prolongs survival, it does not prevent these late complications.

Clonal Transformation

Patients with PNH, similar to those with aplastic anemia and MDS, are at increased risk for clonal transformation; however, the incidence of leukemic transformation in PNH is less than that of MDS. Abnormal cytogenetics can be found in up to 20% of patients with PNH. MDS and acute myeloid leukemia are the most common malignancies to evolve from PNH; the leukemic cells may arise from the GPI anchor–deficient clone in many but not all cases.

NATURAL HISTORY

The natural history of PNH before the era of anticomplement therapy ranged from indolent to severely debilitating and life threatening.[14-16] The ability to pharmacologically interfere with terminal complement appears to have altered the natural history of the disease by markedly decreasing the thrombosis rate. Females and males are equally affected with the median age of diagnosis being 40 years old. Without therapy, the median survival from time of diagnosis is 10 to 20 years. Thrombosis, severe pancytopenia, evolution to MDS or leukemia, older age, and thrombocytopenia at diagnosis portend a poor prognosis. Older literature, in which patients were diagnosed with PNH based on the Ham test or sucrose hemolysis test, reported on the occurrence of spontaneous long-term remissions in up to 10% of PNH cases; however, in patients diagnosed by flow cytometry, the spontaneous remission rate is much less common. In summary, eculizumab, a monoclonal antibody that inhibits terminal complement, appears to have altered the natural history of PNH by reducing the incidence of fatal thrombotic events.

LABORATORY EVALUATION

Blood

Peripheral blood counts in PNH patients vary from severe pancytopenia to normal. Virtually all patients present with anemia, frequently with mild macrocytosis. Thrombocytopenia and neutropenia are also common. A mild to moderate reticulocytosis is usually present in patients with the classical form of the disease; however, in patients with hypoplastic PNH (also referred to as *aplastic anemia/PNH overlap*), the reticulocyte count can be low for the degree of anemia. Similarly, in patients with hypoplastic PNH, the biochemical profile can be normal, but in patients with large PNH clones, the indirect bilirubin and LDH level are significantly elevated. In patients with vigorous hemolysis, it is common for the laboratory to report the specimen as "hemolyzed."

Bone Marrow

Bone marrow cellularity can be hypocellular, normocellular, or hypercellular. In patients with classical PNH (not arising from or coinciding with aplastic anemia), the marrow is usually normocellular to hypercellular with erythroid hyperplasia. Mild to moderate dyserythropoiesis is common. Stainable iron is frequently absent because of iron loss associated with the intravascular hemolysis. Cytogenetic abnormalities can be found in a small number of patients.

DIAGNOSIS

Complement-Based Assays

The Ham test and the sucrose hemolysis test (sugar water test) were two of the first assays used to diagnosis PNH. Both assays are performed on erythrocytes and discriminate PNH cells from normal cells based on a differential sensitivity to the hemolytic action of complement. In the Ham test, complement is activated by acidification of the serum. This results in lysis of PNH erythrocytes but not normal erythrocytes. The Ham test is relatively specific for PNH but is not very sensitive.

Complement is also activated in a low ionic strength sucrose-containing medium. Preferential lysis of PNH erythrocytes through the activation of complement in this sucrose-containing medium forms the basis for the sugar water test. This assay is easier to perform and is more sensitive than the Ham test but not as specific; other hemolytic anemias and even leukemias can produce false-positive results. The complement lysis assay in which complement is activated with antibody also detects PNH erythrocytes. These complement-based RBC assays are important from a historical perspective but should no longer be used to establish the diagnosis of PNH.

GPI Anchor-Based Assays

Most laboratories use monoclonal antibodies against specific GPI-anchored proteins in conjunction with flow cytometry to diagnose PNH.[17,18] Anti-CD59 is most commonly used because it is widely expressed and is displayed on all hematopoietic lineages. Anti-CD55, anti-CD14, anti-CD16, anti-CD67, and a variety of other monoclonal antibodies can also be used to establish the diagnosis. Flow cytometry offers several advantages over complement-based assays for diagnosing PNH: It measures the size of the PNH clone in the various cell lineages, it is more sensitive and specific, and it is less affected by blood transfusions. It is noteworthy that rare congenital deficiencies of CD59 and CD55 can lead to a false-positive test results for PNH if only one monoclonal antibody is used. This, coupled with the variable expression of GPI-anchored proteins on different hematopoietic lineages, accounts for the recommendation that at least two different monoclonal antibodies directed against two different GPI-anchored proteins on at least two different cell lineages should be used to diagnose a patient with PNH. Solely screening patients' RBCs for PNH can lead to falsely negative tests, especially in the setting of a recent hemolytic episode or a recent blood transfusion. Because granulocytes and monocytes have short half-lives and are not affected by blood transfusions, the percentage of PNH cells in these lineages best reflects the size of the PNH stem cell pool.

Aerolysin Assays

A fluorescein-labeled proaerolysin variant, FLAER, is commonly used in conjunction with monoclonal antibodies in a flow cytometric assay to diagnose PNH.[19] Aerolysin is the principal virulence factor of the bacterium *Aeromonas hydrophila*. It is secreted as an inert protoxin termed *proaerolysin* that binds selectively and with high affinity to a GPI anchor. After binding to its receptor (the glycan portion of the GPI anchor), the C-terminal peptide of proaerolysin is cleaved by cell proteases. This activates the toxin and leads to the formation of heptameric channels that insert into the membrane and kill the cell. PNH cells are resistant to aerolysin and proaerolysin because PNH cells lack GPI-anchored proteins.[20] FLAER binds to the GPI anchor without forming channels and gives a more accurate assessment of the GPI-anchor deficit in PNH than anti-CD59. Because the GPI anchor is the major determinant for binding FLAER, it allows for the direct assessment of GPI anchor expression on virtually all cell lineages. RBCs are a notable exception; this may be because both normal and PNH RBCs express large amounts of glycophorin, a protein shown to bind aerolysin weakly. Nevertheless, in mononuclear cells, FLAER eliminates the need for multiple lineage-specific monoclonal antibodies. These properties make FLAER more reliable for detecting the small PNH populations often found in patients with aplastic anemia.

THERAPY

Some PNH patients can be managed conservatively with watchful waiting. The major exceptions are patients with hypoplastic PNH (especially those who also meet criteria for severe aplastic anemia) and patients with life-threatening thromboses or debilitating hemolysis and smooth muscle dystonias.[21] Cytopenias in patients with hypoplastic PNH are usually caused by immune suppression of hematopoiesis; thus, the management of these patients should be similar to those with acquired aplastic anemia. Classical PNH patients manifesting with recurrent thrombosis or severe intravascular hemolysis often require either complement inhibition or sometimes BMT.

Immunosuppressive Therapy

Patients with PNH with hypocellular BM, low reticulocyte count, and pancytopenia (hypoplastic PNH) frequently respond to immunosuppressive therapy. The response rate in this group is more than 50%. In fact, finding a minor population of PNH-like cells in severe aplastic anemia may predict for response to immunosuppressive therapy. The impaired hematopoiesis that occurs in hypoplastic PNH may respond to ATG or cyclosporine, but the PNH clone is usually not affected. In some cases, immunosuppressive therapy has ameliorated the aplasia but with preferential expansion of the PNH clone. Immunosuppressive therapy does not appear to benefit patients with classical PNH.

Management of Anemia

The cause of anemia in PNH is often multifactorial. In patients with hypoplastic PNH, BM failure is the major etiologic factor for anemia. Patients with hypoplastic PNH may respond to immunosuppressive therapy. However, in patients with cellular BM, elevated reticulocyte counts, and high LDH level (classical PNH), intravascular hemolysis is the major mechanism of anemia. Terminal complement inhibition is highly effective for decreasing intravascular hemolysis. Iron deficiency caused by intravascular hemolysis can also contribute to the anemia of PNH; thus, in patients with absent iron stores, iron replacement therapy is indicated. Folic acid supplementation is also recommended in PNH because of the high RBC turnover. Erythropoietin is rarely beneficial in PNH. Often RBC transfusions are required to treat severe anemia. PNH patients should receive group-specific blood and blood products. Washing the RBCs with saline, once advocated to minimize hemolysis after transfusion in PNH, is unnecessary.

Eculizumab

Eculizumab is a humanized monoclonal antibody against C5 that inhibits terminal complement activation (Fig. 29-4).[3,22,23] Because C5 is common to all pathways of complement activation, blockade aborts progression of the cascade regardless of the stimuli. Moreover, prevention of C5 cleavage blocks the generation of the potent proinflammatory and cell lytic molecules C5a and C5b-9, respectively (see Fig. 29-4). Importantly, C5 blockade preserves the critical immunoprotective and immunoregulatory functions of upstream components that culminate in C3b-mediated opsonization and immune complex clearance. In 2007, the U.S. Food and Drug Administration approved eculizumab for use in PNH based pon its efficacy in two phase III clinical trials. Eculizumab is highly effective in reducing intravascular hemolysis in PNH; it does not stop extravascular hemolysis and does not treat BM failure. Thus, eculizumab is most effective in patients with classical PNH. Treatment with eculizumab decreases or

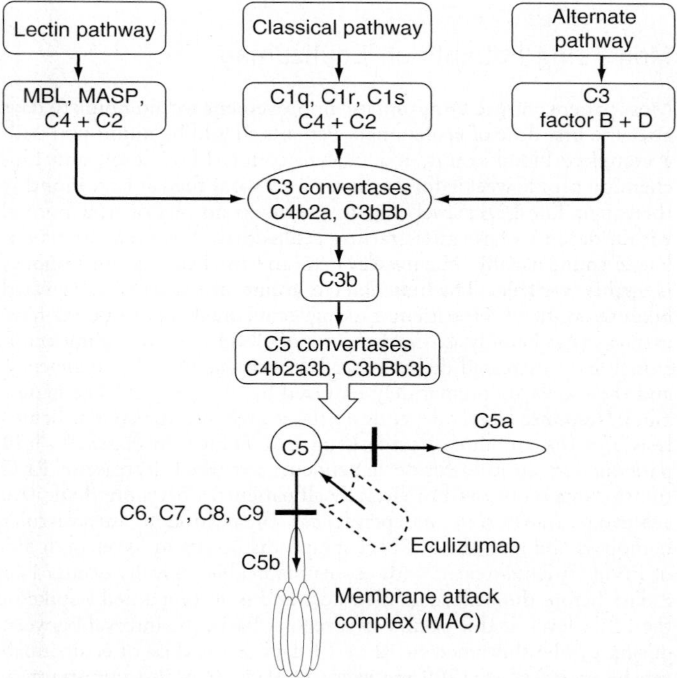

Figure 29-4 OVERVIEW OF THE COMPLEMENT CASCADE. Classic, alternative, and lectin pathways converge at the point of C3 activation. The lytic pathway is initiated with the formation of C5 convertase and leads to the assembly of the C5, C6, C7, C8, (*n*) C9 membrane attack complex. Eculizumab is a monoclonal antibody that binds to C5, thereby preventing the formation of C5a and C5b. C5b is the initiating component of the MAC. *FITC,* Fluorescein isothiocyanate; *MASP,* mannan-binding lectin associated service protease; *MBL,* Mannose binding lectin.

eliminates the need for blood transfusions in most patients, improves quality of life, and reduces the risk of thrombosis. Two weeks before starting therapy, all patients should be vaccinated against *Neisseria meningitides* because inhibition of complement at C5 increases the risk for developing infections with encapsulated organisms, particularly *N. meningitides* and *Neisseria gonorrhoeae*. Eculizumab is administered intravenously at a dose of 600 mg weekly for the first 4 weeks. On week five, the dose is increased to 900 mg IV, and thereafter the drug is dosed at 900 mg intravenously every 14 + 2 days. Rare patients will break through at this dosage and require a higher dose of eculizumab. Eculizumab is generally safe and well tolerated but must be continued indefinitely because it does not treat the underlying cause of the disease. The most common side effect, headache, occurs in roughly 50% of patients after the first dose or two but rarely occurs thereafter. *Neisserial* sepsis is the most serious complication of eculizumab therapy; thus, it is imperative to remind patients that they have a 0.5% yearly risk of acquiring *Neisserial* sepsis even after vaccination. Moreover, patients should be revaccinated against *N. meningitidis* every 3 to 5 years after starting eculizumab.

Indications for Therapy

Not all patients with a diagnosis of PNH require eculizumab therapy. The best candidates for treatment are those with a large PNH clone associated with disabling fatigue, thromboses, transfusion dependence, frequent pain paroxysms, renal insufficiency, or other end-organ complications from disease. Watchful waiting is appropriate for asymptomatic patients and for those with mild symptoms. In patients with hypoplastic PNH, therapy should be directed toward the underlying BM failure with careful monitoring of the PNH clone using flow cytometry. Patients who meet criteria for severe aplastic anemia should be managed with either allogeneic BMT or immunosuppressive therapy depending on the age of the patient and the availability of a suitable donor.

Monitoring Patients on Eculizumab

Most patients notice symptomatic improvement within hours to days after the first dose of eculizumab. Patients should be monitored with a complete blood count, reticulocyte count, LDH level, and biochemical profile weekly for the first 4 weeks and then at least monthly thereafter. The LDH level usually returns to normal or near normal within days to weeks after starting eculizumab; however, the reticulocyte count usually remains elevated, and the hemoglobin response is highly variable. The reticulocyte count often remains elevated because most PNH patients taking eculizumab continue to have extravascular hemolysis. Erythrocytes of PNH patients taking eculizumab have increased deposition of C3 because of CD55 deficiency, and these cells are prematurely removed by the spleen.[4,24] The hemoglobin response largely depends on the degree of extravascular hemolysis and the amount of underlying BM failure. In classical PNH patients who are transfusion dependent, a marked decrease in RBC transfusions is observed in virtually all patients, with more than 50% achieving transfusion independence. Breakthrough intravascular hemolysis and a return of PNH symptoms occurs in fewer than 5% of PNH patients treated with eculizumab. This typically occurs 1 or 2 days before the next scheduled dose and is accompanied a spike in the LDH level. If this occurs on a regular basis, the interval between dosing can be shortened to 12 or 13 days or the dose of eculizumab can be increased to 1200 mg every 14 days. It is also important to recognize that increased complement activation that accompanies infections (e.g., influenza or viral gastroenteritis) or trauma can also result in transient breakthrough hemolysis. These single episodes of breakthrough hemolysis do not require a change in dosing. Patients with continued anemia, a normal or near normal LDH level, and a robust reticulocyte count are likely to be having substantial extravascular hemolysis. In this setting, a direct antiglobulin test will likely be positive for complement and negative for immunoglobulin G.

Thrombosis

Thrombosis is often the most pernicious complication of PNH and is an indication for eculizumab and anticoagulation. In patients with acute onset of abdominal vein thrombosis, thrombolytic therapy has been successfully used. However, in some patients, thrombolytic therapy and anticoagulation are relatively contraindicated because of severe thrombocytopenia. Terminal complement blockade appears to be the most effective way to prevent further thrombotic events and in some patients may allow for the discontinuation of anticoagulation.[25-27] Pregnancy, surgery, or the use of oral contraceptives can increase the risk for thrombosis in PNH and should be considered high risk.

Bone Marrow Transplantation

Bone marrow transplantation is the only curative therapy for PNH, but it is associated with significant morbidity and mortality. The International Bone Marrow Transplant Registry (IBMTR) reported a 2-year survival probability of 56% in 48 recipients of HLA-identical sibling transplants between 1978 and 1995. The median age was 28 years. The majority of the deaths in this study occurred within 1 year of transplantation. One of seven recipients of alternative donor allogeneic transplants reported to the IBMTR during this period was alive 5 years after transplant. The European Blood and Marrow Transplant group reported a 5-year survival rate of 70% after allogeneic BMT for PNH; however, only 54% met criteria for classical PNH. The median age in the study was 30 years. Graft failure occurred in 6% of patients, and acute and chronic graft-versus-host disease (GVHD) occurred in 15% and 20% of patients, respectively.

More recently, the Gruppo Italiano Trapianto Midollo Osseo (GITMO), published a retrospective study of 26 patients (median age, 32 years) who received BMT for PNH in Italy between 1988 and 2006.[28] HLA-matched sibling donors were used as stem cell sources for 22 patients; one patient received stem cells from a matched unrelated donor, and three received stem cells from mismatched donors (two related and one unrelated). A myeloablative conditioning regimen (busulfan + cyclophosphamide) was used for 15 of the patients. The remaining 11 received a variety of different reduced intensity conditioning regimens, most being cyclophosphamide or fludaribine based. GVHD prophylaxis was highly variable but largely cyclosporine based. The 10-year probability of survival was 57% for all patients, with a median follow-up of 131 months. There was one primary graft failure in a patient receiving a myeloablative conditioning regimen and one secondary graft failure in a patient who received a nonmyeloablative BMT; both patients eventually died from complications of a second BMT. Acute GVHD (aGVHD) greater than stage 2 occurred in three of the 26 patients; chronic GVHD (cGVHD) occurred in 10 of 20 evaluable patients with four (16%) experiencing extensive cGVHD. The transplant related mortality at 1 year was 26% in patients receiving a myeloablative conditioning regimen and 63% in the group that received a nonmyeloablative regimen; however, this was likely because all three patients in the nonmyeloablative group received a BMT from a non-identical donor. There was just one patient in the myeloablative group who received a BMT from an unrelated or mismatched donor.

In summary, BMT should not be offered as initial therapy for most patients with classical PNH given the high morbidity and mortality, especially when using unrelated or mismatched donors. Exceptions are PNH patients in countries where eculizumab is not available and patients who do not have a good response to eculizumab therapy. Patients with hypoplastic PNH and life-threatening cytopenias continue to be reasonable candidates for BMT. A myeloablative conditioning regimen is not required to eradicate the PNH clone. Allogeneic BMT after a nonmyeloablative conditioning regimen can cure PNH. Whether or not there is an advantage to one approach over the other will require further study; however, nonmyeloablative regimens may be preferable in young patients seeking to maintain fertility and patients with moderate organ dysfunction who may not tolerate a myeloablative regimen. Last, because BMT is the only curative therapy available for PNH, continued use and investigation of this approach in selected patients is reasonable.[29] Recent advances in mitigating GVHD such as posttransplant high-dose cyclophosphamide may particularly effective in PNH, but further studies are required.[30]

APPROACH TO TREATMENT

The author finds it useful to classify PNH patients as either "classical" or "hypoplastic." This can usually be accomplished by ordering a complete blood count; reticulocyte count; LDH level; peripheral blood flow cytometry for PNH; and BM aspirate, biopsy, and cytogenetics. Patients with classical PNH tend to have mild to moderate cytopenias, a normocellular to hypercellular BM, an elevated reticulocyte count, a markedly elevated LDH level, and a relatively large PNH granulocyte population (>30%). In contrast, hypoplastic PNH patients present with manifestations similar to that of aplastic anemia or hypoplastic MDS. These patients typically present with moderate to severe cytopenias, a hypocellular BM (<25% cellularity), a decreased corrected reticulocyte count, a normal or mildly elevated LDH level, and a relatively small (<20%) PNH granulocyte population. Most, but not all, patients can be readily subdivided into classical versus hypoplastic PNH, a distinction that aids with therapeutic decisions. See Red Box on Approach to Diagnosing Paroxysmal Nocturnal Hemoglobinuria.

Approach to Diagnosing Paroxysmal Nocturnal Hemoglobinuria

Paroxysmal nocturnal hemoglobinuria (PNH) has an estimated incidence of 2 to 5 per million in the United States. This, coupled with its protean manifestations, makes diagnosing PNH a challenge for even the most astute diagnostician. However, given the ease and specificity of modern diagnostic assays, the most important attribute a physician can possess in diagnosing PNH is to maintain a high level of suspicion and to be cognizant of the various presentations of the disease. A small sample of peripheral blood sent to an experienced flow cytometric laboratory is usually sufficient to establish or exclude the diagnosis of PNH. These assays are fast, reliable, and inexpensive. If monoclonal antibodies are used to establish the diagnosis, it is imperative that two or more antibodies be used on at least two different lineages. Assaying granulocytes is the most reliable method of diagnosing PNH because they are not affected by blood transfusions. The author prefers to use FLAER over monoclonal antibodies on granulocytes and monocytes because of the improved sensitivity and specificity; anti-CD59 is the most reliable marker on erythrocytes.

Classical PNH is usually more conspicuous than hypoplastic PNH. Patients typically present with direct antiglobulin-negative hemolytic anemia, hemoglobinuria, and mild to moderate cytopenias. Obscure paroxysms of back pain, abdominal pain, fatigue, or headaches are often present. The BM is typically normocellular to mildly hypercellular with intense erythroid hyperplasia and mild to moderate dyserythropoiesis. BM iron stores are frequently, but not always, absent. PNH patients can also present with abrupt, severe abdominal pain and jaundice caused by thrombosis. All patients presenting with unexplained hepatic vein, portal vein, mesenteric vein, or portal vein thrombosis should be screened for PNH.

It is important to distinguish PNH from myelodysplastic syndrome. Most patients with refractory anemia should be screened for PNH, especially those with moderate to severe cytopenias, an elevated lactate dehydrogenase level, and a hypocellular BM. In addition, all patients diagnosed with aplastic anemia should be screened for PNH. As few as 3% PNH erythrocytes may result in an elevated LDH. In rare instances, idiopathic myelofibrosis or autoimmune hemolytic anemias can mimic PNH. Patients with a history of aplastic anemia—especially those managed with immunosuppressive therapy—should be monitored closely for the outgrowth of PNH.

Hypoplastic Paroxysmal Nocturnal Hemoglobinuria

Because BM failure is the major risk for patients with hypoplastic PNH, I direct my therapy toward the pancytopenia. If, in addition to the PNH, the patient fulfills criteria for severe aplastic anemia (see Chapter 28), appropriate therapeutic options include allogeneic BMT, high-dose cyclophosphamide, or ATG and cyclosporine. Young patients (i.e., <30 years of age) with an HLA-matched sibling should be transplanted; for older patients and for those without an HLA-matched sibling, high-dose cyclophosphamide or antithymocyte and cyclosporine is appropriate. The author prefers to use high-dose cyclophosphamide because of the improved quality and duration of remissions. If the patient's cytopenias do not fulfill criteria for severe aplastic anemia, supportive care or a trial of immunosuppressive therapy is appropriate.

Classical Paroxysmal Nocturnal Hemoglobinuria

Symptoms in patients with classical PNH vary from mild, to severely debilitating, to acutely life threatening. Hence, therapy should be directed toward the specific manifestations (e.g., anemia, thrombosis). Allogeneic BMT, preferably from an HLA-matched sibling, is appropriate for patients with severely debilitating or acutely life-threatening disease. In general, these are patients with recurrent thrombosis or those with clonal evolution to either MDS or acute leukemia. Patients with less severe disease should not be transplanted because of the relatively high morbidity and mortality of the procedure. ATG and cyclosporine or high-dose cyclophosphamide does not appear to benefit patients with classical PNH.

Anemia

All patients with classical PNH should be prescribed folic acid (1-2 mg/day). Patients with absent iron stores, usually because of chronic intravascular hemolysis, should be treated with oral iron supplementation. Eculizumab has become the standard of care to treat selected patients with classical PNH. It is the only drug demonstrated in a randomized study to benefit PNH patients. Eculizumab has been shown to decrease the need for transfusions, decrease paroxysms, and improve quality of life in patients with classical PNH; however, it has not been shown to benefit patients with hypoplastic PNH. In classical PNH, the author recommends eculizumab for patients with disabling fatigue, thromboses, transfusion dependence, frequent pain paroxysms, renal insufficiency, or other end-organ complications from disease. Watchful waiting is appropriate for asymptomatic patients and those with mild symptoms.

If eculizumab is unavailable, a trial of prednisone (0.5-1.0 mg/day) can occasionally decrease hemolysis and increase hemoglobin levels. If a salutary effect is not achieved within 6 to 8 weeks, the steroids should be discontinued. In responding patients, the steroids should be tapered to the lowest dose that still provides a beneficial effect. Alternate-day steroids can help decrease the risk of deleterious long-term side effects. Danazol (400 mg/day) can also decrease hemolysis; if no response is observed after 8 weeks, the drug should be discontinued.

Thrombosis

Patients who present with acute life-threatening or organ-threatening thrombosis should be considered for thrombolytic therapy followed by long-term anticoagulation. Thrombosis is probably the most compelling reason to start eculizumab in PNH patients. Whether or not anticoagulation can be safely discontinued after eculizumab induction is still unknown, but patients who respond well to eculizumab therapy may not need long-term anticoagulation.

REFERENCES

1. Miyata T, Takeda J, Iida Y, et al: The cloning of PIG-A, a component in the early step of GPI-anchor biosynthesis. *Science* 259:1318, 1993.
2. Miyata T, Yamada N, Iida Y, et al: Abnormalities of PIG-A transcripts in granulocytes from patients with paroxysmal nocturnal hemoglobinuria. *N Engl J Med* 330:249, 1994.
3. Hillmen P, Young NS, Schubert J, et al: The complement inhibitor eculizumab in paroxysmal nocturnal hemoglobinuria. *N Engl J Med* 355:1233, 2006.
4. Fridkis-Hareli M, Storek M, Mazsaroff I, et al: Design and development of TT30, a novel C3d-targeted C3/C5 convertase inhibitor for treatment of the human complement alternative pathway-mediated diseases. *Blood* 2011.
5. Takeda J, Miyata T, Kawagoe K, et al: Deficiency of the GPI anchor caused by a somatic mutation of the PIG-A gene in paroxysmal nocturnal hemoglobinuria. *Cell* 73:703, 1993.
6. Hu R, Mukhina GL, Piantadosi S, et al: PIG-A mutations in normal hematopoiesis. *Blood* 105:3848, 2005.
7. Rollins SA, Sims PJ: The complement-inhibitory activity of CD59 resides in its capacity to block incorporation of C9 into membrane C5b-9. *J Immunol* 144:3478, 1990.
8. Rother RP, Bell L, Hillmen P, et al: The clinical sequelae of intravascular hemolysis and extracellular plasma hemoglobin: A novel mechanism of human disease. *JAMA* 293:1653, 2005.
9. Singer AL, Locke JE, Stewart ZA, et al: Successful liver transplantation for Budd-Chiari syndrome in a patient with paroxysmal nocturnal hemoglobinuria treated with the anti-complement antibody eculizumab. *Liver Transpl* 15:540, 2009.
10. Schrezenmeier H, Hertenstein B, Wagner B, et al: A pathogenetic link between aplastic anemia and paroxysmal nocturnal hemoglobinuria is suggested by a high frequency of aplastic anemia patients with a deficiency of phosphatidylinositol glycan anchored proteins. *Exp Hematol* 23:81, 1995.
11. Mukhina GL, Buckley JT, Barber JP, et al: Multilineage glycosylphosphatidylinositol anchor deficient hematopoiesis in untreated aplastic anemia. *Br J Haematol* 115:476, 2001.
12. Luzzatto L, Bessler M, Rotoli B: Somatic mutations in paroxysmal nocturnal hemoglobinuria: A blessing in disguise? *Cell* 88:1, 1997.
13. Savage WJ, Barber JP, Mukhina GL, et al: Glycosylphosphatidylinositol-anchored protein deficiency confers resistance to apoptosis in PNH. *Exp Hematol* 37:42, 2009.
14. de Latour RP, Mary JY, Salanoubat C, et al: Paroxysmal nocturnal hemoglobinuria: Natural history of disease subcategories. *Blood* 112:3099, 2008.
15. Nishimura J, Kanakura Y, Ware RE, et al: Clinical course and flow cytometric analysis of paroxysmal nocturnal hemoglobinuria in the United States and Japan. *Medicine (Baltimore)* 83:193, 2004.
16. Moyo VM, Mukhina GL, Garrett ES, et al: Natural history of paroxysmal nocturnal hemoglobinuria using modern diagnostic assays. *Br J Haematol* 126:133, 2004.
17. Parker C, Omine M, Richards S, et al: Diagnosis and management of paroxysmal nocturnal hemoglobinuria. *Blood* 106:3699, 2005.
18. Borowitz MJ, Craig FE, DiGiuseppe JA, et al: Guidelines for the diagnosis and monitoring of paroxysmal nocturnal hemoglobinuria and related disorders by flow cytometry. *Cytometry B Clin Cytom* 2010.
19. Brodsky RA, Mukhina GL, Li S, et al: Improved detection and characterization of paroxysmal nocturnal hemoglobinuria using fluorescent aerolysin. *Am J Clin Pathol* 114:459, 2000.
20. Brodsky RA, Mukhina GL, Nelson KL, et al: Resistance of Paroxysmal Nocturnal Hemoglobinuria Cells to the Glycosylphosphatidylinositol-Binding Toxin Aerolysin. *Blood* 93:1749, 1999.
21. Brodsky RA: How I treat paroxysmal nocturnal hemoglobinuria. *Blood* 2009.
22. Kelly RJ, Hill A, Arnold LM, et al: Long-term treatment with eculizumab in paroxysmal nocturnal hemoglobinuria: Sustained efficacy and improved survival. *Blood* 117:6786, 2011.
23. Brodsky RA, Young NS, Antonioli E, et al: Multicenter phase 3 study of the complement inhibitor eculizumab for the treatment of patients with paroxysmal nocturnal hemoglobinuria. *Blood* 111:1840, 2008.
24. Risitano AM, Notaro R, Marando L, et al: Complement fraction 3 binding on erythrocytes as additional mechanism of disease in paroxysmal nocturnal hemoglobinuria patients treated by eculizumab. *Blood* 2009.
25. Hillmen P, Muus P, Duhrsen U, et al: Effect of the complement inhibitor eculizumab on thromboembolism in patients with paroxysmal nocturnal hemoglobinuria. *Blood* 2007.
26. Ritis K, Doumas M, Mastellos D, et al: A novel C5a receptor-tissue factor cross-talk in neutrophils links innate immunity to coagulation pathways. *J Immunol* 177:4794, 2006.
27. Emadi A, Brodsky RA: Successful discontinuation of anticoagulation following eculizumab administration in paroxysmal nocturnal hemoglobinuria. *Am J Hematol* 84:699, 2009.
28. Santarone S, Bacigalupo A, Risitano AM, et al: Hematopoietic stem cell transplantation for paroxysmal nocturnal hemoglobinuria: Long-term results of a retrospective study on behalf of the Gruppo Italiano Trapianto Midollo Osseo (GITMO). *Haematologica* 95:983, 2010.
29. Takahashi Y, McCoy JP, Jr, Carvallo C, et al: In vitro and in vivo evidence of PNH cell sensitivity to immune attack after nonmyeloablative allogeneic hematopoietic cell transplantation. *Blood* 103:1383, 2004.
30. Brodsky RA, Luznik L, Bolanos-Meade J, et al: Reduced intensity HLA-haploidentical BMT with post transplantation cyclophosphamide in nonmalignant hematologic diseases. *Bone Marrow Transplant* 42:523, 2008.

CHAPTER 30

ACQUIRED DISORDERS OF RED CELL, WHITE CELL, AND PLATELET PRODUCTION

Jaroslaw P. Maciejewski and Ramon V. Tiu

ACQUIRED PURE RED CELL APLASIA

Acquired pure red cell aplasia (PRCA) is characterized by the presence of an acquired severe normochromic, most frequently normocytic, anemia associated with a complete disappearance of reticulocytes and erythroid precursors in the marrow and normal production of myeloid cells and platelets. Consequently it is presumed that the defect lies within erythroid precursors and not within stem cells as seen in aplastic anemia. Initially described by Kaznelson[1] in 1922, PRCA is a rare bone marrow failure disorder without geographic or racial predilection. All ages can be affected, but, if present in children, it is called transient erythroblastopenia of childhood (TEC) and may be difficult to distinguish from congenital causes of anemia, mainly Diamond-Blackfan anemia (DBA). Former nosology included various terms such as *erythrophthisis, chronic hypoplastic anemia, pure red cell agenesis,* and *primary red cell anemia.*

ETIOLOGY AND CLASSIFICATION

Acquired forms of PRCA must be distinguished from congenital forms of PRCA, which usually manifest themselves early in life (see Chapter 28). Acquired PRCA occurring in childhood may be difficult to distinguish from DBA. As an acquired disease, PRCA may be a primary disorder or secondary to a variety of systemic diseases, including a number of hematologic diseases (Table 30-1).

Pathogenesis

The inciting events in the development of PRCA are not known. However, as with idiopathic aplastic anemia, viruses or exposure to chemicals can serve as potential triggers (Fig. 30-1). Theoretically a viral infection could lead to depletion of erythroid precursors. Studies of B19 parvovirus (see later) suggest such an etiology. Because hematopoietic stem cells are not affected by B19 parvovirus, myeloid cells and platelets are normally produced, and upon clearance of the virus, normal erythroid production can resume. Similarly, in immune-mediated PRCA, the mechanism of erythroid inhibition may vary and may include (1) antibodies to proteins specific to erythroblasts, (2) direct cytotoxic T lymphocyte (CTL)–mediated killing of erythroid precursors, and (3) production of soluble products by CTLs such as inhibitory or proapoptotic cytokines that directly affect the erythroid series.

Historically, initial studies concentrated on examining the effects of soluble serum inhibitors of erythropoiesis. These investigations revealed a decline in erythroid colony formation in the presence of patient serum or failure to induce erythroid colony formation in the presence of erythropoietin.[2,3] Such serum inhibitors can be found in 40% of patients with PRCA.[2-4] In 60% of patients, erythroid colony formation can be induced in vitro with hematopoietic growth factors.[2-4] The inhibitory activity is localized to the immunoglobulin (Ig) G fraction and disappears upon achieving a clinical remission. The antigenic targets for autoantibodies have not been well characterized, but various stages of erythroid differentiation can be affected (also called PRCA type A), as seen in the reduction of burst-forming unit–erythroid (BFU-E) or colony-forming unit–erythroid (CFU-E).[5,6] In certain cases of antibody-mediated PRCA, the involvement of the complement system is a prerequisite to disease causation.[7] Perhaps the exception and a model for antibody-induced red cell aplasia is the identification of PRCA associated with antierythropoietin antibodies (also called PRCA type B) in rare cases.[8,9] Consistent with the specificity of the antibodies, myeloid colony formation is not impaired, making it unlikely that a more ubiquitous inhibitory cytokine mediates the specific erythroid inhibition.

In recent years, experimental and clinical observations have suggested that PRCA may be mediated by CTLs, which specifically recognize and kill erythroid precursors similar to CTL-mediated killing of cells in aplastic anemia.[10-12] Although such a T cell–mediated antierythroid response is likely to be polyclonal, rare instances of T-cell large granular lymphocyte (T-LGL) leukemia associated with PRCA or erythroid inhibition may represent an extreme form of the clonal continuum of CTL responses (see T-Cell Large Granular Lymphocyte–Associated PRCA). In addition to CTLs expressing α/β T-cell receptors (TCRs), T cells with a γ/δ TCR can mediate PRCA.[13,14] The antigens/antigenic peptides triggering such a response have not been well described.[15,16] Similarly, natural killer (NK) cells have also been implicated in mediating cytotoxicity directed against erythroid precursors.[17,18] NK cells, like γ/γ T lymphocytes and unlike α/β CTLs, do not rely on major histocompatibility complex (MHC)–restricted cytotoxicity, but may use killer-cell immunoglobulin-like receptors (KIRs).[19,20] KIRs inhibit cytolysis when they encounter a cell bearing human leukocyte antigen (HLA) class I molecules. A lack of appropriate KIRs may predispose cells to increased attack by NK cells or γ/δ CTLs. Physiologic downregulation of KIRs has been implicated in the pathogenesis of PRCA in a patient with concomitant γ/δ T-LGL clonal proliferation.[13,21] An alternative NK-cell cytotoxic mechanism independent of KIR has been reported in healthy individuals.[22]

Peripheral T-helper lymphocyte polarization has been implicated in the pathogenesis of PRCA.[16,23] Polarization toward the Th2 functional subtype (interleukin [IL]-4) during disease relapse and normalization of Th1/Th2 ratio after effective treatment has been reported in both monoclonal gammopathy of undetermined significance (MGUS) and thymoma-associated PRCA. Further studies have shown increased C-MAF gene expression in relapsed PRCA associated with Th2 polarization, a mechanism that may help explain the alteration in Th1/Th2 balance.[16]

PRIMARY PURE RED CELL APLASIA

Primary PRCA occurs in the absence of any underlying disorder. It may be acute and self-limited or may be a chronic and refractory condition. Acute forms are uncommon. Most cases are protracted and chronic, unlike TEC, which is an acute and self-limited disorder. Most of the cases of classic primary PRCA are autoimmune in origin, but a significant proportion will remain idiopathic in origin in spite of an exhaustive workup.

Table 30-1 Classification of Pure Red Cell Aplasia

Congenital (DBA)		
Primary	Autoimmune Idiopathic	
Secondary	Thymoma[8,9,32-34] Hematologic malignancies	CLL[24,25] T-LGL/chronic NK-LGL leukemia[10,11,17,18,28-31] Myeloma[593] NHL[594,595] MDS[596] ALL[597-599]
	Solid tumors	Renal cell carcinoma[600] Thyroid cancer[601] Various adenocarcinomas[602,603]
	Infections	Parvovirus B19[50] EBV,[39] mumps HIV,[61] HTLV-1[28] CMV[60] Viral hepatitis (hepatitis A,[55,56,604] hepatitis B[57,58]) Leishmaniasis[244] Gram-positive systemic infections (e.g., staphylococcemia) Meningococcemia
	Autoimmune conditions	SLE[74] RA[69] Sjögren syndrome[71,72] Mixed connective tissue disease[66] Autoimmune hepatitis[605] Anti-EPO antibodies[606,607] ABO-incompatible BMT Minor incompatibility[93-98]
	Drugs and chemicals	
	Pregnancy[43,44]	
	Severe nutritional deficiencies[608,609]	
	Renal failure[610]	

ALL, Acute lymphoblastic leukemia; *BMT,* bone marrow transplantation; *CLL,* chronic lymphocytic leukemia; *CMV,* cytomegalovirus; *DBA,* Diamond-Blackfan anemia; *EBV,* Epstein-Barr virus; *EPO,* erythropoietin; *HIV,* human immunodeficiency virus; *HTLV-1,* human T-lymphotrophic virus-1; *MDS,* myelodysplastic syndrome; *NHL,* non-Hodgkin lymphoma; *NK-LGL,* natural killer large granular lymphocyte; *RA,* refractory anemia; *SLE,* systemic lupus erythematosus; *T-LGL,* T-cell large granular lymphocyte.

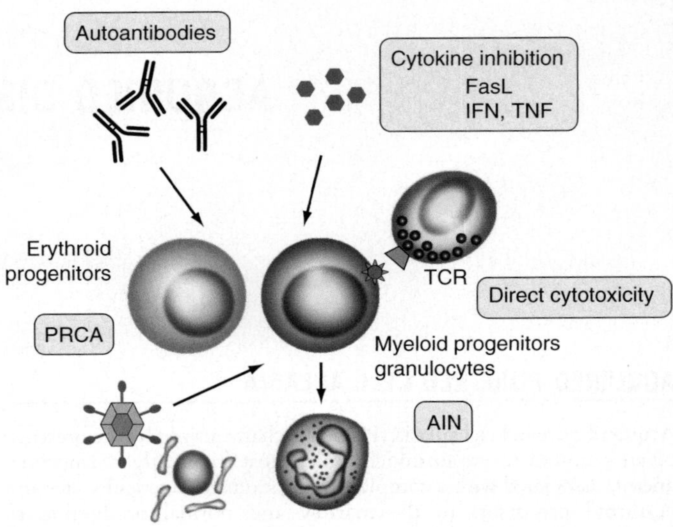

Figure 30-1 PATHOGENESIS OF PURE RED CELL APLASIA. *AIN,* Autoimmune neutropenia; *FasL,* Fas ligand; *IFN,* interferon; *PRCA,* pure red cell aplasia; *TCR,* T-cell receptor; *TNF,* tumor necrosis factor.

SECONDARY FORMS OF PURE RED CELL APLASIA

Clinical Associations

B-Cell Chronic Lymphocytic Leukemia–Associated PRCA

In B-cell chronic lymphocytic leukemia (CLL), PRCA can be observed in up to 6% of cases.[10,24,25] The underlying pathogenetic mechanisms are not clear, and the inhibition of the erythroid series does not appear to be mediated by a soluble factor.[26,27] The distinction between whether the PRCA is a result of the primary B-cell CLL disease or its therapy becomes difficult in circumstances when PRCA presents as a late event. In most cases, PRCA cannot be attributed simply to infiltration of the marrow by the lymphoma.

T-Cell Large Granular Lymphocyte–Associated PRCA

Although neutropenia is a typical finding in T-LGL leukemia, PRCA with varying degrees of erythroblastopenia can also be observed in 10% to 15% of patients with T-LGL leukemia.[11,28-31] In such a setting, PRCA is often accompanied by red cells with an increased mean corpuscular volume. T-LGL leukemia with PRCA may respond to oral cyclophosphamide, cyclosporine A (CsA), methotrexate, and in refractory cases to antithymocyte globulin (ATG) therapy. It is possible that PRCA associated with T-LGL leukemia represents an extreme form of the T cell–mediated disease that, if polyclonal, might be classified as idiopathic PRCA.

Thymoma-Associated PRCA

Thymoma is associated with PRCA; thus a chest x-ray examination or computed tomographic (CT) scan should be included in the workup for PRCA. Antibodies with direct inhibitory effects against erythroid precursors may be present.[8,9,32-34] T cell–mediated inhibition of erythropoiesis has also been implicated in the pathogenesis of PRCA associated with either benign or malignant thymomas.[35-38] Thymectomy is the usual initial treatment approach[34]; however, incomplete responders, nonresponders, and patients who relapse are common,[38] necessitating additional therapies in the form of azathioprine,[39] intravenous immunoglobulins (IVIgs),[40] and CsA.[41]

Pregnancy-Associated PRCA

Pregnancy-associated PRCA is a self-limited syndrome that may occur at any age of gestation.[42] It has a high risk for relapse during subsequent pregnancies and can be safely managed with either blood transfusions or corticosteroids.[43,44] Patients with other forms of PRCA may also be more prone to relapse during pregnancy.[45]

Parvovirus B19 and Other Viral-Induced PRCAs

Parvovirus B19 is a single-stranded deoxyribonucleic acid (DNA) virus, which in normal individuals causes fifth disease (erythema infectiosum) in children and arthropathy in adults.[46-49] The cellular receptor for the virus is the P antigen, a blood group antigen also responsible for the agglutination reaction that occurs in the presence of the virus. Detection of parvovirus B19–specific IgM without anti–parvovirus B19 IgG supports the diagnosis of acute infection, whereas the parvovirus B19–specific IgG suggests immunity.[50] Addition of parvovirus B19 in vitro to cultures of erythroid progenitor cells completely abolishes erythroid colony formation.[47,48] Primary infection causes lifelong immunity; however, it is possible that a latent virus may persist in a healthy individual for years.

A transient aplastic crisis is a typical complication of a primary parvovirus B19 infection in patients with increased red cell turnover (usually chronic hemolysis, e.g., hemoglobinopathies, and hereditary disorders of red blood cell [RBC] membrane, e.g., hereditary spherocytosis).[51-53] In typical cases, the occurrence of acute reticulocytopenia results in a sudden drop in hemoglobin (Hb)/hematocrit (Hct) levels as RBC destruction continues but is unsupported by a suppressed marrow. Occasionally, characteristic giant pronormoblasts may be seen in marrow aspirates (Fig. 30-2). This disorder is often self-limiting with the evolution of a protective IgG response. Viral titers in the serum of affected patients may be high. Supportive transfusions may be needed during the acute phase of the disease.

A more chronic form, parvovirus B19–related PRCA, may develop in immunocompromised patients as, for example, in acquired immunodeficiency syndrome (AIDS). In such cases, IVIg can produce remarkable responses. High doses of IVIg are required (>2 g/kg) because an insufficient dose may not produce the desired effect. DNA dot blot hybridization is the best diagnostic test for the detection of viremia. Parvovirus B19 can also be detected by polymerase chain reaction (PCR), a routinely available test, but this method may provide a high rate of false-positive results. However, if test results are negative, it excludes B19 parvovirus–mediated disease.[50] Improved tests have been developed that allow for the detection of neutralizing antibodies and infectivity of parvovirus B19.[54]

Several other viral infections, including viral hepatitis (A[55,56] and C[57,58]), Epstein-Barr virus (EBV),[59] cytomegalovirus (CMV),[60] human T-lymphotrophic virus-1 (HTLV-1),[28] and human immunodeficiency virus (HIV)[61] have been implicated as causative agents of PRCA. Little is known about the exact mechanisms underlying these disorders, but they likely involve T cell–mediated suppression as observed during HTLV-1 infection[28] and EBV or antibody-mediated destruction of red cell precursors, as in hepatitis C–induced PRCA.[57,58] Frequently the presence of multiple comorbidities and medications makes it difficult to pinpoint the exact causative agent.[61,62]

Connective Tissue Disease--Associated PRCA

The majority of connective tissue diseases associated with PRCA are autoimmune in nature. Several rheumatologic diseases have been associated with PRCA, including adult-onset Still disease,[63,64] dermatomyositis,[65] mixed connective tissue disease,[66] polymyositis,[67] rheumatoid arthritis,[68,69] Sjögren syndrome,[70-72] and systemic lupus erythematosus.[73-75] The pathogenesis of the PRCA in this setting may vary and includes autoantibody-mediated erythroid inhibition,[76] autoantibody directed against erythropoietin,[77] and CTL-mediated killing of erythroid precursors.[73]

Drug-Induced PRCA

Various chemical agents and drugs have been associated with PRCA. The mechanisms responsible for erythroid inhibition may be diverse depending on the offending agent (Table 30-2) but may include induction of antibodies targeting the drugs or drugs bound to cellular and plasma proteins. Another possible mechanism involves drug-mediated triggering of T-cell responses, or direct toxicity to the erythroid series as seen with diphenylhydantoin.[78]

Erythropoietin Antibody–Associated PRCA

Erythropoietin is produced mainly by the kidneys and to a limited extent by the liver. Recombinant erythropoietin is used in the treatment of anemias of various origins, including, for example, anemia of chronic disease, renal disease, and a variety of bone marrow failure syndromes, particularly myelodysplastic syndrome (MDS). Cases of PRCA have developed as a consequence of antibody formation

Table 30-2 Drugs and Chemicals Implicated in Pure Red Cell Aplasia

Alemtuzumab[152]	Isoniazid[631-633]
Allopurinol[611,612]	Lamivudine[62]
α-Methyldopa[613]	Linezolid[634]
Aminopyrine[614]	Maloprim[635]
Azathioprine[615,616]	Mycophenolate mofetil[643]
Benzene[617]	Penicillin[636]
Carbamazepine[618]	Phenylbutazone[637]
Cephalothin[619]	Phenytoin[78,638,639]
Chloramphenicol[620]	Procainamide[640-642]
Chlorpropamide[621,622]	Ribavirin[643,644]
Cladribine[623]	Rifampicin[645]
Cotrimoxazole[624]	Sulfasalazine[646,647]
D-Penicillinamine[625]	Sulfathiozole[648]
Erythropoietin[606,607]	Sulindac[649]
Estrogens[626]	Tacrolimus[650]
Fludarabine[627]	Thiamphenicol[651]
FK506[628]	Ticlopidine[652,653]
Gold[629]	Valproic acid[198,644]
Halothane[630]	Zidovudine[654]
Interferon-α[563,564]	

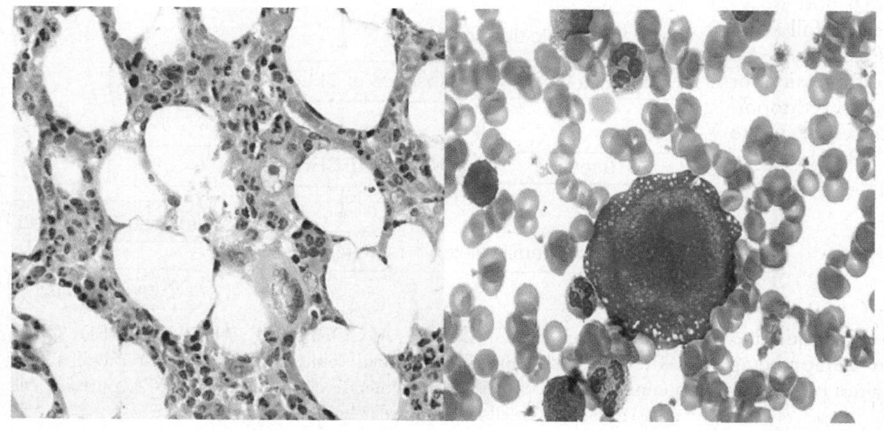

Figure 30-2 PARVOVIRUS B19–MEDIATED PURE RED CELL APLASIA.

against endogenous erythropoietin[79] or while receiving treatment with recombinant erythropoietin.[80-82] The latter condition has been referred to as *epoetin-induced PRCA* or *EPO-PRCA.* The first three cases of EPO-PRCA were reported between 1988 and 1998,[81,83] with 13 cases subsequently reported in France between 1998 and 2000, mainly related to exposure to epoetin alpha (Eprex; 92%) and epoetin beta (NeoRecormon; 8%).[82] The exact pathogenesis remains unclear but may be related to the formation of neutralizing antierythropoietin antibodies. There are several risk factors to the development of EPO-PRCA, including subcutaneous route of administration, use of epoetin alpha stabilized in a human serum albumin (HSA)–free formulation, use of silicone oil as lubricant in prefilled Eprex syringes, and use in patients with chronic renal disease.[84,85] All these factors increase the immunogenic potential of the antierythropoietin antibodies. This observation has lead to modification in the storage, handling, and administration of Eprex favoring intravenous (IV) administration, especially with Eprex stabilized with HSA-free formulation, and avoidance of the subcutaneous non–HSA stabilized Eprex for patients with chronic renal disease. Of note is that cases of EPO-PRCA occurring after IV epoetin administration have been described.[80,86] There are reports of human erythropoietin (HuEPO) neutralizing antibody PRCA related to the use of biosimilar recombinant HuEPO in Thailand.[87] Diagnostic criteria have also been proposed incorporating major features (treatment with epoetin for at least 3 weeks, decrease in Hgb by 0.1 g/dL/day without transfusions or transfusion need of about 1 unit/week to keep hemoglobin level stable, reticulocyte count $<10 \times 10^9$/L, no major drop in white blood cell [WBC] and platelet counts), minor features (skin and systemic allergic reactions), and accessory investigations (e.g., bone marrow showing normal cellularity and <5% erythroblasts with evidence of maturation block, and serum assay showing presence of antierythropoietin antibodies and evidence of neutralizing capacity).[80] All major criteria are required for diagnosis, whereas minor features must be confirmed by additional confirmatory tests, usually in the form of bone marrow biopsy and detection of neutralizing antierythropoietin antibodies. The most commonly used tests to detect antibodies are enzyme-linked immunosorbent assay (ELISA), radioimmunoprecipitation assay, and surface plasmon resonance. Once antibodies are detected, their neutralizing ability is tested using an in vitro bioassay. Following establishment of diagnosis, management should include discontinuation of exogenous erythropoietin, administration of immunosuppressive agents, or, in cases of anemia secondary to renal insufficiency, renal transplantation. It is possible to use and regain response to recombinant erythropoietin once antierythropoietin antibodies have disappeared.[88]

PRCA Postallogeneic Stem Cell Transplantation

In contrast to HLA matching, ABO blood group incompatibility plays a minor role in the success of allogeneic hematopoietic stem cell transplantation (HSCT). However, PRCA may be associated with major ABO incompatibility between the donor and recipient, leading to inhibition of donor erythroid precursors by residual host isoagglutinins. This complication is more commonly observed following the use of nonmyeloablative conditioning regimens. PRCA may also be resistant to the withdrawal or decrease of immunosuppression, or donor lymphocyte infusions. Responses to rituximab,[89,90] erythropoietin,[91] and azathioprine[91] have been reported. A case responsive to purified $CD34^+$ cell infusion has also been reported.[92] Resolution of PRCA is generally associated with decrease and subsequent disappearance of host isoagglutinins.[93-98]

PRCA Postradiation Therapy

In rare circumstances, PRCA may be associated with prior radiation therapy. The cases described usually involve radiation therapy being administered to a patient with an underlying thymoma not previously associated with PRCA.[99,100]

PRCA Associated With Immune Dysregulation, Polyendocrinopathy, Enteropathy, X-Linked Syndrome

Immune dysregulation, polyendocrinopathy, enteropathy, X-linked (IPEX) syndrome is a rare X-linked recessive condition typically seen during infancy. Clinical features may include type 1 diabetes mellitus, eczema, and autoimmune hepatitis. PRCA not associated with parvovirus infections develops at around 39 months of life and is responsive to steroid therapy.[101]

Anemia is the leading symptom of PRCA and can be severe at diagnosis because the fall in hemoglobin occurs over a protracted period of time and patients often exhibit a good degree of adaptation. Arrest of erythropoiesis is obvious with a profound reticulocytopenia. In children, TEC is usually diagnosed during evaluation of a febrile illness. In primary, idiopathic PRCA, physical signs other than those of anemia are usually absent. In secondary PRCA, the physical findings are consistent with the underlying primary disease.

LABORATORY EVALUATION

A complete blood cell count (CBC) with differential, peripheral smear review, reticulocyte count, and a bone marrow examination remain the cornerstone in the diagnosis of PRCA. The classic hematologic picture of PRCA includes a CBC showing a normocytic, normochromic anemia (anemia associated with T-LGL leukemia is often macrocytic) with normal WBC and platelet count. The reticulocyte count is significantly reduced to less than 1% (a reticulocyte level greater than 2% is not compatible with the diagnosis of PRCA; (Fig. 30-3). The bone marrow examination generally shows absence of the erythroid lineage and normal appearance of granulocytic and monocytic precursors and megakaryocytes. Erythroid precursors, if present, are usually less than 1%, and only a few residual proerythroblasts or basophilic erythroblasts may be seen. Blast cell numbers and cellularity are within normal limits. There are no dysplastic changes, ringed sideroblasts, or reticulin fibrosis. Cytogenetic evaluation is normal. In some cases, neutropenia,[102] mild thrombocytopenia, eosinophilia,[16] thrombocytosis,[16] leukocytosis, or relative lymphocytosis may be seen. Cytogenetic abnormalities, if present, may indicate concomitant myelodysplasia and is a poor prognostic marker for both response to treatment and propensity to leukemic

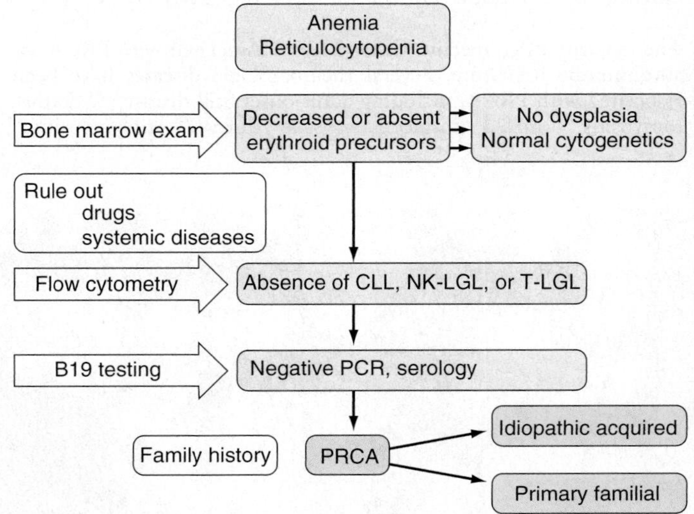

Figure 30-3 DIAGNOSTIC ALGORITHM IN PURE RED CELL APLASIA. *CLL,* Chronic lymphocytic leukemia; *NK-LGL,* natural killer large granular lymphocyte; *PCR,* polymerase chain reaction; *PRCA,* pure red cell aplasia; *T-LGL,* T-cell large granular lymphocyte.

transformation.[103,104] During the natural history of PRCA, ineffective erythropoiesis characterized by maturation arrest at the proerythroblast or basophilic erythroblast stage may be observed and signifies either partial response to treatment or initial recovery from treatment or a prelude to the development of full-blown PRCA.[105]

It is important to exclude vitamin B_{12} and folate deficiencies, and depending on the etiology and associated disease, other blood and bone marrow findings may be seen. The presence of giant and vacuolated pronormoblasts in the bone marrow examination should raise the suspicion for parvovirus B19 infection.[50] The presence of large granular lymphocytosis, neutropenia, and/or thrombocytopenia, expansion of $CD3^+CD8^+CD57^+$ T cells, clonal cytotoxic TCR gene rearrangement, expansion of specific TCR Vβ region family gene segment, and splenomegaly may point toward concomitant T-LGL leukemia,[106,107] B-cell lymphocytosis, especially of the $CD5^+/CD19^+/CD20^+/CD23^+$/cyclin D^-/SmIg^{-dim} phenotype with concomitant lymphadenopathy, hepatosplenomegaly, hypogammaglobulinemia, and thrombocytopenia may be very suggestive of a B-cell CLL. Another laboratory finding that may help point to a secondary cause of PRCA includes the presence of monoclonal gammopathy.[16] Parvovirus B19 DNA titers (DNA hybridization and amplification techniques) may show high levels of the virus at 10^{12} genome copies per milliliter, but it is important to note that serologic (IgM and IgG) titers are usually absent.[50] Erythropoietin antibodies,[82] antinuclear antibodies,[108,109] and/or complement consumption may point toward a specific disease mechanism.[110] A radiographic workup may also be useful in the clinical workup because chest x-ray examination or CT scan may show evidence of a thymoma.

DIFFERENTIAL DIAGNOSIS

PRCA can be easily differentiated from aplastic anemia and other types of bone marrow failure syndromes. A distinction between MDS with erythroid hypoplasia and idiopathic PRCA may be more difficult. In childhood, TEC has to be distinguished from DBA, but a history of normal blood counts, late onset of manifestation, and transient disease course are characteristic of TEC.

THERAPY

The distinction between primary and secondary forms of PRCA is essential because many secondary types have specific and very effective therapies (Table 30-3). All potentially offending drugs should be discontinued, and drug-associated PRCA should remit within 3 to 4 weeks. Nutritional deficiencies (B_{12} and folic acid) should be excluded and treated if present. The therapy of primary and secondary forms of PRCA refractory to the treatment of an underlying disease may be challenging and should include a sequential trial of various immunosuppressive agents until a response is achieved. Spontaneous remissions have been reported.

Surgery or Radiation

In cases associated with thymoma, thymectomy is the usual initial treatment of choice before immunosuppression and may induce remission with return of erythropoiesis in 4 to 8 weeks in about 30% to 40% of patients.[111-113] Patients who remain refractory following surgery should be treated as patients with idiopathic PRCA. The removal of a thymoma may improve responsiveness to immunosuppressive therapy.[112] Thymectomy in the absence of a thymoma in other forms of PRCA is not recommended. In circumstances where surgical resection of thymoma is contraindicated, radiation therapy with or without chemotherapy may be administered.[114]

Medical

Supportive

Supportive care includes blood transfusions and iron chelation with deferasirox (Exjade). Deferasirox is a new once-daily, oral iron chelator developed for treating transfusional iron overload syndromes used in a variety of hematologic disorders, including thalassemia and sickle cell anemia; it works primarily by promoting fecal excretion of iron. Side effects may include diarrhea, renal failure, and rarely agranulocytosis.[115,116]

Immunosuppression

Prednisone therapy at a dose of 0.5 to 1 mg/kg is associated with significant response rates (approximately 40%) and should constitute the initial therapeutic approach.[104] Initial responses are generally observed after 4 to 6 weeks.[103,117] A slow taper of prednisone is suggested over a period of 3 to 4 months. The disease may relapse, and the minimal maintenance dose of corticosteroids may need to be established to maintain the desired hemoglobin levels.[118] Trials of prednisone therapy without clinical response longer than 8 weeks are not warranted.[103,104,117]

Alternative therapies may include cyclosporine, oral cyclophosphamide, azathioprine, antithymocyte globulin (ATG), rituximab, and alemtuzumab (see Table 30-3). Erythropoietin and darbepoietin[119,120] are usually not effective as a sole agent but may hasten recovery following an adequate trial of cyclophosphamide. No randomized trials exist to favor a particular treatment based on efficacy.

Table 30-3 Therapy for Pure Red Cell Aplasia and Its Results

	Study								
Agent	**Chikkappa[143]**	**Means[145]**	**Au[153]**	**Dessypris[117]**	**Zecca[655]**	**Lacy[104]**	**Charles[103]**	**Sloand[149]**	**Abkowitz[147]**
Steroids				18/41		9/29	9/36	—	
Cytotoxic agents				24/54		14/29	8/27	—	
Antithymocyte globulin				2/6		0/1	8/12		6/6
Cyclosporine A	6/7	6/9		3/4		4/5	2/3		
Splenectomy				4/23		0/1	0/1		
Daclizumab (Zenapax)								6/15	
Rituximab					1/1				
Alemtuzumab (Campath)			2/2						
Methotrexate							2/37		

The choice of therapy may be influenced by clinical clues. For example, the presence of large granular lymphocytes (LGLs) may suggest the use of CsA, hypogammaglobulinemia may be corrected with IVIg, whereas detection of hypergammaglobulinemia or monoclonal protein may suggest a choice of rituximab. Most refractory cases may require administration of ATG. The age of the patient may influence the choice of the cytotoxic agent, which may pose a significant risk for the development of secondary leukemias, especially with a prolonged administration.

Danazol is a synthetic attenuated androgen that has been used for many years for the treatment of a variety of hematologic disorders, mainly myelofibrosis.[121] Usually given at 200 mg orally (PO) twice a day, the maximum dose per day is 600 mg. It has been used to treat PRCA either as a single agent or in conjunction with steroids or other agents and has shown efficacy in PRCA of various etiologies.[122-125] The main adverse events reported include liver transaminitis and vascular liver tumors.

IVIg (Gammagard, Octagam, Panglobulin) given at 1 to 2 g/kg IV for 5 days is also effective in several types of PRCA.[126-129] Higher doses of usually 2 g/kg of IVIg for 5 days are necessary for the treatment of parvovirus B19 virus–induced PRCA. In AIDS patients with parvovirus B19 virus–induced PRCA, a regimen consists of induction therapy with 1 g/kg daily for 1 to 2 days followed by 1 g/kg for 2 days. If the patient relapses, then maintenance therapy with IVIg 0.4 to 1.0 g/kg every 4 weeks is recommended.[130]

Azathioprine is an imidazolyl derivative of mercaptopurine that inhibits DNA synthesis by inhibition of purine metabolism. In PRCA, it may be given at a dose of 2 to 3 mg/kg/day IV and has been found to be effective in patients nonresponsive to cyclophosphamide.[39,131]

Oral cyclophosphamide may be started at a dose of 50 mg PO daily, with a maximal dose of no more than 150 mg daily. Blood counts should be monitored, and the dose may be escalated accordingly. Trials of therapy longer than 3 months without signs of response are not warranted. Monitoring of the reticulocyte count may allow for the early assessment of response. Often, a delayed response may be seen when cyclophosphamide is withdrawn, which reflects the fine balance between adequate immunosuppression and cytotoxicity.*

Rituximab given at 375 mg/m^2 IV infusion weekly for 4 weeks has been found to be efficacious in PRCA. PRCA in a variety of settings, including B-cell CLL, EBV-associated posttransplant lymphoproliferative disease (EBV-PTLD), ABO-incompatible allogeneic HSCT for acute myeloid leukemia, and hairy cell leukemia variant, has been successfully treated.[89,134-137] Owing to the fact that rituximab is specific for B cells alone, cases of nonresponders to it have been reported and attributed to an alternative T cell–mediated pathogenesis.[138] In cases of refractory to immunosuppressive agents affecting T-cell function, rituximab or low-dose alemtuzumab constitutes a reasonable option. Rituximab is effective in patients with PRCA owing to ABO incompatibility following bone marrow transplantation.[89,90]

CsA can be administered at a dose of 5 to 10 mg/kg PO daily in divided doses. CsA can be combined with prednisone at doses of 20 to 30 mg PO. The trough levels of CsA should be monitored, and the dose adjusted to achieve a level between 200 and 300 μg/mL. An adequate trial of therapy is considered 3 months of therapy. The response rates may be as high as 60% to 80%. After a response is achieved, the therapy should be continued for 6 months followed by a slow taper.[103,104,139-145]

Horse ATG may be given to refractory cases at a dose of 40 mg/kg IV daily for 4 days with prednisone at 1 mg/kg. Rabbit ATG (Thymoglobulin) may be given a dose of 2.5 to 3.5 mg/kg daily IV for 4 or 5 days with prednisone at 1 mg/kg. Concomitant prednisone should be administered and then tapered over 2 to 3 weeks. A therapeutic response should occur within 3 months posttherapy, although responses at or beyond 6 months may be observed.[8,103,104,117,146-148]

*References 3, 4, 104, 117, 132, 133.

Daclizumab, an anti–IL-2 receptor antibody (Zenapax, anti-CD25 mAb), may constitute a good alternative to ATG because it does not require hospitalization and is well tolerated. In a recent trial, a dose of 1 mg/kg of body weight IV was administered every 2 weeks. The therapy should be given for at least 3 months. It is possible that combination with CsA may increase the response rate, but no data exist as to the observed response rates.[149,150] Unfortunately, this drug was withdrawn from the market in 2009.

Methotrexate, an antimetabolite, at low doses (7.5 to 15 mg/week PO) is useful in treating PRCA, especially in patients with concomitant LGL leukemia. The responses are generally sustained, and therapy is well tolerated. Methotrexate may be given in conjunction with other therapies like CsA.[12,103]

Alemtuzumab (Campath, anti-CD52 mAb) is a recombinant DNA–derived humanized monoclonal antibody directed against the cell surface glycoprotein CD52, which is expressed on the surface of normal and malignant B and T lymphocytes. It can be given IV or subcutaneously every other day with an initial dose of 3 mg, and subsequent doses can be increased until response is obtained. The usual cumulative dose before response is usually between 200 and 400 mg. Alemtuzumab has been tested in a variety of lymphoproliferative disorders, including diffuse large B-cell lymphoma, B-cell CLL, and T-LGL leukemia. Similarly, PRCA occurring in the context of these conditions previously unresponsive to therapy with steroids, CsA, and even cyclophosphamide (Cytoxan) has been shown to be responsive to this agent. Alemtuzumab can be given either intravenously or subcutaneously.[151-153]

Bortezomib (Velcade) is a proteasome inhibitor containing boron that binds to the catalytic site of the 26S proteasome. It is commonly used in the treatment of multiple myeloma and can be given either intravenously or subcutaneously. A patient who developed isohemagglutinin-mediated PRCA after ABO-mismatched allogeneic hematopoietic cell transplant was successfully treated with IV bortezomib given at 1.3 g/m^2 weekly for 4 weeks. Improvement in reticulocyte counts were noted 30 days after therapy accompanied by an increase in Hgb levels. The patient subsequently achieved complete transfusion independence. Anti-A isohemagglutinin titers were undetectable 30 days after the first dose of bortezomib.[154]

Hematopoietic Stem Cell Transplantation

Despite advances in immunosuppressive regimens, subsets of patients with PRCA remain refractory and are very difficult to treat. As with other bone marrow failure disorders with autoimmune pathogenesis like aplastic anemia, HSCT is an important treatment option especially for refractory and relapsed PRCA cases. Matched sibling donor allogeneic HSCT results in restoration of normal hematopoiesis in patients with refractory PRCA.[155-157] In another case, a patient with relapsed PRCA underwent matched sibling donor allogeneic HSCT combined with donor lymphocyte infusions resulting in full donor engraftment and subsequent return of normal hematopoiesis, suggesting a graft-versus-autoimmunity effect as the likely mechanism for response.[158]

PROGNOSIS

The prognosis of secondary PRCA depends upon the underlying disease. Idiopathic PRCA may be very refractory to treatment. Ultimately, remission may be achieved in a significant proportion (approximately 68%) of patients, especially when sequential regimens are used. Spontaneous remissions are observed in 5% to 10% of cases. Relapses are common, especially during the first year postremission but are usually responsive to the same regimen that induced remission.[103,117] Chronic, low-dose immunosuppressive therapy may be needed in certain cases that have relapsed. In one study, median survival was reported to be 14 years.[117] Unlike a megakaryocytic thrombocytopenic purpura, evolution to aplastic anemia is rare[112,159] in PRCA, and, moreover, very few patients (3% to 5%) evolve into acute leukemia.[103,117]

ACQUIRED WHITE BLOOD CELL PRODUCTION DISORDER

Neutropenia is a common condition. The majority of cases are secondary to a variety of causes, including systemic or hematologic diseases. In this chapter we will describe a primary, isolated form of neutropenia in which other hematopoietic lineages are not affected. In such a setting, neutropenia may be the result of peripheral destruction or perhaps less frequently the result of the absence of myeloid progenitors in the marrow. Neutropenia may be initially noted during workup for fever and infections or may be an incidental finding on a routine CBC. The cutoff value for the diagnosis of neutropenia is an absolute neutrophil count (ANC) of less than 1500 cells/μL. This value is generally accepted as a definition for neutropenia for all ages and ethnic backgrounds except for newborn infants.[160] Clinically the most concerning consequence of neutropenia is the propensity to develop infections. ANC is the best parameter to assess the severity of neutropenia; however, the correlation between ANC and the propensity for infection is variable in different circumstances and determined by marrow neutrophil reserves, duration of neutropenia, and clinical context.[161-164] This is best illustrated in patients with chronic benign neutropenia of childhood and infancy, where patients may have an ANC as low as less than 250 cells/μL and yet they may be devoid of infections or only have mild infections.[165-167] Instead of ANC, it is the bone marrow neutrophil pool reserve that serves as the most suitable determinant of risk for infection, best evaluated through a bone marrow biopsy. In the setting of neutropenia, should the bone marrow examination reveal depleted neutrophil reserves, the ANC level correlates with the risk for infection. In contrast, if bone marrow shows adequate neutrophil reserves, then ANC levels are not predictive of the risk for developing a serious infection.

CLASSIFICATION OF ACQUIRED NEUTROPENIAS

Neutropenia as a primary disease should be distinguished from inherited forms of neutropenia, which commonly present during early childhood (see Chapter 27), and secondary forms of neutropenia associated with systemic disorders. In addition, idiopathic neutropenia is distinct from the constitutional or familial benign neutropenia frequently seen in African Americans,[168,169] Yemenites, and Falasha Jews or black Bedouins.[170] The degree of neutropenia is often mild, and there is no propensity to develop infections. Most cases of neutropenia are secondary to a variety of disorders. Primary autoimmune neutropenia (AIN) and idiopathic neutropenia are less common. We will limit our description to isolated forms of neutropenia (Table 30-4).

Table 30-4 Classification of Neutropenia

Congenital	
Primary	Autoimmune neutropenia
	Pure white cell aplasia
	Idiopathic
	Thymoma
	Hematologic malignancies (e.g., T-LGL leukemia)
	Infections/postinfectious
	Viral Measles,[219] mumps, roseola,[220,221] rubella,[656] RSV, influenza[218] Hepatitis A,[213] B,[213,214] and C[58] CMV,[222-224] EBV,[215-217] HIV[228,229] Parvovirus[225-227]
	Bacterial Tuberculosis[239,240] Brucellosis[236-238] Tularemia[235] Typhoid fever [234]
	Rickettsial Rocky Mountain spotted fever[657] Ehrlichiosis.[246,247]
	Fungal Histoplasmosis[241,242]
	Parasitic Malaria,[243] leishmaniasis[244,433]
	Autoimmune conditions, (e.g., SLE[658,659], RA[660])
	Drugs and chemicals
	Neutropenia associated with immunodeficiency[317,323]
	Severe nutritional deficiencies[251,252]
	Neutropenia due to increased margination
	Iatrogenic (e.g., hemodialysis[324,325])

CMV, Cytomegalovirus; *EBV,* Epstein-Barr virus; *HIV,* human immunodeficiency virus; *RA,* refractory anemia; *RSV,* respiratory syncytial virus; *SLE,* systemic lupus erythematosus; *T-LGL,* T-cell large granular lymphocyte.

Primary Neutropenia

Most neutropenias are secondary to various hematologic conditions and systemic diseases. However, in a small proportion of cases, an inciting cause cannot be identified despite intensive testing. Such idiopathic cases are most likely autoimmune in nature.

Chronic Idiopathic Neutropenia in Adults

Chronic idiopathic neutropenia in adults compared with those in infancy and early childhood has less tendency toward spontaneous remission, although it does generally remain clinically benign. There may be concomitant anemia or thrombocytopenia that may portend a higher incidence of splenomegaly, infectious complications, and antineutrophil antibodies (ANAs) that are complement fixing.[171] The bone marrow biopsy may show evidence of arrest in myeloid maturation and mild hypercellularity. ANAs may be seen in 36% of patients, suggesting an immunologic pathogenesis.[171]

Idiopathic neutropenias may be chronic and benign in nature or may be associated with significant morbidity. In certain instances immune neutropenia may be associated with hemolytic anemia or with immune thrombocytopenia, but these forms likely represent a distinct nosologic entity. Idiopathic neutropenia can occur at any age, including early childhood. Such cases may be difficult to distinguish from hereditary neutropenia syndromes. AIN may be associated with moderate and severe depression of neutrophil counts. Monocytosis is frequently present.[162,163] Some cases present with splenomegaly, which is to be distinguished from cytopenias associated with hypersplenism in Felty syndrome.[172] The frequency of infectious complications does not correlate with the severity of neutropenia, and patients with severe depletion of neutrophils may remain asymptomatic for long periods of time. Rare cases of chronic idiopathic neutropenia evolving to acute myeloid leukemia have been reported and were associated with point mutations in granulocyte colony-stimulating factor receptor (CSF3R).[173,174]

Conceptually AIN may be due to peripheral autoimmune destruction of neutrophils due to lineage-specific inhibition of myeloid precursors, with its extreme form being pure white cell aplasia (see Fig. 30-3). Consequently, increased peripheral destruction is associated with marrow hypercellularity and an increased number of myeloid precursors or, if myeloid progenitors are the targets, decreased myeloid precursors and a myeloid maturation arrest. Autoimmune processes have been implicated in the pathogenesis of AIN and could be mediated by both peripheral destruction of neutrophils and inhibition of myelopoiesis.[175,176] The antigens involved in these processes include neutrophil antigens NA1, NA2, ND1, ND2, and NB1 (Table 30-5). Both IgG and IgM antibodies have been implicated. Neutrophil-specific antibodies can be detected using many assays, including specific ELISA, opsonization,[177,178] leukoagglutination,[179] and direct antibody binding.[180] There are several proposed effector mechanisms as to how ANAs can result in neutropenia or affect neutrophil integrity. For example, ANAs may act as opsonins and directly enhance neutrophil destruction.[178] Alternatively, ANAs can indirectly activate, complement, and facilitate opsonization.[181] Immune complexes may also bind to the neutrophil Fc portion, leading to increased neutrophil clearance by the reticuloendothelial system,[182] and finally, ANAs may recognize and damage myeloid precursors.[183] The currently available diagnostic assays used to detect ANAs are generally based on immunofluorescence and agglutination assays. The former allows for the detection of IgM and IgG antibodies from a suspected patient that are attached to normal donor neutrophils detected by flow cytometry performed with the patient's serum and antihuman IgG. The results may be reported as strongly positive, weakly positive, or absent. The second technique, called agglutination assay, uses serum that leads to agglutination of normal neutrophils into either small or large clumps. These tests may help suggest an underlying immunologic process but cannot establish the definite cause. If there is a high index of suspicion that ANAs are the causative factor, some authors suggest that a minimum of two methods be used to detect ANAs, namely, granulocyte agglutination test and granulocyte immunofluorescence test.[184]

In addition to antibodies, T-cell responses may be associated with neutropenia. The most extreme example of such responses is T-LGL leukemia associated with neutropenia and polarized proliferation of CTLs (see later). In AIN, CTL responses are polyclonal and are often accompanied by the simultaneous presence of antibodies. It is likely that specialized CTL clones are capable of recognizing and killing myeloid precursors, interrupting granulocyte production. Consequently some cases of AIN may be amenable to therapy with immunosuppressive agents directed against T cells.

Chronic Benign Neutropenia of Infancy and Childhood

Chronic benign neutropenia of infancy and childhood is considered the most common cause of chronic neutropenia in the pediatric age-group. The majority of cases are autoimmune in nature and show clinical overlap with childhood idiopathic thrombocytopenic purpura and autoimmune hemolytic anemia. It is therefore considered a type of AIN.[185-190] An incidence of 1:100,000 has been reported in a childhood population in Scotland.[189] This form of neutropenia typically presents in children less than 3 years of age, with a median age of 8 to 11 months and with a predominance of girls.[185,187,188] The CBC usually shows an ANC of less than 250 cells/μL with normal morphologic characteristics and normal hemoglobin and platelet count. Occasionally monocytosis, eosinophilia, and mild thrombocytopenia may be present. In this condition, neutropenia is due to chronic depletion of mature granulocytes and is accompanied by a compensatory myeloid left shift in the marrow.[165-167] Most frequent clinical signs and symptoms are oral infections, including bothersome ulcers, but these are often associated with additional functional defects of neutrophils and cellulitis of the labia majora. Of importance is the normal neutrophil count at birth and absence of a history of familial forms of neutropenia. The etiology of this condition is unknown, but the pathogenesis involves ANAs, detectable in the majority of patients.[166,185,187] The antibodies are generally directed against similar antigens seen in adult AIN, especially those involving NA, NB, and ND loci. In about 25% of cases, the antibody is against an allele of neutrophil FcγRIII opsonin receptor called NA1.[185,187,188] Immunosuppressive therapy leads frequently to responses supporting the immune pathogenesis of this disease. Although the neutrophil count can be severely depressed, serious infectious complications are uncommon, and therefore treatment to raise the ANC is generally not indicated except if recurrent infections occur. Antibiotics are useful to treat infections, and granulocyte colony-stimulating factor (G-CSF) has been shown to be effective in elevating neutrophil counts.[191]

Table 30-5 Human Neutrophil Alloantigens and Autoantigens

		Nomenclature
Integrin α M chain	CD11b	HNA-4a (MART)
Integrin α L chain	CD11a	HNA-4a (OND)
Gp50-64	CD177	HNA-2a (NB1) PRV-1
Gp70-95		HNA-3a/5b
Integrin β2 chain	CD18	
FcγIII	CD16	
FCGR3B-01		HNA-1a (NA1)
FCGR3B-02		HNA-1b (NA2)
FCGR3B-03		HNA-1c (SH/NA3)

SECONDARY FORMS OF NEUTROPENIAS

Clinical Associations

Drug-Induced Neutropenia/Agranulocytosis

Drug-induced neutropenia is common.[192] The association was first described by Kracke in 1931 when agranulocytosis was observed in patients taking aminopyrine. The incidence in various studies is 1.0 to 3.4 cases per million per year.[192-197] Drugs may induce granulocytopenia by (1) direct toxicity leading to inhibition of myelopoiesis frequently observed in drugs like valproic acid,[198] carbamazepine,[199] and β-lactam antibiotics[200,201]; (2) immune-mediated (either antibody- or complement-mediated) as seen with penicillin and antithyroid drugs[202-204] or immune complex–mediated (quinidine)[205] destruction of myeloid progenitors and mature neutrophils; and (3) induction of CTL responses.[206] Genetic predisposition due to polymorphisms in various genes coding for cytokine and cytokine receptors as demonstrated for clozapine with tumor necrosis factor (TNF) and HLA polymorphisms as well as possibly variants of genes coding for a variety of metabolizing enzymes also plays a role.[207,208] Of interest are drugs that directly antagonize important vitamin cofactors necessary in normal bone marrow development. Neutropenia observed in patients treated with trimethoprim-sulfamethoxazole is due to the inhibitory effects on granulopoiesis by trimethoprim, owing to its antifolate action, which is reversed by folinic acid.[209] A similar finding can be seen with methotrexate owing to its antifolate action.

Most patients present with either asymptomatic neutropenia discovered on routine examination or symptomatic neutropenia with infectious complications, including fever, angular stomatitis, or pneumonia. The reported mortality rates vary from 1% to 25%. Most patients recover without further complications. It has been estimated that drugs account for 72% of cases of agranulocytosis. The usual time to development of overt neutropenia is around 1 to 2 weeks, and neutropenia resolves upon discontinuation of the offending drug within 10 to 14 days,[210] although time to recovery may vary depending on whether bone marrow hypoplasia is present (10 days) or not (14 days).[211] The recovery in neutrophil counts is usually preceded by increases in peripheral blood monocytes and immature granulocytes.[212] The International Agranulocytosis and Aplastic Anemia Study (IAAAS) has identified the most commonly associated agents and the relative odds ratios for developing agranulocytosis (Table 30-6).[197] In some instances, the severity of neutropenia is related to the dose and duration of the therapy. The therapy includes discontinuation of the potentially offending agents. In some instances associated with infections or prolonged recovery, G-CSF may be administered.

Neutropenia as a Manifestation of Systemic Diseases

Postinfectious Neutropenia

Neutropenia is commonly associated with viral infections, particularly in children. Various mechanisms have been implicated in neutropenia associated with systemic viral infections, including inhibition of hematopoiesis, granulocyte sequestration, margination, and peripheral destruction. Neutropenia generally improves when the viremia resolves. Neutropenia has been associated with hepatitis A,[213] B,[213,214] and C viruses,[58,213] EBV,[215-217] influenza,[218] measles,[219] roseola,[220,221] CMV,[222-224] and parvovirus B19 infections.[225-227] Neutropenia is also frequently encountered in patients with AIDS, with approximately 70% of patients being neutropenic during their illness.[228,229] The mechanisms vary and may include antibody formation against neutrophils,[230-232] direct viral inhibition of hematopoietic progenitor cells, abnormal expression of growth factors and other cytokines, and inhibitory effects exerted by HIV-infected accessory cells.[233] The HIV virus not only suppresses hematopoiesis but also increases the risk for acquiring other infections. Furthermore, therapy with antiretroviral agents may dramatically decrease neutrophil counts (see Table 30-4).

Systemic bacterial, fungal, and parasitic infections can be accompanied by neutropenia, including typhoid fever,[234] tularemia,[235] brucellosis,[236-238] mycobacterial infections,[239,240] histoplasmosis,[241,242] malaria,[243] leishmaniasis,[244,245] and ehrlichiosis.[246,247] The pathogenesis includes margination and sequestration of leukocytes as observed in malaria, in which there is reduction in the circulating polymorphonuclear neutrophil (PMN) pool and enlargement of the marginating PMN pool, primarily in the spleen and lung. Neutropenia can be present during sepsis, especially in newborns or debilitated individuals.[248,249] In such situations, neutropenia may be due to inhibition of hematopoiesis by inflammatory cytokines, exhaustion of marrow reserves, or redistribution.[250]

Table 30-6 Drugs Associated With Agranulocytosis

	Etiologic Fraction	
	Agranulocytosis	*Aplastic Anemia*
Overall	64%	62%
IAAAS	12%	27%
United States	72%	17%
Thailand	70%	2%

Drugs associated with agranulocytosis (IAAAS and other drugs of interest)
Acetyldigoxin[661]
ACE inhibitors[662,663]
Allopurinol[664-666]
Amodiaquine[667]
Benzafibrate[668]
β-Blockers[661,669]
β-Lactam antibiotics[193]
Carbamazepine[670]
Cinepazide[354,671]
Corticosteroids[672]
Cotrimoxazole,[209] other sulfonamides
Dipyridamole[661]
Deferasirox (Exjade)[673]
Dypirone[197,417]
Histamine-2 receptor antagonist[674]
Indomethacin[192]
Isoniazid[675,676]
Macrolides[677,678]
Mefloquine[679]
Nifedipine[680]
Phenytoin[681,682]
Procainamide[683,684]
Salicylates[685]
Sulfasalazine[686,687]
Sulfonylureas[183,688]
Tetracyclines[197]
Thenalidine
Thyrostatics[689-691]
Troxerutine[197]

ACE, Angiotensin-converting enzyme; *IAAAS*, International Agranulocytosis and Aplastic Anemia Study.

Neutropenia in Nutritional Deficiency and Nutritional Excess

Malnutrition, dietary restrictions, malabsorptive states, and concomitant intake of inhibitory drugs are just a few common causes of nutritional deficiencies that may lead to neutropenia. Vitamin B_{12} and folate deficiency, frequently associated with megaloblastic anemia, can also manifest with neutropenia. Lack of these essential vitamin cofactors results in the impairment of normal DNA synthesis, leading to abnormal granulopoiesis. A frequently observed morphologic feature is the presence of hypersegmented neutrophils.

Copper deficiency may also be associated with neutropenia.[251,252] Possible mechanisms may include arrest in maturation of neutrophil development as shown in studies in mice[253] and increased antineutrophil antibody formation.[254] Most cases have been found in malnourished infants, in patients with zinc intoxication[255,256] and malabsorption states,[257,258] and in persons receiving total parenteral nutrition without adequate copper supplementation.[259,260] Copper deficiency is often accompanied by a normocytic anemia, whereas platelet counts are invariably normal.[261] Other clinical and laboratory manifestations associated with copper deficiency include presence of ringed sideroblasts in the bone marrow,[262,263] macrocytic anemia,[264] low ceruloplasmin levels,[262] myeloneuropathy,[265] and skeletal abnormalities.[266]

Zinc intoxication in the absence of concomitant copper deficiency has also been associated with neutropenia generally in conjunction with severe anemia. A dysregulation in calprotectin metabolism has been suggested as a mechanism. Calprotectin, also known as the S100A8/A9 or MRP8/14 complex, is a major calcium-binding protein present in the cytosol of neutrophils, monocytes, and keratinocytes that increases during inflammatory states.[267]

Neutropenia Associated With Metabolic Disorders

Various acquired or inherited metabolic conditions may be associated with neutropenia. For example, neutropenia has been observed in patients with ketoacidosis and hyperglycemia, orotic aciduria, or methylmalonic aciduria.[268-271] Similarly, glycogen storage disease type IB is commonly associated with neutropenia responsive to myeloid growth factors.[272-275]

Acquired Neonatal Neutropenias

Neutropenia has been described in infants of hypertensive mothers. In this syndrome, the ANC can be severely depressed for 1 to 30 days postpartum.[276-278] This type of neutropenia is associated with an increased risk for early-onset sepsis in neonates,[279] a prolonged duration of neutropenia, and an increased risk for neonatal nosocomial infections.[280] Granulocyte kinetic investigations suggested that the neutropenia is the result of diminished neutrophil production. An inhibitor released by the placenta and present in cord blood serum has been shown to play a role in this syndrome.[276,281]

Moderate to severe neutropenia has also been observed secondary to IgG antibodies transferred from mother to infant. This is a condition called *isoimmune neonatal neutropenia* or *neonatal alloimmune neutropenia*. In most cases, antibodies are directed against antigens on neutrophil FcγRIIIb (anti-NA1, anti-NA2, and anti-SH)[282] and NB1,[283,284] but in rare circumstances maternal neutrophil-specific isoantibodies are also produced when there is deficiency of the FcγRIIIb gene.[285-289] The incidence of this condition can be as high as 2:1000 live births.[290] In both neutropenia occurring in hypertensive mothers and isoimmune neonatal neutropenia, differentiation from congenital forms of neutropenia may be difficult. Treatment with G-CSF is usually effective in neutropenia of infants of hypertensive mothers, but higher doses may be needed because preeclampsia-associated inhibitor of rhG-CSF may be present.[278,291,292] IVIg[293] and G-CSF[282,294] are both effective for treatment of isoimmune neonatal neutropenia.

Neutropenia and Hypersplenism

Hypersplenism may be associated with neutropenia, but in most instances other cytopenias will also be present. However, hypersplenism may be a sign of diseases that can result in neutropenia, such as in T-LGL leukemia[106,107,295] and Felty syndrome.[296,297] Other than direct sequestration, another potential mechanism leading to neutropenia may be increased neutrophil apoptosis that normalizes after splenectomy.[298] Recently a high incidence of *Helicobacter pylori* infection has been noted among individuals with neutropenia and splenomegaly. A potential role for the bacterium in the pathogenesis of the splenomegaly is being explored. Conversely one can hypothesize that the bacterium may be the culprit in the development of the neutropenia.[299] Splenectomy either laparoscopically[300] or through laparotomy[301] may be effective in most cases, although in situations precluding splenectomy, intraoperative splenic artery embolization is also effective.[302,303]

Pure White Cell Aplasia

Pure white cell aplasia (PWCA) is a rare condition with pathophysiologic overlap with some forms of AIN associated with myeloid suppression. Similar to PRCA, the pathogenesis may vary and includes antibody-mediated suppression of granulopoiesis,[202,304] T cell–mediated suppression of granulopoiesis, direct myelotoxicity as seen with certain drugs,[305] opsonization of neutrophil precursors in the bone marrow leading to its destruction by macrophages within the bone marrow,[305] and formation of an antibody-drug complex that may damage myeloid progenitors.[306] A bone marrow examination reveals either a total absence of myeloid precursors or arrest at the promyelocyte stage, with megakaryocytes and the erythroid series remaining quantitatively and qualitatively normal. In many cases, a thymoma is present.[307,308] PWCA, if associated with thymoma, has a variable clinical outcome. The complete absence of granulocytic precursors portends a poor response to both immunosuppression and thymectomy and is often fatal, whereas the presence of a maturation arrest at the promyelocyte stage may respond to immunosuppressive therapy.[304,308-311] PWCA has been described in connection with imipenem-cilastatin,[312] ibuprofen,[313] and chlorpropramide.[183] The discontinuation of the offending drug leads to rapid improvement. Recently PWCA has also been associated with primary biliary cirrhosis.[314]

Therapeutic options may include azathioprine,[304] G-CSF combined with plasmapheresis especially if the disease process is antibody mediated,[315] methylprednisolone,[312] IV cyclophosphamide combined with plasmapheresis and G-CSF,[316] and thymectomy.[307] Severe depression of counts may require ATG therapy (see later).

Neutropenia Associated With Immunologic Abnormalities

Acquired and inherited defects of the cellular and humoral immune system may be accompanied by secondary neutropenias. In the inherited immunodeficiency syndromes, the initial presentation is in children and may be associated with failure to thrive. X-linked agammaglobulinemia is a primary immunodeficiency disorder caused by mutations in the gene for Bruton tyrosine kinase (Btk) expressed in both myeloid and B cells that result in the absence of development of B lymphocytes and hypogammaglobulinemia. Neutropenia is seen in 15% to 26% of patients with X-linked agammaglobulinemia, and most suffer from upper respiratory tract infection.[317-319] The exact pathogenetic mechanism is not clear but is believed to be related to the crucial role of Btk in myeloid survival under stress.

Neutropenia is seen in 40% to 50% of patients with X-linked hyper-IgM syndrome[320] and has been associated with defects of myelopoiesis. The most common form of hyper IgM syndrome is due to mutations in the CD40 gene. This defect also leads to a decrease in IgG and IgA. In addition to chronic anemia, children suffer from various infectious complications. They typically lack ANAs and show an arrest at the promyelocyte-myelocyte stage of neutrophil development.[321] Allogeneic HSCT has been curative in some instances.[322]

Common variable immunodeficiency is also frequently associated with neutropenias that can be either chronic or episodic.[323] In addition, hypergammaglobulinemia and hypogammaglobulinemia and T- and NK-cell abnormalities of various causes (both inherited and acquired) can also be associated with neutropenia.

Other Iatrogenic Forms of Neutropenia

Hemodialysis, which is critical in the care of end-stage renal disease patients, can result in neutropenia.[324,325] One important mechanism postulated is through activation of the plasma complement pathway by dialyzer cellophane membranes and generation of C5a (desarg) that causes reversible neutrophil aggregation, resulting in transient neutropenia.[324,326] Similar mechanisms to explain neutropenia have been noted in other clinical settings, including leukapheresis[327] and cardiopulmonary bypass surgery.[328]

LABORATORY EVALUATION

Laboratory studies aim at the identification of the primary causes of neutropenia, as outlined in Fig. 30-4. Idiopathic and autoimmune neutropenia remain, in most instances, diagnoses of exclusion. A careful history, including family history and initial age of first abnormal counts, help to distinguish familial neutropenias (see Chapter 27). Should primary causes such as drugs or systemic diseases be identified, the diagnostic evaluation will concentrate on disease-specific tests. In addition to a CBC and differential, which will help establish the severity of neutropenia, and tests to diagnose a specific disorder such as T-LGL leukemia, a bone marrow examination may be required. Lack of morphologic or cytogenetic signs of primary hematologic diseases (e.g., MDS or aplastic anemia) and peripheral destruction will be supported by the observation of left shift and myeloid predominance. Inhibition of myeloid production is exemplified by an increased erythroid:myeloid ratio.

In some instances, auxiliary tests may help identify the cause of the neutropenia, including vitamin B_{12}, zinc, folate, or copper levels. Determination of immunoglobulin levels may be helpful to establishing the presence of immunodeficiency. Detection of ANAs has a limited significance because most of the currently available routine

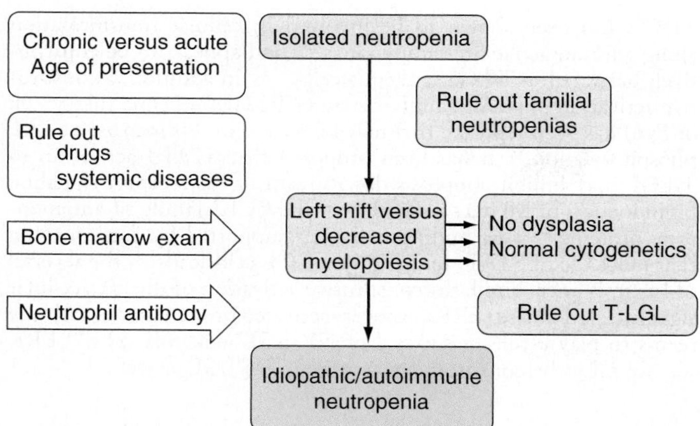

Figure 30-4 EVALUATION OF PRIMARY AND SECONDARY NEUTROPENIA. *T-LGL,* T-cell large granular lymphocyte.

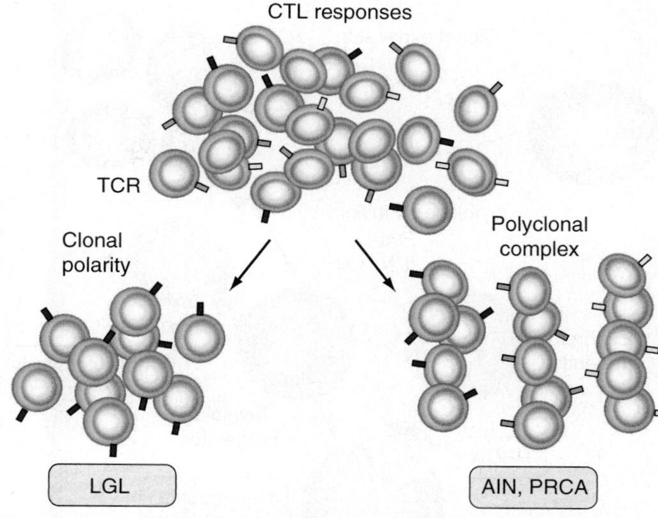

Figure 30-5 PATHOPHYSIOLOGY OF CYTOTOXIC T-LYMPHOCYTE RESPONSES. *AIN,* Autoimmune neutropenia; *CTL,* cytotoxic T lymphocyte; *LGL,* large granular lymphocyte; *PRCA,* pure red cell aplasia; *TCR,* T-cell receptor.

tests are not very sensitive and may not be specific. The presence of antibodies, however, may be helpful and supports the diagnosis of autoimmune forms of neutropenia.

DIFFERENTIAL DIAGNOSIS

Differential diagnostic consideration aims to distinguish primary from secondary forms of neutropenia and to exclude familial hematologic diseases. Suspicion of neutropenia secondary to a primary hematologic disorder requires a bone marrow examination that may be consistent with an early form of aplastic anemia or MDS.

THERAPY

In secondary neutropenias, the therapy is aimed at the primary disease. If potentially offending drugs are present, they should be discontinued. G-CSF (0.5 to 3 μg/kg subcutaneously per day until ANC is above 500 cells/μL) may be used for severe cases of both primary and secondary neutropenias.[275,329,330] It may help to speed up recovery, but if the primary cause persists, it will have only a temporary effect. The use of antibiotics may be useful for the treatment of certain infections. Primary or idiopathic neutropenias most often have an autoimmune cause. Prednisone (1 mg/kg PO daily for 3 months) may be used as first-line therapy,[314] but other B cell–targeted agents may be needed, including rituximab (375 mg/m^2 IV every week for 4 weeks).[331,332] IVIg (2 g/kg IV for 5 days) is effective in certain cases of PWCA.[333] Cytotoxic therapies like cyclophosphamide (Cytoxan) (50 to 100 mg PO daily for 3 to 6 months) may be difficult to administer owing to their inherent myelotoxicity. In cases of neutropenia secondary to lupus or rheumatoid arthritis, such agents may be effective, but the distinction between neutropenia due to the myelosuppressive effects of previous or concurrent treatments for increased activity of the autoimmune disease is necessary. Finally, similar to the treatments applied for T-LGL leukemia, T cell–targeted approaches, such as CsA, can be used (1 to 1.5 mg/kg PO twice a day and titrated to maintain a trough level of 250 to 400 ng/mL).[334,335] A trial of at least 6 weeks is recommended. Similarly use of ATG has also been effective for cases of PWCA[336] and other idiopathic forms of neutropenia.[337] Methotrexate is effective in treating neutropenia related to Felty syndrome[338] and T-LGL leukemia (5 to 7.5 mg/week for 1 to 2 months).[176,339] Of note is that in many instances isolated neutropenias may be asymptomatic, and therapy may not be needed. Alemtuzumab has been used with success in treating thymoma-associated PWCA and other cases of neutropenias.[340-342]

LARGE GRANULAR LYMPHOCYTE LEUKEMIA

Large granular lymphocyte leukemia is a chronic clonal lymphoproliferation of cytotoxic T cells (T-LGL) or NK cells (NK-LGL), often associated with cytopenias, including neutropenia, red cell aplasia, and thrombocytopenia. Pancytopenia is less frequently encountered and may be related to splenomegaly. T-LGL leukemia may be an indolent disorder and present with leukopenia or with lymphocytosis. LGLs observed on a peripheral smear are characteristic of T-LGL leukemia, but their frequency can vary.

T-LGL leukemia results from a proliferation of CTLs and often resembles reactive CTL expansion. It is associated with rheumatoid arthritis (11% to 36%) and B-cell malignancies (5% to 7%)[343] and to a lesser extent with other autoimmune diseases such as Sjögren syndrome,[344] celiac disease,[345] hematologic cancers like MDS, HSCT, and pulmonary hypertension. Most reactive processes are polyclonal, but immunodominant CTL clones may be present, making a distinction between true T-LGL and reactive process difficult (Fig. 30-5). A reduction in the variability of the CTL repertoire can occur in older adults, and clonal or oligoclonal CTL expansions may be more frequent in older individuals. If asymptomatic, this disorder has been termed *monoclonal clonopathy of unclear significance.*

PATHOGENESIS

Inciting Events

T-LGL leukemia frequently arises in the context of a reactive polyclonal CTL expansion undergoing transformation in a manner similar to that proposed for CLL.[346] It is possible also that in T-LGL leukemia one of the effector CTL clones may be initially driven by an exciting antigen, may transform, and consequently the cells fail to undergo apoptosis. The initial or initiating polyclonal response may be a component of the pathophysiologic process associated with infectious agents, rheumatoid arthritis, or other autoimmune disorders.

An initial T cell–mediated process may be responsible for cytopenias in the absence of clonal predominance. In concurrence with this hypothesis, the clinical spectrum of T-LGL is determined by the specificity of the TCR: for example, if myeloid precursors are targets of clonal CTL, neutropenia will be a clinical manifestation. Conversely, if erythroid progenitors are affected, patients will present with anemia (Figs. 30-1 and 30-6). However, unlike the cytopenias that

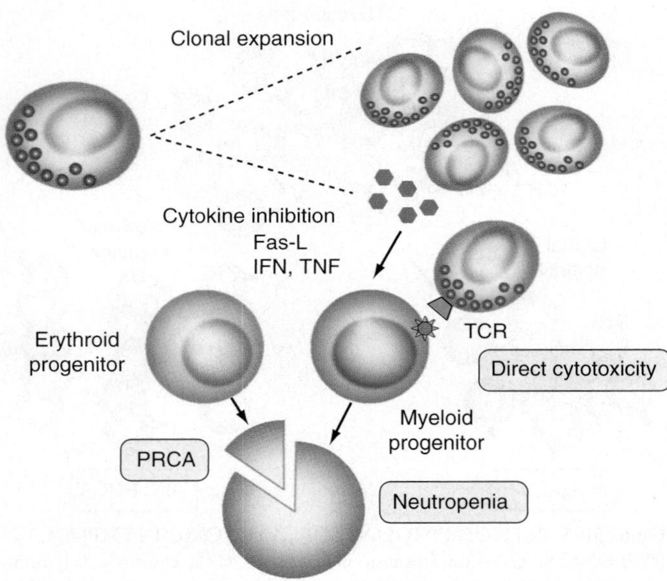

Figure 30-6 PATHOPHYSIOLOGY OF CYTOPENIAS IN T-CELL LARGE GRANULAR LYMPHOCYTE LEUKEMIA. *FasL,* Fas ligand; *IFN,* interferon; *PRCA,* pure red cell aplasia; *TCR,* T-cell receptor; *TNF,* tumor necrosis factor.

resolve following immunosuppression, the CTL clone may persist at a certain level, suggesting that other disease mechanisms involving soluble factors play a role in the development of the cytopenias. Various soluble agents, including Fas ligand (FasL) and perforin, have been implicated in the pathophysiology of the cytopenias in T-LGL leukemia.[347-349]

Clonal Transformation

Clinically T-LGL leukemia does not behave as a typical leukemia: excessive accumulation of malignant cells is often absent, and progression to a more malignant phenotype is rare.[106,350] Instead, the expanded clone in T-LGL leukemia resembles a normal antigen-activated $CD8^+CD57^+$ effector cell; both normal and malignant LGL constitutively express perforin and FasL and can suppress neutrophil development in vitro.[348,351-353] Gene expression studies have shown that the T-LGL leukemia clone exhibits upregulation of cytotoxic proteases and adhesion molecules and downregulation of protease inhibitors.[351,352] Typical clonal LGL cells seem to be terminally differentiated and cannot be effectively expanded in vitro by polyclonal mitogens (unpublished observations).

It is likely that a polyclonal CTL response predates the outgrowth of the immunodominant T-LGL leukemia clone (see Fig. 30-3). The putative transforming event most likely involves a memory cell that feeds into the mature effector CTL compartment.[354] Under normal physiologic circumstances, activated effector T cells are deleted after antigen-driven expansion by Fas-mediated apoptosis. The failure of an activated memory and/or effector clone to undergo apoptosis may result in its persistent expansion.[355-358] LGL leukemia cells express high levels of Fas/FasL, yet themselves are resistant to Fas-mediated apoptosis.[359] It is conceivable that persistent LGL leukemia cell expansion may result from this resistance to homeostatic apoptosis. In addition to the high surface expression of Fas/FasL, soluble FasL has been detected in sera from T-LGL leukemia patients and may contribute to the induction of apoptosis of neutrophil precursors in the bone marrow.[339]

An LGL clone persists mostly in the G_0/G_1 phase of cell cycle,[353] and clonal transformation may also be due to a constitutive overexpression of prosurvival and antiapoptotic transcription factors. STAT3 has been shown to be involved in cellular transformation along with an active Src family kinase[360] and appears to be constitutively activated in T-LGL leukemia cells.[361,362] In addition, a constitutive activation of an Src family kinase in T-LGL leukemia (likely Lck or Fyn) has been reported that may be related to this increased STAT phosphorylation.[363] It has been proposed that STAT3 activation in T-LGL may inhibit apoptosis downstream of Fas receptor signaling by induction of MCL1, a member of the BCL2 family of antiapoptotic proteins.[361] This finding is further supported by data showing that blockade of STAT signaling in T-LGL cells leads to the reversal of Fas resistance. Similarly, constitutive activation of the extracellular signal-related kinase (ERK) mitogen-activated protein kinase pathway seems to play a role in survival of NK-LGL leukemia cells.[364] ERK was found to be constitutively activated in T-LGL as well.[363]

Extreme Clonal Expansion and the Nonrandom Nature of the T-Cell Large Granular Lymphocyte Leukemia Clone

Molecular analysis of the TCR repertoire in T-LGL leukemia has revealed a spectrum of expansion of the T-cell clone in individual patients. In some cases, up to 98% of the peripheral $CD8^+$ repertoire consists of only one clone, a surprising finding given the absence of immunodeficiency among T-LGL leukemia patients. In healthy controls, even the most predominant clones, most likely reactive to ubiquitous antigens, constitute only up to 1.4% of the entire TCR repertoire.[365] Thus detection of an extreme degree of clonal expansion is an important pathologic sign. Similarly, because of the vast diversity of the physiologic TCR repertoire, the probability of isolation of identical CDR3 clonotypes in different individuals is extremely low. We have encountered only a few shared clonotypes even when identical twins were compared. Therefore occurrence of identical and highly similar clonotypes between individual LGL leukemia patients or strikingly homologous clonotypes within the TCR repertoire of an individual patient may lead to the recognition of identical target antigens.[365] This notion might be further supported if patients with identical or highly similar clonotypes share some HLA features, leading to the display of identical antigenic peptides. It is possible that structurally similar clonotypes present in some patients with T-LGL arise in the context of initial polyclonal CTL response and the initial transformation step is not random (see Fig. 30-3). Once a pathogenic immunodominant clonotype is identified and characterized, its sequence can be used for the design of clonotypic TaqMan PCR. This quantitative method may be employed to track the immunodominant clone throughout the course of therapy and thus may potentially predict an impending relapse.[365] Moreover, recent data show that in many cases of T-LGL leukemia the immunodominant clone may change with time as demonstrated by Vβ flow cytometry, suggesting the diversity of the autoimmune process within this disease, and challenges what we know about the leukemic nature of this disease.[366]

Putative Viral Culprits

Although no particular virus has been singled out, according to evidence to date, HTLV-1 (or a related retrovirus) and/or a member of the gammaherpesvirus family are interesting candidates implicated in the pathogenesis of LGL leukemia.[367-371] For instance, patients with NK-cell LGL leukemia are often seropositive for the p21e envelope protein of HTLV-1, known to activate the ERK pathway. HTLV epitope mapping has demonstrated a strong reactivity against env p21e protein, with particular specificity for the BA21 epitope. However, patients seroreactive for this epitope were negative for HTLV-1. HTLV types 3 and 4 were also tested in patients with T-LGL leukemia but results were found to be negative.[372] Consequently it has been hypothesized that a cellular or retroviral protein with homology to BA21 may play a major role in LGL etiology.[367] In addition, rabbit and bovine LGLs infected with alcelaphine herpesvirus 1 or bovine herpesvirus 2, respectively, have been shown to display several properties of human T-LGL leukemia, such as poor proliferation after mitogen stimulation, constitutive ERK activation, and constitutive Lck and Fyn kinase activity.[373]

New Insights Into the Pathogenesis of Large Granular Lymphocyte Leukemia and Potential Therapeutic Targets

IL-15, a cytokine important in survival and proliferation of T and NK cells, is expressed in LGL leukemia. It signals to a heterodimeric receptor that includes IL-15Rα. The exact mechanism by which this cytokine contributes to leukemic transformation in LGLs has recently been tied to its effect on a small subset of NKT cells which expresses NKp46 in both mice and humans.[374] Experimental data also show that IL-15Rα is increased in the serum of patients with T-LGL leukemia and there is upregulation of expression of IL-15Rα in the peripheral blood mononuclear cells in T-LGL leukemia patients. It was proposed that the higher levels of IL-15Rα may lower the IL-15 response threshold and thus contribute to disease pathogenesis.[375] Although T-LGL and NK-LGL leukemias are typically indolent, certain aggressive forms with rapidly progressive and fatal outcomes exemplified by aggressive NK-LGL leukemia are also encountered. This disease entity does not respond to conventional LGL leukemia therapies. A molecule called survivin, which inhibits apoptosis, is highly expressed in the mitochondria of leukemic NK cells in aggressive and indolent forms of NK-LGL leukemia. Efficient knockdown (80%) of survivin has resulted in death of NK-LGL leukemia cells. The upstream activator of survivin is ERK, and a pharmacologic inhibitor of phosphorylated ERK called nanoliposomal C6-ceramide has resulted in dose-dependent inhibition of survivin expression, offering a potential future treatment option.[376] Polymorphisms of the MHC class-I polypeptide-related sequence A (MICA) noted by single-nucleotide polymorphism array analysis may also be important in the pathogenesis of T-LGL leukemia. MICA is the ligand for the receptor NKG2D. MICA*00801/A5.1 polymorphism is found in higher frequency in LGL leukemia patients. Flow cytometric techniques showed that MICA is much more highly expressed in neutrophils of LGL leukemia patients compared to matched controls. Further experiments showed that Ba/F3 lymphocytes transfected with human MICA*019, and neutrophils from patients heterozygous for MICA*008/Af.1 were efficiently killed by large granular lymphocytes.[377]

CLINICAL PRESENTATION AND PHYSICAL FEATURES

Patients with T-LGL leukemia present at a median age of about 55 years, with an equal male/female distribution. The clinical course may be indolent and chronic. Patients are asymptomatic in one-third of cases. The most common clinical presentation is neutropenia (observed in approximately 85% of patients) often accompanied by infections or neutropenic fever.[106,107,295,350,378-380] However, in contrast to neutropenia associated with other hematologic disorders, LGL leukemia patients may remain surprisingly free of infectious complications for extended periods of time regardless of the depressed ANC. Despite the extreme clonality within the T-cell population (suggesting a decreased antigen recognition spectrum), opportunistic infections are rare. Other single-lineage cytopenias, including PRCA and immune-mediated thrombocytopenia, accompany T-LGL leukemia less frequently than neutropenia.[12,378,379,381,382] In some patients, neutropenia, anemia, or pancytopenia may occur at different times throughout the course of the disease.[383] Pancytopenia may be related to splenomegaly reported in 20% to 50% of patients. Hepatomegaly is present in a minority of patients (10% to 20%). Lymphadenopathy and B symptoms may also occur; however, this is uncommon.[350] It has been reported that pregnancy can improve neutropenia in women with LGL leukemia.[384] Clinical transformation to a more malignant form is rare. The clinical presentation of NK-cell LGL lymphocytosis is very similar to that seen in T-LGL leukemia with regard to lymphocyte counts, associated conditions, treatment responses, and survival, although in some reports there is a lower incidence of neutropenia and anemia.[385]

Clinical Overlap and Associations

In some clinical circumstances, natural or pathologic immune responses can resemble T-LGL expansions. For example, responses to viruses such as CMV or EBV, although of an oligoclonal or polyclonal nature, may display a strong clonal dominance mimicking at times a true clonal process.[386] Consequently, polarized CTL responses in the context of infections have to be distinguished from true LGL leukemia.

T-LGL leukemia can occur concomitantly with several autoimmune diseases. Rheumatoid arthritis is likely the most common association, occurring in one-third of patients with T-LGL leukemia, but other diseases such as ulcerative colitis, Sjögren syndrome, systemic lupus erythematosus, multiple sclerosis, and a number of other (auto) immune conditions have been described.[387-394] Felty syndrome is characterized by neutropenia with rheumatoid arthritis and splenomegaly; 80% of cases express the HLA-DR4 allele, a finding also observed in T-LGL leukemia.[395] This common immunogenetic link and similar patterns of cytotoxic clonal expansion with T-cell infiltration suggest that Felty syndrome and T-LGL leukemia represent components of the same disease process.[387,396-398] In addition, PRCA and immune-mediated thrombocytopenia may also be associated with LGL lymphoproliferation. Clonal expansions that characterize T-LGL leukemia can appear similar to oligoclonal CTL responses elicited by strong immunodominant antigens, including certain viruses[398-401]—thus the distinction between T-LGL leukemia and a reactive lymphoproliferative process. LGL leukemia has also been described after bone marrow and solid organ transplantation, perhaps initiated by an alloantigen or an infectious agent such as EBV.[402-407]

LGL-like cell expansions may also be present in other hematologic disorders, including MDS, aplastic anemia, and paroxysmal nocturnal hemoglobinuria,[380,408-412] and may coincide with a number of lymphoproliferative disorders as well.[388,413-415] In MDS the prognosis is usually determined by the presence of MDS, but the presence of LGL may provide a rational target for immunosuppressive therapy. In MDS, T-LGL leukemia has been reported to negatively affect the outcome of therapy directed against the CTL clone.[411] LGL leukemia has also been described in conjunction with hemolytic anemia following bone marrow transplantation, perhaps a process initially driven by an alloantigen or infectious agent such as EBV.[31] As with infections, distinction between an LGL leukemia and reactive lymphoproliferation may be blurred. For example, neutropenia may be associated with various degrees of clonality, with an LGL leukemia representing the most extreme form of this process.

LABORATORY DIAGNOSIS

Diagnostic criteria remain a subject of considerable discussion (Table 30-7). Traditionally LGL lymphocytosis (identified by morphologic characteristics and flow cytometry) is a significant diagnostic criterion.[295,388] However, not all clonal cells display the typical morphologic features, and some patients present with leukopenia. Consequently an LGL count of greater than 2000/μL of blood has been abandoned as a strict diagnostic requirement, and lower numbers such as 0.400/μL of blood have been proposed.[106,416] Most investigators consider the presence of an expanded homogeneous $CD3^+$, TCR-$\alpha\beta^+$, $CD8^+$, $CD16^+$, $CD28^-$, $CD57^+$ cell population as diagnostic of T-LGL leukemia and $CD2^+$, $sCD3^-$, $CD3\varepsilon^+$, TCR-$\alpha\beta^-$, $CD4^-$, $CD8^+$, $CD16^+$, $CD56^+$, $CD57^{(variable)}$ for NK-LGL leukemia. In almost all patients the expanded clone is $CD8^+$ (only very rarely $CD4^+$),[106,417-419] and in the majority of cases this population also expresses CD57, but

LGL leukemia cases without this marker have been observed.[419] Clinical correlations based on immunophenotypic characteristics have been defined; $CD8^{+(dim)}/CD57^{+}$ LGLs are associated with clonal T-LGL leukemia and neutropenia, CD16 expression with complete or partial loss of CD5 is associated with T-LGL leukemia but not cytopenias, and $CD8^{+(dim)}/CD57^{+}$ with loss of CD5 expression is associated with T-LGL leukemia with severe neutropenia.[420] In addition, clinically aggressive T-LGL leukemia is characterized by expression of CD26.[421] In most cases of LGL leukemia, CD94 is expressed at increased levels, and other receptors for class I MHC molecules are abnormally expressed.[422-424] Some investigators have suggested that a pool of $CD8^{+}$ memory cells exists that lack CD57 expression but feed into the mature CD57 effector compartment.[354,417] The size of the abnormal clone defining T-LGL leukemia remains controversial. It is likely that the size of the leukemic T-cell population influences the detection of the clonal TCR γ-chain (G) rearrangement by PCR or Southern blotting; thus such tests are considered mandatory for diagnosis.[425,426] These methods may detect a clonal population that represents 15% of the cell population, but it is also likely that smaller CTL expansions may be consistent with latent T-LGL detected only if more precise methods are used. T-LGL can express CD4, but both $CD4^{+}$ as well as double-positive $CD4^{+}/CD8^{+}$ cases are rare. Cytogenetic analyses are not useful, although cases with chromosomal aberrations have been described.[427,428]

Table 30-7 Immunophenotype and Laboratory Features of T-Cell Large Granular Lymphocyte Leukemia

Laboratory features	
Relative/absolute lymphocytosis	
LGL on peripheral blood smear	
CD4/CD8 ratio reversed	
Vβ family skewing (flow cytometry)	
Immunophenotype	$CD2^{+}$, $CD5^{+}$, $CD3^{+}$
	Majority $CD8^{+}$, few $CD4^{+}/CD8^{+}$ or $CD4^{+}$
	$CD27^{+}CD28^{-}$
	$CD57^{+}CD16^{+}$ perforin/$granzyme^{+}$
	$CD56^{+}$ associated with more aggressive forms
TCR rearrangement	TCR-γ PCR
	Southern blot

LGL, Large granular lymphocyte; *PCR,* polymerase chain reaction; *TCR,* T-cell receptor.

Flow cytometric analysis of Vβ utilization pattern with antibodies directed against most of the Vβ-chain types may be helpful in making the diagnosis. The Vβ family expansion by flow cytometry does not prove clonality, but it may help assess the contribution of the T-LGL clone to the $CD8^{+}$ or $CD4^{+}$ population (Fig. 30-7).

Rare immunophenotypic variants of T-LGL exist that coexpress CD4 and CD8, lack both of these markers, or use γ/δ TCR instead of α/β TCR chains. Vβ flow cytometry has been used to assess the size of the LGL clone and its Vβ use; Vβ use can be identified in 80% of patients. The current Vβ antibody panel does not cover 25% to 35% of the Vβ spectrum. In usual cases, T-LGL does not express CD56 antigen; the presence of this marker has been associated with a more aggressive clinical phenotype.[429] A monotypic expression pattern of KIR can be found with monoclonal antibodies to CD157b, CD158a, and CD158e (corresponding to the most prevalent KIR genes) in about 50% of patients.[430]

Additional supportive tests include a reticulocyte count, which is low in cases presenting with red cell aplasia. The MCV is usually high. Serologic studies or DNA titer to detect evidence of EBV

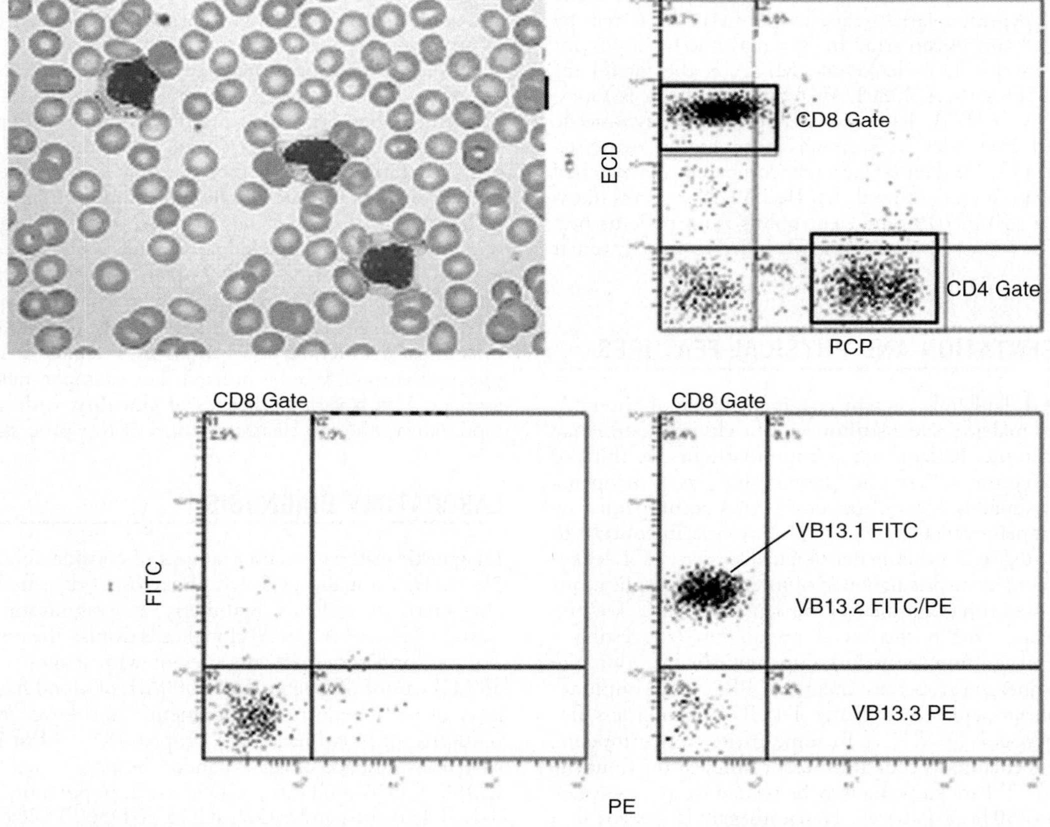

Figure 30-7 MORPHOLOGIC FEATURES AND FLOW CYTOMETRY OF T-CELL LARGE GRANULAR LYMPHOCYTE. *ECD,* Ethyl cysteinate dimer; *FITC,* fluorescein isothiocyanate; *PCP,* phencyclidine hydrochloride; *PE,* phycoerythrin.

Approach to the Diagnosis and Treatment of Acquired Pure Red Cell Aplasia, Acquired Neutropenia, and T-Cell Large Granular Lymphocyte Leukemia

Acquired pure red cell aplasia (PRCA) is characterized by reticulocytopenia, but diagnosis is based on the morphologic absence of erythroid precursors in the bone marrow. Congenital forms of PRCA, including Diamond-Blackfan anemia, need to be distinguished when presenting in young children. In adults, primary idiopathic disease has to be differentiated from secondary forms of red cell aplasia associated with hematologic diseases such as B-cell chronic lymphocytic leukemia, myeloma, T-cell large granular lymphocyte (T-LGL) leukemia, and parvovirus B19–associated chronic reticulocytopenia or acute transient aplastic crisis. The diagnosis of parvovirus B19 infection can be made on the basis of the presence of parvovirus B19–specific immunoglobulin M and by deoxyribonucleic acid (DNA) hybridization techniques. Parvovirus B19–specific polymerase chain reaction can help rule out an ongoing infection. This diagnosis is important because therapy with intravenous immunoglobulin (IVIg) (2 g/kg IV for 5 days) can be curative. The therapy of secondary red cell aplasia includes treatment of the underlying condition. It is also important to distinguish red cell aplasia from myelodysplastic syndromes, which can be associated with erythroid hypoplasia but carry a significantly worse prognosis.

In cases with thymoma, thymectomy is the usual initial treatment approach; however, incomplete responders, nonresponders, and patients who relapse are common, necessitating the addition of immunosuppressive therapy. In patients with idiopathic PRCA, therapy includes immunosuppressive agents such as prednisone (1 mg/kg orally PO for 3 months), cyclosporine A (CsA; 5 to 10 mg/kg PO daily in divided doses for 3 months), or oral cyclophosphamide (50 to 150 mg PO daily for 3 months). Second-line therapies include antithymocyte globulin (ATG; if horse ATG, 40 mg/kg IV daily for 4 days with prednisone at 1 mg/kg, and if rabbit ATG, 2.5 to 3.5 mg/kg daily IV for 4 or 5 days with prednisone at 1 mg/kg) or rituximab (375 mg/m^2 IV every week for 4 weeks).

Neutropenia may be associated with severe infections, but the risk associated with neutropenia depends on its clinical context, severity, and duration. The management of neutropenia must account for its clinical presentation and the risk for possible life-threatening complications and includes supportive care, clinical monitoring, and implementation of prophylactic antibiotics and/or hematopoietic growth factors. Neutropenia in childhood may be due to congenital diseases, be associated with viral infections, or be immune mediated. These three causes are usually self-limiting. In adults, most neutropenias are secondary to other conditions, including hematologic or systemic diseases. In general, drug reactions are a very common cause of neutropenia. Idiopathic or autoimmune neutropenia as a primary disease is a diagnosis of exclusion. The pathogenesis involves T-lymphocyte/natural killer–mediated inhibition of myelopoiesis or antineutrophil antibodies. Immunosuppressive therapy may be employed and includes prednisone (1 mg/kg PO daily for 3 months), methotrexate (5 to 7.5 mg/week PO for 1 to 2 months), CsA (1 to 1.5 mg/kg PO twice a day and titrated to maintain a trough level of 250 to 400 ng/mL), IVIg (2 g/kg IV for 5 days), cyclophosphamide (50 to 100 mg PO daily for 3 to 6 months), or rituximab alone (375 mg/m^2 IV every week for 4 weeks) or in conjunction with myeloid growth factors.

T-LGL leukemia is a chronic, often indolent clonal lymphoproliferation of cytotoxic T cells associated with immune-mediated cytopenias. It may be a part of a continuum of reactive cytotoxic T-cell responses ranging from polyclonal, oligoclonal, to monoclonal expansions as seen in T-LGL leukemia. Persistent antigenic drive or dysfunction of the homeostatic termination of clonal T-cell expansion may be involved, and the abnormal cytotoxic T lymphocyte (CTL) in T-LGL is not entirely autonomous. The pathophysiology of cytopenias includes cytokine effects and direct antigen-specific cytotoxicity. Most patients present with neutropenia. PRCA and pancytopenia are less common. Hemolytic anemia and pancytopenia may be the result of splenomegaly present in a significant minority of patients. B symptoms and lymphadenopathy are uncommon, and many patients remain asymptomatic. The diagnosis is established according to the presence of characteristic LGL lymphocytosis, but in some patients the LGL count may not be very high. The immunophenotype is CD3$^+$, CD8$^+$, CD57$^+$, CD16$^+$, CD56$^-$, and CD28$^-$. CD56 antigen–expressing LGL may be characterized by a more aggressive course. Some cases may coexpress CD4 and CD8. The diagnosis includes detection of T-cell receptor rearrangement. In most instances, expansion of the involved Vβ family may be detected using Vβ flow cytometric clonotyping. T-LGL is often associated with autoimmune diseases, including rheumatoid arthritis and Felty syndrome. T-LGL can accompany myelodysplasia and, in rare instances, aplastic anemia or paroxysmal nocturnal hemoglobinuria. Reactive, often viral infection–associated, CTL proliferation may be difficult to document. Asymptomatic cases are monitored, and development of systemic symptoms or symptomatic cytopenias may prompt therapy. Current treatments include immunosuppressive agents such as prednisone, CsA (1 to 1.5 mg/kg PO twice a day then adjusted to maintain a trough level of 250 to 400 ng/mL for 8 to 10 weeks), oral methotrexate (7.5 mg/m^2 week for 21 months), or cyclophosphamide (50 to 100 mg/day for 3 to 6 months). Chronic long-term therapy may be more effective than high-dose combination chemotherapy applied in B-cell lymphomas. Second-line treatments may involve alemtuzumab or ATG. The prognosis is generally good, and transformation to a more aggressive lymphoproliferative disorder is rare.

infection is usually not needed but may be helpful to distinguish reactive immunologic responses. The rheumatoid factor is frequently positive. Antinuclear antibodies and ANAs may also at times be positive (see box on Approach to the Diagnosis and Treatment of Acquired Pure Red Cell Aplasia, Acquired Neutropenia, and T-Cell Large Granular Lymphocyte Leukemia).[431,432]

Unless additional hematologic diseases, such as MDS, are suspected, bone marrow examination may not be required. Bone marrow biopsy and aspirate should be obtained in cases of pancytopenia or involvement of several lineages. Morphologic hallmarks of MDS and cytogenetic analysis may help establish a diagnosis of MDS.

DIFFERENTIAL DIAGNOSIS

Differential diagnostic considerations include reactive processes such as viral infections. Occasionally MDS may be present simultaneously or serve as an alternative diagnosis; T-cell oligoclonality may accompany MDS.

THERAPY

A significant proportion of patients will be asymptomatic, and the diagnosis may be totally coincidental. Should the patient be asymptomatic, therapy may be delayed. Lymphocytosis may be significant, but absolute lymphocyte counts more than 40,000/μL are unusual. Symptomatic splenomegaly may be an indication for splenectomy. Pancytopenia may be a result of splenomegaly, and the procedure aids in the treatment of a hemolytic anemia that can be present in some patients.

Patients may tolerate significant degrees of neutropenia for many years. Indications for treatment include neutropenic complications or transfusion dependence (Fig. 30-8). G-CSF therapy will increase counts in some patients, but a significant proportion of patients will be refractory or would have delayed response.[229,433-435] Of interest is the observation that high-dose therapy with typical lymphoma regimens such as CVP (cyclophosphamide, vincristine, and prednisone) or CHOP (cyclophosphamide, hydroxydaunomycin, vincristine [Oncovin], and prednisone) may be ineffective and therefore

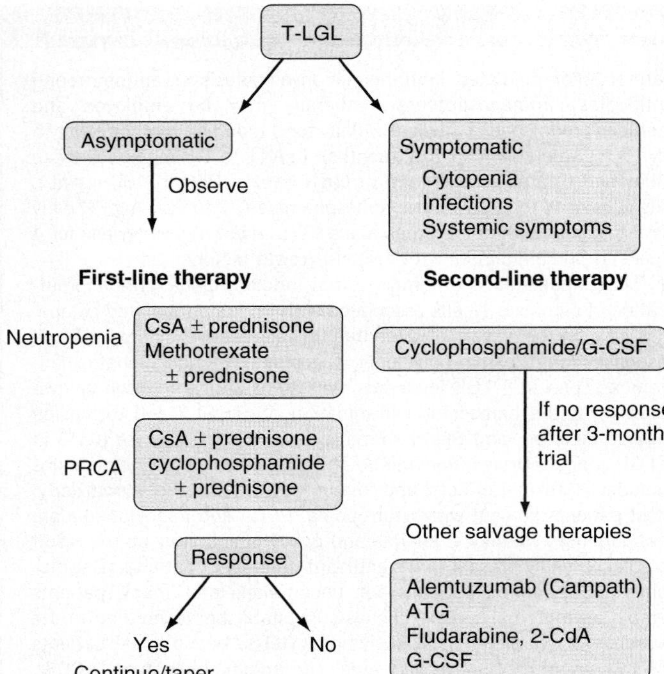

Figure 30-8 THERAPY OF T-CELL LARGE GRANULAR LYMPHOCYTE LEUKEMIA. *ATG,* Antithymocyte globulin; *2-CdA,* 2-chlorodeoxyadenosine; *CsA,* cyclosporine A; *G-CSF,* granulocyte colony-stimulating factor; *PRCA,* pure red cell aplasia; *T-LGL,* T-cell large granular lymphocyte.

should not be used. Cases refractory to bone marrow transplantation have been described.[436] Monotherapy with prednisone may relieve some of the symptoms and improve neutropenia, but remissions are usually not durable. CsA given at 1 to 1.5 mg/kg PO twice a day then adjusted to maintain a trough level of 250 to 400 ng/mL represents a reasonable first-line therapy; however, a course of sufficient duration has to be given, with a response expected after 8 to 10 weeks of therapy.[334,437] Weekly oral methotrexate given at 7.5 to 10 mg/m^2 PO weekly has been used successfully.[437,438] Patients with LGL leukemia–associated PRCA may be better treated with oral cyclophosphamide instead of methotrexate with a dose between 50 and 100 mg/day. In LGL leukemia with associated PRCA, responses may be delayed, and the PRCA may recur after discontinuation of cyclophosphamide therapy, or if insufficient treatment (<6 to 8 weeks) was administered. Therapy with cyclophosphamide in neutropenic patients may be difficult due to myelosuppression. In most refractory cases, ATG has also been used with success.[439] In recent years, successful therapy with alemtuzumab been has reported.[440] CD52 expression determined by flow cytometry is an important predictive factor for response to alemtuzumab.[441] Purine analogues like fludarabine given in combination with mitoxantrone and dexamethasone or with dexamethasone alone have been shown to produce impressive responses of 79%, although these were confined to a small group of patients.[442] Allogeneic HSCT has also been used successfully in some cases.[443,444] Relapses are frequent but usually responsive to the previously effective therapy. Certain patients may require low-dose maintenance therapy with CsA. In some cases, remarkable improvement of cytopenia can be achieved with splenectomy.[445,446]

PROGNOSIS

LGL leukemia is a chronic condition and may be indolent. In general, mortality is low. Transformation to more aggressive forms of lymphomas or leukemias is uncommon. In cases of T-LGL leukemia associated with a primary hematologic disease such as MDS, the prognosis is dependent on the therapy of the underlying problem.

ACQUIRED PLATELET PRODUCTION DISORDER

Megakaryocytes, like all formed elements of the peripheral blood, are ultimately derived from undifferentiated hematopoietic stem cells that exist in a developmental continuum (see Chapter 26).[447] Through a series of still incompletely understood events, stem cells undergo an asynchronous division that gives rise to two daughter cells. One daughter cell remains a stem cell, fulfilling the requirement for self-renewal of the stem cell compartment, and the other commits to developing within a given lineage, likely through the induction of specific transcription factors such as GATA1, FOG-1, and Fli-1, in the case of megakaryocytes,[448,449] and perhaps by downmodulation of other transcription factors, such as c-Myb.[450,451] Lineage-committed progenitor cells are characterized by a loss of "plasticity" and a remarkable capacity for proliferation. The latter is required because approximately 15×10^6 megakaryocytes/kg body weight must be available to produce the roughly 100×10^9 new platelets that are needed daily to maintain a normal platelet count of 150 to 400 × 10^9/L.[452] As progenitor cell divisional activity proceeds, maturation, as defined by the acquisition of lineage-specific proteins, ensues, largely under the control of the hematopoietic cytokine thrombopoietin.[453-455] After a variable number of mitoses, proliferative activity eventually declines, giving rise to many daughter cells, which are known as *precursors.* Precursor cells are essentially postmitotic and are capable of one or two additional cell divisions at most. They are often morphologically identifiable as belonging to a given lineage and are primarily engaged in the terminal maturation steps that allow them to function as competent members of their lineage. In the case of megakaryocytes, precursor cells undergo nuclear endoreduplication to increase their ploidy (to a mean of approximately 16 N), a characteristic unique to cells of the megakaryocyte lineage.[448,456-462] Nuclear endoreduplication is accompanied by an increase in megakaryocyte cytoplasm and thereby the number of platelets that an individual megakaryocyte can produce.[459]

As discussed in Chapter 26, the process of platelet formation, or thrombopoiesis, occurs during megakaryocyte terminal maturation.[463,464] It is initiated by the development of the demarcation membrane system in the megakaryocyte's cytoplasm.[465] Among the functions of the demarcation membrane system is delineation of platelet fields. These fields are filled with the granules and proteins that ultimately make up the contents of mature platelets. The latter are shed from pseudopods that mature megakaryocytes extend through endothelial cell junctions into the lumen of marrow capillaries. The pseudopods fracture, because of shear stress in the lumen of these capillaries, and release shards of megakaryocytic cytoplasm, or proplatelets, that are the immediate antecedents of circulating platelets. A fully mature megakaryocyte is estimated to produce approximately 1 to 1.5 × 10^3 platelets. The molecular regulation of this process is beginning to be better understood. It has been shown, for example, that the apoptosis-stimulating gene Bax promotes platelet production.[466] Interestingly, very recent evidence suggests that the life span of circulating platelets is also regulated by the apoptosis proteins. Using the strategy of ethylnitrosourea-inducted mutations, Mason et al[467] have recently demonstrated that mutations in the Bcl-x_L gene lead to synthesis of a form of the protein that no longer inhibits Bax, and that this in turn leads to accelerated platelet death and a heritable form of thrombocytopenia (Fig. 30-9).

Failure in the process of either megakaryocytopoiesis or thrombopoiesis will result in thrombocytopenia. Under either circumstance, platelet production is characterized as "ineffective," either because there is an absolute decrease in available megakaryocyte cytoplasm (failure of megakaryocytopoiesis) or because cytoplasmic development is defective (failure of thrombopoiesis). Selective impairment of megakaryocytopoiesis may also result from damage to the progenitor cell compartment (the burst-forming units–megakaryocyte [BFU-Mk] or colony-forming units–megakaryocyte [CFU-Mk]; see Chapter 26) or rarely from a compromised ability to synthesize thrombopoietin, the chief cytokine regulator of this compartment (Fig. 30-10).[468] Inherent or acquired defects in megakaryocyte precursor cells may lead to ineffective thrombopoiesis.[468,469] The relative

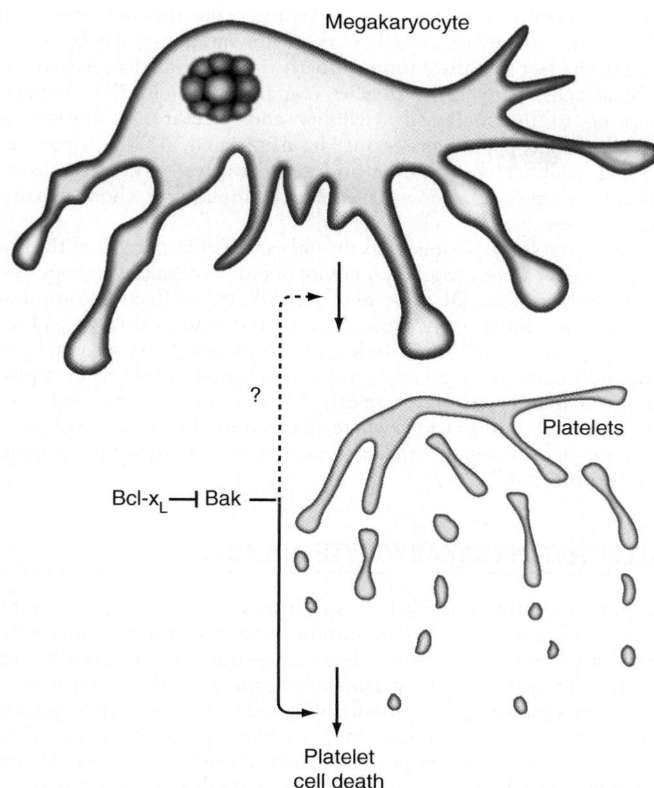

Figure 30-9 Bcl-x$_L$ AND PLATELET LIFE SPAN. Mason et al[467] subjected mice to ethylnitrosourea mutagenesis and screened their first-generation offspring for platelet deficiency. They identified two mutations in the gene encoding the antiapoptotic factor Bcl-x$_L$ that give rise to a dominantly inherited reduction in platelet count. Bcl-x$_L$ appears to promote platelet survival through inhibition of the proapoptotic activity of Bak. Bax promotes production of platelets,[466] and overexpression of antiapoptotic Bcl-x$_L$ impairs the fragmentation of megakayocytes.[592] *(Modified from Qi B, Hardwick JM: A Bcl-x$_L$ timer sets platelet life span.* Cell *128:1035, 2007.)*

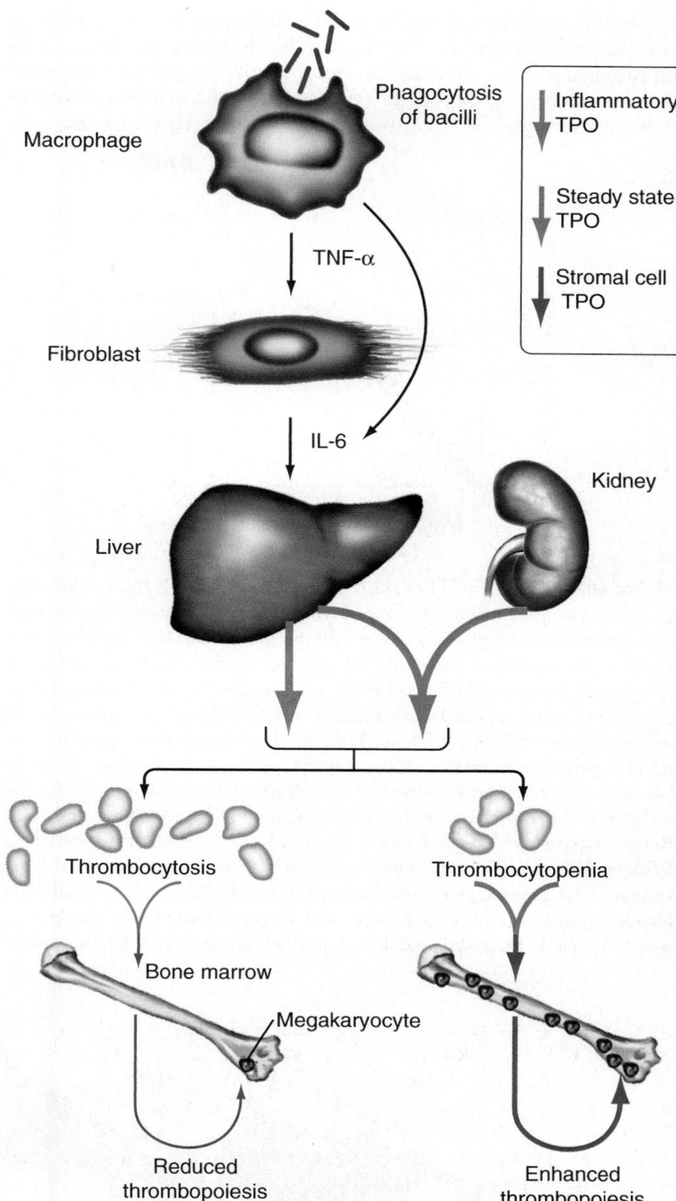

Figure 30-10 THE REGULATION OF THROMBOPOIETIN LEVELS. A steady-state amount of hepatic thrombopoietin (TPO) is regulated by platelet c-Mpl receptor–mediated uptake and destruction of the hormone. Hepatic production of the hormone is depicted. Upon binding to platelet c-Mpl receptors, the hormone is removed from the circulation and destroyed, which reduces blood levels. In the presence of inflammation, interleukin-6 (IL-6) is released from macrophages and, through tumor necrosis factor-α (TNF-α) stimulation, from fibroblasts and circulates to the liver to enhance TPO production. Thrombocytopenia also leads to enhanced marrow stromal cell production of TPO, although the molecular mediator(s) of this effect is not yet completely understood. *(Modified from Kaushansky K: The molecular mechanisms that control thrombopoiesis.* J Clin Invest *115:3339, 2005.)*

effectiveness of platelet production can be calculated by measuring platelet mass turnover, which is defined as the product of the mean megakaryocyte cytoplasmic volume multiplied by the total number of marrow megakaryocytes.[470,470-472] A disparity between cytoplasmic mass and platelet delivery to the peripheral blood (platelet count divided by platelet survival, corrected for splenic pooling) is the hallmark of ineffective platelet production (Fig. 30-11). An examination of the peripheral blood smear is the first step in the initial assessment of patients who present with thrombocytopenia. The presence of platelet clumps, indicative of pseudothrombocytopenia, or abnormally large, or small, platelets can be very useful in generating a differential diagnosis, as can the presence of inclusion bodies in neutrophils. Nevertheless, the current gold standard for diagnosing thrombocytopenia due to ineffective platelet production is a bone marrow aspirate and biopsy. At the moment, direct visualization of the marrow and its cellular contents is the only way to judge the quantity and quality of the megakaryocyte population (Fig. 30-12). However, noninvasive methods for making a diagnosis of ineffective platelet production are being developed. For example, the concentration of serum glycocalicin, the soluble fragment of glycoprotein (GP) Ib, has been shown to be significantly diminished in patients with platelet production abnormalities when compared with normal control subjects.[473] Reticulated platelets, like red blood cell reticulocytes, contain ribonucleic acid (RNA). It has been suggested that as is true for red blood cell reticulocytes, the presence of residual RNA in platelets indicates that they have been newly formed.[473,474] Thus they may be useful for assessing the dynamics of platelet production under baseline conditions and after marrow insults such as chemotherapy or irradiation.[475-478] Platelet RNA can be detected by staining with dyes such as thiazole orange,[474] and it has been suggested that assessing the mean thiazole orange staining can be used to construct a reticulated platelet maturation index.[475] Although appealing in concept, the ultimate usefulness of this assay remains to be determined, because staining artifacts[479] and paradoxically low reticulated platelet counts in cases of disorders characterized by peripheral destruction may complicate the interpretation of such results.[474,479] Yet another approach to assessing platelet production is the measurement of serum thrombopoietin levels. Thrombopoietin is synthesized constitutively in the liver and then binds to its receptor c-Mpl on megakaryocytes and platelets. Accordingly, in patients with disorders in which megakaryocytes are reduced in the marrow, thrombopoietin levels rise.[474,479-482] However, the wide variation in "normal" thrombopoietin concentrations in serum make this determination somewhat problematic as well. Some of this variability may be attributed to the fact that thrombopoietin synthesis is inducible in marrow stromal cells, perhaps by platelet α-granule proteins.[483,484] Reports attesting to the increased reliability and precision of measuring several of these parameters at once have appeared,[484,485] but it remains unclear whether the expense and time involved will prove cost-effective when compared with the relative simplicity of a bone marrow examination.

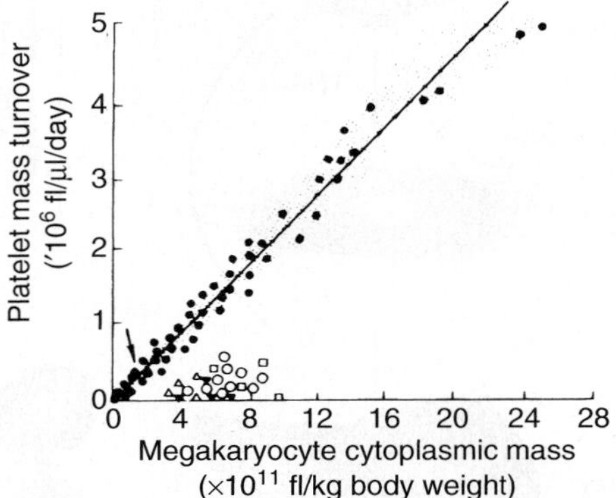

Figure 30-11 INEFFECTIVE PLATELET PRODUCTION. In thrombocytopenia the relationship between marrow megakaryocyte cytoplasmic mass and the turnover of platelet mass in the peripheral blood is usually direct. Platelet mass turnover represents the product of the mean megakaryocyte cytoplasmic volume multiplied by the total number of marrow megakaryocytes. The results in normal subjects are indicated by the *arrow*, and the *stippled area* represents 95% of confidence limits in thrombocytopenic patients with effective production. Ineffective thrombocytopoiesis is identified as a disparity between available marrow substrate (megakaryocyte cytoplasmic mass) and delivery of platelet mass to the peripheral blood (platelet mass turnover). Results in patients with autosomal dominant thrombocytopenia *(open circles)*, Wiskott-Aldrich syndrome *(open triangles)*, megaloblastic anemia *(open squares)*, and preleukemia *(closed triangles)* are characterized by ineffective platelet production. *(Data from Thompson A, Harker L: Quantitative platelet disorders. In* Manual of hemostasis and thrombosis, *Philadelphia, 1983, FA Davis, p 65.)*

As is true for the congenital thrombocytopenias, acquired thrombocytopenia can be caused by a failure of either megakaryocytopoiesis or thrombopoiesis. Of these two possibilities, ineffective thrombopoiesis is the more likely cause, because pure megakaryocyte aplasia or hypoplasia is quite rare. Indeed, thrombocytopenia secondary to decreased marrow megakaryocytes is much more likely to be a prodrome of aplastic anemia, or an early MDS. Clues to these conditions can be found in the marrow, where often subtle abnormalities of other hematopoietic lineages, such as macrocytosis or dyserythropoiesis, can be observed.[486]

SELECTIVE MEGAKARYOCYTE APLASIA

Acquired selective amegakaryocytic thrombocytopenia is quite rare. It is almost always due to an autoimmune mechanism, either antibody or cell mediated. Autoantibodies reacting with megakaryocytes or their progenitor cells, presumably leading to their destruction, have been described.[487] Antibodies directed to cytokines that regulate megakaryocyte development, in particular thrombopoietin, might also play a role in the biogenesis of such disorders. An unusual case of cyclic amegakaryocytic thrombocytopenia due to an antibody to granulocyte-macrophage colony-stimulating factor (GM-CSF) was documented in one patient. Cases of cell-mediated suppression of megakaryocytopoiesis leading to a complete selective megakaryocyte aplasia have also been described.[488] In these cases, suppression was shown in one case to be due to autoreactive T lymphocytes, whereas a macrophage-derived "factor" was implicated in the other. In the

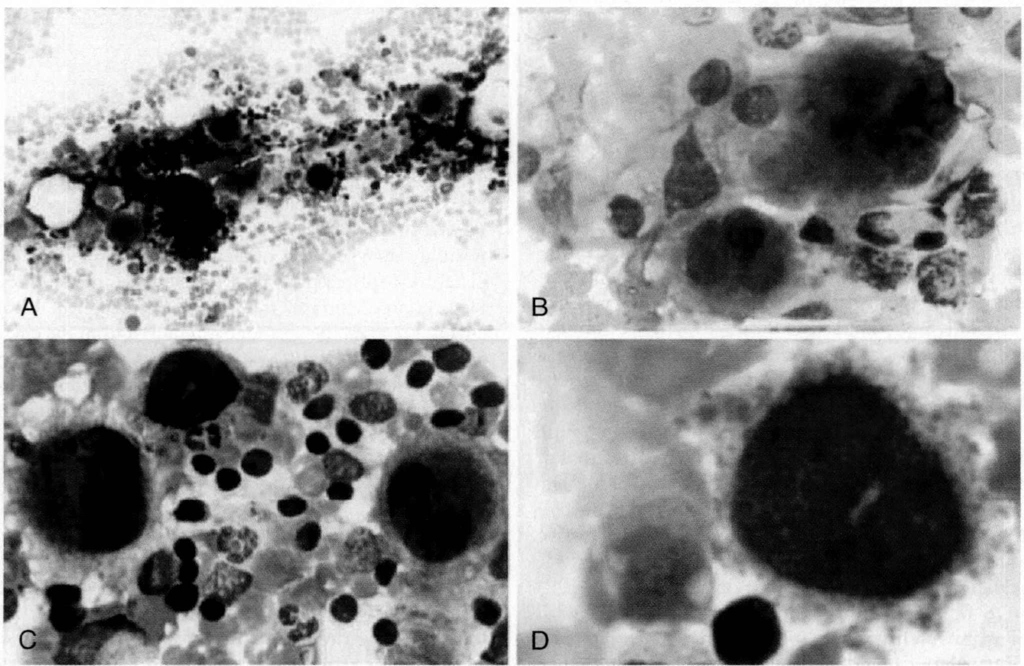

Figure 30-12 MARROW ASPIRATE OBTAINED FROM A CHILD WITH THROMBOCYTOPENIA AND DYSMEGAKARYOCYTOPOIESIS. The megakaryocytes are small and hypolobular, with diminished cytoplasm. Cells are viewed at magnifications of 250× **(A)**, 1000× **(B)**, 200× **(C)**, and 1600× **(D)**. *(From van den Oudenrijn S, Bruin M, Folman CC, et al: Three parameters: Plasma thrombopoietin levels, plasma glycocalicin levels, and megakaryocyte culture, distinguish between different causes of congenital thrombocytopenia.* Br J Haematol *117:390, 2002.)*

latter case, suppression was shown to be specific for megakaryocytes, because no significant effect on BFU-E– or CFU-E–derived colony formation by autologous marrow mononuclear cells was reported.

Patients in whom an autoimmune mechanism is operative may respond to treatment with cyclosporine and ATG, achieving durable remissions.[489] Cytotoxic antibodies directed toward the CFU-Mk may be treated with corticosteroids, plasmapheresis, IV IgG, danazol, cyclosporine, or cyclophosphamide.[490] In a patient in whom an IgG antibody was found to be blocking GM-CSF action, a complete response to cyclophosphamide was observed.[491] Patients with T cell–mediated inhibition of megakaryocytopoiesis may respond to ATG, cyclosporine, or hematopoietic growth factors.[490] If a particular drug or toxin exposure is believed to be responsible, for example. ethanol or a thiazide diuretic, then withdrawal of the offending agent is obviously indicated. If the cause is viral, IV IgG or anti-HIV therapies are indicated.[490] Despite the various causes of ineffective thrombopoiesis, immunosuppressive therapy was found to be effective in 8 of 30 patients in one series.[492] Therefore, although worth trying, most patients do not respond to this form of therapy, and for these individuals, HSCT remains an option. Treatment with intensive immunosuppressive therapy may not prevent progression to aplastic anemia.[491]

INFECTION

Many infectious diseases are associated with thrombocytopenia, and it is likely that infection is the greatest noniatrogenic cause of ineffective platelet production.[493] Infectious agents associated with decreased platelet counts include mycoplasma,[492] mycobacteria,[494] ehrlichiosis,[495] and malaria.[496] In these disorders, the cause of the thrombocytopenia is believed to be diminished platelet production,[497] although immune-mediated thrombocytopenia has also been described in some patients.[494]

Viral infections are by far the most common infectious agents associated with thrombocytopenia due to ineffective megakaryocyte or platelet production. Thrombocytopenia has been reported in cases of mumps, rubella, measles, varicella, CMV, infectious mononucleosis, chickenpox, dengue and other hemorrhagic fevers, hepatitis, and parvovirus infections.[498-501] Live measles virus vaccination can also induce thrombocytopenia due to decreased production.[502] The mechanism responsible for viral suppression of platelet counts is not completely clear. It is known that megakaryocytes are capable of being infected by a variety of viruses. Infected cells may appear dysplastic, with inclusion bodies, vacuoles, or degenerating nuclei. Naked megakaryocyte nuclei may be seen in particular after HIV infection.[497] That such cytopathic cells might have trouble producing platelets is not difficult to imagine.

Perhaps the best studied virally induced thrombocytopenia is that associated with HIV infection.[503] Mild to moderate reduction in platelet counts is quite common in patients with this disease. In a large study (738 patients) of HIV-positive patients with hemophilia, the cumulative frequency of thrombocytopenia 6 years after seroconversion was 16% for children and 18% for adults. At 10 years the frequency increased to 27% in children and 43% in adults.[504] In another study, the frequency of thrombocytopenia was 16% among 103 homosexual men and 37% among 182 IV drug users with a new diagnosis of HIV infection.[505] Thrombocytopenia was also reported to be relatively common in HIV-negative homosexual men (3%) and IV drug users (9%). It was speculated that this might be due to the high rates of hepatitis in these patient groups.[505] Except for patients who acquire HIV in the background of hemophilia, bleeding secondary to thrombocytopenia is unusual, because the counts are rarely less than 50,000/μL. Thrombocytopenia may precede frank immunodeficiency but does correlate with viral load and depletion of the CD4 T-cell population.[490,506]

The principal cause of thrombocytopenia appears to vary with the stage of disease. A retrospective study of 85 patients with HIV and thrombocytopenia suggested that in the early stages of infection, platelet destruction is predominant, whereas in patients with full-blown AIDS, thrombocytopenia is more often due to a production defect.[507,508] Thrombocytopenia due to platelet production abnormalities may be related directly to an HIV infection, to adverse effects of drug therapy, or to secondary malignancy or myelodysplasia. Platelet kinetic studies have shown that patients infected with HIV have a moderate reduction in platelet survival, but all have decreased platelet production regardless of the degree of thrombocytopenia.[507,509] HIV has been shown to infect megakaryocytes directly, as evidenced by finding HIV messenger RNA (mRNA) and p24 antigen in megakaryocyte cytoplasm.[510-512] The portal of entry might be through megakaryocyte surface CD4,[511,512] but more recent studies suggest that CXCR4, which is expressed on megakaryocytes[513] and is a critical coreceptor for viral uptake, is more likely involved.[514] In these studies, infection with HIV-1 env-pseudotyped luciferase reporter viruses indicated that X4 env (CXCR4-using) pseudotypes infected megakaryocytic cells whereas R5 env (CCR5-using) pseudotypes did not.

Examination of a bone marrow aspirate and biopsy specimens may be required to assess whether infiltration by granulomatous infection or a malignancy is contributing to, or causing, the thrombocytopenia in an HIV patient. Assuming no other obvious cause of the thrombocytopenia, and the presence of typical megakaryocytic morphologic abnormalities, antiretroviral therapy is the principal treatment. Zidovudine was the mainstay in the past,[506] but current combination antiretroviral regimens will likely be more effective in increasing platelet counts as well as enhancing CD4 cell counts and reducing HIV viral loads.[502,515,516] For patients with severe and/or symptomatic thrombocytopenia, immune thrombocytopenia purpura (ITP) regimens may well be effective. These include prednisone (1 mg/kg/day) or short courses of dexamethasone.[503] IVIg may be effective in low weekly doses (0.04 g/kg per week),[517] and anti-D has been used extensively in these patients.[503] Splenectomy is quite effective therapy when the therapies described are either ineffective or contraindicated, and it appears to have no adverse effect on HIV progression.[518]

CHEMOTHERAPY AND IRRADIATION

Chemotherapy and irradiation reliably damage bone marrow in a dose-dependent fashion. Megakaryocytes and their progenitors seem to be particularly sensitive to the effects of these agents. As a result, thrombocytopenia is one of the most frequent adverse effects of total body irradiation[519] and chemotherapy. Allogeneic or autologous marrow transplantation is often complicated by prolonged thrombocytopenia, which may persist long after restoration of neutrophil and red blood cell counts. Transplantation of umbilical cord stem cells is also associated with delayed platelet recovery. In one study of 39 pediatric patients receiving such transplants, the median time to platelet count recovery was 49 days (range, 15 to 117 days).[520] The explanation for the tardiness of platelet recovery in these instances is not always clear, but ineffective thrombopoiesis has been shown to be important in at least some cases.[521] Various strategies to ameliorate this problem have been tried, including the use of peripheral blood "stem cells," which may lead to a faster rate of platelet recovery when compared with marrow transplantation. More recently, attempts have been made to expand megakaryocyte progenitor cells, either with a recombinant form of thrombopoietin[522] or other cytokines.[523] The clinical utility of this approach, or the simple administration of recombinant thrombopoietin after transplantation, remains uncertain[524] but might eventually prove useful.[525] Accordingly, posttransplantation thrombocytopenia remains a problem.[526]

Isolated thrombocytopenia with decreased megakaryocytes has been reported after chemotherapy for acute myeloid leukemia. Cyclosporine was reported to augment the platelet count in such patients.[527] Recombinant thrombopoietin has not been shown to be useful in this setting and appears to induce marrow changes suggestive of a myeloproliferative disorder, which is reversed when the thrombopoietin is discontinued.[528]

Alkylating agents in general produce more prolonged thrombocytopenia than antimetabolites. It has been claimed that some alkylating agents spare megakaryocytes (e.g., cyclophosphamide), but this is a relative phenomenon. Agents such as busulfan, the nitrosoureas, or platinum may cause cumulative damage of the more primitive progenitor cells. Other chemotherapeutic agents, such as the vinca alkaloids, may not decrease the platelet count significantly.

Potential mechanisms for the relative sparing of platelet production by certain chemotherapeutic regimens have been investigated.[529] In one study, for example, potential platelet-sparing mechanisms of chemotherapy regimens containing paclitaxel and carboplatin have been explored by examining (1) normal donor- and chemotherapy patient–derived erythroid (BFU-E), myeloid (colony-forming unit–granulocyte-macrophage [CFU-GM]), and megakaryocyte (CFU-Mk) progenitor cell proliferation in vitro; (2) P-glycoprotein and glutathione *S*-transferase (GST) messenger RNA expression; (3) serum thrombopoietin, stem cell factor, IL-6, IL-11, IL-1b, IL-8, and tumor necrosis factor-α levels in patients treated with paclitaxel and carboplatin; and (4) stromal cell production of thrombopoietin and stem cell factor after paclitaxel and carboplatin exposure. It was found that CFU-Mk was more resistant to paclitaxel alone, or in combination with carboplatin, than CFU-GM and BFU-E. Although all progenitors expressed P-glycoprotein and GST mRNA, verapamil treatment significantly, and selectively, increased the toxicity of paclitaxel and carboplatin to CFU-Mk, suggesting an important role for P-glycoprotein in megakaryocyte drug resistance. Compared with normal controls, serum thrombopoietin levels in patients receiving paclitaxel and carboplatin were significantly elevated 5 hours after infusion and remained elevated at day 7 (287% ± 63% increase; $P < 0.001$). Marrow stroma was shown to be the likely source of this thrombopoietin. It was concluded that P-glycoprotein–mediated efflux of paclitaxel, and perhaps GST-mediated detoxification of carboplatin, results in relative sparing of CFU-Mk, which may then respond to locally high levels of stromal cell–derived thrombopoietin. The confluence of these events was hypothesized to bring about the platelet-sparing phenomenon observed in patients treated with this form of combination chemotherapy.

For patients who suffer from severe or prolonged thrombocytopenia, reducing the intensity of the chemotherapy is the most appropriate approach to management. It had been anticipated that the use of recombinant thrombopoietin might significantly ameliorate this problem, but unfortunately this has not yet been demonstrated.[530] The formation of antibodies to a thrombopoietin derivative, with resulting profound thrombocytopenia, has significantly slowed clinical investigations of this cytokine.[531] Administration of the compound intravenously instead of subcutaneously might avoid at least some of this observed immunogenicity.[530] A number of other cytokines have also been reported to raise platelet counts in this setting, including IL-1, IL-3, IL-6, and IL-11, but most are no longer available and their clinical utility was not clearly demonstrated.[532-537] Only IL-11 is currently approved for the treatment of thrombocytopenia following chemotherapy. Newer thrombopoietin mimetic drugs have recently entered clinical trial. It is thought that they will be less immunogenic, and in disorders such as ITP they appear to have activity.[538] Whether they will be of help in patients with impaired thrombopoiesis is undetermined, but this will no doubt be evaluated in the near future.

At the present time, supportive therapy with platelet transfusions and drugs such as ε-aminocaproic acid for patients who have become refractory to platelet transfusions remain the mainstays of therapy. Amifostine, a phosphorylated aminothiol agent used primarily in the treatment of MDS, has been reported to have cytoprotectant value and to ameliorate the neutropenia and thrombocytopenia in patients being irradiated or receiving various types of chemotherapy in a phase III study.[539]

NUTRITIONAL DEFICIENCIES

Thrombocytopenia of various degrees can be observed in patients with either folate or vitamin B_{12} deficiency.[540-542] In some cases, it can be severe.[543,544] The mechanism of thrombocytopenia is ineffective platelet production.[456] Megakaryocyte numbers are normal or increased in the marrow, and platelet survival is normal or slightly shortened.[545] Vitamin B_{12} deficiency was reported to cause a case of amegakaryocytic thrombocytopenia.[546] Folate deficiency is frequently associated with ethanol abuse, and the etiology of the thrombocytopenia in patients who abuse ethanol is often complex.

Examination of a peripheral blood smear will typically show macrocytosis and hypersegmented neutrophils in addition to thrombocytopenia. The bone marrow often, but not always, shows megaloblastic changes in the erythroid and myeloid lineages.[547] Megakaryocytes are normal in number. Some may appear large, and in some cells multiple disconnected nuclear lobulations have been described. Often, however, distinctive morphologic abnormalities of the megakaryocytes are not seen. Rapid recovery of the platelet count can be achieved with administration of the appropriate vitamin.

IRON DEFICIENCY

Patients with iron deficiency typically exhibit thrombocytosis, but rare patients may become thrombocytopenic.[548] In some instances, decreased megakaryocytes are seen in the marrow,[549] but in a study of six children with severe iron deficiency when bone marrow examinations were performed in three patients, all showed increased numbers of megakaryocytes. After treatment with therapeutic doses of oral iron, each of the patients showed rapid increases in their platelet counts. The increased numbers of megakaryocytes and the extremely rapid increase in platelet counts after initiation of iron therapy suggested an essential role for iron in a late stage of thrombopoiesis.[550] Curiously, thrombocytopenia has been caused by iron therapy in a patient with severe iron deficiency. It was suggested, but not addressed experimentally, that the profound anemia caused preferential development of erythroid cells with a consequent decrease in megakaryocytes because they share a common progenitor.[551]

MARROW INFILTRATION

It is not rare for marrow infiltrative diseases of any type to cause ineffective hematopoiesis. Blood cell production disorders are commonly observed when the marrow is involved with metastatic cancer, lymphoma, or leukemia. Table 30-3 categorizes the infiltrative processes associated with thrombocytopenia. Physical replacement of marrow is the cause of the thrombocytopenia in many cases; it is also possible that inhibitory factors produced by the infiltrating cells are toxic to the cells of the megakaryocytic lineage or interfere with normal regulatory mechanisms. The diagnosis of infiltrative disease is made by marrow examination, although diagnostic clues are usually provided by history, physical examination, and a leukoerythroblastic blood smear. The marrow shows decreased megakaryocytes, which may be larger than normal because of a compensatory physiologic response to the thrombocytopenia. The treatment approach is specific to the infiltrative process.

ETHANOL-RELATED DISORDERS

Ethanol abuse is very commonly associated with thrombocytopenia, which may result from several different mechanisms.[542,552-557] These include, most commonly, increased splenic pooling as a result of portal hypertension and ineffective production related to folate deficiency (which may lead to severe thrombocytopenia). Ethanol itself can be directly toxic to the marrow.[555,558,559] In vitro studies have shown that alcohol concentrations achievable in vivo inhibit megakaryocyte maturation but do not inhibit CFU-Mk.[555,558] Megakaryocyte numbers usually are normal, but markedly decreased megakaryocytes have been observed.[555] In one such case, labeling with platelet-specific antibodies demonstrated that numerous, small, unidentifiable cells were immature megakaryocytes.[555] Rarely, marrow panhypoplasia has been observed in association with alcohol ingestion.[559] Anemia and macrocytosis accompanied by megaloblastic changes and ringed sideroblasts in the erythroid marrow are typically observed in the marrows of patients who abuse ethanol. The severity of the anemia shows no correlation with the thrombocytopenia. Treatment consists of withdrawal of ethanol and administration of a normal diet. Recovery of the platelet count, often with a rebound thrombocytosis, usually occurs within 2 weeks.

OTHER DRUG-RELATED DISORDERS

A variety of drugs and toxins have been implicated in isolated platelet production defects. Estrogen, for example, has been reported to decrease platelet counts through an unknown mechanism.[560] Thrombocytopenia due to thiazide diuretics has been reported frequently.[561] Although the cause of the thrombocytopenia in most cases is probably increased clearance, decreased marrow megakaryocyte numbers have been noted.[562] Interferons and IL-2 may induce thrombocytopenia.[563,564] The most likely explanation is an inhibition of CFU-Mk. Anagrelide is a very useful drug for lowering platelet counts in patients with myeloproliferative disorders and appears to work by reducing megakaryocyte size and ploidy and by disrupting maturation.[565]

Paroxysmal Nocturnal Hemoglobinuria

Paroxysmal nocturnal hemoglobinuria (PNH) is a clonal disorder resulting from mutations in the X-linked gene PIGA that encodes for an enzyme required in the initial step of biosynthesis of glycosylphosphatidylinositol anchors (PNH is discussed in Chapter 29).[566] Approximately 25% of patients with PNH have significant marrow aplasia.[567] Thrombocytopenia at diagnosis is a poor prognostic indicator. Because platelet survival is usually normal in cases of PNH,[568] thrombocytopenia is due to decreased or ineffective platelet production. Megakaryocyte progenitors have a decreased proliferative activity and exhibit increased sensitivity to complement.[448,569,570] Treatment with ATG or G-CSF and cyclosporine has ameliorated the thrombocytopenia in some patients,[571,572] whereas marrow transplantation has resulted in long-term remissions in patients with aplasia associated with PNH.[573]

Refractory Thrombocytopenia Due to Myelodysplasia

MDSs may present as isolated thrombocytopenias in a very small number of cases (<1%).[574] The diagnosis of MDS should be considered when there are clonal chromosome abnormalities. Typically they involve chromosomes 3, 5, 8, or 20, but partial deletions of other chromosomes have also been reported.[575] The usual laboratory findings include macrocytosis of platelets and red blood cells. Small dysplastic megakaryocytes, sometimes present in increased numbers, are the most typical abnormalities observed.[574,576,577] Dysplastic erythroblasts or myeloid cells may also be noted.

The clinical course of patients with this type of disorder is progressive. Additional cytopenias invariably develop so that the patient then has a typical MDS. A significant number of cases will evolve into an acute myeloid leukemia.[574] Therapy has not been shown to be beneficial. Some patients with a full-blown MDS associated with marked thrombocytopenia and less than 10% blasts have been reported to experience increases in platelet counts after androgen therapy.[578] As noted earlier, amifostine may be beneficial for some patients. It has been reported that some of these patients have been misdiagnosed as having ITP and treated for this disease. Because such therapy is not useful or helpful, it is important to recognize this entity. Thrombopoietin agonists like romiplostim have also been used in patients with MDS. In an initial study involving 44 patients, a durable platelet response was achieved in 46% of patients with less bleeding events and transfusions seen in patients who achieved a durable response.[579]

Cyclic Thrombocytopenia

Cyclic oscillations in the platelet count have been reported many times in the literature.[491,580-585] The fluctuations in platelet count can be extreme, with thrombocytopenic bleeding being the result.[586] Women are often affected, and in such patients the cycling occurs in association with the menstrual cycle. A study of 10 patients with cyclic thrombocytopenia suggested various causes of the thrombocytopenia, with cyclic variations in platelet production being

Diagnosing Thrombocytopenia Due to Impaired Thrombopoiesis

Compiling a thorough patient history is the first step in a complete workup of a thrombocytopenic patient. Many potential causes will be revealed by a good history, including obtaining a family history of thrombocytopenia, recent infection, medication or substance ingestion, or radiation or chemotherapy.

A careful physical examination could also contribute to making a diagnosis. For example, physical findings suggesting any of the inherited disorders described earlier might be discerned, as might findings suggestive of malignancy such as enlarged lymph nodes. Splenomegaly itself is not indicative of a platelet production abnormality but is often found in patients with lymphoma or other processes associated with marrow infiltration and damage that might cause impaired thrombopoiesis.

The peripheral blood smear is next examined, and this is needed to rule out pseudothrombocytopenia. Moreover, the blood smear provides additional clues to both the pathophysiologic mechanism of the thrombocytopenia and the diagnosis. For example, giant platelets suggest a hereditary or myelodysplastic syndrome; oval macrocytosis and hypersegmented neutrophils suggest a folate or vitamin B_{12} deficiency; and a leukoerythroblastic smear points to an infiltrative process.

Examination of the bone marrow is also required to evaluate megakaryocyte number and morphologic features. A biopsy specimen is more reliable than an aspirate to determine whether megakaryocytes are decreased in number. However, an aspirate showing abundant megakaryocytes in the presence of thrombocytopenia is sufficient to suggest platelet destruction or ineffective production. Megakaryocytes are not evenly distributed throughout the marrow, so examination of many fields is required in order to determine if adequate numbers of cells are present. Megakaryocyte morphologic characteristics are also useful to observe. The normal compensatory response to thrombocytopenia is enlargement of the cells with increased ploidy. Small, microlobulated or hypolobulated megakaryocytes may be seen in myelodysplastic syndromes. Dysmorphic megakaryocytes may be also observed in viral infections, including human immunodeficiency virus. In the future, flow cytometry may provide a more objective analysis of megakaryocytes.

Ultimately a diagnosis of ineffective thrombopoiesis is made by exclusion. The marrow examination reveals quantitatively normal megakaryocytes, and the apparent absence of peripheral platelet destruction together with the appropriate clinical circumstances (e.g., folate or vitamin B_{12} deficiency) often point to this mechanism. Platelet function tests may be helpful in distinguishing ineffective production from platelet destruction. In destructive processes such as immune thrombocytopenia, function is normal, whereas in ineffective platelet production impaired function is not uncommon, as noted earlier. In complex cases, platelet survival studies may be necessary to show that consumption or splenic pooling are not significant contributors to the thrombocytopenia; however, survival studies are rarely required for clinical purposes. In the future, flow cytometric estimation of platelet production rate and measurement of thrombopoietin levels may permit a more facile approach to the differential diagnosis of thrombocytopenia.

responsible for some cases, including the 2 male patients in that group.[587] A case with antibodies toxic to megakaryocytes has also been reported.[482] The possibility that fluctuating cytokine levels may contribute to the pathogenesis of the disorder has been raised by several studies, although it is difficult to distinguish cause from effect.[489,588,589] Cyclic thrombocytopenia may rarely be a presenting manifestation of myelodysplasia.[590] Treatment has been variable; responses to low-dose contraceptives and IV gamma globulin have been reported (see box on Diagnosing Thrombocytopenia Due to Impaired Thrombopoiesis).[582,591]

SUGGESTED READINGS

Boxer LA, Stossel TP: Effects of anti-human neutrophil antibodies in vitro. Quantitative studies. *J Clin Invest* 53:1534, 1974.

Bux J, Behrens G, Jaeger G, et al: Diagnosis and clinical course of autoimmune neutropenia in infancy: Analysis of 240 cases. *Blood* 91:181, 1998.

Casadevall N, Nataf J, Viron B, et al: Pure red-cell aplasia and antierythropoietin antibodies in patients treated with recombinant erythropoietin. *N Engl J Med* 346:469, 2002.

Chen J, Petrus M, Bamford R, et al: Increased serum soluble IL-15Rα levels in T-cell large granular lymphocyte leukemia. *Blood* 119:137, 2012.

Cines DB, Passero F, Guerry D, et al: Granulocyte-associated IgG in neutropenic disorders. *Blood* 59:124, 1982.

Clark DA, Dessypris EN, Krantz SB: Studies on pure red cell aplasia. XI. Results of immunosuppressive treatment of 37 patients. *Blood* 63:277, 1984.

Clemente MJ, Wlodarski MW, Makishima H, et al: Clonal drift demonstrates unexpected dynamics of the T-cell repertoire in T-large granular lymphocyte leukemia. *Blood* 2011.

Conway LT, Clay ME, Kline WE, et al: Natural history of primary autoimmune neutropenia in infancy. *Pediatrics* 79:728, 1987.

Dale DC, Bonilla MA, Davis MW, et al: A randomized controlled phase III trial of recombinant human granulocyte colony-stimulating factor (filgrastim) for treatment of severe chronic neutropenia. *Blood* 81:2496, 1993.

Doron MW, Makhlouf RA, Katz VL, et al: Increased incidence of sepsis at birth in neutropenic infants of mothers with preeclampsia. *J Pediatr* 125:452, 1994.

Greer JP, Kinney MC, Loughran TP Jr: T cell and NK cell lymphoproliferative disorders. *Hematology Am Soc Hematol Educ Program* 259, 2001.

Handgretinger R, Geiselhart A, Moris A, et al: Pure red-cell aplasia associated with clonal expansion of granular lymphocytes expressing killer-cell inhibitory receptors. *N Engl J Med* 340:278, 1999.

Koenig JM, Christensen RD: Incidence, neutrophil kinetics, and natural history of neonatal neutropenia associated with maternal hypertension. *N Engl J Med* 321:557, 1989.

Lalezari P, Khorshidi M, Petrosova M: Autoimmune neutropenia of infancy. *J Pediatr* 109:764, 1986.

Lamy T, Loughran TP Jr: Current concepts: Large granular lymphocyte leukemia. *Blood Rev* 13:230, 1999.

Liu JH, Wei S, Lamy T, et al: Chronic neutropenia mediated by Fas ligand. *Blood* 95:3219, 2000.

Liu X, Ryland L, Yang J, et al: Targeting of survivin by nanoliposomal ceramide induces complete remission in a rat model of NK-LGL leukemia. *Blood* 116:4192, 2010.

Loughran TP Jr: Clonal diseases of large granular lymphocytes. *Blood* 82:1, 1993.

Menke DM, Colon-Otero G, Cockerill KJ, et al: Refractory thrombocytopenia. A myelodysplastic syndrome that may mimic immune thrombocytopenic purpura. *Am J Clin Pathol* 98:502, 1992.

Ohgami RS, Ohgami JK, Pereira IT, et al: Refining the diagnosis of T-cell large granular lymphocytic leukemia by combining distinct patterns of antigen expression with T-cell clonality studies. *Leukemia* 25:1439, 2011.

Perzova R, Loughran TP Jr: Constitutive expression of Fas ligand in large granular lymphocyte leukaemia. *Br J Haematol* 97:123, 1997.

Risks of agranulocytosis and aplastic anemia. A first report of their relation to drug use with special reference to analgesics. The International Agranulocytosis and Aplastic Anemia Study. *JAMA* 256:1749, 1986.

Scadden DT, Zon LI, Groopman JE: Pathophysiology and management of HIV-associated hematologic disorders. *Blood* 74:1455, 1989.

Sood R, Stewart CC, Aplan PD, et al: Neutropenia associated with T-cell large granular lymphocyte leukemia: Long-term response to cyclosporine therapy despite persistence of abnormal cells. *Blood* 91:3372, 1998.

Viny A, Clemente M, Jasek M, et al: MICA polymorphism identified by whole genome array associated with NKG2D-mediated cytotoxicity in T cell large granular lymphocyte leukemia. *Haematologia* 95:1713, 2010.

Young NS, Brown KE: Parvovirus B19. *N Engl J Med* 350:586, 2004.

Yu J, Mitsui T, Wei M, et al: NKp46 identifies an NKT cell subset susceptible to leukemic transformation in mouse and human. *J Clin Invest* 121:1456, 2011.

For complete list of references log on to www.expertconsult.com.

PART

V

RED BLOOD CELLS

CHAPTER 31

PATHOBIOLOGY OF THE HUMAN ERYTHROCYTE AND ITS HEMOGLOBINS

Martin H. Steinberg, Edward J. Benz, Jr., Adeboye H. Adewoye, and Benjamin L. Ebert

Anemia, polycythemia, and functional derangements of the human erythrocyte together represent a common group of human disorders with a significant impact on public health. Although sickle cell disease, hemoglobin E (HbE)–associated disorders, and the thalassemias are humankind's most common single-gene diseases, the relevance of red blood cell (RBC) disorders to general medicine extends beyond their individual clinical severities or the number of patients affected. A critical added dimension of erythrocyte disorders is the extraordinarily detailed knowledge available about the basic biochemistry, physiology, and molecular biology of the human RBC and its membrane; enzymes; and major component, hemoglobin. RBCs are especially abundant, relatively simple, and readily accessible for repeated testing in individual patients. These features have facilitated rapid application of the techniques of cellular and molecular biology to studies of the RBC, its component molecules and structures, and syndromes resulting from abnormalities of these entities. Taken as a group, erythrocyte disorders are better understood at the molecular and cellular levels than disorders of any other cell or tissue. It is for this reason that these conditions merit particularly careful scrutiny by students of hematology.

This chapter reviews concepts about normal RBC homeostasis that form the essential knowledge base for understanding anemias, polycythemias, and functional erythrocyte disorders. The primary focus and the object for detailed discussion within this chapter is hemoglobin, the major component, both quantitatively and qualitatively, of the erythrocyte. Hemoglobin molecules dominate the pathophysiology of many RBC disorders and modulate most of the others, in part because of their sheer quantitative predominance in RBC cytoplasm. The other major relevant aspects of human RBCs—the membrane, the enzymes used for intermediary metabolism, differentiation and development, and the process of destruction—are discussed in detail in the introductory portions of other chapters. This chapter surveys these areas only briefly. Detailed descriptions of the RBC membrane can be found in Chapter 43. RBC enzymes and enzymopathies are described in Chapter 42; differentiation and development are described in Chapter 24; regulation of the RBC mass by erythropoietin is discussed in Chapter 24; and the necessary aspects of RBC destruction are considered in Chapters 32, 41-44.

ESSENTIAL FEATURES OF RED BLOOD CELL HOMEOSTASIS

As discussed in Chapter 24, the mature RBC is the product of a complex and orderly set of differentiation and maturation steps beginning with the pluripotent stem cell. By incompletely understood mechanisms involving hierarchic networks of cytokines, a portion of these cells becomes committed to differentiate along the erythroid pathway. Commitment to erythropoiesis provokes a progressively increasing sensitivity to the stimulatory actions of the hormone erythropoietin. As differentiation proceeds, there is preprogramming of certain genes whose expression at high levels will be required during the maturation phase of erythropoiesis. Genes coding for molecules defining the RBC phenotype (e.g., globin) are poised for activation at later maturation steps.

Intermediate progenitor cells arising during differentiation have been characterized experimentally, including the burst-forming unit-erythroid (BFU-E) and the colony-forming unit-erythroid (CFU-E) stages. BFU-Es are progenitor cells that in culture produce bursts or clusters of erythroid colonies, are relatively less sensitive to erythropoietin, and are more plastic with respect to important gene expression parameters, such as the synthesis of adult or fetal hemoglobin (HbF) by their descendants. CFU-Es produce single colonies, exhibit considerably higher sensitivity to erythropoietin, and appear to be more fixed in their potential to express a particular subset of globin genes. CFU-Es appear to give rise to the first morphologically recognizable erythroid cells, the proerythroblasts. At this "primitive" morphologic stage, the program of erythroid cell expression has already been essentially predetermined. The cell is predestined to undergo only a limited additional number of cell divisions, culminating in formation of the enucleate reticulocyte. The terminal maturation stages are morphologically recognizable as erythroblasts exhibiting progressive hemoglobinization of the cytoplasm, condensation and eventual ejection of the nucleus, and remodeling of the plasma membrane. Actual expression of the preprogrammed genes occurs during the 5- to 7-day period of erythroblast maturation.

As discussed in Chapter 24, the actual reconfiguration of chromatin for activation of the genes and activation itself appear to require the concerted and complex interaction of a diverse but limited group of transcription factors and associated epigenetic regulators. These regulatory proteins recognize a specific array of promoter and enhancer sequences that are embedded as recurrent motifs in and around the appropriate target genes. Even though an enormous amount of information has been gathered about sequences such as the GATA enhancers and their cognate transcription factors (e.g., GATA, FOG, ETS), the precise means by which these sequences and factors cause erythroid differentiation remains mysterious. At this time, this information is of limited clinical relevance to anemias or polycythemias. The orderly 14- to 21-day sequence of differentiation and maturation becomes progressively influenced by the levels of erythropoietin available to the progenitor cells, possibly because of increasing density and affinity of erythropoietin receptors on their cell surfaces. Within 24 hours after enucleation, the reticulocyte traverses the bone marrow–blood barrier membrane and enters the circulation as an immature erythrocyte. These cells retain remnants of nucleated precursors in the form of a relatively small number of polyribosomes actively translating messenger RNA (>90% of which is globin messenger RNA), a cell membrane that retains some molecules and structures reminiscent of its earlier stages of differentiation, and the complement of enzymes, phospholipids, and cytoskeletal proteins that the cell will possess throughout its remaining lifespan.

During its first 24 hours in the circulation, the reticulocyte spends considerable amounts of time in the spleen, during which its membrane is "polished." This is a poorly understood remodeling process by which some lipids and proteins, including adhesive molecules such as fibronectin, are removed. The content of polyribosomes and other nucleic acids progressively declines so that stainability with methylene blue is lost by the end of the first day. At this time, the RBC is regarded as a mature erythrocyte, and it circulates largely unchanged for the remainder of its 120-day lifespan.

Perhaps the most remarkable feature of the human RBC is its durability, given that it is an enucleated cell devoid of organelles that appear to be critical for the survival and function of most other cell types. The RBC has no mitochondria available for efficient oxidative metabolism; no ribosomes for regeneration of lost or damaged proteins; a very limited metabolic repertoire that largely precludes de-novo synthesis of lipids; and no nucleus to direct regenerative processes, adaptation to circulatory stresses, or cell division to replenish itself. Given these handicaps, the 120-day survival of these cells is even more striking considering the multiple and often exceedingly hostile environments they must traverse. Mechanical stresses of the circulation include high hydrostatic pressure and turbulence and the shear stresses inherent in a microcirculation networked with many capillaries having diameters only one-third to one-half that of the normal RBC. Biochemical stresses include osmotic and redox fluxes associated with travel through the collecting system of the kidney; the sluggish vascular beds of the spleen, muscle, and bone; and the rapid changes in ambient oxygen pressures occurring in the lungs. All conspire to damage RBCs. Their 4-month survival is truly remarkable.

The ability of the RBC to persist in the circulation depends on its simple but exquisitely adaptive membrane structures; its pathways of intermediary energy metabolism and redox regulation; and its ability to maintain its largest cytoplasmic component, hemoglobin, in a soluble and nonoxidized state. The membrane and enzymes of the RBC appear to be exquisitely crafted to protect the cell from the external ravages of the circulation and the potential internal assaults of the massive amount of iron-rich and potentially oxidizing protein represented by its complement of hemoglobin molecules. For these reasons, a few basic features of these membrane and enzyme systems merit comment before considering the hemoglobin molecule itself.

MAJOR FEATURES OF THE RED BLOOD CELL MEMBRANE

Chapter 43 describes the RBC membrane in considerable detail using it as a model for understanding membrane structure in general. Only a few major aspects of that discussion bear repeating for the purposes of this chapter. The RBC membrane and its underlying cytoskeleton have evolved to provide mechanical strength and the necessary pliability and resilience to withstand the mechanical, osmotic, and chemical stresses of the circulation. Because the lipid bilayer membrane essentially has the physical properties of a soap bubble, it would rapidly be emulsified in the circulation. Strength and order are provided to the lipid bilayer by the hexagonal arrays of the highly helical protein spectrin, which forms a latticework underlying the membrane.

The spectrin meshwork is held together by adaptor molecules, such as protein 4.1, adducin, p55, and ankyrin, arrayed at defined points along the highly coiled, rodlike structure of the spectrin oligomers. These protein–protein interactions appear to be critical for holding the latticework together in what has been described as the "horizontal" dimension that permits resistance to shear stress. The involvement of intermediate-length actin fibers and the variability of binding affinities by phosphorylation state appear to provide some flexibility and pliability at these points of interaction. Strength in the "vertical" dimension is provided by additional molecules or additional binding functions of the same molecule, whereby the latticework is attached to the lipid bilayer. For the most part, the physiologically important attachments appear to be indirect. Linkage is mediated through the interaction of the adaptor proteins, such as ankyrin and protein 4.1, with the cytoplasmic domains of abundant transmembrane proteins. These proteins traverse and are embedded in the lipid bilayer, providing a firm anchor. The two most critical of these molecules appear to be band 3 (i.e., the anion transport channel) and a glycophorin, probably glycophorin C/D. A possible additional stabilizing role for the Rh protein complex has been suggested. The construction of these attachments by multiple "hinge" or coupling molecules appears to provide for the flexibility and distensibility of the RBC membrane, a property essential to its ability to flow through small capillaries.

As described in Chapter 43, the complex structure of the membrane is exquisitely sensitive to perturbations impinging on any of its components. In particular, the membrane cytoskeleton and phospholipid structures are each highly susceptible to oxidation, particularly by partially proteolyzed molecules of hemoglobin, which denature to form highly toxic compounds called *hemopyrroles*. This interaction of denatured hemoglobin with the RBC membrane is clinically important, as illustrated by its impact on the pathophysiology of sickle cell anemia (see Chapter 40) or of oxidized and precipitated globin inclusion bodies in thalassemia. In this chapter, it is sufficient to note that alterations of proteins of the RBC membrane can contribute to shortening the lifespan of the RBC. Damage can result from direct defects in the cytoskeletal proteins themselves or from susceptibility of these proteins to direct oxidation or attack by oxidized or denatured hemoglobin molecules. Readers are referred to the aforementioned chapters for detailed descriptions of the relevant phenomena.

ENZYMES OF RED BLOOD CELL INTERMEDIARY

Metabolism

Mammalian erythrocytes possess a highly specialized but remarkably simplified set of metabolic pathways. As discussed in Chapter 42, there are essentially three relevant sets of pathways. The first two are interconnected by the enzyme glucose-6-phosphate dehydrogenase (G6PD). Glucose entering the RBC is metabolized by an anaerobic pathway, the Embden-Meyerhof pathway, which terminates with the enzyme lactic dehydrogenase, forming lactate. Despite its inefficiency (a net of only two adenosine triphosphate [ATP]/glucose molecule), this pathway is the sole source of usable ATP in the cell. Moreover, the pathway generates reduced nicotinamide adenine dinucleotide (NADH), a molecule necessary for driving the reduction of methemoglobin to hemoglobin (see Chapter 41). A shunt within this pathway, the Rapoport-Luebering shunt, generates the compound 2,3-bisphosphoglycerate (bis[phosphoglyceric acid]) (2,3-BPG), an important cofactor that, when bound to hemoglobin, reduces the affinity of hemoglobin for oxygen (see Hemoglobin Function). The ATP generated is necessary for kinase reactions controlling phosphorylation of membrane and signaling components, for fueling ion pumps and channels, and for maintaining phospholipid levels.

The anaerobic metabolic pathway generates, as one of its intermediates, glucose-6 phosphate, which is the substrate for G6PD. G6PD appears to be the rate-limiting enzyme for a linked pathway called the *oxidative hexose monophosphate shunt*. This pathway involves a cascade of reactions culminating in the reduction of oxidized glutathione to reduced glutathione. Reduced glutathione is used to reverse oxidation of critical structures, including hemoglobin, cytoskeletal proteins, and membrane lipids. Anaerobic glycolysis generates NADH for methemoglobin reduction, 2,3-BPG for modulation of hemoglobin oxygen affinity, and ATP for metabolic energy requirements. Its end product is lactate. The oxidative glycolysis pathway generates nicotinamide adenine dinucleotide phosphate (NADPH) and reduced glutathione for use as the major erythrocyte antioxidant.

During the past decade, most of the enzymes (or at least the erythroid isoforms of these enzymes) involved in RBC intermediary metabolism have been characterized at the molecular level by cloning of their cDNAs, genomic loci, or both. Some of the more relevant information arising from this progress is discussed in Chapter 42. The erythrocyte possesses membrane-based signaling receptors and cytoplasmic signal transduction elements similar, although perhaps less elaborate, than those of nucleated cells. The relevance of these systems to the pathophysiology of RBC disorders is just becoming apparent.

RED BLOOD CELL SENESCENCE AND DESTRUCTION

Erythrocytes, despite their impressive adaptations to circulatory stresses, eventually wear out and are destroyed. RBC survival in humans appears to be remarkably uniform under normal circumstances, spanning approximately 120 days from release of the reticulocyte into the circulation to sequestration of the senescent RBC in the reticuloendothelial cells of the liver and spleen. The precise signal, or signals, marking RBCs for destruction remain unknown, as does the underlying pathophysiology within the RBC or on its surface. However, several interrelated theories have emerged; these are discussed only briefly because they are mentioned in other chapters.

Red blood cells accumulate surface blemishes during their lives in the circulation. These appear to result in part from the accumulation of small amounts of oxygen damage to membrane structures. The altered regions are sensed by the reticuloendothelial cells during passage of the erythrocytes through the liver and spleen. Removal or pitting of these damaged regions from RBC membranes can be documented microscopically; small amounts of normal membrane are also lost during the process.

The biconcave disk shape of the RBC, so important to its distensibility, depends on a high ratio of surface area to volume. This requires redundant membrane surface area. The membrane surface area of the normal biconcave disk is approximately 140 μm^2. To enclose a sphere containing a normal RBC volume (≈90 fL), only approximately 95 μm^2 would be needed. Progressive loss of membrane surface by means of the pitting phenomenon should ultimately cause the aging erythrocyte to assume a more rigid spherical shape. A sphere is inevitably far less distensible and far less capable of passing through small apertures than a disk, especially in the sluggish and torturous circulation of the spleen. This geometric mechanism can lead to the eventual destruction of the RBC.

Red blood cells progressively lose some of the critical enzymes needed for intermediary metabolism and antioxidant capacity. G6PD levels, for example, progressively decline during the circulating lifespan, as do levels of several other enzymes. The decline of certain enzymes can be used as a crude means of estimating the relative age of different RBC populations. The biochemical or oxidative mechanism of destruction postulates that aged RBCs are eventually depleted of critical enzymes needed for maintenance of redox status. Oxidation of critical membrane proteins, lipids, and hemoglobin would then ensue, causing distortion and rigidity of the RBC membrane, with accelerated loss as previously described. The end product would be spherocytes incapable of traversing the splenic vascular bed and escaping engulfment by the reticuloendothelial cell.

It has been proposed that an immune-type mechanism can contribute to normal and pathologic RBC senescence. This hypothesis is based on the observation that oxidative damage, regardless of cause, promotes a clustering, or *capping,* of oligomers of band 3 on the RBC surface. Under normal circumstances, band 3 molecules form monomers, dimers, or tetramers. Higher order aggregates appear to be recognized by an endogenous isoantibody possessed by all people. Any RBC accumulating oxidative damage from wear and tear in the circulation, from depletion of enzymes, or from internal pathologic processes such as denaturation of hemoglobin in certain hemoglobinopathies can accumulate these aggregates. The aggregates would then be bound by antibody and be removed by the reticuloendothelial cells as antigen–antibody complexes, using the same means used by reticuloendothelial cells to recognize any immune complex. This mechanism could also provide for the pitting or polishing of damaged RBC membranes. All three of the proposed mechanisms are interrelated by their inception with oxidative damage.

Other membrane-related changes might influence RBC destruction. Bcl-X_L, a suppressor of apoptosis, is present in erythrocyte membranes, and its antagonization may promote cell death. This may be mediated by calcium accumulation and phosphatidylserine exposure. Cholesterol and fatty acids accumulate on the aging RBC membrane and might be targets for oxidation induced by reactive oxygen species. RBCs are removed from the circulation by splenic macrophages, probably by several mechanisms. SHPS-1, a surface glycoprotein and a member of the immunoglobulin superfamily that interacts with RBC membrane CD47, is abundant in macrophages. Studies using mice expressing a mutant SHPS-1 suggested that this molecule might negatively regulate phagocytosis, influencing cell lifespan. Increasing phosphatidyl serine exposure and reduced aminophospholipid translocase activity during aging might induced oxidative damage to the cell. It is probable that these mechanisms leading to cell destruction are not mutually exclusive, that no single effect predominates, and that these events occur at different times at different sites of RBC damage.

Regardless of the mechanism(s) fostering eventual senescence and destruction of RBCs, the process itself involves components clinically useful for assessment of anemias associated with accelerated destruction. Chief among these is the generation of indirect or unconjugated bilirubin, the byproduct of heme catabolism occurring within the reticuloendothelial cells. In markedly accelerated states of RBC destruction, hypertrophy of the liver and spleen can also occur, providing a useful physical indicator of hemolytic anemia. These indirect clinical features, coupled with the reticulocyte count, remain more useful for detecting clinical hemolysis than complicated studies of RBC kinetics.

HEMOGLOBIN SYNTHESIS, STRUCTURE, AND FUNCTION

Basic Features

Hemoglobins are the major oxygen-carrying pigments of the body. They are packaged into RBCs in quantities sufficient to carry enough oxygen from the lungs to the tissues to meet the needs of those cells for oxidative metabolism. These quantities are enormous—almost 2 lb of hemoglobin are present in the body of a reasonably sized human at any given time. Because free hemoglobin in the bloodstream is catabolized and excreted renally in a matter of minutes, packaging in erythrocytes is essential to preserve the newly synthesized molecules for the entire 4-month lifespan of the RBC. Otherwise, the caloric and biosynthetic resources needed to replace daily losses of hemoglobin would be prohibitive. The RBC's major function is to encase hemoglobin and protect it so it can function as an oxygen transporter for a prolonged period. An additional function of hemoglobin is to modulate vascular tone by its transport of nitric oxide (NO) and possibly nitrous oxide.

The cellular content of blood influences its viscosity; in particular, the hemodynamics are adversely compromised by the presence of too many circulating erythrocytes because blood viscosity correlates especially with hematocrit. To provide for adequate oxygen transport (i.e., enough hemoglobin molecules) in a number of RBCs compatible with tolerable viscosity, each cell must enclose a high concentration of hemoglobin (32-35 g per 100 mL of cytoplasm). This concentration is close to the solubility limit of hemoglobin in physiologic solutions. It follows that even minor perturbations within these molecules (e.g., oxidation) or in the milieu (e.g., changes in pH or ionic strength) can have potentially devastating effects on the solubility of hemoglobin. Because polymerized or precipitated hemoglobins derange intracellular viscosity, trigger proteolytic reactions that lead to oxidative damage of erythrocytes, and compromise oxygen transport, it is not surprising that the fate of the RBC is inextricably interwoven with the state of its enormous complement of hemoglobin molecules.

Hemoglobin Structure

The hemoglobin tetramer consists of two pairs of unlike globin polypeptide chains, each associated with a heme group. Normal hemoglobin has two α- and two non–α-globin chains; the interaction of these chains is responsible for the quaternary structure of the hemoglobin molecule and normal oxygen transport. Functionally, the second exon of each globin gene encodes the major component of the heme-binding pocket, and the α and non-α contacts are regulated by the third exon.

The behavior of hemoglobin is determined by its primary structure, the covalent linking of amino acids to form the polypeptide globin. The higher order structures of hemoglobin depend on the sequence of amino acid residues that make up the globin chain. The α-globin chains contain 141 residues, and the β-globin–like chains are 146 amino acids long (Fig. 31-1). There is considerable homology among these globins, especially among the non–α-globin chains. Whereas the α-globin genes *(HBA2, HBA1)* result from a very ancient gene duplication, the non–α-globin genes *(HBE, HBG2, HBG1, HBD, HBB)* are the result of more recent gene duplications and are more akin to each other than they are to the α-like globin genes. Gene conversion events also ensure the similarity of duplicated genes.

Elements of the secondary structure of globin are shown in Figs. 31-1 and 31-2. Approximately 75% of the globin polypeptide chain forms an α-helix. There are eight helical segments, A through H, separated by short stretches from which the α-helix is absent. These nonhelical segments permit folding of the polypeptide on itself and are often dictated by the presence of prolyl residues, which are generally unable to participate in the formation of α-helices. Although the helical segments of the α- and non–α-globin chains do not exactly correspond, it is possible to align amino acid residues in all globin peptides by their helical and nonhelical residue numbers, as indicated in Fig. 31-1. This permits greater appreciation of the homology among globins. Some of the amino acids of globin are invariant, or conserved, in the sense that they are preserved during phylogeny. These residues occur at portions of the molecule that are critical for its stability and function, such as heme binding residues, hydrophobic amino acids of the interior of the molecule, and certain subunit contacts at the α_1–β_2 interface. The introduction of prolyl residues into α-helical segments by mutation leads to interruption of the α-helix and instability of the resulting hemoglobin molecule.

The poorly understood laws that govern the folding of proteins are responsible for the tertiary structure of globin, shown in Fig. 31-2. This folding pattern places polar residues exteriorly and provides a hydrophobic niche for the heme ring between the E and F helices. Numerous noncovalent bonds are formed between the heme and surrounding amino acid residues of globin. An iron atom in the center of the porphyrin ring forms an important bond with the F8 or proximal histidine and through the linked oxygen with the E7 or distal histidine residue. Oxygenation and deoxygenation of hemoglobin occur at the heme iron. Folding of globin and association of chains into dimers and tetramers was once thought to occur spontaneously. However, it is now clear that these processes are assisted by chaperone proteins, which are described in Chapters 4 and 5.

Two α-globin chains and two non–α-globin chains fit together specifically to form a hemoglobin tetramer with a molecular mass of approximately 64,000 daltons and with the quaternary structure shown in Fig. 31-3. The motion of individual globin chains, as well

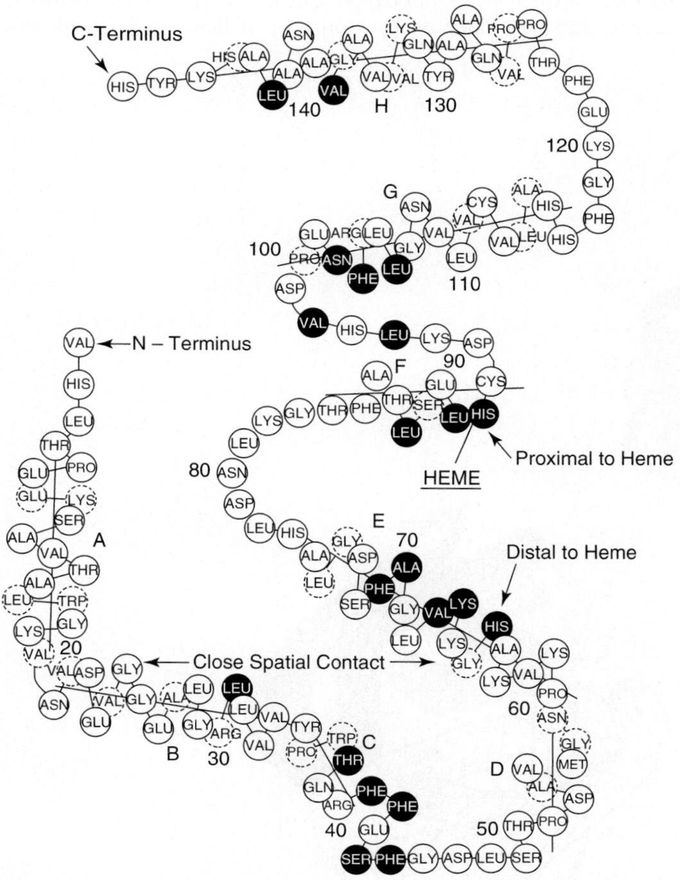

Figure 31-1 THE β-GLOBIN CHAIN SHOWING HELICAL AND NONHELICAL SEGMENTS. The helical segments are labeled A through H, and the nonhelical segments are designated NA for residues between the N terminus and the A helix, CD for residues between the C and D helices, and so forth. *(From Huisman THJ, Schroeder WA:* New aspects of the structure, function, and synthesis of hemoglobin. *Boca Raton, 1971, Fl, CRC Press.)*

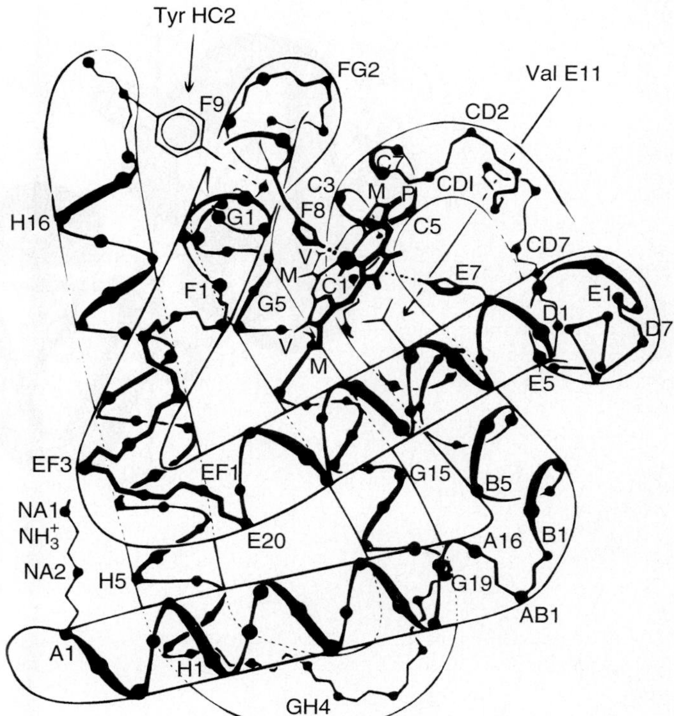

Figure 31-2 TERTIARY STRUCTURE OF A GLOBIN CHAIN. Globin folds into a tertiary structure such that polar or charged amino acids are located on the exterior of the molecule and the heme ring resides in a hydrophobic niche between the E and F helices. Linked to the heme are the proximal (F8) histidine and the distal (E7) histidine. *(From Perutz MF: Molecular anatomy, physiology, and pathology of hemoglobin. In Stamatoyannopoulos G, Neinhuis AW, Leder P, et al, editors:* The molecular basis of blood diseases. *Philadelphia, 1987, Saunders, p 127.)*

as the movement of globin chains relative to each other during oxygenation and deoxygenation, gives hemoglobin its unique usefulness as a respiratory protein.

Hemoglobin Function

Evolution has honed the hemoglobin tetramer into a molecule ideally suited for its tasks. Because human hemoglobin must behave differently than that of altitude dwelling species or species inhabiting hypoxic locales, many different variants of the same basic molecular design have evolved. Because of the exigencies of molecular evolution, we find in the genome of all animals, including humans, attempts by nature to propagate a variety of different globin genes. The crystallographic studies of Perutz and coworkers defined the oxygenated and deoxygenated structures of hemoglobin at Ångström-unit resolution and provided an exquisitely detailed picture of how the globin chains and individual amino acid residues respond to the loading and unloading of oxygen. All of these, however, share the properties of highly reversible oxygen binding and high solubility in cytoplasm. We know more about the function of hemoglobin than about virtually any other protein, and the knowledge of this mechanism provides a beautiful and intellectually satisfying culmination to decades of study by many investigators.

The oxygen dissociation curve of hemoglobin, shown in Fig. 31-4, describes the percent saturation of hemoglobin with oxygen at different oxygen tensions. The sigmoidal shape of this curve is a result of interaction among the subunits of hemoglobin. Communication within the tetramer is called heme–heme interaction or cooperativity. This implies that the four heme groups do not undergo simultaneous oxygenation or deoxygenation but rather that the state of each heme unit with regard to the presence or absence of bound oxygen influences the binding of oxygen to other heme groups. Myoglobin, a heme-containing protein with virtually the same tertiary structure as globin, exists in muscle as a monomer. The oxygen equilibrium curve of myoglobin is a rectangular hyperbola; in physiologic terms, it rapidly becomes fully saturated at low oxygen tensions and remains saturated as the oxygen tension plateaus. The difference in the oxygen equilibrium curves of myoglobin and hemoglobin lies in the tetrameric nature of the hemoglobin molecule and the cooperativity permitted by the association of similar but unlike subunits. Compared with hemoglobin, myoglobin has a very low P_{50} (i.e., oxygen partial pressure at which the molecule is one-half saturated). It therefore has an extremely high oxygen affinity and would not be useful for delivering oxygen to tissues. The oxygen in myoglobin is passed on to the mitochondria, where oxidative metabolism occurs. The sigmoidal shape of the oxygen dissociation curve of hemoglobin indicates that the totally deoxygenated hemoglobin tetramer is slow to become oxygenated, but as oxygenation proceeds, the reaction of heme with oxygen accelerates. Perutz has drawn an analogy in which the "appetite" of heme for oxygen grows with the "eating," and conversely, loss of oxygen by heme lowers the oxygen affinity of the remaining heme groups. The Hill coefficient, *n,* which can be calculated from plots of oxygen equilibrium curves, is a description of heme–heme interaction or cooperativity that explains in part the oxygen-binding properties of hemoglobin and myoglobin. The Hill coefficient for myoglobin is 1, indicating no cooperativity; *n* is approximately 3 for the normal human hemoglobin A molecule.

The oxygen affinity of hemoglobin within the erythrocyte does not depend solely on the intrinsic properties of the tetramer. The position of the hemoglobin oxygen dissociation curve, and therefore the P_{50}, can be influenced by a number of heterotropic modifiers,

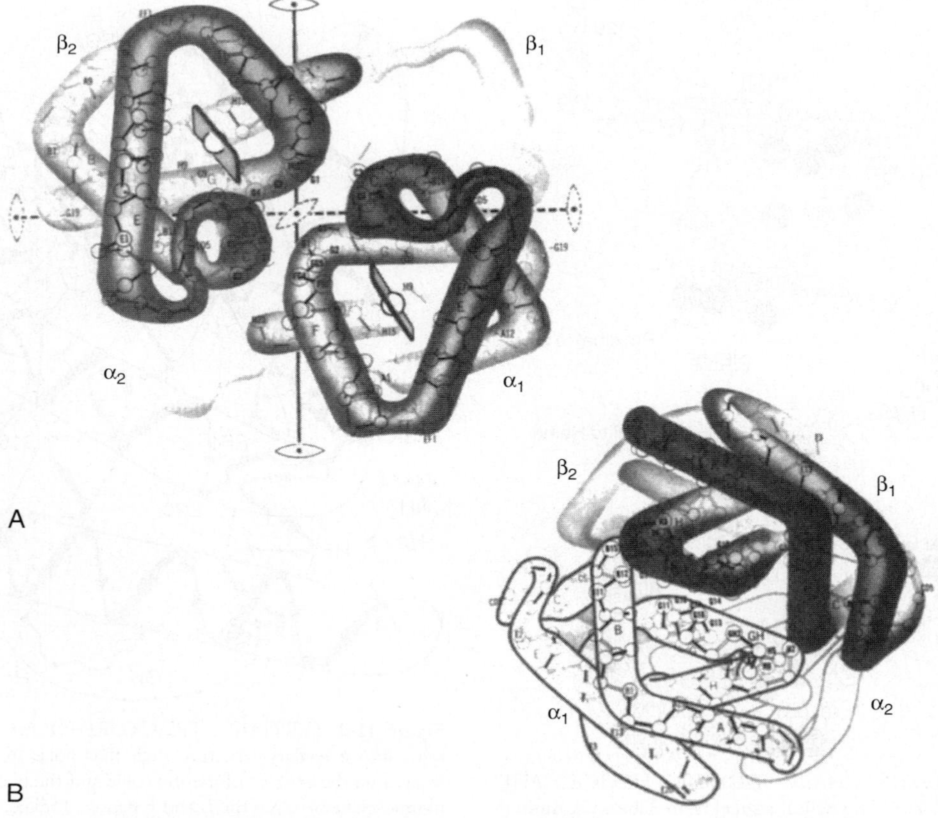

Figure 31-3 QUATERNARY STRUCTURE OF HEMOGLOBIN. The contacts between subunits are shown as circled amino acids. In the front view **(A)**, α_1–β_2 contacts are shown, and in the side view **(B)**, α_1-β–β_1 contacts are depicted. *(From Dickerson RE, Geis I:* Hemoglobin: Structure, function, and evolution pathology. *Menlo Park, Calif, 1983, Benjamin-Cummings.)*

including temperature, pH, and small organic phosphate molecules in the cell. The effects of these modifiers on P_{50} are shown in Fig. 31-4.

Hemoglobin is the prototype of an allosteric protein; its structure and function are influenced by other molecules. The major intracellular modulator of hemoglobin–oxygen affinity in human erythrocytes is 2,3-BPG, an intermediate product of glycolysis that is present within the erythrocyte at concentrations equimolar to hemoglobin. The synthesis of 2,3-BPG is enzymatically regulated, and its levels can change depending on the conditions extant. 2,3-BPG is able to bind stereospecifically within the central cavity of the hemoglobin tetramer. Hemoglobin prepared in the absence of 2,3-BPG has a very high oxygen affinity, but as 2,3-BPG is added to a hemoglobin solution, the oxygen affinity progressively decreases. 2,3-BPG is a polyanion that binds strongly to the deoxygenated form of hemoglobin but poorly to its oxygenated or other liganded forms. Specific amino acids are involved in the binding of 2,3-BPG; these β-chain residues include the N-terminal valines, the H21 histidine (position 143), and the EF6 lysine (position 82). In oxyhemoglobin, the H helices of the β-chains are insufficiently spread to permit firm binding of 2,3-BPG; this, along with other conformational changes, favors the binding of this anion to the deoxygenated rather than the oxygenated form of hemoglobin. The binding of 2,3-BPG stabilizes the T (tense) structure of the deoxygenated form at the expense of the R (relaxed) structure of the oxyhemoglobin tetramer.

Transition from the deoxy (T) to the oxy (R) form of hemoglobin is accompanied by rotation of the αβ dimers along the α_1–β_2 contact region (Fig. 31-5). The T structure is stabilized by salt bridges, which are broken as the molecule switches into the R structure. Some abnormal hemoglobins with an intrinsically high oxygen affinity, or low P_{50}, occur as a result of an amino acid substitution that leads to loss of bonds that stabilize the tetramer in the T conformation. Hydrogen ions, chloride ions, and carbon dioxide all decrease the affinity of hemoglobin for oxygen by strengthening the salt bridges that lock the molecule into its T conformation. The corollary of the lowering of hemoglobin oxygen affinity by protons is the combination of hemoglobin with protons on deoxygenation. This is known as the Bohr effect and is responsible for carbon dioxide transport in blood, another critical function of the hemoglobin molecule. Deoxyhemoglobin binds the hydrogen ion liberated by the reaction of carbon dioxide with water, increasing the concentration of bicarbonate. Within the lungs, hydrogen ions are lost as hemoglobin binds oxygen; therefore, carbon dioxide leaves solution and is excreted from the body through the lungs. Deoxyhemoglobin can also directly bind carbon dioxide; however, this process involves the minority of carbon dioxide exchanged by the RBCs.

Red blood cells containing high levels of hemoglobin F have high oxygen affinity because it binds 2,3-BPG poorly. Physiologically, this predicts that the hemoglobin of fetuses should be oxygenated at the expense of the maternal hemoglobin A. The high oxygen affinity of hemoglobin F is accounted for by a single change in its primary structure, the presence of a serine residue at helical position H21 in place of the histidine found in the β-globin chain. This weakens the binding of 2,3-BPG and leads to stabilization of the molecule in its R state.

Interactions of hemoglobin with NO have been a recent focus of investigation. NO, generated from L-arginine by nitric oxide synthases, activates soluble guanylate cyclase to produce the second messenger cyclic guanosine monophosphate (cGMP). As a potent vasodilator, NO is an important regulator of vascular tone. The reaction of free NO with erythrocytes is diffusion limited. Normally, the primary NO–hemoglobin adduct is nitrosyl (heme) hemoglobin

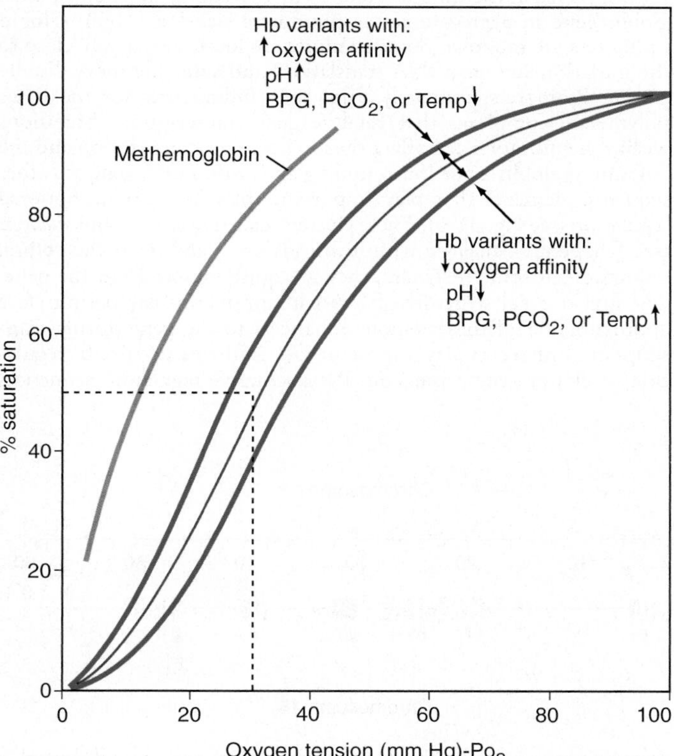

Figure 31-4 OXYGEN DISSOCIATION CURVE OF HEMOGLOBIN. The percent saturation of hemoglobin with oxygen at different oxygen tensions is depicted by the *red sigmoidal curve*. The P50 (i.e., oxygen tension at which the hemoglobin molecule is one-half saturated) is approximately 27 mm Hg in normal erythrocytes *(dotted lines)*. Heterotopic modifiers of hemoglobin function can shift the curve leftward by increasing or rightward by decreasing its oxygen affinity. *PCO_2*, Partial pressure of carbon dioxide; *Po_2*, partial pressure of oxygen. *(From Benz EJ, Jr: Synthesis, structure, and function of hemoglobin. In Kelly WN, DeVita VT, editors:* Textbook of internal medicine, *vol 1. Philadelphia, 1989, JB Lippincott, p 236.)*

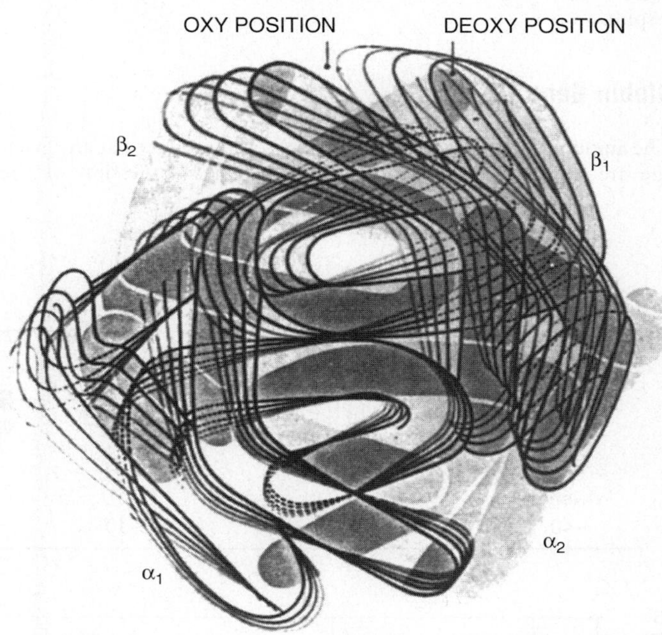

Figure 31-5 SUBUNIT MOTION IN THE HEMOGLOBIN TETRAMER. The relative motion of hemoglobin subunits on oxygenation and deoxygenation is shown. The $\alpha_1\beta_1$ dimer *(black)* is moving relative to the $\alpha_2\beta_2$ dimer *(shaded)*. The oxyhemoglobin tetramer (R state) is more compact than the deoxyhemoglobin configuration (T state). *(From Dickerson RE, Geis I:* Hemoglobin: Structure, function, and evolution pathology. *Menlo Park, Calif, 1983, Benjamin-Cummings.)*

(HbFe[II]NO). Within the erythrocyte, β93 cysteine is reduced and seems incapable of NO storage and delivery by *S*-nitrosohemoglobin as originally proposed. NO was thought to form *S*-nitrosylhemoglobin in the lungs, where hemoglobin is in its R or oxygenated state, and liberate NO in the microcirculation, where the transition of the R to T conformation induced by deoxygenation released NO from hemoglobin. However, studies suggest that NO binding to heme groups is physiologically a rapidly reversible process. This view supports a model of hemoglobin delivery of NO distinct from its dissociation from the β93 cysteine residues. Small nitrosothiol molecules could also be involved in NO transfer. The thiol groups of hemoglobin can exchange NO with small nitrosothiols derived from free cysteine and glutathione. Accordingly, the thiol groups of hemoglobin could bind and transfer NO or exchange NO with small shuttle molecules, increasing perfusion of hypoxic tissues. It has been suggested that cytoskeletal and other erythrocyte proteins slow NO influx into the cell and, coupled with NO heme binding, preserve NO bioactivity. NO–hemoglobin interactions, whether through *S*-nitrosohemoglobin formation at the β93 cysteine or the formation of nitroso intermediates, are likely to be physiologically important. Hemoglobin liberated from the intravascularly hemolyzed RBCs rapidly inactivates NO. As the RBC lyses, arginase is also released and destroys the substrate for NO synthases, L-arginine. Together, this leads to a reduction in biologically active NO. With hemolysis as in sickle cell disease or thalassemia, reduced NO bioavailability is associated with disease complications such as pulmonary hypertension, leg ulcers, priapism, and perhaps increased risk of stroke. Lactic dehydrogenase also released from the RBC in hemolytic anemia is an excellent marker of these complications.

In summary, the primary amino acid structure of α- and non–α-globin chains dictates the inevitable quaternary structure in which resides the ability of hemoglobin to serve as a respiratory protein. Cooperativity ensures rapid binding of oxygen in the lungs and unloading in tissues. Similarly, carbon dioxide is transported from tissues to lungs. The function of hemoglobin may be influenced by mutation and by heterotropic effectors such as protons and 2,3-BPG. The molecule itself changes shape as it provides oxygen for metabolism; it is a lung in miniature, breathing as it allows the body to respire.

Globin Gene Clusters

The amounts and types of human hemoglobin produced at any given age are determined primarily by the selective expression of the individual genes encoding each globin chain. The globin genes of humans are located in two clusters (Fig. 31-6): α-like genes in approximately 30 kb of DNA on the short arm of chromosome 16 between band p13.2 and the telomere and β-like genes in approximately 70 kb of DNA on the terminal portion of the short arm of chromosome 11 (p15). Each gene shares certain basic organizational features. Each contains three exons separated by two introns. Both introns of the α-gene are small (100-300 bp); non–α-genes have one small and one large (1000-1200 bp) intron. The second exon of each globin gene encodes the major components of the heme-binding pocket, and the third encodes the α- and non-α contact points.

Flanking each gene at the 5′ and 3′ ends are groups of conserved nucleotides. In conjunction with protein factors, these influence the promotion of gene transcription, ensure the fidelity of the transcript and its translatability, specify sites for the initiation and termination of translation, and improve the stability of the newly synthesized mRNA (Fig. 31-7). Also encoded within the genes are signals that permit the enzymatic machinery within the nucleus to excise precisely the introns from the mRNA precursor and splice together the exons to form a contiguous "mature" mRNA. The spliced mRNA is transported to the cytoplasm and translated into protein. These conserved signals lie at the junction of the exon and intron and within the introns themselves. They are recognized by small nuclear ribonucleoprotein (RNP) particles, which participate in the formation of a spliceosome, or splicing complex. Their preservation is critical for the splicing process to occur. When mutations occur within splice signal sites, globin synthesis is often impaired. The 5′ end of the mRNA contains a cap structure, and the 3′ end contains a poly(A) tail, as described in Chapter 1.

Conserved nucleotide clusters 5′ to the coding portion of each globin gene in aggregate act as promoters (see Fig. 31-7). Globin promoters are modular. Some modules are located relatively close to the initiation site of mRNA translation, and some are more distally placed. Promoters ultimately form the binding sites for the RNA polymerase complexes that catalyze gene transcription. Mutations within the promoter can affect the level of gene transcription and the amount of globin made. Surrounding and within each gene are other sequence elements that play important roles in its transcriptional regulation (see Fig. 31-6). These clusters, called *enhancers* and *silencers* (see Chapter 1), may lie within introns or 5′ and 3′ to the coding sequences; in some instances, they are quite remote from the gene. The higher order structure of DNA in chromatin may permit close approximation of these remote enhancers to the gene during transcription. Enhancers play important roles in the tissue-specific regulation of globin gene expression. Representative regulatory sequences

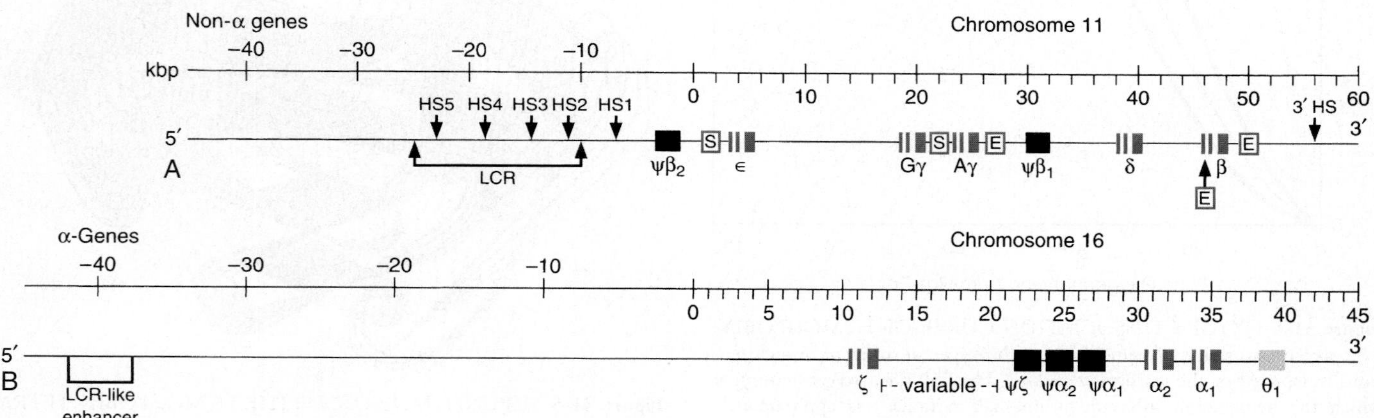

Figure 31-6 Maps of the β-like and α-like globin gene clusters located on chromosome 11 **(A)** and chromosome 16 **(B).** Within each gene cluster are pseudogenes, which are remnants of previously expressed globin genes that have become inactivated as a result of mutation. Active genes are shown in *red boxes* filled with clear introns; inactive or pseudogenes genes are shown in *solid boxes,* and the ζ-globin gene is shown as a *pink box*. Although this gene is transcribed, it is not clear whether it is represented in a cellular protein. The distance between the functional ζ-globin and pseudo-ζ-globin gene is variable because of the presence of repeated elements. *E,* Enhancer; *HS,* DNase hypersensitive site; *LCR,* locus control region; *S,* silencer.

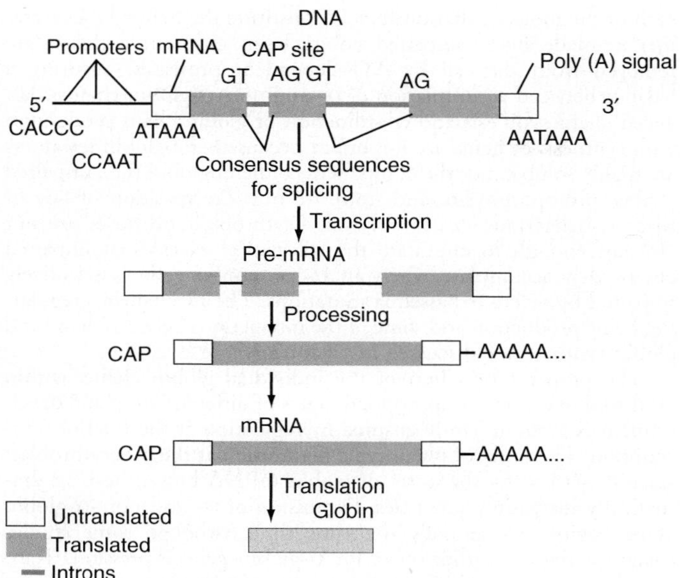

Figure 31-7 PATHWAY OF GLOBIN BIOSYNTHESIS. Transcription of the globin gene results in a large pre-mRNA molecule containing intervening sequences. During intranuclear processing of this molecule, the intervening sequences are excised and the coding sequences ligated to form a contiguous stretch of RNA, which codes for the globin protein. The message is further processed by the addition of a CAP and a poly(A) tail. The mature message is transported from the nucleus to cytoplasm, where it is translated on polyribosomes by the addition of activated amino acids to a growing polypeptide chain. Globin acquires heme and α: non-α dimers are formed and a hemoglobin tetramer is assembled. *(From Steinberg, MH: Hemoglobinopathies and thalassemias. In Stein JH, editor:* Internal medicine, *ed 4, St. Louis, 1994, Mosby-Year Book, p 852.)*

near the globin genes are shown in Fig. 31-6 (locus control region [LCR], LCR-like enhancer). DNA elements controlling globin genes are described in more detail later.

The α-like and β-like globin genes are ordered in the 5′ to 3′ direction in the same sequence expressed during embryonic, fetal, and adult development (Fig. 31-8). The functional significance of this arrangement is unclear. However, evidence suggests that the ordering of the ε, γ, δ, and β genes could be an important factor influencing the ability of each locus to interact with distant control elements at different developmental stages.

The α-like and β-like gene clusters probably are the result of an ancient duplication of a primordial globin gene that existed early in the history of vertebrates, approximately 500 million years ago. Each gene cluster probably developed from the duplication of ancestral genes and subsequent divergence through eons of evolution. Within the α-like gene cluster, the δ-globin gene is expressed only very early in embryogenesis and participates in the formation of embryonic hemoglobins. A μ, α-like globin gene *(HBM),* that codes for a 141 amino acid α-globin–like chain has been recently detected and is expressed in erythroid cells in a highly regulated fashion; however, an associated protein has not been found.

The α-globin genes are duplicated, a characteristic of most globin genes, and their encoded amino acid sequences are identical; therefore, only a single α-globin polypeptide results. Minor differences within the second intervening sequence and the 3′ flanking regions of the α-globin gene permit identification of transcripts from each gene. The 5′ or α_2-gene is expressed more efficiently than the 3′ or α_1-gene, so abnormalities of this gene are more likely to be clinically apparent. Both clusters contain genes that are actively transcribed, as well as pseudogenes whose defective structures prohibit expression at any time.

The gene 3′ to the α_1-gene is the Θ-gene, a somewhat mysterious element of the α-gene cluster. Although Θ-gene transcripts are found in fetal tissue and adult erythroid marrow, it is unclear whether this gene's translation product is able to participate in the formation of a functional tetramer. The Θ-globin protein has been found in vivo, but deletion of the Θ-globin gene does not appear to have any implications for developing fetuses. In vitro, Θ-globin mRNA is correctly spliced, and Θ-globin cDNA can direct synthesis of a translatable mRNA and a Θ-globin protein.

The β-like–globin gene cluster consists of the embryonic ε-gene, transcribed only during the first 6 to 11 weeks of life; the duplicated γ-globin genes that code for the dominant non–α-globin of fetal life; and the δ- and β-globin genes that code for the hemoglobins of adults. The coding sequences of the two γ-globin genes are identical, except at codon 136, where the 5′ or Gγ-gene codes for glutamic acid; the 3′ or Aγ-gene encodes an alanine residue. These genes are unequally expressed during fetal development. A switch in their relative rates of expression leads to a similar disparity between the amounts of Gγ and Aγ chains in adults. Although the Gγ/Aγ switch is interesting from the standpoint of the control of gene expression, it is of little clinical importance. Hemoglobin F in fetuses and adults contains a mixture of Gγ and Aγ chains; the functional qualities of these hemoglobins are identical.

The δ- and β-globin genes are probably the result of a duplication event that occurred more than 40 million years ago. The β-globin gene has become the predominant gene, coding for most non–α-globin chains of adults. The δ-globin gene has undergone mutation in several critical areas, and its expression is greatly curtailed. Its product, a minor fraction of adult hemoglobin (HbA_2), has become functionally insignificant by virtue of its very low level in the erythrocyte. It is likely that the δ-globin gene is a "pseudogene in evolution." HbA_2 is clinically useful, however, for characterizing hemoglobinopathies such as β-thalassemia. In time, its expression may be totally abolished as it acquires an inactivating mutation. The pseudogenes dispersed within both globin gene clusters provide interesting glimpses into the evolutionary history of globin genes. Pseudogenes are inactive remnants of previously expressed genes. As a result of relaxed selection, their mutation rates are higher than those of surrounding active genes.

The expression of the human globin genes is highly regulated. Globin is synthesized in only one tissue—erythroid cells—and only during a narrowly defined stage of erythroid progenitor cell differentiation—the 5 to 7 days that commence with the proerythroblast stage and end when the enucleated reticulocyte loses the last traces of its RNA. Within the confines of these strict tissue-specific and differentiation stage-specific boundaries, the globin genes are extraordinarily active. By the late normoblast and reticulocyte stages, 90% to 95% of all protein synthesis in these cells is globin synthesis.

Individual globin genes are expressed at different levels in developing erythroblasts of human embryos, fetuses, and "adults" (i.e., 37 to 38 weeks of gestation and beyond). Different subsets of α- and non–α-genes are expressed and silenced at each developmental stage. Moreover, the overall balance of non–α-globin, α-globin, and heme production is maintained throughout each of these complex switching events. The complex mechanisms ensuring the proper tissue-specific, differentiation stage—specific, and ontologic stage–specific expression are incompletely defined. Much information about relevant DNA control elements and transcription factors is emerging. These topics are discussed after a review of the ontogeny of hemoglobin.

Ontogeny of Hemoglobin

The hemoglobin composition of the erythrocyte depends on when in gestation or postnatal development it is measured. This is a result of sequential activation and inactivation (i.e., switching) among genes within the α- and non–α-globin gene clusters (see Fig. 31-8). What controls these switches in globin gene transcription is not understood. The two early embryonic hemoglobins consist of ζ- and ε-globin chains (Hb Gower-1) and α- and ε-globin chains (Hb

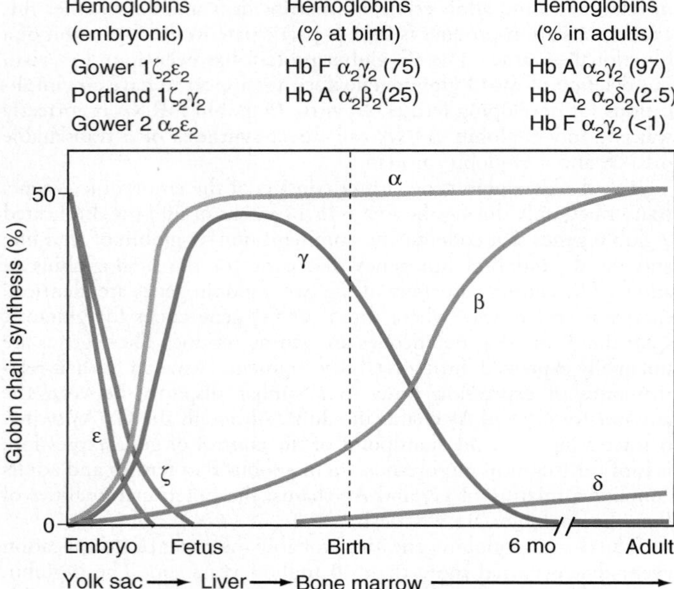

Figure 31-8 HEMOGLOBIN (Hb) SWITCHING DURING EMBRYONIC, FETAL, AND ADULT DEVELOPMENT. The ζ and ε genes are transcribed during embryonic development and are soon replaced by the fetal γ- and adult α-globin gene. At birth, fetal hemoglobin (HbF) forms approximately 75%, and hemoglobin A forms 25% of the total. Transcription of the γ gene begins to decrease before birth, and by 6 months of age, this gene is expressed only at very low levels. Expression of the δ-globin gene begins near birth. In adults, hemoglobin A makes up approximately 97%, hemoglobin A_2 approximately 2.5%, and HbF less than 1% of the total. *(From Steinberg MH: Hemoglobinopathies and thalassemias. In Stein JH, editors:* Internal medicine, *ed 4, St. Louis, 1994, Mosby-Year Book, p 852.)*

Gower-2). The ζ-globin gene is akin to the α-globin genes but is expressed only during early embryogenesis. The ε-embryonic globin chain is a β-like element. The combination of ζ- and γ-globin chains forms hemoglobin Portland. These early hemoglobins are made primarily in yolk-sac erythroblasts and are detectable only during the very earliest stages of embryogenesis except in certain pathologic states, in which they may persist until gestation is complete. The major hemoglobin of intrauterine life is HbF, which consists of two α- and two γ-globin chains. Expression of the γ-globin gene begins early in embryogenesis, peaks during midgestation, and begins a rapid decline just before birth. By 6 months of age in normal infants, only a remnant of prior γ-globin gene expression remains. The level of HbF in the blood declines rapidly thereafter to less than 1% of the total. Expression of the α-globin gene starts early in the first trimester, peaks quickly, and is sustained for life. Expression of the β-globin gene also commences early in gestation and reaches its zenith within a few months after birth. The combination of α-globin with β-globin chains forms hemoglobin A (HbA), the predominant hemoglobin of postnatal life. Adult cells also contain HbA2. The δ-globin gene, which directs synthesis of the non–α-globin chain of HbA2, is very inefficiently expressed. Only low levels of HbA2 are present; defects in the δ-globin gene are of no clinical consequence. In adult blood, HbF is not evenly distributed among erythrocytes and is present in only a very small number of RBCs, called F cells. HbA2 is present in all RBCs, albeit at levels less than 3.5% of the total hemoglobin in adult life.

Hemoglobin Biosynthesis and Its Regulation

Throughout development, genes coding for α-globin, non–α-globin, and heme exhibit coordinated expression. Almost equal amounts of each of the moieties that ultimately constitute the hemoglobin tetramer are made. Excess unpaired globin chains and mutant globins are removed from the cell by ATP-dependent proteases, ensuring a balance between accumulation of α- and non–α-globin chains. Balanced chain synthesis and coordination of globin chain production with synthesis of heme are important because hemoglobin tetramers are highly soluble, but the components of hemoglobin (i.e., unpaired chains, protoporphyrin, and iron) are not. Precipitation of any of these is deleterious to cell survival. Erythroblast proteases are not efficient enough to eliminate the substantial excesses of unpaired chains that accumulate when an α- or non–α-gene is selectively impaired by severe thalassemia mutations. The mechanisms regulating heme production and some of the interactions between heme and globin synthesis are discussed in Chapter 36.

The proper production of the individual globin chains within erythroid tissues at the appropriate states of differentiation and development is predominantly ensured by regulation at the level of transcription. The onset of phenotypic maturation at the proerythroblast stage is marked by the onset of globin mRNA biosynthesis in dramatically increasing quantities. Expression of α- and non–α-globin genes begins at essentially the same time, although some studies suggest a slightly earlier onset for α-globin gene expression. Transcription persists at a high level throughout most of the remainder of erythropoiesis, declines as the nucleus condenses, and is eventually lost in late erythroblasts. Even as the absolute rates of globin gene transcription begin to decrease, however, the relative percentage of total transcriptional activity devoted to globin gene expression continues to increase; this reflects the silencing of transcription of almost every other gene in the erythroblast.

The transcriptional activation of the globin genes is the major event that must be understood to define and manipulate the regulation of hemoglobin biosynthesis and hemoglobin switching. However, posttranscriptional mechanisms contribute to the final distribution of globin and nonglobin mRNAs and to the balance of α- and non–α-globins within the erythroblasts. When compared with many other mRNAs, such as cytokine mRNAs, globin mRNAs are extraordinarily stable. Their half-lives have been estimated at 30 to 50 hours. Most other mRNAs have turnover rates, or half-lives, measured within the range of a few minutes to 5 or 6 hours. The increase in the percentage of total mRNA that is globin mRNA is greatly accentuated because the newly transcribed globin mRNAs accumulate and remain quite stable in the cell, but nonglobin mRNAs, which are no longer being produced, are also disappearing at a faster rate. Consequently, the mRNA content of the reticulocytes consists of 90% to 95% globin mRNA.

The transcription rates of the α- and non–α-globin genes are not precisely equal. (This phenomenon has been studied in detail only in adult erythroid cells expressing the α- and β-globin genes.) A slight, but reproducibly detectable, excess of α-globin mRNA is present in erythroblasts. However, β-globin mRNA is translated somewhat more efficiently than α-globin mRNA. These counterbalancing forces result in almost equal syntheses of α- and β-globin polypeptide chains. There is a very slight excess of α-globin production, resulting in a small pool of free α-globin chains.

Alpha hemoglobin-stabilizing protein (AHSP), a small protein present at high concentrations in RBCs, binds specifically to the α-globin polypeptide, protecting the unstable free α-globin chain by inhibiting heme loss and oxidant-mediated chain precipitation. It remains unclear whether mutations of this protein can modify the phenotype of β-thalassemia by increasing the imbalance in globin chain synthesis. Some α-globin chain variants, because the mutations alter AHSP binding, are associated with mild thalassemia-like features.

Newly synthesized β-globin chains are rapidly and completely incorporated into αβ dimers that spontaneously associate as tetramers. Hemoglobin tetramers are remarkably stable throughout the lifespan of the circulating RBC by virtue of their long half-lives. Only small amounts sustain oxidative or proteolytic damage.

Hemoglobin molecules are exposed for prolonged periods to chemically active compounds in the milieu of the bloodstream. They often become nonenzymatically modified by such processes as glycosylation, acetylation, and sulfation. Glycosylation occurs more extensively during periods of hyperglycemia and leads to elevated levels of the glycosylated form of HbA, HbA_{1c}. This phenomenon is the basis of a useful test for control of the blood sugar in diabetes. Other posttranslational modifications are of little clinical importance except as already noted for 2,3-BPG, carbon dioxide (CO_2), and NO.

Transcriptional Regulation of Globin Gene Expression

Precise regulation of the globin gene clusters involves a complex interplay between trans-acting proteins, such as transcription factors, and cis-acting sequences that act as promoters, enhancers, and silencers of gene activity. DNA-binding proteins interact with sequences in regulatory regions of the globin gene cluster and with other proteins through specific protein–protein interactions, forming DNA—protein complexes that regulate gene transcription. Trans-acting factors mediate the remodeling of chromatin structure, influencing gene expression for the entire globin gene clusters. Mutations in the cis-acting sequences or trans-acting proteins cause dysregulated expression of globin genes, resulting in thalassemia-like syndromes. Elucidating the full extent of sequences required for appropriate expression of globin genes will inform the development of constructs for gene therapy.

The nuclei of erythroid cells contain numerous proteins that have been identified as transcription factors, including GATA1, NFE2, and EKLF. GATA1 is named on the basis of the DNA sequence motif (T/A) GATA (A/G), the GATA motif that it recognizes and binds. It is a zinc finger class DNA-binding protein (see Chapter 24). Activity of GATA1 requires binding to a zinc finger protein cofactor called FOG1 (named for Friend of GATA1). NFE2 recognizes the DNA sequence motif (T/C) GCT GA (C/G) TCA (T/C). It is a member of the B-zip class of transcriptional activators. GATA1 and NFE2 were originally identified and cloned on the basis of their interactions with their cognate sequences in the globin genes. Erythroid Kruppel-like factor (EKLF, also called KLF1) may be the most specific of the erythroid transcription factors yet discovered. EKLF interacts specifically with the β-globin gene promoter and may influence the γ-β switch. Mice homozygous for disruption of the EKLF gene have lethal β-thalassemia. Alone, GATA1, NFE2, EKLF, and FOG1 cannot be the sole determination of tissue specificity of the globin genes. Together, they form a robust transcriptional network that regulates erythroid genes, including the globin genes. Mutations in GATA1 or FOG1 can cause β-thalassemia and thrombocytopenia in patients.

The regions of the globin gene clusters with essential regulatory sequences and erythroid-specific chromatin remodeling extend far beyond the coding sequences of the globin genes. The key regulatory element for the α-globin gene (HS –40) lies in an erythroid-specific DNase I hypersensitive site 40 kb from the α-globin gene. The LCR is critical for high level expression of the β-globin gene cluster, consisting of five sites that are hypersensitive to DNase I (HS 1-5) (see Chapter 1). Patients with deletion of the HS –40 site exhibit α-thalassemia, and patients with deletions of the β-globin LCR develop β-thalassemia; however, the thalassemia can be a result of changes in chromatin caused by the large deletion. Similarly, transgenic mice bearing deletions of these critical regulatory regions have severely restricted expressions of the respective globin genes.

The LCRs contain binding sites for the major erythroid transcription factors, including GATA1, EKLF, and NFE2, as well as sites for transcription factors found more widely distributed in many cell types. The LCRs loop to interact directly with the promoters of individual globin genes, resulting in a complex termed the *active chromatin hub*. The resulting structure enables high level expression of globin genes in erythroid cells at the appropriate developmental stages. Additional elements act as insulators, protecting expressed genes from gene silencing through the regulation of chromatin structure.

BCL11a is a transcriptional repressor that decreases fetal hemoglobin expression in adult tissues. Polymorphisms in the BCL11a gene are powerfully associated with HbF levels, including in patients with sickle cell disease. Inhibition of BCL11a increases HbF levels and attenuates the phenotype of sickle cell disease in a murine model and is therefore an attractive therapeutic strategy for the treatment of sickle cell disease.

Transcription factors recruit enzymes that remodel chromatin structure. "Open" chromatin, or euchromatin, generally appears cytogenetically uncondensed and is associated with hyperacetylated histones, unmethylated CpG dinucleotides, and active transcription. ATRX is a protein that has been implicated in the modulation of chromatin structure at the α-globin locus. Mutations in the *ATRX* gene, located on the X chromosome, cause a syndrome of α-thalassemia, severe mental retardation, facial dysmorphism, and urogenital abnormalities. ATRX, a member of the SNF2 family of helicase/ATPases, localizes to pericentromeric heterochromatin during interphase and mitosis and contains a plant homeodomain (PHD)-like domain that is found in chromatin-associated proteins. Cells with a mutated *ATRX* gene have altered patterns of DNA methylation. The ATRX protein therefore exemplifies the connections among DNA methylation, chromatin remodeling, and expression of the α-globin genes.

Chromatin structure can be manipulated pharmacologically through the influence of drugs on methylation and histone acetylation. Cytidine analogs such as 5-azacytidine and its less toxic derivative, decitabine, inactivate DNA methyltransferases, inducing γ-globin gene expression and increasing HbF levels in patients with sickle cell anemia. Histone deacetylase inhibitors are being studied as agents to increase γ-globin expression.

Posttranscriptional, Translational, and Posttranslational Mechanisms

Processed globin mRNA is exported from the nucleus to the cytoplasm by a mechanism that is not clearly defined. mRNA translation occurs in the cytoplasm (see Fig. 31-7). The triplet codons or mRNA are recognized by the anticodons of specific tRNAs that bring activated amino acid residues to the nascent polypeptide chains. The process of translation, in which an mRNA template directs the synthesis of protein, is typically divided into three phases: initiation, elongation, and termination (see Chapter 1). Each phase is regulated by a variety of protein factors.

The globin mRNA molecule becomes associated with four to six ribosomes, forming the polyribosome. At least 11 eukaryotic translation initiation factors interact with the polyribosome. They mediate stabilization of a preinitiation complex, binding of the initiator methionine tRNA to ribosomal subunits, binding of mRNA to the preinitiation complex, stabilization of mRNA binding, recognition of the cap site at the 5′ end of mRNA, and release of initiation factors from the preinitiation complex. Several elongation and termination factors have also been defined. Initiation or an early step in the elongation process is the rate-limiting factor.

The first posttranslational step in tetramer formation is the combination of α- and non–α-globin chains to form dimers, an event that appears to depend on the relative charge of each globin subunit. The dimers then form tetrameric hemoglobin. Because of charge differences among non–α-globin chains, there is a hierarchy or affinity of these chains for α-globin chains. The combination of α- and β-globin chains is most favored followed by a combination of α-, γ-, and δ-globin chains. Certain mutant hemoglobins that have gained or lost a charge may alter this hierarchic arrangement. This may influence the proportion of variant hemoglobin present, especially when the patient also inherits an α-thalassemia syndrome, in which the synthesis of α-globin chains is reduced. The supply of available α-globin chains is then limited, and non–α-globin chains compete with one another to form tetramers with the limiting α-globin chain pool.

Globin chain biosynthesis and heme synthesis are mutually important. Heme plays a role in the regulation of the initiation complex. A deficiency of heme (e.g., in iron deficiency) is associated with the accumulation of a repressor of translation initiation factors. Translation of β-globin mRNA appears to be initiated more efficiently than α-globin mRNA, conferring on the associated anemia some of the features of mild α-thalassemia. This phenomenon occurs because heme deficiency depresses the availability of initiating factors for which the less efficient α-mRNA must compete with the more efficient β-mRNA.

The identification of genetic mutations that cause congenital and acquired forms of anemia provide further insight into the pathways required for the coordinated production of globin and heme. More than half of patients with Diamond-Blackfan anemia, a disorder characterized by a severe macrocytic anemia and a paucity of erythroid progenitor cells, have heterozygous germline mutations in the *RPS19* gene or other genes encoding ribosomal proteins. Similarly, the macrocytic anemia in patients with myelodysplastic syndrome and a deletion of chromosome 5q is caused by heterozygous deletion of another ribosomal protein gene, *RPS14*. Haploinsufficiency for these ribosomal protein genes activates the p53 pathway, leading to cell cycle arrest and apoptosis selectively in the erythroid progenitor cells.

Table 31-1 Classification of Hemoglobinopathies and Thalassemias

Structural hemoglobinopathies—mutations altering the amino acid sequence of a globin chain and altering physical or chemical properties of the hemoglobin tetramer in such a way that function is deranged
Abnormal Hemoglobin (Hb) Polymerization—Sickle Cell Hemoglobin (HbS); Hemolysis, Vasoocclusion
Abnormal hemoglobin crystallization (e.g., HbC)
High oxygen affinity—polycythemia (Hb Zurich)
Low oxygen affinity—cyanosis (Hb Kansas)
Hemoglobins that oxidize or precipitate too readily—unstable hemoglobins (Hb Köln)
M hemoglobins—methemoglobinemia, cyanosis (e.g., Hb Milwaukee)
Thalassemia—Defective Production of Globin Chains With Hypochromia, Anemia, Hemolysis, Altered Erythropoiesis
α-Thalassemia
β-Thalassemia
δβ-Thalassemias, γδβ-thalassemias, αβ-thalassemias
"Thalassemic" Hemoglobinopathies and Dominantly Inherited Thalassemias—Mutations Altering the Synthesis and Structure or Function of the Hemoglobin Gene Products (e.g., HbE, Hb Terre Haute, Hb Lepore, Hb Constant Spring)
Hereditary persistence of fetal hemoglobin—persistence of high levels of fetal hemoglobin (HbF) into adult life
Pancellular—high HbF levels in all RBCs
Nondeletion forms
Deletion forms
Hb Kenya
Heterocellular—inherited increases in the percentage of F cells
Acquired hemoglobinopathies
Methemoglobinemia Caused by Toxic Exposures
Sulfhemoglobinemia caused by toxic exposures
Carboxyhemoglobinemia caused by toxic exposures
HbH in erythroleukemias
Acquired elevations in F cells and HbF
Erythroid stress (e.g., recovery from BM suppression)
BM dysplasias
Exposure to agents altering stem cells or gene expression (e.g., hydroxyurea, butyric acid)

BM, Bone marrow; *Hb*, hemoglobin; *RBC*, red blood cell.

Refractory anemia with ring sideroblasts (RARS) is a subtype of myelodysplastic syndrome characterized by iron-loaded mitochondria evident on Prussian blue staining. In the majority of RARS cases, somatic mutations are present in the *SF3B1* gene, encoding a core member of the RNA splicing machinery. The precise targets of SF3B1 have not been identified.

NOSOLOGY OF HEMOGLOBINOPATHIES

Inherited abnormalities of the hemoglobin molecules that cause morbidity are called hemoglobinopathies and thalassemias. Many of these conditions produce diseases (e.g., sickle cell anemia, thalassemia, unstable hemoglobins, M hemoglobins) that are especially important to hematologists. A few acquired conditions lead to modifications of hemoglobin (e.g., carbon monoxide exposure, producing carboxyhemoglobinemia, nitrite exposure causing methemoglobinemia) that produce clinical abnormalities. These situations are summarized by the term acquired hemoglobinopathies or dyshemoglobinemias.

Most of the more than 1200 mutations of the globin gene that have been described produce no disease or only trivial clinical effects. The remainder can be classified according to the hematologic and clinical phenotypes that cause reduced solubility with hemolytic anemia (unstable hemoglobins and polymerizing hemoglobins, such as sickle hemoglobin); hemoglobins with altered oxygen affinity; hemoglobins predisposing to methemoglobin formation; and the thalassemias involving abnormal synthesis of one or more globin chains with anemia, hemolysis, and alterations of erythropoiesis. Some mutations, such as that responsible for HbE, can alter the structure and synthesis of the molecule. A classification of hemoglobinopathies and thalassemias is provided in Table 31-1. Individual conditions are discussed in the chapters already cross-referenced in earlier sections of this chapter.

SUGGESTED READINGS

Bank A: Regulation of human fetal hemoglobin: New players, new complexities. *Blood* 107:435, 2006.

Boas FE, Forman L, Beutler E: Phosphatidylserine exposure and red cell viability in red cell aging and in hemolytic anemia. *Proc Natl Acad Sci U S A* 95:3077, 1998.

Burgess-Beusse B, Farrell C, Gaszner M, et al: The insulation of genes from external enhancers and silencing chromatin. *Proc Natl Acad Sci U S A* 99:16433, 2002.

Cantor AB, Orkin SH: Transcriptional regulation of erythropoiesis: An affair involving multiple partners. *Oncogene* 21:3368, 2002.

Chakalova L, Carter D, Debrand E, et al: Developmental regulation of the beta-globin gene locus. *Prog Mol Subcell Biol* 38:183, 2005.

Chiu CH, Schneider H, Slightom JL, et al: Dynamics of regulatory evolution in primate β-globin gene clusters: *cis*-Mediated acquisition of simian gamma fetal expression patterns. *Gene* 205:47, 1997.

Dzierzak E: The emergence of definitive hematopoietic stem cells in the mammal. *Curr Opin Hematol* 12:197, 2005.

Feng L, Zhou S, Gu L, et al: Structure of oxidized alpha-haemoglobin bound to AHSP reveals a protective mechanism for haem. *Nature* 435:697, 2005.

Gibbons RJ, Picketts DJ, Villard L, et al: Mutations in a putative global transcriptional regulator cause X-linked mental retardation with α-thalassemia (ATR-X syndrome). *Cell* 80:837, 1995.

Gladwin MT, Wang X, Reiter CD, et al: *S*-nitrosohemoglobin is unstable in the reductive erythrocyte environment and lacks O_2/NO-linked allosteric function. *J Biol Chem* 277:27818, 2002.

Gow AJ, Stamler JS: Reactions between nitric oxide and haemoglobin under physiological conditions. *Nature* 391:169, 1998.

Hardison R, Riemer C, Chui DH, et al: Electronic access to sequence alignments, experimental results, and human mutations as an aid to studying globin gene regulation. *Genomics* 47:429, 1998.

Higgs DR, Garrick D, Anguita E, et al: Understanding alpha-globin gene regulation: Aiming to improve the management of thalassemia. *Ann N Y Acad Sci* 1054:92, 2005.

Jenuwein T, Allis CD: Translating the histone code. *Science* 293:1074, 2001.

Kato GJ, McGowan V, Machado RF et al: Lactate dehydrogenase as a biomarker of hemolysis-associated nitric oxide resistance, priapism, leg ulceration, pulmonary hypertension, and death in patients with sickle cell disease. *Blood* 107:2279, 2006.

Kihm AJ, Kong Y, Hong W, et al: An abundant erythroid protein that stabilizes free alpha-haemoglobin. *Nature* 417:758, 2002.

Li Q, Peterson KR, Fang X, et al: Locus control regions. *Blood* 100:3077, 2002.

Miller IJ, Bieker JJ: A novel erythroid cell-specific murine transcription factor that binds to the CACCC element and is related to the Kruppel family of nuclear proteins. *Mol Cell Biol* 13:2776, 1993.

Rother RP, Bell L, Hillmen P, et al: The clinical sequelae of intravascular hemolysis and extracellular plasma hemoglobin: A novel mechanism of human disease. *JAMA* 293:1653, 2005.

Stamatoyannopoulos G: Control of globin gene expression during development and erythroid differentiation. *Exp Hematol* 33:259, 2005.

Stamler JS, Jia L, Eu JP, et al: Blood flow regulation by *S*-nitrosohemoglobin in the physiological oxygen gradient. *Science* 276:2034, 1997.

Steinberg MH, Forget BG, Higgs DR, et al: *Disorders of hemoglobin: Genetics, pathophysiology, and clinical management*, Cambridge, 2001, Cambridge University Press.

Viprakasit V, Tanphaichitr VS, Chinchang W, et al: Evaluation of alpha hemoglobin stabilizing protein (AHSP) as a genetic modifier in patients with beta thalassemia. *Blood* 103:3296, 2004.

Walsh M, Lutz RJ, Cotter TG, et al: Erythrocyte survival is promoted by plasma and suppressed by a Bak-derived BH3 peptide that interacts with membrane-associated Bcl-X(L). *Blood* 99:3439, 2002.

Weatherall DJ, Clegg JB: *The thalassaemia syndromes*, ed 4, Oxford, 2001, Blackwell Science Limited, p 818.

Weiss MJ, Zhou S, Feng L et al: Role of alpha-hemoglobin-stabilizing protein in normal erythropoiesis and beta-thalassemia. *Ann N Y Acad Sci* 1054:103, 2005.

CHAPTER 32

APPROACH TO ANEMIA IN THE ADULT AND CHILD

Peter W. Marks

Anemia is one of the most commonly encountered problems in hematology. Although a few entities are responsible for the majority of cases, there are numerous less common causes of anemia in adults and children. A systematic diagnostic approach to the evaluation of anemia, extracting the maximum amount of information available from the complete blood count, reticulocyte count, and peripheral blood smear, can often rapidly point to the appropriate diagnosis and reduce or eliminate the need for additional diagnostic testing.

OVERVIEW OF ERYTHROPOIESIS

Accurate diagnosis of anemia is facilitated by an understanding of red blood cell (RBC) production. Erythropoiesis is the regulated process leading to the production of mature erythrocytes. Stem cells in the bone marrow (BM) are stimulated by the hormone erythropoietin and other factors to proliferate and differentiate along a pathway of recognizable precursors that ultimately leads to extrusion of the nucleus from cells containing a high concentration of hemoglobin and some residual RNA (Fig. 32-1).[1] These cells that are identified as reticulocytes by staining of the residual RNA become mature erythrocytes as the RNA is degraded, which under normal conditions happens in a day. The RBCs then circulate for 100 to 120 days before being removed from the circulation by macrophages in the spleen and other cells of the reticuloendothelial system.[2] At steady state under physiologic conditions, the production and destruction of erythrocytes is equivalent. This process is driven in large part by the hormone erythropoietin, which is produced in a regulated fashion by periglomerular cells in the kidney (≈90%) and constitutively by the liver (≈10%).[3] Because preservation of oxygen delivery to tissues is so important, the oxygen-sensing regulatory proteins located in the kidney respond to decreased oxygen tension from any cause such as blood loss, high altitude, or cardiac shunts with the production of erythropoietin (Fig. 32-2). This hormone then travels through the bloodstream and stimulates RBC production in the BM. Provided that there are adequate nutrients, including folate, vitamin B_{12}, and iron, the precursors in the BM proliferate and mature and are released into the circulation, ultimately expanding the pool of erythrocytes.[4] The increase in oxygen delivery to the kidney then reduces the stimulus for erythropoietin production.

DEFINITION OF ANEMIA

Anemia is defined as a reduction in the RBC mass. Because of a variety of factors, the RBC mass normally changes during the lifespan of an individual and may be different in males and females.[5] Understanding the changes that occur is critical to appropriately identifying what constitutes anemia (Table 32-1). The relatively elevated level of hemoglobin present at birth declines over the first 1 to 2 months of life to levels that are lower than those seen in adulthood. In later childhood, the hemoglobin values are similar and increase modestly over time. Around puberty, girls have reached adult levels of hemoglobin, and androgenic steroids lead to a continued increase in hemoglobin in boys through about age 18 years. This approximately 1.5 g/dL difference between males and females persists through much of adult life until about age 70 years, when the hemoglobin value in men begins to decline. Over the next 2 decades, the hemoglobin value declines by about 1 g/dL in men while decreasing by only approximately 0.2 g/dL in women.[6] Thus, at age 90 years, there is only a modest difference between the mean hemoglobin values observed in men and women (14.1 vs. 13.8 g/dL).

MECHANISMS OF ANEMIA

Although a complete review of all of the mechanisms leading to anemia is beyond the scope of this chapter, an appreciation of some of the mechanisms is useful before approaching the diagnosis of anemia in adults and children. Three broad categories of anemia are blood loss anemia, hypoproliferative anemia, and hemolytic anemia. Blood loss may occur acutely or chronically. When blood is lost acutely through hemorrhage, it may take several hours before a decline in hemoglobin concentration is observed because of the time required for restoration of the plasma volume and equilibration. Several days may elapse before an appropriate reticulocytosis is noted. Chronic blood loss ultimately leads to hypoproliferative anemia because of iron deficiency.

Hypoproliferative Anemia

When used broadly, the term *hypoproliferative anemia* refers to entities that manifest as an inability to produce an adequate number of erythrocytes in response to appropriate signals. Although there are many different causes, the hallmark of hypoproliferative anemia is a low reticulocyte count (Table 32-2). The etiology underlying this class of disorders may relate to the hypoproliferation of precursors within the BM, such as may be seen when there is BM replacement (myelophthisis), or to abnormal maturation of precursors in the BM, such as that which occurs in megaloblastic anemia (folate deficiency, vitamin B_{12} deficiency, myelodysplastic syndromes [MDS], and others). In the latter case of megaloblastic anemia, the BM often is packed. However, intramedullary demise of precursors prevents the formation and release of mature RBCs.

By far, the most common cause of hypoproliferative anemia globally is iron deficiency.[7] It is estimated that about 2% of infants and children may become iron deficient purely because of inadequate dietary intake and that 4% of women ages 20 to 49 years of age in the United States have iron-deficiency anemia primarily because of inadequate dietary intake in the setting of menstruation and childbirth. Iron deficiency is also commonly encountered in older individuals as well (≈2% of individuals older than age 50 years), and it should provoke a thorough search for its etiology, which in both men and nonmenstruating women frequently is gastrointestinal blood loss. After iron deficiency, acute or chronic inflammation and renal disease are common etiologies of anemia.[8,9] BM failure states and BM replacement caused by hematologic malignancies or solid tumors are less common causes of anemia and are often accompanied by other hematologic manifestations, such as leukopenia and thrombocytopenia.

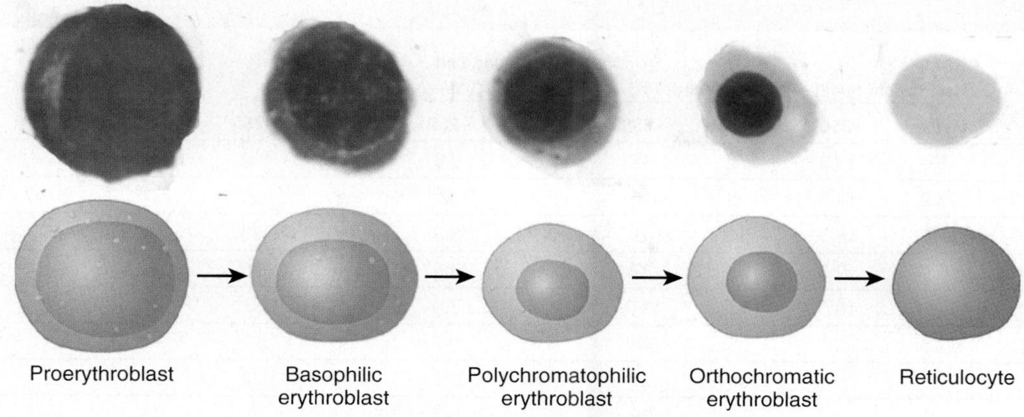

Figure 32-1 OVERVIEW OF ERYTHROPOIESIS.

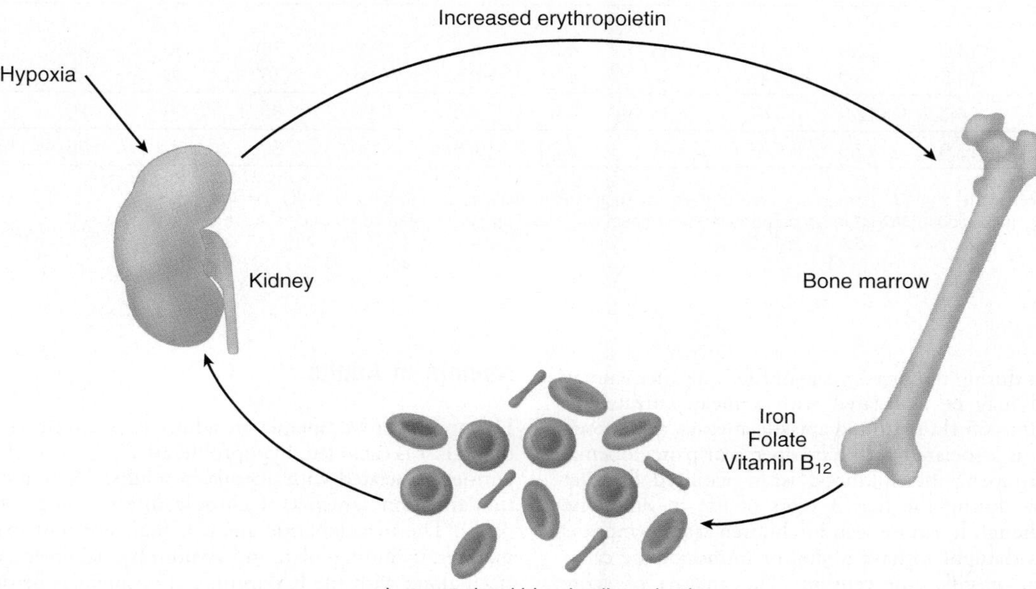

Figure 32-2 REGULATION OF ERYTHROPOIESIS.

Hemolytic Anemia

The causes of hemolytic anemia are quite varied and may be congenital or acquired.[10] The hallmark of hemolytic anemia is an elevated reticulocyte count (see Table 32-2). Other features commonly associated with hemolytic anemia include an elevated lactate dehydrogenase (LDH) level, increased unconjugated (indirect) bilirubin level, and decreased haptoglobin level. Hemolytic anemia also may manifest with distinctive changes on the peripheral blood smear. Congenital causes include the hemoglobinopathies, enzymopathies (predominantly glucose-6-phosphate dehydrogenase [G6PD] deficiency), and membrane disorders.[11] Acquired conditions include autoimmune hemolytic anemia, microangiopathic hemolytic anemia, hemolysis related to infections, and acquired membrane disorders such as those caused by liver disease (spur cell of anemia) and paroxysmal nocturnal hemoglobinuria.[12]

COMPARISON OF ETIOLOGIES OF ANEMIA IN ADULTS AND CHILDREN

As already noted, the designation that anemia is present relies on comparison of the patient's hemoglobin or hematocrit with an age- and sex-appropriate normal range (see Table 32-1). Although many types of anemia may occur across the age spectrum, certain types tend to be identified more commonly in either adults or children, and some are primarily identified in neonates. In children, the most common causes of anemia are related to nutritional deficiency or to a primary hematologic process, either hereditary or acquired. In contrast, in adults, the most common causes of anemia are iron deficiency caused by blood loss or anemia caused by systemic illness or malignancy (Table 32-3).

Anemia in Children

Hypoproliferative anemia in children may be associated with either acquired or congenital etiologies. Acquired cases are most commonly caused by nutritional deficiency but also include those caused by acquired aplastic anemia, transient erythroblastopenia of childhood, the anemia of acute inflammation, and marrow replacement caused by malignancy.[13] Congenital causes include Diamond-Blackfan anemia and other rare syndromes, including refractory sideroblastic anemia and the congenital dyserythropoietic anemias.[14] Iron deficiency may occur in children because of a diet that is rich in cow's milk to the exclusion of other iron-containing foods. This is

Table 32-1 Normal Red Blood Cell Values

Age	Hemoglobin (g/dL)		Hematocrit (%)		Red Blood Cell Count (10^{12}/L)		MCV (fL)		MCH (pg)		MCHC (g/dL)	
	Mean	−2SD	Mean	−2SD	Mean	−2SD	Mean	−2SD	Mean	−2SD	Mean	−2SD
Birth (cord blood)	16.5	13.5	51	42	4.7	3.9	108	98	34	31	33	30
1–3 days (capillary)	18.5	14.5	56	45	5.2	4.0	108	95	34	31	33	29
1 week	17.5	13.5	54	42	3.1	3.9	107	88	34	28	33	28
2 weeks	16.5	12.5	51	39	4.9	3.6	105	86	34	28	33	28
1 month	14.0	10.0	43	31	4.2	3.0	104	85	34	28	33	29
2 months	11.5	9.0	35	28	3.8	2.7	96	77	30	26	33	29
3-6 months	11.5	9.5	35	29	3.8	3.1	91	74	30	25	33	30
0.5-2 years	12.0	11.0	36	33	4.5	3.7	78	70	27	23	33	30
2-6 years	12.5	11.5	37	34	4.6	3.9	81	75	27	24	34	31
6-12 years	13.5	11.5	40	35	4.6	4.0	86	77	29	25	34	31
12-18 years												
Female	14.0	12.0	41	36	4.6	4.1	90	78	30	25	34	31
Male 18-49 years	14.5	13.0	43	37	4.9	4.5	88	78	30	25	34	31
Female	14.0	12.0	41	36	4.6	4.0	90	80	30	26	34	31
Male	15.5	13.5	47	41	5.2	4.5	90	80	30	26	34	31

From Oski FA: Pallor. In Kaye R, Oski FA, Barness LA, editors: Core Textbook of Pediatrics, ed 3, Philadelphia, 1989, Lippincott, p 62.
MCH, Mean corpuscular hemoglobin; *MCHC,* mean corpuscular hemoglobin concentration; *MCV,* mean corpuscular volume.

particularly common during the first 2 years of life. The anemia may be quite severe and may be associated with a mean corpuscular volume (MCV) of 50 to 65 fL. Acquired aplastic anemia, as opposed to pure RBC aplasia, is associated with bicytopenia or pancytopenia. Transient erythroblastopenia of childhood is an acquired disorder that generally occurs during the first 3 years of life in otherwise healthy children, although it can be seen in children from 6 months to 10 years old. It is thought to have a viral or immunologic cause and resolves without specific intervention. The anemia of acute inflammation may be encountered in children who are hospitalized and is generally transient, resolving when the underlying condition has improved. Leukemia may result in BM replacement and is usually associated with abnormalities in other cell lineages in addition to RBCs.

Hemolytic anemia in children is most commonly associated with inherited disorders of hemoglobin or the RBC membrane.[15] However, acquired causes such as autoimmune hemolytic anemia and microangiopathic hemolytic anemia, particularly *Shiga* toxin–associated hemolytic uremic syndrome (HUS), also occur.[16] In older children, many etiologies of hemolytic anemia overlap with those considered in adults, and a similar diagnostic algorithm may be appropriate. However, in newborns, inherited causes of hemolytic anemia must be distinguished from more pronounced cases of the physiologic hyperbilirubinemia that occurs. After true hemolysis has been identified in an infant, the differential diagnosis is relatively limited (Fig. 32-3). Immune-mediated hemolysis may result from ABO, Rh, or minor blood group incompatibility.[17] Other causes include metabolic disorders and disorders of the RBC membrane. Of note, however, is the fact that hemoglobinopathies, such as sickle cell disease and β-thalassemia, are silent during the newborn period and only become manifest at 4 to 6 months of age when the fetal-to-adult hemoglobin transition has been completed. Newborn screening programs in the United States may provide salient information in this regard on the presence or absence of a hemoglobinopathy. Alternatively, ethnic background and family history may be helpful in arriving at the appropriate diagnosis.

Anemia in Adults

Hypoproliferative anemia in adults is relatively common. If acute blood loss is excluded, hypoproliferative causes are the most common entities associated with anemia in adults. These are iron deficiency, inflammation (anemia of chronic disease), and renal disease (Fig. 32-4). The megaloblastic anemias that represent maturation abnormalities, including folate and vitamin B_{12} deficiency, are often categorized along with the hypoproliferative anemias because they present with a low reticulocyte count as well. Drugs and toxins such as ethanol can also be associated with hypoproliferative anemia. Pure RBC aplasia may be associated with other diseases (thymoma) or viral infection (parvovirus B19) or be idiopathic.[18] Finally, MDS may present with hypoproliferative anemia, as may an infiltrative process such as myelofibrosis or acute leukemia. The distinction between the various causes of anemia is facilitated by historical factors, physical findings, and concomitant laboratory abnormalities in conjunction with review of the MCV and RBC distribution width (RDW) along with the peripheral blood smear. In the setting of a low reticulocyte count, MCV values below 70 fL are most commonly associated with iron-deficiency anemia, and those above 120 fL are most commonly associated with folate or vitamin B_{12} deficiency. The differential diagnosis broadens for MCV values that fall just outside of the normal range. For example, in the setting of a low reticulocyte count, MCV values in the range from 75 to 80 fL may be associated with iron-deficiency anemia, the anemia of inflammation, and endocrine causes of anemia. MCV values between 100 and 110 fL may be associated with folate or vitamin B_{12} deficiency, aplastic anemia, MDS, liver disease, and immune hemolytic anemias.

Hemolytic anemia in adults is less common than hypoproliferative anemia, and the differential diagnosis is broad. Congenital causes associated with mild to moderate hemolysis may be clinically silent until detected later in life.[19] This is particularly the case for milder cases of β-thalassemia intermedia, sickle cell-SC disease and sickle-β^+-thalassemia, and hereditary spherocytosis. Additionally, the most common RBC enzymopathy (which is also the one of the most

Table 32-2 Usefulness of the Reticulocyte Count in the Diagnosis of Anemia*

Diagnosis	Value
Hypoproliferative Anemias	**Absolute Reticulocyte Count <75,000/μL**
Anemia of chronic disease	
Anemia of renal disease	
Congenital dyserythropoietic anemias	
Effects of drugs or toxins	
Endocrine anemias	
Iron deficiency	
BM replacement	
Maturation Abnormalities	**Absolute Reticulocyte Count <75,000/μL**
Vitamin B_{12} deficiency	
Folate deficiency	
Sideroblastic anemia	
Appropriate Response to Blood Loss or Nutritional Supplementation	**Absolute Reticulocyte Count ≥100,000/μL**
Hemolytic Anemias	**Absolute Reticulocyte Count ≥100,000/μL**
Hemoglobinopathies	
Immune hemolytic anemias	
Infectious causes of hemolysis	
Membrane abnormalities	
Metabolic abnormalities	
Mechanical hemolysis	

BM, Bone marrow.
*Note that reticulocyte counts in the range of 75,000 to 100,000/μL can sometimes be associated with appropriate response to blood loss or hemolytic anemia.

Table 32-3 Comparison of the More Common Causes of Anemia in Children and Adult

Type of Anemia	Children	Adults
Hypoproliferative	• Nutritional deficiency (most commonly iron deficiency) • Acute inflammation • Transient erythroblastopenia of childhood • Acquired aplastic anemia • Marrow replacement caused by malignancy	• Iron deficiency • Anemia of inflammation (anemia of chronic disease) • Anemia of renal disease • Folate or vitamin B_{12} deficiency • Drugs or toxins • Pure RBC aplasia (viral or idiopathic) • MDS
Hemolytic	• Inherited hemoglobinopathies • Inherited membrane disorders • Autoimmune hemolytic anemia • Microangiopathic hemolytic anemia	• Inherited hemoglobinopathies with milder manifestations • Inherited membrane disorders with milder manifestations • G6PD deficiency • Autoimmune hemolytic anemia • Microangiopathic hemolytic anemia (DIC, TTP, HUS)

DIC, Disseminated intravascular coagulation; *G6PD,* glucose-6-phosphate dehydrogenase; *HUS,* hemolytic uremic syndrome; *MDS,* myelodysplastic syndrome; *RBC,* red blood cell; *TTP,* thrombotic thrombocytopenic purpura.

common human enzyme defect deficiencies), G6PD deficiency, does not present until individuals encounter oxidant stress either because of infection or drugs such as sulfonamides and antimalarials.[20] Acquired hemolytic anemias include autoimmune hemolytic anemia, which is often associated with hematologic malignancies or rheumatologic disorders, and the microangiopathic hemolytic anemias, including disseminated intravascular coagulation (DIC), thrombotic thrombocytopenic purpura (TTP), and HUS.[21] Distinction of the various causes of hemolytic anemia is also facilitated by the associated historical features, physical findings, and laboratory abnormalities of the clinical presentation. For these disorders, review of the peripheral blood smear may be particularly revealing as to the etiology.

SYSTEMATIC APPROACH TO ANEMIA

The correct diagnosis of anemia can often be determined by combining a thorough history and physical examination with review of the complete blood count, concentrating particularly on the MCV and RDW, along with review of the reticulocyte count and the peripheral blood smear.

History and Physical Examination

Because anemia can be a primary disorder or secondary to other systemic processes, a careful history and physical examination provide valuable insight into the potential cause. Fatigue often accompanies anemia, but it is very nonspecific and may be related to systemic illness. Nonetheless, determining the concomitant presence of a systemic inflammatory disorder, infection, or malignancy that may be associated with fatigue can be critical in determining the underlying causes of anemia in both adults and children. The medical history may also be quite informative. For example, a history of diabetes mellitus can be associated with significantly impaired renal production of erythropoietin even in the setting of only a mildly elevated creatinine level. Because certain medications may be associated with BM depression or, alternatively, the development of autoimmune hemolytic anemia, all pharmacologic agents, prescribed and over the counter, including alternative medicines, should be reviewed. Occupational history is occasionally relevant, as in the case of individuals, such as welders, who might have been exposed to lead or other potentially BM toxic agents. Social history can be important. A history of intravenous drug use might suggest the possibility of virally transmitted diseases, such as HIV, which may be associated with anemia. Dietary history is also very important, particularly in young and elderly individuals with anemia. The finding of pica in adults (most commonly ice chips or cornstarch) is well known to be associated with iron-deficiency anemia.[22] Ingestion of paint chips may suggest the need to investigate the possibility of toxic lead ingestion. A family history of anemia is highly relevant in the evaluation of children with anemia. However, it is also relevant in adults because certain congenital anemias, such as milder forms of $S\beta^{+}$-thalassemia and hereditary spherocytosis, occasionally first become clinically apparent in adulthood.

The significance of pallor on physical examination is in many ways similar to the historic feature of fatigue: it is a common but nonspecific finding. More specific findings may be found in certain types of anemia. For example, angular cheilitis (cracking at the edges of the lips) and koilonychia (spooning of the nails) may accompany iron-deficiency anemia. Splenomegaly may be present in patients with anemia arising from a wide variety of different causes. When

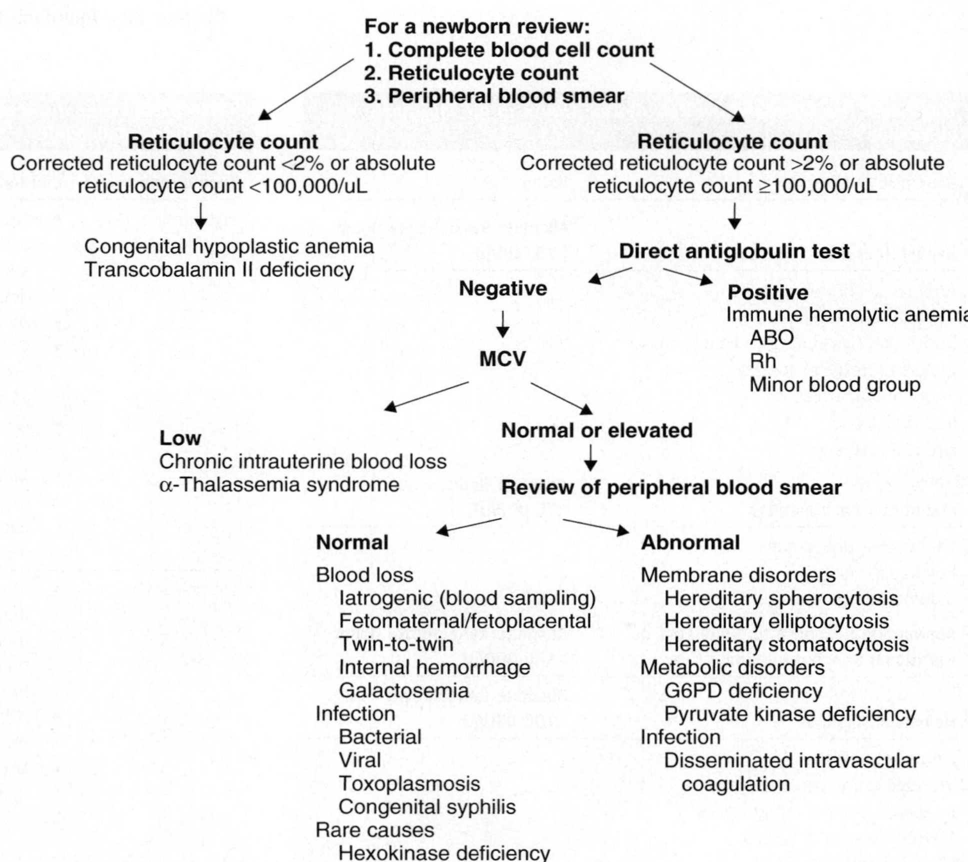

Figure 32-3 APPROACH TO THE DIFFERENTIAL DIAGNOSIS OF ANEMIA IN A NEWBORN. *G6PD,* Glucose-6-phosphate dehydrogenase; *MCV,* mean corpuscular volume.

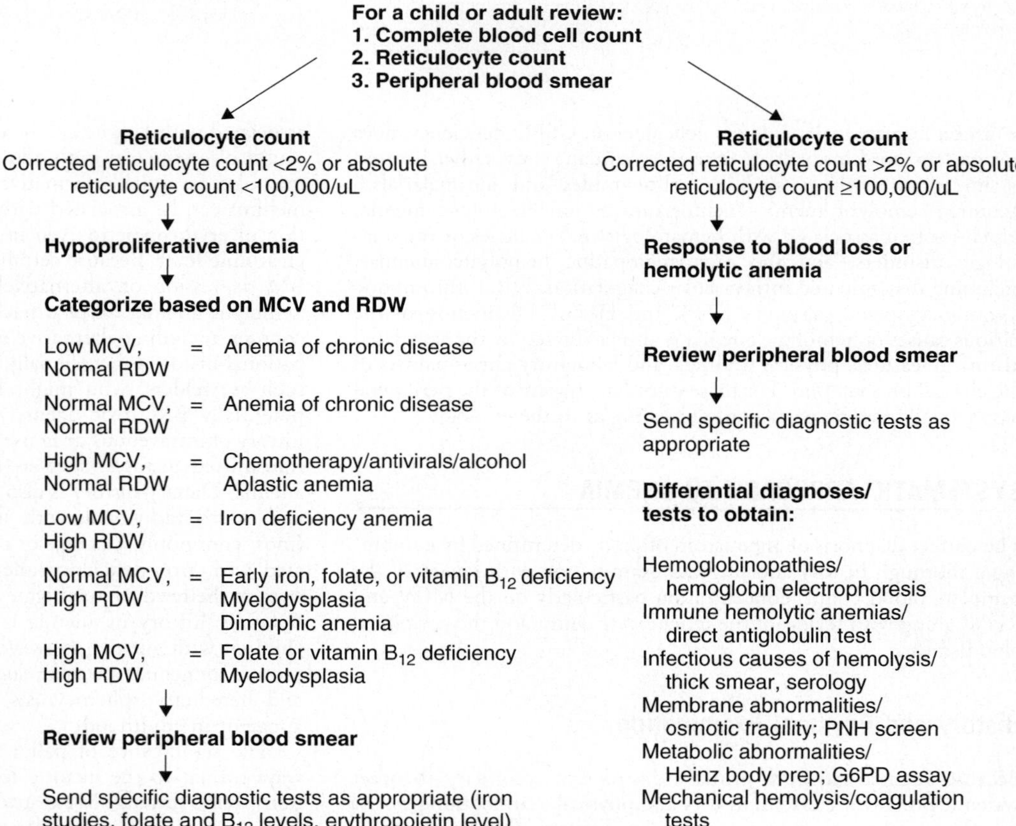

Figure 32-4 APPROACH TO THE DIFFERENTIAL DIAGNOSES OF ANEMIA IN ADULTS AND CHILDREN. *G6PD,* Glucose-6-phosphate dehydrogenase; *MCV,* mean corpuscular volume; *PNH,* paroxysmal nocturnal hemoglobinuria; *RDW,* red blood cell distribution width.

present early in life, it is suggestive of a congenital hemolytic anemia, such as thalassemia, sickle cell disease, or hereditary spherocytosis. When found for the first time later in life, splenomegaly may indicate an acquired disorder, such as autoimmune hemolytic anemia, lymphoproliferative disease, or a myeloproliferative disease such as myelofibrosis. Other physical findings can also sometimes provide insight relevant to the investigation of anemia when combined with historic features and laboratory data. Although anemia itself may lead to the presence of systolic cardiac murmurs, the finding of an increased cardiac murmur in an anemic patient with a prosthetic aortic valve and new microangiopathic change on peripheral smear may indicate that investigation into the possibility of perivalvular leak or prosthetic dysfunction is in order.[23] Finally, because neurologic manifestations can accompany or even predate the anemia associated with vitamin B_{12} deficiency, findings such as loss of vibration or position sense in the extremities may be relevant.[24]

Reticulocyte Count

As a marker of RBC production, the reticulocyte count provides essential information in directing the initial investigation of anemia. Modern flow cytometers accurately determine the reticulocyte count using fluorescent probes that bind to the residual ribonucleic acid present in newly released RBCs.[25] These measurements are useful, are accurate, and reflect the state of erythropoiesis. However, when significant numbers of nucleated RBCs or nuclear debris are present in the peripheral blood, this diagnostic accuracy declines, and manual counting methods are generally preferable.

When the reticulocyte count is reported as a percentage, it needs to be adjusted for the total number of RBCs present. This correction can be made by multiplying the reticulocyte count by the patient's hematocrit divided by an age- and sex-appropriate normal hematocrit. No such correction is necessary when the reticulocyte count is reported as an absolute number or when it is converted to an absolute number by multiplying the percentage by the RBC number (in RBC/μL).

In the absence of anemia, the normal absolute reticulocyte count is between 25,000 and 75,000/μL. In the presence of anemia, an absolute reticulocyte count of less than 75,000/μL is indicative of a hypoproliferative process, and an absolute reticulocyte count of greater than 100,000/μL is indicative of hemolysis or an appropriate erythropoietic response to blood loss (see Table 32-2). Reticulocyte counts between 75,000 and 100,000/μL require interpretation in the context of other available clinical data, including the severity of anemia present.

Mean Corpuscular Volume and Red Blood Cell Distribution Width from the Complete Blood Count

Automated cell counters provide a wealth of information regarding the size, shape, and hemoglobin content of RBCs. The two parameters most useful in classifying anemia are the MCV and the RDW. MCV is reported in femtoliters (fL) and reflects average cell size. RDW is often reported in percent and represents the standard deviation of RBC volume divided by the mean volume. It reflects the variation in cell size in the population of RBCs.[26] These two parameters are useful because relatively reproducible changes in the MCV and RDW are associated with certain types of anemia (Table 32-4). Particularly when combined with the reticulocyte count, the MCV and RDW can significantly narrow the differential diagnosis (Table 32-5).

Examination of the Peripheral Blood Smear

Despite the development and availability of more sophisticated diagnostic testing, review of a well-made peripheral blood smear remains one of the most informative and rewarding diagnostic procedures.[27] It offers the chance to confirm the findings of the automated complete blood cell count, which can be inaccurate in the presence of nucleated RBCs or rouleaux formation. Review of the blood smear also allows for evaluation of other cell lineages, which might suggest a primary BM or infiltrative disease. For example, the finding of hypersegmented neutrophils suggests a megaloblastic process, and this morphologic abnormality can be seen in the blood smear before there are significant changes in the hemoglobin or MCV (see box on Systematic Approach to the Diagnosis of Anemia). Also, only the blood smear reveals the unique morphologic changes occurring with several of the various hemolytic disorders.

Several commonly encountered findings can be seen in RBCs on the peripheral blood smear (Table 32-6 and Fig. 32-5). Whereas microcytic, hypochromic RBCs are suggestive of iron-deficiency anemia or thalassemia (see Fig. 32-5, *F*) macrocytic RBCs with ovalocytes (oval RBCs) are suggestive of megaloblastic anemias (see Fig. 32-5, *G*). Some findings reflect organ dysfunction, such as echinocytes (burr cells) in uremia (see Fig. 32-5, *R*) or acanthocytes (spur cells) in severe liver disease (see Fig. 32-5, *S*), although acanthocytes may also be seen in rare conditions such as abetalipoproteinemia. Target cells may be seen in cases of liver disease but may also be present in hemoglobinopathies, including sickle cell disease and thalassemia (see Fig. 32-5, *W*). The presence of schistocytes or RBC fragmentation often reflects systemic disease, such as DIC, TTP, or HUS (see Fig. 32-5, *P*). Finding spherocytes on a smear is suggestive of autoimmune hemolytic anemia or hereditary spherocytosis (see Fig. 32-5, *H*). Occasionally, the clue to the correct diagnosis of a systemic illness comes in the form of the observation of intraerythrocytic inclusions, such as malarial (see Fig. 32-5, *O*) or babesial forms, and examination of a thick blood smear may be useful for the diagnosis of these disorders when a low parasite burden is suspected.

Bone Marrow Examination

Bone marrow aspiration and biopsy permit evaluation of cellular morphology and BM architecture, respectively. Special stains, flow

Table 32-4 Usefulness of the Mean Corpuscular Value and Red Blood Cell Distribution Width in the Diagnosis of Anemia

	Low MCV (<80 fL)	Normal MCV (80–99 fL)	High MCV (≥100 fL)
Normal RDW	Anemia of chronic disease α- or β-Thalassemia trait Hemoglobin E trait	Acute blood loss Anemia of chronic disease Anemia of renal disease	Aplastic anemia Chronic liver disease Chemotherapy, antivirals, or alcohol
Elevated RDW	Iron deficiency Sickle cell–β-thalassemia	Early iron, folate, or vitamin B_{12} deficiency Dimorphic anemia (for example, iron + folate deficiency) Sickle cell anemia Sickle cell disease Chronic liver disease Myelodysplasia	Folate or vitamin B_{12} deficiency Immune hemolytic anemia Cytotoxic chemotherapy Chronic liver disease Myelodysplasia

MCW, Mean corpuscular value; *RDW*, red blood cell distribution width.

Table 32-5 Combining the Reticulocyte Count and Red Blood Cell Parameters for Diagnosis

MCV, RDW	Reticulocyte Count <100,000/μL	Reticulocyte Count ≥100,000/μL
Low, normal	Anemia of chronic disease	
Normal, normal	Anemia of chronic disease	
High, normal	Chemotherapy, antivirals, or alcohol Aplastic anemia	Chronic liver disease
Low, high	Iron-deficiency anemia	Sickle cell–β-thalassemia
Normal, high	Early iron, folate, vitamin B_{12} deficiency Myelodysplasia	Sickle cell anemia, sickle cell disease
High, high	Folate or vitamin B_{12} deficiency Myelodysplasia	Immune hemolytic anemia Chronic liver disease

MCV, Mean corpuscular volume; *RDW,* red blood cell distribution width.

Table 32-6 Features of the Peripheral Blood Smear

Red Blood Cell Morphology	Definition	Interpretation
Polychromasia	Large, bluish RBCs lacking normal central pallor on peripheral blood smear; bluish stain is the result of residual ribonucleic acid	Rapid production and release of RBCs from BM; elevated reticulocyte count; most commonly seen in hemolytic anemia
Basophilic stippling	Many small bluish dots in portion of erythrocytes; comes from staining of clustered polyribosomes in young circulating RBCs	Seen in a variety of erythropoietic disorders, including acquired and congenital hemolytic anemias and occasionally in lead poisoning (lead inhibits pyrimidine 5′-nucleotidase, which normally digests the residual RNA)
Pappenheimer bodies	Several grayish, irregularly shaped inclusions in a portion of erythrocytes visible on peripheral smear; composed of aggregates of ribosomes, ferritin, and mitochondria	Erythropoietic malfunction in congenital anemias such as hemoglobinopathies, particularly with splenic hypofunction or acquired anemias such as megaloblastic anemia
Heinz bodies	Several grayish, round inclusions visible after supravital staining with methyl crystal violet of the peripheral blood smear, often in the context of bite cells; represent aggregates of denatured hemoglobin	Indicative of oxidative injury to the erythrocyte, such as occurs in G6PD deficiency, or less commonly of unstable hemoglobins
Howell-Jolly bodies	Usually one or at most a few purplish inclusions in the erythrocyte visible on the routine peripheral blood smear; represent residual fragments of nuclei containing chromatin	Associated with states of splenic hypofunction or after splenectomy
Schistocytes	RBCs that are fragmented into a variety of shapes and sizes, including helmet-shaped cells; indicative of shearing of the erythrocyte within the circulation	Associated with microangiopathic hemolytic anemias, including DIC, TTP, or HUS, as well as other mechanical causes of hemolysis, such as prosthetic valves
Spherocytes	RBCs that have lost their central pallor and appear spherical; indicative of loss of cytoskeletal integrity from internal or external causes	Associated with hereditary spherocytosis, autoimmune hemolytic anemia; may also be observed in addition to schistocytes in the presence of microangiopathic hemolytic anemia
Teardrop cells	Pear-shaped erythrocytes visible on peripheral blood smear; indicative of mechanical stress on the RBC during release from the BM or passage through the spleen	Seen in a variety of conditions, including congenital anemias such as thalassemia and acquired disorders such as megaloblastic anemia; may also suggest a more ominous process such as myelophthisis (BM replacement)
Burr cells (echinocytes)	RBCs that have smooth undulations present on the surface circumferentially; pathogenesis unknown	Indicative of uremia when present on a properly made peripheral blood smear
Spur cells (acanthocytes)	RBCs that have spiny points present on the surface circumferentially; reflective of abnormal lipid composition of RBC membrane	Most commonly indicative of liver disease when present in significant numbers; also seen in abetalipoproteinemia and in RBCs lacking the Kell blood group antigen

BM, Bone marrow; *DIC,* disseminated intravascular coagulation; *G6PD,* glucose-6-phosphate dehydrogenase; *HUS,* hemolytic uremic syndrome; *RBC,* red blood cell; *TTP,* thrombotic thrombocytopenic purpura.

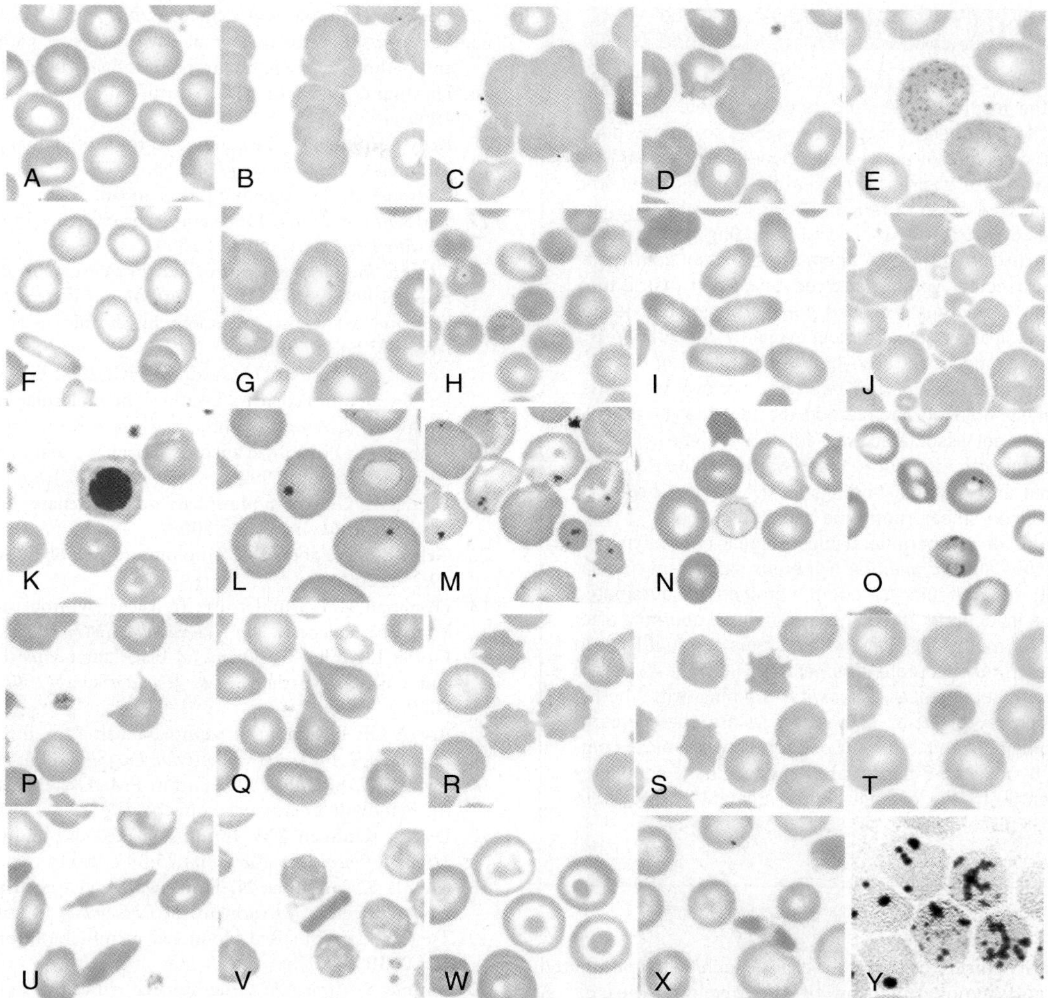

Figure 32-5 USEFUL PERIPHERAL BLOOD AND RED BLOOD CELL FEATURES IN THE EVALUATION OF ANEMIA. **A,** Normal red blood cells (RBCs). Note the central pallor is one-third the diameter of the entire cell. **B,** Rouleaux formation is indicative of increased plasma protein. **C,** Agglutination indicates an antibody-mediated process such as cold agglutinin disease. **D,** Polychromatophilic cell. The gray-blue color is attributable to RNA and the cell is equivalent to a reticulocyte, which must be identified with a reticulocyte stain. **E,** Basophilic stippling. This also is attributable to increased RNA caused either by a left shift in erythroid cells or lead toxicity. **F,** Hypochromic microcytic cells typical of iron-deficiency anemia. Note the widened central pallor and the "pencil" cell in the lower left. **G,** Macroovalocyte as can be seen in either megaloblastic anemia or myelodysplastic syndrome. **H,** Microspherocytes typical of hereditary spherocytosis. **I,** Elliptocytes (ovalocytes) from a patient with hereditary elliptocytosis. **J,** RBC fragments from thermal injury (burn patient). **K,** Nucleated RBC. **L,** Howell-Jolly bodies indicative of splenic dysfunction or absence. **M,** Pappenheimer bodies from a patient with sideroblastic anemia. **N,** Cabot ring, as can be seen in megaloblastic anemia or MDS. **O,** Malarial parasites *(Plasmodium falciparum)*. **P,** Schistocyte typical of a microangiopathic hemolytic anemia. **Q,** Tear-drop form indicates marrow fibrosis and extramedullary hematopoiesis. **R,** Echinocyte (Burr cell) with rounded edges. **S,** Acanthocyte (spur cell) with more irregular pointed ends. This was from a patient with neuroacanthocytosis. They can also be seen in patients with liver disease and lipid abnormalities. **T,** "Bite" cell from a patient with glucose-6-phosphate dehydrogenase (G6PD) deficiency. **U,** Sickle cell, from a patient with homozygous sickle cell disease. **V,** Hemoglobin C crystal. **W,** Target cells. **X,** Hemoglobin C disease. Note that the RBC in center has condensed hemoglobin at each pole. **Y,** Heinz body preparation (supravital stain) from a patient with G6PD deficiency. Note that the cells to the right have increased precipitated hemoglobin.

cytometry, cytogenetic analysis, fluorescence in situ hybridization (FISH), and molecular testing performed on the BM also can provide a wealth of diagnostic information.[28] Because of the discomfort involved in the procedure, however, careful consideration should be given to determining the array of tests required, so that repeated BM aspirates or biopsies need not be performed. If there is any consideration of the possibility of myelodysplasia, leukemia, or lymphoma, an aliquot of anticoagulated aspirate should be set aside at the time of the initial procedure that can be sent, if necessary, for flow cytometry or cytogenetics after review of the aspirate smear. It should be noted that even when properly performed, difficulty obtaining a BM aspirate is commonly observed in certain situations, including myelofibrosis, erythroblastic leukemia (M6), and hairy cell leukemia. In these cases, touch preps of the BM biopsy may help expedite diagnosis.

Diagnostic uncertainty in the setting of hypoproliferative anemia is an indication for BM biopsy. Hematologic disorders such as myelodysplasia, leukemia, lymphoma, or myeloma may be identified. Myelodysplasia in the marrow classically includes megaloblastic change and nuclear budding in maturing erythroblasts, as well as

Systematic Approach to the Diagnosis of Anemia

Integration of historic features and physical findings with thoughtful review of the results of the automated complete blood cell count and of the peripheral smear often serves to narrow down the differential diagnosis of anemia significantly. For example, a patient who has had a gastric bypass eating a normal diet who presents with gradual onset of fatigue accompanied by the more recent onset of distal paresthesias and a finding of decreased vibration sense in the setting of anemia with significantly elevated mean corpuscular volume and red blood cell distribution width values and numerous six-lobed polymorphonuclear leukocytes on peripheral blood smear almost certainly has vitamin B_{12} deficiency. This is suggested even before the return of specific laboratory testing because of the relatively narrow differential diagnosis for megaloblastic anemia and the fact that neurologic abnormalities are not associated with folate deficiency. For the purposes of diagnostic efficiency, the rewards of correlation of historic features and physical findings with a careful review of the peripheral blood smear cannot be overstated.

Special stains of the peripheral blood smear can be helpful in elucidating the cause of anemia. If there is significant nuclear debris present, the reticulocyte count obtained by automated methods can be inaccurate. In such cases, manual counting after staining with new methylene blue, which stains residual RNA in reticulocytes, permits accurate enumeration. If bite cells are detected on peripheral smear, supravital staining with methyl crystal violet can reveal Heinz bodies. These are aggregates of denatured hemoglobin reflecting an oxidative insult, most commonly caused by glucose-6-phosphate dehydrogenase deficiency or, less frequently, by the presence of an unstable hemoglobin (see Fig. 32-5, *H*).

morphologic abnormalities in other lineages, such as hypolobated megakaryocytes and hypogranulation of the myeloid lineage.[29] A variety of infiltrative (myelophthisic) processes may be observed.[30] These include malignancies such as small cell lung, breast, and prostate cancers, which frequently can appear in advanced stages with BM involvement. Alternatively, granulomas may be present, suggesting the possible presence of mycobacterial disease. In children, disseminated neuroblastoma and rhabdomyosarcoma occasionally can appear as a myelophthisic anemia.

FUTURE DIRECTIONS

Anemia may represent a primary hematologic disorder or may represent the manifestation of a systemic process. In children, the former tends to be somewhat more common than the latter, and in adults, the converse is true. However, in both children and adults, a systematic approach to the evaluation of anemia that includes careful review of historic features, the complete blood cell count, and peripheral smear facilitates an efficient diagnosis and minimizes unnecessary testing.

REFERENCES

1. Cantor AB, Orkin SH: Transcriptional regulation of erythropoiesis: An affair involving multiple partners. *Oncogene* 13:3368, 2002.
2. Rosse W: The spleen as a filter. *N Engl J Med* 317:704, 1987.
3. Semenza GL: Involvement of oxygen-sensing pathways in physiologic and pathophysiologic erythropoiesis. *Blood* 114:2015, 2009.
4. Hoffbrand AV, Herbert V: Nutritional anemias. *Semin Hematol* 36:13, 1999.
5. Kelly A, Munan L: Haematologic profile of natural populations: Red cell parameters. *Br J Haematol* 35:153, 1977.
6. Nilsson-Ehle H, Jagenburg R, Landahl S, et al: Blood haemoglobin values in the elderly: Implications for reverence intervals from age 70 to 88. *Eur J Haematol* 65:297, 2000.
7. Centers for Disease Control and Prevention: Iron deficiency—United States, 1999-2000. *MMWR Morb Mortal Wkly Rep* 51:897, 2002.
8. Fishbane S: Anemia treatment in chronic renal insufficiency. *Semin Nephrol* 22:474, 2002.
9. Roy CN, Weinstein DA, Andrews NC: 2002 E. Mead Johnnson Award for Research in Pediatrics Lecture: The molecular biology of the anemia of chronic disease: A hypothesis. *Pediatr Res* 53:507, 2003.
10. Tabbara IA: Hemolytic anemias: Diagnosis and management. *Med Clin North Am* 76:649, 1992.
11. Beutler E: Glucose-6-phosphate dehydrogenase deficiency: A historical perspective. *Blood* 111:16, 2008.
12. Gehrs BC, Freidberg RC: Autoimmune hemolytic anemia. *Am J Hematol* 69:258, 2002.
13. Freedman MH, Saunders EF: Transient erythroblastopenia of childhood: Varied pathogenesis. *Am J Hematol* 14:247, 1983.
14. Lipton JM, Ellis SR: Diamond-Blackfan anemia: Diagnosis, treatment, and molecular pathogenesis. *Hematol Oncol Clin North Am* 23:261, 2009.
15. Atweh GF, DeSimone J, Saunthararajah Y, et al: Hemoglobinopathies. *Hematology Am Soc Hematol Educ Program* 2003:14.
16. Boyce TG, Swerdlow DL, Griffin PM: Escherichia coli O157:H7 and the hemolytic-uremic syndrome. *N Engl J Med* 333:364, 1995.
17. Lee AI, Kaufman RM: Transfusion medicine and the pregnant patient. *Hematol Oncol Clin North Am* 25:393, 2011.
18. Sawada K, Fujishima N, Hirokawa M: Acquired pure red cell aplasia: Updated review of treatment. *Br J Haematol* 142:505, 2008.
19. Tse WT, Lux SE: Red blood cell membrane disorders. *Br J Haematol* 104:2, 1999.
20. Ammus S, Yunis AA: Drug-induced red cell dyscrasias. *Blood Rev* 3:71, 1989.
21. George JN: Evaluation and management of patients with thrombotic thrombocytopenic purpura. *J Intensive Care Med* 22:82, 2007.
22. Moore DF Jr, Sears DA: Pica, iron deficiency, and the medical history. *Am J Med* 97:390, 1994.
23. Lam BK, Cosgrove DM, Bhudia SK, et al: Hemolysis after mitral valve repair: Mechanisms and treatment. *Ann Thorac Surg* 77:191, 2004.
24. Lindenbaum J, Healton EB, Savage DG: Neuropsychiatric disorders caused by cobalamin deficiency in the absence of anemia or macrocytosis. *N Engl J Med* 318:1720, 1988.
25. Corberand JX: Reticulocyte analysis using flow cytometry. *Hematol Cell Ther* 38:487, 1996.
26. Lombarts AJ, Koevoet AL, Leijnse B: Basic principles and problems of haemocytometry. *Ann Clin Biochem* 23:390, 1986.
27. Bain B: Diagnosis from the blood smear. *N Engl J Med* 353:498, 2005.
28. Hyun BH, Stevenson AJ, Hanau CA: Fundamentals of bone marrow examination. *Hematol Oncol Clin North Am* 8:651, 1994.
29. Vardiman JW, Thiele J, Arber DA: The 2008 revision of the World Health Organization (WHO) classification of myeloid neoplasms and acute leukemia: Rationale and important changes. *Blood* 114:237, 2009.
30. O'Keane JC, Wolf BC, Neiman RS: The pathogenesis of splenic extramedullary hematopoiesis in metastatic carcinoma. *Cancer* 63:1539, 1989.

CHAPTER 33

PATHOPHYSIOLOGY OF IRON HOMEOSTASIS

Gary M. Brittenham

Iron is an essential element required for energy production, oxygen utilization, and cellular proliferation. Iron, able to act both as an electron donor and acceptor by readily interconverting between ferric (Fe^{3+}) and ferrous (Fe^{2+}) forms, is an irreplaceable component of oxygen transport (hemoglobin); storage (myoglobin); and sensing molecules, cytochromes, iron-sulfur clusters, and heme and nonheme enzymes. The ease with which iron can gain and lose electrons also makes iron able to catalyze the formation of highly reactive oxygen species that can damage lipids, protein and DNA, and injure subcellular organelles, resulting in cellular dysfunction, apoptosis, and necrosis. Consequently, both the total body iron and the amount within each cell are carefully controlled to assure adequate iron availability but avoid excess iron toxicity. Humans have no regulated means for iron excretion, and obligatory losses are normally minuscule, less than 0.05% of the total body iron each day. As a result, the amount of body iron is determined by control of iron absorption, and human iron homeostasis is distinguished by efficient recycling of iron (Fig. 33-1).

Although all cells require iron, quantitatively, most of the iron in the body is found within erythroid cells, and most of the daily movement of iron cycles through the erythroid compartment. External exchange of iron through absorption of iron from the gastrointestinal tract and from obligatory losses is very limited. Physiologically, iron is carried into the erythroid marrow and incorporated into hemoglobin and enters the circulation within red blood cells (RBCs) dedicated to oxygen transport. At the end of their lifespan, RBCs are phagocytized by a select population of macrophages in the bone marrow, liver, and spleen that then promptly render up most of the catabolized iron for return to the erythroid marrow. Any surplus is stored within macrophages or hepatocytes. After examining the intricate interrelation between intracellular and systemic iron homeostasis, this chapter considers in turn each portion of the pathway of iron transport, utilization, storage, and absorption (see Fig. 33-1). Altogether iron homeostasis is maintained by effective use of iron for erythropoiesis, efficient recycling of iron from senescent erythrocytes, controlled storage of iron by macrophages and hepatocytes, and careful regulation of intestinal iron absorption.[1]

REGULATION OF CELLULAR AND SYSTEMIC IRON HOMEOSTASIS

Each cell in the body needs iron in precise, carefully timed amounts for growth, development, and function. Within the systemic circulation, the varied and varying cellular requirements are met by the transport protein *transferrin*, the physiological carrier of iron through the plasma and extracellular fluid. Each cell obtains its share of circulating transferrin-bound iron by expressing *transferrin receptor 1*, a glycoprotein on cell membranes that binds the transferrin–iron complex and is internalized in an endocytic vesicle, where iron is released and then returns to the cell membrane, liberating apotransferrin into the plasma.[1-4] Within the cell, the iron released from the endosome is either used or sequestered with cytosolic *ferritin*, an iron storage protein that holds iron in a nontoxic form ready for prompt mobilization in time of need.[5] A prime determinant of the iron supply to each cell is the number of transferrin receptors expressed on the cell surface. Within each cell, iron self-regulates its intracellular availability, at least in part, translationally through the iron regulatory proteins (1 and 2) that function as sensors of intracellular iron (Fig. 33-2). The iron regulatory proteins recognize and bind to RNA stem–loop structures called iron responsive elements when iron is absent and dissociate when iron is present.[1-4] When the iron-responsive elements are within the 3′ untranslated region of a mRNA (e.g., transferrin receptor 1 mRNA), binding prevents mRNA degradation, increasing protein expression when iron is lacking. In contrast, when the iron-responsive elements are located in the 5′ untranslated region of an mRNA (e.g., cytosolic ferritin mRNA), binding of the iron regulatory proteins interferes with ribosomal assembly, decreasing protein expression when iron is absent. Accordingly, a *decrease* in intracellular iron availability enhances transferrin receptor 1 protein synthesis, increasing iron import, and reduces cytosolic ferritin protein production and iron storage. Conversely, an *increase* in intracellular iron availability reduces transferrin receptor 1 protein synthesis, inhibiting iron import, and augments cytosolic ferritin protein production and iron storage. In iron-replete cells, F box and leucine-rich repeat protein 5 (FBXL5), a subunit of a ubiquitin ligase complex, monitors cytosolic iron and leads to iron-dependent degradation of iron regulatory proteins.[6] Altogether, *regulation of intracellular iron homeostasis* is provided principally through the iron regulatory proteins by translational control of the synthesis of transferrin receptor and ferritin and, in some cells, other proteins involved in iron homeostasis, such as δ-aminolevulinic acid synthase 2 (eALAS), mitochondrial aconitase (ACO2), hypoxia inducible factor 2α (HIF-2α), intestinal divalent metal transporter 1 (DMT1) isoform I, and ferroportin.[1-4]

Regulation of systemic iron homeostasis is accomplished by control of the entry of iron into plasma for transport by transferrin.[1-4] Circulating transferrin iron is derived from specialized cells that can export iron, primarily reticuloendothelial macrophages that recycle iron from senescent RBCs, hepatocytes that can mobilize iron from stores, and duodenal enterocytes that provide iron absorbed from the diet. To enter plasma, iron in these cells must pass through *ferroportin*, a multitransmembrane-spanning protein that is the sole known cellular iron export channel.[7] *Hepcidin*, a small 25–amino acid peptide hormone secreted principally by the liver, provides post-translational control of ferroportin expression by binding to and inducing its internalization, ubiquitination, and degradation, thereby inhibiting iron entry into plasma (Fig. 33-3).[7,8] Hepatic hepcidin synthesis is stimulated by increases in body iron stores, infection, inflammation, or malignancy and inhibited by hypoxemia and increased erythropoietic demand. Increments in plasma hepcidin reduce the amount of ferroportin in cell membranes, causing a prompt fall in plasma iron concentration. Conversely, decrements in plasma hepcidin concentration increase the amount of ferroportin, producing a rise in plasma iron concentration. Under conditions of iron deprivation, ferroportin can also (1) be posttranscriptionally regulated by iron-regulatory proteins binding to the 5′ iron-regulatory element in ferroportin mRNA and arresting synthesis and (2) be internalized and degraded in a hepcidin-independent manner requiring the E3 ubiquitin ligase Nedd4-2 and the Nedd4-2 binding protein Nfdip-1.[9]

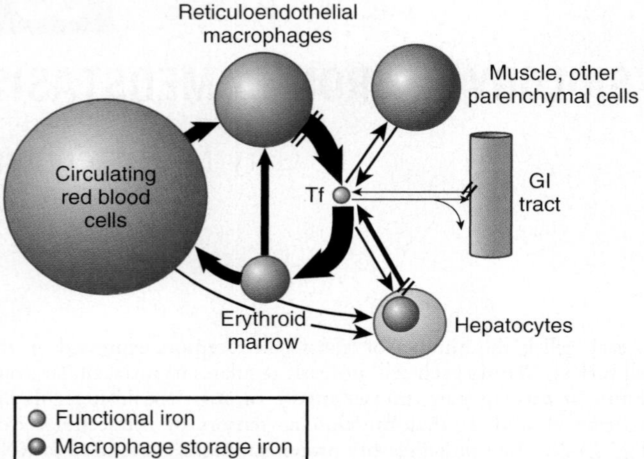

Figure 33-1 BODY IRON SUPPLY AND STORAGE. The figure shows a schematic representation of the routes of iron exchange in an adult. The area of each *circle* is proportional to the amount of iron contained in the compartment, and the width of each *arrow* is proportional to the daily flow of iron from one compartment to another. *Double slashes* indicate the sites of hepcidin action, decreasing macrophage release of iron derived from senescent red blood cells (RBCs), diminishing delivery of iron from duodenal enterocytes absorbing dietary iron, and inhibiting release of iron stored in hepatocytes. The concentration of iron in the human body is normally maintained at about 40 mg Fe/kg in women and about 50 mg Fe/kg in men. The major portion of iron is found in the erythron as hemoglobin iron (28 mg/kg in women; 32 mg/kg in men) dedicated to oxygen transport and delivery. Small amounts of erythron iron (<1 mg/kg) are also present in heme and nonheme enzymes in developing RBCs. The remainder of functional iron is found as myoglobin iron (4 mg/kg in women; 5 mg/kg in men) in muscle and as iron-containing and iron-dependent enzymes (1-2 mg/kg) throughout the cells of the body. Most storage iron (5-6 mg/kg in women; 10-12 mg/kg in men) is held in reserve by hepatocytes and macrophages. The small fraction of transport iron (≈0.2 mg/kg) in the plasma and extracellular fluid is bound to the protein transferrin (Tf). *GI,* Gastrointestinal.

UTILIZATION OF IRON FOR ERYTHROPOIESIS

Each day, almost 200 billion RBCs are produced in a normal adult to replace a similar number reaching the end of their lifespan. Each RBC contains more than a billion atoms of iron, four in each tetrameric molecule of hemoglobin, so that more than 200 quintillion (200×10^{18}) atoms of iron are needed daily for erythropoiesis. Transferrin transports iron in a nonreactive, soluble form in the circulation for delivery to erythroid precursors or other iron-requiring cells (Fig. 33-4). Apotransferrin, transferrin without attached iron, is a single-chain glycoprotein with two structurally similar lobes. Binding of a ferric ion to one of these lobes yields monoferric transferrin; binding of ions to both yields diferric transferrin. The transferrin saturation is the proportion of the available iron-binding sites on transferrin that are occupied by iron atoms, expressed as a percentage. In humans, almost all of the circulating plasma apotransferrin is synthesized by the hepatocyte. After delivering iron to cells, apotransferrin is promptly returned to the plasma to again function as an iron transporter, completing 100 to 200 cycles of iron delivery during its lifetime in the circulation. Apotransferrin is a true carrier that is not lost in delivering iron, so its turnover is unrelated to the plasma iron turnover; the half-life of the protein is about 8 days. In an iron-replete 70-kg man, the amount of transferrin-bound iron in the plasma at any given time is only about 3 mg, but more than 30 mg of iron moves through this transport compartment each day (see Fig. 33-1). Most (≈24 mg Fe/day) of the iron is used for erythropoiesis.

Transferrin receptors on the cell surface selectively bind mono- or diferric transferrin. Two different isoforms of the transferrin receptor exist, encoded by two separate genes. The two glycoproteins have similar extracellular structures but distinct roles in iron homeostasis. Transferrin receptor 1, ubiquitously expressed, functions as the physiologic transferrin iron importer on all iron-requiring cells. Transferrin receptor 2 is predominantly expressed on hepatocytes, functioning in the regulation of hepcidin expression (see later), and in developing erythroid cells, with a role in erythropoiesis (see later).[3,4] Transferrin receptor 1 is a transmembrane glycoprotein dimer composed of two identical subunits linked by a disulfide bond. Each transferrin receptor 1 can bind 2 molecules of transferrin; if each transferrin is diferric, the dimeric receptor can carry a total of 4 atoms of transferrin-bound iron. The affinity of transferrin receptor 1 for transferrin depends both on the iron content of transferrin and on the pH. With amounts of iron-bearing transferrin sufficient to saturate receptors at a physiologic pH of 7.4, transferrin receptor 1 has very little affinity for apotransferrin; an intermediate affinity for monoferric transferrin; and the highest affinity for diferric transferrin, estimated at 2 to 7×10^{-9} M. Under such physiological conditions, the affinity of transferrin receptor 1 for diferric transferrin is more than fourfold greater that for monoferric transferrin. At a pH of about 5, the affinity of transferrin receptor 1 for apotransferrin increases to that of diferric transferrin.

Iron delivery to an erythroid cell (see Fig. 33-4) begins with the binding of one or two molecules of mono- or diferric transferrin to a transferrin receptor 1.[1-4] The efficiency of iron delivery to the cell depends on the amounts of mono- and diferric plasma transferrin available. With normal erythropoiesis and a normal transferrin saturation of about 33%, the higher affinity of the receptor for diferric transferrin results in most of the iron supply to cells being derived from this form, providing four atoms of iron with each cycle. At a transferrin saturation of about 19%, equal amounts of iron are provided by mono- and diferric transferrin; at lower saturations, most of the iron is derived from the monoferric form. Whether mono- or diferric, the fate of transferrin bound to the transferrin receptor is the same. When bound, the iron-bearing transferrin–receptor complex rapidly clusters with other transferrin–receptor complexes in a clathrin-coated pit. When assembled, the clathrin-coated pit is promptly internalized and detaches from the inner membrane. Within the cytoplasm, the coated vesicle is rapidly stripped of clathrin, and the uncoated vesicles fuse to become multivesicular endosomes. Moving to the interior of the cell, a proton pump lowers endosome internal pH to about 5.6. In the acidic environment of the endosome, both transferrin and transferrin receptor 1 undergo conformational changes that enhance the rate and completeness of iron release. After release from transferrin within the acidified endosome as ferric iron, the iron is reduced by the ferrireductase six-transmembrane epithelial antigen of the prostate 3 (STEAP3) to the ferrous form and then transported across the endosomal membrane through the divalent metal transporter 1 (DMT1).[1] A DMT1-independent channel for ferrous iron, mucolipin 1 (TRPML1), has also been identified.[10] Acidification within the endosome increases the affinity of the now iron-free apotransferrin for the transferrin receptor with the result that the apotransferrin-receptor bond remains intact as the complex is transported back to the cell surface within the endosome. On exposure to the neutral pH of the plasma, the apotransferrin loses its affinity for the transferrin receptor and is released from the membrane, making both the apotransferrin and receptor available for reutilization (see Fig. 33-4).

Most of the iron transported across the endosomal membrane is directed to the mitochondria for use in the synthesis of heme (Fig. 33-4). Iron can be imported from the cytosol across the mitochondrial membrane by the transmembrane protein mitoferrin (SLC25A37).[3,4] Transport of iron from endosomes into mitochondria for heme synthesis by direct contact between the organelles, avoiding the cytosol, also has been proposed.[11] Heme (ferrous protoporphyrin

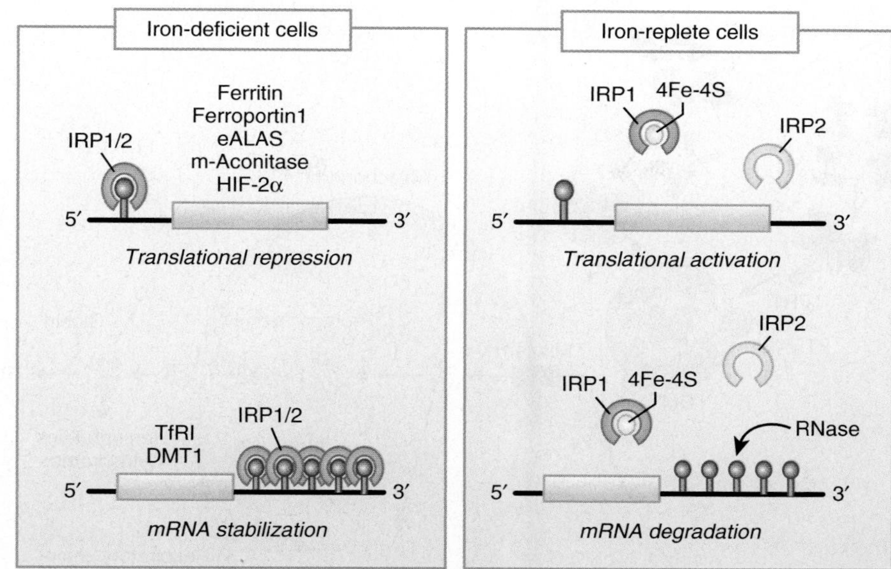

Figure 33-2 REGULATION OF CELLULAR IRON HOMEOSTASIS BY THE IRON REGULATORY PROTEINS (IRP1 AND IRP2). The iron regulatory proteins recognize and bind to RNA stem-loop structures called iron responsive elements (IREs) when iron is absent and dissociate when iron is present. Binding IREs within the 3′ untranslated region of mRNA (e.g., transferrin receptor 1 [TfR1]) and some intestinal divalent metal transporter 1 (DMT1) isoforms increases mRNA stability, increasing protein synthesis. In contrast, binding IREs in the 5′ untranslated region of mRNA (e.g., cytosolic ferritin, ferroportin1 [FPN1A], erythroid aminolevulinic acid synthase [eALAS], mitochondrial aconitase [m-aconitase], and hypoxia-inducible factor 2α [HIF-2α]) inhibits protein expression when iron is absent. In iron-replete cells, IRP1 assembles a cubane Fe/S cluster, acquiring aconitase activity while losing the ability to bind to IREs. In iron-replete cells, IRP2 interacts with F box and leucine-rich repeat protein 5 (FBXL5), a subunit of a ubiquitin ligase complex, leading to its ubiquitination and degradation by the proteasome. See text for details. *(Modified with permission from Wallander ML, Leibold EA, Eisenstein RS: Molecular control of vertebrate iron homeostasis by iron regulatory proteins.* Biochim Biophys Acta *1763:668, 2006.)*

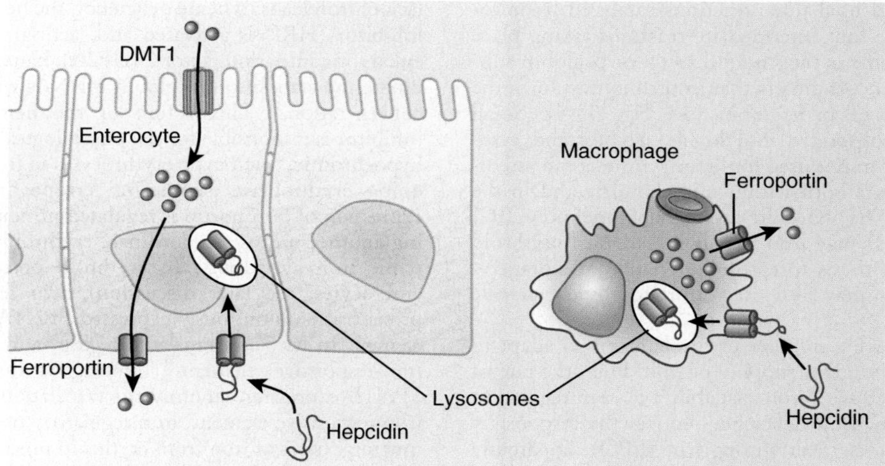

Figure 33-3 CONTROL OF IRON ENTRY INTO PLASMA BY FERROPORTIN AND HEPCIDIN IN THE REGULATION OF SYSTEMIC IRON HOMEOSTASIS. Ferroportin, a multitransmembrane-spanning protein that is the only known iron exporter in humans, is expressed at high concentrations on the basolateral membrane of duodenal enterocytes, reticuloendothelial macrophages, and hepatocytes (not shown). Plasma hepcidin binds to a specific extracellular domain of ferroportin, inducing the binding and then autophosphorylation of cytosolic Janus kinase 2 (JAK2). JAK2 then phosphorylates ferroportin, leading to ferroportin internalization by clathrin-coated pits and its subsequent degradation in the lysosome. See text for details. *DMT1,* Divalent metal transporter 1. *(Modified with permission from Andrews NC: Forging a field: the golden age of iron biology.* Blood *112:219, 2008.)*

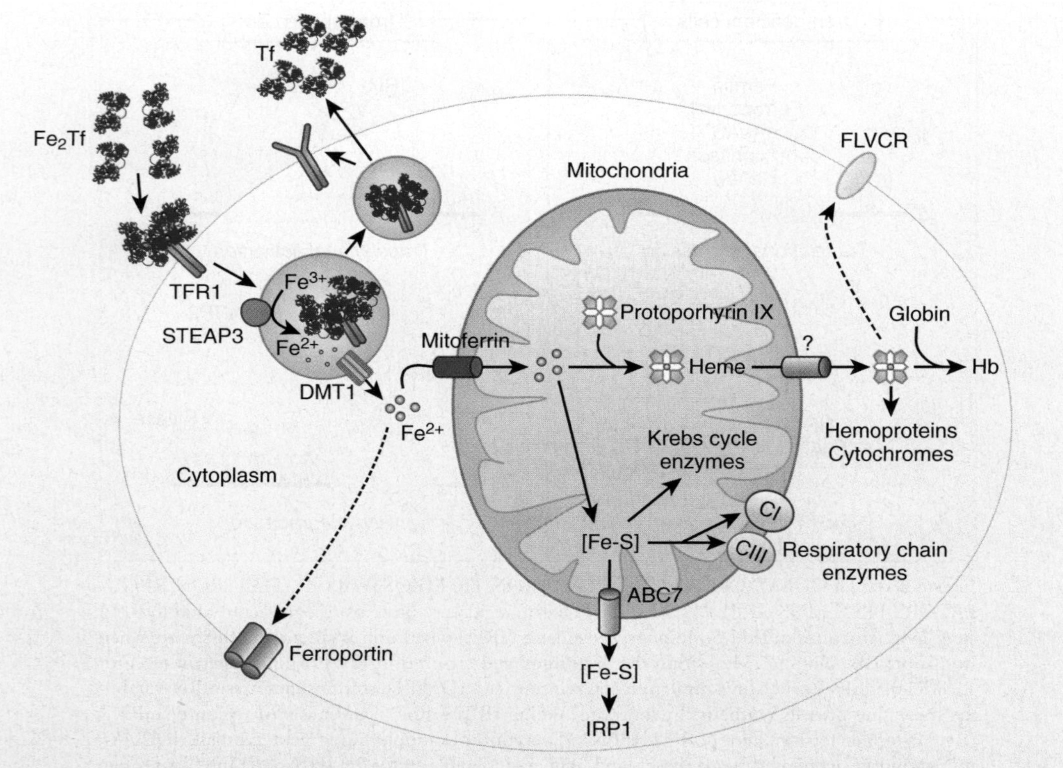

Figure 33-4 ACQUISITION AND UTILIZATION OF IRON BY ERYTHROID PRECURSORS. Iron is imported in the transferrin (Tf) cycle and principally used for the synthesis of heme. See text for details. *ABC7,* Adenosine triphosphate–binding cassette, subfamily B (MDR/TAP), member 7; *DMT1,* divalent metal transporter 1; *Fe_2Tf,* diferric transferrin; *FLVCR,* feline leukemia virus subgroup C cellular receptor; *Hb,* hemoglobin; *IRP1,* iron regulatory protein 1; *STEAP3,* six-transmembrane epithelial antigen of the prostate 3; *TFR1,* transferrin receptor 1. *(Modified with permission from Beaumont C, Delaby C: Recycling iron in normal and pathological states.* Semin Hematol *46:328, 2009.)*

IX), a planar molecule consisting of an atom of ferrous iron in the center of a tetrapyrrole ring, is then synthesized in eight biochemical reactions with the first and final three reactions catalyzed by mitochondrial enzymes and the four intermediate reactions taking place in the cytoplasm. Most heme is then bound to α- or β-globin subunits that combine to form α-β dimers that in turn join to form the functional α_2-β_2-tetramer of hemoglobin (see Fig. 33-4). Small amounts of heme are incorporated into heme enzymes and cytochromes. The fraction of iron not used for heme synthesis can assembled into iron sulfur clusters both within mitochondria and in the cytosol (see Fig. 33-4). The cytosolic iron chaperone poly (rC) binding protein 1 (PCBP1) may iron that is in excess of erythroid requirements for heme synthesis to cytosolic ferritin for storage.[5,12] The same iron chaperone may also carry iron to some cytosolic nonheme enzymes.

Erythroid precursors have a number of mechanisms to adapt to either inadequate or overabundant supplies of iron. First, the rate of erythropoiesis is coordinated with iron availability by iron regulation of erythroid differentiation. Iron deficiency reduces the responsiveness of erythroid progenitors to erythropoietin (EPO), apparently through an iron–aconitase–isocitrate pathway.[13] With a dearth of iron, decreased erythroid utilization for RBC production helps preserve the supply of iron for vital functions in other tissues. Second, transferrin receptor 2 is a component of the EPO receptor complex that is required for efficient erythropoiesis and is involved in the production of growth differentiation factor (GDF-15), a putative regulator of hepatic hepcidin synthesis (see later discussion).[14] Third, heme synthesis is coordinated with iron availability through an iron regulatory element in the 5′ untranslated region of the mRNA for δ-aminolevulinic acid synthase 2 (eALAS), the erythroid-specific initial enzyme in the heme synthetic pathway. If intracellular iron availability is low, binding of an iron regulatory protein will inhibit heme synthesis by preventing translation of the mRNA.[3] Fourth, if a lack of iron leads to heme deficiency, the heme-regulated translational inhibitor (HRI) is activated and, acting through the α-subunit of eukaryotic initiation factor 2 (eIF2α), halts protein synthesis to coordinate the translation of globin mRNAs with the intracellular heme concentration.[15] This action of the heme-regulated translational inhibitor is responsible for the physiological adaptation that produces hypochromic, microcytic erythrocytes in iron deficiency. Fifth, developing erythroblasts synthesize ferroportin to export iron. Their expression of ferroportin is regulated principally by hepcidin, providing another means to coordinate erythroid iron utilization with systemic iron availability. In erythroid precursors (and in duodenal enterocytes; see later discussion), two ferroportin transcripts are present: the ubiquitously expressed FPN1A, with an iron-responsive element in its 5′ untranslated region, and FPN1B, which lacks the iron-responsive element.[16] During erythroid cell differentiation, FPN1B expression circumvents translational repression through the iron responsive element, iron regulatory protein system, thereby permitting export of iron from erythroid precursor cells during the critical time period when cells commit to proliferation and differentiation, express high levels of transferrin receptor 1, and rapidly accumulate iron. As a consequence, erythropoiesis may be partially suppressed when nonerythropoietic tissues risk developing iron deficiency. Iron export from erythroblasts via FPN1B may account for the development of iron deficiency anemia as an initial, early manifestation of systemic iron deficiency.[16] Nonetheless, when the cells begin to produce hemoglobin, FPN1B expression diminishes, and FPN1A predominates, allowing erythroid cells to limit iron export through the iron-responsive element iron regulatory protein system and to efficiently manufacture heme.[16] Sixth, as noted earlier, cytosolic ferritin can be synthesized to sequester surplus iron accumulations in a safe and soluble form.[5] Seventh, a mitochondrial ferritin, consisting of homopolymers of a nuclear gene-encoded H-type ferritin (see later), can be expressed to protect against mitochondrial iron accumulation in sideroblastic anemia and some other disorders.[5] Eighth, erythroblasts have the capacity to export excess heme through the feline leukemia virus subgroup C cellular receptor (FLVCR) and avoid heme toxicity.[17]

Orthochromatic erythroblasts, with nuclei that are unable to synthesize DNA, gradually lose most mitochondria and halt RNA synthesis but continue to produce hemoglobin. The pyknotic nucleus is finally extruded through the erythroblast membrane with the loss of about 5% to 10% of the hemoglobin that had been synthesized previously. The resultant reticulocyte continues to synthesize hemoglobin for another 2 to 3 days until the cellular supply of mRNA is exhausted, producing as much as 30% of the total hemoglobin complement of the RBC. Eventually, the reticulocyte is released from the marrow, remodeled, and pitted of siderotic granules and debris within the spleen to emerge as a mature RBC dedicated to oxygen delivery over its lifespan of 3 to 4 months.

RECYCLING OF ERYTHROCYTE IRON BY MACROPHAGES

The major pathway of iron movement from erythroid cells is to a dedicated population of macrophages in the bone marrow, liver (Kupffer cells), and spleen as RBCs reach the end of their lifespan (Fig. 33-5). Macrophages in the bone marrow also have the responsibilities of culling defective immature erythroid cells to prevent their release into the circulation and of removing some deposits of erythrocyte ferritin from developing RBCs. During their time in the bloodstream, RBCs undergo a multitude of modifications (oxidant damage, metabolic depletion, increasing intracellular calcium concentrations, dehydration, decrease in cell volume, phosphatidylserine exposure, formation of "senescent" antigens, and others) that lead to their recognition and selective removal by specialized macrophages in the bone marrow, liver, and spleen.[18] On average, each of these macrophages can phagocytize one erythrocyte a day. After ingesting the erythrocyte in a phagosomal vacuole known as an erythrophagolysosome, the erythrocyte membrane is lysed. The hemoglobin within then undergoes oxidative precipitation and rapid catabolism into heme (see Fig. 33-5).[2]

A small proportion of aged or damaged erythrocytes undergo intravascular hemolysis. With normal erythropoiesis, this portion of the total iron flux is minor but can increase substantially in disorders with increased ineffective erythropoiesis or intravascular hemolysis. The hemoglobin released into plasma by is then rapidly bound by haptoglobin, a glycoprotein synthesized in the liver.[2] The hemoglobin–haptoglobin complex (M_r 150,000) is too large to be filtered by the kidneys, a feature that helps restrict the renal loss of iron with hemoglobinemia. Macrophages (and hepatocytes; see later) remove the haptoglobin–hemoglobin complex from plasma by binding through the CD163 receptor and after endocytosis digest the complex in lysosomes, liberating heme. In an analogous fashion, any heme released into plasma by intravascular hemolysis complexes with hemopexin and is removed by macrophages (and hepatocytes) expressing the CD91 receptor.[2] In macrophages, heme from all these sources is degraded by an enzymatic complex containing NADPH

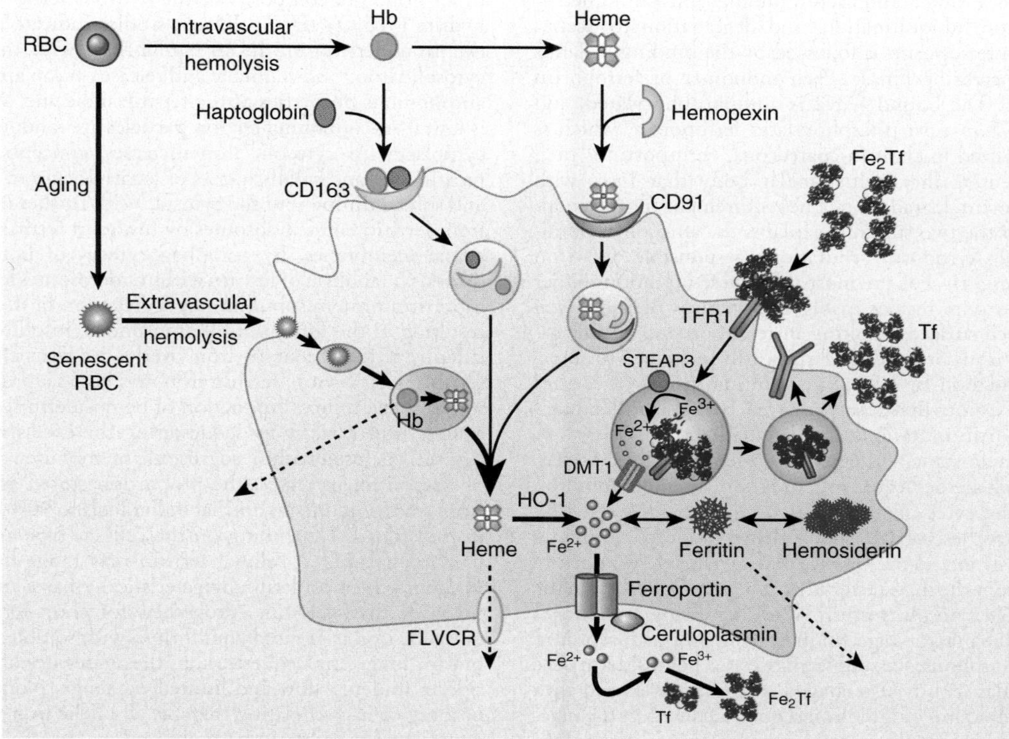

Figure 33-5 RECYCLING OF ERYTHROCYTE IRON BY MACROPHAGES. Most erythrocyte iron is acquired by erythrophagocytosis of senescent red blood cells (RBCs), but smaller amounts are derived from hemoglobin–haptoglobin and heme–hemopexin complexes. Iron derived from plasma transferrin (Tf) is a minor portion of the total iron flux. Heme is catabolized, and the iron exported through ferroportin and oxidized by ceruloplasmin. In the absence of iron deficiency, a portion of the iron is retained as ferritin and hemosiderin. See text for details. *DMT1,* Divalent metal transporter 1; *Fe_2Tf,* diferric transferrin; *FLVCR,* feline leukemia virus subgroup C cellular receptor; *Hb,* hemoglobin; *HO-1,* heme oxygenase-1; *TFR1,* transferrin receptor 1; *STEAP3,* six-transmembrane epithelial antigen of the prostate 3. *(Modified with permission from Beaumont C, Delaby C: Recycling iron in normal and pathological states.* Semin Hematol *46:328, 2009.)*

(nicotinamide adenine dinucleotide phosphate)–cytochrome c reductase, the microsomal enzyme heme oxygenase 1, and biliverdin reductase, yielding carbon monoxide (the sole physiological source in the body), bilirubin, and iron (see Fig. 33-5). Both DMT1 and natural resistance-associated macrophage protein 1 (NRAMP1), a divalent metal transporter expressed within the late endosomal and phagolysosomal membranes of iron-recycling macrophages, seem to be involved in efficient recycling of this iron.[19] Macrophages also can acquire iron from plasma transferrin via the transferrin cycle, but this is a minor portion of their total iron flux.

Ferroportin is the conduit for the outpouring of iron from macrophages in the bone marrow, liver, and spleen to plasma apotransferrin, normally the largest single flux of iron from cells in the body. Ferroportin transcription increases in response to both iron and heme.[9] Ferroportin (FPN1A) levels are also regulated posttranscriptionally through an iron-responsive element in the 5′ untranslated region, with increases in cytosolic iron resulting in increased ferroportin translation. Iron export through ferroportin requires ferroxidase activity, provided by the multicopper oxidase ceruloplasmin in macrophages and by hephaestin in duodenal enterocytes (see later). Ceruloplasmin oxidation may generate a concentration gradient that drives the ferric iron out of the macrophage.[7] In the absence of ceruloplasmin, macrophage ferroportin is rapidly internalized and degraded.[7] Unsaturated transferrin is not required for the release of iron from the macrophages; apotransferrin does not enter the macrophage and accepts iron only after the exit of iron through ferroportin and oxidation by ceruloplasmin. The ferric iron can then be bound by transferrin and transported back to erythroid and other iron-requiring tissues.

Plasma hepcidin regulates iron efflux from macrophages by decreasing the number of ferroportin channels available for iron export. Ferroportin is a dimer, and each monomer must bind hepcidin for internalization, ubiquitination, and degradation to occur.[7] Hepcidin binding to ferroportin is followed by the binding of Janus kinase 2 (JAK2), a tyrosine kinase; each monomer of ferroportin binds a single JAK2. The bound JAK2 is autophosphorylated, and phosphorylated JAK2 in turn phosphorylates ferroportin, which is subsequently internalized in clathrin-coated pits. Ferroportin is then ubiquitinated and enters the multivesicular body that fuses with lysosomes for ferroportin degradation. The requirement for the cooperative interaction of the two subunits explains the autosomal dominant inheritance of ferroportin mutations responsible for iron overload (see Chapter 34).[7] For the most part, these mutations either interfere with iron export by decreasing the amount of functional ferroportin on the cell surface, resulting in retention and accumulation of macrophage iron, or produce ferroportin resistance to internalization and degradation by hepcidin, resulting in loss of control of macrophage iron export that leads to parenchymal iron loading.[7] Homozygous ferroportin mutations are likely lethal.

Under normal circumstances, the macrophages in the liver, spleen, and bone marrow that are dedicated to reprocessing hemoglobin iron from senescent erythrocytes maintain an equilibrium between iron storage and release. Synthesis of cytosolic ferritin is induced in response to erythrophagocytosis and, in the absence of iron deficiency, a portion of the iron derived from the ingested erythrocyte is retained within the macrophage as soluble cytosolic ferritin. With increasing amounts of storage iron within the macrophage, an increasing proportion of iron is stored within amorphous, insoluble masses as hemosiderin (see later). Based on studies with heat-damaged erythrocytes labeled with radioactive iron, the fraction of radioiron sequestered within the macrophage can vary from virtually none in association with iron deficiency to a maximum of almost 80% in the presence of bone marrow aplasia and a fully saturated plasma transferrin.

LIVER IRON STORAGE AND REGULATION OF SYSTEMIC IRON HOMEOSTASIS

The liver is both a major iron storage organ, sequestering iron in cytosolic ferritin and hemosiderin within hepatocytes and macrophages (Kupffer cells), and, as the principal source of plasma hepcidin, the central site for control of systemic iron homeostasis. The dual blood supply of the liver from the portal and systemic circulation may be an important feature, allowing monitoring of both plasma iron in the systemic circulation and newly absorbed iron in the portal circulation.[3] Hepatocytes can acquire iron from plasma transferrin via the transferrin cycle, from hemoglobin–haptoglobin and heme–hemopexin complexes via endocytosis after binding to CD163 and CD91 receptors, respectively; from lactoferrin, apparently by receptor-mediated endocytosis; and from plasma non–transferrin-bound iron (Fig. 33-6). Plasma non–transferrin-bound iron forms when the rate of iron influx into plasma exceeds the rate of iron acquisition by transferrin.[20] Plasma non–transferrin-bound plasma iron enters specific cells independently of the transferrin mechanism, particularly hepatocytes, cardiomyocytes, anterior pituitary cells, and pancreatic β cells, producing toxic accumulations in some forms of iron overload (see Chapter 34).[21] The specific routes for cellular uptake of plasma non–transferrin-bound iron have not been identified with certainty but may include divalent metal transporter 1 (DMT1), ZRT/IRT-like protein 14 (ZIP14), and L-type calcium channels.[3]

Within hepatocytes and other cells, cytosolic iron is present physiologically in low-molecular-weight forms destined for incorporation into functional compounds or, if present in amounts exceeding cellular requirements, for storage. As noted earlier, a cytosolic iron chaperone, poly (rC)-binding protein 1 (PCBP1),[12] delivers excess iron to ferritin, whose structure maintains large amounts of iron in solution in a compact yet bioavailable form, diffusely distributed within the cytosol. Cytosolic ferritin is a heteropolymer consisting of 24 subunits of heavy (H) and light (L) peptides that form a hollow sphere into which as many as 4500 atoms of iron may be deposited in an iron core composed of the hydrous ferric oxide mineral ferrihydrite ($5Fe_2O_3 \cdot 9H_20$).[5] Recent studies indicate that iron entry and exit from ferritin are in an equilibrium with the concentration of cytosolic iron.[22] Both uptake and release of iron appear to be intrinsic, autonomous properties of the ferritin molecule. When cytosolic iron is low, iron-containing ferritin particles are randomly dispersed in the cytoplasm. As cytosolic iron increases, concentrations of dispersed ferritin rise, and small clusters of ferritin begin to appear, still soluble and spread throughout the cytosol. With further increases in cytosolic iron, ferritin enters lysosomes by fusion of ferritin clusters with lysosomal membranes, by autophagocytosis, or both, forming siderosomes. Catabolism of ferritin within siderosomes leads to denaturation of ferritin protein subunits and aggregation of the ferritin iron cores, resulting in the formation of amorphous, insoluble masses of hemosiderin. If the extent of iron overload overwhelms the capacity of ferritin to store iron, ferritin iron may act as a pro-oxidant contributing to tissue injury. Production of hemosiderin seems to help protect against iron toxicity by sequestering the excess iron away from the cytosol, enclosed within siderosome membranes. As the total amount of tissue iron increases, the proportion stored as hemosiderin rises, from trace amounts in normal individuals to 90% or more with severe iron overload. Depending on the cellular type and iron supply and use, the half-life of cellular ferritin may range from less than 20 to 96 hours. Hemosiderin characteristically has a much slower cellular turnover than ferritin. Altogether, for short-term storage of iron, cytosolic iron is in rapid equilibrium with soluble, dispersed ferritin,[22] but for long-term sequestration, the aggregates of iron within hemosiderin undergo slow and limited exchange. Nonetheless, with phlebotomy or iron-chelating therapy, all of the iron within hemosiderin deposits eventually can be mobilized.

The liver functions as the central controller of systemic iron homeostasis by being the predominant synthetic source of hepcidin. The biologically active 25–amino acid peptide is produced by proteolytic processing of an 84–amino acid prepropeptide by furin.[8] After secretion, hepcidin circulates in plasma bound to α2-macroglobulin and is rapidly cleared by the kidneys or degraded after binding to ferroportin. As detailed earlier, hepcidin controls the entry of iron into plasma by decreasing the number of ferroportin channels available for iron export from macrophages, hepatocytes, and

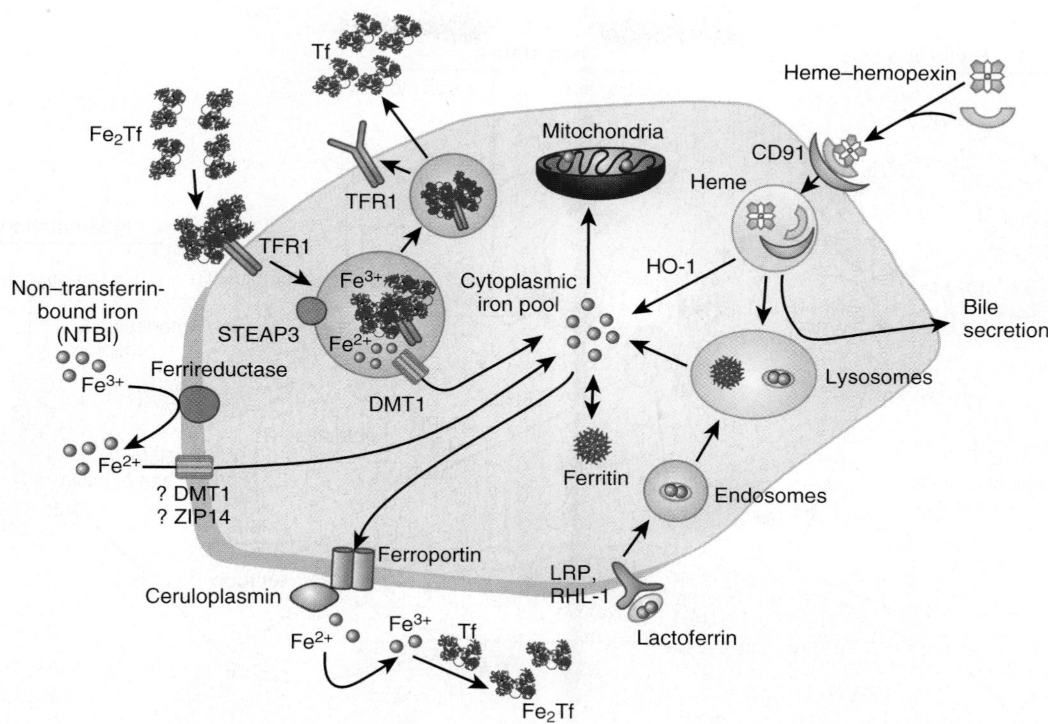

Figure 33-6 ACQUISITION, UTILIZATION, STORAGE, AND EXPORT OF IRON BY HEPATOCYTES. Hepatocytes can acquire iron from plasma transferrin (Tf) via the Tf cycle; from heme–hemopexin complexes via endocytosis after binding to CD91 receptors from lactoferrin, apparently by receptor-mediated endocytosis; and from plasma non–Tf-bound iron (NTBI). Iron is used for synthesis of heme and nonheme enzymes, with any excess stored in ferritin and hemosiderin. Iron is exported through ferroportin and oxidized by ceruloplasmin before being taken up by plasma Tf. See text for details. *DMT1,* Divalent metal transporter 1; *Fe_2Tf,* diferric transferrin; *FLVCR,* feline leukemia virus subgroup C cellular receptor; *HO-1,* heme oxygenase-1; *LRP,* low-density lipoprotein receptor-related protein; *RHL-1,* rat hepatic lectin-1 subunit of the asialoglycoprotein receptor; *STEAP3,* six-transmembrane epithelial antigen of the prostate 3; *TFR1,* transferrin receptor 1; *ZIP14,* Zrt- and Irt-like protein 14 (SLC39A14, solute carrier family 39, member 14). *(Modified from Graham RM, Chua ACG, Herbison CE, et al: Liver iron transport.* World J Gastroenterol *13:4725, 2007.)*

duodenal enterocytes. Plasma hepcidin concentrations increase with elevations in iron in plasma and in hepatocytes, and with infection and inflammation, decreasing plasma iron. Plasma hepcidin concentrations decrease with iron deficiency, hypoxia, and increased erythropoietic requirements for iron, increasing plasma iron.[8] The hepatocyte coordinates the congruent or conflicting influences of iron, infection, and erythropoietic demand to determine hepcidin secretion and thereby the systemic supply of iron. Because the amount of plasma iron is small and is replaced every 2 to 3 hours, changes in plasma hepcidin are followed rapidly by changes in plasma iron.

Regulation of hepcidin seems to be entirely transcriptional,[8] integrating signals for induction and inhibition of synthesis both from within and outside the hepatocyte. Intensive investigation has revealed a complex signaling network for transcriptional regulation of hepcidin[23] (summarized graphically in Fig. 33-7) that remains incompletely characterized and with some features that still require verification in human studies. The available evidence indicates that hepatic hepcidin synthesis is regulated by iron (hepatic iron stores, dietary iron, plasma iron in the systemic circulation), erythropoietic iron requirements, and inflammation and endoplasmic reticulum (ER) stress.[3,7,8,23,24]

Iron Regulation of Hepcidin Expression

Bone morphogenetic protein 6 (BMP6), a member of the transforming growth factor-β (TGFβ) superfamily, is the key endogenous regulator of hepcidin production (see Fig. 33-7). BMP6 seems to be primarily produced (1) by liver nonparenchymal cells in response to hepatocyte iron stores[4] and (2) by duodenal enterocytes in response to dietary iron.[25] BMP6 initiates a signaling cascade by binding to hemojuvelin, a membrane glycophosphatidlyinositol-linked BMP coreceptor essential for effective induction of hepcidin, and to BMP receptors on the surface of hepatocytes. BMP6 binding is followed by phosphorylation of sons of mothers against decapentaplegic (SMAD)1/5/8 and formation of the SMAD1/5/8–SMAD4 complex, which translocates to the nucleus and activates the promoter of the hepcidin gene (*HAMP*).[3,8,23,24] SMAD7 interferes with BMP6-HJV-SMAD–mediated hepcidin activation.[3] Hemojuvelin is a critical potentiator of the BMP6-SMAD regulatory pathway. Mutations in *HJV*, the gene for hemojuvelin, and in *HAMP* almost abolish synthesis of hepcidin, resulting in juvenile forms of hemochromatosis (types 2A and 2B, respectively; see Chapter 34) with severe iron loading. Neogenin, a DCC (deleted in colorectal cancer) family member, seems to stabilize hemojuvelin, thereby enhancing BMP6 signaling and hepcidin expression.[3,23] Furin, a proprotein convertase, cleaves membrane-bound hemojuvelin to produce a soluble form of hemojuvelin that acts as a competitive antagonist of membrane-bound HJV, inhibiting hepcidin activation.[3,23] TMPRSS6, a transmembrane serine protease, inhibits BMP6 induction of hepcidin synthesis by cleaving hemojuvelin from the cell membrane.[26] Inactivating mutations in the gene *TMPRSS6* produce high levels of hepcidin that are responsible for iron-refractory iron-deficiency anemia (see Chapter 34).[27]

Plasma iron, probably as diferric transferrin, is believed to modulate hepcidin synthesis through a distinct pathway that

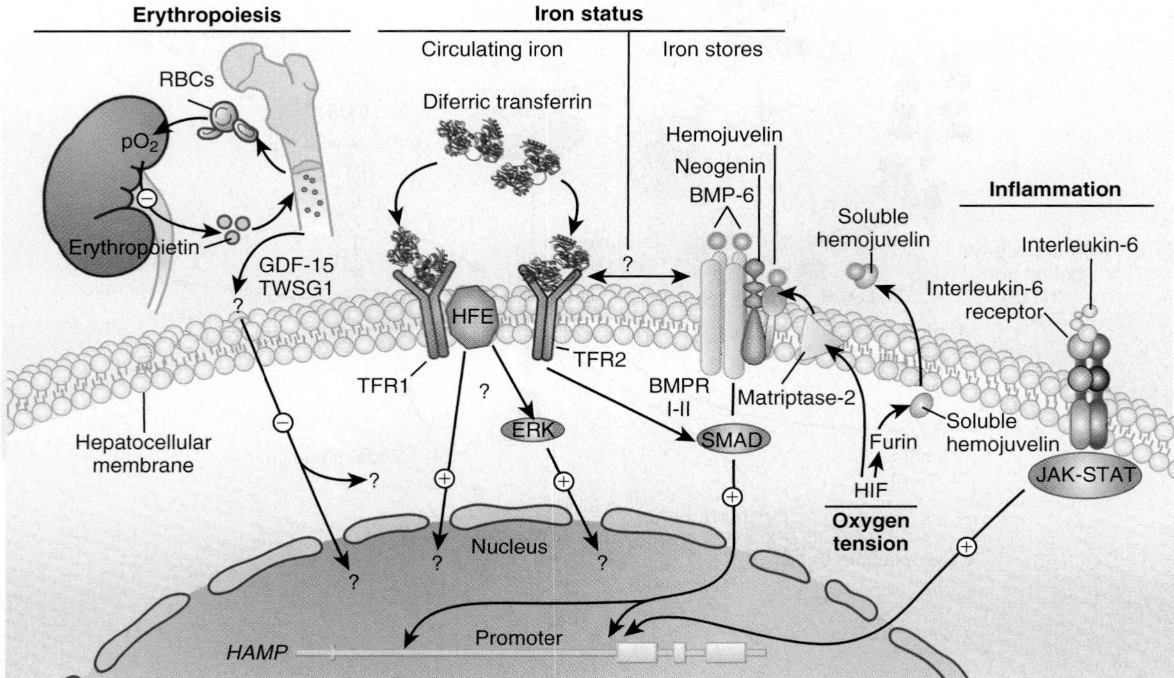

Figure 33-7 TRANSCRIPTIONAL REGULATION OF HEPCIDIN EXPRESSION IN HEPATOCYTES. Hepatic hepcidin synthesis is regulated by iron, erythropoietic iron requirements, inflammation, and endoplasmic reticulum (ER) stress. Bone morphogenetic protein 6 (BMP6) is the key endogenous regulator of hepcidin synthesis. BMP6 initiates a signaling cascade by binding to the BMP coreceptor hemojuvelin and to two type I and two type II BMP receptors (BMPR I-II) on the surface of hepatocytes. Neogenin may act to stabilize hemojuvelin. BMP6 binding is followed by phosphorylation of sons of mothers against decapentaplegic (SMAD)1/5/8 and formation of the SMAD1/5/8–SMAD4 complex, which translocates to the nucleus and activates the promoter of the hepcidin gene (*HAMP*). The soluble form of hemojuvelin, cleaved by furin, seems to compete for BMP binding with membrane-anchored hemojuvelin. SMAD7, stimulated by iron, interferes with SMAD4 hepcidin activation. TMPRSS6 (transmembrane protease, serine 6; matriptase-2) inhibits BMP6 induction of hepcidin synthesis by cleaving hemojuvelin from the cell membrane. HFE (the hemochromatosis protein) interacts with TfR1 and likely also with TfR2 to modulate hepcidin synthesis through the BMP6-HJV-SMAD pathway and, possibly, through alternative routes involving the extracellular signal–regulated kinase 1 and 2 (ERK1/2), mitogen-activated protein (MAP) kinases, and furin. Erythropoietin (EPO), growth differentiation factor15 (GDF15), and twisted gastrulation (TWSG1), have been proposed as mediators of hepcidin suppression by erythropoietic iron demand but the erythroid factors involved remain uncertain. The inflammatory cytokine IL6 induces hepcidin expression through a Janus kinase (JAK) signal transducer and activator of transcription (STAT) signaling pathway. Other cytokines and the BMP6-HJV-SMAD pathway may also be involved along with ER stress (not shown), possibly mediated by the transcription factor cyclic AMP response element–binding protein H (CREBH) or by the stress-inducible transcription factors CCAAT/enhancer-binding protein (C/EBP) homologous protein (CHOP) and CCAAT-enhancer-binding protein-alpha (C/EBPα). See text for details. *HIF,* Hypoxia inducible factor; *RBC,* red blood cell. *(Modified from Fleming RF, Ponka P. Iron overload in human disease.* N Engl J Med *366:348, 2012 and Kroot JJ, Tjalsma H, Fleming RE, et al: Hepcidin in human iron disorders: diagnostic implications.* Clin Chem *57:1650, 2011.)*

involves HFE, an atypical major histocompatibility complex class I protein that forms a complex with β2 microglobulin, and transferrin receptor 2 (see Fig. 33-7).[1,3,4,23] Mutations in the genes encoding these proteins, *HFE* (hemochromatosis gene) and *TFR2* (transferrin receptor 2 gene), respectively, are responsible for adult forms of hemochromatosis (types 1 and 3, respectively; see Chapter 34). In these adult forms of hemochromatosis, hepcidin is expressed but fails to be appropriately upregulated as iron stores increase; iron loading is generally less severe than in the juvenile forms. The means whereby these proteins influence hepcidin synthesis are uncertain but may involve binding of circulating diferric transferrin to transferrin receptor 1, displacing HFE to form a complex with diferric transferrin receptor 2. The complex then acts through the BMP6-HJV-SMAD pathway, alternative routes involving the extracellular signal–regulated kinase 1 and 2 (ERK1/2), mitogen-activated protein kinases, and furin, or some combination of these and other pathways.[3,23] Another level of control has been reported that involves a microRNA, short nucleotide hairpin loops that can interact in a complex with complementary sequences in the 3′- untranslated region of mRNA transcripts. The microRNA miR-122 binds to *HFE* and *HJV* mRNA, apparently increasing hepcidin expression.[28]

Erythropoietic Regulation of Hepcidin Expression

Increased erythropoietic demand for iron decreases hepatic hepcidin synthesis in a dominant manner that can override influences inducing hepcidin expression, such as iron overload and inflammation (see later). Patients with marked ineffective erythropoiesis, such as those with β-thalassemia intermedia, have very low or absent plasma hepcidin, increased iron absorption, and high plasma iron despite severe iron overload. Anemia and hypoxia decrease hepcidin expression, but these effects seem to be principally mediated by erythropoietic activity. In animal models, ablation of the erythroid bone marrow abolishes the effect of anemia. HIF-2 is apparently not involved. EPO, growth differentiation factor15 (GDF15), and twisted gastrulation

(TWSG1) (see Fig. 33-7) have been proposed as mediators of hepcidin suppression, but definitive identification of the erythroid factors involved is lacking.[3,4,23]

Inflammatory and Endoplasmic Reticulum Stress–Related Regulation of Hepcidin Expression

Inflammation increases plasma hepcidin, resulting in retention of iron within macrophages, reduced iron absorption, and hypoferremia.[8] The inflammatory cytokine interleukin-6 (IL-6) induces hepcidin expression (see Fig. 33-7). IL-6 activates the JAK signal transducer and activator of transcription (STAT) signaling pathway, stimulating hepcidin production through STAT3 interactions with a STAT3-binding element in the hepcidin promoter.[8,29] Other cytokines and the BMP6-HJV-SMAD pathway may also be involved. In addition, the acute inflammatory response is linked to endoplasmic reticulum (ER) stress (see Fig. 33-7), resulting from accumulation of unfolded or misfolded proteins with disruption of ER homeostasis. Hepcidin expression is induced by the transcription factor cyclic AMP response element–binding protein H (CREBH) or by the stress-inducible transcription factors CCAAT/enhancer-binding protein (C/EBP) homologous protein (CHOP) and CCAAT-enhancer-binding protein-α (C/EBPα).[3,4,8,29]

INTESTINAL IRON ABSORPTION

Because humans are unable to excrete excess iron, iron balance is physiologically maintained by the control of iron absorption in the proximal portion of the duodenum. Iron overload develops if regulation of iron balance is by passed by parenteral injections of iron or transfusion. Normally, only about 1 to 1.5 mg of iron of the 10 to 20 mg in the adult diet is absorbed to balance obligatory losses. Both nonheme iron and heme iron enter through the microvillous brush border at the apical (luminal) surface of the intestinal enterocytes (Fig. 33-8).[1] Nonheme dietary iron is predominantly ferric (Fe^{3+}) and, before absorption, is converted to ferrous (Fe^{2+}) iron either by the reducing action of other dietary constituents or by the action of brush border ferrireductases, such as membrane-associated duodenal cytochrome B (DCYTB) and likely others.[1] The ferrous iron is then absorbed through divalent metal transporter 1 (DMT1), the same ferrous iron transporter that provides an exit for iron from the endosome (see earlier). The exact means by which heme iron is absorbed are still uncertain, but when inside the enterocyte, inducible heme oxygenase 1 releases the iron from protoporphyrin, apparently into a common pathway with absorbed dietary nonheme iron.[1] In the enterocyte cytosol, the iron can be (1) retained for cellular requirements or stored in cytosolic ferritin and then lost when the enterocyte is exfoliated or (2) exported through ferroportin on the enterocyte basolateral membrane. Iron export through ferroportin requires oxidation by membrane-bound hephaestin or circulating ceruloplasmin to the ferric form for binding by plasma transferrin. Control of duodenal iron uptake is intricate, depending on both local and systemic factors that involving not only hepcidin control of ferroportin but also modulation of iron absorption through HIF-2α and H ferritin expression (see Fig. 33-8).[3] Expression of FPN1B, which lacks the iron-responsive element in its 5′ untranslated region, allows enterocytes to bypass iron regulatory protein repression of ferroportin iron export even when cells throughout the body are iron deficient.[30]

FUTURE DIRECTIONS

Remarkable progress has been made in unraveling the molecular mechanisms underlying systemic iron homeostasis, but much remains to be done. Little is known about developmental changes in the absorption, utilization, and storage of iron. Management of iron disposition within the systemic circulation needs further clarification, especially with respect to the basis for the dominant role of erythropoietic iron requirements and to the integration of intracellular and systemic regulatory elements. Control of iron balance needs more elucidation to determine the basis for individual susceptibilities both to iron deficiency and to iron overload. More insight is needed into organ-specific iron handling and into the iron biology of specific disease states. We need a better understanding of iron homeostasis in the three areas in the body that are outside systemic control: the central nervous system, the testis, and the retina. Nonetheless, a pivotal point has been reached when the advances already made will begin to yield therapeutic benefits from new approaches to biological therapy using agonists and antagonists to the components of the iron regulatory pathways summarized in this chapter.[3,8]

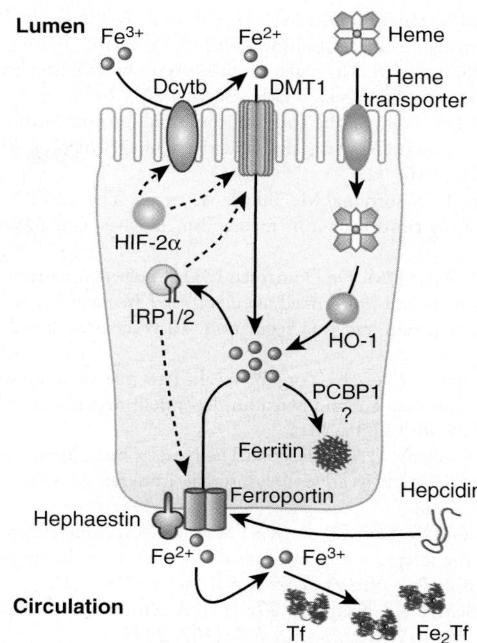

Figure 33-8 ABSORPTION OF DIETARY IRON BY THE INTESTINAL ENTEROCYTE. In the gastrointestinal lumen, dietary iron is presented to the enterocyte as heme or nonheme iron. Heme iron uptake is not well characterized, and the specific membrane transporter remains uncertain. After absorption, heme oxygenase 1 (HO-1) releases iron from heme into a common cytosolic pool. Nonheme dietary iron is predominantly ferric (Fe^{3+}) and, before absorption, is converted to ferrous (Fe^{2+}) iron either by the reducing action of other dietary constituents or by the action of brush border ferrireductases, such as membrane-associated duodenal cytochrome B (DCYTB) and likely others. Ferrous iron is then transported across the apical membrane by the divalent metal transporter 1 (DMT1) into the common cytosolic iron pool. Iron may be transported into plasma through ferroportin, regulated by hepcidin, with hephaestin or circulating ceruloplasmin acting as ferrioxidases. Cytosolic iron in excess of systemic needs may be carried to ferritin by the cytosolic iron chaperone poly (rC) binding protein 1 (PCBP1), retained and then lost when the enterocyte is shed. In addition to regulation by hepcidin, enterocyte iron absorption is modulated by hypoxia inducible factor 2α (HIF-2α), H ferritin and the iron regulatory proteins (IRP1 and 2). The enterocyte also derives iron from plasma transferrin (Tf) via the transferrin cycle (not shown). See text for details. *Fe_2Tf*, Diferric transferrin. *(Modified from Anderson GJ, Frazer DM, McLaren GD: Iron absorption and metabolism.* Curr Opin Gastroenterol *25:129, 2009.)*

REFERENCES

1. Andrews NC: Forging a field: The golden age of iron biology. *Blood* 112:219, 2008.
2. Beaumont C, Delaby C: Recycling iron in normal and pathological states. *Semin Hematol* 46:328, 2009.

3. Hentze MW, Muckenthaler MU, Galy B, et al: Two to tango: Regulation of Mammalian iron metabolism. *Cell* 142:24, 2010.
4. Zhang AS, Enns CA: Molecular mechanisms of normal iron homeostasis. *Hematology Am Soc Hematol Educ Program* 207, 2009.
5. Arosio P, Levi S: Cytosolic and mitochondrial ferritins in the regulation of cellular iron homeostasis and oxidative damage. *Biochim Biophys Acta* 1800:783, 2010.
6. Moroishi T, Nishiyama M, Takeda Y, et al: The FBXL5-IRP2 axis is integral to control of iron metabolism in vivo. *Cell Metab* 14:339, 2011.
7. Kaplan J, Ward DM, De Domenico I: The molecular basis of iron overload disorders and iron-linked anemias. *Int J Hematol* 93:14, 2011.
8. Ganz T: Hepcidin and iron regulation, 10 years later. *Blood* 117:4425, 2011.
9. De Domenico I, Lo E, Yang B, et al: The role of ubiquitination in hepcidin-independent and hepcidin-dependent degradation of ferroportin. *Cell Metab* 14:635, 2011.
10. Dong XP, Cheng X, Mills E, et al: The type IV mucolipidosis-associated protein TRPML1 is an endolysosomal iron release channel. *Nature* 455:992, 2008.
11. Richardson DR, Lane DJ, Becker EM, et al: Mitochondrial iron trafficking and the integration of iron metabolism between the mitochondrion and cytosol. *Proc Natl Acad Sci U S A* 107:10775, 2010.
12. Shi H, Bencze KZ, Stemmler TL, et al: A cytosolic iron chaperone that delivers iron to ferritin. *Science* 320:1207, 2008.
13. Bullock GC, Delehanty LL, Talbot AL, et al: Iron control of erythroid development by a novel aconitase-associated regulatory pathway. *Blood* 116:97, 2010.
14. Forejtnikova H, Vieillevoye M, Zermati Y, et al: Transferrin receptor 2 is a component of the erythropoietin receptor complex and is required for efficient erythropoiesis. *Blood* 116:5357, 2010.
15. Liu S, Bhattacharya S, Han A, et al: Haem-regulated eIF2alpha kinase is necessary for adaptive gene expression in erythroid precursors under the stress of iron deficiency. *Br J Haematol* 143:129, 2008.
16. Zhang DL, Senecal T, Ghosh MC, et al: Hepcidin regulates ferroportin expression and intracellular iron homeostasis of erythroblasts. *Blood* 118:2868, 2011.
17. Keel SB, Doty RT, Yang Z, et al: A heme export protein is required for red blood cell differentiation and iron homeostasis. *Science* 319:825, 2008.
18. Lang KS, Lang PA, Bauer C, et al: Mechanisms of suicidal erythrocyte death. *Cell Physiol Biochem* 15:195, 2005.
19. Soe-Lin S, Apte SS, Mikhael MR, et al: Both Nramp1 and DMT1 are necessary for efficient macrophage iron recycling. *Exp Hematol* 38:609, 2010.
20. Brissot P, Ropert M, Le Lan C, et al: Non-transferrin bound iron: A key role in iron overload and iron toxicity. *Biochim Biophys Acta* 1820:403, 2012;
21. Brittenham GM: Iron-chelating therapy for transfusional iron overload. *N Engl J Med* 364:146, 2011.
22. De Domenico I, Vaughn MB, Li L, et al: Ferroportin-mediated mobilization of ferritin iron precedes ferritin degradation by the proteasome. *EMBO J* 25:5396, 2006.
23. Pietrangelo A: Hepcidin in human iron disorders: Therapeutic implications. *J Hepatol* 54:173, 2011.
24. Camaschella C, Strati P: Recent advances in iron metabolism and related disorders. *Intern Emerg Med* 5:393, 2010.
25. Arndt S, Maegdefrau U, Dorn C, et al: Iron-induced expression of bone morphogenic protein 6 in intestinal cells is the main regulator of hepatic hepcidin expression in vivo. *Gastroenterology* 138:372, 2010.
26. Zhang AS, Anderson SA, Wang J, et al: Suppression of hepatic hepcidin expression in response to acute iron deprivation is associated with an increase of matriptase-2 protein. *Blood* 117:1687, 2011.
27. Finberg KE: Iron-refractory iron deficiency anemia. *Semin Hematol* 46:378, 2009.
28. Castoldi M, Vujic Spasic M, Altamura S, et al: The liver-specific microRNA miR-122 controls systemic iron homeostasis in mice. *J Clin Invest* 121:1386, 2011.
29. Wessling-Resnick M: Iron homeostasis and the inflammatory response. *Annu Rev Nutr* 30:105, 2010.
30. Zhang DL, Hughes RM, Ollivierre-Wilson H, et al: A ferroportin transcript that lacks an iron-responsive element enables duodenal and erythroid precursor cells to evade translational repression. *Cell Metab* 9:461, 2009.

CHAPTER 34

DISORDERS OF IRON HOMEOSTASIS: IRON DEFICIENCY AND OVERLOAD

Gary M. Brittenham

Iron is an essential nutrient required by every human cell. Both decreases and increases in body iron may be clinically important. If too little iron is available (iron deficiency), limitations on the synthesis of physiologically active iron-containing compounds can have harmful consequences. If too much iron accumulates (iron overload) and exceeds the body's capacity for safe transport and storage, iron toxicity may produce widespread organ damage and death. This chapter focuses on the clinical application of recent remarkable progress in understanding the molecular mechanisms underlying iron homeostasis.

Iron disorders are principally abnormalities in the amount or distribution of body iron. A fundamental advance has been the recognition that the interaction of hepcidin, the iron-regulatory hormone, with ferroportin, the cellular iron export channel, is primarily responsible for the quantity and tissue disposition of body iron. Hepcidin controls iron absorption, utilization, and storage by binding to and inducing the degradation of ferroportin, decreasing iron entry into plasma from macrophages, hepatocytes, and intestinal enterocytes (see box on Control of Iron Homeostasis by Hepcidin and Ferroportin and Chapter 33). Hepcidin expression is suppressed with iron deficiency, hypoxia, or increased erythropoietic demand but stimulated with iron overload, inflammation, or infection. Genetic and acquired disorders with a deficiency in hepcidin production or with ferroportin resistance to hepcidin action produce iron overload. Hepcidin excess from genetic causes produces iron-deficiency anemia, but acquired forms, such as those associated with infection or inflammation, result in iron sequestration and anemia.

LABORATORY EVALUATION OF IRON STATUS

Because iron disorders primarily produce quantitative abnormalities in the amount and tissue distribution of iron, laboratory evaluation of iron status relies on indicators of iron supply and storage. The principal routes of iron movement, the amounts and distribution of the major iron pools, and the sites of hepcidin control of iron entry into plasma are shown in Fig. 33-1. The continuum of changes with increased or decreased body iron content is illustrated in Fig. 34-1, showing schematically the amounts of erythroid iron and storage iron together with the division of iron stores between hepatocyte and reticuloendothelial macrophage deposits and with characteristic values for some clinically available indicators of iron status.

Body iron supply and stores can be evaluated by both direct and indirect means, but no single indicator or combination of indicators is ideal for evaluation of iron status in all clinical circumstances. As body iron content decreases from the iron-replete normal to the amounts found in iron-deficiency anemia or as it increases to the magnitudes found in the various forms of iron overload, each available measure reflects in a different manner the continuum of changes shown in Fig. 34-1. In addition, each indicator may be affected by coexisting conditions that modulate hepcidin expression, such as infection, inflammation, malignancy, ineffective erythropoiesis, hypoxemia, liver disease, and malnutrition (see box on Control of Iron Homeostasis by Hepcidin and Ferroportin and Chapter 33).

Direct Measures

The direct measures of body iron status yield quantitative, specific, and sensitive determinations of body or tissue iron stores. Quantitative phlebotomy provides a direct measure of total mobilizable storage iron. Quantitative phlebotomy is inapplicable to most anemic disorders but occasionally is useful in the diagnostic evaluation of some forms of iron overload (e.g., in patients with hereditary hemochromatosis who do not undergo liver biopsy). Bone marrow (BM) aspiration and biopsy can provide information about (1) macrophage storage iron by semiquantitative grading of marrow hemosiderin stained with Prussian blue (Fig. 34-2) or, if needed, by chemical measurement of nonheme iron; (2) iron supply to erythroid precursors by determining the proportion and morphology of marrow sideroblasts (i.e., normoblasts with visible aggregates of iron in the cytoplasm); and (3) general morphologic features of hematopoiesis. BM aspiration and biopsy are useful in studies of iron deficiency but of limited applicability in the evaluation of iron overload because no information about the extent of hepatocyte iron deposition is provided. In the evaluation of iron overload, liver biopsy is the best direct test for assessing iron deposition, permitting quantitative measurement of the nonheme iron concentration and histochemical examination of the pattern of iron accumulation in hepatocytes and macrophages (Kupffer cells).

Direct methods for assessing iron status have the disadvantages of being invasive procedures, with their attendant discomfort, lack of acceptability to patients, and, in the case of liver biopsy, risk. A variety of noninvasive means of measuring tissue iron stores has been developed and applied in clinical studies, including determination of hepatic magnetic susceptibility, computed tomography, and magnetic resonance imaging (MRI). MRI, the most widely available method, can provide information about iron deposition in the liver, spleen, heart, pancreas, and brain.[7] When available as appropriately calibrated and validated techniques, these noninvasive methods are helpful in the diagnosis and management of iron overload but lack the accuracy required to detect iron deficiency.

Indirect Measures

Indirect measures of body iron status have the advantages of ease and convenience but all are subject to extraneous influences and lack specificity, sensitivity, or both. When used to estimate body iron stores, all of the available indirect measures are influenced not only by total body iron stores but also by the effects of acute or chronic changes in plasma hepcidin (see box on Control of Iron Homeostasis by Hepcidin and Ferroportin). Assays for urinary and plasma hepcidin are not yet generally available but are under development and likely to be helpful in the clinical evaluation of patients with disorders of iron homeostasis.[8]

Measurement of the plasma ferritin concentration provides the most useful indirect estimate of body iron stores.[9] The small amounts of ferritin secreted into the circulation can be measured by immunoassay and have a logarithmic relationship to body iron stores in healthy persons. In the absence of complicating factors, plasma ferritin concentrations decrease with depletion of storage iron and

Control of Iron Homeostasis by Hepcidin and Ferroportin

Hepcidin functions as the chief controller of body iron supply and storage by interacting with ferroportin, a transmembrane protein that is the only known iron exporter in humans[1-3] (see Chapter 33). Hepcidin binds to ferroportin, inducing its internalization and degradation, thereby inhibiting iron efflux from the principal sources of plasma iron—macrophages, duodenal enterocytes, and hepatocytes (see Fig. 33-1). Under physiologic conditions, hepatic hepcidin production coordinates body iron supply with iron need.[1-3] If body iron stores expand, hepatic hepcidin production increases. Increments in plasma hepcidin reduce the amount of ferroportin in cell membranes, causing a prompt fall in plasma iron concentration by decreasing macrophage release of iron derived from senescent red blood cells, diminishing delivery of iron from enterocytes absorbing dietary iron, and inhibiting release of iron stored in hepatocytes. Conversely, if body iron stores diminish, hepatic hepcidin production decreases. Decrements in plasma hepcidin concentration increase the amount of ferroportin, producing a rise in plasma iron concentration as a consequence of enhanced delivery from macrophages, increased dietary iron absorption from enterocytes, and mobilization of storage iron from hepatocytes. In addition to the effects of body iron stores, hepcidin production is stimulated by infection, inflammation, or malignancy and inhibited by hypoxemia or increased erythropoietic demand. The influence of infection and inflammation on hepcidin and ferroportin expression link iron sequestration to host defense,[2,4] and the interaction with erythropoiesis connects iron supply to red blood cell production.[2,5] Depending on clinical circumstances, the effects of inflammation or erythropoiesis on hepatic hepcidin synthesis may predominate over those of body iron stores. Liver disease and malnutrition may also impair hepcidin expression. Although hepcidin is the central regulator of iron homeostasis, hypoxia inducible factor 2-α (HIF2-α) and H-ferritin modulate intestinal iron absorption.[6]

increase with storage iron accumulation (see box on Plasma Ferritin Concentrations). Measurement of the plasma transferrin receptor concentration provides a useful means of detecting tissue iron deficiency.[10] A majority of plasma transferrin receptors are derived from the erythroid marrow, and their concentration is determined primarily by erythroid marrow activity. Whereas decreased levels of circulating soluble transferrin receptor are found in patients with erythroid hypoplasia (aplastic anemia, chronic renal failure), increased levels are present in patients with erythroid hyperplasia (thalassemia major, sickle cell anemia, anemia with ineffective erythropoiesis, chronic hemolytic anemia). Iron deficiency also increases soluble transferrin

Plasma Ferritin Concentrations

Plasma ferritin concentrations are helpful in the detection of both iron deficiency and iron overload.[9] Plasma ferritin concentrations decline with storage iron depletion; a plasma ferritin concentration less than 12 mg/L is virtually diagnostic of absence of iron stores. The only known conditions that may lower the plasma ferritin concentration independently of a decrease in iron stores are hypothyroidism and ascorbate deficiency, but these conditions only rarely cause problems in clinical interpretation. Increased plasma ferritin concentrations may indicate increased storage iron, but a number of disorders may increase the plasma ferritin level independently of the body iron store. Plasma ferritin is an acute-phase reactant with increased ferritin synthesis a nonspecific response that is part of the general pattern of the systemic effects of inflammation.[4,9] Thus, fever, acute infections, rheumatoid arthritis, and other chronic inflammatory disorders elevate the plasma ferritin concentration. Both acute and chronic damage to the liver, as well as to other ferritin-rich tissues, may increase plasma ferritin concentration through an inflammatory process or by releasing tissue ferritins from damaged parenchymal cells.[9]

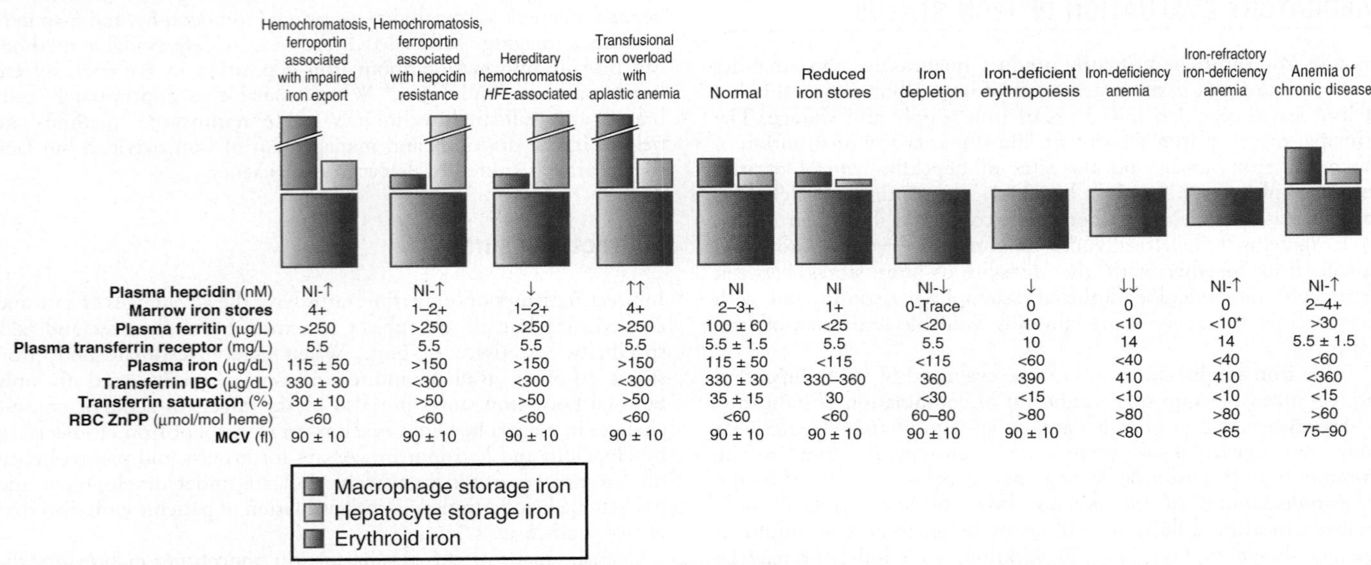

	Hemochromatosis, ferroportin associated with impaired iron export	Hemochromatosis, ferroportin associated with hepcidin resistance	Hereditary hemochromatosis *HFE*-associated	Transfusional iron overload with aplastic anemia	Normal	Reduced iron stores	Iron depletion	Iron-deficient erythropoiesis	Iron-deficiency anemia	Iron-refractory iron-deficiency anemia	Anemia of chronic disease
Plasma hepcidin (nM)	Nl-↑	Nl-↑	↓	↑↑	Nl	Nl	Nl-↓	↓	↓↓	Nl-↑	Nl-↑
Marrow iron stores	4+	1–2+	1–2+	4+	2–3+	1+	0-Trace	0	0	0	2–4+
Plasma ferritin (μg/L)	>250	>250	>250	>250	100 ± 60	<25	<20	10	<10	<10*	>30
Plasma transferrin receptor (mg/L)	5.5	5.5	5.5	5.5	5.5 ± 1.5	5.5	5.5	10	14	14	5.5 ± 1.5
Plasma iron (μg/dL)	115 ± 50	>150	>150	>150	115 ± 50	<115	<115	<60	<40	<40	<60
Transferrin IBC (μg/dL)	330 ± 30	<300	<300	<300	330 ± 30	330–360	360	390	410	410	<360
Transferrin saturation (%)	30 ± 10	>50	>50	>50	35 ± 15	30	<30	<15	<10	<10	<15
RBC ZnPP (μmol/mol heme)	<60	<60	<60	<60	<60	<60	60–80	>80	>80	>80	>60
MCV (fl)	90 ± 10	90 ± 10	90 ± 10	90 ± 10	90 ± 10	90 ± 10	90 ± 10	90 ± 10	<80	<65	75–90

Figure 34-1 CONTINUUM OF CHANGES IN THE AMOUNTS OF ERYTHROID IRON AND OF HEPATOCYTE AND RETICULOENDOTHELIAL MACROPHAGE STORAGE IRON IN THE PRESENCE OF INCREASED OR DECREASED BODY IRON CONTENT. Characteristic values for some clinically available indicators of iron status are shown. In iron overload, the *diagonal lines* are intended to illustrate increases in excess storage iron from the normal range of 1 g or less to as much as 40 to 50 g. *, Plasma ferritin may be normal or increased after administration of parenteral iron; *HFE,* gene for the hemochromatosis protein, HFE; *IBC,* iron-binding capacity; *MCV,* mean corpuscular volume; *RBC,* red blood cell; *ZnPP,* zinc protoporphyrin.

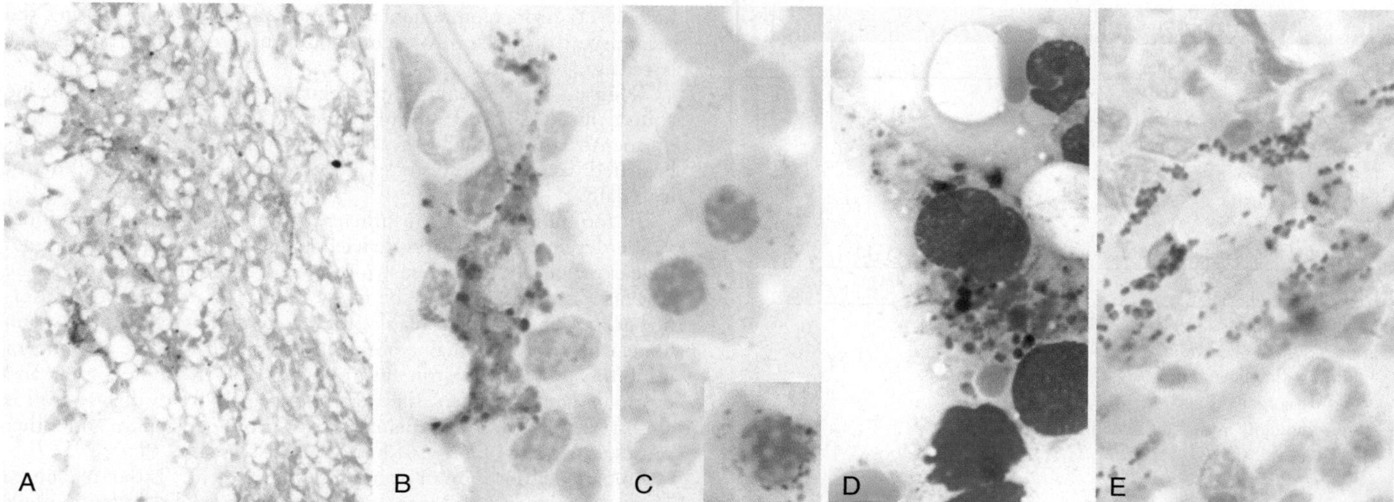

Figure 34-2 ASSESSMENT OF IRON STORES ON A BONE MARROW ASPIRATE. Iron stores are usually assessed on the aspirate as opposed to the biopsy because the decalcification procedure required for processing the biopsy leaches out the iron and can lead to a false conclusion of absent stores. On the aspirate, a Prussian blue stain is usually used to evaluate iron. This can demonstrate iron stores (blue reaction product), particularly in the cytoplasm of macrophages and histiocytes **(A** and **B)**. Iron can also be seen in the cytoplasm of some nucleated red blood cells (tiny blue cytoplasmic specks), which would allow these cells to be designated *sideroblasts* **(C)**. These are in contrast to red blood cell precursors with abnormal iron accumulation around the nucleus, or "ring sideroblasts" **(C,** *insert*). Hemosiderin containing iron can be seen on the Wright-stained aspirate smears as a dark brown or black pigment in histiocytes **(D)**, but generally an iron stain is needed to confirm the presence of iron stores. When parenteral iron therapy is administered, the marrow aspirate can sometimes show coarse iron deposits frequently in long streaks **(E)**. This is most likely iron in endothelial cells; it does not necessarily indicate marrow iron is present.

receptor concentrations. The plasma transferrin receptor concentration reflects the total body mass of tissue receptor; thus, in the absence of other conditions causing erythroid hyperplasia, an increase in plasma transferrin receptor concentration provides a sensitive, quantitative measure of tissue iron deficiency.[10] In particular, measurement of plasma transferrin receptor concentration may help differentiate between the anemia of iron deficiency and the anemia associated with chronic inflammatory disorders. Although the plasma ferritin concentration may be disproportionately elevated in relation to iron stores in patients with inflammation or liver disease, the plasma transferrin receptor concentration seems to be less affected by these disorders and to provide a more reliable laboratory indicator of iron deficiency.[10]

The erythrocyte zinc protoporphyrin provides an indicator of iron supply to erythroid precursors. In heme biosynthesis, the final reaction is chelation of a ferrous ion by protoporphyrin IX. If no iron is available, zinc is chelated instead to form zinc protoporphyrin. Because zinc protoporphyrin formed during development persists throughout the lifespan of the red blood cell (RBC), the blood concentration changes only as new cells are formed and old cells are destroyed, providing a retrospective view of iron supply over the preceding several weeks. Levels also are increased in many sideroblastic anemias and especially with chronic lead poisoning. The test is of no value in detecting iron overload.

Measurements of the proportion of hypochromic circulating RBCs and the hemoglobin content of reticulocytes (CHr) are possible with some hematology analyzers and offer new means of detecting restriction of the iron supply for erythropoiesis.[11] Measurement of urinary iron excretion with chelating agents, usually either deferoxamine or diethylenetriamine pentaacetic acid, offers another means of assessing body iron stores. This test is not helpful for detecting iron deficiency because of the overlap between values in persons with normal and those with decreased iron stores; it is used occasionally for the evaluation of iron overload.

Examination of peripheral blood by measurements of hemoglobin concentration, hematocrit, RBC indices, RBC volume distribution, and reticulocyte count and by inspection of erythrocyte morphology reveals abnormalities only after depletion of iron stores restricts the availability of iron for erythropoiesis. The changes are not specific for iron deficiency and may be found in other conditions with defective hemoglobin synthesis, such as thalassemia, infection, inflammation, liver disease, and malignancy. Iron overload does not produce any diagnostic abnormalities in the peripheral blood.

IRON DEFICIENCY

Iron deficiency is a decrease in the amount of body iron resulting from a sustained increase in iron requirements over iron supply. The continuum of decreased body iron is shown in Fig. 34-1. Three successive stages of iron lack can be distinguished. A decrement in storage iron without a decline in the level of functional iron compounds is termed *iron depletion* (see Fig. 34-1). After iron stores are exhausted, lack of iron limits the production of hemoglobin and other metabolically active compounds that require iron as a constituent or cofactor. Iron-deficient erythropoiesis (see Fig. 34-1) develops, although the effect on hemoglobin production may be insufficient to be detected by the standards used to differentiate normal from anemic states. Further diminution in the body iron produces frank iron-deficiency anemia (see Fig. 34-1). Iron regulation of erythroid differentiation coordinates the rate of erythropoiesis with iron availability. Iron deficiency reduces the responsiveness of erythroid progenitors to erythropoietin, apparently through an iron–aconitase–isocitrate pathway.[5,12] With a lack of iron, decreased erythroid utilization for RBC production helps preserve the supply of iron for vital functions in other tissues.

Epidemiology

Iron deficiency is the most common cause of anemia in the United States and worldwide. In the United States, adequacy of bioavailable iron in the diet, together with food fortification and the widespread use of iron supplements, has reduced the overall prevalence and severity of iron deficiency, but iron nutrition remains a problem in some subpopulations, especially toddlers, adolescent girls, women of childbearing age, and some minority groups. Without iron supplementation, most women will become iron deficient during pregnancy. Globally, 30% to 70% of the populations in developing countries are

Table 34-1 Causes of Iron Deficiency

Increased Iron Requirements
Blood loss
Gastrointestinal tract
Genitourinary tract
Respiratory tract
Blood donation
Growth
Pregnancy and lactation
Inadequate Iron Supply
Dietary insufficiency of bioavailable iron
Impaired absorption of iron
Intestinal malabsorption
Gastric surgery
Iron-refractory iron-deficiency anemia

iron deficient, with the highest prevalence among persons who have diets low in bioavailable iron, who have chronic gastrointestinal blood loss as a result of helminthic infection, or both.

Etiology and Pathogenesis

The foremost task in the evaluation of patients with iron deficiency is identifying and treating the underlying cause of the imbalance between iron requirements and supply that is responsible for the lack of iron (Table 34-1). Overall, the iron requirement for an individual includes not only the iron needed to replenish physiologic losses and meet the demands of growth and pregnancy but also any additional amounts needed to replace pathologic losses. Physiologic iron losses generally are restricted to the small amounts of iron contained in the urine, bile, and sweat; shedding of iron-containing cells from the intestine, urinary tract, and skin; occult gastrointestinal blood loss; and, in women, uterine losses during menstruation and pregnancy. In normal men, the daily basal iron loss is slightly less than 1.0 mg/day. In normal menstruating women, the daily basal iron loss is approximately 1.5 mg/day. The median total iron loss with pregnancy is approximately 500 mg, or almost 2 mg/day over the 280 days of gestation.

The most common pathologic cause of increased iron requirements leading to iron deficiency is blood loss.[13] In men and postmenopausal women, iron deficiency almost inevitably signifies gastrointestinal blood loss. Within the gastrointestinal tract, any hemorrhagic lesion may result in blood loss, and the responsible lesion may be asymptomatic.[13] Iron deficiency often is the first sign of an occult gastrointestinal malignancy or other unrecognized conditions such as coeliac disease, or autoimmune, atrophic, or *Helicobacter pylori* gastritis. Chronic ingestion of drugs such as alcohol, salicylates, steroids, and nonsteroidal antiinflammatory drugs may cause or contribute to blood loss. Worldwide, the most frequent cause of gastrointestinal blood loss is hookworm infection, but other helminthic infections, such as *Schistosoma mansoni* and *Schistosoma japonicum,* and severe *Trichuris trichiura* infection also may be responsible.

In women of childbearing age, genitourinary blood loss with menstruation adds to iron requirements.[13] Other less frequent causes of genitourinary bleeding may be involved, including chronic hemoglobinuria and hemosiderinuria resulting from paroxysmal nocturnal hemoglobinuria or from chronic intravascular hemolysis. Uncommonly, respiratory tract blood loss resulting from chronic recurrent hemoptysis of any cause produces iron deficiency.

In infants, children, and adolescents, the need for iron for growth may exceed the supply available from diet and stores.[14] Premature infants, who have a lower birth weight and a more rapid postnatal rate of growth, are at high risk for iron deficiency unless given iron supplements. With rapid growth during the first year of life, the body weights of term infants normally triple, and iron requirements are at high levels. Iron requirements decline as growth slows during the second year of life and into childhood but rise again with the adolescent growth spurt.

Without supplemental iron, pregnancy entails the net loss of the equivalent of 1200 to 1500 mL of blood.[13] After delivery, resumption of menstruation usually is delayed for months. If the infant is breastfed, lactation necessitates an intake of about 0.5 to 1.0 mg of iron daily.

In some instances, an insufficient supply of iron may contribute to the development of iron deficiency. In infants or in women who have experienced heavy menstrual losses or multiple pregnancies, the risk of iron deficiency may be further increased by diets with insufficient amounts of bioavailable iron, such as those with little or no heme iron and with small amounts of enhancers or large amounts of inhibitors of nonheme iron absorption. For older children, men, and postmenopausal women, the restricted availability of dietary iron is almost never the sole explanation for iron deficiency, and other causes, especially blood loss, must be considered.

Impaired absorption of iron in itself infrequently is the sole source of iron deficiency.[13] Nonetheless, in patients in whom evaluation fails to identify a source of blood loss, as well as in those unresponsive to oral iron therapy, coeliac disease, autoimmune, atrophic, or *H. pylori* gastritis may be responsible. Iron deficiency frequently complicates gastric surgery, such as partial or total gastric resection or gastroenterostomy for bypass of the duodenum.

Increased iron requirements and an inadequate supply of iron often work in concert to produce iron deficiency. Infants fed cow's milk receive a diet that not only contains small amounts of iron of low bioavailability but also increases iron losses by causing gastrointestinal bleeding.[14] Patients with ulcer disease and increased gastrointestinal blood loss may habitually take antacids or proton pump inhibitors, which diminish dietary iron absorption.[13]

An uncommon heritable cause of iron deficiency is iron-refractory iron-deficiency anemia (IRIDA), an autosomal recessive disorder with severe iron-deficiency anemia and increased concentrations of plasma hepcidin.[15] The anemia is unresponsive to orally administered iron and incompletely responsive to parenteral iron. Mutations in *TMPRSS6,* a gene that normally inhibits hepcidin production, are responsible (see Chapter 33).

Clinical Presentation

Patients with iron deficiency may present with (1) no signs or symptoms, coming to medical attention only because of abnormalities noted on laboratory tests; (2) features of the underlying disorder responsible for the development of iron deficiency; (3) manifestations common to all anemias; or (4) one or more of the few signs and symptoms considered highly specific for iron deficiency, namely, pagophagia, koilonychia, and blue sclerae. In addition, a high prevalence of iron deficiency with or without anemia has been reported among patients with the restless legs syndrome, a neurologic disorder characterized by a distressing need or urge to move the legs (akathisia).[16]

An uncomplicated depletion of storage iron generally is not associated with signs or symptoms, although patients without iron reserves will not respond as rapidly to an increased need for iron resulting from blood loss, growth, or pregnancy. Iron-deficiency anemia produces the signs and symptoms common to all anemias, which are pallor, palpitations, tinnitus, headache, irritability, weakness, dizziness, easy fatigability, and other vague and nonspecific complaints. The prominence of these signs depends on the degree and rate of development of the anemia. With greater severity, anemia becomes increasingly debilitating as work capacity and tolerance of physical exertion are restricted and eventually can produce cardiorespiratory failure and even death.

Iron deficiency may produce clinical manifestations independent of anemia. Epithelial tissues have high iron requirements because of rapid rates of growth and turnover and thus are affected in many patients with chronic iron deficiency. Glossitis, angular stomatitis, postcricoid esophageal web or stricture (which may become malignant), and gastric atrophy may develop. Pagophagia, a variant of pica in which ice is the substance obsessively consumed, is a behavioral abnormality that is considered to be a highly specific symptom of iron deficiency, resolving within a few days to 2 weeks after beginning iron therapy. Iron deficiency has other nonhematologic consequences, including impaired immunity and resistance to infection, diminished exercise tolerance and work performance, and a variety of behavioral and neuropsychologic abnormalities. In patients with iron deficiency and heart failure, clinical trials have provided evidence that treatment with intravenous iron improves outcomes.[17]

Laboratory Evaluation

A characteristic sequence of changes in the clinically useful indications of iron status occurs as body iron decreases from the iron-replete normal to the levels found in iron-deficiency anemia. This sequence is illustrated in Fig. 34-1. The patterns shown develop in the absence of complicating factors that increase plasma hepcidin, such as infection, inflammation, liver disease, malignancy, or other disorders (see box on Iron Deficiency and Coexisting Disorders). Initially, as a result of any of the causes listed in Table 34-1, iron requirements exceed the available supply of iron. Iron is mobilized from body stores, and iron absorption is increased. If the amounts of iron available from body reserves and absorption are inadequate, storage iron depletion follows. Exhaustion of iron reserves then results in an inadequate supply of iron to the developing erythroid cell, and iron-deficient erythropoiesis commences. As hemoglobin production becomes restricted, frank iron-deficiency anemia develops (see box on Plasma Iron Concentration and Transferrin Saturation).

Chronic, long-standing iron-deficiency anemia may produce severe microcytosis and hypochromia, with very pale, distorted RBCs and dramatic reductions in the mean corpuscular volume and mean corpuscular hemoglobin (Fig. 34-3). In contrast, some patients with mild iron-deficiency anemia may have erythrocyte morphology and indices indistinguishable from values found in normal, iron-replete individuals. Nonetheless, laboratory evaluation of uncomplicated iron deficiency in otherwise healthy persons usually is not difficult, and the characteristic patterns of indicators of body iron status shown in Fig. 34-1 typically are diagnostic. Diagnostically, early or mild iron deficiency must be considered in the workup of normocytic as well as microcytic anemia.

Iron Deficiency and Coexisting Disorders

Detection of iron deficiency in the presence of chronic infectious, inflammatory, or malignant disorders that increase plasma hepcidin is more problematic than in the absence of such disorders.[4] Even if iron lack contributes to the anemia of chronic disorders, the increase in plasma hepcidin will lead to a fall in the transferrin concentration (or total iron-binding capacity) and an increase in the plasma ferritin concentration.[9,18] Because the serum transferrin receptor concentration is less affected by inflammation, its measurement usually can determine whether iron stores are absent.[10] If uncertainty remains, BM examination is definitive. If iron deficiency is present, iron stores are absent; if the anemia of chronic disorders alone is responsible, iron stores are present and typically increased (see Figure 34-1).

Plasma Iron Concentration and Transferrin Saturation

Plasma iron concentration and transferrin saturation, which equals the ratio of plasma iron to total iron-binding capacity, provide a measure of current iron supply to tissues. After storage iron is depleted, the serum iron concentration falls; a transferrin saturation less than 16% often is used as the criterion for iron-deficient erythropoiesis.[13] In contrast, plasma iron concentration and transferrin saturation are not reliably elevated with increased iron stores within macrophages, as occurs initially with transfusional iron overload, although the transferrin saturation may increase with parenchymal iron loading. Interpretation of the transferrin saturation is complicated by substantial circadian fluctuations in plasma iron concentration with day-to-day variations of 30% or greater. Furthermore, the plasma iron concentration is lowered by ascorbate deficiency and by conditions that increase plasma hepcidin, such as infection, inflammation, malignancy.[4] Plasma iron is raised by iron ingestion and by conditions that decrease plasma hepcidin, such as hypoxemia, erythroid hyperplasia with ineffective erythropoiesis, and liver disease.[3]

Differential Diagnosis

Iron deficiency is the only microcytic hypochromic disorder in which mobilizable iron stores are absent; in all other disorders, storage iron is normal or increased (Table 34-2). In patients with the genetic disorder of iron-refractory iron-deficiency anemia, iron stores may be normal or increased after treatment with parenteral iron.[15] Difficulties in the evaluation of microcytic hypochromic disorders usually arise when direct assessment of BM iron is unavailable and the diagnosis depends on indirect indicators of iron status (see boxes on Iron Deficiency and Coexisting Disorders and Therapeutic Trial of Iron).

Specific entities to be considered in the differential diagnosis of hypochromic microcytic disorders are listed in Table 34-2; in all of these disorders, body iron stores are normal or increased. The anemia of chronic disease (see Chapter 35) is the most common cause of anemia in hospitalized patients and generally is mild to moderate, typically developing over several weeks in patients with chronic infectious, inflammatory, or malignant disorders. In patients treated with erythropoiesis-stimulating agents for the anemia of chronic renal disease or other disorders, the increased iron requirements of the erythroid BM cannot be met by iron mobilization from replete stores, resulting in iron-restricted erythropoiesis.[19] This state, sometimes labeled "functional iron deficiency" despite the presence of storage iron, is a form of iron-restricted erythropoiesis resulting from stimulated erythropoietic demand for iron.[18] Uncommonly, a similar pattern can result from endogenous increases in erythropoietin owing to anemia, hypoxemia, and other conditions. The reticulocyte hemoglobin content (CHr) may be the earliest indicator that stimulated erythropoietic demand for iron exceeds the available supply.[11]

Therapeutic Trial of Iron

The diagnosis of iron deficiency often is confirmed by the outcome of a therapeutic trial of iron. A specific orderly response to, and only to, treatment with iron constitutes the final definitive proof that a lack of iron is the cause of anemia. The unequivocal diagnostic response consists of (1) a reticulocytosis, which begins approximately 3 to 5 days after adequate iron therapy is instituted, reaches a maximum on days 8 to 10, and then declines; and (2) a significant increase in hemoglobin concentration, which should begin shortly after the reticulocyte peak, is invariably present by 3 weeks after iron therapy is begun, and persists until the hemoglobin concentration is restored to normal. The result of a therapeutic trial of iron must be evaluated for possible confounding factors, such as poor compliance with iron therapy; malabsorption of therapeutic iron; continuing blood loss; and the effects of coexisting conditions, especially infectious, inflammatory, or malignant disorders. The therapeutic trial merely aids in establishing the presence of iron deficiency. The search for underlying causes of iron deficiency must continue despite a positive response to iron therapy.

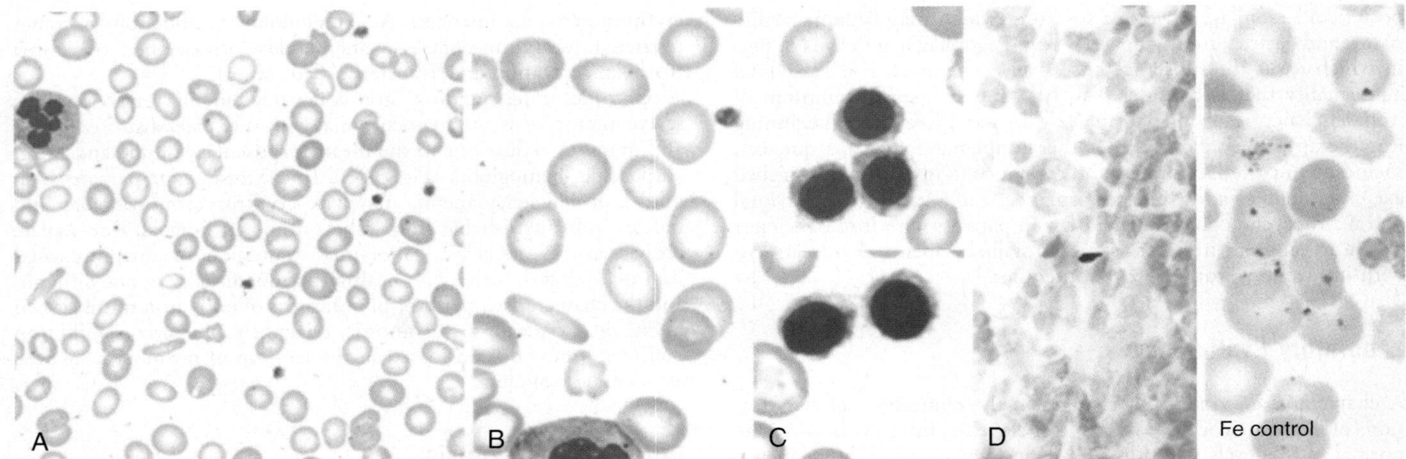

Figure 34-3 IRON-DEFICIENCY ANEMIA. Peripheral blood smear **(A** and **B)**, bone marrow (BM) aspirate **(C)**, and Prussian blue stain of BM aspirate **(D)** with control from a 16-year-old girl with hemoglobin 6.7 g/dL, hematocrit 22.6%, and mean corpuscular volume 59.2 fL. Peripheral smear shows hypochromic microcytic red blood cells **(A)**, with widening of the central pallor and "pencil" cells **(B)**. Polychromatophilic erythroid precursors in the aspirated specimen have scanty cytoplasm that is irregular and vacuolated **(C)**. The Prussian blue–stained aspirate shows no iron stores in multiple spicules **(D)**. Care must be taken not to overinterpret positive staining debris on top of cells *(center)*. Lack of staining on the BM biopsy sample can be misleading because the decalcification process is known to "leach out" iron. An appropriate control should be similar to the patient material. Peripheral blood smears made from a patient with increased iron-containing Pappenheimer bodies and fixed with 100% methanol can serve as an easily accessible control.

Table 34-2 Differential Diagnosis of Microcytic Hypochromic Anemia

Decreased Body Iron Stores
Iron-deficiency anemia
Normal or Increased Body Iron Stores
Anemia of chronic disease
Defective absorption, transport, or use of iron
Iron-refractory, iron-deficiency anemia after parenteral iron
Atransferrinemia
Aceruloplasminemia
Divalent metal transporter 1 (DMT1 or SLC11A2) deficiency
Ferroportin-associated hemochromatosis with impaired iron export (type 4A)
Heme oxygenase 1 deficiency
Disorders of globin synthesis
Thalassemia
Other microcytic hemoglobinopathies
Disorders of heme synthesis: sideroblastic anemias
Hereditary
Acquired

Oral Iron Therapy

Oral iron therapy should begin with a ferrous iron salt[13] taken separately from meals in three or four divided doses and supplying a daily total of 150 to 200 mg of elemental iron in adults or 3 mg of iron per kilogram of body weight in children. Simple ferrous preparations are the best absorbed and least expensive. Ferrous sulfate is the most widely used, either as tablets containing 60 to 70 mg of iron for adults or as a liquid preparation for children. Administration between meals maximizes absorption. In patients with a hemoglobin concentration less than 10 g/dL, this regimen initially provides approximately 40 to 60 mg of iron daily for erythropoiesis, permitting RBC production to increase to two to four times normal and the hemoglobin concentration to rise by approximately 0.2 g/dL/day. An increase in the hemoglobin concentration of at least 2 g/dL after 3 weeks of therapy generally is used as the criterion for an adequate therapeutic response. For milder anemia, a single daily dose of approximately 60 mg of iron per day may be adequate. After the anemia has been fully corrected, oral iron should be continued to replace storage iron, either empirically for an additional 4 to 6 months or until the plasma ferritin concentration exceeds approximately 50 μg/L.

Microcytic hypochromic anemias resulting from disorders of heme synthesis (sideroblastic anemias, congenital and acquired) and disorders of globin synthesis (thalassemias, microcytic hemoglobinopathies) are discussed in Chapters 36 and 38, respectively. Other rare congenital or acquired defects with microcytic hypochromic anemias[6] include atransferrinemia, aceruloplasminemia, divalent metal transporter 1 (DMT1 or SLC11A2) deficiency, some forms of ferroportin disease, heme oxygenase 1 deficiency (mutations in *HMOX1*, encoding heme oxygenase 1), several inherited sideroblastic anemias,[12,20] and a variety of other uncommon disorders.

Therapy

The goal of therapy for iron-deficiency anemia is to supply sufficient iron to repair the hemoglobin deficit and replenish storage iron. Generally, iron therapy for iron deficiency can be deferred until the underlying cause of the lack of iron has been identified. Oral iron is the treatment of choice for most patients because of its effectiveness, safety, and economy and should always be given preference over parenteral iron for initial treatment[13] (see box on Oral Iron Therapy). The risk of local and systemic adverse reactions restricts the use of parenteral iron to patients who are unable to absorb or tolerate adequate amounts of oral iron.[21,22] Rarely, RBC transfusions are needed to prevent cardiac or cerebral ischemia in patients with severe anemia or to support patients whose chronic rate of iron loss exceeds the rate of replacement possible with parenteral therapy.

Most patients are able to tolerate oral iron therapy without difficulty, but 10% to 20% may have symptoms attributable to iron. The most common side effects are gastrointestinal.[13] Decreasing the amount of iron in each dose usually is effective in controlling side effects, but if symptoms persist, a reduction in frequency to a single daily dose may be helpful. Costly iron preparations with other additives, polysaccharide–iron complexes, or enteric coatings or in sustained-release forms do not appear to offer any advantages that

Parenteral Iron Therapy

Five parenteral iron preparations are approved for use in the United States: higher and lower molecular-weight iron dextran, sodium ferric gluconate complex, iron sucrose, and ferumoxytol.[21] Each has been widely used, often in hemodialysis patients receiving recombinant human erythropoietin, but neither prospective, randomized controlled comparisons among the five agents nor long-term safety studies have been done. Although infrequent, immediate life-threatening anaphylactic reactions constitute the most serious risk associated with use of either intramuscular or intravenous iron preparations, may have a fatal outcome, and can occur with all five parenteral iron preparations.[22] Delayed but severe serum sickness–like reactions may also develop, with fever, urticaria, adenopathy, myalgias, and arthralgias.

cannot be achieved by simply reducing the dose of plain ferrous salts. Administering iron with food and decreasing the dose will diminish the amount of iron absorbed daily and thereby prolong the period of treatment, but haste in the correction of iron deficiency is rarely needed.

Parenteral iron therapy (see box on Parenteral Iron Therapy), with the risk of adverse reactions, should be reserved for the exceptional patient who (1) remains intolerant of oral iron despite repeated modifications in dosage regimen; (2) has iron needs that cannot be met by oral therapy because of either chronic uncontrollable bleeding or other sources of blood loss, such as hemodialysis, or a coexisting chronic inflammatory state; or (3) malabsorbs iron.[21,22]

Prognosis

The prognosis for iron deficiency itself is excellent, and the response to either oral or parenteral iron also is excellent.[13] Frequently, both clinical and subjective indications of constitutional improvement are seen within the first few days of treatment, with the patient reporting an enhanced sense of well-being and increased vigor and appetite. Pica may resolve, and soreness and burning of the mouth abate. Mild reticulocytosis begins within 3 to 5 days, is maximal by days 8 to 10, and then declines. The hemoglobin concentration begins to increase after the first week and usually returns to normal within 6 weeks. Complete recovery from microcytosis may take up to 4 months. With oral iron dosage totalling 200 mg/day or less, the plasma ferritin concentration usually remains less than 12 μg/dL until the anemia is corrected and then gradually rises as storage iron is replaced over the next several months. Although epithelial abnormalities begin to improve promptly with treatment, resolution of glossitis and koilonychia may take several months. The overall prognosis depends on the underlying disorder responsible for the iron deficiency.

Failure to obtain a complete and characteristic response to iron therapy necessitates a review of findings and reevaluation of the patient. A common problem is an incorrect diagnosis, with the anemia of chronic disease mistaken for the anemia of iron deficiency. Coexisting conditions, such as other nutritional deficiencies; hepatic or renal disease; or infectious, inflammatory, or malignant disorders, may impede recovery. Occult blood loss may be responsible for an incomplete response. With oral iron therapy, the adequacy of the form and dose of iron used should be reconsidered; compliance with the treatment regimen reviewed; and, finally, the possibility of malabsorption considered.

IRON OVERLOAD

Iron overload is an increase in the amount of body iron resulting from a sustained expansion of iron supply beyond iron requirements. Because requirements are limited and humans lack a physiologic means of excreting excess iron, any persistent increase in iron influx may eventually result in iron overload. The continuum of increased body iron is shown in Fig. 34-1. Whatever the source and the sites of excess iron deposition, when the accumulation overwhelms the cellular capacity for safe storage, potentially lethal tissue damage is the result. The toxic manifestations of iron overload vary with the precise pathogenic defect responsible but are dependent on the amount of excess iron, rate of iron accumulation, cellular pattern of deposition, and presence of complicating factors such as hepatitis or drug or alcohol use.

Epidemiology

The most common form of iron overload in the United States is a genetically determined disorder, the homozygous state for hereditary hemochromatosis, which occurs in approximately 4 to 5 of every 1000 persons of northern European descent.[23-25] In the United States, other forms of iron overload are less frequent but affect thousands of patients with iron-loading or chronically transfused anemias, such as thalassemia major, sickle cell disease, and acquired refractory anemias.[26] Globally, hereditary hemochromatosis is the most common genetic disorder in populations of northern European ancestry.[23-25] Thalassemia major and other iron-loading anemias are important public health problems in countries bordering the Mediterranean and in an area extending from southwest Asia and the Indian subcontinent to southeast Asia.[26] Dietary iron overload resulting from intake of iron in brewed beverages is a common problem affecting many populations in sub-Saharan Africa and may have a genetic component.[24] Other inherited types of systemic iron overload, the various forms of perinatal iron overload, and the syndromes associated with focal sequestration of iron are uncommon or rare disorders.

Genetic Aspects

The varieties of iron overload known to be genetically determined are listed in Table 34-3, and their cardinal features are summarized in Table 34-4. The known forms of hereditary iron overload all involve defects in the interaction of hepcidin and ferroportin (see box on Control of Iron Homeostasis by Hepcidin and Ferroportin and Chapter 33). The autosomal recessive disorders have in common an inappropriately low hepatic hepcidin production that leads to parenchymal iron overload.[1,23,25] *HFE*-associated and transferrin receptor 2–associated hereditary hemochromatosis and hemojuvelin- and hepcidin-associated juvenile hemochromatosis are the consequence, respectively, of mutations in regulatory genes controlling hepcidin expression *(HFE, TFR2, HJV)* and in the structural gene for hepcidin *(HAMP)*. Hepcidin production is also suppressed in three other rare autosomal recessive disorders with distinctive syndromes of iron overload: DMT1-associated hemochromatosis, atransferrinemia, and aceruloplasminemia.[1,23,25] The autosomal dominant disorders have in common mutations in the gene for ferroportin (FPN).[1,23,25] In general, these mutations either (1) interfere with iron export, resulting in reticuloendothelial macrophage iron accumulations with only minor clinical manifestations; or (2) produce resistance to the action of hepcidin, resulting in parenchymal iron loading resembling that in the autosomal recessive forms of hereditary iron overload.

Several of the acquired forms of iron overload involve disorders with a genetic origin or component. The genetically determined iron-loading anemias include the inherited sideroblastic anemias[12,20] (see Chapter 36), some of the hereditary disorders of globin synthesis (see Chapter 38), and some chronic hemolytic anemias (see Chapters 41 to 45). Similarly, some forms of chronic liver disease and porphyria cutanea tarda (see Chapter 36) are inherited disorders. African dietary iron overload[24] and, possibly, susceptibility to iron accumulation with prolonged medicinal iron ingestion may have genetic components. Many of the disorders requiring chronic RBC transfusion are

Table 34-3 Causes of Iron Overload

Hereditary Iron Overload
Autosomal recessive hemochromatosis
Hereditary hemochromatosis
HFE-associated (type 1)
Non–*HFE*-associated: Transferrin receptor 2–associated (type 3)
Juvenile hemochromatosis (type 2)
Hemojuvelin-associated (type 2A)
Hepcidin-associated (type 2B)
DMT1-associated hemochromatosis
Atransferrinemia
Aceruloplasminemia
Autosomal dominant hemochromatosis
Ferroportin-associated with impaired iron export (type 4A)
Ferroportin-associated with hepcidin resistance (type 4B)
Acquired Iron Overload
From increased iron absorption
Iron-loading anemias (refractory anemias with hypercellular erythroid marrow)
Chronic liver disease
Porphyria cutanea tarda
African dietary iron overload*
Medicinal iron ingestion*
From parenteral iron
Transfusional iron overload
Inadvertent iron overload from therapeutic injections
Perinatal Iron Overload
Neonatal hemochromatosis
Trichohepatoenteric syndrome
Cerebrohepatorenal syndrome
GRACILE (Fellman) syndrome
Focal Sequestration of Iron
Idiopathic pulmonary hemosiderosis
Renal hemosiderosis
Associated with neurologic abnormalities
Pantothenate kinase–associated neurodegeneration
Neuroferritinopathy
Friedreich ataxia

GRACILE, Growth retardation, aminoaciduria, cholestasis, iron overload, lactic acidosis, and early death; *HFE,* gene for the hemochromatosis protein, HFE.
*May have a genetic component.

hereditary, including thalassemia major (see Chapter 38), sickle cell disease (see Chapters 39 and 40), and other chronic refractory anemias. Although the exact etiology of some of these conditions is unknown, subsets of the disorders leading to perinatal iron overload or focal sequestration of iron have an established genetic basis.

Etiology and Pathogenesis

Iron overload is caused by conditions that alter or bypass the normal control of body iron content by regulation of intestinal iron absorption. The known forms of hereditary iron overload (see Table 34-3) have a common pathogenic origin in genetically determined abnormalities in the interaction of hepcidin and ferroportin that lead to excessive intestinal iron absorption, resulting in body iron accumulation. The rate, distribution, and harmful effects of tissue iron loading depend on the specific abnormality in the interaction between hepcidin and ferroportin produced by each mutation.

The mechanisms of toxicity in vulnerable iron-loaded cells seem to involve expansion of the pool of cytosolic iron followed by iron-induced generation of reactive oxygen species; damage to lipids, proteins, and deoxyribonucleic acids (DNA); and injury to subcellular organelles, including lysosomes and mitochondria, with cellular dysfunction, apoptosis, and necrosis.[25,26] The pattern of the organs affected, the timing of the onset of toxic manifestations, and the severity of tissue damage are known to be influenced by a variety of factors in both hereditary and acquired varieties of systemic iron overload. Within the systemic circulation, these factors include (1) the specific underlying genetic or acquired abnormality; (2) the magnitude of iron excess; (3) the rate of iron loading; (4) the distribution of iron load among more innocuous storage deposits in reticuloendothelial macrophages and potentially injurious accumulations in parenchymal cells of the liver, pancreas, heart, and other organs; and (5) the extent of internal redistribution of iron between reticuloendothelial macrophage and parenchymal sites. Genetic studies suggest that still unidentified genes have substantial effects on iron accumulation and toxicity.[24] In other forms of iron overload, another level of complexity is introduced because the central nervous system, the testes, and the fetus are functionally separate from the systemic circulation and cannot acquire iron directly from plasma transferrin.[27] Instead, iron must be taken up from the systemic circulation by barrier cells and then exported across the blood–brain and blood–cerebrospinal fluid barriers into the brain interstitial and cerebrospinal fluids, across the blood–testis barrier, and across the placenta to the fetus. As a consequence, disorders affecting the proteins responsible for iron supply to these compartments have distinctive manifestations.

Hereditary Iron Overload

Within the systemic circulation, the specific patterns of iron deposition and damage found in the hereditary disorders of iron overload can be characterized by reference to the pathways of internal iron exchange shown in Fig. 33-1 and the classification given in Table 34-4.

In hereditary *HFE*-associated hemochromatosis, an autosomal recessive disorder, the underlying genetic defect in the regulation of hepcidin production results in an inappropriately elevated iron absorption at any level of body iron, with a chronic progressive increase in body iron stores accompanied by enhanced release of iron from reticuloendothelial macrophages.[23,25] The molecular means whereby mutations in *HFE* produce these effects have not been characterized but result in an impaired increase in production of hepcidin in response to iron loading (see Chapter 33). Patients seem unable to effectively upregulate hepcidin expression as iron stores increase. Intestinal iron absorption, although inappropriately high in hereditary *HFE*-associated hemochromatosis, is still regulated by body iron levels. As the body iron level rises as a consequence of increased absorption, circulating transferrin becomes fully saturated. The excess iron is deposited initially predominantly within hepatocytes (Fig. 34-4), but subsequently the iron accumulates in the pancreas, heart, and other organs.[23,25] By the time symptoms of organ damage develop, usually in the fourth or fifth decade of life, body iron stores typically have increased from the normal range of 1 g or less to 15 to 20 g or more. Further increments in body iron stores may be fatal, although some patients are able to tolerate a total iron accumulation of as much as 40 to 50 g. Patients with autosomal recessive hereditary non–*HFE*-associated hemochromatosis caused by mutations in the gene for transferrin receptor 2 seem to be clinically similar to those with the *HFE*-associated form.[23,25] Patients with autosomal recessive juvenile hemochromatosis have the same pattern of tissue iron deposition found in hereditary *HFE*-associated hemochromatosis but develop severe iron overload much earlier, with hypogonadism and cardiac disease manifesting in the second decade of life.[6,23,25] The rate of iron accumulation is increased substantially and is estimated to be three to four times greater than that in *HFE*-associated disease.

Patients with DMT1-associated hemochromatosis have in common a severe microcytic anemia with low hepcidin, high transferrin saturation, and marked hepatic iron deposition but normal to moderately elevated serum ferritin concentration.[6,23,25] Congenital

Table 34-4 Hereditary Iron Overload Disorders

Disorder	Gene, Chromosome Location	Inheritance	Plasma Transferrin Saturation	Plasma Ferritin	Iron Deposition Sites	Clinical Manifestations
Hereditary hemochromatosis, *HFE*-associated (type 1; OMIM 235200)	*HFE*, 6p21	Autosomal recessive	Early increase; >45%	Later increase after third decade	Parenchymal iron overload affecting hepatocytes, heart, pancreas, other organs	Liver and heart disease, diabetes, gonadal failure, arthritis, skin pigmentation
Hereditary hemochromatosis, TfR2-associated (type 3; OMIM 604250)	*TFR2*, 7q22	Autosomal recessive	Early increase; >45%	Later increase after third decade	Parenchymal iron overload affecting hepatocytes, heart, pancreas, other organs	Liver and heart disease, diabetes, gonadal failure, arthritis, skin pigmentation
Juvenile hemochromatosis, hemojuvelin-associated (type 2A; OMIM 602390)	*HJV*, 1q21	Autosomal recessive	Early increase; >45%	Increased by second decade	Parenchymal iron overload affecting hepatocytes, heart, pancreas, other organs	As for hereditary hemochromatosis, but liver involvement less prominent
Juvenile hemochromatosis, hepcidin-associated (type 2B; OMIM 613313)	*HAMP*, 19q13	Autosomal recessive	Early increase; >45%	Increased by second decade	Parenchymal iron overload affecting hepatocytes, heart, pancreas, other organs	As for hereditary hemochromatosis, but liver involvement less prominent
Hemochromatosis, DMT1-associated (OMIM 206100)	*SCL11A2*, 12q13	Autosomal recessive	Early increase; >45%	Normal to moderately elevated	Hepatic iron overload, predominantly in hepatocytes	Severe microcytic anemia, liver dysfunction
Atransferrinemia (OMIM 209300)	*TF*, 3q22	Autosomal recessive	No plasma transferrin	Increased	Parenchymal iron overload affecting hepatocytes, heart, pancreas; no iron in bone marrow or spleen	Transfusion-dependent iron deficiency anemia, growth retardation, poor survival
Aceruloplasminemia (OMIM 604290)	*CP*, 3q24-q25	Autosomal recessive	Decreased	Increased	Marked iron accumulation in basal ganglia, liver, pancreas	Diabetes, progressive neurologic disease, retinal degeneration
Hemochromatosis, ferroportin-associated, with impaired iron export (type 4A; OMIM 606069)	*SLC40A1*, 2q32	Autosomal dominant	Remains normal or low	Early increase	Predominantly macrophage iron deposition	None
Hemochromatosis, ferroportin-associated, with hepcidin resistance (type 4B; OMIM 606069)	*SLC40A1*, 2q32	Autosomal dominant	Early increase; >45%	Early increase	Parenchymal iron overload affecting hepatocytes, heart, pancreas, other organs	Similar to HFE-associated hemochromatosis

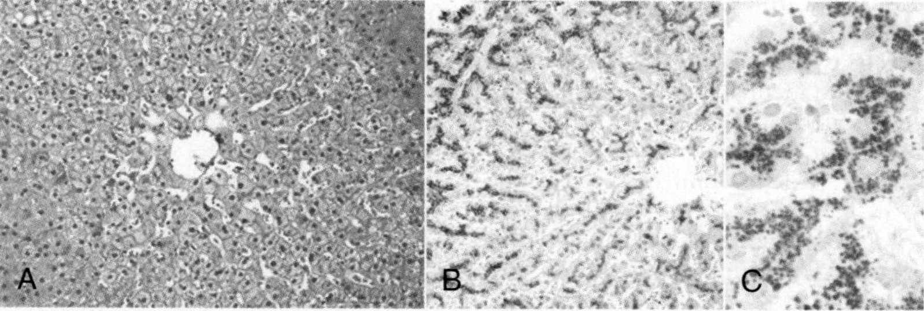

Figure 34-4 HFE-ASSOCIATED HEMOCHROMATOSIS. Liver biopsy sample from a 46-year-old man with homozygous *HFE*-associated hemochromatosis. Hematoxylin and eosin stain of the liver **(A)** shows intact hepatic architecture. Iron stain **(B** and **C)** shows marked diffuse iron deposits in the hepatocytes throughout the lobules. A normal liver would show essentially no iron in the hepatocytes.

atransferrinemia (hypotransferrinemia) is a rare disorder of autosomal recessive inheritance in which plasma transferrin is nearly absent and hepcidin is decreased.[6,23,25] Patients have a severe hypochromic microcytic anemia and die without transferrin infusion or blood transfusions. Hereditary aceruloplasminemia (hypoceruloplasminemia) is a rare disorder of iron homeostasis inherited as an autosomal recessive trait, resulting from absence or severe deficiency of ceruloplasmin occurring as a consequence of mutations in the ceruloplasmin gene.[6,23,25] Patients with aceruloplasminemia typically present in the fourth or fifth decade of life with a triad of diabetes mellitus, progressive neurologic disease (dementia, dysarthria, and dystonia), and retinal degeneration.

Patients with autosomal dominant hemochromatosis resulting from mutations in the ferroportin gene that compromise iron export, such as those resulting in ferroportins that are unable to reach the cell surface to interact with hepcidin, have iron deposition predominantly in macrophages, are almost devoid of clinical manifestations and apparently do not require treatment.[1,23,25] Patients with mutations that result in ferroportins that reach the cell surface but do not respond to hepcidin develop a parenchymal pattern of iron overload that resembles that found in patients with the autosomal recessive forms of hemochromatosis.[1,23,25]

Acquired Iron Overload

Iron-loading anemias may be associated with excessive absorption of dietary iron that can produce severe iron overload. Iron absorption increases dramatically when accelerated erythropoiesis exceeds the ability of transferrin to provide sufficient iron for hemoglobin production[6,26] (see Chapter 33). The iron-loading anemias are characterized by the combination of erythroid hyperplasia with marked ineffective erythropoiesis. Diminished hepcidin production as a result of ineffective erythropoiesis is responsible for the increased iron absorption. These refractory disorders include thalassemia major and intermedia, hemoglobin E/β-thalassemia, congenital dyserythropoietic anemia, pyruvate kinase deficiency, a variety of sideroblastic anemias, and other anemias associated with blocks in the incorporation of iron into hemoglobin. The rate of iron loading is related not to the severity of the anemia but rather to the extent of ineffective erythropoiesis. Patients with nearly normal hemoglobin concentrations may develop massive iron overload and any RBC transfusions will add to the iron burden. Clinical manifestations include liver disease, diabetes mellitus, endocrine disorders, and cardiac dysfunction.

Chronic liver disease with increased absorption of dietary iron may produce mild iron overload in some patients, including individuals with nonalcoholic fatty liver disease (NAFLD), chronic hepatitis C infection, alcohol-related liver disease or portacaval shunts.[28] In porphyria cutanea tarda (see Chapter 36), the most common type of human porphyria, mild hepatic iron overload is found in most patients, and iron depletion by phlebotomy produces clinical and biochemical remission of the disease. African dietary iron overload occurs in sub-Saharan Africa in association with greatly increased dietary iron intake from a traditional fermented beverage with high iron content, but a genetic component not linked to HFE may also be involved.[24] Medicinal iron ingestion can add to the body iron burden of patients with iron-loading disorders, especially iron-loading anemias. In persons without abnormalities affecting iron homeostasis, the extent to which orally administered iron can increase the body iron stores is uncertain.

Parenteral iron overload usually is the result of repeated RBC transfusions in patients with chronic anemia, but occasionally, it is unintentionally produced by repeated injections of iron dextran or other parenteral iron preparations in patients with anemias unresponsive to iron therapy, such as patients undergoing chronic hemodialysis.

Transfusional iron overload progressively develops in patients with chronic refractory anemia who require RBC support (Fig. 34-5).[26] In patients with severe congenital anemias such as thalassemia major (Cooley anemia) or Blackfan-Diamond syndrome, transfusional iron loading begins in infancy. Severe iron loading may develop in transfusion-dependent anemias that appear later in life, namely, aplastic anemia, pure RBC aplasia, hypoplastic or myelodysplastic disorders, and the anemia of chronic renal failure. Patients with sickle cell anemia or sickle cell/β-thalassemia also are at risk for iron overload if chronically given transfusions for prevention of recurrent complications such as stroke, severe infections, and incapacitating painful crises. If ineffective erythropoiesis and erythroid hyperplasia complicate the underlying anemia, increased absorption may contribute to the iron burden. The greater the extent of ineffective erythropoiesis, the greater the suppression of hepcidin synthesis and the greater the magnitude of the increase in iron absorption.

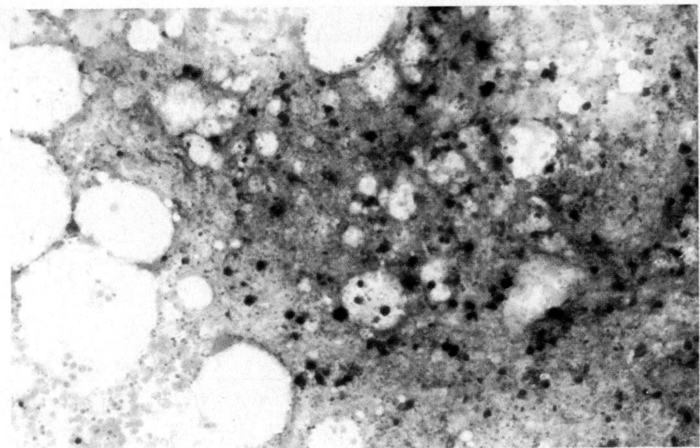

Figure 34-5 ACQUIRED IRON OVERLOAD. Prussian blue–stained bone marrow (BM) aspirate showing excessive iron stores in acquired iron overload. This occurs in a number of instances as discussed in the text, including transfusional iron overload as illustrated here, in the BM of a patient with a myelodysplastic syndrome.

Perinatal iron overload (see Table 34-3) develops in some rare or uncommon metabolic disorders of newborns, apparently as the result of disturbances in the regulation of fetal or maternal–fetal iron balance and in some instances as a result of intrauterine liver disease producing severe hypotransferrinemia.[29] Focal sequestration of iron in other rare disorders produces various patterns of localized iron deposition, in the lung in idiopathic pulmonary hemosiderosis, and in the kidney in renal hemosiderosis. Finally, remarkable progress is being made in elucidating the bases for disorders with specific patterns of brain iron deposition in association with neurologic abnormalities, including Friedreich ataxia, pantothenate kinase-associated neurodegeneration (formerly called Hallervorden-Spatz syndrome), and neuroferritinopathy.[27]

Clinical Presentation

Clinical manifestations of iron toxicity generally develop only in patients with forms of systemic parenchymal iron overload in which the magnitude of iron accumulation is sufficient to produce tissue and organ damage.[23] Individuals at risk include homozygotes for the types of hereditary and juvenile hemochromatosis listed in Table 34-3, some forms of ferroportin-associated hemochromatosis, aceruloplasminemia, and patients with iron-loading anemias, African dietary iron overload, and transfusional iron overload. Patients with forms of iron overload restricted to reticuloendothelial macrophages do not seem to develop clinical complications.[23,25] Specific patterns of neurologic signs and symptoms occur in patients with aceruloplasminemia, pantothenate kinase-associated neurodegeneration, Friedreich ataxia, and neuroferritinopathy that reflect the brain distribution of the excess iron.[27]

In patients with systemic parenchymal iron loading, similar clinical features eventually develop with sufficient iron accumulation to produce organ dysfunction and damage.[23,25,26] At earlier stages, with lower body iron burdens, no distinctive signs or symptoms may be present, and patients may come to attention only because of abnormal laboratory test results. Symptomatic patients may present with any of the characteristic manifestations of parenchymal iron deposition, including liver disease, diabetes mellitus, gonadal insufficiency and other endocrine disorders, cardiac dysfunction, arthropathy, and increased skin pigmentation. Liver disease is the most common complication of systemic iron overload. In all varieties of systemic parenchymal iron overload, the development and severity of liver damage are closely correlated with the magnitude of hepatic iron deposition. Whether derived from increased absorption of dietary iron or from transfused RBCs, progressive parenchymal iron accumulation eventually produces hepatomegaly, functional abnormalities, fibrosis, and, finally, cirrhosis.[23,25,26] Hepatocellular carcinoma seems to be the ultimate complication of cirrhosis in iron overload. The development of cirrhosis increases the risk of hepatoma by more than 200-fold.

Diabetes mellitus is another common complication of all forms of systemic parenchymal iron overload. Virtually all of the secondary manifestations of diabetes may develop, including retinopathy, nephropathy, neuropathy, and vascular disease. Gonadal insufficiency and other endocrine abnormalities occur. During the second decade of life, both growth and sexual maturation usually are retarded in untreated patients with transfusional iron overload.

Iron-induced cardiac disease, occurring as a cardiomyopathy with heart failure, arrhythmias, or both, may be a fatal complication of all varieties of systemic parenchymal iron overload. Heart disease is the most frequent cause of death in patients with thalassemia major.[7] Severe cardiac disease in particular may be the presenting manifestation in young patients with juvenile hemochromatosis.[23]

Increased skin pigmentation, with a bronze hue in some patients and a slate-gray coloration in others, often accompanies iron overload. Chondrocalcinosis and other forms of arthropathy are common complications of hereditary hemochromatosis and may occur in other forms of systemic parenchymal iron overload. An increased susceptibility to infectious disease may be found in patients with transfusional and other forms of iron overload, especially to infections with certain organisms, including *Vibrio vulnificus, Listeria monocytogenes, Yersinia enterocolitica, Escherichia coli, Candida* spp., and *Mycobacterium tuberculosis*.[4]

Laboratory Evaluation

The typical sequences of changes in clinically useful indicators of iron status as body iron increases from the iron-replete normal to the amounts found in hereditary hemochromatosis and transfusional iron overload are shown in Fig. 34-1. Characteristic changes in laboratory measures of iron status in the disorders of hereditary iron overload are listed in Table 34-4.

Screening for iron overload can use phenotypical methods, genotypical methods, or both.[23,25] Phenotypical screening can provide biochemical evidence of iron overload in patients with hereditary or juvenile hemochromatosis but does not identify all persons genetically at risk for iron loading. In populations of northern European ancestry, genotypical screening for the C282Y and H63D mutations in HFE can identify most persons at risk for developing hereditary hemochromatosis but gives no information about the presence or magnitude of iron overload. In most clinical circumstances, a combination of phenotypical and genotypical methods is the best strategy for screening.[24]

In individuals of northern European ancestry, measurement of the serum transferrin saturation usually is the best method for initial phenotypical screening for systemic parenchymal iron overload.[23-25] A persistent value of 45% or greater often is recommended as a threshold value for further investigation. In the absence of complicating factors, elevated concentrations of serum ferritin provide biochemical evidence of iron overload. Genetic testing then should be considered in persons with abnormal transferrin saturation, serum ferritin concentration, or both. Liver biopsy may be indicated for prognostic purposes to detect cirrhosis if the serum ferritin concentration is greater than 1000 μg/L and may be contemplated in the presence of hepatomegaly or abnormalities on liver function testing, or in patients older than 40 years.

Persons with phenotypical evidence of iron overload who are neither C282Y/C282Y homozygotes nor C282Y/H63D heterozygotes can be considered for further genetic testing for less common *HFE* mutations and for non-*HFE* mutations associated with iron loading, for noninvasive assessment of the liver iron concentration, or for diagnostic liver biopsy.

Liver biopsy can establish a definitive diagnosis of hereditary and juvenile hemochromatosis regardless of genotype and can demonstrate the histologic pattern of iron loading found with ferroportin mutations or with chronic liver diseases (NAFLD, chronic hepatitis C infection, and alcohol-related liver disease) (see box on Testing for Iron Overload). A quantitative determination of the nonheme iron concentration in the liver sample should be made, the pattern of iron deposition examined histochemically, and the extent of tissue injury assessed histopathologically. In patients found to have an increased body iron load, additional clinical and laboratory studies should seek evidence of complications of iron overload. Further investigation may include liver function testing; testing for diabetes mellitus; evaluation of hormonal function; cardiac examination; joint and bone radiography examination; and, especially if cirrhosis is present, screening for hepatocellular carcinoma.

Atransferrinemia or hypotransferrinemia is readily demonstrable by measurement of the plasma transferrin concentration. Similarly, aceruloplasminemia or hypoceruloplasminemia can be diagnosed by measurement of the plasma ceruloplasmin concentration. For detection and diagnosis of iron-loading anemias, measurement of the plasma transferrin receptor and examination of the BM may be helpful in demonstrating ineffective erythropoiesis in combination with the erythroid hyperplasia characteristic of these disorders.

Testing for Iron Overload

A direct measure of body iron avoids the uncertainties inherent in the interpretation of indirect indicators of iron status. Liver biopsy is the definitive direct test for assessing iron deposition and tissue damage in iron overload, permitting measurement of the nonheme iron concentration, histochemical determination of the cellular distribution of iron between hepatocytes and Kupffer cells, and pathologic examination of the extent of tissue injury.[23,25] When available as appropriately calibrated and validated techniques, new noninvasive methods using hepatic magnetic susceptibility and magnetic resonance imaging (MRI) may replace liver biopsy when only determination of the liver iron concentration is needed. MRI studies of the heart are particularly useful in patients at risk for cardiac iron deposition.[7] In patients with hereditary hemochromatosis undergoing therapeutic venesection, quantitative phlebotomy provides an accurate retrospective determination of the amount of storage iron that can be mobilized for hemoglobin formation.[24] When liver biopsy is contraindicated in a patient, quantitative phlebotomy occasionally is useful in establishing the diagnosis of hereditary hemochromatosis. BM aspiration and biopsy provide no information about the extent of parenchymal iron loading and are of limited value in the evaluation of iron overload. Iron overload produces no specific abnormalities in the peripheral blood.

Differential Diagnosis

Detection and diagnosis of iron overload are most problematic in the hereditary forms of iron overload (see Table 34-3). A combination of phenotypical and genotypical screening should lead to a definitive diagnosis in most patients. Aceruloplasminemia is a rare disorder, but distinguishing this form of iron overload from hereditary hemochromatosis is important in guiding effective iron-chelating therapy that can prevent or arrest neurologic damage.

In patients with iron-loading anemias who are not transfusion dependent, the severity of anemia provides no indication of the risk of iron loading from increased dietary iron absorption. Patients with only minor degrees of anemia may accumulate major iron loads. The differential diagnosis directed at the remaining causes of iron overload listed in Table 34-3 poses few problems. Porphyria cutanea tarda is discussed more fully in Chapter 36 and is readily diagnosed by the measurement of urinary porphyrins. The source of iron overload in patients with parenteral iron loading is evident, whether from repeated injections of therapeutic iron or from transfusion. The various causes of perinatal iron overload are clearly distinguished by clinical and pathologic findings. The diagnosis of idiopathic pulmonary hemosiderosis should be considered whenever iron-deficiency anemia develops with coexisting pulmonary abnormalities. Previously, the demonstration of iron deposits in the brain of patients with Friedreich ataxia, pantothenate kinase-associated, and neuroferritinopathy was possible only at autopsy, but MRI now provides a means for detecting localized brain iron deposits during life.[27]

Patients with hyperferritinemia but no clinical manifestations or elevated transferrin saturations may have mutations in the ferroportin gene (see Table 34-4) or in the gene for the iron-responsive element in L-ferritin messenger RNA. The latter mutations are responsible for hereditary hyperferritinemia with cataract, a disorder of autosomal dominant inheritance in which affected family members present with early-onset bilateral nuclear cataracts and moderately elevated plasma ferritin concentrations caused by increased concentrations of L-ferritin.[6] Serum iron concentration and transferrin saturation are normal or low, body iron level as evaluated by phlebotomy is not increased, and no hematologic or biochemical abnormalities are evident in affected persons. Molecular studies have identified mutations in the iron-responsive element of the L-ferritin messenger RNA as responsible. The only sign of the mutation seems to be an accumulation of L-type ferritin in the lens, resulting in cataract formation.

Therapy

The goal of therapy for iron overload is reduction and maintenance of body iron at normal or near-normal levels. If possible, phlebotomy is the treatment of choice for hereditary hemochromatosis,[23,25] iron-loading anemia if the hemoglobin concentration is high enough to permit venesection, porphyria cutanea tarda, and African dietary iron overload. After the diagnosis of iron overload has been established, phlebotomy therapy should begin promptly because any delay extends exposure to potentially toxic iron accumulations.

For most patients, phlebotomy should remove 500 mL of blood, containing 200 to 250 mg of iron, once weekly, until storage iron is depleted.[23,25] The regimen should be individualized. For patients with iron-loading anemia, smaller amounts of blood will need to be withdrawn weekly, but for heavily iron-loaded patients with hereditary hemochromatosis, an even more vigorous program of twice-weekly phlebotomy can be used. The hematocrit or hemoglobin concentration should be measured before each phlebotomy procedure. The progress of iron removal can be followed by periodic measurements of plasma ferritin and iron concentrations and transferrin saturation. The plasma ferritin concentration declines progressively as iron is removed, but the plasma iron concentration and transferrin saturation remain elevated until iron stores near depletion. In a patient with porphyria cutanea tarda, a few weeks of phlebotomy will suffice, but in a patient with hereditary hemochromatosis and an initial body iron burden of 25 g, removal of the iron burden may require 2 years or more of phlebotomy. After complete removal of the iron load, lifelong maintenance therapy is needed, usually necessitating phlebotomy of 500 mL every 3 to 4 months or, in some patients, even less frequently.

For patients with transfusion-dependent refractory anemias, most patients with iron-loading anemias, and rare patients with hereditary hemochromatosis in whom phlebotomy is impossible, treatment with an iron chelator is the only means of preventing or removing toxic accumulations of iron[26] (see box on Timing of Chelation Therapy). In patients with hereditary hemochromatosis and cardiac failure, a combination of phlebotomy and chelation therapy has been recommended. In the United States, two iron-chelating agents are available for initial treatment of transfusional iron overload, deferoxamine, given parenterally, and deferasirox, administered orally.[26] A third iron chelator, oral deferiprone, is approved in the United States, the European Union and other countries for patients with thalassemia major when deferoxamine is contraindicated or inadequate.

Timing of Chelation Therapy

In all forms of transfusional iron overload, the most effective means of avoiding complications is to prevent excessive iron accumulation with early iron-chelating therapy.[26] In patients who are transfusion dependent from early infancy (i.e., those with thalassemia major or other congenital refractory anemias), chelation therapy is best started after 10 to 20 transfusions, usually at approximately 3 years of age. In older patients with acquired refractory anemias who become transfusion dependent, it seems advisable to begin chelation early after transfusion of 10 to 20 units of blood. In patients with iron-loading anemias and those with sickle cell disease who are chronically transfused for prevention of complications, early therapy also seems prudent. In each of these disorders, delay in beginning chelation therapy only exposes the patient to a greater risk of iron toxicity.

Over the past 4 decades, clinical experience with deferoxamine, a hexadentate bacterial siderophore purified from *Streptomyces pilosus,* has established the efficacy and safety of this agent in preventing organ dysfunction and prolonging survival in patients with transfusional iron overload.[26] Unfortunately, deferoxamine given orally is poorly absorbed. To be effective, the drug must be administered by prolonged subcutaneous or intravenous infusion with a small portable syringe pump, ideally each day, making compliance a demanding task. In patients with modest iron loads and no evidence of iron toxicity, slow subcutaneous infusion of deferoxamine for 9 to 12 hours daily usually provides adequate therapy. In severely iron-loaded patients and in patients with evidence of iron toxicity, particularly those with cardiac complications, chronic slow intravenous infusions given through an indwelling central venous catheter may permit more rapid reduction of the body iron burden. Deferoxamine is a generally safe and nontoxic drug for iron-loaded patients, but systemic complications have been reported, including allergic anaphylactoid reactions, infectious complications, visual abnormalities, auditory dysfunction, and growth retardation. The risk of many of these complications may be minimized by adjusting the deferoxamine dose to the magnitude of the body iron load. Adequate deferoxamine therapy should produce a progressive decrease in the body storage iron of almost any patient with iron overload. If no decline is observed, blood and deferoxamine use, compliance, ascorbate status, and other features of the therapeutic regimen should be thoroughly reassessed.

Deferasirox, a synthetic orally active tridentate iron chelator, was approved for use by the U.S. Food and Drug Administration in 2005 for treatment of transfusional iron overload in adults and children older than 2 years.[30] Deferasirox has a long plasma half-life, making possible once-daily dosing. Extensive systematic clinical trials in patients with thalassemia major, sickle cell disease, and other transfusion-dependent anemias have provided evidence that the effectiveness of deferasirox in the management of iron overload is comparable to that of deferoxamine.[30] The most common adverse events have been rash, gastrointestinal disturbances, and abnormalities in renal function. Additional clinical studies examining the long-term safety and efficacy of deferasirox are in progress, but the initial 5 years of experience with this drug suggests that this orally active iron-chelating agent is a well-tolerated, once-daily treatment for control of transfusional iron overload.[30] Despite the lack of data on long-term effectiveness, most patients now opt for deferasirox because of the ease of oral administration.

Prognosis

The prognosis in patients with iron overload is influenced by many factors, including the magnitude, rate, and route of iron loading; distribution of iron deposition between reticuloendothelial macrophage and parenchymal sites; amount and duration of exposure to circulating non–transferrin-bound iron; ascorbate status; and coexisting disorders, especially alcoholism.[23,25] The magnitude of iron accumulation seems to be a critical determinant of the risk of cirrhosis of the liver and, in turn, of hepatocellular carcinoma, now the two major causes of death in hereditary hemochromatosis. If the disease is diagnosed before tissue injury occurs, phlebotomy therapy to remove the excess iron can prevent all of the complications of hemochromatosis, including cirrhosis, and return the patient's life expectancy to normal.[23,25] Even if organ damage is present, phlebotomy prevents further progression, and amelioration of some features of the disease is possible. Skin pigmentation diminishes; hepatic function may improve while fibrosis is arrested or sometimes regresses; and cardiac abnormalities, including even cardiac failure, may resolve. Diabetes and other endocrine abnormalities usually are ameliorated only slightly, if at all, although reversal of hypogonadism has occurred. Arthropathy usually does not subside and may even continue to progress despite phlebotomy.

In patients with iron overload who cannot be treated by phlebotomy, chelation therapy is effective in reducing the body iron burden and improving the prognosis. Orally administered deferasirox or chronic infusion of parenteral deferoxamine decreases the hepatic iron concentration, improves hepatic function, promotes growth and sexual maturation, and helps protect against cardiac disease and early death. In all forms of iron overload, the most effective means of preventing complications is prevention of iron accumulation, either by early identification and phlebotomy treatment of hereditary hemochromatosis or by early institution of chelation therapy in patients with iron-loading or transfusion-dependent anemias.

REFERENCES

1. Kaplan J, Ward DM, De Domenico I: The molecular basis of iron overload disorders and iron-linked anemias. *Int J Hematol* 93:14, 2011.
2. Ganz T: Hepcidin and iron regulation, 10 years later. *Blood* 117:4425, 2011.
3. Hentze MW, Muckenthaler MU, Galy B, et al: Two to tango: Regulation of Mammalian iron metabolism. *Cell* 142:24, 2010.
4. Wessling-Resnick M: Iron homeostasis and the inflammatory response. *Annu Rev Nutr* 30:105, 2010.
5. Bullock GC, Delehanty LL, Talbot AL, et al: Iron control of erythroid development by a novel aconitase-associated regulatory pathway. *Blood* 116:97, 2010.
6. Camaschella C, Poggiali E: Inherited disorders of iron metabolism. *Curr Opin Pediatr* 23:14, 2011.
7. Wood JC, Noetzli L: Cardiovascular MRI in thalassemia major. *Ann N Y Acad Sci* 1202:173, 2010.
8. Galesloot TE, Vermeulen SH, Geurts-Moespot AJ, et al: Serum hepcidin: Reference ranges and biochemical correlates in the general population. *Blood* 117:e218, 2011.
9. Knovich MA, Storey JA, Coffman LG, et al: Ferritin for the clinician. *Blood Rev* 23:95, 2009.
10. Skikne BS, Punnonen K, Caldron PH, et al: Improved differential diagnosis of anemia of chronic disease and iron deficiency anemia: A prospective multicenter evaluation of soluble transferrin receptor and the sTfR/log ferritin index. *Am J Hematol* 86:923, 2011.
11. Rehu M, Ahonen S, Punnonen K: The diagnostic accuracy of the percentage of hypochromic red blood cells (%HYPOm) and cellular hemoglobin in reticulocytes (CHr) in differentiating iron deficiency anemia and anemia of chronic diseases. *Clin Chim Acta* 412:1809, 2011.
12. Ye H, Rouault TA: Human iron-sulfur cluster assembly, cellular iron homeostasis, and disease. *Biochemistry* 49:4945, 2010.
13. Goddard AF, James MW, McIntyre AS, et al: Guidelines for the management of iron deficiency anaemia. *Gut* 60:1309, 2011.
14. Baker RD, Greer FR: Diagnosis and prevention of iron deficiency and iron-deficiency anemia in infants and young children (0-3 years of age). *Pediatrics* 126:1040, 2010.
15. Finberg KE: Iron-refractory iron deficiency anemia. *Semin Hematol* 46:378, 2009.
16. Trenkwalder C, Paulus W: Restless legs syndrome: Pathophysiology, clinical presentation and management. *Nat Rev Neurol* 6:337, 2010.
17. van Veldhuisen DJ, Anker SD, Ponikowski P, et al: Anemia and iron deficiency in heart failure: Mechanisms and therapeutic approaches. *Nat Rev Cardiol* 31;8:485, 2011.
18. Goodnough LT, Nemeth E, Ganz T: Detection, evaluation, and management of iron-restricted erythropoiesis. *Blood* 116:4754, 2010.
19. Besarab A, Coyne DW: Iron supplementation to treat anemia in patients with chronic kidney disease. *Nat Rev Nephrol* 6:699, 2010.
20. Camaschella C: Hereditary sideroblastic anemias: Pathophysiology, diagnosis, and treatment. *Semin Hematol* 46:371, 2009.
21. Auerbach M, Ballard H: Clinical use of intravenous iron: Administration, efficacy, and safety. *Hematology Am Soc Hematol Educ Program* 2010:338, 2010.
22. Wysowski DK, Swartz L, Borders-Hemphill BV, et al: Use of parenteral iron products and serious anaphylactic-type reactions. *Am J Hematol* 85:650, 2010.
23. Brissot P, Bardou-Jacquet E, Jouanolle AM, et al: Iron disorders of genetic origin: A changing world. *Trends Mol Med* 17:707, 2011.
24. McLaren GD, Gordeuk VR: Hereditary hemochromatosis: Insights from the Hemochromatosis and Iron Overload Screening (HEIRS) Study. *Hematology Am Soc Hematol Educ Program* 195, 2009.
25. Pietrangelo A: Hereditary hemochromatosis: Pathogenesis, diagnosis, and treatment. *Gastroenterology* 139:393, 408, e1-2, 2010.
26. Brittenham GM: Iron-chelating therapy for transfusional iron overload. *N Engl J Med* 364:146, 2011.
27. Gregory A, Hayflick SJ: Genetics of neurodegeneration with brain iron accumulation. *Curr Neurol Neurosci Rep* 11:254, 2011.
28. Dever JB, Mallory MA, Mallory JE, et al: Phenotypic characteristics and diagnoses of patients referred to an iron overload clinic. *Dig Dis Sci* 55:803, 2010.
29. Knisely AS, Vergani D: "Neonatal hemochromatosis": A re-vision. *Hepatology* 51:1888, 2010.
30. Cappellini MD, Bejaoui M, Agaoglu L, et al: Iron chelation with deferasirox in adult and pediatric patients with thalassemia major: Efficacy and safety during 5 years' follow-up. *Blood* 118:884, 2011.

CHAPTER 35

ANEMIA OF CHRONIC DISEASES

Jane A. Little, Edward J. Benz, Jr., and Lawrence B. Gardner

Anemia is commonly associated with many diverse systemic inflammatory conditions, including infection, rheumatologic disorders, and cancer. The cause of the anemia of chronic disease (ACD) is multifactorial and includes both inhibition of red blood cell (RBC) production (caused by a combination of dysregulated iron metabolism, inhibited hematopoiesis, and relative erythropoietin deficiency) and a mildly decreased RBC lifespan. Teleologically, ACD may serve to decrease infectious virulence by organisms, such as malaria and schistosomiasis, in a nutrient-depleted host.[1-4] Malignancies may also be potentiated in an iron-rich environment in humans.[5-8] Research over the past decade has delineated the important pathophysiological role of inflammatory cytokines in ACD. Once described as a "bag of unsolved questions,"[9] the pathophysiologic underpinnings of ACD have been dramatically illuminated by the recently characterized antimicrobial peptide hepcidin. Hepcidin is both a mediator of innate immunity and an iron regulatory peptide, and it plays a major, although not solo, role in the pathogenesis of ACD.

DESCRIPTION AND EPIDEMIOLOGY

Anemia of chronic disease is an anemia of underproduction that usually is relatively mild, with hemoglobin levels typically greater than 10 g/L, normocytic, and normochromic.[10] However, the anemia can be severe, and the mean corpuscular volume may be reduced, sometimes dramatically, in up to one-third of patients. ACD is one of the most common causes of anemia. Over a 2-month period of observation, 52% of hospitalized patients with anemia who were not iron deficient, hemolyzing, or with a hematologic malignancy met laboratory criteria for ACD.[11] An unselected elderly population (older than 60 years of age), followed prospectively, had a 2.4% 3-year incidence of ACD.[12,13] Anemia (hemoglobin <12 g/dL) is extremely common in cancer, seen in 58% of 420 subjects with nonhematologic malignancies before radiation therapy and in one- to two-thirds of general oncologic populations.[14,15] The presence of anemia may inversely correlate with response to cancer therapy[16] and survival.[17] HIV infection is often associated with anemia, particularly as the infection progresses to clinical AIDS (increasing from a prevalence of one-tenth to one-third).[18] ACD is common in outpatients with rheumatoid arthritis (prevalence of 25%-30%), and the degree of anemia is associated with an elevation in some markers and/or mediators of inflammation, such as sedimentation rate (ESR), C-reactive protein CRP, and interleukin-6 (IL-6).[19-21]

Although most hospitalized patients with ACD have an active infection, inflammatory condition or malignancy, other reported precipitating illnesses include alcoholic liver disease, congestive heart failure, thrombosis, chronic pulmonary disease, diabetes, trauma, and a variety of other medical conditions.[11,22] It is intriguing that diverse diseases, not conventionally considered "inflammatory" in nature, such as congestive heart failure, obesity, renal failure, and diabetes, have been associated both with an ACD-type anemia and with cytokine abnormalities more typically associated with inflammatory condition (e.g., elevated Il-6 and CRP in kidney disease or CRP and fibrinogen in myocardial infarction).[6,11,23-25] Because of the absence of definitive diagnostic criteria or definitive lab tests (as discussed in Diagnosis), however, epidemiologic studies in ACD are at the least confounded by the underlying clinical heterogeneity.

ETIOLOGY AND PATHOGENESIS

Anemia of chronic disease is marked by low serum iron. However, in contrast to iron-deficiency anemia, total iron stores are normal or elevated. In rheumatoid arthritis, this low serum iron and depressed hemoglobin parallel disease activity, not patient age or duration of disease.[26] Because of characteristic abnormalities in laboratory iron studies, initial theories on the etiology of ACD emphasized the role of iron. Recent descriptions of elevated hepcidin levels in ACD and of hepcidin's preeminent role in regulating iron utilization have reinforced an emphasis on the role of iron metabolism in ACD (see Biology and Molecular Aspects). However, iron-centered models do not account for concurrent evidence for the suppression of hematopoiesis, the relative deficiency of erythropoietin (EPO), and the shortened RBC half-life that are also seen in ACD. Interestingly, there is also evidence for a hepcidin-mediated effect on erythroid progenitor proliferation and survival.[13,27] Some inflammatory cytokines may increase hepcidin levels while also suppressing erythropoiesis and shortening RBC half-life. It is clear that the pathogenesis of ACD is multifactorial and complex (Table 35-1).

Although a variety of studies demonstrate that RBC survival in ACD is only mildly decreased, this may be sufficient to depress the hemoglobin concentration when erythropoiesis is concomitantly suppressed (see Biology and Molecular Aspects). A mildly shortened erythrocyte half-life has been observed in patients with rheumatoid arthritis and ACD. Experimentally, rats given endotoxin have a reduced erythrocyte half-life[28] and transgenic mice with elevations in the cytokine interferon-γ (IFN-γ) have a reduced RBC half-life because of removal of RBCs by cytokine-stimulated splenic macrophages.[29] Exogenous administration of IFN-γ in mice likewise increases RBC uptake and hemophagocytosis by macrophages.[30]

Iron metabolism is deregulated in ACD. Early studies in a variety of animal models demonstrated that radiolabeled iron absorption and half-life were diminished in the presence of systemic inflammation.[28,31] Other studies using trace quantities of labeled iron showed no direct impairment of iron incorporation into RBCs, suggesting that inflammation preferentially impairs iron release from storage sites, decreases plasma iron concentration, and limits iron incorporation during hemoglobin synthesis. Sterile inflammation in a dog model impairs only the reuse of iron from senescent RBCs, implying that inflammation primarily leads to a defect in iron release from tissues to the plasma transferrin pool.[32] Studies in patients with rheumatoid arthritis and a diagnosis of ACD also demonstrate decreased iron turnover compared with normal or iron-deficient control participants.[33] As discussed later, hepcidin's molecular mechanism of action (degradation of ferroportin) is consistent with a prominent disruption in release of iron from storage sites.

Abnormal iron turnover in ACD may occur via several mechanisms. Decreased transferrin receptors in the serum[18] and on

Table 35-1 Suspected Causes of Anemia of Chronic Disease

Shortened erythrocyte survival
Block in reuse of iron by erythrocyte
Direct inhibition of erythropoiesis
Relative deficiency of erythropoietin

erythroblasts[34] are seen in patients with ACD. Investigators have suggested that an increased release of lactoferrin from neutrophils[35] or an increased synthesis of apoferritin[36] may lead to a pool of iron trapped in storage form that is unavailable for hemoglobin synthesis. More recently, hepcidin has been implicated in ACD. Hepcidin, a small, circulating antimicrobial peptide, binds to the iron export channel ferroportin, resulting in its phosphorylation, internalization, and degradation.[37] This diminution in ferroportin density on the plasma membrane results in decreased iron absorption from duodenal cells and blocked iron release from ferroportin-expressing macrophages and hepatocytes and leads to a net decrease in the absorption of biologically available iron.[13,38,39] Diminished iron absorption in the duodenum and decreased serum iron coupled with enhanced iron retention in the macrophages (visible on bone marrow examination) cause a redistribution of total body iron. Ferroportin is also present and functional on erythroblasts.[40] Net iron retention in the erythroblast, when ferroportin is degraded by hepcidin, despite decreased serum iron levels may explain the typical normochromic, normocytic nature of ACD. Experimental overexpression of hepcidin leads to a fatal anemia in mice, with a decrease in iron absorption and an increase in reticuloendothelial stores of iron.[41] Hepcidin is increased in inflammatory conditions in mice (see Biology and Molecular Aspects later) and is elevated in a variety of diseases associated with ACD.[42] Together, these data suggest that hepcidin is a major mediator for many of the iron changes seen in ACD.

In addition to a decrease in an important hemoglobin precursor (i.e., iron), a direct inhibition of hematopoiesis and a relative deficiency of EPO are found in ACD. This inhibition of hematopoiesis has been attributed to soluble factors, now known to be cytokines, present in the perturbed bone marrow microenvironment (see Biology and Molecular Aspects later). Studies have shown that removal of bone marrow–adherent cells (mostly macrophages and monocytes) from patients with ACD leads to increased erythroid colony formation. This process can be reversed by co-culture of ACD-adherent cells but not by adherent cells from control bone marrow.[43] Culture with serum from patients with rheumatoid arthritis and anemia produces decreased burst-forming unit-erythroid (BFU-E) proliferation, but serum from nonanemic arthritic patients does not.[44] Peripheral blood mononuclear cells from patients with rheumatoid arthritis also suppress BFU-E growth.[45]

Most of the supporting data for direct inhibition of hematopoiesis are derived from in vitro studies. Data from more clinically relevant studies have clearly documented a relative deficiency of EPO in many chronic diseases associated with anemia. In a study of 81 patients with solid tumors who exhibited laboratory data compatible with ACD and who did not have bone marrow involvement by tumor, EPO levels were higher than in control participants without anemia but were only half the values typical of subjects with similar hematocrits caused by iron deficiency. The normal inverse relationship between hemoglobin and EPO levels also was not seen.[46] In 41 anemic patients with rheumatoid arthritis, 14 of whom had plentiful iron on bone marrow aspirate, serum EPO levels were lower than for those with simple iron-deficiency anemia despite comparable hemoglobin levels.[47] Serum EPO levels have been shown to be inappropriately low in human immunodeficiency virus (HIV)–positive patients with normochromic, normocytic anemia[48] and in lung transplant recipients.[49]

Patients with diabetes with anemia, normal renal function, and lower-than-expected EPO levels have been reported. This condition is hypothesized to be caused by diabetic neuropathy,[50] although there also may be a direct role of insulin on stem cells.[51] Up to 40% of patients with chronic liver disease are anemic. Although this anemia is clearly multifactorial, some studies have found a blunted EPO response to anemia in patients with cirrhosis,[52] but other studies have not.[53] The observation that hepcidin synthesis may be altered in liver disease is likely to provide further insight into ACD in this setting.[54]

Finally, EPO may not function optimally in the presence of inflammatory cytokines. EPO-resistant subjects with end-stage renal disease are more likely to have elevations in inflammatory cytokines.[55] Similarly, peripheral blood mononuclear cells isolated from EPO-refractory subjects with end-stage renal disease are more likely to produce inflammatory cytokines than those isolated from nonrefractory subjects.[56]

BIOLOGY AND MOLECULAR ASPECTS

The role of inflammatory cytokines in many of the underlying diseases associated with ACD has suggested a mechanistic link for much of the pathophysiology of anemia, including decreased erythrocyte survival, decreased access to available iron through upregulation of hepcidin and other mechanisms, direct inhibition of hematopoietic progenitor growth, and inadequate EPO response to anemia.

Increased serum levels of cytokines, particularly IL-1, IL-6, IL-10, tumor necrosis factor (TNF), IFN-α, IFN-β, and IFN-γ, have been observed in many inflammatory diseases, including HIV, hepatitis C, tuberculosis, bacterial and fungal infections, rheumatoid arthritis, inflammatory bowel diseases, and both solid and hematologic malignancies.[57-59] Elevated levels of several cytokines have been found in patients with malarial infections, partly caused by plasmodium-induced stimulation of macrophages.[60] TNF-α synthesis is increased in mucosal T cells in patients with Crohn disease[61] and in blood mononuclear cells from patients with rheumatoid arthritis.[62] High levels of inflammatory cytokines may be concentrated in the bone marrow milieu. Bone marrow of patients with rheumatoid arthritis has increased levels of IL-6 and TNF-α.[63] Bone marrow stromal cells in patients with giant cell arteritis may produce less stem cell factor and granulocyte-macrophage colony-stimulating factor than do control participants.[62]

The fact that cytokines are thought to play such an important role in many of the diseases associated with anemia and that levels of many of these cytokines often correlate with the degree of anemia suggests an association between inflammatory cytokines and anemia. Indeed, serum TNF-α levels correlate with both disease activity and the degree of anemia in rheumatoid arthritis.[64] Experimentally, transgenic mice with endogenous elevations in IFN-γ show increased expression of the proleukocyte transcription factor PU.1 in hematopoietic precursors and diminished BFU-E.[29] Causality is also suggested by the multiple trials of cytokine antagonists in inflammatory diseases that have shown a decrease in anemia.[65-67] Many molecular mechanisms by which cytokines directly or indirectly affect hematopoiesis have been described.

Cytokine-Induced Decreases in Red Blood Cell Survival

Several studies suggest a role for decreased erythrocyte survival in the pathogenesis of ACD. Alterations in RBC rheology (deformability and aggregation) are demonstrably abnormal in intensive care unit patients, especially those with sepsis.[49] In vivo and in vitro experiments have suggested that fever itself can induce rheologic changes in erythrocytes within a few days, leading to increased destruction and up to a 15% decline in RBC mass.[68] Recent studies have shown that cytokines, the cause of fever in many of the diseases associated with ACD, may directly alter RBC kinetics. For example, rats receiving chronic intraperitoneal injections of IL-1 and TNF showed decreased erythrocyte survival, as did mice with high levels of IFN-γ.[42,43] This effect has been postulated to involve cytokine-induced macrophage and reticuloendothelial system activation.[28,42,43]

Cytokine-Induced Abnormalities in Iron Metabolism

Many of the cytokines implicated in ACD have associated effects on iron metabolism. Nude mice inoculated with TNF-α–secreting Chinese hamster ovary cells showed an almost 60% decline in serum iron after 3 weeks while maintaining normal bone marrow stores of iron.[69] Rats injected with IL-1 or TNF experienced a 40% drop in serum iron levels; TNF also caused a significant decrease in iron incorporation into erythrocytes.[28] These findings are consistent with the observation that iron reuse is defective in ACD.[32] TNF has also been shown to increase radiolabeled iron uptake by peritoneal macrophages without an increase in iron release,[32,70,71] suggesting that macrophage sequestration of iron is cytokine induced. In clinical trials, IL-10 led to anemia in patients with Crohn disease and to an increase in ferritin levels, decreasing iron availability to RBC precursors.[59]

Molecular evidence implicates a direct cytokine effect on iron metabolism. IL-1β increases ferritin translation via a 5′ untranslated region, distinct from the well-known iron responsive element but similar to a 38-nucleotide consensus sequence found in other IL-sensitive acute-phase reactants.[72,73] Because this increase in ferritin synthesis occurs without increased cellular transferrin receptor transcription or expression and involves no new iron influx, IL-1 could lead directly to the creation of an intracellular iron pool that is not available for hemoglobin synthesis.[73] IL-10 also appears to increase ferritin translation.[59]

Importantly, more recent data demonstrate that inflammatory cytokines upregulate hepcidin, which, as previously noted, likely mediates many of the iron changes seen in ACD. Hepcidin is primarily regulated transcriptionally. Although IL-1α, IL-1β, IFN-γ, and other inflammatory cytokines upregulate hepcidin expression in vitro,[74,75] compelling experimental data have most closely linked IL-6 (and IL-6–like family members)[50] and the bone morphogenetic proteins (BMPs) as the most important inducers of hepcidin mRNA expression.[76-79]

The association between individual cytokines, hepcidin, iron metabolism, and ACD are more complicated in vivo. In anemia of the elderly, Il-6 and CRP levels, but not urinary hepcidin levels, were inversely correlated with serum iron levels.[31] In 65 subjects with Hodgkin disease, anemia was associated with increased IL-6 and hepcidin levels.[80] In subjects with multiple myeloma, in whom serum IL-6 and BMP levels are often elevated,$_{5,81}$ normochromic, normocytic anemia (absent renal disease) correlates with urinary and serum hepcidin levels, as well as IL-6 levels,[57] but hepcidin elevations were experimentally associated with elevated BMP-2 levels in patients' sera, rather than to alterations in IL-6.[59,81] Furthermore, in animal models of ACD, in vivo antagonists of either hepcidin or of BMP signaling have been shown to prevent IL-6 and inflammation-associated anemia.[82,83]

The transcription factors STAT3 (signal transducer and activator of transcription 3)[79,84] and SMAD4 (Sma and Mad related protein),[85] both of which are upregulated by IL-6 and other inflammatory cytokines via BMP type I receptors,[86] activate the hepcidin promoter and induce hepcidin mRNA. In humans, injection with lipopolysaccharide dramatically increases IL-6 levels by hour 3 followed by an increase in urinary hepcidin by hour 6.[87] Direct administration of IL-6 to humans also leads to increased urinary hepcidin and decreased serum iron.[39] In patients with ACD, increased pro-hepcidin serum concentrations are associated with decreased expression of ferroportin along with increased ferritin accumulation in circulating monocytes.[88]

Finally, the physiological regulation of hepcidin is complicated by a number of experimental studies that have suggested that EPO and its downstream signaling molecules may downregulate hepcidin expression despite the presence of inflammatory cytokines.[89,90] Clinical and experimental data have suggested that EPO and its downstream signaling molecules are better at countervening inflammatory-mediated induction of hepcidin than is hypoxia.[89,91] The signals that regulate hepcidin may be hierarchically determined rather than additive.

Cytokines Leading to Direct Inhibition of Hematopoiesis

Although data demonstrate that cytokines, including IL-1, IFN, and TNF, can have a direct inhibitory effect on hematopoiesis, almost all of the evidence supporting such a role for cytokines is derived from in vitro experiments, and the clinical relevance is unclear. The role of IL-6 in the direct inhibition of hematopoiesis is controversial. Exogenous IL-6 given to monkeys causes a dose-dependent, mild, short-lived anemia within 4 weeks.[92] Some studies have shown that IL-6 has direct inhibitory effects on stem cells.[93] However, other studies have demonstrated that IL-6, which is elevated in rheumatoid arthritis, has no direct effect on bone marrow hematopoiesis.[94] Juvenile-onset chronic arthritis is associated with increased IL-6 levels and anemia, but this anemia is one of iron deficiency.[95] IL-6 also has been shown to cause bleeding in the rat intestinal wall[63] and, as discussed, can also upregulate hepcidin. In vitro studies have demonstrated that colony-forming unit-erythroid (CFU-E) formation is diminished at low EPO conditions when hepcidin is added, which may be attributable to proapoptotic functions of hepcidin.[27]

There is much better evidence for the role of IFN in the direct inhibition of erythropoiesis. IFN-γ can inhibit highly purified CFU-E from mice spleens in a dose-dependent manner.[96-98] Bone marrow stromal cells, retrovirally engineered to secrete IFN-γ, inhibit hematopoiesis in long-term bone marrow cultures by blocking cell cycle progression and inducing apoptosis in CD34 cells to a much greater degree than exogenous IFN.[99] IFN inhibition can be reversed by exogenous addition of murine IFN-γ receptors.[97] Inhibition by IFN-γ can also be reversed in a dose-dependent manner by EPO, a phenomenon seen in ACD,[96,97,100] and partial reversal can be achieved by stem cell factor.[101] The concentration of IFN-γ required to suppress BFU-E is less than that needed to suppress CFU-E, suggesting the suppression occurs at the earlier stages of erythroid development.[98] Similar to IFN-γ, IFN-β appears to act directly on CFU-E, and inhibition does not require accessory T cells or adherent bone marrow cells.[97,102] Inhibition by IFN-α appears to work indirectly. Inhibition by IFN-α or IFN-β is not reversed by EPO.[97]

Tumor necrosis factor serum levels correlate with the degree of anemia in ACD. Erythroid growth is increased in the bone marrow of control and chronically anemic patients by monoclonal antibodies against TNF.[64] Transplantation of a Chinese hamster ovary cell line transfected with the human TNF gene led to anemia in nude mice within 3 weeks, with a significant decrease in BFU-E and CFU-E.[69] Exogenous TNF decreases erythroid colony formation.[64] For example, the inhibition of BFU-E growth sustained by normal bone marrow cultured in the presence of peripheral blood mononuclear cells of patients with rheumatoid arthritis can be reversed by antibodies to TNF-α.[45] However, evidence indicates that the effect of TNF on hematopoiesis is indirect, mediated by the local release of other cytokines, including IFN from accessory cells.[96] The inhibitory effect of TNF on CFU-E was completely abrogated by neutralizing antibodies against IFN-β but not by antibodies to IFN-γ or IL-1.[57] The effects of IL-1 also appear to be indirect. Growth of purified CFU-E is inhibited by recombinant IL-1 only in the presence of adherent T lymphocytes. The inhibition can be reversed by antibodies to IFN-γ, suggesting that IL-1 leads to lymphocyte secretion of IFN.[102]

Cytokines Leading to Decreased Erythropoietin Secretion

Cytokines have been implicated in the blunted, inappropriately low EPO levels seen in ACD. In the EPO-producing human hepatoma cell line HepG2 grown in diffusion-limited oxygen conditions, IL-1α, IL-1β, and TNF-α significantly lowered EPO production. IL-1β also inhibited EPO production in perfused rat kidneys. In these well-controlled experiments, the effect was specific and not secondary to a generalized inhibitory growth effect.[103] Using another hepatoma cell line, Hep3B, hypoxia-driven EPO production was inhibited with IL-1α, IL-1β, and TNF-α in a dose-dependent, additive manner.[93] Other soluble factors, in addition to cytokines, may play a role in directly inhibiting EPO in ACD. Animal models have suggested that vascular endothelial growth factor, which is commonly elevated in cancer, wounds, and ischemia, may act as a negative regulator of EPO synthesis,[104] thus suggesting a potential link between diverse systemic illnesses and EPO deficiency.

Perhaps one of the strongest arguments for a causative role of EPO in ACD is that exogenous EPO can at least partially reverse ACD. However, supraphysiologic levels of EPO may simply overcome a direct inhibition of erythropoiesis (see Treatment later). Inhibition by IFN-γ can be reversed by EPO.[100] Moreover, the capacity of monocytes from patients with inflammatory bowel disease to secrete TNF predicts therapeutic response to exogenous EPO.[105]

DIAGNOSIS

Because ACD is a multifactorial disease and is seen in many clinical settings, an unequivocal diagnosis may be difficult. Many chronic illnesses are associated with other factors leading to anemia, including iron and nutritional deficiency, bleeding, hemolysis, renal failure with absolute EPO deficiency, and bone marrow fibrosis or infiltration. Up to 70% of the anemia associated with rheumatoid arthritis may be multifactorial,[106] including iron deficiency.[107,108] Of 184 patients admitted to intensive care units, most patients with anemia were found to have EPO levels and iron study results consistent with ACD; however, 13% also had iron, folate, or vitamin B_{12} deficiency.[109] The role of frequent phlebotomy in hospitalized patients should be fully appreciated[110] (see box on Diagnosis of Anemia of Chronic Diseases).

Anemia of chronic disease may also be undiagnosed in complicated medical patients. For example, the anemia of renal failure traditionally has not been thought of as an ACD but rather as an anemia of absolute EPO deficiency. However, efficient dialysis leads to an improved response to EPO,[111,112] which suggests that other factors, perhaps including cytokines, play a role. Anemic hemodialysis patients may have occult infections of nonfunctioning arteriovenous grafts with markers of inflammation and EPO resistance; removal of these grafts may correct the anemia.[113] Fifty percent of adults with chronic idiopathic neutropenia have an anemia consistent with ACD.[114] Remarkably, multiply traumatized patients have increased inflammatory cytokines and inappropriately low EPO levels consistent with ACD.[22] In patients with congestive heart failure, TNF is elevated, cytokine levels are proportional to the severity of anemia, and EPO level is not elevated in proportion to the degree of anemia, all consistent with ACD playing a role in the anemia commonly found in patients with heart failure.[115-117]

Although the clinical setting in which the anemia is found helps with the diagnosis of ACD, in 30% of cases, no chronic illness can be identified, and acute illnesses can also lead to anemia.[11] The ACD is primarily a diagnosis of exclusion. This may necessitate evaluation of the bone marrow to ensure adequate iron stores; to rule out infiltration by tumor, fibrosis, or infections; and to exclude myelodysplastic syndromes (MDS) (Fig. 35-1). It should be noted, however, that in a study of mostly older patients with an idiopathic mild anemia (10 ± 0.6 g/dL), a bone marrow aspirate with biopsy was found to add little to an extensive negative serologic workup and physical examination.[111]

The diagnosis of ACD usually is made on the basis of elevated bone marrow iron stores (usually assessed by serum ferritin) and low serum iron level, low transferrin level, and low total iron-binding capacity. Because ACD is a hypoproliferative and sometimes microcytic anemia, the differential diagnosis includes iron deficiency. A low serum ferritin level associated with anemia suggests iron deficiency. A normal or elevated ferritin level is more difficult to interpret because ferritin is an acute-phase reactant. Some investigators argue that a ferritin level higher than 50 ng/mL excludes any component of iron deficiency even in inflammatory states. However, a meta-analysis of iron studies in clinical reports from 1842 subjects with serum ferritin levels above 45 ng/mL showed a prevalence of iron deficiency of 6.7%, but 3.5% of 1368 subjects with a serum ferritin level of greater than 100 ng/mL had iron deficiency.[118] Other researchers have shown that in acute inflammation, serum ferritin levels greater than 3500 ng/mL can coexist with absent bone marrow iron stores tested by aspirate.[119] Nomograms correcting ferritin for the degree of inflammation present have been published.[120] In 120 anemic patients with inflammatory, infectious, or malignant diseases in

Diagnosis of Anemia of Chronic Diseases

The diagnosis of ACD is primarily one of exclusion and often is difficult. Various laboratory tests have been suggested, but few have proven value in the general population because ACD occurs in too large a variety of acute and chronic illnesses. The best way to diagnose ACD, at least provisionally, is to document an anemia of underproduction (i.e., low reticulocyte index) with low serum iron and low transferrin levels and an elevated serum ferritin level in the setting of a systemic, usually inflammatory, illness. A thorough search may be necessary to document the precise underlying illness.

Other causes of anemia, such as hemolysis, nutritional deficiency, or sequestration, should be ruled out, and a component of iron deficiency should be strongly considered in a patient with systemic inflammation and a low or "normal" serum ferritin concentration. These other causes of anemia often accompany ACD. Bone marrow examination usually is not essential for the diagnosis but may be necessary to rule out other diagnoses, including malignancy (including MDS), infection, or iron deficiency.

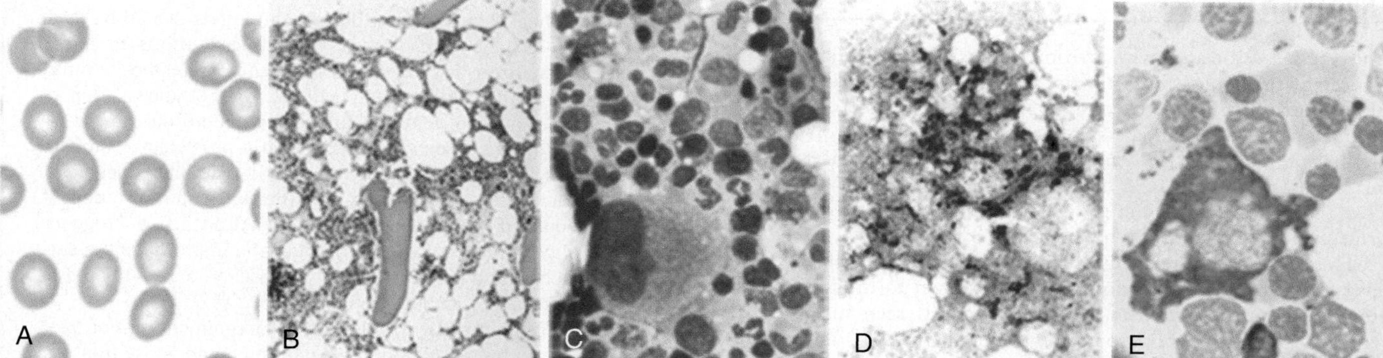

Figure 35-1 ANEMIA OF CHRONIC DISEASE. **A,** Peripheral blood typically exhibits a normochromic, normocytic anemia. **B** and **C,** Bone marrow examination is sometimes performed to rule out other causes of anemia. Typically, the bone marrow is morphologically normal. **D** and **E,** Prussian blue iron stain shows increased iron stores with increased histiocytic iron but decreased sideroblastic iron.

whom bone marrow aspirates were obtained for assessment of iron stores, the serum ferritin level was significantly lower in patients who were iron deficient but was still elevated (63.7 versus 212 ng/mL).[107] A three-step algorithm has been derived for patients with rheumatoid arthritis and serologic evidence of ACD. Male patients with hemoglobin levels less than 11.0 g/dL and serum ferritin concentration less than 40 mg/L have iron deficiency, and those with mean corpuscular volumes greater than 85 fL or an iron saturation level greater than 7% have ACD. This formula led to a correct diagnosis in 89% of patients but has not been independently validated.[108] Most investigators maintain that serum iron studies cannot predictably rule out iron deficiency.[121]

Additional functional tests of iron status have been developed, including soluble transferrin receptors (sTfrs), hemoglobin concentration in reticulocytes (CHr), percent of hypochromic RBCs (% HYPO), and serum hepcidin levels. sTFrs are elevated in iron-deficiency anemia. Several studies have shown that the numbers of transferrin receptors on erythroblasts are lower in rheumatoid arthritis patients with ACD than in patients with iron-deficiency anemia,[34] and some may be decreased even below those without inflammatory conditions.[122] In addition, the levels of sTfr in rheumatoid arthritis and ACD are normal or slighter higher than normal (although generally lower than those with iron-deficiency anemia).[123,124] Patients with rheumatoid arthritis and elevated concentrations of serum transferrin receptors have responded to iron therapy.[124] Algorithms that integrate serum ferritin, sTfr concentration (or a ratio of sTfr to log ferritin, known as an sTfr index), and other markers of inflammation (e.g., ESR or CRP) have been derived in attempts to differentiate iron deficiency from ACD (with or without concomitant iron deficiency).[125-127] A useful strategy, where these tests are available, may be a measured and calculated sTfr index, which reflects iron stores in conventional anemia and in ACD. An sTfr index above 0.8 may discern iron deficiency in subjects with inflammation, and an index above 1.5 may do likewise in subjects without inflammation.[127,128] Recently, the algorithm has been modified to incorporate hepcidin levels, which may increase specificity for iron deficiency in ACD,[129] but this has not yet been prospectively confirmed. Reticulocyte hemoglobin concentration (CHr or Ret he), distinct from indices of mature RBCs, can reflect the recent status of iron stores in normal or EPO-induced erythropoiesis.[130-132] Hepcidin levels, extensively reported based on urinary assays (reported as a hepcidin-to-creatinine ratio), have been shown to mirror hepatic hepcidin mRNA concentrations in patients with a range of inflammatory diseases. A recently developed serum hepcidin immunoassay holds promise.[76] The development of sTfr-, CHr- or Ret he-, and hepcidin-based algorithms for iron-replete and iron-deficient ACD is ongoing.[129] A combination of these newer tests is likely to be useful in diagnosing ACD, but none is fully characterized or yet widely incorporated into clinical practice. Thus, until these assays are reproducibly integrated into clinical care, the diagnosis of ACD remains a clinical one.

TREATMENT

The anemia associated with chronic illness is often mild. In 2120 subjects with rheumatoid arthritis, a classical inflammatory cause of ACD, the annual incidence of anemia less than 10 g/dL, which was proportionate with markers of inflammation, was only 1.5%, with a lifetime prevalence of 13.7%.[35] In 420 subjects with cancer referred for radiation therapy, 16% had Hgb levels of less than 10 g/dL.14 Thus, correction of anemia per se may be unnecessary, especially if contributing factors can be reversed.

There may also be teleologic beneficial contributions of ACD. The fever associated with infections has been shown to inhibit bacterial growth, and decreased iron concentrations (as seen in ACD) act synergistically with pyrexia to inhibit bacterial growth.[133] This attempt by hosts to withhold iron from invaders, called *nutritional immunity*, has been postulated to be an adaptive factor of ACD.[95] Furthermore, elevations in serum iron have been associated with a discernible increase in cancer risk.[6-9] However, ACD can be severe, and almost by definition patients with ACD have comorbidities. Optimizing any reversible process, including hemoglobin and oxygen content and delivery, may have a dramatic beneficial effect because, as discussed, the range of underlying diagnoses in ACD is broad, and therapy precludes a uniform approach. In addition, few randomized, well-controlled, blinded studies are available to support anecdotal therapeutic observations (see box on Treatment of Anemia of Chronic Diseases).

Optimal treatment of ACD is correction of the underlying disease process, if known and if possible. ACD mirrors laboratory[94,106] and clinical[26] correlates of disease activity and duration of disease in rheumatoid arthritis. HIV patients receiving highly active antiretroviral therapy have a mean increase in hemoglobin concentration of more than 3 g/L compared with a decrease in hemoglobin concentration in patients not receiving these medications.[134] Treatment of underlying inflammatory diseases using cytokine antagonists, such as anti–TNF-α therapy, can lead to improvements in anemia.[65-67] Unfortunately, definitive treatment of chronic diseases is the exception.

Serum levels of EPO, although often elevated in ACD, are not elevated appropriately for the degree of anemia. Moreover, inhibition of hematopoiesis by cytokines is reversed in model systems by EPO.[100] Not surprising given the underlying physiology in many cases of ACD, a number of studies have shown responses to EPO, although high doses may be necessary. This strategy may be more cost effective than transfusion. A small, multicenter, placebo-controlled trial monitored the effects of EPO in patients with rheumatoid arthritis and a clinical diagnosis of ACD. The results showed a dose-dependent response to 50 to 150 U/kg of EPO three times each week; 11 of 17 patients had a response rate of almost six hematocrit points.[135] Anemic patients with AIDS who were treated with recombinant EPO had a significantly decreased transfusion requirement, especially if their endogenous EPO level was less than 500 IU/L; however, all of these patients were also receiving zidovudine, a potential bone marrow

Treatment of Anemia of Chronic Diseases

Treating ACD often is unnecessary if the patient is asymptomatic. However, if the anemia is symptomatic or severe, treatment of the anemia itself may be indicated. Epidemiologic studies, such as those in patients with heart failure, HIV, cancer, or kidney disease, suggest physiologic and subjective improvement in signs and symptoms after treatment for anemia.[171,172] However, treatments need to be individualized because the risks of erythropoiesis-stimulating agents or iron therapy in non–iron deficient subjects are theoretically real and practically unknowable given the variety of underlying conditions that are incorporated under the rubric of chronic disease. A trial of ACD-directed therapy may be indicated in symptomatic patients.

The first priority in ACD should be to correct any reversible contributors to the anemia. Because the extent of ACD mirrors the activity of the underlying disease, all efforts should be made to treat the underlying disease. Furthermore, efforts to correct anemia should be modulated by the recognition that the "optimal" target hemoglobin for subjects with ACD is not known. Reports of anemia in subjects without inflammation but religiously opposed to transfusions have suggested a physiologic cutoff for anemia of 5 g/dL, below which increased mortality is seen.[173,174] In addition, acutely ill patients have not been shown to benefit, in randomized, controlled studies, from transfusion "triggers" above 7 g/dL.[174] Nonetheless, symptomatic improvement is seen in subjects with a range of chronic diseases who were treated for anemia of a more modest degree.[171]

Transfusion therapy may be the most common form of treatment of symptomatic ACD, albeit with the potential for transmitting infection; inducing alloimmunization; or, rarely, leading to graft-versus-host disease.

suppressant.[136] Recombinant EPO raised the hemoglobin level in patients with a variety of nonhematologic malignancies, including squamous cell cancer, breast cancer, and colon cancer.[137-140] Large trials enrolling patients undergoing chemotherapy have suggested that once-weekly injections of recombinant EPO are as effective as thrice-weekly injections.[141] Injections of long-lasting EPO analogues have been effective in treating the anemia that occurs with chemotherapy administration[142] and in animal models of ACD[143] and can be used to decrease the frequency of administration.

A starting dose of 20,000 units given subcutaneously each week, anecdotally believed to be a reasonably upper limit in kidney disease patients, can be initiated.[144] If a hemoglobin response is seen, the dose can be decreased and the duration prolonged to titrate the hemoglobin to an asymptomatic level. Careful follow-up and dose titration are essential to minimize expense; the number of injections needed; and, extrapolating from other studies, any potential detriment seen from high hematocrits or high levels of exogenous EPO. This response may take 4 to 8 weeks and should be monitored with objective symptomatic improvements (e.g., exercise tolerance). If after 2 weeks the serum EPO level is higher than 100 mU/mL and the hemoglobin concentration has not increased by at least 0.5 g/dL or if after 2 weeks of treatment the serum ferritin level is higher than 400 ng/mL, a response is very unlikely.[145] In a multivariate analysis of 80 patients with chronic anemia of cancer, only the absolute hemoglobin value, serum EPO level, and ferritin level, but not disease status, bone marrow involvement, or treatment status, were independent predictors of response to EPO treatment.[145] In general, responses by patients with ACD to EPO range from 40% to 80% and can take up to 4 weeks.[135,146,147] Studies suggest that if no effect is seen by 3 months, further treatment is unlikely to be effective.[145]

Functional iron deficiency, even in the setting of normal or elevated total iron stores, is one possible reason for a failed response to EPO.[148] This may be caused by a baseline iron deficiency, depletion of iron stores during hematopoiesis, or an inability to mobilize stored iron; the latter is a hallmark of ACD. Intravenous iron decreased EPO requirements, even compared with oral iron, in several cohorts, including hemodialysis patients[149] and those with inflammatory bowel disease.[150] Intravenous iron improves EPO responses and is a cost-effective measure in dialysis patients, even in those with elevated ferritin levels.[151] In addition, anemia arising from concomitant true EPO deficiency and EPO "resistance" in chronic kidney disease has been successfully managed with supplemental intravenous iron, in short-term studies,[152,153] despite elevated ferritin levels in these subjects. The long-term risks and benefits from such an approach are not known. Paradoxically, iron chelators such as deferoxamine have been shown in some animal studies to have mild effects on ACD, perhaps by decreasing free radicals and inflammation, but other studies have not duplicated this finding.[147,154]

Although EPO administration often leads to an increased hemoglobin concentration, this does not a priori ensure an improvement in morbidity, mortality, or quality of life. Reversal of anemia with EPO in randomized and nonrandomized, open-label studies has been correlated with improvements in functional status, pain, nausea, anxiety, level of activity, and fatigue in large cohorts of patients receiving chemotherapy and smaller studies of cancer patients not undergoing chemotherapy.[137,140,141,155] However, many of these studies have limitations.[115] A thorough examination of the literature led to the suggestion that in cancer patients receiving chemotherapy, the hemoglobin level should be maintained at 12 g/L, and further rigorous studies on the impact on quality of life are necessary.[155] Many studies have shown that pretreatment anemia is a poor prognostic factor for a wide variety of patients with solid tumors undergoing chemotherapy and irradiation, and it is unclear whether correction of this anemia can improve survival.[17]

Most studies and consensus statements on the efficacy of correcting anemia have derived from cancer patients receiving chemotherapy. However, the acute anemia and symptoms associated with myelosuppressive chemotherapy have limited similarities to ACD. Small and preliminary studies of cancer patients with ACD who were not receiving cytotoxic therapy suggest that performance and quality of life may improve with increased hemoglobin concentrations.[140] However, in a large study of critically ill patients, no change in a variety of outcomes were observed when patients were transfused when the hemoglobin level was 10 g/L as opposed to a control group in whom the transfusion trigger was a hemoglobin level of 7 g/L.[156] Although administration of EPO to critically ill patients decreased the number of transfusions, no change in clinical outcome was observed.[157]

Moreover, enthusiasm for EPO use in symptomatic patients with ACD must be tempered by recent observations in individuals with kidney disease and cancer in whom erythropoiesis-stimulating agents (whether short- or long-acting forms of EPO) were associated with increased risks of stroke and thromboembolism, respectively, with a suggestive increase in mortality in large studies.[144,158-163] Studies have also indicated that critically ill patients and those with cancer undergoing chemotherapy may have an increased rate of thromboses and overall death when treated with EPO, particularly if target hemoglobins are higher than 10 to 11 g/dL.[159,163] Increasing the hematocrit to 42% in a large number of hemodialysis patients with cardiac disease led to an increased number of deaths, and the number of cardiac events was increased in patients with chronic renal disease treated with EPO with a goal of complete normalization of hemoglobin (12.0-15.0 g/dL) as opposed to partial normalization (10.5-11.5 g/dL).[164,165] Although low pretreatment hemoglobin levels have been demonstrated repeatedly to be a predictor of good response to chemotherapy and radiation,[166] two studies have demonstrated that patients with breast cancer or head and neck cancer treated with EPO have increased disease progression and worse survival than placebo-treated patients.[167,168] This finding may reflect a direct antiapoptotic effect of EPO on tumors.[169] Not all studies have demonstrated increased risks associated with aggressive EPO treatment in patients with kidney disease or cancer.[159,170] However, based on these studies and interim analyses of several additional studies, in early 2007, the U.S. Food and Drug Administration warned that EPO should be given only in the lowest possible doses necessary to avoid blood transfusions. More recently, consensus agreements have urged that for patients with cancer, erythropoiesis-stimulating agents should only be used in those receiving chemotherapy and only when chemotherapy is with palliative (i.e., not curative) intent.

In summary, although treatment of patients with ACD often increases the hemoglobin level and may improve quality of life and function, data from formal, well-controlled studies are pending, especially for patients not receiving cytotoxic chemotherapy. In particular, high doses of EPO or high hemoglobin levels may be associated with increased risk for cardiac events, thromboses, and tumor progression. Clinicians and patients should be reminded of the unclear benefits and risks in the ACD population of erythropoiesis-stimulating agents and iron. Treatment should be initiated cautiously and followed closely. It is hoped that targeted therapies for ACD, focusing on disrupting cytokine signaling or interfering with hepcidin activity, will be soon available for clinical trials.

SUMMARY AND FUTURE DIRECTIONS

Anemia is common in many chronic inflammatory, infectious, and malignant conditions, and often it is multifactorial. Anemia is exacerbated by inflammatory cytokines, which are thought to be the most important causative factors in ACD. ACD is difficult to diagnose but usually can be strongly suspected based on clinical findings, elimination of other causes of anemia, low serum iron and transferrin levels, and elevated ferritin level. Cytokines such as IFN and TNF have wide-ranging effects, including both direct and indirect inhibition of hematopoiesis. Direct inhibition of hematopoiesis is mediated by both a relative decrease in EPO as well as a decrease in iron available for hemoglobin synthesis. Many of the abnormalities of iron metabolism in ACD are caused by cytokine-induced increases in hepcidin, and appreciation of the role of hepcidin in ACD may aid in the diagnosis and treatment. Anemia, iron deficiency, and hepcidin may have independent antimicrobial and antitumor roles, and this needs further study. Controlled studies, clearly revealing the impact of correction of anemia on quality of life, medical outcomes, and survival of patients with ACD, particularly in those not undergoing chemotherapy, could provide insight into the role of hypoxia on tumors and other disease. The treatment of patients with ACD should be focused on correcting the underlying disease. Although increasing hemoglobin with exogenous EPO can be quite effective, the potential deleterious results of this strategy must be considered. Development of new agents that might stimulate erythropoiesis but not cancer and risk factors for deleterious EPO effects need to be investigated. In addition, the risk of EPO therapy specifically in the ACD, as opposed to in renal disease or as part of chemotherapy, needs to be investigated.

SUGGESTED READINGS

Bohlius J, Wilson J, Seidenfeld J, et al: Recombinant human erythropoietins and cancer patients: Updated meta-analysis of 57 studies including 9353 patients. *J Natl Cancer Inst* 98:708, 2006.

Brower V: Erythropoietin may impair, not improve, cancer survival. *Nat Med* 9:1439, 2003.

Canon JL, Vansteenkiste J, Bodoky G, et al: Randomized, double-blind, active-controlled trial of every-3-week darbepoetin alfa for the treatment of chemotherapy-induced anemia. *J Natl Cancer Inst* 98:273, 2006.

Corwin HL, Gettinger A, Pearl RG, et al: Efficacy of recombinant human erythropoietin in critically ill patients: A randomized controlled trial. *JAMA* 288:2827, 2002.

Dallalio G, Law E, Means RT Jr: Hepcidin inhibits in vitro erythroid colony formation at reduced erythropoietin concentrations. *Blood* 107:2702, 2006.

Detivaud L, Nemeth E, Boudjema K, et al: Hepcidin levels in humans are correlated with hepatic iron stores, hemoglobin levels, and hepatic function. *Blood* 106:746, 2005.

Drueke TB, Locatelli F, Clyne N, et al: Normalization of hemoglobin level in patients with chronic kidney disease and anemia. *N Engl J Med* 355:2071, 2006.

Ganz T: Hepcidin—A peptide hormone at the interface of innate immunity and iron metabolism. *Curr Top Microbiol Immunol* 306:183, 2006.

Nemeth E, Rivera S, Gabayan V, et al: IL-6 mediates hypoferremia of inflammation by inducing the synthesis of the iron regulatory hormone hepcidin. *J Clin Invest* 113:1271, 2004.

Gabrilove JL, Cleeland CS, Livingston RB, et al: Clinical evaluation of once-weekly dosing of epoetin alfa in chemotherapy patients: Improvements in hemoglobin and quality of life are similar to three-times-weekly dosing. *J Clin Oncol* 19:2875, 2001.

Inamura J, Ikuta K, Jimbo J, et al: Upregulation of hepcidin by interleukin-1beta in human hepatoma cell lines. *Hepatol Res* 33:198, 2005.

Kemna E, Pickkers P, Nemeth E, et al: Time-course analysis of hepcidin, serum iron, and plasma cytokine levels in humans injected with LPS. *Blood* 106:1864, 2005.

Kluger MJ, Rothenburg BA: Fever and reduced iron: Their interaction as a host defense response to bacterial infection. *Science* 203:374, 1979.

Lee P, Peng H, Gelbart T, et al: Regulation of hepcidin transcription by interleukin-1 and interleukin-6. *Proc Natl Acad Sci U S A* 102:1906, 2005.

Ludwig H, Crawford J, Osterborg A, et al: Pooled analysis of individual patient-level data from all randomized double-blind, placebo-controlled trials of darbepoetin alfa in the treatment of patients with chemotherapy-induced anemia. *J Clin Oncol* 27:2838, 2009.

Miller CB, Jones RJ, Piantadosi S, et al: Decreased erythropoietin response in patients with the anemia of cancer. *N Engl J Med* 322:1689, 1990.

Nicolas G, Bennoun M, Porteu A, et al: Severe iron deficiency anemia in transgenic mice expressing liver hepcidin. *Proc Natl Acad Sci U S A* 99:4596, 2002.

Obermair A, Petru E, Windbichler G, et al: Significance of pretreatment serum hemoglobin and survival in epithelial ovarian cancer. *Oncol Rep* 7:639, 2000.

Okonko DO, Van Veldhuisen DJ, Poole-Wilson PA, et al: Anaemia of chronic disease in chronic heart failure: The emerging evidence. *Eur Heart J* 26:2213, 2005.

Opasich C, Cazzola M, Scelsi L, et al: Blunted erythropoietin production and defective iron supply for erythropoiesis as major causes of anaemia in patients with chronic heart failure. *Eur Heart J* 26:2232, 2005.

Rizzo JD, Brouwers M, Hurley P. et al: American Society of Hematology/American Society of Clinical Oncology clinical practice guideline update on the use of epoetin and darbepoetin in adult patients with cancer. *Blood* 116: 4045, 2010

Roodman GD, Horadam VW, Wright TL: Inhibition of erythroid colony formation by autologous bone marrow adherent cells from patients with the anemia of chronic disease. *Blood* 62:406, 1983.

Roy CN, Andrews NC: Anemia of inflammation: The hepcidin link. *Curr Opin Hematol* 12:107, 2005.

Roy CN: Anemia of inflammation. *Hematology Am Soc Hematol Educ Program* 2010:276, 2010.

Singh AK, Szczech L, Tang KL, et al: Correction of anemia with epoetin alfa in chronic kidney disease. *N Engl J Med* 355:2085, 2006.

Skikne BS, Punnonen K, Caldron PH, et al: Improved differential diagnosis of anemia of chronic disease and iron deficiency anemia: A prospective multicenter evaluation of soluble transferrin receptor and the sTfR/log ferritin index. *Am J Hematol* 86:923, 2011.

Tam BY, Wei K, Rudge JS, et al: VEGF modulates erythropoiesis through regulation of adult hepatic erythropoietin synthesis. *Nat Med* 12:793, 2006.

Theurl I, Mattle V, Seifert M, et al: Dysregulated monocyte iron homeostasis and erythropoietin formation in patients with anemia of chronic disease. *Blood* 107:4142, 2006.

Vreugdenhil G, Wognum AW, van Eijk HG, et al: Anaemia in rheumatoid arthritis: The role of iron, vitamin B12, and folic acid deficiency, and erythropoietin responsiveness. *Ann Rheum Dis* 49:93, 1990.

Wang RH, Li C, Xu X, et al: A role of SMAD4 in iron metabolism through the positive regulation of hepcidin expression. *Cell Metab* 2:399, 2005.

Zhang DL, Senecal T, Ghosh MC, et al: Hepcidin regulates ferroportin expression and intracellular iron homeostasis of erythroblasts. *Blood* 118:2868, 2011.

For complete list of references log on to www.expertconsult.com.

CHAPTER 36

HEME BIOSYNTHESIS AND ITS DISORDERS: PORPHYRIAS AND SIDEROBLASTIC ANEMIAS

Stephen J. Fuller and James S. Wiley

The porphyrias and the sideroblastic anemias are metabolic disorders that involve defects in heme biosynthesis. Most forms of porphyria are inherited in a mendelian autosomal dominant pattern, but some types are recessive and others are acquired through exposure to porphyrinogenic drugs and chemicals. A linked group of diseases, the porphyrinurias, are not porphyrias but have in common alterations of heme biosynthesis. Porphyrins are tetrapyrroles, which are ubiquitous in nature and exhibit characteristic red fluorescence on exposure to ultraviolet light. The iron-porphyrin complex, called *heme,* is central to all biologic oxidation reactions. In plants, the porphyrin molecule is combined with magnesium to form chlorophyll. Porphyrin biosynthesis is one of the most essential biochemical processes in most life forms.

In humans, mutations affecting the first enzyme of the heme biosynthetic pathway produce sideroblastic anemia. Inborn errors that occur at subsequent sites in this pathway usually result in metabolic disorders known as the *porphyrias* (Fig. 36-1). Historical analysis of the potential presence of acute porphyria in the British royal family has been published,[1-3] as well as a study of the family of Vincent van Gogh.[4]

HEME BIOSYNTHESIS

Biosynthetic Pathways

Heme biosynthesis is an essential pathway and occurs in all metabolically active cells that contain mitochondria. It is most active in erythropoietic tissue, where it is required for hemoglobin synthesis, and in hepatic tissue, where the heme forms the basis of various heme-containing enzymes such as the cytochromes P450, catalase, cytochrome oxidase, and tryptophan pyrrolase. The synthetic pathway starts with the condensation of glycine and succinyl CoA to form 5-aminolevulinate (ALA) under the control of the mitochondrial enzyme ALA synthase (ALAS). This enzyme requires pyridoxal phosphate as a cofactor. A series of enzymes then controls the conversion of ALA first to the monopyrrole porphobilinogen (PBG) and then to the various porphyrins. Iron is inserted into protoporphyrin by the enzyme ferrochelatase to form heme (see Fig. 36-1). During the past 10 years, complementary deoxyribonucleic acid (cDNA) clones have been obtained for all of the enzymes of heme biosynthesis, and the structures of the corresponding genes have been determined. These advances are certain to improve understanding of the pathogenesis of the porphyrias and methods for identification of carriers. The enzymes of the biosynthetic pathway have all been mapped to specific chromosomes (Table 36-1). Heme synthesis and its disorders have been the subject of reviews,[5-10] and advances in our knowledge of mitochondrial iron trafficking and metabolism have recently been reviewed.[11]

Control of Heme Biosynthesis

The overproduction of porphyrins and their precursors in the different porphyrias is mainly hepatic or erythropoietic in origin. In the acute porphyrias and in porphyria cutanea tarda (PCT), the liver is the main source of overproduction; in congenital porphyria, the marrow is the main source; and in erythropoietic protoporphyria, porphyrins are overproduced by the liver and marrow.

Control of hepatic heme biosynthesis is regulated by the rate of the initial enzymatic step, ALAS (now designated ALAS1), which is under negative-feedback control by heme. This occurs by more than one mechanism. Heme represses transcription of the ALAS1 gene and increases the rate of degradation of the messenger ribonucleic acid (mRNA) (Fig. 36-2, *A*). At the posttranslational level, heme blocks the translocation of pre-ALAS1 into the mitochondrion.[12] In the mitochondrion, the molecular mass of ALAS is smaller than that of the cytosolic pre-ALAS[12] because of the removal of the mitochondrial targeting sequence. Finally, heme regulates levels of mature ALAS by activation of a mitochondrial proteolysis system.[13]

The erythroid bone marrow is the major heme-forming tissue in the body, producing 85% of the daily heme requirement. Heme synthesis in erythroid cells varies from that in hepatocytes; it is linked to tissue differentiation, and the half-life of the same end product of the two is quite different. Heme complexed with globin is preserved in circulating red blood cells for approximately 120 days, whereas heme produced in liver for cytochromes and enzymes, such as catalase, is subject to much more rapid turnover, measurable in hours. Regulation in the liver is exquisitely sensitive to fluctuations in intracellular heme levels[14] and responds rapidly to the requirements for synthesis as described in Fig. 36-2, *A*. However, heme synthesis in the bone marrow shows a more leisurely response. This fundamental difference is explained by the finding of two different tissue-specific isoenzymes and two different cDNAs for human liver or "housekeeping" ALAS (ALAS1) and an erythroid ALAS (eALAS or ALAS2), which is expressed exclusively in erythroid cells.[15] The gene for ALAS2 has been mapped to the X chromosome and that for the hepatic enzyme to chromosome 3.[15] The ALAS2 gene has 11 exons; exons 5 to 11 encode the catalytic domain of the enzyme and include a lysine residue that forms a Schiff base with the pyridoxal phosphate cofactor. Exon 1 contributes to the 5′-untranslated region (UTR) whose structure allows iron to regulate ALAS2 mRNA translation, whereas exons 1 and 2 contribute the sequence that targets the enzyme to the mitochondria and is cleaved after import. Succinyl CoA synthetase associates specifically with ALAS2 within the mitochondrion, which helps promote the first step of heme synthesis.[16]

Enzyme levels of ubiquitous and erythroid isoenzymes of ALAS are controlled by different mechanisms. Ubiquitous ALAS1 levels in liver are regulated by negative feedback by heme that inhibits gene transcription and import of pre-ALAS1 (see Fig. 36-2, *A*). More recently ALAS-1 has been shown to be upregulated by peroxisome proliferator-activated receptor-gamma, coactivator 1, alpha (PPAR-γ coactivator 1-α) which regulates mitochondrial biogenesis and oxidative metabolism. Transcription of this coactivator 1-α is controlled by glucose availability. Coactivator 1-α production increases when glucose levels are low, leading to increased levels of ALAS-1 and heme. These conditions are conducive to an acute attack of porphyria. However, the relative contribution of heme and PPAR-γ coactivator 1-α in regulating ALAS-1 expression remains to be resolved.[17,18] In contrast, heme does not affect transcription of the ALAS2 gene, which is under the control of erythroid-specific promoters such as GATA1, a globin transcription factor. Whether heme inhibits import of pre-ALAS2 into the mitochondrial matrix remains to be unequivocally established. Heme may possibly also prevent the accumulation of intracellular iron by controlling the acquisition of iron from transferrin (see Fig. 36-2, *B*). In addition to transport of iron from plasma to the cytosol by the transferrin receptor, a second transport step is required for mitochondrial uptake of iron. This step is fulfilled by mitoferrin,[19] a member of the solute carrier 25 family of proteins located in the inner mitochondrial membrane, which to import iron into the mitochondrion must interact with the adenosine triphosphate (ATP)-binding cassette transporter ABCB10.[20] Levels of intracellular iron regulate the translation of ALAS2 mRNA. Cellular iron homeostasis is maintained through a posttranscriptional regulatory mechanism, which is mediated by iron regulatory proteins that bind to iron-responsive elements in mRNA of target genes to either increase or decrease translation.[21,22] The RNA binding activity of iron-responsive proteins (IRP) is regulated by mitochondrial iron-sulfur cluster synthesis and cytosolic iron levels.[23-25] When iron is available for heme synthesis, translation of ALAS2 is allowed to proceed as a result of decreased IRP binding to the 5′ UTR IRE of ALAS2 mRNA. In contrast, under iron-depleted conditions increased IRP binding to ALAS2 mRNA blocks translation and ensures that ALAS2 and protoporphyrin levels are not produced in excess of available iron. Furthermore, to prevent the cell from becoming iron deficient, increased translation of mRNA from genes that increase cellular iron, such as the transferrin 1 gene, results from stabilization of mRNA by binding of IRPs to mRNA (see Chapter 33). This effect ensures that protoporphyrin synthesis is coupled to iron availability.

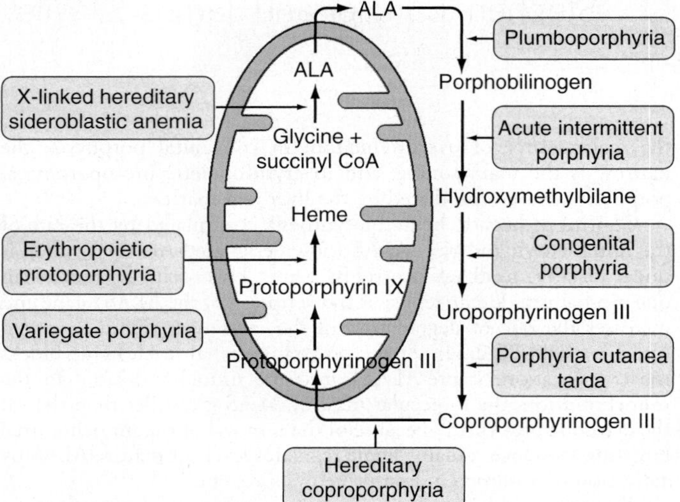

Figure 36-1 PATHWAY OF HEME BIOSYNTHESIS IN MAMMALIAN CELLS. The first step in the pathway is catalyzed by aminolevulinate synthase (ALAS) and occurs within the mitochondrion using pyridoxal 5′-phosphate as a cofactor. 5-Aminolevulinate (ALA) then leaves the mitochondrion and is converted by ALA dehydratase to give a monopyrrole, porphobilinogen. Four molecules of this compound are converted by porphobilinogen deaminase to a linear tetrapyrrole, hydroxymethylbilane. This molecule is then cyclized by uroporphyrinogen III synthase to uroporphyrinogen III, which is decarboxylated to coproporphyrinogen III. This molecule enters the mitochondrion and is oxidized in succession by coproporphyrinogen III oxidase and protoporphyrinogen III oxidase. The product is protoporphyrin IX, a substrate for ferrochelatase, which catalyzes the insertion of Fe^{2+} to form heme. The defective steps associated with specific porphyrias and X-linked hereditary sideroblastic anemias are shown.

A second rate-limiting step in the overall heme synthetic pathway lies at the level of porphobilinogen deaminase (PBGD), which has a low endogenous activity and is inhibited by protoporphyrinogen and coproporphyrinogen. There are also two forms of PBGD. The PBGD gene (HMBS) encodes two enzymes, which arise from alternative splicing of PBGD mRNA. One isoform is expressed in all cells, whereas a second is restricted to red cells.[26] Erythroid PBGD is stimulated by erythropoiesis in vitro and may play a regulatory role in heme biosynthesis during differentiation.[27]

HMBS, the human PBGD gene, has attracted extensive investigation because of the practical importance of detecting carriers of the gene for acute intermittent porphyria.[28] Studies of the genetic locus of PBGD on chromosome 11 show great molecular heterogeneity, with up to 50 mutations resulting either in single amino acid substitutions or premature chain termination listed in the National Center for Biotechnology Information dbSNP database (http://www.ncbi.nlm.nih.gov/snp). Most human mutations have been described in exons 10 and 12,[29] which is consistent with alteration of the binding sites for the dipyrromethane cofactor for the enzyme. The three-dimensional structure of PBGD has been defined by x-ray crystallography, which has allowed study of the structural and functional implications of mutations.[30]

Table 36-1 Porphyrias: Clinical Involvement, Enzymatic Etiology, and Chromosomal Location

Porphyria (Synonym)	Acute Attack, Skin and Organ Involvement	Enzyme of Heme Biosynthesis Affected	Chromosome Location
—	—	Hepatic aminolevulinate synthase-1 (ALAS1)	3p21
X-linked sideroblastic anemia	Bone marrow	Erythroid ALA synthase (ALAS2)	Xp11.21
X-linked dominant protoporphyria	Skin, red cells, liver	Erythroid ALA synthase (ALAS2)	Xp11.21
ALA dehydratase deficiency porphyria (plumboporphyria)	Acute liver	ALA dehydratase (porphobilinogen synthase)	9q33.1
Acute intermittent porphyria (intermittent acute porphyria)	Acute liver	Porphobilinogen deaminase (hydroxymethylbilane synthase)	11q23.3
Congenital erythropoietic porphyria (Günther disease)	Skin, red cells, bone marrow	Uroporphyrinogen III synthase	10q25.2–q26.3
Porphyria cutanea tarda (symptomatic porphyria, cutaneous hepatic porphyria)	Skin, liver	Uroporphyrinogen decarboxylase	1p34
Hereditary coproporphyria	Acute skin, liver	Coproporphyrinogen oxidase	3q12
Variegate porphyria (porphyria variegata)	Acute skin, liver	Protoporphyrinogen oxidase	1q22
Erythropoietic protoporphyria (erythrohepatic protoporphyria)	Skin red cells, liver	Ferrochelatase (heme synthase)	18q21.3

ALA, 5-Aminolevulinate.

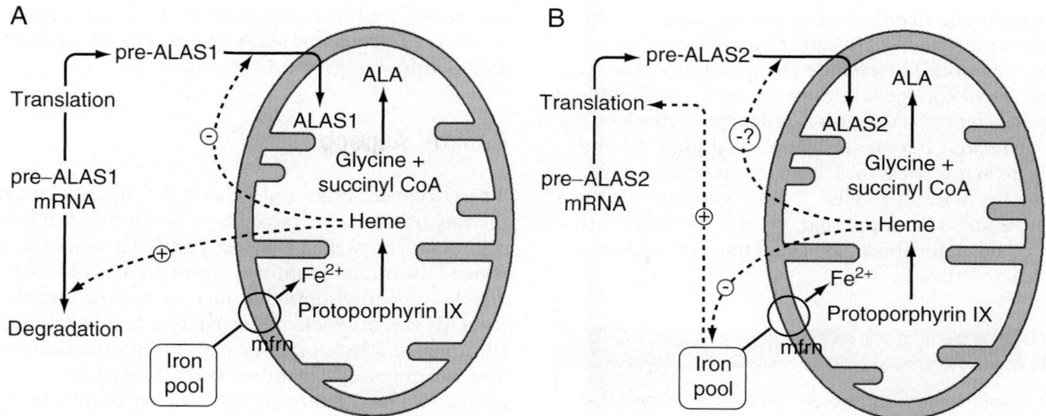

Figure 36-2 A, CONTROL OF HEME SYNTHESIS IN HEPATIC AND OTHER TISSUES. The rate of heme synthesis depends on the first and rate-limiting enzymatic step catalyzed by aminolevulinate synthase-1 (ALAS1). Heme represses transcription of the ALAS1 gene, increases the rate of degradation of its messenger ribonucleic acid (mRNA), and blocks the translocation of the ALAS1 isoenzyme into the mitochondrion. **B,** CONTROL OF HEME SYNTHESIS IN ERYTHROBLASTS. Cytosolic iron enhances the translation of mRNA of the pre-ALAS2 by inhibiting the interaction of a repressor protein with an iron-responsive element in the mRNA. The product of the last step, heme inhibits the uptake of iron from transferrin into the cytosol. Heme also may inhibit translocation of ALAS2 into the mitochondrion. The overall result is that the rate of heme synthesis is tightly linked to the availability of iron for the ferrochelatase reaction. Mitoferrin (mfrn) transports Fe^{2+} into the mitochondrial matrix. *ALA,* 5-Aminolevulinate.

Table 36-2 Classification of Porphyrias

Classification	Disease	Biochemistry	Clinical Features
Acute porphyria	Acute intermittent porphyria	Increased ALA and PBG	Acute attack
	Variegate porphyria	Increased ALA and PBG; increased porphyrin	Acute attack; photosensitivity
	Hereditary coproporphyria	Increased ALA and PBG; increased porphyrin	Acute attack; photosensitivity
	ALA dehydratase deficiency porphyria	Increased ALA; increased porphyrin	Acute and chronic neuropathy
Nonacute porphyria	Porphyria cutanea tarda	Increased porphyrin	Photosensitivity
	Erythropoietic protoporphyria	Increased porphyrin	Photosensitivity
	Congenital porphyria	Increased porphyrin	Photosensitivity
	X-linked dominant protoporphyria	Increased porphyrin	Photosensitivity
Porphyrinurias	Lead, alcohol, iron deficiency anemia, liver disease	Various biochemical manifestations	Various clinical presentations

ALA, 5-Aminolevulinate; *PBG,* porphobilinogen.

PORPHYRIAS

Biologic and Molecular Aspects

The porphyrias are classified as acute or nonacute (cutaneous) according to their clinical and biochemical features (Table 36-2).

Each of the different types of porphyria is linked to a reduced activity or deficiency of a specific enzyme in the heme biosynthetic pathway, with the exception of the recently described X-linked dominant erythropoietic protoporphyria, which results from inheritance of a gain-of-function mutation in the ALAS2 gene[31] (see Fig. 36-1). When porphyria is caused by a loss-of-function mutation, the resulting enzyme deficiency impairs the production of the end-product heme, and there is overproduction and increased excretion of the heme precursors formed by the steps before the enzyme defect. There is also a compensatory increase in activity of the initial and rate-controlling enzyme ALAS. In the acute porphyrias, there is overproduction of all the porphyrins and porphyrin precursors (e.g., ALA, PBG) formed proximal to the enzyme defect. The increased excretion of porphyrin precursors in the acute porphyrias is caused by decreased activity of PBGD in these conditions. The decrease can be caused by genetic mutation of the enzyme (in acute intermittent porphyria) or by inhibition of PBGD by protoporphyrinogen and coproporphyrinogen in variegate porphyria and hereditary coproporphyria, respectively.[32]

In the nonacute porphyrias, there is overproduction of all porphyrins formed before the enzyme defect but no overproduction of porphyrin precursors. The cause of this lack of overproduction of porphyrin precursors in the nonacute porphyrias is unclear, but it may result from a compensatory increase in the activity of the enzyme PBGD in addition to increased activity of ALAS and site-specific heme synthesis.[33] The pattern of overproduction and excretion of porphyrins and porphyrin precursors in the various porphyrias is shown in Table 36-3. A consequence is that each of the different porphyrias is characterized by a different excretion pattern. Quantitative studies of the different porphyrins and precursors in the urine and feces usually identify the particular type of porphyria. The porphyrin precursors ALA and PBG and the more water-soluble porphyrins (with multiple carboxyl groups) are excreted mainly in the urine. Other porphyrins are mainly excreted in the feces by way of the bile (see box on Measurement of Porphyrins and Precursors).

The clinical manifestations of an acute attack of porphyria can be explained by dysfunction of the central, peripheral, and autonomic nervous systems. The mechanism by which altered heme synthesis results in dysfunction is unknown.

Perhaps the most likely hypothesis is that the neurologic and muscular manifestations of acute porphyria arise as a result of heme deficiency within the nerve cells, which causes dysfunction of the energy-dependent Na^+/K^+ ATPase. The proposal that axonal dysfunction results from impaired energy metabolism is supported by the findings of axonal membrane depolarization during acute attacks of porphyric neuropathy and reduction in inward rectification between episodes.[38] However, this does not exclude the possibility that ALA may also act as a pharmacologic agent in these diseases, compounding the effects of heme deficiency.[39] ALA has a prooxidant effect on rat brain tissues and generates free radical species during its autooxidation, and this oxidant stress has been proposed to directly damage myelination by Schwann cells.[40,41] The concept of autooxidation or oxidative stress is supported by the hypothesis that manganese excess could contribute to induction of superoxide dismutase[42] and increased indicators of such stress in lead exposure.[43] There is evidence that ALA enters cells by a pathway common to it and γ-aminobutyric acid (GABA).[44]

Measurement of Porphyrins and Precursors

Fluorescence of urine under ultraviolet (UV) light is recommended as the initial screening test for the acute porphyrias,[34] whereas plasma fluorescent spectroscopy is the best initial test for diagnosis of cutaneous porphyrias.[35] Diverse techniques such as high-pressure liquid chromatography,[36] quantitative extraction, and various forms of fluorometry are used to measure porphyrins and precursors.[37] The International Federation of Clinical Chemistry and Laboratory Medicine presents diagnostic information on the Internet (www.ifcc.org).

Genetic Aspects

The enzymatic links and genetic loci in each of the hereditary porphyrias are shown in Table 36-1. Nearly all are inherited as autosomal dominant traits. The Chester porphyria family pedigree (Fig. 36-3) shows autosomal dominant inheritance of acute porphyria with attacks of neurovisceral dysfunction without cutaneous hypersensitivity. This was originally reported as a dual porphyria[45]; however, identification of a heterozygous truncating mutation in the HMBS gene and no mutations in other heme biosynthesis enzymes in affected individuals has confirmed that Chester porphyria is a variant of acute intermittent porphyria.[46] Few carriers of the abnormal gene show clinical signs of the disease, but most can be identified by intensive biochemical investigation. The rare congenital porphyria shows autosomal recessive inheritance. The mutations producing each of the acute porphyrias are heterogeneous at the molecular level and include complete or partial gene deletions, alterations of splicing or stability of mRNA, and missense mutations. An exception is variegate porphyria in South Africa, in which the founder effect ensures a predominance of the Arg59Tryp mutation in protoporphyrinogen

Table 36-3 Changes in Porphyrins and Their Precursors in the Porphyrias, Porphyrinurias, and Hereditary Sideroblastic Anemia

Porphyrias and Other Conditions	ALA	PBG	Urine Uroporphyrin	Urine Coproporphyrin	Feces Coproporphyrin	Feces Protoporphyrin	Erythrocyte Protoporphyrin
ACUTE PORPHYRIAS							
Acute intermittent porphyria	Raised, very high in attack	Raised, very high in attack	Usually raised*	Sometimes raised	Sometimes raised	Sometimes raised	Normal
Variegate porphyria	Raised in attack	Raised in attack	Usually raised in attack	Usually raised in attack	Raised	Raised	Normal
Hereditary coproporphyria	Raised in attack	Raised in attack	Sometimes raised in attack	Usually raised, always in attack	Raised	Usually normal	Normal
ALA dehydratase–deficiency porphyria	Raised in attack	Normal	Normal	Usually raised in attack	Normal	Normal	Occasionally raised
NONACUTE PORPHYRIAS							
Porphyria cutanea tarda	Normal	Normal	Raised (7-/8- carboxylate porphyrin levels very high in attack)	Slightly raised	Isocoproporphyrin raised in remission	Raised in remission	Normal
Erythropoietic protoporphyria	Normal	Normal	Normal	Normal	Normal	Usually raised	Raised, usually very high
Congenital porphyria	Usually normal	Usually normal	Raised, isomer I	Raised, isomer I	Normal	Usually raised	Usually raised
X-linked dominant protoporphyria	Normal	Normal	Normal	Normal	Normal	Usually raised	Raised, usually very high
OTHER CONDITIONS							
Hereditary sideroblastic anemia	Normal	Normal	Normal	Normal	Normal	Normal	Occasionally raised
Lead poisoning	Raised	Normal	Normal	Sometimes raised	Normal	Normal	Raised when blood lead level >2 μM
Hereditary tyrosinemia	Raised	Normal	Normal	Normal	Normal	Normal	Normal
Iron deficiency anemia	Normal	Normal	Normal	Normal	Normal	Normal	Raised

ALA, 5-Aminolevulinic acid; *PBG,* porphobilinogen.
**PBG* may cyclize to uroporphyrin nonenzymatically.

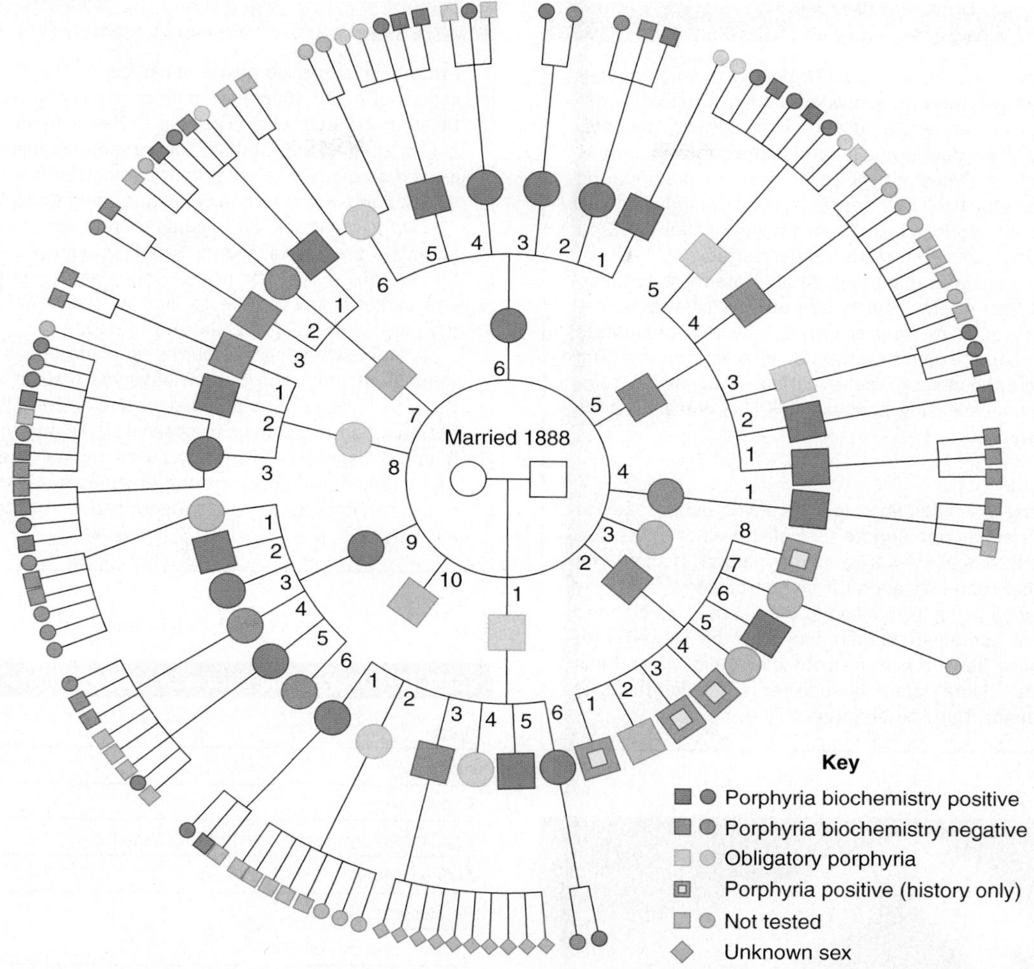

Figure 36-3 THE CHESTER FAMILY PEDIGREE. The propositus, Peter Dobson, was a salmon fisherman from a close-knit community living on the bank of the River Dee, which runs through the city of Chester, UK. Most of the 330 descendants of his marriage in 1888 still live in the city. Many suffered disabling illnesses and psychiatric upsets, which often went unrecognized as porphyria. The family called their illness *Dobson's complaint.* Chester porphyria has recently been confirmed as a variant of acute intermittent porphyria. *(Courtesy Giles R. Youngs.)*

oxidase.[47,48] Homozygotic or compound heterozygotic inheritance has been found in a number of the porphyrias, as has concurrent inheritance of more than one defect. This may present as two types of porphyria in one family[49] or as two types in one patient.[50,51] Dual porphyrias most commonly arise from a combined deficiency of uroporphyrinogen decarboxylase with PBGD, coproporphyrinogen oxidase, or protoporphyrinogen oxidase.[52]

The prevalence of the different forms varies widely. For example, in northern Europe and North America, approximately 1 of 10,000 individuals carries the gene for acute intermittent porphyria, although only about 10% of the affected persons will present with clinical features. It has been suggested that spontaneous mutation accounts for 3% of acute intermittent porphyria cases.[53] Variegate porphyria occurs in 1 of 400 white South Africans. There is a reduction in gene frequency in variegate porphyria from generation to generation that suggests that the allele associated with it is selectively deleterious.[54] The same is probably true of the other porphyrias.

Acute Intermittent Porphyria

Clinical and Laboratory Manifestations

Acute intermittent porphyria is the most severe of the acute porphyrias. During an attack, patients display abdominal and neuropsychiatric or neurovisceral disturbances. Onset occurs in puberty; female patients exhibit a fourfold greater incidence of attacks than males. Attacks occur mainly in young adults and become less frequent after menopause. It is uncommon to see attacks in children.[55] Crises may vary in duration from several days to months. They are most commonly followed by complete remission, although deaths are still reported, especially with acute intermittent porphyria[56] (see box on Precipitating Factors in Acute Porphyria).

Gastrointestinal symptoms occur in 95% of cases; most patients present with acute colicky central abdominal pain. Examination reveals tenderness but little rigidity, and patients may also experience limb pain or generalized muscular aches. Severe vomiting may occur, and constipation is usual. Hyponatremia occurs in severe attacks.

Motor neuropathy complicates two-thirds of porphyric attacks and may be the presenting feature. Motor involvement is most common, but paresthesias may also occur. Paralysis usually starts peripherally and then spreads proximally; however, in some patients, shoulder girdle involvement may be the first manifestation. The neuropathy may progress rapidly, resulting in respiratory insufficiency. Weakness, usually symmetric, involves proximal and distal limb muscles more often than those of the trunk. Upper limbs and proximal muscles are often affected. Involvement of the wrists, ankles, and small muscles of the hand may lead to a permanent deformity (Fig. 36-4), and trunk muscle weakness can lead to respiratory embarrassment. Death is usually caused by respiratory paralysis.

Precipitating Factors in Acute Porphyria

Most patients who have inherited acute porphyria enjoy normal health and go through life without any knowledge of their disorder or ever experiencing an acute attack. All porphyric patients, however, are at risk for developing an attack if exposed to various precipitating factors. Drugs are the most common precipitating agents. Other factors that may trigger attacks include alcohol ingestion, reduced caloric intake (from fasting or dieting), and infection. Smoking can cause more frequent attacks.

Hormonal status is also important. Attacks are more common in females, and they rarely occur before puberty or after menopause. Pregnancy and oral contraceptives may also precipitate attacks. Some women experience regular attacks, commencing in the week before the onset of menstruation. These may require luteinizing hormone–releasing hormone (LH-RH) antagonists for control (Table 36-4).

Drugs for Porphyria

Before prescribing any medication to a porphyric patient, advice must be sought from an appropriate specialist. Full drug lists are available on the Internet (www.drugs-porphyria.org). It should be borne in mind that such lists are far from encyclopedic, that new drugs are constantly being introduced to the pharmacopoeia, and that any form of combined preparation must be viewed with suspicion, because little is known about metabolic interactions in these diseases.[57] More details of such use and side effects of drugs can be sought from the literature.[58]

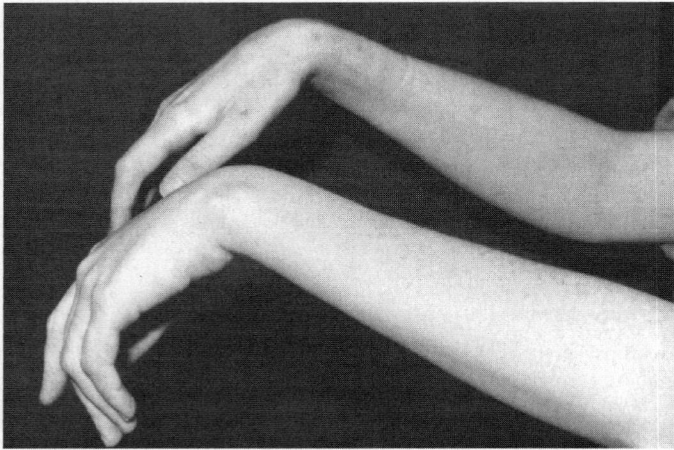

Figure 36-4 BILATERAL WRISTDROP CAUSED BY PERIPHERAL NEUROPATHY IN A PATIENT WITH ACUTE INTERMITTENT PORPHYRIA.

Progressive weakening of the voice may suggest this; treatment requires tracheotomy and intermittent positive pressure ventilation. Paresthesias, numbness, and objective evidence of sensory impairment may occur with loss of pinprick sensation, which is most marked around the shoulder and hip areas; generalized tonic-clonic seizures occasionally occur.

Severe anxiety, depression, and frank psychosis are the main psychiatric manifestations of porphyric attacks. These psychiatric manifestations may result in a patient being misdiagnosed as suffering from a primary psychiatric disorder. Agitation, mania, depression, hallucinations, and schizophrenic-like behavior may occur. Psychiatric manifestations may persist between attacks.[59] Quality of life is severely affected in those suffering from repeated attacks of acute porphyria.[60]

The cardiovascular system is involved in approximately 70% of attacks. Sinus tachycardia (to 160 beats/min) and hypertension can

Differential Diagnosis of Acute Intermittent Porphyria

Attacks of acute porphyria must be distinguished from other causes of acute abdominal pain or peripheral neuropathy sometimes associated with psychosis.[61] Heavy metal poisoning (i.e., lead or arsenic) and Guillain-Barré syndrome must be considered, as well as paroxysmal nocturnal hemoglobinuria with its characteristic early morning hemoglobinuria and abdominal pain.[61]

During an attack, all patients excrete a massive excess of the porphyrin precursors, 5-aminolevulinic acid (ALA) and porphobilinogen (PBG), in their urine. Urine, when first voided, is clear and darkens on exposure to light as the hexa-hydroporphyrins, the porphyrinogens, are oxidized to porphyrins.

A rapid screening test during an acute attack is to mix equal volumes of urine and Ehrlich aldehyde reagent and observe for the pink color of porphobilinogen; alternatively the urine can be left standing in sunlight to observe darkening in color. The differential diagnosis of porphyrias uses qualitative and quantitative measurement of porphyrins and precursors, with subsequent use of enzymatic assay and identification of familial genetic alterations.[62]

Table 36-4 Precipitating Factors in Acute Porphyria

Drugs	Other Stimuli
Alcohol	Fasting or dieting
Barbiturates	Hormones, stress
Angiotensin-converting enzyme (ACE) inhibitors	Smoking
Anticonvulsants	
Antidepressants	
Calcium channel blockers	
Cephalosporins	
Ergot derivatives	
Erythromycin	
Steroids or anabolic steroids	
Contraceptives, hormone replacement therapy	
Sulfonamides	
Sulfonylureas	

occur; these elevations usually revert to normal after an attack. There is evidence that hypertension may occasionally be permanent, even in latent cases of acute intermittent porphyria (see box on Differential Diagnosis of Acute Intermittent Porphyria).

Other Acute Porphyrias

Hereditary Coproporphyria

Hereditary coproporphyria combines the clinical features of acute porphyria with photosensitive skin manifestations. It results from mutations in the gene encoding coproporphyrinogen oxidase, whose activity is decreased,[63,64] leading to overproduction of coproporphyrin.

The porphyrin precursors ALA and PBG and the more water-soluble porphyrins (with multiple carboxyl groups) are excreted mainly in the urine. Other porphyrins are mainly excreted in the feces by way of bile.

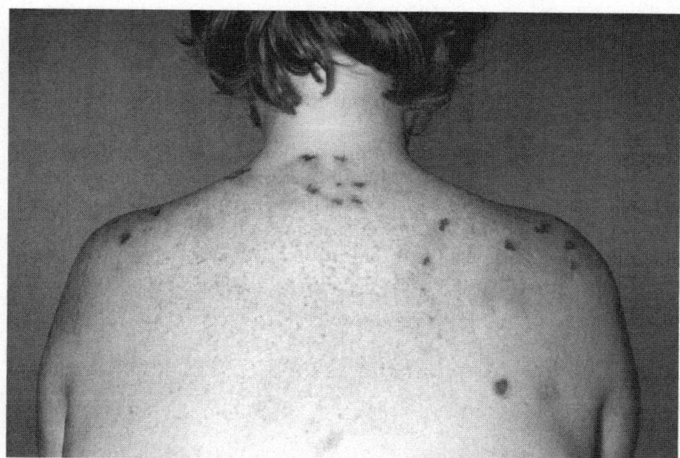

Figure 36-5 CUTANEOUS LESIONS AND SCARRING IN A PATIENT WITH VARIEGATE PORPHYRIA.

Variegate Porphyria

Variegate porphyria is similar to hereditary coproporphyria, except that there are more severe skin lesions, sometimes with scarring (Fig. 36-5). Protoporphyrinogen oxidase is the affected enzyme, and protoporphyrin is the major circulating porphyrin. Conventionally, variegate porphyria is most readily diagnosed by measurement of fecal porphyrin concentrations. However, it has been reported[65] that biliary porphyrin levels may provide a better discriminator from normal patients in the asymptomatic phase. As in erythropoietic protoporphyria, there is a tendency toward cholelithiasis. The mechanism by which gallstones form is not certain, but some studies have suggested that porphyrins are cholestatic.[66] In hereditary coproporphyria and variegate porphyria, the pathway intermediates produced in excess, coproporphyrinogen and protoporphyrinogen, respectively, are inhibitors of the secondary rate-controlling enzyme PBGD.[32,67] Numerous mutations in the protoporphyrinogen oxidase gene have been described leading to 50% reduction in enzyme activity. In a few cases, homozygosity or compound heterozygosity has been described.[68,69]

ALA Dehydratase–Deficiency Porphyria

In this porphyria (also known as plumboporphyria), the ALA dehydratase activity is depressed, as occurs in lead poisoning. The clinical picture resembles acute intermittent porphyria, but very few cases have been described, and the disease only manifests in homozygous cases when there is a precipitating factor.[70,71]

Concurrent Porphyrias

The concurrent porphyrias are a rare group of conditions in which there is concurrent inheritance of two different defects within the heme biosynthetic pathway. There is good precedent for more than one defect within the pathway. Previous descriptions[50-52] have shown the presence of concurrent porphyria within a family, and toxicologically there is good evidence that exposure to poisons such as lead can induce multiple changes within the pathway.[72] The first reported example of concurrent porphyria in a family combined the clinical features of acute and cutaneous porphyria, and biochemical analysis confirmed the segregation of variegate porphyria and PCT as independent inherited traits.[73] In another patient, dual genetic defects involving ALA dehydratase and coproporphyrinogen oxidase have been described[51] (see box on Management of Acute Porphyria).

Management of Acute Porphyria

Treatment of Acute Attack

A carbohydrate intake of 1500 to 2000 kcal/24 hr should be maintained throughout the attack to reduce porphyrin synthesis; give this orally or, for more severe attacks, through a fine-bore Teflon nasogastric tube. If this cannot be tolerated, intravenous dextrose (e.g., 20% solution, 2 L/day) should be given. If early in the attack (2 to 4 days from onset), give intravenous hematin as heme arginate (Normosang, Orphan Europe) at 2 to 4 mg/kg over 30 minutes once or twice each day to further reduce the overproduction of porphyrin and precursors.[74,75] Hematin (Panhematin, Lundbeck) in similar doses may also be used, although it should be reconstituted in human albumin solution to avoid phlebitis and mild transient prolongation of coagulation times. No renal complications have occurred with the standard recommended dosages, and even patients with renal insufficiency tolerate hematin well, although the dosage should be reduced slightly. The action of heme therapy may be extended by heme oxygenase blockers such as tin protoporphyrin.[74] Liver transplantation may be an effective treatment for life-threatening acute intermittent porphyria that fails to respond to medical therapy.[76]

Prophylaxis

Many drugs are contraindicated, and the patient must be warned to avoid precipitating factors. Alcohol should be restricted and smoking discouraged. Dieting (<800 kcal/day) must be avoided. Pregnancy should also be avoided if the disease is active. If a patient requires an anesthetic, nitrous oxide, ether, and cyclopropane are safe, and suxamethonium appears to be a safe muscle relaxant. The opiates and belladonna derivatives can be used for premedication and propofol for maintenance of anesthesia. Infection can precipitate an attack and should therefore be sought and treated. Blood relatives of patients should be screened to see if they carry the gene.

Luteinizing hormone-releasing hormone (LH-RH) antagonists that suppress ovulation are a valuable form of prophylaxis in menstrually related attacks.[77] Estrogens and progestogens such as those in the contraceptive pill must be avoided in acute porphyria. The same applies to most steroids and receptor antagonists such as mifepristone.[78]

Nonacute or Cutaneous Porphyrias

In all cutaneous porphyrias, porphyrins (which are photosensitizing) are deposited in the upper layers of the skin, and they are responsible for the characteristic skin lesions.[79] In the development of these lesions, reactive oxygen species and other radicals are formed and probably induce oxidative membrane damage, particularly to mast cells, which enables complement activation as one part of the inflammatory reaction[80] (see box on Management of Nonacute Porphyria).

Porphyria Cutanea Tarda or Cutaneous Hepatic Porphyria

Biologic and Molecular Aspects

PCT exists in inherited and acquired forms. An inherited, more severe form of this disease, hepatoerythropoietic porphyria (HEP), has been described.[85] Mutations in the uroporphyrinogen decarboxylase are found in around one-third of patients with PCT. In inherited and acquired forms, there is diminution in the activity of hepatic uroporphyrinogen decarboxylase, which converts uroporphyrinogen to coproporphyrinogen by the stepwise decarboxylation of the acetyl

Management of Nonacute Porphyria

Patients should avoid exposure to sunlight and use sunblock and physical barriers such as cotton gloves.

Porphyria Cutanea Tarda

The clinical features are reversed by removing any precipitating agent such as alcohol, halogenated hydrocarbons, and drugs. The patient should be screened for hepatic neoplasm and hepatitis C infection. The mainstay of treatment is to remove liver iron by venesection of 500 mL of blood weekly until clinical remission occurs or until the hemoglobin level falls below 12 g/dL. Chloroquine, at low doses of 125 mg twice per week for several months, has also been helpful because it enhances urinary clearance of porphyrin. When this is not possible, oral cimetidine has been used.[81] When venesection is difficult, parenteral and orally active iron chelators can be used to reduce liver iron stores. It is of value to screen the patient and first-degree relatives for hereditary hemochromatosis.

Erythropoietic Protoporphyria

Oral β-carotene offers effective protection in erythropoietic porphyria (EPP) against solar sensitivity. It does so by quenching the radical formation that is a feature of the skin damage. Yellowing of the skin (i.e., carotenemia) is one side effect. Interruption of the enterohepatic protoporphyrin circulation by bile salt–sequestering agents such as cholestyramine reduces plasma protoporphyrin levels and may retard the development of the liver disease. Liver transplantation has been reported to be an effective measure in preventing the progression of this disease.[82]

Congenital Porphyria

Erythropoiesis should be reduced by means of erythrocyte hypertransfusion and by hematin or heme arginate infusion.[83] Bone marrow transplantation has given encouraging biochemical and clinical results, but insufficient numbers of patients have been treated to be certain of the future prospects of this therapy.[84] Splenectomy and chloroquine therapy (125 mg twice weekly) have an ameliorating effect, as does hypertransfusion, but life expectancy is usually severely shortened.

groups to methyl groups. The mechanism of enzyme inhibition has recently been elucidated, whereby iron-dependent oxidation of uroporphyrinogen generates uroporphomethene, a competitive inhibitor of uroporphyrinogen decarboxylase.[86] Most carriers of mutant uroporphyrinogen decarboxylase are not clinically evident unless precipitating factors are present. Iron alone or chlorinated hydrocarbons can diminish activity of uroporphyrinogen decarboxylase, and this effect is greatly potentiated when both are given together.[87,88] In a murine model, precipitation of uroporphyria by chlorinated hydrocarbons is dependent on hepatic cytochrome P450 1A2 oxidase activity, and inherited variations in enzyme function may modulate susceptibility to PCT in humans.[87]

Patients may have clinical and biochemical evidence of liver disease. Hepatic siderosis invariably occurs, and iron is one of the causative agents in acquired PCT. An association of PCT with hereditary hemochromatosis has been documented, with about 20% of PCT patients being homozygous for the Cys282Tyr mutation in the HFE gene, a defect that characterizes hereditary hemochromatosis.[89-91] These results strongly implicate the HFE gene as a genetic susceptibility factor in acquired PCT. An association between PCT and hepatitis C infection is well documented, and in countries with high prevalence rates, hepatitis C virus may be the dominant risk factor.[92] An apparent association has emerged between human immunodeficiency virus (HIV) infection and PCT.[93] It is possible that therapy for HIV with zidovudine precipitates the disease, but it is more likely that the association is merely coincidental or that the viral infection unmasks the preexisting uroporphyrinogen decarboxylase defect.[94]

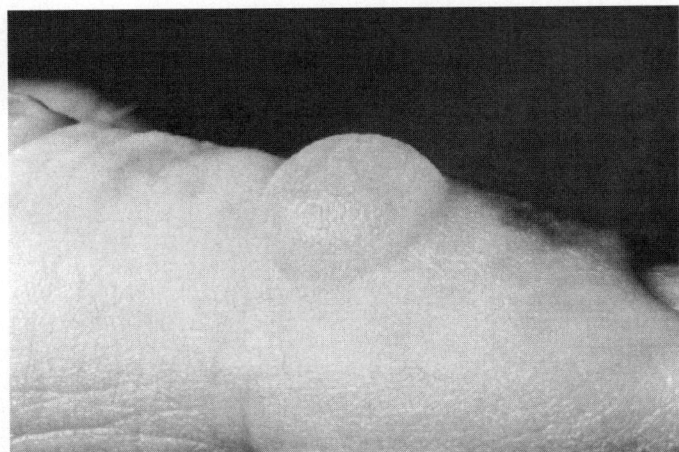

Figure 36-6 A BULLOUS SKIN LESION OF PORPHYRIA CUTANEA TARDA.

Genetics

Whereas familial PCT is inherited in an autosomal dominant mode, HEP is inherited in an autosomal recessive pattern.[95] As in the other genetic lesions in the porphyrias, there is heterogeneity in the mutations causing PCT and HEP phenotypes.[96,97] In the inherited form, more than 40 different mutations (mainly missense) have been identified in uroporphyrinogen decarboxylase, many of which lie near the dimer interface resulting in an unstable protein and reduced enzyme activity.[98] In different population groups, it is difficult to find the relative numbers of acquired and familial disease. In one analysis in Hungary, 77.5% of patients were found to suffer from the acquired form, and of the patients with the familial disease, females were affected more than males, suggesting that inheritance may predispose patients to estrogen-precipitated disease.[99]

Clinical Features

The most striking clinical feature of both forms of PCT is a bullous dermatosis on light-exposed areas. This starts as erythema and progresses to vesicles that become confluent to form bullae (Fig. 36-6), which may hemorrhage and leave scars; pruritus is often troublesome. Milia are common and may precede or follow vesicle formation. Facial hypertrichosis is common and may serve as a diagnostic clue. In less severe cases, increased fragility of the skin may be the only clinical sign. In severe cases, photomutilation can result, usually because of infection of slowly healing lesions.

The thickening and scarring with calcification has been described as pseudoscleroderma. Hyperpigmentation is common, and women often complain of hirsutism. Neurologic change is not observed. Patients may have clinical and biochemical evidence of chronic liver disease, sometimes with cirrhosis. There is an association with hepatocellular carcinoma. Hepatomegaly is particularly common when alcohol intake is excessive.

Precipitating Factors

Many patients with PCT have multiple precipitating factors, including mutations of the HFE gene, hepatitis C infection, or exposure to estrogen.[89,90] Excessive alcohol intake is an important precipitating agent, perhaps because of increased hepatic iron deposition in alcoholics. However, certain halogenated hydrocarbons are sometimes implicated. PCT may also develop in people treated with hemodialysis for kidney failure. An outbreak of cutaneous hepatic porphyria in southeast Turkey in 1956 was traced to seed wheat dressed with the fungicide hexachlorobenzene. A neoplastic subgroup has been identified in which PCT is associated with benign or malignant liver tumors.

Differential Diagnosis

Other causes of bullous or vesicular skin lesions should be excluded, such as a drug reaction (see box on Pseudoporphyria and Renal Dialysis) or chronic renal failure. The distinction between PCT, variegate porphyria, and hereditary coproporphyria rests on biochemical testing of urine and feces, with the highest levels of urinary uroporphyrin found during attacks of PCT (see Table 36-3).

Erythropoietic Protoporphyria

Biologic and Molecular Aspects

Although not described until 1961, this form of erythropoietic porphyria (EPP), also known as erythrohepatic protoporphyria, is much more common than congenital porphyria. Ferrochelatase activity is reduced in peripheral blood, liver, bone marrow, and skin, and protoporphyrin is synthesized in excess.[103] The erythroid progenitor cells (i.e., burst-forming units-erythroid [BFU-E]) in EPP patients show intense fluorescence when viewed under 405-nm light. The gene mutation in EPP shows heterogeneity as in other porphyrias.[104] The last enzyme of the biosynthetic pathway, ferrochelatase, is important because its endogenous activity is relatively low, and it could act as a control point in the pathway. Ferrochelatase ligates iron bound to three cysteine residues in an iron-sulfur cluster,[105] the mutation of which leads to decreased enzyme activity.[106] A multiple-enzyme complex spanning the mitochondrial membrane would allow for channeling of substrate from the cytoplasm to the mitochondrial matrix.[107] Immunologic studies on human protoporphyria show that immunologically reactive ferrochelatase is present, but that enzyme activity in three subjects was on average only 17% of normal.[108] Gain-of-function mutations in the ALAS2 gene have recently been described that result in increased erythrocyte protoporphyrin despite normal ferrochelatase activity. This newly described, X-linked dominant erythropoietic protoporphyria, leads to accumulation of protoporphyrin in amounts sufficient to cause photosensitivity and hepatic damage.[31]

Pseudoporphyria and Renal Dialysis

The term *pseudoporphyria* has been used to describe a bullous dermatosis associated with a number of dermatologic conditions that bear some resemblance to porphyria.[100] This photosensitivity is often induced by drugs such as the tetracyclines, naproxen, furosemide, voriconazole, oxaprozin, and many others. In these conditions, there is no alteration in porphyrin metabolism or excretion. It is therefore incorrect to name any of them porphyria; the term *pseudoporphyria* should not be applied to them, but only to conditions in which alterations of porphyrin metabolism can be found, such as the bullous dermatosis of hemodialysis.[99]

Patients with renal failure can present with many biochemical features of porphyria before hemodialysis. These abnormalities normalize after dialysis, especially when electrolyte abnormalities such as zinc deficiency are also corrected.[101] In a considerable proportion of patients with chronic renal failure, skin changes resembling porphyria cutanea tarda (PCT) develop some months to years after the onset of maintenance hemodialysis. In a minor proportion, genuine PCT can be diagnosed.[102] In such cases, there are elevated total porphyrin levels in plasma and in urine if the patient is not anuric. These patients present a therapeutic dilemma because they are normally anemic and unsuitable for phlebotomy therapy.

Genetics

EPP is inherited as an autosomal dominant disorder with incomplete penetrance, although recessive inheritance has been described.[109,110] Haplotype segregation analysis has shown intronic nucleotide polymorphisms in the ferrochelatase gene (FECH) that produces aberrant splicing of mRNA to a form that degrades more rapidly, resulting in enzyme deficiency.[111] Although these disease-associated polymorphisms are common,[112,113] there is heterogeneity of the molecular defect, including aberrant splicing and loss of function of the mitoferrin protein.[16,103,104,114]

Clinical Features

The clinical features are mainly cutaneous on exposure to sunlight and can occur at any age, including infancy and childhood.[109] They include pruritic urticarial swelling and redness of the skin on exposure to sunlight. The most distressing symptom is an unbearable burning sensation on the affected parts. Remarkably, such features are ameliorated during pregnancy, which has been linked to lowered protoporphyrin levels.[115] Hepatic involvement, which occurs in later life, involves deposition of hepatotoxic protoporphyrin in the liver and can lead to fatal liver failure from an active chronic hepatitis with cirrhosis.[116] Such protoporphyrin deposition may also cause cholelithiasis; the gallstones contain high concentrations of protoporphyrin. The liver disease of EPP seems to correlate with erythrocyte protoporphyrin concentrations.[117] Mild microcytic anemia has been reported,[118,119] as well as mitochondrial iron accumulation and ring sideroblasts, in about 30% of patients.[120] Late onset of EPP has been reported in patients with myelodysplastic syndrome or overlap myelodysplasia/myeloproliferation. In one patient, EPP has been acquired as a result of expansion of hemopoietic cells containing only one allele of the FECH gene.[121] Inactivation of one allele by deletion involving chromosome 18 thus appears to be sufficient for overproduction of protoporphyrin.[120,122]

Differential Diagnosis

EPP should be distinguished from other causes of a photosensitive rash. The distinction can be made by demonstrating fluorescence in a proportion of red cells (i.e., fluorocytes) in the peripheral blood and confirmed by measurement of greatly increased erythrocyte and fecal protoporphyrin. Patients with EPP have a relatively high incidence of ring sideroblasts in the marrow.[120] This can lead to diagnostic difficulty because some patients with idiopathic sideroblastic anemia have increased levels of erythrocyte protoporphyrin.[123-126] However, EPP can be distinguished by the autosomal dominant inheritance pattern, dermal photosensitivity, normal or low serum levels of iron, and levels of protoporphyrin in red blood cells and feces.

Congenital Porphyria (Günther Disease)

Biologic and Molecular Aspects

Congenital porphyria, or Günther disease, although extremely rare, was the first porphyria to be described in 1874.[127] Unlike the other porphyrias, it is inherited in a mendelian autosomal recessive pattern causing reduced activity of uroporphyrinogen III synthase. The onset of solar photosensitivity results from gross overproduction of porphyrins, caused by deficiency of uroporphyrinogen III synthase. Like other porphyrias, the defective enzyme results mainly from point mutations at multiple sites within the gene.[128] Other enzymes are largely normal, although there is an increase in ALAS activity,[129] which in some cases has been shown to result from gain-of-function mutations in the ALAS2 gene.[130] Excess porphyrins, particularly uroporphyrin-1, accumulate in the normoblasts of the bone marrow and are excreted in the urine and feces. They are also deposited in bones and in the teeth, resulting in a pink-brown discoloration that fluoresces bright red in light of wavelengths around 400 nm. Dental restoration has been used to correct the esthetic appearance of the teeth. There are frequently profound changes in bone structure in patients with congenital porphyria. This has been linked to vitamin D deficiency because of light avoidance.[131] However, bone changes can be seen when vitamin D levels are adequate, and it is reasonable to speculate that the porphyrins deposited in bone are cytotoxic because similar bone changes are features of homozygous variegate porphyria and HEP.[132]

Clinical Features

Typically the onset of congenital porphyria is from birth, but occasionally late-onset cases have been reported.[133] The skin reaction is severe and can be devastating, and the teeth become brownish pink because of their high porphyrin content. Severe cutaneous photosensitivity is manifested by blistering of light-exposed areas and fragility of the epidermis. Skin thickening occurs, and there is extensive scarring and hypertrichosis. The recurrent damage associated with scarring on the hand may produce a claw-shaped deformity and loss of digits. Dystrophic nails may curl up and drop off. Lenticular scarring may lead to blindness. Hemolytic anemia often occurs and is associated with increased erythrocyte fragility and splenomegaly. Dyserythropoiesis may contribute to the anemia.[134] One patient who underwent splenectomy at 5 years of age has been described with needle-like inclusions of porphyrin in the circulating red cells (Fig. 36-7).[135]

Differential Diagnosis

The most characteristic feature of congenital porphyria is the excess production of series 1 porphyrins rather than series 3 isomer produced in the other porphyrias. Red blood cells fluoresce in ultraviolet light, as do the brown-stained teeth, because of high porphyrin content (see box on Pseudoporphyria and Renal Dialysis).

SIDEROBLASTIC ANEMIAS

Sideroblastic anemias are a heterogeneous group of disorders characterized by anemia of varying severity and diagnosed by finding ring sideroblasts in the bone marrow aspirate. The peripheral blood shows hypochromic red cells, which are microcytic in the hereditary forms (Fig. 36-8, *A*) but are often macrocytic in the acquired forms of the disease. The red blood cell parameters from automated cell counting may show bimodal volume distribution curves or widened range of cell sizes (see Fig. 36-8, *B*); however, this dimorphic size distribution is not always present. Tiny inclusions may be visible in the red blood cells; these can be confirmed as iron-containing Pappenheimer bodies by Prussian blue staining of the blood smear (see Fig. 36-8, *C*). The diagnostic test is bone marrow examination together with Prussian blue staining of the bone marrow smears.

The presence of ring sideroblasts (see Fig. 36-8, *D*) is defined as erythroblasts containing iron-positive (siderotic) granules arranged in a perinuclear collar distribution around one-third or more of the nucleus. Electron microscopic examination has shown that these siderotic granules are mitochondria containing amorphous deposits of ferric phosphate and ferric hydroxide. Iron is also bound to mitochondrial ferritin, a molecular form of ferritin that can be distinguished from cytoplasmic ferritin and that accumulates in large amounts in the erythroblasts of subjects with impaired heme synthesis.[136,137]

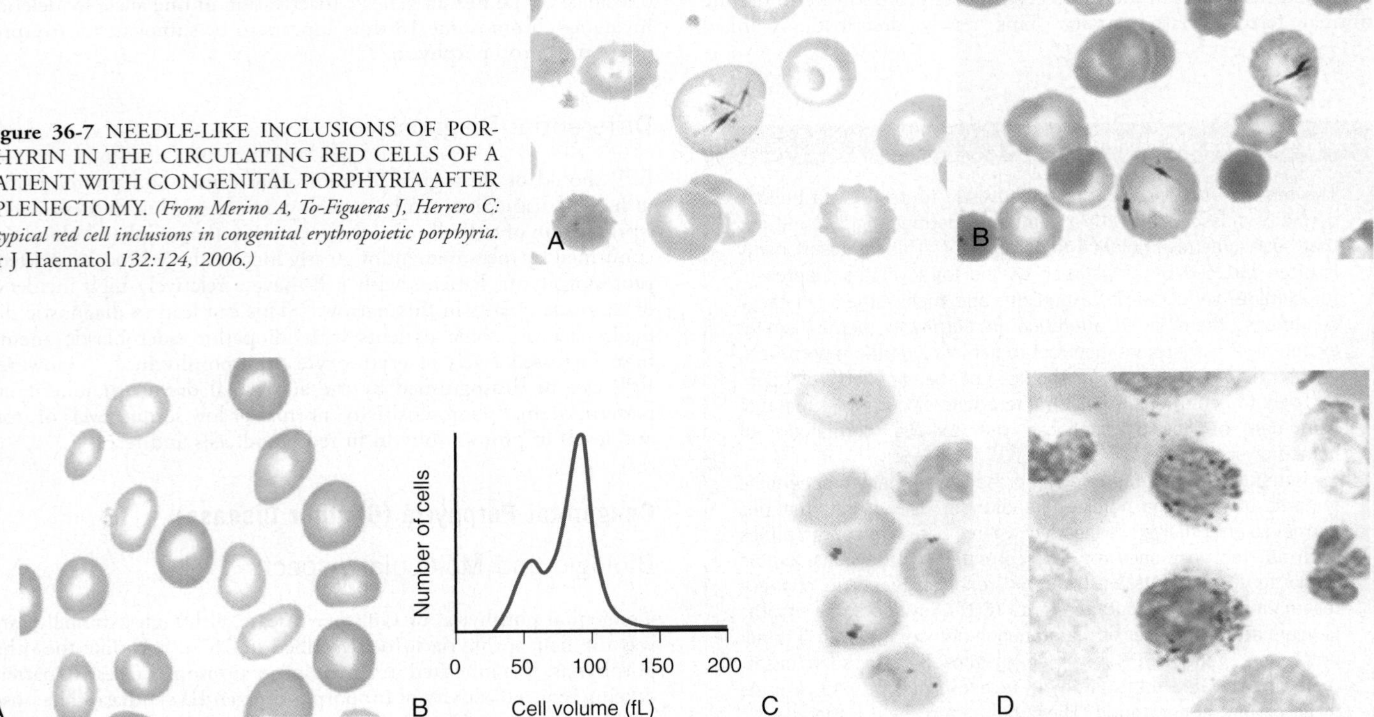

Figure 36-7 NEEDLE-LIKE INCLUSIONS OF PORPHYRIN IN THE CIRCULATING RED CELLS OF A PATIENT WITH CONGENITAL PORPHYRIA AFTER SPLENECTOMY. *(From Merino A, To-Figueras J, Herrero C: Atypical red cell inclusions in congenital erythropoietic porphyria.* Br J Haematol *132:124, 2006.)*

Figure 36-8 A, Peripheral blood smear from a patient with hereditary sideroblastic anemia shows a population of hypochromic and microcytic erythrocytes. **B,** Erythrocyte volume distribution curve of a patient with hereditary sideroblastic anemia. A dimorphic size distribution is evident. **C,** Peripheral blood showing Pappenheimer bodies (Prussian blue stain). **D,** The bone marrow smear stained with Prussian blue shows ring sideroblasts.

Iron overload is a common clinical feature of refractory sideroblastic anemia and, in severe cases, may lead to complications that characterize secondary hemosiderosis (e.g., diabetes, cardiac failure). Marrow examination shows prominent erythroid hyperplasia, which is a sign of the ineffective erythropoiesis and is responsible for increased iron absorption. The sideroblastic anemias have diverse causes but have in common an impaired biosynthesis of heme in the erythroid cells of the marrow. Most sideroblastic anemias are acquired as a clonal disorder of erythropoiesis, with various degrees of myelodysplastic features (Table 36-5). The inherited forms are uncommon and occur predominantly in males with an X-linked pattern of inheritance. A number of drugs have been associated with reversible sideroblastic anemia, and ring sideroblasts may be found in patients who abuse alcohol (see Table 36-5). The first descriptions of ring sideroblasts in association with chronic refractory anemias appeared in the late 1950s,[138,139] after an earlier description of familial X-linked hypochromic microcytic anemia.[140]

Hereditary Sideroblastic Anemia

X-Linked Sideroblastic Anemia

Biologic and Molecular Aspects

Erythroid cells from patients with X-linked forms of hereditary sideroblastic anemia generally exhibit low activity of ALAS[27,141]; however, for a minority of ALAS2 mutations this effect may be difficult to detect in vitro.[142] A defect in this enzyme is firmly established in patients whose anemia responds to pyridoxine therapy, because pyridoxal phosphate is an essential cofactor for ALAS. However, even affected female patients with moderate anemia unresponsive to pyridoxine have been documented to have low levels of ALAS in bone marrow lysates. In some male patients with X-linked pyridoxine-responsive sideroblastic anemia, the low ALAS activity in bone marrow increased to levels above the normal range when the patient took pyridoxine supplements and recovered from the anemia.[143] There are several possible explanations for this enhancement of ALAS activity by dietary pyridoxine supplements. The most likely is that pyridoxine (or its phosphate) may stabilize the ALAS during folding of the mutant enzyme after its synthesis.[141] The gene for the ALAS2 isoenzyme has been localized to the X chromosome, and this gene is known to be the site of most mutations giving rise to X-linked pyridoxine-responsive sideroblastic anemia.[9,144] Approximately three dozen different mutations have been identified in individuals or families with hereditary sideroblastic anemia, and nearly all have resulted from single base alterations in DNA. A frequent mutation affects arginine at residue 452 of ALAS2, which occurs in a quarter of all pedigrees but does not affect enzyme activity measured in vitro.[145] All known mutations lie between exons 5 and 11 of ALAS2, the region that codes for the catalytic domain, with most lying within exon 9, which contains the lysine at which binding of pyridoxal 5′-phosphate occurs.[7] A mutation, Asp190Val, has been described in a pyridoxine-refractory patient and appears to affect the proteolytic processing of the ALAS2 during or after import into the mitochondrion.[146] The variety of different mutations in the erythroid ALAS2 gene responsible for X-linked sideroblastic anemia and their pyridoxine responsiveness have been reviewed recently.[9]

Table 36-5 Classification of Sideroblastic Anemias

HEREDITARY (NONSYNDROMIC)
X-linked
Autosomal dominant or recessive
ACQUIRED
Idiopathic acquired* (refractory anemia with ring sideroblasts)
Associated with previous chemotherapy, irradiation, or in transition myelodysplasia or myeloproliferative diseases
DRUGS
Alcohol
Isoniazid
Chloramphenicol
Other drugs
RARE CAUSES
Erythropoietic protoporphyria
Copper deficiency or zinc overload
Hypothermia
HEREDITARY (SYNDROMIC)
X-linked sideroblastic anemia with ring sideroblasts and cerebellar ataxia
Myopathy, lactic acidosis and sideroblastic anemia
Pearson syndrome
Thiamine-responsive megaloblastic anemia

*Trial of pyridoxine indicated.

Genetic Aspects

In most families with hereditary sideroblastic anemia, males are affected with an X-linked pattern of inheritance (Fig. 36-9). However, female carriers, although usually normal, can develop erythrocyte dimorphism or varying degrees of anemia. The assignment of the gene for erythroid ALAS2 to the X chromosome[144] and the many mutations documented in erythroid ALAS2 provide the genetic basis for this X-linked disease. In several families, coinheritance of other X-linked traits (e.g., glucose-6-phosphate dehydrogenase [G6PD] deficiency, ataxia with sideroblastic anemia) has been described.[147,148] Sporadic and familial cases have been described that affect only females, which has been shown to represent skewed X-chromosome inactivation ("unfortunate skewing") affecting the normal allele for the ALAS2 gene.[149] The absence of affected male members in these pedigrees suggests that the ALAS2 defects identified are lethal in hemizygous males.

Clinical and Laboratory Evaluation

Typically the anemia of X-linked sideroblastic anemia manifests in infancy or childhood, but the milder forms of anemia may not be found until midlife. Even elderly patients have been diagnosed with this anemia.[150] Some cases may be discovered only during family surveys, which should always be undertaken when hereditary

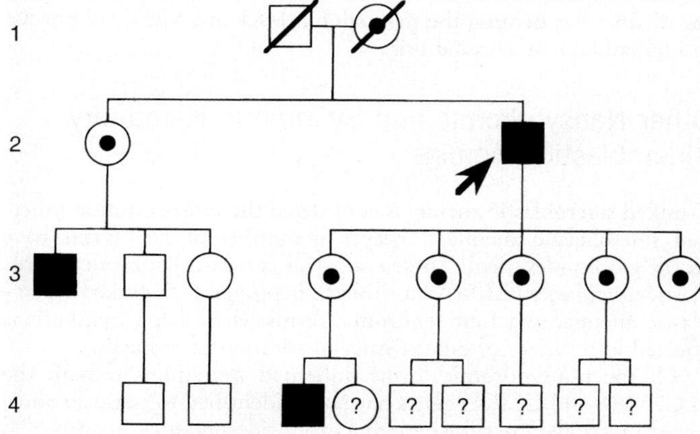

Figure 36-9 PEDIGREE OF A FAMILY WITH PYRIDOXINE-RESPONSIVE SIDEROBLASTIC ANEMIA SHOWING X-LINKED RECESSIVE INHERITANCE. Affected *(filled box),* carrier *(filled circle within open circle),* and unknown status *(question mark within circle or box)* are indicated. Diagonal lines indicate deceased members. This pedigree[143] has been abbreviated to show only the affected branches of the family. The *arrow* indicates the proband.

sideroblastic anemia is diagnosed. Still other patients may present with features of iron overload, such as diabetes or cardiac failure. Iron overload occurs commonly even with mild anemia and may occasionally be seen with female carriers. Enlargement of the liver and spleen may occur with mild abnormalities of liver function tests.

Anemia is extremely variable, but even when little or no anemia is present, the mean corpuscular volume (MCV) is low, and the red cell volume distribution width may be increased. When anemia is severe, the MCV may be as low as 50 fL (50 μm^3). The blood smear shows a population of cells with hypochromic, microcytic morphology (see Fig. 36-8), which contrasts with the other normochromic, normocytic cells (i.e., dimorphism). Anisocytosis, poikilocytosis, elongated cells, and siderocytes may also be seen. The characteristic erythrocyte dimorphism is most prominent in patients with milder anemia, in female carriers, and in patients in whom pyridoxine has corrected the anemia but not restored the MCV to normal. In some pedigrees with only affected females, macrocytosis may be present, which contrasts with the typical microcytosis of male hemizygotes.[126,149] Leukocyte values are normal, whereas the platelet count is normal or increased.

Serum iron concentration is increased, and transferrin shows an increased percentage of saturation with iron. Serum ferritin levels are invariably increased. Ineffective erythropoiesis can be confirmed by ferrokinetic measurements showing that plasma iron clearance is rapid, with subnormal retention of the iron isotope in erythrocytes after 10 to 14 days. Other features of ineffective erythropoiesis may be variably present: a mild increase in bilirubin concentration, decrease in haptoglobin levels, mild increase in lactate dehydrogenase levels, and normal or slight increase in reticulocyte numbers. The magnitude of iron overload correlates poorly with the degree of anemia in patients who are not transfused. The degree of ineffective erythropoiesis is a better predictor of the amount of iron overload. When ferrokinetics are unavailable, the extent of erythroid hyperplasia relative to normal acts as a rough measure of the magnitude of ineffective erythropoiesis. Several studies have shown that the relative increase in erythroid activity multiplied by the patient's age shows a good correlation with the degree of iron overload as measured by plasma ferritin.[151,152] The iron overload does not result from mutations in the HFE gene[153] (see box on Therapy for Hereditary Sideroblastic Anemia).

Differential Diagnosis

Hereditary sideroblastic anemia should be distinguished from idiopathic hemochromatosis, because both have biochemical evidence of iron overload and a similar tissue pattern of iron deposition. Careful hematologic assessment of patient and family members should make the distinction, because the hemoglobin level and MCV are normal in idiopathic hemochromatosis.

Other Nonsyndromic and Syndromic Hereditary Sideroblastic Anemias

X-linked sideroblastic anemia is considered the most common inherited sideroblastic anemia; however, a number of rare forms have recently been identified. These consist of two nonsyndromic sideroblastic anemias, which have a similar phenotype to X-linked sideroblastic anemia, and four syndromic forms where heme synthesis is affected in a variety of other tissues in addition to red cells.

Of the nonsyndromic forms, inherited mutations in both the SLC25A38 and GLRX5 genes have been identified to cause an autosomal recessive pyridoxine-refractory sideroblastic anemia.[156,157] SLC25A38 is located on chromosome 3p22.1 and encodes a mitochondrial carrier protein that may function to import glycine into the mitochondrion or exchange glycine for 5-aminolevulinic acid.[156] Homozygous or compound heterozygote mutations in SLC25A38 result in a similar phenotype to that seen in X-linked sideroblastic anemia, with onset in infancy of a severe microcytic anemia that is refractory to treatment with pyridoxine and folic acid. GLRX5 encodes a mitochondrial protein, glutaredoxin 5, which when deleted in the zebrafish mutant shiraz results in defective iron-sulfur cluster assembly and blocked synthesis of heme.[158] A late-onset pyridoxine-refractory sideroblastic anemia caused by homozygous mutation in GLRX5 has been described in a patient who in middle age developed symptoms of a microcytic hypochromic anemia, type 2 diabetes, cirrhosis, and liver iron overload.[157]

Therapy for Hereditary Sideroblastic Anemia

A trial of pyridoxine (100 to 200 mg/day taken orally) is indicated for 3 months for all patients with hereditary sideroblastic anemia. Response is variable and ranges from complete correction of hemoglobin levels to no effect. Even when pyridoxine completely corrects the anemia (Fig. 36-10), the increase in mean corpuscular volume (MCV) may not reach normal values, and a population of hypochromic, microcytic cells remains.

About 25% to 50% of patients with hereditary sideroblastic anemia show a full or partial response to pyridoxine, and this vitamin should be continued on a lifelong basis in the responders. A lower maintenance dose should be determined for each responding patient by progressive dose reduction, because long-term therapy with pyridoxine at 100 to 200 mg/day has been associated with peripheral neuropathy.[154] The adult nutritional requirement for pyridoxine is 1 to 2 mg/day; some patients have been maintained on as little as 4 mg/day as a supplement.[143] Folic acid supplements should also be administered because the erythroid hyperplasia increases demand for this vitamin.

There is one report of successful allogeneic peripheral blood stem cell transplantation in a 19-year-old man with transfusion-dependent hereditary sideroblastic anemia.[155] Transfusions are the mainstay of treatment for severe anemia unresponsive to pyridoxine. Regular administration of packed red cells using white blood cell filters are given to relieve symptoms and permit normal childhood development. Iron overload and secondary hemosiderosis rapidly progress after transfusions begin; chelation therapy with desferrioxamine or oral deferasirox should be initiated from the onset.

Iron removal may be of great benefit for patients who have mild or moderate anemia and evidence of iron overload.[151,152] These patients can often tolerate intermittent phlebotomy, which is preferable to chelation therapy for iron removal, and should be continued to reduce ferritin levels to less than 300 ng/mL. All patients with iron overload should avoid ingestion of ascorbic acid supplements, which enhance iron absorption and increase the tissue toxicity of elemental iron. Alcohol should also be avoided. Splenectomy is contraindicated in this disease.

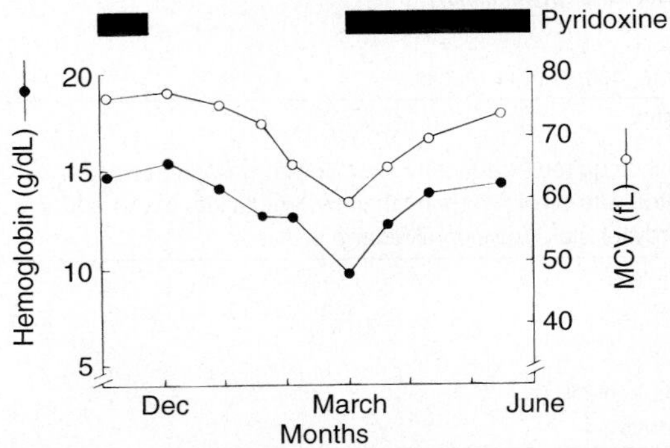

Figure 36-10 RESPONSE OF THE HEMOGLOBIN CONCENTRATION AND MEAN CORPUSCULAR VOLUME (MCV) TO WITHDRAWAL AND REINSTITUTION OF PYRIDOXINE IN A PATIENT WITH RESPONSIVE HEREDITARY SIDEROBLASTIC ANEMIA.

In addition to genetically defined forms of hereditary sideroblastic anemia, four syndromic types have been described, which present with anemia in combination with either muscle, neurologic, or pancreatic tissue involvement. The first of these disorders to be defined by molecular genetics, the Pearson syndrome, is a rare entity that manifests in early infancy with anemia and exocrine pancreatic dysfunction. The anemia is normocytic or macrocytic, reticulocyte counts are low, and variable degrees of neutropenia and thrombocytopenia are present. The bone marrow shows striking vacuolation and ringed sideroblasts.[159] Although usually fatal, milder forms of the anemia are consistent with survival into adult life. The syndrome, which is related to the Kearns-Sayre syndrome, results from deletions, mutations, or duplications of mitochondrial DNA, variably affecting multiple tissues of the body.[160,161]

A second syndromic congenital sideroblastic anemia, X-linked sideroblastic anemia with cerebellar ataxia (XLSA/A), is a rare mitochondrial disease caused by loss-of-function mutations in the ATP-binding cassette transporter ABCB7.[162-164] ABCB7 is localized to the inner mitochondrial membrane and has been proposed to function as an exporter of mitochondrial iron-sulfur clusters to the cytoplasm[165]; however, a direct role in heme synthesis may arise through an interaction with ferrochelatase.[166] Males affected with XLSA/A usually present in infancy with nonprogressive or slowly progressive ataxia and incoordination, which is accompanied by a mild to moderate hypochromic microcytic anemia and the presence of ring sideroblasts on bone marrow examination.

Mutations in the high-affinity thiamine transporter gene SLC19A2, located at 1q24.2, cause the thiamine-responsive megaloblastic anemia (TRMA) syndrome.[167] TRMA has the unusual bone marrow feature of megaloblastic erythroid maturation with ring sideroblasts. TRMA presents with early-onset megaloblastic anemia, diabetes mellitus, and sensorineural deafness, which respond variably to thiamine treatment.

Most recently the genetic variants that cause a fourth syndromic hereditary sideroblastic anemia, myopathy, lactic acidosis, and sideroblastic anemia (MLASA), have been reported.[168,169] A missense mutation in the PUS1 gene coding for pseudouridine synthase-1 causes the rare autosomal recessive disease, MLASA.[168,170] Mitochondrial and cytoplasmic transfer RNAs (tRNAs) from affected patients lack tRNA pseudouridylation at sites normally modified by PUS1; however, the mechanism by which this affects oxidative phosphorylation and iron metabolism in skeletal muscle and bone marrow are yet to be elucidated.[170] MLSA displays genetic heterogeneity such that an identical phenotype is caused by a homozygous mutation in the mitochondrial tyrosyl-tRNA synthetase gene, YARS2.[169] The homozygous mutation in YARS2, identified in three patients from two consanguineous Lebanese families, causes defective mitochondrial synthesis and, similar to mutations in PUS1, results in defective oxidative phosphorylation.[169] MLASA1 and MLASA2 usually present with progressive exercise intolerance commencing in childhood followed by later development of sideroblastic anemia, basal lactic acidemia, and mitochondrial myopathy.

Acquired Sideroblastic Anemia

Acquired sideroblastic anemia is categorized within the myelodysplastic syndromes and may appear de novo or occur after chemotherapy or irradiation (see Table 36-5). The clonal nature of hemopoiesis in this condition was first suggested by Dacie et al.[139] Nearly all cases show evidence of dyserythropoiesis in the marrow, and there may also be dysplastic changes in the myeloid precursors or megakaryocytes, or both. Acquired idiopathic sideroblastic anemia falls within the diagnostic category of refractory anemia with ring sideroblasts as defined by the French-American-British group and World Health Organization classification.[171,172] Acquired sideroblastic anemia has also been a rare finding in myeloproliferative disorders such as idiopathic myelofibrosis or essential thrombocythemia. Distinguishing between idiopathic myelofibrosis and myelodysplasia is sometimes difficult, and there is increasing recognition for an overlap or transitional entity, myelodysplasia/myeloproliferative disease, unclassifiable.[172-174] Thus many patients with refractory anemia with ring sideroblasts and thrombocytosis have a point mutation in the Janus kinase 2 gene (changing valine-617 to phenylalanine), which is a feature usually associated with the myeloproliferative disorders.[175] This latter group have a clinical phenotype that includes normal MCV, marrow fibrosis, and splenomegaly (see Chapter 59).[175]

Biologic and Molecular Aspects

Clonal hematopoiesis has been demonstrated in acquired idiopathic sideroblastic anemia and in the related myelodysplastic syndromes. Specific evidence was first provided by finding a single G6PD isoenzyme in erythrocytes, granulocytes, platelets, and B lymphocytes in a woman who was heterozygous for G6PD and carried two isoenzymes in her skin and T lymphocytes.[176] This technique is applicable only to the few women who have G6PD heterozygosity, but restriction fragment length polymorphism analysis can be applied to most women using probes directed at other X-chromosome genes such as that for phosphoglycerate kinase or to an X-linked, variable-copy-number tandem repeat sequence (see Chapter 1).[177] The results show uniform monoclonality of hematopoiesis in acquired sideroblastic anemia with or without associated myelodysplastic features. Some indirect evidence exists for a primary mitochondrial lesion, perhaps in the mitochondrial respiratory chain, which impairs the reduction of Fe^{3+} because Fe^{2+} is essential for heme synthesis.[178-180] Recurrent mutations in the SF3B1 gene have recently been described in acquired sideroblastic anemia and are found in 65% of patients with refractory anemia and ring sideroblasts.[181] The product of SF3B1 is associated with mRNA splicing, and mutations in this gene may influence a number of mitochondrial gene networks resulting in iron-laden mitochondria during erythroid development.

Etiology

Clonal chromosomal changes are found in bone marrow cells in approximately 60% of patients with acquired sideroblastic anemia. Characteristic changes are monosomy 7; trisomy 8; deletions involving chromosomes 5, 7, 11, or 20; and a number of balanced translocations.[182] When sideroblastic anemia is acquired after chemotherapy or irradiation, chromosomal changes are usually found and tend to be multiple.[182] Among these changes, the loss of an entire chromosome (5 or 7, or both), deletion of a long arm [del(5), del(7), or del(13)], and an unbalanced translocation are typical.[183,184] When karyotype shows loss of material from chromosomes 5 or 7, or both, a detailed occupational history may show exposure to potentially mutagenic chemical agents in a proportion of patients.[185] However, the development of visible chromosomal changes is probably a late event in acquired sideroblastic anemia and may be preceded by the expansion of a clone of genetically unstable stem cells. This concept is in accord with the view that multiple genetic events underlie the pathogenesis of other myelodysplastic syndromes and acute myeloid leukemia[176,186] (see box on Clinical and Laboratory Evaluation of Sideroblastic Anemia).

Differential Diagnosis

Ring sideroblasts are not limited to acquired sideroblastic anemia; they also occur in other myelodysplastic conditions, such as refractory anemia with excess blasts, in which the blast count is higher than 5%.[195] Careful examination of peripheral blood and bone marrow can distinguish acquired idiopathic sideroblastic anemia from these related myelodysplastic conditions. Family surveys are very useful in distinguishing acquired from hereditary forms of sideroblastic anemia, because the latter may present in late adult life.

Clinical and Laboratory Evaluation of Sideroblastic Anemia

Typically, sideroblastic anemia develops insidiously in a middle-aged or elderly patient with normal or increased mean corpuscular volume (MCV) and a blood smear showing a population of hypochromic red cells. Hepatosplenomegaly may be present. Leukocyte and platelet counts are usually normal, but some patients have thrombocytosis that occasionally exceeds 1000×10^9/L.[187] If leukopenia or thrombocytopenia is present, a careful search should be made for myelodysplastic features, which lead to the more descriptive term of *refractory cytopenia* for the condition.[188,189] An iron stain of the bone marrow aspirate shows ring sideroblasts, which should total more than 15% of all erythroblasts to make the diagnosis of acquired sideroblastic anemia.[171,189-191] Iron cannot be assessed in the marrow trephine biopsy core because it may leach out during decalcification.

The bone marrow also shows erythroid hyperplasia. Although mild dyserythropoiesis (e.g., multinuclearity, nuclear budding) and megaloblastoid changes are present, myelopoiesis and megakaryopoiesis are usually normal. When changes are confined to dyserythropoiesis, the condition has been called *pure sideroblastic anemia*.[189,192] However, dysplasia of myelopoietic and megakaryopoietic elements may be present (i.e., trilineage dysplasia) with the following features: Pelger-Huët–like anomaly, hypersegmentation or hypogranularity of neutrophils, micromegakaryocytes, large mononuclear megakaryocytes, and megakaryocytes with multiple small nuclei (see Chapter 59).[189] Dysmegakaryopoiesis is more easily detected in trephine biopsies than in marrow smears, although the trephine may also show unsuspected islands of myeloblasts characteristic of myelodysplasia.[193] The overall blast count in marrow smears is, by definition, less than 5%, and the peripheral blood monocyte count is less than 1.0×10^9/L. Cytogenetic analysis of marrow aspirates provides important information, because a normal karyotype predicts long survival in any type of acquired sideroblastic anemia.[194]

Prognosis

Acquired idiopathic sideroblastic anemia and the related entity of refractory anemia have the most favorable outlook among the myelodysplastic syndromes, with a median survival of 42 to 76 months and 3% to 12% incidence of leukemic progression in different series.[182,196,197] The prognosis can be correlated with three factors. First is the severity of the anemia, because repeated transfusions markedly increase iron overload and invariably lead to the organ dysfunction characteristic of secondary hemosiderosis (e.g., heart and liver failure, diabetes). The second factor is whether neutropenia and thrombocytopenia are associated with the anemia. These cytopenias form the basis of a simple prognostic scoring system in which two or more of the following place the patient in a poor prognostic category: hemoglobin level less than 10 g/dL, neutrophil count less than 2.5×10^9/L, platelet count less than 100×10^9/L, and blasts more than 5% of the total.[196,197] Thirdly, karyotypic analysis of marrow aspirates provides valuable information, because a normal karyotype carries a more favorable prognosis. Conversely, monosomy 7 or a partial loss of the long arm of chromosome 7 as a single defect imparts a high probability of transformation to acute myeloid leukemia. Multiple chromosomal abnormalities and del(20q) are also associated with an increased risk for progression to leukemia; in contrast, trisomy 8 has no adverse prognostic significance.[182] Evolution of acquired idiopathic sideroblastic anemia to other myelodysplastic conditions, such as refractory anemia with excess blasts, has been described[198] (see box on Therapy for Acquired Sideroblastic Anemia).

Therapy for Acquired Sideroblastic Anemia

Transfusions are indicated for relief of symptomatic anemia. A trial of pyridoxine at 100 to 200 mg/day for 3 months is worthwhile in patients who have anemia but who do not display neutropenia or thrombocytopenia. However, few patients with acquired idiopathic sideroblastic anemia respond to this vitamin. If any response is achieved, maintenance therapy with pyridoxine at lower dosage is indicated. Cyclosporin (5 to 6 mg/kg/day) has been reported to benefit the anemia of the closely related myelodysplastic condition of refractory anemia, although the response appeared limited to those with hypoplastic bone marrows.[199]

SIDEROBLASTIC ANEMIA AND PORPHYRINURIA CAUSED BY DRUGS

Alcohol

Ring sideroblasts may be found in the bone marrow of malnourished anemic alcoholics, usually in the presence of associated folate deficiency.[200-202] In contrast, binge drinking or chronic alcohol ingestion in subjects with good nutrition is not associated with sideroblastic abnormality. Sideroblastic change is never the sole cause for the anemia of alcoholism. Alcohol has a direct toxic effect on hematopoiesis.[203] An increased or high-normal MCV and vacuolation of red blood cell precursors is often seen in addition to the ring sideroblast abnormality. Red blood cells show dimorphic morphology; evidence in the marrow of folate deficiency is present in half of cases.[203] Transferrin saturation and marrow iron stores tend to be increased but may be low if gastrointestinal bleeding is present. The ring sideroblasts gradually disappear over 4 to 12 days when alcohol is withdrawn[202]; during this period, there may be a rebound erythroid hyperplasia, reticulocytosis, and thrombocytosis. Folic acid should be given for the associated megaloblastic changes after blood is taken for vitamin B_{12} and folate assays.

Alcohol consumption lowers the plasma concentration of pyridoxal phosphate, a cofactor for ALAS, needed in the first step in heme synthesis.[204] Conversion of ethanol to acetaldehyde is necessary for this effect, and acetaldehyde acts by accelerating the degradation of intracellular pyridoxal phosphate in the liver, lowering plasma levels of this coenzyme.[205]

Chronic alcoholics have an altered heme metabolism with increased urinary excretion of coproporphyrin, mainly isomer III, but normal urinary excretion of uroporphyrin, ALA, and porphobilinogen. Acute and chronic ethanol ingestion markedly depresses the activity of ALA dehydratase in peripheral blood. Ethanol administration to normal subjects results in increased activity of leukocyte ALAS and erythrocyte PBGD, the two rate-controlling enzymes of the pathway. The activities of each of the other four enzymes are depressed. Ferrochelatase, the enzyme that inserts iron into protoporphyrin to form heme, shows the most marked depression, and in alcoholism there is prolonged depression of uroporphyrinogen decarboxylase, which provides a rationale for the role of ethanol in the etiology of PCT.[206,207] As earlier, ethanol is a major precipitating factor in acute porphyria.[208]

Isoniazid

Administration of the antituberculous drug isoniazid occasionally has been associated with development of a sideroblastic anemia after 1 to 10 months of therapy. The anemia is hypochromic and microcytic, with a dimorphic blood smear and ring sideroblasts in the marrow. This complication is thought to occur only in slow acetylators of isoniazid, allowing this drug to react nonenzymatically with pyridoxal and to form a hydrazone that is rapidly excreted in the urine. The anemia can be fully reversed by coadministration of pyridoxine (25 to 50 mg/day) with isoniazid or by withdrawing isoniazid.[209] Another antituberculous drug, pyrazinamide, may also cause a sideroblastic anemia, which is caused by inhibition of ALAS2 and responds to pyridoxine therapy.[210]

Chloramphenicol

Chloramphenicol is an antibiotic that produces a reversible suppression of erythropoiesis after several days of therapy (plasma levels of 10 to 15 mcg/mL). This effect is predictable and separate from the rare idiosyncratic side effect of aplastic anemia in approximately 1 of 20,000 exposed persons. Nearly all patients given chloramphenicol (>2 g/day) develop vacuolation of the erythroid precursors and ring sideroblasts. These effects are thought to arise from suppression of mitochondrial respiration. Chloramphenicol inhibits mitochondrial protein synthesis and reduces cytochrome a, a_3, and b levels.[211] Serum iron concentrations are increased, and reticulocyte numbers are subnormal; these changes revert on stopping the antibiotic.

Other Drugs

A reversible acquired sideroblastic anemia has been described with penicillamine therapy and with the use of triethylene tetramine hydrochloride, a copper-chelating agent used in the treatment of Wilson disease.[212] Acquired sideroblastic anemia has also been precipitated by progesterone given to a patient on two separate occasions 15 years apart, and this anemia promptly reversed on withdrawal of the drug.[213]

PRESENTATIONS ASSOCIATED WITH SIDEROBLASTIC ANEMIA OR PORPHYRINURIA

Copper Deficiency or Zinc Overload

The copper content of a Western diet averages 0.9 to 1.6 mg each day, which is only a few times greater than the amount needed to maintain homeostasis of this essential element.[214] Copper deficiency has been described in malnourished premature infants,[215] in patients receiving long-term parenteral or enteral hyperalimentation,[216] after gastrectomy,[217] with copper-chelating agents,[212] or on an idiopathic basis.[218] The syndrome of copper deficiency consists of sideroblastic anemia with hypochromic cells in the blood smear, accompanied by ring sideroblasts and vacuolated erythroid and myeloid precursors in the marrow, and of neutropenia with an absence of late myeloid forms in the marrow (Fig. 36-11). In some reports, patients present with neurologic symptoms such as paresthesias, weakness, or ataxia; and demyelination is seen on the magnetic resonance image of the brain.[218] In infants, additional features may be seen, such as osteoporosis and long bone changes, depigmentation of skin and hair, and central nervous system abnormalities. The platelet counts remain normal. Serum copper and ceruloplasmin levels are low, whereas serum iron and transferrin saturation levels are normal. The serum zinc concentration may be increased.[218] Prompt reversal of the hematologic changes follows therapy with 2 to 5 mg/day of copper sulfate taken orally or 100 to 500 mcg/day of copper supplement to the intravenous alimentation formula.

Large quantities of ingested zinc interfere with copper absorption and produce the neutropenia and sideroblastic anemia characteristic of copper deficiency.[219] Zinc sulfate is freely available from health food stores, and as little as 450 mg/day for 2 years is sufficient for this effect. Sideroblastic anemia has also been ascribed to zinc toxicity arising from the ingestion of coins over a period of many years.[220] Serum zinc levels are high, whereas serum copper and ceruloplasmin levels are low. Zinc must be discontinued for 9 to 12 weeks for full reversal of the anemia and neutropenia.

Iron Deficiency Anemia

In iron deficiency anemia, there is an accumulation of protoporphyrin in erythrocytes that rarely reaches the level found in EPP. The zinc complex of protoporphyrin is produced because ferrochelatase uses Zn^{2+} during iron-deficient erythropoiesis.[221] Erythrocyte protoporphyrin may be raised before changes appear in peripheral blood and may be helpful in diagnosing iron deficiency when serum iron and ferritin levels are rising as a result of patients having started iron therapy. In iron-deficient erythropoiesis, erythroid ALAS activity is reduced below normal.[222]

Hypothermia

Thrombocytopenia, erythroid hypoplasia, and ring sideroblasts have been described in patients with hypothermia associated with neurologic disease.[223] These changes reverse slowly as body temperature returns to normal.

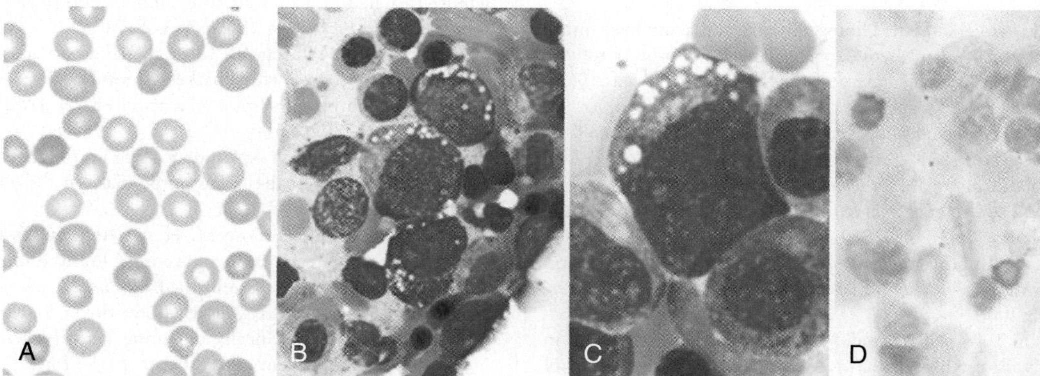

Figure 36-11 THIS 70-YEAR-OLD MAN WAS BEING TREATED WITH ZINC SUPPLEMENTATION AND WAS FOUND TO HAVE ANEMIA AND NEUTROPENIA (HEMOGLOBIN, 8.3 G/DL; HEMATOCRIT, 23.9%; AND WHITE BLOOD CELL COUNT, 1200/μL). His peripheral smear **(A)** showed a biphasic erythroid population with some small slightly hypochromic cells and increased anisocytosis (red blood cell distribution width [RDW], 23.9%). The bone marrow aspirate showed a left shift in granulopoiesis with vacuolization of immature granulocytic and erythroid precursors (**B** and **C**). A Prussian blue–stained aspirate revealed ring sideroblasts **(D).** The patient's copper level was less than 0.1 mcg/mL (normal reference range, 0.75 to 1.45 mcg/mL).

Other Conditions

In hereditary tyrosinemia, excess urinary ALA is excreted because ALA dehydratase is inhibited by succinyl acetone. Like acute porphyria and lead poisoning, this disease is associated with neurobehavioral disturbance (see box on Lead Poisoning). In liver disease, there may be increased urinary excretion of coproporphyrin, predominantly isomer I. In the Dubin-Johnson syndrome, the ratio of coproporphyrin isomer I to isomer III is markedly increased in the urine (>80%), possibly as a result of deficiency of hepatic uroporphyrinogen III cosynthase and increased activity of PBGD. In Rotor syndrome, total urinary excretion of coproporphyrin is markedly increased and consists predominantly of coproporphyrin isomer I. In the unconjugated hyperbilirubinemia of Gilbert syndrome, depressed activity of protoporphyrinogen oxidase and increased activity of ALAS has been found in peripheral leukocytes.[226]

Environmental Intolerances

It has been hypothesized that several otherwise-unexplained chemical-associated illnesses, such as multiple chemical sensitivity syndrome, may represent mild chronic cases of porphyria or other acquired abnormalities in heme synthesis. However, evidence for this concept is lacking.[225,227]

Lead Poisoning

It has been known for some time that patients suffering from lead poisoning have an accumulation of protoporphyrin in erythrocytes and increased urinary excretion of ALA and coproporphyrin.[224] There are sex-related differences in the porphyrin synthetic response to lead, with females showing a more profound coproporphyrinuria than men.[225] The elevated protoporphyrin chelated by zinc is retained in the erythrocyte, which may explain the absence of photosensitivity. This accumulation of porphyrins and precursors is caused by the inhibition by lead of the heme biosynthetic enzymes: 5-aminolevulinate (ALA) dehydratase, coproporphyrinogen oxidase, and ferrochelatase. An increase in the activity of the rate-controlling enzyme ALA synthase (ALAS) results.

Many of the clinical manifestations of lead poisoning may be the result of altered heme biosynthesis.[72] A mild to moderate anemia that can be hypochromic and microcytic occurs in a minority of patients, whereas basophilic stippling is prominent due to inhibition of pyrimidine 5′-nucleotidase in the maturing reticulocyte. Ring sideroblasts have not been reported. The abdominal pain, constipation, and peripheral neuropathy that occur in lead poisoning are also seen in acute attacks of hepatic porphyria. Neuropathy, seen in lead poisoning, may also be the result of disorders of heme biosynthesis, as in the porphyrias.[224] Alterations in porphyrin metabolism have provided a useful means of detecting and assessing the severity of lead exposure and poisoning. The diminution in activity of erythrocyte ALA dehydratase and elevated erythrocyte protoporphyrin levels are the most sensitive measures.

SUGGESTED READINGS

Aivado M, Gattermann N, Rong A, et al: X-linked sideroblastic anemia associated with a novel ALAS2 mutation and unfortunate skewed X-chromosome inactivation patterns. *Blood Cells Mol Dis* 37:40, 2006.

Ajioka RS, Phillips JD, Weiss RB, et al: Down-regulation of hepcidin in porphyria cutanea tarda. *Blood* 112:4723, 2008.

Anderson KE, Bloomer JR, Bonkovsky HL, et al: Recommendations for the diagnosis and treatment of the acute porphyrias. *Ann Intern Med* 142:439, 2005

Bergmann AK, Campagna DR, McLoughlin EM, et al: Systematic molecular genetic analysis of congenital sideroblastic anemia: Evidence for genetic heterogeneity and identification of novel mutations. *Pediatr Blood Cancer* 54:273, 2010.

Chen W, Dailey HA, Paw BH: Ferrochelatase forms an oligomeric complex with mitoferrin-1 and Abcb10 for erythroid heme biosynthesis. *Blood* 116:628, 2010.

Furuyama K, Harigae H, Heller T, et al: Arg-452 substitution of the erythroid-specific 5-aminolaevulinate synthase, a hot spot mutation in X-linked sideroblastic anaemia, does not itself affect enzyme activity. *Eur J Haematol* 76:33, 2006.

Goodwin RG, Kell J, Laidler P, et al: Photosensitivity and acute liver injury in myeloproliferative disorder secondary to late-onset protoporphyria caused by deletion of a ferrochelatase gene in hematopoietic cells. *Blood* 107:60, 2006.

Guernsey DL, Jiang H, Campagna DR, et al: Mutations in mitochondrial carrier family gene SLC25A38 cause nonsyndromic autosomal recessive congenital sideroblastic anemia. *Nat Genet* 41:651, 2009.

Lin CS, Krishnan AV, Lee MJ, et al: Nerve function and dysfunction in acute intermittent porphyria. *Brain* 131:2510, 2008.

Macours P, Cotton F: Improvement in HPLC separation of porphyrin isomers and application to biochemical diagnosis of porphyrias. *Clin Chem Lab Med* 44:1438, 2006.

Nakano H, Nakano A, Toyomaki Y, et al: Novel ferrochelatase mutations in Japanese patients with erythropoietic protoporphyria: High frequency of the splice site modulator IVS3-48C polymorphism in the Japanese population. *J Invest Dermatol* 126:2717, 2006.

Phillips JD, Bergonia HA, Reilly CA, et al: A porphomethene inhibitor of uroporphyrinogen decarboxylase causes porphyria cutanea tarda. *Proc Natl Acad Sci U S A* 104:5079, 2007.

Pondarre C, Campagna DR, Antioches B, et al: Abcb7, the gene responsible for X-linked sideroblastic anemia with ataxia, is essential for hematopoiesis. *Blood* 109:3567, 2007.

Puy H, Gouya L, Deybach JC: Porphyrias. *Lancet* 375:924, 2010.

Rand EB, Bunin N, Cochran W, et al: Sequential liver and bone marrow transplantation for treatment of erythropoietic protoporphyria. *Pediatrics* 118:1896, 2006.

Richardson DR, Lane DJ, Becker EM, et al: Mitochondrial iron trafficking and the integration of iron metabolism between the mitochondrion and cytosol. *Proc Natl Acad Sci U S A* 107:10775, 2010.

Sarkany RP, Ross G, Willis F: Acquired erythropoietic protoporphyria as a result of myelodysplasia causing loss of chromosome 18. *Br J Dermatol* 155:464, 2006.

Schultz IJ, Chen C, Paw BH, et al: Iron and porphyrin trafficking in heme biogenesis. *J Biol Chem* 285:26753, 2010.

Szpurka H, Tiu R, Murugesan G, et al: Refractory anemia with ringed sideroblasts associated with marked thrombocytosis (RARS-T), another myeloproliferative condition characterized by JAK2 V617F mutation. *Blood* 108:2173, 2006.

Thunell S, Pomp E, Brun A: Guide to drug porphyrogenicity prediction and drug prescription in the acute porphyrias. *Br J Clin Pharmacol* 64:668, 2007.

Whatley SD, Ducamp S, Gouya L, et al: C-terminal deletions in the ALAS2 gene lead to gain of function and cause X-linked dominant protoporphyria without anemia or iron overload. *Am J Hum Genet* 83:408, 2008.

Ye H, Jeong SY, Ghosh MC, et al: Glutaredoxin 5 deficiency causes sideroblastic anemia by specifically impairing heme biosynthesis and depleting cytosolic iron in human erythroblasts. *J Clin Invest* 120:1749, 2010.

For complete list of references log on to www.expertconsult.com.

CHAPTER 37

MEGALOBLASTIC ANEMIAS

Aśok C. Antony

The term *megaloblastic anemia* is used to describe a group of disorders characterized by a distinct morphologic pattern in hematopoietic cells. A common feature is a defect in deoxyribonucleic acid (DNA) synthesis, with lesser alterations in ribonucleic acid (RNA) and protein synthesis, leading to a state of unbalanced cell growth and impaired cell division. Most megaloblastic cells are not resting but vainly engaged in attempting to double their DNA, with frequent arrest in the S phase and lesser degrees of arrest in other phases of the cell cycle. An increased percentage of these cells have DNA values between 2 N (N is the amount of DNA in the haploid genome) and 4 N because of delayed cell division. This increased DNA content in megaloblastic cells is morphologically expressed as larger-than-normal "immature" nuclei with finely particulate chromatin, whereas the relatively unimpaired RNA and protein synthesis results in large cells with greater "mature" cytoplasm and cell volume. The net result of megaloblastosis is a cell whose nuclear maturation is arrested (immature) while its cytoplasmic maturation proceeds normally independently of the nuclear events. The microscopic appearance of this nuclear-cytoplasmic asynchrony (or dissociation) is morphologically described as megaloblastic. Each cell lineage has a limited but unique repertoire of expression of defective DNA synthesis. This is significantly influenced by the normal patterns of maturation of the affected cell line. Additional variables that affect RNA and protein synthesis can lead to the attenuation or modification of megaloblastic expression (see Masked Megaloblastosis).

Megaloblastic hematopoiesis commonly manifests as anemia, but this feature is only a manifestation of a more global defect in DNA synthesis that affects all proliferating cells. The peripheral blood picture is characteristic and reflective of megaloblastic hematopoiesis within the bone marrow. The diagnosis is therefore usually straightforward, but because any condition that specifically perturbs DNA synthesis may lead to megaloblastosis, determination of the precise cause is necessary before institution of therapy. Inappropriate therapy can lead to disastrous consequences for the patient. The biochemical basis for megaloblastosis needs to be understood within the context of evaluation of potential and real variables affecting DNA, RNA, and protein synthesis in a given patient. The most common causes of megaloblastosis are true cellular deficiencies of vitamin B_{12} (cobalamin) or folate, vitamins that are essential for DNA synthesis.

Because of the imperative for conservation of cobalamin within the body, there is a finely tuned mechanism in place to ensure a sequential handover of this precious cargo from one protein to another—from the point of its entry into the mouth through the gut, across the enterocyte, into the circulation with specialized uptake into cells, passage through lysosomes into cytoplasm, and even into mitochondria. Throughout this odyssey cobalamin is accompanied by several chaperones that sequentially bind, sequester, and thereby ensure that cobalamin does not participate in side reactions. This ensures its fitness for service for critical enzymes.

Despite the greater abundance of folate in the diet relative to cobalamin, there are also specialized means to ensure that the natural folates in food are first chopped and diced before being ushered across the enterocyte through specialized pathways. After passage from the portal blood into the general circulation, folate is extracted by cell surface folate receptors, undergoes endocytosis, and is then shunted together with a proton across another channel into the cytoplasm. It is then received by an overabundance of high-affinity multifunctional enzymes that channel the folate across set pathways to support critical synthesis of thymidine for DNA.

Indeed, the care with which cobalamin and folate is handled is analogous to the swarm of Secret Service agents escorting a president as he walks by a crowd of well-wishers, their sole aim being to prevent him from getting too close to the public—to shake hands, or hug and kiss a baby, and the like, which could also expose him to potential harm by an ill-wisher—and detract him from doing his primary job as chief executive.

The pathophysiology of cellular cobalamin and folate deficiency is most readily discerned by the clinician who approaches megaloblastosis with a clear understanding of the physiology of these vitamins. A detailed discussion of cobalamin and folate therefore follows.

COBALAMIN

The term *cobalamin* refers to a family of compounds with the structure shown in Fig. 37-1. Details of the chemistry, nomenclature, and in vivo substitutions of cobalamin are shown in Figs. 37-1 to 37-3, and excellent reviews are available on the colorful history, chemistry, and biology of cobalamin.[1-4]

Nutrition

Cobalamin is produced in nature only by microorganisms, and humans receive cobalamin solely from the diet.[5] Cobalamin is synthesized and used by some microorganisms (e.g., bacteria, fungi). Some strains produce cobalamin in excess of their requirements, making them excellent and cheap commercial sources for cobalamin used in therapy. Herbivores obtain their dietary quota of cobalamin from plants contaminated with cobalamin-producing soil bacteria (rhizobia) that grow in roots and nodules of legumes. Because rhizobia-related organisms are also found in the large intestine of animals (and humans), volitional or inadvertent coprophagy can lead to intake of cobalamin by herbivores; however, cobalamin from manure that contaminates plants is not likely to be a significant source for humans.[5] Nevertheless, colonic cobalamin-producing bacteria—like *Klebsiella pneumoniae* that are related to rhizobia—can be found in the small intestine of some individuals from which cobalamin can be absorbed. Because microscopic insects found in vegetables (cabbage, lettuce, spinach) can be unwittingly consumed, in theory, "organically grown" leafy vegetables may have higher cobalamin than those exposed to chemical fertilizers, but this awaits confirmation.[6] For all practical purposes, there is *no* unfortified plant food, including fermented soy products, tempeh/*tempe,* seaweed—(which are actually multicellular algae, such as nori [red algae], chlorella [green algae], spirulina [blue-green algae]—or other organic produce that can consistently provide a sufficient amount of active cobalamin to support daily requirements.

Animal protein is the major dietary cobalamin source for nonvegetarians. Meats from parenchymal organs are richest in cobalamin (over 10 mcg/100 g wet weight); fish and muscle meats, milk

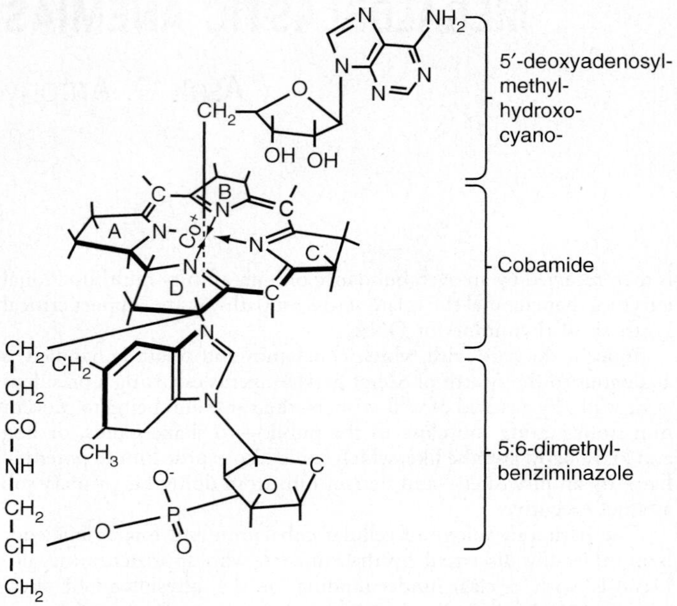

Figure 37-1 COBALAMIN (VITAMIN B_{12}) CHEMISTRY AND NOMENCLATURE. The central cobalt atom of cobalamin forms the focal point of this large complex organometallic molecule (approximately 1300 to 1500 Da). There are up to six ligands that can bind to this cobalt; of these, four involve nitrogen atoms of the planar corrin ring that surround the cobalt atom. The lower α-axial ligand, extending perpendicular below the corrin ring, links to nitrogen of a 5,6-dimethylbenzimidazole phosphoribosyl moiety that is also attached back to the corrin ring through one of its propionamide side chains (this is analogous to the hand guard on the handle on a sabre that covers the knuckles of the hand). The upper or β-axial ligand varies and can exist in the fully oxidized Co^{+++} state, which is referred to as cob(III)alamin; in the Co^{++} state, called cob(II)alamin (which can be used for the synthesis of methylcobalamin or adenosylcobalamin); or the fully reduced Co^{+} state (cob[I]alamin). These upper axial ligands include cyano- (cyanocobalamin), hydroxyl- (hydroxocobalamin), methyl- (methylcobalamin), or 5′-deoxyadenosyl- (adenosylcobalamin) and confer a distinct identity to cobalamin for participation in one-carbon metabolism. All these forms with substituted upper axial ligands are cob(III)alamins, which adopt a configuration in which the 5,6-dimethylbenzimidazole nitrogen base is coordinated to the cobalt in the lower axial position. This is referred to as the "base-on" position. However, when cobalamin is bound to the enzymes methionine synthase and methylmalonyl-CoA mutase, another conformational change results in the replacement of the 5,6-dimethylbenzimidazole by a histidine donated by the enzyme; this is the "His-on" position. Thus shifts from "base-on/His-off" conformation to an alternative "base-off/His-on" conformation have an important bearing on the catalytic activity of these enzymes. Conversion of cyanocobalamin to its active cofactor forms requires a decyanation step. *(From Chanarin I:* The megaloblastic anemias, *Oxford, UK, 1979, Blackwell Scientific Publications.)*

products, and egg yolk have 1 to 10 mcg/100 g of wet weight. An average nonvegetarian Western diet contains 5 to 7 mcg/day of cobalamin, which adequately sustains normal cobalamin equilibrium. A vegetarian diet supplies between 0.25 and 0.5 mcg/day of cobalamin, so most vegetarians *do not* receive adequate dietary cobalamin and are at risk for cobalamin deficiency.[7] The recommended daily allowance is 2.4 mcg for men and nonpregnant women, 2.6 mcg for pregnant women, 2.8 mcg for lactating women, and 1.5 to 2 mcg for children 9 to 18 years old.[6]

Food cobalamin is stable to high-temperature cooking but is readily converted to inactive cobalamin analogues by ascorbic acid. Cobalamin is exceptionally well stored in tissues in its coenzyme forms. Of the total-body content of 2 to 5 mg in adults, about 1 mg is in the liver. There is an obligatory loss of 0.1% per day (1.3 mcg) regardless of total-body cobalamin content. It takes about 3 to 4 years to deplete cobalamin stores when dietary cobalamin is abruptly malabsorbed, but it may take longer to develop nutritional cobalamin deficiency, because of an efficient enterohepatic circulation, which accounts for turnover of 5 to 10 mcg/day of cobalamin.[8]

Absorption

Cobalamin in food is usually in coenzyme form (5′-deoxyadenosylcobalamin [adenosylcobalamin] and methylcobalamin), nonspecifically bound to proteins (see Fig. 37-2). In the stomach, peptic digestion at low pH is a prerequisite for cobalamin release from food protein.[8] Once released by proteolysis, cobalamin preferentially binds a high-affinity, 150-kDa, cobalamin-binding protein called *R protein* (a haptocorrin) from gastric juice and saliva that has higher affinity for cobalamin than gastric intrinsic factor (IF). The cobalamin–R protein (holo-R protein) complex, along with excess unbound (apo)-R protein and IF, pass through into the second part of the duodenum, where pancreatic proteases degrade holo-R and apo-R proteins (but not IF). This results in the transfer of cobalamin to IF, a 45-kDa glycoprotein with high-affinity binding ($K_a = 1.5 \times 10^{10}\ M^{-1}$), 1:1 molar stoichiometry, stability, and resistance to proteolysis over a pH range of 3 to 9.[8] Failure to degrade holo-R proteins by pancreatic protease precludes the involvement of IF in cobalamin absorption because the downstream ileal IF-cobalamin receptors only interact with IF-bound cobalamin.[8] Although R proteins bind cobalamin and most cobalamin analogues with comparably high affinity, IF only binds cobalamin.

IF is produced in parietal (oxyntic) cells in the fundus and cardia of the stomach[8] and is released by membrane-associated vesicular transport.[8] IF has two binding sites: one for cobalamin and another for the ileal IF-cobalamin receptor. IF is produced in far greater excess than is actually required for absorption,[8] and the IF in only 2 to 4 mL of normal gastric juice can reverse cobalamin deficiency in adults who lack IF. In the absence of IF, less than 2% of ingested cobalamin is absorbed, whereas in its presence, approximately 70% is absorbed.

IF is secreted in response to food in the stomach in a manner analogous to secretion of acid (i.e., by vagal and hormonal stimulation). IF binds biliary cobalamin and newly ingested cobalamin following its transfer from R protein.[8,9] Because biliary cobalamin analogues are not transferred from R protein to IF, this is an efficient method for fecal excretion of cobalamin analogues while allowing for reabsorption of biliary cobalamin. The stable IF-cobalamin complex passes through the jejunum to the ileum, where specific membrane-associated IF-cobalamin receptors for IF-cobalamin are located on microvilli of ileal mucosal cells.[8]

The functional IF-cobalamin receptors are composed of a complex of two proteins collectively known as cubam—composed of *cub*ilin[10] and *am*nionless[11]—that is essential to complete transport of the IF-cobalamin complex from the intestinal lumen into the enterocyte. Cubilin is the large 400-kDa extracellular portion of the cubam complex; it is anchored to the membrane by amnionless, which is nearly one-tenth its size; both are however dependent on one another for proper localization as cubam in the membrane. Dysfunction of cubam is the basis for Imerslund-Gräsbeck syndrome. These IF-cobalamin receptors (cubam) require Ca^{2+} for binding at pH above 5.4; they do not bind free IF, cobalamin, or R protein–bound cobalamin; so these receptors are highly specific and have a high affinity for IF-cobalamin ($K_a = 1 \times 10^9\ M^{-1}$). The human ileum contains enough cubam receptors to bind up to 1 mg of IF-bound cobalamin; this is the rate-limiting factor in cobalamin absorption.[8]

After the cobalamin-IF complex is internalized by cubam receptor for subsequent processing, cubam is recycled to the cell surface, whereas cobalamin enters the cytoplasm. Subsequent physiologic events are unclear. Although multidrug resistance–associated protein 1 (MRP1) may act as the molecular gate for the cellular export of cobalamin across the basolateral membrane of intestinal epithelium

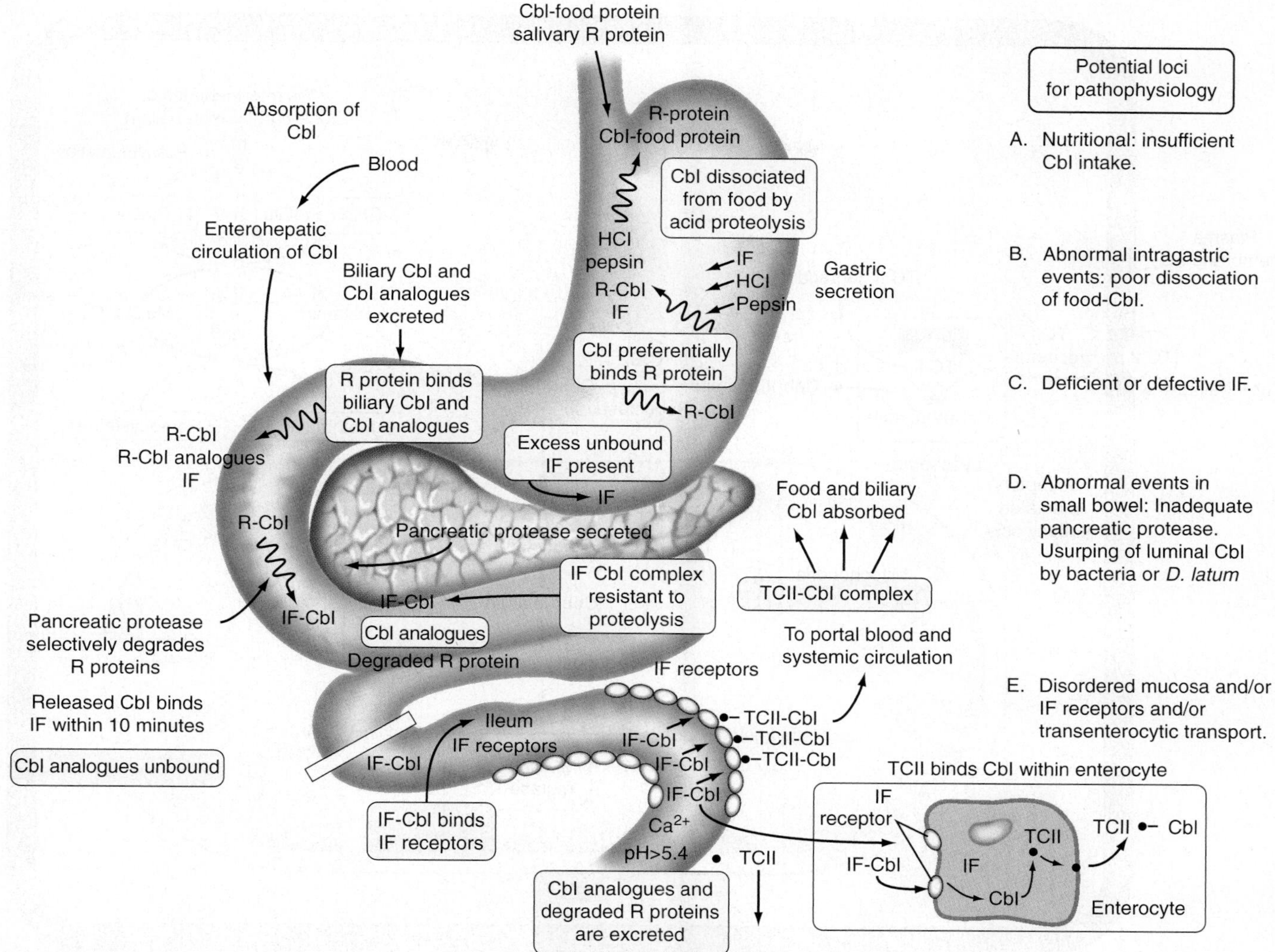

Figure 37-2 COMPONENTS AND MECHANISM OF COBALAMIN ABSORPTION. *Cbl,* Cobalamin; *D. latum, Diphyllobothrium latum; HCl,* hydrochloric acid; *IF,* intrinsic factor; *R-Cbl,* R-protein bound cobalamin; *TCII,* transcobalamin II.

and in other cells,[12] studies on mutated MRP1 fail to identify defects in cobalamin absorption[13]; so a physiologic role for MRP1 is still unclear. The next step involves interaction with transcobalamin II (TCII), which is secreted unidirectionally across the basolateral surface, and cobalamin apparently binds TCII within or at the basal surface of the ileal enterocyte.[8] TCII, which is abundant in the microvascular endothelium, is also available to bind cobalamin. After 3 to 5 hours, cobalamin appears in portal blood largely (over 90%) bound to TCII and reaches peak levels in about 8 hours.[8]

Cobalamin in large doses can also passively diffuse through buccal, gastric, and jejunal mucosa so that less than 1% of a large dose of oral cobalamin appears in the circulation within minutes. This property is used to advantage in individuals with cobalamin malabsorption in lieu of parenteral replacement (discussed later).[8]

Transport

More than 90% of recently absorbed or injected cobalamin is bound to TCII, which is the specific transport protein for delivery of cobalamin to tissues. TCII, a 38-kDa polypeptide synthesized in many tissues, binds cobalamin with 1:1 molar stoichiometry and high affinity ($K_a = 1 \times 10^{11}\ M^{-1}$).[9] The TCII-cobalamin complex is rapidly cleared from the circulation in less than an hour. TCII-bound cobalamin binds to specific cell surface TCII-cobalamin receptors present on several cells.[14,15] High-affinity TCII-cobalamin binding to TCII receptors is specific only for holo- and apo-TCII ($K_a = \sim 5 \times 10^{10}\ M^{-1}$). Because some cobalamin analogues can bind TCII with high affinity, these also have the same potential for cellular uptake as cobalamin.[8]

Circulating cobalamin, which is predominantly in the form of methylcobalamin, is not found free in plasma. Binding to TCII accounts for only 10% to 30% of the total serum cobalamin, with the majority (approximately 75%) of remaining cobalamin being bound to another protein, transcobalamin I (TCI). TCI (another haptocorrin) binds biologically active cobalamins as well as biologically inactive cobalamin derivatives. Because TCI is not a transport protein, it is best viewed as a plasma-storage form of cobalamin; indeed, cobalamin-bound TCI has a slow clearance rate (half-life of 9 to 12 days).[9] A third transport protein, transcobalamin III (TCIII), is closely related to TCI but has a half-life in minutes because it is an asialoglycoprotein. TCIII binds a wide spectrum of cobalamin analogues with high affinity and delivers them via hepatic asialoglycoprotein receptors to hepatic cells, and thence into bile for fecal excretion. Between 0.5 and 9 mcg of cobalamin taken up by hepatic TCII receptors is secreted into bile, of which approximately 75% is reabsorbed, analogous to food cobalamin,[8] reflecting an efficient enterohepatic circulation of cobalamin.

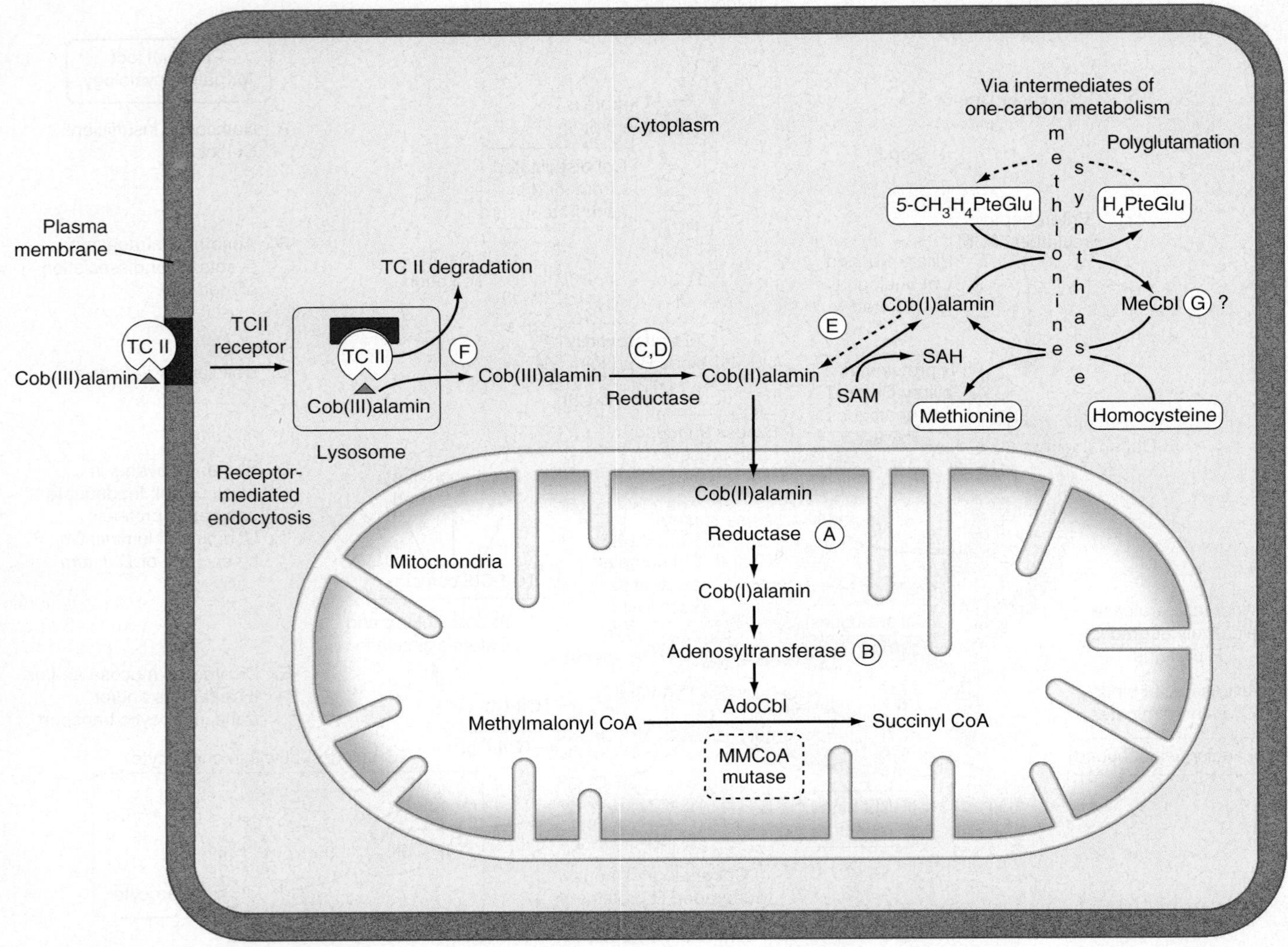

Figure 37-3 CELLULAR UPTAKE AND INTRACELLULAR REACTIONS INVOLVING COBALAMIN. A large family of natural and synthetic cobalamins can be generated when the cyanide (CN) moiety (upper axial ligand in cyanocobalamin) is replaced. On exposure to light, CN is gradually lost from cyanocobalamin, with the production of hydroxocobalamin. In vivo substitutions include the replacement of hydroxocobalamin or cyanocobalamin by a 5′-deoxyadenosyl group attached by a covalent bond, giving rise to adenosylcobalamin (AdoCbl). Methylcobalamin (MeCbl) is the main form in plasma. In vivo, 5-methyl-tetrahydrofolate readily donates its methyl group to cob(I)alamin in a reaction involving methionine synthase to form methylcobalamin. The approximate loci for defects in cobalamin mutants, cblA to cblG, are shown. See text for details. *MMCoA mutase,* Methylmalonyl-CoA mutase; *SAH, S*-adenosylhomocysteine; *SAM, S*-adenosylmethionine.

Cellular Processing

Once bound to TCII receptors, the TCII-cobalamin complex is internalized by conventional receptor-mediated endocytosis (see Fig. 37-3).[8] At the low pH extant in lysosomes, TCII dissociates from cobalamin and is degraded, whereas cobalamin is transported by the lysosomal transporter, LMBRD1 protein,[16] into the cytosol as a mixture of cob(III)alamin and cob(II)alamin. LMBRD1 is missing in cblF mutation (see Fig. 37-3). Cob(III)alamin, the most “oxidized” form of cobalamin, must be converted to cob(II)alamin and cob(I)-alamin by two sequential reductase steps (see Fig. 37-3). Once in the cytoplasm, cobalamin is bound to MMACHC, an enzyme that catalyses removal of the cyano or methyl or adenosyl groups that are bound to cobalt in the cobalamin molecule.[17] From here, cobalamin is moved to target enzymes in the mitochondria or the cytoplasm.

More than 95% of intracellular cobalamin is bound to two intracellular enzymes, methylmalonyl-CoA mutase and methionine synthase.[8] When cobalamin interacts with its target enzymes, it exists in a “base-off/His-on” conformation, which reflects a very close relationship with these enzymes (see legend for Fig. 37-1).

In mitochondria, cob(I)alamin is converted to its coenzyme form, adenosylcobalamin, which acts as a coenzyme with methylmalonyl-CoA mutase to mediate the intramolecular exchange of a hydrogen atom attached to one carbon atom with a group attached to an adjacent carbon atom; in this way, methylmalonyl-CoA is converted to succinyl-CoA. (Methylmalonyl-CoA is normally generated during the catabolism of branched-chain amino acids, odd-chain fatty acids, and cholesterol. When formed, succinyl-CoA can then enter the Krebs tricarboxylic acid cycle.)

In the cytoplasm, cobalamin, as methylcobalamin, functions as a coenzyme for methionine synthase, a critical enzyme for which both folates and cobalamin are required for normal one-carbon metabolism (see Fig. 37-3). Methionine synthase is a modular protein with four distinct and separate regions for binding homocysteine, 5-methyl-tetrahydrofolate (5-methyl-THF; 5-methyl-H_4PteGlu), the cobalamin prosthetic group, and *S*-adenosylmethionine (SAM).[9] The reaction proceeds by methyl transfer from 5-methyl-tetrahydrofolate to methionine synthase–bound cob(I)alamin to form methylcobalamin, followed by transfer of this methyl group to homocysteine to form methionine and regeneration of cob(I)alamin. In this process,

5-methyl-tetrahydrofolate is converted to tetrahydrofolate. During this reaction, spontaneous oxidation of cob(I)alamin (which has no axial ligand) to the catalytically inactive cob(II)alamin form can occur about once in every 1000 to 2000 catalytic cycles[18]; this requires reduction back to cob(I)alamin before it can accept a methyl group. There is a specific redox regulator known as methionine synthase reductase that restores enzyme activity in the presence of SAM and NADPH[19]; this enzyme is mutated in patients with cblE mutations.

The physiologic importance of the key cofactor roles of the two forms of cobalamin (i.e., adenosylcobalamin and methylcobalamin) in methylmalonyl-CoA mutase and methionine synthase, respectively, is that the products and by-products of these enzymatic reactions are critical for DNA, RNA, and protein biosynthesis.

FOLATES

Nutrition

Folates (the anionic forms of folic acid, also called vitamin B_9), are synthesized by microorganisms and plants, including leafy vegetables (spinach, lettuce, broccoli), beans, fruits (bananas, melons, lemons), yeast, and mushrooms, and are also found in animal meats[8]; see Fig. 37-4 for chemistry and nomenclature.

Among natural folates, which are predominantly in polyglutamylated form, only one-half are bioavailable; by contrast, 85% of folic acid that is added to food or ingested as a supplement is bioavailable. Several factors can influence the bioavailability of folates. These include the following: (1) The stability of the food folate affects its bioavailability. Natural reduced folates are labile and susceptible to oxidative cleavage by nitrates or light exposure, but folic acid is much more stable. Prolonged boiling or cooking for over 30 minutes reduces natural folates by 50% to 80%, whereas ascorbate increases bioavailability, and refrigeration of leafy foods exposed to artificial fluorescent light in supermarkets can double the folate content.[21] (2) Pureed foods allow easier access to the glutamate carboxypeptidase II (also known as folate-polyglutamate hydrolase), which converts folate polyglutamates to simpler folate monoglutamates before absorption[22]; any perturbation of this enzyme by organic acids (orange juice), sulfasalazine, or ethanol can preclude absorption; conversely, folate-binding proteins in human or cow's milk can increase folate absorption for infants and women.[23] (3) Interference with folate absorption across the proximal jejunum from intestinal diseases will affect the bioavailability of food folate. (4) Drugs that interfere with the proton-coupled folate transporter (PCFT) can also compromise folate absorption.

The recommended daily allowance of folate is as follows: adult men and nonpregnant women, 400 mcg; pregnant women, 600 mcg; lactating women, 500 mcg; children 9 to 18 years, between 300 and 400 mcg.[6] A balanced Western diet contains adequate amounts of folate, but the net dietary intake of folate in many developing countries is often insufficient to sustain folate balance.[8,9,24,25]

Absorption

After dietary folate polyglutamates are converted to folate monoglutamates at the enterocyte brush border, they are transported through the duodenal and jejunal brush border by physiologically relevant, high-affinity membrane-associated, luminal surface–facing proton-coupled folate transporters (PCFT), which are most efficient in an acidic milieu. At pH 5.5, there is equivalent affinity for transport of physiologic reduced folates and folic acid, but at pH 6.5, reduced 5-methyl-tetrahydrofolate is transported more efficiently.[26] PCFT is a folate-hydrogen symporter, so with each folate molecule transported, there is a net translocation of positive charge. Loss-of-function mutations in PCFT in the enterocyte and choroid plexus result in (congenital) hereditary folate malabsorption,[27,28] a condition associated with an inability to transport folate across the intestine and the

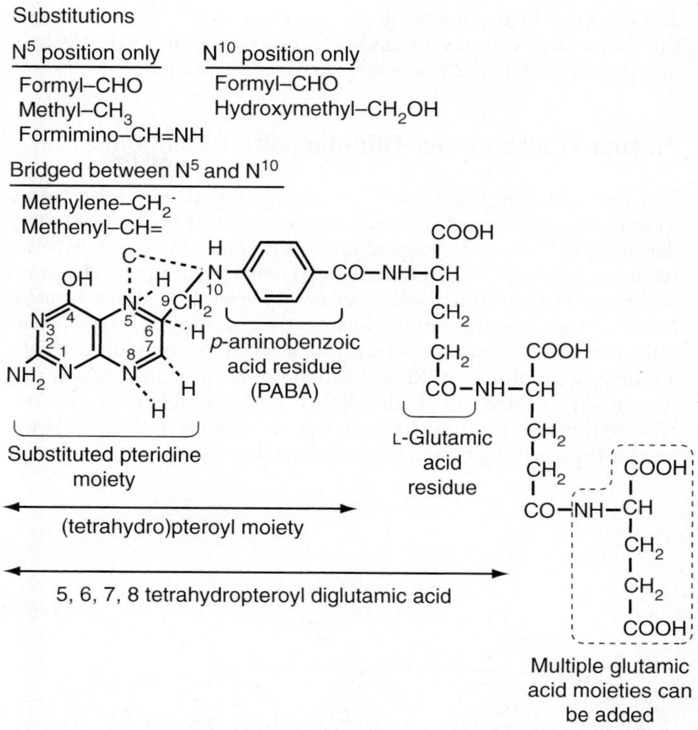

Figure 37-4 FOLATE CHEMISTRY AND NOMENCLATURE. Folic acid (pteroylmonoglutamate [PteGlu]) is the commercially available parent compound for more than 100 compounds collectively referred to as *folates*. PteGlu consists of three basic components: a pteridine derivative, a *p*-aminobenzoic acid residue, and an L-glutamic acid residue. Before PteGlu can play a role as a coenzyme, it must first be reduced at positions 7 and 8 to dihydrofolic acid (H_2PteGlu) and then to 5,6,7,8-tetrahydrofolic acid (THF; H_4PteGlu), and one to six additional glutamic acid residues must then be added by means of γ-peptide bonds to the l-glutamate moiety (for which the subscripted *n* in PteGlu$_n$ denotes polyglutamation). Folate coenzymes donate or accept one-carbon units in numerous reactions in amino acid and nucleotide metabolism. The various substitutions in H_4PteGlu$_n$ occur at positions 5 or 10, or both; position 5 can be substituted by methyl (CH_3), formyl (CHO), or formimino (CHNH), and position 10 can be substituted by formyl or hydroxymethyl (CH_2OH). Positions 5 and 10 can be bridged by methylene (–CH_2–) or methenyl (–CH=). For an engaging account of the history of folic acid, see reference 20.

choroid plexus. The expression of PCFT is increased in folate-deficient mice, suggesting a physiologic regulatory mechanism. Proton pump inhibitors can reduce expression, and blocking the function of PCFT by sulfasalazine and pyrimethamine can lead to acquired folate malabsorption.[28,29] Within the enterocyte, folates are reduced to tetrahydrofolate and methylated before release into plasma as 5-methyl-tetrahydrofolate. Most of the folic acid taken up by the PCFT in the proximal small intestine is also converted within the enterocyte to 5-methyl-tetrahydrofolate.

The flux of folate from the basolateral membrane of the enterocyte to the portal blood is mediated through multidrug resistance–associated protein 3 (MRP3).[28] MRP proteins have low affinity but high capacity and are best visualized as cellular "sump pumps" that eject excess folates (and antifolates) out of cells. Together with MRP2, which mediates folate transport into the bile,[30] these MRPs maintain an efficient enterohepatic circulation, which helps the body retain folate.[28]

Some bacterially produced folate can be absorbed across the large intestine,[31] but this accounts for no more than about 5% of the average folate requirement and likely supports the nutrition of colonocytes.

Passive diffusion of folic acid (pteroylmonoglutamate [PteGlu]) is probably the primary mechanism of intestinal mucosal folate absorption at high pharmacologic concentrations.[8] The small intestine has a large capacity to absorb folate, with peak folate levels in plasma achieved 1 to 2 hours after oral administration.

Plasma Transport and Enterohepatic Circulation

The normal serum folate level is maintained by dietary folate and a substantial enterohepatic circulation that amounts to about 90 mcg/day of folate.[8] Biliary drainage results in a dramatic fall in serum folate (to about 30% of basal levels in 6 hours), whereas abrupt interruption of dietary folate leads to a fall in serum folate levels in about 3 weeks. In the plasma, one-third of the folate is free, two-thirds is nonspecifically bound to serum proteins, and a small fraction binds high-affinity, hydrophilic 40-kDa folate-binding proteins, which are structurally related to hydrophobic (native) folate receptors.[32] However, in contrast to cobalamin uptake, there is no specific *serum* transport protein that enhances cellular folate uptake.

Cellular Folate Uptake

Folate Receptors

Plasma 5-methyl-tetrahydrofolate and folic acid are rapidly transported into proliferating cells by specialized, high-affinity, glycosyl-phosphatidylinositol-anchored (membrane) folate receptor-α, which takes up these folates at physiologic concentrations found in serum.[28,32] The plasma membrane containing the folate–folate receptor complex then invaginates and forms an endosomal vesicle that moves into the cytoplasm along microtubules. The perinuclear endosomal compartment then gets acidified to pH 6, which dissociates folate from folate receptors. The released folate then passes across the acidified endosome into the cytoplasm by a transendosomal pH gradient, which is mediated by the PCFT or related moiety[27,28] (Fig. 37-5).

Folate receptor-α is critical to mediating the cellular uptake of folates in proliferating malignant and normal cells and in transport

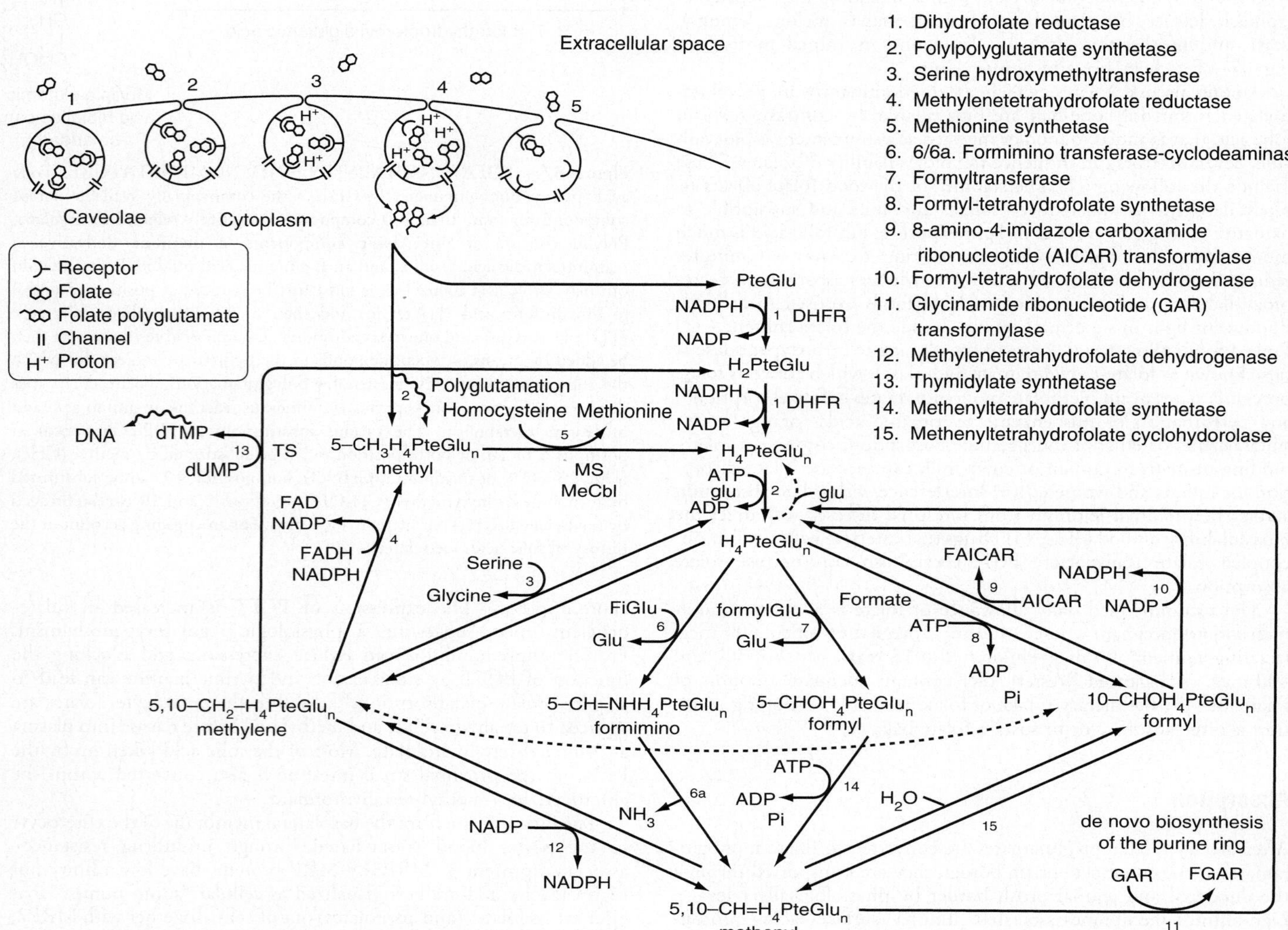

Figure 37-5 FOLATE RECEPTOR-COUPLED FOLATE UPTAKE AND INTRACELLULAR ONE-CARBON METABOLISM INVOLVING FOLATES. See text for details. The channel within the caveolae/endocytotic vesicle is related to the proton-coupled folate transporter (PCFT). The contribution of the reduced folate carrier–mediated transport and passive diffusion of folate into cells is not shown. *ADP,* Adenosine diphosphate; *ATP,* adenosine triphosphate; *DHFR,* dihydrofolate reductase; *DNA,* deoxyribonucleic acid; *dTMP,* deoxythymidine monophosphate; *dUMP,* deoxyuridine monophosphate; *FAD,* flavin adenine dinucleotide; *FADH,* the reduced form of flavin adenine dinucleotide; *FiGlu,* formimino glutamic acid; *Glu,* glutamic acid; *NADP,* nicotinamide adenine dinucleotide phosphate; *NADPH,* the reduced form of nicotinamide adenine dinucleotide phosphate. *(Modified from Shane B, Stokstad EL: Vitamin B_{12}-folate interrelationships.* Annu Rev Nutr *5:115, 1985; and Rothberg KG, Ying Y, Kolhouse JF, et al: The glycophospholipid-linked FR internalizes folate without entering the clathrin-coated pit endocytic pathway.* J Cell Biol *110:637, 1990.)*

of folate across the placenta to the fetus,[33] into the brain,[27,32,34] and in renal conservation of folates. Folate receptor-α is expressed in several types of cancer cells, whereas folate receptor-β is expressed most in monocytes and macrophages[35]; hence these folate receptors are under intense scrutiny for potential clinical use in detecting (and treating) occult malignancy and inflammation.[35]

The physiologic role of the reduced-folate carrier is less clear; it is a "low-affinity" but "high-capacity" system that can also mediate the uptake of 5-methyl-tetrahydrofolate and pharmacologic folates (like methotrexate and folinic acid well, but folic acid poorly) into a variety of cells at physiologic pH.[28]

Folate Receptor Regulation and Cellular Folate Homeostasis

Cell surface folate receptor-α is upregulated in response to low extracellular and intracellular folate concentrations through transcriptional, translational, and posttranslational mechanisms.[32,36-38] Poised in this location facing the external milieu of cells, upregulated folate receptor-α can bind all available folate and thereby restore cellular folate homeostasis.

The answer to the more fundamental question—how do cells sense the existence of folate deficiency in the first place so that folate homeostasis can be subsequently restored by upregulating folate receptors?—has finally been discovered.[39] It so happens that the accumulation of intracellular homocysteine during cellular folate deficiency leads to the covalent binding (by homocysteine) of a protein known as heterogeneous nuclear ribonucleoprotein-E1 (hnRNP-E1), which is already known to mediate the translational upregulation of folate receptor-α.[37,40] Homocysteinylation of hnRNP-E1 at specific cysteine–cysteine disulfide bonds leads to the unmasking of an underlying messenger RNA (mRNA)-binding pocket for which folate receptor-α mRNA has a high affinity. This RNA-protein interaction then triggers the biosynthesis of folate receptors, which soon results in a net increase of cell surface folate receptors that are able to bind more available folate and thereby normalize cellular folate levels. In this context, hnRNP-E1 fulfils criteria as a cellular sensor of physiologic folate deficiency (Fig. 37-6) because this protein is able to sense folate deficiency (by interacting with homocysteine) and respond by increasing RNA-protein interaction that triggers the biosynthesis and upregulation of folate receptors.

The broader significance of this mechanism is that *homocysteinylated hnRNP-E1 actually orchestrates a nutrition-sensitive posttranscriptional RNA operon during folate deficiency*. This means that during folate deficiency, the mRNA-binding pocket within homocysteinylated-hnRNP-E1 is actually highly promiscuous, in that it allows the binding of a variety of very diverse mRNAs (perhaps over 100), all of which have a common password composed of short RNA sequences; these RNA-protein interactions can, in turn, trigger the modulation up or down of a variety of several otherwise entirely unrelated proteins that contribute to the biologic features of reduced cell proliferation, differentiation, and apoptosis, which are a hallmark of folate deficiency.[39]

Folate Receptors and Placental Folate Transport

Because fetal and newborn blood folate is invariably more elevated than maternal blood folate, this suggested the existence of a placental mechanism for preferential maternal-to-fetal folate transport. Placental folate receptors[43,44] are abundant and polarized to the maternal-facing microvillous membrane of the syncytiotrophoblast; they are not present on the basement membrane.[45] Poised in this location, these folate receptors are the first to bind maternal folate at physiologic concentrations and pH; they are critical to transplacental maternal-to-fetal folate transport. This was shown experimentally when irreversible occupancy of the folate-binding site of placental folate receptors led to complete inhibition of transplacental folate transport in an isolated human placental cotyledon perfusion model.[33]

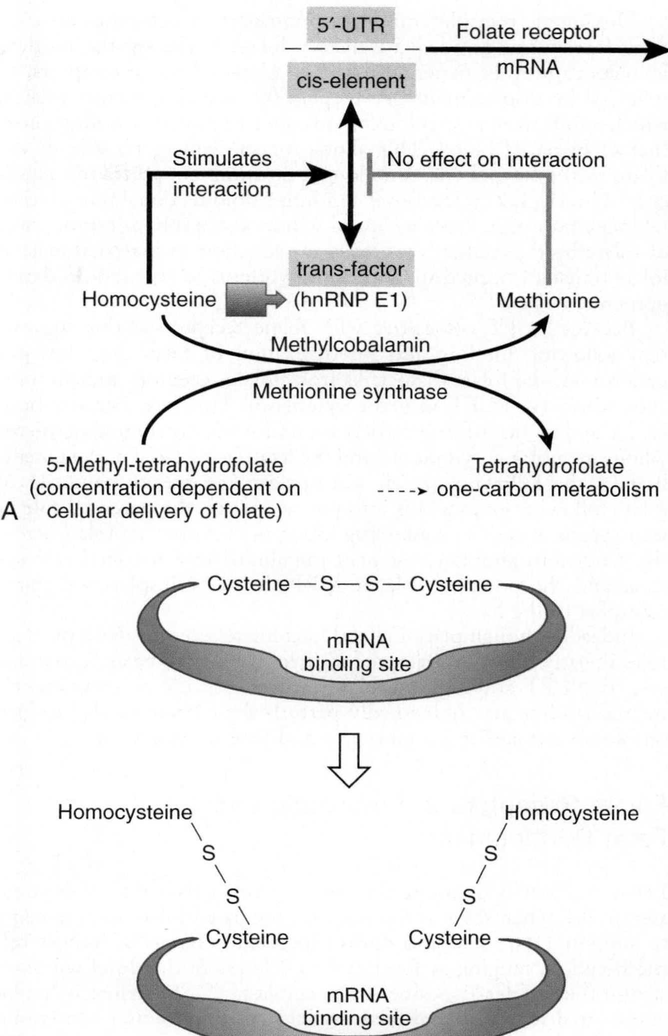

Figure 37-6 MODEL FOR HOW THE CELL SENSES FOLATE DEFICIENCY AND RESPONDS BY UPREGULATING FOLATE RECEPTORS. Note how this model links perturbed folate metabolism, ribonucleic acid (RNA)–protein interaction, and coordinated translational regulation of folate receptor to optimize cellular folate uptake and restore folate homeostasis. The prominent red arrow highlights the critical role of heterogeneous nuclear ribonucleoprotein E1 (hnRNP-E1) as a candidate sensor of cellular folate deficiency. **A,** Reduced folate availability results in inactivation of methionine synthase and intracellular homocysteine buildup, which induces a direct posttranslational homocysteinylation of hnRNP-E1 via targeted homocysteine-S-S-cysteine mixed disulfide bonds; this results in the unmasking of a high-affinity folate receptor messenger RNA (mRNA) cis-element binding site and leads to increased translation of folate receptor-α. The net effect is a homeostatic response that aims to restore intracellular folate concentrations to normal by upregulating cell surface folate receptor. Folate repletion reactivates methionine synthase, which converts homocysteine to methionine. Methionine has no effect on the RNA-protein interaction that leads to reduced folate receptor-α synthesis and its downregulation.[37] (Note: Other metabolic pathways involving homocysteine[41,42] are not included.) **B,** A proposed mechanism for the unmasking of a cryptic mRNA binding site in hnRNP-E1 following the covalent binding of L-homocysteine, through the replacement of one (of many potential) cysteine disulfide bonds by protein-cysteine-S-S-homocysteine mixed disulfide bonds. *5′-UTR,* 5′ Untranslated region. *(From Tang YS, Khan RA, Zhang Y, et al: Incrimination of heterogeneous nuclear ribonucleoprotein E1 (hnRNP-E1) as a candidate sensor of physiological folate deficiency.* J Biol Chem *286:39100, 2011.)*

Physiologic transplacental folate transport, which relies on continued provision of adequate dietary folate intake by the mother, involves capture of maternal folate by placental folate receptors,[43,46] followed by displacement of this pool by incoming dietary folates, which results in an intervillous blood concentration that is three times that of maternal blood. This allows for subsequent transfer of the folate to the fetal circulation along a downhill concentration gradient.[33] This elegant cycle ensures continued unidirectional transplacental folate transport. From a clinical standpoint, a suboptimum intake of folate by the mother that leads to reduction in maternal-to-fetal folate transfer can predispose the embryo/fetus to very serious developmental defects.[47,48]

Because PCFT colocalizes with folate receptor-α, this suggests that following binding and internalization of folate into low-pH endosomes, the folate dissociates from folate receptors and presumably passes via PCFT into the cytoplasm. However, because both PCFT and reduced-folate carriers are uniformly distributed in microvillous membrane, cytoplasm, and the fetal-facing basal plasma membrane,[45] the following are all still unclear: the precise handover of folate following endocytosis into the cytoplasm, the potential role of transcytosis of vesicles containing folate, the transport of folate across the syncytiotrophoblast basement membrane into the fetal vasculature, and the potential role of MRPs in net transplacental folate transport to the fetus.

Indeed, although placental and fetal folate receptors have primary roles in early human development, there is likely to be an important role for PCFT and reduced-folate carriers, because ongoing experimental studies that individually perturb these proteins also induce serious abnormalities in embryonic and fetal development.

Folate Receptors in Embryonic and Fetal Development

Folate receptor-α is among the earliest genes activated in embryonic stem cells[49] when there is the need for increased folate requirements to support DNA synthesis during spectacular bursts of intense cell proliferation, ranging as short as 2 to 3 hours during brief windows within the proliferative zone in the epiblast.[47,50,51] Therefore it can be appreciated why maternal folate deficiency compromises embryonic and fetal development—and perhaps even accounts for an as-yet-uncharacterized number of early miscarriages, as suggested from experimental studies in mice.[48]

Both early-stage neural tube cells and neural crest cells abundantly express folate receptor-α. Experimental perturbation of folate receptor-α can lead to profound abnormalities in neural tube closure and in heart, facial, and eye development.[34,47,52-54] Such studies are consistent with a physiologic role for folate receptor-α and the importance of its functioning normally to prevent the development of neural tube defects (NTDs) and neurocristopathies (the latter involve abnormal proliferation and/or migration and/or differentiation of neural crest cells that can result in cleft lip or cleft palate, endocardial cushion defects, and other midline defects).[34,47,52] Indeed, as predicted,[47] brief experimental perturbation of folate receptor-α expression in these neural crest cells within a short window during embryonic development can impair the mitosis and the migration of these cells into the pharyngeal arches, leading to abnormal development of the pharyngeal arch arteries as well as the outflow tract, predisposing to abnormal heart development.[55] Thus congenital heart defects, which occur at a rate of approximately 1% of live births, and NTDs, the second most common congenital neurologic birth defects, are both dependent on the fidelity of folate receptor-α expression, precisely at the right time and in the right cells during early cardiac and neurologic development. The finding of a significant increase in blocking autoantibodies against placental folate receptor-α in women with pregnancy complicated by neural tube defects[56] is a striking human correlate of the experimental studies.[54]

Folate receptor-α is also involved in providing sufficient folate during neuronal regeneration and repair after injury where DNA methylation is also involved.[57]

Folate Receptors and PCFT in Cerebral Folate Transport Across the Choroid Plexus

Folate receptor-α and PCFT are found in the basolateral membranes of the choroid plexus. After folate binds first to folate receptor-α in the choroid plexus, the PCFT assists in transporting folates into the cerebrospinal fluid, which accounts for the normal cerebrospinal fluid–to blood-folate ratio in healthy humans of 3:1. There are documented individuals with abnormalities in either folate receptor-α or PCFT that limit transport of folate to the cerebrospinal fluid. The following are examples: (1) A syndrome of cerebral folate deficiency can arise from a mutation in folate receptor-α, which perturbs folate transport into the cerebrospinal fluid, leading to severe developmental regression in early childhood associated with movement disturbances, epilepsy, and leukodystrophy that is reversed by folinic acid.[58,59] In addition, anti–folate receptor-α antibodies can prevent uptake of folate into the cerebrospinal fluid and lead to either infantile acute cerebral folate deficiency[60] or one of two autism spectrum disorders (Rett syndrome and infantile low-functioning autism with neurologic abnormalities). High doses of oral folinic acid can normalize the cerebrospinal fluid folate and lead to partial or complete clinical recovery in 12 months.[61] (2) Mutations in PCFT result in hereditary folate malabsorption with low to undetectable cerebrospinal fluid folate values,[26,28] which is also evidence that these proteins have a role in mediating folate transport across the choroid plexus.

Renal Retention of Folates (and Cobalamin)

After glomerular filtration, luminal folate binds folate receptor-α in the brush border membranes of proximal renal tubular cells[9] and is internalized rapidly by folate receptor-α–mediated endocytosis; in the low pH of endocytotic vesicles, there is dissociation of folates and slow transport across basolateral membranes into the blood, with recycling of apo-folate receptor-α back to the luminal brush border membrane.[8] A large 550-kDa membrane protein called megalin, which interacts with cubulin and is found in renal proximal epithelial cells, functions as a multiligand receptor for a variety of macromolecules.[62] Megalin also specifically binds to and mediates endocytosis of TCII-cobalamin complexes as well as filtered folate bound to soluble folate-binding proteins in kidney proximal tubules.[63]

INTRACELLULAR ONE-CARBON METABOLISM AND COBALAMIN–FOLATE RELATIONSHIPS

Cellular Folate Retention and One-Carbon Metabolism

Polyglutamylation of folate by the enzyme folylpolyglutamate synthase catalyzes the addition of multiple glutamate equivalents to their γ-carboxyl residue[9] (see Figs. 37-4 and 37-5). In most eukaryotic cells, the pentaglutamate and hexaglutamate forms predominate. Polyglutamylation is needed to retain folates (and antifolates) within cells; in addition, polyglutamylated folates are more efficient substrates for folate-dependent enzymes. In human erythrocytes (red blood cells [RBCs]), folate is accumulated at earlier stages within the marrow by folate receptors[8]; on maturation, more than 90% of $H_4PteGlu_{(n)}$ molecules interact with hemoglobin, which, because of its high capacity, assists in intracellular folate retention.[8] Folate turnover and catabolism in the cytoplasm can be experimentally accelerated by heavy chain ferritin,[64] but the clinical significance is still unclear.

Compartmentalization and Channeling of Folate Metabolism

In an elegant example of conservation of resources, metabolic pathways involving folate are compartmentalized within cells as multienzyme complexes that shuttle one-carbon units along set paths toward key reactions leading to pyrimidine and purine biosynthesis. The major form of folate transported into the cell is 5-methyl-tetrahydrofolate (5-methyl-THF; 5-methy-H_4PteGlu) (see Fig. 37-5); folic acid, which is formally called pteroylmonoglutamate (PteGlu), requires reduction to tetrahydrofolate by dihydrofolate reductase in a two-step reaction (PteGlu to *dihydro*pteroylglutamate [H_2PteGlu] to *tetrahydro*pteroylglutamate [H_4PteGlu, or THF]). After cellular uptake, 5-methyl-THF must first be converted to THF via methionine synthase (in the methylation cycle). This is a key reaction because THF is the preferred physiologic substrate for folylpolyglutamate synthase, which adds multiple glutamate moieties to THF (see Fig. 37-4). Only then can the polyglutamylated form of THF participate in one-carbon metabolism[41] where it can be converted to either 10-formyl-THF—used in de novo biosynthesis of purines, or to 5,10-methylene-THF—used for synthesis of thymidylate. Moreover, 5,10-methylene-THF and 10-formyl-THF can be interconverted by intermediates (see Fig. 37-5).

Folate metabolism and folate-dependent enzymes are compartmentalized: approximately 40% are in the mitochondrial matrix, 50% in the cytoplasm, and 10% in the nucleus.[65] The mitochondrial compartment *not* shown in Fig. 37-5 contains its complement of folate cofactors, and homologues of the major cytosolic enzymes. For example, cytoplasmic 5-methyl-THF and 5-formyl-THF can enter mitochondria by a mitochondria-specific reduced-folate carrier,[66] whereas SAM, which is also required for mitochondrial methylation reactions, enters mitochondria by a specific transporter.[67] Other one-carbon donors like serine, glycine, dimethylglycine, and sarcosine also enter mitochondria and ultimately generate formate that crosses back into the cytoplasm. In the cytoplasm, C1-THF synthase, a trifunctional enzyme, uses this mitochondria-derived formate with THF to form 10-formyl-THF, which is required for the de novo synthesis of purines (see Fig. 37-5); this enzyme can also catalyze the interconversion of THF, 10-formyl-THF, 5,10-methenyl-THF, and 5,10-methylene-THF. In this way, the continued delivery of mitochondrial formate helps perpetuate cytoplasmic one-carbon metabolism.[65] Another major entry point of one-carbon units into cytoplasmic folate metabolism is through the formation of 5,10-methylene-THF from serine (which is derived from glycolytic intermediates); here the enzyme serine hydroxymethyltransferase catalyzes the addition of carbon 3 from serine to THF to give rise to the key intermediate coenzyme 5,10-methylene-THF.[65] After 5,10-methylene-THF is converted to 5-methyl-THF by the enzyme methylenetetrahydrofolate reductase, it can be used in the methylation cycle that involves methylation of homocysteine via methionine synthase to form methionine and tetrahydrofolate. After 5,10-methylene-THF is converted (via intermediates) to 10-formyl-THF, it can be used for purine nucleotide biosynthesis involving de novo synthesis of purine nucleotides for DNA and RNA. 5,10-Methylene-THF can also be used in the thymidylate cycle via the enzyme thymidylate synthase, which generates thymidylate for DNA synthesis (see Fig. 37-5). Parenthetically, this nuclear one-carbon metabolism compartment is activated during S phase of the cell cycle, following a posttranslational modification of folate-dependent enzymes like thymidylate synthase, serine-hydroxymethyltransferase, and dihydrofolate reductase by specialized small ubiquitin-like modifier (or SUMO) proteins; this modification allows the entry of these sumoylated enzymes into the nucleus[68] so they can generate thymidylate (by converting deoxyuridine monophosphate [dUMP] to deoxythymidine monophosphate [dTMP) close to where DNA is synthesized.

Methylation

After methionine is generated, it can be converted to a methyl donor through its adenosylation to SAM. SAM is a universal donor of methyl groups for critically important biologic methylation reactions involving over 80 proteins, membrane phospholipids, the synthesis of neurotransmitters, RNA, DNA, and histones. Among these, DNA methylation is a major epigenetic mechanism that is central to the regulation of several cellular functions such as gene transcription, chromatin structure, imprinting, development, and genomic instability. DNA is highly methylated in CpG sequences (over 50%); here a methyl group is targeted to the DNA base cytosine in the context of a CpG dinucleotide by DNA methyltransferases. Methylation confers a condensed structure and transcriptional repression, whereas does the opposite. Altered patterns of DNA methylation, particularly hypomethylation involving growth-promoting genes, or hypermethylation of tumor suppressor genes, are popular contemporary themes in our understanding of the epigenetic changes in DNA and the genesis of cancer. In addition, histone hypomethylation can alter gene expression. After these transmethylation reactions that use SAM, the immediate product of these reactions is *S*-adenosylhomocysteine (SAH), which is converted to homocysteine by SAH hydrolase. The SAM to SAH ratio regulates the balance of such cellular methylation reactions.

Dietary folate deficiency can lead to hypomethylation in experimental animals, whereas folate consumption supports normal patterns of methylation. However, analysis in humans has not yielded consistent results, nor has the correlation of folate status and DNA methylation been rigorously studied clinically.

Consequences of Perturbed One-Carbon Metabolism

Methyl-Folate Trapping

Because of the critical role of methylcobalamin for methionine synthase, a deficiency of cobalamin inactivates methionine synthase and results in the accumulation of the substrate 5-methyl-THF; this so-called methyl-folate trap results because the upstream enzyme reaction involving methylenetetrahydrofolate reductase (which converts 5,10-methylene THF to 5-methyl-THF in preparation for the methionine synthase reaction) is irreversible. Because 5-methyl-THF accumulates and cannot be converted to THF, it leaks out of the cell. (This explains why patients with cobalamin deficiency can have normal to high serum folate values). The ensuing intracellular THF deficiency compromises one-carbon metabolism and initiates the pathophysiologic cascade leading to perturbed DNA synthesis and megaloblastosis.

Hyperhomocysteinemia

Similarly, when methionine synthase is inhibited during either cobalamin or folate deficiency, there is a buildup of the thiol amino acid, homocysteine, which can also leak out of the cell and have multiple deleterious effects on the body through a variety of molecular and biochemical pathways. Indeed, measurement of serum homocysteine is a sensitive measure of clinical folate and cobalamin deficiency in nutritional anemias. The clinical significance of hyperhomocysteinemia is discussed later.

Thymidylate Deficiency and Perturbed DNA Synthesis

With either cobalamin or folate deficiency, there will be a net decrease in 5,10-methylene-THF that interrupts the thymidylate synthase–mediated conversion of dUMP to dTMP. (Although salvage pathways for purine synthesis can compensate for reduced generation of purines through one-carbon metabolism, salvage pathways cannot compensate for reduced thymidine). This results in a high dUMP/dTMP ratio and an increase in deoxyuridine triphosphate (dUTP), which can get misincorporated into DNA. At this juncture, an editorial enzyme recognizes this faulty misincorporation and excises dUTP. However, with a continued inadequate supply of deoxythymidine triphosphate (dTTP), there is a failure to repair this break in DNA, leading to several (similar) additional DNA strand breaks that develop over time; this eventually results in fragmentation of DNA and leakage of DNA fragments out of the cell, leading to megaloblastic changes.

Chromosome and Cell Cycle Defects

Defective DNA synthesis is reflected by numerous chromosomal abnormalities. There is excessive chromosomal elongation with despiralization associated with random breaks and exaggerated centromere constriction, expression of folate-sensitive fragile sites in hematopoietic cells, and reduced biosynthesis, acetylation, and methylation of arginine-rich histone.[8,9] All this leads to perturbation of the cell cycle with an increased proportion of cells in prophase of the mitotic cycle and G_2 that leads to apoptosis of erythroid precursors and anemia.[9]

MORPHOLOGIC EXPRESSION OF MEGALOBLASTOSIS

There is widening disparity in nuclear-cytoplasmic asynchrony as a cobalamin- or folate-deficient cell divides, until the more mature generations of daughter cells die in the marrow or are arrested (as megaloblastic cells) at various stages of the cell cycle.[8] The plethora of bone marrow morphologic changes can lead an untrained observer to the diagnosis of erythroleukemia.[9] All proliferating cells exhibit megaloblastosis, including the luminal epithelial mucosal cells of the entire gastrointestinal tract, cervix, vagina, and uterus.[8] However, megaloblastic changes are most striking in the blood and bone marrow. Ineffective hematopoiesis extends into long bones, and the bone marrow aspirate (which is superior to the biopsy for observing megaloblastosis) exhibits trilineal hypercellularity, especially of the erythroid series. The appearance of exuberant cell proliferation with numerous mitotic figures is misleading because these cells are actually proliferating very slowly (see box on Morphology in Megaloblastosis From Cobalamin and Folate Deficiency Is the Same).

Erythroid hyperplasia reduces the myeloid-to-erythroid ratio from 3:1 to 1:1. Proerythroblasts are not as obviously abnormal as later forms; they may simply be larger (promegaloblasts). Megaloblastic changes are most strikingly displayed in intermediate and orthochromatic stages, which are larger than their normoblastic counterparts. In contrast to the normally dense chromatin of comparable normoblasts, megaloblastic erythroid precursors have an open, finely stippled, reticular, sieve-like pattern (Fig. 37-7). The orthochromatic megaloblast, with its hemoglobinized cytoplasm, continues to retain its large sieve-like immature nucleus, in sharp contrast to the clumped chromatin of orthochromatic normoblasts. The nucleus is often

Morphology in Megaloblastosis From Cobalamin and Folate Deficiency Is the Same

Peripheral Smear

- Increased mean corpuscular volume (MCV) with macro-ovalocytes (up to 14 μm), which is variously associated with anisocytosis and poikilocytosis
- Nuclear hypersegmentation of polymorphonuclear neutrophils (PMNs) (one PMN with six lobes or 5% with five lobes)
- Thrombocytopenia (mild to moderate)
- Leukoerythroblastic morphology (from extramedullary hematopoiesis)

Bone Marrow Aspirate

- General increase in cellularity of all three major hematopoietic elements
- Abnormal erythropoiesis—orthochromatic megaloblasts
- Abnormal leukopoiesis—giant metamyelocytes and "band" forms (pathognomonic), hypersegmented PMNs
- Abnormal megakaryocytopoiesis—pseudo hyperdiploidy

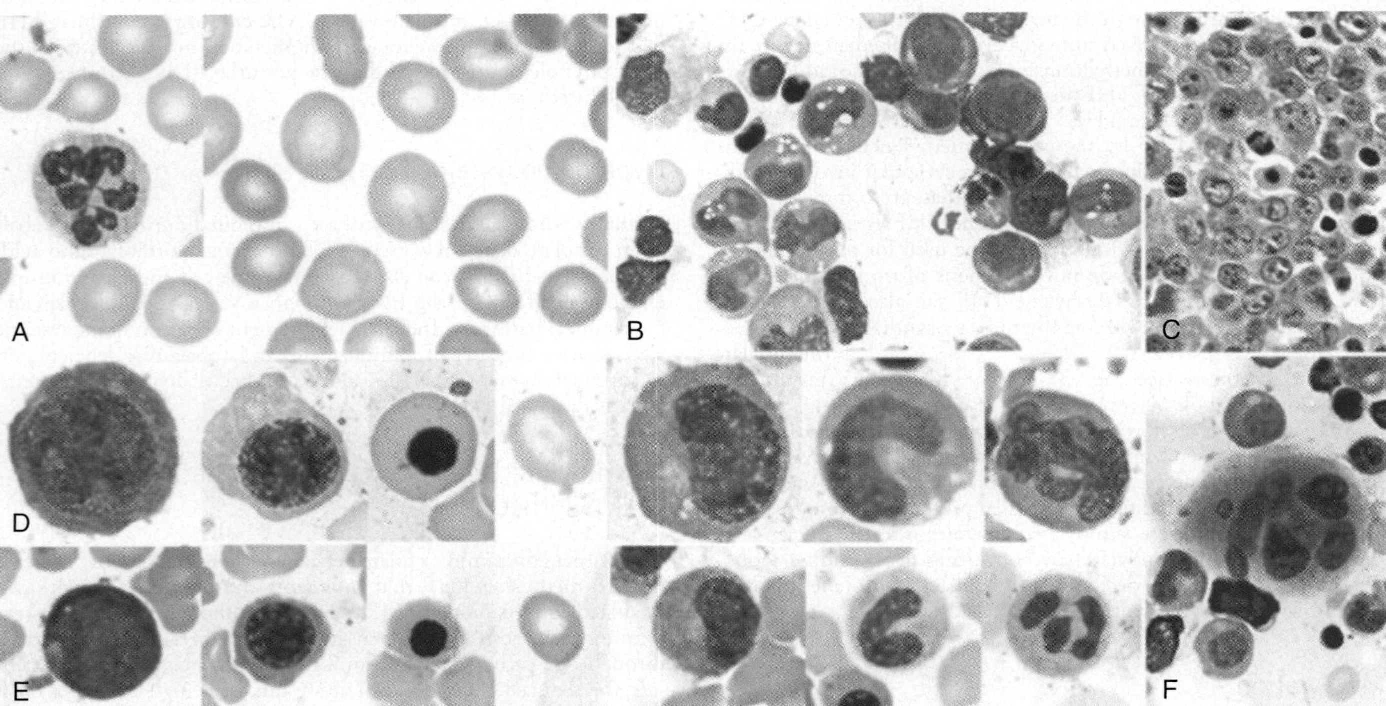

Figure 37-7 MEGALOBLASTIC ANEMIA. The peripheral smear **(A)** exhibits macro-ovalocytosis and hypersegmented polys (inset). The bone marrow aspirate **(B)** shows megaloblastic changes in both granulopoiesis and erythropoiesis. The biopsy **(C)** is hypercellular and shows sheets of immature erythroid precursors with the appearance of a high mitotic rate. These can mimic acute erythroleukemia or even metastatic tumor cells. Details from the cells in the aspirate **(D)** compared with normal hematopoiesis at same magnification **(E)**. Note the giant metamyelocyte and band form. In megaloblastic anemia, megakaryocytes also have nuclear atypica, including abnormal nuclear segmentation **(F)**.

eccentrically placed in these large oval or oblong cells, and lobulation or indentation of nuclei with bizarre karyorrhexis is often seen. In cells destined for the circulation as macro-ovalocytes, the nucleus may occasionally not be completely extruded. Of the potential progeny of proerythroblasts that develop into later megaloblastic forms, 80% to 90% dies in the bone marrow. Marrow macrophages effectively scavenge dead or partially disintegrated megaloblasts. This is the basis for ineffective erythropoiesis (intramedullary hemolysis).

Leukopoiesis is also abnormal. There is an absolute increase in these cells, which are large and have similar sieve-like chromatin. Spectacular giant (20 to 30 μm) metamyelocytes and "band" forms that are often seen are pathognomonic for megaloblastosis (see Fig. 37-7). There may be bizarre nucleoli with small cytoplasmic vacuoles. It is probable that giant metamyelocytes cannot easily traverse marrow sinuses, and their maturation into circulating hypersegmented polymorphonuclear neutrophils (PMNs) is unlikely. Granulation of the cytoplasm remains unaffected.

Megakaryocytes may be normal or increased in numbers and may exhibit additional complexities in megaloblastic expression (see Fig. 37-7). Complex hypersegmentation (i.e., pseudo hyperdiploidy) is associated with liberation of fragments of cytoplasm and giant platelets into the circulation. The net output of platelets is decreased in severe megaloblastosis, and abnormal but reversible platelet dysfunction has been documented.[9]

In early cobalamin or folate deficiency, normoblasts may dominate the marrow with only a few megaloblasts seen. Complete transformation to megaloblastic hematopoiesis is observed in florid cases and is reflected by various degrees of pancytopenia.

The earliest manifestation of megaloblastosis is an increase in mean corpuscular volume (MCV) with macro-ovalocytes (up to 14 μm) (see Fig. 37-7). Because these cells have adequate hemoglobin, the central pallor, which normally occupies about one-third of the cell, is decreased. In severe anemia, poikilocytosis and anisocytosis are evident. Cells containing remnants of DNA (i.e., Howell-Jolly bodies), arginine-rich histone, and nonhemoglobin iron (i.e., Cabot rings) may be observed. Extramedullary megaloblastic hematopoiesis may also result in a leukoerythroblastic picture.

Nuclear hypersegmentation of DNA in PMNs strongly suggests megaloblastosis when associated with macro-ovalocytosis (see Fig. 37-7). Normally less than 5% of PMNs have more than five lobes, and no cells have more than six lobes in the peripheral blood. If megaloblastosis is suspected (greater than 5% PMNs with more than five lobes or a single PMN with more than six lobes), a formal lobe count/PMN (i.e., lobe index) above 3.5 may be obtained.

Ineffective use of iron results in an increased percentage of saturation of transferrin and increased iron stores. If there is associated iron deficiency, the MCV may be normal, and only iron therapy can unmask the megaloblastic manifestations in the peripheral blood. In thalassemia, the entire erythrocyte morphology normally expected in megaloblastosis is masked[8]; however, megaloblastic leukopoiesis is still observed. Significant intramedullary hemolysis (ineffective erythropoiesis) involving more than 90% of megaloblastic precursors is reflected by a lowered absolute reticulocyte count, increased bilirubin (up to 2 mg/dL), decreased haptoglobin, and increased lactate dehydrogenase (LDH) often above 1000 units/mL. There is also a modest decrease in the circulating RBC life span.

Megaloblastosis in rapidly proliferating cells of the gastrointestinal tract leads to a variable degree of morphologic changes and atrophy of luminal epithelial cells. This leads to functional defects, which can include malabsorption of cobalamin and folate in some patients. A vicious cycle whereby megaloblastosis begets more megaloblastosis is established that can be interrupted only by specific therapy with cobalamin or folate.

NEUROLOGIC DYSFUNCTION WITH COBALAMIN DEFICIENCY

Because megaloblastosis due to folate or cobalamin deficiency leads to a functional folate coenzyme deficiency, the morphologic manifestations of both deficiencies are understandably indistinguishable. However, only cobalamin deficiency results in a patchy demyelination process, which is expressed clinically as cerebral abnormalities and subacute combined degeneration of the spinal cord.[8] The precise role of cobalamin in maintaining the integrity of the central nervous system has not been completely defined (see box on Clues for Distinguishing Cobalamin and Folate Deficiencies).

The demyelinating process involves patchy swelling of the myelin sheath followed by its breakdown (demyelination), leading to axonal degeneration. Microscopic foci coalesce with one another, giving the surface of the spinal cord (on cross section) a spongy appearance; later there is secondary Wallerian degeneration of long tracts. Patchy demyelination usually begins in the dorsal columns in the thoracic segments of the spinal cord (Fig. 37-8) and then spreads contiguously to involve corticospinal tracts. These lesions spread throughout the length of the cord and ultimately involve spinothalamic and spinocerebellar tracts. There is also degeneration of the dorsal root ganglia, celiac ganglia, the Meissner plexus, and the Auerbach plexus. Although demyelination may also extend to the white matter of the brain, it is unclear whether the peripheral neuropathy is caused by a distinct lesion or results from spinal cord disease; the clinical manifestations may be extremely varied.[8,9]

Clues for Distinguishing Cobalamin and Folate Deficiencies

Although the megaloblastic manifestations of cobalamin and folate deficiencies are clinically indistinguishable, certain distinct patterns in mode of presentation provide clues to the type and cause of deficiency. In general, the cause of folate deficiency can be found in the patient's recent past (within 6 months), primarily discerned from the history and physical examination. In contrast, the cause of cobalamin deficiency can remain obscure until specific tests to define the cause are carried out. In the past, by the time anemia was symptomatic, more than 80% of patients had neurologic manifestations, and in 50% this led to some incapacity. Perhaps as a result of widespread use of multivitamins containing folic acid among patients and even in the food given livestock in the West, the hematologic expression of cobalamin deficiency is often substantially attenuated, leading to pure neurologic presentations. Studies highlight the apparent inverse correlation between hematologic and neurologic presentations such that in a third of patients with cobalamin deficiency, the earliest signs are often purely neurologic, and symptoms related to paresthesias and diminished proprioception may cause the patient to see the physician. Based on the multiple potential causes (see box on Etiopathophysiologic Classification of Cobalamin Deficiency or box on Etiopathophysiologic Classification of Folate Deficiency), the warning that "what the mind does not know, the eyes do not see" is a caveat that cannot be taken lightly; failure to recognize cobalamin deficiency as the cause of neurologic disease and treatment of cobalamin deficiency with folate, or misdiagnosis of megaloblastosis as erythroleukemia represent significant extremes of deviation from the dictum *primum non nocere*. Areas of overlap in the symptoms of cobalamin or folate deficiency are related to megaloblastosis (i.e., common cardiopulmonary and some gastrointestinal manifestations). Although pure folate deficiency in the alcoholic with thiamine deficiency (i.e., Wernicke encephalopathy) and peripheral neuropathy is almost indistinguishable from and may mimic cobalamin deficiency, the remaining neurologic manifestations are uniquely characteristic of cobalamin deficiency. Folate deficiency in adults has not been unequivocally shown to give rise to neurologic findings. Coexistence of folate deficiency with neurologic disease should prompt investigations to rule out cobalamin and other nutrient deficiencies arising from dietary insufficiency or malabsorption.

Etiopathophysiologic Classification of Cobalamin Deficiency

I. Nutritional cobalamin deficiency (insufficient cobalamin intake)—vegetarians, poverty-imposed near-vegetarians, breastfed infants of mothers with pernicious anemia
II. Abnormal intragastric events (inadequate proteolysis of food cobalamin)—atrophic gastritis, hypochlorhydria, proton pump inhibitors, H_2 blockers
III. Loss/atrophy of gastric oxyntic mucosa (deficient intrinsic factor [IF] molecules)—total or partial gastrectomy, adult and juvenile pernicious anemia, caustic destruction (lye)
IV. Abnormal events in the small bowel lumen
  A. Inadequate pancreatic protease (R factor–cobalamin not degraded, cobalamin not transferred to IF)
    1. Insufficient pancreatic protease—pancreatic insufficiency
    2. Inactivation of pancreatic protease—Zollinger-Ellison syndrome
  B. Usurping of luminal cobalamin (inadequate binding of cobalamin to IF)
    1. By bacteria-stasis syndromes (blind loops, pouches of diverticulosis, strictures, fistulas, anastomosis), impaired bowel motility (scleroderma), hypogammaglobulinemia
    2. By *Diphyllobothrium latum* (fish tapeworm)
V. Disorders of ileal mucosa/IF-cobalamin receptors (IF-cobalamin not bound to IF-cobalamin receptors [cubam receptors])
  A. Diminished or absent cubam receptors—ileal bypass/resection/fistula
  B. Abnormal mucosal architecture/function—tropical/nontropical sprue, Crohn disease, tuberculous ileitis, amyloidosis
  C. Cubam receptor defects—Imerslund-Gräsbeck syndrome
  D. Drug-effects—metformin, cholestyramine, colchicine, neomycin
VI. Disorders of plasma cobalamin transport (transcobalamin [TCII]-cobalamin not delivered to TCII receptors)—congenital TCII deficiency, defective binding of TCII-cobalamin to TCII receptors (rare)
VII. Metabolic disorders (cobalamin not used by cell)
  A. Inborn enzyme errors—cblA to cblG disorders
  B. Acquired disorders (cobalamin inactivated by irreversible oxidation)—nitrous oxide

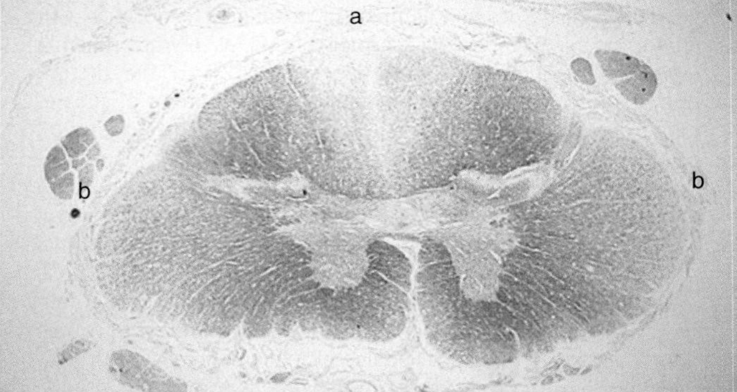

Figure 37-8 SPINAL CORD IN COBALAMIN DEFICIENCY. The cross section of the spinal cord stained with Luxol blue shows demyelination of the dorsal columns *(a)* and early demyelination of the lateral columns *(b)*.

Etiopathophysiologic Classification of Folate Deficiency

I. Nutritional causes
  A. Decreased dietary intake—poverty and famine, institutionalized individuals (psychiatric/nursing homes)/chronic debilitating disease, prolonged feeding of infants with goat's milk, special slimming diets or food fads (folate-rich foods not consumed), cultural/ethnic cooking techniques (food folate destroyed)
  B. Decreased diet and increased requirements
    1. Physiologic—pregnancy and lactation, prematurity, hyperemesis gravidarum, infancy
    2. Pathologic
      a. Intrinsic hematologic diseases involving hemolysis with compensatory erythropoiesis, abnormal hematopoiesis, or bone marrow infiltration with malignant disease
      b. Dermatologic disease—psoriasis
II. Folate malabsorption
  A. With normal intestinal mucosa
    1. Drugs—sulfasalazine, pyrimethamine, proton pump inhibitors (via inhibition of proton-coupled folate transporter [PCFT])
    2. Hereditary folate malabsorption (mutations in PCFTs) (rare)
  B. With mucosal abnormalities—tropical and nontropical sprue, regional enteritis
III. Defective cerebral spinal fluid folate transport—cerebral folate deficiency (mutation or autoantibodies to folate receptors) (rare)
IV. Inadequate cellular utilization
  A. Folate antagonists (methotrexate)
  B. Hereditary enzyme deficiencies involving folate
V. Drugs (multiple effects on folate metabolism)—alcohol, sulfasalazine, triamterene, pyrimethamine, trimethoprim-sulfamethoxazole, diphenylhydantoin, barbiturates

Vegetarians with cobalamin neuropathy in India[69] had cognitive impairment in nearly one-half of 36 patients; it was mostly global with impaired recall and serial sevens (which are useful bedside tests of attention); impaired naming was found among one-quarter of the patients. Nearly one-half had abnormal evoked potential (using the oddball auditory paradigm), which revealed P300 latency that was reversible within 3 months of cobalamin replacement; (in one-fifth P300 was unrecordable). Objective tests to document cobalamin neuropathy[69] include nerve conduction studies and motor- and sensory-evoked potentials,[70,71] visual pathway abnormalities (in 60%[72]), and magnetic resonance imaging (MRI) that shows T2 hyperintensity and atrophy.

Recent studies confirm that among elderly patients with mild cognitive impairment, lowering the homocysteine level by a cocktail that includes cobalamin and folate over 2 years did slow the rate of brain atrophy by almost 30%.[73] This issue is further discussed in Subclinical Cobalamin Deficiency.

Among another cohort of patients with cobalamin neuropathy from the United States, 65% had mild, about 25% had moderate, and about 10% had severe neurologic deficits.[9] Paresthesias or ataxia were most commonly the first symptoms, and diminished vibratory sensation and proprioception in the lower extremities were the most common objective early signs. Although multiple neurologic syndromes were often seen in the same patient, the spectrum of objective signs could include loss of fine or coarse touch, decreased or increased deep tendon reflexes with spasticity or muscle weakness, urinary or fecal incontinence, orthostatic hypotension, amaurosis, dementia, psychosis, or mood disturbances.[9] Overall, although the neurologic deficits were mild in most cases, the severity was judged related to the duration of symptoms before diagnosis; not unexpectedly, those with the shorter duration of symptoms responded most to appropriate replacement.

OTHER EFFECTS OF COBALAMIN AND FOLATE DEFICIENCY

Cobalamin deficiency more often than folate deficiency can also result in sterility from the effects on the gonads. An unexplained finding is generalized melanin pigmentation that is reversible by specific nutrient replenishment.

SPECTRUM OF CLINICAL PRESENTATIONS WITH COBALAMIN DEFICIENCY

The age-specific presentations with cobalamin deficiency are discussed in Nutritional Cobalamin Deficiency. Classical presentations of nutritional cobalamin deficiency in developing countries are often accompanied by iron deficiency, and among malnourished populations, many will also have folate deficiency. Among vegetarians in developing countries, cases with nutritional cobalamin deficiency may present in the second and third decades with pancytopenia, mild hepatosplenomegaly, fever, and occasionally thrombocytopenic bleeding.[9] Alternatively, a neurologic and psychiatric syndrome may develop with or independent of anemia. Because neuropsychiatric presentations may dominate the clinical picture and the patient may not have anemia, careful review of the peripheral smear may reveal macrocytosis.[9] In over a quarter of patients with cobalamin neuropathy in the United States, there was no reduction in the hematocrit despite neurologic disease, and only a minority of patients had combined hematologic and neurologic disease. Indeed, the higher the hematocrit, the more severe the neurologic disorder! Conversely, anemic patients may have no neurologic deficits, and the level of cobalamin may have no correlation with the existence or severity of neurologic disease.

BIOCHEMICAL INDICATORS OF EVOLVING DEFICIENCY

Early manifestations of negative cobalamin balance are increased serum methylmalonic acid (MMA) and total homocysteine levels (Table 37-1).[9] This occurs when the total cobalamin in serum is still in the low-normal range. Continued negative cobalamin balance leads to an absolute decrease in serum cobalamin level. Normal levels of MMA and homocysteine rule out clinically significant cobalamin deficiency with virtually 100% certainty.[9]

Likewise, metabolic evidence for folate deficiency (i.e., increased serum total homocysteine level) is often found when serum folates are still in the low-normal range.

Laboratory tests are more likely to be accurate when there is a high pretest probability of a particular disease. This can however be more vexing in the case of diagnosis of early cobalamin deficiency when symptoms are subtle, nonspecific, or not yet fully manifest. If there is macrocytosis and cobalamin levels are borderline or just below the normal, unequivocal elevation of MMA will support the diagnosis. However, in elderly patients with anemia, there may be several other causes for anemia, and depending on the population studied, cobalamin deficiency may be only one among several possible causes in the differential diagnosis. This is when a modified therapeutic trial—in which a patient is treated with full doses of both cobalamin and folate for 10 days—and the lack of objective response to cobalamin would effectively rule out cobalamin deficiency as a cause (see box on Modified Therapeutic Trials). Alternatively, attribution of the cause of anemia to cobalamin deficiency would be reasonably confirmed retrospectively if there was evidence for resolution of anemia following such therapy with cobalamin. Although reductions from high serum MMA and homocysteine values to baseline following therapy would also be confirmatory, this is impractical due to the expense of multiple testing.

Table 37-1 Stepwise Approach to the Diagnosis of Cobalamin and Folate Deficiency

MEGALOBLASTIC ANEMIA OR NEUROLOGIC-PSYCHIATRIC MANIFESTATIONS CONSISTENT WITH COBALAMIN DEFICIENCY *PLUS* TEST RESULTS ON SERUM COBALAMIN AND SERUM FOLATE

Cobalamin* (pg/mL)	Folate† (ng/mL)	Provisional Diagnosis	Proceed With Metabolites?‡
>300	>4	Cobalamin or folate deficiency is unlikely	No
<200	>4	Consistent with cobalamin deficiency	No
200-300	>4	Rule out cobalamin deficiency	Yes
>300	<2	Consistent with folate deficiency	No
<200	<2	Consistent with (1) combined cobalamin plus folate deficiency or (2) isolated folate deficiency	Yes
>300	2-4	Consistent with (1) folate deficiency or (2) an anemia unrelated to vitamin deficiency	Yes

TEST RESULTS ON METABOLITES: SERUM METHYLMALONIC ACID AND TOTAL HOMOCYSTEINE

Methylmalonic Acid (Normal, 70-270 nM)	Total Homocysteine (Normal, 5-14 μM)	Diagnosis
Increased	Increased	Cobalamin deficiency confirmed; folate deficiency still possible (i.e., combined cobalamin plus folate deficiency possible)
Normal	Increased	Folate deficiency is likely
Normal	Normal	Cobalamin and folate deficiency is excluded

*Serum cobalamin levels: abnormally low, less than 200 pg/mL; clinically relevant low-normal range, 200 to 300 pg/mL.
†Serum folate levels: abnormally low, less than 2 ng/mL; clinically relevant low-normal range, 2 to 4 ng/mL.
‡Any frozen-over sample from serum folate/cobalamin determination can be subjected to metabolite tests.

BIOCHEMICAL EVALUATION OF COBALAMIN AND FOLATE DEFICIENCIES

Total Serum Homocysteine and Methylmalonic Acid Levels

Cellular nutrient *deficiency* of cobalamin or folate is reflected by decreased intracellular concentrations. Cobalamin deficiency perturbs methionine synthase activity; this results in substrate (homocysteine) buildup and elevated serum levels of homocysteine, which can be measured by a sensitive assay.[9] In addition, cobalamin

Modified Therapeutic Trials

The traditional therapeutic trial using physiologic doses of vitamins (100 mcg of folate or 1 mcg of cobalamin given daily while monitoring the reticulocyte response)[8] has given way to a modified therapeutic trial. Rather than making the diagnosis of a deficiency, *the intention is often to confirm the clinical suspicion that the patient does not have deficiency.* This can be demonstrated by lack of response to full replacement doses of both vitamins (1 mg of folic acid orally for 10 days and 1 mg of cobalamin intramuscularly or subcutaneously daily for 10 days). Clinical scenarios in which such trials may be applicable (after drawing blood for serum cobalamin and folate levels) are as follows:

1. There is a clinical suspicion that the underlying disease is not caused by a vitamin deficiency, but this idea is not supported by results of clinical, morphologic, and biochemical evaluations. Such conditions include anemia with a megaloblastic bone marrow that may be secondary to chemotherapy, myelodysplastic syndromes, or acute leukemia; when time is of the essence in making the diagnosis; when the levels of cobalamin are likely to be falsely abnormal because of these diseases; or when there is underlying dehydration or renal dysfunction that predictably gives falsely high levels of metabolites.
2. In other situations (i.e., pregnancy, acquired immunodeficiency syndrome [AIDS], or alcoholism) with a multifactorial basis for anemia, the response or lack thereof to full replacement doses can eliminate cobalamin or folate deficiency and thereby narrow the (often extensive) differential diagnosis.
3. In instances when severe anemia with megaloblastosis is clinically obvious and so serious that the physician cannot wait for the results of specific tests for deficiency. Full doses of both vitamins are administered, and if there is a response manifested by brisk reticulocytosis by days 5 to 7, retrospective assignment of the deficiency is based on the results of blood samples drawn before beginning the trial.

In all therapeutic trials, if there is no evidence of response within 10 days, bone marrow aspiration is indicated to identify another primary hematologic disease.

deficiency perturbs the activity of methylmalonyl-CoA mutase, which leads to elevated serum MMA levels. Thus homocysteine and MMA are sensitive tests for cobalamin deficiency (see Table 37-1).

Folate deficiency also results in elevated levels of homocysteine due to reduced activity of the methionine synthase–catalyzed reaction.[9] Total homocysteine concentration, which comprises the sum of all homocysteine species in plasma/serum, including free and protein-bound forms, can be measured in plasma or serum.[9,74] In general, plasma levels are slightly lower. Thus an elevation of both homocysteine and MMA, while consistent with cobalamin deficiency, cannot rule out a combined cobalamin and folate deficiency (see Table 37-1); see box on Serum Homocysteine and Methylmalonic Acid Levels in Cobalamin and Folate Deficiencies.

Both homocysteine and MMA levels are elevated in patients with dehydration and renal failure; propionic acid derived from anaerobic fecal bacterial metabolism can also substantially contribute to methylmalonate production.[6] In this setting, the fraction of gut flora contribution to MMA can be reduced by treatment with metronidazole.

The normal value for serum homocysteine is 5.1 to 13.9 μM and serum MMA is 73 to 271 nM, and in general the higher the values, the more severe the clinical abnormalities.[9] However, there is a fairly wide range of "normalcy" in homocysteine values because of age-, creatinine-, gender-, diet-, and race-dependent variables.[74] Basal levels of MMA are usually less than 500 nM, and in renal failure, it rarely

Serum Homocysteine and Methylmalonic Acid Levels in Cobalamin and Folate Deficiencies

The combined use of homocysteine and methylmalonic acid (MMA) levels can differentiate cobalamin from folate deficiency, because most patients with folate deficiency have normal MMA levels, and the remainder have only mild elevations.[9] These two tests are useful diagnostically. The abnormally high levels of metabolites return to normal only when the patient receives replacement with the appropriate (deficient) vitamin. A positive response to cobalamin, documented by falling levels of homocysteine and MMA, is evidence of cobalamin deficiency. Conversely, therapy with folate results in a decrease in the isolated homocysteine level if folate deficiency is present.[9] Indeed, because several variables that are not related to vitamin deficiency (such as age, mild renal dysfunction) can falsely elevate serum homocysteine and MMA levels, if there is ambiguity, proof of vitamin deficiency would require clear-cut demonstration of a reduction in metabolite levels after specific vitamin supplementation.[9,75]

increases by more than 1000 nM.[9] If unseparated blood stands at room temperature, homocysteine levels will *increase* over 4 to 24 hours. Frozen serum (from measurements of serum folate or cobalamin) can be used for serum MMA and homocysteine determinations.

Serum Cobalamin Levels

For the most part, a low serum cobalamin level is an established biochemical indicator of cobalamin deficiency. In general, in patients with clinical cobalamin deficiency and megaloblastic anemia or neurologic disease consistent with cobalamin deficiency, the sensitivity of cobalamin concentration less than 200 pg/mL (or less than 148 pmol/L) exceeds 95%[76]—when the pretest probability is high. However, up to 10% of adults with true cobalamin deficiency have cobalamin values in the low-normal (200 to 300 pg/mL) range and only metabolite testing with homocysteine and MMA will reveal the deficiency (see Table 37-1).

Thus a serum cobalamin concentration is less than 300 pg/mL in 99% of patients with clinical hematologic or neurologic manifestations of cobalamin deficiency,[9] and a cobalamin level of more than 300 pg/mL predicts folate deficiency or another hematologic or neurologic disease (see Table 37-1). However, a low serum cobalamin concentration is not synonymous with cobalamin deficiency, and several associated diseases and conditions can falsely raise or lower cobalamin levels (Table 37-2). Studies have also identified patients with true cobalamin deficiency who have cobalamin levels in the low-normal range. Among 173 unambiguously cobalamin-deficient patients,[9] about 5% had normal cobalamin levels. In addition, a high titer of anti-IF antibody can interfere with the measurement of cobalamin and result in a falsely normal serum cobalamin level.[76]

If the serum cobalamin test is broadly used as a screening test without clinical context, by virtue of the way normalcy is defined, 2.5% of nondeficient individuals will have low levels, which reflects our definition of the lower limit of normal for this test.[9] However, the finding that the same blood sample can give different cobalamin results (one below normal versus one above normal) using different commercial assays is of significant concern.[76] The more recent assays have periodically had such problems, apparently arising from a lack of transparency related to these tests, poor validation using low-cobalamin sera, and poor track record of continuous proficiency testing and tracking of assay performance.[76]

So in the absence of availability of metabolite tests, if there are hematologic or neurologic findings that are consistent with clinical cobalamin deficiency, and the serum cobalamin level is normal or borderline low, it is entirely appropriate to treat as for a cobalamin deficiency. If there is no improvement in hematologic parameters

Table 37-2 Serum Cobalamin: False-Positive and False-Negative Test Results

FALSELY LOW SERUM COBALAMIN IN THE ABSENCE OF TRUE COBALAMIN DEFICIENCY
Folate deficiency (one-third of patients)
Multiple myeloma
TCI deficiency
Megadose vitamin C therapy
FALSELY RAISED COBALAMIN LEVELS IN THE PRESENCE OF A TRUE DEFICIENCY*
Cobalamin binders (TCI and II) increased (e.g., myeloproliferative states, hepatomas, and fibrolamellar hepatic tumors)
TCII-producing macrophages are activated (e.g., autoimmune diseases, monoblastic leukemias and lymphomas)
Release of cobalamin from hepatocytes (e.g., active liver disease)
High serum anti-IF antibody titer

IF, Intrinsic factor; *TC*, transcobalamin.
*Although a low serum cobalamin level is not synonymous with cobalamin deficiency, 5% of patients with true cobalamin deficiency have low-normal cobalamin levels, a potentially serious problem because the patient's underlying cobalamin deficiency will progress if uncorrected.

within a couple of months, provided there are no other conditions that limit a full response to cobalamin (e.g., iron deficiency or underlying thalassemia trait, hypothyroidism, renal disease, infection, alcoholism, or intrinsic hematologic disease in the bone marrow), cobalamin deficiency would be unlikely.

Cobalamin deficiency can falsely raise serum folate by 20% to 30% via methyl-folate trapping. Folate deficiency can also reduce serum cobalamin, but the mechanism is unclear.

Serum Folate Levels

The serum folate level is clinically relevant and widely used. Microbiologic assays for folate, which measure all biologically active forms equally, have been replaced in the West by competitive folate-binding protein assays (from various commercial sources) that are indirect immunoassays, which rely on chemiluminescence methods. These tests are notorious for considerable lack of agreement with one another (see box on Diagnosing Folate Deficiency). Alignment with a new higher-order precision isotope-dilution liquid chromatography–tandem mass spectrometry assay—which demonstrates excellent agreement with the traditional *Lactobacillus casei* method[77]—will allow better standardization of the current competitive folate-binding protein assays.[78]

When negative folate balance continues, hepatic folate stores are depleted in about 4 months.[8] This leads to tissue folate deficiency, which clinically correlates with a decrease in RBC folate (less than 150 ng/mL) by the microbiologic assay.[8] However, current RBC folate tests using different commercial kits have major limitations in sensitivity and specificity and are notoriously unreliable in alcoholics and in pregnancy; furthermore, a reduction of RBC folate also occurs in about 60% of patients with cobalamin deficiency.

The use of red-cell folates as a measure of long-term folate status is valid during clinical trials in which a single kit is used for a cohort of patients; however, it is *not* valuable for routine clinical diagnosis because of the significant variability of performance between different commercial kits and lack of clinical validation. Because of these reasons, the serum folate level, although labile, is a good initial choice.[41]

Other Tests

The use of low holo-transcobalamin II (holo-TCII) levels, a test that was developed to provide information on the extent of saturation of

Diagnosing Folate Deficiency

When combined with a clinical picture of megaloblastic anemia and additional results of cobalamin levels, the serum folate concentration is the cheapest and most useful initial biochemical test to diagnose folate deficiency[9] (see Table 37-1). The serum folate level is highly sensitive to folate intake, and a single hospital meal may normalize it in a patient with true folate deficiency. Rapidly developing nutritional folate deficiency first leads to a decline in the serum folate level below normal (less than 2 ng/mL) in about 3 weeks; it is a sensitive indicator of negative folate balance.[8] However, isolated reduction of serum folate level in the absence of megaloblastosis (i.e., false-positive result) occurs in one-third of hospitalized patients with anorexia, after acute alcohol consumption, during normal pregnancy, and in patients on anticonvulsants[9]; unfortunately, these are the very groups at high risk for folate deficiency and the people who exhibit low serum folate levels when they become folate deficient.[8] Conversely, in 25% to 50% of cases (predominantly alcoholics) with folate-deficient megaloblastosis, the serum folate levels may be low normal or borderline (2 to 4 ng/mL).[9] The serum folate level alone should never dictate therapy. It is important to consider the clinical picture, peripheral smear, and bone marrow morphology and also to rule out underlying cobalamin deficiency.

Summary of the Clinical Usefulness of Tests for Cobalamin and Folate Deficiencies

Within the clinical context of hematologic or neurologic features that suggest the diagnosis of cobalamin deficiency, if the cobalamin levels are suggestive but not definitive, then the MMA and homocysteine tests are an excellent gold standard test to confirm a clinical diagnosis. Patients with clinical cobalamin deficiency usually have MMA values over 1000 nM and homocysteine values that are over 25 μM. The MMA and homocysteine test results are much more sensitive than cobalamin levels and progressively increase much earlier than the drop in cobalamin levels; one or both metabolites was increased in 99.8% of more than 400 patients with proven cobalamin deficiency.[9]

Based on the lower costs of serum cobalamin and folate compared with serum MMA and homocysteine levels, it is recommended (see Table 37-1) to first use the cheaper tests that can assist in the diagnosis of cobalamin and folate deficiency.[9] Clinicians should also restrict use of serum MMA and homocysteine to patients with borderline cobalamin and folate levels; to patients with existing conditions associated with difficulties in the interpretation of test results; to situations in which cobalamin and folate levels are low, when a high MMA level is useful in confirming cobalamin deficiency (rather than attributing the condition to folate deficiency alone); and to patients with clearly low serum levels but for whom there is an alternative explanation for the findings that caused an unusual serum cobalamin level to be obtained (e.g., a diabetic or alcoholic with peripheral neuropathy, an alcoholic with a high MCV and a low serum cobalamin without anemia). In these cases, serum levels of metabolites can assist in the diagnosis of vitamin deficiency.

Diagnostic algorithms consistently stress the value of clinical data to improve the pretest probability of serum cobalamin and serum folate tests.[9] Without detailed clinical information, the combined test results for serum cobalamin, folate, and metabolite (homocysteine and MMA) are not sufficiently unambiguous to diagnose and distinguish cobalamin deficiency from combined cobalamin-plus-folate deficiency. In combined cobalamin-plus-folate deficiency, both vitamins would be needed to restore baseline values, particularly of homocysteine.[9]

serum TCII as an early marker of cobalamin homeostasis,[79] as a surrogate for the Schilling test, or to diagnose cobalamin deficiency in lieu of serum cobalamin values, is still unclear. This test has not yet been clinically validated[76] among groups with various established causes of cobalamin deficiency (to define sensitivity, specificity, and other clinical confounders that can alter results). Although an increase in holo-TCII level has been used to show that cobalamin can be absorbed normally in vegetarians,[80] a cheaper option could be to treat a vegetarian with full replacement doses of cobalamin up front and then move to smaller doses; assuming there are no symptoms, a simple reassessment of cobalamin levels a year later could suffice to ensure that there is no problem. Because even mild renal dysfunction elevates MMA and homocysteine levels, and both the serum cobalamin and holo-TCII rise with only advanced renal disease, they could be useful in mild to moderate renal insufficiency. There is still insufficient clinical data to support the routine use of a urinary MMA test.[9]

PATHOGENESIS OF COBALAMIN DEFICIENCY

Nutritional Cobalamin Deficiency

Vegetarian diets can be classified as lactovegetarian, ovovegetarian, lacto-ovovegetarian, or vegan, respectively, if they include dairy products, eggs, dairy products and eggs, or no animal products at all.[7] Vegan diets have a very low cobalamin content, mandating cobalamin supplementation. Likewise, we now know that asymptomatic lacto-ovovegetarians and lactovegetarians[7,81] and those with low dietary consumption of animal source foods (like dairy products, eggs, or animal meats) must be routinely supplemented with cobalamin.

The fetus is dependent on the mother's cobalamin stores for a sufficient quota of cobalamin at birth; a close correlation exists between low maternal serum- and breast milk–cobalamin concentrations and cobalamin insufficiency in the infant.[82] Therefore when mothers do not consume sufficient amounts of animal-source foods, they themselves are at risk for nutritional cobalamin deficiency, and their infants will have smaller stores of the vitamin at birth.[83] In one study, among breastfed infants 6 to 11 months of age in a middle- to low-income community in New Delhi, one-third had cobalamin deficiency.[84] Thus maternal cobalamin stores exert a strong effect on the infant's cobalamin status[85] for up to 12 months,[86] especially in areas where vegetarianism or poverty-imposed near-vegetarianism is common and prolonged breastfeeding is the norm.[7]

Cobalamin-deficient infants can present with a spectrum of clinical findings, ranging from feeding difficulties and refusal of both breast milk and complementary food by regurgitation (which results in failure to thrive) and motor and social retardation, reflecting a developmental delay. The child is persistently drowsy and rarely sits up or makes eye contact.[87] There may be lemon-tint jaundice with hypotonia, insufficient head control, and delayed spontaneous turning. There can be brownish black areas of hyperpigmentation in the dorsal fingers and toes as well as over the medial thighs, arms, and axillae (which usually resolve within 3 months of therapy). Evidence of megaloblastic anemia may be masked with superimposed iron deficiency. If left untreated, there is growth retardation with reduced height and weight, and reduced head circumference with cranial MRI showing delayed myelination and frontoparietal cortical atrophy in affected infants[88]; these can also be reversed within 3 months of cobalamin replacement. Treatment results in a dramatic increase in alertness and responsiveness of the child, who is now miraculously transformed into a normal child who, within a few days, rolls over spontaneously, makes eye contact with its mother, and is much more interested in the surroundings. Any previous abnormal movements (tremors, chorea, or myoclonus) may regress but transiently return within a few days to affect the face or tongue; however, these will resolve in 2 to 3 months.[89] Cobalamin deficiency often resurfaces during wartime, which invariably leaves women and their infants malnourished.[90]

Infants in the West fed a macrobiotic diet (vegan-like with occasional servings of fish) must be rapidly replenished with cobalamin before switching to a cobalamin-rich diet. Otherwise, up to 20% continue to have low cobalamin status, which can lead to impaired psychomotor functioning well into youth and later adolescence with compromise in faculties related to reasoning, abstract thinking, and learning ability.[91]

Reports on nutritional macrocytic anemia identified cobalamin deficiency as the basis for anemia in up to 50% of cases of Indian children 6 months to 12 years of age, and one-fifth of anemic children 3 months to 3 years of age in an urban Indian slum had cobalamin deficiency based on low serum cobalamin levels. Metabolite testing would have picked up many more asymptomatic cobalamin-deficient children because only anemic children were studied. It is also likely that there is widespread deficiency of iron, folate, and cobalamin among children in India.[7,75] Parallel results come from studies on Guatemalan schoolchildren.[92]

Among schoolchildren in Embu, Kenya, who subsist on restricted monotonous diets,[93,94] there was a similar striking influence of (cobalamin-rich) meat supplementation on performance on tests of fluid intelligence that taps into on-the-spot reasoning and problem-solving ability when compared to controls. This speaks volumes on the sheer inadequacy of these children's diets in most developing countries. The number of affected children in developing countries is staggering: There are tens of millions of breastfed infants, whose mothers have borderline or low cobalamin status, who need aggressive cobalamin supplementation to avoid the risk for permanent neurologic and psychologic stigmata from severe deficiency in infancy.

The prevalence of cobalamin deficiency among older children and adolescents is also high, ranging from 40% to 80% in various communities, because of monotonous diets low in animal-source foods (reflecting poverty-imposed near-vegetarianism). Without any intervention, these adolescent girls with low to borderline cobalamin stores fall next in line as a new generation of prospective mothers who will give birth to infants with low or borderline cobalamin stores. And so this vicious cycle continues from one generation to another.

Recent longitudinal studies from the West among women who apparently consume a balanced nonvegetarian diet confirm that pregnancy places an additional stress on the mother's cobalamin stores and can lead to metabolic evidence of cobalamin deficiency.[95-97] This can negatively affect their breastfed infants' cobalamin status at 6 weeks; indeed, over two-thirds of Norwegian infants of otherwise healthy mothers had a metabolic profile consistent with cobalamin deficiency, which reverted to normal after cobalamin replenishment.[96,97] This emphasizes that many more breastfed infants may need cobalamin supplements early in life than previously realized. Such studies raise new questions as to whether the optimal intake of cobalamin in women should be much higher than 2.4 mcg/day, perhaps increased to between 4 and 7 mcg/day.[98]

There is dual significance of cobalamin deficiency for mothers and their infants: Inadequate cobalamin status among women is associated with adverse pregnancy outcomes, including NTDs,[99,100] preterm births,[101] intrauterine growth-retardation,[102,103] and even recurrent miscarriage.[104] For the infant, there is a critical time in prenatal and early postnatal neurodevelopment when sufficient folate and cobalamin is required for the proper formation of neurologic circuits; indeed, perturbation of neurodevelopment can give rise to subtle changes that can manifest in behavioral abnormalities long after the folate and cobalamin deficiency is reversed.

Pregnant adolescents are more generally likely than adults to consume energy-dense, micronutrient-poor diets containing suboptimal folate[105] and thereby experience adverse pregnancy outcomes with small-for-gestational-age babies.[106] And as more young girls recognize that adoption of vegetarian diets can help them to keep slim—a not uncommon practice among high-profile Hollywood celebrities and supermodels—cobalamin deficiency could be on the rise even in Western countries.

Intragastric Events Leading to Cobalamin Malabsorption

Inadequate Dissociation of Cobalamin From Food Protein

Dietary cobalamin is bioavailable only after proteolytic digestion of food by gastric acid and pepsin. Failure to release cobalamin from food protein can lead to food-cobalamin malabsorption and frank cobalamin deficiency despite the presence of IF.[9]

Congenital Intrinsic Factor Deficiency

Congenital IF deficiency due to mutations in gastric IF,[107] resulting in complete loss of IF, can be transmitted as an autosomal recessive trait and expressed in homozygotes by the age of 2 years as severe megaloblastic anemia (less than 100 cases reported).[108] Dysfunctional IF may lead to only a mild abnormality in binding to cobalamin and result in a delayed presentation into the second decade.

Loss or Atrophy of Gastric Oxyntic Mucosa

IF deficiency, which arises from atrophy of gastric parietal (oxyntic) mucosal cells, can be caused by total or partial gastrectomy; by autoimmune destruction, as observed in adult Addisonian pernicious anemia or, rarely, in a similar disease in children (juvenile pernicious anemia); and after destruction of gastric mucosa by caustic (lye) ingestion.

Total gastrectomy invariably leads to cobalamin deficiency in about 5 years (range, 2 to 10 years). This condition is often associated with iron deficiency (leading to a dimorphic anemia),[8] warranting routine cobalamin and iron replacement prophylactically.

Cobalamin deficiency can eventually develop in 10% to 20% of patients 8 years after partial gastrectomy; a minority (about 5%) develop frank clinical manifestations of cobalamin deficiency with megaloblastic anemia. The cause is multifactorial, and contributing factors include decreased IF secretion, hypochlorhydria, intestinal bacterial overgrowth of cobalamin-consuming organisms, and associated iron deficiency. The degree of cobalamin deficiency depends on the size of the remaining gastric remnant. It is more common in Bilroth II than in Bilroth I surgery, and in subtotal than in partial gastrectomy. Morbidly obese patients treated surgically with gastric bypass also have more food-cobalamin malabsorption than patients treated with vertical banded gastroplasty.[9] Even after laparoscopic Roux-en-Y gastric bypass, and despite multivitamin supplementation, iron deficiency was seen in one-half of patients and cobalamin deficiency seen in one-quarter at 3 years[109]; therefore these patients probably need higher oral cobalamin (or addition of parenteral) therapy.

Absent Intrinsic Factor Secretion and Pernicious Anemia

A common cause of cobalamin malabsorption is pernicious anemia, an autoimmune disease in which the fundamental defect is atrophy of the gastric (parietal cell) oxyntic mucosa that eventually leads to the complete absence of IF and HCl secretion (Fig. 37-9). The autoimmune gastritis (leading to chronic atrophic gastritis) associated with pernicious anemia involves the fundus and body of the stomach, and the histologic appearance of the gastric mucosa (infiltration with plasma cells and lymphocytes) is strongly reminiscent of the autoimmune type of lesions. Because cobalamin is absorbed only by binding to IF and uptake by ileal IF-cobalamin receptors, the net consequence is severe cobalamin malabsorption leading to cobalamin deficiency.

The annual incidence of pernicious anemia is approximately 25 new cases per 100,000 persons older than 40 years. Although the average age of onset is about 60 years, pernicious anemia is no respecter of age, race, or ethnic origin. The predisposition to developing pernicious anemia may have a genetic basis, but neither the mode of inheritance nor the initiating events or primary mechanism is precisely understood. There is a positive family history for about 30% of patients, among whom the risk for familial pernicious anemia is 20 times as high as in the general population; about 20% of siblings of patients are projected to develop pernicious anemia by the age of 90 years. And pernicious anemia has developed concordantly in identical twins.

There is a significant association of pernicious anemia with other autoimmune diseases,[8] including Graves disease (30%), Hashimoto thyroiditis (11%), vitiligo (8%), Addison disease, idiopathic hypoparathyroidism, primary ovarian failure, myasthenia gravis, type 1 diabetes mellitus, and adult hypogammaglobulinemia.[8,9]

Anti-IF antibodies are found in the serum of about 60% of patients with pernicious anemia and in the gastric juice of 75%; about 90% of patients with pernicious anemia have anti-IF antibodies in serum or gastric juice.[8] Among African American women with pernicious anemia, 95% have high titers of anti-IF antibodies. Similar IF antibodies are quite rare in the general population. Thus anti-IF antibodies are highly specific and confirmatory for pernicious anemia, but their absence does not rule out the condition. Despite the high incidence of anti–parietal cell immunoglobulin G (IgG) antibodies in the serum of 90% of patients with pernicious anemia, this test is nonspecific and not useful clinically to diagnose pernicious anemia.

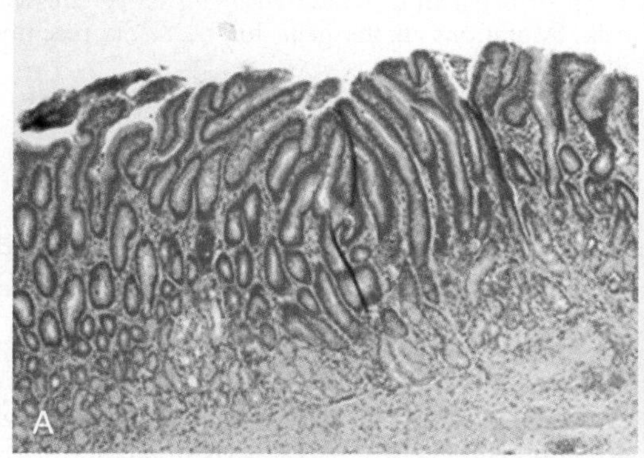

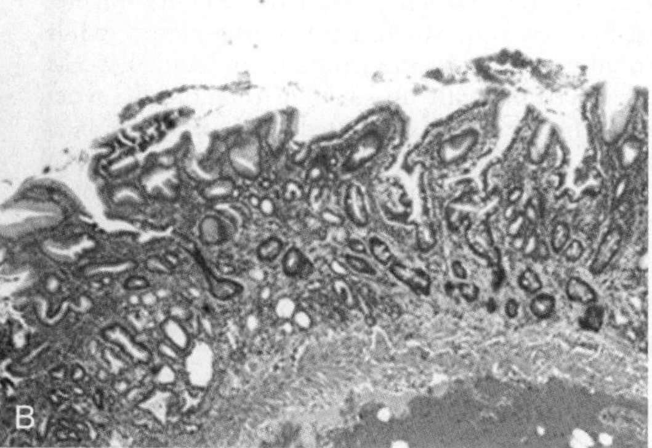

Figure 37-9 HISTOLOGIC FEATURES OF STOMACH IN PERNICIOUS ANEMIA COMPARED TO NORMAL. The normal gastric mucosa **(A)** is contrasted to that seen in pernicious anemia **(B)**, in which there is atrophy of gastric glands, intestinal metaplasia with goblet cells, and loss of parietal cells (not visible at this magnification).

Juvenile pernicious anemia can manifest in the second decade with severe cobalamin deficiency in conjunction with many of the associated endocrinopathies and autoantibodies observed in adults.[8]

Undiagnosed pernicious anemia is common among free-living elderly persons (over 60 years of age)[9] who have only minimal clinical manifestations of cobalamin deficiency (i.e., 1.9% of the Southern California survey population had unrecognized and untreated pernicious anemia). The prevalence was 2.7% in women and 1.4% in men; but 4.3% of the African American women and 4.0% of the white women had pernicious anemia.

Abnormal Events in the Small Bowel Lumen

Insufficient Pancreatic Protease

About 30% of patients with severe pancreatic insufficiency fail to degrade R proteins, which will lead to impaired transfer of cobalamin from R protein to IF. Pancreatic extract will normalize cobalamin malabsorption.[8]

Inactivation of Pancreatic Protease

Pancreatic protease can be inactivated by massive gastric hypersecretion arising from a gastrinoma in Zollinger-Ellison syndrome.[8] The continued low pH of the luminal contents reaching the ileum may also perturb interaction of the IF-cobalamin complex with IF-cobalamin receptors (which requires a pH above 5.4).

Usurpation of Luminal Cobalamin

The near-sterile condition of the small bowel is maintained by a combination of the mechanical cleansing action of peristalsis and the chemical action of gastric acid. Disorders conducive to relative stasis, impaired motility, and hypogammaglobulinemia are predisposing factors that favor colonization by bacteria. Many of these bacteria can take up free cobalamin, but not IF-bound cobalamin. However, if colonization extends proximally to the locus at which IF and cobalamin interact, significant cobalamin may be usurped before it can bind to IF.[8] This cobalamin malabsorption can be corrected to some extent by a 7- to 10-day course of antibiotic therapy; definitive surgical correction may be indicated if the patient has significant symptoms (weight loss and diarrhea) that are only partially relieved by antibiotics. The malabsorption of food-cobalamin in patients with atrophic gastritis has also been normalized with antibiotics, thereby incriminating bacterial usurpation of food cobalamin at a very proximal level.[9]

Approximately 3% of individuals infested with the fish tapeworm *Diphyllobothrium latum,* which avidly usurps cobalamin for growth,[8] can develop frank cobalamin deficiency. Humans become infected when they eat partially cooked or raw fish containing plerocercoids, which develop into adult worms in the jejunum in about 6 weeks, growing to a length of 10 m, with up to 4000 proglottids[8]; when these worms lay eggs, the life cycle is repeated. After ova have been identified in the stools, expulsion of the worms by praziquantel (10 to 20 mg/kg as a single dose taken orally) and cobalamin replenishment is curative.

Disorders of Ileal Intrinsic Factor–Cobalamin Receptors or Mucosa

Absence of Intrinsic Factor–Cobalamin Receptors

The distal ileum has the greatest density of IF-cobalamin receptors. Disease or removal of only 1 to 2 feet of terminal ileum by resection or bypass reduces ileal IF-cobalamin receptor numbers for interaction with IF-cobalamin, resulting in cobalamin malabsorption.[8,9]

Defective Intrinsic Factor–Cobalamin Receptors or Post–Intrinsic Factor–Cobalamin Receptor Defects

Imerslund-Gräsbeck syndrome is a term used collectively for a heterogeneous group of congenital (autosomal recessive) disorders in children arising from biallelic mutations (in 80% of cases) involving either the cubulin (CUBN) or amnionless (AMN) genes that constitute the functional IF-cobalamin receptor (i.e., cubam).[110-112] This results in selective cobalamin malabsorption. Children present between 3 and 10 years of age with megaloblastic anemias and neurologic presentations with low serum cobalamin levels associated with mild, persistent, benign proteinuria (in 90% of cases). Because cubam also participates in the renal tubular absorption of several other proteins, this is the basis for proteinuria found in Imerslund-Gräsbeck syndrome. Diagnosis requires analysis of mutational status of gastric IF, CUBN and AMN genes.[113]

Drug-Induced Defects

Long term use of H_2 antagonists or proton pump inhibitors may interfere with the handover of food-cobalamin to IF, especially in those with preexisting borderline cobalamin stores. Long-term treatment with metformin can interfere with IF-cobalamin binding to ileal cubam receptors[114] and progressively increases the risk for cobalamin deficiency over time.[115] In some individuals the serum cobalamin will dip down to such sufficiently low levels by 3 to 4 years that many physicians would consider cobalamin replacement. Cumulative metformin dose has been correlated strongly with clinically worsening diabetic peripheral neuropathy and increase in MMA and homocysteine levels.[116] Therefore if a patient is not regularly taking at least 1.2 g/day of calcium (to reverse the metformin effect on IF-cobalamin interaction with the cubam receptor[114]), a prudent approach would be to preemptively screen for cobalamin deficiency after about 3 to 4 years of metformin therapy; additional confirmation of metabolic evidence of cobalamin deficiency (elevated MMA) can reasonably trigger replacement therapy with cobalamin. Other drugs (e.g., cholestyramine, colchicine, neomycin) probably also impair transepithelial transport of cobalamin.[8]

Disorders of Plasma Cobalamin Transport

Polymorphism or absence of TCI can be associated with low cobalamin levels, but the MMA and homocysteine levels are normal. By contrast, either deficiency or defective TCII can present with megaloblastic anemia in infancy; this can be associated with normal cobalamin levels (because TCI, which binds over 75% of serum cobalamin is normal). However, there will be metabolic evidence of cobalamin deficiency that can be reversed by daily or biweekly injections of 1 mg of cobalamin, which ensures passive cobalamin delivery into cells. Mutations in the gene for the TCII receptor have also been identified.[117]

Disorders of Intracellular Cobalamin Use

Congenital Metabolic Defects of Cobalamin Metabolism: Cobalamin Mutants A to G

Given the multitude of chaperones or transporters involved in escorting cobalamin intracellularly to their destination to function as coenzymes for methionine synthase and methylmalonyl-CoA mutase, it is not difficult to envision that there would invariably be inborn errors of cobalamin metabolism where one of these escorts or transporters is missing. The combination of megaloblastic anemia with increased levels of homocysteine or MMA, or both, in serum and urine despite normal cobalamin and folate levels should suggest an inborn error of cobalamin metabolism.[9,108] The inherited defects of cobalamin use (see Fig. 37-3) are heterogeneous and are empirically defined as cobalamin mutations A to G (cblA to cblG).[118]

Among these conditions, the cblC metabolic disease warrants special mention because it is the most common of these inborn errors of metabolism (more than 400 patients have been reported). Patients with cblC are usually diagnosed within the first year of life. These infants must be differentiated from those with nutritional cobalamin deficiency who could have similar clinical features. Some patients with cblC disorder may have a later onset of presentation, even in the fourth decade of life, with neurologic manifestations, cognitive and psychiatric problems, and megaloblastic anemia with a *normal* cobalamin level but *high* homocysteine and MMA levels.[119] Patients suspected of having an inborn error of metabolism should be evaluated by specialized laboratories, such as the McGill University laboratory of Professor David Rosenblatt—a premier diagnostic center.[118]

Functional Cobalamin Deficiency After Nitrous Oxide Exposure

Nitrous oxide (N_2O) inactivates coenzyme forms of cobalamin by oxidizing the fully reduced cob(I)alamin to cob(III)alamin; this results in a state of functional intracellular cobalamin deficiency. This syndrome was first identified in patients with tetanus given nitrous oxide for up to 6 days.[8] Subsequently, persons exposed to nitrous oxide for open heart surgery and through chronic (surreptitious, accidental, or occupational) exposure have been recognized as being at high risk for developing megaloblastosis and cobalamin-deficient neuromyelopathy.[8] The slang word for recreational use of nitrous oxide is *nanging;* capsules that are used for making whipped cream are a cheap and easy source of nitrous oxide in the community. Megaloblastosis develops within 24 hours and lasts less than 1 week after a single exposure. The neurologic syndrome is usually seen with chronic intermittent exposure. Severe neurologic deficits have been reported after prolonged intraoperative exposure to nitrous oxide in patients with unsuspected cobalamin deficiency.[9]

Subclinical Cobalamin Deficiency

The issue of subclinical cobalamin deficiency has been a vexing problem and a semantic dilemma. Many elderly persons may have various symptoms consistent with aging (including fatigue, cognitive changes, lower quality-of-life measures, and subtle symptoms of neuropathy) that cannot be directly attributed to cobalamin deficiency, despite the fact that these very symptoms are often seen in symptomatic cobalamin deficiency; often this triggers testing with a serum cobalamin test, and a borderline result generates a new set of problems, including the need to label this entity and thereby make clinical decisions.

Although dependent on the population studied, the frequency of (silent) subclinical cobalamin deficiency in the United States is likely to be 10 times higher than classical (overt) cobalamin deficiency that is found in 1% to 2% of the population. This is best shown in populations in India, where many individuals had low cobalamin levels and no apparent symptoms of clinical hematologic or neurologic evidence of cobalamin deficiency.[7] Today, with the ability to demonstrate an increase in metabolites (i.e., serum homocysteine and MMA test results), many of these individuals (with elevated metabolite test values) would be characterized as having subclinical cobalamin deficiency, provided they had no subtle cognitive abnormalities (discussed further later). If such cognitive tests were positive, such patients would have to be reclassified as having overt clinical cobalamin deficiency.

A cutoff value of 148 pmol/L (less than 200 pg/mL) is consistent with 3 standard deviations (SDs), and using this cutoff, about 3% to 5% of patients with clinical cobalamin deficiency will be missed.[76] Of course, those patients with low cobalamin values without clinical or metabolic evidence of cobalamin deficiency clearly do not have deficiency. In this context, abnormal MMA values that are less than 800 nM are considered borderline and probably not of clinical significance because true cobalamin deficiency results in values that are more than 1000 nM and more often in the thousands of nM.

Other patients may have low-normal cobalamin levels that spontaneously revert to normal, or minimally fluctuate above or below the cutoff value, or remain stable without change over many years. For these patients, the history and physical findings can identify existing disease conditions and drugs that may predispose to cobalamin deficiency, and follow-up is an important mandate. In this cohort, unless the MMA is above 1000 nM on initial testing, the cobalamin can be repeated a year later, and without further change, repeated testing would be required only if new symptoms attributable to cobalamin deficiency were to develop in the future.

However, in other patients, on subsequent testing, the previously equivocal cobalamin level will have dropped further and the MMA result will rise well over 1000 nM, supporting the likelihood of a more ominous progression toward frank cobalamin deficiency with potential for developing overt clinical symptoms.

It should be noted that the literature is ambiguous about how to manage the entity of subclinical cobalamin deficiency, defined when there is biochemical evidence for cobalamin deficiency—reflected by a low cobalamin value (and increased MMA and homocysteine) but without overt clinical manifestations. Although some experts do not feel obliged to treat, preferring to wait until there are overt symptoms, others feel ethically bound to treat even without overt clinical manifestations. Indeed, the issue of "overt clinical manifestations" poses a new problem because some patients with low cobalamin levels plus elevated metabolites with cognitive impairment (when formally tested) can respond to replacement therapy. And upon improvement, these individuals would then have to be recategorized (in retrospect) as having had overt clinical manifestations. On the other hand, patients without cognitive abnormalities (upon formal testing) would be categorized as having subclinical cobalamin deficiency and not require cobalamin replacement. Therefore the central issue here is whether the patient has had formal cognitive testing. However, not all clinicians can reliably diagnose cognitive abnormalities in the clinic; therefore formal cognition testing requires specialized neurocognitive studies, like P300 testing. Thus unless we do formal cognitive testing for patients with low cobalamin and elevated metabolites, we will not know with certainty that a given patient does, or does not, have subclinical versus clinical evidence of cobalamin deficiency. Parenthetically, because cognitive changes are best measured using specialized tests, a related question is whether such testing belongs to the realm of clinical medicine; a strong case can be made that this does, in the same way a computed tomographic (CT) scan or positron emission tomographic (PET) scan is used today, and with far less risk to the patient.

Should all such patients with low cobalamin and high MMA values be subjected to formal P300 cognition testing and/or MRI for brain atrophy[73] to confirm that they do not have organic disease? The answer depends on whether any intervention can make a difference. Because there was a slowing of the rate of brain atrophy among a cohort of patients with mild cobalamin impairment who were given a cocktail of B vitamins, including cobalamin,[73] then using the principle of *primum non nocere,* any biochemical evidence of cobalamin deficiency with cognitive or MRI-imaging evidence of abnormality should, in theory, be characterized as overt disease that warrants cobalamin replacement therapy.

Assuming that sending all patients with metabolic evidence of cobalamin deficiency for MRI imaging or formal neurocognitive P300 testing would be too expensive or impractical, are there heuristic methods that can be used to ensure a satisfactory outcome for these patients? A minimalist approach with substantially reduced costs would be to preemptively treat all patients with low cobalamin and high MMA values on the assumption that we were potentially treating (some or many) patients with *cobalamin-responsive* cognitive dysfunction and thereby possibly preventing their morbidity, whereas those without cognitive dysfunction or MRI abnormalities would not be harmed. In this context, after replenishing potentially depleted cobalamin stores with parenteral cobalamin therapy, oral supplementation for 4 to 6 months on and 4 to 6 months off may afford an adequate cobalamin status in most patients[120] as an alternative to continuous therapy. A key factor is the cost of cobalamin (and the lack of side effects associated with cobalamin therapy); for example, parenteral cobalamin, which can be purchased on the Internet for $15 for each 10 mg/10 mL vial, would last a year after replenishing stores. The additional purchase of 30-gauge ½-inch insulin U100 syringes for monthly subcutaneous injection would be less cost than even generic tablets of 1 mg taken daily.

In the case of evolving metformin-induced cobalamin deficiency,[115,116] an even stronger case can be made to prevent harm and to therefore treat early documented biochemical evidence of cobalamin deficiency on the basis that this is not going to get better with continued intake of a valuable drug for diabetes.

Some experts have suggested that randomized trials are needed to define the best approach to manage such patients with subclinical cobalamin deficiency.[76] However, the new information on preventing brain atrophy with combined B vitamins[73] could force many institutional review boards and/or institutional research ethics committees to issue a mandate that all patients with subclinical cobalamin deficiency who were to enter such trials (to define the natural history of this condition) should have prior clearance of normal cognitive function and evidence of no brain atrophy by MRI imaging. However, this would still not obviate the need for these tests for the majority of patients with subclinical cobalamin deficiency if a watch-and-wait approach were to be adopted. Hence the better (and cheaper) option may be that which empirically treats all patients using the principle of beneficence and thereby not harming those with cobalamin-reversible brain disease.[73]

Table 37-3 Clinical Conditions Not to Be Confused With Megaloblastosis

MACROCYTOSIS* WITHOUT MEGALOBLASTOSIS†
Reticulocytosis
Liver disease
Aplastic anemia
Myelodysplastic syndromes (especially 5q-)
Multiple myeloma
Hypoxemia
Smokers
SPURIOUS INCREASES IN MCV WITHOUT MACRO-OVALOCYTOSIS‡
Cold agglutinin disease
Marked hyperglycemia
Leukocytosis
Older individuals

MCV, Mean corpuscular volume.
*The central pallor that normally occupies about one-third of the normal red blood cell is decreased in macro-ovalocytes. This contrasts with the finding of thin macrocytes, in which the central pallor is increased.
†Although megaloblastosis implies that a bone marrow test has been performed, with the addition of highly sensitive tests for the specific diagnosis of cobalamin and folate deficiency, the need for a bone marrow test is often dictated by the urgency to make the diagnosis.
‡When the Coulter counter readings of a high MCV are not confirmed by looking at the peripheral smear.

PATHOGENESIS OF FOLATE DEFICIENCY

Folate deficiency is usually recognized in the course of certain clinical presentations that predispose to negative folate balance and subsequent deficiency. It is instructive therefore to conceptualize cellular folate deficiency as arising from etiologic categories of decreased supply (i.e., reduced intake, absorption, transport, or use) or increased requirement (i.e., metabolic consumption, destruction, or excretion). However, in the same patient more than one mechanism may result in net folate deficiency. The precise contribution of one mechanism over the other is often not obvious, and specific tests to define each mechanism are not routinely available for clinical use. Thus the clinical context is especially important. Megaloblastic manifestations of folate deficiency (Table 37-5) are discussed within the context of the history and physical examination (discussed later). Cases of neuropathy in adults attributed to folate deficiency are rarely encountered; when they are, the possibility of alcoholism with thiamine deficiency must be considered. In any case, every patient with neuropathy, myelopathy, or psychiatric manifestations associated with megaloblastosis must be investigated in detail to rule out cobalamin deficiency. Gastrointestinal megaloblastosis begets further folate malabsorption, which propagates a vicious cycle of folate deficiency in the short term and cobalamin deficiency in the long term. With the exception of drug-induced defects or inborn errors of folate metabolism that result in decreased use of intracellular folates, all causes, irrespective of mechanism, result in reduced net delivery of folates to normal proliferating cells.

Nutritional Causes of Folate Deficiency

The body stores of folate are adequate for only about 4 months.[8] Individuals who are chronically in negative folate balance may only require a brief "nudge"—from superimposition of an associated illness that leads to hemolysis, anorexia, or folate malabsorption—to "tip" them into frank folate deficiency. The incidence of folate deficiency varies from country to country and even within regions in the same country. This is highly influenced by the economic status and ethnic diet where cooking and choice of foods vary from region to region. For example, in Benin, central Africa, the prevalence of folate deficiency anemia was 20%, and in Zimbabwe, 30% had low folate levels, whereas in Sudan it was nearly 60%.[121] In Sri Lanka, one-half of schoolchildren had low-folate status, but less than 1% had folate deficiency in Thailand, which likely relates to the abundant consumption of greens and meats by Thais. Even in the United States, before folate fortification of food, about 20% of the population had low-folate status, and in Venezuela, 30% had low-folate status before such fortification. Decreased availability of folate-rich foods (in winter, after natural disasters, or during the wet season in central Africa), poverty, various cultural or ethnic diets (consisting of maize, rice, or well-cooked beans and vegetables), and cooking techniques that destroy food folate, coupled with the anorexia that accompanies chronic illnesses, are just a few of the reasons for rapid development of folate deficiency.[8,9]

In Western countries food faddism, alcoholism, or unbalanced slimming diets usually lead to decreased folate intake in young to middle-age individuals.[8] Edentulous or infirm persons or neglected older adults who are too ill to prepare their meals, as well as psychiatric patients, are particularly at risk for nutritional folate deficiency[8] (see box on Etiopathophysiologic Classification of Folate Deficiency).

Pregnancy and Infancy

Pregnancy and lactation are associated with significantly higher folate requirements (over 400 mcg/day) for growth of the fetus, placenta, breast, and other maternal tissues.[122] Folate requirement increases throughout pregnancy and is maximal near term. There is also increased urinary loss of folate in pregnancy (about 14 mcg/day versus approximately 4.2 mcg/day in nonpregnant women) because of a lower renal threshold. Poor preparation for pregnancy—with a poorly balanced diet and preexisting multifactorial nutritional anemia that remains unaddressed—is a major factor accounting for serious pregnancy complications and adverse birth outcomes. Therefore additional folate during pregnancy is required to prevent both pregnancy complications (preeclampsia, placental abruption or infarctions, recurrent miscarriage) and poor pregnancy outcomes (preterm delivery, NTDs, congenital heart defects, and intrauterine growth retardation).[123] Low-folate status associated with short interpregnancy intervals or twin pregnancies also predisposes to preterm births.[124,125] All this demand for folate must somehow be met by increased folate intake.

However, the vast majority (over 90%) of pregnant women in resource-poor countries consume less than the estimated average requirement of folate[126]; in addition, a substantial number also consume less than optimum amounts of several other minerals, such as iron, and micronutrients, including cobalamin, as noted earlier. For example, studies on women from groups with low socioeconomic status from North India[24,25] have estimated that the daily intake of folic acid ranged between 75 mcg and 167 mcg, which is far lower than the 400 mcg/day required to prevent birth defects. This is simple to remedy. When given daily or even twice weekly, the combination of iron (100 mg elemental iron) and folic acid (0.5 mg) has been shown to significantly improve several cognitive abilities of schoolgirls in India,[87] which renders them better prepared for pregnancy in the future. This is all the more important because of results from experimental studies designed to define the influence of gestational folate deficiency on the fetus (discussed later). Thus pregnancy with poor folate intake is the most common cause of megaloblastic anemia in the world.

As noted earlier, the placenta has a large number of folate receptors,[44] which facilitate binding and transport of folates to the developing fetus.[44] Preferential delivery of folate to the fetus can cause or aggravate folate deficiency in the mother.[8] This is observed clinically when a mother with severe folate deficiency gives birth to a baby who has normal folate stores.[43]

The rapidly proliferating tissues in children also have an absolute requirement for exogenously supplied folate. Although human milk can maintain folate balance in breastfed infants, the breast milk content of folate is low when the mother's folate status is poor.

Before the advent of routine folate supplementation during pregnancy, the incidence of megaloblastic marrows in the United States, Canada, and the United Kingdom during late pregnancy was about 25%, but in South India, it was about 55%.[8] Folate deficiency is eight times as high in twin pregnancies. Multiparity (multiple frequent pregnancies with a prolonged state of negative folate balance) and hyperemesis gravidarum commonly lead to folate deficiency. Because the anemia of pregnancy is most frequently caused by iron deficiency, combined iron and folate deficiency (dimorphic anemia) is the more frequent clinical presentation. Increased use of folates by the newborn leads to a drop in serum folate levels by about 6 weeks of age. This drop is exaggerated in premature infants (who have feeding difficulties, infection, or hemolytic disease leading to pure folate deficiency); hence supplementation is routine for them.[8]

Folates and Neurodevelopment

All inborn errors of folate metabolism, which result in reduced folate availability to the developing brain, give rise to mental retardation and related mental health problems. The fetal brain is dependent on sufficient provision of maternal folate during embryogenesis. Thus it has been predicted that, under conditions where maternal folate deficiency can compromise the delivery of folate to the developing fetal brain, and depending on the degree of deficiency, there could be a spectrum of neurologic abnormalities; this could range from full-blown NTDs to more subtle changes that manifest in childhood as behavioral abnormalities.[47,48,127] Because routine folate supplementation is now the norm for women, we must rely on experimental studies in animals to clarify the pathologic effects of folate deficiency in pregnancy. Such studies[48] indicate that folate deficiency will significantly compromise early pregnancy outcomes (including the rates of pregnancy, rate of implantation, and effects on the number of live births). Even lesser degrees of folate deficiency to only one-third of optimum dietary folate for 2 months before and throughout gestation in dams—which coincidentally mimics the extent of insufficient dietary folate availability among women in vast areas of Northern India[44]—also resulted in subtle histologic aberrations and defects during murine fetal development.[48] These included increased apoptotic cell loss involving nearly every organ and fine architectural anomalies, as well as adverse influences on fetal brain development and unexpectedly profound abnormalities in the white matter, reflecting perturbed neuronal development.[48] Surprisingly, despite postnatal folate replenishment, these mice exhibited an anxiety phenotype in adulthood.[128] The latter studies indicate a new paradigm for the developmental origin of neuropsychiatric disease that points to poor maternal folate nutrition during pregnancy. These data also suggest the existence of a sensitive window during fetal neurodevelopment when folate deficiency dysregulates the expression of certain genes and/or proteins, which leads to the imprinting of abnormal neural circuits in utero that predispose to anxiety in adulthood. In concordance with these studies in mice, a recent prospective cohort human study has reported that lower maternal folate status in early pregnancy was associated with childhood hyperactivity/inattention and peer problems in early childhood.[129] The associations between low maternal folate and head circumference at birth[129] are similar to murine studies in which a net reduction in the number of cells (by approximately 20%) in the brains of murine fetuses that experienced gestational folate deficiency[48,127] was observed; this increased brain cell loss was due to apoptosis arising from megaloblastosis of folate-deficient cells during development.

There is additional clinical support for a relationship between suboptimal folate delivery to the developing fetal brain and abnormal behavior. For example, 18-month-old children of mothers who took folate supplements had less "internalizing" patterns of behavior (emotionally reactive, anxious/depressed, somatic complaints, withdrawn) and less "externalizing" syndromes involving attention problems and aggressive behavior compared to offspring of women who did not take folate supplements.[130] Thus it appears that we are likely peering through the mist into a new field whereby nutritional sensitivity during fetal neurodevelopment predisposes to neuropsychiatric illness!

The long-lasting benefit to the offspring of women who take iron and folic acid during the early stages of pregnancy appears to be a consistent theme; in Nepalese women, such supplementation provided significant benefits to the proper neurodevelopment of their babies in utero.[131] Children of these women exhibited improved brain function, manifest by improvement in both general intellectual ability and some aspects of executive functions as well as fine motor skills when tested at ages 7 to 9 years. Although this clinical study was unable to assign whether iron or folic acid was the more important, there is sufficient supporting experimental evidence in the literature for both being critically important. Indeed, these human parallels to murine studies are consistent with the Barker hypothesis on developmental origins of disease. Finally, there is also evidence to suggest that suboptimal folate intake that leads to low-folate status during adolescence can affect cognition, which will negatively affect academic achievements, quite independent of socioeconomic status.[132] And another recent large observational study has also identified that maternal use of folic acid supplements in early pregnancy was associated with a reduced risk for severe language delay in children at age 3 years.[133] Collectively these clinical and experimental studies strongly support the importance of folate during neurodevelopment.

The new finding that homocysteinylated-hnRNP-E1 orchestrates a nutrition-sensitive posttranscriptional RNA operon that includes mRNAs that are important for the integrity of myelin and neuronal intermediate neurofilament-middle molecular mass proteins, as well as tyrosine hydroxylase, which generates dopamine and norepinephrine, provides insight into how folate and cobalamin deficiency during pregnancy can influence neurodevelopment.[39,48,128] Indeed, the activation of multiple members of the hnRNP family by high intracellular homocysteine—via folate or cobalamin deficiency in pregnancy—may in fact activate several such nutrition-sensitive posttranscriptional RNA operons, which, acting together in concert as a higher-order nutrition-sensitive (homocysteine-responsive) posttranscriptional RNA regulon, would lead to the modulation of several diverse mRNAs that exert a profound effect on fetal neurodevelopment.[39]

Folate-Responsive Neural Tube Defects and Neurocristopathies

NTDs are the most common major congenital malformation of the central nervous system. They arise from disturbances in neurulation that involve incomplete closure of neural tissues, leading to major midline defects. The neural tube, which begins as a tiny ribbon of tissue, normally folds inward to form a tube by the 28th day after conception. Thus NTDs originate in the first month of pregnancy (before many women know they are pregnant). The expression of folate receptors on embryonic neural tube and neural crest cells as well as the critical bursts of proliferative activity and the need for folate to support cell proliferation have been discussed earlier. Thus it is critical for a woman to have enough folic acid in her body before conception (periconceptionally) to ensure sufficient availability for the embryo. Anencephaly and spina bifida, the commonest NTDs, are important factors in fetal mortality (Fig. 37-10). Worldwide, the risk in the general population ranges from less than 1 to 9 cases per 1000 births; for example, a recent population-based study in the least-developed area in India identified that the incidence of NTDs was up to 8.21 per 1000 live births, which is among the highest worldwide.[134] Landmark studies have established the preventive role of periconceptional folates in both the *recurrence* of NTD (using folic acid 4000 mcg/day) and the *first occurrence* of NTD (using folic acid 400 mcg/day). Of significance, the greatest protection by folates occurs in those regions with the highest rates of NTDs. Conversely, the use of folic acid antagonists (trimethoprim, triamterene, carbamazepine, phenytoin, phenobarbital, and primidone) during pregnancy increases the risk for these birth defects by twofold.[135]

Because 50% of pregnancies in the United States and elsewhere are unplanned and compliance with taking folic supplements to prevent NTD is only at about 50%, a consensus developed that fortification of food with folic acid in the United States was the best way to improve overall folate status in women at risk for NTD occurrence. By January 1998, fortification of foods (i.e., rice, flour, pasta, macaroni, breads, and cake with folic acid at 140 mcg/100 g of food) was part of American law. This level was chosen to ensure that women of childbearing age would have an increase in folic acid intake of at least 100 mcg a day, which is about 25% of the recommended daily intake. Subsequent evaluation has clearly demonstrated that fortification of food with folic acid has had multiple salutatory effects during human development and that major congenital abnormalities can be prevented.[122] Table 37-4 shows several documented collateral benefits identified through population-based studies.

There remain questions about the effectiveness of the folic acid fortification program for women in the 15- to 35-year-old age-group

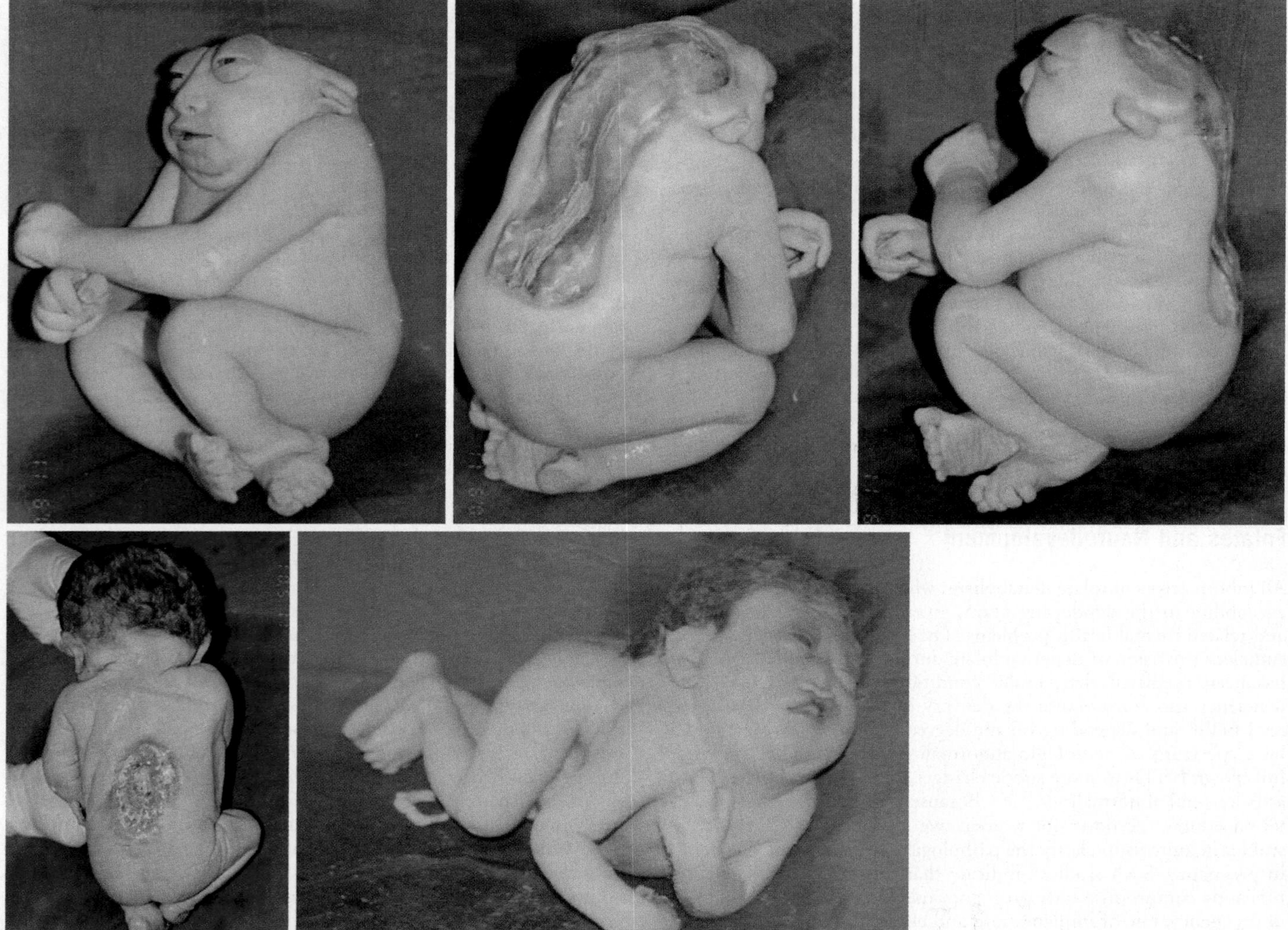

Figure 37-10 FOLATE-RESPONSIVE NEURAL TUBE DEFECTS. Anencephaly with complete rachischisis *(top panel),* open infected meningomyelocele *(bottom left),* and iniencephaly with cleft lip *(bottom right). (Courtesy Prof Molly Paul, Anatomy Department Museum, Christian Medical College and Brown Memorial Hospital, Ludhiana, Punjab, India.)*

Table 37-4 Beneficial Effects of Homocysteine-Lowering Therapy on Nonhematopoietic Systems

USING FOLIC ACID, COBALAMIN, PYRIDOXINE SUPPLEMENTATION (GRADE A STUDIES)
Reduction in hip fracture[136,*]
Reduction in the progression of carotid intima media thickness[137,*] (a surrogate marker of early subclinical arteriosclerosis)
Reduction in age-related macular degeneration[138,*]
Reduction in rate of brain atrophy[73,*]
USING FOLIC ACID SUPPLEMENTATION (GRADE A STUDIES)
Reduction in stroke[139,*]
Reduction in the rate of cognitive decline among healthy older adults[140,*]
Reduction in age-related (sensorineural) hearing loss[141,*]
Reduction in first occurrence of NTDs[142,143]
Reduction in recurrence of NTDs[144,*]
Reduction in phenytoin-induced gingival hyperplasia[145,*]
BENEFICIAL EFFECTS OF FOLIC ACID FORTIFICATION OF FOOD (POPULATION-BASED STUDIES)
Reduction in NTDs[146-148] (anencephaly, spina bifida, encephalocele, meningocele, iniencephaly)
Reduction in cleft lip with or without cleft palate[149]
Reduction in severe congenital heart disease[149,150] (endocardial cushion defects, conotruncal defects)
Reduction in congenital pyloric stenosis, stenosis of the ureteropelvic junction, limb reduction defects[149]
Reduction in stroke mortality[151]
Decreased risk for preterm births,[152] low birth weight, and small-for-gestational-age babies

NTD, Neural tube defect.
*Paper with randomized controlled trial data; grade A studies.

in preventing NTDs. Because of an incomplete knowledge base among some women[9,153] and their tendency to consume low-carbohydrate foods (which are the very foods that are fortified), there is continued concern that this group is still not getting adequate amounts of dietary folate. This is the basis for recommendations to continue to educate women of childbearing age to take folate supplements at 400 mcg/day (beyond what they are already receiving through folate fortification of food).

Indeed, a recent large U.S. study suggests that preconceptional folate supplements (1 year or longer)—*over and above* the folate present in folate-fortified foods—reduced spontaneous preterm delivery between 20 to 28 weeks by 70%, with 50% reduction between 28 and 32 weeks.[152] However, because folate fortification of food—which was operative 2 years before this study also likely afforded small reductions in preterm delivery, the magnitude of benefit by folic acid[152] is likely underestimated.[123] Hence all women capable of becoming pregnant, particularly those women in the periconceptional period, are advised to consume 400 mcg folate daily from folic acid supplements, folate-fortified foods, or both.

Contrary to the assertion in the American Dietetic Association's position paper on vegetarianism,[154] there is an insufficient body of evidence to confidently assert that women in the United States of childbearing age who consume a balanced vegetarian diet with abundant green leafy vegetables will obtain sufficient folate and therefore not be at risk for giving birth to babies with NTDs. Until robust evidence from clinical trials is available to support this association's position paper,[154] all women who are vegetarians must take cobalamin and folate supplements.

Folates and Intrinsic Hematologic Disease

Because folate is necessary for hematopoiesis, folate requirements are increased when there is significant compensatory erythropoiesis in response to peripheral RBC destruction, abnormal hematopoiesis, or infiltration by abnormal cells in marrow. The recognition that folate deficiency developing in hemolytic disorders can lead to an acute aplastic crisis has led to routine prophylactic administration of folate. An unexpected increase in transfusional requirement or a fall in platelets can also suggest folate deficiency.[8] The case of a patient with sickle cell disease on long-term folate who developed pernicious anemia and presented with neuropsychiatric dysfunction is a valuable reminder that those on folate prophylaxis need periodic follow-up for symptoms and signs of supervening cobalamin deficiency.[155]

Folate Malabsorption With Normal Intestinal Mucosa

Hereditary Folate Malabsorption

Hereditary folate malabsorption, which is due to a mutation in PCFT, is associated with inability to transport folate across the intestine and into the brain, resulting in low serum and cerebrospinal fluid folate values with megaloblastic anemia, chronic diarrhea, and neurodevelopmental defects with seizures and mental retardation; this syndrome responds to high-dose parenteral folinic acid that bypasses and overcomes the transport defects. Affected patients can also present with a syndrome of reversible subacute combined immunodeficiency syndrome with hypogammaglobulinemia and recurrent infections.[156] If diagnosed early in infancy, hereditary folate malabsorption responds well to parenteral 5-formyltetrahydofolate and can allow normal development into adulthood.[157]

Folate Malabsorption With Intestinal Mucosal Abnormalities

Tropical Sprue

Residents of, and visitors to, endemic areas in the tropics can acquire a disorder characterized by small intestinal malabsorption.[8] Generalized, nonspecific small bowel malabsorption leads to a wide spectrum of clinical manifestations arising from defective absorption of fat, carbohydrate, albumin, calcium, folate, and in later stages, cobalamin.[8] There is abrupt onset of explosive, intermittent, or continuous diarrhea, abdominal distention, and pain, associated with anorexia, vomiting, and extreme fatigue. Stools are fluid or semisolid and frequently contain mucus and blood. This stage is followed weeks to months later by nutrient deficiency. Later, as steatorrhea continues, megaloblastosis dominates the clinical picture. In the short term, malabsorption leads to folate deficiency, but later in the chronic (longer than 3 years) phase of the disease, cobalamin malabsorption contributes additional clinical manifestations of cobalamin neuropathy.[8] There is some degree of villous atrophy and loss of intestinal functional surface. Although less severe than in nontropical sprue, it is more extensive, involving the entire small intestine.

After investigations for associated iron, cobalamin, and folate deficiencies, therapy with folate and a broad-spectrum antibiotic (e.g., tetracycline) is indicated together with symptomatic treatment of diarrhea and vomiting; fluid, mineral, and electrolyte imbalance; and other associated nutritional deficiencies.[8]

The endemic nature of this disorder in the tropics (and in certain households)[8] and the beneficial response to antibiotics all suggest an infectious origin. However, the dramatic response to folate, which is curative in the first year in about 60% of cases (this cure is cited to be almost diagnostic of the disease), has not been explained.[8] It is unlikely that pure folate deficiency is the primary cause, because nutritional folate deficiency does not result in tropical sprue; the clinical response to antibiotics suggests a close interplay between a pathogenic infectious agent, endogenous flora, and the folate status of the enterocyte.

Nontropical Sprue

Nontropical sprue (i.e., celiac disease, gluten-induced enteropathy) is the most common cause of intestinal malabsorption in temperate zones. It results from a possibly inherited sensitivity to gluten (a glutamine-rich protein found in wheat, barley, rye, and other grains) and a related substance, gliadin.[8] The intestinal lesion (i.e., villous atrophy with hypertrophied crypts and lymphocytic and plasma cell infiltrate of the lamina propria) is more florid than that seen in tropical sprue but occurs to a greater extent in the proximal small intestine with relative ileal sparing; as a result, cobalamin malabsorption is less common. The consequences of malabsorption are otherwise the same. Patients present between the ages of 30 and 50 years with intermittent or persistent diarrhea (abrupt in 20%), weight loss, abdominal distention with discomfort, glossitis, and megaloblastic anemia. Iron deficiency may also be prominent. Diagnosis is established by demonstration of sensitive and specific serum antiendomysial antibodies IgA type or anti–tissue transglutaminase antibodies, malabsorption, and jejunal biopsy. The megaloblastosis responds well to folate therapy.[8]

Regional Enteritis and Other Small Intestinal Disorders

The distal small intestine is involved in 80% of individuals with Crohn disease, but folate is efficiently absorbed in other more proximal areas. Only with extensive involvement or fistulas do these patients develop folate deficiency. Even in this case, the blood picture is more that of an iron deficiency or anemia of chronic disease. Frank, pure megaloblastic anemia occurs rarely enough in this setting to suggest another cause for folate or cobalamin malabsorption.

Cerebral Folate Deficiency

Infants fed cow's milk can develop autoantibodies to milk folate-binding proteins, which have close homology to folate receptors.[32,158] These anti–folate receptor antibodies can bind folate receptors in the choroid plexus and block folate receptor–mediated folate transport across the cerebrospinal fluid to induce cerebral folate deficiency[60] or one of two autism spectrum disorders.[61]

Infantile-onset cerebral folate deficiency[159,160] usually develops 4 to 6 months after birth and is characterized by agitation, insomnia, delayed development with deceleration of head growth, psychomotor retardation, cerebellar ataxia, pyramidal tract signs in the legs, dyskinesias (such as choreoathetosis and ballismus), a severe polyneuropathy, and in some cases, seizures. Untreated, central visual disturbances can become manifest and lead to optic atrophy and blindness by the third year.

Affected children have normal serum folate but low cerebrospinal fluid folate levels. The folate receptor autoantibody titer decreases with restriction of bovine milk intake but promptly increases upon rechallenge. Cerebral folate deficiency responds to high doses of folinic acid and a bovine milk–free diet.[61]

Anti–folate receptor antibodies are also associated with neural tube defects,[161-163] infertility,[164] and orofacial clefts[165]; however, more information is required to confidently assign causality with these conditions.

Polymorphisms and Inborn Errors of Folate Metabolism

Several genetic polymorphisms involve genes that participate in one-carbon metabolism. These genetic polymorphisms merely reflect variants that are more frequent than the expected 1% allelic variation that could be found in any population. Whereas some polymorphisms impinge on normal physiology of folate and explain abnormal laboratory levels of folate, cobalamin, or metabolites, others may redistribute folate toward thymidylate synthesis and be "DNA protective." Predictably, two or more polymorphisms in the same individual (a combined heterozygote) can be associated with an increased risk for certain congenital diseases in offspring such as Down syndrome[166] or other birth defects. However, because disease association is not equivalent to disease causation, much more study is required to strengthen such relationships. A listing of the spectrum of these polymorphisms can be found in specialized texts.[167] Excellent reviews of these and other inborn errors of folate metabolism are available.[9,108]

MEGALOBLASTIC ANEMIA NOT CAUSED BY FOLATE OR COBALAMIN DEFICIENCY

Several chemotherapeutic agents (e.g., antimetabolites, alkylating agents) kill malignant cells primarily by interfering with DNA synthesis; megaloblastosis is therefore an expected side effect. Hereditary orotic aciduria usually manifests in the first year of life because of a deficiency or absence of enzymes that convert orotic acid to uridine monophosphate via orotidine monophosphate. The net cellular deficiency of uridine monophosphate leads to perturbed synthesis of DNA as well as RNA[8] (see box on Miscellaneous Megaloblastic Anemias Not Caused by Cobalamin or Folate Deficiency).

CLINICAL PRESENTATIONS AND EVALUATION FOR FOLATE AND COBALAMIN DEFICIENCY

Clinical presentations and evaluations for folate and cobalamin deficiency are shown in Table 37-5.

The Interview

The patient's general demeanor and answers to questions may reveal a blunted affect with evidence of depression, irritability, forgetfulness, and sleep deprivation (common in pure folate deficiency). Alternatively, cobalamin deficiency may present with paranoid ideation, dementia, cognitive dysfunction, delusions, or lack of energy manifested by slowed responses. Hallucinations or even obtundation may preclude obtaining an adequate history. The family may indicate the progressive evolution of a marked personality change and may be able to help trace the evolution of symptoms and deviations from the time when the patient was last well. Intermittent therapy with multivitamins, liver pills, or injections (often given by a well-meaning family member or unregistered practitioner) is a common quick fix in many cultures. Family members are a good source for details on the patient's

Miscellaneous Megaloblastic Anemias Not Caused by Cobalamin or Folate Deficiency

I. Congenital disorders of deoxyribonucleic acid (DNA) synthesis
   A. Orotic aciduria
   B. Lesch-Nyhan syndrome
   C. Congenital dyserythropoietic anemia
II. Acquired disorders of DNA synthesis
   A. Deficiency—thiamine-responsive megaloblastic anemia (thiamine transporter 1 mutation)
   B. Erythroleukemia, refractory sideroblastic anemias
   C. Drugs—all antineoplastic drugs that inhibit DNA synthesis (including antinucleosides used against human immunodeficiency virus [HIV] and other viruses), alcohol

Table 37-5 Similarities of Clinical Manifestations and Megaloblastic Sequelae of Folate and Cobalamin Deficiency*

System	Manifestations
Hematologic	Pancytopenia with megaloblastic marrow
Cardiopulmonary	Congestive heart failure
Gastrointestinal	Beefy-red tongue and added stigmata of broad-spectrum malabsorption in folate deficiency†
Dermatologic	Melanin pigmentation and premature graying
Genital	Cervical or uterine dysplasia
Reproductive	Infertility or sterility
Psychiatric	Depressed affect and cognitive dysfunction
Neuropsychiatric‡	Unique to cobalamin deficiency with cerebral, myelopathic, or peripheral neuropathic disturbances, including optic and autonomic nerve dysfunction

*However, the neurologic spectrum of dysfunction in cobalamin deficiency is distinct. Inadequate hemoglobinization (from inadequate iron stores or globin synthesis) can mask the expected erythroid megaloblastic morphologic findings in the bone marrow and peripheral smear, and only specific therapy (i.e., iron) can unmask classic megaloblastic manifestations (i.e., masked megaloblastosis). Megaloblastic leukopoiesis is unchanged.
†If folate deficiency is uncorrected for 2 to 3 years, cobalamin deficiency will supervene.
‡Dorsal tract involvement is earliest manifestation in more than 70% of patients with cobalamin deficiency. Neuropsychiatric manifestations are not associated with megaloblastosis in up to 30% of patients.

dietary habits (food faddism, vegetarianism, alcohol intake) and family history of medical problems (blood diseases, gluten sensitivity, autoimmune diseases).

A medical history of epilepsy or alcoholism with seizure disorder (anticonvulsant therapy) is important. Rarely, patients with autoimmune hemolytic anemias may be lost to follow-up and return with acute aplastic crises when they run out of folate. A surgical history of total or partial gastrectomy, anastomosis, fistula, or bowel resection can reveal the potential for perturbation of physiologic absorption (loss of IF, bypassing or loss of absorptive surface, blind loop syndromes). Surreptitious or accidental inhalation of nitrous oxide in an occupational setting (dental or anesthesiology professionals) and deliberate inhalation of nitrous oxide (nanging) using cartridges attached to whipped cream dispensers or visits to "houses of laughter," where nitrous oxide can be inhaled for a small fee can be revealed only on direct questioning. Visits to tropical countries and the development of intermittent episodic diarrhea may give a clue to tropical sprue; prolonged (over 3 years) chronic gastrointestinal symptoms followed by insidious development of neurologic problems predicts a combined (folate followed by cobalamin) deficiency (see box on Drugs That Perturb Folate Metabolism).

Systemic review of symptoms may range from none (i.e., incidental increased MCV or PMN hypersegmentation) to severe (i.e., unstable angina from severe anemia). With slow development of anemia, the patient often does not develop cardiopulmonary symptoms until there is a 50% reduction in hemoglobin concentration, which leads to dyspnea on exertion, palpitation, and generalized fatigue or lethargy. Only when the hemoglobin concentration is below 5 g/dL does the patient develop dyspnea at rest and angina on modest exertion or even at rest. Congestive heart failure is heralded by pedal edema, nocturia, orthopnea, and tender hepatomegaly.

Upper gastrointestinal symptoms with anorexia associated with intrinsic gastrointestinal disease or anemia with heart failure must be distinguished from symptoms due to glossitis. The latter may lead to inability to wear dentures, tolerate hot drinks or spicy foods because of burning, and even odynophagia, which may compromise further food intake (seen in cobalamin and folate deficiencies). The patient may volunteer that glossitis is relieved by multivitamin ingestion. Weight loss in cobalamin deficiency is not as severe as in folate deficiency arising from intrinsic gastrointestinal disease. Episodic or chronic diarrhea with steatorrhea is commonly caused by tropical sprue, although it may be brought on by gluten-containing foods. Although these symptoms may be accompanied by abdominal pain, pain in the absence of diarrhea could be caused by tabetic crisis (vomiting, abdominal rigidity, absence of leukocytosis, or fever) accompanying spinothalamic involvement in cobalamin-deficient myelopathy.

The patient with pernicious anemia may have two or three semisolid bowel movements per day; although this may be construed as

Drugs That Perturb Folate Metabolism

Ethanol. Although beer has a higher folate content than other alcoholic beverages, alcoholism may lead to neglect of healthy dietary practices in favor of alcohol. Patients who have one nutritious meal each day tend to stave off the eventual development of folate deficiency. Alcohol consumption leads to a relatively rapid (2- to 4-day) fall in serum folate levels. Excess alcohol consumption is possibly the most common cause of folate deficiency in the United States.[8]

Trimethoprim and *pyrimethamine* bind to bacterial and parasitic dihydrofolate reductase with much greater affinity than to human dihydrofolate reductase, but patients with underlying folate deficiency appear to be more susceptible to the effects of these drugs. The megaloblastosis can be reversed by folinic acid (5-formyl-tetrahydrofolate [5-formyl-THF]; leucovorin).

Methotrexate binds with high affinity to human dihydrofolate reductase and leads to trapping of folate as a metabolically inert form (dihydrofolate). This leads to a true depletion of THF within hours and consequently to functional deficiency of 5,10-methylene-THF and reduced thymidylate synthesis. Although megaloblastosis can develop rapidly, the toxic effects of methotrexate can be avoided by rescue with 5-formyl-THF (leucovorin).

Sulfasalazine produces megaloblastosis in up to two-thirds of patients taking full doses (over 2 g/day) by decreasing absorption of folates and induction of Heinz body hemolytic anemia (i.e., increased requirements).

Anticonvulsants can induce NTD, and consensus guidelines have stressed the importance of ensuring that pregnant women[9] and children[168-171] with epilepsy be prescribed folates together with anticonvulsants. Whereas folates protect against spontaneous abortion,[172] folic acid supplementation of women receiving antiepileptic drugs, which are known to interfere with folate absorption, also led to a significant reduction of spontaneous abortion.[173] Now there is new clinical data on phenytoin-induced gingival hyperplasia, which is a cosmetically undesirable side effect that affects a large percentage of patients, usually between 2 and 6 months of initiating therapy. A recent randomized controlled trial among children 6 to 15 years of age who were initiated on phenytoin has provided incontrovertible evidence that taking folic acid 0.5 mg daily can largely prevent phenytoin-induced gingival hyperplasia[145]; whereas 88% in the placebo group developed gingival hyperplasia, only 21% in the folic acid group developed this side effect. The data from this paper provides more "ammunition" to encourage young women on antiepileptic drugs to keep taking folic acid to prevent them from getting cosmetically unsightly gingival hyperplasia (particularly if reducing the risk for having a baby with NTD is too nebulous a concept for them). The only caveat is that before initiating long-term folic acid supplements, the cobalamin status must be normalized.

Although *antineoplastics* and *antiretroviral antinucleosides* such as azidothymidine lead to megaloblastosis, the temporal sequence and investigations to rule out cobalamin or folate deficiency should easily lead to a correct causal assignment.

a normal pattern, it may represent a change since the last time the patient was well. Constipation may be related to obstipation arising from involvement of the Meissner plexus and the Auerbach plexus within the gastrointestinal tract. Similarly, incipient loss of bladder or bowel control due to cobalamin myelopathy may present with urgency or nocturia.

In contrast to musculoskeletal symptoms (arthralgia or frank arthritis) of autoimmune diseases, nocturnal cramps or pain in upper and lower extremities may indicate spinothalamic tract involvement. Hypoparathyroidism or systemic lupus erythematosus, alone or associated with pernicious anemia, leads to significant overlap of cerebral, musculoskeletal, and neurologic presentations.

Review of skin symptoms may elicit a history of increased diffuse or blotchy generalized brownish skin pigmentation, especially of nail beds and skin creases. This is common in cobalamin and folate deficiency; associated vitiligo suggests autoimmune disease.

Although symptoms related to neurologic dysfunction may be volunteered, a complete detailed questionnaire should be formulated during the interview. Questions should be directed to perversions in taste or smell, decreased visual acuity, changes in color vision, and eye pain (neuritis), tinnitus, or headache. Dizziness with orthostatic hypotension and "blacking out" may be related to severe anemia. Vertigo or difficulty in walking in the dark (loss of proprioception and position sense), difficulty in ambulation (which may feel like "walking on cotton wool"), stiffness of extremities (corticospinal tracts), or ataxia (spinocerebellar tracts) may be indicative of a serious cobalamin myelopathy. Early symptoms are symmetrical tingling ("pins and needles"), extending from the tips of the toes to a glove and stocking distribution in later stages. "Burning feet" syndrome, or more commonly, complaints of difficulty in performing simple tasks such as buttoning clothes, may also be a presenting symptom. When loss of bladder and bowel control brings the patient to the physician, advanced neurologic dysfunction is invariably present.

Genitourinary symptoms such as impotence or recurrent cystitis from bladder dysfunction can suggest cobalamin neuropathy. Multiple pregnancies with short intervals between delivery and conception predispose to a high risk for overt folate deficiency and contribute to fetal growth restriction in babies (cobalamin deficiency is more often associated with infertility).

The Physical Examination

Physical examination may reveal different features in well-nourished patients (cobalamin-deficient vegetarians or pernicious anemia) and poorly nourished (folate-deficient) individuals. The latter show evidence of significant weight loss or other stigmata of multiple deficiencies due to "broad-spectrum" malabsorption. Associated deficiency of vitamins A, D, and K and protein-calorie malnutrition may give rise to angular cheilosis, bleeding mucous membranes, dermatitis, osteomalacia, and chronic infections. Various degrees of pallor with lemon-tint icterus (i.e., a combination of pallor and icterus best observed in fair-skinned individuals) are common features of megaloblastosis.

When anemia is severe, the patient may have a low-grade fever. The skin may reveal a diffuse, brownish pigmentation or abnormal blotchy tanning.[174] A macular hyperpigmentation with follicular accentuation may be observed in the axilla and groin; hyperpigmentation can also involve the dorsal acral distal interphalyngeal joints and a reticular pigmentation in the mid–upper back can develop slowly over a year (but resolves within 2 months of cobalamin replacement).[174] Special emphasis should be given to pigmentation of skin creases and nail beds. (Mucous membrane pigmentation is not observed, in contrast to Addison disease.) Premature graying, observed in light- and dark-haired individuals, is reversible within 6 months of cobalamin therapy.

A blunted masklike facies is extremely common in folate deficiency. Alternatively, there may be evidence of classic hyperthyroid or hypothyroid facies (associated with pernicious anemia). Special attention should be given to the eyes and eyebrows for signs of thyroid dysfunction.

Examination of the mouth may reveal glossitis with a smooth (depapillated), beefy red tongue with occasional ulceration of the lateral surface or gingival hyperplasia (antiepileptics). The neck may reveal thyromegaly (diffuse or with nodules) if there is associated disease. Increased jugular venous distention should alert the examiner to cardiovascular failure, with its attendant gallop, cardiomegaly (with or without pericardial effusions), pulmonary basal crepitations, pleural effusion, tender hepatomegaly, and pedal edema. Nontender hepatomegaly, but more often mild splenomegaly, may rarely be caused by extramedullary hematopoiesis in severe anemia, but a midepigastrium mass raises the ominous possibility of gastric carcinoma, which is three times as likely in patients with pernicious anemia.

An inverse correlation has been identified between the extent of anemia and neurologic dysfunction. Patients with normal complete blood count values often have neurologic signs and symptoms. In prolonged cobalamin deficiency, the neurologic examination reveals clear-cut evidence of involvement of posterior and pyramidal, spinocerebellar, and spinothalamic tracts. Among the earliest signs of posterior column dysfunction are loss of position sense in the index toes (before great toe involvement), which is elicited by passive movement, and loss of the ability to discern vibration of a high-pitched (256 cycles/sec) tuning fork. This is a very early elicitable, objective sign, which invariably precedes by many months the loss of ability to sense the vibration of a lower-pitched (128 cycles/sec) tuning fork. Usually the patient loses vibration sense to 256 cycles/sec from toe to hip before loss of 128 cycles/sec vibration sense even begins. Because of the slow coalescence of contiguous spinal cord lesions, a constellation of elicitable signs may be obtained. Upper motor neuron disease is indicated by weakness and progressive spasticity with increased muscle tone, exaggerated deep tendon reflexes with clonus, extensor plantar response, and incoordinate or scissor gait, which may progress to spastic paraplegia. The involvement of peripheral nerves may markedly modify these signs to include flaccidity and the absence of deep tendon reflexes. A positive Romberg sign is not uncommon, and a positive Lhermitte sign may be elicited. Loss of sphincter and bowel control, altered cranial nerve dysfunction with altered taste, smell, and visual acuity or color perception, and optic neuritis (unexplained predominance in males) may be other physical signs indicating cobalamin deficiency. Inability to carry out serial subtraction of 7 from 100 is a valuable test to document reduced cerebral function (the electroencephalogram often reveals slow wave frequency) in pernicious anemia.

Diagnostic Issues: Information From the Peripheral Smear and Bone Marrow Aspirate

Although not specific for megaloblastic anemia, macro-ovalocytes are the hallmark of megaloblastosis (see Fig. 37-7). However, only one-half with MCV values greater than 105 fl may have vitamin deficiency. In almost one-half of all cases, macrocytosis per se is not associated with megaloblastosis, and additional tests are necessary for complete diagnosis.

The frequency of hypersegmented PMNs (5% with five lobes or 1% with six-lobed PMNs) in patients with megaloblastic hematopoiesis is 98%. The sensitivity decreases to 78% in alcoholics, although the specificity of this finding is approximately 95%. With a combination of hypersegmented PMNs and macro-ovalocytosis, the specificity is 96% to 98%, and the positive predictive value of folate or cobalamin deficiency is about 94%.[9] Hypersegmentation of PMNs is insufficiently sensitive, when compared with metabolite levels, to be used as a clinical tool in the diagnosis of mild cobalamin deficiency[9] (see box on Diagnostic Bone Marrow Aspiration).

Masked Megaloblastosis

The term *masked megaloblastosis* is reserved for conditions in which true cobalamin or folate deficiency with anemia is not accompanied

Diagnostic Bone Marrow Aspiration

Is bone marrow aspiration always necessary to diagnose cobalamin- or folate-deficient megaloblastosis? With the addition of highly sensitive serum tests for the specific diagnosis of cobalamin and folate deficiency, the need for a bone marrow test is often dictated by the urgency to diagnose megaloblastosis (with results available in an hour). For example, in the case of florid hematologic disease with or without neurologic disease suggestive of cobalamin or folate deficiency, bone marrow aspiration carried out as soon as possible is invaluable in assisting the rapid diagnosis of megaloblastosis. However, in the outpatient setting, when the patient has a characteristic peripheral smear, or for a patient with a primary neuropsychiatric presentation, a case can be made to initiate the sequence of diagnostic tests without bone marrow aspiration by proceeding with measurement of serum levels of vitamins or metabolites (see Table 37-1). In a pregnant patient with pancytopenia with macro-ovalocytes, hypersegmented PMNs, and reticulocytopenia with a history of noncompliance with prenatal supplements (and no neurologic findings suggestive of cobalamin deficiency), bone marrow aspiration may not be necessary to initiate therapy for a strong presumptive diagnosis of folate deficiency. If there is no evidence of response within 10 days, bone marrow aspiration is indicated.

by classic findings of megaloblastosis in the peripheral blood and bone marrow. This occurs when there is a coexisting condition that neutralizes the tendency to generate megaloblastic cells (usually involving reduction in RBC hemoglobinization, as in iron deficiency or thalassemia).[9] A wide RBC distribution width (RDW) on the Coulter counter readout in the presence of a "normal" mean corpuscular hemoglobin or MCV may reflect megaloblastic anemia[9] or dimorphic anemia (macro-ovalocytes plus microcytic hypochromic RBCs). Because megaloblastic white blood cells and precursors are unaffected by deficient hemoglobinization, these pathognomonic findings (giant myelocytes and metamyelocytes, and hypersegmented PMNs) remain; the latter may persist for up to 2 weeks after replacement with cobalamin or folate.[8] The recognition of masked megaloblastosis should initiate investigations to rule out iron deficiency, anemia of chronic disease, or hemoglobinopathies. Appropriate replacement with cobalamin or folate elicits a maximal therapeutic benefit only when iron deficiency is corrected. Conversely, if combined iron and cobalamin deficiency (total gastrectomy or pernicious anemia) or iron and folate deficiency (pregnancy) is treated with iron alone, megaloblastosis will be unmasked.

APPROACH TO DIAGNOSIS AND THERAPY OF MEGALOBLASTOSIS

In general there are three stages in approaching a patient: *recognizing* that megaloblastic anemia is present; *distinguishing* whether folate, cobalamin, or combined folate and cobalamin deficiencies have led to the anemia; and diagnosing the *underlying disease* and *mechanism* causing the deficiency. Establishing that the patient does have megaloblastosis is, in theory, straightforward. This is easily done by first evaluating the complete blood count, the MCV, and the peripheral smear, followed by a bone marrow aspiration. Clues to whether cobalamin or folate deficiency is responsible for megaloblastosis can be obtained by serum cobalamin and serum folate levels; if these levels are borderline, additional testing of serum MMA and serum homocysteine can define the true nature of the deficiency.[9,175] However, this ideal and orderly workup is not always feasible in clinical practice, because the patient may present for the first time with megaloblastosis with or without associated neurologic disease; may be referred after a variable workup has already been initiated for possible megaloblastosis; may present with symptoms primarily attributed to a disease predisposing to cobalamin or folate deficiency; may present with a disease associated with hyperhomocysteinemia (discussed later), in which case anemia or neurologic dysfunction may only be a minor symptom; may present with isolated neurologic disease in the absence of anemia; or may be referred after empirical therapy has been given for presumed cobalamin or folate deficiency. The immediate question therefore pertains to the overall status of the patient.

If the patient is decompensated or decompensation is imminent, obtain serum folate and cobalamin levels and bone marrow aspiration to confirm megaloblastosis and proceed with transfusion of 1 unit of packed RBCs *slowly,* with vigorous diuretic therapy to obviate further congestive heart failure from fluid overload; this mandates close monitoring and correction of fluid and electrolyte imbalance. Cobalamin and folate should be administered simultaneously in full doses. Transfusion does not alter serum folate or cobalamin levels.

If the patient is moderately symptomatic (but not in heart failure), the strong likelihood of a dramatic response (in the sense of well-being and relief of sore tongue) within 2 to 3 days even before hematologic improvement argues against immediate blood transfusion.[9] Therefore (and provided the patient is unlikely to decompensate in the short-term) proceed with appropriate diagnostic workup as for the well-compensated patient.

If the patient is well compensated and in the outpatient setting, the physician has time to develop an orderly sequence of diagnostic tests. First, check the peripheral smear and rule out other macrocytic anemias (thin macrocytes with a normoblastic marrow in contrast to macro-ovalocytes) (see Fig. 37-7). Draw blood for cobalamin and folate levels (*before* the patient's first hospital meal) to sort out whether the problem is caused by a deficiency of folate or cobalamin, or both, or some other deficiency (see Table 37-1). Assuming that there is no urgency to make the diagnosis, the physician can elect to wait for the results of these tests before proceeding with the next test in the diagnostic workup. If making the diagnosis is urgent, a cost-effective test is the bone marrow aspirate; results indicating megaloblastosis (or not) can be available within an hour. If bone marrow aspiration is performed, samples are sent for special stains and flow cytometry (megaloblastic erythropoiesis can resemble erythroleukemia) and cytogenetic analysis (myelodysplastic syndromes can exhibit some megaloblastic changes in the erythroid series, but megaloblastic granulopoiesis is not seen). If the marrow is not obviously megaloblastic but the iron stain reveals absent stores, review the morphologic evaluation again with special emphasis on granulocytic precursors and promegaloblasts, and look for more subtle megaloblastic changes.

If the patient refuses bone marrow aspiration and serum cobalamin and folate levels are equivocal (i.e., in the low-normal range), a strong case can be made to test for serum homocysteine and MMA. Serum MMA and homocysteine levels are ordered together (the same sample remaining from the serum sent for cobalamin and folate levels may be used if it was frozen). Integrating the results for serum MMA and homocysteine levels (which will be available after a week or more) with those for serum cobalamin and folate levels can help distinguish cobalamin and folate deficiencies (see Table 37-1). A normal MMA and homocysteine level eliminates cobalamin deficiency with 100% confidence, and normal homocysteine levels suggest that megaloblastic anemia is not caused by folate deficiency. These tests are particularly useful if the patient has pure neurologic disease or if there are associated conditions such as iron deficiency or thalassemia that can mask megaloblastosis. Administration of folate or cobalamin will reduce elevated serum homocysteine and MMA levels to basal values by 1 week, so there is only a narrow window to clinch the diagnosis using metabolite tests.[9] In the rare situation when a defect in cobalamin or folate metabolism is suspected, early consultation with experts who have published in this area is advised.[108,118]

A reticulocyte count is useful to follow the patient's response to appropriate replacement therapy. Additional supporting studies to document increased serum LDH, haptoglobin, and bilirubin (evidence for intramedullary hemolysis) may be performed.

When the megaloblastic state is established, try to determine the underlying mechanism of cobalamin or folate deficiency. The cause of folate deficiency is usually sorted out by this time from the history,

Practicing Classical Medicine Without the (Classical) Schilling Test

The Schilling test was used to identify the locus of cobalamin malabsorption and, in some instances such as pernicious anemia or bacterial overgrowth, the cause of cobalamin deficiency. However, this test has been unavailable since 2003 in the United States. Because only 50% of patients with pernicious anemia have serum anti–intrinsic factor (IF) antibodies, there are limitations in differentiating the other one-half without measurable anti-IF antibodies from those with food-bound cobalamin malabsorption and others with an intestinal cause for cobalamin malabsorption. A minimalist approach is to work around the nonavailability of the Schilling test and use a classical clinical approach to rule out potential differential diagnoses of cobalamin deficiency (see box on Etiopathophysiologic Classification of Cobalamin Deficiency). For example, most conditions predisposing to cobalamin deficiency should be clinically manifest by the time cobalamin deficiency is evident. It should therefore be possible to identify several conditions through a detailed dietary history or past medical history, travel history, and drug history to suggest a dietary cause, esophagogastroduodenal disease, pancreatic insufficiency, impaired bowel motility, or other autoimmune diseases. The history and physical examination could provide further leads and suggest additional focused laboratory testing for rare conditions (stool for ova, anti–tissue transglutaminase antibodies, lipase, gastrin, intestinal biopsy, or radiographic contrast studies for stasis, strictures, fistulas). With no further leads, and therefore by default, one can assume that the diagnosis is either pernicious anemia or food-cobalamin malabsorption, which are both treated with similar replacement doses of cobalamin. For the younger patient with megaloblastic anemia, differentiating juvenile pernicious anemia and congenital IF deficiency would warrant measurement of gastric juice for IF and achlorhydria, deoxyribonucleic acid (DNA) for gastric IF can identify hereditary megaloblastic anemia, and DNA for mutations in cubam receptor (amnionless/cubulin genes) could identify Imerslund-Gräsbeck syndrome.

Thus the history, physical findings, and focused laboratory tests with careful clinical follow-up can potentially identify the cause of the majority of cases of cobalamin deficiency and bypass the need for a Schilling test.

physical examination, and the clinical setting. If pure folate deficiency has been prolonged, expect associated cobalamin deficiency to ensue (special emphasis should be given to identifying subtle manifestations of neurologic disease). If cobalamin deficiency is suspected, test for serum anti-IF antibodies (highly specific for pernicious anemia).

See box on Practicing Classical Medicine Without the (Classical) Schilling Test.

THERAPY

Routinely, treatment with full doses of parenteral cobalamin (1 mg/day) and oral folate (folic acid) (1 to 5 mg) before knowledge of the type of vitamin deficiency is established should be reserved for the severely ill patient. An appropriate regimen for conditions in which cobalamin replenishment can correct cellular cobalamin deficiency (but not correct the underlying problem that led to the deficiency, such as pernicious anemia) is 1 mg of intramuscular or subcutaneous cyanocobalamin per day (week 1), 1 mg twice weekly (week 2), 1 mg/week for 4 weeks, and then 1 mg per month for life (about 15%, or 150 mcg, is retained 48 hours after each 1-mg cobalamin injection). *Ideally, this protocol for rapid correction of cobalamin deficiency and complete replenishment of cobalamin stores should be used in the beginning for all patients with cobalamin deficiency, regardless of the etiology* (see box on Modified Therapeutic Trials).

Parenteral hydroxocobalamin should be reserved for all inborn errors of cobalamin metabolism. There is no major advantage of other preparations over generic cyanocobalamin. There is equivalence between oral 2-mg cobalamin tablets consumed daily (where cobalamin is passively absorbed at high doses) and traditional monthly parenteral treatment with 1 mg of intramuscular/subcutaneous cobalamin among those requiring long-term cobalamin. So for patients who refuse monthly parenteral therapy, or prefer daily oral therapy, or in those with disorders of hemostasis, cobalamin (1 to 2 mg/day as tablets) can be recommended for all those patients with cobalamin malabsorption.[8,9] The physician must ensure that the patient is compliant and demonstrates adequate cobalamin levels as well as resolution of hematologic and neurologic abnormalities on follow-up. For nutritional cobalamin deficiency (e.g., vegetarians) when the entire circuitry in cobalamin absorption is intact, daily oral cobalamin of 5 to 10 mcg (found in conventional multivitamin tablets in the United States) taken for a lifetime of vegetarianism will suffice. However, if malabsorption of food-bound cobalamin is suspected (especially in the elderly with achlorhydria), higher doses of daily oral cobalamin (equal to or greater than 1000 mcg/day) is required.[176]

The bioavailability of oral cobalamin can be reduced by about 40% when it is taken with a meal; so taking cobalamin on an empty stomach will lower losses in the stool. More than 98% of all the cobalamin in feces is in the form of cobalamin analogues, and about 80% of the ingested cobalamin is converted to analogues by microorganisms in the gut.[177]

Oral folate (folic acid) at doses of 1 to 5 mg/day results in adequate absorption (even where intestinal malabsorption of physiologic food folate is present). Therapy should be continued until complete hematologic recovery is documented. If the underlying cause leading to folate deficiency is not corrected, folate may be continued. Folinic acid (i.e., 5-formyl-THF [leucovorin]) should be reserved *only* for rescue protocols involving antifolates (methotrexate or trimethoprim-sulfamethoxazole), for 5-fluorouracil modulation protocols, after nitrous oxide toxicity, or in pediatric cases involving cerebral folate deficiency or inborn errors of folate metabolism. It is too expensive for conventional repletion in folate-deficient states in adults.

Response to Replenishment

The response of the patient to appropriate replacement is reversion of megaloblastic hematopoiesis to normal hematopoiesis within the first 12 hours; by 48 hours normal hematopoiesis is reestablished, and the only evidence for a prior megaloblastic state may be the persistence of a few giant metamyelocytes. Because megaloblastosis caused by cobalamin or folate deficiency can be reversed in 24 hours by administration of folate (i.e., a nutritious hospital meal), delay of a diagnostic bone marrow aspirate should be avoided. Clinically the first 36 to 48 hours are often highlighted by the awakening of an occasional semistuporous individual whose "chief complaint" is amazement at the remarkably improved sense of well-being experienced, with increased alertness and appetite and reduced soreness of the tongue. The elevated serum MMA and homocysteine levels will return to normal by the end of the first week.

Accelerated turnover of normal DNA in erythroid precursors is associated with an increase in serum urate level, which usually peaks by the fourth day, and with increased cellular phosphate uptake for nucleotide synthesis. This may precipitate an attack of gout if the patient has a "gouty predisposition." The reticulocyte count increases by the second to third day and peaks by the fifth to eighth day (the peak reticulocyte count is directly proportional to the degree of preexisting anemia). This is followed by a rise in RBC count, hemoglobin, and hematocrit by the end of the first week, which normalizes in approximately 2 months, regardless of the initial degree of anemia. By the end of the third week, the RBC count should be above $3 \times 10^6/mm^3$; if it is not, additional causes of underlying iron deficiency, hemoglobinopathy, chronic disease, or hypothyroidism should be considered (Table 37-6).

Table 37-6 Causes of Megaloblastosis Not Responding to Therapy With Cobalamin or Folate

WRONG DIAGNOSIS
Combined folate and cobalamin deficiencies being treated with only one vitamin
Associated iron deficiency
Associated hemoglobinopathy (e.g., sickle cell disease, thalassemia)
Associated anemia of chronic disease
Associated hypothyroidism

Table 37-7 Indications for Prophylaxis With Cobalamin or Folate

PROPHYLAXIS WITH COBALAMIN
Infants on specialized diets*
Premature infants
Infants of mothers with pernicious anemia*
Infants and children of mothers with nutritional cobalamin deficiency
Vegetarianism and poverty-imposed near-vegetarianism*
Total gastrectomy[†]
PROPHYLAXIS WITH FOLIC ACID[‡]
All women contemplating pregnancy (at least 400 mcg/day)[§]
Pregnancy and lactation, premature infants
Mothers at risk for delivery of infants with neural tube defects[‖,¶]
Hemolytic anemias/hyperproliferative hematologic states
Patients with rheumatoid arthritis or psoriasis on therapy with methotrexate[#]
Patients on antiepileptic drugs
Patients with ulcerative colitis

*For vegetarians, prophylaxis with cobalamin (5- to 10-mcg tablet/day) orally should suffice. In all other conditions involving any abnormality of cobalamin absorption, cobalamin tablets of 1000 mcg/day should be administered orally to ensure that cobalamin transport by passive diffusion across the intestine is sufficient to meet daily needs.
†Consider late development of cobalamin deficiency and iron malabsorption (prophylaxis with oral cobalamin and iron).
‡Ensure that the patient does not have a cobalamin deficiency before initiating long-term folate prophylaxis.
§For prevention of first occurrence of neural tube defects.
‖Previous delivery of a child with neural tube defects (e.g., anencephaly, spina bifida, meningocele) imparts a 10-fold greater risk for subsequent delivery of infant with neural tube defects.
¶Folic acid (4 mg/day) administered periconceptionally and throughout the first trimester.
#To reduce toxicity of the antifolate.

Hypersegmented PMNs continue to remain in the blood for 10 to 14 days; however, the number of normal PMNs and platelets rises and normalizes within the first week. During this process, there may be a transient left shift to include myeloid precursors. The reduced intramedullary hemolysis (as a result of normalized hematopoiesis) leads to a gradual reduction in the serum bilirubin level by the end of the first week, and LDH levels will drop concomitantly.

In response to cobalamin, progression of neurologic damage and dysfunction is inhibited. In general the degree of functional recovery is inversely related to the extent of disease and duration of signs and symptoms. As a rough estimate, signs and symptoms that have been present for less than 3 months are usually completely reversible; with longer duration, there is invariable residual neurologic dysfunction. The reversibility of neurologic damage is slow (a maximal response may take 6 months). Substantial increments (in recovery) are unlikely to be gained after the first 12 months of appropriate therapy. However, most neurologic abnormalities have improved in up to 90% of patients with documented subacute combined degeneration.

Follow-Up

Patients with neurologic dysfunction from cobalamin deficiency have traditionally been given more frequent doses of cobalamin (biweekly rather than monthly therapy for the first 6 months), despite the lack of evidence that this form of therapy is more beneficial. This approach nevertheless serves a purpose in that improvement in neurologic status can be carefully documented. Once maximal responses have been established, most patients can be treated with life-long cobalamin with a dose that is appropriate for the underlying cause of cobalamin deficiency. Follow-up outpatient visits every 6 months should be instituted to ensure adequate maintenance of hematopoiesis, as well as early diagnosis of other diseases commonly associated with the cobalamin- or folate-deficient state. Follow-up of patients with pernicious anemia suggest that individuals older than 60 years are prone to developing iron deficiency that arises from poor iron absorption from achlorhydria.[9] All patients with pernicious anemia should be screened for iron deficiency at the beginning and during follow-up.

Patients with pernicious anemia have a twofold increase in proximal femur and vertebral fractures and a threefold increase in distal forearm fractures. Finally, three studies (from Sweden, the United States, and Denmark) on a total of nearly 15,000 patients with pernicious anemia have identified an excess risk for gastric cancers within the first few years of diagnosis[178]; so it is prudent to recommend upper endoscopy for these patients.

ROUTINE SUPPLEMENTATION OF COBALAMIN AND FOLATE

Routine periconceptional supplementation of folate for normal women[9] and in 10 times higher doses for women at risk for delivery of subsequent babies with NTDs[9] provides effective prophylaxis against the development of NTDs (Table 37-7). Food fortification with folic acid (140 mcg/100 g flour) has nearly eliminated folate deficiency[179,180]—the prevalence of low serum folate level decreased from 18.4% to 0.8% with a small (0.3 g/dL) increase in hemoglobin (for men an increase from 15.1 to 15.4 g/dL and for women from 13.3 to 13.6 g/dL)[181]; it has consistently reduced NTDs[143,182]; and it is a cost-effective intervention.[183] Food fortification was intended to provide only one-quarter of the recommended dietary allowance of folate. A very brief focused interaction involving physician advice combined with a booster phone call and starter bottle of folic acid tablets can markedly increase a woman's regular intake of folic acid (increase by 68% versus 20% in the control group).[184] Distressingly, however, two decades after the landmark studies showed the way to prevention of first occurrence of NTDs, women in large areas of North India continue to subsist on monotonous and largely vegetarian diets containing only one-third to one-fifth of the RDA of folate required,[25,44] which can well explain the shockingly high incidence of NTDs.[134] Folic acid supplements during early pregnancy appear to reduce the risk for isolated cleft lip (with or without cleft palate) by about one-third.[185]

The administration of folate and cobalamin in addition to the standard administration of intramuscular iron to premature infants less than 36 weeks of gestation significantly improved hemoglobin values.[186] For the anemia of prematurity, addition of cobalamin and folate to erythropoietin and orally and intravenously administered iron appeared more effective in stimulating erythropoiesis among premature infants, when compared with erythropoietin, iron, and low-dose folate alone[187]; so this should be the standard of care.

Supplementation with folate during pregnancy also helps to prevent premature delivery of low-birth-weight infants,[8] and routine supplementation for premature infants and lactating mothers is also recommended.

In addition to hematologic diseases leading to increased folate requirements (e.g., autoimmune hemolytic anemia, β-thalassemia), folic acid supplements reduce the hepatotoxicity and gastrointestinal intolerance of methotrexate in psoriasis[9,188] and rheumatoid arthritis[189] without impairing the efficacy of methotrexate.

Supplementation with folic acid protects against the development of colorectal neoplasia in high-risk patients with ulcerative colitis.[9]

A recent innovative large-scale universal program to harness more efficient ways to use existing public health structures has been described. This program, which involved weekly iron–folic acid supplementation combined with a regular deworming program, was able to successfully improve the hemoglobin and iron status among 52,000 Vietnamese women of reproductive age.[190] Similar approaches are applicable for thousands of women of reproductive age in Southeast Asia and Africa. Anemia with a hemoglobin value of less than 11 g/dL is found in 75% of children[191]; although this is primarily related to low iron stores, there is also an association with low folate stores. There would be additional benefit of cobalamin supplements for women who are already at risk for cobalamin deficiency because of poverty-imposed near-vegetarianism or for those who are vegetarians. For schoolchildren, simple community-level interventions, such as micronutrient fortification (using a premix added to school lunch meals), that build upon the infrastructure of an existing program have proven to be contextually acceptable and efficacious in improving folate and cobalamin (in addition to vitamin A and iron) status in Himalayan villages of India.[192] Such programs are critically important to the health of both women and their children (discussed later). Table 37-7 summarizes conditions that warrant routine folate or cobalamin supplementation.

Studies have shown that iron plus folic acid supplementation was beneficial to young children in a low-income area in Nepal where there was no malaria risk but iron deficiency was common[193]; therefore in this setting, routine iron plus folic acid supplementation is likely to have long-term benefits on several areas of physical growth and development, including cognitive performance. However, in areas where malaria is very common, widespread control of iron (and folate) deficiency anemia among children should be accompanied by intermittent preventive malaria therapy.[194,195] This is relevant to very young children in Africa who invariably have a multifactorial basis for severe anemia (hemoglobin less than 5 g/dL)—which includes malaria, bacteremia, hookworm, human immunodeficiency virus (HIV), glucose-6-phosphate dehydrogenase deficiency, and vitamin A, as well as 30% who have cobalamin deficiency.[196] There was an apparently lower incidence of folate deficiency in this cohort; however, because of cobalamin deficiency–associated methyl-folate trapping and the associated malaria-induced hemolysis in these children, there could well have been an artificial increase in serum folate. This is because red cells contain 30 times more folate than that which is found in the serum. Therefore the serum folate level may be falsely elevated, leading to an underestimation of the extent of folate deficiency. Of course the use of metabolite assays would have doubtless increased the prevalence of both cobalamin and folate deficiency in these populations.[7,75,197] However, this is impractical in resource-poor areas, so the prudent approach is to assume that these children also have folate deficiency and treat them with full replacement doses of cobalamin and folate. Only with correction of underlying deficiency of iron, cobalamin, and folate deficiency, together with other causes for anemia, will normal hematopoiesis be initiated.

Following food fortification, the total folate intake of most U.S. children 1 to 13 years of age does meet the estimated average requirement,[198] but children given supplements are at risk for exceeding the tolerable upper intake level; this remains a concern because the long-term effects are unknown. Whereas folic acid supplements consumed in excess of 1 mg/day can mask hematologic symptoms of cobalamin deficiency, it has been found that 94% of U.S. adults who do not consume supplements, or who consume less than 400 mcg of folic acid per day from supplements, do not exceed the upper limit in intake for folic acid.[199] There is also no evidence that taking high-folate supplements or consuming large amounts of folate-fortified foods places individuals at risk for exacerbating any underlying cobalamin deficiency.[200]

Is there a role for cobalamin fortification of foods? A strong case can to be made to consider the fortification of flour (or other contextually relevant food vehicle in developing countries) with small amounts of cobalamin to serve the majority of the population whose dietary intake of animal-source foods is poor. However, this type of fortified food will not benefit those (in developed countries) with food-cobalamin malabsorption; these individuals usually need the equivalent of 1 mg of oral cobalamin daily, an amount that could not possibly be achieved by the small amount of cobalamin added to fortify foods. Other issues related to cobalamin analogue formation upon exposure to light or mixing with other food ingredients and other stability issues during storage have not been resolved; hence this topic remains a work in progress.

HYPERHOMOCYSTEINEMIA

Normally homocysteine is metabolized by the methylation reaction (discussed earlier) and by a second trans-sulfuration pathway, which essentially eliminates homocysteine as a potential source of methionine. In the trans-sulfuration pathway, cystathionine β-synthase catalyzes the condensation of homocysteine with serine in the presence of pyridoxyl phosphate (vitamin B_6) to form cystathionine, which is further cleaved by a vitamin B_6–dependent γ-cystathionase to form cysteine and α-ketobutyrate. The cysteine that is formed can be used for synthesis of the antioxidant glutathione, a key component that defends against oxidative stress within cells. In some tissues like liver, homocysteine can also be remethylated to methionine by the transfer of a one-carbon moiety from betaine by the enzyme, homocysteine methyltransferase, which is restricted to the liver and kidney. Thus the level of plasma homocysteine depends on genetically regulated levels of essential enzymes in one-carbon metabolism, the intake of folic acid or food folates, vitamin B_6, cobalamin, and other acquired conditions (dehydration, renal dysfunction, antifolates, and nitrous oxide).

Chronic hyperhomocysteinemia is established as a major risk factor in occlusive vascular diseases.[41] These include myocardial infarctions from coronary atherosclerosis, extracranial carotid artery stenosis, vascular disease in end-stage renal failure, thromboangiitis obliterans, aortic atherosclerosis, venous thromboembolism, placental abruption or infarction, and recurrent stillbirths. Hyperhomocysteinemia is also associated with reduced bone mineral density and increased incidence of fractures,[201] increased small-vessel cerebrovascular disease–related strokes,[202,203] dementia and Alzheimer disease.[204]

There is more than one mechanism for transport of homocysteine across the microvillous membrane of the human placenta.[205] Raised maternal plasma levels of homocysteine primarily from cobalamin and folate deficiency are associated with various pregnancy complications. These include preeclampsia and spontaneous pregnancy loss,[172,206-209] placental abruption,[206,208,210] recurrent pregnancy loss,[206,208,211] fetal growth restriction[207,208] preterm birth,[212] and stillbirth.[207] The adverse outcomes for the baby include NTDs and congenital malformations.[207,208] Normalization of maternal homocysteine level with cobalamin and folate and improvement of these pregnancy outcomes for some complications[208,211] indicate that some of these risks can be reduced with good nutrition.

Homocysteine-Lowering Trials and Primary Versus Secondary Prevention

Most homocysteine-lowering intervention trials have been underpowered; they have looked at populations in which the serum homocysteine level has been borderline elevated rather than being elevated to the higher level (over 20 μM); and they have only had a follow-up of less than 5 years. Moreover, many of the intervention trials have been compromised by the advent of food fortification with folate or by enrolled patients who were consuming multivitamins containing folic acid. A recent review of this "homocysteine controversy"[213] has noted that the duration of follow-up in most studies has been too short (and likely dictated by the dramatic results from the use of antihypertensives and statins, which required only short follow-up to demonstrate positive effects). The point made is that such expectations are unrealistic for atherosclerosis because the atherosclerotic plaque commonly takes 30 to 40 years to develop into a full-blown clinical event. Moreover, there is a distinct difference between primary prevention of the earliest stages of a disease process and attempts to intervene after demonstrated vascular damage (secondary prevention). (Indeed, it was only longer follow-up for 10 to 15 years that established the primacy of blood glucose control in management of patients with diabetes).

Despite the failure of homocysteine-lowering therapy in several trials related to secondary prevention of atherosclerotic disease, this has not eliminated the possibility of a beneficial role of lowering homocysteine in primary prevention of diseases. Indeed, clinical trials that used folates have suggested that folate also has a role in reduction in strokes,[139] reduction in the rate of cognitive decline among healthy older adults,[140] and a reduction in age-related (sensorineural) hearing loss.[141] There is also grade A evidence from randomized controlled trials for a role of folate in combination with cobalamin for reduction of hip fractures,[136] subclinical atherosclerosis,[137] and stroke prevention.[139] In addition, the value of a triple combination of folate, pyridoxine, and cobalamin to reduce age-related macular degeneration in women is also established[138] (see Table 37-4).

By inference, in addition to clinical presentation with nutritional anemia, patients can also present with any of these additional clinical conditions, as well as a variety of pregnancy complications with or without poor pregnancy outcomes (affecting the newborn), when they have long-standing untreated hyperhomocysteinemia.

Homocysteine and Mild Cognitive Impairment

All inherited diseases involving a severe elevation of homocysteine are associated with cognitive deficit and poorer neurocognitive performance. Accelerated brain atrophy is often a characteristic among those with mild cognitive impairment who then go on to develop Alzheimer disease. Now a randomized controlled trial from the UK—where folate fortification of food is not mandatory—among elderly patients with mild cognitive impairment has identified that lowering of homocysteine level by B vitamins over 2 years did slow the rate of brain atrophy by almost 30%.[73] This is consistent with another randomized controlled trial (in a region without folate fortification of food) that demonstrated beneficial effects of folates on cognition over 3 years.[140] While awaiting larger confirmatory trials, these studies suggest that homocysteine-lowering therapy can slow down the accelerated rate of brain atrophy that is found with mild cognitive impairment.

Homocysteine Lowering and the Progression of Diabetic Nephropathy

Even though patients with diabetic nephropathy have elevated levels of homocysteine, attempts to use a combination of high doses of oral B vitamins (folic acid, pyridoxine, cobalamin) to reduce homocysteine concentrations have now been shown to *worsen* their kidney disease and place them at greater risk for dying from serious vascular events.[214] Hence there is *no* justification for using high-dose B vitamins in this setting or outside the framework of properly conducted clinical research.

FOLATE FORTIFICATION OF FOOD AND THE RISK FOR CANCER

Three large prospective studies[215-217] suggest that long term folate intake actually *decreases the risk* for initiation or early development of colorectal cancer[217]; in addition, there appears to be a diminished to nonexistent influence on (precancerous) adenomas. Collectively, these papers provide reassurance that the fortification of food to prevent NTDs in women of childbearing age has not led to harm among the remaining "nontargeted" population of adults. There also could be long-term benefits in primary prevention (see Table 37-4).

FUTURE DIRECTIONS

In this age of spiraling costs for health care delivery, and the ongoing debate on ways to reduce these costs, few instances in internal medicine and hematology yield more satisfying dividends than diagnosing and treating cobalamin and folate deficiency using generic vitamins that are "dirt-cheap"—costing only one or two cents a day. These conditions are devastating when undiagnosed or misdiagnosed or when cobalamin deficiency is treated with folate alone. Recognition of various populations at risk and the clinical scenarios in which folate and cobalamin deficiency are likely to be present, and the availability of sensitive and specific tests, should reduce uncertainty in diagnosis. The studies on folate supplementation during pregnancy that identified new folate-responsive NTDs and neurocristopathies are a paradigm for identification of hitherto unrecognized roles for other nutrients in human development. The significant impact of supplemental folates in relieving human suffering consonant with reducing costs for intensive and long-term care of infants with prematurity or NTDs is a major achievement and outstanding example of cost-effective preventive medicine. Other recent advances from randomized controlled studies indicate beneficial effects of supplemental folate and cobalamin in the prevention of diverse diseases. The newest information related to the influence of folates and cobalamin during development in utero—especially on behavioral neuroscience—allows us to peer into a new field where groundbreaking discoveries will be made in the coming decade. Finally in early 2012, we identified a molecular link between folate deficiency and Human Papillomavirus (type 16)-induced cancer.[218] Because this virus is the most common cause of cervical cancer worldwide (and also responsible for a significant number of vulvar, vaginal, penile, anal, and oropharyngeal cancers), such studies open the door to new investigations into the potential role of these vitamins in the field of preventive oncology.

SUGGESTED READINGS

Antony AC: Vegetarianism and vitamin-B12 (cobalamin) deficiency. *Am J Clin Nutr* 78:3, 2003.

Antony AC: In utero physiology: Role of folic acid in nutrient delivery and fetal development. *Am J Clin Nutr* 85:598S, 2007.

Bjorke-Monsen AL, Ueland PM: Cobalamin status in children. *J Inherit Metab Dis* 34:111, 2010.

Calis JC, Phiri KS, Faragher EB, et al: Severe anemia in Malawian children. *N Engl J Med* 358:888, 2008; and 358:2291, 2008; author reply 2291.

Carmel R: Biomarkers of cobalamin (vitamin B-12) status in the epidemiologic setting: A critical overview of context, applications, and performance characteristics of cobalamin, methylmalonic acid, and holotranscobalamin II. *Am J Clin Nutr* 94:348S, 2011.

Cherian A, Seena S, Bullock RK, et al: Incidence of neural tube defects in the least-developed area of India—a population based study. *Lancet* 366:930, 2005.

Christen WG, Glynn RJ, Chew EY, et al: Folic acid, pyridoxine, and cyanocobalamin combination treatment and age-related macular degeneration in women: The Women's Antioxidant and Folic Acid Cardiovascular Study. *Arch Intern Med* 169:335, 2009.

Czeizel AE: Periconceptional folic acid and multivitamin supplementation for the prevention of neural tube defects and other congenital abnormalities. *Birth Defects Res A Clin Mol Teratol* 85:260, 2009.

de Jager J, Kooy A, Lehert P, et al: Long term treatment with metformin in patients with type 2 diabetes and risk of vitamin B-12 deficiency: Randomised placebo controlled trial. *BMJ* 340:c2181, 2010.

De Wals P, Tairou F, Van Allen MI, et al: Reduction in neural-tube defects after folic acid fortification in Canada. *N Engl J Med* 357:135, 2007.

Durga J, van Boxtel MP, Schouten EG, et al: Effect of 3-year folic acid supplementation on cognitive function in older adults in the FACIT trial: A randomised, double blind, controlled trial. *Lancet* 369:208, 2007.

Durga J, Verhoef P, Anteunis LJ, et al: Effects of folic acid supplementation on hearing in older adults: A randomized, controlled trial. *Ann Intern Med* 146:1, 2007.

Froese DS, Gravel RA: Genetic disorders of vitamin B metabolism: Eight complementation groups—eight genes. *Expert Rev Mol Med* 12:e37, 2010.

Gordon N: Cerebral folate deficiency. *Dev Med Child Neurol* 51:180, 2009.

Hodis HN, Mack WJ, Dustin L, et al: High-dose B vitamin supplementation and progression of subclinical atherosclerosis: A randomized controlled trial. *Stroke* 40:730, 2009.

House AA, Eliasziw M, Cattran DC, et al: Effect of B-vitamin therapy on progression of diabetic nephropathy: A randomized controlled trial. *JAMA* 303:1603, 2010.

Ionescu-Ittu R, Marelli AJ, Mackie AS, et al: Prevalence of severe congenital heart disease after folic acid fortification of grain products: Time trend analysis in Quebec, Canada. *BMJ* 338:b1673, 2009.

Lee JE, Chan AT: Fruit, vegetables, and folate: Cultivating the evidence for cancer prevention. *Gastroenterology* 141:16, 2011.

Quadros EV: Advances in the understanding of cobalamin assimilation and metabolism. *Br J Haematol* 148:195, 2010.

Ramaekers VT, Blau N, Sequeira JM, et al: Folate receptor autoimmunity and cerebral folate deficiency in low-functioning autism with neurological deficits. *Neuropediatrics* 38:276, 2007.

Ramaekers VT, Rothenberg SP, Sequeira JM, et al: Autoantibodies to folate receptors in the cerebral folate deficiency syndrome. *N Engl J Med* 352:1985, 2005.

Sato Y, Honda Y, Iwamoto J, et al: Effect of folate and mecobalamin on hip fractures in patients with stroke: A randomized controlled trial. *JAMA* 293:1082, 2005.

Sayed AR, Bourne D, Pattinson R, et al: Decline in the prevalence of neural tube defects following folic acid fortification and its cost-benefit in South Africa. *Birth Defects Res A Clin Mol Teratol* 82:211, 2008.

Smith AD, Smith SM, de Jager CA, et al: Homocysteine-lowering by B vitamins slows the rate of accelerated brain atrophy in mild cognitive impairment: A randomized controlled trial. *PLoS One* 5:e12244, 2010.

Smulders YM, Blom HJ: The homocysteine controversy. *J Inherit Metab Dis* 34:93, 2011.

Stabler SP, Allen RH: Vitamin B12 deficiency as a worldwide problem. *Annu Rev Nutr* 24:299, 2004.

Tamura T, Picciano M: Folate and human reproduction. *Am J Clin Nutr* 83:993, 2006.

Wang X, Qin X, Demirtas H, et al: Efficacy of folic acid supplementation in stroke prevention: A meta-analysis. *Lancet* 369:1876, 2007.

Xiao S, Tang YS, Khan RA, et al: Influence of physiologic folate deficiency on human papillomavirus type 16 (HPV16)-harboring human keratinocytes in vitro and in vivo. *J Biol Chem* 287:12559, 2012.

Yang Q, Botto LD, Erickson JD, et al: Improvement in stroke mortality in Canada and the United States, 1990 to 2002. *Circulation* 113:1335, 2006.

Zhao R, Matherly LH, Goldman ID: Membrane transporters and folate homeostasis: Intestinal absorption and transport into systemic compartments and tissues. *Expert Rev Mol Med* 11:e4, 2009.

For complete list of references log on to www.expertconsult.com.

CHAPTER 38

THALASSEMIA SYNDROMES

Patricia J. Giardina and Stefano Rivella

The thalassemia syndromes are a heterogeneous group of inherited anemias characterized by defects in the synthesis of one or more of the globin chain subunits of the hemoglobin tetramer. The clinical syndromes associated with thalassemia arise from the combined consequences of inadequate hemoglobin production and imbalanced accumulation of globin subunits. The former causes hypochromia and microcytosis; the latter leads to ineffective erythropoiesis (IE) and hemolytic anemia. Clinical manifestations are diverse, ranging from asymptomatic hypochromia and microcytosis to profound anemia, which can be fatal in utero or in early childhood if untreated. This heterogeneity arises from the variable severities of the primary biosynthetic defects and coinherited modifying factors, such as increased synthesis of fetal globin subunits or diminished or increased synthesis of α-globin subunits. Palliative treatment of the severe forms by blood transfusion is eventually compromised by the concomitant problems of iron overload, alloimmunization, and bloodborne infections.

As a group, the thalassemias represent the most common single genetic disorder known. In many parts of the world, they constitute major public health problems. Laboratory analysis of these disorders has been one of the most productive and enlightening endeavors of biomedical research. Study of the molecular defects underlying the thalassemia syndromes has led to fundamental advances in our understanding of eukaryotic gene structure and function. For each of these reasons, a thorough understanding of thalassemia and its related disorders is essential to hematologists. This chapter reviews the major features of these syndromes. Readers wanting more detailed information than can be included here are referred to more comprehensive monographs elsewhere.[1,2]

The classification, genetic basis, and pathophysiology of the thalassemia syndromes are based on a thorough understanding of the human hemoglobins, their biosynthesis, their encoding globin gene families, and their roles as soluble oxygen-carrying molecules. Therefore, readers of this chapter should first familiarize themselves with the material presented in Chapter 31. The material presented in this chapter is also substantially clarified by prior reading of Chapters 33 and 34 because the principles underlying the pathophysiology of and therapy for thalassemia draw heavily on knowledge of iron metabolism.

DEFINITIONS AND NOMENCLATURE

The term *thalassemia* is derived from a Greek term that roughly means "the sea" (Mediterranean) in the blood.[1] It was first applied to the anemias frequently encountered in people from the Italian and Greek coasts and nearby islands.[3-5] The term is now used to refer to inherited defects in globin-chain biosynthesis. Individual syndromes are named according to the globin chain whose synthesis is adversely affected. Thus, α-globin chains are absent or reduced in patients with α-thalassemia, β-globin chains in patients with β-thalassemia, δ-globin and β-globin chains in patients δβ-thalassemia, and so forth. In some contexts, it is also useful to subclassify the syndromes according to whether synthesis of the affected globin chain is totally absent (e.g., β°-thalassemia) or only partially reduced (e.g., β^{+}-thalassemia).

The most common forms of thalassemia arise from total absence of structurally normal globin chains or a partial reduction in their synthesis. In contrast to the "structural" hemoglobinopathies (e.g., sickle cell anemia), which are characterized by the production of normal amounts of mutant globin chains having deranged physical or chemical properties, the thalassemias are quantitative disorders: the primary lesion lies in the amount of globin produced. However, some rare forms of thalassemia are characterized by the production of structurally abnormal globin chains in reduced amounts. These thalassemic hemoglobinopathies share features of thalassemia as well as those of structural hemoglobinopathies.[6]

Some mutations alter the patterns of fetal to adult hemoglobin switching. These conditions, called *hereditary persistence of fetal hemoglobin,* are not generally associated with clinical symptoms; nonetheless, they merit consideration in this chapter. Their importance lies in their role as modulating factors when coinherited with other hemoglobinopathies; in their usefulness as models for investigating the molecular basis for globin gene regulation during human development; and as paradigms for rational therapy for the major β-chain hemoglobinopathies, namely, sickle cell anemia and β-thalassemia.

ETIOLOGY, EPIDEMIOLOGY, AND PATHOPHYSIOLOGY

The thalassemias are inherited as pathologic alleles of one or more of the globin genes located on chromosomes 11 and 16 (see Chapter 31). These lesions range from total deletion or rearrangement of the loci to point mutations that impair transcription, processing, or translation of globin mRNA. The precise nature of the defects is summarized in a later section.

Thalassemias have been encountered in virtually every ethnic group and geographic location. They are most common in the Mediterranean basin and tropical or subtropical regions of Asia and Africa. The "thalassemia belt" extends along the shores of the Mediterranean and throughout the Arabian peninsula; Turkey; Iran; India; and southeastern Asia, especially Thailand, Cambodia, and southern China.[7-10] The prevalence of thalassemia in these regions is in the range of 2.5% to 15%. Similar to sickle cell anemia, thalassemia is most common in areas historically affected by endemic malaria. Malaria seems to have conferred selective survival advantage to thalassemia heterozygotes in which infection with the malarial parasite is believed to result in milder disease and less impact on reproductive fitness.[1,2,11] Therefore, the gene frequency for thalassemia has become fixed and high in populations exposed to malaria over many centuries.

PATHOPHYSIOLOGY: GENERAL PRINCIPLES

The pathophysiology and molecular genetics of individual forms of thalassemia are closely intertwined. Therefore, detailed consideration of these syndromes is best deferred to their individual subsections. This section considers only mechanisms common to the pathogenesis of all of these syndromes.[1-5,12]

The primary lesion in all forms of thalassemia is reduced or absent production of one or more globin chains. For all practical purposes, the major impact on clinical well-being occurs only when these lesions affect the α- or β-globin chains necessary for the synthesis of hemoglobin (Hb A; $\alpha_2\beta_2$). (Severe impairment of γ-, ε-, or ζ-globin production is presumably lethal in utero.) One consequence of reduced globin-chain production is immediately apparent: reduced production of functioning hemoglobin tetramers. As a result, hypochromia and microcytosis are characteristic of virtually all patients with thalassemia. In the milder forms of the disease, this phenomenon may be barely detectable.

The second consequence of impaired globin biosynthesis is unbalanced synthesis of the individual α- and β-subunits. Hemoglobin tetramers are highly soluble and have reversible oxygen-carrying properties exquisitely adapted for oxygen transport and delivery under physiologic conditions. Free or "unpaired" α-, β-, and γ-globin chains are either highly insoluble or form homotetramers (Hb H and Hb Bart) that are incapable of releasing oxygen normally and are relatively unstable and precipitate as the cell ages. For poorly understood reasons, no compensatory regulatory mechanism exists whereby impaired synthesis of one globin subunit leads to a compensatory downward adjustment in the production of the other (partner) globin chain of the hemoglobin tetramer. Thus, whereas useless excess α-globin chains continue to accumulate and precipitate in β-thalassemia, excess β-globin chains form Hb H in α-thalassemia. During uterine development, excess γ-globin chains form Hb Bart in individuals with α-thalassemia.

The abnormal solubility or oxygen-carrying properties of these chains lead to a variety of physiologic derangements. Indeed, in the severe forms of thalassemia, it is the behavior of the unpaired globin chains accumulating in relative excess that dominates the pathophysiology of the syndrome rather than the mere underproduction of functioning hemoglobin tetramers. The precise complications of this pathophysiologic phenomenon are diverse and depend on the amount and the identity of the globin chain accumulating in excess. For the moment, the fundamental principle that must be appreciated is that thalassemias cause symptoms by underproduction of hemoglobin and by accumulation of unpaired globin subunits. The unpaired subunits are usually the major sources of morbidity and mortality.

The predominant circulating hemoglobin at the moment of birth is fetal hemoglobin (Hb $F^{\alpha 2\gamma 2}$) (see Chapter 31). Although the switch from γ- to β-globin biosynthesis begins before birth, the composition of hemoglobin in the peripheral blood changes much later because of the long life span of normal circulating red blood cells. Hb F is thus slowly replaced by adult hemoglobin (Hb A) so that infants do not depend heavily on normal amounts and function of Hb A until they are between 4 and 6 months old. The pathophysiologic consequences of these considerations are that whereas α-chain hemoglobinopathies tend to be symptomatic in utero and at birth, individuals with β-chain abnormalities are asymptomatic until 4 to 6 months of age. These differences in the onset of phenotypic expression arise because α-chains are needed to form Hb F and Hb A, but β-chains are required only for Hb A.

β-THALASSEMIA SYNDROMES

Nomenclature

Many different mutations cause β-thalassemia and its related disorders, such as δβ-thalassemia and the silent carrier state. They are inherited in a multitude of genetic combinations responsible for a heterogeneous group of clinical syndromes. β-Thalassemia major, also known as Cooley anemia or homozygous β-thalassemia, is a clinically severe disorder that results from the inheritance of two β-thalassemia alleles, one on each copy of chromosome 11. As a consequence of diminished Hb A synthesis, the circulating red blood cells (RBCs) are very hypochromic and abnormally shaped; they contain markedly reduced amounts of hemoglobin. Accumulation of free α-globin chains leads to the deposition of precipitated aggregates of these chains to the detriment of the erythrocyte and its precursor cells in the bone marrow (BM). The anemia of thalassemia major is so severe that long-term blood transfusions are usually required.

The term *β-thalassemia intermedia* is applied to a less severe clinical phenotype in which significant anemia occurs but chronic transfusion therapy is not absolutely required. It usually results from the inheritance of two β-thalassemia mutations, one mild and one severe; the inheritance of two mild mutations; or, occasionally, the inheritance of complex combinations, such as a single β-thalassemia defect and an excess of normal α-globin genes, or two β-thalassemia mutations coinherited with heterozygous α-thalassemia (in this last form, known as αβ-thalassemia, the α-thalassemia allele reduces the burden of unpaired α-chains).[13-15] Simple heterozygosity for certain forms of β-thalassemic hemoglobinopathies can also be associated with a thalassemia intermedia phenotype, sometimes called *dominant β-thalassemia*.[16,17]

Thalassemia minor, also known as β-thalassemia trait or heterozygous β-thalassemia, is caused by the presence of a single β-thalassemia mutation and a normal β-globin gene on the other chromosome. It is characterized by profound microcytosis with hypochromia but mild or minimal anemia.

β-Thalassemia is also called by several other names, including Cooley anemia, Mediterranean anemia, von Jaksch anemia,[1] target cell anemia, erythroblastic anemia, and familial microcytosis.

Molecular Pathology

Forms of β-thalassemia arise from mutations that affect every step in the pathway of globin gene expression: transcription, processing of the mRNA precursor, translation of mature mRNA, and posttranslational integrity of the β-polypeptide chain (Fig. 38-1 and Table 38-1).[18-20] Large deletions removing two or more non–α-genes are found in rare cases, as are smaller partial or total deletions of the β-gene alone (see Fig. 38-1). Most types of β-thalassemia are caused by point mutations affecting one or a few bases. (The original literature for this section is extensive; it is summarized in various publications and databases.[18-25]) Of the more than 200 mutations causing β-thalassemia, approximately 15 account for the vast majority of affected patients, with the remainder responsible for the disorder in only relatively few patients. It has been determined that five or six mutations usually account for more than 90% of the cases of β-thalassemia in a given ethnic group or geographic area (see Table 38-1).[22]

Table 38-1 Common β-Thalassemia Mutations in Different Racial Groups

Racial Group	Description
Mediterranean	IVS-1, position 110 (G → A)
	Codon 39, nonsense (CAG → TAG)
	IVS-1, position 1 (G → A)
	IVS-2, position 745 (C → G)
	IVS-1, position 6 (T → C)
	IVS-2, position 1 (G → A)
Black	-34 (A → G)
	-88, (C → T)
	Poly(A), (AATAAA → AACAAA)
Southeast Asian	Codons 41/42, frameshift (-CTTT)
	IVS-2, position 654 (C → T)
	-28 (A → T)
Asian Indian	IVS-1, position 5 (G → C)
	619-bp deletion
	Codons 8/9, frameshift (++G)
	Codons 41/42, frameshift (–CTTT)
	IVS-1, position 1 (G → T)

Data from Kazazian HH Jr, Boehm CD: Molecular basis and prenatal diagnosis of beta-thalassemia. *Blood* 72(4):1107, 1988; and Kazazian HH Jr, Boehm CD: personal communication, 1993.

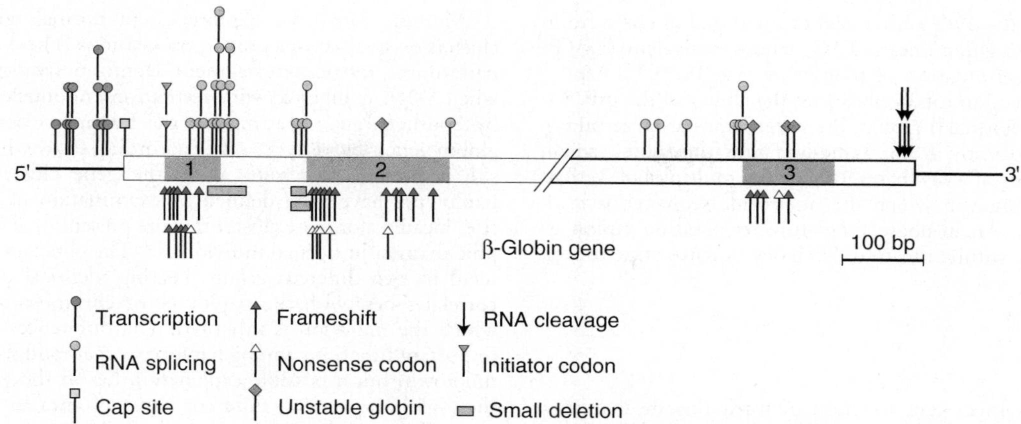

Figure 38-1 MODEL OF THE HUMAN β-GLOBIN GENE SHOWING SITES AND TYPES OF VARIOUS MUTATIONS CAUSING β-THALASSEMIA. *(Adapted from Kazazian HH Jr: The thalassemia syndromes: Molecular basis and prenatal diagnosis in 1990.* Semin Hematol *27:209, 1990.)*

Transcription

Whereas several mutations alter the promoter region upstream of the β-globin mRNA-encoding sequence, impairing mRNA synthesis, mutations that derange the sequence used as the signal for the addition of the poly-(A) tail of the mRNA (polyadenylation signal[21] have been shown to result in abnormal cleavage and polyadenylation of the nascent mRNA precursor, with resulting reduced accumulation of mature mRNA.[19-21]

Processing

Many forms of β-thalassemia are caused by mutations that impair splicing of the mRNA precursor into mature mRNA in the nucleus or that prevent translation of the mRNA in the cytoplasm. The molecular pathology of splicing mutations is complex (see Fig. 38-1). Some base substitutions ablate the donor (GT) or acceptor (AG) dinucleotides, which are absolutely required at the intron–exon boundaries for normal splicing and thereby completely block production of mature functional messenger RNA. Thus, no β-globin can be synthesized (β^0-thalassemia). Other mutations alter the consensus sequences that surround the GT- and AG-invariant dinucleotides and decrease the efficiency of normal splicing signals by 70% to 95%, resulting in β^+-thalassemia; some consensus mutations even abolish splicing completely, causing β^0-thalassemia. A third type of splicing aberration results from mutations that are not in the immediate vicinity of a normal splice site. These alter regions within the gene, called *cryptic splice sites,* which resemble consensus splicing sites but do not normally sustain splicing (Fig. 38-2). The mutations activate the site by supplying a critical GT or AG nucleotide or by creating a sufficiently strong consensus signal to stimulate splicing at that site 60% to 100% of the time. The activated cryptic sites generate an abnormally spliced, untranslatable mRNA species. Only 10% to 40% of the mRNA precursors are thus spliced at the normal sites, which causes β^+-thalassemia of variable severity. The mutation responsible for the most common form of β-thalassemia among Greeks and Cypriots (see Fig. 38-2) activates a cryptic splice site near the 3′ end of the first intron (position 110).[26,27] The determinants that dictate the degree to which each mutation alters splice site use remain largely unknown.

Translation

Mutations that abolish translation occur at several locations along the mature mRNA and are very common causes of β^0-thalassemia (see Fig. 38-1 and Table 38-1). The most common form of β^0-thalassemia in Sardinians results from a base substitution in the gene that changes

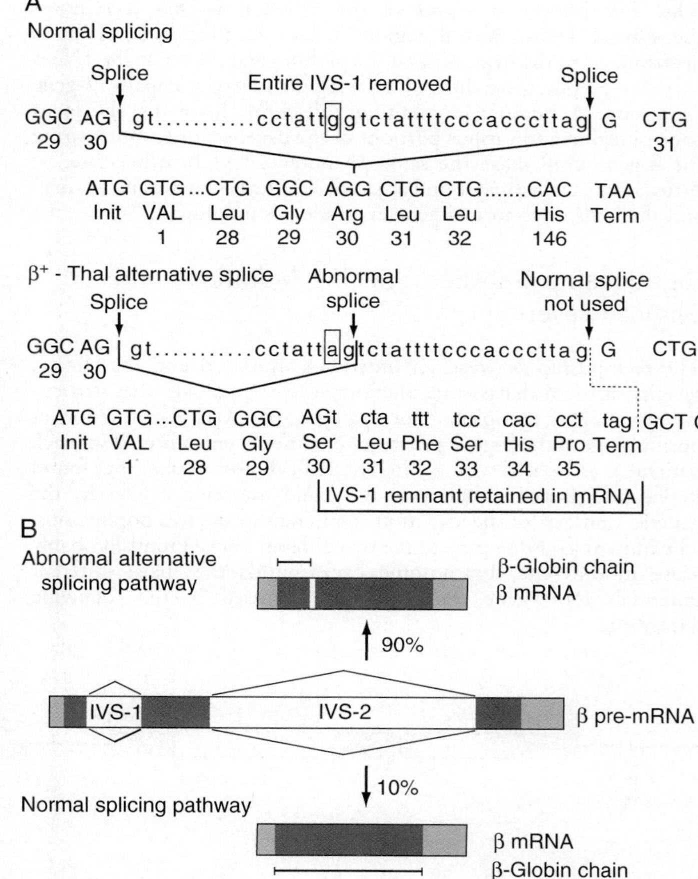

Figure 38-2 β^+-THALASSEMIA ARISING FROM ALTERNATIVE MRNA SPLICING CAUSED BY A MUTATION ACTIVATING A CRYPTIC SPLICING SITE. **A,** The G→A mutation is shown enclosed in *squares* located near the 3′ end of intron 1 (IVS-1); it creates a sequence motif closely mimicking a pre-mRNA acceptor splice site. The product of the alternative splicing event is also shown. Note that use of the activated cryptic site generates a mature mRNA that contains an in-frame termination codon and therefore does not encode a functional β-globin chain. (From Benz EJ Jr: The hemoglobinopathies. In Kelly WN, DeVita VT, editors: *Textbook of Internal Medicine,* Philadelphia, 1988, JB Lippincott, p 1423.) **B,** Diagram of the means by which use of the cryptic splice site 90% of the time results in only 10% of the mRNA precursor molecules to be spliced normally into translatable mature mRNA, thus causing β^+-thalassemia. *(Adapted from Bunn HF, Forget BG:* Hemoglobin: molecular, genetic and clinical aspects. *Philadelphia, WB Saunders, 1986.)*

the codon encoding the 39th amino acid of the β-globin chain from CAG, which encodes glutamine to TAG, whose equivalent (UAG) in mRNA specifies termination of translation (Fig.38-3).[28,29] A premature termination codon totally abrogates the ability of the mRNA to be translated into normal β-globin. Premature translation termination also results indirectly from frameshift mutations (i.e., small insertions or deletions of a few bases, other than multiples of 3, that alter the phase or frame in which the nucleotide sequence is read during translation).[29] An in-phase premature termination codon is usually encountered within the next 50 bases downstream from a frameshift.

Other Sites

Rare mutations that affect gene function by intriguing mechanisms have been described. An extremely large deletion of the β-globin gene cluster has been described that removes the ε-, γ-, and δ-genes.[30] The patient has a severe β-thalassemia phenotype, but the β-globin gene and 500 bases of adjacent 5′ and 3′ DNA have an entirely normal nucleotide sequence. The β-gene functions normally in surrogate cells. The important aspect of this deletion is that it removes the critical locus control region[18,31] located thousands of bases upstream from the beginning of the globin gene cluster at the 5′ end of the ε-globin gene; loss of this region severely impairs β-gene expression. A number of additional deletions involving the locus control region and various portions of the β-gene cluster, but sparing the β-gene itself, have the same phenotype.[1,2,19-21] In other cases of β-thalassemia, the β-gene and adjacent DNA are structurally normal, and the basis of abnormal gene expression is unknown.[22]

Relationship Between Specific Mutations and Clinical Severity

The relationship between an individual mutation and the clinical severity of the β-thalassemia phenotype associated with that particular mutation is complex.[22] For example, the A to G mutation at position -34 of the β-gene promoter commonly encountered in black patients is associated with a different clinical severity than that found in Chinese patients inheriting the same mutation.[32] Clearly, the genetic "context" of the mutation is different in the two populations. The mutant β-globin gene in the two different racial groups probably arose in different chromosome backgrounds that have different potentials for γ-gene expression, as discussed in the following paragraph.

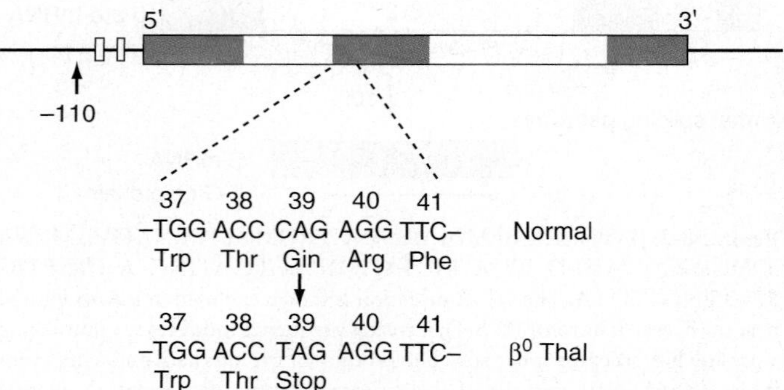

Figure 38-3 β°-THALASSEMIA ARISING FROM A MUTATION CHANGING AN AMINO ACID CODON TO A TERMINATION CODON (NONSENSE MUTATION). *(Adapted from Takeshita K, Forget BG, Scarpa A, Benz EJ Jr: Intranuclear defects in b-globin mRNA accumulation due to a premature translation termination codon.* Blood *64:13, 1984.)*

Multiple forms, or haplotypes, of normal non–α-globin gene clusters exist in various human populations. These are defined by the patterns of restriction fragment length polymorphisms[28] detected when DNA is digested with restriction endonucleases and analyzed by Southern gene blotting for the fragments bearing the non–α-globin genes. Haplotypes differ according to whether each restriction site is present or absent along the gene cluster. More than 12 haplotypes have been defined by examination of several restriction sites located along the cluster that are present or absent in a polymorphic manner in normal individuals.[28] The clinical variability encountered in two different groups bearing identical primary mutations correlates best with the haplotype or chromosome background on which the mutation is inherited. The differences in physiologically important functions among haplotypes that modulate severity remain unknown, but a possible explanation lies in the variable abilities of the γ-globin genes on different chromosomes to respond to severe erythroid stress by increased expression during postnatal life. The β-globin genes carried on some haplotypes differ in the degree to which they can respond in this manner.[33] Because Hb F synthesis reduces the severity of β-chain hemoglobinopathies,[1] the level of γ-gene expression from a given chromosome can play an important modulating role.

Pathophysiology

The biochemical hallmark of β-thalassemia is reduced biosynthesis of the β-globin subunit of Hb A ($\alpha_2\beta_2$). In β-thalassemia heterozygotes, β-globin synthesis is about half-normal (β/α synthetic ratio, 0.5-0.7). In homozygotes for β°-thalassemia, who account for approximately one-third of patients, β-globin synthesis is absent. β-globin synthesis is reduced to 5% to 30% of normal levels in β^+-thalassemia homozygotes or β^+/β°-thalassemia compound heterozygotes, who together account for approximately two-thirds of cases.[1]

Because the synthesis of Hb A ($\alpha_2\beta_2$) is markedly reduced or absent, the RBCs are hypochromic and microcytic. γ-Chain synthesis is partially reactivated so that the hemoglobin of the patient contains a relatively large proportion of Hb F.[1] However, these γ-chains are quantitatively insufficient to replace β-chain production.

In heterozygotes (β-thalassemia trait), relatively little α-globin accumulation occurs. Output from the single normal β-globin gene supports substantial Hb A formation, thus preventing harmful accumulation of excess α-globin chains. Thus, one encounters hypochromia with microcytosis but relatively little evidence of anemia, hemolysis, or IE.

Individuals inheriting two β-thalassemic alleles experience a more profound deficit of β-chain production. Little or no Hb A is produced; more importantly, the imbalance of α- and β-globin production is far more severe (Fig. 38-4). The limited capacity of RBCs to proteolyze the excess α-globin chains, a capacity that probably exerts a protective effect in heterozygous β-thalassemia, is overwhelmed in homozygotes. Free α-globin accumulates, and unpaired α-chains aggregate and precipitate to form inclusion bodies, which cause oxidative membrane damage within the RBC[34] and destruction of immature developing erythroblasts within the BM IE.[35] Consequently, relatively few of the erythroid precursors undergoing erythroid maturation in the BM survive long enough to be released into the bloodstream as erythrocytes. The occasional erythrocytes that are formed during erythropoiesis bear a burden of inclusion bodies. The reticuloendothelial cells in the spleen, liver, and BM remove these abnormal cells prematurely, producing a hemolytic anemia.

Defective β-globin synthesis exerts at least three distinct yet interrelated effects on the generation of oxygen-carrying capacity for the peripheral blood (see Fig. 38-4): (1) IE, which impairs production of new RBCs; (2) hemolytic anemia, which shortens the survival of the few RBCs produced; and (3) hypochromia with microcytosis, which reduces the oxygen-carrying capacity of the few RBCs that do survive.

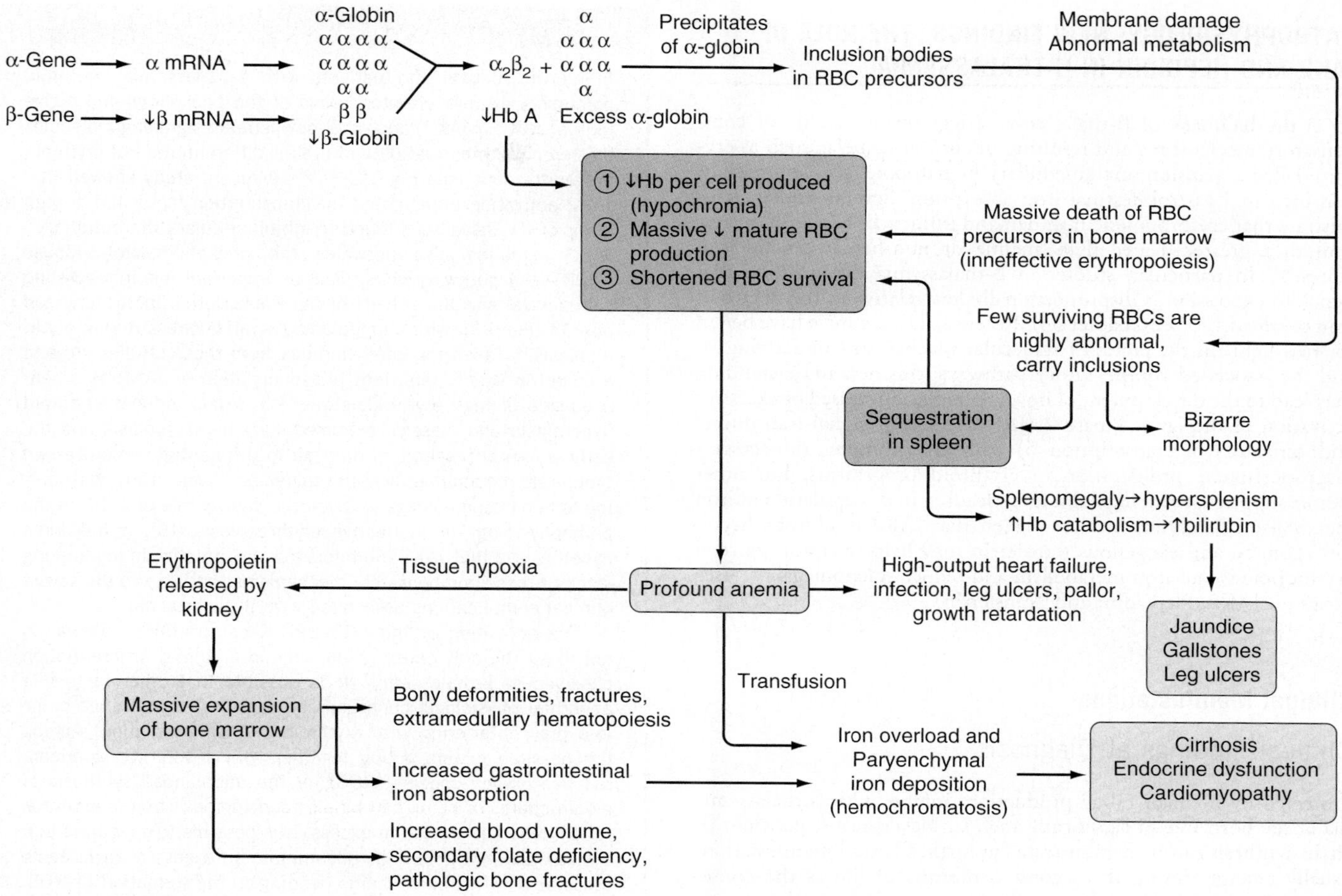

α-Globin
α α α α
α α α α
α α
β β
↓β-Globin
α-Gene → α mRNA
β-Gene → ↓β mRNA
$\alpha_2\beta_2$ + α α α
↓Hb A
α
α α α
α
Excess α-globin
Precipitates of α-globin
Inclusion bodies in RBC precursors
Membrane damage
Abnormal metabolism
① ↓Hb per cell produced (hypochromia)
② Massive ↓ mature RBC production
③ Shortened RBC survival
Massive death of RBC precursors in bone marrow (inneffective erythropoiesis)
Few surviving RBCs are highly abnormal, carry inclusions
Sequestration in spleen
Bizarre morphology
Splenomegaly→hypersplenism
↑Hb catabolism→↑bilirubin
Jaundice
Gallstones
Leg ulcers
Erythropoietin released by kidney
Tissue hypoxia
Profound anemia
High-output heart failure, infection, leg ulcers, pallor, growth retardation
Transfusion
Massive expansion of bone marrow
Bony deformities, fractures, extramedullary hematopoiesis
Increased gastrointestinal iron absorption
Increased blood volume, secondary folate deficiency, pathologic bone fractures
Iron overload and Paryenchymal iron deposition (hemochromatosis)
Cirrhosis
Endocrine dysfunction
Cardiomyopathy

Figure 38-4 PATHOPHYSIOLOGY OF SEVERE FORMS OF β-THALASSEMIA. The diagram outlines the pathogenesis of clinical abnormalities resulting from the primary defect in β-globin chain synthesis. *RBC,* Red blood cell.

In the most severe forms of the disorder, these three factors conspire to produce a catastrophic anemia complicated by the effects of exuberant hemolysis.

The profound deficit in the oxygen-carrying capacity of the blood stimulates production of high levels of erythropoietin in an attempt to promote compensatory erythroid hyperplasia. Unfortunately, the ability of the BM to respond positively is markedly impaired by IE. Massive BM expansion does occur, but very few erythrocytes are actually supplied to the circulation. The BM becomes packed with immature erythroid precursors, which die from their burden of precipitated α-globin chains before they reach the reticulocyte stage. Profound anemia persists, driving erythroid hyperplasia to still higher levels. In some cases, erythropoiesis is so exuberant that masses of extramedullary erythropoietic tissue form in the chest, abdomen, or pelvis.

As described in the following section, massive BM expansion exerts numerous adverse effects on the growth, development, and function of critical organ systems and creates the characteristic facies caused by maxillary BM hyperplasia and frontal bossing (Fig. 38-5). Hemolytic anemia results in massive splenomegaly and high-output congestive heart failure. In untreated cases, death occurs during the first 2 decades of life. Treatment with RBC transfusions sufficient to maintain hemoglobin levels above 9.0 to 10.0 g/dL improves oxygen delivery, suppresses the excessive IE, and prolongs life. Unfortunately, as discussed in more detail later, complications of chronic transfusion therapy, including iron overload, can be fatal before 30 years of age. The addition of iron chelation therapy to regular transfusion therapy now prolongs survival and improves the quality of life.

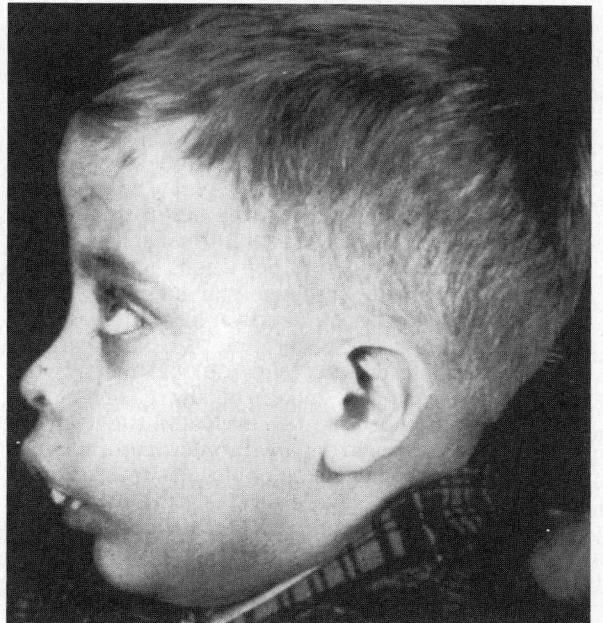

Figure 38-5 THALASSEMIC FACIES. See text for description. *(From Jurkiewicz MJ, Pearson HA, Furlow LT Jr: Reconstruction of the maxilla in thalassemia.* Ann N Y Acad Sci *165:437, 1969.)*

PATHOPHYSIOLOGY: NEW FINDINGS, THE ROLE OF JAK2 AND HEPCIDIN IN β-THALASSEMIA

IE is the hallmark of β-thalassemia, triggering a cascade of compensatory mechanisms and resulting in clinical sequelae such as erythroid BM expansion, extramedullary hematopoiesis, splenomegaly, and increased gastrointestinal iron absorption. Several studies demonstrate that erythropoietic iron demand influences hepcidin expression to a greater degree than anemia or non-hematopoietic iron stores.[36,37] In particular, studies in β-thalassemia demonstrate that hepcidin expression is disproportionally low relative to the degree of iron overload.[38-40] (see Chapter 33). Recent studies in mice have begun to shed light on the complex molecular mechanisms underlying IE and the associated compensatory pathways; this new understanding may lead to the development of novel therapies. Increased or excessive activation of the Janus kinase 2 (JAK2)–STAT5 (signal transducers and activators of transcription 5) pathway promotes unnecessary disproportionate proliferation of erythroid progenitors, but other factors suppress serum hepcidin levels leading to dysregulation of iron metabolism. Preclinical studies suggest that JAK2 inhibitors, hepcidin agonists, and exogenous transferrin may help to restore normal erythropoiesis and iron metabolism and reduce splenomegaly[41-51] (see boxes on JAK2, Hepcidin, and Transferrin).

Clinical Manifestations

Clinical Findings at Diagnosis

Protected by prenatal Hb F production, infants with β-thalassemia major are born free of significant anemia. Nevertheless, deficient β-chain synthesis can be demonstrated at birth. Clinical manifestations usually emerge during the second 6 months of life as the consequences of defective β-globin synthesis on overall hemoglobin production become more pronounced. The diagnosis is almost always evident by 2 years of age.[90] Pallor, irritability, growth retardation, abdominal swelling caused by enlargement of the liver and spleen, and jaundice are the usual presenting features.[91] Facial and skeletal changes caused by BM expansion develop later.

Clinical Findings in Untreated or Undertreated Patients

Untreated patients die in late infancy or early childhood as a consequence of severe anemia. In a retrospective review from Italy, the average survival of children with untreated thalassemia major was less than 4 years; approximately 80% died in the first 5 years of life.[92] Patients who receive transfusions sporadically may live somewhat longer than untransfused patients, but their quality of life is extremely poor as a result of both the chronic anemia and the IE. The low hemoglobin level and massive organomegaly are usually disabling, and the changes in the facial bones are disfiguring. After 10 to 20 years of weakness, stunted growth, and impaired activity, the undertransfused patients usually succumb to congestive heart failure.

This disastrous symptom constellation, so prevalent in the past, is now rare in North America and most industrialized countries. Nonetheless, the clinical manifestations and complications of untreated or undertreated β-thalassemia major illustrate the principles of the pathophysiology. Furthermore, these descriptions accurately characterize the disease that is still prevalent in many parts of the world.

Initial Laboratory Findings

The anemia of thalassemia major is characterized by severe hypochromia and microcytosis. The hemoglobin level decreases progressively

JAK2

In murine models and patients with β-thalassemia, erythroid precursors express elevated levels of the phosphorylated active form of JAK2 (pJAK2) and other downstream signaling molecules that promote proliferation and inhibit differentiation of erythroid progenitor cells (see Fig. 38-3).[52,53] A recent study showed that JAK2 activation upregulated the transcription factor ID1[54]; high levels of ID1 have been found to inhibit cellular differentiation.[53] JAK2 signaling also activates the phosphoinositol-3-kinase (PI3K)–AKT pathway, which plays an important role in regulating cell survival and the activity of the transcription factor forkhead box O3 (FOXO3), which modulates oxidative stress during erythropoiesis.[53] Taken together, findings from these studies suggest a model in which persistent phosphorylation of JAK2 as a consequence of high erythropoietin (EPO) levels induces erythroid hyperplasia and massive extramedullary hematopoiesis and the early erythroid progenitors that fail to differentiate colonize and proliferate predominantly in the spleen and liver,[52] thus contributing to hepatosplenomegaly. Given the central role of JAK2 in the pathophysiology of ineffective erythropoiesis (IE), it has been hypothesized that JAK2 inhibitors may be effective in modulating some of these compensatory mechanisms that lead to the severe clinical complications associated with β-thalassemia.

The activation of the EPO–EPO-Receptor–JAK2 pathway is not likely the only cause of the limited erythroid differentiation observed in β-thalassemia. It is possible that other factors or abnormal physiologic conditions present in β-thalassemia come into play, interfering with erythroid cell differentiation. Among the possible factors acting together with JAK2, iron overload, reactive oxygen species (ROS), or the unbalanced synthesis of globin chains or heme can be also considered.[55] Iron is essential for all cells but is toxic in excess. It is possible to speculate that thalassemic erythroid cells accumulate an excess of toxic heme associated with free α-chains, leading to the formation of ROS, which has been involved with cell RBC hemolysis and altered differentiation.[56,57]

Serum iron is bound to transferrin and enters erythroid cells primarily via receptor-mediated endocytosis of the transferrin receptor (TfR1). TfR1 is essential for developing erythrocytes, and reduced TfR1 expression is associated with anemia. *STAT5*-null mice are severely anemic and die perinatally. Two studies associated STAT5 to iron homeostasis showing that ablation of STAT5 leads to a dramatic reduction in the iron regulatory protein 2 (IRP-2) and *Tfr1* mRNA and protein.[58,59] Both genes were demonstrated to be direct transcriptional targets of STAT5, establishing a clear link between EPO-R–JAK2–STAT signaling and iron metabolism. Therefore, it is possible that activation of JAK2 might increase erythroid iron intake and that this might be detrimental in thalassemic cells, in which part of the iron ends up in toxic hemichromes (α-chain/heme aggregates), triggering ROS formation.

The persistent phosphorylation of JAK2 leads to an increased number of surviving erythroid precursors, contributing to the IE. Therefore, suppression of JAK2 activity may modulate IE. Based on this hypothesis, a JAK2 inhibitor was utilized for 10 days in mice affected by thalassemia intermedia (Hbbth3/+) and demonstrated a reduction in splenomegaly ("nonsurgical splenectomy").[52] This study also demonstrated that JAK2 inhibitors decreased the number of cells expressing cell cycle–related genes and partially reversed the IE, ameliorating the ratio between erythroid precursors and enucleated RBCs.[52,60] Thus, although a complete understanding of how JAK2 inhibitors achieve this effect is unavailable, modulation of cell cycle and differentiation are likely involved.

Hepcidin

Iron absorption and recycling are regulated by the peptide hormone hepcidin, the main regulator of body iron flows. Hepcidin exerts its function by binding to the only known iron export protein, ferroportin (FPN-1), found on all cells involved in iron metabolism; binding FPN-1 results in its internalization, degradation, and cessation of iron export.[61] Regulation of hepcidin is influenced by iron, hypoxia, inflammation, and erythropoiesis, possibly through distinct mechanisms. In the recent past, major advances have been made in understanding the molecular mechanism of hepcidin regulation.[62] In short, in the liver, the bone morphogenic protein (BMP) pathway plays a central role in hepcidin regulation by iron.[63,64] When BMP6 and hemojuvelin (HJV) interact with BMP receptors type I/II, phosphorylation and activation of the small mothers against decapentaplegic (SMAD) complex results in increased hepcidin expression.[65] Additionally, holo-Tf regulates hepcidin expression through TfR2 and HFE. Holo-Tf binds both TfR1 and TfR2, although it has a stronger affinity for TfR1. In a proposed model, HFE associates with TfR1 under low iron conditions and is displaced when TfR1 binds holo-Tf.[66-68] As serum iron and holo-Tf concentrations rise, the ratio of TfR2 to TfR1 expression increases. Together, this leads to TfR2/holo-Tf membrane stabilization and induces HFE/TfR2 binding and hepcidin expression.[69,70] Mutations in many of these genes are central to the pathophysiology of hereditary hemochromatoses (HH) in which insufficient hepcidin expression is a common feature (reviewed elsewhere).[71]

Several studies demonstrate that erythropoietic iron demand influences hepcidin expression to a greater degree than anemia or nonhematopoietic iron stores.[36,37] In particular, studies in β-thalassemia demonstrate that hepcidin expression is disproportionally low relative to the degree of iron overload.[38-40] These and previous studies proposed that an “erythroid factor” suppresses hepcidin synthesis.[72] This “erythroid regulator” is likely a factor secreted either from immature and proliferating or dying erythroid precursors. If this factor is secreted by immature erythroid precursors, it would be present in all conditions in which erythroid precursor expansion occurs (e.g., after recovery from phlebotomy and transient anemia in blood donors).[73,74] Twisted gastrulation-1 (TWSG1) has been isolated from immature erythroid precursors in β-thalassemic mice.[75] As a small secreted cysteine-rich protein able to influence BMPs signaling, the expression of TWSG1 is increased in β-thalassemic mice and represses hepcidin in vitro.[75,76] However, whether this factor is present in other conditions and how efficiently TWSG1 represses hepcidin in physiologic conditions are still unclear. If the proposed “erythroid factor” is secreted by dying erythroid precursors, it would be present only in conditions in which large numbers of erythroid precursors undergo apoptosis. Growth differentiation factor-15 (GDF15) has been isolated from the sera of β-thalassemic patients and in other individuals exhibiting features of IE, such as MDS and congenital dyserythropoietic anemia type I and II and an inverse correlation with hepcidin levels has been demonstrated.[77-79] GDF15 is a member of the TGF-β superfamily of proteins, which are known to control cell proliferation, differentiation, and apoptosis in numerous cell types. However, it is possible that in conditions such as β-thalassemia, multiple “erythroid factors” suppress hepcidin expression.[80,81] The mechanisms of action of GDF15 and TWSG1 in repressing hepcidin expression remain undefined but are likely to alter the function of proteins that modulate hepcidin production.

Based on these and previous observations, it has been postulated that in β-thalassemic patients, more iron is absorbed than required for erythropoiesis. Thus, decreasing dietary iron intake or hepcidin administration might prevent iron overload. In fact, mice affected by thalassemia intermedia (Hbb*th3*/+) avoid iron overload when placed on a low-iron diet or are engineered to overexpress a moderate level of hepcidin.[82] Reversal of iron overload results in reduced erythroid iron intake, limiting the synthesis of heme and the formation of hemichromes and reactive oxygen species.[82] Because hemichromes and ROS cause IE in ß-thalassemia, iron restriction and decreased erythroid iron intake result in more effective erythropoiesis, normalize RBC morphology and lifespan, increase circulating Hb, and reverse splenomegaly.[60,82] Thus, the use of hepcidin agonists or drugs that increase hepcidin expression decreases iron uptake from the diet, reduces iron overload, and improves erythropoiesis in TI.[82] In TM, repeated blood transfusions are the principal cause of iron overload. Despite iron overload, hepcidin concentrations are low; transfusion also suppresses endogenous erythropoiesis and, as a consequence, results in a transient increase in hepcidin.[38,83,84] Although intestinal iron absorption contributes part of the total iron load in these patients, hepcidin therapy may be effective in conjunction with transfusion to prevent intestinal iron uptake when endogenous hepcidin falls.

Transferrin

Iron directed to the erythroid compartment is restricted to Tf-bound iron, and its relationship with TfR1 is well established.[85] Tf takes up iron from duodenal enterocytes (when it is absorbed) and from macrophages (when iron is recycled from senescent RBCs). The amount of iron delivered to each erythroid precursor depends on the amount of monoferric- and holo-Tf found in circulation as well as the density of TfR1 on the cell surface. Typically, each erythroid precursor has more than 1 million TfR1s on its membrane because of its large iron requirement, greater than all other cell types.[86] Iron uptake starts when holo-Tf binds TfR1. Under normal circumstances, the affinity of TfR1 for holo-Tf is greater than for monoferric-Tf. However, this greater affinity wanes as the iron supply is diminished.[87] Monoferric-Tf is the predominant form of Tf in circulation when Tf saturation is lowered.[88] Each molecule of monoferric-Tf delivers less iron to erythroid precursors than holo-Tf.[87] This enables a greater number of erythroid precursors to receive a smaller portion of the iron pool to offset developing anemia and is consistent with a low MCV and MCH.

Transferrin receptor takes up iron from duodenal enterocytes where iron is absorbed and from macrophages when iron is recycled from senescent RBCs and delivers it to cells by binding TfR1. Tf saturation is the main player in determining the rate of erythroid iron intake, modulating erythropoiesis. In turn, erythropoiesis influences hepcidin expression in the liver. Therefore, reducing the saturation levels of Tf might have beneficial effects in β-thalassemia, decreasing formation of hemichromes in the RBCs as well as the florid erythropoiesis that suppresses hepcidin expression in the liver. In fact, chronic treatment with apo-Tf injections in *Hbbth1/th1* mice (another murine model of thalassemia intermedia) results in increased Hb production, decreased reticulocytosis and serum EPO levels, reverses splenomegaly, and elevates hepcidin expression.[89] Apo-Tf injections reduce hemichrome formation and change the proportion of erythroid precursors to more mature relative to immature precursors, lower the rates of apoptosis in mature erythroid precursors, and reduce the amount of extramedullary erythropoiesis in the liver and spleen in *Hbbth1/th1* mice. These observations suggest that addition of exogenous apo-Tf results in decreased Tf saturation and likely a shift toward more monoferric-Tf molecules with more Tf molecules available to deliver smaller amounts of iron to more erythroid precursors, resulting in further decreased MCH and fewer hemichromes. However, how additional apo-Tf is able to improve erythropoiesis in *Hbbth1/th1* mice is incompletely understood.

during the first months of life. When the child becomes symptomatic, the hemoglobin level may be as low as 3 to 4 g/dL. RBC morphology is strikingly abnormal, with many microcytes, bizarre poikilocytes, teardrop cells, and target cells (Fig. 38-6). A characteristic finding is the presence of extraordinarily hypochromic, often wrinkled and folded cells (leptocytes) containing irregular inclusion bodies of precipitated α-globin chains (see box on Clinical Heterogeneity of Thalassemia).

Nucleated RBCs are frequently present. The reticulocyte count is 2% to 8% lower than would be expected in view of the extreme erythroid hyperplasia and hemolysis. The low count reflects the severity of intramedullary erythroblast destruction. The white blood cell count is elevated. A moderate polymorphonuclear leukocytosis and normal platelet count are typical unless hypersplenism has developed. The BM exhibits marked hypercellularity caused by erythroid hyperplasia. The RBC precursors show defective hemoglobinization and reduced amounts of cytoplasm.

Clinical Heterogeneity of Thalassemia

The severity of β-thalassemia is remarkable for its variability in different patients. Two siblings inheriting identical thalassemia mutations sometimes exhibit markedly different degrees of anemia and erythroid hyperplasia. Many factors contribute to this clinical heterogeneity. Individual alleles vary with respect to severity of the biosynthetic lesion. Other modifying factors ameliorate the burden of unpaired α-globin. High levels of Hb F expression persist to widely various degrees in β-thalassemia. Because γ-globin can substitute for β-globin, simultaneously generating more functional hemoglobins and reducing the α-globin inclusion burden, this is a powerful modulating factor. Theoretically, patients may also vary in their ability to solubilize unpaired globin chains by proteolysis. Occasional heterozygous patients have had more severe anemia than expected, possibly because of defects in these proteolytic systems or because of the type of thalassemic mutation. Inheritance of more than the usual complement of α-globin genes may also increase with severity of β-thalassemia because of additional production of unpaired α-globin chains. All of these factors emphasize the essential role of α-globin inclusions in the pathophysiology of β-thalassemia.

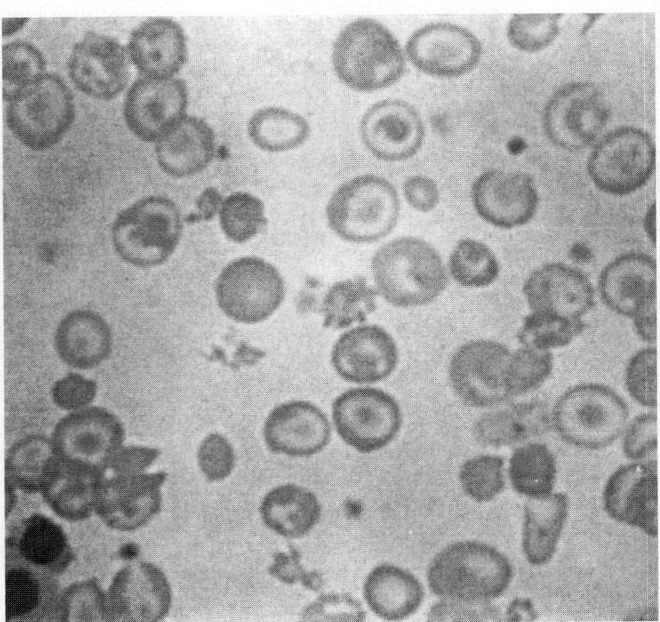

Figure 38-6 MORPHOLOGIC APPEARANCE OF THE PERIPHERAL BLOOD FILM IN A CASE OF SEVERE β-THALASSEMIA. Note the many bizarre cells, the hypochromia, nucleated red blood cells, target cells, and leptocytes. *(From Pearson HA, Benz EJ Jr: Thalassemia syndromes. In Miller DR, Baehner RL, McMillan CW, editors:* Smith's blood diseases of infancy and childhood, *ed 5, St. Louis, 1984, CV Mosby, p 439.)*

The osmotic fragility is strikingly abnormal. The RBCs are so markedly resistant to hemolysis in hypotonic sodium chloride solution that some are not entirely hemolyzed even in distilled water. Before transfusion therapy is initiated, the serum iron and transferrin saturation are already increased as a result of increased iron absorption.[93]

The hemoglobin profile reveals predominantly Hb F. In patients with homozygous β°-thalassemia, no Hb A is found throughout life. Hb A may be undetectable in the newborn with β^+-thalassemia and is present in reduced amounts in later life. The levels of Hb A_2 in thalassemia major are variable, probably because of increased numbers of F cells that have a decreased Hb A_2 content.[1] Other biochemical abnormalities of the RBC in cases of thalassemia major include a postnatal persistence of the i antigen and a decrease of RBC carbonic anhydrase; these findings are probably also caused by the elevated levels of circulating F cells.

The intraerythrocytic inclusions in the peripheral blood cells of patients with thalassemia, first described by Fessas,[94] are especially prominent after splenectomy. These inclusions, best seen by staining with methyl violet or by phase microscopy, are aggregates of precipitated, denatured α-chains.[95] They are also found in large numbers within erythroid precursors in the BM.

The serum is icteric; unconjugated bilirubin levels are in the range of 2.0 to 4.0 mg/dL at the time of diagnosis but may rise substantially as the anemia worsens in the absence of transfusion. RBC survival in cases of thalassemia major is variable but usually markedly decreased. The ^{51}Cr half-life ranges between 6.5 and 19.5 days compared with the normal half-life of 25 to 35 days.[35] Increased plasma iron turnover and poor use of radiolabeled iron indicate IE.[35] Serum aspartate aminotransferase levels are frequently increased at diagnosis because of hemolysis. Alanine aminotransferase levels are usually normal before transfusion therapy but may rise subsequently because of iron-induced hepatic damage or viral hepatitis. Lactate dehydrogenase levels are markedly elevated as a consequence of IE. Haptoglobin and hemopexin are reduced or absent.[96]

Later Laboratory Findings

Serum zinc levels may fall to abnormally low levels. A relationship between this finding and growth failure has been postulated but not established.[97,98] Low levels of plasma and leukocyte ascorbic acid are common in thalassemic patients because of increased metabolism of the vitamin to oxalic acid in the presence of iron overload.[99,100] Biochemical evidence of folic acid deficiency may occur as a result of excessive consumption secondary to increased requirements.[101,102] The serum levels of α-tocopherol are often reduced to less than 0.5 mg/dL, and increased RBC membrane lipid peroxidation has been described.[103-105]

Coagulation abnormalities consistent with liver disease (i.e., lowered levels of factors II, V, VII, IX, and X) may occur in older patients with hepatitis or iron-induced hepatic injury.[106] Only rarely are the abnormalities sufficient to require specific therapy. However, the combination of mild thrombocytopenia from hypersplenism and low coagulation factors and platelet dysfunction from liver disease may cause or aggravate bleeding.[107]

Numerous laboratory abnormalities reflect the accumulation of excessive iron and the consequences of iron-induced organ damage, and they are described in the following sections.

Treatment

The advent of modern therapy has had a major impact on the clinical and laboratory features of thalassemia major. Transfusion and chelation therapy, described subsequently in detail, have ameliorated many of the most striking manifestations of the disease. Bone marrow transplantation (BMT) has allowed for the cure of a select few. However, these therapies have created their own complications; therefore, this section addresses the treatment of the complications of thalassemia and its therapy. Current clinical management and associated clinical manifestations and complications have been reviewed in a number of publications.[108-113]

Transfusion Therapy

Transfusion therapy for thalassemia was once sparingly administered as a palliative measure when patients became symptomatic. These periodic transfusion regimens were unsatisfactory even for those limited purposes; symptoms of anemia and the cosmetic and other consequences of overgrowth of erythropoietic tissue rendered life unpleasant and uncomfortable for patients. Consequently, several centers initiated transfusion programs in which patients received regular transfusions to keep their hemoglobin levels high enough to ameliorate these symptoms,[114,115] but the median survival time of patients transfused to maintain hemoglobin levels of 7 to 8 g/dL in the United States in the 1960s was only 17 years of age.[115,116] These "hypertransfusion" programs were designed initially to maintain hemoglobin levels above 8 g/dL. In the more modern application of hypertransfusion therapy, hemoglobin levels are usually maintained above 9 to 10.5 g/dL.

The clinical benefits of hypertransfusion programs are dramatic. The growth of younger children follows normal percentiles for height and weight.[117] Erythropoiesis is partially but substantially suppressed as evidenced by decreased numbers of reticulocytes and normoblasts and transferrin receptor levels.[118,119] Hypertransfusion reduces or prevents the enlargement of the liver and spleen. Abnormal facies and bone fractures occur less frequently. The overall sense of well-being allows normal age-appropriate activities[120,121] (see box on Guidelines for Transfusion Therapy).

A more vigorous transfusion program (supertransfusion) aimed at keeping hemoglobin levels above 12.0 g/dL is no longer recommended.[122] This approach rested on the assumption that the benefits of further suppression of erythropoiesis and gastrointestinal iron absorption will offset the increased need for RBCs. However, several, although not all, studies have demonstrated that transfusion requirements (and therefore the rates of transfusional iron loading) increase as the hemoglobin level is raised (Fig. 38-7).[117,123,124] As a result, the consistent maintenance of hemoglobin levels above 11 or 12 g/dL is generally reserved for patients with poor tolerance of lower hemoglobin levels because of cardiac disease or other reasons.

Alternative approaches to conventional transfusion therapy have been proposed in an effort to reduce the rate of transfusion iron loading. These approaches have generally relied on the concept that younger RBCs (neocytes) will circulate longer in the recipient than older RBCs. Preclinical experiments based on the difference in density between younger and older RBCs established the validity of this approach.[125,126] However, in prospective clinical trials, blood requirements were reduced only by 13% to 20%.[127-129] This reduction in iron loading did not outweigh the disadvantages of neocyte transfusions that included increased cost, wastage of 50% of the donor RBCs, and increased donor exposures. The use of automated exchange transfusion has been proposed as another approach to reducing iron loading in patients with thalassemia.[130] With this method, RBCs are removed from the patient at the same time that new donor RBCs are transfused. This approach has been applied successfully to transfusion therapy for sickle cell disease. However, the goal of transfusion therapy in sickle cell disease is the replacement of Hb S–containing RBCs with Hb A–containing RBCs irrespective of the total hemoglobin level. In contrast, the goal of transfusion therapy in patients with thalassemia is to maintain a specific total hemoglobin level. Despite these different goals, studies of automated exchange transfusion in patients with thalassemia have demonstrated a reduction in net RBC requirements of 30% to 50%, either by reducing the amount of blood administered at the usual transfusion interval or by prolonging the interval between transfusions.[130,131] The benefits of this approach are probably attributable to the removal of previously transfused RBCs from the patients and replacement with younger, recently donated RBCs, reducing the overall age of the circulating RBC population. Further clinical trials of automated exchange transfusion in thalassemia are currently underway.

The decision to initiate transfusion therapy should take into account the overall clinical condition of the patient as well as the hemoglobin level. Patients with severe and persistent anemia (hemoglobin <6-7 g/dL) usually also have failure to thrive, decreased activity level, and irritability. For these patients, transfusion therapy should begin after confirmation of the diagnosis of thalassemia and after demonstration that acute factors such as a febrile illness or folic acid deficiency are not confounding the assessment of the severity of anemia. For patients with higher hemoglobin levels, the decision to begin transfusion depends on the careful assessment of the child's clinical findings. For example, some children with thalassemia have early and pronounced facial bone deformities caused by BM expansion despite a hemoglobin level of 8 g/dL or higher. For such children, the benefits of transfusion therapy may outweigh the risks. In contrast, some patients with thalassemia have little or no clinical difficulty despite a persistent hemoglobin level of 7 to 8 g/dL, and the benefits of transfusion therapy may be small. Determination of

Guidelines for Transfusion Therapy

Although some of the details of a transfusion program for patients with thalassemia major vary from center to center, the following guidelines are important for achieving the benefits while controlling the risks of a transfusion program. The rationales for these guidelines are discussed in the text.

1. Obtain a complete RBC antigen profile before the first transfusion.
2. Administer 10 to 15 mL/kg of RBCs every 2 to 4 weeks to maintain the pretransfusion hemoglobin level above 9 to 10.5 g/dL.
3. Use leukoreduced RBCs that have been stored for less than 7 to 10 days.
4. Avoid the use of first-degree relatives as blood donors.
5. For patients who come to a new center after receiving transfusions elsewhere, contact the previous blood bank for information about alloantibodies.

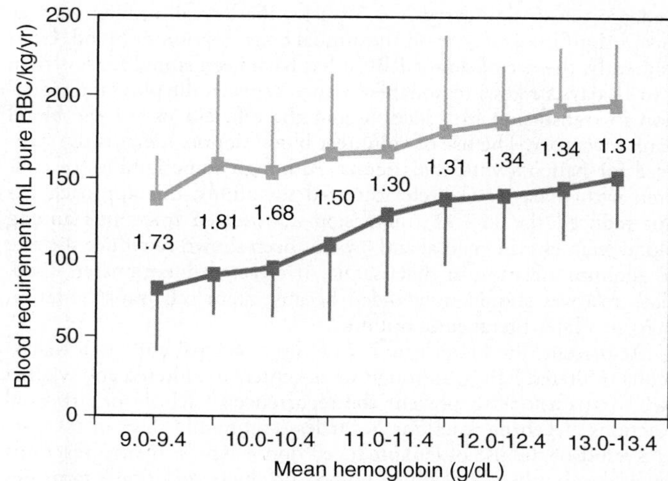

Figure 38-7 Relationship between transfusion requirements and mean hemoglobin level maintained by patients with thalassemia major. *(Adapted from Rebulla P, Modell B: Transfusion requirements and effects in patients with thalassemia major.* Lancet *337:277, 1991.)*

Deciding to Begin Transfusion Therapy in Patients With Thalassemia

The decision to initiate regular RBC transfusions is one of the most important—and sometimes most difficult—steps in the management of patients with thalassemia. Regular RBC transfusions not only distinguish thalassemia major from thalassemia intermedia but also commit the patient to long-term chelation therapy to control the transfusional iron loading. The decision should include consideration of both clinical and laboratory findings. Children who are growing poorly and developing disfiguring bone changes will benefit from regular transfusions even if their hemoglobin levels are 8 to 9 g/dL. On the other hand, children who are asymptomatic at hemoglobin levels of 7 to 8 g/dL may have little to gain from transfusions. Hemoglobin levels below 7 g/dL are usually associated with problems related to both the anemia and the compensatory erythropoiesis. When the hemoglobin level is consistently less than 7 g/dL, there is usually little to be gained from delaying transfusion.

genotype may provide some guidance by distinguishing patients with more severe defects in β-globin production from those with less severe defects, but the overlap between genotype and phenotype in thalassemia still requires reliance on clinical assessment (see box on Deciding to Begin Transfusion Therapy in Patients With Thalassemia).

Before the first blood transfusion is given to a child with thalassemia major, a complete RBC antigen profile should be obtained. This information is valuable for identifying minor blood group incompatibility if alloimmunization develops later and helps to distinguish alloantibodies from autoantibodies. The value of extended matching of donor RBCs has not been established in cases of thalassemia, but experience with sickle cell disease suggests that matching for the full Rh system as well as the Kell antigen may reduce the rate of alloimmunization.

In practice, the goal of maintaining the hemoglobin level above 9 to 10.5 g/dL is usually achieved by administration of approximately 15 mL/kg/mo or 1 to 2 units of donor RBCs every 2 to 5 weeks. Patients with heart disease may need smaller aliquots of RBCs at more frequent intervals to prevent problems related to volume overload. In general, patients can receive the entire unit of donor packed RBCs. However, fractional units are appropriate for infants, small patients, and older patients with heart disease. With the use of current additive solutions, the duration of storage of donor RBCs has only a small effect on the 24-hour recovery and the survival of the RBCs in each transfused unit. However, for patients with thalassemia major who undergo transfusion every 2 to 5 weeks, these small differences may have a significant impact on the annual consumption of blood. Consequently, the use of donor RBCs that have been stored for less than 7 to 10 days strikes a reasonable balance between the potential reduction in transfusion iron loading and the efficient use of the blood bank inventory. The use of volunteer blood donors remains the standard for patients with thalassemia. Although some families of children with thalassemia prefer directed donations, this approach has not reduced the rate of transfusion-transmitted infections among blood recipients in general and has not been shown to reduce the rate of alloimmunization in thalassemia. If directed donations are used, close relatives should be avoided because stem cell transplantation may be a later therapeutic option.

At present, the blood product of choice for patients with thalassemia is filtered RBCs, although some centers use filtered and washed RBC transfusions to prevent the recurrence of febrile or urticarial reactions.[132] Febrile reactions occur less commonly than in the past as a result of the use of leukoreduced donor RBCs. If such reactions occur despite the use of filtered blood products, additional measures include pretransfusion therapy with acetaminophen and the use of washed or frozen-thawed RBCs. Urticarial and other allergic reactions can usually be managed with antihistamine therapy or, when persistent, pretransfusion administration of corticosteroids. Frozen-thawed RBCs are primarily useful for patients with multiple antibodies who require donor RBCs with rare phenotypes that must be collected and stored well in advance of the actual transfusion.

Red blood cell alloimmunization occurs in 3% to 23% of patients with thalassemia major.[124,132-135] If blood donors and recipients come from different ethnic backgrounds with different RBC antigen profiles, as in some North American thalassemia centers, the risk of alloimmunization is increased.[136] New alloantibodies may be clinically silent, associated with increasing transfusion requirements, or accompanied by signs of active hemolysis such as increasing jaundice and dark urine. As noted earlier, the use of extended antigen matching may help prevent alloimmunization. Initiation of transfusion therapy before the age of 3 years may also be associated with a lower risk of this complication.[124,135,137] Patients with a history of alloantibodies require particular attention when receiving a transfusion at a new hospital because the serologic studies may fail to detect a clinically significant antibody that is present in low amounts. A review of the blood bank records from the previous institutions is essential in choosing the appropriate RBC product.

Autoantibodies also occur in patients with thalassemia major, usually, but not always, after the development of an alloantibody.[138] A subset of patients with autoantibodies has a clinically important autoimmune hemolytic anemia that leads to the premature destruction of donor cells as well as destruction of the patient's own RBCs. Transfusion requirements are markedly increased, and further transfusion therapy may be impossible for some patients. Treatment with corticosteroids, other immunosuppressive therapy, or intravenous gamma globulin may improve RBC survival in some cases.

A syndrome of posttransfusion hypertension, convulsions, and cerebral hemorrhage has also been reported.[139] The mechanism underlying this complication is uncertain but is possibly related to large changes in hemoglobin level at the time of transfusion. These reactions are uncommon in conventional transfusion programs.

The potential impact of transfusion-transmitted infections on patients with thalassemia major is demonstrated by the high prevalence of human immunodeficiency virus (HIV) infection in certain thalassemia centers during the 1980s and the nearly universal problem with hepatitis C infection in patients who began transfusion therapy before the 1990s. A 1987 study found that 17% of patients with thalassemia major in one center in New York City were positive for HIV antibody.[140] The prevalence of hepatitis C infection among patients with thalassemia major is 12% to 91%, with a higher rate among older patients.[141,142] Improvements in donor screening and testing have markedly reduced the risk of transmission by transfusion of known viruses,[143] but patients with thalassemia, because of the frequency of their transfusions, remain at risk not only for viruses that are transmitted infrequently but also for new agents such as hepatitis A, babesiosis, and West Nile virus.[144] Hepatitis B vaccine, if not administered as part of the routine childhood immunization program, should be given to patients with thalassemia before transfusion therapy begins.[145] Hepatitis A vaccine should also be administered when age appropriate. The cytomegalovirus (CMV) status of patients who are potential candidates for stem cell transplantation should be ascertained prior to transfusion and every attempt should be made to provide them with CMV-negative blood products. Current studies of pathogen-inactivated RBC products hold forth the promise of a means for preventing transfusion-transmitted infections even when the donor's infection escapes detection or when new agents enter the blood supply.[146,147]

Progressive iron overload is the life-threatening complication of transfusion therapy that accounts for the most important long-term morbidity and mortality in patients with thalassemia major.

Chelation Therapy

The clinical effects of iron overload in patients with thalassemia major depend on the amount and the duration of excessive iron accumulation. Transfusion hemosiderosis is the major cause of late morbidity and mortality in patients with thalassemia major. Establishment of therapeutic strategies to achieve iron balance should lead to improved survival. Various strategies to reduce the rate of transfusion iron loading have included modifying the pretransfusion hemoglobin level, adjusting the intervals between transfusions and splenectomy as well as with methods to enhance the rate of iron removal through chelation therapy. Historically, efforts were focused on identifying methods to enhance parenteral iron chelation by adjusting the frequency of daily use, the hours of administration, and the route of parenteral administration. These have optimized the use of iron chelation with deferoxamine (Desferal, DFO). More recently, efforts are focused on addressing the safety and efficacy of new U.S. Food and Drug Administration (FA) approved oral iron chelators, deferasirox (Exjade) and deferiprone (L1), combination use of parenteral and oral iron chelators, and new ways to assess iron excess by magnetic resonance imaging (MRI).

Each unit of packed RBCs contains approximately 200 to 250 mg of iron. Based on usual blood requirements in patients with thalassemia major, the rate of transfusional iron accumulation is approximately 0.30 to 0.60 mg/kg/day. The massive IE associated with the intermedia and major thalassemias leads to excessive gastrointestinal iron absorption that adds to the transfusional iron burden, although absorption is reduced when a hemoglobin level above 9 g/dL is maintained.[148,149] Humans have no physiologic mechanism to induce significant excretion of excess iron. Phlebotomy, the most efficient method of removing iron in other situations, is precluded in severely anemic patients with thalassemia owing to transfusion dependence. Phlebotomy may be only applicable in a very few select patients with thalassemia intermedia and constitutes an important part of the management of patients with thalassemia major who have successfully undergone stem cell transplantation (see box on Benefits of Iron Chelation Therapy).

A pharmacologic approach using specific iron-chelating agents remains the only strategy for removing excess iron in transfusion-dependent patients.

Several drugs with chelating properties have been synthesized or recovered from microorganisms. Many lack iron specificity or are inefficient; others cause significant toxicity. To chelate iron, the chelating agent must complex with all of the iron atom's six available coordination sites. Three general classes of iron chelators occur or have been synthesized: hexadentate (deferoxamine), bidentate (deferiprone), and tridentate (deferasirox). Only one hexadentate molecule is necessary to bind one atom of iron, but three molecules of a bidentate iron chelator bind one iron atom and two molecules of a tridentate chelator are required to bind one atom of iron.

Chelatable iron is thought to be derived from the intracellular "labile iron pool"[150,151] and from non–transferrin-bound plasma iron.[152,153]

Benefits of Iron Chelation Therapy

More than 30 years of experience using iron chelation therapy with deferoxamine in thalassemia major patients have demonstrated that:

1. Liver iron concentrations can be maintained at normal or mildly elevated levels.
2. Hepatic fibrosis is slowed or prevented.
3. The risk of iron-induced cardiac disease, including heart failure and serious arrhythmias, is markedly decreased.
4. Normal growth and sexual development are common but not universal.
5. Long-term survival is substantially improved. These benefits are directly related to compliance and generally require the prolonged administration of deferoxamine at least five times per week.
6. Long-term safety and efficacy studies of the oral iron chelators deferiprone and deferasirox are ongoing.

Deferoxamine

Deferoxamine mesylate is a naturally occurring hexadentate siderophore isolated from cultures of *Streptomyces pilosus* introduced in 1960. Deferoxamine has a high molecular weight of approximately 600 g/mol, is poorly absorbed by the gastrointestinal tract, and is rapidly removed from the plasma. It has a relatively short half-life of 8 to 10 minutes, which necessitates intravenous or subcutaneous parenteral administration. It is a hexadentate iron chelator that binds iron in a one-to-one complex. It is highly specific for iron and is associated with relatively low toxicity.[154] Deferoxamine enters cells; chelates iron; and appears in the serum and bile as the iron chelate product, ferroxamine.[155] Deferoxamine chelates iron released by the reticuloendothelial systems (RES) after the catabolism of senescent RBCs and is excreted in the urine.[156] Unbound deferoxamine is absorbed by the hepatic parenchymal cells and chelates iron from the intracellular pool which is excreted in bile. Approximately one-half to two-thirds of the iron excreted in response to deferoxamine is in the stool, with the remainder in the urine.[157] These proportions vary from patient to patient and at different levels of iron overload, dose of deferoxamine, and endogenous erythropoietic activity.[158]

Iron excretion after the administration of deferoxamine is proportional to body iron stores. To achieve negative iron balance, the chelating agent must cause the daily excretion of 0.3 to 0.6 mg/kg of iron. In the 1960s, deferoxamine was initially administered by daily intramuscular injections of 0.5 g, which led to reduced rates of hepatic iron accumulation and hepatic fibrosis in patients with thalassemia.[159,160] However, intramuscular injections proved to be too painful and were insufficient to achieve negative iron balance. In the mid-1970s, it was demonstrated that iron excretion with deferoxamine at 20 to 60 mg/kg/day was markedly enhanced and negative iron balance was attained by continuous, prolonged 24-hour intravenous or 8- to 12-hour subcutaneous infusions administered via a lightweight battery-operated or balloon-driven pump.[161,162] In addition, maintaining normal ascorbic acid levels optimizes iron excretion because it increases tissue iron turnover in the plasma.

Continuous, slow deferoxamine infusions allow for a longer exposure of the drug to the relatively small nontransferrin iron or labile iron pool that is in equilibrium with a nearly nonchelatable iron pool.[163]

A pump infuses an aqueous solution of deferoxamine through a small 27-gauge butterfly needle placed under the skin of the abdomen, thigh, or extremities. Most patients use the pump during sleep.[164] Bolus subcutaneous injections of deferoxamine used twice daily induce levels of urinary iron excretion comparable with subcutaneous infusions and may prove helpful as a respite from overnight infusions in some patients not adherent to prolonged infusions.[165,166] In patients who are poorly compliant with subcutaneous therapy, administration of deferoxamine in normal or higher doses can be accomplished intravenously by means of a deep line indwelling catheter, externalized venous catheter, or subcutaneous port. Continuous intravenous administration of deferoxamine is particularly useful for rapidly lowering the total iron burden and is used for reversal of cardiac morbidity (e.g., cardiac arrhythmias or left ventricular dysfunction). Complications of indwelling catheters, including infection and thrombosis rates, have been reported at 1.2 and 0.5 per 1000 catheter days, respectively, in patients treated over 1 to 5 years.

Prolonged infusions of deferoxamine achieve negative iron balance in most transfusion-dependent patients older than 4 or 5 years of age.[116,167-171] This approach to chelation therapy involves daily 8- to 12-hour subcutaneous infusions of 20 to 60 mg/kg of deferoxamine that should result in 20 to 50 mg/day of iron loss in the urine and stool.[116]

The optimal age for beginning parenteral or oral iron chelation therapy in patients with thalassemia has not been established with certainty. The surprisingly high liver iron concentrations that have been found in some patients with thalassemia within the first 2 to 3 years of transfusion therapy, occasionally accompanied by histologic finding of fibrosis, provided the rationale for the early initiation of deferoxamine iron chelation.[172,173] On the other hand, iron excretion in response to deferoxamine is relatively low during the first few years of iron accumulation, and the pharmacokinetics and clearance of iron chelators in children is being further evaluated. Regular deferoxamine chelation therapy begun after the age of 3 to 5 years seems capable of removing previously stored iron and preventing iron-induced liver disease.[116] Data show that deferoxamine started by the age of 2 to 4 years forestalls significant iron overload; however, it also promotes elimination of excess iron in patients if started after significant transfusional iron burden has already developed.[174-184] Moreover, deferoxamine may adversely affect bone development and growth in some young patients and the effect of newer oral chelators on growth has yet to be addressed.[185-187] Some investigators have recommended the baseline and annual assessment of liver iron concentration of greater than 3 mg Fe/g dry weight as a guide for determining the appropriate time to begin iron chelation therapy[173] or a test infusion of deferoxamine to determine if mobilizable iron is present.[188] Others have based this decision on the number of transfusions administered to the patient, that is, approximately 10 to 25 units of blood and a serum ferritin level above 1000 ng/mL, a level that usually occurs after 1 to 2 years of transfusions.[189] Still others wait until the patient is older than 3 years of age, when significant iron excretion can be accomplished and patient cooperation is better[116,187] (see box on Assessment of Iron Stores).

The most common side effect of subcutaneous deferoxamine therapy is inflammation and induration at the site of infusion. Painful lumps may occur despite rotation of infusion sites, appropriate dilution of the drug, and proper placement of the needle. Some investigators have recommended the addition of small amounts of hydrocortisone to the infusion to prevent local reactions. Patients receiving aggressive chelation therapy with lower iron burdens may be more susceptible to toxicity. Neurosensory toxicity of deferoxamine is dose related and inversely correlated with body iron burden. Impairments of visual and auditory acuity are associated with high doses of deferoxamine relative to the iron load.[194] The ototoxicity is characterized by bilateral high-frequency hearing loss. The retinal toxicity is characterized by the loss of night and color vision, retinal atrophy, and cataract formation.[195] Patients receiving deferoxamine should undergo baseline and annual audiograms and ophthalmologic examinations. Deferoxamine should be discontinued if such abnormalities arise, with cautious reinitiation at lower doses when abnormalities improve or resolve. The risk of visual and auditory side effects can be minimized by adjusting the daily deferoxamine dose to the patients' serum ferritin level.[194] Impaired growth associated with growth plate deformities or metaphyseal rickets-like changes in the long bones and histologic evidence of cartilage dysplasia may occur in young children receiving deferoxamine.[185-187] Regular monitoring with plain radiographs of the extremities and vertebral column allows early detection of this complication and reduction in the dose of deferoxamine or temporary interruption of chelation therapy.

Other, less common complications of deferoxamine include anaphylaxis, hypotension, allergic reactions, acute pulmonary disease, impairment of renal function, and infection.[196-202] Severe allergic reactions are rare, and desensitization has been achieved successfully in some patients.[198,199] Acute pulmonary disease and renal failure have occurred in a few patients receiving unusually high doses of deferoxamine by intravenous infusion.[200] The mechanism of this toxicity is unclear. One of the most serious complications of deferoxamine is an increased risk of infection with *Yersinia* and mucormycosis, which uses the deferoxamine iron chelate as a siderophore, whereby enhancing their growth and presenting as colitis, abdominal abscess, or sepsis.[201,202] The safety of deferoxamine during pregnancy has been inferred from case reports rather than formal studies. A summary of these case reports identified 11 women who received deferoxamine beginning in the first trimester and 33 women who used the chelator beginning in the second or third trimester.[202] None of the infants showed evidence of drug-related toxicity.[203]

Regular chelation with deferoxamine has proven remarkably effective in reducing the transfusional iron burden of thalassemia patients. Increasing evidence indicates that endocrine dysfunction is improved and cardiac disease is delayed or prevented with standard deferoxamine regimens.[204] Cardiac arrhythmias and congestive heart failure have reversed in some patients with standard or aggressive deferoxamine regimens, and life expectancy is significantly prolonged.[205-207] Intense 24-hour intravenous deferoxamine regimens of no more than 15 mg/kg/hr have been reported to reverse early

Assessment of Iron Stores

Because excess transfusional iron cannot be actively excreted it is deposited in the macrophages of the RES. When the RES is overwhelmed, iron spills over into parenchymal tissue, generating free radical damage with cellular membrane lipid peroxidation and leading to end-organ dysfunction, especially of the liver, endocrine system, and myocardium.

The best strategy for monitoring iron accumulation in patients with thalassemia remains controversial. Multiple approaches should be considered to assess iron stores, including transfusion requirements, ongoing transfusion burdens, serum ferritin, and liver and cardiac iron concentration. Before chelation therapy is begun, careful recording of transfusion volumes provides an accurate assessment of iron loading. Each milliliter of RBCs contains approximately 1.1 mg of iron. Therefore, each unit of blood contains approximately 200 mg of iron. The total transfusional iron intake can be calculated from the transfusion record and should be as useful in determining the need to begin chelation therapy as indirect or direct measures of body iron stores. Chelation therapy is initiated after approximately 10 to 25 units of blood have been transfused, serum ferritin levels are above 1000 mg/mL, and liver iron concentration is greater than 3 mg Fe/g dry weight. However, when chelation therapy has been initiated, iron is going out as well as coming in. Under these circumstances, regular assessment of iron stores is needed to determine the severity of iron overload and to achieve an optimal treatment program.

Measurement of liver iron concentration by biopsy provides a direct assessment of tissue iron loading and reflects total body iron stores but liver biopsy requires a skilled technician, at least 1 mg of tissue at least 2.5 cm in length with five portal tracts and has the risk of hemorrhage. MRI changes in R2 reflects liver iron concentration comparable to that on liver biopsy. The use of MRI to estimate hepatic and cardiac iron in patients with transfusional siderosis has largely replaced liver biopsy for liver iron concentration quantification at the start of chelation therapy and with annual assessments. Future MRI use may involve the quantification of iron concentration of endocrine glands to predict or monitor dysfunction.[190-192] Levels between 3 and 7 mg Fe/g dry weight appear to be associated with minimal toxicity. Levels greater than 15 mg Fe/g dry weight are associated with an increased risk of heart disease. Recent experience with cardiac magnetic resonance imaging suggests that changes in T2* reflect levels of iron in the heart and may predict adverse changes in cardiac function.

Serum ferritin levels are safe, inexpensive, and readily available, and serial measurements are predictive both of critical complications such as iron-induced heart disease and of adverse effects of chelation therapy such as impairment of vision and hearing. However, single ferritin levels may correlate poorly with liver iron concentration because it is an acute phase reactant and may be influenced by inflammation, vitamin C deficiency, hepatitis, and other infectious states. Transferrin saturation is not very useful in evaluating the severity of iron overload in patients with thalassemia because the massive IE usually results in a transferrin saturation greater than 60% even in the absence of iron overload.[193]

Noninvasive hepatic MRI of liver iron by R2 changes correlates with liver iron concentration by biopsy but cannot be used in patients with pacemakers or those who are claustrophobic.

cardiac hemosiderosis, but even more conventional doses of 50 mg/kg/day have improved left ventricular ejection fractions and prevented death in some patients.[208,209]

Before subcutaneous deferoxamine therapy, estimated survival was approximately 16 to 17 years of age, with rare patients surviving into their mid-20s.[116,206,210,211] Since regular subcutaneous deferoxamine regimens have been in use, life expectancy has extended into the fourth decade of life.[212-214] The increasing widespread use of deferoxamine has steadily increased survival probabilities worldwide.[213,214] However, long-term European studies have demonstrated that improved survival times are clearly related to the degree of compliance with chelation regimens and are associated with lower serum ferritin levels (<1000 mg/mL).[215] Deferoxamine chelation regimens are clearly cumbersome, inconvenient, and costly. More tolerable approaches are required, and investigations for alternative oral iron-chelating agents have been ongoing and recently more successful.

Although the prevalence of endocrine disturbances, for example, glucose intolerance and diabetes have reduced since the regular use of subcutaneous deferoxamine,[109,112,204] they persist, especially in those in whom deferoxamine was initiated late in their first decade of life.[179] Growth hormone deficiency, hypothyroidism, hypoparathyroidism, vitamin D deficiency, diabetes, and osteoporosis are still observed, and there is little evidence that deferoxamine can reverse established endocrine dysfunctions. The North American Thalassemia Clinical Research Network Registry reported that 96% of thalassemia patients with median age of 20 years were free of hypoparathyroidism, 91% were free of thyroid disease, 90% were free of diabetes mellitus, and overall 62% were free of any endocrinopathy.[216]

It remains to be determined if starting chelation at a very young age or more easily administered use of oral iron chelation will diminish the endocrine morbidities and further prolong survival associated with iron overload. Direct and indirect measures of iron stores reflect the progress of chelation therapy and help determine appropriate changes in the dose or frequency of chelator use. The serum ferritin level generally declines during regular chelation therapy and may decline rapidly in the first year of treatment in patients with very large iron stores.[167,169] Serum ferritin levels measured over time with use of deferoxamine have predicted the risk of iron-induced heart disease in patients with thalassemia major, and the ratio of the dose of deferoxamine to the ferritin level has identified patients at risk for auditory and visual complications of chelation therapy.[194,207] Although easy to obtain and relatively inexpensive, the serum ferritin level may be increased in the presence of inflammation and may be decreased when iron overload is accompanied by vitamin C deficiency.[217] For these and other reasons, serum ferritin levels frequently correlate poorly with liver iron concentrations, and clinicians and patients may have a false sense of security when the ferritin level is below 2000 μg/L. Some studies using deferoxamine suggest ferritin levels lower than 1000 μg/L are associated with better survival times and less cardiac disease as well as hepatic histology and pathology.[215,218,219]

Liver biopsy with biochemical measurement of iron concentration provides a more direct assessment of iron overload, and some investigators recommend such testing yearly. Hepatic iron levels of 15 mg/g dry weight have been associated with a greater risk of iron-induced heart disease.[174] The meaning of lower hepatic iron levels has generally been inferred from experience with primary hemochromatosis.[220] Further studies are needed to determine the clinical usefulness of liver iron concentration in the overall management of thalassemia. Noninvasive techniques using magnetic susceptometry and MRI for assessing tissue iron offer the possibility of serial measurements without substantial risk to the patient. The noninvasive measurement of iron in the liver, heart, and other target organs is in development. Measurements of liver iron concentration by magnetic susceptometry using a superconducting quantum interference device (SQUID) correlate well with biochemical measurements of tissue iron.[221,222] At present, measurement of tissue iron by SQUID is limited to the liver, and the instruments are available in only two sites in the United States and two sites in Europe. The ability to use MRI to measure iron stores would dramatically extend the availability of noninvasive tissue iron measurements. Investigators have reported success using proton transverse relaxation rates (R2) with spin-echo imaging, signal intensity ratios, and gradient-echo T2* to assess liver iron concentration.[223-227] The latter two techniques also yield information that appears and to reflect cardiac iron loading. Direct comparisons with hepatic tissue samples demonstrate significant correlations ($r = 0.97$ vs. 0.95) with biopsy-measured liver iron concentrations in two separate studies.[224,226-230] These noninvasive technologies to measure liver, cardiac, and other tissue iron concentration may prove useful in the future to refine therapeutic strategies. Current needs include the further refinement of MRI techniques and a better understanding of the relationship between liver iron, iron in other organs (particularly the heart), and clinical complications of iron overload.

A relationship between iron overload and ascorbic acid depletion, first suggested by the epidemiology of scurvy among the Bantu, exists in thalassemia major.[99,217] For thalassemia patients with low levels of ascorbic acid, daily supplementation with 100 to 200 mg of this vitamin increases urinary iron excretion in response to deferoxamine by approximately twofold.[100,163] Ascorbic acid may retard the conversion of ferritin to hemosiderin and therefore allow more iron to remain in the chelatable form.[231,232] However, it can also enhance iron-mediated peroxidation of membrane lipids[233,234] as well as membrane damage in cultured myocardial cells.[235] Cardiac toxicity manifested as arrhythmias and decreased ventricular contractility has been attributed to vitamin C therapy.[236] Ascorbic acid should be used only while deferoxamine is being administered and only in patients who are ascorbate depleted.

Chelation therapy with deferoxamine is expensive and cumbersome because of the need for daily or nightly subcutaneous infusions. Regular infusions require a great deal of dedication and persistence from the patient and family. Noncompliance is common, particularly in the teenage and young adult years, and failure to follow prescribed treatment regimens is the major cause of mortality in patients with thalassemia major.[215] The cost and complexity of deferoxamine administration prevents its availability worldwide, especially in developing countries. The search for a less expensive iron chelator that can be more easily orally administered led to the identification of compounds such as deferiprone and deferasirox.

Deferiprone

One such oral agent is 1,2-dimethyl-3-hydroxypyrid-4-one (L1, deferiprone), a synthetic compound with a low molecular weight of approximately 200 g/mol. It is an orally active bidentate iron chelator that requires three molecules to bind one iron atom. Deferiprone is absorbed by the gastrointestinal tract and has a plasma half-life of approximately 90 minutes (2-3 hours). Chelated iron is excreted predominantly in the urine (90%) and far less in the stool (10%). It was synthesized in the late 1980s and was first tested in uncontrolled clinical trials at the Royal Free Hospital in London, hence the eponym L1.[237,238] Subsequent clinical efficacy studies appeared initially encouraging,[239-241] but its long-term efficacy and safety have not been totally established.[240,242-246] Retrospective studies have shown reduced cardiac morbidity and mortality and lower cardiac iron deposition in patients treated with deferiprone compared with deferoxamine.[247,248] A large observational study demonstrated improvement in cardiac iron deposition with deferiprone treatment.[249] Unfortunately, deferiprone was not subjected to phase III studies in which its safety and efficacy were directly compared with those of deferoxamine. Nonetheless, at doses of 75 mg/kg/day, deferiprone administered in three divided doses with meals reduces or maintains iron stores, thereby achieving negative iron balance or iron balance in many regularly transfused patients for the most part, particularly those with more severe transfusional iron overload.[239,240,242-246,250,251] However, some patients remain in positive iron balance and continue to accumulate iron during long-term therapy with this dose of deferiprone.[240,244,252] Some studies have shown the reduction of serum ferritin levels and liver iron concentration in most, but not all, patients with transfusional iron overload.[247] Regimens using higher doses up to 100 mg/kg/day of deferiprone may be more effective.[248] Combination regimens with deferoxamine may also reduce iron stores or prove effective in restoring negative iron balance in some of these patients.[253-255] Enhanced urine and stool iron excretion in thalassemia patients using both deferoxamine and deferiprone have suggested an additive effect postulated by the shuttle hypothesis, that is, deferiprone may chelate intracellular labile iron and shuttle it to deferoxamine.[256] Some studies have also suggested that deferiprone alone or in combination with deferoxamine may be more effective than deferoxamine in removing iron from the heart, improving cardiac function, and preventing iron-induced cardiac disease.[230,251,257-260] Schedules for combination therapy vary but have usually included 5 to 7 days of deferiprone and 2 days of subcutaneous deferoxamine weekly. Intensive combined chelation therapy has been reported to reverse both cardiac and endocrine complications of thalassemia major.[261]

Side effects of deferiprone include gastrointestinal complaints, mostly nausea and some vomiting that occur in approximately 33% of patients and usually resolve without specific intervention. Arthropathy with arthralgias and some joint effusions occur in approximately 15% of patients. The incidence of joint symptoms varies widely among various studies but may be severe enough to require reduction or interruption of chelation therapy. Abnormal liver function tests may occur gradually or suddenly and in the absence of other causes of hepatic dysfunction. These elevations may return to baseline values with the interruption of deferiprone followed by reinitiation beginning with lower doses and close monitoring of liver function tests. Progressive liver disease attributed to deferiprone has not been reported, and concerns about drug-induced hepatic fibrosis have not been substantiated by subsequent studies.[240,243,262,263] However, in vitro evidence shows that deferiprone may potentiate oxidative DNA damage in iron-loaded liver cells that could occur when the concentration of iron is low relative to the iron chelator (Fig. 38-8).[264] Agranulocytosis occurs in 1% of patients and, although rare, remains the principal concern for patients receiving deferiprone. Milder neutropenia is more common and occurs in approximately 8% of patients. Severely depressed neutrophil counts represent a significant risk of sepsis and hospitalizations, and in some cases, administration of granulocyte colony-stimulating factor (G-CSF) is required. Some reported deaths have been related to deferiprone-induced agranulocytosis or neutropenia. Regular weekly monitoring of blood counts during deferiprone therapy is essential to detect the rare but important deferiprone-induced complications of neutropenia and agranulocytosis.[244-246,265]

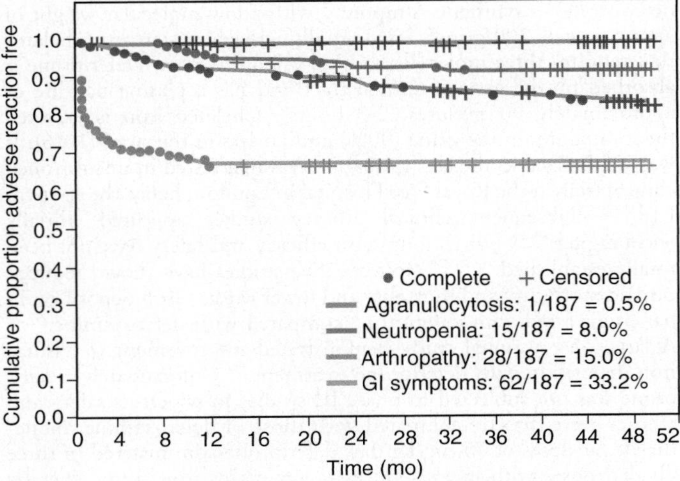

Figure 38-8 KAPLAN-MEIER CURVES SHOWING THE TIME TO FIRST OCCURRENCE OF IMPORTANT ADVERSE EVENTS IN PATIENTS TREATED WITH DEFERIPRONE. The only case of agranulocytosis occurred in the first year, and gastrointestinal complaints were very uncommon after the first year. Neutropenia and joint problems occurred throughout the 4-year study period but were more common in the first year than in each of the subsequent years. *(Adapted from Cohen AR, Galanello R, Piga A, et al: Safety and effectiveness of long-term therapy with the oral iron chelator deferiprone.* Blood *102:1583, 2003.)*

Several clinical studies of deferiprone speak to its relative safety and utility demonstrated by a decline in serum ferritin levels in the majority of patients.[230,243-246,250,251,257,258,260] Retrospective studies have suggested that deferiprone might be more effective than deferoxamine in chelating cardiac iron. Two multicenter studies have further supported the theory that combination therapy increases total iron excretion and selectively reduces organ iron burden.[258,260] Longitudinal clinical studies using innovative MRI technology to measure cardiac (T2*) and liver iron concentration have demonstrated higher estimated liver iron concentration but lower myocardial iron concentration in deferiprone-treated thalassemia patients compared with those treated with deferoxamine.[257] In another study, thalassemia patients using deferiprone did not experience any cardiac events or any cardiac-related deaths compared with thalassemia patients taking deferoxamine who experienced both cardiac events and some deaths.[258] In another 1-year prospective trial of cardiac iron and function, thalassemia patients treated with deferiprone or deferoxamine had improved myocardial T2* values but more so in the deferiprone-treated group, who also showed a greater improvement in left ventricular ejection fraction. Liver iron concentration fell significantly in the deferoxamine-treated patients but not in the patients receiving deferiprone. A prospective randomized study comparing the combination of deferiprone at 75 mg/kg/day and deferoxamine at 40 to 50 mg/kg/day with deferoxamine alone demonstrated that the combination therapy more rapidly reduced hepatic and cardiac iron stores than deferoxamine alone.[266] Further prospective studies are warranted, especially with the combination of deferiprone with deferoxamine. Deferiprone may play a role in shuttling iron from within intracellular pools and enhance the available iron pool to bind with deferoxamine.[243,267-269] Deferiprone continues to be tested in clinical trials alone and in combination with deferoxamine to address its impact on cardiac function.[260] The safety profile of deferiprone has been largely defined by single-center studies, multicenter trials, and postmarketing surveillance largely in European and Asian continents. Deferiprone is currently licensed in both Europe and the United States of America as of 2011 as alternative iron chelation therapy for those who are unable to be successfully treated with deferoxamine.

Deferasirox

Deferasirox (ICL670, ExJade) is an orally active iron chelator that was identified by computer technology at Novartis Pharmaceuticals in the 1990s. It is a tridentate compound known as 4-(3,5-bis[2-hydroxyphenyl]-1*H*-1,2,4-triazol-1-yl)-benzoic acid,[270] wherein two molecules of deferasirox are required to bind one atom of iron. It has a high affinity for iron and a much lower affinity for copper and zinc. Deferasirox is orally bioavailable with a low molecular weight of 373 g/mol and is absorbed by the gastrointestinal tract. It has a dose-dependent plasma half-life of 12 to 18 hours that allows for once-daily oral administration after fasting on an empty stomach.[271] Deferasirox is given as a suspension in water or apple or orange juice.[272] Iron excretion in response to deferasirox is largely in the stool (90%) and far less in the urine (10%).[272] The pharmacodynamic effects of deferasirox tested in a phase I clinical iron balance metabolic study measuring stool and urine iron excretion demonstrated increasing iron excretion at doses of 10, 20, and 40 mg/kg/day, which induced a mean net iron excretion (0.119, 0.329, and 0.445 mg Fe/kg/day, respectively) within the clinically relevant range of the rate of transfusion iron loading for most patients.

The phase III worldwide multicenter open-label randomized active comparator control study of deferasirox compared with deferoxamine was conducted in 65 sites with 586 regularly transfused patients 2 years or more of age with β-thalassemia. Results indicated that chronic daily use of deferasirox, via a single oral dose of 20 to 30 mg/kg/day, induced decreases in liver iron concentration by biopsy comparable to that achieved with deferoxamine. Patients with liver iron concentrations greater than 7 mg/g dry weight receiving deferasirox at 20 to 30 mg/kg/day had a mean decrease of 5.3 mg/g dry weight that did not differ significantly from a mean decrease of 4.3 mg/g dry weight in patients receiving 35 mg/kg/day or more deferoxamine. Changes in serum ferritin were dose dependent in both treatments, paralleling trends in liver iron content.[273] Doses of 5 and 10 mg/kg/day of deferasirox were unlikely to achieve negative iron balance and did not maintain or reduce absolute liver iron concentration and serum ferritin levels increased at these lower doses. The rate of transfusional iron loading may also influence the effectiveness of deferasirox in controlling liver iron concentration.[274] Using a dose of 20 to 30 mg/kg/day of Deferasirox to reduce liver iron concentration has been demonstrated in several additional studies.[274-276] Deferasirox was given orphan drug status and was approved by the FDA in 2005 in the United States.

Higher doses of Deferasirox at 30 to 50 mg/kg/day have been demonstrated to significantly improve cardiac T2* iron deposition over 2 years of treatment in two groups of thalassemia patients with normal ventricular function but with either moderate to mild siderosis (T2* = 10 to <20 ms) or severe (T2* >5 to <10 ms) cardiac siderosis.[277] Failure of T2* cardiac siderosis to respond to deferasirox has been predicted by higher baseline liver iron concentrations and ferritin levels.[278] Deferasirox has also been shown to prevent cardiac iron accumulation in thalassemia patients without evidence of cardiac siderosis as well as improvement in left ventricular function.[279]

Deferasirox was generally well tolerated in these clinical trials. Mild gastrointestinal complaints and skin rashes were the most common adverse events. Discontinuation of deferasirox was rarely required, but abdominal discomfort occurred in 14% of patients, 12% with diarrhea, 10% nausea, and 9% vomiting. Mild increases in serum creatinine occurred in 38% of patients, and a small number exceeded the upper limits of normal; intermittent proteinuria was also observed in 19% of patients. Duplicate serum creatinine level should be assessed before initiating therapy. Close monthly monitoring of serum creatinine needs to be maintained because of nephropathy in animal studies and cases of acute renal failure that were reported after postmarketing use of deferasirox. Severe renal complications may occur in patients with preexisting renal disease. Dose reduction, interruption, or discontinuation should be considered for elevations in serum creatinine. Elevations in serum transaminases also occurred in a small number of patients (6%). Rare reports of fulminant hepatic liver failure have resulted in the recommendation to obtain liver function tests every 2 weeks for 1 month after starting therapy and then monthly thereafter with interruptions or discontinuations of deferasirox if unexplained or progressive transaminase increases occur. Skin rashes also occurred in 15% of patients usually within the first 2 weeks of treatment. The maculopapular eruptions often resolved spontaneously, but severe rashes may require interruption of deferasirox with antihistamine support and possible steroid administration after which deferasirox may be reintroduced at a lower dose with gradual dose escalation. Minimal (<1%) auditory and ophthalmologic toxicity occurred in the preliminary 1-year safety and efficacy trial. No agranulocytosis was observed in thalassemia subjects during the 1-year primary efficacy trial. Reports of pancytopenia have occurred in postmarketing reports, but mostly in patients with preexisting hematologic disorders such as myelodysplastic syndromes (MDS) that are frequently associated with BM failure.

Future Iron Chelation Research Strategies

Other approaches to improved chelation therapy have looked to both oral and parenteral therapy. The compound N, n'-Bis-(2-Hydroxybenzyl)ethylenediamine-N, n'-Dipropionic Acid (HBED), originally developed as a potential oral agent, has been shown in primate studies to be more effective when administered as a subcutaneous injection than deferoxamine administered by subcutaneous infusion.[280] The attachment of deferoxamine to a backbone of starch (S-DFO) extends the circulation time of the chelator, and early studies suggest that this novel form of deferoxamine may reduce the frequency of infusions required to achieve negative iron balance.[281] Another promising oral desferithiocin derivative, FBS0701, a member of the desazadesferrithiocin class of siderophore-related tridentate chelators, has been modified to limit nephrotoxicity and is entering phase II studies.[282]

Specific Complications and Their Management

Skeletal Changes

Skeletal abnormalities (Fig. 38-9) are less common in patients receiving regular RBC transfusions but may still occur as a result of partially unchecked IE and expansion of the erythroid BM.[283] These cause widening of the BM space and thinning of the cortex, with consequent osteoporosis.[284,285] Changes in the skull and facial bones, including expansion of the frontal bone with prominent frontal bossing, may occur before the initiation of transfusion therapy. Radiographs reveal the diploic spaces to be widened. At first, the skull has a granular appearance, but later perpendicular bony trabeculae appear, giving the classic "hair on end" or "crewcut" appearance. Marked overgrowth of the maxilla results in severe malocclusion, jumbling of the upper incisors, and prominence of the molar eminences.[286] These bone changes produce the classic facies. Additional skeletal changes are observed in the metacarpals, metatarsals, and phalanges, where expanded medullary cavities produce a rectangular and then a convex shape (see Fig. 38-9). Irregular fusion of the epiphyses of the proximal humerus results in characteristic shortening of the upper arms.[287,288] Marked osteoporosis and cortical thinning may predispose to pathologic fractures of the extremities and compression fractures of the vertebrae (Fig. 38-10).

Several abnormalities in the ribs may occur, including notching and osteolytic lesions.[283,289] The ribs become very wide, especially at the points of their attachment to the vertebral column. BM masses may extrude from these sites, creating the appearance of paravertebral masses and compressing the spinal cord.[290] Although bone deformities and extramedullary hematopoiesis are uncommon in properly transfused patients with β-thalassemia major, it is frequently observed in patients with thalassemia intermedia whose BM is not suppressed by regular transfusions (see the section Thalassemia Intermedia).

The character and degree of the bone lesions change significantly with age. In older children, the bone lesions regress in the more distal portions of the skeleton (hands, arms, and legs), a feature correlating with the normal developmental replacement of red BM by fatty BM. The characteristic changes of the hands and other peripheral areas are thus diminished and may disappear in later life.[109,291] However, in the skull, spine, and pelvis (which are sites of active, persistent erythropoiesis), the radiographic changes become more conspicuous.[129]

Growth and Endocrine Status

Growth retardation, including skeletal and dental deformities,[292] was common even in young children until the use of hypertransfusion regimens restored relatively normal growth during the first decade. Without iron chelation therapy, the adolescent growth spurt is often delayed or absent; most patients, even those well maintained by transfusion, may not attain normal stature, partly because of iron-induced damage to the hypothalamic–pituitary axis.[90,293,294] Menarche is frequently delayed. Breast development may be poor, and many female patients have primary or secondary amenorrhea. Boys are frequently immature, with sparse facial and body hair. Although spermatogenesis may be normal, libido is often decreased. A multicenter study of 250 adolescent patients in northern Italy showed that despite hypertransfusion and 7 to 10 years of deferoxamine iron chelation therapy, two-thirds of male patients and one-third of female patients older than 14 years of age were 2 standard deviations or more below the mean for height.[295] Many adolescents between 12 and 18 years of age lacked any secondary sexual changes of puberty. However, the mean serum ferritin level in the entire group was 3500 ng/mL, indicating persistence of a high level of excess iron burden in most of this group.

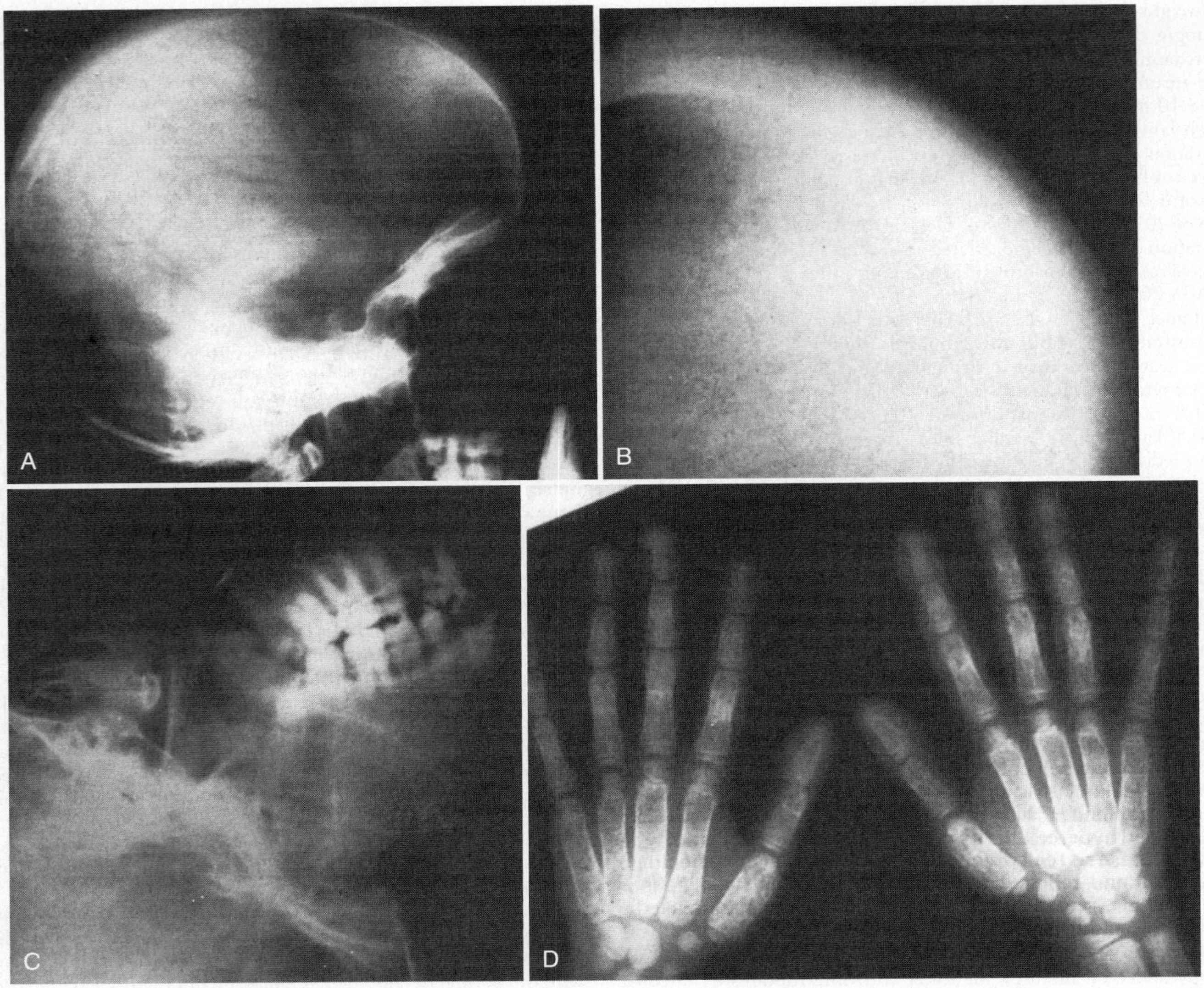

Figure 38-9 BONY ABNORMALITIES IN A PATIENT WITH SEVERE β-THALASSEMIA. **A** and **B**, "Hair-on-end" appearance of the skull, especially obvious in the close-up view shown in part **B**. **C**, Distortion of the maxillary bones, as well as poor development of the sinus cavities caused by opaque masses of extramedullary erythropoiesis. **D**, Squaring and convexity abnormalities of the hands. *(From Pearson HA, Benz EJ Jr: Thalassemia syndromes. In Miller DR, Baehner RL, McMillan CW, editors:* Smith's blood diseases of infancy and childhood, *ed 5, St. Louis, 1984, CV Mosby, p 439.)*

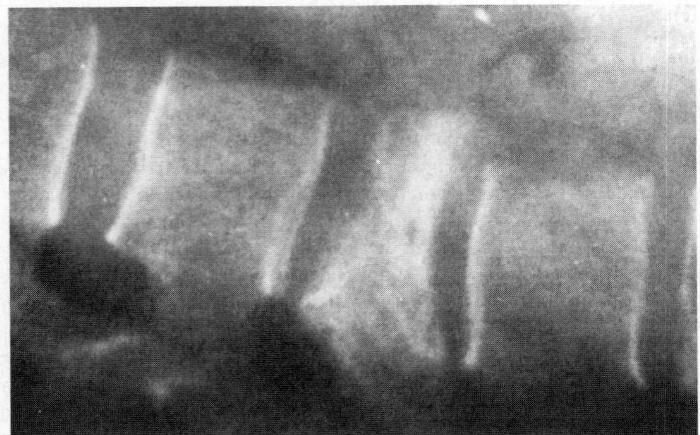

Figure 38-10 COMPRESSION FRACTURE OF L2 VERTEBRA IN A PATIENT WITH SEVERE β-THALASSEMIA. *(From Pearson HA, Benz EJ Jr: Thalassemia syndromes. In Miller DR, Baehner RL, McMillan CW, editors:* Smith's blood diseases of infancy and childhood, *ed 5, St. Louis, 1984, CV Mosby, p 439.)*

Regular chelation therapy started early in the first decade of life frequently allows a normal onset of puberty and development of secondary sexual changes.[296] Administration of recombinant human growth hormone in conventional doses increases height velocity in patients with growth hormone deficiency.[297,298] Normal or higher doses of recombinant human growth hormone increase growth velocity in patients with normal growth hormone reserve but low levels of insulin-like growth factor I.[299,300] For patients with a functional hypothalamic–pituitary axis, treatment with gonadotropin-releasing hormone may induce pubertal changes.[301] In others, administration of sex steroids is necessary to induce secondary sexual characteristics.

More than 100 pregnancies either have been achieved spontaneously in patients with normal menstrual function or have been induced in patients with primary or secondary amenorrhea.[302-307] Transfusion requirements frequently increase during pregnancy, especially during the third trimester.[302] Diminished ventricular contractility during pregnancy and the death from heart disease of at least one mother within 1 year of delivery argue strongly for the careful consideration of the overall clinical condition and degree of iron loading before planning a pregnancy.[305,308] The safety of chelation therapy during pregnancy is discussed earlier. At least one successful pregnancy has occurred in a woman with thalassemia after BMT that included ablative therapy with busulfan and cyclophosphamide.[309]

Abnormal carbohydrate metabolism is common in older patients with thalassemia major. Prepubertal children usually have normal glucose metabolism, but pubertal patients exhibit impaired responses to glucose load. Higher than normal insulin levels despite normal glucose levels are also encountered during puberty.[310] The defect in these patients appears to be related to insulin resistance, with insulin deficiency developing later in the progression to diabetes. Rates of diabetes are reported close to 6% to 8%.[214] Diabetes occurs more frequently in patients with hepatitis C and hepatic dysfunction.[311-313] Oral hypoglycemic agents have been used to regulate hyperglycemia and may reduce the rate of further deterioration of glucose metabolism.[314]

Laboratory findings of hypothyroidism and hypoparathyroidism are present in approximately 14% of patients with thalassemia major.[315-319] Clinical findings associated with these deficiencies are uncommon.[320]

Low Bone Mass

With improved survival in patients with thalassemia major, the problem of osteoporosis has assumed greater importance. The widespread prevalence of osteoporosis in patients with thalassemia major was first observed across all ages in 1995.[285] Subsequently, others reported a high frequency of abnormal *Z* scores in pediatric, adolescent, and adult patients. Abnormal bone mineral density has been reported in pediatric and adolescent patients with thalassemia major.[321-323] The Thalassemia Clinical Research Network has identified the overall fracture prevalence of 12% in a contemporary sample of 702 patients with α- and β-thalassemia. The fractures occurred more frequently in thalassemia major (17%) and intermedia (12%) compared with β-E (7%) and α-thalassemia (2%). Facture prevalence increased with age and with sex hormone replacement therapy.[324] More recently an observational study by the Thalassemia Clinical Research Network has demonstrated a high prevalence of low bone mass across all the thalassemia syndromes, including β-thalassemia major, intermedia, β-E, hemoglobin H, H-Constant Spring, and homozygous α-thalassemia, which progresses with aging. Low bone mass is associated with high prevalence of fractures, hypogonadism, and increased bone turnover.[324,325] Bone resorption is usually increased, and new bone formation is decreased.[326] Treatment with some, but not all, bisphosphonates improves bone mineral density.[327-330] Vitamin D and calcium supplementation with age-appropriate hormone replacement therapy are important preventive measures, although low bone mass may still occur in treated patients. Gonadal steroid replacement of hypogonadal patients has been shown to improve bone mass in some studies.[325,331]

Liver and Gallbladder

Hepatomegaly occurring before the initiation of transfusion therapy in severely affected patients is primarily a consequence of extramedullary hematopoiesis. With the amelioration of the anemia, the liver diminishes in size. However, as transfusion therapy continues, iron accumulation provides a new reason for hepatomegaly and resultant liver injury. Iron deposition, first present in the Kupffer cells, ultimately engorges the parenchymal cells, resulting in an appearance that is indistinguishable from that of idiopathic hemochromatosis.[332-334] The hepatocellular injury of iron overload may be attributable to the liberation of hydrolases resulting from initiation by the ferrous form of iron and peroxidative damage of lysosomal membrane lipids.[335] Fibrosis is usually followed by cirrhosis and an increased risk of hepatocellular carcinoma. The risk of liver damage and the rate of progression may be increased by the concomitant presence of excessive iron with viral hepatitis. The concentration of liver iron that constitutes a threshold for liver damage in patients with thalassemia is similar to that found in patients with hereditary hemochromatosis. In contrast to hereditary hemochromatosis, however, death from liver failure or liver cancer is much less common than death from cardiac failure in patients with thalassemia.[213]

Regular chelation therapy is the key to maintaining normal or near-normal hepatic iron concentrations and preventing iron-induced hepatic fibrosis and cirrhosis. Treatment with deferoxamine slows or prevents iron-induced liver damage and may reduce the severity of preexisting fibrosis in some cases.[159,179,336] Results of treatment of hepatitis C in patients with thalassemia major are similar to those found in other patients. Sustained viral responses occur in 28% to 40% of patients treated with interferon alone and, in two smaller series, 46% to 72% of patients treated with interferon and ribavirin.[337-341] Transfusion requirements increase by 30% to 40% in patients treated with ribavirin as a result of drug-induced hemolysis.[338,340,341] Lower levels of viral RNA and non-1 genotypes are associated with better responses. Higher iron levels adversely affect the response to antiviral therapy in some studies but not in others.[337,339,342] The Thalassemia Clinical Research Network studied the use of pegylated interferon and ribavirin in 16 thalassemia patients. Fifty percent genotype 1 patients had sustained viral response as well as 25% of genotype 2 and 3 patients; median transfusion requirements increased by 44% after 24 weeks of treatment, and liver iron concentration increase of more than 5 mg/g dry weight occurred in 29% of patients, but overall liver iron concentration remained stable over the course of the study. In addition, neutropenia occurred in 52% of patients.[341] Interferon therapy in patients with hepatitis C who have previously undergone BMT is as effective and safe as in nontransplanted patients.[343]

Pigmentary gallstones caused by high levels of bilirubin production are found in an increasing number of patients older than 4 years old. Two-thirds of patients have multiple calcified bilirubinate calculi after the age of 15 years.[344] Gallbladder surgery is not usually indicated unless biliary colic or obstructive jaundice has occurred.

Heart

Cardiac abnormalities are important causes of morbidity and mortality in patients with thalassemia major. Cardiac enlargement secondary to anemia is almost always present in untransfused children (see Fig. 38-9). Before the availability of chelation therapy, myocardial hemosiderosis and serious iron-induced cardiac diseases were inevitable during the second decade. These problems still occur often in older patients with thalassemia who are poorly compliant with chelation therapy, and heart disease, usually in the form of cardiac failure or serious arrhythmias, remains the most common cause of death in patients with thalassemia major.[213,215]

Left-sided heart failure predominates in patients with thalassemia major and is characterized by dyspnea and orthopnea.[345] Right-sided heart failure is less common but may be the presenting cardiac finding in older patients with more severe iron overload. Symptoms include hepatic pain, abdominal discomfort, and peripheral edema. Acute myocarditis, which occurs in approximately 5% of patients with thalassemia, is frequently followed by acute or chronic heart failure.[346]

Early electrocardiographic abnormalities include a prolonged P–R interval, first-degree heart block, and premature atrial contractions. Later, ST-segment depression and ventricular ectopic beats constitute ominous indicators of myocardial damage. Periodic evaluation of cardiac function is essential to detect iron-induced heart disease and to identify patients who will benefit from more intensive chelation therapy (see later discussion). Unfortunately, by the time cardiac results of studies such as echocardiography and 24-hour rhythm monitoring become abnormal, clinical heart disease is imminent. Whether assessment of cardiac iron by MRI using T2* or other measures can better anticipate the development of clinical heart disease is currently under investigation.

In the absence of intensified chelation therapy, ventricular dysfunction progresses rapidly to chronic refractory congestive heart failure, and arrhythmias become increasingly difficult to control. In the past, death usually occurred within 1 year of onset of heart failure.

More recent data demonstrate a survival rate of 48% at 5 years.[345] Survival is notably poorer in patients with heart failure after myocarditis or with heart failure accompanied by arrhythmias.[346]

In addition to standard therapy for heart failure and arrhythmias, including angiotensin-converting enzyme inhibitors, β-blockers, diuretics, and antiarrhythmic agents, the pretransfusion hemoglobin level should be maintained between 10 and 12 g/dL. The volume of transfused RBCs should be reduced as needed to prevent acute fluid overload. Because the iron-overloaded myocardium has little capacity to improve its performance unless excess iron is removed, intensive chelation therapy is a critical part of the management of heart disease in patients with thalassemia. Several studies have shown that heart failure can be reversed in many patients with the use of continuous treatment with deferoxamine.[205,347,348] The benefits of this approach may derive from the reduction in cardiac iron stores, the prevention of acute toxicity from non–transferrin-bound iron, or a combination of these two mechanisms. Recent data suggest that deferiprone may be more effective than deferoxamine in reducing the cardiac iron load and treating iron-induced cardiac disease, perhaps because of deferiprone's ability to enter cardiac cells more rapidly than deferoxamine.[230,257] Different iron chelators seem to have different accessibility to hepatic and extrahepatic iron stores. Deferoxamine works more rapidly and efficiently in removing liver iron than cardiac iron.[209,348] Deferiprone seems to remove iron from the heart effectively[349] despite its relative inefficiency in controlling hepatic iron content.[230,257] In the gerbil animal model, deferasirox and deferiprone were equally effective in removing cardiac iron and deferasirox removed even more hepatic iron for a given cardiac iron burden.[350] Deferasirox treatment for 1 to 2 years has also been shown to reduce cardiac iron and improve cardiac MRI T2* in patients with transfusional iron overload.[351,352] Additional studies are needed to confirm these observations and to establish the relative roles of deferiprone, deferasirox, and deferoxamine or a combination thereof in the management of patients with established iron-related heart disease.[353] In patients who have undergone BMT, improvements in left ventricular contractility and diastolic function accompany the removal of excess iron by phlebotomy.[354] Heart transplantation and combined heart–liver transplantation have been performed successfully in patients with end-stage cardiac disease.[355-357]

Sterile pericarditis occurs in some patients with massive iron overload.[358] Although pericarditis is most often attributed to hemosiderosis, an association with β-hemolytic streptococcal infection and other infectious agents has also been suggested.[359] Therapy usually consists of bed rest, treatment of infection, management of superimposed congestive heart failure, and the use of salicylates or corticosteroids. Occasionally, pericardectomy may be indicated.

Lungs

Mild abnormalities of pulmonary function are common in patients with thalassemia but rarely cause clinical problems. Some patients exhibit primarily restrictive defects[360,361]; others experience mild to moderate small airway obstruction and hyperinflation.[362-364] Most patients have a decreased maximal oxygen uptake and anaerobic threshold; these do not normalize after transfusion.[365] Postsplenectomy thrombocytosis and other prothrombotic changes can predispose to pulmonary vascular occlusion and pulmonary hypertension.[366-369] Treatment with high doses of the iron chelator deferoxamine may also be associated with acute deterioration of pulmonary function.[200,201]

Kidneys

The kidneys are frequently enlarged, partly because of extramedullary hematopoiesis and partly because of marked dilation of the renal tubules.[370] The urine is often dark brown, reflecting the excretion of products of heme catabolism.[371] The urine also contains large amounts of urates and uric acid.

Recently, the Thalassemia Clinical Research Network studied the prevalence of renal abnormalities in patients with thalassemia major and thalassemia intermedia receiving deferoxamine chelation. One-third of thalassemia patients who were not regularly transfused had abnormally high creatinine clearance. Regular transfusions were associated with a decrease in clearance (P =004). Almost one-third of patients with thalassemia had hypercalciuria, and regular transfusions were associated with an increase in the frequency and degree of hypercalciuria (P <0001). Albuminuria was found in more than half of patients but was not consistently associated with transfusion therapy. In summary, renal hyperfiltration, hypercalciuria, and albuminuria are common in patients with thalassemia. Higher transfusion intensity is associated with lower creatinine clearance but more frequent hypercalciuria.[372]

Spleen and Splenectomy

Massive splenomegaly is unusual in regularly transfused patients, but even mild or moderate splenomegaly may be associated with findings of hypersplenism, including thrombocytopenia, neutropenia, and increasing anemia. The usual indication for splenectomy is a progressive increase in transfusion requirements caused by hypersplenism. The transfusion requirements, and therefore the rates of iron loading, of splenectomized patients are often considerably less than those of patients whose spleens are intact.[278,349,373,374] A transfusion requirement of more than 180 to 200 mL/kg/yr of packed RBCs usually represents excessive RBC requirements.[373,374] For such patients, a 25% to 60% reduction in transfusion requirements after splenectomy is generally predictable. Before attributing increased transfusion requirements to hypersplenism, it is important to look for other causes, such as RBC alloimmunization or a change in the hematocrit of the units of donor blood. RBC survival studies using ^{50}Cr-labeling are not usually of value for predicting response to splenectomy. Because of the greater risk of postsplenectomy sepsis in younger patients, surgery should be deferred until after 5 years of age whenever possible. For well-transfused and well-chelated patients, splenectomy may have little benefit, and some centers have noted a significant decline in the number of patients undergoing splenectomy in recent years.

Laparoscopic splenectomy has proved safe for patients with thalassemia and has dramatically shortened the recovery time compared with open procedures.[375] Partial splenectomy and partial dearterialization of the spleen have been suggested as alternative approaches to reducing blood requirements without incurring the risk of sepsis.[376-378] The long-term benefits of this approach remain uncertain. Therapeutic embolization of the spleen avoids the need for surgery,[379-381] but this approach is frequently associated with postprocedure pain and fever and does not permit the removal of accessory spleens.

After splenectomy, striking thrombocytosis may occur, which may require thrombophilia prophylaxis or platelet deaggregating agents.[382] Increased numbers of nucleated RBCs appear in the blood, and the presence of many RBCs containing inclusion bodies composed of precipitated α-globin chains can be demonstrated by staining with methyl violet or brilliant cresyl blue.

A period of observation without transfusion after splenectomy may be helpful in identifying patients who can now maintain an acceptable hemoglobin level without regular transfusions. This approach may be particularly useful for patients whose thalassemia mutations would predict a milder clinical course. Hemoglobin levels should be monitored weekly to determine whether transfusion therapy should be reinstituted.

Patients with thalassemia major are at significant risk for the development of overwhelming, often fatal, infection after splenectomy (postsplenectomy sepsis syndrome).[383] The problem is most common in young children. *Streptococcus pneumoniae* causes two-thirds of cases; *Hemophilus influenzae* type B and *Neisseria meningitidis* account for most of the remaining infections. Typically, there is a fulminant clinical course, proceeding from mild fever and headache to hyperpyrexia, prostration, shock, and death within 6 to 12 hours. Immunization against the most common pathogens before splenectomy, prophylaxis with antibiotics, and early assessment of fever after splenectomy have dramatically reduced the incidence of fatal postsplenectomy sepsis.

Splenectomy should generally be reserved for patients with excessive transfusion requirements from hypersplenism and difficulty controlling iron overload. A large spleen alone does not usually cause significant clinical problems and should rarely, if ever, be the sole reason for splenectomy. If possible, splenectomy should be delayed until children with thalassemia are at least 5 years old. By this time, children are more likely to have developed humoral immunity to a broad range of bacteria. Before splenectomy, polyvalent pneumococcal, meningococcal, and *H. influenzae* vaccines should be administered if they have not been given earlier in life.[384,385] Oral penicillin therapy, 250 mg twice daily, is generally used as prophylaxis against postsplenectomy infection in patients with thalassemia. However, the optimal duration of penicillin prophylaxis remains unknown, and compliance is frequently inadequate.[386] Although the risk of postsplenectomy sepsis decreases with age, it does not disappear, and fatal pneumococcal sepsis has occurred many years after removal of the spleen.[387]

Pneumococcal sepsis is not totally preventable because not all pneumococcal strains are represented in the available vaccines. In addition, penicillin-resistant strains of *S. pneumoniae* have emerged with a prevalence in the United States of 5% to 10% or even higher in some localities. Therefore, it is particularly important that patients and families be instructed to seek medical attention immediately if significant fever or other signs of infection develop.

Vitamin Supplementation

Although folic acid deficiency is uncommon in patients receiving regular transfusions, daily supplementation with 1.0 mg of folic acid is reasonable, especially if dietary intake is not optimal. Therapy with large doses of vitamin E neither improves survival of transfused RBCs nor decreases transfusion requirements.[388] Whether vitamin E supplementation decreases the toxic effects of iron overload on specific tissues remains uncertain. Zinc supplementation is appropriate for patients with clinical or laboratory findings of zinc deficiency, usually a result of intensive iron chelation therapy. One center has reported an enhancement of linear growth in children with thalassemia receiving zinc for 1 to 7 years.[389]

Survival in Patients with Thalassemia Major

Improved transfusion therapy and the consistent use of iron chelation therapy have extended the life span of patients with thalassemia major.[115,213,215,390] In a multicenter study of 1079 patients in Italy, the probability of survival to age 20 years was 96% for patients born between 1975 and 1979, the time at which chelation therapy became a regular part of the overall management of thalassemia major (Table 38-2).[213] In contrast, the probabilities of survival at 20 years of age were only 61% and 69% for those born in the periods of 1960 through 1964 and 1965 through 1969, respectively. Other investigators have shown that survival or prevention of life-threatening complications is strongly related to good chelation therapy, assessed either by compliance or by control of iron stores (Fig. 38-11).[174,207,215] The importance of good compliance with chelation therapy is further demonstrated by data from the United Kingdom showing that the probability of survival for the 1975 through 1984 birth cohort is to date not substantially different than the probability of survival for the 1965 through 1974 birth cohort.[390] The researchers attribute this poorer than expected survival rate, despite the availability of deferoxamine, to a lack of adherence to the recommended schedule of treatment with this chelator.

Table 38-2 Survival by Birth Cohort at Different Ages of Patients With Transfusion-Dependent Thalassemia

Patient Age (Years)	Cohort 1970-1974	Cohort 1975-1979	Cohort 1980-1984
10	98% (96-99)	98% (96-99)	99% (95-100)
15	95% (92-97)	97% (94-98)	98% (93-100)
20	89% (85-92)	96% (93-98)	
25	82% (77-86)		

Data from Borgna Pignatti C, Rugolotto S, De Stefano X, et al: Survival and disease complications in thalassemia major. *Ann N Y Acad Sci* 850:227, 1998.

Hematopoietic Stem Cell Transplantation

The first transplantation of allogeneic hematopoietic stem cells (HSCs) derived from the BM of a human leukocyte antigen (HLA)–identical sibling donor was reported in 1982.[391] There is now extensive experience with transplantation, with well over 3000 patients having undergone transplantation.[392] The pioneering work of Lucarelli's group in Pesaro, Italy, has allowed for the prognostic classification of patients younger than the age of 17 years who receive an HLA-identical sibling donor with a preparative regimen, including busulfan, cyclophosphamide, and cyclosporine. This risk classification is based on hepatomegaly, the degree of portal fibrosis, and the regularity of prior iron chelation therapy.[393] In class 1 without adverse factors, the overall survival rate is 95%, and the event-free survival rate (without thalassemia) is 90%; class 2 patients with one or two risk factors have an 85% survival and an 81% event-free survival; and class 3 patients with all three risk factors have only 64% and 62% overall and event-free survival rates, respectively (Fig. 38-12).[393] Advances in conditioning regimens have considerably improved the outcome of class 3 patients who are younger than 17 years of age. Preparatory chemotherapeutic regimens to enhance immunosuppression and eradicate thalassemic clones using hydroxyurea, azathioprine, fludarabine, busulfan, and cyclophosphamide have increased the survival rate of class 3 patients to 93%; the rejection rate fell to 8%.[394] These favorable results have not been reproduced in the older,

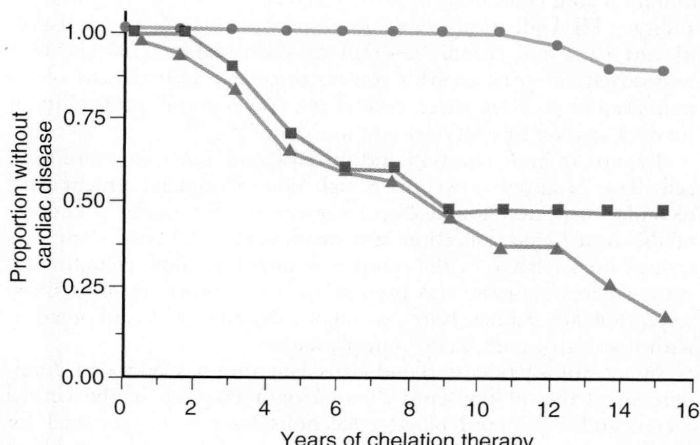

Figure 38-11 SURVIVAL WITHOUT CARDIAC DISEASE IN PATIENTS WITH THALASSEMIA MAJOR TREATED WITH DEFEROXAMINE ACCORDING TO THE PROPORTION OF SERUM FERRITIN MEASUREMENTS GREATER THAN 2500 NG/ML. The *circles* show cardiac disease-free survival among patients in whom less than 33% of ferritin measurements exceeded 2500 ng/mL; *squares* show survival among patients in whom 33% to 67% of ferritin measurements exceeded 2500 ng/mL; and *triangles* show survival among patients in whom more than 67% of ferritin measurements exceeded 2500 ng/mL. *(Adapted from Olivieri NF, Nathan DG, MacMillan JH, et al: Survival in medically treated patients with homozygous beta-thalassemia.* N Engl J Med *331:574, 1994.)*

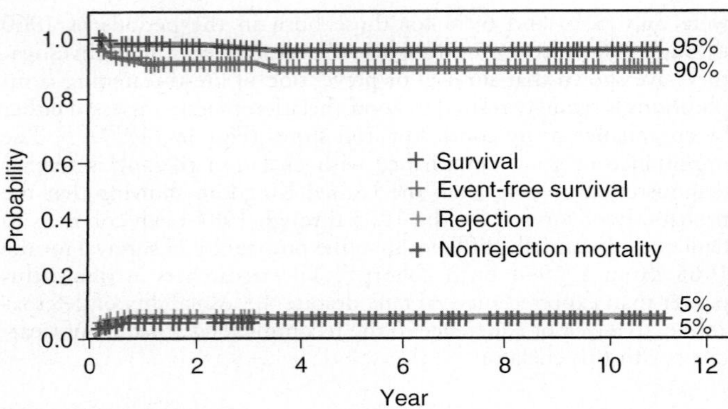

Figure 38-12 Kaplan-Meier probabilities of survival, event-free survival, rejection, and nonrejection mortality for 121 class 1 thalassemic patients younger than 17 years receiving bone marrow transplants from human leukocyte antigen–identical donors after preparation with busulfan (14 mg/kg), cyclophosphamide (200 mg/kg), and cyclosporine alone, from January 2, 1986, through April 10, 1997, and calculated on May 15, 1997. *(Adapted from Lucarelli G, Galimberti M, Giardini C, et al: Bone marrow transplantation in thalassemia.* Ann N Y Acad Sci *850:270, 1998.)*

more heavily iron-overloaded patients who remain high risk for transplant-related mortality.[395] Stem cell transplantation can fail or be lethal owing to its immunologic complications. The overall incidence of acute graft-versus-host disease (GVHD) is 17% to 32% depending on the prophylaxis regimen, and the incidence of chronic GVHD is 27% in patients receiving BM HSCs from a parental or sibling HLA-identical donor.[396]

Although HSC transplantation is the only curative therapy available, its use has been limited by cost and the rarity of HLA-identical related donors.

Building on the success of BMT for patients with thalassemia major using HLA-identical related donors, investigators have explored alternative strategies to increase the safety and availability of transplantation. In pediatric patients, transplantation of stem cells from umbilical cord blood has been associated with a reduced risk of GVHD compared with BMT.[397,398] Stem cells derived from sibling umbilical cord collections have increased in part the safety and availability of HLA-identical related donor transplantation. The probabilities of acute and chronic GVHD are decreased to 11% and 6%, respectively, in patients who receive allogeneic related cord blood transplantation.[397] However, despite the 100% overall probability of survival, disease-free survival rate was only 79%.[398]

Reports of graft rejection and mixed chimerism using cord stem cells have occurred as well as a high rate of nonengraftment with secondary rejection at a median follow-up of 49 months.[398] The size of the cord blood collection and small number of cord stem cells transplanted relative to the number required to allow engraftment, sustain hematopoiesis, and prevent graft rejections are most likely responsible for failures. Rare case reports describe successful outcome with nonrelated cord blood transplantation.

Successful use of cord blood transplantation has led to the development of the Sibling Cord Blood Donor Program in the United States, and 1617 cord blood collections have been processed for families with thalassemia. Some patients have received cord blood transplantation either alone or in combination with BM or peripheral progenitor cells.[399] In addition, BM donor registries have also developed worldwide to identify HLA-compatible unrelated donors with more that 10 million volunteers registered.

In an effort to increase the pool of potential recipients of stem cell transplantation for thalassemia, investigators have also explored the use of matched unrelated donor BMT. Extended haplotype and family segregation studies may identify suitable unrelated donors using HLA closely matched unrelated donor transplantation in thalassemia using high-resolution molecular HLA typing. La Nasa et al[400] reported 79% disease-free and 66% event-free survival, but 19% died of transplant-related complications, 41% developed grade II to IV acute GVHD, and 25% had chronic GVHD. Most of the deaths occurred in patients with heavy iron overload or hepatic complications. The results suggested that engraftment and less GVHD occurred when the recipient and donor were identical for one or two extended haplotypes.[400] Other reports also using unrelated HSCs selected according to stringent criteria of compatibility and using high-resolution molecular typing have indicated that unrelated donor transplantation may offer results comparable to those obtained with HLA-identical family donors for patients with limited iron overload.[400,401] Otherwise, the overall disease-free survival rate is only 60%, with a significant risk of chronic GVHD. The results obtained with cord blood stem cell transplantation are encouraging, but too little experience exists for definitive conclusions.[402]

Alternative unrelated matched or mismatched related donor transplantation is associated with a greater risk of immune complications. The only well-established curative therapy is allogeneic stem cell transplantation from a matched related donor. Transplantation is an important consideration in management for young thalassemia patients who have yet to accumulate excessive iron and those who have successfully controlled iron stores with chelation and who have an HLA-identical matched related donor.

The options of cord blood stem cell collection and cord blood or BMT discussions with families of the newly diagnosed are warranted as is a discussion of the long-term outcomes.

After a successful stem cell transplantation, some patients remain iron overloaded and require phlebotomy to prevent the risks of progressive hepatic fibrosis; other previously affected patients with hepatitis C require antiviral treatment[220,403] that may improve hepatic fibrosis and cirrhosis.[404]

After transplantation, some patients develop a state of mixed chimerism that may persist in 10% to 30% of patients with a predominance of host cells in the BM even though transfusion dependence may have dissipated.[405] However, 30% of patients with early mixed chimerism subsequently reject their graft.[406] Those patients with mixed chimerism and falling hemoglobin who require supportive transfusion may successfully undergo a second transplant with nonmyeloablative conditioning to restore normal hemoglobin levels.[407,408]

Subsequent investigations to evaluate the effect of nonmyeloablative conditioning regimens as a primary approach to transplantation with the objective of causing a chimeric outcome have been attempted and are of questionable benefit.[401,409,410]

Allogeneic HSC transplantation from a partially HLA-matched relative has also been investigated, with much less encouraging results. Gaziev et al[395] reported early or late graft-versus-host and graft failure in 55% of partial HLA familial matched without significant correlation between the degree of antigen disparities and graft failure. GVHD was a major factor contributing to death (50%) followed by infection (30%). The probability of overall survival and transfusion dependence were 65% and 21%, respectively, with a median follow-up at 2.5 years for surviving patients.[395]

In view of the available evidence, stem cell transplantation from a partially HLA-matched relative is not routinely advisable, although it may be considered in extreme situations when transfusion support is impossible or life threatening when a patient is completely noncompliant with any type of iron chelation therapy.

The excellent results of BMT in young patients with thalassemia who have yet to accumulate excessive iron or who have successfully controlled iron stores have made transplantation an important consideration in their management. The option of BM or umbilical cord blood transplantation should be discussed with families of newly diagnosed patients with thalassemia major and should be compared with long-term transfusion and chelation therapy. Both approaches should be addressed in terms of currently identified risks and benefits, the likelihood of future improvements, and the potential for new treatments such as gene therapy. In some centers, tissue typing of immediate family members is undertaken routinely, but in others, this evaluation is performed only if the family wishes to consider transplantation as a treatment option. On the basis of the positive results with umbilical cord blood transplantation, parents of children with thalassemia should be encouraged to collect and store cord blood with future pregnancies.[399,411] The use of preimplantation diagnosis to identify an HLA-identical embryo unaffected with the sibling's blood disorder poses significant ethical dilemmas but has been used to create suitable donors for cord blood or BMT in cases of other hematologic diseases.[412-416] A related and also controversial approach is the use of both fetal and family HLA typing in pregnancies at risk of homozygous thalassemia to determine whether an HLA-identical sibling is available as a potential BM donor if the fetus is affected and carried to term.[417,418]

The rate of success for BMT in children with more significant iron overload, in adults, and in patients without an HLA-identical sibling or parent suggests caution in the use of this approach. Transplantation has been recommended for such patients if they show progressive deterioration with conventional transfusion and chelation therapy. The availability of new chelating agents may significantly affect this balance, as may improvements in transplantation.

Long-term complications of stem cell transplantation have also been reported, including gonadal dysfunction and fertility as well as growth failure and other endocrinopathies.[419,420]

In conclusion, HSC transplantation with the use of matched related or unrelated donors is an alternative to standard transfusion and chelation therapy and generally results in excellent outcomes for low-risk patients. However, there are small risks of serious complications including death, graft failure or rejection, GVHD as well as growth failure, infertility, and other endocrinopathies. Stem cell transplantation should be considered for class 1 and 2 children who have suitable donors. Unrelated HLA-matched donors, although an acceptable source of allogeneic stem cell for other conditions, are not yet considered suitable for children with thalassemia because of the relatively long-term survival associated with conventional therapy. Owing to the considerable risks and experiences of transplantation as well as the prospect of 2 or 3 decades of life with conventional management, discussions with the families of children who are potential candidates for transplant should be thorough.

Transplantation for those class 3 older patients and adults fare less well[421-423] and should be considered only for those who have a suitable donor or deteriorate with conventional treatment.[113]

Experimental Therapies

Enhancement of β and γ Gene Expression

For many years, much effort has focused on stimulation of γ-globin gene expression or replacement of defective β-globin genes. Enhanced γ-globin gene expression would ameliorate the unbalanced globin chain synthesis and replace the missing adult hemoglobin with fetal hemoglobin.

Active γ-globin genes are hypomethylated in utero but are methylated and inactive after birth. Hypomethylation of the γ-globin genes can be induced by the drug 5-azacytidine; indeed, short-term administration of this drug produced the predicted effect in vivo.[424-426] Despite much subsequent experimental work, it remains unclear whether the effect was attributable to direct stimulation of fetal genes by demethylation or to recruitment and accelerated differentiation of primitive burst-forming unit–erythroid (BFU-E) progenitor cells, which have greater potential to produce Hb F.[427-429] Hydroxyurea has an effect on BFU-E similar to that of 5-azacytidine and is a safer drug for long-term use.[428,430] Short-term as well as longer trials with hydroxyurea have been reported in a number of patients with thalassemia.[431-438] Hb F levels frequently increase without a proportionate increase in total hemoglobin level. A small improvement in total hemoglobin level occurs in some patients with thalassemia intermedia but usually does not exceed 1 to 2 g/dL.[435,436] Some patients report improvement in their overall sense of well-being even in the absence of an improvement in the anemia.[435] This may be a result of suppression of abnormal erythropoiesis, an effect that may also explain the value of hydroxyurea in the treatment of extramedullary hematopoietic masses (see later discussion).[439] Although one patient with thalassemia major had sufficient improvement in his hemoglobin level to end his dependency on regular transfusions,[437] most transfusion-dependent patients have shown no clinical benefit. In a review of hydroxyurea therapy, Steinberg and Rodgers[438] identified 52 patients with β-thalassemia who were treated with a variety of regimens. They concluded that hydroxyurea alone had only a modest effect in thalassemia intermedia and did not look promising for thalassemia major.[440]

Recombinant erythropoietin has produced inconsistent responses in patients with thalassemia intermedia.[441-445] When the series are combined, approximately 40% of patients have an increase in hemoglobin level of 2 to 3 g/dL. Fetal hemoglobin levels are unchanged. The potentially adverse consequences of further stimulation of an already hyperactive BM are uncertain. Erythropoietin has shown little benefit overall in patients with thalassemia major, although there are occasional reports of patients whose transfusion requirements were reduced or eliminated.[444,446]

Butyrate and other short-chain fatty acids have been demonstrated to augment Hb F production in various animal model systems as well as in humans.[447-449] These compounds are believed to act by altering chromatin configuration, perhaps because of inhibition of histone deacetylatase.[450-454] Short-term treatment with intravenous infusions of arginine butyrate in a limited number of cases[451,452] resulted in a marked increase in γ/α-globin chain synthetic ratios,[450,455] but others did not have a sustained hematologic response.[456] In yet another trial, administration of arginine butyrate intravenously in pulsed fashion to patients with sickle cell anemia and thalassemia resulted in favorable hematologic responses, raising the possibility of hematologic toxicity and suboptimal responses with continuous infusions of the drug.[457] Orally absorbable butyric acid compounds, including sodium phenylbutyrate and isobutyramide, also have been reported to result in an increase in F-cell and γ-globin chain production, but the effect was not as sustained or as quantitatively comparable to that originally obtained with intravenous arginine butyrate.[430,439,458-464] A study of isobutyramide in cases of thalassemia major found a reduction in transfusion requirements in two of eight patients. No severe toxic side effects were observed in these relatively short-term trials in humans, but the infusion of high doses of butyrate into baboons did result in significant neurologic toxic effects. Further studies will be required to assess the long-term safety and efficacy of therapy with butyrate. Most recently, a new fetal hemoglobin inducer, HQK-1001, has been identified, and its erythropoietic stimulatory efforts are being studied.[465]

Various combinations of hydroxyurea, butyrate, and erythropoietin have been used to try to achieve hematologic benefits that cannot be achieved with a single agent.[450] The addition of hydroxyurea to therapy with sodium phenylbutyrate led to a further increase in hemoglobin level in a patient with homozygous Lepore. However, the combination of sodium phenylbutyrate and hydroxyurea was no better than hydroxyurea alone in other patients with thalassemia intermedia.[436] Combined therapy with hydroxyurea and erythropoietin produced marginally higher hemoglobin levels than either drug alone in only two of seven patients with thalassemia intermedia.[442] A more dramatic rise in hemoglobin level occurred in a patient with thalassemia major, but the relative contributions of pharmacologic therapy and splenectomy are unclear.

Decitabine has been shown to result in a considerable sustained increase of Hb F and total hemoglobin in patients with sickle cell disease with the low likelihood of neutropenia and may have a similar effect in thalassemia but its therapeutic efficacy remains to be proven.[466,467] A pilot study of subcutaneous decitabine in β-thalassemia intermedia has shown somewhat favorable changes in hemoglobin levels ($P = .004$) and absolute fetal hemoglobin levels ($P = .003$).[468]

Although the pharmacologic enhancement of fetal hemoglobin production remains an attractive strategy in the management of thalassemia, the results to date strongly suggest the need for new agents or new combinations of agents. At present, the primary clinical application of this approach is in the management of severely affected patients who are unable to be transfused because of multiple alloantibodies or because of autoantibodies. This approach might also be used for patients with thalassemia intermedia who develop a need for frequent transfusions. However, studies suggest that the current approaches to fetal hemoglobin enhancement will usually be unsuccessful in either of these situations.

Another potential strategy is to develop techniques to silence HbF suppression. Recently, the knock down of BCL11A expression resulted in the reactivation of HbF expression.[469] Other important molecular targets to induce HbF include KLF1, MYB, SOX6, MiRNAs, and histone acetylase, which may lead to other targeted approaches to enhance HbF.[470-478] BCL11A is a zinc-finger transcriptional repressor active in erythroid cells and in other hematopoietic lineages.[479] Several studies indicate that BCL11A silences γ-globin.[479-481] BCL11A does not bind the γ-globin promoter but the LCR and different intergenic regions in the globin locus that were previously tied with γ-globin repression.[479,482-485] KLF1 (also known as EKLF) is an erythroid transcription factor activating BCL11a and playing a major role in the switch from fetal to adult hemoglobin.[486-489] Thalassemia intermedia patients with mutations in the CACCC box of the β-globin promoter (which is recognized by KLF1) demonstrate significant elevation of HbF.[490,491] An additional locus highlighted by GWAS is the intergenic interval between HBS1L and MYB.[492-495] More recently, it has been demonstrated that knockdown of c-Myb was associated with decreased expression of KLF1.[496] In conclusion, new key regulators of the globin switch have been identified that may be used to develop new and more powerful drugs aimed at increasing fetal hemoglobin synthesis.

β-Globin Gene Transfer

Cure of thalassemia by genetic transfer of the normal β-globin gene into the pluripotent HSC awaits further advances in molecular biology but is a goal of the foreseeable future.[497] β-Globin gene transfer and expression has been accomplished in thalassemia murine models, which have demonstrated that retroviral vectors, specifically lentiviral vectors, are capable of transferring the human β-globin gene sequences and its promoter regions into murine stem cells[498,499] and into long-term repopulating hematopoietic cells of primates and humans.[500,501] Studies of safe and efficient specific targeting vectors in humans are ongoing.[502] Techniques for obtaining long-term expression of human globin genes after transfer into murine HSCs have been developed.[503,504] Thus, there has been remarkable success in the use of globin gene transfer for "therapy" of murine models of β-thalassemia and sickle cell anemia.[497,498,503,505-507] However, clinical trials have suffered from problems of vector instability, low viral titers, and variable expression of globin genes.[508] Additional safety modifications to prevent potential genotoxic effects have been studied, including the use of insulators or genetic elements with enhancer-blocking properties to increase the safety of clinical trials.[509-511] Genetic elements with enhancer-blocking properties, such as insulators, could increase the safety of the clinical trails. These elements have been investigated to shelter the vector from the repressive influence of flanking chromatin by blocking interactions between regulatory elements within the vector and chromosomal elements at the site of integration.[509-511] This property of insulators can also be harnessed to diminish the risk that the vector will activate a neighboring oncogene.[508,512] These formidable problems need to be solved before it becomes routinely possible to transfer and effectively express globin genes in human HSCs; ensure their safe and active expression at effective levels; and preserve normal growth, differentiation, and proliferation of the genetically transformed stem cell.[513-517] Nevertheless, protocols have been developed to carry out gene transfer experiments in humans.[518] A phase I human gene therapy clinical trial for hemoglobinopathies was initiated in France in 2007.[519] To date, one compound heterozygote patient with β-E thalassemia received a lentiviral vector with a normal β-globin gene who after gene transfer is transfusion independent and is producing the "therapeutic" vector hemoglobin as well as fetal and embryonic hemoglobins.[519] This trial used a lentiviral vector that expresses an adult β-globin gene flanked by two copies of the 250-base-pair core of the cHS4 chromatin insulator implanted in the U3 region of the 3′ long terminal repeat. After gene transfer, the patient became transfusion independent. However, the therapeutic hemoglobin in this patient contributed only one-third of the total hemoglobin synthesized; the embryonic and fetal hemoglobins accounted equally for the remaining hemoglobin. Therefore, the success of this first trial was made possible by the additive effect of transgenic β-globin chains synthesized by the vector and those (fetal and adult) made by the patient's cells. Thus, without the support of endogenous hemoglobins, the gene transfer would not have allowed this patient to become transfusion independent. Further work is currently planned, and studies are being conducted to better predict the outcome of gene transfer.[518]

iPS Cells and Gene Correction

Alternatively, somatic cells reprogrammed to induced pluripotent stem cells (iPSCs) might also provide a possible new approach to treat β-thalassemia and sickle cell disease.[520] Currently, robust generation of iPSCs requires the introduction and integration of genes encoding the transcriptional factors OCT3/4, SOX2 with either KLF4 and c-MYC or NANOG and LIN28.[521-523] Ye and coworkers[520] have shown that iPSCs can be generated from cells derived from skin fibroblasts, amniotic fluid, or chorionic villus sampling of patients with β-thalassemia and subsequently differentiated into hematopoietic cells that synthesized hemoglobin.

However, these iPS cells will need to be corrected for the β-globin mutation before they can be redifferentiated to HSC hemoglobin producing RBCs. Homologous recombination (HR) in embryonic and iPSCs for the cure of hemoglobinopathies has several potential advantages over conventional gene therapy, including eliminating the need for immunosuppression, avoiding the risk of insertional mutagenesis by therapeutic vectors, and maintaining expression of the corrected gene by endogenous control elements rather than a constitutive promoter. Wu et al[524] and Chang et al[525]'s laboratories used HR to generate iPSCs from, respectively, a β-thalassemic patient and sickle mice and correct their mutations. Moreover, using a humanized sickle cell disease (SCD) mouse model, Jaenisch's laboratory demonstrated that mice can be rescued after transplantation with hematopoietic progenitors obtained in vitro from autologous iPSCs. This was achieved after correction of the human sickle hemoglobin allele by gene-specific targeting.[526] Furthermore, proof of principle that the β-globin gene can be repaired in human iPSCs was provided by two groups.[527,528] They achieved correction of the β-globin gene by HR in iPSCs derived from a SCD patient using specific β-globin zinc finger nucleases engineered to specifically stimulate HR at the β-globin locus. Importantly, this work strongly supports the rationale to generate corrected iPSCs using HR, showing that this technique is feasible and can lead to the production of corrected iPSCs. However, additional studies need to be done before this approach can be used for humans.

Thalassemia Intermedia

Approximately 10% of patients with homozygous β-thalassemia exhibit a phenotype characterized by intermediate hematologic severity.[1-4] The balance of globin chain synthesis is better than in typical thalassemia major because of a less severe defect in β-globin chain synthesis, a decrease in α-globin chain synthesis as well as β-globin chain synthesis, or an increase in γ-globin chain synthesis. For example, homozygous β-thalassemia in African Americans, Portuguese, and other populations may be relatively mild, at least for the first 2 decades of life.[529-531] Homozygotes or mixed heterozygotes for forms of β-thalassemia associated with normal Hb A_2 and normal Hb F (silent carrier state) also tend to have mild to moderate disease.[532,533] Certain patients have a milder clinical phenotype because they have co-inherited a form of α-thalassemia[13-15] or because they carry one (or two) β-thalassemia chromosome(s) with a greater than usual potential for high levels of γ-globin gene expression.

The ability to maintain a hemoglobin level compatible with comfortable survival in the absence of regular transfusions is the generally accepted criterion for the diagnosis of thalassemia intermedia. In other words, distinguishing between thalassemia major and thalassemia intermedia, which in turn is the distinction between initiating a regular transfusion program or not, requires consideration of the hemoglobin level and the quality of life. These two parameters do not have a predictable relationship. Patients with thalassemia and hemoglobin levels of 7 g/dL may be relatively symptom free, but patients with hemoglobin levels of 9 g/dL may have numerous problems related to ineffective erythropoiesis. Thus, the assessment of the patient rather than the hemoglobin level alone is essential in deciding who does not require regular transfusions and therefore, by definition, has thalassemia intermedia. Some nontransfused patients have normal growth and sexual development, few medical problems, and normal or near-normal survival rates. However, others develop disfiguring facial changes, markedly delayed growth and sexual maturation, heart failure, severe osteoporosis, repeated fractures, arthritis, and massive splenomegaly. Calling the condition of this latter group "thalassemia intermedia" implies a milder disease than thalassemia major but, in fact, the patients' quality of life does not compare favorably with the quality of life of patients with thalassemia major. Nonetheless, many families and physicians are reluctant to initiate a chronic transfusion program because of concern about the risks of long-term transfusion therapy and the inevitable need for iron chelation therapy. If the decision is made to manage the patient initially without regular transfusions, regular reassessments of the patient's clinical condition, including appearance, growth, and development, and bone expansion are crucial.[534] Short-term transfusion therapy may be useful during pregnancy or in the management of cardiac and other serious complications. The need for regular transfusions often develops in adults with thalassemia intermedia because of a further decline in the hemoglobin level or a growing intolerance of the anemia.[535]

Even in the absence of regular transfusions, many patients develop progressive iron overload because of increased absorption of dietary iron induced by ineffective erythropoiesis and, in many cases, the intermittent administration of RBC transfusions. By the third or fourth decade, the total iron burden may attain the levels seen in transfusion-dependent patients.[536] Ferritin levels may underestimate the degree of tissue iron loading in thalassemia intermedia, and assessment of liver iron concentration is more helpful in determining the need for chelation therapy. Deferoxamine as well as the orally active iron chelator deferiprone (L1) has proved effective in thalassemia intermedia.[537,538]

Splenectomy raises the hemoglobin level by 1 to 3 g/dL in many patients with thalassemia intermedia.[539,540] Removal of the spleen should receive careful consideration as a potential alternative to beginning transfusion therapy. As noted earlier, for patients who undergo splenectomy while on a chronic transfusion program, a period of careful monitoring of the hemoglobin level after surgery may occasionally identify individuals who are no longer transfusion dependent and who can therefore be reclassified as having thalassemia intermedia.

Thromboembolic events represent a major complication of thalassemia intermedia, occurring in 10% to 34% of patients.[369,541] These events include stroke, pulmonary embolism, portal vein thrombosis, and deep vein thrombosis of the legs. A hypercoagulable state may also contribute to the pulmonary hypertension that commonly occurs in patients with thalassemia intermedia and is the primary cause of congestive heart failure.[542] Splenectomy is a risk factor for thromboembolic events in patients with thalassemia intermedia, resulting in thrombocytosis and allowing the prolonged circulation of damaged RBCs that generate increased amounts of thrombin.[369] Some investigators consider the risk of thromboembolic events after splenectomy for thalassemia intermedia to be sufficiently high to warrant short-term anticoagulation in the perioperative period and during pregnancy.[369] Oral contraceptives should be used with extreme caution, if at all.

Extension of hematopoietic tissue beyond the confines of the bones occurs in patients with thalassemia intermedia as a result of the intense erythropoiesis. This complication occurs less frequently in patients with thalassemia major because of the partial suppression of erythropoiesis by regular transfusions. Masses of extramedullary hematopoietic tissue develop in the spinal epidural space, thorax, cranium, pelvis, and elsewhere.[439,543-553] These masses may be detected as incidental findings on imaging studies of the chest or abdomen.[544-550] In other instances, the masses produce symptoms by compressing neighboring structures. For example, patients with extramedullary hematopoietic masses may develop paraplegia from spinal cord compression or loss of visual acuity or visual fields caused by optic nerve compression.[543,546,552,553] Additional clinical presentations of hematopoietic masses include pleural effusions and upper airway obstruction.[548,549,551] Initiation of regular transfusions for patients with thalassemia intermedia or intensification of the ongoing transfusion program for patients with thalassemia major reduces the size of extramedullary hematopoietic masses and helps to prevent recurrences. Therapy with hydroxyurea has also been associated with shrinkage of hematopoietic masses.[439] Low-dose radiation therapy provides more immediate relief and may be particularly useful for acute neurologic complications.[554]

Reconstruction of the maxilla may be needed for some patients with thalassemia intermedia to provide cosmetic improvement of facial asymmetry and malocclusion.[555] Gallstones regularly occur by the second decade of life.[556] Leg ulcers often occur in late adolescence or afterward and may require RBC transfusions as well as local measures for healing. Because of the marked BM hyperplasia, supplementation with folic acid is necessary to prevent megaloblastic anemia. Aplastic crises associated with parvovirus or other infections may result in exacerbations of the anemia.

Some patients with heterozygous β-thalassemia will have a moderately severe clinical disorder, with anemia, hemolysis, and splenomegaly. Some of these patients carry a greater than normal number of α-globin genes as a result of triplication of one of the α-globin gene loci: ααα/αα.[34,404,557,558] However, most heterozygous patients with triplicated α-globin gene loci are clinically similar to those with the simple β-thalassemia trait. Most patients with severe heterozygous β-thalassemia have so-called dominant β-thalassemia, which is attributable to the inheritance of a gene for a β-thalassemia hemoglobinopathy associated with a structurally abnormal, unstable, β-globin chain that may form inclusion bodies.[16,17] For heterozygotes with disease of unusual clinical severity, splenectomy may be beneficial.

β-Thalassemia Minor (Thalassemia Trait)

Inheritance of a single β-thalassemia allele usually results in a mild hypochromic microcytic anemia. The hemoglobin level averages 1 or 2 g/dL lower than that seen in normal persons of the same age and gender. Hb F levels decline more slowly than usual in the first year of life, and the diagnostic elevated Hb A_2 levels are established by approximately 6 months of age.[559-561] Strong intrafamilial correlations of both Hb A_2 and mean corpuscular volume (MCV) are noted.[562,563] Osmotic fragility is decreased; indeed, a one-tube osmotic fragility test has been used in the past for mass screening.[560] The RBC count is increased or normal. The RBCs are characteristically hypochromic (mean corpuscular hemoglobin <26 pg) and microcytic (MCV <75 fL). The smear shows varying numbers of target cells, poikilocytes, ovalocytes, and basophilic stippling (Fig. 38-13). The reticulocyte count is normal or slightly elevated. RBC survival is normal, iron utilization is decreased, and slight IE is present.[561] Most patients are asymptomatic. Many patients who have thalassemia trait are erroneously believed to have iron deficiency. Testing to distinguish these two disorders is important for genetic counseling of carriers of thalassemia trait, for the avoidance of unnecessary investigations in patients incorrectly assumed to have iron deficiency and to prevent unwarranted supplementation with iron. Although a variety of indices calculated from blood count parameters have been suggested to differentiate thalassemia from iron deficiency, each has some degree of inaccuracy; most are no better than the MCV alone.[563,564] In general, the MCV is rarely greater than 75 fL or the hematocrit less than 30 in patients with β-thalassemia trait. In cases of iron

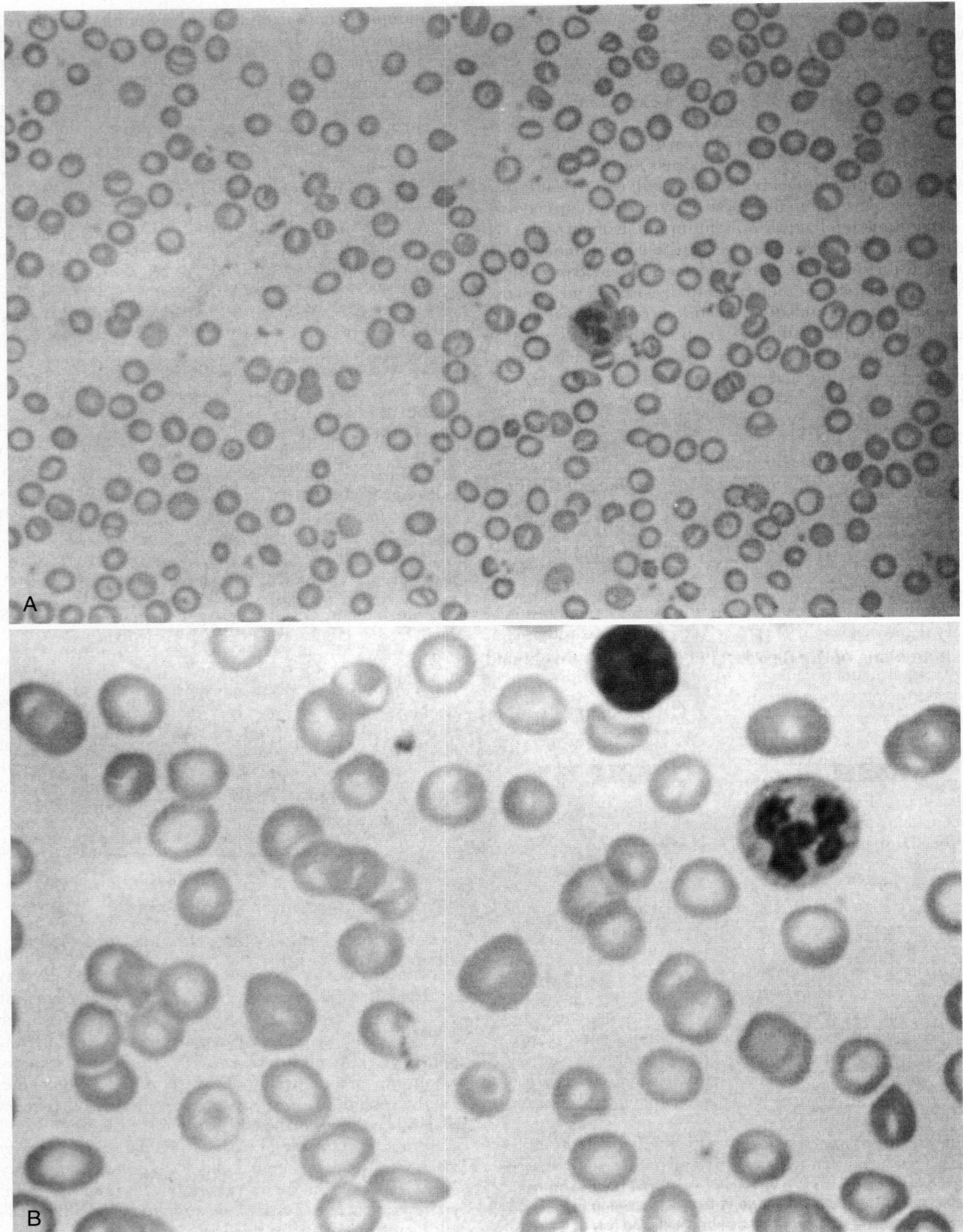

Figure 38-13 MORPHOLOGY OF THE PERIPHERAL BLOOD FILM IN A PATIENT WITH HETEROZYGOUS β-THALASSEMIA (**A**) AND A PATIENT WITH HETEROZYGOUS α-THALASSEMIA (**B**). Note the profound hypochromia and microcytosis and the many target cells. *(From Pearson HA, Benz EJ Jr: Thalassemia syndromes. In Miller DR, Baehner RL, McMillan CW, editors:* Smith's blood diseases of infancy and childhood, *ed 5, St. Louis, 1984, CV Mosby, p 439.)*

deficiency, the hematocrit level usually falls to less than 30 before the MCV falls to less than 80 fL. Free erythrocyte porphyrin levels are normal in patients with thalassemia trait but are elevated in patients with iron deficiency (see Chapter 34).[1] Specific studies for iron deficiency, such as the serum iron level and total iron-binding capacity or the serum ferritin level, help to prevent misdiagnosis.

During pregnancy, the anemia of thalassemia trait often becomes more severe, but transfusions are rarely necessary. Because iron deficiency may occur during pregnancy, iron supplementation has been advised to avoid compounding the causes of anemia.[565,566]

There may be characteristic racial differences in the hematologic severity of β-thalassemia trait. In African Americans, the condition is invariably milder, RBC morphologic abnormalities are less marked, and β/α synthetic ratios are higher than in whites and Asians with the trait.[567]

The diagnosis of β-thalassemia trait is established in most instances by the demonstration of altered proportions of Hb A_2. The level of Hb A_2 in β-thalassemia trait averages 5.1% (range, 3.5%-7.0%), approximately twice the normal level (1.5%-3.5%); the Hb A_2 to Hb A_1 ratio is 1 : 20 instead of the normal 1 : 40. This increase is probably attributable to a posttranslational (assembly) phenomenon with increased opportunity for δ-globin chains to combine with α-globin chains in the face of β-globin chain deficiency. If concomitant iron-deficiency anemia occurs, Hb A_2 levels may fall, sometimes into the normal range.[568]

The Hb F levels are inconsistently elevated in β-thalassemia. In approximately half of cases, Hb F is within the normal range (<2.0%); in the remainder, it is moderately elevated (2.1%-5.0%). However, in almost every instance, a minor population of RBCs (F cells) containing substantial amounts of Hb F can be demonstrated by the Kleihauer technique.[1] Rarely, an individual with heterozygous thalassemia, as evidenced by a reduced β/α synthetic ratio or by virtue of having a child with thalassemia intermedia or major, has normal Hb A_2, Hb F, and hemoglobin electrophoresis, with minor (quiet carrier) or no (silent carrier) hematologic changes.[533] Rare individuals have been encountered who exhibit characteristically abnormal RBC morphology but normal levels of Hb A2 and Hb F.[1] Such individuals are probably carriers of γδβ-thalassemia.[1] Iron deficiency must be excluded and globin-chain synthesis or molecular studies done to establish a diagnosis with certainty.

The diagnosis of thalassemia trait assumes particular importance in women who are pregnant or considering pregnancy because of the potential for having a child with thalassemia major. The presence of a low MCV should be investigated further with levels of Hb A_2 and Hb F, as well as a hemoglobin electrophoresis to look for thalassemic variants such as Hb E and Hb Lepore (see later discussion). If either the father or the mother is known to have thalassemia trait, the other person should be assessed using these more definitive studies rather than the MCV alone.

Prenatal Diagnosis of β-Thalassemia

Thalassemia mutations can now be routinely and reliably diagnosed by using fetal DNA obtained between the 8th and 18th weeks of gestation. The most reliable methods are based on identification of the abnormal gene by direct DNA analysis.[22,569,570] Both amniocentesis and chorionic villus sampling have been used with success. In experienced hands, the latter method is preferable because adequate amounts of DNA can be obtained safely at an earlier gestational age. New techniques have been developed for obtaining fetal DNA for prenatal diagnosis either directly from maternal plasma or by the isolation of fetal nucleated RBCs from maternal peripheral blood.[566,571,572] The DNA is analyzed by a variety of polymerase chain reaction (PCR)–based or other methods for the presence of the thalassemia mutation.

The heterogeneity of thalassemia mutations complicates the approach to antenatal diagnosis. More than 175 independent mutations can cause β-thalassemia. However, a number of factors have improved the speed, efficacy, and reliability of DNA diagnosis. Extensive surveys of most populations in which these alleles are frequent have revealed that approximately 15 β-thalassemia mutations account for more than 90% of individuals affected worldwide. Within any given ethnic group, three to six mutations usually account for the vast majority of severe cases (see Table 38-1).[22] One can thus customize the search for mutations according to the ethnic origins of the family at risk. PCR techniques and exquisitely precise hybridization assays (allele-specific oligonucleotide hybridization), which detect single-base changes with great reliability, can now be combined to permit screening of minute DNA samples for several mutations very rapidly (Fig. 38-14). This procedure can also be done using nonradioactive oligonucleotide probes immobilized to filters, so-called reverse dot blot analysis.[573,574] Single-base mutations can also be detected by the PCR technique called amplification refractory mutation system (ARMS).[570,575] An amplification and direct sequencing of the β-globin genes (in cases in which the mutation is unknown) can also be carried out rapidly by use of PCR techniques.

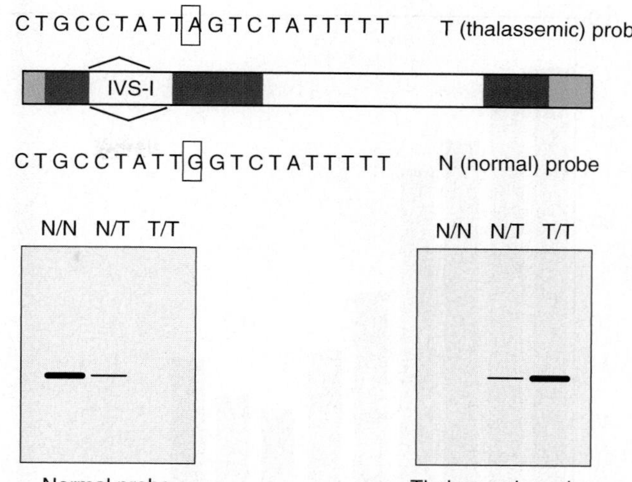

Figure 38-14 EXAMPLE OF THE USE OF ALLELE-SPECIFIC OLIGONUCLEOTIDE PROBES FOR DIAGNOSIS OF A COMMON FORM OF β-THALASSEMIA. The mutation shown is that discussed in Figure 38-2 and the text. Two oligonucleotide probes are synthesized, differing only at the position of the mutation. When hybridized under sufficiently stringent conditions, each probe will anneal only to the gene that is perfectly complementary by Watson-Crick base pairing. Thus, a homozygous normal fetal DNA sample (N/N) will anneal only to the normal probe, homozygous β-thalassemic DNA (T/T) only to the thalassemic probe, and DNA from a heterozygote (N/T) to both probes but with a reduced intensity to each. *(Adapted from High KA, Benz EJ Jr: The ABCs of molecular genetics: A haematologist's introduction. In Hoffbrand AV, editor:* Recent advances in haematology, *New York, 1985, Churchill Livingston, p 25.)*

Genetic counseling and antenatal diagnosis should be offered to all families at risk for severe α- or β-thalassemia. Prenatal diagnosis is one component of large-scale screening, education, and genetic counseling programs that are active in Italy, Greece, Cyprus, and other areas where the frequency of thalassemia is very high.[576] In some countries, particularly those with a high rate of consanguineous marriages, screening efforts can be refined to gain further efficiency in identifying at-risk couples.[577] Comprehensive programs of education, screening, and diagnosis have dramatically decreased the incidence of thalassemia major births in several countries (Fig. 38-15),[576,578,579] but they require a critical mass of expert professionals and laboratory backup. Voluntary informed participation, confidentiality of results, and meaningful counseling must be ensured.

α-THALASSEMIA SYNDROMES

The α-thalassemias are more difficult to diagnose because characteristic elevations in Hb A_2 or Hb F, seen in many cases of β-thalassemia, do not occur. However, the gene deletions responsible for the most common varieties are readily detectable by molecular biology methods.[580]

Molecular Pathology and Pathophysiology

The four classic α-thalassemia syndromes are α^+-thalassemia trait, in which one of the four α-globin genes fails to function; α°-thalassemia trait, with two dysfunctional genes; Hb H disease, with three affected genes; and hydrops fetalis with Hb Bart, in which all four genes are defective. In the older literature, α°- and α^{++}-thalassemia are referred

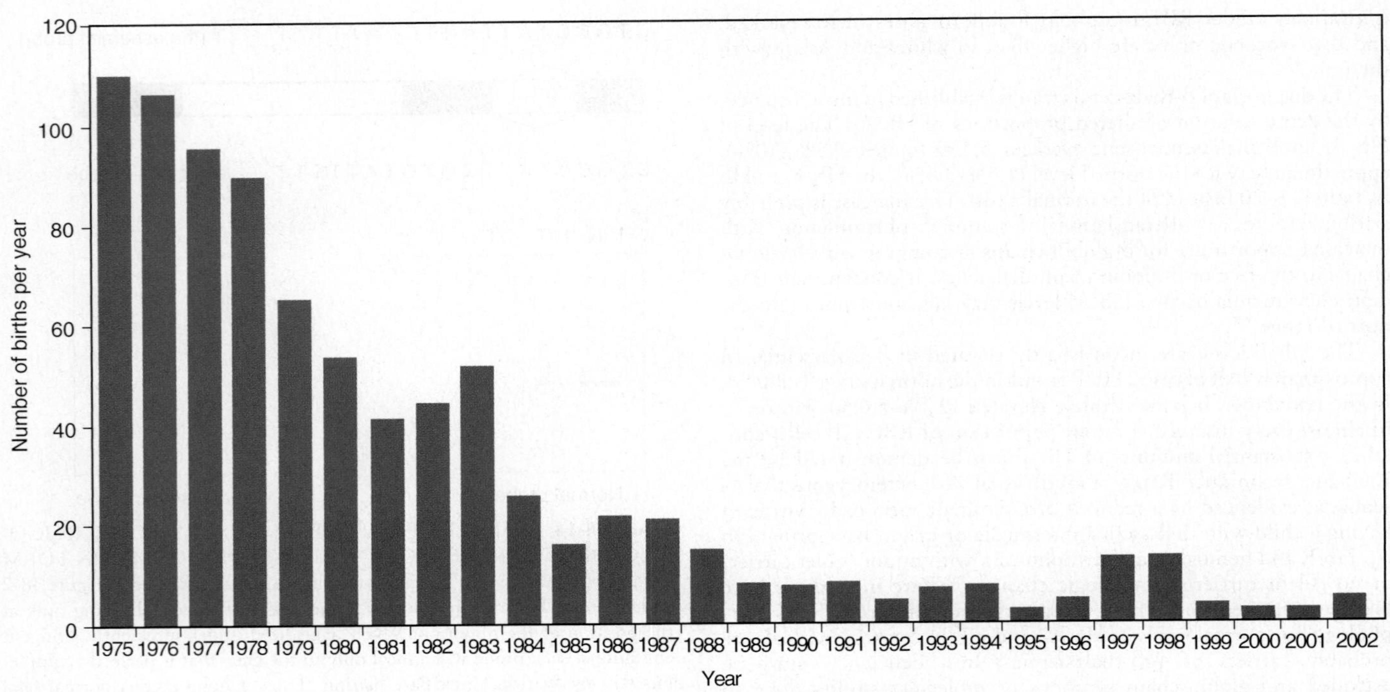

Figure 38-15 DECLINING RATE OF BIRTH OF INFANTS HOMOZYGOUS FOR β-THALASSEMIA IN SARDINIA SINCE 1975, WHEN A COMPREHENSIVE SCREENING PROGRAM BEGAN. *(Adapted from Cao A, Galanello R: Effect of consanguinity on screening for thalassemia.* N Engl J Med *347:1200, 2002.)*

to as α-thalassemia-1 and α-thalassemia-2, respectively. These syndromes are usually caused by deletion of one, two, three, or all four of the α-globin genes, respectively (Fig. 38-16). Nondeletional forms of α-thalassemia, which account for 15% to 20% of patients, arise from mutations similar to those described for β-thalassemia.[581,582] Fig. 38-17 illustrates the different α-thalassemia mutations and phenotypes. Structurally abnormal hemoglobins have also been associated with α-thalassemia. The Quong Sze α-globin chain ($\alpha^{125\text{Leu}\rightarrow\text{Pro}}$) is exceedingly labile and is destroyed so rapidly after its synthesis that no hemoglobin tetramers containing the mutant α chain can be formed.[583]

α^+-Thalassemia trait is an asymptomatic silent carrier state that is commonly associated with the deletion of a single α-globin gene. Offspring of an individual with α^+-thalassemia whose spouse has α°-thalassemia trait can inherit a form of α-thalassemia more severe than either of these, namely Hb H disease.

α°-Thalassemia trait results from deletion or nonfunction of two α-globin alleles. In Asian and Mediterranean populations, a deletion that removes both loci from the same chromosome (*cis* deletion) is common[581,582]; homozygosity for α^+-thalassemia (*trans* deletion) is also seen. In African Americans, both α-globin genes are only rarely deleted in *cis,* but homozygosity for α^+-thalassemia (*trans* deletion) is quite common.[584] Both genotypes produce asymptomatic hypochromia and microcytosis. Hb H disease usually results from coinheritance of the *cis* α°-thalassemia deletion and α^+-thalassemia trait. α-Globin chain production is only 25% to 30% of normal; excess γ-globin chains accumulate during gestation and excess β-globin chains during adult life (see Fig. 38-17). The unpaired β-globin chains are somewhat more soluble than the excess α-globin chains that accumulate in cases of β-thalassemia, forming recognizable β4 tetramers designated as Hb H. Hb H forms relatively few inclusions in erythroblasts; rather, it precipitates slowly within mature circulating RBCs. Patients with Hb H disease thus have a moderately severe hemolytic anemia but relatively little IE. Patients usually survive into adult life. These clinical observations illustrate the central role of unpaired globin chains and IE as determinants of clinical severity.

Hydrops fetalis with Hb Bart results from the homozygous state for the α°-thalassemia *cis* deletion. The α-globin genes are totally absent; no α-globin is produced, so no physiologically useful hemoglobin accumulates beyond the embryonic stage. Free γ-globin chains accumulate, forming γ_4 tetramers called Hb Bart (see Fig. 35-13). Hb Bart has an extraordinarily high oxygen affinity comparable with that of myoglobin. It binds oxygen delivered to the placenta but releases almost none of it to fetal tissues. Severe hypoxia occurs at the tissue level, causing profound edema (hydrops); congestive heart failure; and, in most cases, death in utero. These fatal complications do not occur in fetuses with Hb H disease because enough Hb F is made to sustain life.

α^+-Thalassemia trait is very common in black patients, having a genetic frequency of 20% to 30% in some populations. However, the *cis* α°-thalassemia deletion is rare in black patients. Thus, even though α^+-thalassemia trait and the *trans* deletion form of α°-thalassemia are very common, Hb H disease is rarely encountered, and hydrops fetalis has not yet been reported in black patients.[584,585]

Clinical Manifestations

Silent Carrier (α^+-Thalassemia Trait)

α^+-Thalassemia trait has no consistent hematologic manifestations. The RBCs are not microcytic, and Hb A_2 and Hb F are normal. During the newborn period, small amounts (≤3%) of Hb Bart (γ_4) can be seen by electrophoresis or other techniques. This condition is most often recognized when an apparently normal individual becomes the parent of a child with Hb H disease after mating with a person with α°-thalassemia trait. The mild excess of β-globin chains is probably removed in erythroblasts by proteolysis.[586] α^+-Thalassemia is particularly common in Melanesia, as well as in Southeast Asia and in African Americans, reaching a prevalence of more than 80% in north coastal Papua New Guinea. At the molecular level, α^+-thalassemia has been found to be associated with two common gene deletions resulting from different nonhomologous crossing-over events between the two linked α-globin genes: a 3.7-kb rightward deletion ($-\alpha^{3.7}$) resulting in a fused α2α1-globin gene and a 4.2-kb leftward deletion ($-\alpha^{4.2}$) resulting in loss of the 5′ (α2) gene.[581,582,587] The level of α-globin gene expression differs in the two conditions, as discussed in the following section.

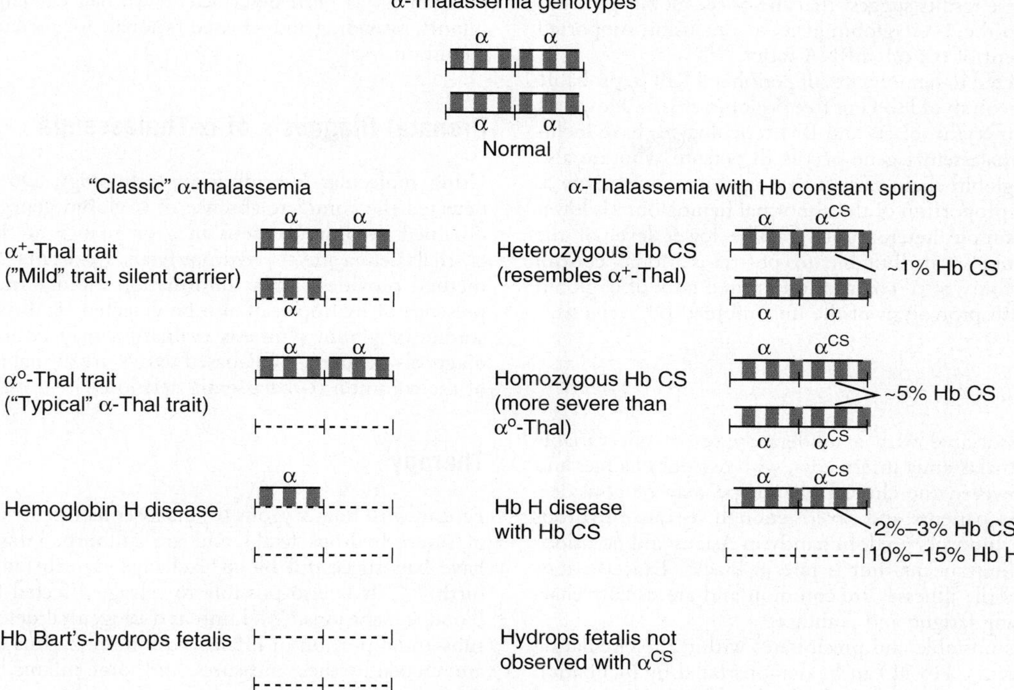

Figure 38-16 GENETIC ORIGINS OF THE "CLASSIC" α-THALASSEMIA SYNDROMES CAUSED BY GENE DELETIONS IN THE α-GLOBIN GENE CLUSTER. Hemoglobin (Hb) Constant Spring (CS) is an α-globin chain variant synthesized in such small amounts (1%-2% of normal) that it has the phenotypic impact of a severe nondeletion α-thalassemia allele; however, the α^{cs} allele is always linked to a functioning α-globin gene, so it has never been associated with hydrops fetalis.

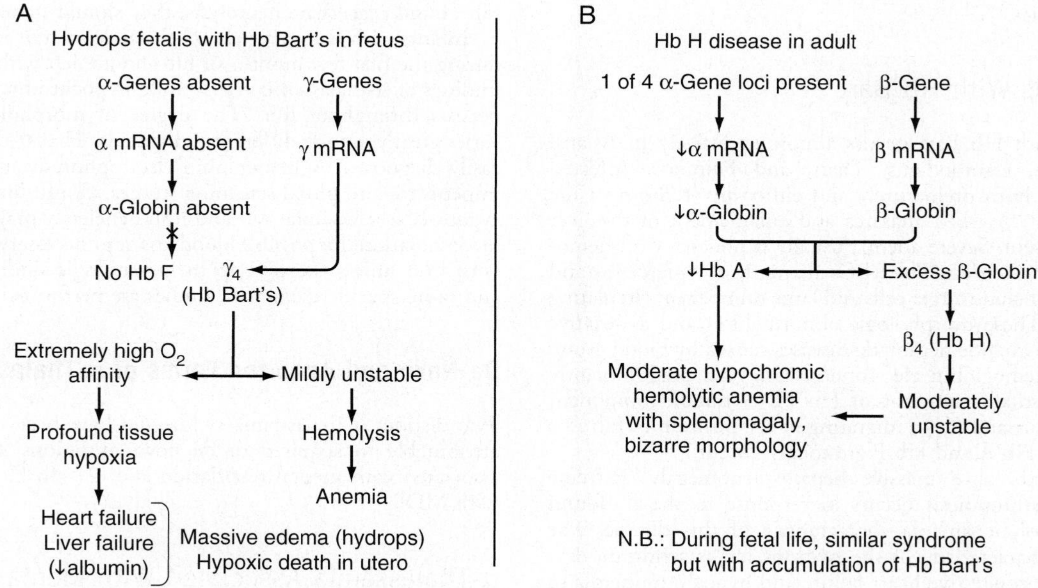

Figure 38-17 PATHOPHYSIOLOGY OF HEMOGLOBIN (HB) H DISEASE AND HYDROPS FETALIS WITH HB BART. *(Adapted from Benz EJ Jr: The hemoglobinopathies. In Kelly WN, DeVita VT, editors:* Textbook of internal medicine, *Philadelphia, 1988, JB Lippincott, p 1423.)*

α-Thalassemia Trait (α°-Thalassemia Trait)

Levels of Hb A_2 in the low to low normal range (1.5%-2.5%) and β/α synthetic ratios averaging 1.4 : 1 characterize α°-thalassemia trait. During the perinatal period, elevated amounts of Hb Bart are noted (3%-8%). Microcytosis is present in cord blood erythrocytes.

Studies of newborns from the archipelago of Vanuatu in the southwest Pacific and from Papua New Guinea indicate that homozygotes for the rightward -$\alpha^{3.7III}$ deletion (where only a fused α2α1-globin gene, mostly of the α2 type, remains) have lower Hb Bart levels (3.5% ± 0.8%) than those of infants homozygous for the leftward -$\alpha^{4.2}$ deletion (in whom only the α1-globin gene remains)

(6.0% ± 1.4%). These results suggest that the 5′ α2-globin gene has a higher output than the 3′ α1-globin gene, a conclusion supported by direct measurement of α2/α1 mRNA ratios.[588,589]

Hb H is not detected in hemolysates of peripheral RBCs, probably because of rapid proteolysis of Hb H or free β-globin chains. However, approximately 1% of erythroblasts and BM reticulocytes have inclusions. When an α-thalassemia gene occurs in persons who are also heterozygous for α-globin chain variant hemoglobins, such as Hb S, Hb C, or Hb E, the proportion of the abnormal hemoglobin is lower than that seen in simple heterozygotes.[590] The lower level of the abnormal hemoglobin is attributable to posttranslational control because of higher affinity of β^A chains for a limited pool of α-globin chains[591] coupled with proteolysis of the uncombined $\beta^{variant}$ chains.

Hb H Disease

Hb H disease is associated with a moderately severe but variable anemia resembling thalassemia intermedia, with osseous changes and splenomegaly.[592] However, the clinical phenotype may be considerably milder in some patients and severe enough to cause hydrops fetalis in others.[593,594] It occurs predominantly in Asians and occasionally in whites (Mediterraneans) but is rare in blacks. Exacerbations of anemia during febrile illnesses are common and are usually characterized by increasing fatigue and jaundice.

Because Hb H is unstable and precipitates within the circulating RBCs, hemolysis occurs. Hb H can be demonstrated by incubation of blood with supravital oxidizing stains such as 1% brilliant cresyl blue. Multiple small inclusions form in the RBCs (see Fig. 38-17). Electrophoresis of a freshly prepared hemolysate at alkaline or neutral pH demonstrates a fast-moving component amounting to 3% to 30% of the total hemoglobin. Concomitant iron deficiency may reduce the amount of Hb H in the patient's RBCs.[595] A syndrome of Hb H disease associated with mental retardation, other congenital anomalies, and large deletions on chromosome 16 has been noted in several white families.[596,597]

Hydrops Fetalis With Hb Bart

Hydrops fetalis with Hb Bart occurs almost exclusively in Asians, especially Chinese, Cambodians, Thais, and Filipinos. Affected fetuses usually are born prematurely and either are stillborn or die shortly after birth.[1-4] Marked anasarca and enlargement of the liver and spleen are present. Severe anemia usually is present, with hemoglobin levels of 3 to 10 g/dL. The RBCs are markedly microcytic and hypochromic and include target cells and large numbers of circulating nucleated RBCs. These morphologic abnormalities and a negative Coombs test result exclude hemolytic diseases caused by blood group incompatibility. Hemoglobin electrophoresis reveals predominantly Hb Bart, with a smaller amount of Hb H. A minor component identified as Hb Portland ($\zeta_2\gamma_2$) migrating in the position of Hb A is also seen. Normal Hb A and Hb F are totally absent.[598]

Hydropic infants have massive hepatosplenomegaly. Extreme extramedullary erythropoiesis occurs in response to the profound hypoxia and hemolytic anemia characteristic of this disease. The universal edema characteristic of the hydrops fetalis syndrome is a reflection of severe congestive heart failure and hypoalbuminemia in utero. This is partly a consequence of anemia, but the strikingly abnormal oxygen affinity of the tetrameric Hb Bart is probably the most important determinant of the severe tissue hypoxia. The oxygen dissociation curve of Hb Bart lacks the normal sigmoid form because of noncooperativity during oxygen loading and unloading and is markedly shifted to the left. The shift is so great that little oxygen is released under conditions of low oxygen concentration in the tissues.

Infants with this syndrome do not die in an earlier trimester of pregnancy because of the presence of Hb Portland ($\zeta_2\gamma_2$). This hemoglobin does display cooperativity in a manner similar to that of Hb F and therefore has a much more favorable oxygen dissociation pattern than that of Hb Bart. A high incidence of toxemia of pregnancy has been described in women carrying severely affected infants, providing an increased rationale for prenatal diagnosis of this condition.

Prenatal Diagnosis of α-Thalassemia

Using molecular hybridization technology, Dozy and associates[599] detected the complete absence of α-globin genes in fetal fibroblasts obtained by amniocentesis in a pregnancy at risk of homozygous α°-thalassemia and the hydrops fetalis syndrome. A quantitative PCR method provides similar information rapidly and accurately.[600] The presence of hydrops can also be detected by ultrasonography. DNA studies or globin synthesis evaluation may be used to confirm the diagnosis in utero. PCR-based assays are available for the detection of the common α-thalassemia deletions.[600-603]

Therapy

Fetuses with homozygous α°-thalassemia usually die in utero because of severe hydrops fetalis and are stillborn. However, some infants have had successful blood exchange transfusion immediately after birth.[604-608] It is also possible to salvage affected fetuses by in utero blood transfusions.[609,610] Limb and urogenital defects are present in a substantial portion of infants with homozygous α°-thalassemia who are rescued by these measures, and some infants have developmental delay or other neurologic abnormalities. Management after the perinatal period is similar to the management of patients with thalassemia major and includes transfusion and chelation therapy as well as the possibility of BMT.[611]

Many patients with Hb H disease do not require RBC transfusions. For patients with more severe disease, characterized by lower hemoglobin levels or frequent exacerbations of the anemia, splenectomy can be helpful. Oxidant drugs can accelerate precipitation of Hb H and exacerbate hemolysis; they should therefore be avoided.

Infants with heterozygous α°-thalassemia trait lose their Hb Bart during the first few months of life and are left with the hematologic findings of α-thalassemia trait, a mild hypochromic microcytosis that persists throughout life.[1] The degree of morphologic abnormality varies greatly among different individuals. That α-thalassemia can be easily diagnosed by hemoglobin electrophoresis at birth gives some impetus to cord blood screening studies. Confusion between heterozygous α°-thalassemia trait and iron deficiency may lead to unnecessary evaluations for possible blood loss or unnecessary supplementation with iron unless the overlap in hematologic findings is recognized and more specific diagnostic studies are performed.

De Novo and Acquired Forms of α-Thalassemia

Two distinct α-thalassemia syndromes have been described that are attributable to acquired or de novo mutations: (1) α-thalassemia associated with mental retardation and (2) Hb H disease associated with MDS.

α-Thalassemia Associated With Mental Retardation

α-Thalassemia or Hb H disease can occur as a de novo abnormality in a rare disorder called the α-thalassemia with mental retardation syndrome (ATR).[596,597] In this disorder, affected patients have mental retardation and a number of other developmental abnormalities in association with α-thalassemia trait or Hb H disease that is inherited in a nontraditional manner. Two distinct types of the ATR syndrome have been identified. In some cases, there is the de novo appearance of large (2000 kb or so) deletions involving the entire α-globin gene cluster and adjacent DNA at the tip of chromosome 16, the so-called ATR-16 syndrome. In some of these patients, the deletion produces detectable cytogenetic abnormalities of chromosome 16, indicating that a very large segment of the chromosome is deleted, sometimes because of unbalanced chromosomal translocations involving the telomeres of the affected chromosomes. In some cases, one parent is heterozygous for α^+-thalassemia by various criteria and the other parent is completely normal; in such cases, the child has Hb H disease (- -/- α). In other cases, both parents are normal and the affected child has the hematologic phenotype of heterozygous α^o-thalassemia (- -/- α) without Hb H disease. In this form of ATR, the clinical findings, such as the degree of mental retardation and associated congenital abnormalities, are variable.

The second type of ATR syndrome is not associated with detectable deletions of the α-globin gene complex. The molecular basis of the disorder consists of mutations of a gene on the X chromosome, and the condition has been called the ATR-X syndrome.[612] In contrast to patients with the ATR-16 syndrome who have a varied phenotype of developmental abnormalities, patients with the ATR-X syndrome have a more uniform or consistent phenotype, particularly severe mental retardation (with IQs of 50-70) and a characteristic dysmorphic facial appearance.[597]

The affected gene in this syndrome encodes a *trans*-acting factor, called ATRX, that is thought to influence the expression of the α-globin genes as well as that of other genes.[613,614] The structure of this large (280 kd) DNA-binding protein is complex and contains two major functional domains: an *N*-terminal cysteine-rich zinc finger–containing domain, called the ADD domain, that has structural features similar to those of DNA methyl transferases, and a C-terminal helicase/ATPase domain. The majority of the mutations associated with the ATR-X syndrome are located in the ADD domain or the helicase domain. The ATRX protein is widely expressed in many different tissues and its intracellular localization is within three different nuclear subcompartments: heterochromatin, ribosomal DNA arrays, and PML bodies. It has been shown to interact with other proteins such as the heterochromatin-associated protein HP1 and Daxx, one of the proteins localized in PML bodies. The prevailing opinion is that the ATRX protein is part of a large chromatin-remodeling complex of the SWI2/SNF2 family. It also has ATPase activity and has translocase activity, that is, it can move along DNA as a "molecular motor." The precise mechanism(s) by which ATRX influences the expression of α-globin (and other) genes remains unknown.

Acquired Hb H Disease Associated With Myelodysplastic Syndrome or ATMDS

Hb H disease has occasionally been observed to develop during the course of different types of MDS and more rarely in patients with other hematologic malignancies.[615] The disorder usually affects elderly men older than the age of 60 years. The degree of imbalance of globin chain synthesis and of α-globin mRNA deficiency in erythroid cells of affected patients is greater than that observed in the hereditary type of Hb H disease. It is conceivable that erythroid cells of the abnormal clone synthesize no α-globin chains at all and that the expression of all four α-globin genes is suppressed or silenced,[616] but this phenomenon is difficult to document in total blood as long as some normal erythroid cells are being produced.

Until recently, the molecular basis of this fascinating disorder remained unknown. Cytogenetic, gene mapping, gene sequencing, and gene or chromosome transfer studies failed to detect any deletion or mutation in the α-globin gene cluster or functional abnormality of α-globin gene of affected patients. The results of all of these prior studies suggested that the defect responsible for this disorder probably involved the abnormal expression or function of a *trans*-acting factor capable of influencing α-globin gene expression and, indeed, such a factor was recently identified. The discovery of the factor responsible for Hb H disease in MDS results from cDNA microarray analysis of RNA isolated from granulocytes of an affected patient. One of the genes that was found to be markedly underexpressed, compared with results obtained with RNA of normal granulocytes, was the *ATRX* gene,[617] the same gene that is mutated in the α-thalassemia with mental retardation syndrome of the ATR-X type. Sequence analysis of the *ATRX* gene in the DNA of blood cells of affected individuals has identified a number of different mutations. It is noteworthy that the mutations of the *ATRX* gene associated with acquired Hb H disease associated with MDS (ATMDS) occur in the same regions of the gene as the mutations associated with the ATR-X syndrome, that is, in the ADD or helicase domains. In fact, some of the *ATRX* gene mutations identified in ATMDS are identical or similar in expected functional consequences to various mutations found in the ATR-X syndrome.

The hematologic features in the syndrome are characterized by the presence on blood smear of a dimorphic RBC population, one of which is hypochromic, microcytic, hypochromic, and poikilocytic. Incubation of the blood with the supravital stain brilliant cresyl blue results in the detection of typical Hb H inclusions. Hemoglobin electrophoresis or HPLC detects the presence of Hb H, usually in greater quantities than that typically observed in inherited Hb H disease. In typical MDS, the MCV of the erythrocytes is normal or elevated, frequently higher than 100 fL. However, in ATMDS, the MCV and mean corpuscular hemoglobin (MCH) are low: MCV usually less than 80 fL and MCH usually less than 26 pg.[615] The amount of Hb H usually remains stable but may actually decrease during the course of the disease and no longer persists after transformation of MDS to acute leukemia. This finding suggests that the Hb H–producing clone does not have a selective survival or growth advantage.

The hematologic phenotype, as reflected by the amount of Hb H present in blood, of ATMDS is much more severe than that of the ATR-X syndrome.[613] Some of this difference in severity may be due to the nature of the ATMDS mutations, some of which are null mutations that are likely to be lethal when present in germline DNA of ATR-X embryos. However, the difference in severity is also observed in the case of mutations found in both syndromes that are identical or similar in expected functional consequences. This finding suggests that additional abnormalities in gene expression in ATMDS contribute to the severity of the deficit in α-globin gene expression observed in this syndrome. Perhaps the responsible defective cofactor(s) is one or more of the proteins that interact with the ATRX protein to produce a fully functional macromolecular complex that can act as a transcriptional cofactor or that can influence the epigenetic control of α-globin gene expression.

THALASSEMIC STRUCTURAL VARIANTS

Certain structural hemoglobin variants are characterized by the presence of a biosynthetic defect as well as abnormal structure.[6] Thalassemic hemoglobinopathies are unusual forms of thalassemia caused by such structural variants.

Hb Lepore

Hb Lepore ($\alpha_2\beta\delta$) is the prototype of a group of hemoglobinopathies characterized by fused globin chains.[1-4] The chains begin with a normal δ-chain sequence at their N-terminus and end with the normal β-chain sequence at their C-terminus. These hemoglobinopathies arise by unequal or nonhomologous crossover or recombination events that fuse the proximal end of one gene with the distal end of a closely linked structurally homologous gene (Fig. 38-18). During meiosis, mispairing and crossover of the highly homologous δ- and β-globin genes can occur, resulting in a Lepore chromosome, which contains (in addition to γ-globin genes) only the fused δβ gene, and an anti-Lepore chromosome, which contains the reciprocal fusion product (δβ), as well as intact δ- and β-globin genes.[1]

Lepore globin is synthesized in low amounts, presumably because it is under the control of the δ-globin gene promoter, which normally sustains transcription at only 2.5% the level of the β-globin gene.[618] Patients with Hb Lepore have the phenotype of β-thalassemia, distinguished by the added presence of 5% to 15% Hb Lepore. In

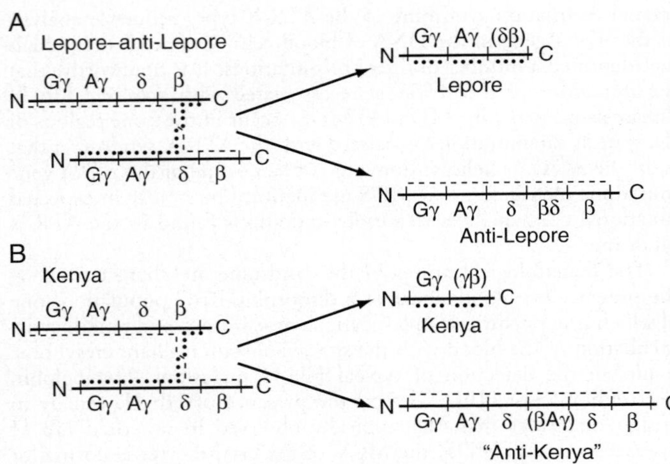

Figure 38-18 GENETIC ORIGINS OF HEMOGLOBIN (HB) LEPORE, ANTI-LEPORE HB, AND HB KENYA. *(Adapted from Benz EJ Jr: The hemoglobinopathies. In Kelly WN, DeVita VT, editors:* Textbook of internal medicine, *Philadelphia, 1988, JB Lippincott, p 1423.)*

contrast, the anti-Lepore globin (Miyada) is not associated with a β-thalassemia phenotype because of the presence of an intact and functionally normal β-globin gene on the same chromosome.

Heterozygotes for Hb Lepore have the clinical phenotype of β-thalassemia trait; homozygotes are usually similar to patients with homozygous β-thalassemia. Compound heterozygotes for Hb Lepore and a "classic" β-thalassemia allele usually have severe thalassemia. Hb Lepore thus interacts with thalassemia in the same way that a severe β-thalassemia gene does, although occasional cases have a milder phenotype of the thalassemia intermedia variety, perhaps because of an associated higher than usual level of γ-globin gene expression. The presence of Hb Lepore should be suspected in individuals with a microcytic, hypochromic anemia who also have a small amount of an abnormal hemoglobin migrating in the position of Hb S on routine hemoglobin electrophoresis. Hb Lepore accounts for 5% to 10% of the β-thalassemias seen in Greek and Italian populations. Several forms of Hb Lepore have been described that differ in the position at which the transition from δ to β DNA and amino acid sequence occurs.

An analogous but rare variant, Hb Kenya $[\alpha_2(^A\gamma\beta)_2]$, arises from nonhomologous crossing over between the $^A\gamma$- and β-globin genes[619] (see Fig. 38-14) and is associated with the phenotype of $^G\gamma$ hereditary persistence of fetal hemoglobin (HPFH). A DNA sequence approximately 600 bases downstream from the β-globin gene acts as a strong enhancer, promoting the erythroid-specific expression of the β-globin genes in adult cells.[3,4,21] The fused $^A\gamma$ β gene as well as the linked upstream $^G\gamma$ gene are believed to come under the influence of the enhancer because of its abnormal proximity and thus are expressed at high levels in adult life.

Hb E

Hb E $(\alpha_2\beta_2^{26Glu\rightarrow Lys})$ is a common variant (15%-30% of the population) in Cambodia, Thailand, parts of China, and Vietnam. Hb E is very mildly unstable, but this instability does not significantly alter the life span of RBCs. Hb E trait resembles very mild β-thalassemia trait. Homozygotes exhibit more microcytosis but are still asymptomatic.[620] Compound heterozygotes for Hb E and a β-thalassemia gene (Hb E-β-thalassemia) resemble patients with β-thalassemia intermedia or β-thalassemia major. However, some problems such as infection and pulmonary hypertension may occur more commonly in Hb E-β-thalassemia than in homozygous β-thalassemia.[621]

The only nucleotide sequence abnormality found in the β^E-gene is a base change in codon 26 that causes the amino acid substitution. This mutation, which occurs in a potential cryptic RNA splice region, alters the consensus sequence surrounding a potential GT donor splice site and thus activates the cryptic site. Alternative splicing at this position occurs approximately 40% to 50% of the time, generating a structurally abnormal globin mRNA that cannot be translated appropriately.[622] The other mRNA precursors are spliced at the normal site, generating functionally normal mRNA, which is translated into β^E-globin because the mature mRNA retains the base change that encodes lysine at codon 26.

Hb E is important because it is so common in Southeast Asian populations. With increased emigration of Southeast Asians to North America, Hb E syndromes are being seen there with increased frequency.[623,624] Genetic counseling of these individuals should emphasize the potential consequences of the interaction of Hb E with β-thalassemia. Hb E is also an instructive example of the pleiotropic effects that point mutations can have on the amounts and types of gene products derived from a single mutant gene.

Hb Constant Spring

Hb Constant Spring (see Fig. 38-16) is an elongated α-globin variant resulting from a mutation that alters the normal translation termination codon.[625] Polyribosomes read through the usual translation stop site and incorporate an additional 31 amino acids until another in-phase termination codon is reached within the 3′ untranslated sequence. The amount of α^{cs} mRNA is markedly reduced, and α^{cs}-globin is synthesized in only minute amounts.[587,626] Six possible mutations of the normal translation termination codon (UAA) in α-globin mRNA could result in the generation of a "sense" codon.[627] Of these, five variants have been identified, each having a markedly underproduced abnormal variant, indicating that disruption of normal translation termination is in some way associated with abnormal mRNA accumulation, presumably because of instability of the mRNA.[587] The output of α-globin from the α^{cs} allele is only approximately 1% of normal, and the gene is thus rendered α-thalassemic. The α^{cs} allele has been identified only on chromosomes containing a *cis*-linked functionally normal α-globin gene.[1-4] Thus, α^+-thalassemia trait and Hb H disease–(- $/\alpha^{cs}\alpha$) associated with Hb Constant Spring are common, but hydrops fetalis caused by four abnormal α-globin genes cannot occur in association with this variant. Homozygosity for the variant is associated with a relatively mild form of Hb H disease.[1]

EXTRAORDINARILY UNSTABLE HEMOGLOBINS

Rare cases of α-thalassemia (e.g., Hb Quong Sze)[583] and β-thalassemia (e.g., Hb Indianapolis, recently renamed Hb Terre Haute)[628,629] arise from mutations that produce extremely labile globin chains. The chains fail to pair with the complementary chain, or they precipitate and are degraded so rapidly that they never form tetramers. These posttranslational lesions have the same pathophysiologic effects on hemoglobin biogenesis as reduction of globin mRNA production or function. Another group of β-globin chain variants, usually caused by mutations in exon 3 of the β-globin gene, are associated with inclusion body formation and a phenotype of dominant β-thalassemia intermedia.[16,17,630]

HEREDITARY PERSISTENCE OF FETAL HEMOGLOBIN

Hereditary persistence of fetal hemoglobin consists of a group of rare conditions characterized by continued synthesis of high levels of Hb F in adult life.[1,631-633] No deleterious effects on patients are observed even when 100% of the hemoglobin produced in HPFH homozygotes is Hb F. These patients thus demonstrate convincingly that prevention or reversal of the Hb F–to–Hb A switch would provide efficacious therapy for β-thalassemia.

Two major types of HPFH have been described. Very high levels of fetal hemoglobin synthesis and uniform distribution of Hb F among all RBCs characterize pancellular HPFH. Heterocellular HPFH results from inherited increases in the number of F cells.

HPFH shows ethnic differences. In black patients with heterozygous pancellular deletional HPFH, the Hb F is within a range of 15% to 35% and contains $^{G}\gamma$ and $^{A}\gamma$ chains in a ratio of two to three. In Greeks with pancellular nondeletional HPFH, Hb F levels are lower, 10% to 20%, and the Hb F is 90% of the $^{A}\gamma$ type. Hb A_2 levels are lower than normal. There are usually no other hematologic abnormalities in these persons, although β/α-globin chain synthesis ratios may be lower in some black heterozygotes.

A few black patients have been described with homozygous HPFH. All hemoglobin within the RBCs of these patients is Hb F. Mild microcytosis and hypochromia of the RBCs are present without anemia. In fact, hemoglobin levels are mildly elevated, presumably because of increased erythropoiesis stimulated by the left-shifted oxygen dissociation curve of RBCs rich in Hb F. Globin chain synthesis reveals a γ/α synthetic ratio of approximately 0.5.

Pancellular HPFH can be divided into two classes. The deletional forms arise from large deletions within the β-globin gene cluster that remove the δ- and β-globin genes, part of the γδ intergenic DNA, and DNA downstream (to the 3′ side) from the β-globin genes.[1,631-633] The deletions appear to bring enhancer sequences into the proximity of the remaining γ-globin genes, promoting their high expression. Homozygotes for this condition produce only Hb F. In nondeletional HPFH, the β- and δ-globin genes are present. Single-base changes have been shown to occur in the promoter regions of either the $^{A}\gamma$- or $^{G}\gamma$-globin gene, resulting in overexpression of that form of Hb F.[1,631-633] In these individuals, Hb F levels rarely account for more than 20% of total hemoglobin.

A case of HPFH/β-thalassemia resembles β-thalassemia trait except for a higher proportion and regular distribution of Hb F in the RBCs.[1]

In δβ-thalassemia and HPFH patients, persistence of Hb F after the period of perinatal Hb F to Hb A switching is more marked than in patients with the "classic" (high Hb A_2) forms of thalassemia. Indeed, δβ-thalassemia and HPFH represent various degrees of the same genetic phenomenon. Both conditions frequently arise from deletions of DNA that remove or inactivate the β-globin gene.[1,631-633]

Heterocellular HPFH appears to result in many cases from mutations outside the β-globin gene cluster.[633] One controlling locus resides on the X chromosome.[634,635] Patients with these conditions probably represent the extreme end of a distribution of polymorphic capacities to produce F cells in adult life. Hb F levels are usually much lower than those in the pancellular forms. In some situations, elevated levels of Hb F are seen in otherwise normal individuals. In others, the high levels of Hb F become apparent only when other factors producing erythroid stress are present.

SUGGESTED READINGS

Angelopoulos NG, Goula A, Rombopoulos G, et al: Hypoparathyroidism in transfusion-dependent patients with beta-thalassemia. *J Bone Miner Metab* 24:138, 2006.

Borgna-Pignatti C, Cappellini MD, De Stefano P, et al: Cardiac morbidity and mortality in deferoxamine- or deferiprone-treated patients with thalassemia major. *Blood* 107:3733, 2006.

Boulad F: Hematopoietic stem cell transplantation for the treatment of beta thalassemia. In Kline R, editor: *Pediatric hematopoietic stem cell transplantation,* New York, 2006, Informa Healthcare, p 383.

Cappellini MD, Cohen A, Piga A, et al: A phase 3 study of deferasirox (ICL670), a once-daily oral iron chelator, in patients with beta-thalassemia. *Blood* 107:3455, 2006.

Cohen A, Glimm E, Porter JB: Effect of transfusional iron intake on response to chelation therapy in β-thalassemia major. *Blood* 111:583, 2008

Dodd RY: Current safety of the blood supply in the United States. *Int J Hematol* 80:301, 2004.

Gilfillan CP, Strauss BJ, Rodda CP, et al: A randomized, double-blind, placebo-controlled trial of intravenous zoledronic acid in the treatment of thalassemia-associated osteopenia. *Calcif Tissue Int* 79:138, 2006.

Harmatz P, Olivieri N, Kwiatkowski J, et al: Safety and efficacy of peginterferon alfa-2a and ribavirin for hepatitis C in thalassemia. *Blood* 108:558, 2006.

Harmatz P, Grady R, Dragsten P, et al: Phase Ib clinical trial of starch-conjugated deferoxamine (40SD02): A novel long-acting iron chelator. *Br J Hematol* 138:374, 2007.

Hongeng S, Pakakasama S, Chuansumrit A, et al: Outcomes of transplantation with related- and unrelated-donor stem cells in children with severe thalassemia. *Biol Blood Marrow Transplant* 12:683, 2006.

Kattamis A, Ladis V, Berdousi H, et al: Iron chelation treatment with combined therapy with deferiprone and deferioxamine: A 12-month trial. *Blood Cells Mol Dis* 36:21, 2006.

Kolnagou A, Economides C, Eracleous E, et al: Low serum ferritin levels are misleading for detecting cardiac iron overload and increase the risk of cardiomyopathy in thalassemia patients: The importance of cardiac iron overload monitoring using magnetic resonance imaging T2 and T2*. *Hemoglobin* 30:219, 2006.

Kolnagou A, Kontoghiorghes GJ: Effective combination therapy of deferiprone and deferoxamine for the rapid clearance of excess cardiac iron and the prevention of heart disease in thalassemia. The Protocol of the International Committee on Oral Chelators. *Hemoglobin* 30:239, 2006.

Neufeld EJ: Oral chelators deferasirox and deferiprone for transfusional iron overload in thalassemia major: New data, new questions. *Blood* 107:3436, 2006.

Pennell DJ, Berdoukas V, Karagiorga M, et al: Randomized controlled trial of deferiprone or deferoxamine in beta-thalassemia major patients with asymptomatic myocardial siderosis. *Blood* 107:3738, 2006.

Rachmilewitz ER, Giardina PJ: How I Treat Thalassemia. *Blood* Sept 29; 118:3479.

Tanner M, Galanello R, Dessi C, et al: A randomized placebo controlled double blind trial of the effect of combination therapy with deferoxamine and deferiprone on myocardial iron in thalassemia major using cardiovascular magnetic resonance. *Blood* 106:1017A, 2006.

Vogiatzi MG, Macklin EA, Fung EB, et al: Prevalence of fractures among the Thalassemia syndromes in North America. *Bone* 38:571, 2006.

Voskaridou E, Anagnostopoulos A, Konstantopoulos K, et al: Zoledronic acid for the treatment of osteoporosis in patients with beta-thalassemia: Results from a single-center, randomized, placebo-controlled trial. *Haematologica* 91:1193, 2006.

Wood JC, Otto-Duessel M, Gonzalez I, et al: Deferasirox and deferiprone remove cardiac iron in the iron-overloaded gerbil. *Transl Res* 148:272, 2006.

For complete list of references log on to www.expertconsult.com.

CHAPTER 39

PATHOBIOLOGY OF SICKLE CELL DISEASE

Robert P. Hebbel

Since it was recognized as the "first molecular disease," sickle cell anemia caused by homozygosity for the mutant sickle hemoglobin (HbS) has provided the classic paradigm for single-gene disorders. Predominant clinical features include hemolytic anemia, episodic painful events, chronic organ deterioration, disparate acute complications, and a foreshortened life span. However, the genesis of clinical sickle cell disease is complicated, and an understanding of its pathophysiology integrates concepts from multiple disciplines, includes contributions from the red blood cell (RBC) membrane and the vascular wall endothelium, and recognizes the likely participation of multiple genetic influences. This chapter addresses the pathophysiology that underlies the sickle cell disease syndromes described in Chapter 40.

EARLY YEARS OF SICKLE CELL DISEASE RESEARCH

Sickle cell disease syndromes were known in folk medicine for centuries in parts of Africa, but the disease was first reported in the medical literature in 1910 when Herrick described a young Grenadan man with recurrent pain, anemia, and sickle-shaped red corpuscles in the blood (Fig. 39-1, *A*). Early milestones in elucidating this disorder included discovery that deoxygenation induces reversible RBC sickling (Fig. 39-1, *B* to *E*) and recognition of genetic transmission. In 1940, Ham and Castle described a pO_2 threshold for concomitant induction of sickling and hyperviscosity, postulating that sickle cell pathophysiology resulted from a "vicious cycle of erythrostasis" involving mutually promotive sickling and viscosity changes. In 1949, Neel validated the Mendelian autosomal dominant inheritance of sickle cell anemia, and Pauling demonstrated presence of an abnormal hemoglobin in patients and carriers. This was followed by observation of the reversible sol-gel transformation of Hb solutions and the poor solubility of deoxygenated HbS, and in 1957 Ingram identified the underlying amino acid substitution. Thereafter, increasingly detailed investigations began to reveal the striking complexities of sickle cell disease pathobiology.

GENETIC CONSIDERATIONS

Molecular Context

The sickle mutation in the *HBB* gene is a GAG→GTG conversion that creates a $\beta^{6Glu\rightarrow Val}$ substitution and thereby forms β^S globin chains. Genes for other β-globin variants are allelic to the β^S gene and have a codominant impact on the hemoglobin phenotype. Examples include genes for the normal β chain (β^A), β mutants (e.g., β^C, β° or β^+ thalassemia), and deletional hereditary persistence of fetal hemoglobin (HPFH). Compound heterozygosity for β^S and each one of these results in well-defined clinical syndromes, such as HbAS (i.e., sickle trait), HbSC disease, HbS–β-thalassemia, and HbS-HPFH. Eight percent of African Americans have a β^S gene, 3% have β^C, 1.5% have β-thalassemia, and 0.1% have HPFH. Among African Americans, about one in 600 births results in the homozygous state, sickle cell anemia (HbSS), and about one in 400 results in some form of "sickle cell disease," which additionally includes the compound heterozygous variants other than sickle trait.

The *HBB* gene resides in a cluster of β-like genes within which are various nonexonic polymorphic sites. Different combinations of these define discrete β-locus background haplotypes, referred to as the Senegal, Benin, Bantu, Cameroon, and Arab–India haplotypes (Fig. 39-2). Each designation refers to an ethnographic region in which the sickle gene arose and achieved high frequency (typically peaking at 0.10-0.15 and perhaps even 0.20 in West Africa), which diminishes as distance from the regional center increases. The proportion of individuals having the mutation is about twice the gene frequency. In most cases, the sickle gene resides on one of these five major haplotypes, but there are other less common ones.

Origin, Selection, and Dispersion of the Sickle Gene

The residence of both β^A and β^S alleles on the distinct regional β cluster haplotype suggests that the sickle mutation arose independently in the five regions. The β^C mutation arose only once. Historical and biologic data argue that frequency of the β^S gene greatly expanded in Africa about 3000 years ago and in Asia about 4000 years ago. Its high prevalence suggests positive selection that is believed to have occurred after the introduction of iron tools. This led to adoption of an agricultural system that promoted both increased human habitation density and favorable breeding conditions for the mosquito vector, *Anopheles,* which in turn allowed development of endemic *Plasmodium falciparum*. In this context, high fixed β^S gene frequencies were reached because of a balanced polymorphism, such that heterozygotes (HbAS) have an adaptive advantage over either homozygote. Thus the Old World geographic distributions of the sickle gene and historical endemic malaria are notably concordant (see Fig. 39-2), suggesting that the sickle gene represents "a biologic solution to a cultural problem."

In hyperendemic areas, falciparum malaria uniformly infects the young and is the primary killer of children with sickle cell anemia. However, those with sickle trait are less likely to develop high-level parasitemia, to have severe malaria, or to die, an effect exerted early in childhood. At the level of the RBC, this protection probably reflects steps after initial parasite invasion. A mechanism that seems particularly plausible links protection to the instability of HbS, immune status, and splenic function. Infection of sickle trait RBCs with *P. falciparum* leads to augmented hemoglobin denaturation, clustering of membrane protein band 3, attraction of band 3 autoantibody, complement binding, and enhanced erythrophagocytosis, even of the early ring forms. This should result in accelerated clearance by the spleen. Indeed, in mice, the protective effect of HbS is lost after splenectomy, possibly suggesting that the "autosplenectomized" state may contribute to malarial virulence in HbS homozygotes. However, the timing of this scenario vis à vis appearance of immune mechanisms of protection is not yet defined.

Eventually, the sickle gene spread geographically by means of commerce, migration, and the Atlantic slave trade. This dispersion has

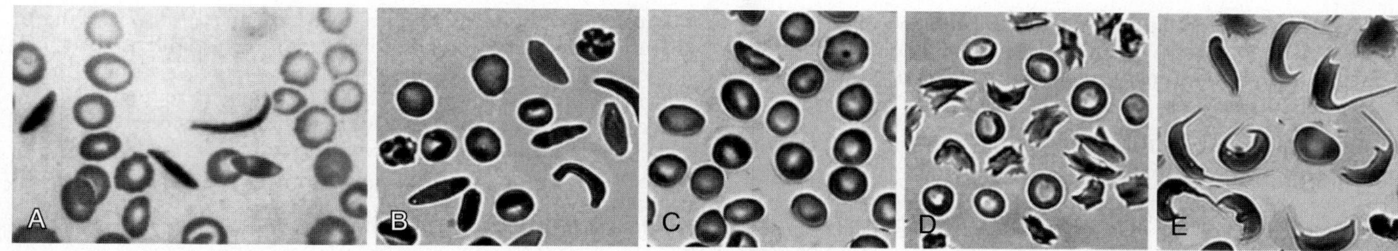

Figure 39-1 SICKLE RED BLOOD CELL (RBC) MORPHOLOGIES. **A,** Blood smear from the first patient report on sickle cell disease. **B** to **E,** Blood smears prepared under differing conditions from the same sickle cell anemia patient. **B,** Antecubital venous blood was fixed immediately at a pO_2 of approximately 40 mm Hg to document RBC shapes in vivo. Several RBC morphologies are evident, including two granular (raisinlike) cells, five somewhat elongated cells, and two highly elongated and curved cells. **C,** The mixed venous blood **(B)** was then fully oxygenated. Most cells have resumed normal shape, but one irreversibly sickled cell is present. **D,** The oxygenated cells **(C)** were then partially deoxygenated and assumed classical holly-leaf forms typical of rapid deoxygenation. **E,** The already partially deoxygenated mixed venous cells **(B)** were then fully deoxygenated (pO_2 = 0 mm Hg) and display the more elongated shape having fewer spikes that is assumed by slowly deoxygenated sickle RBC. The physical–chemical basis for these shapes is presented in Fig. 39-5. *(**B** to **E** from Obata K, Mattiello J, Asakura K, et al: Exposure of blood from patients with sickle cell disease to air changes the morphological, oxygen-binding, and sickling properties of sickled erythrocytes.* Am J Hematol *81:26, 2006. **A** from Herrick JB. Peculiar elongated and sickle-shaped red blood corpuscles in a case of severe anemia.* Arch Intern Med *5:517, 1910).*

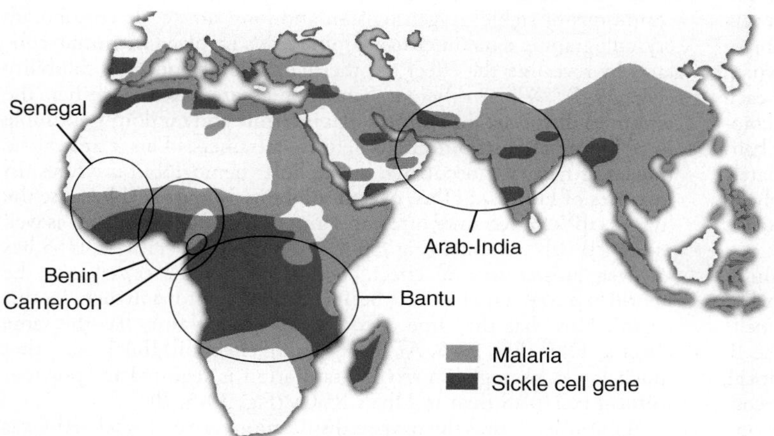

Figure 39-2 SICKLE GENE AND MALARIA. The five regions in which the sickle gene achieved high allelic frequency are superimposed on shading that identifies the Old World distribution of the sickle gene and of historical, endemic malaria. *(Adapted from Friedman MJ, Trager W: The biochemistry of resistance to malaria.* Sci Am *244:154, 1981 and from Nagel RL, Steinberg MH: Genetics of the β^S gene: Origins, epidemiology, and epistasis in sickle cell anemia. In Steinberg MH: Forget BG, Higgs DR, Nagel RL, eds:* Disorders of hemoglobin: Genetics, pathophysiology, and clinical management, *Cambridge, 2001, Cambridge University Press, p 711.)*

been tracked by analyses of regional β haplotypes, a biologic marker that largely corroborates predictions of gene flow derived from historical records. As a generalization, it spread on the Benin haplotype to North Africa and then across the Mediterranean. All three major African haplotypes are present in the western Arabian Peninsula, but on the eastern side, the sickle gene tends to be on the Arab-India haplotype, as it is in south Asia. In the Americas, the β^S gene is mostly found on the Benin, Senegal, and Bantu haplotypes.

ABNORMAL MOLECULAR BEHAVIORS OF SICKLE HEMOGLOBIN

Because the $\beta^{6Glu \rightarrow Val}$ substitution entails a loss of negative charge and gain in hydrophobicity, HbS exhibits three abnormal molecular behaviors of direct relevance to pathophysiology.

Hemoglobin S Charge and Tetramer Assembly

Formation of hemoglobin tetramers requires proximate assembly of stable dimers from unlike monomers (e.g., $\alpha + \beta \rightarrow \alpha\beta$), an event governed by electrostatic attraction. The normal α and β chains are positively and negatively charged, respectively. In heterozygous states for β-globin mutants, β-chain competition for dimer assembly is a determinant of the relative proportions of the hemoglobin variants.[1] Mutant β chains with lowered negative charge form αβ dimers more slowly; the relative rates for dimer association are $\alpha\beta^A > \alpha\beta^S > \alpha\beta^C$, with $\alpha\beta^A$ dimers formed about twice as rapidly as $\alpha\beta^S$ dimers. This explains why those with sickle trait typically have only 40% HbS and why the proportion of HbS is higher in HbSC disease than in HbAS. It also explains the effect of concurrent α-thalassemia on the proportion of HbS in sickle trait; as availability of α chains becomes limiting, the percentage of HbS typically drops from 40% to 35% (one α deletion), 30% (two α deletions), or less than 25% (three α deletions).

Hemoglobin S Stability and Oxidant Formation

HbS is modestly unstable, observed in vitro as instability to various applied stresses. Two stresses that are most clearly physiologic involve hemoglobin oxidation.[2] HbS has an abnormal redox potential compared with HbA that may underlie its modestly (≈40%) increased auto-oxidation rate. On the other hand, HbS exhibits markedly (≈340%) augmented instability upon interaction with aminophospholipids characteristic of the membrane's inner leaflet. Although the

Relationship of HbS Molecular Behaviors to Disease Features

Dimer assembly → RBC Hb composition
- Hb phenotype and diagnosis
- Polymerization risk

HbS instability → Membrane defects
- Sickling
- Hemolysis
- Malaria resistance

HbS polymerization → Sickling
- Vasoocclusion
- Hemolysis

physical-chemical mechanism of the destabilizing role of the β^6 valine in HbS is not known, this instability leads to accumulation of various hemoglobin and iron forms at the cytosol–membrane interface.[2]

Hemoglobin S Solubility and Hemoglobin S Polymerization

Oxy-HbS, oxy-HbA, and deoxy-HbA have very high solubilities, but deoxy-HbS aggregates into densely packed polymers, a process that is fully reversible on reoxygenation.[3,4] This abnormal property causes the eponymous RBC shape change from polymer-mediated distortion, the fundamental basis for disease promotion in sickling disorders.

Polymer Structure

Deoxygenation causes transformation of soluble HbS to a highly viscous and semisolid gel that behaves thermodynamically similar to a crystal in equilibrium with a solution of individual tetrameric Hb molecules. Even complete deoxygenation does not convert all deoxy-HbS to polymer. The insoluble phase is a collection of domains of aligned polymers, the basic unit of which is a double strand in which two strings of deoxy-Hb tetramers make multiple contacts with each other (Fig. 39-3). In the physiologic form of the polymer, the component strings of hemoglobin molecules in a double strand are half-staggered and have a slight twist, creating a fiber that is approximately 21 nM in diameter and is composed of one central and six peripheral double strands. The crystal formed in vitro lacks the twist, but its molecular structure is known in great detail.

Each HbS tetramer has two β chains, the β_1 and β_2 subunits. Deoxy-HbS undergoes a slight structural shift so that the A helix β^{6Val} "donor" site of the β_2 subunit in one tetramer can contact an EF helix "acceptor" site (formed mainly by β^{85Phe}, β^{88Leu}, and β^{70Ala}) in the β_1 subunit of a tetramer in the neighboring single string. This critical, lateral association can be made only when HbS is in its deoxy conformation; the EF helix hydrophobic pocket is not a favorable acceptor site for the charged β^{6Glu} of HbA. The β^{6Val} in the β_1 subunit is located so it cannot participate in such contacts. However, the β_2 subunit of the second single string can form chemically similar β^{6Val}-dependent contacts with the β_1 subunit of the first single string. There are multiple additional axial and lateral contacts, but these are largely the same for deoxy-HbA and deoxy-HbS and are not themselves sufficient to stabilize a polymeric structure.

Role of Hemoglobin S Solubility

The RBC's hydration state dominates the physical-chemical behavior of HbS. The solubility of deoxy-HbS, approximately 16 g/dL, is so much lower than the mean cell hemoglobin concentration (MCHC) that deoxy-HbS polymerization can occur even during partial cellular deoxygenation, which can raise the deoxy-HbS concentration above its solubility limit. The biophysical effect of macromolecular crowding (boosting activity far above that predicted from concentration alone) confers non-ideal behavior on cytoplasmic constituents, augmenting likelihood for polymerization.

In vitro studies carried out under (nonphysiologic) equilibrium conditions of stable oxygen tension and long time scale corroborate crystallographic data on critical amino acids involved in atomic contacts by revealing the effect of other hemoglobins on HbS solubility (Fig. 39-4).[3] When different hemoglobins are mixed together, the tetramers dissociate into dimers that intermix and randomly assemble in a binomial distribution to reform tetramers. This clarifies the impact of naturally occurring, intracellular hemoglobin mixtures. In mixtures of HbS and HbA, overall solubility is improved because the hybrid $\alpha\beta^S/\alpha\beta^A$ tetramer integrates into polymer only one half as well as the $\alpha\beta^S/\alpha\beta^S$ tetramer (Fig. 39-4, A). Addition of HbF to HbS has an even greater sparing effect because neither the $\alpha\gamma/\alpha\gamma$ nor the hybrid $\alpha\beta^S/\alpha\gamma$ tetramer can be incorporated into polymer. In this regard, HbC has the same effect as HbA, and HbA_2 has the same effect as HbF (Fig. 39-5, A). This sparing effect of HbA is such that much lower hemoglobin oxygen saturation is required for polymer to form in HbAS than in HbSS RBCs (Fig. 39-5, *B*).

A curiosity is that the oxygen dissociation curve of sickle RBCs is right shifted, which increases in proportion to the MCHC. This is

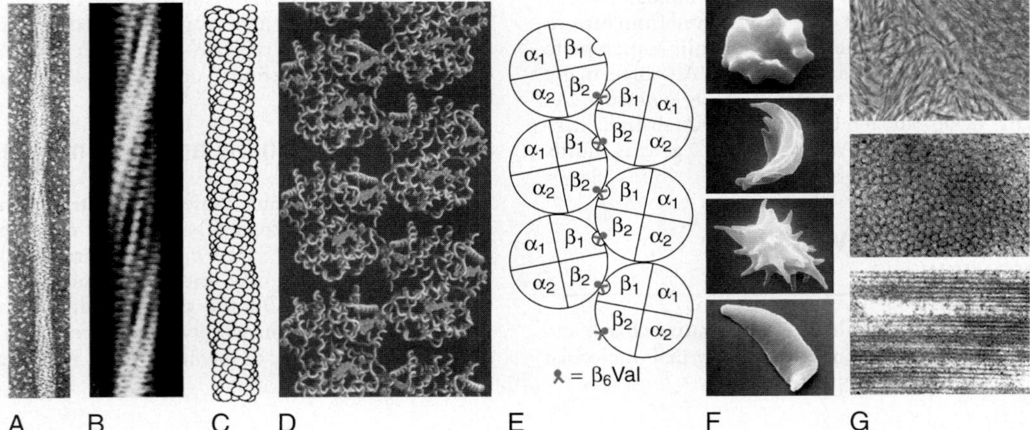

Figure 39-3 DEOXYGENATED HEMOGLOBIN S (HbS) POLYMER. **A,** Electron micrograph of a fiber of polymerized HbS obtained from a sickled red blood cell. **B,** Electron density surface map, modeled from authentic HbS fibers, shows pairings that create double strands plus a helical twist. **C,** Model of the HbS fiber, with Hb tetramers rendered as solid spheres. **D,** Protein backbone shows tetramer staggering in the HbS crystal. **E,** Schematic, two-dimensional representation of a double strand, demonstrating that only one of the two β^6 valine residues in each given tetramer participates in critical lateral contacts. **F,** Sickled red blood cells, showing various morphologies *(top to bottom):* granular, holly leaf shaped, classically sickled, and smoother and irreversibly sickled. **G,** Electron microscopy of sickled red blood cells reveals highly ordered polymer domains, as seen from the side *(bottom)* and on end *(middle),* or highly disorganized domains *(top). (**A** and **C** from Dykes G, Crepeau RH, Edelstein SJ: Three-dimensional reconstruction of the fibres of sickle cell hemoglobin.* Nature *272:506,1978; **B** from Carragher B, Bluemke DA, Becker M, et al: Structural analysis of polymers of sickle cell hemoglobin.* J Mol Biol *199:315,1988; **D** from Harrington DJ, Adachi K, Royer WE, Jr: The high resolution crystal structure of deoxyhemoglobin S.* J Mol Biol *272:398, 1997; **F** and **G** courtesy of Dr. James G. White and from White JG: Ultrastructural features of erythrocyte and hemoglobin sickling.* Arch Intern Med *133:545, 1974.)*

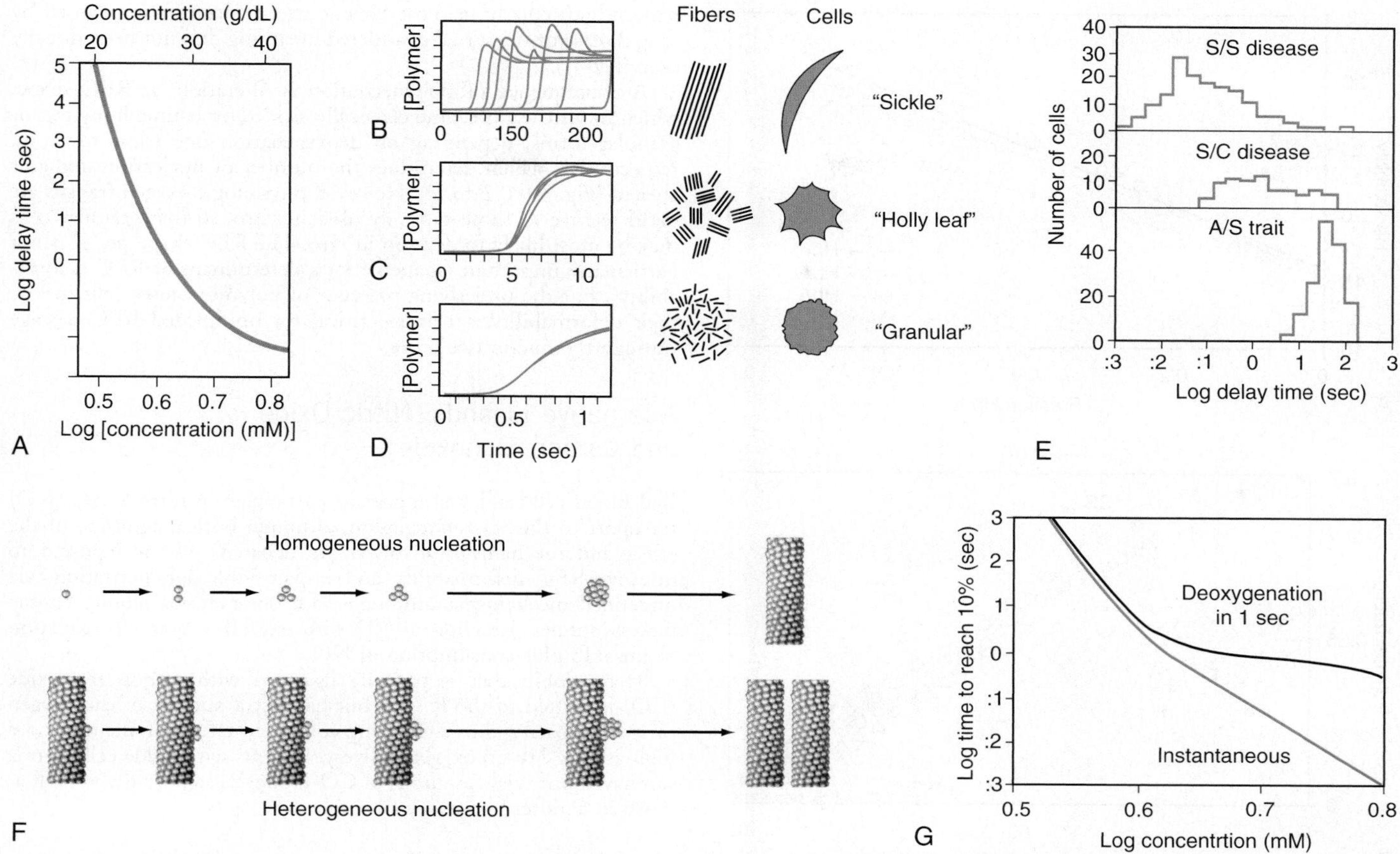

Figure 39-4 KINETICS OF HEMOGLOBIN S POLYMERIZATION, STUDIED BY NEAR-INSTANTANEOUS AND COMPLETE DEOXYGENATION. **A,** Extreme dependence of delay time on hemoglobin concentration. **B** to **D,** Kinetic progress curves for polymer formation show that long delay times are highly variable **(B),** but very short delay times are highly reproducible **(D).** *To the right* is a representation of domains and corresponding red blood cell morphology postulated to result from these different scales of polymerization rate (see Fig. 39-1, **B** to **E** and Fig. 39-3, **F**). **E,** Delay times for individual red blood cells are influenced by substituent hemoglobins. **F,** A double nucleation process is hypothesized to underlie polymer formation. **G,** Physiologically, the finite rate of deoxygenation effectively caps the polymerization rate and eliminates the relevance of delay times that are short relative to deoxygenation rate (<1 sec). *(**A** to **E**, Data from Eaton WA, Hofrichter J: Hemoglobin S gelation and sickle cell disease.* Blood *70:1245, 1987;* ***F*** *adapted from Ferrone FA, Hofrichter J, Eaton WA: Kinetics of sickle hemoglobin polymerization II. A double nucleation mechanism.* J Mol Biol *183:611, 1985;* ***G,*** *Data from Ferrone FA: Oxygen transits and transports. In Embury S, Hebbel RP, Mohandas N, Steinberg MH, eds:* Sickle cell disease: basic principles and clinical practice, *New York, 1994, Raven Press.)*

caused by the vanishingly low oxygen affinity of extant deoxy-HbS polymer, and it should promote neither hemoglobin polymerization (it results from it) nor tissue oxygenation (polymer is nonfunctional in oxygen delivery).

Kinetics of Polymerization

In vitro measurements of polymerization kinetics, allowed by inducing (nonphysiologic) instantaneous and complete conversion of HbS from R (oxy) to T (deoxy) state, reveal a delay before onset of polymerization, which then occurs explosively.[4] Under in vitro conditions, this delay time is inversely related to an extremely high power of the initial Hb concentration; it is approximately 10 msec at Hb of 40 g/dL, but it is 100,000 seconds at 20 g/dL (Fig. 39-4, *A*). HbS solutions and sickle RBCs behave similarly in this regard. Delay times must then vary enormously from cell to cell because they are dominated by marked heterogeneity in MCHC (i.e., shorter delay for more dehydrated cells) and are influenced by the presence of any non-S Hb (i.e., longer delay for presence of HbA, C, or F) (Fig. 39-4, *E*). Admixture of 20% to 30% HbA with HbS (simulating HbS-β^+-thalassemia) increases the delay time 10^1- to 10^2-fold, and admixture of 20% to 30% HbF with HbS increases it by 10^3- to 10^4-fold.

Actual polymer formation is hypothesized to proceed by a two-step, double-nucleation mechanism (Fig 39-4, *F*). Accordingly, the initial homogeneous nucleation takes place in bulk solution, during which small numbers of tetramers associate, with accumulation not favored until a critical nucleus size develops (estimated to be 30-50 tetramers). Then new tetramers can be added lengthwise to form a very large polymer. After this occurs, heterogeneous nucleation of new fibers takes place on the surface of the preexisting polymers, resulting in explosive, autocatalytic polymer formation. It is believed that the striking irreproducibility of long delay times (Fig. 39-4, *B*) reflects stochastic formation of a single (or at least very few) homogeneous nucleation event(s) in cells that slowly polymerize and that very short delay times (Fig. 39-4, *D*) reflect simultaneous formation of multiple nucleation sites in cells that polymerize rapidly.

The two central features of the polymerization process, governance by MCHC and the delay time, are highly dependent on the RBC membrane's control of cellular hydration. Whether the RBC membrane itself has any influence on polymerization remains under investigation. The good qualitative correspondence between polymerization in solution and in RBCs argues that the fundamental mechanism (Fig. 39-4, F) is not altered by membranes. Yet emerging evidence suggests that the abnormal sickle RBC membrane may even be able to contribute nucleation sites, thereby shortening delay times.

Polymerization Under (Patho)physiologic Conditions

Under physiologic conditions, sickle RBCs are not at equilibrium with a constant oxygen tension, and venous blood typically contains

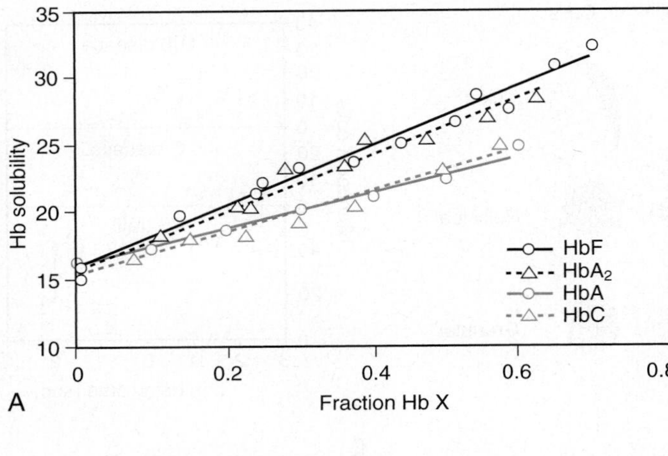

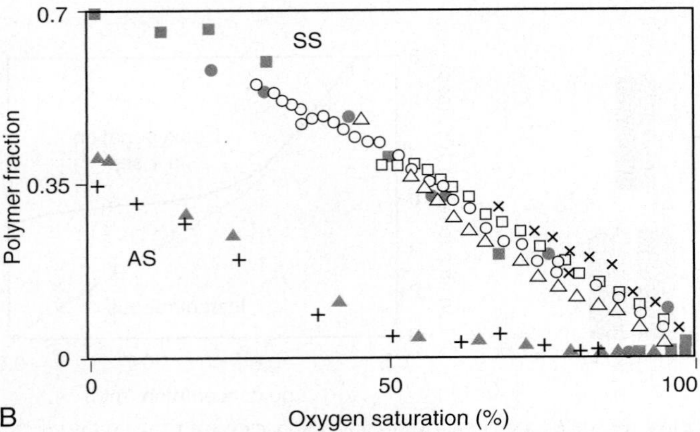

Figure 39-5 DEOXYHEMOGLOBIN S SOLUBILITY, DEFINED BY STUDIES UNDER EQUILIBRIUM CONDITIONS. **A,** Admixture of other hemoglobins with hemoglobin S raises overall solubility in absence of oxygen. **B,** The hemoglobin oxygen saturation required to initiate intracellular polymer formation (i.e., polymer fraction) is much lower for sickle trait than for normal red blood cells. *(**A,** Data from Poillon WN, Kim BC, Rodgers GP, et al: Sparing effect of hemoglobin F and hemoglobin A_2 on the polymerization of hemoglobin S at physiologic ligand saturations.* Proc Natl Acad Sci U S A *90:5039, 1993; **B,** Data from Schechter AN, Noguchi CT: Sickle hemoglobin polymer: Structure-function correlates. In Embury SH, Hebbel RP, Mohandas N, Steinberg MH, eds:* Sickle cell disease: Basic principles and clinical practice, *New York, 1994, Raven Press.)*

only about 20% sickled cells instead of the 90% predicted by equilibrium studies. Likewise, pathophysiologic deoxygenation is neither instantaneous nor complete. Indeed, HbS polymerization in vivo would be limited by the finite rate of physiologic RBC deoxygenation, and this effectively imposes a limit on what delay times are likely to be relevant in vivo: only those 1 second or longer (Fig. 39-4, G).[4] In aggregate, kinetic considerations argue that most RBCs in patients with sickle cell anemia are unlikely to sickle during their passage through the microcirculation unless something such as RBC–endothelial adhesion slows their transit time. Predictability, however, is complicated by the marked heterogeneity among RBCs in MCHC and HbF content, such that individual RBCs vary enormously in their likelihood of sickling.

The presence in RBCs of any preexisting polymer that did not completely melt during pulmonary transit would eliminate the delay time requirement because nucleation is already completed. Given the expected rapid RBC transit time through the lung (<1 second), fewer than 1% of RBCs should reach the arterial circulation still containing polymer. Despite it being critical to understanding in vivo pathophysiology, the practical balance of these considerations in the patient, particularly in those having arterial desaturation caused by lung disease or nocturnal disordered breathing, has not been directly examined.

A consequence of polymerization is alteration in RBC shape, which in vitro can become classically sickled or assume holly leaf or granular forms, depending on deoxygenation rate (slow to rapid, respectively), which determines the number of nucleation domains created (Fig. 39-4, *B* to *D*). However, physiologic oxygen transits are rapid relative to those typically used in vitro, so that granular cells may be most likely to develop in vivo. The RBC shape per se is not particularly important (shape is not a determinant of RBC deformability), but the underlying presence of polymer causes cells to lose their deformability, a feature critical for unimpeded RBC passage through the microvasculature.

Alternative Ligands: Nitric Oxide and Carbon Monoxide

Red blood cells and Hb appear to participate in nitric oxide (NO) transport to the microcirculation, although both magnitude of the effect and mechanisms involved are debated. NO is reported to improve RBC deformability and impair HbS polymerization, via undefined mechanisms, although both observations require confirmatory studies. Reaction of NO with oxy-Hb causes Hb oxidation to met-Hb plus consumption of NO.

Hemoglobin that is partially liganded with carbon monoxide (CO) is shifted to the R state but has lost a portion of the oxygen carrying capacity, thus simulating combined effects of anemia and a high-affinity Hb on oxygen delivery. Patients with sickle cell anemia can have nontrivial elevations of CO-Hb levels (reportedly as high as 7.6% in children) because of hemolysis.

ABNORMALITIES OF SICKLE RED BLOOD CELLS

Even oxygenated sickle RBCs exhibit a variety of membrane abnormalities that contribute to pathophysiology. Some are the consequence of proximate polymer formation, and others result from oxidative biochemistry. The integrated pathogenic context in which these abnormalities reside is presented below in sections on hemolysis and vascular biological disturbances.

Membrane Iron and Oxidant Generation

An abnormal oxidative biochemistry takes place at the cytosol–membrane interface of the sickle RBC.[2] The modest oxidation of HbS in solution and especially its avidity for bilayer lipid result in formation of superoxide and met-Hb, the proximate step in hemoglobin denaturation. Denatured hemoglobin can lose its heme to the lipid bilayer, where it is easily destroyed to liberate "free" iron. Membrane-associated iron is catalytically active, using cytosolic reducing substances (e.g., ascorbate, superoxide) to redox cycle and generate highly reactive oxidants. Also, it can form a redox couple with soluble oxy-Hb to promote further hemoglobin oxidation and denaturation. It is probable that this scenario underlies the various iron forms found at the cytosol–membrane interface of sickle RBC: hemoglobin, denatured hemichrome, free heme, and nonheme iron.

These processes may lead sickle RBCs to spontaneously generate excessive oxidant. Most importantly, however, the membrane location of catalytic iron establishes unique oxidant risk because it effectively targets oxidative damage to membrane components. In sickle RBCs, this is evidenced by oxidation of membrane protein thiols and peroxidation of membrane lipids. The unique juxtaposition of heme and iron with bilayer lipid is a critical feature because it effectively bypasses vitamin E, allowing reinitiation of peroxidative chain reactions. It is likely that deficient levels of RBC antioxidants (e.g., vitamin E, glutathione, ascorbic acid) caused by oxidative consumption or dietary insufficiencies contribute to this oxidative stress state. Among the many sickle membrane defects, evidence for an oxidative origin or contribution is strongest for band 3 clustering, abnormal membrane microrheology, irreversibly sickled cell (ISC) formation, aberrant cation homeostasis, microvesiculation tendency, abnormal mechanosensitivity, and erythrophagocytosis.[2]

Cation Homeostasis and Dehydrated Cells

For normal RBCs, the MCHC averages about 32 g/dL and varies from 27 to 38 g/dL, with fewer than 1% of cells having an MCHC greater than 38 g/dL. In contrast, the MCHC of sickle RBCs averages about 34 g/dL and varies from 23 to 50 g/dL, with up to 40% of cells having an MCHC greater than 38 g/dL. This extreme density heterogeneity results from reticulocytosis (low-density, low-MCHC cells) and dehydrating mechanisms (higher density, high-MCHC cells) (Fig. 39-6).[5,6]

The most dramatic ion-handling abnormality of the sickle RBC is sickling-induced permeabilization of the RBC membrane to cations (Na^+, K^+, Ca^{2+}). This depends on cell deformation, so it probably partly reflects the sickle RBCs' exaggerated leak susceptibility to deformation (mechanosensitivity).[7] Sickling induces calcium influx and a slight acidification, occurring stochastically and only in some cells at any one time. This results in net potassium and water loss mediated mostly by activation of a Ca^{2+} activated (Gardos) K^+ channel and K-Cl cotransport. The latter can be activated by lowered pH, endothelin-1, thiol oxidation, and a membrane interaction effect of hemoglobins that are relatively positively charged (HbC >HbS). It is influenced by macromolecular crowding of cytosolic proteins caused by the high MCHC. Even at steady state, sickle RBCs contain increased Ca^{2+} because it is sequestered in cytoplasmic inside-out membrane vesicles, providing evidence of prior cytosolic Ca^{2+} transients.

These aberrancies lead to decremental changes in RBC hydration and deformability. However, hyper-dense RBCs—mostly ISCs—are not older cells with longer histories of sickling and unsickling but rather can develop via a rapid reticulocyte-to-ISC transformation, with the RBC having lower HbF levels being particularly susceptible. Dehydrated RBCs have very diminished deformability and increased propensity for polymerization, the mutually promotive effects of dehydration and sickling comprising a vicious cycle. RBC dehydration is particularly likely to be exaggerated by the hypoxic and acidotic renal medullary environment, the greatest focus of disease in persons with sickle trait, and very probably by nocturnal arterial desaturation.

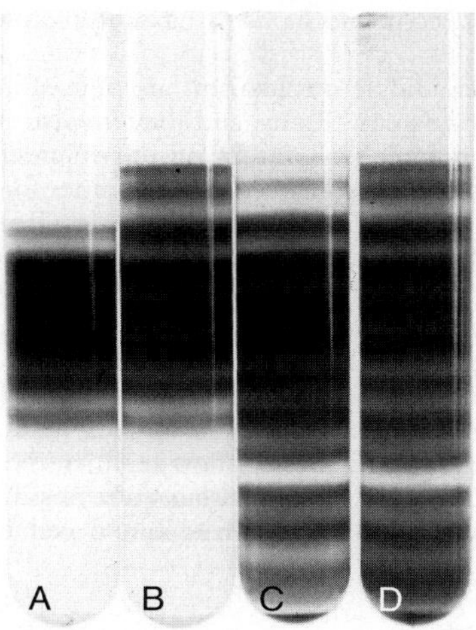

Figure 39-6 MARKED HETEROGENEITY IN SICKLE RED BLOOD CELL (RBC) HYDRATION. Compared with normal RBCs **(A)** studied by discontinuous density-gradient centrifugation, RBCs from a sickle subject with four α genes **(D)** include cells of unusually low density (usually reticulocytes) and abnormally high density (dehydrated cells). Sickle subjects with three and two α genes are shown in **C** and **B,** respectively. *(From Embury SH, Clark MR, Monroy G, Mohandas N: Concurrent sickle cell anemia and a-thalassemia.* J Clin Invest *73:116, 1984.)*

Deformability, Fragility, and Vesiculation

Even oxygenated sickle RBCs are poorly deformable.[8] The dominant cause of this is the high MCHC that imposes increased cytoplasmic viscosity and a poorly understood, hemoglobin-induced effect on membrane stiffness. There may also be a smaller oxidation-related component to membrane stiffness. Upon RBC deoxygenation in vitro, there is a temporal correspondence between appearance of polymer-induced shape change and deterioration of deformability, as measured by micropipette and laser diffractometer. On the other hand, filtration studies found decreased deformability before morphologic change, and viscometry reveals a large deterioration in bulk viscosity caused by deoxygenated dense discocytes that show little shape change.

Sickle RBCs are somewhat mechanically fragile, which may be a consequence of dehydration and a weakening of critical skeletal associations caused by oxidative protein damage. The tendency of sickled RBCs to lose membrane microvesicles reflects separation of the bilayer from the underlying skeleton by spicules of polymerized hemoglobin, with enhanced susceptibility caused by protein thiol oxidation and dysfunction.

Membrane Proteins and Lipids

Sickle RBC membrane protein function is adversely affected by thiol oxidation and possibly other oxidative protein modifications.[2] Ankyrin interactions with spectrin and band 3 are abnormal, glycophorin and band 3 exhibit decreased mobility, and thiol-oxidized β-actin displays abnormal associations in the spectrin–actin-4.1

Major Sickle RBC Membrane Defects

- Membrane iron deposits →
  - Band 3 clumping → Ig attraction → erythrophagocytosis
  - Oxidative reactions targeted at membrane →
    - Thiol oxidation →
      - ISC formation
      - ↓ Deformability and ↑ fragility
      - Cation leak
      - Microvesiculation
    - Lipid peroxidation →
      - Enhanced mechanosensitivity
      - Erythrophagocytosis
- Abnormal cation homeostasis →
  - RBC dehydration → ↓ deformability
- Abnormal microrheology →
  - ↓ Deformability
- PS externalization →
  - Coagulation acceleration
  - Erythrophagocytosis
- Enhanced mechanosensitivity → ↑ deformability responses →
  - Cation loss
  - Microvesiculation → PS-positive microparticles
  - Fragility
  - PS externalization
- Abnormal RBC adhesion to endothelium
- Abnormal RBC adhesion to monocytes and macrophages

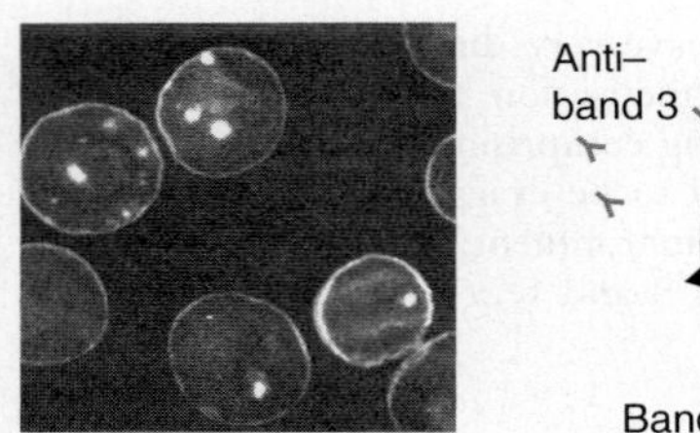

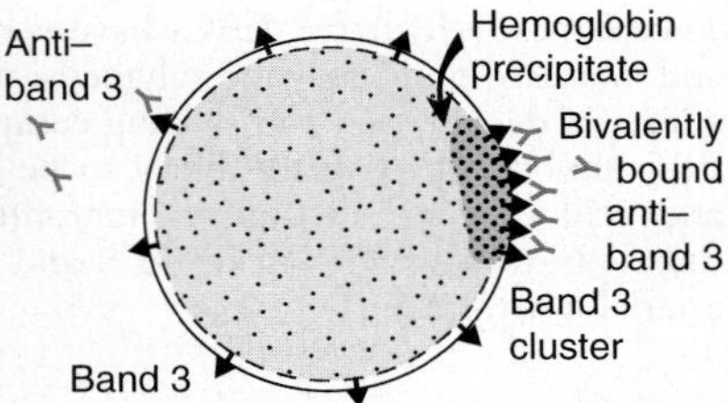

Figure 39-7 BAND 3 AND IMMUNOGLOBULIN COCLUSTERING. Denatured hemoglobin on the RBC membrane, is associated with clumping of band 3, and opsonization by naturally occurring anti-band 3 antibody. Clusters of band 3 are colocalized with immunoglobulin on the membranes of sickle red blood cells *(left)*. The drawing shows the colocalization scheme *(right)*. *(From Schluter K, Drenckhahn D: Co-clustering of denatured hemoglobin with band 3: Its role in binding of autoantibodies against band 3 to abnormal and aged erythrocytes.* Proc Natl Acad Sci U S A *83:6137, 1986.)*

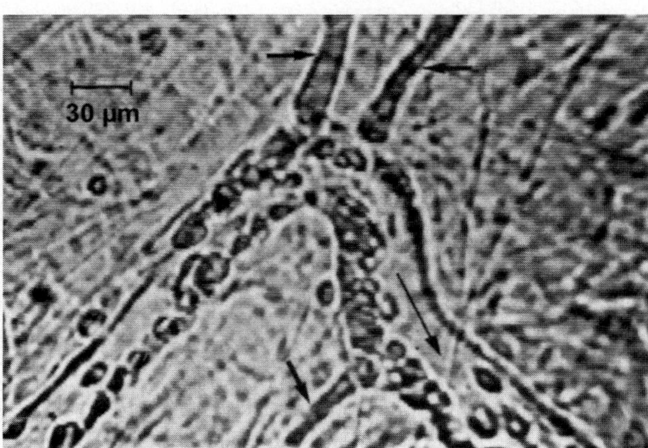

Figure 39-8 RBC ADHESION TO ENDOTHELIUM. RBCs adhere to the vascular wall endothelium under flow conditions in the microcirculation of a rat infused with human cells. Immobile RBCs are on walls of the post-capillary venule, and the smaller feeder microvessels *(small arrows)* have no flow because of the logjam of RBC. *(From Kaul DK, Fabry ME, Nagel RL: Microvascular sites and characteristics of sickle cell adhesion to vascular endothelium in shear flow conditions: Pathophysiological implications.* Proc Natl Acad Sci U S A *86:3356, 1989.)*

complex. Band 3 is abnormally clumped because of binding of denatured HbS to its cytosolic portion, which causes binding of naturally occurring anti–band 3 immunoglobulin (Fig. 39-7).

The processes that normally enforce bilayer phospholipid asymmetry are impaired in sickle RBCs: a scramblase that moves phosphatidylserine (PS) outward and is activated by calcium transits, and a translocase that moves PS inward can be inhibited by thiol oxidation. RBC sickling promotes PS externalization, a permanent feature of ISCs, but a substantial portion of reticulocytes also exhibits this because of impaired translocase activity. Other changes include presence of peroxidation byproducts such as malondialdehyde that can crosslink proteins and thereby promote erythrophagocytosis.

Notably, the increased presence of bilayer lipid hydroperoxides appears to account for the sickle RBC membranes' enhanced responsiveness to deformation-induced cation loss[7] and possibly other features promoted by the deformation of sickling.

Irreversibly Sickled Cells

The sickled RBCs seen on a typically-obtained blood smear are mostly ISCs (see Fig 39-1). Their permanent shape abnormality is caused not by retained polymer but rather by membrane retention of an elongated shape. This is explained by thiol oxidation of β-actin such that the spectrin–actin-4.1 complex exhibits abnormally slow dissociation and hence retention of elongation. Otherwise, ISCs are similar to other equally dense RBC: high MCHC, poor deformability, externalized PS, and low HbF content. ISC counts on average are higher in male patients, perhaps reflecting their average lower levels of HbF. The fundamental requirements for ISC formation seem to be RBC dehydration, prolonged deoxygenation, and assumption of a fixed membrane shape. This perhaps implies a prior "conditioning" residence in the microcirculation.

The clinical importance of ISCs lies in their ability to prompt diagnosis of a sickling disorder when seen on blood smear and in their short life span that contributes to overall hemolytic rate. They presumably would contribute to the RBC logjam involved in occlusion, but it is unclear whether ISC count correlates with vasoocclusive manifestations. Although still adhesive to endothelium, ISCs are less so than other sickle subpopulations, but they exhibit greater adherence to macrophages.

Endothelial Adhesivity

Oxygenated sickle RBCs are abnormally adhesive to vascular endothelial cells (Fig. 39-8). In vitro studies have identified about 20 candidate mechanisms involving adhesion molecules on endothelium, adhesive structures restricted to reticulocytes or present on all RBCs, with or without involvement of bridging by adhesogenic plasma proteins.[9] A central, unanswered question is whether in vivo this process occurs via a single, dominant mechanism. Alternatively, there may be mechanistic heterogeneity, with multiple mechanisms varying over time, in different vascular regions, among individuals, or even associated with different clinical contexts. For example, platelet activation releases α granule thrombospondin (TSP), a plausible adhesogenic intermediary bridge, so variation in the former could affect TSP-mediated RBC/endothelial adhesion. Likewise, adhesion mediated by endothelial vascular cell adhesion molecule 1 (VCAM1) (pairs with RBC $\alpha_4\beta_1$), $\alpha_v\beta_3$ (pairs with intercellular adhesion molecule 4 [ICAM4] and plasma TSP), and P-selectin (binds to sialylated RBC structures) are activated by tumor necrosis factor (TNF), platelet activating factor (PAF), and thrombin, respectively. Each of these stimulants is elevated in sickle blood. Only the $\alpha_v\beta_3$ and P-selectin mechanisms have been studied and verified in vivo so far.

Most of the candidate mechanisms are high affinity and demonstrable under flowing conditions, and they involve adhesive reticulocytes. Yet in the biologic context of the microcirculation where spatial constraints create enhanced opportunities for receptor–ligand contacts, even the low-affinity adhesive mechanisms observable for more dense RBC probably are relevant. This pathophysiology undoubtedly is governed by the plethora of biologic modifiers of endothelial activation state. Indeed, some adhesion mechanisms are relevant only if the endothelium is activated. Others become relevant if internal RBC signaling is triggered. Additional governing factors include the reticulocyte count, flow and shear rates, vessel diameter and geometry, and disturbances of flow regimens because of marginated white blood cells (WBCs). It also is quite possible that pathobiologic RBC adhesivity involves mixed blood cell interactions with endothelium.

Macrophage Interaction

Sickle RBCs are readily phagocytosed by macrophages because of RBC membrane modifications by malondialdehyde, PS externalization, and opsonization by immunoglobulin. The latter process probably is triggered mainly by clustering of membrane protein band 3 caused by denatured hemoglobin at the cytosol–membrane interface (see Fig. 39-7). The most dense cells have the most surface immunoglobulin and higher PS externalization, and they exhibit the greatest interaction with macrophages and potential for erythrophagocytosis.

THE ROLE OF SICKLE RED BLOOD CELLS IN DISEASE PATHOGENESIS

Vascular Occlusion

Notwithstanding the conceptual simplicity of the sickling phenomenon, it is likely that development of microvascular occlusion is a complex process having an evolving genesis. Insofar as sickling is responsible, risk factors would comprise anything that would increase MCHC and RBC dehydration (e.g., insufficient clinical hydration, injudicious use of diuretics), foster arterial oxygen desaturation (e.g., lung disease, sleep-disordered breathing), prolong microvascular transit time (e.g., inflammation), increase blood viscosity (e.g., transfusion, clinical dehydration), right shift the oxygen binding curve (e.g., acidosis), disturb vascular dynamics (e.g., cold, aberrant neurochemical responses, abnormal vasomotive rhythms), or reduce HbF level. The latter is complicated, however, because in sickle RBCs, HbF is located mostly in a subpopulation of F cells. Variations in the percentage of F cells, therefore, have a large impact on the overall HbF level.[10] Yet RBCs pass through the microcirculation single file, and behavior of every individual RBC depends on its specific HbF content. This inherent contrariety has not been adequately studied, defined, or reconciled vis à vis mechanisms of vasoocclusion. Nonetheless, at the sensitivity of epidemiology, HbF level is inversely related to frequency of vasoocclusive painful crises.[11]

Sickle RBC adhesion to endothelium can slow microvascular flow, thus overcoming the delay time requirement for HbS polymerization. Indeed, experimental studies in sickle mice revealed that occlusion is a two-step process.[9] The current (although not necessarily definitive) model holds that adhesion of less dense (reticulocyte-enriched) sickle RBCs in the postcapillary venule initiate vasoocclusion, after which logjamming by dense and poorly deformable cells provides retrograde propagation (see Fig. 39-8). This predicts that determinants of RBC adhesivity and endothelial activation or dysfunction would help govern pathobiology. Consistent with this, clinical vasoocclusive severity does correlate with the endothelial adhesivity of sickle RBCs in vitro.

Diminished RBC deformability can additionally impair microvascular flow, and dense sickle RBC (especially ISC) appear to have difficulty entering the microvasculature (e.g., at bifurcations). Within the smaller vessels, RBC adhesivity and deformability would be predicted to exert combined—possibly synergistic—effects, although this has not been sufficiently studied. However, in humans with sickle disease, clinical vasoocclusive severity correlates with preservation of RBC deformability rather than degradation thereof.

Consequences of Vasoocclusion

Microvascular vasoocclusion has long been assumed to underlie the acute painful episode and chronic organ deterioration in sickle cell disease, although there are associated enigmas.[12] However, both microvascular and macrovascular disease are features of sickle pathobiology. These may well be linked because localized vasoocclusion can exert adverse systemic effects on vascular biology.[13] In addition, a new concept has questioned whether occlusive disease really underlies all complications of this disease.

Hemolytic Anemia

RBC life span in SCA averages about 15 days but with marked interindividual variability (from ≈7 to ≈30 days); in HbSC disease, the average is about 30 days.[14] All four fundamental mechanisms that can underlie RBC removal in hematologic disease—erythrophagocytosis, fragmentation, trapping, and osmotic lysis probably contribute (Fig. 39-9, *bottom*). These are consequences of the proximate aberrancies of the sickle RBC discussed earlier (Fig. 39-9, *middle*) that result from the specific molecular behaviors of the mutant HbS (Fig. 39-9, *top*). This integrated synthesis of research data presents the most plausible mechanistic blueprint.[14]

Although complex, the routes to accelerated RBC removal resolve into two basic pathogenic cascades: one from polymer formation that underlies the three mechanisms (trapping, fragmentation, osmotic lysis) that cause intravascular hemolysis and one from HbS instability that leads to erythrophagocytosis and extravascular hemolysis. Notably, intravascular hemolysis accounts for only one-third of overall sickle hemolysis; two-thirds is explained by extravascular hemolysis.[14]

Because these distinct destructive processes would contribute differentially to appearance of serum lactate dehydrogenase (LDH), it is unlikely to be a *quantitative* biomarker of hemolytic rate in the sickle context. The only biomarkers that have been documented to correlate strongly and quantitatively with measured RBC life span in sickle cell anemia are the (uncorrected) reticulocyte percentage and HbF level.[14]

The shortest survival is exhibited by the sickle RBC that are most dehydrated and that have the lowest amounts of HbF.[15,16] This is consistent with the polymerization-based cascade of abnormalities (see Fig. 39-9). Whether these two features fully explain the very wide range of hemolytic rates is not known; the precise mechanism by which sickling leads to direct lysis is also unknown. Presumably, the sickle RBCs' fragility is related, and sickled RBCs lose Hb via microvesiculation when sickling is reversed in vivo. Improved RBC hydration caused by concurrent α-globin gene deletion improves RBC survival,[17] as does the increment in HbF level in patients taking hydroxyurea.[10] The reason that sickle RBC survival drops substantially in association with acute vasoocclusive crises[14] has not been defined, nor is it known whether this precedes or follows crisis onset.

The influence of the instability-based cascade is evident in enhanced erythrophagocytosis of sickle RBC, promoted by denatured Hb causing band 3 clumping and attraction of immunoglobulin, membrane modification by the lipid oxidation product malondialdehyde, and PS externalization.

Consequences of Hemolysis

The presence of hemolysis-derived cell-free oxy-Hb in sickle plasma can consume NO,[18] but how substantially this contributes to the overall diminished bioavailability of NO is not known.[14] Hemolysis causing this precise consumptive process has been asserted to be the proximate cause of certain specific clinical complications,[19] but supporting data are only correlative (e.g., association of stroke with elevated LDH). In fact, hemolytic release of free Hb in sickle disease would be paralleled by several additional potentially injurious products that presumably would also correlate with the same clinical events. Two are perhaps most notable.[14] Sickle hemolysis causes robust generation of PS-positive microparticles that can adversely impact endothelium; these also accelerate coagulation activation,[20] thrombin being an additional potential perturbant. Also, the likely release of free heme caused by HbS instability in the context of severely depleted levels of haptoglobin and hemopexin would exert toxic effects on endothelium. Heme also would stimulate monocyte production of TNF, yet another endothelial perturbant. Thus hemolysis as a proximate cause of events seems perfectly plausible, but this has not been unambiguously demonstrated and its mechanism is debatable.

INFLAMMATION AND ENDOTHELIAL DYSFUNCTION

Sickle cell disease is a chronic, systemic inflammatory state.[13,14] Characteristic features include elevated leukocyte counts; activation of granulocytes and monocytes; elevation of proximate inflammatory mediators, acute-phase reactants, and soluble adhesion molecules; activation of hemostatic systems; and excess oxidant generation.

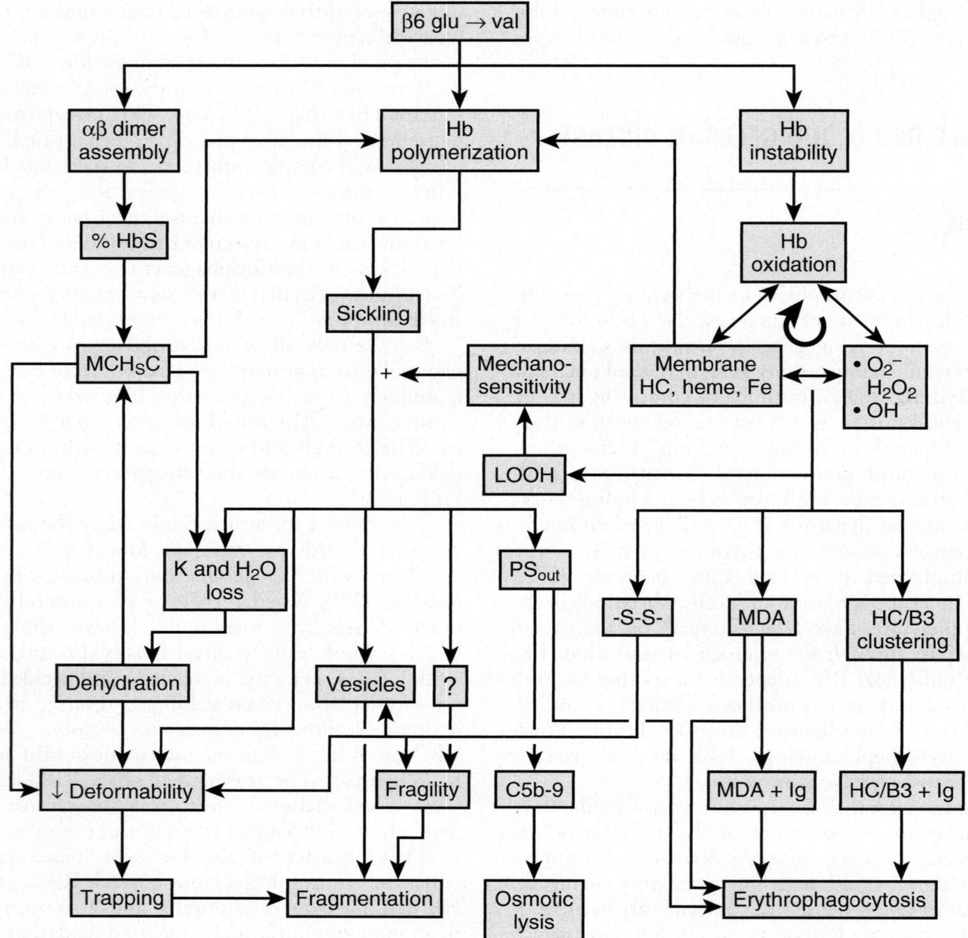

Figure 39-9 MECHANISMS LEADING TO HEMOLYSIS IN SICKLE CELL DISEASE. This integrated synthesis shows how the molecular behaviors of hemoglobin S (HbS) *(top)* cause development of multiple red blood cell (RBC) abnormalities *(middle)* that lead to the four mechanisms of accelerated RBC destruction *(bottom)*. *(Modified with permission from* The American Journal of Hematology *from Hebbel RP: Reconstructing sickle cell disease: A data-based analysis of the "hyperhemolysis paradigm" for pulmonary hypertension from the perspective of evidence-based medicine.* Am J Hematol *86:123-154, 2011.)*

Clinically, leukocytosis in sickle cell disease is a risk factor for mortality, clinical and silent stroke, and acute chest syndrome, and it helps predict which babies will develop a severe clinical course. Sickle transgenic mice share with humans an inflammatory phenotype. The most prominent consequences of this state are endothelial activation and dysfunction and enablement of vasoocclusion (via adhesion molecule expression).

Experimental data from sickle transgenic mice, clinical data from sickle patients, and a vast relevant general medical literature suggest that this inflammatory state is best understood as a consequence of recurrent ischemia/reperfusion injury physiology (Fig. 39-10).[13,14] This well-understood, postocclusive cascade causes oxidative stress, intense inflammatory responses, and endothelial dysfunction that is systemic, not localized.

Endothelial Dysfunction

The most plausible hierarchical relationships between the multiple vascular biological abnormalities in sickle disease illustrate the probable centrality of endothelial dysfunction in their genesis (see Fig. 39-10).[13,14] In this construct, recurrent RBC sickling comprises the system input, reperfusion injury provides the incessant driving force, and systemic inflammation causing endothelial dysfunction comprises the executor of clinical disease. In a dysfunctional state, the endothelium has a proinflammatory and prothrombotic phenotype, it exhibits excessive superoxide generation (typically via endothelial NADPH [nicotinamide adenine dinucleotide phosphate-oxidase] oxidase and uncoupled endothelial nitric oxide synthase [eNOS]), and it causes diminished NO bioavailability caused by the eNOS uncoupling (itself predominantly caused by tetrahydrobiopterin oxidation). Sickle transgenic mice exhibit all of these features; the few relevant data available from humans with sickle cell anemia are consistent with this. Additional features of sickle cell anemia can help promote endothelial dysfunction: elevated asymmetric dimethylarginine, oxidized lipids, aberrant wall shear stress, microparticles, and others.[14] A state of NO deficiency is an inevitable consequence of endothelial dysfunction, but it does not cause it.[14]

Diminished Nitric Oxide Bioavailability and Vasoregulation

Sickle cell disease is such a state of diminished NO bioavailability, as evidenced in humans primarily by abnormal endothelial-dependent, flow-mediated arterial dilation.[21,22] In addition to the presumably dominant role of endothelial dysfunction with eNOS uncoupling, other contributing processes could include NO consumption by both excess superoxide and plasma oxyHb, limited NO generation from impaired L-arginine availability resulting from elevations of plasma

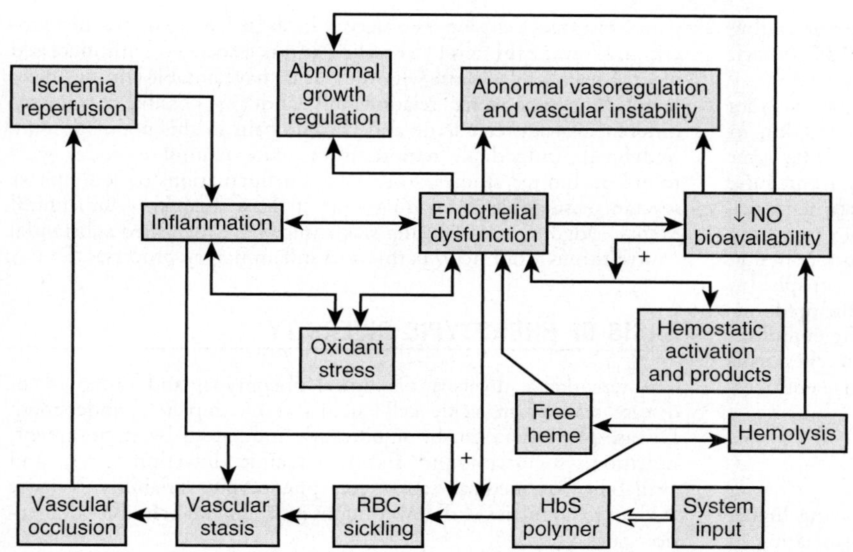

Figure 39-10 THE CENTRALITY OF ENDOTHELIAL DYSFUNCTION IN SICKLE CELL DISEASE. Sickle hemoglobin (HbS) polymerization provides the system input, ischemia–reperfusion provides the incessant driving force, and the resulting systemic inflammation is the executor of the HbS affect on vascular biology, which is realized by the disparate consequences of endothelial dysfunction. *NO,* nitric oxide; *RBC,* red blood cell. *(Modified from Hebbel RP: Reconstructing sickle cell disease: A data-based analysis of the "hyperhemolysis paradigm" for pulmonary hypertension from the perspective of evidence-based medicine.* Am J Hematol *86:123, 2011).*

and endothelial arginase (the latter being a consequence of TNF stimulation), and others.[14] The proportionate contributions of these disparate causes is unknown. NO bioavailability seems to be higher for females than males, who exhibit substantial non-NO regulation of flow.[22]

Perfusion patterns are complex in sickle disease but can generally be described as impaired microvascular flow and augmented macrovascular flow.[21] The systemic nature of the inflammation and endothelial dysfunction consequent to the ischemia–reperfusion paradigm provides a likely resolution to the enigma presented by concurrent microvascular occlusive disease (vasoocclusion) and macrovascular clinical disease (e.g., pulmonary hypertension, circle of Willis disease). In turn, this predicts dominance of different proximate determinants of the two vascular perturbations: blood cell–endothelial adhesion, deformability and polymerization for microvascular disease; and cellular and humoral endothelial stressors, and possibly aberrant wall shear stress, for macrovascular disease.

Aberrancy of both endothelial-dependent (NO-mediated) and endothelial-independent vasoregulation is apparent. Also, a state of vascular instability is emerging as a disease feature, with sickle mice exhibiting tonic upregulation of both vasoconstrictive and vasodilatory systems, as well as exaggerated α_1-adrenergic vessel wall responsiveness. Sickle humans reveal disruption of autonomic regulation (e.g., with augmented risk for hypoxia-induced perfusion decrements).[23] Notably, the underlying endothelial dysfunction in sickle disease would comprise a state of enhanced susceptibility to transient pulmonary vasoconstrictive stressors.

Systemic blood pressure in subjects with sickle cell disease is lower than in nonanemic control participants yet is higher than in comparably anemic β-thalassemic patients.

Coagulation Activation

Sickle cell anemia involves chronic activation of plasmatic coagulation, fibrinolysis, and platelets. This is accompanied by increased whole blood tissue factor (TF) and its increased expression on blood monocytes and endothelial cells, liberation of PS-positive and TF-positive microparticles, thrombin generation, consumption of antithrombotic proteins, and presence of antiphospholipid antibodies. That the abnormally externalized PS on sickle RBCs and microparticles plays a significant accelerating role for lipid-dependent coagulation reactions.[20] Notably, consequent generation of thrombin is a major endothelial cell perturbant. The biodeficiency of NO would enable TF expression and augmented platelet activation because it normally inhibits these.

Chronic Vasculopathy

The macrovascular component of sickle vascular disease appears to be a chronic inflammatory vasculopathy.[13] Most available information is obtained from the large and medium vessels at the circle of Willis, where some sickle children develop occlusive pathology characterized by intimal hyperplasia, fibrotic and proliferative changes, and damage to internal elastic lamina. Similar pathologic changes have been observed in arteries in other organs. Sickle vascular lesions do include a fatty streak and foam cells, but they do seem nonrandom in location. Clearly, this is an incompletely evaluated aspect of sickle cell anemia.

CLINICAL PHENOTYPES AND COMPLICATIONS

Some clinical complications (pulmonary hypertension, leg ulcers, priapism, stroke) are more common in patients with higher serum LDH, but others (acute chest syndrome, acute painful episodes) occur more commonly in those having lower serum LDH.[19] On this basis, it has been assumed by some that hemolytic rate per se is the etiologic factor via degree of NO consumption caused by cell-free Hb. Certainly, the basic concept that different processes underlie different clinical complications is entirely plausible. However, support for this concept of dichotomous phenotype is based solely on statistical association focusing upon outlier quartiles of serum LDH level. Corresponding differences in Hb are small, reticulocyte counts are not different, and actual correspondence with measured RBC survival has not been examined.[19] In any case, it is evident that about half of patients are in an overlap group, and the prognostic value of serum LDH has not been tested at the level of the individual patient.

Pulmonary Disease

Around 6% of adults with sickle cell anemia have pulmonary hypertension, as documented by catheter measurement of pulmonary vascular resistance or mean pulmonary artery pressure.[24] Reports of higher prevalence were based on use of a faulty diagnostic criterion.[14] The hypothesis that consumption of NO by plasma Hb causes this complication is intriguing but unproven, as the supporting data to date are amenable to alternative interpretations. For example, placental growth factor generated by erythropoietic activity also correlates with pulmonary hypertension in sickle disease, and additional features of sickle vascular pathobiology, in particular endothelial dysfunction, are known risk contributors. It seems possible that the never-ending perfusion of the pulmonary arterial tree with sickled RBC (which induce an endothelial injury response in vitro) could play a role.

The spectrum of sickle pulmonary complications also includes chronic restrictive lung disease, pulmonary hypertension, infection, in situ and embolic thrombosis, and acute chest syndrome.[25] The latter is a life-threatening event and a predictor of subsequent chronic lung disease and stroke. Risk factors include leukocytosis, lower hemoglobin levels, and a lower level of HbF. Multiple proximate triggering events may lead to this syndrome in which inflammation, adhesion biology, NO deficiency, and endothelial permeability conspire to augment the deleterious effects of hypoxia on the lung. The predominant apparent triggers are infection in children and fat embolism (probably caused by marrow infarction) in adults. Acute chest syndrome does tend to occur after onset of acute vasoocclusive episodes.

Mortality and Sudden Death

The mortality rate is increased in sickle cell patients having higher rates of acute painful episodes,[26] perhaps revealing an association of clinically evident severity with extent of subclinical disease. Notable risk factors for mortality are a low HbF level and a high WBC count, implicating sickling and inflammation. In 1994, a large study in the United States reported a median age at death of 42 years for men and 48 years for women with sickle cell anemia; the comparable ages were 60 and 68 years, respectively, for HbSC disease.[26] This reflected a large improvement in mean life span after the introduction of prophylactic penicillin for children, revealing the earlier dominance of pneumococcal sepsis in disease natural history. Recently, further improvement has derived from chronic use of hydroxyurea for more severely affected individuals, an agent that boosts HbF level, lowers WBC count, and improves RBC hydration and survival.

The cause of death in this disease is from multiple complications, with cardiopulmonary disease being the most prominent category.[25-27] A striking incidence of sudden death is accounted for only partly by undiagnosed histopathologic pulmonary hypertension. It has been hypothesized that transient (possibly even ballistic) elevations of pulmonary artery pressure could be responsible because the state of underlying endothelial dysfunction would substantially exaggerate the vessel wall's constrictive response to potential vasoconstrictors (e.g., from nocturnal hypoxia, augmented hemolytic rate, inflammatory signaling).[14]

Stroke

Several stroke syndromes occur in sickle disease and may have differing pathogeneses. Ischemic stroke develops in about 85 of children with sickle cell anemia, with occlusive disease at the circle of Willis being the strongest risk factor; completion of the clinical stroke tends to involve thrombosis at the site of vessel wall disease. Other identified risk factors include greater anemia, a higher WBC count, systolic blood pressure at the higher end of the sickle range, acute development of hypoxia, a prior neurologic event, presence of moyamoya, low pain crisis rate, and concurrent or antecedent inflammatory conditions. Concurrent α-thalassemia or HbSC disease lower the risk; HbF level is not protective. The chronic inflammatory state may be a significant pathogenic factor.

The other sickle stroke syndromes are even less well understood; these include silent strokes during childhood associated with degradation of IQ, hemorrhagic stroke in young adults, and microvascular stroke that increases with age.

Pain

Pain signaling in sickle disease appears to be multimodal and complex, and inflammatory mediators play a major role. In adults, a higher frequency of classical acute painful episodes, assumed to be ischemic pain from vasoocclusion, is observed in those having higher hematocrit and lower HbF level at baseline and is associated with increased mortality.[11] Many of those with the disease have notable chronic, daily pain.[28] The pathogenic relationship—and any possible risk factor differences—between acute and chronic pain in this population are undefined. Individuals remote from acute painful episodes were found, in limited studies, to still exhibit fluctuations of acute phase reactants, suggesting ongoing—or at least frequent—subclinical events. Ongoing studies using sickle mice have identified substantial contributions from neuropathic and inflammatory processes.[29]

BASIS OF PHENOTYPIC DIVERSITY

The remarkable diversity of clinical phenotypes and variability of disease severity in sickle cell anemia is incompletely understood. Disease phenotype can be significantly influenced by environment, nutrition, socioeconomic status, endemic infection rates, and availability of medical care. Thus phenotypic variability is more evident in countries with lower infant mortality and childhood infection rates.

Level of Hemoglobin F

After the decline in HbF level over the first 6 months of life, most of the antisickling protection from its high level at birth is lost, but its level still varies among adults over a 20-fold range. HbF level reflects the number of F cells, the amount of HbF per F cell, and the preferential survival of F cells.[10] Known determinants account for perhaps one-half of its variance: a polymorphic *XmnI* site 5′ to the Gγ gene in the Senegal and Arab-India β-globin haplotypes, the HBS1L-Myb intergenic region, and polymorphisms of BCL11A (a transcriptional silencer of the *HBG* gene).[30] A putative "F-cell production locus" on the X chromosome has so far escaped being identified.

α-Thalassemia

The normal genotype is αα/αα, but about 30% of African Americans have a single α deletion (–α/αα), so concordance with sickle cell disease is common; and homozygosity for the allele is seen (–α/–α). Its prevalence elsewhere varies regionally. An α-gene deletion has minimal effect on the HbF level but results in improved RBC hydration (see Fig. 39-6), a lower ISC count, improved RBC survival, and less severe anemia.[17] Yet there is no amelioration of pain severity, and some complications (osteonecrosis, retinopathy) increase, possibly because of the increased blood viscosity.

β-Globin Alleles

Compound heterozygosity for the sickle gene and another β allele can affect clinical phenotype, generally as predicted by the extent to which they admix $β^A$ or γ chains with $β^S$, as presented earlier. HbSC disease presents a unique case.[31] Rather than simulating sickle trait (see Fig. 39-5A), the presence of HbC stimulates of K–Cl cotransport and causes RBC dehydration, thereby increasing the MCHC and RBC HbS concentration. Combined with a concurrent augmentation of HbS proportion (≈50% versus ≈40% in HbAS), this yields a sickling disorder only somewhat less severe than sickle cell anemia, but with an increased propensity for retinopathy and osteonecrosis. Other less common alleles can likewise interact with HbS and affect clinical phenotype via impact on polymerization.

Unexplained Phenotypic Diversity

Beyond these well-defined influences, there is still a substantial, unexplained variability in the clinical phenotype of sickle cell anemia. The disparate biological processes that participate in vasoocclusion, macrovascular vasculopathy, hemolysis, and specific complications highlights the probability that phenotypic heterogeneity will be influenced by underlying genetic variations affecting adhesion molecules, cation homeostasis, inflammatory signaling, vasoregulation, and so on. Multiple single-nucleotide polymorphisms (SNP) associations have been detected in association with specific clinical complications, with SNPs in transforming growth factor-β–related genes emerging as a prominent feature.[30] Exaggerated endothelial cell signaling response to inflammation, apparently genetically based, has been implicated in childhood ischemic stroke. It is likely that the contribution of such additional genetic influences will begin to be identified now that modern molecular approaches are being applied to the problem of phenotypic diversity in sickle cell disease.

REFERENCES

1. Bunn HF: Subunit assembly of hemoglobin: An important determinant of hematologic phenotype. *Blood* 69:1, 1987.
2. Browne P, Shalev O, Hebbel RP: The molecular pathobiology of cell membrane iron: The sickle red cell as a model. *Free Radic Biol Med* 24:1040, 1998.
3. Noguchi CT, Schechter AN: The intracellular polymerization of sickle hemoglobin and its relevance to sickle cell disease. *Blood* 58:1057, 1981.
4. Ferrone FA: Polymerization and sickle cell disease: A molecular view. *Microcirculation* 11:115, 2004.
5. Joiner CH: Cation transport and volume regulation in sickle red blood cells. *Am J Physiol* 264:C25, 1993.
6. Lew VL, Bookchin RM: Ion transport pathology in the mechanism of sickle cell dehydration. *Physiol Rev* 85:179, 2005.
7. Sugihara T, Rawicz W, Evans EA, et al: Lipid hydroperoxides permit deformation-dependent leak of monovalent cation from erythrocytes. *Blood* 77:2757, 1991.
8. Ballas SK, Mohandas N: Sickle red cell microrheology and sickle blood rheology. *Microcirculation* 11:209, 2004.
9. Kaul DK, Finnegan E, Barabino GA: Sickle red cell-endothelium interactions. *Microcirculation* 16:97, 2009.
10. Steinberg MH, Lu ZH, Barton FB, et al: Fetal hemoglobin in sickle cell anemia: Determinants of response to hydroxyurea. Multicenter study of hydroxyurea. *Blood* 89:1078, 1997.
11. Platt OS, Thorington BD, Brambilla DJ, et al: Pain in sickle cell disease. Rates and risk factors. *N Engl J Med* 325:11, 1991.
12. Embury SH: The not-so-simple process of sickle cell vasoocclusion. *Microcirculation* 11:101, 2004.
13. Hebbel RP, Vercellotti G, Nath KA: A systems biology consideration of the vasculopathy of sickle cell anemia: The need for multi-modality chemo-prophylaxis. *Cardiovasc Hematol Disord Drug Targets* 9:271, 2009.
14. Hebbel RP: Reconstructing sickle cell disease: A data-based analysis of the "hyperhemolysis paradigm" for pulmonary hypertension from the perspective of evidence-based medicine. *Am J Hematol* 86:123, 2011.
15. Franco RS, Yasin Z, Lohmann JM, et al: The survival characteristics of dense sickle cells. *Blood* 96:3610, 2000.
16. Franco RS, Yasin Z, Palascak MB, et al: The effect of fetal hemoglobin on the survival characteristics of sickle cells. *Blood* 108:1073, 2006.
17. Embury SH, Clark MR, Monroy G, et al: Concurrent sickle cell anemia and alpha-thalassemia. Effect on pathological properties of sickle erythrocytes. *J Clin Invest* 73:116, 1984.
18. Reiter CD, Wang X, Tanus-Santos JE, et al: Cell-free hemoglobin limits nitric oxide bioavailability in sickle-cell disease. *Nat Med* 8:1383, 2002.
19. Taylor JG, 6th, Nolan VG, Mendelsohn L, et al: Chronic hyper-hemolysis in sickle cell anemia: Association of vascular complications and mortality with less frequent vasoocclusive pain. *PLoS One* 3:e2095, 2008.
20. Setty BN, Kulkarni S, Rao AK, et al: Fetal hemoglobin in sickle cell disease: Relationship to erythrocyte phosphatidylserine exposure and coagulation activation. *Blood* 96:1119, 2000.
21. Nath KA, Katusic ZS, Gladwin MT: The perfusion paradox and vascular instability in sickle cell disease. *Microcirculation* 11:117, 2004.
22. Gladwin MT, Schechter AN, Ognibene FP, et al: Divergent nitric oxide bioavailability in men and women with sickle cell disease. *Circulation* 107:271, 2003.
23. Sangkatumvong S, Khoo MC, Kato R, et al: Peripheral vasoconstriction and abnormal parasympathetic response to sighs and transient hypoxia in sickle cell disease. *Am J Respir Crit Care Med* 184:474, 2011.
24. Parent F, Bachir D, Inamo J, et al: A hemodynamic study of pulmonary hypertension in sickle cell disease. *New Engl J Md* 365:4, 2011.
25. Gladwin MT, Vichinsky E: Pulmonary complications of sickle cell disease. *New Engl J Med* 359:2254, 2008.
26. Platt OS, Brambilla DJ, Rosse WF, et al: Mortality in sickle cell disease. Life expectancy and risk factors for early death. *New Engl J Med* 330:1639, 1994.
27. Fitzhugh CD, Lauder N, Jonassaint JC, et al: Cardiopulmonary complications leading to premature deaths in adult patients with sickle cell disease. *Am J Hematol* 85:36, 2010.
28. Smith WR, Penberthy LT, Bovbjerg VE, et al: Daily pain assessment of pain in adults with sickle cell disease. *Ann Intern Med* 15:94, 2008.
29. Kohli DR, Li Y, Khasabov SG, et al: Pain-related behaviors and neurochemical alterations in mice expressing sickle hemoglobin: Modulation by cannabinoids. *Blood* 116:456, 2010.
30. Fertrin KY, Costa FF: Genomic polymorphisms in sickle cell disease: Implications for clinical diversity and treatment. *Expert Rev Hematol* 3:443, 2010.
31. Bunn HF, Noguchi CT, Hofrichter J, et al: Molecular and cellular pathogenesis of hemoglobin SC disease. *Proc Natl Acad Sci U S A* 79:7527, 1982.

CHAPTER 40

SICKLE CELL DISEASE: CLINICAL FEATURES AND MANAGEMENT

Yogen Saunthararajah and Elliott P. Vichinsky

Hemoglobinopathies are the most common genetic diseases in humans. In sickle cell disease (SCD), a mutated β-globin gene produces sickle hemoglobin (Hb S). This mutation has been positively selected during human evolution because one copy of the sickle gene and one normal β-globin gene (sickle cell trait) confers a survival advantage in malaria-endemic regions. With two copies of the sickle gene (Hb SS or sickle cell anemia) or the sickle mutation and another mutated β-globin gene, for example, sickle cell–β°-thalassemia (Hb S–β thal) or Hb SC disease (Hb SC), the less soluble Hb S can polymerize in deoxygenated regions of the circulation, resulting in red blood cell (RBC) rigidity, RBC adhesion to endothelium, and hemolysis. These events activate inflammation and coagulation pathways and cause vasoocclusion.[1] These processes manifest clinically as chronic hemolytic anemia, recurrent painful episodes, and chronic organ damage from vasoocclusion. This chapter presents the diagnosis and natural history, describes overall clinical management, and as specific management by organ complications. Clinical interventions are founded on an understanding of underlying pathophysiologic processes. The exigency of living with a painful, life-threatening chronic disease in an ethnically diverse society adds complexity to the psychosocial aspects of this illness. A comprehensive management approach directed at preventing pain crises, chronic organ damage, and early mortality while effectively managing acute complications is recommended. For a full discussion of the fascinating history and molecular pathology of this disease, please see Chapter 42. Normal Hb synthesis, structure, and function are described in Chapter 33, and the thalassemias are considered in Chapter 41.

PREVALENCE

The distribution and frequency of the sickle cell gene in different areas of the world have been influenced by natural selection and transmission of the gene via trade routes and the slave trade.[2] Among African Americans,[3] the prevalence of sickle cell trait is 8% to 10% among newborns,[4] and in this population, the frequencies of the sickle cell (0.045), Hb C (0.015), and β-thalassemia (0.004) genes[4] indicate that there are 4000 to 5000 pregnancies a year at risk for SCD. The burden of this disease in the United States is dwarfed by that in the rest of the world, as evidenced by a prevalence of the sickle cell gene as high as 25% to 30% in western Africa and an estimated annual birth of 120,000 babies with SCD in Africa.[5]

DIAGNOSIS

The diagnosis of a sickle cell syndrome is suggested by characteristic findings on the complete blood count (CBC) and peripheral smear, that prompt Hb electrophoresis. If a diagnosis of SCD is confirmed, evaluation of the various organ systems at risk is required. These evaluations are discussed in the section on clinical management.

Complete Blood Count and Peripheral Blood Smear

The chronic hemolytic anemia of SCD presents with mild to moderately low hematocrit and Hb levels and a reticulocytosis of approximately 3% to 15%. Additional laboratory features of hemolysis are unconjugated hyperbilirubinemia, elevated lactate dehydrogenase (LDH), and low haptoglobin levels. The reticulocytosis accounts for high or high-normal mean corpuscular volume (MCV). If the age-adjusted MCV is not elevated, the possibility of sickle cell–β-thalassemia, coincident α-thalassemia, or iron deficiency must be considered.

In the peripheral smear (Fig. 40-1), there may be sickled forms, target cells, polychromasia indicative of reticulocytosis, and Howell-Jolly bodies demonstrating hyposplenia. The RBCs are normochromic unless there is coexistent thalassemia or iron deficiency. Sickled forms (irreversibly sickled cells [ISCs]) occur in the peripheral smear only in the SCDs and not in sickle cell trait. In Hb SS disease, ISCs predominate, and target cells may be few; in sickle cell–β-thalassemia, ISCs, target cells, and hypochromic microcytic discocytes are prominent; in Hb SC disease, target cells predominate, and ISCs are rare.

White blood cell (WBC) counts are higher than normal in Hb SS disease, particularly in patients under age 10 years. Mean WBC counts tend not to be elevated in Hb SC disease or sickle cell–β^+-thalassemia. Mean platelet counts are elevated in Hb SS disease, particularly in patients younger than age 18 years, but are usually normal in those with Hb SC disease and sickle cell–β^+-thalassemia.

Solubility Tests and Hemoglobin Electrophoresis

Solubility test results (e.g., Sickledex) are positive in both SCD and sickle cell trait. All patients require definitive diagnosis with Hb electrophoresis (which separates Hb species according to amino acid composition) (Fig. 40-2) or high performance liquid chromatography (HPLC).[6] Cellulose acetate electrophoresis at a pH of 8.4 is a standard method of separating Hb S from other variants. However, Hb S, G, and D have the same electrophoretic mobility with this method. Using citrate agar electrophoresis at pH 6.2, Hb S has a different mobility than Hb D and G, which comigrate with Hb A in this system.

Results from electrophoresis or thin-layer isoelectric focusing are similar in Hb SS disease and sickle cell–β°-thalassemia: nearly all of the Hb consists of Hb S. Although differences in the fetal Hb (Hb F) (see Variant Sickle Cell Syndromes) and Hb A_2 levels may be useful in distinguishing these syndromes, the presence of microcytosis or of one parent without sickle cell trait is a more useful indicator of sickle cell–β°-thalassemia. The diagnosis of Hb SC disease is straightforward; nearly equal amounts of Hb S and Hb C are detected. Sickle cell–β^+-thalassemia and sickle cell trait both have substantial amounts of Hb A and Hb S. This superficial electrophoretic similarity does not provide an obstacle to diagnosis: whereas sickle cell trait is associated with neither anemia nor microcytosis and has an Hb A fraction more than 50%,[7] sickle cell–β^+-thalassemia is associated with anemia, microcytosis, and an Hb A fraction that ranges from 5% to 30%.

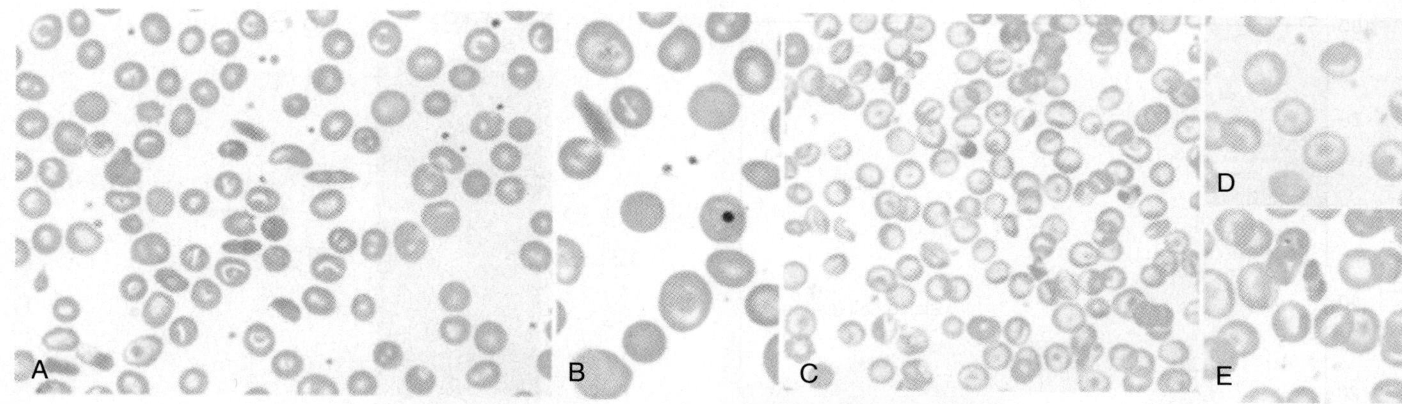

Figure 40-1 SICKLE CELL DISEASE AND HEMOGLOBIN SC PERIPHERAL BLOOD SMEARS. The peripheral smear in sickle cell disease **(A)** shows sickle cells that are mostly irreversibly sickled and sometimes referred to as "cigar forms." Higher power detail **(B)** shows a sickle cell *(upper left)*, red blood cell containing a Howell-Jolly body *(middle right)*, and polychromatophilic cell *(lower center)*. These indicate sickle cell anemia and splenic dysfunction but marrow response with reticulocytosis, respectively. A peripheral smear of a patient with Hgb SC **(C)** shows no sickled cell, but there are target forms **(D)** and occasional cells **(E)** with hemoglobin condensed at each pole of the cell.

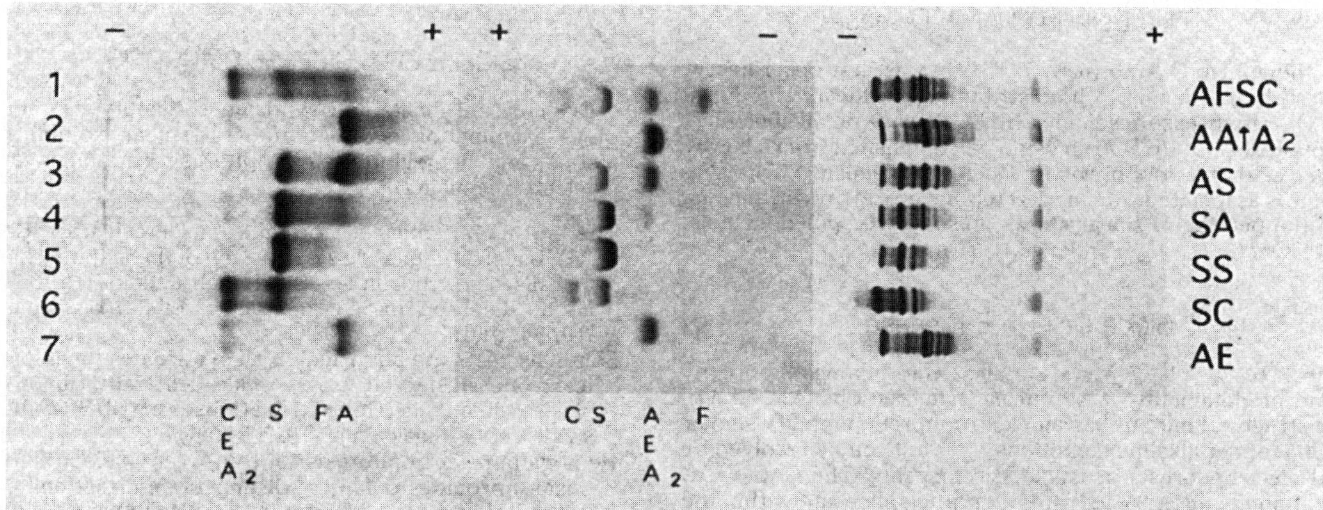

Figure 40-2 COMPARATIVE ANALYSES OF SEVERAL MUTANT HEMOGLOBINS USING ALKALINE ELECTROPHORESIS, ACID ELECTROPHORESIS, AND THIN-LAYER ISOELECTRIC FOCUSING. On the *right* are shown the components of the standard *(top)* and the phenotypes of the other six samples. Their analyses are shown by alkaline hemoglobin electrophoresis in the *left panel*, acid electrophoresis in the *center panel*, and thin-layer isoelectric focusing in the *right panel*. Locations of the various hemoglobin bands are shown *below the left and center panels*. *(Courtesy M.H. Steinberg.)*

The Hb F level is usually slightly to moderately elevated; the degree varies among patients. The amount of Hb F present is a function of the number of reticulocytes that contain Hb F, the extent of selective survival of Hb F–containing reticulocytes that become mature Hb F–containing erythrocytes (F cells), and the amount of Hb F per F cell.[8] The Arab–Indian and Senegal haplotypes are associated with higher levels of Hb F than the others.[9]

Newborn Screening

The use of prophylactic penicillin[10] and the provision of comprehensive medical care during the first 5 years of life have reduced the mortality rate from approximately 25% to less than 3%, thereby underlining the importance of early identification of infants with SCD. Based on its economy and superiority of detection, universal screening of all newborns is preferred over ethnically targeted approaches.[11,12] Blood samples for testing are obtained by heel stick and spotted onto filter paper for stable transport and subsequent HPLC. (Solubility testing is unreliable because of the large amount of Hb F present.)

As Hb S increases and Hb F declines in the first months of life (Fig. 40-3), the clinical manifestations of SCD, including anemia, emerge.[13] ISCs can be seen on the peripheral blood smear (Fig. 40-4) of children with sickle cell anemia at 3 months of age, and by 4 months of age, moderately severe hemolytic anemia is evident.

A requirement for tests used in newborn screening is the capability to distinguish among Hb F, S, A, and C. The Hb distribution pattern is described in descending order according to the quantities detected. Therefore, a newborn with sickle cell anemia who has predominantly Hb F with a small amount of Hb S and no Hb A is described as having an FS pattern. An FS pattern is obtained also in newborns who have sickle cell–β°-thalassemia, sickle cell–hereditary persistence of Hb F (HPFH), and sickle cell–Hb D or sickle cell–Hb G (i.e., Hb D and E have the same electrophoretic mobility as Hb S). A newborn with sickle cell trait will have Hb F, Hb A, and Hb S (FAS pattern).

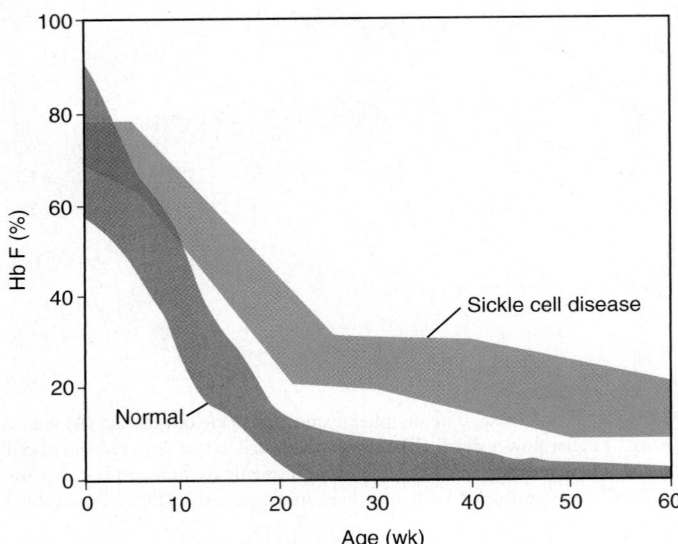

Figure 40-3 FETAL HEMOGLOBIN (HB F) DECLINE IN CHILDREN WITH HEMOGLOBINS AA AND SS. *(Data from O'Brien, Mclatosh S, Aspnes AT, et al: Prospective study of sickle cell anemia in infancy.* J Pediatr *89:205, 1976.)*

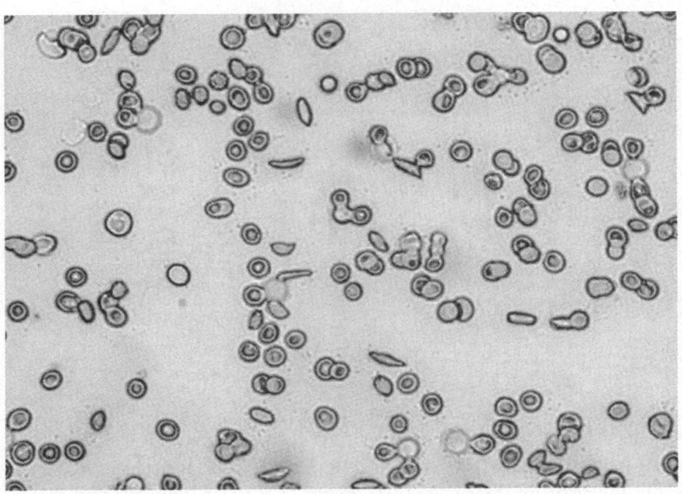

Figure 40-4 The peculiar elongated shapes of the erythrocytes is what Herrick's intern Ernest E. Irons noted, and together with a report from the German literature of *sichel formen* blood cells, inspired the name by which this condition is now known.

The quantity of Hb A is greater than that of Hb S. If the quantity of Hb S exceeds that of Hb A, the presumptive diagnosis is sickle cell–β^+-thalassemia (FSA pattern). It may not be possible to distinguish FAS and FSA patterns in newborns, so DNA-based testing or repeat Hb testing at age 3 to 6 months is recommended.

Prenatal Diagnosis

One large survey found that parents at risk for having a child with SCD were interested in prenatal diagnosis and would consider termination of pregnancy for an affected fetus.[14] Community acceptance of reproductive genetic services depends on the effectiveness of education and counseling. One major ethical issue pertains to our diagnostic skills' having outstripped our ability to predict the severity of diagnosable conditions.

Fetal DNA samples are obtained by chorionic villus sampling at 8 to 10 weeks' gestation. Polymerase chain reaction (PCR)–based

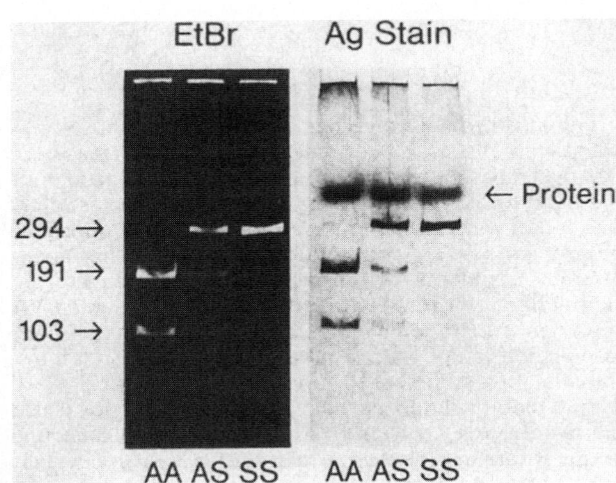

Figure 40-5 POLYMERASE CHAIN REACTION (PCR)–BASED RESTRICTION ANALYSIS FOR THE SICKLE CELL GENE. The genotypes of the DNA samples tested are shown *below*. The size in base pairs for the undigested PCR product and the products resulting from Oxa NI are shown at the *left* in base pairs. The fragments from normal β-globin DNA (AA) shows complete Oxa NI cleavage, from sickle cell trait DNA (AS) shows partial cleavage, and from sickle cell anemia (SS) shows no cleavage.

methods for detecting the sickle gene include restriction analysis (Fig. 40-5), allele-specific hybridization, reverse dot blotting, and allele-specific fluorescence PCR. PCR-based diagnosis for Hb SC disease is possible using specific molecular methods for detecting the Hb C gene, and the diagnosis of sickle cell–β-thalassemia can be made using reverse dot-blot methodology to screen the many African American β-thalassemia mutations, as well as the Hb S and Hb C mutations, in a single hybridization reaction.

CLINICAL PRESENTATION AND MANAGEMENT

The cardinal clinical manifestations of SCD are chronic hemolytic anemia; recurrent painful episodes; and chronic organ damage, particularly of the spleen, bones, brain, kidneys, lungs, skin, and heart. The pattern of disease manifestation varies among the major genotypes of Hb SS, Hb SC, and Hb S–β-thalassemia but also within the same genotype. Some of this variability results from additional inherited genotypes, for example, α-thalassemia or HPFH (discussed at the end of this chapter).

Typically, patients are anemic but lead a relatively normal life punctuated by painful episodes. However, it is important to realize that chronic organ damage and decreased survival occur even in patients who do not have recurrent pain. This section begins with a brief overview of natural history and survival followed by a discussion of basic management that has as its aim improving this natural history (disease modification) and then a discussion of management of organ-specific complications.

Natural History and Life Expectancy

The manifestations of disease begin after the first few months of life as Hb F levels decline and Hb S levels increase. Certain complications predominate in particular age groups. Between the ages of 1 and 3 years, affected individuals have splenomegaly and splenic sequestration (Fig. 40-6), pneumonia, and meningitis from *Streptococcus pneumoniae* and other encapsulated organisms (because of functional hyposplenism), and hand–foot syndrome; in early childhood, they have stroke, acute chest syndrome, and osteonecrosis; in midchildhood, they have pain crises, osteonecrosis, and acute chest syndrome; between ages 12 and 20 years, they have strokes, priapism, and pain

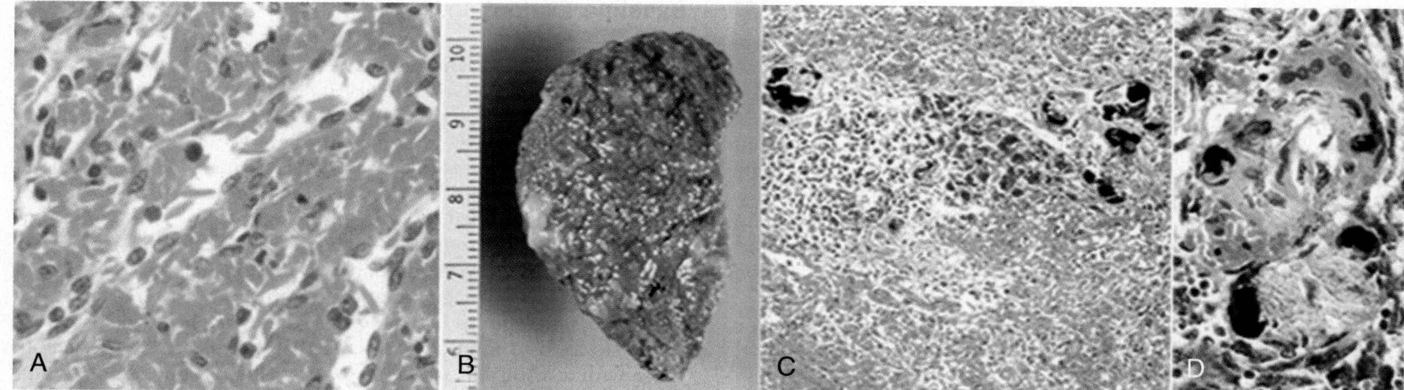

Figure 40-6 THE SPLEEN IN SICKLE CELL DISEASE. Histologic section **(A)** of the splenic red pulp shows engorgement of the splenic cords with sickled cells. In infants, excessive pooling in cords can lead to a splenic sequestration crisis. Later in life, the spleen undergoes autoinfarction. The gross pathology **(B)** shows a tiny 4.5-cm spleen with rough external surface caused by scarring from repeated infarcts. Histologic section reveals classic Gamna-Gandy bodies (**C** and **D**) also caused by repeated infarction. These are composed of hemosiderin-laden macrophages, calcium deposits, and foreign body giant cells.

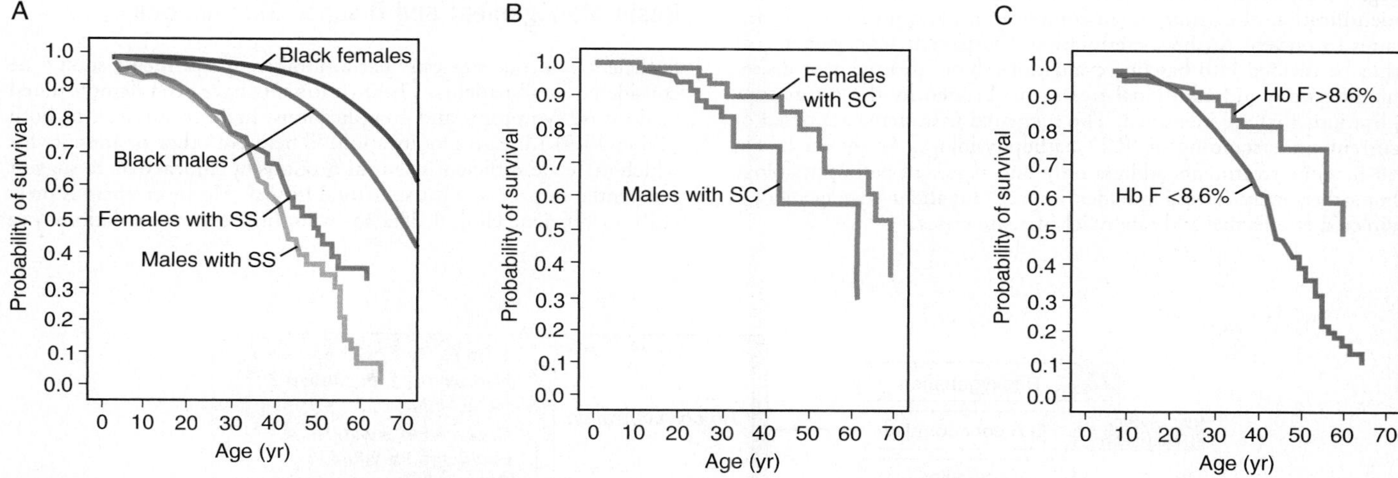

Figure 40-7 Life expectancy in patients with sickle cell disease for patients with Hb SS disease **(A)**, Hb SC disease **(B)**, and with different levels of fetal hemoglobin (Hb F) **(C)**. *(From Platt OS, Brambilla DJ, Rosse WF, et al: Mortality in sickle cell disease. Life expectancy and risk factors for early death.* N Engl J Med *330:1639, 1994.)*

crises; between ages 20 and 30 years, they have renal insufficiency, pulmonary hypertension, disabling osteonecrosis, retinopathy, leg ulcers, and pain crises; and at age older than 30 years, they have renal failure, congestive heart failure, and pain crises.

Life expectancy is decreased, although in the past 30 years, this has dramatically improved for patients in the West. In 1973, Diggs[15] reported that the mean survival was 14.3 years; in 1994, Platt et al[16] reported that life expectancy was 42 years for men and 48 years for women with sickle cell anemia (Fig. 40-7). This improvement in survival is most likely the result of improved general medical care, including prophylactic penicillin therapy and vaccination against *S. pneumoniae*.[9] These survival profiles are likely to be relevant even today, although a cohort of patients followed since 1975 show improvement in the probability of survival to age 20 years compared with patients born before 1975 (89% versus 79%).[17] The poor survival and litany of chronic organ damage in survivors emphasize the need for disease-modifying interventions to prevent vasculopathy.[17] There are indications that disease-modifying agents such as hydroxyurea (HU) can improve survival.[18,19]

Table 40-1 Effect of α-Thalassemia on the Level of Anemia in Sickle Cell Anemia

Reference	αα/αα*	–α/αα	–α/–α
Embury et al[241]	7.8[†] (*n* = 25)[‡]	9.7 (*n* = 18)	9.2 (*n* = 4)
Higgs et al[242]	7.8 (*n* = 88)	8.1 (*n* = 44)	8.8 (*n* = 44)
Steinberg et al[243]	8.0 (*n* = 73)	9.0 (*n* = 39)	9.5 (*n* = 13)
Felice et al, age 5 years[244]	8.6 (*n* = 88)	8.4 (*n* = 52)	8.3 (*n* = 50)
Felice et al, age 11 years[244]	7.9 (*n* = 40)	8.5 (*n* = 34)	9.6 (*n* = 2)

*The different α-globin genotypes indicate the presence of four (αα/αα), three (–α/αα), or two (–α/–α) α-globin genes.
†The mean hemoglobin level (g/dL) for each group is shown.
‡The number of subjects in each group is denoted by n.

Predictors of Disease Severity

The ability to predict clinical course would allow more rational tailoring of therapy to individual patients (e.g., selection of patients for high-risk but effective options such as stem cell transplant). Higher Hb F levels and the coinheritance of an α-thalassemia trait have been identified as favorable disease modifiers in multiple studies (Table 40-1).[20-22] The level of chronic anemia (which is influenced by the presence of an α-thalassemia trait and by Hb F levels) is of considerable predictive value. Patients with more severe anemia are more likely to develop infarctive and hemorrhagic stroke,[23] to have glomerular dysfunction,[24,25] and perhaps to give birth to low-birthweight babies.[26,27] Conversely, they have fewer episodes of acute chest syndrome[28] and (after age 20 years) a lower mortality rate.[28] Progressive anemia from renal endocrine deficiency or a decrease in bone marrow function from vasoocclusion is associated with early death.[18,19]

A number of other genetic polymorphisms may be relevant to disease severity, for example, with regards to the risk of stroke. However, most of these markers are not widely used to guide decision making.[21]

Principles of Management

The twin pillars of therapy are disease modification (prevention of crises, complications, chronic organ damage, and early mortality) and compassionate, prompt, effective, and safe relief of acute crises, including pain episodes. Therefore, outpatient clinic management is mostly directed at initiating measures to prevent pain crises, prevent organ complications, and improve survival. This effort should include identification of existing organ complications and initiation of measures to prevent further deterioration. Outpatient management can thus be divided into baseline evaluations, basic treatment or disease modification, and additional treatment dictated by the organ complications that are identified. The suggested treatments are based on current understanding of SCD pathophysiology. As shown in Fig. 40-8, some treatments address only one aspect of pathophysiology, but others may have a broader impact. Inpatient management is directed at effective and safe relief of acute crises.

Baseline Evaluations

Baseline blood, urine, and other evaluations are directed at quantifying the chronic hemolytic anemia and organ-specific complications (Table 40-2). They also provide baseline parameters that can be followed to assess response to therapeutic interventions.

In pediatric patients, at least annual assessment of cerebral blood flow in the internal carotid artery and the middle or anterior cerebral artery using transcranial Doppler ultrasonography (TCD) is recommended. This evaluation is a validated predictor of stroke risk. Primary prevention with chronic transfusion is effective in such patients.[29] In adults, magnetic resonance imaging (MRI) or magnetic resonance angiography (MRA) of the brain can be used instead of TCD[30] to assess thrombotic or hemorrhagic stroke risk, especially in those with a history of stroke or seizure. The recognition of cardiopulmonary complications as a cause of early mortality in SCD warrants evaluation for this condition with either echocardiogram or brain natriuretic peptide (BNP) levels. Retinal evaluation is begun at school age and continued on an annual basis. More frequent retinal evaluations are necessary if retinopathy is noted.

Basic Management and Disease Modification

Sufficient evidence suggests that a number of treatments should be considered in all patients. These treatments have been demonstrated to decrease symptoms and complications, increase survival, or both (Table 40-3) (disease modification). There are other treatments for which there are sufficient scientific grounds or clinical data to suggest a potential impact on disease natural history. However, there is presently insufficient clinical data to make firm recommendations (see

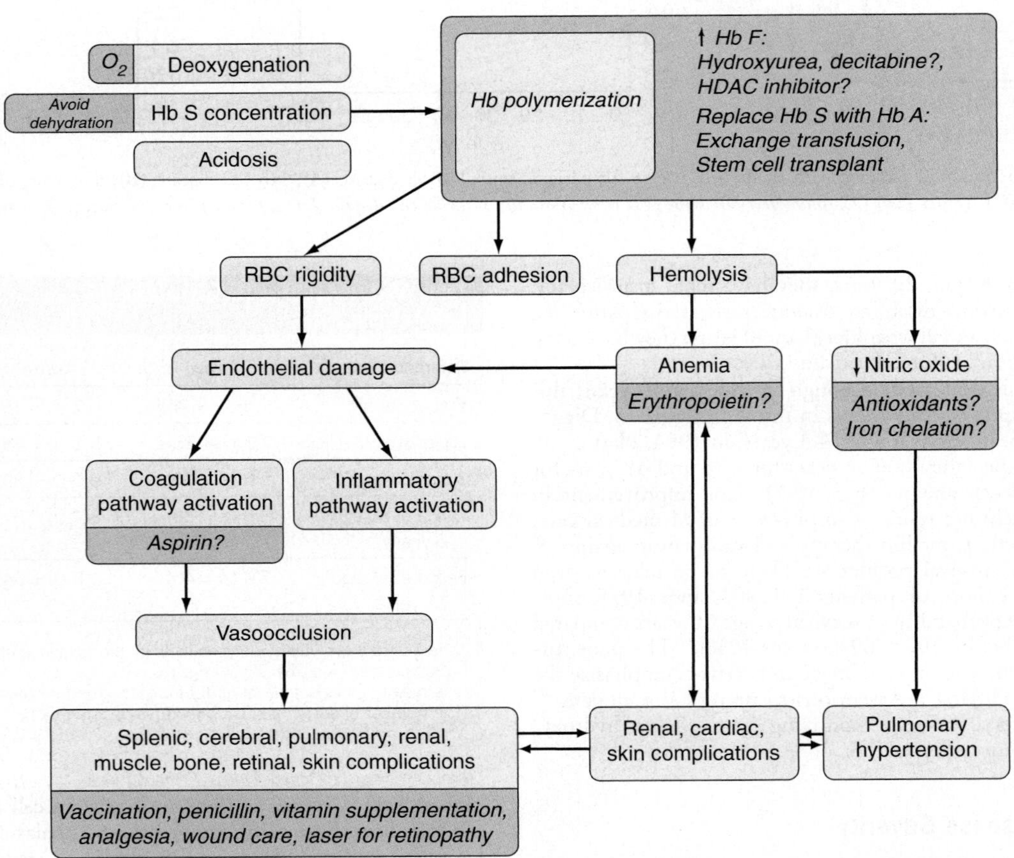

Figure 40-8 WHERE THERAPEUTICS INTERVENE IN THE PATHOPHYSIOLOGICAL CASCADE. *Hb*, Hemoglobin; *RBC*, red blood cell.

Table 40-2 Baseline Evaluations to Consider

	Tests
Blood tests	CBC with differential Reticulocyte count Hemoglobin electrophoresis LDH Renal function tests Liver function tests Mineral panel Serum iron, ferritin, TIBC Hepatitis B sAg Hepatitis C antibody RBC alloantibody screen RBC typing D-dimer* C-reactive protein* Brain natriuretic peptide
Urine and kidney tests	Urinalysis Renal ultrasonography†
Radiology	MRI or MRA brain (adults)‡ or transcranial Doppler ultrasonography starting at age 2 years (children) Chest radiography§ Hip or shoulder radiograph or MRI (or both)‡ Bone density in teenagers and adults
Cardiology and pulmonary	Echocardiogram
Neurocognitive	Neurocognitive testing§

LDH, lactate dehydrogenase; *MRA*, magnetic resonance angiography; *MRI*, magnetic resonance imaging; *RBC*, red blood cell; *sAg*, surface antigen; *TIBC*, total iron-binding capacity.
*Consider following as surrogate markers after initiation of disease-modifying intervention.
†If hematuria with red blood cells in urine.
‡As clinically indicated.
§If the patient has poor school performance, an abnormal memory, or abnormal MRI findings.

Table 40-3 Disease-Modifying Treatments to Consider*

Robust clinical data	Penicillin prophylaxis *Streptococcus pneumoniae* vaccination Hydroxyurea Chronic exchange transfusion Iron chelation for chronic iron overload†
Limited clinical data	Folate supplementation‡ *Haemophilus influenzae* vaccination Influenza vaccination Erythropoietin Phlebotomy
Experimental	Hb F reactivation with decitabine, histone deacetylase inhibitors, or imids Erythropoietin for chronic relative reticulocytopenia Nutritional supplements and antioxidants (e.g., glutamine, zinc, multivitamins) N-acetylcysteine

Hb F, Fetal hemoglobin.
*See text for specific indications and limitations.
†Best data from thalassemia patient experience.
‡Risks minimal (however, can mask vitamin B_{12} deficiency). Therefore, it is generally done.

Fig. 40-8 and Table 40-3). Although treatments such as vaccination and penicillin prophylaxis do not directly affect the sickling process or vasculopathy, they have had an impact on survival and therefore are included under the umbrella of disease-modifying therapies.

Therapeutic options are further discussed in the sections describing organ-specific complications.

Vaccination and Penicillin Prophylaxis

Children should be immunized against *S. pneumoniae, Haemophilus influenzae,* hepatitis B, and influenza.[31] Vaccination and penicillin prophylaxis can reduce the risk of serious pneumococcal infections.[9,32] Vaccination schedules recommend inoculation with heptavalent pneumococcal conjugated vaccine (PCV_7) at 2 months followed by two more doses 6 to 8 weeks apart (primary series) and a booster at 12 months. This is followed by Pneumovax at age 2 and 5 years. In adults, the Pneumovax should be readministered every 5 years (http://www.cdc.gov/vaccines/pubs/vis/default.htm).

For children younger than age 5 years, prophylactic penicillin recommendations are 125 mg penicillin V orally twice daily until age 2 to 3 years and 250 mg thereafter.[31] Penicillin prophylaxis begins at 2 months. Randomized, double-blind, placebo-controlled studies of prophylactic penicillin beginning in infancy, including the prophylactic penicillin or placebo study (PROPS), have found that this therapy reduced the incidence of *S. pneumoniae* bacteremia by 84% in children younger than 3 years.[9,32] A randomized, double-blind, placebo-controlled study, the PROPS II study concluded that it is safe to stop prophylactic penicillin therapy at age 5 years in children who have not had prior severe pneumococcal infection or splenectomy and are receiving regular follow-up care.[33] However, the power of the study was restricted by the limited number of *S. pneumoniae* systemic infection events. In an analysis of a patient population receiving penicillin prophylaxis and the Pneumovax, the rate of severe *S. pneumoniae* infections was 2.4 per 100 patient-years. This was favorable compared with the historical pre-penicillin prophylaxis rate of 3.2 to 6.9 per 100 patient-years.[34] These measures reduce risk but do not remove it. The risk of recurrent *S. pneumoniae* sepsis and death in patients who have had previous sepsis is much increased; all patients having a history of pneumococcal sepsis should remain on penicillin prophylaxis indefinitely and are not candidates for outpatient management of febrile episodes.[35] Parents must be aggressively counseled to seek medical attention for all febrile events.

Hydroxyurea and Fetal Hemoglobin Reactivation

The level of Hb F in erythrocytes plays a critical role in determining patient outcomes. Individuals who have SCD and another condition called HPFH have 70% Hb S in their RBCs but are neither anemic nor symptomatic.[36] The uniform distribution of Hb F among their RBCs interferes with Hb S polymerization, increases its solubility, and prevents RBC sickling.[37,38] Even at lower levels of Hb F seen in patients without HPFH, crisis rate and mortality are inversely proportional to Hb F level.[19-22] These findings prompted the idea that pharmacologic reactivation of Hb F production might be of benefit to patients.

Hydroxyurea is an inhibitor of ribonucleotide reductase and a cytotoxic agent that can elevate Hb F levels via an unknown pathway. A double-blind, placebo-controlled, intention-to-treat multicenter study of HU as treatment of pain crisis in SCD found that HU produced definite hematologic changes. HU was started at 0.15 mg/kg/day and escalated to 0.30 mg/kg/day as tolerated and to maintain an absolute neutrophil count no lower than $2000 \times 10^9 L^{-1}$. There were significant increases in the levels of Hb, Hb F, F cells, F reticulocytes, packed cell volume (PCV), and MCV and declines in the mean level of leukocytes, polymorphonuclear leukocytes, reticulocytes, and dense sickle cells (Table 40-4).[39] The significant clinical changes were decreased rate of acute painful episodes, longer interval to first and second acute painful episode, fewer episodes of acute chest

Table 40-4 Hematologic Effects of Hydroxyurea Therapy

Variable	Hydroxyurea	Placebo	P
Leukocytes (103 cells/μL)	9.9	12.2	.0001
PMNs (103 cells/μL)	4.9	6.4	.0001
Reticulocytes (103 cells/μL)	231	300	.0001
Hemoglobin (g/dL)	9.1	8.5	.0009
PCV (%)	27.0	25.1	.0007
MCV (fl)	103	93	.0001
Hb F (%)	8.6	4.7	.0001
F cells (%)	48	35	.0001
(10^3 cells/μL)	17	15	.0036
Dense sickle cells (%)	11	13	.004

Adapted from Charache S, Terrin ML, Moore RD, et al: Effect of hydroxyurea on the frequency of painful crises in sickle cell anemia. Investigators of the Multicenter Study of Hydroxyurea in Sickle Cell Anemia. *N Engl J Med* 332:1317, 1995, with permission.

Shown are mean values after 2 years of study. Baseline values, which were not significantly different, are not shown.

Hb F, Fetal hemoglobin; *MCV,* mean corpuscular volume; *PCV,* packed cell volume; *PMN,* polymorphonuclear leukocyte.

Table 40-5 Clinical Effects of Hydroxyurea Therapy

Variable	Hydroxyurea	Placebo	P
Acute pain crisis rate	2.5/yr	4.5/yr	<.001
Hospitalization rate for acute pain crisis	1.0/yr	2.4/yr	<.001
Interval to first pain crisis	3.0 mo	1.5 mo	<.001
Interval to second pain crisis	8.8 mo	4.6 mo	<.001
Acute chest syndrome	25	51	<.001
Subjects transfused	48	73	.001
Blood units transfused	336	586	.004

Adapted from data in Charache S, Barton FB, Moore RD, et al: Hydroxyurea and sickle cell anemia. Clinical utility of a myelosuppressive "switching" agent. The Multicenter Study of Hydroxyurea in Sickle Cell Anemia. *Medicine (Baltimore)* 75:300, 1996.

syndrome, and diminished number of subjects and units transfused (Table 40-5).[40] In follow-up analysis, higher pre- or posttreatment Hb F levels were associated with a reduction in mortality rate (although no significant changes were observed in the incidence of stroke, hepatic sequestration, or death in the initial study).[18] No short-term toxicity caused by HU was observed. One child born to a patient taking HU and two born to partners of patients taking HU were normal at birth. Although the follow-up analyses suggest the importance of Hb F to better outcomes, it is possible that some HU-induced changes in sickle cell erythrocytes, such as increased water content and decreased Hb S concentration,[41] may be independent of Hb F.

In the original study, only patients with two or more pain crises per year requiring hospitalization were eligible. However, other at-risk patients should be considered for HU therapy. These include patients with evidence of chronic organ damage, patients with severe anemia (unless the reticulocyte count is <250,000 μL^{-1}, in which case consider erythropoietin [EPO] deficiency from renal damage or bone marrow suppression that may require alternative treatment), and patients with indications for chronic transfusion but who have alloantibodies. After obtaining the baseline evaluations per Table 40-2, HU is usually started at 500 to 1000 mg/day with monitoring of the CBC every 4 to 8 weeks to ensure that neutropenia (absolute neutrophil count <2×10^9 L^{-1}) is not produced. Lower doses may be required in patients with renal insufficiency and/or relative reticulocytopenia. The dose is increased to a stable maximum HbF response or neutropenia, but most patients receive between 1000 and 2000 mg/day. Response is defined by clinical symptoms, by a persistent and significant (>0.5 g/dL) increase in total Hb or Hb F, and a decrease in LDH. These improvements in symptomatology and hematologic indices may require at least 3 to 4 months of therapy but can be seen as soon as week 6.

In studies of HU as a therapy for children with SCD, the drug was well tolerated and produced favorable hematologic changes similar to those seen in the adult population.[42] In approximately 10% of the children treated, the increase in Hb F was less than 2%. Baseline Hb F levels, baseline total Hb levels, and compliance were associated with the final Hb F level.[43] Other studies in children have documented a decrease in the number of days of hospitalization and suggest a decreased incidence of vasoocclusive crises.[44] The favorable changes in hematologic indices suggest that HU therapy might be an alternative to blood transfusions for the prevention of recurrent stroke in children with SCD.[45,46] HU therapy appears to lower transcranial Doppler velocities in children with SCD.[47] Studies in the United States and in Belgium support the potential role of HU in the prevention of cerebrovascular accidents.[46,48,49] HU was found to improve, but not correct, the abnormal cerebral oxygen saturation associated with SCD.[50]

A persistent concern pertaining to the use of HU in SCD is its putative leukemogenic effect. This concern derives from reports on HU treatment of myeloproliferative diseases, conditions associated with an inherent propensity for leukemic conversion. Although the use of HU combined with ^{32}P or alkylating agents is associated with increased leukemic conversion in patients with myeloproliferative disease,[51] reports claiming a leukemogenic effect for HU alone in polycythemia vera either lacked control subjects[52] or were not designed to assess this issue.[53] In children with the nonmalignant underlying condition of erythrocytosis secondary to inoperable cyanotic congenital heart disease, no leukemic conversion was observed.[54]

Vitamin or Nutritional Supplementation

Chronic hemolysis results in increased utilization of folic acid stores. Megaloblastic crises from folic acid deficiency have been reported.[55,56] Pediatric patients with SCD had higher homocysteine levels than age-matched control African American patients.[57] Folic acid, 1 mg/day orally, is administered as a standard of care.[58] Vitamin B_{12} deficiency can also be seen in patients with SCD. Folate replacement can mask and possibly exacerbate vitamin B_{12} deficiency.[59]

A growing body of research indicates that sickle cell patients have widespread mineral and vitamin deficiencies, including zinc, vitamin C, vitamin E, acetylcysteine, calcium, vitamin D, vitamin A, and others.[60] Fifty percent of children with SCD have evidence of osteoporosis or osteopenia that is associated with inadequate calcium and vitamin D intake.[61-63] Recently, zinc supplementation in a prospective trial documented significant improvement in linear growth and weight gain in children with SCD.[64]

Despite increased intestinal absorption of iron in SCD, the combination of nutritional deficiency and urinary iron losses results in iron deficiency in 20% of children with SCD.[65] The diagnosis of iron deficiency may be obscured by the elevated serum iron levels associated with chronic hemolysis, necessitating the detection of a low serum ferritin level or an elevated serum transferrin level for the diagnosis.

Transfusion Therapy

The two main approaches to transfusion in SCD are simple transfusion and exchange transfusion. These transfusions can be administered in an episodic fashion or in a chronic fashion. Therefore, transfusion therapy in SCD is of the following types: episodic simple, episodic partial exchange, or chronic partial exchange. In both simple and exchange transfusion, the target Hb level is 10 to 11 g/dL (hematocrit, 30%).[66,67] Transfusing to a higher Hb or hematocrit level is avoided because a hematocrit level greater than 30% is associated with hyperviscosity if there is a substantial proportion of Hb S in the blood. In exchange transfusion, an additional objective is to achieve an Hb S percentage of less than 30% (or sometimes <50%). In partial-exchange transfusion, a proportion of the patient's diseased RBCs are removed before transfusion of normal donor RBCs; this can be done manually through phlebotomy followed by transfusion or concurrently using an automated device. In patients who need chronic transfusions, partial exchange is recommended because of the reduced iron burden of this approach. Partial exchange is also indicated if the baseline Hb level is more than 10 g/dL. Simple transfusion in this instance risks exacerbating the clinical condition through increased viscosity. For critical illness, exchange transfusion is also preferred. Although the target Hb S level should be less than 30% in exchange transfusion, decreasing Hb S levels to less than 50% may suffice depending on the severity of the complication being treated.

The volumes required for simple and exchange transfusions (Table 40-6) are particularly important for transfusing children. For normal-size adults, the general rule is that each unit of RBCs infused increases the Hb level approximately 1 g/dL.[68]

Episodic simple transfusion should be considered for blood volume replacement in aplastic crisis and splenic sequestration crises and for protection when there is a more than 20% decrease in Hb from baseline from severe illness such as septicemia or severe vasoocclusive crisis or hyperhemolysis or Hb levels of less than 5 g/dL. Episodic simple or exchange transfusion should be considered for acute chest syndrome, priapism, and preoperatively. The choice of simple versus exchange transfusion is determined by the pretransfusion total Hb level and the severity of the illness.

In the preoperative setting, simple transfusion to increase the total Hb level to 10 g/dL was effective in preventing perioperative complications and was associated with fewer transfusion-associated complications than an aggressive exchange transfusion regimen to decrease Hb S levels to less than 30%.[69] The efficacy of preoperative partial-exchange transfusion in patients with Hb SC disease undergoing abdominal surgery suggests that this type of transfusion be performed preoperatively in this group of patients.

Chronic partial-exchange transfusion is indicated in primary and secondary prevention of cerebral thrombosis as discussed in the section on neurologic complications.

Transfusion complications include alloimmunization, delayed hemolytic transfusion reactions (discussed in Exacerbations of Anemia), iron overload, and transmission of viral illness. The incidence of alloimmunization is between 19% and 30% and usually occurs with fewer than 15 transfusions.[70] Some patients seem to tolerate multiple transfusions without developing alloantibodies, but others are readily allosensitized. The high rate of alloimmunization in transfused sickle cell patients is partly attributable to minor blood group incompatibilities between the recipient and donor pool, which often differ in ethnicity.[70,71] Antibodies against the C and E antigens of the Rh group, Kell (K) and Lewis, Duffy (Fya, Fyb), and Kidd (Jk) are common.[70] In the Stroke Prevention Trial in Sickle Cell Anemia, the routine use of WBC-reduced RBCs matched for E, C, and Kell decreased the allosensitization rate compared with historical data from 3% to 0.5% per unit transfused and decreased the rate of hemolytic transfusion reactions by 90%.[72] Therefore, the recommended approach to preventing alloimmunization is to reduce leukocytes and perform limited phenotype matching for all patients (ABO, C, D, E, and Kell) and extended phenotype matching for patients with alloantibodies.[67] The management of a delayed hemolytic transfusion reaction and transfusional iron overload are discussed under Exacerbations of Anemia later.

Transmission of HIV, hepatitis B and C, and human T-cell leukemia/lymphoma virus-1 has diminished with improved screening of banked units but remains an issue. In addition to better screening programs, the use of leukocyte-depleted RBC transfusions can reduce this hazard.[73]

Table 40-6 Transfusion Formulas

Dilutional effects of transfusion on Hb S: PRBC volume (PRBCV) (mL) = $(Hct_d - Hct_i) \times TBV \times Hct_{rp}B$

Manual partial-exchange transfusion:* Hb Sf = $1 - (PRBCV \times Hct_{rp})(TBV \times Hct_i) + (PRBCV \times Hct_{rp}) \times Hb\ S_iC$

Automated exchange transfusion: Exchange volume (mL) = $(Hct_d - Hct_i) \times TBVHct_{rp} - (Hct_i + Hct_d)2D$

RBC volume (mL) = $Hct_i \times TBV$

From Nieburg and Stockman, with permission. Copyright 1977, American Medical Association.

[†]From Linderkamp et al, with permission. Copyright 1977, Springer-Verlag.

Hct_d, desired hematocrit; *Hct_i*, initial hematocrit; *Hct_{rp}*, hematocrit of replacement cells (usually 0.75); *Hb S_i*, initial Hb S; *Hb S_f*, final Hb S; *PRBC*, packed red blood cells; *TBV*, estimated total blood volume in milliliters (children, 80 mL/kg; adults, 65 mL/kg; nomograms are available).[†]

*In these formulas, Hct and Hb S are fractions (e.g., 40% = 0.4).

Stem Cell Transplantation

At this time, allogeneic stem cell transplantation remains the only curative option for SCD. The largest series to date has been in a pediatric population with severely symptomatic SCD failing to respond to HU. Using myeloablative conditioning and human leukocyte antigen (HLA)–matched or one-mismatch (two cases) sibling donors, with bone marrow as the source of stem cells in the majority, there was a 10% mortality rate with 90% overall survival and 82% event-free survival at a median follow-up of 54 months.[74] Similar results were obtained when related, HLA-matched umbilical cord blood was used as the source of stem cells.[75] According to these results, stem cell transplant is a therapeutic option for the severely symptomatic child with an HLA-matched sibling donor. In adults, incorporation of rapamycin (to induce immunologic tolerance) into nonmyeloablative stem cell transplant protocols has enabled stable mixed hematopoietic chimerism with associated full-donor erythroid engraftment and normalization of blood counts. The attainment of tolerance may allow extension of these potentially curative approach to alternative donor sources, an active area of research.[76,77] The issue of the cost-effectiveness of bone marrow transplantation (BMT) gains perspective from the comparative costs in the United States of $150,000 to $200,000 for an uncomplicated BMT versus up to $112,000 annually for conventional medical care of a chronically transfused, iron-overloaded patient.[78]

Education

Education regarding the nature of the disease, genetic counseling, and psychosocial assessments of patients and their families are best accomplished during routine visits. Parents of small children are instructed regarding early detection of infection and palpating enlarging spleens.

Phlebotomy

As mentioned, an Hb level of more than 10 to 11 g/dL (hematocrit 30%) in the presence of substantial amounts of Hb S (>30%) is associated with hyperviscosity. Some data indicate that phlebotomy to reduce the hematocrit and viscosity (and which may also address iron-overload) can decrease the frequency of crises in Hb SC or Hb S–β^+ disease.[79] In Hb SS disease, phlebotomy has successfully been used in combination with HU (which increases the Hb level) in secondary stroke prevention in patients previously treated with chronic transfusion.[80] Phlebotomy alone has also been used in Hb SS disease with baseline Hb levels of more than 9.5 g/dL with favorable results on the frequency and duration of pain crises. This benefit may have resulted from decreased hematocrit and viscosity and from a decrease in intracellular Hb concentration from iron deficiency.[81] One approach to phlebotomy is to remove approximately 10 mL/kg of blood over 20 to 30 minutes followed by infusion of an equal volume of normal saline. This is repeated every 2 weeks until the target Hb level of 9 to 9.5 g/dL is achieved.

Erythropoietin or Darbepoetin

The chronic hemolytic anemia of SCD is partially compensated by vigorous reticulocytosis. A decrease in compensatory reticulocytosis will exacerbate already existent anemia and can be expected to increase clinical risk. Accordingly, chronic relative reticulocytopenia (defined as Hb <9 g/dL and absolute reticulocyte count <250,000 × 10^9 L^-) was identified as a significant risk factor for early mortality in a prospective cohort study of SCD patients.[82]

In the general population, evaluation of EPO levels is usually prompted by the combination of anemia and abnormal serum creatinine level. EPO levels are then interpreted in relationship to the Hb level to assess for the possibility of EPO deficiency. In patients with SCD, this approach to diagnosis has pitfalls. Patients with SCD are already anemic; therefore, gradual anemia exacerbation is easily missed, and clinicians must weigh many possible causes in the context of complex, multisystem SCD pathology. Furthermore, patients with SCD have low serum creatinine levels at baseline. Therefore, a substantial increase in serum creatinine from baseline may nonetheless remain below the threshold defined as abnormal for the general population, potentially disguising the presence of renal damage that is sufficient to decrease renal endocrine function. Furthermore, EPO levels are not readily interpreted in the individual SCD patient: EPO levels in SCD are generally low for the level of hemoglobin.[83] One contributing factor could be increased uptake by the massive compensatory reticulocytosis. However, EPO levels are lower in SCD adults than in children,[83] and EPO levels are inappropriately lower in patients with chronic relative reticulocytopenia.[19] Hence, EPO deficiency should be considered as a possible cause of progressive anemia in patients with absolute reticulocyte counts below 250,000 × 10^9 L^- even if their serum creatinine levels are in the normal range. The cumulative published experience of EPO use in SCD is limited (52 patients).[84] Although EPO by itself has been reported to increase Hb F levels, the most important role for EPO may be as replacement therapy for EPO deficiency that causes relative reticulocytopenia and progressive anemia. EPO replacement can also facilitate enhanced HU dosing and Hb F augmentation.[84] In using recombinant human EPO, caution must be exercised not to elevate the hematocrit to levels that result in hyperviscosity. Also, the reticulocyte fraction is the most adhesive, and it is possible that EPO could exacerbate or trigger sickle cell crises.[84] Patients with SCD may be relatively resistant to EPO and require doses higher than those used in other patients with chronic renal failure. The reasons for EPO resistance are unclear but may include increased inflammation-mediated suppression of erythropoiesis.[85]

Erythropoietin therapy is probably not indicated in patients receiving chronic transfusion therapy in whom encouraging endogenous Hb S containing erythropoiesis may be counterproductive.

Iron Chelation

Early death is well described in association with iron overload from β-thalassemia and hereditary hemochromatosis.[86,87] Similarly, iron overload is likely to be a problem in chronically transfused SCD patients, although the clinical significance may critically depend on the degree and duration of overload. Chelation guidelines for patients with SCD are similar to those for other chronically transfused, iron-overloaded patients; iron chelation is indicated when the total body iron level is elevated (ferritin >2000 mcg/L, quantitative liver iron of 2000 mcg/g dry weight, transfusion history >1 year of monthly transfusions).[88] Notably, the serum ferritin level may underestimate clinically significant iron overload.[89,90] Iron chelation options in the United States are deferoxamine (via continuous intravenous or subcutaneous infusion) or deferasirox (orally), both of which appear to have similar efficacy, although the oral route of administration and toxicity profile may favor deferasirox.[91,92]

Newer U.S. Food and Drug Administration (FDA)–approved methods of quantitating iron burden by Ferriscan of the liver[93] can avoid the need for liver biopsies. T2-weighted MRI of the heart indicates hemosiderosis of cardiac tissue, and when the results are abnormal, aggressive chelation is mandated.[94]

Alternatives to Hydroxyurea for Hb F Induction

Alternatives to HU for pharmacologic induction of Hb F that are being studied in clinical trials include the methyltransferase inhibitor 5-aza-2′-deoxycytidine (decitabine) and histone deacetylase inhibiters.[95] These classes of agents act on chromatin processes that regulate gene transcription.

The methyltransferase inhibitors 5-azacytidine and 5-aza-2′-deoxycytidine have produced the largest increases in Hb F of any of the pharmacologic reactivators of Hb F that have been tested.[96,97] Responding patients include those who did not respond to HU, consistent with a different mechanism of action. Although improvements in a number of surrogate clinical endpoints have been demonstrated, larger studies to confirm safety and clinical effectiveness with chronic use are required. In the United States, 5-azacytidine and decitabine have been approved by the FDA for the treatment of myelodysplastic syndrome.

The efficacy of the class of agents known as histone deacetylase inhibitors in Hb F reactivation has been reviewed.[97-99] However, the absence of large clinical trial data, practical issues with administration and stability of some agents, and the lack of FDA approval for many drugs in this class are limitations.

Preclinical studies suggest that the "imid" class of drugs (analogues of thalidomide such as pomalidomide) could have a potential role in Hb F reactivation.[100]

Preventing Red Blood Cell Dehydration With Ion Channel Inhibitors

Polymerization of Hb S is related to the Hb S concentration within the cell. Therefore, a therapeutic strategy could be to reduce the intracellular Hb S concentration by improving cellular hydration. Potential therapeutic options to maintain RBC hydration for which there are preliminary clinical data include cetiedil citrate, imidazole inhibitors of the Gardos pathway,[101] novel Gardos channel inhibitors,[102] or magnesium supplements, which inhibit potassium chloride cotransport.[103]

It also is possible to reduce the Hb concentration by reducing the Hb content with iron deficiency. It has been observed that spontaneous or induced iron deficiency (see Phlebotomy above) sufficient to reduce the serum ferritin, MCV, and mean cell Hb concentration (MCHC) resulted in variably improved Hb S polymerization, RBC survival, level of anemia, and clinical status.[104]

Anticoagulation or Antiplatelet Therapy

Although there is clear evidence of activation of the coagulation system in SCD, the role of thrombogenesis in vasoocclusive crisis remains unclear.[105] Similarly, there have been no thorough evaluations of the role of antiplatelet or antithrombotic agents for the treatment of SCD. D-dimer levels (a degradation product of cross-linked fibrin) increase during acute vasoocclusive crisis.[106]

Minidose heparin, 5000 to 7500 units every 12 hours, administered to four patients for 2 to 6 years reduced hospitalization and emergency department time by 75%, and pretreatment pain frequency recurred after heparin was discontinued.[107] Larger clinical studies will be required to better understand the risks and benefits of heparin therapy for acute vasoocclusive crisis in SCD. Heparin has not been studied for acute arterial stroke in patients with SCD but has a role in SCD-associated dural venous sinus thrombosis.[108] The management of stroke is fully discussed under Specific Complications and Their Management.

Acenocoumarol was administered in low doses that achieved a mean international normalized ratio (INR) of 1.64 and reduced the elevated levels of prothrombin activation fragment (fragment 1+2) to 50% of pretreatment levels.[109] Clinical endpoints were not measured. In a crossover study, 29 patients were treated with acenocoumarol to target an INR of 1.6 to 2.0. No effect on crisis frequency was noted, although again, there were significant reductions in markers of coagulation system activation.[110] In 37 acutely ill sickle cell patients with elevated D-dimers, the effect of low-dose warfarin therapy (1 mg without a target INR) in 12 of them was examined. In multivariate analysis, low-dose warfarin was the only variable associated with a significant decrease in D-dimer levels, suggesting a warfarin-induced decrease in thrombin activity.[106] Therefore, oral anticoagulation, even at low doses, is associated with a decrease in laboratory markers of coagulation pathway activation in SCD; however, further clinical trials are required to understand the clinical risks and benefits.

Aspirin was compared with placebo in 49 pediatric SCD patients in a double-blind crossover study. The frequency and severity of crises were not affected by aspirin therapy.[111] Cerebral thrombosis, which accounts for 70% to 80% of all cerebrovascular accidents (CVAs) in SCD, results from large-vessel occlusion (Fig. 40-9) rather than the more typical microvascular occlusion of SCD. In the United States, there is an ongoing clinical trial testing the safety and efficacy of aspirin in diminishing the incidence and progression of cognitive defects and overt or silent stroke in pediatric patients.

The management of stroke risk and stroke is fully discussed under Specific Complications and Their Management.

Experimental Therapies

A number of therapies are in the early stages of clinical evaluation and could have a role in disease modification of SCD. These include agents that directly address sickle erythrocyte adhesion to endothelium (recombinant P-selectin glycoprotein ligand-1 [PSGL]–immunoglobulin G conjugate), agents that increase the production of nitric oxide (NO) (glutamine), and herbal extracts with unknown mechanisms of action (Niprisan).[112]

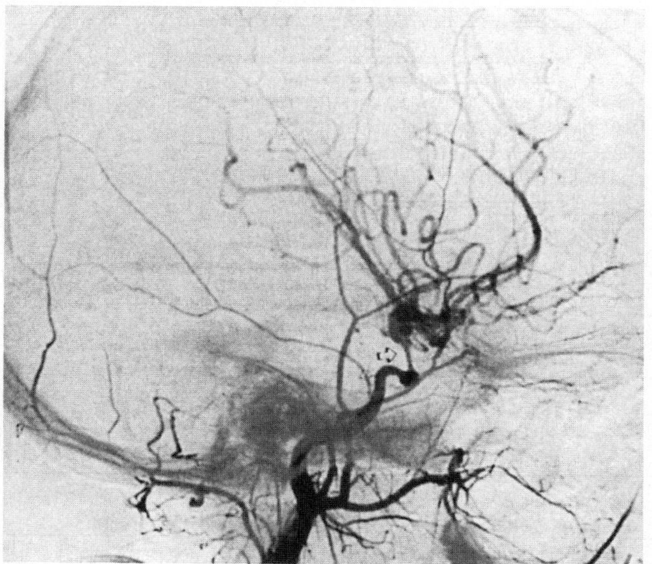

Figure 40-9 Right common carotid arteriogram taken in anteroposterior projection demonstrating complete occlusion of the origin of the right anterior cerebral artery *(arrowhead). (From Stockman JA, Nigro MA, Mishkin MM, Oski FA: Occlusion of large cerebral vessels in sickle-cell anemia.* N Engl J Med *287:846, 1972.)*

Specific Complications and Their Management

Pain Crisis

Acute Pain Episode or Crisis

Acute pain is the first symptom of disease in more than 25% of patients and is the most frequent symptom after age 2 years.[113] Pain is the complication for which patients with SCD most commonly seek medical attention.[114] An episode of acute pain was originally called a "sickle cell crisis" by Diggs, who used the expression "crisis" to refer to any new rapidly developing syndrome in the life of a patient with SCD.[115] The basic mechanism is believed to be vasoocclusion of the bone marrow vasculature causing bone infarction, which in turn causes release of inflammatory mediators that activate afferent nociceptors.[116]

Although a general correlation of vasoocclusive severity and genotype has been posited,[117] there is tremendous variability within genotypes and in the same patient over time. In one large study of patients with Hb SS disease, one-third rarely had pain, one-third were hospitalized for pain approximately two to six times per year, and one-third had more than six pain-related hospitalizations per year.[118] Over a 5-year period in the National Cooperative Study of SCD, 40% of patients had no painful episodes, and 5% of patients accounted for one-third of the emergency department visits. Pain is more frequent with the Hb SS genotype, low levels of Hb F, higher Hb levels,[28] and sleep apnea.[119] The frequency of pain peaks between ages 19 and 39 years. After the age of 19 years, more frequent pain correlates with a higher mortality rate.[28] Medical personnel who see patients only in the emergency department gain a biased view of SCD skewed by a frequently affected minority with severe disease.[120,121]

Pain may be precipitated by events such as cold, dehydration, infection, stress, menses, and alcohol consumption. Any underlying cause should be searched for and corrected, but the majority of painful episodes have no identifiable cause. Pain can affect any area of the body, most commonly the back, chest, extremities, and abdomen; may vary from trivial to excruciating; and is usually endured at home without a visit to the emergency department. There may be premonitory symptoms.[121] The duration averages a few days, with hospital admissions typically lasting between 4 and 10 days. Painful episodes are biopsychosocial events caused by vasoocclusion in an area of the body having nociceptors and nerves.[116] Pain is an effect and, as such, consists of sensory, perceptual, cognitive, and emotional components. Frequent pain generates feelings of despair, depression, and apathy that interfere with everyday life and promote an existence that revolves around pain. This scenario may lead to a chronic debilitating pain syndrome; fortunately, this is rare.

There is no specific clinical or laboratory finding pathognomonic of pain crisis. The diagnosis is established by history and physical examination. Changes in steady-state Hb values, sickled cells on blood smear, WBC counts, and so on are not reliable indicators. Numerous laboratory tests, leukocytosis, D-dimer fragments of fibrin, and markers of platelet activation have been found to lack specificity as indicators of acute vasoocclusion. Often patients can tell if they are having a typical pain crisis or something more sinister. It is thus good practice to ask the patient if it feels like usual pain crisis pain.

Initial medical assessment should focus on detection of triggers or medical complications requiring specific therapy, which include infection, dehydration, acute chest syndrome (fever, tachypnea, chest pain, hypoxia, and chest signs), severe anemia, cholecystitis, splenic enlargement, neurologic events, and priapism.[122] Pain management should be aggressive to make the pain tolerable and enable patients to attain maximum functional ability. To make the patient pain free is an unrealistic goal and risks oversedation and hypoventilation, which must be avoided. A pain chart should be started and analgesia titrated against the patient's reported pain together with medical assessment of the patient's overall clinical status, paying particular attention to avoiding oversedation. When clinicians consistently observe a disparity between patients' verbal self-report of their pain and their ability to function, further assessment should be performed to ascertain the reason for disparity. Patients are often undertreated for pain because many physicians and other health care providers are overly concerned with the potential for addiction. Undertreatment of pain is no more desirable than overtreatment and oversedation; undertreatment can prolong the duration of a painful episode and can poison the relationship between the patient and the health care system. In assessing patient responses to conventional doses of analgesia, it must be remembered that individuals with SCD metabolize narcotics rapidly.[123]

The pain pathway should be targeted at different points with different agents, avoiding toxicity with any one class (Table 40-7). The mainstays are nonsteroidal antiinflammatory drugs (NSAIDs), acetaminophen, and opioids. NSAIDs can be used to control mild to moderate pain and may have an additive role in combination with opioids for severe pain. The most potent NSAID is ketorolac. NSAIDs should be used with caution in those with a history of peptic ulcer, renal insufficiency, asthma, or bleeding tendencies. Within limits, use the agents that the patients know work for them and avoid meperidine (Demerol), which should only be used under very exceptional circumstances. Sedatives and anxiolytics alone should not be used to manage pain because they can mask the behavioral response to pain without providing analgesia.

Treatment of persistent or moderate to severe pain should be based on increasing the opioid strength or dose.[122] One approach is to administer morphine 0.1 mg/kg intravenously or subcutaneously every 20 minutes until pain is controlled. The patient should be checked at 20-minute intervals for pain; respiratory rate, depth, and quality; and sedation until the patient is stable with adequate pain control. Subsequently, the patient should receive a maintenance dose of 0.05 to 0.15 mg/kg intravenously or subcutaneously every 2 to 4 hours. A rescue dose of 50% of the maintenance dose can be considered on an as-needed basis every 30 minutes for breakthrough pain.

During maintenance with opioids, pain control; respiratory rate, depth, and quality; and oxygen saturation should be monitored approximately every 2 hours. If respiratory depression is noted, omit the maintenance dose of morphine. For severe respiratory depression or oxygen desaturation, administer naloxone. Incentive spirometry and mandatory time out of bed are helpful in patients with chest pain to decrease the risk for hypoventilation. Adjuvant medications to consider include NSAIDs, acetaminophen, antiemetics, and antihistamines. Laxatives or stool softeners should be prescribed in keeping with close monitoring for constipation.

After 2 to 3 days, consider decreasing the dose and switching from parenteral to oral administration of opioids. For adult patients whose pain requires several or many days to resolve, a sustained-release opioid preparation is appropriate and provides a more consistent analgesia.

Hydration is a critical part of management. However, cardiac function may be significantly impaired, especially in adult patients, and standard discipline must be followed with intravenous fluid management to avoid iatrogenic fluid overload. SCD patients cannot

Table 40-7 Recommended Dose and Interval of Analgesics Necessary to Obtain Adequate Pain Control in Patients With Sickle Cell Disease

	Dose/Rate	Comments
	Severe to Moderate Pain	
Morphine	Parenteral: 0.1-0.15 mg/kg every 3-4 hr Recommended maximum single dose, 10 mg PO: 0.3-0.6 mg/kg every 4 hr	Drug of choice for pain; lower doses in elderly adults and infants and in patients with liver failure or impaired ventilation
Meperidine	Parenteral: 0.75-1.5 mg/kg every 2-4 hr Recommended maximum dose, 100 mg PO: 1.5 mg/kg every 4 hr	Increased incidence of seizures; avoid in patients with renal or neurologic disease and those who receive MAOIs
Hydromorphone	Parenteral: 0.01-0.02 mg/kg every 3-4 hr PO: 0.04-0.06 mg/kg every 4 hr	
Oxycodone	PO: 0.15 mg/kg/dose every 4 hr	
Ketorolac	IM: Adults: 30 or 60 mg initial dose followed by 15-30 mg; children: 1 mg/kg load followed by 0.5 mg/kg every 6 hr	Equal efficacy to 6 mg MS; helps narcotic-sparing effect; not to exceed 5 days; maximum, 150 mg first day, 120 mg maximum on subsequent days; may cause gastric irritation
Butorphanol	Parenteral: Adults: 2 mg every 3-4 hr	Agonist–antagonist; can precipitate withdrawal if given to patients who are being treated with agonists
	Mild Pain	
Codeine	PO: 0.5-1 mg/kg every 4 hr Maximum dose, 60 mg	Mild to moderate pain not relieved by aspirin or acetaminophen; can cause nausea and vomiting
Aspirin	PO: Adults: 0.3-6 mg every 4-6 hr; children: 10 mg/kg every 4 hr	Often given with a narcotic to enhance analgesia; can cause gastric irritation; avoid in febrile children
Acetaminophen	PO: Adults: 0.3-0.6 g every 4 hr; children: 10 mg/kg	Often given with a narcotic to enhance analgesia
Ibuprofen	PO: Adults: 300-400 mg every 4 hr; children: 5-10 mg/kg every 6-8 hr	Can cause gastric irritation
Naproxen	PO: Adults: 500 mg/dose initially and then 250 every 8-12 hr; children: 10 mg/kg/day (5 mg/kg every 12 hr)	Long duration of action; can cause gastric irritation
Indomethacin	PO: Adults: 25 mg every 8 hr; children: 1-3 mg/kg/day given 3 or 4 times	Contraindicated in psychiatric, neurologic, renal diseases; high incidence of gastric irritation; useful in gout

Adapted from Charache S, Terrin ML, Moore RD, et al. Effect of hydroxyurea on the frequency of painful crises in sickle cell anemia. Investigators of the Multicenter Study of Hydroxyurea in Sickle Cell Anemia. *N Engl J Med* 332:1317, 1995.
IM, Intramuscular; *MAOI,* monoamine oxidase inhibitor; *MS,* morphine sulphate; *PO,* oral.

concentrate their urine and are at risk for dehydration when not taking adequate fluids (60 mL/kg/24 hr in adults). Intravenous hydration is indicated when the patient is not taking oral fluids adequately. Ideally, the urine specific gravity should be kept under 1.010 by daily testing when in the hospital. Hb may decrease by 1 to 2 g/dL in an uncomplicated pain crisis; blood transfusion is not routinely indicated for an uncomplicated pain crisis.

Equianalgesic doses of oral opioids should be prescribed for home use when necessary to maintain the relief achieved in the emergency department or hospital ward. Care should be taken to appropriately taper opioids in patients who have received daily opioids over many days. In these patients, there may be physical opiate dependence, which is characterized by the onset of acute withdrawal symptoms upon cessation of opioid administration. For patients at risk for physical dependence, opiates should be titrated downward by 15% to 20% per day to zero. Physical dependence is a physiological problem, but addiction is a psychological problem characterized by craving—behavior that is overwhelmingly directed at obtaining the drug; use of the drug for purposes other than pain control; and use of the drug despite negative physical, social, legal, or psychological consequences.

If the patient is not taking a disease-modifying agent such as HU, consideration should be given to initiating such therapy either as an inpatient or during follow-up in the outpatient setting.

Chronic Pain

Chronic pain in SCD usually (but not always) has an identifiable basis such as vertebral fractures, femoral head necrosis, early degenerative changes or osteoarthritis, or chronic skin ulcers. Most patients without such identifiable complications do not require chronic pain medications similar to those used for terminal cancer because the pain from a typical vasoocclusive crisis is episodic. Inappropriately maintaining patients without chronic musculoskeletal degeneration on long-acting opiates can impair their overall psychosocial functioning. On the other hand, adequate analgesia with long-acting opiates (e.g., long-acting morphine preparations similar to those used in cancer patients) is important to maintain the psychosocial functioning of patients who do have complications that cause chronic pain. Also consider agents such as amitriptyline or antiseizure medications[124] that can address neuropathic components and help decrease the sleep impairment and depression that can occur with chronic pain. If the patient is not taking a disease-modifying agent such as HU, consideration should be given to initiating such therapy.

Chronic Anemia

Chronic hemolytic anemia is one of the hallmarks of SCD. Sickle erythrocytes are destroyed randomly, with a mean life span of 17 days.[125] The overall hemolytic rate reflects the number of ISCs.[126] The degree of anemia is most severe in sickle cell anemia, and Hb S–β^{o}-thalassemia, milder in Hb S–β^{+}-thalassemia and Hb SC disease,[127] and, among patients with sickle cell anemia, less severe in those who have coexistent α-thalassemia (Tables 40-8 and 40-1).[128]

As already noted, EPO deficiency from otherwise subclinical chronic renal damage may also contribute to a decline in Hb levels below baseline. The level of chronic anemia is a significant prognostic marker.[19]

The treatment options for the chronic anemia of SCD have already been mentioned. These strategies attempt to decrease hemolysis by increasing Hb F (HU and the experimental approaches with EPO, decitabine, and histone deacetylase inhibitors) or decreasing the intracellular Hb S concentration by preventing RBC dehydration (Gardos channel inhibitors).

Exacerbations of Anemia

The rather constant level of hemolytic anemia may be exacerbated by additional events such as aplastic crises, acute splenic

Table 40-8 Bacteria and Viruses That Most Frequently Cause Serious Infection in Patients With Sickle Cell Disease

Microorganism	Type of Infection	Comments
Streptococcus pneumoniae	Septicemia Meningitis Pneumonia Septic arthritis	Common despite prophylactic penicillin and pneumococcal vaccine Less frequent than in years past Rarely documented except in infants and young children Uncommon
Haemophilus influenzae type b	Septicemia	
Meningitis		
Pneumonia	Much less common in recent years because of immunization with conjugate vaccine	
Salmonella species	Osteomyelitis	
Septicemia	Most common cause of bone and joint infection	
Escherichia coli and other gram-negative enteric pathogens	Septicemia	
Urinary tract infection		
Osteomyelitis	Focus sometimes inapparent	
Staphylococcus aureus	Osteomyelitis	Uncommon
Mycoplasma pneumoniae	Pneumonia	Pleural effusions; multilobe involvement
Chlamydia pneumoniae	Pneumonia	
Parvovirus B19	Bone marrow suppression (aplastic crisis)	High fever common; rash and other organ involvement infrequent
Hepatitis viruses (A, B, and C)	Hepatitis	Marked hyperbilirubinemia

Data from Buchanan GR, Glader BE: Benign course of extreme hyperbilirubinemia in sickle cell anemia: Analysis of six cases. *J Pediatr* 91:21, 1977.

sequestration, acute hepatic sequestration, chronic renal disease, or renal endocrine deficiency that may be present without overt renal failure, bone marrow necrosis, deficiency of folic acid or iron, delayed hemolytic transfusion reactions, autoimmune hemolytic anemia, or hyperhemolysis (hemolytic exacerbations) of unknown etiology. Laboratory evaluations that are very useful in the evaluation of a patient with anemia exacerbation are the reticulocyte count, LDH, alloantibody screening, the direct antiglobulin (Coombs) test, and EPO level.

Aplastic Crises

Aplastic crises are transient arrests of erythropoiesis characterized by abrupt falls in Hb levels, reticulocyte number, and RBC precursors in the bone marrow without necessarily an increase in the LDH. Although these episodes typically last only a few days, the level of anemia may be severe because the hemolysis continues unabated in the absence of RBC production. Although the mechanisms that impair erythropoiesis in inflammation are operative in infections of all types (see Chapter 24), human parvovirus B19 specifically invades proliferating erythroid progenitors, which accounts for its importance in SCD (see Chapters 19 and 24).[129] Parvovirus B19 (Fig. 40-10) accounts for 68% of aplastic crises in children with SCD,[130] but the high incidence of protective antibodies in adults makes parvovirus a less frequent cause of aplasia in this age group (see also Infections later in this chapter). Other reported causes of transient aplasia are infections by *S. pneumoniae,* salmonella, streptococci, and Epstein-Barr virus. Bone marrow necrosis, which also may be the result of parvovirus infection, characterized by fever, bone pain, reticulocytopenia, and a leukoerythroblastic response, also causes aplastic crisis.[131,132]

Inhaled oxygen therapy also causes transient RBC hypoproduction; supraphysiologic oxygen tensions curtail EPO production promptly and suppress reticulocytosis within 2 days.[133]

The mainstay of treating aplastic crises is RBC transfusion. When transfusion is necessitated by the degree of anemia or cardiorespiratory symptoms, a single transfusion usually will suffice because reticulocytosis resumes spontaneously within a few days. Transfusion may be avoided by keeping severely anemic patients on bed rest to prevent symptoms and by avoiding supraphysiologic oxygen tensions. A useful guideline for transfusion in the context of an aplastic crisis is the reticulocyte count. A patient having an aplastic crisis with a reticulocyte count that is recovering is less likely to require urgent transfusion than one with a normal or low absolute reticulocyte count.

Sequestration Crisis (Spleen or Liver)

Acute splenic sequestration of blood is characterized by acute exacerbation of anemia; persistent reticulocytosis; a tender, enlarging spleen; and sometimes hypovolemia.[134] The LDH level may remain stable or increase. Patients susceptible to this complication are those whose spleens have not undergone fibrosis—young patients with sickle cell anemia and adults with Hb SC disease or sickle cell–β⁺-thalassemia. Sequestration may occur as early as a few weeks of age and may cause death before SCD is diagnosed. In one study, 30% of children had splenic sequestration over a 10-year period and 15% of the attacks were fatal.[135]

The basis of therapy is to restore blood volume and RBC mass. Because splenic sequestration recurs in 50% of cases, splenectomy is recommended after the event has abated. Alternatively, chronic transfusion therapy is used in young children to delay splenectomy until it can be tolerated safely. Because recurrence is possible during transfusion therapy, parents should be trained to detect a rapidly enlarging spleen and to seek immediate medical attention in this event. Less common sites of acute sequestration include the liver and possibly the lung.[136,137]

Delayed Hemolytic Transfusion Reaction and Autoimmune Hemolytic Anemia

Approximately 30% of patients are predisposed to develop alloantibodies, in part because of minor blood group incompatibilities in racially mismatched blood.[71,72] The corollary is that the other patients can receive multiple transfusions without demonstrating alloantibodies. After alloimmunization, there is a subsequent decrease in antibody titer that can fall below serologically detectable levels. Therefore, antigen-positive RBCs appear compatible in cross-matching and are transfused. This can result in a delayed hemolytic transfusion reaction produced by the amnestic response of the immune system (as opposed to the immediate hemolytic reaction that occurs with preformed antibody). The delayed hemolytic transfusion reaction consists of an unexplained fall in Hb, elevated LDH level, elevated bilirubin above baseline, and hemoglobinuria, all occurring between 4 and 10 days after the RBC transfusion. Delayed hemolytic reactions and hyperhemolysis have been shown to occur in 11% of pediatric patients with SCD and a history of alloantibodies.[138] In SCD, the delayed hemolytic transfusion reaction can be particularly devastating because it can be accompanied by reticulocytopenia, which together with a bystander effect of destruction of recipient blood (not just donor blood) can result in unanticipated worsening of anemia to levels below that seen before transfusion.[139] In addition to the manifestations of a delayed hemolytic transfusion reaction as listed, patients may develop acute congestive heart failure, acute renal failure, or acute chest syndrome (accompanied by vasoocclusive pain crisis). Subsequent transfusions may further exacerbate the anemia.

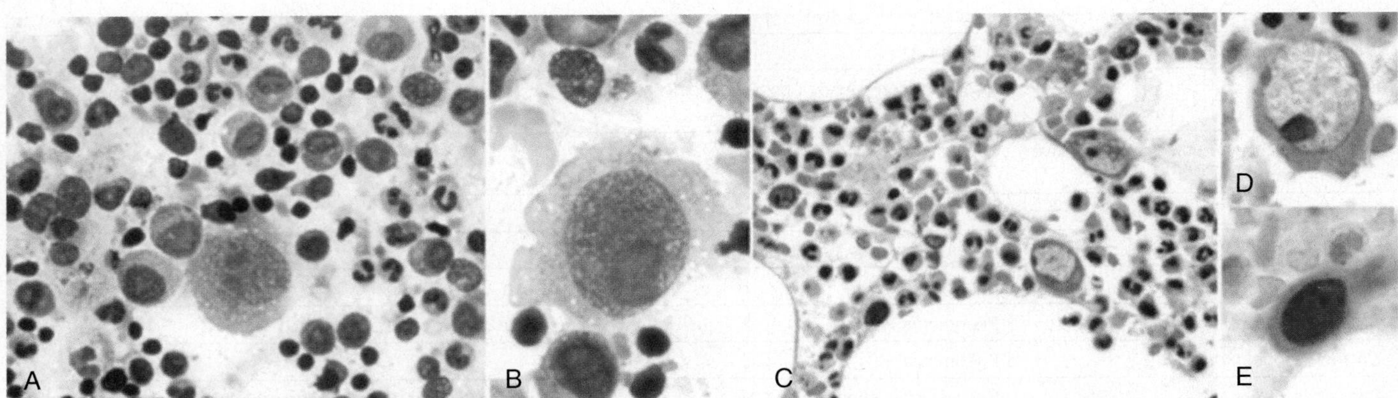

Figure 40-10 PARVOVIRUS. Bone marrow aspirate in a patient with sickle cell disease and aplastic crisis **(A)**. Note the absence of red blood cell precursors except for the single, large degenerating pronormoblast *(lower center)*. Such pronormoblasts contain large nuclear inclusions **(B)** as a result of replication of parvovirus B19. The same can be seen in the tissue sections of a bone core biopsy (**C** and **D**). The parvovirus can now be recognized immunohistochemically with an immunostain **(E)**.

Resolution of severe anemia may only occur after withholding further transfusions with subsequent reticulocyte count recovery. Corticosteroids at high doses (e.g., intravenous methylprednisolone 500 mg/day for 2 to 3 days) should be considered if the anemia is life threatening or if further transfusion is deemed necessary to save the patient's life. Intravenous immunoglobulin can also be considered, with proper attention paid to avoiding iatrogenic fluid overload. Approaches to minimizing this complication include transfusing extended-matched (see Basic Management and Disease Modification), phenotypically compatible blood.[70-72] This syndrome may or may not recur with further transfusions after a recovery period.[140]

Hyperhemolytic Crisis

Hyperhemolytic crisis is the sudden exacerbation of anemia with increased reticulocytosis and bilirubin level. If suspected, the approach to management should first be to look for an underlying etiology, which may be one of the events listed earlier: aplastic crisis (during the recovery phase when the reticulocyte count may not be decreased), sequestration crisis, delayed hemolytic transfusion reaction, or autoimmune hemolysis. Another possible cause is G6PD deficiency.[141]

Erythropoietin Deficiency

This entity is discussed under Basic Management and Disease Modification.

Nutritional Deficiencies: Folate, Iron, or Vitamin B_{12} Deficiency

This entity is discussed under Basic Management and Disease Modification.

Hypothyroidism

Iron overload in SCD can result in hypothyroidism.[142] Therefore, hypothyroidism is another etiology to consider in a SCD patient with an otherwise unexplained decrease in Hb below baseline.

Infections

Immune Deficit

The propensity of children with SCD to contract *S. pneumoniae* infection is related to impaired splenic function[143] and diminished serum opsonizing activity. Even before the anatomic autoinfarction of the spleen in patients with sickle cell anemia, defective splenic function is demonstrable by Howell-Jolly bodies on the peripheral blood smear, visible "pits" on the surface of RBCs, and abnormal results of radionuclide spleen scanning.[144] Specific syndromes exhibiting greater rates of hemolysis cause loss of splenic function at earlier ages—sickle cell anemia earlier than Hb SC disease earlier than sickle cell–β^+-thalassemia.

Infectious complications of SCD are a major cause of morbidity and mortality[145] even with current vaccination and prophylactic antibiotic regimens. The infections caused by particular organisms are shown in Table 40-8, and the specific organisms affecting different target organs are shown in Table 40-9. By 5 years of age, almost all patients are functionally asplenic, contributing to infectious susceptibility. Historically, pneumococcal sepsis has been the predominant cause of death in those younger than 20 years of age.[146]

Evaluation

The most critical aspect of infectious illness in SCD is the evaluation and treatment of febrile children. Routine evaluation includes a physical examination, a CBC, blood and urine cultures, a lumbar puncture if meningitis is suspected, and chest radiography to evaluate for pneumonia. Results of the CBC are compared with baseline values. A left shift in the differential count suggests bacterial infection.

Penicillin Prophylaxis and Pneumonia Vaccination

Data and recommendations regarding penicillin prophylaxis and pneumonia vaccination are discussed under Basic Management and Disease Modification.

Streptococcus Pneumoniae, Haemophilus Influenzae, Atypical Mycobacteria, and Acute Febrile Illness

Streptococcus pneumoniae bacteremia is accompanied by leukocytosis, a left shift, aplastic crisis, sometimes disseminated intravascular coagulation, and a 20% to 50% mortality rate.[145] Although concerns about *S. pneumoniae* sepsis are largely for young children, this complication also occurs in adults, often with devastating results.[147] *S. pneumoniae* is the major cause of meningitis in infants and young children with SCD, and it occurs in the setting of bacteremia.

The second most common organism responsible for bacteremia in these children, *H. influenzae* type b, accounts for 10% to 25% of episodes. *H. influenzae* bacteremia affects older children and is less fulminant than *S. pneumoniae* bacteremia, but it may be fatal.[145]

Table 40-9 Organ-Related Infection in Sickle Cell Disease

Primary Sites of Infection	Most Common Pathogen(s)	Other Pathogens	Pathophysiology	Prevention	Management
Septicemia	*Streptococcus pneumonia*	*Haemophilus influenza* type b *Escherichia coli* *Salmonella* spp.	Defective splenic function; deficiency of opsonic antibody	Vaccines* Prophylactic penicillin	Empiric intravenous antibiotics for fever
Meningitis	*S. pneumoniae*			Same as for septicemia	
Osteomyelitis and septic arthritis	*Salmonella* spp. *S. pneumonia*	*E. coli* *Proteus* spp. *Staphylococcus aureus*		—	Surgical drainage, intravenous antibiotics
Pneumonia	*Mycoplasma pneumoniae* Respiratory viruses	*Chlamydia pneumoniae* *S. pneumoniae*		Vaccines*	See pulmonary and therapy sections for management of acute chest syndrome.

Data from Buchanan GR, Glader BE: Benign course of extreme hyperbilirubinemia in sickle cell anemia: Analysis of six cases. *J Pediatr* 91:21, 1977.
*Against *Streptococcus pneumoniae* and *Haemophilus influenzae* type b.

Conjugated *H. influenzae* type b vaccines produce excellent antibody responses in children with SCD and now are administered in early infancy (http://www.cdc.gov/vaccines/recs/schedules/child-schedule.htm).

Owing to the high mortality rate of bacteremia, hospitalization, blood and cerebrospinal fluid cultures, and parenteral antibiotics have been the standard of care for children with fevers higher than 38.5° C. Prompt attention to fever can reduce the risk of severe pneumococcal sepsis. Rapid administration of antibiotics has resulted in a lower incidence of meningitis among patients with bacteremia than 20 years ago when the incidence was 50%.[148] The efficacy of ceftriaxone therapy for *S. pneumoniae* and *H. influenzae* infection[149] has led to new treatment algorithms that recommend outpatient therapy for most patients. However, resistant *S. pneumoniae* have emerged, necessitating a thorough knowledge of local resistance patterns to guide the choice of alternate antibiotics (particularly vancomycin, to which resistance has not been observed).

Please see Pulmonary Complications for further discussions regarding pneumonia and acute chest syndrome.

Meningitis

Meningitis therapy should cover *S. pneumoniae* and probably *H. influenzae* type b and should be continued for at least 2 weeks.

Salmonella and Osteomyelitis

In this patient population, osteomyelitis is commonly caused by *Salmonella* spp.[150] *Staphylococcus aureus,* the most common etiology in patients without SCD, accounts for less than 25% of SCD cases. Infection usually affects long bones, often at multiple sites.

The diagnosis is confirmed by culture of blood or infected bone. Parenteral antibiotics that cover *Salmonella* spp. and *S. aureus* are given, and antibiotic therapy is based on culture results. Parenteral antibiotics are continued for 2 to 6 weeks.[150] Surgical drainage or sequestrectomy may be required. Most patients are cured by this approach, but there may be recurrences.[150]

Articular infection is less common and is often caused by *S. pneumoniae.*[150]

Parvovirus B19

The specificity of the parvovirus B19 (see also Aplastic Crisis) for erythroid precursor cells, coupled with the accelerated erythropoiesis in hemolytic anemias, leaves sickle cell patients vulnerable to infection by this agent.[151] In SCD, parvovirus infection is a common cause of aplastic crisis, especially in children. It has been reported to cause bone marrow necrosis, acute chest syndrome, pulmonary fat embolism, hepatic sequestration, and glomerulonephritis.[129-132]

Urinary Tract Infections

Patients with SCD are at a higher risk for urinary tract infections and pyelonephritis than the general population. *Escherichia coli* is the most common uropathogen and can cause septicemia in these patients. Persistent urinary tract infections may be secondary to renal papillary necrosis. All urinary tract infections in this patient population should be considered complicated, requiring 10 to 21 days of appropriate antibiotic therapy.

Neurologic Complications

Neurologic complications occur in 25% or more of patients with SCD.[152] Neurologic complications include CVAs (consisting of transient ischemic attacks [TIAs], overt and silent cerebral infarction, cerebral hemorrhage), seizures (which can be a presenting feature of CVA), unexplained coma, spinal cord infarction or compression, central nervous system infections, vestibular dysfunction, and sensory hearing loss.[153]

Cerebrovascular Accidents, Pathophysiology, Incidence, Risk Factors, and Presentation[154]

Histopathologic evaluation of large-vessel involvement in SCD shows a pattern of smooth muscle proliferation with overlying endothelial damage and fibrosis. Smaller arterioles and capillaries demonstrate distension, thrombosis, and vessel wall necrosis.[155,156] Aneurysmal dilation associated with hemorrhagic stroke occurs at regions of intimal hyperplasia.[157] The vessel wall changes are likely multifactorial in origin related to endothelial injury from high and turbulent flow, RBC adherence, and hypoxia. But in addition, it has been speculated that depletion of NO by the free Hb released through intravascular hemolysis may also play a role.[157] The age-specific pattern of stroke risk in SCD may be related to the higher cerebral flow rates in early childhood.[157] Cerebral thrombosis, which accounts for 70% to 80% of all CVAs in patients with SCD, results from large-vessel occlusion (see Fig. 40-9) rather than the more typical microvascular occlusion of SCD.[158] Silent infarcts are thought to result from microvascular vasoocclusion or thrombosis or chronic hypoxia in the periphery stemming from large-vessel disease.[159] In 30% of patients with SCD, major vessel stenosis results in the formation of friable collateral vessels that appear as puffs of smoke (*moyamoya* in Japanese) on angiography.[160] Moyamoya disease predisposes to thrombotic and hemorrhagic strokes, seizures, and cognitive disability.[161]

The relative risk for stroke is 200 to 400 times higher in children with SCD compared with the children without SCD. The prevalence of clinically overt stroke is 11%. Clinically silent infarction detectable by MRI affects 17% to 20% of patients by age 20 years.[162] Silent infarcts are associated with cognitive impairment. Even in patients without silent or overt cerebral infarction, cognitive functioning can be impaired.[163] Almost 50% of the children with "silent" infarcts eventually require lifelong support or custodial care because of neuropsychologic deficits.[164] Whereas infarctive strokes were common in children and those older than 30 years of age, hemorrhagic stroke was most common between ages 20 and 30 years.[23]

Sickle cell–specific risk factors for CVA include increased cerebral blood flow velocity[165] (discussed further under Primary Prevention of Cerebrovascular Accidents), a history of overt or silent cerebral infarction,[166] nocturnal hypoxemia,[167] more severe anemia, higher reticulocyte counts, lower Hb F levels, higher WBC counts, the Hb SS genotype (rather than Hb SC disease or sickle cell–β-thalassemia), nocturnal hypoxemia or sleep apnea, migraines, elevated homocysteine levels, "relative" systolic hypertension (i.e., those at the high end of the lower-than-normal range characteristic of SCD).[23,168] Genetic markers of increased risk are the Central African Republic haplotype and the absence of α-thalassemia.[157,169] Both small- and large-vessel thrombosis can occur. Specific HLA alleles separately correlate with small- versus large-vessel stroke risk, suggesting that different pathologic processes may be involved.[157]

In addition to these sickle cell–specific predictors of stroke, one must also consider the well-documented modifiable risk factors for stroke that are operational in the general population; these are hypertension, exposure to cigarette smoke (active smoking or passive exposure), diabetes, atrial fibrillation, dyslipidemia, carotid artery stenosis, postmenopausal hormone therapy, poor diet, physical inactivity, obesity, and fat distribution. Less well-documented but potentially modifiable risk factors include alcohol or drug use, oral contraceptive use, and sleep-disordered breathing.[162]

Cerebrovascular accidents are heralded by focal seizures in 10% to 33% of cases and by TIAs in 10%. CVAs are fatal in approximately 20% of initial cases, recur within 3 years in nearly 70%, and are the cause of motor and cognitive impairment in the majority. Intracranial hemorrhage results in the same signs as thrombosis, but in addition, neck stiffness, photophobia, severe headache, vomiting, and altered consciousness may occur. Coma suggests hemorrhage rather than thrombosis. A typical presentation is coma and seizures without hemiparesis. Although the mortality rate may be as high as 50%, the morbidity of survivors is low. Hemorrhage may be subarachnoid, intraparenchymal, or intraventricular, which can be differentiated by angiography. The favorable neurosurgical outcome in subarachnoid hemorrhage caused by ruptured aneurysm justifies an aggressive approach to diagnosis, transfusion, vasodilatory therapy, and surgery.

Primary Prevention of Cerebrovascular Accidents

The overall risk of stroke in pediatric patients with SCD is 1% per year; however, in the subset of patients with transcranial Doppler evidence of a high (>200 cm/sec) cerebral blood flow velocity in the internal carotid artery or middle cerebral artery the stroke risk is in excess of 10% per year (although this is still much lower than the risk of recurrent stroke in a sickle cell patient after a first event, which is approximately 70%). In the Stroke Prevention Trial in Sickle Cell Disease (STOP), 130 children diagnosed as having clinically silent cerebral artery stenosis on the basis of high cerebral flow rates were randomized to receive chronic transfusion therapy or not. Over a period of more than 2 years, the risk of stroke was reduced to less than 1% per year in the transfused group[165] (a risk reduction of >90%). The ability of transfusion to curtail progression of large-vessel stenosis has also been proven with angiography.[170]

Because of the risks of iron overload and allosensitization with chronic transfusion, a randomized controlled trial of withdrawal of transfusion was conducted (STOP 2). This trial evaluated discontinuation of transfusion after at least 30 months in children who had not had an overt stroke and in whom the cerebral flow rates decreased to low risk (<170 cm/sec) with transfusion. This study was terminated early because of a high rate of reversion to high-risk TCD flow rates (34%) and stroke (5%) in the patients taken off transfusion compared with the group who continued transfusion.[171]

In children, MRI can also be used to assess stroke risk: 8.1% of children with an asymptomatic MRI lesion versus 0.5% of those with a normal MRI had a stroke during the ensuing 5 years.[166] A randomized trial of MRI-guided prophylactic transfusion is in progress (Silent Infarct Treatment Trial [SITT]). In adults, MRI or MRA of the brain should be used[30] to assess thrombotic or hemorrhagic stroke risk.

Chronic transfusion is associated with a significant complication rate. Therefore, there is a need for alternatives, especially because some patients and physicians believe that the 10% annual stroke risk does not warrant the risks and burdens of chronic transfusion.[154] The role of aspirin in ischemic stroke prevention in SCD is being evaluated (see Basic Management and Disease Modification). HU significantly lowered the TCD velocity values in a group of 24 children with Hb SS disease compared with an age-matched control group.[47] The role of HU is being formally evaluated in secondary stroke prevention (see Secondary Prevention). Stem cell transplantation has resulted in stabilization of cerebral vasculopathy[172] but there is a mortality risk with this procedure of between 6% and 10%.

Other modifiable risk factors for stroke (see Cerebrovascular Accidents, Pathophysiology, Incidence, Risk Factors, and Presentation) should be identified and treated. Notably, in the general population, hypertension is particularly associated with a risk for hemorrhagic stroke, and effective treatment of hypertension can produce a relative risk reduction of 26% for ischemic stroke and 49% for hemorrhagic stroke.[173] In patients with SCD followed through the Cooperative Study of Sickle Cell Disease, both diastolic and systolic blood pressures were noted to be lower than for matched control participants. Patients with systolic pressures in the higher range for the sickle cell group, even with systolic pressures less than 140 mm Hg, had an increased risk of first ischemic stroke (there were insufficient events to make firm conclusions regarding hemorrhagic stroke).[23] Therefore, at a minimum, it seems reasonable to follow population-wide recommendations for blood pressure control in patients with SCD.

Evaluation and Management of Acute Cerebrovascular Accidents

Patients with symptoms and signs of CVA should be evaluated immediately using computed tomography (CT) scanning or MRI to distinguish among TIA, cerebral thrombosis, and hemorrhage. In those with hemorrhage, angiography or MRA is indicated after partial-exchange transfusion is performed to avoid complications associated with the injected contrast material. In both thrombosis and hemorrhage, prompt partial-exchange transfusion is performed, and chronic direct transfusion to maintain the Hb S level below 30% is instituted to prevent recurrent events (see also Basic Management and Disease Modification) and promote resolution of arterial stenoses.[170]

Secondary Prevention of Cerebrovascular Accidents

The risk of recurrent stroke is approximately 70%, a risk that is reduced to around 13% with chronic transfusion.[174] Although recurrent CVAs during chronic transfusion have been reported, this therapeutic modality provides the best means of preventing recurrence (Fig. 40-11). This treatment also provides incidental protection against pain crises, bacterial infections, acute chest syndrome, and hospitalization.

Based on the data from STOP 2 (see Primary Prevention of Cerebrovascular Accidents), chronic transfusion is continued indefinitely. This may not be feasible for administrative reasons or because of allosensitization or iron overload for which the patient is unable or unwilling to undergo treatment. Therefore, clinical trials to determine if disease modifiers such as HU or decitabine can reduce stroke risk are indicated. In patients with a history of CVA transitioned from chronic transfusion to HU, the recurrent stroke rate remained stable and in the range seen with continued transfusion.[80]

Per primary prevention, all other identified modifiable risk factors for stroke should be identified and treated.

In patients with moyamoya disease, surgical approaches to therapy, such as extracranial–intracranial bypass, have been useful in improving the perfusion of affected regions of the brain.

Stem cell transplantation has resulted in stabilization of cerebral vasculopathy,[172] but the risk of a second neurologic event is higher in the peritransplant period, and the mortality rate with this procedure is between 6% and 10%.[172]

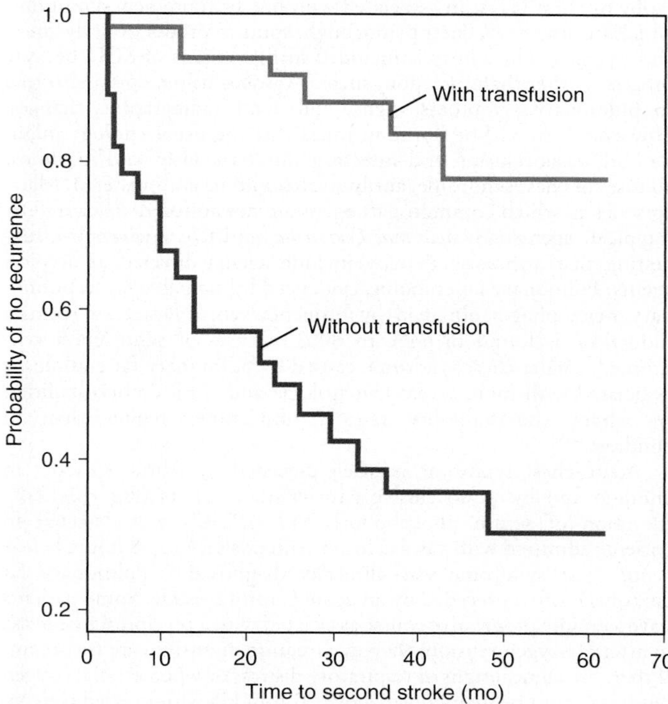

Figure 40-11 COMPARISON OF STROKE RECURRENCE OVER 62 MONTHS IN A TRANSFUSED GROUP AND IN UNTRANSFUSED HISTORICAL CONTROL GROUPS. *(Adapted with permission from Pegelow CH, Adams RJ, McKie V, et al: Risk of recurrent stroke in patients with sickle cell disease treated with erythrocyte transfusions.* J Pediatr *126:896, 1995.)*

Seizures

Seizures occur more commonly among patients with SCD. In one study, 21 of 152 patients in a pediatric clinic had seizures, four of which were related to meperidine therapy. Most had nonfocal CT and MRI studies but focal electroencephalographic changes.[175] CVAs are heralded by focal seizures in 10% to 33% of cases. Therefore, seizures in SCD ultimately may be related to the underlying vasculopathy.

Pulmonary Complications

Pulmonary disease is the leading cause of death in patients with SCD.[16] Both acute and chronic pulmonary complications are common. The common acute complications are pneumonia and acute chest syndrome, and the common chronic complication is pulmonary hypertension.

Pneumonia

Pneumonia is defined as chest infiltrates on chest radiography or chest CT scan associated with fever and an identified infectious etiology.

The risk for and increased frequency of *S. pneumoniae* infections is discussed under Infections earlier. In addition, *Mycoplasma pneumoniae, Chlamydia pneumoniae,* and *Legionella* spp. are also relatively common causes of pneumonia in patients with SCD. Antibiotic therapy for pneumonia or acute chest syndrome should cover these agents in addition to pneumococcus and *H. influenzae.*

When antibiotics are used to treat the acute chest syndrome, they should cover *S. pneumoniae, H. influenzae* type b, *M. pneumoniae,* and *C. pneumoniae*. The combination of cefuroxime and erythromycin is recommended.

Acute Chest Syndrome

Acute chest syndrome occurs in approximately 30% of patients.[176] Acute chest syndrome is defined as a new infiltrate on chest radiography or chest CT scan associated with one or more new symptoms, which include fever, chest pain, cough, sputum production, dyspnea, and hypoxia. This entity is included in discussions of SCD because processes other than infection, such as vasoocclusion, could also lead to pulmonary symptoms, signs, and chest radiographic changes. However, it should be borne in mind that the usual etiology might be both vasoocclusion and infection simultaneously, and in almost all cases of chest syndrome, antibiotics should be administered. Many episodes in which common pathogens are not cultured are caused by "atypical" agents (*Mycoplasma, Legionella,* and *Chlamydia* spp.), suggesting that antibiotic therapy include agents directed at atypical agents. Pulmonary fat embolus, evidenced by stainable fat in pulmonary macrophages obtained by bronchoalveolar lavage or sputum induction, is found in 44% to 60% of cases of acute chest syndrome.[177] Acute chest syndrome caused by pulmonary fat embolus is associated with more severe hematologic and clinical abnormalities. In adults, the mortality rate is four times higher than in children.[3,178]

Acute chest syndrome is often preceded by febrile episodes in children and by vasoocclusive pain crisis in adults (Fig. 40-12).[178] Elevation of serum phospholipase A2 (sPLA2) was detected in patients admitted with vasoocclusive pain crisis 24 to 48 hours before acute chest syndrome was clinically diagnosed.[179] Pulmonary fat embolus is often preceded by an acute painful episode. Some patients have a rapidly progressive course associated with a precipitous decrease in arterial oxygen tension; they may require intensive care treatment. If there are clinical signs of respiratory distress or when arterial oxygen tension cannot be maintained above 70 mm Hg with inhaled oxygen, partial-exchange transfusion is indicated. Artificial ventilation may be required.

In patients with pneumonia or chest syndrome, antibiotics should cover *S. pneumoniae, M. pneumoniae, Chlamydia pneumoniae, H. influenzae,* and *Legionella* spp.

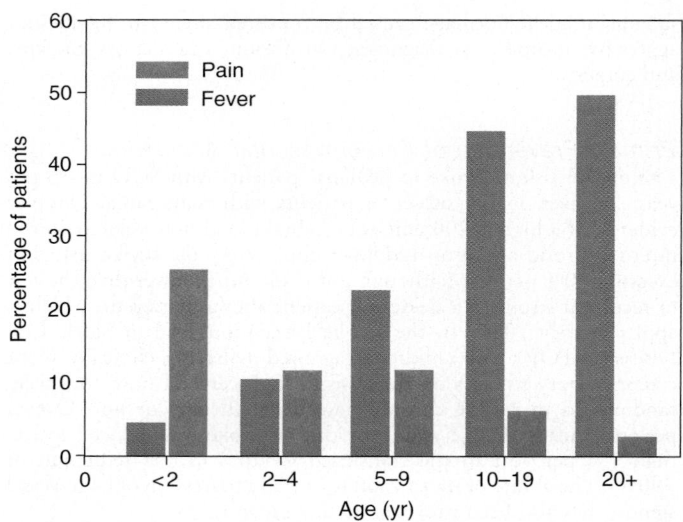

Figure 40-12 AGE-SPECIFIC ASSOCIATED EVENTS WITHIN 2 WEEKS PRECEDING ACUTE CHEST SYNDROME. *(Adapted with permission from Vichinsky EP, Styles LA, Colangelo LH, et al: Acute chest syndrome in sickle cell disease: Clinical presentation and course. Cooperative Study of Sickle Cell Disease.* Blood *89:1787, 1997.)*

Pulmonary Hypertension

Chronic complications such as pulmonary hypertension occur in as many as 60% of patients.[180-182] There does not appear to be an association with the occurrence of acute chest syndrome,[181] emphasizing that the pathophysiology of these two conditions may differ in some key features. The pathophysiology may involve thrombi in large and small arteries,[183,184] cardiac decompensation from progressive anemia, and potentially reversible increases in vascular tone from NO depletion and medial and intimal hypertrophy.[184] The recognition that pulmonary hypertension is a feature of hemolytic syndromes other than sickle cell and that markers of hemolysis correlate with the risk of pulmonary hypertension supports the idea that depletion of NO through scavenging by free Hb may have an important role in the pathophysiology of this disease.[181,185] Pulmonary hypertension usually occurs in adults and carries a poor prognosis.[186]

The association with early death and the emerging availability of candidate treatments suggest that efforts should be made to diagnose this condition in all patients with SCD.[181,185] The feasibility of an echocardiogram determined tricuspid regurgitant jet (TR-jet) velocity measurement of 2.5 m/sec to make the diagnosis was suggested by selective cardiac catheterization in a cohort of 195 patients[180]; however, the sensitivity and specificity of this test may have limitations.[185] Elevations in BNP levels correlate with an increased TR-jet and risk of early death.

In a 16-week, double-blind, placebo-controlled trial of sildenafil to treat patients with SCD with increased TR-jet velocity and a low exercise capacity, sildenafil increased hospitalization rates for pain without evidence of improvement in TR-jet velocity or BNP levels.[187] If such patients have chronic relative reticulocytopenia, measures to increase total hemoglobin could be a consideration requiring evaluation in clinical trials (see Basic Management and Disease Modification).

Other Pulmonary Complications

Other findings include restrictive and obstructive lung disease and hypoxemia.[188] High-resolution, thin-section CT scanning of the lungs may show chronic interstitial fibrosis. Airway hyperreactivity occurs in nearly two-thirds of children with SCD not diagnosed as having asthma. Thirty-six percent of 53 children with SCD were found to have sleep-related upper airway obstruction, 16% had hypoxemia, and all 15 who underwent adenotonsillectomy were symptomatically improved and had improved hypoxemia.[189] Sleep apnea may be associated with surgically reversible exacerbations of painful episodes and strokes. Blood gas and pulmonary function measurements should be obtained as baseline data for all patients.

Hepatobiliary Complications

Hepatobiliary complications in patients with SCD include cholelithiasis, cholecystitis, acute hepatic cell crisis, acute hepatic sequestration crisis, and sickle cell intrahepatic cholestasis.[190] Chronic transfusion also places patients at risk for infection with hepatitis viruses and for transfusional hemosiderosis. Non–transfusion-related hepatic hemosiderosis can also be seen.

The serum bilirubin level is higher in sickle cell anemia (Hb SS) than in Hb SC disease or sickle cell–β^+-thalassemia as a result of a greater hemolytic rate. The level rises after the first decade, possibly as a result of chronic hepatobiliary dysfunction. The aspartate aminotransferase (AST) and alanine aminotransferase (ALT) levels are often elevated, particularly in adult patients with sickle cell anemia, but mean levels are normal. Alkaline phosphatase levels are elevated in all genotypes until puberty, which occurred later in males and in those with sickle cell anemia. Percutaneous liver biopsy is associated with a high risk of severe complications and death in SCD patients with acute hepatic syndromes.[191]

Cholelithiasis and Cholecystitis

The prevalence of pigmented gallstones in SCD is directly related to the rate of hemolysis.[192] In sickle cell anemia, gallstones occur in children as young as 3 to 4 years of age and are eventually found in approximately 70% of patients. Some have recommended the surgical removal of asymptomatic gallstones to avoid subsequent difficulty in distinguishing gallbladder pain from acute painful episodes. This approach has become more feasible with the availability of laparoscopic cholecystectomy.[193]

Acute Hepatic Cell Crisis

Acute hepatic cell crisis presents with tender hepatomegaly, worsening jaundice, and fever.[190] The likely etiology is hepatocellular cell ischemia. The AST and bilirubin are elevated, but rarely above 300 IU/L and 255 μM, respectively. This syndrome usually resolves within 3 to 14 days with supportive care alone but can progress to liver failure and fatal outcome; therefore, patients should be monitored closely and exchange transfusion initiated if they show signs of progressive liver dysfunction (e.g., increasing AST).

Acute Hepatic Sequestration Crisis

Acute hepatic sequestration crisis presents with acute hepatic enlargement and a dramatic fall in Hb concentration, the most likely mechanism being sequestration of sickled erythrocytes in the liver. Management is with supportive care and transfusions.

Intrahepatic Cholestasis

Sickle cell intrahepatic cholestasis results in severe, asymptomatic hyperbilirubinemia without fever, pain, leukocytosis, hepatic failure, or death.[194] Asymptomatic hyperbilirubinemia without signs of progressive liver dysfunction (e.g., increasing AST) does not require specific therapy. Evidence of progressive liver dysfunction should prompt consideration of acute hepatic cell crisis and exchange transfusion.

Hepatitis C Infection

Chronic hepatitis C infection in SCD occurs with a prevalence that is related to the number of transfusions received; it may be a leading cause of cirrhosis. Liver transplantation has been used successfully as therapy for this complication.[195] If indicated, interferon-ribavirin can be used to treat hepatitis C in SCD patients.[196]

Obstetric and Gynecologic Issues

Gynecologic complications (delayed menarche, dysmenorrhea, ovarian cysts, pelvic infection, and fibrocystic disease of the breast) are more common in women with SCD. Pregnancy entails increased risks to the mother and child compared with the general population.

Pregnancy

Pregnancy in patients with SCD is associated with increased risks to both the mother and fetus, although these risks are not so great as to prohibit continuation of pregnancy.[197,198] The fetal complications of pregnancy, most of which are related to compromised placental blood flow, are the increased incidence of spontaneous early abortion, intrauterine growth retardation, low birthweight, and fetal death. Maternal complications include increased rates of painful episodes, severe anemia caused by iron or folate deficiencies, exaggeration of the physiologic "anemia of pregnancy," increased infections (urinary tract infections, pneumonias, endometritis), preeclampsia, and death.[198] It is controversial whether the degree of anemia predicts the birth of babies with low birthweight. The occurrence of a perinatal death in a previous pregnancy and the presence of twins in the present pregnancy are two major risk factors for an unfavorable outcome. The course of pregnancy is more benign in Hb SC disease than in sickle cell anemia.

Better fetal and maternal outcomes in recent years are largely attributable to generally improved antenatal and obstetric care. Patients should be followed in a high-risk obstetric clinic in addition to the hematology clinic and receive the usual vitamin, mineral, and folate supplements. A high-calorie, high-protein diet can be considered. There is no specific therapeutic or preventive treatment for intrauterine growth retardation. Some experts recommend prophylactic transfusion, but a large controlled study showed no improvement in fetal outcome from this management option, although maternal symptoms are reduced. In addition to the usual indications for transfusion therapy in SCD, transfusion therapy is indicated for patients with cardiac or respiratory compromise, in preparation for cesarean section, preeclampsia, twin pregnancy, acute chest syndrome, Hb levels more than 20% below steady state or less than 5 g/dL, and previous history of perinatal mortality. If the Hb is between 8 and 10 g/dL and transfusion is indicated for any of the reasons above, partial exchange should be performed (e.g., phlebotomy of 400-500 mL and transfusion of 2 units of packed RBCs).[197] The type of delivery does not appear to represent a problem, and both spontaneous delivery and cesarean section are well tolerated.

Some experts advise that hypertonic saline injections are contraindicated for elective termination of pregnancy because of the risk of sickling-induced vasoocclusion. However, most methods of abortion are well tolerated. There are anecdotal reports of a higher incidence of acute painful episodes after therapeutic abortion; inpatient intravenous hydration before and for the 24 hours after the procedure is recommended.

Birth Control

Modern non–estrogen-containing intrauterine devices should be considered. Although depot injections of medroxyprogesterone (Depo-Provera) given every 3 months may be safe with regards to stroke risk,[199] there is a risk of bone loss, a consideration in patients with SCD and their propensity to skeletal complications. Oral contraceptives containing low doses of estrogen can be considered with no clear evidence of increased stroke demonstrated to date, although the patients' overall stroke risk should probably still be taken into consideration until there is more phase IV follow-up on the clinical experience. Another caution with low-dose estrogen oral contraception is the risk of contraceptive failure with less than excellent compliance. There may be risks to contraception, but against this must be weighed the risks of unintended pregnancy. Sexually active women should have routine pelvic examinations and birth control instructions.

Renal Complications

Hypertension, proteinuria, hematuria, increasing anemia, and nephrotic syndrome reliably predict progression to renal failure, which are clinical indices to pay attention to because the serum creatinine may be misleading. Patients with sickle cell anemia exhibit an increased proximal tubular secretion of creatinine. Thus, patients may have a significant decline in renal function before it is detectable by measuring creatinine clearance.[200] The mean age at presentation with end-stage renal disease is 41 years.[201] Serum creatinine levels are low in all genotypes until age 18 years, when young men experience a rise, apparently related to increasing muscle mass. Creatinine levels increase with age in all genotypes, presumably because of declining renal function (see also organ-specific complications, kidney in Clinical Presentation and Management, later).

Other risk factors for the development of chronic renal failure include use of NSAIDs[202] and a genetic predisposition associated with the Central African Republic (CAR) β-globin haplotype; the latter has been suggested as an indication for BMT to prevent this outcome.[203] Acute renal failure from infarction may result from hypovolemia, sepsis, hepatorenal syndrome, cardiac failure, renal vein thrombosis, and rhabdomyolysis. These patients typically survive and recover their renal function with no increased risk of developing chronic renal failure.

There are seven well-described nephropathies that affect patients with either sickle cell trait or disease. These are gross hematuria, papillary necrosis, nephrotic syndrome, renal infarction, inability to concentrate urine, pyelonephritis, and renal medullary carcinoma.[200]

Renal transplantation is recommended for patients with sickle cell and end-stage renal diseases.

Renal Endocrine (Erythropoietin) Deficiency

This is discussed under Basic Management and Disease Modification.

Gross Hematuria

Hematuria may result from microthrombi formation in the peritubular capillaries of the renal medulla or from frank papillary necrosis. Significant hematuria may resolve with high urinary flow through oral hydration and bed rest. Hematuria that lasts longer than 1 to 2 weeks or the need for transfusion may require maintenance of a high urinary flow using a combination of hypotonic fluids and loop diuretics and urinary alkalinization using sodium bicarbonate and acetazolamide. These therapies are aimed at changing the acidic, hypertonic environment of the renal medulla that favors erythrocyte dehydration, increased Hb S concentrations, and Hb S polymerization. If bleeding persists for 72 hours despite these measures, then alternative treatment should be considered. These may include oral urea,[204] ε-aminocaproic acid, and vasopressin. Embolization or nephrectomy should be reserved for prolonged, life-threatening cases of hematuria that require multiple transfusions.

Increased hematuria can also be seen as a consequence of delayed hemolytic transfusion reactions (discussed in Exacerbations of Anemia).

Papillary Necrosis

Papillary necrosis is most often detected incidentally by imaging or microscopic examination of urine in asymptomatic patients. Sloughed papilla may cause ureteral obstruction and urinary tract infection. In addition to broad-spectrum antibiotics, this occurrence requires emergent relief of the obstruction with a retrograde ureteral stent or placement of a percutaneous nephrostomy tube. NSAIDs should be avoided in patients with papillary necrosis. Otherwise treatment is as for hematuria.

Proteinuria

Proteinuria has been found in 20% to 30% of patients with SCD. Increasing age and low Hb levels correlate with proteinuria. Proteinuria can progress to nephrotic syndrome characterized by proteinuria, hypoalbuminemia, edema, and hyperlipidemia. Angiotensin-converting enzyme (ACE) inhibitors produce a significant reduction in sickle proteinuria, although it is unclear if ACE inhibitors might slow or halt the progression of proteinuria to nephrotic syndrome and renal failure.[205,206] Angiotensin II inhibitors are being studied for a potential role in decreasing sickle cell–related proteinuria and renal function deterioration.

Hyposthenuria and Other Abnormalities of Tubular Function

The inability to maximally concentrate urine (hyposthenuria) in response to water deprivation is an early finding of sickle cell nephropathy. Both sickle cell trait and SCD patients may be affected. Hyposthenuria is the cumulative result of recurrent microinfarcts in the vasa recta caused by sickling (Fig. 40-13). When water deprived, these patients cannot maximally concentrate their urine and develop hypovolemia and dehydration.

Other abnormalities of renal tubular dysfunction found in sickle cell anemia include an incomplete form of distal renal tubular acidosis with hyperchloremic metabolic acidosis and hyperkalemia.[207] The hyperkalemia may respond to oral sodium bicarbonate.

Urinary Tract Infections

Urinary tract infections and pyelonephritis are discussed under infectious complications.

Renal Medullary Carcinoma

Sickle cell trait has been reported to be associated with renal medullary carcinoma.[208] Presentation is with gross hematuria, abdominal or flank pain, or significant weight loss. The disease may be metastatic at diagnosis, and the prognosis is poor. There is a weak association of renal medullary carcinoma with Hb SC disease but no identified association with sickle cell anemia. The reason for these patterns of disease is unknown.

Priapism

Priapism is a condition that is characterized by a sustained erection that does not result from sexual desire and is not relieved by sexual activity. Stuttering priapism is a separate entity that is characterized by multiple, brief episodes of sustained unwanted erection. It has been reported to affect 6.4% to 42% of boys and men with SCD[209] and can also occur in sickle cell trait. Its peak frequencies are between ages 5 and 13 years and 21 and 29 years. Priapism is most likely to develop in patients with lower Hb F levels and reticulocyte counts, increased platelet counts, and the Hb SS genotype. Priapism caused by SCD is usually ischemic, or low-flow, priapism. (High-flow priapism is caused by unregulated arterial flow and can be distinguished from low-flow priapism by a blood gas obtained from the corpora.) Most likely, priapism begins with a physiologic erection. The relative stasis of blood within the corpora leads to a decrease in oxygen tension and development of acidosis, predisposing to Hb S polymerization in the corporal sinusoids, venous occlusion, and low-flow priapism. Pain develops as the corpora become increasingly ischemic after approximately 4 hours of erection. In a minority of patients, usually postpubertal, the engorgement also affects the corpus spongiosum and glans. The mild acidosis that accompanies hypoventilation during sleep may also contribute to the pathophysiology. Impotence is the primary complication of priapism, although patients with a history of multiple episodes of priapism and significant corporeal fibrosis may report fair erections and maintain active sex lives. Corporeal ischemia during priapism may induce local inflammation, causing the fibrosis responsible for impotence.

The goal of treatment is to relieve priapism and maintain potency. Patients should be educated to seek medical attention for unrelenting

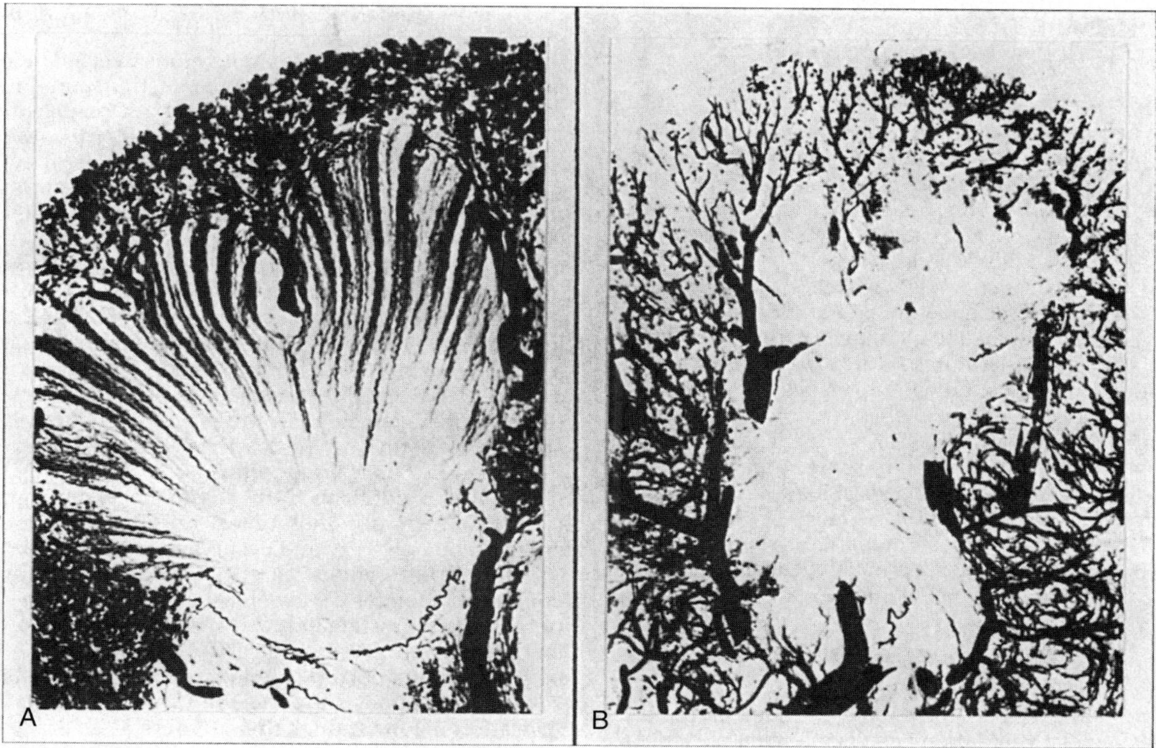

Figure 40-13 Postmortem microangiographic studies of the vasa recta in a normal individual **(A)** and a patient with sickle cell anemia **(B)**. *(With permission from Bertles JF, Döbler J: Reversible and irreversible sickling: A distinction by electron microscopy.* Blood *33:884, 1969.)*

erection of more than 2 hours' duration. Detumescence within 12 hours is optimal to retain potency. After 72 hours, impotence is more likely. The strategy is prompt initiation of supportive medical therapy with intravenous hydration and analgesia and involvement by a urology consultant if the priapism persists for more than 4 hours; aspiration of blood from the corpora with or without irrigation and injection of an α-adrenergic agonist should be considered (Guidelines of the American Urological Association, guidelines.gov/content.aspx?id=3741). If priapism persists 12 hours, options include partial-exchange transfusion to reduce the Hb S level to less than 30% with a total Hb of less than 10 g/dL or irrigation as outlined above. The latter procedure is less effective after 36 hours of priapism. Irrigation should be performed using penile anesthesia (dorsal nerve block; circumferential penile block; or subcutaneous, local, penile shaft block). All irrigation in boys should be performed under conscious sedation. There is anecdotal evidence for the use of hydralazine to treat acute priapism.[210]

Preventing recurrent priapism is an important component of management. Strategies include HU administration; chronic transfusion; the antiandrogen bicalutamide;[211] self-administration of the α-adrenergic agent etilefrine orally and for episodes lasting over 1 hour, by intracavernous injection; and monthly administration of intramuscular gonadotropin-releasing hormone analogue.[212,213] Prophylactic pseudoepinephrine (Sudafed) appears beneficial in preventing recurrent mild episodes.

Surgical creation of shunts is reserved for severe cases resistant to the above interventions. As many as 45% of patients who have priapism develop some degree of impotence.[214] When impotence persists for 12 months, a semirigid penile prosthesis may be implanted.

Ocular Complications[215]

The retina is particularly vulnerable to vasoocclusion, and annual retinal examination is part of routine health care maintenance for patients with SCD. Superficial retinal hemorrhages have a pink "salmon patch" appearance. Deeper retinal hemorrhages have a "black sunburst" appearance. Other manifestations of sickle cell retinopathy include iridescent spots, retinal neovascularization, and retinal detachment. More subtle signs of sickle cell retinopathy are optic nerve head vascular changes, vascular tortuosity, macular changes (e.g., microaneurysms and vascular loops), and peripheral arteriovenous anastomoses. Other ophthalmologic complications are anterior chamber ischemia, tortuosity of conjunctival vessels, retinal artery occlusion, and angioid streaks. Sickle cell retinopathy is best seen by fluorescein angiography (Fig. 40-14). The earlier onset and greater frequency of proliferative retinopathy in Hb SC disease and sickle cell–β^+-thalassemia compared with sickle cell anemia and sickle cell–β^0-thalassemia suggest that retinal vessels are more susceptible to occlusion by more viscous blood than by more rigid individual cells. Peripheral sickle retinopathy may require vision-saving therapy with laser photocoagulation. Orbital compression syndrome caused by vasoocclusion of the periorbital marrow space and subperiosteal hemorrhage has been observed to result in headache, fever, and palpebral edema. In this situation, culture, CT scan, and MRI should be used to rule out infectious, neoplastic, and other hemorrhagic etiologies. Conservative therapy, including local measures, analgesia, fluids, transfusion, and careful ophthalmologic surveillance, is recommended unless compression of the optic nerve ensues, in which case surgical decompression should be considered.

Bone Complications

Chronic tower skull, bossing of the forehead, and fish-mouth deformity of the vertebrae are the result of extended hematopoietic bone marrow, causing widening of the medullary space, thinning of the trabeculae and cortices, and osteoporosis. Osteonecrosis may cause a steplike depression of the vertebrae, selected shortening of the cuboidal bones of the hands and feet, and acute aseptic or avascular

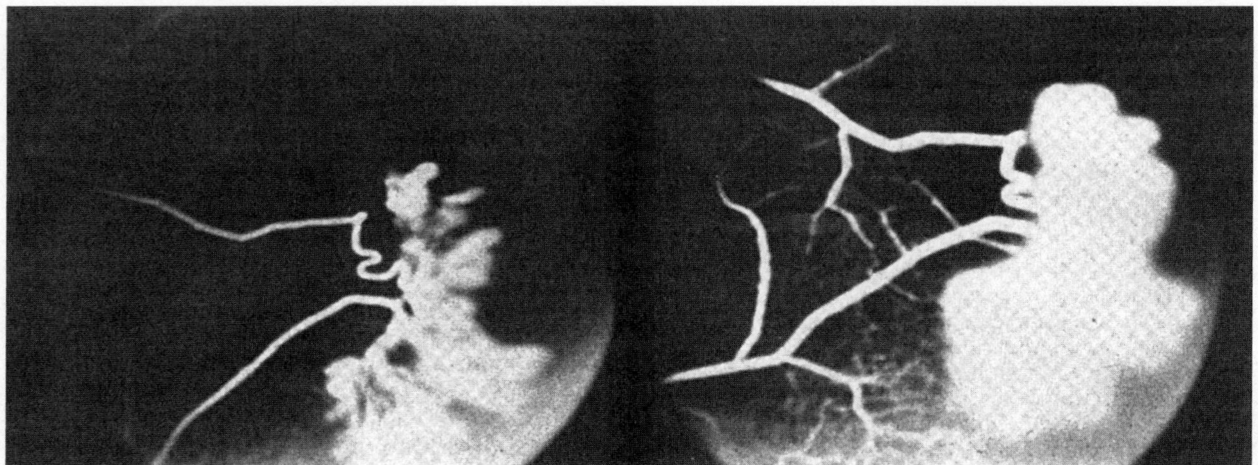

Figure 40-14 FLUORESCEIN ANGIOGRAPHY DEMONSTRATING A "SEA FAN" APPEARANCE OF SICKLE PROLIFERATIVE RETINOPATHY. *(Courtesy W.C. Mentzer.)*

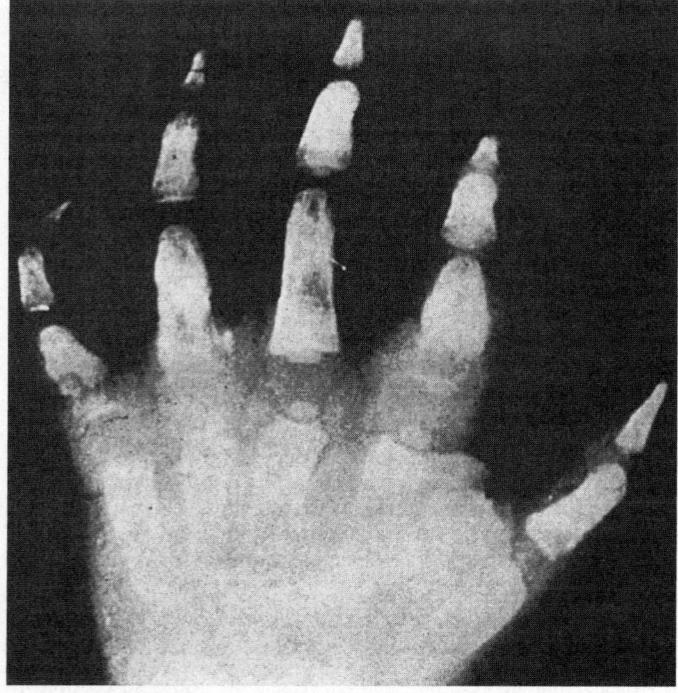

Figure 40-15 RADIOGRAM SHOWING THE BONE INFARCTIONS IN THE HANDS OF A CHILD WITH THE "HAND–FOOT SYNDROME" DACTYLITIs. *(Courtesy W.C. Mentzer.)*

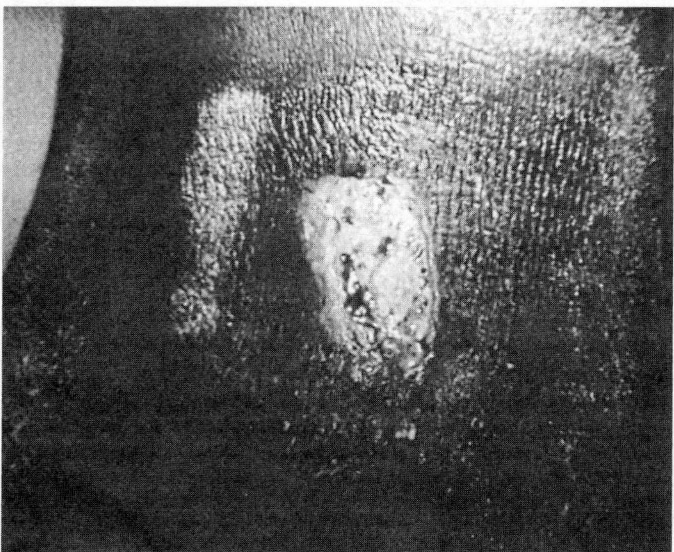

Figure 40-16 CHRONIC LEG ULCER NEAR THE MEDIAL MALLEOLUS. *(Courtesy W.C. Mentzer.)*

necrosis. The excruciating pain of bone infarction in the "hand–foot syndrome" that occurs around age 2 years of age is often the first symptom of SCD (Fig. 40-15).[216] This dactylitis resolves spontaneously and is treated with hydration and analgesia. Bone infarcts are demonstrable using nuclear medicine scintigraphy or MRI. Serial scans specific for bone osteoclasts, bone marrow macrophages, and inflammatory cells may be useful adjuncts for distinguishing bone marrow infarction from osteomyelitis, but it is essential to obtain cultures directly from the affected tissue before starting antibiotics. Treatment of osteomyelitis is addressed in the Infection sections.

Bone necrosis occurs with equal frequency in the femoral and humeral heads, but the femoral heads more commonly undergo progressive joint destruction as a result of chronic weight bearing. The process is associated with increased intraosseous pressure and is most sensitively detected by MRI. Aggressive physical therapy appears to prevent progression in mild cases and should be considered in the therapy of avascular necrosis. Core decompression surgery to relieve increased intraosseous pressure can be used in early-stage osteonecrosis (i.e., no radiographic evidence of bone collapse) to prevent disease progression. In more advanced disease, joint replacement can be considered. There is a 30% likelihood that a second hip revision will be required within 4 to 5 years of prosthetic hip placement in patients with SCD.[217]

Arthritic pain, swelling, and effusion may be related to periarticular infarction or gouty arthritis.

Bone marrow infarction causes reticulocytopenia, exacerbation of anemia, a leukoerythroblastic picture, and sometimes pancytopenia.[131,132] Pulmonary fat embolism is a rare complication of bone marrow infarction.[218] It is associated with fat globules in the sputum and refractile bodies visible in the optic fundi. It is a life-threatening event that may require prompt exchange transfusion and perhaps the use of heparin and corticosteroids.[218]

Dermatologic Complications

Leg ulcers are major causes of morbidity in SCD as a result of their frequency, chronicity, and resistance to therapy. Most occur near the medial or lateral malleolus (Fig. 40-16), may be associated with venous hypertension[219] and hemolytic rate,[220] and are frequently bilateral.[221] They may begin spontaneously or as a result of trauma and may become infected, most commonly by *S. aureus, Pseudomonas* spp., streptococci, or *Bacteroides* spp. Systemic infection, osteomyelitis, and tetanus are rare complications. Ulcers are resistant to healing and tend to be recurrent in well over half of cases. Their incidence has been reported to vary from 25% to 75%.[222] Ulcers rarely occur in patients younger than age 10 years and are most common in sickle cell anemia, less common in sickle cell–β°-thalassemia, and nonexistent in Hb SC disease and sickle cell–β^+-thalassemia.[221] The incidence in sickle cell anemia patients declines substantially in those who have coexistent α-thalassemia.[221] Low steady-state Hb levels and low Hb F levels are associated with an increased risk of leg ulceration.[223] Males have a threefold greater risk for developing leg ulcers than females. Treatment of leg ulcers requires persistence and patience; healing usually takes weeks. Therapy[224] begins with gentle debridement to remove nonviable, superficial tissue from more vital areas. Wet-to-dry dressings and DuoDerm hydrocolloid dressings facilitate devitalization. When debridement is complete, zinc oxide–impregnated Unna boots are used to promote healing. Bed rest speeds healing,[225] and topical antibiotics may be required. It may be necessary to use elastic wraps or leg elevation to control edema. Rapid healing of leg ulcers has been reported in patients treated with intravenous arginine butyrate.[226] Oral zinc, local hyperbaric oxygen, chronic transfusion, recombinant EPO, propionyl-L-carnitine, skin grafts, pentoxifylline, and becaplermin (platelet-derived growth factor) may have therapeutic roles and should be considered in individual cases but have not been formally tested for their effectiveness in accelerating resolution of sickle cell–associated leg ulcers.

Myofascial syndromes consist of soft tissue swelling in subcutaneous edema that may have a *peau d'orange* appearance. These may be large or discrete lesions a few centimeters in diameter. These lesions are probably the result of dermal or subdermal vasoocclusion. Treatment is symptomatic.

Cardiac Complications

The chronic anemia of SCD is compensated by high cardiac output, which results in chronic chamber enlargement and cardiomegaly, and mild to moderate mitral and tricuspid regurgitation even in young children. The electrocardiogram shows evidence of left ventricular hypertrophy and less often first-degree block and nonspecific ST-T wave changes. Left ventricular dilation correlates with age and inversely correlates with total Hb.[227] An age-dependent loss of cardiac reserve may predispose to heart failure in adult patients stressed by fluid overload, transfusion, exacerbation of anemia, hypoxia, or hypertension. Cardiac function can be improved by transfusion.[228] Acute myocardial infarction in the absence of coronary disease has been reported, and in one autopsy series, 9.7% of 72 consecutive patients with SCD had myocardial infarction.[229] It appears that myocardial infarction may occur with normal coronary arteries as a result of increased oxygen demand exceeding limited oxygen-carrying capacity or as a result of microcirculatory impairment. As mentioned earlier, pulmonary hypertension (>30 mm Hg) is a relatively common finding in patients with SCD and can be associated with right ventricular hypertrophy. It has been suggested that the increased rate of sudden death observed in SCD may be related to cardiac autonomic dysfunction, as detected by abnormal heart rate variability in response to selected postural maneuvers.[230]

Multiorgan Failure

This disastrous acute event involves multiple organ systems, including the lungs, brain, kidneys, liver, hematologic system, and heart, and usually leads to death.[231] It may be precipitated by infection, vasoocclusion, or fat embolus and consists of a constellation of life-threatening processes, including hypoxemia, acidosis, inflammation, vascular permeability, severe anemia, disseminated intravascular coagulation, renal failure, and hepatic failure. In addition to therapy specific for these processes, exchange transfusion, plasma infusion or exchange, and corticosteroids should be considered.

Psychosocial Issues

Modern insights into the psychosocial adjustment of patients with SCD have provided a level of understanding that allows interventional therapy. Although most patients with SCD are generally well adjusted,[232] there are risks of depression, low self-esteem, social isolation, poor family relationships, and withdrawal from normal daily living.[232] Particular stressors are recurrent and unpredictable pain and the response to it, curtailed activity because of pain, misinterpretation of the meaning of pain, and depression leading to learned helplessness. Although some patients with SCD become addicted to narcotics, this is uncommon and usually is the result of social influences rather than pain therapy. Well-adjusted patients have active coping strategies, family support, and support from the extended family unit common in African American society. Interventional approaches should emphasize recognizing and reinforcing individual strengths; confronting pathologic behavior; and establishing coping skills through reinterpreting pain, diverting attention from pain, and using support systems.[233] Attention to psychosocial concerns is vital to the psychosocial well-being and integration into society of patients with SCD (see Chapter 93).

Growth and Development

By age 2 years, children with SCD have detectable growth retardation that affects weight more than height and has no clear gender difference.[234] By adulthood, normal height is achieved, but weight remains lower than that of control participants. More severe growth delay is noted in children with sickle cell anemia and sickle cell–β°-thalassemia; Hb SC disease is associated with a less severe growth delay. Girls with SCD have retarded sexual maturation that is greater in those with sickle cell anemia and sickle cell–β°-thalassemia than those with Hb SC disease and sickle cell–β^+-thalassemia[234]; it is associated with elevated gonadotropin levels for the stage of sexual development and delayed menarche. Boys also have delayed sexual maturation, which is more severe in those with sickle cell anemia than those with Hb SC disease.[234] Retarded sexual maturation in boys can be attributable to primary hypogonadism, hypopituitarism, or hypothalamic insufficiency. The etiology of these multiple endocrine deficiencies may relate to underlying sickle cell pathophysiology or iron overload and emphasizes the importance of a comprehensive basic management and disease modification approach as outlined earlier in this chapter. Improved growth has been reported with HU,[235] transfusion,[235] folic acid supplementation, zinc supplementation,[236] and nutritional supplementation.[237] When children have both SCD and hypersplenism, splenectomy may result in improved protein turnover, metabolic rate, and growth parameters.[238]

VARIANT SICKLE CELL SYNDROMES

The sickle cell syndromes that result from inheritance of the sickle cell gene in simple heterozygosity or in compound heterozygosity with other mutant β-globin genes are sickle cell trait, Hb SC disease, and sickle cell–β-thalassemia. These and other less common compound heterozygosity syndromes are reviewed.

Sickle Cell Trait

The prevalence of sickle cell trait is approximately 8% to 10% in African Americans and as high as 25% to 30% in certain areas of western Africa.[4] Approximately 2.5 million people in the United States and 30 million in the world are heterozygous for the sickle cell gene.

Sickle cell trait is largely a benign carrier condition with no obvious laboratory hematologic manifestations under basal conditions: RBC morphology, RBC indices, and the reticulocyte count are normal, and sickle forms (ISCs) are not seen on the peripheral blood smear. The usual partition of Hb A and Hb S in sickle cell trait is 60:40 owing to a greater posttranslational affinity of α chains for β^A than for β^S chains.[6] When α-thalassemia is coinherited with sickle cell trait, the preferential affinity results in a decreased percentage of Hb S relative to the number of α-globin genes deleted (i.e., αα/αα 40% Hb S; −α/αα 35% Hb S; −α/−α 29% Hb S; —/−α 21% Hb S).[127]

There are a few clinical complications of sickle cell trait; splenic infarction occurs at high altitude.[239] It is a cause of hematuria and hyposthenuria.[240] The frequency of urinary tract infection may be increased. There is an association with renal medullary carcinoma.[208] There is an increased risk for venous thrombosis with an approximately twofold increase in risk and sickle trait explaining 7% of thrombotic episodes in African Americans.[241] Armed forces recruits in basic training with the sickle-cell trait have a substantially increased, age-dependent risk of exercise-related sudden death.[242]

Despite the known complications, past experiences with discrimination in the employment market and health insurance industry provide reminders that the rare clinical events in sickle cell trait provide no real justification for regarding it as anything but a benign carrier condition.[243] Newborn screening programs detect a large number of infants with sickle cell trait; for these parents, genetic counseling is essential. Parents should understand that their child has a benign hereditary condition with some risks as above but that there is a risk for a subsequent child to be born with SCD.

In individuals who appear to have sickle cell trait but are symptomatic, the laboratory diagnosis must be verified. Hemoglobins other than S that polymerize may account for reports of "sickle cell trait" associated with clinical problems. Examples are heterozygous Hb S Antilles and Hb Quebec-CHORI. In the latter case, the Hb variant was distinguished from Hb A using mass spectroscopy.

Hb SC Disease

The gene for Hb C ($\alpha_2\beta_2{}^{6}$Glu→Lys) is approximately one-fourth as frequent among African Americans as the sickle cell gene.[8] Although oxygenated Hb C forms crystals, Hb C does not participate in polymerization with deoxy-Hb S. However, HbC sustains potassium chloride cotransport and RBC dehydration, raising the intraerythrocytic concentration of Hb S to levels that support polymerization, sickling, and clinical symptoms. As a result of a longer circulatory survival of Hb SC RBCs compared with Hb SS cells (i.e., 27 versus 17 days),[124] the degree of anemia and reticulocytosis is frequently mild: 75% of the patients have a milder level of anemia (hematocrit level >28%) than is usually seen in sickle cell anemia. The predominant RBC abnormality on the peripheral smear is an abundance of target cells; folded ("pita bread") cells, ISCs, "billiard ball" cells, and crystal-containing cells may also be seen.

Splenomegaly may be the only physical finding, and the frequency of acute painful episodes is approximately half that in Hb SS disease, with a life expectancy two decades longer.[16] Nonetheless, significant morbidity can occur. The incidence of fatal bacterial infection is less than in sickle cell anemia, but there is still an increased risk of *S. pneumoniae* and *H. influenzae* infection. Osteonecrosis occurs in approximately 15% of patients.[244] There is a higher incidence of peripheral retinopathy in Hb SC disease than in sickle cell anemia. Coexistent α-thalassemia reduces risk of chronic organ complications.[244] There is an association between renal medullary carcinoma and Hb SC disease.

Sickle Cell–β-Thalassemia

The gene frequency of β-thalassemia among African Americans is 0.004, one-tenth that of the sickle cell gene,[8] and hence there is one-tenth the prevalence of compound heterozygous sickle cell–β-thalassemia in this population. Sickle cell–β-thalassemia is divided into sickle cell–β^+-thalassemia and sickle cell–β°-thalassemia, which have, respectively, reduced or no amounts of Hb A present. Most β-thalassemia mutations among African Americans result in β^+-thalassemia. Sickle cell–β^+-thalassemia is subclassified according to the percentage of Hb A present: type I has 3% to 5%, type II has 8% to 14%, and type III has 18% to 25%. Eighty percent of African American α-thalassemia mutations are attributable to the promoter region mutations [−88 (C to T) and −29 (A–G)] that result in a type III phenotype. Compound heterozygous sickle cell–β°-thalassemia occurs infrequently.

In sickle cell–β-thalassemia, the RBCs are hypochromic and microcytic. The ISCs present on the peripheral blood smear are more numerous in sickle cell–β°-thalassemia than in sickle cell–β^+-thalassemia. The hematologic and clinical severity is a function of the amount of Hb A inherited (Table 40-10).

Additional mitigating influences in sickle cell–β-thalassemia are elevated levels of Hb A_2 and, in sickle cell–β^+-thalassemia, levels of Hb A up to 30%. These affect both the solubility and polymerization of Hb S. Hb F is a more active inhibitor of polymerization than Hb A, as shown by Hb S solutions with 15% to 30% Hb A (resembling sickle cell–β^+-thalassemia) having delay times 10 to 100 times longer than pure Hb S solutions, and Hb S solutions with 20% to 30% Hb F (resembling Hb S–HPFH) having delay times 1000 to 1,000,000 times longer. A further influence mitigating the polymerization, sickling, and clinical aspects of sickle cell–β-thalassemia is the reduced MCHC, which retards Hb S polymerization. Hematologic values for sickle cell anemia, the sickle cell–β-thalassemias, and Hb S–HPFH are found in Table 40-10.

Sickle Cell–Hb Lepore Disease

The Hb Lepore gene is a crossover fusion product of the δ- and β-globin genes, the product of which, in the case of Hb Lepore Boston, has the same alkaline electrophoretic mobility as Hb S. Therefore, patients with the Hb Lepore trait can appear to have sickle cell trait but with only 12% Hb S from thalassemic expression of the abnormal fusion gene. Again, because of the electrophoretic similarity with Hb S, compound heterozygous Hb S–Hb Lepore Boston resembles sickle cell anemia or sickle cell–β°-thalassemia electrophoretically but clinically have less severe anemia, resembling that of sickle cell–β^+-thalassemia. The diagnosis is also suggested by the low to low-normal Hb A_2 levels that result from the incapacitation of one δ-globin gene by the crossover. Hb F levels vary. The peripheral smear shows microcytosis, hypochromia, and ISCs. Vasoocclusive complications occur, and splenomegaly is common.

Sickle Cell–Hb D Disease[245]

Because Hb D Punjab or Hb D Los Angeles ($\alpha_2\beta_2{}^{121}$Glu→Gln) has a similar electrophoretic mobility to Hb S under alkali conditions, Hb SD disease was first reported as an unusual case of sickle cell anemia. Hb D can be distinguished from Hb S by acid electrophoresis or isoelectric focusing. There is moderately severe hemolytic anemia, and the peripheral smear shows marked anisocytosis and poikilocytosis, target cells, and ISCs. The clinical manifestations of this syndrome are similar to those of sickle cell anemia.

Sickle Cell–Hb O Arab Disease[246]

Although Hb O Arab ($\alpha_2\beta_2{}^{121}$Glu→Lys) was first described in an Israeli Arab family, its distribution is widespread. Sickle cell–O Arab disease resembles Hb SC disease on alkaline electrophoresis, but Hb O Arab can be distinguished from Hb C by acid electrophoresis or isoelectric focusing. This syndrome is associated with moderately severe hemolytic anemia, and the peripheral smear shows anisocytosis, poikilocytosis, and ISCs.

Table 40-10 Hematologic Variables Associated With Sickle Cell Anemia and the Different Sickle Cell–β-Thalassemia Syndromes

Genotype	Hb*	%Hb A†	%Hb F†	%Hb A_2*	MCV*	Reticulocytes*	n
Hb SS‡	7.83	0	4.56	2.87	85.9	10.18	≈123
Hb S–β°-thalassemia‡	8.85	0	5.86	5.02	69.3	7.2	≈41
Hb S–β+-thalassemia, type I§	8.37	3-5	6.8	4.90	63.7	9.7	3
Hb S–β+-thalassemia, type II§	10.28	8-14	5.2	4.68	70.0	6.6	14
Hb S–β+-thalassemia, type III¶	11.55	18-25	5.1	4.66	73.3	1.27	76
Hb S-HPFH¶	14.6	0	25.8	1.95	81.7	2.4	4

*The mean data for each variable are shown. Units of measure are grams per deciliter for Hb, percentage of total hemoglobin for Hb F and A2, fl for MCV, and percentage of total red blood cells for reticulocytes.
†Percentage Hb A that defines the Hb S-β+-thalassemia type.[245]
‡Data from Serjeant et al.[247]
§Data from Christakis et al.[246]
¶Data from Serjeant et al.[248]
¶Data from Friedman et al.[249]
Hb, Hemoglobin; *HPFH,* persistence of fetal hemoglobin; *MCV,* mean corpuscular volume.

Sickle Cell–Hb E Disease[247]

Hb E ($\alpha_2\beta_2{}^{26}$Glu → Lys) is a β-thalassemic hemoglobinopathy found predominantly in southeast Asia (see Chapter 41). The structural mutant has an electrophoretic mobility similar to Hb C under alkaline conditions but can be resolved by acid electrophoresis or isoelectric focusing. The GAG→AAG mutation in codon 26 activates a cryptic splice site within the first intron of the β^E gene, causing alternate splicing and decreased expression of the structural mutant. As a result, Hb E makes up only 30% of the total Hb in compound heterozygosity for the sickle cell and Hb E genes. Hb SE disease is essentially benign in at least 50% and possibly most patients, with only mild hemolysis, no vasoocclusive complications, and no remarkable abnormality of RBC morphology. However, vasoocclusive complications and manifestations of chronic hemolytic anemia such as pain crisis, splenic infarction, recurrent pneumonia, and frontal bossing have been reported.

Coinherited Hemoglobin Abnormalities That Interact With Sickle Cell Disease: Hereditary Persistence of Fetal Hemoglobin and α-Thalassemia Trait

Sickle Cell–Hereditary Persistence of Fetal Hemoglobin

Adult Hb (or in the case of sickle cell anemia Hb S) replaces Hb F as a result of the switch from γ- to β-globin synthesis that occurs in fetuses. Because of the inhibitory effect of Hb F on Hb S polymerization and cellular sickling (see Chapter 42), the high fraction of Hb F at birth masks the expression of SCD until Hb S levels increase to 75% at approximately 6 months of age (see Fig. 40-3). Conditions that preserve elevated levels of Hb F into adulthood similarly modulate the course of SCD. The compound heterozygous conditions sickle–HPFH (Hb SS–HPFH) and sickle cell–β°-thalassemia–HPFH both have higher Hb F levels and milder clinical courses than are characteristic of sickle cell anemia.[117]

Hereditary persistence of Hb F results from one of several large deletions of the δ- and β-globin genes that retard the switch from the production of Hb F to adult Hb. A more recently discovered variety of HPFH is not caused by a deletion but by one of many point mutations that upregulate the expression of the γ-globin gene. The clinical expression of deletional and nondeletional HPFH differs in that the 15% to 35% Hb F in the former is distributed in a pancellular fashion, the 1% to 5% Hb F in the latter is distributed in a heterocellular fashion, and certain mild types of nondeletional HPFH express high Hb F levels not in simple heterozygosity but only in conditions of erythropoietic stress, such as compound heterozygosity with the sickle cell gene. It is likely that many cases of apparent sickle cell anemia with unexplained elevations of Hb F are the result of a nondeletion HPFH mutation.

The gene frequency of the deletional HPFH locus is 0.0005 among African Americans, resulting in a calculated incidence for compound heterozygous sickle cell–deletional HPFH of 1/100 that of sickle cell anemia. Sickle cell–deletional HPFH provided the first evidence that Hb F was a potent inhibitor of Hb S polymerization: individuals with pancellular distribution of 25% Hb F were generally neither anemic nor affected with vasoocclusive manifestations (see Table 40-10).[248] Hb electrophoresis revealed only Hb S, F, and A_2, which resembles sickle cell anemia, sickle cell–β°-thalassemia, and sickle cell–δβ°-thalassemia. Notable differences, however, are the pancellular distribution of 15% to 35% Hb F, Hb A_2 levels less than 2.5%, and the absence of anemia.[249] The generally benign course of sickle cell–deletional HPFH is uncommonly associated with vasoocclusive complication.

Sickle Cell Anemia With Coexistent α-Thalassemia

Prevalences of the silent carrier of α-thalassemia syndrome (genotype -α/αα) and α-thalassemia trait (genotype –α/–α) among African Americans are approximately 30% and 2%, respectively.[250] The peripheral blood smear contains less polychromasia and fewer sickle forms and more hypochromia and microcytosis, commensurate with the numbers of α-globin genes deleted. Increased Hb A_2 levels are associated with increasing α-globin gene deletions; the Hb F levels are not consistently affected.

Clinically, the impact of α-globin gene deletions on sickle cell is not as consistent as that of high Hb F.[21] Because of the powerful effect of Hb S concentration on the kinetics and extent of Hb S polymerization (see Chapter 42), the lower MCHC from α-globin gene deletions decreases the hemolytic rate, and anemia is milder in subjects with both α-thalassemia syndrome (genotype -α/αα) and trait (genotype –α/–α) (see Table 40-1). There is a decreased incidence of leg ulcers but an increased incidence of osteonecrosis. The frequency of retinal vessel closure is higher but not the incidence of retinopathy. Complications related to hemolysis (e.g., leg ulcers, chronic renal damage) may be decreased, but the heterogeneity of the patients in previous studies and mixed results make conclusions difficult. Similarly, the influence of α-gene deletions on survival in patients with SCD is not well understood.[21]

SUGGESTED READINGS

Austin H, Key NS, Benson JM, et al: Sickle cell trait and the risk of venous thromboembolism among blacks. *Blood* 110:908, 2007.

Goldstein LB, Adams R, Alberts MJ, et al: Primary prevention of ischemic stroke: A guideline from the American Heart Association/American Stroke Association Stroke Council: Cosponsored by the Atherosclerotic Peripheral Vascular Disease Interdisciplinary Working Group; Cardiovascular Nursing Council; Clinical Cardiology Council; Nutrition, Physical Activity, and Metabolism Council; and the Quality of Care and Outcomes Research Interdisciplinary Working Group. *Circulation* 113:e873, 2006.

Karam LB, Disco D, Jackson SM, et al: Liver biopsy results in patients with sickle cell disease on chronic transfusions: Poor correlation with ferritin levels. *Pediatr Blood Cancer* 50:62, 2008.

Knox-Macaulay HH, Ahmed MM, Gravell D, et al: Sickle cell-haemoglobin E (HbSE) compound heterozygosity: A clinical and haematological study. *Int J Lab Hematol* 29:292, 2007.

Machado RF, Anthi A, Steinberg MH, et al: N-terminal pro-brain natriuretic peptide levels and risk of death in sickle cell disease. *JAMA* 296:310, 2006.

Maggio A: Light and shadows in the iron chelation treatment of haematological diseases. *Br J Haematol* 138:407, 2007.

Manchikanti A, Grimes DA, Lopez LM, et al: Steroid hormones for contraception in women with sickle cell disease. *Cochrane Database Syst Rev* CD006261, 2007.

Pakbaz Z, Fischer R, Fung E, et al: Serum ferritin underestimates liver iron concentration in transfusion independent thalassemia patients as compared to regularly transfused thalassemia and sickle cell patients. *Pediatr Blood Cancer* 49:329, 2007.

Schleucher R, Gaessler M, Knobloch J: Rapid healing of a late diagnosed sickle cell leg ulcer using a new combination of treatment methods. *J Wound Care* 16:197, 2007.

Zimmerman SA, Schultz WH, Burgett S, et al: Hydroxyurea therapy lowers transcranial Doppler flow velocities in children with sickle cell anemia. *Blood* 110:1043, 2007.

For complete list of references log on to www.expertconsult.com.

CHAPTER 41

HEMOGLOBIN VARIANTS ASSOCIATED WITH HEMOLYTIC ANEMIA, ALTERED OXYGEN AFFINITY, AND METHEMOGLOBINEMIAS

Edward J. Benz, Jr., and Benjamin L. Ebert

Hemoglobinopathies are inherited diseases caused primarily by mutations affecting the globin genes. Nearly 1000 mutations that alter the structure, expression, or developmental regulation of individual globin genes, and the hemoglobins they encode, have been described; most do not produce clinical disease. Many are highly instructive for students of gene structure, function, and regulation, but further consideration of most is not warranted in a clinically oriented textbook. The gene mutations that cause sickle cell anemia and the thalassemia syndromes are by far the most important mutations that cause clinical morbidity, in terms of both the complexity of the clinical syndromes they cause and the number of patients affected. These conditions are considered in detail in other chapters (see Chapters 38, 39, and 40). This chapter reviews other abnormalities of the hemoglobin molecule that produce clinical syndromes. Each variant is uncommon. In the aggregate, however, hemoglobinopathies represent important problems for hematologists because they must be considered as possible causes for conditions about which hematologists are often consulted: hemolytic anemia, cyanosis, polycythemia, jaundice, rubor, splenomegaly, and reticulocytosis.

The major hemoglobinopathies producing clinical symptoms, other than sickle cell anemia and thalassemias, can be classified as those hemoglobins exhibiting altered solubility (unstable hemoglobins), hemoglobins with increased oxygen affinity, hemoglobins with decreased oxygen affinity, and methemoglobins (Table 41-1). A few acquired conditions in which toxic modifications of the hemoglobin molecule are important (e.g., carbon monoxide poisoning) are also considered briefly.

The sections that follow emphasize hemoglobinopathies that produce the most severe or dramatic alterations in clinical phenotype and those in which a single clinical abnormality (e.g., hemoglobin precipitation) predominates. It is important to emphasize at the outset, however, that although more than 100 mutations affect solubility or affinity, only a few are clinically important. The abnormal functional properties of most mutant hemoglobins can be detected readily in sophisticated research laboratories, but only a few mutant hemoglobins produce laboratory or clinical abnormalities relevant to clinical practice. Moreover, many mutations are pleiotropic, affecting several functional properties of the hemoglobin molecule. Thus a single mutation can increase oxygen affinity and reduce solubility, or produce methemoglobinemia and reduce solubility.

Table 41-2 summarizes the major forms of structurally abnormal hemoglobin, with examples. This table serves as a point of reference for the remaining sections of the chapter.

UNSTABLE HEMOGLOBINS

Unstable hemoglobins are hemoglobins exhibiting reduced solubility or higher susceptibility to oxidation of amino acid residues within the individual globin chains. More than 100 unique unstable hemoglobin mutants have been documented. Most exhibit only mild instability in in vitro laboratory tests and are associated with minimal clinical manifestations. Both α- and β-globin variants can cause this condition. Approximately 75% of the mutations described, however, are β-globin variants. This probably reflects the potential for α-globin variants to exert pathologic effects in utero. Clinical symptoms of unstable hemoglobins also depend in part on the quantitative proportion of the abnormal hemoglobin. Because the α-globin genes are duplicated, mutations in an individual locus generally produce only 25% to 35% abnormal globin. By contrast, a simple heterozygote at the single β-globin locus usually produces approximately 50% of the abnormal variant.

The mutations that impair hemoglobin solubility usually disrupt hydrogen bonding or the hydrophobic interactions that either retain the heme moiety within the heme-binding pockets or hold the tetramer together (Fig. 41-1). Some alter the helical segments (e.g., hemoglobin [Hb] Geneva [$\beta^{28\text{Leu}\rightarrow\text{Pro}}$]), others weaken contact points between the α and β subunits (e.g., Hb Philadelphia [$\beta^{35\text{Tyr}\rightarrow\text{Phe}}$]), and still others derange interactions of the hydrophobic pockets of the globin subunits with heme (e.g., Hb Köln [$\beta^{98\text{Val}\rightarrow\text{Met}}$]). The common pathway to reduced solubility invariably involves weakening of the binding of heme to globin. Actual loss of heme groups can occur, for example, in Hb Gun Hill, in which five amino acids, including the F8 histidine, are deleted. In other cases, mutations that introduce prolines into helical segments disrupt the helices and interfere with normal folding of the polypeptide around the heme group. Another feature of these mutations is disruption of the integrity of the tetrameric structure of globin chains. Only the intact hemoglobin tetramer can remain dissolved at the high concentrations that must be achieved within the circulating red blood cell (see Chapters 31 and 43).

Pathophysiology of Unstable Hemoglobin Disorders

The mechanisms by which unstable hemoglobin mutations produce hemoglobin precipitation remain incompletely understood. However, the major outlines of the process have been described (Fig. 41-2). The fundamental step in pathogenesis appears to be derangement of the normal linkages between heme and globin. Loss of appropriate globin chain folding and interaction may ultimately destabilize the heme-globin linkage or lead to partial proteolysis of the chain, thereby releasing heme from that linkage. Once freed from its cleft, heme probably binds nonspecifically to other regions of the globin molecule, forming precipitated hemichromes, which lead to further denaturation and aggregation of the globin subunits. These form a precipitate containing α- and β-globin chains, globin fragments, and heme, called the *Heinz body*.

Heinz bodies interact with delicate red blood cell membrane components (see Chapters 31 and 43), thereby reducing red blood cell deformability. These rigid cells tend to be detained in the splenic microcirculation and "pitted," reflecting attempts by the splenic macrophages to remove the Heinz bodies. Red blood cell damage can be aggravated by the release of free heme into the red blood cell. Several biochemical perturbations correlate with the presence of free heme, such as generation of reactive oxidants (i.e., hydrogen peroxide, superoxide, and hydroxyl radicals). The end result of this process is premature destruction of the red blood cell, producing hemolytic anemia.

Individual unstable hemoglobins vary in their propensity to generate Heinz bodies and hemolysis. For example, Hb Zurich exhibits relatively mild insolubility. Hemolysis is minimal in nonstressed patients with this variant and becomes clinically apparent only in the

Table 41-1 Classification of Hemoglobinopathies

Structural hemoglobinopathies—hemoglobins with altered amino acid sequences that result in deranged function or altered physical or chemical properties

ABNORMAL HEMOGLOBIN POLYMERIZATION—HBS

ALTERED OXYGEN AFFINITY

High affinity—polycythemia
Low affinity—cyanosis, pseudoanemia

HEMOGLOBINS THAT OXIDIZE READILY

Unstable hemoglobins, hemolytic anemia, jaundice
M hemoglobins—methemoglobinemia, cyanosis

THALASSEMIAS—DEFECTIVE PRODUCTION OF GLOBIN CHAINS

α-Thalassemias
β-Thalassemias
δβ-, γδβ-, αβ-Thalassemias
Structural hemoglobinopathies—structurally abnormal Hb associated with coinherited thalassemia phenotype
HbE
Hb Constant Spring
Hb Lepore

HEREDITARY PERSISTENCE OF FETAL HEMOGLOBIN—PERSISTENCE OF HIGH LEVELS OF HBF INTO ADULT LIFE

Pancellular—all red blood cells contain elevated HbF levels
Nondeletion forms
Deletion forms
Hb Kenya
Heterocellular—only specific subpopulation of red blood cells contain elevated levels of HbF

"ACQUIRED HEMOGLOBINOPATHIES"

Methemoglobin due to toxic exposures
Sulfhemoglobin due to toxic exposures
Carboxyhemoglobin
HbH in erythroleukemia
Elevated HbF in states of erythroid stress and bone marrow dysplasia, usually heterocellular

Hb, Hemoglobin.

presence of additional oxidant stresses, such as infection, fever, or the ingestion of oxidant agents. Because of the propensity of unstable hemoglobins to be hypersensitive to oxidation, some patients with unstable hemoglobins can exhibit episodic hemolysis in response to many of the same oxidative stressors as those exacerbating the clinical phenotype of glucose-6-phosphate dehydrogenase (G6PD)–deficient patients (see Chapter 42).

Patterns of Inheritance and Clinical Manifestations

Unstable hemoglobins are usually inherited as autosomal dominant disorders. However, the rate of spontaneous mutation appears to be high, so the absence of affected parents or siblings does not rule out the presence of an unstable hemoglobin in an individual family. Nonetheless, the presence of a positive family history can be a useful adjunct to diagnosis and should provoke consideration of an unstable hemoglobin as the cause of the familial hemolytic diathesis.

The clinical syndrome associated with unstable hemoglobin disorders is often called *congenital Heinz body hemolytic anemia.* This term derives from the fact that only the most severe cases were detected before the widespread availability of sophisticated methods for detecting and characterizing abnormal hemoglobins. Clinical manifestations are highly variable, ranging from a virtually asymptomatic state in the absence of environmental stressors to severe

Table 41-2 Mutations Producing Abnormal Hemoglobin Molecules*

Residue	Mutation	Common Name(s)	Molecular Pathology
ABNORMAL SOLUBILITY			
β6	Glu→Val	S	Polymerization
β6	Glu→Lys	C	Crystallization
β121	Glu→Gln	D-Los Angeles, D-Punjab	Increases polymer in S/D heterozygote
β121	Glu→Lys	O-Arab	Increases polymer in S/O heterozygote
INCREASED OXYGEN AFFINITY			
α92	Arg→Gln	J-Capetown	Stabilizes R state
α141	Arg→His	Suresnes	Eliminates bond to Asn 126 in T state
β89	Ser→Asn	Creteil	Weakens bonds in T state
β99	Asp→Asn	Kempsey	Breaks T state intersubunit bonds
DECREASED OXYGEN AFFINITY			
α94	Asp→Asn	Titusville	Alters R state intersubunit bonds
β102	Asn→Thr	Kansas	Breaks R state intersubunit bonds
β102	Asn→Ser	Beth Israel	Breaks R state intersubunit bonds
METHEMOGLOBIN			
α58	His→Tyr	M-Boston, M-Osaka	Heme liganded to Tyr not His
α87	His→Tyr	M-Iwate	Heme liganded to both His and Tyr
β28	Leu→Gln	St Louis	Opens heme pocket
β63	His→Tyr	M-Saskatoon	Tyr ligand stabilizes ferriheme
β67	Val→Glu	M-Milwaukee-I	Negative charge stabilizes ferriheme
β92	His→Tyr	M-Hyde Park	Bond of His to heme disrupted
UNSTABLE			
α43	Phe→Val	Torino	Loss of heme contact
ν94	Asp→Tyr	Setif	Alters subunit contacts
β28	Leu→Gln	St Louis	Polar group in heme pocket
β35	Tyr→Phe	Philadelphia	Loss of dimer bond favors precipitation
β42	Phe→Ser	Hammersmith	Loss of heme
β63	His→Arg	Zurich	Opens heme pocket
β88	Leu→Pro	Santa Ana	Disrupts helix
β91	Leu→Pro	Sabine	Disrupts helix
β91-95	Deletion	Gun Hill	Shortens F helix
β98	Val→Met	Köln	Alters heme contact

Modified from Dickerson RE, Geis I: *Hemoglobin: Structure, function, evolution, and pathology.* Menlo Park, Calif, 1983, Benjamin-Cummings. Copyright Irving Geis.
*Partial list includes some of the most widely studied hemoglobin structural mutations.

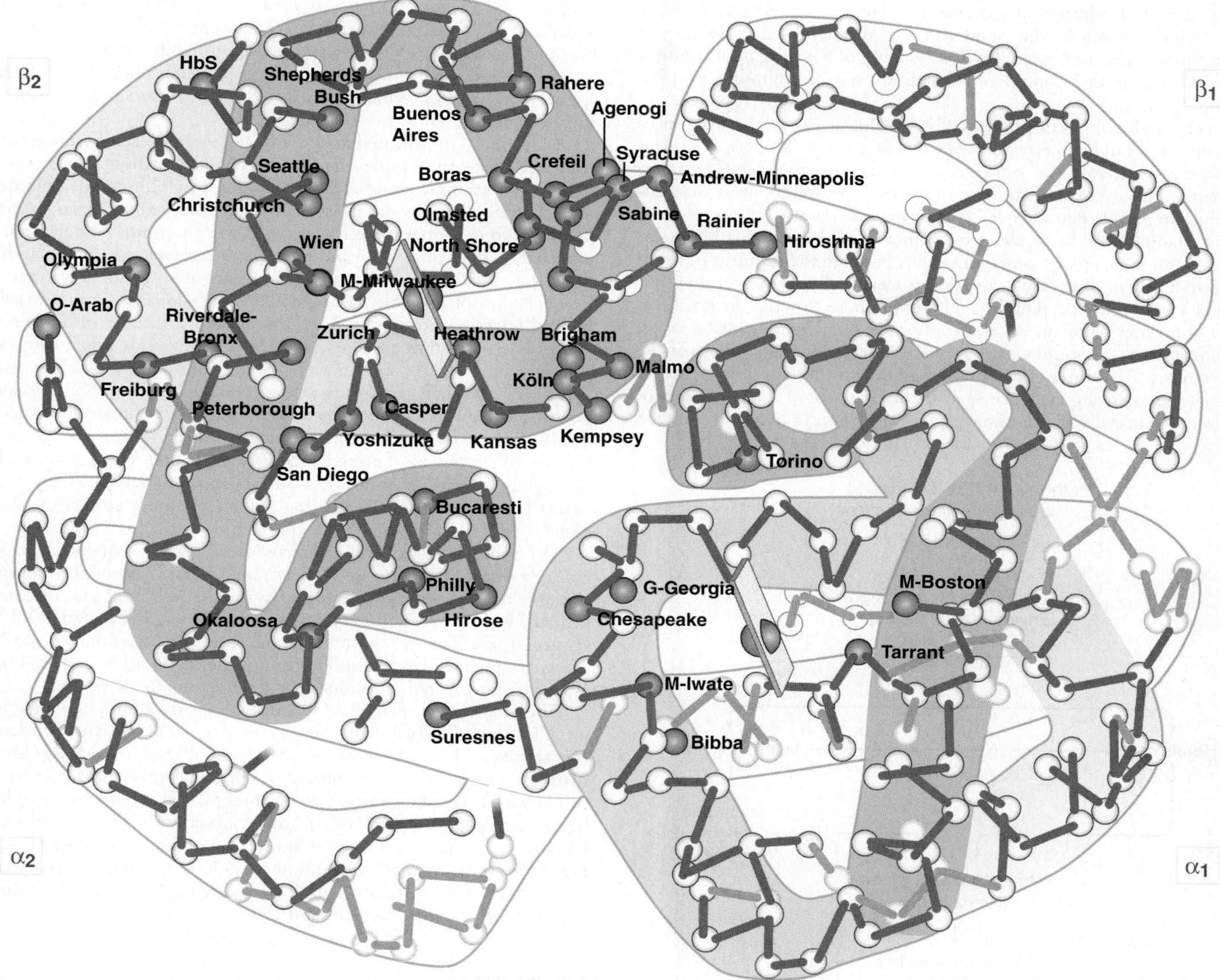

Figure 41-1 HEMOGLOBIN TETRAMER SHOWING THE POSITION OF THE MORE COMMON, CLINICALLY SIGNIFICANT HEMOGLOBIN MUTANTS. Most of those that have been described occur on the β-chain at invariant residue sites, near critical intermolecular contacts, or in proximity to the prosthetic heme-binding site. *(Modified from Dickerson RE, Geis I:* Hemoglobin: Structure, function, evolution, and pathology, *Menlo Park, Calif, 1983, Benjamin-Cummings. Copyright Irving Geis.)*

hemolytic anemia manifesting at birth. Patients with chronic hemolysis present with variable degrees of typical symptoms, including anemia, reticulocytosis, hepatosplenomegaly, jaundice, leg ulcers, and a propensity toward premature biliary tract disease.

For hemoglobin variants with a given degree of reduced solubility, the degree of anemia may fluctuate because some of these variants also exhibit altered oxygen affinity. Thus Hb Köln has increased oxygen affinity, resulting in relatively higher levels of tissue hypoxia and erythropoietin stimulation at any given level of hematocrit (see Diagnosis); therefore patients with Hb Köln tend to have higher hematocrit levels than expected on the basis of hemolytic severity because of increased erythropoietin stimulation. By contrast, Hb Hammersmith exhibits decreased oxygen affinity, improving oxygen delivery and allowing patients to function at a lower hematocrit level. Hb Zurich possesses, for complex molecular reasons, a higher-than-normal affinity for carbon monoxide. A high hemoglobin carbon monoxide level develops in patients with Hb Zurich who also smoke. Binding of carbon monoxide protects Hb Zurich from denaturation, thus reducing hemolysis, so these people tend to exhibit lesser degrees of hemolytic anemia than do nonsmoking relatives.

Diagnosis

The presence of an unstable hemoglobin should be suspected in patients with one or more stigmata of accelerated red blood cell destruction: chronic or intermittent hemolytic anemia or jaundice, premature development of bilirubin gallstones or biliary tract disease (as a result of accelerated red blood cell turnover), unexplained reticulocytosis, or bouts of intermittent symptoms that can be related to exposure to oxidant drugs or infections. Other suggestive symptoms include dark urine, transient jaundice, and leg ulcers.

Laboratory diagnosis depends on identification of a mutant hemoglobin that precipitates more easily than normal hemoglobin. The peripheral blood smear may or may not show evidence of hemolysis (i.e., poikilocytosis, polychromasia, or shift cells; Fig. 41-3, *A*). The morphologic evidence for precipitated hemoglobin is the Heinz body, the intraerythrocytic inclusion body detected by staining the peripheral blood smear with a supravital dye, such as brilliant cresyl blue or new methylene blue (see Fig. 41-3, *B, C*). The spleen removes Heinz bodies efficiently, especially if hemolysis is not particularly acute or brisk. Thus Heinz bodies may not be demonstrable at all times. Two provocative laboratory maneuvers are used to aid detection, both of which unmask the tendency of unstable hemoglobins to precipitate: the heat instability test (heating of a hemoglobin solution to 50° C) or the isopropanol instability test (insolubility in 17% isopropanol).

Hemoglobin electrophoresis or hemoglobin analysis by mass spectrometry should be performed but *should not be relied on as the major diagnostic criterion for ruling in or ruling out a hemoglobinopathy.* Many amino acid substitutions that have a profound effect on solubility do not change the overall charge on the hemoglobin molecule. For example, Hb Köln, the most common of the unstable hemoglobin mutations, arises from a mutation changing the valine at position 98 to a methionine. This mutation is electrically neutral; it does not alter electrophoretic mobility. Therefore these variants do not form an abnormal band on an electrophoresis gel. Demonstration of an abnormal band would clearly add strong evidence in support of the diagnosis. A normal electrophoretogram, however, should never be regarded as strong evidence against the presence of a mutant hemoglobin, especially if the clinical picture or family history otherwise supports the diagnosis. Mass spectrometry analysis of hemoglobin and direct globin gene sequencing are supplanting electrophoresis as diagnostic strategies. They usually provide unambiguous identification of the sequence abnormality. However, electrophoresis is still in use in many clinical settings. Thus the aforementioned precautions in interpretation are still worth noting.

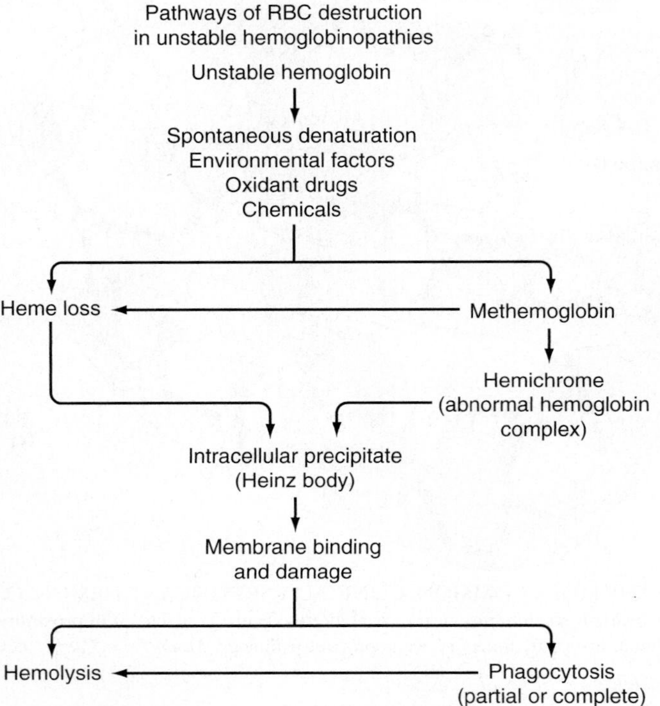

Figure 41-2 PRESUMED MECHANISMS BY WHICH DENATURATION OF HEMOGLOBIN LEADS TO ERYTHROCYTE DESTRUCTION. The rate of travel through the various pathways probably differs for the different hemoglobin variants and for a variety of stresses to which the protein is subjected. *RBC,* Red blood cell. *(From Wynngaarden JB, Smith LH Jr, Bennett JC, editors:* Cecil textbook of medicine, *Philadelphia, 1992, WB Saunders.)*

Additional sophisticated analyses of hemoglobin can be obtained from reference laboratories if detailed characterization seems warranted. For example, abnormal hemoglobin or globin bands migrating to novel positions on an isoelectric focusing gel can result from hemoglobin or globin moieties lacking heme in groups. When heme is added to the sample and the proteins are reanalyzed, these bands disappear. This behavior is nearly diagnostic of an unstable variant.

Detection of unstable hemoglobins is occasionally compromised by the selective precipitation of the unstable variant into Heinz bodies. Because most patients are heterozygotes, this phenomenon greatly reduces the apparent percentage of the variant in soluble form. Thus even a variant possessing altered electrophoretic mobility may be very difficult to detect. Indeed, some unstable hemoglobins, such as Hb Geneva or Hb Terre Haute, are so unstable that no mutant gene product can be detected in the steady state. These abnormal hemoglobins actually produce a thalassemic phenotype. They are detectable only by isotope labeling studies or direct analysis of the globin genes.

The amino acid sequence predicted from genetic sequencing may rarely be inaccurate because of posttranslational conversion into an unstable hemoglobin. For example, in the first reported case of congenital Heinz body hemolytic anemia due to Hb Bristol, the DNA sequence predicts a valine-to-methionine substitution at β67. Through posttranslational modification, the methionine is altered to aspartate, a hydrophilic residue that disrupts the heme pocket.

The differential diagnosis of unstable hemoglobin variants is usually straightforward if the general category of hemolytic disorders is suspected. The most common form of G6PD deficiency can also manifest with bouts of intermittent or chronic hemolysis exacerbated by oxidant drugs or infection (see Chapter 42). This diagnosis should be considered, as should other causes of chronic or intermittent hemolytic anemia, such as red blood cell membrane disorders (e.g., hereditary spherocytosis) or immune hemolytic anemias. Spherocytes are relatively rare in patients with unstable hemoglobin disorders; this is sometimes a useful discriminant.

Management

The severity of the clinical complications of unstable hemoglobins varies enormously. Many patients can be managed adequately by observation and education to avoid agents that provoke hemolysis. Some patients require transfusions during bouts of severe acute hemolytic anemia. Patients who have significant morbidity because of chronic anemia or repeated episodes of severe hemolysis should be considered candidates for splenectomy, especially if hypersplenism has developed. Children with severe hemolysis may require transfusion support until they are old enough (at least 3 or 4 years of age) to undergo splenectomy without unacceptable immunologic compromise. Splenectomy is usually effective for abolition or reduction

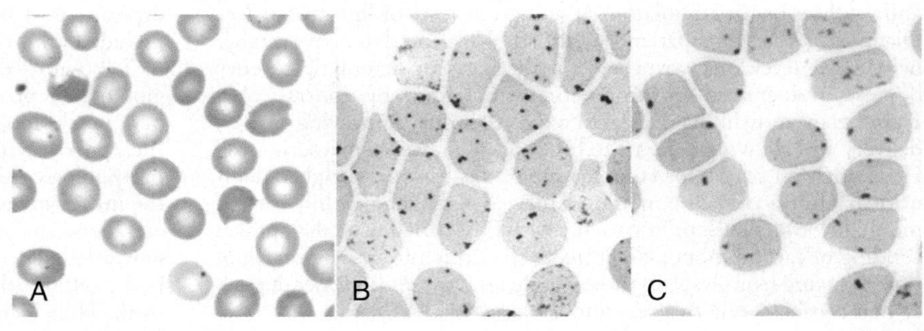

Figure 41-3 UNSTABLE HEMOGLOBINS; PERIPHERAL BLOOD SMEAR AND HEINZ BODY PREPARATION. The peripheral smear **(A)** shows "bite" cells with pitted-out semicircular areas of the red blood cell membrane as a result of removal of Heinz bodies by macrophages in the spleen. The Heinz body preparation **(B)** shows increased Heinz bodies in the same specimen, when compared to a control **(C)**.

of anemia. However, splenectomy should be used only as a last resort because of the long-term risks of overwhelming sepsis and thrombosis. Infection often exacerbates hemolysis. Fever should therefore prompt close monitoring of patients for evidence of hemolysis or infection.

HEMOGLOBINS WITH INCREASED OXYGEN AFFINITY

Efficient oxygen delivery by hemoglobin depends on the sigmoid shape of the hemoglobin-oxygen affinity curve. During the transition from the fully deoxygenated to the fully oxygenated state, the initial oxygenation steps occur with difficulty. In fact, the act of binding the first oxygen molecule increases the affinity of the molecule for subsequent oxygen-binding events, thus creating the sigmoid shape of the curve. The necessary intramolecular reorganization occurs only when the precise arrangement of hydrogen bonds, hydrophobic interactions, and salt bridges is broken and formed in the proper sequence.

Mutant hemoglobins exhibiting altered oxygen affinity arise from amino acid substitutions at the interface between α- and β-chains or in regions affecting the hydrogen bonds, hydrophobic interactions, or salt bridges that influence the interaction of heme with oxygen. A second major class of mutations alters binding to 2,3-diphosphoglycerate (2,3-DPG), which in turn alters oxygen affinity when bound to hemoglobin.

Pathogenesis and Pathophysiology

High-affinity hemoglobins exhibit higher avidity for oxygen, causing the oxygen dissociation curve to shift to the left; an example is Hb Kempsey ($\beta^{99Asp\rightarrow Asn}$) (Fig. 41-4). These hemoglobins bind oxygen more readily than normal and retain more oxygen at lower partial pressure of oxygen (Po_2) levels. They thus deliver less oxygen to tissues at normal capillary oxygen pressures. The PO_2 in the normal lung (90 to 100 mm Hg) is well above that needed to saturate hemoglobin fully with oxygen (60 mm Hg). These variant hemoglobins cannot acquire any additional oxygen in the lung despite their higher affinity. At capillary PO_2 (35 to 45 mm Hg), however, high-affinity hemoglobins deliver *less* oxygen. At normal hematocrit levels, a mild tissue hypoxia results, triggering increased production of erythropoietin and red blood cells, thus resulting in polycythemia. In extreme cases, hematocrit levels of 60% to 65% can be encountered.

Many types of mutations can increase oxygen affinity. Some alter interactions within the heme pocket, others disrupt the Bohr effect or the salt-bond site, and still others impair the binding of HbA to 2,3-DPG. Loss of 2,3-DPG binding results in increases in oxygen affinity. These and numerous other examples that have been analyzed at the molecular level have greatly aided our understanding of the molecular basis for reversible oxygen binding.

Diagnosis

High-affinity hemoglobins are a cause of familial unexplained erythrocytosis (see Chapters 24 and 67). Functional testing of the hemoglobin is the key to diagnosis. Oxygen affinity is usually measured as P_{50}, the Po_2 at which hemoglobin is 50% saturated with oxygen (see Fig. 41-4). The hemoglobin preparation is exposed to increasing oxygen pressures, and the relative percentages of oxyhemoglobin and deoxyhemoglobin are determined. The values are plotted on a curve, and the 50% saturation point is determined. A shift to the left means that the hemoglobin reaches 50% saturation at a lower Po_2. High-affinity variants are thus associated with a lower-than-normal P_{50} value. Hemoglobin electrophoresis can, but may not, reveal an abnormal band.

The most common cause of a low P_{50} value is carbon monoxide. Carbon monoxide stabilizes hemoglobin in the R "oxy" state without the need for oxygen binding. The oxygen affinity curve is therefore

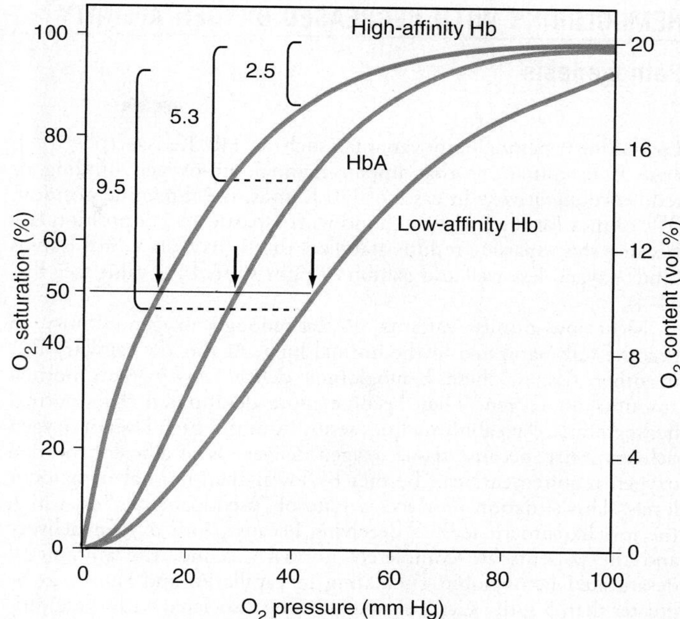

Figure 41-4 HEMOGLOBIN-OXYGEN DISSOCIATION CURVES ARE ILLUSTRATED FOR NORMAL HEMOGLOBIN (HBA) AND FOR MODEL ABNORMAL HEMOGLOBINS WITH HIGH AND LOW OXYGEN AFFINITIES. On the abscissa, the partial pressure of oxygen (Po_2) is indicated in millimeters of mercury. On the left ordinate, the saturation of hemoglobin with oxygen is indicated as a percentage; on the right ordinate, the oxygen content of the hemoglobin is expressed as volume percent. The three inverted arrows show the Po_2 at which the hemoglobin is 50% saturated (P_{50}) for the three hemoglobins. This value is lowest for the high-affinity hemoglobin. As the Po_2 drops from 100 (arterial) to 40 (tissues) mm Hg, hemoglobin desaturates, giving up a portion of its bound oxygen; the numbers on the brackets indicate the amount of oxygen unloaded by the three hemoglobin types expressed as volume percent. Note that the high-affinity hemoglobin delivers less than one-half the oxygen that HbA gives to the tissues, resulting in tissue anoxia, increased erythropoietin secretion, and erythrocytosis. Conversely, the low-affinity hemoglobin is even more efficient than HbA in supplying tissues with oxygen, resulting in diminished erythropoietin production and anemia. *(From Wynngaarden JB, Smith LH Jr, Bennett JC, editors:* Cecil textbook of medicine, *Philadelphia, 1992, WB Saunders.)*

extremely left shifted and is hyperbolic, rather than sigmoidal, in shape. The clinical consequences of mild chronic carbon monoxide poisoning are the same as those seen with high-affinity hemoglobin variants. The most common cause of carbon monoxide toxicity is cigarette smoking, although chronic carbon monoxide exposure can elevate the hematocrit level in people such as caisson workers or tunnel toll collectors. Severe acute carbon monoxide poisoning can cause rapid death as a result of tissue hypoxia.

Management

Most patients with high-affinity hemoglobins have mild erythrocytosis; they do not require intervention. Very rarely, the hematocrit level is very high (>55% to 60%). The blood viscosity is then sufficiently elevated to require therapeutic phlebotomy. Carbon monoxide poisoning is treated with supplemental oxygen. When a patient breathes room air, the half-life of carboxyhemoglobin is 4 to 6 hours, but the half-life is 40 to 80 minutes with the use of normobaric oxygen and 15 to 30 minutes with the use of hyperbaric oxygen. Carbon monoxide detectors, designed to detect occult carbon monoxide poisoning, are now required in many municipalities and are predicted to prevent numerous fatalities from occult carbon monoxide poisoning.

HEMOGLOBINS WITH DECREASED OXYGEN AFFINITY

Pathogenesis

Low-affinity hemoglobin variants, such as Hb Kansas ($\beta^{102Asn\rightarrow Thr}$), arise from mutations that impair hemoglobin-oxygen binding or reduce cooperativity. In cases of Hb Kansas, the threonine position, β^{102}, cannot form a hydrogen bond with aspartic acid at position α^{94}. Because this aspartate residue stabilizes the R (oxy) state, Hb Kansas binds oxygen less well and exhibits a right-shifted P_{50} value (see Fig. 41-4).

Most low-affinity variants possess enough oxygen affinity to become fully saturated in the normal lung. At the low capillary PO_2 in other tissues, these hemoglobins deliver *higher* than normal amounts of oxygen. They become more desaturated than normal hemoglobins. Two abnormalities result from this high level of oxygen delivery. First, because tissue oxygen delivery is so efficient, normal oxygen requirements can be met by lower-than-normal hematocrit levels. This situation produces a state of "pseudoanemia," in which the low hematocrit level is deceiving because both oxygen delivery and the patients are completely normal. Second, the amount of desaturated hemoglobin circulating in capillaries and veins can be greater than 5 g/dL. Cyanosis may thus be associated with these variants. This usually ominous finding is entirely misleading in these individuals, because it reflects no morbidity.

Diagnosis

Patients with unexplained anemia or cyanosis who appear to be entirely well in all other respects should be evaluated, especially if there is a positive family history. Testing for the abnormal variant follows the same reasoning as that just described for high-affinity variants. The oxygen dissociation curve will be shifted to the right, and the numeric value of the P_{50} will be higher than normal.

Management

Patients with low-affinity hemoglobins are usually asymptomatic. No treatment is required. It is important to document that a low-affinity hemoglobin is the cause of an apparent anemia or cyanosis to preempt inappropriate workups and provide reassurance to the patient. Cyanosis in some patients can pose a cosmetic problem, but correction with transfusions is rarely justified.

METHEMOGLOBINEMIAS

Methemoglobin results from oxidation of the iron moieties in hemoglobin from the ferrous (Fe^{2+}) to the ferric (Fe^{3+}) state. Normal oxygenation of hemoglobin causes a partial transfer of an electron from the iron to the bound oxygen. Iron in this state thus resembles ferric iron and the oxygen resembles superoxide (O_2^-). Deoxygenation returns the electron to the iron, with release of oxygen. Methemoglobin forms if the electron is not returned. Methemoglobin constitutes 3% or less of the total hemoglobin in normal humans. Under normal circumstances, these levels in humans are maintained at 1% or less by the methemoglobin reductase enzyme system (the reduced form of nicotinamide adenine dinucleotide [NADH]–dehydratase, [NADH]-diaphorase, erythrocyte cytochrome b_5).

Pathogenesis and Clinical Manifestations

Methemoglobinemias of clinical interest arise by one of three distinct mechanisms: (1) globin chain mutations that result in increased formation of methemoglobin, (2) deficiencies of methemoglobin reductase, and (3) "toxic" methemoglobinemia, in which normal red blood cells are exposed to substances that oxidize hemoglobin iron to such a degree that normal reducing mechanisms are subverted or overwhelmed (see Chapter 42; Table 41-3).

Table 41-3 Types of Methemoglobinemia

CONGENITAL
Defective enzymatic reduction of Fe^{3+}-hemoglobin to Fe^{2+}-hemoglobin
NADH-methemoglobin reductase (cytochrome-b_5 reductase) deficiency
Cytochrome b_5 deficiency
Abnormal hemoglobins resistant to enzymatic reduction (M hemoglobins)
ACQUIRED
Excessive (toxic) oxidation of Fe^{2+}-hemoglobin
Environmental chemicals
DRUGS

NADH, Reduced form of nicotinamide adenine dinucleotide.

Abnormal hemoglobins producing methemoglobinemia (M hemoglobins) arise from mutations that stabilize the heme iron in the ferric state. Classically a histidine in the vicinity of the heme pocket is replaced by a tyrosine; the hydroxyl group of the tyrosine forms a complex that stabilizes the iron in the ferric state (Fig. 41-5). The oxidized heme iron is relatively resistant to reduction by the methemoglobin reductase system.

Methemoglobin has a brownish to blue color that does not revert to red on exposure to oxygen. Patients with methemoglobinemia thus appear to be cyanotic. In contrast to truly cyanotic people, however, aterial partial pressure of oxygen (PaO_2) values are usually normal. Patients with these hemoglobins are otherwise asymptomatic because methemoglobin is rarely greater than 30% to 50%, the levels at which symptoms becomes apparent.

Hereditary methemoglobinemia resulting from methemoglobin reductase deficiency (cytochrome-b_5 reductase deficiency) is very rare. Mutations in the b_5 reductase gene cause two distinct phenotypes. In cases of type I methemoglobin reductase deficiency, patients suffer solely from cyanosis; in cases of type II disease, patients manifest both cyanosis and severe mental retardation. One isoform of the b_5 reductase gene is expressed in diverse tissues for participation in a variety of cellular processes. A second isoform, produced by alternative splicing, is expressed in erythrocytes, producing a soluble protein that reduces methemoglobin. Mutations causing type I methemoglobin reductase deficiency occur throughout the gene and result in an unstable protein. Such mutations are primarily significant in erythrocytes that, without nuclei, cannot replace the degraded protein. Mutations causing type II disease occur in the critical NADH or flavin adenine dinucleotide (FAD)–binding domains, causing inactivation of the protein in all tissues and the more severe clinical phenotype.

Like patients with M hemoglobins, patients with methemoglobin reductase deficiency exhibit slate-gray "pseudocyanosis." Even homozygotes, however, rarely accumulate more than 25% methemoglobin, a level compatible with minimal symptoms. Heterozygotes can have normal methemoglobin levels but are especially sensitive to agents causing methemoglobinemia.

A third toxic form of methemoglobinemia is caused by exposure to certain chemical agents and drugs that accelerate the oxidation of methemoglobin (Table 41-4). Some compounds directly oxidize hemoglobin, whereas other compounds produce reactive oxygen intermediates that oxidize hemoglobin. Nitrite compounds are especially notorious and common. Some of these compounds also have a propensity to exacerbate G6PD deficiency and the precipitation of unstable hemoglobins.

Nitrates are a frequent environmental cause of toxic methemoglobinemia. Nitrates do not directly interact with either hemoglobin or the reductase pathway but are converted to nitrites in the gut. Well

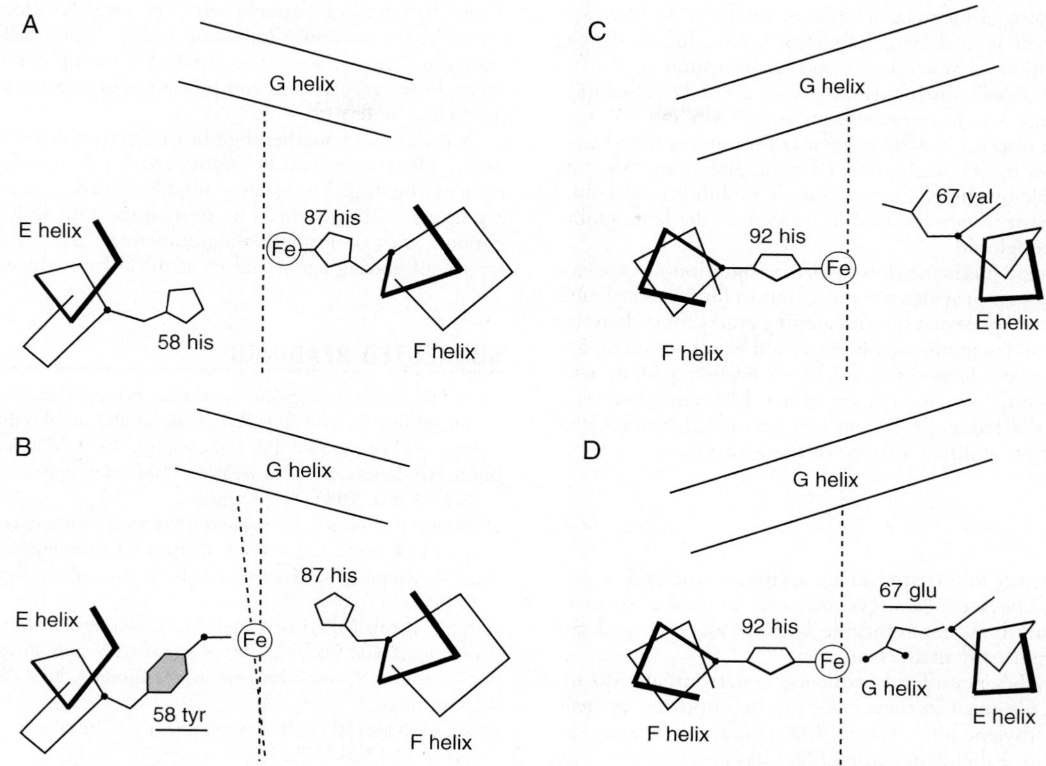

Figure 41-5 MODIFICATIONS OF THE HEME AND ITS ENVIRONMENT THAT ACCOUNT FOR TWO COMMON M HEMOGLOBINS. **A,** Hemoglobin A has a His residue at the α58(E7) position. **B,** In hemoglobin M-Boston, the histidine is replaced by a tyrosine, the phenolic side chain of which is capable of covalently binding to the heme iron, resulting in stabilization in the oxidized form. **C,** HbA has a Val residue at position β67(E11). **D,** Hb M-Milwaukee has a glutamic acid substitution for the β67 valine. The carboxylic side chain of the Glu forms a bond with iron, shifting the equilibrium toward the ferric state. *(Modified from Dickerson RE, Geis I:* Hemoglobin: Structure, function, evolution, and pathology, *Menlo Park, Calif, 1983, Benjamin-Cummings. Copyright Irving Geis.)*

Table 41-4 Drugs and Chemicals Having Toxic Effects on Hemoglobin Molecule

	Observed Hemoglobin Derivative	
Agent	***Methemoglobin***	***Sulfhemoglobin***
Acetanilid, phenacetin	+	+
Nitrites (ferryic, amyl, sodium, potassium, nitroglycerin)	+	+
Trinitrotoluene, nitrobenzene	+	+
Aniline, hydroxylamine dimethylamine	+	+
Sulfanilamide	+	+
p-Aminosalicylic acid	+	
Dapsone	+	
Primaquine, chloroquine	+	
Prilocaine, benzocaine, lidocaine	+	
Menadione, naphthoquinone	+	
Naphthalene	+	
Resorcinol	+	
Phenylhydrazine	+	+

water is a frequently encountered source of excessive nitrates. In general, substantial intake of these agents is required before significant amounts of methemoglobin are generated. Very young infants have lower levels of methemoglobin reductase in erythrocytes and are therefore more susceptible to these agents than are adults. However, all age-groups are at risk, given sufficient exposure. Systemic acidosis, particularly in young infants suffering from diarrhea and dehydration, can also cause clinically significant methemoglobinemia.

Acquired methemoglobinemia is virtually the only situation in which life-threatening amounts of methemoglobin accumulate. In general the only symptom produced when methemoglobin constitutes less than 30% of total hemoglobin is the cosmetic effect of cyanosis. As levels of methemoglobin rise to greater than 30%, however, patients begin to exhibit symptoms of oxygen deprivation, such as malaise, giddiness, and other alterations of mental status. The symptoms reflect a true lack of oxygen availability at the tissue level. Methemoglobin is a markedly left-shifted hemoglobin that delivers little oxygen to the tissues. When methemoglobin accounts for more than 50% of total hemoglobin, loss of consciousness, coma, and death can rapidly ensue. At this level the blood is chocolate brown.

Diagnosis

Methemoglobinemia should be suspected in patients with unexplained cyanosis. It is obviously a medical emergency when any patient has cyanosis and altered mental status; a normal PaO_2 should trigger a consideration of methemoglobinemia. The ingestion of nitrites as a suicidal gesture, especially in people knowledgeable with respect to chemistry, medicine, or pharmacology, should be considered. Methemoglobinemia can be suspected from the brownish color of blood when it is drawn. Laboratory detection is simple; methemoglobin exhibits characteristic peaks of absorption at 630 and 502 nm, rendering it easily distinguishable from normal hemoglobin. Pulse oximetry, using a ratio of absorption at 660 nm and 940 nm, gives an inaccurate reading of 85% oxygen saturation for blood with 100% methemoglobin. The inherited M hemoglobin mutants are frequently detectable by altered electrophoretic mobility, especially if ferricyanide treatment in vitro is used to convert all the hemoglobin solution to methemoglobin.

In the case of toxic methemoglobinemia, recognition of exposure to an appropriate agent provides the most important historical clue. Acute poisoning can represent a life-threatening emergency; therefore laboratory evaluation for methemoglobin should be requested for any person displaying atypical cyanosis or cyanosis occurring along with more normal than anticipated blood gas values. Methemoglobin due to deficiencies of the reductase system can be further evaluated in reference laboratories by direct analysis of these enzymes.

Management

Patients with M hemoglobins are usually asymptomatic and require no management. The secondary cyanosis can present a cosmetic problem. The cyanosis is not reversible because ascorbic acid and methylene blue are usually ineffective.

Patients with deficiency of the reductase system usually do not require treatment. Cyanosis in these cases can be improved by treatment with oral methylene blue, 100 to 300 mg/day, or 500 mg/day of oral ascorbic acid. Riboflavin (20 mg/day) has also been reported to be effective and may be the preferred agent, because methylene blue produces discolored (blue) urine, and ascorbic acid can cause sodium oxalate stones.

Emergency treatment of high levels of toxic methemoglobinemia begins with 1 to 2 mg/kg of intravenous methylene blue as a 1% solution in saline. It is usually infused rapidly (over 3 to 5 minutes); the dose can be repeated at 1 mg/kg after 30 minutes if necessary. This treatment is usually effective. Methylene blue acts through the reduced form of nicotinamide adenine dinucleotide (NADPH) reductase system, which in turn requires G6PD activity. The method is therefore ineffective in patients who also have G6PD deficiency. These patients, or patients who are severely affected, may require exchange transfusion. Oral ascorbic acid is not useful for emergency situations because it acts too slowly. Follow-up maintenance management, however, can be accomplished with either ascorbic acid or oral methylene blue.

Mild cases of methemoglobin intoxication do not require treatment. The patient can be monitored for 1 to 3 days, during which time methemoglobin levels gradually return to normal if the offending agent is eliminated. The most important follow-up therapy for patients with toxic methemoglobinemia involves a thorough search for the offending agent and its removal from the environment.

SUGGESTED READINGS

Bunn HF: Sickle hemoglobin and other hemoglobin mutants. In Stamatoyannopoulos G, Nienhuis AW, Majerus PO, et al, editors: *The molecular basis of blood disease,* ed 2, Philadelphia, 1993, WB Saunders.

Bunn HF, Forget BG: *Hemoglobin: Molecular, cellular and clinical aspects,* Philadelphia, 1985, WB Saunders.

Dickerson RE, Geis I: *Hemoglobin: Structure, function, evolution, and pathology,* Menlo Park, Calif, 1983, Benjamin-Cummings.

Ernst A, Zibrak J: Carbon monoxide poisoning. *N Engl J Med* 339:1603, 1998.

Fermi G, Perutz MF: *Atlas of molecular structures in biology. Vol. 2: Hemoglobin and myoglobin,* Oxford, 1981, Oxford University Press.

Ho C, editor: *Hemoglobin and oxygen binding,* New York, 1982, Elsevier Biomedical.

Park CM, Nagel RL: Sulfhemoglobinemia: Clinical and molecular aspects. *N Engl J Med* 310:1579, 1984.

Perutz MF: Molecular anatomy, physiology, and pathology of hemoglobin. In Stamatoyannopoulos G, Nienhuis AW, Leder P, et al, editors: *The molecular basis of blood diseases,* Philadelphia, 1987, WB Saunders, p 127.

Smith RP, Olson MV: Drug-induced methemoglobinemia. *Semin hematol* 10:253, 1973.

Wishner BC, Ward KB, Lattman EE, et al: Crystal structure of sickle-cell deoxyhemoglobin at 5Å resolution. *J Mol Biol* 98:179, 1975.

Wright RO, Lewander WJ, Woolf AD: Methemoglobinemia: Etiology, pharmacology, and clinical management. *Ann Emerg Med* 34:646, 1999.

Wynngaarden JB, Smith LH, Jr, Bennett JC, editors: *Cecil textbook of medicine,* Philadelphia, 1992, WB Saunders.

CHAPTER 42

RED BLOOD CELL ENZYMOPATHIES

Elizabeth A. Price, Stavroula Otis, and Stanley L. Schrier

When evaluating the patient with hemolytic anemia, it is good practice to determine whether the hemolysis is due to an intracorpuscular or extracorpuscular defect. With the exception of paroxysmal nocturnal hemoglobinuria, intracorpuscular causes of hemolysis are all hereditary and involve the three major compartments of the red blood cell (RBC): hemoglobin, the plasma membrane, and the RBC's metabolic machinery. Abnormalities of hemoglobin and the plasma membrane are covered elsewhere. This section is devoted to an analysis of the abnormalities of the RBC's enzymatic-metabolic machinery. The study of human RBCs has afforded numerous insights into cellular enzymatic pathways. Defects in the enzymes of these pathways can be categorized according to which essential functions of RBC metabolism are crippled by their deficiency. The following functions, when impaired, are deleterious to RBC survival:

1. **Maintenance of RBC reducing power:** The RBC's reducing power is of paramount importance to its survival. Red cells are loaded with the oxygen they carry to the tissues and are constantly bombarded with reactive oxygen species. The erythrocyte has a remarkable ability to absorb extreme oxidative stress by virtue of the enzymes involved in glutathione metabolism and generation of the reduced form of nicotinamide adenine dinucleotide phosphate (NADPH). These enzymes provide the red cell with tremendous reducing power by serving as a large reservoir of electrons that can be donated to hemoglobin, lipoproteins, and other intracellular proteins damaged by oxidative stress.
2. **Generation of adenosine triphosphate (ATP):** The RBC uses energy in the form of ATP to energize the pumps and membrane transport mechanisms that allow the red cell to maintain its stable internal environment. The mature red cell is incapable of oxidative phosphorylation because it has lost its mitochondria and mitochondrial enzymes. As such, the red cell must rely on the less efficient, classic Embden-Meyerhof pathway of glycolysis for ATP generation. The glycolytic enzymes catalyzing this evolutionarily conserved pathway are critical for the production of the ATP requisite for the pumps and transport mechanisms, as well as the production of the reduced form of nicotinamide adenine dinucleotide (NADH) needed for cytochrome-b_5 reductase (Cb5R), the major methemoglobin reductase.
3. **Maintenance of hemoglobin in a functional state:** The enzymes that catalyze the formation of NADH and NADPH play a critical role in maintaining hemoglobin in its reduced state by supplying Cb5R (the major methemoglobin reductase) and the alternative methemoglobin reductase with its cofactors. The enzymes that catalyze the formation of 2,3-bisphosphoglycerate (2,3-BPG) via the Rapoport-Luebering shunt also play an important role in hemoglobin function because 2,3-BGP binds to the end of the β-globin chain and facilitates the off-loading of oxygen from hemoglobin to the tissues.
4. **Degradation of ribosomal proteins:** The RBC is unique in that it transitions from a typical nucleated cell capable of protein synthesis and oxidative and anaerobic metabolism to a cell devoid of organelles, incapable of protein synthesis, and dependent on glycolysis for energy production. The RBC must modify its membrane and volume accordingly and expel ribosomal proteins, which could otherwise prove deleterious. Pyrimidine 5′-nucleotidase is effective in degrading the ribosomal contents into smaller components that can pass through the RBC membrane.

For the most part, these enzyme deficiencies are exceedingly rare, with a few notable exceptions. The more prevalent enzyme deficiencies presumably offer an evolutionary advantage, whereas the rare deficiencies likely represent spontaneous mutations that offer no selective advantage.

ENZYMOPATHIES OF GLUTATHIONE METABOLISM

Glutathione Metabolism

Glutathione is a key player in numerous cellular functions, including free radical scavenging, redox reactions, and biosynthesis of deoxyribonucleic acid (DNA), proteins, and leukotrienes. GSH also plays a role in neurotransmission and neuromodulation. In the RBC, glutathione is present in extremely high concentrations, higher than any other cell in the body, and plays a critical role in protecting the RBC from oxidant injury. The ratio of reduced glutathione (GSH) to oxidized glutathione (GSSG) is maintained at high levels in the red cell by two mechanisms: (1) GSSG is converted to GSH by glutathione reductase, and (2) GSSG is actively transported out of the erythrocyte.

GSH is a tripeptide composed of glutamate, cysteine, and glycine. γ-glutamylcysteine synthetase catalyzes the first and rate-limiting step in the synthesis of GSH (Fig. 42-1). The product of this reaction, γ-glutamylcysteine, is then converted to GSH in the presence of glycine via glutathione synthetase, the enzyme that catalyzes the second and final step in GSH synthesis (see Fig. 42-1). Oxidation of GSH by glutathione peroxidase or other free radicals leads to the formation of glutathione disulfide (GSSG) and other mixed disulfides of proteins that contain free –SH groups (like hemoglobin). GSSG is rapidly restored to reduced glutathione via glutathione reductase and its cofactor NADPH. NADPH is maintained at high levels by glucose-6-phosphate dehydrogenase (G6PD). Defects in each of these enzymes have been described and are extremely rare, with the notable exception of G6PD deficiency.

G6PD Deficiency

History

G6PD deficiency was first recognized in the early 1950s during the Korean War when approximately 10% of African American soldiers given the antimalarial drug primaquine developed a self-limited hemolytic anemia. This phenomenon led to further investigations on healthy volunteers who were given 30 mg of primaquine daily. Most subjects tolerated the drug well, but a minority developed a self-limited hemolytic anemia. Pursuant studies showed that ^{51}Cr-labeled RBCs from primaquine-sensitive subjects transfused into nonsensitive subjects were rapidly destroyed, whereas RBCs from nonsensitive subjects transfused into primaquine-sensitive subjects

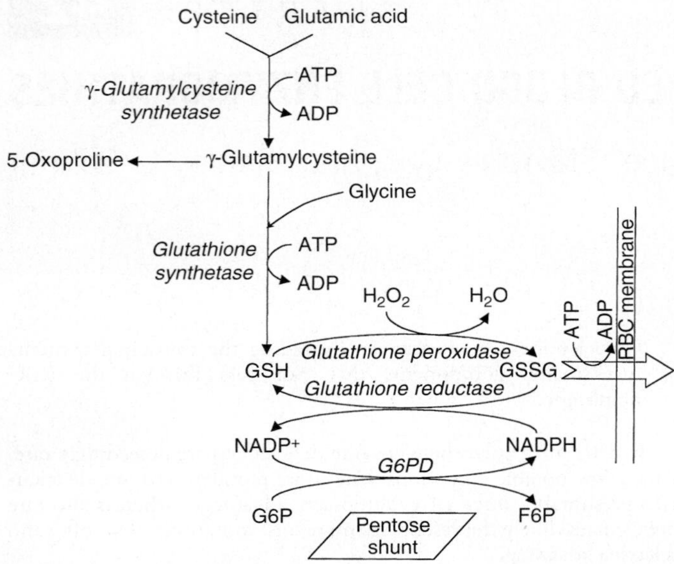

Figure 42-1 GLUTATHIONE PATHWAY. *ADP,* Adenosine diphosphate; *ATP,* adenosine triphosphate; *F6P,* fructose 6-phosphate; *G6P,* glucose 6-phosphate; *G6PD,* glucose-6-phosphate dehydrogenase; *GSH,* reduced glutathione; *GSSG,* oxidized glutathione; *NADP+,* oxidized form of nicotinamide adenine dinucleotide phosphate; *NADPH,* reduced form of nicotinamide adenine dinucleotide phosphate; *RBC,* red blood cell.

survived normally even when the host's RBCs were rapidly destroyed.[1,2] These findings established clearly that primaquine sensitivity was due to an intrinsic defect of the erythrocyte. Subsequent studies showed that younger, more metabolically active RBCs were resistant to destruction, whereas older RBCs were being destroyed, suggestive of an underlying metabolic defect.[3] By 1956, researchers had systematically deduced that the primary defect was in the G6PD enzyme.[4-8] In 1961 the G6PD gene was discovered to be X-linked, due to its linkage to red-green color blindness.

Epidemiology

G6PD deficiency is the most prevalent human enzyme deficiency in the world, affecting an estimated 350 to 400 million people. The geographic distribution of G6PD deficiency coincides with the geographic distribution of endemic malaria, implicating a survival benefit. The highest prevalence of G6PD deficiency is in sub-Saharan Africa, followed by the Middle East, Mediterranean Europe, and Southeast Asia.[9,10]

The most common allelic variants of G6PD are G6PD A- and G6PD Mediterranean. In fact, these two variants coexist at polymorphic frequencies in several populations, most notably in countries surrounding the Persian Gulf.[11] G6PD A- accounts for approximately 90% of G6PD in Africa but is also prevalent in North and South America, the West Indies, Italy, the Canary Islands, Spain, Portugal, and the Middle East.[12-16] G6PD Mediterranean is prevalent in all countries surrounding the Mediterranean Sea, as well as the Middle East, India, and Indonesia.[14,17]

In addition to geographic overlap, numerous studies support the premise that polymorphic variants of G6PD confer a survival benefit in malaria-endemic regions. Ruwende et al[18] showed that the G6PD A- allele is associated with a substantial reduction in the risk for severe *Plasmodium falciparum* malaria for female heterozygotes (46% risk reduction) and male hemizygotes (58% risk reduction). In addition, several in vitro studies comparing the growth of malarial parasites in G6PD-B (wild type) erythrocytes to growth in G6PDA- and G6PD Mediterranean erythrocytes have shown protracted growth in the G6PD-deficient cells.[19-24] Growth is also blunted in G6PD-deficient RBCs taken from female heterozygotes, whose cells have undergone random X-chromosome inactivation, when compared to parasite growth in RBCs with normal G6PD activity from the same individuals.[25]

Oxidant injury to the parasite itself appears to be one mechanism by which G6PD deficiency confers its protective effects. Due to the host cell's impaired ability to restore intracellular NADPH and GSH, malarial parasites in G6PD-deficient RBCs may be more vulnerable to the reactive intermediates they generate (particularly oxidized iron) when they break down hemoglobin.[26,27] Other studies have shown that malaria-infected, G6PD-deficient RBCs undergo phagocytosis by macrophages at an earlier stage of parasite maturation than do normal malaria-infected RBCs, which could be another means by which G6PD-deficient cells offer a selective advantage.[20]

The prevalence of G6PD deficiency in the United States ranges from 0.5% to 7% and is most common among African American males, affecting approximately 10%.[10,28] Screening for G6PD deficiency is generally reserved for individuals at increased risk, such as human immunodeficiency virus (HIV)–infected individuals from susceptible racial and ethnic groups. The overall prevalence rate of G6PD deficiency among HIV-infected patients is estimated to be approximately 6.8%.[29] Because HIV patients are more likely to be exposed to oxidant drugs like dapsone, primaquine, and sulfonamides, primary care guidelines for management of HIV recommend screening patients from higher prevalence ethnic or racial groups (e.g., African and Mediterranean descent) for G6PD deficiency either at baseline or before initiating therapy with an oxidant drug.[30]

Pathobiology

G6PD is a cellular housekeeping enzyme that catalyzes the first step in the hexose monophosphate shunt, wherein glucose 6-phosphate (G6P) is converted to ribose 5-phosphate (Fig. 42-2), a precursor of many important molecules like ribonucleic acid (RNA), DNA, ATP, coenzyme A, nicotinamide adenine dinucleotide (NAD), flavin adenine dinucleotide (FAD). Another major role of the hexose monophosphate shunt is to maintain high levels of NADPH, which acts as a cofactor for GSH. Most cells have alternate enzymatic pathways that can generate NADPH, but RBCs lack a nucleus, mitochondria, and other organelles necessary to produce these enzymes and are therefore particularly dependent on G6PD and the hexose monophosphate shunt for maintaining high levels of NADPH and GSH to protect against oxidative stress.

G6PD is encoded by a gene located on the telomeric region of the long arm of the X chromosome (Xq28) that spans 18 kb, and consists of 13 exons and 12 introns. The G6PD gene product comprises 515 amino acids with a molecular weight of 59 kDa.[31] The enzyme is active as a tetramer or dimer. Stability of the active quaternary structure is crucial for normal G6PD activity.

Within the RBC, oxidant injury leads to the oxidation of sulfhydryl groups on the hemoglobin molecule, resulting in the formation of disulfide bridges, which in turn leads to decreased hemoglobin solubility and ultimately the irreversible precipitation of oxidized hemoglobin.[32,33] Under normal conditions oxidized hemoglobin is reduced by GSH, which itself is oxidized in the process but restored to its reduced form by intracellular NADPH, whose levels are maintained by G6PD. In the G6PD-deficient RBC, GSH is not restored to adequate levels under oxidative stress, leading to a buildup of free radicals and insoluble hemoglobin within the cell, which can be visualized under the microscope as Heinz bodies. Precipitated hemoglobin is disruptive to the structure and function of the RBC membrane and leads to increased membrane permeability, osmotic fragility, and cell rigidity. The compromised integrity of the cell membrane results in both intravascular hemolysis and rapid removal of these cells within the splenic pulp.[34]

Over 400 variants of the G6PD enzyme have been identified by biochemical methods, 100 of which reach polymorphic levels. Most variants are due to point mutations and, to a lesser extent, small in-frame deletions that result in missense mutations. Gross deletions, nonsense mutations, frame-shift mutations, and splicing defects are

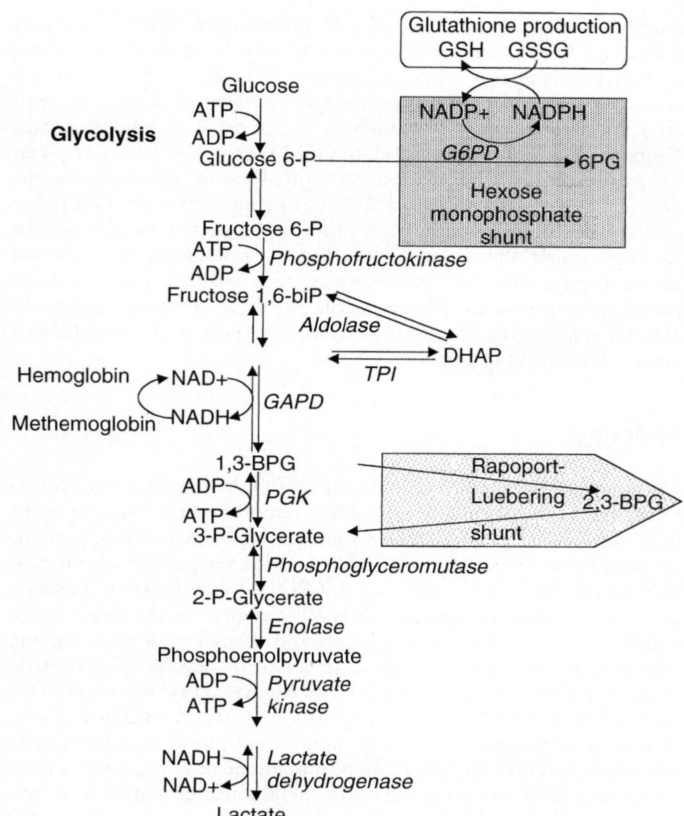

Figure 42-2 GLYCOLYSIS (EMBDEN-MEYERHOF PATHWAY). *ADP,* Adenosine diphosphate; *ATP,* adenosine triphosphate; *1,3-BPG,* 1,3- bisphosphoglycerate; *2,3-BPG,* 2,3-bisphosphoglycerate; *DHAP,* dihydroxyacetone phosphate; *GAPD,* glyceraldehyde phosphate dehydrogenase; *G6PD,* glucose-6-phosphate dehydrogenase; *GSH,* reduced glutathione; *GSSG,* oxidized glutathione; *NAD+,* nicotinamide adenine dinucleotide; *NADP+,* oxidized form of nicotinamide adenine dinucleotide phosphate; *NADPH,* reduced form of nicotinamide adenine dinucleotide phosphate; *6PG,* 6-phosphogluconate; *PGK,* phosphoglycerate kinase; *TPI,* triose-phosphate isomerase.

not reported for this gene, because mutants showing 100% deficiency of the G6PD enzyme would presumably be incompatible with life.[35-37]

The World Health Organization classifies the G6PD variants based on their enzymatic activity and the degree of associated hemolysis (Table 42-1).[38,39]

Wild-type G6PD is referred to as G6PD B (Western). It is the most common worldwide normal isoenzyme and is the ancestral human sequence, as demonstrated by showing that G6PD B matches the sequence of G6PD in the chimpanzee, our nearest relative, and by analysis of linkage disequilibrium.[12,40] The numerous G6PD variants differ in molecular stability and enzymatic activity. The degree of hemolysis associated with each isoenzyme is dependent on the type of defect and severity of oxidant injury. Class I variants are severe, occur sporadically, and lead to chronic hemolytic anemia. Class II and III variants are found at much higher frequencies than class I variants, and are implicated in providing protection against malaria. Class IV and V variants are of no clinical significance.

In normal erythrocytes the G6PD enzyme operates at 1% to 2% of its maximum potential, leaving a large reserve of reductive potential for times of severe oxidative stress.[41] This potential is variably decreased in G6PD-deficient erythrocytes. Under normal conditions a mild to moderate deficiency in the activity of G6PD is not deleterious, and there are no clinical or laboratory signs of hemolysis in these individuals. Under conditions of oxidative stress, however, the reductive potential of G6PD-deficient erythrocytes is overwhelmed, resulting in acute hemolysis. Oxidative stress may be due to exogenous agents like drugs, fava beans, chemicals (e.g., naphthalene, antifungal sprays), and herbs (e.g., *Coptis sinensis,* calculus bovis), or the result of a systemic process like infection, liver injury, and diabetic ketoacidosis.[35]

Table 42-1 World Health Organization Classification of G6PD Variants

Class	Enzymatic Activity	Degree of Associated Hemolysis
I	Severely deficient	Chronic hemolysis
II	Severely deficient (<10% residual activity)	Acute, episodic
III	Moderately to mildly deficient (10%-60% residual activity)	Acute, episodic
IV	Mildly deficient to normal (60%-150%)	Absent
V	Increased (>150%)	Absent

From WHO Working Group: Glucose-6-phosphate dehydrogenase deficiency. *Bull World Health Organ* 67:601, 1989.
G6PD, Glucose-6-phosphate dehydrogenase.

Clinical Manifestations

Most people with G6PD deficiency have no clinical symptoms and are not anemic. In fact, the majority of affected individuals live out their lives unaware of their status. Diagnosis typically occurs when an episode of acute hemolysis is triggered by exposure to oxidant drugs, infection, or ingestion of fava beans. Unusual presentations include hemolysis precipitated by complications of diabetes, myocardial infarction, and strenuous physical exercise.[42-44]

The symptoms are characteristic of acute hemolysis and include fatigue, jaundice, pallor, dark urine, and abdominal and low back pain. In the case of drug-induced hemolysis, symptoms occur 2 to 4 days after drug ingestion and are associated with a 3 to 4 g/dL drop in hemoglobin level. The bone marrow responds appropriately by generating a reticulocytosis that peaks approximately 7 to 10 days after the onset of hemolysis.[1]

Depending on the G6PD variant, hemolysis can be self-limited despite continuation of the offending drug, or it can be protracted despite discontinuation of the offending drug. Class III G6PD variants have a moderately shortened half-life (e.g., the half-life of G6PD A- is approximately 13 days) when compared to the half-life of wild-type G6PD (approximately 62 days).[45,46] Consequently, hemolysis is restricted to older RBCs that are more deficient in G6PD. As the older RBCs are eradicated, they are replaced by reticulocytes with higher concentrations of G6PD. The concentration of G6PD in these younger cells is sufficient to overcome the oxidative stress induced by the offending agent, and the hemolytic process is thereby self-limited, even when the offending agent is continued. In contrast, individuals with a Class II variant of G6PD (such as G6PD Mediterranean) experience a more severe drug-induced hemolysis because the half-life of these variants is on the order of hours,[45] making all erythrocytes, young and old, more vulnerable to oxidant injury. In these individuals, hemolysis continues well after discontinuation of the culprit drug.[47,48]

Favism

For centuries fava beans have been associated with the clinical sequelae of acute hemolysis.[49] The beans are a staple food in the Mediterranean, Middle East, and Far East, and their ingestion results in acute hemolysis in susceptible individuals. Only a minority of G6PD-deficient individuals develop hemolytic anemia after ingestion of the bean, suggesting other genetic factors at play.[50-52] Two components of the fava bean, divicine and isouramil, may play a role in driving hemolysis by further impairing the reductive capacity of the G6PD-deficient RBC.[53] Favism develops within 5 to 24 hours of bean ingestion and is characterized by the typical symptoms of acute intravascular hemolysis: headache, nausea, back pain, chills, fever, hemoglobinuria, and jaundice. Favism has also been reported in breastfed babies whose mothers consumed fava beans.[54]

Neonatal Jaundice

Among the clinical manifestations associated with G6PD deficiency, neonatal jaundice now carries the highest risk for potentially devastating clinical consequences, namely, kernicterus.[55] Contrary to what is commonly believed, jaundice in neonates with G6PD deficiency is not the result of hemolysis. In fact, most neonates have normal hemoglobin and reticulocyte levels, and the RBC life span is only modestly shortened, if at all.[56] Rather, the hyperbilirubinemia is secondary to the newborn liver's inability to adequately conjugate bilirubin.[57] This problem is compounded when the newborn also inherits a mutation of the uridine diphosphate-glucuronosyltransferase 1 (UGT1A1) gene promoter that is associated with Gilbert syndrome, increasing the risk for neonatal jaundice.[58] Over 30% of kernicterus cases are associated with G6PD deficiency,[59] raising the question of whether G6PD deficiency should be included in routine newborn screening programs.

Congenital Nonspherocytic Hemolytic Anemia

As mentioned earlier, class I G6PD variants have very low enzymatic activity and/or marked instability, resulting in lifelong hemolysis due to the everyday oxidative stresses encountered by the circulating erythrocyte. These variants are sporadic, and almost all arise from independent mutations clustering in exons 10 and 11, which are close to the substrate binding domain in the folded protein.[60] The disorder is first suspected when affected infants develop severe neonatal jaundice, or it is discovered later when the typically mild anemia is exacerbated by oxidant drug exposure, infection, or parvovirus-induced aplastic crisis.

Laboratory Manifestations

Under normal conditions, most G6PD-deficient individuals (class II and III variants) are not anemic and have no laboratory evidence of hemolysis. In the setting of oxidative stress, the laboratory findings are those of any acute hemolytic process and include anemia, reticulocytosis, hyperbilirubinemia, increased lactate dehydrogenase (LDH), decreased haptoglobin, and hemoglobinuria. The peripheral blood smear is notable for Heinz bodies (precipitated sulfhemoglobin), and on occasion for "bite cells" (also known as *hemiblister cells, eccentrocytes,* and *cross-bonded cells*), which occur when denatured hemoglobin binds to the cell membrane, creating a puddling of hemoglobin to one side of the cell with an adjacent membrane-bound clear zone.[61,62]

Diagnosis

The enzymatic activity of G6PD can be quantitated by measuring the rate of NADPH production in red cell hemolysates that contain G6P and NADP+ (the enzyme's substrates); this is done using a spectrophotometer, which can measure the rate of NADPH formation at wavelength 340 nm. This method is used to make a biochemical definitive diagnosis. For more rapid screening of at-risk populations, there are several semiquantitative methods available. The most simple, sensitive, and inexpensive screening test is the fluorescent spot test.[63] In this procedure, NADPH production is detected by virtue of its fluorescence under ultraviolet light. As with the quantitative test, G6P and NADP+ are added to a hemolysate of the patient's red cells, and fluorescence under ultraviolet light indicates enzyme activity, whereas absence of fluorescence indicates enzyme deficiency. Other semiquantitative tests have been used but require definitive testing to confirm an abnormal result.[64,65] False negatives are a concern when diagnostic tests are performed during or right after an acute hemolytic episode in the midst of a reticulocytosis. Younger RBCs have higher levels of G6PD than older RBCs, so when the patient's red cell population is weighted toward younger cells, the deficiency may go undetected. Females heterozygous for G6PD are particularly difficult to diagnose due to the natural mosaicism for X-chromosome enzymes. Heterozygotes with extremely skewed X-inactivation can have enzymatic activity ranging anywhere from hemizygote to normal. Molecular diagnostic methods are more reliable for making the diagnosis of females suspected of being heterozygous for G6PD deficiency.

Therapy

Treatment of the clinical sequelae of G6PD deficiency is straightforward. In the case of acute hemolysis, removal of the inciting agent (e.g., drug, fava beans) is recommended. This maneuver is of particular importance in patients with Class I and II variants, in whom even the young RBCs lack adequate G6PD activity to resist ongoing exposure to oxidative agents. Class III variants, on the other hand, usually undergo a self-limited hemolysis that resolves despite ongoing exposure to the inciting agent. In cases of severe, symptomatic anemia, blood transfusion may be necessary, especially in patients with a blunted erythropoietic response (e.g., HIV, infection, drug-related myelosuppression). Very rarely, congenital nonspherocytic hemolytic anemia is severe enough to mandate ongoing transfusions, which may lead to iron overload in the absence of appropriate iron chelation. Folic acid supplementation is also recommended for patients with congenital nonspherocytic hemolysis. Antioxidants like vitamin E and selenium may also be beneficial in these patients, but there are no consistent data to support their use.[66]

In the event of neonatal jaundice, the treatment is the same as that recommended for neonatal jaundice arising from other causes. Mild cases do not require treatment, intermediate cases require phototherapy, and severe cases require exchange transfusion (total bilirubin >20 mg/dL). The true key to management of G6PD is prevention of its clinical sequelae, which requires awareness of the disorder on the part of both the physician and the patient. The disease should always be suspected in patients with a nonimmune hemolytic anemia and patients with an otherwise unexplained personal or family history of recurrent jaundice, splenomegaly, or cholelithiasis. G6PD deficiency should be considered in any neonate with hyperbilirubinemia, especially those of high-risk ethnic descent. There has been considerable debate in recent years as to whether testing for G6PD deficiency should be a routine part of neonatal screening tests. Interestingly, in a study done in Cleveland, Ohio, investigators found that the routine cord blood screening protocol for isoimmune hemolytic disease had a lower yield and higher cost than their pilot protocol for cord blood G6PD deficiency screening,[67] both of which are considered major risk factors for neonatal jaundice. One caveat to routine screening of all newborns is that heterozygous females and hemizygous males with residual enzyme activity greater than 20% are likely to be erroneously classified as "normal" due to the limitations of the fluorescent spot test,[68,69] instilling a false sense of security and subverting the prevention of complications.

Once the diagnosis of G6PD deficiency is established, patients must be counseled to avoid drugs, chemicals, and foods known to precipitate hemolysis. Although there are some medications classically connected to hemolysis in G6PD patients, there are a number of medications for which there is considerable confusion as to whether they are safe in G6PD-deficient patients. In an attempt to better clarify which are truly high-risk drugs, investigators in Israel performed a comprehensive literature search and categorized drugs according to how much evidence there is in the literature to contraindicate their use.[70] They found only seven medications for which there is solid evidence to prohibit their use in G6PD-deficient patients: dapsone, methylthionine chloride (methylene blue), nitrofurantoin, phenazopyridine, primaquine, rasburicase, and tolonium chloride (toluidine blue). Their review found no substantial evidence to absolutely contravene the use of other medications in normal therapeutic doses.

Prognosis

Except for rare cases of severe congenital nonimmune hemolytic anemia and severe neonatal jaundice, the prognosis of patients with G6PD deficiency is excellent with no apparent impact on life expectancy.

Future Directions

Current screening tests for G6PD deficiency do not reliably identify female heterozygotes or male hemizygotes with greater than 20% residual enzyme activity. This is problematic because these groups remain at risk for hemolytic complications. It would be useful to devise a rapid and inexpensive screening test that could detect patients with moderately reduced enzymatic activity (20% to 60%), so they too may be counseled on avoiding exogenous agents that could precipitate a hemolytic crisis. It would also be useful to devise a simple in vitro method to determine whether new drugs will cause hemolysis. Simply incubating RBCs with the drug in question is unreliable, most likely because drug metabolites are often the culprits, rather than the original drug. And finally, the value of G6PD screening of all newborns must be flushed out, because this is a major cause of neonatal kernicterus, even in first world countries.[71-73]

γ-Glutamylcysteine Synthetase Deficiency

As described earlier, γ-glutamylcysteine synthetase catalyzes the first step in glutathione synthesis. Deficiency of this enzyme is exceedingly rare. Only nine patients in seven families have been reported worldwide.[74] All nine patients developed a relatively mild hemolytic anemia, and four of the nine manifested neurologic problems, including spinocerebellar degeneration, peripheral neuropathy, and mental retardation.[75-78]

Glutathione Synthetase Deficiency

Glutathione synthetase deficiency is the most common of the inborn errors of GSH metabolism, with more than 70 patients in over 50 families reported worldwide.[74] Patients are homozygous or compound heterozygous for mutations in the glutathione synthetase gene. The clinical presentation is variable, and patients are categorized as mildly, moderately, or severely affected.[79] Mildly affected patients have an isolated hemolytic anemia, whereas moderately affected patients develop a metabolic acidosis within the first few days of life due to the buildup of 5-oxoproline, a metabolite of γ-glutamylcysteine (the substrate of glutathione synthetase). Under normal circumstances GSH negatively feeds back on γ-glutamylcysteine synthetase, but in patients with moderate to severe glutathione synthetase deficiency there is loss of negative feedback, leading to the accumulation of 5-oxoproline in body fluids, resulting in metabolic acidosis and massive 5-oxoprolinuria. Severely affected patients may also develop recurrent bacterial infections and progressive dysfunction of the central nervous system (CNS). The mechanism behind CNS involvement remains unclear. Autopsy of the first patient described with glutathione synthetase deficiency revealed selective atrophy of the granule cell layer of the cerebellum, focal lesions in the frontoparietal cortex, and bilateral focal lesions in the thalamus and visual cortex.

The diagnosis of glutathione synthetase deficiency is suspected in patients with a nonimmune hemolytic anemia, elevated levels of 5-oxoproline in the urine, and markedly reduced RBC glutathione content. The diagnosis is confirmed by demonstrating low levels of glutathione synthetase in cultured skin fibroblasts and/or RBCs or by demonstrating mutations in the glutathione synthetase gene.[74] Treatment involves correcting the metabolic acidosis with bicarbonate and protecting the cells against further oxidant injury by administering antioxidants like vitamin C and vitamin E. N-acetylcysteine was used in the past to protect against oxidant damage but is no longer recommended because studies have shown that cysteine, which is known to be neurotoxic at high concentrations, accumulates in the tissues of patients with glutathione synthetase deficiency.[80,81] Patients with glutathione synthetase deficiency should avoid the same agents known to precipitate acute hemolysis in patients with G6PD deficiency.

Glutathione Reductase Deficiency

Glutathione reductase restores intracellular GSH by reducing GSSG in the presence of NADPH and FAD, a derivative of the water-soluble vitamin riboflavin. Consequently, malnourished patients, or patients who are otherwise deficient in riboflavin, develop an acquired partial deficiency of glutathione reductase. Riboflavin deficiency can be demonstrated by testing the in vitro activity of glutathione reductase with and without exogenously added FAD. Acquired glutathione reductase deficiency has no documented hematologic phenotype and is easily corrected by administration of physiologic quantities of riboflavin.

Congenital deficiency of glutathione reductase has been reported in two Dutch families. In the first family, the eldest of three siblings from a consanguineous marriage developed a hemolytic crisis after ingesting fava beans.[82] All three siblings (one male, two female) were found to be homozygous for a large deletion in the glutathione reductase gene encoding almost the entire dimerization domain of the enzyme.[83] In the second family, an infant was born with severe neonatal jaundice and found to be a compound heterozygote for a nonsense and missense mutation in the glutathione reductase gene.[83] There was no evidence of enhanced hemolysis in this infant, which is consistent with the neonatal jaundice associated with G6PD deficiency.

Glutathione Peroxidase Deficiency

Glutathione peroxidase is a selenium-containing enzyme that catalyzes the oxidation of GSH by hydrogen peroxide, producing GSSG and water. Although rare cases of glutathione peroxidase deficiency have been described in association with hemolysis,[84-86] a causative relationship between the two has not been clearly established. There are several reported cases of normal individuals with reduced glutathione peroxidase activity and no evidence of hemolysis.[87,88]

ENZYMOPATHIES OF THE GLYCOLYTIC PATHWAY

Pyruvate Kinase Deficiency

Epidemiology

Pyruvate kinase (PK) deficiency is the most common red cell enzymopathy leading to congenital nonspherocytic hemolytic anemia. The prevalence has been estimated by gene frequency studies to be 51 cases per million in the general white population.[89] However, recognized clinical cases in the Northern United Kingdom based on a registry study initiated in 1974 had a much lower prevalence,[90] suggesting premature disease-related death, clinically mild disease, or diagnostic error.[91] Conversely, the prevalence of homozygous PK deficiency was found to be quite high (1 in 830) in a small, remote town in the Western United States,[92] likely due to consanguinity within the community. Common mutations have well-defined geographic associations. Mutation 1529A is frequently seen in the United States[93] and central Europe,[94] 1456T is commonly found in Southern Europe,[95-97] and 1468T is the most common mutation found in Asia.[89,98] PK deficiency is an autosomal recessive disease, and affected patients are typically double heterozygotes, or, less commonly, homozygous for the same mutation. Homozygous mutations are usually seen in groups with marked consanguinity, and homozygous PK deficiency has been well described in the Amish populations of Pennsylvania and Ohio.[99,100]

Pathobiology

PK catalyzes the irreversible transfer of phosphate from phosphoenolpyruvate to adenosine diphosphate (ADP), forming ATP and pyruvate in the second ATP-generating step of the glycolytic pathway. There are four distinct PK isoforms, M_1, M_2, L, and R types, encoded by two separate genes (PKM and PKLR).[101] PKM_1 and PKM_2 are produced from the PKM gene by alternative RNA splicing.[102] The M_2 isoform is expressed in early fetal and proliferating tissues and remains the dominant form in adults in leukocytes and platelets. PKM_1 is found in skeletal muscle, heart, and brain.[103] PKL, found in the liver, and PKR, in red cells, are both encoded by the PKLR gene on chromosome 1q21 through the use of alternate promoters.[104] PKM_2 is expressed in normal erythroid precursors[105] and is gradually replaced during maturation by the PK-R isoform. The functional enzyme is a tetramer, and each isoform has characteristic kinetic properties,[103] although all isoforms except M_1 are allosterically activated by fructose 1,6-diphosphate (FDP).[106,107] More than 190 mutations in the PKLR gene encoding the red cell PK have been identified, most of which are missense mutations (www.pklrmutatinodatabase.com). Mutations may alter the stability of the enzyme or the enzyme's affinity for its substrate, phosphoenolpyruvate (PEP), or its allosteric activator, FDP.[106,108] There appears to be some correlation with the location of the mutation and the severity of the hemolytic anemia, with more severe disease being associated with disruptive mutations and with missense mutations directly involving the active site or protein stability.[92,101]

The mechanism of hemolysis in PK deficiency is not fully understood. Reticulocytes are preferentially destroyed in the spleen and the liver,[109] and following splenectomy a striking reticulocytosis may be seen.[110,111] It has been suggested that the higher metabolic requirement of reticulocytes renders them more vulnerable to PK deficiency than mature erythrocytes, leading to increased destruction.[109] The defect in ATP generation may contribute to the anemia, although it is likely not the sole cause, because other disorders with more severe ATP deficiency do not have significant hemolytic anemia.[112] The metabolic derangements found in PK deficiency may also lead to increased apoptosis and ineffective erythropoiesis, as seen in the spleen of a patient with PK deficiency[113] and in a mouse model.[114] The metabolic defect is distal to the Rapoport-Leubering shunt, and thus the concentration of 2,3-BPG is increased. Although accumulation of 2,3-BPG may lead to further impairment in glycolysis through inhibition of hexokinase,[101] the resultant shift in the oxyhemoglobin dissociation curve to the right[115] leads to improved tolerance of the anemia.[116]

Clinical and Laboratory Manifestations

Clinical severity in patients with PK deficiency is widely variable, ranging from fully compensated hemolysis to a transfusion-dependent anemia. Newborns may present with severe hemolytic anemia and pronounced jaundice, requiring exchange transfusion.[117] In the worst cases, hydrops fetalis[118] with intrauterine or neonatal death may rarely occur.[119] Severe liver dysfunction has also been reported as an unusual cause of death in infants with PK deficiency.[120] Early onset of symptoms is typically associated with a more severe clinical course.[121] Heterozygotes for PK deficiency who are heterozygotes or homozygotes for the Gilbert syndrome polymorphism may have neonatal jaundice that persists in childhood.[92] The anemia is relatively stable in adults,[121] although transient worsening may occur with infection,[122] pregnancy, or the use of certain medications, including oral contraceptives.[123] Gallstones may be present. Extramedullary hematopoiesis can occur even in patients who are transfusion independent[124] and may lead to characteristic bone deformities.[125] Extradural extramedullary hematopoiesis leading to spinal cord compression and neurologic deficits has been reported,[126] with good response to surgical excision and radiation therapy.[126] Leg ulcers are seen rarely.[127] Recurrent venous thromboembolic disease was reported in one adult patient who underwent splenectomy as a young child,[110] and idiopathic pulmonary arterial hypertension was reported in another patient who had undergone splenectomy at age 5.[128]

Iron overload has been reported in nontransfused[129,130] and transfusion-dependent patients and may be severe, leading to cirrhosis and cardiac and endocrine dysfunction.[131] Splenectomy and the presence of hemochromatosis-related genes may increase the risk for iron overload.[132] Serum levels of the iron regulatory protein hepcidin were lower in PK-deficient patients compared to controls, and growth differentiation factor 15 (GDF15) levels were higher, suggesting suppression of hepcidin as a contributing mechanism of iron overload in some PK-deficient patients.[133]

Although PK deficiency does not localize to geographic areas of malarial endemicity, PK deficiency may be protective against malaria.[134] In a mouse model of infection with *Plasmodium chabaudi,* mice carrying a loss-of-function mutation in the PKLR gene had reduced blood-stage parasite replication and improved survival compared to control mice.[135] In vitro, erythrocytes from homozygous PK-deficient patients have decreased invasion by *P. falciparum* compared to normal or heterozygous PK-deficient control erythrocytes.[136] In addition, phagocytosis of ring-stage infected erythrocytes from patients with homozygous and heterozygous mutations was increased compared to control subjects.

Laboratory findings are those typical for hemolytic anemia, including low hemoglobin, increased reticulocyte count, high LDH, low haptoglobin, and elevated indirect bilirubin. Reticulocytosis may be suppressed in the context of the normal hypoplastic phase of erythropoiesis following birth, making the diagnosis more challenging.[137] The bilirubin is usually less than 6 mg/dL: if higher, the patient may have coexisting Gilbert syndrome.[101,138] Red cells are commonly without characteristic morphologic abnormalities; however, following splenectomy they may become markedly abnormal, with numerous crenated cells, lobulated cells, and target cells.[125] Establishing the diagnosis requires the demonstration of low enzyme activity.[112] Care must be taken in interpreting in vitro test results, because contamination with transfused red cells or leukocytes can increase measured enzyme activity.[101] Specialized laboratories can assess for kinetically abnormal mutant PKs.[112] Molecular diagnostic methods can be used if the likely mutation is known, as in the case of prenatal diagnosis.

Therapy

Treatment for PK deficiency remains supportive. Exchange transfusion and/or intense phototherapy may be required in the neonatal period to prevent kernicterus and its resultant sequelae, including permanent hearing loss.[92] Patients with more severe disease may require periodic or even regular red cell transfusions. Increased transfusion may be needed during pregnancy both for maternal supportive care and to prevent miscarriage.[100] Splenectomy typically leads to an increase in hemoglobin by 1 to 3 g/dL[121] and can lead to transfusion independence. In one reported case, partial splenectomy failed to ameliorate transfusion needs secondary to rapid regeneration of the spleen.[139] General recommendations include, where possible, delaying splenectomy until the patient is 3 years of age or older to reduce the risk for postsplenectomy sepsis.[112] If iron overload occurs, both pharmacologic iron chelation therapy[140] and, if the anemia is not too severe, phlebotomy,[141] can successfully reduce excess iron. Hematopoietic stem cell transplant was reportedly successful in one 5-year-old boy with PK deficiency and hemoglobin E trait.[142]

Glucose Phosphate Isomerase Deficiency

Glucose phosphate isomerase (GPI) catalyzes the interconversion of G6P and fructose 6-phosphate in the second step of glycolysis. GPI deficiency is an autosomal recessive disorder and is one of the four most common erythrocyte enzymopathies, including deficiencies of G6PD, PK, and pyrimidine 5′-nucleotidase.[143] The hemolytic anemia is of variable severity and may require chronic transfusions.[144] Hydrops fetalis has been reported.[143] Splenectomy can improve the anemia, eliminating transfusion requirements.[143,145] GPI deficiency can also be associated with neurologic impairment, including myopathy and mental retardation.[146]

Hexokinase Deficiency

Hexokinase catalyzes the initial step of glycolysis, the phosphorylation of glucose to G6P (see Fig. 42-2) and is one of the rate-limiting steps of this pathway.[107] Hexokinase deficiency is a rare cause of congenital nonspherocytic anemia. Hemolytic anemia may occur as a sole manifestation or as part of a constellation of abnormalities that can include other cytopenias, diabetes mellitus, skeletal malformations, hypogonadism, and abnormal pigmentation.[147] Severe iron overload can occur.[148] Most patients are of European descent, although an affected Chinese kindred has also been described.[147] A mouse model of generalized hexokinase deficiency has been described, with manifestations of severe hemolytic anemia, marked reticulocytosis, and extensive tissue iron deposition.[149] Splenectomy may provide benefit.[150] In contrast to PK deficiency, the defect occurs proximal to the Rapoport-Leubering shunt, and thus the concentration of 2,3-BPG is reduced, shifting the oxyhemoglobin dissociation curve to the left[115] and decreasing patient tolerance to the anemia.[116]

Phosphofructokinase Deficiency

Phosphofructokinase (PFK) catalyzes the phosphorylation of fructose 6-phosphate to fructose-1,6-bisphosphate (see Fig. 42-2).[151,152] Two of the three identified isoenzymes (muscle type [PFKM] and liver type [PFKL]) are expressed in erythrocytes. Mutations in the muscle-type PFKM isoenzyme cause type VII glycogen storage disease (Tarui disease), a rare autosomal recessive disorder. Such mutations lead to an almost complete loss of PFK activity in muscle, but only partial loss of activity in erythrocytes. Clinical manifestations of type VII glycogen storage disease may present in infancy or older adulthood and include hypotonia, exercise intolerance, and weakness.[152] The severity of the hemolytic anemia is highly variable, ranging from a mild, compensated hemolysis[153] to severe chronic nonspherocytic hemolytic anemia.[152]

ALDOLASE DEFICIENCY

Aldolase catalyzes the interconversion of fructose 1,6-diphosphate to glyceraldehyde 3-phosphate and dihydroxyacetone phosphate.[107] One of the three distinct isoenzymes, aldolase A, is present in erythrocytes, muscle, and brain. Aldolase deficiency is a very rare cause of nonspherocytic hemolytic anemia, and clinical manifestations may also include myopathy and mental retardation.[154]

Phosphoglycerokinase Deficiency

Phosphoglycerate kinase catalyzes the reversible conversion of 1,3-bisphosphoglycerate to 3-phosphoglycerate. Deficiency of this X chromosome–encoded enzyme is associated with an array of findings that can variably include hemolytic anemia, myopathy, rhabdomyolysis, mental retardation, and other neurologic symptoms.[155] Splenectomy may improve the anemia.[156]

Triose-Phosphate Isomerase Deficiency

Triose-phosphate isomerase (TPI) catalyzes the reversible interconversion of the triose phosphate isomers, dihydroxyacetone phosphate, and glyceraldehyde 3-phosphate. TPI deficiency is a rare, autosomal recessive, multisystemic disease, characterized by chronic nonspherocytic hemolytic anemia, frequent bacterial infections, and progressive neuromuscular disease.[157-159] Cardiomyopathy may also be present. Hemolytic anemia manifests before 14 months of age[157] and may be severe enough to require ongoing red cell transfusions.[160] In cases with a milder degree of anemia, intermittent transfusions may be required during acute exacerbations triggered by bacterial infection.[161] Hydrops fetalis can rarely occur.[143] The typical course involves progressive neurologic degeneration with frequent early death; however, rare adult cases with less severe involvement are reported.[162] A high prevalence of heterozygous TPI deficiency has been found in African American newborns.[163] No specific therapy for this disorder is available.

Pyrimidine 5′-Nucleotidase Deficiency

Pathobiology

Red cell pyrimidine 5′-nucleotidase type 1 (P5′NT-1) deficiency, initially described in 1974,[164] is the third most common red cell enzymopathy causing hemolytic anemia, after G6PD deficiency and PK deficiency.[91] It is transmitted as an autosomal recessive trait. Maturation of the reticulocyte results in degradation of ribosomal RNA into pyrimidine 5′ nucleoside monophosphates, which must be dephosphorylated in order to freely diffuse across the cell membrane. P5′NT-1 is a member of a family of enzymes that catalyze this dephosphorylation.[165] Two main types of 5′NT, P5′NT-1 and P5′NT-2, have been isolated from RBCs.[166] Only deficiency of P5′NT-1, encoded by a gene found on chromosome 7, is associated with hemolytic anemia. P5′NT-1 is dependent on Mg^{2+} for activity and is readily inhibited by lead[167] and other heavy metals.[168] P5′NT-1 activity levels are highest in the youngest cells.[169] Mutations in P5′NT-1 lead to the accumulation of pyrimidine nucleotides, which impede RNA breakdown. The resultant ribosomal aggregates are visible as the characteristic coarse basophilic stippling seen on the peripheral smear.[164] Characterized mutations in P5′NT-1 lead to decreased thermal stability and/or impaired catalytic ability of the enzyme,[170] although residual measured enzyme activity in some cases suggests that enzyme deficiency is at least in part compensated by other nucleotidases. Acquired P5′NT deficiency occurs in the instance of lead intoxication, manifesting as hemolytic anemia, reticulocytosis, and striking basophilic stippling.[167]

Clinical and Laboratory Manifestations

P5′NT-1 deficiency is inherited in an autosomal recessive manner, and patients are usually homozygotes, or, less commonly, compound heterozygotes.[166] The disease is characterized by mild to moderate hemolytic anemia, reticulocytosis, indirect hyperbilirubinemia, and variable hepatosplenomegaly.[171,172] The anemia is occasionally severe. Gallstones may be present, and ulcers are seen rarely.[171] Learning disabilities have been described in a few cases.[171] Iron overload occurs in both severe transfusion-dependent cases and mild cases.[173] Conversely, iron deficiency secondary to intravascular hemolysis was described in one case.[174] Homozygous P5′NT-1 deficiency inherited in combination with homozygous hemoglobin E in one described case led to a particularly severe hemolytic anemia, which responded well to splenectomy.[175]

The laboratory hallmark of the disorder is the pronounced basophilic stippling seen on the peripheral smear.[164] Thus in contrast to most cases of congenital nonspherocytic hemolytic anemia, the peripheral smear provides a rapid, inexpensive diagnostic clue to the underlying disorder. This is a sensitive but not specific finding, because basophilic stippling can also be seen in other causes of anemia, including lead poisoning, some hemoglobin variants,[176] and sideroblastic anemia. Confirmation of the diagnosis requires demonstration of decreased P5′NT-1 activity and high concentrations of pyrimidine nucleotides in red cells.[166]

Therapy

There is no targeted therapy for this disorder. In the atypical case with severe anemia, patients may be red cell transfusion dependent.[177] In other cases, transfusions may be needed sporadically, such as during pregnancy or acute infections.[178] Splenectomy in a few cases has provided benefit,[179] but in other cases has not led to any significant improvement in the anemia.[177] Patients should be monitored for iron overload, and iron chelation may be required.

Red Cell Enzymopathies Causing Methemoglobinemia

Pathobiology

Normal hemoglobin A is composed of two α-chains and two β-chains, and each one of the globin chains carries a heme group in the center of which is a molecule of ferrous iron (Fe^{2+}). In oxyhemoglobin, each ferrous atom links reversibly to a molecule of oxygen. As is shown in the sigmoidal oxyhemoglobin association curve, the binding of oxygen is cooperative, such that the binding of the first molecule of oxygen facilitates the binding of the second molecule of oxygen. Methemoglobin occurs when the ferrous molecule is oxidized to ferric (Fe^{3+}), either in the usual course of events (Fig. 42-3) or due to inadequately controlled oxidant attack. Methemoglobin causes two sorts of problems: methemoglobin cannot bind oxygen, and, further, if a methemoglobin becomes part of the hemoglobin tetramer, the oxygen affinity is increased with a left shift in the oxyhemoglobin dissociation curve and a biologically important fall in the partial pressure of oxygen at which hemoglobin is 50% saturated with oxygen (P_{50}).[180] The combined effect of decreased oxygen-carrying capacity and decreased oxygen release may lead to a profound functional impairment,[181] particularly in the patient with underlying cardiopulmonary disease.

Methemoglobin is being formed continuously, but there are mechanisms in place that normally keep the methemoglobin level at about 1% of the total hemoglobin.[182] The most important of these is the NADH-dependent Cb5R (also known as methemoglobin reductase).[183,184] The electrons from NADH are transferred first to FAD, reducing it to $FADH_2$, which is a prosthetic group of the enzyme. $FADH_2$ then transfers these electrons to the enzyme Cb5R, which completes the transfer of electrons to Fe^{3+}, completing the reduction of methemoglobin to Fe^{2+} hemoglobin (Fig. 42-4).

There is a backup flavin-dependent methemoglobin reductase that uses the electrons catalyzed by G6PD when it reduces NADP+ to NADPH. This flavin NADPH methemoglobin reductase, lacking a physiologic electron acceptor, is of minimal physiologic importance, but becomes important when methylene blue is used in the treatment of toxic causes of methemoglobinemia, where the normal Cb5R system is inadequate. In that case the flavin NADPH-dependent methemoglobin reductase reduces methylene blue as an electron acceptor to leukomethylene blue, which then directly reduces methemoglobin (Fig. 42-5).[185]

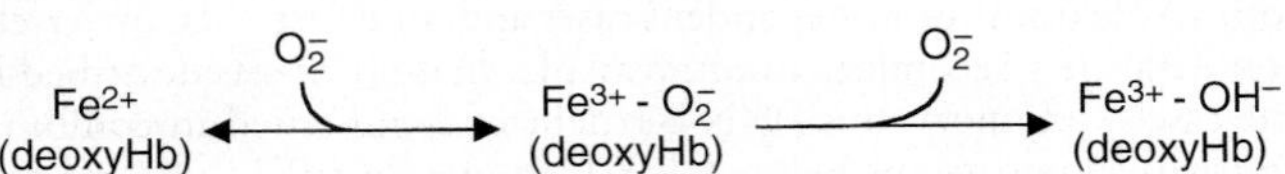

Figure 42-3 AUTO-OXIDATION OF HEMOGLOBIN. Iron is in the ferrous state (Fe^{2+}) in deoxyhemoglobin (deoxyHb). When oxygen is bound, an electron is partially transferred from the iron moiety to the bound oxygen, forming a ferric-superoxide anion complex (Fe^{3+}-O_2^-). During deoxygenation, some of the oxygen leaves as a superoxide (O_2^-) radical. The partially transferred electron is not returned to the iron moiety, leaving the iron in the ferric state (Fe^{3+}) and forming methemoglobin (metHb).

Acquired or Acute Toxic Methemoglobinemia

Most cases of methemoglobinemia are acquired, resulting from either exposure to oxidizing agents or from pathologic underlying conditions. Oxidizing agents may accelerate the rate of formation of methemoglobin up to 1000-fold[182] and eventually overwhelm the capacity of the methemoglobin reduction pathways. Numerous toxins and drugs or their metabolites have been implicated in causing methemoglobinemia (see box on Substances Associated With Methemoglobinemia), including the more common culprits, dapsone, local anesthetics (benzocaine, lidocaine, prilocaine), and derivatives of the anesthetic phenacetin. In a retrospective study of pediatric oncology patients who were treated with dapsone for the prevention of *Pneumocystis carinii* pneumonia, methemoglobinemia was documented in 32 of 167 (19.2%) patients.[186] In this study, higher dapsone dosing was associated with increased risk. In another retrospective study of 138 cases of acquired methemoglobinemia, 42% of cases were due to dapsone.[181] In this series, methemoglobinemia was mild (<8% of total hemoglobin) in the majority of cases. Five of the most severe cases were caused by topical 20% benzocaine spray. In 2006 the U.S. Food and Drug Administration (FDA) issued a public health advisory regarding the risk for methemoglobinemia with the use of benzocaine sprays.[187] In a follow-up safety announcement in 2011, the FDA reported a total of 319 cases of methemoglobinemia due to topical benzocaine sprays, including 32 life-threatening and 7 fatal cases.[188] A single spray of benzocaine, and doses well below the maximum standard allowable dose of prilocaine, particularly in the presence of predisposing factors, have been reported to lead to methemoglobinemia.[189] The FDA has recommended that benzocaine products not

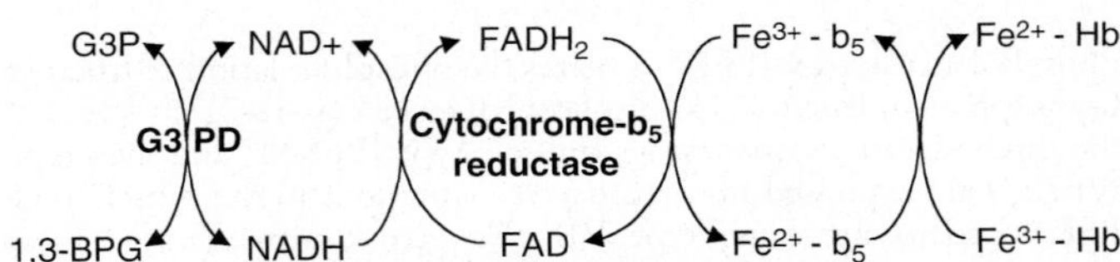

Figure 42-4 NADH-DEPENDENT METHEMOGLOBIN REDUCTION. The reduced form of nicotinamide adenine dinucleotide (NADH) is generated during glycolysis in the reaction mediated by glucose-3-phosphate dehydrogenase (G3PD). A pair of electrons from NADH is transferred to the flavin adenine dinucleotide (FAD) prosthetic group of cytochrome-b_5 reductase, reducing it to $FADH_2$. Two molecules of ferric (Fe^{3+}) cytochrome b_5 are then sequentially bound and reduced, forming ferrous (Fe^{2+}) cytochrome b_5. An ionic complex between ferrous (Fe^{2+}) cytochrome b_5 and a ferric (Fe^{3+}) subunit of a hemoglobin (methemoglobin) tetramer is formed and an electron transferred between the two hemes, creating ferrous (Fe^{2+}) hemoglobin. *1,3-BPG,* 1,3- Bisphosphoglycerate; *G3P,* glyceraldehyde 3-phosphate; *Hb,* hemoglobin; *NAD+,* nicotinamide adenine dinucleotide.

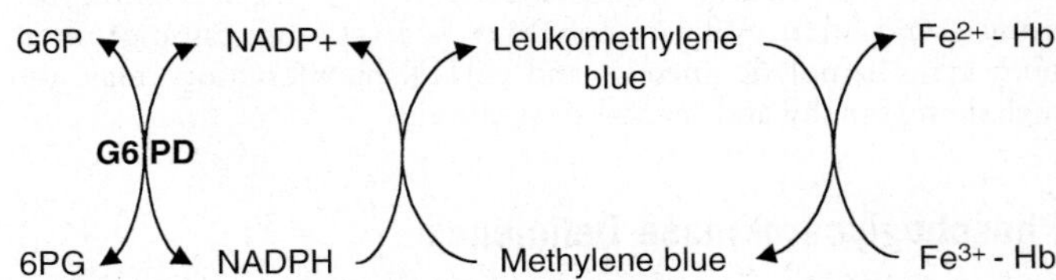

Figure 42-5 NADPH-DEPENDENT METHEMOGLOBIN REDUCTION. NADPH methemoglobin reduction can be activated by exogenously administered methylene blue. *G6P,* Glucose 6-phosphate; *G6PD,* glucose-6-phosphate dehydrogenase; *6PG,* 6-phosphogluconate; *NADP+,* oxidized form of nicotinamide adenine dinucleotide phosphate; *NADPH,* reduced form of nicotinamide adenine dinucleotide phosphate.

Substances Associated With Methemoglobinemia

- Acetaminophen (nitrobenzene derivative)
- Acetanilide
- Local anesthetics
  - Benzocaine
  - Lidocaine
  - Prilocaine
- Aniline dyes
- Celecoxib
- Dapsone
- Flutamide
- Ifosfamide
- Metoclopramide
- Nitric oxide
- Nitrites
  - Amyl nitrite
  - Isobutyl nitrite
  - Sodium nitrite
  - Nitrates (bacterial conversion to nitrites)
- Nitrobenzenes/nitrobenzoates
- Nitroethane (nail polish remover)
- Nitrofurans
- Nitroglycerin
- Paraquat/monolinuron
- Phenacetin
- Phenazopyridine (Pyridium)
- Primaquine
- Rasburicase
- Sulfamethoxazole

be used on children less than 2 years of age, such as in use of over-the counter teething medicine,[190] except under the advice and supervision of a health care professional.[188] The offending agent may be hidden, as is seen when local anesthetics are used in the preparation of cocaine.[191,192] Inhalation and/or ingestion of volatile nitrites is another recreational drug practice that can cause methemoglobinemia.[192]

Exposure to nitrates and nitrites, widely used as food preservatives and found in well water,[193] can also cause methemoglobinemia.[194] Infants less than 6 months of age may have increased susceptibility to methemoglobinemia due to low gastric pH, which allows proliferation of intestinal flora that reduces ingested nitrates to nitrites. Neonates are at particularly increased risk due to decreased Cb5R activity (50% to 60% of adult activity).[195] Homemade baby food purees of high-nitrate-containing foods such as carrots, spinach and silver beets may cause methemoglobinemia, as can acquired illnesses, including diarrheal disease in infants and sepsis.

Clinical Manifestations

Clinical manifestations develop secondary to impaired tissue oxygenation. Typical "cyanotic" slate-blue coloring of the skin and mucous membranes will be visible when 5% to 15% of the total hemoglobin is methemoglobin.[189,196] Although methemoglobin levels up to 20% or even higher may be well tolerated in some individuals, others may experience tachypnea, shakiness, altered consciousness, and signs of myocardial ischemia at methemoglobin levels of 10% to 20%.[189,190] As methemoglobin levels rise above 20% to 30%, patients can experience progressive respiratory compromise, myocardial ischemia, seizures, and coma.[189] Death typically ensues at methemoglobin levels above 70%[197] but can occur at lower levels.[189] Signs and symptoms may be potentiated by factors such as concomitant use of other oxidizing agents, age less than 6 months, anemia, or significant underlying comorbid disease. The onset of disease may be abrupt, and the clinician must maintain a high index of suspicion in at-risk situations (i.e., procedures in which topical anesthetics are used).

Laboratory Manifestations and Diagnosis

Methemoglobinemia should be suspected when the patient appears cyanotic but has a normal PaO_2 as measured by arterial blood gas assessment. The blood will typically be a dark purple to chocolate color, and the blood will not become more red on exposure to oxygen. The diagnosis of methemoglobinemia relies on analysis of its absorbance spectrum. Pulse oximetry is unreliable in the presence of methemoglobinemia, due to its light absorbance properties[198]; however, cooximetry can determine the methemoglobin fraction.[199] The presence and percentage of methemoglobin can be confirmed by use of the Evelyn-Molloy method.[200]

Therapy

Treatment is guided by the level of methemoglobinemia and patient symptoms. In the case of acute onset due to oxidizing agents or disease states, any potential offending agents should be immediately discontinued. The asymptomatic patient with methemoglobin levels of less than 20% may only need observation. If the patient is symptomatic or if methemoglobin levels are greater than 20%, intervention with methylene blue is indicated. Methylene blue is given in a dose of 1 to 2 mg/kg intravenously over 5 minutes, and the dose may be repeated after 60 minutes if necessary. Cumulative doses greater than 4 to 7 mg/kg (or even lower in infants) may cause cyanosis, dyspnea, and acute hemolysis.[201,202] Methemoglobinemia generally resolves promptly with treatment, and within 20 hours in those who receive no treatment.[189] Rebound methemoglobinemia[189] has been reported to occur after methylene blue administration, in one case several days following intentional massive nitrobenzene ingestion.[203] Therefore treated patients should be carefully monitored for recurrence of methemoglobinemia. The therapeutic effect of methylene blue is dependent on the NADPH generated by G6PD. As such, methylene blue will probably not be effective in treating toxic methemoglobinemia in patients who are also G6PD deficient and may even cause hemolysis due to its oxidant effects.[204] Patients with G6PD deficiency who require therapy can be treated with exchange transfusion.[205] Hyperbaric oxygen has also been used successfully in severe cases of methemoglobinemia.[206]

Hereditary Methemoglobinemia

Hereditary causes of methemoglobinemia are secondary to deficiency of Cb5R, very rarely described deficiency of cytochrome b_5,[207] or inheritance of an abnormal hemoglobin in hemoglobin M disease (see Chapter 41).

Cytochrome-b_5 Reductase Deficiency

Cb5R deficiency is the most common cause of congenital methemoglobinemia and is inherited in an autosomal recessive manner.[208] Cb5R is present in two forms, a soluble form present mainly in red cells[183] and a membrane-bound form found in the endoplasmic reticulum and outer mitochondrial membrane.[209,210] Type I Cb5R deficiency is characterized by a deficiency of the soluble, red cell form of Cb5R and manifests as cyanosis, fatigue, and dyspnea. This is the more common form of hereditary methemoglobinemia and is endemic in certain populations, including Navajo[211] and Athabasca[212] Native Americans and natives of Yakutsk, Siberia.[213] Compensatory polycythemia is seen only rarely. Methemoglobinemia, even up to levels of 40%, may be well tolerated.[208] The less common type II Cb5R deficiency, characterized by deficiency of the enzyme in all tissues, has a devastating clinical course, characterized, in addition to cyanosis, by progressive microcephaly, severe mental retardation, dystonia, and early death.[208,214] The types can be differentiated by the clinical phenotype, as well as by assaying enzyme activity in erythroid and nonerythroid tissues. The cyanosis can be treated with oral doses of methylene blue (100 to 300 mg/day) or ascorbic acid (300 to 1000 mg/day in divided doses). There is currently no treatment for the neurologic manifestations of type II Cb5R deficiency.

POLYCYTHEMIA DUE TO CONGENITAL RED BLOOD CELL ENZYME DEFICIENCY

Polycythemia is defined as an absolute increase in RBC mass. Primary polycythemia refers to an inherent defect (acquired or inherited) within the RBCs that results in increased proliferation, whereas secondary polycythemia refers to a reactive process that is usually driven by elevated levels of serum erythropoietin (EPO) as a consequence of chronic tissue hypoxia or EPO-secreting tumors. The vast majority of primary and secondary polycythemias are acquired. The congenital secondary polycythemias are extremely rare and occur when germline mutations alter hemoglobin oxygen affinity or decrease the concentration of 2,3-BPG, resulting in impaired oxygen delivery to the tissues. The latter condition is a result of a congenital deficiency of the erythrocyte enzyme bisphosphoglycerate mutase (BPGM).

Epidemiology and Clinical Manifestations

Only two families with complete BPGM deficiency have been comprehensively studied because of the rarity of the condition. The first case of complete BPGM deficiency was described in 1978 in a family in France.[215] The propositus was a 42-year-old male with a hemoglobin level of 19 g/dL. He had a ruddy complexion but was otherwise clinically well. His 2,3-BPG levels were 3% of normal, and BPGM activity was undetectable.[215] Both the patient and three of his sisters were found to be compound heterozygotes for mutations in the BPGM gene.[216] A second family with complete BPGM deficiency was described in 2004 and included the first and only reported instance (to date) of a patient homozygous for a mutation in the BPGM gene. The mutation was determined to be a missense mutation near the active binding site of the enzyme.[217]

Pathobiology

2,3-BPG is an important modifier of oxygen delivery by RBCs. It binds to a central cavity of the hemoglobin tetramer and allosterically converts hemoglobin to a low oxygen affinity state, resulting in a rightward shift of the oxygen dissociation curve. Patients with chronic hypoxia have elevated levels of 2,3-BPG to facilitate oxygen unloading and increase oxygen delivery to the tissues (Fig. 42-6). BPGM is the enzyme responsible for the synthesis of 2,3-BPG via the Rapoport-Luebering shunt. BPGM is a homodimer with both synthase and phosphatase activity; its synthetic function converts 1,3-bisphosphoglycerate to 2,3-BPG, and its phosphatase activity metabolizes 2,3-BPG to 3-phosphoglycerate, an intermediate of the glycolytic pathway. A deficiency of BPGM leads to a decrease in 2,3-BPG. The ensuing increase in hemoglobin oxygen affinity results in a decrease in oxygen delivery to the tissues, which in turn leads to a compensatory polycythemia.

Diagnosis and Therapy

The diagnosis of BPGM deficiency is first suspected when a patient with an otherwise unexplained polycythemia is noted to have a decreased P_{50} on the oxygen dissociation curve and a normal hemoglobin electrophoretic profile. These studies should be followed by an assay measuring 2,3-BPG activity and, if decreased, an assay measuring BPGM activity. The condition is confirmed by demonstrating a mutation in the BPGM gene.

Due to the rarity of the condition, there is limited experience to guide treatment. Presumably the reactive polycythemia compensates for the diminished oxygen delivery to the tissues and thereby

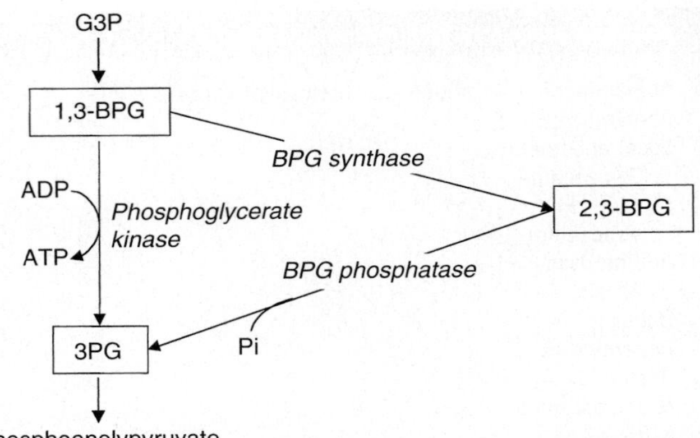

Figure 42-6 RAPOPORT-LUEBERING SHUNT. 2,3-BPG metabolism is regulated by a multifunctional enzyme, bisphosphoglycerate mutase, with both synthase (BPG synthase) and phosphatase (BPG phosphatase) activity. This reaction bypasses the formation of adenosine triphosphate (ATP) in the glycolytic pathway. *ADP,* Adenosine diphosphate; *1,3-BPG,* 1,3-bisphosphoglycerate; *2,3-BPG,* 2,3-bisphosphoglycerate; *G3P,* glyceraldehyde 3-phosphate; *3PG,* 3-phosphoglycerate; *Pi,* inorganic phosphate.

circumvents frank tissue hypoxia. These patients may, however, be more sensitive to decreases in hemoglobin and become symptomatic from what would otherwise be deemed a mild anemia.

SUGGESTED READINGS

Aberg, JA., Kaplan JE, Libman H, et al: Primary care guidelines for the management of persons infected with human immunodeficiency virus: 2009 update by the HIV Medicine Association of the Infectious Diseases Society of America. *Clin Infect Dis* 49:651, 2009.

Ash-Bernal R, Wise R, Wright SM: Acquired methemoglobinemia: A retrospective series of 138 cases at 2 teaching hospitals. *Medicine* 83:265, 2004.

Baronciani L, Beutler E: Molecular study of pyruvate kinase deficient patients with hereditary nonspherocytic hemolytic anemia. *J Clin Invest* 95:1702, 1995.

Beutler E: G6PD deficiency. *Blood* 84:3613, 1994.

Beutler E: PGK deficiency. *Br J Haematol* 136:3, 2007.

Beutler E: Glucose-6-phosphate dehydrogenase deficiency: A historical perspective. *Blood* 111:16, 2008.

Cappadoro M, Giribaldi G, O'Brien E, et al: Early phagocytosis of glucose-6-phosphate dehydrogenase (G6PD)-deficient erythrocytes parasitized by *Plasmodium falciparum* may explain malaria protection in G6PD deficiency. *Blood* 92:2527, 1998.

Cappellini MD, Fiorelli G: Glucose-6-phosphate dehydrogenase deficiency. *Lancet* 371:64, 2008.

Clark IA, Hunt NH: Evidence for reactive oxygen intermediates causing hemolysis and parasite death in malaria. *Infect Immun* 39:1, 1983.

Delivoria-Papadopoulos M, Oski FA, Gottlieb AJ: Oxygen-hemoglobulin dissociation curves: Effect of inherited enzyme defects of the red cell. *Science* 165:601, 1969.

Esbenshade AJ, Ho RH, Shintani A, et al: Dapsone-induced methemoglobinemia: A dose-related occurrence? *Cancer* 117:3485, 2011.

FDA: FDA Drug Safety Communication: FDA continues to receive reports of a rare, but serious and potentially fatal adverse effect with the use of benzocaine sprays for medical procedures. 2011 August 1. Available from: http://www.fda.gov/Drugs/DrugSafety/ucm250040.htm#data, 2011.

Friedman, MJ: Oxidant damage mediates variant red cell resistance to malaria. *Nature* 280:245, 1979.

Gaetani, GD, Parker JC, Kirkman HN: Intracellular restraint: A new basis for the limitation in response to oxidative stress in human erythrocytes containing low-activity variants of glucose-6-phosphate dehydrogenase. *Proc Natl Acad Sci U S A* 71:3584, 1974.

Guay J: Methemoglobinemia related to local anesthetics: A summary of 242 episodes. *Anesth Analg* 108:837, 2009.

Kaplan M, Hammerman C: The need for neonatal glucose-6-phosphate dehydrogenase screening: A global perspective. *J Perinatol* 29:S46, 2009.

Kwiatkowski, DP: How malaria has affected the human genome and what human genetics can teach us about malaria. *Am J Hum Genet* 77:171, 2005.

Lenzner C, Nürnberg P, Jacobasch G, et al: Molecular analysis of 29 pyruvate kinase-deficient patients from central Europe with hereditary hemolytic anemia. *Blood* 89:1793, 1997.

Miller J, Golenser J, Spira DT, et al: *Plasmodium falciparum:* Thiol status and growth in normal and glucose-6-phosphate dehydrogenase deficient human erythrocytes. *Exp Parasitol* 57:239, 1984.

Nkhoma ET, Poole C, Vannappagari V, et al: The global prevalence of glucose-6-phosphate dehydrogenase deficiency: A systematic review and meta-analysis. *Blood Cells Mol Dis* 42:267, 2009.

Nock ML, Johnson EM, Krugman RR, et al: Implementation and analysis of a pilot in-hospital newborn screening program for glucose-6-phosphate dehydrogenase deficiency in the United States. *J Perinatol* 31:112, 2011.

Percy MJ, Lappin TR: Recessive congenital methaemoglobinaemia: Cytochrome b(5) reductase deficiency. *Br J Haematol* 141:298, 2008.

Ruwende C, Khoo SC, Snow RW, et al: Natural selection of hemi- and heterozygotes for G6PD deficiency in Africa by resistance to severe malaria. *Nature* 376:246, 1995.

Serpa JA, Villarreal-Williams E, Giordano TP: Prevalence of G6PD deficiency in a large cohort of HIV-infected patients. *J Infect* 61:399, 2010.

Tantular IS, Kawamoto F: An improved, simple screening method for detection of glucose-6-phosphate dehydrogenase deficiency. *Trop Med Int Health* 8:569, 2003.

Valentine WN, Fink K, Paglia DE, et al: Hereditary hemolytic anemia with human erythrocyte pyrimidine 5'-nucleotidase deficiency. *J Clin Invest* 54:866, 1974.

Youngster I, Arcavi L, Schechmaster R, et al: Medications and glucose-6-phosphate dehydrogenase deficiency: An evidence-based review. *Drug Saf* 33:713, 2010.

Zaffanello M, Rugolotto S, Zamboni G, et al: Neonatal screening for glucose-6-phosphate dehydrogenase deficiency fails to detect heterozygote females. *Eur J Epidemiol* 19:255, 2004.

Zanella A, Bianchi P, Fermo E, et al: Hereditary pyrimidine 5′-nucleotidase deficiency: From genetics to clinical manifestations. *Br J Haematol* 133:113, 2006.

Zanella A, Fermo E, Bianchi P, et al: Pyruvate kinase deficiency: The genotype-phenotype association. *Blood Rev* 21:217, 2007.

For complete list of references log on to www.expertconsult.com.

CHAPTER 43

RED BLOOD CELL MEMBRANE DISORDERS

Patrick G. Gallagher

Characterization of the structure and function of red blood cell membrane proteins and their genes (Fig. 43-1) has led to considerable advances in our understanding of the molecular pathology of membrane-associated disorders, including the definition and characterization of mutations of membrane proteins as a well-defined cause of hereditary hemolytic disease. Likewise, knowledge of the molecular mechanisms underlying changes in red blood cell deformability, structural integrity, and shape has advanced. Red blood cell shape abnormalities often provide a clue to the pathobiology and diagnosis of the underlying disorder. This chapter categorizes red blood cell membrane disorders according to the following morphologic and clinical phenotypes: (1) hereditary spherocytosis (HS); (2) hereditary elliptocytosis (HE), hereditary pyropoikilocytosis (HPP), and related disorders; (3) Southeast Asian ovalocytosis (SAO); (4) hereditary and acquired acanthocytosis; and (5) hereditary and acquired stomatocytosis (Tables 43-1 and 43-2).

VERTICAL AND HORIZONTAL INTERACTIONS OF MEMBRANE PROTEINS AND DISORDERS OF RED BLOOD CELL SHAPE

Palek et al first proposed dividing membrane protein-protein and protein-lipid interactions into two categories, vertical and horizontal interactions. Vertical interactions, which are perpendicular to the plane of the membrane, stabilize the lipid bilayer. These interactions include spectrin-ankyrin–band 3 interactions, spectrin–protein 4.1R–junctional complex proteins linkage, spectrin-ankyrin–Rh multiprotein complex linkage, and the weak interactions between the skeletal proteins and the negatively charged lipids of the inner half of the membrane lipid bilayer. Horizontal interactions, which are parallel to the plane of the membrane, support the structural integrity of erythrocytes after their exposure to shear stress. Horizontal interactions involve the spectrin heterodimer association site, where spectrin heterodimers assemble into tetramers, the principal building blocks of the membrane skeleton, and the contacts of the distal ends of spectrin heterodimers with actin and protein 4.1R within the junctional complex. Although interactions between proteins of the erythrocyte membrane are significantly more complex than can be classified by this model of horizontal and vertical interactions, the model serves as a useful starting place for understanding erythrocyte membrane protein interactions, particularly in reference to membrane-related disorders.

According to the vertical/horizontal model, HS is considered a disorder of vertical interactions (Fig. 43-2). Although the primary molecular defects in HS are heterogeneous (including deficiencies or dysfunctions of α- and β-spectrin, ankyrin, band 3, and protein 4.2), one common feature of HS red blood cells is a weakening of the vertical contacts between the skeleton and the overlying lipid bilayer membrane together with its integral proteins. Consequently the lipid bilayer membrane is destabilized, leading to release of bilayer lipids from the cells in the form of skeleton-free lipid vesicles. This lipid loss, in turn, results in membrane surface area deficiency and spherocytosis.

In most patients with HE and the related disorder HPP (see Hereditary Elliptocytosis and Related Disorders), the principal lesion involves horizontal membrane–protein associations, primarily spectrin dimer-dimer interactions. In a subset of HE patients with a deficiency or a dysfunction of protein 4.1R or glycophorin C (GPC), the horizontal defect resides in the junctional complex, where the distal ends of spectrin tetramers connect to actin, in conjunction with protein 4.1R. In patients with severely dysfunctional spectrin mutations, the weakened spectrin dimer-dimer self-association disrupts the skeletal lattice, leading to a marked skeletal instability and cell fragments. In patients with mildly dysfunctional spectrins, red blood cell shape is that of biconcave elliptocytes. It is speculated that elliptocytes are permanently deformed cells because the weakened horizontal interactions facilitate a shear stress–induced rearrangement of skeletal proteins, precluding recovery of the normal biconcave shape. This hypothesis is not applicable to all forms of elliptocytosis. For example, in SAO, the elliptocytic/ovalocytic cells containing mutant band 3 protein are rigid and "hyperstable" rather than unstable.

Acanthocytosis, Stomatocytosis, and the Bilayer Couple Hypothesis

The mechanism of acanthocytosis and stomatocytosis associated with defects of membrane proteins is much less clear. Most forms of acanthocytosis are associated with either acquired or inherited abnormalities of membrane lipids (e.g., acanthocytosis in end-stage liver disease or abetalipoproteinemia). In rare subjects with acanthocytosis, membrane protein abnormalities have been detected, but the associated mechanisms leading to acanthocyte formation are unknown. These abnormalities occur in the McLeod phenotype, the chorea-acanthocytosis syndrome, and other rare disorders. In acanthocytosis erythrocytes, agents that interact with the lipids of the inner lipid bilayer leaflet normalize the shape. These studies suggest that the shape abnormalities reflect an asymmetry in the distribution of membrane lipids between the two halves of the red blood cell lipid bilayer as predicted by the bilayer couple hypothesis. According to the bilayer hypothesis, the shape of the red blood cell reflects the ratio of the surface areas of the two hemileaflets of the bilayer. The preferential expansion of the outer leaflet leads to red blood cell crenation (echinocytosis or acanthocytosis), whereas expansion of the inner lipid bilayer produces a cup shape (stomatocytosis) and surface invaginations.

Hereditary Spherocytosis

Introduction and Epidemiology

The typical features of HS include a dominantly inherited hemolytic anemia of mild to moderate severity, spherocytosis on the peripheral blood film, and a favorable response to splenectomy. The clinical spectrum of HS is variable and includes both mild and asymptomatic forms, as well as severe forms that appear in infancy. The previously

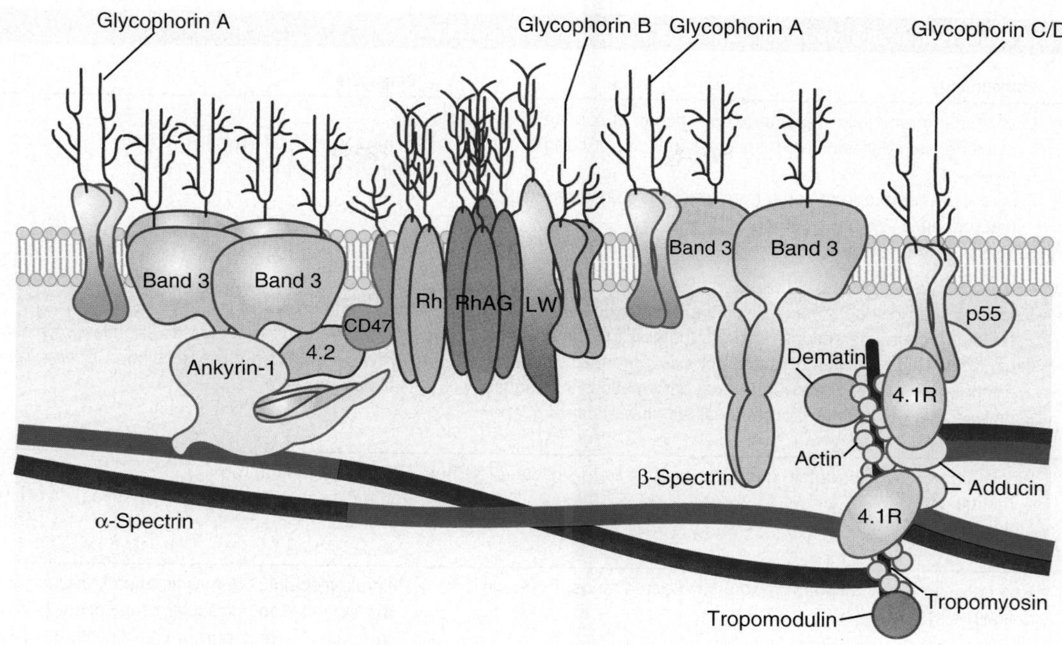

Figure 43-1 A SIMPLIFIED CROSS-SECTION OF THE ERYTHROCYTE MEMBRANE. The lipid bilayer forms the equator of the cross-section with its polar heads *(small circles)* turned outward. *4.1R,* Protein 4.1R; *4.2,* protein 4.2; *Rh,* Rhesus polypeptide; *RhAG,* Rh-associated glycoprotein; *LW,* Landsteiner-Wiener glycoprotein. *(From Perrotta S, Gallagher PG, Mohandas N: Hereditary spherocytosis.* Lancet *372:1411, 2008.)*

Table 43-1 Erythrocyte Membrane Abnormalities in Hereditary Spherocytosis, Hereditary Elliptocytosis, and Related Disorders

Gene	Disorder	Comment
α-Spectrin	HS, HE, HPP, NIHF	Location of mutation determines clinical phenotype. α-Spectrin mutations are most common cause of typical HE.
Ankyrin	HS	Most common cause of typical dominant HS.
Band 3	HS, SAO, NIHF	In HS "pincer-like" spherocytes on smear presplenectomy. SAO erythrocytes have transverse ridge or longitudinal slit.
β-Spectrin	HS, HE, HPP, NIHF	Location of mutation determines clinical phenotype. In HS, acanthrocytic spherocytes on smear presplenectomy.
Protein 4.2	HS	Common in Japanese HS.
Protein 4.1	HE	
Glycophorin C	HE	Concomitant protein 4.1 deficiency is basis of HE in glycophorin C defects.

HE, Hereditary elliptocytosis; *HPP,* hereditary pyropoikilocytosis; *HS,* hereditary spherocytosis; *NIHF,* nonimmune hydrops fetalis, *SAO,* Southeast Asian ovalocytosis.

reported HS prevalence in Western populations of 1 in 5000 persons is an underestimation, because milder forms of HS might be asymptomatic, suggesting a prevalence of 1 in 2000 individuals. HS has been reported worldwide, particularly in Japanese and African populations, but its prevalence in other ethnic groups is unknown.

Pathobiology

Two major factors are involved in HS pathophysiology: (1) an intrinsic red blood cell defect and (2) an intact spleen that selectively retains and damages abnormal HS erythrocytes. An inherited deficiency or dysfunction of proteins of the erythrocyte membrane leads to a multistep process of accelerated HS red blood cell destruction. Destabilization of the lipid bilayer facilitates a release of lipids from the membrane, leading to surface area deficiency and formation of poorly deformable spherocytes that are selectively retained and damaged in the spleen (see Fig. 43-2).

Molecular Pathology

The molecular basis of HS is heterogeneous. Based on densitometric quantitation of membrane proteins separated by polyacrylamide gel electrophoresis, HS can be divided into the following subsets: (1) isolated deficiency of spectrin, (2) combined deficiencies of spectrin and ankyrin, (3) deficiency of band 3 protein, (4) deficiency of protein 4.2, and (5) no abnormality identified.

Isolated Spectrin Deficiency

The reported mutations of isolated spectrin deficiency include defects of both α- and β-spectrin. Mutations of the β-spectrin gene have been identified in a number of patients with dominantly inherited HS associated with spectrin deficiency. A few cases have been associated with de novo β-spectrin gene mutations. With a few exceptions, these mutations are private and may be associated with decreased β-spectrin messenger ribonucleic acid (mRNA) accumulation. Mutations in the highly conserved region of β-spectrin involved in the interaction with protein 4.1R likely lead to dysfunctional binding to protein 4.1R and thereby the linkage of spectrin to actin.

In nondominantly inherited HS associated with isolated spectrin deficiency, the defect involves α-spectrin. In normal erythroid cells, α-spectrin is synthesized in large excess of β-spectrin. Thus subjects

Table 43-2 Peripheral Blood Film Evaluation in a Patient With Red Cell Membrane Disorder

Shape	Pathobiology	Diagnosis
Microspherocytes	Loss of membrane lipids leading to a reduction of surface area resulting from deficiencies of spectrin, ankyrin, or band 3 and protein 4.2 Removal of membrane material from antibody-coated red cells by macrophages Removal of membrane-associated Heinz bodies, with the adjacent membrane lipids, by the spleen	HS Immunohemolytic anemias Heinz body hemolytic anemias
Elliptocytes	Permanent red cell deformation resulting from a weakening of skeletal protein interactions (such as the spectrin dimer-dimer contact). This facilitates disruption of existing protein contacts during shear stress–induced elliptical deformation. Subsequently, new protein contacts are formed that stabilize elliptical shape Unknown	Mild common HE Iron deficiency, megaloblastic anemias, myelofibrosis, myelophthisic anemias, myelodysplastic syndrome, thalassemias
Poikilocytes/ Fragments	Weakening of skeletal protein contacts resulting from skeletal protein mutations Unknown	Hemolytic HE/HPP Iron deficiency, megaloblastic anemias, myelofibrosis, myelophthisic anemias, myelodysplastic syndrome, thalassemias
Schistocytes, fragmented red cells	Red cells "torn'' by mechanical trauma (fibrin strands, turbulent flow)	"Microangiopathic" hemolytic anemia associated with disseminated intravascular coagulation, thrombotic thrombocytopenic purpura, vasculitis, heart valve prostheses
Acanthocytes	Uptake of cholesterol and its preferential accumulation in the outer leaflet of the lipid bilayer Selective accumulation of sphingomyelin in the outer lipid leaflet Unknown	Spur cell hemolytic anemia in severe liver disease Abetalipoproteinemia Chorea-acanthocytosis syndrome, malnutrition, hypothyroidism McLeod phenotype
Echinocytes	Expansion of the surface area of the outer hemileaflet of lipid bilayer relative to the inner hemileaflet Unknown	Hemolytic anemia associated with hypomagnesemia and hypophosphatemia in malnourished patients, pyruvate kinase deficiency; in vitro artifact of low blood storage (ATP depletion), contact with glass or elevated pH Hemolysis in long-distance runners, renal failure
Stomatocytes	Expansion of the surface area of the inner hemileaflet of the bilayer relative to the outer leaflet Unknown	Exposure of red cells to cationic anesthetics in vitro; in vivo the drug concentrations may not be sufficient to produce similar effect Alcoholism, inherited disorders of membrane permeability (hereditary stomatocytosis)
Target cells	Absolute excess of membrane lipids (both cholesterol and phospholipids: "symmetric" lipid gain), followed by an increase of cell surface area Relative excess of surface area because of a decrease in cell volume	Obstructive jaundice, liver disease with intrahepatic cholestasis Thalassemias and some hemoglobinopathies (C, D, E)

ATP, Adenosine triphosphate; *HE,* hereditary elliptocytosis; *HPP,* hereditary pyropoikilocytosis; *HS,* hereditary spherocytosis.

with one normal and one defective α-spectrin allele are asymptomatic, because α-spectrin production remains in excess of β-spectrin synthesis, allowing normal amounts of spectrin heterodimers to be assembled on the membrane. Patients who are homozygotes or compound heterozygotes for α-spectrin defects suffer from moderate to severe HS.

A number of patients with atypical HS associated with karyotypic abnormalities involving deletions or translocations of the ankyrin gene locus on chromosome 8p have been described. Ankyrin deletions may be part of a contiguous gene syndrome with manifestations of spherocytosis, mental retardation, typical facies, and hypogonadism.

Combined Deficiency of Spectrin and Ankyrin

The biochemical phenotype of combined spectrin and ankyrin deficiency is the most common abnormality found in the erythrocytes of HS patients. Ankyrin represents the principal binding site for spectrin on the membrane; thus it is not surprising that ankyrin deficiency is accompanied by a proportional decrease in spectrin assembly on the membrane despite normal spectrin synthesis. Similar to HS associated with β-spectrin mutations, most ankyrin defects are private point mutations associated with decreased mRNA accumulation. In some cases, mutations of the ankyrin promoter leading to decreased ankyrin expression have been found. Approximately 15% to 20% of ankyrin gene mutations reported are de novo mutations.

Deficiency of Band 3 Protein

Deficiency of band 3 protein is found in a subset of HS patients who present with a phenotype of a mild to moderate dominantly inherited HS. Most, if not all, of these patients also have concomitant protein 4.2 deficiency. Numerous band 3 mutations associated with HS have been reported, spread throughout both the cytoplasmic and the membrane-spanning domains.

A number of band 3 mutations clustered in the membrane-spanning domain that replace highly conserved arginines have been described. These arginines, which are all located at the cytoplasmic end of a predicted transmembrane helix, exhibit defective cellular trafficking from the endoplasmic reticulum to the plasma membrane.

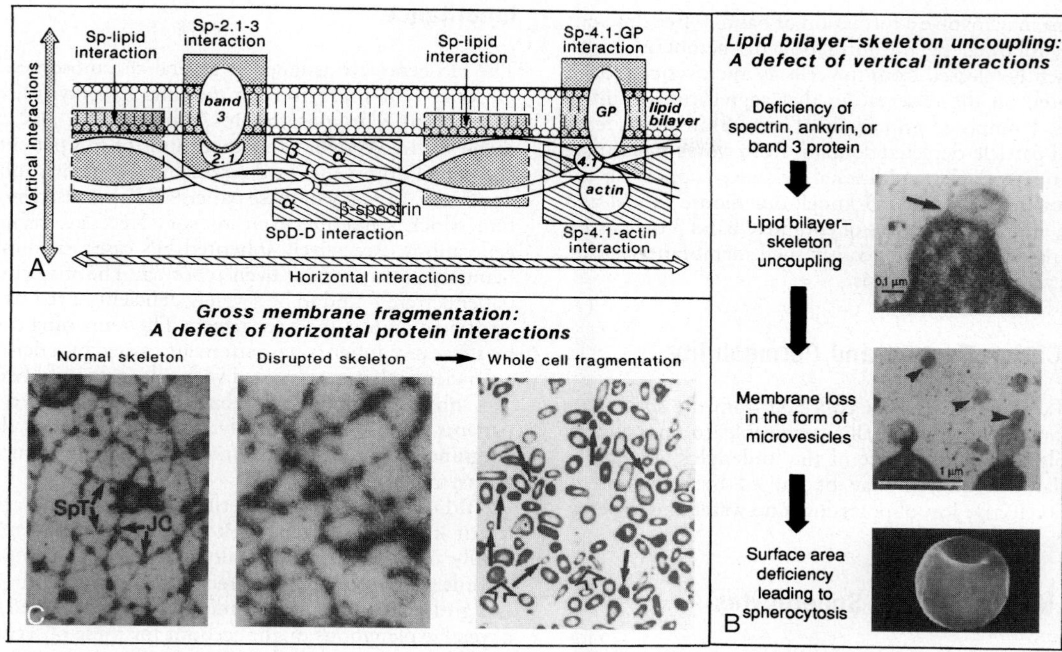

Figure 43-2 VERTICAL AND HORIZONTAL INTERACTIONS OF MEMBRANE PROTEINS AND THE PATHOBIOLOGY OF THE RED CELL LESION IN HEREDITARY SPHEROCYTOSIS AND HEREDITARY ELLIPTOCYTOSIS. **A,** In one model of the erythrocyte membrane, proteins interact in a series of horizontal and/or vertical interactions. Perturbation of these interactions leads to disorders of erythrocyte shape. **B,** A defect of vertical interactions as exemplified by the membrane lesion in hereditary spherocytosis. Deficiency of spectrin, ankyrin, or band 3 protein leads to uncoupling of the membrane lipid bilayer from the underlying skeleton *(top panel),* followed by a formation of spectrin-free microvesicles of about 0.2-0.5 mm in diameter *(arrowheads, middle panel)*. These vesicles can be visualized by transmission electron microscopy, but they are not seen on examination of a peripheral blood film. The subsequent loss of cell surface area and a decrease in the surface/volume ratio lead to spherocytosis *(bottom panel).* **C,** Defect of horizontal interactions of membrane skeleton proteins as exemplified by the membrane lesion in hemolytic forms of hereditary elliptocytosis and hereditary pyropoikilocytosis. The molecular lesion of weakened self-association of spectrin heterodimers to tetramers (SpT) leads to decreased linkage of spectrin to junctional complexes (JC), representing a horizontal defect of shear stress-resisting protein interactions. It leads to a disruption of the membrane skeletal lattice and, consequently, to destabilization of the whole cell, followed by cell fragmentation, as seen as seen on peripheral blood smear.

Alleles have been identified that influence band 3 expression and that, when inherited in trans to a band 3 mutation, aggravate band 3 deficiency and worsen the clinical severity of the disease.

Deficiency of Protein 4.2

Recessively inherited HS caused by mutations in protein 4.2 is relatively common in Japan. In these cases, an almost total absence of protein 4.2 from the erythrocyte membranes of homozygous patients is detected. Protein 4.2–deficient erythrocytes can also have a decreased content of ankyrin and band 3. Protein 4.2 deficiency also occurs in association with band 3 mutations, probably as a result of abnormal binding of protein 4.2 to the cytoplasmic domain of band 3.

A detailed listing of HS mutations is available (http://research.nhgri.nih.gov/RBCmembrane/) in a mutation database maintained by the National Human Genome Research Institute and Yale University.

Molecular Basis of Surface Area Deficiency

Hereditary spherocytes are intrinsically unstable, releasing lipids under a variety of in vitro conditions, including adenosine triphosphate (ATP) depletion or exposure of cells to shear stress. The loss of membrane material occurs through the release of vesicles containing integral proteins devoid of spectrin. During in vitro incubation, the loss of membrane material is sufficient to augment the surface area deficiency, as evidenced by increased osmotic fragility of the cells after incubation. It is assumed but not proved that a similar process takes place in vivo.

The molecular basis of HS is heterogeneous; thus it is likely that surface area deficiency is a consequence of several distinct molecular mechanisms whose common denominator is either a weakening of the vertical connections between the skeleton and the lipid bilayer membrane or a weakening of the stabilizing effect of transmembrane proteins on adjacent lipid molecules of the plasma membrane. Three distinct hypothetic pathways that can lead to surface area deficiency are depicted in Fig. 43-2. In patients with isolated spectrin deficiency or a combined deficiency of spectrin and ankyrin, the loss of red blood cell surface may be caused by an uncoupling of the lipid bilayer membrane from the underlying skeleton. In normal red blood cells, the skeleton forms a nearly monomolecular submembrane layer occupying more than one-half of the inner surface of the membrane. Consequently spectrin deficiency leads to a decreased density of this network. As a result, areas of the lipid bilayer membrane that are not directly supported by the skeleton are susceptible to release from the cells in the form of microvesicles.

In HS associated with a deficiency of band 3 protein, two hypothetic pathways may lead to a loss of surface area. One mechanism may involve a loss of band 3 protein from the cells. Because band 3 protein spans the lipid bilayer membrane many times, it is likely that a substantial amount of "boundary" lipids are released together with the band 3 protein, thus leading to surface area deficiency. Another possible mechanism may involve a formation of band 3–free domains in the membrane, followed by the formation of membrane blebs, which are subsequently released from the cells as microvesicles. Such a hypothesis is based on the observation that aggregation of intramembrane particles (composed principally of band 3) in ghosts leads to the formation of particle-depleted domains from which membrane lipids bleb off as microvesicles. Additional evidence supporting the latter model comes from the band 3 knock-out mouse model and from human, cow, and zebrafish cases of complete band 3 deficiency. Erythrocytes lacking band 3 spontaneously shed membrane vesicles, leading to spherocytosis and hemolysis.

Alterations in Cation Content and Permeability

HS red blood cells, particularly those collected from the spleen, are somewhat dehydrated and abnormally permeable to monovalent cations, presumably as a consequence of the underlying membrane defect. The cellular dehydration may be caused by activation of pathways causing a selective loss of potassium and water or a hyperactive Na^+/K^+ pump.

Entrapment of Nondeformable Spherocytes in the Spleen

The importance of the spleen in the pathophysiology of hemolysis in HS was appreciated in the original description of the disease and has been substantiated by subsequent studies. HS cells are selectively destroyed in the spleen because of their poor deformability and because of the unique anatomy of the splenic vasculature that acts as a microcirculation filter.

The poor red blood cell deformability is principally a consequence of a decreased cell surface/cell volume ratio resulting from the loss of surface material. Normal discocytes have an excess surface, which allows them to deform and pass through narrow microcirculation openings. In contrast, HS red blood cells lack this extra surface, and their poor deformability may be further impaired by cellular dehydration.

The principal sites of red blood cell entrapment in the spleen are fenestrations in the wall of splenic sinuses, where blood from the splenic cords of the red pulp enters the venous circulation. In rat spleen, the length and width of these fenestrations, 2 to 3 μm and 0.2 to 0.5 μm, respectively, are approximately half the red blood cell diameter. Electron micrographs show that very few HS red blood cells traverse these slits. Consequently the nondeformable spherocytes accumulate in the red pulp, which becomes grossly engorged.

Splenic Conditioning and Destruction

Once trapped in the spleen, HS erythrocytes undergo additional damage or conditioning with further loss of surface area and an increase in cell density, as is evident in cells removed from the spleen at splenectomy. Some of these conditioned red blood cells reenter the systemic circulation, as revealed by the "tail" of the osmotic fragility curve, indicating the presence of a subpopulation of cells with a markedly reduced surface area. After splenectomy, this red blood cell population disappears.

Contributions to conditioning may include a relatively low pH in the spleen as well as in the sequestered red blood cells that may further compromise the poor HS red blood cell deformability, and contact of red blood cells with macrophages that may inflict additional damage on the red blood cell membrane. The conditioning effect of the spleen appears to represent a cumulative injury. The average residence time of HS red blood cells in the splenic cords is between 10 and 100 minutes compared with 30 to 40 seconds for normal red blood cells, and only 1% to 10% of blood entering the spleen is temporarily sequestered in the congested cords, whereas the remaining 90% of blood flow is rapidly shunted into the venous circulation.

Inheritance

The HS genes are assigned to several chromosomes, including chromosome 1 (α-spectrin), chromosome 8 (ankyrin), chromosome 14 (β-spectrin), chromosome 15 (protein 4.2), and chromosome 17 (band 3). In approximately two-thirds of HS patients, inheritance is autosomal dominant. In the remaining patients, inheritance is nondominant. In many of these patients, HS is caused by a de novo mutation, which is inherited in an autosomal recessive fashion in subsequent generations. Recessively inherited HS cases manifesting with severe hemolytic anemia have been reported. The majority of the affected patients were found to be severely deficient in red blood cell spectrin, associated with α-spectrin defects. The remaining cases characterized by a recessive inheritance pattern are caused by a defect in protein 4.2, a deficiency that is associated with relatively mild hemolysis.

Only a few cases of homozygous HS have been reported. These patients have a severe hemolytic anemia, whereas their mostly consanguineous parents have a mild to moderate form of the disease or are asymptomatic.

Although the clinical severity of HS is highly variable among different kindreds, in general it is relatively uniform within a given family, in which HS is typically inherited as an autosomal dominant disorder. However, HS kindreds have been described in which there was great variability in the clinical severity of affected family members. Several explanations might account for these observations, including variable penetrance of the genetic defect, a de novo mutation, presence of a mild recessive HS in the kindred, presence of a modifier allele that influences the expression of a membrane protein, or a tissue-specific mosaicism of the defect.

Clinical Manifestations

Typical Forms

The typical HS patient is relatively asymptomatic. As noted in the earliest descriptions of HS, mild jaundice can be the only symptom of the disease. Splenomegaly gradually develops in most patients, with the spleen occasionally reaching large dimensions. Anemia is usually mild to moderate but may be absent because of compensatory bone marrow hyperplasia.

Mild Forms and Carrier State

In some families, anemia is absent, the reticulocyte count is normal or only minimally elevated, laboratory evidence of hemolysis is minimal or absent, and the changes in red blood cell shape can be mild, escaping detection on the peripheral blood film. The presence of HS is detected only by osmotic fragility testing or during evaluation of a relative with a more symptomatic form of the disease. Some patients are first diagnosed during transient viral infections such as infectious mononucleosis or parvovirus infection, during pregnancy, or even in the seventh to ninth decades of life as the bone marrow's ability to compensate for hemolysis wanes.

Severe and Atypical Forms

The relatively uncommon patients with nondominant forms of HS can present with a severe life-threatening hemolysis early in life. Some patients can be transfusion dependent during early infancy and childhood. The underlying molecular defects include severe spectrin or band 3 deficiency.

Hereditary Spherocytosis and Nonerythroid Manifestations

In most HS cases, the clinical manifestations are confined to the erythroid lineage, probably because many of the nonerythroid counterparts of the red blood cell membrane proteins (e.g., spectrin and ankyrin) are encoded by separate genes or because some proteins (e.g., protein 4.1R, β-spectrin, ankyrin) are subject to tissue-specific alternative splicing. However, several HS kindreds have been reported with a cosegregating neurologic or muscular abnormality, such as a degenerative disorder of the spinal cord, cardiomyopathy, or mental retardation. The observation that both erythrocyte ankyrin and β-spectrin are also expressed in muscle, brain, particularly the cerebellum, and spinal cord raises the possibility that these HS patients may have a defect in one of these proteins. This hypothesis is further supported by studies of nb/nb mice, a mouse model of HS caused by an ankyrin mutation. These mice develop a neurologic syndrome with a progression that coincides with the loss of ankyrin from the Purkinje cells of the cerebellum.

Mutations of band 3 without HS have been described in patients with distal renal tubular acidosis. With a few rare exceptions, most patients with heterozygous mutations of band 3 and HS have normal renal acidification.

Laboratory Manifestations

Most HS patients have either a mild to moderate anemia or no anemia at all, reflecting the facts that the hemolytic rate can be very mild and that the hemolysis is fully compensated for by increased red blood cell production, as evidenced by reticulocytosis. Some patients, however, particularly those with nondominantly inherited HS, are severely anemic, with hemoglobin concentrations as low as 4 to 6 g/dL.

Despite the increased percentage of reticulocytes with a larger volume than mature red blood cells, the mean corpuscular volume (MCV) of HS red blood cells is often low normal or even slightly decreased, and the mean corpuscular hemoglobin concentration (MCHC) is usually increased (>35 g/dL), together reflecting mild cellular dehydration.

The finding of an MCHC greater than 35.4 g/dL combined with a red blood cell distribution width (RDW) of less than14% has been found to be an excellent screening test for HS. Another screening method measures MCV by light scattering and provides a histogram of hyperdense erythrocytes (MCHC >40 g/dL) claimed to identify nearly all HS patients. These hyperdense erythrocytes can be detected with newer laser-based blood counters or using aperture impedance analysis available in many clinical laboratories.

Evidence of accelerated red blood cell destruction, as indicated by increased lactate dehydrogenase and unconjugated bilirubin levels and by decreased haptoglobin, as well as by reticulocytosis, is present in typical HS patients. However, these abnormalities can be absent in individuals with a mild form of the disease.

Blood Film

In a typical case of HS, spherocytes are readily identified by their characteristic shape on the peripheral blood film (Fig. 43-3). They lack central pallor, their mean cell diameter is decreased, and they appear more intensely hemoglobinated, which reflects both altered red blood cell geometry and increased cell density. In a three-dimensional view, some spherocytes have a spherostomatocytic shape that is occasionally appreciated on the peripheral blood film. In mild forms of the disease, the peripheral blood smear can appear normal because the loss of surface area can be too small to be appreciated by blood smear evaluation; the cells appear as "fat" disks rather than as true spherocytes.

Additional morphologic features have been described in some HS patients (see Fig. 43-3). A subset of HS patients whose red blood cells are deficient in band 3 protein have some pincer-like red blood cells on the peripheral blood film, a finding that is both sensitive and specific for this HS subset. These pincer-like cells disappear after splenectomy. Surface spiculations or acanthocytic spherocytes have been described in cases of HS associated with defects in β-spectrin. Frequent sphero-ovalocytes and stomatocytes have been reported in Japanese patients with protein 4.2 deficiency.

Osmotic Fragility

The osmotic fragility test (Fig. 43-4) measures the in vitro lysis of red blood cells suspended in solutions of decreasing osmolarity. The normal red blood cell membrane is unstretchable and is virtually freely permeable to water. Thus the cell behaves as a nearly perfect osmometer in that it increases its volume in hypotonic solutions progressively until a "critical hemolytic volume" is reached. At this point, the red blood cell membrane ruptures, and hemoglobin escapes into the supernatant solution. As a result of the loss of membrane and the ensuing surface area deficiency, the critical hemolytic volume of spherocytes is considerably lower than that of normal red blood cells. Consequently these cells hemolyze more than normal red blood cells when suspended in hypotonic sodium chloride solutions. However, a finding of increased osmotic fragility is not unique to HS and is also present in other conditions associated with spherocytosis on the peripheral blood film, such as autoimmune hemolytic anemia.

The slight dehydration of hereditary spherocytes (which in other conditions is associated with decreased osmotic fragility) has no appreciable effect on HS osmotic fragility because of the overriding effect of the markedly diminished cell surface area. In fact, the densest, most dehydrated cells exhibit the greatest increase in osmotic fragility.

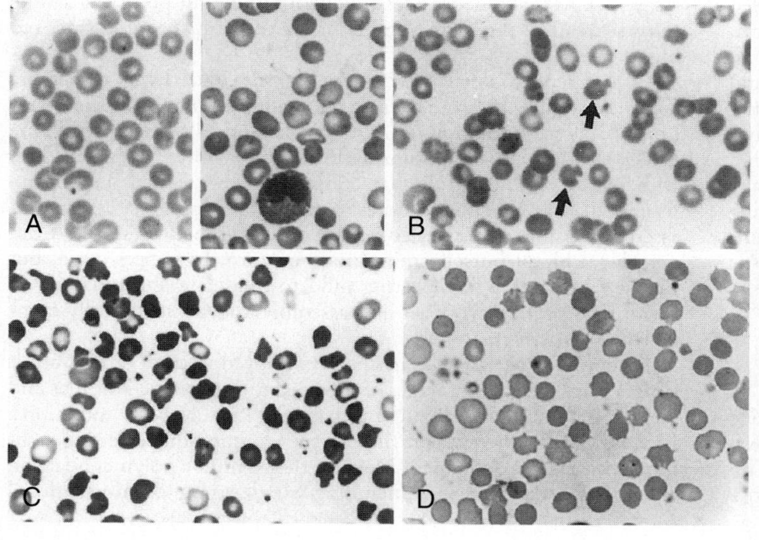

Figure 43-3 BLOOD FILMS FROM PATIENTS WITH HEREDITARY SPHEROCYTOSIS (HS) OF VARYING SEVERITY. **A,** Two blood films of typical moderately severe HS with a mild deficiency of red blood cell spectrin and ankyrin. Although many cells have a spheroidal shape, some retain a central concavity. **B,** HS with pincer-like red blood cells *(arrows),* as typically seen in HS associated with band 3 deficiency. Occasional spiculated red blood cells are also present. **C,** Severe atypical HS caused by a severe combined spectrin and ankyrin deficiency. In addition to spherocytes, many cells have irregular contour. **D,** HS with isolated spectrin deficiency caused by a β-spectrin mutation. Some of the spherocytes have prominent surface projections resembling spheroacanthocytes.

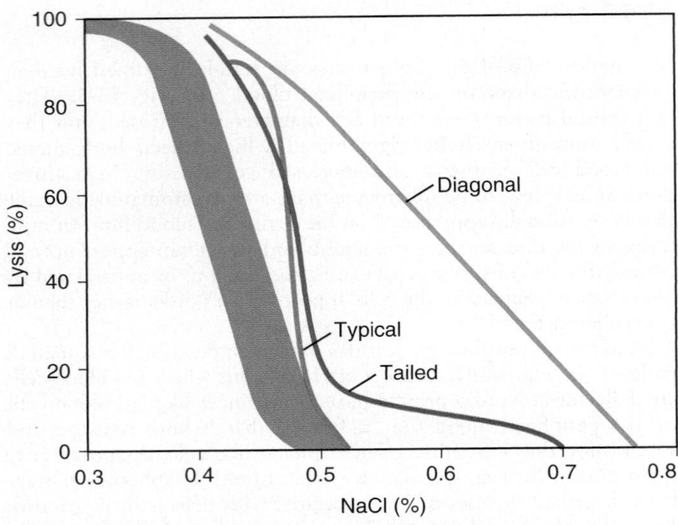

Figure 43-4 CHARACTERISTIC OSMOTIC FRAGILITY CURVES IN HEREDITARY SPHEROCYTOSIS (HS). The typical curve of increased osmotic fragility is the most common finding. The tailed curve reveals a second population (a tail) of very fragile erythrocytes conditioned by the spleen. This tail disappears after splenectomy. The diagonal curve is seen in patients with severe HS. *(Modified from Dacie J: Hereditary spherocytosis (HS). In* The haemolytic anaemias, *ed 3, vol 1, Edinburgh, 1985, Churchill Livingstone, p 134.)*

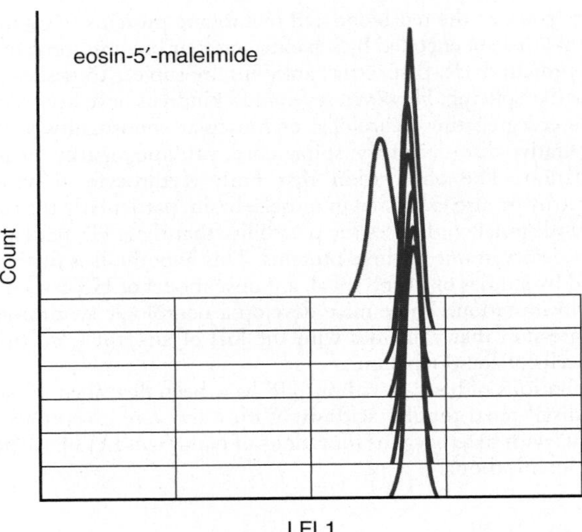

Figure 43-5 A flow cytometric test that measures the fluorescence intensity of intact red blood cells labeled with the dye eosin-5′-maleimide, which reacts with band 3 protein, has been shown to be useful as a first-line test for the diagnosis of hereditary spherocytosis. Shown is log fluorescence (LFL1) versus count with six normal controls *(green)* and a patient with hereditary spherocytosis *(red)*.

The osmotic fragility curve often reveals uniformly increased osmotic fragility. A "tail" of the osmotic fragility curve can be present in nonsplenectomized HS subjects, indicating a subpopulation of particularly fragile red blood cells conditioned by splenic stasis. This subpopulation of cells disappears after splenectomy. In subjects with mild HS, osmotic fragility can be normal and abnormalities can be found only after incubation that further augments the loss of surface area; however, the sensitivity of the incubated osmotic fragility test can be outweighed by a loss of its specificity. The relative contributions of cell dehydration and surface area deficiency can be accurately determined by osmotic gradient ektacytometry, available only in specialized laboratories.

Eosin-5′-Maleimide Binding

The observation that most spherocytes are deficient in band 3 and that eosin-5′-maleimide (EMA) covalently binds band 3 and Rh-related proteins with a 1:1 stoichiometry has been used as the basis for a screening test for HS. The binding of fluorescently-labeled EMA to erythrocytes is followed by flow cytometric quantitation. The intensity of EMA binding is decreased in HS erythrocytes (Fig. 43-5). This technique appears to have both high sensitivity and specificity. Like osmotic fragility, other erythrocyte abnormalities such as abnormalities of erythrocyte hydration and variants of dyserythropoietic anemia can also yield abnormal results. In cases of mild HS (e.g., most of the patient's erythrocytes are phenotypically normal), results may be normal or indeterminate. EMA binding studies are relatively straightforward to perform and provide results within a few hours. The test is gaining popularity as more diagnostic laboratories obtain experience with its use.

Autohemolysis and Other Tests

Red blood cell autohemolysis, the spontaneous hemolysis of red blood cells incubated under sterile conditions without glucose, was previously advocated as a sensitive test for the detection of HS. This test is being used less frequently and is probably no more sensitive than the incubated osmotic fragility test. Other tests described in the literature such as the glycerol lysis test, the pink test, hypertonic cryohemolysis, and the skeleton gelation test, are infrequently performed in diagnostic laboratories in the United States. The former two tests, which employ glycerol to retard the osmotic swelling of red blood cells, are preferred by some laboratories because they are easy to perform and can be adapted to microsamples. Cryohemolysis testing in particular remains popular in Europe.

Detection of the Underlying Molecular Defect

Because the most common finding in erythrocytes of patients with HS is a deficiency of one or more of the membrane proteins, initial studies often include sodium dodecyl sulfate–polyacrylamide gel electrophoresis (SDS-PAGE) solubilized red blood cell membrane proteins followed by densitometric quantitation. The results are expressed as ratios of individual red cell membrane proteins to band 3. This technique reveals abnormalities in approximately 70% to 80% of patients, defining the distinct biochemical phenotypes discussed previously. Direct quantitation of membrane proteins by radioimmunoassay is superior to densitometric quantitation and permits accurate measurement of the copy number of the individual proteins per red blood cell.

Subsequent strategies to search for the underlying defect are complex. Studies of protein function, readily employed in the detection of spectrin mutations in cases of HE and HPP (see Membrane Effects), have been disappointing in detecting abnormalities in HS, with the exception of HS characterized by a weakened β-spectrin–protein 4.1R interaction. Studies of membrane protein synthesis and assembly, using either reticulocytes or erythroblasts derived from peripheral blood burst-forming units in vitro, have been used, but they are insensitive in detecting mild to moderate abnormalities in membrane protein synthesis and assembly and are technically cumbersome to perform.

Genetic linkage analysis has been employed in cases of HS, but it suffers from the disadvantages of the need to study large kindreds and its lack of usefulness in studying patients with de novo mutations. Because of the large sizes of the HS genes, mutation-screening techniques have been developed. Many of these employ polymerase chain reaction–based strategies, including single-strand conformational polymorphism analyses, denaturing high-performance liquid chromatography, and direct nucleotide sequence analyses. Application of recently developed ultrahigh throughput sequencing techniques will overcome these technical obstacles to HS genetic diagnosis.

Complications

Gallstones

Bilirubin stones are found in approximately 50% of patients with HS, often even in those with a very mild form of the disease. Gallstones have occasionally been detected during infancy, but they are most likely to occur in children and young adults. The coinheritance of Gilbert syndrome markedly increases the risk for gallstones in HS patients. Because of the high incidence of gallstones, HS patients should be periodically examined by ultrasonography for the presence of gallstones, beginning early in childhood.

Crises

True hemolytic crises are relatively rare and only occasionally reported in association with infections. Aplastic crises during viral infections are largely attributable to infection by parvovirus B19. This infection (erythema infectiosum, fifth disease) manifests with fever, chills, lethargy, malaise, nausea, vomiting, abdominal pain with occasional diarrhea, respiratory symptoms, muscle and joint pains, and a maculopapular rash on the face (slapped cheek appearance), trunk, and extremities. The virus selectively infects erythroid precursors and inhibits their growth. The ensuing anemia, often profound, can be the first manifestation of HS. Multiple family members with undiagnosed HS who are infected with parvovirus have developed aplastic crises at the same time. Infection with parvovirus is a particular danger to susceptible pregnant women because it can infect the fetus, leading to fetal anemia, hydrops fetalis, and fetal demise.

Rarely, at least in developed countries, patients present with megaloblastic crises caused by folate deficiency. This typically occurs in patients with increased folate demands, such as those recovering from an aplastic crisis, pregnant women, and older adults. Megaloblastic crisis in pregnancy has been reported as the first manifestation of HS. Folate supplementation is recommended for patients with moderate to severe HS.

Other Complications

In patients with more severe forms of HS, other complications include gout, leg ulcers, or chronic dermatitis of the legs that heal after splenectomy. Symptoms of expanded erythroid space, including paravertebral or renal pelvic masses of extramedullary hematopoiesis, which can mimic an underlying neoplasm, may occur. Several cases of hemochromatosis in HS patients have been reported. In some, iron overload resulted from repeated transfusions; in others, the patients had two genetic defects, one involving HS and the other involving a hemochromatosis carrier state. Other rare complications include thrombosis, pulmonary hypertension, spinocerebellar degenerative syndromes, movement disorders, myopathy, and hypertrophic cardiomyopathy.

More than a dozen cases of HS and hematologic malignancy, including myeloproliferative disorders, multiple myeloma, and leukemia, have been reported. It is unknown if long-standing hematopoietic stress predisposes to the development of these secondary disorders or if they occurred randomly.

Differential Diagnosis

Because of the relatively asymptomatic presentation of HS, this diagnosis should be considered during an evaluation for unexplained splenomegaly, unconjugated hyperbilirubinemia of unknown cause, gallstones at a young age, severe anemia during pregnancy, or transient anemia during acute infections. The diagnosis of HS can be missed in mild forms of the disease, because spherocytosis might not be apparent on the peripheral blood film. Autoimmune hemolytic anemia should be ruled out by negative results of a Coombs test.

More typical forms of HS, characterized by relatively uniform spherocytosis with increased MCHC, are usually easily distinguished from other disorders manifesting with spherocytosis, such as immune hemolytic anemias and unstable hemoglobins. In some patients, the spherostomatocytes in the rare Rh-null syndrome and the intermediate syndromes of hereditary stomatocytosis can be confused with HS red blood cells.

Spherocytosis is transiently improved, and both the osmotic fragility and hemolysis are normalized in patients with obstructive jaundice. This is because of an expansion of red blood cell surface area that follows an increased uptake of phospholipids and cholesterol from the abnormal plasma lipoproteins. In normal red blood cells, this leads to target cell formation; in HS, spherocytes are transformed to discocytes. Spherocytosis and the increased osmotic fragility of HS red cells are likewise improved by iron deficiency, but the red blood cell life span remains shortened. In addition, coexistence of β-thalassemia trait and HS partially corrects the HS phenotype.

Therapy and Prognosis

Splenectomy

Splenectomy is curative in almost all patients with typical forms of HS, because red blood cell survival is normalized, and anemia and hyperbilirubinemia are corrected. Spherocytosis and the increase in osmotic fragility persist, but the tail of the osmotic fragility curve, indicating the presence of a subpopulation of cells conditioned by the spleen, disappears. In patients with severe, nondominantly inherited HS, splenectomy produces a dramatic clinical improvement, but hemolysis is only partially corrected.

Several weeks to months before splenectomy, patients should be immunized with polyvalent vaccine against pneumococcus as well as vaccines against *Haemophilus influenzae* type b and meningococcus.

Indications for Splenectomy

Risks and benefits should be considered carefully in HS patients before splenectomy is performed (see box on Splenectomy for Hereditary Spherocytosis). A multitude of factors influence the decision for splenectomy in HS patients, including the risk for overwhelming postsplenectomy sepsis, the emergence of penicillin-resistant pneumococci, and the potentially increased risk for cardiovascular disease and pulmonary hypertension later in life. Indications for splenectomy include growth retardation, skeletal changes, symptomatic hemolytic disease, anemia-induced compromise of vital organs, the development of leg ulcers, or the appearance of extramedullary hematopoietic tumors. Whether to perform splenectomy in patients with moderate HS without any of these factors remains controversial.

Because of an increased frequency of postsplenectomy infection in young children, most practitioners avoid splenectomy in infancy and early childhood.

Operative Considerations

When splenectomy is warranted, laparoscopic splenectomy has become the procedure of choice in many centers. Laparoscopic splenectomy has been associated with less postoperative discomfort, a quicker return to preoperative diet and activities, a shorter hospitalization time, decreased costs, and smaller scars. Early complications of splenectomy include local infection, bleeding, and pancreatitis. In general, the morbidity rate of splenectomy is lower in patients with HS than with other hematologic diseases. However, the benefits of

Splenectomy for Hereditary Spherocytosis

Splenectomy is a permanently curative treatment in most cases of hereditary spherocytosis (HS). Thus for years splenectomy was recommended for all HS patients regardless of the severity of anemia, gall bladder disease, or other symptoms. However, increasing concerns regarding overwhelming postsplenectomy infection (OPSI), the emergence of penicillin-resistant pneumococci, and increased risk for cardiovascular diseases have tempered these recommendations. When considering splenectomy, health care providers, the patient, and the patient's family should review and consider the risks and benefits. Individual factors that may pose additional risk, such as distance from medical care in case of febrile illness and residence in or travel to areas where parasitic diseases such as malaria or babesiosis occur, should be considered. Expert opinions vary on indications for splenectomy. There are no studies to guide practice. However, because the risk for OPSI is highest in infancy and childhood, most agree it is best to avoid total splenectomy in early childhood.

Benefits

Anemia ameliorated
Risk for hemolysis-associated gall bladder disease eliminated
Risk for aplastic crisis eliminated

Risks

OPSI—especially with encapsulated organisms (*Streptococcus pneumoniae, Neisseria meningitides,* and *Haemophilus influenzae*)
Increased risk for thrombotic complications
Increased risk for vascular complications (pulmonary hypertension, cardiovascular disease)

Indications for Splenectomy

Expert opinions vary
Severe, symptomatic spherocytosis
Growth failure, skeletal changes, leg ulcers, and extramedullary hematopoietic tumors (signs of severe anemia)
Older patients with vascular compromise of vital organs
Moderate HS with compensated, asymptomatic anemia: controversial; decision should be individualized

surgery must be weighed against possible complications, such as postsplenectomy infections. Although these complications are rare and their frequency is likely to diminish further with appropriate vaccinations, the indiscriminate performance of splenectomy in all HS patients with splenomegaly is unwarranted.

Subtotal (Partial) Splenectomy

Partial splenectomy was developed for infants and young children with severe HS, anemia, and poor growth with the goals of palliating anemia and decreasing transfusion requirements while preserving splenic function. More recently some have advocated expanding the procedure to all patients being splenectomized for HS. The goal of the operation is to decrease hemolysis while maintaining splenic phagocytic function. In initial cohorts of patients treated with partial splenectomy, stable increases in hemoglobin levels with decreased reticulocyte counts have been observed. The volume of splenic tissue left behind ranges from 10 to 30 mL. Although initial data are promising, it is not clear whether the remaining splenic tissue will effectively prevent postsplenectomy sepsis. In addition, regrowth of the splenic remnant has been reported in many patients, which can eventually lead to recurrence of HS and another operative procedure.

There are no specific data to support the use of prophylactic antibiotics postsplenectomy. Some practitioners avoid the prescription of prophylactic antibiotics, others recommend prophylactic antibiotics for at least 5 years postsplenectomy, and others recommend their use for life.

Postsplenectomy Failures

Postsplenectomy failures are caused either by the presence of an accessory spleen missed during surgery (accessory spleens were found in 17% to 39% of all patients) or by the presence of another superimposed red blood cell disorder such as pyruvate kinase deficiency. The recurrence of hemolytic anemia several years after splenectomy should raise the suspicion of development of splenunculi, resulting from autotransplantation of splenic tissue during surgery. The presence of an accessory spleen or splenunculus is suggested by the absence of both Howell-Jolly bodies and the "pitted" cells with crater-like surface indentations readily seen by interference contrast microscopy. A definitive confirmation of splenosis is made by a radiocolloid liver-spleen scan or by a scan using chromium (Cr)-labeled heated red blood cells, which are taken up by the ectopic splenic tissue.

Genetic Counseling

After a patient is diagnosed with HS, family members should be examined for the presence of HS. A history, physical examination for splenomegaly, complete blood count with indices, reticulocyte count, examination of the peripheral blood smear for spherocytes, and biochemical evaluation including bilirubin and haptoglobin levels should be obtained for available close relatives.

Future Directions

Advances in ultrahigh throughput deoxyribonucleic acid (DNA) sequencing methodology will greatly facilitate precise genetic diagnosis in cases of suspected inherited membrane-associated disorders. The technique of exome sequencing has rapidly developed into an effective tool for the identification of disease-causing variants in genetic disease, particularly monogenic disorders. It can be applied to disorders with recessive or dominant inheritance or de novo occurrence, and it obviates the need for linkage analysis in large numbers of individuals. As more patients are studied, it is likely that new HS-associated loci will be discovered, specific mutations will provide insight into the structure and function of associated membrane protein genes, and our understanding of genotype-phenotype relationships, particularly those with variable influence on disease severity, will be extended.

HEREDITARY ELLIPTOCYTOSIS AND RELATED DISORDERS

Introduction and Epidemiology

Hereditary elliptocytosis designates a group of inherited disorders that have in common the presence of elliptical red blood cells on peripheral blood films. Elliptocytosis was first described by Dresbach in 1904, and its heritability was firmly established by Hunter. Subsequent reports have revealed a considerable heterogeneity of clinical expression and have defined several distinct syndromes, including HPP and SAO.

Hereditary elliptocytosis is common in people of African and Mediterranean ancestries. In the U.S. population, the prevalence of HE is approximately 3 to 5 per 10,000. The true incidence of HE is unknown because its clinical severity is heterogeneous and most patients are asymptomatic without anemia. HE is considerably more frequent in areas of endemic malaria. In equatorial Africa, the prevalence of common HE has been estimated at between 0.6% and 1.6%.

Worldwide, HE appears to be more common among people of African origin. In Southeast Asian populations, the prevalence of SAO, a variant of HE, is as high as 30%.

The molecular basis of HE remained obscure until a defect of membrane skeletal proteins was suggested. Subsequently defects in the erythrocyte membrane proteins α-spectrin, β-spectrin, protein 4.1R, GPC, and band 3 were described.

On the basis of red blood cell morphologic characteristics, HE can be divided into three major groups (Fig. 43-6). Common HE, a dominantly inherited condition, is morphologically characterized by biconcave elliptocytes and, in some patients, rod-shaped cells. The clinical severity of common HE is highly variable, ranging from an asymptomatic condition to a severe recessively inherited hemolytic anemia, including hemolytic HE and HPP, in which the blood film reveals numerous red blood cell fragments, microspherocytes, and poikilocytes. Spherocytic HE, also called hemolytic ovalocytosis, is a much less common condition in which both round "fat" ovalocytes and spherocytes are present on the blood film. SAO, a disorder highly prevalent in the malaria belt of Southeast Asia and the Pacific, is characterized by rigid, spoon-shaped cells that have either a longitudinal slit or a transverse ridge.

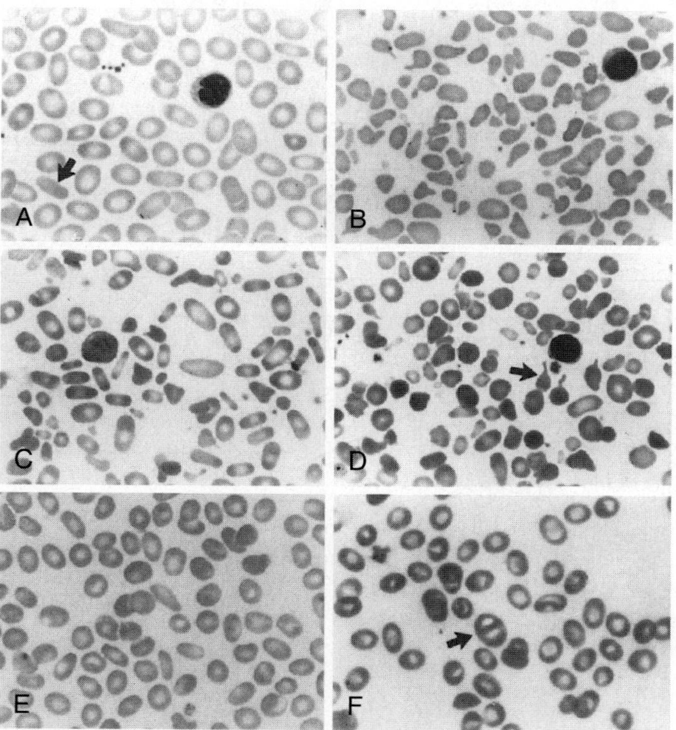

Figure 43-6 BLOOD FILMS OF SUBJECTS WITH VARIOUS FORMS OF HEREDITARY ELLIPTOCYTOSIS (HE). **A,** Simple heterozygote with mild common HE. Note the predominant elliptocytosis with some rod-shaped cells *(arrow)* and virtual absence of poikilocytes. **B,** Simple heterozygote with severe common hemolytic elliptocytosis. Note the numerous small fragments and poikilocytes. **C,** "Homozygous" common HE because of doubly heterozygous state for two mutant α-spectrins. Both parents have mild HE. Note the many elliptocytes as well as numerous fragments and poikilocytes. **D,** Hereditary pyropoikilocytosis. The patient is a double heterozygote for a structural α-spectrin mutant and a presumed α-spectrin synthetic defect. Note the prominent microspherocytosis, micropoikilocytosis, and fragmentation. Only few elliptocytes are present. Some poikilocytes are in the process of budding *(arrow)*. **E,** Spherocytic HE (hereditary ovalocytosis). Most red blood cells are oval rather than truly elliptical. Many oval cells are "fat," lacking a central concavity, the feature distinguishing spherocytic HE from common HE. **F,** Southeast Asian ovalocytosis. Most cells are oval, some containing either a longitudinal slit or a transverse ridge *(arrow)*.

Pathobiology of Common Hereditary Elliptocytosis

The possibility that the primary lesion of HE and HPP erythrocytes resides in the proteins of the red blood cell membrane skeleton was first raised by the findings of thermal instability of HPP spectrin, retention of the elliptical shape in HE membrane skeletons, disintegration of membrane skeletons after exposure to shear stress, defective self-association of spectrin dimers to tetramers, altered susceptibility of spectrin to tryptic digestion, and a deficiency of the membrane skeleton proteins spectrin and protein 4.1R. Gene cloning and determination of the primary structure of these proteins was soon followed by reports of mutations in the genes encoding erythrocyte membrane proteins.

Spectrin Mutations

The most common defects in HE, found in approximately two-thirds to three-quarters of all patients, are mutations of α- or β-spectrin. Both α- and β-spectrin are elongated flexible molecules consisting of triple-helical repeats connected by nonhelical segments. These polypeptides are associated side to side in an antiparallel position, forming a flexible, rod-like αβ heterodimer in which the NH_2-terminal of α-spectrin and the COOH-terminal of β-spectrin form the head region of the heterodimer. Spectrin heterodimers associate head to head to form spectrin tetramers, the major structural subunits of the membrane skeleton. Spectrin tetramers in turn are interconnected into a highly ordered two-dimensional lattice through binding, at their distal ends, to actin oligomers with the aid of protein 4.1R.

The contact site between the α- and β-spectrin chains of the opposed heterodimers is a combined "atypical" triple-helical repetitive segment in which the first two helices are contributed by the COOH-terminal of β-spectrin, whereas helix 3 is the first helical segment of α-spectrin. Spectrin dimer-tetramer interconversion is governed by a simple thermodynamic equilibrium that under physiologic conditions strongly favors spectrin tetramers. Most α-spectrin defects are at or near the NH_2-terminal of α-spectrin, which is involved in the heterodimer contact (the αI domain defined by limited tryptic peptide mapping; see the discussion under Laboratory Manifestations), and impair the self-association of spectrin into tetramers. Most α-spectrin mutations are point mutations. These mutations create abnormal proteolytic cleavage sites that typically reside in the third helix of a repetitive segment and give rise to abnormal tryptic peptides on two-dimensional tryptic peptide maps of spectrin.

Elliptocytogenic β-spectrin mutations are COOH-terminal point mutations or truncations that disrupt the formation of the combined β triple-helical repetitive segment and consequently the self-association of spectrin heterodimers to tetramers. All of these mutations open a proteolytic cleavage site residing in the third helix of the combined repetitive segment, which gives rise to a 74-kDa αI peptide.

Although most spectrin mutations reside in the vicinity of the αβ-spectrin self-association site, a few mutations remote from the self-association site have been described. These mutations are asymptomatic in the simple heterozygous state but cause hemolytic anemia, which can be severe, in homozygous patients. Unlike mutations located in the self-association contact site, which are predicted to disrupt the conformation of the local protein structure, mutations outside this region are predicted to perturb long-range protein-protein interactions, disrupting the positively coupled, cooperative interactions of αβ spectrin self-association, spectrin-ankyrin interactions, and ankyrin–band 3 interactions. One HE-associated mutation in a linker region remote from the self-association contact site disrupted the stability propagated from one spectrin repeat to the next.

Protein 4.1R Mutations

Another group of elliptocytogenic mutations, although much less common than spectrin mutations, are quantitative or qualitative defects of protein 4.1R. Protein 4.1R is a multifunctional protein that contains several important sites of protein interactions, including the spectrin-binding domain, where 4.1R binds to the distal end of the spectrin αβ heterodimer, markedly increasing the binding of spectrin to oligomeric actin, and the basic NH_2-terminal domain, where 4.1R interacts with GPC, phosphatidylinositol, and phosphatidylserine, facilitating the attachment of the distal end of spectrin to the membrane.

Studies of 4.1R mRNA from normal red blood cells revealed 4.1R isoforms resulting from complex tissue- and developmental stage–specific patterns of alternate mRNA splicing. Alternate translation initiation sites are present in the protein 4.1R mRNA. When an upstream AUG is used, isoforms greater than 80 kDa are synthesized. During erythropoiesis, this upstream AUG is spliced out and a downstream AUG is used, leading to the production of the 80-kDa mature erythroid protein 4.1R isoform. On SDS-PAGE, protein 4.1R is resolved into two bands of different sizes: 4.1a and 4.1b. The larger band, 4.1a, is typically found in normal red blood cells, whereas the shorter one, 4.1b, represents the major isoform of reticulocytes. The 4.1b isoform is converted into the 4.1a isoform by deamidation of Asn 502.

A partial deficiency of protein 4.1R is associated with mild, dominantly inherited HE, whereas a complete deficiency (a homozygous state) leads to a severe hemolytic disease. Homozygous protein 4.1R(–) erythrocytes fragment more rapidly than normal at moderate sheer stresses, an indication of their intrinsic instability. Membrane mechanical stability can be restored by reconstituting the deficient red blood cells with protein 4.1R or the protein 4.1R/spectrin/actin-binding site. Homozygous protein 4.1R(–) erythrocytes also lack p55 and have only 30% of the normal content of GPC. These homozygous protein 4.1R(–) erythrocytes, as well as GPC-deficient Leach erythrocytes, demonstrate decreased invasion and growth of *Plasmodium falciparum* in vitro.

Mutations associated with protein 4.1R deficiency have included deletions that include the exon encoding the erythroid transcription start size and mutations of the transcription initiation codon. Qualitative defects of protein 4.1R protein include deletions and duplications of the exons encoding the spectrin-binding domain, leading either to truncated or elongated forms of protein 4.1R. Electron microscopic studies of homozygous protein 4.1R(–) erythrocyte membranes revealed a markedly disrupted skeletal network with disruption of the intramembrane particles, suggesting that protein 4.1R plays an important role in maintenance not only of the skeletal network but also of the integral proteins of the membrane structure.

Glycophorin C Deficiency

GPC has been found absent because of a variety of molecular defects. In contrast to other forms of HE, which are dominantly inherited, heterozygous carriers are asymptomatic, with normal red blood cell morphology, and homozygous subjects have no anemia and only mild elliptocytosis apparent on the peripheral blood film.

GPC deficiency with elliptocytosis, the so-called Leach phenotype, caused by reduced expression of GPC, should be distinguished from the immunochemically defined phenotypes Gerbich and Yus, in which abnormal glycoproteins are formed that can functionally substitute for normal GPC and preserve the normal red blood cell shape. The Leach phenotype is usually caused by a large deletion of genomic DNA (~7 kb) that removes exons 3 and 4 from the GPC/glycophorin D locus. In one patient, the Leach phenotype was caused by a frameshift mutation.

GPC-deficient subjects are also partially deficient in protein 4.1R and lack p55, presumably because these proteins form a complex and recruit or stabilize each other on the membrane. It has been speculated that the protein 4.1R deficiency in Leach erythrocytes is the cause of the elliptocytic shape. In contrast, subjects deficient in glycophorin A, the major transmembrane glycoprotein, are asymptomatic.

Membrane Effects

Most of the elliptocytogenic mutations of spectrin reside within, or in the vicinity of, the spectrin heterodimer self-association site, disrupting this region and consequently disrupting the two-dimensional integrity of the membrane skeleton (Fig. 43-7). These defects are detected by ultrastructural examination of the membrane skeleton, which reveals disruption of a normally uniform hexagonal lattice. Consequently membrane skeletons are mechanically unstable, as are whole cell membranes and the cells. In patients with severely dysfunctional spectrin mutations or patients homozygous or doubly heterozygous for spectrin mutations, the membrane instability is sufficient to cause red blood cell fragmentation with hemolytic anemia under conditions of normal circulatory shear stress.

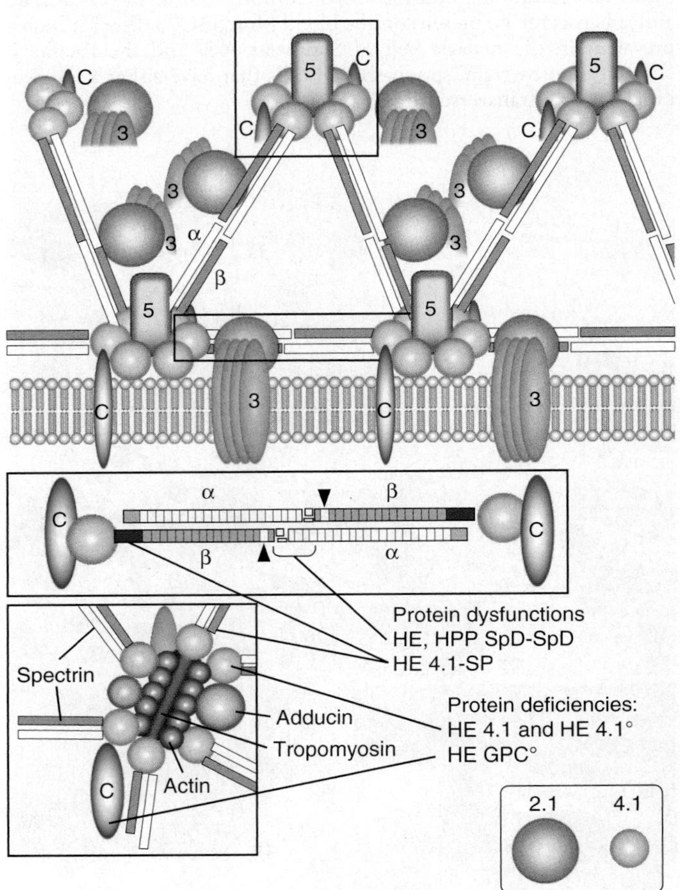

Figure 43-7 SCHEMATIC REPRESENTATION OF THE MOLECULAR ASSEMBLY OF THE MEMBRANE SKELETON AND THE MOLECULAR DEFECTS IN HEREDITARY ELLIPTOCYTOSIS (HE) AND HEREDITARY PYROPOIKILOCYTOSIS (HPP). Spectrin is composed of α- and β-spectrin heterodimers (SpD) that associate in their head regions into tetramers. At their distal ends, SpD bind to the junctional complexes of oligomeric actin (band 5 *[5]*) and protein 4.1. Additional proteins found in the junctional complex, such as adducin and tropomyosin, are shown in the lower enlarged area. The membrane skeleton is attached to transmembrane proteins by interactions of β-spectrin with ankyrin (protein 2.1; *[black arrowhead]* designates the ankyrin-binding site in β-spectrin), which in turn binds to the cytoplasmic domain of band 3 *(3)*, and by linkage of protein 4.1 to glycophorin C (GPC). The known protein dysfunctions in HE and HPP include (1) defects of the SpD head region because of a mutation of either α- or β-spectrin, causing impaired assembly of SpD into tetramers, and (2) defects of proteins of the junctional complex such as a qualitative or quantitative defect of protein 4.1R or GPC. *SP,* Spectrin.

The pathobiology of the elliptocytic shape is less clear. Red blood cell precursors in common HE are round, and the cells become progressively more elliptical as they age in vivo. Red blood cells subjected to shear stress in vitro, or red blood cells flowing through microcirculation in vivo, have an elliptical or parachute-like shape, respectively. It is possible that elliptocytes and poikilocytes are permanently stabilized in their abnormal shape because the weakened spectrin heterodimer contacts facilitate skeletal reorganization, which follows axial deformation of cells resulting from application of a prolonged or excessive shear stress. This reorganization is likely to involve breakage of the unidirectionally stretched protein connections followed by the formation of new protein contacts that preclude the recovery of a normal biconcave shape. This process has been shown to account for permanent deformation of irreversibly sickled cells.

In HPP, the recessively inherited form of HE characterized by severe hemolysis, red blood cells have two abnormalities. They contain a mutant spectrin that characteristically disrupts spectrin heterodimer self-association, and they are also partially deficient in spectrin, as evidenced by a decreased spectrin/band 3 ratio. In some HPP cases, this biochemical phenotype is a consequence of a double heterozygous state for an elliptocytogenic α-spectrin mutation and a defect involving reduced α-spectrin synthesis. Such synthetic defect of α-spectrin is fully asymptomatic in the heterozygous carrier, because under normal conditions, the synthesis of α-spectrin is approximately three to four times greater than that of β-spectrin.

When present in conjunction with an elliptocytogenic mutation of α-spectrin, such a synthetic defect augments the expression of the mutant spectrin. Because the elliptocytogenic α-spectrin mutants are often unstable, the combination of the two defects leads to spectrin deficiency in the cells. Other HPP subjects are homozygous or doubly heterozygous for one or two elliptocytogenic spectrin mutations, respectively. In such cases, the spectrin deficiency may be a consequence of spectrin instability that reduces the amount of spectrin available for membrane assembly. Furthermore, in red blood cells containing a high fraction of unassembled dimeric spectrin, the spectrin deficiency may in part be related to the stoichiometric ratio of one ankyrin copy per one spectrin tetramer (i.e., two spectrin heterodimers). Consequently only approximately one-half of spectrin heterodimers succeed in attaching to the ankyrin-binding sites. The phenotype of HPP, characterized by the presence of fragments and elliptocytes, together with evidence of red blood cell surface area deficiency (as reflected by the presence of microspherocytes on the peripheral blood film), suggests that the membrane dysfunction involves both vertical interactions (a consequence of spectrin deficiency) and horizontal interactions involving the elliptocytogenic spectrin mutation.

The red blood cell lesion in protein 4.1R deficiency shows similarities in regard to cell shape and membrane stability to the elliptocytogenic mutations of spectrin, suggesting that the deficiency principally affects the spectrin-actin contact (see Fig. 43-7) rather than the skeleton attachment to GPC via protein 4.1R (a vertical interaction).

The molecular basis of elliptocytosis and the mechanical instability of GPC-deficient red blood cells are not fully understood. However, recent studies suggest that the deficiency of GPC is not directly responsible for the altered mechanical properties. Instead, the mechanical instability appears to be related to a concomitant partial deficiency of protein 4.1R, as evidenced by a full correction of membrane instability by introduction into the cells of protein 4.1R or its spectrin-binding peptide, which facilitates the contact of β-spectrin to actin. The superimposed deficiency of protein 4.1R is likely to be related to the fact that GPC serves as an attachment site for protein 4.1R to the membrane, recruiting protein 4.1R to the red blood cell membrane. The effects of these defects on the mechanical stability of GPC–deficient cells appear to be relatively minor, because GPC–deficient subjects have no detectable hemolytic anemia and the mechanical properties of the red blood cells are normal when tested by micropipette aspiration.

Inheritance

In most patients, HE is inherited as an autosomal dominant disorder. The clinical severity is highly variable among different kindreds (reflecting heterogeneous molecular lesions) and, to a lesser extent, within a given kindred, presumably because of other genetic or acquired defects that modify disease expression. Occasionally HE is inherited as an autosomal recessive condition from an asymptomatic parent who carries the same molecular defect of spectrin as the HE offspring. In one kindred with a submicroscopic chromosome X deletion, inheritance was X-linked.

The inheritance of the related disorder HPP is autosomal recessive: one of the parents carries the α-spectrin mutation and either is asymptomatic or has mild HE, whereas the other parent is fully asymptomatic and has no abnormalities detectable by current biochemical approaches. However, several HPP patients have recently been studied who were doubly heterozygous for two α-spectrin mutations; in the heterozygous parents, these mutations were either silent or expressed as mild HE.

Clinical Manifestations

In view of the striking molecular heterogeneity of common HE, it is not surprising that the clinical spectrum of this disorder is variable, ranging from an asymptomatic trait without hemolysis to a life-threatening hemolytic anemia.

Mild Hereditary Elliptocytosis and Asymptomatic Carrier State

In most of these subjects, HE is found accidentally during evaluation of the peripheral blood film. Although some HE subjects have a mild compensated hemolytic anemia, others do not have any evidence of hemolysis, their red blood cell survival is normal, and the peripheral blood film may reveal only modest (≥15%) elliptocytosis. The molecular basis of mild HE is heterogeneous, and the reported molecular defects include both α- and β-spectrin mutations, partial deficiency of the 4.1R protein, and the absence of GPC. Some individuals carrying the spectrin mutation are completely asymptomatic, including normal red blood cell morphologic features; this is often the case in one of the parents of a patient with HPP.

Hereditary Elliptocytosis With Sporadic Hemolysis

Worsening of hemolysis together with the appearance of poikilocytes on the peripheral blood film has been reported in patients with hypersplenism, infections, or vitamin B_{12} deficiency, as well as in those with microangiopathic hemolysis such as disseminated intravascular coagulation or thrombotic thrombocytopenic purpura. In the latter two conditions, worsening hemolysis can be caused by microcirculatory damage superimposed on the underlying mechanical instability of the red blood cells.

Hereditary Elliptocytosis With Neonatal Poikilocytosis

Neonatal offspring of parents with mild HE present with symptomatic hemolytic anemia and a marked poikilocytosis. During the first year of life, the hemolysis and poikilocytosis abate, and the clinical picture transforms into that of mild HE. Such patients typically carry one mutant α-spectrin allele. The severity of the molecular defect, in terms of the percentage of spectrin dimers and the amount of mutant spectrin in the cells, is the same in the neonatal period as it is later in life. The worsening of hemolysis in the neonatal period has been attributed to the presence of fetal hemoglobin, which binds poorly to 2,3-diphosphoglycerate (2,3-DPG). The ensuing elevation of free

2,3-DPG levels has a marked destabilizing effect on the spectrin–protein 4.1R–actin interaction, thereby further destabilizing the membrane skeleton.

Hereditary Elliptocytosis With Chronic Hemolysis

Patients with HE with chronic hemolysis present with moderate to severe hemolytic anemia with elliptocytes and poikilocytes on peripheral blood film; some require splenectomy. In some of the kindreds, the hemolytic HE has been transmitted through several generations. In some kindreds, not all of the HE subjects have chronic hemolysis; some have a mild hemolysis only, presumably because of another genetic factor modifying the disease expression.

Homozygous and Compound Heterozygous Hereditary Elliptocytosis

Several HE individuals have been described who were apparent homozygotes for the HE gene. These individuals were found to be either homozygotes or compound (double) heterozygotes for one or two α- or β-spectrin mutations. The clinical severity is variable, from a relatively mild hemolytic anemia to a severe, life-threatening disease, depending on the severity of the underlying molecular defect, and in some cases is indistinguishable from HPP.

Hereditary Pyropoikilocytosis

It is now established that HPP represents a subtype of common HE, as evidenced by the coexistence of both HE and HPP in the same family and by the presence of the same molecular defect of spectrin. Unlike HE subjects carrying the spectrin mutation, the red blood cells of HPP subjects are also partially deficient in spectrin. Typically one parent of the HPP offspring carries an α-spectrin mutation, whereas the other parent is fully asymptomatic and has no detectable biochemical abnormality. In many such patients the asymptomatic parent carries a silent "thalassemia-like" defect of spectrin synthesis, enhancing the relative expression of the spectrin mutant and leading to a superimposed spectrin deficiency in the HPP offspring. Subsequent studies of the original HPP kindred revealed that defective spectrin synthesis from the null allele was caused by a splicing mutation of the α-spectrin gene. Some HPP subjects inherited two α-spectrin mutations; either their parents were hematologically normal or one had mild HE. In these HPP subjects, spectrin deficiency may be related to instability of the mutant spectrin. The thermal instability of spectrin originally reported as diagnostic of HPP is not unique for this disorder; it is also found in HE subjects carrying this α-spectrin mutation, in the homozygous and in the heterozygous states. HPP is seen predominantly in black subjects, but it has also been diagnosed in Arabs and whites.

Molecular Determinants of Clinical Severity

The severity of hemolysis in common HE often varies not only among different kindred but within a given family as well. The two principal determinants of severity of hemolysis are the spectrin content of the cells and the percentage of dimeric spectrin in the crude spectrin extract. The fraction of dimeric spectrin in such extracts in turn depends on several factors. The first of them is the degree of dysfunction of the mutant spectrin. Typically mutations that are either within or near the combined αβ triple-helical repetitive segment representing the spectrin heterodimer self-association site produce a more severe clinical phenotype and a more severe defect of spectrin function than those seen with point mutations in the more distant triple-helical repeats. Second, the percentage of the dimeric spectrin depends on the fraction of the mutant spectrin in the cells, which in turn is determined by the gene dose (e.g., simple heterozygote versus homozygote or double heterozygote) or the presence of other genetic defects such as the presence, in trans, of a defect leading to a reduced α-spectrin synthesis in some subjects with HPP.

The low-expression α-spectrin allele α^{LELY} is the best-characterized abnormality affecting spectrin content and clinical severity. Initially a polymorphism of the αV domain, $\alpha^{V/41}$, was identified in HE patients who, when they inherited $\alpha^{V/41}$ in trans, had more severe HE than expected. Subsequently an amino acid substitution of exon 46, Leu1857Val, and partial skipping of exon 46, linked to the $\alpha^{V/41}$ polymorphism, were identified as the characteristics of the α^{LELY} allele. These abnormalities are located within the site at which spectrin monomers assemble into heterodimers (the spectrin heterodimer nucleation site). In vitro studies suggest that the inability of α-spectrin chains to assemble into the mature membrane skeleton is because of a combination of decreased αβ dimer-binding affinity and increased proteolytic cleavage of the mutant α-spectrin chains. The presence of α^{LELY} in trans diminishes the propensity of the otherwise normal allele to associate with the corresponding β-chain, favoring the attachment of the elliptocytogenic α-spectrin allele. Conversely, coexistence of the α-spectrin mutation in cis and the mutation involving the α-spectrin nucleation site diminishes the propensity of the mutant allele to be incorporated into the spectrin heterodimer, thereby ameliorating the clinical severity of this mutation. The α^{LELY} allele is clinically silent by itself, even when inherited in the homozygous state, probably because α-spectrin is normally synthesized in threefold to fourfold excess.

Laboratory Manifestations

Blood Film and Laboratory Evidence of Hemolysis

A careful blood smear evaluation is essential for the diagnosis of HE and for the classification of the disorder into the three major subtypes outlined earlier (see Hereditary Elliptocytosis and Related Disorders, Introduction and Epidemiology and Fig. 43-6). In patients in whom elliptocytosis is the only morphologic abnormality, hemolysis is characteristically minimal or absent, with the exception of spherocytic elliptocytosis, in which the presence of round "fat" ovalocytes is associated with accelerated red blood cell destruction. In patients with hemolytic forms of common HE, poikilocytosis is characteristically found on the blood film. In severe forms of HE, particularly in homozygous HE, many red blood cells circulate as cell fragments, producing a marked decrease in MCV. The finding of red blood cell fragments together with a striking microspherocytosis and often only occasional elliptocytes is characteristic of HPP (see Fig. 43-6).

Osmotic and Thermal Fragility

Osmotic fragility is increased in HPP, in spherocytic elliptocytosis, and in HE subjects with poikilocytosis apparent on the peripheral blood film. In patients with a mild common HE without poikilocytosis on the peripheral blood film, osmotic fragility is normal.

Thermal instability of red blood cells was originally reported as a characteristic feature of HPP. It reflects thermal instability of the mutant spectrin: In normal red blood cells, spectrin is denatured and red blood cells fragment at 50° C. HPP red blood cells fragment and their spectrin denatures at 41° C. However, the diagnostic value of this test is limited, because thermal instability of red blood cells is also noted in HE red blood cells containing mutant spectrin. In contrast, an occasional patient with otherwise typical HPP may have normal thermal stability of red blood cells and spectrin. Red blood cells in common HE have unstable membranes and membrane skeletons when subjected to shear stress.

Electrophoretic Separation of Solubilized Membrane Proteins

In HE and HPP, SDS-PAGE can reveal proteins of abnormal mobility, the origin of which can be subsequently identified by Western blotting (e.g., truncated α- or β-spectrins in HE and HPP, or elongated or truncated forms of the 4.1R protein, and a partial or, rarely, complete deficiency of the 4.1R protein in HE). In HPP, SDS-PAGE reveals a partial deficiency of spectrin, as indicated by a decreased spectrin/band 3 ratio. Spectrin deficiency, in conjunction with an elliptocytogenic spectrin mutation affecting the spectrin heterodimer contact, is invariably found in cases of HPP.

Nondenaturing Gel Electrophoresis of Low-Ionic-Strength Spectrin Extract

Analysis of the ratio of tetrameric and dimeric spectrin in the low-ionic-strength extracts reveals the most common functional abnormality in HE (i.e., weakened self-association of spectrin heterodimers into tetramers). Because the spectrin dimer-tetramer interconversion has a high activation energy, it is kinetically immobilized at near 0° C. Consequently the percentage of spectrin dimers and tetramers in the 0° C crude spectrin extract reflects the relative distribution of these species in the red blood cell membrane in situ. Mutations of α- or α-spectrin residing within or near the αβ-spectrin heterodimer self-association site invariably lead to an increase in the fraction of dimeric spectrin in the crude 0° C spectrin extract.

Tryptic Peptide Mapping of Spectrin and the Detection of the Underlying DNA Defect

Tryptic digestion of spectrin followed by electrophoretic separation gives rise to highly reproducible tryptic peptide patterns. Among these peptides, the 80-kDa αI domain peptide representing the self-association site of the normal α-spectrin is among the most prominent. Nearly all α- or β-spectrin mutations reported are associated with a formation of tryptic peptides of abnormal size and mobility that are generated from the normal 80-kDa αI domain peptide. The cleavage sites of the most common abnormal tryptic peptides are found in the third helix of a given triple-helical repetitive segment. The reported mutations reside in the vicinity of these cleavage sites either in the same helix or, less commonly, in helix 1 or 2 of a given repetitive segment. Consequently tryptic peptide mapping remains a powerful tool with which to map the site of the underlying spectrin mutation, which can be subsequently defined by polymerase chain reaction amplification and sequencing of the respective region of the genomic DNA or complementary DNA (cDNA).

Differential Diagnosis

Various acquired and inherited conditions can be associated with elliptocytosis and poikilocytosis, including iron deficiency, thalassemias, megaloblastic anemias, myelofibrosis, myelophthisic anemias, myelodysplastic syndromes, and pyruvate kinase deficiency. The percentage of elliptocytes in these conditions is seldom greater than 60%. However, this is not diagnostically useful, because some HE subjects can have a relatively low percentage of elliptocytes. In normal subjects the percentage of elliptocytes is not greater than 5%, although in earlier reports it was listed as high as 15%. Previous diagnostic criteria of HE, based on the percentage of elliptocytes, such as 25%, 33%, or 40%, and their axial ratio, do not appear useful. The most reliable differentiation of HE from the other conditions mentioned is based on a positive family history rather than on the percentage of elliptocytes.

Therapy and Prognosis

As in the case of HS, red blood cells from patients with more severe forms of HE are retained by the spleen, producing a marked engorgement of splenic pulp. Consequently patients with symptomatic hemolysis benefit from splenectomy. This procedure is virtually never indicated in heterozygotes with autosomal dominant HE because most do not have clinically significant hemolytic anemia. If hemolysis is still active after splenectomy, folate should be administered daily. Recommendations for antibiotic prophylaxis, immunizations, and monitoring for intercurrent illnesses are similar to those noted earlier for HS patients before and after splenectomy. Serial interval ultrasonographic investigations to detect gallstones should be performed in patients with significant hemolysis.

Spherocytic Elliptocytosis

Spherocytic elliptocytosis, which shares features of HS and HE, has been designated spherocytic HE, HE with spherocytosis, or hereditary hemolytic ovalocytosis. The diagnosis is based on the simultaneous presence of elliptical red blood cells and spherocytes or "fat," round sphero-ovalocytes in the peripheral blood film (see Fig. 43-6). In contrast to common HE, cells of other shapes, such as rod-shaped cells, poikilocytes, and fragments, are absent. Importantly, hemolysis, despite relatively mild alterations in red blood cell morphologic features, and increased osmotic fragility are the main diagnostic features distinguishing this disorder from common HE.

The molecular basis of spherocytic HE is unknown. However, patients with mutations, particularly truncations at the C-terminal of β-spectrin, have many of the clinical features of spherocytic HE and probably represent an example of this disorder. Patients who lack GPC have rounded, smooth elliptocytes and could be classified as having a mild, recessively inherited variant of spherocytic HE. Finally, some patients with recessively inherited defects of protein 4.2 can display some features of spherocytic HE, particularly mild ovalostomatocytosis.

Southeast Asian Ovalocytosis

Southeast Asian ovalocytosis is characterized by the presence of oval red blood cells, many containing one or two transverse ridges or a longitudinal slit (see Fig. 43-6). The condition is widespread in certain ethnic groups of Malaysia, Papua New Guinea, the Philippines, and Indonesia. Numerous functional abnormalities of ovalocytes have been reported, including increased red blood cell rigidity, decreased osmotic fragility, increased thermal stability, resistance to shape change by echinocytogenic agents, and a reduced expression of many red blood cell antigens. A remarkable feature of ovalocytes is their resistance to in vitro invasion by several strains of malaria parasites, including *Plasmodium falciparum* and *Plasmodium knowlesi*. Moreover, in areas of endemic malaria, the ovalocytic subjects have reduced numbers of intracellular parasites in vivo. In these regions there is a decrease in the prevalence and in the disease severity of malaria in patients with SAO compared with control subjects.

All SAO individuals are heterozygotes for two band 3 gene mutations in cis: the deletion of nine codons encoding amino acids 400 through 408 from the boundary of the cytoplasmic and membrane domains of band 3, and the 56 Lys to Glu substitution. The 56 Lys to Glu substitution represents an asymptomatic polymorphism known as band 3 Memphis. The SAO phenotype is associated with a tighter binding of band 3 to ankyrin, increased tyrosine phosphorylation of the band 3 protein, inability to transport sulfate anions, and a markedly restricted lateral and rotational mobility of band 3 protein in the membrane.

Laboratory Manifestations

The finding of 30% or greater of oval red blood cells on the peripheral blood film, some containing a central slit or a transverse ridge, in the context of a notable absence of clinical and laboratory evidence of hemolysis in a subject from the ethnic groups noted earlier is highly suggestive of the diagnosis. A useful screening test is the demonstration of the resistance of ovalocytes or their ghosts to changes in shape produced by treatments that produce spiculation in normal cells, such as metabolic depletion or exposure of ghosts to salt solutions. In contrast to normal red blood cells, which form spicules in response to such stimuli, SAO red blood cells or ghosts do not change shape after these treatments. The mechanism of this resistance to changes in shape is not clear, and it may reflect the high rigidity of the red blood cell membrane.

Because the underlying cause of SAO is the deletion of 27 bases from the band 3 gene, isolation of genomic DNA or reticulocyte cDNA with subsequent amplification of the deletion-containing region appears to be the most specific test for establishing the diagnosis of SAO. Interestingly, this mutation appears to be lethal in the homozygous state, because large screens of individuals from indigenous areas have only identified heterozygotes.

Molecular Basis of Southeast Asian Ovalocytosis Membrane Rigidity and Malaria Resistance

The red blood cells of SAO are unique among axially deformed cells in that they are rigid and hyperstable rather than unstable. The SAO mutation is the first example of a defect of an integral membrane protein leading to red blood cell membrane rigidity, an observation previously attributed to properties of the membrane skeleton. The basis of the increased rigidity is unclear.

The molecular basis of malaria resistance of SAO red blood cells is likely related to altered properties of the band 3 protein, which serves as one of the malaria receptors, as evidenced by the inhibition of in vitro invasion by band 3–containing liposomes. In normal red blood cells, the invasion process is associated with a marked membrane remodeling that involves redistribution of intramembrane particles that contain band 3 protein. Such particles cluster at the site of parasite invasion, forming a ring around the orifice through which the parasite enters the cell. The invaginated red blood cell membrane, which surrounds the invading parasite, is free of intramembrane particles. The reduced lateral mobility of band 3 protein in SAO red blood cells may preclude band 3 receptor clustering, thereby preventing the attachment of the parasites to the cells. Decreased exchange of anions across the red blood cell membrane has also been proposed to contribute to the resistance of ovalocytes to malaria invasion. In addition, SAO red blood cells consume ATP at a higher rate than normal cells, and the partial depletion of ATP levels in ovalocytes has been suggested to account, at least in part, for the resistance of these cells to malaria invasion in vitro.

Acanthocytosis and Related Disorders

Acanthocytes (from the Greek *acantha,* "thorn") or spur cells are red blood cells with prominent thorn-like surface protrusions that vary in width, length, and surface distribution. Spur cells must be distinguished from echinocytes (Greek *echinos,* "sea urchin") or burr cells, characterized by multiple small projections that are uniformly distributed throughout the cell surface (Fig. 43-8). Acanthocytes should also be distinguished from keratocytes ("horn" red cells) that have few massive protuberances.

Acanthocytosis was first described in cases of abetalipoproteinemia and subsequently in severe liver disease, the chorea-acanthocytosis syndrome, the McLeod blood group phenotype, and other

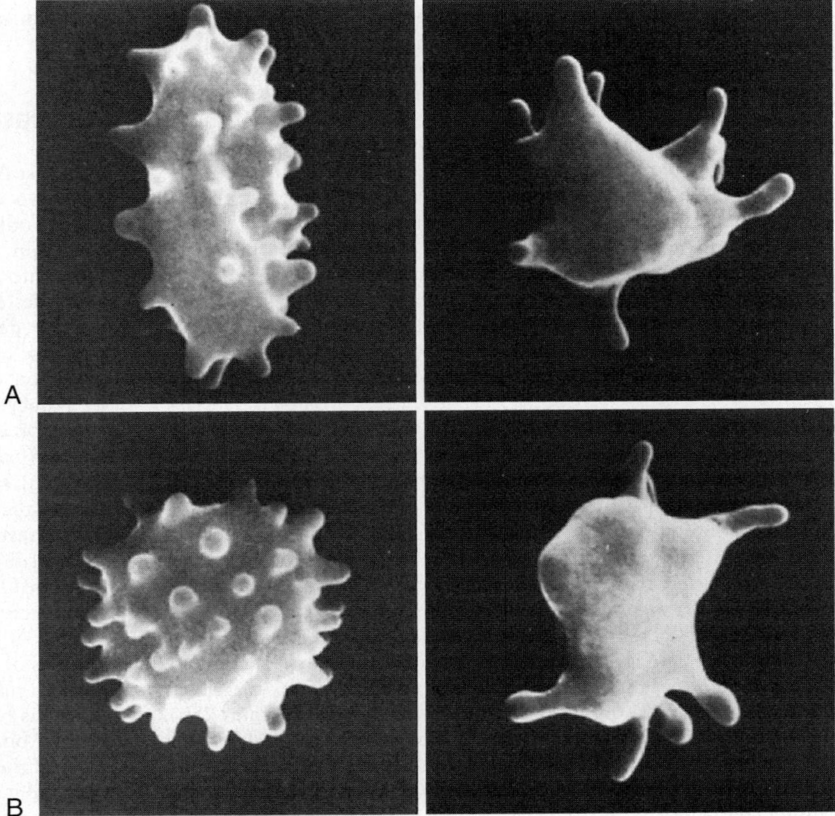

Figure 43-8 MORPHOLOGIC DIFFERENCES BETWEEN ACANTHOCYTES **(A)** AND ECHINOCYTES **(B)** AS DEMONSTRATED BY SCANNING ELECTRON MICROSCOPY. *(Modified from Bessis M:* Red cell shapes: An illustrated classification and its rationale, *New York, 1973, Springer-Verlag.)*

conditions. The molecular mechanisms leading to acanthocytosis in abetalipoproteinemia and severe liver disease have been extensively studied and have been attributed to changes in composition of membrane lipids and their altered distribution between the two hemileaflets of the lipid bilayer.

Spur Cell Hemolytic Anemia of Severe Liver Disease

Spur cell hemolytic anemia is an uncommon ominous complication of severe liver disease that is manifested by rapidly progressive hemolytic anemia and acanthocytes on the peripheral blood smear.

Pathobiology

The human red blood cell membrane contains nearly equal amounts of free (unesterified) cholesterol and phospholipids. The free cholesterol in the plasma readily equilibrates with the red blood cell membrane cholesterol pool. This is in contrast to esterified cholesterol, which cannot be transferred from plasma into the red blood cell membrane. The plasma of patients with severe liver disease contains abnormal lipoproteins that have a high free cholesterol/phospholipid ratio. The excess free cholesterol readily partitions into the red blood cell membrane, leading to a marked increase in free cholesterol in the cells. Consequently normal cells can develop a spur cell shape after their transfusion into a patient with severe liver disease or after incubation with the liver disease patient's plasma or cholesterol-enriched liposomes.

Spur cell formation involves two steps (Fig. 43-9). The first step is evident in red blood cells of splenectomized subjects with spur cell hemolytic anemia: Red blood cells have an expanded surface area with irregular contour and targeting, reflecting accumulation of free cholesterol in the membrane. This extra cholesterol accumulates preferentially in the outer bilayer leaflet, as suggested by findings of increased accessibility of cholesterol to cholesterol oxidase and a selective decrease in lipid fluidity of the outer hemileaflet of the lipid bilayer.

The second step in acanthocyte formation involves red blood cell remodeling by the spleen. As a result, red blood cells become spheroidal, and the surface projections are considerably longer and more irregular (see Fig. 43-9). The end result of these processes is poorly deformable red blood cells with long bizarre projections that are readily trapped in the spleen, which is often markedly enlarged because of passive congestion as a result of underlying portal hypertension. Cholesterol also alters membrane permeability and interacts with several membrane skeletal proteins, but the role of these changes in spur cell lesions is unclear.

Clinical Manifestations

Most patients with chronic liver disease have a mild to moderate anemia related to gastrointestinal blood loss, iron and folic acid deficiencies, or hemodilution or as a direct effect of alcohol on red blood cell precursors. Peripheral blood smears from these patients often reveal target cells that are particularly prominent in obstructive jaundice.

In some patients, particularly those with end-stage liver disease, anemia rapidly worsens and spur cells appear in high percentage in the peripheral blood. This is accompanied by worsening jaundice, rapid deterioration of liver function, hepatic encephalopathy, and hemorrhagic diatheses. A similar clinical syndrome has been described in patients with advanced metastatic liver disease, cardiac cirrhosis, Wilson disease, fulminant hepatitis, and infantile cholestatic liver disease. The development of spur cell hemolytic anemia is an ominous sign in most patients, predicting a survival seldom exceeding weeks to months. In theory, splenectomy could provide a marked improvement, because the spleen is the major sequestration site of nondeformable acanthocytes; in reality, splenectomy is seldom considered because of severity of the underlying liver disease.

Abetalipoproteinemia

Bassen and Kornzweig first described an association of acanthocytosis with atypical retinitis pigmentosa, progressive ataxic neurologic disease, and a "celiac disease" later attributed to fat malabsorption. Subsequently several investigators reported a congenital absence of β-lipoprotein, accounting for the diverse manifestations of the disorder.

Pathobiology

Abetalipoproteinemia is an autosomal recessive disorder found in people of diverse ethnic backgrounds. The primary molecular defect involves a congenital absence of β-apolipoprotein in plasma. The B apoproteins (B100 and B48) are generated by alternate transcription of a single gene residing on the short arm of chromosome 2. Their

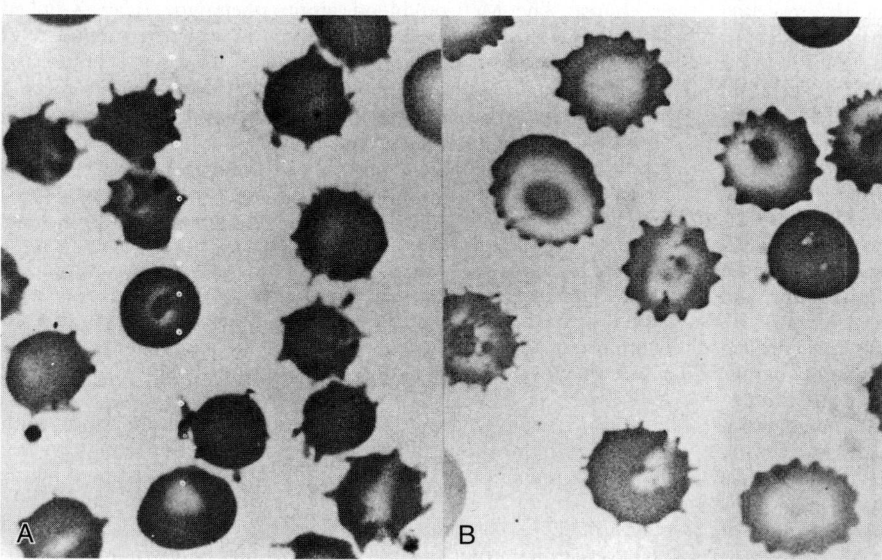

Figure 43-9 BLOOD FILM OF A PATIENT WITH LIVER CIRRHOSIS AND SPUR CELL ANEMIA BEFORE **(A)** AND AFTER **(B)** SPLENECTOMY. The latter smear demonstrates the effect of cholesterol acquisition leading to targeting (indicating increase in surface area) and irregularities in cell contour. The conditioning effect of the spleen **(A)** is demonstrated by the spheroidal shape of the cells and the remodeling of the spicules. *(From Cooper RA, Kimball DB, Durocher JR: The role of the spleen in membrane conditioning and hemolysis of spur cells in liver disease.* N Engl J Med *290:1279, 1974.)*

deficiency is secondary to defective cellular secretion of the apoprotein by liver cells, caused either by aberrant posttranslational processing or by defective aposecretion. In some patients this is because of qualitative or quantitative defects in the microsomal triglyceride transfer protein, which catalyzes the transport of triglyceride, cholesterol ester, and phospholipid from phospholipid surfaces. Microsomal triglyceride transfer protein is the only tissue-specific component, other than apolipoprotein B, required for secretion of apolipoprotein B–containing lipoproteins. As a result, apoprotein B is absent in plasma, as are the individual lipoprotein fractions that contain this apoprotein. These lipoprotein fractions include chylomicrons and very-low-density lipoproteins that transport triglycerides, as well as the low-density lipoproteins that are products of very-low-density lipoproteins and transport cholesterol. Consequently, preformed triglycerides are not transported from the intestinal mucosa, and they are nearly absent in the plasma. Plasma cholesterol and phospholipids are markedly reduced, with a relative increase in sphingomyelin at the expense of lecithin.

As is the case in acanthocytosis of liver disease, the acanthocytic lesion is acquired from the plasma. Erythrocyte precursors are of normal shape, and the acanthocytic lesion develops as the cells mature and age in the circulation. Normal cells acquire this shape when transfused into the recipient.

The most striking abnormality of red blood cell membrane lipids involves a net increase in sphingomyelin. Because plasma lipids readily exchange with the lipids of the red blood cell membrane, it is likely that this change simply mirrors the alterations in plasma lipid composition. In contrast to red blood cells in spur cell anemia of severe liver disease, the content of membrane cholesterol is normal or only slightly increased.

The role of membrane lipids in the acanthocyte shape transformation was first established by findings of restoration of biconcave shape after extraction of lipids from the cell membrane by detergents. The molecular basis of the acanthocytic shape is unknown, but several indirect observations suggest that it is related to an increase of the surface area of the outer hemileaflet of the lipid bilayer relative to the inner leaflet. Several other abnormalities have been noted in abetalipoproteinemia, including a decrease in plasma lecithin cholesterol transferase activity and an increased susceptibility of membrane and plasma lipids to oxidation as a result of malabsorption-induced deficiency of vitamin E. The contributions of these abnormalities to the acanthocyte red cell lesions are unknown.

Clinical Manifestations

This autosomal recessive disease can become evident in the first few months of life, manifested by fat malabsorption with normal absorption of other nutrients. Intestinal biopsy is diagnostic, revealing engorgement of mucosal cells with lipid droplets. Other features include retinitis pigmentosa and a progressive ataxia with intention tremors that usually develops at 5 to 10 years of age, progressing to death in the second or third decade of life. The hematologic manifestations are mild and include mild normocytic anemia with acanthocytosis (50% to 90%) and normal or slightly elevated reticulocyte counts. Occasional patients can have more severe anemia resulting from the nutritional deficiencies (iron and folate) that accompany fat malabsorption. The treatment includes dietary restriction of triglycerides and supplementation with the lipid-soluble vitamins A, K, D, and E. Vitamin E can stabilize or even improve both the retinal and neuromuscular abnormalities.

Autosomal recessive abetalipoproteinemia should be distinguished from the homozygous form of familial hypobetalipoproteinemia. Although the clinical presentation of both disorders is similar, the latter disorder is milder, and the parents have occasional acanthocytes on the peripheral blood film, and their plasma low-density lipoprotein levels are decreased. The molecular lesions in familial hypobetalipoproteinemia involve a variety of apoprotein B gene mutations, leading to aberrant apoprotein B gene transcription or translation.

Varying degrees of acanthocytosis without anemia have also been described with isolated deficiency of apoprotein B100.

Neuroacanthocytosis Syndromes

The neuroacanthocytosis syndromes are a group of degenerative neurologic disorders with phenotypic and genetic heterogeneity that share the feature of acanthocytes on peripheral blood smear. These disorders include chorea-acanthocytosis, the X-linked McLeod syndrome (see McLeod phenotype), and several other neurodegenerative diseases, including Huntington disease-like 2 caused by mutations in junctophilin-3 and pantothenate kinase–associated neurodegeneration (formerly known as Hallervorden-Spatz syndrome and its allelic variant syndrome—hypobetalipoproteinemia, acanthocytosis, retinitis pigmentosa, pallidal degeneration [HARP]) caused by mutations in pantothenate kinase 2.

Chorea-acanthocytosis syndrome is an autosomal recessive syndrome of adult onset that is manifest by multiple neurologic abnormalities, including limb chorea, progressive orofacial dyskinesia with tics, tongue-biting neurogenic muscle hypotonia, and atrophy. The hematologic manifestations are minimal and include a variable percentage of acanthocytes on the peripheral blood film without anemia and normal or only slightly decreased red blood cell survival. The mechanism of acanthocytosis in this syndrome is unknown. Studies of plasma and red blood cell membrane lipids have revealed a high content of unsaturated fatty acids, presumably accounting for reduced red blood cell membrane fluidity. Additional abnormalities of uncertain significance include an uneven distribution of intramembrane particles, impaired phosphorylation of the erythrocyte actin-bundling protein dematin, abnormal accumulation of transglutaminase products, and altered function and structure of band 3.

Mutations have been identified in the chorein gene (also known as CHAC or VPS13A—vacuolar protein sorting 13 homolog A) in many affected patients. Chorein does not belong to any known human gene family, and computer searches have not identified any known structural motifs or domains. The function of the chorein gene product remains unknown in either erythrocytes or the brain. In yeast, a chorein homologue is involved in protein sorting and transport.

McLeod Phenotype

The McLeod syndrome is characterized by a mild compensated hemolytic anemia with a variable percentage of acanthocytes on the peripheral blood film and, in some patients, late-onset myopathy or chorea. The McLeod blood group phenotype is an X-linked anomaly of the Kell blood group system in which red blood cells, white blood cells, or both react poorly with Kell antisera. The affected cells lack Kx, the product of the XK gene, which appears to be a membrane precursor of the Kell antigens. The XK gene encodes a novel 444–amino acid integral membrane transporter. As expected, Kx is defective in McLeod patients. Male hemizygotes who lack Kx have variable acanthocytosis (8% to 85%) and mild, compensated hemolysis. Because of the red blood cell mosaicism predicted by the Lyon hypothesis of X chromosome inactivation, female heterozygote carriers can have occasional acanthocytes on the peripheral blood film. Lyonized women with more severe symptoms have been described. Because of the susceptibility to alloimmunization, it is important to diagnose affected patients because if they are transfused, they can develop antibodies compatible only with McLeod red cells.

The McLeod syndrome has been reported in association with chronic granulomatous disease of childhood, retinitis pigmentosa, and Duchenne muscular dystrophy. This association is caused by the close proximity of the genetic loci for these disorders in the p21 region of the X chromosome (Xp21), suggesting the occurrence of various manifestations because of contiguous gene syndromes. This may explain the occasional findings of either echinocytes or stomatocytes in Duchenne dystrophy, or a choreiform disorder in some subjects with the McLeod phenotype.

The Kell antigen consists of two protein components: a 37-kDa protein that carries the Kx antigen, a precursor molecule necessary for the Kell antigen expression, and a 93-kDa protein that carries the Kell blood group antigen. Red blood cells with the McLeod phenotype have no detectable Kx antigen, and they have a marked deficiency of the 93-kDa protein that carries the Kell antigen. McLeod red blood cells should be distinguished from Kell null (K_0) red blood cells, which have a normal shape. In K_0 cells, only the Kell antigen carrying the 93-kDa glycoprotein is absent, whereas these cells have twice the amount of the Kx antigen. As in the other acanthocytic disorders, the surface projections of acanthocytes may be related to asymmetry of the surface area of the two lipid bilayer hemileaflets, as indicated by correction of the acanthocytosis by agents that expand the inner lipid layer, as well as the finding of an increased rate of exchange of phosphatidylcholine (localized preferentially in the outer lipid hemileaflet) with an exogenous source.

Acanthocytosis in Other Conditions

Acanthocytes have also been noted in malnourished patients, including those with anorexia nervosa and cystic fibrosis. In these patients, red blood cell shape normalizes after restoration of the nutritional status. Likewise, a small number of cells with long spicules resembling acanthocytes are found in patients with hypothyroidism, after splenectomy, and with myelodysplasia.

Differentiation of Acanthocytes From Other Spiculated Red Blood Cells

Echinocytes (Burr Cells)

In contrast to acanthocytes, echinocytes, also called burr cells, have rather uniform surface projections. Although early echinocytic forms have a regularly scalloped cell contour, advanced forms of echinocytes have a spheroidal shape and the surface projections appear as short, narrow spikes (see Fig. 43-8). Although the finding of echinocytes on a peripheral blood film is often an artifact related to blood storage, contact with glass, or an elevated pH, several hemolytic anemias have been reported in association with echinocytosis on peripheral blood films. These conditions include mild hemolytic anemia in long-distance runners and in patients with hypomagnesemia and hypophosphatemia (presumably because of decreased intracellular ATP stores), uremia because of an unknown plasma factor, and pyruvate kinase deficiency.

Inspection of wet blood preparations (but not dried blood films) reveals echinocytosis in most patients with liver disease. In contrast to spur cells in patients with severe liver disease, these echinocytes have a normal cholesterol content, and the molecular abnormality may be related to the binding of abnormal echinocytogenic high-density lipoproteins to the red blood cell surface.

The mechanisms of echinocytosis in these diverse disorders are likely to be heterogeneous, as suggested by findings that many diverse factors, such as exposure of red blood cells to certain drugs, calcium loading, or ATP depletion, can induce the transformation of discocytes to echinocytes in vitro. However, in vitro studies of the discocyte-echinocyte-stomatocyte equilibrium have suggested a possible common denominator. As discussed earlier, the lipid bilayer of normal red blood cells is asymmetric in lipid composition: The outer half of the lipid bilayer is relatively enriched in sphingomyelin and phosphatidylcholine, whereas the inner half is preferentially enriched in the negatively charged phosphatidylserine and phosphatidylethanolamine. Agents that preferentially bind to one or another class of these phospholipids dramatically influence red blood cell shape. Consequently agents that preferentially accumulate in the outer half of the red blood cell lipid bilayer, expanding this lipid bilayer, produce an echinocytic shape, presumably by creating an asymmetry between the two surface areas of the two halves of the lipid bilayer. Conversely, agents that asymmetrically expand the inner half of the lipid bilayer, such as chlorpromazine, lead to stomatocytic shape transformation. In the case of echinocytes produced by ATP depletion or calcium loading, the altered phospholipid distribution between the two bilayer hemileaflets may be a consequence of calcium-induced phospholipid scrambling or a decrease in the activity of aminophospholipid translocase, an ATP-dependent enzyme that actively translocates aminophospholipids from the outer leaflet to the inner hemileaflet.

Keratocytes, Bizarre Poikilocytes, and Schistocytes

Mechanical trauma of circulating red blood cells has occasionally produced bizarre shapes resembling acanthocytes, such as cells with horny projections (keratocytes). Some acanthocyte-like cells are also seen in splenectomized HE and HS subjects. Similar shape changes are seen in heated red blood cells, in which spectrin has been damaged by thermal denaturation, suggesting that these cells are bizarre poikilocytes rather than true acanthocytes.

RED BLOOD CELL MEMBRANE DISORDERS MANIFESTED BY TARGET CELL FORMATION

The common feature of target cells is an increase in the ratio of the cell surface area to cell volume. In microcytic red blood cells of patients with various forms of thalassemia and hemoglobinopathies, the increased surface to volume ratio, and consequently the target cell shape, reflect at least in part the relative abundance of cell surface area. In liver disease and other disorders discussed subsequently, the target cell formation reflects an absolute expansion of the cell surface area because of a net accumulation of membrane phospholipids and cholesterol.

Liver Disease

The presence of target cells in association with either normal or slightly increased cell volume is characteristically found in patients with obstructive jaundice, including various forms of liver disease associated with intrahepatic cholestasis. These target cells have a normal survival in the peripheral circulation and do not typically account for the anemias often encountered in patients with liver disease.

In these patients, target cell formation is a consequence of a net uptake of both free cholesterol and phospholipids into the red blood cell membrane from the plasma because of abnormalities in the cholesterol/phospholipid/protein ratios of low-density lipoproteins. Target cells have a decreased osmotic fragility, because the excess of membrane surface area leads to an increase in the critical hemolytic volume.

Lecithin-Cholesterol Acyltransferase Deficiency

The lecithin-cholesterol acyltransferase (LCAT) enzyme catalyzes the transfer of fatty acids from phosphatidylcholine to cholesterol. It circulates in plasma as a complex with components of high-density lipoproteins. LCAT deficiency is a rare autosomal dominant disorder manifested by hyperlipidemia, premature atherosclerosis, corneal opacities, chronic nephritis, proteinuria, mild anemia, and the presence of target cells on the blood film. The anemia is caused by mild hemolysis together with a diminished compensatory erythropoiesis. As in obstructive jaundice, the target cells in LCAT deficiency have a marked increase in both cholesterol and phospholipids. In addition, the membrane phosphatidylcholine is increased at the expense of sphingomyelin and phosphatidylethanolamine. Bone marrow aspiration and biopsy reveal the presence of sea-blue histiocytes. Analysis of plasma lipoproteins reveals multiple abnormalities secondary to the underlying enzyme deficiency. Inherited LCAT deficiency should be distinguished from an acquired deficiency of this enzyme, which is found in patients with severe liver disease.

Stomatocytosis and Related Disorders

Stomatocytes were first described in a girl with dominantly inherited hemolytic anemia. On blood films, her red blood cells contained a wide transverse slit or stoma (Fig. 43-10). In a three-dimensional view, these cells have a shape of a cup or a bowl. The slit-like appearance is an artifact that results from folding of the cells during blood smear preparation.

Stomatocytes are seen in a variety of acquired and inherited disorders. The latter are often associated with abnormalities in red blood cell cation permeability that lead to changes in red blood cell volume, which can be either increased (hence the designation hydrocytosis or overhydrated stomatocytosis) or decreased (desiccytosis [dessicate] or xerocytosis), or in some cases near normal.

There is no unifying theory to explain this morphologic abnormality. In vitro, stomatocytes can be produced by drugs that preferentially intercalate into the inner half of the asymmetric lipid bilayer, expanding its surface area relative to that of the outer half of the bilayer.

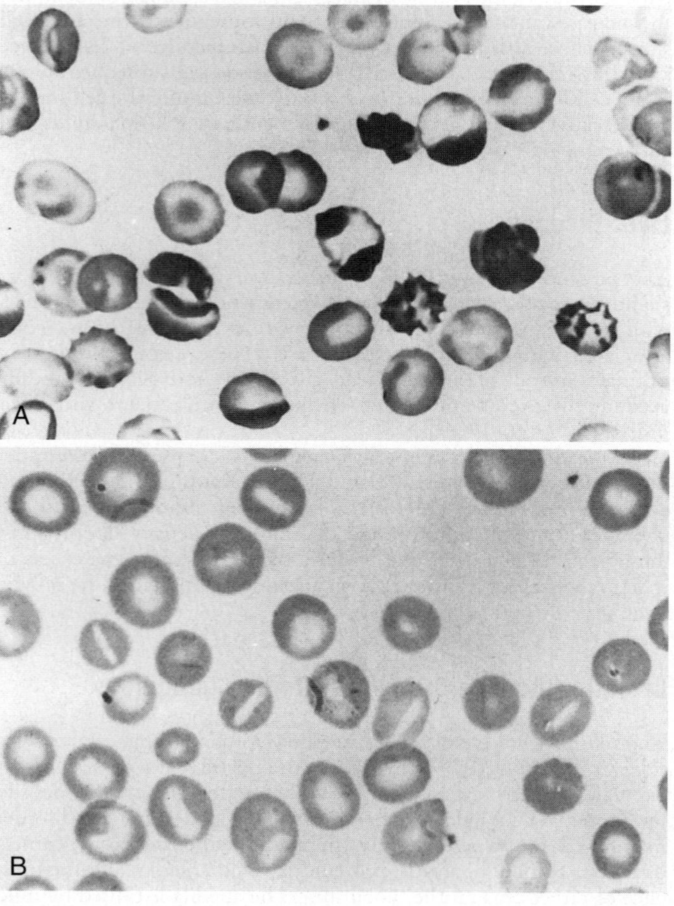

Figure 43-10 PERIPHERAL BLOOD SMEAR OF A PATIENT WITH HEREDITARY XEROCYTOSIS (DESICCYTOSIS) **(A)** AND STOMATOCYTOSIS (HYDROCYTOSIS) **(B)**. *(From Lande WM, Mentzer WC: Haemolytic anaemia associated with increased cation permeability.* Clin Haematol *14:89, 1985.)*

Hereditary Stomatocytosis-Hydrocytosis

Hereditary hydrocytosis designates a heterogeneous group of hereditary hemolytic anemias that are transmitted in an autosomal dominant manner. The disorder is characterized by a moderate to severe hemolytic anemia with 10% to 30% stomatocytes (see Fig. 43-10), an elevated MCV, and a reduced MCHC. Osmotic fragility of red blood cells is markedly increased, as some of the swollen red blood cells approach their critical hemolytic volume. For unexplained reasons, red blood cell membrane lipids and consequently membrane surface area are also increased, but this increase in surface area is insufficient to correct the osmotic fragility of the red blood cells. Red blood cell deformability is decreased.

The principal cellular lesion involves a marked increase in intracellular sodium and water content with a mild decrease in intracellular potassium as a result of a marked sodium influx into the red blood cells. Despite a marked compensatory increase in active transport of sodium (Na) and potassium by the Na^+/K^+-ATPase (which normally maintains the low sodium and high potassium concentrations in the cells) and an ensuing increase in glycolysis, the pump hyperactivity is unable to compensate for the vastly increased sodium leak. Stomatin (also known as band 7.2b), an integral membrane protein, is decreased or absent from the erythrocyte membranes of most affected patients. This deficiency appears to be a maturational loss in the bone marrow and in the circulation, perhaps because of a defect in cellular trafficking. Stomatin gene mutations have not been found in unrelated stomatocytosis patients deficient in this protein.

In some patients with hereditary hydrocytosis, missense mutations in RhAG, I61R or F65S have been found. In oocytes these mutations induce a monovalent cation leak, possibly opening the pore of an ammonium transporter. Additional studies suggest that the F65S mutation exhibits a gain-of-function phenotype with increased cation conductance/permeability.

Splenectomy can improve, but not fully correct, the hemolysis. In some patients, splenectomy can be deleterious or even contraindicated (see later), perhaps because of altered endothelial cell adherence and membrane phospholipid asymmetry.

Hereditary Xerocytosis and the Intermediate Syndromes

Hereditary xerocytosis or desiccytosis describes an autosomal dominant hemolytic anemia characterized by red blood cell dehydration and decreased osmotic fragility. Affected individuals have characteristically moderate to severe hemolysis with an increased MCHC, reflecting cellular dehydration. Hydrops fetalis with fetal anemia or fetal ascites has been reported in a number of xerocytosis kindreds. Frequently the MCV is mildly increased. In Coulter-type electronic counters, the conversion of pulse height (from the resistance of a cell passing through an electric field) to a cellular volume is dependent on cell shape. Xerocytes do not deform to the same degree as normal cells, which causes the MCV to be approximately 10% too high. The peripheral blood film (see Fig. 43-10) does not always reveal stomatocytes (which are more prominent on wet films), but frequently target cells, dessicytosis (dessicate), and spiculated cells are seen. In some of the cells, hemoglobin is concentrated ("puddled") in discrete areas on the cell periphery.

The mechanism of cellular dehydration is unclear and complex, involving a net potassium loss from the cells that is not accompanied by a proportional gain of sodium. Consequently the net intracellular cation content and cell water are decreased. In some reports a decrease in red blood cell 2,3-DPG has also been noted. The gene for xerocytosis has been mapped to 16q23-q24. A clinical syndrome of xerocytosis, perinatal ascites, and pseudohyperkalemia has been described. Genetic studies of patients with this constellation of disorders and with isolated pseudohyperkalemia also show linkage to this region.

Some of the reported cases of hereditary stomatocytosis share features of both hereditary stomatocytosis and xerocytosis categorized as "intermediate" syndromes. These patients characteristically have both stomatocytes and some target cells on the peripheral blood smear. Osmotic fragility is either normal or slightly increased. Sodium and potassium permeability is somewhat increased, but the intracellular cation concentration and the red blood cell volume are either normal or slightly reduced. These cells were reported to have subnormal glutathione content. In some patients, red blood cells undergo in vitro hemolysis at 5° C, hence the designation *cryohydrocytosis.* A similar susceptibility to cold-induced cation permeability in which potassium and water loss predominates and xerocytes instead of hydrocytes are present, has also been described.

A study of stomatocytosis, spherocytosis, and spherostomatocytosis patients whose erythrocytes demonstrated significant cation leaks at 0° C and in some cases, band 3–deficient membranes, revealed a series of missense mutations located in an intramembrane domain of band 3. In vitro studies suggest that these mutations convert band 3 from an anion exchanger to a nonselective cation leak channel.

Several investigators have also reported a dominantly inherited hemolytic anemia with stomatocytosis, occasional target cells, spherocytes, and a decreased osmotic fragility in which the main red blood cell membrane abnormality involved a nearly 50% increase in phosphatidylcholine and a corresponding decrease in phosphatidylethanolamine. Because abnormalities in membrane phospholipid composition have not been systematically investigated, it is uncertain whether the disorder represents a distinct disease entity.

The results of splenectomy in this group of disorders are variable. In some patients the hemolytic anemia is improved, although often not fully corrected, by splenectomy, whereas in others the severity of the hemolysis is unchanged. Splenectomy should be carefully considered in patients with hereditary stomatocytosis. Several patients with stomatocytosis (both hydrocytosis and xerocytosis) have developed hypercoagulability after splenectomy, leading to catastrophic thrombotic episodes or chronic pulmonary hypertension. Fortunately, the majority of persons with hereditary stomatocytosis are able to maintain an adequate hemoglobin level, so that splenectomy is not required.

Rh Deficiency Syndrome

Rh deficiency syndrome designates rare individuals who have either absent (Rh_{null}) or markedly reduced (Rh_{mod}) Rh antigen expression, mild to moderate hemolytic anemia associated with the presence of stomatocytes, and occasional spherocytes on the peripheral blood film. Hemolytic anemia is improved by splenectomy.

The Rh antigens are present in approximately 20,000 to 30,000 copies per cell and reside on minor transmembrane proteins with an electrophoretic mobility of 28 to 33-kDa on SDS-PAGE. The Rh gene locus encodes two closely linked genes, one encoding the D polypeptide and the other encoding the CcEe proteins, the antigenic expression of which is a consequence of alternate splicing of their pre-mRNA.

Rh proteins are part of a multiprotein complex that includes two Rh proteins and two Rh-associated glycoproteins (RhAG). Other proteins that associate with this complex include CD47, LW, glycophorin B, and protein 4.2. The Rh-RhAG complex interacts with ankyrin to link the membrane skeleton to the lipid bilayer. The Rh proteins share sequence homology to the Mep/Amt family of ammonium transporters in lower organisms and may participate in ammonium transport.

Rh_{null} erythrocytes have no Rh antigen and have reduced or absent LW, Fy5, Ss, U, and Duclos antigens. Rh, RhAG, LW, glycophorin B, CD47, and protein 4.2 are also reduced or absent. Rh_{null} erythrocytes have increased osmotic fragility, reflecting a marked reduction in membrane surface area. These cells are also dehydrated, as indicated by decreased cell cation and water content and increased cell density. The potassium transport and the Na^+/K^+ pump activity are increased, possibly because of reticulocytosis. Phospholipid asymmetry is also altered.

Although the clinical syndromes are the same, the genetic basis of the Rh deficiency syndrome is heterogeneous, and at least two groups have been defined. The amorph type is caused by defects involving the RH30 locus encoding the RhD and RhE polypeptides. The regulatory type of Rh_{null} and Rh_{mod} phenotypes results from suppressor or modifier mutations at the RH50 locus. When one chain of the Rh-RhAG complex is absent, the complex either is not transported to or is assembled at the membrane.

Familial Deficiency of High-Density Lipoproteins

Familial deficiency or absence of high-density lipoproteins (Tangier disease) because of mutations in ABCA1, a protein involved in cellular export of cholesterol, leads to accumulation of cholesterol esters in many tissues. Clinical manifestations include large orange tonsils, hepatosplenomegaly, lymphadenopathy, cloudy corneas, and peripheral neuropathy. Reported hematologic manifestations include a moderately severe hemolytic anemia with stomatocytosis and thrombocytopenia. Erythrocyte membrane lipid analyses reveal a low free cholesterol content, leading to a decreased cholesterol/phospholipid ratio and a relative increase in phosphatidylcholine at the expense of sphingomyelin.

Sitosterolemia

Sitosterolemia or phytosterolemia is a recessive disorder associated with elevated plasma levels of plant sterols. Affected patients exhibit xanthomatosis and early-onset premature cardiovascular disease. Reported hematologic manifestations include hemolytic anemia with stomatocytosis and macrothrombocytopenia. Mutations in the transporters ABCG5 or ABCG8 lead to gastrointestinal hyperabsorption and decreased biliary elimination of plant sterols as well as altered cholesterol metabolism. Plant sterols are not synthesized endogenously in humans but are passively absorbed in the intestine. ABCG5 and ABCG8 actively pump plant sterols out of the intestinal cells back into the intestine and out of liver cells into bile ducts. It has been hypothesized that the stomatocytic phenotype is caused by intercalation of plant sterols into the inner leaflet of the lipid bilayer.

Acquired Stomatocytosis

Stomatocytes have been noted in diverse acquired conditions, including neoplasms, cardiovascular and hepatobiliary disease, alcoholism, and therapy with drugs, some of which are known to be stomatocytogenic in vitro. In some of these conditions, the percentage of stomatocytes on the peripheral blood smear can approach 100%. However, the clinical significance of this observation is unclear because stomatocytes are absent in most patients with the conditions listed. Furthermore, some stomatocytes can be found in normal individuals (3% to 5%). The most consistent association is that of stomatocytosis and heavy alcohol consumption.

RED CELL MEMBRANE VARIANTS AND INFECTIOUS DISEASE

Viral, bacterial, and parasitic infection can all cause anemia. Multiple mechanisms leading to hemolysis have been described. As mentioned earlier in this chapter, parvovirus B19 selectively infects erythroblasts through interaction with globoside, which encodes the P blood group antigen and temporarily shuts down erythropoiesis. Although this infection is tolerated well by healthy subjects, it can lead to severe, at times life-threatening, aplastic crises in patients with anemias because of premature erythrocyte destruction. As one might predict, parvovirus cannot invade erythroblasts of the rare P-negative individuals.

Most infections cause hemolytic anemias triggered by several distinct, and at times overlapping, mechanisms. *Plasmodium, Babesia,* and *Bartonella* species directly attack the membrane and lyse the red cells. Some bacteria, such as *Clostridium perfringens,* elaborate hemolytic toxins or phospholipases that damage the membrane. Other infectious agents trigger occasional production of autoantibodies against red cell membrane components, which in turn leads to autoimmune hemolytic anemia. Finally, many sepsis syndromes are associated with anemia because of disseminated intravascular coagulation.

Malaria and the Erythrocyte Membrane

The red cell membrane defects described earlier in this chapter cause mild to severe hemolytic anemias. At the same time, many red cell membrane alterations have developed as a defense against microorganisms and parasites invading and lysing red cells. This is especially true for malarial parasites. Although four different species of the malaria parasite *Plasmodium,* including *P. falciparum, P. ovale, P. vivax,* and *P. malariae,* infect humans, almost all of the 1.5 to 2 million annual deaths caused by malaria are attributable to *P. falciparum.*

Because malaria coexisted with humans over the course of human evolution, it comes as no surprise that multiple erythroid genotypes were selected that confer some level of resistance to infection or mitigate disease severity. The ensuing heritable phenotypes include, among others, resistance to red cell adhesion and/or invasion, slower intraerythrocytic growth, decreased or increased adhesion of infected red cells to vascular endothelium, and increased phagocytosis of parasitized red cells.

Malaria and other infections causing hemolytic anemias are described in more detail in Chapter 160, which also discuss hemoglobinopathies and red cell enzyme variants that reduce invasion and/or retard parasite growth. Consequently we focus here on the heritable erythrocyte membrane alterations that developed as a defense against malaria.

Erythrocyte Preference

Two parasites, *P. vivax* and *P. ovale,* selectively infect reticulocytes, whereas *P. malariae* infects older erythrocytes. In contrast, *P. falciparum* infects red cells of all ages. This fact and the tendency of *P. falciparum*–infected erythrocytes to sequester in circulation explain the markedly higher severity of *P. falciparum* malaria.

Attachment and Invasion

Duffy Antigen

The *P. vivax* merozoite is completely dependent on attachment to the Duffy blood group antigen (also known as the *Duffy antigen receptor for chemokines [DARC]*) for erythrocyte invasion, and consequently it cannot invade Duffy-negative red blood cells. It has been hypothesized that this is why the Duffy-negative phenotype is common in large areas of Africa. The Duffy-negative phenotype is caused by mutation in a GATA1 motif in the Duffy antigen gene promoter, preventing its expression in erythroid cells, leaving its expression in other tissues intact. Elucidation of this mutation explained a longstanding conundrum of transfusion medicine: why individuals with the Duffy-negative phenotype never develop antibodies against the Duffy antigen.

Glycophorins

All major erythrocyte glycophorins, A, B, and C/D, are involved in attachment of *P. falciparum* to the red blood cell membrane. Consequently invasion of *P. falciparum* into red cells from subjects lacking glycophorin A (En(a−)), glycophorin B (S-s-U−), or glycophorins C and D (Gerbich negative, Ge−) is diminished. As noted earlier, the Gerbich-negative phenotype is associated with mild, asymptomatic ovalocytosis.

Protein 4.1R and Spectrin

Deficiency of protein 4.1R or self-association defects of spectrin are associated with elliptocytosis of varying severity. Both phenotypes appear to reduce the burden of red blood cell invasion.

Band 3 and Southeast Asian Ovalocytosis

Conflicting explanations of the basis of the protective phenotype of Southeast Asian ovalocytosis (described earlier) from malaria have been described. Initial reports suggested that SAO erythrocytes were resistant to malarial invasion. These results were repeatedly questioned until recent studies demonstrated SAO cells to be resistant to invasion by the more virulent *P. falciparum* strains. This may explain the apparent contradiction with the reports of comparable parasitemias in SAO carriers and subjects with a normal red cell phenotype from Papua New Guinea.

The protection from cerebral malaria afforded by SAO erythrocytes is likely because of reduced cytoadherence of SAO red cells to the cerebral vasculature. Under conditions of flow, *P. falciparum*-infected ovalocytes adhere more strongly than normal infected red cells to the endothelial receptor CD36. Because this receptor is not expressed in the brain, this raises a possibility that ovalocytosis protects from cerebral malaria by diminishing the number of parasitized red cells available for adhesion to the cerebral vasculature via alternative receptors. Moreover, ovalocytes appeared resistant to invasion by parasite strains that tend to bind to intracellular adhesion molecule I (ICAM1), the likely receptor for cytoadherence in the brain, but the exact mechanism is not yet known.

Knops Blood Group System

Severe malaria, particularly cerebral malaria, has been associated with the formation of rosettes, clumps of cells formed by the adhesion of malaria-infected erythrocytes to complement receptor 1 (CR1) on uninfected erythrocytes. Identification of the Knops blood group antigens on CR1, followed by observations that frequencies of various Knops antigens varied significantly in whites and individuals of African ancestry, led to the hypothesis that some Knops group antigens might be protective from rosetting and severe malaria. Case control studies with genotyping and/or flow cytometry have yielded conflicting results, but several have linked low-expression CR1 alleles with malaria resistance. Further studies have shown that the expression of CR1 and other complement proteins increases with age. Together these data suggest that genetic and age-related differences in complement protein expression contribute to the variability observed in individuals with severe malaria.

Although these erythrocyte membrane polymorphisms offer fascinating insight into natural defenses against one of the most serious diseases affecting humans, the mechanism of resistance to malaria has not been fully elucidated for any of them. Malaria has clearly had a profound impact on the genetic makeup of populations living in endemic areas and provided us with multiple clues about the host-parasite relationship. Better understanding of these natural defenses might eventually be converted into effective therapeutic interventions.

SUGGESTED READINGS

An X, Mohandas N: Disorders of red cell membrane. *Br J Haematol* 141:367, 2008.

Anstee DJ: The functional importance of blood group-active molecules in human red blood cells. *Vox Sang* 100:140, 2011.

Barcellini W, Bianchi P, Fermo E, et al: Hereditary red cell membrane defects: Diagnostic and clinical aspects. *Blood Transfus* 9:274, 2011.

Barneaud-Rocca D, Pellissier B, Borgese F, et al: Band 3 missense mutations and stomatocytosis: Insight into the molecular mechanism responsible for monovalent cation leak. *Int J Cell Biol* 2011:136802, 2011.

Bennett V, Healy J: Organizing the fluid membrane bilayer: Diseases linked to spectrin and ankyrin. *Trends Mol Med* 14:28, 2008.

Bolton-Maggs PH, Langer JC, Iolascon A, et al: Guidelines for the diagnosis and management of hereditary spherocytosis—2011 update. *Br J Haematol* 2011.

Bruce LJ: Red cell membrane transport abnormalities. *Curr Opin Hematol* 15:184, 2008.

Bruce LJ: Hereditary stomatocytosis and cation-leaky red cells—Recent developments. *Blood Cells Mol Dis* 42:216, 2009.

Bruce LJ, Guizouarn H, Burton NM, et al: The monovalent cation leak in overhydrated stomatocytic red blood cells results from amino acid substitutions in the Rh-associated glycoprotein. *Blood* 113:1350, 2009.

Bruce LJ, Robinson HC, Guizouarn H, et al: Monovalent cation leaks in human red cells caused by single amino-acid substitutions in the transport domain of the band 3 chloride-bicarbonate exchanger, AE1. *Nat Genet* 37:1258, 2005.

Casale M, Perrotta S: Splenectomy for hereditary spherocytosis: Complete, partial or not at all? *Expert Rev Hematol* 4:627, 2011.

Daniels G: The molecular genetics of blood group polymorphism. *Transplant Immunol* 14:143, 2005.

Darghouth D, Koehl B, Heilier JF, et al: Alterations of red blood cells metabolome in overhydrated hereditary stomatocytosis. *Haematologica* 2011.

Dhermy D, Schrevel J, Lecomte MC: Spectrin-based skeleton in red blood cells and malaria. *Curr Opin Hematol* 14:198, 2007.

Flatt JF, Guizouarn H, Burton NM, et al: Stomatin-deficient cryohydrocytosis results from mutations in SLC2A1: A novel form of GLUT1 deficiency syndrome. *Blood* 118:5267, 2011.

Gallagher PG: Hereditary elliptocytosis: Spectrin and protein 4.1R. *Semin Hematol* 41:142, 2004.

Genetet S, Ripoche P, Picot J, et al: The human RhAG ammonia channel is impaired by the Phe65Ser mutation in overhydrated stomatocytic red cells. *Am J Physiol Cell Physiol* 2011.

Guizouarn H, Borgese F, Gabillat N, et al: South-east Asian ovalocytosis and the cryohydrocytosis form of hereditary stomatocytosis show virtually indistinguishable cation permeability defects. *Br J Haematol* 152:655, 2011.

Houston BL, Zelinski T, Israels SJ, et al: Refinement of the hereditary xerocytosis locus on chromosome 16q in a large Canadian kindred. *Blood Cells Mol Dis* 47:226, 2011.

Iolascon A, Avvisati RA: Genotype/phenotype correlation in hereditary spherocytosis. *Haematologica* 93:1283, 2008.

Ipsaro JJ, Harper SL, Messick TE, et al: Crystal structure and functional interpretation of the erythrocyte spectrin tetramerization domain complex. *Blood* 115:4843, 2010.

Mariani M, Barcellini W, Vercellati C, et al: Clinical and hematologic features of 300 patients affected by hereditary spherocytosis grouped according to the type of the membrane protein defect. *Haematologica* 93:1310, 2008.

Perrotta S, Gallagher PG, Mohandas N: Hereditary spherocytosis. *Lancet* 372:1411, 2008.

Salomao M, Chen K, Villalobos J, et al: Hereditary spherocytosis and hereditary elliptocytosis: Aberrant protein sorting during erythroblast enucleation. *Blood* 116:267, 2010.

Satchwell TJ, Shoemark DK, Sessions RB, et al: Protein 4.2: A complex linker. *Blood Cells Mol Dis* 42:201, 2009.

Schilling RF: Risks and benefits of splenectomy versus no splenectomy for hereditary spherocytosis—A personal view. *Br J Haematol* 145:728, 2009.

Stewart AK, Kedar PS, Shmukler BE, et al: Functional characterization and modified rescue of novel AE1 mutation R730C associated with overhydrated cation leak stomatocytosis. *Am J Physiol Cell Physiol* 300:C1034, 2011.

Tracy ET, Rice HE: Partial splenectomy for hereditary spherocytosis. *Pediatr Clin North Am* 55:503, 2008.

Wilder JA, Stone JA, Preston EG, et al: Molecular population genetics of SLC4A1 and Southeast Asian ovalocytosis. *J Hum Genet* 54:182, 2009.

Williamson RC, Toye AM: Glycophorin A: Band 3 aid. *Blood Cells Mol Dis* 41:35, 2008.

CHAPTER 44

AUTOIMMUNE HEMOLYTIC ANEMIA

Ulrich Jäger and Klaus Lechner

Autoimmune hemolytic anemia (AIHA) is caused by autoimmune-mediated destruction of red blood cells (RBCs) by autoantibodies with various properties and target specificities. Exact laboratory diagnosis is often difficult; therefore, experienced diagnostic reference centers play an important role. The disease can be primary (idiopathic) or caused by an underlying condition (secondary), including autoimmune diseases, infections, drugs, or neoplasms. The clinical course of the disease as well as treatment decisions are influenced by the type of antibody involved. Success in treatment and the evaluation of therapies have lagged behind the achievements in laboratory diagnosis but will hopefully improve with the introduction of new effective drugs. Currently, almost all treatments in AIHA are based on experience and opinion but not on evidence. There are no established guidelines. Thus, management of the disease requires general hematologic skills and critical evaluation of treatment recommendations.

HISTORY

The history of diagnostic and therapeutic progress in AIHA has been described by Dacie,[1] one of the great pioneers in this field. Milestones were the discovery of the first RBC autoantibody (Donath-Landsteiner antibody) in 1904, the introduction of the Coombs test in 1945, the establishment of splenectomy as effective treatment of AIHA in the 1950s, and the finding that rituximab is an effective treatment in the past decade. The diagnosis and treatment of patients with AIHA were recently reviewed by several authors.[2-8]

EPIDEMIOLOGY

The incidence of primary AIHA is 0.8% per year. Secondary AIHA has at least the same frequency. Because only a low proportion of patients have spontaneous or treatment-induced long-term remissions and the death rate is low, the prevalence of AIHA is relatively high and has been estimated as 17 in 100.00 (in Denmark). The incidence of AIHA in children and teenagers is 0.2 to 1.0 per million per year.[9] There is some evidence of a familial clustering of AIHA in children, but no hereditary genetic background has been identified. Warm antibodies (WAIHAs) are found in 87% and cold antibodies (CAIHAs) in 13% of patients with AIHA.

Primary AIHA and Evans syndrome are slightly more prevalent in women and in children.[10] In secondary AIHA, the female-to-male ratio is very high in systemic lupus erythematosus, but low in chronic lymphocytic leukemia (CLL)–associated AIHA. The incidence of chronic cold agglutinin disease (CAD) is estimated to be one per million per year with a female prevalence. Geographical differences have been suggested with a higher incidence of CAD in Northern climates.

PATHOBIOLOGY

Hemolysis is initiated when an autoantibody binds to the RBC membranes and recruits complement. Destruction of the RBC can occur directly in the circulation (intravascular hemolysis) or by removal of the cell by macrophages in spleen, liver, or both (extravascular hemolysis) (Fig. 44-1). Several immunoglobulin subclasses can fix complement: immunoglobulin (Ig) G, IgA, and IgM. Macrophages recognize opsonized erythrocytes via receptors specific for the Fc fragment of IgG and for C3d. RBCs coated with IgG or complement alone are destroyed in spleen and liver, IgG-coated cells in the spleen, and IgM-coated cells in the liver. This has major implications for treatment, particularly for the effect of steroids and splenectomy.

Warm Antibody Hemolytic Anemia

About 70% to 80% of cases of AIHA are caused by warm antibodies. The RBC antibodies in WAIHA are mostly polyclonal IgG (IgG_{1-4}), which have a low capacity to activate the complement system (Table 44-1). The direct antiglobulin test (DAT) in WAIHA is positive either with IgG (37%) or IgG + C3d (43%). Rarely, the DAT is only positive with C3d (when the amount of IgG on the RBCs is very small). Patients with IgG antibodies may have also IgA antibodies, but IgA antibodies without IgG antibodies are a very rare cause of WAIHA. Warm antibodies are often directed against Rh antigens but also against other blood group antigens (non–Rh-related autoantibodies) such as band 3 protein or glycophorin A. The antibodies fix complement and bind tightly to the RBCs at 37° C. Therefore, there is only a small amount of antibody detectable in the serum. The antibody coated RBCs are removed from the circulation by splenic (to a lesser degree also by hepatic) macrophages via $F_{c\gamma}RIII$ receptors. IgG_3 and IgG_1 have the highest affinity for the Fc receptors of macrophages. Erythrocytes that are only partially phagocytosed by the macrophages become spherocytes, which are removed in the splenic cords because of their rigid structure. Destruction of RBCs may also be caused by other mechanism such as antibody-dependent cellular cytotoxicity.[11]

Immunoglobulin M warm antibodies are a very rare cause of AIHA. This type of AIHA can be suspected if a RBC autoagglutination occurs at room temperature. The DAT result is positive with C3d alone (65%) or with IgG (24%). Using sensitive methods, IgM on the RBCs can be detected in 71%.[12] Non-Hodgkin lymphoma (NHL) is the underlying disease in some of these cases. This AIHA is severe, often fatal and refractory to steroids and splenectomy.

Cold Antibody Hemolytic Anemia

Cold antibodies in primary or secondary CAIHA are usually monoclonal IgM. The IgM has two binding sites for C1q and fixes complement easily. The targets are polysaccharides (I, I^T, i or Pr antigens). The "i" antigen is a nonbranched polysaccharide in the cord blood, and the "I" antigen is a similar but branched molecule expressed in the RBCs of adults. The cold antibodies bind to the RBCs at low temperatures and cause their lysis at temperatures above 22° C. The DAT is typically positive with C3d alone. When cold antibodies are present at high titers, they may activate the complement system directly and produce a membrane attack complex (MAC) and intravascular hemolysis with hemoglobinuria. Usually the complement-coated RBCs are sequestered by liver macrophages.

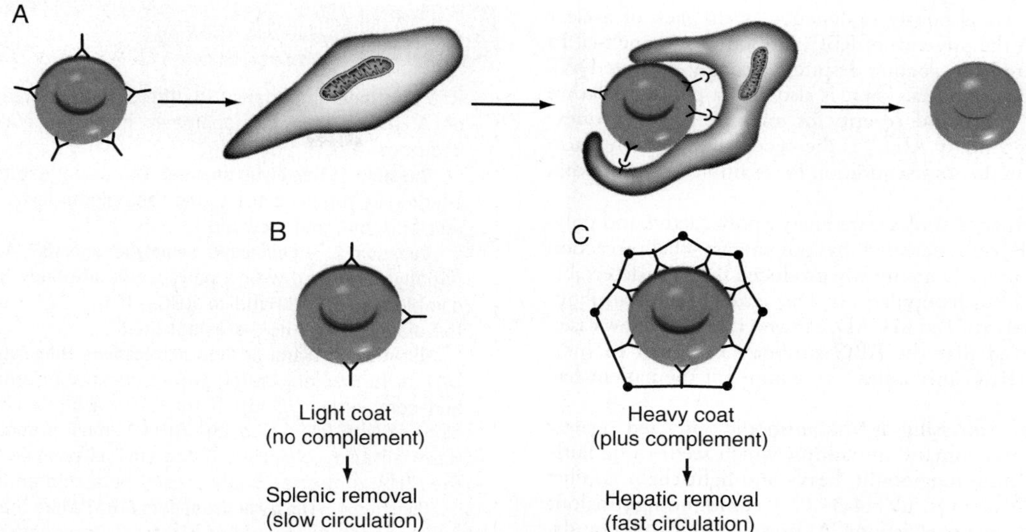

Figure 44-1 MECHANISM OF EXTRAVASCULAR HEMOLYSIS IN AUTOIMMUNE HEMOLYTIC ANEMIA. **A,** Macrophage encounters an IgG-coated erythrocyte and binds to it via its Fc receptors. Thus entrapped, the red blood cell (RBC) loses bits of its membrane as a result of digestion by the macrophage's ectoenzymes. The discoid erythrocyte transforms into a sphere. **B,** RBC lightly coated with IgG (and therefore incapable of activating the complement cascade) is preferentially removed in the sluggish circulation of the spleen. **C,** RBC with a heavy coat of IgG; thus, C3b *(black circles)* can be removed both by the spleen and the liver. *(From Cunningham MJ, Silberstein LE: Autoimmune Hemolytic Anemia. In Hoffman R, Benz EJ Jr, Shattil SJ, et al, eds:* Hematology: Basic principles and practice, *ed 4, 2005, Philadelphia, Elsevier.)*

Table 44-1 Properties and Specificities of Red Blood Cell Autoantibodies

	Immunoglobulin (Subclass)	Type of Antibody	Clonality	Specificity	Hemolysis	Site of Removal of Red Blood Cells
WAIHA	$IgG_{(1-4)}$, IgA	Incomplete	Mostly polyclonal	Rh- and non–Rh- antigens	Extravascular	Spleen (liver)
CAIHA	IgM	Complete	Mostly clonal	Anti-i, -I^{T}, -I, -Pr	Intravascular	Liver
Donath-Landsteiner antibody	IgG	—	Polyclonal	P antigen	Intravascular	—

CAIHA, Cold autoimmune hemolytic anemia; *Ig,* immunoglobulin; *WAIHA,* warm autoimmune hemolytic anemia.

Paroxysmal cold hemoglobinuria (PCH) is caused by the Donath-Landsteiner antibody. This is a rare, usually polyclonal IgG cold antibody to P antigen (glycosphingolipid globoside), which binds to the RBCs at 4° C. The cells are lysed at higher temperatures. The DAT is positive with C3d, and the diagnosis is made by the Donath-Landsteiner test. In this test, normal RBCs and patient and normal serum are incubated at 4° C. Agglutination occurs after warming to 37° C. The prominent clinical feature of PCH is a brisk, immediate but sometimes also delayed hemoglobinuria after cold exposure even in patients with low antibody titers. In the past, it has been associated with secondary or tertiary syphilis. Now, two types can be distinguished clinically[13]: (1) an acute, severe form (often associated with hemoglobinuria) but self-limiting AIHA after (respiratory) infections in children and (2) a rare chronic AIHA in nonsyphilitic persons with various underlying conditions, including NHL. Patients with chronic PCH respond poorly to steroids and splenectomy.

ETIOLOGY AND PATHOPHYSIOLOGY

Our knowledge about the etiology of AIHA is still limited. Factors that may play a role are antigen mimicry; immune deficiency; and to a lesser extent, probably genetic factors. AIHA, similar to other autoimmune diseases, is a consequence of the loss of immunologic (self-) tolerance against antigens expressed on the erythrocyte surface. Production of RBC antibodies is a result of the interaction of T and B cells as well as regulatory factors (e.g., T regulatory cells, cytokines).[14] Disturbances of the Th1/2 T-cell subset balance as well as the occurrence of clonal regulatory T cells specific for a RBC autoantigen have been described. This may be linked to the fact that AIHA does not only occur in immunocompetent individuals but frequently occurs in patients with acquired T-cell defects such as HIV infection or immunosuppressive therapy, particularly after organ transplantation. Polymorphisms or altered expression of negative regulators of T-cell responses such as CTLA-4 (cytotoxic T lymphocyte antigen 4) or interleukin-10 (IL-10) may also play a role. Mouse models (New Zealand black mice) have revealed an association of genetic loci with antierythrocyte antibody production or cold agglutinin escape tolerance after *Mycoplasma* infection.

Various target antigens have been described, with Rhesus polypeptides, glycophorin, and erythrocyte band 3 being the most prominent in WAIHA. Cold reactive antibodies frequently target the I or i blood group–specific antigens. Events linked to the development of secondary AIHA by induction of cross-tolerance (molecular mimicry) are infections (*Mycoplasma pneumoniae* [I antigen target], parvovirus, herpes viruses), neoplastic diseases (paraneoplasia), and drugs by various mechanisms. There are important differences in the pathogenesis of WAIHA and CAIHA. The pathogenesis of primary WAIHA is largely unknown. Secondary WAIHA is a complication of several congenital or acquired immune deficiencies. Both moderate (for example in CLL) and severe (HIV, posttransplant, congenital severe T-cell deficiencies) T-cell and humoral immune deficiency predispose to WAIHA, but no correlation between the type and severity of immune deficiency and the risk of AIHA has been established.

One phenomenon that is poorly understood is the lack of a clear relationship between the presence of RBC antibodies and anemia. In many instances, there is no anemia despite a strongly positive DAT or high titers of cold antibodies. There is also only a poor correlation between antibodies titers and severity of anemia. Another unexplained finding in secondary AIHA is the occurrence of both warm and cold antibodies in the some condition for example in lymphomas or infections.

Antibodies in primary AIHA are frequently polyreactive and polyclonal (no clonal B cells detected by polymerase chain reaction [PCR]). Antibodies in CAD are mostly produced by PCR-detectable oligo- or monoclonal B-cell populations. The nature of these antibodies has been extensively studied in CAD. However, in only a few cases, it has been established that the RBC antibody is clonal. In most reports, clonality of RBC antibodies was assumed if the patient had a paraproteinemia.

B-cell neoplasms expressing IgMκ antibodies directed against RBC antigens have few somatic mutations, which seem to be fairly restricted to certain immunoglobulin heavy and light chain families (VH4-34, VκIV).[15] Moreover, a VH4-34 CLL confounding subclone was shown to arise from a preexisting CAD-producing B-cell population. The restricted clonality of CAD producing B cells is further corroborated by the detection of recurrent chromosomal aberrations (trisomy 3).[16] CLL cells may also drive AIHA by presenting the autoantigen (e.g., erythrocyte protein band 3) to T cells.

Four Important Questions for the Diagnosis and Management of Autoimmune Hemolytic Anemia

It is of utmost importance to differentiate between various types of AIHA. A stepwise approach helps in making the right decisions:

Question 1: Hemolytic anemia? The basic features of hemolytic anemia are reticulocytosis, low haptoglobin levels, elevated indirect bilirubin, and elevated LDH.

Question 2: Autoimmune hemolytic anemia? A direct DAT is initially performed with a polyspecific antibody to detect IgG or complement C3d bound to RBCs. If the DAT result is positive, the diagnosis of AIHA is established.

Question 3: Warm or Cold Autoimmune Hemolytic Anemia? The DAT is further elaborated with monospecific antibodies to IgG and complement (C3d). If the DAT result is positive with IgG alone or with IgG + C3d, the AIHA is most probably caused by a warm antibody (WAIHA). If the DAT is positive with C3d only, the AIHA is most probably caused by a cold antibody (CAIHA).

Question 4: Primary or secondary AIHA? More than half of AIHAs are secondary to underlying diseases. Secondary AIHA should be suspected in patients with additional findings or who are refractory to initial steroid treatment. In this case, the underlying disease has to be diagnosed (e.g., by serologic tests, CT scan, or bone marrow biopsy).

SYMPTOMS, CLINICAL FINDINGS, AND RISKS

The symptoms of AIHA depend on the type of antibody, the mode of onset, and the severity of anemia. In patients with WAIHA, the onset is mostly gradual or subacute, and the symptoms (i.e., tiredness, reduction of physical activity, and shortness of breath in elderly patients) are attributable only to anemia. However, patients with postinfectious, drug-induced AIHA or patients with Donath-Landsteiner or Pr antibodies often present with acute severe symptoms such as malaise, fever, jaundice, abdominal pain, shortness of breath, and hemoglobulinuria. The course in such patients may be fulminant and even fatal. Patients with chronic cold antibody AIHA (CAD) often have an indolent course. Symptoms suggestive for CAIHA are cold sensitivity, cold-dependent acrocyanosis, acral numbness, and rarely livedo reticularis or organ ischemia. Anemia worsens after cold exposure or conditions associated with an acute phase reaction.

During clinical examination, a subicterus may be seen. Lymphadenopathy, palpable splenomegaly, or any organomegaly is rare in patients with primary AIHA. Its presence suggests secondary AIHA.

Patients with WAIHA are at an increased risk of venous thromboembolism, particularly when the AIHA is associated with a lupus anticoagulant (LA).[17] Older patients with AIHA are at an increased risk of cardiovascular complications, which may also be partly caused by the treatment.

LABORATORY DIAGNOSIS OF AUTOIMMUNE HEMOLYTIC ANEMIA

Autoimmune hemolytic anemia is essentially a laboratory diagnosis. The diagnostic pathway of AIHA should proceed in a stepwise fashion answering the following questions:

Step 1: Hemolytic Anemia?

The first step is to establish the diagnosis of hemolytic anemia (see box on Four Important Questions for the Diagnosis and Management of Autoimmune Hemolytic Anemia). This diagnosis is established by the presence of the following pentad of findings: normocytic or macrocytic anemia (male hemoglobin < 13.0-14.0 g/dL; female <12.0 g/dL), reticulocytosis (corrected reticulocyte count >2% or absolute reticulocyte count >100.000-120.000/μL), low haptoglobin, elevated lactate dehydrogenase (LDH), and elevated unconjugated (indirect) bilirubin. Haptoglobin is an α2-globuline that binds hemoglobin. This hemoglobin–haptoglobin complex is degraded in the liver. Hemopexin is another plasma protein with a very high binding affinity to hemoglobin. It scavenges heme released from RBCs and protects the organisms from the adverse effects of circulating hemoglobin. The determination of hemopexin is not essential for the diagnosis of AIHA. Indirect bilirubin is usually not more than 5 mg/dL except in associated liver disease (Epstein-Barr (EBV)–associated AIHA). Additional findings are increased urobilinogen in the urine and spherocytes in the blood smear. Leukoerythroblastosis occurs only in peracute AIHA, but microangiopathic hemolytic anemia should always be suspected in such cases. Bone marrow examination is usually not necessary except in patients in whom secondary AIHA, in particular lymphoma, is suspected. RBC survival is shortened, but its measurement with radioisotopes has no diagnostic value, not even for the prediction for the efficacy of splenectomy.

Among methodologic diagnostic problems, reticulocyte counting is the biggest because in many laboratories, low-precision microscopic counts are still performed. Automatic flow cytometric methods are more precise, reliable, and convenient. With flow cytometry, the number of highly fluorescent reticulocytes (which are increased in AIHA but are low in hereditary spherocytosis) can also be measured. Falsely very high mean corpuscular volume and mean corpuscular hemoglobin concentration occur in some cases of CAIHA because RBC counts are falsely low because of agglutination of RBC at room temperature. If a CAIHA is suspected, blood samples should be sent to the laboratory in warmed containers.

All of the findings of the pentad are not always present. Reticulocytosis is often (in ≈25%) not present at the onset of AIHA. This is mostly because of a delayed initial bone marrow response of erythropoiesis. After 1 week, most of these patients have reticulocytosis. In other patients (particularly in secondary cases), absence of reticulocytosis may be attributable to impairment of erythropoiesis caused by bone marrow infiltration or blunted erythropoiesis caused by an acute phase reaction. If the reticulocyte count is very low, pure RBC aplasia (PRCA), either immune mediated or induced by a parvovirus (or HHV6) infection, should be suspected. Haptoglobin may be falsely normal or even increased, particularly in patients with malignant or immune diseases, because haptoglobin is an acute phase protein. Haptoglobin may be falsely low in patients with a haplotype H_0H_0 and in patients with severe liver disease. Both increased bilirubin and elevated LDH have a limited sensitivity and specificity for AIHA.

Step 2: Autoimmune Hemolytic Anemia?

The next step is to find out whether the hemolytic anemia is an AIHA. This is best done by the DAT (Fig. 44-2). In this test, washed RBCs of the patient (obtained from an EDTA [ethylenediaminetetraacetic acid] blood sample) are incubated in a tube with a polyspecific antibody to IgG and complement (C3d). If the RBCs agglutinate, the test result is positive. In many laboratories, the tube test has been replaced by the tube gel test, which is easier to perform, more reliable, and probably more sensitive. In the indirect antiglobulin test (IAT), patient plasma or serum is incubated with test RBCs, and (after washing) RBC-bound IgG is detected with the DAT. IAT is usually not required for the diagnosis of AIHA except when a drug-dependent antibody is suspected. For the differentiation of drug-dependent antibodies and autoantibodies, an acid eluate of the patient's RBCs should be made and tested in the IAT. If the IAT result is positive, the patient has autoantibodies. The severity of AIHA does not correlate with the strength of the DAT but rather with the immune globulin subclass of the antibody (IgG_1 or IgG_3). The result of the DAT is not a reliable marker of treatment success because patients with a complete hematologic remission may remain DAT positive, and DAT positivity or negativity has only limited value to predict the duration of hematologic remission.

Falsely Negative and Positive Direct Antiglobulin Test Results without Hemolysis or Anemia

If the conventional DAT test result is negative, hemolytic anemia is defined as DAT negative. However, AIHA cannot be definitely excluded because about 5% (2%-11%) of AIHA patients are DAT negative. If AIHA is suspected for clinical grounds despite a negative DAT result, more sensitive quantitative tests are required to determine the amount of IgG on the RBCs. The threshold of positivity of the conventional DAT is 100 to 200 IgG molecules per RBCs, but in some AIHA patients, the RBC IgG is less than this amount. In about one-third of DAT-negative cases, one of the more sensitive test results (e.g., immunoradiometric tests) will be positive. However, the relationship between the amount of RBC IgG and hemolysis is not clearcut, and there is no "hemolysis threshold."[18] The reasons for these discrepancies between the in vitro and in vivo activity of RBC antibodies are largely unknown. Differences in macrophage activity may be one possible explanation. A search for antibodies in the RBC eluate in which antibodies are more concentrated is also useful. IgA antibodies are rare and sometimes not included in the analysis. Finally, there is the possibility of low-affinity antibodies. Such antibodies are washed out when the washes are made with 37° C saline. A high rate of DAT-negative AIHA has been observed in AIHA induced by nucleoside analogues but also in other secondary AIHA.

The DAT result is positive in one in three to 10,000 normal persons and 10% of hospital patients without anemia or signs of hemolysis.

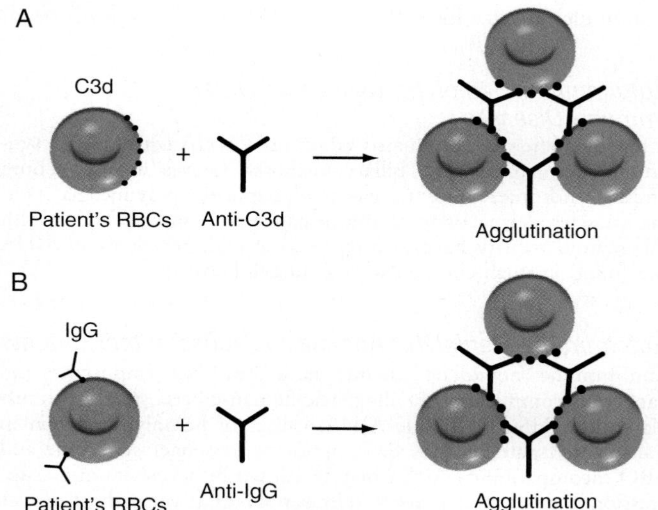

Figure 44-2 DIRECT ANTIGLOBULIN TEST (DAT) FOR DETECTION OF **(A)** ERYTHROCYTE-BOUND C3D OR **(B)** IGG. Hemagglutination occurs when anti-C3d or anti-IgG can create a lattice structure by bridging sensitized red blood cells (RBCs). *(From Cunnigham MJ, Silberstein LE: Autoimmune hemolytic anemia. In Hoffman R, Benz EJ Jr, Shattil SJ, et al, eds:* Hematology: Basic principles and practice, *ed 4, 2005, Philadelphia, Elsevier.)*

Step 3: Warm or Cold Autoimmune Hemolytic Anemia?

In a further step, the DAT is done with monospecific antibodies to IgG and complement (C3d) to find out whether a warm or cold antibody is the cause of hemolysis. If the DAT result is positive with IgG alone or with IgG plus C3d, the AIHA is most probably a WAIHA. If the DAT result is positive with only C3d, the AIHA is most probably a CAIHA. The differentiation between WAIHA and CAIHA is extremely important for the choice of treatment.

There are some special diagnostic problems in CAIHA. If cold antibodies are suspected, it must be taken care that the blood that is sent to the laboratory is kept at 37° C to get reliable results. Patients with only RBC C3d may (rarely) have WAIHA when the amount of RBC IgG is very small. In patients with C3d positivity, the cold agglutinin titer should be determined. If it is greater than 1:512, the diagnosis of a CAD is established. There is no threshold titer that separates normal from abnormal. If the titer is less than 1:512 the thermal amplitude of the antibody must be determined. If the thermal amplitude is above 22° C, the diagnosis is CAD. Mixed-type AIHA is probably rare. The criteria are a positive IgG DAT result and a positive eluate (WAIHA) result plus a C3d-positive DAT result and the presence of cold antibodies with a thermal amplitude of greater than 30° C (CAIHA). Many published cases of mixed-type antibodies do not fulfill these criteria.[19]

Step 4: Primary or Secondary Autoimmune Hemolytic Anemia?

In the last diagnostic step, it must be determined whether the AIHA is primary or a complication of an underlying disease (secondary). The decision regarding which diagnostic procedures should be used for this purpose depends mainly on the type of AIHA (WAIHA or CAIHA) and should include history, physical examination, laboratory tests, and imaging procedures if indicated. In children and younger patients with WAIHA, evidence for an infection should be sought. A list of all recent medication should be made. A history of weight loss, fever, or poor general condition and arthritis points to a malignancy or immune disease as the underlying condition. Palpable lymphadenopathy and splenomegaly do not belong to the clinical picture of primary WAIHA. In this case, lymphoma (particularly splenic marginal zone lymphoma [SMZL]) should be suspected. Laboratory tests should include acute phase proteins, LDH, quantitative determination of immune globulins, and other tests guided by the clinical history. A bone marrow examination is not obligatory except when lymphoma is suspected. Abdominal ultrasonography is reasonable in all cases to exclude splenomegaly, the remote (but important) possibility of an ovarian teratoma (in women), lymphadenopathy, or solitary extranodal lymphomas. Some experts recommend computed tomography (CT) of the abdomen or thorax in all cases, but there is concern of radiation exposure. An activated partial thromboplastin time (aPTT) with a lupus-sensitive reagent may reveal a LA. Fluorescence activated cell sorting (FACS) or PCR for the detection of monoclonal lymphocytes may be done, but the clinical usefulness of such tests to guide treatment decisions is uncertain.

In CAIHA, a history of a febrile illness should prompt a thoracic radiography, and if results are positive, a serologic test for mycoplasma pneumoniae is required. The quantitative determination of serum immunoglobulins and a search for a clonal immune globulin by immune fixation are important. If immune fixation findings are positive, a search for lymphoma is necessary, which may include bone marrow biopsy even when there is no lymphadenopathy.

Other tests, including blood glucose, Hba_{1c}, renal and hepatic function tests, HIV serology, hepatitis B antigen, and exclusion of latent tuberculosis are necessary to avoid complications of steroids (in WAIHA) or rituximab (in CAIHA and WAIHA).

IMMUNOLOGIC PHENOMENA ASSOCIATED WITH AUTOIMMUNE HEMOLYTIC ANEMIA

Evans syndrome is the combination of WAIHA with autoimmune thrombocytopenia (ITP), a typical but rare association. Platelet antibodies are usually directed against glycoprotein IIB/IIIA. Neutropenia occurs in 25% of patients. There is no sex predilection; about half of the cases are secondary. Evans syndrome is relatively more common in patients with systemic lupus erythematosus (SLE), antiphospholipid antibodies (APAs), and autoimmune lymphoproliferative syndrome (ALPS).[20] A search for an ALPS is mandatory in younger patients with Evans syndrome. In roughly 50% of the cases, AIHA and ITP occur simultaneously; in 25%, the disease starts with ITP; and in 16%, the disease starts with AIHA. There may be an interval of several years between the onset of AIHA and ITP.[10]

WAIHA, CAIHA, or a positive DAT result without anemia may be associated with PRCA. PRCA may be either immune mediated such as in T-cell neoplasms (particularly T-cell large granulocytic leukemia) or may be caused by an infection with parvovirus. Patients with parvovirus-associated AIHA often present with PRCA.

Autoimmune hemolytic anemia is definitely associated with APAs and LA. In one single centre prospective study, LA was found in 30% predominantly idiopathic AIHA. AIHA (4%) and Evans syndrome (10%) are frequent in patients with APA. It is well established that patients with AIHA have a significantly (2.8- to3.8-fold) elevated risk of venous thromboembolism.[17] It is likely but not proven that patients with AIHA associated with LA are at a higher risk.

In lymphomas, some cases of AIHA are associated with C1-esterase inhibitor deficiency and mixed cryoglobulinemia.

SECONDARY AUTOIMMUNE HEMOLYTIC ANEMIA

About half of cases of AIHA (or probably even more) are secondary. The main causes are immune diseases and malignancies. Other underlying conditions are infections, drugs, transplantation, and congenital defects.

Temporal Relationship of Secondary Autoimmune Hemolytic Anemia to the Underlying Condition

The temporal relationship of AIHA to an underlying condition is complex. AIHA antedates the diagnosis of malignancy in many cases—in NHL, sometimes for years. In population-based studies, clonal B cells have been detected in some patients with seemingly idiopathic AIHA. In most instances, AIHA occurs concurrently with the malignancy. In some other cases, AIHA occurred only at the recurrence and rarely in complete remission after successful treatment. In CLL, AIHA occurs in a late phase of the disease. The patients have poor prognostic factors and often have been treated with various agents.

In immune diseases, particularly SLE, AIHA is a complication of the early phase of the disease. Infection-related AIHA occurs shortly after the onset of symptoms except in HIV infection, in which AIHA is a complication in the late advanced stage of the disease.

Serologic Type of Autoimmune Hemolytic Anemia in Secondary Autoimmune Hemolytic Anemia

It is an interesting phenomenon that in underlying diseases associated with AIHA, all serologic types of AIHA may occur, but usually one serologic type (WAIHA, CAIHA, or Donath-Landsteiner (DL) antibody) prevails. The only exception is ovarian teratoma, which is only associated with WAIHA.

Autoimmune Hemolytic Anemia in Immune Diseases

Autoimmune Hemolytic Anemia in Systemic Lupus Erythematosus and Primary Antiphospholipid Syndrome

The prevalence of AIHA in patients with SLE is 7.5% (average of seven studies; range, 5.2%-12.5%). AIHA may occur at any time during the course of SLE, but two-thirds of cases of AIHA occur at diagnosis or soon thereafter. Almost half of the patients are already taking steroids. Most patients are women and have WAIHA. Evans syndrome is common. Compared with SLE patients without AIHA, those with AIHA are younger; have a higher prevalence of thrombocytopenia, APAs, renal disease, serositis, and central nervous system involvement; and have a higher risk of venous thrombosis.[21]

The prevalence of AIHA in primary antiphospholipid syndrome (PAPS) is about 10%. AIHA precedes PAPS in 25% of cases, but in others occurred after a median time of 4.4 years after the diagnosis of PAPS. Patients with PAPS and AIHA have an increased risk for the development of SLE.[22]

Autoimmune Hemolytic Anemia in Inflammatory Bowel Disease

In the only larger study the prevalence of AIHA in ulcerative colitis was 1.7%. The mean time from diagnosis of colitis to AIHA was 17 months. Three-quarters of these patients had a total colitis. AIHA may also be associated with Crohn disease, but the prevalence is lower than in ulcerative colitis.

Autoimmune Hemolytic Anemia in Other Immune Diseases

A few or single cases of an association of WAIHA with Sjögren syndrome, dermatomyositis, biliary cirrhosis, Graves disease, Churg Strauss syndrome, crescentic glomerulonephritis, polymyalgia rheumatica, scleroderma, or autoimmune pancreatitis and of CAIHA with rheumatoid arthritis have been reported. A high prevalence of AIHA was found in small children with giant cell hepatitis.

Autoimmune Hemolytic Anemia in Transplanted Patients

Autoimmune hemolytic anemia is a rare but important and dangerous complication of allogeneic hematopoietic stem cell transplantation (HSCT). Beside AIHA, causes of hemolytic anemia in transplanted patients may be lymphocyte passenger syndrome and ABO incompatibility. AIHA may be caused by severe immune suppression by drugs to prevent rejection or graft-versus-host-disease (GVHD), viral infections, EBV lymphoproliferative disorder (LPD), or the recurrence of an immune disorder after transplantation (biliary cirrhosis).

The highest rate of AIHA occurred in small children after unrelated cord HSCT for inborn metabolic defects (44%) and in children with severe combined immune deficiency after haploidentical HSCT with T cell–depleted stem cell grafts.

In adults, the incidence of AIHA ranges from 3.0% to 4.4% after allogeneic HSCT.[23] The median time from HSCT to AIHA is 4 to 10 months. Most patients have warm antibodies. Risk factors for AIHA are unrelated donor, T-cell depletion, and extensive GVHD. In most cases, AIHA occurred in patients in complete remission of the underlying disease, but in one study, AIHA was associated with a relapse of chronic myeloid leukemia in the majority of patients.

After transplantation of solid organs, the highest risk of AIHA was in patients with pancreatic transplantation. A number of patients with AIHA or CAIHA were observed after liver transplantation but only a small number after cardiac, lung, intestinal, and renal transplantation. The most likely cause of AIHA in these patients is severe drug-induced immunosuppression.

Autoimmune Hemolytic Anemia in Pregnancy and After Blood Transfusion

Very few cases of AIHA and Evans syndrome occurred during pregnancy, all with warm antibodies. In these patients, there seems to be a higher risk for preeclampsia. AIHA responds well to steroids and resolves in most cases after delivery. In two cases, the newborns had mild hemolysis.

Development of RBC autoantibodies is common in multitransfused patients and is associated with presence of alloantibodies. However, anemia is rare.

Autoimmune Hemolytic Anemia in Malignancies

Autoimmune Hemolytic Anemia in Lymphoproliferative Disorders

Autoimmune hemolytic anemia is a typical, relatively common immune-mediated paraneoplastic syndrome in LPD. It occurs in almost all histologic subtypes of NHL, but there is no correlation between the frequency of lymphoma and the risk of AIHA. AIHA is relatively most common in SMZL and angioimmunoblastic T-cell lymphoma (Table 44-2). In most LPD WAIHA is predominant. Most warm antibodies, particularly in CLL, seem to be polyclonal. The proportion of patients with WAIHA is highest in CLL and Hodgkin disease; in other malignancies, the ratio of WAIHA to CAIHA is two to one. In lymphoplasmacytic lymphoma (LPL), almost all antibodies are clonal cold antibodies.

Table 44-2 Secondary Autoimmune Hemolytic Anemia in Malignancies

Malignancy	Prevalence	WAIHA	CAIHA
MGUS	Very low	None	All
All NHL	0.23-2.6%		
CLL	4.3%-9%	90%	10%
SMZL	10%	2/3	1/3
LPL	3%-5%	None	Most
Angioimmunoblastic T-cell lymphoma	13%	One-third	Two-thirds
Hodgkin disease	0.19%-1.7%	All	None
Ovarian teratoma	Very low	All	None
Solid tumors	Very low	Two-thirds	One-third

CLL, Chronic lymphocytic leukemia; *LPL,* lymphoplasmacytic lymphoma; *MGUS,* monoclonal gammopathy with unknown significance; *NHL,* non-Hodgkin lymphoma; *SMZL,* splenic marginal zone lymphoma.

Autoimmune Hemolytic Anemia As a Risk Factor for Lymphoproliferative Disorder

In various population-based studies, AIHA emerged as a risk factor for subsequent development of diffuse large B-cell lymphoma, LPL, CLL, monoclonal gammopathy with unknown significance (MGUS), and multiple myeloma. Data regarding the type of AIHA and a possible influence of treatment were not available in these studies. It is uncertain whether autoimmune disorder per se is the causal factor or whether these patients had a clinically silent clonal disorder at the time of AIHA.

Autoimmune Hemolytic Anemia in Chronic Lymphocytic Leukemia

The prevalence of AIHA is highest in CLL, ranging from 4.3 to 9%. The prevalence is highest in poor-risk patients (Binet stage B or C, increased ZAP70 expression, unmutated IgVH status, and CD38 positivity) and patients who had already been treated. However, AIHA may also occur in very early stages of CLL, including B-cell monoclonal lymphocytosis. In a large group of nontreated CLL patients, the prevalence of positive DAT result (with or without anemia) was 14%.[24] Most CLL patients with AIHA are men. The vast majority of patients have (presumably) polyclonal warm antibodies, but in all studies, there is small number of cases with CAIHA (specificity anti-I), often with IgM paraproteinemia.

Autoimmune Hemolytic Anemia in Monoclonal Gammopathy With Unknown Significance and Lymphoplasmacytic Lymphoma

The clinical picture of primary chronic CAD suggests the presence of an "idiopathic" CAIHA, but in fact, most of these patients have a clonal disease with either only clonal IgM (IgM-MGUS) or LPL with IgM paraproteinemia and bone marrow infiltration (or Waldenström macroglobulinemia). Traditionally, the latter category would be classified as secondary AIHA. More than 90% of patients with "CAD" have a monoclonal IgMκ; 7% had IgG or IgA monoclonal immune globulin with λ chains. The course of CAD is usually indolent. Fewer than half of patients require transfusions, and the risk for progression to highly malignant lymphomas is small.

Autoimmune Hemolytic Anemia in Other Lymphoproliferative Diseases and Myeloma

The prevalence of AIHA is low in NHL, ranging from 0.23% to 2.6%. AIHA has been described in all histologic subtypes of NHL. Based on the prevalence of NHL, the association with AIHA is highest with SMZL, LPL, angioimmunoblastic T-cell lymphoma, and γ heavy chain disease. The antibody may be either a warm (two-thirds) or a cold (one-third) antibody. In NHL, there seems to be a relatively frequent association of AIHA with LA, C1-esterase deficiency, or essential cryoglobulinemia.

A number of predominantly WAIHAs have been described in IgG and IgA myelomas.

Autoimmune Hemolytic Anemia in Myeloid Disorders

Generally, AIHA is rare in patients with myeloid malignancies. A number of cases have been reported in myelodysplastic syndromes, particularly chronic myelomonocytic leukemia. Very few cases were described in acute myelogenous and lymphoblastic leukemia, myelofibrosis, and polycythemia.

Autoimmune Hemolytic Anemia in Solid Tumors

A special, rare, but highly interesting cause of WAIHA is ovarian dermoid cyst. These patients respond very poorly to drug therapies, but the AIHA resolves completely, and the DAT result becomes negative a few weeks after ovariectomy. The same behavior has been described in microcystic adenoma of the pancreas and dermoid cyst of the mesentery associated with AIHA.

Autoimmune hemolytic anemia is rarely but definitely associated with solid tumors. It is a very rare complication of lung, renal cell, and ovarian cancer. In some cases of renal cell cancer, AIHA resolved after curative surgery.

Infection-Related Autoimmune Hemolytic Anemia

In immune-competent patients, AIHA may occur after viral, bacterial, or parasitic infections (Table 44-3). Virus-associated AIHA occurs mostly in newborns and children; bacterial AIHA occurs more often in adults. The onset of AIHA is often shortly after signs of infection but sometimes after a latency time up to weeks. After some specific infections, patients may develop preferentially a warm or a cold antibody (sometimes with specific targets such as I, i, P, or Pr antigen), but in almost all instances beside the dominant antibody (cold or warm), there are a few cases of another antibody (see Table 44-3). Of particular interest is varicella-zoster virus– and rubella-associated CAIHA because the cold antibody is mostly directed to the Pr antigen and the AIHA is clinically severe. In *Mycoplasma*-associated AIHA, the antibody target is almost always "I". After *Mycoplasma* infection, the DAT result is positive in 50% to 60% of cases, but anemia is rare. In some specific infections, the antibody was a DL antibody, but in a large study, most DL antibodies were found after unspecific respiratory infections.[13] In many cases, the course of AIHA is short, uncomplicated, und self-limited, but some cases with a severe, even fatal, course, particularly in patients with Pr antibodies and in *Mycoplasma*-associated AIHA, have been reported. In AIHA associated with bacterial infections or in leishmaniasis, treatment of the infection seemed to be beneficial.

Autoimmune hemolytic anemia has been described in a few cases of acute hepatitis A, B, C, or E and in a number of cases of untreated chronic hepatitis C. However, in a large study, an increased prevalence of AIHA has only been found in interferon (INF)-treated hepatitis C patients.[25]

Anecdotal reports have described patients in whom WAIHA was associated with measles, *Chlamydia pneumoniae*, or miliary tuberculosis and CAIHA with adenovirus, measles, leptospiral pneumonia, *Escherichia coli* infection (all anti-I), pneumococcal pneumonia (anti-Pr), *Haemophilus influenzae*) (DL), or *Bartonella henselae* (DAT negative).

Some cases of AIHA have been described after vaccination against hepatitis B, influenza (MF59 adjuvanted), diphtheria–tetanus–pertussis, or rubella. Such associations could not be confirmed in systematic studies.

Table 44-3 Autoimmune Hemolytic Anemia After Infections

	Infection	WAIHA	CAIHA (Specificities)
Respiratory tract infections (unspecified)	–	–	+ (DL)/PCH
Viral infections (specific)	EBV	+/–	+ (anti-i)
	CMV	+	+/– (anti-i)
	Parvovirus (B19)	+ (often with PRCA)	+/– (DL)
	Varicella	+/–	+ (anti-Pr, anti-I, anti-DL)
	Rubella	–	+ (anti-Pr1) Monotypic IgM
	HIV	+	+ (anti-I, anti-i, anti-Pr)
Bacterial infections (specific)	Mycoplasma	+/–	+ (anti-I, anti-Pr)
	Brucellosis	+/–	+ (anti-I)
	Haemophilus influenzae		+ (DL)
Parasitic infections (specific)	Visceral leishmaniosis	+	–

–, not reported; +, predominant type of autoimmune hemolytic anemia; +/–, single or few cases reported; *CMV,* cytomegalovirus; *DL,* Donath-Landsteiner antibody; *EBV,* Epstein-Barr virus; *PCH,* paroxysmal cold hemoglobinuria; *PRCA,* pure red blood cell aplasia.

Drug-Induced Autoimmune Hemolytic Anemia

Historically, methyldopa, an antihypertensive drug, was the first known drug to induce AIHA. The prevalence of methyldopa induced AIHA is 1% with 10 to 20% DAT-positive patients without anemia, indicating that DAT positivity is not always followed by overt disease. Currently, INF-α and purine nucleoside analogues are the most common causes of drug-induced AIHA (Table 44-4). The diagnosis of drug-induced AIHA in a patient with AIHA after drug exposure can only be made if the *indirect* DAT result is positive and the RBC eluate contains a RBC antibody. Such tests have not been performed in all patients in whom drug-induced AIHA was claimed.

The temporal relationship between drug exposure and AIHA is complex. In some instances, AIHA may occur after long-term exposure to a drug (INF or targeted antibodies). In AIHA caused by purine analogues, AIHA occurs typically after a few cycles of therapy of CLL and is probably dose related (lower incidence and severity at reduced doses of fludarabine). Chlorambucil is said to induce AIHA, particularly after the end of treatment. This has not been found in all studies.

Interferon-induced AIHA has been described in various diseases (particularly hepatitis C and malignant diseases). It is caused by warm antibodies, occurs usually after long exposure to the drug, and disappears spontaneously after cessation of the drug within weeks. AIHA induced by purine analogues (fludarabine, cladribine) occurs mostly during or immediately after the end of drug treatment, but the onset is delayed in some cases. The antibodies are warm or mixed antibodies. This complication occurs predominantly in patients with CLL but seems to be very rare in lymphoma patients treated with these drugs. The incidence of AIHA in patients with CLL after fludarabine or cladribine monotherapy ranges from 2% to 11%. When fludarabine is combined with cyclophosphamide (and rituximab), AIHA is less frequent and probably less severe, but this may be attributable to the lower fludarabine dose in these protocols. Patients with a positive DAT result before treatment have a higher risk of purine analogue–induced AIHA. With steroids alone, about half of the patients achieve a lasting complete remission. So far no cases of AIHA have been reported after treatment of CLL with bendamustine.

An interesting and as yet unexplained phenomenon is the fact that some patients with CLL-associated AIHA may achieve remissions after fludarabine or cladribine treatment. However, it is general practice to avoid purine analogues in patients with AIHA.

Other drugs that have been associated with WAIHA (in single case reports) were INF-ß, the monoclonal anti-CD 11 antibody efalizumab, and lenalidomide.

A peculiar type of CAIHA has been described in some patients with paroxysmal nocturnal hemoglobinuria who had been treated with the anti C5 antibody ecuzulimab. These patients had an incomplete response to ecuzulimab. The RBCs of these patients accumulate C3d on their surfaces.

Table 44-4 Drug-Induced Autoimmune Hemolytic Anemia

Drug	Risk Factors	AIHA Onset	Type of AIHA	Response to Treatment	Diseases Treated
Methyldopa	Not known	Delayed	WAIHA	Resolution after withdrawal	Hypertension
INF-α	Pretherapeutic positive DAT	Delayed (8-11 mo)	WAIHA	Resolution spontaneous or after steroids	Hepatitis C Hematologic malignancies
Efazulimab	Not known	Many months	WAIHA	Resolution after withdrawal	Arthritis (rare)
Etanercept	Not known	Delayed	CAIHA	Resolution after rituximab	Rheumatoid arthritis (rare)
Fludarabine Cladribine Pentostatin	CLL Pretherapeutic positive DAT result	Early (median, 3-4 cycle) or delayed	WAIHA Mixed AIHA	Half of AIHA resolve after steroids	CLL Lymphomas* AML*
Bendamustin	CLL	No or only very low risk of AIHA			CLL Lymphomas
Chlorambucil	CLL	Delayed onset	WAIHA		CLL
Eculizumab	Patients with incomplete response	After treatment	CAIHA		PNH
Lenalidomide		During treatment	WAIHA	Resolution after withdrawal	One case treated for lymphoma

AML, Acute myeloid leukemia; *CAIHA*, cold autoimmune hemolytic anemia; *CLL*, chronic lymphocytic leukemia; *INF*, interferon; *PNH*, paroxysmal nocturnal hemoglobinuria; *WAIHA*, warm autoimmune hemolytic anemia.
*No or very low risk.

Autoimmune Hemolytic Anemia in Immune Deficiency States

Autoimmune hemolytic anemia is one of the classical complications of common variable immune deficiency (CVID). The prevalence of AIHA was 4% to 5.5% in large studies. AIHA preceded the diagnosis of CVID in more than half of the cases (median time from diagnosis of AIHA to CVID, 5.5 years). Evan syndrome is common.

Autoimmune hemolytic anemia (often combined with thrombocytopenia) occurs in 23% to 51% of patients with ALPS. The diagnosis of ALPS is made by the demonstration of a high number of circulating $TCR\alpha\beta^+$ double-negative ($CD4^-$ $CD8^-$) T lymphocytes. The basic defect of ALPS is a disturbance of apoptosis.[20]

Autoimmune hemolytic anemia is also common in deficiency of purine nucleoside phosphorylase (a T-cell deficiency with almost normal B cells). At least 15% of patients with Wiskott-Aldrich syndrome have AIHA. AIHA occurs before the age of 5 years and is associated with high serum IgM levels. These patients are candidates for allogeneic stem cell transplantation.

DIFFERENTIAL DIAGNOSIS

In patients with DAT-positive hemolytic anemia, the distinction from drug-dependent immune hemolytic anemia is important. In recipients of ABO- or D-incompatible allografts, anti-RBC antibodies are probably produced by immunocompetent memory B cells from the donor. This so-called passenger lymphocyte syndrome (PLS) is frequent in heart and lung transplantation (≤68%). A difficult problem is differential diagnosis of DAT-negative AIHA or Evans syndrome. In younger patients with isolated hemolytic anemia with or without symptoms, hereditary diseases such as hereditary spherocytosis, sickle cell anemia, and thalassemia must be considered. Family history and RBC morphology are most helpful in these cases. In patients with drug-induced hemolytic anemia, nonimmune hemolysis caused by glucose-6-phosphate-dehydrogenase deficiency should be considered. Babesiosis or other infections may cause nonimmune hemolytic anemia. In severely ill patients with hemolytic anemia and thrombocytopenia, idiopathic or cancer-related thrombotic thrombocytopenic purpura, hemolytic uremic syndrome, or disseminated intravascular coagulation should prompt a search for schistocytes in the blood smear.

Paroxysmal nocturnal hemoglobinuria is diagnosed by a deficiency of glycosylphosphatidylinositol (GPI)-anchor proteins on the cell surface caused by a mutation of the *PIG-A* gene. Type II mixed cryoglobulinemia is a condition caused by a monoclonal IgM autoantibody with anti-IgG activity with rheumatoid factor properties frequently associated with hepatitis C. The clinical picture is characterized by a systemic vasculitis syndrome but not by anemia.

TREATMENT

For man years, drugs and procedures routinely used in the treatment of AIHA were not subjected to studies that today are regarded as the gold standard for approval and recommendation. No randomized studies have ever been performed, and even the phase II studies were usually not prospective, small, and often with a heterogeneous population of patients and with a short observation time. Thus, the treatment recommendation in this chapter should be viewed critically.[8]

Goals of Treatment

As in all diseases, the goal of treatment of AIHA is the achievement of a complete clinical and laboratory sustained remission without any residual signs of the disease. Such results can be obtained not only in primary AIHA but also in a substantial number of secondary cases when the underlying disease disappears spontaneously (infection), when the causative drug is withdrawn, or after (curative) treatment (surgery or chemoimmunotherapy) of an underlying malignancy). In most patients with primary WAIHA, the expectations for success must be tempered. Therefore, a practical goal is the achievement of a good clinical response with freedom from symptoms in the absence of side effects of treatment. Remission of AIHA after treatment is often defined by laboratory values, but there is no consensus on the definition of complete (CR) or partial (PR) remission regarding hemoglobin concentration. Formally, one could define CR as absence of transfusion requirement, a normal hemoglobin value (according to the age and sex of the patient), and absence of signs of hemolysis (normal reticulocyte counts, haptoglobin, and LDH; negative DAT result). Such CR is sometimes seen in secondary AIHA. In primary AIHA, CR is often defined as hemoglobin above 11.0 g/dL without sign of hemolysis, but the DAT result may remain positive. A minimal requirement for PR is the absence of transfusion requirement and a satisfactory clinical condition (usually hemoglobin >9 g/dL). Thus, in AIHA, the treatment goals must be defined individually and tailored to the patient's needs.

Blood Transfusions

Blood transfusions may be necessary for emergency treatment of AIHA. The problem is to find well-matched RBC concentrates. In critical cases, transfusions should not be avoided or delayed because of uncertainty in matching (see box on Transfusion Therapy in Selected Patients With Severe Autoimmune Hemolytic Anemia). The decision is made on an individual basis depending on the speed of development and severity of anemia, the type and cause of hemolytic anemia (the highest acute death rates were observed in patients with fludarabine associated AIHA, IgM WAIHA, and DL antibodies), and the age and clinical condition of the patient. Because the antibody in WAIHA is directed against blood group antigens, no truly matched blood transfusions are possible, but RBCs can be safely given if alloantibodies are excluded.[3] However, some precautions have to be taken. In patients without a history of previous transfusions or pregnancy, the risk of alloantibodies is low, allowing for transfusion of only ABO- and RhD-matched RBCs. In all other patients, extended phenotyping with respect to Rh subgroups (C, c, E, e), Kell, Kidd, and S/s using monoclonal IgM antibodies should be performed for selection of compatible RBC concentrates. Warm autoadsorption or allogeneic adsorption procedures for detection of alloantibodies may be used in exceptional cases. In patients with CAIHA, transfused blood must be prewarmed using commercial warming coils. In all instances, an important precaution is a biological in vivo compatibility test, which includes rapid infusion of 20 mL of blood; 20 minutes observation; and, if there is no reaction, further transfusion at usual speed.

Treatment of Primary Warm Antibody Hemolytic Anemia

First-Line Treatment with Steroids

Newly diagnosed severe WAIHA should be treated immediately with glucocorticoids (steroids) (Fig. 44-3 and Table 44-5; see also box on Initial Steroid Therapy). Therapy starts with an initial dose of 1 mg/kg/day of prednisone orally or an equivalent dose of methylprednisone intravenously. It is recommended to continue with this dose until a hematocrit of greater than 30% or a hemoglobin level of greater than 10 g/dL is achieved. Complete or partial remission is obtained in approximately 80% of patients. Failure to achieve this goal after 3 weeks should result in a switch to second-line therapy. In responding patients, prednisone dose is gradually reduced to 20 to 30 mg/day within a few weeks. Subsequently, the dose is tapered slowly by 2.5 mg to 5 mg/day per month guided by hemoglobin and reticulocyte counts. If the patient is still in remission after 3 to 4 months at a dose of 5 mg/day, withdrawal of steroids can be attempted. The exact rate of patients remaining in CR after the end of steroid therapy is not known but is estimated to be around 20%. Most responders require maintenance steroids to keep the hemoglobin above 9 to 10g/dl\L. About 40% to 50% of patients need 15 mg/day or less prednisone (regarded as the highest tolerable dose for long-term treatment). However, 15% to 20% need higher maintenance prednisone doses.

Great concerns are osteoporosis, osteonecrosis, and bone fracture, particularly of the lumbar spine. About 30% to 50% of patients on long-term steroid treatment experience fractures. The highest loss of bone density occurs early, even at smaller steroid doses, and the risk of fracture increases by 75% during the first months of treatment.

Thus, patients on steroid therapy should receive bisphosphonates, vitamin D, and calcium from the beginning. Folic acid is also recommended. Steroid-induced diabetes is a major risk factor for treatment-related deaths from infections. Although heparin treatment is not recommended for all patients, the possibility of pulmonary embolism must be considered, particularly in patients with AIHA and LA or recurrent AIHA after splenectomy. Previous studies have also found a beneficial effect of standard heparin on AIHA.

Second-Line Treatment

Second-line treatment is considered in patients (1) refractory to initial steroids as defined earlier, (2) in need of a maintenance dose of more than 15 mg/day of prednisone (absolute indications) or (3) who need between 15 mg/day and 0.1 mg/kg/day (relative indication) (Fig. 44-4). Patients with prednisone requirement of 0.1 mg/kg/day or less are potential candidates for long-term low-dose prednisone. Patients refractory to steroid treatment should be reevaluated for underlying diseases or warm IgM antibodies.

Currently, there are two major second-line options for primary WAIHA with proven short- (and long-) term efficacy these ae splenectomy (preferentially laparoscopic) and therapy with the

Transfusion Therapy in Selected Patients With Severe Autoimmune Hemolytic Anemia

Immediate blood transfusion should not be withheld from patients with severe anemia. Small amounts of RBCs may be lifesaving in patients with acute cardiac or cerebral dysfunction caused by anemia. However, precautions have to be taken to avoid transfusion reactions. This requires close cooperation between clinicians and the blood bank. The exclusion of alloantibodies is most important. Patients with a low risk for severe reactions caused by an alloantibody are those without a history of previous transfusions or pregnancy. In high-risk patients, extended RBC phenotyping should be performed for selection of compatible RBC concentrates. In all instances, a biologic in vivo compatibility test has to be performed at the beginning of the transfusion.

Initial Steroid Therapy

Steroid therapy is initiated with oral prednisone (or intravenous methylprednisone) at a dose of 1 mg/kg/day. It is important to keep this dose up until a stable response (hemoglobin >10 g/dL or hematocrit >30%) is achieved. When response is achieved, the prednisone dose should be reduced to 20 to 30 mg/day within a few weeks. The dose is then tapered slowly by 2.5 mg to 5 mg/day per month guided by hemoglobin and reticulocyte counts. If the patient is still in remission after 3 to 4 months at a dose of 5 mg/day, withdrawal of steroids can be attempted. Most responders require maintenance steroids to maintain hemoglobin of greater than 9 to 10 g/dL. Second-line treatment is indicated if the AIHA does not respond within 3 weeks of initial treatment or if high steroid doses are needed for maintenance.

Therapeutic management should include blood glucose monitoring, prophylaxis against osteoporosis (commence early), supplementation with folic acid, and heparin treatment in selected cases.

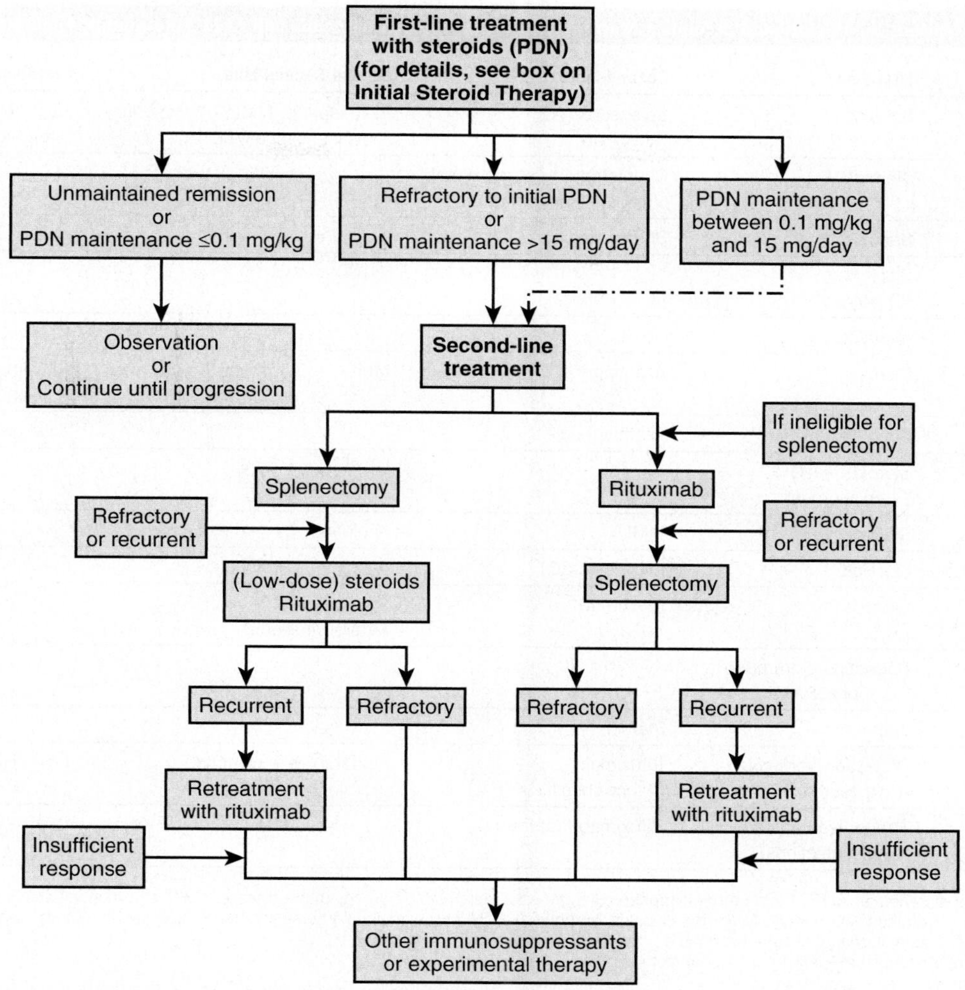

Figure 44-3 PROPOSED ALGORITHM FOR THERAPY OF WARM AUTOIMMUNE HEMOLYTIC ANEMIA. *PDN,* Prednisone. *(Modified from Lechner K, Jäger U: How I treat autoimmune haemolytic anemias in adults.* Blood *116:1831, 2010.)*

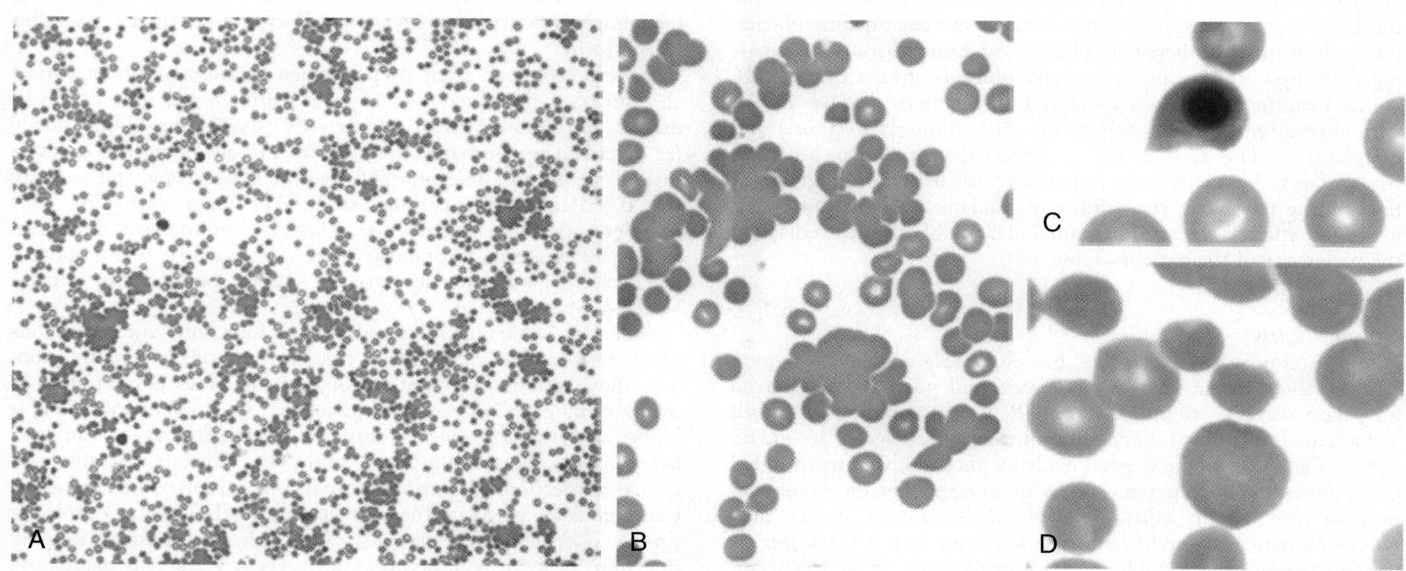

Figure 44-4 PERIPHERAL SMEAR IN COLD AGGLUTININ DISEASE. Low-power scan shows uneven distribution of red blood cells (RBCs) **(A),** which at slightly higher power **(B)** shows the RBCs to be clumped together or agglutinated. This must be distinguished from rouleaux formation. High-power scan shows nucleated RBCs **(C),** polychromatophilia, and microspherocytes **(D).**

Table 44-5 Treatment Options for Primary and Secondary Warm Autoimmune Hemolytic Anemia and Cold Autoimmune Hemolytic Anemia

Disease or Condition	First Line	Second Line	Beyond Second Line	Last Resort
Primary AIHA	Steroids	Splenectomy Rituximab	Azathioprine, MMF, cyclosporine, cyclophosphamide	High-dose cyclophos-phamide, alemtuzumab
B- and T-cell NHL	Steroids	Chemotherapy +/– rituximab (splenectomy in SMZL)		
Hodgkin's lymphoma	Steroids	Chemotherapy		
Solid tumors	Steroids Surgery			
Ovarian dermoid cyst	Ovariectomy			
SLE	Steroids	Azathioprine	MMF	Rituximab Autologous SCT
Ulcerative colitis	Steroids	Azathioprine		Total colectomy
CVID	Steroids + IgG replacement			
ALPD	Steroids	MMF	Sirolimus	
Wiskott Aldrich syndrome	Steroids	Allogeneic SCT		
Allogeneic SCT	Steroids	Rituximab*	Splenectomy T-cells infusion	
Organ transplantation	Reduction of immune suppression, steroids			
Drug induced	Withdrawal	Steroids		
Primary CAD	Protection from cold exposure	Rituximab Chlorambucil	Fludarabine + rituximab	Ecuzulimab,† bortezomid†
PCH	Supportive treatment (postinfectious)	Rituximab* (chronic)		

AIHA, Autoimmune hemolytic anemia; *ALPD,* autoimmune lymphoproliferative disorders; *CAD,* cold agglutinin disease; *CVID,* common variable immune deficiency; *IgG,* immunoglobulin G; *MMF,* mycophenolate mofetil; *NHL,* non-Hodgkin lymphoma; *PCH,* paroxysmal cold hemoglobinuria; *SCT,* stem cell transplantation; *SLE,* systemic lupus erythematosus; *SMZL,* splenic marginal zone lymphoma.
*Early second-line treatment because of known poor response to steroids.
†Off-label use in single cases.

monoclonal anti-CD20 antibody rituximab. From the scientific point of view on the basis of published data, no definite preference for one these treatments is possible because of the insufficient quality of data. For both treatments, there have been no randomized studies comparing these two options, no prospective phase II studies of the individual treatments, and not even high-quality retrospective studies with unselected consecutive patients with uniform diagnosis and pretreatment. The decision for the preferred treatment in a specific patient has to be made on an individual basis based on judgment of the treating physician, the validity of available data on short- and long-term efficacy, the assumed individual risk of adverse events, and the preference of the patient (Table 44-6).

Splenectomy

For splenectomy, there are more, but older data on the short- term efficacy, few data on long-term efficacy, and good recent data on long-term adverse events. CR or PR is achieved in two-thirds of patients (38%-82%), depending on the percentage of secondary cases. In addition, there is good evidence that a substantial number of patients will remain in remission without need of medical intervention for years. In the initial series by Chertkow and Dacie,[26] only two of 28 patients were in remission for more than 5 years, but six patients remained in a stable PR for up to 7 years. In 52 splenectomized patients (percentage of primary AIHA unknown), Coon[27] found that 63% had a hematocrit of 30% or greater without steroids after a mean follow-up of 33 months and 21% had a hematocrit of 30% or greater with a prednisone requirement of 15 mg/day or less after a mean follow up of 73 months. In a study by Allgood and Chaplin,[28] 44% of patients were in CR after more than 1 year after splenectomy.

Splenectomy can safely be performed laparoscopically in almost all patients with primary AIHA with normal-sized spleens. Withdrawal of steroids after splenectomy should be done slowly (as described for primary treatment) to prevent hemolytic crises in case of recurrence. The mortality rate of laparoscopic splenectomy was 0.5% in a large national study. The main short-term risks of splenectomy (in general) are infections, pulmonary embolism, and splenic-portal thrombosis (rare in patients with normal-sized spleen), but these risks have not studied specifically in primary WAIHA.

There is a lifelong increased risk of infections and of venous thrombosis and a very small risk of pulmonary hypertension. The most serious, often fatal, but rare infectious complication is overwhelming pneumococcal septicemia). The risk of infections is highest shortly after splenectomy and decreases after 1 year. In a Scandinavian population-based study, the adjusted relative risk of major infections (requiring hospital contact) in a matched indication comparison 1 year after splenectomy for ITP (with a probably similar risk as AIHA) was 1.4. Although fatal postsplenectomy infections seem to be less common in recent years, it is mandatory to take all measures to reduce this risk. There is good but not definite evidence that preoperative vaccination reduces the risk of severe infections. Vaccination for pneumococci, meningococci, and

Table 44-6 Second-Line Treatment Options After Steroids

Treatment	Dosing and Application	Side Effects	Precautions
Splenectomy (acute)	Preferentially laparoscopic	Infections, thrombosis	Postoperative thromboprophylaxis
Splenectomy (long term)	—	Infections Venous thrombosis	Vaccination, patient information
Rituximab	375 mg/m² on days 1,8, 15, and 22 IV	Infusional reactions Infections	Premedication with antihistamines (and steroids)
Danazol	200-400/day PO	Hepatotoxicity	None
Cyclophosphamide	PO or IV Dose adjusted to neutrophil count	Neutropenia Mutagenesis	Neutrophil count monitoring, bladder protection after high doses
Azathioprine	2.0-3.mg/kg/day PO Dose adjusted to neutrophil count	Neutropenia	Neutrophil count monitoring; avoid interaction with other drugs (e.g., allopurinol)
Mycophenolate mofetil	1-2 × 1 g/d PO	Gastrointestinal	
Cyclosporine	PO Dose adjusted to blood levels of CyA Target level, 200-400 ng/mL	Nephrotoxicity Gum hyperplasia	Monitoring of CyA levels and creatinine
Alemtuzumab	SC (variable doses)	Neutropenia	Anti-infectious prophylaxis

CyA, Cyclosporine A; *IV*, intravenous; *PO*, oral; *SC*, subcutaneous.

Haemophilus influenzae should be done before splenectomy. Pneumococcal vaccination should be repeated regularly. Long-term antibiotic prophylaxis is probably not required in adults, but patients should be informed about this risk and should take immediately antibiotics in case unexplained fever. Risk in children maybe reduced by subtotal splenectomy. The long-term risk of venous thrombosis is moderate. Information for patients about short- and long-term risks is required and may be one of the reasons for the fact that surgical treatment is underused. However, splenectomy is the only therapy so far which may provide freedom from treatment in a substantial number of patients for more than 2 years and possibly cure in about 20%.

Rituximab

Rituximab is currently the best available drug option for second-line treatment. Given at a standard induction dose of 375 mg/m² intravenously on days 1, 8, 15, and 22, it induces an overall response rate of 82% with a range 17% to 100%. Half of the remissions were reported to be CR. The rituximab schedule and dose are empirically derived from lymphoma treatment, and it is not known whether other schedules including maintenance are equal or better. There are limited data on short-term and almost no data on long-term efficacy and no data on long-term adverse effects. With regard to short-term efficacy, there seems to be no much difference between rituximab and splenectomy. However, in all rituximab studies, the patient population was heterogeneous and included primary and secondary cases, recurrences after splenectomy, and sometimes multiply pretreated patients with WAIHA or CAIHA. In only one study, almost all patients (10 of 11) had steroid-refractory primary WAIHA, but four patients received additional therapies.[29] Eight patients achieved CR and three PR, but six patients had still moderate signs of hemolysis and therefore did not formally fulfill the criteria for a complete remission. Thus, the true response rates for steroid-refractory WAIHA are still unclear. The efficacy and toxicity of rituximab monotherapy was tested in several additional retrospective studies in a mixed population of refractory primary or secondary AIHA. Response usually occurs within 3 weeks. Patients taking steroids before initiation of rituximab should continue on steroids until response to the CD20 antibody. In the D'Arena et al study,[28] at a mean follow-up of 604 days, all patients were still in CR or PR. The longest remission duration was 2884 days. Because of the small patient number, data on long-term efficacy of rituximab should be regarded with caution. Predictors of long-term response are achievement of a CR, conversion to a negative DAT result, and previous splenectomy. Retreatment with rituximab is feasible and may be necessary after 1 to 3 years. Rituximab has been given to children without apparent safety problems.

The caveats of rituximab therapy are that the drug is not licensed for the indication and that infectious complications are rare but sometimes life threatening, particularly with repeat or maintenance treatment. There is a small long-term risk of progressive multifocal leukodystrophy. Nevertheless, rituximab is the preferred option for patients who are not eligible for splenectomy. If one explains the benefits and risks of the two second-line treatments to a patient, he or she usually favors rituximab because it is a noninvasive outpatient treatment, and splenectomy remains still an option in case of failure.

Treatment of Patients with Refractory or Recurrent Disease After Splenectomy or Rituximab

In patients failing splenectomy, an accessory spleen should be excluded. Patients who are refractory to splenectomy or with recurrence after splenectomy can be retreated with steroids, assuming that the disease has become more responsive. This may work well in patients with previous requirement of lower steroid doses (<15 mg/day of prednisone). The other option is to initiate treatment with rituximab immediately.

Patients who are refractory to rituximab should undergo splenectomy, if eligible. There are no data on the influence of initial remission duration on the efficacy of retreatment. In patients relapsing late (>1 year) after rituximab, retreatment with the antibody maybe a good option.

A potentially interesting drug for second-line treatment (which has also been used as first-line treatment along with steroids) is danazol, an attenuated androgen (see Table 44-6).[14] It has established efficacy in C1 esterase deficiency, and efficacy has been claimed in several immune diseases, including WAIHA. Initial very promising results (overall response rate [ORR] 60%-70%) in AIHA could not be confirmed in subsequent studies, but it may worthwhile to do further studies because the toxicity seems to be relatively low with the exception of a potentially increased risk for hepatocellular carcinoma.

The advantage of high-dose immunoglobulins is low toxicity. Remission rates are low, and routine use in patients with AIHA is not recommended in a recent guideline.

Treatment Options Beyond Second-Line Therapy in Primary Warm Autoimmune Hemolytic Anemia

Given the nature of the disease, the use of immunosuppressive treatment of all kinds seems logical. Response rates of up to 60% have been reported, but data are frequently based on low patient numbers or anecdotal reports. Cyclophosphamide was very effective in two studies. Other published data of treatment with azathioprine or cyclophosphamide are less favorable with only about one-third of patients having any response. Evaluation is even more complicated by the fact that patients frequently received concomitant treatment with steroids. Dosing of azathioprine is difficult because of the narrow therapeutic window, hypersensitivity because of genetic defects, and interaction with other drugs. Cyclophosphamide may have long-term mutagenic effects. Other immunosuppressive drugs such as cyclosporine or mycophenolate mofetil (MMF) have shown high response rates in very small series.

Repeated cycles of high-dose cyclophosphamide (50 mg/kg/day for 4 days) remain an option in selected, highly refractory patients. In a pilot study, six of nine patients received a CR with a median duration of 15 months or more. Alemtuzumab has also been effective at a dose of 10 mg/day for 10 days. Promising results were recently published for a combination of low-dose rituximab (100 mg on days 1, 8, 15, and 22) with alemtuzumab (10 mg on days 1-3). The results of autologous stem cell transplantation were disappointing, but allogeneic transplantation may be used as treatment of last resort in patients with Evans syndrome.

In general, second-line treatment should be selected taking into account severity of AIHA, age, comorbidity, and patient preference. Because of the low curative potential of all treatment options, patient safety remains the major concern.

Treatment of Secondary Warm Autoimmune Hemolytic Anemia

In secondary AIHA, the treatment goal depends on the type and severity of the underlying disease. The treatment goal may vary from palliative treatment of AIHA to cure by eradication of the underlying disease. Preferred treatment options are listed in Table 44-6.

Warm Autoimmune Hemolytic Anemia Associated With Systemic Lupus Erythematosus

Steroids used similar as in primary WAIHA induce high response rates. Maintenance treatment with azathioprine, cyclophosphamide, or both may be required. Rituximab is effective against WAIHA and SLE but may be associated with a higher risk of progressive multifocal leukoencephalopathy in this setting.

Warm Autoimmune Hemolytic Anemia Associated With Chronic Lymphocytic Leukemia

In previously untreated CLL with isolated DAT-positive anemia but no other treatment indication, treatment with prednisone as in primary WAIHA is the first choice. In case of refractoriness or relapse, rituximab monotherapy is moderately effective but produces response rates of more than 80% in combination with cyclophosphamide and dexamethasone. Cyclosporine also has good activity. In refractory AIHA or in AIHA with advanced or progressive CLL, treatment of the underlying disease with a rituximab-containing regimen according to International Workshop on Chronic Lymphocytic Leukemia guidelines is recommended.[30] In elderly or comorbid patients with active CLL, chlorambucil with prednisone with or without rituximab is a good choice. In general, fludarabine-containing regimens should be used with caution in the presence of a positive DAT result or overt AIHA. In this case, bendamustine with (or without) rituximab is a good alternative. Alemtuzumab has proven activity against CLL and AIHA and is a good second-line option, particularly in patients with associated pure RBC aplasia.

Warm Autoimmune Hemolytic Anemia in Other Non-Hodgkin Lymphomas

AIHA in NHLs does not respond well to steroids in general and splenectomy is only effective in splenic marginal zone lymphomas. Sustained responses in most other lymphoma subtypes have been obtained with lymphoma-specific treatment with or without rituximab.

Drug-Related Warm Autoimmune Hemolytic Anemia

Cessation of the drug may be effective in many cases, and further use of the drug should be avoided. Fludarabine-induced AIHA may be life threatening but responds to steroid therapy.

Treatment of Warm Autoimmune Hemolytic Anemia in Congenital and Acquired Immune Deficiency States and Special Serologic Types

The treatment of WAIHA in patients with CVID is very similar to that of those with primary WAHA. Additional regular prophylactic treatment with IgG concentrates reduces the risk of recurrence. Splenectomy is effective, but the risk of serious infections is high.

In ALPS, treatment should be started with steroids and then switched to MMF, but sirolimus has the highest efficacy improving not only AIHA but also lymphadenopathy. AIHA associated with IgM hypergammaglobulinemia in Wiskott-Aldrich syndrome is an indication for allogeneic stem cell transplantation.

Patients with AIHA after allogeneic stem cell transplantation respond poorly to steroids but often do respond to rituximab. An early switch to rituximab may be reasonable in these patients. AIHA in drug-related severely immunesuppressed patients after transplantation of solid organs responds best to reduction of immune suppression. Patients with IgM WAIHA respond poorly to steroids. These patients are candidates for early rituximab treatment. The same is true for chronic AIHA caused by DL antibodies.

Treatment of Cold Autoimmune Hemolytic Anemia

Primary Chronic Cold Agglutinin Disease

Primary CAD is defined as a CAIHA in patients with IgM MGUS or in lymphoma without overt clinical signs but with bone marrow infiltration. All patients should be advised to avoid cold exposure. Drug treatment is required in only half of the patients. Treatment is initiated in symptomatic patients or when hemoglobin levels drop below 9 to 10 g/dL. Because IgM-coated RBCs are mainly destroyed in the liver, CAIHA does not respond to splenectomy and poorly to steroids. The most effective and best evaluated treatment is rituximab in a standard lymphoma dose. Two studies have provided similar results. In a prospective phase II study, 20 of 27 patients responded, but most responses ($n = 19$) were partial. The median response duration was 11 months, but most patients responded to retreatment with rituximab. A combination of rituximab and oral fludarabine induced higher overall response rates (76%) with a longer duration (median, 66 months).[31] Remarkable responses have recently been obtained with the terminal complement inhibitor ecuzulimab and the proteasome inhibitor bortezomib in single rituximab-refractory patients. Preparation of patients with high-titer cold antibodies for surgery by cryofiltration may be required in rare instances.

Secondary Cold Autoimmune Hemolytic Anemia

In CAIHA associated with lymphomas or solid tumors, treatment of the underlying disease by chemo(immuno)therapy or curative resection results in good responses. Cases of infection related CAIHA usually resolve spontaneously, but antibiotic therapy may accelerate the process.

FUTURE DIRECTIONS

Future research should mainly be directed toward generation of better treatment options. The generation of international guidelines is still hampered by the lack of evidence from randomized trials. Every effort should be made to initiate valid comparisons of major treatment options such as steroids, splenectomy, and rituximab, potentially through registries or randomized trials.

Novel therapeutic options may be provided by next-generation anti-CD20 antibodies or antibodies against other targets such as complement factors. Insights into the way T cells drive and control the immune reaction could lead to novels immunotherapeutic approaches. Synthetic peptides modulating Th1 responses via regulatory T cells may be developed into therapeutic tools. Another option would be to target structures on macrophages responsible for RBC destruction (e.g., the CD47–SIRP-α interaction). There is hope that novel targeted therapies will replace splenectomy and even steroid treatment of patients with AIHA.

REFERENCES

1. Dacie SJ: The immune haemolytic anaemias: A century of exciting progress in understanding. *Br J Haematol* 114:770, 2001.
2. Packman CH: Hemolytic anemia due to warm autoantibodies. *Blood Rev* 22:17, 2008.
3. Garratty G: Immune hemolytic anemia-a primer. *Semin Hematol* 42:119, 2005.
4. Petz LD: Immune hemolysis associated with transplantation. *Semin Hematol* 42:145, 2005.
5. Pirofsky B: Clinical aspects of autoimmune hemolytic anemia. *Semin Hematol* 13:251, 1976.
6. Berentsen S, Ulvestad E, Langholm R, et al: Primary chronic cold agglutinin disease: A population based clinical study of 86 patients. *Haematologica* 91:460, 2006.
7. King KE, Ness PM: Treatment of autoimmune hemolytic anemia. *Semin Hematol* 42:131, 2005.
8. Lechner K, Jäger U: How I treat autoimmune haemolytic anemias in adults. *Blood* 116:1831, 2010.
9. Aladjidi N, Leverger G, Leblanc T, et al: New insights into childhood autoimmune hemolytic anemia: A French national observational study of 265 children. *Haematologica* 96:655, 2011.
10. Michel M, Chanet V, Dechartres A, et al: The spectrum of Evans syndrome in adults: New insight into the disease based on the analysis of 68 cases. *Blood* 114:3167, 2009.
11. Garratty G: The James Blundell Award Lecture 2007: Do we really understand immune red cell destruction? *Transfusion Med* 18:321, 2008.
12. Arndt PA, Leger RM, Garratty G: Serologic findings in autoimmune hemolytic anemia associated with immunoglobulin M warm autoantibodies. *Transfusion* 49:2352, 2009.
13. Sokol RJ, Booker DJ, Stamps R, et al: Autoimmune hemolytic anemia caused by warm-reacting IgM-class antibodies. *Immunohematol* 14:53, 1998.
14. Barros MM, Blajchman MA, Bordin JO: Warm autoimmune haemolytic anemia: Recent progress in understanding the immunobiology and the treatment. *Transfus Med Rev* 24:195, 2010.
15. Silberstein LE, Litwin S, Carmack CE: Relationship of variable region genes expressed by a human B cell lymphoma secreting pathologic anti-Pr2 erythrocyte autoantibodies. *J Exp Med* 169:1631, 1989.
16. Michaux L, Dierlamm J, Wlodarska L, et al: Trisomy 3q11-q29 is recurrently observed in B-cell non-Hodgkin's lymphomas associated with cold agglutinin syndrome. *Ann Hematol* 76:201, 1998.
17. Ramagopalan SV, Wotton CJ, Handel AE, et al: Risk of venous thromboembolism in people admitted to hospital with selected immune-mediated diseases: Record-linkage study. *BMC Med* 9:1, 2011.
18. Garratty G: Immune hemolytic anemia associated with negative routine serology. *Semin Hematol* 42:156, 2005.
19. Mayer B, Yürek S, Kiesewetter H, Salama A: Mixed-type autoimmune hemolytic anemia: Differential diagnosis and a critical review of reported cases. *Transfusion*, 48:2229, 2008.
20. Teachey DT, Seif AE, Grupps SA: Advances in the management and understanding of autoimmune lymphoproliferative syndrome (ALPS). *Br J Haematol.* 148:205, 2010.
21. Kokori SI, Ioannidis JP, Voulgarelis M, et al: Autoimmune hemolytic anemia in patients with systemic lupus erythematosus. *Am J Med* 108:198, 2000.
22. Gómez-Puerta JA, Martín H, Amigo MC, et al: Long-term follow-up in 128 patients with primary antiphospholipid syndrome: Do they develop lupus? *Medicine (Baltimore)* 84:225, 2005.
23. Sanz J, Arriaga F, Montesinos P, et al: Autoimmune haemolytic anemia following allogeneic hematopoietic stem cell transplantation in adult patients. *Bone Marrow Transplant* 39:555, 2007.
24. Dearden C, Wade R, Else M, et al: The prognostic significance of a positive direct antiglobulin test in chronic lymphocytic leukemia: A beneficial effect of the combination of fludarabine and cyclophosphamide on the incidence of hemolytic anemia. *Blood* 111:1820, 2007.
25. Chao TC, Chen CY, Yang YH, et al: Chronic hepatitis C virus infection associated with primary warm-type autoimmune hemolytic anemia. *J Clin Gastroenterol* 33:232, 2001.
26. Chertkow G, Dacie JV: Results of splenectomy in auto-immune haemolytic anaemia. *Br J Haematol* 2:237, 1956.
27. Coon WW: Splenectomy in the treatment of hemolytic anemia. *Arch Surg* 120:625, 1985.
28. Allgood JW, Chaplin H Jr: Idiopathic acquired autoimmune hemolytic anemia. A review of forty-seven cases treated from 1955 through 1965. *Am J Med* 43:254, 1967.
29. D'Arena G, Laurenti L, Capalbo S, et al: Rituximab therapy for chronic lymphocytic leukemia-associated autoimmune hemolytic anemia. *Am J Hematol* 81:598, 2006.
30. Hallek M, Cheson BD, Catovsky D, et al: Guidelines for the diagnosis and treatment of chronic lymphocytic leukemia: A report from the International Workshop on Chronic Lymphocytic Leukemia updating the National Cancer Institute-Working Group 1996 guidelines. *Blood* 111:5446, 2008.
31. Berentsen S, Randen U, Vågan AM, et al: High response rate and durable remissions following fludarabine and rituximab combination therapy for chronic cold agglutinin disease. *Blood* 2010:3180, 2010.

CHAPTER 45

EXTRINSIC NONIMMUNE HEMOLYTIC ANEMIAS

Elizabeth A. Price and Stanley S. Schrier

By definition, extrinsic causes of hemolysis are abnormalities in the environment in which the red blood cells (RBCs), usually normal themselves, circulate. These abnormalities can be acute or chronic in nature. They can arise from congenital lesions but usually result from acquired lesions. Inherited anomalies of glucose-6-phosphate dehydrogenase (G6PD) deficiency, which reduces the RBCs' ability to deal with oxidative insults, can leave RBCs more vulnerable to environmental insults. Determination of hemolysis with various levels of compensation as the cause of an anemia is accomplished using the approaches described in Chapter 32. Signs of extrinsic hemolysis with minimal or no anemia can be valuable clues to diseases of other organ systems. Among the most important forms of extrinsic hemolytic anemia are those caused by immune mechanisms; these are discussed in Chapter 44.

Clinical and morphologic findings suggest the many misfortunes that can befall RBCs in their travels. They can be trapped in an abnormal bone marrow stroma network, sheared by jets in an abnormal heart, cut and fragmented by fibrin strands stretched across damaged areas in the microvasculature, or attacked by parasites. They can undergo stasis and perhaps metabolic depletion in giant hemangiomas or in an enlarged spleen. An abnormally functioning liver or kidney can cause a buildup of substances in plasma that alter RBC shape and metabolism. Drugs can cause oxidation or other metabolic damage. Oxidant injury provokes degradation of hemoglobin with the formation of hemichromes (see Drug-Induced Oxidative Hemolysis later). Degraded hemoglobin and hemichromes bind avidly to the cytoplasmic tail of the major transmembrane protein band 3 (see Chapter 43) and cause clustering of band 3 oligomers. Immunoglobulins and complement then bind to the external membrane face over clusters of band 3, promoting immune destruction. Other membrane proteins may be subject to oxidative attack. Toxins, venoms, heat, and mechanical trauma can directly destroy the membrane. These agents may cause an alteration in the asymmetry of the phospholipid bilayer, causing phosphatidylserine to move from the inner leaflet of the membrane bilayer to the outer leaflet, where it can be recognized by macrophages.

In general, only the most devastating damage leads to direct intravascular destruction. Usually, the initial insult leads to an eventual change in the external portion of the RBC membrane, which causes macrophages to retard, hold, remove, or otherwise modify RBCs. Infection or inflammation can activate these macrophages. Some RBC changes are accompanied by a decrease in RBC deformability, which retards flow and thereby facilitates the action of macrophages on the affected RBC. All of these changes lead to extravascular hemolysis.

FRAGMENTATION HEMOLYSIS: MICROANGIOPATHY

Clinical Manifestations

Patients present with various degrees of hemolytic anemia and compensation, with evidence of RBC fragmentation on smear (Fig. 45-1; see box on Differential Diagnosis of Extrinsic Nonimmune Hemolytic Anemias). RBC removal is generally extravascular, with minimal or moderately decreased levels of haptoglobin. If RBC damage is sufficiently severe, signs of intravascular hemolysis may be present. Because of the underlying pathology, some of these syndromes show evidence of platelet removal, leading to thrombocytopenia. Occasionally, the underlying cause produces activation and depletion of procoagulant factors with consequent activation of the fibrinolytic system, consistent with disseminated intravascular coagulation (DIC) (see box on Causes of Red Blood Cell Fragmentation Hemolysis).

Pathophysiology

Fragmentation hemolysis occurs when mechanical forces disrupt the physical integrity of the RBC membrane. In vitro shear stresses in excess of 3000 dynes/cm^2 cause RBC fragmentation. In vivo studies in patients with mitral prosthetic regurgitation and hemolysis show high peak shear stresses of 4500 dynes/cm^2, very rapid acceleration or deceleration, or both.

Research suggests alternative mechanisms of producing microangiopathic hemolysis that involve platelets and small vessel thrombi. The platelet-rich, fibrin-poor microvascular thrombi found in many patients with thrombotic thrombocytopenic purpura (TTP) now are thought to be caused by abnormally decreased ADAMTS-13 activity.[1] This metalloprotease is responsible for converting the highly thrombogenic ultra large multimers of von Willebrand factor made by platelets and endothelial cells into the smaller forms normally found in circulation. Mutations in or antibodies against ADAMTS-13 result in unusually large multimers of von Willebrand factor attached to endothelial cell surfaces, where platelets may excessively aggregate, leading to formation of microvascular thrombi even in the absence of endothelial damage. In the case of disseminated cancer, the cause of microangiopathy may be microvascular tumor emboli.

Whatever the mechanism of mechanical trauma, the RBC membrane is viscoelastic and has self-sealing properties (see Chapter 43) so that little hemoglobin leaks out as the cell is being cut. However, prolonged distortion of the membrane produces a plastic change; therefore, the smaller RBC fragments usually do not become microspheres or microdisks but continue to display evidence of the shearing

Differential Diagnosis of Extrinsic Nonimmune Hemolytic Anemias

There is no simple approach to the differential diagnosis of hemolysis caused by extrinsic nonimmune hemolytic anemia. The physician must pay close attention to the clinical finding. Useful clues come from a determination of whether RBC breakdown is predominantly extravascular or intravascular, but most important in the analysis is the observation of RBC morphology, which can focus the differential diagnosis. Unhelpful terms such as *aniso* and *poik* should be discarded. RBCs are spherocytic, stomatocytic, fragmented, echinocytic, acanthocytic, spurred, or bite cells or can be mixtures of these types.

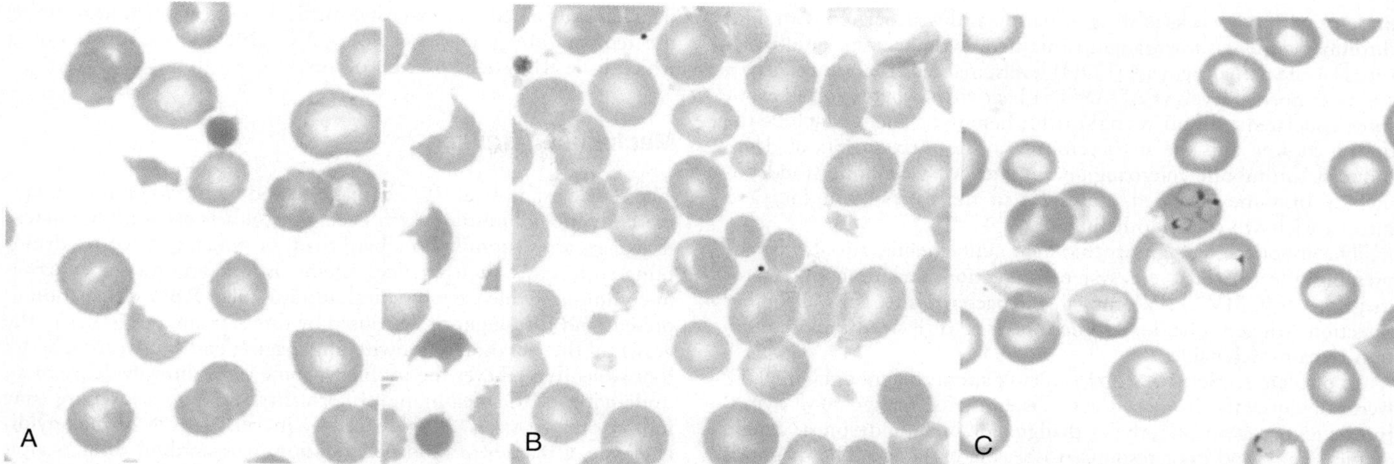

Figure 45-1 PERIPHERAL BLOOD SMEARS FROM EXAMPLES OF EXTRINSIC NONIMMUNE HEMOLYTIC ANEMIA. **A**, Microangiopathic hemolytic anemia. Note the schistocytes, fragmented cells, spherocyte, and polychromasia. More examples of damaged red blood cells (RBCs), including classic "helmet cell" *(top)*, are seen to the immediate *right insert*. **B**, Thermal injury from a burn. Thermally damaged RBCs form numerous microspherocytes and tiny RBC fragments. **C**, Malaria infestation. RBCs containing *Plasmodium falciparum* malaria. Note the high rate of infestation, the presence of only ringed forms, and the multiply infested RBC *(center)*.

Causes of Red Blood Cell Fragmentation Hemolysis

- Damaged microvasculature
- Thrombotic thrombocytopenic purpura–hemolytic uremic syndrome (TTP–HUS)
- Associated with pregnancy: preeclampsia or eclampsia; hemolysis plus elevated liver enzymes plus low platelets (HELLP syndrome)
- Associated with malignancy, with or without mitomycin C treatment
- Vasculitis: polyarteritis, Wegener granulomatosis, acute glomerulonephritis, or *Rickettsia*-like infections
- Systemic lupus erythematosus
- Abnormalities of renal vasculature: malignant hypertension, acute glomerulonephritis, scleroderma, or allograft rejection with or without cyclosporine treatment
- Disseminated intravascular coagulation
- Malignant hypertension
- Catastrophic antiphospholipid antibody syndrome
- Atrioventricular malformations
- Kasabach-Merritt syndrome
- Hemangioendotheliomas
- Atrioventricular shunts for congenital and acquired conditions (e.g., stents, coils, transjugular intrahepatic portosystemic shunt, Levine shunts)
- Cardiac abnormalities
  - Replaced valve, prosthesis, graft, or patch
  - Aortic stenosis or regurgitant jets (e.g., in ruptured sinus of Valsalva)
- Drugs: cyclosporine, mitomycin, ticlopidine, clopidogrel, tacrolimus, or cocaine
- Systemic infection: bacterial endocarditis, brucellosis, cytomegalovirus, HIV, ehrlichiosis, Rocky Mountain spotted fever

event or distortion in the form of typical irregular shapes. These irregular shapes and the rigidity that they reflect subsequently interfere with the ability of RBCs to fold, elongate, and deform sufficiently to pass through 3-µm capillaries and even smaller slits in the walls of the sinusoids of the reticuloendothelial system. This sequence leads to their destruction.

Differential Diagnosis

Generally, the differential diagnosis of fragmentation hemolysis can be deduced from the clinical findings. The presence of a prosthetic heart valve or a regurgitant jet that fragments or accelerates (i.e., Waring blender syndrome) can be readily discerned. The clinical picture of thrombotic thrombocytopenic purpura–hemolytic uremic syndrome (TTP–HUS) is generally dramatic and acute (see Chapter 136). Atrioventricular malformations may be associated with DIC and platelet removal; the diagnosis requires a high index of suspicion and imaging studies. The presence of preeclampsia in a pregnant woman with microangiopathic hemolysis usually is obvious, but the HELLP (hemolysis, elevated liver enzymes, and low platelet count) syndrome is a serious complication of pregnancy that can occur without other signs of preeclampsia or hypertension. This syndrome can produce hepatic rupture, visual failure, DIC, seizures, and congestive heart failure and requires treatment by prompt delivery of the fetus. Cancer can be an underlying cause of microangiopathy. Vessels supplying malignant tumors are thought to be structurally abnormal. They exhibit the same sort of fibrin stranding that produces fragmentation hemolysis in DIC and TTP–HUS.

Continued use of invasive diagnostic and therapeutic procedures with insertion of foreign bodies into the circulation has been complicated by microangiopathic hemolysis. A transjugular intrahepatic portosystemic shunt can cause the syndrome in approximately 10% of patients. The hemolysis usually disappears after 12 to 15 weeks. Similarly, use of coil embolization to seal off a patent ductus arteriosus may also cause significant hemolytic anemia. Vasculitis has also been implicated as a cause.

Multiple drugs are associated with microangiopathic hemolysis, most commonly quinine.[2] Cyclosporine, tacrolimus, and mitomycin C have been implicated as causing an HUS picture that typically develops within weeks to months of exposure. Total body irradiation and bone marrow transplantation also are associated with microangiopathic hemolysis. Both chemotherapeutic agents and targeted cancer agents, including immunotoxins, monoclonal antibodies, and tyrosine kinase inhibitors, are associated with thrombotic microangiopathy.[3] The thienopyridines ticlodipine and clopidogrel are both capable of producing a significant thrombotic microangiopathy that differs somewhat in presentation. Ticlodipine-associated TTP typically occurs between 2 and 12 weeks after initiation of therapy and presents with severe thrombocytopenia, microangiopathic hemolytic anemia, highly elevated lactate dehydrogenase, and normal renal function and is associated with severe deficiency of plasma ADAMTS13 activity.[4] In contrast, clopidogrel-associated TTP usually presents within 2 weeks of drug initiation and is associated with mild thrombocytopenia, microangiopathic hemolytic anemia, mildly elevated lactate dehydrogenase (LDH) levels, marked renal insufficiency, and near-normal levels of ADAMTS13 activity. Other reported exposures associated with microangiopathic hemolytic anemia include the use of cocaine and the herb echinacea, The mechanisms of drug-induced thrombotic microangiopathy are not well understood but include immune-mediated causes (as in the case of quinine) and direct toxicity to the endothelium.[5]

Thrombotic microagniopathic hemolytic anemia can also be the presenting feature of severe, systemic infection, including viral (cytomegalovirus [CMV], HIV), fungal, and bacterial infections.[6] Whether infection "triggers" the development of TTP or instead the presentation remains debatable.

In one large series, 10 of 351 (2.8%) patients diagnosed with TTP were subsequently diagnosed with disseminated malignancy.[7] Symptoms suggesting an underlying malignancy include dyspnea, cough, atypical pain, and poor response to plasma exchange. The diagnosis was made by bone marrow biopsy in six of the 10 patients, and all patients died shortly after the diagnosis of malignancy was made.

Therapy

Management is primarily directed toward the underlying disease or event. Compensation of RBC production should be optimized by replacing iron or folic acid if the patient is deficient in these nutrients. Occasionally, removal or repair of a damaged native or prosthetic heart valve is necessary when the hemolysis produces a disabling transfusion requirement. Treatment of TTP with plasma exchange has been found to be superior to plasma infusions, with fresh-frozen plasma and cryo-free plasma appearing to have equal efficacy. Thrombotic microangiopathy associated with cyclosporine often is reversible with cessation of cyclosporine.

OTHER FORMS OF MECHANICAL DAMAGE TO RED BLOOD CELLS

Heat Denaturation

Normal RBCs undergo budding and fragmentation when exposed to a temperature of 49°C (120°F) in vitro (Fig. 45-1, *B*). In some of the hereditary hemolytic anemias, this process occurs at temperatures as low as 46°C (115°F) (see Chapter 43). Under some clinical circumstances, temperatures sufficient to cause heat denaturation of RBCs have been generated. Occasionally, cell warmers used with transfusions in cold agglutinin disease have malfunctioned and cooked the RBCs about to be transfused. In one case, a patient's mother warmed the RBCs with a hot water bottle, reasoning that such cells would cause less vein irritation to her child. Such transfusion was followed by evidence of intravascular and extravascular hemolysis, and the peripheral smear showed RBC budding and fragmentation (Fig. 45-2). Presumably, similar events can lead to hemolysis in patients who have sustained very extensive burns. In patients with heat stroke, the temperature usually is below 42°C (108°F), a temperature at which little RBC denaturation occurs.

Mechanical Trauma

The classic example of RBC damage caused by mechanical trauma is march hemoglobinuria, which occurs in soldiers after a long march, in joggers after running on a hard road, or in karate or conga drumming enthusiasts after practice. Anemia is rare, and reticulocytosis is uncommon. Evidence of typical intravascular RBC destruction is present and is thought to be caused by direct trauma to RBCs in the vessels of the feet or hands. Switching jogging paths or wearing better footwear often relieves the problem. Some cases show evidence of an underlying RBC membrane abnormality. Strenuous exercise may induce oxidant stress, as evidenced by increased levels of malonyldialdehyde, a marker of lipid peroxidation, in marathon runners after a race. Occasionally, malfunction of the cell savers used during abdominal or thoracic surgery mechanically injures RBCs.

Cardiopulmonary Bypass

Postperfusion syndrome occurs in some patients after cardiopulmonary bypass. The syndrome includes acute intravascular hemolysis and leukopenia as part of a febrile, inflammatory clinical picture. Affected patients may develop pulmonary distress and even adult or acute respiratory distress syndrome. Visible hemoglobinemia occurs, with rising plasma hemoglobin levels, and is associated with an increase in lysed RBC ghosts seen in the whole blood and plasma. These ghosts are coated with the complement complex C5bC9 (see Chapter 22). Presumably, the complement pathway is activated as the blood passes through the oxygenator. The reason why complement activation results in lytic attack on RBCs (and granulocytes) is unknown. Free hemoglobin released into the plasma secondary to intravascular hemolysis may contribute to acute kidney injury after cardiopulmonary bypass.[8] Treatment involves knowledge of the process and requisite support until the situation corrects itself.

Osmotic Attack

Abrupt changes in osmolality can cause hemolysis. Freshwater drowning may be associated with so much water in the lungs that the RBCs swell as they undergo an in vivo osmotic fragility test in the pulmonary vasculature. Conversely, saltwater drowning can cause profound dehydration of RBCs, producing a situation analogous to xerocytosis (see Chapter 43). Rarely, acute hemolysis occurs from mistaken infusion of or exposure to concentrated hypertonic solutions such as those used in hemodialysis. To manage such an event, the physician must recognize its cause, appreciate the shrunken RBCs on a peripheral smear, and restore isotonicity as quickly as possible. In these cases, use of a hemodialysis device, if available, may be helpful.

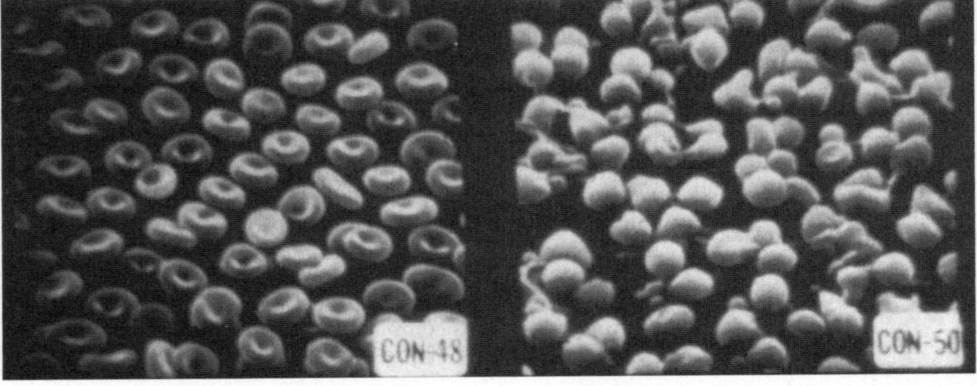

Figure 45-2 MORPHOLOGIC CHANGES ARE PRODUCED BY HEATING NORMAL RED BLOOD CELLS AT THE INDICATED TEMPERATURES. Budding begins abruptly at 50°C (122°F) and eventually leads to spherocytosis.

Hypersplenism

In all organs of the monocyte–macrophage system (i.e., reticuloendothelial system), blood cells leaving the arterial bed are generally unloaded into channels such that the RBCs must pass through the wall of the sinus to reenter the circulation. The sinusoidal wall has slits 2 to 3 μm long and usually is endothelialized on one side and has a macrophagic lining on the other side. The normal human adult RBC is a discocyte with a surface area 40% larger than a sphere of that volume (see Chapter 31). This excess surface area allows an RBC with a diameter of approximately 8 μm to twist, elongate, and deform sufficiently to squeeze through these 2- to 3-μm slits. The excess surface area, occasionally referred to as the ratio of surface area to volume (SA:V), is critical and normally is approximately 1.4. Any condition that reduces SA:V reduces the ability of RBCs to traverse these sinusoidal slits because plump spheres cannot deform sufficiently.

Factors that interfere with interaction of the cytosol and the membrane also impair the ability of the RBC to deform. Oxidant attack may produce Heinz bodies that come to lie adjacent to the membrane. They interfere with the smooth movement of the membrane over the cytosol, a process called *tank treading*. Such cells are selectively blocked from leaving the splenic cords and entering the sinuses. Inflammation or infection may enhance the ability of splenic macrophages to attack and ingest RBCs. Although not strictly a mechanism of hypersplenism, Kupffer cell erythrophagocytosis is a prominent finding in patients undergoing graft-versus-host hemolysis seen after liver transplantation.

The spleen is more complicated than other reticuloendothelial organs in that the afferent arterioles pass through lymphoid nodules (i.e., white pulp) and then terminate in the cords of Billroth (i.e., red pulp), into which blood cells are discharged. In the slow flow of the cords of Billroth, blood cells are selectively attacked by macrophages and are in direct contact with several classes of lymphocytes. The blood cells then must pass through the cordal walls before they can approach the sinus wall, which they must pass through to reenter the circulation. The spleen provides a double filter, and the blood cells must be remarkably deformable to pass through it. This slow passage permits highly selective action by macrophages, which have receptors that can detect several sorts of alterations in these blood cells. These receptors include the Fc receptor for the appropriate portion of the immunoglobulin molecule, receptors for complement components such as C3b, and perhaps receptors that detect alterations in the outer portion of the phospholipid bilayer or in the externally oriented glycopeptides. The macrophage then holds, retards, modifies (i.e., pitting function), or removes (i.e., culling function) the blood cells identified. Normally, the pitting function of the spleen allows it to remove Howell-Jolly bodies and normally occurring endocytic vacuoles (called *pocks* because of their appearance on phase interference or Nomarski microscopy). The normal culling function of the spleen is exemplified by its removal of senescent RBCS.

All the activities of the spleen presumably are markedly accentuated in a large spleen, and if the increased activity is sufficiently extensive, hypersplenism ensues. The size of the spleen, not the portal pressure, is important in determining the degree of RBC sequestration. Other factors that may play a role are the state of activation of the splenic macrophages and the size of the small slits between the splenic cords and sinuses. The macrophages and slits seem to be under a degree of control, as evidenced by variations in splenic removal of RBCs in patients with malaria.

The clinical picture of hypersplenic hemolysis is dominated by the specific cause of the splenomegaly. Although the causes of splenomegaly are legion, there are several general mechanisms (Table 45-1). Usually some degree of anemia is seen, with evidence of a compensatory increase in RBC production. Because stasis and trapping in the spleen are associated with macrophagic attack and remodeling of the RBC surface, the reduction in SA:V leads to spherocytosis. If the RBCs undergo a prolonged period of distortion when traversing the cordal–sinus barrier, tailed RBCs will be present as the RBC membranes undergo a plastic change (see Chapter 43). Because the enlarged spleen can trap and remove platelets and white blood cells, variable thrombocytopenia and leukopenia may occur. The bone marrow may show normal to increased cellularity with erythroid hyperplasia.

Table 45-1 Causes of Splenomegaly

Cause	Example
Neoplasia	Lymphoma, hairy cell leukemia
Infection	Bacterial endocarditis, malaria, schistosomiasis, tuberculosis
Portal bed obstruction	Alcoholic cirrhosis, splenic vein thrombosis
Collagen vascular disease	Systemic lupus erythematosus, malignant phase of rheumatoid arthritis
Chronic inflammatory disease	Rheumatoid arthritis
Chronic hereditary or acquired hemolytic anemia	Severe β-thalassemia, autoimmune hemolytic anemia
Lipoidosis	Gaucher disease
Amyloidosis	AL and AA types
Tropical splenomegaly syndrome	Hyperreactive malarial splenomegaly syndrome

Management depends on the cause of splenic enlargement. The anemia or pancytopenia usually is not profound; however, splenectomy may be contemplated if the anemia is severe. In most situations, recognition of the possibility of hypersplenism is most important in guiding the approach to diagnosis of an unexplained anemia. Massive splenomegaly frequently is associated with expansion of the plasma compartment, and measurement of hemoglobin, hematocrit, or RBC levels may give a falsely low value of the RBC mass present. In that circumstance, the true RBC mass can be determined by ^{51}Cr assay.

A good example of massive splenomegaly causing plasma volume expansion is tropical splenomegaly syndrome, also known as *hyperreactive malarial splenomegaly syndrome*. Diagnostic criteria include massive splenomegaly more than 10 cm below the costal margin with no other cause identified; immunity to malaria; elevated serum immunoglobulin M (IgM) levels; and clinical response to treatment with antimalarial drugs such as chloroquine, proguanil, or pyrimethamine and folic acid. The pathophysiology of the splenomegaly seems to be poorly controlled B-lymphocytic production of antibodies, and IgM stimulation may be a response to malarial antigens or an unidentified mitogen. Malarial parasites are almost never found. The apparent anemia is in large part caused by plasma volume expansion, although RBC survival is reported to be slightly attenuated. Antimalarial therapy for several months reduces spleen size, so splenectomy is unnecessary.

Infection

Infection can cause hemolytic anemia via several pathophysiologic mechanisms (Table 45-2).

Parasite Infections

The classic example of direct parasitization is infection by *Plasmodium falciparum* (Fig. 45-1, *C*), *Plasmodium vivax,* or *Plasmodium malariae.* Infection with malaria, primarily *P. falciparum,* is a major health problem in the developing world, causing an estimated 300 to 500 million infections and 1 to 3 million deaths annually.[9] The burden of disease rests most heavily on young children and pregnant women. *Falciparum* malaria can cause a life-threatening anemia, with severe anemia defined as hemoglobin less than 5 g/dL associated with parasitemia and a normocytic blood film.[9] Malaria is primarily a

Table 45-2 Mechanisms by Which Infection Can Cause Hemolysis

Mechanism	Example
Direct parasitization of red cells	Malaria, babesiosis
Immune mechanisms	Cold agglutinin hemolysis after infectious mononucleosis or mycoplasmal pneumonia (see Chapter 44)
Induction of hypersplenism	Malaria, schistosomiasis
Altered red cell surface topology	*Haemophilus influenzae* infection
Release of toxins and enzymes	Clostridial infection causing thrombotic thrombocytopenic purpura–hemolytic uremic syndrome, *Escherichia coli* 0197, human immunodeficiency virus infection

disease of the tropical developing world but is still seen in the United States and its territories, primarily as an import from outside the United States.[10] Of the 1298 cases reported in the United States in 2008, 117 (9%) were classified as severe, two of which were fatal. In each of the malarias, sporozoites injected by the mosquito in its saliva make their way to liver cells. After 1 to 2 weeks, they become merozoites, which burst out of the liver cells and into the bloodstream. Then, in a remarkable process, the parasite, by means of its apical end and related organelles called rhoptries, attaches to a specific receptor on the RBC surface. For *P. vivax,* the Duffy blood group antigen appears to be involved.

Plasmodium falciparum binds to sialic acid residues on the RBC surface that are on glycophorin A. After specific attachment, a convulsive movement occurs during which the RBC engulfs the parasite by a process resembling receptor-mediated endocytosis. Upon invasion of the RBC, the malarial parasite starts digesting the hemoglobin, depositing the undigested heme in the form of hemozoin. Knobs appear on the RBC surface, and the RBC becomes a sphere. Many proteins of parasitic origin are inserted into the RBC membrane, and some appear to cluster underneath these knobs. A parasite protein called mature-parasite-infected erythrocyte surface antigen (MESA) binds to membrane protein 4.1, and another parasite protein called ring-infected erythrocyte surface antigen (RESA) binds to β spectrin. Both spectrin and protein 4.1 are integral components of the membrane skeleton, and the consequence of the binding of malarial proteins is RBC membrane stabilization. Thus stabilized, the parasitized RBC can continue to survive while the parasite continues to digest its contents.[11]

The parasite recruits the RBC's metabolic machinery, degrades and ingests hemoglobin, and grows, eventually bursting out of the RBC, and the cycle begins again. The RBCs are lysed intravascularly as a consequence of direct parasitic destruction, extravascularly as a consequence of changes in the splenic microvasculature and in the activation state of the monocyte–macrophage system. Treatment consists of the use of appropriate antimalarials and the support of erythropoiesis, including the use of RBC transfusion or exchange (or both) when indicated.

The anemia of malarial infections also involves mechanisms distinct from lysis of parasitized RBCs. Erythropoiesis is suppressed, leading to suppression of erythroid precursors and inadequate reticulocytosis during acute infection.[12] This inadequate hematopoietic response may be exacerbated by underlying iron deficiency, hemoglobinopathies, or concomitant infection (e.g., HIV), all potential contributors to the severity of anemia. In addition, loss of uninfected erythrocytes plays a major role in the development of anemia, with an eight- to 10-fold greater loss of unparasitized RBCs compared with parasitized cells. Uninfected RBCs have reduced deformability, and the degree of reduced deformability correlates with the severity of infection. Poorly deformable RBCs likely are cleared by the spleen. Evidence of in vivo removal of immature malarial forms prompts the question of whether "uninfected" cells that are lost represent previously infected cells that nevertheless remain abnormal. Insertion of a merozoite rhoptry protein, ring surface protein 2, on RBCs in which infection was aborted has been implicated in the clearance of unparasitized erythrocytes and erythroid progenitors. In addition, uninfected RBCs demonstrate increased binding of immunoglobulins that probably are nonspecific immune complexes. Acute malarial infection, particularly with *P. falciparum,* also leads to alteration in splenic function that incites premature destruction of uninfected RBCs.[13]

The lifespan of transfused RBCs is likewise decreased. ^{51}Cr-labeled normal RBCs infused into patients infected with malaria demonstrate a shorter lifespan than in normal control participants; this effect may persist after clearance of the parasitemia. Alternatively, parasites can be removed from RBCs along with RBC membrane by the process of pitting, producing parasite-free spherocytes. This mechanism potentially explains the observed disparity between anemia and parasitemia.

Other infections that have somewhat similar pathophysiologies include Carrión disease (i.e., bartonellosis), in which a bite from the sandfly injects *Bartonella bacilliformis,* which attaches to the RBC surface of up to 80% of erythrocytes and causes lysis, leading to the massive hemolysis that characterizes acute infection. It appears that invasion of RBCs partly depends on the flagella of *Bartonella* spp. Incubation with antiflagellin antiserum reduces invasion of RBCs. The bacteria also secrete deformin, a factor that leads to deep pitting on the surface of RBCs, presumably providing a portal of entry into the erythrocyte. There also may be a role for splenic clearance of infected cells, and prior splenectomy appeared to protect a patient from hemolysis during acute infection.

Babesia organisms also directly invade RBCs, producing fever and hemolytic anemia. The parasite is transmitted by ticks and transfusions of infected blood products[14] and can be transmitted vertically. Most tickborne cases occur on the West Coast, particularly in Washington and California, and in the northern portion of the Midwest; cases occurring on the East Coast are concentrated in Massachusetts and Nantucket Island. However, transfusion-associated cases have been reported throughout the United States.[14] In one report of transfusion-associated babesiosis, the median interval from transfusion to onset of clinical manifestations was 37 days. The organisms can be seen invading RBCs on smear examination, somewhat like *P. falciparum* malaria, but these organisms produce no pigment. The highest risk of death from babesiosis occurs in individuals who are older than 50 years or are immunocompromised because of acquired immunodeficiency syndrome (AIDS), drugs, transplantation, or asplenism. Sporadic reports indicate that acquired chronic toxoplasmosis occasionally is associated with hemolytic anemia.

Alteration of the Red Blood Cell Surface by Bacterial Products

Infection can produce hemolysis by altering the RBC surface. An example is the hemolysis caused by *Haemophilus influenzae* type b. Severely affected patients, particularly those with meningitis, have developed hemolytic anemias requiring RBC transfusions. The capsular polysaccharide of the bacterium, composed of polyribosyl ribitol phosphate (PRP), is released during infection and binds to the RBC surface. Infected patients develop antibodies to PRP. When the balance between PRP-coated RBCs and anti-PRP antibodies is correct, an immune-type hemolysis occurs and requires complement. RBC destruction is thought to be both intravascular and extravascular.

Bacterial Products Causing Hemolysis by Direct Damage to Red Blood Cells

The most dramatic example of hemolysis caused by bacterial action is clostridial infection, during which the organism releases enzymes that acutely degrade the phospholipids of the membrane bilayer and the structural membrane proteins. The resulting spherocytes are extremely sensitive to osmotic lysis. The setting can be any infection, but our experience is limited to acute cholecystitis, surgery of the biliary tree, and infections surrounding an obstetric event, including criminal or self-induced abortion or other infection of the gravid uterus. Patients may also have an underlying gastrointestinal, genitourinary, neuroendocrine, or hematologic malignancy.[15] The signs of infections may be obvious, but fever may be unimpressive. Signs of collapse appear acutely, and the clue is profound intravascular hemolysis, with a spherocytic anemia developing with shocking suddenness. The blood smear characteristically has numerous spherocytes with little evidence of microangiopathy, may be tinged red because of marked hemoglobinemia, and may have ghost cells. A clue to the severity of the process may be the inability of the laboratory to perform chemical determinations or to type and cross-match the blood because the sample is hemolyzed. With even the slightest suspicion of hemolysis caused by bacterial action, the physician immediately starts full doses of penicillin and clindamycin; evaluates the patient for DIC (see Chapter 141); and prepares to support the patient for shock, DIC, acute renal failure, and hemolytic anemia. Whether hysterectomy is lifesaving in the case of septic abortion is unclear.

Hemolysis Caused by Less Well Understood Infections

HIV infection can cause Coombs-positive autoimmune hemolytic anemia, a TTP-like syndrome, and microangiopathic hemolysis. Primary HIV infections manifested as an acute hemolytic crisis in a patient with G6PD deficiency.[16] CMV infection has been reported to cause severe Coombs-negative hemolytic anemia in immunocompetent adults.[17] Case reports of autoimmune hemolytic anemia and HUS associated with CMV infection have emerged. The hemolytic anemia in visceral leishmaniasis may be caused in part by generation of oxidative metabolic products. Severe microangiopathic hemolytic anemia has been described in cases of cutaneous anthrax.

Hemolysis Associated with Liver Disease

Hemolysis in liver disease by itself usually is not of overwhelming clinical importance, but it may contribute to the severity of anemia when coupled with defects in RBC production and the type of gastrointestinal blood loss that occurs in several forms of liver disease. Hemolysis in patients with liver disease has several causes. The spleen may be enlarged as a consequence of portal hypertension and produce a hypersplenic picture, a phenomenon seen commonly in hepatic cirrhosis.

The literature on RBC shape change in liver disease is considerable. The target cell in cirrhosis has an increased SA:V that appears to be a consequence of increased cholesterol and phospholipid content of the membrane bilayer. The cholesterol increase usually is proportionately greater, resulting in an increased cholesterol-to-phospholipid ratio. This increase in lipid probably accounts for the increased RBC surface area, such that more membrane than usual is present in relation to cellular contents. These RBCs probably circulate as bell-shaped RBCs called *codocytes*. However, on dried blood films, they assume the appearance of target cells. Target cells do not have a shortened survival. The RBCs of patients with liver disease frequently are echinocytes when wet preparations are examined, but these echinocytes are not easily apparent on dried blood smears. The echinocytes seem to be produced by a material in the patient's plasma that causes normal RBCs to become echinocytic; this material is an abnormal echinocytogenic high-density lipoprotein. Echinocytes do not necessarily have a shortened survival. Some forms of echinocytic RBCs are normally deformable when studied in the ektacytometer or rheoscope.

A brisk, clinically important hemolysis can occur in some patients with severe liver disease. The peripheral smear in these individuals usually shows acanthocytes (i.e., distorted RBCs). Extreme forms are called *spur cells,* which probably are acanthocytes additionally remodeled by an enlarged spleen (see box on Reduction of Dangerous Methemoglobin Levels) and are considerably enriched in cholesterol. They are rapidly removed in the spleen, which usually is enlarged.

> **Reduction of Dangerous Methemoglobin Levels**
>
> Levels of methemoglobin in excess of 20% to 30% can be dangerous, but they can be easily treated with methylene blue (1-2 mg/kg) infused intravenously over 5 minutes as 0.1 to 0.2 mL/kg of a 1% solution. In the presence of a functioning, intact NADPH–methemoglobin reductase system, methylene blue is reduced to leukomethylene blue, which reduces methemoglobin to hemoglobin.

Increased RBC membrane proteolytic activity may be a partial explanation for the differences between acanthocytosis and spur cells, and additional pathophysiologic mechanisms may be involved. Although the adult RBC cannot synthesize phospholipids de novo, it can identify and remove peroxidized fatty acid chains that interfere with normal membrane lipid fluidity. When the fatty acid is removed, a lytic lysoderivative remains; therefore, the missing fatty acid chain must be replaced. A store of acyl groups in the form of acylcarnitine exists in RBC membranes. When needed, the fatty acid (i.e., acyl group) is transferred to acyl-coenzyme A and then inserted into the potentially lytic lysophospholipid by the enzyme lysophosphocholine acyltransferase. Lysophosphocholine acyltransferase is inhibited in spur RBCs, and the same inhibition can be produced by heavily loading RBCs with cholesterol in vitro.

In a case of almost fatal oxidative hemolysis, hydrogen peroxide was injected directly into the Hickman catheter of a patient with AIDS because some persons infected with HIV had circulated a pamphlet suggesting that hydrogen peroxide could be used therapeutically to control HIV infection. We now are seeing AIDS patients with dapsone-induced methemoglobinemia and hemolytic anemia (see Chapter 42). Methemoglobinemia, if severe, is treated as described in the preceding paragraph and in Chapter 42.

In spur cell anemia, the RBCs have an abnormal membrane SA:V ratio, their membrane fluidity is impaired, and they are unable to remove and repair peroxidatively damaged fatty acids. Occasionally, spur cell hemolytic anemia is severe enough to necessitate consideration of splenectomy. Operative morbidity in such cases is considerable because the underlying liver disease usually produces problems with thrombocytopenia and leukopenia as well as with procoagulants and intolerance to anesthesia. Spur cell anemia is typically associated with alcoholic cirrhosis, but can also be seen in patients with nonalcoholic cirrhosis. The anemia tends to be severe and portends a poor prognosis. Transfusions are of limited efficacy because the membrane abnormalities are acquired by transfused RBCs.[18] In one case, spur cell anemia occurred in a pediatric patient after orthotopic liver transplantation and resolved after retransplantation.[19]

Acute alcoholism can be associated with hypophosphatemia, defined as levels less than 0.2 mg/dL. Such hypophosphatemia presumably interferes with RBC intermediary metabolism (see Chapters 31 and 42), and RBC adenosine triphosphate (ATP) levels fall. Very low ATP levels are associated with RBC rigidity, which leads to fragmentation, loss of surface area, and spheroidicity. The RBCs then are further trapped in the spleen. This hypophosphatemia syndrome can also cause neuromuscular disorders, including weakness, paresthesias, tremors, and seizures. It should be treated aggressively with orally and intravenously administered phosphate supplements. Hypophosphatemia also occurs in patients with cirrhosis, patients receiving total parenteral nutrition whose phosphate intake is not carefully monitored, and patients taking large amounts of phosphate-binding antacids.

Stomatocytosis can occur in severe liver disease and is thought to be a sign of acute alcoholic intoxication. The change in RBC shape can also be seen in acute pancreatitis. The stomatocyte is a cell well on its way to becoming a spherocyte. The reduction in SA:V leads to trapping in the microvasculature of the spleen and other organs of the monocyte–macrophage system, producing various degrees of hemolysis.

Renal Disease

The anemia in renal disease is multifactorial. A major component is impaired RBC production, which can be well controlled with erythropoietin. Renal disease also impairs platelet function, which may lead to occult blood loss. However, hemolysis also can occur and is multifactorial. Disease of the small renal arterioles can produce fragmentation hemolysis of the sort seen in TTP–HUS, preeclampsia, and malignant hypertension (see the box on Causes of Red Blood Cell Fragmentation Hemolysis). Otherwise, whether uremia produces significant shortening of RBC survival is not clear. Patients with chronic renal failure who are undergoing hemodialysis may be particularly susceptible to oxidative damage to their RBCs. RBC glutathione (GSH) is reduced in some patients, and the activity of the enzymes G6PD and glutathione peroxidase is relatively low. The ability of these RBCs to deal with generation of peroxides probably is impaired.

Venoms, Bites, Stings, and Toxins

The best-known example of toxin-caused hemolysis is discussed in the earlier section on Bacterial Products Causing Hemolysis by Direct Damage to Red Blood Cells.

Insect, Spider, and Snake Bites

Hemolysis occurs after bee and wasp stings, snake bites, and spider bites. Isolated cases of acute intravascular hemolysis after bee and wasp stings have been reported. Two kinds of dangerous spiders live in the United States: the southern black widow and the brown recluse spider. Both sexes of the black widow produce the venom, but only the female has fangs capable of penetrating human skin. Black widow spider bites produce generalized muscle pain and muscular rigidity. Hemolysis is not common. Brown recluse spider bites cause a considerable local reaction, called the *volcano lesion*. DIC and hemolysis may occur after a lag of 24 to 48 hours. Envenomation results in cleavage of RBC glycophorins, presumably making the RBCs more susceptible.[20] Corticosteroids may be beneficial. The hemolysis appears to be self-limiting, but RBC transfusion support may be needed.

In some parts of the world, cobra bites can cause intravascular hemolysis because the venom contains phospholipases. In the United States, the two classes of venomous snakes are pit vipers (e.g., rattlesnakes, cottonmouths, moccasins, and copperheads) and coral snakes. Pit viper venom affects hemostasis and may produce DIC with bleeding but rarely hemolysis. Coral snake venom produces severe neurologic impairment. Therapy consists of support and use of the appropriate antivenin and prophylactic antimicrobials and tetanus injections.

Drugs and Chemicals Exclusive of Those Producing Oxidative Hemolysis

Potassium Chlorate

Potassium chlorate ingestion is listed as a cause of hemolysis, but this compound is no longer available in hospital pharmacies and has no currently recognized medical use. Arsine gas (AsH3) is generated in industrial plants that engage in lead plating, galvanizing, etching, and soldering. Inhalation of a toxic amount produces a severe intravascular hemolysis of unknown pathogenesis and may require urgent RBC and plasma exchange.

Copper

The idea that copper can produce human hemolytic disease is best supported by observations of episodes of severe hemolysis and acute liver failure in patients with Wilson disease. The patient usually is a child, adolescent, or young adult for whom the diagnosis of Wilson disease has not yet been made. The initial clinical presentation usually is dominated by Coombs-negative hemolytic anemia accompanied by weakness and dark urine. Associated findings include coagulopathy, a rapid progression to renal failure, relatively modest rises in serum aminotransferases, and a low alkaline phosphatase level. In addition to the presence of a brisk reticulocytosis, the typical findings of intravascular hemolysis may be present, including elevated LDH, low haptoglobin, and markedly elevated bilirubin levels.[21] Review of the peripheral smear may not reveal any specific morphologic findings, although both stomatocytosis and blister cells consistent with oxidant injury have been described. In one reported patient with concomitant transfusion-dependent hemoglobin E/β thalassemia, the acute hemolysis led to a severe unexpected drop in the post-transfusion hemoglobin level.[22] Because of the hereditary deficiency in the copper-binding protein ceruloplasmin, urine and serum non–ceruloplasmin-bound copper levels in patients with hemolysis are very high.

Free copper can interfere with glucose metabolism by hexokinase inhibition and alternatively can generate oxidative hemolysis, perhaps by acting as a Fenton reagent. It is important to establish the diagnosis promptly. When this condition is suspected, the practitioner should look for Kayser-Fleischer rings on physical examination and measure serum and urine copper and ceruloplasmin levels. Treatment with penicillamine[23] or trientine plus zinc reduces the serum copper level and stops the hemolysis. In the case of acute liver failure, the treatment is urgent liver transplantation. Plasmapheresis and hemofiltration may be beneficial in reducing the copper level and can serve as a bridge to transplant. In some cases, plasmapheresis in combination with chelation therapy or the use of a fractionated plasma separation and adsorption dialysis system may avert the need for transplant in impending acute liver failure. Other forms of copper poisoning may cause hemolysis in patients who do not have underlying Wilson disease. The amount of copper ingested would have to exceed the copper-binding capacity of normal ceruloplasmin levels.

Lead

There are at least two general forms of lead intoxication. One type is chronic, slow cumulative poisoning (i.e., saturnism). An example is occupational exposure. Symptoms are predominantly neurologic and nephrologic, with variable degrees of anemia, which may be caused by a production defect combined with hemolysis. Relatively acute poisoning occurs when lead inadvertently finds its way into a food source or is consumed as part of an exotic medication. Subacute lead poisoning leads to central nervous system symptoms, hepatitis, nephrotoxicity, hypertension, and abdominal colic along with seizures and severe hemolytic anemia. Physical examination may reveal a lead line on the gums. Peripheral smear shows extensive coarse basophilic stippling and reticulocytosis; however, RBC morphology is not otherwise characteristic. Some researchers state that intravascular destruction occurs, but no proof has been provided. Bilirubin levels are not significantly elevated.

The diagnosis of lead-related hemolysis can be made from the history and findings on physical examination, which include a lead line on the gingiva and coarse basophilic stippling on RBCs, which reflects the pathologic aggregation of ribosomes. The diagnosis is confirmed by measuring blood and urine lead levels. The level of acuity determines the therapy.

The cause of the anemia is complex. Lead interferes with several steps in heme synthesis, particularly those involving heme synthetase and δ-aminolevulinic acid dehydratase (see Chapter 36). The inhibition of heme synthetase probably accounts for the elevation in free erythrocyte protoporphyrin, which provides a useful corroborative diagnostic test for lead toxicity. Inhibition of heme synthesis also probably accounts for the elevated urinary levels of δ-aminolevulinic acid and coproporphyrin. Lead poisoning mimics the basophilic stippling and accumulation of pyrimidines seen in hereditary deficiency of the enzyme pyrimidine 5′-nucleotidase, probably because lead attacks the enzyme (see Chapter 42).

Ribavirin

Current treatment of chronic hepatitis C virus (HCV) infection consists of combination therapy with pegylated interferon (INF) and ribavirin, a nucleoside analogue. Ribavirin's activity against HCV includes inhibition of inosine monophosphate dehydrogenase, a key step in de novo guanine synthesis. Treatment with ribavirin may produce a dose-dependent hemolytic anemia, which typically is reversible 1 to 2 months after discontinuing treatment.[24] The hemoglobin drops by an average of 2 to 3 g/dL and may fall below 11 g/dL in one third or more of patients. The anemia may necessitate a dose reduction of ribavirin or may be treated with recombinant erythropoietin at 40,000 units weekly. A decrease in the total cumulative dose of ribavirin may be associated with decreased sustained virologic response, which would suggest that dose reduction secondary to anemia would have an adverse impact on treatment efficacy. However, in one retrospective study, a drop in hemoglobin of greater than 3 g/dL was instead associated with improved sustained viralogic response rate compared with those with a drop in hemoglobin 3 g/dL or less,[25] suggesting conversely that the degree of hemolytic anemia may serve as a biomarker of efficacy. Ribavirin is transported into the erythrocytes and accumulates as ribavirin monophosphates, diphosphates, and triphosphates.[24] The steady-state concentration of ribavirin in erythrocytes is approximately 100-fold higher than that of plasma, and higher erythrocyte ribavirin levels correlate with worsened anemia during therapy. Accumulation of phosphates leads to a decrease in ATP levels compared with control erythrocytes. Because ATP is required to generate the glucose-6-phosphate needed for glycolysis and the hexose monophosphate shunt, reduced levels of ATP may lead to oxidative damage, as evidenced by increased aggregates of band 3, which bind anti–band 3 immunoglobulin G (IgG) and complement. The ribavirin prodrug viramidine induces less anemia than ribavirin, although efficacy was decreased when used at fixed-doses compared with a ribavirin-containing regimen. Fellay et al[26] have detected two polymorphisms in the inosine triphosphatase (ITPA) gene, which encodes a protein that hydrolyses inosine triphosphate, and were protective against severe anemia in patients treated with HCV. These two polymorphisms were associated with reduced ITPA activity and accumulation of inosine triphosphate in red blood cells. The mechanism of this protective effect is not yet fully understood. The anemia in patients treated with ribavirin may be exacerbated by concomitant treatment with pegylated INF, which suppresses hematopoiesis, and may also be associated with autoimmune hemolytic anemia. Anemia may also be exacerbated when ribavirin and INF are used in combination with the protease inhibitor,[27] a regimen which is efficacious in the treatment of genotype 1 disease.

DRUG-INDUCED OXIDATIVE HEMOLYSIS

General Concepts

The potential for normal RBCs to undergo auto-oxidative destruction is great because the cell is loaded with 20-mM hemoglobin, most of which is bonded to oxygen at the iron(II) atom in heme. The bond that allows the reversible association and dissociation of oxygen from the heme moiety of hemoglobin involves partial transfer of an electron from iron(II) to oxygen. That oxygen then has an extra electron, which makes it a superoxide radical. Ordinarily, when oxygen leaves hemoglobin, it returns the electron. If it does not, a highly reactive superoxide ion is released, leaving behind it an iron(III) moiety called *methemoglobin*.

$$\text{Hb Fe}^{2+}\text{O}_2 \rightarrow \text{Hb Fe}^{3+} + \text{O}_2^{-1}$$

Methemoglobin cannot reversibly bind oxygen. Methemoglobin in itself is not harmful to RBCs, but if the oxidative assault persists, methemoglobin is converted to hemichromes, which are variably denatured hemoglobin intermediates in which the distal histidine unit binds to the oxidized heme. This step is associated with conversion from a high to a low spin state, as measured by electron spin resonance. Continued oxidation leads to irreversibility of hemichrome oxidation, precipitation, and eventually formation of Heinz bodies. Hemichromes and Heinz bodies can destroy membrane function directly or by causing oxidation of membrane proteins and lipids.[28] Approximately 3% of hemoglobin is converted to methemoglobin each day, but the finding that only 1% of hemoglobin normally is in the form of methemoglobin indicates that a mechanism preventing oxidation in RBCs is in effect. These mechanisms are limited because RBCs lack the ability to either efficiently generate ATP or synthesize enzymes. The primary means for preventing or addressing oxidant injury are the generation of the reduced form of nicotinamide adenine dinucleotide (NADH) via the Embden-Meyerhof glycolytic pathway and the generation of nicotinamide adenine dinucleotide phosphate (NADPH) via the hexose monophosphate shunt. NADH is used to reduce methemoglobin by cytochrome b5 reductase, and NADPH is used to reduce glutathione and for catalase activity. Defects in this defense system against oxidation lead to an enhanced tendency to oxidative hemolysis. Examples are G6PD deficiency states. G6PD catalyzes the initial rate-limiting step in the hexose monophosphate shunt. Deficiencies lead to a reduced ability to generate NADPH in response to oxidant stress. Any agent or event that interferes with the smooth offloading of oxygen enhances the generation of O_2^{-1} and methemoglobin, as indicated in the equation. If the reducing power of the RBC is inadequate, hemichromes and Heinz bodies are generated. Many agents appear to cause oxidative hemolysis by interfering with the smooth functioning of the heme cleft.

Pathophysiology

After the oxidative attack has been initiated, the sequence proceeds along a recognizable track. The oxidative attack is directed at hemoglobin and the RBC membrane. However, these structures are not clearly separable because the precipitated hemichrome and Heinz bodies come to lie against the cytosolic face of the membrane. Methemoglobin may be detectably elevated, with levels as high as 50% to 60% of total hemoglobin. The hemichromes, by themselves or with their iron portions acting as a Fenton reagent, mediate the generation of hydroxyl free radicals, which add their effect to that of superoxide and hydrogen peroxide. Lipid peroxidation may take place, leading to membrane blebbing and cell lysis as well as loss of asymmetry of the phospholipid membrane bilayer. Movement of phosphatidylserine and phosphatidylethanolamine to the outer bilayer of the membrane results in increased recognition by macrophages in the reticuloendothelial system. Membrane proteins may be cross-linked, with binding of denatured, oxidized hemoglobin to the membrane cytoskeleton, which may increase splenic macrophage recognition. In addition, the RBCs are rigid and susceptible to trapping in sinusoidal structures, whether or not they have Heinz bodies lying against the membrane. In vitro evidence suggests that oxidized RBCs are increasingly susceptible to phagocytosis by macrophages. These features may account for extravascular destruction. The oxidative lesions can be severe enough to cause intravascular destruction as well, producing hemoglobinemia and hemoglobinuria.

Agents that Cause Oxidative Hemolysis

Therapeutic agents
- Nitrofurantoin (Furadantin)
- Sulfasalazine (Azulfidine)
- *p*-Aminosalicylic acid
- Phenazopyridine (Pyridium)
- Phenacetin
- Dapsone and other sulfones
- Primaquine

Recreational drugs
- Isobutyl nitrate
- Amyl nitrite

Miscellaneous agents
- Naphthalene mothballs
- Paraquat
- Hydrogen peroxide

The smear may show bite cells, which look as if a macrophage had taken a bite, removing a Heinz body–containing segment of membrane. RBC rigidity may result in irregularly shaped cells because these undeformable cells are unable to undergo elastic recoil after fighting their way through the sinus wall. Recurrent loss of membrane material may produce spherocytes. Severe hemolysis may produce the kind of circulating ghost or hemighost called a *blister cell* or *bite cell*. These RBCs have an empty veil of membrane on one side and puddled hemoglobin on the other. A Heinz body preparation may be positive. However, the absence of bite cells does not rule out the diagnosis.

The clinical picture is determined by the specific agent used. Screening for G6PD deficiency or a related disorder using an enzyme assay or the ascorbate cyanide test may be useful. Although any defect in the antioxidant defense mechanisms, such as G6PD deficiency, considerably increases the susceptibility to hemolysis, many agents can produce oxidant hemolysis even in persons with normal defense mechanisms (see box on Agents That Cause Oxidative Hemolysis). Paraquat ingestion has occurred inadvertently and in suicide attempts. Profound cyanosis with methemoglobinemia can occur within hours, with levels of 120% or higher. The condition may be succeeded by hemolysis, with Heinz bodies seen in appropriate preparations of RBCs.

Toxic ingestion or inhalation of nitrites may occur in suicide attempts from industrial exposures; via diets high in pickled or smoked foods; through intentional recreational use; or in infants from formulas prepared using well water high in nitrates, which are reduced to nitrites in the infant gut.[29] Nitrites bind to hemoglobin, producing methemoglobinemia, which may be so profound as to produce coma. If methylene blue infusion does not quickly turn the chocolate color of blood back to normal, the physician must consider the possibility that the patient is G6PD deficient and therefore unable to generate adequate amounts of NADPH (discussed earlier under Drug-Induced Oxidative Hemolysis: General Concepts). In that case, exchange transfusion may be lifesaving. Benzocaine topical anesthesia in the form of a spray or cream can cause severe methemoglobinemia, with cyanosis and dyspnea requiring methylene blue treatment.

Pyridium (phenazopyridine) can cause oxidative hemolysis even in the absence of renal disease. This agent is commonly used for treatment of bladder irritation. The *Physician's Desk Reference* recommends maximum therapy of 2 days. However, patients not uncommonly are given a prescription for 1 to 4 weeks of therapy.

It has been recognized for more than 130 years that therapy with dapsone causes oxidative hemolysis. In the past, dapsone was used primarily to treat leprosy and dermatitis herpetiformis and was not often encountered as a cause of oxidative hemolysis. Dapsone has come into more widespread use in some communities as a very effective prophylactic agent against *Pneumocystis carinii* pneumonia in patients with AIDS. The reduced levels of GSH reported in patients with AIDS may enhance dapsone toxicity. Some clinics screen potential recipients for G6PD deficiency (see Chapter 42) and, if results are negative, proceed with dapsone therapy. However, dapsone can cause oxidative attack on normal RBCs, leading sequentially to methemoglobinemia, Heinz bodies, and hemolysis, all occurring at generally accepted standard doses. Dapsone is metabolized to a hydroxylamine derivative that is directly toxic to RBCs.

Hemolytic Anemia in Chronic Large Granular Lymphocytic Leukemia

Although large granular lymphocytic leukemia usually manifests as neutropenia and a rheumatoid-like picture, several patients with a severe Coombs-negative hemolytic anemia in the absence of splenomegaly have been described. Large granular lymphocytic leukemia has occurred in a splenectomized subject. The mechanism is unknown, but one report identified direct cytotoxicity against RBCs by the large granular lymphocytic cell lines.

There have been no formal studies on therapy for large granular lymphocytic leukemia–related hemolysis, although immunosuppressive therapy with prednisone or methotrexate has been reported as being partially or wholly successful.

MISCELLANEOUS, POORLY CHARACTERIZED CAUSES OF EXTRINSIC HEMOLYTIC ANEMIAS

Interferon-α as a Cause of Hemolytic Anemia

Both microangiopathic and autoimmune hemolysis have been reported with INF-α use. Zuber et al[30] reported eight patients with chronic myeloid leukemia who developed thrombotic microangiopathy confirmed by renal biopsy. Seven of these patients had identifiable hemolysis, and three had thrombocytopenia. They also reviewed 13 other cases of microangiopathy associated with INF-α reported in the literature and observed that most cases occurred in the setting of prolonged therapy in chronic myeloid leukemia. Two cases of chronic hepatitis with microangiopathy were notable for having received unusually high doses of INF for this indication. Cases of autoimmune hemolysis have been reported with INF-α therapy in the setting of chronic myeloid leukemia or chronic hepatitis C.

Hemolysis With Intravenous Immunoglobulin G

Strictly speaking, hemolysis with intravenous IgG is a form of immune hemolysis. However, preparations of IgG contain anti-A and anti-B antibodies and rarely cause an alloimmune hemolytic anemia, as described in two young women undergoing treatment for idiopathic thrombocytopenic purpura. If this situation occurs and more intravenous IgG is needed, performing a minor cross-match and choosing a preparation of intravenous IgG that gives no reaction is recommended. In addition to isoantibody production, anemia has been reported with intravenous IgG because of immune complex–mediated complement activation.

For hemolytic anemia with large granular lymphocyte leukemia, see box on Hemolytic Anemia in Chronic Large Granular Lymphocytic Leukemia.

REFERENCES

1. Moake J: Thrombotic microangiopathies: Multimers, metalloprotease, and beyond. *Clin Transl Sci* 2:366, 2009.
2. George JN: How I treat patients with thrombotic thrombocytopenic purpura: 2010. *Blood* 116:4060, 2010.
3. Blake-Haskins JA, Lechleider RJ, Kreitman RJ: Thrombotic microangiopathy with targeted cancer agents. *Clin Cancer Res* 17:5858, 2011.

4. Zakarija A, Kwaan HC, Moake JL, et al: Ticlopidine- and clopidogrel-associated thrombotic thrombocytopenic purpura (TTP): Review of clinical, laboratory, epidemiological, and pharmacovigilance findings (1989-2008). *Kidney Int Suppl* S20, 2009.
5. Zakarija A, Bennett C: Drug-induced thrombotic microangiopathy. *Semin Thromb Hemost* 31:681, 2005.
6. Booth KK, Terrell DR, Vesely SK, et al: Systemic infections mimicking thrombotic thrombocytopenic purpura. *Am J Hematol* 86:743, 2011.
7. Francis KK, Kalyanam N, Terrell DR, et al: Disseminated malignancy misdiagnosed as thrombotic thrombocytopenic purpura: A report of 10 patients and a systematic review of published cases. *Oncologist* 12:11, 2007.
8. Vermeulen Windsant IC, Snoeijs MG, Hanssen SJ, et al: Hemolysis is associated with acute kidney injury during major aortic surgery. *Kidney Int* 77:913, 2010.
9. Casals-Pascual C, Roberts DJ: Severe malarial anaemia. *Curr Mol Med* 6:155, 2006.
10. Mali S, Steele S, Slutsker L, et al: Malaria surveillance — United States, 2008. *MMWR Surveill Summ* 59:1, 2010.
11. An X, Mohandas N: Red cell membrane and malaria. *Transfus Clin Biol* 17:197, 2010.
12. Chang KH, Tam M, Stevenson MM: Inappropriately low reticulocytosis in severe malarial anemia correlates with suppression in the development of late erythroid precursors. *Blood* 103:3727, 2004.
13. Looareesuwan S, Ho M, Wattanagoon Y, et al: Dynamic alteration in splenic function during acute falciparum malaria. *N Engl J Med* 317:675, 1987.
14. Herwaldt BL, Linden JV, Bosserman E, et al: Transfusion-associated babesiosis in the United States: A description of cases. *Ann Intern Med* 155:509, 2011.
15. McArthur HL, Dalal BI, Kollmannsberger C: Intravascular hemolysis as a complication of clostridium perfringens sepsis. *J Clin Oncol* 24:2387, 2006.
16. Schulze Zur Wiesch J, Wichmann D, Hofer A, et al: Primary HIV infection presenting as haemolytic crisis in a patient with previously undiagnosed glucose 6-phosphate dehydrogenase deficiency. *Aids* 22:1886, 2008.
17. Veldhuis W, Janssen M, Kortlandt W, et al: Coombs-negative severe haemolytic anaemia in an immunocompetent adult following cytomegalovirus infection. *Eur J Clin Microbiol Infect Dis* 23:844, 2004.
18. Cooper RA, Kimball DB, Durocher JR: Role of the spleen in membrane conditioning and hemolysis of spur cells in liver disease. *N Engl J Med* 290:1279, 1974.
19. Alkhouri N, Alamiry MR, Hupertz V, et al: Spur cell anemia as a cause of unconjugated hyperbilirubinemia after liver transplantation and its resolution after retransplantation. *Liver Transpl* 17:349, 2011.
20. Tambourgi DV, Morgan BP, de Andrade RM, et al: Loxosceles intermedia spider envenomation induces activation of an endogenous metalloproteinase, resulting in cleavage of glycophorins from the erythrocyte surface and facilitating complement-mediated lysis. *Blood* 95:683, 2000.
21. Mehta AR, Salaru G, Harrison JS: Stomatocytosis heralding a case of acute Wilsonian crisis. *Ann Hematol* 89:527, 2010.
22. Thapa R, Mukherjee K: Acute Wilson disease associated with E β-thalassemia. *J Pediatr Hematol Oncol* 30:925, 2008.
23. Roberts EA, Schilsky ML: Diagnosis and treatment of Wilson disease: An update. *Hepatology* 47:2089, 2008.
24. McHutchison JG, Manns MP, Longo DL: Definition and management of anemia in patients infected with hepatitis C virus. *Liver Int* 26:389, 2006.
25. Sulkowski MS, Shiffman ML, Afdhal NH, et al: Hepatitis C virus treatment-related anemia is associated with higher sustained virologic response rate. *Gastroenterology* 139:1602, 2010.
26. Fellay J, Thompson AJ, Ge D, et al: ITPA gene variants protect against anaemia in patients treated for chronic hepatitis C. *Nature* 464:405, 2010.
27. Jacobson IM, McHutchison JG, Dusheiko G, et al: Telaprevir for previously untreated chronic hepatitis C virus infection. *N Engl J Med* 364:2405, 2011.
28. Hebbel RP, Eaton JW: Pathobiology of heme interaction with the erythrocyte membrane. *Semin Hematol* 26:136, 1989.
29. Greer FR, Shannon M: Infant methemoglobinemia: The role of dietary nitrate in food and water. *Pediatrics* 116:784, 2005.
30. Zuber J, Martinez F, Droz D, et al: Alpha-interferon-associated thrombotic microangiopathy: A clinicopathologic study of 8 patients and review of the literature. *Medicine (Baltimore)* 81:321, 2002.

PART VI

NON-MALIGNANT LEUKOCYTES

CHAPTER 46

NEUTROPHILIC LEUKOCYTOSIS, NEUTROPENIA, MONOCYTOSIS, AND MONOCYTOPENIA

Lawrence Rice and Moonjung Jung

Abnormalities of leukocyte number are commonly encountered in medical practice. The clinical significance of leukocytosis or leukopenia varies from none at all to being an early clue to a life-threatening process, whether a primary hematologic or secondary reactive process. Potential causes of leukocytosis or leukopenia are myriad. This chapter considers disorders faced by adult practitioners in hospital and outpatient clinics, where the predominant hematologic abnormality is neutrophilic leukocytosis, neutropenia, monocytosis, or monocytopenia; other chapters consider lymphocytosis, lymphopenia, eosinophilia, pancytopenia, and hematologic neoplasms.

The normal range for leukocyte count in most laboratories is from about 4500 to 11,000/mm^3. Neutrophils (and band forms) comprise the majority of circulating leukocytes (1800-7700); monocytes are about 4% of cells (mean absolute count, 300/mm^3). The physician must always think in terms of absolute counts of leukocyte subpopulations (total leukocyte count multiplied by the differential percentage). Thus, in a patient presenting with a normal white blood cell (WBC) count of 5000/mm^3 and an elevated lymphocyte percentage of 65%, the differential diagnosis to be considered is that of neutropenia, not lymphocytosis, because the absolute neutrophil count (ANC) is decreased but absolute lymphocytes are normal (only relatively increased).

When approaching a patient with abnormal leukocyte number, several factors impact heavily on the differential diagnosis and the vigor with which diagnosis and therapy should be pursued. Diagnostic considerations are vastly different when the abnormality first manifests **in the hospital versus in the outpatient clinic.** Also crucial is the **degree of the abnormality,** providing guidance to its likely cause and consequence. For example, agranulocytosis is a life-threatening disorder in which neutrophils are at or near zero, has a limited spectrum of underlying causes (drug reactions being paramount), and demands immediate interventions. **Duration** has major implications; determining the onset of changes and whether they are stable or progressive informs as to etiology and significance. Whether the abnormality is **symptomatic**—for example, whether a neutropenic or monocytopenic patient has or has had infectious complications—bears on likely etiologies and need for therapy. If there are known or suspected **comorbid conditions,** such as autoimmune or inflammatory disorders, this can crystallize the approach; occasionally, the leukocyte abnormality may be the first sign of a previously unrecognized disorder or may provide important confirmation (e.g., neutropenia in a patient with systemic lupus erythematosus [SLE]). If the leukocyte abnormality is accompanied by **additional hematologic abnormalities** (unexplained abnormalities of red blood cells [RBCs], platelets, or cell morphology), this would point away from disorders considered in this chapter and often toward a primary hematologic disease. Beyond *history and physical examination,* the peripheral blood smear is key to establish the direction of further evaluation.

NEUTROPHILIC LEUKOCYTOSIS (NEUTROPHILIA)

A high WBC count, particularly high neutrophil count, is common with any infectious or inflammatory disorder. In the emergency department, leukocytosis is often equated with significant bacterial infection or at least a sign of illness severe enough to warrant hospital admission rather than outpatient management. Leukocytosis can also be a prominent presenting feature of leukemias and myeloproliferative disorders (MPDs). The presence of increased neutrophils assures that acute leukemia is not present. When leukocytosis is extreme, it indicates chronic myeloid leukemia (CML), other MPDs, or a leukemoid reaction.

Leukemoid reaction has been defined as a reactive (nonclonal) neutrophilic leukocytosis with a WBC count above 50,000/mm^3. The clinician must differentiate this from a neoplastic proliferation.

Leukoerythroblastosis refers to the presence in the peripheral blood of immature myeloid cells (generally myelocytes) and nucleated RBCs, often with giant platelets as well. This is always abnormal. Patients with leukoerythroblastosis do not necessarily have leukocytosis, but they usually do. Most patients (two-thirds) with leukoerythroblastosis have an underlying myelophthisic process, such as primary or secondary myelofibrosis, metastatic tumor, necrosis, or granulomas in the bone marrow (BM). Therefore, BM examination is indicated when leukoerythroblastosis is unexplained. Teardrop poikilocytes and elliptocytes on blood smear would strengthen concerns for myelophthisis. In 20% of patients with leukoerythroblastosis, the cause is hemolytic anemia, and miscellaneous other causes consist mainly of those with shock (septic, hemorrhagic, cardiogenic, anaphylactic) when hypoperfusion of areas of BM disrupt the microenvironment and permit disorderly egress of precursor cells.

Left-shifted neutrophils refers to relative immaturity of circulating cells, often manifest as an increased percentage of band neutrophils. Marked left shift includes less mature precursor forms, myelocytes and metamyelocytes. Left shift is nonspecific and may occur with infection or any cause of marked neutrophilia.

Detailed directed history and physical examination are indispensible to the evaluation of neutrophilia (Table 46-1). Fever and chills suggest infection (or inflammation), mandating a search for more specific symptoms that could pinpoint the focus. Examples include a sore throat, pharyngeal erythema, and exudate in pharyngitis; productive cough and abnormal lung auscultation in pneumonia; and dysuria and flank tenderness in urinary tract infection. Medication history mainly explores glucocorticoid use. With mild chronic neutrophilia, smoking habits and obesity become considerations. Recent vigorous exercise, emotional stress, burns, shock, or trauma can increase circulating neutrophils because of catecholamine-induced demargination. A positive family history may suggest hereditary neutrophilia. Often neglected are attempts to delineate the time course of the leukocyte abnormality by seeking prior medical contacts and blood count results at the time. On the physical examination, care should be directed to lymph node palpation because this can be an important clue for infection or malignancy. Palpable splenomegaly may not only direct the evaluation toward hematologic disorders but can be a cardinal sign of a variety of infectious and inflammatory disorders.

Blood smear should always be a part of initial evaluation when there are abnormalities of blood counts. BM aspirate or biopsy morphology may be helpful when pathophysiology and diagnosis are unclear. When appropriate, essential information can be gained by sending BM for microbiologic cultures, cytogenetic or molecular, or other ancillary studies.

Table 46-1 Causes of Neutrophilia

1. Hematologic malignancy (CML, CNL, CMML)
2. Infection
3. Inflammation, physiologic stress, hemorrhage, hemolysis
4. Hereditary or congenital neutrophilias
5. Smoking
6. Drugs: colony-stimulating factors, glucocorticoids, epinephrine, lithium
7. Nonhematologic malignancy
8. Asplenia
9. Obesity
10. Recovery from neutropenia

CML, Chronic myeloid leukemia; *CMML*, chronic myelomonocytic leukemia; *CNL*, Chronic neutrophilic leukemia.

Leukemoid Reaction Versus Chronic Leukemia

A relatively common reason for hematologic consultation is for very high WBC count. CML is reviewed elsewhere in this text, as are chronic myelomonocytic leukemia (CMML) and a rarer, more difficult disorder to pinpoint, chronic neutrophilic leukemia. Marked neutrophilic leukocytosis or overt leukemoid reaction (WBC count >50,000/mm^3) can represent an overly exuberant reaction to any stimulus associated with neutrophilia. In patients with leukemoid reaction, a disproportionate number have infection with *Clostridium difficile*, an organism that elicits a vigorous neutrophil response. Leukemoid reactions are commonly associated with solid tumors, particularly lung cancers and aggressive tumors with necrotic areas. It can be important to quickly differentiate a reactive neutrophilic leukocytosis from a clonal leukemic proliferation.

The history and clinical context are usually quite different between leukemoid reaction and CML. Most patients with leukemoid reaction are encountered very ill in the hospital with obvious underlying illnesses (e.g., sepsis, organ rejection). Prior WBC counts, which are often available, demonstrate normal WBC counts until the recent onset of acute illness. This contrasts with CML, typically presenting in outpatients with hypermetabolism (weight loss, sweats, low-grade fever), symptoms referable to splenomegaly, or frequently asymptomatic. On physical examination, the spleen is palpable (occasionally massive) in the great majority of patients with CML but is unusual with leukemoid reaction (in the absence of comorbidities such as liver disease).

Laboratory findings reliably differentiate CML from leukemoid reaction. The total leukocyte count is commonly extremely high with CML (median, 100,000/mm^3), but with leukemoid reaction, counts above 100,000/mm^3 are rare and are virtually unheard of above 150,000/mm^3. Circulating myelocytes and even a few blasts are more typical of CML but can be seen in both disorders. Similarly, changes in platelet number and morphology can be seen with both but point to CML when changes are extreme. RBC changes do not reliably separate the disorders except in a few cases with prominent teardrops, which point toward MPD. More helpful is the leukocyte differential: patients with CML almost always have some degree of absolute basophilia and eosinophilia, but infection and glucocorticoid excess induce eosinopenia. (When the leukocyte count is 100,000/mm^3, realize that 2% to 3% basophils is a substantial absolute increase.)

The leukocyte alkaline phosphatase (LAP) score, which is high with leukemoid reaction and classically low with CML, has limited utility now that more sensitive and specific tests for CML have emerged. When CML is reasonably considered, testing should be done for the Philadelphia chromosome (t[9;22];bcr/abl) generally by chromosome banding or FISH. When other MPDs are judged reasonably possible, *JAK2* mutational status may be informative.

Infection

To protect against the ever-present threat to health and longevity, evolution has armed us with reactant cytokine cascades designed to increase the number of phagocytes and dispatch them to threatened locales. Neutrophilia is classically seen as a response to bacterial infection, responding to such cytokines as interleukin-6 (IL-6), tumor necrosis factor (TNF), and granulocyte colony-stimulating factor (G-CSF). Neutrophilia is also a frequent response to other infections, including fungal, parasitic, mycobacterial, and sometimes viral.

Changes in neutrophil morphology may be useful in predicting whether bacterial or other infection underlie a neutrophilic response. The authors have confirmed some published reports that prominent neutrophil vacuolization is highly specific and has moderate sensitivity for serious bacterial infection, as do prominent Dohle bodies (in the absence of a primary hematologic disorder). The authors blindly scored blood smears from 50 patients with serious bacterial infection (half bacteremic), 25 with influenza, 25 with noninfectious fever, and 25 control smears. Toxic granulation of neutrophils, touted as a sign of bacterial infection, was found useless in distinguishing infections from other febrile illnesses.

Inflammation and Stress

Acute or chronic inflammation can cause neutrophilia by mechanisms similar to infection, mediated by the proinflammatory cytokines G-CSF, granulocyte macrophage colony-stimulating factor (GM-CSF), TNF, IL-1, IL-6, IL 8, and others. Diseases such as rheumatoid arthritis (RA), vasculitis, inflammatory bowel disease, thyrotoxicosis, eclampsia, and many others are commonly accompanied by neutrophilia. Another rare but notable example is familial Mediterranean fever in which an inherited *MEFV* mutation leads to dysfunctional pyrin downregulation of neutrophil activation, leading to chronic inflammatory serositis and secondary AA amyloidosis.

Physiologic stresses, including exercise and emotional stress, lead to endogenous catecholamine and glucocorticoid release in addition to inflammatory cytokines. This causes a rapid doubling of circulating neutrophils caused by demargination and by more rapid BM egress of maturing neutrophils. Paulsen found early peaks in M-CSF, growth hormone, and cortisol after exercise followed by increases in G-CSF, IL-6, and monocyte chemoattractant protein 1. Acute hemorrhage and hemolytic anemia are other physiologic stresses. This contributes to increased steady-state neutrophil counts recorded in patients with sickle cell anemia, and the degree of elevation correlates with pain crisis frequency, other complications, and mortality; leukocyte reduction has been postulated to be one mechanism of hydroxyurea's beneficial actions. The stress of acute myocardial infarction is commonly accompanied by mild neutrophilia, and the early magnitude of rise has correlated with poor outcomes.

Hereditary and Congenital Neutrophilias

In newborns, neutrophilia and leukoerythroblastosis are among the hematologic abnormalities associated with trisomy 13, trisomy 18, and trisomy 21 (Down syndrome). A transient clonal MPD can be seen in children with Down syndrome and is usually self-limited, but it does put patients at increased risk for later acute megakaryoblastic leukemia.

Very rare hereditary neutrophilias sometimes are first appreciated in adults. In 1971, Herring reported a mother and three of her four children with lifelong neutrophilia (WBC, 14,000-164,000/mm^3; granulocytes, 9000-62,000/mm^3), unusual bleeding, thickened calvariae, and hepatosplenomegaly. They had no increase in infections. LAP score was high, BM revealed few Gaucher-like histiocytes, karyotype was normal by routine banding, but chromatid breaks and gaps were increased. In 2009, French investigators identified a mutation in the *CSF3R* gene in a kindred with hereditary chronic neutrophilia. The point mutation led to constitutive activation of the

G-CSF receptor, driving neutrophil proliferation and differentiation. One of 12 affected individuals in this kindred developed overt myelodysplastic syndrome (MDS). The frequency of this and other mutations are unknown with hereditary neutrophilias.

Smoking

Smoking has been well associated with mild neutrophilia in epidemiologic and animal studies. Perry et al found a 27% higher WBC count in smokers. Sunyer et al correlated the degree of leukocytosis and percentage of neutrophils with the number of cigarettes smoked. The effect can persist up to 5 years in those who stop smoking. A suggested mechanism was chronic inflammation because inflammatory markers, including C-reactive protein (CRP) and fibrinogen, are elevated. In a rodent model, cigarette smoke caused overexpression of hematopoietic growth factor genes IL-6, G-CSF, and GM-CSF. Thus, mild neutrophilia without other symptoms in an active smoker or recent smoker could be attributed to this practice without further evaluation.

Drugs

Systemic glucocorticoids cause neutrophilia mainly by interfering with neutrophil adhesion to the capillary wall and decreasing neutrophil turnover rate. Maximal neutrophil count occurs 4 to 6 hours after dexamethasone use in normal volunteers. G-CSF increases circulating neutrophils by increasing BM production and mobilization. Epinephrine increases proinflammatory cytokines and demargination. Suggested mechanisms for lithium-induced neutrophilia are induction of G-CSF and downregulation of CXCR4, thus facilitating egress from the BM.

Malignancy

Leukocytosis is frequently associated with solid tumors without direct BM involvement. Some malignant tumors have been reported to produce G-CSF or GM-CSF, occasionally producing leukocytosis in the range of a leukemoid reaction.

Asplenia

Whereas neutrophilia is classically observed early after splenectomy, lymphocytosis predominates in the long run. Nevertheless, chronic mild neutrophilia can also be seen in functionally asplenic individuals. Furthermore, there may be an exaggerated neutrophil response to infections or other stresses. On the blood smear, Howell-Jolly bodies are a very sensitive and specific (when numerous) sign of functional asplenia.

Obesity

Recent studies have documented chronic mild neutrophilia with obesity. Fat tissue can release inflammatory cytokines, creating a state of low-grade inflammation manifest by elevated CRP. Leptin is a key hormone elevated with obesity, and it has been found to act on $CD34^+$ cells to promote neutrophil differentiation. In an obese patient with chronic mild neutrophilia and no obvious other underlying disorder, this can be assumed to be the cause.

NEUTROPENIA (AND AGRANULOCYTOSIS)

The risk of neutropenia-related infection begins to rise at an ANC near $1000/mm^3$, rising dramatically below $500/mm^3$ and more so below $100/mm^3$; thus, an ANC of 500 to $1000/mm^3$ is considered moderate neutropenia, and below $500/mm^3$ is considered severe. This corresponds to NCI criteria for adverse hematologic event reporting: grade 1 toxicity is $1500/mm^3$ to lower limit of normal, grade 2 is 1000 to $1500/mm^3$, grade 3 is 500 to $1000/mm^3$, and grade 4 is less than $500/mm^3$. Beyond the ANC, the risk for infection is greatly influenced by the nature of the underlying problem, the BM myeloid reserve, and whether other risk factors for infection are present (e.g., immunoglobulin deficiency or breaks in mucosal barriers). The course with mild and moderate neutropenia is often benign.

The history focuses on the severity and duration of neutropenia, whether infectious complications have occurred (including severe stomatitis or gingivitis), and whether prior blood counts can be obtained. A history of drug exposures and their timing is especially relevant, not only for prescribed medications but also for over-the-counter, herbal, and illicit drugs. Symptoms of systemic inflammatory illness, such as arthritis, skin rash, and photosensitivity, can bear on the etiology and significance of the low WBC count. Fevers, weight loss, and sweats could be clues to many disorders, including malignancy. Liver disorders commonly present with cytopenias, so a history of hepatitis, jaundice, hepatitis risk factors, and HIV risks should be specifically questioned. Symptoms of anemia or bleeding could be clues to more general hematologic disorders. As with most hematologic problems, physical examination should devote extra attention to lymph node areas and the spleen. Oropharynx and skin examination also take on added importance.

Peripheral blood smear review is irreplaceable to direct the workup. MDS does not characteristically present with isolated neutropenia, but this is occasionally the predominant finding in this relatively common syndrome affecting older patients. Specific blood smear findings should be sought, which could suggest MDS, such as pseudo-Pelger Huet neutrophils, hypogranularity, Dohle bodies, macrocytosis, and dimorphic RBCs with a hypochromic population. Megaloblastic processes, such as vitamin B_{12} and folic acid deficiency, similarly do not characteristically present with isolated neutropenia, but this occasionally predominates (especially in the presence of acute infection). Hypersegmentation of neutrophils is always present with megaloblastic processes, including those that are drug induced (e.g., methotrexate, hydroxyurea), and can also be seen with uremia, as an autosomal dominant benign polymorphism, and in MDS and MPD. In a neutropenic patient, one should always specifically look for large granular lymphocytes (LGLs). A modest increase could indicate a reactive T-cell natural killer (NK) cell process, and a more dramatic increase could alert to clonal T-NK or NK cell proliferations. Hairy cells, other morphologic types of circulating lymphoma cells, and blasts are obvious indicators of hematologic malignancy. Morphologic suspicions for such processes could be confirmed by flow cytometry. Reactive lymphocytes may suggest viral infection but could also be present with drug reactions and other processes.

Further laboratory testing in patients with neutropenia may often be unnecessary. Especially in mild or moderate cases, the lack of specific diagnostic tests has created some overlap and confusion among what have been called chronic idiopathic neutropenia, chronic benign neutropenia, ethnic neutropenia, and autoimmune neutropenia. Autoimmune neutropenia is a relatively common cause of both mild and more severe neutropenia, so serologic tests for antinuclear antibodies and rheumatoid factor can be informative when this is considered. Positive results may raise suspicion for a previously undiagnosed collagen vascular disorder or just be supportive of a less specific autoimmune problem. Direct antiglobulin test and antiphospholipid antibodies can be supportive when there is very high suspicion of this diagnosis. Quantitative immunoglobulin levels may reveal an underlying immunodeficiency when there is evidence of autoimmunity or when infectious complications are disproportionate. Serologic tests for some viral infections (HIV, hepatitis, Epstein-Barr virus [EBV]) may be appropriate for many. Flow cytometry finds its main utility when peripheral blood smear suggests an abnormal lymphocyte population (e.g., LGLs or hairy cells). BM examination may not be helpful or warranted with mild or even moderate isolated neutropenia or in straightforward cases of severe neutropenia (e.g., after drug exposure) but can be essential when the diagnosis is in doubt and especially if other cell lines are compromised.

Severe Congenital Neutropenias

It is beyond the scope of this chapter to review in detail the heterogeneous genetic disorders that manifest in early childhood as severe congenital neutropenia; nevertheless, consultant hematologists should have some familiarity with the problem because modern therapy has extended survival for many into adulthood, and there may be milder forms of disease that go undiagnosed until young adulthood. The more severe of these disorders present with severe stomatitis and recurrent bacterial infections in infancy. The molecular bases have been greatly elucidated in recent years. Kostmann syndrome and Schwachman-Bodin-Diamond syndrome (SBDS), both associated with mental retardation and other congenital defects, have been linked to mutations in *HAX1* and *SBDS,* respectively. Several other severe congenital neutropenic disorders and their genetic bases have been defined. In young children, the differential diagnosis often includes transient postinfectious neutropenia, alloimmune neutropenia, or hematologic malignancy. BM examination often shows a pattern of maturation arrest. The majority of affected patients are responsive to G-CSF, although high doses may be required, and this has had favorable impact on infectious morbidity and mortality; allogeneic stem cell transplant is another therapeutic option. An intrinsic risk of acute myeloid leukemic transformation, 15% at 20 years, accompanies many of these disorders.

Cyclic neutropenia is often considered a variant of congenital neutropenia. Neutrophil counts vary from mildly to severely low with predictable periodicity, usually every 21 days. The vast majority of cases are autosomal dominant mutations in the elastase gene (ELA2, ELANE). G-CSF, often at low dosage, has reduced the risk of serious infections.

Benign Ethnic Neutropenia

Americans of African descent may have chronic mild neutropenia not associated with infectious complications. The 1999 to 2004 National Health and Nutrition Survey found that blacks had mean leukocyte counts 900/mm^3 lower than whites, with ANCs below 1500/mm^3 in 4.5% (compared with 0.8% of whites). The neutropenia correlates in some individuals with a polymorphism in the Duffy antigen receptor chemokine (DARC), a cytokine receptor also responsible for a Duffy-negative RBC phenotype. Some report this neutropenia more common in males, but others can sometimes demonstrate autosomal dominant inheritance. Marrow granulocyte reserve or release (or both) may be compromised. Benign neutropenia has also been seen in other ethnic populations, including those of Middle Eastern or Japanese descent. Thus, an asymptomatic mildly neutropenic person of appropriate ethnicity without abnormalities on blood smear may require no further diagnostic workup. It may be reassuring to the patient (and the doctor) if prior blood counts can be retrieved to document the chronic, nonprogressive, and complication-free course of the neutropenia.

Autoimmune Neutropenia (Primary and Secondary)

Autoimmune neutropenia can be primary or secondary to an autoimmune disorder such as SLE or RA. Neutropenia can be mild or severe. Classically, it caused by antineutrophil autoantibodies, although autoreactive cytotoxic lymphocytes are also known to cause this problem. When performed, BM examination most often is normocellular or hypercellular with a late "maturation arrest" picture. Severe cases can display pure WBC aplasia (similar to drug-induced agranulocytosis, which may also be antibody mediated). There are several challenges in making the diagnosis. One is that the maturation arrest BM picture is actually nonspecific with regard to mechanism: it could indicate a true stem cell differentiation defect or early release of later precursors (as with sepsis or splenic sequestration), or it could be a true sign of immune attack aimed at antigens borne by later myeloid precursors. Another problem is the lack of validated, clinically reliable neutrophil antibody tests. Experimentally, several methods have been used, generally suffering from high false-negative rates and also false-positives results from the detection of antibodies or immune complexes that bind to neutrophil Fc receptors nonspecifically. In the absence of a definitive test, diagnosis of autoimmune neutropenia must rest largely on clinical judgment.

Neutropenia caused by antineutrophil antibodies has been seen in infants about 1 year old, usually running a benign clinical course with spontaneous remissions in 95% within 2 years. Newborns are at risk of alloimmune neutropenia in the first months of life, but this is not generally accompanied by infectious complications. Secondary autoimmune neutropenias are most common in adults, related to disorders such as SLE, RA, Sjogren Syndrome, thymoma, and common variable immunodeficiency. In SLE, neutrophil counts correlate with disease activity and have been related to the induction of TRAIL, a ligand that increased myeloid apoptosis and killing by autologous T cells. Treatment of the SLE with immunosuppression or the use of G-CSF can improve the WBC count.

Felty syndrome was classically described as severe neutropenia and splenomegaly complicating RA, and has been attributed to antineutrophil antibodies, but the distinction between this syndrome and other causes of neutropenia with RA have become blurred, in particular, classic Felty syndrome and LGL syndrome probably are representative of a disease continuum. About 1% of patients with RA develop Felty syndrome, and it predisposes many to serious infections. Effective therapies have often included methotrexate, gold salts, and rituximab. Because of some risk of exacerbating underlying inflammatory problems, G-CSF should be used cautiously at the lowest effective dose.

Large Granular Lymphocyte Syndrome and Natural Killer Cell Proliferations

Proliferations of LGLs, T-NK cells, and NK cells are covered elsewhere, but mention is required here because they are common considerations in adults with neutropenia. These are extremely heterogeneous disorders, varying from nonclonal reactive processes to indolent clonal proliferations to highly aggressive neoplasms. Both reactive and clonal increases in T-NK cells can be seen with RA, representing a form of Felty syndrome. Reactive LGLs can be seen with other autoimmune disorders, after organ transplantation, or with tyrosine kinase inhibitor therapy, or they may be idiopathic. These proliferations are associated with variable degrees of neutropenia, commonly splenomegaly, and increased infectious risks. The diagnosis is suggested on blood smear by large lymphocytes with mature chromatin, excessive cytoplasm, with or sometimes without prominent cytoplasmic granules. Flow cytometry demonstrates increased CD3$^+$CD57$^+$ lymphocytes with the more common T-NK proliferations or may show CD3-CD56$^+$ clones with "pure" NK cell proliferation. Variably effective treatments for indolent proliferations are corticosteroids, methotrexate, cyclosporine, intravenous immunoglobulin, purine nucleoside analogs, and G-CSF.

Neutropenia With Infectious Diseases

Leukocytosis is the expected response to most bacterial infections, but leukopenia is also well-known to occur and is actually characteristic of infection by certain organisms. Viral infections often cause transient mild leukopenia, so restraint is in order in the diagnostic approach to a newly recognized moderate leukopenia in a febrile, modestly ill patient. Nonbacterial infections in which neutropenia is frequent or even characteristic include HIV, EBV, cytomegalovirus (CMV), hepatitis A and B, measles, rubella, varicella, rickettsia, and anaplasmosis (ehrlichiosis). Bacterial infections with characteristic leukopenia include typhoid fever and brucellosis, but granulomatous infections (tuberculosis, histoplasmosis) cause neutropenia, especially when the BM is directly involved. In patients with poor BM reserve (e.g., prior chemotherapy, malnutrition, myelodysplasia), an acute infection quite commonly lowers, rather than raises, the neutrophil count. Profound neutropenia is a known consequence of overwhelming sepsis and has been associated with poor outcomes.

Hypersplenism

Hematologists are frequently consulted for cytopenias, only to find an unappreciated large spleen as the etiology (and this is most often caused by liver disease with portal hypertension). Splenic enlargement can lead to sequestration and reduction of circulating WBCs, RBCs, platelets, or any combination of these. The degree of cytopenia is somewhat proportional to the degree of splenic enlargement. Substantial neutropenia out of proportion to depletion other cell lines and to the size of the spleen likely involves other factors, such as an autoimmune component (as can be seen with hepatitis C or autoimmune hepatitis) or medication effect (e.g., interferon).

Chemotherapy-Induced Neutropenia

The major dose-limiting toxicity of most cancer chemotherapy regimens continues to be neutropenia. This results in hospitalizations, antibiotic costs, reduced quality of life, infectious morbidity, and dose reductions and treatment delays that compromise efficacy and outcomes. Infectious complications have been blamed for 75% of chemotherapy-related mortality. Febrile neutropenia is defined as an ANC less than 500/mm^3 (or expected to decrease to <500/mm^3 over the next 48 hours) with fever (>38.3° C or sustained >38° C).

Principles of empiric antibiotic coverage for acute febrile episodes in severely neutropenic patients are covered in detail elsewhere. Basically, there is a high risk of sepsis (even when the source is occult), and a favorable outcome depends on prompt effective antimicrobial coverage, so empiric administration of broad-spectrum antibacterial agents is considered medically emergent. These must cover the aerobic gram-negative rods that were the traditional culprits, yet vigilance must be maintained for the gram-positive organisms that have emerged as major pathogens. With prolonged or repeated episodes of neutropenia, invasive fungi become common threats to survival, particularly *Aspergillus, Candida, Mucor,* and *Fusarium* spp. Published guidelines can aid in the choice of empiric antimicrobials. Because of difficulty demonstrating favorable impact, enthusiasm for granulocyte transfusion support has waned substantially in the past 30 years; clinical studies are readdressing this in the modern era.

The utility of prophylactic antibiotics is problematic because of the wide array of potential pathogens and because of concerns of inducing antibiotic resistance. A role of prophylactic quinolones has been shown in very high-risk patients after therapy for acute leukemia or stem cell transplant.

G-CSF is widely used for either primary or secondary prevention of neutropenia to decrease morbidity and mortality of febrile neutropenia. Primary prophylaxis is recommended by various guidelines if the risk of developing febrile neutropenia is greater than 20%, with this risk calculated from age, extent of primary cancer, comorbidities, and the known myelotoxicity of the chemotherapy regimen. G-CSF is begun 24 to 72 hours after the completion of myelotoxic chemotherapy. Pegfilgrastim allows prophylaxis to be given more conveniently (one subcutaneous injection per cycle).

Drug-Induced Neutropenia

Drug reactions account for a high percentage of acquired neutropenias, both mild but more so severe cases (agranulocytosis) (Table 46-2). Development of neutropenia is often abrupt, commonly within 4 weeks of initiation of a causative agent. Pathophysiology may involve immune mechanisms or more direct toxicity such as enhancement of reactive oxygen species made by NADPH (nicotinamide adenine dinucleotide phosphate) oxidase or myeloperoxidase of neutrophil precursors. The diagnosis is generally strongly suspected from an accurate history that plots leukocyte numbers against the time course of drug exposure; confirmation is leukocyte recovery after drug withdrawal. More specific confirmatory testing, such as for drug-dependent antibodies, is mainly an area of research laboratory investigation. BM examination is not usually required but may be helpful when pathophysiology and diagnosis are in doubt, when the course is atypical, and to provide prognostic information (earlier recovery anticipated with a picture of "maturation arrest" than one of myeloid aplasia). Treatment demands discontinuation of suspected offending drugs. Although the efficacy of myeloid growth factors (G-CSF) has been questioned by some, most recommend this therapy because even a modest shortening of the duration of severe neutropenia can occasionally be lifesaving. Mortality of drug-induced agranulocytosis is generally reported to be 10%.

Table 46-2 Drugs Commonly Associated With Neutropenia

1. Antibiotics: vancomycin, semisynthetic penicillins, chloramphenicol, sulfa, linezolid
2. Antithyroid drugs: methimazole, propylthiouracil
3. Cardiovascular: ticlopidine, procainamide
4. Antipsychotics: clozapine, olanzapine, chlorpromazine
5. Anticonvulsants: phenytoin, carbamazepine, valproic acid
6. Antiinflammatory agents: indomethacin, sulfasalazine, phenylbutazone
7. H2 blockers: cimetidine, ranitidine
8. Analgesics: dipyrone
9. Antineoplastic: rituximab
10. Anthelminthic: levamisole

The most commonly implicated drugs are listed in Table 46-2. Some merit additional comments. Some drugs have a direct myelotoxic effect rather than induce an idiosyncratic immune-based reaction. Neutropenia has more gradual onset related to dose and duration and may be accompanied by suppression of other hematologic cell lines. Linezolid and most instances of chloramphenicol myelosuppression are examples.

Beginning 2007, an epidemic of agranulocytosis was found among intravenous cocaine users. The adulterant levamisole was found in 71% of confiscated cocaine by the Drug Enforcement Agency, with the incidence of agranulocytosis 2.5% to 13% in those exposed. Nadir BM showed severe myeloid hypoplasia. Levamisole had long been linked to agranulocytosis, having been used as an antihelminth and as an adjuvant immune modulator in patients with autoimmune disorders and colorectal cancer.

Increasingly, severe neutropenia is recognized in patients treated with rituximab. The decrease in WBC count is unusual for its late onset, generally about 3 months after the last rituximab dose. It occurs with underlying autoimmune disorders, B-cell malignancies, and stem cell transplants—basically in all situations in which rituximab is used—usually occurring while the underlying illness is in complete remission. Moderate or severe neutropenia has been reported in about 5% of rituximab-treated patients, although much higher incidences have been reported in some series. Most patients recover quickly, usually after G-CSF therapy, but some protracted cases have been encountered. The authors and others have reported a high risk of relapse if rituximab is reinitiated. The mechanism is not definitively established, but an intriguing report implicates imbalanced recovery of B-cell clones with a deficiency of stromal-derived factor 1.

MONOCYTOSIS

Monocytosis is extremely nonspecific, usually not requiring investigation per se. Monocytosis has been defined as a sustained absolute increase in monocyte count greater than 800 to 1000/mm^3 (Table 46-3). Transient monocytosis, relative or absolute, is common with recovery from myelosuppression, such as after chemotherapy. Relative or absolute monocytosis may occur in other myelosuppressed states,

Table 46-3 Changes in Monocyte Number

MONOCYTOSIS
Infections: tuberculosis, granulomatous infection, brucellosis, subacute bacterial endocarditis
Connective tissue disorder
Recovery from myelosuppression
Hematologic malignancies
1. MDS, MPD, MDS–MPD overlap, CMML
2. Acute and chronic monocytic leukemia, myelomonocytic leukemia
3. Hodgkin and non-Hodgkin lymphomas
MONOCYTOPENIA
Hairy cell leukemia
MonoMAC syndrome
Aplastic anemia
Drugs: chemotherapy, IFN-α, glucocorticoids (transient)
Radiation therapy

CMML, Chronic myelomonocytic leukemia; IFN, interferon; *MDS,* myelodysplastic syndrome; monoMAC, Monocytopenia and mycobacterium avium complex syndrome; *MPD,* myeloproliferative disorder.

such as aplastic anemia. This is a favorable factor associated with a lower risk of neutropenic infection, perhaps because some phagocytic capacity is maintained. On the other hand, monocytosis is very common with hematologic dysplasias. In a patient with unexplained cytopenia, monocytosis can be an important clue to an underlying MDS.

Infectious Diseases

Mycobacterial infection is a common cause of monocytosis worldwide related to its propensity for intracellular infection and tissue granuloma formation. Brucellosis and subacute bacterial endocarditis have also been associated with monocytosis. Certain viral infections, such as influenza virus, varicella-zoster, CMV, and Dengue hemorrhagic fever, are reported to cause monocytosis.

Connective Tissue Disorder

Connective tissue disorders, such as SLE and RA, have been reported to be associated with monocytosis in the context of chronic inflammation.

Hematopoietic Malignancies

Monocytosis is common with MDS. CMML is defined as persistent peripheral blood monocytosis greater than 1000/mm^3, absent Philadelphia chromosome, and evidence of dysplasia in one or more hematopoietic cell lineages. Juvenile myelomonocytic leukemia (JMML), a disease of children that shares pathologic features with CMML, results from defective RAS signaling. Acute myeloid leukemias involving the monocyte line (acute myelomonocytic and acute monoblastic leukemias) may release substantial amounts of lysozyme (muramidase), which is toxic to renal tubules. Serum lysozyme has actually been used to aid in the diagnosis of these leukemia subtypes. Other myeloid leukemias and MPDs can cause monocytosis, as can lymphomas, particularly Hodgkin disease.

MONOCYTOPENIA

Monocytopenia frequently accompanies granulocytopenia with chemotherapy, aplastic anemia, or other BM suppressive insults. Isolated or disproportionate monocytopenia is rarely recognized, but observations suggest that this can have serious clinical sequelae when it occurs. In hairy cell leukemia and monoMAC syndrome, there is a clear association with often severe opportunistic infections, particularly those normally engendering a granulomatous response.

Hairy Cell Leukemia

This disorder, considered in detail elsewhere, classically presents with pancytopenia and splenomegaly, most often in middle-aged men. The WBC count may sometimes be high because of hairy cell proliferation, but monocytes are invariably severely depressed. (Monocytopenia is not seen with "variant hairy cell leukemia.") Neutropenia only partly explains the very high infectious morbidity and mortality. An extraordinary incidence of opportunistic granulomatous infections used to be encountered, including atypical mycobacteria, tuberculosis, histoplasmosis, and other fungi. These were linked to the monocytopenia, with demonstration of impaired granuloma formation. With remission induced by modern therapies, (e.g., 2-chlorodeoxyadenosine), the monocytopenia and infectious risks have been abrogated.

MonoMAC Syndrome

In 2010, investigators at the National Institutes of Health described an immunodeficiency syndrome characterized by decreased or absent monocytes, NK cells, B cells, and dendritic cells. This was largely diagnosed in young adults (median age, 33 years). All patients have opportunistic infections, particularly *Mycobacterium avium* complex, and other mycobacteria, opportunistic fungi, and viruses. Both autosomal dominant and sporadic cases are described, all linked to mutations in the hematopoietic stem cell regulator GATA-2. BM examination findings are always abnormal, usually hypocellular, with reticulin fibrosis and multilineage dysplasia. Clonal cytogenetic abnormalities are seen in most patients, particularly deletion 7 and trisomy 8. All cases have met criteria for MDS. Because leukemic progression with or without death from infection is high, stem cell transplantation is recommended when feasible.

SUGGESTED READINGS

Aapro MS, Bohlius J, Cameron DA, et al: 2010 Update of EORTC guidelines for the use of granulocyte-colony stimulating factor to reduce the incidence of chemotherapy-induced febrile neutropenia in adult patients with lymphoproliferative disorders and solid tumours. *Eur J Cancer* 47:8, 2011 Jan.

Akhtari M, Curtis B, Waller E: Autoimmune neutropenia in adults. *Autoimmun Rev* 9:62, 2009.

Aster RH: Adverse drug reactions affecting blood cells. *Handb Exp Pharmacol* 57, 2010.

Bhatt V, Saleem A: Review: Drug-induced neutropenia: Pathophysiology, clinical features and management. *Ann Clin Lab Sci* 34:131, 2004.

Calvo KR, Vinh DC, Maric I, et al: Myelodisplasia in autosomal dominant and sporadic monocytopenia immunodeficiency syndrome: Diagnostic features and clinical implications. *Hematologica* 96:1221, 2011.

Dale DC, Bolyard AA, Schwinzer BG, et al: The severe chronic neutropenia international registry: 10-Year follow-up report. *Support Cancer Ther* 3:220, 2006.

Dale DC, Link DC: The many causes of severe congenital neutropenia. *N Engl J Med* 360:3, 2009.

Donadien J, Fenneteau O, Beaupain B, et al: Congenital neutropenia: Diagnosis, molecular bases and patient management. *Orphanet J Rare Dis* 6:26, 2011.

Freifeld AG, Bow EJ, Sepkowitz KA, et al: Clinical practice guideline for the use of antimicrobial agents in neutropenic patients with cancer: 2010 Update by the Infectious Diseases Society of America. *Clin Infect Dis* 52:e56, 2011.

Gasche C, Reinisch W, Schwarzmeimer JD: Evidence of colony suppressor activity and deficiency of hematopoietic growth factors in hairy cell leukemia. *Hematol Oncol* 11:97, 1993.

Haas P, Straub R, Beoui S, et al: Peripheral but not central leptin treatment increases numbers of circulating NK cells, granulocytes and specific monocyte subpopulations in non-endotoxaemic lean and obese LEW-rats. *Regulatory Peptides* 51:26, 2008.

Herishanu Y, Rogowski O, Polliack A, et al: Leukocytosis in obese individuals: Possible link in patients with unexplained persistent neutrophilia. *Eur J Haematol* 76:516, 2006.

Hsieh MM, Everhart JE, Byrd-Holt DD, et al: Prevalence of neutropenia in the U.S. population: Age, sex, smoking status, and ethnic differences. *Ann Intern Med* 146:486, 2007 Apr 3.

Kroft SH: Infectious diseases manifested in the peripheral blood. *Clin Lab Med* 23:253, 2003.

Marchetti M, Falanga A: Leukocytosis, JAK2V617F mutation, and hemostasis in myeloproliferative disorders. *Pathophysiol Haemost Thromb* 36:148, 2008.

Neureiter D, Kemmerling R, Ocker M, et al: Differential diagnostic challenge of chronic neutrophilic leukemia in a patient with prolonged leukocytosis. *J Hematopathol* 1:23, 2008.

Plo I, Zhang Y, Couedic JL, et al: An activating mutation in the CSF3R gene induces a hereditary chronic neutrophilia. *J Exp Med* 206:1701, 2009.

Rice L, Harris RL, Lynch EC, et al: Utility of peripheral blood changes in discriminating causes of fever and infection. *Blood* 70:94A, 1987.

Rice L, Shenkenberg T, Wheeler T, et al: Opportunistic granulomatous infections in hairy cell leukemia. *Cancer* 49:1924, 1982.

Seshadri RS, Brown EJ, Zipursky A: Leukemic reticuloendotheliosis. A failure of monocyte production. *N Engl J Med* 22295:181, 1977.

Tesfa D, Keisu M, Palmblad J: Idiosyncratic drug-induced agranulocytosis: Possible mechanisms and management. *J Hematol* 84:428, 2009.

Weick JK, Hagedorn AB, Linman JW: Leukoerythroblastosis. Diagnostic and prognostic significance. *Mayo Clin Proc* 49:110, 1974 Feb.

Wolach O, Bairey O, Lahav M: Late-onset neutropenia after rituximab treatment: Case series and comprehensive review of the literature. *Medicine* 89:308, 2010.

CHAPTER 47

LYMPHOCYTOSIS, LYMPHOCYTOPENIA, HYPERGAMMAGLOBULINEMIA, AND HYPOGAMMAGLOBULINEMIA

Martha P. Mims

Any discussion of quantitative abnormalities of lymphocytes and immunoglobulins is necessarily linked because the B-cell compartment is responsible for immunoglobulin production, and the T-cell compartment helps provide the stimulus. Nevertheless, clinicians are often consulted when a quantitative disorder of one or the other is recognized. Thus, although overlapping, the defects are presented separately.

QUANTITATIVE DISORDERS OF LYMPHOCYTES

The normal number and distribution of lymphocyte subtypes in the peripheral blood varies with age, but no careful study has demonstrated gender or ethnic differences in lymphocyte count. In general, circulating T cells exceed B cells by a ratio of approximately four to one with that ratio increasing slightly with age (Table 47-1). Natural killer cells are grouped with lymphocytes but comprise only about 10% of the lymphocyte population. Infants have total lymphocyte counts between 5500 and 7000/μl, but this number declines beginning at about 1 year of age to reach 2000 to 2400/μl in adults. At birth, the total number of circulating B cells is approximately 1000/μl but decreases over the first 10 years of life to approximately 200 to 300/μl by the age of 18 years. A slow decline in circulating B cells continues throughout adulthood and is primarily accounted for by a decline in transitional and naive B cells with a stable or mild increase in circulating memory B-cell numbers with age. Circulating naïve B cells represent about two-thirds of the entire naive B-cell pool, and circulating memory B cells represent only about one third of the entire memory B-cell pool.[1]

T cells dominate the circulating lymphocyte population with approximately 3500/μl in infancy declining to 1500/μl on average in young adults, with even lower numbers (≈1200/μl) in elderly adults. In both children and adults, CD4 cells outnumber CD8 cells. Naive CD4 and CD8 T cells decline with age by two- to fourfold. In one large study, CD4 memory T cells significantly increased with age, but no such trend was seen for CD8 memory T cells.[2]

Against this background, *lymphocytosis* is defined as lymphocyte count greater than 8000/μl in young children and greater than 4000/μl in teenagers and adults. Lymphocytopenia has been defined as a total lymphocyte count of less than 1000/μl. Given the composition of the circulating lymphocyte pool, it is critically important to define which lymphocyte subsets are over- or underrepresented when there is a quantitative disorder.[2]

Lymphocytosis

As in any clinical disorder, a careful history is critical to defining the origin of lymphocytosis. Inherited causes of lymphocytosis are essentially nonexistent (with the exception of some inherited predispositions to clonal lymphoid disorders); thus the issue is usually to determine whether a lymphocyte disorder is clonal/malignant or benign and related to infection, drugs, or physiologic stress. Rarely, neither a malignancy nor an underlying condition can be identified, in which case the lymphocytosis is termed *persistent polyclonal B-cell lymphocytosis*. When an excess of B cells exists, clonality can usually be defined by examining cell surface expression of κ- and λ-light chains using antibody techniques; with T-cell proliferation, it may be important to define clonality by examining T-cell receptor gene rearrangement using molecular procedures. In the case of natural killer (NK) cell disorders, clonality can be quite difficult to determine.

Clonal Disorders

Malignant causes of peripheral blood lymphocytosis are covered in Chapters 76 to 80, 84, and 86 and include chronic lymphocytic leukemia (CLL), hairy cell leukemia, splenic marginal zone lymphoma, lymphoplasmacytic lymphoma, follicular lymphoma, mantle cell lymphoma, adult T-cell leukemia or lymphoma, and Sézary syndrome. Occasionally, precursor T-cell or precursor B-cell leukemia presents with circulating small cells, which morphologically appear more similar to mature lymphocytes than blasts.

A recently identified clonal disorder causing lymphocytosis is monoclonal B-cell lymphocytosis (MBL), an accumulation of clonal B lymphocytes that does not meet the criteria for CLL (>5000 clonal B cells/μl), but is nevertheless defined by the presence of a clonal population of B cells. Data demonstrate that up to 10% to 15% of patients with lymphocytosis have MBL. Three major subtypes of MBL exist: the CLL immunophenotype ($CD5^+$, $CD23^+$), which is by far the most common; the atypical CLL type ($CD5^+$, $CD23^-$); and non-CLL lymphoproliferative disorder ($CD5^-$). Similar to the relationship between monoclonal gammopathy of uncertain significance and multiple myeloma, only a small proportion of patients with MBL (1%-4% per year) with CLL-type MBL go on to develop progressive disease requiring treatment. Epidemiologic studies of MBL patients have demonstrated strong familial risk for CLL, and the first reports of MBL came from studies of "unaffected" CLL family members. Studies of CLL families suggest that there is an inherited abnormality that increases the risk of developing CLL, and some families exhibit anticipation with the disease occurring earlier in successive generations. The supposition that MBL is a progenitor lesion for CLL is strengthened by the observation that 6 of 10 germline single nucleotide polymorphisms known to confer increased risk of CLL are also significantly associated with MBL. MBL has been identified in up to 30% of individuals infected with HCV, and up to 50% of the HCV-associated cases demonstrate the atypical CLL immunophenotype. The presence of MBL correlates with more advanced liver disease, suggesting that the persistence of viral infection is crucial to development of the B-cell clone. Follow-up for MBL patients is not clearly defined, although it is probably reasonable to evaluate lymphocyte counts with complete blood counts and follow the clone with flow cytometry at periodic intervals depending on the pace of the lymphocyte rise, the clinical scenario, the family history, and the age of the patient.[3]

Infectious Causes

The most common infections causing lymphocytosis are Epstein-Barr virus (EBV) and cytomegalovirus (CMV). In young children, EBV infection frequently presents as an upper respiratory infection, but in

Table 47-1 Normal Lymphocyte Subsets with Age*

	Cord Blood	2 Days-11 Months	1-6 Years	7-17 Years	18-70 Years
Total lymphocyte count (× 10^3 cells/ml)	5.4 (4.2-6.9)	4.1 (2.7-5.4)	3.6 (2.9-5.1)	2.4 (2.0-2.7)	2.1 (1.6-2.4)
$CD4^+$T cells (%)	35 (28-42)	41 (38-50)	37 (30-40)	37 (33-41)	42 (38-46)
$CD45Ra^+$ in $CD4^+$ (naive T cells)†	91 (82-97)	81 (66-88)	71 (66-77)	61 (55-67)	40 (32-49)
$CD8^+$ T cells (%)	29 (26-33)	21 (18-25)	29 (25-32)	30 (27-35)	35 (31-40)
B cells (%)	20 (14-23)	23 (19-31)	24 (21-28)	16 (12-22)	13 (11-16)
NK cells (%)	20 (14-30)	11 (8-17)	11 (8-15)	12 (9-16)	14 (10-19)

NK, Natural killer.
*Values are median, with ranges from the 25th to 75th percentiles.
†Naive T cells expressed as a percentage of $CD4^+$ T cells.

adolescents and young adults, it can result in acute glandular fever with pharyngitis, splenomegaly, lymphadenitis, and profound reactive lymphocytosis. Lymphocytosis is less prominent in older adults. Although the B cells are targeted by EBV, the lymphocytosis consists of $CD8^+$ lymphocytes reacting to neoantigens expressed on the surface of infected B cells. The massive T-cell response usually clears the infection in a matter of days to one week, and the lymphocytosis resolves. CMV infection can produce a similar lymphocytosis. In the case of CMV, however, the macrophages are the target of infection, and the T-cell lymphocytosis results from a response to the macrophage neoantigen. CMV infection and lymphocytosis are more common in older adults. In both viral infections, lymphocytosis can be profound with 50% or more of the circulating white blood cells (WBCs) identified as lymphocytes. Examination of the peripheral smear reveals that up to 10% of the circulating lymphocytes are atypical and larger than normal lymphocytes with open chromatin and increased cytoplasm. It is particularly important to recognize lymphocytosis caused by these two viruses in pregnant women because congenital infection can cause fetal death and birth defects. In addition to EBV and CMV, primary infection with HIV can cause lymphocytosis and should be suspected in the presence of a viral syndrome in the proper clinical circumstance. In children, infection with Coxsackie A and B6 viruses, echovirus, and adenovirus can cause a brief but profound lymphocytosis. Infections with other viruses, including human herpesvirus 6 (HHV-6) and HHV-8 as well as rubella virus, varicella, human T-lymphotropic virus type 1 (HTLV-1), and hepatitis viruses, can cause a lymphocytosis, although much less frequently than CMV and EBV.

Important nonviral infections causing lymphocytosis include *Toxoplasma gondii* and *Bordetella pertussis*. In an immune competent host, *Toxoplasma* infection is often asymptomatic, but patients can have fever, chills, and lymphadenopathy. Mild lymphocytosis with atypical lymphocytes can be observed. As in the case of EBV and CMV, infections during pregnancy can lead to adverse effect on the fetus. In children and adults, infection with *B. pertussis* can lead to lymphocytosis with the absolute lymphocyte count frequently greater than 10,000/μl. In more severe cases, lymphocytosis is more pronounced.[4] Unlike viral infections and *Toxoplasma* infection, the lymphocytosis observed in *B. pertussis* infection is caused by increases in all lymphocyte subsets, and it appears that the pertussis toxin blocks migration of the lymphocytes from the bloodstream into lymph nodes.[4] Tuberculosis, rickettsial infection, brucellosis, and shigellosis may also cause lymphocytosis.

Physiologic Stress

Lymphocytosis related to physiologic stress is a poorly studied phenomenon. After strenuous physical exercise, subjects develop lymphocytosis, which returns to preexercise levels within 15 minutes to 1 hour of ceasing the activity. The exercise-induced rise is thought to be attributable to catecholamine and steroid hormones and their effect on expression of cell adhesion molecules and on cardiac output and shear stress.[5] Exposure to catecholamines increases the expression of β_2-adrenergic receptors on lymphocytes influencing cell trafficking. Reports suggest that a number of other physiologic stresses increase lymphocyte counts, including surgery, trauma, cardiac conditions, sickle cell crises, abdominal pain, and obstetric emergencies. In these cases, all lymphocyte subsets appear to increase, but the increase is most profound for CD4 and CD8 memory T cells. Neutrophil counts also rise in these patients, but in most cases, the lymphocytosis resolves before the peak of the neutrophil count.[6]

Drug Reactions

Drug-induced lymphocytosis can occur as part of a hypersensitivity syndrome. In these cases, the lymphocytosis is usually part of a systemic condition that includes a fever, rash, and lymphadenopathy. Elevation in other WBC counts, including eosinophils and monocytes, is common, and atypical lymphocytes are seen. The time period between drug introduction and the syndrome is usually about 3 weeks with the commonest implicated drugs being aromatic anticonvulsants and sulfonamides.[7] Some studies differentiate this syndrome from drug-induced cutaneous pseudolymphomas in which collections of nonclonal lymphocytes appear in the skin after longer periods of drug exposure, but there is no peripheral lymphocytosis.

Polyclonal B-Cell Lymphocytosis

A final entity causing lymphocytosis is persistent polyclonal B-cell lymphocytosis (PPBL). This rare disorder is seen primarily in young to middle-aged smoking women and results in mild polyclonal lymphocytosis. The lymphocytes are medium sized with abundant cytoplasm; a variable proportion is binucleate. A polyclonal increase in serum immunoglobulin M (IgM) is also observed, and there is an association with the human leukocyte antigen (HLA) DR7 phenotype. Examination of the B cells reveals that most are $CD19^+$, $CD5^-$, and $CD23^-$ with a normal kappa-to-lambda ratio and a variety of heavy chain rearrangements. Adenopathy, hepatomegaly, or splenomegaly has been observed in some, but not all, patients. Genetic analysis has demonstrated the presence of isochromosome 3q in a proportion of B cells as well as the presence of multiple *BCL2-Ig* gene rearrangements. Similar gene rearrangements have been identified in family members of PPBL patients along with increases in serum IgM, suggesting that there may be an underlying genetic defect. Cessation of smoking does not appear to resolve the lymphocytosis. Overall, the clinical course of this disorder is benign, and the lymphocytosis is not usually progressive; however, clonal B-cell disorders have been seen in a few patients with the disorder, suggesting that it may represent a preneoplastic state.[8]

Lymphocytopenia

Inherited Disorders

Although there are few, if any, inherited causes of lymphocytosis, such is not the case for lymphocytopenia, in which the genetic bases of a number of inherited immunodeficiency disorders have been identified. Chief among these disorders is severe combined immunodeficiency (SCID), which is characterized by the absence of functional T lymphocytes. T lymphocytes, B lymphocytes, and NK cells share progenitors, signaling pathways in development and function, and metabolic pathways; thus B lymphocytes, NK cells, or both are often severely affected in SCID. Moreover, in the absence of functional $CD4^+$ T-helper lymphocytes, B lymphocytes cannot function properly, and hypo- or agammaglobulinemia is observed. In most cases of SCID, the absence of T lymphocytes leads to an extremely low absolute lymphocyte count. As detailed in Chapter 49, SCID can be grouped based on the cellular pathway that is affected. In general, whereas SCID is characterized by complete loss of function of the affected gene, hypomorphic mutations of the same genes lead to quite different phenotypes (Omenn syndrome and atypical SCID). Defects in more than 30 genes are known to lead to SCID. Inheritance is primarily X-linked or autosomal recessive, but in a few cases, such as the DiGeorge anomaly and some cases of Hoyeraal-Hreidarsson syndrome (defects in telomerase), inheritance is autosomal dominant. Deficiency in cytokine-mediated signaling (*IL2RG, JAK3,* and *IL7RA* mutations) leads to T^-B^+ SCID, defects in V(D)J recombination (*RAG1, RAG2 DCLRE1C, PRKDC, LIG4, and NHEJ1* mutations) leads to T^-B^- SCID, and absent signaling through the pre-T cell receptor (*CD3D, CD3E, CD3Z, CD3G, PRPRC, ZAP70, LCK* mutations) leads to T^-B^+ SCID. Defects that lead to increased lymphocyte apoptosis (*AK2, ADA,* and *PNP* gene mutations) lead to TB^- SCID and are often associated with anomalies outside of the immune system. Defects in thymic embryogenesis and calcium flux as well as a collection of other abnormalities, including defects in telomerase activity, can also lead to SCID and are usually associated with abnormalities of other organ systems.[9]

In addition to SCID, other inherited disorders can also perturb T- and B-cell numbers. Patients with Wiskott-Aldrich syndrome, caused by mutations in *WASP* (which encodes a cytoplasmic protein responsible for transducing cell surface signals to the actin cytoskeleton), can present with low T-cell counts early in life and become profoundly lymphopenic over time. Abnormalities in immunoglobulins are also noted in this syndrome with low levels of IgM and high levels of IgA and IgE.[10] Immunodeficiency affects more than half of all patients with ataxia telangiectasia. Patients with ataxia telangiectasia have homozygous or compound heterozygous mutations in the *ATM* gene, which encodes a protein kinase with functions in the cellular response to DNA damage. Lymphopenia, especially of naive CD4 cells, is observed in about half of patients with ataxia telangiectasia with mutations leading to absent expression of ATM kinase activity.[11] Recently, a new syndrome known as monoMAC has been described.[12] Affected patients demonstrate monocytopenia; B-cell and NK-cell lymphopenia; and mycobacterial, fungal, and viral infections and alveolar proteinosis. Over time, monoMAC patients develop myelodysplasia, acute myeloid leukemia (AML), or chronic myelomonocytic leukemia (CMML). Studies indicate that this disorder is caused by mutations in *GATA2*, which appears to regulate features of monocyte, macrophage, dendritic cell, B-cell, and NK-cell development and function.

Infections

A variety of viral and nonviral infections can lead to lymphopenia. HIV is most common virus associated with lymphopenia. The target of HIV is the CD4 receptor, and the virus selectively targets and infects activated expanding CD4 T cells. Large studies in HIV-infected patients have shown that peripheral blood CD4 T-cell counts fall most rapidly in the year after seroconversion (from ≈1000/μl before seroconversion to 670/μl at 1 year after infection) and then decline more slowly by about 50/μl per year.[13] In a subset of untreated patients, viremia is absent or well controlled, and lymphocytopenia develops very slowly if at all; particular HLA class I alleles are overrepresented in this group. Lymphopenia is an early and reliable laboratory observation in adult influenza A infection and is also detected in infections caused by swine influenza (H1N1) and the highly pathogenic avian influenza (H5N1).[14] Lymphopenia has been reported in patients with severe acute respiratory syndrome (SARS) caused by the SARS-coronavirus. In children, respiratory syncytial virus (RSV) infection is associated with a reduction in lymphocyte count, which is most extreme in the sickest patients; similar effects on lymphocyte counts are seen in measles infections (also a paramyxovirus). In West Nile virus encephalitis, lymphopenia is profound and prolonged, and the initial degree of lymphopenia is predictive of outcome. A variety of other viruses can also cause lymphopenia, including herpes viruses (herpes simplex, HHV-6, HHV-8), parvovirus B19, and Dengue virus. In many viral infections, the degree of lymphopenia is correlated with the severity of the disease.[14]

A variety of nonviral infections cause lymphopenia. Infections with *Ehrlichia* (a tickborne obligate intracellular gram negative bacteria), *Salmonella typhi*, and *Leptospira* have all been reported to cause lymphocytopenia during the acute illness. $CD4^+$ T-cell depletion has been described in a subset of HIV-negative patients with tuberculosis and low albumin levels, low body weight, and more extensive disease. Recovery of CD4 count after treatment of tuberculosis suggests that the lymphopenia is caused by the tuberculosis infection.[15] Lymphocytopenia is often observed in sepsis and is thought to occur as a result of cytokine-mediated apoptosis of B cells and $CD4^+$ T cells. In fact, autopsy series have demonstrated that most deaths from sepsis occur during the prolonged hypoimmune state, and the more prolonged the sepsis, the more profound the loss of splenic lymphocytes. Retrospective studies of emergency department patients suggest that lymphopenia is a better predictor of bacteremia than leukocyte count, neutrophil count, or C-reactive protein level.[16]

Collagen Vascular Disorders

Autoimmune diseases frequently exhibit decreases in circulating lymphocytes. In systemic lupus erythematosus (SLE), lymphopenia (usually decreases in T cells but occasionally in B cells as well) is not only one of the diagnostic criteria but also a parameter used to assess disease activity. Lymphopenia in SLE seems to be more frequent in patients of African descent. Deficient expression of CD55 and CD59 has been observed in SLE-induced lymphopenia, and data suggest that acquired deficiency of these complement regulatory molecules may contribute to the destruction of lymphocytes. Antigalectin 8 antibodies have been described in patients with SLE, rheumatoid arthritis, and sepsis. In SLE, these autoantibodies are associated with lymphopenia.[17] CD4-T cells may also be decreased in rheumatoid arthritis, and increasing evidence suggests that deficiencies in DNA repair enzymes such as ATM render rheumatoid arthritis T cells sensitive to apoptosis.[18] Apoptotic loss of naive T cells results in lymphopenia-induced proliferation to preserve T-cell homeostasis; this proliferation is now thought to lead to both premature immune aging and an autoimmune-biased T-cell repertoire. In Sjögren syndrome, a minority of patients has been noted to have deficient CD4 counts, and this has been correlated with the presence of anti-CD4 antibodies. Similarly, low lymphocyte counts have been observed in patients with primary vasculitides, type I diabetes, and Crohn's disease.[17]

Malignancies

Lymphopenia is found in a variety of systemic illnesses; chief among them are cancers. In hematologic malignancies, including Hodgkin lymphoma, diffuse large B-cell lymphoma, and peripheral T-cell lymphoma, patients with lymphopenia have a worse prognosis.

Lymphopenia has also been observed in solid tumors, including breast and colon cancer, and soft tissue sarcomas, in which its presence before treatment predicts decreased overall survival. Which specific lymphocyte subsets are involved and the cause(s) of lymphopenia in these tumor types has not been described.

Systemic Disorders

End-stage renal disease (ESRD) has also been associated with lymphopenia, an observation not thought to be exclusively attributable to an effect of dialysis alone. Naive and central memory CD4 and CD8 T cells are significantly reduced in the blood of ESRD patients apparently because of increased susceptibility of these cells to apoptosis. Lymphopenia occurs in more than 50% of sarcoidosis patients and is associated with chronic disease. Sarcoidosis patients with severe organ system involvement, including neurologic, cardiac, ocular, and advanced pulmonary disease, have lower lymphocyte counts than patients with less severe manifestations. Older studies suggest that burn victims have profound decreases in T-cell counts, which may contribute to the infection risk in these patients. Interestingly, lymphopenia is a characteristic of both protein-energy malnutrition and zinc deficiency. Both of these deficiencies perturb the hypothalamic-pituitary-adrenocorticoid axis and increase glucocorticoid levels, which results in increased apoptosis of B and T cells.[19] Intestinal lymphangiectasia, which may be either congenital or secondary to processes that obstruct lymphatic drainage of the gastrointestinal tract, can cause lymphopenia because of loss of lymph fluid into the gut along with lymphocytes.

A rare cause of lymphopenia is idiopathic $CD4^+$ lymphocytopenia (ICL), which is defined as a CD4 count less than 200/μl or less than 20% of the T-cell count on two occasions that is not caused by HIV (or HTLV) infection, drug therapy, or a known immunodeficiency. Patients usually come to clinical notice when they present with opportunistic infections. CD4 T-cell counts typically remain low, but counts do not continue to drop or do not fall rapidly after diagnosis. In one large series, only about 20% of patients recovered from lymphopenia within 3 years of diagnosis. Opportunistic infections plague these patients, and autoimmune diseases occur both before and after the diagnosis of ICL. In ICL, unlike HIV infection, increased activation and turnover are observed in CD4 but not CD8 T lymphocytes.[20]

Drug Effects

A number of drugs are known to cause lymphopenia. Glucocorticoids inhibit production of a number of cytokines and rapidly deplete circulating T cells by enhancing emigration from the circulation, inducing apoptosis, interfering with growth signaling, and inhibiting release from lymphoid tissues. B cells are less affected acutely by glucocorticoid administration, but prolonged administration may result in decreased IgG levels. Antimetabolite chemotherapeutic agents such as methotrexate, azathioprine, and 6-mercaptopurine lower lymphocyte as well as neutrophil counts, and alkylating agents such as cyclophosphamide have more profound effects on lymphocytes. Purine nucleoside analogs, including cladribine, fludarabine, pentostatin, nelarabine, clofarabine, and others, inhibit DNA synthesis and repair and cause accumulation of DNA strand breaks. All of these agents are associated with profound lymphopenia, which may persist for several years after completion of treatment. In general, T cells are more affected than B cells. Nelarabine in particular is a prodrug of ara-G and is converted to ara-GTP that accumulates at higher levels in T cells.[21]

Monoclonal and polyclonal antibodies directed against lymphocytes are useful in clinical practice and can induce profound and long-lasting lymphopenia. Whereas antithymocyte globulin and alemtuzumab produce depletion of both T and B cells, the monoclonal antibodies OKT3, daclizumab, and basiliximab produce a more pronounced decrease in T cells. The drugs rituximab and ofatumumab are monoclonal antibodies directed against distinct epitopes on B cells. These drugs deplete peripheral B cells but do not routinely produce lymphopenia.

Finally, radiation exposure commonly results in lymphopenia, which occurs before depression of other cell counts. In fact, lymphopenia can develop within the first 24 hours of exposure if the dose of radiation is great enough, and a drop of 50% or more predicts an increased risk of death. B cells are more sensitive to radiation than T cells and recover more slowly than T-cell numbers.[22]

QUANTITATIVE DISORDERS OF IMMUNOGLOBULINS

In practice, there are several methods for determining serum immunoglobulin levels; thus in evaluating immunoglobulin levels, it is critical that age-adjusted normal reference ranges are provided by the laboratory. Children first achieve adult levels of IgM around 2 years of age, of IgG by 6 years of age, and of IgA during puberty. Hypogammaglobulinemia is defined as an IgG less than 2 standard deviations from normal, and agammaglobulinemia is usually defined as an IgG level less than 100 mg/dL. Low levels of IgA, IgG, and IgM are characteristic of most forms of SCID.

Hypogammaglobulinemia

Causes of hypogammaglobulinemia can be divided into primary causes related to genetic deficiencies and secondary causes related to malignancies or their treatment, infections, medications, and protein-losing states that deplete antibody.

Secondary Causes

Before embarking on a search for a primary disorder causing hypogammaglobulinemia, it is important to rule out secondary causes. Malnutrition, malabsorption, and any disease state in which large amounts of protein are lost, such as nephrotic range proteinuria, severe burns, lymphangiectasia, or protein-losing enteropathy, can overwhelm the capacity of the B cells to provide adequate immunoglobulin to maintain normal serum levels. Aside from chemotherapeutic agents, a number of medications can produce hypogammaglobulinemia; these include captopril, antiseizure medications (carbamazepine, phenytoin), gold salts, antimalarials, fenoclofenac, penicillamine, and sulfasalazine, as well as glucocorticoids. Infection with HIV and EBV and congenital infection with rubella, CMV, and *T. gondii* can produce very low immunoglobulin levels and should be ruled out as appropriate. A host of lymphoid malignancies produce hypogammaglobulinemia, but the defect is most profound in CLL, in which up to 85% of patients are said to possess hypogammaglobulinemia even in the absence of treatment.[23]

Primary Immunodeficiencies

The International Union of Immunological Societies has classified the primary immunodeficiency diseases into eight groups, including one class called *predominantly antibody deficiencies.* These disorders present in both adults and children, although some are very rare. Table 47-2 provides a simple grouping of these antibody disorders, some of which are discussed in greater detail in Chapter 49.

The first group is characterized by a severe reduction in all serum immunoglobulin isotypes with absence or profound reduction in B cells. Patients with these disorders, particularly those with a well-defined genetic basis, present with severe bacterial infections, most commonly in the respiratory tract (pneumonia, sinusitis, otitis media) as well as diarrhea caused by bacteria, parasites, and viruses. The prototypic member of this group is X-linked agammaglobulinemia (XLA) caused by a mutation in the Bruton tyrosine kinase (*Btk*) gene, which produces a block in B-cell maturation. Female carriers of *Btk*

Table 47-2 Predominant Antibody Deficiencies

	Disease	Mode of Inheritance/Genetic Locus	Clinical Features
Severe reduction in all serum immunoglobulin isotypes with absent B cells	Bruton tyrosine kinase deficiency	XL/Xq21.3-22	Severe bacterial infections (especially of the respiratory tract), absent lymphoid tissue
	μ Heavy chain deficiency	AR/14q32.3	Severe bacterial infections
	λ5 deficiency	AR/22q11.21	Severe bacterial infections
	Igα deficiency	AR/19q13.2	Severe bacterial infections
	Igβ deficiency	AR/17q23	Severe bacterial infections
	BLNK deficiency	AR/10q23.2	Severe bacterial infections
	Thymoma with immunodeficiency (Good syndrome)	None	Recurrent infection with encapsulated bacteria and diarrhea, autoimmune phenomena
	Myelodysplasia	Variable/monosomy 7, trisomy 8, dyskeratosis congenita	Recurrent infections and pancytopenia
Severe reduction in at least two serum immunoglobulin isotypes with low or normal B-cell numbers	Common variable immunodeficiency syndromes	≈10% with family history AR or AD AD and AR/17p11.2 AR/22q13	Recurrent respiratory tract infections leading to chronic sinusitis, hearing loss, bronchiectasis, autoimmune disease, lymphoproliferation, malignancy (especially non-Hodgkin lymphoma and gastric carcinoma)
	TACI alterations	Unk/6p22.1-p21.3	
	BAFFR alterations		
	MSH5 alterations		
	ICOS deficiency	AR/2q33	Recurrent infections
	CD19 deficiency	AR/16p11.2	Recurrent infections
	X-linked lymphoproliferative disease (mutation in SH2 domain protein 1A)	XL/Xq25-q26	Fulminant infection with EBV, lymphoma, dysgammaglobulinemia
Severe reduction in serum IgG and IgA with increased IgM and normal B-cell numbers (disorders of immunoglobulin class switching)	CD40 ligand deficiency	XL/Xq26.3-Xq27.1	Recurrent infections with bacteria and opportunistic pathogens, neutropenia, autoimmune disease
	CD40 deficiency	AR/20q11-20q13.2	Recurrent infections with bacteria and opportunistic pathogens, neutropenia, autoimmune disease
	NF-κB essential modulator (*NEMO*) hypomorphic mutations	XL/Xq28	Recurrent infections with bacteria and opportunistic pathogens, neutropenia, autoimmune disease
	AID deficiency	AR/12p13	Recurrent bacterial infections and diarrhea, marked enlargement of lymphoid organs
	UNG deficiency	AR/12q23-q24.1	Recurrent bacterial infections and diarrhea, marked enlargement of lymphoid organs
Isotype or light-chain deficiencies with normal B-cell numbers	Ig heavy-chain deficiency	AR/14q32	Most patients are healthy
	κ-Chain deficiency	AR/2p11.2	Most patients are healthy
	Isolated IgG subclass deficiency	Variable/unknown	Most patients are healthy
	IgA deficiency associated with IgG subclass deficiency	Variable/unknown	Most patients are healthy
	Selective IgA deficiency	Variable/unknown	Most patients asymptomatic, but increased prevalence of infections, autoimmune disease, atopy, and celiac disease
Specific antibody deficiency with normal immunoglobulin level and B-cell number	Inability to make antibodies to specific antigens	Variable/unknown	Recurrent sinopulmonary infection, bronchiectasis, diarrhea, autoimmune disease
Transient hypogammaglobulinemia of infancy	IgG and IgA deficiency	Variable/unknown	More likely to be male (60%–80%), mild infections and diarrhea, atopy

λ5, immunoglobulin lambda-like polypeptide (a surrogate light chain subunit that is part of the pre–B-cell receptor); *AID,* activation induced cytidine deaminase (thought to be essential for initiation of the DNA cleavage required for class switch recombination and somatic hypermutation); *BAFF-R,* B cell–activating factor receptor; *BLNK,* B linker (a cytoplasmic linker or adaptor protein that plays a critical role in B-cell development); *EBV,* Epstein-Barr virus; *ICOS,* inducible T-cell costimulator (belongs to CD28 family of costimulatory surface molecules); *Igα,* immunoglobulin-associated α (necessary for expression and function of the B-cell antigen receptor); *Igβ,* immunoglobulin-associated β (necessary for expression and function of the B-cell antigen receptor); *MSH5,* mutS homolog 5 (a protein involved with DNA mismatch repair and meiotic recombination); *NF-κB,* nuclear factor kappa-B; *TACI,* transmembrane activator and CAML-interactor; *UNG,* uracil DNA glycosylase (allows creation of single-stranded breaks essential to class switch recombination and somatic hypermutation).

mutation are generally asymptomatic, but most boys with XLA come to clinical attention by the age of 1 year. In addition to low-serum immunoglobulins, a clue to the diagnosis is the absence of lymphoid tissue, including tonsils. Autosomal recessive mutations in the μ heavy chain as well as defects in *λ5, Igα, Igβ,* and *BLNK* produce a similar phenotype. In a small percentage of patients, no clear molecular defect can be identified. Also included in this group are thymoma with immunodeficiency (Good syndrome) and myelodysplasia. Good syndrome is a poorly understood disorder that presents primarily in middle-aged adults. Immunodeficiency can precede or follow the diagnosis of thymoma and does not resolve with thymectomy. In addition to infections, patients experience autoimmune phenomena, including myasthenia gravis, immune thrombocytopenia purpura, pure red blood cell aplasia, and pernicious anemia. Myelodysplastic syndromes can also mimic XLA and generally present with low B cells and pancytopenia with monosomy 7, trisomy 8, or dyskeratosis congenita.[24]

A second group is characterized by severe reduction of at least two serum immunoglobulin isotypes with normal or low numbers of B cells. Most patients in this group can be categorized as having common variable immune deficiency (CVID), a heterogenous disorder characterized by recurrent infection and failure to make antibody to vaccine antigens. Both males and females are affected, and patients can have autoimmune and gastrointestinal disease as well as lymphoproliferative disorders. Autoimmune disease can precede the hypogammaglobulinemia. About 10% of patients with a CVID phenotype have a family history of immunodeficiency and can be shown to have mutations in one of five genes expressed on both T and B cells. Homozygous or compound heterozygous mutations in *ICOS* (inducible costimulator), which is expressed on activated T cells and plays a role in activating T-helper cells and providing B-cell help, and *CD19*, a B-cell surface molecule that participates in signaling after antigen binding to the B-cell receptor, have been shown to result in recurrent infections in childhood and hypogammaglobulinemia. Mutations in *TACI* (transmembrane activator and CAML-interactor) and *BAFF-R* (B cell–activating factor receptor) members of the tumor necrosis factor receptor superfamily, which play roles in B-cell survival and antibody production, and *MSH5*, a mismatch repair gene, are thought to predispose to CVID and IgA deficiency but are not sufficient to independently cause their onset. X-linked lymphoproliferative syndrome caused by mutation in the signaling lymphocyte activation molecular-associated protein SAP (gene, *SH2D1A*) can present atypically or later in life with a CVID phenotype.[25]

Class switch recombination defects encompass a third group of antibody deficiencies and result in hyper-IgM syndrome characterized by reductions in serum IgG and IgA with normal or elevated IgM. Mutations in the gene for CD40 ligand make up about 30% of these syndromes. CD40L on the surface of T cells interacts with CD40 on B cells, which is required for immunoglobulin class switching, and CD40 on monocytes, which is required for T-cell response. Patients with *CD40L* mutations and rarer mutations in *CD40* itself and in nuclear factor kappa-B (NF-κB) essential modulator (*NEMO*) required for CD40-induced signaling have combined antibody and cellular immune deficits, resulting in hypogammaglobulinemia and recurrent bacterial infection as well as opportunistic infections with organisms similar to those observed in acquired immune deficiency syndrome. Defects in the activation-induced cytidine deaminase gene (*AID*) produce hypogammaglobulinemia with recurrent bacterial infections and diarrhea as well as enlarged lymphoid organs filled with proliferating B cells. A similar clinical picture is produced by homozygous defects in uracil-DNA glycosylase (*UNG*). AID is thought to deaminate cytosine to uracil, and UNG subsequently deglycosylates and removes the uracil residue, creating an abasic site, which allows for creation of single-stranded DNA breaks. Deficiencies in these enzymes result in defective class switching and somatic hypermutation. Patients with similar phenotypes but without defects in *AID* or *UNG* have been described and probably have mutations in other essential genes involved in class switching.[26]

Additional groups of antibody deficiencies exist in which overall antibody levels are normal, but there are defects in specific isotypes, light chains, or specific antibodies with normal numbers of B cells; the majority of patients with these deficiencies are healthy. The commonest member of these groups is selective IgA deficiency, which occurs in about one in 500 whites. The molecular mechanisms underlying this deficiency are unknown, but there is an association with CVID. Finally, an entity termed *transient hypogammaglobulinemia of infancy* has been described in which the normal decline in immunoglobulins after maternal transfer is prolonged. This entity is poorly understood and usually affects boys who have mild infections and diarrhea. Recovery usually, but not always, occurs by 3 years of age.[27]

Hypergammaglobulinemia

Hypergammaglobulinemia results from an overproduction of immunoglobulins by plasma cells, either monoclonal and reflective of a plasma cell or lymphoproliferative disorder or polyclonal and accompanying other disease states. The distinction between polyclonal and monoclonal disorders is made by inspection of the serum protein electrophoretic pattern. Detection of one or several monoclonal bands within a polyclonal background is not unusual, and the literature suggests that small bands frequently disappear and do not become clinically relevant. No data are available to suggest that polyclonal gammopathy drives development of monoclonal gammopathy; however, if a clonal plasmaproliferative disorder is suspected, immunofixation or immunoelectrophoresis should be performed.

Disorders Producing Polyclonal Gammopathy

Polyclonal gammopathy usually reflects one of five major disorders, including liver disease, connective tissue disorders, infections, hematologic disorders, and solid tumors.[28] Interleukin-6 (IL-6) and IL-10 have been implicated in polyclonal gammopathy as have defects in T cells and chronic antigenic stimulation, but the exact sequence of events leading to polyclonal B-cell activation is not known. In general, treatment is directed at the underlying disease, but there are reports of polyclonal gammopathy leading to symptomatic hyperviscosity. In these cases, plasmapheresis and/or corticosteroids seem to be effective. It should also be noted that polyclonal elevations in serum immunoglobulins can sometimes interfere with the direct Coombs test, possibly via nonspecific antibody binding to red blood cells. The degree of gamma globulin elevation does not seem to be helpful in defining the underlying disease state.

In the largest recent review of polyclonal gammopathy, the majority of patients had liver disease, which covered the spectrum from autoimmune disorders (autoimmune hepatitis, primary biliary cirrhosis, primary sclerosing cholangitis) to viral hepatitis and alcoholic liver disease. In fact, elevation of serum gamma globulins is a distinguishing characteristic of autoimmune hepatitis, and the levels usually correlate with activity of disease. The commonest etiology for polyclonal gammopathy related to liver disease in the United States is likely infection with hepatitis C, but in any particular clinical setting, the exact distribution likely depends on the population demographic. Other diseases affecting the liver such as α-1 antitrypsin deficiency and hemochromatosis are also accompanied by increases in serum immunoglobulins.

Connective tissue diseases, including Sjögren syndrome, SLE, ankylosing spondylitis, and rheumatoid arthritis, are also accompanied by polyclonal gammopathy. In many of these diseases, the degree of gamma globulin elevation may reflect disease activity, although a causative link between the autoimmune phenomena and immunoglobulin levels has not been determined. Several of the periodic fever syndromes, which are sometimes classified with the connective tissue disorders, have elevated immunoglobulin levels as a part of their manifestations. Hyperimmunoglobulinemia D is one such syndrome and is linked to mutations in the mevalonate kinase gene. Patients with this disorder present in the first year of life with febrile attacks, lymphadenopathy, abdominal symptoms, arthritis, and oral and genital ulcers. The hallmark finding is elevated levels of polyclonal

IgD often accompanied by elevated IgA levels. Tumor necrosis factor receptor 1–associated periodic syndrome (TRAPS) results from mutation in the gene for the TNF receptor 1 (*TNRF1*) and can cause prolonged febrile attacks with abdominal pain, arthralgias, and myalgias. During attacks, polyclonal elevation of immunoglobulins (primarily IgA) is observed.[29]

Infections, usually chronic in nature, are frequently accompanied by polyclonal gammopathy. HIV infection is a common cause, and immunoglobulin levels tend to increase slowly until the diagnosis of AIDS and then decline over the ensuing 6 to 18 months. Polyclonal gammopathy can be a clue to occult infections such as subacute bacterial endocarditis, tuberculosis, perinephric abscess, Lyme disease, and a variety of parasitic infections.

Malignant B- and T-cell disorders can cause polyclonal hypergammaglobulinemia. These diseases include CLL; large granular lymphocytic leukemia; hairy cell leukemia; and angioimmunoblastic T-cell lymphoma (AITL), a rare disease characterized by rash, widespread lymphadenopathy and extranodal involvement, autoimmune phenomena, and polyclonal gammopathy. Interestingly, despite the elevated levels of immunoglobulins observed in AITL, patients exhibit immunodeficiency and a propensity to develop opportunistic infections. Patients with myeloid disorders can also have polyclonal gammopathies; in one large series, nearly 40% of patients with myelodysplastic syndrome had hypergammaglobulinemia, and patients with immunologic abnormalities had inferior survival.[30] The incidence of hypergammaglobulinemia is reported to approach 50% in CMML. Hypergammaglobulinemia has been reported in AML both in adults and children, but it appears to be a rare phenomenon. Among solid tumors, ovarian and hepatocellular cancers are the commonest associated with polyclonal gammopathy. There are case reports of cancers, particularly lung and breast tumors, producing and releasing the secretory component of IgA into the bloodstream with the binding of SC to polyclonal IgA, producing hypergammaglobulinemia of serum sIgA.[30]

A variety of other diseases, including asbestos exposure and several subtypes of hypersensitivity pneumonitis and idiopathic interstitial pneumonia, are associated with polyclonal gammopathy. In general, these disorders represent diffuse activation of B cells.

Table 47-3 Diseases Associated With Monoclonal Gammopathy

Category	Disease	Comment
Plasma cell and related disorders	MGUS	See Chapters 85 to 87
	Solitary plasmacytoma:	
	Bone	
	Soft tissue	
	Multiple myeloma	
	Waldenström macroglobulinemia	
	Primary amyloidosis (AL)	
Lymphoid disorders	Non-Hodgkin lymphoma	Monoclonal protein observed in CLL (>20% of cases with IgM, ≈50% with IgG, light chains also observed), extranodal marginal zone lymphomas (>30% of cases and correlated with BM involvement), follicular, mantle cell, and diffuse large B-cell lymphomas also reported with serum M proteins as has AITL
	Hodgkin lymphoma	Rare but reported
	Castleman disease	<2% with monoclonal gammopathy
Other hematologic disorders	Acquired von Willebrand disease	IVIG more effective than factor concentrate in increasing factor VIII coagulant and VWF levels
	Gaucher disease	Observed in 25% in one study; M protein declined after splenectomy
	Pernicious anemia, pure RBC aplasia, hereditary spherocytosis, MPD, MDS	
Connective tissue disorders	SLE	IgG, IgM, and IgA have been observed, no difference in disease activity or outcome
	Inclusion body myositis	80% with IgG M protein
	Polymyositis, RA, scleroderma	
Neurologic disorders	POEMS syndrome	Most have M-protein of λ light chain
	Peripheral neuropathy	Most common is IgM followed by IgG and IgA In half, IgM protein binds to myelin-associated glycoprotein Size of M protein not correlated with severity of neuropathy Some benefit from plasma exchange for those with IgG and IgA Fludarabine and rituximab with some benefit for IgM
	Myasthenia gravis, ALS, Alzheimer disease	
Dermatologic disorders	Schnitzler syndrome	Neutrophilic urticarial dermatitis, monoclonal IgM protein and two of: lymphadenopathy, fever, hepatosplenomegaly, joint pain, increased ESR, increased neutrophils, or abnormal bone imaging
	Scleredema	
	Pyoderma gangrenosum	Frequently an IgA protein
Infections	HIV	Both IgG and IgM M proteins observed
	HCV	M protein present in up to 10% of patients
Immunosuppression	Renal transplant	In children CMV infection associated with M protein
	Liver and heart transplant	Most patients with posttransplant lymphoproliferative disorders have M proteins
	BM transplant	Observed in both autologous and allogeneic transplants Appearance of M protein correlated with GVHD

AITL, Angioimmunoblastic T-cell lymphoma; *ALS,* amyotrophic lateral sclerosis; *BM,* bone marrow; *CLL,* chronic lymphocytic leukemia; *CMV,* cytomegalovirus; *ESR,* erythrocyte sedimentation rate; *GVHD,* graft-versus-host disease; *HCV,* hepatitis C virus; *Ig,* immunoglobulin; *IVIG,* intravenous immunoglobulin; *MGUS,* monoclonal gammopathy of uncertain significance; *MPD,* myeloproliferative disorder; *POEMS,* polyneuropathy, organomegaly, endocrinopathy, monoclonal gammopathy, and skin changes; *RA,* rheumatoid arthritis; *RBC,* red blood cell; *SLE,* systemic lupus erythematosus.

Disorders Producing Monoclonal Gammopathy

The differential diagnosis of monoclonal gammopathy includes monoclonal gammopathy of undetermined significance (MGUS), multiple myeloma, solitary plasmacytoma of bone or extramedullary plasmacytoma, Waldenström macroglobulinemia, lymphoma, CLL, and primary systemic amyloidosis. These individual disorders are described elsewhere in this text; however, there are a few points to be made about the M protein itself and MGUS. These disorders can produce intact immunoglobulins (IgG, IgM, IgD, or IgE), κ- or λ-light chains alone or in combination with intact immunoglobulins and rarely heavy chains only. The monoclonal protein is usually detected as a discrete band in the γ or β region in serum or urine protein electrophoresis (M spike) and then characterized and confirmed by immunofixation electrophoresis (IFE). Monoclonal antibodies have been associated with a wide variety of bacterial antigens as well as various antigens, including thyroglobulin, von Willebrand factor, and lactate dehydrogenase; however, for most M proteins, the antigen is not recognized. A variety of other disorders are also associated with an M protein (Table 47-3), including connective tissue disorders, neurologic disorders (including POEMS [polyneuropathy, organomegaly, endocrinopathy, monoclonal gammopathy, and skin changes] syndrome), renal disorders, and some infections such as hepatitis C and HIV. Patients undergoing bone marrow and solid organ transplants in which there is immune suppression are also occasionally observed to have M proteins, but these are usually transient and disappear with recovery of the immune system. Acquired immune disorders such as acquired C1 inhibitor deficiency, type 2 acquired angioedema, and acquired von Willebrand syndrome have also been associated with M proteins.

REFERENCES

1. Morbach H, Eichhorn EM, Liese JG, et al: Reference values for B cell subpopulations from infancy to adulthood. *Clin Exp Immunol* 162:271, 2010.
2. Erkeller-Yuksel FM, Deneys V, Hulstaert F, et al: Age-related changes in human blood lymphocyte subpopulations. *J Pediatr* 120:216, 1992.
3. Lanasa MC, Weinberg JB: Immunologic aspects of monoclonal B-cell lymphocytosis. *Immunol Res* 49:269, 2011.
4. Hudnall SD, Molina CP: Marked increase in L-selectin-negative T cells in neonatal pertussis: The lymphocytosis explained? *Am J Clin Pathol* 114:35, 2000.
5. Walsh NP, Gleeson M, Shephard RJ, et al: Position statement. Part one: Immune function and exercise. *Exerc Immunol Rev* 17:6, 2011.
6. Karandikar NJ, Hotchkiss EC, McKenna RW, et al: Transient stress lymphocytosis: An immunophenotypic characterization of the most common cause of newly identified adult lymphocytosis in a tertiary hospital. *Am J Clin Pathol* 117:819, 2002.
7. Choi TS, Doh KS, Kim SH, et al: Clinicopathological and genotypic aspects of anticonvulsant-induced pseudolymphoma syndrome. *Br J Derm* 148:730, 2003.
8. Cornet E, Lesesve JF, Mossafa H: Long-term follow-up of 111 patients with persistent polyclonal B-cell lymphocytosis with binucleated lymphocytes. *Leukemia* 23:419, 2009.
9. Kalman L, Lindegren ML, Kobrynski L, et al: Mutations in genes required for T-cell development: IL7R, CD45, IL2RG, JAK3, RAG1, RAG2, ARTEMIS, and ADA and severe combined immunodeficiency: HuGE review. *Genetics in Medicine* 6:16, 2004.
10. Notarangelo, LD, Miao CH, Ochs DH: Wiskott-Aldrich syndrome. *Curr Opin Hematol* 15:30, 2008.
11. Staples ER, McDermott EM, Reiman A: Immunodeficiency in ataxia telangiectasia is correlated strongly with the presence of two null mutations in the ataxia telangiectasia mutated gene: *Clin Exp Immunol* 153:214, 2008.
12. Hsu AP, Sampaio EP, Khan J: Mutations in GATA2 are associated with the autosomal dominant and sporadic monocytopenia and mycobacterial infection (MonoMAC) syndrome. *Blood* 118:2653, 2011.
13. Stein DS, Korvick JA, Vermund SH: $CD4^+$ lymphocyte cell enumeration for prediction of clinical course of human immunodeficiency virus disease: A review. *J Infect Dis* 165:352, 1992.
14. Yuen KY, Chan PK, Peiris M, et al: Clinical features and rapid viral diagnosis of human disease associated with avian influenza A H5N1 virus. *Lancet* 351:467, 1998.
15. Turett GS, Telzak EE: Normalization of $CD4^+$ T-lymphocyte depletion in patients without HIV infection treated for tuberculosis. *Chest* 105:1335, 1994.
16. de Jager CP, van Wijk PT, Mathoera RB, et al: Lymphocytopenia and neutrophil-lymphocyte count ratio predict bacteremia better than conventional infection markers in an emergency care unit. *Crit Care* 14:R192, 2010.
17. Kyttaris VC, Juang Y-T, Tsokos GC: Immune cells and cytokines in systemic lupus erythematosus. *Curr Opin Rheumatol* 17:518, 2005.
18. Shao L, Fujii H, Colmegna I, et al: Deficiency of the DNA repair enzyme ATM in rheumatoid arthritis. *J Exp Med* 206:1435, 2009.
19. Fraker PJ, King, LE: Reprogramming of the immune system during zinc deficiency. *Annu Rev Nutr* 24:277, 2004.
20. Zonios DE, Falloon J, Bennett JE, et al: Idiopathic $CD4^+$ lymphocytopenia: Natural history and prognostic factors. *Blood* 112:287, 2008.
21. Robak T, Lech-Maranda E, Korycka A, et al: Purine nucleoside analogs as immunosuppressive and antineoplastic agents: Mechanism of action and clinical activity. *Curr Med Chem* 13:3165, 2006.
22. Juks Z, Strober S, Bobrove AM: Long term effects of radiation of T and B lymphocytes in peripheral blood of patients with Hodgkin's disease. *J Clin Invest* 58:803, 1976.
23. Hamblin AD, Hamblin TJ: The immunodeficiency of chronic lymphocytic leukaemia. *Br Med Bull* 87:49, 2008.
24. Geha RS, Notarangelo LD, Casanova JL, et al: Primary immunodeficiency diseases: An update from the International Union of Immunological Societies Primary Immunodeficiency Diseases Classification Committee. *J Allergy Clin Immunol* 120:776, 2007.
25. Deane S, Selmi C, Naguwa SM, et al: Common variable immunodeficiency: Etiological and treatment issues. *Int Arch Allergy Immunol* 150:311, 2009.
26. Durandy A, Peron S, Fischer A: Hyper-IgM syndromes. *Curr Opin Rheumatol* 18:369, 2006.
27. Moschese V, Graziani S, Avanzini MA, et al: A prospective study on children with initial diagnosis of transient hypogammaglobulinemia of infancy: Results from the Italian Primary Immunodeficiency Network. *Int J Immunopathol Pharmacol* 21:343, 2008.
28. Dispensieri A, Gertz M, Therneau T, et al: Retrospective cohort study of 148 patients with polyclonal gammopathy. *Mayo Clin Proc* 76:476, 2001.
29. Wurster VM, Carlucci JF, Edwards KM: Periodic fever syndromes. *Pediatr Ann* 40:48, 2011.
30. Alizadeh AA, Advani RH: Evaluation and management of angioimmunoblastic T-cell lymphoma: A review of current approaches and future strategies. *Clin Adv Hematol Oncol* 6:899, 2008.

CHAPTER 48

DISORDERS OF PHAGOCYTE FUNCTION

Mary C. Dinauer and Thomas D. Coates

Phagocytic leukocytes are an essential component of the innate immune system that has evolved to rapidly respond to the presence of invading bacteria, fungi, and parasites. This first line of host defense also includes natural killer (NK) lymphocytes, complement, and other plasma proteins. As reviewed in Chapters 17 and 25, phagocytes are responsible for ingesting, killing, and digesting pathogens. Granulocytic phagocytes (neutrophils and eosinophils) circulate in the bloodstream until they sense chemotactic signals from infected tissues, resulting in adhesion to the vascular endothelium and subsequent migration into the site of infection. Mononuclear phagocytes (macrophages and their circulating precursor, the monocyte), on the other hand, function primarily as resident cells in a variety of tissues such as the lungs, liver, peritoneal cavity, and spleen, where they perform a surveillance role and also interact closely with lymphocytes to promote specific immune responses. Microbial killing is accomplished by two types of mechanisms: (1) de novo synthesis of highly toxic and often unstable derivatives of molecular oxygen by an enzyme known as the respiratory burst oxidase and (2) preformed polypeptide "antibiotics" and proteases stored within several types of lysosomal granules that are delivered into phagocytic vacuoles containing the ingested microbes.

This chapter reviews the major congenital and acquired disorders of phagocyte function, which from the clinical standpoint largely involve neutrophils. As would be predicted, these disorders manifest clinically by recurrent bacterial and fungal infections, often with atypical pathogens or unusual presentations. Interestingly, the converse of this is only rarely observed. Most patients with recurrent infections do not have any identifiable abnormality in their phagocytes. There are at least two explanations for the clinical rarity of phagocyte disorders. First, given their critical role in host defense, nature may be quite intolerant of major abnormalities in phagocytes. Before the modern antibiotic era, patients with severe disorders probably did not survive into their childbearing years. Second, there is a remarkable redundancy in the antimicrobial machinery of the phagocytes that permits one system to compensate for a defect in another. For example, the host does not rely on a single chemotactic signal or neutrophil membrane receptor to ensure that phagocytes accumulate at sites of infection. Instead, multiple chemotactic signals and receptors are used. A similar phenomenon is seen in the reactions that kill microbes as both oxidative and nonoxidative systems are used.

This chapter is organized according to the cellular functions outlined above: disorders of the respiratory burst microbicidal pathway, abnormalities of phagocyte adhesion and chemotaxis, and defects in the structure and function of lysosomal granules. The chapter is not meant to be an encyclopedic review of the numerous papers published on phagocyte abnormalities. It is important to note that many of these reports describe marginal in vitro defects, with little evidence that they are responsible for a clinical problem. Comprehensive reviews offering additional information on phagocyte disorders are available.[1,2]

APPROACH TO DIAGNOSIS OF PHAGOCYTE FUNCTION DISORDERS

Inherited and acquired clinical disorders of phagocyte function result from defects in one or more of the major steps leading to microbial killing—adhesion, chemotaxis, ingestion, degranulation, and production of microbicidal oxidants (Fig. 48-1). Patients with inherited disorders typically present in infancy or childhood with recurrent, unusual, or recalcitrant bacterial and fungal infections, and it is usually not difficult to determine that these are outside the range of normal. The presentation of these different inherited disorders can overlap, so that a specific diagnosis cannot be made on clinical grounds alone. Infections commonly seen include those of skin or mucosa, lung, lymph node, deep tissue abscesses, or childhood periodontitis. These can often have an indolent presentation with only low-grade fevers. Bacterial sepsis is an unusual initial symptom and usually reflects dissemination from an infected site. Inherited defects in phagocyte function are rare and represent only about 20% of the primary immunodeficiencies.[1] Thus, children with suspected disorders of host defense should also be screened for defects in humoral, cellular, and complement-mediated immunity. An approach to evaluating the patient with significant recurrent infections is shown in Figure 48-2. Patients in whom a defect is identified should be referred to a center specialized in care of such patients.

In clinical practice, although nearly all patients with well-characterized phagocyte abnormalities have recurrent or unusual infections, the majority of individuals with histories of persistent or recurrent infections do not have identifiable phagocyte disorders or other immune defects. In some cases, these reflect another underlying medical condition or nonimmunologic problem related to an anatomic or obstructive defect. This chapter focuses largely on disorders in which a good correlation exists between the clinical condition and an identifiable defect in phagocyte function.

DISORDERS OF THE RESPIRATORY BURST PATHWAY

Reactive oxygen species generated by the phagocyte respiratory burst are critical for microbial killing. The enzyme responsible for the initial reaction in this pathway is a nicotinamide adenine dinucleotide phosphate (NADPH) oxidase found in plasma and phagolysosomal membranes. Upon activation by inflammatory stimuli, the NADPH oxidase catalyzes the transfer of an electron from NADPH to molecular oxygen, thereby forming superoxide (as the O_2^- ion) (Fig. 48-3, reaction 1).[2-4] This NADPH oxidase, along with enzymes and reactions that are directly involved in the production or metabolism of O_2^-, constitutes the respiratory burst pathway as depicted in Fig. 48-3. Superoxide is the precursor to numerous microbicidal oxidants, including hydrogen peroxide and hypochlorous acid. Five clinically significant defects have been identified in the respiratory burst, involving the following enzymes: NADPH oxidase (reaction 1), leukocyte glucose-6-phosphate dehydrogenase (G6PD) (reaction 8), myeloperoxidase (MPO) (reaction 4), glutathione reductase, and glutathione synthetase (reaction 9). These reactions are involved in the production of O_2^- (reactions 8 and 1) in the conversion of O_2^- and hydrogen peroxide to other toxic derivatives (reaction 4) or in the detoxification of excess hydrogen peroxide needed to protect the phagocyte during the respiratory burst (reactions 7 and 9). Of note, NOX homologues to the leukocyte NADPH oxidase have recently been discovered in the gut, vascular cells, and other tissues, which may generate oxidants for local host defense or for regulation of other cellular functions.[5]

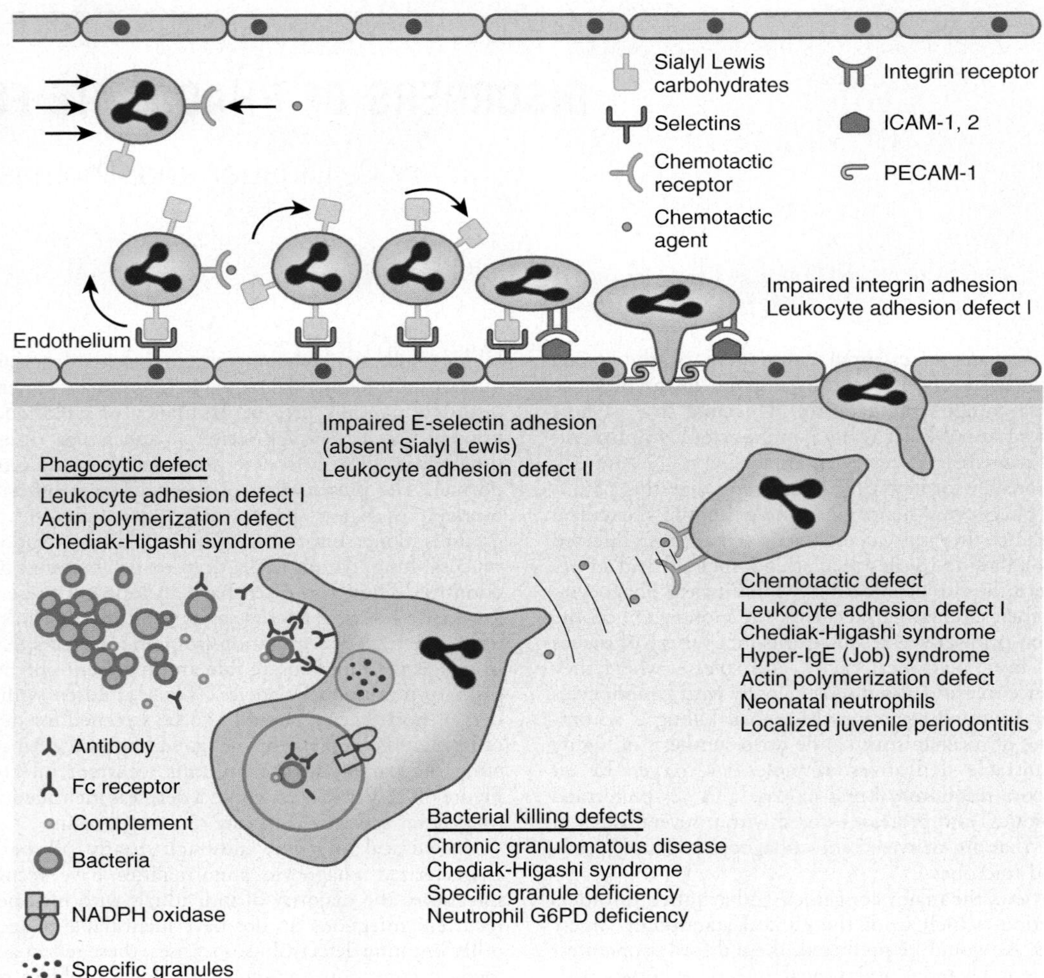

Figure 48-1 STEPS IN THE RESPONSE OF CIRCULATION NEUTROPHILS TO INFECTION. The adhesion molecule E-selectin is upregulated on endothelial cells in response to inflammatory mediators (interleukin-1 [IL-1], endotoxin, tumor necrosis factor-α [TNF-α]), resulting in rolling attachment and margination through interaction with sialyl Lewis carbohydrates on its surface. Chemoattractants such as IL-8 cause upregulation of neutrophil $\beta 2$ integrins that, in turn, mediate tight adhesion to intercellular adhesion molecule 1 (ICAM-1) and platelet endothelial cell adhesion molecule 1 (PECAM-1) on endothelial cells. Activated neutrophils can detect as little as a 2% change in the chemoattractant gradient and move to the site of infection. Neutrophils phagocytose bacteria opsonized by antibody and complement. Both oxidative and nonoxidative antimicrobial mechanisms are then used to kill bacteria. Disorders of phagocyte function associated with each of these steps are noted. *G6PD,* Glucose-6-phosphate dehydrogenase; *NADPH,* nicotinamide adenine dinucleotide phosphate. *(Modified from Kyoto W, Coates TD: A practical approach to neutrophil disorders.* Pediatr Clin North Am *49:929, 2002, with permission.)*

Chronic Granulomatous Disease

Chronic granulomatous disease (CGD) is a genetically heterogeneous group of defects that share in common the failure of neutrophils, monocytes, macrophages, and eosinophils to undergo a respiratory burst and generate O_2^-.[2,6,7] CGD is relatively rare, having an estimated incidence of between one in 200,000 and one in 250,000 live births based on data from the United States CGD Registry,[7] although it is still the most common inherited phagocyte disorder of clinical significance (MPO deficiency is more common, but affected patients are rarely symptomatic). The absence of respiratory burst-derived oxidants results in recurrent, often life-threatening bacterial and fungal infections and is also associated with formation of inflammatory granulomas.[2,6-9] The disease was first described in 1957 as a syndrome characterized by severe recurrent infections in boys who also had visceral granulomas containing pigmented histiocytes. The disease was termed *fatal granulomatous disease* owing to this distinguishing histologic feature and the grim clinical course in most patients. It was not until the late 1960s and early 1970s that the defect in oxygen consumption and O_2^- production was identified and a convenient diagnostic assay, the nitroblue tetrazolium (NBT) test, was developed. In the 1980s a combination of biochemical and molecular genetic approaches led to the identification of four critical subunits of the NADPH oxidase and the recognition that mutations in the corresponding genes are responsible for four different genetic subgroups of CGD (Fig. 48-4). Recently, a fifth genetic subgroup was identified in a single patient.[10] Databases for the main four genetic subgroups of CGD have been developed that are accessible through the website http://bioinf.uta.fi/idr. Recent publications on disease manifestations and genotypes in large patient registries are also available (see references 9, 11, and 12) and support earlier reports.[7]

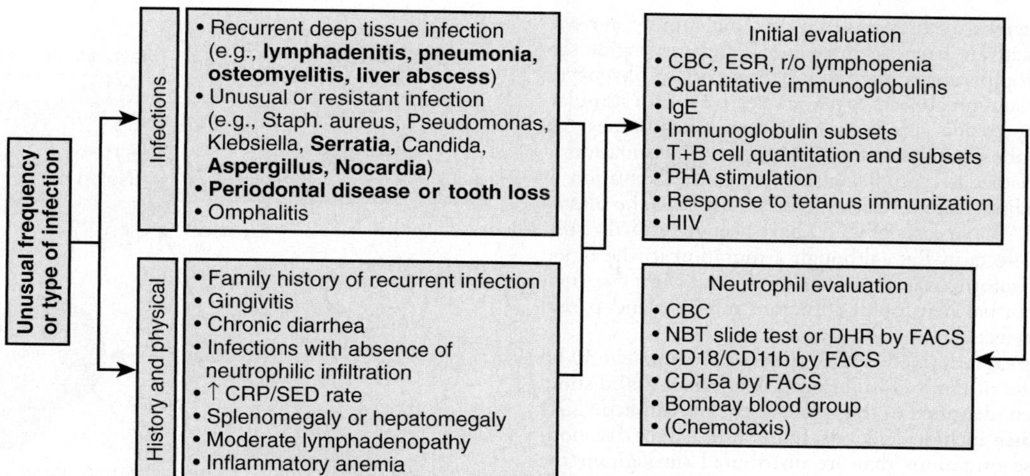

Figure 48-2 EVALUATION OF PATIENTS WITH RECURRENT BACTERIAL OR FUNGAL INFECTIONS. The history, physical examination, and infections episodes in patients with a possible primary neutrophil dysfunction syndrome are noted. The initial evaluation can be done in most clinical laboratories. A qualified reference laboratory with special expertise in this area should do the neutrophil evaluations. Chemotaxis is very difficult to evaluate clinically and should only be attempted in a qualified research laboratory with extensive experience.
CBC, Complete blood count; *DHR,* dihydrorhodamine; *ESR,* erythrocyte sedimentation rate; *FACS,* Fluorescence activated cell sorter; *PHA,* phytohemagglutinin; *r/o,* rule out.

Clinical Approach to Patients With Disorders of Phagocyte Function

Index of Suspicion

Patients with disorders of phagocyte function usually present at a young age with recurrent, deep-seated bacterial and fungal infections. Unlike patients with severe neutropenia caused by bone marrow failure, these patients usually do not have sepsis. Blood cultures are often negative. The major diagnostic problem faced by the clinician is to determine if the history of infection is unusual enough to warrant consideration of an underlying neutrophil dysfunction defect. The first point to remember is that primary immunodeficiency disorders are rare and primary neutrophil dysfunction syndromes form only a small percentage of all primary immunodeficiency syndromes. The patient is more likely to have recurrent community-acquired *Staphylococcus* infection than chronic granulomatous disease.

Specific features that may suggest a phagocytic defect are shown in Figure 48-2. Excellent discussions of this problem have been published (see Kyono and Coates[1] and Dinauer and Newburger[2]). Four aspects of each patient's infection history should be considered: frequency, severity, location, and responsible pathogen. Patients with unusual features in at least one of these aspects should alert the clinician to a possible underlying phagocyte disorder. When considering frequency, the patient's age and associated medical conditions must be taken into account. For example, recurrent otitis media in a 2-year-old patient is far less worrisome than a similar history in a 40-year-old patient. The more unusual or severe the infections, the less frequently these have to occur before a phagocyte evaluation is indicated. Infections in unexpected anatomic locations, such as hepatic, pulmonary, and rectal abscesses, may indicate an underlying phagocyte defect. Childhood periodontal disease or gingivitis is distinctly uncommon, and in the absence of neutropenic conditions, strongly suggests underlying neutrophil dysfunction. The identification of certain pathogens (e.g., *Serratia marcescens, Klebsiella* spp., *Aspergillus* spp., *Nocardia* spp., *Burkholderia cepacia,* invasive candidiasis) in children and young adults can provide the strongest indications for pursuing further studies. A history of delayed separation of the umbilical cord is often mentioned as a sign of phagocytic defect. This is fairly common as an isolated finding and is usually of no significance. However, this is in conjunction with omphalitis or other pyogenic infections raises the possibility of LAD or chemotactic defects. A child with nystagmus, fair skin, and recurrent staphylococcal infections should be evaluated for CHS.

Evaluation

Performing a good history and physical examination to eliminate common causes of recurrent infection is important before looking for rare syndromes. For example, is the recurrent pneumonia caused by an aspirated foreign body in the bronchus? In general, patients should first be evaluated for lymphocyte or complement defects. A useful algorithm is presented in Figure 48-2. Note that testing described in this algorithm is not exhaustive, and patients with truly striking histories of unusual kinds of infections should be referred for further evaluation by specialized research laboratories.

Molecular Genetics of Chronic Granulomatous Disease

Chronic granulomatous disease results from mutations in any of the five genes encoding essential subunits of the NADPH oxidase (Table 48-1).[11,12] In turn, the biochemical and genetic analysis of CGD has been instrumental in characterizing this complex enzyme. The oxidase subunits are referred to by their apparent molecular mass (kDa) and have been given the designation *phox,* for *ph*agocyte *ox*idase. A b-type cytochrome known as flavocytochrome b_{558}, a membrane bound heterodimer composed of gp91^{phox} and p22^{phox}, is the redox center of the oxidase. Approximately two-thirds of CGD cases result from defects in the X-linked gene encoding the gp91^{phox} subunit of flavocytochrome b_{558}, which contains both the flavoprotein and heme-binding domains responsible for electron transport. A rare autosomal recessive (AR) form of CGD is caused by mutations in the gene encoding p22^{phox}, the smaller subunit of flavocytochrome b_{558}, which provides a critical docking site for p47^{phox}, a regulatory subunit. The remaining cases of AR CGD involve genetic defects in p47^{phox}, p67^{phox}, or p40^{phox}, three regulatory proteins associated with each other in the cytosol of unstimulated cells but rapidly move to the membrane to activate flavocytochrome b_{558} and superoxide formation when neutrophils are exposed to inflammatory or phagocytic stimuli. The p40*phox* subunit appears to play a selective role in stimulating high-level superoxide production within phagosomes via membrane-bound phosphatidylinositol-3-phosphate.[10] Formation of the active NADPH oxidase complex also involves the activation of the small GTP-binding protein Rac, which then binds to the plasma membrane and p67*phox*.[2] No cases of CGD have been identified resulting from genetic defects in Rac, although a mutation in the blood cell-specific Rac2 isoform was found in an infant with recurrent infections and abnormal neutrophil adhesion, motility, and partial NADPH oxidase defects.[2]

The gene for gp91*phox*, termed *CYBB*, spans approximately 30 kb in the Xp21.1 region of the X chromosome. More than 600 distinct mutations have been identified in the gp91*phox* gene in X-linked CGD (MIM306400), which include deletions, frameshifts, splice site, nonsense, and missense mutations that are distributed throughout the gene (Table 48-2).[11] Approximately 10% to 15% of X-linked CGD

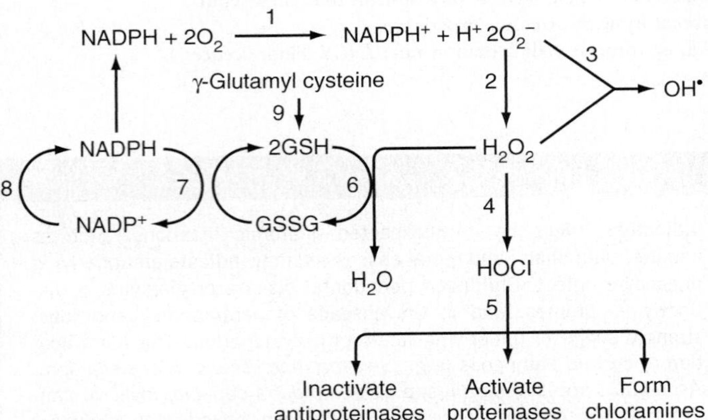

Figure 48-3 Reactions of respiratory burst pathway. *GSH,* glutathione; *GSSG,* oxidized glutathione; *HOCl,* hypochlorous acid *NADPH,* nicotinamide adenine dinucleotide phosphate.

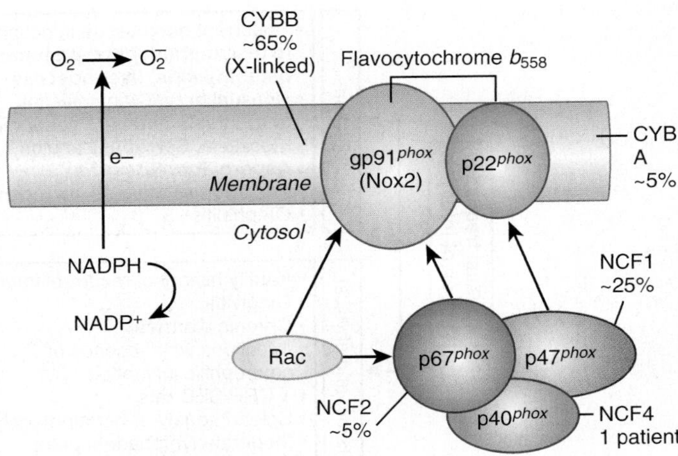

Figure 48-4 NICOTINAMIDE ADENINE DINUCLEOTIDE PHOSPHATE (NADPH) OXIDASE AND MOLECULAR GENETICS OF CHRONIC GRANULOMATOUS DISEASE (CGD). Shown are the membrane and soluble subunits of the NADPH oxidase, indicating how these correspond to the five different genetic subgroups of CGD and their approximate incidence. Flavocytochrome b_{558} is the redox center of the enzyme and is located in plasma, specific granule, and phagolysosomal membranes. This heterodimer is composed of the gp91*phox* and p22*phox* subunits of the NADPH oxidase, which are affected in X-linked and an autosomal recessive form of CGD, respectively. The soluble regulatory proteins p47*phox*, p67*phox*, and p40*phox* are found in the cytosol until phagocyte activation by soluble or particulate inflammatory stimuli, after which they move to the membrane where p47*phox* and p67*phox* bind flavocytochrome *b558,* binds Rac, and p40*phox* binds phosphatidylinositol-3-phosphate, a phosphoinositide present on phagosome membranes. Mutations in the genes encoding p47*phox*p67*phox* and p40*phox* account for other autosomal recessive forms of CGD. Another essential regulatory component of the NADPH oxidase is the small GTPase, Rac, which in its active guanosine triphosphate–bound state, becomes membrane bound, and associates with the oxidase. By a mechanism that is not fully understood, binding of these multiple regulatory subunits activates the flavocytochrome to catalyze the transfer of electrons from cytosolic NADPH across the membrane via the FAD and heme redox centers to molecular oxygen, thereby forming superoxide in the extracellular or intraphagosomal compartment. No cases of CGD have been described owing to mutations in Rac.

Table 48-1 Classification of Chronic Granulomatous Disease

Component Affected	Gene Symbol	Gene Locus	Inheritance	Subtype*	NBT Score (% Positive)	O_2^- Production (% Normal)	Flavocytochrome *b* Spectrum (% Normal)	Defect in Cell-Free NADPH Oxidase Assay	Frequency (% of Cases)†
Gp91*phox*	*CYBB*	Xp21.1	X	X91°	0	0	0	Membrane	68
				X91⁻	80-100 (weak)	3-30	Low	Membrane	5
				X91⁻	5-10	5-10	Low	Membrane	<1
				X91⁺	0	0	N	Membrane	1
P22*phox*	*CYBA*	16p24.3	AR	A22°	0	0	0	Membrane	4
				A22⁺	0	0	N	Membrane	<1
P47*phox*	*NCF1*	7q11.23	AR	A47°	0	0-1	N	Cytosol	17
P67*phox*	NCF2	1q25.3	AR	A67°	0	0	N	Cytosol	5
p40*phox*‡	NCF4	22q13.1	AR	A40⁺	100	<10 (intracellular)	N	n/a	1

AR (or A), Autosomal recessive inheritance; *N,* normal; *NADPH,* nicotinamide adenine dinucleotide phosphate; *NBT,* nitroblue tetrazolium; *X,* X-linked inheritance.
*In this nomenclature, the first letter represents the mode of inheritance (X-linked [X] or autosomal recessive [A]), and the number indicates the *phox* component that is genetically affected. The superscript symbols indicate whether the level of protein of the affected component is undetectable (°), diminished (–), or normal (+) as measured by immunoblot analysis.
†Combined data from 209 kindreds evaluated at the Scripps Research Institute/Stanford University CGD Clinic and a cooperative European study representing 57 kindreds and 63 patients. (Modified from Casimir C, Chetty M, Bohler MC, et al: Identification of the defective NADPH-oxidase component in chronic granulomatous disease: A study of 57 European families. *Eur J Clin Invest* 22:403, 1992; and Curnutte JT: Chronic granulomatous disease: The solving of a clinical riddle at the molecular level. *Clin Immunol Immunopathol* 67:S2, 1993.) These frequencies remain similar to those in more recent reports from Europe and the United States.
‡A single patient reported to date who was a compound heterozygote for a frameshift mutation and a nonfunctional form of p40*phox* caused by a point mutation. (Matute JD, Arias AA, Wright NA et al: A new genetic subgroup of chronic granulomatous disease with autosomal recessive mutations in p40 phox and selective defects in neutrophil NADPH oxidase activity. *Blood* 114:3309, 2009.)

Table 48-2 Summary of Mutations in the *CYBB* Gene Encoding gp91*phox* in 261 Kindreds With X-linked Chronic Granulomatous Disease

Type of Mutation	Number of Kindreds	Frequency (%)	Phenotype
Deletions	63	24.2	X91°
Insertions	27	10.3	X91°
Splice-site mutations	42	16.1	X91°
Missense mutations	59	22.6	X91°, X91–, X91+
Nonsense mutations	70	26.8	X91°

Data from Roos D, Curnutte J, Hossle JP, et al: X-CGDbase: A database of X-CGD-causing mutations. *Immunol Today* 17:517, 1996.

is caused by new germline mutations. In most X-linked CGD, gp91*phox* is completely absent, and there is no measurable flavocytochrome *b* or superoxide production (the X91° subtype). In about 5% of X-linked cases, gp91*phox* can be present in normal levels but be nonfunctional (X91+), mutated in such a way that gp91*phox* is poorly functional (X91–), or expressed in only a small fraction of phagocytes (X91+). The first two "variant" forms of X-linked CGD result from coding sequence mutations, and the latter are caused by mutations in the regulatory portion of the gp91*phox* gene. Some X-linked CGD patients have large deletions that affect not only the gene encoding gp91*phox* but also portions of or all the flanking gene loci for the McLeod hemolytic anemia syndrome (absence of the Kell erythrocyte antigen, Kx), Duchenne muscular dystrophy, and X-linked retinitis pigmentosa. Two kindreds with point mutations in *CYBB* leading to marked impairment of flavocytochrome b expression and activity in macrophages with less effect on neutrophils were recently reported.[13] Affected patients were susceptible to mycobacterial infections but did not have other bacterial and fungal infections characteristic of CGD, highlighting the importance of macrophages for controlling mycobacteria.

Autosomal recessive CGD involving p22*phox* (MIM 233690) occurs in approximately 5% of CGD patients and usually involves the complete absence of cytochrome *b* (A22°), encoded by CYBA. Mutations in A22 CGD are heterogeneous and range from large interstitial gene deletions to point mutations associated with missense, frameshift, or RNA splicing defects.[12] Because the full expression of flavocytochrome *b* in the membrane requires the production of both subunits, a primary deficiency of either component leads to a secondary loss of the other. Thus, neither subunit can be detected on immunoblot analysis in either X91° or A22° CGD. A single patient with A22+ CGD has been described, who has a missense mutation disrupting the binding site for p47*phox*.

Autosomal recessive patients with p47*phox* deficient CGD (MIM 233700) account for approximately one-fourth of cases in the United States and Europe but only about 7% of cases in Japan. The p47*phox* subunit is encoded by the NCF1 gene. A limited number of mutations have been identified in the p47*phox* gene.[12] Virtually all patients are either homozygotes or compound heterozygotes for a mutant allele with a GT deletion at the beginning of exon 2 that predicts a premature stop codon following amino acid residue and results in absence of the p47*phox* protein. The high frequency of the p47*phox* GT deletion mutation appears to reflect the existence of at least one closely linked highly conserved p47*phox* pseudogene(s) that contains this GT deletion. This close physical proximity leads to recombination events between the wild-type gene and pseudogene(s).

A heterogenous group of mutations in the p67*phox* gene, NCF2, are responsible for A67 CGD, a rare AR form of CGD (MIM233710) accounting for about 5% of cases overall.[12] Almost all of mutations identified to date in A67 CGD lead to absent expression of the p67*phox* protein. However, one A67+ patient has been reported in which a nonfunctional form of p67*phox* with an amino acid deletion is expressed but is unable to translocate to the membrane or bind to Rac.

Finally, a boy with AR p40*phox* defects (MIM613960) was recently reported.[10] This patient was a compound heterozygote for two null alleles in NCF4. Although NADPH oxidase activity on the plasma membrane was normal, phagosome oxidant production was markedly impaired. The main clinical manifestation in this patient was chronic granulomatous inflammation of the intestinal tract rather than opportunistic infections characteristic of CGD, perhaps related to the more selective role of p40*phox* in regulating NADPH oxidase activity.

Even though more than 90% of patients with CGD have respiratory burst defects that result in undetectable levels of O_2^- production, there is a surprising heterogeneity in the clinical manifestations of the disease.[7] At one end of the spectrum are patients who begin to have severe bacterial and fungal infections during infancy and who rarely have more than 4 to 12 months between such serious infections. At the other end of the spectrum are patients who are well for many years and then unexpectedly develop a serious infection typical of CGD, such as a staphylococcal hepatic abscess or *Aspergillus* pneumonia. After their first major infection, some of these patients may be relatively healthy again for another 3 to 10 years before the next severe infection occurs. As a group, patients with X-CGD, A22 CGD, and A67 CGD seem to have a more severe clinical course compared with patients with A47 CGD,[7,9] who have a small amount of detectable oxidant production even in the complete absence of this subunit (Fig. 48-5, *G*). Individuals with partial respiratory burst activity less than 10% of normal (most X91– patients; see Table 48-1) also tend to have disease of intermediate severity. Polymorphisms in oxygen-independent antimicrobial systems or other components[9] regulating the innate immune response are also likely to play an important role in modifying disease severity. Specific polymorphisms in the MPO, mannose binding lectin, and FcγRIIa genes are associated with a higher risk for granulomatous or autoimmune or rheumatologic complications.[2,8] Because of this heterogeneity, the diagnosis of CGD should be entertained, not only in young children with recurrent severe infections, but also in adolescents and young adults who experience exceptionally severe or unusual infections.

Clinical Manifestations

In approximately two-thirds of patients, the first symptoms of CGD appear during the first year of life with the onset of recurrent, purulent bacterial and fungal infections.[7] Table 48-3 summarizes the types of infections and infecting organisms most frequently encountered in CGD. The most common types of infections are those that involve sites in contact with the outside world, which is consistent with the role of neutrophils as a first line of defense against infection. *Staphylococcus aureus,* enteric gram-negatives, *Serratia marcescens, Burkholderia cepacia, Nocardia* spp., and *Aspergillus* spp. represent the most frequently encountered pathogens in North American patients, but *Burkholderia* and *Nocardia* spp. are less frequently seen in Europe.[8] *S. aureus* is the most frequently isolated organism overall. The most common causes of death have been pneumonia or sepsis caused by *B. cepacia* and *Aspergillus* spp., although use of newer azole antifungals has markedly improved the outcome of the latter in recent years.[7,8]

Most CGD pathogens share the property of being catalase negative and as such inadvertently "lend" H_2O_2 secreted from the pathogen to the peroxide-starved CGD phagocyte, which in turn uses it (after being converted to hypochlorous acid [HOCl] by MPO; see Fig. 48-3) to kill the microbe. It also appears that at least some of the CGD pathogens are resistant to the nonoxidative killing mechanisms of the phagocyte. It is somewhat surprising how often one fails to identify the infecting organism in CGD—perhaps greater than half the time despite aggressive culturing. In this situation, one treats empirically with the antibiotic that should work and if it fails, one then aggressively pursues more invasive diagnostic procedures looking for one (or more) of the less commonly seen microbes such as *Nocardia* spp., *Candida* spp., mycobacteria, and a host of other bacteria and fungi (see Table 48-3). Other unusual organisms that cause infection in CGD include other members of the Burkholderia family,

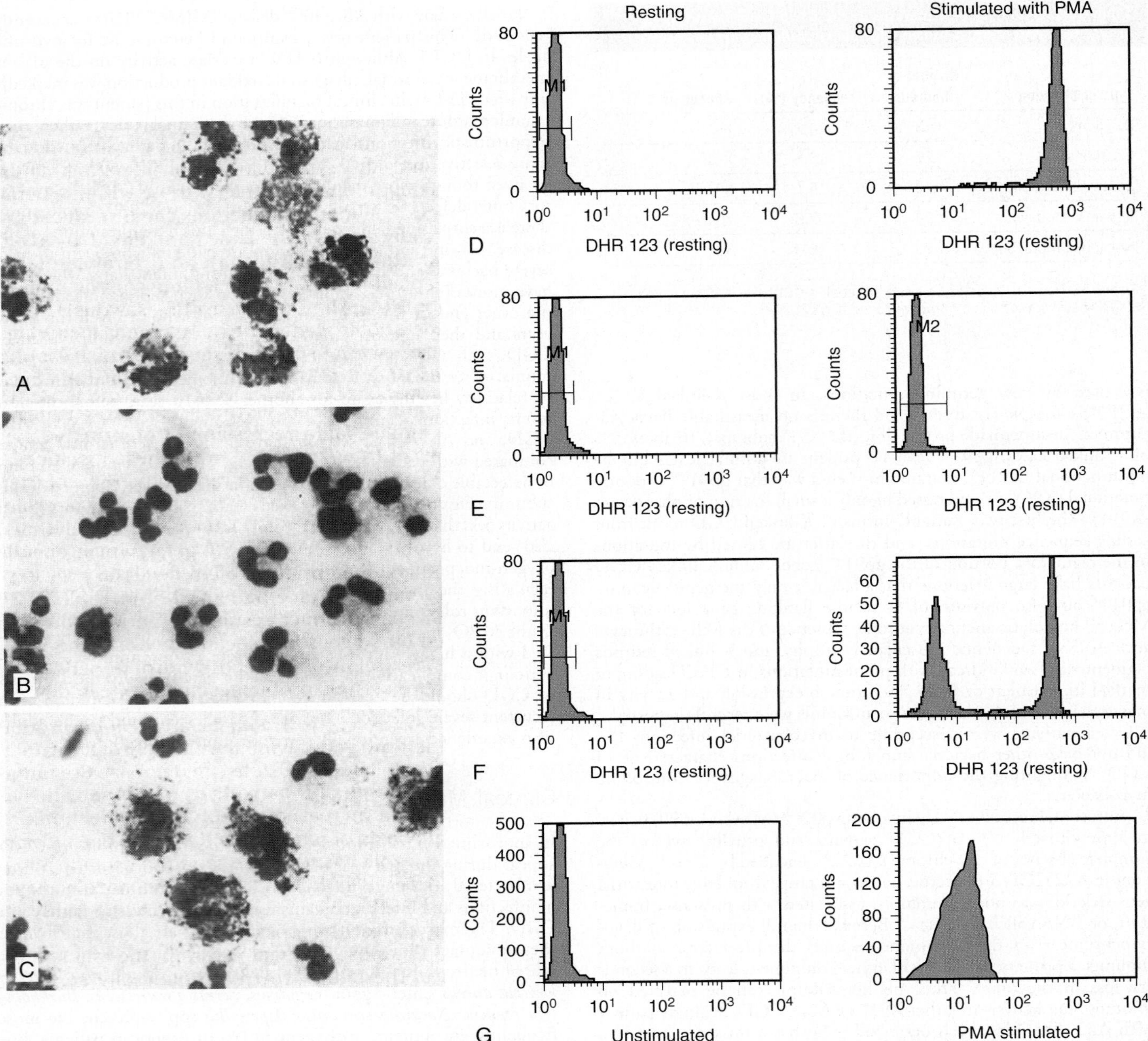

Figure 48-5 ANALYSIS OF NEUTROPHIL NICOTINAMIDE ADENINE DINUCLEOTIDE PHOSPHATE (NADPH) OXIDASE ACTIVITY FOR THE DIAGNOSIS OF CHRONIC GRANULOMATOUS DISEASE (CGD). **A** to **C,** Nitroblue tetrazolium (NBT) slide test. Peripheral blood neutrophils and monocytes from a drop of fresh whole blood were made adherent to glass slides and stimulated with phorbol myristate acetate. **A,** Normal neutrophils and monocytes, all of which are NBT positive. **B,** Neutrophils and monocytes from an X-linked CGD patient, which are all NBT negative. **C,** A mixture of NBT-positive and NBT-negative neutrophils from the X-linked carrier mother of the patient in part **B. D** to **G,** Dihydrorhodamine (DHR) 123 flow cytometry test. Nonfluorescent DHR 123 is taken up by neutrophils and become fluorescent after reaction with reactive oxygen species produced in the respiratory burst. **D,** Normal neutrophils. **E,** Neutrophils from an X-linked CGD patient, which do not fluoresce after stimulation. **F,** A mixture of nonfluorescent and fluorescent neutrophils from an X-linked CGD carrier. **G,** Neutrophils from a $p47^{phox}$-deficient patient, which show weak fluorescence after stimulation.

including *Burkholderia cenocepacia, Burkholderia Gladioli,* and *Burkholderia mallei* (the causative agent in melioidosis, a septic illness common in East Asia) and *Chromobacterium violaceum,* found in brackish fresh water and that can cause a febrile illness with bacteremia in CGD. A previously unknown gram-negative bacteria, *Granulobacter bethesdensis,* was recently identified in a CGD patient with recurrent fevers associated with chronic necrotizing deep lymphatic infection. This organism is a member of the *Acetobacteraceae* family, which has previously not been linked to invasive human disease.

Pneumonia is the most common type of infection seen in CGD with *S. aureus, Aspergillus* spp., *B. cepacia,* and enteric gram–negative organisms as the major pathogens. It is noteworthy that *B. cepacia* has emerged as a particularly lethal organism in CGD. This organism often is not covered with the first line of antibiotics used for *S. aureus* and most gram–negative organisms and can quietly proliferate (with persistent fevers) to the point of quick, explosive collapse caused by endotoxic shock. Intravenous trimethoprim–sulfamethoxazole (TMP-SMX) has been most effective in treating patients if given

Table 48-3 Infections in Chronic Granulomatous Disease

Infections	Percent of Infections	Infecting Organisms
Pneumonia	70-80	*Aspergillus, Staphylococcus, Burkholderia cepacia, Pseudomonas, Nocardia, Mycobacterium* (including atypical), *Serratia, Candida, Klebsiella, Paecilomyces*
Lymphadenitis	50-60	*Staphylococcus, Serratia, Candida, Klebsiella, Nocardia*
Cutaneous infections/ impetigo	50-60	
Hepatic or perihepatic abscesses	20-30	*Staphylococcus, Serratia, Streptococcus viridans, Nocardia, Aspergillus*
Osteomyelitis	20-30	*Serratia, Aspergillus, Paecilomyces, Staphylococcus, B cepacia, Pseudomonas, Nocardia*
Perirectal abscesses or fistulae	15-30	Enteric gram-negatives organisms, *Staphylococcus*
Septicemia	10-20	*B. cepacia, Pseudomonas, Salmonella, Staphylococcus, Serratia, Klebsiella*
Urinary tract infections or pyelonephritis	5-15	Enteric gram-negative organisms
Brain abscesses	<5	*Aspergillus, Staphylococcus*
Meningitis	<5	*Candida lusitaniae, Haemophilus influenzae, B. cepacia*

The relative frequencies of different types of infections in chronic granulomatous disease are estimated from data pooled from several large series of patients in the United States, Europe, and Japan: (1) Mouy R, Fischer A, Vilmer E, et al: Incidence, severity, and prevention of infections in chronic granulomatous disease. *J Pediatr* 114:555, 1989; (2) Bemiller LS, Roberts DH, Starko KM, et al: Safety and effectiveness of long-term interferon gamma therapy in patients with chronic granulomatous disease. *Blood Cells Mol Dis* 21:239, 1995; (3) Forrest CB, Forehand JR, Axtell RA, et al: Clinical features and current management of chronic granulomatous disease. *Hematol Oncol Clin North Am* 2:253, 1988; (4) Hitzig WH, Seger RA: Chronic granulomatous disease, a heterogeneous syndrome. *Hum Genet* 64:207, 1983; (5) Tauber AI, Borregaard N, Simons E, et al: Chronic granulomatous disease: A syndrome of phagocyte oxidase deficiencies. *Medicine (Baltimore)* 62:286, 1983; (6) Cohen MS, Isturiz RE, Malech HL, et al: Fungal infection in chronic granulomatous disease. The importance of the phagocyte in defense against fungi. *Am J Med* 71:59, 1981; (7) Hayakawa H, Kobayashi N, Yata J: Chronic granulomatous disease in Japan: A summary of the clinical features of 84 registered patients. *Acta Paediatr Jpn* 27:501, 1985; and (8) Johnston RB, Newman SL. Chronic granulomatous disease. *Pediatr Clin North Am* 24:365, 1977. These series encompass approximately 550 patients with CGD after accounting for overlap between reports. Unpublished data from the United States CGD Registry encompassing 368 patients was also used to estimate the relative frequencies of infections and the responsible organisms. The infecting organisms are arranged in approximate order of frequency for each type of infection. Note: *B. cepacia* was previously classified as *Pseudomonas cepacia.*

Table 48-4 Chronic Conditions Associated With Chronic Granulomatous Disease*

Condition	Relative Frequency (%)
Lymphadenopathy	98
Hypergammaglobulinemia	60-90
Hepatomegaly	50-90
Splenomegaly	60-80
Anemia of chronic disease	Common†
Underweight	70
Chronic diarrhea	20-60
Short stature	50
Gingivitis	50
Dermatitis	35
Hydronephrosis	10-25
Granulomatous ileocolitis	10-15
Gastric antral narrowing	10-15
Ulcerative stomatitis	5-15
Granulomatous cystitis	5-10†
Pulmonary fibrosis	<10†
Esophagitis	<10†
Granulomatous cystitis	<10
Chorioretinitis	<10
Glomerulonephritis	<10
Discoid lupus erythematosus	<10

*The relative frequencies of chronic conditions associated with chronic granulomatous disease (CGD) were estimated from the series of reports listed in Table 48-3.
†The incidence is estimated from the 50 cases of CGD followed at Scripps Research Institute and Stanford University (unpublished data).

before widespread dissemination of the infection. Proven or suspected *Aspergillus* infections were treated with amphotericin B therapy, but new azole antifungal agents are now typically used.

Lymphadenitis is the second most common infection and is usually caused by gram-negative organisms, *S. aureus,* or *Serratia marcescens.* Incision and drainage should not be delayed if the lesion fails to respond to parenteral antibiotics. Cutaneous abscesses should be similarly managed. Recurrent perinatal impetigo is almost a signature infection in CGD and often requires months of therapy (mostly oral antibiotics) to clear. Hepatic (and perihepatic) abscesses are also common in CGD and are usually, but not always, caused by *S. aureus.* Most lesions require drainage (needle or surgical) to permit efficient healing to occur. Bone infections, most commonly caused by *Serratia* spp. or *Aspergillus* spp., are particularly problematic in CGD and arise from either hematogenous or contiguous spread (as often is the case with *Aspergillus* infections in the lung invading ribs, vertebral bodies, or the diaphragm). Perirectal abscesses are difficult to treat, even with months of therapy, and can lead to fistula formations.

Chronic inflammation with granuloma formation is a distinctive hallmark of CGD and contributes to some of its more problematic complications.[8,14] In some cases, this results from imperfectly controlled infections in which stalemates develop between the pathogen and the patient's leukocytes. These lesions become granulomas as the host uses lymphocytes and activated macrophages to assist in containing the pathogens. However, this complication is not always clearly linked to persistent infection and in these cases has been speculated to involve a dysregulated inflammatory response, inefficient degradation of debris, or both. In the absence of oxidant production, excessive production of cytokines and delayed neutrophil apoptosis at inflammatory sites appear to contribute as underlying mechanisms.

As a result of persistent inflammatory stimulation, CGD patients can have from a variety of more chronic complications (Table 48-4). Lymphadenopathy, hepatosplenomegaly, eczematoid dermatitis, and anemia of chronic disease (hemoglobin levels usually 8-10 g/dL) are common manifestations of this process and are most prominent in the first 5 to 10 years of life in those with CGD. Throughout the body, granuloma formation can lead to dysfunction and obstruction in the esophagus, urinary bladder, and kidneys. In the stomach, the gastric antral narrowing can be severe enough in infants and children to resemble pyloric stenosis. Inflammatory involvement of the gastrointestinal tract can be seen in up to one-third of CGD patients, typically in association with the X-linked form. A chronic ileocolitis resembling Crohn disease occurs in about 10% of patients and can range from mild diarrhea to a debilitating syndrome of bloody diarrhea and malabsorption that can necessitate a colectomy. Interestingly, antigliadin antibodies suggesting Crohn disease are positive in more than 50% of CGD patients. Other types of chronic inflammation include gingivitis, chorioretinitis, destructive white matter lesions in the brain, and glomerulonephritis. Discoid lupus has been reported in 10% to 20% of patients, and occasional patients may develop systemic lupus erythematosus, sarcoidosis, or rheumatoid arthritis. The underlying mechanisms are poorly defined, although recent studies suggest that these manifestations may be partly related to subtle defects in the absence of the NADPH oxidase in memory B or T cells.

Carriers of CGD, whether the X-linked form or any one of the AR forms, are usually asymptomatic with two important exceptions. First, about one-fourth of X-linked carriers are at risk of developing mild to moderately severe discoid lupus erythematosus characterized by discoid skin lesions and photosensitivity.[2,14] The onset is usually in the second decade of life. The disease does not progress to systemic lupus nor does one find serologic evidence of even subclinical disease. Those with severe discoid lupus can be treated with Plaquenil. Recurrent stomatitis, significant gingivitis, or both have also been noted in as many as half of X-CGD carriers. A few also have from arthralgias, polyarthritis, and Raynaud phenomenon. The second important complication of the X-linked CGD carrier state is serious infection in women who have a usually high degree of inactivation of the normal X chromosome in their myeloid cells. If the circulating neutrophil population is skewed to the point that fewer than 10% to 15% of the cells function, then the carrier has an increased risk of bacterial infections that in some cases have been severe.[2] Those with fewer than 5% oxidase positive cells have full-blown CGD.

Diagnosis

The diagnosis of CGD is usually suggested by the unusual clinical histories outlined earlier or by a family history of CGD. The NBT slide test on fresh blood is the classic diagnostic test. A typical result is shown in Fig. 48-5. Fig. 48-5, *A* shows the normal positive staining of a group of seven neutrophils and one monocyte. Fig. 48-5, *B* shows the complete absence of NBT staining in a patient with X91° CGD, the classic X-linked form of the disease. Fig. 48-5, *C* shows the mixed population of NBT-positive and -negative cells observed in that patient's mother, reflecting random X chromosome inactivation. Because nearly 100% of the normal cells in this test are positive, the carrier state in X-linked CGD can be detected when as few as 5% of the cells are NBT negative. This test also permits detection of diffuse populations of weakly positive cells such as those seen in $X91^-$ CGD, which are characterized by a partial deficiency of flavocytochrome *b*. Because X-linked CGD can arise by new mutations in the maternal germ line, one does not always see NBT-negative cells in the mother. Flow cytometric assays of oxidase activity, such as those based on the conversion of dihydroxyrhodamine (DHR) 123 to rhodamine 123, can also provide both quantitative measurements of oxidant generation and the cell-by-cell distribution of activity (see Fig. 48-5, *D* to *G*). The DHR 123 assay for oxidase activity is now available in many referral centers and through reference laboratories. In addition to $X91^-$ CGD neutrophils, weak staining in the NBT test or a small but measurable level of DHR fluorescence can be seen in $A47^0$ cells (see Fig. 48-5, *H*) because of a small amount of residual oxidant production. Regardless of diagnostic assay used, is important to have these tests performed on appropriately handled blood samples and by experienced laboratories to avoid inconclusive or false normal results.

Genetic classification is useful primarily for purposes of genetic counseling and prenatal diagnosis. With the exception of classic X-linked disease in a male whose mother is a carrier, determining the

Diagnosis of Chronic Granulomatous Disease

The diagnosis of CGD is easily established by doing an NBT slide test or flow cytometry of DHR 123 fluorescence to detect neutrophil NADPH oxidase activity. The NBT slide test is very easy to set up, as is DHR flow cytometry. However, because the probability of getting an abnormal result is very low, there may be confusion in interpretation because of a lack of experience. In the authors' experience, incorrect positive and negative results have been reported for both assays. Thus, if the index of suspicion is high, consultation should be obtained from a center with extensive experience with the test and with the disorder.

Neutrophil respiratory burst activity is preserved in anticoagulated blood maintained at room temperature for several days; thus, DHR testing can be done 1 to 2 days later after shipping to a commercial laboratory. A normal control should always be shipped with the patient specimen to eliminate problems in specimen handling during transport.

NBT Slide Test

- No NBT reduction (absence of cells with dark blue formazan deposits) in both X-linked and AR forms of CGD (see Fig. 48-5, *B*).
- Usually no reduction in 50% of cells and normal in 50% for X-linked carrier. The percent positive cells can vary if there is unequal X inactivation and may appear normal or like CGD with extreme lyonization (see Fig. 48-5, *C*).
- False-positive results can occur (i.e., apparent failure to reduce NBT supporting the diagnosis of CGD) if the neutrophils do not adhere to the slide. This happens with greasy slides or with some cases of LAD. Using PMA to stimulate the cells will avoid this.

DHR Flow Cytometry

- This approach has replaced the NBT slide test in many laboratories. It has the advantage of assessing large numbers of cells and can give quantitation of the amount of oxidant production.
- The change in fluorescence channel number with stimulation is the critical number and not the percent positive cells.
- X-linked CGD patients will not respond at all and show no increase in fluorescence with stimulation (see Fig. 48-5, *F*).
- X-linked carriers will show about 50% of the cells that respond with a normal increase in fluorescence, and the other half will have no response. Degrees of unequal X inactivation are much more accurately quantified by this assay (see Fig. 48-5, *G*).
- AR patients, particularly those with absent $p47^{phox}$, have some response to stimulation and show a small increase in fluorescence (see Fig. 48-5, *H*). This level of oxidant production is usually not visible on the NBT test.
- AR carriers have a good response, but the histogram may be broader than normal and may even appear bimodal with a weakly fluorescent peak and a strongly fluorescent peak. This is not distinguishable on the NBT slide test.
- Falsely negative results not supporting the diagnosis of CGD have been reported in specimens that have been run a few days after phlebotomy.
- Falsely abnormal results suggesting CGD can be seen in patients with MPO deficiency because MPO is required to generate strong DHR fluorescence.

Genetic Analysis

- Genetic analysis for X-linked and AR CGD is clinically available and should be performed on at least the proband in each kindred.

specific oxidase gene affected in a given CGD patient (see Table 48-1) requires additional laboratory studies. Genetic testing for the four most common genetic subgroups is commercially available. Laboratories specializing in neutrophil biochemistry can also perform immunoblot analysis of neutrophil extracts, flavocytochrome *b* spectroscopy, or functional analysis of membrane and cytosol fractions in the cell-free oxidase assay. In a male with absent flavocytochrome *b* without clear evidence for a maternal carrier, it is necessary to search for the mutation in both the gp91^{phox} and p22^{phox} genes by DNA sequencing or another method of analysis.

Testing for the McLeod red cell phenotype should be done in all patients diagnosed with X-linked CGD. This causes a mild hemolytic anemia. More importantly, there can be serious problems with development of hemolytic antibodies if these patients are transfused.

Prognosis and Treatment

The cornerstones of therapy in CGD are currently (1) prevention and early treatment of infections, (2) aggressive use of parenteral antibiotics for most infections, (3) use of prophylactic TMP-SMX (5 mg/kg/day of trimethoprim) or dicloxacillin (25-50 mg/kg/day) for sulfa-allergic patients, (4) prophylactic itraconazole (200 mg/day if 13 years of age or older or if weighing at least 50 kg or 100 mg daily if younger than 13 years of age or weighing less than 50 kg), and (5) use of prophylactic recombinant human interferon-γ (rIFN-γ) (0.05 mg/m^2 or 0.0015 mg/kg if less than 0.5 m^2 three times per week).[6,8] Using these guidelines, the prognosis for patients with CGD has improved dramatically since the disorder was first described in the 1950s, when almost all patients died in childhood. In a large study based on data collected by a CGD registry in the United States in the 1990s, the overall mortality rate was estimated to be 5% per year for X-CGD and 2% per year for AR CGD,[7] and a more recent single-institution study on 76 patients reported an overall mortality rate of 1.5% per year.[8] There is a general consensus that a large majority of newly diagnosed children should survive well into their adult years with aggressive and careful management. As already noted, patients with deficiency of p47^{phox} have a tendency for milder disease compared with those with flavocytochrome-negative CGD. On the other hand, some patients (usually X-linked) prove to have more frequent serious infections or inflammatory complications (or both), likely because of the effects of modifier genes; these patients may warrant more aggressive treatment such as bone marrow transplantation (BMT; see later).

Several approaches can be used to prevent infections. Patients with CGD should receive all their routine immunizations on schedule (including live virus vaccines), with influenza vaccine administered each year as well. Cuts and skin abrasions should be cleansed promptly with soap and water and a topical antiseptic applied (2% hydrogen peroxide, Betadine ointment, or both). Frequent brushing, flossing, use of antibacterial mouthwash, and professional cleaning of teeth can help prevent gingivitis. Constipation should be avoided because it can lead to rectal or anal fissures and abscesses. Early anal infections can be treated with soaking in soapy water (with or without Betadine). The frequency of pulmonary infections can be reduced by not using commercially available bedside humidifiers; avoiding smoking (cigarettes and marijuana); and refraining from handling decaying plant materials (e.g., hay, mulch, rotting sawdust), which often contain numerous *Aspergillus* spp. Avoidance of construction sites, especially demolition of old buildings that may harbor fungi, is recommended. There have been clear outbreaks of *Aspergillus* pneumonias in immunosuppressed children visiting hospitals undergoing renovation.

There is clear evidence that chronic prophylactic TMP-SMX can decrease the number of bacterial infections in CGD patients by more than half without a concomitant increased risk of fungal infection. In addition, itraconazole is an effective agent for prophylaxis for fungal infections in CGD. Liver function tests should be monitored in patients receiving itraconazole.

Prophylactic rIFN-γ has been another mainstay of current management of CGD.[2,8] The clinical benefit of rIFN-γ is probably related to generally enhanced phagocyte function and killing by nonoxidative mechanisms because its use is not accompanied by any measurable improvement in NADPH oxidase activity in the vast majority of CGD patients. In the original multicenter trial, patients were randomized in a double-blind fashion to receive either placebo or rIFN-γ (0.05 mg/m^2 three times per week). As summarized in Table 48-5, there was a substantial decrease in the number of serious infections in the rIFN-γ arm. Side effects were observed in some of the patients but typically were restricted to mild fever and flulike symptoms. No additional adverse reactions, including any increased incidence of chronic inflammatory complications, have been noted with more prolonged courses of prophylactic rIFN-γ (more than 10 years), and the patients continued to have a substantial benefit with fivefold fewer serious infections compared with the placebo group in the phase III study in Table 48-5. On average, this group of patients averaged one serious infection per patient every 4 to 5 years. However, rIFN-γ is used less frequently in Europe as nonrandomized data did not suggest much benefit, and the usage in a cohort followed at the National Institutes of Health was recently reported to be only 36% because of either lack of access or because of side effects (fever, myalgia); the availability of more potent antifungals and oral antibiotics may be a mitigating factor for reducing serious infectious complications in the absence of prophylactic rIFN-γ.

Table 48-5 Efficacy of Interferon-γ in Preventing Serious Infections in Chronic Granulomatous Disease

	Clinical Study				
Variable	**Phase III Placebo***	**Phase III IFN-γ***	**Phase IV (U.S.) IFN-γ†**	**Phase IV (Europe) IFN-γ‡**	**Phase IV IFN-γ§**
Patients (*n*)	65	63	30	28	76
Average duration of therapy on study (years)	0	0.83	1.03	2.4	4.3
Patient-years in study	50.9	52.1	31.10	67.2	328
Serious infections per patient-year	1.1	0.38	0.13	0.4	0.30
Number of hospital days per patient-year	28.2	8.6	2.2	15.0	Not reported

IFN, Interferon.

*Results from The International Chronic Granulomatous Disease Cooperative Study Group: A controlled trial of interferon gamma to prevent infection in chronic granulomatous disease. *N Engl J Med* 324:509, 1991.

†Results from Weening RS, Leitz GJ, Seger RA: Recombinant human interferon-gamma in patients with chronic granulomatous disease—European follow up study. *Eur J Pediatr* 154:295, 1995.

‡Results from Bemiller LS, Roberts DH, Starko KM, et al: Safety and effectiveness of long-term interferon gamma therapy in patients with chronic granulomatous disease. *Blood Cells Mol Dis* 21:239, 1995.

§Results from Marciano BE, Wesley R, De Carlo ES, et al: Long-term interferon-gamma therapy for patients with chronic granulomatous disease. *Clin Infect Dis* 39:692, 2004.

One of the most frequent errors in the management of CGD patients is the failure to treat potentially serious infections promptly and aggressively with appropriate parenteral antibiotics. Even the best antibiotics can be rendered ineffective if given too late in the course of an infection in CGD. Therefore, early intervention is advisable. Although many of the minor infections and low-grade fevers in CGD patients can be managed on an outpatient basis, episodes of consistently high fever over a 24-hour period or clearly established infections (e.g., pneumonia or lymphadenitis) should be treated with parenteral antibiotics that cover, at least initially, *S. aureus* and enteric gram-negative organisms. Reasonable attempts to define the source of the infection and the responsible microbe should also begin promptly. Monitoring markers of inflammation such as the erythrocyte sedimentation rate (ESR) or C-reactive protein (CRP) can be very useful, both as a clue to the presence of a significant infection as well as following the patient's response to therapy. If the patient fails to respond, then more aggressive diagnostic procedures should be instituted (computed tomography, bone, and gallium scans; open biopsies if indicated) and empirical changes in the antibiotics used to broaden coverage to *Pseudomonas cepacia*. If fungus is identified or strongly suspected, amphotericin B has been the drug of choice in the past, but newer azole antifungal agents such as voriconazole are supplanting its use. Even with appropriate antibiotics, certain types of infections respond slowly and may require many months of therapy. Surgical drainage or resection can sometimes play a key role in accelerating healing of certain types of infection such as lymphadenitis, osteomyelitis, and abscesses of visceral organs such as the liver or lung. Finally, granulocyte transfusions may be of benefit in the treatment of stubborn or life-threatening infections.[7]

Recurrent fever in CGD always raises the possibility of infection in these patients; however, the macrophage activation syndrome (MAS)–hemophagocytic lymphohistiocytosis (HLH) spectrum of disorders should be considered, especially if the patient has splenomegaly, leukopenia, or thrombocytopenia. As in inflammatory disorders like rheumatoid arthritis, secondary MAS-HLH has been reported in CGD and is probably often overlooked. Specific treatment may be indicated, especially if the patient has significant cytopenias or evidence of hepatic dysfunction.

Use of corticosteroids should generally be avoided, including extensive topical use, except in cases of severe asthma, esophageal strictures, gastric antral narrowing, granulomatous cystitis, inflammatory bowel disease, or certain cases of pneumonia. Clear evidence shows that corticosteroids are beneficial in these clinical settings because the steroids induce rapid regression of obstructive symptoms at low oral doses (e.g., 1 mg/kg/day of prednisone). Steroids can be lifesaving in young children with airway obstruction because of inflammation. Because of the exaggerated inflammatory reaction seen in CGD, there can be significant swelling in the airway and compression by pulmonary nodes that can block air movement and impede drainage. In these cases, the physician and patient should be aware of the risks of the additional immunosuppression caused by the corticosteroids.

Rare patients with X91° CGD have genomic deletions that span the gp91^{phox} gene and the Xk gene, which encodes a membrane protein necessary for expression of the Kell genes.[2] Absence of the Xk gene product results in the McLeod syndrome, in which red blood cells have weak Kell antigens and variable acanthocytosis along with nerve and muscle disorders related to its expression in nonerythroid tissues. Transfusion of patients with McLeod syndrome poses a serious problem because they can develop alloantibodies of wide specificity that can preclude any further transfusions except with Kell-negative blood products. McLeod-matched blood is extremely rare, and patients with this syndrome should have their own blood frozen in case it is needed. Note that use of maternal blood does not solve the problem because only 50% of the mother's blood will match. Because of the difficulty in finding blood, transfusion with non-McLeod blood is likely to occur. Although management is difficult and use of steroids is necessary, the hemolytic anemia can be managed successfully.

Allogeneic BMT can be used to treat CGD, including using matched unrelated donors.[6,8] Because of the risks associated with this procedure, BMT had generally considered only for patients who have a fully human leukocyte antigen–matched sibling and frequent and severe infections despite aggressive medical management. However, reduced-intensity conditioning regimens for allogeneic transplantations have now been successfully used for BMT in CGD, including several cases with ongoing fungal infections.[6,8] Despite improved success rates and decreased complications, which patients with CGD should undergo transplantation remains an individualized decision, particularly for those with residual NADPH oxidase activity and little or no history of serious infection or other complications.[8] Finally, genetic therapies aimed at correcting the defective gene in bone marrow (BM) stem cells hold promise for the future if obstacles can be solved to achieve effective and safe gene delivery and their transplantation.[6] Observations on female carriers of X-linked CGD with skewed X-inactivation and preclinical studies in murine CGD models suggest that complete correction of NADPH oxidase activity in 10% of circulating neutrophils will lead to clinically relevant improvements in host defense.

Neutrophil Glucose-6-Phosphate Dehydrogenase Deficiency

NADPH, the primary substrate for the respiratory burst oxidase, is generated by the first two reactions of the hexose monophosphate shunt pathway, which are catalyzed by G6PD (see Fig. 48-3, reaction 8) and 6-phosphogluconate dehydrogenase (6PGD).[15] The leukocyte and erythrocyte G6PD are encoded by the same gene. Thus, a severe deficiency of G6PD in neutrophils can result in a greatly attenuated respiratory burst because of low levels of NADPH. However, the vast majority of individuals with inherited G6PD deficiency do not have problems with a decreased respiratory burst or recurrent infections. A CGD-like syndrome has very rarely been observed in G6PD-deficient patients who have congenital nonspherocytic hemolytic anemia (CNSHA), in whom hemolysis occurs in the absence of redox stress.[2,15] Even in CNSHA, most G6PD mutations cause the enzyme to decay over a period of days and weeks, so that levels in the short-lived neutrophil usually do not become critically low even in some of the most unstable G6PD variants. A few rare and poorly understood G6PD mutations that cause CNSHA are associated with extremely low (<5% of normal) levels of G6PD in the neutrophil, resulting in a deficient respiratory burst and CGD-like symptoms. The combination of chronic, severe hemolytic anemia, recurrent infections, and the laboratory demonstration of extremely low G6PD levels in neutrophils and erythrocytes serves to distinguish this disease from CGD. The treatment for neutrophil G6PD deficiency is the same as for CGD except that the efficacy of rIFN-γ has not been demonstrated in the former. The chronic hemolytic anemia is treated by supportive means, including transfusions.

Disorders of Glutathione Metabolism

As depicted in Fig. 48-3 (reaction 6), the reduced form of glutathione (GSH) serves to protect the neutrophil from the harmful effects of hydrogen peroxide on NADPH oxidase and other neutrophil proteins. Adequate intracellular levels of reduced glutathione are maintained by recycling oxidized glutathione (GSSG) to GSH by glutathione reductase (see Fig. 48-3, reaction 7) as well as by de novo synthesis of glutathione by glutathione synthetase (see Fig. 48-3, reaction 9). Severe deficiencies in either of these enzymes are extremely rare and are apparently inherited in an AR manner.[2] In the case of glutathione reductase deficiency, the respiratory burst terminates prematurely, presumably owing to the toxic effects of accumulating hydrogen peroxide on NADPH oxidase. This brief burst of O_2X91^-, however, appears to be sufficient for adequate microbial killing because the few patients reported have not had problems with recurrent infections. However, they do have a congenital hemolytic anemia during periods of oxidant stress caused by diminished levels of glutathione reductase in erythrocytes. In glutathione synthetase deficiency, the respiratory burst proceeds normally. Patients have a severe metabolic acidosis caused by elevated levels of 5-oxoproline, which is the product of the first step in glutathione synthesis and is present in increased levels because of a lack of feedback of GSH on the synthetic pathway. Patients with glutathione synthetase deficiency also have intermittent neutropenia (perhaps caused by the acidosis) as well as oxidant-induced hemolysis. There are mild problems with recurrent infections. Therapy with vitamin E (400 IU/day) has been found to be beneficial in patients with severe glutathione synthetase deficiency with hemolysis and infections.

Myeloperoxidase Deficiency

Myeloperoxidase deficiency is the most common inherited disorder of phagocytes but is almost always asymptomatic.[16] MPO is present in azurophilic granules of neutrophils and monocytes and catalyzes the production of a potent antimicrobial agent, HOCl from chloride and hydrogen peroxide (see Fig. 48-3, reaction 4).[3,4] HOCl in turn reacts with a variety of primary and secondary amines to form chloramines, some of which can be toxic. Moreover, HOCl is capable of activating latent metalloproteinases (e.g., collagenase) and inactivating antiproteinases.

Complete MPO deficiency is seen in approximately one in 4000 individuals, and partial deficiency is even more common (one in 2000 persons). The key features of MPO deficiency are summarized in Table 48-6. The disorder is inherited in an AR manner. In the few cases reported, several different mutations have been identified, which generally appear to affect the posttranslational processing of a precursor polypeptide for MPO. Acquired forms of MPO deficiency are also seen. The gene that encodes for MPO is located on chromosome 17 at q22-q23 near the breakpoint for the 15 to 17 translocation of promyelocytic leukemia. Subpopulations of MPO-deficient cells can be seen not only in the M3 (promyelocytic) form of acute myeloid leukemia but also in the M2 and M4 forms. MPO-deficient cells are also seen in approximately 25% of patients with chronic myeloid leukemia and myelodysplastic syndromes.

One of the most curious features of MPO deficiency is the remarkable lack of clinical symptoms in affected persons, given the prediction that severe MPO deficiency would cripple important antimicrobial reactions catalyzed by HOCl. In vitro, an impressive defect in killing *Candida albicans* and hyphal forms of *Aspergillus fumigatus* is observed.[16] Bacterial killing in vitro is also abnormal in being somewhat slower than normal, but eventually it is complete. MPO-deficient mice also exhibit abnormalities in host defense against *Candida* and *Klebsiella* spp. Excessive or unusual infections in MPO-deficient patients, however, are uncommon, except for rare individuals who also have diabetes mellitus.[16] In these individuals, disseminated fungal infections (usually candidiasis) are seen.

The discrepancy between the in vitro and in vivo manifestations of MPO deficiency in most patients can be explained in several ways. First, the respiratory burst in MPO-deficient neutrophils is substantially augmented, presumably from the absence of HOCl-mediated toxic effects on the NADPH oxidase. Second, other products of the respiratory burst, together with the oxygen-independent antibacterial proteins, appear to have sufficient potency to compensate for the loss of MPO-dependent reactions. Finally, residual amounts of MPO coupled with the normal levels of eosinophil peroxidase may provide at least some degree of peroxidative activity at the sites of infection.

Treatment is usually not required for MPO deficiency except in those individuals with fungal infections. In these patients, aggressive use of antifungal antibiotics is indicated. The prognosis is excellent in the majority of patients with MPO deficiency.

Table 48-6 Summary of Myeloperoxidase Deficiency

Incidence	On in 2000 (partial deficiency) On in 4000 (total deficiency)
Inheritance	Autosomal recessive with variable expression; MPO gene on chromosome 17 at q22-q23
Molecular defect	Defective posttranslational processing of an abnormal MPO precursor polypeptide; eosinophil peroxidase encoded by different gene and levels normal
Pathogenesis	Partial or complete MPO deficiency leads to diminished production of HOCl and HOCl-derived chloramines; MPO products are necessary for rapid killing of microbes (especially *Candida* spp.) but not absolutely required
Clinical manifestations	Usually clinically silent Disseminated candidiasis or fungal disease (rare; usually in conjunction with diabetes mellitus) Acquired deficiency in M2, M3, and M4 AMLs and myelodysplasia
Laboratory evaluation	Deficiency of neutrophil and monocyte peroxidase by histochemical analysis (eosinophil peroxidase normal) Delayed, but eventually normal, killing of bacteria in vitro Failure to kill *Candida albicans* and hyphal forms of *Aspergillus fumigatus* in vitro
Differential diagnosis	Acquired partial MPO deficiency seen in M2, M3, and M4 AML; MDS; and Batten disease
Therapy	None in asymptomatic patients Aggressive treatment of fungal infections when they occur Control of blood glucose levels in diabetics
Prognosis	Usually excellent

AML, Acute myeloid leukemias; *HOCl,* hypochlorous acid; *MDS,* myelodysplastic syndromes; *MPO,* myeloperoxidase.

DISORDERS OF PHAGOCYTE ADHESION AND CHEMOTAXIS

Since 1970, numerous investigators have found in vitro chemotactic abnormalities in neutrophils from patients with a wide variety of clinical disorders associated with increased susceptibility to bacterial and fungal infections.[2] In most circumstances, the chemotactic abnormality identified was only marginal and not always clearly related to the clinical status of the patient. In other instances, clear and major defects were identified in vitro that correlated with the in vivo propensity for infection. Extensive classification systems have been devised to categorize the numerous acquired defects in chemotaxis. The problem in many of these reports is that it is unclear whether the infections were caused by the in vitro chemotactic abnormality or by the medical complications of the underlying disorder (e.g., acidosis, malnutrition, or exposure to nosocomial infections). A further complicating factor is that there are inherent limitations in the in vitro chemotaxis assay, which is subject to laboratory artifacts both as a result of neutrophil purification procedures as well as the assay itself. Furthermore, the extent to which these in vitro chemotactic assay systems faithfully reflect prevailing in vivo conditions is not known. Our understanding of chemotactic disorders has been hampered by the limitations of these assays, just as the elucidation of respiratory burst defects was obscured when the major available assay was in vitro bacterial killing. In this section, the most important and best characterized of the chemotactic disorders, leukocyte adhesion deficiency (LAD), is discussed in detail. A brief discussion of several other clinically significant chemotactic disorders is also provided.

Leukocyte Adhesion Deficiency Type I

Leukocyte adhesion deficiency type I (LAD I) is a rare AR disorder of leukocyte adhesion, chemotaxis, and ingestion of C3bi-opsonized microbes as a result of decreased or absent expression of the leukocyte β_2 integrins (Table 48-7).[17,18] The hallmark of LAD I is the occurrence of repeated, often severe bacterial and fungal infections without the accumulation of pus despite persistent granulocytosis (see Table 48-7). The molecular basis for LAD was first suggested by Crowley and colleagues, who found that neutrophils from a patient with this clinical syndrome lacked a high-molecular-weight membrane glycoprotein (see Dinauer and Newburger[2]). The patient's neutrophils could not be made to adhere to plastic surfaces or to respond to serum-opsonized particles in terms of ingestion and respiratory burst activity.

The molecular basis of LAD I is now known to result from mutations in the gene for the common CD18 β2 subunit for these three leukocyte glycoproteins, now termed *β2 integrins,* that belong to the integrin superfamily of adhesion molecules. Integrins are noncovalently linked heterodimeric glycoproteins consisting of an α and a β subunit. Within each of the eight known integrin subfamilies the β subunit is identical (and defines the subfamily), but the α subunit varies and confers the functional specificity on the integrin. The molecular defect in LAD involves all members of the β2 integrin subfamily: αL β 2 (CD11a/CD18), αm β 2 (CD11b/CD18), and αx β 2 (CD11c/CD18). CD11a/CD18 is often referred to as LFA-1 while CD11b/ CD18 is also called Mac-1, Mo1, or CR3. LAD I patients have an absent, diminished, or structurally abnormal β 2 subunit (CD18) (see later), and as a result, the three types of α chains in the β 2 integrin subfamily cannot assemble into normal α-β heterodimers. Thus, all three β 2 integrins are moderately to severely deficient on all leukocytes in LAD.

Table 48-7 Summary of Leukocyte Adhesion Deficiency Type 1

Incidence	More than 60 patients described in literature
Inheritance	AR
Molecular defect	An absent, diminished, or structurally abnormal β subunit (CD18) caused by one of several types of mutations in the β gene; in the absence of a normal β subunit, the three types of α chains in the β_2 integrin subfamily (CD11a, b, c) cannot assemble into normal α-β heterodimers
Pathogenesis	All three β_2 integrins (CD11a/CD18, CD11b/CD18, and CD11c/CD18) are deficient on all leukocytes, causing multiple abnormalities in cell function: adherence; chemotaxis; and C3bi-mediated ingestion, degranulation, and respiratory burst
Clinical manifestation	Persistent granulocytosis (neutrophil count, 12,000-100,000/mm^3) Severe or moderate phenotypes depending on severity of deficiency Recurrent pyogenic infections with absent neutrophil infiltration Delayed umbilical cord separation Severe gingivitis or periodontitis
Laboratory evaluation	Flow cytometric measurement of surface CD11b in stimulated neutrophils with monoclonal anti-CD11b
Differential diagnosis	CGD May be associated with severe neutrophil actin dysfunction
Therapy	Hematopoietic stem cell transplant in clinically severe patients (CD11b < 0.3% of normal) Aggressive use of parenteral antibiotics Possible benefit of prophylactic TMP-SMX
Prognosis	Severe: high incidence of death before age 2 years unless transplantation is performed Moderate: can survive into 20s and 30s but with recurrent infections

AR, Autosomal recessive; *CGD,* chronic granulomatous disease; *TMP-SMX,* trimethoprim–sulfamethoxazole.

The β2 integrins serve as receptors for the opsonic complement fragment C3bi, the intercellular adhesion molecules 1 and 2 (ICAM-1 and ICAM-2) that are expressed on endothelial cells and leukocytes, and fibrinogen. The diminished or absent expression of β2 integrins in LAD I leukocytes results in the failure of phagocytes to emigrate from the blood stream to sites of infection. The early interactions with the endothelium, termed *rolling,* are normal in LAD I because these are mediated by a different family of adhesion molecules known as selectins. However, β2 integrins are responsible for the subsequent tight binding of neutrophils and monocytes to cytokine-activated endothelium, and this step is therefore severely defective in LAD I. Transendothelial migration is also impaired. A second major functional defect in LAD is the failure of phagocytes to bind C3bi opsonized microbes. Because CD11b/CD18 is the predominant phagocyte receptor for this complement fragment, C3bi-mediated ingestion, degranulation, and respiratory burst activity are severely affected in LAD. Finally, β2 integrin-dependent signals play a key role in activating neutrophils for enhanced migration, phagocytosis of antibody-opsonized microbes, and degranulation.

Despite in vitro defects in lymphocyte responses dependent on LFA-1 (CD11a/CD18), patients with LAD I rarely have clinical manifestations related to impaired lymphocyte function. It is believed that the role CD11a/CD18 plays in lymphoid cell function can be compensated by other adhesion proteins (CD2, CD4, CD8, and so on).

Molecular Genetics of Leukocyte Adhesion Deficiency Type I

The fact that LAD I involves a deficiency of all leukocyte β2 integrins focused attention on the common β2 chain (CD18), and mutations in the corresponding gene, *ITGB2,* have been identified in all LAD I patients who have been analyzed at the molecular level to date.[17,18] Although expression of the leukocyte integrin α subunits is normal in LAD I, these are not transported to the cell surface because the β2 chain is absent or contains mutations that disrupt its structure or its interaction with the α subunit. Mutations in the α subunits have not been found thus far in patients with LAD I. The CD18 glycoprotein has a large extracellular domain at the N terminus, a single transmembrane domain, and a 46-residue cytoplasmic tail. As with X-linked CGD, CD18 mutations in LAD I are heterogeneous in nature and family specific and can lead to either undetectable or low (9%-20% of normal) levels of α-β dimer expression that correlates with the clinical severity of the disease. More than 50 different mutations have now been characterized in more than 100 families.[17] These include missense mutations, mRNA splicing defects, small deletions, and a premature termination signal. Many patients are compound heterozygotes and have two different mutant alleles for CD18. About half of patients with LAD I in whom the genetic defect has been identified have point mutations in a stretch of 250 amino acids in the extracellular domain of CD18. This region is highly conserved among all β subunits and appears to be important for interaction with the α subunit.

Clinical Features

The key features of LAD I are summarized in Table 48-7. The clinical presentation of LAD is heterogeneous and is related to the severity of the deficiency of the β2 integrins. The severe clinical phenotype is associated with less than 0.3% of the normal amount of these glycoproteins on the leukocyte surface; the moderate phenotype has 2.5% to 6% of normal levels. In both the severe and moderate forms of the disease, persistent granulocytosis (neutrophil count of 12,000-100,000/mm^3) is a constant finding, as are recurrent cutaneous abscesses and aggressive periodontitis and gingivitis. Additional clinical features seen more often in the severe clinical phenotype include delayed umbilical cord separation, omphalitis, perirectal cellulitis, severe ulcerative stomatitis, and bacterial sepsis. A striking finding in LAD I is that abscesses and other sites of infections are devoid of pus despite the marked neutrophilia because neutrophils are unable to emigrate to tissues. *S. aureus* and gram-negative enteric bacteria cause the majority of infections in LAD I. Fungal infections can also occur, particularly from *C. albicans* and *Aspergillus* spp.

Note that infants with delayed separation of the umbilical cord who are healthy and have normal blood counts are very unlikely to have LAD I. Although the mean age of cord separation ranges from 7 to 15 days, 10% of healthy infants can have cord separation at 3 weeks of age or later.

Diagnosis

The diagnosis of LAD I is made by flow cytometric measurement of surface CD11b (Mac1) (or the shared CD18 subunit) in unstimulated and stimulated neutrophils using commercially available monoclonal antibodies directed against CD11b or CD18 (see Fig. 48-6). Neutrophils contain an intracellular pool of CD11b/CD18 in their secondary (specific) and tertiary granules, which can be mobilized to the cell surface during stimulation. Therefore, the deficiency of CD11b can be more dramatically demonstrated by using stimulated neutrophils. Carriers of LAD I can be identified by this method because they have been found to express approximately 50% of normal levels of CD11b on the surface of their stimulated neutrophils (see Fig. 48-6).

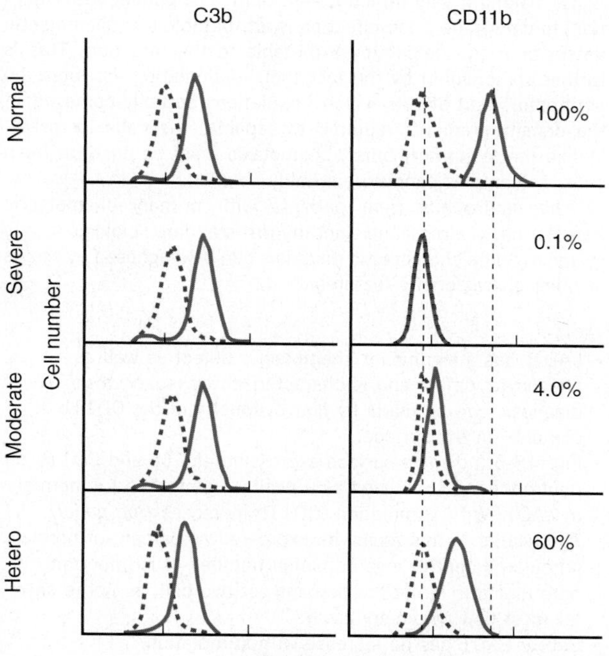

Figure 48-6 EVALUATION OF ADHESION MOLECULE EXPRESSION FOR DIAGNOSIS OF LEUKOCYTE ADHESION DEFICIENCY (LAD). Fluorescence of C3b specific antibody labeled neutrophils *(solid line)* increases compared with a nonspecific control *(dashed line)* after 30-minute exposure to 10-nM fMLP in healthy donors, subjects with severe and moderate forms of LAD-I, and a heterozygous LAD-1 carrier. However, the increase in CD11b fluorescence *(solid line)* is markedly diminished in LAD-1 patients. The respective percent of normal stimulated mean channel number is shown in the *right column*. Note that these results are expressed as percent of normal fluorescence intensity, not as percent of positive cells as is the case in most flow cytometry assays.

Prognosis and Treatment

Treatment for LAD I depends on the clinical severity of the disorder. In patients with the moderate clinical phenotype, cutaneous and oral infections can be managed as they occur. The use of prophylactic antibiotics such as TMP-SMX appears to be beneficial, as does aggressive prophylactic treatment of periodontal disease. It is important to note that even patients with the moderate phenotype can die of overwhelming infection. In patients with severe LAD I, aggressive management is indicated because of the high incidence of death before the age of 2 years, and hematopoietic stem cell transplantation is recommended. LAD I should also be amenable to gene replacement therapy in the future.

Leukocyte Adhesion Deficiency Types II and III

Leukocyte adhesion deficiency type II is a very rare clinical syndrome closely related to LAD I but caused by a defect in selectin-mediated adhesion events from a deficiency in leukocyte Siayl-Lewis X ligands.[17,18] It was first reported by Etzioni and colleagues in two unrelated boys of Muslim Arab origin and has since described in a total of five individuals (four Arab and one Turkish). The disease is inherited in an AR manner. Patients presented with neutrophilia, recurrent bacterial infections, and periodontitis, similar to LAD I, although these symptoms were generally not as severe. In addition, LAD II is associated with dysmorphic features and psychomotor retardation. LAD II neutrophils express normal levels of CD18. A clue as to the molecular cause of LAD II came from the observation that LAD II red cells were Lewis antigen negative and also had the rare Bombay (hh) erythrocyte phenotype, in which red blood cells express a nonfucosylated variant of the H antigen. These antigenic defects share in common the failure to form certain fucose carbohydrate linkage. The defect in fucose metabolism in LAD II has now been shown to result from mutations in the Golgi guanosine diphosphate–fucose membrane transporter. This leads to a generalized loss of expression of fucosylated glycans on the surface of cells, particularly the sialylated and fucosylated tetrasaccharide, SleX (CD15a), on the neutrophil surface. As a result, LAD II neutrophils are unable to bind to E- and P-selectin receptors on endothelium and therefore have an impairment in the early steps of rolling and loose binding to blood vessel walls before tight adhesion and emigration into infected tissues. Fucose supplementation has been partially successful in increasing expression of SLeX and decreasing clinical problems.

Leukocyte adhesion deficiency type III has recently been described in a handful of patients with severe, recurrent infections similar to LAD I as well as a bleeding tendency similar to Glanzmann thrombasthenia (a β3 integrin-related disorder).[17,18] This disorder results from AR defects in KINDLIN-3, a regulatory protein required for "inside-out" activation of multiple classes of integrins in blood cells. Because the clinical manifestations are typically severe, early BMT may be indicated for patients with LAD III (see Etzioni[18]).

Hyperimmunoglobulin E Syndrome

The hyperimmunoglobulin E syndrome (HIES) is a complex disorder characterized by markedly elevated serum IgE levels, serious recurrent staphylococcal infections, mucocutaneous candidiasis, chronic dermatitis, and skeletal and dental abnormalities.[19,20] Although not a primary phagocyte defect, neutrophils from patients with this syndrome exhibit a variable and at times profound chemotactic defect. HIES was first described in 1966 and was called Job syndrome, in reference to the biblical description of Job as being affected by "sore boils from the soles of his feet unto his crown." The skin abscesses in patients with HIES lack the erythema that is typical of such lesions and are referred to as *cold abscesses*. The key features of HIES are described in Table 48-8.

Most cases of HIES result from inherited or sporadic autosomal dominant (AD) mutations in signal transducer and activator of transcription 3 (STAT3), a Janus kinase (JAK)–activated transcription factor activated in response to many cytokines and growth factors. These mutations, which are located primarily in regions of the protein that interact with other proteins or with DNA, inhibit the activity of the wild-type STAT3 allele and result in a complex pattern of altered cytokine signaling and impaired T helper type 17 (Th17) cell differentiation. Mutations in *DOCK8*, a guanine nucleotide exchange factor, or *TYK2*, a JAK family member, result in the more rare AR forms of HIES that have more profound impairments in lymphocyte function, leading to a broader risk of infection and other immune dysregulation.

Insights into how STAT3 signaling defects lead to the clinical syndrome characteristic of AD HIES are now emerging. Defective responses to IL-6 may account for the minimal inflammatory responses characteristic of HIES, and the enhanced IgE production may reflect dysregulated immune responses secondary to impaired signaling by IL-10, a negative regulator. TH17 cells are important for control of mucocutaneous *Candida* infection, which is problematic in many patients. In addition, keratinocytes and bronchial epithelial cells are particularly dependent on TH17 cytokines to produce chemokines and antimicrobial peptides, which may explain the predilection for skin and lung infections. The dental and skeletal abnormalities may be related to defective STAT3 signaling in osteoblasts and osteoclasts.

Clinical Manifestations

The clinical manifestations of HIES are at times dramatic. Onset is generally in the first 2 months of life and is manifested by chronic dermatitis. By 5 years of age, patients have a history of recurrent skin abscesses, pneumonias, chronic otitis media, and sinusitis. As patients grow older, recurrent staphylococcal pneumonia is a common problem and can be complicated by the formation of pneumatoceles. Septic arthritis, cellulitis, and osteomyelitis are also observed and are

Table 48-8 Summary of Hyperimmunoglobulin E Syndrome

Incidence	More than 200 patients reviewed in the literature
Inheritance	AD with incomplete penetrance; sporadic forms, AR (rare)
Molecular defect	Dominant-negative mutations in STAT3 (AD inheritance; sporadic), Dock8 or Tyk2 kinase (AR)
Clinical manifestations	Staphylococcal pneumonia Pneumatoceles Fungal superinfection of lung cysts "Cold" cutaneous skin abscesses and furuncles Chronic eczematoid dermatitis Mucocutaneous candidiasis Chronic cutaneous viral infections (AR) Severe allergies (AR) Coarse facies, growth retardation (AD) Osteopenia, recurrent fractures (AD) Sinusitis, keratoconjunctivitis Scoliosis (AD) Hyperextensible joints (AD) Delayed shedding of primary teeth (AD) Vascular disease (AD)
Laboratory evaluation	Serum IgE > 2,500 IU/mL Peripheral blood eosinophilia
Differential diagnosis	Atopic dermatitis Wiskott-Aldrich syndrome, DiGeorge syndrome Hypergammaglobulinemia Chronic granulomatous disease
Therapy	Prophylactic anti–*Staphylococcus aureus* antibiotics Aggressive treatment of acute infections with parenteral antibiotics Surgical drainage of deep infections and resection of lung cysts Monitor for scoliosis, fractures, vascular disease
Prognosis	Generally good if managed aggressively Some patients develop lymphoid malignancies; patients with AR HIES have an increased risk and broader spectrum of cancer susceptibility

AD, Autosomal dominant; *AR*, autosomal recessive; *HIES*, hyperimmunoglobulin E syndrome; *IgE*, immunoglobulin E.

Diagnosis of Chemotactic Disorders

The direct measurement of neutrophil chemotaxis in a clinical setting is very difficult and requires a specialized research laboratory. Because the assays are biologic assays, the laboratory must run the tests at least monthly to maintain competence and have acceptable normal ranges. Neutrophil chemotaxis is significantly affected by inflammation, complement activation, and medications, making it very difficult, especially in a patient with infection, to determine if the infection is attributable to a chemotactic defect or if the defect is attributable to the infection. This is further complicated by the fact that inflammation activates the neutrophils and affects which populations actually come off of the density gradients required to separate the cells for assay. Unlike the respiratory burst, chemotaxis must be done on fresh cells, so samples cannot be reliably shipped.

The neutrophils from patients with primary chemotactic defects have almost no motility in standard biologic assay systems. Some chemotactic disorders can be diagnosed by assays of other characteristic features.

LAD-1

- LAD-1 has a significant chemotactic defect as well as phagocytic defect and is characterized by leukocytosis. The diagnosis can be made by flow cytometry of the CD11b complex on the surface.
- Fig. 48-6 indicates surface expression of C3b and CD11b on neutrophils. C3b is used as a positive control and is normal in LAD1. With stimulation, CD11b increases *(top panel)*.
- The results in this assay are expressed as percent of normal stimulated control mean channel number. It is important to note that this is not the percent positive cell, as is the case for most flow cytometry assays.
- Severe LAD1 has no increase with stimulation.
- Moderate LAD1 shows some shift of fluorescence with stimulation.
- Genetic analysis for this disorder is clinically available.

Other chemotactic disorders: Genetic analysis is available for several primary neutrophil defects, and this approach should be pursued before attempting assay of chemotaxis in a clinical setting.

No other primary chemotactic defects are readily diagnosed by a routine clinical laboratory. Measurement of neutrophil chemotaxis itself to look for secondary defects for any kind of clinical decision making is difficult if not impossible to interpret.

usually caused by *S. aureus,* although other bacterial pathogens have also been found. Patients can have chronic mucocutaneous candidiasis and occasionally exhibit keratoconjunctivitis, sometimes complicated by corneal scarring. One feature noted in the majority of patients by the time they reach the teenage years is the presence of coarse facial features (broad nasal bridge, prominent nose). Dental and bone abnormalities are also common features of HIES. Delayed or failure to shed primary teeth occur in the majority. Hyperextensible joints and scoliosis are frequent. Osteopenia of unknown etiology is observed in most patients, and there is an increased risk of fractures to the long bones and vertebral bodies even in the absence of osteopenia. Vascular disease, including aneurysms, tortuosity of middle-sized arteries, and hypertension is also frequently seen.

Patients with the AR form of HIES, the majority of whom have defects *DOCK8,* which is also referred to as *DOCK8* immunodeficiency syndrome, also have recurrent sinopulmonary infections, skin abscesses, and dermatitis, with the latter often the first symptom and developing in infancy. Unlike AD HIES, patients with *DOCK8* defects can develop asthma; severe allergies, including to foods, and chronic cutaneous viral infections with human papilloma virus, molluscum contagiosum virus, and herpes family viruses is a distinctive feature seen in approximately 90% of patients. These patients are also at high risk for a variety of malignancies in late childhood to early adulthood, believed to be caused by loss of immune surveillance for tumors.[19] AR HIES patients do not have the nonimmunologic skeletal and dental abnormalities characteristic of AD HIES.

Diagnosis

The diagnosis of HIES should be entertained in any child or young adult who has the above-described clinical picture or simply a history of recurrent infections. The hallmark laboratory finding is a marked elevation of serum immunoglobulin E (IgE), almost always greater than 2500 IU/mL. Levels can be as high as 150,000 IU/mL. Most patients also have peripheral eosinophilia. However, there is no correlation of clinical disease activity with the level of either IgE or peripheral eosinophilia. Atopic dermatitis is the major differential diagnosis because comparably high serum levels of IgE can be seen in patients in this disorder, as well as superficial skin infections. The severe and recurrent nature of the staphylococcal furuncles and pneumonias usually seen in HIES can help distinguish these patients from those with atopic dermatitis. Patients with other primary immunodeficiency syndromes may also manifest elevated IgE levels. Scoring criteria predictive of STAT3 mutations, including recurrent pneumonia, pathologic bone fractures, and lack of Th17 cells, are helpful.[19] DNA testing should be used to make a definitive diagnosis.

Therapy

The therapy for AD HIES is largely supportive.[19] Prophylactic antibiotics (e.g., dicloxacillin or TMP-SMX) can be effective in preventing *S. aureus* infections. Dermatitis can be treated with topical steroids. Bathing in diluted bleach can diminish colonization by *S. aureus.* Prophylactic antifungals can be helpful in patients with chronic mucocutaneous candidiasis. Intravenous antibiotics are used for deep-seated infections or for resistant cutaneous infections. Surgical resection of persistent pneumatoceles is sometimes indicated to prevent superinfection by fungal and gram-negative organisms. Intravenous Ig infusions have shown some success in the management of HIES. Attention should also be paid to blood pressure and other vascular complications. Although a role for hematopoietic stem cell transplantation in AD HIES is unclear, two children with STAT3 mutations who underwent transplantation for non-Hodgkin lymphoma are alive 10 and 14 years later with resolution of all immunologic and nonimmunologic features of HIES.[20] Patients with AR HIES may need prophylaxis for viral infections, and hematopoietic stem cell transplant may be a consideration in selected patients.

Miscellaneous Chemotactic Disorders

It is extremely rare to have primary defects in neutrophil actin polymerization as a cause of abnormal chemotaxis and recurrent infections.[1,2] In one case, neutrophils had diminished actin polymerization, chemotaxis, and phagocytosis of serum opsonized particles. Family members had decreased CD11b/CD18 expression and a partial decrease in actin polymerization, which suggested that this disorder might be a variant of LAD I; however, no similar cases have otherwise been described. An apparent AR disorder of actin polymerization has been described in a male infant of Tongan descent who presented with severe skin infections, recurrent pulmonary infiltrates, thrombocytopenia, and invasive *Candida tropicalis* infection. Neutrophil actin polymerization was markedly abnormal and associated with increased expression of an actin binding protein. Finally, a heterozygous point mutation in β-actin affecting binding to actin-regulatory proteins was discovered in a female patient with recurrent infections, photosensitivity, and mental retardation. Neutrophils had a marked impairment in chemotaxis and in the formyl peptide-induced respiratory burst.

A new syndrome of severe neutrophil dysfunction caused by a dominant-negative mutation in Rac2, a small GTPase expressed in blood cells that acts in many signal transduction pathways, was recently described in an infant boy born to unrelated parents (see Dinauer and Newburger [2]). This baby presented with rapidly progressive and deep-seated soft tissue infections, along with neutrophilia and poor formation of pus but normal expression of β2 integrins and fucosylated proteins. Neutrophils had marked defects in actin polymerization, chemotaxis, degranulation, and the respiratory burst in response to chemoattractants. Neutrophil responses to other agonists were normal, suggesting that the dominant negative Rac2 mutation produces a selective intracellular signaling defect.

Localized juvenile periodontitis (LJP) is a heterogeneous disorder of unknown etiology characterized by chronic and recurrent periodontal infections and severe alveolar bone loss with onset at the time of puberty.[21] Many patients with LJP have been reported to have defective neutrophil chemotaxis in vitro. At present, it appears that LJP is an acquired disorder in some patients and a genetic disorder in others. It may also be a combination of both in certain patients because they may inherit an unusual sensitivity to the chemotactic inhibitors released by certain periodontal microorganisms. The diagnosis of the disorder is made on the basis of severe periodontal disease and destructive alveolar bone loss involving the first molars and incisors developing during adolescence. It is important to note that many qualitative and quantitative neutrophil disorders are also associated with severe periodontal disease. Therefore, the differential diagnosis should include neutropenia (both chronic and cyclic), LAD, CGD, and Chédiak-Higashi syndrome (CHS).

One of the most consistently observed chemotactic abnormalities is seen in neonatal neutrophils.[22] These cells exhibit impaired chemotaxis in vitro in response to a wide variety of chemotactic factors. It appears as though this abnormality is caused, at least in part, by defects in cellular adhesion as a result of diminished mobilization of intracellular adhesion-promoting molecules to the cell surface. Defective neutrophil chemotaxis can be seen in normal neonates between birth and 5 days of age. In severely ill infants, the defect may persist for a longer time.

DEFECTS IN THE STRUCTURE AND FUNCTION OF LYSOSOMAL GRANULES

Two major disorders of neutrophil granules have been described, CHS and specific granule deficiency (SGD). A great deal has been learned about the structural and functional abnormalities of neutrophils from patients with these conditions. Although rare, these disorders are also obligatory components in the differential diagnosis for any patient with recurrent bacterial and fungal infections.

Chédiak-Higashi Syndrome

Chédiak-Higashi syndrome is a rare AR, multisystem disease resulting from widespread defects in granule morphogenesis, with giant lysosomes in leukocytes and other cells throughout the body.[23,24] The disorder is characterized by partial oculocutaneous albinism, frequent (and sometimes fatal) bacterial infections, a mild bleeding diathesis, and peripheral as well as cranial neuropathies associated with defects at the optic chiasm. Those who survive the recurrent infections develop an "accelerated phase" of the disease; one of the hereditary forms of HLH, which, if untreated, is eventually fatal because of a profound pancytopenia that develops.

The most dramatic granule defects are manifested in the various blood cells. Neutrophils contain a highly inhomogeneous population of huge granules derived from coalescence of azurophilic (primary) granules. The giant granules are often more prominent in the BM than in the peripheral blood because many of the abnormal myeloid precursors are apparently destroyed before they leave the BM, resulting in moderate neutropenia with absolute neutrophil counts ranging from 500 to 2000 cells/mm^3. Granules are also markedly deficient in antimicrobial granule enzymes such as cathepsin G and elastase, consistent with a defect in granule morphogenesis. Degranulation is delayed and incomplete in Chédiak-Higashi neutrophils, resulting in impaired bacterial killing. Chemotaxis is also defective, perhaps related to poor deformability because of the presence of the large granules. Monocytes and macrophages exhibit similar giant cytoplasmic granules, with resultant abnormalities in their phagocytic functions. Giant granules are also seen in lymphocytes and are associated with defects in cytotoxic T-lymphocyte and NK cell function. Eosinophils contain large granules, the functional significance of which is not known. Platelets in this disorder have a storage pool deficiency of adenosine diphosphate and serotonin, presumably caused by the abnormal granule morphogenesis in megakaryocytes, leading to a defect in platelet aggregation.

Abnormal giant granules are also present in other cell types. These include melanocytes, which contain abnormal melanosomes that cannot transfer their contents to adjacent keratinocytes; Schwann cells; astrocytes; and certain cells in the liver, spleen, pancreas, gastric mucosa, kidney, adrenal gland, and pituitary gland.

Table 48-9 Summary of Chédiak-Higashi Syndrome

Incidence	More than 200 cases described
Inheritance	AR
Molecular defect	A defect in granule morphogenesis in multiple tissues resulting from mutations in the *CHS1 (LYST)* gene encoding a lysosomal trafficking regulator protein
Pathogenesis	Giant coalesced azurophil granules in neutrophils, resulting in ineffective granulopoiesis and neutropenia, delayed and incomplete degranulation, and defective chemotaxis; abnormal granules in other cells (NK cells, cytotoxic T cells, platelets, melanocytes, neurons)
Clinical manifestations	Partial oculocutaneous albinism Recurrent severe bacterial infections (usually *Staphylococcus aureus*) Cranial and peripheral neuropathies (muscle weakness, ataxia, sensory loss) HLH (accelerated phase)
Laboratory evaluation	Giant granules in peripheral blood granulocytes and in BM myeloid progenitor cells Widespread lymphohistiocytic infiltrates in accelerated phase
Differential diagnosis	Other genetic forms of partial albinism Giant granules can be seen in acute and CMLs
Therapy	Prophylactic TMP-SMX Parenteral antibiotics for acute infections Ascorbic acid (200 mg/day for infants; 6 g/day for adults) HSCT before or at beginning of HLH
Prognosis	Most patients die from infection or complications of HLH during the first or second decade of life unless transplantation is performed

AR, Autosomal recessive; *BM,* bone marrow; *CML,* chronic myeloid leukemia; *HLH,* hemophagocytic lymphohistiocytosis; *HSCT,* hematopoietic stem cell transplant; *NK,* natural killer; *TMP-SMX,* trimethoprim–sulfamethoxazole.

Molecular Genetics

A gene termed *CHS1* or *LYST* (for its presumed function as a lysosomal trafficking regulatory protein) affected in the majority of CHS cases has recently been identified and is on the long arm of chromosome 1.[24] The encoded protein is very large (3801 amino acids); its specific function is unknown, but recent studies suggest that it may inhibit lysosome fusion with other intracellular membrane vesicles. A variety of frameshift and nonsense mutations that predict synthesis of truncated forms of the protein have been identified in most, but not all, CHS patients studied to date. There is no correlation between the length of the truncated CHS1 protein and the severity of the disease. Disorders similar to human CHS have also been described in many mammalian species, including Aleutian mink, *beige* mice, blue foxes, cats, killer whales, and Hereford cattle. Identification of the human CHS1 gene was aided by positional cloning of the mouse *lyst* homolog affected in *beige* mice.

Clinical Manifestations

The key features of CHS are summarized in Table 48-9. The disease usually presents in infancy or early childhood, with infections involving the lungs, skin, and mucous membranes being most commonly encountered. Dental caries and periodontal disease are also common. The most frequent offending organism is *S. aureus*. Gram-negative bacteria, *Aspergillus* spp. and *Candida* spp. also are responsible for many infections. Platelet granule defects result in easy bruising and epistaxis. There is partial oculocutaneous albinism and photosensitivity. Patients may have a white forelock or an ashen or grayish silver sheen to the hair, which can vary from blond to dark brown. In younger patients, there may be a cartwheel distribution of pigment in the iris and an abnormal red reflex. Neurologic manifestations include peripheral or cranial neuropathies, gait abnormalities, muscle weakness, sensory loss, seizures, or spinocerebellar degeneration. Neurologic symptoms worsen with age.

Approximately 85% of children surviving into the second decade of life develop an accelerated phase of the disease, with fever, lymphadenopathy, and progressive pancytopenia, that is now recognized to be a genetic form of HLH caused by impaired lymphocyte and NK cell function.[25] The development of HLH can sometimes be precipitated by Epstein-Barr virus infection. A reactive-appearing lymphohistiocytic proliferation occurs in the liver, spleen, lymph nodes, and BM, and the prognosis is uniformly fatal unless patients undergo BMT.

Diagnosis

The diagnosis of CHS is made on the basis of the giant peroxidase-positive lysosomal granules in the peripheral blood granulocytes or in BM myeloid cells. Identification of large, acid phosphatase–positive lysosomes in amniocytes and chorionic villus cells has been used to diagnose CHS prenatally. Other clinical features characteristic of CHS can support the diagnosis, including mild oculocutaneous albinism; silvery hair, in which microscopic examination reveals giant melanin granules; and a bleeding diathesis. The development of HLH is characterized by diffuse infiltrates of lymphohistiocytic cells seen on biopsy and by pancytopenia. Occasionally, giant granules that resemble those of CHS can be seen in both acute and chronic myelogenous leukemias.

Therapy

The treatment for the stable phase of CHS is similar to that for other neutrophil disorders. Prophylactic antibiotics such as TMP-SMX appear to be beneficial. Parenteral antibiotics are indicated for acute infections, and responses are often slow. Treatment with high-dose ascorbic acid (200 mg/day for infants; 6 g/day for adults) has been found to improve the clinical status of some patients. Although there is some controversy regarding the efficacy of ascorbic acid, given the safety of this medication, it seems prudent to administer it to all patients. The treatment of HLH (accelerated phase) includes combinations of drugs that suppress the function of activated macrophages and T cells followed by allogeneic hematopoietic stem cell transplantation.[25] Indeed, transplantation is ideally performed before or at the beginning of the accelerated phase. Note that transplantation does not prevent the progressive neuropathy of CHS.

Specific Granule Deficiency

Neutrophil SGD is an extremely rare congenital disorder characterized by recurrent bacterial and fungal infections, primarily involving the skin, ears, and lungs.[2,26] Infections are often indolent and smoldering, and *S. aureus, P. aeruginosa,* enteric gram-negative bacteria, and *C. albicans* are the major pathogens. Family studies suggest that it is inherited in an AR manner. Neutrophils from patients with SGD have atypical bilobed nuclei, absent specific granules, and multiple deficiencies of secondary and tertiary granule mRNAs and proteins, including lactoferrin, vitamin B_{12}-binding protein and gelatinase B; although azurophil granules in this disorder are present and contain MPO and lysozyme, they are markedly deficient in defensins. Monocytes display cell surface and functional defects, eosinophils lack eosinophil-specific granule proteins such as eosinophil cationic protein and platelets have abnormal α granules, suggesting that the underlying defect may be related to regulation of the synthesis of certain granule and membrane proteins. This defect in synthesis is confined to BM-derived cells because lactoferrin secretion is normal in the glandular epithelia of SGD patients despite the severe deficiency in the neutrophils.

The recurrent skin and pulmonary infections characteristic of SGD appear to be caused by two fundamental defects in the neutrophils. One defect is the marked deficiency of at least two important microbicidal granule proteins, lactoferrin and defensins. The other defect is a relatively severe chemotactic abnormality presumably caused by the absence of the intracellular pool of leukocyte adhesion molecules that normally reside in the specific granules. As discussed earlier, these $\beta 2$ integrins play a key role in phagocyte chemotaxis.

The molecular defect responsible for most cases of SGD has recently been shown to involve a myeloid transcription factor known as C/EBPε that regulates expression of certain genes activated during granulocyte differentiation.[2,26] This came about serendipitously when it was recognized that mice with a targeted deletion in the C/EBPε gene characteristics similar to those of SGD patients, including neutrophils with bilobed nuclei, absent secondary granules, and impaired chemotaxis along with increased susceptibility to bacterial infections. To date, mutations in the C/EBPε gene have been identified in two SGD patients that encode truncated, nonfunctional proteins. However, DNA sequencing of the C/EBPε gene of several other SGD patients has not revealed abnormalities, suggesting that SGD is a genetically heterogeneous disorder.

The diagnosis of SGD can be readily made by microscopic examination. Wright-stained neutrophils are devoid of specific granules but contain normal numbers of azurophilic granules. Electron microscopy reveals small peroxidase-negative vesicles, which presumably represent empty specific granules. The diagnosis of SGD can also be established by demonstrating a severe deficiency in either lactoferrin or vitamin B_{12}-binding protein. An acquired form of SGD can be seen in burn patients or in individuals with various myeloproliferative disorders. The treatment for SGD is similar to that for other neutrophil disorders. If medical management is aggressive, the prognosis appears quite good, with patients surviving into their adult years.

MISCELLANEOUS INHERITED AND AQUIRED DISORDERS OF PHAGOCYTE FUNCTION

Rare inherited defects in phagocyte production or response to inflammatory cytokines are manifested as recurrent infections.[27,28] HIES also falls into this category (see earlier discussion). A distinctive group of disorders referred to as *Mendelian susceptibility to mycobacterial diseases* (MSMD) involve inherited defects in macrophage IL-12/23–dependent IFN-γ–mediated immunity. Macrophage production of IL-12 and IL-23 after ingestion of mycobacteria triggers IFN-γ production by T and NK lymphocytes, which in turn activates crucial genes in macrophages. MSDM (MIM 20990) can be caused by inherited AR, AD, or X-linked defects leading to impaired T-cell production of IFN-γ, expression of the IFN-γ receptor, or downstream signaling, which results in a spectrum of recurrent and severe atypical mycobacterial infections, as well as susceptibility to *Salmonella* and, in some subgroups, viral infections.[27,28] A variety of genetic defects in a scaffolding protein known as IKK-γ or NEMO that is important for activation of the nuclear factor kappa-B (NFκB) signaling pathway have been reported in patients with anhydrotic ectodermal dysplasia and immunodeficiency; affected children have recurrent pyogenic infections with a minimal systemic inflammatory response and can also develop opportunistic infections with atypical mycobacteria or *Pneumocystis carinii.*[28] Several other kindreds have been described with genetic deficiency of another protein, IRAK-4, important for NFκB activation by pyogenic bacteria via the Toll-like receptor/IL-I receptor superfamily. Affected children also had recurrent infections with *S. pneumonia* and *S. aureus* and a poor inflammatory response but no dysmorphic features or opportunistic infections.

Patients with glycogen storage disease type Ib (GSD-Ib), which results from absence of a glucose-6-phosphate transporter, have impaired neutrophil functions and neutropenia.[29] Neutrophil defects include depressed chemotaxis, phagocytosis, and NADPH oxidase activity. Although neutropenia appears to result from increased neutrophil apoptosis, how impaired glucose homeostasis leads to abnormal neutrophil function is uncertain. Interestingly, the BM in the face of neutropenia shows marked hypercellularity with increased mature neutrophils in some patients. The neutrophil count increases within hours of granulocyte colony-stimulating factor (G-CSF) administration, suggesting it is acting in part by releasing neutrophils from the BM. GSD-Ib patients can have infections as well as inflammatory bowel disease. Therefore, in addition to management of the metabolic disruption, these patients are also often treated with G-CSF to improve neutropenia.

There are a variety of noncongenital defects in phagocyte function that can be associated with an increased risk of bacterial or fungal infection. Several have already been mentioned, including neonatal neutrophil dysfunction manifested as poor adhesion and chemotaxis. Patients with myelodysplastic syndromes and acute nonlymphoblastic lymphoma can have subpopulations of neutrophils variably defective in adhesion, migration, production of reactive oxidants, and microbicidal activity that has correlated with an increased risk of infection. Similar defects have been described in diabetes mellitus, Gaucher disease, and renal failure. Severe bacterial infections, surgical trauma, and severe burns can also result in transient depression of a variety of neutrophil functions. The underlying mechanism(s) are incompletely defined and may be related to effects of high levels of inflammatory mediators produced in response to infection or trauma or to products released by bacteria.

Management of Infections

The management of infections in patients with primary neutrophil dysfunction syndromes is quite different than in the normal population and for the most part different from patients with neutropenias.

- Patients tend to present with relatively low fevers and chronic inflammatory processes associated with marked elevation of ESR and CRP. Unless they have untreated abscesses or inflammatory masses, they tend not to present with frank sepsis and positive blood cultures.
- The frequency of infections decreases somewhat with age in children as their normal T and B cell-mediated immunity develops.
- Although one should always attempt to obtain culture proof of an infection, more often than not, it is not possible to identify an organism, and it is necessary to treat empirically.
- Because these patients tend to develop deep seated tissue infections, the ESR can be of great value even though it is quite nonspecific. Elevation in the ESR suggests deep tissue inflammation; CRP is more acute and suggests monocyte activation. Persistent significant elevation of the ESR (>15-20 mm/hr) even in the absence of fever or other symptoms may warrant radiologic search for deep-seated infection.
- The authors advocate an "antibiotic sensitivity by ESR response" approach to empiric therapy in stable patients. One can start at parenteral anti-staphylococcus and gram-negative therapy and monitor the ESR daily. A monotonic decrease in the ESR within several days that is clear-cut suggests the process is sensitive to the antibiotic selected. Although complete resolution of inflammatory response may take many weeks, usually there is some clear change in the ESR within 1 week. If there is worsening or no clear response, then an antifungal can be added and the ESR monitored in the same fashion. Return of an elevated ESR can be a sign of development of organism resistance.
- If a patient with CGD is particularly ill appearing or febrile, it is important to make sure that *B. cepacia* complex bacteria are covered.
- There is no fixed duration of therapy for any infections in these patients. If the infections are not completely extinguished, they will return and will contribute to development of chronic pulmonary and hepatic fibrosis. Parenteral antibiotics or antibiotics that can deliver very high tissue levels should be continued significantly past normalization of the ESR and disappearance of any radiographic evidence of deep tissue infection. This can take many months for some pneumonias and liver abscesses.
- Short pulses of steroids (4-6 days) can be lifesaving, particularly for pulmonary infections in young children with CGD. They reduce airway inflammation and promote drainage.
- Young children are susceptible to infections with routine childhood viruses and infections and tend to do well with standard therapeutic approaches and courses of treatment that are 2 to 3 times longer than the usual recommended course. Again, monitoring with the ESR can be a guide.
- All standard childhood immunizations and influenza vaccinations are strongly recommended. Prophylactic antibiotics may be appropriate (see text).

ACKNOWLEDGMENT

This work was partially supported by the National Institutes of Health Grant R01HL45635 (MCD).

REFERENCES

1. Kyono W, Coates TD: A practical approach to neutrophil disorders. *Pediatr Clin North Am* 49:929, viii, 2002.
2. Dinauer MC, Newburger PE: The phagocyte system and disorders of granulopoiesis and granulocyte function. In: Nathan DG, Orkin SH, Ginsburg D, et al, editors: *Nathan and Oski's Hematology of infancy and childhood*, ed 7, Philadelphia, 2009, WB Saunders Company, p 1109.
3. Hampton MB, Kettle AJ, Winterbourn CC: Inside the neutrophil phagosome: Oxidants, myeloperoxidase, and bacterial killing. *Blood* 92:3007, 1998.
4. Nauseef WM: How human neutrophils kill and degrade microbes: An integrated view. *Immunol Rev* 219:88, 2007.
5. Al Ghouleh I, Khoo NK, Knaus UG, et al: Oxidases and peroxidases in cardiovascular and lung disease: New concepts in reactive oxygen species signaling. *Free Rad Biol Med* 51:1271, 2011.
6. Seger RA: Modern management of chronic granulomatous disease. *Br J Haematol* 140:255, 2008.
7. Winkelstein JA, Marino MC, Johnston RB, Jr, et al: Chronic granulomatous disease. Report on a national registry of 368 patients. *Medicine* 79:155, 2000.
8. Kang EM, Marciano BE, DeRavin S, et al: Chronic granulomatous disease: Overview and hematopoietic stem cell transplantation. *J Allergy Clin Immunol* 127:1319; quiz 27-28, 2011.
9. Kuhns DB, Alvord WG, Heller T, et al: Residual NADPH oxidase and survival in chronic granulomatous disease. *N Engl J Med* 363:2600, 2010.
10. Matute JD, Arias AA, Wright NA, et al: A new genetic subgroup of chronic granulomatous disease with autosomal recessive mutations in p40 phox and selective defects in neutrophil NADPH oxidase activity. *Blood* 114:3309, 2009.
11. Roos D, Kuhns DB, Maddalena A, et al: Hematologically important mutations: X-linked chronic granulomatous disease (third update). *Blood Cells Mol Dis* 45:246, 2010.
12. Roos D, Kuhns DB, Maddalena A, et al: Hematologically important mutations: The autosomal recessive forms of chronic granulomatous disease (second update). *Blood Cells Mol Dis* 44:291, 2010.
13. Bustamante J, Arias AA, Vogt G, et al: Germline CYBB mutations that selectively affect macrophages in kindreds with X-linked predisposition to tuberculous mycobacterial disease. *Nat Immunol* 12:213, 2011.
14. Schappi MG, Jaquet V, Belli DC, et al: Hyperinflammation in chronic granulomatous disease and anti-inflammatory role of the phagocyte NADPH oxidase. *Semin Immunopathol* 30:255, 2008.
15. Beutler E: G6PD deficiency. *Blood* 84:3613, 1994.
16. Lanza F: Clinical manifestation of myeloperoxidase deficiency. *J Mol Med (Berl)* 76:676, 1998.
17. van de Vijver E, Maddalena A, Sanal O, et al: Hematologically important mutations: Leukocyte adhesion deficiency (first update). *Blood Cells Mol Dis* 48:53, 2012.
18. Etzioni A: Genetic etiologies of leukocyte adhesion defects. *Curr Opin Immunol* 21:481, 2009.
19. Zhang Q, Su HC: Hyperimmunoglobulin E syndromes in pediatrics. *Curr Opin Pediatr* 23:653, 2011.
20. Sowerwine KJ, Holland SM, Freeman AF: Hyper-IgE syndrome update. *Ann N Y Acad Sci* 1250:25, 2012.
21. Oh TJ, Eber R, Wang HL: Periodontal diseases in the child and adolescent. *J Clin Periodontol* 29:400, 2002.
22. Koenig JM, Yoder MC: Neonatal neutrophils: The good, the bad, and the ugly. *Clin Periodontol* 31:39, 2004.
23. Introne WJ, Westbroek W, Golas GA, et al: Chediak-Higashi syndrome. In: Pagon RA, Bird TD, Dolan CR, et al, editors: *GeneReviews*, Seattle (WA), 2010.
24. Kaplan J, De Domenico I, Ward DM: Chediak-Higashi syndrome. *Curr Opin Hematol* 15:22, 2008.

25. Janka GE: Familial and acquired hemophagocytic lymphohistiocytosis. *Ann Rev Med* 63:233, 2012.
26. Gombart AF, Koeffler HP: Neutrophil specific granule deficiency and mutations in the gene encoding transcription factor C/EBP(epsilon). *Curr Opin Hematol* 9:36, 2002.
27. Rosenzweig SD, Holland SM: Recent insights into the pathobiology of innate immune deficiencies. *Curr Allergy Asthma Rep* 11:369, 2011.
28. Zhang SY, Boisson-Dupuis S, Chapgier A, et al: Inborn errors of interferon (IFN)-mediated immunity in humans: Insights into the respective roles of IFN-alpha/beta, IFN-gamma, and IFN-lambda in host defense. *Immunol Rev* 226:29, 2008.
29. Chou JY, Jun HS, Mansfield BC: Glycogen storage disease type I and G6Pase-beta deficiency: Etiology and therapy. *Nat Rev Endocrinol* 6:676, 2010.

CHAPTER 49

CONGENITAL DISORDERS OF LYMPHOCYTE FUNCTION

Sung-Yun Pai and Luigi D. Notarangelo

More than 150 molecular defects that result in impairment of T- and B-cell development or function have been identified in the past several decades. Although the existence of the most severe disorders, such as severe combined immunodeficiency (SCID) and Wiskott-Aldrich syndrome (WAS), was known since the 1930s and 1950s, the definition of the genes responsible for primary immunodeficiencies (PIDs) has occurred mostly in the past 2 decades. Moreover, characterization of the molecular basis of these diseases has also revealed unanticipated heterogeneity of the clinical and immunologic phenotype. The study of patients with PIDs has illustrated the critical role played by many of these genes for immune system development and function. This chapter reviews disorders of thymus organogenesis, SCID, other combined immunodeficiencies and disorders of T-cell regulation, and disorders of humoral immunity.

DEFECTS OF THYMUS ORGANOGENESIS

The thymus is the primary organ where T lymphocytes are generated and educated. Endoderm-derived thymic stem cells derived from the third pharyngeal pouch differentiate into cortical and medullary epithelial cells, which in turn induce the differentiation of hematopoietic precursors into T cells. Thus defects of thymus organogenesis have important consequences on immune function.

DiGeorge Syndrome

DiGeorge syndrome (DGS) is attributable to developmental anomalies of the third and fourth pharyngeal pouches and is characterized by thymic hypoplasia, hypoparathyroidism, conotruncal heart malformations, and facial dysmorphisms.

Between 50% and 90% of patients with DGS carry a hemizygous deletion of chromosome 22q11, which occurs in about one in 3000 newborns, most arising de novo. More rarely, DGS is associated with CHARGE (coloboma of the eye, heart defects, atresia of the nasal choanae, retardation of growth or development, genital or urinary abnormalities, and ear abnormalities and deafness) syndrome; chromosome 10p deletion; or mutations of the *TBX1* gene, contained within the 22q11 interval.

Typical cases of DGS are diagnosed at birth because of the association of heart defect (especially interrupted aortic arch type B or truncus arteriosus) with hypocalcemic seizures. Micrognathia, hypertelorism, an antimongoloid slant of the eyes, cleft palate, and ear malformations are also common. Feeding problems, microcephaly, speech delay, neurobehavioral problems (including bipolar disorders, autistic spectrum disorders, and schizophrenia later in life), and scoliosis are frequently observed. Fluorescent in situ hybridization (FISH) readily identifies the 22q11del in most cases.

Immunologic investigations should include analysis of T-lymphocyte subsets and function. Most patients have "partial DGS," manifested by mild T-cell lymphopenia and immunodeficiency. Such patients may be asymptomatic; may have oral thrush and recurrent infections; or may develop autoimmune disease such as juvenile idiopathic arthritis, immune thrombocytopenic purpura, and Raynaud phenomenon. Approximately 1% of DGS patients have "complete DGS" with absence of circulating T cells. Some DGS patients may develop few oligoclonal T lymphocytes that undergo activation in vivo and infiltrate target tissues, causing skin rash, liver dysfunction, and lymphadenopathy. This condition is known as "complete atypical DGS."

Treatment of DGS includes correction of severe heart defects and supplementation with calcium and vitamin D for hypocalcemia. If a significant immune defect is present, prophylaxis against *Pneumocystis jiroveci* pneumonia with trimethoprim–sulfamethoxazole (TMP-SMZ) is indicated. Live-attenuated vaccines can be safely administered to patients with partial DGS who have good cellular immunity (with $CD8^+$ count >300 cells/μL); however, these vaccines are contraindicated in patients with complete DGS. Use of immunosuppressive drugs is indicated in patients with the complete atypical form of the disease.

Ultimately, survival in patients with complete DGS requires immune reconstitution. Bone marrow transplantation from human leukocyte antigen (HLA)–identical donors may allow engraftment of mature T cells contained in the graft. However, because of the absence of thymic tissue, no newly developed T cells are generated, and the patient may remain susceptible to pathogens that are not recognized by donor-derived T cells contained in the graft.

By contrast, thymic transplantation represents the treatment of choice for patients with complete DGS, including the atypical variant. The thymus is obtained as discarded tissue from unrelated infants undergoing heart surgery. It is sliced and cultured in vitro; sterility and viability tests are performed before implanting the thymus slices in the quadriceps muscles of the infant. Using this approach, 36 of 50 infants with complete DGS treated by Markert at Duke University were reported to survive. In most cases, naive T cells appear at around 4 to 7 months; these cells are tolerant to donor thymic cells, display a polyclonal repertoire, and have normal proliferative capacity. Although the number of $CD3^+$ T cells in transplanted patients often remains lower than normal, their diversity and function are sufficient to prevent life-threatening infections.

FOXN1 Deficiency

The transcription factor FOXN1 (whose gene is mutated in the *nude* mouse) plays a critical role in thymus and eccrine glands development. *FOXN1* mutations in humans cause athymia, profound T-cell lymphopenia, alopecia totalis, and nail dystrophy. Similar to DGS, reconstitution of T-cell immunity can be achieved with thymic transplantation.

SEVERE COMBINED IMMUNODEFICIENCY CAUSED BY EARLY DEFECTS IN T-LYMPHOCYTE DEVELOPMENT

Severe combined immunodeficiency includes a heterogeneous group of genetic disorders that affect development of T, and in some cases also of B or natural killer (NK) lymphocytes. The presence or absence of the main lymphocyte subsets serves as the basis for SCID classification. The frequency of SCID is estimated to be one in 50,000 to one in 100,000 live births.

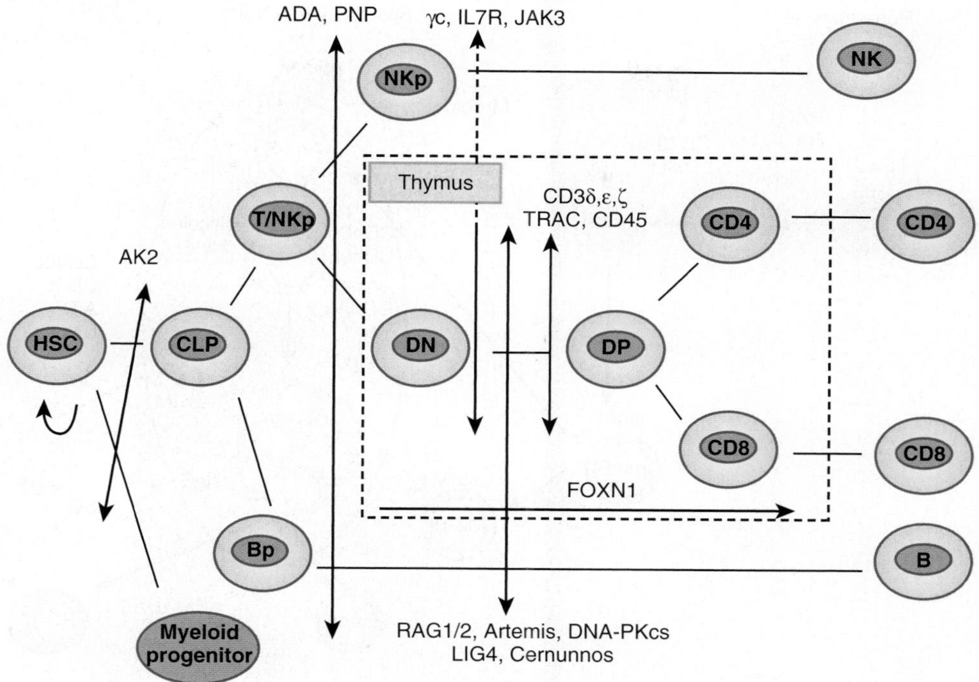

Figure 49-1 GENETIC DEFECTS ASSOCIATED WITH SEVERE COMBINED IMMUNODEFICIENCY (SCID). Schematic representation of blocks *(arrows)* in lymphoid development associated with genetic defects responsible for SCID. *Dashed line* indicates that generation of natural killer (NK) lymphocytes is compromised in γc and Janus-activated kinase 3 (JAK3) deficiency but not in interleukin-7 receptor (IL7R) deficiency. *ADA,* Adenosine deaminase; *AK2,* adenylate kinase 2; *Bp,* B-cell progenitor; *CLP,* common lymphoid progenitor; *DN,* double-negative thymocyte; *DNA-PKcs,* DNA protein kinase catalytic subunit; *DP,* double-positive thymocyte; *γc,* common gamma chain; *HSC,* hematopoietic stem cells; *LIG4,* DNA ligase IV; *NKp,* natural killer cell progenitor cell; *PNP,* purine nucleoside phosphorylase; *RAG,* recombinase activating gene; *T/NKp,* common progenitor of T and NK lymphocytes; *TRAC,* T-cell receptor α constant chain.

Pathobiology and Genetics

Genetic defects that cause SCID affect various stages in T-cell development (Fig. 49-1) and can be grouped in three major categories: (1) defects in cytokine receptor signaling, (2) defects in lymphocyte survival, and (3) defects of expression and function of the pre–T-cell receptor (TCR).

Cytokine Receptor Signaling Defects

The most common form of SCID in humans is the X-linked form caused by mutations of the *IL2RG* gene that encodes for the common gamma chain (γc). This protein is shared by receptors for interleukin-2 (IL-2), IL-4, IL-7, IL-9, IL-15 and IL-21 and signals through the intracellular kinase Janus-activated kinase 3 (JAK3). Patients with mutations in *IL2RG* or *JAK3* lack both T and NK cells because development of these subsets depends on IL-7– and IL-15–mediated signaling, respectively. B lymphocytes are present, but antibody production is impaired because of the lack of T cells and of defective signaling through IL-21R.

Defects in Lymphocyte Survival

Proliferation and survival of lymphoid progenitor cells are essential to permit generation of a normal number of mature lymphocytes. Some forms of SCID are associated with increased apoptosis. Adenosine deaminase (ADA) converts adenosine to inosine (and deoxyadenosine to deoxyinosine). In patients with ADA deficiency, accumulation of toxic phosphorylated derivatives of deoxyadenosine causes cell death and results in extreme lymphopenia, with virtual absence of T, B, and NK lymphocytes. Reticular dysgenesis (RD) is a form of SCID characterized by the association of severe lymphopenia, agranulocytosis, and sensorineural deafness. RD is due to defects in adenylate kinase 2 (AK2), resulting in increased apoptosis.

Defects of Expression and Signaling Through the Pre–T-Cell Receptor and the T-Cell Receptor

Rearrangement of the TCR genes by means of VDJ recombination allows expression of the pre-TCR (composed of the pre-Tα and the TCRβ chain) and of mature TCRs (either as TCRαβ or TCRγδ).

The lymphoid specific recombinase activating gene (RAG) 1 and RAG2 proteins initiate VDJ recombination by recognizing recombination-specific sequences that flank the variable (V), diversity (D) and joining (J) elements of the TCR and of immunoglobulin genes, introducing DNA double-strand breaks. These are then repaired through the ubiquitously expressed nonhomologous end-joining (NHEJ) pathway. Mutations of the *RAG1* and *RAG2* genes, and of genes that encode for Artemis, DNA ligase IV, and DNA-PKcs (all components of the NHEJ pathway), result in SCID with lack of T and B lymphocytes (Figs. 49-1 and 49-2) but a normal number of NK lymphocytes. Mutations of Cernunnos/XLF, another component of the NHEJ pathway, severely impair but do not completely abrogate T- and B-cell development. Because NHEJ is involved in general mechanisms of DNA repair also in nonlymphoid cells, patients with defects of this pathway also show increased cellular radiation sensitivity, are at higher risk of tumors, and may present with neurological problems.

Signaling through the pre-TCR is essential to promote progression from $CD4^-$ $CD8^-$ double-negative (DN) thymocytes to $CD4^+$ $CD8^+$ double-positive (DP) cells and is mediated by the CD3

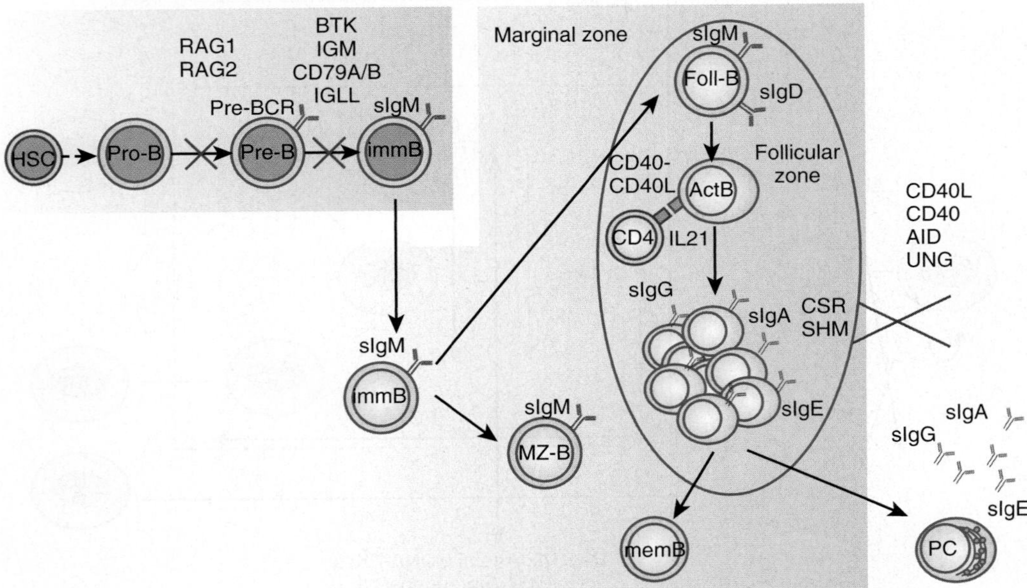

Figure 49-2 GENETIC DEFECTS ASSOCIATED WITH HYPOGAMMAGLOBULINEMIA. Schematic of B-cell development in bone marrow and secondary lymphoid organs, including migration of B cells into the follicular zone, where they undergo activation, class switch recombination (CSR), and somatic hypermutation (SHM). *X* denotes maturation steps at which the genes indicated are required, resulting in a block in differentiation at that stage when the gene is deficient. *ActB,* Activated B cell; *AID,* activation-induced cytidine deaminase; *BTK,* Bruton tyrosine kinase; *HSC,* hematopoietic stem cell; *IL-21,* interleukin-21; *immB,* immature B cell, also termed transitional B cell; *memB,* memory B cell; *MZ-B,* marginal zone B cell; *pre-B,* precursor B cell; *pre-BCR,* pre–B cell receptor; *pro-B,* progenitor B cell; *RAG,* recombination activating gene; *sIgA,* surface IgA; *sIgD,* surface IgD; *sIgG,* surface IgG; *sIgM,* surface IgM; *UNG,* uracil-DNA glycosylase.

complex. Mutations of the CD3δ, CD3ε, and CD3ζ chains interfere with this process and result in SCID. In contrast, mutations of *CD3G* are more often associated with a milder phenotype that includes autoimmunity. Finally, mutations of the CD45 phosphatase, also involved in cell signaling, cause T^- B^+ SCID.

Clinical Manifestations

Typical clinical features of SCID include early-onset severe infections caused by bacteria, viruses, fungi, and opportunistic pathogens (including *P. jiroveci* pneumonia) along with protracted diarrhea, candidiasis, and failure to thrive. Engraftment of maternally derived T lymphocytes is common in SCID, occurring in 40% to 56% of infants with the disease. It may be asymptomatic or may manifest similarly to graft-versus-host disease (GVHD), including skin rash, elevation of liver enzymes, diarrhea, cytopenias. Hypomorphic mutations in SCID-causing genes may lead to residual development of T cells that undergo peripheral expansion and infiltrate target organs, causing various symptoms (erythroderma, diarrhea, hepatosplenomegaly, lymphadenopathy, diarrhea). This clinical phenotype is also known as Omenn syndrome.

Some forms of SCID may present with additional clinical features (see earlier section on defects in thymic development). In patients with ADA deficiency, accumulation of toxic metabolites may cause cupping and flaring of the ribs, liver dysfunction, sensorineural deafness, and neurobehavioral problems. Microcephaly is typically seen in forms of SCID associated with cellular radiosensitivity and impairment of DNA double-strand break repair. Sensorineural deafness is observed in RD.

Diagnostic Approach and Laboratory Manifestations

A thorough family history (including investigation of consanguinity, deaths in infancy, and genders of other affected family members) should be part of the diagnostic approach to infants with possible SCID. Absolute lymphocyte counts (ALCs) should be measured and compared with the normal range for infants (2000–10,000 cells/μL). Lymphopenia is common. Analysis of the distribution and absolute number of $CD3^+$ T lymphocytes, $CD4^+$ and $CD8^+$ T-cell subsets, $CD19^+$ B lymphocytes, and NK ($CD16^+/CD56^+$ NK lymphocytes) will not only confirm the diagnosis of SCID in most cases but will also orient toward specific gene defects. Most SCID patients have profound T-cell lymphopenia; however, $CD3^+$ cells are present in infants with maternal T-cell engraftment or with hypomorphic mutations that allow residual T-cell development. In both of these situations, the T cells have an activated or memory ($CD45RO^+$) phenotype; T cells in normal infants are predominantly naive ($CD45RA^+$). In vitro proliferative response to mitogens is drastically reduced in patients with SCID but may be partially preserved in infants with Omenn syndrome.

Other diagnostic tests that may support the diagnosis of SCID include lack of a thymic shadow in chest radiography and low or undetectable serum IgA and IgM. IgG serum levels may be normal early in life, reflecting the transplacental passage of maternally derived antibodies.

Severe combined immunodeficiency can be diagnosed at birth by measuring levels of TCR excision circles (TRECs). TRECs are a byproduct of V(D)J recombination and are present as circularized DNA fragments in newly generated naive T lymphocytes that express the αβ form of the TCR. Levels of TRECs in circulating lymphocytes are particularly high in newborns and infants and can be detected by PCR amplification of DNA extracted from the Guthrie card.

Diagnostic Approach to Severe Combined Immune Deficiency

- SCID presents early in life with severe infections of bacterial, viral, or fungal origin.
- Opportunistic infections are common in infants with SCID.
- Respiratory infections, protracted diarrhea, and failure to thrive are typical signs at presentation.
- Lymphopenia is present in 50% to 70% of infants with SCID. Age-specific norms must be used in evaluating the ALC because infants and children have much higher ALCs than adults (3500–13,000 cells/mcL in very young infants versus 1000–2800 cells/mcL in adults).
- T-cell lymphopenia is the hallmark of the disease; abnormalities of the absolute count of B and NK lymphocytes are observed in some forms of SCID. However, T lymphocytes may be present in SCID infants with maternal T-cell engraftment or with hypomorphic mutations in SCID-associated genes that allow residual T-cell development. Thus a normal ALC does not rule out SCID.
- Maternally engrafted T cells proliferate in the infant with SCID in vivo, but the vast majority of the time do not proliferate in vitro when stimulated with traditionally used mitogens such as concavalin A and phytohemagglutinin, as measured by thymidine incorporation. Thus, if SCID is suspected but T cells are detectable, maternal engraftment studies and proliferation to mitogens must be done.
- Universal newborn screening has now been piloted in a growing number of states since 2009. The analyte is detection of TRECs by quantitative polymerase chain reaction. TRECs are high in newly generated T cells and low when T cells are absent or when maternally engrafted T cells are present.
- SCID is genetically heterogeneous. The most common form in Western countries is inherited as an X-linked trait and is $T^- B^+ NK^-$.
- The lack of all lymphocytes ($T^- B^- NK^-$ SCID) is highly suspicious for the ADA form of SCID in which toxic metabolites result in death of all lymphocytes. Testing for ADA enzyme level is critical because if confirmed to be absent, treatment with PEG-ADA can often result in sufficient reconstitution of T-cell immunity to protect the baby from infection.

Ultimately, infants with SCID should be evaluated for specific gene defects. However, definitive treatment of SCID (typically, by hematopoietic cell transplantation [HCT]) should not await demonstration of a specific gene defect because this may take some time. An exception to this general principle is ADA deficiency that can be easily diagnosed by measuring enzyme activity in red blood cells, allowing prompt initiation of enzyme replacement therapy (ERT).

Prognosis, Therapy, and Future Directions

Supportive Management

Management of patients with SCID includes observance of strict hygiene measures, prevention of *P. jiroveci* pneumonia with TMP-SMZ, prompt investigation and aggressive treatment of infections, immunoglobulin replacement, and adequate support with enteral or parenteral nutrition. Infections caused by cytomegalovirus (CMV) (causing interstitial pneumonia, hepatitis, or gastroenteritis) and Epstein-Barr virus (EBV) (responsible for lymphoproliferative disease) require active surveillance and preemptive therapy. To prevent transmission of viral infection, blood products from CMV-seronegative donors or leukofiltered products should be used and must be irradiated to prevent transfusion-associated GVHD. Immunosuppression with steroids and cyclosporine A may be needed to treat GVHD-like manifestations associated with Omenn syndrome or maternal T-cell engraftment. Administration of live vaccines must be avoided in infants with SCID. Despite these measures, SCID is inevitably fatal within the first few years of life unless immune reconstitution is achieved with treatment.

Weekly intramuscular injection of pegylated bovine ADA (PEG-ADA) is another therapeutic approach for infants with ADA deficiency. PEG-ADA acts extracellularly to transform adenosine and deoxyadenosine into inosine and deoxyinosine, respectively, thus preventing accumulation of toxic phosphorylated derivatives. ERT for ADA-SCID allows immune reconstitution but is very expensive and must be continued indefinitely. Therapeutic effect may wane over time, and some patients have developed neutralizing antibodies to PEG-ADA.

General Principles of Hematopoietic Cell Transplantation for Severe Combined Immunodeficiency

Hematopoietic cell transplantation is the treatment of choice to obtain long-term immune reconstitution in infants with SCID. HCT for other conditions is generally performed with chemotherapy or radiation conditioning to prevent graft rejection and eliminate or reduce host hematopoietic stem cells (HSCs), favoring donor hematopoiesis. Because of the lack of T lymphocytes, infants with SCID (especially the NK^- forms) are generally considered to have inherent inability to reject the graft and may therefore receive HCT from an HLA-identical related donor without conditioning. T-cell reconstitution in this case is generally prompt, with initial reconstitution in the first 1 to 3 months mediated by expansion of mature T cells present in the donor bone marrow and later reconstitution derived from newly generated T cells that mature in the thymus from donor HSC and progenitors. GVHD prophylaxis is not needed. Unconditioned HCT may also be performed from mismatched related donors, with T-cell depletion of the graft to avoid fatal GVHD. Here the reconstitution is slower because the generation of T cells is entirely dependent on thymic ontogeny and can take 4 to 6 months. Engraftment of T cells may not always occur in this setting, and up to 25% of patients may require repeat transplantation. GVHD prophylaxis is not needed if the T-cell depletion is sufficiently rigorous. These approaches to HCT without conditioning can lead to sustained T-cell immune reconstitution because of the selective advantage for donor cells differentiating into the T lineage. However, this approach rarely results in significant donor HSC engraftment, which is generally less than 1%, and thus may fail to correct impairment of humoral immunity.

Hematopoietic cell transplantation from matched unrelated adult or cord blood donors has been generally performed with myeloablative conditioning, similar to that used for other nonmalignant disorders. In the case of unrelated donor adult HCT, memory T cells present in the graft can expand in the host similarly to the matched related donor situation and can already provide some protection against infection (according to their antigen specificity) in the first few weeks after transplantation. In contrast, cord blood contains mostly naive T lymphocytes and is therefore less efficient in providing antigen-specific immunity early after HCT. Conditioning before unrelated donor HCT or before mismatched related HCT improves the rate of HSC engraftment but exposes the patient to short- and long-term toxicity and to an increased risk of GVHD. Reduced-intensity conditioning regimens have been proposed, with the aim to facilitate stem cell engraftment while reducing the risk of treatment-related toxicity; however, there is no clear evidence that such regimens are associated with better outcomes in patients with SCID treated by HCT.

Survival and Long-Term Outcome After Hematopoietic Cell Transplantation for Severe Combined Immunodeficiency

Survival after HCT for SCID has improved with time because of advances in early diagnosis and supportive care for infants with SCID, as well as in prevention and treatment of GVHD and other complications, including infections and posttransplant lymphoproliferative disease. The type of donor remains the most important determinant of survival. In the largest series of SCID patients treated by HCT in Europe in from 1968 to 2005, 10-year survival was 84% for recipients of HCT from HLA-identical related donors, 66% for those treated with HCT from unrelated donors, and 54% for patients who had received HCT from related HLA-mismatched donors. A single-center study from Buckley and collaborators showed that 16 of 16 recipients of HLA-identical related donors (100%) and 108 out of 145 recipients of HLA-mismatched related donors (74%) with SCID were alive after HCT, with a median follow-up of 10 years. Thus survival remains best for recipients of transplant from HLA-identical related donors.

Respiratory infections at the time of transplant are associated with a poorer outcome. Consistent with this, transplantation at a young age is associated with improved survival, which may be a proxy for the lack of infection at the time of diagnosis or the inherent capacity of the thymic epithelium to support T-cell neogenesis. In the series by Buckley and collaborators, 94% of SCID infants who received HCT during the first 3.5 months of life survived. Use of a protected environment and prophylaxis of infections with TMP-SMZ are also associated with better outcomes after HCT for SCID include. The specific type of SCID may also affect the outcome: survival after HCT for SCID is better in patients with B^+ than B^- SCID.

Complications may occur after HCT for SCID. Acute GVHD (aGVHD) occurs in 35% to 45% of the patients and is more common after HCT from unrelated and HLA-mismatched donors. Limited or extensive chronic cGVHD occurs in approximately 10% of the patients and is more common after haploidentical and unrelated donor transplantation; typical target organs include the skin, gastrointestinal (GI) tract, and liver. The long-term requirement for nutritional support has been reported in up to 20% of patients with SCID who survived at least 2 years after HCT. Certain forms of SCID are associated with a higher risk of long-term complications and sequelae, including nutritional problems, poor growth and development, and cGVHD in patients with Artemis deficiency and neurologic complications (mental retardation, motor dysfunction, sensorineural hearing deficits) in patients with ADA deficiency.

In infants with SCID, donor-derived stem cells present a strong selective advantage versus autologous stem cells during T-cell development, and long-term T-cell reconstitution may also be achieved from committed lymphoid progenitors that seed to the thymus even in the absence of engraftment of bona fide stem cells. Consistent with this, donor T-cell chimerism and T-cell reconstitution after HCT are achieved in more than 90% of infants with SCID, and the majority have a polyclonal repertoire. Some reports have indicated that in the absence of donor stem cell engraftment, there is a progressive decline of thymic function after HCT for SCID. Others have shown that the decline of TREC levels (hence of thymic function) with age follows a similar rate as in normal individuals. Patients with poor T-cell reconstitution are at risk for viral and opportunistic infections; autoimmunity (especially cytopenias and hypothyroidism) has been reported in 10% to 20% of these patients, particularly in those with cGVHD.

Reconstitution of humoral immunity after HCT for SCID is less uniform. Engraftment of donor B cells is usually associated with humoral immune reconstitution. Inadequate B-cell function (requiring immunoglobulin replacement therapy) is often observed in patients with γc and JAK3 deficiency who remain with autologous B cells, because of intrinsic defects in the host B cells to respond to γc-dependent cytokines such as IL-4 and IL-21.

Therapeutic Approach to Severe Combined Immune Deficiency

- HCT is the mainstay of treatment. Optimal survival is achieved when the transplant is performed early in life. This is now possible with newborn screening.
- Transplantation for SCID can be performed without conditioning because of the profound absence of T cells and inability to reject. Thus the bone marrow of a fully HLA-matched sibling can be infused without manipulation and without giving any conditioning to the baby. GVHD prophylaxis is also not necessary. Haploidentical bone marrow from a parent can also be infused without conditioning but must first be T-cell depleted.
- Such transplants without conditioning can result in T-cell reconstitution that lasts for decades. In the case of a matched sibling graft, initial T-cell reconstitution is rapid, generally within the first 1 to 3 months, because of proliferation of mature T cells. In the case of a haploidentical graft, mature T cells are removed, so 4 to 6 months is required for HSCs to develop and emerge from the thymus as mature T cells.
- Without conditioning, few long-lived HSCs from the donor engraft, which may lead to a lack of donor B-cell reconstitution and a lack of humoral immunity. With conditioning, donor HSCs are more likely to engraft and give rise to donor B cells. Currently, matched unrelated donor transplants are performed with conditioning.
- Enzyme replacement may be used in patients with adenosine deaminase deficiency. Gene therapy has offered promising results, but it is also associated with an increased risk of leukemic proliferation because of insertional mutagenesis.

The number of circulating NK lymphocytes often remains low in patients with γc and JAK3 deficiency and may contribute to the increased risk of warts.

Gene Therapy for Severe Combined Immunodeficiency

Gene therapy, in which the gene of interest is introduced into the patient's own cells, is an attractive therapeutic option for SCID, particularly for infants who do not have an HLA-identical related donor. Expression of the normal copy of the gene in $CD34^+$ stem cells confers a selective advantage to the gene-corrected cells during T-cell differentiation. Furthermore, there is no risk of GVHD. Gene therapy has been used successfully to correct SCID in patients with ADA deficiency and with X-linked SCID. Since 2000, more than 30 patients with ADA-deficient SCID have been treated with gene therapy worldwide. The largest experience reported from Milan, Italy, describes 15 patients, all alive, with progressive reconstitution of T-cell counts and sufficient T-cell function in 13 of the 15 patients to stop ERT. In the Milan protocol, engraftment of gene-corrected stem cells has been facilitated by use of a reduced-intensity chemotherapy regimen with low-dose busulfan.

Twenty patients with X-linked SCID have been treated by gene therapy in Paris and London. In both protocols, no chemotherapy was used. Eighteen patients are alive, and 17 of them show normalization of T-cell count and function, with demonstration of reconstituted thymic output, diversified T-cell repertoire, and ability to mount antigen-specific T-cell responses. In some cases, improvement of humoral immunity has also been observed. However, leukemic T-cell proliferation caused by insertional mutagenesis has been observed in five of 20 patients. Novel and potentially safer vectors for gene therapy in X-linked SCID have been recently developed, and a new multicenter trial with a self-inactivating γ-retroviral for X-linked SCID started in 2010.

LATE DEFECTS IN T-CELL DEVELOPMENT

Upon expression of a functional TCR, double-positive thymocytes migrate to the thymic medulla and continue their differentiation into single-positive ($CD4^+$ or $CD8^+$) cells that eventually egress from the thymus and are exported to the periphery. Several genetic defects have been identified that affect late stages in T-cell development. At variance with classical forms of SCID, these disorders are characterized by residual number or function of T cells, consistent with partially preserved thymic architecture and function. Because these patients' thymuses are not empty, use of chemotherapy is required to facilitate engraftment and T-cell differentiation with donor-derived cells.

ZAP-70 Deficiency

This autosomal recessive disease is caused by mutations of the zeta-associated protein of 70 kDa (ZAP-70) tyrosine kinase, that phosphorylates the CD3 chains and thus participates at TCR-mediated signaling. The immunologic phenotype of ZAP-70 deficiency in humans is characterized by virtual lack of $CD8^+$ lymphocytes; the number of $CD4^+$ cells is preserved, but they are unable to proliferate in response to mitogens and antigens. In contrast, both $CD4^+$ and $CD8^+$ lymphocytes are absent in *Zap70*$^{-/-}$ mice; an inability of the T cells to respond to antigens in patients with ZAP-70 deficiency causes increased susceptibility to severe infections, resulting in a clinical phenotype that is indistinguishable from that of SCID. Rarely, ZAP-70 deficiency has been associated with clinical features of Omenn syndrome. Prevention of infections is based on antimicrobial prophylaxis and use of intravenous immunoglobulins; however, ultimate treatment requires HCT.

Human Leukocyte Antigen Class II Deficiency

Expression of HLA class II molecules on the surfaces of thymic epithelial and dendritic cells is essential to promote positive selection of $CD4^+$ lymphocytes. HLA class II deficiency includes a group of autosomal recessive disorders in which mutations in transcription factors (CIITA, RFXAP, RFX5, and RFXANK) that regulate HLA class II gene expression result in a profoundly reduced number of $CD4^+$ lymphocytes. The clinical phenotype consists of recurrent infections since infancy that may also be caused by opportunistic pathogens. Treatment is based on antimicrobial prophylaxis and regular use of immunoglobulins, but the prognosis remains severe. HCT does not correct defective expression of HLA class II molecules by thymic epithelial cells, causing persistence of CD4 lymphopenia in a large fraction of transplanted patients. However, HCT from HLA-matched donors may allow reconstitution of the $CD4^+$ cell compartment by mature cells contained in the graft, with little or no contribution by newly generated $CD4^+$ cells.

Human Leukocyte Antigen Class I Deficiency

Presentation of antigens in association with major histocompatibility class I molecules is important for thymic development of $CD8^+$ lymphocytes and for the development of antigen-specific cytotoxic T-cell responses. In addition, HLA class I molecules also modulate the function of NK cells that express several HLA class I–binding molecules. HLA class I molecules are assembled and loaded with peptides in the endoplasmic reticulum by a transporter associated with antigen presentation (TAP) proteins (TAP1 and TAP2) and the Tapasin protein. Mutations of TAP1, TAP2, or Tapasin cause defective expression of HLA class I molecules, associated with a severe reduction in the number of circulating $CD8^+$ $TCR\alpha\beta^+$ lymphocytes. NK cells expressing killer inhibitory receptors may not receive HLA class I–dependent inhibitory signals and hence may mount cytotoxic responses to uninfected cells, causing inflammatory lesions in the lungs and in the skin. There is no definitive treatment for this disease, and management is based on supportive care.

OTHER COMBINED IMMUNODEFICIENCIES

Several other conditions are known that affect the ability of T lymphocytes to respond to activating signals or to interact with other cells during immune responses. Despite the presence of peripheral T cells, these conditions often have a poor prognosis, and use of HCT should be carefully considered.

CD40LG Deficiency

CD40 ligand (CD40LG) is expressed by activated $CD4^+$ cells. Interaction of CD40LG-expressing $CD4^+$ cells with B lymphocytes that constitutively express CD40 delivers a signal for B-cell proliferation and class switch recombination in combination with appropriate cytokines (see Fig. 49-2). Furthermore, interaction between CD40LG-expressing $CD4^+$ lymphocytes and $CD40^+$ dendritic cells and macrophages promotes secretion of IL-12 and thus enables development of Th1 responses against intracellular pathogens.

The *CD40LG* gene is located on the X chromosome (at Xq26). Males with *CD40LG* mutations have a combined immunodeficiency characterized by recurrent infections. Opportunistic infections are common. *P. jiroveci* pneumonia may mark the clinical onset of the disease in the first year of life. *Cryptosporidium parvum* infection may cause chronic watery diarrhea and is often responsible for sclerosing cholangitis. Chronic or intermittent neutropenia has been frequently observed. Patients with CD40LG deficiency are also uniquely prone to peripheral neuroectodermal tumors, especially of the GI tract.

Levels of serum IgG and IgA are markedly reduced or undetectable; IgM may be normal or increased, and for this reason, the disease is also known as X-linked hyper-IgM syndrome. The number of memory B cells is also markedly reduced.

In vitro activation of T cells with phorbol myristate acetate and ionomycin fails to induce expression of CD40LG on the surface of $CD4^+$ cells, but other activation markers (e.g., CD69) are normally expressed.

The prognosis is severe. Death may occur early in life secondary to infections or during late childhood and young adulthood because of severe liver disease and tumors. Clinical management is based on continuous prophylaxis of *Pneumocystis* infection with TMP-SMZ, regular use of intravenous immunoglobulins, and hygiene measures to limit the risk of exposure to *Cryptosporidium* spp. HCT represents the only definitive cure. In a series of 38 patients transplanted in Europe, 26 (68.4%) survived. Preexisting pulmonary disease and *Cryptosporidium* infection are risk factors for a less favorable outcome.

CD40 Deficiency

This is a rare autosomal recessive disorder whose clinical and immunologic phenotype is indistinguishable from CD40LG deficiency (see Fig. 49-2). The diagnosis is based on the lack of expression of CD40 on the surface of circulating B lymphocytes. Management is as for CD40LG deficiency.

Wiskott-Aldrich Syndrome

Wiskott-Aldrich syndrome is an X-linked disorder characterized by thrombocytopenia with small-sized platelets, eczema, and immunodeficiency. Autoimmune manifestations are common, and there is an increased risk of hematologic malignancies (primarily non-Hodgkin lymphoma [NHL], sometimes EBV driven). This X-linked disease is estimated to occur in one in 100,000 births. The defect is caused by mutations in the *WAS* gene that encodes for an intracytoplasmic protein (WASp) expressed in hematopoietic cells and involved in cytoskeleton reorganization and immune synapse formation. Deficiency of WASp results in impaired T-cell activation; poor production of antibodies, particularly to carbohydrate antigen; defective NK function; impaired phagocytic cell migration; and defective antigen presentation, thus explaining the immunodeficiency of the disease.

Boys with WAS typically present in infancy with bleeding, prompting the discovery of low numbers of small platelets, with mean platelet volume typically 4 to 5 fL. Bleeding manifestations can range from petechiae and bruising to severe GI and intracranial hemorrhages. Eczema can be mild to severe. Common infections in patients with WAS include otitis, sinusitis, pneumonia, and cellulitis. Viral infections (especially from herpesviruses, including CMV, EBV, and herpes simplex virus 1 [HSV-1]) and opportunistic infections, such as *P. jiroveci* pneumonia, are also frequent. Approximately 40% of patients with WAS develop autoimmunity, including autoimmune hemolytic anemia, autoimmune thrombocytopenia, thyroiditis, colitis, vasculitis, nephropathy, and arthritis. In addition to thrombocytopenia, typical laboratory findings include an inability to mount responses to polysaccharide antigens, low or absent isohemagglutinin titers, high IgE, and poor proliferation of T cells when stimulated with anti-CD3 antibody. Other immune findings are more variable, including progressive T lymphopenia with age, low IgM, and high IgA. Analysis of WASp protein expression and demonstration of *WAS* gene mutations confirm the diagnosis.

Supportive treatment for WAS consists of monitoring and treatment for bleeding, antimicrobial prophylaxis, immunoglobulin replacement therapy, and treatment of eczema and of autoimmune manifestations with immunosuppressive drugs. Splenectomy can be effective in many to correct thrombocytopenia but leads to increased risk of sepsis.

Allogeneic HCT (typically with myeloablative regimens) for WAS has become standard at many institutions and may be indicated early in life, especially in patients with severe mutations that abrogate protein expression.

Hematopoietic cell transplantation is usually associated with robust T-cell engraftment, but some patients develop mixed chimerism in the B and myeloid lineages, indicating differential requirement for normal WAS protein to promote lineage-specific development or survival. Poor myeloid chimerism is associated with the risk of persistent thrombocytopenia, and mixed chimerism may favor autoimmune manifestations.

Survival after HCT for WAS is influenced by donor type and age at transplantation. An international retrospective review of 170 boys transplanted from 1968 to 1996 showed that survival after HLA-identical sibling HCT recipient (87%) was similar to that of matched unrelated donor HCT recipients who were transplanted before the age of 5 years, but those transplanted after age 5 years had a high relative risk of death. In a multi-institutional retrospective survey of 194 patients transplanted from 1980 to 2009, this trend was confirmed, although the absolute survival of these high-risk patients has improved substantially.

Because outcome after HCT is not uniformly good and many patients lack matched related or unrelated donors, somatic gene therapy is an attractive treatment option for WAS. The results of the first two of a total of 10 boys treated with gene therapy by transduction of CD34$^+$ selected peripheral blood stem cells using an MFG-based γ-retroviral vector after low-dose busulfan conditioning has recently been reported. These two patients achieved successful reconstitution of immune function, control of eczema, and rise in platelets. However, this treatment has been associated with insertional mutagenesis and development of leukemia. Therefore, efforts are underway to develop safer strategies, and trials using a lentiviral self-inactivating vector have been recently opened.

NEMO Deficiency

A rare syndrome in which boys were affected by hypohidrotic ectodermal dysplasia and immunodeficiency (EDA-ID) was described in 2002 to be attributable to hypomorphic mutations in the *IKGBG* gene. The *IKGBG* gene encodes for the protein nuclear factor kappa-B (NFκB) essential modulator (NEMO), also known as IKK-γ, the regulatory subunit of the IκB kinase complex. This disorder was the first example of an immunodeficiency caused by defects in the NFκB signaling pathway in humans.

The NFκB signaling pathway is ubiquitous to all tissues and stages of development, playing critical roles in cell proliferation, oncogenesis, cell survival, and inflammatory responses. All described patients have partial expression of NEMO. Complete lack of NEMO expression is embryonically lethal in males; females who are heterozygous for null NEMO mutations have incontinentia pigmenti.

Phenotypic manifestations of EDA-ID are largely restricted to epithelial tissues and the immune system, with sparse hair, shiny skin, lack of sweat glands and other appendages, and rare conical shaped teeth. There is often frontal bossing and a characteristic facies. Typical infections are due to bacteria, including sepsis and meningitis, especially *Streptococcus pneumoniae, Staphylococcus* spp. and *Haemophilus influenzae;* DNA viral infections such as CMV and HSV; and atypical mycobacterial infection. Pneumocystis and other opportunistic infections can occur but less frequently. Other manifestations of the disease that are present in some, but not all, patients include inflammatory colitis, lymphedema, and osteopetrosis. Furthermore, some patients do not have prominent features of ectodermal dysplasia, adding to phenotypic heterogeneity.

T- and B-cell numbers in general are normal, but variable defects in T-cell proliferation to mitogen and antigens are seen. Hypogammaglobulinemia with normal or high IgM and defective antibody production (especially against polysaccharides) are common. Defects in NK cell cytotoxicity have been reported. Finally, monocytes from patients with NEMO fail to elaborate inflammatory cytokines such as tumor necrosis factor-α (TNF-α) in response to stimulation by a variety of TLR ligands.

The prognosis and natural history of NEMO mutation is not well known, but these patients have an increased risk of sepsis, mycobacterial disease, and inflammatory complications. Aside from supportive therapy with intravenous immunoglobulin (IVIG) replacement, antibiotic prophylaxis, and treatment of infections, HCT has been used to treat patients with severe cases of NEMO deficiency with variable results. Because of the expression of NEMO in nonhematopoietic tissues, certain manifestations such as colitis may not be immediately ameliorated by HCT.

DISORDERS WITH T CELL-MEDIATED IMMUNE DYSREGULATION

Along with generation of a diversified repertoire of T and B lymphocytes, purging of self-reactive cells is essential to maintain immune homeostasis and prevent autoimmune diseases. We have already reported how autoimmune manifestations are common in severe forms of immunodeficiency characterized by oligoclonal expansion of T lymphocytes (e.g., Omenn syndrome, complete atypical DGS) or by defective intracellular signaling (e.g., calcium flux defects). Here we describe other forms of PID with faulty control of central or peripheral T-cell tolerance.

Autoimmune Polyendocrinopathy Candidiasis Ectodermal Dystrophy Syndrome

Also known as autoimmune polyglandular syndrome type 1 (APS1), autoimmune polyendocrinopathy candidiasis ectodermal dystrophy (APECED) is an autosomal recessive disorder characterized by autoimmune endocrine manifestations (hypoparathyroidism, Addison disease), candidiasis, and nail dystrophy. The disease is caused by mutations of the autoimmune regulator *(AIRE)* gene, which encodes for a transcription factor expressed by medullary thymic epithelial cells (mTECs), where it regulates expression of tissue-specific antigens that are presented to nascent T cells, thereby promoting clonal deletion of self-reactive T lymphocytes or their conversion to natural regulatory T cells (nTreg cells).

In patients with APECED, mucocutaneous candidiasis usually develops first (in infancy or early childhood) followed by autoimmune hypoparathyroidism with hypocalcemia and adrenal failure. Around 15% to 20% of the patients may develop insulin-dependent diabetes. Other autoimmune manifestations (hepatitis, ovarian failure) are also common. Hyposplenism has been reported in one study. Candidiasis may reflect elevated levels of antibodies to IL-17 and IL-22 that play an important role in the defense against *Candida* spp.

Management of patients with APECED is based on regular follow-up and search for autoantibodies, which should be repeated every 6 months. Hormone replacement therapy is indicated for the endocrinopathies. Aggressive management and prevention of candidiasis is important to avoid persistent or recurrent infections that may favor development of squamous cell carcinoma.

Immune Dysregulation Polyendocrinopathy Enteropathy X-linked Syndrome

Immune dysregulation polyendocrinopathy enteropathy X-linked (IPEX) syndrome is an X-linked disorder of systemic autoimmunity. Males with IPEX present early in life with skin rash, intractable watery diarrhea, insulin-dependent diabetes mellitus, lymphadenopathy, splenomegaly, and failure to thrive. Other autoimmune manifestations include thyroid disease, nephropathy, cytopenias, and vasculitis. In addition, patients with IPEX show elevated levels of IgE.

IPEX is caused by mutations of the *FOXP3* gene that encodes for a transcription factor that plays a critical role in the development and function of Treg lymphocytes. These cells have suppressive functions; they have a distinctive phenotype ($CD4^+$ $CD25^{hi}$ $FOXP3^+$) and normally represent 5% to 15% of $CD4^+$ circulating lymphocytes. Most patients with IPEX lack Treg cells; activated self-reactive T lymphocytes infiltrate target tissues and secrete cytokines, causing tissue damage.

IPEX has a severe prognosis. Death often occurs within the first few years of life because of severe malabsorption, failure to thrive, metabolic derangement, or severe infections secondary to immune suppression. Use of immunosuppressive drugs (steroids, sirolimus, tacrolimus, rituximab) is necessary to treat the disease. However, the only definitive treatment is allogeneic HCT. Mixed chimerism is sufficient to control the disease; therefore, reduced-intensity conditioning has been used with good results.

CD25 Deficiency

IL-2 plays an important role in T-lymphocyte proliferation and in immune homeostasis by increasing expression of FOXP3 and enhancing the suppressive activity of Treg cells. Autosomal recessive mutations of the *IL2RA (CD25)* gene that encodes for the α chain of the IL-2 receptor cause a disease that associated IPEX-like manifestations (lymphadenopathy, hepatosplenomegaly, autoimmune cytopenias, inflammatory bowel disease) and increased susceptibility to severe viral infections. The number of circulating T cells may be normal or slightly reduced, and in vitro proliferative response to mitogens is decreased. The patients' T cells produce reduced amounts of the immunosuppressive cytokine IL-10 upon in vitro activation. HCT represents the only definitive treatment.

Autoimmune Lymphoproliferative Syndrome

Interaction between FAS (CD95) on activated T and B lymphocytes and FAS ligand (FAS-LG) on activated T cells triggers the extrinsic pathway to activation of the caspase cascade, culminating in apoptosis. In addition, cellular stress (including cytokine deprivation) may activate the intrinsic pathway of apoptosis, leading to disruption of mitochondrial membrane permeability, release of cytochrome c, activation of caspase 9, and apoptosis. Defects of FAS- or mitochondrial-dependent apoptosis are responsible for the autoimmune lymphoproliferative syndrome (ALPS, also known as Canale-Smith syndrome), characterized by early-onset, chronic (>6 months), nonmalignant lymphoproliferation; autoimmunity; and an increased risk of lymphoma.

The majority of patients with ALPS carry heterozygous dominant-negative mutations in the *FAS (CD95, TNFRSF6)* gene (ALPS-FAS). Somatic mutations of the *FAS* gene are the second most common cause of the disease (ALPS-sFAS). More rarely, ALPS is caused by mutations of the *FASLG* gene (ALPS-FASLG), of caspase 8, caspase 10, Fas-associated death domain (FADD) protein, or somatic activating mutations of N-RAS or K-RAS. Both caspase 8 and caspase 10 deficiency are inherited as autosomal dominant traits.

Lymphoproliferation, manifesting as lymphadenopathy, splenomegaly, or hepatomegaly, is the most common clinical manifestation, with a trend toward progressive remission in adulthood. More than 70% of ALPS patients develop autoimmune disease, most commonly immune cytopenias and less frequently organ-specific autoimmunity. There is an increased risk of malignancies, especially EBV-associated NHL.

An immunologic signature of ALPS is the increased number of DN circulating T lymphocytes that express the αβ form of the TCR but do not express CD4 or CD8 molecules. There is defective in vitro apoptosis of lymphocytes through FAS-mediated or intrinsic pathway (depending on the genetic variant). Elevated levels of soluble FAS ligand, vitamin B_{12}, and IL-10, hypergammaglobulinemia, and antiphospholipid antibodies are often present in patients with ALPS-FAS. Patients with caspase 8 deficiency and with FADD deficiency have recurrent infections, and the latter have functional hyposplenism. The number of DN T cells may be normal in patients with *NRAS* or *KRAS* mutations.

Treatment is based on immunosuppression (with steroids, rituximab, mycophenolate mofetil, or sirolimus) and surveillance against lymphoma. Splenectomy may improve cytopenias; however, relapse of autoimmunity has been observed in 50% of splenectomized patients. Furthermore, severe, invasive bacterial infections have been reported in 30% of splenectomized patients, and the mortality rate for invasive bacterial infection after splenectomy is as high as 13.3%.

DEFECTS OF CELL-MEDIATED CYTOTOXICITY

Mechanisms of immune defense against viral infections are largely dependent on responses mediated by $CD8^+$ cytotoxic T lymphocytes (CTLs) and NK lymphocytes. Multimers of perforin, a protein contained in cytolytic granules, form pores through which CTL and NK cells release cytotoxic proteins (granzyme B, granulolysin) into virus-infected target cells, causing activation of caspases and apoptosis. In resting CTL and NK lymphocytes, cytotoxic proteins are contained in endosomal secretory lytic granules. After interaction of CTL or NK cells with the target cell, lytic granules are transported, dock, and fuse with the cell membrane, permitting release of cytotoxic proteins into the target cells.

Defects along this process are responsible for various forms of familial hemophagocytic lymphohistiocytosis (FHL). Defective cell-mediated cytotoxicity is also observed in Chédiak-Higashi syndrome (CHS). Finally, selective susceptibility to EBV infection is at the basis of various forms of lymphoproliferative syndrome.

Chédiak-Higashi Syndrome

Chédiak-Higashi syndrome is an autosomal recessive disease caused by mutations of the *LYST* gene, which encodes for a protein involved in the sorting of proteins to secretory endosomes. This defect affects not only cytotoxic lymphocytes (accounting for FHL-like clinical features) but also melanocytes (that are unable to transfer melanin to keratinocytes and other epithelial cells) and peripheral neurons. Clinical features of CHS include partial albinism (with silvery hair), progressive peripheral neuropathy, recurrent bacterial infections, and a mild tendency to bleeding. Patients with CHS are prone to accelerated phases of hemophagocytic lymphohistiocytosis (HLH) because of uncontrolled macrophage activation in response to viral infections. Neutropenia is often present and may cause bacterial infections. Giant lysosomes can be identified in circulating leukocytes.

Treatment is based on prophylactic antibiotics and aggressive treatment of infections. HCT may restore hematologic and immunologic abnormalities; however, progressive neurologic dysfunction is not affected by treatment.

X-Linked Lymphoproliferative Disease

In normal individuals, primary infection with the EBV causes infectious mononucleosis, a self-limiting disease. EBV establishes latency in B lymphocytes, salivary glands, and some epithelial cells and is maintained under control by $CD8^+$ CTL and NK lymphocytes. Males with X-linked lymphoproliferative disease type 1 (XLP1) are uniquely susceptible to life-threatening complications of EBV infections. XLP1 is caused by mutations of the *SH2D1A* gene that encodes for a small adaptor molecule, signaling lymphocyte activation molecule (SLAM)-associated protein (SAP). In the absence of SAP, cytotoxic responses to EBV-infected cells are markedly reduced. Persistence of EBV triggers continuous activation of $CD8^+$ CTLs that hyperproliferate and release high amounts of interferon-γ. Ultimately, this condition ensues in a macrophage activation syndrome. After EBV infection, patients with XLP1 are also at high risk of B-cell lymphoma. SAP is also important for the function of follicular helper T cells (T_{FH}) that promote maturation of antibody responses. Consistent with this, males with XLP1 often develop hypogammaglobulinemia with a lack of memory B lymphocytes. Finally, XLP1 is also associated with impaired development of NK T lymphocytes. Flow-cytometric analysis of SAP expression and mutation analysis at the *SH2D1A* locus confirm the diagnosis.

A minority of patients with XLP carry defects in another gene *(BIRC4)* that encodes for the X-linked inhibitor of apoptosis (XIAP). Consistent with this, lymphocytes from patients with this disease (XLP2) show increased susceptibility to activation-induced apoptosis. Compared with XLP1, patients with XLP2 have a higher incidence of HLH (with or without EBV infection) but do not show an increased risk of lymphoma. Hypogammaglobulinemia is often present. Flow cytometric analysis of XIAP expression and mutation analysis at the *BIRC4* locus are used to confirm the diagnosis.

Both XLP1 and XLP2 are life-threatening disorders. Administration of immunoglobulins may be beneficial, but the only curative approach is HCT.

Diagnostic and Therapeutic Approach to Cytotoxicity Defects

- PID with defects of cell-mediated cytotoxicity includes a heterogeneous group of disorders characterized by increased susceptibility to severe viral infections.
- Typical clinical features include high fever, liver and spleen enlargement, lymphadenopathy, coagulation defects, abnormalities of liver function, and cytopenias after viral infections.
- Two major groups of cell-mediated cytotoxicity defects include familial forms of hemophagocytic lymphohistiocytosis (fHLH) and X-linked lymphoproliferative disease. In the former, diagnosis is based on demonstration of abnormal cytotoxic function of T and NK lymphocytes. Defective expression of CD107a on activated lymphocytes or reduced expression of perforin may help define the nature of the underlying disorder causing fHLH.
- Prompt recognition and treatment of the underlying infection is essential. Immunosuppression is also required to block exaggerated inflammatory responses. However, the only curative approach to defects of cell-mediated cytotoxicity is represented by HCT. Mixed chimerism is sufficient to allow immune reconstitution. This goal can be achieved with reduced-intensity conditioning, with a lower risk of treatment-related toxicity.

DEFECTS OF B-CELL DEVELOPMENT AND FUNCTION

The previous section covered defects that predominantly affect T lymphocytes' development and/or function. This section covers PIDs in which abnormalities of B cell development or function are the main feature (Figs. 49-2 and 49-3).

X-linked Agammaglobulinemia

X-linked agammaglobulinemia (XLA), also known as Bruton agammaglobulinemia, is the most common monogenic cause of failure of B-cell development and affects approximately one in 390,000 individuals in central Europe. Males with XLA lack circulating B cells because of mutations of the Bruton tyrosine kinase or *BTK* gene, which encodes for a tyrosine kinase involved in signaling through various receptors, including the pre–B-cell receptor (BCR) and the BCR. Impaired signaling through the pre-BCR causes a severe, but incomplete, block at the pre–B cell stage in the bone marrow (see Fig. 49-2).

Approximately 1000 mutations have been reported in the BTKbase (http://bioinf.uta.fi/BTKbase). Milder mutations that are permissive for BTK protein expression are associated in vivo with higher levels of serum IgM and later age at diagnosis.

Clinical manifestations of XLA include recurrent sinopulmonary infections (pneumonia, bronchitis, sinusitis, otitis), particularly with encapsulated organisms such as pneumococcus and *H influenza;* bacterial skin infections (cellulitis, impetigo, pyoderma gangrenosum, perirectal abscess); and sepsis with *Pseudomonas* spp. or staphylococcus. Symptoms typically begin after 3 to 6 months of age when maternally derived antibodies disappear. The proportion of circulating B cells is markedly reduced (typically 0.05%–0.3% of lymphocytes), and there is profound deficiency of all immunoglobulin isotypes. Neutropenia, secondary to severe infections, is observed in approximately 10% to 25% of patients; typically, it resolves with antibiotics and immunoglobulin replacement therapy.

In addition to bacterial infections, patients with XLA are uniquely susceptible to enteroviral infections (including chronic meningoencephalitis) caused by poliovirus, Coxsackie, and others; infections with *Mycoplasma* and *Ureaplasma* spp. affecting joints, the prostate, or lungs; and *Giardia lamblia* infection, causing protracted diarrhea and malabsorption. Increased incidences of lymphoma, colorectal cancer, and gastric adenocarcinoma have been reported in patients with XLA.

Therapy is based on lifelong regular administration of immunoglobulins intravenously or subcutaneously and on prompt and aggressive treatment of infections. With this regimen, survival approaches that of the general population. Antibiotic prophylaxis may be beneficial, but its role has not been firmly established. Treatment of enteroviral meningoencephalitis is more problematic; some success has been reported with high-dose immunoglobulins and the antiviral agent pleconaril. Patients on immunoglobulin replacement therapy should be monitored for side effects and adverse reactions and for liver and renal function.

Autosomal Recessive Agammaglobulinemia

Although the majority of agammaglobulinemia cases are caused by the X-linked form, about 15% of cases are presumed to be autosomal recessive (see Fig. 49-2). Mutations of the immunoglobulin μ heavy chain gene *(IGHM)* are the second most common cause of agammaglobulinemia. Other cases are caused by defects in other

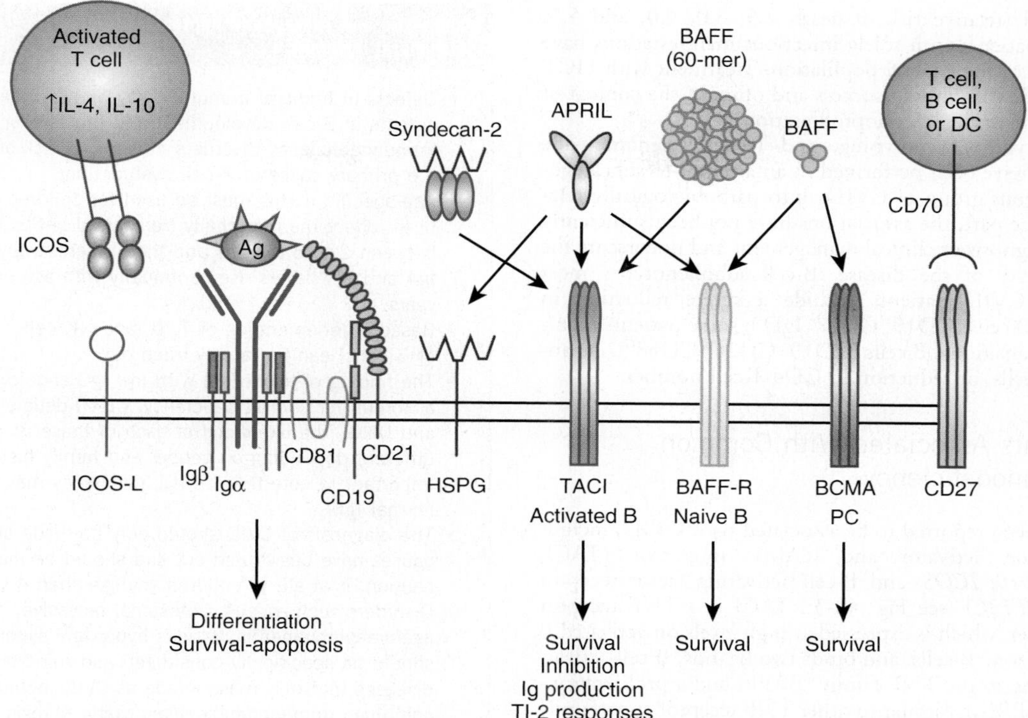

Figure 49-3 GENETIC DEFECTS ASSOCIATED WITH COMMON VARIABLE IMMUNODEFICIENCY (CVID). Schematic of cell surface molecules expressed on B cells and their ligands, highlighting those in which defects have been shown to be associated with CVID. *Ag,* Antigen; *APRIL,* a proliferation-inducing ligand; *BAFF,* B-cell activating factor; *BAFFR,* B-cell activating factor receptor; *BCMA,* B-cell maturation antigen; *DC,* dendritic cell; *HSPG,* heparin sulfate proteoglycan; *ICOS,* inducible T-cell costimulator; *ICOS-L,* inducible T-cell costimulator ligand; *IL,* interleukin; *PC,* plasma cell; *TACI,* transmembrane activator and calcium modulator and cyclophilin ligand interactor; *TI-2,* T-cell independent type 2.

components of the pre-BCR–BCR complex, including the signaling moieties Igα (CD79A), Igβ (CD79B), and λ5 (IGLL1), the surrogate light chain that pairs with Vpre-B. Finally, mutation in the scaffold protein B cell linker (BLNK), which brings BTK into the signaling complex, was reported in a single patient. Aside from the genetics, the clinical phenotype and treatment of all of these patients is similar to XLA.

Common Variable Immunodeficiency

Common variable immunodeficiency (CVID) is the most common PID severe enough to require treatment, with a prevalence estimated to be one in 25,000 to 30,000 whites and accounting for approximately 10% to 20% of humoral immunodeficiencies. Although a growing number of genetic defects have been found to be associated with a CVID phenotype, these defects account for a minority of cases. The "variable" nature of the clinical manifestations of CVID patients could reflect genetic heterogeneity but also refers to distinct clinical and immunologic features that distinguish subgroups of CVID patients. However, the most common genetic variant described to date (mutations in *TACI*) can be found in asymptomatic individuals and more likely represents a predisposition to CVIDs than primary cause. Thus the genetic causes of the majority of cases of CVIDs remain obscure and are not clearly monogenic in nature.

Diagnostic criteria for CVIDs were established in 1999 by consensus of European and Pan-American societies and include the presence of hypogammaglobulinemia (<2 standard deviations below the mean for age of IgG, IgA, or IgM) and lack of specific antibody responses in individuals with onset of symptoms after 2 years of age for whom other causes of humoral immunodeficiency have been ruled out. The number of circulating B cells detected is variable. Specific antibody responses should be assessed to more than one antigen. Because an increasing number of gene defects causing hypogammaglobulinemia early in life have been identified, many experts would recommend limiting the diagnosis of CVID to patients in whom symptoms appeared after 4 years of age.

Consistent with the antibody deficiency, CVID patients have recurrent bacterial infections of the respiratory tract; sepsis with encapsulated organisms; and infections from *Ureaplasma urealyticum, Giardia* spp., and enteroviruses. However, variable derangement of T-cell numbers and function often results in noninfectious manifestations, including autoimmunity, lymphoid infiltration or proliferation, and malignancy. In one survey, only 26% of CVID patients had infections as the only manifestation of disease. Autoimmune cytopenias are quite common (≈12%) and may be the presenting feature. Other autoimmune complications include rheumatoid arthritis, systemic lupus erythematosus, hypothyroidism, vitiligo, psoriasis, diabetes, and autoimmune gastritis with pernicious anemia. Polyclonal lymphocytic granulomatous infiltrates are common and may involve the lungs, liver, or gut (causing enteropathy that is resistant to gluten withdrawal). Finally, both lymphoid (NHL, chronic lymphocytic leukemia) and nonlymphoid (gastric cancer) malignancies are more frequent in patients with CVID, although the latter may be related to *Helicobacter* pylori infection.

Replacement of immunoglobulins and treatment and prevention of infection remain the mainstays of management of CVID. Immunosuppression may be needed for inflammatory and autoimmune manifestations. Analysis of the European CVID registry containing 334 patients observed over 25 years revealed that disease manifestations such as autoimmunity, polyclonal lymphocytic infiltrative disease, enteropathy, and malignancy have differential and increasing impact on survival (relative risk of death 2.5, 3.0, 4.0, and 5.5, respectively), but patients with solely infectious manifestations have equivalent survival to the general population. Treatment with HCT has been performed with limited success and often in the context of consolidative treatment for lymphoproliferation.

Immunophenotyping, genotyping, and recently genome-wide association studies have been performed in an attempt to subcategorize the heterogeneous group of CVIDs into pathobiologically relevant groups. In large part, the associations have not been sufficiently robust to direct diagnosis or clinical management and underscore the genetic heterogeneity of the disease. B-cell subphenotypes most common among CVID patients include a severe reduction in switched memory B cells ($CD19^+$ $CD27^+$ IgD^-); some patients manifest expansion of transitional B cells ($CD19^+$ $CD24^{hi}$ $CD38^{hi}$), expansion of $CD21^{lo}$ B cells, or reduction in CD4 T-cell number.

Genetic Variants Associated With Common Variable Immunodeficiency

A few genes have been reported to be associated with CVID, including transmembrane activator and CAML interactor (TACI, *TNFRSF13B*), *CD19, ICOS,* and B-cell activating factor receptor (BAFF-R, *TNFRSF13C*) (see Fig. 49-3). TACI is a TNF receptor superfamily member, which is expressed at high levels on activated B cells and marginal zone B cells, and binds two ligands, B cell activating factor belonging to the TNF family (BAFF) and a proliferation-inducing ligand (APRIL). Similar to other TNF receptor superfamily members, TACI assembles as a trimer or higher order multimer. Heterozygous and homozygous mutations in TACI have been documented in 10% to 15% of CVID patients; however, they are also found at lower frequency in the general population. Thus the presence of TACI mutations is considered to be a predisposing factor to CVID rather than a disease-causing factor.

Mutations of CD19, CD81, and CD21, which are all components of the B-cell coreceptor, have been reported in few individuals. These defects do not affect B-cell development but impair signaling, causing hypogammaglobulinemia, a low number of switched memory B cells, and poor antibody response to T-independent antigens.

Mutations of inducible T cell co-stimulator (ICOS), a molecule expressed by activated T cells, account for rare cases of CVID. Most patients present during early adulthood with increased rates of respiratory infections. Autoimmune phenomena and lymphoproliferative disorders have been described.

One family with two affected older adult members exhibited homozygous mutation in BAFFR, with a 24–base pair deletion in the transmembrane region. One sibling was diagnosed at age 57 years with CVID; the other was 80 years old and essentially asymptomatic. Both exhibited hypogammaglobulinemia and normal response to T-dependent antigen but defective response to carbohydrate antigen. Peripheral B-cell numbers and percentage of memory B cells were low.

Finally, mutations of CD27, a molecule expressed by T, B, and NK lymphocytes, and an important costimulator of plasma cell differentiation, were identified in two individuals with hypogammaglobulinemia, defective antibody response to T-dependent antigens, and persistent EBV viremia (see Fig. 49-3).

Diagnostic and Therapeutic Approach to Defects in Humoral Immunity

- Defects in humoral immunity may be attributable to intrinsic defects in B-cell development and function or combined immunodeficiency disorders in which a lack of T-cell help is the primary cause of B-cell dysfunction.
- Age-specific norms must be used for children. IgG levels at birth reflect the maternally transferred antibody, which nadir between 2 to 6 months and then progressively rise with age. IgA and IgM levels rise continually with age until the teenage years.
- Based on enumeration of T, B, and NK cells, XLA (absence of B cells) can be rapidly ruled out.
- The finding of hyper-IgM with low IgG should prompt a workup for CD40L deficiency, CD40 deficiency, AID, and UNG. The likelihood of each of these is, of course, different depending on gender and family history. It is important to note that CD40L deficiency may present with a normal IgM.
- The diagnosis of CVID should only be made after other causes have been ruled out and should be made with caution, if at all, in children younger than 4 years of age. Disorders such as XLA, autosomal recessive agammaglobulinemia, various hyper-IgM syndromes, and XLP should be specifically considered and ruled out. Other diseases that may masquerade as CVID include other combined immunodeficiencies, cystic fibrosis, HIV, and conditions leading to immunoglobulin loss such as protein-losing enteropathy. Medications may cause a picture that looks like CVID. Finally, in adults, hypogammaglobulinemia may herald the development of thymoma or lymphoid malignancies and therefore may be secondary to evolving neoplasia.
- Treatment of patients with XLA and the hyper-IgM syndromes other than CD40L deficiency is long-term IVIG replacement, which is very effective.
- Experts disagree on whether patients with CD40L deficiency should be treated with early HCT, and currently, there are no clear predictors to determine who is likely to experience opportunistic infections. A patient with CD40L deficiency who has developed *Cryptosporidium* infection and sclerosing cholangitis generally has a much worse outlook with HCT.
- Treatment of patients with CVID with HCT is generally reserved for those with an alternate reason for allogeneic transplant such as lymphoid malignancy or lymphoproliferation that requires continual immunosuppression.

B-CELL–INTRINSIC DEFECTS OF CLASS SWITCH RECOMBINATION: DEFECTS OF ACTIVATION-INDUCED CYTIDINE DEAMINASE AND URACIL-N-GLYCOSYLASE

Maturation of the antibody response is associated with class switch recombination (CSR), whereby the μ heavy chain is replaced by other immunoglobulin heavy chains and somatic hypermutation (SHM), with introduction of mutations in the immunoglobulin variable region that allow affinity maturation. After CD40LG–CD40 interaction and activation of the NFκB signaling pathway, expression of activation-induced cytidine deaminase (AID) and of uracil-DNA-glycosylase (UNG) occurs in germinal center B lymphocytes (see Fig. 49-3). AID acts on the DNA of immunoglobulin heavy chain switch regions and converts cytidine to uridine, which is recognized and removed by UNG. The abasic sites are cleaved by a DNA endonuclease. DNA repair then brings together two different switch regions allowing CSR.

Mutations of AID and of UNG are inherited as autosomal recessive traits. Patients have recurrent bacterial infections. Autoimmune manifestations have been observed in several patients. Circulating B cells are present, but there is a severe reduction of all immunoglobulin isotypes with the exception of IgM, which are often elevated. Lymphadenopathy is common and is associated with expansion of germinal centers. SHM is severely compromised in patients with AID deficiency and follows an abnormal pattern in patients with UNG deficiency.

Treatment is based on regular administration of immunoglobulins and prompt recognition and therapy of infections.

SUGGESTED READINGS

Al-Herz W, Bousfiha A, Casanova JL, et al: Primary immunodeficiency diseases: An update on the classification from the International Union of Immunological Societies Committee for Primary Immunodeficiency. *Frontiers Immunol* 2:54, 2011.

Buckley RH: Transplantation of hematopoietic stem cells in human severe combined immunodeficiency: Longterm outcomes. *Immunol Res* 49:25, 2011.

Chapel H, Cunningham-Rundles C: Update in understanding common variable immunodeficiency disorders (CVIDs) and the management of patients with these conditions. *Br J Haematol* 145:709, 2009.

Chase NM, Verbsky JW, Routes JM: Newborn screening for T-cell deficiency. *Current Opinion in Allergy and Clinical Immunology* 10:521, 2010.

Conley ME, Dobbs AK, Farmer AK, et al: Primary B cell immunodeficiencies: Comparisons and contrasts. *Annu Rev Immunol* 27:199, 2009.

de Saint Basile G, Ménasché G, Latour S: Inherited defects causing hemophagocytic lymphohistiocytic syndrome. *Ann N Y Acad Sci* 1246:64, 2011.

Feske S: Immunodeficiency due to defects in store-operated calcium entry. *Ann N Y Acad Sci* 1238:74, 2011 Nov.

Fischer A, Hacein-Bey-Abina S, Cavazzana-Calvo M: Gene therapy for primary adaptive immunodeficiencies. *J Allergy Clin Immunol* 127:1356, 2011.

Fischer A, Le Deist F, Hacein-Bey-Abina S, et al: Severe combined immunodeficiency. A model disease for molecular immunology and therapy. *Immunol Rev* 203:98, 2005.

Gennery AR, Slatter MA, Grandin L, et al: Transplantation of hematopoietic stem cells and long-term survival for primary immunodeficiencies in Europe: Entering a new century, do we do better? *J Allergy Clin Immunol* 126:602, 2010.

Hanson EP, Monaco-Shawver L, Solt LA, et al: Hypomorphic nuclear factor-kappaB essential modulator mutation database and reconstitution system identifies phenotypic and immunologic diversity. *J Allergy Clin Immunol* 122:1169, 2008.

Hoernes M, Seger R, Reichenbach J: Modern management of primary B-cell immunodeficiencies. *Pediatr Allergy Immunol* 22:758, 2011.

Kisand K, Peterson P: Autoimmune polyendocrinopathy candidiasis ectodermal dystrophy: Known and novel aspects of the syndrome. *Ann N Y Acad Sci* 1246:77, 2011.

Kracker S, Gardes P, Mazerolles F, et al: Immunoglobulin class switch recombination deficiencies. *Clin Immunol* 135:193, 2010.

Markert ML, Devlin BH, McCarthy EA: Thymus transplantation. *Clin Immunol* 135:236, 2010.

McDonald-McGinn DM, Sullivan KE: Chromosome 22q11.2 deletion syndrome (DiGeorge syndrome/velocardiofacial syndrome). *Medicine* 90:1, 2011.

Nadeau K, Hwa V, Rosenfeld RG: STAT5b deficiency: An unsuspected cause of growth failure, immunodeficiency, and severe pulmonary disease. *J Pediatr* 158:701, 2011. Epub 2011 Mar 17. Review. Erratum in: *J Pediatr* 159:356, 2011.

Notarangelo LD, Roifman CM, Giliani S: Cartilage-hair hypoplasia: Molecular basis and heterogeneity of the immunological phenotype. *Curr Opin Allergy Clin Immunol* 8:534, 2008.

Ochs HD, Filipovich AH, Veys P, et al: Wiskott-Aldrich syndrome: Diagnosis, clinical and laboratory manifestations, and treatment. *Biol Blood Marrow Transplant* 15:84, 2008.

Oliveira JB, Blesing JJ, Dianzani U, et al: Revised diagnostic criteria and classification for the autoimmune lymphoproliferative syndrome (ALPS): Report from the 2009 NIH International Workshop. *Blood* 116:e35, 2010.

Oliveira JB, Fleisher TA: Laboratory evaluation of primary immunodeficiencies. *J Allergy Clin Immunol* 2:S297, 2009.

Pai SY, Notarangelo LD: Hematopoietic cell transplantation for Wiskott-Aldrich syndrome: Advances in biology and future directions for treatment. *Immunology and Allergy Clinics of North America* 30:179, 2010.

Picard C, Fischer A: Hematopoietic stem cell transplantation and other management strategies for MHC class II deficiency. *Immunol Allergy Clin North Am* 30:173, 2010.

Railey MD, Lokhnygina Y, Buckley RH: Long-term clinical outcome of patients with severe combined immunodeficiency who received related donor bone marrow transplants without pretransplant chemotherapy or post-transplant GVHD prophylaxis. *J Pediatr* 155:834, 2009.

Rezaei N, Mahmoudi E, Aghamohammadi A, et al: X-linked lymphoproliferative syndrome: A genetic condition typified by the triad of infection, immunodeficiency and lymphoma. *Br J Haematol* 152:13, 2011 Jan.

Roifman CM, Dadi H, Somech R, et al: Characterization of ζ-associated protein, 70 kd (ZAP70)-deficient human lymphocytes. *J Allergy Clin Immunol* 126:1226, 2010.

Szabolcs P, Cavazzana-Calvo M, Fischer A, et al: Bone marrow transplantation for primary immunodeficiency diseases. *Pediatr Clin North Am* 57:207, 2010.

Su HC: Dedicator of cytokinesis 8 (DOCK8) deficiency. *Current Opinion in Allergy and Clinical Immunology* 10:515, 2010.

Torgerson TR, Ochs HD: Regulatory T cells in primary immunodeficiency diseases. *Current Opinion in Allergy and Clinical Immunology* 7:515, 2007.

Zimmer J, Andrès E, Donato L, et al: Clinical and immunological aspects of HLA class I deficiency. *QJM* 98:719, 2005.

CHAPTER 50

HISTIOCYTIC DISORDERS

Michael B. Jordan and Alexandra Hult Filipovich

The histiocytic disorders comprise a broad grouping of hematologic diseases united by the observation that monocyte/macrophages or dendritic cells appear to be the principal pathologic protagonists. The term *histiocyte* refers to phagocytic cells, historically identified on tissue sections but now more precisely defined as cells of the monocyte/macrophage lineage (Fig. 50-1). The ontogeny of these cells continues to be actively studied and debated, and their role(s) in pathogenesis is an active area of investigation. The characteristic cells seen in various histiocytic lesions can, in general, be differentiated by a variety of functional and phenotypic markers. The modern classification of the histiocytoses mirrors this biology (Table 50-1). Although malignant disorders involving monocyte/macrophages or dendritic cells were originally included in this classification, this chapter focuses solely on nonmalignant disorders in this category.

Of the dendritic cell–related histiocytoses, the most clinically prominent and common is Langerhans cell histiocytosis (LCH). This chapter also briefly discusses other dendritic cell–related histiocytic disorders, including juvenile xanthogranuloma (JXG); Erdheim-Chester disease (ECD); and sinus histiocytosis with massive lymphadenopathy (SHML), also referred to as Rosai-Dorfman disease.

The prominent monocyte/macrophage–related histiocytic disorder, hemophagocytic lymphohistiocytosis (HLH), is discussed in detail later in this chapter. In HLH, activated macrophages, activated T cells, and defective natural killer (NK) cells are the dysfunctional interactive partners.

Table 50-1 lists a currently accepted classification of histiocytic disorders. These disorders are a diverse grouping, ranging from benign skin lesions to rapidly life-threatening systemic disorders. Tables 50-2 and 50-3 list clinical features and commonly used pathological markers or features that may be used to help distinguish some of these disorders. The clinical diversity of histiocytic disorders is underscored by recent discoveries related to their pathogenesis. Studies dating to the late 1990s have demonstrated that HLH (at least in its familial form) is a primary immune deficiency, albeit a very unique one. Demonstrations of clonality as well as genetic abnormalities of B-Raf now suggest that LCH is a benign neoplasm despite its variable clinical phenotype. The pathogeneses of less common dendritic cell– and macrophage-related histiocytic disorders are still unknown.

LANGERHANS CELL HISTIOCYTOSIS

Langerhans cell histiocytosis is the most common of the histiocytoses. The central cell of LCH, the Langerhans dendritic cell, was first described in 1868 by 21-year-old Paul Langerhans. Between 1893 and 1920, Hand, Schüller, and Christian described the various nonfatal presentations of LCH, which include bony lesions, skin rash, and diabetes insipidus (DI). Letterer and Siwe (1924 and 1933, respectively) added to the list of clinical presentations by describing cases with liver and spleen involvement in infants and toddlers. These disorders were later grouped under the term *histiocytosis X* (denoting the uncertainty about disease pathogenesis) by Lichtenstein. It was eventually theorized by Nezelof (1973) that histiocytosis X is due to a proliferation of pathologic Langerhans cells. At present, the term *LCH* has been adopted to refer to all of the varied manifestations of this protean disorder. It is now well recognized that LCH can present at any time in life from the neonatal period to old age. LCH lesions may spontaneously regress or repeatedly "reactivate," contributing to long-term disabilities such as DI or a neurodegenerative disease. Life-threatening forms of LCH, previously referred to as Letterer-Siwe disease, typically present in infancy and clearly require intensive therapy and sometimes salvage treatment such as allogeneic bone marrow transplantation (BMT) to cure the children.

Epidemiology

The incidence of LCH has been estimated to be between five and 15 cases per million children, per year. The incidence of LCH in adults is believed to be lower than in children but is likely underestimated because of a lack of recognition of LCH in adult medicine. Notably, LCH does not appear to have significant geographic or ethnic predilections. Although families with multiple cases of LCH have been reported, these kindreds are extremely rare. One notable clinical or epidemiologic association reported thus far involves an unexplained coincidence of both LCH and leukemia (of various subtypes) in rare patients.

Pathobiology

The understanding of the pathobiology of LCH is currently undergoing significant evolution driven by new insights into both normal and disease-associated Langerhans cells. Over the years, LCH has been classified as a neoplasm, a reactive disorder, or an aberrant immune response. LCH cells are pathologic in that they bear heterogeneous characteristics not normally identified in healthy Langerhans cells that are typically resident in the skin. The granulomatous lesions of LCH, which can be found in nearly any organ, represent an accumulation of normal inflammatory cells, including eosinophils, lymphocytes (especially T cells), and macrophages, in addition to the LCH cells. The clinically benign behavior of most cases, including spontaneous remissions and lack of aggressive disease evolution with recurrences, as well as the benign histopathologic appearance of lesions, have suggested a nonmalignant etiology. The failure of many laboratories to culture pathologic Langerhans cells has reinforced this impression. Thus LCH has been hypothesized to be a reactive or immunologic disorder by many. On the other hand, lesional Langerhans cells have been demonstrated by several investigators to be clonal. This observation, combined with the clinical utility of antineoplastic drugs, has bolstered the opinion that LCH may be a neoplastic disorder.

A recent report (which has been independently confirmed) of highly prevalent B-Raf mutations in lesional Langerhans cells has again shifted thinking and strongly supports a neoplastic etiology. The mutation in question (B-Raf, V600E) is well described in both malignant melanomas and in benign nevi, among other neoplasms. This mutation leads to activation of the extracellular signal-related kinase (ERK) pathway. Along with these disease-specific findings, understanding of the biology of normal Langerhans cells has advanced. Cutaneous Langerhans dendritic cells have been shown to arise from in situ precursors, but during inflammation or stress, to arise from circulating myeloid precursors. Therefore, a picture is emerging in

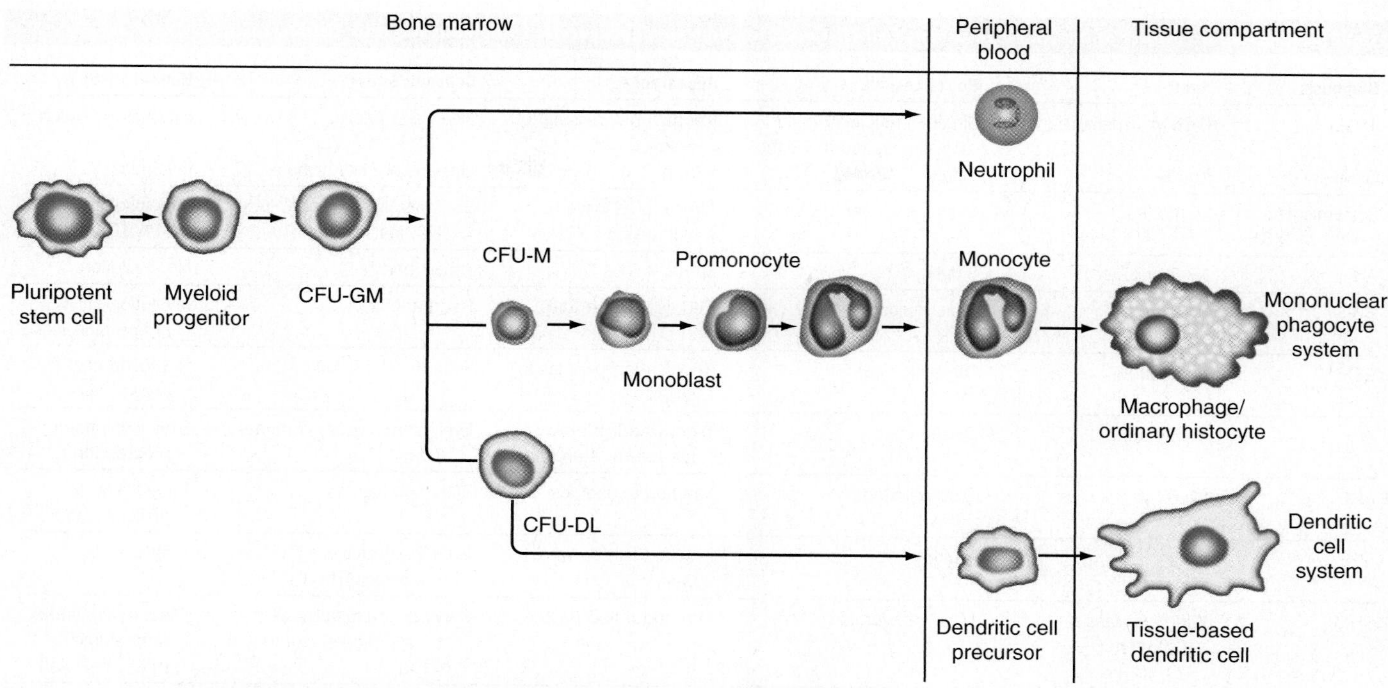

Figure 50-1 DEVELOPMENT OF CELLS OF THE MONOCYTE/MACROPHAGE LINEAGE. *CFU-DL,* Colony-forming unit–dendritic Langerhans cell; *CFU-GM,* colony-forming unit–granulocyte-macrophage; *CFU-M,* colony-forming unit–macrophage.

Table 50-1 Classification of Histiocytic Disorders: Benign Disorders of Varying Biologic Behavior

A. Dendritic cell related
   Langerhans cell histiocytosis
   Juvenile xanthogranuloma and related disorders including:
   - Erdheim-Chester disease
   - Solitary histiocytomas with juvenile xanthogranuloma phenotype
   - Secondary dendritic cell disorders

B. Monocyte/macrophage-related
   Hemophagocytic lymphohistiocytosis: familial and sporadic
   Secondary hemophagocytic syndromes
   - Infection-associated
   - Malignancy-associated
   - Autoimmune-associated

   Sinus histiocytosis with massive lymphadenopathy (Rosai-Dorfman disease)
   Solitary histiocytoma of macrophage phenotype

which the acquisition of mutation(s), such as B-Raf V600E, in myeloid precursors may cause a neoplastic proliferation of a terminally differentiated clone that colonizes a distinct anatomic location. Similar to a cutaneous nevus, this neoplasm is a benign one because lesional cells are not fully transformed. Thus recent findings support the hypothesis that LCH is a benign hematopoietic neoplasm, or a hematopoietic "mole." Thus far, there has been no compelling insight into why LCH has such diverse manifestations, ranging from solitary to widely disseminated disease.

Clinical Manifestations

Clinical involvement with LCH can be highly variable but most often involves bony lesions (present in ≈80% of cases), which may be painful or painless; the latter is common with skull lesions. Skin involvement, typically papulosquamous lesions, often affecting the scalp (and frequently mistaken for cradle cap, seborrhea) is reported in 30% to 60% of patient series. Soft tissue swelling, often in proximity to bony lesions, external ear drainage, enlargement of lymph nodes and thymus, and gum hypertrophy with premature eruption of baby teeth are also well-recognized manifestations. More serious systemic involvement occurs when there is hepatosplenomegaly, liver dysfunction, lung scarring, and hematopoietic failure with or without intestinal involvement. The latter findings are more typical of the widely disseminated form of LCH seen in young infants, which carries a high mortality rate.

Bony Involvement

Solitary or multifocal bony lesions are found predominantly in older children and young adults, usually within the first 3 decades of life. Such lytic bone lesions are commonly referred to as *eosinophilic granuloma* because of their pathologic appearance. The incidence of bone lesions peaks between 5 and 10 years of age. Solitary or multifocal eosinophilic granuloma (with or without involvement of other organ systems) represents approximately 60% to 80% of all instances of LCH. Patients with systemic involvement frequently have bone lesions in addition to other manifestations of disease. Patients often cannot bear weight and may have tender swelling caused by tissue infiltrates overlying the bone lesions. Radiographically, the lesions are sharply marginated, round, or oval and usually have a beveled edge on radiography that gives the appearance of depth. Hand-Schüller-Christian disease, referring to the triad of bony involvement, skin lesions, and DI, is most commonly described in younger children, ages 2 to 5 years. It represents 15% to 40% of these patients, although this type of involvement can be observed in patients of all ages. Signs and symptoms include bony defects with exophthalmos, with a tumor mass in the orbital cavity being characteristic. This condition usually occurs from involvement of the roof and lateral wall of the orbital bones. In addition, teeth are often lost because of gum infiltration or mandibular involvement (Fig. 50-2).

The most frequent sites of skeletal involvement include the flat bones of the skull, ribs, pelvis, and scapula. There may be extensive involvement of the skull, with irregularly-shaped, lucent lesions giving rise to the so-called geographic skull. Long bones and lumbosacral vertebrae, usually the anterior portion of the vertebral body, are involved less frequently. Involvement of the vertebral bodies may lead to collapse *(vertebra plana)* as the principal or only presenting

Table 50-2 Clinical Features of the Non–Langerhans Cell Histiocytosis, Non–Hemophagocytic Lymphohistiocytosis Histiocytoses

Diagnosis	Ages	No. of Lesions	Appearance	Common Sites	Natural History
JXG	0-18 yr (median, 2 yr)	Single: multiple 9:1 (disseminated in <6 mo)	Reddish progressing to yellow brown	Head and neck	Gradual involution
Giant JXG	Young	Single	>2 cm	Upper extremity or back	Involution
Systemic JXG (4% of JXG)	(3 mo*)	Single, multiple	Almost 50% have no skin lesions	Subcutis, liver, spleen, lung, CNS, iris	May involute (4%-10% fatal)
Adult XG	18-80 (35 yr*)	Single	Same as JXG	Upper body	No involution
BCH	Young child	Few, multiple	Reddish-tan papules	Head and neck	Involution or progression to XG
GEH	Young adult	Disseminated	Reddish-tan papules in crops	Face, trunk, arms	Involution or progression
XD	Young adult	Disseminated	Yellow/reddish-brown plaques and nodules	Eyelids, mucosae, viscerae, CNS	Slow involution or progression
PNH	40-60 yr	Disseminated	Xanthoma, nodules	Skin, subcutis	Progression to disfigurement
MRH	40 yr+	Multiple	Pink/reddish-brown or yellow	Head, extremities with erosive polyarthritis	Progression
SHML	Wide age range (20 yr*)	Mainly systemic	Firm indurated papules	Cervical adenopathy, 80% "B" symptoms, extranodal (43%)	Exacerbations and remissions (5%-11% fatal)
ECD	7-84 yr (53 yr*)	Mainly systemic	Xanthelasma, xanthoma	Long bone sclerosis, retroperitoneal fibrosis	Highly fatal

Adapted from Weitzman S, Jaffe R: Uncommon histiocytic disorders: The non-Langerhans cell histiocytoses. *Pediatr Blood Cancer 45:256,* 2005.
BCH, Benign cephalic histiocytosis; *CNS,* central nervous system; *DI,* diabetes insipidus; *ECD,* Erdheim-Chester disease; *GEH,* generalized eruptive histiocytosis; *JXG,* juvenile xanthogranuloma; *MRH,* multicentric reticulohistiocytosis; *PNH,* progressive nodular histiocytosis; *SHML,* sinus histiocytosis with massive lymphadenopathy; *XD,* xanthoma disseminatum.

Table 50-3 Biopsy Markers or Features of Various Histiocytic Disorders

Clinical Entity	LCH	JXG Family	HLH	SHML
Cell type involved	LC	DD	M/M	M/M
HLA-DR	++	–	+	+
CD1a	++	–	–	–
CD14	–	++	++	++
CD68	+/–	++	++	++
CD163	–	–	++	++
Factor XIIIa	–	++	–	–
Langerin	++	–	–	–
Fascin	–	++	+/–	+
S100	+	–	+/–	+
Lysozyme	–	–	++	++
Birbeck granules	+	–	–	–
Hemophagocytosis			+/–	
Emperipolesis				+

Adapted from Weitzman, Egeler, eds: *Histiocytic disorders of children and adults.* Cambridge, 2005, Cambridge University Press.
DD, dermal dendrocyte; *HLA-DR,* human leukocyte antigenDR; *HLH,* hemophagocytic lymphohistiocytosis; *JXG,* juvenile xanthogranuloma; *LC,* Langerhans cell; *LCH,* Langerhans cell histiocytosis; *M/M,* monocyte/macrophage; *SHML,* sinus histiocytosis with massive lymphadenopathy.

manifestation. In such cases, the diagnosis may be problematic, although biopsy is typically not advisable unless a soft tissue mass is present. In long bones, growth of lesions in the medullary cavity leads to pressure that may result in erosion through the cortex, stimulating the formation of periosteal new bone accompanied by soft tissue extension. The differential diagnosis includes Ewing and osteogenic sarcoma, bone lymphoma, benign bone tumor and cyst, and infection. Involvement of the wrists, hands, knees, feet, or cervical vertebrae is less common. Orbital involvement may result in vision loss or strabismus caused by optic nerve or orbital muscle involvement, respectively, and may mimic preseptal cellulitis. Oral involvement commonly affects the gums, palate, or both. Erosion of the lamina dura gives rise to the characteristic "floating tooth" seen on dental radiographs. The entire mandible may be involved (see Fig. 50-2), with loss of bone leading to diminished height of the mandibular rami. Erosion of gingival tissue causes premature eruption, decay, and tooth loss. Parents of affected children, particularly infants, frequently report precocious eruption of teeth when, in fact, the gums are receding leading to exposure of immature dentition. Chronic otitis media caused by involvement of the mastoid and petrous portion of the temporal bone, leading to otitis externa is common.

Cutaneous Involvement

Cutaneous involvement by LCH is both common (occurring in 20%-40% of patients) and highly variable. The rash is typically a scaly seborrheic, eczematoid, sometimes purpuric rash involving the scalp, ear canals, abdomen, and intertriginous areas of the neck, face, trunk and groin (Fig. 50-3). The rash may be maculopapular or nodulopapular. Ulceration may result, especially in intertriginous areas, and may be painful. Mild, isolated cutaneous involvement is relatively common in young infants. Rarely, LCH may present as deep subcutaneous skin nodules only (formerly described as Hashimoto-Pritzker syndrome), typically in young infants.

Involvement of Other Organ Systems

A subset of infants and toddlers with LCH have involvement of the spleen, liver, or bone marrow (BM), usually in addition to prominent skin involvement and variable bony disease. This clinical phenotype, previously referred to as Letterer-Siwe disease, is the most severe manifestation of LCH and the only form that is likely to be life threatening. Involvement of the BM, usually as evidenced by cytopenias, is an especially poor prognostic factor. Of note, unlike with other tissues, biopsy of the BM in these patients does not typically reveal an obvious infiltrate with CD1a$^+$ cells but rather tends to have a dysplastic appearance. Liver involvement may be severe, leading to significant cholestasis, hypoproteinemia, and diminished synthesis of clotting factors.

Langerhans cell histiocytosis can have a strictly nodal presentation, not to be confused with SHML, also known as Rosai-Dorfman disease. This presentation is characterized by significant enlargement of multiple lymph node groups with little or no other signs of disease. Thymic involvement is relatively common in children with multisystem involvement. Pancreatic and thyroid involvement have also been reported. Gastrointestinal tract disease has rarely been identified. It is sometimes associated with severe symptoms of diarrhea, malabsorption, and hypoproteinemia.

Isolated pulmonary involvement usually is seen in young adults in their third or fourth decades of life and occasionally in adolescents. It may follow a severe and often chronic debilitating course; patients may present with pneumothorax. Cigarette smoking has been strongly implicated in primary pulmonary histiocytosis. In contrast, pulmonary involvement in younger patients with systemic disease frequently is mild, although fulminant pulmonary disease may occur. Findings on chest radiographs vary from a diffuse infiltrate consistent with bilateral interstitial pneumonia to a "honeycomb lung" appearance (Fig. 50-4).

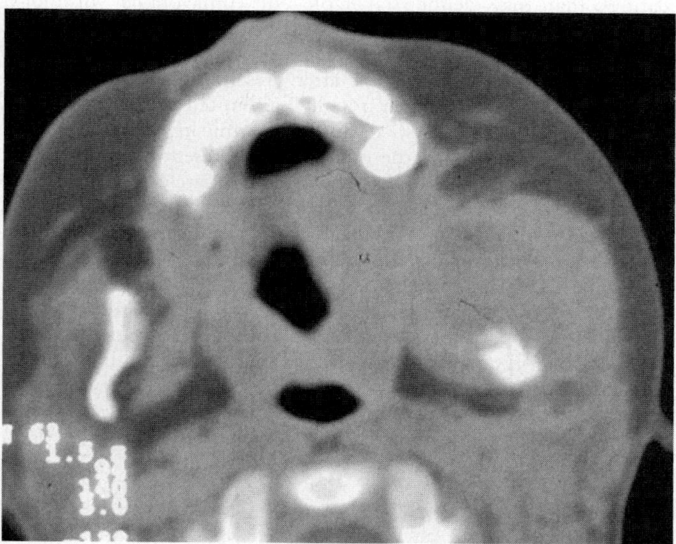

Figure 50-2 COMPUTED TOMOGRAPHIC SCAN OF A DESTRUCTIVE LANGERHANS CELL HISTIOCYTOSIS MANDIBULAR LESION IN A CHILD.

Other Clinical Features

Diabetes insipidus affects 5% to 40% of patients with LCH, depending on the report. Most instances of DI occur in children who present with systemic disease and involvement of the orbit and skull. Fewer than one-third of children who ultimately develop DI have polydipsia and polyuria as presenting symptoms of LCH. Most cases of DI present within 4 years of diagnosis. DI is caused by infiltration by Langerhans cells and macrophages into the hypothalamus with or without involvement of the posterior pituitary gland (Fig. 50-5). DI may occur at any time during the course of LCH. Patients should be instructed to report signs of DI as soon as they develop because dehydration and electrolyte imbalance may be quite serious. In addition, definitive documentation of DI with measurement of serum and urine electrolytes and osmolality before and after a several-hour water deprivation period should be performed. Vasopressin levels can be measured to document a deficiency. The effectiveness of LCH treatment for reversal of new-onset DI is controversial.

Short stature has been found in up to 40% of children with systemic LCH. Chronic illness and steroid therapy are believed to play an important role in this phenomenon. However, short stature also may be a consequence of anterior pituitary involvement and growth hormone deficiency, which can occur in up to half of patients with initial anterior pituitary dysfunction. Other endocrine manifestations include hyperprolactinemia and hypogonadism caused by hypothalamic infiltration.

A severe complication or manifestation of LCH is the development of a delayed central nervous system (CNS) neurodegenerative syndrome. This CNS involvement is typically seen in children who had classic lytic bony involvement or soft tissue mass lesions in or

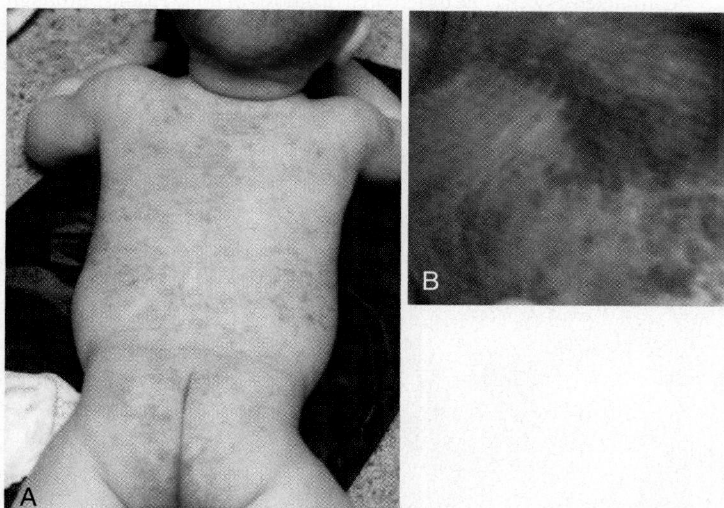

Figure 50-3 SKIN INVOLVEMENT IN LANGERHANS CELL HISTIOCYTOSIS. **A,** Diffuse maculopapular rash. **B,** Hemorrhagic scalp rash.

around the CNS years earlier. Delayed CNS involvement is typically diagnosed after a prolonged, sometimes insidious, decrease in school function. Magnetic resonance imaging (MRI) reveals diffuse or polymorphic lesions involving the white matter of the cerebellum, pons, and cerebral hemispheres. Limited biopsy studies have revealed an inflammatory infiltrate, predominated by $CD8^+$ T cells. Such findings suggest that this form of CNS involvement is analogous to a paraneoplastic syndrome. However, the timing (usually years after disease resolution) and the lack of concurrently active LCH in most patients are unique to this syndrome. Currently, there are no agreed upon diagnostic criteria for CNS LCH, but neurologic involvement (as evidenced by neuropsychiatric testing) with or without MRI findings is essential. Of note, although abnormal MRI findings (with white matter lesions) may precede clinical manifestations, such findings do not always correlate with clinical disease (even in retrospect). Lesions involving the CNS itself or bony lesions of the skull base and facial bones (but not the calvarium or mandible) are thought to confer the greatest risk for subsequent development of this complication.

Laboratory Manifestations

Langerhans cell histiocytosis is the most common and prominent of numerous dendritic cell–related histiocytic disorders. Tables 50-2 and 50-3 list the clinical and pathologic features that help to describe and distinguish LCH from other, much rarer, histiocytic disorders (as well as SHML and HLH, discussed in the next section). The typical histologic appearance of LCH varies with the age of the lesion examined (Fig. 50-6). The Langerhans cell is the essential diagnostic feature in the histology of LCH. Early lesions often are locally destructive, with proliferation and accumulation of phenotypically and functionally immature Langerhans cells. Mitoses usually are not present in great numbers but when found are of no known prognostic significance. Multinucleated giant cells are commonly noted. Other inflammatory cells, such as granulocytes, eosinophils, macrophages, and lymphocytes, are also present. Giant cells and macrophages may be phagocytic and, over time, may accumulate cholesterol. As lesions mature or show signs of regression, fewer Langerhans cells are present, and development of fibrotic reaction is less. The diagnosis of LCH relies on the immunohistochemical identification of the presence of Langerhans cells by cell surface CD1a or by the presence of Birbeck granules by electron microscopy in biopsied lesions. Pathologic criteria for the diagnosis of LCH have been established and were formalized by the Histiocyte Society in 1987. With the availability of antibodies to CD1a for use in routinely processed paraffin-embedded specimens, electron microscopy is rarely needed. Of note, $CD1a^+$ Langerhans cells are known to accumulate at the sites of inflammation and may be seen at the margins of malignant lesions. Thus care should be taken that an adequate biopsy specimen has been obtained to observe the full context of a putative lesion.

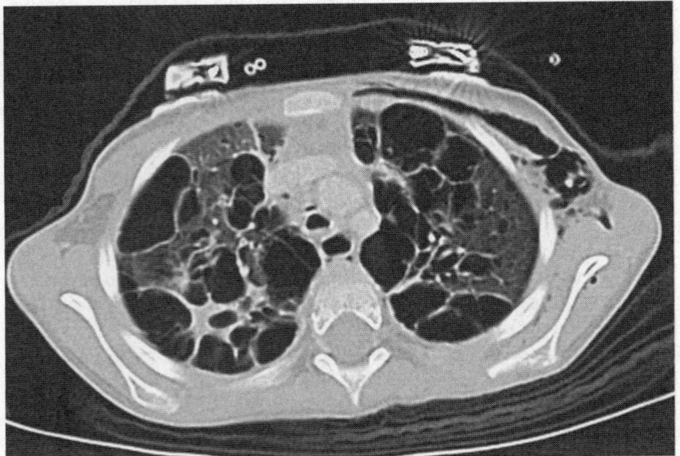

Figure 50-4 COMPUTED TOMOGRAPHIC SCAN OF THE LUNGS SHOWING CYSTIC CHANGES ASSOCIATED WITH LANGERHANS CELL HISTIOCYTOSIS. *(Courtesy Dr. Melanie Committo.)*

Unlike with many malignancies, there are no predictive pathologic features that may define "favorable" or "unfavorable" histology. Although patients are grouped based on their organ system involvement, untreated patients generally do not progress to a different grouping. Within a few months after presentation, it will become apparent that the lesions seen initially are limited to the skeleton or were the "heralding lesion(s)" of diffuse systemic involvement. When cutaneous involvement is the only obvious presenting sign, several months may be required to determine the ultimate extent of disease.

Patients who are suspected to have LCH or who have a new biopsy-proven diagnosis of LCH should have a screening positron emission tomography (or plain radiography and bone scan, although this has been demonstrated to be less sensitive) to help determine the extent of disease involvement. All patients should be evaluated with a complete blood count, chemistries including liver function tests, coagulation workup, and urine osmolality. Dental examination and radiographs should also be considered. The occurrence of cytopenias, particularly thrombocytopenia, in the presence of liver or spleen involvement may be diagnostic of BM involvement.

Differential Diagnosis

The differential diagnosis of LCH depends on the clinical presentation and is typically clarified with a tissue biopsy. Skin involvement frequently mimics seborrheic dermatitis, albeit with a severe or refractory course. Immunodeficiency syndromes or viral infection must be considered as well. The differential diagnosis of bony lesions, although typically quite distinctive, may include bone cyst, lymphoma, sarcoma, or metastatic solid tumor. Chronically draining ears from

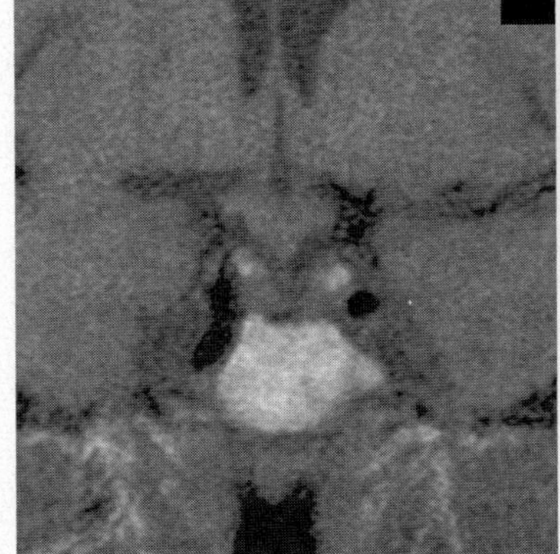

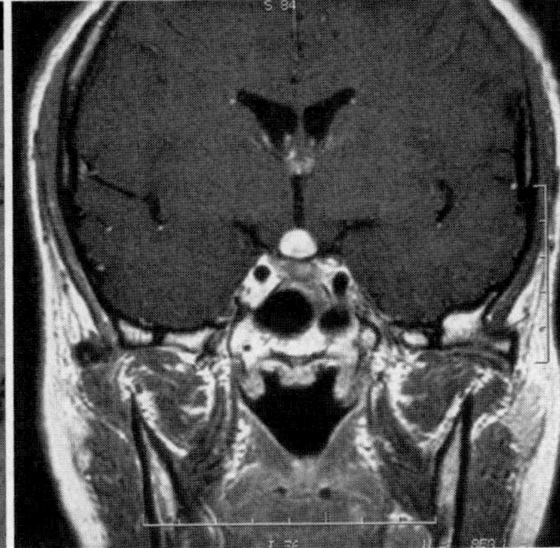

Figure 50-5 MAGNETIC RESONANCE IMAGING CONTRAST CORONAL VIEWS SHOWING TWO PATIENTS WITH DIABETES INSIPIDUS AND PITUITARY INVOLVEMENT CAUSED BY LANGERHANS CELL HISTIOCYTOSIS.

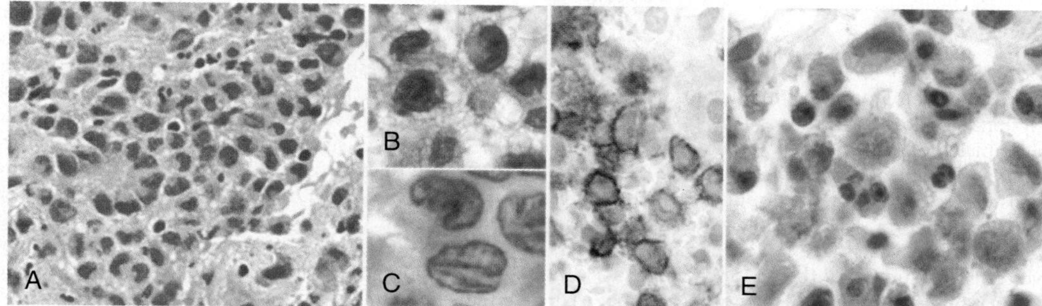

Figure 50-6 A to **E,** LANGERHANS CELL HISTIOCYTOSIS. **A** and **B,** Biopsy sample showing sheets of histiocytes with abundant pink cytoplasm and folded nuclei with prominent nuclear grooves. **C,** Cell with a central longitudinal nuclear groove giving the cell a coffee-bean appearance. **D,** Immunohistochemical stain for CD1A showing the histiocytic cells are positive. **E,** Some cases of Langerhans histiocytosis are associated with prominent eosinophilia. Another term for such cases is *eosinophilic granuloma.*

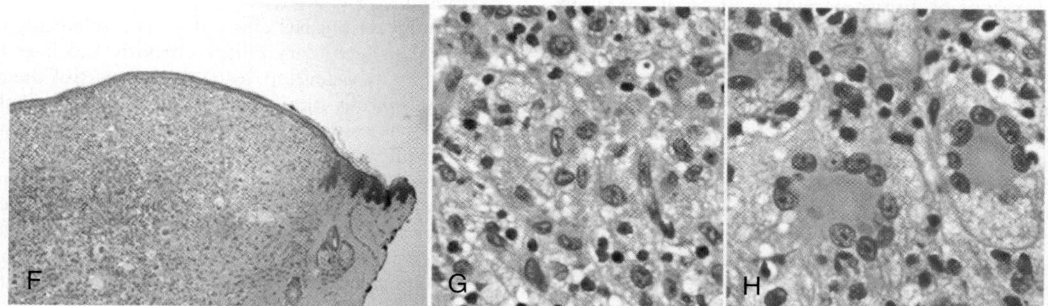

Figure 50-6, cont'd F to **H,** JUVENILE HISTIOCYTOSIS. Histologic features of juvenile xanthogranuloma vary. **F,** In this case, low-powermagnification shows a dome-shaped lesion with an attenuated epidermis. **G,** At higher power, the bulk of the lesion is composed of a proliferation of histiocytes with abundant pink cytoplasm. Sometimes these histiocytes show more vacuolization or xanthomatization. **H,** Scattered Touton-type giant cells are present.

temporal bone involvement is often diagnosed as chronic otitis media. Liver and spleen involvement must be distinguished from leukemia and storage diseases.

Prognosis

The prognosis of patients with LCH is largely determined by the nature of their disease presentation and their response to initial therapies. In general, the only patient population with significant mortality rates are those with visceral, or so-called "risk organ," involvement (e.g., liver, spleen, or BM). Furthermore, the international Histiocyte Society conducted a clinical trial (LCH-II) that identified the response after an initial 6 weeks of therapy with weekly vinblastine and daily prednisolone as the single most important factor in predicting mortality in patients with risk organ involvement. Of the approximately 79% of patients who responded to initial therapy, 94% were alive at 5 years, but only 11% of the nonresponders survived. These important data suggest that alternative therapies should be tested early during the course of therapy for patients with poor early responses. Based on early clinical trials, a staging system was developed for the LCH-III trial that will be further modified in the upcoming LCH-IV trial.

Therapy

A generally accepted standard for initial treatment of patients with LCH is use of an appropriate amount of the least toxic therapy to treat the disease. In patients with potentially morbid or life-threatening disease at presentation or in those who develop morbid or life-threatening disease during the course of treatment, alternative and sometimes more aggressive treatment should be implemented. This approach emphasizes the need for treatment protocols based on careful prognosis-based risk stratification. Whether more intense upfront therapy in lower risk patients can reduce disease sequelae such as DI, CNS degeneration, sclerosing cholangitis, or disease recurrence is currently under evaluation. For the majority of patients with localized or limited systemic disease, the goal of therapy should be minimizing loss of function and preventing cosmetic deformity. Seborrhea-like dermatitis of the scalp may improve with use of a selenium- or phenol-based shampoo. Topical steroids can be effective, but prolonged exposure or use on the face should be avoided. Topical nitrogen mustard has been used for problematic focal skin lesions. In patients with particularly refractory and extensive skin involvement, psoralen ultraviolet A (PUVA) can be effective. These topical therapies have not been studied in clinical trials.

Surgery and Radiotherapy

Patients with disease involving a single bone usually can be managed with local therapy. This most often involves surgical curettage for patients whose lesions are in easily accessible, noncritical locations. Complete "cancer operation" resections are not considered necessary and should be avoided to reduce cosmetic and orthopedic deformities as well as loss of function. Local soft tissue disease (e.g., scalp, thymus, lymph nodes) generally recurs despite surgery; thus additional treatment with antiinflammatory or cytoreductive drugs is usually required. Because of concerns about the development of secondary malignancies, systemic therapy usually is favored over radiation. However, local radiotherapy is indicated under certain circumstances, for example, when patients are at risk for visual or hearing loss, skeletal deformity, spinal cord injury, or severe pain when systemic therapy is not rapidly effective.

Chemotherapy

Historically, drugs used in therapy for classic malignant diseases have been used for the systemic or local treatment of LCH. A variety of drugs, including vinblastine, vincristine, cytarabine, nitrogen mustard, cyclophosphamide, procarbazine, chlorambucil, etoposide, methotrexate, corticosteroids, and 6-mercaptopurine (6-MP), have been used, alone or in combination, with variable success. Therapeutic advances for LCH in recent years have largely come from international cooperative trials conducted by the Histiocyte Society. The Histiocyte Society is currently developing the next international trial, LCH-IV, which has strata allowing for the enrollment of all patients with LCH, either as a treatment or as a registry study. For patients not enrolled on LCH-IV, detailed treatment recommendations are available on the Histiocyte Society's website (http://www.histio.org).

A reasonable therapeutic approach to systemic therapy is to observe patients with limited, single-system disease who respond to local (i.e., surgery, radiation) or nonsystemic (i.e., topical steroids) therapy and look for signs of disease resolution. If persistent symptomatic lesions or evidence of progressive disease is seen, systemic treatment should be pursued. Patients with disease that is localized to skin, bone, and lymph nodes (defined as "non-risk" organs) generally have a good prognosis and may require only minimal treatment. Extensive refractory skin disease may warrant systemic therapy with low-dose oral methotrexate, vinblastine–prednisone, or low-dose cytarabine or with topical therapy such as nitrogen mustard.

Multisystem disease or multifocal bony disease usually warrants treatment with systemic chemotherapy. The current standard of care is a risk-adapted approach, largely using vinblastine, prednisone, and 6-MP, based on the LCH-III trial. This approach has evolved in a stepwise fashion from previous multicenter trials conducted by international groups (DAL-HX 83/90 protocols [Austria, Germany, Switzerland, Netherlands], LCH-I, and LCH-II). All of these protocols were risk adapted and were based on different combinations of prednisone, vinblastine, etoposide, methotrexate, and 6-MP. The Histiocyte Society has stratified patients with LCH into "low-" (LR) and "high-" (HR) risk groups based on outcomes related to the extent and location of the LCH lesions. LR patients include patients with skin, bone, lymph node, and pituitary involvement. Patients with liver, spleen, or BM involvement usually have a worse prognosis and are considered higher risk. Children with lung LCH, without involvement of other HR organs, are generally not considered to be HR. Additionally, LR patients believed to have lesions that may increase their future risks of CNS degenerative disease (lesions within the CNS, skull base, or facial bones) are designated as "CNS risk."

Alternative treatment has not been standardized for patients with recurrent or refractory disease. Patients with recurrent disease (i.e., disease that reappears after a period of remission) often respond well to the drugs with which they initially were treated. Several studies, including an international phase II trial, have demonstrated significant activity of 2-chlorodeoxyadenosine (2-CdA) against recurrent and refractory LCH. In addition, the combination of 2-CdA and high-dose cytarabine has been used in refractory, high-risk patients. BMT for high-risk or refractory patients warrants further evaluation in the context of a controlled clinical trial.

Long-Term Follow-Up

Retrospective analysis of "CNS risk" patients treated with only surgery, steroid injection, radiation therapy, or a single chemotherapy drug have a 40% incidence of DI. If they receive vinblastine and prednisone for 6 months the incidence of DI is 20%. Complications of developing DI include a significant incidence of anterior pituitary hormone deficiencies or neurodegenerative syndrome. Patients with neurodegenerative syndrome may have ataxia, dysarthria, dysmetria, and learning and behavior difficulties. The diagnosis may be aided by brain MRI, in which T2 hyperintense signals in the cerebellum, basal ganglia, or pons may be present, but such abnormalities do not always correlate with clinical disease or vice versa. Treatment with intravenous immunoglobulin (IVIG) or low-dose cytarabine has anecdotally resulted in stabilization of these symptoms.

A retrospective analysis by Willis et al of 71 patients from a single institution followed for a median of 8.1 years from diagnosis revealed the presence of significant late sequelae in 64% of patients followed for more than 3 years. Skeletal defects were found in 42%, dental problems in 30%, DI in 25%, growth failure in 20%, sex hormone deficiency in 16%, hypothyroidism in 14%, hearing loss in 16%, and CNS dysfunction in 14%. The risk of malignancy in patients with LCH undergoing radiation and chemotherapy is well documented. Thus judicious use of radiotherapy, avoidance of potentially carcinogenic chemotherapeutic agents, and good supportive care are recommended. Leukemia in LCH patients treated with etoposide as a single agent and in combination with other agents has been reported. Because etoposide was not shown to be any more effective than vinblastine in both the LCH-I and LCH-II trials for patients without risk organ involvement, there does not appear to be reason to include this leukemogenic agent in the treatment of these patients with newly diagnosed LCH.

Another serious late effect of LCH is sclerosing cholangitis, which may lead to secondary biliary cirrhosis and liver failure. Sclerosing cholangitis may develop years after successful therapy for LCH and does not typically signify disease recurrence. The only successful treatment of sclerosing cholangitis has been liver transplantation. Other late complications of LCH are pulmonary cyst formation, fibrosis, and chronic pneumothoraces. No effective treatment is available, and progression to cor pulmonale and respiratory failure may occur. Lung transplantation has been used for treatment of such patients. Thus all patients with LCH require long-term follow up. In addition to late malignancies, patients should be monitored for signs of long-term disabilities, including cosmetic, orthopedic, and cutaneous deformities that may lead to loss of function and emotional disorders, loss of permanent dentition, endocrinologic disorders and growth failure, hearing impairment, CNS abnormalities and neurocognitive function, sclerosing cholangitis with biliary cirrhosis, and pulmonary fibrosis and cor pulmonale.

Future Directions

The treatment of LCH has undergone significant refinement over the past decade. However, therapy remains empirically defined. With the recent insights into the pathophysiology of LCH, such as B-Raf mutations, new possibilities for more intelligently designed, targeted therapies are conceivable. Future clinical trials for such targeted therapies will likely focus on patients with therapy-resistant risk organ involvement because these children have the least satisfactory outcomes.

JUVENILE XANTHOGRANULOMATOUS DISEASE

Juvenile xanthogranuloma (or more broadly, the full spectrum of juvenile xanthogranulomatous diseases) is a dendritic cell–related histiocytic disorder. JXG most commonly affects infants and young children and presents as a solitary or a few "fleshy nodules." These red-yellowish, benign-appearing lesions are sometimes mistaken for molluscum. However, when biopsied, these lesions reveal a distinctive pathology (see Fig. 50-6). Multinucleated, Touton giant cells are usually found, and lesional histiocytes are positive for CD14, CD68, CD163, factor XIIIa, and fascin, suggesting that they are dermal dendrocytes. The cells are usually negative for CD1a, S100, and the plasmacytoid monocyte antigen CD123.

Juvenile xanthogranuloma most commonly presents as a single skin lesion in infants and young children. The lesions are nodular and usually yellowish to reddish purple. Lesions may vary significantly in size and number but often are several millimeters to 1 cm in size and solitary. However, in some patients, the lesions become widespread and quite disfiguring (Fig. 50-7). Furthermore, JXG may

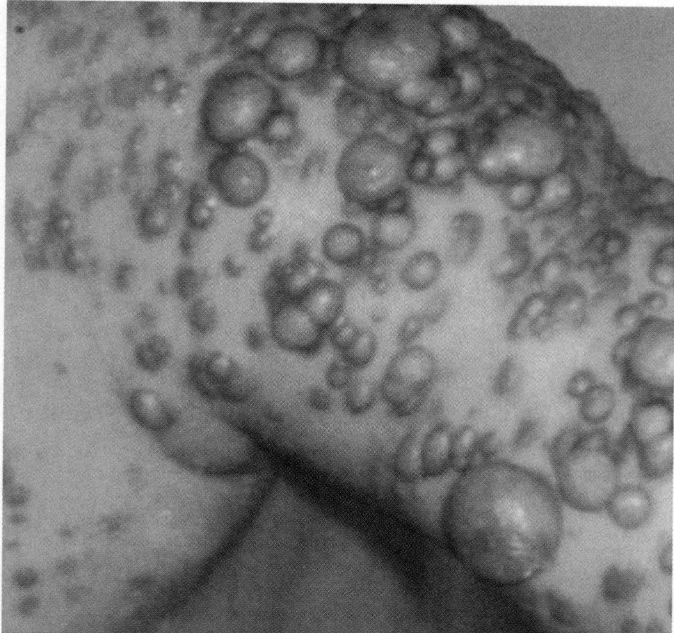

Figure 50-7 EXTENSIVE JUVENILE XANTHOGRANULOMATOUS DISEASE IN AN INFANT.

become systemic, involving multiple organs, including the liver, lungs, heart, and CNS. CNS involvement can present with seizures, hemiplegia, and increased intracranial pressure. Patients diagnosed with JXG, particularly multifocal JXG, may benefit from screening CT scans to rule out disseminated involvement, particularly if clinical history suggests this. However, regardless of clinical symptoms, all patients with JXG should have ophthalmologic examination to rule out anterior chamber involvement and prevent potentially blinding complications.

Cutaneous JXG lesions usually resolve over several months and require no treatment. Of note, residual pigmented areas may persist indefinitely even after lesions have regressed. In patients in whom JXG becomes systemic and involves multiple organs, systemic chemotherapy similar to that for patients with LCH has been used. In patients who do not respond to initial treatment with vinblastine and steroids, use of other agents, such as methotrexate, steroids, and 2-CdA, has led to responses, according to anecdotal reports.

ERDHEIM-CHESTER DISEASE

Erdheim-Chester disease is a rare, non-Langerhans form of histiocytosis first described in 1930 with a wide range of manifestations. The number of new cases has dramatically increased over the past 10 years because of the better recognition of this condition. The natural evolution is variable, but the prognosis in the absence of effective therapy is poor.

Erdheim-Chester disease is seen most commonly in patients 50 years or older. It usually presents with xanthoma-like skin nodules and bilateral lower limb bone pain. Patients with more disseminated disease may have cardiopulmonary insufficiency; renal failure caused by characteristic retroperitoneal and perinephric infiltrative or constrictive changes; and CNS involvement manifested by ataxia, DI, and altered mental status. They may also have periorbital involvement with exophthalmos and impingement on the optic nerves. The disease may be progressive and fatal. The pathophysiology of ECD remains a mystery, although a plasma cytokine profile consisting of elevated interferon-α (IFN-α), interleukin-12 (IL-12), monocyte chemotactic protein-1 (MCP-1), IL-4, and IL-7 in these patients suggests a systemic immune perturbation.

Table 50-4 Diagnostic Criteria for Hemophagocytic Lymphohistiocytosis, Established for the Conduct of the Hemophagocytic Lymphohistiocytosis-2004 Trial

The diagnosis of HLH may be established by:*

A. A molecular diagnosis consistent with HLH: Pathologic mutations of *PRF1, UNC13D, Munc18-2, Rab27a, STX11, SH2D1A,* or *BIRC4*
or

B. Five of the eight criteria listed below are fulfilled:
1. Fever ≥38.3° C
2. Splenomegaly
3. Cytopenias (affecting at least two of three lineages in the peripheral blood)
4. Hemoglobin <9 g/dL (in infants <4 weeks: hemoglobin <10 g/dL)
Platelets <100 × 10^3/mL
Neutrophils <1 × 10^3/mL
5. Hypertriglyceridemia (fasting >265 mg/dL) or hypofibrinogenemia (<150 mg/dL)
6. Hemophagocytosis in BM, spleen, lymph nodes, or liver
7. Low or absent NK cell activity
8. Ferritin >500 ng/mL
9. Elevated soluble CD25 (soluble IL-2 receptor α)

BM, Bone marrow; *HLH,* hemophagocytic lymphohistiocytosis; *IL-2,* interleukin-2; *NK,* natural killer.
*Additionally, in the case of familial HLH, no evidence of malignancy should be apparent.

First-line treatment for ECD consists of IFN-α. Other effective treatments have been limited, although responses have been observed with steroids, vinblastine plus steroids, methotrexate, 2-CdA, and bisphosphonates, in addition to IFN-α. Autologous hematopoietic BMT has been reported as a therapeutic modality.

HEMOPHAGOCYTIC LYMPHOHISTIOCYTOSIS

In the broad classification of histiocytic disorders (see Table 50-1), HLH is categorized as a monocyte/macrophage–related histiocytic disorder. HLH derives its name from its sometimes distinctive pathology (hemophagocytosis) in which macrophages appear to be widely infiltrating tissues and engulfing blood and BM cells in a nonspecific fashion. However, HLH is best conceptualized as an immune regulatory disorder, which is characterized by clinical signs and symptoms of extreme inflammation and the development of cytopenias, hepatitis, and CNS dysfunction which are severe and life threatening.

Hemophagocytic lymphohistiocytosis was first described as a familial disease by Farquhar and Claireux in 1952, which they named *familial haemophagocytic reticulosis*. Through the years, the syndrome of HLH has been recognized as both a sporadic and familial disorder and in various clinical contexts. Although we prefer to lump each of these clinical variations into a single syndrome (HLH), the medical literature has used a plethora of names: familial erythrophagocytic lymphohistiocytosis (FEL), viral-associated hemophagocytic syndrome (VAHS), and malignancy-associated hemophagocytic syndrome (MAHS), among others. Furthermore, macrophage activation syndrome (MAS), the systemic inflammatory syndrome observed in association with rheumatologic disorders, is likely a variant of the HLH syndrome because both "classic" HLH and MAS have similar clinical phenotypes and appear to share some underlying mechanisms. The International Histiocyte Society formally adopted the name of HLH in 1998 and defined criteria for its diagnosis, which were updated in 2004 (Table 50-4).

Epidemiology

The true incidence and prevalence of HLH are unknown and remain difficult to ascertain accurately. The diagnosis of HLH is challenging because of its variable presentation and the many nonspecific clinical features it shares with other disease processes. HLH is considered to be rare, but increasing awareness and recognition of the syndrome is leading to more frequent diagnoses. Currently, it is estimated that the autosomal recessive forms of familial HLH have a prevalence of one in 50,000 live births. A recent report estimated the incidence of HLH in tertiary care pediatric hospitals at one case of HLH per 3000 inpatient admissions. Because of the typically autosomal recessive nature of familial HLH, this disorder is reported to occur more frequently in isolated populations or kindreds with consanguinity.

Pathobiology

The immunologic basis of HLH was long suspected because of its inflammatory nature and the finding of cytotoxic deficiencies and other immune abnormalities in patients with HLH. The first confirmation that HLH is an immunodeficiency came in 1999 with the discovery of perforin mutations in affected patients. However, unlike other immunodeficiencies, the principal clinical characteristic of HLH is one of intense, prolonged, systemic inflammation rather than unusual or severe infections. Although this inflammation may be triggered by infection or vaccination, the inflammation itself (and not apparently the sometimes benign or transient infection) appears to drive the clinical features of HLH. Thus familial HLH appears to be a deficiency of immune regulation. Animal studies have begun to detail how this immune regulation functions and how deficiencies may lead to HLH. In brief, cytotoxic lymphocytes kill not only infected cells but also antigen-presenting cells (APCs). These APCs promote T-cell activation during infection. This persistence of activating signals leads to excessive or prolonged acute T-cell activation. Abnormal T-cell activation, in turn, leads to activation of macrophages and the development of disease pathology. In animal models, INF-γ appears to be the critical nexus between T-cell activation and disease development. In several published series, INF-γ appears to be elevated in patients with HLH. However, clinical data appear mixed, and it remains uncertain whether INF-γ is critical for HLH development in all patients. An underlying lesion of immune regulation and the associated pathophysiology is less clear in apparently sporadic cases of HLH, sometimes referred to as *secondary HLH*. However, the traditional dichotomy between primary (familial) HLH and secondary HLH (associated with infections, malignancy, or autoimmunity) is becoming increasingly murky.

Hemophagocytic lymphohistiocytosis may present in a variety of clinical contexts and with a variety of etiologic associations. Patients are often categorized as having either "primary" or "secondary" HLH. Patients in the primary HLH category are those with clear familial inheritance or genetic causes, are usually infants or younger children, and are thought to have fixed defects of cytotoxic function (although this is not always the case). These patients have a clear risk of HLH recurrence and will not survive long term without hematopoietic cell transplantation (HCT). Although HLH in these patients can be associated with infections (e.g., cytomegalovirus [CMV] or Epstein-Barr virus [EBV]) or vaccination, the immunologic trigger is often not apparent. The term *secondary HLH* generally refers to older children (or adults) who present without a family history or known genetic cause for their HLH. These patients typically have concurrent infections or medical conditions that appear to trigger their HLH, such as EBV infection, malignancy, or rheumatologic disorders. The list of triggering stimuli for both familial and apparently nonfamilial HLH is extensive. Patients with presumed secondary HLH are sometimes reported as having immune studies that normalize with disease resolution, although in the authors' experience, this is variable or unclear. Although the mortality rate from HLH may be significant, the risk of recurrence in cases of secondary HLH is poorly defined. Recurrence of HLH in the absence of autoimmune disease or malignancy is generally considered to be good evidence that a patient has primary HLH, regardless of the other clinical features. Absent a known genetic defect or family history, it is often not possible to make an initial diagnosis of "primary" or "secondary" HLH. Further obscuring this dichotomy, a recent report by Zhang et al described a large series of adults with HLH who were found to have genetic mutations typically seen in children with familial HLH.

A variety of genetic causes of familial HLH have been identified, all either autosomal recessive or X-linked (Table 50-5). Most of these genetic lesions affect a biologic pathway referred to as *granule-dependent,* or *perforin-dependent, cytotoxicity* (Fig. 50-8). This pathway is used by T cells and NK cells to kill target cells, typically those infected by viruses. When triggered, specialized lysosomal granules containing perforin, granzymes, and other proteins are released, leading to apoptotic death of target cells. The first genetic lesions

Table 50-5 Hemophagocytic Lymphohistiocytosis–Associated Gene Mutations

Gene	Location	Disease
PRF1	10q21-22	FHL2
UNC13D	17q25	FHL3
STX11	6q24	FHL4
RAB27A	15q21	Griscelli syndrome
STXBP2	19p13	FHL5
Unknown	9q21.3-22	FHL1
SH2D1A	Xq24-26	XLP1
XIAP	Xq25	XLP2/X-linked HLH

FHL, Familial hemophagocytic lymphohistiocytosis; *XLP,* X-linked lymphoproliferative syndrome.

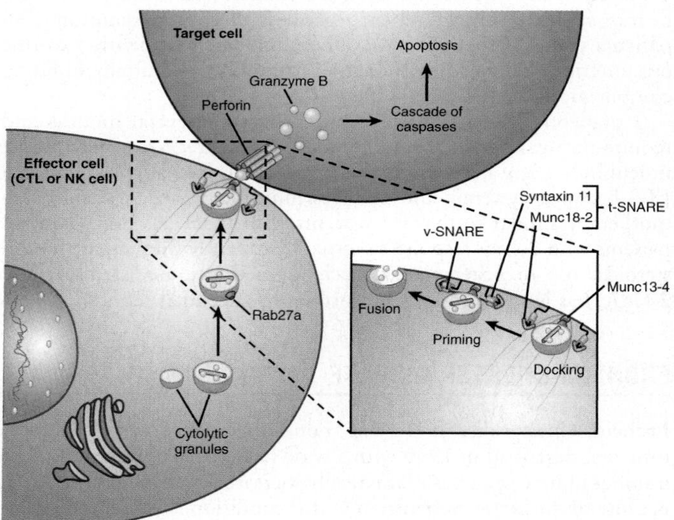

Figure 50-8 MECHANICS OF CYTOTOXIC FUNCTION REVEALED BY HEMOPHAGOCYTIC LYMPHOHISTIOCYTOSIS (HLH)–ASSOCIATED GENE MUTATIONS. HLH-associated genetic abnormalities (in the indicated genes) may affect granule-dependent lymphocyte cytotoxicity by impairing trafficking, docking, priming for exocytosis, or membrane fusion of cytolytic granules. The function of this pathway may also be severely impaired by loss of functional perforin, the key delivery molecule for proapoptotic granzymes. Diverse mutations in this pathway all give rise to similar clinical phenotypes (albeit of variable severity). Lyst (the gene affected in Chédiak-Higashi syndrome) is not portrayed because its function is not entirely clear, although it appears to play an important role in the maintenance of normally-sized (and functional) cytolytic granules. *(Adapted from Jordan MB, Allen CE, Weitzman S, Filipovich AH, McClain KL: How I treat hemophagocytic lymphohistiocytosis.* Blood *118:4041, 2011.)*

identified in patients with HLH were mutations in *prf1*, the gene encoding the protein perforin. *Prf1* mutations account for about 15% to 20% of HLH in certain geographic areas and are known as familial HLH 2 (FHL2). FHL2 has mild and severe phenotypes that correlate with the degree of mature perforin protein that is produced. Abnormalities of granule formation, mobilization, and extrusion are also identified as causes of HLH. MUNC 13-4, a protein essential to the exocytotic process, is mutated in FHL3. FHL3 has a worldwide distribution and accounts for 15% to 20% of all hereditable HLH. However, recent discoveries of previously unappreciated intronic mutations in this gene may expand the proportion of patients with FHL3. FHL4 is caused by mutations in the protein syntaxin 11, a member of the SNARE (soluble N-ethylmaleimide-sensitive fusion attachment receptor protein) family of proteins, which is necessary for the fusion of cytotoxic vesicles with the plasma membrane to release their granules. Mutations in the syntaxin-binding protein 2, also important for this process, have been designated FHL5. The genetic defect responsible for FHL1 has not been identified, and no mutations in granzyme proteins have been associated with HLH.

Two X-linked causes of HLH are known. The first, called X-linked lymphoproliferative syndrome 1 (or XLP1), is caused by defects in SH2D1A or SAP. This disorder is a complex one characterized by lymphoproliferation, hypogammaglobulinemia, excess risk of lymphoma, and development of HLH. It appears to share some of the pathophysiology with classic familial HLH, although other abnormalities (of B cells and other cells) make this disorder distinctive. The second X-linked cause of HLH, sometimes called XLP2 (although this is disputed), are abnormalities of a gene/protein called BIRC4 (baculoviral inhibitor of apoptosis protein repeat-containing protein 4)/XIAP (X-linked inhibitor of apoptosis protein). The apparently unique pathophysiology of HLH caused by XIAP deficiency is not understood. Other immunodeficiency syndromes caused by defects in lysosomal trafficking have been linked to life-threatening episodes of HLH. These include Chédiak-Higashi syndrome; Griscelli syndrome; and Hermansky-Pudlak syndrome, type II.

Taken together, the nine genetic disorders described above still account for fewer than half of the diagnosed cases of HLH in children, including many familial cases still awaiting molecular definition. Until recently, it was widely believed that symptoms of HLH caused by genetic causes arose during infancy and early childhood. With the more widespread availability of genetic testing, it is apparent that the first significant episode of HLH can occur throughout life from prenatal presentations through the seventh decade of life. Distinctions between primary (genetically determined) and secondary (acquired) forms of HLH become increasingly blurred together as new genetic causes are identified and patients who develop HLH beyond early childhood or in the contexts of EBV infection or autoimmune disease are being found to share some of the same genetic etiologies.

Clinical Manifestations

The classic presentation of HLH consists of prolonged, hectic fevers (usually present for 1-2 weeks before diagnosis), hepatosplenomegaly, and cytopenias. Neurologic symptoms are common and distinctive features of these patients; these include symptoms of irritability, ataxia, hypo- or hypertonia, evidence of increased intracranial pressure, meningismus, depressed mental status, cranial nerve palsies, and seizures. Standard diagnostic criteria have been defined by the Histiocyte Society for the conduct of the now closed HLH2004 trial (see Table 50-4). Although imperfect, these criteria are widely accepted for the diagnosis of HLH. However, because HLH is a clinical syndrome, it may present in many forms, including fever of unknown origin (FUO); hepatitis or acute liver failure; and sepsis-like, Kawasaki-like, and primary neurologic abnormalities. Not all of the HLH diagnostic criteria may be present initially, so it is important to follow clinical signs and laboratory markers of pathologic inflammation repeatedly to identify the trends. Typical clinical features seen in patients with HLH, grouped by organ system, are described below.

Prolonged Fever

Fever of unknown origin is a very common diagnosis on general pediatric wards, and differentiating HLH from other causes of FUO may be challenging. In one series, patients ultimately diagnosed with HLH presented with fevers above 102° F for a median of 19 days (range, 4-41 days). In patients with FUO, cytopenias, highly elevated ferritin (>3000 g/dL), or sCD25 significantly above age-adjusted normal ranges generally suggest that a complete HLH diagnostic evaluation should be pursued.

Liver Disease and Coagulopathy

Most patients with HLH have variable evidence of hepatitis at presentation. HLH should be considered in the differential diagnosis of acute liver failure, especially if lymphocytic infiltrates are noted on biopsy. Autopsy evaluation of the liver has shown chronic persistent hepatitis with periportal lymphocytic infiltration in the majority of patients. Neonates with HLH may present with hydrops fetalis and liver failure. Most patients have evidence of disseminated intravascular coagulation (DIC) and are at high risk for acute bleeding. Furthermore, patients with HLH caused by degranulation defects may have intrinsic platelet dysfunction.

Bone Marrow Failure

Anemia and thrombocytopenia occur in more than 80% of patients at the time of presentation with HLH. The cellularity of BM aspirates varies from normocellular to hypo- or hypercellular. The prevalence of hemophagocytosis in association with HLH diagnosis ranges from 25% to 100%. Although hemophagocytosis in BM is associated with HLH, the morphologic phenomenon may also be induced by more common events, including blood transfusions, infection, autoimmune disease, and other forms of BM failure or causes of red blood cell destruction. Despite the nomenclature of HLH, diagnosis of HLH should never be made or excluded solely on the presence or absence of hemophagocytosis. Infiltration of BM or liver by CD^{163+} macrophages, along with global clinical evaluation, may distinguish HLH from other causes of hemophagocytosis.

Skin Manifestations

Patients may have a variety of skin manifestations, including generalized maculopapular erythematous rashes, generalized erythroderma, edema, panniculitis, inflamed papular lesions, petechiae, and purpura. The incidence of skin manifestations ranges from 6% to 65% in published series with highly pleomorphic presentations. Some patients may present with features suggestive of Kawasaki disease, including erythematous rashes, conjunctivitis, red lips, and enlarged cervical lymph nodes. Rashes may correlate with lymphocyte infiltration on skin biopsy, and hemophagocytosis may also be found.

Pulmonary Dysfunction

Patients may develop pulmonary dysfunction that leads to urgent admission to the intensive care unit. In a review of the radiographic abnormalities in 25 patients, 17 had acute respiratory failure with alveolar or interstitial opacities, with fatal outcomes in 88% of those cases.

Brain, Ophthalmic, and Neuromuscular Symptoms

More than one-third of patients present with neurologic symptoms, including seizures, meningismus, decreased level of consciousness, cranial nerve palsy, psychomotor retardation, ataxia, irritability, or hypotonia. The cerebrospinal fluid (CSF) is abnormal in more than 50% of HLH patients with findings of pleocytosis, elevated protein, or hemophagocytosis. MRI findings are highly variable and include discrete lesions, leptomeningeal enhancement, or global edema, and images correlate with neurologic symptoms. Retinal hemorrhages, swelling of the optic nerve, and infiltration of the choroid have been reported in infants with HLH. Diffuse peripheral neuropathy with pain and weakness secondary to myelin destruction by macrophages may also occur.

Laboratory Manifestations

Laboratory manifestations are a critical component of diagnosing HLH. Biochemical abnormalities noted on clinical laboratory assessment include anemia, thrombocytopenia, neutropenia, elevated liver transaminases, hyperbilirubinemia, hypofibrinogenemia, coagulation abnormalities, hypoalbuminemia, hyponatremia, hypertriglyceridemia, elevated soluble CD163, elevated soluble CD25 (sCD25, also called soluble IL-2 receptor), and hyperferritinemia. Specialized immunologic testing may reveal low or absent NK cell or CTL function (although this is not always seen), low levels of perforin or other disease-associated proteins (e.g., SAP or XIAP), and decreased degranulation (observed with mutations affecting granule trafficking). Additionally, pathologic examination of BM biopsy, liver biopsy, CSF, spleen or lymph node, or even occasionally peripheral blood may reveal hemophagocytosis and infiltration with CD^{163+} macrophages and activated T cells (Fig. 50-9). Examination of CSF reveals pleocytosis, elevated protein, and elevated neopterin levels with CNS involvement. Brain MRI often reveals polymorphic white or grey matter abnormalities in such cases.

Elevations in sCD25 are a particularly useful and notable laboratory feature of HLH. In the authors' experience, this marker is dynamically associated with "active" HLH, and patients with active HLH rarely, if ever, have normal levels of sCD25. Of note, the interpretation of soluble IL-2 receptor levels must be undertaken with care because normal levels change with age and the method of analysis. Despite a few small reports of increased soluble IL-2 receptor levels in sepsis, significant elevations of this marker are rarely observed outside the context of HLH. However, the clinical utility of sCD25 is often compromised by delays because most institutions must send patient samples to referral laboratories. Because of its ready availability in most hospitals, the serum ferritin level can serve as an important adjunct to the decision-making process. The HLH diagnostic guidelines define a cutoff at greater than 500 µg/L, which may be observed in sepsis or other hyperinflammatory conditions. Ferritin levels in HLH are usually dramatically higher, with some series finding mean levels near 45,000 µg/L. A recent review of elevated ferritin values at a large pediatric academic tertiary care hospital demonstrated that a ferritin level greater than 10,000 was 90% sensitive and 96% specific for HLH.

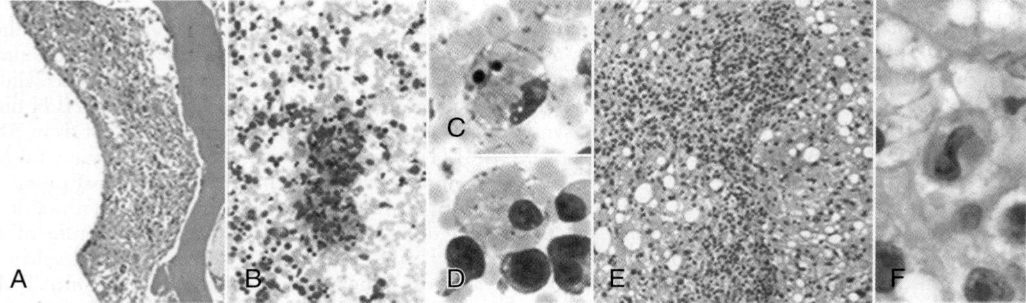

Figure 50-9 A to **F**, FAMILIAL HEMOPHAGOCYTIC LYMPHOHISTIOCYTOSIS. Illustrations from a 3-month-old girl who presented with diarrhea, pancytopenia, hepatomegaly, and liver failure. Bone marrow (**A** and **B**) showed left-shifted granulopoiesis and increased histiocytes, which at high power (**C** and **D**) were undergoing prominent phagocytosis of erythrocytes, platelets, and other cells. Liver biopsy sample **(E)** showed a lymphohistiocytic infiltrate also associated with hemophagocytosis **(F).** The patient was shown to harbor a mutation of the perforin gene in exon 2.

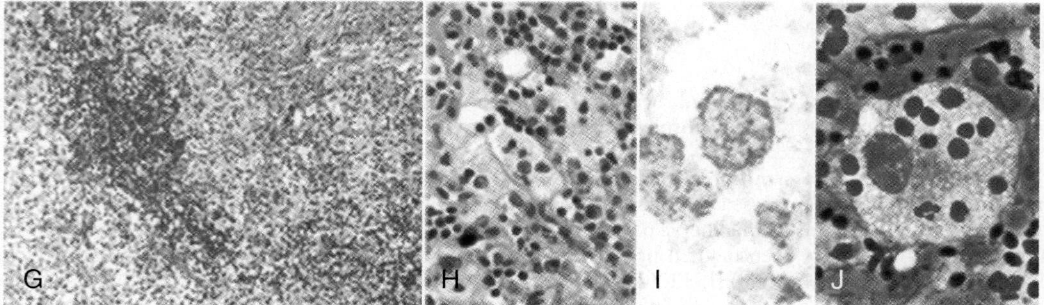

Figure 50-9, cont'd G to **J**, SINUS HISTIOCYTOSIS WITH MASSIVE LYMPHADENOPATHY (ROSAI-DORFMAN DISEASE). Low-power magnification of the biopsy sample **(G)** shows a mottled appearance of the lesion caused by dark areas containing small lymphocytes and lighter areas containing histiocytes. At higher magnification **(H),** the histiocytes have abundant pale cytoplasm with scattered cells within. This is emperipolesis, a process of cells traveling through the cytoplasm but not apparently becoming phagocytized or degraded. Note the plasma cells in the background. The emperipolesis can be better visualized with a CD68 stain for histiocytes **(I).** This process delineates the cell boundary and the cells within the histiocyte cytoplasm. The emperipolesis can also be seen on a Wright-stained touch preparation **(J).**

Differential Diagnosis of Hemophagocytic Lymphohistiocytosis

Because HLH presents as an inflammatory syndrome, the differential diagnosis of this disorder is a broad one. Infection must be considered as either a mimic of HLH or as an underlying trigger of the disorder. The list of infections reported as associated with HLH is extensive. If the patient presents with acute multiorgan failure, then sepsis is generally considered first before a diagnosis of HLH is considered. Viral infections, including EBV, CMV, dengue, severe influenza, and so on, should always be considered and treated. Protozoan infections, including malaria, toxoplasmosis, and leishmaniasis, may be a consideration in endemic areas. Visceral leishmaniasis, in particular, may be clinically indistinguishable from primary HLH. In addition to infectious disorders, rheumatologic disorders, including systemic onset juvenile idiopathic arthritis (soJIA) and Kawasaki syndrome, should be considered. Finally, as either a mimic or trigger, malignancy should be considered, particularly lymphoma and leukemia.

Diagnosis

Because of the severe nature of this disorder and the existence of disease-altering therapies, it is crucial to identify patients early in their course. The Histiocyte Society established diagnostic criteria for the HLH-2004 trial, which is widely used for patients not treated on this trial, using both clinical and laboratory findings (see Table 50-4). Laboratory verification of a known genetic defect confirms the diagnosis independent of the presence or absence of any clinical signs or symptoms. However, genetic diagnosis is not usually available in a timely fashion for patients with acute clinical presentations. In the absence of a genetic diagnosis, five of the eight clinical criteria must be met to make a diagnosis. It is important to note that NK cell dysfunction is only present in about 50% of patients with HLH. Additionally, hemophagocytosis may not be present early in the HLH disease process; therefore, serial assessments may be required if that diagnostic criterion is to be met.

Therapy

Without therapy, survival of patients with active familial HLH is historically reported to be approximately 2 months. The first international treatment protocol for HLH was organized by the Histiocyte Society in 1994 and led to reported survival of 55%, with a median follow-up of 3.1 years. The HLH-94 protocol, as illustrated in Fig. 50-10, included an 8-week induction therapy with dexamethasone, etoposide, and intrathecal methotrexate. The principal goal of induction therapy is to suppress the life-threatening inflammatory process that underlies HLH. At the end of 8 weeks, patients are either weaned off of therapy or transitioned to continuation therapy, which is intended only as a bridge to transplantation.

The Histiocyte Society opened a new trial in 2004, HLH-2004, which is now closed. The major modifications from HLH-94 were to move cyclosporine dosing to the beginning of induction and add hydrocortisone to intrathecal therapy. Results of this trial are not reported at this time. An alternative approach to etoposide-based regimens with comparable survival was published as a single center retrospective experience over 14 years in which all patients were treated with corticosteroids and antithymocyte globulin (ATG) followed (rapidly) by HCT. Until this immunotherapy approach can be compared with etoposide–dexamethasone in the setting of a clinical trial and until the results of the HLH-2004 study are published, the standard of care therapy for patients not enrolled in a clinical trial should be based on HLH-94.

Often, the principal challenge for treating patients with HLH is making a timely and accurate diagnosis. It is critical to search for and treat underlying triggers of HLH and institute specific antimicrobial therapy. Rituximab is often helpful in controlling EBV infection. IVIG is an appropriate adjunct for most viral infections. If the patient is stable and not severely ill, consideration can be given to treating the underlying trigger with disease-specific therapy with or without corticosteroids and close follow-up. However, in most cases, an aggressive therapeutic approach is warranted and may reasonably be initiated before obtaining final results for all diagnostic studies. Specifically, HLH therapy should not be withheld while awaiting results of genetic testing because our understanding of HLH-associated gene defects remains incomplete and testing typically takes weeks to complete. With the exception of autoimmune disease and malignancy, initial therapy for patients with suspected familial or reactive HLH does not differ.

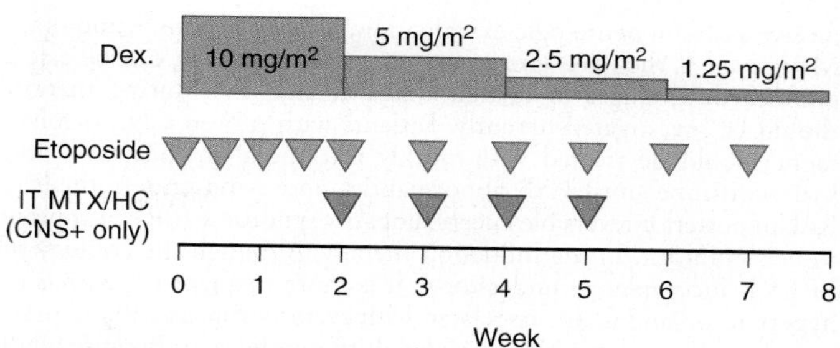

Figure 50-10 INDUCTION THERAPY FOR HEMOPHAGOCYTIC LYMPHOHISTIOCYTOSIS (HLH). Based on the HLH-94 study, this approach should be considered standard of care for all patients not enrolled in clinical trials based on published evidence of efficacy. Etoposide is dosed as 150 mg/m^2 per dose. Alternatively, for patients weighing less than 10 kg, consideration may be given to dosing etoposide as 5 mg/kg per dose. Dexamethasone (Dex.) is dosed as indicated and may be given orally or intravenously, although the latter is preferred at therapy initiation. Intrathecal methotrexate and hydrocortisone (IT MTX/HC) should be given to patients with evidence of central nervous system (CNS) involvement as early as lumbar puncutre (LP) may be safely performed (which may vary from the diagram) and dosed as follows: age younger than 1 year, 6/8 mg (MTX/HC); age 1 to 2 years, 8/10 mg; age 2 to 3 years, 10/12 mg; and age older than 3 years, 12/15 mg. Weekly intrathecal therapy is generally continued until at least 1 week after resolution of CNS involvement (both clinical and cerebrospinal fluid indices). *(Adapted from Jordan MB, Allen CE, Weitzman S, Filipovich AH, McClain KL: How I treat hemophagocytic lymphohistiocytosis.* Blood *118:4041, 2011.)*

Induction Therapy

The current standard of care consists of a decrescendo course of etoposide and dexamethasone with or without intrathecal therapy (see Fig. 50-10). Ideally, critically ill patients should be treated at facilities familiar with care of cancer and BMT patients. It is important to initiate therapy promptly even in the face of unresolved infections, cytopenias, or organ dysfunction. After starting therapy, patients should be monitored closely for signs of improvement as well as potential complications and toxicities, and therapy may need to be customized. For patients who respond well, with resolution of symptoms and normalization of inflammatory markers, therapy may be weaned per protocol. However, dexamethasone doses and etoposide frequency may need to be increased in response to disease reactivation (see Salvage Therapy below). Deterioration of liver function and blood counts as well as steady increases in serum ferritin, sCD25, and sCD163 tests may signal relapse of HLH disease activity. If patients do not display at least a partial response within 2 to 3 weeks of therapy initiation, salvage therapy should be considered. Recurrence of fever and increased inflammatory markers after an apparent response should also prompt a careful search for opportunistic infection.

Central Nervous System Disease

Patients may present with CNS involvement or may have recurrent disease as treatment doses are being tapered. All patients should receive a careful neurologic examination, lumbar puncture, and brain MRI, even if they are asymptomatic, as soon as they can be safely performed. Changes in mental status at any time during therapy should be investigated urgently. Patients with proven CNS involvement should be treated with weekly intrathecal methotrexate and hydrocortisone until CSF abnormalities and symptoms normalize. Risk of posterior reversible encephalopathy syndrome (PRES) appears to be significant during induction therapy. Although the etiology of PRES is incompletely understood, it is more frequent in settings of hypertension and is also associated with cyclosporine use. Blood pressure should be aggressively managed during induction. Because CNS involvement suggests a familial etiology and because this disease feature is associated with substantial risks for long-term morbidity, HCT should be considered for patients with this complication.

Supportive Care

Supportive care guidelines for patients on therapy for HLH should be similar to standard practice for patients undergoing HCT, including acute care nursing, *Pneumocystis jiroveci* prophylaxis, fungal prophylaxis, IVIG supplementation, and neutropenic precautions. Any new fever should be evaluated for HLH reactivation, as well as opportunistic infection, and empiric broad-spectrum antibiotic therapy should be initiated. Because of inflammation, consumptive coagulopathy, and intrinsic platelet defects in some patients, they are at very high risk of spontaneous bleeding. The authors aim to maintain platelet count greater than 50×10^9/L and do not recommend prophylactic heparin, which is sometimes used in acutely ill patients. Platelets, fresh-frozen plasma, cryoprecipitate, and occasionally activated factor VII are required for acute bleeding.

Continuation Therapy

Patients who can be weaned off of dexamethasone and etoposide without recurrence, recover normal immune function, and have no identified HLH-associated gene defects may stop therapy after the 8-week induction course. HCT is generally recommended in patients with age younger than 2 years, CNS involvement, recurrent or refractory disease, persistent NK cell dysfunction, or proven familial or genetic disease. Continuation according to HLH-94 consists of pulses of dexamethasone and etoposide (etoposide, 150 mg/m^2 every 2 weeks alternating with dexamethasone 10 mg/m^2/day for 3 days every 2 weeks). Cyclosporine may be added in patients with stable blood pressure and adequate liver and kidney function. Patients on continuation therapy should proceed to HCT as quickly as possible because of the ongoing risks of infection, disease reactivation, or leukemia or myelodysplastic syndrome related to prolonged use of etoposide.

Salvage Therapy

A significant number of patients with HLH either fail to respond adequately to current therapies or relapse before HCT. Approximately 50% of patients treated in the HLH-94 study experienced a complete resolution of HLH, 30% experienced a partial resolution, and approximately 20% died before HCT. Notably, most deaths occurred during the first few weeks of treatment and may reflect either preexisting morbidities or primary refractory disease. Although it is hoped that some patients will fare better with more prompt diagnosis of HLH, others remain unresponsive to standard therapy. Initial treatment with ATG (thymoglobulin, rabbit ATG) has been reported to give higher complete response rates, but partly because of higher relapse rates, long-term outcomes do not appear superior. Although current therapy is effective, there is a need for new treatments for patients with refractory HLH. At present, there are few data regarding potential second-line therapies. Case reports exist describing the use of infliximab, daclizumab, alemtuzumab, anakinra, vincristine, and other agents as salvage therapies for HLH. A recent report found that alemtuzumab has significant activity against refractory HLH in a larger series of patients. Although refractory HLH appears to have a dismal prognosis, approximately 70% of patients in this series survived. Because of its immunoablative qualities, alemtuzumab should be used with caution and by those with experience caring for profoundly immune compromised patients. CMV reactivation and adenoviremia were frequent complications of this therapy. In contrast to refractory patients, those patients who initially respond well to standard therapy but then relapse as treatment is tapered or withdrawn often respond to reintensification of therapy with standard agents. Because of the variability in patient responses, a critical aspect of initial or salvage therapy is close monitoring of the patients for improvement and potential toxicities such as BM suppression or infection.

Hematopoietic Cell Transplantation

Because the time to transplant is a factor in morbidity and mortality from the disease, a donor search should begin at the time of diagnosis even though the precise etiology of HLH (e.g., genetic defect) has not yet been defined. Generally, HCT is recommended in cases of documented familial HLH, recurrent or progressive disease despite intensive therapy, and CNS involvement. Long-term disease-free survival after HCT was approximately 50% to 65% before 2000, regardless of whether a matched sibling or closely matched unrelated donor was used. Most patients transplanted during that era succumbed to "transplant-related" complications during the first 100 days after infusion. A significant proportion of fatal complications involved inflammatory conditions termed acute respiratory distress syndrome, veno occlusive disease (VOD), and multisystem organ failure, unspecified. In rare cases, residual HLH was identified at autopsy despite the use of myeloablative conditioning therapy.

During the past decade, the use of reduced-intensity conditioning (RIC) regimens before HCT has been investigated after encouraging results from an institutional series. Most cases of RIC pretreatment have included alemtuzumab and demonstrated superior early posttransplant survival. In a single-center analysis directly comparing HCT outcomes after myeloablative conditioning versus RIC, a statistically significant improvement was observed after RIC conditioning, with all patients surviving at 6 months after transplant. At present, published data regarding outcome of RIC transplants using umbilical cord blood is not sufficient to draw conclusions regarding safety or efficacy. Donor choice should also take into account the possibility of an occult predisposition to HLH in siblings of patients without identified gene defects. Much remains to be learned and refined regarding the optimal application of alemtuzumab as well as other agents used before HCT. The timing of pretransplant alemtuzumab impacts the probability of graft-versus-host disease; mixed chimerism; and in rare cases, rejection. Other factors, such as donor source, human leukocyte antigen match, cell dose, and patient condition with regard to HLH disease activity at time of conditioning, may all play roles in determining the likelihood of success after RIC HCT.

Patients with CNS HLH need close posttransplant follow-up. The authors recommend examination of CSF within 100 days of HCT even in asymptomatic patients. Follow-up MRIs are recommended if pretransplant abnormalities were present. In some patients with mixed or full hematopoietic donor chimerism, HLH disease activity in the CSF can be effectively treated with intrathecal therapy during the early posttransplant months. CNS disease is subsequently controlled as donor immune reconstitution progresses.

Prognosis

Significant strides have been made in the treatment of HLH with survival now generally ranging from 50% to 70%. In children with nonfamilial HLH, overall survival has been reported at 72%, but only

20% of the patients did not require HCT. Survival is increased in children, irrespective of genetic status, who receive HSCT from matched rather than unmatched donors. RIC pretransplant regimens appear to further decrease mortality. The best outcomes in HSCT are seen in children who have a rapid and complete response to pretransplant therapies and who do not exhibit significant neurologic involvement. Prompt initiation of HSCT in familial patients after disease remission is obtained is also likely to increase survival. Patients with significant neurologic involvement may experience severe and permanent sequelae even if they survive.

MACROPHAGE ACTIVATION SYNDROME

Macrophage activation syndrome is the name commonly given to a severe, potentially fatal, inflammatory condition seen in the context of rheumatologic disorders such as soJIA or systemic lupus erythematosus (SLE). The syndrome of MAS shares many similarities with classic HLH, and many investigators view it as a special form of HLH. The main manifestations of MAS include fever, hepatosplenomegaly, lymphadenopathy, severe cytopenias, serious liver disease, and coagulopathy consistent with DIC. Hemophagocytosis is often seen in the BM of patients with MAS. The true incidence of MAS may be underestimated because relatively mild cases of MAS often remained unrecognized. Recent evidence suggests that mild subclinical MAS occurs in as many as one-third of patients with active soJIA and may be the first manifestation of soJIA. Infections or change in medications may precede the diagnosis of MAS; in most patients, MAS is triggered by a flare-up of the underlying rheumatologic disease. Published observations suggest that as in HLH, MAS patients have profoundly depressed NK cell function, sometimes associated with abnormal perforin expression, and these abnormalities are associated with specific perforin and MUNC13-4 polymorphisms.

Diagnosis and Treatment

There are no validated diagnostic criteria for MAS, and early diagnosis is often difficult. Thus, in a patient with persistently active underlying rheumatologic disease, a fall in the erythrocyte sedimentation rate (ESR) and platelet count, particularly in combination with persistently high C-reactive protein and increasing levels of ferritin, should raise a suspicion of impending MAS. The diagnosis of MAS is usually confirmed by the demonstration of hemophagocytosis in the BM. Assessment of the levels of sCD25 and sCD163 in serum may help with the timely diagnosis of MAS. Although mild elevation of sCD25 has been reported in many rheumatic diseases, including JIA and SLE, a several-fold increase in the levels of sIL2Rα in these diseases is highly suggestive of MAS. The application of the HLH diagnostic criteria to systemic JIA patients with suspected MAS is problematic. Some of the HLH markers, such as lymphadenopathy, splenomegaly, and hyperferritinemia, are common features of active systemic JIA itself and therefore do not distinguish MAS from a conventional systemic JIA flare. Patients with systemic JIA often have increased white blood cell and platelet counts as well as serum levels of fibrinogen as a part of the inflammatory response seen in this disease. Therefore, when they develop MAS, they reach the degree of cytopenias and hypofibrinogenemia seen in HLH only at the late stages of the syndrome when medical management becomes challenging. This is even more problematic for the diagnosis of MAS in patients with SLE in whom autoimmune cytopenias are common and difficult to distinguish from those caused by MAS.

Early recognition of this syndrome and immediate therapeutic intervention to produce a rapid response are critical. Prompt administration of more aggressive treatment in these patients may, in fact, prevent development of the full-blown syndrome. To achieve rapid reversal of coagulation abnormalities and cytopenias, most clinicians start with intravenous methylprednisolone pulse therapy (30 mg/kg for 3 consecutive days) followed by 2 to 3 mg/kg/day divided in four doses. After normalization of hematologic abnormalities and resolution of coagulopathy, steroids are tapered slowly to avoid relapses of MAS. Commonly, however, MAS appears to be corticosteroid resistant, with deaths being reported even among patients treated with massive doses of steroids. Parenteral administration of cyclosporine A has been shown to be highly effective in patients with corticosteroid-resistant MAS. The utility of biologic drugs in MAS treatment remains unclear. Although tumor necrosis factor–inhibiting agents, biologics that neutralize IL-1 and IL-6, have been reported to be effective in occasional MAS patients, other reports describe patients in whom MAS occurred while they were receiving these agents. Based on some success with IVIG administration in virus-associated HLH, this treatment might be effective in MAS triggered by viral infection. If MAS, however, is driven by EBV infection, rituximab, a monoclonal antibody that depletes B lymphocytes (the main type of cells harboring the EBV virus) may be considered.

Future Directions

As an alternative approach to etoposide-based approaches, ATG–prednisone has been used for a number of years in some centers. These two approaches appear to have unique strengths and weaknesses. Although a significant number of patients fail to respond adequately or completely to etoposide-based regimens, ATG-based regimens are complicated by relatively frequent and early relapse (median time to relapse reported by Ouachee-Chardin et al, 5.5 weeks). Thus a rational combination of these approaches may improve outcomes by increasing initial responses and maintaining them until HCT can be obtained. Currently, a multicenter clinical trial, called *hybrid immunotherapy for HLH* (HIT-HLH) is underway in North America testing the potential of this idea. A sister trial is being conducted in Europe. In this approach, ATG and etoposide are incorporated into one regimen, but the etoposide dose intensity is decreased to minimize potential myelosuppression. No data are available yet regarding the usefulness of this approach. Alternative strategies using anticytokine antibodies for induction therapy are also being developed.

Although HLH appears to be a disease of excessive immune activation, the ideal form of immune suppression and antiinflammatory therapy remains unknown. Although somewhat responsive to corticosteroids and clearly responsive to anti–T-cell serotherapy, such as ATG or alemtuzumab, HLH remains difficult to treat. In the foreseeable future, a variety of new, rationally designed immunosuppressive agents are likely to come into clinical use for transplantation and autoimmune disorders. Future studies will likely focus on defining which sort of immune suppression displays the best balance of safety and efficacy.

SINUS HISTIOCYTOSIS WITH MASSIVE LYMPHADENOPATHY OR ROSAI-DORFMAN DISEASE

First described in 1969, sinus histiocytosis with massive lymphadenopathy, or Rosai-Dorfman disease, is clinically characterized as a benign, frequently chronic, painless massive lymphadenopathy usually involving cervical lymph nodes and, less frequently, axillary, hilar, peritracheal, and inguinal nodes. Extranodal disease is present in approximately 30% of patients. The upper respiratory mucosa is involved in 20% of patients, bone in 25%, and orbit or eyelid in 10%. Occasionally, there is involvement of skin, CNS (meninges), lung, liver, and kidney. Ocular manifestations, such as uveitis, have been observed. Although SHML is a histologically reactive and molecularly polyclonal disorder, significant morbidity and death have been associated with massive tissue invasion of the liver, kidney, lung, brain, and other critical structures. In these instances, the disease may have a rapid downhill course.

Eighty percent of patients are diagnosed in the first or second decade of life; however, the disorder also can affect elderly adults. Typically, patients are of African descent; the incidence of SHML is greatest in Africa and the West Indies. Males and females are equally affected.

Laboratory evaluation frequently reveals an elevated ESR, moderate polyclonal hypergammaglobulinemia, anemia, and granulocytosis. Subtle abnormalities of immune indices may also be seen. Involved lymph nodes (see Fig. 50-9) show marked sinusoidal dilation with proliferation of foamy histiocytes within the sinuses. Eosinophils usually are low in number, but plasma cells are abundant. A characteristic finding, referred to as *emperipolesis,* demonstrates lymphocytes surrounded by the membranes of histiocytes as observed best by electron microscopy. The proliferating histiocytes appear to be macrophages. These large, pale cells show variable expression of S100. They can be distinguished from Langerhans cells found in the lymph nodes of patients with classic LCH by the absence of Birbeck granules, the presence of α1-antichymotrypsin, and the absence of CD1a expression.

The etiology of Rosai-Dorfman disease is unknown, but disordered immune regulation has been proposed as a significant contributor. It was originally thought that Rosai-Dorfman disease represented an unusual response to herpesviruses, but this has not been confirmed. Although patients frequently are febrile, infectious agents are not commonly implicated, and the fever is presumed to be a manifestation of systemic disease.

Disease manifestations can subside over several months to years. Of 215 cases in a patient registry, 21% had complete resolution of disease. However, 14 patients died. Five died of "immunologic" causes, such as severe hemolysis; three died of infections; and six probably died as a direct consequence of disease infiltration. As the disease resolves, extranodal disease regresses before nodal disease. Corticosteroids, vinblastine, and low-dose cyclophosphamide are sometimes effective; however, the results with these agents have been inconsistent. Attempts at treatment should be reserved for special circumstances, such as tracheal or epidural compression or invasion of other vital structures, as well as for significant cosmetic disfigurement. Local excision may be useful in selected patients, although the lesions may reappear.

SUGGESTED READINGS

Allen CE, Li L, Peters TL, et al: Cell-specific gene expression in Langerhans cell histiocytosis lesions reveals a distinct profile compared with epidermal Langerhans cells. *J Immunol* 184:4557, 2010.

Aricò M, Janka G, Fischer A, et al: Hemophagocytic lymphohistiocytosis. Report of 122 children from the International Registry. FHL Study Group of the Histiocyte Society. *Leukemia* 10:197, 1996.

Arnaud L, Gorochov G, Charlotte F, et al: Systemic perturbation of cytokine and chemokine networks in Erdheim-Chester disease: A single-center series of 37 patients. *Blood* 117:2783, 2011.

Badalian-Very G, Vergilio JA, Degar BA, et al: Recurrent BRAF mutations in Langerhans cell histiocytosis. *Blood* 116:1919, 2010.

Côte M, Ménager MM, Burgess A, et al: Munc18-2 deficiency causes familial hemophagocytic lymphohistiocytosis type 5 and impairs cytotoxic granule exocytosis in patient NK cells. *J Clin Invest* 119:3765, 2009.

Fahrner B, Prosch H, Minkov M, et al: Long-term outcome of hypothalamic pituitary tumors in Langerhans cell histiocytosis. *Pediatr Blood Cancer* 58:606, 2012.

Farquhar JW, Claireaux AE: Familial haemophagocytic reticulosis. *Arch Dis Child* 27:519, 1952.

Feldmann J, Callebaut I, Raposo G, et al: Munc13-4 is essential for cytolytic granules fusion and is mutated in a form of familial hemophagocytic lymphohistiocytosis (FHL3). *Cell* 115:461, 2003.

Gadner H, Grois N, Pötschger U, et al: Improved outcome in multisystem Langerhans cell histiocytosis is associated with therapy intensification. *Blood* 111(5):2556, 2008.

Grom, AA, Mellins ED: Macrophage activation syndrome: Advances towards understanding pathogenesis. *Curr Opin Rheumatol* 22:561, 2010.

Grom AA, Villanueva J, Lee S, et al: Natural killer cell dysfunction in patients with systemic-onset juvenile rheumatoid arthritis and macrophage activation syndrome. *J Pediatr* 142:292, 2003.

Haroche J, Arnaud L, Amoura Z: Erdheim-Chester disease. *Curr Opin Rheumatol* 24:53, 2012.

Henter JI, Horne A, Aricó M, et al: HLH-2004: Diagnostic and therapeutic guidelines for hemophagocytic lymphohistiocytosis. *Pediatr Blood Cancer* 48:124, 2007.

Jordan MB, Allen CE, Weitzman S, et al: How I treat hemophagocytic lymphohistiocytosis. *Blood* 118:4041, 2011.

Jordan MB, Hildeman D, Kappler J, et al: An animal model of hemophagocytic lymphohistiocytosis (HLH): CD8+ T cells and interferon gamma are essential for the disorder. *Blood* 104:735, 2004.

Marsh RA, Jordan MB, Filipovich AH: Reduced-intensity conditioning haematopoietic cell transplantation for haemophagocytic lymphohistiocytosis: An important step forward. *Br J Haematol* 154:556, 2011.

Marsh RA, Madden L, Kitchen BJ, et al: XIAP deficiency: A unique primary immunodeficiency best classified as X-linked familial hemophagocytic lymphohistiocytosis and not as X-linked lymphoproliferative disease. *Blood* 116:1079, 2010.

Marsh RA, Vaughn G, Kim MO, et al: Reduced-intensity conditioning significantly improves survival of patients with hemophagocytic lymphohistiocytosis undergoing allogeneic hematopoietic cell transplantation. *Blood* 116:5824, 2010.

Minkov, M: Multisystem Langerhans cell histiocytosis in children: Current treatment and future directions. *Paediatr Drugs* 13:75, 2011.

Minkov M, Steiner M, Pötschger U, et al: International LCH Study Group: Reactivations in multisystem Langerhans cell histiocytosis: Data of the international LCH registry. *J Pediatr* 153:700, 705, e701-702, 2008.

Phillips M, Allen C, Gerson P, et al: Comparison of FDG-PET scans to conventional radiography and bone scans in management of Langerhans cell histiocytosis. *Pediatr Blood Cancer* 52:97, 2009.

Ravelli A, Grom AA, Behrens EM, et al: Macrophage activation syndrome as part of systemic juvenile idiopathic arthritis: Diagnosis, genetics, pathophysiology and treatment. *Genes Immun*, 2012.

Rigaud S, Fondanèche MC, Lambert N, et al: XIAP deficiency in humans causes an X-linked lymphoproliferative syndrome. *Nature* 444:110, 2006.

Risma K, Jordan MB: Hemophagocytic lymphohistiocytosis: Updates and evolving concepts. *Curr Opin Pediatr* 24:9, 2012.

Stepp SE, Dufourcq-Lagelouse R, Le Deist F, et al: Perforin gene defects in familial hemophagocytic lymphohistiocytosis. *Science* 286:1957, 1999.

Trottestam H, Horne A, Aricò M, et al: Histiocyte Society: Chemoimmunotherapy for hemophagocytic lymphohistiocytosis: Long-term results of the HLH-94 treatment protocol. *Blood* 118:4577, 2011.

Weitzman, S, Jaffe R: Uncommon histiocytic disorders: The non-Langerhans cell histiocytoses. *Pediatr Blood Cancer* 45:256, 2005.

Zhang K, Jordan MB, Marsh RA, et al: Hypomorphic mutations in PRF1, MUNC13-4, and STXBP2 are associated with adult-onset familial HLH. *Blood* 118:5794, 2011.

zur Stadt U, Schmidt S, Kasper B, et al: Linkage of familial hemophagocytic lymphohistiocytosis (FHL) type-4 to chromosome 6q24 and identification of mutations in syntaxin 11. *Hum Mol Genet* 14:827, 2005.

CHAPTER 51

LYSOSOMAL STORAGE DISEASES: PERSPECTIVES AND PRINCIPLES

Edward H. Schuchman and Melissa P. Wasserstein

The lysosomal storage diseases (LSDs) are a diverse group of inherited disorders caused by the defective function of specific lysosomal proteins (Table 51-1). Originally described by DeDuve and colleagues,[1] lysosomes are ubiquitous organelles required to metabolize macromolecules. This includes molecules internalized by cells through the process of endocytosis, as well as those produced during the natural turnover of endogenous cell components (autophagocytosis). More than 50 hydrolytic enzymes have been found within the lysosome, as well as several membrane-embedded transport proteins, ion pumps, and other specialized components. Unique to the lysosome is a highly acidic pH, and the enzymes and proteins found within this organelle have evolved to optimally function within this unique environment. Hers[2] was the first to describe enlarged and abnormally shaped lysosomes in a patient with Pompe disease (α-glucosidase deficiency), thus delineating the first LSD. To date, more than 50 disorders have been attributed to defective lysosomal proteins. Most are inherited as autosomal recessive traits, although two are X-linked (Fabry disease and mucopolysaccharidosis [MPS] type II [Hunter disease]). In general, LSDs are categorized according to the type of macromolecule(s) that accumulate (e.g., lipidoses, mucopolysaccharidoses). The pathophysiology of these diseases is directly related to these accumulating material(s), although as the diseases progress many secondary abnormalities also occur and contribute to the disease pathology. There is also considerable cell and organ specificity related to the location and function of the specific macromolecules affected.

PATHOBIOLOGY OF LYSOSOMAL STORAGE DISEASES

Biology of the Lysosome and Lysosomal Enzymes: Basic Principles

Lysosomes are formed through the fusion of enzyme-containing vesicles produced in the trans-Golgi network (TGN) with other vesicles such as endosomes or autophagosomes. Central to the formation of a mature lysosome is the establishment of an acidic pH. Mature lysosomes have a pH below 5, which is maintained by a proton pump found within the lysosomal membrane. Acidification of the compartment is required for proper activation of the hydrolytic enzymes and the release of macromolecules from their membrane receptors, providing access to the fully active hydrolytic enzymes. Although lysosomes have been historically considered discrete organelles, it is now known that the lysosomal system is highly dynamic and consists of a series of digestive vesicles with varying pH, hydrolytic enzyme activities, and cellular location.[3]

Key to the formation of the lysosome is the delivery of the hydrolytic enzymes to the acidified vesicles in the TGN. This is accomplished through a series of specific targeting mechanisms unique to these proteins[4] (see box on Lysosomal Protein Biosynthesis and Sorting). All lysosomal enzymes are glycoproteins that are synthesized in the rough endoplasmic reticulum (ER) with typical amino-terminal hydrophobic leader or signal peptides. Within the ER, they are glycosylated on select *N*-glycosylation sequences through the en block transfer of a core mannosyl oligosaccharide chain from a lipid intermediate, dolichophosphate.

After the completion of their synthesis and *N*-glycosylation, the lysosomal enzymes in the ER generally undergo additional proteolytic processing and are assembled into transport vesicles for delivery and further processing in the cis-Golgi apparatus. At this stage, all proteins destined for the lysosomes contain only branched mannosyl oligosaccharide chains that terminate with short-chain α-glucosyl moieites. During transport through the Golgi apparatus, they acquire additional, complex oligosaccharide modifications that result in their sorting to lysosomes. A series of glycosyl hydrolases and transferases within specific regions of the cis-, mid-, and trans-Golgi participate in these sequential modifications. For example, in the cis-Golgi, α-glucosidase and α-mannosidases remove terminal glucose and mannose residues to produce mannose-terminated core oligosaccharides. Within the mid-Golgi, additional sugars are added, including β-*N*-acetylglucosamine and β-galactoside. The addition of terminal sialic acid residues occurs in the trans-Golgi.

Coincident with the addition of the β-*N*-acetylglucosamine moiety is the addition of a phosphate group to this sugar by the enzyme *N*-acetylglucosaminyl-1-phosphotransferase. This modification is essential for lysosomal targeting, and mutations in the gene encoding this enzyme lead to a severe LSD (I-cell disease) characterized by the abnormal targeting and secretion of many lysosomal enzymes.[5] The glucosaminyl residues are subsequently cleaved, exposing terminal mannose-6-phosphate residues (M6P) on the

Lysosomal Protein Biosynthesis and Sorting

More than 50 distinct LSDs have been described that are caused by the deficient function of specific lysosomal enzymes or transport proteins. All lysosomal enzymes are cotranslationally *N*-glycosylated in the rough ER through en block transfer of the carbohydrate chain from a lipid intermediate (dolichol). In the Golgi apparatus, the carbohydrate chains are modified to acquire M6P residues, allowing sorting of these proteins to newly formed lysosomes by interaction with M6P receptors embedded in the membrane. Interaction of the M6P-containing proteins with the receptors occurs in the trans-Golgi, where the newly formed vesicles bud from the Golgi membrane and undergo sequential acidification to become mature lysosomes. These vesicles also may fuse with endosomal vesicles that deliver materials from the cell surface. Most lysosomal proteins undergo this sorting mechanism, although a small number are delivered to lysosomes by non–M6P-mediated pathways. Two enzymes localized in the Golgi are responsible for the creation of the M6P residues, and a deficiency of one can lead to a rare inherited disorder (I-cell disease) in which many of the lysosomal proteins are abnormally sorted and secreted from cells. Within the mature acidified lysosomes, additional proteolytic and carbohydrate modifications may occur, leading to full activity of the proteins. Acidification also triggers the release of the M6P-containing proteins from the receptors. In addition, within lysosomes, the active and mature proteins may associate into higher order molecular scaffolds that function to degrade the macromolecules.

Table 51-1 Examples of Lysosomal Storage Diseases

Category	Disease	Protein Abnormalities
Lipidoses	Fabry	α-Galactosidase A
	Farber	acid ceramidase
	Gaucher (types 1, 2, and 3)	β-Glucosidase
	GM_1 gangliosidosis	β-Galactosidase
	GM_2 Gangliosidosis	β-Hexosaminidase A
	Tay-Sachs	β-Hexosaminidase A and B
	Sandhoff	
	Metachromatic leukodystrophy	Arylsulfatase A
	Niemann-Pick	
	Types A and B	Acid sphingomyelinase
	Type C	
	Type 1	NPC1
	Type 2	NPC2/HE1
	Wolman disease (cholesterol ester storage disease)	Acid lipase
Mucopolysaccharidoses	MPS I (Hurler and Scheie)	α-Iduronidase
	MPS II (Hunter)	Iduronidase sulfatase
	MPS III (Sanfilippo)	
	Type A	Heparan *N*-sulfatase
	Type B	*N*-Acetyl-α-D-glucosaminidase
	Type C	Acetyl-CoA-α-glucosaminide acetyltransferase
	Type D	*N*-Acetylglucosamine-G-sulfate sulfatase
	MPS IV (Morquio)	
	Type A	Galactosamine-6-sulfatase
	Type B	β-Galactosidase
	MPS VI (Maroteaux-Lamy)	*N*-Acetylgalactosamine-4-sulfatase (arylsulfatase B)
	MPS VII (Sly)	β-Glucuronidase
	MPS IX	Hyaluronidase
Others	Aspartylglycosaminuria	Aspartylglycosaminidase
	Cystinosis (Fanconi syndrome)	Cystinosin
	Fucosidosis	Fucosidase
	I-cell disease (MLII)	*N*-Acetylglucosamine-I-phosphotransferase
	Pompe	α-Glucosidase
	Mannosidosis	α-Mannosidase
	Schindler disease	α-Galactosidase B

oligosaccharides. Importantly, for any given lysosomal enzyme, the oligosaccharide chains may be highly heterogeneous, containing varying amounts of M6P, sialic acid, and glucosaminyl sugars.

In addition to targeting the lysosomal enzymes to the organelle, the oligosaccharide side chains also participate in the tertiary structure and folding of the proteins and are in many cases necessary for their activity. Proteolytic processing within the lysosome is also sometimes required for activity, as well as assembly into macromolecular "scaffolds" that may include protector proteins, activators, and so on. These events may be driven, at least in part, by pH. Finally, although most lysosomal enzymes use the M6P targeting system, it is also important to recognize that non-M6P targeting systems have been described and may function alone or in combination with M6P.[6] For example, the lysosomal membrane proteins (LIMPs or LAMPs) are sorted to the lysosomal membrane through tyrosine residues located near the carboxyl-terminal end of the proteins.

Pathogenesis of Lysosomal Storage Diseases: General Concepts

The majority of LSDs result from mutations in genes encoding individual lysosomal enzymes, leading to the intralysosomal accumulation of the enzyme's substrate. A small number of the diseases also result from mutations in genes encoding defective transport proteins that reside within the lysosomal membrane or other nonhydrolytic enzymes required for lysosomal enzyme biosynthesis (e.g., I-cell disease). Two main categories of LSDs are distinguished by the type of primary macromolecules that accumulate: those that accumulate mucopolysaccharides (i.e., the mucopolysaccharidoses; MPS diseases), and those that accumulate lipids (i.e., the lipidoses) (see Schulze et al[7] and Giugliani et al[8] for reviews). With only a few exceptions (e.g., Wolman disease), the lipid substrates stored in the lipidoses share a common structure that includes a ceramide backbone (2-*N*-acylsphingosine, i.e., the sphingolipids). More than 100 sphingolipids are known, and because many of these molecules are essential components of cell membranes,[9] their abnormal metabolism and accumulation in the LSDs results in a wide range of physiologic and morphologic alterations, as well as characteristic clinical manifestations. For example, progressive lysosomal accumulation of glycosphingolipids in the central nervous system leads to neurodegeneration, and storage in visceral cells can lead to organomegaly, skeletal abnormalities, pulmonary infiltration, and other manifestations.

For the MPS diseases, the mucopolysaccharides (also known as glycosaminoglycans [GAGs]) are the primary accumulating macromolecules and are found predominately within connective tissues. The accumulation of these materials results in severe cartilage and bone abnormalities that affect the skeletal system, trachea, and other organs, which are characteristic of the disorders. In some cases, the brain also may be affected.

In general, the storage of a substrate in a specific tissue of an LSD patient is dependent on its normal distribution in the body, and this tissue-specific storage pattern is responsible for the organ-specific pathology. For example, in Hurler syndrome (MPS type I), two GAGs, dermatan and heparan sulfate, accumulate, resulting in severe skeletal and neurologic manifestations. In contrast, in Maroteaux-Lamy disease (MPS type VI), only dermatan sulfate accumulates. Because this GAG is not normally found in the brain, neurologic disease does not occur in MPS VI. Similarly, in Tay-Sachs and Sandhoff diseases, the deficiencies of β-hexosaminidase A, or β-hexosaminidases A and B, respectively, results either in primary CNS disease or in combined CNS and visceral disease caused by the different accumulated substrates. Whereas β-hexosaminidase A cleaves the glycosphingolipid (ganglioside) GM2, which is very abundant in the brain, β-hexosaminidase B cleaves primarily sialic acid containing gangliosides and globosides. Globosides, in particular, are synthesized in visceral tissues, resulting in visceral storage in Sandhoff disease.

Although the primary pathogenic mechanisms leading to most LSDs is clear (i.e., a single genetic lesion results in a primary protein defect and the resultant accumulation of a specific substrate or substrates), in recent years, the complexity of these diseases has been recognized. For example, in the MPS diseases, although GAGs are the primary accumulating macromolecules, other compounds, including the neural-specific gangliosides, also accumulate, contributing to disease pathogenesis. In addition, in Niemann-Pick disease (NPD) type C, the primary protein abnormalities affect cholesterol transport, although sphingolipids also accumulate and are responsible, in part, the cellular dysfunction and death. In fact, an approved therapy for NPD type C, Miglustat (see below), is based on the principle of reducing ganglioside storage in the brain rather than correcting the primary cholesterol transport defect. Similarly, in NPD types A and B, the sphingolipid sphingomyelin is the primary accumulating substrate, although cholesterol storage also is a major contributory factor.

Indeed, for any individual LSD, the pattern of macromolecule accumulation may be extremely heterogeneous and, importantly, also may be tissue and cell specific.[10] Although the mechanism(s) leading to this heterogenous storage pattern is not always known, it presumably relates to a global dysfunction of the lysosomal system, providing a connection between seemingly distinct metabolic pathways. For example, the accumulation of cholesterol in NPD type C is known to have a secondary, inhibitory effect on acid sphingomyelinase (ASM) activity. The resultant loss of functional ASM leads to the secondary accumulation of sphingomyelin, which has a major impact on cell function. Recovery of ASM activity in type C NPD cells also leads to a reduction in cholesterol storage and restoration of normal cellular function. In addition, because most lysosomal enzymes are likely assembled in higher order molecular scaffolds in which their activities are tightly and coordinately controlled, this also likely contributes to the multiple effects of the single enzyme deficiencies.

As the macromolecules accumulate, the lysosomes become distended and destabilized and eventually may fail to carry out their normal functions related to phago- and autophagocytosis. In turn, this may result in cell senescence or death or at the very least cell dysfunction. In addition, because of the progressive cell and organ disease that occurs in the LSDs, inflammatory pathways are frequently activated in an attempt to repair the damage. However, because the inflammatory cells themselves are dysfunctional, the diseases progress, and the inflammatory changes may become chronic. Inflammation is therefore also an important contributory factor to the pathogenesis of LSDs. For example, in the MPS diseases, GAG storage is known to activate the Toll-like receptor 4 signaling pathway, leading to the release of tumor necrosis factor-α (TNF-α) and other inflammatory cytokines.[11] TNF-α, in turn, causes the elevation of the toxic lipid ceramide within cartilage cells (chondrocytes), contributing to the cell death. Treatment of animal models of MPS with anti-TNF-α drugs alone has resulted in the reduction of chondrocyte death, and the combination of enzyme replacement and anti–TNF-α therapies can have substantial clinical benefits in animal models.

GENETICS AND DIAGNOSIS OF LYSOSOMAL STORAGE DISEASES

All LSDs except for two, Fabry disease and MPS type II (Hunter disease), are inherited as autosomal recessive traits. Fabry and Hunter diseases are inherited as X-linked recessive traits. Most mutations causing individual LSDs result in single amino acid changes in the enzyme's polypeptide chain, resulting in absent or defective function. The genes encoding most lysosomal proteins have been cloned, and there is no obvious clustering of these genes within the genome. In some cases, nonfunctional pseudogenes also have been described, which may or may not be transcribed or translated into a nonfunctional protein. Although there is no clustering of the lysosomal genes, it has recently been shown that most of these genes exhibit coordinated transcriptional behavior and are regulated by the transcription factor EB (TFEB).[12] In LSDs, TFEB is translocated from the cytoplasm to the nucleus to "turn on" expression of other lysosomal proteins and enhance lysosomal biogenesis. However, because the newly formed lysosomes in these diseases will retain the same primary metabolic defect, this may lead to amplification of the disease pathology.

In some cases, mutations in a lysosomal gene may lead to abnormal biosynthesis of the enzymes or delivery to lysosomes or may affect the individual gene's expression or mRNA stability. The mutant proteins in LSD patients may be stable and delivered to lysosomes, but with reduced function, or may be unstable with only partial or absent delivery to lysosomes. The effect of these individual mutations also may be cell and tissue specific. In general, heterozygous "carriers" of single mutations in a lysosomal gene do not develop clinical symptoms of the disorder, except in the X-linked disorders (Fabry and Hunter diseases), where X-inactivation patterns can lead to clusters of cells without enzyme activity that develop disease related pathology.[13] In addition, one lysosomal gene, *SMPD1,* encoding ASM, is known to be "paternally imprinted" (i.e., preferentially expressed from the maternal chromosome), suggesting that type A and B NPD individuals who inherit "severe" *SMPD1* mutations on the maternal chromosome may be more severely affected than those who inherit the same mutations from the paternal chromosome.[14] This also suggests that some NPD carrier individuals (with maternally-derived mutations) might exhibit clinical or laboratory manifestations of the disorder, and there is at least one report documenting very low serum high-density lipoprotein levels in such carrier individuals.

Although all LSDs are caused by DNA abnormalities in the genes encoding lysosomal proteins, as already noted, the disease pathogenesis is more directly related to the individual effect of these mutations on the proteins themselves and the resultant biology of the accumulating macromolecules. Diagnostic assays for patients suspected of having an LSD generally rely on the measurement of specific enzymatic activities in isolated leukocytes or cultured fibroblasts. For some disorders, carrier identification and prenatal diagnosis are available as well. However, because the detection of individual enzyme activities in these cell sources must use in vitro assay conditions and nonnatural substrate analogues (e.g., fluorescently conjugated), the enzymatic confirmation of suspected cases should be carried out in specialized laboratories experienced in these methods. In addition, because in most LSDs, leukocytes and skin fibroblasts are not clinically relevant cell types, these assay methods are at best indirect measures of the defective lysosomal protein's function at the pathological sites. For this reason, predicting the clinical outcome from these analyses is generally not reliable.[15] For example, cells from patients with the infantile, neurologic form of ASM deficient NPD (type A) and the later-onset, non-neurologic form (type B) often have similar residual enzymatic activities, although their clinical course is markedly different. This likely reflects the function of the individual mutant ASM polypeptides in the brain.

As already noted, many genetic abnormalities have been identified as causing individual LSDs. For most diseases, multiple mutations have been found, and the majority of these are unique (i.e., private) to individual families. However, for some LSDs, there are specific populations that may have recurrent mutations caused by founder effects or consanguinity, facilitating the use of DNA-based screening methods for the detection of the LSD. This has been most effectively translated into clinical use in the Ashkenazi Jewish population, in which relatively small number(s) of mutations account for several LSDs (and several other genetic disorders).[16] This has led to the establishment of a DNA-based "Jewish Genetic Disease" screening panel and the population-based identification of carrier individuals for the same disorder. Such individuals are referred for genetic counseling to assist with family planning and pregnancy outcome choices. The implication of such screening has led to a dramatic reduction in the incidence of some diseases within this population (e.g., infantile Tay-Sachs disease), and will likely lead to the prevention of other disorders as well. The rapid evolution of cost-effective, high-throughput sequencing methods is also likely to open other populations and disorders to these DNA-based approaches.[17] However, it is important to note that the functional consequences of most DNA abnormalities on the protein function have not been confirmed, and thus DNA-based methods alone should not be used to predict clinical outcome unless the biochemical consequences of these abnormalities is fully established. In general, confirmation of a suspected LSD case should be confirmed by both enzymatic and DNA-based studies, and in only rare cases can the laboratory results be used to predict clinical outcomes.

THERAPY OF LYSOSOMAL STORAGE DISEASES: AN OVERVIEW

Since the first recognition that LSDs resulted from the defective function of lysosomal proteins, the concept of simply "replacing" the missing protein in individual patients was put forward[18] (see box on Treatment of Lysosomal Storage Diseases). This concept was further strengthened in the 1970s by the identification of the M6P targeting system for lysosomal enzymes and the finding that the secreted forms of many lysosomal enzymes could be rapidly internalized, or "taken up," by cell surface M6P receptors and delivered into the lysosomal system.[19]

Initial attempts at replacing the normal protein in LSD patients were accomplished by cell and organ transplantation. The premise of this approach is that transplanted cells expressing the normal lysosomal proteins would release some of these proteins into the circulation and locally at the sites of pathology and that these proteins would be taken up by the diseased cells, leading to metabolic "cross-correction." "Proof-of-principle" for this approach was documented by Neufeld,[20] who showed that metabolic cross-correction of MPS cells could be achieved by co-culture of these cells with normal cells or by replacing the media in MPS cells with "conditioned" media obtained from the normal cells. In addition to these proof-of-principle experiments, there also was an early recognition that very low levels of residual enzymatic activities in the individual LSDs could have an important impact on the clinical presentation of the individual patients. This suggested that low levels of enzyme release and re-uptake were likely required to achieve metabolic cross-correction in vivo.

The majority of the clinical experience using cell-based therapy in LSDs comes from bone marrow transplantation (BMT).[21] Bone marrow has several advantages as a cell source, including the fact that it contains multiple stem and progenitor cell lineages that can lead to repopulation of various organs and tissues. Thousands of individual LSD patients have received BMTs over the past 3 decades, and the results have been mixed. First, aggressive immunosuppressive preconditioning is required to achieve effective engraftment in the transplanted patients, leading to high morbidity and, in some cases, mortality. In addition, graft-versus-host disease may occur. These deleterious effects can be severe and may lead to clinical complications in patients that are worse than the disorders themselves. The availability of cord blood repositories and improved transplant methods have reduced these risks, but the possibility of high morbidity remains.

In patients who have successfully undergone BMT and achieved a high level of engraftment, the clinical results have been variable. A number of factors account for this. First, repopulation after BMT is not uniform throughout the body, and depending on the organ systems affected in the patients, clinical improvement may or may not occur. For example, the hematopoietic system is particularly amenable to BMT repopulation, but the skeletal system (cartilage and bone) is not. In the nervous system, some bone marrow–derived cells may cross the blood–brain barrier and repopulate the microglial population, but the number of these cells is small and the repopulation efficiency low.[22] A second factor accounting for the variable clinical results after BMT is the age at which the transplant is undertaken. Many of the disease manifestations that occur in LSDs lead to permanent tissue damage (e.g., fibrosis, apoptosis) and are not reversible. Thus, not only must efficient engraftment be achieved after transplantation, but the procedure must also be undertaken before irreversible damage sets in.

Other than BMT, liver transplantation also has been undertaken in various LSDs, also with variable success (e.g., see Ayto et al[23]). Because the liver is a natural secretory organ, the concept underlying liver transplantation is that even partial repopulation of this organ with healthy cells will lead to secretion of these proteins into the circulation and widespread metabolic cross-correction. As with BMT, however, the uptake and distribution of the secreted enzymes will be limited by physiologic barriers (e.g., blood–brain barrier) and dependent on the vascular supply to the tissue. Unlike BMT, there also will no circulating stem cells available for organ engraftment other than in the liver. It is also of interest that early attempts at cell therapy for LSDs used amniotic cells for transplantation. Although the engraftment of these cells was extremely low and the clinical outcomes poor, these studies represented the first embryonic stem cell–based approach for these disorders.

Simultaneous with the development of cell and organ transplantation for LSDs, investigators also began to isolate and study the normal lysosomal proteins involved in the individual disorders and

Treatment of Lysosomal Storage Diseases

The principle underlying the treatment of most LSDs is replacement of the missing or defective protein. This can be accomplished by stem cell transplantation, protein replacement therapy, or gene therapy. In some cases, treatments also have been developed that are either aimed at slowing the accumulation of undegraded materials (substrate reduction therapy) or enhancement of the mutant protein function (chaperone therapy). BMT has been undertaken in more than 1000 LSD patients with varying results. The premise of this approach is that stem cells in the bone marrow will repopulate in the transplanted individual and provide a source of secreted and normal lysosomal proteins that can be taken up by neighboring cells for metabolic correction (cross-correction). This approach is most effective for soluble lysosomal proteins and diseases in which cells of the monocyte–macrophage system are primary sites of pathology. However, despite the availability of cord blood registries, such cell transplantation is still limited by a high morbidity and the lack of suitable donors. Enzyme replacement therapy is also available for six LSDs and under development for several others. This approach, although effective, requires lifelong weekly or biweekly infusions of the recombinant proteins, and the costs are very high. Gene therapy approaches have been evaluated in numerous LSD animal models but are not yet available for patients. This approach, however, has also proven very effective in some disease models and could be evaluated in the clinic during the upcoming years. In general, the efficacy of any of these approaches is dependent on the cellular and tissue sites of pathology and the ability of the therapeutic proteins, stem cells, or gene therapy vectors to access these sites.

to explore the idea of protein (enzyme) replacement therapy (ERT). Because this work originated before the development of recombinant DNA technology, it relied on discarded human materials as the enzyme source, usually urine or placentas. The first short-term experience with ERT in human patients took place in the early 1970s by Brady,[18] Desnick, and others, and revealed (1) that the enzymes were generally well tolerated, (2) that the half-life of the enzymes in the circulation was short lived, and (3) that the sugar moieties on the enzymes had an important influence on their clearance from the circulation. In general, enzymes with terminal sialic acid residues had longer half-lives in the circulation than those with exposed mannose or M6P residues.

Despite these early successes, the further development of ERT was limited by the inability of the academic-based research laboratories to produce enough of the enzymes for long-term treatment. In the 1980s, a small biotechnology company took on this challenge and began to commercially prepare β-glucocerebrosidase, the enzyme deficient in Gaucher disease, from human placentas. This led to the first long-term experience with ERT in patients with non-neurologic (type 1) Gaucher disease.[24] Importantly, the purified enzyme was chemically modified to expose terminal mannose residues, leading to preferential uptake by macrophages, the major cellular site of pathology in this disease.

The results of ERT in type 1 Gaucher disease were life changing and led to remarkably reduced organomegaly and improved hematologic findings. Although the therapy required biweekly intravenous infusions, it led to substantially improved quality of life and was approved by the international regulatory authorities. By the early 1990s, DNA technologies had evolved to the point where human recombinant β-glucocerebrosidase could be produced (in overexpressing Chinese hamster ovary cells), and this eventually replaced the use of placental enzyme.

In addition, based on the outstanding success in Gaucher disease, several other ERTs began to be developed, including therapies for Fabry disease (α-galactosidase), Pompe disease (α-glucosidase), and several of the MPS disorders. ERT is now commercially available for Fabry, Pompe, and three MPS diseases (MPS I, II, and VI) and under development for others. With these developments came the recognition that the effects of ERT were disease specific and could be complicated by immune reactions to the infused recombinant proteins. In addition, the costs of these therapies were extremely high, placing a very high burden on the reimbursement systems.

These realizations have led researchers to explore other therapies as well, and this research has been greatly aided by the use of DNA technologies to develop animal models for most of the LSDs. Considerable effort has been directed towards gene therapies, which have been extensively evaluated in the animal models.[25] Clinical and pathological improvements have been obtained, although the translation of these technologies into the clinic has been slow because of safety concerns and issues with large-scale vector production. Recently, the first gene therapy clinical trials for LSDs have been approved in Europe, and over the next decade, results should be forthcoming regarding the efficacy of these approaches.

Other investigators have sought alternative therapeutic approaches for these diseases, focusing on inhibiting the production of substrate in order to reduce glycosphingolipid production and accumulation (substrate reduction therapy [SRT]). Miglustat (OGT 918, *N*-butyldeoxynojirimycin; trade name, Zavesca) is a low–molecular-weight compound that inhibits glucosylceramide synthase, which catalyzes the first step in the biosynthesis of glucosylceramide and other glycosphingolipids. Miglustat is an oral compound that has been shown to effectively decrease organ volume and improve hematologic parameters in patients with type 1 Gaucher disease. However, gastrointestinal side effects are fairly common, so the use of Miglustat is limited to Gaucher disease patients for whom ERT is not suitable. Miglustat has also been used in patients with type C NPD, which causes progressive and severe neurologic disease. Most patients with type C NPD have mutations in an integral membrane protein involved in cholesterol transport (NPC1). However, because the deficiency in NPC is a nonsoluble transporter, protein replacement therapy is not a therapeutic option at the present time. Using animal models, investigators showed that the neurologic pathology in type C NPD was associated with the secondary accumulation of a particular glycolipid, GM_2 ganglioside. Based on this finding, studies were carried out in the type C NPD animal models using SRT to inhibit glycolipid biosynthesis, resulting in reduction of GM_2 storage and partial neurologic improvements. Clinical trials of Miglustat in type C NPD patients revealed stabilization or improvement of some clinical markers.

Another small molecule approach under development for the LSDs is based on the use of enzyme-specific inhibitors that can act as "chaperones" of the corresponding mutant proteins, thereby facilitating their delivery to lysosomes and enhancing their residual enzymatic activities. Such "chaperone" therapy is currently being evaluated in clinical trials for several LSDs. Numerous other approaches also have been or are being evaluated in the various LSD animal models, including targeting of inflammatory pathways and stem cell–based therapies, and in the future, patients should have access to various therapeutic choices. As with ERT, the effects of these individual therapies are likely to be disease and organ specific, and it is expected that in the future effective treatment of LSD patients will require a combination of these approaches.

HEMATOLOGIC MANIFESTATIONS OF LYSOSOMAL STORAGE DISEASES

Hematologic findings are associated with several LSDs, but in two, Gaucher disease and types A and B NPD, hematologic abnormalities are among the common presenting features. Hematologic findings should be considered in the differential diagnosis of both disorders, and patients with Gaucher disease or NPD may be seen by hematologists to manage their symptoms. In the section below, the hematologic features of these disorders are discussed, as well as several other relevant issues related to hematologic manifestations and LSDs.

Gaucher Disease: β-Glucosidase Deficiency

Cells of the monocyte–macrophage system are the primary sites of pathology in this disorder. In general, these cells are enriched for lysosomes and highly active in phagocytosis. As such, disruption of lysosomal function may have a profound effect on their function. An important diagnostic hallmark of Gaucher disease is the presence in a variety of tissues of lipid-filled cells derived from the monocyte–macrophage system, referred to as *Gaucher cells*. These cells are readily evident in the bone marrow but also can be seen in blood smears and histologically in other tissues, including liver, spleen, lung, and others. As the disease progresses, the deposition of Gaucher cells in these organs increases.

Bleeding is a common presenting symptom of patients with Gaucher disease and is primarily caused by thrombocytopenia. The major sites of bleeding are mucocutaneous, including epistaxis, easy bruising, and gingival hemorrhage. Thrombocytopenia in Gaucher disease is generally thought to be caused by splenic sequestration of platelets. Spleen enlargement is present in all symptomatic patients and is a common presenting sign of the disease. Splenic enlargement in Gaucher disease may be massive, up to 75-fold normal.[26]

Some patients with type 1 Gaucher disease have excessive bleeding that is disproportionate to their platelet counts and coagulation profiles. Abnormal platelet function has been described in patients with type 1 Gaucher disease with abnormal bleeding tendencies.[27] These defects have been attributed to defects in platelet adhesion as well as aggregation. Coagulation deficiencies, particularly low factor levels of factor XI, also have been described.[28] Because both factor XI deficiency and type 1 Gaucher disease are relatively common in the Ashkenazi Jewish population, this finding may reflect concurrence of the two disorders. However, a report describing Egyptian type 1 Gaucher disease patients with deficiencies in factors II, V, VII, VIII, X, XI, and XII supports the concept that the coagulopathy is not

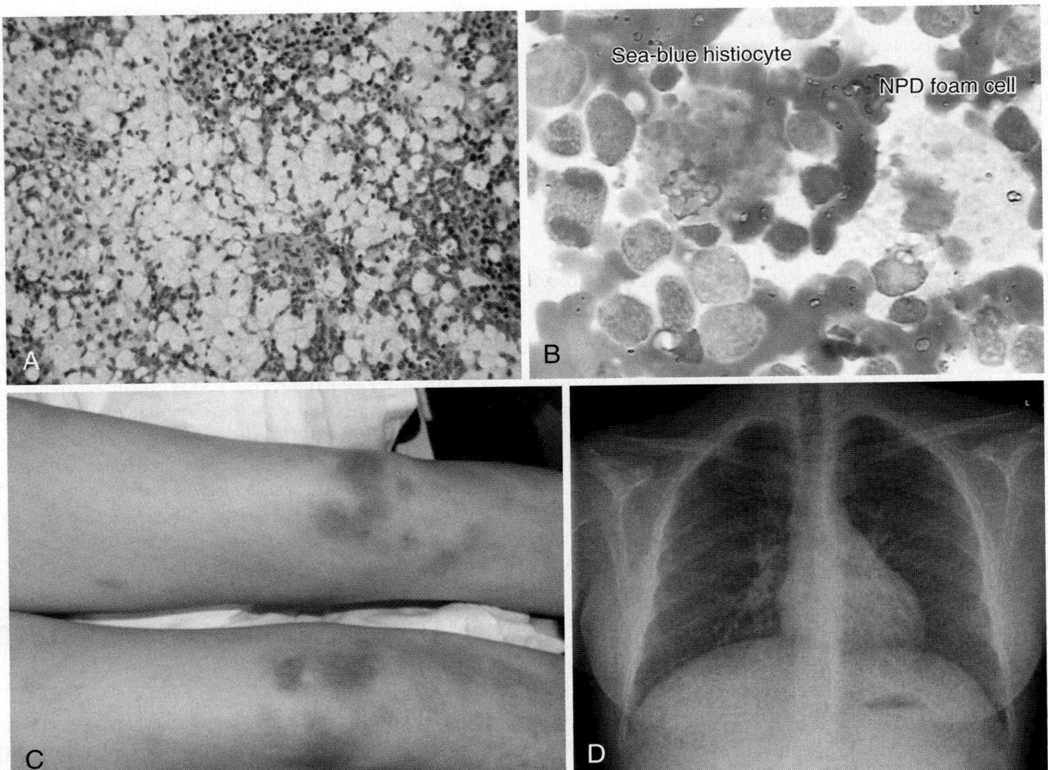

Figure 51-1 **A,** Typical histopathology (hematoxylin and eosin E staining) of a liver section from a patient with type B Niemann-Pick disease (NPD). Note the lipid-filled macrophages (Niemann-Pick cells) that are characteristic of this disorder. **B,** Micrograph of the bone marrow from the same patient with type B NPD showing the presence of an NPD cell, as well as a sea-blue histocyte. Both cells may be characteristically found in the bone marrow of these patients. **C,** Bruising that may be seen in type B NPD and is associated with thrombocytopenia. **D,** Chest radiograph of a patient with type B NPD showing the diffuse reticulonodular interstitial changes in this disorder.

limited to Ashkenazi Jewish patients and may have a distinct pathophysiology.[29] In fact, many patients with Gaucher disease have significant deficiencies (<50%) of multiple coagulation factors.[28] This is associated with elevations of coagulation activators, suggesting ongoing activation of the coagulation cascade with a resultant consumption of coagulation factors.[28]

Anemia in patients with Gaucher disease is usually mild but occasionally may be severe and can be associated with leukopenia. These findings are also probably attributable to sequestration of cells in the spleen, as well as dysfunctional bone marrow production of cells as the disease progresses. The mainstay of treatment for the hematologic abnormalities in Gaucher disease is ERT. ERT typically produces a remarkable improvement in the platelet count, hemoglobin, and white blood cell count, as well as a reduction in spleen size.[24] ERT may also partially improve the coagulation profile.[28]

In patients with massive splenomegaly, splenectomy is often approached as a treatment option with the expectation that it will improve the platelet count and reduce the risk of splenic rupture. However, the spleen is an important reservoir for storage material, and its removal can displace lipid deposition to other organs, accelerating the rate and severity of disease.

Types A and B Niemann-Pick Disease: Acid Sphingomyelinase Deficiency

The hematologic findings in types A and B NPD are similar to those in Gaucher disease and may include thrombocytopenia and anemia. Splenic enlargement is also a common presenting feature of this disorder, and sequestration of cells in the spleen is thought to be the underlying cause of the low platelets, low hemoglobin, or leukopenia (Fig. 51-1, *A* and *B*). Some patients with type B NPD have excessive bleeding without significant thrombocytopenia or coagulopathy. Frequent and prolonged epistaxis can be particularly problematic and in some extreme cases may require cauterization, packing, and blood transfusions.

As with Gaucher disease, a primary cellular site of pathology in types A and B NPD is the monocyte–macrophage system, and the characteristic pathological cells are referred to as *Niemann-Pick cells*. These can be distinguished from Gaucher cells by an experienced pathologist but are frequently missed, leading to misdiagnosis. They are also readily evident in blood smears, bone marrow, and other organs and increase as the disease progresses. As noted earlier, there is another form of NPD (type C) that is caused by primary defects in cholesterol transport. These patients also may present with mild hematologic findings and an enlarged spleen, although in general, the hematologic findings are less severe than in patients with types A and B NPD (Fig. 51-1, *C* and *D*)

Fabry Disease: α-Galactosidase Deficiency

Unlike Gaucher and NPD diseases, in Fabry disease, the monocyte–macrophage system is not primarily affected. In this disorder, the primary site of accumulation of glycolipids occurs in the vascular endothelial and smooth muscle cells that surround blood vessels. As such, constriction of blood vessels occurs, leading to skin lesions, strokes, and kidney dysfunction. It is noteworthy that several of the accumulating glycolipids in Fabry disease also are blood group lipids. For example, a number of blood group B glycolipids may contain terminal α-galactosyl moieties, and as such, patients with Fabry disease who have blood groups B and AB will accumulate four glycolipid substrates as opposed to those with A or O blood groups, who will only accumulate two. The clinical consequence of this differential accumulation of blood group lipids in Fabry disease is unknown.

Sea Blue Histiocytosis and Lysosomal Storage Diseases

Sea-blue histocytes are lipid-laden macrophages detectable by May-Giemsa staining of the bone marrow, blood cells, or other organs (Fig. 51-1, *B*). The appearance of these cells may be secondary in many disorders, but for the LSDs, they are principally associated with NPD, Gaucher, Fabry, or ceroid storage diseases. For NPD and Gaucher disease specifically, there are several reports in the literature of patients with these disorders being misdiagnosed with primary sea-blue histocytosis and only later being found to have the primary lysosomal enzyme defect. Thus, the appearance of sea-blue histocytes should be considered as part of the differential diagnosis of these disorders.

CONCLUSIONS AND FUTURE DIRECTIONS

The LSDs comprise a diverse group of genetic disorders that may present from infancy through adulthood. Most LSDs are caused by single enzyme deficiencies, but these single protein defects can result in a complex array of metabolic abnormalities, leading to a wide range of clinical presentations. The pathophysiology of individual LSDs depends on the specific cells and tissues in which these metabolic abnormalities occur. Phenotypic heterogeneity among patients may be caused by different mutations in the enzyme-encoding gene, resulting in varying levels of residual enzyme activity. Hematologic abnormalities occur in several LSDs, although two diseases, type 1 Gaucher disease and types A and B NPD, primarily affect cells of the monocyte–macrophage system, and hematologic complications can be common and severe in some cases. Several treatment options are available for some of the LSDs, including ERT, and in the case of Gaucher disease, ERT is very effective at correcting the hematologic findings. ERT is also under development for type B NPD. Other treatment options, including small molecule approaches, also are actively being developed for many LSDs, and in the future, most LSD patients are likely to be treated by a combination of these methods. These efforts, together with the development of population-wide enzyme and DNA-based screening for the LSDs, should lead to better medical management and improved quality of life for most patients.

REFERENCES

1. de Duve C: Lysosomes revisited. *Eur J Biochem* 137:391, 1983.
2. Hers HG: Inborn lysosomal diseases. *Gastroenterology* 48:625, 1965.
3. Hasilik A, Wrocklage C, Schroder B: Intracellular trafficking of lysosomal proteins and lysosomes. *Int J Clin Pharmacol Ther* 47:S18, 2009.
4. Kornfeld R, Kornfeld S: Assembly of asparagine-linked oligosaccharides. *Annu Rev Biochem* 54:631, 1985.
5. Reitman ML, Varki A, Kornfeld S: Fibroblasts from patients with I-cell disease and pseudo-Hurler polydystrophy are deficient in uridine 5′-diphosphate-N-acetylglucsamin: Glycoprotein N-acetylglucosaminylphosphotransferase activity. *J Clin Invest* 67:1574, 1981.
6. Bonifacino JS, Traub LM: Signals for sorting of transmembrane proteins to endosomes and lysosomes. *Annu Rev Biochem* 72:395, 2003.
7. Schulze H, Sandhoff K: Lysosomal lipid storage diseases. *Cold Spring Harb Perspect Biol* 1:3, 2011.
8. Giugliani R, Federhen A, Rojas MV, et al: Mucopolysaccharidosis I, II and VI: Brief review and guidelines for treatment. *Genet Mol Biol* 33:589, 2010.
9. Hannun YA, Bell RM: Functions of sphingolipids and sphingolipid breakdown products in cellular regulation. *Science* 243:500, 1989.
10. Walkley SU, Vanier MT: Secondary lipid accumulation in lysosomal disease. *Biochim Biophys Acta* 1793:726, 2009.
11. Simonaro CM, Ge Y, Eliyahu E, et al: Involvement of the Toll-like receptor 4 pathway and the use of TNF-alpha antagonists for treatment of the mucopolysaccharidosis. *Proc Natl Acad Sci U S A* 107:222, 2010.
12. Settembre C, Di Malta C, Polito VA, et al: TFEB links autophagy to lysosomal biogenesis. *Science* 332:1429, 2011.
13. Germain DP: General aspects of X-linked disease. In Mehta A, Beck M, Sunder-Plassman G, editors: *Fabry Disease: Perspectives from 5 yers of FOS,* Oxford, 2006, Oxford ParmaGenesis, Chapter 7.
14. Simonaro CM, Park JH, Eliyahu E, et al: Imprinting at the SMPD1 locus: Implications for acid sphingomyelinase-deficient Niemann-Pick disease. *Am J Hum Genet* 78:865, 2006.
15. Balwani M, Grace ME, Desnick RJ: Gaucher disease: When molecular testing and clinical presentation disagree—the novel c. 1226A>G(p. N370S)-RecNcil allele. *J Inherit Metab Dis* 34:789, 2011.
16. Dolgin E: Jewish genetic screening grows despite questions about breadth. *Nat Med* 17:639, 2011.
17. Bell CJ, Dinwiddie DL, Miller NA, et al: Carrier testing for severe childhood recessive diseases by next-generation sequencing. *Sci Transl Med* 3:65ra4, 2011.
18. Brady RO: Enzyme replacement for lysosomal diseases. *Annu Rev Med* 57:283, 2006.
19. Sly WS, Fischer HD, Gonzalez-Moriega A, et al: Role of the 6-phosphomannosyl-enzyme receptor in intracellular transport and adsorptive pinocytosis of lysosomal enzymes. *Methods Cell Biol* 23:191, 1981.
20. Neufeld EF: The uptake of enzyme into lysosomes: An overview. *Birth Defects Orig Artic Ser* 16:77, 1980.
21. Prasad VK, Kurtzberg J: Cord blood and bone marrow transplantation in inherited metabolic diseases: Scientific basis, current status and future directions. *Br J Haematol* 148:356, 2010.
22. Krivit W, Sung JH, Shaprio EG, et al: Microglia: The effector cell for reconstitution of the central nervous system following bone marrow transplantation for lysosomal and peroxisomal storage diseases. *Cell Transplant* 4:385, 1995.
23. Ayto RM, Hughs DA, Jeevaratnam P, et al: Long-term outcomes of liver transplantation in type 1 Gaucher disease. *Am J Transplant* 10:1934, 2010.
24. Barton NW, Furbish FS, Murray GJ, et al: Therapeutic response to intravenous infusions of glucocerebrosidase in a patient with Gaucher disease. *Proc Natl Acad Sci U S A* 87:1913, 1990.
25. Seregin SS, Amalfitano A: Gene therapy for lysosomal storage disorders: Progress, challenges and future prospects. *Curr Pharm Des* 17:2558, 2011.
26. Sibille A, Eng CM, Kim SJ, et al: Phenotype/genotype correlations in Gaucher disease type I: Clinical and therapeutic implications. *Am J Hum Genet* 52:1094, 1993.
27. Gillis S, Hyam E, Abrahamov A, et al: Platelet function abnormalities in Gaucher disease patients. *Am J Hematol* 61:103, 1999.
28. Hollak CE, Levi M, Berends F, et al: Coagulation abnormalities in type 1 Gaucher disease are due to low-grade activation and can be partly restored by enzyme supplementation therapy. *Br J Haematol* 96:470, 1997.
29. Deghady A, Marzouk I, El-Shayeb A, et al: Coagulation abnormalities in type 1 Gaucher disease in children. *Pediatr Hematol Oncol* 23:411, 2006.

CHAPTER 52

INFECTIOUS MONONUCLEOSIS AND OTHER EPSTEIN-BARR VIRUS–ASSOCIATED DISEASES

Carl Allen, Cliona M. Rooney, and Stephen Gottschalk

The initial clinical descriptions of primary Epstein-Barr virus (EBV) infections are credited to Filatov and Pfeiffer at the end of the 19th century. Pfeiffer coined the term *glandular fever,* which described an illness consisting of fever, malaise, sore throat, and lymphadenopathy. In 1920, Sprunt and Evans introduced the term *infectious mononucleosis (IM)* to describe a series of patients with fatigue, fever, lymphadenopathy, and prominent mononuclear lymphocytosis (Fig. 52-1). Serologic diagnosis of IM became available in the 1930s with the heterophile agglutination test developed by Paul and Bunnel and later modified by Davidson (see box on EBV-Associated Clinical Syndromes).

The identification of EBV as the causative agent of IM was impeded for many years by the inability to transmit the disease to animals or to grow the virus ex vivo. In 1958 Burkitt described a lymphoma in African children and investigators suspected an infectious etiology because the lymphoma's geographic distribution pattern coincided with the African mosquito belt.[1] In 1964 Epstein, Achong, and Barr described herpesvirus-like particles in tumor biopsies from Burkitt lymphoma patients. Werner and Gertrude Henle developed an indirect immunofluorescent antibody assay to this new virus, now called *Epstein-Barr virus,* and showed that Burkitt lymphoma patients, as well as 90% of American adults, had antibodies against EBV. In 1965 the Henles documented seroconversion to EBV of an individual who presented with clinical symptoms of IM. This initial observation was corroborated by larger studies confirming the association of EBV and IM.

Since then, EBV has been linked to a heterogeneous group of diseases.[2] EBV was the first human virus implicated in oncogenesis, and the biology of the virus has been studied extensively on a cellular and molecular level.[3] Because primary EBV infection is a self-limiting disease in almost all individuals, therapeutic strategies have focused on the treatment of rare, potentially fatal EBV-associated diseases. Over the last decade, successful immunotherapeutic approaches have been developed for EBV-associated lymphoproliferative disease, using either monoclonal antibodies or the adoptive transfer of EBV-specific T cells[4,5] (see box on EBV-Associated Clinical Syndromes).

BIOLOGY OF EBV

EBV belongs to the family of herpesviruses, which has almost 100 members. Membership is based on the architecture of the virion that is 120 to 300 nm in size and contains (a) a core of linear, double-stranded DNA, (b) an icosadeltahedral capsid with 162 capsomers, (c) an amorphous material between the capsid and envelope designated tegument, and (d) an envelope containing viral glycoproteins.

EBV-Associated Clinical Syndromes

- Infectious mononucleosis
- Chronic active EBV infection
- Hemophagocytic lymphohistiocytosis
- X-linked lymphoproliferative disease
- Oral hairy leukoplakia

Besides EBV, designated human herpesvirus 4, seven other herpesviruses have been isolated from humans: herpes simplex viruses 1 and 2, cytomegalovirus, varicella-zoster virus, human herpesvirus 6, human herpesvirus 7, and the Kaposi sarcoma–associated herpesvirus (KSHV, human herpesvirus 8). Herpesviruses are further divided into subfamilies to reflect evolutionary relatedness and similar biologic properties. EBV and KSHV belong to the human gamma herpesvirus subgroup and have a limited tissue tropism to B and T lymphocytes and certain types of epithelial cells. Several variants of EBV have been identified by genomic polymorphisms. Initially, two EBV types were distinguished by sequence changes in EBV nuclear antigens 2 and 3 (EBNA2 and EBNA3). However, using polymorphisms in the latent membrane protein 1 (LMP1), further subtypes have been described. EBV strains vary by geography and have not been linked to a particular EBV-associated disease.

PRIMARY EBV INFECTION

Primary EBV infection usually occurs through the oropharynx, where mucosal epithelial cells and/or B cells become productively infected (Fig. 52-2). Infection of B cells by EBV is initiated by binding of the dominant viral glycoprotein gp350/220 to CD21, the C3d complement receptor; subsequent cell entry is mediated by a complex of three viral glycoproteins, gH, gL, and gp42. Gp42 binds to HLA class II, which functions as a coreceptor, and gH is most likely involved in virus-cell fusion. The entry of EBV into epithelial cells may occur through multiple mechanisms because the majority of epithelial cells are CD21 negative. After viral entry, the capsid is dissolved and the EBV genome is transported into the nucleus, where it circularizes. Infection of epithelial cells results in lytic or abortive infection, and whereas B-cell infection results predominantly in latency, the lytic infection also occurs, resulting in the release of infectious virus into the saliva and other secretions. During primary infection, EBV establishes lifelong latency in B cells and it is estimated that 1 to 50 cells per 1×10^6 B cells in the peripheral circulation are infected with EBV. The number of latently infected B cells within a person remains stable over years; however, intermittent reactivation of EBV in B cells into the lytic cycle at mucosal sites is probably responsible for the observed shedding of infectious virus into the saliva of asymptomatic carriers (see Fig. 52-2).

Although EBV can infect any B cell and express the full spectrum of latency proteins, extensive studies by the group of Thorley-Lawson have suggested that only infection of naive B cells results in persistent infection (see Fig. 52-2). EBV infection pushes the naive B cell into a memory state independent of an antigen-dependent germinal center reaction by upregulation of cytosine deaminase, which induces both class switching and somatic hypermutation. The former also requires the expression of EBV-encoded LMP1, a constitutively activated CD40 molecule, or CD40 ligation, most likely provided by germinal center Th3 cells that can provide T-cell help for B-cell differentiation by provision of CD40 ligand, IL-4, and IL-10 while preventing antigen-dependent effector T cell–mediated B-cell elimination by expression of TGF-β. This reaction occurs within the lymph node and also involves downregulation of latency proteins and expression of latency type II. On exit from the lymph node,

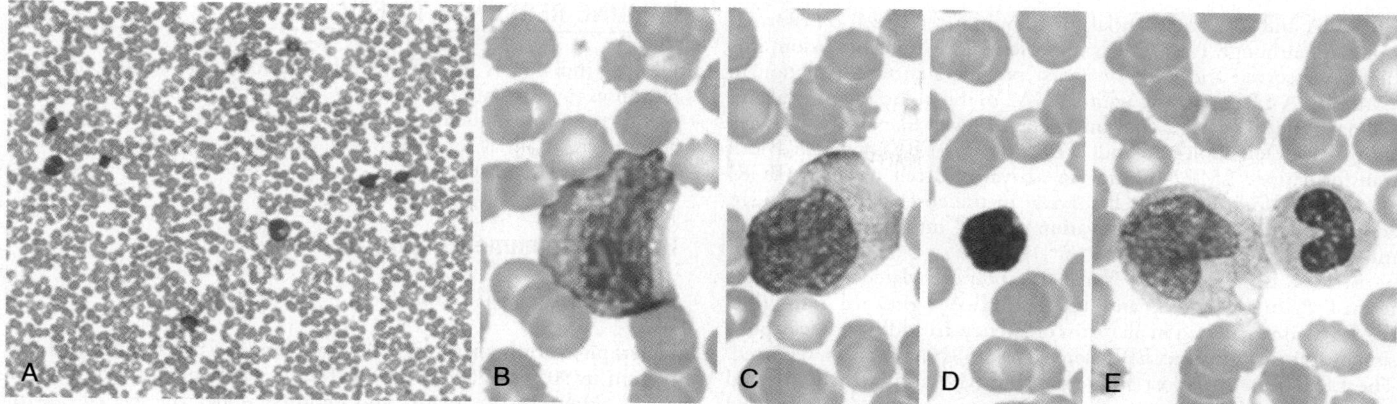

Figure 52-1 PROMINENT MONONUCLEAR LYMPHOCYTOSIS IN MONONUCLEOSIS. Low power **(A)** illustrates the leukocytosis, mainly due to activated lymphocytes (**B** and **C**), which are contrasted with a normal small lymphocyte **(D)** and a monocyte and granulocyte **(E)**. The large reactive lymphocytes are frequently confused with monocytes because of their morphologic resemblance and the term *mononucleosis*. Monocytes usually have a finer, lacy chromatin and a gray cytoplasm with small granules and vacuoles when compared with the large activated lymphocytes.

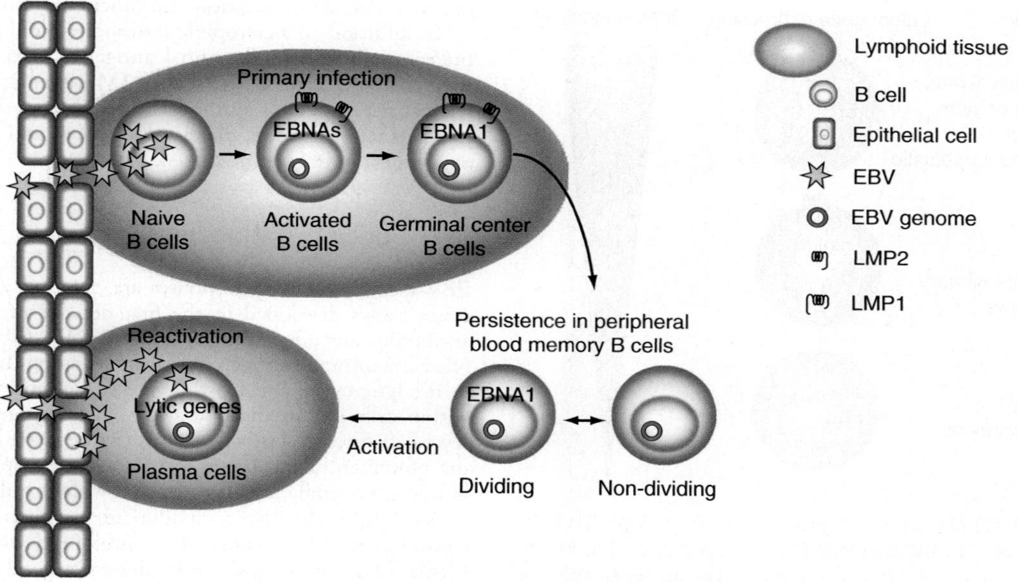

Figure 52-2 INFECTIOUS LIFE CYCLE OF EPSTEIN-BARR VIRUS.

expression of latency proteins is completely inhibited. In this way infected B cells can evade immune elimination. By contrast, primarily infected memory B cells enter and remain in latency type III and are rapidly eliminated by effector T cells and therefore do not contribute to virus persistence.

LATENT EBV INFECTION

During latent infection, EBV persists episomally in resting memory B cells. Initially, it was thought that EBNA1 and LMP2 were expressed in memory B cells; however, more recent studies indicate that the majority of infected cells do not express viral proteins and that of the almost 100 viral proteins, only EBNA1 is expressed during memory B-cell division (see Fig. 52-2).[3] This extremely limited expression of viral proteins allows EBV to persist long term despite a robust cellular EBV-specific immune response.

Three other distinct types of EBV latency have been characterized in a heterogeneous group of malignancies (Fig. 52-3). Latency type III, which can be readily produced by infecting B cells in vitro with EBV, is expressed in lymphoblastoid cell lines (LCL). These cells express the entire array of nine EBV latency proteins: EBNA1, -2, -3A, -3B, and -3C, EBNA leader protein (LP), and the two viral membrane proteins LMP1 and LMP2. This pattern of EBV gene expression characterizes the EBV-associated lymphoproliferative diseases (EBV-LPD) that occur in individuals severely immunocompromised by solid organ or hematopoietic stem cell transplantation, congenital immunodeficiency, or human immunodeficiency virus (HIV) infection. Latency type II is the hallmark of EBV-positive Hodgkin disease and non-Hodgkin lymphomas (NHL), as well as nasopharyngeal carcinomas (NPC). EBV proteins expressed in these malignancies are EBNA1, LMP1, and LMP2. In addition, BARF1 is expressed in subsets of latency type II associated malignancies. In latency type I, found in EBV-positive Burkitt lymphoma and gastric adenocarcinomas, only EBNA1 is expressed. However, variants in which all EBNAs are expressed in the absence of LMP1 have also been described.

The EBV proteins expressed during type III latency are involved in the transformation and growth of EBV-infected B cells. EBNA1 binds to the origin of replication of the latent viral genome and is responsible for the maintenance of the EBV episome in host B cells. EBNA2 upregulates the expression of the viral proteins LMP1 and LMP2 and cellular proteins that contribute to transformation.

EBNA3A and -3C are essential for EBV-induced B-cell transformation, and although EBNA3B is not essential for transformation, it is highly conserved and therefore must provide a survival function in vivo. EBNA-LP cooperates with EBNA2 in the induction of viral and cellular genes. LMP1, a viral oncogene, behaves like a constitutively activated CD40 molecule and is essential for EBV-mediated B-cell transformation. LMP2 mimics an activated B-cell receptor (BCR) allowing for long-term B-cell survival in the absence of antigen. In addition, it prevents the reactivation of EBV into the lytic phase of infection.

Besides EBV proteins, small nonpolyadenylated viral RNAs termed *EBERs 1* and *2* and the BamHI-A rightward transcripts (BARTS) are expressed in all forms of latency. In addition, the expression of at least 17 distinct EBV-derived microRNAs has been reported. The EBERs are the most abundant viral RNAs in latently infected cells. They enhance the oncogenic phenotype of EBV-transformed cells but are nonessential for EBV-mediated transformation. The expression pattern of the microRNAs depends on the latency type, and it is therefore likely that they play an important role during the life cycle of the virus.

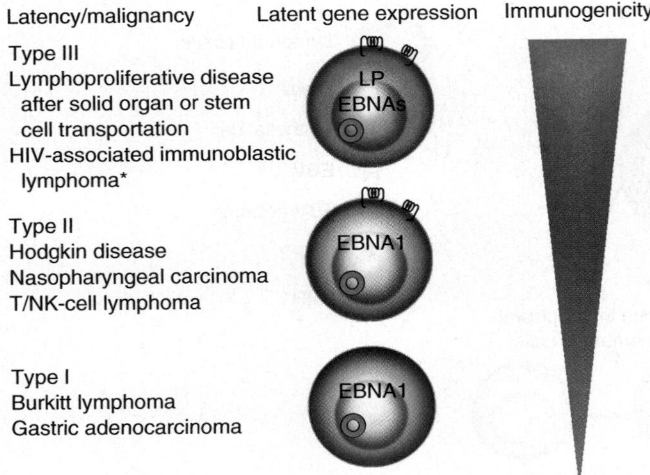

Figure 52-3 EBV-LATENT GENE EXPRESSION AND IMMUNOGENICITY OF COMMON EBV-ASSOCIATED MALIGNANCIES. *EBNA,* Epstein-Barr nuclear antigen; *LP,* leader protein. For an explanation of symbols, see Fig. 52-1. *Not all lymphomas are latency type III.

IMMUNE RESPONSE TO EBV

Healthy individuals mount vigorous humoral and cellular immune responses to primary EBV infection.[6] Although antibodies to the viral membrane proteins neutralize virus infectivity, the cellular immune response is essential for controlling virus-infected cells during both lytic and latent phases.

Humoral Immune Responses

Heterophile Antibodies

Heterophile antibodies, originally described by Paul and Bunnell, are present in 90% to 95% of EBV infections at some point during the illness. However, in infants and children under the age of 4 with primary EBV infection, heterophile antibody responses are often not detected. Heterophile antibodies are IgM antibodies, which agglutinate erythrocytes from different species, including bovine, camel, horse, goat, and sheep. EBV-induced heterophile antibodies have no reactivity against guinea pig kidney cells in contrast to naturally occurring antibodies (Forssman antibodies) or antibodies present in patients with serum sickness and other conditions.

In addition to heterophile antibodies, cold agglutinins directed preferentially against the anti-I antigen on red cell membranes are frequently detected in the sera of IM patients; however, hemolytic anemia is rare. Other antibodies (including anti-I, anti-N, Donath-Landsteiner antibodies, platelet antibodies, and anti–smooth muscle antibodies) have been described.

EBV-Specific Antibodies

EBV-specific antibody responses are detected with immunofluorescence assays developed in the first decades of EBV research. EBV antibodies are directed against (a) EBNA, (b) early antigen (EA), (c) the membrane antigen (MA) expressed on the surface of cells late in the lytic cycle, and (d) the viral capsid antigen (VCA) expressed within cells late in the lytic cycle. Each antigen is a composite of several distinct viral proteins, and attempts have been made to replace the aforementioned assays with tests using specific viral proteins; however, no single test has attracted widespread use.

VCA-IgM and -IgG antibodies are usually present at the onset of clinical symptoms because of the prolonged viral incubation period (Table 52-1). VCA-IgM antibodies are a good marker for an acute infection because they rapidly disappear within 4 to 8 weeks.

Table 52-1 Frequently Determined EBV-Specific Antibodies

Antibody Specificity	Positive in IM (%)	Time of Appearance in IM	Persistence	Comments
VIRAL CAPSID ANTIGEN				
VCA-IgM	100	At clinical presentation	4-8 weeks	Highly sensitive and specific; of major diagnostic utility
VCA-IgG	100	At clinical presentation	Lifelong	Useful for documentation of past EBV infection
EARLY ANTIGEN (EA)				
Anti-D	70	Peaks 3-4 weeks after onset	3-6 months	Correlates with disease severity; seen in NPC patients
Anti-R	Low	2 weeks to several months after onset	2 months to >3 years	Occasionally seen with unusually severe cases; seen in patients with African Burkitt lymphoma
EBNA	100	3-4 weeks after onset	Lifelong	Presence excludes primary EBV infection

Modified from Schooley RT: Epstein-Barr virus (infectious mononucleosis). In Mandell GL, Bennett JE, Dolin R, editors: *Principles and practice of infectious diseases,* Philadelphia, 2000, Churchill Livingstone, p 1599.

VCA-IgG antibodies persist for life and are commonly used to document prior EBV infection. IgG antibodies against EA are present at the onset of the clinical illness in approximately 70% of patients. EA antibodies are divided into methanol-sensitive (anti-D) and methanol-resistant (anti-R) antibodies, and the majority of EA antibodies detected are anti-D antibodies. The presence of anti-D antibodies is consistent with recent infection, because titers disappear after recovery. IgG antibodies to EBNA appear late in the course of almost all cases of EBV infection and persist throughout life; their presence early in a suspected case of primary EBV infection excludes the diagnosis. Aberrations in this pattern of serum reactivity are observed in many EBV-associated diseases and will be discussed under the specific disease sections. For example, the absence of EBNA antibodies despite previous EBV infection is one of the serologic markers suggestive for chronic active EBV infection (see CAEBV, later).

Cellular Immune Responses

In normal individuals, primary EBV infection often results in a massive expansion of activated, antigen-specific T cells. Using tetramer technology to enumerate antigen-specific T cells, it has been documented that the CD8 positive T-cell response may be dominated by T cells specific for a limited number of epitopes, as seen with T-cell responses against other herpesviruses. T cells specific for epitopes derived from immediate early and several early EBV proteins of the lytic cycle are dominant during the acute phase of IM, and long-term persistence of EBV-specific, CD8-positive T cells has been documented after primary EBV infection. As many as 5.5% of the circulating CD8-positive T cells in a healthy virus carrier may be positive for a single EBV epitope, illustrating how persistent EBV infection can influence the composition of the host's T-cell pool. Besides EBV-specific CD8-positive T cells, EBV-specific CD4-positive T cells play an important role in the control of EBV infections, and EBNA1-specific CD4-positive T cells have been implicated in the control of newly infected B cells. As for CD8-positive T-cell responses, there is a marked hierarchy of immunodominance, with the majority of CD4-positive T cells' responses directed against EBNA1 and to a lesser extent against EBNA3C.

EBV-Associated Malignancies

Malignancy	EBV Frequency
Hodgkin disease	≈40%
Non-Hodgkin lymphomas	
Burkitt lymphoma	20%-95%
Diffuse large B-cell lymphoma and CD30⁺ Ki-1⁺ anaplastic large cell lymphoma	10%-35%
Lymphomatoid granulomatosis	80%-95%
T cell–rich B-cell lymphoma	20%
Angioimmunoblastic lymphoma	>80%
T-cell, NK cell, and T/NK-cell lymphomas	30%-90%
Nasopharyngeal carcinoma	>95%
Gastric adenocarcinoma	5%-10%
Pyothorax-associated lymphoma	>95%
Leiomyosarcoma in immunocompromised patients	>95%

EBV VACCINE DEVELOPMENT

At present there is only limited experience with human EBV vaccines. In one study, nine seronegative children in Southern China were vaccinated with a recombinant vaccinia virus expressing the major EBV viral glycoprotein gp350. All nine patients developed neutralizing antibodies, and six patients remained EBV-negative over a 16-month period in contrast to none of the 10 controls. Another vaccine trial with a gp350 subunit vaccine has been completed, but efficacy data are not yet available. Although potentially ideal for preventing EBV-associated malignancies, vaccines providing life long immunity against primary EBV infection may not be feasible because the type of immunity required to avoid repeated infection through mucosal surfaces is not clearly defined. Moreover, a recent study suggests that the natural immune response to EBV is not sufficient to protect healthy EBV-positive individuals from repeated infections with different EBV strains.

Vaccine strategies for the immunotherapy of EBV-associated malignancies should seek to elicit or boost the EBV-specific cellular immune response against EBV latency. Individuals likely to benefit from this approach are EBV-seronegative patients scheduled to undergo solid organ transplantation or patients who have an EBV-associated malignancy with a low tumor burden or are in remission (see box on EBV-Associated Malignancies). Three vaccine studies have been conducted in EBV-positive NPC patients. In two studies patients with advanced disease were vaccinated with either dendritic cells (DCs) loaded with peptides derived from LMP2 or DCs transduced with an adenoviral vector encoding full-length LMP2 and an inactive form of LMP1. Administration of DC vaccines was safe, and a transient increase in the frequency of LMP2-specific T cells was observed on the DC/peptide vaccine trial. However, the clinical benefit in both studies was limited. Thus future studies should focus on DC vaccines with greater potency administered to subjects with less tumor burden. In another phase I clinical study, after frontline therapy, NPC patients were vaccinated with a vaccinia virus encoding the c-terminal portion of EBNA1 and LMP2. Induction of CD4- and CD8-positive antigen-specific T-cell responses was observed in the majority of patients after vaccination, and a Phase II clinical study is currently being planned.

In another trial, EBV-seronegative, HLA-B8 positive individuals were vaccinated with an MHC class I-restricted EBV peptide epitope derived from EBV latent viral protein EBNA3A; the peptide vaccine was well tolerated, but immunologic and virologic studies are pending.

In the past, EBV vaccine development was impeded by the lack of a suitable animal model. Most vaccination studies so far have been done in cottontop tamarins, a species of New World monkeys that develop B-cell lymphomas after intraperitoneal injection of EBV. This model lacks key features of human EBV disease such as oral transmission and long-term viral persistence, which are considered to be important for vaccine development. Since 1997 a rhesus monkey model for acute and persistent EBV infection is available that takes advantage of the rhesus lymphocryptovirus, which belongs to the same herpes virus subgroup as EBV. This animal model reproduces the salient features of human EBV infection, such as oral transmission, lymphadenopathy, atypical lymphocytosis, serologic responses to EBV proteins, and viral latency in B cells. In the future, this model has the potential to become a useful platform to test different vaccination strategies.

INFECTIOUS MONONUCLEOSIS

Epidemiology

EBV infections occur worldwide and in most populations 90% to 95% of adults have antibodies against EBV. Depending on geographic and socioeconomic factors, there is a wide variation in the age of primary EBV infections. Early, asymptomatic primary EBV infection occurs in individuals from lower socioeconomic groups and in third world countries. In higher socioeconomic groups in industrialized countries, the age of primary infection is often delayed until the second decade of life and clinically apparent IM is more prevalent.

Humans are the only source of EBV. EBV is present in the saliva of IM patients. A majority of EBV-positive adults shed virus into their saliva, and this percentage is increased in immunocompromised patients such as solid organ transplant recipients. EBV is viable outside the body for 2 weeks at 4° C but is susceptible to drying; the virus has not been recovered from environmental sources, suggesting that close contact is needed for viral spread. The incubation period of IM is estimated to be 30 to 50 days.

Clinical Manifestations

Primary EBV infection in infants and young children either is asymptomatic or accompanied by mild, nonspecific symptoms and signs such as fever, upper respiratory tract infection, pharyngitis with or without tonsillitis, and cervical lymphadenopathy. In contrast, approximately 50% of adolescents and young adults present with the clinical picture of IM. Frequently, a prodrome consisting of fatigue, malaise, and low-grade fever is present for 1 to 2 weeks. Prominent pharyngitis with exudative tonsillitis is often the cardinal sign of IM; other signs and symptoms are listed in Table 52-2. The adenopathy in IM most commonly affects the posterior cervical lymph nodes, although diffuse adenopathy can occur. The enlarged lymph nodes are not fixed, may be tender to palpation, and lack overlying skin erythema. Hepatomegaly is uncommon; however, splenomegaly develops in more than 50% of patients and is more prominent in the second to fourth week of the illness. Skin manifestations include a faint, morbilliform rash reminiscent of rubella and less commonly erythema multiforme and erythema nodosum. Most patients with primary EBV infection have symptoms for 2 to 4 weeks and recover without significant complications or sequelae.

Complications of Primary EBV Infections

The incidence of complications associated with primary EBV infection is low, although any organ system can be affected.

Hematologic Complications

Patients with IM may present with a wide range of hematologic findings besides the atypical lymphocytosis (Fig. 52-4). These include anemia, neutropenia, thrombocytopenia, and rare cases of aplastic anemia.

Anemia

Autoimmune hemolytic anemia occurs in approximately 3% of patients with IM. It presents in the first 2 weeks of the illness, and the majority of patients recover within 1 to 2 months. Patients usually have a positive direct Coombs test. Most common anti-I antibodies are present; however, anti-I, anti-N, and Donath-Landsteiner antibodies have also been reported. In addition to hemolysis, IM-associated anemia can be caused by erythroblastopenia.

Neutropenia

Mild, self-limiting neutropenia is a common finding during the first 4 weeks of the disease. However, severe neutropenia associated with fatal bacterial infections has been reported.

Thrombocytopenia

Mild thrombocytopenia (50,000 to 150,000/mm^3) is a common finding in patients with IM. It usually occurs within the first 2 weeks of presentation and resolves within 2 months. Severe

Table 52-2 Clinical Manifestations of Infectious Mononucleosis

Manifestation	Percentage (Range)
SYMPTOMS	
Sore throat	82 (70-88)
Malaise	57 (43-76)
Headache	51 (37-55)
Anorexia	21 (10-27)
Myalgias	20 (12-22)
Chills	16 (9-18)
Abdominal discomfort	9 (2-14)
SIGNS	
Lymphadenopathy	94 (93-100)
Pharyngitis	84 (69-91)
Fever	76 (63-100)
Splenomegaly	52 (50-63)
Hepatomegaly	12 (6-14)
Palatal enanthem	11 (5-13)
Rash	10 (0-15)
Jaundice	9 (4-10)

Modified from Schooley RT: Epstein-Barr virus (infectious mononucleosis). In Mandell GL, Bennett JE, Dolin R, editors: *Principles and practice of infectious diseases*, Philadelphia, 2000, Churchill Livingstone, p 1599.

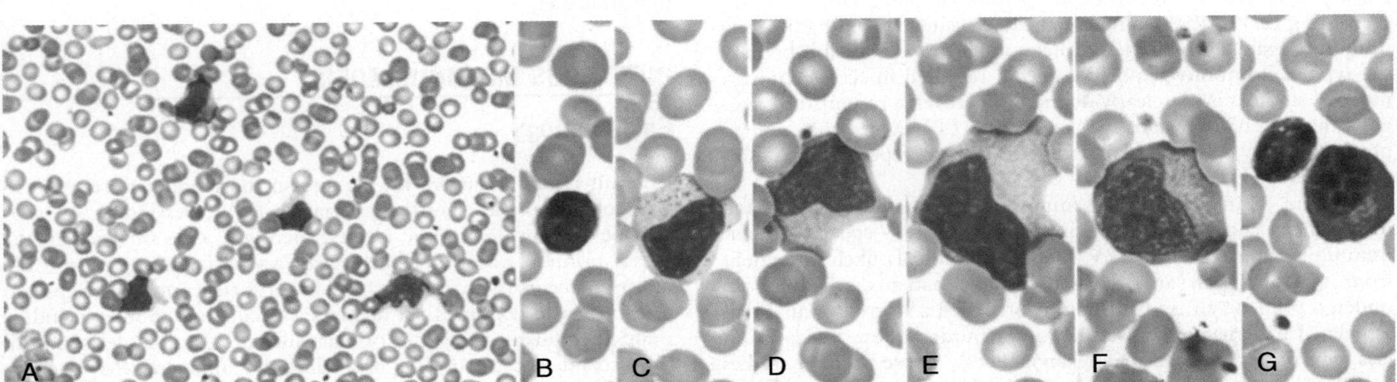

Figure 52-4 PERIPHERAL BLOOD SMEAR IN INFECTIOUS MONONUCLEOSIS. Low power **(A)** shows moderately high white blood cell count and high number of reactive, or "atypical" lymphocytes. Higher power **(B** to **G)** illustrates spectrum of lymphoid morphology, including small resting lymphocyte **(B)** for comparison, large granular lymphocyte **(C)**, atypical forms **(D** to **F)**, also referred to as "reactive" lymphs, and circulating plasma cell **(G)**.

thrombocytopenia with overt bleeding is rare; however, death from intracranial hemorrhage has been described. The etiology of the thrombocytopenia is not completely understood, and a variety of explanations have been suggested. Because bone marrow examination shows normal or increased numbers of megakaryocytes, peripheral platelet destruction is most likely due to the presence of antiplatelet antibodies or platelet pooling and destruction within an enlarged spleen.

Splenic Rupture

Splenic rupture (Fig. 52-5) occurs predominately in males, with an incidence of 1/1000 to 1/3000. The incidence of rupture is highest in the second and third week of illness and can be the first sign of IM. Clinical symptoms include abdominal pain or pain referred to either shoulder. Because abdominal pain is an unusual symptom of uncomplicated IM, a splenic rupture should be strongly considered in IM cases whenever abdominal pain is reported. Although it is a life-threatening complication, with current management, the mortality rate is very low.

Neurologic Complications

Neurologic complications develop usually during the first 2 weeks of IM and may be the only manifestation of IM. EBV infection can cause a wide spectrum of neurologic diseases, including encephalitis, meningitis, Guillain-Barré syndrome, acute transverse myelitis, and peripheral neuritis. Patients with neurologic complications have an excellent outcome, with most patients recovering completely.

Other Organ Involvement

Although symptomatic heart disease with IM is uncommon, in one cohort of patients, unspecific ST- and T-wave abnormalities were found in 6% of patients. Renal involvement manifested as microscopic hematuria, and proteinuria is seen in 10% to 15% of patients; however, significant renal dysfunction is rare. Airway compromise due to hypertrophy of the adenoids and tonsils or mucosal inflammation and edema is uncommon but potentially fatal.

Diagnosis

Atypical lymphocytosis is the cardinal hematologic finding in IM (see Fig. 52-4). It develops during the first week of the illness and peaks between the second and third week. Atypical lymphocytes represent 60% to 70% of the total white cell count, which ranges between 12,000/mm^3 and 18,000/mm^3. In general, the atypical lymphocytes are large and vary in size. Nuclei are large and eccentrically placed; the cytoplasm is basophilic, and vacuoles are often present. The variable morphologic pattern of atypical lymphocytes in IM distinguishes them from the monotonous appearance of immature leukemic blasts. Atypical lymphocytosis is not pathognomonic for IM and is associated with other diseases such as acute viral hepatitis, cytomegalovirus infections, mumps, toxoplasmosis, rubella, roseola, and drug reactions.

The diagnosis of EBV infection depends on serologic testing. Tests for heterophile antibodies, including the monospot test and slide agglutination tests, are routinely available. The results of these tests are often negative in children less than 4 years of age, but they identify 90% of cases in older children and adults. Of the available EBV-specific serologic tests, VCA-IgM antibodies are most commonly determined to diagnose primary EBV infection in heterophile-negative IM cases; determining antibodies against EA may also be helpful (Table 52-1). VCA-IgG antibodies are positive during acute infections as well as the convalescent period. The presence of anti-EBNA antibodies excludes an acute infection. Isolation of EBV from throat washings is feasible; however, it is of little diagnostic value because 10% to 20% of healthy adult EBV carriers may shed the virus.

Differential Diagnosis

In the majority of cases, the diagnosis of IM is straightforward. The differential diagnosis includes streptococcal and nonstreptococcal pharyngitis, acute infections with cytomegalovirus, human herpesvirus 6, hepatitis viruses, and toxoplasma. Depending on the presentation, other diseases may be considered such as HIV, rubella, and leukemia or lymphoma.

Treatment

Supportive therapy should include rest and analgesia in the acute stage of IM. Contact sports should be avoided until the patient has fully recovered and the spleen is no longer palpable. The use of corticosteroids is not indicated for uncomplicated IM; however, a trial of corticosteroids is warranted in patients with marked tonsillar inflammation and hypertrophy resulting in impending airway obstruction. Although acyclovir reduces EBV shedding into oral secretions, treatment of IM with acyclovir has resulted in no clinical benefit.

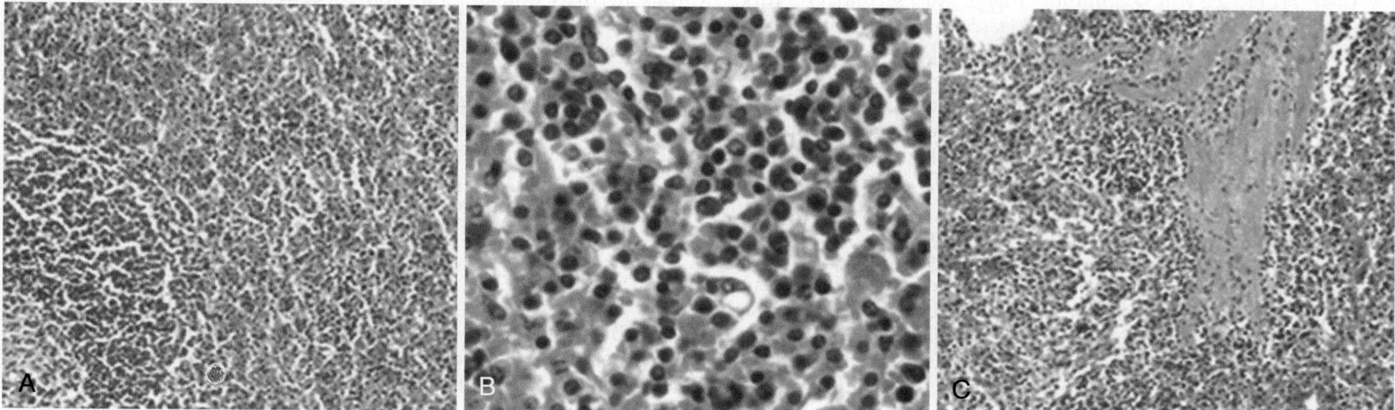

Figure 52-5 RUPTURED SPLEEN FROM PATIENT WITH INFECTIOUS MONONUCLEOSIS. Sections from the spleen show increased white cells in the red pulp (**A** and **B**). These correspond to the proliferating activated lymphocytes seen in the blood. The lymphocytes can infiltrate into the splenic trabeculae (**C**), weakening the integrity of the spleen and making it more prone to rupture.

OTHER EBV-ASSOCIATED DISEASES

Most individuals recover from the acute phase of primary EBV infection with no long-term sequelae. However, a minority of patients with intrinsic defects in immune function may respond with potentially lethal uncontrolled pathologic inflammation with fever and multisystem organ failure, meeting diagnostic criteria for hemophagocytic lymphohistiocytosis (HLH). Others may develop chronic active EBV infections (CAEBV) with persistent fever, arthralgia, myalgia, and lymphadenopathy. Additional long-term consequences of EBV infection include lymphoproliferative and malignant disorders.

Hemophagocytic Lymphohistiocytosis

HLH is a syndrome characterized by uncontrolled inflammation (see Chapter 50). Diagnostic criteria defined by the Histiocyte Society reflect the clinical features of pathologic immune activation, including persistent fever, splenomegaly, cytopenias, hyperferritinemia, decreased fibrinogen or increased triglycerides, hemophagocytosis (in bone marrow, spleen, or lymph nodes), increased soluble interleukin-2 receptor alpha, and decreased or absent natural killer (NK) cell function. The diagnosis of HLH can also be established by a pattern of familial inheritance or proven gene defects. It was first characterized as an inherited disorder in infants in the 1950s, referred to as "familial hemophagocytic reticulosis."

Gene defects resulting in impaired cytotoxic NK and T-cell function have been associated with autosomal recessive inheritance of HLH, including PRF1, UNC13D, Munc18-2, STX11, Rab27a (Griscelli syndrome, type 2), LYST (Chédiak-Higashi syndrome), and AP3B1 (Hermansky-Pudlak syndrome, type II).[7] EBV infection may trigger HLH in patients with any form of familial disease. Gene defects are identified in only 50% of patients with family history consistent with inherited HLH. Therefore, although a diagnosis "primary" or "familial" HLH may be proven, it is impossible to exclude. Familial HLH commonly presents in young children, but there are reports of new onset of HLH in adults as old as 62 years with mutations in HLH-associated genes. Patients with familial HLH typically require prompt treatment with chemotherapy and immune suppression (etoposide/dexamethasone) followed by hematopoietic stem cell transplant (HSCT).[8] Without therapy, survival of patients with active familial HLH is approximately 2 months. The first international treatment protocol for HLH organized by the Histiocyte Society in 1994 reported long-term survival of over 50%. More recently, survival rates of greater than 90% have been reported with reduced intensity conditioning regimens.[9]

The term *secondary HLH* generally refers to older children (or adults) who present without a family history or known genetic cause for their HLH. EBV is a common trigger for "secondary HLH," ranging from inflammation that resolves spontaneously to unrelenting disease requiring HSCT. Differentiating infectious mononucleosis from EBV-associated HLH (EBV-HLH) is challenging. Clinical criteria for HLH should be evaluated in patients with persistently high cell-free EBV genome copy numbers in plasma, persistent symptoms of inflammation, or severe symptoms. Patients who initially meet clinical criteria for HLH may occasionally improve spontaneously. Patients with less severe presentations may also respond to corticosteroids, intravenous immunoglobulins or cyclosporine. However, in patients with progressive or severe disease, early initiation (within 4 weeks of onset of symptoms) of etoposide is associated with significant improvement in survival.[10] Because it can eliminate EBV-infected B cells, rituximab may be a beneficial addition to other therapies in patients with progressive EBV-HLH. Some patients with apparently self-resolving HLH after primary EBV infection later develop recurrent HLH requiring immunochemotherapy and HSCT. Therefore it remains important to follow patients beyond resolution of initial symptoms. Alemtuzumab has also been reported to be effective in patients with recurrent or refractory disease.[8]

X-Linked Lymphoproliferative Diseases

XLP1

Mutations or deletions in SH2D1A (Src homology 2 domain protein 1A) results in X-linked lymphoproliferative disease (XLP1; Duncan disease), an immunodeficiency characterized by fatal IM meeting the diagnostic criteria for HLH, agammaglobulinemia, or B-cell lymphoma. SH2D1A interacts with SLAM (signaling lymphocyte activation molecule), which plays a central role in the stimulation of B and T cells. SH2D1A controls several distinct key T-cell signaling pathways, and mutant SH2D1A does not bind SLAM, suggesting that it is a natural SLAM inhibitor. SAP association with SLAM receptors is crucial for development of normal NKT cells, formation of normal germinal centers, and NK- and T-cell killing of EBV-infected B cells. T cells from patients with XLP1 are also resistant to apoptosis by reactivation-induced cell death (RICD). Immune hyperactivation induced by primary EBV infection may be due to specific defects in NK- and CD8-positive T-cell cytotoxicity rather than from decreased or absent cytotoxic proteins. Resistance to apoptosis may exacerbate the inflammatory response due to persistence of ineffective activated NK and T cells.

Following infection with EBV, XLP1 patients mount a vigorous, uncontrolled polyclonal expansion of T and B cells. Infiltrating T cells cause extensive tissue destruction of the liver and bone marrow, resulting in death in 50% of XLP1 patients during primary EBV infection. Approximately 30% of patients have acquired hypogammaglobulinemia and 25% of patients develop malignant B-cell lymphomas that are often extranodal, involving the intestinal ileocecal region. It is important to realize that some patients with SH2D1A mutations may only present with hypogammaglobulinemia mimicking common variable immunodeficiency, and a diagnosis of XLP1 should be considered when more than one male patient with hypogammaglobulinemia is encountered in the same family. Patients with fulminant immunologic responses to primary EBV infection may be treated with HLH treatment strategies (steroids and etoposide) and/or rituximab. However, the only curative therapy for XLP1 is hematopoietic stem cell transplantation.

XLP2

A second X-linked immune deficiency characterized by recurrent HLH (with or without EBV infection) is XLP2, caused by BIRC4 mutations and XIAP deficiency.[11] Unlike patients with XLP1, those with XLP2 have less pleotropic clinical manifestations. It rarely results in lymphoproliferation or lymphoma and may be more accurately characterized as "X-linked familial HLH." XIAP is a ubiquitously expressed member of a family of proteins defined by baculovirus IAP repeat (BIR) domains that inhibit apoptosis through inhibition of caspases. The mechanism of XIAP-induced HLH remains uncertain. Paradoxically, unlike in cases of XLP1, in which lymphocytes are resistant to apoptosis, XIAP deficiency in XLP2 confers increased sensitivity to radiation-induced cell death. The clinical manifestations of HLH in XLP2 patients with primary EBV infections appear less severe than in patients with XLP1. However, data remain insufficient to make specific therapy recommendations for XLP1 versus XLP2 or other forms of familial HLH.

CAEBV

CAEBV represents a range of clinical manifestations resulting from persistent, uncontrolled infection of B, T, and/or NK cells by EBV (Table 52-3).[12] Inability to control infection is likely due to defects in cytotoxic immune function. CAEBV has considerable pathologic and clinical overlap with HLH, and immune dysfunction is likely due to a variety of causes. Early descriptions of CAEBV primarily reported disease in Asian patients, and almost all cases were due to

Table 52-3 Classification of Chronic Active EBV Infection

EBV-Infected Lymphocyte	Geography	Clinical Symptoms: General	Clinical Symptoms: Skin	Clinical Course
B cell	Predominant in Western hemisphere	Fever, adenopathy, organomegaly, hepatic, cardiac, or pulmonary dysfunction	None	Chronic
T cell	Predominant in Asia: *Japan, Taiwan, Korea* Also in Native Americans: *Mexico, Central and South America*		Hydroa vacciniforme	Risk for aggressive lymphoma/leukemia
NK cell			Hypersensitivity to mosquito bites	

proliferation of EBV-infected T or NK cells. A recent review of several centers in the United States found a predominance of B cell–associated CAEBV in the western hemisphere.

To establish the diagnosis of CAEBV, patients must have (a) signs and symptoms for at least 6 months and (b) an abnormal EBV serology with high antibody titers of VCA-IgG and EA-IgG and little or no antibodies against EBNA. Affected individuals may also have measurable EA-messenger-RNA or EBV-DNA in the peripheral blood, serum, or affected tissues. The life-threatening form of CAEBV is characterized by high fevers, hepatosplenomegaly, and extensive lymphadenopathy, followed by hepatic, cardiac, or pulmonary dysfunction. These patients have very high EBV-VCA titers and EBV-DNA levels in their peripheral blood. Although EBV usually resides in B cells, in severe CAEBV, either T cells or NK cells are often infected, predisposing the patient to lethal T-cell or NK-cell lymphomas. Severe, often fatal CAEBV is more common in Japan, whereas mild/moderate CAEBV is more common in the Western hemisphere and is predominantly associated with B-cell infection. These patients do not have XLP-associated SH2D1A or BIRC4 mutations, and the etiology of CAEBV remains poorly understood. Severe allergy to mosquito bites is associated with EBV-infected NK cells, whereas hydroa vacciniforme is associated with EBV-infected T cells. The proposed classification scheme of CAEBV-associated lymphoproliferative disease (LPD) includes three categories: (1) polymorphic LPD without clonal proliferation of EBV-infected cells, (2) polymorphic LPD with clonality, and (3) monomorphic LPD (T- or NK-cell lymphoma/leukemia) with clonality.[13] In the 2008 *WHO Classification of Tumours of the Haematopoietic and Lymphoid Tissues,* LPDs associated with EBV-infected T cells are classified as systemic EBV-positive T-cell LPDs of childhood; LPDs associated with EBV-infected NK cells, as hydroa vacciniforme–like lymphoma.

Although sporadic clinical improvements of mild/moderate CAEBV have been reported after infusion of interleukin 2, high-dose immunoglobulin, antiviral drugs, anti–tumor necrosis factor (TNF)-α antibodies, or steroids, the only curative option for severe CAEBV is HSCT. Survival rates vary between 50% and 95%, with better outcomes for patients who (a) are transplanted early after diagnosis, (b) have fewer complications before transplant, and (c) have received a reduced intensity.[14] Besides HSCT, the adoptive transfer of autologous EBV-specific cytotoxic lymphocytes (CTL) has been explored in five patients with mild or moderate CAEBV. Infusion of EBV-specific CTL resulted in resolution of fatigue, malaise, fever, lymphadenopathy, and splenomegaly lasting for 6 to 36 months. For severe CAEBV in which EBV resides in the T- or NK-cell compartment, the use of EBV-specific CTL has been investigated anecdotally. For example, we have infused donor-derived LMP2-specific T cells with a good partial response as judged by decreasing EBV-DNA load.

Oral Hairy Leukoplakia

Oral hairy leukoplakia (OHL) develops frequently, although not exclusively, in HIV-positive patients. It is a nonmalignant hyperplasia of epithelial cells, and most patients present with white, corrugated lesions on the tongue. Besides IM, OHL is the only EBV-associated disease in which active viral replication is apparent, and multiple strains are often present within the same lesion. Inhibiting EBV replication in vivo with antivirals such as valacyclovir results in resolution of OHL. However, after valacyclovir treatment, EBV replication recurs in normal tongue epithelial cells, indicating that productive EBV replication is necessary but not sufficient to induce OHL.

EBV-Associated Malignancies

Over the past decades, EBV has been associated with a heterogeneous group of malignancies.[15] Although there is strong circumstantial evidence linking EBV to these malignancies, the potential causative relationship between EBV and these tumors remains to be firmly established. The following section focuses on EBV-associated lymphoproliferative disease, Hodgkin disease, NHL (including Burkitt lymphoma), and nasopharyngeal carcinoma (Fig. 52-6 and Fig. 52-7). All EBV-associated malignancies are associated with viral latency, and spontaneous viral replication occurs at a very low frequency. Because antiviral agents, like acyclovir, only prevent viral replication and do not affect latency, these agents are of limited therapeutic value.

Lymphoproliferative Disease

EBV-LPD develops in patients with congenital or acquired immunodeficiencies, including severe combined immunodeficiency, XLP, HIV infection, and immunosuppression in recipients of solid organ transplants (SOT) (see Fig. 52-6, *A, B*) or HSCT.[16] Besides EBV and a dysfunctional cellular immune system, genetic alterations in B cells have also been implicated in the pathogenesis of posttransplant lymphoproliferative disorder (PTLD), especially in SOT recipients, including microsatellite instability, DNA hypermethylation, aberrant somatic hypermutation, and mutations in specific genes such as *MYCC, BCL-6, N-ras,* and *p53.* Most cases of EBV-LPD are lymphomas of B-cell origin, histologic high-grade NHL of the immunoblastic or undifferentiated large cell type that respond poorly to cytotoxic therapy. In the setting of solid organ transplantation, the reported incidence of EBV-LPD ranges from 1% to 25%, with the highest risk in seronegative recipients, patients receiving intensive immunosuppressive therapy, and patients receiving grafts with a high lymphoid content. After HSCT the incidence of EBV-LPD varies with the transplant regimen and may be as high as 25%. Risk factors for the development of EBV-LPD include the use of stem cells from an HLA-mismatched family member or closely HLA-matched unrelated donor, T-cell depletion of the donor cells, intensive immunosuppression, and an underlying diagnosis of primary immunodeficiency. The incidence is much lower when methods that also deplete B cells are employed. The onset of EBV-LPD seems to be preceded by a large increase in virus load as well as the proliferation of

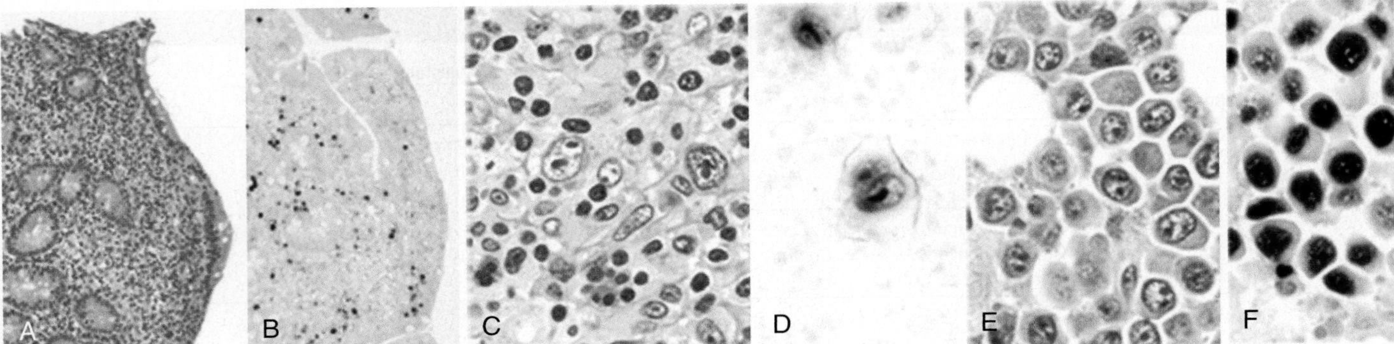

Figure 52-6 EXAMPLES OF EBV-POSITIVE LYMPHOID MALIGNANCIES: Posttransplant lymphoproliferative disorder, Hodgkin lymphoma, and large B-cell lymphoma. PTLD in the duodenum of a 15-month-old **(A)** with history of liver transplant. The PTLD was classified as a polymorphic type and was EBV-positive **(B)**. Hodgkin lymphoma **(C)** and EBV-positive Reed-Sternberg cells **(D)**. Large B-cell lymphoma (plasmablastic type) in an HIV-positive patient **(E)**, diffusely EBV-positive **(F)**. Note, all EBV studies are in situ hybridizations for EBV mRNA, EBER.

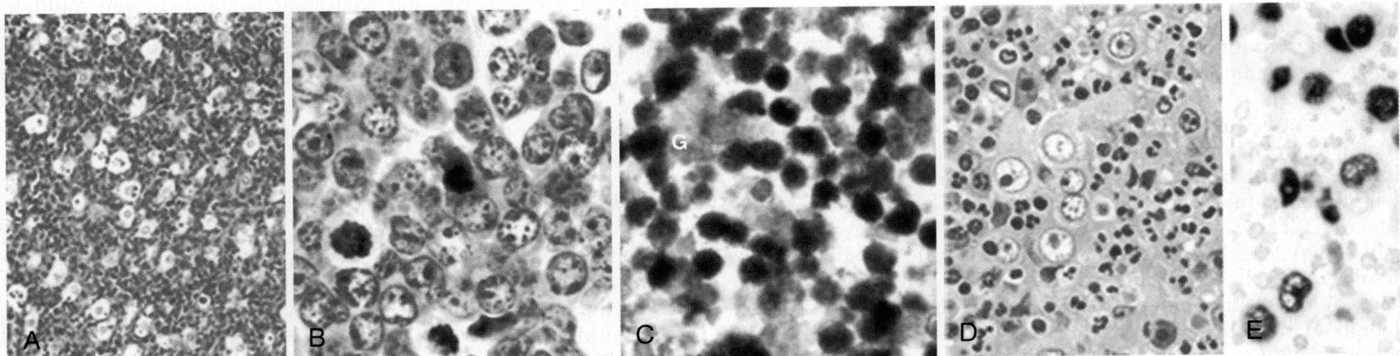

Figure 52-7 FURTHER EXAMPLES OF EBV-POSITIVE MALIGNANCIES: Burkitt lymphoma and nasopharyngeal carcinoma **(A** to **E)**. Low power of Burkitt lymphoma showing the classic "starry sky" appearance **(A)** and higher power illustrating the highly proliferative lymphoma cells **(B)**, which are uniformly EBV$^+$ **(C)**. Nasopharyngeal carcinoma **(D)** with EBV-positive cells **(E)** demonstrated by in situ hybridization for EBV mRNA.

EBV-infected B cells. Frequent monitoring of the EBV-DNA load in peripheral blood is a valuable diagnostic test for early detection of EBV-LPD after HSCT or SOT. The threshold level of EBV-DNA suggestive of impending EBV-LPD varies according to the PCR method of quantifying viral DNA. However, it should be emphasized that not all patients with high EBV-DNA levels, especially those with a solid organ transplant, develop EBV-LPD. Several distinct patterns of EBV latent gene expression have been identified in the memory B cells of high-load EBV carriers, with type III latency conferring the highest risk for EBV-LPD development. Besides EBV-DNA levels, determining the frequency of EBV-specific T cells or the functionality of T cells in patients with high EBV-DNA load might also assist in identifying patients who are at increased risk for developing EBV-LPD. In addition, host factors such as polymorphisms in the promoter regions of cytokines have been implicated in increasing the risk for developing EBV-LPD. Thus an elevated EBV-DNA load can lead to early diagnosis of EBV-LPD, with consequent reductions in mortality and treatment-related morbidity, although additional results such as clinical signs and symptoms, as well as radiographic findings, must be taken into account before therapy is initiated (Fig. 52-8).[17,18]

Treatment of Lymphoproliferative Disease

A variety of treatment approaches have been explored for EBV-LPD (Fig. 52-9). These include reduction or withdrawal of immunosuppression, conventional chemotherapy, radiation for localized disease, monoclonal antibodies, adoptive transfer of T cells or EBV-specific cytotoxic T lymphocytes (CTL), and autologous or allogeneic HSCT for refractory cases.[16,19] Other potential strategies include the use of hydroxyurea to eradicate EBV episomes or inducing the lytic cycle of EBV so that the lymphoma cells become sensitive to ganciclovir. In SOT recipients simple withdrawal of immune suppression can result in the regression of localized EBV-LPD by allowing recovery of the suppressed cellular immune system. This approach is limited by the risk for graft rejection, and it is not useful after HSCT because of the profound immunosuppression and the risk for inducing graft-versus-host disease (GVHD).

Monoclonal Antibody Therapy

The CD20 monoclonal antibody rituximab is currently widely used as prophylaxis and as therapy for EBV-LPD. A comprehensive review of the literature that included articles and abstracts published between 1999 and 2008 reported that the use of rituximab as preemptive therapy prevented the development of EBV-LPD in 90% of 341 HSCT recipients, while therapy was associated with a response rate of 63% in 126 HSCT patients.[20] However, response rates varied widely, likely reflecting heterogeneity in patient populations and the fact that early diagnosis and treatment leads to better outcomes. For EBV-LPD after SOT, a recent multicenter analysis of 80 patients reported that rituximab-based therapy had a 3-year progression-free survival of 70% compared with 21% for patients treated without rituximab.[21] Half of the patients treated with rituximab also received chemotherapy, most of them having bulky disease and a high International Prognostic Index. A recent prospective multicenter study suggests that sequential therapy of rituximab followed by chemotherapy results in excellent disease control and overall survival. However, at present it remains unclear for which group of patients rituximab monotherapy is sufficient. Retrospective studies have identified risk factors including extralymphatic disease, high LDH, low albumin, and poor performance status, but these risk factors need to

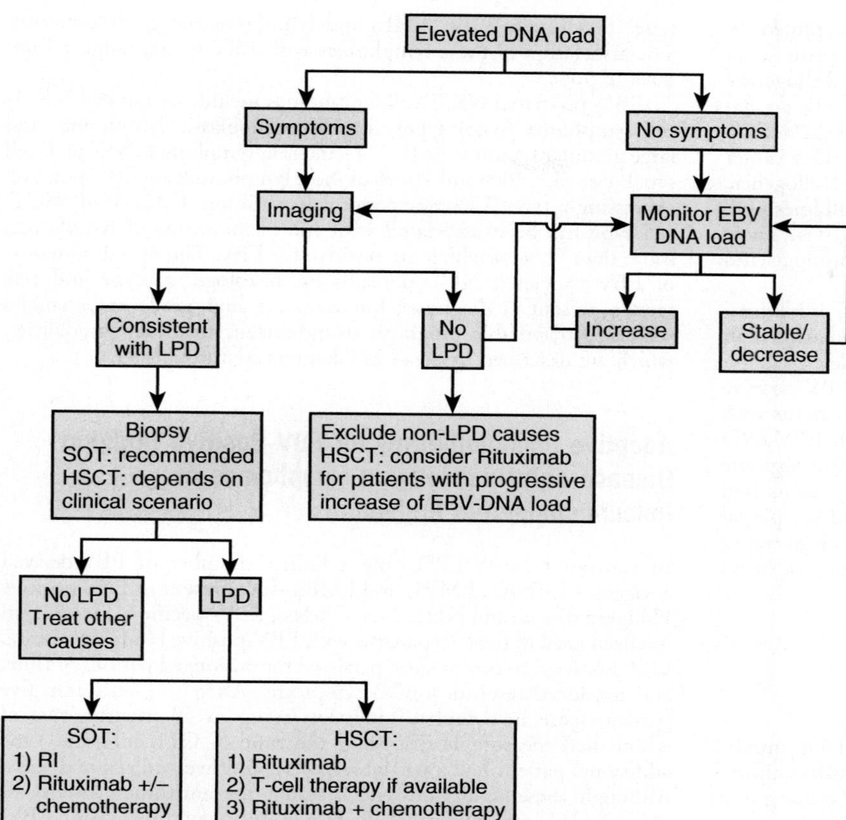

Figure 52-8 RECOMMENDED ALGORITHM FOR FOLLOWING PATIENTS WITH INCREASED EBV-DNA LOAD. *HSCT,* Hematopoietic stem cell transplant; *RI,* reduction of immunosuppression; *SOT,* solid organ transplant.

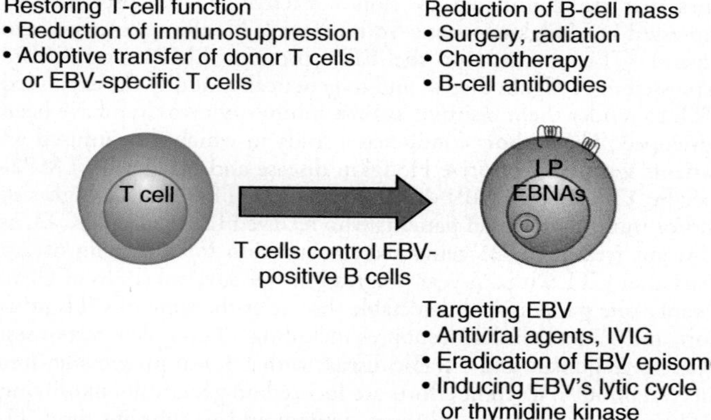

Figure 52-9 TREATMENT STRATEGIES FOR EPSTEIN-BARR VIRUS–ASSOCIATED LYMPHOPROLIFERATIVE DISEASES (EBV-LPD). For an explanation of symbols, see Fig. 52-1.

be validated in prospective studies.[22] In summary, rituximab has led to a dramatic improvement in outcome of EBV-LPD. However, rituximab does not restore the cellular immune response to EBV, which may be crucial for the long-term control of EBV-mediated B-cell proliferation. EBV-infected B cells may therefore increase with B-cell recovery, and EBV-LPD may recur. Although rare, the recurrence of CD20-negative lymphomas with the use of rituximab has been reported. Patients who fail to respond to chemo-immunotherapy strategies may respond to high-dose chemotherapy with HSC rescue.

T-Cell Therapies

Donor T-cell infusions have been used successfully to treat EBV-LPD post-HSC transplantation but carry the inherent risk for GVHD. One strategy to prevent GHVD after T-cell infusion is the administration of donor-derived ex vivo expanded polyclonal EBV-specific CTL. To determine whether adoptive transfer of donor-derived EBV-specific CTL is effective prophylaxis for EBV-LPD, EBV-specific CTL lines were infused into approximately 100 recipients of HSC transplant. Patients infused with CTL experienced no GVHD, survived long-term, and developed reconstituted immunity against EBV, and no infused patient developed EBV-LPD compared with an incidence of 11.5% in a comparable untreated control group.[5] Immunotherapy with EBV-specific CTL was also used to treat 13 HSC transplant recipients who developed overt lymphoma. Eleven of these patients responded well with complete regression of bulky tumors, although infused CTL caused inflammation at the tumor site. One of the responders had central nervous system (CNS) PTLD, indicating that EBV-specific CTL can cross the blood-brain barrier to eradicate CNS lesions. One patient died of progressive disease, a failure attributed to a deletion in the EBV protein EBNA3B in the tumor virus causing resistance to killing by the infused CTL.

In solid organ transplant recipients who develop EBV-LPD, donor-derived T cells are of limited value, because the tumor almost always arises in recipient B cells, and donor T cells are unlikely to survive in the recipient's hematopoietic system. Initial studies using autologous or partly HLA-matched EBV-specific CTL for the treatment or prevention of EBV-LPD after SOT have shown promising results but need further investigation.[23] In our study, 12 SOT recipients at high risk for EBV-LPD, or with active disease, received autologous CTL infusions without toxicity. None of the treated patients developed PTLD. One patient with liver PTLD showed a complete response, and one with ocular disease has had a partial response stable for more than 1 year. However, the expansion and persistence of adoptively transferred EBV-specific CTL was limited in the presence of continued immunosuppression. Drawbacks of EBV-specific T-cell therapies are the facilities needed and the time required (3–4 months) for CTL production using standard methods. Although rapid CTL production protocols are being developed, the use of readily available "banked" allogeneic EBV-specific CTL is actively being explored. In one multicenter clinical trial 31 SOT and 2 HSCT recipients with EBV-LPD, who had failed conventional therapies, received allogeneic EBV-specific CTL.[24] CTL infusions were well tolerated with no evidence of graft rejection. The overall response rate was 52% at 6 months, including 14 patients with a complete response. Our center has conducted a multicenter clinical trial with banked allogeneic multivirus-specific CTL in 41 HSCT recipients. Eight cell lines were infused because of EBV-LPD with a response rate of 75%. These studies document the feasibility of using banked CTL products and warrant further active exploration.

Several preclinical studies have shown that HDAC inhibitors, proteosome inhibitors, and chemotherapy and/or radiation can induce the EBV lytic cycle, which is associated with the expression of the EBV-encoded thymidine kinase rendering the EBV-positive cancer cells sensitive to acyclovir or ganciclovir. Fifteen patients with refractory EBV-positive malignancies including six with EBV-LPD were treated on one clinical trial with the HDAC inhibitor arginine butyrate followed by ganciclovir.[25] Ten out of fifteen patients had significant antitumor responses with four complete and six partial responses. Three patients experienced complications from rapid tumor lysis. Nevertheless, the encouraging antitumor responses warrant further active exploration of this approach.

EBV-Positive Hodgkin Disease and Non-Hodgkin Lymphomas

EBV is associated with Hodgkin disease as well as NHLs in immunocompetent patients. An increased incidence of EBV-positive diffuse large B-cell lymphomas has been seen in older adults,[26] leading to a separate entity in the 2008 *WHO Classification of Tumours of the Haematopoietic and Lymphoid Tissues.* All EBV lymphomas are associated with the virus latent cycle (see Fig. 52-3).[15] The majority of EBV-associated lymphomas in immunocompetent patients are latency type II and express EBNA1, LMP1, and LMP2, except for Burkitt lymphoma, which is latency type I and only expresses EBNA1.

Hodgkin Disease

Hodgkin disease is a malignant neoplasm of lymphoreticular cell origin, and 40% to 50% of cases in immunocompetent individuals are associated with expression of EBV-derived antigens in malignant Hodgkin and Reed-Sternberg (HRS) cells and their variants (see Fig. 52-6, *B, C*). EBV-positive Hodgkin disease is more commonly seen in young children and in less developed countries. EBV association with Hodgkin disease differs by histologic subtype, being highest with the mixed-cellularity subtype. Evidence linking EBV to the pathogenesis of Hodgkin disease includes the findings that (a) every HRS cell in an EBV-positive tumor mass carries the virus, and (b) the EBV genome is clonal, indicating that the malignant HRS cells originated from a single EBV-infected cell. In addition, LMP1, one of the EBV proteins expressed in HRS cells, activates the transcription factor NF-κB, which is thought to play an important role in the pathogenesis of Hodgkin disease. EBV-positive HD patients also differ in their antibody response to the major EBV-associated antigens in comparison with healthy controls. The overall outcome of EBV-positive and EBV-negative Hodgkin disease is similar; with combination chemotherapy and radiation, the prognosis is excellent for low-stage disease, and overall survival rate for advanced-stage disease is between 65% and 80% (see Chapter 74). Depending on age and histologic subtype, the presence of EBV might be associated with better survival.

Non-Hodgkin Lymphomas

NHLs expressing type II latency include diffuse large B-cell lymphoma, CD30$^+$ Ki-1 anaplastic large cell lymphoma (ALCL) of B-cell type, T cell–rich B-cell NHLs and lymphomatoid granulomatosis. The association of these lymphomas with EBV varies, ranging from 10% to 95%.

EBV-associated NK/T-cell lymphomas include extranodal NK/T-cell lymphoma (nasal type), angioimmunoblastic lymphoma, and large granular lymphocyte (LGL) leukemia/lymphoma (NK- or T-cell type). Between 30% and 100% of these lymphomas are EBV-positive, expressing a type II latency pattern. In addition, CAEBV of NK/T-cell type has been associated with fulminant forms of lymphoma, more than 95% of which are positive for EBV. The overall outcome of EBV-associated NHL depends on histologic subtype and risk factors present at diagnosis, but most are high-grade malignancies with an unfavorable prognosis using current treatment modalities, which are described in detail in Chapters 81 through 84.

Adoptive Immunotherapy for EBV-Positive Hodgkin Disease and Non-Hodgkin Lymphomas in Immunocompetent Individuals

In contrast to EBV-LPD only a limited number of EBV-derived antigens—EBNA1, LMP1, and LMP2—are present in EBV-positive Hodgkin disease and NHL. Nevertheless, EBV-specific CTL infusion has been used to treat 20 patients with EBV-positive Hodgkin disease. CTL localized to tumor sites, persisted for prolonged periods of time, and produced resolution of B symptoms. After CTL infusion, five patients were in complete remission at up to 40 months, two of whom had measurable disease at the time of CTL infusion. One additional patient had a partial response, and five had stable disease. Although these results are encouraging, the antitumor activity of infused CTL was lower than in HSCT recipients treated for EBV-LPD. This lack of efficacy could be due in part to immunosuppressive factors secreted by HRS cells or may simply be quantitative in that the method used for EBV-specific CTL generation produces CTL lines that are dominated by clones reactive to viral proteins not expressed in Hodgkin disease. To improve CTL efficacy, methods to expand CTL specific for the EBV proteins LMP1 and LMP2 expressed in Hodgkin disease and to genetically modify the expanded CTL to render them resistant against inhibitory cytokines have been developed. The authors conducted a study in which they infused 43 patients with EBV-positive Hodgkin disease and NHL with LMP2-specific CTLs[27] or LMP1-/LMP2-specific CTLs. Of 22 high-risk and/or multiply relapsed patients who received LMP-specific CTL as adjuvant treatment, 21 remained in remission for a median of 2.5 years after CTL with a 3-year progression-free survival (PFS) of 80%. Twenty-one patients had detectable disease at the time of CTL infusion, and 17 had clinical responses including 13 complete responses, 3 partial responses, and 1 stable disease with a 3-year progression-free survival of 60%. Current efforts are focused on genetically modifying CTLs to increase their antitumor activity and to simplify the CTL production process in preparation for a definitive efficacy study.

EBV-Associated Non-Hodgkin Lymphoma in HIV Patients

Patients infected with HIV are at high risk to develop NHL. The incidence increases with age, and the male-to-female ratio is approximately 2 : 1. Depending on certain histologic features, the EBV association ranges from 30% in systemic HIV-related Burkitt lymphoma (HIV-BL) to 70% to 80% in HIV-related immunoblastic lymphoma (HIV-IBL), and virtually all cases of primary central nervous system lymphoma (PCNSL) are EBV positive. In biopsies of EBV-associated HIV-NHL, there is considerable variation in the number of EBV-positive cells, and the pattern of EBV latent gene expression varies among tumor types as in immunocompetent individuals (see Fig. 52-6, *E, F*). In HIV-infected patients, the development of EBV-associated HIV-NHL is preceded by a loss of functional EBV-specific CTL, suggesting that strategies to boost the endogenous EBV-specific

T-cell response might prevent lymphomas. Restoring CD4-positive T-cell counts in HIV patients with highly active antiretroviral therapy (HAART) has decreased the incidence of PCNSL and HIV-NHL. The clinical experience with T-cell therapy for EBV-associated HIV-NHL is limited.

Burkitt Lymphoma

Burkitt lymphoma (BL) is a high-grade malignant small noncleaved B-cell lymphoma. Histology usually reveals a "starry-sky" pattern resulting from numerous benign macrophages that have ingested apoptotic tumor cells (see Fig. 52-7, *A-C*). Although almost all endemic BLs in equatorial Africa are associated with EBV, the virus has been implicated less often in sporadic cases, and in the United States only 20% of BL are EBV positive. In developing countries, an intermediate type of BL has been described, both in its clinical presentation and association with EBV, which varies from 25% to 80%. As with NPC and Hodgkin disease, there is strong circumstantial evidence linking EBV to BL. The EBV genome is clonal as in other EBV-associated malignancies. The majority of BLs carry a translocation between the long arm of chromosome 8, the site of the MYCC oncogene (8q24), and the Ig heavy chain region on chromosome 14, t(8;14). Although the t(8;14) translocation is seen in endemic as well as sporadic BLs, the exact location of the chromosomal breakpoints on chromosome 8 and 14 differ. Other chromosomal translocations seen in BLs are between MYCC and the κ-light chain locus on chromosome 2, t(2;8), or the λ-light chain locus on chromosome 22, t(8;22).

Current treatment strategies rely on intensive chemotherapy, and overall survival depends on extent of disease at presentation, being 90% to 100% for local and 60% to 70% for advanced disease. The prospect for the development of an EBV-specific immunotherapy for BLs is problematic because lymphoma cells evade the immune system by downregulating the expression of EBV latency antigens, cell adhesion molecules, and MHC class I molecules. EBNA1, the only EBV protein expressed in BL, autoregulates its own translation and inhibits HLA class I presentation because of an internal glycine-alanine repeat region. However, the characterization of EBNA1-specific CD4-positive T cells, as well as rare CD8-positive T cells that can recognize BL through EBNA1, has provided impetus to explore the role of CD4-positive T cells in the control and therapy of BL. In addition, EBNA1-specific CD4-positive T cells had potent antitumor activity in a murine model of Burkitt lymphoma. As discussed in the EBV-LPD section, induction of the lytic EBV cycle is another attractive EBV-targeted approach for Burkitt lymphoma.

Nasopharyngeal Carcinoma

Nasopharyngeal carcinoma (NPC) arises from the epithelial cells of the nasopharynx. The WHO classifies NPC into keratinizing squamous cell carcinoma (type 1), nonkeratinizing carcinoma (type 2), and undifferentiated carcinoma (type 3, most common). Type 2 and 3 carcinomas are associated with EBV (see Fig. 52-7, *D, E*)[28]; however, environmental and genetic factors play an important role in oncogenesis, because the incidence of NPC varies 50- to 100-fold from Southern China to Western countries. EBV was initially linked to NPC by the observation that patients had elevated levels of VCA-IgG, VCA-IgA, and EA-IgG antibodies. Further studies showed that EBV-DNA is present in every tumor cell of type 2 and 3 carcinomas with remarkable consistency. As in Hodgkin disease, the EBV episome in an individual tumor is clonal.

EBV antibody responses have been used to follow tumor burden in NPC patients; in addition, VCA-IgA antibodies and antibodies against EBV DNase are predictive for NPC in high-risk populations. More recently, detection of EBV-DNA in serum by different PCR methods has shown to be useful for the diagnosis, prognosis, and monitoring of NPC patients. Most NPC patients are treated with radiation. Other modalities such as surgery, chemotherapy, and combined approaches may be appropriate in selected circumstances, but a detailed discussion is beyond the scope of this chapter. In NPC, as for EBV-positive lymphomas, only a limited number of EBV latent antigens are expressed. Three therapeutic vaccine studies targeting LMP2, LMP1 and LMP2, or EBNA1 and LMP2 have been conducted, and the results of these trials were discussed in the earlier section EBV Vaccine Development.

The adoptive transfer of autologous EBV-specific CTL is being actively explored.[29] Several groups have reported that the infusion of CTLs is safe and has resulted in clinical responses, especially in patients with locoregional disease.[30] Clinical outcome correlated with the presence of LMP2-specific T cells in the CTL product. As for EBV-positive Hodgkin disease and NHL, current research studies are focused on improving the antitumor activity of EBV-specific CTL, simplifying CTL production, and determining how to best integrate the adoptive transfer of EBV-specific CTL with conventional therapy.

FUTURE DIRECTIONS

Since its discovery in 1964, EBV has been linked to a heterogeneous group of diseases. EBV was the first human virus implicated in oncogenesis, and the biology of the virus has been studied extensively on a cellular and molecular level. Over the last decade, successful immunotherapeutic approaches have been developed for EBV-associated lymphoproliferative disease using either monoclonal antibodies or the adoptive transfer of EBV-specific T cells. Further insights into the function of EBV proteins and host-virus interactions hold the promise of improving the outcome of patients with EBV-associated diseases in the future.

REFERENCES

1. Young LS, Rickinson AB: Epstein-Barr virus: 40 years on. *Nat Rev Cancer* 4:757, 2004.
2. Cohen JI: Epstein-Barr virus infection. *N Engl J Med* 343:481, 2000.
3. Rickinson AB, Kieff E: Epstein-Barr virus. In Knipe DM, Howley PM, editors: *Fields virology*, Philadelphia, 2001, Lippincott Williams & Williams, p 2575.
4. Choquet S, Oertel S, Leblond V, et al: Rituximab in the management of post-transplantation lymphoproliferative disorder after solid organ transplantation: Proceed with caution. *Ann Hematol* 86:599, 2007.
5. Heslop HE, Slobod KS, Pule MA, et al: Long-term outcome of EBV-specific T-cell infusions to prevent or treat EBV-related lymphoproliferative disease in transplant recipients. *Blood* 115:925, 2010.
6. Hislop AD, Taylor GS, Sauce D, et al: Cellular responses to viral infection in humans: Lessons from Epstein-Barr virus. *Annu Rev Immunol* 25:587, 2007.
7. Filipovich AH: Hemophagocytic lymphohistiocytosis (HLH) and related disorders. *Hematology Am Soc Hematol Educ Program* 127, 2009.
8. Jordan MB, Allen CE, Weitzman S, et al: How I treat hemophagocytic lymphohistiocytosis. *Blood* 118:4041, 2011.
9. Marsh RA, Vaughn G, Kim MO, et al: Reduced-intensity conditioning significantly improves survival of patients with hemophagocytic lymphohistiocytosis undergoing allogeneic hematopoietic cell transplantation. *Blood* 116:5824, 2010.
10. Imashuku S: Treatment of Epstein-Barr virus–related hemophagocytic lymphohistiocytosis (EBV-HLH); update 2010. *J Pediatr Hematol Oncol* 33:35, 2011.
11. Filipovich AH, Zhang K, Snow AL, et al: X-linked lymphoproliferative syndromes: Brothers or distant cousins? *Blood* 116:3398, 2010.
12. Cohen JI, Kimura H, Nakamura S, et al: Epstein-Barr virus–associated lymphoproliferative disease in non-immunocompromised hosts: A status report and summary of an international meeting, 8-9 September 2008. *Ann Oncol* 20:1472, 2009.
13. Ohshima K, Kimura H, Yoshino T, et al: Proposed categorization of pathological states of EBV-associated T/natural killer–cell lymphoproliferative disorder (LPD) in children and young adults: Overlap with

chronic active EBV infection and infantile fulminant EBV T-LPD. *Pathol Int* 58:209, 2008.
14. Kawa K, Sawada A, Sato M, et al: Excellent outcome of allogeneic hematopoietic SCT with reduced-intensity conditioning for the treatment of chronic active EBV infection. *Bone Marrow Transplant* 46:77, 2011.
15. Thorley-Lawson DA, Gross A: Persistence of the Epstein-Barr virus and the origins of associated lymphomas. *N Engl J Med* 350:1328, 2004.
16. Gottschalk S, Rooney CM, Heslop HE: Post-transplant lymphoproliferative disorders. *Annu Rev Med* 56:29, 2005.
17. Heslop HE: How I treat EBV lymphoproliferation. *Blood* 114:4002, 2009.
18. Weinstock DM, Ambrossi GG, Brennan C, et al: Preemptive diagnosis and treatment of Epstein-Barr virus–associated post-transplant lymphoproliferative disorder after hematopoietic stem cell transplant: An approach in development. *Bone Marrow Transplant* 37:539, 2006.
19. Nourse JP, Jones K, Gandhi MK: Epstein-Barr virus–related post-transplant lymphoproliferative disorders: Pathogenetic insights for targeted therapy. *Am J Transplant* 11:888, 2011.
20. Styczynski J, Einsele H, Gil L, et al: Outcome of treatment of Epstein-Barr virus–related post-transplant lymphoproliferative disorder in hematopoietic stem cell recipients: A comprehensive review of reported cases. *Transpl Infect Dis* 11:383, 2009.
21. Evens AM, David KA, Helenowski I, et al: Multicenter analysis of 80 solid organ transplantation recipients with post-transplantation lymphoproliferative disease: Outcomes and prognostic factors in the modern era. *Journal of Clinical Oncology* 28:1038, 2010.
22. Knight JS, Tsodikov A, Cibrik DM, et al: Lymphoma after solid organ transplantation: Risk, response to therapy, and survival at a transplantation center. *J Clin Oncol* 27:3354, 2009.
23. Savoldo B, Goss JA, Hammer MM, et al: Treatment of solid organ transplant recipients with autologous Epstein-Barr virus–specific cytotoxic T lymphocytes (CTLs). *Blood* 108:2942, 2006.
24. Haque T, Wilkie GM, Jones MM, et al: Allogeneic cytotoxic T-cell therapy for EBV-positive posttransplantation lymphoproliferative disease: Results of a phase 2 multicenter clinical trial. *Blood* 110:1123, 2007.
25. Perrine SP, Hermine O, Small T, et al: A phase 1/2 trial of arginine butyrate and ganciclovir in patients with Epstein-Barr virus–associated lymphoid malignancies. *Blood* 109:2571, 2007.
26. Dojcinov SD, Venkataraman G, Pittaluga S, et al: Age-related EBV-associated lymphoproliferative disorders in the Western population: A spectrum of reactive lymphoid hyperplasia and lymphoma. *Blood* 117:4726, 2011.
27. Bollard CM, Gottschalk S, Leen AM, et al: Complete responses of relapsed lymphoma following genetic modification of tumor antigen–presenting cells and T-lymphocyte transfer. *Blood* 110:2838, 2007.
28. Raab-Traub N: Epstein-Barr virus in the pathogenesis of NPC. *Semin Cancer Biol* 12:431, 2002.
29. Comoli P, Pedrazzoli P, Maccario R, et al: Cell therapy of stage IV nasopharyngeal carcinoma with autologous Epstein-Barr virus–targeted cytotoxic T lymphocytes. *J Clin Oncol* 23:8942, 2005.
30. Louis CU, Straathof K, Bollard CM, et al: Adoptive transfer of EBV-specific T cells results in sustained clinical responses in patients with locoregional nasopharyngeal carcinoma. *J Immunother* 33:983, 2010.

PART VII

Hematologic Malignancies

CHAPTER 53

PROGRESS IN THE CLASSIFICATION OF MYELOID NEOPLASMS: CLINICAL IMPLICATIONS

John Anastasi and Ronald Hoffman

The myeloid neoplasms are a heterogeneous group of diseases. In general terms, they are clonal hematopoietic malignancies that can arise in or affect a single myeloid lineage (e.g., monocytic) or they can be derived from a pluripotent progenitor cell and can affect multiple or even all myeloid cell types (erythroid, megakaryocytic, monocytic, neutrophilic, basophilic, eosinophilic, and mast cells). The myeloid neoplasms include chronic and acute diseases and those that evolve from an indolent process to a more aggressive state. As such, they can manifest as proliferative disorders, mostly involving primary mature hematopoietic elements, they can predominately affect immature or blastic cells, or sometimes they can be a combination of the two. Also, indolent disorders can evolve to more aggressive forms over time. The diseases can be proliferative, resulting in excess production of blood cells, or they can proliferate in the bone marrow (BM) and exhibit ineffective hematopoiesis, resulting in peripheral cytopenias. Because the diseases range from indolent to acute, they exhibit a wide variation in prognosis. Some disorders are fairly indolent and require only supportive care and transfusional support; others slowly progress but have no successful treatment option; and others are acute and life threatening, even within days or weeks after presentation, but are often curable if appropriately managed. Accurate, timely diagnosis and correct classification can have a tremendous clinical impact on outcome.

The diagnosis of the myeloid neoplasms typically requires a multifaceted team approach that relies on cooperation among the clinician, laboratory personnel, and a skilled pathologist. The precise diagnosis requires compiling accurate historical data, clinical information, general laboratory findings, and carefully interpreted observations from the peripheral blood smear, bone core biopsy, and aspirate merged with information from immunophenotyping, cytogenetic analysis, and molecular studies (Table 53-1). Although in some cases a diagnosis can be made with a quick examination of the blood smear, with a single molecular test, or with a simple immunophenotype, in general, careful assessment of a large body of information gives the most accurate and clinically relevant diagnosis. Future routine diagnostic modalities may include next-generation sequencing, single-nucleotide polymorphism array karyotyping, gene expression arrays, and genome-wide epigenetic studies.

The myeloid neoplasms are grouped and understood as different categories of diseases. These categories seem to constantly be changing in name and in the component disorders, but the refinements have evolved with more understanding of the clinical, pathologic, and genetic basis of the diseases and ultimately serve, or at least strive to, improve diagnosis, treatment, and outcome. Currently, the categories of myeloid neoplasms include the myeloproliferative neoplasms (MPNs), acute myeloid leukemias (AMLs), myelodysplastic syndromes (MDS), and a category of entities with features intermediate between MDS and MPN, the MDS/MPNs (Table 53-2). This generally accepted classification system was derived historically from a number of earlier classification systems,[1-4] with recent revisions from the World Health Organization (WHO) committee working on hematopoietic and lymphoid tumors. The latter was undertaken in conjunction with input from a panel of clinicians with expertise in the specific areas.[5-7] It is likely that newer information from the more recent molecular testing modalities will provide additional insight into the molecular pathogenesis that will further impact the classification and categorization of these neoplasms (Fig. 53-1).[8]

THE MYELOPROLIFERATIVE NEOPLASMS

The MPNs (Table 53-3), formerly referred to as the myeloproliferative disorders (MPDs), are a group of clonal multipotential hematopoietic stem cell disorders that have a proliferative nature, frequently with hypercellular BMs, and an elevation of one or more cell types in the blood. They are insidious in onset, and chronic in course but have a variable tendency to terminate in BM failure or acute leukemia.[9] The MPNs include the model disease, chronic myeloid leukemia (CML) (see Chapter 66). This has become a prototype in medicine because it illustrates how the elucidation of pathways involved in the molecular pathogenesis of a process (i.e., dysregulation of *ABL1* tyrosine kinase signaling) can lead to the rational development of targeted therapy for the disease (i.e., imatinib and other tyrosine kinase inhibitors).[10]

The MPNs also include the rare myeloid (and lymphoid) neoplasms with eosinophilia (listed separately in the WHO schema) (see Chapter 70). Although quite uncommon, these are noteworthy, because similar to CML, they have also been found to be caused by dysregulation of TK signaling (caused by mutations in *PDGFRA, PDGFRB,* or *FGFRA*) and, at least partly, can also be successfully treated with TK inhibition.[11] The other MPNs include the more common *BCR-ABL1*–negative entities, essential thrombocythemia, polycythemia vera (PV), and primary myelofibrosis (see Chapters 67 to 69). These are related biologically, with multipotential hematopoietic stem cell origin, clonal proliferation, and chronic nature. Although they seem to be distinctive because there is very little transformation from one to another, early in their course they can present a diagnostic challenge, and they can be difficult to distinguish from one another because more characteristic features have not yet developed. Recent discoveries in the underlying molecular pathology of these entities have demonstrated that similar to CML and the eosinophilic disorders, they too share TK signaling dysregulation, at least to some degree. This is attributable to an associated mutation in the TK, *JAK2* (*JAK2* V617F), which is present in about 50% to 95% of cases.[12] This association has led to significant revisions in the criteria for diagnosis of these entities but has raised questions of how a single mutation can be associated with such heterogeneous phenotypic characteristics.[13] Unfortunately, the *JAK2* V617F discovery has not yet led to a successful therapeutic approach[14] but has focused attention on issues such as clone size, mutational load, and clonal dynamics that will likely be of clinical importance.[15] Mutations in other genes may also provide a more complete picture of additional pathways involved in these disorders.[16]

Chronic neutrophilic leukemia (CNL) and mast cell disease (see Chapter 71) are also included in the category of MPNs. Although it is surrounded by some controversy as to whether it is truly neoplastic, CNL is a rare entity that is not well understood at either the clinical or molecular level.[17] Mast cell disease is yet another disease related to

Table 53-1 Components in the Routine Clinical Evaluation of the Myeloid Diseases

CURRENT

- Accurate clinical history, including family history and physical examination findings
- General laboratory findings, including CBC, and other specific tests (e.g., EPO) when appropriate
- Evaluation of well-prepared and stained peripheral blood smear with 200 cell differential count
- Review of BM aspirate, including iron stain, and 500 cell differential count
- Evaluation of H&E sections of BM biopsy of sufficient length and reticulin stain
- Phenotyping studies, including cytochemical reactions (nonspecific and specific esterase reactions and myeloperoxidase) and flow cytometric analysis of peripheral blood or BM for phenotype of blasts or other cells when appropriate
- Cytogenetic analysis, including karyotype, and FISH for specific abnormalities when appropriate
- Genetic analysis for particular genetic rearrangements or mutations, including gene sequencing when appropriate

POTENTIAL FUTURE CLINICAL STUDIES

- Next-generation sequencing
- Single-nucleotide polymorphism array karyotyping
- Gene expression arrays
- Genome-wide epigenetic studies

BM, Bone marrow; *CBC,* complete blood count; *EPO,* erythropoietin; *FISH,* fluorescence in situ hybridization; *H&E,* hematoxylin and eosin.

Table 53-2 The Myeloid Neoplasms

The myeloproliferative neoplasms (MPN), including the myeloid and lymphoid neoplasms with eosinophilia and abnormalities of *PDGFRA, PDGFRB,* and *FGFRA*
The acute myelogenous leukemias (AML)
The myelodysplastic syndromes (MDS)
The myelodysplastic/myeloproliferative ("overlap") syndromes (MDS/MPN)

abnormal TK signaling, in this case the *KIT* gene.[18] It has a complex classification system, including one type that is a mast cell proliferation associated with a clonal non–mast cell hematopoietic malignancies that can be another myeloid disorder or, less commonly, a lymphoid malignancy.

It is important to emphasize that the diagnosis of the MPNs does not rest solely with the routine microscopic examination of cells and tissues on slides. The diagnostic workup is more far reaching and must include reviewing the clinical history and pertinent physical findings, as well as obtaining and assessing laboratory values, including recent complete blood cell counts. Examination of a well made peripheral blood smear and both BM aspirate and biopsy specimens are still crucial. However, ancillary studies, such as cytogenetic and molecular analysis, as well as other more specific laboratory evaluations, are just as important in formulating the correct diagnosis, and in particular, in distinguishing them from reactive myeloid proliferations. This is particularly true, for example, regarding the *JAK2*

Table 53-3 The Myeloproliferative Neoplasms

Disease	Tyrosine Kinase Involvement
Chronic myeloid leukemia, *BCR-ABL1+*	*ABL1* (100%)
Myeloid and lymphoid neoplasms with eosinophilia TK abnormalities	*PDGFRA, PDGFRB,* or *FGFRA* (100%)
Polycythemia vera	*JAK2* V617F (≈95%), *JAK* exon 12 (≈4%)
Primary myelofibrosis	*JAK2* V6174 (≈50%), *MPL* W515 K/L (5%-9%)
Essential thrombocythemia	*JAK2* V617F (≈50%), *MPL* W515 K/L (≈1%)
Chronic neutrophilic leukemia	—
Chronic eosinophilic leukemia, not otherwise specified	—
Mastocytosis	*KIT* D816V (≈95%)
MPN, unclassified	—

MPN, Myeloproliferative neoplasm; *TK,* tyrosine kinase.

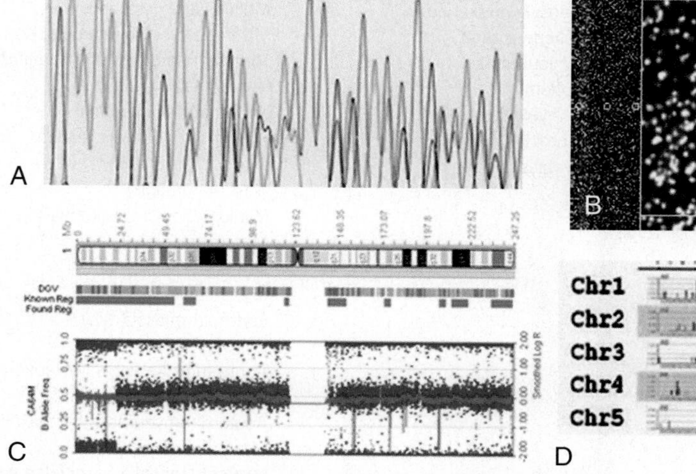

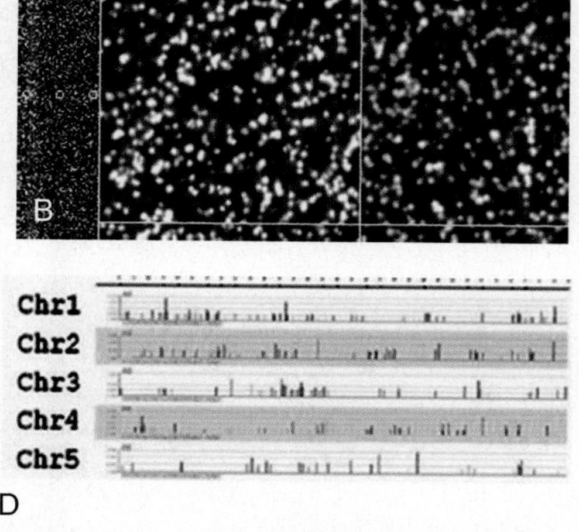

Figure 53-1 Molecular testing modalities such as sequencing **(A)**, next-generation sequencing **(B)**, single nucleotide polymorphism array karyotyping **(C)** and epigenetic studies such as whole-genome methylation analysis **(D)** will provide additional insight into the molecular pathogenesis that will undoubtedly further impact the classification and categorization of these neoplasms. *(Courtesy Drs. Loren Joseph, Megan McNerney, and Gordana Raca, University of Chicago, and Jason Cheng, University of Michigan.)*

V617F mutation and its impact on diagnosis of PV and the other more common entities in which the findings of the mutation establishes that the proliferation is clonal and not a physiologic response. Perhaps future testing with deep sequencing and epigenetic studies will become the next level of ancillary evaluations for diagnosis and classification.[19]

THE ACUTE MYELOID LEUKEMIAS

The historical and emerging classifications systems for AML dramatically illustrate the marked heterogeneity of the acute diseases within this category (Chapters 57 and 58). Despite this heterogeneity, however, decisions regarding specific initial treatment seem limited to only a few types of leukemias (e.g., acute promyelocytic leukemia).[20] Perhaps this may change as newer agents targeting molecularly or genetically defined AML become available (e.g., FLT3 inhibitors for FLT3 mutated cases).[21] It is anticipated that the gap between the growing number of unique or genetically defined acute leukemia types and the somewhat limited treatment options may begin to close.

The French–American–British (FAB) classification of AML in 1976 with its subsequent revision provided the first real framework for classifying the AMLs.[2,3] It also provided definitions of diseases that were fairly reproducible. The classification was mainly based on morphologic and cytochemical features of the leukemic blasts in the BM. In general, the FAB scheme required that 30% of the BM nucleated elements be blasts and then defined cases based on the presence of maturation in the granulocytic series, the presence of a monocytic component, and the presence of an erythroid component. Later, as immunophenotyping allowed better identification of myeloid precursors, acute megakaryoblastic leukemia and AML with minimal differentiation were added.[3] The types of AML noted in the revised FAB scheme included one with minimal differentiation (MO), a type without maturation (M1), a type with maturation (M2), acute promyelocytic leukemia (M3), a type with combined monocytic and myeloid (neutrophilic) components (M4), a pure monocytic or monoblastic type (M5A, M5B), a type with a prominent erythroid component (M6), and (as noted) a megakaryoblastic type (M7) (Table 53-4).

Although the FAB provided a framework and defined criteria for different types of acute leukemia, genetic changes associated with the leukemias that began to be recognized in the 1980s seemed to provide more important prognostic information and did not always correlate well with the FAB-defined entities. As the cytogenetic abnormalities became more widely appreciated and their prognostic implications better understood, classification schemes based solely on the "favorable," "intermediate," and "adverse" prognostic cytogenetic findings were introduced and used along with or as an alternative to the FAB scheme (see Table 53-4).[22]

The WHO classification of the acute leukemias published in 2001 provided a different strategy than the FAB in two important ways: it redefined AML as requiring only 20% blasts in the BM or blood and emphasized the importance of the associated cytogenetic abnormalities.[5] The change in blast percentage came from the recognition that patients with 20% to 30% blasts who previously were classified as having MDS (refractory anemia with excess of blasts in

Table 53-4 Classification Schemes for the Acute Myelogenous Leukemias

French–American–British (FAB, 1985)	Cytogenetic	WHO (2001)	WHO (2008)
M0: AML with minimal differentiation	**Favorable**	**Genetic**	**With recurrent genetic abnormalities**
M1: AML without maturation	t(8;21)	t(8;21)	With t(8;21)(q22;q22)
M2: AML with maturation	inv(16)/t(16;16)	t(inv(16)/t(16;16)	With inv(16)/t(16;16)(p13.1;q22)
M3: APL	t(15;17)	t(15;17)	With t(15;17)(q22;q12)
M3v: microgranular variant	**Intermediate**	t(v;11q23)	With t(9;11)(p22;q23)
M4: AMML	Normal	**AML with dysplasia therapy related AML**	With t(6;9)(p23;q34)
M4eo: AMML with abnormal eosinophils	+8	Etoposide	With inv(3)/t(3;3)(q21;q26.2)
M5A: acute monoblastic leukemia	t(v;11q23)	Cytotoxic or radiation	With t(1;22)(p13;q13)
M5B: acute monocytic Leukemia	del(7q)	**Not otherwise specified**	With mutated NPM1 (provisional)
M6: erythroleukemia	+21	With minimal differentiation	With mutated CEBPA (provisional)
M7: acute megakaryoblastic leukemia	+22	Without maturation	**With myelodysplasia related changes**
	Other	With maturation	Previous history of MDS
	Adverse	Myelomonocytic leukemia	Multilineage dysplasia
	del(5q)	Monoblastic leukemia	MDS-related cytogenetic abnormalities
	-5	Monocytic leukemia	**Therapy-related myeloid neoplasms**
	-7	Erythroleukemia	t-AML/t-MDS (t-MN)
	Complex	Erythroid myeloid type	**Not otherwise specified**
	abn (3q)	Pure erythroid	With minimal differentiation
		Megakaryoblastic	Without maturation
			With maturation
			Myelomonocytic leukemia
			Monoblastic leukemia
			Monocytic leukemia
			Erythroleukemia
			Erythroid myeloid type
			Pure erythroid
			Acute megakaryoblastic leukemia
			Acute basophilic leukemia
			Acute panmyelosis with myelofibrosis
			Myeloid sarcoma
			Myeloid leukemia associated with Down syndrome
			Blastic plasmacytoid dendritic cell tumor

AML, Acute myeloid leukemia; *AMML,* acute myelomonocytic leukemia; *APL,* acute promyelocytic leukemia; *WHO,* World Health Organization.

transformation [RAEB-T] in the FAB MDS classification) often had outcomes similar to those of AML and frequently required treatment as AML. Furthermore, the inclusion of cytogenetics recognized the important prognostic information associated with these abnormalities, as well as the fact that cytogenetics could point to the underlying molecular pathogenesis, which is critical in developing new drugs and treatment strategies as learned with CML experience. However, the WHO classification recognized that not all acute leukemias could be defined by cytogenetic abnormalities and that some needed to be defined clinically or even still based on morphologic findings. In this regard, the 2001 classification recognized four major subclasses of AML, and these included AML with recurring cytogenetic abnormalities; therapy-related AML (subclassified further as those with etoposide treatment and those with history of cytotoxic drug therapy or radiation); AML with multilineage dysplasia; and cases that did not fit into the other categories, referred to as AML, not otherwise categorized (see Table 53-4).

A revision of this 2001 classification scheme in 2008 made a number of changes (see Table 53-4).[6] In particular, it expanded the cytogenetic abnormality-associated cases to those with some less common translocations. It added provisional entities defined by mutations often occurring in cytogenetically normal cases, namely those with *NPM1* and *CEBPA* mutations. It combined the different types of therapy-related MDS/AML and renamed this category therapy-related myeloid neoplasm (t-MN). It also redefined the dysplasia-associated cases by allowing the cases to be identified by history (of previous MDS), morphology (with multilineage dysplasia) or by cytogenetics (with defined chromosomal changes associated with dysplasia). Additional categories were also added, including AML associated with Down syndrome, acute panmyelosis with myelofibrosis, granulocytic sarcoma, and blastic plasmacytoid dendritic cell tumor. In the end, the current classification defines more than 25 different types of AML. Newer technologies, such as single nucleotide polymorphism array karyotyping,[23] that will likely facilitate the recognition of many of these, may also identify additional variants. Recognizing unique entities, it is hoped will prove beneficial for understanding the diseases and common affected pathways and for developing sorely needed and successful targeted treatments.

Table 53-5 Evolving Classifications of the Myelodysplastic Syndromes (MDS)

FAB 1982	WHO 2001	WHO 2008	
RA	RA	RCUD RA RN RT	Uni- or bilineage dysplasia,* <1% PB blasts,† <5% BM blasts, <15% RS
RARS	RARS	RARS	No PB blasts, at least 15% RS, <5% BM blasts
	RCMD RCMD-RS	RCMD (-RS)	<1% PB blasts,† dysplasia >10% in two cell lines, <5% BM blasts, +/– RS, no AR§
RAEB	RAEB-1	RAEB-1	Cytopenia, <5% PB blasts, <1000/μL monocytes; dysplasia in 1 or more lines 5%-9% blasts, no AR§
	RAEB-2	RAEB-2	Cytopenia, 5%-19% blasts, <1000/μL monocytes, +/– AR; dysplasia in one or more lines, 10-19% BM blasts
		MDS-U	Cytopenia, <1% PB blasts; <10% dysplasia in any one cell line; cytogenetic abnormalities present, <5% BM blasts
		MDS with 5q-	Anemia, normal or increased platelets; isolated 5q, hypolobated megakaryocytes, no AR
		RCC (provisional)	
RAEB-T			
CMML			

AML, Acute myeloid leukemia; *AR,* Auer rods; *BM,* bone marrow; *CMML,* chronic myelomonocytic leukemia; *FAB,* French–American–British classification; *MDS-U,* myelodysplastic syndrome, unclassified; *PB,* peripheral blood; *RA,* refractory anemia; *RARS,* refractory anemia with ring sideroblasts; *RAEB,* refractory anemia with excess blasts; *RAEB-T,* refractory anemia with excess blasts in transformation; *RCC,* refractory cytopenia of childhood; *RCMD,* refractory cytopenia with multilineage dysplasia; *RCUD,* refractory cytopenia with unilineage dysplasia; *RS,* ring sideroblasts (% indicates percent RS of total nucleated erythroid precursors); *WHO,* World Health Organization classification.
*If pancytopenia, change to MDS-U.
†If 1% blasts, change to MDS-U.
‡If 2% to 4% PB blasts, upgrade to RAEB-1.
§If AR present, upgrade to RAEB-2.

THE MYELODYSPLASTIC SYNDROMES

The earliest recognition of myelodysplastic disorders came with the identification of an anemia that was long-standing and refractory to vitamin replacement followed by the recognition that these were sometimes preleukemic (see Chapters 59 and 62).[24] The classic MDS is exemplified by pancytopenia in the blood and by a hypercellular BM with ineffective hematopoiesis characterized by multilineage dysplasia, with or without an increase in blasts. Although this is fairly typical, it belies the wide pathologic spectrum of MDS, which includes cases that are diagnostically challenging and difficult to distinguish on one hand from benign causes of cytopenias in elderly patients and, on the other hand, from AML and other more aggressive clonal myeloid neoplasms.

The first real classification of MDS was proposed by the FAB group in 1982.[4] In this classification scheme, the myelodysplastic disorders were divided into four subtypes with increasing blast percentage or as chronic myelomonocytic leukemia (CMML). The four entities included refractory anemia (RA), refractory anemia with ring sideroblasts (RARS), refractory anemia with excess of blasts (RAEB), and refractory anemia with excess of blasts in transformation (RAEB-T). These entities differed mainly by the percentage of blasts seen in the BM (see Table 53-5). In the FAB scheme, as noted earlier, AML was defined by the presence of 30% or more blasts in the blood or BM.

Chronic myelomonocytic leukemia was included by the FAB in the MDS category, although it was well recognized that CMML differs in that it has a proliferative component with increased circulating monocytes.[25] At times, the peripheral leukocytosis was increased in the so-called myeloproliferative type of CMML, but the process was considered to be a dysplastic type and included in the MDS category when the white blood cell count was less than 13,000/μL.[26]

The classification of MDS presented by the WHO committee in 2001 resulted in significant changes to the classification of both MDS (Table 53-5), as well as in AML as discussed earlier.[5] As mentioned, the most notable change was the reduction in the blast percentage required for a diagnosis of AML from 30% to 20%, leading to the elimination of the RAEB-T category. The new classification also included a new subtype of MDS that, despite the lack of increased blasts (<5%), had a more aggressive course, probably owing to the presence of more pronounced multilineage dysplasia.[27] This category was called refractory cytopenia with multilineage dysplasia (RCMD), and it comprised a substantial proportion of cases previously grouped in the low-grade RA and RARS categories. Although the recognition of RCMD as a relatively more aggressive MDS served to deemphasize

Table 53-6 The Myelodysplastic/Myeloproliferative Neoplasms

- Chronic myelomonocytic leukemia (CMML)
- "Atypical" chronic myeloid leukemia ("aCML"), *BCR-ABL1* negative
- Juvenile myelomonocytic leukemia (JMML)
- Refractory anemia with ring sideroblasts and thrombocytosis (RARS-T) (provisional)

the importance of the blast percentage for prognosis, the new classification subdivided the RAEB category into two types, with 5% to 9% blasts (RAEB-1) and 10% to 19% blasts (RAEB-2), paradoxically emphasizing the prognostic significance of blast percentage in this category.[28]

A further significant change in the WHO 2001 classification scheme for MDS included the exclusion of CMML from the MDS category and the development of a separate nosologic group for CMML and other diseases in which there were features at diagnosis of both myelodysplasia and myeloproliferation.[29] These "overlap" disorders are mentioned briefly below.

Further refinements in the WHO classification scheme for MDS were made most recently in 2008 (see Table 53-5).[6,30] These included expanding low-grade MDS from refractory anemia to refractory cytopenia with unilineage dysplasia (RCUD), which recognized that the megakaryocyte or granulocyte lineage could be equally affected. The 2008 WHO classification scheme also placed emphasis on the key role of cytogenetic analysis in the diagnosis of MDS, particularly in cases with otherwise insufficient morphologic evidence to substantiate a diagnosis of MDS. This is reflected in the inclusion of the subtype, MDS unclassified (MDS-U), defined by the presence of cytopenia, less than 1% peripheral blasts, less than 10% dysplastic cells in any lineage, and less than 5% BM blasts with the presence of specific cytogenetic abnormalities commonly seen in MDS. In addition, the WHO 2008 classification now includes "MDS with an isolated del(5q)" including the "5q- syndrome".[30] This syndrome had been well known for some time and is characterized typically by its presentation in middle-aged women with macrocytic anemia, splenomegaly, normal to elevated platelet counts, hypolobated megakaryocytes in the BM, and an isolated del(5q). Thus, similar to AML, the specific types of MDS have also been increased and now account for more than 10 different entities.

THE OVERLAP MYELODYSPLASTIC/ MYELOPROLIFERATIVE NEOPLASMS

The overlap syndromes—that is, the MDS/MPNs (Table 53-6)—were introduced by the WHO committee in 2001 because there was no agreement among committee members as to whether CMML was an MDS, as suggested by the FAB, or an MPN, as suggested by a number of investigators. This group of diseases was defined to include disorders that share features of the MPNs and the MDS at the time of initial presentation but do not fit well into either group.[30] Some of the entities in the MPD/MPN category are not well understood and may represent a disease in transition from MDS or MPN, although a case should not be placed in this group if initially diagnosed as MDS or MPN. However, without the complete knowledge of the historical pathology of each individual patient, it is useful to have this category for a more reasonable classification. The overlap syndromes consist of CMML, including the juvenile type and juvenile myelomonocytic leukemia (JMML) (see Chapter 62) in addition to "atypical" chronic myeloid leukemia (atypical CML, *BCR-ABL1* negative) and an "unclassifiable" category that includes refractory anemia with ring sideroblasts and thrombocytosis (RARS-T). The MDS/MPNs share proliferative features in some cell lineages but also have dysplastic features, including ineffective hematopoiesis in others. Similar to the MPNs, the overlap syndromes require a full evaluation of clinical and morphologic findings and evaluation of ancillary studies before a firm diagnosis can be rendered.

REFERENCES

1. Dameshek W: Some speculations on the myeloproliferative syndromes. *Blood* 6:372, 1951.
2. Bennett JM, Catovsky D, Daniel MT, et al: Proposals for the classification of the acute leukaemias. French-American-British (FAB) co-operative group. *Br J Haematol* 33:451, 1976.
3. Bennett JM, Catovsky D, Daniel MT, et al: Proposed revised criteria for the classification of acute myeloid leukemia. A report of the French-American-British Cooperative Group. *Ann Intern Med* 103:620, 1985.
4. Bennett JM, Catovsky D, Daniel MT, et al: Proposals for the classification of the myelodysplastic syndromes. *Br J Haematol* 51:189, 1982.
5. Jaffe ES, Harris NL, Stein H, et al, editors: *WHO classification of tumours of haematopoietic and lymphoid tissues*, ed 3, Lyon, France, 2001, International Agency for Research on Cancer (IARC).
6. Swerdlow SH, Campo E, Harris NL, et al, editors: *WHO Classification of tumours of haematopoietic and lymphoid tissues,* ed 4, Lyon, France, 2008, IARC Press.
7. Vardiman JW, Thiele J, Arber DA, et al: The 2008 revision of the World Health Organization (WHO) classification of myeloid neoplasms and acute leukemia: Rationale and important changes. *Blood* 114:937, 2009.
8. Maciejewski JP, Haferlach T: Introduction: Molecular pathogenesis of hematologic malignancies. *Seminars Oncol* 39:9, 2012.
9. Anastasi J: The myeloproliferative and overlap, myeloproliferative/myelodysplastic neoplasms. In Hsi ED, editor: *In Hematopathology,* ed 2, St. Louis, 2012, Elsevier, p 479.
10. Druker BJ, Talpaz M, Resta DJ, et al: Efficacy and safety of a specific inhibitor of the BCR-ABL tyrosine kinase in chronic myeloid leukemia. *N Engl J Med* 344:1031, 2001 5.
11. Gotlib J: World Health Organization-defined eosinophilic disorders: 2011 Update on diagnosis, risk stratification, and management. *Am J Hematol* 86:677, 2011.
12. Campbell PJ, Baxter EJ, Beer PA, et al: Mutation of JAK2 in the myeloproliferative disorders: Timing, clonality studies, cytogenetic associations, and role in leukemic transformation. *Blood* 108:3548, 2006.
13. James C: The JAK2V617F mutation in polycythemia vera and other myeloproliferative disorders: One mutation for three diseases? *Hematology Am Soc Hematol Educ Program* 69, 2008.
14. Tefferi A: Challenges facing JAK inhibitor therapy for myeloproliferative neoplasms. *N Engl J Med* 366:844, 2012.
15. Jadersten M, Saft L, Smith A, et al: TP53 mutations in low-risk myelodysplastic syndromes with del(5q) predict disease progression. *J Clin Oncol* 29:1971, 2011.
16. Abdel-Wahab O: Genetics of the myeloproliferative neoplasms. *Curr Opin Hematol* 18:117, 2011.
17. Elliott MA, Hanson CA, Dewald GW, et al: WHO-defined chronic neutrophilic leukemia: A long-term analysis of 12 cases and a critical review of the literature. *Leukemia* 19:313, 2005 Feb.
18. Chiu A, Orazi A: Mastocytosis and related disorders. *Semin Diagn Pathol* 29:19, 2012 Feb.
19. Zhang S-J, Abdel-Wahab O: Disordered epigenetic regulation in the pathophysiology of myeloproliferative neoplasms. *Curr Hematol Malig Rep* 7:34, 2012.
20. Ablain J, de The H: Revisiting the differentiation paradigm in acute promyelocytic leukemia. *Blood* 117:5795, 2011.
21. Pratz K, Levis M: Incorporating FLT3 inhibitors into acute myeloid leukemia treatment regimens. *Leuk Lymphoma* 49:852, 2008.
22. Grimwade D, Walker H, Oliver F, et al: The importance of diagnostic cytogenetics on outcome in AML: Analysis of 1,612 patients entered into the MRC AML 10 trial. The Medical Research Council Adult and Children's Leukaemia Working Parties. *Blood* 92:2322, 1998.
23. Bullinger L, Frohling S: Array-based cytogenetic approaches in acute myeloid leukemia: Clinical impact and biological insights. *Semin Oncol* 39:37, 2012.
24. Lichtman MA: Myelodysplasia or myeloneoplasia: Thoughts on the nosology of clonal myeloid diseases. *Blood Cells Mol Dis* 26:572, 2000.
25. Germing U, Gattermann N, Minning H, et al: Problems in the classification of CMML–dysplastic versus proliferative type. *Leuk Res* 22:871, 1998.

26. Voglova J, Chrobak L, Neuwirtova R, et al: Myelodysplastic and myeloproliferative type of chronic myelomonocytic leukemia: Distinct subgroups or two stages of the same disease? *Leuk Res* 25:493, 2001.
27. Rosati S, Mick R, Xu F, et al: Refractory cytopenia with multilineage dysplasia: Further characterization of an 'unclassifiable' myelodysplastic syndrome. *Leukemia* 10:20, Jan 1996.
28. Germing U, Strupp C, Kuendgen A, et al: Prospective validation of the WHO proposals for the classification of myelodysplastic syndromes. *Haematologica* 91:1596, 2006.
29. Foucar K: Myelodysplastic/myeloproliferative neoplasms. *Am J Clin Pathol* 132:281, 2009.
30. Brunning RD, Orazi A, Germing U, et al: Myelodysplastic syndromes/neoplasms, overview. In Swerdlow SH, Campo E, Harris NL, et al, Editors: *WHO classification of tumors of haematopoietic and lymphoid tissues,* Lyons, France, 2008, IARC: 2008.

CHAPTER 54

CONVENTIONAL AND MOLECULAR CYTOGENETIC BASIS OF HEMATOLOGIC MALIGNANCIES

Vesna Najfeld

Dedicated to the loving memory of Eta Najfeld, MD, a holocaust survivor and an amazing mother.

Over the past 53 years, cytogenetic analysis of cells belonging to the array of hematologic malignancies has been an area of prolific growth. Chromosome studies and karyotype information provide information of both biologic and clinical significance. Refinements in cell culture methods and the application of chromosome banding techniques have advanced our understanding of disease-specific abnormalities, and molecular cytogenetic methods now have made possible the identification of genes involved at translocation breakpoints in specific chromosomal rearrangements. These advances in molecular cytogenetic methods permit mapping of structural rearrangements within a single gene and fundamentally contribute to our knowledge of the biology of leukemia. This evolution in our understanding of cancer genetics has resulted in distinct terminology (Table 54-1). Application of conventional and molecular cytogenetic methods has identified almost 600 fusion genes involving 250 different genes and approximately 1000 recurrent balanced translocations in human cancers.[1] Application of these methods has played a pivotal role in the diagnosis, treatment, and prognosis of the hematologic malignancies. This chapter discusses specific cytogenetic events and delineates molecular phenotypes that are important in order to understand the molecular pathogenesis of hematologic malignancies and provides several genetic testing algorithms. The remarkable hypothesis put forward by Boveri at the turn of the 20th century—namely, that an abnormal chromosome pattern is intimately associated with the malignant phenotype of a tumor cell—has proven correct. Knowledge of the molecular cytogenetic phenotype of hematologic malignancies has led to innovative and specifically tailored treatments. The first example of such gene-targeted therapy has already been successfully applied to chronic myelogenous leukemia (CML).

METHODS

Cytogenetic Analysis

Cells arrested in metaphase are obtained by exposing marrow cells sequentially to mitotic inhibitors, hypotonic KCl, and fixative. Chromosomes obtained from leukemic marrow are then subjected to the most widely used banding method, trypsin-Giemsa banding (Fig. 54-1). The criteria used to define clonal abnormalities are listed in Table 54-1 and described in the International System for Human Cytogenetic Nomenclature.[7]

Fluorescence In Situ Hybridization

Fluorescence in situ hybridization (FISH) is a molecular method that allows detection of the number, size, and location of DNA and RNA segments within individual cells in a tissue sample. It is based on the ability of single-stranded DNA to anneal to complementary DNA. In hematologic disorders, the target DNA is the marrow or peripheral blood DNA present in interphase cells or the DNA of metaphase chromosomes that is fixed on a microscope slide. Other biologic material that may be involved in the leukemic process, such as spleen cells, ascites, and spinal fluid, are particularly useful for FISH studies. In lymphoma, the target DNA is present in lymph nodes, and FISH studies are performed on touch preparations, frozen sections, or paraffin-embedded tissue.

Fig. 54-2 shows four types of FISH probes that are used alone or in combination to determine both numerical and structural rearrangements: (a) centromere enumeration probes, which, as the name implies, are used most frequently in interphase nuclei for detection of numerical chromosome anomalies, (b) whole chromosome painting probes, which are used only on metaphase cells and are very useful in delineating complex rearrangements or the origin of a marker chromosome, (c) subtelomeric probes, and (d) unique gene loci probes applied to both interphase and metaphase cells in single, dual, triple, or multiple colors to determine specific chromosomal rearrangements, deletions, or amplifications.

The four FISH probe strategies are used in probe design for detection of chromosomal translocations in hematologic malignancies (Figs. 54-3 and 54-4): (a) conventional strategy, (b) extrasensitive strategy, (c) dual-fusion strategy, and (d) "breakapart strategy." The first application of FISH technology for detection of chromosomal translocations in hematologic malignancy was when the BCR-ABL hybrid gene was identified using two-color FISH in interphase cells as well as in metaphase marrow-derived CML cells. In the standard strategy for interphase evaluation of chromosomal translocation, a DNA probe comprising sequences mapped proximally to the breakpoint in one of the chromosomes involved in reciprocal translocations is combined with a differentially labeled DNA probe that includes sequences mapped distantly to the breakpoint in the other chromosome. Positive nuclei for the translocation display one dual-color fusion signal, representing one of the derivative chromosomes generated by the translocation, and two single-color signals, one for each of the normal alleles. This standard FISH strategy has been used for detection of translocations in hematologic disorders at diagnosis.

For detection of minimal residual disease, the conventional strategy lacks specificity because cells with random spatial co-localization of normal signals with different colors, found at a frequency from 1% to 10% of scored nuclei, are seen as false positive. To minimize this problem, an extrasensitive method was developed in which a probe for one abnormal chromosome is designed to generate extra, smaller signals in positive nuclei. Hybridization using this strategy results in abnormal cells with co-localization of two signals in dual colors, an additional two signals in one single color and one signal in another single color. Application of the extrasensitive probe has been useful in discriminating between BCR-ABL fusion-positive blast crisis of CML and de novo acute lymphoblastic leukemia (ALL).

A dual-fusion strategy was developed not only to minimize false-positivity but also to detect additional deletions at translocation breakpoints. The dual-color/dual-fusion strategy includes a probe set with DNA sequences that encompasses proximally and distally the translocation breakpoints on both chromosomes involved in the translocation. The sequences for each chromosome are labeled with a specific color, and the translocation generates fused signals in both derivative chromosomes. Positive nuclei exhibit two copies of fusion

Table 54-1 Glossary of Cytogenetic and Fluorescence In Situ Hybridization Terminology

Term	Definition
Aneuploidy	Abnormal chromosome number, either gain or loss.
Balanced translocation	Exchange of chromosomal material that creates no extra or missing DNA.
Banding	Set of dark and pale segments along the length of chromosomes, resulting from treatment with enzyme before staining. Each chromosome identified by its unique set of bands.
Breakpoint	Specific site on a chromosome containing a break in the DNA that is involved in chromosomal structural rearrangement, such as translocation or deletion.
Centromere	Constriction on the chromosome at the spindle site attachment. During cell mitosis two copies of the DNA in each chromosome are separated by shortening of the spindle fibers attached to opposite sides of the dividing cell. Position of the centromere determines whether the chromosome is metacentric (X-shaped; e.g., 1, 3, 19, 20), submetacentric (centromere positioned more toward the short arms; e.g., 2, 4, 5, 6-12, 16-18, X), or acrocentric (inverted V-shaped; e.g., 13-15, 21, 22, Y).
Centromere enumeration probe (CEP)	Highly repetitive α (or β) satellite DNA, located in the heterochromatin of the centromeric area of chromosomes. CEP targets repetitive α (or β) sequences and produces bright compact signals; particularly useful for detection of numerical loss or gain of chromosomes.
Comparative genomic hybridization (CGH)	Molecular cytogenetic technique that provides a copy-number karyotype at the chromosome and band level. Array CGH is a higher-level CGH technology that provides gene copy information. Variety of arrays include disease specialized, chromosome arm specific, and others.
Chromosomal rearrangement	Aberration in which chromosomes are broken and rejoined.
Clonal abnormality	In cytogenetic analysis, two cells showing the same additional or structural abnormality or three cells with loss of the same chromosome. In FISH analysis, any abnormality present after the probe has been validated and normal reference range established, above the normal reference range. Cytogenomics is the application of molecular biology to determine genomic copy number.
Deletion	Segment of chromosome that is missing (terminal) or segment of chromosome missing between two breakpoints (interstitial).
DNA sequence	Order of nucleotides in a DNA segment, usually displayed from the 5′-triphosphate (5′ end) to the 3′-hydroxyl (3′ end) nucleotides.
Enhancer	DNA sequence that increases the rate of transcription.
Exon	Portion of gene that encodes protein.
Fiber FISH	Application of FISH technology to extended DNA or free DNA fibers.
FISH	Fluorescence in situ hybridization, a method for detection of the number and location of DNA sequences (genes) in tissue section or cell population.
Fluorochrome	Fluorescence molecule that, when conjugated to a molecule, binds to a hapten to facilitate detection of the chromosomal probe. By definition, a fluorochrome is a molecule that will become excited by the light of one wavelength.
Gene construct	Recombinant DNA containing a gene of interest surrounded by sequences engineered to promote a measure of its expression.
Gene map	Order of genes within a chromosome or entire genome.
Genotype	Genetic constitution, usually with reference to particular alleles at a locus.
Haploid	Half of a normal complement (i.e., 23 chromosomes).
Haploinsufficiency	Deletion or inactivation of one allele producing disease due to inadequate activity of the remaining allele.
Hybrid gene	Fusion of two different genes as a result of a structural chromosomal rearrangement that functions as one transcriptional unit.
Hybridization	Method for rejoining (reannealing) complementary DNA or RNA strands.
Hyperdiploid	Additional chromosomes (e.g., 47 or 48 chromosomes).
Hypermetaphase FISH	Application of FISH to accumulated large number of metaphase cells.
Hypodiploid	Loss of chromosomes (e.g., 45 or 44 chromosomes).
I-FISH	Interphase fluorescence in situ hybridization, application of FISH to nondividing (resting) cells.
Interphase	Stage of mitosis in which the cell is not dividing.
Inversion	Structural chromosomal rearrangement as a result of two breaks occurring in the same chromosome. Paracentric inversion refers to both breaks occurring on the same side of the centromere. Pericentric inversion refers to breaks occurring on the opposite side of the centromere.
Isochromosome	Structural chromosomal rearrangement that consists of doubling of one of the two chromosome arms (connected by the centromere) and loss of the other arm.

Continued

Table 54-1 Glossary of Cytogenetic and Fluorescence *In Situ* Hybridization Terminology—cont'd

Karyotype	Arrangement of metaphase chromosomes from a particular cell according to size and banding so that the largest chromosome is placed first and the smallest one last (see Fig. 54-1).
kb (kilobase)	Unit of DNA/RNA length = 1000 base pairs of DNA.
Locus	Unique location of a gene on a chromosome.
Locus (sequence)-specific probe (LSI)	Probe targeted to unique sequence region of the chromosome. Useful for localization of genes on normal chromosomes (gene mapping) and for detection of gene amplification, deletion, inversion, or translocation.
Marker chromosome	Chromosome whose morphology cannot be identified using banding method. Marker chromosomes are frequent in hematologic neoplasms.
M-FISH	Multicolor FISH karyotyping, which allows identification of 24 different human chromosomes (22 autosomes, and the X and Y chromosomes) (see text for details).
Oncogene	Locus that is activated in association with tumor growth. One abnormal allele is sufficient to cause tumor formation or cancer.
PCR	Polymerase chain reaction, by which individual gene segments are amplified through sequential cycles of polymerization, heat denaturation, and reannealing.
Pseudodiploid	Diploid number of chromosomes (46) accompanied by structural rearrangement.
Recurrent abnormality	Structural or numerical abnormality observed in multiple patients with the same or similar disease. Recurrent chromosome abnormalities in hematologic neoplasms have prognostic significance.
Telomeric probe	Used to detect repeated DNA sequences present at the end of the chromosome, which is called the *telomere*. Telomeric DNA contains 10-15 kb of TTAGGG repeats. Adjacent to the telomere is a region called the *proximal subtelomeric region,* and centromeric to it is a unique chromosome telomeric region. Chromosome-specific telomeric probes are useful for detection of cryptic translocations involving ends of chromosomes.
Translocation	Structural chromosome abnormality resulting from a break in at least two chromosomes with an exchange of material. In reciprocal or balanced translocation, no loss of chromosomal material occurs. In unbalanced translocation, loss of chromosomal DNA occurs.
Tumor suppressor gene	Locus that prevents tumor growth when at least one allele is functional. Loss of both alleles, first through constitutional and then through somatic mutation, is associated with tumor formation or cancer.
Whole chromosome painting probe (WCP)	Spans the entire length of chromosomal DNA sequences and, as the name implies, targets the entire length of DNA sequences. Useful for identification of complex or cryptic structural rearrangements as well as for identification of marker chromosomes.
	Nomenclature
p	= Short arm
q	= Long arm
+	When placed before the chromosome, denotes a gain of a whole chromosome (e.g., +8)
–	When placed before the chromosome, indicates a loss of a whole chromosome (e.g., –7); in rare situations, when placed after the chromosome, as in 5q–, indicates loss of a part of the long arms of chromosome 5
t	translocation
del	deletion
der	derivative
inv	inversion
i	isochromosome
mar	marker chromosome
con	connected
nuc ish	nuclear in situ hybridization
nuc ish 21q22 (D21S65X2)	two copies of D21S65 DNA segment on chromosome 21
nuc ish 9q34 (ABL x2), 22q11.2 (BCRx2) (ABL con BCRx1)	two ABL and two BCR loci, but one of each locus is juxtaposed on one chromosome as a result of t(9;22)

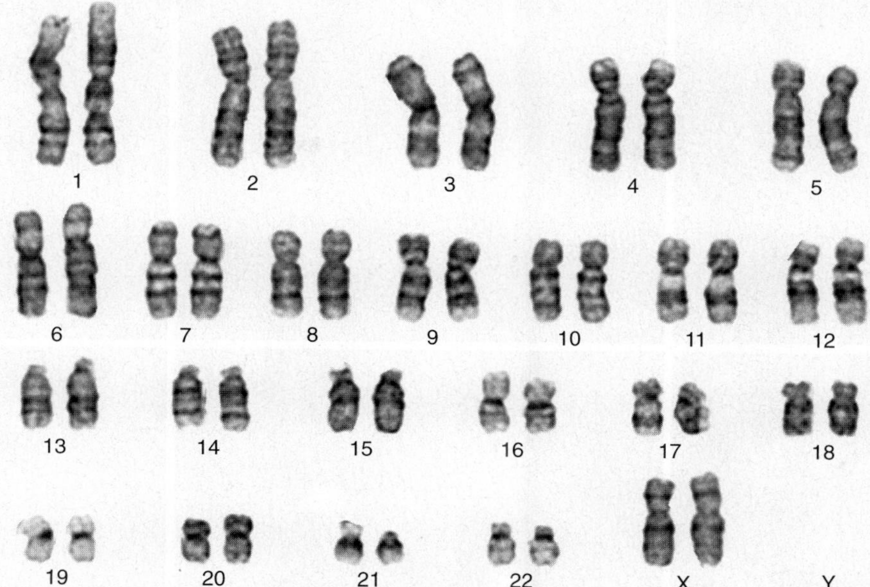

Figure 54-1 NORMAL ARRANGEMENTS OF CHROMOSOMES IN A KARYOTYPE FROM A BONE MARROW METAPHASE CELL SHOWING A SLIGHTLY FUZZY MORPHOLOGY COMPARED WITH A NORMAL KARYOTYPE OBTAINED FROM PHYTOHEMAGGLUTININ-STIMULATED PERIPHERAL BLOOD CELLS.

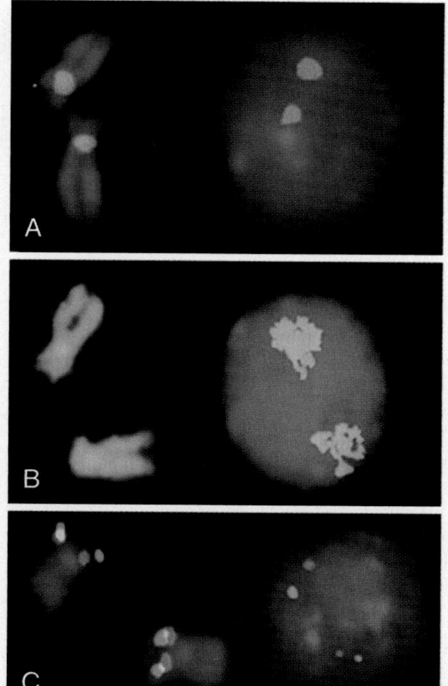

Figure 54-2 TYPES OF CHROMOSOMAL PROBES (SEE TEXT FOR DETAILS). **A,** Pair of chromosome 12 *(left)* and interphase cell *(right)* after FISH study with centromere enumeration probe (CEP) showing two hybridization signals *(red)* in the centromeric area of chromosome and two tight signals in interphase cell consistent with disomy (normal copy number). CEP probes are most useful for detection of numerical abnormalities. **B,** Hybridization with whole chromosome 8 painting probe showing the hybridization signal *(green)* along the length of the entire chromosome 8 *(left)* and hybridization domains in interphase cell *(right)*. Whole chromosome painting probes are useful for identifying unknown chromosomes in metaphase cells. **C,** Target of locus-specific indicators (LSI) are specific gene sequences such as P53 seen after hybridization as two small signals *(red)* on chromosome 17, band p13. The main applications of LSI probes are gene mapping, numerical enumeration in interphase cells, and detection of translocations. Telomeric probe, shown in green for the short arms of chromosome 17, are repetitive probes and are useful for detection of cryptic translocations involving ends of chromosomes. Chromosomes and nuclei are counterstained with DAPI *(blue)*.

signals and one copy of each of the signals representing the normal alleles. If a third color is added for detection of particular sequences, such as deletion of chromosome 9 at the site of the Philadelphia (Ph) translocation (Figs. 54-5, *C* and 54-6; see also Fig. 54-4), the lack of one copy with the third color is consistent with sequence deletion at the site of the translocation of one derivative chromosome. Dual-color/dual-fusion probes are very useful in differentiating various leukemia and lymphoma-associated translocations.

Multiple translocation partners are well known for genes commonly associated with leukemias such as mixed-lineage leukemia (MLL), the retinoic acid receptor α (RARA) gene, and the anaplastic lymphoma kinase (ALK) gene. The fourth FISH strategy, with break-apart probes, was developed to address this issue. The breakapart probe includes DNA sequences mapped proximally and distally to the breakpoint within a critical gene (the 3′ end and the 5′ end) labeled with two different fluorochromes. The fused fluorescence signals represent a normal gene, whereas nuclei with rearrangements within the target gene show one single-color signal and one for each derivative chromosome, regardless of which chromosome is the partner in translocation.

One of the most significant advances in diagnostic leukemia cytogenetics has been the application of interphase FISH. Interphase

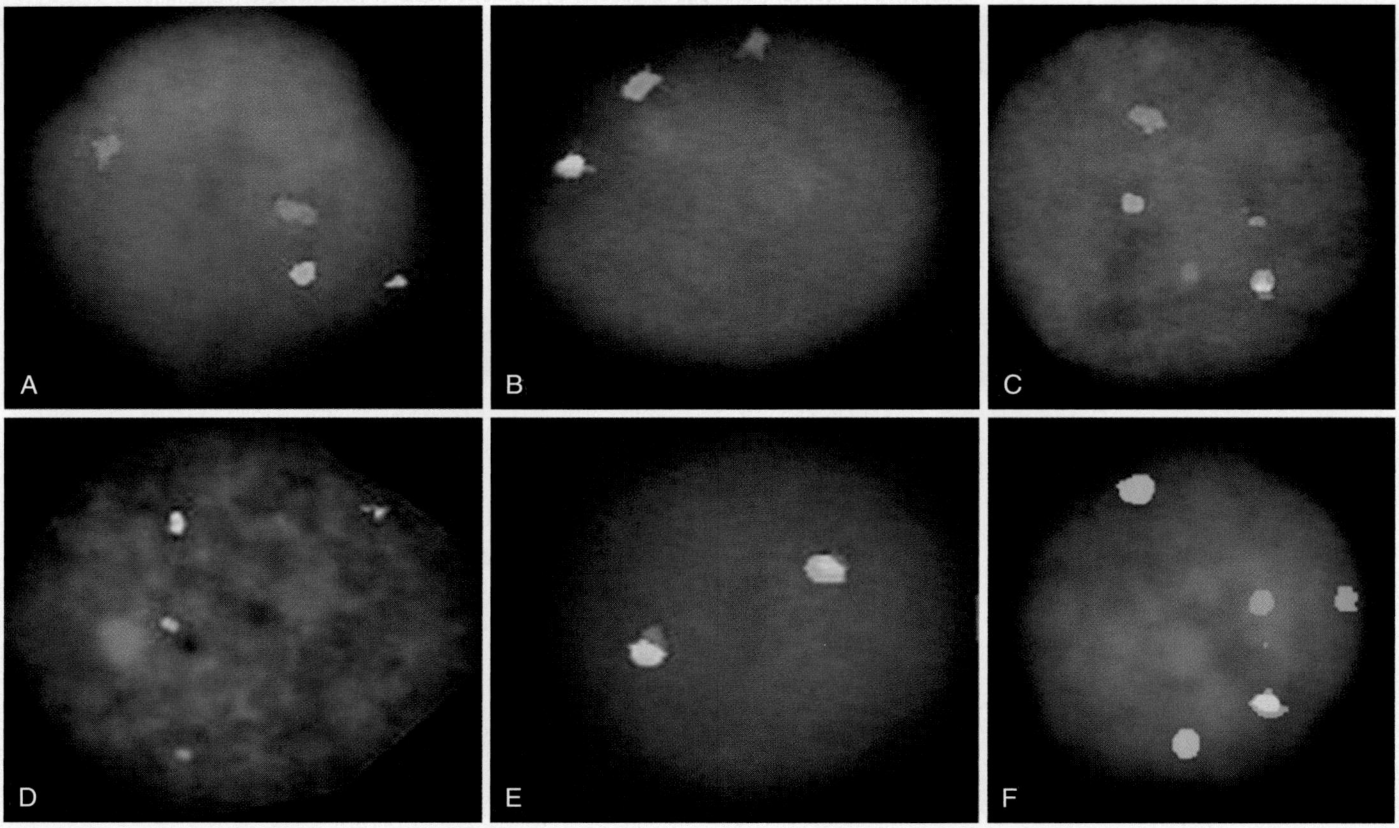

Figure 54-3 FOUR DIFFERENT PROBE STRATEGIES FOR DETECTION OF CHROMOSOMAL TRANSLOCATIONS (SEE TEXT FOR DETAILS). **A,** Normal cell after in situ hybridization with BCR *(green)* and ABL *(red)* showing a normal distribution of two red and two green single signals. **B,** Conventional fusion strategy after in situ hybridization shows one fusion *(yellow)* signal representing derivative chromosome generated by the translocation and one single-color signal, red and green, for normal homologues in positive nuclei. **C,** An extrasensitive fusion approach generates an extra small *(red)* signal, as well as a fusion signal *(yellow)* and one signal in single color *(green and red)* on normal homologues. **D,** Dual-fusion strategy generates two fusion signals *(yellow)* on two derivative chromosomes and one single-color signal on each of two normal chromosomes. **E,** Breakapart approach in a normal cell appears as two fusion signals *(yellow)*. In this strategy, the 3′ end and the 5′ part of the gene are labeled in two colors. **F,** When the rearrangement occurs, the normal chromosome shows co-localization of red and green *(yellow)* as a result of the proximity of the sequences on the chromosome, whereas abnormal derivative chromosomes each have one single red and single green signal, indicating that the rearrangement occurred between the two ends of the gene separating the green and red signals on two different chromosomes. The third-color probe *(blue)* can be used as an internal control (usually CEP probe) to determine the disomic number of chromosomes.

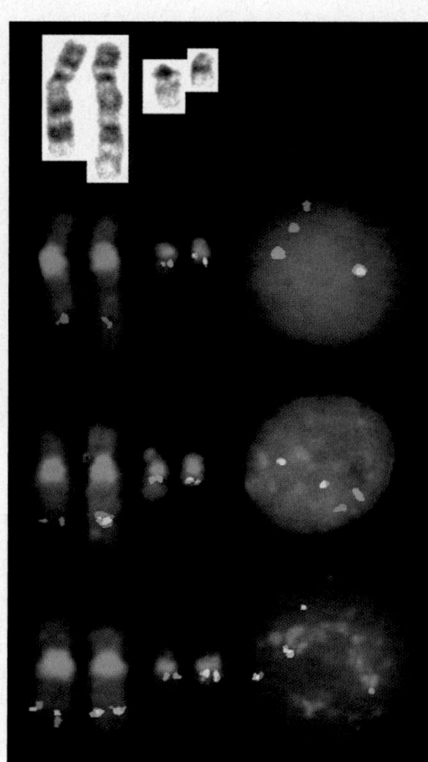

Figure 54-4 CURRENT FISH PROBE STRATEGIES FOR DETECTING BCR-ABL1 FUSION. Partial karyotype showing the Philadelphia chromosome as a result of t(9;22)(q34;q11.2) *(top row)*. The same chromosomes 9 and 22, as well as a bone marrow nucleus, after hybridization with BCR *(green)* and ABL1 *(red)* using an extrasensitive (ES) dual-color, single-fusion FISH strategy *(second row)*. Chromosomes and a nucleus are counterstained with DAPI *(blue)*. In the ES strategy, a part of ABL1 *(red)* remains on der(9) and is shown in interphase nucleus as a smaller red signal, whereas the normal-size ABL1 hybridization signal is seen on normal homolog 9. The other part of ABL1 is on the Ph chromosome and is seen co-localized with BCR as yellow in interphase nucleus. Therefore interphase nuclei will have one normal-size red signal, one smaller-size red signal, one normal-size BCR signal, and co-localization of BCR and ABL1, producing a yellow signal both in interphase cells and metaphase chromosomes. In the dual-color, dual-fusion strategy *(third row)*, there are two co-localized signals on both der(9) and the Ph chromosome, as well as one red signal of ABL1 on chromosome 9 and one green signal of BCR on normal chromosome 22. In the triple-color, dual-fusion strategy, ASS gene *(aqua)* is added. It is used to determine whether sequences from der(9) are deleted at the time of the Ph formation. As shown in the fourth row, ASS is localized centromeric from ABL1 on 9q34, and in patients without deletion, ASS is present as two signals in nucleus and on the chromosome 9 (see Fig. 54-6).

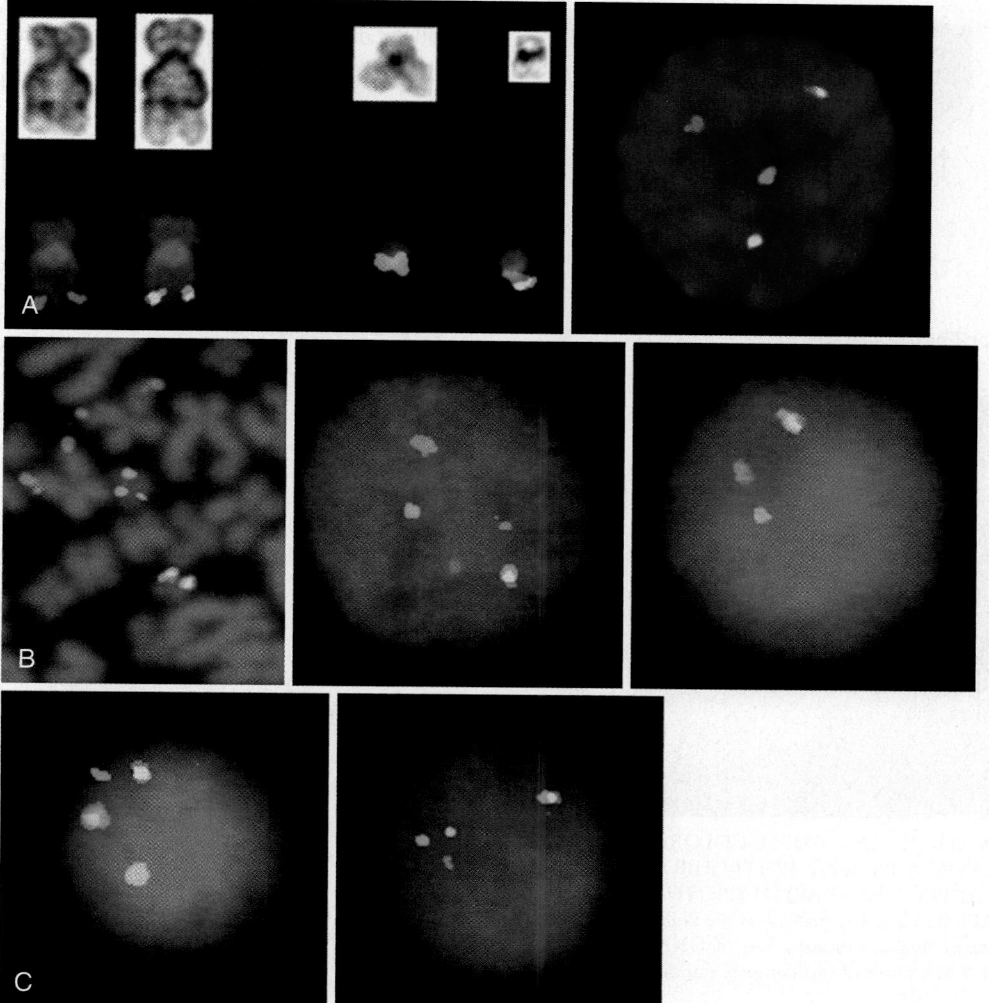

Figure 54-5 IDENTIFICATION OF THE PHILADELPHIA (PH) CHROMOSOME. **A,** Conventional cytogenetics *(left)* shows t(9;22)(q34;q11.2), and metaphase FISH with dual-color/dual-fusion BCR-ABL probe *(underneath)* shows two fusion signals *(yellow)* on abnormal chromosomes 9 and 22, one red single signal on normal homologue 9, and one single green signal on normal chromosome 22. *Right,* Nucleus after hybridization with dual-color/dual-fusion probe, indicating two fusion signals. **B,** Metaphase cell *(left)* and interphase cell *(middle)* after hybridization with BCR-ABL extrasensitive probe, indicating a fusion signal *(yellow)* on the Ph chromosome, BCR *(green)* on normal chromosome 22, ABL *(red)* signals on normal chromosome 9, and part of ABL on der(9) to reduce the number of false-positive cells. The interphase nuclei on the right are hybridized with a single-fusion BCR-ABL probe showing one fusion signal *(yellow)* and one single red and green signal on normal homologues. **C,** Two interphase nuclei after hybridization with triple-color BCR-ABL-ASS probe in which ASS is aqua. The left nuclei indicate a BCR-ABL fusion and disomy for ASS. The right nucleus shows deletion for ASS locus, consistent with deletion of der(9) (see Fig. 54-11).

cytogenetics is the term used to describe detection of chromosomal abnormalities in nondividing, interphase nuclei (Fig. 54-7). Six aspects of interphase FISH are particularly useful. (1) Interphase cytogenetics allows screening of a large number of cells. This permits investigation of hematologic malignancies with a low mitotic yield, such as chronic lymphocytic leukemia (CLL) or multiple myeloma (MM). (2) Interphase cytogenetics permits detection of chromosomal rearrangements in peripheral blood samples, thus obviating the need for marrow aspiration. For instance, in CML, which rarely yields a large number of dividing cells in peripheral blood, conventional cytogenetics usually is uninformative. However, detection of BCR-ABL, a molecular equivalent of the Ph, in peripheral blood using interphase FISH provides reliable, fast, quantitative results (see the section on Chronic Myelogenous Leukemia later in this chapter). (3) Interphase FISH offers a quantitative assay for monitoring disease progression or detection of minimal residual disease after ablative chemotherapy or hematopoietic cell transplantation (HCT). (4) Use of specific probe sets allows detection of specific disease-associated abnormalities such as t(8;21), which denotes the M2 subtype of acute myeloid leukemia (AML), or t(15;17), which is associated with acute promyelocytic leukemia, in a very short time period, allowing for timely and appropriate therapy. (5) Abnormalities can be detected accurately in archival specimens stored to 15 years. (6) Simultaneous use of interphase FISH and immunophenotyping is a powerful tool for investigation of lineage involvement in diseases such as myelodysplasia and to determine which cell population carries the specific chromosome abnormality. FISH nomenclature is described in the International System for Human Cytogenetic Nomenclature.

Higher resolution of chromosomal abnormalities can be achieved when fluorescently labeled probes are hybridized to extended DNA

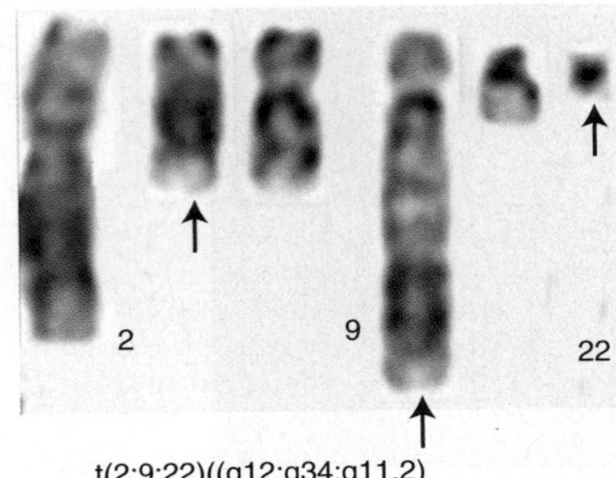

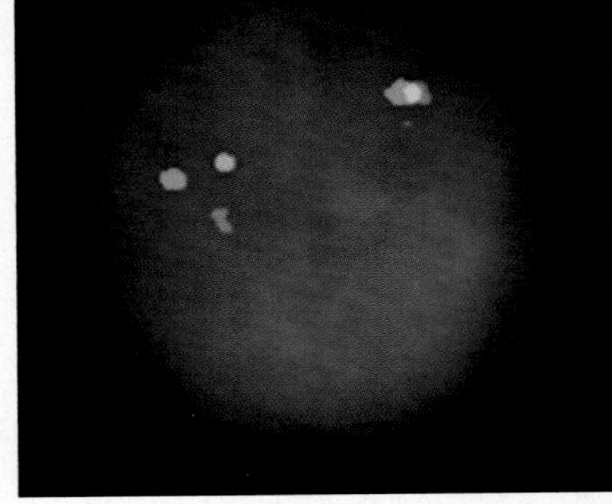

Figure 54-6 APPLICATION OF TRIPLE-COLOR BCR-ABL-ASS PROBE TO CELLS FROM A PATIENT WITH CHRONIC MYELOGENOUS LEUKEMIA AND T(2;9;22) KARYOTYPE *(TOP).* Interphase cell *(bottom)* shows BCR-ABL fusion signal *(yellow)* on the Philadelphia chromosome and one ASS *(aqua)* signal, indicating loss of DNA sequences from derivative chromosome 9 as a result of this complex translocation.

or free chromatin (chromatin strands released from their chromosomal scaffold) or free DNA fibers. This approach is termed *fiber FISH* (Fig. 54-8, *top*). The hybridized signals have the appearance of a "string of pearls" along the fiber rather than tight fluorescing spots observed in interphase cells. Although at the present time fiber FISH has limited clinical applicability because it requires special techniques of target DNA preparation on a glass slide, it has been successfully applied to map chromosomal breakpoints of the cyclin D gene in mantle cell lymphoma and for detailed mapping of the breakpoint site region in the BCL2 gene in follicular lymphoma.[10,11]

Multicolor karyotyping permits examination of the entire genome in a single analysis (Fig. 54-9). In 1996 it became possible to identify 24 different human chromosomes (12 autosomes and the X and the Y sex chromosomes), each with a unique color, with the help of fluorochrome-specific optical filters. This method is called *multicolor FISH (M-FISH)*. When interferometer-based spectral imaging is used, the method is called *spectral karyotyping*. The starting point in both methodologies is the use of whole chromosome painting probes for each chromosome. Thus each chromosome is labeled with a different combination of fluorescent dyes. The fluorochrome colors are not distinct enough for the unaided human eye to distinguish the combination with which the chromosome is labeled. In M-FISH, images are sequentially obtained using five different fluorochrome-specific optical filters. A computer program combines the data and displays each chromosome as if it were stained with a distinct color. Spectral karyotyping is based on the use of an interferometer (used by astronomers to measure the light spectra of distant stars) to determine the full spectrum of light emitted by each stained chromosome. A computer program then displays all the chromosomes simultaneously, each with its own unique color. These methods are applied with increasing frequency to resolve complex karyotypes, to detect cryptic translocations in patients with normal karyotype, and to define karyotypes with deletions. Their clinical use may be limited because the cost of equipment and probes is beyond what can be afforded by most clinical laboratories. The M-FISH technology cannot be used to discriminate structural intrachromosomal rearrangements such as duplications, deletions, and inversions.

Another powerful method used for identifying the location of chromosomal gains, losses, deletions, or amplifications, without prior knowledge of the chromosomal target that may be altered, is comparative genomic hybridization (CGH). Briefly, isolated DNA from leukemic marrow or tumor tissue is labeled with a one-color fluorochrome (e.g., red), whereas DNA isolated from normal control tissue is labeled with a different color (e.g., green). These differently labeled DNAs are hybridized against each other in a competitive hybridization reaction onto normal metaphase spreads. Computer-assisted image analysis detects colors generated after hybridization, which indicate equal hybridization, relative excess, or deficiency of the target DNA (relative to control). The ratio of color intensity provides a "copy number" karyotype. CGH has been successfully applied to study many leukemias, but its clinical use remains limited because it cannot detect balanced translocations, which are the hallmark of many hematologic malignancies. Nevertheless, CGH is an efficient approach to scanning the entire genome for variations in DNA copy number.

A particularly useful investigational approach is a "microchip array" in which labeled DNA or RNA from the sample of interest is hybridized with defined target sequences immobilized on a solid support (see Chapter 2).[2] The advantage of this method is its ability to screen genes that are amplified or deleted from the genome on a large scale or, in the case of RNA, to learn whether such genes are expressed at a particular stage of disease. The first example of successful RNA application of the microchip array technique was the differentiation of AML from ALL based solely on gene expression. As shown in Fig. 54-8 *(bottom panel),* in the "array CGH" procedure, large-insert genomic clones, oligonucleotides, or single-nucleotide polymorphisms (SNPs) have replaced metaphase chromosomes used in the regular CGH. Array CGH is a higher-resolution CGH technology and provides diagnostic information for diseases associated with DNA dosage. It also can be used to discover previously unexpected sites of gene dosage associated with specific hematologic malignancy type. The concept of obtaining gene copy number from multiple genome locations in a single measurement has been used to characterize numerous hematologic malignancies over the last 5 to 6 years, and its clinical utility is demonstrated throughout this chapter (see also Chapter 2).[3]

These modern cytogenomic methods have increased the resolution at which chromosomal rearrangements can be identified. Whereas in conventional cytogenetics the targets are whole chromosomes in metaphase spreads at a resolution of approximately 5 Mb, molecular cytogenetics methods may be used to analyze interphase nuclei at a resolution of 50 kb to 2 Mb or fiber FISH analysis of chromatin strands at a resolution of 5 kb to 500 kb. Moreover, the current resolution of array CGH is restricted only by clone size and by the density of clones on the array, some of which may contain resolution at the level of a single nucleotide.

Conventional cytogenetics and FISH methodologies are complementary. Each has its own advantages and limitations in investigating genomic rearrangements of malignant cells. Although conventional cytogenetics is the comprehensive study of all chromosomes, it requires a large number of dividing cells, which, in some diseases, such as myelofibrosis, is difficult to obtain. Furthermore, many small deletions or structural rearrangements are beyond the microscopic level of detection. FISH can be used in conjunction with conventional cytogenetics with both interphase and metaphase cells. It is a more sensitive method and can detect rearrangements smaller than 1 kb. The main disadvantage of interphase FISH is that it cannot be used unless a known abnormality is suspected. When the abnormality is known, interphase FISH can pinpoint the clonal aberration at the single-cell level in a very short period of time.

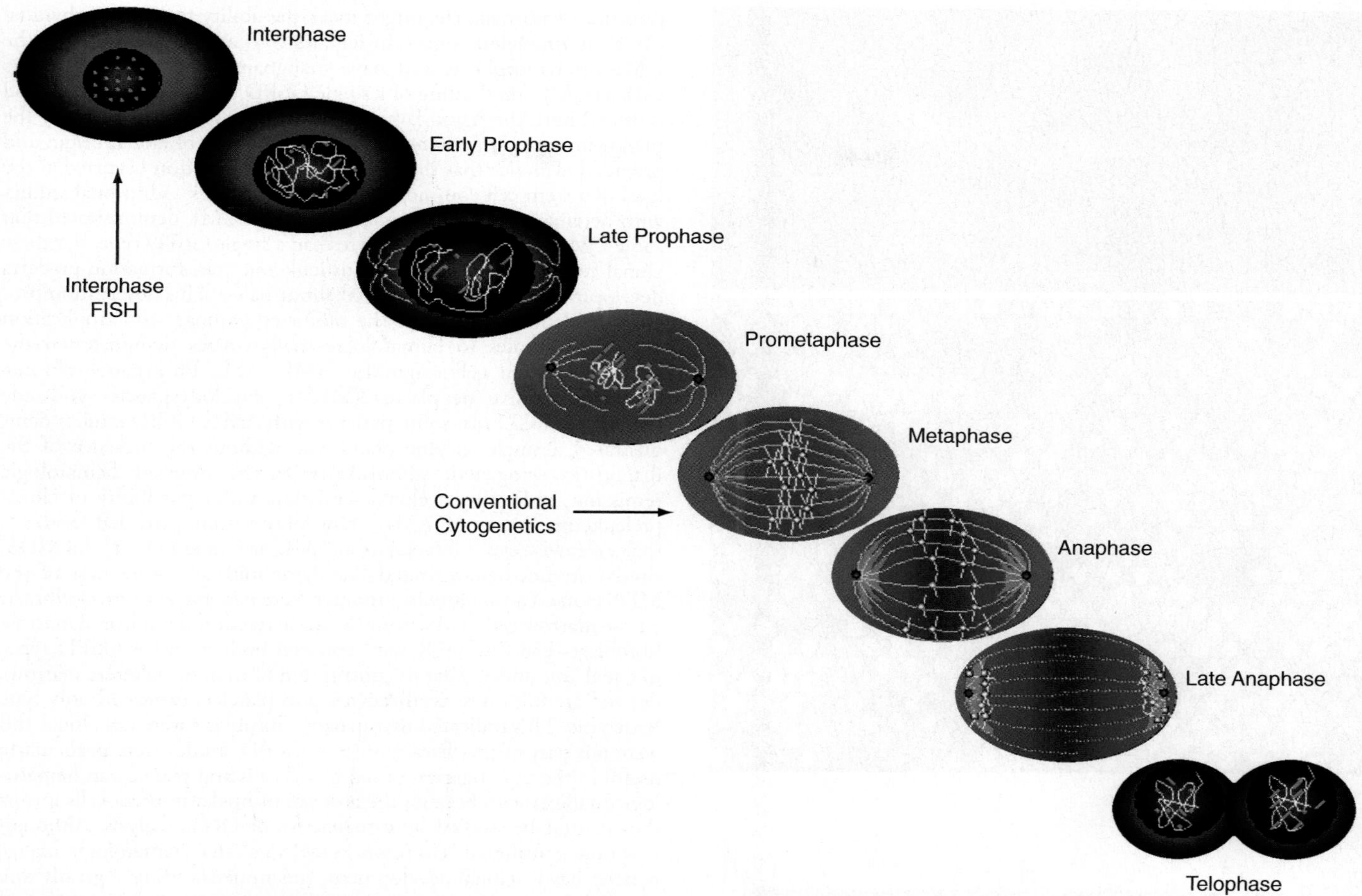

Figure 54-7 SCHEMATIC REPRESENTATION OF CELL DIVISION. Most clinical FISH studies are performed on nondividing interphase cells, whereas conventional cytogenetics is performed at the metaphase stage of cell division. *(Courtesy Dr. Ari Melnik, Mount Sinai Medical Center, New York.)*

Clonal Origin of Leukemia

The question of whether cell proliferation is monoclonal or polyclonal is fundamental to understanding the underlying etiology of hematologic malignancies. Markers of clonality are used to determine the origin of disease; to differentiate malignant from nonmalignant populations; to establish hematopoietic hierarchy, clonal evolution, and clonal remission; and to delineate steps involved in the multistep pathogenesis of hematologic malignancies.

The clonal origin of leukemias and lymphomas can be assessed by either intrinsic or extrinsic cellular markers. Intrinsic cellular markers are specific for a cell population, arising either during normal differentiation or as a part of disease process. For instance, cell surface-associated immunoglobulin (Ig) markers such as the λ or κ light chain or idiotypes and T-cell receptors (TCRs) can be useful for evaluating lymphoid diseases. Application of Ig markers demonstrated for the first time that MM was of clonal origin. Somatic cytogenetic alterations are useful intrinsic markers for identifying abnormal clones and following disease progression. Thus the observation of identical chromosome anomalies in different cells of the same tumor is evidence of clonality. Since the discovery of the Philadelphia chromosome (Ph) in 1960, it is well established that nonrandom, recurrent chromosomal abnormalities characterize many hematopoietic malignancies. The finding of the Ph in different CML-derived hematopoietic cell lineages led to the hypothesis that CML might originate in a single precursor cell and may have a clonal development. Moreover, the presence of additional recurrent chromosomal abnormalities in the Ph-positive clone (such as trisomy 8, duplication of the Ph, or trisomy 19) not only indicates the clinical progression of the disease and the occurrence of the accelerated phase or blast crisis, but also demonstrates the subclonal evolution of the Ph-positive clone. Currently, disease-associated somatic genomic mutation, such as rearrangements of MLL, AML1, TEL/ETV6, PML-RARA, and many others, can be identified by polymerase chain reaction (PCR)–based assays or by FISH assay and may serve, with or without conventional cytogenetics, as intrinsic marker of disease processes.

On the other hand, extrinsic marker systems use cellular mosaicism that is completely independent of the disease being studied and is not restricted to the cell lineages. Individuals with Turner or Klinefelter syndrome are mosaic for XX or XY and X cells or XXY and XY cells, respectively. The mosaicism created by X-chromosome inactivation in females is much more widely applicable and has provided fundamental insights into the pathogenesis of hematologic malignancies. Original studies with X-linked glucose-6-phospate dehydrogenase (G6PD) as a marker of clonality were based on the Lyon hypothesis, which asserts that early in embryogenesis, one X chromosome in females is inactivated in somatic cells and the activation status is stably transmitted to daughter cells during mitosis (Fig. 54-10)[4]. The choice of maternal versus paternal X-chromosome inactivation is random; however, once it occurs, it is maintained in all daughter cells.[37] Random X inactivation occurs by embryonic day 6.5 around the start of gastrulation and results in a mosaic pattern that characterizes adult females.[38-40] Therefore an adult female is a mosaic for two-cell populations, one expressing genes from an active X chromosome and the other expressing genes from the inactive X chromosome. Incidentally, mammalian X-chromosome inactivation is a mechanism that equalizes the dosage of X-linked genes between sexes. Although the exact mechanism of X-chromosome inactivation

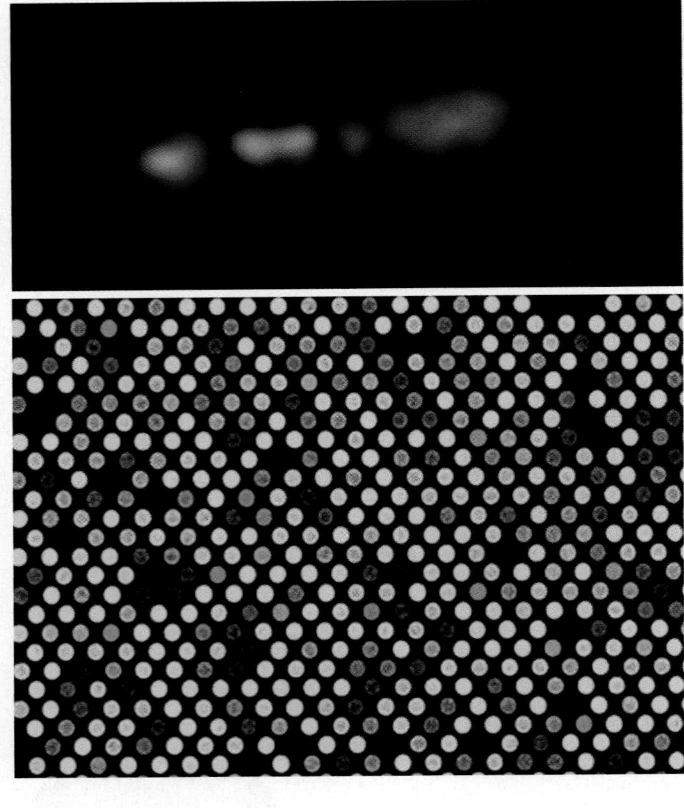

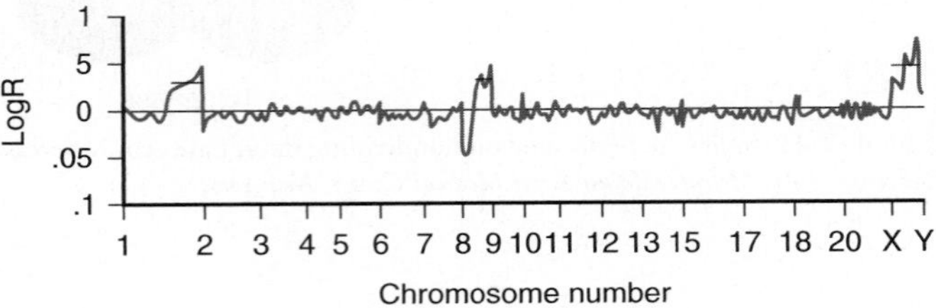

Figure 54-8 *Top panels,* Application of higher-resolution FISH (fiber FISH) to extended DNA fibers. The hybridization signals have the appearance of a "string of pearls" along the fiber, rather than tight fluorescing spots observed in interphase nuclei. *Bottom panel,* Portion of array CGH image. The tumor or normal cell fragmented DNA sample was labeled with Cy5 or CY3, respectively. Yellow spot indicates the intensity signal of the genomic element on that spot in the tumor equals that of the normal cell reference. Red or green spot indicates intensity of the tumor is greater or less than the reference, suggesting copy-number change for the genomic element on that spot. Graph underneath is the copy-number change profile. Y-axis is the log2 ratio of the intensity of each gene in the order of its position on the genome in tumor sample versus that of normal liver sample. Gained or lost regions are marked by red or green line, respectively. Gains of 1q and 8q and loss of 8p were observed in this tumor. *(Courtesy Dr. D. Weijia Zhang, Mount Sinai School of Medicine, New York.)*

remains to be elucidated, the process of X inactivation starts with methylation of CpG islands. The inactivation process is believed to occur before differentiation of embryonic stem cell into various cell lineages. Hematopoietic cells do not originate from a single embryonic stem cell but from several progenitors, thereby allowing for mosaic expression from both X chromosomes.

The observation that human females are heterozygous for the G6PD variant A and A^- and that two mosaic cell populations may be distinguishable by electrophoretic mobility was reported in the 1960s. The X-inactivation G6PD mosaic system was then applied to the study of clonality in human tumors in 1964 by Gartler and Linden. They studied uterine leiomyomas and recognized that the presence of normal cells might mask the ability to detect individual clonal uterine leiomyomas. In females who are heterozygous for the G6PD polymorphism and have malignant hematologic disorders such as CML, the finding of a single G6PD type in marrow or blood cells and both the A and B type G6PD in tissues not involved by the malignant process demonstrated that CML was of clonal origin and provided evidence that the malignant transformation occurred at the level of a stem cell common to most cell lineages. Additional studies with heterozygous G6PD females who had CML demonstrated that some CML-derived B lymphocytes had a single G6PD type, but these clonal cells were Ph-negative; thus leukemic transformation predates development of the chromosomal abnormality. This observation provided evidence that CML has a multistep pathogenesis. Application of G6PD studies to hematologic malignancies demonstrated the clonal and stem cell origin for AML, ALL, Ph-negative chronic myeloproliferative neoplasms (MPNs), myelodysplastic syndrome (MDS), and CLL. In some patients with AML, G6PD studies demonstrated a single-enzyme phenotype without the presence of the diagnostic cytogenetic abnormality at the time of hematologic remission, indicating a clonal remission and a possibility of clonal preleukemic phase of AML. This observation provided evidence that a stepwise evolution occurs in AML, as it does in CML. In MDS, similar studies demonstrated that lymphoid cells were part of the MDS clone. Particularly informative were patients with myelofibrosis whose marrow cells had trisomy 8. In sharp contrast, cultured marrow fibroblasts had disomy 8 and expressed both B and A G6PD types in equal amounts similar to control skin fibroblasts, whereas marrow-derived granulocytes, erythrocytes, and platelets expressed only type A enzyme. This indicated that marrow fibroblasts were not clonal and were not part of the disease process. G6PD studies were particularly useful in the investigation of red blood cells and platelets in hematologic malignancies because the absence of nuclei in these cells means they cannot be studied by cytogenetics or DNA analysis. Although it is now considered "common knowledge" that hematologic malignancies have a clonal development, this understanding is greatly due to what is now known as classic Fialkow's work, whose profound insight contributed much to current concepts and understanding.

Despite the importance of the G6PD approach, it is limited by the rarity of females who are heterozygous for the G6PD isoenzyme. An alternative and more extensive DNA-based X-chromosome clonal assay uses common polymorphic markers that are caused by changes in DNA methylation patterns that accompany inactivation of the X chromosome.[5] These X-linked loci, such as phosphoglycerine kinase, hypoxanthine phosphoribosyltransferase, DXS25 (M27β), and human androgen receptor (HUMARA), have been extensively used in assessment of clonality, and now it is possible to identify clonal cell populations in virtually all females. DNA-based marker systems rely on a sequence polymorphism that has adjacent differences in methylation on the active and inactive X chromosomes. The inactive X chromosome is more highly methylated than its active homologue, but this is only true for certain regions of genes as 10% to 20% of X-linked genes escape inactivation and can be found both in clusters and in isolation. The most widely used HUMARA assay appears to maintain the stringent methylation differences. The number of CAG tandem repeats differentiates the maternal from the paternal X chromosome.

The DNA-based X-chromosome clonal assay is limited to females younger than 60 years because they usually have 1 : 1 distribution of two-mosaic–cell population. A ratio greater than 3 : 1 is found in women older than 60 years, probably as a result of stem cell kinetics influenced by X-linked genetic factors. When the ratio of two cell populations is greater than 3 : 1, this phenomenon is called a *skewed X-inactivation pattern.* With the HUMARA assay, acquired unequal or skewed X-chromosome inactivation (excessive lyonization) is found in 35% to 40% of women older than 60 years. Thus X-chromosome–based clonality studies must incorporate age-matched controls. Despite the enormous contribution of clonality assays to the understanding of disease processes, they are usually performed in research investigations and are rarely used as diagnostic tools.

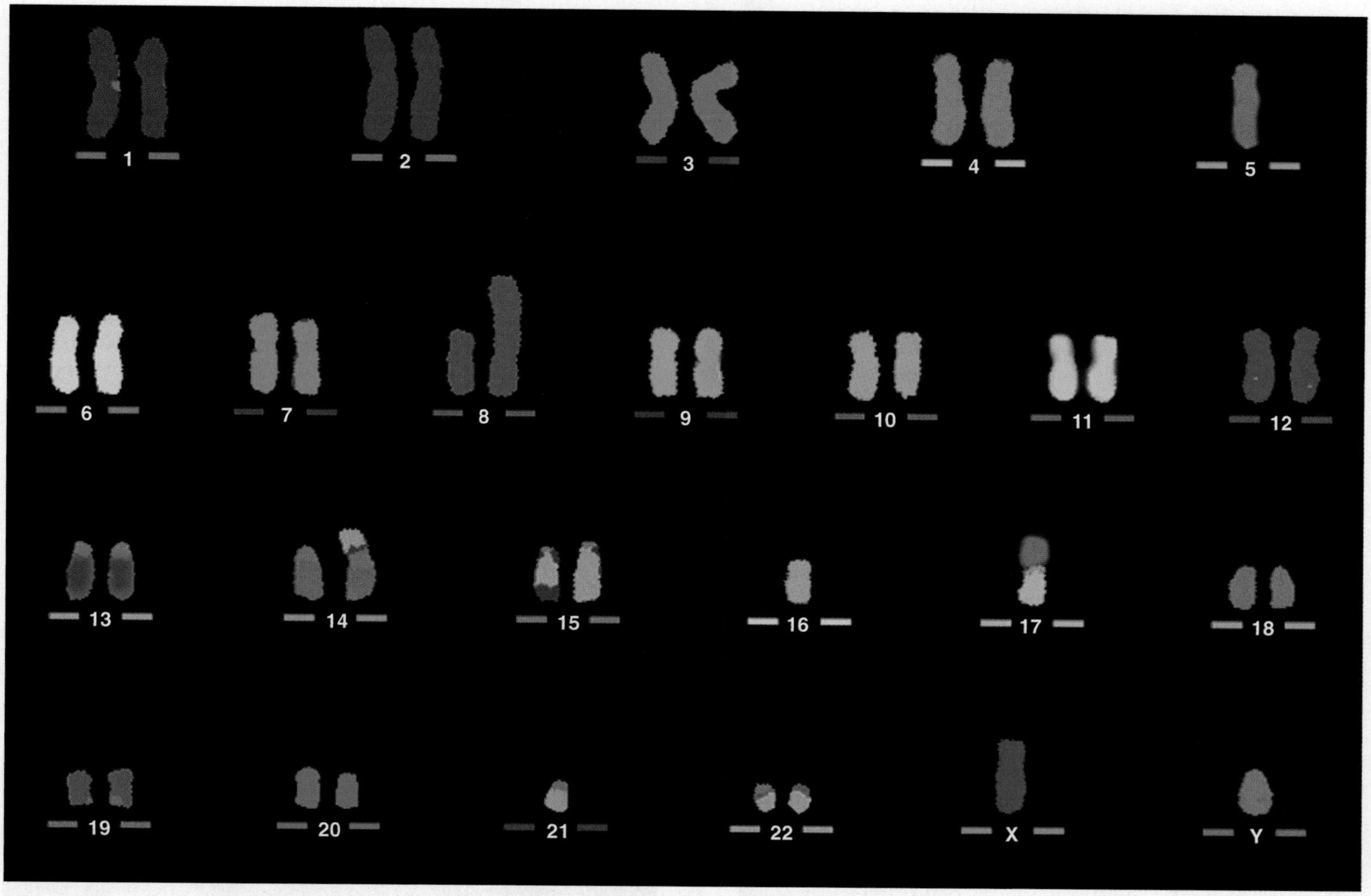

Figure 54-9 Multicolor metaphase FISH of a bone marrow cell from a patient with myelodysplastic syndrome documenting 43,XY, −5, der(8)t(8;8)(p23;q11.2), der(14;16)(p12;p11.1), inv(15)(q21;q24), der(17)t(5;17)(p13;p13), −21 karyotype. The origin of t(8;8) and der(14;16) could not have been determined by conventional cytogenetic study alone.

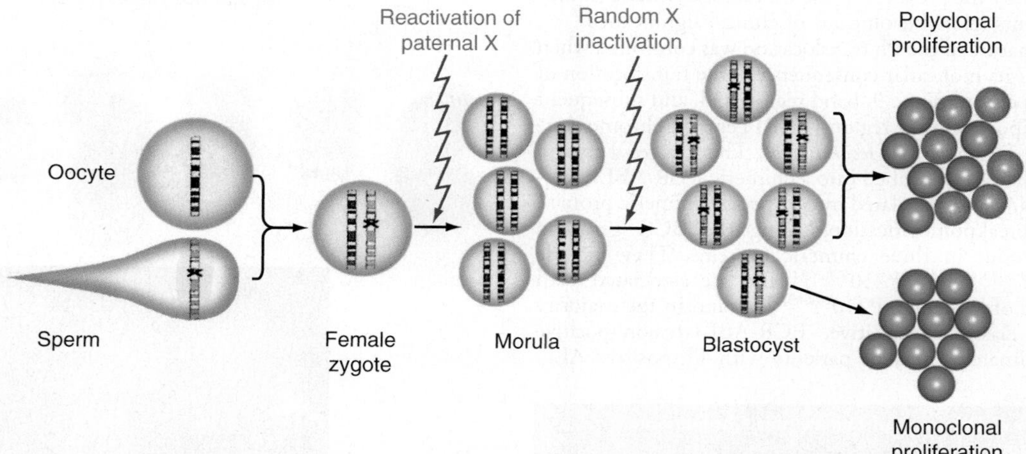

Figure 54-10 X-CHROMOSOME–LINKED ENZYME GLUCOSE-6-PHOSPHATE DEHYDROGENASE (G6PD) AS A MARKER TO INVESTIGATE CLONAL DEVELOPMENT OF HUMAN HEMATOPOIETIC DISORDERS. Early in embryogenesis, regions of all but one X chromosome are inactivated in each cell containing two or more X chromosomes. The choice of maternal versus paternal X chromosome for inactivation is random. Once the inactivation occurs, it is fixed and is stably transmitted to daughter cells during mitosis (Lyon hypothesis). Females who are heterozygous for the common B type and the less frequent A type, G6PD (localized on Xq27), are mosaic. This cellular mosaicism is used to study monoclonal versus polyclonal cell proliferation and development of malignant hematopoietic diseases. *(Courtesy Dr. W Raskind, University of Washington, Seattle.)*

CHRONIC MYELOPROLIFERATIVE NEOPLASMS

The World Health Organization (WHO) characterizes MPNs as clonal stem cell disorders. CML has a unique place among hematologic malignancies and is described separately from the other Ph-negative MPNs. CML is characterized by the t(9;22) or the BCR-ABL1 fusion confirmed by cytogenetic, FISH (see Figs. 54-4 and 54-5), or PCR analysis.

Chronic Myelogenous Leukemia

Knowledge of the origins of CML has accumulated over the last 52 years and serves as a classic example of the fruits of molecular medicine (Table 54-2). The Ph chromosome is the first example of a specific chromosomal abnormality associated with a malignant disease. ABL1 and BCR genes are the first oncogenes (see Chapter 66) localized at the site of a chromosomal breakpoint in t(9;22)(q34;q11). The BCR-ABL1 fusion leads to a "hybrid" gene, resulting in the production of a dysregulated tyrosine kinase protein. Finally, imatinib mesylate, a specific tyrosine kinase inhibitor, was the first rationally designed gene-targeted form of cancer therapy.

The Ph, named in honor of Philadelphia, the city of its discovery, was described for the first time in 1960.[6] It represents a signature genomic rearrangement occurring in more than 95% of patients with CML. Approximately 3% of all pediatric leukemias are Ph-positive CML. The Ph results from a balanced translocation t(9;22)(q34;q11.2)[7] (see Fig. 54-5, *A*). The Ph arises postzygotically, being found only in hematopoietic tissue. The findings of the Ph in myeloid cells, erythroid cells, eosinophils, monocytes/macrophages, basophils, and B lymphocytes, along with the absence of the Ph in cultured marrow fibroblasts, support the concept that the Ph results from a specific rearrangement in a multipotent hematopoietic stem cell and that it is an acquired rather than an inherited abnormality.[8] Of interest, the Ph is rarely identified in T cells. T lymphocytes are long-lived cells and may antedate the development of CML. These observations combined with G6PD heterozygotes and have CML provide further evidence for the concept that CML is a clonal disease arising in a stem cell capable of differentiation into most of the hematopoietic cell lineages.

In a review of 1129 Ph-positive patients, the 9;22 translocation was identified in 1036 (92%) cases. Karyotypic analysis of marrow cells in patients with CML is a time-consuming task. However, it demonstrates not only the presence of the Ph but also other chromosomal rearrangements (clonal evolution) of clinical significance.

The reciprocal nature of the Ph translocation was confirmed when studies showed that its molecular consequence is the translocation of the ABL gene from chromosome 9, band region q34, and subsequent fusion to the breakpoint cluster region (BCR) gene on chromosome 22, band q11 (see Fig. 54-5, *A, second row*). This creates a hybrid BCR-ABL1 gene that is transcribed into a chimeric BCR-ABL1 messenger RNA (mRNA) and translated into a specific chimeric protein.

Three major breakpoint locations along the BCR gene on chromosome 22 result in three chimeric proteins. They include $P210^{BCR\text{-}ABL1}$, $P190^{BCR\text{-}ABL1}$, and $P230^{BCR\text{-}ABL1}$ and are associated with three distinct types of leukemia. $P210^{BCR\text{-}ABL}$ is found in the majority of patients with classic Ph-positive, BCR-ABL1-fusion–positive CML and approximately 30% of patients with Ph-positive ALL.

Table 54-2 History of Discovery of Philadelphia Chromosome and BCR-ABL Fusion

1960	Philadelphia chromosome (Ph) is identified.
1973	Ph is t(9;22)(q34;q11.2).
1983	ABL is translocated from chromosome 9 to chromosome 22.
1984	BCR is localized to 22q11.
1987	Ph′ is BCR-ABL fusion.

Expression of $P190^{BCR\text{-}ABL1}$ is seen in 20% to 30% of adults and 80% of children with ALL, in rare CML patients, and in the majority of patients with rare Ph-α–positive AML, whereas expression of $P230^{BCR\text{-}ABL1}$ is associated with a rare indolent chronic neutrophilic leukemia variant and up to 1.6% of CML (approximately 50 patients in the worldwide literature have been described).

The BCR-ABL1 fusion is present in both standard and variant forms, in cases where chromosome 9 involvement is cytogenetically not detectable, and when a masked Ph is present. In the majority of patients, the fusion of ABL1 and BCR takes place on chromosome 22 (Fig. 54-11; see also Fig. 54-4). However, in a small group of patients the BCR gene is translocated to chromosome 9, and the fusion of the two genes is localized to 9q34. The prognosis of these patients may be inferior, but the number of reports is too small for a definitive conclusion. The BCR-ABL1 fusion transcript is present

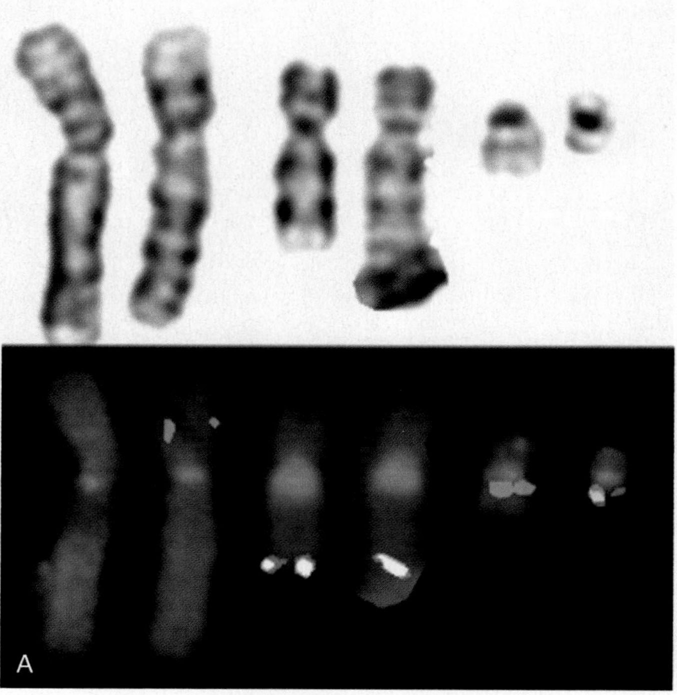

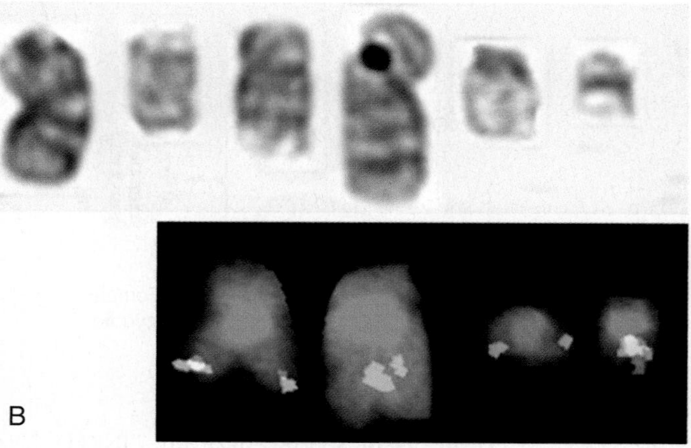

Figure 54-11 IDENTIFICATION OF BCR-ABL1 FUSION IN PATIENTS WITH COMPLEX KARYOTYPEs. Partial karyotype from a patient with chronic myelogenous leukemia showing t(2;9;22)(p21;q34;q11.2) **(A)** and from a patient showing a four-way translocation with t(7;9;22;22) karyotype **(B)**, indicating the BCR-ABL 1 is on the Philadelphia chromosome even in complex chromosomal translocations.

in neutrophils, monocytes, eosinophils, erythrocytes, B cells, rarely in T cells, and in CD34 cells and is associated with increased proliferation of CD34 myeloid progenitor cells but not of other more mature myeloid precursors. These observations confirm the hypothesis that CML originates in a multipotent stem cell capable of differentiating to all hematopoietic cell lineages with the exception of T cells. Studies provide evidence for the existence of clonal BCR-ABL1 fusion–negative stage. The formation of BCR-ABL1 and Ph occurs in an already abnormal and genetically unstable clone of pluripotent hematopoietic cells. Thus it is the preexisting genetic instability that predisposes to formation of BCR-ABL1 and Ph. Once Ph formation occurs, it has a further selective growth advantage over normal cells, resulting in overwhelming BCR-ABL1–positive, Ph-positive marrow cells at the time of diagnosis of CML.

In the 5% of patients with CML who are Ph-negative by cytogenetic studies, clonal and stem cell origin of these hematologic malignancies can still be demonstrated, and molecular analysis reveals the BCR-ABL fusion in approximately 2% to 3% of these patients (Fig. 54-12). In the majority of Ph-negative patients, an ABL insertion from chromosome 9 to 22q11.2 results in a BCR-ABL1–fusion product without reciprocal translocation of sequences from chromosome 22 to chromosome 9. Approximately 2% of patients truly are Ph negative, BCR-ABL fusion negative. These patients may not have CML but rather another myeloproliferative neoplasm. The concept that the BCR-ABL fusion plays a central role in the pathogenesis of CML is strongly supported by two lines of evidence: (a) retroviral transduction experiments in which $P210^{BCR\text{-}ABL1}$ is expressed in murine marrow cells, resulting in a myeloproliferative disorder resembling CML, and (b) the fact that imatinib, a tyrosine kinase inhibitor, selectively inhibits the BCR-ABL fusion protein in mice and specifically inhibits the growth of human Ph-positive cells in vitro and in vivo. Although considered necessary, BCR-ABL may not be initial or sufficient to cause the malignant transformation in CML.

Genomic PCR and Southern blot analysis can determine the exact breakpoints of DNA fusion products. Reverse transcriptase PCR (RT-PCR) and Northern blot analysis allows detection of BCR-ABL transcripts at the RNA level. Current FISH studies for detection of BCR-ABL1 fusion at diagnosis use a dual-color BCR-ABL ES probe or BCR-ABL1 dual-fusion probe (Fig. 54-13; see also Figs. 54-4 and 54-5, *A* and *B*). A triple-color BCR-ABL1-ASS probe is used for detection of deletions on both chromosomes 9 and 22 (see Fig. 54-13). Approximately 12% to 15% of patients with CML have large deletions adjacent to the Ph translocation breakpoint on the derivative 9 chromosome, and initial reports demonstrated inferior survival in these patients (see Fig. 54-5, *C*). Subsequent quantitative PCR and FISH studies have demonstrated that deletions are heterogeneous and may involve both chromosomes 9 and 22 (majority of cases), only chromosome 9 (8% of patients with deletions) (see Fig. 54-13), or only chromosome 22 (4% of cases with deletions). FISH analysis using multiple large genomic probes along the length of chromosomes 9 and 22 show that the deletion size is variable ranging from 0.5 Mb to greater than 10 Mb. A more refined recent study, applying genomic SNP microarrays revealed three common deletion regions: (1) a 162 kb loss at 9q34, (2) a 138 kb deletion at 22q11.2, and (3) a 102 kb deletion at 22q11.2. It appears that the partial deletion of the ABL1-BCR fusion (not the pathogenetic form) on derivative 9 chromosome occurs as a part of the same process as the formation of the BCR-ABL1 translocation. Before imatinib therapy, these deletions were associated with adverse prognosis, inferior survival, and higher probability of relapse after hematopoietic cell transplantation. A multivariate analysis of 339 patients, with a median observation of 7 years, confirms that deletions involving 9q alone, spanning the ABL1-BCR breakpoint, were significant independent predictors of an adverse prognosis. However, in a recent study of 521 CML patients, including 60 with the del(9q) during the early chronic phase of imatinib treatment, the cumulative incidence of complete cytogenetic response and major molecular response and the overall survival are comparable at the 5-year follow-up between CML patients with and without the del(9q). These results indicate that 9q deletions have a negative impact only on those patients with large deletions or one involving both BCR and ABL1, which may be overcome in the majority of patients with TKI therapy.

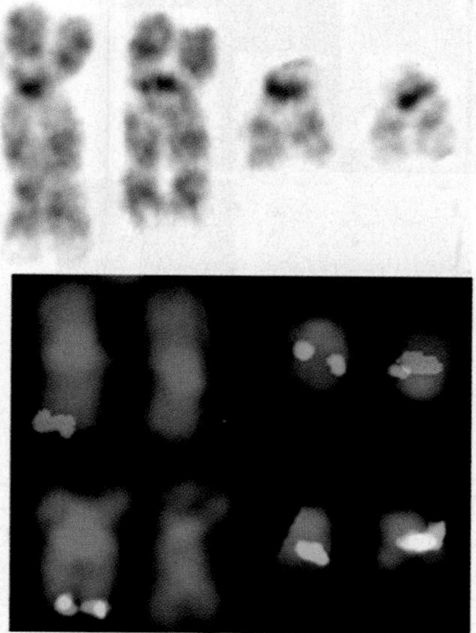

Figure 54-12 PARTIAL KARYOTYPE FROM A PATIENT WITH PH-NEGATIVE CHRONIC MYELOGENOUS LEUKEMIA *(TOP)* SHOWING NORMAL CHROMOSOMES 9 AND 22. Two pairs of chromosomes 9 and 22 after hybridization with dual color *(middle)* and triple color *(bottom)* demonstrating BCR-ABL fusion on the Ph chromosome without apparent t(9;22). Tricolor strategy showed ABL and ASS in close proximity and appearing as fusion on normal 9 (*bottom left* chromosome) and BCR-ABL-ASS fusion *(white)* on normal 22.

At diagnosis, conventional cytogenetics remains the gold standard because the chromosome analysis will identify not only the t(9;22) but also other chromosomal abnormalities that may indicate accelerated or blast phase of the disease or clonal proliferation of Ph-negative cells. The current international recommendation is that FISH studies should be performed at diagnosis in conjunction with conventional cytogenetics to determine deletion status on der(9q) and to identify patients who are BCR-ABL1 but lack the Ph- karyotype.

Imatinib mesylate (Gleevec, formerly known as STI-157) has revolutionized therapy for CML and, for many patients, has transformed a deadly disease into a chronic disorder that is compatible with normal life.[10] The standard method for monitoring a patient's response to therapy is conventional cytogenetic analysis of cells obtained from a marrow aspirate. In the phase III International Randomized Interferon and STI-571 (IRIS) study, 89% of patients had Ph-negative marrow aspirates as determined by conventional cytogenetics at 5 years. However, conventional cytogenetics has limited sensitivity. The degree of tumor load reduction is determined to be an important prognostic factor for patients with CML on therapy. CML patients without discernible Ph detected by conventional cytogenetics analysis may still harbor up to 10^{10} leukemic cells.

Hypermetaphase FISH has greater sensitivity compared with conventional cytogenetics and may detect 31% of BCR-ABL1 metaphase cells in patients who are Ph-negative as assessed by conventional cytogenetics. Interphase FISH does not depend on the cycling status of cells, and use of double-fusion probes has reduced false-positive results to approximately 1%. However, if peripheral blood cells rather than marrow aspirate cells are used to monitor residual disease, the high percentage of BCR-ABL1 fusion-negative lymphoid cells may underrepresent actual residual tumor load. In most direct comparison studies, interphase FISH of peripheral blood compared with conventional cytogenetics of marrow in patients who are treated with imatinib showed good correlations ($r = 0.91\text{-}0.97$). Real-time quantitative PCR (RQ-PCR) is by far the most sensitive method. It provides an accurate measure of the total leukemia cell mass and the degree to which BCR-ABL1 transcripts are reduced by therapy, and it correlates with progression-free survival.[9]

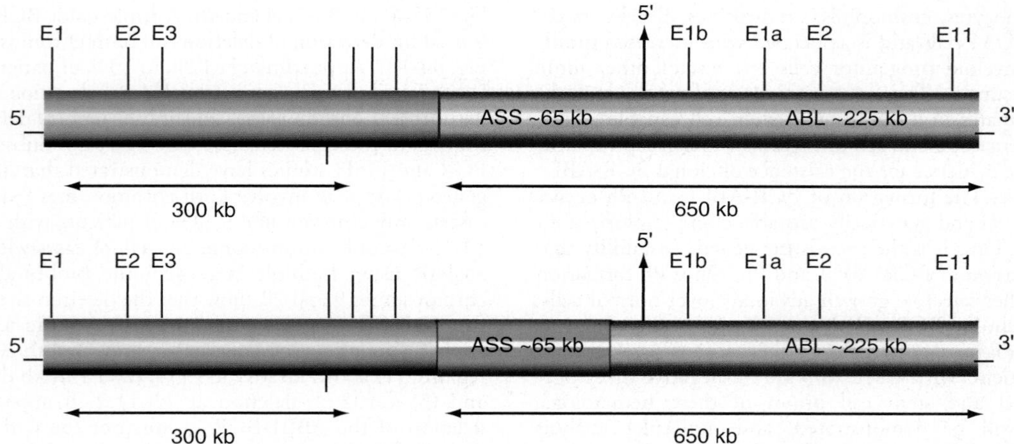

Figure 54-13 SCHEMATIC REPRESENTATION OF THE MOST FREQUENTLY USED BCR-ABL PROBES. Dual-color/single-fusion extrasensitive probe strategy, as indicated in text, uses a 650-kb probe in which two loci, ABL and ASS, both are labeled in red. BCR-ABL fusion-positive nuclei show three red signals: one small red signal on der(9), one red signal on normal homologue 9, and a third red signal in fusion with BCR. When a triple-color probe is applied, the ASS locus usually is labeled in aqua and the BCR-ABL fusion-positive cells show two aqua signals, unless there is deletion of der(9). The most useful application of triple-color probe is documentation of deletion of derivative chromosome 9.

The goal of therapy in CML is to achieve a molecular remission as measured by the reduction or elimination of BCR-ABL1 transcripts. In IRIS, at 5-year follow-up, complete cytogenetic response combined with major molecular response at 12 months is associated with a 97% progression-free survival rate. This compares with an 89% progression-free survival for those with complete cytogenetic response but without major molecular response. Current international recommendations for optimal molecular monitoring of patients receiving imatinib treatment includes an RQ-PCR assay expressing the BCR-ABL1 transcript levels on an internationally agreed scale.[9] The term *major molecular response (MMR)* corresponds to ≤0.1% BCR-ABL1, whereas the designation *CMR (complete molecular response)* should be used only for patients with undetectable BCR-ABL1, where the limit of detection is confirmed to be at least ≈4.5 log reduction from IRIS baseline response. The two major obstacles to successful imatinib-based therapy for patients with Ph-positive, BCR-ABL1 fusion-positive CML are the persistence of BCR-ABL fusion-positive cells and relapse of the disease due to emergence of resistance to imatinib. Acquired resistance to imatinib treatment is manifested in two ways: amplification of BCR-ABL1 fusion product (Fig. 54-14) and mutations in the ABL kinase domain. Currently, 100 different ABL1 kinase domain mutations have been described, although only about 15 are common and they account for more than 85% of all mutations detected.

Between 5% and 8% of patients undergoing treatment with imatinib will develop chromosomal abnormalities such as trisomy 8, monosomy 7, del(20q), and other anomalies in BCR-ABL1 fusion-negative cells. Imatinib may induce chromosomal abnormalities in BCR-ABL1$^-$ cells. Alternatively, imatinib may uncover chromosomal abnormalities present before therapy after significant reduction of overlying Ph-positive cells (Fig. 54-15). Presence of +8 and other chromosomal anomalies in Ph-negative cells in patients treated with imatinib suggests that CML has a multistep pathogenesis and that clonal Ph-negative cells precede the development of the Ph-positive clone (Fig. 54-16).[11] This important observation about the pathogenesis of CML demonstrates the power of conventional cytogenetics, even in the era of molecular assays, and should be used at least annually while patients are undergoing imatinib treatment.

CML patients who cannot tolerate or are resistant to imatinib may benefit from the second and now third generation of tyrosine kinase inhibitors, such as dasatinib and nilotinib. These agents bind to the

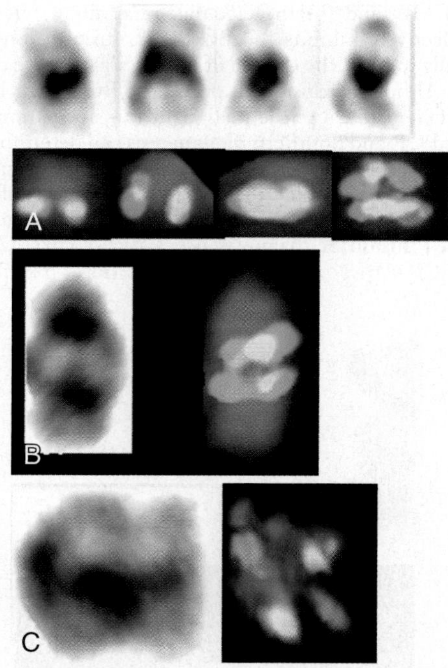

Figure 54-14 EXAMPLES OF UNUSUAL Ph CHROMOSOMES ASSOCIATED WITH IMATINIB RESISTANCE AND BLAST CRISIS OF CHRONIC MYELOGENOUS LEUKEMIA. **A,** Amplification of the Ph chromosome *(top row)* and the BCR-ABL fusion in a patient treated for 3 months with imatinib. The patient developed five copies of the Ph chromosome and 5 copies of the BCR-ABL fusion *(yellow)*. **B,** G banding of dicentric Ph chromosome *(left)* dic der(22)t(9;22)(q34;q11.2) and after FISH studies *(right)* showing two copes of BCR-ABL fusion. **C,** G-banding of isoderivative Ph, ider(22)t(9;22)(q34;q11.2) *(left)* and after FISH studies showing two copies of BCR-ABL fusion *(yellow)* on the end of both arms.

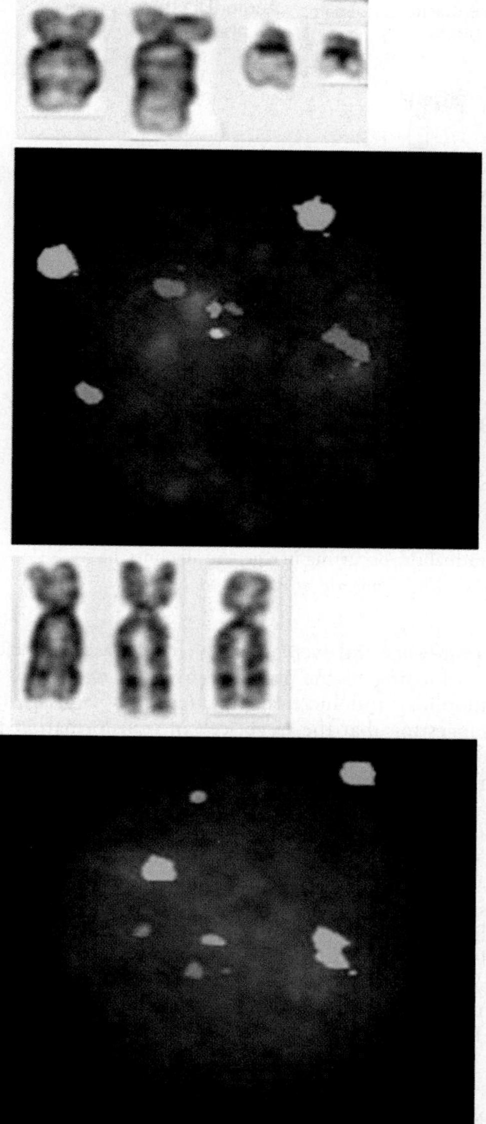

Figure 54-15 TWO DIFFERENT CELL POPULATIONS FROM A PATIENT TREATED WITH IMATINIB. One population shows t(9;22) (*top row,* partial G-banded karyotype) and the BCR-ABL fusion signal *(yellow, second row)* as well as disomy 8 *(aqua).* In contrast, the second population shows trisomy 8 (*third row,* partial G-banded karyotype) in the BCR-ABL fusion-negative cells *(fourth row),* showing disomy for the *BCR (green),* ABL *(red)* as well as trisomy for chromosome 8 *(aqua)* (see text for details).

ABL kinase domain in a matter distinct from that of imatinib and thereby retain activity against nearly all imatinib-resistant mutations (see Chapter 66).

The mechanism of transformation to advanced-phase CML is heterogeneous and poorly understood. In blast crisis of CML, 80% to 85% of patients show karyotypic evolution, that is, new chromosomal abnormalities in very distinct patterns are present in addition to the Ph. The most common changes include gain of chromosome 8 (33%) or +19 (12%), gain of a second Ph (30%), i(17q)(20%), alone or in combination, to produce modal chromosome numbers of 47 to 50 (Fig. 54-17). Isochromosome 17q occurs almost exclusively in myeloid blast crisis. Others less frequently observed include monosomies of chromosomes 7 and 17, loss of Y, and trisomies of chromosomes 17 and 21. In addition to these common karyotypic evolutions, additional chromosomal aberrations specific for acute myelogenous leukemia—for example, t(8;21) (Fig. 54-18), inv(16),

Genetic Testing for Chronic Myelogenous Leukemia

At diagnosis of CML, perform quantitative cytogenetic analysis of bone marrow aspirate, which is sine qua non because peripheral blood cells rarely contain blast cells at the time of presentation. If the bone marrow aspirate is a "dry tap," perform interphase FISH using either a BCR-ABL extrasensitive or BCR-ABL dual-fusion color probe. Triple-color BCR-ABL-ASS is particularly useful for identifying patients with deletion on either chromosome 9 or chromosome 22. To monitor patients with CML during therapy, use FISH to study blood or bone marrow to track changes in the percentage of cells with BCR-ABL fusion at 3-month intervals. Once the patient is in complete cytogenetic and FISH remission, the international recommendation is to perform real-time quantitative polymerase chain reaction and to follow the patient at 3-month intervals until molecular remission is achieved. At relapse, perform a chromosome study to assess the karyotype of the malignant clone and to determine whether a new chromosomally abnormal clone has developed or a new subclone in the Philadelphia chromosome (Ph)–positive clone.

t(3;21)(q26;q22), and most frequently, inv(3q)/t(3;3), resulting in the overexpression of EVI1—have been observed. Complete cytogenetic remission for patients in accelerated phase or blast crisis CML treated with imatinib is rarely accompanied by a normal karyotype; however, 6% to 17% of these patients may have some cytogenetic response (see box on Genetic Testing for Chronic Myelogenous Leukemia).

High-resolution cytogenomic studies have demonstrated that in contrast to the chronic phase (which is characterized only by genomic imbalances in or around BCR and ABL1, specifically deletions), during the blast phase, many additional genomic imbalances occur. Using aCGH, 44 patients in chronic phase of CML (11 in myeloid and 1 in lymphoid blast crisis) were investigated, and a spectrum of recurrent genomic imbalances were associated with disease progression, including losses at 1p36, 5q21, 9p21, and 9q34 and gains at 1q, 8q24, 9q34, 16p, and 22q11. Moreover, analysis of 78 CML patients in lymphoid blast crisis found a unique signature of genomic deletions within the immunoglobulin heavy-chain and T-cell receptor genes, indicating that their presence is essential for the development of a malignant clone with the lymphoid phenotype. The most common mutations in myeloid blast phase occur at tumor suppressor gene TP53 (≈25% of cases) and runt-related transcription factor gene (RUNX1) in about 40% of cases. In lymphoid blast crisis, 50% of patients have mutation in cycline-dependent kinase inhibitor CDKN2A. Recently, mutations in genes frequently found in Ph-negative MPNs such as CBL, TET2, ASXL11, and IDH1/2 were also identified in patients in accelerated/blast phase. Moreover, deletions of RB1, gain of function mutations in GATA-2 and RAS are just some of the spectrum of cytogenomic changes characterizing progression of CML. The current thinking is that progression of CML is the result of increased genomic instability combined with defective or insufficient ability to repair DNA.

Ph-Negative Chronic Myeloproliferative Neoplasms

Ph-negative MPNs are disorders arising in a single clone of multipotent precursor cells in which one or all myeloid lineages are abnormally amplified. Classic and more frequently encountered Ph-negative MPDs include polycythemia vera (PV), primary myelofibrosis (PMF), and essential thrombocytopenia (ET). Their cytogenetic profiles are included in Chapters 67, 68 and 69

Less frequently encountered are neutrophilic leukemia, hypereosinophilic syndrome/chronic eosinophilic leukemia, systemic mast cell proliferations, atypical CML, and unclassifiable myeloproliferative neoplasms. Rare recurrent balanced abnormalities in

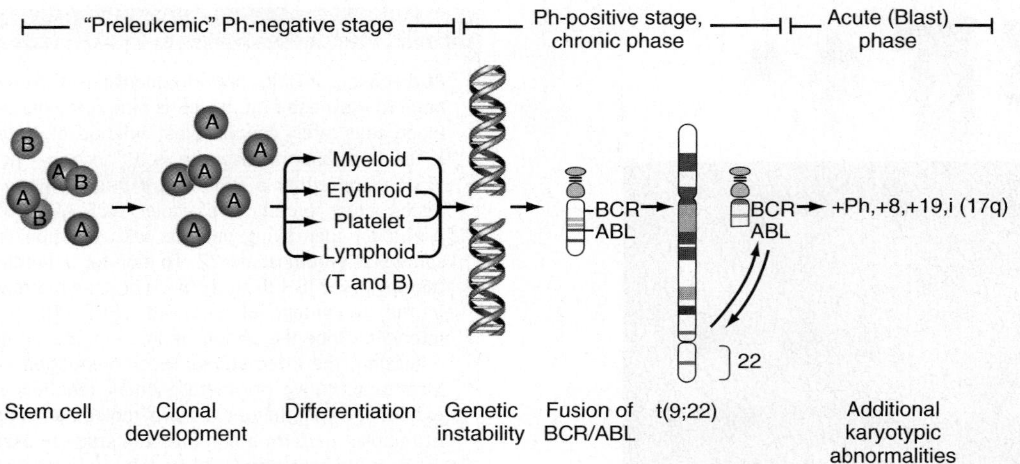

Figure 54-16 HYPOTHETICAL MODEL OF MULTISTEP PATHOGENESIS OF PH-POSITIVE CHRONIC MYELOGENOUS LEUKEMIA. The first detectable event is a clonal proliferation of cells that are capable of differentiating to all hematopoietic lineages. These cells are genetically unstable and give rise to BCR-ABL fusion and the Ph chromosome. The blast crisis is characterized by nonrandom abnormalities occurring in a genetically unstable Ph-positive clone. At least six events can be delineated. *(Courtesy Dr. W Raskind, University of Washington, Seattle.)*

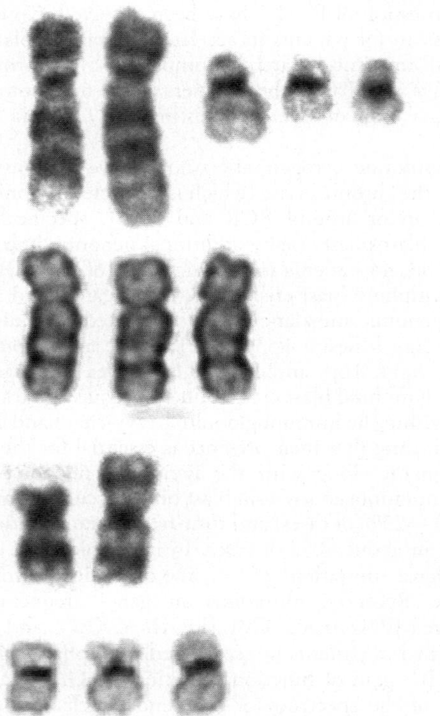

Figure 54-17 THE FOUR MOST FREQUENT ABNORMALITIES ASSOCIATED WITH THE BLAST CRISIS OF CHRONIC MYELOGENOUS LEUKEMIA. Duplication of the Ph chromosome *(top row)* is identified in ≈30% of patients, trisomy 8 *(second row)* is found in 30%, isochromosome of the long arms of chromosome 17 *(third row)* is found in 20% and gain of chromosome 19 *(fourth row)* is seen in approximately 12% patients with blast crisis of chronic myelogenous leukemia.

atypical Ph-negative MPN generally involve the PDGFRB gene found at 5q33, FGFR1 gene on 8p11 (these disorders are referred to as *myeloproliferative syndrome* or *stem cell leukemia syndrome*), and PDGFRA gene on 4q12. The best described are t(5;12)(q33;p13), resulting in ETV6-PDGFRB fusion protein, and t(8;13)(p11;q12), resulting in the ZNF198-FGFR1 fusion gene. These disorders are also known as *8p11 myeloproliferative syndrome* (EMS) or *stem cell leukemia/lymphoma* and were recently recognized and classified by WHO as belonging to the group of myeloid neoplasms associated with eosinophilia and increased incidence (≈30%) of T-cell lymphoma, suggesting that the target cell of transformation is a multipotent progenitor cell (Table 54-3).

The most frequent recurrent abnormality is the cryptic deletion on 4q12 as a result of FIP1L1-PDGFRA fusion gene reported to occur at frequencies ranging from 3% to 56% in patients with chronic eosinophilic leukemia/hypereosinophilic syndrome (see Chapters 7 and 71). The disparity in frequencies reflects differing levels of stringency criteria in the diagnosis of disorders with hypereosinophilia as well as different methodology used for detection of FIP1L1-PDGFRA fusion. The most recent investigation of 376 patients with persistent unexplained hypereosinophilia revealed an 11% incidence of FIP1L1-PDGFRA fusion detected using highly sensitive RQ-PCR. Patients with FIP1L1-PDGFRA fusion are characterized by male predominance, marrow fibrosis, increased number of mast cells, elevated serum tryptase levels, and a favorable response to low doses of imatinib. Most of these patients have a normal karyotype because a cryptic deletion of CHIC2 locus on 4q12 is only 800 kb in size, but a more sensitive FISH technology and RQ-PCR will detect the majority of cases with this deletion at diagnosis. Moreover, the most recent commercially available tricolor FISH probe will detect not only deletion 4q12 as a result of FIP1L1-PDGFRA but also a rare BCR-PDGFRA fusion resulting from the t(4;22)(q12;q11.2) rearrangement (Fig. 54-19). Serial monitoring with RQ-PCR demonstrates exquisite sensitivity of FIP1L1-PDGFRA–positive patients to low-dose imatinib treatment.

Although translocations involving PDGFRB at 5q32 region were identified with 22 different fusion partners, they are indeed very rare, and any patient with a 5q31-q33 chromosomal abnormality with or without eosinophilia should be investigated by FISH testing for PDGFRB rearrangements. At the molecular level, EMS is characterized by various translocations fusing at least 11 different 5′ partner genes to the 3′ part of the FGFR1 gene (8p11) that encodes the tyrosine kinase domain. They include LRRFIP1 (2q37), FGFR10P (6q27), TRIM24 (7q34), CUX1 (7q22), CEP110 (9q33), Nup98 (11p15), FGFR1OP2 (12p11), CPSF6 (12q15), ZMYM2 (13q12), MYO18A (17q11), HERVK (19q13), and BCR (22q11). The most frequent translocation is t(8;13), and cases with the submicroscopic deletion of the 5′ part of the FGFR1 gene were also reported, similar to the formation of t(9;22) with deleted sequences from der(9q) and/or 22q identified in CML.

Once the PDGFRA, PDGFRB, and FGFR1 rearrangements are excluded, the only other recurrent secondary abnormalities

Table 54-3 Chromosomal Translocations in Ph-Negative MPN

Chromosomal Abnormality	Genes Involved	MPD Entity
t(9;12)(q34;p13)	ETV6-ABL	CML-like, T-ALL
5q32	PDGFRB	**Associated Translocations**
t(1;5)(q25;q32)	TPM3-PDGFRB	Atypical MPN
t(2;5)(p21;q32)	SPTBN1-PDGFRB	Atypical MPN
t(4;5)(q21;q32)	PRKG2-PDGFRB	Atypical MPN
t(5;7)(q32;q11)	HIP1-PDGFRB	CMML-like
t(5;10)(q32;q21)	CCDC6-PDGFRB	Ph-negative MPN
t(5;12)(q32;p13)	ETV6-PDGFRB	CEL, CMML
t(5;12)(q32;p13.3)	ERC1-PDGFRB	Atypical MPN
t(5;14)(q33;q24)	NIN-PDGFRB	Atypical MPN
t(5;14)(q32;q32)	KIA1509-PDGFRB	Atypical MPN
t(5;14)(q32;q32)	TRIP11-PDGFRB	AML
t(5;15)(q23;q15)	TP53BP1-PDGFRB	CEL
t(5;15)(q32;q22)	TPS3BP1-PDGFRB	Atypical MPN
t(5;16)(q32;p13)	NDE1-PDGFRB	Atypical MPN
t(5;17)(q32;p11)	HCMOGT1-PDGFRB	Juvenile CMML
t(5;17)(q32;p11,2)	MYO18A-PDGFRB Atypical MPN	
t(5;17)(q32;p13)	RABEP1-PDGFRB	CMML
t(5;17)(q32;q21)	COL1A1-PDGFRB Atypical MPN	
8p11	FGFR1	**Associated Translocations**
t(2;8)(q37;8p11)	LRRFIP1-FGFR1	MPN Syndrome
t(6;8)(q27;p11)	FGFR1OP-FGFR1	Stem cell MPD
t(7;8)(q32;p11)	TRIM24-FGFR1	MPN
t(7;8)(q22;p11)	CUX1-FGFR1	MPN syndrome
t(8;9)(p11;q22)	CEP110-FGFR1	MPN syndrome
t(8;11)(p11;p15)	Nup98-FGFR1	MPN syndrome
t(8;12)(p11;p11)	FGFR1OP-FGFR1	MPN syndrome
t(8;12)(p11;q12)	CPSF6-FGFR1	MPN syndrome
t(8;13)(p11;q12)	ZMYM2-FGFR1	MPN syndrome, leukemia, lymphoma
t(8;17)(p11;q11)	MYO18A-FGFR1	MPN syndrome
t(8;19)(p11;q13) *HERVK-FGFR1* MPN syndrome		
t(8;22)(p11;q11.2)	BCR-FGFR1	Lymphoproliferative disorder
4q12	PDGFRA	
del(4)(q12;q12)	FIP1L1-PDGFRA	CEL
t(4;22)(q12;q11.2)	BCR-FGFR1	Atypical CML
4q12	KIT	SM
9p24	JAK2	
t(9;22)(p24;q11.2)	BCR-JAK2	CML-like
t(9;12)(p24;p13)	JAK2-ETV6	CML-like
der(9)t(9;12)(p24;q13)	JAK-NF-E2	MDS
t(8;9)(p22;p24)	PCM1-JAK2	CMPD, AL,
der(9;18)t(p13;p11)	Not reported	PV, PV→MF
der(9;18)(p10;q10)	Not reported	PV, PV→MF, ET→AML
der(9)t(1;9)(q12;q12)	Not reported	PV, MF
der(1;7)(q10;p10)	Not reported	ET
t(12)(q21 or q21)	Not reported	MF

Modified from De Keersmaecker K, Cools J: Chronic myeloproliferative disorders: A tyrosine kinase tale. *Leukemia* 20:200, 2006.
AL, Acute leukemia; *ALL*, acute lymphoblastic leukemia; *AML*, acute myelogenous leukemia; *CEL*, chronic myeloproliferative disorder; *CML*, chronic myelogenous leukemia; *CMML*, chronic myelomonocytic leukemia; *CMPD*, chronic eosinophilic leukemia; *ET*, essential thrombocytopenia; *MDS*, myelodysplastic syndrome; *MF*, myelofibrosis; *MPD*, myeloproliferative disorder; *T-ALL*, T-cell acute lymphoblastic leukemia.

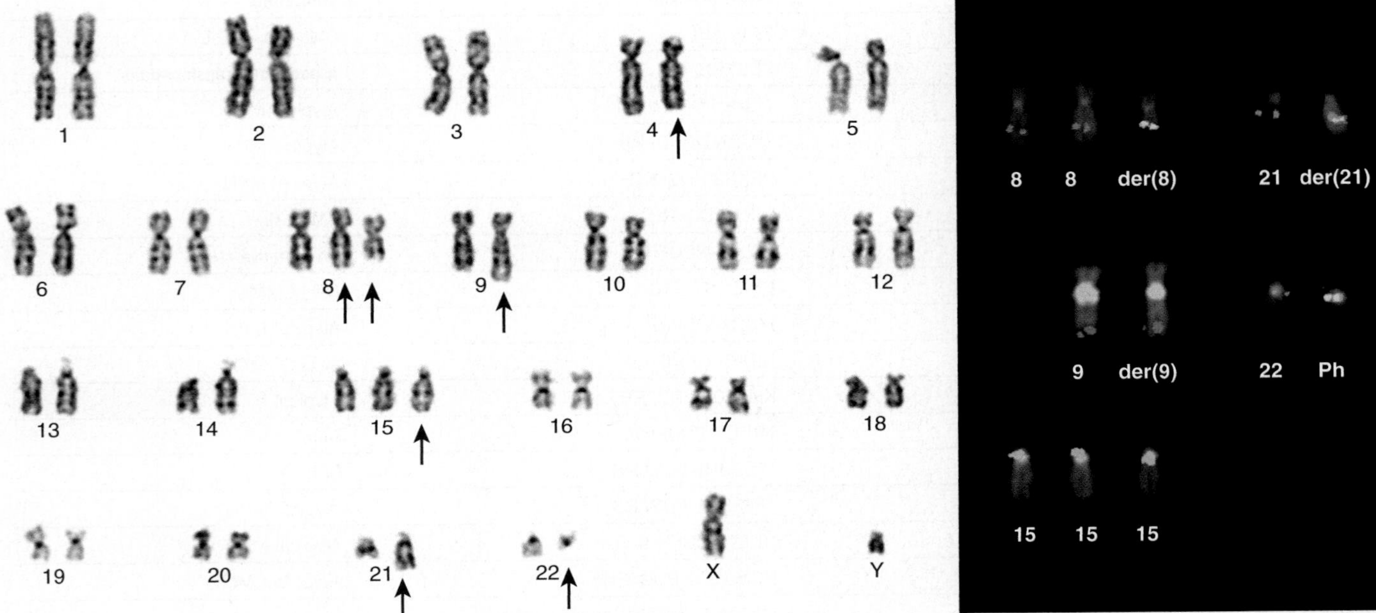

Figure 54-18 A karyotype *(left)* from a patient with chronic myelogenous leukemia who failed three tyrosine kinase inhibitors treatment and progressed into blast crisis showing 46,XY, del(4)(q31q33),t(8;21)(q22;q22),+8,t(9;22)(q34;q11.2),+15. Metaphase FISH studies *(right panel)* confirmed that in the BCR-ABL1 fusion–positive cells (*middle row, yellow* co-localization), the patient had RUN1-RUNXT1 fusion as a result of t(8;21) [*yellow* signals on der(8) and der(21)] and a gain of chromosome 8 *(top row)* as well as trisomy 15 *(bottom row)* as shown using centromeric FISH probe specific for chromosome 15 *(aqua)*.

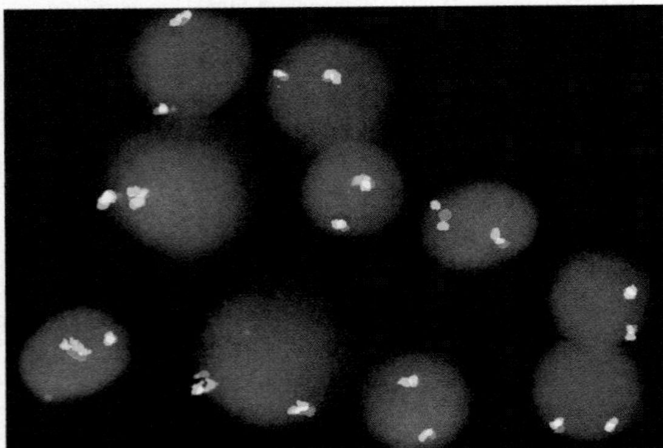

Figure 54-19 BONE MARROW INTERPHASE NUCLEI AFTER FISH STUDIES USING TRICOLOR PROBE FOR CHROMOSOME 4, BAND REGION q12. The *green* color covers an approximately 750-kb region centromeric from FIP1L1. The *red* probe is telomeric of the FIP1L1 gene. The *aqua* color probe begins between exons 15 and 16 of the PDGFRA gene and extends toward the 4q telomere. In normal nuclei, as shown here, the probe appears as two tricolor fusions because of close proximity of probes in interphase DNA. Patients with hypereosinophilic syndrome (HES) have fusion of FIP1L1 and PDGFRA genes by interstitial deletion and produce one signal with *green-aqua* fusion and a missing orange signal. If the translocation involves the PDGFRA gene with loci on other chromosomes, the expected signal pattern is one *orange–green* fusion and one separate aqua signal.

include trisomy 8 and trisomy 21. Once the patient transforms to acute leukemia, various other abnormalities have been reported. Conventional and molecular cytogenetic findings in atypical Ph-negative MPNs, as well as the presence of the JAK2 V617VF mutation in typical Ph-negative MPNs, provide support that abnormalities in tyrosine kinase genes are central to the molecular pathogenesis of these disorders (see box on Genetic Testing for Ph-Negative Myeloproliferative Neoplasms).

Genetic Testing for Ph-Negative Myeloproliferative Neoplasms

At diagnosis, perform JAK2V617F real-time alleles-specific polymerase chain reaction, as well as cytogenetic analysis of marrow cells. Unstimulated peripheral blood can be used instead of marrow aspirate for patients with primary myelofibrosis. Perform FISH studies with BCR-ABL1 for patients with essential thrombocythemia. FISH studies can be performed when cytogenetics is uninformative for detection of most frequent abnormalities: +8, +9, +9p, del(13)(q14), and del(20)(q11q13). The panel of five probes include CEP9, P21 at 9p21, D8Z2 as a centromeric probe for chromosome 8, RB1 for deletion 13q, and D20S108 for deletion of 20q12. At diagnosis and to monitor patients with hypereosinophilic syndrome, perform FISH using triple-color FIP1L1 probe. For 5q32 rearrangements perform FISH with PDGFRB FISH probe.

MYELODYSPLASTIC SYNDROMES

The MDSs (see Chapter 59) are a clinically heterogeneous group of hematologic neoplasms with differing biology and clinical manifestations. They have in common a clonal origin, dysplastic cellular morphology, abnormalities of cellular maturation, increased propensity to develop acute leukemia (20%-40%), and multistep pathogenesis. Cytogenetic studies are important for patients with these disorders because the results can provide both diagnostic and prognostic information. A chromosomally abnormal clone can be detected in 40% to 60% of patients with de novo MDS and in approximately 90% of patients with therapy-related MDS. There appears to be a correlation between the frequency of chromosomal abnormalities and the severity of disease. Approximately 35% of patients with less aggressive MDS, such as refractory anemia and refractory anemia with ring sideroblasts, have clonal chromosomal rearrangements, whereas approximately 60% to 70% of patients with refractory anemia with excess blasts in transformation have such chromosomal abnormalities. A single or complex chromosomal abnormality may be present

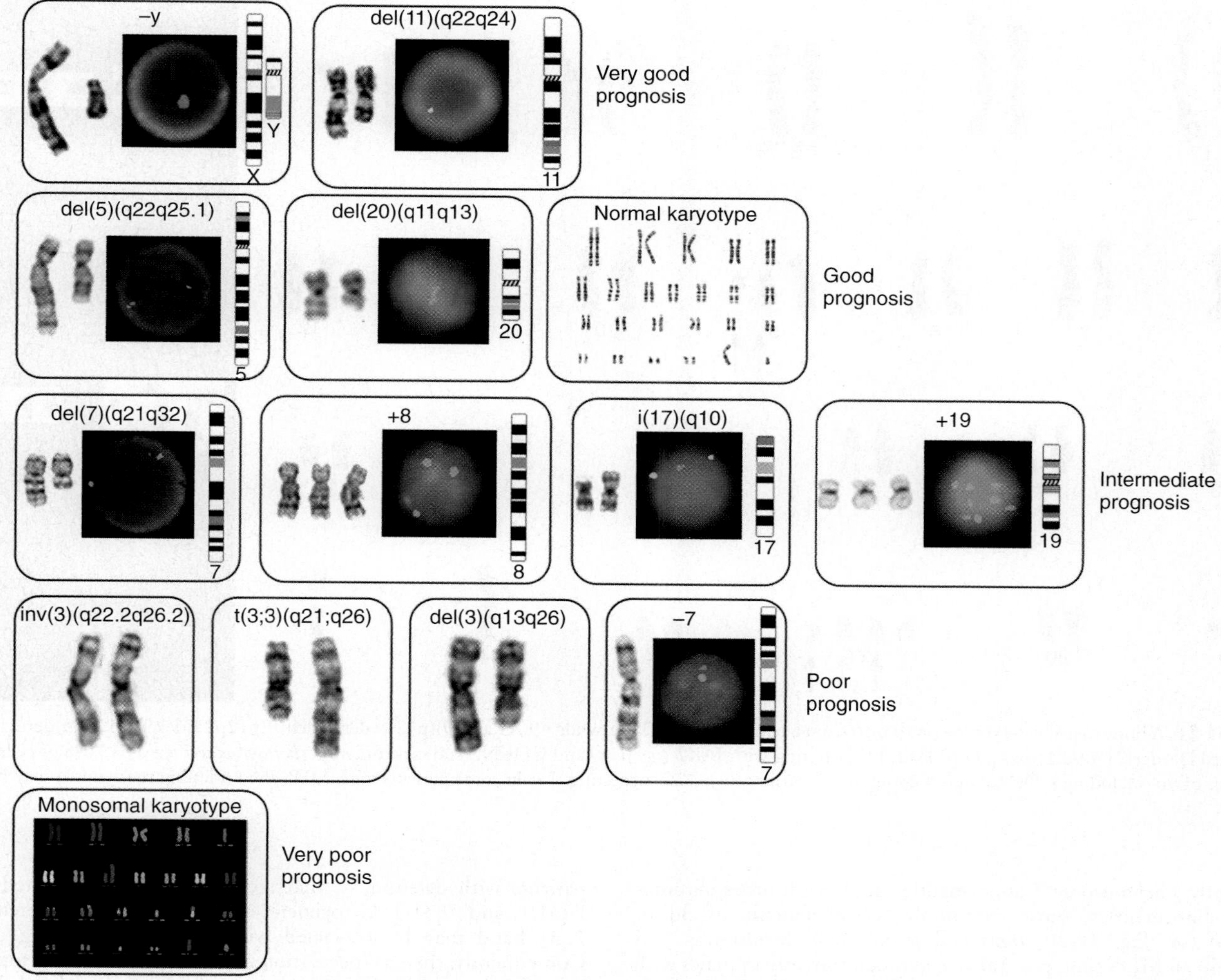

Figure 54-20 PROGNOSTIC SIGNIFICANCE OF THE RECURRENT CHROMOSOMAL ABNORMALITIES IN MYELODYSPLASTIC SYNDROME, ACCORDING TO THE NEW COMPREHENSIVE CYTOGENETIC SCORING SYSTEM.

initially, and evolutionary change may occur during the course of the disease. Even at diagnosis of MDS, complex genomic lesions involving five or more different chromosomes are not unusual. Despite heterogeneity of chromosomal defects (gain, loss, deletion, amplification, rare balanced translocations, transcriptional silencing via methylation or point mutation), the unifying concept of genetic instability in MDS is hemizygosity of specific genes or chromosomal regions. The most common chromosome anomalies in MDS involve gain of 1q, del(5q)/−5, del(7q)/−7, trisomy 8, del(11)(q23), del(12p), +13/del(13q), t(11q23), del(12p), del(17p), del(20)(q11q13), +21, and idic(X)(q13) (Figs. 54-20 and 54-21).

The clinical relevance and the power of conventional cytogenetics in MDS were recognized by the WHO classification for hematologic malignancies, which accepted a strong association between del(5)(q13q33) and 5q− syndrome, and idic(X)(q13) and refractory anemia with ring sideroblasts. The 5q− syndrome is a unique subtype of low-risk MDS with a favorable prognosis, lack of other cytogenetic abnormalities, low rate of leukemic transformation, and more common occurrence in older adult females (Fig. 54-20, *second row*).

Among patients who do not have 5q− syndrome (with or without other chromosome abnormalities), interstitial deletions of the long arms of chromosome 5 occur in 10% to 15% and are among the most frequent chromosomal abnormalities in MDS (see Fig. 54-20, *second row*). The finding of del(5q) in CD34CD38$^-$ cell indicates its occurrence in a stem cell capable of differentiating into myeloid and lymphoid cell lineages and represents an early event in the pathogenesis of MDS. Data on 1432 patients with del(5q) show a significant amount of heterogeneity in breakpoints. FISH methods delineated the commonly deleted segment, currently estimated to be 1.5 Mb in size, on 5q31.1. The clustering of genes responsible for growth and differentiation of hematopoietic cells and the recurrent nature of −5/del(5q) in MDS caused many investigators to speculate that a tumor suppressor gene(s) was located in the 5q31 or 5q22-23 band region. Despite numerous efforts for more than 20 years, mutations in genes located in the chromosomal regions affected by del(5q) have been unsuccessful, in part because no homozygous deletion has been detected and because 5q31 is a very gene-rich region. To date, the tumor suppressor gene responsible for MDS on 5q has not been identified. Because the mechanism causing the interstitial del(5q) is elusive, perhaps haploinsufficiency or inactivation due to methylation, rather than a typical tumor suppressor gene, is involved in these patients.

Patients with isolated del(5q) have a more favorable prognosis and live longer than patients with additional chromosomal abnormalities. Specifically, patients with del(5)(q13q31) have significantly longer survival than do patients with other 5q deletions, indicating that the type of 5q deletion may significantly affect prognosis and therapy. Indeed, a normal marrow karyotype is achieved in 44% of 148 patients with interstitial del(5q) treated with lenalidomide. The sensitivity of del(5q) to lenalidomide remains to be elucidated.

In de novo MDS, isolated monosomy 7 or 7q deletion (Fig. 54-22; see also Fig. 54-20, *third row*) occurs with a frequency of 20%.

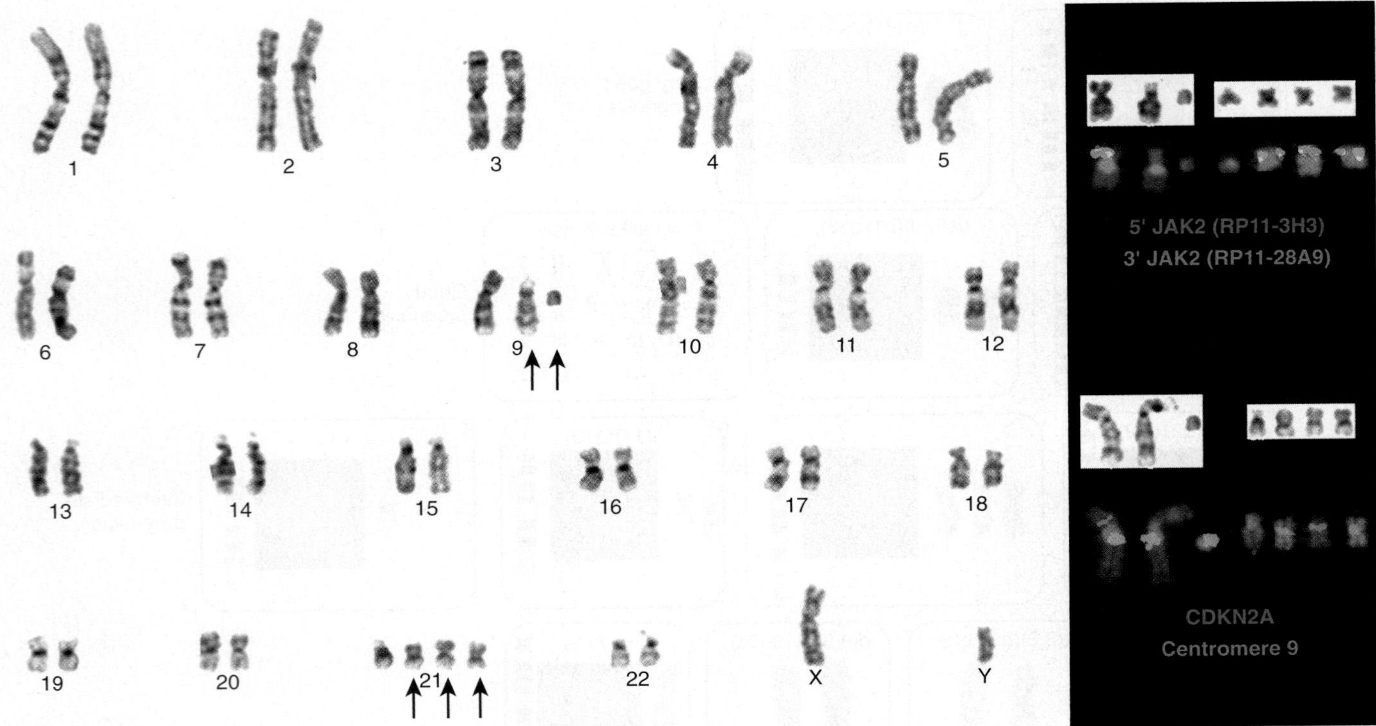

Figure 54-21 A bone marrow karyotype *(left panel)* from a patient with MDS showing 49,XY,add(9)(p12),+der(9)del(9)(p12p24)del(9)(q12q34)der(21)t(9;21)p21p24;p11),+der(21)t(9;21)(p21p24;p11)x2. FISH testing with JAK2 *(top part)* and CDKN2 and centromere 9 *(bottom panel)* revealed 70% of cells to have a deletion of 9p, including CDKN2 and 4 copies of unrearranged JAK2, suggesting that in some patients with MDS the underling mechanism may be a gain of JAK2.

Frequently, chromosome 7 abnormalities occur with other chromosomal abnormalities, most commonly rearrangements of 3q or del(12p) (see Fig. 54-20, *third* and *fourth row*). Monosomy 7 is present in all MDS subtypes and is seen predominantly in males with clinical characteristics similar to those of juvenile CMML. In pediatric patients with constitutional disorders associated with a predisposition to development of myeloid leukemia, such as individuals with Fanconi anemia, congenital neutropenia, neurofibromatosis type 1, Down syndrome, or Kostmann syndrome, −7/del(7q) may be seen as an isolated abnormality. Therefore the question as to whether these patients have genetic imprinting and preferentially lose chromosome 7 from one parent is relevant to understanding the origin of the genetic abnormality. Unequivocal evidence shows that preferential parental origin of the missing chromosome 7 is not present because approximately half of patients have loss of either the maternal or paternal homologue, excluding the genomic imprinting phenomenon as a cause for monosomy 7. Embryonic origin of partial chromosome 7 deletion in monozygotic twins with juvenile chronic myelomonocytic leukemia has been reported.

According to the IPSS, patients with chromosome 7 abnormalities present either as a single anomaly or in combination with other anomalies and are considered a high-risk karyotype group.[12] However, more recent results have indicated that patients with del(7q) as a single abnormality have a distinct clinical–pathologic profile with an overall better prognosis than seen in patients with an isolated monosomy 7. Isolated del(7q) is more frequent in patients with less advanced MDS according to the WHO classification or the International Prognostic Scoring System. Their characteristics include association with fewer blasts in bone marrow than other cytogenetic groups and significantly superior survival when compared with patients with isolated monosomy 7. The presence of additional chromosomal abnormalities in patients with del(7q) shortened the overall survival. The current recommendation is that isolated del(7q) should not be considered in the same prognostic category as monosomy 7 (see Fig. 54-20). Allele typing studies implicated three regions in patients with deletion 7q that are most frequently deleted: 7q22, 7q31.1, and 7q31.3. Cytogenetic results indicated that retention of 7q31 band may be associated with longer survival (Fig. 54-22). Consequently, there is speculation that a putative myeloid suppressor gene(s) is located in the regions that are frequently deleted. Because prototypic tumor suppressor genes have not been identified in patients with 7q deletions, an alternative explanation may be haploinsufficiency whereby the level of protein is critical, or a complex of two cooperating proteins is affected as a result of inactivation due to methylation.

Trisomy 8 (see Fig. 54-20, *third row*) is the third most frequent chromosomal abnormality in MDS. As a sole abnormality, it is found in 11% of patients with MDS and overall is found in 17%. A significantly higher incidence of trisomy 8 occurs in males than in females. Trisomy 8 is present in all age groups of patients with MDS. Although trisomy 8 is detected in hematopoietic stem cell of patients with MDS, a sizable fraction of stem cells is disomic but functionally abnormal, suggesting that trisomy 8 is a secondary event in MDS pathogenesis. These findings provide evidence for a multistep pathogenesis of MDS, whereby gain of chromosome 8 is not an early event in stepwise evolution. Although trisomy 8 carries an intermediate risk when detected at diagnosis, findings suggest that MDS patients treated with the hypomethylating agent 5-azycytidine have a significantly better survival than patients with other chromosomal abnormalities.

The first series of patients with MDS or MDS/MPN associated with trisomy 11 as a sole abnormality or as a part of noncomplex karyotype was recently reported. This rare recurrent abnormality has an overall frequency of approximately 0.3% and is associated with a significantly inferior survival in patients with IPSS intermediate-risk disease (P = 0.0002) but comparable to the poor-risk group (P = 0.97). Trisomy 11 correlates with clinical aggressiveness and represents a high-risk cytogenetic abnormality.

Deletions of 17p are seen in 3% to 4% of MDS and AML patients. These patients often display several other chromosomal

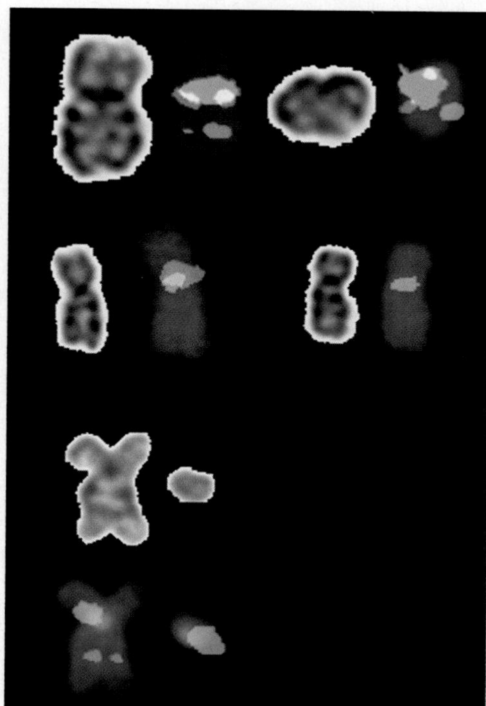

Figure 54-22 EXAMPLES OF CHROMOSOME 7 ABNORMALITIES IN MYELODYSPLASTIC SYNDROME (MDS). Ring chromosome 7 is a recurrent but rare formation. In the case shown in the *top row,* FISH study *(right)* demonstrates retention of centromeric region *(aqua),* 7p12 (*red*), and 7q31 *(green)* regions. Retention of 7q31 region is associated with longer survival. Deletion 7p *(second row)* is less frequent than del(7q) and may be missed by conventional cytogenetics. Note loss of 7p12 band in the patient with MDS by FISH study *(right),* showing only the centromeric *(green)* signal and no red signal for the EGFR gene, localized at 7p12. Loss of both the short and long arms of chromosome 7 in pediatric and adult patients with MDS often may appear as a marker chromosome *(third row),* but FISH study with dual-color probes for centromere *(green)* and 7q31 *(red)* revealed the presence of only the centromeric region on the minute chromosome *(fourth row).*

rearrangements, including monosomy 17, isochromosome 17q (see Fig. 54-20, *third row*), and unbalanced translocations between chromosome 17 and another chromosome. Approximately 30% of these deletions are related to therapy. Most patients who develop MDS or AML are treated with hydroxyurea, usually for a prolonged period of time. The extent of 17p deletion in all cases involves the p53 gene. There appears to be a close correlation between dysgranulopoiesis (e.g., pseudo–Pelger-Huet hypolobulation) and small vacuoles in neutrophils with 17p abnormalities and p53 deletion. Median survival of these patients is poor.

An isodicentric X chromosome in Xq13-idic(X) is a rare but recurrent abnormality that has been suggested to be specifically associated with refractory anemia with ringed sideroblasts. All MDS patients with idic(X)(q13) are females, most likely because formation of idic(X) would result in nullisomy for Xq13-qter in males. Median age at the time of diagnosis is 73.5 years. The outcome of idic(X)-positive cases is variable; some investigators report aggressive and rapidly fatal disease and others a relatively favorable clinical course with survival for several years despite the generally advanced age of the patients. The fact that idic(X) most often occurs as the sole cytogenetic abnormality suggests that it may in itself be sufficient for leukemogenesis. Using a high-resolution SNP array, the breakpoints on idic(X)(q13) were mapped into two distinct breakpoint clusters, at approximately 70.9 MB (five cases) and 72.1MB (seven cases) on the X chromosome. None of the 11 breakpoints occurred in a gene, strongly indicating that the idic(X)(q13) does not result in a fusion gene. Instead, the functional outcome of the abnormality is a gene dosage effect due to the concurrent gain of Xpter-q13 and loss of Xq13-qter. This region of X chromosome is enriched for repeated sequences and most likely, these repeats may facilitate the formation of idic(X). The isodicentric X chromosome was inactive in some patients and active in other patients; hence idic(X) appears to be leukemogenic regardless of X_a or X_i involvement.

Gain of 1q, usually in the form of unbalanced translocation, is a recurrent abnormality in MDS and appears to be a marker of disease progression. Specifically, the gain of 1q in the form of jumping translocations either at diagnosis or the subsequent acquisition of jumping 1q translocations appears to be associated with imminent transformation to AML in patients after an average of 9 months (Fig. 54-23). Once acquired, prognosis tended to be dependent on a copy number of 1q, indicating that gain of jumping 1q translocations was associated with both disease progression and poor prognosis. In MDS, the average time to develop jumping 1q was less than 2 years. Treatment (azacitidine, chemotherapy, or stem cell transplant) may temporarily reduce or eradicate the clone, but the responses were not durable. These findings did not provide any common pattern as to the role of the partner chromosomes in unbalanced jumping 1q translocations. However, 81% of recipient breakpoints were localized in pericentric regions whereas the remaining 19% were telomeric fusions. Decondensation of pericentromeric heterochromatin of chromosome 1 together with centromere and repeat DNA sequences interspersed with histones and acetylated sequences may favor illegitimate recombinations leading to jumping 1q translocations. Moreover, exposure to azacitidine has been shown to be associated with alterations of pericentromeric heterochromatin of chromosome 1, as well as an increase in Alu DNA repeats amplification. The most frequent rearrangement of chromosome 3 involves two bands on chromosome 3—band 3q21 and 3q26 simultaneously—which produces either t(3;3)(q21;q26) or inv(3)(q21q26) (see Fig. 54-20, *fourth row*). These chromosomal rearrangements are present in de novo and therapy-related MDS, as well as in AML and megakaryoblastic crisis of CML. The incidence of the 3q rearrangements is 2% to 5%. Characteristic clinical features include an elevated platelet count, marked hyperplasia with dysplasia of megakaryocytes, and a poor prognosis with minimal or no response to chemotherapy and a short survival. In addition to similar clinicopathologic features, patients with 3q21q26 chromosomal abnormalities share molecular heterogeneity in both the breakpoints and the expression pattern of the genes near these breakpoints. The chromosomal breakpoints, defined by FISH, in 3q26 are scattered over several hundred kilobases in either the 5′ or the 3′ region of the EVI1 gene, whereas the breakpoints in the 3q21 region are restricted to two smaller different genomic clusters approximately 100 kb downstream of the RPN1 gene. EVI1 overexpression is observed in the majority of patients, but some patients with the 3q21q26 rearrangement do not have detectable EVI1 expression, and at least 9% of AML patients without 3q26 abnormalities overexpress EVI1. Therefore the poor prognosis in these patients may be independent of EVI1 expression, despite the fact that extensive 3q26 breakpoint FISH mapping on both metaphases and interphase nuclei suggests EVI1 involvement in numerous novel sporadic and recurrent 3q26 rearrangements. A fusion transcript of RPN1-EVI1 is rarely observed in patients with 3q21q26 rearrangements. However, evidence suggests that overexpression of GATA2 at 3q21 may be responsible for erythroid and megakaryocytic dysplasia observed in patients with 3q21q26 chromosomal abnormalities.

A monosomal karyotype (MK), a new cytogenetic category, is defined as a karyotype showing two or more distinct autosomal chromosome monosomies or one single autosomal monosomy (excluding isolated loss of X or Y) in the presence of a structural abnormality (see Fig. 54-20, *bottom row*). Initial reports indicated that the MK in MDS, with or without monosomy for chromosomes 5 and 7, was prognostically worse than other complex karyotype, although later reports could not confirm these results. The reason may be that treatment with azacitidine may have reduced the negative impact of MK in high-risk patients with MDS.

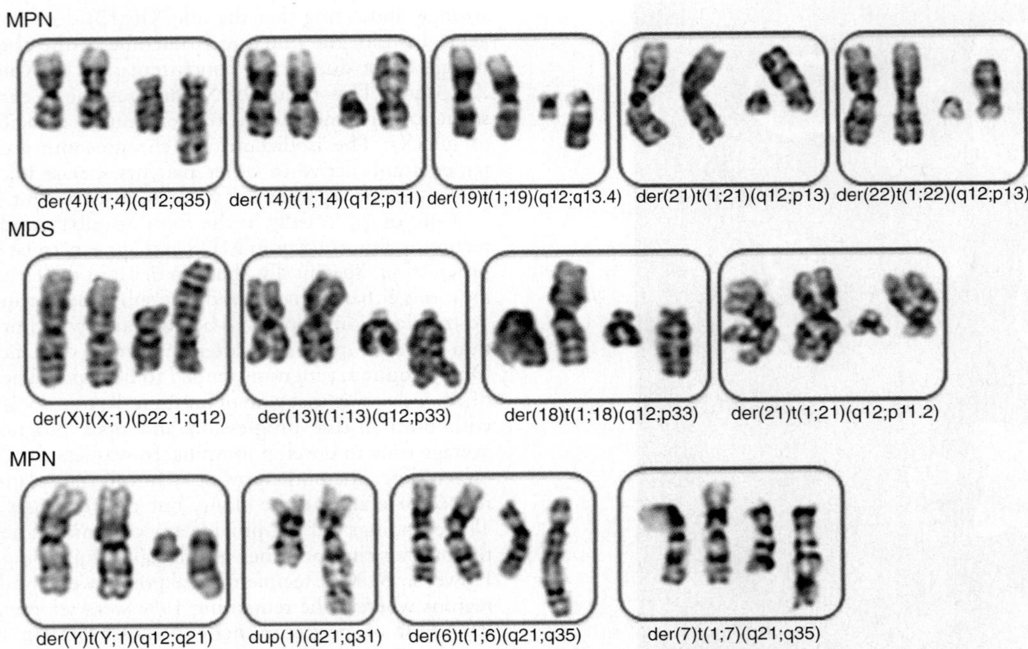

Figure 54-23 JUMPING 1q TRANSLOCATIONS FROM TWO PATIENTS WITH MPN AND ONE PATIENT WITH MDS. The *top row* shows five different clones created as a result of a gain of 1q translocated to chromosomes 4, 14, 19, 21, and 22. The *middle row* shows four different cell populations identified in a patient with MDS, all characterized by trisomy 1q translocated to X chromosome as well as to chromosomes 13, 19 and 21. The *bottom row* shows a follow up bone marrow from a patient with MPN that at diagnosis had i(9)(p10) and with progression of disease acquired jumping 1q to Y chromosome, to chromosome 6 and 7, as well as an insertion within the long arms of 1, resulting in duplication of 1q.

The clinical significance of loss of the Y chromosome, observed in 10% of MDS patients and approximately 7% of older adult males without MDS, is undefined, although older adult males with MDS and loss of Y chromosome who achieve complete hematologic remission show the Y chromosome in their marrow cells.

The prognosis of patients with MDS is very heterogeneous. In 1997, based on the cytogenetic abnormalities identified in 816 patients with MDS, as well as percentage of blasts and number of cytopenia, an International Prognostic Scoring System (IPSS) was proposed.[12] According to the IPSS, 86% of all cytogenetic findings can be explicitly classified according to their prognostic impact. The system is highly reproducible and very simple to use, but it has certain limitations. Moreover, the remaining 14% of patients with cytogenetic abnormalities have unknown prognostic significance. This limitation underscores two major cytogenetic classification problems in MDS: the profound heterogeneity of acquired cytogenetic aberrations in MDS and the associated challenge of designing a comprehensive cytogenetic scoring system that predicts the prognostic impact of rare abnormalities. A new and comprehensive cytogenetic scoring system based on an international data collection of 2902 patients was recently proposed (see Fig. 54-20). Patients included were from the German-Austrian MDS Study Group (n = 1193), the International MDS Risk Analysis Workshop (n = 816), the Spanish Hematological Cytogenetics Working Group (n = 849), and the International Working Group on MDS Cytogenetics (n = 44) databases.[13] In total, 19 cytogenetic categories were defined, providing clear prognostic classification in 91% of all patients. All abnormalities were arranged according to overall survival and development of AML in order to classify their prognostic impact. The abnormalities were classified into five prognostic subgroups: very good (n = 81) included del(11q) and loss of Y chromosome (median OS, 61 months); good (n = 1809) included normal karyotype, del(5q),del(12p), and del(20q) (all as single anomaly) and double abnormalities including del(5q) (median OS 49 months); intermediate (n = 529) included del(7q), +8, i(17q)(q10), +19, +21, any other single abnormality, independent clones, and double abnormalities not harboring del(5q) or −7/del(7q) (median OS 26 months); poor (n = 148) included inv(3)/t(3q)/del(3q), −7, and double abnormalities including −7/del(7q) and complex (three abnormalities; OS of 16 months); and very poor (n = 197) included complex with more than three abnormalities (OS of 6 months) (see Fig. 54-20). Both internal and external validation of the new scoring system was performed, and results confirmed that the score efficiently predicts outcome in patients with MDS. This new scoring system proposed should be viewed as a dynamic model, open to further refinement as the knowledge in karyotypic abnormalities of MDS continues to evolve.

Cytogenetic and FISH studies have relatively similar sensitivities in detecting an abnormal clone among patients with MDS. A FISH test for MDS should use probes to detect numerical and structural anomalies of chromosome regions 1q, 3q, 5q, 7q, 7q31, 8, 11q, 12p, 13q, 17p, 20q, and 21. Occasional patients with normal chromosomes show an occult neoplastic clone by FISH. On the other hand, in conventional cytogenetic studies, some patients exhibit a neoplastic clone that is not detected by FISH (see box on Genetic Testing for Myelodysplastic Syndrome and Fig. 54-20).

Genetic Testing for Myelodysplastic Syndrome Disorder

The best genetic test at diagnosis is conventional cytogenetic studies. FISH is useful for some clinical situations, such as marrow samples lacking analyzable metaphases, or to follow the percentage of abnormal cells with known cytogenetic anomalies for patients undergoing treatment (see Fig. 54-20 for selection of appropriate fluorescence in situ hybridization probes).

In contrast to the wealth of genetic profiling data for most leukemias, MDS has not been analyzed extensively, probably as a result of MDS heterogeneity both on the clinical and genomic level.

Familial MDS is very rare. However, a recent description of four families with telomerase mutations, both in the RNA component (TERC) and in the reverse transcriptase (TERT), has raised the awareness of the pathologic role of telomerase mutations in development of MDS/AML. The telomerase activity of the mutations identified in the 4 of 20 families with familial MDS/AML was between 0% and 11% of the wild-type levels. Patients with telomerase mutations have short telomeres. The recognition of familial MDS/AML arising from constitutional mutations in TERC or TERT is important because these mutations probably act as initiating mutations. Moreover, next generations present with increasingly more severe phenotypes at an earlier age so that each successive generation inherits progressively shorter telomeres, which increasingly promote genomic instability and may lead to earlier development of marrow failure, MDS, or AML. The recommendation is that inherited lesions always be considered in a young patient presenting with MDS, even in the absence of preexisting morphologic or hematologic abnormalities. Another constitutional abnormality that appears to predispose to MDS/AML is a deletion of band region q22.1-q22.2 of chromosome 21 with a complex phenotype (dysmorphic features, organ malformations, growth delay, and mental retardation), germline RUNX1 deletion, and congenital thrombocytopenia. Three of nine reported patients subsequently developed MDS/AML.

ACUTE MYELOID LEUKEMIA

AML refers to a group of heterogeneous diseases with respect to clonality, chromosomal aberrations, and response to treatment (see Chapters 57 and 58). AML develops clonally and has a multistep pathogenesis. In adults, at the time of diagnosis all hematopoietic cell lineages are clonal. In children younger than 16 years, erythroid cells and platelets often are not part of the leukemic clone. Observations made by the International Workshop on Chromosomes in Leukemia asserted that cytogenetics findings provide the single most important factor in AML; these observations were subsequently validated through studies conducted by the Medical Research Council (MRC), the Cancer and Leukemia Group B (CALGB), and the Southwest Oncology Group. Finally, in 2008 the WHO incorporated cytogenetic analysis of leukemic blasts along with morphology, immunologic markers, and molecular genetics into the classification system for AML. Cytogenetics is the most powerful independent prognostic factor in AML and provides the framework for risk stratification schemes that have been generally adopted to guide treatment approach. Based on karyotype status, two major groups of AML can be distinguished: (a) those with an abnormal karyotype, which accounts for approximately 52% of patients, and (b) those who demonstrate a normal karyotype by conventional cytogenetics, which accounts for 48% of AML patients.[14]

AML patients with a normal karyotype who present between the ages of 16 and 60 years carry an intermediate prognosis. However, cytogenetically normal AML is highly heterogeneous at the molecular level, both mutations and overexpression of single genes have been identified, and their complex interactions are frequently refined to provide more accurate risk stratification. Within the normal cytogenetic category, 45% to 62% of patients with AML have NPM1 mutations (localized on chromosome 5, band q35), 23% to 33% show FLT3 (localized on chromosome 13, band q12), 5% to 10% have MLL tandem duplications (localized on chromosome 11, band q23), and 8% to 15% have CEBPA mutations (localized on chromosome 19, band q13.1). The prognosis of patients with normal karyotype differs in the presence of each of these mutations (Table 54-4 and Fig. 54-24). Patients with NPM1 mutations alone have a

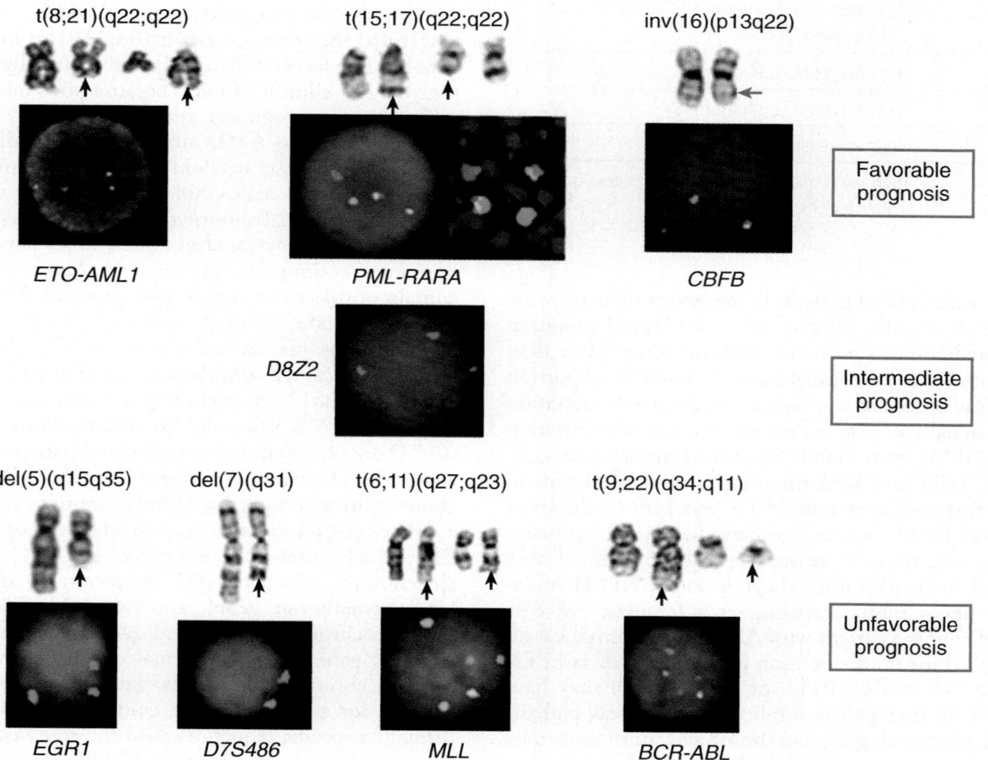

Figure 54-24 PROGNOSTIC CYTOGENETIC RISK CATEGORIES IN ACUTE MYELOID LEUKEMIA. Favorable prognosis includes t(8;21) and ETO-AML1 fusion, t(15;17) and PML-RARA fusion, and inv(16) and rearrangements of *CBFB* on 16q22. Trisomy 8 is associated with intermediate prognosis. Unfavorable cytogenetic risk categories include monosomy 5/del(5q), −7/del(7q), and translocations of 11q23 and MLL, represented here by t(6;11), and the Philadelphia chromosome.

Table 54-4 Gene Mutations in Patients With Acute Myelogenous Leukemia and Normal Karyotype

Gene	Frequency (%) of Patients With a Normal Karyotype	Prognosis
NPM1	45-62	Favorable, increased CR rates and prolonged OS in the absence of FLT3 mutation
FLT3-IDT	30	Unfavorable, specifically when the mutant to WT allelic ratio is high
FLT3-TKD	7-10	Controversial
CEBPA	15	Favorable
MLL-PTD	10	Not known
WT1	10	Not known (possibly favorable)
RAS	10-15	Not known
IDH1	15-20	Most likely unfavorable
IDH2	20	Most likely unfavorable
DNMT3A	36	Most likely unfavorable
TET2	5	Likely unfavorable

Table 54-5 Over-Expression of Single Genes in Acute Myelogenous Leukemia and Normal Karyotype

	Prognostic Implications	
Gene	**Frequency (%)**	**Prognosis**
BAALC	50-60	High expression, inferior EFS, and shorter OS
ERG	30	High expression, inferior CR rates, and decreased DFS
MN1	Variable	High expression, shorter OS
AFq1	80-90	High expression, shorter OS
EVI1	10	High expression, shorter OS
Id1	65	High expression, decreased CR rates, and shorter OS

favorable prognosis, with 60% of patients living longer than 11 years. Even in patients age 70 or older, the presence of an NPM1 mutation is an independent predictor of a more favorable outcome. More than 20 different mutations have been described in the C-terminal portion of the protein that lead to loss of tryptophan residues and generation of a nuclear export signal that acts in concert to cause delocalization of nucleophosmin (NPM) from the nuclei to the cytoplasm. In contrast, the presence of FLT3 and MLL mutations is associated with an adverse prognosis, and coexistence of FLT3 and NPM1 does not improve the prognosis. NPM1 mutation is considered to be a primary lesion in the pathogenesis of AML, being very stable over the disease course. In childhood AML with normal cytogenetics, NPM1 mutations are relatively uncommon, occurring at a frequency of 8%. Currently, a newly diagnosed patient with AML and a normal karyotype should be checked for more common mutations such as FLT3, NPM1, CEBPA, RUNX1, MLL-PTD, or EVI1, which may have prognostic and possibly therapeutic implications, whereas patients with overexpression of other single genes should stay, until more data are collected, in a research setting of clinical trials (Table 54-5).

Among patients with an abnormal karyotype, 25% have balanced translocations [t(8;21),t(15;17),inv(16)], and 27% showed unbalanced abnormalities [–5/del(5q), –7/del(7q), or complex karyotype].

The pretreatment karyotype in AML constitutes an independently prognostic determinant for attainment of complete remission and

Table 54-6 Cytogenetic/Molecular Risk Categories in Acute Myelogenous Leukemia

Category	Abnormality
Favorable (45%)	t(8;21)/RUNX1-RUNXT1 (8%),* t(15;17)/PML-RARA (11%), inv(16)/CBFB-MYH11 (5%) with or without other abnormalities Normal karyotype with NPM1+, FLT3-ITD Neg/WT1 wt (18%)
Intermediate (17%)	+6, +8, +21, +22, Y, del(9q) Normal karyotype with CEBPA+ biallelic/FLIT3-IDT Neg (3%)
Unfavorable (38%)	–5/del(5q), –7/del(7q), abn(3q) t(9;22),t(6;9), abn(11q), 20q, or 21q, abn(17p), complex karyotype, RUNX1 mut, MLL-PTD, FLT3-IDT/NPM1 wt

*Without deletion 9q or complex karyotype.

risk for relapse and survival.[15] Four broad cytogenetic risk categories of AML are applied in clinical practice: favorable, intermediate, unfavorable, and unknown (see Fig. 54-24 and Table 54-5). It is important to perform appropriate cytogenetic and FISH studies to establish the correct cytogenetic risk category. Tables 54-6 and 54-7 list 166 of approximately 200 recurrent chromosomal translocations in leukemia, including AML (Fig. 54-25; see also Fig. 54-24). Because of their specific association with distinct subtypes of leukemia, some AML-specific translocations have been incorporated into the WHO classification as the criteria for subclassification of AML, including t(8;21), t(15;17), inv(16), and 11q23 rearrangements, regardless of the morphology or percentage of blast cells.

Two specific cytogenetic types of AML—t(8;21)(q22;q22) and inv(16)(p13q22) or t(16;16)(p13;q22) (see Fig. 54-24)—are called core-binding factor (CBF) AML and are usually grouped and reported together in clinical studies because of similarities between their molecular and prognostic features. However, the morphologic features of these two AML subtypes are very different. Patients with t(8;21) exhibit large myeloid blasts with abundant basophilic cytoplasm, numerous azurophilic granules, and occasional Auer rods. Patients with 16q22 abnormalities show a variable number of eosinophils, usually in increased numbers, in all stages of maturation. The immature eosinophilic granules are larger than normal and may contain purple-violet cytoplasmic granules. The t(8;21) subtype may be present alone, although 30% to 35% of patients also display loss of Y chromosomes in males and loss of X chromosome in females (see Fig. 54-24, *top left*). Another 20% of patients with t(8;21) show deletion of 9q12-23, including a commonly deleted segment that spans 7 to 8 Mb. Trisomies for chromosomes 4 and 8 together with t(8;21) are observed in 6% to 10% of patients. Virtually all patients with t(8;21) achieve complete remission. Additional cytogenetic abnormalities, irrespective of their nature or complexity, do not have a deleterious effect on remission, relative risk, and overall survival. The t(8;21) interrupts two genes—RUNX1 (AML1, CBFA2) on chromosome 21, band q22, in intron 5, and RUNX1T1 (ETO [eight, twenty-one gene], also called MTG8-myeloid translocated gene) on chromosome 8, band q22—and joins them to form a new chimeric gene on the abnormal der(8) chromosome. RUNX1 is a gene on chromosome 21, also known as CBFA2/AML1 because it encodes for a DNA-binding component of CBF and binds DNA through a specific sequence called the *runt domain*. The AML1 gene locus on chromosome 21 spans 120 kb; the RUNX1T1 (ETO) gene on chromosome 8 is distributed over 87 kb.

The RUNX1 (AML1) gene has been identified in more than 39 chromosomal translocations in leukemia and plays a critical role during hematopoiesis. The fusion gene is located on the partner chromosome in the majority of AML1 translocations. Its disruption

Table 54-7 Recurring Chromosome Translocations in Leukemia and the Genes Involved

Translocations	Genes Involved	Associated Diseases	Translocations	Genes Involved	Associated Diseases
CBF (AML1/CBFA AND CBFB)- AND TEL/ETV6-ASSOCIATED TRANSLOCATIONS/INVERSIONS			**E2A-ASSOCIATED TRANSLOCATIONS**		
t(X;21)(p22;q22)	PRDX4-AML1	AML	t(1;19)(q23;p13)	PBX1-E2A	B-ALL
t(3;21)(q26;q22)	EVI1-MDS1-EAP-AML1	t-AML/CML-ACC/BC	t(17;19)(q23;p13)	HLF-E2A	B-ALL
t(8;21)(q22;q22)	ETO-AML1	AML	**TYROSINE KINASE–ASSOCIATED TRANSLOCATIONS**		
t(8;21)(q23;q22)	FOG2-AML1	MDS	del(4)(q12;q12)	FIP1L1-PDGFRA	HES
t(8;21)(q24;q22)	TRPS1-AML1	ALL/AML	t(4;22)(q12;q11)	PDGFRA-BCR	
t(16;21)(q24;q22)	MTG16-AML1	t-AML	t(1;5)(q23;q33)	Myomegalin-PDGFRB	MPD
t(19;21)(q13;q22)	AMP19-AML1	t-AML	t(5;7)(q33;q11.2)	PDGFRB-HIP1	CMML
t(12;21)(p12;22)	ETV6-AML1	ALL	t(5:10)(q33;q21)	PDGFRB-H4	MPD
t(21;21)(q11;q22)	UPS25-AML1	MDS	t(5;12)(q33;p13)	PDGFRB-ETV6	CMML, CEL
inv(16)/t(16;16)(p13;q22)	MYH11-CBFB	AML-M4	t(5;14)(q33;q32)	PDGFRB/-AV14	AML
t(1;12)(p36;p13)	MDS2-ETV6	CML/MDS	t(5;14)(q33;q24)	PDGFRB/-IN	MPD
t(1;12)(q21;p13)	ARNT-ETV6	AML	t(5;15)(q33;q15)	PDGFRB/-P53BP1	MPD
t(1;12)(q25;p13)	ARG-ETV6	AML	t(5;17)(q33;p13)	PDGFRB-RABEPI	CMML
t(3;12)(q26;p13)	MDS1-EV1-ETV6	MPD	t(5;17)(q33;p11.2)	PDGFRB-HCMOGT	JMML
t(4;12)(p11;p13)	BTL-TV6	AML	t(q;22)(p24;q11.2)	BCR-JAK2	CML–
t(5;12)(pq31;p13)	ACS2-ETV6	AML	t(q;12)(p24;q13)	JAK2-ETV6	CML–
t(5;12)(q33;p13)	PDGFRB-ETV6	CMML	t(8;9)(p22;p24)	PCMI-JAK2	MPD, AL
t(6;12)(q23;p13)	STL-ETV6	ALL	**NUP98/NUP214-ASSOCIATED TRANSLOCATIONS**		
t(7;12)(q36;p13)	HLXB9-ETV6	AML	t(1;11)(q23;p15)	PMX1/Nup98	AML
t(9;12)(p24;p13)	JAK2/-ETV6	ALL, aCML	t(2;11)(q31;p15)	HOXD13/Nup98	t-AML
t(9;12)(q22;p13)	SYK-ETV6	MDS	t(4;11)(q21;p15)	RAP1GDS1/Nup98	T-ALL
t(9;12)(p34;p13)	ABL-ETV6	CMML	t(5;11)(q35;p15)	NSD/Nup98	AML
t(12;13)(p13;q12)	ETV6-CSX2	AML	t(7:11)(p15;p15)	HOXA9/Nup98	AML
t(12;13)(p13;q14)	ETV6-TTL	ALL	t(9;11)(p22;p15)	LEDGF/Nup98	AML
t(12;15)(p13;q25)	ETV6-NTRK3	AML	inv(11)(p15;q22)	Nup98/DDX10	t-AML
t(12;17)(p13;p12)	ETV6-PER1	AML	t(11;20)(p23;q34)	Nup98/TOP1	t-MDS
t(12;21)(p13;q11)	ETV6-MN1	AML	t(6;9)(p23;q34)	DEK/Nup214(CAN)	AML
t(12;16)(p13;p11)	CHOP-TLS/FUS	AML	Normal Karyotype	SET/Nup214(CAN)	AML
t(16;21)(p11;q22)	TLS-FUS/-RG	AML, MDS	**FGFR1-ASSOCIATED TRANSLOCATIONS**		
RARA-ASSOCIATED TRANSLOCATIONS			t(8;13)(p11;q12)	ZNF198-FGFR1	CMML, MPD
t(15;17)(q22;q21)	PML-RARA	APL	t(7;8)(q32;P11)	TRIM24-FGFR1	
t(5;17)(q32;q21)	NPM-RARA	APL	t(6;8)(q27;P11)	FGFR1OP-FGFR1	
t(11;17)(q23;q21)	PLZF-RARA	APL	ins(12;8)(p11;p11p22)	FGFR1OP2-FGFR1	
t(11;17)(q13;q21)	NuMA-RARA	APL	t(8;17)(p11;q11)	MYO18A-FGFR1	
der(17)	STAT5-RARA	AML	t(8;22)(p11;q11,2)	BCR-FGFR1	
t(3;5)(q25;q35)	MLF1-NPM	AML/MDS			

AL, Acute leukemia; *ALL*, acute lymphoblastic leukemia; *AML*, acute myelogenous leukemia; *APL*, acute promyelocytic leukemia; *B-ALL*, B-cell acute lymphoblastic leukemia; *CEL*, chronic eosinophilic leukemia; *CML*, chronic myelogenous leukemia; *CMML*, chronic myelomonocytic leukemia; *HES*, Hypereosinophilic syndrome; *JMML*, juvenile myelomonocytic leukemia; *MDS*, myelodysplastic syndrome; *MPD*, myeloproliferative disorder; *T-ALL*, T-cell acute lymphoblastic leukemia; *t-AML*, therapy-related AML; *t-MDS*, therapy-related MDS.

is associated with the development of myeloid and lymphoid leukemias. Therefore AML1 is viewed as a master regulatory switch that controls development of a definitive hematopoietic lineage. Moreover, the RUNX1T1 (AML1) transcription factor is critical for proliferation and differentiation of hematopoietic stem cells. Haploinsufficiency of AML1 has been linked to a propensity to develop AML, and biallelic nonsense mutations in the AML1 gene have been identified in most immature AMLs of the FAB M0 subtype. The RUNX1 (ETO) protein belongs to the ETO family of proteins involved in protein–protein interactions but not in protein-DNA interactions.

In the hybrid RUNX1-RUNXT1 (AML1-ETO) protein, the C-terminus of RUNX1 (AML1) is replaced by the entire ETO protein. A main functional characteristic of RUNX1-RUNX1T1 (AML1-ETO) chimeric protein is its ability to bind DNA containing AML1 binding sites and thereby exert a dominant negative inhibition of the

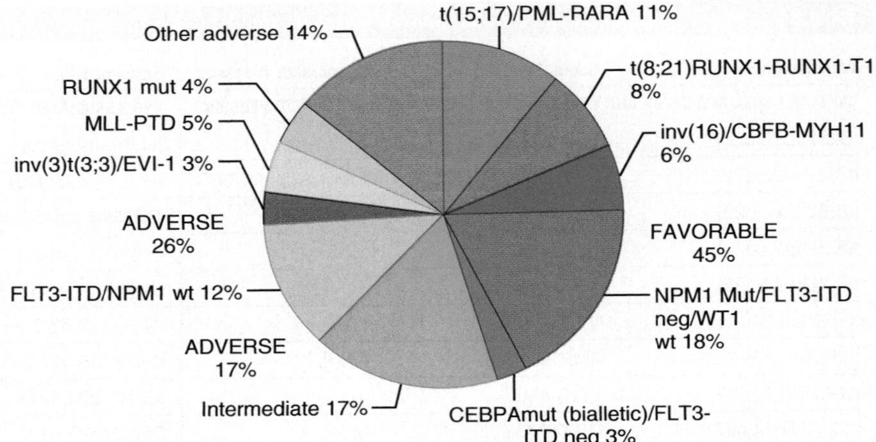

Figure 54-25 INTEGRATION OF CYTOGENETIC ABNORMALITIES AND MOLECULAR MARKERS TO REFINE RISK GROUPS IN AML. *(Reprinted from Smith ML, Hills RK, Grimwade D: Independent prognostic variables in acute myeloid leukemia.* Blood Rev *25:39, 2001; with permission.)*

endogenous AML1 protein. The exact function of the RUNX1-RUNX1T1 (AML1-ETO) fusion protein in the onset and progression of AML is not fully understood; however, accumulating evidence indicates that even a point mutation in the AML1 protein, responsible for assembling and organizing the machinery for hematopoietic gene expression at multiple sites in target genes, results in a block of differentiation of myeloid progenitors to granulocytes. AML1/RUNX1 mutations are present in 46% of AML patients with the M0 subtype and in 80% of AML patients with trisomy 13. As mentioned earlier, FLT3 is localized on chromosome 13, and quantitation of FLT3 transcript levels is associated with a fivefold increase in patients with AML1/RUNX1 mutations and trisomy 13 compared with patients without trisomy 13. The exact cooperation of FLT3 and AML1/RUNX1 in leukemogenesis remains unknown. Multiple copies of ETO-AML1 fusion have been demonstrated (Fig. 54-26). The t(8;21) is the most common translocation in pediatric AML patients (10%-20%). Prenatal origin of t(8;21) was established for approximately 50% of pediatric patients using Guthrie card analysis.

Although 60% to 70% patients with t(8;21) achieve complete and long-term remission, monitoring minimal residual disease is important in identifying patients with a high risk for relapse. Multiparametric approaches, such as flow cytometry, RQ-PCR, and interphase FISH, are complementary methods and provide useful clinical information on relapse kinetics, although each has limitations. It should be noted that 18% of healthy individuals have RUN1-RUNXT1 transcript by PCR and the fusion transcript was also detected in 40% of cord blood samples, suggesting that RUNX1-RUNXT1 by itself may not have overt clinical manifestations.

In patients with 16q22 abnormalities such as inv(16)(p13;q22) and t(16;16)(p13;q22) (Fig. 54-27), the marrow contains an increased percentage of abnormal eosinophils. Combined May-Grünwald-Giemsa staining with FISH demonstrates that the abnormal eosinophils have inv(16) and are therefore part of the leukemic clone. Trisomy 22 is a frequent accompanying abnormality. Both inv(16) (see Fig. 54-24, *top right*) and t(16;16) (see Fig. 54-27) are abnormalities of the core-binding factor β (CBFβ) gene at 16q22 and are associated with M4Eo subtype, according to the French-American-British classification of AML. Both rearrangements result in fusion of CBFβ and MYH11 (myosin heavy-chain) gene on 16p13. The exact role of the resulting hybrid protein, CBFβ-SMMHC (smooth muscle myosin heavy chain), is unknown, but it probably is involved in impaired hematopoietic differentiation. Both t(8;21) and inv(16) rearrangements result in abnormal repression of CBF target genes. CBF is a heterodimeric transcription factor complex that consists of three distinct DNA-binding CBFα subunits (RUNX1, RUNX2, and RUNX3) and a common CBFβ subunit, which is non–DNA-binding. The binding affinity of RUNX1 subunit to the DNA promoter sequences is significantly increased by association with CBFβ, which does not directly interact with DNA and protects RUNX1 subunit from proteolysis. The breakpoints in t(8;21) affect RUNX1 exon 5

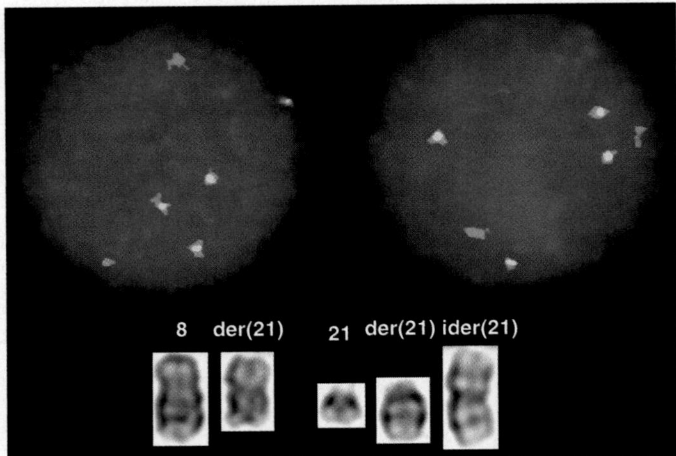

Figure 54-26 Four copies of ETO-AML1 (RUNX) fusion *(yellow)* shown in two interphase cells *(top)* from a patient with acute myeloid leukemia and t(8;21) *(bottom)* karyotype, as well as ider(21). This formation is equivalent to the Ph duplication in the blast crisis of chronic myelogenous leukemia because of duplication of der(21) without accompanying t(8;21).

and RUNX1T1 exon 2. The breakpoint in MYH11 involved in aberrations inv(16) and t(16;16) is variable and gives rise to at least 10 different fusion variants. In contrast, the breakpoints in CBFB at 16q22 are in intron 5. Both translocations are associated with a favorable prognosis, but they exhibit different leukemic cell morphology.

Approximately 4% of patients with CBFB-MYH11 rearrangement do not have a cytogenetically detectable inv(16) or t(16;16). Cytogenetic detection of inv(16) may be difficult, and interphase FISH with a dual-color CBFβ probe at diagnosis is a crucial genetic test. Detection of CBFβ-MYH11 fusion by either RT-PCR or FISH is found in patients without eosinophilia; therefore CBFβ testing should be included in the standard testing panel for genomic rearrangement in AML. The presence of additional abnormalities, such as trisomy 8, does not adversely affect clinical outcome. The CBFβ-MYH11 chimeric fusion is detected in utero with approximately 10 years of postnatal latency before development of childhood leukemia. This observation suggests that formation of CBFβ-MYH11 is not sufficient to cause leukemia and that subsequent genetic events must occur before clinically recognizable leukemia is identified.

Most clinical studies have found that the CBF AML group is associated with a better complete remission rate, overall survival, and lower relapse risk than patients with cytogenetically normal AML. However, a recent retrospective analysis of 113 patients with CBF AML demonstrated that at diagnosis, patients with inv(16) karyotype are less likely to have any normal metaphases when compared with patients showing t(8;21) karyotype. Moreover, an increasing number of cells with normal metaphases increased the risk for relapse and negatively affected survival of patients with inv(16); identifying at least one normal metaphase at diagnosis [as well as 19 with inv(16)] had a significant impact on 5-year survival (60% versus 14%, $P = 00005$). These factors, along with age, were the only independent variables associated with refractory disease and higher relapse.

Risk-adapted stratification based on the genomic makeup of each individual patient is used. Patients with CBF AML and mutations in KIT gene (exon 17) have a higher risk for relapse. KIT mutations represent not only a prognostic indicator but also a potential therapeutic target for tyrosine kinase inhibitors. RUNX1 mutations present in patients with AML, usually M0 in about 5% to 15%, are mutually exclusive when t(8;21) and inv(16) are present. As mentioned earlier, there are 39 recurrent abnormalities involving the 21q22 chromosomal site where RUNX1 is localized. Some of the more frequent rearrangements are discussed here.

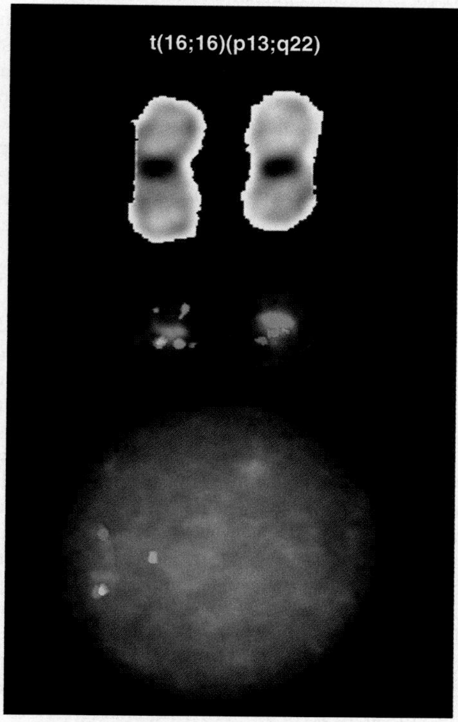

Figure 54-27 Partial G-banded karyotype from a patient with M4 acute myeloid leukemia showing t(16;16) *(top)*, after FISH study using a breakapart CBFB probe (at 16q22), demonstrating that the 5′ end *(red)* of the gene remains on 16q of one chromosome 16, whereas the 3′ end *(green)* translocated to the short arms of the other chromosome 16. Separation of 5′ and 3′ ends as single signals is indicated in the bone marrow nucleus *(bottom)*.

t(16;21)(q24;q22) is a rare but recurrent chromosomal abnormality associated with therapy-related AML. Studies using FISH and RT-PCR methods have demonstrated fusion of AML1 on 21q22 and MTG16 (myeloid translocation gene on chromosome 16) on chromosome 16, which produces an AML1-MTG16 fusion gene on chromosome 16. The breakpoints of both t(8;21) and t(16;21) occur within the same intron of the AML1/RUNX1 gene. AML1/RUNX1-MTG16 gene fusion results in the production of a protein that is very similar to the RUNX1/RUNX1T1 (AML1-ETO) protein in t(8;21).

(16;21)(p11;q22) is a rare chromosomal rearrangement associated with M1-M2 AML. A proportion of patients may have additional abnormalities. This translocation fuses the TLS/FUS gene on chromosome 16, band p11, to the ERG gene on chromosome 22, band q22. The ERG gene is a member of the ETS family of transcription factors and is a sequence-specific transcriptional activator. The presence of a fusion transcript is detected by RT-PCR, at the time of diagnosis, at relapse, and during remission. These observations are consistent with the impression that patients with t(16;21) have a poor prognosis and may benefit from early detection of this chimeric gene in order to determine the need for more aggressive therapy.

t(15;17)(q22;q21) involves the PML (promyelocytic leukemia) gene on chromosome 15, band q22, and RARA on chromosome 17, band q21. This abnormality constitutes the genetic basis for approximately 94% of all cases of acute promyelocytic leukemia (Fig. 54-28, *middle panels*).[16] The remaining 6% of cases include eight rare variant translocations: t(11;17)(q23;q21) (including two different genes on 11q23 MLL and ZBTB10), t(11;17)(q13;q21), t(5;17)(q35;q21), t(2;17)(p21;q21), dup(17)(q21.3-q21), t(4;17)(q12;q21), and t(X;17)(p11q21). Therefore acute promyelocytic leukemia is associated with several different genetic rearrangements fusing the RARA gene with a different partner gene in each case. Variant RARA fusion partners include PLZF (promyelocytic leukemia zinc finger) gene on 11q23, NPM gene on 5q35, NuMA (nuclear matrix-associated) gene on 11q13, STATb5 gene on 17q11, and BCOR (BCL6 corepressor) gene on Xp11. Based on these genomic rearrangements, a FISH assay, using a breakapart probe strategy with dual-color RARA, can identify two different clinical syndromes. These syndromes occur in patients who are not responsive to all-trans retinoic acid (ATRA) therapy and carry the RARA-PLZF fusion gene, as well as in patients whose promyelocytes have exquisite sensitivity to differentiate in response to ATRA treatment and have one of the other six RARA fusion rearrangements (Fig. 54-29). FISH study also identifies patients with cryptic translocations and unusual chromosomal variants (see Fig. 54-29). It is important to recognize patients who will or will not respond to ATRA so that appropriate therapy can be administered.

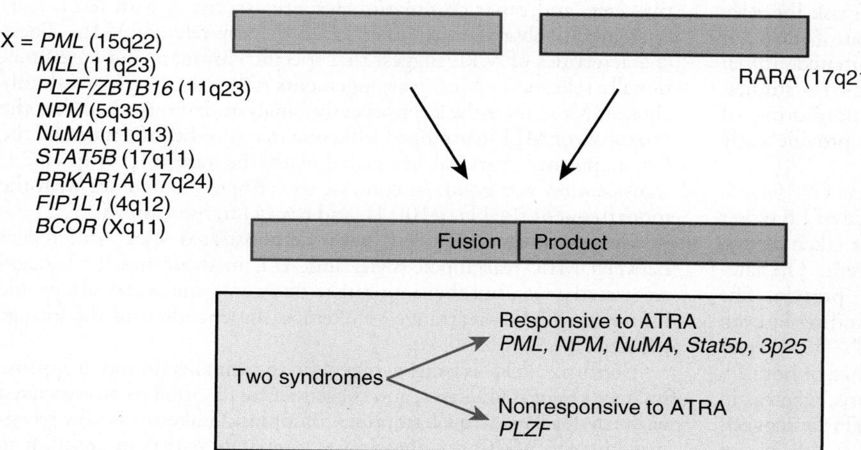

Figure 54-28 MOLECULAR CYTOGENETIC DEFECTS IN ACUTE PROMYELOCYTIC LEUKEMIA ARE RESPONSIBLE FOR DIFFERENT RESPONSE TO ALL-TRANS RETINOIC ACID DIFFERENTIATION THERAPY. Patients with t(11;17)(q23(q22) and PLZF(ZBTB16)-RARA fusion do not respond to all-trans retinoic acid differentiation therapy, whereas patients with classic t(15;17) and other four cytogenetic variants have exquisite sensitivity to differentiate in response to all-trans retinoic acid.

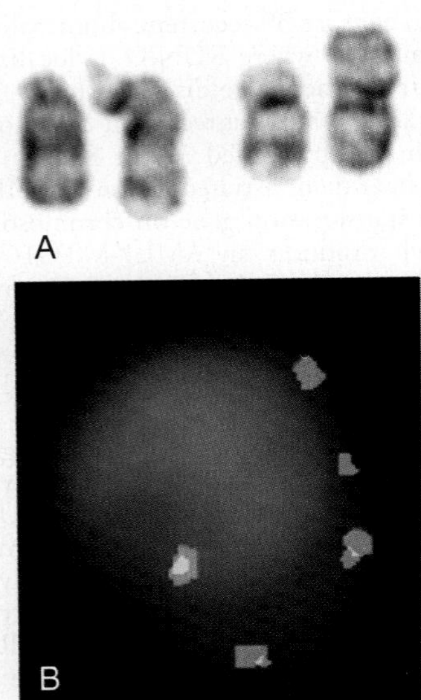

Figure 54-29 Partial karyotype from a patient with acute promyelocytic leukemia, showing ider(17)t(15;17)(q22;q21) *(top)*. The karyotype shows isochromosome for the long arms of chromosome 17 and deletion of the short arms. FISH studies revealed three copies of PML-RARA fusion in bone marrow nucleus *(bottom)*, confirming that the first event in the pathogenesis was PML-RARA fusion and the subsequent event was a structural rearrangement of isochromosome. *(From Cheng L, Zhang DY, editors:* Molecular genetic pathology, *Totowa, NJ, 2008, Humana Press, a part of Springer Science.)*

Acute promyelocytic leukemia is a disease characterized by accumulation of blasts blocked at the promyelocytic stage of granulocytic differentiation. APL accounts for only 5% to 8% of pediatric AML, and 95% of children with APL show a classic t(15;17). However, almost 35% of pediatric APL have FLT3-ITD mutations. The clinical impact of these mutations on relapse rate and overall survival is not yet clear.

Our current understanding of the molecular pathogenesis of acute promyelocytic leukemia is that PML-RARA behaves as a potent transcriptional repressor and that supraphysiologic doses of retinoic acid can overcome this repression. In the presence of retinoic acid, PML-RARA behaves as a transcriptional activator. In patients with variant PLZF-RARA, an additional corepressor complex binding site is present, and histone deacetylase inhibitors are used to restore sensitivity to retinoic acid. It appears that PML-RARA fusion-induced differentiation arrest of leukemic blasts and increased self-renewal of progenitors are two distinct features of APL and are probably driven by two different gene programs. Accurate identification of the acute promyelocytic leukemia-associated genomic lesion at diagnosis is important because acute promyelocytic leukemia is a medical emergency that frequently presents with abrupt onset, high risk for early death (10% to 20%), and potential for high cure rate (>80%) if appropriate treatment, based on genetic profile, is initiated. Initial workup may include conventional karyotyping, FISH studies, RT-PCR, and anti-PML antibodies. Longitudinal monitoring of disease with RQ-PCR is currently recommended to provide early intervention if relapse should occur.

Less than 1% of patients with AML have Ph (see Fig. 54-24, *bottom left*). In rare patients with AML, late appearance of Ph either as a sole abnormality or in a clone showing t(8;21) is taken as evidence that the Ph in these patients is a secondary event. The late-appearing Ph in AML is characterized by $P190^{BCR\text{-}ABL1}$ protein. The coexistence of Ph and inv(16) is a rare but recurrent finding in both CML and AML. In CML the fusion transcript is $P210^{BCR\text{-}ABL1}$, whereas in AML the fusion transcript is $P190^{BCR\text{-}ABL1}$. The presence of both Ph and inv(16) in AML seems to have a favorable prognosis, whereas in CML, the coexistence of BCR-ABL and CBFB-MYH11 suggests rapid transformation to blast crisis.

The MLL (also referred to as ALL1 or HRX) gene at 11q23 is responsible for 95% of all 11q23 translocations, including AML and ALL (Fig. 54-30 and Table 54-8). Approximately 20% of all translocations in human neoplasia involve the MLL gene. The MLL abnormalities are found in approximately 15% of patients with AML and ALL. To date, 88 partner genes participate in MLL translocations, and 74 of these are characterized at the molecular level. The most common translocation involving the MLL gene in AML (see Table 54-7) is t(9;11)(p23;q23), occurring in ≈2% of cases (see Fig. 54-30, *M*) and resulting in MLL-MLLT3 (AF9) fusion, and t(11;19)(q23;p13.1) (see Fig. 54-30, *E*), producing the MLL-ELL fusion. The t(9;11), which has been associated with a more favorable outcome in adult and pediatric studies, is distinguished as a separate entity in the latest WHO classification. Other frequent MLL translocations are t(6;11)(q27;q23) involving MLLT4(AF6) and t(11;19)(q23;p13.3) involving MLLT1 (ENL). A partial tandem duplication of the amino-terminus region of the MLL gene is associated in patients with or without trisomy 11 (see Figs. 54-24 and 54-30, *B, C, F,* and *G*). MLL is an epigenetic regulator that plays a critical role in hematopoiesis, modulating HOX gene expression. The MLL gene is encoded by 37 exons. The MLL-binding protein possesses multiple recognizable protein motifs, including DNA-binding domain, transcriptional and repression domains, and a COOH-terminal SET domain that contains histone H3 lysine 4 (H3K4) methyltransferase activity. Recent biochemical evidence has identified MLL as a member of a large multiprotein complex that contains protein involved in chromatin modification/remodeling. In addition, MLL is recruited to the promoters of select cell-cycle regulatory genes, suggesting its role in cell-cycle control. The current understanding is that MLL protein regulates gene expression and cell cycle control via chromatin modification. 11q23 translocations cluster within an 8.3-kb region that encompasses exons 8 to 14 of MLL and fuses the N-terminal portion of MLL, which contains the AT hook and methyltransferase domains, to numerous different proteins. In infant and in therapy-related AML, the MLL genomic breakpoints cluster in the 3′ end, near exon 12. In childhood and adult de novo AML, the breakpoints usually occur in the 5′ end, between exons 9 and 10. AML patients with MLL rearrangements have a poor prognosis despite treatment with aggressive multiagent chemotherapy. Identical MLL rearrangements have been detected in three pairs of infant monozygotic twins, raising the possibility of in utero MLL rearrangements.

The contribution of various MLL fusion partners to transformation was not previously known.[17] The partner genes in the translocations did not appear to have any unifying characteristics that would clarify their role in leukemogenesis. However, two observations suggest that MLL fusion partners are not randomly chosen. First, a precise localization of genomic MLL breakpoints in 414 samples with MLL rearrangements, using a novel long-distance inverse PCR method, showed that the most frequent translocation fusion partners (AF4, MLLT3, MLLT1, AF10) belong to the same nuclear protein network involved in histone methylation. Second, several chromatin structural elements, such as topoisomerase II cleavage sites, DNase I hypersensitive sites, and other chromatin sites, are associated with MLL rearrangements observed in infant and therapy-related AML. These characteristics of MLL suggest that specific chromatin sites are functionally selected in MLL rearrangements rather than being randomly chosen. More recently, a retrospective analysis demonstrated that the prognosis of MLL-rearranged leukemia may also be influenced by the fusion partner. Survival associated with the rare t(1;11)(q21;q23) translocation was good, in contrast to very poor outcomes with the more frequent t(4;11), t(10;11), and t(6;11) translocations.

Gene expression studies have demonstrated clear differences between MLL-rearranged AML and ALL in expression of lineage-associated genes, but there appears to be a core gene expression profile found in all MLL-rearranged leukemias, independent of the lineage markers.

t(6;9)(p23;q34) is a rare cytogenetic abnormality, found in approximately 1% of AML cases, and subsequently reported to be associated with AML and marrow basophilia. Basophilic leukemia is now recognized by the WHO classification as a separate entity. In addition to

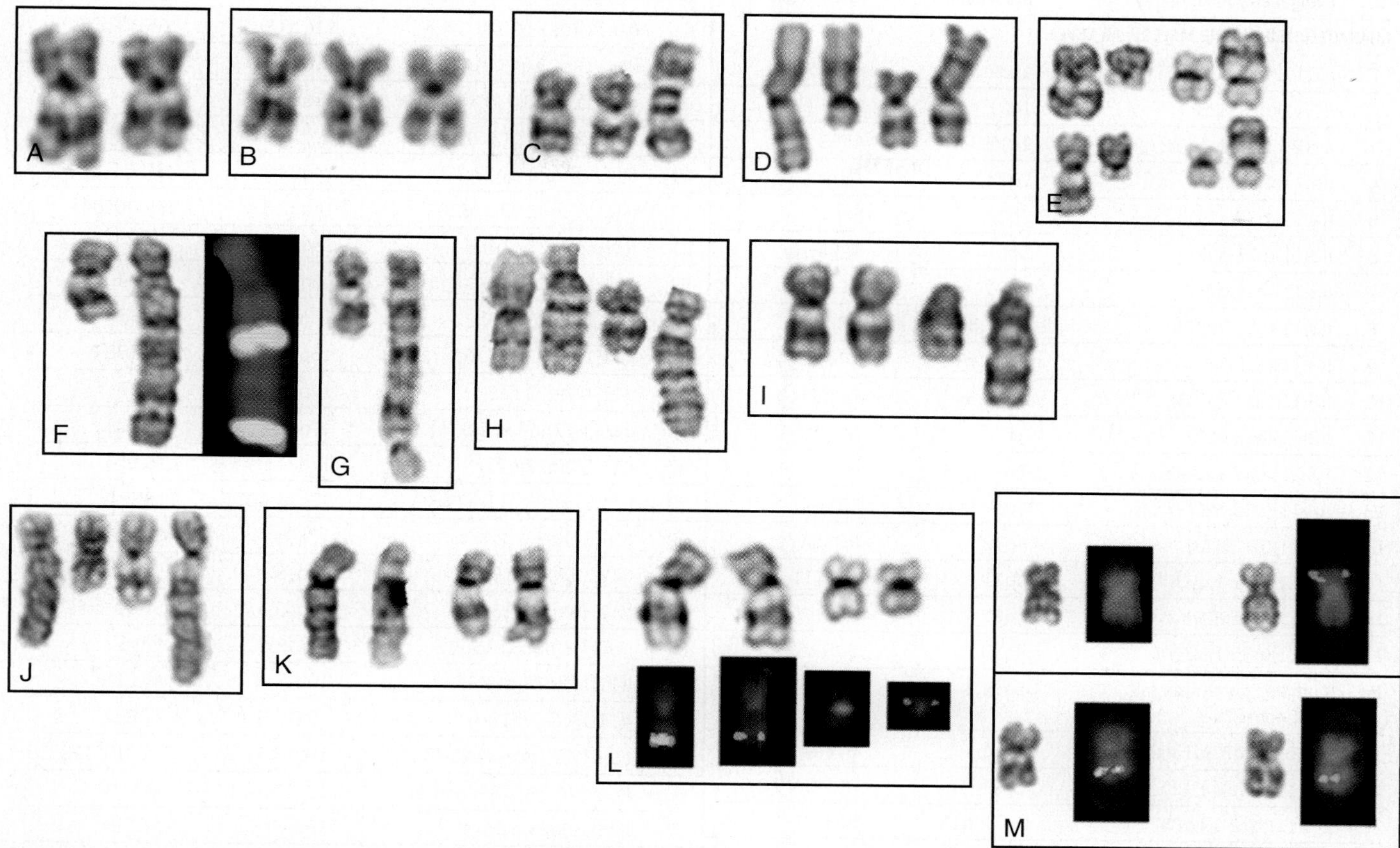

Figure 54-30 EXAMPLES OF CHROMOSOME 11 ABNORMALITIES. **A**, Deletion of chromosome 11 at band q23. **B**, Gain (trisomy) of chromosome 11. **C**, Gain of isodicentric, idic(q11) in myelodysplastic syndrome (MDS). **D**, Balanced t(1;11)(q13;p15) in MDS. **E**, t(11;19)(q13;p13) in a pediatric patient with acute myeloid leukemia. **F**, Duplication of the long arms of chromosome 11 and FISH image of MLL duplication. **G**, Duplication (11;22) in the form of dicder(11;22)dup(11)(q13q14)t(11;22)(q23;p11) in a patient with MDS. **H**, der(11)dic(1;11)(q12;q23) in a patient with myelofibrosis transforming to acute myeloid leukemia. **I**, der(14)t(11;14)(q23;q23), resulting in trisomy for part of the long arms of chromosome 11. **J**, t(4;11)(q23;q23) in pediatric acute lymphoblastic leukemia. **K**, t(6;11)(q27;q23) in pediatric acute lymphoblastic leukemia. **L**, t(11;19)(q23;p13) in pediatric acute lymphoblastic leukemia and after FISH study, showing separation of MLL breakapart probe where the 5′ end of the MLL *(green)* remains on der(11), and the 3′ end *(red)* is translocated to 19p. **M**, t(9;11)(p22;q23) in pediatric acute myeloid leukemia and after metaphase FISH study *(right)*, showing that the 3′ end of the MLL *(red)* is translocated to 9p but the 5′ end *(green)* remains on der(11).

t(6;9), other chromosomal abnormalities [such as t(8;21)(q22;q22), del(12)(p11-13), t(X;6),(p11;q23), and t(2;6)(q23;p22)] may be found in basophilic leukemia. As a result of t(6;9), the 3′ part of the CAN (Nup214, nuclear pore complex protein 214 kd) gene located on chromosome 9, band q34, is fused to the 5′ part of the DEK gene located on chromosome 6, band p23. The resulting DEK-CAN/Nup214 fusion gene is a derivative of chromosome 6. The translocation breakpoints occur in a single intron of 8 kb in the CAN gene and in a single intron of 12 kb in the DEK gene. As a result, the presence of the DEK-CAN fusion can be identified in blood or marrow cells by Southern blot analysis and PCR methods. Dual-color commercial FISH probes are not available for this translocation.

The nuclear pore complex is a massive structure that extends across the nuclear envelope, forming a gateway that regulates the flow of macromolecules between the nucleus and the cytoplasm. Nup214 may serve as a docking site in the receptor-mediated import of substrates across the nuclear pore complex and plays a role in nuclear protein import, mRNA export, and cell cycle progression. The hybrid protein contains almost the entire DEK protein fused to the C-terminal two-thirds of the CAN protein. The role of DEK-CAN/Nup214 hybrid protein in leukemogenesis awaits elucidation.

inv(3)(q21q26.2) or t(3;3)(q21;q26.2) (see Fig. 54-20) occurs in ≈1% of AML; each is associated with upregulation of the zinc finger transcription factor EVI1. Both rearrangements may present de novo or secondary to prior MDS and are characterized by normal or increased platelet counts and abnormal megakaryopoiesis.

The presence of hyperdiploid karyotype in acute erythroleukemia is found in 47% to 56% of patients, along with a loss of genetic material occurring in chromosomes 5, 7, and 18. A monosomal karyotype was identified in 43% in one series. Balanced translocations are rare in erythroleukemia, although rare cases of MLL rearrangements have been reported. The frequent occurrence of complex karyotype and abnormalities of chromosomes 5 and 7 may be one reason for poor prognosis associated with acute erythroleukemia. Mutations frequently seen in other subgroups of AML (such as FLT3, KIT or RAS mutations) have not been reported in acute erythroleukemia. In pediatric patients acute erythroleukemia is very rare, present in 2.3% of all patients with AML. Congenital erythroleukemia is exceedingly rare with only six cases reported in the literature.

The M7 or megakaryocytic subtype of AML is a clonal disease, arising in a multipotent stem cell capable of differentiating along the megakaryocytic and granulocytic pathway.[18] This acute leukemia subtype has a variety of genetic and morphologic characteristics. The M7 subtype has an estimated frequency of 3% to 14% of all AML and is more frequent in children than in adults. In adults, megakaryocytic leukemia is frequently observed as a secondary leukemia after chemotherapy or leukemic transformation of several chronic MPDs, including CML. Approximately 65% of acute megakaryocytic leukemia is associated with myelofibrosis. No specific chromosomal abnormality is associated with the adult form of megakaryocytic leukemia. Approximately 50% of M7 AML patients have chromosomal

Table 54-8 MLL Translocations and Rearrangements

#	Cytogenetic Abnormality	Breakpoint	HUGO Name
CHARACTERIZED ON THE MOLECULAR LEVEL			
1	t(1;11)(p32;q23)	1p32	EPS15
2	t(1;11)(q21;q23)	1q21	MLLT11
3	ins(2;11)(q11.2-q12;q23)	2q11.2-q12	AFF3
4	t(2;11)(q33;q23)	2q33	ABI2
5	t(2;11)(q37;q23)	2q37	SEPT2
6	t(3;11)(p21;q23)	3p21	SACM1L
7	t(3;11)(p21;q23)	3p21	NCKIPSD
8	t(3;11)(p21.3;q23)	3p21.3	DCP1A
9	t(3;11)(q12-13;q23)	3q13.13	KIAA1524
10	t(3;11)(q21.3;q23)	3q21.3	EEFSEC
11	t(3;11)(q24;q23)	3q24	GMPS
12	t(3;11)(q27-q28;q23)	3q27-q28	LPP
13	t(4;11)(p12;q23)	4p12	FRYL
14	t(4;11)(p12;q23)	4p12	PDS5A
15	t(4;11)(q21.1;q23)	4q21.1	SEPT11
16	t(4;11)(q21;q23)	4q21	AFF1
17	t(4;11)(q35.1;q23)	4q35.1	SORBS2
18	complex chromosomal abnormalities	5q12.3	CENPK
19	ins(5;11)(q31;q13q23)	5q31	AFF4
20	t(5;11)(q31;q23)	5q31	ARHGAP26
21	t(6;11)(q12-13;q23)	6q12-q13	SMAP1
22	t(6;11)(q13;q23)	6q15	CASP8AP2
23	t(6;11)(q21;q23)	6q21	FOXO3
24	t(6;11)(q27;q23)	6q27	MLLT4
25	t(7;11)(p22.1;q23)	7p22.1	TNRC18
26	t(7;11)(q21;q23)	7q21	RUNDC3B
27	t(9;11)(p22;q23)	9p22	MLLT3
28	t(9;11)(q33.1-q33.3;q23);	9q33.1-q33.3	DAB2IP
29	ins(11;9)(q23;q34)inv(11)(q13)(q23)	9q34	FNBP1
30	t(9;11)(q31-q34;q23)	9q31-34	LAMC3
31	t(10;11)(p11.2;q23)	10p11.2	ABI1
32	ins(10;11)(p12;q23q13)	10p12	MLLT10
33	ins(10;11)(p12;q23)	10p12	NEBL
34	t(10;11)(q21;q23)	10q21	TET1
35	inv(11)(p15.3;q23)	11p15.3	NRIP3
36	INV(11)(q12;q23)	11q12.1	BTBD18
37	t(11;11)(q13.4;q23)	11q13.4	ARHGEF17
38	inv(11)(q13.4;q23)	11q13.4	C2CD3
39	inv(11)(q14;q23)	11q14	PICALM
40	inv(11)(q21;q23)	11q21	MAML2
41	t(11;15)(q23;q21)inv(11)(q23;q23)	11q23	LOC100131626
42	inv(11)(q23q23)	11q23	BUD13
43	del11q23	11q23.3	CEP164
44	del(11)(q23;q23.3)	11q23.3	CBL
45	del(11)(q23;q23.3)	11q23.3	ARHGEF12
46	del(11)(q23;q23.3)	11q23.3	BCL9L
47	del(11))(q23;q24.2)	11q24.2	DCPS
48	t(11;12)(q23;q13.2)	12q13.2	SARNP
49	t(11;14)(q23.3;q23.3)	14q23.3	GPHN
50	t(11;14)(q32.33;q23.3)	14q32.33	KIAA0284
51	t(11;15)(q23;q14)	15q14	CASC5
52	t(11;15)(q23;q14)	15q14	ZFYVE19
53	t(11;17)(q23;p13)	17p12-p11.2	TOP3A
54	t(11;16)(q23;p13.3)	16p13.3	CREBBP
55	t(11;17)(q23;p13.1)	17p13.1	GAS7
56	ins(11;17)(q23;q21)	17q21	ACACA
57	t(11;17)(q23;q21)	17q21	MLLT6
58	t(11;17)(q23;q11-q21.3)	17q11-q21.3	LASP1
59	t(11;17)(q23;q25)	17q25	SEPT9
60	t(11;19)q23;p13.1)	19p13.1	ELL
61	t(11;19)q23;p13)	19p13.3	SH3GL1
62	ins(11;19)q23;p13.2)	19p13.2	VAV1
63	t(11;19)(q23;p13.3)	19p13.3	MLLT1
64	t(11;19)q23;p13.3)	19p13.3	ACER1
65	t(2;11;19)(p23.3;q23;p13.3)	19p13.3	LOC100128568
66	t(11;19)q23;p13.3-p13.2)	19p13.3-p13.2	MYO1F
67	t(11;19)q23;q13)	19q13	ACTN4
68	t(11;20)q23;q11)	20q11	MAPRE1
69	t(11;22)(q23;q11.21)	22q11.21	SEPT5
70	t(11;22)(q23;q13.2)	22q13.2	EP300
71	t(X;11)(q13.1;q23)	Xq13.1	FOXO4
72	ins(X;11)(q24;q23)	Xq24	SEPT6
73	ins(X;11)(q24;q23)	Xq26.3	CT45A2
74	ins(11;X)(q23;q28;q13.1)	Xq28	FLNA
1	No partner gene is directly fused to the MLL gene		
2	t(1;11)(p13.1;q23)	1p13.1	
3	t(9;11)(p13.3;q23)	9p13.3	
4	del(11)(q23;q23.3)	11q23.3	
5	t(11;21)(q23;q11.21)	21q22	
6	INV(11)(q23;q23.3)	11q23.3	
NOT CHARACTERIZED ON THE MOLECULAR LEVEL			
1	t(1;11)(p36;q23)		
2	t(1;11)(q31;q23)		
3	t(1;11)(q32;q23)		
4	t(2;11)(p21;q23)		
5	t(2;11)(q37;q23)		
6	t(3;11)(p13;q23)		
7	t(4;11)(p11;q23)		
8	t(6;11)(q13;q23)		

Courtesy C Meyer and R Marschalek, Diagnostic Center of Acute Leukemia, Institute of Pharmaceutical Biology, JWG University of Frankfurt, Germany, May 16, 2012.
ALL, Acute lymphoblastic leukemia; *AML*, acute myelogenous leukemia; *CML*, chronic myelogenous leukemia; *CMML*, chronic myelomonocytic leukemia; *JMML*, juvenile myelomonocytic leukemia; *t-AL*, therapy-related acute; *t-ALL*, therapy-related ALL; *t-AML*, therapy-related AML; *t-CML*, therapy-related CML; *t-MDS*, therapy-related MDS; *t-T-ALL*, therapy-related T-cell ALL.

abnormalities at diagnosis. Observed diverse abnormalities include 3q21-3q26 rearrangements, partial or total deletion of chromosomes 5 and 7, gain of chromosomes 8 and 19, and t(9;22). In multivariate analysis, M7 diagnosis in adults is an independent adverse prognostic factor for overall survival. Three manifestations of childhood megakaryocytic leukemia are observed. First is the t(1;22)(p13;q13) with constitutional trisomy 21 associated with GATA1 mutation. Children with constitutional trisomy 21 have a 10- to 20-fold increased risk for developing leukemia. The incidence of developing M7 leukemia is up to 500 times higher in children with constitutional trisomy 21 than in children without it. However, children with constitutional trisomy 21 and megakaryocytic leukemia have a more favorable prognosis compared with patients without constitutional trisomy 21. Somatic mutation of transcription factor GATA1 in these patients leads to exclusive expression of a truncated form of GATA1. The second form of childhood acute megakaryocytic leukemia involves t(1;22)(p13;q13) encoding the OTT-MAL (RBM15-MKL1) fusion protein in infants without constitutional trisomy 21 (Fig. 54-31). It is a very rare abnormality, described in about 40 cases worldwide (≈5% of infant AML cases), and associated with infantile M7 and with children younger than 3 years of age. Detection of t(1;22) is diagnostic. Adults with t(1;22)(p13;q13) encoding the OTT-MAL fusion protein are not reported to date. Third, approximately 19% of infants with constitutional trisomy 21 (or mosaic trisomy 21C) and transient myeloproliferative disorder subsequently develop M7 leukemia at a mean age of 20 months. With development of leukemia, these children acquire diverse chromosomal abnormalities, most notably tetrasomy 21 and trisomy 8. The t(1;22) rearrangement has been observed in a set of monozygotic twins, suggesting an in utero origin in some cases.

Preliminary results using gene expression profiling (GEP) are providing the first insight into the molecular pathogenesis of M7 leukemia in children with and without constitutional trisomy 21. These two groups of patients have distinct molecular phenotypes, with increased expression of chromosome 21 genes in patients with constitutional trisomy 21 compared with M7 leukemia patients without constitutional trisomy 21. The AML1 (RUNX1) gene, localized on chromosome 21 and essential for normal megakaryopoiesis, is expressed at lower levels in children with constitutional trisomy 21 and M7 leukemia, indicating a mechanism that may contribute to a block in differentiation in megakaryocytic leukemia.

In a recent study of 1058 patients with AML and abnormal karyotype, 30% had monosomal karyotype (see Fig. 54-20, *bottom row*). AML with MK is frequently associated with other adverse risk cytogenetic abnormalities, such as inv(3), −5 or del(5q), −7 or del(7q), abnormal (12p), −18/del(18q), abnormal (17p), and complex karyotype. Response to induction therapy and overall survival of patients who have AML with MK is dismal—complete remission rates of 32% and a 4-year survival of 9%. Monosomal karyotype in

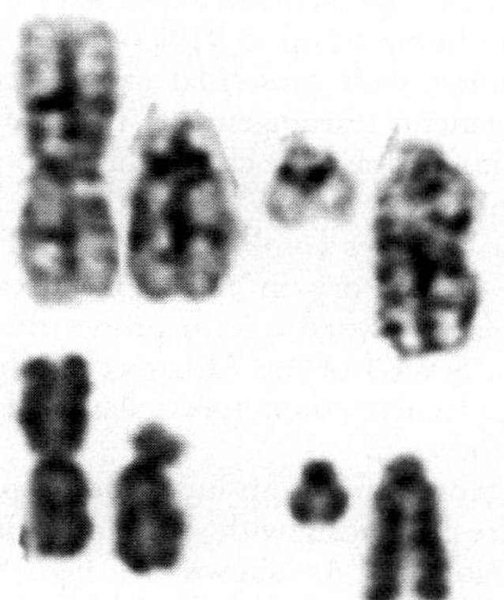

Figure 54-31 Partial bone marrow karyotype from two metaphase cells from a 4-week-old baby with M7 megakaryocytic leukemia showing a diagnostic t(1;22)(p13;q13) abnormality.

a study of 248 patients with AML was found to be associated in more than 50% of these patients with deletion of P53, whereas in another study of newly diagnosed 369 patients with AML, MK predicted adverse treatment outcome and was associated with multidrug-resistance functional activity of leukemic blasts.

Approximately 15% to 20% of patients with AML have a numerical gain or loss of a single chromosome as the sole primary karyotypic abnormality. Each of the autosomes and sex chromosomes contributes to the numerical changes. The most common trisomies in decreasing order of frequency are gain of chromosome 8, 22, 13, 21, and 11. The gain of chromosome 8, the most frequent abnormality seen in AML, is found as a sole abnormality in 6.3% and overall in 16%. The incidence of +8 detected by FISH varies between 19% and 25%. The prognosis of AML with +8 depends on whether +8 occurs as an isolated abnormality or accompanies other cytogenetic aberrations. In the latter situations, +8 does not appear to adversely affect the favorable outcome of patients with t(15;17), inv(16)t(16;16), and t(8;21). In contrast, patients with +8 and a complex karyotype and/or an unfavorable aberration such as del(5q) or −7 usually have very poor outcome. Isolated +8 has been considered to be associated with either intermediate or unfavorable prognosis.

Deletion of 17p often results in the loss of tumor suppressor TP53 gene on band p13.1, which has been reported in 5% to 9% of adult AML. The abnormalities of 17p are often associated with other chromosomal aberrations such as del(5q), −5, −7, but it is also an independent poor-risk prognostic factor for disease-free survival, relapsed risk, and OS. Patients with p53 mutations are more common in older patients and those who have previously received alkylating agents. These patients were found to have an increase in the number of $CD34^+$ cells, suggesting that the loss of p53 function could cause cell cycle arrest at an immature stage.

Whether PCR-based molecular screening, conventional cytogenetics, or both, should be used at diagnosis of AML is an important question with major consequences for treatment strategy, monitoring therapy, and overall genetic risk assessment. A prospective comparison study demonstrated approximately 20% discrepancy between broad molecular screening using a multiplex RT-PCR system and cytogenetic testing. This discrepancy has the potential to influence treatment strategies. Cryptic translocations detected as submicroscopic genetic lesions detected by RT-PCR may have no influence on prognosis or treatment strategy. In contrast, cytogenetic results influence treatment decisions by conferring unfavorable risk assignment on patients with negative broad molecular screening. These methodologies provide complementary genetic information for diagnosis, treatment, and follow-up.

Cytogenetic studies are valuable in assessing the effectiveness of therapy (see box on Genetic Testing for Acute Myeloid Leukemia and Fig. 54-24). In most patients with AML, a clonal cell population cannot be detected during remission. However, in some cases, hematopoiesis remains clonal, with normal karyotype showing only a single G6PD enzyme type—hence the fourth aspect of AML heterogeneity. When disease relapses, cells with the original chromosome anomalies are observed. If an appropriate FISH or RT-PCR test is available, these are the genetic tests of choice for predicting relapse because these methods are less expensive and more sensitive than chromosome studies.

The striking clinical, cytogenetic, and biologic heterogeneity of AML is only partly explained by the known chromosomal or molecular rearrangements. DNA microarray technology (cytogenomics) provides a higher resolution and has been demonstrated to detect cryptic copy number alterations (CNA) and UPD (uniparental disomy) that occurs in commonly in AML. The clinical implications of array CGH and SNP microarray analyses in AML are still limited. However, it has been demonstrated that in cases with UPD, gene mutations precede mitotic recombination, resulting in loss of the remaining wild-type allele, which can act as a "second hit" mutation. Evidence suggests that the association of UPD with a more advanced disease is also reflected in clinical outcome because UPD has been shown to be predictive of poor event-free and overall survival. For example, SNP microarray analysis of AML patients with a normal karyotype

Genetic Testing for Acute Myeloid Leukemia

At diagnosis, the recommended general practice should be FISH studies using the panel of chromosomal probes for acute myeloid leukemia, including RUNX1-RUNXT1,PML-RARA, CBFB, BCR-ABL and MLL. Conventional cytogenetic studies must be also performed at diagnosis. Patients with CBF AML subtype should be tested for KIT exon 17 mutations because these mutations adversely affect the prognosis. These tests are performed at diagnosis to establish a benchmark for the percentage of neoplastic cells and are used in follow-up studies to help assess the effectiveness of therapy. In patients with a normal karyotype, mutation studies for the most common genes (NPM1, FLT3, CEBPA, and TET2) are recommended.

The impact of cytogenetics on outcome in a pediatric group of patients with AML (excluding APL) demonstrated ≈80% overall survival for 10 years in patients with CBF AML. In contrast, patients with MLL abnormalities had an intermediate prognosis (61% OS at 10 years) with no evidence of heterogeneity according to the translocation partner of MLL. Additional abnormalities among the 11q23 leukemia have diverse prognoses; trisomy 8 is an independent favorable, whereas trisomy 19 is considered an adverse prognostic factor in MLL rearranged group of pediatric patients.

demonstrated UPD of chromosome 13q, leading to duplication of a mutant FLT3 allele at band 13q12, which was associated with significantly inferior overall survival. Approximately 20% of patients with AML and a normal karyotype have UPD. The most common chromosomal regions of UPD are 1p, 2p, 2q, 4q (TET2), 6p, 7q (EZH2), 11p (WT1), 11q, 13q (FLT3), 14q, 16p, 17p (TP53), 19q (CEBPA), 21q (RUNX1), and Xq. Analysis of genes located within UPD chromosomal region showed a copy-neutral loss of heterozygosity with duplication of gene mutations that has been already implicated in AML pathogenesis and a loss of corresponding normal allele.

Numerous studies using cytogenomics have uncovered a broad range of cryptic CNAs in patients with AML and a normal karyotype, as well as in patients exhibiting balanced translocations or chromosomal imbalances. Not only did these studies reveal a tremendous genetic diversity of AML; they also showed that the estimated average number of CNAs per genome is 2 to 2.5. This finding implies either that most AML genomes are relatively stable or that at the current level of resolution provided by the modern cytogenomics (≈35 kb), more sensitive methods are required (e.g., complete genome sequences) to capture the whole spectrum of genetic alterations. Genomic imbalances (and their associated target genes) include gains of regions 4q25-26 (PRDM5), 8p11.21 (ZMAT4), 8q24.21 (CCDC26), 13q32 (ABCC4), 14q23.1 (PRKCH), 16q24.1 (USP10, CRISPLD2), and 21q22.3 (PRMT2), as well as losses of regions 6q27 (RPS6KA2), 7p22.3 (FAM20C), 8q24.12 (TRPS1), 9p21.2 (TISCI), 10q11,21 (HNRNPF), 15q21.3 (RFX7), Xp11.4 (BCOR), and XP25 (STAG2). The biologic consequences of these small genomic imbalances are not fully understood. In some cases submegabase-sized CNAs may uncover cryptic rearrangements, as has been shown for NSD1-Nup98 and MALT4 -MLL fusion genes. The systemic analysis of CNAs and regions of UPD in AML in future may fully uncover genomic changes that contribute to AML pathogenesis.

The biology of AML changes with age. The spectrum of cytogenetic abnormalities in older adults includes a higher percentage of patients with abnormalities involving −5/del(5q), −7/del(7q), and 17p and a lower incidence of translocations associated with favorable prognosis and treatment outcome. Older patients with a complex karyotype have an extremely poor prognosis, with 26% achieving CR because of high rates of resistant disease. Multidrug resistance is demonstrated in 57% of patients older than 75 years but in 33% of AML patients younger than 56 years. The overall survival rate in older adult

Genetic Testing for Therapy-Related Neoplasms

The best genetic test for therapy-related myelodysplastic syndrome or acute myeloid leukemia is a conventional cytogenetic study. FISH studies with probes for loci on chromosomes 5 and 7, MLL, and RUNX1 should be performed if therapy-related leukemia is suspected. This approach is useful for t(8;21), t(9;22), t(11;var), t(15;17), inv(16), −5/del(5q), −7/del(7q), rearrangements of ETV6 on 12p, and some others.

patients with AML is only 2% at 5 years. The different biology of AML in older patients may be a consequence of the age of hematopoietic stem cells, shortened telomere length (associated with older cells), and presence of fewer normal stem cells to compete with malignant clones and repopulate marrow following chemotherapy.

Therapy-related AML and therapy-related MDS are distinct clinical syndromes occurring as late complications after high-dose chemotherapy, radiation therapy, or autologous HCT. A normal karyotype is observed in 8%, and abnormal karyotype is detected in 92%. From the cytogenetic point of view, two different categories of therapy-related AML and therapy-related MDS can be distinguished. The first is found in patients exposed to alkylating agents who developed therapy-related approximately 5 years after therapy. These leukemias are associated with the presence of monosomy 5/del(5q) or monosomy 7/del(7q). Many of these patients initially develop myelodysplastic features before transforming into a frank AML. Recurrent abnormalities of chromosomes 5, 7, or both account for 70% of all abnormalities observed in therapy-related leukemia. These patients have a poor response to therapy and poor overall survival. A second group of patients develop therapy-related AML without prior MDS. Leukemia cells in these patients often exhibit 11q23 (3%) and 21q22 (3%) balanced rearrangements, attributed to late effects of topoisomerase II inhibitors combined with alkylating agents and radiation. The leukemia may develop within a few months to 3 years after therapy. Polysomy (tetrasomy, pentasomy, hexasomy) of chromosome 8 defines a clinicocytogenetic entity associated with therapy-related myeloid malignancies and poor overall survival (see box on Genetic Testing for Therapy-Related Neoplasms).

ACUTE LYMPHOBLASTIC LEUKEMIA

ALL (see Chapters 63, 64, and 65) is a clonally derived disease involving progenitor cells with differentiation expression detected only in the lymphoid lineage. ALL accounts for at least 85% of acute leukemias in children and 20% of acute leukemias in adults. Most published series of patients with acute ALL indicate that 70% to 75% have an abnormal clone by conventional cytogenetic studies (Fig. 54-32). Genomic rearrangements detected with intensive interphase FISH screening are found in up to 91% of cases. The application of contemporary genome-wide molecular analysis continues to reveal many additional genetic rearrangements that are not detectable by chromosome studies. At least one clonal aberration has been detected in 60% to 79% of adults and 57% to 82% of children with ALL. Today, cytogenetic analyses combined with FISH and/or RT-PCR investigations are mandatory in most ALL treatment trials, and genetic findings play a pivotal role in proper risk stratification and treatment options. Several of the ALL-specific chromosome aberrations and their molecular counterparts have been included in the 2008 WHO classification.

Pretreatment cytogenetics is an independent prognostic factor in children and adults presenting with ALL and is important in determining risk categories.[19] As shown in Fig. 54-32 and Tables 54-9 and 54-10, the risk categories in children include (a) low risk: high hyperdiploidy (trisomies for chromosomes 4, 10, and 17) and t(12;21)/TEL-AML1; (b) high risk: t(1;19)/E2X-PBX1; and (c) very high risk: t(9;22)/BCR-ABL and 11q23/MLL rearrangements. In

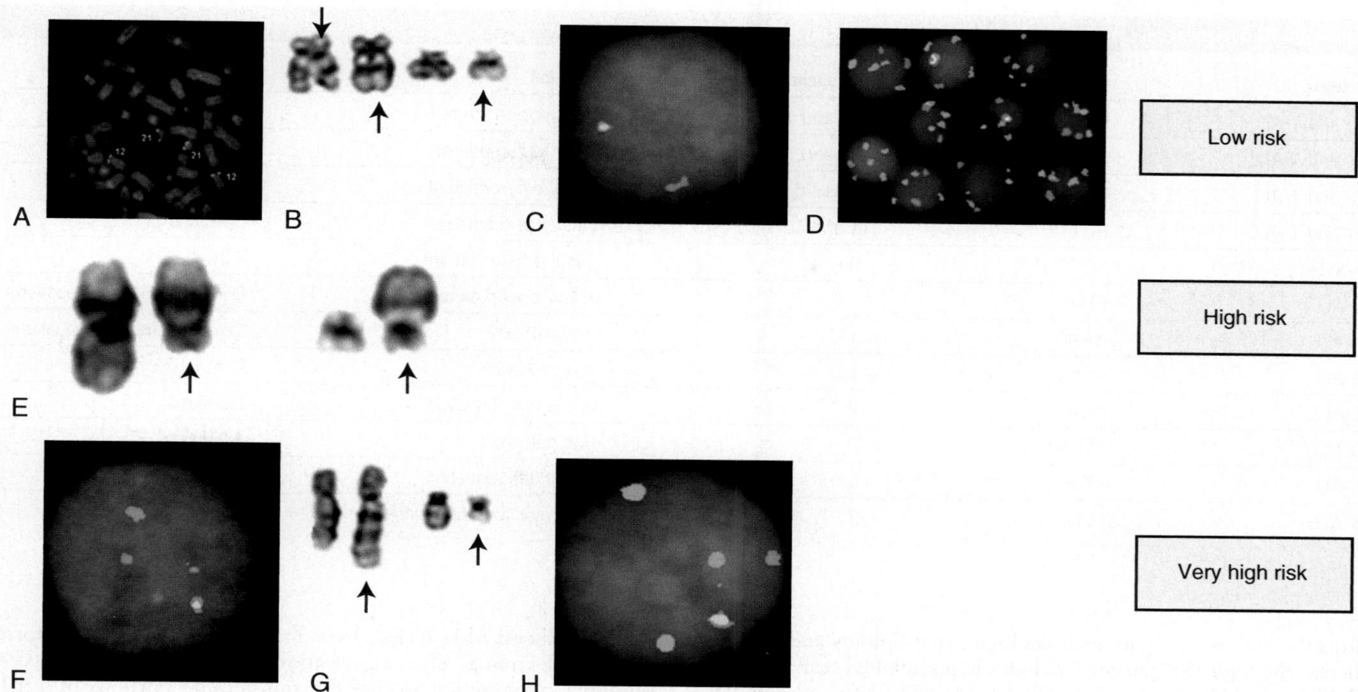

Figure 54-32 PROGNOSTIC CYTOGENETIC CATEGORIES IN ACUTE LYMPHOBLASTIC LEUKEMIA. **A,** Localization of TEL/ETV6 and AML1 fluorescence probes to chromosomes from a normal bone marrow metaphase cell. TEL/ETV6 is on 12p13 *(green)* and AML1 is on 21q *(red)*. **B,** Partial karyotype showing t(12;21)(p13;q22) *(arrows)*. The short arrow at 12p indicates a possible TEL deletion from normal chromosome 12. **C,** FISH study showing loss of TEL *(green)* from normal 12 homologue in interphase nucleus, a frequent subclonal evolution in patients with t(12;21). **D,** Hyperdiploidy [specifically trisomies for chromosomes 4 *(green)*, 10 *(red)*, and 17 *(aqua)*] is associated with low-risk cytogenetic category (see text for details) and is present in disomy in interphase cells *(top left)*. **E,** Partial G-banded karyotype showing t(1;19)(q23;p13.3), which occurs in approximately 6% of patients with B-cell precursor childhood acute lymphoblastic leukemia. **F,** FISH hybridization to bone marrow nucleus showing BCR-ABL fusion *(yellow)*. **G,** as a consequence of t(9;22), occurring in 5% of children and 20% to 25% of adults with acute lymphoblastic leukemia. **H,** Interphase nucleus after FISH study with tricolor probe. Dual-color/breakapart MLL shows separation of the 3′ end and the 5′ end as a result of 11q23 rearrangement. CEP11 *(aqua)* indicates disomy for chromosome 11, used as internal control. MLL rearrangements in acute lymphoblastic leukemia are associated with unfavorable prognosis.

Table 54-9 Frequencies of Cytogenetic Aberrations in Adult and Childhood ALL and Their Prognostic Relevance

		Adults		Children	
Cytogenetic Abnormality	**Genes Involved**	***Frequency (%)***	***Prognosis***	***Frequency (%)***	***Prognosis***
Normal karyotype	NA	15-34	Intermediate-good	31-42	Favorable
High hyperdiploidy (>55)	NA	7-8	Good-intermediate	23-30	Good
Low hyperdiploidy (>50)	NA	10-15	Poor	10-11	Intermediate
Near haploidy (<35)	NA	Rare	NA	1-4	Poor
Pseudodiploidy	NA	31-50	Poor	18-26	Intermediate
Hypodiploidy (35-44)	NA	4-9	Poor	6	Poor to intermediate
t(9;22)(q34;q11.2)	BCR-ABL1	11-29	Poor	1-3	Poor
t(4;11)(q21;q23)	MLL-AFF1	4-9	Poor	2	Poor
t(1;19)(q23;p13.3)	TCF3-PBX1	1-3	Poor, intermediate favorable	1-6	Intermediate, favorable
t(12;21)(p12;q22)	ETV6 (TEL)-RUNX1 (AML1)	0-3	Not known	22-26	Good
Abnormal 9p	P16 (CDKN2A, MTS1)	5-15	Intermediate	7-11	Adverse
Abnormal 12p	ETV6	4-5	Favorable-unfavorable	3-9	Not prognostic
del(6q)	Not known	3-6	Not prognostic	6-9	Not prognostic
del(7p)/del(7q)/–7	Not known	6-11	Not prognostic	4	Adverse
del(5q)	Not known	<2	Not prognostic	1	Adverse
Trisomy 8	NA	10-12	Poor	2	Not known
14q11	TCRα	5-7 (26% in T-ALL)	Excellent	3-4 (17-22% in T-ALL)	Not Prognostic
t(10;14)(q24;q11)	TRD-TLX1	1-3	Excellent, intermediate	Rare	Not known

Table 54-10 Frequent and Activating Mutations in Acute Lymphoblastic Leukemia

Disease	Gene	Frequency (%)	Function	Type of mutation
B- and T-ALL	CDKN2A/2B	30 and 70	Cell cycle modulator	Deletions
B- and T-ALL	PAX5	30 and 10	B-cell differentiation	Deletions
B- and T-ALL	EBF	4 and 6	B-cell differentiation	Deletions
B- and T-ALL	RB1	4 and 12	Cell cycle modulator	Deletions
T-ALL	NOTCH1	56	T-cell differentiation	Activating
B-ALL	ETV6		Transcription factor	Deletions and translocations
B-ALL	NRAS	17	Ras pathway	Deletions and translocations
B-ALL	KRAS	16	Ras pathway	Activating
B-ALL	IKZF1	8	B-cell differentiation	Deletions
B-ALL	PTPN11	7	Ras pathway	Activating
B-ALL	E2-2	6	B-cell differentiation	Deletions
B-ALL	FLT3	3	Receptor tyrosine kinase	Activating ITD

adults the low-risk category includes high hyperdiploidy and del(9p), whereas the high-risk category includes hypodiploidy/near triploidy, t(9;22)(q34;q11), t(4;11)(q21;q23), t(8;14)(q24;q32), and complex karyotype (five or more chromosomal abnormalities).

Approximately 20% of children and 26% of adults with B-cell ALL have a hyperdiploid number of chromosomes. Two groups are distinguished based on cytogenetics: (a) those with 51 to 55 chromosomes whose prognosis is poorer, and (b) those with 56 to 67 chromosomes whose prognosis is excellent. Both groups have a more favorable prognosis than do children with hypodiploidy or near-haploid ALL. In a study of 1880 children with ALL, patients with 45 chromosomes have an outcome similar to that of ALL patients with pseudodiploid or low hyperdiploid (47-50 chromosomes).[20] Children and adolescents with ALL and hypodiploidy with fewer than 44 chromosomes have a poor outcome despite contemporary therapy. The distribution of specific chromosome gains is not random, with the most often gained chromosomes being 21, X, 14, 6, 18, 4, 17, and 10, each of which is gained in more than 50% of hyperdiploid ALL patients, followed by chromosomes 8, 5, 11 and 12, gains that occur more often in patients with 57 or more chromosomes. Prognosis of children with high hyperdiploidy is excellent with 5-year event-free survival rates of between 71% and 83% and a 5-year overall survival rate of approximately 90% being reported. Pretreatment cytogenetic analysis of more than 5400 children with ALL unequivocally shows that simultaneous trisomies for chromosomes 4, 10, and 17 are associated with long-term event-free survival (see Fig. 54-32, *D*). In contrast to children who have a favorable prognosis when a hyperdiploid karyotype is present, such a favorable constellation has not been found in patients with adult ALL. The reason for this discrepancy may be that adults often have poor-risk chromosomal translocations, such as the Ph. Approximately 50% of the high hyperdiploid patients harbor other structural abnormalities, such as gains of 1q, del(6q), which do not appear to influence prognosis, with a possible exception of prognostically adverse isochromosome for the long arms of chromosome 17. Frequently, hyperdiploid leukemic cells fail to proliferate in culture; therefore, in the face of unsuccessful chromosome analyses or in those with normal karyotype interphase FISH with an ALL panel of FISH, it is strongly recommended that probes be performed to determine cytogenetic risk category before initiation of therapy.[21]

Modal chromosome numbers of 45 or less occur in less than 1% of cases (specifically, the near-haploid numbers of 24-36) and confer a poor prognosis. Similarly, ALL in adults presenting with low hyperdiploid/near-triploidy is associated with poor outcome. Loss of chromosome 7 is frequent in adult ALL. The majority of these patients also have t(9;22).

In childhood ALL, t(12;21) was first reported in 1994 as a fortuitous FISH finding. This translocation is difficult to detect by conventional cytogenetics because the translocated portions of 12p13 and 21q22 have virtually identical G-banding patterns. In contrast, the ETV6-RUNX1(AML1) fusion product of t(12;21) is detected using PCR or FISH in 17% to 41% of pediatric patients with ALL (see Fig. 54-32, *A* to *C*). The ETV6-RUNX1 (AML1) fusion, found almost exclusively in children 1 to 15 years old with B-precursor ALL, represents the most frequent molecular rearrangement in childhood cancer. Children with the ETV6-RUNX1 (AML1) fusion gene have significantly lower rates of relapse than do ETV6-AML1–negative patients. ETV6-RUNX1 (AML1)–positive B-precursor ALL is characterized by a prolonged duration of first remission and excellent cure rates. Prospective analyses have demonstrated that the survival rate in t(12;21)–positive patients is significantly better when compared with negative cases; however, this abnormality in multivariate analysis is not found to be an independent predictor of outcome. The ETV6-RUNX1 (AML1) fusion is rare in adult ALL. t(12;21)(p13;q22) fuses the helix-loop-helix domain of the ETV6 gene, located on chromosome 12, band p13, to the DNA-binding and transactivation domain of the RUNX1 (AML1) gene, located on 21q22. FISH studies allow visualization of the fusion gene on 21q22. Fusion with ETV6 converts RUNX1 (AML1) from an activator to a repressor of transcription. The ETV6-RUNX1 fusion is accompanied in 55% to 70% patients by the loss of the other normal nonrearranged TEL/ETV6 allele. This deletion probably represents a subclonal evolution. ETV6-AML1 has been detected in utero, probably in a committed B-cell progenitor, and is present in normal cord blood and peripheral blood samples at frequencies 100-fold greater than the risk for corresponding leukemia. The current view of development of ETV6-RUNX1 (AML1)–positive leukemia is that these early events are followed by a long "preleukemic" phase followed by loss of the normal ETV6 homologue, which appears to be an important event in the multistep pathogenesis of this leukemia. Currently, of the 397 children with ETV6-RUNX1–positive leukemia reported, approximately 60% harbor additional karyotypic abnormalities that contribute to the pseudodiploid or near-diploid karyotype in these cases. The most common secondary change, which occurs in approximately 50% of cases with additional abnormalities, is trisomy 21.

A rare group of patients with B-precursor ALL lack fusion of TEL and AML1 but have 3 to 15 copies of the q22 band of chromosome 21, including the RUNX1 (AML1) locus. Amplification of the 21q22 band of chromosome 21 is a clonal marker of the leukemic cells (Fig. 54-33, *A*). Following this initial observation, the British Childhood Leukemia Working Party prospectively screened 1630 patients with childhood ALL and identified 28 children with

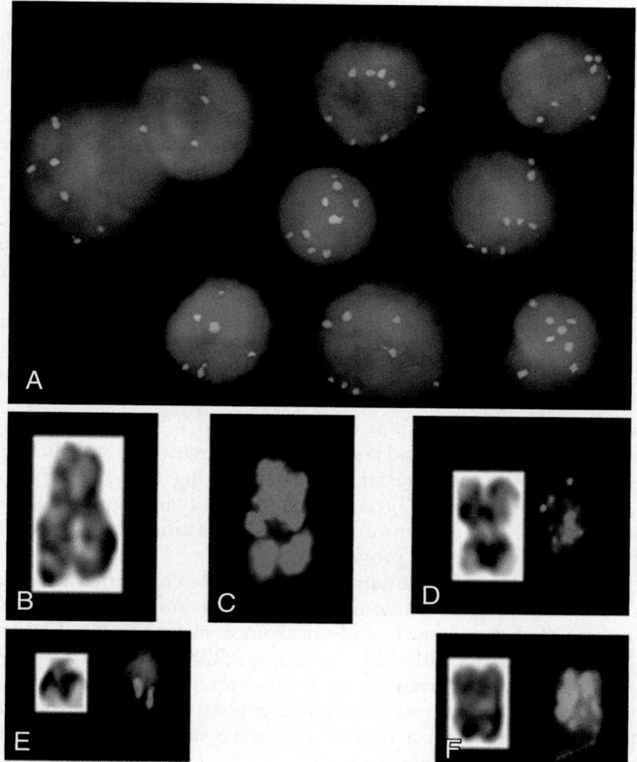

Figure 54-33 DETECTION OF AML1 AND 21q22 AMPLIFICATION. **A,** Intrachromosomal amplification of AML1 *(red)* (TEL *[green]*, present in disomy) in a pediatric patient with pre–B-cell acute lymphoblastic leukemia. This finding is associated with poor prognosis. **B,** G banding of der(18) chromosome and after FISH study **(C)** with WCP 18 *(green)* and LSI 21q22.13 *(red)*, documenting der(18)t(18;21) and amplification of 21q22 region in a patient with myelodysplastic syndrome/acute myeloid leukemia. **D,** Amplification of 21q22 region in myelodysplastic syndrome may be present in another formation: der(21) (G banding, *left*). FISH study shows amplification of 21q22.13 locus *(red)* and identified der(21) as t(5;21) with 5p15.2 probe *(green)*. **E,** Localization of 21q22.13 LSI probe on normal chromosome 21. **F,** Homogeneous staining region (hsr)(21), G banding *(left)*, and after FISH study *(right)* with locus-specific probe for 21q22.13 *(red)* consistent with 21q22.13 band amplification in a patient with myelodysplastic syndrome.

intrachromosomal amplification of chromosome 21 (iAMP21) (see Fig. 54-33, *D*). Approximately 2% of children and less than 0.5% of adults display iAMP21. Children with iAMP21 have a common or pre–B-cell immunophenotype, median age of 9 years, and significantly inferior event-free and overall survival at 5 years compared with children exhibiting other cytogenetic subgroups. Even children with Ph-positive ALL, known for its poor prognosis, have a better 5-year event-free survival compared with children with iAMP21. These children have a threefold increased risk for relapse and are twice as likely to die than are their counterparts without iAMP21.

ETV6 or TEL (for translocation, ETS, leukemia) transcription factor gene, most frequently found in translocations, was first identified as a part of a TEL–platelet-derived growth factor receptor β fusion (TEL-PDGFRB) created by t(5;12)(q33;p13) in chronic myelomonocytic leukemia. It was detected using FISH because, as mentioned earlier, of difficulties in detecting cytogenetic rearrangements at the 12p13 site. As a result of this translocation, the helix-loop-helix domain of TEL/ETV6 is fused in frame to the PDGFRB transmembrane and tyrosine kinase domain. Fusion of TEL/ETV6 to a tyrosine kinase also occurs as a result of t(9;12)(q34;p13), leading to the ABL-TEL(ETV6) fusion that has been observed in patients with ALL,

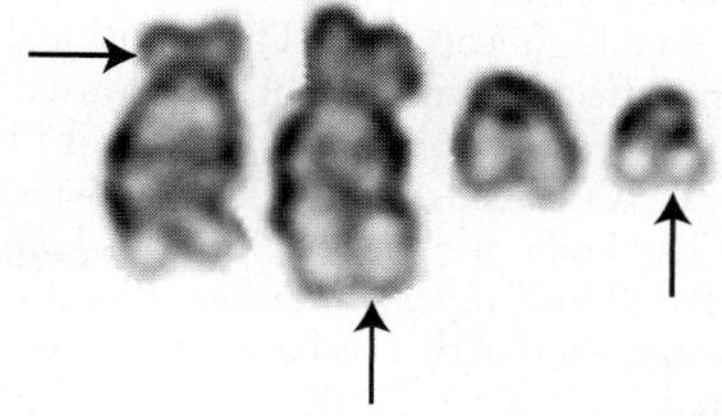

Figure 54-34 t(9;22)(q34;q11) *(arrows)* in a patient with acute lymphoblastic leukemia. Note that the first chromosome 9 has deletion of the short arms, a frequent finding in both adult and pediatric acute lymphoblastic leukemia patients.

AML, and atypical CML. More than 39 partner genes are known to participate in fusions with ETV6/TEL, primarily in ALL and less frequently in myeloid malignancies.

Other rearrangements involving 12p include deletions, duplications, and translocations and are observed most often as part of a complex karyotype, frequently associated with chromosome 5 and/or 7 abnormalities. Deletion of 12p13 is much more frequent in children than in adults with ALL and is observed in patients with myeloid disorders, specifically in adults with MDS. Two other genes residing on 12p also are rearranged: CCND2 is frequently amplified, and CDKN1B is often deleted.

Approximately 5% of children and 20% to 25% of adults with ALL have Ph, making it the most common structural rearrangement in adult ALL (Fig. 54-34). The breakpoint on Ph is more centromeric than in CML (see Chronic Myelogenous Leukemia section, earlier). It includes the 5′ breakpoint on chromosome 22, distal to the first exon (falling between exon e1 and e2) of the BCR gene, resulting in the $P190^{BCR\text{-}ABL1}$ variant, providing a diagnostic distinction between lymphoid blast crisis of CML and de novo ALL. Ph-positive ALL is characterized by the smallest BCR-ABL1 (P190) protein, containing less BCR than the P210 and P230 fusion proteins. Among Ph-positive patients with ALL, approximately 58% to 70% of adults and 80% of children have this genomic breakpoint variant. Up to 19% of Ph-positive ALL patients may express both the P190 and the P210 BCR-ABL1 fusions. A number of earlier studies indicated that the P190 type of the BCR-ABL1 breakpoint is associated with a more aggressive form of disease, with higher tyrosine kinase transforming ability than the P210 protein associated with CML. Ph-positive ALL has been classified as a stem cell disorder because of the presence of the BCR-ABL transcript in both the myeloid and lymphoid lineages. More recent reports suggest that the presence of the P190 protein does not confer a poorer prognosis.

The BCR-ABL1 fusion variants are easily detectable by FISH testing using the extrasensitive probe strategy, and BCR-ABL1 leukemia can be identified in up to 10% of Ph-negative cases. Moreover, FISH testing will identify ABL rearrangements in BCR-ABL1 fusion-negative ALL patients. The role of imatinib used alone or in combination with conventional chemotherapy in older adult patients with de novo Ph-positive ALL is being studied. Initial GEP studies have failed to identify specific genes associated with differences in overall survival of adult patients with P190 or P210 ALL.

Reactivation of BCR-ABL kinase activity is most commonly associated with the emergence of point mutation in the ABL kinase domain implicated in resistance to imatinib treatment (see Chronic Myelogenous Leukemia section, earlier). Retrospective analysis reveals that 40% of newly diagnosed and imatinib-naive Ph-positive ALL patients have kinase domain mutations, and 83% to 90% have identical mutation at relapse or at the time of hematologic or cytogenetic resistance to imatinib. The frequency of the mutant allele is always below the level of detectability by direct cDNA sequencing method at diagnosis, and use of more sensitive methods, such as denaturing high-performance liquid chromatography, is recommended.

More than 60% of adult patients with Ph-positive ALL show additional chromosomal abnormalities in the Ph-positive clone. Most frequent are gain of Ph, monosomy 7, +8, +X, del(9p) (see Fig. 54-34), and high triploidy. The additional chromosomal abnormality has no effect on survival of Ph-positive patients. High hyperdiploidy is detected in approximately 15% of Ph-positive ALL. According to the WHO classification, 1% of all leukemia are mixed phenotype acute leukemia with t(9;22)(q34;q11.2) and leukemic blasts showing a B-cell and myeloid lineage. Occasional T-cell phenotype and trilineage BCR-ABL1 mixed phenotype leukemia have been rarely reported.

t(1;19)(q23;p13.3) occurs in 5% to 6% of patients with B-cell precursor childhood ALL. However, among patients with a pre-B (cytoplasmic immunoglobulin–positive) immunophenotype, t(1;19) is found in approximately 25%. t(1;19) occurs in 2% to 3% of adults (see Fig. 54-32, *E*). Cytogenetically, two forms of t(1;19) can be identified: 25% of cases have a balanced reciprocal t(1;19), whereas 75% of cases have a more common rearrangement of unbalanced der(19)t(1;19)(q23;p13.3). The unbalanced der(19)t(1;19) arises from the initial trisomy of chromosome 1 followed by the t(1;19) translocation, with subsequent loss of the derivative chromosome 1. More than 95% of t(1;19) is associated with the E2A (TCF3)–PBX1 fusion gene. The E2A gene (originally identified by binding of E2A proteins to the kE2DNA sequence motif contained in the Ig κ light-chain enhancer) on chromosome 19, band p13.3, is fused to the PBX1 (homeobox) gene on chromosome 1, band q23. Approximately 1% of pediatric B-ALL patients have a variant t(17;19)(q21-q22;p13) translocation resulting in two different genomic rearrangements. The first is the fusion between the HLF gene (breakpoint in intron 3) on chromosome 17 and the E2A gene (within intron 13) on chromosome 19, associated with disseminated intravascular coagulation. The second is the breakpoint in intron 12 of E2A and intron 3 of HLF associated with hypercalcemia. In contrast to ETV6-RUNX1 rearrangements, which have a prenatal origin, current evidence suggests a postnatal etiology for t(1;19) translocations.

Currently, it is thought that an unbalanced der(19) in pediatric patients with ALL is associated with significantly improved outcome compared with patients with balanced t(1;19), which remains an adverse prognostic factor. In adults the prognostic relevance of t(1;19) is unclear, and both favorable and unfavorable outcomes have been reported. In contrast, a variant t(17;19) rearrangement is associated with poor prognosis. A recent study of adult ALL has suggested that prognosis of patients with t(1;19) can be substantially improved by the hyper-CVAD regimen. Both t(1;19) and t(17;19) are easily identifiable by conventional cytogenetics, FISH, and RT-PCR, and the latter two methodologies are particularly useful in posttreatment specimens that are cytogenetically normal.

In ALL, the most frequent MLL translocations include t(4;11) (see Fig. 54-30, *J*) leading to MLL-AFF1(AF4) fusion and t(11;19) (q23;p13.3) (see Fig. 54-30, *L*) resulting in MLL-MLLT1(ENL) fusion. These abnormalities are present in more than 80% of infant leukemia and 10% of childhood and adult leukemia. MLL rearrangements are associated with poor outcome in both children and adults (see Acute Myelogenous Leukemia, earlier, and T-Cell Lymphoproliferative Diseases, later). t(4;11) is one of the most common 11q23 abnormalities, occurring in 2% of children and approximately two-thirds of adults with MLL-associated translocations. The outcome of patients with t(4;11) is generally poor. One-third of patients with t(4;11) have secondary abnormalities; the most frequent are +X, i(7q), abnormalities of 9p, including i(9q), and +8. The outcome of patients with t(11;19) is also generally poor, especially in children younger than 1 year of age. The most frequent additional abnormalities in patients with t(11;19) are +X, +8, and del(6q). Other less common MLL translocations include t(9;11)(p22;q23)/MLL-MLLT3,t(10;11)(p13-15;q23)/MLL-MLLT10 and others. A large multiinstitutional study has determined that secondary aberrations do not affect prognosis of children with ALL and t(4;11),t(11;19) or other MLL translocations.

t(8;14)(q24;q32) is seen in fewer than 5% of all ALL patients (children and adults). Variant translocations t(8;22)(q24;q11) and t(2;8)(p12;q24) are seen in less than 1% of children and adults. These patients have CD10, CD19, CD20, surface IgM immunophenotype, and extremely poor prognosis. The same translocation is found in Burkitt lymphoma, and both entities likely represent the same disease with different manifestations. It has been reported that the majority of adult patients with t(8;14) die within 1 year of diagnosis.

Approximately 2% of children and 8% of adult pre–B-cell precursor ALL show recurrent IGH translocations usually identified by FISH as t(8;14)(q11;q32), t(14;19)(q32;q13), inv(14), (q11q32/t(14;14)(q11;q32), and t(14;20)(q32;q13). These five recurrent IGH translocations have in common deregulated expression of unmutated CEBP genes (CCAAT enhancer–binding protein transcription factors), and approximately 1% of all B-cell precursor ALL are characterized by novel CEBP-IGH fusions.

Abnormalities of the short arms of chromosome 9 (p21-22) occur at a frequency of 7% to 13%. In adults the presence of del(9p) appears to be associated with improved outcome, whereas in children with ALL, del(9p) is associated with poor outcome. The most frequent abnormalities are codeletions of two genes, $p15^{INK4B}$ and $p16^{INK4A}$, as well as the interferon α and β genes found in many, but not all, cases. Among the structural rearrangements involving the short arms of chromosome 9, t/dic(9;12)(p11-12;p11-13) is a rare recurrent abnormality associated with L1 morphology (FAB classification), pre–B-cell phenotype, and excellent prognosis.

Other chromosomal abnormalities detected in nonrandom fashion in adult ALL include deletions, both terminal and interstitial, of the long arm of chromosome 6, and isochromosomes of 7q, 9q, 17q, and 21q. Adult patients with ALL showing t(9;22), t(4;11), t(8;14), −7, +8 chromosomal aberrations have a poorer prognosis and significantly lower probability of long-term complete remission and survival than do patients with a normal karyotype or patients with other chromosomal rearrangements.

Gene expression profiling in childhood ALL suggests that ALL segregates according to cell lineage and primary genomic defects. However, some clues about the genes that participate in drug resistance and influence treatment are provided by a comparison between GEP and response to therapy. In this study of 187 children with ALL, 14 functionally related genes with roles in regulation of cell proliferation were independently associated with risk for relapse. Retrospective studies have demonstrated that expression profiling can be effective in classifying ALL into recognized, prognostically important subtypes such as those mentioned earlier; these studies have also identified a new subtype of ALL without the BCR-ABL1 fusion, but with a similar expression profile to BCR-ABL1 leukemia. Moreover, GEP has shown that ALL with MLL rearrangements has a unique expression profile separate from other types of AML and ALL.

Epidemiologic and twin studies indicate a multistep pathogenesis of B-cell ALL in infants and children, with initial leukemogenic event(s) occurring in utero and subsequent genomic changes occurring postnatally. Twin studies provide insight into the pathogenesis of pediatric leukemia because most common chromosomal translocations and their resultant gene fusions can be documented by molecular analysis of neonatal blood spots or Guthrie cards. If a unique gene fusion sequence is present in at least one cell per 30,000 in peripheral blood, it will be detected by a sensitive PCR-based assay. The first observations of in utero origin of an acute leukemia were demonstrated for MLL rearrangements in three children with ALL, in monozygotic twins who shared the identical TEL(ETV6)–AML1 (RUNX1) fusion, and in a pair of twins diagnosed at age 3 with B-precursor ALL. The concordance rate of twins who share a monochorionic placenta and develop leukemia is probably 100%, whereas older twins have a discordance rate of 90%, indicating that additional postnatal leukemic events are needed. The frequency of in utero origin of B-cell precursor ALL in nontwins as measured by clonal IGH rearrangements is reported to be 71%, supporting the notion that in the majority of infants older than 1 year, the development of ALL occurs during fetal hematopoiesis. Subsequent physiologic postnatal switch may eliminate these abnormal clones in the vast majority of the cases; however, a small number of children have a "preleukemic" clone for some time, with later emergence of leukemia (see box on Genetic Testing for Acute Lymphoblastic Leukemia).

B-CELL CHRONIC LYMPHOCYTIC LEUKEMIA

Approximately 40% to 50% of CLL patients have clonal abnormalities identified by conventional cytogenetics (see Chapter 76). This may be an underestimation because chromosomal changes may occur in one or more cell subsets of the malignant clone. Classic cytogenetic analyses of B-CLL has remained difficult because of the low mitotic yield of neoplastic B cells despite the use of B-cell mitogens, such as 12-O-tetradecanoylphorbol-13-cetate (TPA) and stimulation with CD40 ligand and interleukin 4. Molecular cytogenetics, such as interphase FISH, CGH, and array CGH, have raised the detection rate to 80% to 90%. Analysis of clinically relevant chromosomal loci, combined with immunophenotyping, mutational analyses of the immunoglobulin heavy-chain variable region (IgV_H), and ZAP-70 overexpression, are of prognostic importance, even though oncogenic events that lead to the origin of B-CLL remain unknown (Table 54-11 and Fig. 54-35; see also box on Genetic Testing for B-Cell Chronic Lymphocytic Leukemia). Although microarray and high-density SNP array studies have not identified genes involved in the pathogenesis of CLL, they clarify that CLL, despite its heterogeneous nature, is one disease entity with a common genetic phenotype resembling memory B lymphocytes. Genetic testing is strongly recommended for all CLL patients, particularly in the context of novel therapeutic trials for CLL.

Genetic Testing for Acute Lymphoblastic Leukemia

At diagnosis, conventional cytogenetic studies should be performed, especially for pediatric patients in whom solely numerical anomalies occur in 25%. FISH and molecular genetic methods are valuable to detect certain cryptic chromosome anomalies, such as TEL/AML1 fusion associated with t(12;21)(p12;q22). The panel of FISH probe at the diagnosis of pediatric acute lymphoblastic leukemia includes TEL(ETV6)-AML1 (RUNX1), MLL, BCR-ABL, P21 at 9p, and centromeric probes for chromosomes 4, 10, and 17. In adults, the role of hyperdiploidy as it relates to prognosis is uncertain; thus FISH testing with centromeric probes is not useful. Establishing benchmarks with FISH and/or molecular testing is crucial for follow-up of patients during and after therapy.

Genetic Testing for B-Cell Chronic Lymphocytic Leukemia

Interphase FISH is used in lieu of chromosome studies because FISH detection of abnormalities in chronic lymphocytic leukemia correlates with clinical risk groups and prognosis. FISH studies should be performed on blood for detection of trisomy 12, deletions of 11q22.3, 13q14.3, and P53 loci, as well as rearrangement of 14q32.3, IGH locus. The FISH test can distinguish between patients with B-cell chronic lymphocytic leukemia and those with the leukemic phase of certain lymphomas, such as mantle cell lymphoma and follicular lymphoma.

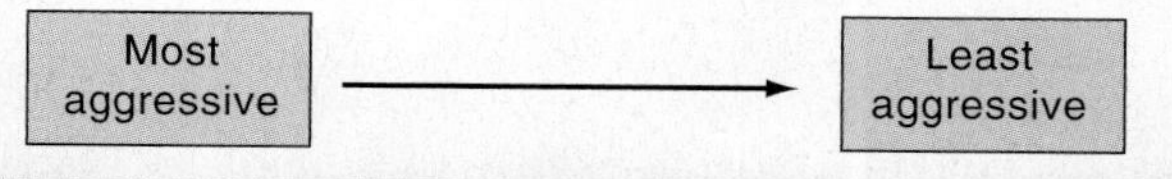

Figure 54-35 SURVIVAL OF PATIENTS WITH SPECIFIC GENOMIC DEFECTS IN CHRONIC LYMPHOCYTIC LEUKEMIA.

Table 54-11 Recurrent Chromosomal Translocations in B-Cell Lymphoproliferative Disorders

Translocations	Genes Involved	Associated Diseases
IMMUNOGLOBULIN (*IG*)-RELATED TRANSLOCATIONS		
t(1;14)(p22;q32)	CNN3-IGH	B-cell ALL, NHL
t(1;14)(q21;q320)	BCL9-IGH	pre–B-ALL
t(1;14)(q21;q32)	MUC1-IGH	Multiple myeloma
t(1;14)(q24;q32)	LHX4-IGH	
t(2;14)(p13;q32)	BCL11A-IGH	CLL/SLL, ALL, NHL
t(2;8)(p12;q32)	IGK-cMYC	ALL (Burkitt)
t(4;14)(p16.3;q32.3)	FGFR3-IqH	Multiple myeloma
t(5;14)(q31;q32)	IL3-IGH	B-CLL
t(6;14)(p25;q32)	IRF-IGH	Multiple myeloma
t(6;14)(p22;q32)	ID4-IGH	Plasma cell leukemia
t(6;14)(p21;q32)	CCND3-IGH	B-ALL
t(7;14)(q21;q32)	IGH/-CDK6	B-CLL
t(8;14)(q24;q32)	IGH/-cMYC	ALL (Burkitt)
t(8;22)(q24;q11)	IGL-CMYC	ALL (Burkitt)
t(10;14)(q24;q34)	NFKB2-IGH	T-cell ALL, CLL, NHL
t(11;14)(q13;q32.3)	CCND1-IGH	Multiple myeloma
t(11;14)(q23;q32)	DDX6-IGH	
t(11;14)(q23;q32)	PAFAH1B2-IGH	
t(11;14)(q23;q32)	PCSK7-IGH	
t(12;14)(p13;q32)	ETV6-IGH	pre–B-ALL
t(14;14)((q11;q32)	TCRA-IGH	T-PLL
t(14;16)(q32.3;q23)	IGH-MAF	Multiple myeloma
t(14;19)(q32;p13)	IGH-BCL-3	B-CLL
t(14;20)(q32;q11)	IGH-MAFb	Multiple myeloma
t(14;20)(q32;q13)	IGH-CEPBP B-ALL	
LYMPHOMA-ASSOCIATED TRANSLOCATIONS		
t(1;14)(p22;q32)	BCL10-IGH	MALT
t(3;14)(q14;q32)	FOXP1-IGH	MALT
t(5;14)(q35;q32)	ODZ2-IGH	MALT
t(11;14)(q13;q32.3)	CCNDI-IGH	Mantle cell
t(14;18)(q32.3;q21)	IGH-BCL2	Follicular
t(3;14)(q27;q32)	BCL6-IGH	Follicular
t(11;18)(q21;q21)	API2-MALTI	MALT
t(14;18)(q32.3;q21)	IGM-MALT	MALT
t(1;14)(p22;q32.3)	BCL10-IGH	MALT
3q27 rearrangements	BCL 6	Diffuse large B cell
t(14;15)(q32.3;q11-13)	IGH-BCL8	Diffuse large B cell
t(3;14)(p14;q32.3)	FOXPIF-IGH	MALT
t(9;14)(p13;q32.3)	PAX5-IGH	LPL

ALL, Acute lymphoblastic leukemia; *B-CLL*, B-cell chronic lymphocytic leukemia; *LPL*, lymphoplasmacytoid lymphoma; *MALT*, mucosa-associated lymphoid tissue.

Chromosome abnormalities in CLL detected by FISH are of prognostic significance.[22] Four genomic aberrations, as well as normal findings, are independent predictors of disease progression and survival. Genomic aberrations of prognostic significance include 17p deletion, 11q deletion, trisomy 12, and 13q deletion. Survival in these groups was 32, 79, 114, and 133 months, respectively, and the treatment-free interval was 8, 12, 33, and 92 months, respectively (see Fig. 54-35). Survival of patients with a normal karyotype was 111 months, and the treatment-free interval was 49 months. The deletion of 17p13 affects the tumor suppressor gene TP53. In 80% to 90% of the cases, a deletion of 17p is associated with the mutated TP53 on the remaining copy. This is considered one reason why p53 pathway-based therapies such as fludarabine or its combinations are not effective in patients with 17p deletion. TP53 genes have been found in 4% to 15% of patients in early-stage CLL and are associated with poorer outcome. Deletion of 11q and deletion of the ATM gene on 11q23.1 are found in 18% of CLL patients. In about one-third of 11q-deleted patients, a simultaneous mutation of the ATM has been found. The overall survival of these patients is shorter.

A comparison of known prognostic features of B-CLL with interphase FISH results indicates that FISH-detected anomalies are frequent in B-CLL cases, even in Rai stages 0 to 1, but are more frequent among patients with progressive disease (88%) than in those with stable disease (66%). Two risk groups are recognized: (a) low risk includes patients with a normal karyotype or isolated del(13q); (b) high risk includes patients with del(11q) and del(17p). Patients with +12 are high risk, but in contrast to del(11q) and del(17p), they respond to fludarabine-based therapies (Fig. 54-36). Comparison of a quantitative PCR method with FISH for assessment of the four most frequent aneuploidies revealed a tight correlation in 103 of 110 patients examined, with FISH being more sensitive in detecting subclonal genetic evolution.

The frequency of abnormalities of chromosome 13 in CLL detected by conventional cytogenetics is 10% to 15%. However, with the application of FISH, smaller or larger deletions of band q14.3 are detected in up to 60% of patients over time. When multiple DNA probes are used, D13S319 and D13S25 DNA markers are deleted more frequently in B-CLL than is RB1. Molecular analyses have detected deletions of 13q in cells that are cytogenetically normal as well as abnormal. Homozygous deletion of D13S25 and/or D13S319 DNA segments from the 13q14.3 band region is a rare but consistent finding in a subset of patients with B-cell CLL. In a study examining loss of heterozygosity and subchromosomal copy losses on chromosome 13, two types of deletions were defined: type 1 aberrations occurred in 60% of del(13)(q14) cases and had loss of Rb1 and breaks close to the miR16/15a locus; and type 2 aberrations that included Rb1 occurred in 40%. As mentioned earlier, the 13q14.3-deleted segment contains micro-RNA (miRNA) genes. Micro-RNAs are normally made by cells, including B lymphocytes, and they regulate the function of many genes. Preliminary findings demonstrate that all patients with homozygous 13q deletion have dramatic miRNA15a downregulation, whereas patients with hemizygous 13q deletions are indistinguishable from controls, providing the first molecular clues for the genetic basis and pathogenesis of CLL.

Trisomy 12 or 13q rearrangements are found separately in a substantial proportion of patients with CLL. They coexist in only 2% to 5% of patients, suggesting that each change may have a distinct pathogenetic route. The presence of del(13q) as the sole abnormality in CLL is associated with the most favorable prognosis, with a median survival of 11 years.

Among the first-degree relatives of patients with familial CLL, population studies have demonstrated a sevenfold increased risk for developing CLL and a twofold increased risk for developing lymphoproliferative disorders. More than 80 families with CLL affecting multiple family members have been reported. Linkage studies suggest a region of interest in band q22.1 of chromosome 13 (marker D13S156). Fine FISH mapping of six CLL-prone families (63 individuals) reveals deletion of 13q14 in 85% of patients with familial CLL, and four CLL families shared a 3.6-Mb minimal region in 13q21.33-q22.2. This region included 12 candidate genes, but thus far informative candidates have not been identified.

Trisomy 12 was the first reported recurrent abnormality in CLL. It is detected by classic cytogenetics in 7% to 15% of all cases. FISH assessment detects +12 in 15% to 20% of patients with CLL. FISH studies are more representative of the true incidence of trisomy 12 because the interphase FISH methodology provides information on cells independent of their cycling status. Trisomy 12 may be present as the sole abnormality or in combination with other chromosomal rearrangements. Because only a proportion of cells are trisomic, normal cells or disomic neoplastic cells also may be present. Follow-up analysis over a 4-year period demonstrates clonal expansion of cells with trisomy 12 as the disease progresses. These observations suggest that trisomy 12 might be relevant in the cell activation process in CLL. The observation that trisomy 12 is documented in B cells and is absent from T lymphocytes and CD34 cells in the majority of patients is consistent with the original hypothesis that CLL has a clonal origin and that trisomy 12 arises in a progenitor cell already committed to the B-cell pathway. Routine FISH testing identifies patients with trisomy 12 because it uses the probe that is hybridized only to the centromeric area of chromosome 12. More sophisticated molecular cytogenetic methods may be useful. Increased expression of the CLLU1 gene on 12q22 has been observed in CLL samples from patients with or without trisomy 12. Overexpression of CLLU1 in CLL patients without IgV_H hypermutation combined with restricted and CLL-unique expression pattern suggests that CLLU1 is among the first disease-specific genes identified in CLL.

Three recent studies utilizing whole genome sequencing detected NOTCH1 mutations in 42% of patients with trisomy 12. Almost all

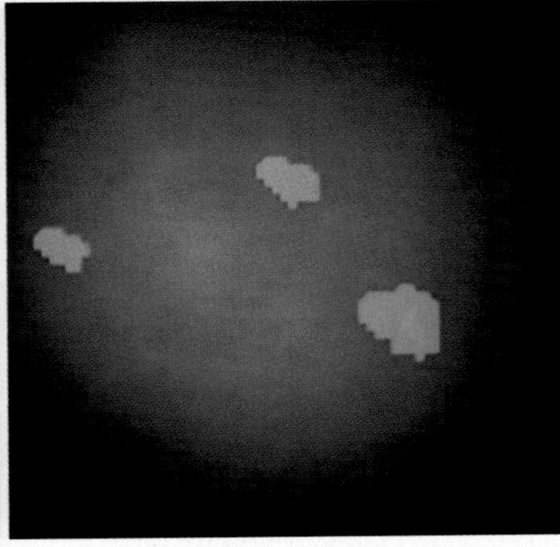

Figure 54-36 PANEL OF CHROMOSOMAL PROBES USED FOR DETECTION OF GENOMIC DEFECTS IN CHRONIC LYMPHOCYTIC LEUKEMIA. They include 13q14.3 *(red),* 13q34 *(aqua),* and CEP12 (all present in disomy; *left*) and 11q22.3 (ATM, *green*) and 17p13.1 (P53*; red, right*). Note only one copy of the ATM gene *(green, right)* consistent with deletion of sequences from the 11q22.3 band region, which is associated with unfavorable prognosis.

NOTCH1 mutations resulted in a truncated protein, lacking the C-terminal PEST degradation domain, rendering it constitutively active. Deletions of the long arm of chromosome 11 in CLL as detected by conventional cytogenetics have been reported in 5% to 8% of cases. An interphase FISH study identified a clinical subset of B-cell CLL defined by deletion of 11q22.3-23.1 in 7% to 10% of these cases. FISH characterization of aberrations involved in 11q21-q23 demonstrate a minimal consensus deletion segment of 2 to 3 Mb, containing a number of genes including ATM at 11q22.3 (see Fig. 54-36, *right*). Up to 12% of patients have simultaneous deletions of ATM and MLL at 11q23. The ATM gene is responsible for ataxia-telangiectasia and functions as a cell-cycle checkpoint regulator. Somatic disruptions of both alleles of the ATM gene by deletion or point mutation are detected in 25% to 34% of cases. This finding strongly suggests the pathologic role of ATM in some patients with B-CLL. A study revealed discontinuous deletions at 11q23.1-q23.3, indicating that genes in this region may have pathogenic significance because they constitute independent targets for amplification or deletion in cases of B-CLL. Patients with 11q deletion exhibit extensive lymphadenopathy, more rapid disease progression, a shorter treatment-free interval, inferior molecular remission, and reduced overall survival. Structural aberrations of chromosome 17 are observed in 4% of cytogenetically evaluable B-CLL cases. This abnormality frequently affects the short arm of chromosome 17, the site of the P53 tumor suppressor gene. Monoallelic deletions of P53, detected by FISH, are present in 7% to 20% of patients and represent the strongest predictor of survival in B-cell CLL. The median survival time of these patients is only 32 months. A novel recurrent dic(8;17)(p11;p11) abnormality also leads to loss of TP53, and low copy repeats in 17p12 and 8p11 may the origin of the translocation by nonallelic homologous recombination on one chromosome 17. B-CLL in patients with deletion of the P53 gene is associated with refractory advanced disease, resistance to treatment, and shorter survival. A comprehensive assessment of genetic and molecular features predicting outcome in previously untreated CLL patients receiving either fludarabine or fludarabine plus cyclophosphamide identified del(17)(p13) along with del(11q), but not IgV_H, CD38 expression, or ZAP-70 status, as significant risk factors for early relapse. Because the leukemic phase of certain lymphomas can clinically mimic B-CLL, FISH testing for translocation using an IgH probe is important. Fewer than 5% of patients with CLL/prolymphocytic leukemia have t(11;14)(q13;q32), and these conditions usually transform into prolymphocytic leukemia. Moreover, IGH testing in CLL is important for detecting patients with recurrent del(14)(q24.1) associated with unmutated IgV_H status (66%) and trisomy 12 (47%).[23]

Solid evidence exists that chromosomal translocations detected by conventional cytogenetics independently predict treatment failure, treatment-free survival, and overall survival in untreated and cladribine-treated B-cell CLL patients. When CLL-derived metaphase cells are obtained with systematic stimulation using B-cell mitogens and activators, balanced and unbalanced translocations are seen in 34% to 42% of patients. In multivariate analysis, unbalanced translocations are independently associated with risk for treatment failure. Because del(13q) usually is cryptic by conventional cytogenetics but easily detected with FISH studies, both conventional cytogenetics and interphase FISH should be performed at baseline in patients with advanced CLL. Comparison of the performance between the custom made 44K oligonucleotide array platform with results obtained by FISH panel (including ATM at 11q22.3, D13S319 at 13q14,3 TP53 at 17p13.1 chromosomal site, and centromere 12 in 100 CLL samples) showed 89% concordance rate. The genomic imbalances and LOH, investigated by different resolution SNP arrays, showed 66% to 82% of genomic lesions including uniparental disomy. Currently, the 250K NSP array was validated for routine clinical use in the diagnosis of CLL and demonstrated 98.5% concordance with the standard CLL FISH panel.

The most novel gene mutation implicated in more rapid disease progression and poorer overall survival is a somatic mutation of SF3B1. The somatic mutations of SF3B1 gene, encoding a small nuclear RNA-splicing protein, were uncovered using the whole-exome sequencing of matched tumor and normal samples from 105 patients at a frequency of ≈10%. SF3B1 mutations were associated with more rapid disease progression and poor overall survival.

The validity of hierarchical interphase FISH categories at diagnosis in predicting overall survival of CLL patients is confirmed by long-term follow-up studies. Interphase FISH testing can identify approximately 27% of patients with clonal chromosomal evolution occurring after 5 or more years of follow-up, with approximately two-thirds of patients acquiring del(13q) and del(17p). These observations have important clinical implications for management of patients with highest-risk early-stage CLL.

In 2011, using next generation sequencing technique, a new phenomenon called *chromothripsis* (from the Greek *chromos,* meaning "chromosomes," and *thripsis,* meaning "shattering into pieces") was described for the first time and was identified in CLL. Chromothripsis describes a process whereby hundreds of genomic rearrangements have been acquired in a single catastrophic event. A chromosomal region or a chromosome or telomere of other chromosomes gets shattered into hundreds of pieces, some but not all are stitched together by the DNA repair machinery in a mosaic patchwork of genomic fragments. Cells not only survive this crisis but emerge with a genomic landscape that confers selective advantage, thereby promoting further malignant evolution. Subsequent evidence of chromothripsis has been described in other types of malignancies, including multiple myeloma, where it is accompanied by a poor outcome.

MULTIPLE MYELOMA

Multiple myeloma (MM) is a malignancy of terminally differentiated B cells (see Chapter 85). These plasma cells have a very low proliferative rate, a characteristic that has limited their application in cytogenetic studies. Conventional karyotyping reveals chromosome abnormalities in 25% to 30% of newly diagnosed patients, especially in cases with exceptionally high plasma cell proliferative rates. Karyotypes obtained from these cells usually are complex and exhibit more than 20 aberrations in approximately 10% of cases.

When reassessed by FISH, CGH, and multicolor karyotyping using a large panel of centromere-specific and translocation-specific probes, interphase plasma cell nuclei revealed chromosomal aneuploidy in almost all patients with MM or monoclonal gammopathy of unknown significance. Even during complete clinical remission, 12% to 71% of cells still show a numerical gain or loss of chromosomes 3, 7, 8, 9, 11, 13, 15, 21, and X.

Analysis of numerical abnormalities reveals two broad groups of MM patients: hyperdiploid and nonhyperdiploid. Approximately 55% to 60% of newly diagnosed MM patients are characterized by a hyperdiploid karyotype with a number of chromosomes ranging from 48 to 74 and trisomies of odd-numbered chromosomes including 3, 5, 7, 9, 11, 15, 19, and 21 and fewer IGH translocations (Fig. 54-37). The remaining patients are cases of hyperdiploid MMs that include tumors with hypodiploid, near diploid, pseudodiploid, or near-tetraploid chromosome numbers (fewer than 48 or more than 74 chromosomes), which are characterized by a high frequency of IGH translocations (>85%). Both these groups are also present in monoclonal gammopathy of unknown significance, suggesting that they occur early in the evolution of disease. The prognostic relevance of numerical abnormalities is difficult to ascertain because frequently, other adverse genetic changes are present in the same clone.

Nevertheless, patients with hyperdiploid MM tend to have a better prognosis than do those with nonhyperdiploid disease. A recent array-comparative genomic hybridization-based classification schema has identified a subset of patients who present with additional gains of 1q and/or losses of chromosome 13. These patients have a worse prognosis than do patients in the nonhyperdiploid group. More detailed analysis using genome-wide CNAs revealed numerical aberrations in 98% of cases and identified amplification of 1q and deletions of 1p, 12p, 14q, 16q, and 20p to be associated with poor

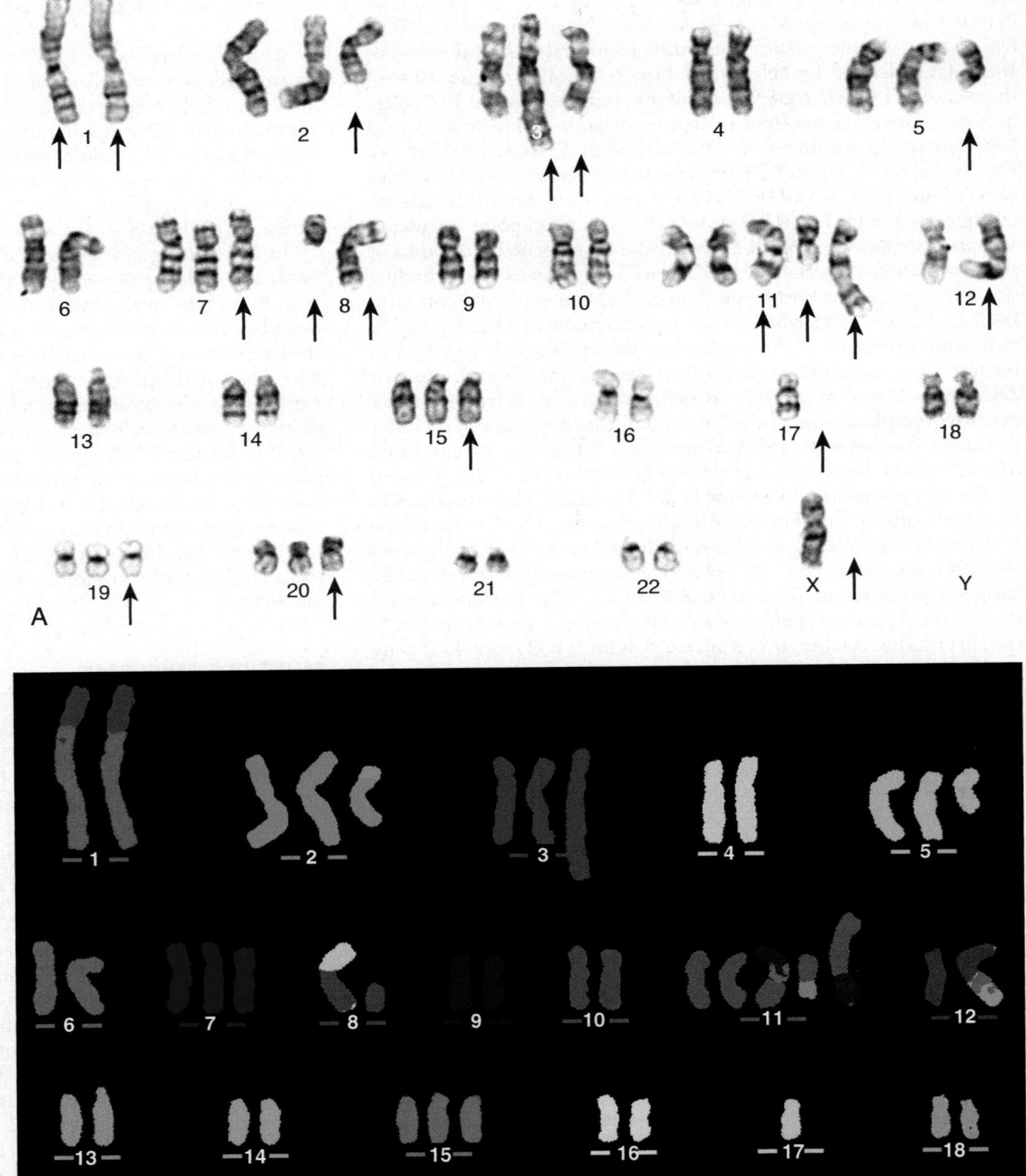

Figure 54-37 A complex hyperdiploid karyotype from a patient with multiple myeloma **(A)** and after multicolor FISH **(B)**, which was used to resolve a number of complex derivative chromosomes: 54, X, −X, der(1)t(1;8)(q34;q21q24)×2, der(2)del(2)(p13p25)t(X;2)(p21p22.3;p13), t(3;8)(q27;q22q24), +i(5)(p13p15), +7, der(8;17)(p23;q11.2q25), +der(11)t(1;9;11(?p36;q21q31;p15), t(11;20)(q13;q11.2, der(11)t(9;11)(q13q34;q25), t(12;13)9(p13;q14q34), +15, +19, +20.

prognosis, whereas amplification of chromosomes 5, 9, 11, 15, and 19 conferred a superior outcome. The Arkansas Multiple Myeloma Group pioneered the use of GEP as a highly sensitive method to stratify multiple myeloma patients in terms of outcome and to more fully characterize an individual's tumor at the molecular level. This group identified a distinctive 70-gene molecular signature (GEP70) for high-risk myeloma that correlated with a strong probability of early recurrence and shorter overall survival compared with patients with low-risk MM who had much greater probability of maintaining a longer-term remission[24] (Fig. 54-38). These 70 genes have overlapping functions and are involved in cell-cycle regulation, angiogenesis, cell adhesion, cell migration, and proliferation. When compared with standard metaphase and interphase FISH, the GEP70 gene signature significantly reduces the number of patients traditionally classified with a poor prognosis, while at the same time identifying those patients who may be at increased risk for relapse. The marked increase of GEP70 high-risk patients from 13% at diagnosis to 76% at relapse provides strong molecular evidence of disease evolution. GEP studies require plasma cell purifications and highly specific dedicated platforms (including very sophisticated bioinformatics), which are presently not widely available to the majority of physicians. However, GEP70 analysis and numerous other reports have demonstrated

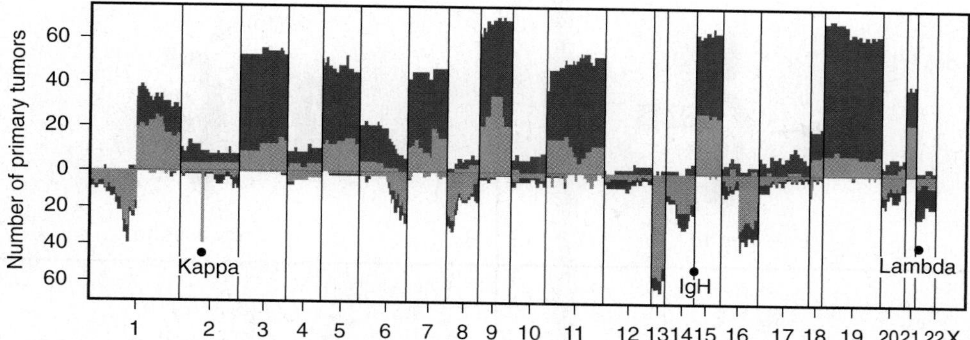

Figure 54-38 Summary of genomic profiles and recurrence of chromosomal alterations in primary tumors demonstrated by array comparative genomic hybridization. The recurrence plot mirrors the frequencies of previously reported chromosomal gains and losses, including the deletions of 1p and amplifications of 1q. Integer-value recurrence of copy number aberrations across the samples in segmented data is plotted on the y-axis. The x-axis is in chromosomal order. *Dark red* or *green* bands denote the number of samples with gain or loss of chromosome material, and *bright red* or *green* bars represent the number of samples showing amplification or deletion. *Black dots* show focal deletions of the kappa (2p12), IgH (14q32), and lambda (22q11) loci physiologic in B-cell postgerminal center neoplasms. *(Reprinted with permission from Carasco DR, Tonon G, Huang Y, et al: High resolution genomic profiles define distinct clinic pathogenic subgroups of multiple myeloma patients.* Cancer Cell *4:313, 2006.)*

that gains of 1q12-q44 are an independent marker associated with disease progression and that deletion of TP53 defines a group of patients with ultra high-risk MM (Figs. 54-39 and 54-40). Hence testing with FISH for 1q21 and/or 1q25 loci, as well for deletion of 17p13.1 chromosomal region, will identify patients with unfavorable prognoses (Fig. 54-41).[25]

Even with the application of GEP and SNP arrays, MM-specific oncogenes associated with hyperdiploidy have not been identified. However, in such a genetically heterogeneous group, it is anticipated that the application of novel cytogenomic technologies for detection of copy number aberrations may provide more precise and predictive tools.

It is believed that primary translocations occur early in the pathogenesis of MM, whereas secondary translocations occur late and are involved in tumor progression.[26,27] Most primary translocations are simple balanced translocations and juxtapose an oncogene and one of the immunoglobulin enhancers. An IGH rearrangement on 14q32.3 is found in most patients with MM. The rearrangement consists of complex and heterogeneous translocations with the breakpoint involving either the switch region of IGH or the V, D, or J gene (see Table 54-10). The primary translocations are due to somatic hypermutation or errors in the VDJ portion of the switch region recombination. The translocations include a promiscuous array of at least 20 nonrandom chromosomal partners, and the characterization of these translocations has led to the identification of critical dysregulated oncogenes (e.g., BCL2, cyclin D). In each translocation, a potent enhancer is juxtaposed to dysregulated oncogenes. The five most frequent IGH translocations are t(4;14)(p16.3;q32.3), t(6;14)(p21;q32.3), t(11;14)(q13;q32.3), t(14;16)(q32.3;q23), and t(14;20)(q32.3;q12) (Table 54-12 and Fig. 54-42).

Patients with a recurrent CCND1-IGH have an overexpression of cyclin D1. In contrast to mantle cell lymphoma, breakpoints on 11q13 in MM are not clustered but are scattered over a relatively large genomic region. Virtually all MM and MGUS tissues have cyclin D dysregulation, suggesting an early and unifying pathogenetic event. (see Fig. 54-40, *bottom left*). In contrast to other abnormalities involving the IGH locus, clonal t(11;14) MM cells, which occur in 15% to 20% of MM patients, tend to be diploid. There appears to be an association of the t(11;14) with oligosecretory or light chain only, CD20 expression, and lymphoplasmacytic morphology.

Approximately 15% of patients have a recurrent t(4;14)(p16.3;q32.3) abnormality. This cytogenetic abnormality is associated with IgA subtype, λ light chain, immature plasma cell morphology, and poor response to therapy. This abnormality is cytogenetically cryptic

Table 54-12 Most Frequent Chromosomal Abnormalities in Multiple Myeloma and Their Frequencies

Genetic Lesion	Frequency (%)	Oncogenes/Fusion Genes
TRANSLOCATIONS		
t(4;14)(p16.3;q32.3)	15	FGFR3, MMSET-IGH
t(11;14)(q13;q32.3)	15-20	CCND1-IGH
t(14;16)(q13;q23)	5-10	MAF-IGH
t(8;14)(q24;q32.3)	<10	MYC-IGH
t(14;20)(q32.3;q11)	5	IGH-MAFB
GAIN OF CHROMOSOMAL REGION		**CANDIDATE ONCOGENES**
1q21-q22	55	BCL9, IL6R
3q27.1-3q27.2	47	POLR2H, EIF4G1
5p12	44	?
7p11.2	44	?
9q34.11-9q34.3	54	ABL1, ANAPC2
11q13.4-11q14.1	52	SPCS2
15q24.2	44	IMP3
19q13.1	47	PDCD5
21q22.3	37	MCM3AP, HRMT1L1
LOSS OF CHROMOSOMAL REGION		**CANDIDATE TUMOR SUPPRESSOR GENE**
1p13.1-1p12	41	DENND2D
8p23.3-8p21.3	28	DLC1
10q26,2-10q26.3	18	PTPRE
13q34	49	RFP2, micro RNA 15/16
1432.13-13q32.2	33	?
16q11.2-16q12.3	31	CYLD

Modified from Anderson KC, Carrasco RD: Pathogenesis of myeloma. *Ann Rev Pathol* 6:249, 2011.

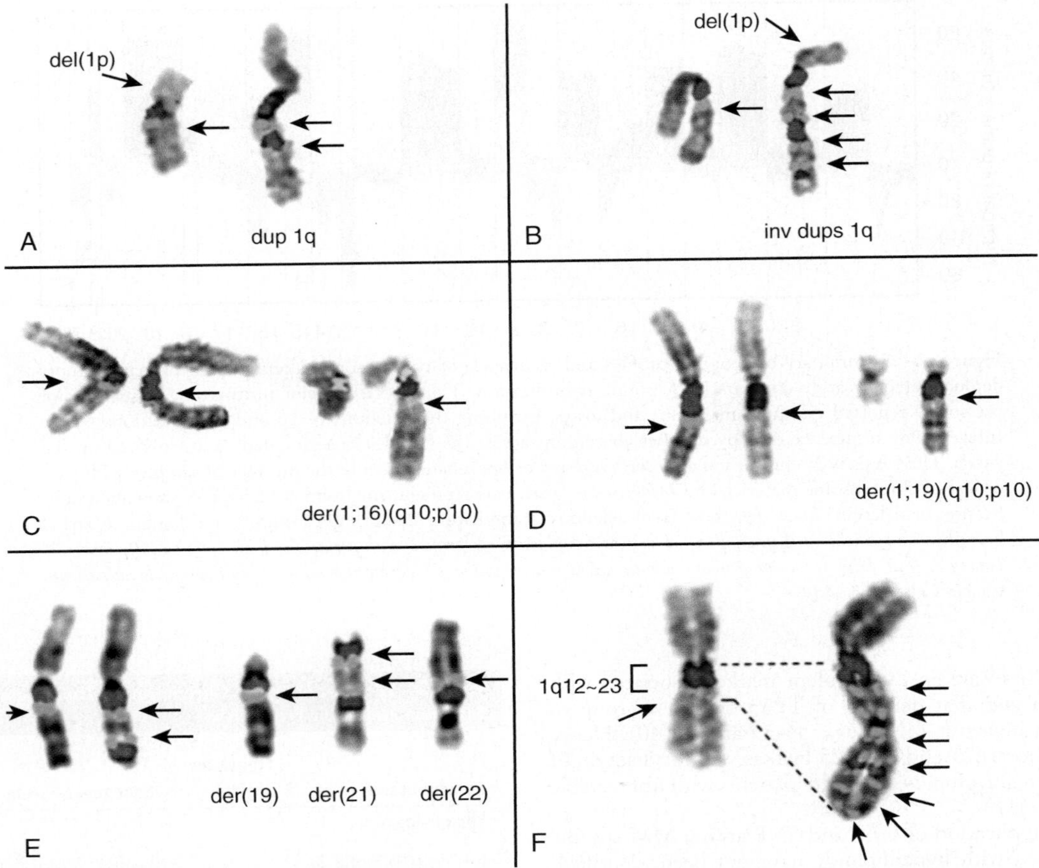

Figure 54-39 REPRESENTATIVE PARTIAL KARYOTYPES OF METAPHASE CHROMOSOMES DEMONSTRATING THE DIFFERENT TYPES AND DEGREE OF AMPLIFICATION OF CHROMOSOME 1. FISH probes for 1q12 *(red),* 1q21 *(green),* and 16q11 *(aqua)* are shown on inverted DAPI images of chromosomes. **A,** Interstitial deletion of 1p *(arrow)* in the homolog on the left and a direct dup1q12-q23 on chromosome on the right. **B,** Normal homolog 1 on the left and the abnormal homolog on the right, demonstrating both an interstitial deletion of 1p and the amplification of 1q in the same chromosome. Note four copies of 1q21 *(arrows)* in an inverted duplication pattern. **C,** Examples of an unbalanced whole-arm translocation of 1q to chromosome 16q. Chromosomes 1 are on the left, and chromosomes 16 are on the right. Aqua probe denotes 16q11 heterochromatin. Note the loss of 16q distal to the aqua probe on the der(1;16)(q10;p10). The entire long arm 1q is translocated to the pericentromeric region of 16q, and a total of three copies of 1q21 *(arrows)* are present. **D,** Examples of an unbalanced whole-arm translocation of 1q to 19q. Note that the result of this translocation is the der(1;19)(q10;p10) chromosome, which shows an extra copy of 1q21 *(arrows)* and loss of the entire 19q. **E,** Examples of jumping 1q, in which all or a part of 1q is translocated to three copies of 1q *(arrows)* on the three different nonhomologous chromosomes. The whole-arm der(19)(q10;p10) in this case is the same type seen in patient in **D.** The der(21) results from the segmental translocation of the inverted dup of 1q to the short arm of 21. The der(22) results from the whole-arm 1q translocated to the short arm of 22. **F,** Homologous of chromosome 1 demonstrating amplification of 1q12-q23 by breakage-fusion-bridge (BFB) cycles. Note multiple copies of 1q21 *(arrows)* on the abnormal homologue on the right. The copies of the 1q12-q23 amplicon occur in an inverted repeated pattern, with a deletion of the 1q distal to the amplified region. Dotted lines between normal homologue 1 *(left)* and abnormal homologue denote the size of expansion of the 1q12-q23 region by BFB cycles. *(Reprinted from Sawyer JR: The prognostic significance of cytogenetics and molecular profiling in multiple myeloma.* Cancer Genetics *204:3, 2011; with permission.)*

and is detected by FISH and other molecular cytogenetic methods. Two genes on chromosome 4p16.3 and the IGH switch region on 14q32.3 are involved. The fibroblast growth factor receptor 3 gene (FGFR3) is detected on der(14), where it is overexpressed along with a fusion of the multiple myeloma set domain (MMSET) gene, located on 4p16.3. This is the first example of a translocation that simultaneously deregulates two genes with oncogenic potential: the FGFR3 gene detected on der(14) and the MMSET gene detected on der(4). FGFR3 is 50 to 100 kb telomeric to MMSET. Loss of FGFR3 on der(14) is detected in approximately 20% of cases. A significant number of these patients display del(13q) in the same clone and are hypodiploid.

Translocation (14;16)(q32.3;q23) had never been cytogenetically detected because of the telomeric positions of both loci. However, with FISH studies the incidence of t(14;16) has been estimated to be approximately 2% to 8% of cases. In this translocation, the MAF protooncogene is translocated from its normal position on 16q23 to chromosome 14, band q32.3, and it is overexpressed. Rare variants t(14;20) and t(8;20) are included in this group because they share a similar gene expression signature and clinical outcome. The clinical outcome of patients with t(14;16) is significantly shorter compared with a t(14;16)-negative cohort.

A large number of secondary chromosomal aberrations are found during tumor progression, but four main aberrations include

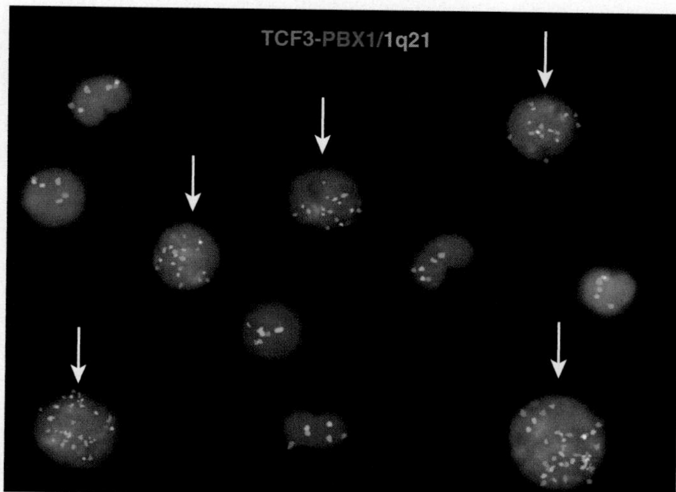

Figure 54-40 Bone marrow nuclei from a patient with multiple myeloma after hybridization using three probes 1q21 *(aqua),* PBX1 *(red)* localized on 1q25 and TCF3 *(green)* localized on 19q13. Note amplification (up to 17 copies) of 1q21 an2 1q25 *(white arrows),* as well as multiple copies of 19q loci. Amplification of 1q21-q25 is associated with disease progression and very poor prognosis in multiple myeloma despite novel therapies.

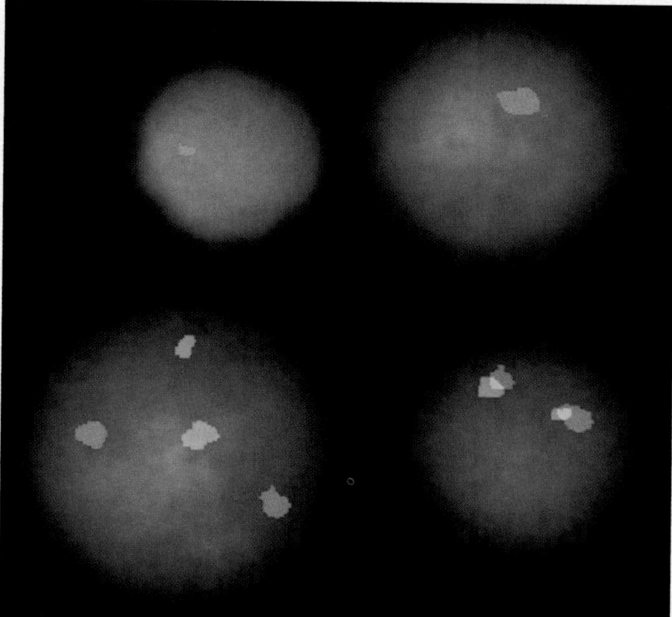

Figure 54-41 COMPOSITE IMAGE OF MARROW NUCLEI FROM A PATIENT WITH MULTIPLE MYELOMA AFTER HYBRIDIZATION WITH FIVE PROBES. The following probes are the most frequently used for detection of genomic structural rearrangements in clinical testing of multiple myeloma. *Top left cell* has 17p13.1 deletion (one red signal). *Top right nucleus* also shows a single red signal after hybridization with D13S319 probe, consistent with deletion of 13q14.3 locus. The patient had co-deletion of both loci, which is associated with unfavorable prognosis. *Bottom left cell* shows two green and two red signals after FISH study with CCND1 and IGH, indicating disomy for both probes and lack of CCND1-IGH fusion. Also shown are confirmatory results *(bottom right)* obtained after application of breakapart IGH probe, showing lack of separation of green and red signals, consistent with intact IGH gene.

translocations of MYC, the loss or deletion of chromosome 13, deletions of short arms and amplification of long arms of chromosome 1, and deletion of short arms of chromosome 17 predominates.

Translocations and/or amplification of MYC (8q24) may involve up to 45% of patients with an advanced MM, and they are frequently very complex and involve nonreciprocal rearrangements, duplications, and amplifications.

Deletion of either band q14 or q14.3 (RB1, DNA marker D13S319) on chromosome 13 is detected in 10% to 20% of patients by conventional cytogenetics and in 50% by FISH (see Fig. 54-40, *top right*). Microarray CGH data of the critical region on chromosome 13 are consistent with previous findings. Loss of the entire chromosome 13 (82%) is more frequent than is deletion of the long arms of chromosome 13. The most commonly deleted region has not been delineated. The median percentage of plasma cells carrying del(13q), identified by FISH, ranges from 75% and 90%. Deletion of 13q is associated with specific clinicopathologic features, including a higher frequency of λ-type MM, high plasma cell-labeling index, female predominance, and inferior survival after standard chemotherapy.

Numerous earlier studies have demonstrated that del(13q) represents an adverse prognostic marker in patients with MM treated with conventional low- and high-dose chemotherapy. However, more recent studies have demonstrated that del(13q) no longer has adverse prognostic significance in patients treated with bortezumib. However, molecular cytogenetics analyses revealed that del(13q) is present in 90% of patients showing t(4;14) or t(14;16); therefore the apparent adverse impact of del(13q) may not be the only genomic defect influencing unfavorable prognosis in these patients.

Deletion of TP53 at 17p13.1, which occurs in 10% of MM patients, is a powerful independent predictor of shortened survival and is associated with clonal evolution, drug resistance, and genetic instability (see Fig. 54-41, *top left*). This deletion is not found in patients with other high-risk abnormalities such as t(4;14) or t(14;16), and it appears mutually exclusive. Patients characterized by P53 deletion have significantly shorter overall survival regardless of therapy. The 17p deletion, identified by FISH as deletion of P53, is considered the most important molecular cytogenetic factor for prognosis.

The gain of 1q21 locus is identified in 45% of cases of monoclonal gammopathy of unknown significance, 43% of newly diagnosed MM, and 72% of relapsed MM, and it represents one of the most frequent recurrent chromosomal abnormalities in MM (see Figs. 54-40 and 54-41). Gain of 1q can be detected cytogenetically as isochromosome, duplications, or jumping translocations or detected with a 1q21-specific FISH probe. Among 479 patients with newly diagnosed MM, 43% with amplq21 also have either a hypodiploid and hyperdiploid karyotype, del(13q) by FISH, immunoglobulin A predominance, and poor prognosis compared with patients lacking amp1q21. A recent study of 92 patients treated with lenalidomide and dexamethasone demonstrated that del(17p) and gain of 1q21 are associated with a dismal overall survival, whereas the presence of t(11;14) or del(13q) as exclusive abnormalities had no impact on outcome. In the most comprehensive expression profiling survey of MM, reported by the Arkansas Multiple Myeloma Group using the previously mentioned GEP70, 30% of these genes were located on chromosome 1, with most of the downregulated genes located on the short arms of chromosome 1 and most of the upregulated genes on 1q. The clinical implication and significance of this finding is difficult to determine because of the lack of highly focal lesions and the lack of consensus of any critical genes on 1q21-q23. The mechanism for the amplification of 1q is believed to involve 1q12 pericentromeric instability, which most commonly increases the copy number of 1q by a direct and/or inverted duplication. Further instability can result in adding a whole-arm segment of 1q to nonhomologous chromosomes by jumping translocations of 1q. Two recurrent whole-arm unbalanced pericentromeric translocations are der(1;16)(q10;p10) and the der(1;19)(q10;p10). The 1q12-q23 amplicon has been reported to be formed by breakage-fusion-bridge (BFB) cycles of the 1q12 pericentromeric heterochromatin and the adjacent bands of 1q, resulting in an inverted repeat pattern of amplification of the

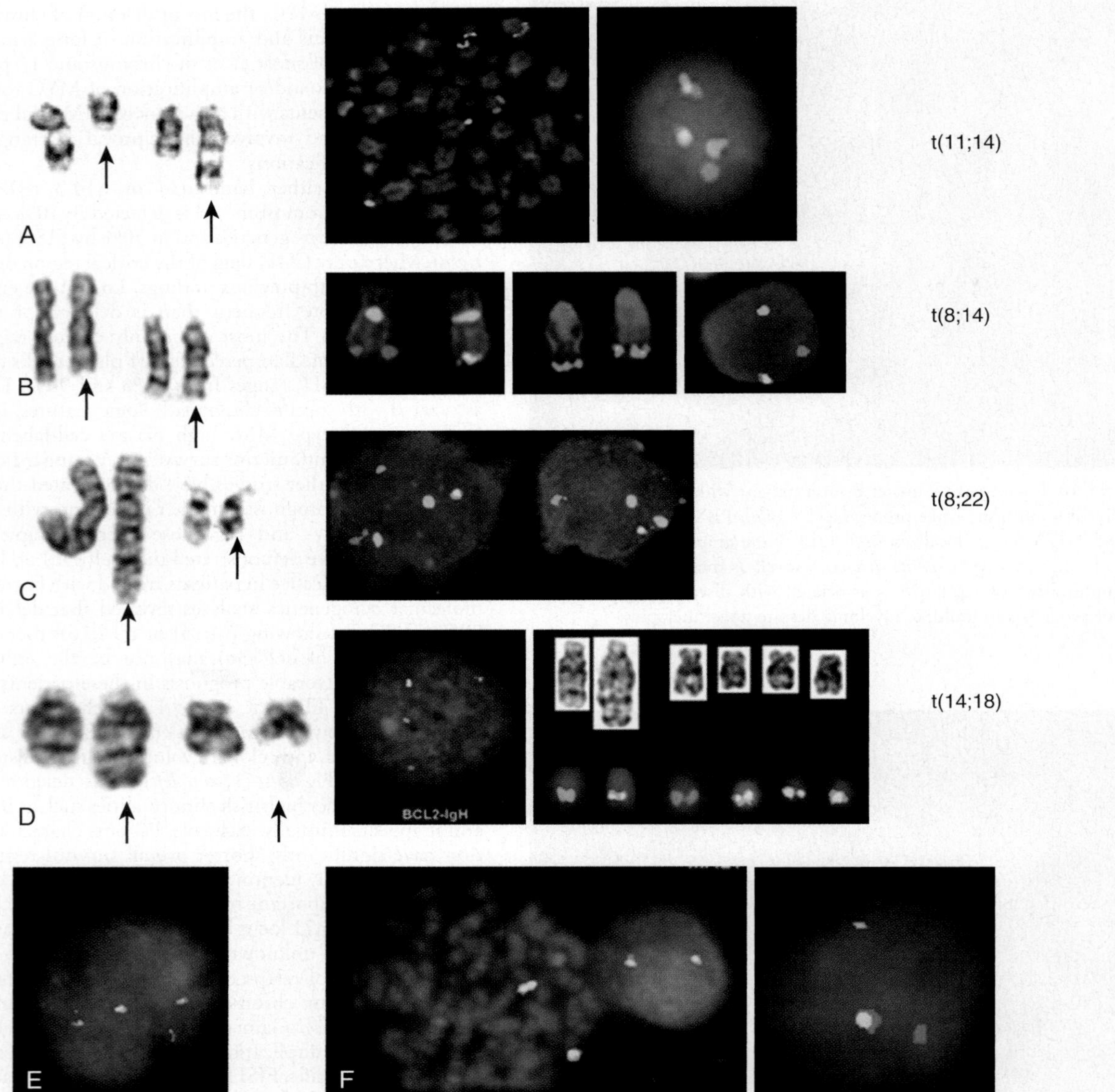

Figure 54-42 MOST FREQUENT CHROMOSOMAL ABNORMALITIES IN NON-HODGKIN LYMPHOMA. **A,** Partial G-banded karyotype of t(11;14)(q13;q32.3) *(left),* resulting in CCND1-IGH fusion *(yellow)* on metaphase *(middle)* and in interphase cell *(right)* present in the majority of patients with mantle cell lymphoma. **B,** Partial G-banded karyotype of t(8;14)(q24;q32.3) *(left),* resulting in MYC-IGH fusion [*yellow* on der(8) on isolated chromosomes]. Application of *MYC* breakapart probe shows separation of red and green signals consistent with MYC rearrangement. Approximately 80% of Burkitt lymphomas are characterized by t(8;14); **C,** Partial G-banded karyotype of t(8;22)(q24;q11), a variant of Burkitt lymphoma *(left).* Two interphase lymph node cells after hybridization with MYC breakapart probe and CEP8 *(aqua).* Separation of green and red signals is consistent with MYC relocation from 8q24 to 22q11: **D,** Partial G-banded karyotype of t(14;18)(q32.3;q21.3) *(left),* resulting in IGH-BCL fusion (two yellow signals, *middle*). A composite image on the right shows both a partial karyotype and FISH study of triplicated der(18) t(14;18) and three copies of *IGH-BCL2* fusion *(yellow),* as well as normal chromosome 14 and 18. Multiple copies of abnormal der(18) chromosome are associated with progressive disease similar to a duplication of the Philadelphia chromosome in the blast crisis of chronic myelogenous leukemia. **E,** Lymph node cell from a patient with diffuse large B-cell lymphoma (DLBCL), showing four copies of *BCL6* (breakapart probe). BCL6 is localized at 3q27 and is numerically or structurally rearranged in 35% of DLBCL. **F,** Bone marrow metaphase and interphase cell hybridized with breakapart MALT1 gene at 18q21 *(left)* indicating two fusion *(yellow)* signals when MALT1 gene is intact. In contrast, rearrangement of the MALT1 gene in MALT lymphoma usually is the consequence of t(11;18)(q21;q21.1)m as shown in the cell *(right)* with clear separation of the 3′ end *(green)* and the 5′ end *(red).*

1q12-q23 region. Copies of the 1q12-q23 amplicon can become integrated in complex multichromosome translocations during tumor progression.

The molecular basis of MM is slowly emerging, but the precise role of oncogenes is not yet defined. In order to address this issue and to understand the molecular basis of aneuploidy, work has evaluated the role of centrosome amplification in plasma cell neoplasms. Preliminary evidence indicates that centrosome amplification is common in all stages of plasma cell neoplasms, including monoclonal gammopathy of unknown significance, and probably is integral to disease

Genetic Testing for Multiple Myeloma

Chromosome studies of isolated plasma cells from the marrow are very useful at diagnosis. Perform interphase FISH and molecular genetic studies for detection of CCND1-IGH [t(11;14)], del(13)(q14.3)/D13S319, del(17)(p13.1)/P53, IGH/14q32.3, and 1q21 locus. If IGH rearrangements are detected using a breakapart IGH locus and CCND-IGH fusion is not identified, refine the partner and use the following set of probes: MAF-IGH for detection of t(14;16) and FGFR3-IGH for detection of t(4;14).

pathogenesis and genomic instability of MM. Dickkopf-1 (DKK1) may be associated with the presence of lytic bone lesions in patients with MM.

Molecular abnormalities such as CCND1-IGH, IGH-MAF, and FGHR3-IGH are found in approximately 40% of patients presenting with MM. In the remaining 60% of cases, chromosomal translocations cannot be identified, but hyperdiploidy is present. These presenting features are followed by further karyotypic instability and often include deletions/monosomy of chromosome 13 or chromosome 17, band region p13.1 (P53) (see Fig. 54-41). Amplification of 1q21 represents a late event in this multistep process and is associated with a malignant phenotype. From a practical point of view (see box on Genetic Testing in Multiple Myeloma and Fig. 54-40), the report of the International Myeloma Workshop Consensus Panel 3 provided recommendations for standard investigative workup at diagnosis of MM. These recommendations included the standard metaphase cytogenetics, despite the low mitotic yield (<20%), in order to separate hyperdiploid from nonhyperdiploid patients and to capture uncommon structural chromosomal rearrangements. Patients should undergo FISH testing, preferably after sorting of plasma cells, with probes that include 1q21, 17p13, t(4;14), and t(14;16).

LYMPHOMA

Non-Hodgkin lymphoma (NHL) is a heterogeneous group of disorders characterized by localized proliferation of lymphocytes (see Chapters 78 through 84). Analogous to other hematopoietic disorders, the pathogenesis of these malignancies is attributable to a multistep process involving progressive and clonal accumulation of genetic lesions. The majority of NHLs are of B-cell origin and involve translocations of immunoglobulin loci (see Table 54-10 and Fig. 54-42). IGH translocations usually are detected by cytogenetics, often in conjunction with FISH probes that span the IGH loci and/or PCR-based technologies. These molecular abnormalities exhibit enormous complexity with multiple and complex translocations, deletions, and amplifications within one clone. The WHO recognizes that genetic anomalies represent one of the most reliable criteria for classification of malignant lymphomas. The most common associations between chromosome anomalies and specific lymphomas include t(14;18)(q32;q21) and follicular lymphoma; t(8;14)(q24;q32) and Burkitt lymphoma; t(11;14)(q13;q32) and mantle cell lymphoma; and t(11;18)(q21;q21) and mucosa-associated lymphoid tissue (MALT) lymphoma (see box on Genetic Testing for Non-Hodgkin Lymphoma and Fig. 54-42). However, identification of a specific translocation is not diagnostic of a specific lymphoma subtype. Chromosome studies are difficult and expensive for the study of lymphomas. Thus many investigators use FISH and/or molecular genetic methods to study touch preparations or paraffin-embedded lymphoid tissue to detect important genetic anomalies in lymphomas.

Approximately 85% to 90% of patients with follicular lymphoma and some patients with large cell lymphoma exhibit t(14;18)(q32.3;q21.3), which results in fusion of BCL2 on 18q21 and IGH on 14q32 and represents one of the most common abnormalities in NHL (Fig. 54-43, *D*). Although the exact underlying mechanism is not known, t(14;18) results from a mistake of VDJ recombination

Genetic Testing for Non-Hodgkin Lymphoma

FISH testing can be performed on touch preparations, paraffin-embedded tissue, or bone marrow cells if bone marrow is involved. Peripheral blood cells are not appropriate for genetic testing of non-Hodgkin lymphoma. Bone marrow cytogenetics at diagnosis is not useful but may be important for staging in some cases. Fig. 54-42 lists the most useful FISH probes for detection of genomic defects in non-Hodgkin lymphoma. They include CCND1-IGH, IGH-BCL2, MYC-IGH, BCL6, MYC breakapart for detection of Burkitt variant not associated with t(8;14), and MALT1 breakapart for detection of t(11;18). For patients with suspected anaplastic large cell lymphoma, ALK breakapart probe should be informative.

and juxtaposes the BCL2 oncogene with the nonexpressed IGH allele. As a consequence, the BCL2 gene comes under the control of IGH enhancer, causing dysregulated expression of BCL2 protein, one of the proteins involved in regulation of apoptosis. The breakpoints within BCL2 occur mostly within the 3′ region of the gene, whereas the breakpoints in IGH fall within the D_H and J_H regions. Although 75% of breakpoints are clustered within a remarkably narrow region of 15 to 20 bp at the 3′ end of the BCL2 gene, they are frequently missed by standard PCR. With regular and fiber FISH methods using BCL2 breakpoint flanking probes, individual 5′ and 3′ breakpoints can be detected. BCL2 rearrangements are detected with immunohistochemical staining for BCL2 protein. With disease progression, 100% of patients have BCL2 overexpression. Variant translocations, such as t(2;18)(p12;q21) and t(18;22)(q21;q11) involving the IGK or IGL gene, respectively, rather than IGH, also show overexpression of BCL2.[28]

Numerous secondary chromosomal abnormalities are identified by conventional cytogenetics, and at least five recurrent anomalies, each occurring in at least 20% of follicular lymphomas, may distinguish two subgroups of follicular lymphoma patients. Patients with t(14;18) showing additional trisomy for chromosome 2, 7, or 8 are associated with a more favorable course of disease compared with patients with additional del(1p), del(1q), del(6q), der(18), del(22q), or gain of chromosome 12 and X, which are associated with inferior outcome. Unfavorable outcome of patients with loss of X chromosome is confirmed by CGH, and del(6)(q25-q27) is identified as the strongest predictor of poor prognosis and shorter survival time. Rearrangements of chromosome 1, such as del(1)(p32-36), +1(p11-q44), and unbalanced translocations of der(1)(1;1)(p36;q11-23) regions are among the most frequent secondary chromosomal abnormalities in follicular lymphoma. Progression of follicular lymphoma to diffuse large B-cell lymphoma (DLBCL) occurs in 60% to 80% and is accompanied by accumulation of secondary abnormalities, of which homozygous del(9p) might be associated with histologic progression.

The combination of BCL-2 and MYC rearrangements resulting from t(8;14)(q24;q32) and t(14;18)(q32;q21) or variants in the same karyotype is characteristic of high-grade B-cell lymphoma/leukemia, which occurs in fewer than 2% of patients and is associated with aggressive histology and poor prognosis. In these cases, a translocation within a single IGH allele separates the 3′ from the 5′ IGH enhancer element, with relocation of the BCL2 5′ IGH enhancer fusion to the der(8) and translocation of MYC adjacent to the 3′ IGH enhancer element that is retained on the der(14). The ISCN cytogenetic description der(8)t(8;14)(q24;q32)t(14;18)(q32;q21), der(14)t(8;14)(q24;q32), der(18)t(14;18)(q32;q21) does not reflect the complexity of the underlying molecular rearrangements (see Fig. 54-43). Because one of the translocation may be cryptic, a combination of three FISH probes, labeled in three colors, is especially useful in identifying these complex translocations.

The IGH-BCL formation is believed to represent a very early event in the pathogenesis of follicular lymphoma. This notion is

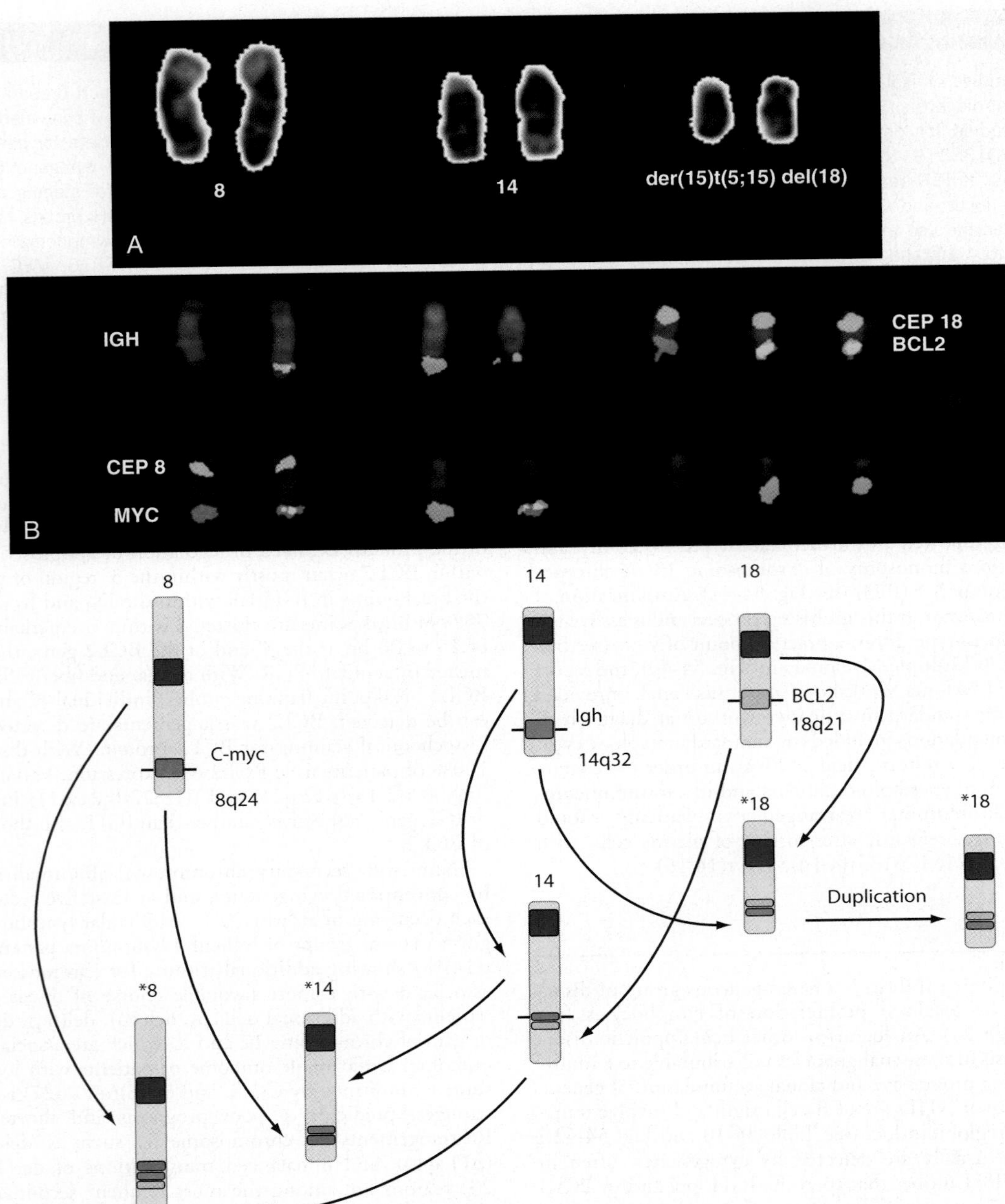

Figure 54-43 IDENTIFICATION OF SIMULTANEOUS BCL2 AND MYC REARRANGEMENTS IN HIGH-GRADE B-CELL LYMPHOMA LEUKEMIA (SEE TEXT FOR DETAILS). Partial G-banded karyotype **(A)** of chromosomes 8 and 14 and what is initially identified as der(15)t(5;15) and der(18). Partial karyotype of the same chromosomes after FISH study **(B)** with probes for IGH *(green)*, CEP8 *(aqua)*, and MYC *(red)* indicating IGH-MYC fusions *(yellow)* on both chromosomes 8 and 14. Sequential hybridization with CEP18 *(aqua)*, BCL2 *(red)*, and IGH *(green)* also revealed IGH-BCL2 fusion *(yellow)* on both der(15) and der(18), indicating that der(15) actually is a duplication of rearranged chromosome 18. **C,** Schematic representation of genomic events leading to duplication 18. Rearrangements of both *MYC* and *BCL2* show a complex molecular array.

supported by the observation that t(14;18) is also found in peripheral blood in more than 50% of healthy individuals and may persist for at least 3 years without overt disease. Because the incidence of follicular lymphoma in the United States is approximately 1 case per 24,000 persons per year, the occurrence of follicular lymphoma is relatively rare. GEP shows a distinct pattern associated with an indolent form of disease (median survival 11.1 years) and a more aggressive form (median survival 3.9 years), indicating that these different conditions may represent distinct stages in the evolution of follicular lymphoma. These and other observations point to an immune response that may regulate the pace of the malignant process and may restrain the proliferation of t(14;18)-positive B cells in healthy individuals. The molecular pathogenesis of follicular lymphoma may include formation of t(14;18) in a naive B cell. If stimulated by an exogenous agent such as a virus or autoantigen, a germinal center reaction may occur. Upon further stimulation by an antigen on the surface of a follicular dendritic cell, together with the T cell, a memory cell may form. This type of cell represents the majority of t(14;18)-positive cells identified in the peripheral blood of normal individuals. Further oncogenic events and accumulation of different, recurrent chromosomal abnormalities in a stepwise pathogenesis may transform this cell into clinically recognizable follicular lymphoma.

Three translocations, all affecting the MYC gene at 8q24, have been recognized in Burkitt lymphoma. In 80% of patients a reciprocal translocation t(8;14)(q24; q32) is observed between the MYC gene and the IGH locus (Fig. 54-44). In the remainder of patients, the reciprocal translocation t(8;22)(q24;q11) or t(2;8)(p12;q24) is observed juxtaposing MYC to one of the light-chain loci (κ on 2p12 and λ on 22q11). The t(8;14) translocation originally was described in Epstein-Barr virus (EBV) tumor cells obtained from

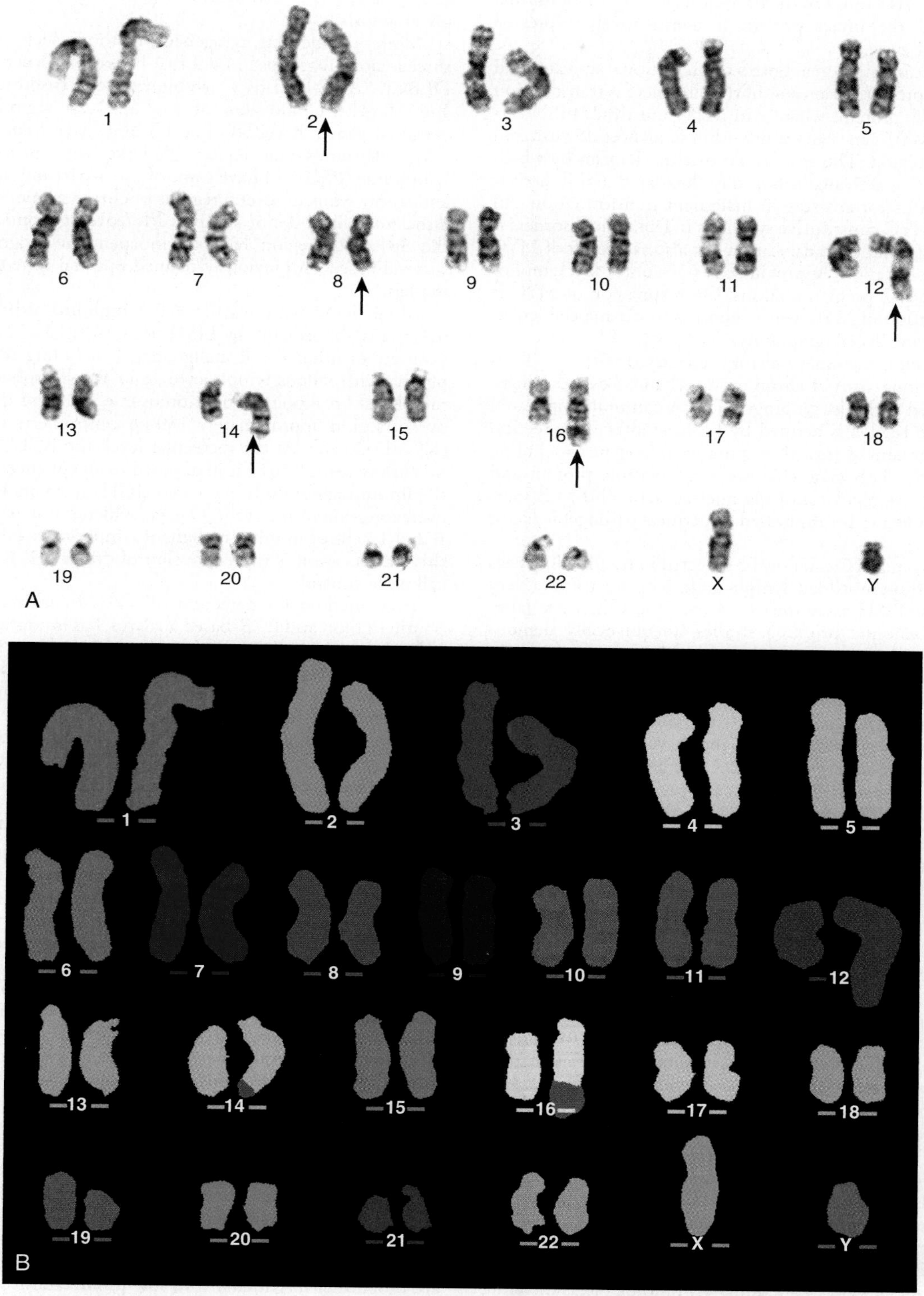

Figure 54-44 Bone marrow karyotype of a patient diagnosed in an advanced stage of Burkitt lymphoma **(A)** and after application of the multicolor FISH **(B)** to resolve complex derivative chromosomes, showing 46,XY, del(2)(p21p23), t(8;14)(q24;q32), dup(12)(q13q24.3), der(16)(t(11;16)(p11.2;q24) karyotype. *Arrows* indicate abnormal chromosomes. In addition to the classic t(8;14), both duplications of 11q and 12q were identified with multicolor FISH technology.

patients in Africa (see Fig. 54-44, *B* and *C*). Variant translocations involving MYC with a variety of other non-IG loci subsequently have been reported. In most patients with sporadic Burkitt lymphoma, the breakpoints on 8q24.1 are located on 5′ of the coding region of the MYC gene. In contrast, in most cases of endemic Burkitt lymphoma and in variant translocations, the MYC breakpoints are a considerable distance centromeric or telomeric from the MYC coding exons. As a result of the translocation, control of normal MYC is lost, and the intact protein is constitutively expressed throughout the cell cycle.

The MYC gene can function as both a transcriptional activator and a transcriptional repressor. As a result of t(8;14), there is transcription of a truncated MYC protein, whereas in t(2;8) and t(8;22) the rearrangement of the MYC gene can occur within sequences downstream of the transcribed region. The exact molecular mechanism by which the rearranged MYC is activated is not fully elucidated, but its activation constitutes an important step in malignant transformation. An increased level of MYC constitutive synthesis in leukemic disorders is found not only as a result of translocation but also as a result of MYC mutations and amplification. Approximately 65% of Burkitt lymphomas demonstrate MYC point mutations. Overexpression of MYC is linked to amplification of MYC genes reported in plasma cell leukemia, AML, CML, and T-cell lymphoma.

The most common secondary change associated with t(8;14) is duplication of the long arms of chromosome 1, and these rearrangements are associated with disease progression. A common duplicated region of 93 kb at 1q21.2 is defined by FISH studies. This section of chromosome contains at least three putative oncogenes, including the OTUD7B gene. This gene encodes a cytoplasmic protein and functions as a negative regulator of the nuclear factor (NF)-κB transcription factor, known to be implicated as a critical pathogenic factor in lymphoma.

Rearrangements of MYC can now be detected in nondividing cells as well as in paraffin-embedded lymph node biopsies using a very sensitive interphase FISH assay for t(8;14), with less than 2% false-positive results. Genomic profiling studies unequivocally demonstrated that the majority of patients with MYC rearrangements should be classified as Burkitt lymphoma, even though pathologists called some of the cases *diffuse large cell lymphoma*. However, these studies also indicate that rare cases with the Burkitt signature gene expression lack MYC rearrangements and have BCL2 rearrangements, suggesting that in rare cases MYC rearrangement alone may not be sufficient for diagnosis of Burkitt lymphoma.

According to the WHO classification, a Burkitt-like lymphoma is a separate entity characterized by one of the Burkitt lymphoma translocations. However, many such cases fail to show Burkitt lymphoma translocations but do exhibit increased MYC expression.

Approximately 35% of patients with diffuse DLBC and approximately 5% to 10% of patients with follicular lymphoma have rearrangements in the BCL6 gene normally residing at 3q27. Translocation of 3q27 is the third most frequent translocation in NHL, and at least 33 different partners have been described as participating in these rearrangements (see Fig. 54-42, *E*). The most frequent chromosomal band partners are 2p13, 4p13, 6p22, 7p12, 8q24, 13q14, 14q32, 18p11.2, and 22q11. These translocations juxtapose different promoters derived from other chromosomes, with the BCL6 coding domain causing persistent expression of BCL6.

Most of the breakpoints in 3q27 occur within a 10-kb region. The fact that the 3q27 region is affected in different lymphomas, irrespective of the translocation partner chromosomes, strongly suggests that alterations of BCL6, and not the reciprocal loci, are important in the pathogenesis. The alterations in 3q27 are too small for microscopic detection, so most of these rearrangements are detected by Southern blot analysis, PCR-based assay, or FISH. BCL6 functions as a transcriptional repressor of genes containing its binding sites; therefore the mechanism responsible for the malignant phenotype is transcriptional deregulation. The prognostic significance of BCL6 rearrangements is not clear, and different outcomes have been reported.

Approximately 3% to 4% of DLBCLs have t(14;15)(q32;q11-13), which results in fusion of the BCL8 gene on chromosome 15 to the V_H segment of the IGH locus. The most common secondary abnormalities are trisomies of chromosomes 3, 5, 7q, 11, 12p, 18q, and Xq, which are observed in greater than 10% of cases. Amplification of REL (2p12-16), MYC (8q24), BCL2 (18q21), GLI, CDK4, and MDM2 (12q13-14) genes, identified by a combination of molecular cytogenetic methods, are most frequently associated with advanced-stage disease. The most frequent monosomies include chromosomes 13, 14, and 15. A complex karyotype may have an adverse impact on prognosis.

Modern molecular cytogenetic methods such as CGH identify three major subgroups in DCLBC. Patients with activated B cell–like DLBCL (ABC-DCLBC) exhibit frequent trisomy 3, gains of 3q and 18q21-23, and loss of the 6q21-23 region. Patients with germinal center B (GCB)–like DLBCL have frequent gains of the 12q12 chromosomal region. Patients with primary mediastinal lymphoma (PMBCL) have gains of 2p14-p16 and 9p21-pter. Apparently, only gains in several regions of chromosome 3 are significantly associated with inferior survival. Moreover, genomic gains involving the 3p11-p12 region have an independent prognostic power for survival based on previously defined optimal gene expression–based models.

All patients with mantle cell lymphoma exhibit the t(11;14)(q13;q32) abnormality by FISH. t(11;14)(q13;q32) is also found in a variety of other B-cell malignancies, including MM, splenic lymphoma with villous lymphocytes, and B-cell prolymphocytic leukemia. Most breakpoints on chromosome 11, band q13, are dispersed over a region approximately 130 kb centromeric to the cyclin D1 (CCND1) gene. At the molecular level, the BCL1 locus (CCND1) on chromosome 11q13 is juxtaposed to an enhancer sequence within the immunoglobulin heavy-chain (IGH) gene on 14q32, leading to overexpression of the cyclin D gene, which is not expressed in normal B and T cells or in other malignant lymphomas. The consequence of this translocation is overexpression of cyclin D1, a gene involved in cell cycle control.

Each method for detection of t(11;14), including cytogenetics, Southern blot, and PCR-based analyses, has limitations. Cytogenetics is hampered by a low mitotic index of neoplastic B cells. Southern blot and PCR-based analyses for 11q13 rearrangements are positive in only 50% to 60% of patients with mantle cell lymphoma because the breakpoints within 11q13 are scattered along a 130-kb distance. In practical terms, dual-color FISH has proved to be the most sensitive assay for detection of IGH-CCND1 fusion, which is found in 100% of cases. Furthermore, the CCND1 fusion rearrangement can be detected in formalin-fixed, paraffin-embedded samples, making this method rapid, reliable, independent of cell cycle, and applicable to all cases of mantle cell lymphoma (see Fig. 54-42, *A*).

Gene expression studies have identified a subset of patients with D1-negative mantle cell lymphoma, so called because of the lack of cyclin D1 expression and t(11;14). However, both cyclin D1–positive and cyclin D1–negative patients have the same secondary genomic alterations when assessed with conventional cytogenetics, CGH, and array-based CGH. These secondary chromosomal alterations include gains of 3q, 8q, and 15q and losses of 1p, 8p23-pter, 9p21-pter, 11q21-23, and 13q. Some of the genes residing in these chromosomal regions are dysregulated and involved in cell proliferation, DNA repair mechanism of chromosome stability, and cellular homeostasis and apoptosis mechanisms. Unlike other lymphomas, in mantle cell lymphoma, DNA amplifications of several chromosomal regions appear to be associated with a blastoid variant. Loss of 9p21-pter, inactivation of TP53, gain of 3q, and high cyclin D expression are reported molecular and cytogenetic markers of shorter survival and a more aggressive clinical evolution. The prognostic value of 3q27-qer gains and loss of 9q21-32 region is determined to be independent of the gene expression-based signature. Extra copies of 3q are prognostic in patients with low proliferation, whereas loss of 9q has improved clinical value in a subgroup of patients with high proliferation.

Marginal zone lymphoma and MALT lymphoma are considered the third most frequent NHL subtype. According to the WHO classification, they are subdivided into splenic marginal zone lymphoma, nodal marginal zone lymphoma, and MALT lymphoma. An etiologic link between low-grade gastric MALT lymphoma and the lymphoid reaction associated with *Helicobacter pylori* infection is well established. Growing evidence suggests that chronic antigenic stimulation in autoimmune diseases, such as Hashimoto thyroiditis, contributes to an increased risk for developing MALT lymphoma.

The most frequent and specific aberration occurring in MALT lymphomas is t(11;18)(q21;q21.1). Although it has been described in other B-cell lymphomas, t(11;18) in MALT lymphoma is usually the only genetic lesion and does not show additional chromosomal anomalies. It is the only recurrent translocation that does not involve IG genes, even though it presents as a B-cell lymphoma. As a consequence of t(11;18), API2 gene on chromosome 11, band q21, which encodes an inhibitor of apoptosis (also known as IAP2, HIAP1, and MIHC), and a novel gene MALT1 on chromosome 18, band q21, characterized by several Ig-like C2-type domains, are often rearranged. The resultant chimeric transcript consists of 5′-API2 and 3′-MAT located on der(18). More than 90% of breakpoints in the API2 locus occur in intron 7, whereas the breakpoints within MALT1 are variable and occur in four different introns. The API2-MALT1 fusion is easily identified using a dual-color API2-MALT1 FISH probe or the breakapart strategy of dual-color MALT1 probe on lymph node biopsies (see Fig. 54-42, *F*). However, detection of deletions and duplications occurring at high frequencies in both the API2 and MALT1 genomic sequences requires more precise molecular cytogenetic methods.

t(1;14)(p22;q32) and its variant t(1;2)(p22;p12) occur in less than 5% of MALT lymphomas, typically display other chromosomal abnormalities, and are associated with an advanced stage of disease at diagnosis (see reference list for more information). This translocation relocates the entire BCL10 gene from 1p22 to chromosome 14, bringing it under the control of an IGH enhancer. Currently, a specific probe for detecting BCL10-IGH fusion is not available, but IGH dual-color breakapart FISH strategy may determine IGH rearrangements without identifying the partner chromosome. The t(3;14)(p13;q32) abnormality, which results in fusion of the FOXP1F gene on chromosome 3 to IGH, is a rare rearrangement that causes FOXP1F overexpression. Its significance in lymphoma remains unknown. t(14;18)(q32;q21), which occurs in 2% to 18% of all MALT lymphomas, results in fusion of IGH-MALT. The 18q21 breakpoint involving the MALT1 gene is 5 Mb centromeric from the BCL2 breakpoint on chromosome 18 associated with follicular lymphoma. In contrast to API2-MALT1 cases, patients with IGH-MALT1 fusion have disease outside the gastrointestinal tract, usually presenting with ocular, skin, liver, or salivary gland tumors. FISH studies are useful for detecting the IGH-MALT fusion in paraffin-embedded lymph node biopsies. Although a unifying concept linking MALT-associated translocations to the pathogenesis of MALT lymphoma is not available, compelling evidence links these translocations to constitutive activation of the NF-κB pathway.

Lymphoplasmacytoid lymphoma (LPL) is a small lymphocytic lymphoma with plasmacytoid differentiation ($CD5^-CD10^-$) characterized by t(9;14)(p13;q32) in approximately 50% of cases. As a result of this translocation, the paired homeobox 5 (PAX5) gene on 9p13 moves to the IGH locus on der(14), causing dysregulation of PAX5. Molecular characterization of t(9;14) revealed that the coding region of the PAX5 gene remains intact in some patients. In those individuals, t(9;14) should be considered a regulatory mutation in which the PAX5 gene is brought under the control of the IGH locus. In other cases, molecular studies of t(9;14) reveal that the breakpoint occurs upstream of the PAX5 promoter, leading to insertion of the IGH enhancer upstream of the PAX5 gene.

Waldenström macroglobulinemia (see Chapter 86) is a plasma cell dyscrasia characterized by a CD138, CD19 phenotype, with a lympho/plasmacytic clonal expansion in the marrow. The biologic nature is different from lymphoplasmacytoid lymphoma because patients do not display t(9;14)(p13;q32). Recurrent chromosomal abnormalities include deletion of the long arms of chromosome 6 in 55% of cases by cytogenetics and in 21% of cases by FISH. Trisomy 4 is present in approximately 20% of cases. In contrast to other B-cell disorders, abnormalities of IGH at 14q32 as measured by FISH and Southern blot are rarely identified in Waldenström macroglobulinemia.

Not much progress has been made in delineating recurrent chromosomal abnormalities in Hodgkin lymphoma (HL) (see Chapters 72 and 73). Less than 1% of the cells in HL are Reed-Sternberg cells, of B-cell origin, and the paucity of dividing tumor cells for karyotype analysis has represented a major obstacle for conventional cytogenetics. In one study, simultaneous fluorescence, immunophenotyping, and interphase FISH (FICTION) demonstrated numerical aberrations of CD30 cells in all HL patients. The most specific chromosomal abnormalities in HL are hyperdiploidy/tetraploidy with tremendous variations in chromosome number, indicating heterogeneity from patient to patient. Even with use of nine different centromeric probes, no specific numerical chromosomal abnormality has been identified. Deletions of 1p, 4q, 6q, and 7q are recurrent, and JAK2, located on 9p21, frequently is amplified in patients with HL. Another gene, c-REL, on chromosome 2, band region p14-p15, is amplified in 50% of patients. Of note, c-REL is under the influence of NF-κB transcription factor, and constitutive NF-κB activation is a critical prerequisite for HL/Reed-Sternberg cell survival and proliferation. Thus it appears that constitutive NF-κB activation is the unifying concept and the hallmark of HL.

T-Cell Lymphoproliferative Diseases

This is a diverse group of hematologic disorders. The group includes T-cell ALL and T-cell CLL/promyelocytic leukemia, as well as several indolent or small T-cell disorders, large granular lymphocyte leukemia, natural killer leukemia/lymphoma, and anaplastic large cell lymphoma (ALCL).

T-cell ALL represents 15% of childhood ALL cases and 25% of adult ALL cases. At diagnosis, approximately 50% of patients have a normal karyotype. Table 54-11 lists recurrent cytogenetic and molecular genomic changes associated with T-cell ALL. Immunophenotypic and gene expression analyses are consistent with genetic heterogeneity in T-cell ALL, reflecting, to some degree, distinct stages of T-cell maturation arrest.

One of the common themes in T-lymphoid malignancies is the juxtaposition of T-cell receptor (TCR) gene enhancer element adjacent to a variety of transcription factors located at or near breakpoints on the partner chromosome. The chromosomal bands most frequently involved are 14q11, where TCRA and TCRD are located; 7q35, the site of TCRB; and 7p15, the site of the TCRG. TCR translocations are found in approximately 35% of T-cell ALL cases (see Table 54-12). The rearrangements of TCRB and TCRG are relatively rare, whereas 14q11 rearrangements involving both TCRA and TCRD are frequent in T-lymphoid neoplasms[29] (Table 54-13).

In children, the overall frequency of T-cell ALL translocations is 40% to 50%, and several molecular/cytogenetic abnormalities have prognostic relevance (Table 54-14). TAL1 rearrangements include t(1;14)(p32;q11), t(1;7)(p32;q35), rare t(1;3)(p32;p21), and t(1;5)(p32;q31). Generally, TAL1 rearrangements are submicroscopic and

Table 54-13 Frequency of TCR Rearrangements Using Conventional Cytogenetics Versus FISH

Locus	Conventional Cytogenetics (%)	FISH (%)	
		Total Karyotype	Abnormal Karyotype
TCR-αδ	9.5	17.4	24.7
TCR-β	3.1	19	26.9
TCR-γ	0	0	0

FISH, Fluorescence in situ hybridization; *TCR*, T-cell receptor.

Table 54-14 Frequent Translocations and Mutations in T-Cell ALL

Translocations	Genes Involved	Children	Frequency (%)	Adults
TCR-ASSOCIATED TRANSLOCATIONS				
t(7;10)(q34;q24) and	TCRB-TLX1 (HOX11)	7		31
t(10;14)(q24;q11)	TCRA-TLX1			
t(5;14)(q35;q32) (cryptic)	TLX3 (HOX11L2)	20		13
inv(7)(p15q34), t(7;7)	HOXA cluster		5	
t(1;14)(p32;q11) and t(1;7)(p32;q34)	TCRA-TAL1		3	
t(7;9)(q34;q32)	TCRB-TAL2		<1	
t(7;19)(q34;p13)	TCRB-LYL1		<1	
t(9;14)(p21;q11)	TCRA_TAL1		<1	
t(14;21)(q11.2;q22)	TCRA-HLHB1		<1	
t(11;14)(p15;q11)	TCRA-LMO1		2	
t(11;14)(p13;q11) and	TCRA-LMO2		3	
t(7;11)(q35;p13)	TCRB-LMO1			
t(1;7)(p32;q34)	LCK		<1	
t(7;9)(q34;q34.3)	NOTCH1		<1	
t(7;12)(q34;p13) and t(12;14)(p13;q11)	CCND2		<1	
FORMATION OF FUSION GENES				
1p32 deletion (cryptic)	SIL-TALI	9-30		Decreases with age
t(10;11)(p13;q14) (often cryptic)	CALM-AF10		10	
t(11;19)(q23;p13)	MLL		8	
t(6;11)(q27;q23)	MLL-AF6			
t(10;11)(p13;q23)	MLL/AF10			
t(X;11)(p13;q23)	MLL-AFX1			
t(4;11)(q21;q23)	MLL-AF4			
t(9;9)(q34;q34) (episomal or hsr)	Nup214-ABL1		<6	
t(9;14)(q34;q32) (cryptic)	DML1-ABL1		<1	
t(9;12)(q34;p13)	ETV6(TEL)-ABL1		<1	
t(9;12)(p24;p13)	ETV6(TEL)-JAK2		<1	
t(9;22)(q34;q11)	BCR-ABL1		<1	
t(4;11)(q21;p15)	Nup98-RAP1GDS1		<1	
t(10;11)(q25;p15)	Nup98-ADD3		<1	
(CRYPTIC) DELETIONS				
9p21 (homozygous/hemizygous)	P16		65/15	
del (6q)	Unknown		20-30	
MUTATIONS				
NOTCH1	NOTCH1		56	
FLT3-ITD and m835	FLT3		5	
N-RAS	N-RAS	<10		?

Modified from Graux C, Cools J, Michaux L, et al: Cytogenetics and molecular genetics of T-cell acute lymphoblastic leukemia: From thymocytes to lymphoblast. *Leukemia* 20:1496, 2006.
ALL, Acute lymphoblastic leukemia; *TCR*, T-cell receptor.

best identified with FISH. They are observed in approximately 3% of patients with T-cell ALL and are more frequent in pediatric ALL than in adult ALL. In children, rearrangements involving the TAL1 gene occur at a frequency of 20% and tend to be associated with better outcome. TAL2, residing at 9q32, is detected in rare t(7;9)(q34;q32) as a result of juxtaposition of TAL2 to TCRB. LYL1, originally described as a fusion partner of TCRB in rare (7;19)(q34;p13), is associated with poor prognosis. Rearrangements of HOX11L2, which include cryptic t(5;14)(q35;q32), t(5;7)(q35;q21), and other variants, occur at a frequency of 24% in children and represent a predictor of poor outcome, regardless of treatment strategies. Similarly, the presence of t(10;11)(p13;q14), which results in the CALM-AF10 fusion gene and occurs at a frequency of 2% to 5% in children, may be associated with poor outcome. Abnormalities of

HOX11 are more common in adults (31%) than in children (7%) and are associated with t(10;14)(q34;q24) and t(7;10)(q34;q24). According to the French collaborative study, t(10;14) is the most frequent chromosomal translocation in patients with T-cell ALL. It is associated with excellent outcome in both children and adults. In t(10;14) the homeobox gene HOX11 (TCL3) is fused with TCRD. The coding regions of HOX11 are not disturbed by the translocation. In the variant translocation t(7;10)(q35;q24), HOX11 is juxtaposed to TCRB, which results in overexpression of normal HOX11 mRNA by bringing HOX11 under the influence of TCR promoter sequences.

MLL rearrangements are present in 8% of T-cell ALL cases. The most frequent MLL translocation partners in T-cell ALL include ENL, which results from t(11;19)(q23;p13.3) and is associated with better prognosis than are other fusion partners. Gene expression profiling data characterized T-cell ALL with MLL rearrangements as a distinct molecular subtype with specific molecular signature. Homeobox genes, regulators of embryonic development, are known targets of MLL and are overexpressed in patients with T-cell ALL and MLL rearrangements.

Deregulation of NOTCH, tyrosine kinase genes (ABL1, JAK2), and LIM domain genes (LMO1, LMO2) is also common in T-cell ALL. NOTCH1 has been discovered to be a fusion partner of TCRB in t(7;9)(q34;q34.3). These mutations are present in 56% of T-cell ALL cases. The NOTCH1 gene is important in lymphocyte lineage specification, and resequencing of functional domains of NOTCH1 revealed that activating NOTCH1 mutations are present in most primary pediatric and adolescent molecular subtypes of T-ALL. Three types of NOTCH1 mutations have been described: those in the heterodimer domain, those in the PEST domain, and rarely, as internal tandem duplications of the juxtamembrane portion (7 of 210 of pediatric T-ALL). Mutations in heterodimer domain and internal tandem duplication result in constitutive ligand-independent activation of NOTCH1.

The LIM family of genes is found at the breakpoint of rare but consistent chromosomal translocations in T-cell ALL. LMO1, located at 11p15, is involved in t(11;14)(p15;q11). LMO2, located at 11p13, is involved in t(11;14)(p13;q11) and t(7;11)(q35;p13). As an oncogenic transcription regulator, LMO2 overexpression in erythroid and T cells leads to differentiation arrest, which is a prerequisite for development of T-cell malignancies 30.

The C-MYB gene, which is localized on chromosome 6, band q23.3, in normal cells, is rearranged in rare T-cell ALL subtype observed in young patients (median 2.2 years). Two types of recurrent C-MYB genomic alterations are found in T-cell ALL: (a) a reciprocal t(6;7)(q23;q34) that results in juxtaposition of C-MYB near to TCRB regulatory sequences on chromosome 7 and (b) a short genomic tandem duplication, identified using genome-wide copy-number analysis. Both rearrangements are cytogenetically cryptic. The breakpoints in t(6;7) are subtelomeric and usually missed. The translocation was discovered using a locus-specific FISH probe for C-MYC. The tandem MYB duplication is cryptic using both conventional cytogenetics and locus-specific FISH. It is mapped using high-density oligonucleotide array CGH. Discovery of MYB highlights the strength of high-density array CGH in identifying cryptic copy-number abnormalities associated with leukemia.

Although only 1% of Ph-positive ALL consist of patients with T-cell ALL, the ABL1 gene, which is involved in BCR-ABL1 fusion-positive B-cell ALL and CML, is also involved in fusion with Nup21, creating the Nup214-ABL1 chimeric gene, which is identified in up to 6% of T-cell ALL cases. Additionally, this fusion gene is found amplified only in T-cell ALL. When identified with FISH using ABL1 probe, it appears as an amplified episome between the chromosomes in metaphase cells. RT-PCR also can be used for its detection. Nup214-ABL1 is a constitutively activated tyrosine kinase activating similar pathways as BCR-ABL1 and is sensitive to inhibition with tyrosine kinase inhibitors, especially nilotinib and disatinib. These patients usually have homozygous or heterozygous deletion of CDKN2A at 9p21 chromosomal site and trisomy 8, t(7;10)(q35;q24), or t(10;14)(q24;q11) abnormalities. The estimated 5-year overall survival rate of these patients in one study was 49%. In rare cases of T-cell ALL, JAK2 has been identified as a partner chromosome with ETV6 in t(9;12)(p24;q13) (Fig. 54-45), one of the three JAK2 fusion transcripts seen in hematologic malignancies (see Ph-Negative Myeloproliferative Neoplasms, earlier, and Table 54-13).

Numerical changes are rare except for tetraploidy, which occurs in less than 5% of cases and is of unknown prognostic significance. In contrast, cryptic cytogenetic abnormalities revealed by FISH are frequent in ALL. They include deletion of 9p21 (INK4/ARF) and 1p32 regions. Deletion of 6q is less common, and the region 6q16 appears to be the common deletion band region.

In contrast to childhood B-cell ALL, the majority of childhood T-cell ALL cases develop after birth. In utero origin of this leukemia is rare. Dramatic treatment advances have been achieved in children with T-cell ALL in the last four decades. Initial results with GEP to determine specific molecular prognostic markers for children with T-cell ALL who may benefit from more intense therapy identified that expression of three genes, CFLAR, NOTCH2, and BTG 3, at the time of diagnosis may accurately predict disease outcome. All three genes are involved in regulation of apoptosis and cellular proliferation. Expression of NOTCH2, but not of the other two gene abnormalities, is implicated in T-cell ALL. Genome-wide expression profiling at the time of diagnosis can likely identify novel molecular markers that may be used to predict the clinical outcome of patients.

T-cell CLL and prolymphocytic leukemia are characterized by T-cell leukemia 1 (TCL1) gene rearrangements. These include inv(14)(q11q32.1), t(14;14)(q11;q32.1), and t(7;14)(q35;q32.1). In patients showing these karyotypic changes, TCL1 is found to be dysregulated.

Adult T-cell leukemia/lymphoma is associated with human T-cell lymphotropic virus type 1. The most frequent genetic lesions include altered expression of CDKN2 (cyclin-dependent kinase inhibitor) gene on 9p21 (15% to 20%) and loss of heterozygosity at 6q15 to q21. The most frequent chromosomal abnormalities are gain of 3p, 7q, and 14q and loss of 6q and 13q. Translocations involving 14q32 or 14q11 are frequently observed. Patients with more chromosomal gains than losses show significantly shorter survival.

Natural killer lymphoma/leukemia, a group of highly aggressive hematolymphoid malignancies of natural killer cell lineage, exhibit chromosomal rearrangements in greater than 80% by conventional karyotyping. The most frequent abnormalities include del(6)(q21-23) and gain of the X chromosome. FISH, CGH, and spectral karyotyping confirmed the presence of del(6) in $CD3^{-}CD56$ tumor cells. Other less common but recurrent karyotypic changes include isochromosome 1q, 6p, and 17q, as well as del(11q), 13q, and 17p, and trisomy 8.

Angioimmunoblastic T-cell lymphoma and unspecified peripheral T-cell lymphoma are the most frequent nodal T-cell lymphomas.

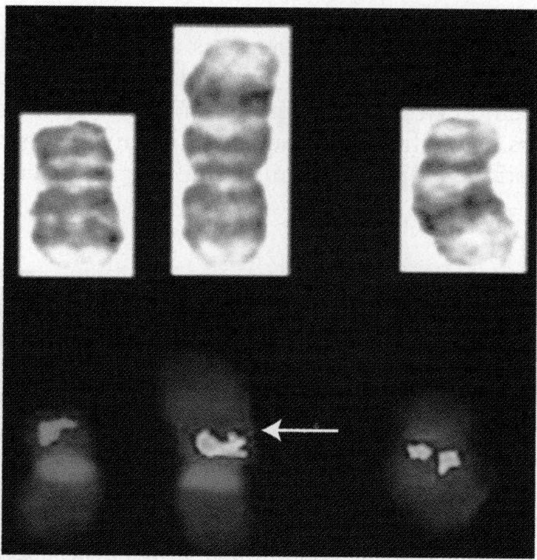

Figure 54-45 Partial karyotype of t(9;12)(p24;q23) *(top)* and after FISH study *(bottom)* with JAK2 *(red)* and TEL/ETV6 *(green)*, showing JAK2-TEL fusion *(yellow)* at 9p24.

Losses of 5q/10q/12q, identified by CGH, characterize a subtype of peripheral T-cell lymphoma associated with a better prognosis. Gain of 11q13 may represent a primary change in angioimmunoblastic T-cell lymphoma. In general, chromosomal imbalances are more common in unspecified peripheral T-cell lymphoma than in angioimmunoblastic T-cell lymphoma. Both disorders may share similar genomic imbalances.

The molecular basis of ALCL is the result of t(2;5)(p23;q35), which fuses part of the NPM gene on 5q35 with part of the ALK receptor tyrosine kinase gene on 2p23 to produce a chimeric NPM-ALK gene. This encodes a chimeric NPM-ALK protein that has a constitutively activated kinase. ALK is thought to play a direct role in the malignant transformation of lymphoid cells, probably by aberrant phosphorylation of intracytoplasmic substrates because accumulation of the ALK protein is observed only in cytoplasm. The WHO classification of lymphoid tumors considers ALCL a distinct clinical entity, with t(2;5) detected by cytogenetics in 60% to 85% of patients. The NPM-ALK fusion is identified by FISH (Fig. 54-46) and by RT-PCR assay in 88% of pediatric patients and 60% of adult patients. The other cases of ALCL have variant translocations. These include rearrangements of the 2p23 region: t(1;2)(q25;p23), t(2;5)(q37;q31), t(2;19)(p23;p13), and inv(2)(p23q35), all associated with ALK gene expression. They also include rearrangements of the 5q35 region: t(1;5)(q32;q35), t(3;5)(q12;q35), and t(3;5)(q25;q34-35). Detection of ALK rearrangements by FISH corresponds to a cytoplasmic staining pattern associated with translocations other than t(2;5).

As a result of these variant rearrangements, three new fusion genes have been identified. ATTIC-ALK is a fusion gene resulting from inv(2)(p23q35). This translocation fuses ALK and 5-aminoimidazole-4-carboxamide ribonucleotide formyltransferase/IMP cyclohydrolase (ATIC). This molecular variant is detected by RT-PCR and is the most common ALK variant. TFG-ALK is a consequence of t(2;3)(p23;q21), which fuses TRK-fused gene (TFG) with ALK at the same breakpoint as found in t(2;5). In t(1;2)(q25;p23), the TPM3 gene on chromosome 1, which encodes nonmuscular tropomyosin, is fused to ALK, producing the TPM3-ALK fusion gene.

The prognosis of patients with t(2;5) or variant translocations is excellent but is clearly different from that of patients with ALK-negative ALCL. The true nature of ALK-negative ALCL remains obscure. GEP showed that ALK ALCL and ALK$^-$ ALCL have different GEZPS, indicating that different, as yet unknown, oncogenic mechanisms may be associated with each type. Of interest, C/EBPβ transcription factor, which is implicated in leukemogenesis of AML, is constitutively active and overexpressed in patients with ALK ALCL but not in ALK$^-$ patients or other lymphomas. C/EBPβ expression is transcriptionally induced through the kinase activity of NPM-ALK, which provides insight into the molecular pathogenesis of ALK ALCL.

A variety of genomic rearrangements are seen in the T lymphocytes of patients with mycosis fungoides and Sézary syndrome. However, specific cytogenetic abnormalities are not associated with these disorders. Most frequent abnormalities involve loss of chromosome 10, deletion of 1p, isochromosome 17q, additions of 17p and 19p, and translocations involving 1p, 10q, and 14q. Both CGH and M-FISH identify chromosome 10, region 10q22-26, as the most frequent abnormality in these disorders.

Posttransplant lymphoproliferative disorder (PTLD) is a morphologically diverse group of lymphoid disorders that occurs in immunosuppressed organ transplant recipients. Chromosomal abnormalities are detected in 51% to 72% of B-cell diseases and in almost all T-cell proliferations, as measured by CGH, FISH, and conventional karyotyping. Although a number of recurrent genomic imbalances are observed, the unfavorable prognostic effect on survival is observed in two main WHO morphologic groups—monomorphic PTLD (M-PTLD) and polymorphic PTLD (P-PTLD)—and can be correlated with the grafted organ. Generally, three groups of nonrandom abnormalities are of importance. The pathogenetic roles of abnormalities known to be involved in lymphomas, such as 8q24 and MYC, 17p13 and P53, and 18q21 associated with BCL2 and MALT1, and those associated with large genomic imbalances, such as 2p24-25, 9q22-34, 12q22-24, and 14q32, await elucidation. Trisomy for chromosomes 9 and 11 appears to be associated with EBV PTLD and prolonged survival. In contrast, PTLD patients showing MYC rearrangements are associated with Burkitt lymphoma and an aggressive clinical course. PTLD associated with T cells develops late after transplantation. These disorders are EBV$^-$ and are associated with poor outcome and short survival.

ALLOGENEIC HEMATOPOIETIC CELL TRANSPLANTATION

Molecular and cytogenetic analyses can be used to characterize the origin of engrafted cells and the development and evolution of recurrent malignancies after allogeneic HCT. Newly developed hematopoietic cells that emerge after allogeneic HCT may be of host origin, donor origin, or both. Genetic studies of posttransplant hematopoiesis are called *chimerism analysis*. This term was introduced into medicine by Anderson and others in 1951 to indicate an organism whose cells are derived from two or more distinct zygote lineages. Chimerism should be distinguished from mosaicism, which is characterized by two or more different cell populations originating from one zygote. Monitoring chimerism in recipients of allogeneic HCT is essential to identify early engraftment, monitor residual disease in leukemia patients, predict relapse, and optimize posttransplantation therapy in case of graft failure.

Historically, karyotype analysis was used to evaluate engraftment after sex-mismatched allogeneic HCT. Polymorphism of chromosomes 1, 9, and 16, as well as satellite polymorphism of chromosomes 13, 14, 15, 21, and 22, were used to differentiate donor from recipient cells in sex-matched allogeneic HCT. Karyotype analysis could identify not only chimerism but also recurrence of hematologic malignancies. However, this is a time-consuming process and has low sensitivity (5%). In the past two decades, many methods for detection of chimerism have been developed. All follow the basic principle of using the differences in polymorphic genetic markers to distinguish donor from patient hematopoiesis. These methods, such as restriction fragment length polymorphism, red cell phenotyping, and interphase FISH, do not offer the possibility to study all patients. The most

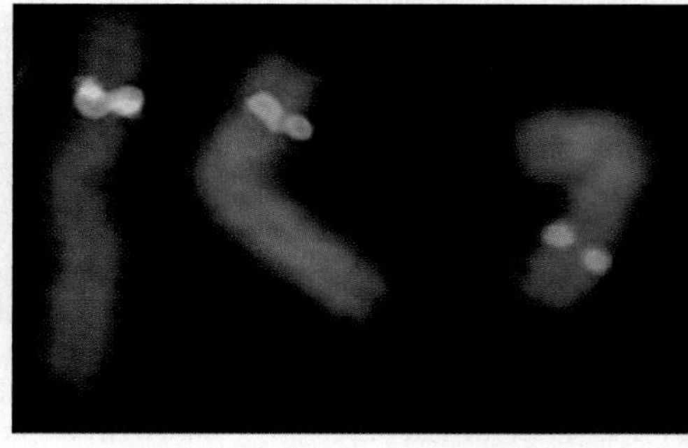

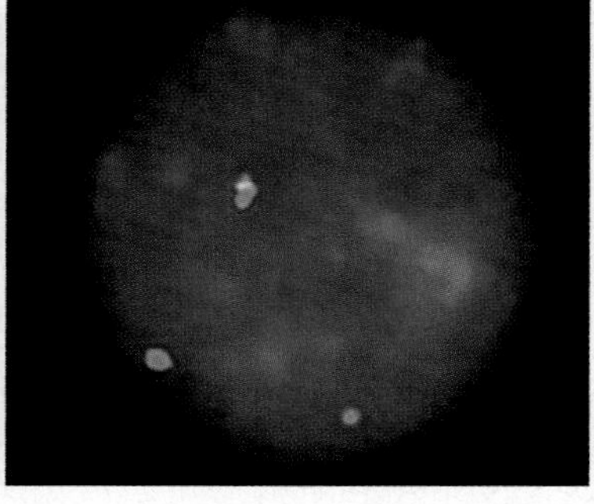

Figure 54-46 FISH STUDY WITH BREAKAPART ALK GENE AT 2p23 IN A PATIENT WITH ANAPLASTIC LARGE CELL LYMPHOMA. Partial karyotype shows a normal chromosome 2 *(left)* with yellow signal, as the 3′ end and the 5′ end of ALK gene are in close proximity on chromosome 2. The other chromosome 2 homologue *(middle)* has only a single green signal (5′ end) as a result of t(2;5)(p23;q35), the most frequent translocation in anaplastic large-cell lymphoma. The 3′ end *(red)* of the ALK gene is translocated to 5q35. Abnormal ALK gene is also shown in interphase cell *(right)*.

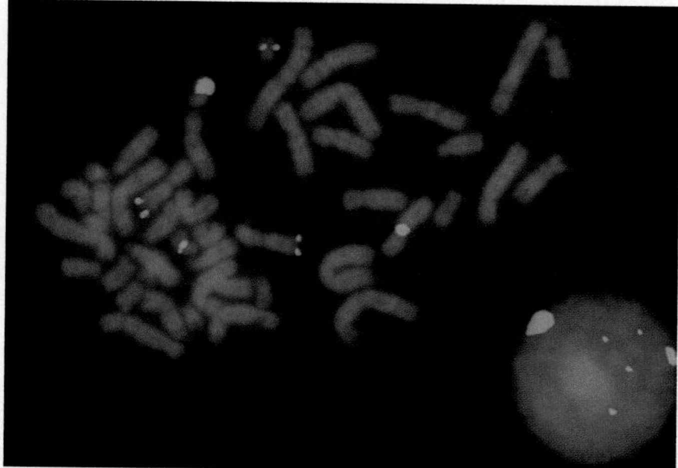

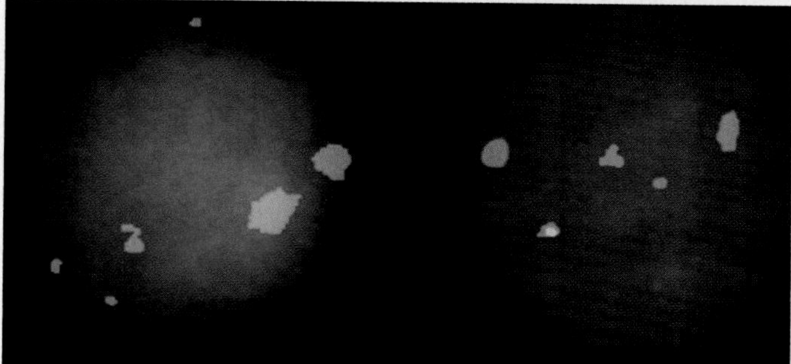

Figure 54-47 DETECTION OF ENGRAFTMENT AND RESIDUAL DISEASE WITH FISH IN SEX-MISMATCHED HEMATOPOIETIC CELL TRANSPLANTATION. Metaphase and nondividing cell *(blue)* after DAPI counterstaining, hybridized with X *(large red)* and Y *(large green)* for detection of engraftment and with ABL *(small red)* and BCR *(small green)* for detection of residual chronic myelogenous leukemia *(top panel)*. Left nucleus *(bottom panel)*, is showing a donor male (XY) cell origin and lack of BCR-ABL fusion. In contrast, a host female (XX), BCR-ABL fusion *(yellow)*–positive cell is shown on the *right*. Combination of XY FISH probes with diagnostic genomic markers is a powerful and fast FISH method for simultaneous detection of chimerism and minimal residual disease.

widely used technique is PCR for a variable number of tandem repeats/short tandem repeats (VNTR/STR-PCR). This technique has a moderate sensitivity of 3% to 5%, and the quantitation of donor and recipient cells may be cumbersome. The method that allows study of chimerism in all patients involves fluorescence labeling of the primers and resolution of PCR products with capillary electrophoresis. It provides high quantitative accuracy with 1% to 5% sensitivity. Real-time PCR or RQ-PCR for analysis of the SRY gene on the Y chromosome allows identification of male cells in the background of 100,000 female cells, providing a high sensitivity for mixed chimerism. However, this approach is limited to the 50% of patients who receive sex-mismatched transplants. Nevertheless, it remains the most sensitive and fastest method of chimerism analysis, providing reliable quantitative results within 2 hours.

Detection of SNPs by chimerism analysis (SNP-PCR) is highly sensitive. In one study using 11 different SNP loci, SNP-PCR analysis identified independent predictors of relapse after HCT. The two most commonly used methods for detection of chimerism after HCT are fluorescence-based PCR amplification of short tandem repeats (STR-PCR) and interphase FISH (Fig. 54-47). Both methods have high quantitation accuracy and reproducibility. The sensitivity of both methods approaches 1%; however, STR-PCR is sex independent and can be applied to all patients. FISH analysis, on the other hand, permits simultaneous evaluation of chimerism and residual disease in the same cell when high sensitivity is not a requirement.

Genetic Testing for Hematopoietic Cell Transplantation

Testing consists of either variable number of tandem repeats/short tandem repeats PCR for detection of engraftment in patients with sex-matched HCT or single-nucleotide polymorphism PCR, which has a high sensitivity. In sex-mismatched HCT, both interphase FISH with XY probes and real-time quantitative PCR for analysis of SRY gene on the Y chromosome can be used for detection of engraftment. Detection of both engraftment and minimal residual disease is best accomplished by FISH, simultaneously using probes for XY and the probe for diagnostic genetic defect, such as XY and BCR-ABL.

FISH analysis for diagnostic genomic abnormalities in conjunction with conventional cytogenetics remains useful and reliable in determining the presence of residual disease (see Fig. 54-47).

Leukemia relapse occurring in donor cells after allogeneic HCT is a rare complication reported in 0.12% to 5% of cases. It was first described in 1971, and more than 60 cases have been reported. Careful genetic analysis of relapse cells is essential. VNTR, restriction fragment length polymorphism, STR analysis, or FISH XY analysis alone may not definitively assign the origin of the leukemic clone because genomic deletions or amplifications of chromosomal segments may occur during the transplantation or disease process. The increased use of unrelated cord blood as a source of stem cells for allogeneic HCT raises the concern that hematopoietic progenitors containing preleukemic clonal molecular rearrangements may be inadvertently transplanted. Systematic screening of unselected cord blood samples revealed putative preleukemic rearrangements such as ETV6-RUNX1 and RUNX1-RUNXT1. However, a recent study including 1417 umbilical cord blood samples revealed no positive findings for the ETV6/(TEL) or RUNX1/RUNXT1 fusions. Kaplan-Meier analysis of pooled data on 13 cases of donor-derived leukemia after unrelated cord blood HCT appears to show an increased risk for donor-derived leukemia when compared with other sources of stem cells. The reason for an increased risk for leukemia or myelodysplasia in donor cells is not understood and may be a function of the conditioning regimen used or the less stringent HLA matching required for unrelated cord blood SCT. Specific mechanisms that result in development of donor cell leukemia are unknown. Proposed mechanisms include the following: (a) sustained host-origin antigenic stimulation, (b) impaired hematopoietic microenvironment and defective stromal support system, (c) immune surveillance escape secondary to posttransplant immunosuppressive therapy, (d) similar genetic susceptibility in cases of related donors, (e) viral driven pathogenesis (CMV, EBV), (f) delayed effects of conditioning regimen, and (g) transfection of host cell oncogene into donor cells. Most likely, the underlying cause is a combination of these mechanisms active in individual cases. A very compelling hypothesis for the mechanisms leading to the development of donor-derived leukemia HCT is the "2-hit hypothesis." A donor HSC that has an inherent susceptibility to malignant transformation (hit 1) is placed within a defective stromal structure elaborating a microenvironment that applies repeated stress signals (hit 2), inducing additional genetic or even epigenetic mutations promoting malignant transformation. A common cytogenetic abnormality has not been recognized, and almost half of cases are associated with a normal karyotype. Nevertheless, these patients must be carefully evaluated using an array of molecular methods for determination of leukemia in donor cells (see box on Genetic Testing for Hematopoietic Cell Transplantation).

FUTURE DIRECTIONS

The question of how initial genetic damage in hematopoietic stem cell disorders causes a cascade of other genetic events that leads to the development of malignancy is unresolved for many diseases. However, major advances have been made, and molecular unraveling of the Philadelphia chromosome led to the rationally designed imatinib treatment that has transformed CML from a fatal disease into a chronic disorder compatible with normal life in many patients. Precise molecular characterization of leukemic cells not only provides more insight into the pathogenesis of disease but allows patients to be stratified as having high or low risk for recurrence and adverse outcome. The ultimate goal is to translate this basic knowledge into increasingly better treatment outcomes. Molecular diversity is currently the genetic hallmark of many leukemias, even within a single disease entity such as AML or T-cell ALL. We are at the threshold of understanding other genetic events and common genetic pathways. Such an understanding is crucial to designing molecular interventions for specific abnormalities of genetic pathways underlying hematologic malignancies. It is clear that genetic revolution has already changed the clinical hematology practice.

REFERENCES

1. Mitelman F, Johannsson B, Mertens F: The impact of translocations and gene fusions on cancer causation. *Nature* 7:233, 2007.
2. Golub TR, Slonim DK, Tamayo P, et al: Molecular classification of cancer cells discovery and class prediction by gene expression monitoring. *Science* 286:531, 1999.
3. Pinkel D, Segravers R, Sudar D, et al: High resolution analysis of DNA copy number variation using comparative genomic hybridization in microarrays. *Nat Genetics* 20:207, 1998.
4. Novelli M, Cossu A, Oukrif D, et al: X-inactivation patch size in human female tissue confounds the assessment of tumor clonality. *Proc Natl Acad Sci U S A* 100:3311, 2003.
5. Vogelstein B, Fearon ER, Hamilton SR, et al: Use of restriction fragment length polymorphisms to determine the clonal origin of human tumors. *Science* 227:642, 1985.
6. Nowell PC, Hungerford DA: A minute chromosome in human chronic granulocytic leukemia. *Science* 132:1497, 1960.
7. Rowley JD: A new consistent chromosomal abnormality in chronic myelogenous leukemia identified by quinicrine fluorescence and Giemsa staining. *Nature* 243:290, 1973.
8. Martin PJ, Najfeld V, Hansen JA, et al: Involvement of the B-lymphoid system in chronic myelogenous leukemia. *Nature* 287:49, 1980.
9. Cross NCP, White H, Muller MC, et al: Standardized definitions of molecular response in chronic myeloid leukemia. *Leukemia* 2012 Apr 16. doi: 10.1038/leu.2012.104. [Epub ahead of print].
10. Hochhaus A: Managing chronic myeloid leukemia as a chronic disease. *Hematol AM Soc Hematol Educ Program* 1:128, 2011.
11. Feldman E, Najfeld V, Schuster M, et al: The emergence of Philadelphia negative, trisomy 8 positive cells in patients with chronic myeloid leukemia treated with imatinib mesylate. *Experimental Hematol* 31:702, 2003.
12. Greenberg P, Cox C, LeBeau MM, et al: International Scoring System for evaluating prognosis in myelodysplastic syndromes. *Blood* 89:2079, 1997.
13. Schanz, J, Tuchler H, Sole F, et al: New comprehensive cytogenetic scoring system for primary myelodysplastic syndromes (MDS) and oligoblastic acute myeloid leukemia after MDS derived from an international database merge. *J Clin Oncol* 30:820, 2012.
14. Baldus CD, Mrozek K, Marcucci G, et al: Clinical outcome of de novo acute myeloid leukaemia patients with normal cytogenetics is affected by molecular genetic alterations: A concise review. *Br J Haematol* 137:387, 2007.
15. Grimwade D, Mrózek D: Diagnostic and prognostic value of cytogenetics in acute myeloid leukemia. *Hematol Oncol Clin North Am* 25:1135, 2011.
16. Melnick A, Licht JD: Deconstructing a disease: RARα, its fusion partners, and their roles in pathogenesis of acute promyelocytic leukemia. *Blood* 93:3167, 1999.
17. Meyer C, Kowartz E, Schneider B, et al: Genomic DNA of leukemic patients: Target for clinical diagnosis of MLL rearrangements. *Biotech J* 1:656, 2006
18. Dastugue N, Lafage-Pochitaloff M, Pages MP, et al: Cytogenetic profile of childhood and adult megakaryoblastic leukemia (M7): A study of the Groupe Francais de Cytogenetique Hematologique (GFCH). *Blood* 15:618, 2002.
19. Moorman AV, Harrison CJ, Buck GAN, et al: Karyotype is an independent factor in adult acute lymphoblastic leukemia (ALL): Analysis of cytogenetic data from patients treated on the Medical Research Council (MRC) UKALLXII/Eastern Cooperative Oncology Group (ECOG) 2993 trial. *Blood* 109:3189, 2007.
20. Sutcliffe MJ, Shuster JJ, Sather HN, et al: High concordance from independent studies by the Children's Cancer Group (CCG) and Pediatric Oncology Group (POG) associating favorable prognosis with combined trisomies 4, 10, 17 in children with NCI standard-risk B-precursor acute lymphoblastic leukemia: A Children's Oncology Group (COG) initiative. *Leukemia* 19:734, 2005.
21. Mrozek K, Harper DP, Aplan PD: Cytogenetics and molecular genetics of acute lymphoblastic leukemia. *Hematol Oncol Clin N Am* 23:991, 2009.
22. Dohner H, Stilgenbauer S, Benner A, et al: Genomic aberrations and survival in chronic lymphocytic leukemia. *N Engl J Med* 343:1910, 2000.
23. Schnaiter A, Mertens D, Stilgenbauer S: Genetics of chronic lymphocytic leukemia. *Clin Lab Medicine* 31:649, 2011.
24. Shaughnessy JD, Jr, Zhan F, Burington BE, et al: A validated gene expression model of high-risk multiple myeloma is defined by deregulated expression of genes mapping to chromosome 1. *Blood* 109:2276, 2007.
25. Munshi NC, Avet-Loiseau H: Genomics in multiple myeloma. *Clinical Cancer Research* 17:1234, 2011.
26. Dimopoulos M, Kyle R, Fermand J-P, et al: Consensus recommendation for standard investigative work up: Report of International Myeloma Workshop Consensus Panel 3. *Blood* 117:4701, 2011.
27. Anderson KC, Carrasco RD: Pathogenesis of myeloma. *Annu Rev Pathol Mech Dis* 6:249, 2011.
28. Staud LM: A closer look at follicular lymphoma. *N Eng J Med* 356:741, 2007.
29. Cauwelier B, Dastugne N, Cools J, et al: Molecular cytogenetic study of 126 unselected T-ALL cases reveals high incidence of TCR beta locus rearrangements and putative new T-cell oncogenes. *Leukemia* 20:1238, 2006.
30. Graux C, Cools J, Michaux L, et al: Cytogenetics and molecular genetics of T-cell acute lymphoblastic leukemia: From thymocytes to lymphoblast. *Leukemia* 20:1496, 2006.

CHAPTER 55

PHARMACOLOGY AND MOLECULAR MECHANISMS OF ANTINEOPLASTIC AGENTS FOR HEMATOLOGIC MALIGNANCIES

Stanton L. Gerson, Paolo F. Caimi, Erica Campagnaro, Kapil N. Bhalla, Steven Grant, and Richard J. Creger

The treatment of patients with several hematologic malignancies has been revolutionized over the past decades as new therapeutic targets have been identified through studies of the molecular and cell biology of these malignancies. These studies have spawned the discovery, clinical evaluation, and Food and Drug Administration (FDA) approval of new mechanistic-based therapeutic agents. A surprising number of these agents have progressed from discovery, validation, animal modeling, and successful clinical testing. In addition, there has been a wider spectrum of agents, including small molecules, peptides, antibodies, radiolabeled molecules, drug immunoconjugates, immunotoxins, and complex delivery systems. This chapter provides information on several new therapeutic agents available for the treatment of patients with hematologic malignancies. The chapter reviews the "classic" agents as well as the newly developed, targeted agents. Both cytotoxic and growth-inhibitory agents are covered; however, the use of therapeutic antibodies and antibody conjugates is reviewed within the chapters dealing with specific diseases.

CELL KINETICS, THE CELL CYCLE, AND TUMOR GROWTH

Malignant hematopoietic cells proliferate more than their normal counterparts. It is important to recognize that this characteristic of hematologic malignancies is exploited in developing treatment strategies. The cell cycle consists of a series of stages through which normal and neoplastic cells proceed during the course of cellular replication (shown schematically in Fig. 55-1). The cell cycle is divided into G_1 (pre-DNA synthetic phase), S phase (in which DNA replication takes place), G_2 (post-DNA synthetic phase), and mitosis (M), during which chromosomal division and segregation occur. In addition, nonproliferating, resting cells reside in G_0, a phase that may theoretically last for an indefinite period. Such cells remain in G_0 until they are induced to cycle (at G_1) by specific triggers (e.g., hematopoietic growth factors). The *growth fraction* of a tumor represents the percentage of cycling cells relative to the total cell population. The *generation* time represents the time required for a cell to proceed through a single cell cycle (generally 24-36 hours for hematopoietic tissues). Surprisingly, in the case of acute myeloid leukemia (AML), the generation time of leukemic blasts is not shorter than that of normal hematopoietic progenitors and may in fact be longer. The proliferative advantage of malignant hematopoietic cells (and of many nonhematopoietic tumors) stems, at least in part, from the fact that a higher percentage of cells are in cycle at any one point in time (i.e., the growth fraction is higher). The *doubling time* represents the period required for a tumor to double in mass and is, in general, inversely related to the tumor's growth fraction. Tumor-doubling times range from longer than 120 days in the case of some solid tumors (e.g., lung and colon) to less than 2 weeks (in some leukemias and lymphomas). Tumor-doubling times are influenced by multiple other factors, including the rate of spontaneous cell death (or apoptosis) and the availability of appropriate nutrients. The importance of these considerations stems from the fact that tumors with high growth fractions and short doubling times tend to be more sensitive to chemotherapy than slowly growing neoplasms with low growth fractions and long doubling times. It is unlikely to be a coincidence that many advanced neoplasms that are potentially curable by chemotherapy (e.g., hematologic malignancies such as leukemia, lymphoma, and testicular cancer) fall into the former group; conversely, most incurable advanced malignancies (e.g., non–small cell lung cancer, colon cancer) fall into the latter.

The transition of normal as well as neoplastic cells through the cell cycle is governed by a complex network of proteins consisting of cyclins, cyclin-dependent kinases (CDKs), and CDK inhibitors. The progression through S phase is regulated primarily by CDK2 in association with cyclins A and E; the progression through G_2M is regulated by CDK1 ($p34^{cdc2}$) and cyclin A and cyclin B; and progression through G_1 involves CDKs 4 to 6 in conjunction with cyclin D. CDK inhibitors fall into two major categories: the low-molecular-weight inhibitors (pINK14, -15, -16, -17, and -18), which primarily inhibit cyclin D (and to some extent, CDK2) complexes, and the higher-molecular-weight inhibitors, p21, p27, and p57, which are more universal in their actions and inhibit most or all CDKs. Signals for the progression of cells through G_1S are essential for maintenance of the neoplastic phenotype. In the commonly accepted model of G_1S progression, inactivation of the retinoblastoma protein (PRB) is required. In quiescent cells, PRB is in an active dephosphorylated state and bound to the transcription factor E2F. Phosphorylation of PRB by CDK4 and CDK6 and CDK2 leads to release of E2F, which is then free to activate diverse genes essential for S-phase progression, such as *MYC* (also known as c-Myc), *TYMS* (thymidylate synthetase), and *DHFR* (dihydrofolate reductase). Conversely, induction of CDK inhibitors (e.g., by transforming growth factor β [TGFβ] or differentiation-inducing agents) results in inactivation of CDK4 and CDK6 and CDK2, dephosphorylation of PRB, inactivation of E2F, and inhibition of the progression through S phase. Aberrant expression of cyclins and CDK inhibitors is commonly encountered in human malignancies, and it has been postulated that the resultant cell cycle dysregulation contributes to the neoplastic phenotype.

In addition to growth control, cell cycle proteins are intimately involved in the regulation of programmed cell death (apoptosis) and checkpoint control mechanisms. Consequently, cell cycle regulatory proteins can exert a major influence on the response of neoplastic cells to cytotoxic agents. For example, when cells undergo DNA damage, they may arrest in G_2M or G_1, during which repair occurs, or if the damage is too severe, the cells undergo apoptosis. In particular, the tumor suppressor gene *TP53* and its downstream inducible target p21 have been implicated in the G_1 arrest process after genotoxic insult. Dysregulation of various cell cycle regulatory proteins can have a major impact on the sensitivity of neoplastic cells to chemotherapeutic agents. Loss of the *TP53* gene renders cells resistant to diverse chemotherapeutic agents, presumably by preventing cells from undergoing repair in G_1 and thereby inhibiting the cell death processes and allowing DNA damage to accumulate, culminating in cellular transformation. Conversely, transfection of P53-negative cells with wild-type P53 restores responsiveness to most drugs. Dysregulation of the CDK inhibitors p21 (a downstream target of P53) and p27 increases the sensitivity of neoplastic cells to various cytotoxic agents, possibly by uncoupling S-phase progression and mitosis. In this model, loss of the CDK inhibitors p21 or p27 prevents cells that have sustained DNA damage from arresting in G_1 and allows them to progress inappropriately through S and ultimately G_2M, eventually

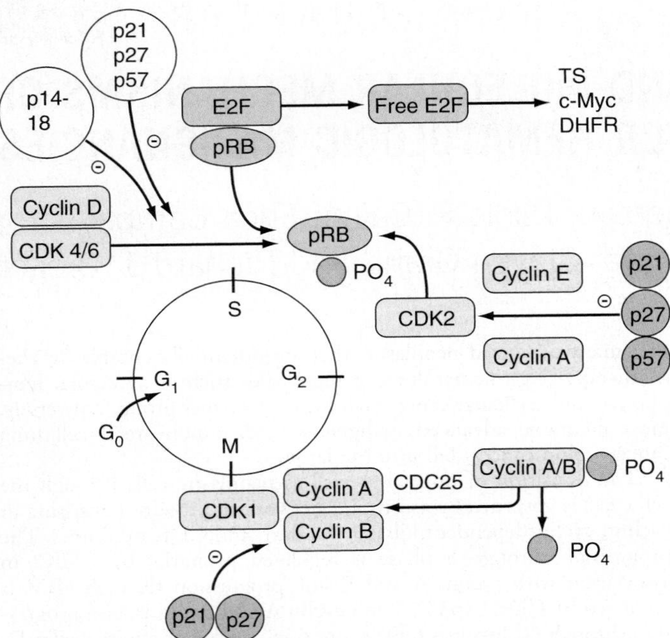

Figure 55-1 PROGRESSION THROUGH THE CELL CYCLE IS CONTROLLED THROUGH COMPLEX INTERACTIONS AMONG CYCLINS, CYCLIN-DEPENDENT KINASES (CDKs), AND CDK INHIBITORS. Progression across the G_1S interface and through S phase involves the E2F transcription factor, which activates numerous enzymes (e.g., thymidylate synthase, dihydrofolate reductase) required for DNA replication. The retinoblastoma protein (pRb) in its dephosphorylated state binds to and inactivates E2F in conjunction with DP proteins, thereby inhibiting S-phase progression. Conversely, phosphorylation of pRb antagonizes binding to E2F, allowing S-phase events to proceed. Phosphorylation of pRb results from activation of (1) cyclin-dependent kinase-2 (CDK2):cyclin A/E and (2) CDK4/6:cyclin D complexes. The former complexes are inhibited by the CDK1s p21, p27 (and p57), and the latter are inhibited by the low-molecular-weight CDK inhibitors (p14-18) but also by p21 and p27. The complex formed by CDK1 ($p34^{cdc2}$) and cyclins A and B regulates G_2M progression and is inhibited by the "universal" CDK inhibitor, p21. Moreover, its phosphorylation status, which plays a major role in determining activity, is regulated by the phosphatase cdc25. Proteins such as pRb, E2F, p21, and p27 can influence the response of cells to chemotherapeutic agents by controlling cell cycle progression and possibly via cell cycle—unrelated actions.

leading to cell death. Mutations in the E2F protein have been shown to lengthen S phase and increase the sensitivity of malignant cells to S phase–specific agents. Furthermore, cells lacking functional PRB have been shown to be significantly less sensitive to the actions of antimetabolites, including methotrexate. Aside from regulating cell cycle status and the susceptibility of neoplastic cells to cell cycle–specific agents, cell cycle regulatory proteins can actively contribute to the cell death response.

The growth of tumors is best described by Gompertz's law rather than classic exponential kinetics. For neoplasms that grow exponentially, the tumor growth rate remains constant as the number of cells increases. However, in vivo, the growth of tumors is limited by various factors such as vascular supply, nutritional requirements, and possibly physical restraints. Consequently, the rate of tumor growth declines as the number of cells increases. To the extent that tumor-doubling times are inversely correlated with drug responsiveness, large, late-stage tumors would be anticipated to be less susceptible to cytotoxic drugs than early stage tumors, with higher growth fractions. Most chemotherapeutic drugs kill by *first-order kinetics*. This results in a given drug dose killing a constant fraction, rather than number, of tumor cells. The implication of this phenomenon is that it requires the same drug dose to reduce the number of tumor cells from 10^4 to 10^1 cells as it does to reduce the tumor burden from 10^{10} to 10^7 cells.

Recent emphasis on leukemic and lymphoma stem cells has raised a new potential cellular target for therapeutics and provides another level of analysis of the efficacy of available agents both in clinical and preclinical settings. The value of targeting leukemia, lymphoma, and myeloma stem cells either in clinical trial design or therapeutic development is unclear at present. However, for neoplasms now considered incurable with chemotherapy, a focus on the stem cell subpopulation might lead to curative therapies. Regardless of the availability of targeted therapies, the ability to identify and track cancer stem cells will likely lead to more sensitive and precise measurement of minimal residual disease. One factor in common for most malignant stem cells is the overexpression of the ABC transporters. Adenosine triphosphate (ATP)–binding cassette transporters are often highly expressed in early hematopoietic stem cells and other tissue stem cells that are CD44 positive. Inhibition of these transporters is a logical approach to therapeutically targeting leukemic stem cells. Progress in this area is discussed in the section on multidrug resistance protein (MRP) and the ABC transporters.

Cytotoxic agents may be divided into several categories with respect to their effects on the cell cycle or the cell cycle specificity of their actions or both.

1. *Non–cycle-active drugs* kill both cycling and noncycling cells in all phases of the cell cycle. Examples include steroids and antitumor antibiotics (except bleomycin).
2. *Cycle-active, non–phase-specific drugs* are more active against cycling cells and can kill cells in each phase of the cell cycle. However, such drugs may preferentially kill cells in a particular phase of the cell cycle. Examples include alkylating agents, cisplatin, and 5-fluorouracil.
3. *Cycle-active, phase-specific drugs* primarily kill cells in a specific phase of the cell cycle. Examples include most antimetabolites, which are active against cells engaged in DNA synthesis (S-phase cells), and microtubule-active drugs (e.g., vinca alkaloids, taxanes), which kill cells in G_2M.

An example of a cytokinetically rational approach to chemotherapy involves the combination of a non–cycle-active agent (e.g., daunorubicin) with a cycle- and a phase-specific agent (e.g., cytosine arabinoside [ara-C], fludarabine, decitabine, clofarabine and nelarabine). From a theoretical standpoint, administration of a non–cycle-active agent may reduce tumor mass, leading in turn to an increase in the growth fraction caused by recruitment of cells into cycle. Such cells would then be more susceptible to a cycle- and phase-specific agent, particularly one administered over a prolonged interval. In the case of hematopoietic malignancies, attempts have been made to recruit neoplastic cells into the more susceptible S phase of the cell cycle through the use of *hematopoietic growth factors*. The success of such a strategy has been limited because of several factors, including the inability of growth factors to increase the S-phase fraction significantly, the lack of selectivity of this strategy, and the theoretical possibility that growth factors may protect neoplastic cells from apoptosis.

Unfortunately, cytokinetic differences between normal and neoplastic tissues have been difficult to exploit. Both normal hematopoietic stem cells and hematologic malignant stem cells have a low proportion of cells in G1. However, prolonged dosage schedules can provoke these malignant cells into cell cycle and may explain their efficacy. Consequently, rapidly dividing normal tissues such as gastrointestinal epithelium and normal hematopoietic progenitors tend to be very sensitive to most chemotherapeutic agents. As a result, mucositis and myelosuppression represent frequent dose-limiting toxicities for many cytotoxic drugs.

TUMOR CELL HETEROGENEITY OF HEMATOLOGIC MALIGNANCIES

Whereas hematologic malignancies are of *clonal* origin (i.e., they are derived from a single transformed cell), individual neoplastic cells from a patient's malignancy exhibit a great deal of phenotypic diversity and acquire secondary mutations that affect proliferation, drug sensitivity, and resistance. This diversity likely arises from the progeny of clonal populations and subsets of stem cells. In animal models, it has been shown that the clones themselves can give rise to progeny that can transmit the clonal malignancy after transplantation into secondary recipients, suggesting that stem cells are not required to transmit the malignant phenotype.

New evidence indicates that leukemia stem cells are more quiescent, have higher levels of protective proteins such as efflux pumps for drugs, and have higher levels of DNA repair proteins or antiapoptosis proteins than the more abundant cell making up the circulating population of cells. Tumor cell heterogeneity arises as a consequence of spontaneous mutational events, changes in gene promoter methylation, impact of abnormal expression of transcription factors, lymphoid reactivity, and cytokine responsiveness. In fact, these can be reinforced if they provide a survival, tissue homing, or including homing to bone marrow (BM) niches for preferential engraftment and metastasis or a proliferative advantage for the affected cells and their progeny. For example, a mutation or change in expression that renders a hematopoietic cell clone autonomous or growth factor–independent would be expected to render such cells less susceptible to adverse environmental conditions (e.g., growth factor withdrawal). Similarly, one would also predict that a genetic change facilitating cell cycle entry or disruption of cellular maturation would ultimately lead to overgrowth of affected clones. For obvious reasons, mutations that interfere with drug metabolism or the cell death pathway itself would provide a net survival advantage, particularly under the selection pressure of cytotoxic drug treatment.

Malignant myeloid and lymphoid cells have many reasons to have increased mutational rates. Genomic instability can arise from dysregulation of the cell cycle machinery because of a number of events, including pertubations of cyclins leading to MYC overexpression; AKT activation; disruption of replication sequences; loss of DNA repair enzymes such as mismatch repair; enzymes' loss of proper homologous recombination from a defect in the BRCA–Fanconi pathways; and loss of ATM/ATR, which can give rise to chromosomal recombination, loss and microsatellite instability, and loss of checkpoint regulation. These events can give rise to intraclonal emergent point mutations, translocations, and intragenic losses that might not only result in malignant transformation but also lead to disruption of genomic stability and selection in favor of proliferative and apoptosis-resistant subclones. Leukemic clonal evolution favors drug resistance.

Common mechanisms may be involved in events associated with malignant transformation and the development of mutations that result in tumor heterogeneity. For example, the cell cycle checkpoint and tumor suppressor gene, *TP53,* is induced during DNA damage, leading to G_1 arrest and, if the damage is too severe to repair, cell death by apoptosis occurs. The presumed goal of this process is to eliminate cells that develop deleterious mutations as a result of damage to the genome. Loss of *TP53* may not only increase cellular survival by inhibiting the cell death process but may also promote the transmission of mutations that would otherwise be deleted. In this manner, a defect of the cell death pathway can have multiple consequences, including (1) selection of cells exhibiting a growth advantage over their normal counterparts, (2) development of drug resistance, and (3) promotion of mutations that result in either (1) or (2) as well as neoplastic cell heterogeneity. Age-dependent changes in these processes may explain the more favorable behavior of leukemias and lymphomas in response to chemotherapy in young patients than older patients.

A model of the relationship between tumor growth rate, the occurrence of spontaneous mutations, and the development of drug resistance was first described by Goldie and Coldman and is referred to as the Goldie and Coldman hypothesis. In this model, the size of a tumor depends on a complex interaction between tumor growth rate and cell loss, the latter stemming from the status of the cell death process, exhaustion of available nutrients, and outstripping of the blood supply. As tumors increase in size, the cell death rate tends to increase. The heterogeneous nature of additional mutations makes it likely that multiple mechanisms of resistance will develop as well. From an operational standpoint, this model has clear implications for the rational design of therapeutic strategies and provides a basis for early and intensive combination drug therapy. The successful implementation of this strategy is exemplified by the administration of dose-intensive multidrug regimens (i.e., the BEACOPP [bleomycin, etoposide, Adriamycin, cyclophosphamide, vincristine—Oncovin—procarbazine, and prednisone] regimen in Hodgkin disease, CODOX-M-IVAC in Burkitt lymphoma [non-Hodgkin lymphoma or NHL]) and combinations of cytotoxic agents with monoclonal antibodies, such as CHOP (cyclophosphamide, hydroxydaunorubicin, vincristine [Oncovin], and prednisone)–rituximab, which are potentially curative when given early in the course of the disease. Other examples include combined use of multitargeted agents such as lenalidomide and bortezomib for myeloma, fludarabine and rituximab for chronic lymphocytic leukemia (CLL), or maneuvers to overcome resistance of pretreated disease outside of cell-based therapies. However, as predicted by the model, administration of these or other intensive regimens in patients with relapsed or late-stage disease generally fails because of a generalized resistance of tumor cells to all classes of chemotherapeutic agents.

DEVELOPMENT OF CHEMOTHERAPEUTIC AGENTS

The quest for anticancer agents for hematologic malignancies began with the nitrogen mustard class of compounds developed from the chemical warfare agent sulfur mustard gas used in World War I. Since that time, the National Cancer Institute (NCI) and the pharmaceutical industry have developed complex approaches to drug development, screening, and evaluation. Initial screening consisted of toxicity assessment against murine tumor cell lines. Currently, screening is directed toward numerous cell targets, including receptor and downstream signaling kinases; inducers of cell death pathways, including those at the cell surface, mitochondrial DNA, and nuclear DNA; DNA processing and repair proteins, including topoisomerases and telomerase; and inhibitors of histone deacetylase (HDAC) cell cycle proteins, proteasomes, and the mitosis and spindle machinery. Although killing cells remains the backbone of chemotherapeutic approaches to human malignancies, the field of antineoplastic agent development is at a tipping point moving toward novel targeted and highly effective compounds that block the function of specific kinases with surprising efficacy even at late stages of disease. Examples include Bruton tyrosine kinase and phosphatidylinositol 3-kinase (PI3K) inhibitors in lymphoid malignancies as well as Janus kinase (JAK) inhibitors for treatment of myelofibrosis. A number of differentiating agents, kinase inhibitors, and immunomodulatory and cytostatic agents have now entered the antineoplastic armamentarium. In addition, agents that target tumor angiogenesis have been evaluated. Although "conventional" cytotoxic agents cause myelosuppression and mucositis because of their effect on rapidly dividing normal cells, newer agents cause more diverse systemic side effects. Secondary leukemias induced by hematopoietic progenitor cell damage incurred by alkylating agents, topoisomerase inhibitors, and combination chemotherapy and radiation are not associated with the newer classes of compounds. The emphasis on targeted therapeutics in recent drug development has focused in several areas, including recognized fusion or mutant proteins specific to the malignant cell, such as Bcr-Abl in chronic myeloid leukemia (CML) (see Chapter 66), PML-RARα in promyelocytic leukemia (see Chapter 65), and the JAK2V617F mutation present in myeloproliferative neoplasms (see Chapters 67 to 69); cellular signaling pathways such as B-cell receptor signaling, PI3 kinase, mammalian target of rapamycin (mTOR), bcl-2, and nuclear factor kappa-B (NFκB); and monoclonal antibodies and immunoconjugates, antibody–toxin conjugates, antibody–drug conjugates, and radioimmunoconjugates (see Chapter 81).

Screening for Antitumor Activity Among Chemotherapeutic Agents

While in the past, discovery of new agents to treat hematologic malignancies relied on the NCI Division of Cancer Treatment initiative to maintain a large cell bank of malignancies for drug testing, newer approaches are using high-throughput drug screening with either cell-based or specific mechanism–based assays. For instance, to screen for a kinase inhibitor, cells overexpressing an activated kinase may be used. The NCI has evaluated more than 60,000 compounds for cytotoxic and growth inhibitory activity using a standard human tumor cell line screen, and this database remains the most comprehensive even as both pharmaceutical companies and academic laboratories develop their independent screening programs. After an initial in vitro screen, human tumor cell activity is evaluated using a series of athymic mouse xenograft studies targeting tumors from tissues that show promise in in vitro assays. Drugs with promising efficacy and novel mechanisms of action then go on to formulation and toxicology testing and ultimately are developed for phase I clinical testing through industry or the NCI Cancer Therapy Evaluation Program. Cell lines are being used, along with cell line banks of human hematologic malignancies for high-throughput screening efforts that are especially useful for screening for noncytotoxic agents that affect gene expression, differentiation, migration, and other cell-based assays. In addition, drug discoveries that start as a survey of specific pathway inhibition, such as signaling kinases (Bcr-Abl, JAK2, platelet-derived growth factor [PDGF], kit, and FLT3) and Src kinases, represent new approaches validated by the discovery of agents such as imatinib, dasatinib, nilotinib, and ruxolitinib.

Human tumor xenografts have been used as a requisite screen in preclinical testing of new chemotherapeutic agents. For leukemia and lymphoma cell lines, prolongation of life span is used as an end point measured at the percent increased life span (ILS), $((T - C/C) \times 100)$, where T is the life span after drug treatment and C untreated. The best predictive mouse systems for this purpose are primary malignancies grown in immunodeficient mice and mice with specific chromosomal translocations and oncogenes that mimic human disease. In mice with severe combined immune deficiency (SCID), the RPMI 8226 human myeloma cell line and the multidrug-resistant subline, 8226-C1N inoculated intraperitoneally led to a life span that was numbered in days, and the tumor cells in vivo were completely resistant to treatment with doxorubicin. Investigators established a human acute promyelocytic leukemia (APL) ascites model in the SCID mice and found responses to all-trans retinoic acid (ATRA). Other investigators have used the SCID leukemia model to test antisense oligonucleotide strategies directed against such tumor-specific genes as *BCR-ABL* in CML. Use of primary and serially passaged human leukemias and myelomas in the SCID model have facilitated drug screening. In both instances, infusion of antisense constructs increased the ILS significantly and led to clinical studies with these agents. Others have used the SCID model for B-cell lymphomas to study chemotherapy or lymphotoxins. Although these models have not entered the NCI drug screen, they represent significant systems to test new agents.

Phase I Clinical Trial Design

New anticancer agents are assessed through a series of clinical trials termed *phase I, phase II,* and *phase III* (Table 55-1). The purpose of phase I clinical trials is to establish the safe and optimal biochemically active dose of the compound in question with acceptable toxicity that can be used in disease-targeted phase II testing. During phase I development, pharmacokinetics and pharmacodynamic measures are studied in detail so that appreciable information can be forthcoming from the very first set of patients targeted for treatment and to allow confirmation of these observations in larger phase II disease-focused trials. Dose schedule and route of administration are key considerations in early phase I development. Numerous considerations have guided dose escalation strategies that accompany phase I trial development. The starting dose is typically 10% of the lethal dose (LD10) in animals adjusted for species dose equivalency. In classic phase I development, a modified Fibonacci dose schedule is used. Groups of three patients are treated at each of the following doses until the maximum tolerated dose is observed: 1N (the starting dose), 2N, 5N, 7N, 9N, 12N, and 16N. Typically, the maximum tolerated dose is defined as the maximum dose not causing irreversible toxicity of any type and causing less than grade 4 toxicity in any organ. Newer agents often have off-target toxicities, and these complicate drug evaluation because the dose-dependent toxicities are replaced by rashes, cardiac effects from prolonged QT intervals, activation or inhibition of other pathways, and unusual side effect profiles such as pleural and pericardial polyserositis. Typically, if one dose-limiting toxicity is observed, the patient cohort is expanded to six patients, and if two patients develop dose-limiting toxicity, typically defined as grade 4 toxicity except as previously noted, then further entry at this dose is not pursued, and the next lower dose level is used to establish the maximum tolerated dose with a total of six patients accrued at that dose level.[1]

Table 55-1 Clinical Trial Design

Phase I
Evaluate safety by dose escalation and multiple dose schedules.
Establish maximum tolerated dose and dose-limiting toxicity.
Consider use of hematopoietic support if myelosuppression is dose limiting.
Phase II
Establish response (complete, partial, objective) in specific diseases.
Phase III
Compare new treatment with established regimen for the disease in randomized trials.

Alternative strategies of drug escalation have included the use of toxicity grades to enhance dose escalation in early drug development, allowing that if no toxicity is observed, fewer patients might be accrued to each dose. Using the modified Fibonacci scheme, one patient is entered at each dose level until grade 2 toxicity is observed, at which point cohorts of three patients are entered at each level. Early in drug development, level skipping may take place if no toxicity is observed. The overall impact of this is to reduce the number of patients treated at suboptimal doses of therapy and to increase the number of patients evaluated at biologically active doses.

More importantly, biomarker driven studies can be used to optimize inhibition of the target rather than treating to toxicity. This can then be extended in phase 2 to determine whether the drug effects on its biochemical target correspond to efficacy and tolerance.

Phase II Drug Development

Phase II drug development uses the established phase I dose to define therapeutic efficacy, typically in a two-stage design. If an expectant response rate in excess of 20% is deemed clinically significant, 15 patients are accrued, and if two or more responses are seen, accrual is continued to a total of 26 patients to establish the definite response rate. At this point, combination therapies are instituted in an effort to optimize therapeutic efficacy. For instance, topotecan was found in phase I testing to have efficacy against refractory leukemias leading to combinations of topotecan with ara-C and other agents. Likewise, fludarabine was initially evaluated as a single agent for activity against low-grade lymphomas and acute and chronic leukemias and is now used in combination with ara-C for the treatment of acute lymphocytic leukemia and with chlorambucil for the treatment of CLLs. In the past, strategies for combination chemotherapeutic agents have included the use of non–cross-resistant agents with non-overlapping toxicities. However, more recently, mechanism-based therapeutics has become the focus of drug development. For instance, with the combination of fludarabine and cisplatin, fludarabine may inhibit nucleotide excision repair and enhance persistence of cisplatin-induced DNA adducts, resulting in increased antitumor efficacy in CLL. Likewise, combining a receptor kinase inhibitor with a cell cycle inhibitor might potentiate efficacy in leukemias.

Most phase III trials randomize patients between an established standard therapy and a new therapy that has appeared promising in the phase II setting. These studies are usually multi-institutional and many involve large national and international cooperative groups. The end point of these studies is disease response, survival, and patient tolerance. Linking multiple centers removes the vagaries of reports from single centers, which remain the focus of phase II trials. Phase III trials are important for positive and negative results.[2]

PHARMACOLOGY OF CHEMOTHERAPEUTIC AGENTS

As noted earlier, although cytotoxic anticancer agents may be divided into several categories based on the cell cycle specificity of their action, in keeping with traditional classification, they are more appropriately divided into alkylating agents, antimicrotubule agents, antimetabolites, topoisomerase I or II inhibitors, platinum analogs, and miscellaneous agents. The pharmacology and cellular mechanisms of action of these agents are schematically presented in Fig. 55-2. Targeted therapeutics such as imatinib and bortezomib are discussed in later sections.

Alkylating Agents

Drug treatment for cancer began with the use of the mustard class of alkylating agents, initially mechlorethamine (nitrogen mustard),

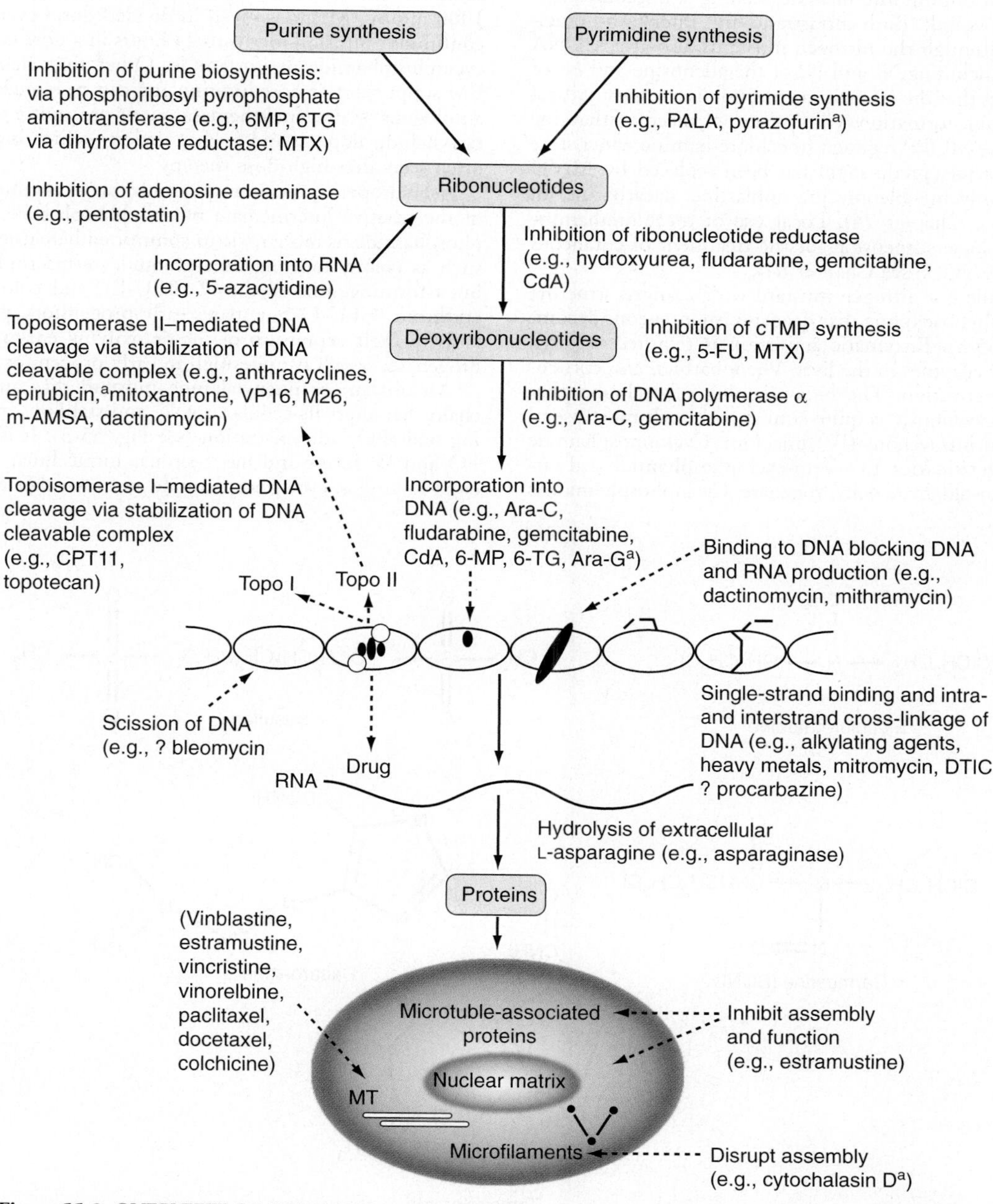

Figure 55-2 OVERVIEW OF SITES AND MECHANISMS OF ACTION OF THE MOST USEFUL CHEMOTHERAPEUTIC AGENTS.

which entered into clinical use in the mid-1940s. Alkylating agents are used in many regimens but are rapidly being supplanted by newer classes of agents.

Nitrogen Mustard

The nitrogen mustard class includes mechlorethamine, cyclophosphamide, 4-hydroperoxy cyclophosphamide, ifosfamide, chlorambucil, and melphalan. These drugs all share a common bischloroethyl group attached to nitrogen and a substituted "R" group that provides drug specificity (Fig. 55-3). All nitrogen mustards react with DNA in an SN_2 reaction, a bimolecular nucleophilic displacement reaction, also called a second-order reaction. Although numerous sites are targeted for alkylation, nucleophiles in DNA, including nitrogen (N), oxygen (O), and phosphate (P), attract the chloroethyl moiety attached to the R-N backbone, and the chlorine is displaced by the nucleophilic atom to form an aziridinium moiety. The remaining chloroethyl group is then attracted to a second nucleophilic atom, forming a second aziridinium intermediate, leading to a second alkylation, forming a cross-link. Both intrastrand and interstrand cross-links are formed. Although the nitrogen mustards also attack DNA at other nitrogens, including N^1 and N^3 of the adenosine and N^3 of thymidine, it appears that the N^7 guanine position is the most critical for cytotoxic cross-link formation. Clinical use of mechlorethamine is limited because the MOPP regimen (mechlorethamine, vincristine [Oncovin], procarbazine, prednisone) has been replaced by ABVD (doxorubicin [Adriamycin], bleomycin, vinblastine, dacarbazine) in Hodgkin disease (see Chapter 74). Local use of mechlorethamine occurs in a dermatologic suspension for the treatment of cutaneous T-cell lymphomas (CTCLs; see Chapter 84).

Cyclophosphamide is a nitrogen mustard with a ringed structure off the end-chloroethyl backbone that decreases spontaneous decomposition (see Fig. 55-3). Enzymatic activation is required through multifunction P450 enzymes in the liver. Phenobarbital and corticosteroids may alter activation. The bioavailability of cyclophosphamide orally and intravenously is quite similar, although most use of the drug is by bolus intravenous (IV) injection. Cyclophosphamide is detoxified through oxidation to 4-keto-cyclophosphamide and carboxyphosphamide by aldehyde dehydrogenase. Cyclophosphamide is used in doses as little as 50 to 100 mg/day orally and in bolus doses of 400 to 700 mg/m^2 for solid tumors and 750 mg/m^2 in combination with doxorubicin and vincristine and prednisone as part of the CHOP regimen for NHLs. It is also used at doses of up to 60 mg/kg/day for 4 days in autologous and allogeneic BM transplantation (BMT) protocols. Cyclophosphamide is used in numerous treatment protocols for NHLs and high-dose therapy regimens designed to eradicate tumor and BM in patients with lymphomas and leukemias and those undergoing BMT. It is commonly used with granulocyte colony-stimulating factor (G-CSF) for mobilizing hematopoietic stem cells to be collected before autologous transplantation.

Cyclophosphamide is metabolically activated by cytochrome P450 mixed function oxidases in the liver to 4-hydroxycyclophosphamide. 4-Hydroxycyclophosphamide is further converted to aldophosphamide and then to phosphoramide mustard, the alkylated species, and acrolein. Acrolein is a highly reactive aldehyde and the cause of hemorrhagic cystitis. Mercaptoethane sulfonate (Mesna) is used to prevent recurrence and to provide prophylaxis against hemorrhagic cystitis caused by cyclophosphamide and ifosfamide and is now standard for doses of cyclophosphamide and ifosfamide above 1000 mg/m^2. Mesna is given in divided doses every 4 hours or as a continuous infusion for 18 to 24 hours in a dose equivalent to either cyclophosphamide or ifosfamide. Other than hemorrhagic cystitis, BM suppression is dose limiting and can be rescued by reinfusion of autologous or allogeneic hematopoietic progenitor cells. Other toxicities include alopecia and cardiac toxicity, which is unusual and most often seen after high-dose therapy.

4-Hydroperoxycyclophosphamide is a chemically stable form of the reactive intermediate of cyclophosphamide, 4-hydroxycyclophosphamide, is more toxic to committed hematopoietic progenitors such as colony-forming unit–granulocyte/macrophage (CFU-GM), burst-forming unit–erythroid (BFU-E), and colony-forming unit–erythroid (CFU-E) but spares early progenitors, presumably on the basis of their expression of the detoxifying enzyme aldehyde dehydrogenase, which is quite high in early progenitor populations.

Melphalan, or phenylalanine mustard, has an amino acid side chain that alters its cellular uptake and stabilizes its structure, allowing oral (PO) administration (see Fig. 55-3). It is available in both PO and IV forms and has a similar intracellular pathway to DNA cross-linking as cyclophosphamide and the other nitrogen mustards.

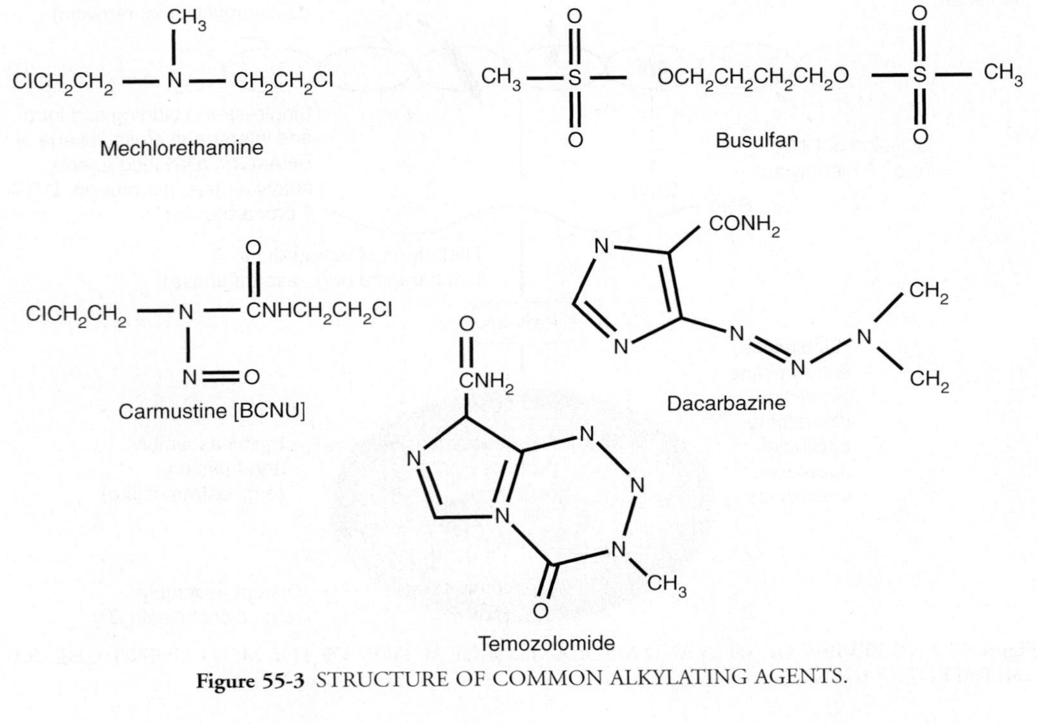

Figure 55-3 STRUCTURE OF COMMON ALKYLATING AGENTS.

Melphalan uptake by cells is by means of a neutral amino acid transporter. Its rate of cross-link formation is much slower than that of mechlorethamine, presumably because of delayed metabolism. PO melphalan is used predominantly for the standard treatment of multiple myeloma and intravenously in high-dose regimens in preparation for stem cell transplantation (see Chapter 85) for multiple myeloma patients.

Chlorambucil has been used for more than 40 years for the treatment of CLL. Chlorambucil is the phenylbutyric acid derivative of nitrogen mustard and is very stable, entering the cell by diffusion rather than by a specific uptake mechanism. It is typically administered orally on a daily basis or intermittently. It appears to have greater bioavailability than melphalan and a more consistent half-life of approximately 2 hours.

Busulfan is an alkylsulfonate, unique among alkylating agents because of two sulfur groups and the lack of a chloroethyl moiety (see Fig. 55-3). Busulfan, similar to the nitrogen mustards, reacts predominantly at the N^7 position of guanine and produces an N^7–N^7 biguanyl DNA cross-link, although the precise nature of this cross-link appears different than that of the nitrogen mustards. This may explain the different clinical effects of busulfan compared with the nitrogen mustards. The pharmacokinetics of busulfan is important for its use in high-dose therapy for ablation of the BM in patients undergoing autologous transplantation for acute leukemia or allogeneic stem cell transplantation (see Chapters 104 and 105). Busulfan clearance does not appear to be accurately predicted by creatinine clearance. Because the incidence of venoocclusive disease is lower in patients receiving high-dose busulfan with predosing pharmacokinetics performed, this is now recommended in high-dose regimens, the target being an area under the curve (AUC) of 800 to 1200 ng hr/mL. Busulfan is a potent stem cell toxin, killing both early and late hematopoietic progenitor cells and damaging the BM stroma. Other toxicities of busulfan include nausea and vomiting and pulmonary interstitial and intraalveolar edema leading to fibrosis. The pulmonary fibrosis is distinct from the interstitial pneumonitis, which accompanies allogeneic stem cell transplantation and is not related to cytomegalovirus or other viral infections.

Nitrosoureas

Four chloroethyl nitrosoureas and one methyl nitrosourea are in clinical use. These agents are different from the nitrogen mustards in that they alkylate through an SN^1 reaction, forming a highly reactive intermediate in the presence of N, O, and P nucleophiles in DNA. The commonly used clinical agent is (2-chloroethyl)-*N*-nitrosourea (BCNU). *N*-[(4-amino-2-methyl-5-pyrimidinyl) methyl]-*N*-(2-chloroethyl)-*N*-nitrosourea (ACNU) is commonly used in Japan. A third agent, *N*-(2-chloroethyl)-*N*-cyclohexyl-*N*-nitrosourea (CCNU), is used predominantly as an PO nitrosourea in children with brain tumors. All of these compounds have high hydrophobicity, actively penetrating the blood–brain barrier.

The DNA alkylation sites include N^7 and O^6 of guanine. Chloroethylation at the O^6 position of guanine appears critical to cytotoxicity. DNA cross-linking by chloroethyl nitrosoureas include at 1-(3-cytosinyl), 2-(1-guanyl) ethane, and 1-2-bis(7-guanyl) ethane. The former is responsible for much of the cytotoxicity observed with the chloroethyl nitrosoureas. It is formed after alkylation at the O^6 position of guanine. This adduct undergoes intramolecular rearrangement to a circular intermediate, N^1. O^6 ethanoguanine is formed, which can then rearrange by attack at the opposite hydrogen-bonded base N^3 of cystine forming the interstrand cross-link. This is a unique DNA cross-link and is poorly recognized by DNA repair processes, leading to marked cytotoxic potency of this cross-link.

The pharmacokinetics of the chloroethyl nitrosoureas have been evaluated in both conventional and high-dose schedules. A very short half-life has been detected, which is quite variable, but an association between the AUC of BCNU and pulmonary toxicity has been observed. BCNU is predominantly used for high-dose treatment of recurrent lymphomas. In both settings, it is an effective form of therapy with sustained complete remission (CR) rates of approximately 40% to 60%. Doses of between 600 and 1000 mg/m^2 have been safely administered. The chloroethyl nitrosoureas cause profound and cumulative BM suppression at conventional doses of 120 to 150 mg/m^2, limiting treatment to three to five cycles at 6-week intervals.

Complications of high-dose BCNU therapy include pulmonary toxicity and renal toxicity at doses higher than 600 mg/m^2. Pulmonary toxicity, as evidenced by a decrease in the DL_{CO} (diffusing capacity of the lung for carbon monoxide), occurs in up to 40% of patients and is symptomatic in 10% to 15% of patients. It can be managed with steroids during the inflammatory but not during the fibrotic phase and is lethal in some cases. Fibrosis is associated with an early interstitial infiltrate followed by evidence of hyaline membrane formation and replacement of the chronic inflammatory cells by fibrosis over a 4- to 6-week period. Renal dysfunction associated with nitrosourea therapy occurs less frequently than severe cumulative myelosuppression and pulmonary fibrosis and is typically seen at doses above 1000 mg/m^2. Interstitial nephritis with glomerulosclerosis, interstitial fibrosis, and dropout of tubules has been reported with BCNU or CCNU.

Methylating Agents

Four methylating chemotherapeutic agents are available for clinical use. These include procarbazine, dacarbazine (DTIC), streptozotocin, and temozolomide. Procarbazine and DTIC are triazines. Streptozotocin is a monofunctional methyl nitrosourea derivative with an attached sugar moiety, and temozolomide is an imidazotetrazine synthesized in England in the 1960s, reaching clinical trials in the late 1980s. All react with DNA by undergoing SN^1 reactions forming a methyldiazonium ion, resulting in methylation of N^7 guanine, O^6 guanine, O^4 and O^2 thymine, and N^3 adenine. None form DNA cross-links. However, all induce high levels of DNA methylation. N^7 methylguanine is unstable, leading to ring opening and both spontaneous and enzymatically mediated depurination. Repair proceeds through the base excision repair system. Recognition by the *N*-methylpurine glycosylase results in removal of the adducted base with formation of an abasic site that is recognized by the apurinic (AP) endonuclease, which then cleaves the backbone at the AP site. Subsequently, the free 5′ sugar is released by DNA lyase with repair initiated by β-polymerase and DNA ligase. Base excision repair effectively removes N^7 methylguanine and N^3 methyladenine and restores DNA to normal. These lesions appear to contribute little to cytotoxicity and appear to be up to 500-fold less potent as cytotoxic adducts than O^6 methylguanine.

O^6 methylguanine mispairs with thymine during DNA synthesis, resulting in a lesion recognized by the mismatch repair system. This system consists of two sets of enzyme homologs of mismatch repair in prokaryotes, mutS and mutL. Mispair recognition proteins are MSH6, MSH3, and MSH2, homologs of the mutS system in bacteria. MSH2 and MSH3 form a stable heterodimer with MSH6. Recognition of the mispair recruits additional proteins to the complex, including MLH1 and PMS1/PMS2, which are homologs of mutL in bacteria. These proteins initiate exonuclease cleavage of a long patch in the newly synthesized strand of DNA. This is then repaired by polymerases delta and epsilon. Unfortunately, if the O^6 methylguanine adduct is not removed before repair synthesis, a thymine is again inserted opposite the O^6 methylguanine and the repair process begins again, resulting in an aberrant episode of repair and multiple single-strand breaks. Cell protection from methylating agents arises either by removal of O^6 methylguanine (vide infra) or inactivation of the mismatch repair system. Cells expressing high levels of the DNA repair protein for O^6 methylguanine, O^6 alkylguanine DNA alkyltransferase are approximately 10-fold more resistant to methylating agents than alkyltransferase-negative cells. Mismatch repair-mediated single-strand patches promote chromosomal aberrations, homologous and nonhomologous recombination, and induction of apoptosis in a p53-dependent and -independent manner. Absence of one or more protein components responsible for mismatch repair, leads to the phenotype of replication error repair (RER), which is commonly observed in hereditary colon cancer as well as endometrial cancer, gastric cancer, and approximately 15% of lymphomas. Cells lacking mismatch repair are up to 100-fold more resistant to methylating agents than cells with mismatch repair, regardless of alkyltransferase activity. Acquisition of mismatch repair defects is associated with acquired resistance to methylating agents and cisplatin, which is also recognized by this protein complex.

Procarbazine was synthesized as a monoamine oxidase inhibitor and has been used since the 1950s for the treatment of Hodgkin lymphoma and NHL, as well as a component of combination therapies for gliomas. Recent use has been superseded by newer agents. Patients receiving procarbazine form O^6 methylguanine DNA adducts with depletion of the alkyltransferase enzyme, a suicide protein that removes the methyl group in irreversible stoichiometric reaction. Chromosomal breaks, single-strand breaks, and chromosomal aberrations and sister chromosome exchanges observed after procarbazine treatment support its association with treatment-related myelodysplasia and leukemia.

DTIC is metabolically activated by cytochrome P450 microsomal oxidoreductases, ultimately leading to formation of the methyldiazonium ion and DNA methylation. DTIC is used in combination with doxorubicin, vinblastine, and bleomycin (ABVD) for treating Hodgkin disease (see Chapter 74) and is also used for metastatic malignant melanoma in combination with BCNU, cisplatin, and tamoxifen. Activation of DTIC requires hydroxylation of one terminal methyl group caused by demethylation forming 5(3-methyltriazeno)-imidazole-4-carboxamide (MTIC), with spontaneous decomposition to the methyldiazonium ion, which alkylates the DNA, as noted earlier. Similar to procarbazine, DTIC has been shown to form N^7 methylguanine and O^6 methylguanine DNA adducts in human peripheral blood lymphocytes and to deplete alkyltransferase through repair of O^6 methylguanine DNA adducts. A correlation has been documented between tumor response and formation of O^6 methylguanine DNA adducts, indicating their importance in clinical antitumor effects. Maximum tolerated doses of DTIC are approximately 1000 mg/m^2, with myelosuppression and gastrointestinal toxicity (including severe watery diarrhea) as the most common side effects.

Temozolomide represents an imidazotetrazinone. It differs from DTIC in that it is chemically degraded to the monomethyl triazine, MTIC, at neutral pH and does not require P450 enzymatic demethylation. Compared with DTIC, temozolomide has much more consistent pharmacokinetic parameters, including peak serum concentrations, volume of distribution and clearance, and conversion to MTIC. Clinical studies found considerable activity in acute leukemias. Dose-limiting toxicity was thrombocytopenia and, less frequently, neutropenia, with maximum tolerated doses of 1000 mg/m^2 given over 5 days on a daily or twice daily regimen. Nausea and vomiting were the other common side effects, easily controlled with antiemetics. Formation of O^6 methylguanine has been documented in clinical trials with temozolomide with much more rapid depletion of the alkyltransferase, suggesting that temozolomide may be more effective than the other methylating agents because of its ability to form higher levels of toxic O^6 methylguanine DNA adducts. Early phase clinical trials using temozolomide in patients older than 60 years with AMLs indicated that the drug is well tolerated and has a modest response rate. A second study has shown that combination therapy including temozolomide, which may induce neoantigens, is also effective.

Bendamustine

Bendamustine is comprised of a 2-chloroethylamine nitrogen mustard alkylating group, a benzimidazole ring, and a butyric acid side chain. Its mechanism of action is unknown but appears to be different than other alkylating agents, causing DNA damage that is repaired predominantly by the base–excision repair system and has activity against lymphoid cell lines resistant to alkylating agents.[3] Myelosuppression with leukopenia and thrombocytopenia is the most frequent side effect, with mild nonhematologic side effects, including nausea, fatigue, constipation and diarrhea. In vitro studies demonstrated synergy between bendamustine and rituximab. This observation led to several phase II trials of the combination for treatment of relapsed CLL and low-grade lymphoma patients, with high response rates observed. Phase III studies comparing standard treatment with bendamustine and rituximab in frontline treatment of CLL[4] and indolent lymphomas (see Chapter 76) have been completed, with demonstrated efficacy in this setting. Bendamustine is also active against multiple myeloma, and combinations with steroids and bortezomib or the immunomodulatory agents thalidomide and lenalidomide have been reported to result in high response rates in patients with relapsed or refractory disease.

Alkylating Agent–Induced Leukemias

Alkylating agents induce dose-limiting myelosuppression and cause sublethal DNA damage to hematopoietic progenitors, causing mutational events that lead to malignant transformation to preleukemic and leukemic states. A concern exists about the use of hematopoietic growth factors after exposure to alkylating agents (see Chapter 59). There is evidence of increased cytotoxicity to hematopoietic progenitors during simultaneous exposure to these agents and growth factors. Treatment-related AML (T-AML) accounts for approximately 15% of all adult AML. Approximately 50% of T-AML patients have a preleukemic phase compared with only 10% of patients with de novo AML. CRs are achieved in 15% to 30% of patients with T-AML and a mean remission duration of 2 months. Chromosomal abnormalities are common in T-AML, with more than 90% of cases expressing a chromosomal rearrangement, loss, or addition.

Historically, patients with Hodgkin disease treated with mechlorethamine and procarbazine in the MOPP regimen or with CCNU were at the highest risk if exposed to radiation as well as an alkylating agent combination. Patients with polycythemia vera treated with chlorambucil were at much higher risk than patients treated with phlebotomy alone, which can contribute to a shift in treatment strategy. Patients with myeloma and ovarian cancer have developed T-AML, especially after prolonged exposure to alkylating agents. The introduction of temozolomide for the treatment of glioblastoma multiforme is of concern given its use as a 5 day per month or daily regimen for an extended period of time. There have been a number of reports of secondary leukemia in this patient population indicating that the mutagenic effect of temozolomide seen preclinically will need to be monitored in treated patients. Patients treated with alkylating agents for benign diseases such as nephritis, lupus, psoriasis, rheumatoid arthritis, and Wegener granulomatosis also have an increased risk of T-AML. The mean latency between exposure and T-AML from alkylating agents is 4 to 5 years, in contrast to T-AML from etoposide, which has a latency period as short as 1 year. The cumulative risk of developing T-AML is between 10% and 17% at 4 to 6 years for myeloma patients treated with melphalan and between 2% and 10% at 7 to 10 years in patients with Hodgkin disease. Alkylating agent–associated T-AML has also been recognized in patients with breast and colon cancer. A series of nonrandom chromosomal aberrations associated with T-AML has been identified. Loss or deletion of all or part of the long arm [q] of chromosomes 5 or 7 is common, as are trisomy chromosome 8 and deletions of the short arm of chromosomes 12, 17, and 21.

Antimicrotubule Agents

The antimicrotubule drugs include the vinca alkaloids (e.g., vincristine, vinblastine, vinorelbine and vindesine), taxanes (e.g., paclitaxel and docetaxel), and novel epothilones (ixabepilone).

The vinca alkaloids are naturally occurring (vincristine and vinblastine) or semisynthetic (vinorelbine) nitrogenous bases derived from the pink periwinkle plant, *Catharanthus roseus*. Paclitaxel was originally isolated from the bark of the Pacific yew, *Taxus brevifolia*. Paclitaxel can also be isolated from other members of the *Taxus* genus and from a fungal endophyte that grows on the Pacific yew. Docetaxel is derived semisynthetically from 10-deacetyl-baccatin III, which is obtained from the needles of the European yew, *Taxus baccata*.

The vinca alcaloids bind to the protein tubulin at a site distinct from that of the taxanes and, at low concentrations, inhibit microtubule dynamics. At higher concentrations, these vinca alkaloids disrupt microtubules and mitotic spindle, resulting in cell cycle mitotic arrest and apoptosis of cells (see Fig. 55-3). In contrast, after binding to a-tubulin, taxanes kinetically stabilize microtubule dynamics at their plus ends and shift the equilibrium toward tubulin polymerization into micrutubule bundles. This also causes mitotic arrest and apoptosis of cells. The mitotic arrest caused by antimicrotubule drugs is associated with phosphorylation of the BCL2 protein and increased intracellular levels of the BCL2-associated X protein (BAX), which promote apoptosis.

Antimicrotubule agents, particularly the vinca alkaloids, are used in the management of lymphomas and leukemias and continue to be used in the mainstay of clinical chemotherapeutic regimens. Because of their mechanism of action, they are best used in multiagent combinations, in which potentiation of efficacy with other classes of agents, such as antimetabolites and DNA-damaging agents, provide better therapeutic responses and well-tolerated treatments.

Antimetabolites

The antimetabolites consist of low-molecular-weight compounds that interfere with micromolecular synthesis. As a group, they may be contrasted with agents such as the anthracycline antibiotics, which interfere with macromolecular synthesis. The nucleoside analogs exhibit structural similarities to naturally occurring nucleosides and are incorporated into either DNA or RNA with lethal consequences. Alternatively, they block key enzymes in de novo purine or pyrimidine biosynthesis. The antimetabolites in use in hematologic disorders can be divided into the following broad categories:

1. Inhibitors of de novo purine or pyrimidine synthesis (e.g., hydroxyurea)
2. Folic acid analogs (e.g., methotrexate)
3. Pyrimidine analogs (e.g., cytosine arabinoside [ara-C], 5-azacytidine, gemcitabine)
4. Purine analogs (e.g., 6-thioguanine, 6-mercaptopurine, fludarabine, chlorodeoxyadenosine, deoxycoformycin, clofarabine, nelarabine)

These categories are not mutually exclusive; for example, some nucleoside analogs (e.g., ara-C and 6-thioguanine) also inhibit enzymes involved in DNA or deoxyribonucleotide biosynthesis. The antimetabolites are predominantly cycle-active agents and in most cases are phase specific, being primarily active against cells in S phase. Because the growth fraction of hematologic malignancies tends to be higher than that of nonhematologic malignancies, antimetabolites are particularly useful in the former disorders. In contrast to alkylating agents, antimetabolites have limited carcinogenic and leukemogenic potential. The fluorinated pyrimidines (e.g., 5-fluorouracil) are generally not used in treating hematologic disorders and are not discussed further in this chapter.

Clofarabine (2-chloro-2′-arabino-flouro-2′-deoxyadenosine) is a purine analog with activity in patients with relapsed acute leukemia. Its activation requires cellular uptake and conversion to the triphosphate nucleotide. It then decreases ribonucleotide reductase; alters nucleotide precursors; inhibits and reduces the function of antiapoptotic proteins such as Bcl-X(L), Mcl-1, and Bax with dephosphorylation of akt; and inhibits DNA synthesis. It appears more active against B-cell than T-cell lymphomas but also has activity in AML and myelodysplastic syndromes (MDS). Reversible liver toxicity and myelosuppression can be dose limiting (see Chapter 58).

Nelarabine (9-β-D-arabinofuranosylguanine) is another FDA-approved purine analog for the treatment of refractory T-cell leukemias and lymphomas. It preferentially accumulates in T cells and is incorporated into DNA, causing chain termination and inhibiting DNA synthesis. The FDA approved this drug after analyzing the results of two phase II clinical trials, one in pediatric T-cell acute lymphoblastic leukemia (ALL) and the other in adults with T-cell lymphoblastic lymphoma. In both cases, patients had relapsed after at least two induction regimens. Because CRs were seen in 13% of the 39% of pediatric patients and in 18% of the 28 adult patients, the FDA granted approval. Neurologic toxicity is dose limiting. Good response rates, including CRs, have been seen in patients with refractory T-cell leukemias.

Inhibitors of DNA Topoisomerase I and II

The inhibitors of DNA topoisomerases I and II include such drugs as doxorubicin, daunorubicin, mitoxantrone, etoposide, and topotecan. Before describing the specific inhibitors, a brief review of the drug targets (topoisomerase enzymes) will be presented (Table 55-2).

DNA Topoisomerase I

Topoisomerase I is a ubiquitous enzyme whose function in vivo is to relieve the torsional strain in DNA, specifically to remove positive supercoils generated in front of the replication fork and to relieve negative supercoils occurring downstream of RNA polymerase during transcription. Topoisomerase I is catalytically active as a 100-kd monomer and is concentrated in nucleoli, although smaller amounts are found in a diffuse nuclear distribution. The gene for this enzyme is located on human chromosome 20q12-13.2. Topoisomerase I does not require ATP for catalytic activity. It binds double-strand DNA over 15 to 25 bp (with a preference for supercoiled or bent DNA) followed by cleavage of one DNA strand and forming a transient covalent phosphotyrosyl bond at the 3′-end of DNA. DNA torsional strain is then relieved by a "controlled rotation" mechanism (see Fig. 55-1) subsequent to which the cleaved DNA is religated. The three-dimensional crystal structure of human topoisomerase I, both in covalent and noncovalent complexes with DNA, has defined the structural elements of the enzyme that contacts DNA. The association between topoisomerase I and the 3′-end of cleaved DNA has been termed the *cleavable complex,* which is stabilized by topoisomerase I inhibitors.

DNA Topoisomerase II

Two isoforms of human topoisomerase II (α and β) exist. They act as homodimers to cleave double-stranded DNA and require ATP for full activity. Their role in vivo is to relieve torsional strain in DNA, and their cellular distribution is determined by nuclear localization signals contained in the C-terminal domain. These isoforms are distinct in that they have different-size monomers (see Table 55-2), their genes are located on separate chromosomes, their nuclear distribution is different, and only the α-isoform shows cell cycle variations in amount and activity (with maximal activity being in G_2/M). The mechanism of action of topoisomerase II involves several steps (Fig. 55-4): DNA recognition and binding (curved and supercoiled DNA, as well as DNA crossovers, are preferred), the sequential cleavage of the two strands of DNA with covalent attachment of a monomer to each 5′-end of the cleaved DNA, passage of another DNA duplex through the break site (e.g., to relieve DNA torsional strain or decatenate daughter chromosomes at the end of replication), religation of the cleaved DNA, and ATP hydrolysis-dependent enzyme turnover. The binding of ATP by topoisomerase II is required for the strand passage reaction. Again, the association between topoisomerase II monomers and the 5′-end of the cleaved DNA has been termed the *cleavable complex,* the stabilization of which generally correlates with the cytotoxic activity of specific topoisomerase II inhibitors.

Table 55-2 Characteristics of Mammalian DNA Topoisomerases

	Topoisomerase I	Topoisomerase IIα and Topoisomerase IIβ	
Size of monomer (kd)	100	170	180
mRNA (kb)	4.2	6.2	6.5
Chromosome	20q12-13.2	17q21-22	3p24
DNA cleavage	Single-strand breaks	Double-strand breaks	Double strand
Covalent intermediate	3′PO$_4$-Tyr^{723}	5′PO$_4$-Tyr^{804}	5′PO$_4$-Tyr^{821}
ATP requirement	No	Yes	Yes
Nuclear location	Nucleoli, diffuse	Nuclear matrix and scaffold, nucleoli	Nucleoli Nuclear matrix
Cell cycle dependence	None	Yes, maximum in G$_2$/M	None
Nuclear localization signal	NH$_2$-end	COOH-end	COOH-end
Phosphorylation	By CK II and PKC (increases activity)	By CK II, PKC, p34^{cdc2}, MAPK	Increases mass to 190 kd
Role	In replication, transcription, and recombination	In replication, transcription, chromosome condensation/segregation, and recombination	rRNA transcription
Inhibitors	Camptothecins	(see Table 55-3)	

ATP, Adenosine triphosphate; *MAPK*, mitogen-activated protein kinase; *PKC*, protein kinase C.

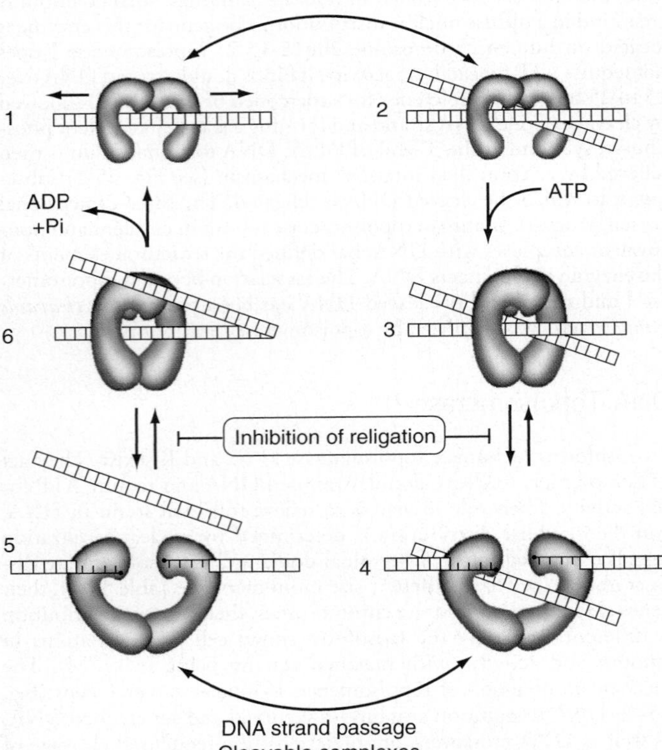

Figure 55-4 DNA TOPOISOMERASE II CATALYTIC CYCLE. (1) Noncovalent binding of DNA by the topoisomerase II homodimer. (2) DNA recognition and preferential binding to crossovers by topoisomerase II. (3) Binding of adenosine triphosphate (ATP) promotes the formation of a topologic complex. (4) DNA cleavage with covalent linkage of each topoisomerase II monomer to the 5′-DNA terminus of the break. (5) Poststrand passage cleavable complex. (6) Religation of the cleaved DNA is followed by ATP hydrolysis and enzyme turnover. DNA topoisomerase II inhibitors generally increase cleavable complexes by inhibiting the religation activity.

Because topoisomerase I and II inhibitors convert their respective enzymes into DNA-damaging agents, it is usually true that the more enzyme target a cell contains (provided it is in the nucleus), the more cytotoxic is the specific inhibitor. An exception to this generalization is CLL cells, which have abundant topoisomerase I but are not very sensitive to topoisomerase I inhibitors because topoisomerase I inhibitors are S phase–specific and CLL cells have very few cells in S phase. Finally, in addition to topoisomerase I and II, a mammalian DNA topoisomerase III has been described and found to be essential for early embryogenesis in the mouse. In addition to the presumed lethality of a homozygous deletion of the topoisomerase II gene, topoisomerases I and III appear to be essential for cell growth and division in mammals. The specific role of topoisomerase III in humans is unknown at present.

DNA Topoisomerase I Inhibitors

Camptothecin is a plant alkaloid first identified in 1966 from the tree *Camptotheca acuminata.* Early clinical studies with camptothecin were stopped primarily because of hemorrhagic cystitis, resulting from conversion of the sodium salt form to the active lactone form owing to its acidic pH in the bladder. Renewed interest in camptothecin occurred in 1985 when topoisomerase I was identified as the target of this drug and as new more water-soluble analogs became available. At present, two topoisomerase I inhibitors have been approved by the FDA as second-line agents for the treatment of ovarian carcinoma and colorectal cancer; these are topotecan and irinotecan (CPT-11) (Fig. 55-5). Topotecan has been shown to be active in the treatment of MDS and inactive in the treatment of CLL. Responses to topotecan have also been seen in refractory multiple myeloma, refractory large cell lymphoma, and refractory acute leukemia.

The lactone forms of topotecan and SN-38 (the active form of CPT-11 generated in vivo by the action of a carboxylesterase) are as much as 1000-fold more active inhibitors of DNA topoisomerase I than are their carboxylate forms. The lactone form predominates at an acidic pH. Topoisomerase I inhibitors stabilize the DNA–enzyme cleavable complex and thus inhibit DNA religation, but the production of DNA double-strand breaks results from a collision of the DNA replication fork with the ternary drug–enzyme–DNA complex that is the lethal event (see Fig. 55-4). Topoisomerase I inhibitors are considered S phase–specific agents because they require ongoing DNA synthesis to exert their cytotoxic effect.

DNA Topoisomerase II Inhibitors

Inhibitors of DNA topoisomerase II are commonly used for the treatment of hematologic malignancies. Three general types of topoisomerase II inhibitors (Table 55-3) exist. The first are the topoisomerase II *poisons,* typified by etoposide, which results in the stabilization of cleavable complexes. The second group are the *catalytic inhibitors,* represented by aclarubicin, merbarone, and the bis-2,6-dioxopiperazine derivatives (ICRF-193, ICRF-159, ICRF-187); these are drugs that, except for aclarubicin, do not bind DNA and do not stabilize cleavable complexes but rather interfere with some aspect of topoisomerase II catalytic activity (e.g., ICRF-187 inhibits topoisomerase II adenosine triphosphatase [ATPase] activity). The final class includes drugs that can inhibit both DNA topoisomerases I and II and are represented by intoplicine and saintopin.

DNA topoisomerase II poisons (see Fig. 55-5 for structures) are most likely cytotoxic because they trap DNA topoisomerase II complexes on nascent DNA in the nuclear matrix. The topoisomerase II poison-stabilized enzyme–DNA complex likely acts as a replication fork barrier and leads to the generation of irreversible DNA damage and cell death in proliferating cells. Whereas experiments in yeast show that although DNA synthesis is a major determinant for cell killing by topoisomerase I inhibitors, topoisomerase II poisons are also cytotoxic during other phases of the cell cycle.

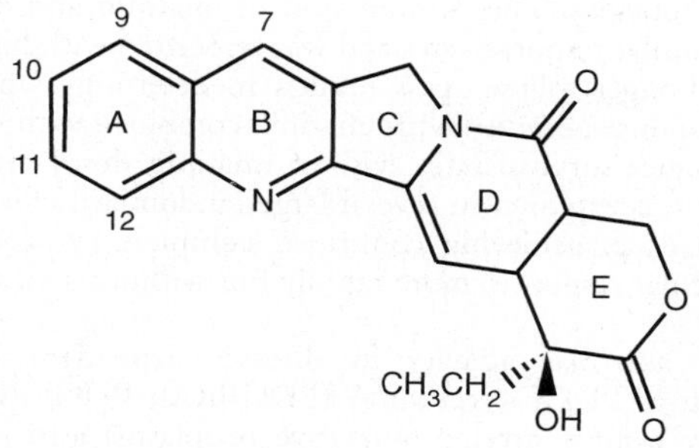

	C-10	C-9	C-7
Camptothecin	H	H	H
Topotecan	OH	$(CH_3)_2NCH_2$	H
9-Aminocamptothecin	H	NH_2	H
SN-38	OH	H	CH_3CH_2
CPT-11	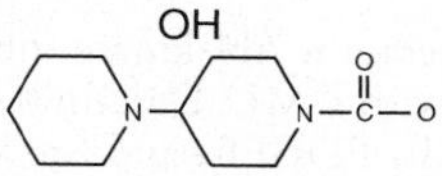 N–(piperidinyl)–N–C(=O)–O	H	CH_3CH_2

Figure 55-5 STRUCTURE OF CAMPTOTHECIN ANALOGS.

Drug Resistance to Topoisomerase Inhibitors

Essentially all of the topoisomerase II poisons (see Tables 55-2 and 55-3) are substrates for the drug efflux pump P-glycoprotein (PGP), and many are substrates for MRP and lung resistance–related protein. In addition, several point mutations and gene deletions have been defined in the gene for topoisomerase II, resulting in the production of an enzyme with altered catalytic or cleavage activity. The third mechanism of resistance is a decrease in expression of the enzyme such that there is less target for the inhibitor to "convert" to a DNA-damaging agent. This can result from a proliferation-dependent or cell cycle–dependent decrease in topoisomerase II, from a specific attenuation of topoisomerase II or from an intrinsic absence of topoisomerase II (identified in some acute and chronic leukemias). The fourth resistance mechanism involves alterations in the subcellular distribution of the enzyme. Truncation of the COOH-end of topoisomerase II has resulted in the cytoplasmic distribution of enzyme caused by a loss of nuclear localization signals, so that the enzyme cannot interact with DNA in the presence of an inhibitor and the cell is resistant. However, mutations in the gene for topoisomerase II do not appear to be common because only a single patient with AML has been found to have a point mutation. By contrast, CLL cells are resistant to topoisomerase II inhibitors because they express very low levels of the protein.

Table 55-3 Mechanism(s) of Action of Antineoplastic Agents That Are Primarily Topoisomerase II Inhibitors

Drug	Topoisomerase II Inhibition Poison	DNA Suppressor	Free Radical Intercalation	Formation
Epipodophyllotoxins	+++	–	–	+
VP-16				
VM-26				
Anthracyclines				
Doxorubicin				
Daunorubicin	++	++	++	+
Idarubicin				
Epirubicin				
Anthracenedione				
Mitoxantrone	++	++++	++	+
Acridine				
m-AMSA	+++	+	+	–
Catalytic inhibitors				
Aclarubicin	–	+++	+	–
Others (merbarone, fostriecin, bis-2,6-dioxopiperazines)	–	+++	–	–

m-AMSA, Amsacrine.

Platinum Analogs

During a study of the effects of electric current on growing bacteria, the antibacterial and, later, the antitumor activities of the platinum compounds were fortuitously discovered. The antitumor agent cisplatin, its cis-carboxylester analog, carboplatin, and the diaminocyclohexane-containing oxaliplatin, are heavy metal platinum complexes. They are activated when one of their ligands (cisplatin; chloride and carboplatin; carboxylester) is displaced by water, leading to the formation of positively charged aquated platinum complexes, allowing platinum to stably bind DNA, RNA, proteins, or other critical biomacromolecules (see Fig. 55-2). With DNA, platinum complexes form covalent links to the N^7 position of guanine and adenine. The N^7 adducts at d(GpG) or d(ApG) result in intrastrand or interstrand DNA cross-links that bend the DNA helix and inhibit DNA synthesis. The cytotoxicity of platinum analogs correlates with the total platinum binding to DNA, as well as with the intrastrand or interstrand cross-links. This results in DNA damage, which triggers apoptosis of sensitive cells.

Cisplatin, carboplatin, and oxaliplatin are used in the treatment of refractory lymphomas as part of high-dose and intensification therapy.

Miscellaneous Agents

Among the agents included in this category, only plicamycin, bleomycin, procarbazine, L-asparaginase, gallium nitrate, and glucocorticoids are of current interest to hematologists; these are discussed in Appendix 55-6.

Targeted Agents

Imatinib Mesylate and Other BCR/ABL Kinase Inhibitors

Imatinib mesylate (formerly CFP57148; Gleevec; STI571) is a phenylaminopyrimidine developed as an inhibitor of the aberrant tyrosine kinase BCR-ABL, expressed in the leukemic cells of most patients with CML (see Chapter 66). The role of the BCR-ABL kinase in the pathogenesis of CML and its use in CML treatment are discussed in further detail in Chapter 69.

Imatinib mesylate represents the prototypical molecularly targeted agent belonging to the class of signal transduction inhibitors and exerts its action through direct inhibition of the BCR-ABL kinase, expressed in CML but not in normal cells. Imatinib mesylate is not absolutely specific for the BCR-ABL kinase because it also inhibits other kinases, including KIT (formerly designated c-KIT), PDGF, stem cell factor (SCF), and TEL-ARG. Radiographic crystallography studies revealed that imatinib mesylate competitively binds to the ATP-binding site of the Abl kinase and stabilizes it in an inactive conformation. The 50% inhibitory concentration (IC_{50}) of imatinib mesylate for BCR-ABL is in the submicromolar range and is substantially lower than the supramicromolar levels achievable in the plasma of patients receiving the drug by the PO route.

Exposure of BCR-ABL$^+$ leukemic cells to imatinib mesylate not only blocks their proliferation but also induces apoptosis. This finding suggests that CML cells have become "addicted" to constitutive activation of BCR-ABL for their survival. This is believed to be secondary to activation of a large number of downstream survival pathways, including those related to STAT5A (signal transducer and activator of transcription 5A, previously designated STAT5), MEK/extracellular signal-regulated kinase (ERK), NFκB, AKT, and Bcl-xL, among others. In addition to promoting survival in BCR-ABL$^+$ cells, activation of these pathways also confers resistance to conventional cytotoxic drugs.

Despite the success of imatinib mesylate in the treatment of chronic phase CML and, to a lesser extent, accelerated or blast phase CML, the preexistence or development of resistance represents a major therapeutic challenge that can occur at any stage of the disease. Primary or secondary resistance can develop through a variety of mechanisms.[5] BCR-ABL–dependent mechanisms correspond to the emergence of mutations in ABL kinase domain, which can be located in the imatinib-binding site, the P loop, the catalytic domain, or the activation loop. Many of these mutations are present at the time of diagnosis, and resistant clones emerge after exposure to imatinib. Resistance mechanisms independent of BCR-ABL include development of multidrug resistance mechanisms (e.g., P-gp related); decreased levels of human organic cation transporter (hOCT-1); acquisition of additional genetics abnormalities (clonal evolution), including acquisition of an additional Philadelphia chromosome, trisomy 8, and isochromosome 17q; increased expression of the BCR-ABL protein; and SRC kinase overexpression.

One logical approach to enhancing imatinib mesylate activity or overcoming resistance, or both, is to combine it with more conventional cytotoxic agents, including ara-C, interferon, and others. The combination of imatinib mesylate with pegylated interferon resulted in higher rates of major molecular response (MMR) than standard dose imatinib, albeit with increased toxicity, including rash, depression, and cytopenias. The combination of imatinib and cytarabine resulted in similar response rates and was associated with higher rates of toxicity. Longer follow-up is needed to determine whether the improved response observed with imatinib combined with interferon results in higher survival rates. Use of imatinib doses higher than 400 mg/day was explored in several large randomized clinical trials, with higher doses achieving confirmed complete cytogenetic and major molecular responses more rapidly but without a clear survival benefit.

Imatinib also has activity in diseases dependent on other kinases, such as PDGF receptor A (PDGFRA), PDGFRB, or Kit, and is active against myeloproliferative neoplasms associated with eosinophilia and FIP1L1/PDGFRA or PDGFRB fusion genes, as well as against systemic mastocytosis without KIT^{D816V} mutation (see Chapter 66).

Dasatinib

Dasatinib is a second-generation Abl kinase inhibitor approved for the treatment of patients with CML. Dasatinib is a PO multikinase inhibitor, affecting Abl, Kit, PDGFR, and Src kinases. It binds the ATP-binding site of Abl in opposite direction than imatinib, can inhibit active and inactive forms of the kinase, and requires fewer points of contact. Compared with imatinib, dasatinib is several hundred times a more potent inhibitor of Abl. Initial studies demonstrated dasatinib induced responses in patients who had developed resistance to imatinib who are treated in the chronic, accelerated and blast phase of CML. A recent large phase III randomized trial compared dasatinib and imatinib as initial therapy for chronic phase CML and observed that dasatinib therapy led to deeper and more rapid responses, albeit with no differences in survival outcomes.[6] As a multikinase inhibitor, it has a broader and alternative toxicity profile, with pulmonary edema, pleural effusions, and thrombocytopenia being the more frequent adverse effects. Recently, higher rates of pulmonary hypertension have been observed in patients receiving dasatinib. There is a high response rate in patients with wild-type sequences of BCR-ALB and in patients with mutations in the Abl protein, conferring resistance to imatinib, with the exception of the T315I mutation. Dasatinib is approved in two doses: 70 mg twice daily and 100 mg once daily for chronic phase and 70 mg twice daily or 140 mg once daily for accelerated phase. Once-daily dosing achieved comparable efficacy with less toxicity (see Chapter 66).

Nilotinib

Nilotinib is the other second-generation Abl kinase inhibitor approved for treatment of patients with CML (see Chapter 66). Nilotinib has increased affinity for the Abl kinase compared with imatinib, binding with an improved topologic fit to the kinase site in its inactive form.[7] Nilotinib is active in chronic and accelerated phase CML patients who have developed resistance to imatinib. As with dasatinib, nilotinib was compared with imatinib in a phase III randomized trial as initial therapy for chronic phase CML patients, with nilotinib achieving higher rates of complete cytogenetic and major molecular responses and with fewer cases of disease progression or clonal evolution in the nilotinib-treated cohorts. Survival outcomes were similar in all arms. Common adverse events with nilotinib included rash, gastrointestinal disturbances (nausea, vomiting, diarrhea), neutropenia, and thrombocytopenia. Pleural effusion and peripheral edema are less common than with dasatinib. In addition, QT prolongation and a risk of pancreatitis are serious side effects of nilotinib.

Bruton Tyrosine Kinase Inhibitors

Bruton tyrosine kinase (Btk) is a cytoplasmic tyrosine kinase with a well-defined role in B-cell receptor signaling that is fundamental in B-lymphocyte development, differentiation, and signaling. Btk is a member of the Tec family of kinases (see Chapter 76). Activation of Btk triggers a cascade of signaling events that culminates in the generation of calcium mobilization and fluxes, cytoskeletal rearrangements, and transcriptional regulation of NFκB and nuclear factor of activated T cells (NFAT).[8] Ibrutinib (PCI-32765) is a first-in-class, selective, irreversible, small molecule inhibitor of Btk. Ibrutinib binds covalently to a cysteine (Cys 481) in the Btk active site, with potent and irreversible enzymatic activity. Early clinical trials have demonstrated a favorable toxicity profile with remarkable clinical activity in patients with relapsed CLL.

An early transient phase of lymphocytosis followed by resolution was associated with response in CLL and mantle cell lymphoma patients. Serious adverse events associated with PCI-32765 occurred in approximately 10% of patients, with rash and febrile neutropenia as reported events. Rare cases of serious bleeding were reported. Dosing has not yet been established, and ibrutinib has not to date received FDA approval. Tested doses were 420 mg and 840 mg/day, with both doses having similar efficacy.

PI3K/AKT Inhibitors

The PI3K/AKT (PKB) pathway is involved in the regulation of diverse cellular functions, including cell growth, protein synthesis, cell cycle regulation, glucose metabolism, and motility. PI3K catalyzes the conversion of phosphatidylinositol diphosphate to phosphatidylinositol triphosphate, which activates, through PDK1, the phosphorylation and activation of the serine/threonine kinase AKT. The dual-specific phosphatase and tensin homologue (PTEN) opposes the actions of PI3K and is mutated in many cancers. Activation of AKT signals to multiple downstream targets, and generally results in prosurvival actions. Targets of AKT involve proteins involved in cell survival (e.g., Bad, procaspase 9, CREB, forkhead transcription factors [FHKR], IB), cell cycle regulation ($p21^{CIP1}$, $p27^{KIP1}$, cyclin D_1), glycogen synthesis (GSK3), and protein synthesis (FRAP1, $p70^{S6K}$). Because of the frequency of PTEN mutations in transformed cells and the dependence of numerous cancers on an intact PI3K/AKT pathway for survival, the PI3K/AKT cascade has become an attractive target for therapeutic intervention.

In addition, evidence indicates that dysregulation of the PI3K/AKT pathway is a key proliferative pathway in hematologic malignancies. For example, the fusion protein nucleophosmin/anaplastic large cell lymphoma (NP-ALK) constitutively activates the PI3K/AKT cascade and has been shown to play a functional role in NP-ALK–related transformation. Constitutive activation of AKT plays a pathogenetic role in mantle cell lymphoma.[9] In vitro studies with the AKT inhibitors wortmannin and LY294002 have resulted in apoptosis of mantle cell lymphoma cell lines.

PI3K Inhibitors

CAL-101 (GS 1101) is a highly selective inhibitor of the p110d isoform of PI3K (PI3Kδ), an isoform of PI3K that is expressed selectively in hematopoietic cells. CAL-101 has been shown to have in vitro activity against lymphoid cell lines and primary CLL cells (see Chapter 76). CAL-101 inhibits not only B-cell receptor signaling pathway–induced survival signals but also appears to disrupt the effects of microenvironmental signals on neoplastic cells,[10] affecting chemotaxis of tumor cells, which could explain the transient lymphocytosis observed after treatment of CLL patients with CAL-101. Clinical trials have shown that CAL-101 is active in treating patients with relapsed CLL and other relapsed lymphoid malignancies. The most common dose-limiting toxicity was elevation of tests measuring liver function. Dose escalation and dose response assessments support use of the 150 mg twice daily dose schedule. Ongoing trials include combinations of CAL-101 and rituximab or bendamustine.

AKT Inhibitors

The frequent presence of AKT abnormalities in human neoplasms makes this enzyme an attractive target for potential novel treatment strategies. Several drugs have been developed using dephosphorylation of the active enzyme, ATP competition, or allosteric inhibition of the enzyme as strategies for targeting AKT. These agents have, however, shown modest activity and some have been associated with significant toxicity. Perifosine, a synthetic PO alkylphospholipid, inhibits AKT by targeting the lipid-binding domain of AKT, which is essential for membrane translocation and subsequent activation of the enzyme. Early trials showed that perifosine had modest clinical activity as a single agent in patients with Waldenström macroglobulinemia and in patients with myeloma alone or in combination with bortezomib. A phase III study of perifosine plus bortezomib and dexamethasone for treatment of plasma cell myeloma is underway.

Janus Kinase 2 Inhibitors

Janus kinase 2 is a nonreceptor tyrosine kinase that plays a central role in the transduction of differentiation and proliferation signals in hematopoietic progenitor cells. Ligand-binding to surface receptors for hematopoietic growth factors leads to phosphorylation of JAK2 with subsequent activation of transcription factors in the JAK/STAT pathway, including STAT3 and STAT5 (see Chapters 67 to 69). Identification of the JAKV617F mutation in patients with myeloproliferative neoplasms, including polycythemia vera, essential thrombocytosis, and primary myelofibrosis (PMF), represented a fundamental step in understanding the pathophysiology of these disorders. The genetic abnormality corresponds to a point mutation in nucleotide 1849 of the molecule, where guanine replaces thiamine, resulting in substitution of a valine for phenylalanine in the JH2 pseudokinase autoinhibitory domain of the molecule. The result is either hypersensitivity to cytokine signals or constitutive activation of the kinase. Development of JAK2 inhibitors followed as a rational, targeted therapeutic strategy for these neoplasms (see Chapters 67 to 69).

Ruxolitinib (INCB018424) is a small molecule inhibitor of JAK1 and JAK2, and the first-in-class JAK inhibitor to receive FDA approval for treatment of intermediate and high-risk myelofibrosis[11,12] (see Chapters 67 to 69). It exerts its inhibitory activity through competitive inhibition of the kinase's ATP-binding catalytic site. In preclinical studies, JAK1/2 inhibition with ruxolitinib decreased STAT3/5 signaling both in wild-type cells and those carrying JAKV617F. In the initial phase I/II study, the maximum tolerated dose was 25 mg when given twice daily and 100 mg on once-daily dosing. The most common side effect was myelosuppression, primarily thrombocytopenia. After only 3 months of therapy, 44% of patients with splenomegaly experienced a reduction of more than 50%. Responses were observed in patients with carriers of the JAKV617F mutation as well as those with wild-type JAK2. Importantly, the majority of patients experienced a decrease in constitutional symptoms and improved exercise tolerance and performance status as well as weight gain. Of concern are subsequent observation of rapid redevelopment of splenomegaly as well as the reported development of life-threatening syndromes when the agent was discontinued abruptly.

The COMFORT I and II randomized controlled clinical trials compared the efficacy of ruxolitinib for treatment of patients with intermediate- and high-risk myelofibrosis with either placebo or best available therapy, respectively. Both trials reached their primary end point with spleen volume reduction rates markedly superior with ruxolitinib (see Chapters 67 to 69). A survival benefit was observed when compared with placebo, but no progression-free survival (PFS), overall survival (OS), or leukemia-free survival was observed when compared with the best available therapy. Of note, treatment with ruxolitinib was not effective in reversing histologic, cytogenetic, or molecular abnormalities in peripheral blood or BM, suggesting that this agent may not be curative. Longer follow-up is needed to determine whether a survival benefit is present when ruxolitinib is used instead of other conventional agents. An ongoing phase III trial is comparing ruxolitinib with the best available treatment in patients with hydroxyurea-resistant polycythemia vera requiring phlebotomy.

A phase II trial from MD Anderson Cancer Center examined the role of ruxolitinib at a dose of 25 mg orally twice daily for the treatment of patients with relapsed or refractory AML (de novo or secondary to myeloproliferative neoplasms), MDS, ALL, or CML either in blast phase or resistant to tyrosine kinase inhibitors (TKIs). Ruxolitinib was very well tolerated, with only 4 out of 38 patients experiencing grade 3 or greater toxicities. Three patients achieved CR (CR = 08032; CRi = 1); these patients all had AML secondary to myeloproliferative neoplasms, and two were positive for the JAKV617F mutation. Further studies of combinations of ruxolitinib with hypomethylating agents are planned.

Other JAK2 Inhibitors

SB1518, also known as ONYX, is a JAK2 inhibitor with activity against the wild-type kinase as well as the JAKV617F mutated kinase; it also inhibits FLT3. It achieves high rates of reduction in spleen volume. The tested dose is 400 mg/day. The main side effects are gastrointestinal, predominantly diarrhea, nausea, and vomiting, with no hematologic toxicity observed.

CYT387 is a PO multikinase inhibitor, affecting JAK1/2, TYK2, TBK1, PRKD1, ROCK2, PRKCN, MAPK8 (mitogen-activated protein kinase 8), and CDK2/cyclin A. Early trials in myelofibrosis patients resulted in decreased splenomegaly and improvement in symptoms in the majority of patients treated. Of note, more than one-third of patients with improved splenomegaly had previously been treated with ruxolitinib. The most common side effects included myelosuppression (grade 3/4 thrombocytopenia in 22%; anemia in 3%). Nonhematologic side effects included headache, QTc prolongation, and abnormal liver test results. The maximum tolerated dose has been established at 300 mg/day given continuously in 28-day cycles.

TG 01348 is a multikinase inhibitor with activity against JAK2, FLT3, and RET. The maximum tolerated dose has been established at 680 mg/day. In a phase I study performed in intermediate- and high-risk PMF patients, a large proportion achieved spleen volume reduction, with symptom improvement as well as normalization of thrombocytosis and leukocytosis. Hematologic toxicities, including anemia and thrombocytopenia, were common. The most frequent nonhematologic toxicities were gastrointestinal disturbances.

Hypomethylating Agents

Promoter methylation within CpG islands regulates gene expression in all cells. Disruption of normal gene expression profiles accompanies malignant transformation, giving rise to complex patterns of gene expression. As a consequence, promoters of many genes have an altered pattern of methylation, resulting in either gene activation or gene repression. The link between these concepts and the interest in agents that alter promoter methylation began with the realization that azacytidine, an agent used sparingly for treating myeloid leukemias, had efficacy when given at low doses either intravenously or subcutaneously for extended periods of time and that in these cases, altered gene expression accompanied responses. Both azacytidine and 5-aza-2′-deoxycytidine (decitabine) act by irreversible inhibition of the DNA methyltransferases responsible for methylation of the cytidine in CpG islands and are thus S phase–specific agents. Wijermans et al first described that a related compound, 5-aza-2′-deoxycytidine, was effective when given as a continuous infusion to elderly patients with high-risk MDS, with a 54% response rate. The mechanism of action included both a direct change in promoter methylation and independent changes, with up to 70% genome-wide demethylation, suggesting either that genes with altered expression either up- or downregulated a second set of genes through altered pathways such as induction of WAFp21, p15, and p16 or in a more direct fashion through altered transcription factor expression. More recent studies have identified activity of these agents in both AML and CML. Most often, partial responses or short-lived complete responses are seen in AML with complete responses more common in MDS. Recent studies also describe a number of extended therapy regimens. Kantarjian et al reported a comparison of 20 mg/m^2 decitabine intravenously for 5 days with 20 mg/m^2 subcutaneously daily for 5 days and 10 mg/m^2 intravenously for 10 days. The 5-day IV dose schedule was judged superior on the basis of clinical outcome with 39% CR, a higher proportion of reactivation of p15, and achievement of a hypomethylation state as well as clinical tolerance.

Ubiquitin–Proteasome Inhibitors

The 26S proteasome is the central proteolytic machinery of the highly conserved ubiquitin proteasome system. In eukaryotic cells, whereas the lysosomal pathway degrades extracellular proteins imported into the cell through endocytosis or pinocytosis, the proteasome controls the degradation of intracellular proteins. Numerous studies have demonstrated that the ubiquitin–proteasome system controls basic cellular functions such as cell cycle progression, signal transduction, and programmed cell death, hence the interest in therapeutic interventions that manipulate proteasomal activity and potentially restore cellular homeostasis into transformed cells (see Chapter 85).

Ubiquitin is a highly conserved 76-amino-acid polypeptide that is expressed in all eukaryotic cells. Under the sequential action of E1 (ubiquitin-activating enzyme), E2 (ubiquitin-conjugating enzyme), and E3 (ubiquitin ligase), ubiquitin is activated and covalently conjugated to potential proteasome substrates via an isopeptide bond between the C-terminal glycine residue of ubiquitin and the ε-amino group of internal lysine residues in target proteins. The same set of enzymes also catalyzes the formation of the isopeptide bond between G76 and the lysine residue (K48) of previously conjugated ubiquitin, leading to formation of a polyubiquitin chain. Polyubiquitinated substrates are usually targeted for proteasomal degradation.

The 26S proteasome is a large (2000-kd) threonine protease present in the nucleus and cytoplasm of all eukaryotic cells. This ATP-dependent, multicatalytic protease eliminates damaged or misfolded proteins and regulates cyclins and CDK inhibitor cell cycle regulatory proteins as well as other proteins that govern the transcription factor activation, apoptosis, and cell trafficking. Its structure consists of two parts: the 20S core and the 19S cap regulatory particle (Fig. 55-6). The 19S cap is involved in the recognition, binding, and unfolding of ubiquitinated proteins and in the regulation of the opening of the 20S core. The 20S core is a cylinder composed of four stacked heptameric rings, each containing seven different α or β subunits ($\alpha7\beta7\beta7\alpha7$) (Figs. 55-6 and 55-7). Three different active sites are located inside the cylindrical core within the β-subunit rings. At least three distinct proteolytic activities are associated with the proteasome: chymotryptic, tryptic, and peptidylglutamyl. After release from the substrate, the polyubiquitin chain is hydrolyzed into single ubiquitin moieties, and tagged proteins are degraded to small peptides. Both the assembly of the 26S proteasome and the degradation of protein substrates are ATP dependent.

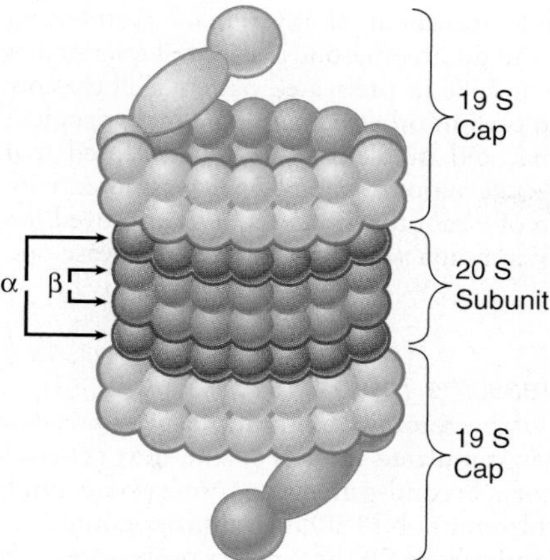

Figure 55-6 26S PROTEASOME.

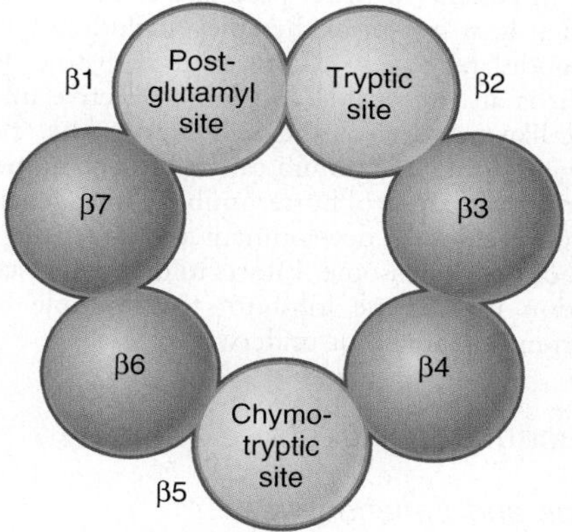

Figure 55-7 CROSS SECTION OF BETA RING OF THE 20S CORE OF THE 26S PROTEASOME.

Transformed cells are much more sensitive to blockade of the proteasome than are normal cells; the exact mechanism of this selective susceptibility is not fully understood. Early studies revealed that proteasomes are abnormally highly expressed in rapidly growing metazoan embryonic and human neoplastic cells but not in their well-differentiated and normal proliferating cells. The selectivity of proteasome inhibitors is not solely dependent on proliferative status because both transformed and normal fibroblasts have similar growth rates, although proteasome inhibitors are selectively toxic to SV-40–transformed cells. Cyclins A, B, D, and E; CDK inhibitors (p21, p27); inhibitory proteins (I-kB); oncogenes *(FOS, MYC);* and tumor suppressors (e.g., cyclin B1, p21WAF1/CIP1, p27, p53) are known substrates for the ubiquitin–proteasome pathway. The specificity of the ubiquitin proteasome is such that the degradation of individual substrates can be upregulated without affecting the proteolysis of others. Different classes of proteasome inhibitors have been identified and include peptide aldehydes (MG132, PSI, LLnV, ALLN, CEP1612, Z-LLF), streptomyces metabolite (lactacystin), dipeptidyl boronic acid bortezomib, vinyl sulfone tripeptides (NLVS), and natural products such as epoxomycin.

Proteosome Targeted Agents (Bortezomib)

Bortezomib (pyrazylcarbonyl-Phe-Leu-boronate), the first in this class of agents to enter clinical trials, is a dipeptidyl boronic acid that is a specific and selective inhibitor of the 26S proteasome. The Boron atom interacts reversibly with the catalytic threonine residue of the proteasome, primarily inhibiting its chymotrypsin-like activity. The inhibition of the ubiquitin–proteasome pathway with bortezomib was demonstrated to arrest the growth of malignant cells (breast, colon, prostate tumor cell lines, Burkitt lymphoma, adult T-cell leukemia, Lewis lung carcinoma, CLL, and myeloma cell lines) and sensitize them to chemotherapeutic agents (5-fluorouracil, cisplatin, taxol, doxorubicin, CPT-11, and gemcitabine). Bortezomib mediates these effects through multiple mechanisms by regulating the expression of proteins involved in cell cycle progression ($P21^{cip1}$, $P27^{Kip1}$), oncogenesis (P53, I-kB), apoptosis (BCL2, BIRC2, BIRC3, BIRC4, BAX), and more recently DNA repair (DNA-PKcs, ATM). Loss of I-kB destabilizes NFκB, reducing expression of a critical plasma cell cytokine stimulatory molecule, interleukin-6 (IL-6) (see Chapter 85). The process of cell death appears to be p53-independent and to result in mitotic catastrophe, although the classical caspase 8–dependent apoptosis pathway has also been implicated. A recent study found a strong correlation between immunoglobulin production and apoptotic sensitivity to bortezomib, suggesting that the active requirement for protein folding in the endoplasmic reticulum (ER) provides a direct target and explains sensitivity to proteasome inhibition. It also suggests a selective mechanism that could explain the emergence of less differentiated myeloma cells with decreased immunoglobulin production during treatment. These processes also increase oxidative stress and contribute to apoptotic signaling, explaining the sensitivity of myeloma cells to proteasome inhibition.

Preclinical Studies With Bortezomib. Screening of the NCI tumor cell lines revealed that bortezomib is active against a broad range of tumor types. The average growth inhibition of 50% (GI_{50}) value for bortezomib across the entire NCI cell panel (60 human-derived cell lines) was 7 nM. Among solid tumor cell lines, those of the prostate, breast, colon, and pancreas were exquisitely sensitive to proteasomal inhibition. PC-3 prostate carcinoma cells, treated with bortezomib, underwent growth arrest in G2-M phase with a parallel increase in P21 levels and decreased activity but not the levels of CDK-4. Bortezomib treatment also led to caspase activation, PARP cleavage, and apoptotic cell death with an IC_{50} of 20 nM. Bortezomib exhibited synergistic effects when combined with SN-38 and radiation against colon tumor cells and in mouse xenografts. Similarly, pancreatic tumor xenografts were sensitive to the cytotoxic effect of bortezomib, particularly when combined with gemcitabine or CPT-11. Cytotoxic activity was reported as well against Lewis lung carcinoma cells and nasopharyngeal squamous cell carcinoma cells. In most of these studies, an increase in the cellular levels of P21WAF1, P27KIP1, P53, and I-kB was observed.

In hematologic malignancies, proteasome inhibitors exhibited cytotoxic activity in a wide range of cell lines, including multiple myeloma, U937 human monocytic leukemia, HL-60 promyelocytic leukemia, Jurkat T-cell leukemia, K562 CML, Ramos Burkitt lymphoma, and primary B-cell CLL. In multiple myeloma cells, bortezomib induced p53 and MDM2 protein expression, induced phosphorylation (Ser15) of p53 protein, and activated JUN NH2-terminal kinase (JNK), which in turn activated caspase 8 and caspase 3. Bortezomib was also shown to activate the intrinsic (mitochondria–cytochrome C–caspase 9) and extrinsic (JNK–death receptor-activated caspase 8) apoptotic pathways of the myeloma cells. Bortezomib blocked tumor necrosis factor (TNF)–induced NFκB activation through inhibition of IkB degradation. TNF-induced intracellular adhesion molecule (ICAM)-1 expression on RPMI8226 and MM.1S cells was also inhibited. The unfolded protein response not only is increased in plasma cells producing large quantities of immunoglobulin but also induces a stress apoptosis response. Bortezomib also induces osteoblast activity through the Runx2/Cbfa2 pathway. Furthermore, bortezomib inhibits RANKL-induced osteoclastogenesis through inhibition of P38 kinase. Increased osteoblast activity has the potential to restore the clinical osteoporosis associated with multiple myeloma when used with or without bisphosphonates. Moreover, it prevented the adherence of myeloma cells to BM stromal cells and the NFκB-dependent production of IL-6. Importantly, bortezomib demonstrated synergistic activity with dexamethasone, thalidomide, melphalan, and doxorubicin and did not appear to be a substrate for multidrug-resistance transporters. However, the NFκB blockade could not account for all of the antimyeloma activity of bortezomib, and other mechanisms clearly contribute to its antineoplastic effects. Finally, an IC_{50} concentration of bortezomib in myeloma cells had no effect on peripheral blood mononuclear cells from healthy volunteers and did not affect cultured BM stromal cells. This did not preclude the observation of myelosuppression during treatment of patients with bortezomib as a single agent.

Pharmacology of Bortezomib. Bortezomib is primarily metabolized through cytochrome P450 (CYP) and not via phase II pathways (e.g., glucuronidation and sulfation). In vitro studies indicated that the primary metabolic pathway is deboronation mediated by CYP3A4. Bortezomib was also metabolized by CYP2D6, but the rate of metabolism was slower than that observed with CYP3A4. Deboronated metabolites have been shown to be inactive in the 20S proteasome assay. Bortezomib rapidly exits the plasma compartment with more than 90% cleared within 15 minutes of IV administration. In whole-body autoradiography of [^{14}C] boretezomib-treated rats, the central nervous system, testes, and eyes appeared to be protected from bortezomib. Bortezomib specifically and selectively inhibits proteasome function by binding tightly (K_i >0.6 nM) and reversibly to the enzyme's chymotrypsin-like site. In ex vivo 20S proteasome activity bioassays, the proteasome was inhibited within 1 hour of bortezomib administration, and baseline proteasome activity was restored within 48 to 72 hours. Intermittent but high inhibition (>70%) of proteasome activity was better tolerated than sustained inhibition. Thus a twice-weekly clinical dosing regimen is better tolerated. Nonetheless, this dose schedule is often associated with significant myelosuppression and onset of peripheral neuropathy. Reducing the dose schedule to a weekly regimen ameliorates these toxicities and appears to increase patient tolerance without jeopardizing clinical efficacy.

Clinical Studies With Bortezomib. In several phase I clinical studies, antitumor activity was reported in patients with squamous cell carcinoma of the nasopharynx, bronchoalveolar carcinoma, renal cell carcinoma, prostate cancer, NHL, and multiple myeloma. Richardson and coworkers reported on the activity of bortezomib in the treatment of relapsed and refractory myeloma patients. In a large, multicenter, nonrandomized phase II study, 202 patients were treated with a bolus IV infusion of bortezomib (1.3 mg/m^2). Of the 202 patients, 27% achieved a complete or partial response as defined by the Blade criteria; an additional 7% achieved a minimal response. The median time to response was 1.3 months, and the median time to progression among patients who achieved a partial or complete response was 13 months. The median survival time among all patients was 16 months. In a multivariate analysis, only age and the percentage of plasma cells in the BM at the time of enrollment predicated response to bortezomib. A recent study further defines the safety of using bortezomib in older patients with myeloma. The most common grade 3 to 4 adverse events were thrombocytopenia (31%), fatigue (12%), neuropathy (12%), and neutropenia (14%). The thrombocytopenia, although significant with a mean decrease of more than 60%, was rapidly reversible and associated with a shortened platelet survival rather than a direct toxic effect on megakaryocytes. The randomized phase III clinical trial compared bortezomib with dexamethasone and indicated that there was a significant advantage for bortezomib-treated patients. A response rate of 38% was seen with a greater than median 6-month time to progression. A second trial added dexamethasone after 2 cycles of bortezomib with an overall response rate of 88%. Additional clinical trials have shown the efficacy of bortezomib in multiple myeloma in combination with other cytotoxic agents, including dexamethasone, melphalan, liposomal doxorubicin, lenalidomide, and thalidomide (see Chapter 85). A recent study showed a significantly prolonged time to disease progression in patients with myeloma who had undergone at least one prior treatment regimen of bortezomib plus liposomal doxorubicin (Doxil) compared with bortezomib alone. The combination of melphalan and bortezomib is well tolerated, with an overall response rate of 68% in pretreated patients, and based on positive results from a phase III study by San Miguel et al, the combination of bortezomib with melphalan and prednisone has received FDA approval for use in the frontline treatment of myeloma.[13] Combining bortezomib, thalidomide, and dexamethasone is also well tolerated, with an overall response rate of 53% in pretreated patients. These combinations are also being explored in other hematologic malignancies (CLL, mantle cell lymphoma, and indolent NHL). In relapsed mantle cell lymphoma, an overall response rate of 33% was noted with a mean time to progression of 9 months; its use is FDA approved for patients with mantle cell lymphoma who have received at least one prior line of therapy.

Newer Proteasome Inhibitors

The success of bortezomib in multiple myeloma and mantle cell lymphoma has stimulated interest in the next generation of proteasome inhibitors. Second-generation proteasome inhibitors include PR-171 (carfilzomib), NPI-0052 (salinosporamide A, marizomib), MLN 9708, and others. Of these newer proteasome inhibitors, carfilzomib (see Chapter 85) is furthest along in clinical development and based on positive results of two phase II trials, was approved by the FDA for use in patients with relapsed and refractory myeloma who have received at least two prior therapies, including bortezomib and an immunomodulatory agent. Carfilzomib is distinct from bortezomib in that it is an irreversible and more selective inhibitor of the chymotryptic-like protease of the 26S proteasome. Because it has fewer off-target effects, carfilzomib causes little or no neuropathy, an often dose-limiting toxicity of bortezomib.[14] Third-generation proteasome inhibitors are now in development and target the regulatory, or 19S subunit, of the proteasome. Efforts to define the activity of these next generation proteasome inhibitors in multiple myeloma and NHL are currently planned or underway.

Immunomodulatory Agents

Thalidomide and Lenalidomide

The related compounds thalidomide and lenalidomide provide effective PO immunomodulatory (see Chapters 69 and 85) therapy for patients with multiple myeloma. They have complex mechanisms of action. Further details on their therapeutic impact are found in Chapters 69 and 85.

Thalidomide has been in clinical use for more than 50 years and has well-documented and sometimes serious side effects, including severe birth defects, somnolence, an axonal length-dependent peripheral neuropathy, orthostatic hypotension, neutropenia, bradycardia and occasional heart block, and increased HIV load in HIV-positive patients. The risk of developing thrombotic events is elevated in patients taking either agent, giving rise to the recommended use of an anticoagulant regimen such as aspirin, low-molecular-weight heparin or Coumadin. Experimental studies have identified that thalidomide reduces expression of the cellular inhibitor of apoptosis protein and potentiates proapoptotic processes such as TRAIL (TNF-related apoptosis-inducing ligand)/po2L. Thalidomide also reduces NFκB and I-kB expression, thereby reducing IL-6 expression. In addition, thalidomide decreases vascular endothelial growth factor (VEGF) and reduces angiogenesis and vessel density in the BM of patients with multiple myeloma. The lack of a simple mechanism of action has been confusing because it is unclear which, if any, biomarker is an appropriate correlate for clinical success or toxicity. Nonetheless, efficacy is certainly seen clinically and validated in SCID models of human myeloma. Data also point to its potential clinical efficacy in patients with solid tumors and MDS.[15]

Lenalidomide was identified as an analog of thalidomide with more potent immunomodulatory functions but fewer side effects, and it has emerged as a more potent agent. Both have similar anti-angiogenic properties, block IL-6 production, and reduce NFκB and I-kB levels. Lenalidomide also induces caspase 8–mediated apoptosis and mitochondrial-mediated cell death. In addition, lenalidomide induces T-cell activation and NK activity, providing some measure of anticancer immune response. It leads to a similar and dose-dependent peripheral neuropathy as thalidomide and more significant BM suppression, which can be dose limiting. It is also associated with a significant increased risk of thrombosis, leading to recommendations for the use of anticoagulation in this population.[16] Hypersensitivity rash occurs in up to 10% of patients. However, a variety of dose schedules provide a flexible therapeutic approach and a high response rate in relapsed myeloma patients with an overall response rate of 25% and median OS of 28 months. Excellent results were seen, with 31 of 34 patients achieving an objective response combining lenalidomide 25 mg/m^2 for 21 days and dexamethasone 40 mg daily for 4 days on days 1, 9, 17, of the 28-day cycle. Both thalidomide and lenalidomide are under evaluation for the treatment of primary amyloidosis, MDS, CLL, and solid tumors. In amyloidosis, the combination of lenalidomide and dexamethasone is a well-tolerated regimen with an overall response rate of 67%, including complete hematologic remissions. Lenalidomide has been approved by the FDA for the treatment of 5q minus MDS based on studies indicating more than a 40% response rate owing to the rate of transfusion independence that occurred in this group of patients (see Chapter 59). In a randomized trial of patients with relapsed or refractory multiple myeloma comparing dexamethasone and lenalidomide with dexamethasone alone, a much higher and sustained response rate of 58% was observed. Effective dose ranges appear to be 5 to 25 mg daily for 21 days of a 4-week cycle, with a range of patient tolerance and adverse reactions that in large part are dose dependent.

Agents in Development

The newer drugs in the class of immunomodulatory agents have been designed to increase efficacy and improve the toxicity profile.

The newest drug immunomodulatory agent to enter development is pomalidomide (see Chapters 69 and 85). Pomalidomide has a mechanism of action similar to those of thalidomide and lenalidomide but demonstrates efficacy in treating relapsed and refractory myeloma patients, including patients who have previously failed treatment with thalidomide, lenalidomide, and bortezomib. Phase I studies have shown the drug to be well tolerated in doses ranging from 1 to 5 mg/day orally. Interrupted dosing may help with mitigating drug-induced cytopenias. Results of a phase II study combining pomalidomide with dexamethasone in patients with relapsed myeloma showed an encouraging overall response rate of 63% (partial response or better), including 60% of patients who were refractory to bortezomib and 40% of patients who were refractory to lenalidomide.[17]

TARGETING APOPTOSIS SIGNALING IN HEMATOLOGIC MALIGNANCIES

The processes of cell division and cell death are tightly coupled so that a net increase in cell numbers does not occur. Alterations in the expression or function of the genes controlling cell division and cell death can upset this delicate balance and are hallmarks of cancer. Although conventional anticancer drugs cause cell cycle perturbation or DNA damage, they do not directly interact with the intracellular machinery involved in apoptosis. Tumor selectivity of conventional agents is largely caused by the increased sensitivity to apoptosis of tumor cells after DNA damage or cell cycle perturbation. Novel therapeutic agents or strategies that target critical regulators or effectors of apoptosis are under development and clinical testing, and these agents or strategies have the potential to exert selective cytotoxicity against cancer cells.

Caspases are the "executioners" for apoptosis. They are proteases that exist as inactive zymogens and are activated by proteolytic cleavage of their proforms in response to a variety of death stimuli (explained in the next section). This processing occurs at conserved aspartic acid residues, thus generating the enzymatically active caspases. Caspase activation is organized as a cascade, with an upstream initiator and downstream effector caspase. Upstream initiator caspases contain large prodomains that interact with specific proteins involved in triggering the cascade. The downstream caspases, which function as the ultimate effectors of apoptosis, possess small prodomains and are activated predominantly by proteolytic cleavage by upstream caspases. The irreversible cleavage of specific protein death substrates by the downstream effector caspases directly or indirectly accounts for the biochemical and morphologic changes that are recognized as apoptosis.

At least three pathways of caspase activation leading to apoptosis have been identified (Fig. 55-8): (1) the receptor-initiated apoptosis pathway, where the TNF family of cytokine receptors activate initiator caspases such as caspase 8; (2) the mitochondria-initiated apoptosis pathway, where cytochrome C and other pro-death effectors are released from mitochondria into cytosol that results in activation of caspase 9; and (3) a pathway of caspase activation, which involves a serine protease, granzyme B, that directly cleaves and activates several caspases, including procaspase 3.

Proapoptotic Targets of Anticancer Agents

Most cancer cells have active antiapoptotic pathways that prevent cell death in response to growth, checkpoint, DNA damage, and metabolic stimuli. A number of current anticancer agents in development target these pathways and are designed to be effective alone or in combination with other agents that disrupt the cell cycle, DNA synthesis, invoke DNA damage, and so on.

Death Receptor–Initiated Apoptotic Signaling

Several TNF family receptors are known to transduce signals that result in apoptosis. These include TNFRSF1A (also known as CD120a and previously designated TNFR1), TNFRSF6 (also known as CD95, APO-1, or FAS), TNFRSF25 (also designated TRAMP and known as DR3 or APO3), TNFRSF10A (also known as DR4 or TRAIL-R1), and TNFRSF10B (also known as DR5 or TRAIL-R2). These receptors, also called *death receptors,* are characterized by the presence of a death domain within their cytoplasmic region, and have been shown to trigger apoptosis upon binding to their cognate ligands or specific agonist antibody. The activating ligands for these death receptors are structurally related molecules that also belong to the TNF gene superfamily such as TNFSF6 (also known as Fas ligand), TNF, and TRAIL.

Ligation of death receptors produces receptor trimerization and formation of a death-inducing signaling complex (DISC). This is composed of TNFRSF6, FADD (Fas [TNFRSF6]-associated via death domain), and procaspase 8, an apical signaling complex that mediates receptor-induced apoptosis. FADD binds directly to FasR, TNFRSF10A, or TNFRSF10B and indirectly to TNFRSF1A via TRADD (TNFRSF1A-associated via death domain protein). FADD is essential for cell death signaling from all three receptors. FADD interacts through its C-terminal death domain to cross-link TNFRSF6, TNFRSF10A, or TNFRSF10B receptors and recruits procaspase 8 and procaspase 10, or TRADD, through its N-terminal death effector domain (DED) to the DISC (see Fig. 55-8). Oligomerization of caspase 8 within the DISC results in a high local concentration of the zymogen. The induced proximity under these crowded conditions generates low levels of intrinsic proteolytic activity of caspase 8, enough to allow the various proenzymatic molecules to mutually cleave each other. Processing of caspase 8 removes the DED-containing prodomain, thus releasing the activated protease into the cytosol, where it can cleave and activate other downstream procaspases. In certain types of cells (type I), enough caspase 8 is activated by the activation of the death receptor to cause apoptosis. In other cell types, such as hepatocytes (type II), a high level of caspase 8 activation is not achieved and the apoptotic signal is amplified by the mitochondrial pathway. The active caspase 8 cleaves the cytosolic p 22 Bid into a BH3-only domain containing, proapoptotic, truncated p15 tBid fragment, which translocates to the mitochondria and triggers the release of cyt c into the cytosol. Cleavage by caspase 8 has been shown to cause exposure of a glycine residue on p 15 Bid

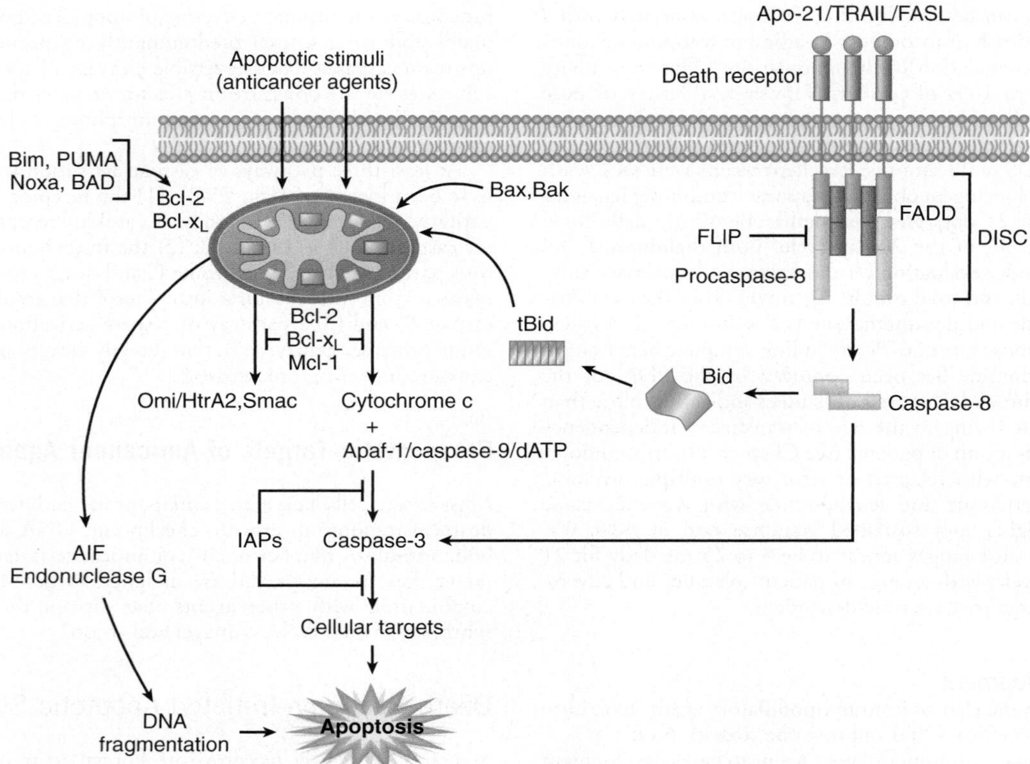

Figure 55-8 SCHEMATIC REPRESENTATION OF APOPTOTIC PATHWAYS.

that is myristoylated, thereby targeting p 15 Bid to the mitochondria. Thus N-myristoylation acts as an activating switch that enhances tBid-induced release of cyt c and apoptosis. The ability to cleave Bid may not be limited to caspase 8. Other caspases, such as caspase 3, as well other proteases, such as granzyme B and lysosomal proteases, have been shown to activate Bid. This indicates that Bid probably serves to amplify the caspase cascade rather than to initiate it (see Fig. 55-8).

Fas ligation has also been shown to initiate an alternative pathway leading to apoptosis, involving activation of c-Jun N-terminal kinase/stress-activated protein kinase (JNK/SAPK). After ligation, Fas recruits an adaptor protein called Daxx that interacts with the apoptosis signal-regulating kinase 1 (ASK1), activating the transcription factors AP-1 and ATF-2. After activation, ASK-1 launches a phosphorylation cascade that culminates in the activation of c-Jun N-terminal kinase (JNK). Activated JNK phosphorylates substrates such as c-Jun, p53, and a pro-death Bcl-2 member Bim. This, in turn, has been shown to trigger the mitochondrial or death receptor–initiated apoptotic signaling.

Mitochondria-Initiated Apoptotic Signaling

Mitochondria sequester a potent cocktail of proapoptotic proteins. These proteins promote apoptosis by activating caspases (e.g., by Cyt c), by inducing DNA fragmentation (e.g., by endonuclease G or apoptosis-inducing factor [AIF]), or by neutralizing cytosolic inhibitors of apoptosis or IAPs (e.g., by SMAC or Omi/HtrA2). On induction of apoptosis, unlike other proapoptotic proteins, mitochondrial AIF translocates to the nucleus to induce DNA fragmentation and apoptosis. Cyt c is a well-known component of the mitochondrial electron transfer chain. Cyt c is released from the mitochondria during apoptosis. After release into the cytosol, cyt c binds to Apaf-1 (apoptosis-activating factor), a cytosolic adapter protein that contains a caspase recruitment domain (CARD), a nucleotide-binding domain, and multiple WD-40 repeats. Binding of Cyt c to Apaf-1 increases its affinity for dATP or ATP by approximately 10-fold. It also triggers the oligomerization of Apaf-1 into a multimeric Apaf-1–Cyt c complex, also called the apoptosome. This exposes the CARD domain of Apaf-1, which recruits several molecules of procaspase 9, inducing their autoactivation. Only the caspase 9 bound to the apoptosome is able to efficiently cleave and activate downstream executioner caspase, caspase 3.

SMAC/DIABLO is a 25-kd mitochondrial protein that is released by mitochondria into the cytosol during apoptosis. SMAC contains a mitochondria-targeting sequence at its N-terminus. This sequence is removed on import into the mitochondria, generating the mature SMAC protein. In the mitochondria-initiated and common effector pathways of apoptosis, the processing and proteolytic activity of caspase 9 followed by caspases 3 and 7 are inhibited by the inhibitor of apoptosis (IAP) family of proteins. IAP family members include X-linked IAP (XIAP), cIAP1, cIAP2, and survivin. All IAPs contain at least one BIR domain, although some contain three. Another region, the RING domain, has ubiquitin ligase activity and promotes the self-degradation of IAPs through proteasomes in response to some apoptotic stimuli. Furthermore, during Fas death receptor–mediated apoptosis, XIAP is cleaved by activated caspase 3 into the amino-terminal BIR1 and 2 and BIR3-RING finger fragments. BIR3 domain binds and sequesters the monomeric and inactive caspase 9, thereby inhibiting its activation. Overexpression of XIAP inhibits anticancer drug (including Ara-C)–induced caspase activity and apoptosis. In contrast, downregulation of XIAP sensitizes cancer cells to apoptosis induced by chemotherapeutic drugs. The antiapoptotic activity of NFκB has also been shown to be mediated by the induction of IAPs. The first four amino acids of the mature Smac, Ala-Val-Pro-Ile (AVPI), bind to the BIR (baculovirus repeat) domain of IAP (inhibitor of apoptosis protein) proteins. The four amino acids (AVPI) of Smac that bind to the BIR3 domain of XIAP are similar to the XIAP-binding sequence of active caspase 9. In addition, Smac has been shown to form a stable complex with the BIR2 domain of XIAP. Smac binds to the linker-BIR2 domain and presumably disrupts its inhibition of the active caspase 3 and caspase 7 by steric hindrance. On induction of apoptosis, another mitochondrial protein, Omi/HtrA2 (a serine protease), is released from mitochondria and can induce caspase-independent cell death. Additionally, like Smac, the mature Omi protein contains a conserved IAP-binding motif (AVPS) at its N-terminus. Omi complexes with XIAP at high stoichiometry and promotes apoptosis by neutralizing the caspase-inhibitory effect of XIAP. Recently, Omi has also been shown to process XIAP and promote its proteasomal degradation.

The Bcl-2 family of proteins is divided into three subfamilies. Members of the subfamily that include Bcl-2, Bcl-x_L, and Mcl-1 inhibit apoptosis (see Fig. 55-8). The Bax subfamily members that promote apoptosis, including Bax and Bak, share with Bcl-2 three of the four Bcl-2 homology domains, BH1 to BH3. A C-terminus hydrophobic tail is responsible for the localization of these proteins to the outer membranes of the mitochondria and ER. The third BH3-only subfamily of proteins that includes Bid, Bim, and Bad also promotes apoptosis by binding and inactivating prosurvival Bcl-2 family members. The prosurvival Bcl-2 family members, to a variable degree, are bound to the membranes of the mitochondria, ER, and the nuclear envelope. In the event of an apoptotic stimulus, BH3-only proteins require Bax and Bak to trigger mitochondrial apoptotic signaling. For example, the exposed BH3 domain of tBid oligomerizes with Bak and Bax, causing their mitochondrial membrane insertion and Cyt c release. In response to apoptotic stimuli, Bax and Bak undergo conformational change and form membrane-associated homooligomers, disrupting the outer membrane of the mitochondria and ER and releasing the pro-death molecules into the cytosol. Besides tBid, Humanin peptide has been shown to activate Bax. Bcl-2 can block these events involving Bax activation by titrating tBid or Bim and/or heterodimerization with Bax and preventing mitochondrial permeabilization.

Induction of $P53^{wt}$ in cells triggers apoptosis by transcriptional activation of pro-death effectors, including Bax, Noxa, Puma, Apaf-1, and DR5, and by transcriptional repression of Bcl-2 and IAPs. P53-dependent apoptosis has also been shown to occur in the absence of any gene transcription or translation. In response to apoptotic stimulus such as irradiation, p53 translocates to the mitochondria, where it directly induces permeabilization of the outer membrane by forming complexes with the protective Bcl-2, resulting in the release of cyt c into the cytosol. The E2F transcription factor, normally restrained by the Rb tumor suppressor to inhibit cell proliferation, has been shown to induce apoptosis though p53-dependent and p53-independent mechanisms. These mechanisms include transcriptional activation of ARF (the alternate reading frame product of the INK4a/ARF tumor suppressor locus) or p73 (a member of the p53 family), repression of Mcl-1, and inducing the levels of caspase proenzymes.

Selective Antitumor Agents or Strategies

BCL2 Family of Proteins as Targets for Anticancer Drug Design

The antiapoptotic protein BCL2 was originally identified during the process of the discovery of the t(14;18) in human follicular lymphoma. Since this elucidation, overexpression of BCL2 has been shown in both hematologic and solid malignancies and to mediate resistance to traditional chemotherapeutic agents, radiation, and other antitumor treatments (Table 55-4).

Table 55-4 Effectors of Apoptosis Pathways as Targets for Cancer Therapy

Receptor-Mediated Pathway	Mitochondrial Pathway Targets or Agents
At the death receptors	Antisense oligos to BCL2 (Genasense)
TNFSF10	BH3 mimetic (peptides)
Anti-DR5 and anti-DR4	BCL2/BCL2L1 small molecule
Antibodies	Antagonists
CDDO	Tea polyphenols

Bcl-2 Antisense

Liposomal antisense Bcl-2 oligonucleotide (Bcl-ASODN) has been created and shown to cause apoptosis of many types of cancer and leukemia cells. Bcl-2-ASODN also sensitized tumor cells in vitro and in vivo to chemotherapeutic drugs. The most promising agent to target Bcl-2 is Genasense (oblimersan sodium; G3139), an 18-mer phosphorothioate oligodeoxynucleotide antisense compound. Clinical studies suggest safety and efficacy in solid and hematologic malignancies. In a phase III trial, 241 patients were randomly assigned to receive oblimersan 3 mg/kg/day as a 7-day continuous infusion in addition to fludarabine–cyclophosphamide versus fludarabine–cyclophosphamide. This study met its primary objective by demonstrating a significantly superior CR or nodular partial remission (CR/nPR) (17% vs. 7%; $P = .025$); however, no significant differences in overall response rates as well as time to progression were found. However, at 5-year follow–up, a significant improvement in survival was noted, with a hazard ratio of 0.6 for those treated with Oblimersen. Results of another phase III study were reported in which the addition of Oblimersan to high-dose dexamethasone did not improve OS or time to progression in myeloma patients.

BH3 Peptide/Mimetics or Bcl-2/Bcl-xL Small Molecule Antagonists

Another strategy to create Bcl-2 inhibitors has focused on developing small molecules that mimic the action of the endogenous Bcl-2-binding death agonists. Compounds that mimic the BH3-only class of death agonists such as Bad inhibit the survival proteins Bcl-2 and Bcl-x_L but do not appear to have independent proapoptotic activity. Two classes of novel small molecule cell-permeable inhibitors of the Bcl-x_L-BH3 domain (BH3I) have been identified. Studies have demonstrated that BH3Is induce apoptosis by preventing BH3 domain–mediated interaction between proapoptotic and antiapoptotic members of Bcl-2 family. Two natural products have been suggested to antagonize the antiapoptotic function of Bcl-2 or Bcl-x_L. Tetrocarcin A was reported to inhibit mitochondrial functions of Bcl-2 and suppress its antiapoptotic activity. In another report, Antimycin-A was shown to mimic activity of BH3 peptides and selectively induce apoptosis in cell lines overexpressing Bcl-x_L. Certain green tea catechins and black tea theaflavins were identified as potent inhibitors (K_i in the nanomolar range) of the antiapoptotic Bcl-2 family of proteins. On the basis of the high-resolution three-dimensional structure of the target receptor, small organic molecules that bind to this interface have been designed. ABT-737, is a BH3 mimetic that binds to Bcl-2, Bcl-xL, and Bcl-w with high affinity (K_i <1 nM) but not to Mcl-1. Preclinical data demonstrate cytotoxic activity in B lymphoid tumor cell lines, human follicular lymphoma, myeloma, and CLL cells as well as synergism with other chemotherapeutic agents. Also, ABT-737 effectively kills AML blast, progenitor, and stem cells without disturbing normal hematopoietic cell development. However, the clinical utility of ABT-737 is limited, as it undergoes rapid metabolism and is not orally bioavailable. Targeted modifications of ABT-737 led to synthesis of Navitoclax (ABT-263), an orally bioavailable BH3 mimetic. In the initial phase I trial[18] more than half of patients had a decrease in their lymphocytosis, with 35% achieving partial remission. The main toxicity was dose-dependent thrombocytopenia, which occurred early in the treatment cycle (days 2-5 of a 21-day cycle). Neutropenia occurred at higher dose levels. Other adverse events included gastrointestinal side effects and fatigue. The remarkable activity of this agent in early trials validates Bcl-2 as a target for the treatment of CLL. Trials of Navitoclax in combination with rituximab are ongoing.

Cyclin-Dependent Kinase Inhibitors as Therapeutic Targets

Orderly progression through the cell cycle is regulated by the coordinated expression of a variety of genes and proteins, and the decision of a cell to progress through the cell cycle is determined by the activity of cyclins, levels of which fluctuate throughout the cell cycle, CDKs (e.g., CDKs 1-9), and several endogenous small molecule CDK inhibitors (e.g., $p21^{CIP1}$, $p27^{KIP1}$, and $p57^{KIP2}$) (see Fig. 55-1). In general, whereas CDK1, in association with cyclins A and B, is involved in G_2M progression, CDK2, CDK4, and CDK6, in association with cyclins A, D, and E, are involved in G_1S progression. Activation of CDKs results in phosphorylation of the retinoblastoma protein (PRB), which leads to its dissociation from the E2F transcription factor. Once freed, E2F triggers the transcription of diverse genes involved in cell cycle progression (thymidylate synthase and dihydrofolate reductase, among numerous others). Endogenous small molecule inhibitors such as $P21^{CIP1}$ and $P27^{KIP1}$ bind stoichiometrically to CDKs and inhibit their activity. Activity of CDKs can also be regulated through inhibitory phosphorylation of these proteins (e.g., on threonine 14 or tyrosine 15 residues) or, conversely, activating phosphorylation on threonine 160 or 161 (mediated by CDK5 or cyclin-dependent activating kinase [CAK]). Interference with the activation of CDKs results in dephosphorylation of PRB, leading in turn to binding and inactivation of E2F and inhibition of cell cycle progression.

Cell cycle dysregulation is a cardinal characteristic of cancer in general and hematologic malignancies in particular. A classic example of this phenomenon is the regular association of increased expression of cyclin D_1 in mantle cell lymphoma. Regulation of the cell cycle has been found to be closely related to apoptosis. Disruption of the cell cycle transit has been shown to be a potent cell death stimulus in a wide variety of neoplastic cell types, including those of hematopoietic origin. A corollary of this observation is that agents that interfere with the cell cycle, in addition to blocking cell cycle progression, can be potent inducers of programmed cell death. For these reasons, inhibitors of the cell cycle have become logical targets for therapeutic intervention in hematologic and other malignancies. Cell cycle inhibitors can be subdivided into several categories. For example, they can act directly, as in the case of CDK inhibitors, or indirectly, as in the case of HDAC inhibitors, compounds that block cell cycle progression by inducing endogenous cell cycle inhibitors such as $P21^{CIP1}$. The latter agents are discussed later in this chapter. CDK inhibitors can also be classified as specific (i.e., directed against a particular CDK, such as CDK2) or those that nonspecifically inhibit most CDKs (e.g., flavopiridol). The development of cell cycle inhibitors has primarily focused on CDK inhibitors, several of which have entered clinical trials, including those involving hematologic malignancies. A brief summary of the status of CDK inhibitors, with an emphasis on hematologic malignancies, follows.

Flavopiridol

Flavopiridol (L86-8275) is a semisynthetic flavonoid derived from the Indian plant *rohitukine* (see Chapter 76). It was the first CDK inhibitor to enter clinical trials in humans. Flavopiridol binds to the ATP-binding site of CDKs, resulting in reversible, competitive enzyme inhibition at concentrations of less than 100 nM. As noted earlier, flavopiridol is a relatively nonspecific CDK inhibitor and inhibits all CDKs, although it is less effective against CDK7. Flavopiridol induces G_1S or G_2M arrest, presumably a consequence of inhibition of CDK1 and CDK2. Flavopiridol may also act to block cell cycle progression by downregulating cyclin D_1 levels, inhibiting the CDK-activating complex (CDK7), or both.

In addition to blocking cell cycle progression, flavopiridol has been shown to be a potent inducer of apoptosis in malignant hematopoietic cells (e.g., acute and chronic leukemia) at low concentrations (e.g., u100 nM). Moreover, flavopiridol has shown activity against multiple myeloma cell in vitro.

The proapoptotic actions of flavopiridol have been attributed to its capacity to inhibit the positive transcription elongation factor-β (PTEF-β), cyclin T/CDK9 complex by inhibiting phosphorylation of the carboxy-terminal domain of RNA polymerase II. This leads to downregulation of several antiapoptotic proteins, including BIRC4; P_{21}^{CIP1}; and, in the case of multiple myeloma cells, Mcl-1. Flavopiridol has also recently been shown to block the antiapoptotic actions of the IAP family member survivin.

In clinical studies, flavopiridol was initially administered as a 72-hour continuous infusion every 2 weeks, with a maximally tolerated dose of 40 mg/m^2. Steady-state plasma levels in excess of those necessary to inhibit CDKs and induce apoptosis in leukemia cells (e.g., 350 nM) were achieved. Dose-limiting toxicities were fatigue, diarrhea, nausea, and myelosuppression. However, the occurrence of thromboembolic phenomena and the general lack of single-agent activity have limited enthusiasm for administering flavopiridol by this schedule. Flavopiridol has also been administered as a daily IV bolus for 1, 3, or 5 days every 3 weeks with manageable toxicity, and other schedules are being examined, including a hybrid schedule with half the dose administered as an IV bolus and the other half as a more prolonged infusion. When administered as a daily bolus infusion for 3 days every 3 weeks, flavopiridol exhibited modest activity in patients with mantle cell lymphoma. A novel pharmacologically directed schedule of flavopiridol has been developed in which half of the dose (e.g., 30 mg/m^2) is administered as a 30-minute bolus loading infusion and 30 mg/m^2 as a 4-hour infusion. In a phase I study, objective response rates of 45% were obtained with this schedule in patients with progressive CLL, including some with high-risk disease.[19] Because of the rapidity of response, particularly in patients with high white blood cell counts, aggressive measures designed to avoid tumor lysis syndrome (e.g., hydration, alkalinization of the urine, administration of rasburicase) are advisable. Efforts are now underway to use this novel flavopiridol schedule in combination with other agents and in other hematologic malignancies.

Because of limited single-agent activity, combination regimens involving flavopiridol are being explored in hematologic malignancies. On the basis of preclinical evidence of synergism with the antimetabolite ara-C, a regimen combining flavopiridol on a daily IV bolus schedule followed by high-dose ara-C has been initiated in patients with acute leukemia and has shown some activity. In a successive phase II study, flavopiridol was administered as a 1-hour bolus infusion of 50 mg/m^2 daily for 3 days before administration of high-dose ara-C (day 6) and mitoxantrone (day 9). Complete response rates of 67% were obtained in patients with high-risk AML and more than half were durable. More recently, evidence of synergism between flavopiridol and other signal transduction modulators has become the focus of considerable attention. For example, the observation that flavopiridol interacts synergistically with imatinib mesylate against CML cells, including some that are imatinib mesylate resistant, has prompted the initiation of a phase I trial of flavopiridol and imatinib mesylate in patients with progressive BCR-ABL$^+$ hematologic malignancies. Four of 21 patients responded. Evidence that flavopiridol interacts synergistically with HDAC and proteasome inhibitors in human leukemia cells has appeared, and clinical trials combining flavopiridol with the HDAC inhibitor vorinostat or the proteasome inhibitor bortezomib in patients with refractory AML/MDS and multiple myeloma/indolent NHL are currently underway.

SNS032

SNS032 is a small molecule CDK inhibitor discovered through high-throughput screening that is primarily active against CDK2. In preclinical studies, SNS032 has shown potent antiproliferative activity against ovarian and breast cancer cells in vitro. As is the case with other CDK inhibitors, SNS032 induces cell-cycle arrest; PRB dephosphorylation; and, under some circumstances, apoptosis in CLL and myeloma cell lines. At least in some tumor cell lines, however, CDK2 may be dispensable for cell cycle progression. In CLL cells, SNS-032 was cytotoxic in vitro in untreated and refractory cell lines. RNA synthesis was suppressed after treatment, with evidence of CDK 2 and 7 inhibition.[20]

Several phase I trials of SNS032 have been initiated. SNS032 has been administered as either a 24-hour or 1-hour infusion every 3 weeks. Dose levels of 4 to 59 mg/m^2 have proven to be tolerable; the maximum tolerated dose for either of these schedules has not been reached. Toxicities have been mild and include rash, nausea and vomiting, diarrhea, and fatigue. In a clinical trial in patients with CLL (19 patients) and myeloma (18 patients), Cdk7 and -9 inhibition was observed, but responses as a single agent were modest.

Farnesyltransferase Inhibitors: Zarnestra

RAS proteins represent low-molecular-weight proteins that bind guanosine triphosphate (GTP) and are located at the cell membrane. They are critically involved in the regulation of signal transduction pathways implicated in the control of cell proliferation, differentiation, and survival. One of the key effectors of RAS proteins is the serine-threonine kinase RAF1, which is recruited to the cell membrane by activated RAS, and in turn activates the survival- and proliferation-associated kinases MEK1/2 (mitogen-activated kinase 1/2) and ERK (extracellular signal-regulating kinase). RAS is also involved in regulation of the AKT pathway, which exerts multiple antiapoptotic functions.

There are four separate RAS proteins: H-RAS, N-RAS, K-RAS4A, and K-RAS4B. Of these, H-RAS mutations are most commonly encountered in hematologic malignancies (i.e., myeloid leukemia). Because of the frequency of RAS mutations in human neoplasia and the importance of RAS downstream targets (e.g., RAF1/MEK/ERK and AKT) in the survival of neoplastic cells, the RAS pathway is a logical target for therapeutic intervention.

To function, Ras must be localized to the cell membrane. This in turn requires posttranslational modifications of the RAS protein, most notably farnesylation. This primarily involves addition of a 15-carbon isoprenoid farnesol to the C terminus of RAS following recognition of a CAAX motif. This process is catalyzed by the enzyme farnesyl transferase. Inhibitors of farnesyl transferase (FTIs) thus block RAS farnesylation, preventing the protein from associating with the plasma membrane and subsequently participating in downstream signaling events.

Initial preclinical studies suggested that FTIs inhibited the proliferation and survival of several tumors driven by RAS mutations. However, it soon became clear that tumors with H-RAS mutations were more sensitive to FTIs than those with N-Ras or K-RAS mutations. Furthermore, the antiproliferative effects of FTIs did not always correlate well with their effects on RAS farnesylation or the presence of Ras mutations. Two possible explanations may account for these findings. First, alternative prenylation events (e.g., geranylgeranylation of the RAS protein) may also promote its membrane localization, particularly in cells bearing N-RAS or K-RAS mutations, and could theoretically confer resistance to FTI lethality. Second, several other non-RAS candidate proteins have been identified in which interference with farnesylation might contribute to FTI-associated lethality. These include small GTPases (e.g., RHO family members) and a variety of nuclear proteins (e.g., CENP-E and CENP-F).

Zarnestra is an orally active FTI that has undergone extensive evaluation in patients with solid tumors and hematologic malignancies. In patients with hematologic malignancies, the generally accepted dose and schedule is 600 mg/m^2 orally twice daily for 21 days repeated at monthly intervals or for 28 days repeated at 6-week intervals. Dose-limiting toxicities include myelosuppression, nausea, vomiting, diarrhea, rash, neurotoxicity, and fatigue. In a series of phase I and II studies, promising activity was observed in patients with AML, ALL, CML, and MDS. For example, in one study, six of 22 patients with CML achieved complete or partial responses, and two of eight patients with myelofibrosis achieved objective responses. In a study in refractory leukemia, a response rate with 1200 mg/m^2 of about 15% was reported. In patients with AML, the combination with idarubicin cytarabine and escalating doses of Zarnestra, the combination was well tolerated with expected pancytopenia and a CR rate of more than 60% with a median duration of response of more than 17 months. A study in elderly patients with AML the combination of Zarnestra and etoposide generated an overall response rate of 25% in 84 patients. However, leukemias that expressed high RASGRP1 and low aprataxin (APTX), with a ratio of over 5.2 had a CR rate of 78%.[21] Responses in patients with multiple myeloma have also been observed but have been modest. Interestingly, blasts obtained from a number of leukemic patients who responded did not exhibit RAS mutations, suggesting that the lethal effects of Zarnestra may proceed, at least in part, through RAS-independent pathways.

Inhibitors of the RAF1/Mek/ERK Pathway

The MAPK pathways consist of three parallel serine-threonine kinase modules that are intimately involved in the control of cell survival, proliferation, and differentiation. Two of these, JNK and p38 MAPK, are activated in response to environmental stresses, including DNA damage and osmotic stress, but p42/44 MAPK (also known as ERK; extracellular signal-regulating kinase) is primarily induced by growth factors and other mitogenic stimuli. Although exceptions exist, JNK and p38 MAPK primarily exert proapoptotic functions, but ERK activation is generally associated with cell survival. The only well-defined activator of ERK is the serine-threonine kinase MEK1/2 (mitogen-activated protein kinase kinase 1/2), but numerous ERK targets have been identified, including ELK-1, CREB, BCL2, BAD, FRAP1 (also known as mTOR), and caspase 9, among numerous others. The activating effects of MEK1/2 on ERK are opposed by phosphatases that dephosphorylate and inactivate the enzyme (e.g., MAP kinase phosphatase 1/2 [MKP1/2]).

The major activator of MEK1/2 is the serine-threonine kinase RAF, of which three forms exist: RAF1, B-RAF, and A-RAF. RAF can be activated by Ras (discussed earlier) as well as through various RAS-independent pathways, including PKC, KSR, as well as the SRC and JAK family of kinases among others. The activation of RAF involves several processes, including recruitment to the plasma membrane, phosphorylation on serine and threonine residues, and dimerization. Interference with any of these processes can lead to inhibition of Raf activation as well as downstream targets.

Dysregulation of the RAF/MEK/ERK pathway has been observed in most hematopoietic malignancies, including acute leukemia, CLL, multiple myeloma, and lymphomas. Consequently, there has been considerable interest in the development of pharmacologic inhibitors of the RAF/MEK/ERK pathway in these disorders. In addition to their potential intrinsic activity against malignant hematopoietic cells, evidence indicates that such agents might also enhance the activity of conventional cytotoxic drugs.

Sorafenib

Initial approaches to RAF inhibition focused on efforts to destabilize the protein. For example, geldanamycin and the related compound 17-AAG act as inhibitors of HSPCA, a chaperone protein necessary for Raf processing and stabilization. Interference with HSPCA results in destabilization and proteasomal degradation of RAF as well as numerous other proteins, including AKT. More recently, however, a Raf kinase inhibitor, sorafenib, which is approved for use in kidney cancer, has been developed and has entered phase I and II clinical trials in humans for leukemias. In preclinical studies, induction of leukemic cell death by sorafenib has been shown to stem from inhibition of translation and downregulation of the short-lived antiapoptotic protein Mcl-1 and induction of ER stress with bim-mediated apoptosis. In the clinical setting, modest response rates of 10% were observed in two studies, suggesting the need to consider combination therapy.

Inhibitors of the Mammalian Target of Rapamycin

The first mTOR inhibitor discovered was the naturally occurring macrolide rapamycin (sirolimus), widely used as an immunosuppressant (see Chapter 109). The importance of mTOR in cancer suggested this agent would have antineoplastic activity. Improvements in solubility and pharmacokinetic properties led to development of rapamycin analogs (rapalogs), of which everolimus and temsirolimus are available as antineoplastic agents.[22] The mechanism of rapamycin and its analogs is similar: after complexing with the small protein FKBP12, they bind irreversibly to the FKBP12-rapamycin binding site on the mTOR protein. Acute rapamycin treatment only affects mTORC1 because the FKBP12-rapamycin is occluded in mTORC2. Prolonged rapalog exposure may result in decreased mTOR availability and therefore indirectly decreased mTORC2 activity through limited mTORC2 complex formation. It is well recognized that growth factor signaling initiated through the receptor tyrosine kinases (RTKs) or caused by the activity of cytosolic tyrosine kinases (TKs), such as BCR-ABL, results in the activation of the PI3K/AKT signaling. AKT has been shown to phosphorylate and inactivate TSC2 (tuberous sclerosis 2; also known as tuberin), thereby disrupting its interaction with TSC1 (or hamartin) (Fig. 55-9). Inhibition of TSC1-TSC2 complex de-represses RHEB, which is a small G protein that activates mTOR. When RHEB is in an active GTP-bound state, its localization to the membrane stimulates mTOR-mediated phosphorylation of the downstream eukaryotic initiation factor 4E (eIF4E)–binding protein 1 (4E-BP) and ribosomal protein S6 kinase 1 (S6K1) (see Fig. 55-9). However, the association of mTOR with the 150-kd Raptor (regulatory associated protein of mTOR) is necessary for the phosphorylation of 4E-BP and S6K1. mTOR-mediated phosphorylation and activation of S6K1 results in the phosphorylation of the ribosomal S6 protein and eIF4B (see Fig. 55-9). AKT has also been shown to directly activate S6K1. S6K1 activity is involved in regulating the translation of a group of mRNAs that have highly structured 5′UTR, including mRNAs that have a 5′TOP (terminal oligopyrimidines, a stretch of 4-14 pyrimidines).[23]

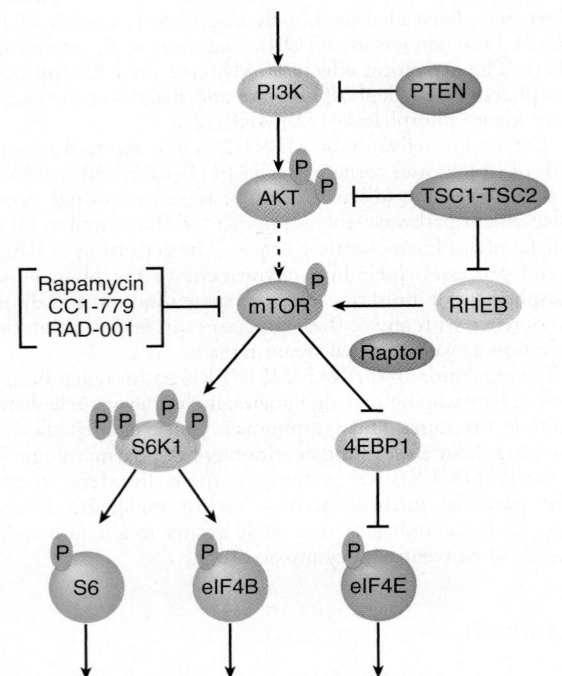

Figure 55-9 RAPAMYCIN OR ITS ANALOGS INHIBIT MAMMALIAN TARGET OF RAPAMYCIN (MTOR) AND THE DOWNSTREAM PHOSPHORYLATION OF S6K1 AND 4EBP1, THEREBY ATTENUATING THE TRANSLATION INITIATION OF MRNAS WITH HIGHLY STRUCTURED 5′UTR. Activation of the receptor (FLT-3) or cytosolic tyrosine kinase (e.g., Bcr-Abl) can lead to increased activity of phosphatidylinositol 3-kinase (PI3K)/AKT. Although it can directly phosphorylate mTOR, AKT activity inhibits the TSC1-TSC2 complex, thereby derepressing RHEB and activating mTOR. The phosphorylation and activation of S6K1, and phosphorylation and inactivation of 4E-BP through Raptor, results in the phosphorylation of S6, eIF4B, and eIF4E, which are involved in the cap-dependent translation of mRNAs with highly structured 5′URT.

The rapalogs temsirolimus and everolimus have been tested in lymphoid malignancies, and as single agents, they have demonstrated activity, although modest, against a variety of lymphomas (see Chapter 81). In the initial phase II study in patients with mantle cell lymphoma, temsirolimus was administered at a dose of 250 mg based on a phase II study done in renal cell carcinoma patients. A modest response rate was noted (overall response rate (ORR) 38%), but the majority of patients required a dose reduction because of myelosuppression, particularly thrombocytopenia. A second trial in relapsed refractory mantle cell lymphoma patients was conducted to determine if a lower dose of temsirolimus could be used. In a follow-up phase II study, temsirolimus was given at a dose of 25 mg IV weekly and was found to be as effective as the 250-mg IV dose, with a modest improvement in the side effect profile and dose reductions. This dose and schedule were also noted to be efficacious in non–mantle cell NHL with again thrombocytopenia being the main dose-limiting toxicity. A recent phase III study in relapsed refractory mantle cell lymphoma patients evaluated two different dosing regimens of temsirolimus, 175 mg weekly for 3 weeks followed by 75 mg weekly versus 175 mg weekly for 3 weeks followed by 25 mg weekly versus the investigator's choice.[24] At the conclusion of this study, it was determined that the temsirolimus regimen with 175/75 mg dosing had a significant improvement in PFS and objective response rate compared with the investigator's choice. Everolimus, given orally at a daily dose of 10 mg, has single-agent activity against Hodgkin lymphoma (PMI, Waldenström macroglobulinemia, DLBCL, CLL, and other relapsed lymphomas).

The most common side effect of rapalogs is myelosuppression; other common side effects include fatigue, oral ulcers, and dermatologic abnormalities. Metabolic abnormalities are common, including hyperglycemia, hypercholesterolemia, and hypertriglyceridemia. An uncommon pulmonary toxicity manifested as interstitial lung disease has also been observed with rapalogs.

Histone Deacetylase Inhibitors

Histone acetyl transferases (HATs) control gene expression through the modification of chromatin structure through acetylation of chromatin-bound histones. Regulation of acetylation is through histone deacetylation. Without the ability to fine tune histone binding to chromatin regions, gene expression is perturbed. Inhibition of this process by a group of agents termed *histone deacetylation inhibitors* alters gene expression in both normal and malignant cells. Often the result is differentiation of malignant cells or induction of apoptosis. Given the long history of the use of differentiating agents in leukemias, for APL (retinoids), low-dose ara-C and azacytidine, it is not surprising that newer HDAC inhibitors have undergone extensive evaluation in leukemias.

Posttranslational Histone and Nonhistone Protein Modifications and Gene Transcription

Nucleosomes are regularly repeating, structural units of chromatin, which are essential in packaging eukaryotic DNA. Each unit is composed of 146 base pairs of DNA tightly wrapped around a core histone octamer. Each histone octamer consists of 2 units each of histones H2A, H2B, H3, and H4, and each nucleosome in turn is connected to its neighbor by a short segment of linker DNA, approximately 10 to 80 base pairs in length. Histone H1 binds and stabilizes linker DNA. Each core histone has an amino (N) terminal tail, which is lysine rich and positively charged. Specific amino acid residues at the N-terminal undergo a variety of enzymatic posttranslational modifications. Modifications can also occur within the globular domain of histones that make extensive contacts with DNA. *Histone code* is the name given to the combination of biochemical modifications affecting different histone residues that specify chromatin function. However, it has been suggested that various postsynthesis histone modifications be considered an epigenomic alphabet. Each modification is a letter, and the combination of modifications at a specified genomic region is a word that may have different functional meanings depending on the context.

Histone acetyl transferases and HDACs are two classes of enzymes that mediate the acetylation and deacetylation, respectively, at evolutionarily conserved N-terminal lysine residues. Acetylated histones are negatively charged and do not bind as tightly to negatively charged DNA, thereby facilitating gene transcription. In contrast, deacetylated histones bind closely to DNA, preventing transcription. Acetylation status of chromatin and hence gene transcription is dictated by balanced activity of HATs and HDACs. Acetylation of core histone bases has also been implicated in chromatin assembly, DNA repair, and replication timing of specific genomic regions. Crosstalk also exists between acetylation and ubiquitination. Thus HDACs can decrease the half-lives of substrates by exposing the lysine residue for ubiquitination. Other crucial functions affected by the delicate balance between HATs and HDACs include activation of the apoptotic program via interaction between Ku70 and BAX; protein localization (nuclear vs. cytoplasm); and DNA binding of transcription factors such as p53, E2F1, GATA1, RelA, YY1, and hormone receptors. There is a growing list of nonhistone proteins that are modulated by HATs or HDACs. These include hypoxia-inducible factor-1α (HIF-1α), β-catenin, α-tubulin, Ku70, importin-α 7, cortactin, and most recently heat shock protein (hsp) 90. HATs and HDACs can be classified into subfamilies according to the presence of highly conserved structural motifs. Please refer to Table 55-5 for details.

Aberrant Histone Acetyl Transferase and Histone Deacetylase Activity in Hematologic Malignancies

Aberrant activity of HATs and HDACs resulting in aberrant gene transcription is a hallmark of many cancers, including many hematologic malignancies. Several chromosomal translocations in leukemia that produce chimeric fusion oncoproteins have been shown to recruit HDACs to promoters and repress genes involved in cell cycle growth inhibition and differentiation. For example, PML-RARα in APL and AML1-ETO generated by t(8;21) translocation in AML recruit HDACs to their target genes, resulting in chromatin modification and repression of genes, leading to blocked differentiation and inhibition of apoptosis. HDACs have also been found in complexes with proteins that regulate cell cycle checkpoints such as Rb and its family members. Resistance to chemotherapy can occur because of increased levels of thioredoxin, a thiol reductase, and decreased levels of thioredoxin-binding protein (TBP-2) in many cancers; HDAC inhibitors (HDIs) can reverse this phenomenon. These effects create a strong rationale for developing inhibitors of HDAC activity that would correct transcriptional deregulation of genes involved in cell-cycle regulation and apoptosis as cancer therapeutic agents.

Mechanisms of Anticancer Activity of Histone Deacetylase Inhibitors

Treatment with HDIs modulates expression of 2% to 10% of a selective, but variable, subset of genes in various cell types with as many genes upregulated as are downregulated. Normal cells are more resistant than cancer cells to the effects of HDIs. HDI-induced cell cycle arrest, and apoptosis is usually correlated with upregulation of p21, p27, and p16 and attenuation of cyclin A and D levels, leading to decreased activity of CDK4 and CDK2. Induction of GADD45α and -β and upregulation of TGF-β, which inhibits c-Myc, may also contribute to the cell cycle arrest in G1 or G2. Promoter regions of p21 and the telomerase catalytic unit TERT have been shown to contain SP1 sites that bind HDAC-recruiting transcription complexes. HDIs also activate the mitochondrial apoptotic pathway by transcriptional activation of apoptotic proteins such as TBP2, Bad, Bim, Bid, BAK, Bax, and caspases 3 and 9 and repression of anti-apoptotic proteins such as thioredoxin, bcl-2, XIAP, and Mcl-1. HDIs have also been shown to upregulate Fas and the Apo-2L/TRAIL receptors DR4 and DR5, downregulate c-FLIP, and enhance Apo-2L/TRAIL-induced death-inducing signaling complex (DISC) and apoptosis.

Treatment of leukemias with HDI alone or in combination with other agents such as ATRA has been shown to overcome the inhibition of differentiation caused by chimeric fusion oncoproteins such as PML-RARα, PLZF-RARα, or AML-ETO. HDIs have also been shown to induce the expression of gelsolin, an actin-binding protein involved in morphologic and cytostructural changes associated with differentiation. Several HDIs have been shown to induce acetylation of hsp90 and inhibit its chaperone association with important pro-survival client proteins such as AKT and c-Raf. This directs these

Table 55-5 Human Histone Deacetylases

Characteristics	Class I	Class IIa	Class IIb	Class III
Members	HDAC1, 2, 3, 8, 11	HDAC4, 5, 7, 9	HDAC6, 10	SIRT1, 2, 3, 4, 5, 6, 7
Localization	Nuclear	Nucleo-cytoplasmic	Nucleo-cytoplasmic	Nuclear/cytoplasmic/mitochondrial
Substrates	Histones p53 (HDAC1) NFκB (HDAC3)	Histones Hsp90	Histone Tubulin Hsp90?	Histones Tubulin (SIRT2) p53 (SIRT1) TAF(I)68 (SIRT1)
Binding site inhibitors	Zn^{++} TSA SAHA/LAQ824 Depsipeptide Trapoxin Butyrate VPA	Zn^{++} TSA SAHA/LAQ824 Trapoxin Butyrate VPA	Zn^{++} TSA SAHA/LAQ824 Tubacin	NAD^+ Nicotinamide

HDAC, Histone deacetylase; *NFκB*, nuclear factor kappa-B; *SAHA*, suberoylanilide hydroxamic acid; *TSA*, tricostatin A; *VPA*, valproic acid.

client proteins to polyubiquitylation and proteasomal degradation, thus contributing to the lowering of the threshold for apoptosis in cancer cells. Inhibition of HDAC6 results in marked accumulation of ubiquitinated proteins (inhibition of the aggresome), via acetylation of α-tubulin, which in turn results in increased cellular stress and cytotoxicity.

Histone deacetylase inhibitors may also act by exerting antiangiogenic and immune modulatory effects via downregulation of HIF-1α and epidermal growth factor (EGF). HDIs also affect cancer cell migration, invasion, and metastasis by altering expression of extracellular matrix proteins and metastasis genes in favor of reduced cell invasion.

Classes of Histone Deacetylase Inhibitors

Several structurally diverse classes of naturally occurring and synthetic compounds have been investigated for their ability to inhibit HDAC activity (Table 55-6). These include short-chain fatty acids (e.g., valproic acid), hydroxamic acid derivatives (e.g., vorinostat, panobinostat), synthetic benzamides (e.g., entinostat), and cyclic tetrapeptides (e.g., romidepsin). All of these have undergone clinical evaluation.

Short-Chain Fatty Acid Histone Deacetylase Inhibitors

Sodium butyrate (SB), a well-studied member of this class of compounds, induces in vitro growth arrest and differentiation of human leukemia cells at millimolar concentrations. Its clinical development has been hampered by its short half-life and difficulty in achieving millimolar levels in vivo. Phenylbutyrate, another derivative of butyric acid, is able to induce in vitro growth arrest and differentiation of leukemia cells at clinically achievable submillimolar concentrations. Importantly, at these levels, phenylbutyrate is able to synergize with retinoids in inducing cell cycle arrest, differentiation, and apoptosis of myeloid leukemia cells and with ara-C in myeloid leukemias. Valproic acid (VPA), a well-tolerated antiepileptic, was shown to be effective as an HDI at levels ranging between 0.5 and 2.5 mM.

Two phase I trials have examined the therapeutic effects of phenylbutyrate in patients with AML and MDS. No responses were noted in either study, with neurotoxicity being the dose-limiting toxicity. Several studies have used valproic acid as monotherapy or in combination with other agents in hematologic malignancies. As monotherapy in MDS, response rates have been as high as 16% using the IWG criteria. Neurotoxicity has been the major side effect. Other side effects of VPA include thrombocytopenia, weight gain, asthenia, and rarely hepatic failure and pancreatitis. Given the low response rate, emphasis has shifted to newer HDIs.

Vorinostat and Other Hydroxamic Acid Derivative Histone Deacetylase Inhibitors

Members of this class are some of the most potent HDIs. They contain a functional group that interacts with the critical zinc atom at the base of the catalytic pocket of the class I and II HDACs. These HDIs also possess a hydrophobic cap and an aliphatic side chain that interacts with the edge and fits into the hydrophobic catalytic pocket, respectively, of the HDACs. Members of this class inhibit both class I and II HDACs. Vorinostat (SAHA, Zolinza) is a second-generation polar–planar compound that induces in vitro growth arrest, differentiation, or apoptosis of a variety of cancer, leukemia, and multiple myeloma cells by restoring function of aberrantly silenced genes among other effects. In phase I studies, vorinostat was administered intravenously to patients with solid tumors or hematologic malignancies daily × 3 or daily × 5 for up to 3 weeks. The maximum tolerated dose of vorinostat in patients with hematologic malignancies was 300 mg/m^2 daily × 5 for 3 weeks; thrombocytopenia and leukopenia were the notable toxicities, but induced no significant responses as a single agent in refractory AML. In sequential treatments in vitro, a schedule-dependent synergy was seen with other agents used to treat AML, but in some instances, antagonistic activity was observed. In a phase II study of vorinostat combined with gemtuzumab ozogamicin as induction therapy for elderly AML patients, a complete response rate of more than 20% was observed. In a phase I trial of relapsed AML, vorinostat with idarubicin induced a 17% response rate with modification of histone acetylation patterns.

More impressive responses have been seen in patients with lymphoma. Specifically, treatment of patients with progressive, persistent, or recurrent T-cell cutaneous lymphoma showed strong evidence of significant responses, resulting in rapid FDA approval (see Chapter 84). In the pivotal study, 74 patients with stage IB and higher T-cell cutaneous lymphoma who had failed two systemic therapies were treated with vorinostat at a dose of 400 mg orally once daily.

Table 55-6 Histone Deacetylase Inhibitors*

Name	Type of Compound	Cell Culture (Activity)	Animal Tumor Models	Clinical Trial
Butyrates	Short-chain fatty acids	Yes (uM)	Yes	Phase I/II
Valproic acid	Short-chain fatty acid	Yes	Yes	Phase I/II
Trichostatin A	Hydroxamic acid	Yes (nM)	Yes	—
Pyroxamide	Hydroxamic acid derivative	Yes (nM)	Yes	Phase I
Oxamflatin	Hydroxamic acid derivative	Yes (uM)	Yes	—
Suberoylanilide hydroxamic acid (SAHA)	Hydroxamic acid derivative	Yes (nM)	Yes	Phase I/II
TPX-HA analog (CHAP)	Hydroxamic acid derivative	Yes (nM)	Yes	—
LAQ824	Hydroxamic acid derivative	Yes (nM)	Yes	Phase I
MS-275	Benzamide derivative	Yes (uM)	Yes	—
CI-994 (N-acetyl dinaline)	Benzamide derivative	Yes	Yes	Phase I
Depsipeptide (FR901228, FK-228)	Cyclic tetrapeptides	Yes (nM)	Yes	Phase I/II
Trapoxin	Cyclic tetrapeptides	Yes (nM)	—	—
Apicidin	Cyclic tetrapeptides	Yes (nM)	Yes	—

*Activity reported as "Yes" indicates that the compound has been shown to inhibit histone deacetylase (HDAC) activity, that is, growth of transformed cells in culture and in vivo tumor growth in animal studies. (—) indicates no data reported. CI-994 is reported to inhibit histone deacetylation but does not directly inhibit HDAC.

Sixty-one patients (82%) had stage IIB or higher CTCL and 30 patients (41%) had Sézary syndrome. The objective response rate was 30% based on a standardized scoring system, and the median time to tumor progression was 202 days. In these studies, the common toxicities were diarrhea (52%), fatigue (52%), nausea (41%), and anorexia (24%). Although the definitive mechanism of action of this high degree of response is not known, a recent review outlines the current hypotheses. Furthermore, highly significant synergy has been observed in preclinical models combining vorinostat with bortezomib.

Progress with other lymphomas has been more complex. Thirty-nine patients with advanced hematologic malignancies were enrolled in a trial composed of two cohorts examining IV and PO formulations of vorinostat. Up to 70% of patients had diffuse large B-cell lymphoma. The median numbers of prior treatments were seven and five in the IV and PO cohorts, respectively. A substantial number of patients had undergone a prior stem cell transplant. Most patients tolerated vorinostat well. Responses were seen in about 15% of patients.

In patients with refractory follicular lymphoma, NHL, or mantle cell lymphoma, overall response rates of 47% were seen, and responses were observed in two of nine patients with marginal zone lymphoma. The duration of response was longer than 1 year. The largest recent study, by the Southwest Oncology Group (SWOG), in NHL, showed a very low response rate as a single agent, which resulted in combination therapy studies. A number of such studies are underway, but none to date has generated significant results showing combined agent clinical synergy.

Panobinostat is a second-generation hydroxamic acid-based hybrid polar HDI tested both in vitro and in vivo tumor models and in clinical trials. Panobinostat induces apoptosis in a dose-dependent manner on human CML blast crisis K562 cells and acute leukemia MV4-11 cells with the activating length mutation of FLT-3. Exposure to panobinostat is associated with hyperacetylation of H3, H4, and Hsp 90; increase in p21; and induction of cell cycle G1 phase accumulation.

Fifteen patients with a median age of 63 years and refractory AML, ALL, or MDS received IV panobinostat in a phase I trial at the following dose levels (mg/m^2): 4.8, 7.2, 9.0, 11.5, and 14.0. Grade III QTc prolongation was observed in four patients at the 14.0 mg/m^2 level and in one patient at the 11.5 mg/m^2 level. QTc prolongation was asymptomatic and reversible on drug discontinuation. Other toxicities included nausea, diarrhea, vomiting, hypokalemia, and thrombocytopenia. Eight of 11 patients with peripheral blasts had transient reductions in blast counts, which increased shortly after drug discontinuation. Panobinostat has also been shown to be highly effective in CTCL[26] but not more effective than vorinostat. However, unlike vorinostat, single-agent activity has been seen, with response rates of almost 40% in refractory Hodgkin lymphoma. Even more impressive have been recent results in patients relapsing after autologous transplantation, in which overall responses of greater than 70% and objective and durable responses were seen in 27% in a large cohort of 129 patents.[27] This agent also synergizes with everolimus in blocking bcl-6 and mTOR. Panobinostat is being tested as a single agent or in combination with conventional chemotherapy or novel agents in NHL, myeloma, myeloid malignancies, and solid tumors.

Synthetic Benzamide Derivative Histone Deacetylase Inhibitors

Although structurally diverse, these compounds contain a benzamide moiety. Two important members of this class of HDIs are entinostat, which exerts antiproliferative effects at micromolar levels against pancreas, breast, colorectal, lung, and ovarian cancer cell types and in Hodgkin lymphoma cell lines. It has been shown to induce TGF-β receptor, which may enhance the antitumor effects of TGF-β. DLT was reached with the starting dose of 2 mg/m^2 daily for 28 days in a 42-day cycle. Pharmacokinetic data revealed a 30- to 50-fold longer half-life in humans than that predicted from animal models.

Cyclic Tetrapeptide Histone Deacetylase Inhibitors

The principal members of this class of agents are depsipeptide (Romidepsin). Romidepsin has recently been approved by the FDA as an IV agent for the treatment of patients with relapsed or refractory CTCL. It is a potent HDI that exerts in vitro antitumor effects at nanomolar levels against several cancer cell types. It also induces apoptosis of human acute leukemia and CLL cells. It is a natural product derived from *Chromobacterium violaceum,* a bacterium isolated from Japanese soil samples. Additionally, Romidepsin was shown to exert antiangiogenic effects by modulating the expression of genes involved in angiogenesis. In the pivotal study, 130 patients with confirmed peripheral T-cell lymphoma received Romidepsin at 14 mg/m^2 as a 4-hour IV infusion weekly for 3 weeks every 28 days. Objective responses were seen in 25% and complete responses in 15%, with a duration of response of 17 months. A second study in 47 peripheral T-cell lymphoma patients had a 38% objective response rate. A phase I study of romidepsin in patients with CLL and AML at a dosage of 13 mg/m^2 IV on days 1, 8, and 15 of a 4-week cycle showed antitumor activity in several patients, although no CRs or partial responses (PRs) were observed. Response was greater in patients with CLL than AML. There were no life-threatening toxicities, but constitutional symptoms characteristic of HDAC inhibition were observed in the majority of patients.

Depsipeptide shows substantial activity against CTCL and has recently been approved by the FDA for treatment of CTCL patients who have received at least one prior line of systemic therapy at a dose of 14 mg/m^2 intravenously over 4 hours on days 1, 8, and 15 of a 28-day cycle. Another phase II study of depsipeptide as a single agent has shown an encouraging 38% response rate in PTCL. In relapsed myeloma, no objective responses have been observed.

Combinations of Histone Deacetylase Inhibitors With Other Agents

Histone Deacetylase Inhibitors With Cell Cycle and Cell-Signaling Modulators

Both vorinostat and SB have also been combined with the cell cycle–dependent kinase (CDK) inhibitor flavopiridol. The combination of HDI and flavopiridol dramatically increased apoptosis of cultured and primary AML cells, resulting in a synergistic cytotoxic response. Because treatment with flavopiridol also transcriptionally downregulates several antiapoptotic gene expressions, this may be responsible for the synergistic effect observed with the combination. Recent studies have shown that treatment with vorinostat or LAQ824 attenuates the mRNA level of *BCR-ABL* and promotes polyubiquitylation and proteasomal degradation of BCR-ABL. In addition, a combined treatment with LAQ824 and imatinib or PD180970 was shown to induce apoptosis of imatinib-sensitive or imatinib-refractory CML cells. Similarly, the combination of vorinostat and dasatinib on cultured human, primary CML, or murine pro-B BaF 3 cells expressing unmutated or mutated form of BCR-ABL showed enhanced apoptosis. The more potent TKI, nilotinib, has also been studied with the HDI, panobinostat, in cells with ectopic expression of *BCR-ABL* and mutated clones (T315I, E255K) that are imatinib resistant. Taken together, these preclinical findings support the rationale to study the safety and efficacy of the combinations of these HDIs with specific inhibitors of pro-growth and survival signaling triggered by oncoprotein tyrosine kinases.

Heat Shock Protein Inhibitors

The "heat shock response" was first described in 1962. Crucial observations were made indicating that certain regions of the chromosomes of the fruit fly *Drosophila* puffed out in response to a sudden increase in temperature. The gene products encoded on these chromosomes were later termed *heat-shock proteins* (HSPs). Contrary to most cellular proteins, HSP production increases several-fold in response to environmental stresses, including heat shock, nutrient deprivation, oxidative stresses, heavy metals, and alcohol exposure. They form multimolecular complexes with variable cellular proteins, regulating their correct folding, repair, degradation, and function; hence the HSPs' more accurate designation is "molecular chaperones." A number of multigene families of HSPs exist, and their individual products vary in cellular expression, function, and localization. They are classified according to their molecular weight (e.g., HSP90, HSP70, HSP27). Exceptions to this rule are the chaperones identified as glucose-regulated proteins (GRP94 and GRP75).

HSP90 regulates the function and stability of many key signaling proteins that allow cancer cells to escape the inherent toxicity of their environment, to evade the effects of chemotherapy, and to protect themselves from their own genetic instability. In humans, HSP90 consists of four genes, cytosolic HSP90α and HSP90β, GRP94, and HSP75/TNF-associated protein 1 (TRAP1). The monomer HSP90 consists of conserved 25-kd N-terminal and 55-kd C-terminal domains. The N-terminus contains a highly conserved ATP-binding domain. Dimerization of these nucleotide-binding domains is essential for ATP binding and hydrolysis. Phosphorylation leads HSP90 to interact with co-chaperones such as HSP70 and p23 to form heteroprotein complexes, which are essential for various protein functions. Such proteins include several transcription factors (e.g., steroid hormone receptor, retinoid receptors, and HIF-1α) serine/threonine and tyrosine kinases (e.g., c-SRC/v-SRC, RAF-1, ERB2, EGFR, MEK, CDK4, AKT, BCR-ABL, LCK, FAK, c-MET), and other proteins with various functions (e.g., mutant p53, catalytic subunit of telomerase hTERT, TNFR1, and RB). HSP90 inhibition leads to misfolded client proteins that are involved in malignancy to be polyubiquitinated and degraded by proteosomes. Significant interest in HSP90 inhibition has led to the following compounds.

Benzoquinone Ansamycins (Herbamycin A, Geldanamycin, and Tanespimycin)

The first class of HSP90 inhibitors to be discovered was the benzoquinone ansamycins, which include herbamycin A and geldanamycin. These natural products were first isolated from the actinomycete broths in the 1970s. Hemamycin A was later shown to reverse the malignant phenotype of *v-Src*–transformed fibroblasts, with potent antitumor activity in vitro and in vivo animal models. The effects of this drug on other tyrosine kinases, including $p210^{bcr\text{-}abl}$, were also described, leading to the frequent use of herbimycin A as a general TKI. However, Whitesell and colleagues later identified HSP90 as the prominent benzoquinone ansamycin-binding protein, and they described the ability of these drugs to disrupt the complex between v-Src and HSP90, resulting in destabilization of v-Src protein and its eventual loss from treated cells. Subsequent immunoprecipitation and x-ray crystallography studies showed that geldanamycin competes at the ATP-binding site and inhibits the intrinsic ATPase activity of HSP90, preventing the formation of mature multimeric HSP90 complexes capable of chaperoning client proteins (Fig. 55-10). As a result, the client proteins are ubiquitinated and targeted for proteasomal degradation. Although clearly active in human tumor xenograft models, preclinical evaluation of geldanamycin demonstrated significant hepatotoxicity at therapeutic levels. Screening for geldanamycin analogs resulted in the discovery of 17-allylamino-17-demethoxygeldanamycin, or tanespimycin (17-AAG), a semisynthetic geldanamycin derivative in which an allylamino group replaces the methoxy in the 17 position (see Fig. 55-10). Tanespimycin has a significantly improved toxicity profile but similar to geldanamycin retains the ability to inhibit HSP90. In addition, tanespimycin has been shown to have greater affinity for binding to HSP90 from cancer versus normal host cells.

Preclinical Studies of Tanespimycin

Preclinical studies of tanespimycin exhibited significant antiproliferative and cytotoxic effects against a wide panel of transformed cell

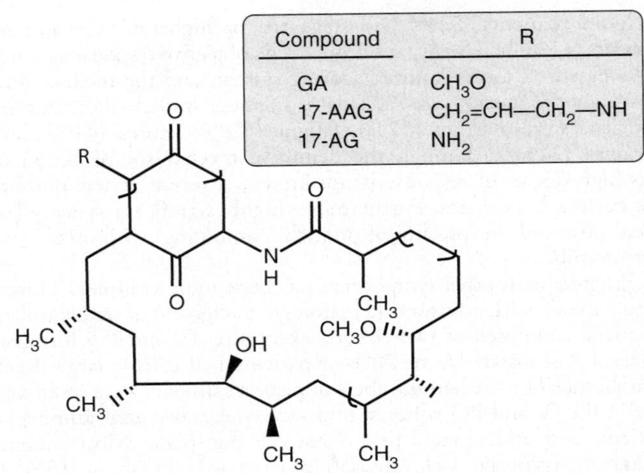

Figure 55-10 CHEMICAL STRUCTURE OF GELDANAMYCIN (GA), 17-ALLYLAMIN-17-DEMETHOXYGELDANAMYCIN (17-AAG), AND 17-AMINO-GELDANAMYCIN (17-AG).

lines, inhibiting pathways that regulate cell cycle progression, apoptosis, invasion, and angiogenesis. In the NCI in vitro cancer screen, the mean GI_{50} for tanespimycin was 0.19 μM, with greater than average sensitivity in melanoma, leukemia, non–small cell lung, ovarian, breast, prostate, and renal cancer panels.

Benzoquinone ansamycins have been reported to induce G1 as well as G2/M block. In a panel of breast cancer cell lines, 17-AAG and geldanamycin caused a G1 arrest. This G1 block resulted from downregulation of signaling pathways controlling cyclin D or CDK4/cyclin D1 activity, particularly depletion of tyrosine kinases (ERBB2, EGF receptor), and degradation of c-RAF-1 with reduced phosphorylation of ERK. A G2/M block has been reported in RB-deficient cells treated with tanespimycin; however, the requirement for RB deficiency appears to be cell dependent. A number of G2 checkpoint kinases such as WEE1 and MYT1 have also been identified as HSP90 client proteins.

HSP90 plays a crucial role in regulating apoptosis. Tanespimycin induced cytosolic accumulation of cytochrome C and cleavage and activation of caspases 9 and 3, triggering apoptosis in HL-60/Bcr-Abl with ectopic expression of p185-Bcr-Abl and K562 with endogenous p210-Bcr-Abl cells. Tanespimycin treatment leads to proteasomal degradation of Bcr-Abl along with AKT depletion. However, high ectopic expression of HSP70 inhibits 17-AAG–induced Bax conformation change, mitochondrial localization, and apoptosis. This is important because of tanespimycin and other analogs of geldanamycin (17-DMAG and IPI504) or radicicol induce HSP70 levels. Therefore, strategies leading to abrogation of HSP70 induction would further antileukemic effects of HSP90 inhibitors.

In addition to their modulation of the cell cycle and programmed cell death, geldanamycin and tanespimycin have been implicated in the regulation of invasion, metastasis, and angiogenesis. Tanespimycin treatment of H322 and H358 cells enhanced E-cadherin expression and inhibited secretion of MMP-9 and VEGF. Geldanamycins have also been shown to inhibit the HGF/SF-MET signaling pathway, resulting in decreased cell motility and invasion of c-MET transformed cells. HSP90 inhibitors also significantly reduce VEGF secretion by decreasing HIF1α expression as well as inducing degradation of all three VEGF receptors.

Combination studies incorporating tanespimycin have shown promise. In lung and colorectal cell lines, combinations of tanespimycin with cisplatin, doxorubicin, or paclitaxel have been synergistic or additive. In addition, tanespimycin is synergistic with novel agents, including imatinib, bortezomib, ERK inhibitors, and SAHA. Combined treatment of panobinostat, a histone deacetylase inhibitor, with tanespimycin exerted synergistic effects in AML and CML cells with decreased Bcr-Abl, p-AKT, AKT, and p-STAT5 levels.

Metabolism of Tanespimycin

In human and murine microsome assays, three metabolites of tanespimycin (17-AAG) were identified: 17-aminogeldanamycin (17-AG), a diol, and an epoxide. The 17-AAG diol is the major metabolite in human hepatic microsomes followed by 17-AG. Cytochrome P450 (3A4) was identified as the enzyme responsible for 17-AAG metabolism. Acrolein, a known nephrotoxin, is a byproduct of 17-AG. Also, the 17-AG metabolite has biological activity equivalent to that of the parent compound. The quinone-metabolizing enzyme DT-diaphorase has been shown to alter tanespimycin's antitumor properties. A positive correlation between DT-diaphorase expression levels and growth inhibition by tanespimycin has been established. Transfection of an active DT-diaphorase gene NQO1 into a human carcinoma cell line increased tanespimycin's growth-inhibitory activity 32-fold. Polymorphisms of the NQO1 gene, which is found in 5% to 20% of the population, as well as acting as a substrate for PGP efflux pump may limit its clinical efficacy.

Clinical Investigation With Tanespimycin

Several phase I trials in adults have explored different scheduling regimens of tanespimycin. Administration of tanespimycin daily for 3 days or for 5 days has been associated with dose-limiting toxicities, namely, hepatotoxicity, diarrhea, and thrombocytopenia at substantially lower doses (40-56 mg/m^2). Grade III GI toxicity, including nausea, vomiting, and diarrhea, is associated with the formulation of tanespimycin, which contains 4% DMSO. No objective clinical responses were reported with either schedule; however, in xenograft models, the effects of tanespimycin on HSP90 client proteins lasted up to 72 hours, suggesting that twice-weekly dosing might be more effective. Thus additional trials have evaluated twice weekly and weekly for 3 weeks out of 4. A recent study recommended phase II doses of 175 to 200 mg/m^2 given twice weekly. This schedule was associated with a persistent increase of HSP70; however, no consistent changes in PBMC phosphorylated Akt, HSP90, or Raf-1 during treatment. Combination phase I studies of tanespimycin with docetaxel, irinotecan, imatinib, trastuzumab, and bortezomib are currently ongoing.

Clinical Investigation With IPI-504

Because tanespimycin has poor aqueous solubility and must be administered with DMSO or newer Cremophor formulations, synthesis of HSP90 inhibitors with more favorable pharmaceutical properties is required. IPI-504, the highly soluble hydroquinone hydrochloride derivative of tanespimycin, has been shown to be 4000-fold more soluble than tanespimycin. In preclinical studies, single-agent IPI-504 as well as in combination with bortezomib has shown antitumor effects in xenograft models of multiple myeloma. Also, treatment with IPI-504 resulted in BCR-ABL protein degradation, decreased numbers of leukemia stem cells, and prolonged survival of leukemic mice bearing the T315I mutation. A phase I study has been initiated in relapsed myeloma patients. IPI-504 is administered over 30 minutes on days 1, 4, 8, and 11 every 21 days. Thus far, 15 patients have been treated, with doses ranging from 90 to 300 mg/m^2. No dose-limiting toxicities have been observed to date.

Clinical Investigation With Alvespimycin (KOS-1022)

Alvespimycin (KOS-1022) is a second-generation HSP90 inhibitor that has begun phase I trials with IV and PO schedules. Escalating doses of alvespimycin were given intravenously over 1 hour twice weekly every 3 weeks. Alvespimycin demonstrated antileukemic activity with tolerable toxicity at 24 mg/m^2 twice weekly. In 23 patients with AML, 3 patients experienced complete response and 1 patient demonstrated stable disease while on study for 9 cycles. Clinical trials of alvespimycin in combination with trastuzumab in solid malignancies are also ongoing.

17-DMAG

The water-soluble stable geldanamycin derivative, 17-(dimethylaminothylamino)-17-demethoxygeldanamycin (17-DMAG), has demonstrated more potent in vitro and in vivo antitumor activity than 17-AAG. In addition, 17-DMAG offers three potential advantages over 17-AAG: (1) aqueous solubility eliminates formulation problems associated with 17-AAG, (2) 17-DMAG undergoes limited metabolism, and (3) it has higher PO bioavailability. Phase I studies evaluating 17-DMAG have been recently initiated.

Other HSP90 Inhibitors

In addition to benzoquinone ansamycins and the semisynthetic analog tanespimycin, several other compounds were found to bind HSP90 and disrupt its chaperone function.

Radicicol

Radicicol, a macrocyclic antibiotic isolated from *Monosporum bonorden,* binds the N-terminal domain of HSP90, competing with its natural ligand, ATP. Although a more potent inhibitor of HSP90 ATPase compared with geldanamycin, radicicol lacks antitumoral activity in vivo owing to its unstable chemical nature. Oxime-derivative compounds, which retain the HSP90 inhibitory activity and have a more stable chemical structure, were developed.

Novobiocin

Novobiocin, a coumarin antibiotic, binds the C-terminus domain of HSP90, as opposed to N-terminus binding with geldanamycin and radicicol. However, it was shown to retain inhibitory activity against HSP90 and degrade its client-signaling proteins. Thus it appears that N- and C-terminal domains are both essential for HSP90 chaperone functions.

Bryostatin 1

Bryostatin 1 (NSC339555) is a macrocyclic lactone isolated from the marine bryozoan *Bugula neritina.* It originally attracted attention because of its activity against a wide variety of tumor types in an NCI screen. In hematopoietic cells, bryostatin 1 displays the unique capacity to inhibit the growth of human leukemia cells while stimulating the growth of their normal counterparts.

Bryostatin 1 has been shown to act like the phorbol ester phorbol myristate acetate (PMA) in that it binds to and activates the serine-threonine kinase protein kinase C. However, in contrast to PMA, it is a weak inducer of leukemic cell maturation and in fact blocks PMA-mediated differentiation. This may reflect the ability of bryostatin 1, on chronic administration, to downregulate PKC activity.

In preclinical studies, bryostatin 1 has shown activity against continuously cultured and primary human leukemia and lymphoma cells when administered at nanomolar concentrations. In addition, bryostatin lowers the threshold for leukemic and lymphoma cell apoptosis in response to conventional cytotoxic agents. The latter include ara-C, fludarabine, vincristine, paclitaxel, and chlorodeoxyadenosine. It is postulated, although not definitively established, that such actions may reflect bryostatin 1–mediated downregulation of PKC, which exerts antiapoptotic actions. More recently, bryostatin 1 has been shown to interact synergistically with more novel agents, including flavopiridol, through a process that may involve induction of TNF. In clinical studies, bryostatin 1 has been administered according to a variety of schedules. Dose-limiting toxicity consists of myalgias, which are cumulative and which do not respond well to standard analgesic therapy. Other toxicities include fatigue, hepatotoxicity, nausea and vomiting, and phlebitis.

Bryostatin 1 as a single agent has shown some, although limited, activity. For example, when administered as a 120-hour continuous infusion every 2 weeks at a dose of 120 μg/m^2, three of 25 patients with CLL or NHL achieved a CR or objective PR. On the other hand, of nine patients with multiple myeloma, none responded to this bryostatin 1 dose and schedule.

Results have been somewhat more promising when bryostatin 1 was combined with established cytotoxic drugs. For example, administration of bryostatin 1 as a 24-hour infusion (50 μg/m^2) immediately before and after a split course of high-dose ara-C resulted in four CRs in 23 patients with highly refractory disease. Administration of escalating doses of bryostatin 1 as a 1-hour infusion immediately before or after a 5-day course of fludarabine (doses of 16-25 mg/m^2/day) resulted in 17 of 53 objective responses, including six in patients who had progressed on fludarabine previously. Neither sequence was clearly superior to the other.

Finally, in a phase I study, patients with B-cell malignancies were treated with a 24-hour continuous infusion of bryostatin 1 followed by a bolus injection of vincristine every 2 weeks. The maximally tolerated dose of bryostatin 1 was 50 μg/m^2. Of the 24 evaluable patients, five patients had durable CRs or PRs, and an additional five patients had stable disease. Collectively, these findings suggest that bryostatin 1 may have a role in hematologic malignancies when combined with established cytotoxic agents.

DRUG RESISTANCE TO CHEMOTHERAPEUTIC AGENTS OR MULTIDRUG RESISTANCE

Although many hematologic malignancies develop resistance to a specific class of chemotherapeutic agents, especially to targeted therapeutics, through the development of kinase region point mutations, emergence of resistance to multiple cytotoxic chemotherapeutic agents is also common among hematologic malignancies. The basis for resistance includes specific drug resistance mechanisms, overexpression of the ABC transports such as MDR-1 for drug efflux, and overexpression of antiapoptotic proteins. The Goldie–Coldman hypothesis predicts that drug-resistant tumor cell clones survive because of a favorable spontaneous mutation, which occurs in approximately one in a million cells. Because 1 g of tumor contains 1×10^9 cells, it becomes obvious that high tumor burden states have a tremendous number of mutations, which can contribute to drug resistance. This is the rationale for using combination chemotherapy at specific dose intervals to maximize dose intensity.

Drug resistance mechanisms have been discovered and subsequently defined at the molecular level by investigators working in vitro with tumor cell lines selected in the presence of specific antitumor agents, by analysis of primary samples of untreated and treated hematologic malignancies, and through screening of tumor banks. Classes of resistance include acquired protein deficiency, loss of sensitivity to apoptotic signals, and age-related defects in the cellular pathways that normally lead to apoptosis.

P-Glycoprotein (ABC-B1 Transporter)

Structure and Function

The ABC superfamily of membrane transporters mediates the cross membrane flux of xenobiotics, naturally occurring toxic compounds, drugs, peptides, and ions. *ABC* stands for ATP-binding cassette transporter family. They have profound impact on homeostasis and are critically important to proliferation and differentiation signals in normal progenitor cells. They also mediate drug sensitivity. The terminology remains challenging because many earlier works referred to PGP and MRP, but the more recent consensus on the ABC superfamily has created a more simple approach going forward. PGP (ABC B1 transporter) has been the subject of intense biochemical and clinical studies since it was first discovered in drug-resistant cell lines more than 20 years ago. The biochemistry of PGP has been reviewed in detail by several investigators. This phosphorylated glycoprotein has a molecular mass of approximately 170 kd and is localized to the plasma membrane, where it functions as a drug efflux pump (Table 55-7). The ATP-dependent extrusion of antineoplastic agents confers a relative level of resistance to the cell that overexpresses PGP. Recently, the family of drug-transporting proteins has been more carefully characterized, leading to the use of the terms *ATP-binding cassette transporters*. The observation of double minute chromosomes and homogeneously staining regions in several MDR cell lines suggested that gene amplification is involved in PGP-mediated MDR. The human *MDR1* gene, which codes for PGP and is involved in antitumor drug resistance, and the human *MDR2* gene (the product of which is expressed by hepatocytes) are located very near each other on human chromosome 7q21.1. The human *MDR1* gene has 28 exons and codes for a protein of 1280 amino acids. The PGP molecule has two homologous halves, each with a hydrophobic region containing six transmembrane domains and a hydrophilic region containing an ATP-binding site. The N-linked glycosylation occurs on the extracellular side (Fig. 55-11). PGP is a member of the ABC superfamily, which includes, among more than 100 others, the multidrug resistance–associated protein (MRP); the pf*mdr* pump in *Plasmodium falciparum*, which results in chloroquine resistance; STE6, the transporter of the "a" peptide mating factor in yeast; the cystic fibrosis transmembrane conductance regulator (CFTR); and the TAP-1 and TAP-2 proteins that transport antigenic peptides for association with class I molecules and surface antigen presentation. MRP has been demonstrated in several MDR mammalian cell lines and in human tumors (see later), but a recent study in human tumor cell lines has shown TAP overexpression associated with MRP as well as drug resistance resulting from transfection of the *TAP* genes.

P-glycoprotein has a broad specificity for hydrophobic compounds and can both reduce the influx of drugs into the cytosol and increase efflux from the cytosol. To accomplish the former, this "hydrophobic vacuum cleaner" must detect drugs and expel them while they are still in the plasma membrane. Drugs are thought to be effluxed from the cytosol through a single barrel of the PGP transporter, although an exact mechanism has been lacking. A recent study has used electron microscopy to generate an initial structure of PGP to 2.5-nm resolution. The structure was further refined by three-dimensional reconstructions from single particle image analysis of detergent-solubilized PGP and by Fourier projection maps of small crystalline arrays of PGP. This demonstrates that PGP is monomeric, with the shape of a cylinder 10 nm in diameter with a maximum height (in the plane of the membrane) of 8 nm (see Fig. 55-11). Approximately half of the PGP molecule is within the membrane because the lipid bilayer is approximately 4 nm in depth. When viewed from the extracellular surface of the membrane, PGP is pteroidal with a large central pore 5 nm in diameter. This large aqueous chamber in the membrane that is open to the extracellular space is closed on the cytoplasmic side presumably by the two 3-nM intracellular lobes (putative nucleotide-binding domains) and the hydrophilic cytoplasmic loops between the transmembrane domains. Thus this large pore has a "gate" on the cytoplasmic side of the membrane that can regulate the transport of different-sized substrates.

Substrates of PGP include (see Table 55-7) anthracyclines (doxorubicin, daunorubicin, epirubicin, and idarubicin), anthracenediones (mitoxantrone), aminoacridines (*m*-AMSA), taxanes (taxol and taxotere), epipodophyllotoxins (VP-16 and VM-26), vinca alkaloids (vincristine, vinblastine, and vinorelbine), bortezomib, and actinomycin D. Mitomycin C and one of the topoisomerase I inhibitors (topotecan) are both weak substrates for PGP. Several drugs reverse the resistance mediated by PGP overexpression and sensitize cells to the cytotoxic effects of antineoplastic agents. These drugs compete with antitumor agents for efflux from the cell, effectively increasing the intracellular concentration of the cytotoxic drug, and include immunosuppressants (cyclosporin A, FK 506, rapamycin, PSC 833), calcium channel blockers (verapamil, nifedipine), antiarrhythmics (quinidine), and other miscellaneous agents. Several of these MDR-modulating agents have been used in clinical trials in an effort to sensitize resistant tumor cells (see later).

Table 55-7 Characteristics of Three Mechanisms of Multidrug Resistance That Result From Overexpression of P-Glycoprotein (PGP), Multidrug Resistance-Associated Protein (MRP), or Lung Resistance-Related Protein (LRP)

	PGP	MRP	LRP
Gene on chromosome	7q21.1	16p13.1	16p11.2
Protein			
Molecular mass	170 kd	190 kd	110 kd
Cellular location	Plasma membrane	Plasma membrane	Cytoplasm » nuclear membrane
Function	Efflux pump, chloride channel	Drug transporter	Major vault protein (nucleocytoplasmic transport?)
Energy source	ATP	ATP	
Post-translational modifications	N-glycosylation, phosphorylation	N-glycosylation, phosphorylation	*No* N- or O-glycosylation
Analogs	Member ABC superfamily	Member ABC superfamily; GS-X pump, MOAT, LTC_4 transport	
Drug Resistance Phenotype			
Antitumor agents	Act-D, AMSA, dauno, dox, epi, ida, mito-C	Act-D, chlor, CDDP-GSH, dauno, dox, epi, mel, tax (low), vbl (low), vcr, VM-26, VP-16	Carbo, CDDP, dox, mel, vcr, VP-16
	(Low), mtz, nav, tax, txtr, tpt (low), vbl, vcr, VM-26, VP-16	As, Cd, colch (low), GSH	
Other drugs	Colch, rhod	Conjugates, GSSG, LT_4, Sb	
Reversing agents	CSA, FK506, nifed, PSC833, quin, rap, verap	CSA, gnstn, indo, nicard, prbn, PSC833, verap, VX-710	
Normal hematopoietic tissues with increased expression	NK ($CD56^+$) T cells, suppressor T cells ($CD8^+$), B cells, $CD34^+$ stem cells	PBMNs (especially T cells), rbc membranes; liver and spleen low level	Macrophages
Prognostic significance	AML, MM, NHL	AML (inv 16)	AML, ALL

ABC, ATP-binding cassette; *act-D,* actinomycin D; *ALL,* acute lymphoblastic leukemia; *AML,* acute myeloid leukemia; *As,* arsenicals; *ATP,* adenosine triphosphate; *carbo,* carboplatin; *Cd,* cadmium; *CDDP-GSH;* cisplatin glutathione conjugate; *chlor,* chlorambucil; *colch,* colchicine; *CSA,* cyclosporin A; *dauno,* daunomycin; *dox,* doxorubicin; *epi,* epirubicin; *gnstn,* genistein; *GS-X,* glutathione conjugate; *GSSG,* oxidized glutathione; *ida,* idarubicin; *indo,* indomethacin; *LTC_4,* cysteinyl leukotriene; *mel,* melphalan; *mito-C,* mitomycin C; *MM,* multiple myeloma; *MOAT,* multispecific organic anion transporter; *mtz,* mitoxantrone; *nav,* navelbine; *NHL,* non-Hodgkin lymphoma; *nicard,* nicardipine; *NK,* natural killer; *nifed,* nifedipine; *prbn,* probenecid; *quin,* quinidine; *rap,* rapamycin; *rhod,* rhodamine; *Sb,* antimonials; *tax,* taxol; *tpt,* topotecan; *txtr,* taxotere; *vbl,* vinblastine; *vcr,* vincristine; *verap,* verapamil; *VM-26,* teniposide; *VP-16,* etoposide.

Methods of Detection

Several monoclonal antibodies that recognize PGP and are commercially available for routine analyses have been described. Monoclonal antibodies C219 and JSB-1 recognize internal epitopes of PGP, whereas antibodies MRK16 and UIC2 detect external antigens and are more suited for FACS analysis.

P-Glycoprotein Expression in Normal Human Tissue

High levels of expression of *MDR1*/PGP have been found in the epithelium of several human tissues with excretory function, suggesting that PGP is normally involved in transporting both exogenous toxic compounds and endogenous metabolites. These tissues include the adrenal cortex, renal proximal tubule epithelium, biliary hepatocytes, small and large intestinal mucosa, pancreas, and endothelial cells of the brain and testis. Normal human hematopoietic tissues with high levels of *MDR1*/PGP include $CD34^+$ progenitor cells, $CD56^+$ (NK) cells, and $CD8^+$ (T-suppressor) cells. Lower levels of expression have also been observed in $CD4^+$ (T-helper) cells, $CD19^+$ B cells, and $CD14^+$ cells (monocytes).

P-Glycoprotein Expression in Human Malignancies

Increased expression of PGP has been observed in several human tumors, especially those malignancies that arise in tissues that normally have high levels of PGP expression. An analysis of 61 human tumor cell lines (from leukemia, CNS tumors, melanoma, breast cancer, ovarian cancer, colon cancer, lung cancer, and kidney cancer), which were not selected for resistance to antitumor agents, demonstrated coexpression of two or three of the MDR proteins (PGP, LRP, or MRP) in 64% of the cell lines. PGP and LRP were overexpressed in 3% of the tumors; MRP and LRP in 43%; and PGP, LRP, and MRP in 18%. The cell lines with the highest levels of drug resistance were found to overexpress all three proteins. Whether this is true in primary human tumors awaits further investigations.

Acute Myeloid Leukemia

An earlier meta-analysis of studies that examined the expression of *MDR1*/PGP in blasts of patients with AML found that 40% (105 of 261 patients) who were PGP positive achieved a CR, but 81% (192 of 238) of PGP-negative patients obtained a CR. An analysis of 96 untreated patients with AML showed that PGP expression predicted induction failure (P<.0001) and decreased OS (P<.001), as did unfavorable cytogenetics. PGP expression was not detected in patients with favorable cytogenetic abnormalities [t(15;17), inv(16), t(8;21)], was found in 29% of those samples with a normal karyotype, and expressed in 62% of patients with an unfavorable cytogenetic abnormality. PGP was also detected in 63% of those with secondary AML compared with 25% of those with de novo disease. PGP analysis with the MRK16 antibody in 211 elderly patients (older than 55 years) with untreated AML again showed that PGP expression is significantly associated with a decreased CR rate and

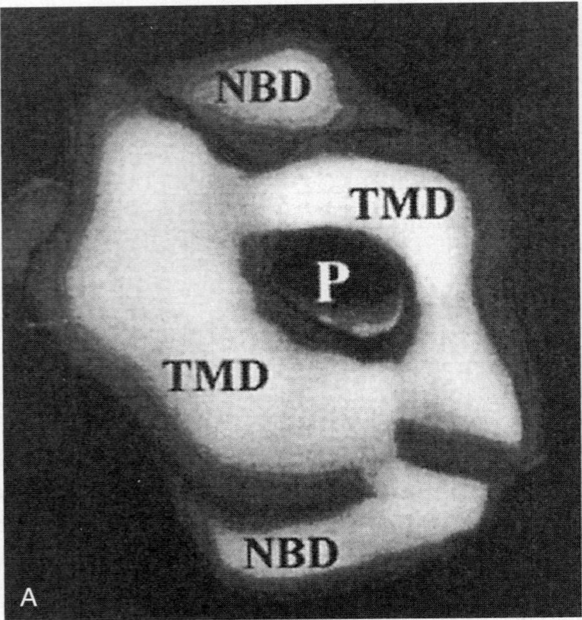

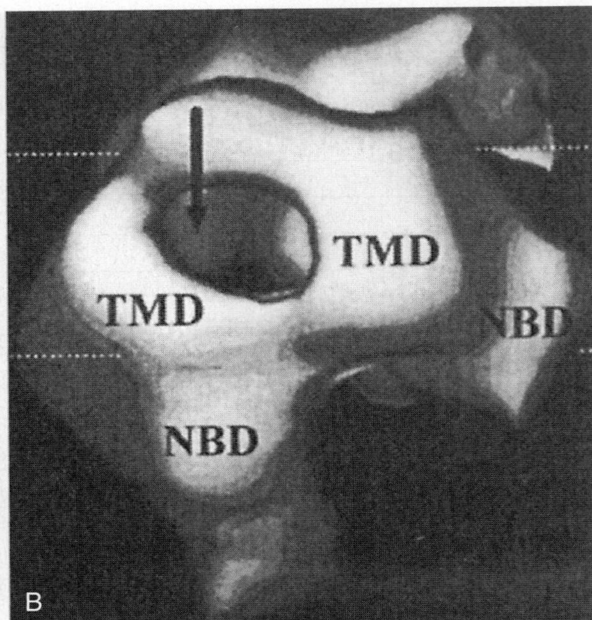

Figure 55-11 STRUCTURE OF P-GLYCOPROTEIN (PGP) DETERMINED BY ELECTRON MICROSCOPY; A COMPUTER GRAPHIC REPRESENTATION OF THE THREE-DIMENSIONAL RECONSTRUCTION IS SHOWN AS A SHADED SURFACE REPRESENTATION OF THE STRUCTURE. The straight arrow shows the putative adenosine triphosphate (ATP)–binding domains. P represents the aqueous pore open at the extracellular face of the membrane. TMD, two thumbs, each of which probably corresponds to one of the two transmembrane domains. NBD, 3-nm lobes projecting from the structure at the cytoplasmic face of the membrane, probably corresponding to the two nucleotide-binding domains. **A,** View perpendicular to the extracellular surface of the lipid bilayer; **B,** side view of PGP in which the approximate position of the lipid bilayer is indicated by the two horizontal *dashed lines. Arrow* indicates asymmetric opening providing access from the lipid phase to the aqueous core of the protein. *(Reproduced with permission from Rosenberg MF, Callaghan R, Ford RC, et al: Structure of the multidrug resistance P-glycoprotein to 2.5 nm resolution determined by electron microscopy and image analysis.* J Biol Chem *272:10685, 1997.)*

resistant disease. Patients in this report with de novo PGP-negative AML with favorable cytogenetics have a CR rate of 81% compared with 12% for those with secondary AML, which is PGP positive and has unfavorable cytogenetics. Clinical trials using the PGP substrate PSC833 acting as a competitive inhibitor did not show the dramatic benefit expected, especially in older patients with acute leukemias.

Impact of P-Glycoprotein in Other Hematologic Malignancies

The role of PGP in the drug resistance of NHL, myeloma, and ALL is ill-defined. CLL is another chronic leukemia in which few PGP-related antineoplastic agents are used. However, a single study has shown a correlation between *MDR1* expression and survival, in which the 10 B-CLL patients who were *MDR1* positive had a median survival of 19 months compared with 46 months for the 17 patients who were *MDR1* negative (P <.01). Nonetheless, a recent study identified bortezomib as a substrate for PGP, raising the possibility that myeloma PGP levels affect clinical response. There have not been recent studies of the role of PGP in drug resistance in NHL in the past 5 years. With the newer kinase inhibitors, it has recently been noted that Nilotinib and dasatinib are high-affinity substrates of ABCG2. These agents appear to inhibit the function of this transporter, but whether this will translate into clinical impact has not received prospective attention.

Clinical Studies With Modulators of P-Glycoprotein

The clinical trials that have used various modulators of PGP have been reviewed by several investigators. An early study in VAD-refractory multiple myeloma resulted in short-lived partial responses to VAD plus racemic verapamil in five of 22 patients. Four of the five responders overexpressed PGP; however, cardiac side effects precluded further dose escalation of IV *R,S*-verapamil. Continuous IV infusion of cyclosporin A (CSA) with VAD in VAD-resistant myeloma patients resulted in seven of 15 responses, which were more common in those who overexpressed PGP. A randomized SWOG phase III study of VAD and PO verapamil in 120 patients with refractory myeloma demonstrated a 41% and 36% response in the VAD and VAD/verapamil arms, respectively, with median survival times of 10 and 13 months. Continuous-infusion CSA has been dose escalated in combination with daunorubicin and ara-C. A transient hyperbilirubinemia was seen in 62% of the patients; these same patients had increased serum daunorubicin levels and a higher response rate. A complete response was seen in 26 of 42 patients; however, the MDR phenotype was not found to influence the response. A study of PSC833 in patients with acute leukemia treated with cytarabine, daunorubicin, and etoposide showed a modest benefit in patients younger than 45 years of age, raising the potential of developing an effective strategy in patients older than 60 years of age in whom PGP expression in leukemic cells is more common. Zosuquidar, a PGP inhibitor, was tested for efficacy in a phase 3 trial through ECOG in 449 patients older than the age of 60 years. No benefit in response rate or survival was noted. Likewise, in a CALGB study, in adults with untreated leukemia younger than the age of 60 years, PSC-833 also did not improve survival or response rates. Thus the future role of modulation of PGP in leukemia management remains ill defined.

Multidrug Resistance–Associated Protein (ABC G2 Transporter)

Structure and Function

The MRP was first described in 1992 in the doxorubicin-selected small cell lung cancer cell line, and its biochemical characteristics and biologic properties have been reviewed. It has now been classified within the larger context of ABC transporters, termed *ABC G2 transporters*. Because much of the literature uses the MRP nomenclature, we refer to this herein except for the studies using the ABC terminology. This N-glycosylated plasma membrane phosphoprotein has a molecular mass of 190 kd (1531 amino acids) and is a member of the ABC transporter superfamily (see Table 55-7 and Fig. 55-12). This transporter has 18 transmembrane domains (12 in the amino end and six in the carboxyl end) and is coded on human chromosome 16p13.1.

The overexpression of MRP has been shown in vitro to result in different levels of drug resistance to several classes of antineoplastic agents, represented by actinomycin D, chlorambucil, melphalan, CDDP, daunomycin, doxorubicin, epirubicin, VM-26, VP-16, and vincristine. Low levels of resistance have also been reported to taxol, vinblastine, and colchicine. In addition to antitumoral agents, MRP (and its isoforms) are capable of transporting heavy metals (arsenicals, cadmium, and antimonials) as well as glutathione conjugates and cysteinyl leukotriene. Compounds reported to modulate MRP-mediated drug resistance in vitro include the calcium channel blocker verapamil nocardipine; the protein kinase C inhibitor GF109203X; the cyclosporin analog PSC 833; the TKI genistein; the gyrase-inhibiting antibiotic difloxacin; and amiodarone VX-710 Amiodarone VX-710, a nonmacrocyclic ligand of the FK506-binding protein FKBP12 and a potent modulator of PGP-mediated MDR, has been found to restore sensitivity of MRP-expressing HL60/ADR cells to the cytotoxic action of doxorubicin, VP-16, and vincristine. Other investigational agents include Danusertib, a potent pan-aurora and ABL kinase inhibitor being developed for CML. The nonsteroidal antiinflammatory drug indomethacin has also been shown to significantly increase the sensitivity of HL60/ADR cells to doxorubicin and vincristine and may be a specific inhibitor of MRP.[29]

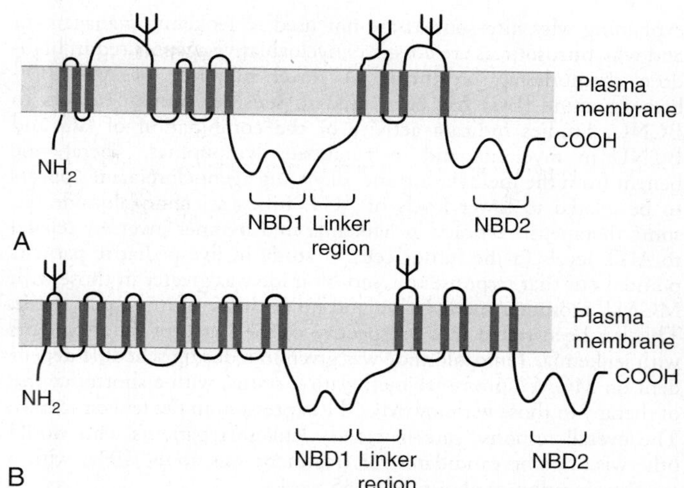

Figure 55-12 MODELS OF MULTIDRUG RESISTANCE PROTEIN (MRP) MEMBRANE TOPOLOGY. MRP possesses features common to all members of the adenosine triphosphate (ATP)–binding cassette transporter superfamily in that each half of the protein is predicted to consist of several transmembrane domains followed by a cytosolic nucleotide-binding domain (MBD). The first model **(A)** is based on computer-assisted hydropathy analyses of the human MRP amino acid sequence and predicts that MRP is composed of 12 transmembrane domains *(solid bars),* eight of which are within the NH-2 proximal half of the protein. The second model **(B),** based on a comparison of human and murine MRP with other ATP-binding cassette transporters, suggests that there are up to four additional transmembrane domains in the NH2-proximal half of the protein. *(Adapted from Loe DW, Deley RG, Cole SPC: Biology of the multidrug resistance-associated protein, MRP.* Eur J Cancer *32A:945, 1996.)*

Multidrug Resistance Protein Expression in Hematologic Malignancies

The expression of MRP mRNA or the level of MRP protein has been assessed in 148 patients with hematopoietic malignancies. MRP mRNA expression was found to be significantly increased in 84% of patients with CLL and in 30% of those with AML. The vast majority of patients with ALL, CML, multiple myeloma, hairy cell leukemia, and NHL were found to have low levels of MRP mRNA expression. MRP protein was assayed using monoclonal antibody MRPr1, and the results were generally similar with increased expression in most patients with CLL. A study of 40 patients with refractory lymphoma and 16 with newly diagnosed lymphoma suggests a limited role for MRP mRNA expression in drug resistance in NHL because 15 paired samples in the refractory group showed no difference in MRP expression pre- and post-EPOCH treatment. In addition, the untreated patients had MRP mRNA levels that were no different from the pre- or post-EPOCH patient levels. A study of 49 patients with AML and 29 with ALL demonstrated significantly higher expression of MRP in ALL ($P < .007$) and in secondary AML ($P < .016$) but not in de novo AML. Combining overexpression of ABC G2 and FLT3-ITD, an Italian group identified that in adult AML, overexpression of ABC G2 was detected in 83 (50%) and of FLT3-ITD in 47 (28%) patients. Although the response rate was not affected, the duration of remission was much shorter when these proteins were overexpressed. In a small study of 14 patients with relapsed AML, relapse was associated with a twofold increase in blast MRP mRNA relative to 29 patients with newly diagnosed AML ($P < .01$). Paired blast samples (obtained at diagnosis and at relapse) from 13 AML and four ALL patients showed a twofold increase in 80% of the patients at relapse, suggesting that the expression of the MRP transporter at relapse may be involved in drug resistance. Because purine nucleoside antimetabolites may be exported by ABC G2, as noted earlier, it is of note that the recently released antileukemia agent clofarabine is also a substrate but its function is mediated inversely by levels of deoxycytidine kinase. Also of note is the recent finding that drug treatment can demethylate and thus activate the ABC G2 exporter, thereby increasing its protective tumor impact.

The larger family of transporters, the ABC group that includes ABC G2 and ABC B1, are overexpressed in leukemic cells and in many malignant stem cells. In fact, in addition to CD44, high levels of ABC transporters assist in the characterization and isolation of the transplantable subpopulation of malignant stem cells. Brendel and coworkers found that both imatinib and nilotinib used to block the abl kinase in CML were effectively blocking the ABC transporter in CML cells. This suggested both that these agents might function in part by blocking expression of an important leukemic stem cell protein and that they would sensitize CML cells to other agents transported by the ABC system.

DNA Repair Pathway Mechanisms of Drug Resistance

O6-Alkylguanine-DNA Alkyltransferase (MGMT)

As noted previously, the nitrosoureas and methylating agents are cytotoxic largely because of formation of DNA adducts at the O^6 position of guanine. The most efficient means of protection from the cytotoxicity of adducts at the O^6 position of guanine is rapid repair by the O^6-alkylguanine-DNA alkyltransferase (AGT or MGMT). This protein serves as the stoichiometric acceptor protein for O^6-alkylguanine DNA monoadducts, transferring the alkyl group from DNA to the active site of the protein, inactivating the protein, and restoring DNA to normal. However, the N^1G-N^3C DNA cross-link that follows chloroethylation is not a substrate for AGT. There is a striking correlation between drug resistance and alkyltransferase activity. Of interest, high levels of AGT are found in many leukemias, but low AGT is observed in normal human CD34 cells, perhaps explaining why nitrosoureas are not used in leukemia management and why nitrosoureas are effective myeloablative agents used in high-dose chemotherapy regimens. A novel inhibitor of AGT, O^6-benzylguanine (BG) has been used to sensitize human tumors to BCNU. Studies indicate activity of the combination of BG and BCNU in myeloma and in cutaneous lymphomas. Therapeutic benefit from the methylating and alkylating agent cloretazine appears to be related to lower levels of AGT. Likewise, temozolomide has some therapeutic efficacy in leukemia in a manner inversely related to AGT levels in the tumor cells. A study in five pediatric patients pointed out that response to temozolomide was greater in those with MGMT promoter methylation and no evidence of mismatch repair. This has been tested in a prospective phase 2 trial of older patients with leukemia. Temozolomide was given in a dosing schedule dependent on MGMT promoter methylation status, with a shorter course of therapy in those with low MGMT expression in the leukemic cells. The overall response rate in elderly leukemia patients who would otherwise not be candidates for treatment was about 40%, with a median duration of about 29 to 35 weeks.

Mismatch Repair

The spectrum of drug resistance and sensitivity to methylating agents does not end with AGT. Evidence suggests that methylating agent–induced cell death involves an aborted effort at mismatch repair. Karran and others, in mammalian systems, have shown that the replicative DNA polymerase and the repair polymerase pauses at O^6-mG and preferentially inserts a thymine (T) at the site. The O^6-mG:T base pair is recognized by the mismatch repair (MMR) system, which initiates base excision repair (BER; see later). In human cells, the MMR complex consists of at least six proteins involved in the recognition and repair of mismatch lesions: HMLH1, hMSH2, hMSH3, hPMS1, hPMS2, and GTBP (GT-binding protein, also called MSH6), all of which appear to be homologs of MMR proteins found in *Escherichia coli* and in yeast. After binding recognition, an endonuclease removes a patch of approximately 100 to 1000 bp containing the T mismatch, DNA polymerase δ or γ fills in the patch, with reinsertion of a T opposite the O^6-mG, and a DNA ligase closes the strand break. Because the O^6-mG:T is re-formed, cytotoxicity ensues as a result of repetitive efforts at DNA repair and induction of chromosomal breakage, rearrangements, energy depletion, and apoptosis. Drug resistance based on mutation or loss of expression of an MMR protein, owing to mutation within one of the gene coding regions, or promoter methylation leading to loss of gene expression, has been noted in solid tumors and in leukemias and lymphomas. The mutator phenotype was originally described in cells with acquired resistance to methylnitrosourea, methylmethanesulfonate, or *N*-methyl-*N*-nitroso-*N*-nitrosoguanidine, which were tolerant to G→A point mutations according to the inability to repair O^6-mG and are cross-resistant to 6-thioguanine (6-TG) used in childhood leukemia maintenance regimens, which form the 6-TG:T mismatch.

Major Molecular Response Mutations and Methylating Agent Resistance

Mismatch repair defects in humans were initially described in hereditary nonpolyposis colon cancer, which comprises approximately 15% of all colon cancer, lymphomas, and relapsing acute leukemias. The genetic defect results in a high rate of spontaneous mutations within microsatellite DNA, resulting in the RER phenotype arising as the expansion or contraction of mono-, di-, or tri-nucleotide repeats within the microsatellites. Tumor cells defective in MMR are remarkably resistant to temozolomide regardless of AGT activity or its inhibition by BG, confirming the importance of MMR in sensitivity to methylating agents. Of interest, MMR mutant cells are also two- to threefold resistant to cisplatin, perhaps because the cisplatin DNA adduct is bound by the MMR complex, slowing its recognition and repair by the nucleotide repair pathway and increasing its cytotoxicity. Such MMR-deficient cells also exhibit microsatellite instability, a measure of genomic instability and the propensity to develop further mutations during therapy leading to subclones of resistant cells. Loss of PMS2 has been identified in a family of childhood lymphomas. Microsatellite instability is seen in acute leukemias and in T-cell leukemias, suggesting both that these malignancies have lost MMR function and that they are more prone to drug resistance and acquisition of additional mutations that give rise to further drug resistance. Evidence of microsatellite instability and loss of MMR is present in some leukemias but is much more common in treatment-related leukemias, again providing a mechanism of drug resistance.

Base Excision Repair

Methylating agents such as procarbazine and temozolomide form large numbers of N^3-A and N^7-G adducts in addition to O^6-mG (with TMZ, the relative amounts are 72 N^7mG : 8 O^6mG : 5 N^3mA). Thus, under normal circumstances, cells process many more N^7mG and N^3mA lesions than O^6mG lesions even though the latter appear much more cytotoxic except in MMR-defective cells. Repair of N^3-A and N^7-G adducts through BER is efficient and normally leads to cell survival rather than cell death. Adducts are recognized by the methylpurine glycosylase (MPG) with removal of the base, generating an abasic (or AP) site. The AP site is then cleaved by the class II hydrolytic endonuclease (or AP endonuclease) generating a single strand break with a 5′ PO_4, which becomes the substrate for DNA polymerase-β, and to a lesser extent, polymerases δ and γ, followed by DNA ligase (reviewed by Sancar). Other compounds induce nucleotide pool imbalance leading to misincorporation of bases that become substrates for BER. These compounds include folate antagonists such as methotrexate, 5-ourouracil (5-FU), and to a lesser extent, nucleoside analogs such as fludarabine. Misincorporation of uracil after 5-FU inhibition of thymidilate synthase also leads to BER. Compounds to disrupt BER, such as methoxyamine, are now being developed and may lead to combination therapy for hematologic malignancies. An initial phase 1 trial with methoxyamine has been completed with pemetrexed, and a second trial with temozolomide continues. A third trial using the combination of fludarabine and methoxyamine (TRC-102) in patients with CLL has found remarkable efficacy in the first cohorts after relapsing from fludarabine (unpublished).

DRUG RESISTANCE TO ANTIMETABOLITES

Although overlap exists, antimetabolites can be classified into nucleoside analogs that are incorporated into RNA or DNA (or both) and agents that inhibit de novo purine and pyrimidine biosynthetic pathways. Mechanisms of resistance to these agents fall into several broad categories. For example, many antimetabolites are prodrugs in that they must be converted intracellularly into active nucleotide forms to exert their cytotoxic actions. Consequently, events that interfere with cellular accumulation of drug or nucleotide formation will reduce activity. Examples include decreased transport of methotrexate or decreased nucleotide formation of Ara-C and 6-thioguanine by reductions in activity of deoxycytidine kinase or HGPRT, respectively. Alternatively, enhanced drug catabolism reduces cytotoxicity. Examples include the deamination of Ara-C (to inactive Ara-U) by cytidine deaminase or catabolism of 6-TG by thiopurine methyltransferase. A third mechanism of resistance stems from the presence of increased intracellular levels of a competing metabolite (e.g., dCTP in the case of Ara-C, or hypoxanthine or guanine in the case of 6-TG). Fourth, alterations in the level of activity of a target enzyme or the presence of a mutant form that is a poor target of inhibition will also confer resistance. Examples include increased activity or a mutant form of DHFR (in the case of methotrexate), an altered DNA polymerase α (in the case of Ara-C), or increased activity of ribonucleotide reductase (through overexpression of either subunit). Finally, cytokinetic factors represent a common theme in the case of most (but not all) antimetabolites in that a reduction in the S-phase fraction generally leads to reduced drug sensitivity. Note that these resistance mechanisms are agent specific and are distinct from the more general modes of resistance (e.g., increased expression of BCL2) associated with defects in the distal cell death pathway.

FUTURE DIRECTIONS

Future treatment strategies for hematologic malignancies are directed against cellular targets that are responsible for the altered biology and transformed phenotype of cancer versus normal cells. This altered biology results from the accumulation of genetic mutations and alterations secondary to the unique genomic instability of cancer cells. A major advance has occurred with the targeting of protein kinases, fusion proteins, promoter demethylation and histone deacetylation, immunomodulatory proteins such as lenazolid, and inhibitors of cytokines such as IL-6 that are overexpressed in hematologic malignancies. Defects in the DNA repair pathway and in cell cycle checkpoints that cause inappropriate progression through the cell cycle facilitate the genomic instability of cancer cells. These are also critical for transformation, and agents that overcome these abnormalities are potential targets for drug development.

Because dysregulated cell cycle progression is a common feature of neoplastic cells, several strategies are being developed and tested to exploit this therapeutic strategy. These approaches include the use of drugs that inhibit the function of the mitotic kinase $p34^{cdc\text{-}2}$ (CDK1), for example, flavopiridol or inhibitors of the dual-specific phosphatase cdc25, which dephosphorylates and activates $p34^{cdc\text{-}2}$. Flavopiridol also inhibits CDK2 and CDK4 by binding to the hydrophobic, adenine-binding pocket of the ATP site of these G_1-S kinases, thereby inducing G_1 arrest. An additional strategy is to inhibit mitogenic signaling mediated by oncogene products such as activated Ras, Raf, and BCR-ABL. Antisense oligonucleotides to RAF, BCR-ABL, MYB, RAS, and BCL2 are being tested for their antitumoral effects alone or in combination with other cytotoxic drugs. Inhibitors of Ras farnesylation exert their antitumoral effects by, as yet, unclear mechanisms.

The growth of tumors and leukemia also requires the delivery of nutrients and growth factors through new blood microvessels (angiogenesis). Inhibitors of angiogenesis have potential use in treating patients with cancer and leukemia. Such agents target the vascular endothelial growth factors (e.g., VEGF, bFGF, and PDGF) or their receptor-mediated signaling (e.g., SU 5416).

REFERENCES

1. LoRusso PM, Boerner SA, Seymour L: An overview of the optimal planning, design, and conduct of phase I studies of new therapeutics. *Clin Cancer Res* 16:1710, 2010. Epub 2010 Mar 9. Review. PubMed PMID: 20215546.
2. Seymour L, Ivy SP, Sargent D, et al: The design of phase II clinical trials testing cancer therapeutics: Consensus recommendations from the clinical trial design task force of the National Cancer Institute Investigational Drug Steering Committee. *Clin Cancer Res* 16:1764, 2010. Epub 2010 Mar 9. PubMed PMID: 20215557; PubMed Central PMCID: PMC2840069.
3. Cheson BD, Rummel MJ: Bendamustine: Rebirth of an old drug. *J Clin Oncol* 27:1492, 2009. Epub 2009 Feb 17.
4. Knauf WU, Lissichkov T, Aldaoud A, et al: Phase III randomized study of bendamustine compared with chlorambucil in previously untreated patients with chronic lymphocytic leukemia. *J Clin Oncol* 27:4378, 2009. Epub 2009 Aug 3. PubMed PMID: 19652068.
5. Milojkovic D, Apperley J: Mechanisms of resistance to imatinib and second-generation tyrosine inhibitors in chronic myeloid leukemia. *Clin Cancer Res* 15:7519, 2009. PubMed PMID: 20008852.
6. Kantarjian HM, Shah NP, Cortes JE, et al: Dasatinib or imatinib in newly diagnosed chronic-phase chronic myeloid leukemia: 2-year follow-up from a randomized phase 3 trial (DASISION). *Blood* 119:1123, 2012. Epub 2011 Dec 9. PubMed PMID: 22160483.
7. Deremer DL, Ustun C, Natarajan K: Nilotinib: A second-generation tyrosine kinase inhibitor for the treatment of chronic myelogenous leukemia. *Clin Ther* 30:1956, 2008. Review. PubMed PMID: 19108785.
8. Mohamed AJ, Yu L, Bäckesjö CM, et al: Bruton's tyrosine kinase (Btk): Function, regulation, and transformation with special emphasis on the PH domain. *Immunol Rev* 228:58, 2009. Review. PubMed PMID: 19290921.
9. Rudelius M, Pittaluga S, Nishizuka S, et al: Constitutive activation of Akt contributes to the pathogenesis and survival of mantle cell lymphoma. *Blood* 108:1668, 2006. Epub 2006 Apr 27. PubMed PMID: 16645163; PubMed Central PMCID: PMC1895501.
10. So L, Fruman DA: PI3K signalling in B- and T-lymphocytes: New developments and therapeutic advances. *Biochem J* 442:465, 2012. PubMed PMID: 22364281.
11. Mascarenhas J, Hoffman R: Ruxolitinib: The first FDA approved therapy for the treatment of myelofibrosis. *Clin Cancer Res* 2012. [Epub ahead of print] PubMed PMID: 22474318.
12. Harrison C, Kiladjian JJ, Al-Ali HK, et al: JAK inhibition with ruxolitinib versus best available therapy for myelofibrosis. *N Engl J Med* 366:787, 2012. PubMed PMID: 22375970.
13. San Miguel JF, Schlag R, Khuageva NK, et al: VISTA Trial Investigators: Bortezomib plus melphalan and prednisone for initial treatment of multiple myeloma. *N Engl J Med* 359:906, 2008. PubMed PMID: 18753647
14. Appel A: Drugs: More shots on target. *Nature* 480:S40, 2011. doi: 10.1038/480S40a. PubMed PMID: 22169800.
15. Vallet S, Witzens-Harig M, Jaeger D, et al: Update on immunomodulatory drugs (IMiDs) in hematologic and solid malignancies. *Expert Opin Pharmacother* 13:473, 2012. Epub 2012 Feb 13. PubMed PMID: 22324734.
16. Larocca A, Cavallo F, Bringhen S, et al: Aspirin or enoxaparin thromboprophylaxis for patients with newly diagnosed multiple myeloma treated with lenalidomide. *Blood* 119:933, 2012; quiz 1093. Epub 2011 Aug 11. PubMed PMID: 21835953.
17. Lacy MQ, Hayman SR, Gertz MA, et al: Pomalidomide (CC4047) plus low-dose dexamethasone as therapy for relapsed multiple myeloma. *J Clin Oncol* 27:5008, 2009. Epub 2009 Aug 31. PubMed PMID: 19720894.
18. Roberts AW, Seymour JF, Brown JR, et al: Substantial susceptibility of chronic lymphocytic leukemia to BCL2 inhibition: Results of a phase I study of navitoclax in patients with relapsed or refractory disease. *J Clin Oncol* 30:488, 2012. Epub 2011 Dec 19. PubMed PMID: 22184378
19. Tong WG, Chen R, Plunkett W, et al: Phase I and pharmacologic study of SNS-032, a potent and selective Cdk2, 7, and 9 inhibitor, in patients with advanced chronic lymphocytic leukemia and multiple myeloma. *J Clin Oncol* 28:3015, 2010. Epub 2010 May 17. PubMed PMID: 20479412.
20. Chen R, Wierda WG, Chubb S, et al: Mechanism of action of SNS-032, a novel cyclin-dependent kinase inhibitor, in chronic lymphocytic leukemia. *Blood* 113:4637, 2009. Epub 2009 Feb 20. PubMed PMID: 19234140; PubMed Central PMCID: PMC2680368.
21. Karp JE, Vener TI, Raponi M, et al: Multi-institutional phase 2 clinical and pharmacogenomic trial of tipifarnib plus etoposide for elderly adults with newly diagnosed acute myelogenous leukemia. *Blood* 119:55, 2012: Epub 2011 Oct 14. PubMed PMID: 22001391; PubMed Central PMCID: PMC3251236.
22. Zaytseva YY, Valentino JD, Gulhati P, et al: mTOR inhibitors in cancer therapy. *Cancer Lett* 319:1, 2012. Epub 2012 Jan 17. Review. PubMed PMID: 22261336.
23. Liu Q, Thoreen C, Wang J, et al: mTOR mediated anti-cancer drug discovery. *Drug Discov Today Ther Strateg* 6:47, 2009. PubMed PMID: 20622997; PubMed Central PMCID: PMC2901551.
24. Hess G, Herbrecht R, Romaguera J, et al: Phase III study to evaluate temsirolimus compared with investigator's choice therapy for the treatment of relapsed or refractory mantle cell lymphoma. *J Clin Oncol* 27:3822, 2009. Epub 2009 Jul 6. PubMed PMID: 19581539.
25. Mann BS, Johnson JR, Cohen MH, et al: FDA approval summary: Vorinostat for treatment of advanced primary cutaneous

T-cell lymphoma. *Oncologist* 12:1247, 2007. PubMed PMID: 17962618.

26. Ellis L, Pan Y, Smyth GK, et al: Histone deacetylase inhibitor panobinostat induces clinical responses with associated alterations in gene expression profiles in cutaneous T-cell lymphoma. *Clin Cancer Res* 14:4500, 2008. PubMed PMID: 18628465.
27. Younes A, Sureda A, Ben-Yehuda D, et al: Panobinostat in patients with relapsed/refractory Hodgkin's lymphoma after autologous stem-cell transplantation: Results of a phase II study. *J Clin Oncol* 2012. [Epub ahead of print] PubMed PMID: 22547596.
28. Mo W, Zhang JT: Human ABCG2: Structure, function, and its role in multidrug resistance. *Int J Biochem Mol Biol* 3:1, 2012. Epub 2011 Mar 30. PubMed PMID: 22509477; PubMed Central PMCID: PMC3325772.
29. Tiwari AK, Sodani K, Wang SR, et al: Nilotinib (AMN107, Tasigna) reverses multidrug resistance by inhibiting the activity of the ABCB1/Pgp and ABCG2/BCRP/MXR transporters. *Biochem Pharmacol* 78:153, 2009. Epub 2009 Apr 11. PubMed PMID: 19427995.

APPENDIX 55-1

CLINICAL PHARMACOLOGY OF ALKYLATING AGENTS

MECHLORETHAMINE (MUSTARGEN)

Chemistry: Mechlorethamine, also called nitrogen mustard, is a water-soluble and alcohol-soluble analog of sulfur mustard gas. It is a bifunctional chloroethylating agent that alkylates DNA, RNA, and protein.

Absorption, Fate, and Excretion: The parent compound is highly reactive and has a biologic half-life of approximately 15 minutes. The principal route of degradation is spontaneous hydrolysis, but some enzymatic demethylation also occurs.

Preparation and Administration: Mechlorethamine is supplied in vials of 10 mg with 100 mg of sodium chloride and is reconstituted with 10 mL of sterile water to yield a 1-mg/mL solution, ideally prepared immediately before use. However, the manufacturer considers the drug expired 1 hour after reconstitution. The drug is injected over a few minutes through a tubing as a freely running IV infusion. For topical application (e.g., in mycosis fungoides), 10 mg of drug is dissolved in 60 mL of tap water. Alternatively, a 10 mg% ointment has been used by dissolving the drug in 95% ethyl alcohol and petrolatum (Aquaphor). Mechlorethamine is a powerful vesicant. In the event of extravasation, vigorous irrigation followed by 0.25% sodium thiosulfate injection at the site of extravasation should be attempted. Ice packs may be placed for 6 to 12 hours to minimize the local reaction.

Toxic Effects: Myelosuppression is the dose-limiting systemic side effect. This worsens with each additive cycle. Severe nausea and vomiting, infertility, alopecia, and pain at the site of injection, which can sometimes spread to involve the venous system (tracking), are also common. Occasionally, a macular papular rash is observed, but this does not appear to be allergic in nature and does not contraindicate continuation of therapy. Infertility is common but may be reversible. Infrequent adverse effects include alopecia, anorexia, weakness, and diarrhea. The drug has also been shown to induce chromosomal abnormalities and may contribute to the development of secondary leukemias, as seen in patients treated with this agent as part of the MOPP (mechlorethamine, vincristine, procarbazine, prednisone) regimen.

Potential Drug Interactions: None reported.

Therapeutic Indications in Hematology: Mechlorethamine is incorporated in many chemotherapy combinations used in the treatment of Hodgkin disease (MOPP and MOPP/ABV [Adriamycin, bleomycin, and vinblastine] hybrid) and in some NHLs (prednisone, etoposide, methotrexate, doxorubicin [Adriamycin], cyclophosphamide, Leucovorin [PROMACE]/MOPP). However, its use has largely been supplanted by other agents.

CYCLOPHOSPHAMIDE (CYTOXAN)

Chemistry: Cyclophosphamide is a cyclic phosphamide ester of mechlorethamine. After being metabolically activated, it alkylates DNA, forming cross-links.

Absorption, Fate, and Excretion: The drug is relatively well absorbed orally, with approximately 75% oral bioavailability. The parent compound is not active. The drug is metabolized by the hepatic CYP system, which ultimately generates at least two active compounds, phosphoramide mustard and acrolein. The latter appears to be responsible for cyclophosphamide's bladder toxicities. The plasma half-life of cyclophosphamide varies from 4 to 6.5 hours. Approximately 15% of the drug is excreted unchanged in the urine. Dose reduction should be considered in patients with severe renal failure.

Preparation and Administration: Cyclophosphamide is supplied as 25- and 50-mg tablets and as a powder for parenteral administration in 100-, 200-, and 500-mg and 1- and 2-g vials. It is dissolved by adding 5 mL of preservative-free sterile water for every 100 mg of drug. Cyclophosphamide is chemically stable for 24 hours at room temperature and for 6 days if refrigerated.

Toxic Effects: Bone marrow suppression is the major side effect. The myeloid series is primarily affected, although thrombocytopenia also occurs at high doses and alopecia is common. Nausea and vomiting can be severe and are usually delayed, occurring 6 to 8 hours after administration. Hemorrhagic cystitis occurs in 10% of patients receiving nontransplant doses and is apparently caused by the formation of the urotoxin acrolein. Because of this potential side effect, patients should be well hydrated. Mesna disulfide (sodium 2-mercaptoethanesulfonate disulfide) has also been used on a weight-equivalent basis to ameliorate cyclophosphamide-induced bladder toxicity. Other potential toxic effects include stomatitis, skin and nail hyperpigmentation, interstitial pulmonary fibrosis, and the syndrome of inappropriate secretion of antidiuretic hormone. Rare episodes of acute congestive heart failure have been reported. After bone marrow transplant doses, hemorrhagic cystitis is common, and cardiac toxicity (cardiomyopathy) may be seen. Late sequelae include bladder fibrosis (more common with daily [oral] therapy), bladder cancer, leukemogenesis, and infertility.

Potential Drug Interactions: Corticosteroids may increase P450 enzyme–induced metabolism and is often avoided in high-dose therapy. When combined with doxorubicin, it may increase cardiac toxicity. This may be prevented by amifostine. In animal studies, conflicting results were reported when the P450 enzyme inducer phenobarbital was given with cyclophosphamide. Most investigators, however, have observed a reduction in the amounts of active metabolites. Conversely, when cimetidine (but not ranitidine) was administered in leukemia-bearing mice before treatment with cyclophosphamide, a significant prolongation of their survival and higher plasma concentrations of alkylating metabolites were observed. Although one should remain alert for these potential drug interactions, none has been demonstrated in humans. Cyclophosphamide reduces serum pseudocholinesterase levels, which may prolong the neuromuscular blocking effects if given simultaneously. Caution must be exercised when administering high doses of these two drugs to critically ill patients. Life-threatening hyponatremia may develop when used in conjunction with indomethacin, although the precise incidence is unknown.

Therapeutic Indications in Hematology: Cyclophosphamide is a key drug in the treatment of lymphomas and myeloma. It is incorporated in many chemotherapy regimens, including CHOP, MACOP-B, PROMACE/CYTABOM, CVP, and VMCP (see Chapters 81 and 85 for details). In addition, cyclophosphamide is the drug most commonly used in preparatory regimens for bone marrow transplantation. It is also used in solid tumors and as an immunosuppressant in nonmalignant conditions such as glomerulonephritis and systemic lupus erythematosus.

IFOSFAMIDE (IFEX)

Chemistry: Ifosfamide is an oxazaphosphine nitrogen mustard that differs from cyclophosphamide by the placement of chloroethyl groups.

Absorption, Fate, and Excretion: As in the case of cyclophosphamide, the parent compound is inactive and is metabolized by the cytochrome P450 system in the liver. The metabolism of ifosfamide is influenced by the dose and schedule of administration. When administered as a single bolus, 60% is eliminated into the urine, 53% as unchanged inactive drug. When administered daily for 5 consecutive days, 56% is excreted into the urine, 15% as the inactive parent compound. The half-life is 7 hours when administered daily for 5 consecutive days and 15 hours when given as a single bolus dose. There is poor penetration across the blood–brain barrier. Its longer half-life and slower metabolic activation allow higher doses to be given.

Preparation and Administration: The drug is provided in 1-g vials and should be reconstituted in sterile water or bacteriostatic water to a final concentration of 50 mg/mL. Ifosfamide can be diluted further in 5% dextrose, normal saline, or Ringer solution for injection to achieve concentrations of between 0.6 and 20 mg/mL. The solution should be infused over 30 minutes. To prevent hemorrhagic cystitis, patients must receive Mesna disulfide for protection against urotoxicity and must be kept well hydrated (2 L/day). Mesna is a thiol compound that is rapidly oxidized to dimesna in vivo. Mesna and dimesna are filtered by the glomeruli, reabsorbed in the proximal tubule, and finally secreted back into the tubular lumen of the kidney. In the tubules, approximately one-third of the filtered dimesna is readily converted back to Mesna. The free sulfhydryl group of this compound reacts with the urotoxic metabolite acrolein produced by both ifosfamide and cyclophosphamide (see Fig. 55-6). This reaction creates a nontoxic acrolein–Mesna thioether that is safely eliminated in the urine. Mesna has also been shown to inhibit the degradation of ifosfamide or cyclophosphamide to acrolein.

Mesna has been given in combination with ifosfamide in different doses and schedules. One recommended schedule uses IV bolus injection in a dosage equal to 20% of the ifosfamide dose (on a milligram-to-milligram basis) at the time of ifosfamide administration and 4 and 8 hours after each dose of ifosfamide. Mesna has also been given by continuous infusion with excellent results. The two agents may be mixed together in the same IV solution; however, Mesna is not compatible with cisplatin.

Toxic Effects: With the use of Mesna to protect against urotoxicity, myelosuppression—especially leukopenia and, to a lesser extent, thrombocytopenia—is the dose-limiting side effect. Renal tubular acidosis can occur. Central nervous system effects, observed in approximately 10% of patients treated, include somnolence, confusion, depressive psychosis, and hallucinations. Less commonly, dizziness, disorientation, and cranial nerve dysfunction occur. Nausea and vomiting are common. Low serum albumin and elevated serum creatinine may enhance central nervous system toxicity. As with cyclophosphamide, such side effects as alopecia, leukemogenesis, and infertility also occur. Cardiac toxicity is rare.

Potential Drug Interactions: Because ifosfamide is also metabolized by the P450 system, physicians should remain alert for the same type of potential drug interactions that have been reported with cyclophosphamide. A recent report advises close monitoring of warfarin anticoagulant control in patients receiving ifosfamide/Mesna.

Therapeutic Indications in Hematology: Ifosfamide was recently approved for treatment of patients with refractory testicular cancer. In hematologic malignancies, its major indication is in the treatment of refractory lymphomas.

MELPHALAN (MELPHALAN)

Chemistry: Melphalan is synthesized from nitrogen mustard and phenylalanine. It is a bifunctional chloroethylating agent that forms DNA cross-links.

Absorption, Fate, and Excretion: The oral bioavailability of melphalan is quite variable, 20% to 50% of the drug being excreted in the stool. Some patients show virtually no oral absorption. This fact is particularly pertinent in the treatment of myeloma patients, in whom a lack of response to melphalan may simply be caused by poor oral absorption. Melphalan has a half-life of approximately 90 minutes. It is extensively metabolized, with only approximately 10% to 15% of an administered dose excreted unchanged in the urine.

Preparation and Administration: Melphalan is commercially available in 2-mg tablets and in IV formulation for high-dose therapy.

Toxic Effects: The dose-limiting toxicity is myelosuppression, manifested by leukopenia and thrombocytopenia and generally occurring 2 to 3 weeks after therapy. Recovery may take 6 weeks, however, in patients who have been heavily pretreated with chemotherapy drugs, radiotherapy, or both. Nausea, vomiting, and alopecia are uncommon side effects and are usually mild. Occasionally, amenorrhea and azoospermia, pulmonary fibrosis, dermatitis, and secondary malignancies (e.g., leukemia) occur, especially in patients receiving the drug over the long term. At cumulative doses of less than 600 mg, the incidence of second hematologic malignancy is probably less than 2% but may be greater than 15% at higher doses. Higher doses used in transplant patients result in gastrointestinal toxicity that is dose limiting. At these doses, the syndrome of inappropriate secretion of antidiuretic hormone, pneumonitis, and hepatic venoocclusive disease have been observed.

Potential Drug Interactions: Administration of high-dose IV melphalan with cyclosporine increases the risk of cyclosporine nephrotoxicity.

Therapeutic Indications: The major use of melphalan is for the treatment of multiple myeloma, either as a single agent or in combination with other alkylating agents and prednisone (e.g., the MP and VMCP regimens). The IV formulation has been approved for isolated limb perfusion in melanoma. It is used in high-dose protocols for myeloma and solid tumors at doses of 140 to 200 mg/m^2.

CHLORAMBUCIL (CHLORAMBUCIL)

Chemistry: Chlorambucil is an aromatic derivative of mechlorethamine.

Absorption, Fate, and Excretion: Chlorambucil is well absorbed after oral administration. It is extensively metabolized in the liver to its major metabolite, phenylacetic acid mustard (PAAM), which also has bifunctional alkylating activity. The half-lives of chlorambucil and PAAM are 1.5 and 2.5 hours, respectively; less than 1% of either chlorambucil or PAAM is excreted in the urine.

Preparation and Administration: Chlorambucil is commercially available as 2-mg tablets.

Toxic Effects: Treatment is usually well tolerated, with myelosuppression the dose-limiting toxic effect. Patients on a daily oral schedule should have biweekly complete blood counts (CBCs). Nausea and vomiting are uncommon, but mild alopecia and skin rashes occasionally occur. As with the other alkylating agents, azoospermia (especially above a cumulative dose of 400 mg), amenorrhea, and secondary leukemia are potential risks of prolonged therapy. Rare cases of pulmonary fibrosis have also been reported.

Potential Drug Interactions: None reported.

Therapeutic Indications in Hematology: The major uses are in the treatment of Waldenström macroglobulinemia, low-grade lymphomas, chronic lymphocytic leukemia (CLL), and Hodgkin disease. Except for CLL, chlorambucil has been supplanted by newer agents.

BUSULFAN (MYLERAN)

Chemistry: Busulfan is an alkylsulfonate bifunctional alkylating agent not chemically related to mechlorethamine. It forms DNA intrastrand and interstrand cross-links.

Absorption, Fate, and Excretion: Busulfan is well absorbed after oral administration. When given by the IV route, greater than 90% is cleared from the plasma after 3 minutes. The drug is extensively metabolized to inactive compounds that are excreted renally. The major metabolite is methane sulfonic acid, although more than 10 other not fully identified metabolites exist. Virtually no intact busulfan is found in the urine. The biologic half-life of busulfan is approximately 2.5 hours.

Preparation and Administration: The drug is commercially available as 2-mg tablets.

Toxic Effects: Although at low doses the major effect of busulfan is on the granulocytic series, at high doses, all three hematologic series are affected. Compared with the other alkylating agents, its nadir of myelosuppression may be relatively late, in a range of 11 to 30 days. Hematologic recovery is also prolonged and may take approximately 54 days. A relatively common side effect is an Addisonian-like syndrome characterized by skin hyperpigmentation and weakness but without abnormalities in adrenal function. Cumulative pulmonary toxicity has been well described and consists of a mixed alveolar and interstitial pneumonitis. As with the other alkylating agents, infertility and leukemogenesis can occur. Nausea and vomiting are rare. At high doses, it is associated with hepatic venoocclusive disease in up to 19% of patients. Seizures may also occur and are controlled by diphenylhydration.

Potential Drug Interactions: A metabolic interaction may take place between busulfan and various anticonvulsant medications; however, further description of the specific effects is awaited.

Therapeutic Indications in Hematology: Busulfan is used mainly in the treatment of chronic myeloid leukemia. More recently, high-dose busulfan has been incorporated into preparatory regimens for bone marrow transplantation. Blood level monitoring with adjustment for higher dose levels improved therapeutic outcome and reduced toxicity.

CARMUSTINE (BCNU)

Chemistry: Carmustine, also called BCNU (1,3[bis]-2-chloroethyl-nitrosourea), decomposes spontaneously into a chloroethyl hydroxide that can alkylate the DNA and into an isocyanide molecule, which may produce carbamylation of proteins. Cytotoxicity is caused by DNA cross-links.

Absorption, Fate, and Excretion: Intravenously administered carmustine is rapidly metabolized, with a half-life of 70 minutes. Approximately 30% to 80% of metabolites are eliminated in the urine within 24 hours. The drug, its metabolites, or both readily cross the blood–brain barrier, resulting in cerebrospinal fluid concentrations within the range of 15% to 70% of plasma levels. Peak serum levels vary widely in patients treated at 200 to 600 mg IMF.

Preparation and Administration: Carmustine is commercially available in 100-mg vials as a white lyophilized powder. The drug is reconstituted with 3 mL of absolute alcohol provided by the manufacturer and 27 mL of sterile water and can be further diluted with normal saline or 5% dextrose in water. It should be used immediately after reconstitution and can be infused over 1 to 2 hours.

Carmustine is chemically stable for 3 hours at room temperature and for 24 hours when refrigerated.

Toxic Effects: Myelosuppression is the dose-limiting toxic effect and tends to increase with successive cycles of therapy. Leukopenia and thrombocytopenia are characteristically delayed and reach their maximum between the third and sixth weeks after drug administration. Nausea and vomiting can be severe. Abnormal liver function test results may be found, but the abnormalities are usually mild and reversible. Two rare but serious toxic effects include cumulative pulmonary or interstitial pneumonitis progressing to fibrosis and progressive renal damage, which are dose related. Secondary leukemias can also occur 5 to 10 years after treatment. Patients who receive greater than 1100 mg/m^2 are at increased risk of pulmonary fibrosis. Carmustine is not a vesicant, but rapid infusion often produces a burning sensation at the injection site.

Potential Drug Interactions: Cimetidine may enhance the myelosuppressive effect of carmustine. Carmustine may decrease the pharmacologic effects of phenytoin. In rats with intracerebrally implanted tumors, pretreatment with phenobarbital eliminated the antitumor activity of carmustine. The reduction in carmustine antitumor activity correlated with increased carmustine metabolism, which is apparently the result of hepatic microsomal enzyme induction.

Therapeutic Indications in Hematology: Carmustine in combination with other cytotoxic agents may be used in the initial treatment of Hodgkin disease (BCVPP regimen) and multiple myeloma (VBAP regimen). In high-dose therapy, it appears in BEP for relapsed lymphomas.

LOMUSTINE (CCNU)

Chemistry: Lomustine, also called CCNU, is a nitrosourea derivative with choloroethyl and cyclohexyl side chains.

Absorption, Fate, and Excretion: The drug is rapidly absorbed from the gastrointestinal tract and is rapidly and completely metabolized. Its active metabolites have prolonged plasma half-lives, within a range of 16 to 48 hours. Approximately 50% of an administered dose is detectable (as metabolites) in the urine within 24 hours, and 75% is detectable within 4 days. Active metabolites cross the blood–brain barrier and can be detected in significant concentrations in the cerebrospinal fluid.

Preparation and Administration: The drug is commercially available in 10-, 40-, and 100-mg capsules.

Toxic Effects: The toxicity profile of lomustine is similar to that of carmustine. Because lomustine can produce vomiting and the drug is given orally, special attention should be directed to emesis control. If the patient vomits soon after ingestion, the vomitus should be inspected for the presence of intact capsules. The drug should be given again if capsules are identified with certainty. Secondary leukemias are reported 3 to 10 years after use.

Potential Drug Interactions: These are similar to those of carmustine.

Therapeutic Indications in Hematology: Lomustine is occasionally used as second-line treatment for patients with Hodgkin disease and non-Hodgkin lymphoma (NHL) and for childhood gliomas.

STREPTOZOCIN (ZANOSAR)

Chemistry: Streptozocin is a naturally occurring nitrosourea derived from *Streptomyces acromogenes*. The drug is a glucosamine-1-methyl-nitrosourea, which, unlike the other nitrosoureas, methylates DNA and is cytotoxic owing to induced mismatch repair.

Absorption, Fate, and Excretion: After IV administration, the drug is rapidly metabolized, with no intact drug detectable in the plasma after 3 hours. Its half-life is 40 hours. Within the first 24 hours after administration, approximately 10% of the parent compound is excreted in the urine.

Preparation and Administration: The drug is commercially available in 1-g vials and is reconstituted with either 9.5 mL of normal saline or 5% dextrose in water for injection to form a 100-mg/mL solution. IV infusion of the drug over 30 to 45 minutes usually prevents discomfort at the injection site. Patients should be kept well hydrated to preclude renal tubular toxicity.

Toxic Effects: Although nausea and vomiting have been considered by some investigators to be the limiting toxic effects, in most phase I trials, nephrotoxicity was the principal dose-limiting effect. Nausea and vomiting are severe and require aggressive antiemetic support. Streptozocin may also aggravate duodenal ulcers. Renal toxicity frequently occurs and includes mild proteinuria, glycosuria, hypophosphatemia, renal tubular acidosis, and occasionally irreversible azotemia. Although the myelosuppressive effect of streptozocin is mild, it can potentiate the bone marrow suppression of other cytotoxic drugs. Slight increases in hepatic enzymes can also occur. Occasionally, patients (primarily those with insulinomas) may experience transient alterations in glucose metabolism.

Potential Drug Interactions: Streptozocin can potentiate the hyperglycemic effect of glucocorticosteroids. Phenytoin therapy decreases the cytotoxic effect of streptozocin on the pancreatic β cells, leading to potential interference with its therapeutic effect in patients with pancreatic islet cell tumors. Streptozocin is a potent renal toxin, and every effort should be made to avoid concomitant administration of other nephrotoxins.

Therapeutic Indications in Hematology: Streptozocin has been used in the initial treatment of Hodgkin disease and, less commonly, in NHLs.

DACARBAZINE (DTIC)

Chemistry: Dacarbazine is also called DTIC [5-(3,3-dimethyl-1-triazeno)imidazole-4-carboxamide]. After undergoing metabolic activation by microsomal enzymes in the liver, it acts primarily as an alkylating agent.

Absorption, Fate, and Excretion: After IV administration, the drug is extensively metabolized. Activated DTIC has an elimination half-life of 5 to 7 hours. Approximately 40% to 50% of the parent drug is found in the urine within the first 24 hours after administration.

Preparation and Administration: DTIC is commercially available in 100- and 200-mg vials, which must be protected from light and stored at a temperature of 2° to 8° C. The drug is reconstituted with normal saline or sterile water to produce a 10-mg/mL solution. It can be administered as a slow IV push or by infusion over 15 to 30 minutes.

Toxic Effects: Myelosuppression, primarily represented by leukopenia, is the dose-limiting toxic effect. Use of the drug leads to considerable problems with emesis and requires aggressive antiemetic support. A flulike syndrome consisting of fever, malaise, and myalgias may occur. Direct sunlight during the first 2 days after drug administration may result in facial flushing, facial paresthesias, and lightheadedness. Hepatotoxicity and diarrhea have also been reported. Pain along the injection site can occur if the drug is rapidly infused but can usually be lessened by prolonging the infusion rate. Secondary leukemias are reported between 3 and 10 years after use.

Potential Drug Interactions: DTIC activation may be enhanced by phenytoin or phenobarbital, although the clinical significance of this potential interaction remains uncertain. There may be a potential (as yet poorly characterized) drug interaction with levodopa, whereby the response to levodopa is diminished.

Therapeutic Indications in Hematology: DTIC is used primarily in the treatment of Hodgkin disease as part of the ABVD (doxorubicin [Adriamycin], bleomycin, vinblastine, and DTIC) regimen and for melanoma.

PROCARBAZINE

Chemistry and Mechanism of Action: Procarbazine is a substituted hydrazine derivative with a chemical structure similar to that of the monoamine oxidase inhibitors (MAOIs). Accordingly, procarbazine exhibits weak MAOI effects. Procarbazine itself is inert and must undergo metabolic activation to generate cytotoxic reactants, the mode of action of which is not clear. They may inhibit transmethylation of methyl groups of methionine into tRNA or may also directly damage DNA. Hydrogen peroxide, formed during the autooxidation of procarbazine, may attack protein sulfhydryl groups contained in residual proteins tightly bound to DNA.

Absorption, Fate, and Excretion: Procarbazine is rapidly and completely absorbed by the oral route, with peak plasma levels occurring within 60 minutes. It penetrates well into the cerebrospinal fluid. The drug is readily metabolized in the liver and has a plasma half-life of 10 minutes after IV injection. The major sites of elimination are the kidneys, where approximately 70% of the drug is excreted as *N*-isopropylterephthalamic acid and less than 5% is excreted unchanged.

Preparation and Administration: Procarbazine is commercially available as 50-mg capsules.

Toxic Effects: The usual dose-limiting toxic effect is myelosuppression. Occasionally, nausea and vomiting may be dose limiting, although tolerance to those effects may develop during continued administration. Other less common side effects include paresthesias, headache, dizziness, depression, apprehension, insomnia, nightmares, hallucinations, drowsiness, ataxia, foot drop, decreased reflexes, tremors, coma, confusion, convulsions, skin rash, alopecia, myalgia, and arthralgia. Procarbazine may possibly be leukemogenic.

Potential Drug Interactions: Combination chemotherapy that includes procarbazine may result in a decrease in digoxin plasma levels. Because procarbazine is a weak MAOI, hypertensive reactions could theoretically occur after concurrent ingestion of sympathomimetics, levodopa, tricyclic antidepressants, or foods with high tyramine content (e.g., dark beer, yogurt, cheeses, and red wines). However, such reactions have not been reported. Concomitant use of narcotics or other strong sedatives may result in exaggerated depressant effects, leading to coma and possibly death. Procarbazine also interacts with alcohol, causing a disulfiram-like reaction.

Therapeutic Indications in Hematology: Procarbazine is often used in combination with other cytotoxic agents in the treatment of Hodgkin disease (MOPP and MOPP derivatives) and to a lesser extent in the treatment of non-Hodgkin lymphoma (PROMACE-MOPP).

TEMOZOLOMIDE

Chemistry and Mechanism of Action: Temozolomide is not active but undergoes rapid nonenzymatic conversion at physiologic pH to the reactive compound monomethyl 5-triazino imidazole carboxamide (MTIC), which is also the active methyl group–donating metabolite of dacarbazine. Unlike dacarbazine, formation of MTIC from temozolomide does not require metabolic activation (liver); thus there is much more consistent conversion from temozolomide to the methyl-donating MTIC. The cytotoxicity of MTIC is thought to be primarily caused by alkylation of DNA. Alkylation (methylation) occurs mainly at the O6 and N7 positions of guanine. Cytotoxicity results from processing of these lesions by methylguanine methyltransferase, mismatch repair, and base excision repair.

Absorption, Fate, and Excretion: Temozolomide is rapidly and completely absorbed after oral administration; peak plasma concentrations occur in 1 hour. Food reduces the rate and extent of temozolomide absorption.

Temozolomide exhibits a mean elimination half-life of 1.8 hours and exhibits linear kinetics over the therapeutic dosing range. Temozolomide is spontaneously hydrolyzed at physiologic pH to the active species, 3-methyl-(triazen-1-yl)imidazole-4-carboxamide (MTIC) and to temozolomide acid metabolite. MTIC is further hydrolyzed to 5-amino-imidazole-4-carboxamide (AIC), which is known to be an intermediate in purine and nucleic acid biosynthesis and to methylhydrazine, which is believed to be the active alkylating species. Approximately 38% of the administered temozolomide total radioactive dose is recovered over 7 days, 37.7% in urine and 0.8% in feces. The majority of the recovery of radioactivity in urine is as unchanged temozolomide (5.6%), AIC (12%), temozolomide acid metabolite (2.3%), and unidentified polar metabolite(s) (17%). Overall clearance of temozolomide is approximately 5.5 L/hr/min.

Preparation and Administration: Temozolomide is given orally with each capsule containing either 5, 20, 100, 140, 180, or 250 mg of temozolomide. The inactive ingredients for TEMODAR capsules are lactose anhydrous, colloidal silicon dioxide, sodium starch glycolate, tartaric acid, and stearic acid.

Toxic Effects: Bone marrow depression, including neutropenia, lymphopenia, anemia, and thrombocytopenia, occurs frequently with temozolomide. Mild transaminase elevations of up to 40% of patients and hyperbilirubinemia of up to 19% are seen. Mild to moderate headache is among the most commonly reported adverse effects along with moderate nausea and vomiting, although these may be secondary to the use of antiemetics.

Drug Interactions: None described.

Therapeutic Indications in Hematology: Temozolomide may have some activity in both acute myeloid leukemia and acute lymphocytic leukemia, but the correct dose is presently unknown. Temozolomide has no activity in non-Hodgkin lymphoma.

BENDAMUSTINE

Chemistry and Mechanism of Action: Bendamustine is a bifunctional alkylating agent (mechlorethamine analogue) Its structure is characterized by a nitrogen mustard group linked to a benzimidazole nucleus, which forms covalent bonds with electron-rich nucleophilic moieties, resulting in interstrand DNA crosslinks. Bendamustine is active against both quiescent and dividing cells.

Absorption, Fate, and Excretion: Although absorbed well orally, bendamustine is only administered intravenously. It is highly protein bound, averaging approximately 95%. The half-life of bendamustine is approximately 40 minutes. Bendamustine is primarily metabolized in the liver via hydrolysis, and little is excreted in urine unchanged, but the pharmacokinetics in patients with significant renal failure are unknown.

Preparation and Administration: Bendamustine is available for IV use in single-use vials containing either 25 mg or 100 mg of bendamustine HCl. Sterile water for injection is added to each vial to obtain a 5-mg/mL solution. The lyophilized powder should completely dissolve in 5 minutes. After being diluted with either 0.9% sodium chloride injection, USP, or 2.5% dextrose/0.45% sodium chloride injection, USP, the final admixture is stable for 24 hours when stored refrigerated or for 3 hours when stored at room temperature.

Toxic Effects: Bendamustine frequently causes anemia, severe neutropenia, and thrombocytopenia. Infusion reactions presenting as fever, chills, pruritus, and rash have been seen. Antihistamines, antipyretics, and corticosteroids have been effective in preventing these reactions. Tumor lysis syndrome has been seen with the first dose of bendamustine, so appropriate precautions should be taken. Local reactions are seen with extravasation, and care should be taken when administering the drug in a peripheral site. Headache, nausea, and vomiting as well as skin reactions, including rash, toxic skin reactions, and bullous exanthema, have occurred with bendamustine. Acute myeloid leukemia has been reported in patients after use of bendamustine hydrochloride.

Drug Interactions: Although their clinical significance is unknown, ciprofloxacin, fluvoxamine, and omeprazole may increase bendamustine levels and decrease levels of active minor metabolites.

Therapeutic Indications in Hematology: Bendamustine has been effective in treating chronic lymphoid leukemia, multiple myeloma, Hodgkin disease, non-Hodgkin lymphoma, and indolent B cell lymphomas.

APPENDIX 55-2

CLINICAL PHARMACOLOGY OF ANTIMICROTUBULE AGENTS

VINCRISTINE (ONCOVIN) AND VINBLASTINE (VELBAN)

Chemistry and Mechanism of Action: Both vincristine and vinblastine are asymmetric dimeric compounds that bind to the protein tubulin at a site distinct from that for the taxanes. At low concentrations, vincristine and vinblastine inhibit microtubule dynamics. At higher concentrations, they disrupt microtubules that constitute the mitotic spindle, resulting in metaphase arrest. They are relatively M-phase specific. Owing to their lipophilicity, vinca alkaloids are rapidly taken into cells and achieve several-hundred-fold higher intracellular than extracellular concentrations. Whereas overexpression of the multidrug resistance transporters P-glycoprotein or multidrug resistance protein can reduce the intracellular accumulation, alterations in the α or β tubulins can affect drug–target interaction for vinca alkaloids.

Absorption, Fate, and Excretion: After IV injection, both drugs are rapidly distributed to the body tissues, especially the red blood cells and platelets. Their elimination follows a triphasic pattern. The elimination half-lives are as follows: α, less than 5 minutes; β, 50 to 155 minutes; and γ, 20 to 85 hours. Both vinca alkaloids are primarily eliminated through the liver into the bile and feces, making patients with obstructive liver disease more susceptible to toxic effects. A 50% reduction in the dose is recommended for serum bilirubin concentrations of 1.5 to 3.5 mg/dL. Dose modification for renal dysfunction is not indicated. After brief IV bolus administration, peak plasma vincristine concentrations of 100 to 400 mM are achieved, which decline to less than 10 mM in 2 to 4 hours. Continuous infusion doses of 1.0 mg/m^2/day produce vincristine plasma concentrations ranging from 1 to 10 nM.

Preparation and Administration: Vincristine is commercially available in 1-, 2-, and 5-mg vials. Each milliliter contains 1 mg of vincristine sulfate, 100 mg of mannitol, 1.3 mg of methylparaben, and 0.2 mg of propylparaben. Vincristine is a powerful vesicant that should be administered only intravenously into a freely running infusion of normal saline or dextrose solution. If the drug is given by continuous infusion, it must be infused through a central IV line. In case of extravasation, infusion should be discontinued and any residual drug aspirated through the line. The manufacturer also recommends infiltrating the area with 1 to 2 mL of hyaluronidase, 150 U/mL, and then applying warm compresses for 72 hours to facilitate dispersion of the drug. Vinblastine is commercially available as a lyophilized powder and a 1-mg/mL solution in 10-mg vials. The lyophilized drug is reconstituted by adding sodium chloride for injection (which may be preserved with either phenol or benzyl alcohol) to the 10-mg vial. Administration of vinblastine should follow the same guidelines described for vincristine.

Toxic Effects: Vincristine's dose-limiting toxic effect is neurotoxicity, which appears to be related to its relative polarity. Peripheral neurotoxicity usually manifests as sensory impairment, decreased deep tendon reflexes, and paresthesias. Less commonly, severe painful dysesthesias, ataxia, foot drop, and cranial nerve palsy (e.g., affecting the extraocular and laryngeal muscles) can occur. Autonomic neurotoxicities include constipation, abdominal cramps, and ileus, which may be prevented by use of mild laxatives. Alopecia occurs frequently, but myelosuppressive effects are minimal. Rare side effects include inappropriate secretion of antidiuretic hormone and ischemic cardiac toxicity. Vinblastine's dose-limiting toxic effect is myelosuppression, with leukopenia more pronounced than thrombocytopenia. Anemia is uncommon. Neurotoxicity can also occur but is significantly less common than with vincristine. Vinblastine is also a vesicant.

Potential Drug Interactions: Both vinca alkaloids have been reported to increase the accumulation of methotrexate and etoposide in tumor cells. Acute shortness of breath and bronchospasm can occur when vincristine or vinblastine is given in conjunction with mitomycin C. Because asparaginase may impair the hepatic clearance of vincristine, it is preferable to administer the vincristine 12 to 24 hours before L-asparaginase. Vincristine may decrease the absorption and plasma levels of orally administered drugs such as digoxin. Dilantin may increase the cytotoxicity of vincristine in multidrug-resistant tumor cells; however, this remains to be demonstrated in the clinic. When concurrently administered, erythromycin may increase the toxicity of vinca alkaloids, especially vinblastine.

Therapeutic Indications in Hematology: The vinca alkaloids are among the most important drugs in the treatment of hematologic malignancies. They have a broad spectrum of activity and are often incorporated into many chemotherapy regimens used in the treatment of ALL, Hodgkin disease, non-Hodgkin lymphoma, chronic lymphocytic leukemia, and multiple myeloma.

VINORELBINE (NAVELBINE)

Chemistry and Mechanism of Action: Vinorelbine is a semisynthetic derivative of vinblastine (5′-nor-hydrovinblastine) with an eight-member catharanthine ring. Similar to other vinca alkaloids, it also binds to tubulin, inhibits microtubule assembly, and produces a mitotic arrest of cells. These occur at concentrations that relatively spare axonal microtubules, which may reduce neurotoxicity.

Absorption, Fate, and Excretion: Short (6-10 minutes) IV infusions of 30 mg/m^2 produce peak plasma concentrations approximately 1.0 μg/mL with a triphase decay. Rapid α (<5 minutes) and β (49-168 minutes) half-lives result in a rapid decline in the plasma concentration in the first hour posttreatment followed by a prolonged terminal half-life of 18 to 49 hours, reflecting slow efflux from the peripheral compartment. The volume of distribution at steady state is 20 to 75.6 L/kg. The drug is extensively bound to platelets, lymphocytes, and plasma proteins. The major site of metabolism is the liver, with 33% to 80% of the drug excretion in feces and approximately 20% in urine.

Preparation and Administration: Vinorelbine is available for injection in single use as 10 mg/mL in 1- or 5-mL vials without preservatives. The calculated dose is diluted to 1.5 to 3.5 mg/mL for a slow injection (6-10 minutes) by a syringe with 5% dextrose or

0.9% saline or between 0.5 or 2.0 mg/mL in an IV bag. Because vinorelbine is a strong vesicant, it should be administered through a freely flowing IV access avoiding all extravasation.

Toxic Effects: Vinorelbine shares many of the principal toxicities of vinblastine. Myelosuppression is dose limiting but not cumulative, with nadirs occurring 7 to 10 days after administration.

Anemia and thrombocytopenia occur infrequently. Because of lower affinity for axonal versus spindle microtubules, neurotoxicity is less prominent with vinorelbine. Mild to moderate peripheral neuropathy and constipation occur in approximately 30% of patients, and the incidence of neuropathy increases with the duration of treatment. Mild to moderate nausea and vomiting is seen in 33% of patients. Stomatitis and diarrhea are less frequent. Transient elevations of transaminases have been reported. Among the miscellaneous side effects noted are chest pain with or without electrocardiographic changes (6%, most with underlying cardiac disease), as well as bronchospasm and dyspnea (5%). Alopecia is seen in 10% of patients.

Therapeutic Indications in Hematology: Objective responses have been observed in approximately 33% of patients with Hodgkin disease or non-Hodgkin lymphoma.

PACLITAXEL (TAXOL) AND DOCETAXEL (TAXOTERE)

Chemistry and Mechanism of Action: Both paclitaxel and docetaxel are complex diterpene alkaloid esters consisting of a taxane system linked to an oxetane ring and a C-13 side chain that is necessary for their cytotoxic effects in mammalian cells. After binding to the N-terminal 31 amino acids of the β-tubulin subunit in the tubulin oligomers or polymers, these taxanes kinetically stabilize microtubule dynamics at plus ends. They also decrease the lag time and shift the equilibrium toward tubulin polymerization into microtubule bundles. The disequilibrium of tubulin–microtubule polymerization results in mitotic arrest and apoptosis of cells. Taxane-induced mitotic arrest is associated with phosphorylation of BCL2 protein and increased intracellular levels of free BAX protein, which promote apoptosis. Compared with paclitaxel, docetaxel demonstrates 1.9-fold greater affinity for tubulin-binding sites and greater potency in mediating BCL2 phosphorylation.

Absorption, Fate, and Excretion: Taxanes generally are administered by IV infusion lasting over 3, 24, or 96 hours (paclitaxel) or 1 hour (docetaxel). Depending on the dose and schedule, peak plasma concentrations of paclitaxel range between 0.05 and 15.0 mM. Its steady-state volume of distribution ranges between 48 and 182 L/m^2, with rapid uptake in almost all tissues except the central nervous system and 98% plasma protein binding. Plasma decay for paclitaxel is biphasic, with α and β half-lives of 0.34 and 5.8 hours, respectively. Saturable distribution and elimination appear to be responsible for paclitaxel's nonlinear pharmacokinetics. This means that paclitaxel dose escalation in shorter schedules may result in disproportionate increases in area under the concentration–time curve and peak plasma concentration. It is metabolized to 6 hydroxy paclitaxel by the CYP3A isoform of the PU_{50} mixed-function oxidases in the hepatic microsomes. Total fecal and urinary excretion of paclitaxel and its metabolites is approximately 70% and 10%, respectively. Although dose modification is not necessary for renal insufficiency, a 50% reduction in dose is recommended even for moderate hyperbilirubinemia or significant elevations in hepatocellular enzymes. When administered as a 1-hour IV infusion, docetaxel has linear pharmacokinetics that fit a three-compartment model. Similar to paclitaxel, docetaxel also has a high clearance rate (0.36 L/hr), steady-state volume of distribution (67.3 L/m^2), and terminal half-life of 12 hours. Docetaxel also has high protein binding (97%) and extensive tissue distribution. The drug or its metabolites also have high fecal (80%) and low urinary elimination (5%). Metabolism of docetaxel also primarily occurs in hepatic microsomal P450 mixed-function oxidases, CYP3A, CYP2B, and CYP1A.

Preparation and Administration: Paclitaxel is available as a 30-mg/5 mL single-dose vial in polyoxyethylated castor oil (Cremophor EL) 50% and dehydrated alcohol, USP 50%. The contents of the vial must be diluted before use. Docetaxel for injection is available as a concentrate in polysorbate 80 in two vial contents (23.6 mg/0.59 mL or 94.4 mg/2.36 mL) along with the appropriate diluent (1.83 or 7.33 mL) in separate vials. Adding diluent that is 13% (w/w) ethanol in water for injection to the concentrate produces a final premix concentration of 10 mg docetaxel/mL. The required amount of premix is transferred by a calibrated syringe into 0.9% saline or 5% dextrose to produce a final concentration of 0.3 or 0.9 mg/mL. The IV infusion is administered over 1 hour.

Toxic Effects: Hypersensitivity reaction (HSR) was noted in up to 30% of patients in the early phase I studies. HSR occurs early in the first or second infusion and may be caused by vehicle Cremophor EL or paclitaxel itself. HSR consists of dyspnea, bronchospasm, urticaria, and hypotension. Most HSRs regress completely after stopping the infusion and treatment with antihistamines, fluids, and vasopressors. Prolonged infusions (>3 hours) and premedication (dexamethasone 20 mg orally, 12 and 6 hours before treatment, diphenhydramine 50 mg, and ranitidine 150 mg IV 30 minutes before treatment) have reduced the incidence of major HSRs to less than 3%. Patients with a history of HSR may be rechallenged with paclitaxel at a markedly slower infusion rate, 20 mg dexamethasone IV every 6 hours for four doses before treatment. Although not formulated in Cremophor EL, HSRs can occur in up to 25% of patients receiving docetaxel. Most HSRs are minor, consisting of flushing, chest tightness, and low back pain. Premedication with dexamethasone 8 mg orally twice daily for 3 days starting 1 day before treatment with docetaxel considerably reduces the incidence of HSRs and fluid retention. Neutropenia is the main toxicity of paclitaxel and docetaxel, but it is not cumulative. With higher doses of paclitaxel (250 mg/m^2 over 24 hours), this can be ameliorated with subsequent administration of granulocyte colony-stimulating factor. Severe thrombocytopenia and anemia are rare. Symmetric, distal, peripheral sensory neuropathy is usually seen with higher doses or multiple doses of paclitaxel. This often limits chronic use of paclitaxel. Diffuse areflexia and neuronopathy are less commonly seen. Higher doses can also cause motor and autonomic neuropathy as well as myalgias, especially in patients with preexisting neuropathy or when paclitaxel is used with cisplatin. Severe peripheral neuropathy or myalgias are less common after repetitive docetaxel at 100 mg/m^2. Cardiac rhythm abnormalities, especially bradyarrhythmias and (rarely) heart blocks, have been reported secondary to paclitaxel treatment. A direct causal link between paclitaxel and myocardial ischemic episodes and tachyarrhythmias has not been established. Although noted, a direct link has also not been established between the occurrence of cardiac conductance abnormalities or ischemia and docetaxel treatment. Nausea, vomiting, diarrhea, and stomatitis are uncommon and generally mild to moderate. Alopecia is universal with both drugs. Skin toxicity is more severe and common with docetaxel. It is characterized by an erythematous pruritic maculopapular rash affecting the forearms and hands. Onychodystrophy with discoloration, ridging, and brittleness of fingernails also occurs. Docetaxel can cause cumulative fluid retention, resulting in peripheral edema, third-space fluid collection, and weight gain, which usually resolves slowly after stopping docetaxel. Concurrent treatment with dexamethasone, as noted earlier, delays the onset and decreases the incidence of these side effects.

Potential Drug Interaction: When paclitaxel infusion (24 hours) is administered after cisplatin, there is a 33% reduction in the clearance rate of paclitaxel. This produces suboptimal antitumor cytotoxicity and more profound neutropenia. Hence, the sequence of paclitaxel followed by cisplatin is commonly recommended. The use of carboplatin after paclitaxel has been reported to cause less thrombocytopenia than carboplatin alone. Mucositis is more pronounced when paclitaxel is used before doxorubicin, a sequence that reduces the clearance of doxorubicin. Hematologic toxicity is more prominent with the sequence of cyclophosphamide followed by paclitaxel compared with the reverse sequence of administration. Anticonvulsants such as phenytoin and phenobarbital induce the metabolism of paclitaxel and docetaxel by the P450 mixed-function oxidases. Conversely, in vitro studies have shown that inhibitors of the P450 system can interfere with the metabolism of both drugs. These inhibitors include erythromycin, testosterone, ketoconazole, and fluconazole.

Therapeutic Indications in Hematology: Both paclitaxel and docetaxel have significant activity against previously treated patients with non-Hodgkin lymphoma. Paclitaxel is also very active against HIV-associated Kaposi sarcoma.

APPENDIX 55-3

CLINICAL PHARMACOLOGY OF ANTIMETABOLITES

CYTOSINE ARABINOSIDE

Chemistry and Mechanism of Action: Cytosine arabinoside (1′-β-D-arabinofuranosylcytosine; ara-C) is a nucleoside analog that differs from its naturally occurring counterpart (2′-deoxycytidine) by virtue of the presence of a hydroxyl group in the 2′-β configuration. The altered reactivity of the resulting arabinosyl sugar moiety confers on ara-C its cytotoxic activity. Ara-C enters the cell by a facilitated nucleoside diffusion mechanism and is converted to its nucleoside monophosphate form, ara-CMP, by the pyrimidine salvage pathway enzyme, deoxycytidine kinase. This represents the rate-limiting step in ra-C metabolism. Ara-C may also be catabolized intracellularly to an inactive form, ara-U, by the enzyme cytidine deaminase. Ara-C is ultimately converted to its lethal triphosphate derivative, ara-CTP, by a mono- and diphosphate kinase. Ara-CTP is an inhibitor of DNA polymerases α, β, and γ and is also incorporated into replicating DNA strands, leading to inhibition of chain initiation and elongation and premature chain termination. The extent of incorporation of ara-C into DNA closely correlates with lethality in leukemic cells. Although ara-C is generally thought of as a prototypical S phase–specific agent, its ability to interfere with DNA repair polymerases (e.g., β and γ) as well as lipid biosynthetic enzymes may account for lethal effects in noncycling cells.

Absorption, Fate, and Excretion: After IV administration, ara-C is rapidly deaminated to an inactive form, ara-U, by cytidine deaminase. This enzyme is present in the plasma, liver, and kidney but is present at very low levels in the central nervous system (CNS). The initial plasma half-life of ara-C has been estimated to be 10 to 12 minutes. Approximately 90% of the administered ara-C dose is excreted by the kidneys as ara-U or other inactive metabolites. The terminal half-life of ara-C is approximately 2 to 3 hours. CNS ara-C levels after a 2-hour infusion approximate 50% of plasma concentrations. Steady-state plasma concentrations after standard-dose therapy (e.g., 100-200 mg/m^2/day as a continuous infusion) approximate between 10^{-7} and 10^{-6} M. When ara-C is given as a high-dose bolus infusion (e.g., 1-3 g/m^2 over 1-3 hours), plasma levels as high as 100 μM can be achieved.

Preparation and Administration: Ara-C is provided as a sterile, lyophilized powder for reconstitution in vials containing 100 mg, 200 mg, 1 g, or 2 g of material. The powder is reconstituted with sterile bacteriostatic water for injection with benzyl alcohol (0.945%) added as a preservative. When reconstituted in this way, solutions are stable for up to 48 hours under controlled temperatures (e.g., between 15° C and 30° C or 60°-86° F). Material reconstituted without preservative should be used immediately. For intrathecal injection, ara-C should be reconstituted in a diluent that does not contain preservative (e.g., preservative-free 0.9% sodium chloride, USP) and used immediately.

Toxic Effects: Ara-C is primarily toxic to rapidly dividing tissues; consequently, myelosuppression and gastrointestinal toxicity represent the major side effects of this agent. Patients receiving ara-C regularly experience leukopenia, anemia, and thrombocytopenia, with nadirs appearing 7 to 14 days after drug administration. Gastrointestinal toxicity includes nausea and vomiting, abdominal pain, mucositis, and a chemical hepatitis characterized by elevation of liver function enzymes. The latter is generally reversible. Patients receiving ara-C as a high-dose infusion (e.g., 1-3 g/m^2 repeated every 12 hours for a total of 6-12 doses) experience standard toxicities and several unique ones. These include alopecia, an exfoliative dermatitis, a chemical conjunctivitis (generally ameliorated by the prophylactic administration of a steroid or saline ophthalmic solution), a respiratory distress–like syndrome (characterized by the appearance of rales, abnormal radiography findings, and pulmonary insufficiency), and cerebellar toxicity. The latter, which is characterized by nystagmus, ataxia, and other cerebellar signs, may be irreversible, and its appearance mandates discontinuation of therapy. Intrathecal administration of ara-C has been rarely associated with toxicities described below for methotrexate.

Potential Drug Interactions: None reported.

Therapeutic Indications in Hematology: Ara-C represents a mainstay in the treatment of AML (e.g., as part of the "7 and 3" regimen in which it is given in conjunction with daunorubicin). It is also incorporated into some induction regimens for ALL. High-dose ara-C (HIDAC), either alone or in combination with anthracycline antibiotics, is frequently used in the treatment of refractory or relapsed acute myeloid leukemia or acute lymphoblastic leukemia. HIDAC has also been used in some salvage regimens for non-Hodgkin lymphoma (e.g., ESHAP). Chronic low-dose ara-C has been used in the treatment of patients with the myelodysplastic syndrome.

METHOTREXATE

Chemistry and Mechanism of Action: Methotrexate (*N*-4-[[(2,4-diamino-6-pteridinyl)methyl]methylamino]benzoyl]-L-glutamic acid) represents a member of a class of compounds referred to as antifolates. Methotrexate is a potent inhibitor of dihydrofolate reductase, an enzyme responsible for the reduction of dihydrofolates to tetrahydrofolates. The latter are required in 1-carbon transfer reactions involved in de novo purine and pyrimidine biosynthesis, including conversion of deoxyuridylate (dUMP) to thymidylate (dTMP) by thymidylate synthase. As in the case of most antimetabolites, methotrexate is primarily active against S-phase cells. Methotrexate is transported across cell membranes by an energy-dependent, temperature-sensitive, concentrative process involving folate-binding proteins, after which it is polyglutamylated by the enzyme folylpolyglutamyl synthetase. Polyglutamylation of methotrexate enhances its intracellular retention and in some studies has been shown to correlate with the sensitivity of leukemic cells to this agent. The mechanism by which methotrexate kills cells may stem from interference with DNA synthesis (leading to a "thymine-less death") secondary to DHFR inhibition, disruption of purine biosynthesis, or a combination of these actions. The lethal actions of methotrexate may be reversed by reduced folates such as 5-formyltetrahydrofolate (leucovorin). The possibility that tumor cells may exhibit impaired transport of such reduced folates serves as the basis for strategies involving administration of high-dose methotrexate in conjunction with leucovorin rescue.

Absorption, Fate, and Excretion: In adults, oral absorption is dose dependent, with mean bioavailability approximating 60% at doses of 30 mg/m^2 or less. At higher doses (e.g., ≥80 mg/m^2), bioavailability is less. Peak plasma concentrations occur 1 to 2 hours after oral administration. Methotrexate bioavailability approximates 100% for parenteral routes of administration; with these routes, peak plasma methotrexate levels are achieved within 30 to 60 minutes after administration. For each route, the steady-state volume of distribution ranges from 40% to 80% of body weight. Methotrexate tends to accumulate in third-space fluids (e.g., ascites or pleural effusions) and can result in prolonged release and accompanying toxicity. Consequently, it is generally not advisable for patients with fluid accumulations to receive methotrexate. Methotrexate competes with reduced folates for transport across cell membranes; however, at high doses (e.g., ≥100 mg/m^2), passive diffusion is the primary mechanism through which intracellular accumulation occurs. Methotrexate is approximately 50% protein bound and does not penetrate the CNS barrier when administered orally or parenterally at conventional doses. However, when given by the intrathecal route, high CNS levels are achieved. Administration of high-dose methotrexate with leucovorin rescue can also result in therapeutic CNS levels.

The primary route of excretion is renal, with 80% to 90% of the drug appearing unchanged in the urine within 24 hours after IV administration. The terminal half-life of methotrexate is 4 to 10 hours for patients receiving low-dose therapy and 8 to 15 hours for those receiving high-dose therapy. Because of the primary renal rate of excretion and the possibility of nephrotoxicity, methotrexate should be withheld or administered at reduced doses in patients with impaired renal function. Patients receiving high-dose methotrexate therapy should be hydrated and their urine alkalinized before administration to reduce the risks of toxicity.

Preparation and Administration: Methotrexate is available in multiple formulations: (1) tablets, containing 2.5 mg methotrexate and inactive ingredients (lactose, magnesium stearate, and pregelatinized starch; (2) methotrexate sodium injection, available in vials of 25, 50, and 250 mg, containing benzyl alcohol as a preservative, sodium chloride, and water for injection (preservative-containing solutions should not be used for intrathecal or high-dose administration); (3) methotrexate sodium injection without preservative, which can be used for intravenous, intraarteriolar, intrathecal, and high-dose administration; and (4) lyophilized powder, which is provided in 20-mg vials and is reconstituted with preservative-free sodium chloride or 5% dextrose in water to a final concentration not exceeding 25 mg/mL.

For intrathecal administration, solutions of 1 to 1.5 mg/mL should be prepared using preservative-free 0.9% sodium chloride as the diluent. For high-dose therapy, leucovorin rescue is required to prevent significant toxicity. Leucovorin is administered 12 to 24 hours after methotrexate at a dose of between 15 and 25 mg intravenously, intramuscularly, or orally every 6 hours until the methotrexate dose declines to levels of less than 5×10^{-7} M.

For patients receiving intermediate or high-dose methotrexate (e.g., ≥500 mg/m^2), serum methotrexate and creatinine levels should be monitored at 24-hour intervals. If, after 48 hours, serum methotrexate levels are greater than 5×10^{-7} M but less than 1×10^{-6} M, leucovorin is continued at a dose of 25 mg/m^2 every 6 hours for eight doses until methotrexate levels decline to below 5×10^{-7} M. If levels are greater than 1×10^{-6} M but less than 2×10^{-6} M at 48 hours, the dose of leucovorin is increased to 100 mg/m^2 every 6 hours for eight doses. For methotrexate levels $\geq 2 \times 10^{-6}$ M at 48 hours, the dose of leucovorin is 200 mg/m^2 every 6 hours for eight doses.

Toxic Effects: Methotrexate primarily exhibits its toxic effects toward proliferating tissues. Consequently, dose-limiting toxicities include bone marrow suppression (leukopenia, thrombocytopenia, anemia), mucositis, and diarrhea. High-dose therapy is occasionally accompanied by transient elevations in liver function test results, but chronic low-dose therapy is more often associated with hepatic fibrosis. Standard-dose therapy is rarely associated with nephrotoxicity, but acute renal failure can be seen with high-dose therapy secondary deposition of 7-*OH*-methotrexate in the renal tubules. The risk of methotrexate nephrotoxicity is significantly reduced by ensuring adequate hydration and alkalinization of the urine. Other reported toxicities include a maculopapular rash and an idiosyncratic pulmonary toxicity characterized by cough, fever, dyspnea, hypoxia, and interstitial infiltrates.

A necrotizing leukoencephalopathy has been reported in patients receiving methotrexate who have had prior cranial irradiation. Intrathecal methotrexate has been associated with several toxicities, including (1) chemical arachnoiditis; (2) motor paralysis accompanied by cranial nerve dysfunction, seizures, and coma; and (3) chronic demyelinating syndrome. Each of these may be exacerbated by prior craniospinal irradiation.

Potential Drug Interactions: Methotrexate exhibits many potential drug interactions that are related to plasma protein binding. For example, many compounds are known to displace methotrexate from serum albumin, potentially increasing its bioavailability. These agents include sulfonamides, salicylates, tetracyclines, chloramphenicol, and phenytoin. However, the clinical implications of such interactions are not clear. Nonsteroidal antiinflammatory drugs should not be administered in conjunction with methotrexate when the latter is given at intermediate or high doses owing to the potential for elevation and prolongation of methotrexate plasma concentrations. Penicillins can reduce renal clearance of methotrexate and should be used with caution in this setting. Probenecid may also reduce renal transport of methotrexate. Administration of methotrexate can also reduce the clearance of theophyllines, and concomitant use of these agents requires careful monitoring. Increases in methotrexate toxicity have been observed in some patients receiving trimethoprim–sulfamethoxazole, possibly as a consequence of enhanced antifolate effects. Administration of folates in vitamin preparations may reduce the efficacy of methotrexate by bypassing dihydrofolate reductase inhibition. Methotrexate may increase the toxicity (and potentially the activity) of various antineoplastic agents in a schedule-dependent manner (e.g., when given before 5-fluroracil).

Therapeutic Indications in Hematology: Methotrexate is widely used in the treatment of acute lymphoblastic leukemia (ALL), particularly in the maintenance phase. Methotrexate is frequently administered intrathecally in patients with CNS leukemia and prophylactically in certain patients with ALL. It also represents a component of various multidrug regimens used in the treatment of non-Hodgkin lymphoma (e.g., M-BACOD, PROMACE-CYTABOM).

HYDROXYUREA

Chemistry and Mechanism of Action: Hydroxyurea is an inhibitor of the ribonucleotide reductase system that catalyzes the rate-limiting step in the de novo biosynthesis of purine and pyrimidine deoxyribonucleotides, that is, the conversion of ribonucleotide diphosphates to their deoxyribonucleoside diphosphate derivatives. Ribonucleotide reductase consists of two subunits: a binding and allosteric effector component and an iron-binding catalytic component. Hydroxyurea binds to and inactivates the catalytic subunit of the enzyme. Similar to most antimetabolites, hydroxyurea is an S phase–specific agent and blocks cells in the G_1S phase of the cell cycle. Exposure of cells to hydroxyurea leads to a depletion of deoxyribonucleotide triphosphate (dNTP) pools, the extent of which correlates with DNA synthesis inhibition and cell death. Two consequences of hydroxyurea administration include potentiation of the metabolism or cytotoxicity of nucleoside analogs (e.g., ara-C) as a result of dNTP pool depletion and elimination of amplified genes present extrasomally in double minute chromosomes.

Absorption, Fate, and Excretion: Hydroxyurea is generally administered orally, although IV regimens are currently being investigated. The drug is readily absorbed from the gastrointestinal tract, with peak plasma levels as high as 2.0 mM occurring approximately 2 hours after oral administration. Serum concentrations decline to undetectable levels after 24 hours. The drug is primarily excreted via the renal route, with 75% to 80% of the drug appearing in the urine 12 hours later. The drug penetrates the cerebrospinal fluid, although it has not been established that therapeutic levels are achieved after standard oral administration.

Preparation and Administration: Hydroxyurea is provided as 500-mg capsules. The drug is stored at room temperature in tightly capped containers and protected from heat.

Toxic Effects: The most common adverse reactions include myelosuppression (leukopenia, thrombocytopenia, anemia), gastrointestinal symptoms (e.g., nausea and vomiting, stomatitis, anorexia, appetite disturbances), and dermatologic toxicity (e.g., rashes, skin ulcerations, facial erythema). Rarer toxicities, generally seen at high doses include neurologic disturbances, such as drowsiness, dizziness, headache, and convulsions; altered renal function; and alopecia. The mutagenic potential of hydroxyurea is unknown, and the drug should be avoided when possible in pregnant women.

Potential Drug Interactions: As noted earlier, hydroxyurea may increase the toxicity of certain nucleoside analogs. Hydroxyurea may also serve as a radiosensitizing agent; consequently, patients receiving concurrent radiation therapy may experience enhanced toxicity.

Therapeutic Indications in Hematology: Hydroxyurea has become, along with interferon-α, the mainstay of therapy in patients with chronic or accelerated phase chronic myeloid leukemia (CML). It is currently recommended for initial therapy of CML over busulfan and may prolong the chronic phase of this disease compared with the latter agent. Hydroxyurea has also been successfully used in the treatment of other myeloproliferative disorders, including myeloid metaplasia and myelofibrosis, polycythemia vera, and essential thrombocytosis. Its leukemogenic potential is uncertain, however, and it should be used with caution, particularly in younger patients. Hydroxyurea has also been shown to reduce the incidence of painful crises in individuals with sickle cell anemia in a subset of patients, a phenomenon that may result from increases in red blood cell fetal hemoglobin levels.

FLUDARABINE

Chemistry and Mechanism of Action: Fludarabine phosphate is a fluorinated derivative of the nucleotide analog 9′-β-D-arabinofuranosyladenine (ara-A) that is resistant to deamination by the degradative enzyme cytidine deaminase. It is converted intracellularly to its triphosphate derivative, which inhibits ribonucleotide reductase, as well as DNA polymerase α and DNA primase. Fluoro-ara-ATP is also incorporated into DNA, a process that appears to be essential for the induction of apoptosis in leukemic cells. Fludarabine is toxic to S-phase cells, but its ability to interfere with DNA repair may contribute to lethality in their noncycling counterparts.

Absorption, Fate, and Excretion: After IV injection, fludarabine phosphate is rapidly deaminated (i.e., within minutes) in the plasma to its nucleoside derivative, 2′-fluoro-ara-A, which is then converted intracellularly to its nucleotide form, 2′-fluoro-ara-AMP by the pyrimidine salvage pathway enzyme, deoxycytidine kinase. The half-life of 2′-fluoro-ara-A is approximately 10 hours; the primary mode of elimination is renal, with 25% of the total dose appearing in the urine as unchanged 2-fluoro-ara-A. Total body clearance of fludarabine is inversely correlated with serum creatinine.

Preparation and Administration: Fludarabine is supplied as a sterile powder in 50-mg vials containing 50 mg of mannitol and sodium hydroxide to adjust the pH to 7.7. Material is reconstituted in 2 mL of sterile water to yield a 25 mg/mL solution for injection. The material may be stored at 4° C (40° F); because the reconstituted solution contains no antimicrobial preservative, the drug should be administered within 8 hours of formulation.

Toxic Effects: The most common dose-limiting toxicity is myelosuppression (neutropenia, thrombocytopenia, and anemia). Other toxicities include fever, chills, infection, nausea, and vomiting. Rarer toxicities include malaise, fatigue, anorexia, and weakness. Patients with chronic lymphocytic leukemia (CLL) receiving fludarabine have experienced serious opportunistic infections and tumor lysis syndrome. The most serious toxicity of fludarabine when administered at high doses (>40 mg/m^2/day for 5 days) is irreversible neurotoxicity, including cortical blindness, necrotizing leukoencephalopathy, and death. This phenomenon has rarely, if ever, been seen in patients receiving conventional doses (e.g., 25 mg/m^2/day for 5 days). Rare reports of interstitial pneumonitis have appeared.

Potential Drug Interactions: Fludarabine has been shown to potentiate the intracellular metabolism and activity of ara-C, although the toxicity of this combination may also be enhanced. No other interactions have been reported.

Therapeutic Indications in Hematology: Fludarabine has shown marked activity in both untreated CLL and in disease refractory to standard alkylating agent therapy. Fludarabine has also shown activity as a single agent, and particularly in combination with others (e.g., mitoxantrone, Cytoxan) in indolent non-Hodgkin lymphoma.

2′-CHLORODEOXYADENOSINE

Chemistry and Mechanism of Action: 2′-Chlorodeoxyadenosine (CdA; cladribine) is a derivative of deoxyadenosine that differs from its parent compound by the presence of a chlorine moiety at the 2′-position of the purine ring. It is transported intracellularly by facilitated nucleoside diffusion and phosphorylated by the pyrimidine salvage pathway enzyme deoxycytidine kinase. CdA is relatively resistant to deamination by cytidine deaminase. CdA is readily converted to its triphosphate derivative, 2′-chlorodeoxyadenosine-5′-triphosphate, particularly in cells of lymphoid origin, and is incorporated into tumor cell DNA by DNA polymerase α. CdATP is also an effective inhibitor of ribonucleotide reductase, which may contribute to lethal effects. CdA induces cell death (apoptosis) in both cycling and noncycling cells, possibly by promoting DNA fragmentation and by depleting cells of adenosine triphosphate or NAD, or both.

Absorption, Fate, and Excretion: Relatively little pharmacokinetic information concerning CdA is available. The drug is most commonly administered as a 7-day continuous infusion or as a 2-hour infusion over 5 days. The bioavailability of CdA after subcutaneous administration approximates that of the IV route but is less than that after oral administration. Renal excretion appears to be the major route of elimination. When given as a 2-hour infusion, CdA has a relatively long terminal half-life (e.g., ≈6 hours), and plasma concentrations after such a schedule may approximate those associated with the continuous infusion. Cerebrospinal fluid levels are approximately 25% of plasma concentrations.

Preparation and Administration: For daily infusions, CdA is diluted under sterile conditions in bags containing 500 mL of 0.9% sodium chloride injection, USP. The use of 5% dextrose solutions is not recommended because of enhanced degradation of the drug. For preparation of longer infusions (e.g., 7 days) the use of bacteriostatic sodium chloride injection, USP, is recommended. After being prepared, solutions of CdA should be refrigerated at a temperature between 4° C (40° F) and 8° C (47° F) for no more than 8 hours before administration.

Toxic Effects: The major toxicity of CdA is myelosuppression, which is primarily observed after intermittent rather than continuous infusion. Other toxicities include fever, generally beginning several days after initiation of therapy, and increased susceptibility to opportunistic infections. Rare side effects include nausea and hepatic and renal toxicity.

Potential Drug Interactions: None reported.

Therapeutic Indications in Hematology: CdA has shown significant activity in CLL and hairy cell leukemia. However, response rates in the former disorder appear to be somewhat less than those obtained with fludarabine; moreover, patients who have progressed on fludarabine therapy infrequently respond to CdA. Other diseases in which CdA has shown activity include non-Hodgkin lymphoma and Waldenström macroglobulinemia.

2′DEOXYCOFORMYCIN (PENTOSTATIN; DCF)

Chemistry and Mechanism of Action: 2′-Deoxycoformycin is an adenosine analog that is a highly effective inhibitor of the purine biosynthetic enzyme adenosine deaminase (ADA). It is transported across cell membranes by facilitated nucleoside diffusion, where it binds tightly to ADA. Inhibition of ADA results in accumulation of deoxyadenosine metabolites, most notably dATP. dATP exerts its toxic effects through inhibition of ribonucleotide reductase and induction of global imbalances in deoxyribonucleotide triphosphate pools. These result in interference with DNA synthesis and repair. 2′-Deoxycoformycin is particularly toxic to certain lymphoid cells with low levels of ADA activity. It is also toxic to both cycling and resting cells; the mechanism underlying its cytotoxicity toward quiescent cells is unknown.

Absorption, Fate, and Excretion: After IV injection of 2′-deoxycoformycin, the plasma clearance follows a biphasic pattern, with a terminal elimination half-life of 3 to 15 hours. Protein binding is limited. The drug is only partially metabolized, with approximately 60% to 80% of the drug appearing unchanged in the urine after 24 hours. The total body clearance of 2′-deoxycoformycin correlates well with creatinine clearance. Patients with impaired renal function may require reductions in the 2′-deoxycoformycin dose.

Preparation and Administration: 2′-Deoxycoformycin is unstable when reconstituted in solutions of pH less than 5.0. Consequently, it is customarily reconstituted in normal saline. 2′-Deoxycoformycin is provided in vials containing 10 mg of drug, 50 mg of mannitol, and sodium hydroxide to adjust the pH to less than 7.0. It is administered as an IV infusion over 20 to 30 minutes. Hydration is recommended before and after 2′-deoxycoformycin administration.

Toxic Effects: The major toxicities of 2′-deoxycoformycin include myelosuppression, nausea and vomiting, immunosuppression, acute renal failure, keratoconjunctivitis, fever, and elevations of liver function enzymes. At high doses, neurologic toxicity, including somnolence, seizures, and coma, have been reported, although these are seen infrequently in patients receiving standard dose therapy. When administered at such doses (e.g., 4 mg/m^2 biweekly), side effects are relatively minor.

Potential Drug Interactions: 2′-Deoxycoformycin may augment the toxicity of ara-A (vidarabine) as a consequence of inhibition of ADA.

Therapeutic Indications in Hematology: 2′-Deoxycoformycin is primarily used in the treatment of hairy cell leukemia, in which response rates of up to 90% have been reported, even in patients refractory to other therapy, including α-interferon. Activity has also been reported in other lymphoid malignancies, such as T-cell lymphoma, chronic lymphocytic leukemia, prolymphocytic leukemia, and Waldenström macroglobulinemia, although its precise role in the treatment of these disorders remains to be fully evaluated.

6-THIOGUANINE

Chemistry and Mechanism of Action: Thioguanine (6-TG) is a guanine analog in which the 6′-hydroxyl group is replaced by a sulfhydryl group. It interferes with de novo purine biosynthesis at multiple levels. After transport across the cell membrane by facilitated diffusion, 6-TG competes with hypoxanthine and guanine for phosphorylation by hypoxanthine–guanine phosphoribosyltransferase (HGPRT) and is converted to its nucleotide form, 6-thioguanylic acid (TGMP), which accumulates within cells. TGMP inhibits several purine biosynthetic enzymes, including glutamine-5-phosphoribosylpyrophosphate aminotransferase and IMP dehydrogenase. 6-TG nucleotides are also incorporated in DNA and RNA, where they function as fraudulent bases. It is presently unknown which of these actions (interference with purine interconversions, blockade of de novo purine biosynthesis, or nucleic acid incorporation) is primarily responsible for 6-TG cytotoxicity, although DNA incorporation appears to play a significant role. 6-TG is considered to be an S phase–specific agent.

Absorption, Fate, and Excretion: After oral administration, the bioavailability of 6-TG is variable, ranging from 14% to 46% of the administered dose (mean, 30%). Peak plasma levels are achieved 8 hours after administration and decline slowly thereafter. The average plasma disappearance of 6-TG is approximately 80 minutes, with a range of 25 to 240 minutes. Relatively little unchanged material appears in the urine; the major excreted product is the methylated derivative 2-amino-6-methyl thiopurine. Central nervous system penetrance after parenteral administration is minimal.

Preparation and Administration: 6-TG is available in tablet form for oral administration. Each tablet contains 40 mg of 6-TG and inactive ingredients, including gum acacia, lactose, magnesium stearate, potato starch, and stearic acid. IV preparations are available only in experimental settings.

Toxic Effects: The major dose-limiting toxicity of 6-TG is myelosuppression. Other less common toxicities include gastrointestinal disturbances (nausea and vomiting, anorexia, diarrhea), jaundice, and elevated liver function test results.

Potential Drug Interactions: In contrast to 6-MP, the metabolism of 6-TG is not modified by allopurinol; consequently, dose adjustments do not have to be made when these agents are administered concurrently.

Therapeutic Indications in Hematology: The primary indication for 6-TG is in the treatment of acute myeloid leukemia, generally in conjunction with other agents (e.g., daunorubicin and ara-C). However, it has not been firmly established that addition of 6-TG to such regimens improves therapeutic efficacy. 6-TG also has activity in chronic myeloid leukemia, although it has been supplanted by other agents (e.g., hydroxyurea, interferon-α) in this disorder.

6-MERCAPTOPURINE

Chemistry and Mechanism of Action: 6-Mercaptopurine (1,7-dihydro-6*H*-purine 6-thione monohydrate; 6-MP; purinethol) is an analog of the purine bases adenine and hypoxanthine. It is both an antineoplastic and immunosuppressive agent. Similar to 6-TG, 6-MP and its metabolites act at multiple levels to interfere with purine biosynthesis and interconversions. It competes with hypoxanthine and guanine for HGPRTase, and after conversion to thioinosinic acid (TIMP), blocks conversion of IMP to xanthylic acid and IMP to AMP. Both TIMP and another metabolite, 6-methylthioinosinate (MTIMP) inhibit glutamine-5-phosphoribosylpyrophosphate aminotransferase. 6-MP is also incorporated into RNA and DNA, thereby functioning as a fraudulent base. It is unknown which of these actions is primarily responsible for the lethal actions of 6-MP, although available evidence points to DNA incorporation as a prime determinant of cytotoxicity.

Fate, Absorption, and Excretion: After oral administration, the bioavailability of 6-MP is highly variable, presumably because of interpatient differences in gastrointestinal absorption, which averages 50% of the administered dose. Extensive catabolism by hepatic xanthine oxidase also contributes to drug elimination. Approximately 50% of the administered 6-MP or its metabolites are recovered in the urine. The volume of distribution generally exceeds the total body water. After IV administration, the plasma disappearance half-life was 47 minutes in adults. Plasma protein binding is modest (≅19%), and central nervous system penetrance is minimal.

Preparation and Administration: 6-MP is supplied as tablets for oral administration. Each tablet contains 50 mg of 6-MP and the inactive ingredients corn and potato starch, lactose, magnesium stearate, and stearic acid. An IV preparation containing 500 mg of 6-MP per vial is available for investigational use.

Toxic Effects: The major dose-limiting toxicity of 6-MP is myelosuppression. This is dose related and is manifested by leukopenia, thrombocytopenia, and anemia. The hematologic effects of 6-MP may be delayed, so it is important to withdraw the medication temporarily at the first sign of unusual hematologic toxicity. Individuals with an inherited disorder of thiopurine methyltransferase deficiency may be particularly susceptible to 6-MP–mediated hematopoietic suppression. Other toxicities include hepatotoxicity (elevated liver function test results, cholestasis, hepatic necrosis, ascites), nausea, vomiting, mucositis, fever, rash, and diarrhea. The hepatotoxicity, which occurs in 10% to 40% of patients, requires close monitoring and discontinuation of therapy until recovery occurs. Patients receiving 6-MP uniformly experience immunosuppression.

Potential Drug Interactions: Allopurinol, an inhibitor of xanthine oxidase, significantly reduces the catabolism of 6-MP when the latter is given orally, leading to major increases in plasma concentrations. Allopurinol does not alter the pharmacokinetics of IV 6-MP, presumably because of the absence of first-pass metabolism of 6-MP when administered by this route. When administered in conjunction with allopurinol, the dose of 6-MP should be reduced by one-third to one-fourth. Increased toxicity has been reported in patients receiving concurrent 6-MP and trimethoprim–sulfamethoxazole. 6-MP may also modify the effects of warfarin.

Therapeutic Indications in Hematology: The major use for 6-MP is in the maintenance phase of treatment for acute lymphoblastic leukemia. 6-MP has also been used in the treatment of patients with immune thrombocytopenia purpura or autoimmune hemolytic anemia refractory to all other forms of therapy.

5-AZACITIDINE

Chemistry and Mechanism of Action: 5′-Azacitidine is an analog of the nucleoside cytidine, differing from the parent compound by virtue of the presence of nitrogen at the 5′ position of the heterocyclic ring. 5′-Azacytidine is transported across the cell membrane by facilitated nucleoside diffusion and is converted to its nucleotide monophosphate form, 5′-aza-CMP, by the pyrimidine salvage pathway enzyme uridine–cytidine kinase. 5′-Azacytidine is also a substrate for the degradative enzyme cytidine deaminase. It is ultimately converted to its lethal derivative, 5′-aza-CTP, which is incorporated into RNA, and to a lesser extent, DNA. The lethal actions of 5′-azacytidine are believed to result from its ability to interfere with protein synthesis through disruption of RNA processing. The chemical instability of the 5′-azacitidine ring structure is also believed to contribute to the cytotoxicity of this compound.

Absorption, Fate, and Excretion: The drug distributes into a volume corresponding to the total body water after IV administration and is also well absorbed after subcutaneous injection.

It is extensively deaminated in the plasma and liver and displays minimal plasma binding. Peak plasma concentrations after IV injection approximate 1.0 mM. The initial half-life of 5′-azacitidine (or its metabolites) is approximately 4 hours, although the drug is rapidly converted to various derivatives within minutes of administration. There is minimal cerebrospinal fluid penetrance.

Preparation and Administration: Azacitidine is available in 100-mg vials and can be administered both intravenously and subcutaneously When given subcutaneously, it should be reconstituted with 4 mL of sterile water for injection. The diluents should be injected slowly into the vial. Vigorously shake or roll the vial until a uniform suspension is achieved. The suspension will be cloudy. The resulting suspension will contain azacitidine 25 mg/mL. Do not filter the suspension after reconstitution. Doing so could remove the active substance. Azacitidine reconstituted for subcutaneous administration may be stored for up to 1 hour at 25° C (77° F) or for up to 8 hours between 2° C and 8° C (36° F and 46° F).To provide a homogeneous suspension, the contents of the dosing syringe must be resuspended immediately before administration. To resuspend, vigorously roll the syringe between the palms until a uniform, cloudy suspension is achieved. When given intravenously, reconstitute each vial with 10 mL of sterile water for injection. Vigorously shake or roll the vial until all solids are dissolved. Withdraw the required amount of solution to deliver the desired dose and inject into a 50- to 100-mL infusion bag of either 0.9% sodium chloride injection or lactated Ringer solution.

Toxic Effects: The major toxicity of 5′-azacitidine has been leukopenia and, to a lesser extent, thrombocytopenia. Nausea and vomiting, which are often refractory to standard antiemetic therapy, have also been encountered, most frequently in patients receiving bolus infusions. Gastrointestinal toxicity is ameliorated by administering 5′-azacitidine as a continuous infusion. Other potential side effects include diarrhea, fever, hepatotoxicity (most frequently in patients with preexisting hepatic disease), neuromuscular toxicity, rash, and hypotension.

Drug Interactions: None reported.

Therapeutic Indications in Hematology: 5′-Azacitidine is primarily used in the treatment of refractory acute myeloid leukemia, with response rates ranging from 17% to 30% when used as a single agent. 5′-Azacitidine has also yielded clinical responses in a subset of patients with the myelodysplastic syndrome when administered as a low-dose continuous infusion. In early trials, low-dose 5′azacytidine has increased fetal hemoglobin levels in some patients with sickle cell anemia and thalassemia; however, its mutagenic potential has limited the use of this agent in nonmalignant conditions.

DECITABINE

Chemistry and Mechanism of Action: Decitabine is a synthetic nucleoside analog of 2′-deoxycytidine, a cytotoxic S-phase pyrimidine analogue that induces hypomethylation of DNA at concentrations that do not cause major suppression of DNA synthesis. It also causes cellular differentiation or apoptosis. This is accomplished by intracellular phosphorylation of decitabine to its triphosphate form, which is incorporated into DNA and blocks methylation of newly synthesized DNA by binding to DNA methyltransferase. Nonproliferating cells seem relatively insensitive to decitabine.

Absorption, Fate, and Excretion: Decitabine is widely distributed with less than 1% protein binding and is tolerated after subcutaneous injection. There is some central nervous system penetration after subcuaneous injection with cerebrospinal fluid concentrations in patients with meningeal leukemia that were approximately 20% of corresponding steady-state plasma levels. The mean half-life is 0.5

to 0.6 hours. The route of metabolism appears to be deamination by cytidine deaminase, principally found in the liver but also in granulocytes, intestinal epithelium, and whole blood.

Preparation and Administration: Decitabine is available in 50-mg vials, which are reconstituted with 10 mL of sterile water for injection (USP); upon reconstitution, each milliliter contains approximately 5.0 mg of decitabine at a pH of 6.7 to 7.3. Immediately after reconstitution, the solution should be further diluted with 0.9% sodium chloride injection, 5% dextrose injection, or lactated Ringer solution injection to a final drug concentration of 0.1 to 1.0 mg/mL. Unless used within 15 minutes of reconstitution, the diluted solution must be prepared using cold (2°-8° C) infusion fluids and stored at 2° to 8° C (36°-46° F) for up to a maximum of 7 hours until administration.

Toxic Effects: The major toxicity of decitabine has been bone marrow suppression, including leukopenia, thrombocytopenia and anemia. Nausea and vomiting are mild. Other potential side effects include diarrhea; fever; and hepatotoxicity, including hyperbilirubinemia, transamination elevations, and electrolyte abnormalities.

Drug Interactions: None reported.

Therapeutic Indications in Hematology: Decitabine is indicated for treatment of patients with myelodysplastic syndromes (MDS) including previously treated and untreated, de novo, and secondary MDS. It has also been used as salvage therapy both alone and in combination for acute myeloid leukemia, chronic myeloid leukemia, and acute lymphoid leukemia.

GEMCITABINE

Chemistry and Mechanism of Action: Gemcitabine (2′,2′-difluorocytidine monohydrochloride) is a nucleoside analog that differs from 2′-deoxycytidine by virtue of the presence of fluorine atoms in the 2′α and 2′β positions of the cytidine ring. It is transported across the cell membrane by facilitated nucleoside diffusion, phosphorylated by deoxycytidine kinase, and ultimately converted to its lethal metabolites, dFdCDP and dFdCTP. The diphosphate form (dFdCDP) inhibits ribonucleotide reductase, leading to disruption of dNTP pools and resultant interference with DNA synthesis and repair. The triphosphate form (dFdCTP) competes with dCTP for incorporation into DNA. Reductions in dCTP pools (secondary to ribonucleotide reductase inhibition) result in self-potentiation of gemcitabine action. Incorporation of gemcitabine into DNA in S phase inhibits elongation of the replicating strand, leading to DNA chain termination. The lethal actions of gemcitabine in leukemia cells have been related to the induction of apoptosis and are not restricted to cells actively engaged in DNA synthesis. Gemcitabine has been shown to be considerably more potent in inducing apoptosis in cultured human leukemia cells than ara-C.

Absorption, Fate, and Excretion: In studies involving intravenously administered labeled gemcitabine, up to 98% of the drug was recovered in the urine after 1 week. The excreted dose was composed of a minor fraction (gemcitabine; <10%) and inactive metabolites (e.g., 2′-deoxy-2′,2′-difluorouridine). Plasma protein binding was minimal. In studies involving both short and long gemcitabine infusions, the pharmacokinetics were found to be linear and best described by a two-compartment model. Plasma half-life and clearance are influenced both by age and gender. For short infusions, half-lives varied from 32 to 94 minutes; for longer infusions, half-lives varied from 245 to 638 minutes. The volume of distribution was approximately 50 L/m^2 for short infusions and 370 L/m^2 for long infusions.

Preparation and Administration: Vials of gemcitabine contain 200 mg or 1 g of the HCl derivative formulated with mannitol (200 mg or 1 g) and sodium acetate (12.5 mg or 62.5 mg) as a sterile lyophilized powder. HCl or NaOH has been used for pH adjustment.

Toxic Effects: The major dose-limiting toxicity of gemcitabine is myelosuppression, although anemia and thrombocytopenia have also been encountered. Other toxicities include nausea and vomiting, transient elevations in liver function test results, mild hematuria, proteinuria (and in rare cases, hemolytic uremic syndrome), fever, rash, dyspnea, edema, and a flulike syndrome. Other infrequent toxicities included alopecia, paresthesias, and bronchospasm.

Potential Interactions: Gemcitabine may function as a radiosensitizing agent and can increase the toxicity of ionizing radiation. No other interactions are known.

Indications in Hematology: The primary indication for gemcitabine is in the treatment of patients with pancreatic carcinoma. However, as an experimental agent, gemcitabine is being evaluated for the treatment of acute lymphoblastic leukemia and chronic lymphocytic leukemia.

NELARABINE

Arabinofuranosylguanine (Ara-G)

Chemistry and Mechanism of Action: Nelarabine is a pro-drug of the deoxyguanosine analog 9′-β-D-arabinofuranosylguanine also known as ara-G. Accumulation of a metabolite ara-GTP in leukemic blasts allows for incorporation into deoxyribonucleic acid (DNA), leading to inhibition of DNA synthesis and cell death.

Absorption, Fate, and Excretion: Nelarabine is demethylated by adenosine deaminase (ADA) to ara-G; then monophosphorylated by deoxyguanosine kinase and deoxycytidine kinase; and subsequently converted to the active 5′-triphosphate, ara-GTP. Nelarabine is only available in an IV formulation. Nelarabine and ara-G are both partially eliminated by the kidneys. Approximately 5% to 10% of nelarabine is excreted by the kidneys compared with 20% to 30% of ara-G. Nelarabine exhibits a half-life of 30 minutes, and ara-G, the active metabolite, has a half-life of 3 hours.

Preparation and Administration: Nelarabine for injection is supplied as a clear, colorless, sterile solution in glass vials. Each vial contains 250 mg of nelarabine (5 mg of nelarabine per milliliter) and sodium chloride (4.5 mg/mL) in 50 mL of water for injection, USP. Nelarabine is not diluted before administration. The dose is transferred into polyvinylchloride (PVC) infusion bags or glass containers and administered as a 2-hour infusion in adult patients or as a 1-hour infusion in pediatric patients.

Toxic Effects: Bone marrow suppression encompassing all cell lines causing anemia, leucopenia, thrombocytopenia, and neutropenia occurs in all patients. Neurologic complications of nelarabine, include asthenia, altered mental states, including severe somnolence; central nervous system (CNS) effects, including convulsions, and peripheral neuropathy ranging from numbness and paresthesias to motor weakness and paralysis. Demyelinating disease of the CNS may occur when combining nelarabine with other drugs that may have CNS toxicity. Nausea and vomiting are seen and antiemetics are necessary.

Drug Interactions: Pentostatin has been shown to be a strong inhibitor of adenosine deaminase (ADA) in vitro. Concurrent administration of nelarabine and pentostatin may result in reduced ADA-dependent conversion of nelarabine to its active moiety, thereby potentially decreasing nelarabine efficacy or altering nelarabine's adverse event profile. Therefore, concomitant administration of nelarabine and pentostatin is not recommended.

Therapeutic Indications in Hematology: Nelarabine is effective in T-cell acute lymphoblastic leukemia, T-cell lymphoma, and T-cell lymphoblastic lymphoma. The dosage in adults of nelarabine is 1500 mg/m^2 administered intravenously over 2 hours on days 1, 3, and 5 repeated every 21 days. The pediatric dosage of nelarabine is 650 mg/m^2 administered intravenously over 1 hour daily for 5 consecutive days repeated every 21 days. The proper number of cycles for adult and pediatric patients has not been determined.

CLOFARABINE

Chemistry and Mechanism of Action: Clofarabine is a purine nucleoside antimetabolite formulated in unbuffered normal saline with a pH range of 4.5 to 7.5. It inhibits DNA synthesis by decreasing cellular deoxynucleotide triphosphate pools by inhibiting ribonucleotide reductase, terminating DNA chain elongation, and inhibiting repair through incorporation into the DNA chain by competitive inhibition of DNA polymerases.

Absorption, Fate, and Excretion: Clofarabine is 47% bound to plasma proteins, primarily albumin. Clofarabine is phosphorylated intracellularly to the cytotoxic active form (clofarabine triphosphate) by deoxycytidine kinase. The terminal half-life is estimated to be 5.2 hours with the metabolite clofarabine triphosphate, yielding a half-life greater than 24 hours, and 49% to 60% of the dose is excreted in the urine unchanged. Systemic clearance and volume of distribution at steady state were estimated to be 28.8 L/hr/m^2 and 172 L/m^2, respectively.

Preparation and Administration: Clofarabine is supplied in a 20-mL, single-use vial that contains 20 mg of clofarabine in 20 mL of unbuffered normal saline at a concentration of 1 mg/mL. Clofarabine should be filtered through a sterile 0.2-μm syringe filter and diluted with 5% dextrose injection, USP, or 0.9% sodium chloride injection, USP, before IV infusion to a final concentration between 0.15 and 0.4 mg/mL.

Toxic Effects: Bone marrow suppression encompassing all cell lines causing anemia, leucopenia, thrombocytopenia and neutropenia occurs in all patients. A capillary leak syndrome, also known as systemic inflammatory response syndrome (SIRS), thought related to cytokine release leading to respiratory distress, hypotension, pleural effusions, pericardial effusions, and multiorgan failure may occur in a small number of patients. Elevations of liver transaminases are seen and are transient (typically, less than 2 weeks' duration) and occurred within 1 week of clofarabine initiation. Elevations in bilirubin may also occur.

Drug Interactions: None described.

Therapeutic Indications in Hematology: Clofarabine is effective in treating acute lymphocytic leukemia. The recommended pediatric dose is 52 mg/m^2 administered by IV infusion over 2 hours daily for 5 consecutive days. Treatment cycles are repeated after recovery or return to baseline organ function, approximately every 2 to 6 weeks. Clofarabine has been used in adults at a dosage of 40 mg/m^2 administered by IV infusion over 2 hours daily for 5 consecutive days. Clofarabine has also been used in combination with cytarabine. Because this drug is excreted to a major extent by the kidneys, extreme caution should be used in patients with renal dysfunction.

APPENDIX 55-4

TOPOISOMERASE I INHIBITORS AND TOPOISOMERASE II INHIBITORS

TOPOISOMERASE II INHIBITORS

Etoposide (Vepesid), Etoposide Phosphate (Etopophos), Teniposide (Vumon)

Chemistry and Mechanism of Action: Etoposide (VP-16), etoposide phosphate, and teniposide (VM-26) are semisynthetic derivatives of epipodophyllotoxin. The mechanism of action of these drugs appears to be related to their ability to stabilize a topoisomerase II–DNA cleavable complex, which acts as a replication fork barrier and leads to the generation of irreversible DNA damage and cell death in proliferating cells.

Absorption, Fate, and Excretion: *Etoposide* has an oral bioavailability of 25% to 75%. Its terminal half-life is 6 to 8 hours, with approximately 30% to 40% excreted in the urine, two-thirds as unchanged drug. There is no accumulation with consecutive daily administration, but cytotoxicity has strict schedule dependency. Clinical studies suggest that in patients with a plasma creatinine level greater than 130 mol/L, the etoposide dose should be reduced by more than 25%.

Etoposide phosphate is rapidly and completely converted in vivo to VP-16 by the activity of phosphatase and has been shown to have the same pharmacokinetics as VP-16. Because of its increased water solubility, etoposide phosphate can be given intravenously in much less volume. In addition, the metabolic acidosis and hypotension seen with the infusion of VP-16 are not seen with this prodrug.

Teniposide has a multiphasic pattern of clearance from plasma with a terminal half-life of 9.5 to 21 hours. Unlike those of etoposide, metabolites of teniposide account for greater than 80% of the drug excreted in the urine. Similar to etoposide, there is significant interpatient and intrapatient variation in clinical pharmacokinetics. There are currently no formal recommendations for dose modification in patients with renal insufficiency.

Preparation and Administration: *Etoposide* is commercially available as 50-mg capsules and in vials of 50 and 100 mg at a concentration of 20 mg/mL. When the drug is diluted with normal saline or 5% dextrose in water to a concentration of 0.2 or 0.4 mg/mL, it is stable for 96 or 48 hours, respectively. Etoposide must be administered slowly over more than 30 minutes to prevent hypotension.

Etoposide phosphate is available commercially as single-dose vials containing etoposide phosphate equivalent to 100 mg of etoposide. When it is diluted with water, 5% dextrose, or normal saline to a concentration of 10 to 20 mg/mL, it can be administered without dilution over 5 to 10 minutes. When reconstituted, etoposide phosphate is stable for 24 hours at room temperature or under refrigeration.

Teniposide is supplied in 50-mg vials for IV use only. The IV solution may be taken orally but is unpalatable. Currently, no oral preparation is available in the market; however, for investigational purposes, each 50-mg vial may be dissolved in 50 to 100 mL of syrup or juice. To achieve optimal absorption, a single oral dose of 60 mg/m^2, which may be repeated at 6-hour intervals, is advised. As with etoposide, rapid infusion can produce hypotension.

Toxic Side Effects: Myelosuppression, especially leukopenia, is the dose-limiting toxic effect of *etoposide* and *teniposide*. Nausea and vomiting are usually mild and easily prevented with antiemetics. Rapid infusion of etoposide (<30 minutes) may cause hypotension. Anaphylactoid reactions (e.g., bronchospasm) occur in fewer than 2% of patients and may be related to the Cremophor vehicle. Alopecia occurs in approximately 20% of patients treated with etoposide. This side effect is more common with teniposide. When the drug is given in bone marrow transplantation doses, mucositis and diarrhea are prominent and may be dose limiting.

Potential Drug Interactions: Theoretically, any drug that increases the S-phase fraction will increase the cytotoxicity of epipodophyllotoxins and other topoisomerase inhibitors. Conversely, drugs that inhibit DNA synthesis antagonize the effect of *etoposide* and *teniposide* (e.g., 5-fluoro-2′-deoxyuridine given before etoposide in some human cancer cell lines decreases the cytotoxicity of the latter). More recent in vitro data suggest that synergistic cytotoxic effects are seen when VP-16 is given after a topoisomerase I inhibitor, which appears to upregulate the amount of topoisomerase II enzyme. Antagonistic effects have been reported when a topoisomerase II inhibitor is given before a topoisomerase I inhibitor. In hematology, etoposide and teniposide may inhibit the intracellular ara-CTP formation leading to reduced ara-C cytotoxicity. Potentiation of teniposide activity has been seen with methotrexate and dipyridamoles. There is at least a twofold increase in the clearance of teniposide with concomitant administration of phenobarbital or phenytoin. Cyclosporine and other P-glycoprotein antagonists (PSC 833) potentiate the cytotoxic effects of etoposide.

Therapeutic Indications: *Etoposide* is used in the treatment of non-Hodgkin lymphoma (NHL) and as a second-line treatment for Hodgkin disease. It is also incorporated in the preparatory regimens for bone marrow transplantation of refractory lymphomas (CBV) and acute leukemia. *Teniposide* has been approved as a front-line agent with combination chemotherapy for childhood acute lymphoblastic leukemia (ALL). Combination chemotherapy with teniposide has been used successfully in some cases of refractory adult ALL and acute monocytic leukemia, but the duration of remission is not significantly different from that with other standard salvage regimens. In NHL, teniposide has shown comparable activity to vincristine. *Etoposide phosphate* has been given in both standard-dose and high-dose (as a single agent) chemotherapy regimens and appears to have the same pharmacokinetics and antitumor activity as VP-16.

Daunorubicin

Chemistry and Mechanism of Action: Daunorubicin is an anthracycline that inhibits DNA topoisomerase II, acting as a poison at lower concentrations and a suppressor of cleavable complex formation at higher doses. Daunorubicin is also a DNA intercalator and generates reactive oxygen intermediates.

Absorption, Fate, and Excretion: After IV injection, daunorubicin undergoes rapid tissue uptake and concentration. It is rapidly metabolized in the liver, where approximately 25% of the drug concentrates and has a half-life of 20 to 50 hours. The principal metabolite is daunorubicinol, which also displays antineoplastic activity. Biliary excretion accounts for approximately 75% of the drug and metabolite elimination. Patients with significant hepatic dysfunction should receive an attenuated dose of daunorubicin.

Preparation and Administration: Daunorubicin is supplied with 100 mg of mannitol in 20-mg vials, from which it is reconstituted with 4 mL of sterile water for injection. The vial should be protected from sunlight. Daunorubicin is a powerful vesicant that should be administered into the tubing of a freely flowing IV infusion of either 5% dextrose in water or normal saline. In the event of extravasation, as much infiltrated drug as possible should be aspirated from the tissue, and cold compresses should be maintained on the site for several hours. Despite these measures, skin grafting may be necessary. Daunorubicin is not physically compatible with heparin, and the two drugs should not be coadministered in the same IV tubing. The patient should be informed that daunorubicin may impart a red color to the urine for up to 72 hours after administration.

Toxic Effects: Myelosuppression, predominantly leukopenia, is the dose-limiting toxic effect. Mucositis, nausea and vomiting, and alopecia are common. Facial flushing, conjunctivitis, and lacrimation may occur in rare cases. Erythematous streaking near the site of injection occurs as a benign local allergic reaction and should not be confused with extravasation. The drug can produce a severe local reaction (e.g., pneumonitis, esophagitis) in previously irradiated areas, even when both therapies are not administered concomitantly (radiation recall). Cardiac toxicity is a unique characteristic of the anthracycline antibiotics and can be acute or chronic. In the acute form, abnormal ECG changes such as ST-T wave elevation and arrhythmias may be seen. Transient reduction in the ejection fraction can also occur acutely and is often associated with pericarditis (pericarditis-myocarditis syndrome). The chronic form of anthracycline cardiac toxicity is related to the cumulative dose. The dose limit of doxorubicin is generally considered to be 450 to 500 mg/m^2, where the risk of clinical cardiotoxicity is between 1% and 10%. The corresponding cumulative dose limit for daunorubicin is 900 to 1000 mg/m^2. The cardiac toxicity is clinically characterized by congestive heart failure, usually refractory to medical therapy. Cardiac irradiation or the administration of cyclophosphamide may increase the risk of cardiotoxicity. The cardiotoxic effects appear to be related to the formation of free radicals and not to the inhibition of DNA topoisomerase II. The cardioprotective agent dexrazoxane (Zinecard) is now available and recommended to be started at a doxorubicin cumulative dose greater than 350 mg/m^2.

Potential Drug Interactions: Daunorubicin is not physically compatible with heparin or dexamethasone. The drug interactions described for doxorubicin (description follows) probably occur with daunorubicin as well.

Therapeutic Indications in Hematology: Daunorubicin is used in combination with other drugs in the treatment of acute myeloid leukemia and ALL.

Doxorubicin (Adriamycin)

Chemistry and Mechanism of Action: Doxorubicin is also an anthracycline glycoside antibiotic. It differs from daunorubicin at C-8, in which a hydroxyacetyl group replaces an acetyl group. Because of this, doxorubicin is also called hydroxyl daunorubicin. Its mechanisms of action also involve stabilizing DNA–topoisomerase II complexes, DNA intercalation, and free radical formation.

Absorption, Fate, and Excretion: Doxorubicin has a triphasic plasma clearance with a half-life of approximately 30 hours. The drug is extensively metabolized in the liver to yield an active metabolite (doxorubicinol) and a number of inactive metabolites (aglycones). Within 7 days, more than 50% of an injected dose is excreted in the bile, but only 5% to 10% of the drug is excreted in the urine. Penetration into the cerebrospinal fluid is poor.

Preparation and Administration: Doxorubicin is commercially available in vials of 10, 20, 50, 150, and 200 mg. The lyophilized powder is reconstituted with either normal saline or sterile water for injection to yield a 2-mg/mL solution. The reconstituted solution must be protected from sunlight. The drug should be injected slowly into the tubing of a freely running IV infusion of normal saline or 5% dextrose in water. Erythematous streaking along the vein is often an indication that the administration rate is too rapid. The drug is a powerful vesicant, and in case of extravasation, the measures described for daunorubicin should be followed.

Toxic Effects: The toxic effects are similar to those of daunorubicin. It is important to emphasize that weekly low-dose regimens or administration by continuous infusion can decrease the risk of cardiotoxicity with doxorubicin.

Potential Drug Interactions: When used in combination with other drugs as treatment for leukemia or lymphoma, doxorubicin may decrease the oral bioavailability of digoxin. It is not physically compatible with heparin or 5-fluorouracil. Barbiturates may increase the plasma clearance of doxorubicin and decrease its cytotoxic effect. Doxorubicin is compatible with vincristine, and the two drugs can be administered together in the same IV solution.

Therapeutic Indications in Hematology: Doxorubicin is one of the most important drugs in the treatment of hematologic malignancies. It is used in the treatment of Hodgkin disease (ABVD regimen), non-Hodgkin lymphoma (CHOP, MACOP-B), and multiple myeloma (VBAP, VAD).

Idarubicin (Idamycin)

Chemistry and Mechanism of Action: Idarubicin, also called 4′-demethoxydaunorubicin (4-DMDR), is an analog of daunorubicin in which the methoxy group from the aglycone has been replaced with hydrogen. Idarubicin is also a topoisomerase II inhibitor and generates free radicals.

Absorption, Fate, and Excretion: The elimination half-life of the parent compound is 11.3 hours and that of the primary metabolite, 13-epirubicinol, is 40 to 60 hours. The major metabolite is as active as idarubicin. The oral bioavailability of this drug is approximately 30%; 80% of the drug is excreted in the urine as 13-epirubicinol.

Preparation and Administration: Idarubicin is supplied in 5- and 10-mg vials from which it is reconstituted with sterile water or normal saline to obtain a 1 mg/mL solution. The drug should be infused from 10 to 15 minutes through the tubing of a freely running IV infusion. Extravasation precautions should be instituted during administration. The oral formulation remains investigational.

Toxic Effects: The side effects of idarubicin are similar to those of daunorubicin and doxorubicin but are of lesser intensity at equal myelosuppressive doses.

Potential Drug Interactions: None reported.

Therapeutic Indications in Hematology: Idarubicin in combination with ara-C is equivalent, if not superior, to combination chemotherapy with daunorubicin in the treatment of adult acute myeloid leukemia (AML) and myelodysplastic syndromes. Idarubicin has been approved for use in combination therapy for adult AML.

Mitoxantrone (Novantrone)

Chemistry and Mechanism of Action: Mitoxantrone is a synthetic anthracenedione. Its mechanism of action appears to involve primarily the inhibition of DNA topoisomerase II. Its reduced potential for free radical formation may explain the decreased cardiotoxicity of this drug.

Absorption, Fate, and Excretion: Mitoxantrone is excreted via the renal and hepatobiliary systems, but the hepatobiliary elimination accounts for approximately 30% of active drug elimination and appears to be of greater importance. The half-life is quite variable, with a range of 23 to 42 hours. Patients with severe hepatic dysfunction have been shown to eliminate the drug more slowly.

Preparation and Administration: Mitoxantrone is commercially available as a 2 mg/mL solution in 10-mL, 12.5-mL, and 15-mL vials (20, 25, and 30 mg per vial, respectively). The drug is further diluted in normal saline or 5% dextrose in water for injection and is administered for approximately 15 to 30 minutes into the tubing of a freely running IV infusion. As with the anthracyclines, erythema or streaking along the vein of infusion indicates that the drug is being infused too rapidly. Although mitoxantrone is not a vesicant, there have been rare reports of tissue necrosis after extravasation.

Toxic Effects: Myelosuppression, principally leukopenia, is the dose-limiting toxic effect. Thrombocytopenia is relatively mild. Nausea, vomiting, and alopecia are usually mild and occur in fewer than 30% of patients treated. Rarely, mucositis and elevation of liver enzymes occur. The drug imparts a blue color to the urine of patients treated. One of the primary advantages of mitoxantrone, compared with doxorubicin, is its reduced incidence of cardiac toxicity. Occasionally, patients develop congestive heart failure after treatment with mitoxantrone in the absence of prior anthracycline exposure, although the incidence appears to be less than 5%.

Potential Drug Interactions: None reported.

Therapeutic Indications in Hematology: Mitoxantrone is approved for induction therapy of acute myeloid leukemia in adults.

Amsacrine

Chemistry and Mechanism of Action: Amsacrine, or 4′-(9-acridinylamino) methanesulfon-*m*-anisidide (AMSA) is a synthetic aminoacridine derivative. Amsacrine is a DNA intercalator and inhibits the activity of DNA topoisomerase II.

Absorption, Fate, and Excretion: When given intravenously, this drug has an initial half-life of 30 minutes and a terminal half-life of 7.9 hours. It is 50% protein bound after 2 hours. It is metabolized by conjugation with glutathione, and approximately 50% of the drug is eliminated in the bile. The remainder of the drug is eliminated via the urinary route as metabolites and parent drug.

Preparation and Administration: Amsacrine is an investigational agent supplied by the National Cancer Institute as a group C drug. It is provided in a dual pack containing two sterile liquids that must be combined before use. One vial contains 1.5 mL of 50 mg/mL of AMSA in anhydrous *N,N*-dimethylactamide, and the other contains 13.5 mL of 0.0353 mL lactic acid diluent. When these are combined, the resulting orange-red solution contains 5 mg/mL of AMSA. Because of the *N,N*-dimethylactamide solvent, plastic syringes should not be used with the undiluted AMSA solution.

Toxic Effects: The dose-limiting toxic effect is myelosuppression, predominantly affecting granulocytes. Alopecia is common, and nausea, vomiting, and mucositis can occur. Cardiotoxicity, manifested as a decrease in ejection fraction, acute arrhythmias, or electrocardiographic changes was reported in 2.3% of 3200 patients, but most of these patients had been heavily pretreated with anthracyclines. Hypokalemia seems to enhance amsacrine cardiotoxicity and if present should be corrected before administration of the drug.

Potential Drug Interactions: The reconstituted solution is physically incompatible with chloride-containing solutions.

Therapeutic Indications in Hematology: Amsacrine is a group C investigational drug approved for the treatment of refractory acute myeloid leukemia, although it is being evaluated in combination with other cytotoxic agents in the initial treatment of this disease. As a group C drug, amsacrine must be administered as a single agent.

TOPOISOMERASE I INHIBITORS

Topotecan (Hycamtin)

Chemistry and Mechanism of Action: Topotecan is a semisynthetic derivative of camptothecin that stabilizes a complex between DNA topoisomerase I and DNA. The cytotoxic effect of this drug is believed to result from the collision of DNA replication forks with a ternary complex of topoisomerase I, DNA, and topotecan. The resulting double-strand DNA breaks are lethal. The lactone form of topotecan, which predominates at an acidic pH, is a much more potent inhibitor of DNA topoisomerase I.

Absorption, Fate, and Excretion: At neutral or physiologic pH, the carboxylate form of topotecan is favored, and at a pH of less than 7, the lactone form is favored. Topotecan has been given as a bolus or by continuous infusion. In less than 1 hour after infusion, most of the circulating drug in the plasma is in the carboxylate form as a result of the physiologic pH. Whereas the terminal half-life of the lactone form of this S phase–specific agent is 2.6 hours, the terminal half-life of the total drug is 3.3 hours. In an IV dose, 36% is excreted unchanged in the urine, and there is a 1.5-fold concentration of the drug in bile. Cerebrospinal fluid levels of topotecan lactone reach approximately 32% of plasma levels. Dose adjustment is required for a creatinine clearance less than 60 mL/min, but no adjustment is necessary for a bilirubin up to 10 mg/dL.

Preparation and Administration: Topotecan is commercially available as 4-mg vials that are reconstituted with 4 mL of sterile water. This solution can be further diluted in normal saline or 5% dextrose in water and should be used immediately.

Toxic Effects: The dose-limiting toxicity for topotecan for all schedules is neutropenia. Thrombocytopenia and anemia are less common, although there is an increase in thrombocytopenia with continuous infusion schedules. Other less common and mild toxicities include nausea, vomiting, diarrhea, fever, fatigue, alopecia, skin rash, and increased liver function tests. Mucositis has been seen with prolonged infusion schedules over 5 days or when topotecan is given in higher doses.

Potential Drug Interactions: In vitro data suggest that there may be some synergism if a topoisomerase I inhibitor is given before a topoisomerase II inhibitor. In vitro data also suggest that synergism may be seen if a topoisomerase I inhibitor (topotecan) is given after an alkylating agent, suggesting that topoisomerase I may be involved in the repair of alkylator-induced DNA damage.

Therapeutic Indications in Hematology: Phase II studies suggest that topotecan has activity in myelodysplastic syndromes, acute myeloid leukemia, and multiple myeloma.

Irinotecan (Camptosar or CPT-11)

Chemistry and Mechanism of Action: CPT-11 is a prodrug that has a bulky piperidino side chain at C-10 that is cleaved in vivo by a carboxylesterase-converting enzyme to generate SN-38. SN-38 is approximately 1000-fold more potent a topoisomerase I inhibitor than CPT-11. The lactone forms of both SN-38 and CPT-11 are more potent inhibitors of topoisomerase I than the carboxylate forms, which is felt to be the mechanism of action of these drugs as described for topotecan.

Absorption, Fate, and Excretion: The terminal half-life of the lactone form of CPT-11 is 7 hours, and that of the total drug is 10.5

hours. The terminal half-life of SN-38 lactone is 8.7 hours, and that of the total drug is 14.7 hours. Of a dose of irinotecan, 22% is excreted unchanged in the urine. SN-38 is excreted into the bile and can undergo glucuronidation. Whereas the plasma protein binding of CPT-11 is reported to be between 30% and 68%, that of SN-38 is 95%.

Preparation and Administration: Irinotecan is available as a 100-mg single-dose vial with 20 mg/mL of irinotecan. This preparation also contains 45 mg of sorbitol per milliliter and 0.9 mg of lactic acid per milliliter with the pH adjusted to 3.5. This solution can be diluted with 5% dextrose in water (preferred) or in normal saline to a final concentration of 0.1 to 1.2 mg/mL. The solution is stable for up to 24 hours at room temperature or 48 hours when refrigerated. The dose should be modified for severe diarrhea.

Toxic Effects: The major toxic effect of irinotecan is diarrhea. This can be early-onset diarrhea, occurring within hours of administration, or during the infusion, which can be associated with cramping, vomiting, flushing, and diaphoresis. These side effects are attributable to the cholinergic effects of CPT-11 and can be managed with atropine. Severe later onset diarrhea can be treated with high-dose loperamide, which has been found to decrease the incidence of grade 4 diarrhea from 20% to 2%. Diarrhea has been found to be the dose-limiting toxicity when irinotecan is given on a weekly schedule, and neutropenia is the dose-limiting toxicity when the drug is given every 3 weeks. Also seen are alopecia, nausea, vomiting, mucositis, fatigue, increased liver function test results, and rare cases of pulmonary toxicity.

Potential Drug Interactions: As described for topotecan, in vitro data suggest some synergism when topoisomerase I inhibitors precede topoisomerase II inhibitors or follow alkylating agent administration.

Therapeutic Indications in Hematology: Phase I and phase II studies have shown responses in refractory leukemia and lymphoma.

APPENDIX 55-5

CLINICAL PHARMACOLOGY OF PLATINUM ANALOGS

CISPLATIN (PLATINOL)

Chemistry and Mechanism of Action: Cisplatin [cisdiamined ichloroplatinum(II)] is an inorganic heavy metal complex. This complex can have *cis-* and *trans-*isomers; the *cis-*isomer is the active antitumor drug. In the relatively higher chloride concentrations of plasma, cisplatin is uncharged in the dichloroform and passes through plasma membranes. Intracellularly, the low chloride concentrations allow the displacement of the chloride ligands by water to form the positively charged aquated complex. This forms covalent cross-links between two nucleophilic atoms of macromolecules such as the N^7 positions of guanine and adenine in DNA. The cytotoxicity of cisplatin correlates closely with total platinum binding to DNA, to interstrand cross-links and to the formation of intrastrand bidentate N^7 adducts at d(GpG) and d(ApG), resulting in intrastrand cross-links that bend the DNA helix and inhibit DNA synthesis. Cisplatin damage to DNA induces apoptosis of sensitive cells.

Absorption, Fate, and Excretion: After IV injection, the drug concentrates in the liver, kidneys, and bowel. Plasma levels of cisplatin decay in a biphasic manner, with an initial half-life of 25 to 49 minutes and a terminal half-life of 58 to 73 hours. Although 15% of the administered cisplatin is excreted unchanged in the urine, up to 90% of the administered dose of the drug can be recovered from the urine.

Preparation and Administration: Cisplatin is commercially available as a lyophilized powder, supplied in 10- and 50-mg vials also containing mannitol, sodium chloride, and hydrochloric acid and as an aqueous solution in 50- and 100-mg vials. Reconstitution of the powder for injection is achieved by adding sterile water to make a 1-mg/mL solution. The reconstituted solution should be further diluted in normal saline (usually 500 mL to 1 L) and administered over 1 to 3 hours. To prevent nephrotoxic effects, 25 to 50 g of mannitol is often added to the saline solution, and patients are aggressively hydrated before and after cisplatin infusion. Magnesium sulfate (12-24 mEq) is commonly added to the saline solution to preclude the development of hypomagnesemia.

Toxic Effects: Nephrotoxicity is the dose-limiting toxic effect. Cisplatin produces a dose-dependent impairment of renal tubular function manifested by an increase in serum creatinine as well as potassium and magnesium wasting. The renal dysfunction is usually reversible, but repeated treatments may produce a cumulative and permanent mild to moderate impairment of renal function. Administration of other nephrotoxic agents such as aminoglycosides, even between courses, can potentiate its toxicity. Nausea and vomiting are usually severe and require the use of aggressive antiemetic support. When doses greater than 70 mg/m^2 are used, it is also important to protect against delayed nausea and vomiting by administering antiemetic agents (e.g., prochlorperazine plus dexamethasone) for 3 days after therapy. Myelosuppression is usually mild. High-frequency hearing loss, tinnitus, and frank deafness may occur. Peripheral neurotoxicity, characterized by paresthesias or sensory loss in a glove-and-stocking distribution or as muscular weakness, is relatively common in patients who receive total cumulative doses of greater than 500 mg/m^2. The peripheral neuropathy may take many months to resolve, if it does at all. Vestibular toxicity and anaphylactic reactions may occur rarely.

Potential Drug Interactions: Aminoglycosides and amphotericin may enhance cisplatin nephrotoxicity. Caution should be exercised when cisplatin is administered with bleomycin and methotrexate because cisplatin-induced renal damage may delay the excretion and thus increase the toxicity of these agents.

Therapeutic Indications in Hematology: Cisplatin is used in the treatment of refractory lymphomas, usually in combination with ara-C and high-dose dexamethasone.

CARBOPLATIN (PARAPLATIN)

Chemistry and Mechanism of Action: Carboplatin is a second-generation platinum (II) complex. Its mechanism of action is very similar to that of cisplatin. However, the carboxyl ester groups in this platinum complex are less easily displaced and less chemically reactive. The peak levels of DNA cross-linking also occur 6 to 12 hours later for carboplatin than for cisplatin.

Absorption, Fate, and Excretion: Carboplatin is primarily eliminated through the kidneys. Its elimination is slower than cisplatin with a terminal half-life between 2 and 6 hours. After IV injection, approximately 60% of the total drug is excreted within 24 hours.

Preparation and Administration: Carboplatin is commercially available as a lyophilized powder in 50- and 150-mg vials containing carboplatin and mannitol. It is reconstituted with sterile water to a final concentration of 10 mg/mL. For injection, further dilution with 5% dextrose and water or normal saline to a concentration of 0.5 or 2 mg/mL, in which it is stable for 8 hours at room temperature. Carboplatin is often administered by IV injection over 15 to 30 minutes. Patients with reduced renal function (creatinine clearance of <60 mL/min) should have the dose of carboplatin decreased according to the formula described by Egorin et al.

For previously untreated patients:

$$\text{Dosage (mg/m}^2) = (0.091)\,(\text{Creatinine clearance/Body surface area}) \times [\text{Pretreatment platelet count} - \text{Platelet nadir desired/Pretreatment platelet count} \times 100] + 86$$

For heavily pretreated patients:

$$\text{Dosage (mg/m}^2) = (0.091)\,(\text{Creatinine clearance/Body surface area}) \times [(\text{Pretreatment platelet count} - \text{Platelet nadir desired/Pretreatment platelet count} \times 100) - 17] + 86$$

A formula developed by Calvert and colleagues also takes into account the patient's pretreatment renal function, as follows:

$$\text{Dose (mg)} = \text{Target AUC (mg/mL} \times \text{min) H [GFR (mL/min)} + 25]$$

where the dose in mg (not mg/m^2 body surface area) equals target AUC (area under the plasma clearance curve) × GFR (glomerular filtration rate) + 25.

In previously untreated adults, the AUC can be estimated at 7 when carboplatin is used alone and 4.5 when used in combination. If AUC is set lower, less toxicity is expected.

Toxic Effects: The dose-limiting toxic effect is myelosuppression, thrombocytopenia being more significant than leukopenia. Carboplatin leads to less emesis than cisplatin. Although nausea and vomiting are common, they can be easily controlled with antiemetics. At high doses such as those used for bone marrow transplantation, hepatotoxicity, renal dysfunction, and moderate to severe cytotoxicity can occur.

Potential Drug Interactions: None reported.

Clinical Indications in Hematology: Carboplatin has been recently approved for the treatment of ovarian cancer. It is also used to treat small cell lung, testicular, head and neck, and genitourinary cancers. High-dose carboplatin is presently under evaluation in acute leukemias and lymphomas.

APPENDIX 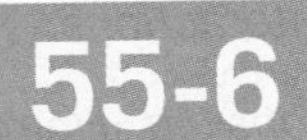

CLINICAL PHARMACOLOGY OF MISCELLANEOUS AGENTS

THALIDOMIDE

Chemistry and Mechanism of Action: The mechanism of action of thalidomide is not fully understood. Thalidomide has immunomodulatory, antiinflammatory, and antiangiogenic properties. The immunologic effects vary substantially under differing conditions but seem to suppress tumor necrosis factor-α production and downmodulate cell surface adhesion molecules. Other antiinflammatory and immunomodulatory properties include suppression of macrophage involvement in prostaglandin synthesis and modulation of interleukin-10 and interleukin-12 production by peripheral blood mononuclear cells. Angiogenesis inhibition is described, but the exact mechanism is not yet definitively defined.

Absorption, Fate, and Excretion: Thalidomide absorption is slow after oral administration, and the bioavailability of capsules has not yet been determined, but based on radiolabeled thalidomide, greater than 90% is recovered in urine, suggesting good oral absorption. The mean elimination half-life of thalidomide ranges from 3 to 6.7 hours, but the exact metabolic fate of thalidomide is unknown. Protein binding is 55% to 66%.

Preparation and Administration: Thalidomide is available as 50-, 100-, 150-, and 200-mg oral capsules. A 20-mg/mL oral suspension may be prepared with capsules and a 1 : 1 mixture of Ora-Sweet and Ora-Plus by emptying the contents of twelve 100-mg capsules into a glass mortar. Add small portions of the vehicle and mix to a uniform paste; mix while adding the vehicle in incremental proportions to almost 60 mL; transfer to an amber calibrated bottle and add quantity of vehicle sufficient to make 60 mL. Stable for 35 days refrigerated.

Toxic Effects: Thalidomide frequently may cause deep venous thrombosis and pulmonary embolism. Thalidomide causes birth defects in humans. It must not be given during pregnancy. Leucopenia along with thrombocytopenia is observed. Pruritus and rash as well as constipation are seen.

Drug Interactions: Thalidomide increases cyclosporine A metabolism and clearance. An increase in the thrombogenic state in patients with myelodysplastic syndrome (MDS) has been observed in patients receiving darbepoetin alfa and thalidomide. The addition of docetaxel to thalidomide increases the risk of venous thromboembolism.

Therapeutic Indications in Hematology: Thalidomide has been used to treat multiple myeloma and MDS.

LENALIDOMIDE

Chemistry and Mechanism of Action: Lenalidomide, a thalidomide analog, is an immunomodulatory agent with antineoplastic and antiangiogenic activity. Lenalidomide affects ligand-induced responses (angiogenesis, inflammation, cell adhesion, immune response), inhibits production of tumor necrosis factor, increases production of interleukin-2 and interferon-γ, and increases cytolytic T-cell and natural killer (NK) cell responses. It inhibits trophic signals to angiogenic factors in cells. and inhibits growth of myeloma cells by inducing cell cycle arrest and apoptosis.

Absorption, Fate, and Excretion: Lenalidomide is rapidly absorbed after oral administration. Lenalidomide has a half-life of 3 hours with 67% of the drug excreted unchanged in the urine. Adjustment to the initial dosage is recommended in patients with moderate or severe renal impairment. Compared with patients with normal renal function, those with moderate and severe renal impairment have a 66% to 75% decrease in drug clearance, and patients on hemodialysis have an 80% decrease in clearance. Although the drug is 30% protein bound, lenalidomide is partially removed by hemodialysis and should be given after dialysis. Food does not alter the extent of absorption nor the AUC of lenalidomide.

Preparation and Administration: Lenalidomide is available in 2.5-, 5-, 10-, 15-, and 25-mg capsules for oral administration. Each capsule contains lenalidomide as the active ingredient along with lactose anhydrous, microcrystalline cellulose, croscarmellose sodium, and magnesium stearate.

Toxic Effects: Lenalidomide frequently may cause deep venous thrombosis and pulmonary embolism. Severe myelosuppression across all cell lines is common. Pruritus and rash as well as constipation and hypokalemia are seen. Lenalidomide is an analogue of thalidomide and may cause birth defects in humans. It must not be given during pregnancy.

Drug Interactions: Lenalidomide increases digoxin plasma concentrations. Dexamethasone increases the thrombogenic effect of Lenalidomide.

Therapeutic Indications in Hematology: Lenalidomide has activity in multiple myeloma when used in combination with dexamethasone, Chronic lymphoid leukemia as well myelodysplastic syndrome with deletion 5q abnormality. It also has shown some efficacy in myelofibrosis and refractory non-Hodgkin lymphoma.

POMALIDOMIDE

Chemistry and Mechanism of Action: Pomalidomide is structurally and functionally related to thalidomide. Its mechanism is not fully understood but has effects on angiogenesis, alters inflammatory and regulatory cytokines, and may affect T cells.

Absorption, Fate, and Excretion: Pomalidomide is administered orally. Pharmacokinetic data are still being elucidated.

Preparation and Administration: Pomalidomide is an investigational agent administered orally.

Toxic Effects: Pomalidomide has extensive bone marrow toxicity affecting all three cell lines, peripheral neuropathy, orthostasis, rashes, pulmonary toxicity and clotting abnormalities.

Drug Interactions: Data not available.

Therapeutic Indications in Hematology: Pomalidomide has been studied in multiple myeloma.

TEMSIROLIMUS

Chemistry and Mechanism of Action: Temsirolimus is an inhibitor of mTOR (mammalian target of rapamycin) and binds to an intracellular protein (FKBP-12). This protein–drug complex inhibits the activity of mTOR and results in G1 growth arrest. When mTOR is inhibited, its ability to phosphorylate p70S6k and S6 ribosomal protein, which are downstream of mTOR in the PI3 kinase/AKT pathway, was blocked.

Absorption, Fate, and Excretion: Temsirolimus is predominately metabolized in human liver microsomes by cytochrome P450 3A4 (CYP3A4). Temsirolimus is extensively metabolized to sirolimus. Four other metabolites account for less than 10% in the plasma. The mean half-life of temsirolimus is 17.3 hours, and the mean half-life of sirolimus, the active metabolite, is 54.6 hours. Neither the parent drug nor its metabolite is dialyzable. Dosage reduction or discontinuance may be warranted in patients with hepatic impairment to reduce the potential for toxicity.

Preparation and Administration: Temsirolimus is supplied as a kit consisting of 2 vials, temsirolimus injection (25 mg/mL) and a diluent of 1.8 mL. Temsirolimus is mixed with 1.8 mL of the diluent. The resultant solution contains 10 mg/mL The concentrate–diluent mixture is stable below 25° C for up to 24 hours. To administer, withdraw the required amount of concentrate–diluent mixture and further dilute into an infusion bag containing 250 mL of 0.9% sodium chloride injection, USP. Patients should receive prophylactic IV diphenhydramine 25 mg before the start of each dose.

Toxic Effects: Temsirolimus causes a decreased lymphocyte count, leucopenia, decreased hemoglobin, and thrombocytopenia. Hyperglycemia, edema, and rash (which may progress to Stevens-Johnson syndrome) have also been seen.

Drug Interactions: The concomitant use of strong CYP3A4 inhibitors (e.g., ketoconazole, itraconazole, clarithromycin, atazanavir, indinavir, nefazodone, nelfinavir, ritonavir, saquinavir, telithromycin, and voriconazole) may increase plasma concentrations of sirolimus (a major metabolite of temsirolimus). The use of concomitant strong CYP3A4 inducers (e.g., dexamethasone, phenytoin, carbamazepine, rifampin, rifabutin, rifampicin, phenobarbital) may decrease plasma concentrations of sirolimus (a major metabolite of temsirolimus).

Therapeutic Indications in Hematology: Temsirolimus has been shown to have activity in mantle cell lymphoma.

EVEROLIMUS

Chemistry and Mechanism of Action: Everolimus is an analogue of rapamycin (sirolimus) with immunosuppressive and antiproliferative activity. Everolimus is an inhibitor of rapamycin (mTOR), a serine-threonine kinase, downstream of the PI3K/AKT pathway. After binding and forming a complex with the cytoplasmic FK506–binding protein 12 (FKBP-12), the complex binds to and inhibits the mammalian mTOR and phosphorylates P70 S6 ribosomal protein kinase (a substrate of mTOR). Everolimus reduces the activity of S6 ribosomal protein kinase (S6K1) and eukaryotic elongation factor 4E–binding protein (4E-BP1). In addition, everolimus inhibits the expression of hypoxia-inducible factor 1 and reduces the expression of vascular endothelial growth factor.

Absorption, Fate, and Excretion: Peak everolimus concentrations are reached 1 to 2 hours after oral administration with protein binding of 74%. Everolimus is extensively metabolized by the liver with everolimus being a substrate of CYP3A4 and P-glycoprotein. Metabolism involves demethylation, hydroxylation, and ring degradation. There are six main metabolites of everolimus, which have approximately 100 times less activity than the parent everolimus compound, including three monohydroxylated metabolites, two hydrolytic ring-opened metabolites, and a phosphatidylcholine conjugate of everolimus. The elimination half-life is 30 hours and is prolonged to a mean of 79 hours in patients with moderate hepatic impairment.

Preparation and Administration: Everolimus is available in 2.5-, 5-, 7.5- and 10-mg nonscored tablets.

Toxic Effects: Everolimus causes bone marrow suppression across all cell lines, hyperglycemia, rash, and mucositis along with pulmonary toxicity.

Drug Interactions: Everolimus concentrations are increased when administered with CYP3A4 or P-glycoprotein Inhibitors such as ketoconazole, itraconazole, clarithromycin, atazanavir, nefazodone, saquinavir, telithromycin, ritonavir, indinavir, nelfinavir, voriconazole, amprenavir, fosamprenavir, aprepitant, erythromycin, fluconazole, verapamil, diltiazem, grapefruit, grapefruit juice, or St. John's wort. Everolimus concentrations are decreased when administered with strong CYP3A4 inducers such as phenytoin, carbamazepine, rifampin, rifabutin, rifapentine, or phenobarbital.

Therapeutic Indications in Hematology: Everolimus has been used in mantle cell lymphoma, diffuse large B-cell lymphoma, and Hodgkin lymphoma.

ARSENIC TRIOXIDE

Chemistry and Mechanism of Action: The mechanism of action of arsenic trioxide is not completely understood. Arsenic trioxide causes morphologic changes and DNA fragmentation characteristic of apoptosis in NB4 human promyelocytic leukemia cells in vitro possibly mediated by activation of cysteine-proteases (caspases). Arsenic trioxide also causes damage or degradation of the fusion protein PML/RARβ.

Absorption, Fate, and Excretion: The metabolism of arsenic trioxide involves reduction of pentavalent arsenic to trivalent arsenic by arsenate reductase and methylation of trivalent arsenic to monomethylarsinic acid and monomethylarsinic acid to dimethylarsinic acid by methyltransferases. The main site of methylation reactions appears to be the liver. The pharmacokinetics of trivalent arsenic, the active species, have not been characterized.

Preparation and Administration: Arsenic trioxide is available in 10-mL, single-use ampules containing 10 mg of arsenic trioxide. It is formulated as a sterile, nonpyrogenic, clear solution of arsenic trioxide in water for injection using sodium hydroxide and dilute hydrochloric acid to adjust to pH 8. Trisenox should be diluted with 100 to 250 mL of 5% dextrose injection, USP, or 0.9% sodium chloride injection, USP. Arsenic trioxide should be administered intravenously over 1 to 2 hours. The infusion duration may be extended up to 4 hours if acute vasomotor reactions are observed. A central venous catheter is not required.

Toxic Effects: Arsenic trioxide has electrocardiographic abnormalities, including QT interval prolongation, T-wave flattening, and atrioventricular block. Nonspecific edema and weight gain have been reported. Dry skin, pruritus, and rashes have occurred relatively frequently. Anemia, thrombocytopenia, and neutropenia are also observed.

Drug Interactions: Arsenic trioxide can cause QT interval prolongation and complete atrioventricular block. QT prolongation can lead to a torsade de pointes–type ventricular arrhythmia. The risk of torsade de pointes is related to the extent of QT prolongation, and concomitant administration of QT-prolonging drugs may exacerbate this phenomenon.

Therapeutic Indications in Hematology: Arsenic trioxide is effective in newly diagnosed acute promyelocytic leukemia, FAB M3.

Moreover, in patients who are refractory to or have relapsed from retinoid and anthracycline chemotherapy, arsenic trioxide has some activity as a single agent for relapsed or refractory multiple myeloma. Arsenic trioxide produced hematologic improvement in a subset of patients with myelodysplastic syndrome.

BORTEZOMIB (VELCADE)

Molecular Formula: The mlecular formula is $C_{19}H_{25}BN_4O$ molecular weight 384.24 g/mol bortezomib (*N*-pyrazinecarbonyl-L-phenylalanine-L-leucine boronic acid).

Absorption, Fate, and Excretion: After IV administration of 1.3 mg/m^2 dose, the median estimated maximum plasma concentration of bortezomib was 509 ng/mL (range, 109-1300 ng/mL). The mean elimination half-life of bortezomib after first dose ranged from 9 to 15 hours at doses ranging from 1.45 to 2.00 mg/m^2 in patients with advanced malignancies. In vitro studies with human liver microsomes and human cDNA-expressed cytochrome P450 isozymes indicate that bortezomib is primarily oxidatively metabolized via cytochrome P450 enzymes, 3A4, 2D6, 2C19, 2C9, and 1A2. The major metabolic pathway is deboronation to form two deboronated metabolites that subsequently undergo hydroxylation to several inactive metabolites.

Preparation and Administration: Bortezomib for injection is supplied as a lyophilized powder for reconstitution. Each sterile single-use vial contains 3.5 mg of bortezomib and 35 mg of mannitol USP. Each vial is reconstituted with 3.5 mL normal (0.9%) saline such that the reconstituted solution contains bortezomib at a concentration of 1 mg/mL. The pH of the reconstituted solution is between 5 and 6. The drug is given without any further dilution as an IV bolus over 3 to 5 seconds. Intact vials of lyophilized bortezomib for injection are stored in a refrigerator at 2° to 8° C (35°-47° F) and protected from light. Stability studies are ongoing to monitor each clinical lot. Product should be administered immediately after reconstitution. The solution as reconstituted is stable for 43 hours at room temperature. Bortezomib is administered as an IV bolus (over 3-5 sec) twice weekly for 2 weeks followed by a 1-week rest period.

Toxic Effects: The most commonly reported adverse events were asthenic conditions (including fatigue, malaise, and weakness; 65%), nausea (64%), diarrhea (51%), decreased appetite (including anorexia; 43%), constipation (43%), thrombocytopenia (43%), peripheral neuropathy (including peripheral sensory neuropathy and peripheral neuropathy aggravated; 37%), pyrexia (36%), vomiting (36%), and anemia (32%). Fourteen percent of patients experienced at least one episode of grade 4 toxicity, with the most common being thrombocytopenia (3%) and neutropenia (3%).

Potential Drug Interactions: No formal drug interaction studies have been conducted with bortezomib. In vitro studies with human liver microsomes indicate that bortezomib is a substrate of cytochrome P450 3A4, 2D6, 2C19, 2C9, and 1A2. Bortezomib may inhibit 2C19 activity (IC_{50} = 18 μM, 6.9 μg/mL) and increase exposure to drugs that are substrates for this enzyme. Patients who are concomitantly receiving bortezomib and drugs that are inhibitors or inducers of cytochrome P450 3A4 should be closely monitored for either toxicities or reduced efficacy. Patients on oral antidiabetic agents receiving bortezomib treatment may experience hypo- or hyperglycemia and require close monitoring of their blood glucose levels and adjustment of the dose of their antidiabetic medication. Finally, patients should be cautioned about the use of concomitant medications that may be associated with peripheral neuropathy (e.g., amiodarone, antivirals, isoniazid, nitrofurantoin, or statins), or with a decrease in blood pressure.

Therapeutic Indications in Hematology: Bortezomib is approved by the Food and Drug Administration for the treatment of multiple myeloma patients who have received at least two prior therapies and have demonstrated disease progression on the last therapy.

CARFILZOMIB

Chemistry and Mechanism of Action: Carfilzomib is an epoxomicin derivate that irreversibly binds to and inhibits the chymotrypsin-like activity of the 20S proteasome. Inhibition of proteasome-mediated proteolysis results in an accumulation of polyubiquinated proteins, which may lead to cell cycle arrest, induction of apoptosis, and inhibition of tumor growth.

Absorption, Fate, and Excretion: Carfilzomib is an investigational product. It has rapid clearance with an elimination half-life of less than 30 minutes and a clearance higher than liver blood flow that suggests there are multiple clearance pathways.

Preparation and Administration: Carfilzomib currently is available investigationally as an intravenous product.

Toxic Effects: Carfilzomib has shown to produce mild to moderate nausea and diarrhea. Respiratory symptoms occur and include cough, dyspnea, and exertional dyspnea. Neurologic symptoms include hypoesthesia, headache, and paresthesia. Additional adverse events seen are fatigue, pyrexia, and peripheral edema.

Drug Interactions: Data not available.

Therapeutic Indications in Hematology: Carfilzomib has been used in multiple myeloma, Hodgkin lymphoma, and non-Hodgkin lymphoma.

IBRUTINIB

Chemistry and Mechanism of Action: Ibrutinib is a first-in-class oral therapy that is a selective, irreversible inhibitor of Bruton tyrosine kinase (BTK) and inhibits BTK activity, preventing B-cell activation and B cell–mediated signaling and inhibiting the growth of malignant B cells that overexpress BTK.

Absorption, Fate, and Excretion: No data available.

Preparation and Administration: Ibrutinib is an investigational agent available as an oral dose.

Toxic Effects: Ibrutinib may cause diarrhea, fatigue, nausea, and skin bruising. Also. transient high lymphocyte count are frequently seen.

Drug Interactions: No data available.

Therapeutic Indications in Hematology: Ibrutinib is used in chronic lymphocytic leukemia/small lymphocytic lymphoma, mantle cell lymphoma, diffuse large B-cell lymphoma, and multiple myeloma.

DASATINIB

Chemistry and Mechanism of Action: Dasatinib is an orally active tyrosine kinase inhibitor against BCR-ABL, SRC family, c-KIT, EPHA2, and PDGFR-β. The primary mechanism of resistance to dasatinib is the T315I mutant clone.

Absorption, Fate, and Excretion: Dasatinib is orally absorbed and extensively metabolized in human liver microsomes, primarily by cytochrome P450 CYP3A4 to an active metabolite. CYP3A4 is the primary enzyme responsible for the formation of the active metabolite. Flavin-containing monooxygenase 3 and uridine diphosphate-glucuronosyltransferase enzymes are also involved in the formation of dasatinib metabolites. In human liver microsomes, dasatinib was a weak time-dependent inhibitor of CYP3A4. The exposure of the active metabolite, which is equipotent to dasatinib, represents approximately 5% of the dasatinib AUC.

Preparation and Administration: Dasatinab is an oral agent usually taken twice daily without regard to meals.

Toxic Effects: Treatment with dasatinib is associated with severe thrombocytopenia, neutropenia, anemia, and platelet dysfunction. Also seen is fluid retention, including pleural and pericardial effusion, pulmonary edema, severe ascites, and generalized edema. A prolonged QT interval has been observed as well as extensive skin rashes.

Drug Interactions: Dasatinib is a CYP3A4 substrate. Administration with drugs that are CYP3A4 inhibitors may cause increased dasatinib plasma concentrations and subsequent increase in toxicities. Drugs that induce CYP3A4 activity may decrease dasatinib plasma concentrations and decrease its effectiveness. The solubility of dasatinib is pH dependent. Simultaneous administration of SPRYCEL with antacids should be avoided, and there should be 2 hours' separation in the administration of dasatinib and antacids. Long-term suppression of gastric acid secretion by H_2 blockers or proton pump may reduce dasatinib exposure, and antacids are preferred. Dasatinib is a time-dependent inhibitor of CYP3A4; therefore, CYP3A4 substrates may have their plasma concentration altered by dasatinib.

Therapeutic Indications in Hematology: Treatment with dasatinib results in hematologic and cytogenetic responses in patients with lymphoid blast crisis, Philadelphia chromosome-positive (Ph^+), chronic myeloid leukemia, and Ph+ acute lymphoblastic leukemia as initial treatment and in disease-resistant or intolerant to imatinib.

NILOTINIB

Chemistry and Mechanism of Action: Nilotinib is a selective tyrosine kinase inhibitor active against Bcr-Abl kinase Nilotinib binds to and stabilizes the inactive conformation of the kinase domain of ABL protein. Nilotinib is 30-fold more potent than imatinib.

Absorption, Fate, and Excretion: Nilotinib is rapidly absorbed and reaches its peak concentration in 3 hours. Nilotinib AUC was increased by 82% when given 30 minutes after a high-fat meal compared with a fasting state. Its elimination half-life is approximately 17 hours. It is metabolized by oxidation and hydroxylation as well as undergoing metabolism by CYP3A4. None of the nilotinib metabolites have significant pharmacologic activity.

Preparation and Administration: Nilotinib is available in capsules for oral use, containing a 150- or 200-mg nilotinib base, anhydrous (as hydrochloride, monohydrate) with the following inactive ingredients: colloidal silicon dioxide, crospovidone, lactose monohydrate, magnesium stearate, and polyoxamer 188.

Toxic Effects: Nilotinib may cause anemia, neutropenia and thrombocytopenia. Prolonged QT interval and sudden death has occurred. Pruritus, rash, and nausea are common. Also seen with nilotinib are arthralgias and myalgias. Cough has also been associated with nilotinib.

Drug Interactions: Nilotinib is a competitive inhibitor of cytochrome P-450 (CYP) isoenzymes 3A4, 2C8, 2C9, and 2D6 and has the potential to increase concentrations of drugs metabolized by these enzymes. Nilotinib plasma concentration is increased during concomitant use with potent CYP3A4 inhibitors (e.g., atazanavir, clarithromycin, indinavir, itraconazole, ketoconazole, nefazodone, nelfinavir, ritonavir, saquinavir, telithromycin, voriconazole). Decreased nilotinib plasma concentration occurs during concomitant use with potent CYP3A4 inducers (e.g., dexamethasone, carbamazepine, phenobarbital, phenytoin, rifabutin, rifampin, and St. John's wort). Drugs that increase the pH of the upper gastrointestinal tract may decrease the solubility of nilotinib and reduce its bioavailability. The oral administration of esomeprazole resulted in a 34% reduction in the AUC of nilotinib.

Therapeutic Indications in Hematology: Nilotinib has demonstrated activity in the case of chronic myeloid leukemia CML resistance resulted from Bcr-Abl kinase mutations from treatment with imatinib. This includes accelerated phase chronic myeloid leukemia, resistant or intolerant to prior therapy. Acute lymphoid leukemia, Philadelphia chromosome-positive, relapsed/refractory. Blastic phase chronic myeloid leukemia, Resistant or intolerant to imatinib. Chronic phase, Philadelphia chromosome-positive, newly diagnosed. Chronic phase chronic myeloid leukemia, resistant or intolerant to prior therapy.

PLICAMYCIN

Chemistry and Mechanism of Action: Plicamycin, also called mithramycin, forms complexes with DNA and inhibits DNA-directed synthesis of RNA. Plicamycin also inhibits the effect of parathyrin on osteoclasts. The hypocalcemic effect is independent of the antitumor effect.

Absorption, Fate, and Excretion: The pharmacology of plicamycin has been poorly described. Within 15 hours of IV administration, 40% is excreted in the urine. The elimination half-life has been estimated to be approximately 2 hours.

Preparation and Administration: Plicamycin is commercially available as a lyophilized powder in 2.5-mg vials, from which it is reconstituted with 4.9 mL of sterile water for injection. This dose should be further diluted in 1 L of 5% dextrose in water or normal saline and infused over 4 to 6 hours.

Toxic Effects: When plicamycin is used as an antitumor agent, its most common side effects include myelosuppression; elevated liver enzymes; increased serum creatinine and proteinuria; and coagulopathy caused by decreased clotting factors II, V, VII, and X. The drug also causes nausea and vomiting, diarrhea, stomatitis, headache, and irritability. Cutaneous toxicity may occur in up to one-third of patients, manifested by progressive blushing of the face and thickening and coarsening of the skinfolds. The drug can produce severe local irritation if extravasation occurs.

Potential Drug Interactions: None reported.

Therapeutic Indications in Hematology: Plicamycin is primarily used to treat hypercalcemia of malignancy. Claims of antitumor activity in the blast phase of CML have been made but have not been confirmed.

BLEOMYCIN

Chemistry and Mechanism of Action: Bleomycin is a glycopeptide. Its antitumor effect correlates with its ability to cause scission of both double- and single-stranded DNA via activated oxygen formed by the iron–bleomycin complex. Bleomycin also affects DNA repair by inhibiting DNA ligase.

Absorption, Fate, and Excretion: Bleomycin is rapidly distributed throughout the body and concentrates in the skin, lung, kidney, peritoneum, and lymph nodes. Its plasma half-life is 2 to 4 hours. Within 24 hours of injection, approximately 50% of an administered dose is excreted unchanged in the urine. Bleomycin elimination correlates well with creatinine clearance; accordingly, patients with renal failure should receive reduced doses. In the tissues, bleomycin is inactivated by bleomycin hydrolase. Tissues lacking this enzyme, such as the lungs and skin, are more susceptible to the drug's toxic effects.

Preparation and Administration: Bleomycin is commercially available in vials containing 15 U (approximately equivalent to 15 mg), from which it is reconstituted for injection with 3 to 5 mL of sterile water, normal saline, 5% dextrose in water, or bacteriostatic water. For IV infusion, the reconstituted solution can be further diluted with either normal saline or 5% dextrose in water and administered over 5 minutes. Bleomycin can also be administered by the subcutaneous, intravenous, intramuscular, intracavitary, and intraarterial routes. Because patients with lymphomas are at an increased risk of anaphylactoid reactions, which may not occur until 12 hours after administration, the first two doses should be intramuscular "test doses" of 1 to 2 mg. If no reactions occur, full doses may be given.

Toxic Effects: The most serious toxic effect is interstitial pneumonitis, which is dose related and occurs in approximately 10% of patients treated with cumulative doses of greater than 350 to 400 U. The interstitial pneumonitis may evolve into life-threatening pulmonary fibrosis. Pulmonary toxicity is more common in patients older than 70 years, in those receiving a total dose of greater than 400 U, and in those who received prior radiotherapy to the lung. It is important to emphasize, however, that the pulmonary toxicity is unpredictable; it has been reported in patients who had none of these risk factors and has occurred in a patient after administration of only 20 U. Some reports suggest that an increased concentration of inspired oxygen acts synergistically with bleomycin to produce pulmonary fibrosis. During critical illness and perioperatively, therefore, an attempt should be made to maintain the inspired oxygen concentration at 21%. The early phases of the pulmonary toxicity are clinically manifested by dyspnea and fine rales. Although corticosteroids are often used in this setting, it is not clear that they are of benefit.

Mucocutaneous toxicity occurs in 50% of patients treated and is manifested by hyperpigmentation, pruritic erythema, mucositis, desquamation of the plantar surface skin of the hands or feet, ridging of the nails, and alopecia. The mucositis can be severe and is the acute dose-limiting toxic effect. Febrile reactions, which occur a few hours after bleomycin administration and may last 4 to 12 hours, are also common. Fever becomes less frequent with continued use of the drug and can usually be prevented by concurrent administration of glucocorticosteroids (e.g., 100 mg of hydrocortisone). Bleomycin has virtually no myelosuppressive effect. Anaphylactoid reactions are observed in approximately 1% (up to 8% in some series) of patients with lymphomas treated with bleomycin.

Potential Drug Interaction: Bleomycin, administered with other drugs for the treatment of lymphorrhea, can decrease the oral bioavailability of digoxin and the pharmacologic effect of phenytoin and certain anesthetic drugs.

Therapeutic Indications in Hematology: Bleomycin is often incorporated in the chemotherapy regimens of Hodgkin disease (ABVD and MOPP-ABV hybrid regimens) and non-Hodgkin lymphoma (MACOP-B, PROMACE-CYTABOM, M-BACOD, and CHOP-Bleo).

ASPARAGINASE

Chemistry and Mechanism of Action: Asparaginase contains the high-molecular-weight enzyme L-asparaginase amidohydrolase, type EC-2, derived from *Escherichia coli*. Asparaginase hydrolyzes serum asparagine to nonfunctional aspartic acid and ammonia, depriving tumor cells of a required amino acid; thus tumor cell proliferation is blocked by the interruption of asparagine-dependent protein synthesis. The drug appears to be most active in the G_1 phase.

Absorption, Fate, and Excretion: Asparaginase is not absorbed orally. Its plasma half-life varies from 8 to 30 hours and is not influenced by dosage, age, sex, surface area, or renal or hepatic function.

Preparation and Administration: Asparaginase is commercially available in vials containing 10,000 IU of asparaginase in 80 mg of mannitol. For IV use, the drug should be reconstituted with 5 mL of either sterile water or sodium chloride for injection and injected in the tubing of a freely running infusion of either normal saline or 5% dextrose in water over 30 minutes. For intramuscular or subcutaneous use, each vial should be reconstituted with 2 mL of sodium chloride for injection to obtain a 5000-U/mL solution. For dosages that exceed 2 mL, use of two injection sites is recommended. For both IV and intramuscular administration, the drug must be used within 8 hours of reconstitution, and only if it is clear. Because of the possibility of hypersensitivity reactions (particularly in patients with lymphomas), an intradermal skin test is recommended before initial administration of asparaginase or when 1 week has elapsed between doses. For this test, 2 IU should be injected intradermally and observed for a wheal or erythema for 1 hour. A negative skin test result, however, does not preclude possible development of a hypersensitivity reaction. It is recommended that oxygen, epinephrine, and corticosteroids be available at the bedside during administration of the drug. For allergic patients, the *E. coli* form of asparaginase should be replaced by the asparaginase derived from *Erwinia carotovora,* provided by the National Cancer Institute as an investigational group C agent.

Toxic Effects: The toxicity of asparaginase is reported to be greater in adults than in children. Anorexia, nausea, or vomiting occurs in approximately one-third of patients. Most of the other side effects can be divided into two main groups, those related to hypersensitivity reactions to the foreign protein and those resulting from decreased protein synthesis. The hypersensitivity reaction is characterized by urticaria, laryngeal edema, bronchospasm, or hypotension and may occur with the initial dose of the drug even if the skin test result is negative. More commonly, however, allergic phenomena are observed after multiple courses of treatment. Adverse effects related to the inhibition of protein synthesis include hypoalbuminemia and decreases in serum fibrinogen, prothrombin, antithrombin III, and other coagulation factors, which may lead to both clotting and hemorrhagic complications; decreased serum insulin with hyperglycemia; and decreased serum lipoproteins. In 25% or fewer of patients, cerebral dysfunction, characterized by confusion, stupor, and frank coma, can occur. Although the neurotoxic effects resemble those of ammonia toxicity, they are apparently caused by low concentrations of either L-asparagine or L-glutamine in the brain. Acute pancreatitis, which may progress to severe hemorrhagic pancreatitis, may occur in 15% of patients. Elevation of liver enzymes and serum bilirubin is almost universal and is histologically represented by fatty metamorphosis. Liver toxicity, although usually not clinically significant, has resulted in occasional fatalities. Asparaginase can occasionally produce renal functional impairment with oliguric renal failure.

Potential Drug Interactions: When asparaginase is administered immediately before or concurrent with methotrexate, it decreases the cytotoxic effect of the latter. When administered to patients with acute leukemia 9 to 10 days before or shortly after methotrexate, however, asparaginase appears to enhance the cytotoxic effect of methotrexate. Concurrent administration of asparaginase with vincristine may increase vincristine's neurotoxic effects, but this effect appears to be less pronounced when asparaginase is given after vincristine. The effects of asparaginase on liver function may potentially interfere with the activation or metabolism of other cytotoxic agents.

Therapeutic Indications in Hematology: Asparaginase is used in combination therapy for remission induction of acute lymphocytic leukemia.

GLUCOCORTICOIDS

Chemistry and Mechanism of Action: Glucocorticoids are synthetic compounds derived from the natural adrenal hormone cortisol. Glucocorticoids mediate their biologic actions predominantly by binding to their cytosolic receptor, which then translocates to the nucleus. There, as a homodimer, it binds to specific DNA sequences located in the regulatory regions of a number of genes. Gene transcription can be upregulated or downregulated by glucocorticoids. They can also inhibit binding of the AP-1 transcription factor to its DNA consensus sequence site. Lymphocytes treated with glucocorticoids undergo apoptosis mediated by glucocorticoid receptors. An early cytostatic phase is marked by growth inhibition and cessation of proliferation caused by inhibition of cellular uptake of glucose, amino acids, and nucleosides as well as inhibition of macromolecular synthesis. This is followed by a cytolytic phase characterized by chromatin condensation and internucleosomal DNA cleavage.

Absorption, Fate, and Excretion: Many synthetic glucocorticoids are available, the three most commonly used in hematology being prednisone, dexamethasone, and methylprednisolone. The glucocorticoids are well absorbed orally and are primarily metabolized in the liver. Unlike the other two glucocorticoids, the activity of prednisone depends on hepatic conversion to the 11-hydroxy form (prednisolone). Whereas the biologic half-lives of prednisone and methylprednisolone are approximately 12 to 36 hours, dexamethasone has a biologic half-life of 36 to 72 hours. Plasma half-lives for all three drugs are within the range of 3 to 4 hours. Compared with cortisol, the relative antiinflammatory potencies of dexamethasone, methylprednisolone, and prednisone are 25, 5, and 4, respectively, for equivalent doses.

Preparation and Administration: Prednisone is available only for oral administration, but methylprednisolone and dexamethasone are available in oral and parenteral dosage forms.

Toxic Effects: When glucocorticoids are used for less than 14 days, as is often done when they are used in combination with other cytotoxic agents, the most common side effects include euphoria, insomnia, psychosis, hyperglycemia, hypokalemia, increased appetite, metabolic alkalosis, proximal muscular weakness, and fluid retention with edema formation and hypertension. When used on a chronic basis, glucocorticoids also may induce a "Cushingoid" appearance, easy bruisability, peptic ulcers, osteoporosis, subcapsular cataracts, and an increased susceptibility to infections related to impaired cellular immunity. Because of this, H_2 blockers, antifungal agents (e.g., ketoconazole), and sulfamethoxazole–trimethoprim have been used in certain glucocorticoid chemotherapy combinations.

Potential Drug Interactions: Glucocorticoids interact with a variety of drugs, including barbiturates, oral contraceptives, erythromycin, hydantoins, rifampin, isoniazid, and salicylates. Given the wide range of doses of glucocorticoids used, however, these interactions are of no major clinical relevance.

Clinical Indications in Hematology: Glucocorticoids have direct anticancer activity in many hematologic malignancies, including acute lymphoblastic leukemia, chronic lymphocytic leukemia, Hodgkin disease, non-Hodgkin lymphoma, and plasma cell neoplasms. Because of their efficacy and toxic profiles, which do not overlap with the toxic effects of the other cytotoxic agents, glucocorticoids are used in many chemotherapy regimens. In addition, they are useful in the management of hypercalcemia secondary to myeloma and lymphomas and are of paramount importance in the treatment of autoimmune hematologic disorders.

BRYOSTATIN

Chemistry and Mechanism of Action: Bryostatin is a macrocyclic lactone that activates protein kinase C by causing translocation of the enzyme from the cytoplasmic to the membrane-associated active fraction during short-term exposure and protein kinase C membrane depletion and inactivation at long-term exposure.

Absorption, Fate, and Excretion: There is no reliable assay for determining the fate of bryostatin in humans.

Preparation and Administration: Bryostatin is supplied and prepared as a two-part formulation. Vial one contains 0.1 mg of lyophilized bryostatin as a white powder and is combined with 1 mL of a PET diluent (60% polyethylene glycol 400, 30% dehydrated ethyl alcohol, and 10% polysorbate 80). This solution must be further diluted with 9 mL of 0.9% sodium chloride injection and yields a 10-μg/mL solution of bryostatin. Polyvinyl chloride (PVC) bags should not be used because there may be leaching of a plasticizer and some limited adsorption. The drug may be further diluted with 0.9% sodium chloride or dextrose 5% in water to a concentration of 0.15 μg/mL to 0.75 μg/mL in a glass or polyolefin container. Non-PVC tubing is recommended.

Toxic Effects: Dose-limiting myalgias, eye pain, and photophobia are frequently seen. Phlebitis is common with peripheral administration. Fatigue, headache, nausea and vomiting, and diarrhea are also seen. Thrombocytopenia, neutropenia, and anemia occur, although infrequently.

Drug Interactions: No known reports.

Therapeutic Indications in Hematology: Bryostatin has activity against myeloid leukemia, chronic lymphocytic leukemia, non-Hodgkin lymphoma, and multiple myeloma. Enhanced tumor effect has occurred with the combination of bryostatin with vincristine, cisplatin, and cytarabine.

FLAVOPIRIDOL

Chemistry and Mechanism of Action: Flavopiridol is a semisynthetic flavone and selective inhibitor of CDKs 1, 2, 4-7, PKC, PKA, and platelet-derived growth factor causing cell cycle arrest. It also may inhibit CDK9/TEFb, which causes downregulation of Mcl-1, BIRC4, cyclin D1, and p21CIP1.

Absorption, Fate, and Excretion: Flavopiridol is 94% protein bound and is metabolized by the UDP glucuronyltransferase isoenzymes. Its half-life varies with infusion duration and ranges from 3.5 hours (1-hour infusion) to 27 hours (72-hour infusion).

Preparation and Administration: Flavopiridol is supplied as a 10 mg/mL yellow-greenish solution in a 5-mL vial. Contents may be diluted in either 5% dextrose injection or 0.9% sodium chloride injection to achieve a final concentration of 0.09 to 1 mg/mL. If the drug is administered through peripheral IV access, a concentration of less than 0.5 mg/mL is thought to decrease thrombotic complications. Flavopiridol has been administered as a 1-, 24-, and 72-hour infusion.

Toxic Effects: Grade 4 neutropenia and grade 3 lymphocytopenia occur and are more common with shorter durations of infusion. Thrombocytopenia is seen infrequently. Secretory diarrhea is a dose-limiting toxicity and may last for up to 3 days. Orthostatic hypotension is a frequently seen occurrence. Thrombosis with the 72-hour infusion duration was far more common than in the shorter infusion durations. A fatigue rate approaching 75% has been reported. Other toxicities include pleuritic chest pain, hyperbilirubinemia, and nausea.

Potential Drug Interactions: Paclitaxel in combination with flavopiridol has been associated with severe dose-limiting neutropenia.

Therapeutic Indications in Hematology: Flavopiridol's place in therapy is still being assessed. It has activity and use in hematologic malignancies, including mantle cell lymphoma, leukemias, and multiple myeloma. It may cause potential solid tumors in combination with other agents.

TANESPIMYCIN (17-AAG, GELDANAMYCIN, NSC 330507)

Chemistry: Tanespimycin is a water-soluble benzoquinone ansamycin antibiotic that binds to heat shock protein 90.

Fate, Absorption, and Excretion: Tanespimycin has a mean terminal half-life of 2.3 hours and is primarily metabolized by liver microsomal enzymes, specifically CYP3A4. One metabolite, 17-AG, is known to be active and has a mean terminal half-life of 4.6 hours. Peak plasma concentrations of 17-AAG and 17-AG occur at 30 and 60 minutes, respectively. 10.6% of 17-AAG and 7.8% of 17-AG is recovered in the urine over a 72-hour period.

Preparation and Administration: Tanespimycin is available as a single use amber vial containing 50 mg of tanespimycin in 2 mL of dimethylsulfoxide. Before administration, the tanespimycin concentrate must be completely thawed at room temperature (over ≤1 hour). Incomplete thawing affects the concentration of the drug because of changes in volume. Tanespimycin concentrate must be diluted to 1 mg/mL by withdrawing 2 mL and adding it to 48 mL of EPL diluent 2% egg phospholipids with 5% dextrose in water. A clear solution should be obtained with gentle mixing. Shaking should be avoided to prevent foaming. No further dilution is required and the final solution should be dispensed in a glass bottle. A 0.45 micron filter may be used, but is not required. The infusion should be completed within 8 hours of mixing. Intact vials of Tanespimycin should be stored in the freezer (−10° to −20° C). EPL diluent should be stored in the refrigerator (2°-8° C) and not frozen. Administration is by IV infusion.

Toxicity: Anemia, diarrhea, nausea, vomiting, fatigue, transaminitis, and muscle pain.

Drug Interactions: Tanespimycin is metabolized by CYP3A4. Agents that alter CYP3A4 activity may affect drug levels and metabolism, although this has not been shown to affect clinical use.

Therapeutic Uses: Lymphoma and leukemia in clinical trials.

IMATINIB (GLEEVEC)

Chemistry and Mechanism of Action: Imatinib, a phenylaminopyrinadine derivative, is a selective protein tyrosine kinase inhibitor effecting BCR-ABL tyrosine kinase. This enzyme is found commonly in chronic myeloid leukemia and in some clones of acute lymphoblastic leukemia. Imatinib also inhibits the kinases for platelet-derived growth factor, stem cell factor, and KIT.

Absorption, Fate, and Excretion: Imatinib is well absorbed and achieves peak levels within 2 to 4 hours and follows linear pharmacokinetics at the standard doses. The cytochrome P450 is the major route of metabolism with CYP3A4 being the primary pathway. An *N*-desmethyl piperazine is the main metabolite and is active. Pediatric patients follow the same pharmacokinetics as in adults.

Preparation and Administration: Imatinib is available in a film-coated tablet. In its pure form, it is a white to brownish to yellowish powder and is soluble in aqueous buffers of less than 5.5.

Toxic Effects: Gastrointestinal effects are common and include nausea and diarrhea. Muscle cramps are seen in one-third of patients receiving imatinib. Myelosuppression reflected as thrombocytopenia, anemia, and neutropenia occurs, with thrombocytopenia and neutropenia seen more frequently in patients in accelerated phase or blast crisis. Fluid retention is dose related and is exhibited as edema and weight gain, but pleural and pericardiac effusions are also seen. Fatigue and headache, although low grade, occur in 25% of patients.

Potential Drug Interactions: Drugs that inhibit CYP3A4 may increase imatinib plasma concentrations; these include ketoconazole, itraconazole, erythromycin, and clarithromycin. CY3A4 inducers that may decrease plasma concentration of CY3A4 are dexamethasone, rifampin, phenytoin, and carbamazepine. Imatinib increases concentrations of simvastatin, cyclosporine, and warfarin, along with other medications that are metabolized by CYP3A4.

Therapeutic Indications in Hematology: Imatinib is considered first-line therapy in Philadelphia-positive CML and has activity in accelerated or blast-phase CML. Some effect has been shown in ALL as well as hypereosinophilic syndrome and polycythemia vera.

TOPOTECAN (HYCAMTIN)

Chemistry and Mechanism of Action: Topotecan is a semisynthetic derivative of camptothecin that stabilizes a complex between DNA topoisomerase I and DNA. The cytotoxic effect of this drug is believed to result from the collision of DNA replication forks with a ternary complex of topoisomerase I, DNA, and topotecan. The resulting double-strand DNA breaks are lethal. The lactone form of topotecan, which predominates at an acidic pH, is a much more potent inhibitor of DNA topoisomerase I.

Absorption, Fate, and Excretion: At neutral or physiologic pH, the carboxylate form of topotecan is favored, and at a pH less than 7, the lactone form is favored. Topotecan has been given as a bolus or by continuous infusion. In less than 1 hour after infusion, most of the circulating drug in the plasma is in the carboxylate form because of the physiologic pH. The terminal half-life of the lactone form of this S phase–specific agent is 2.6 hours, and the terminal half-life of the total drug is 3.3 hours. Thirty-six percent of an IV dose is excreted unchanged in the urine, and there is a 1.5-fold concentration of the drug in bile. Cerebrospinal fluid levels of topotecan lactone reach approximately 32% of plasma levels. Dose adjustment is required for a creatinine clearance less than 60 mL/min, but no adjustment is necessary for a bilirubin up to 10 mg/dL.

Preparation and Administration: Topotecan is commercially available as 4-mg vials that are reconstituted with 4 mL of sterile water. This solution can be further diluted in normal saline or 5% dextrose in water and should be used immediately.

Toxic Effects: The dose-limiting toxicity for topotecan for all schedules is neutropenia. Thrombocytopenia and anemia are less common, although there is an increase in thrombocytopenia with continuous infusion schedules. Other less common and mild toxicities include nausea, vomiting, diarrhea, fever, fatigue, alopecia, skin rash, and increased liver function test results. Mucositis has been seen with prolonged infusion schedules over 5 days or when topotecan is given in higher doses.

Potential Drug Interactions: In vitro data suggest that there may be some synergism if a topoisomerase I inhibitor is given before a topoisomerase II inhibitor. In vitro data also suggest that synergism may be seen if a topoisomerase I inhibitor (topotecan) is given after an alkylating agent, suggesting that topoisomerase I may be involved in the repair of alkylator-induced DNA damage.

Therapeutic Indications in Hematology: Topotecan has activity in myelodysplastic syndromes, acute myeloid leukemia, chronic myeloid leukemia, and multiple myeloma.

VORINOSTAT (ZOLINZA)

Chemistry and Mechanism of Action: Vorinostat is a histone deacetylase (HDAC) inhibitor. It inhibits HDAC 1, HDAC2, HDAC3, and HDAC6 at nanomolar concentrations. Inhibition prevents removal of the acetyl groups from lysine residues in target histones and transcription factors. Loss of deacetylase function results in persistence of acetyl groups on histones, resulting in larger segments of open chromatin and a general increase in gene expression. Often this promotes differentiation and cell cycle arrest with apoptosis. The number of genes affected continues to grow so that the impact of vorinostat is complex.

Absorption, Fate, and Excretion: Reported pharmacokinetics after a 400-mg oral administration are an AUC of 5.5 micromolar-hours, a C_{max} of 1.2 micromolar, and T_{max} of 2 to 10 hours. Fatty meals decrease the rate of absorption but increase overall drug levels. There is no recommended dosing relative to meals. Vorinostat is heavily plasma protein absorbed. It undergoes glucuronidation hydrolysis, and later β-oxidation to inactive metabolites. Little is excreted unchanged.

Preparation and Administration: Oral dosing of 400 mg with food is standard. If side effects are noted, reduce the dose to 300 mg. There is no approved pediatric dosing.

Toxic Effects: Many side effects are noted. Common are fatigue, thrombocytopenia, muscle spasms, and anorexia. Serious reported adverse effects in clinical trials included pulmonary embolism in 4.7% and anemia in 2.3%.

Potential Drug Interactions: Vorinnostat can prolong Coumadin effect, raising the international normalized ratio. It can also induce glucose intolerance.

Therapeutic Indications in Hematology: Vorinostat is approved for cutaneous manifestations of cutaneous T-cell lymphoma in patients who have become refractory to standard treatments. It is being tested in other disorders such as myeloma and leukemias to determine whether it works through the HDACs or through altered expression of numerous proteins.

CHAPTER 56

RADIATION THERAPY IN THE TREATMENT OF HEMATOLOGIC MALIGNANCIES

Andrea K. Ng and Peter M. Mauch

In 1895, x-rays were first described by the German physicist Wilhelm Conrad Röntgen. Shortly after, in 1898, Antoine Henri Becquerel discovered radioactivity, and in the same year, the Curies isolated radium. The therapeutic potential of x-rays was first demonstrated in 1897, when the German surgeon Wilhelm Alexander Freund reported the disappearance of a hairy mole after x-ray treatments. In the early part of the century, radiation therapy consisted of primitive equipment, crude dosimetry, and little knowledge of normal tissue or tumor radiation biology. Although initial tumor shrinkage was achieved, the superficial characteristics of the radiation therapy deposited high doses in the skin and subcutaneous tissues, causing burns and ulceration, and underdosed deeper tumors, resulting in suboptimal long-term control. By 1930, the development of reliable orthovoltage machines enabled treatment of deeper tumors. The concept of fractionated radiation therapy was also developed in the 1930s. However, even with the more penetrating beams, adequate treatment of tumors deep in the abdomen or chest frequently was associated with complications involving the skin, muscles, heart, or bowel. Modern high-energy megavoltage equipment became available in the 1950s with cobalt 60 (^{60}Co). The linear accelerator, designed from microwave technology developed for radar during World War II, was first used in the United States by Kaplan and his group at Stanford University in the late 1950s.

Many of the principles and early techniques of radiation therapy for hematologic malignancies came from pioneering work in Hodgkin lymphoma. Vera Peters, in 1950, was the first physician to present definitive evidence that radiation therapy was a curative modality for patients with early-stage Hodgkin lymphoma. She did this by treating patients with limited-stage disease who were cured with high-dose, fractionated radiation therapy. Patients received 1800 to 5000 R to areas of involvement, with the highest dose given to patients with early-stage disease. She reported 5-year and 10-year survival rates of 88% and 79%, respectively, for patients with stage I Hodgkin lymphoma, rates that were incredibly high for a disease at that time in which virtually no one survived 10 years. The early success of radiation therapy in the treatment of lymphoma and Hodgkin lymphoma provided encouragement for the treatment of other tumors. These developments in radiation therapy are detailed in the next sections.

TYPES OF RADIATION

Electromagnetic Radiation

The ionizing radiation (photons) used during clinical treatment strategies is part of the electromagnetic spectrum. The energy of x-rays, described in terms of electron volts (eV), eject an electron from the target tissue, thus the term *ionizing radiation.* High-energy radiation is produced by linear accelerators by radioactive decay. The photons produced from radioactive decay are called gamma rays; they are identical to the x-rays produced by linear accelerators. Radioactive isotopes can be produced that emit gamma rays at sufficient energy and the dose to be used in clinical external-beam therapy. The most common isotope for external-beam irradiation is ^{60}Co (half-life 5.26 years). This isotope was in use before the availability of linear accelerators. The decay of ^{60}Co to nickel produces two gamma rays of energy that are 1.17 and 1.33 MeV. Linear accelerators generate photon beams by bombarding a target with electrons. Higher energy and thus more penetrating x-rays can be produced. Furthermore, linear accelerators have a smaller source and as a result can produce a much sharper beam edge compared with a cobalt machine.

Particle Radiation

High-energy electrons are one of the most frequently used forms of particle radiation in cancer treatment. They can be produced directly from a linear accelerator with the proper extraction technique. The typical energy range for electrons is 6 to 20 MeV, which allows treatment of superficial tumors up to a depth of 5 cm, with a characteristic sharp drop-off in dose beyond the prescribed depth.

Neutrons, protons, helium, carbon ions, and pi-mesons are other particles used for experimental radiation therapy. Because of their mass and charge, these particles can be sharply localized in tissue (Bragg peak), allowing precise localization, and potential sparing of normal tissues. In recent years, comparative dosimetry studies have been reported using proton beam therapy for treating mediastinal lymphoma, although uncertainty in radiologic path lengths of the proton beam may result in the only benefit in selected cases depending on the disease location.

RADIATION TREATMENT PLANNING AND DELIVERY

Radiation treatment requires a precise knowledge of normal anatomy and a detailed knowledge of growth patterns of tumors. Patient treatment plans are developed using a simulator before commencement of radiation therapy. Historically, in the two-dimensional (2D) planning era, fluoroscopy, bony landmarks, or other anatomic structures visible fluoroscopically were typically used to guide treatment field design. Three-dimensional conformal radiation therapy (3D CRT), which provides a 3D model of the patient's anatomy and tumor, allows more accurate tumor targeting while sparing neighboring critical normal organs. Beam's eye view display is used to select optimal beam directions and design beam apertures. Intensity-modulated radiation therapy (IMRT), an advanced form of 3D CRT, is increasingly incorporated into treatment of selected cases of lymphoma.[1-5] It is based on the use of optimized nonuniform radiation beam intensities incident on the patient, allowing dose "sculpting" and dose "painting," and has the potential to further improve the therapeutic ratio and reduce radiation toxicity. IMRT may especially benefit treatment to head and neck sites eliminate and where treatment is required.

Positron emission tomography (PET) scanning using ^{18}F-fluorodeoxyglucose is currently used in the staging, restaging, and follow-up of most lymphoma patients. In addition, for radiation treatment planning, the accuracy of tumor targeting can be improved by incorporating information from the PET scan into the planning process. The fusion of prechemotherapy PET data with computed tomography (CT) simulation information has been shown to lead to significant modifications of the treatment strategy and the

Table 56-1 Ongoing Randomized Trials Evaluating Elimination of Radiation Therapy After Complete Response to Chemotherapy as Assessed by Positron Emission Imaging

	Eligibility	Treatment Arms	Results
EORTC/ GELA H10	Stage I-II Favorable*	ABVD × 3 → INRT 30 Gy versus ABVD × 2 → if PET CR → ABVD × 2, no RT → if PET pos → BEACOPPesc × 2 → INRT 30 Gy ABVD × 4 → INRT 30 Gy versus ABVD × 2 → if PET CR → ABVD × 4, no RT → if PET pos → BEACOPPesc × 2 → INRT 30 Gy	Experimental arm of omitting RT by PET response closed early based on interim analysis
RAPID Trial	Stage I-IIA	ABVD × 3 → if PET CR†: IFRT versus No RT	Pending
GHSG HD16	Stage I-II Favorable‡	ABVD × 2 → PET → IFRT 30 Gy versus ABVD × 2 → if PET CR → no RT → If PET pos → IFRT 30 Gy	Pending

ABVD, Doxorubicin (Adriamycin), bleomycin, vinblastine, and dacarbazine; *BEACOPP,* bleomycin, etoposide, doxorubicin (Adriamycin), cyclophosphamide, vincristine (Oncovin), procarbazine, and prednisone; *CR,* complete response; *EORTC/GELA,* European Organization for Research and Treatment of Cancer/ Groupe d'Etude des Lymphomes de l'Adulte; *GHSG,* German Hodgkin Study Group; *IFRT,* involved-field radiation therapy; *INRT,* involved-node radiation therapy; *PET,* positron emission tomography; *RT,* radiation therapy.
*Age <60, <4 sites, no large mediastinal adenopathy, and no B symptoms/ESR <50 or B symptoms/ESR <30.
†If PET positive then one additional cycle of ABVD followed by IFRT.
‡<3 sites, no large mediastinal adenopathy, no extranodal sites, and no B symptoms/ESR <50 or B symptons/ESR <30.

radiotherapy planning in lymphoma patients (Table 56-1). As radiation treatment fields evolve toward involved-node radiation therapy (discussed later), where accurate delineation of prechemotherapy tumor volume is critical, PET-CT fusion planning will likely be increasingly used.

RADIATION BIOLOGY

Four R's of Radiation Biology

The laboratory and clinical findings of classic radiation biology have been defined in terms of the four R's of repair, redistribution, repopulation, and reoxygenation.

Repair

Two basic types of repair have been defined operationally: sublethal damage repair and potentially lethal damage repair. A radiation cell survival curve is characterized by a shoulder region and a terminal exponential portion (Fig. 56-1). In the shoulder region, a minimum number of targets must be hit before cell death occurs. This is defined

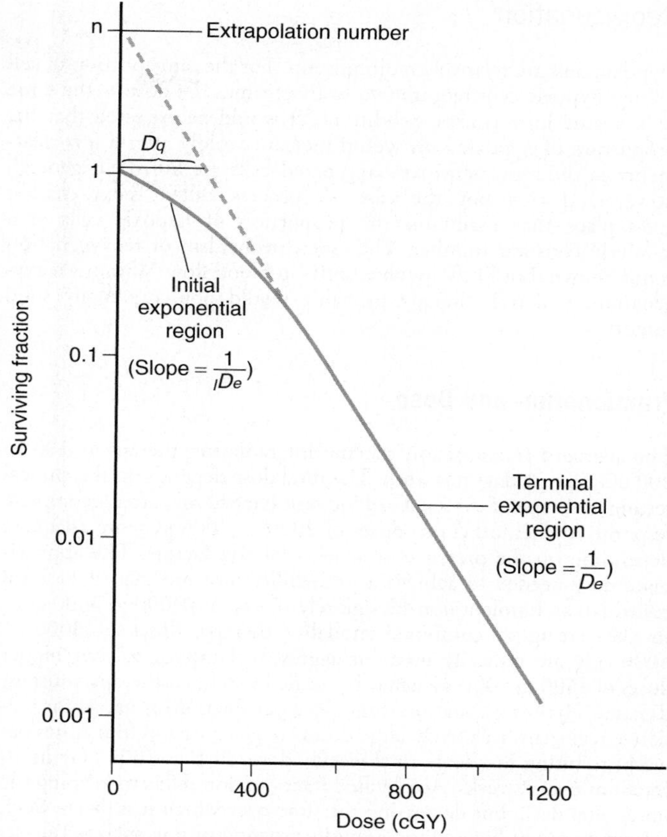

Figure 56-1 CELL SURVIVAL CURVE. D_e, Dose required to reduce the fraction of surviving cells by 37%; D_q, quasi-threshold dose. *(Modified from Withers HR: Biologic basis of radiation therapy. In Perez CA, Brady LW, editors:* Principles and practice of radiation oncology, *ed 2, Philadelphia, 1992, JB Lippincott, p 72.)*

as sublethal injury. Sublethal damage repair refers to the repair that occurs within the shoulder region, with the reappearance of another shoulder during that time. Potentially lethal damage repair refers to the increase in survival over time after a single treatment. If the cells remain in situ for a number of hours posttreatment, the proportion of surviving cells will increase. It is likely that similar biochemical mechanisms are involved to some extent for both, although the importance to clinical outcome of each of these repair processes is not completely understood.

Redistribution

Redistribution refers to the synchronization of the cell cycle that occurs after a single dose of radiation. Cells have decreasing radiosensitivity as from M/G2 to G1, to early S to late S phase. The relative radioresistance of S phase has prompted the combined use of radiation with S phase–specific drugs. An example is the delivery of radiation therapy concurrently with cycle active agents such as 5-fluorouracil (5-FU) in gastrointestinal malignancies.

Repopulation

Tumors and normal tissues repopulate during a course of irradiation. Normal tissue repopulation is observable with the healing of mucosal and skin reactions that takes place despite continuing radiation. The repopulation of tumors has been inferred from split-course radiation regimens in which there are a few weeks of no treatment between treatment segments. In settings in which the total dose is the same, local control is worse for split-course than for continuous treatment.

Reoxygenation

Hypoxic cells are relatively radioresistant. For the same portion of cell killing, hypoxic cells require two to three times the dose as the same cells treated in normoxic conditions. It would be expected that the proportion of hypoxic cells would increase rapidly after a few treatments as the more sensitive oxygenated cells are killed. In general, however, this is not the case. A process called reoxygenation takes place that maintains the proportion of hypoxic cells at a relatively constant number. The exact mechanism of reoxygenation is not known, but likely involves shifts in blood flow. Without reoxygenation, radiation therapy probably would not cure many solid tumors.

Fractionation and Dose

The standard fractionation scheme for radiation therapy is 180 to 200 cGy/day, 5 days per week. The total dose depends on the clinical setting and type of tumor. For Hodgkin lymphoma, after a complete response to chemotherapy, doses of 2000 to 3000 cGy are adequate depending on the presence or absence of risk factors. The approximate dose needed to achieve a probability of more than 95% local control of an indolent non-Hodgkin lymphoma is 3000 to 3600 cGy. In the setting of combined modality therapy, doses of 3000 to 4000 cGy are typically used for aggressive lymphomas, but higher doses of 4500 to 5000 cGy may be needed for chemotherapy-resistant diseases. Hypofractionation (high dose per fraction) is useful for palliative regimens. Relatively large doses are given one to four times per week, resulting in a large total weekly dose, such as 3000 cGy in 10 fractions over 2 weeks. Accelerated fractionation refers to keeping the same total dose, but decreasing the time over which it is given. Such a regimen might be used for a rapidly growing tumor, such as Burkitt lymphoma or refractory lymphoma. Hyperfractionation uses a small single dose given two to three times per day such that the total time is about the same as with standard fractionation, but the total dose must be higher to obtain the same effect. The lower dose per fraction spares late-responding tissues relative to tumor. Accelerated hyperfractionation is a hybrid regimen of delivering small doses two to three times per day over a shortened time period. In considering the total dose received by a patient, it is imperative to consider the dose per fraction, the number of doses per week, the total dose, the total treatment time, and when considering retreatment, the time elapsed since completion of the previous course of therapy.

Clinical Radiation Tolerance

The extent and frequency of injury to normal tissues depend on both radiation dose and volume treated. The risk can be enhanced by surgery and chemotherapy. Specific organ tolerance is not known, but estimates can be derived from reports of small numbers of patients.

Central Nervous System

Brain tolerance is about 5500 to 6000 cGy in small fractions, but small volumes can tolerate higher doses. Radiation myelitis can occur at doses in excess of 5000 cGy. The combined use of certain cytotoxic agents may increase the risk for spinal cord injury. The peripheral nervous system has a higher tolerance, and injury is uncommon unless fields overlap.

Heart

Radiation injury to the heart may involve a number of different cardiac tissues. Cardiac injury is rare unless the entire heart is treated with more than 3000 cGy. Anthracycline therapy enhances the risk for myocardial injury, and the total cardiac dose is limited to 1500 cGy in patients who have received anthracycline-containing chemotherapeutic regimens.

Lung

Fractionated doses as low as 2000 cGy or single doses as low as 800 cGy can cause radiation pneumonitis. Acute radiation pneumonitis can occur up to 6 months after treatment and is characterized by a dry cough, dyspnea and low-grade fever, and radiographic changes within the radiation fields. Long-term fibrosis and loss of pulmonary function depends on the presence of underlying lung pathologic conditions and the use of chemotherapeutic agents, in particular bleomycin, which may lower the threshold for clinical radiation lung injury. Using 3D radiation planning, dose-volume histograms of the lungs can be generated. In a typical mantle field, 25% to 30% of lungs may receive up to 2000 cGy, but most patients remain asymptomatic in this dose range.

Kidney

A portion of the kidney that receives a total dose in excess of 2000 cGy will permanently lose function. The development of late hypertension or renal failure depends on the volume of kidney irradiated. Even if a portion of one kidney is treated to a high dose, it is rare to see any clinical signs or symptoms. If cisplatin is administered after kidney irradiation, the toxicity of the platinum may be increased.

Liver

The irradiation of a large segment of liver to a dose in excess of 3000 cGy produces a clinical syndrome of hepatomegaly, ascites, and elevated liver function test results. Radiation injury is similar to that of venoocclusive disease, a syndrome that occurs with high-dose alkylating agent therapy used in some marrow transplantation conditioning regimens. If not fatal, radiation liver injury completely resolves.

Gastrointestinal Tract

The gastrointestinal tract is modestly sensitive to irradiation, with small bowel tolerance lower than that of the esophagus or large bowel. During radiation therapy, patients who receive large abdominal or pelvic fields get some degree of bowel irritation. Permanent gastrointestinal injury occur at doses above 4500 cGy and may require surgical excision of the damaged bowel segment, but this should be done only after a trial of conservative management.

Other Organs

Virtually all organs are susceptible to injury. The following are the lower limits for a permanent injury for some other organs: bone marrow stroma, 4000 cGy; spleen with functional asplenia, 4000 cGy; ovary, 2000 cGy; skin, 5500 cGy; salivary and endocrine glands, 4500 cGy; bladder, 6000 cGy; peripheral nerve, bone, and muscle, 6000 cGy; oral cavity mucosa, 6000 cGy. Acute reactions (e.g., bowel, skin, mucous, hair loss, blood count depression) occur 2 to 3 weeks after the start of treatment. These systems may recover despite an early decrease in function and the continuation of therapy. Conservative management helps a patient get through treatment with a minimum interruption of treatment. As a rule, the presence or extent of an acute reaction does not predict the likelihood of a delayed reaction. A major concern after treatment with radiation or chemotherapy is the development of secondary malignancies. The risk is especially well documented in long-term survivors of Hodgkin lymphoma and has been shown to be directly related to radiation dose and size of the treatment field. The trend toward reducing radiation dose and field size in the treatment of Hodgkin lymphoma will hopefully reduce the future risk for radiation-related second malignancies.

SPECIFIC USES OF RADIATION THERAPY FOR TREATMENT OF HEMATOLOGIC AND LYMPHOID MALIGNANCY

Early-Stage Hodgkin Lymphoma

The current standard therapy for stage I-II Hodgkin lymphoma is doxorubicin (Adriamycin), bleomycin, vinblastine, and dacarbazine (ABVD) chemotherapy followed by involved-field radiation therapy, yielding 5-year freedom-from-treatment-failure rates of approximately 95% and 85% in patients with favorable-prognosis and unfavorable-prognosis early-stage disease, respectively.[6,7] For patients with early-stage disease without any risk factors according to the German Hodgkin Study Group (GHSG) criteria (lack of large mediastinal adenopathy, extranodal disease, elevated sedimentation rate/B symptoms and three or more sites of disease), the GHSG HD10 trial showed that reduced treatment with only two cycles of ABVD followed by involved-field radiation therapy to 20 Gy is adequate in these patients.[6] In patients with risk factors, however, after four cycles of ABVD, results of the GHSG HD11 trial showed that a dose of 30 Gy is needed.[6]

In addition to a reduction of radiation dose, there is also increasing interest in further reducing radiation field size, from involved-field to involved-node radiation therapy, based on the known patterns of disease relapse after chemotherapy. In the ongoing GHSG HD17 trial the standard arm of involved-field radiation therapy following chemotherapy, regardless of response, is compared against the experimental arm of involved-node radiation therapy in patients who have achieved a complete response to chemotherapy.

Finally, the question of omitting radiation therapy has been addressed by several randomized trials, most of which showed a benefit in disease-free survival but not overall survival benefit with the addition of radiation therapy. However, a meta-analysis conducted by the Cochrane Haematological Malignancies Group[8] included five randomized controlled trials that compared chemotherapy alone with identical chemotherapy combined with radiotherapy for patients with stage I-II Hodgkin lymphoma and found a highly significant overall survival benefit with the addition of radiation therapy (hazard ratio [HR], 0.4; $P < 0.00001$). Picardi et al[9] conducted a randomized trial that included patients with stage I-IV disease with disease sites of greater than 5 cm, evaluating whether radiation therapy can be safely eliminated if a complete response by PET scan is achieved after six cycles of vinblastine, etoposide, bleomycin, epirubicin, and prednisone (VEBEP). A significant event-free survival benefit was found with the addition of radiation therapy in this carefully selected group of patients (96% versus 86%, $P = 0.03$). One key criticism of this trial is the use of suboptimal chemotherapy rather than the standard ABVD. Several ongoing randomized trials are addressing the question of whether radiation therapy can be eliminated in early-stage Hodgkin lymphoma patients with a complete response or early complete response by PET to ABVD, including the European Organization for Research and Treatment of Cancer/Groupe d'Etude des Lymphomes de l'Adulte (EORTC/GELA) H10 trial, the RAPID trial, and the GHSG HD16 trial. Details of the trial designs are summarized in Table 56-1.

Early-Stage Non-Hodgkin Lymphoma

Non-Hodgkin Lymphoma is a heterogeneous disease. The two most common histologic subtypes are diffuse large B-cell lymphoma and follicular lymphoma, accounting for three-quarters of all cases of non-Hodgkin lymphoma. Radiation therapy plays an important role in both of these subtypes of non-Hodgkin lymphoma in patients with limited-stage disease. Another subtype of non-Hodgkin lymphoma in which the role of radiation therapy is increasingly recognized is marginal zone lymphoma or mucosa-associated lymphoid tumor (MALT).

Stage I-II Diffuse Large B-Cell Lymphoma

Historically patients with localized diffuse large-cell lymphoma, many of whom were staged surgically, were treated with radiation therapy alone, with a cure rate of less than 50%. Since 1980, a doxorubicin-based combination chemotherapy regimen with or without radiation therapy has become the treatment of choice, yielding significantly improved relapse-free survival and overall survival rates (see box on Preferred Treatment for Early-Stage Non-Hodgkin Lymphoma). Table 56-2 summarizes randomized trials that compare chemotherapy alone versus combined modality therapy in patients with stage I-II aggressive non-Hodgkin lymphoma. These trials vary considerably in baseline patient and disease characteristics[10-13] and are associated with a number of limitations. Two of the trials used

Preferred Treatment for Early-Stage Non-Hodgkin Lymphoma

Early-Stage Diffuse Large B-Cell Lymphoma Treated With Combined Modality Therapy
Use of Involved Fields

- After a complete remission achieved with six to eight cycles of CHOP or R-CHOP: 36 Gy if initial bulky disease; 30 Gy for the remainder of patients
- After three to four cycles of CHOP or R-CHOP: 35 to 40 Gy
- After a partial remission: 40 Gy

Early-Stage Follicular Grade 1 and 2 Lymphoma
Use of Involved or Regional Fields

Carefully planned radiation therapy to limited fields with modest doses can significantly reduce the risk for significant damage to the marrow reserve, the risk for developing a treatment-related malignancy, and the risk for long-term toxicity to other normal tissues such as the salivary glands, lungs, heart, kidneys, and bowel.

The recommended dose is 30 to 36 Gy with a boost to areas of initial involvement to 36 to 40 Gy. Bulky disease should be treated to the upper end of the range; 30 to 36 Gy should suffice for smaller-volume disease.

Early-Stage Mucosa-Associated Lymphoid Tumor or Extranodal Marginal Zone Lymphoma
Use of Radiation Therapy to Involved Nodal Regions or Extranodal Sites

Doses of 30 Gy result in a near 100% local control rate. Although there are limited data with lower doses such as 25 Gy (except for orbital MALT), local control rates can also be high with this dose. This should allow for modification of dose in settings where the risk for injury to normal tissue is higher (orbit, salivary glands).

Although there are high complete response rates with chemotherapy for marginal zone lymphoma, there is little evidence that it is curative. Therefore, outside of clinical trials, chemotherapy should be reserved for patients with stage III-IV disease. Asymptomatic individuals with generalized disease may be considered for observation, similar to patients with generalized follicular lymphoma.

CHOP, Cyclophosphamide, hydroxydaunomycin, vincristine (Oncovin), and prednisone; *MALT,* mucosa-associated lymphoid tumor; *R-CHOP,* rituximab-CHOP.

Table 56-2 Randomized Trials Comparing Chemotherapy Alone and Chemotherapy Followed by Radiation Therapy in Localized Diffuse Large B-Cell Lymphoma

Trial	Patient Characteristics	No.	Treatment Arms	Results	P Value
SWOG[10,*]	Median age: 59 yr Extranodal involvement: 37% PS 0-1 97%; no bulky stage II	401	201: CHOP × 8 200: CHOP × 3 + RT (40-55 Gy)	5-yr PFS: 64% 5-yr OS: 72% 5-yr PFS: 77% 5-yr OS: 82%	.03 .02
ECOG[11]	Median age: 59 yr PS 0-1 92% Stage II: 68%; bulky disease: 31%	352	CHOP × 8 If CR (n = 215) → RT (30 Gy) / No RT If PR (n = 71) → RT (40 Gy)	6-yr FFS: 70% 6-yr OS:79% 6-yr FFS: 53% 6-yr OS: 67% 6-yr FFS: 63% 6-yr OS; 69%	.05 .23
Reyes et al[12]	Median age: 47 yr Stage II: 32% Bulky disease: 32%	647	309: ACVBP × 3 321: CHOP × 3 + RT (40 Gy)	5-yr EFS: 82% 5-yr OS: 90% 5-yr EFS: 74% 5-yr OS: 81%	<.001 .001
Bonnet et al[13]	Median age: 68 yr Bulky disease: 8% Extranodal involvement: 50% Most with nl LDH, PS 0-1	576	277: CHOP × 4 299: CHOP × 4 + RT (40 Gy)	5-yr EFS: 61% 5-yr OS: 72% 5-yr EFS: 64% 5-yr OS: 68%	.6 .5

ACVBP, Doxorubicin (Adriamycin) cyclophosphamide, vindesine, bleomycin, prednisone; *CHOP,* cyclophosphamide, hydroxydaunomycin, vincristine (Oncovin), and prednisone; *CR,* complete response; *ECOG,* Eastern Cooperative Oncology Group; *EFS,* event-free survival; *FFS,* failure-free survival; *nl LDH,* normal lactate dehydrogenase; *OS,* overall survival; *PFS,* progression-free survival; *PR,* partial response; *PS,* performance status; *RT,* radiation therapy.
*2001 Abstract update: Median follow-up of 8.2 years: OS and PFS of two arms overlapped.

abbreviated chemotherapy in the radiotherapy-containing arms[10,12] and are thus more suited to address alternatives to intensive chemotherapy alone, rather than to specifically address the role of radiation therapy after chemotherapy. Other shortfalls of these trials include inadequate chemotherapy,[13] limited power,[11] poor compliance to assigned treatment arms,[11] and suboptimal radiotherapy quality control. Most importantly, none of the trials included the use of rituximab in combination with doxorubicin-based chemotherapy and therefore did not address the role of consolidation radiation therapy when used in conjunction with current standard systemic therapy.

More recently retrospective studies that included mostly patients treated with rituximab, cyclophosphamide, hydroxydaunomycin, vincristine (Oncovin), and prednisone (R-CHOP) chemotherapy have shown a significant advantage to the addition of consolidation radiation even in patients with a complete response to chemotherapy.[14] An ongoing prospective randomized trial conducted by the German High-Grade Non-Hodgkin's Lymphoma Study Group (DSHNHL) may clarify the role of radiation therapy in the rituximab era and identify the subgroup of patients who may benefit from consolidation radiation therapy. In this study, patients with nonbulky disease are randomized to R-CHOP-21 alone versus R-CHOP-14 alone. Patients with bulky disease and/or extranodal disease are randomized to one of four arms: R-CHOP-21 alone, R-CHOP-14 alone, R-CHOP-21 followed by radiation therapy if a complete response is achieved, and R-CHOP-14 followed by radiation therapy if complete response is achieved.

Stage I-II Follicular Lymphoma

A number of studies have shown that radiation therapy alone can result in long-term cure in 30% to 40% of patients with stage I-II follicular grade 1-2 lymphoma. Several large series showing the treatment for limited-stage follicular lymphoma are shown in Table 56-3.[15-24] The median radiation doses vary from 30 to 40 Gy in eight of the nine series with the two largest series reporting a median dose of 35 Gy.[15,16] Recurrences within the treatment field range from 0% to 13.8% with higher percentages occurring in patients with bulky disease or who receive a radiation dose of less than 30 Gy. A variety of field sizes have been used, ranging from total-nodal, extended-field, regional-field, to involved-field irradiation. A recent retrospective explored further reducing the size of the radiation field to involved-node radiation therapy, defined as coverage of the involved lymph node(s) with margins of 5 cm or less, compared with regional-field radiation therapy for patients with stage I-II follicular lymphoma.[25] After multivariable analysis, the treatment field size did not significantly predict for disease specific–, progression free–, and overall survival outcome. As discussed later under Radiation Treatment Fields in Hematologic Malignancies, the definition of involved-node radiation therapy varies from group to group and currently remains in evolution.

Although radiation therapy alone is considered potentially curative therapy for patients with stage I-II follicular lymphoma, a multicenter, longitudinal, observational study from the United States showed that only 23% of patients with stage I disease at presentation received radiation therapy alone, suggesting that this well-established, potentially curative treatment approach is currently underutilized.

Stage I-II Mucosa-Associated Lymphoid Tumor Lymphoma

The indolent extranodal marginal zone or MALT lymphomas most commonly involve the gastrointestinal tract, salivary glands, breast, thyroid, orbit, conjunctiva, skin, and lungs. Because this subtype of lymphoma tends to remain localized for long periods of time, local treatment (surgery or local/regional irradiation) is effective at achieving long-term control and possible cure. Tsai et al[26] reported 77 patients with stage I-II marginal zone lymphoma. The majority were treated with radiation therapy, and the remaining patients were treated with surgery with or without systemic therapy. For those who received radiation therapy, the median radiation dose was 30 Gy. After a median follow-up of 61 months, the 5-year progression-free survival, freedom from treatment failure, and overall survival rates were 76%, 78%, and 91%, respectively. Patients who received radiation therapy had significantly greater local control (100% versus 50%, $P = 0.001$), freedom from treatment failure (81% versus 50%, $P = 0.0004$), and progression-free survival (79% versus 50%, $P = 0.002$)

Table 56-3 Large Series (>50 Patients) of Radiation Therapy for Localized Follicular Lymphoma

Institution	No.	Median f/u (yr)	Median RT Dose (Gy)	RT Field	Infield Relapses	10-yr FFTF	10-yr OS
PMH*,†	573	10.6	35	IF	NR	48%	>60%
BNLI*	208	NR	35	NR	NR	47%	64%
Stanford*,†	177	7.7	35-50	IF/RF/EF (77%) TLI (23%)	13.8%	44%	64%
Foundation Bergonie†	103	8.3	35-40	IF (54%) RF (46%)	NR	49%	56%
Edinburg	64	5	30-40	NR	Nonbulky: 0% at 30-40 Gy Unk/bulky: 9% at 30-40 Gy, 11% at 40 Gy	49%	78%
U. Florida†	72	8.5	NR	IF (53%) EF (43%) TNI (4%)	<30 Gy: 10% ≥30 Gy: 0%	46%	59%
NCI†	54	9	36	IF (38%) EF (48%) TLI/TBI (14%)	2%	48%	69%
Royal Marsden	58	NR	40	IF (52%) EF (48%)	9%	43%	79%
Harvard	106	12	36.7	IF (60%) RF (34%) EF (6%)	7%	46%	75%
GHSG‡	65	9.1	40	IF (3%) RF (11%) EF (54%) TNI (10%) Consolidative (23%)	7%	37%	55%

BNLI, British National Lymphoma Investigation; *EF*, extended field; *FFTF*, freedom from treatment failure; *f/u*, follow-up; *GHSG*, German Hodgkin Study Group; *IF*, involved field; *NCI*, National Cancer Institute; *NR*, not reported; *OS*, overall survival; *PMH*, Princess Margaret Hospital; *RF*, regional field; *RT*, radiation therapy; *TBI*, total body irradiation; *TLI*, total lymphoid irradiation; *TNI*, total nodal irradiation; *unk*, unknown.
*Included patients with follicular grade 3.
†Included patients who received chemotherapy.
‡Included patients who received chemotherapy; 12% had advanced-stage disease.

rates. More recent data suggest that doses lower than 30 Gy may be adequate, especially to the orbit, where the use of limited doses may avoid damage to the lacrimal glands. Goda et al,[27] from Princess Margaret Hospital, reported the long-term results of 167 patients with stage I-II MALT lymphoma who received involved-field radiation therapy. The median dose to nonorbital sites was 30 Gy and that to the orbit was 25 Gy. After a median follow-up of 7.4 years, the 10-year rate of local control was 95%, cause-specific survival was 98%, disease-free survival was 68%, and overall survival was 87%. Nine of 31 (29%) patients developed disease recurrence in the contralateral paired organ. These results suggest that local control can be achieved with lower doses of radiation such as 25 Gy, which should allow for modification of the dose in settings where the risk for damaging normal tissues is especially high (orbit, salivary glands).

Leukemia and Myeloma

The primary means of treating the leukemias and multiple myeloma is systemic therapy. The role of radiation therapy in the overall management of these patients in complex and depends on the overall treatment plan. Therefore only a few of the principles of radiation therapy are discussed.

Acute Lymphoblastic Leukemia and Lymphoma

The predominant role for radiation therapy is for central nervous system prophylaxis of leukemia and lymphoma patients given the pattern of relapse in particular disease types. The standard dose for adult patients is 1800 cGy, although in the pediatric population, lower doses are being evaluated, because of concerns of delayed neurocognitive dysfunction. Radiation therapy doses of 2400 to 3000 cGy are occasionally used for palliation or for salvage therapy in patients with central nervous system or testicular relapses.

Solitary Plasmacytomas and Multiple Myeloma

Solitary plasmacytomas may occur in bone or in soft tissue. Radiation therapy produces long-term local control of over 80%. The precise dose needed has been debated, but at least 4000 to 5500 cGy should be administered.

Radiation therapy is often used as palliation for patients with bony lesions from multiple myelomas. A typical palliative regimen might be 3000 cGy over 2 weeks. The dose and fractionation must be tailored to the clinical setting. A patient with newly diagnosed multiple myeloma who is expected to live many years should be treated with a higher total dose and a lower dose per fraction. Lesions near the spinal cord should be treated with a dose equivalent to 4000 cGy because a local failure would be difficult to retreat.

RADIATION TREATMENT FIELDS IN HEMATOLOGIC MALIGNANCIES

The radiation field designs that have been used in the past or are currently employed in lymphoma therapy include the following:

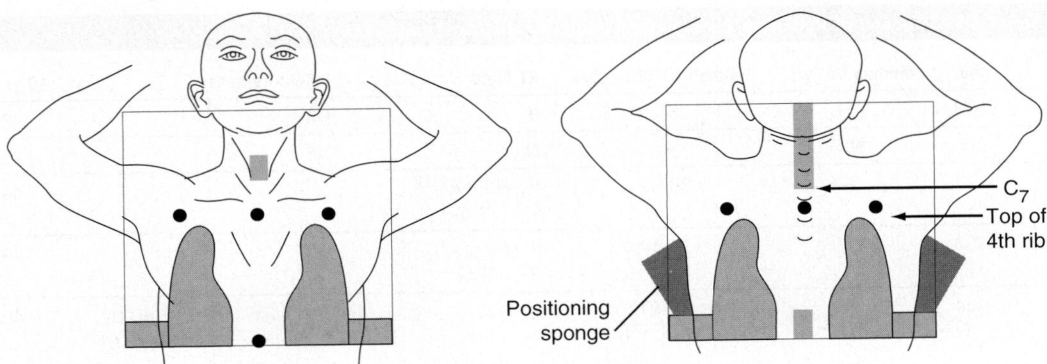

Figure 56-2 A TYPICAL MANTLE IRRADIATION FIELD.

1. Mantle field: This treatment field and its variations have been the most commonly used treatment field in patients with supradiaphragmatic Hodgkin lymphoma. It includes the submental, cervical, supraclavicular and infraclavicular, axillary, hilar, and mediastinal lymph nodes (Fig. 56-2). The dose inhomogeneity in a mantle field is a result of variation in separation of a patient's upper body and the irregularly contoured lung blocks that affect the scatter doses to different areas within the field. For instance, the dose to the cervical and axillary regions tends to be higher because of decreased patient thickness in the soft tissue of the neck and axilla, whereas the dose toward the inferior border of the mantle field tends to be lower, because of the thicker separation in that region of the body as well as loss of scatter doses due to the adjacent lung blocks. Some of the techniques that are employed to minimize dose inhomogeneity include the use of an extended source-to-node distance of 110 cm or greater, and by the use of higher-energy megavoltage machines. However, the energy used is limited by the need to ensure adequate doses to superficial nodes, which can fall within the "build-up" regions of the radiation beams and be potentially underdosed if energy higher than 6 MV is used.
2. Mantle and para-aortic (MPA) ± splenic field: Also known as subtotal nodal or lymphoid irradiation, the para-aortic lymph nodes in addition to the mantle field are treated. The spleen is included in the treatment field in patients who do not undergo surgical staging and splenectomy.
3. Total nodal irradiation (TNI) or total lymphoid irradiation: This encompasses most of the lymphoid tissue, with the addition of a pelvic field to the mantle and para-aortic field. However, other nodal groups, such as the brachial, epitrochlear, popliteal, sacral, and mesenteric nodes are not specifically included in the TNI field. MPA radiation therapy and TNI are used less frequently today because of the widespread use of chemotherapy.
4. Inverted-Y field: This is used in patients presenting with infradiaphragmatic lymphoma and includes treatment to the para-aortic and pelvic lymph nodes.
5. Involved-field radiation: By definition, this includes at least the entire lymph node group but may also contain the contiguous nodes. For example, in a patient presenting with an enlarged cervical lymph node, an involved-field treatment would include the entire ipsilateral cervical chain and the supraclavicular region, because these nodes are considered one region (Fig. 56-3). In a patient with mediastinal involvement, the field would include the mediastinal, hilar, subcarinal, and medial supraclavicular nodes. Although the hilar nodes are scored separately traditionally, the hilar and subcarinal nodes are included in the mediastinal field (Fig. 56-4). In addition, the medial supraclavicular nodes are included in order to cover the upper mediastinum (top of T1).

The radiation field designs employed in lymphoma therapy have evolved substantially over the last several decades, from total nodal irradiation to subtotal nodal irradiation (or MPA radiation therapy) to involved-field radiation therapy. The definition of involved-field radiation therapy was described in detail with site-specific examples by Yahalom and Mauch in 2002, although this was mostly based on 2D planning, relying on the use of bony landmarks to determine field setup. In recent years, there has been an increasing effort to further reduce radiation field size to include nodes. However, the definition of involved-node radiation therapy differs from group to group,[28-30] including inconsistencies on the expansion from clinical target volume to planning target volume, which ranges from 1 cm to 5 cm, on the requirement of use of prechemotherapy PET scanning to determine the clinical target volume, and treatment techniques. As summarized in Table 56-4, there is considerable variation in the definition of involved-node radiation therapy by the EORTC/GELA,[28] GHSG,[29] and British Columbia group,[30] and there is a need to standardize this definition. Outside of a clinical trial, the optimal treatment field may be a modified form of involved-field treatment, tailored to the tumor site and the surrounding normal tissues. For example, in patients with low cervical and supraclavicular involvement, the upper neck can be excluded to spare salivary gland function; in patients with mediastinal involvement only, the hila can be excluded to limit exposure to the heart, lungs, and breasts.

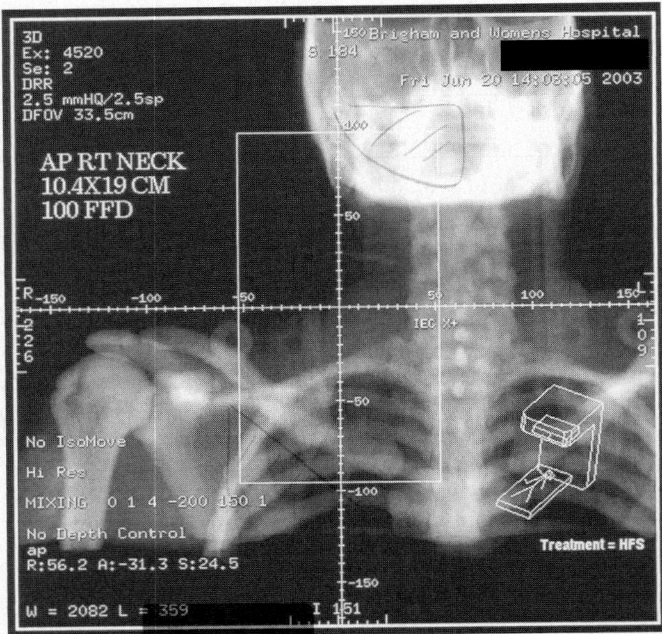

Figure 56-3 INVOLVED FIELD TO THE CERVICAL AND SUPRACLAVICULAR NODAL CHAIN IN A PATIENT WITH CERVICAL NODE INVOLVEMENT ONLY.

Table 56-4 Definitions of Involved-Node Radiation Therapy

Pretreatment Evaluation	CTV	GTV	PTV	Technique
EORTC/GELA				
CT in treatment position if possible PET in treatment position strongly recommended	If CR/CRu, initial volume of LN with exclusion of normal displaced structures (e.g., muscles, blood vessels) For mediastinum, CTV is normal mediastinum with length of CTV based on prechemotherapy volume If PR, CTV definition same as CR/CRu	If CR, not applicable If PR, postchemotherapy volume	If CR/CRu, 1 cm isotropic margin of CTV If PR, PTV1: CTV + 1 cm isotropic margin PTV2: GTV + 1 cm isotropic margin PTV should receive 95%-107% of prescribed dose	3D, 4D, IMRT, if APPA, field size needs to be ≥5 × 5 cm If LN >5 cm apart, use separate fields; if ≤5 cm, then encompass in same field
GHSG				
Examination by radiation oncologist CT of neck/C/A/P in treatment position PET/CT in treatment position if possible	Same as EORTC/GELA	Not specified	2-cm axial and 3-cm cranial caudal expansion of CTV (if necessary, can be reduced to 1-1.5 cm if close proximity to critical structures) For mediastinum, 1 cm axial and 2 cm cranial caudal)	Not specified
BCCA (INRT≤5 CM)				
Not specified	Prechemotherapy and postchemotherapy nodal volume, restricted by postchemotherapy anatomic limits	Not specified	Margin from CTV to field edge: 1.5-5 cm	CT planning not mandatory

APPA, Anterior-posterior; *BCCA,* British Columbia Cancer Agency; *C/A/P,* chest/abdomen/pelvis; *CR/CRu,* complete response/complete response unconfirmed; *CT,* computed tomography; *CTV,* clinical target volume; *3D,* three-dimensional; *4D,* four-dimensional; *EORTC/GELA,* European Organization for Research and Treatment of Cancer/Groupe d'Etude des Lymphomes de l'Adulte; *GHSG,* German Hodgkin Study Group; *GTV,* gross target volume; *IMRT,* intensity-modulated radiation therapy; *INRT,* involved-node radiation therapy; *LN,* lymph node; *PET,* positron emission tomography; *PR,* partial response; *PTV,* planning target volume.

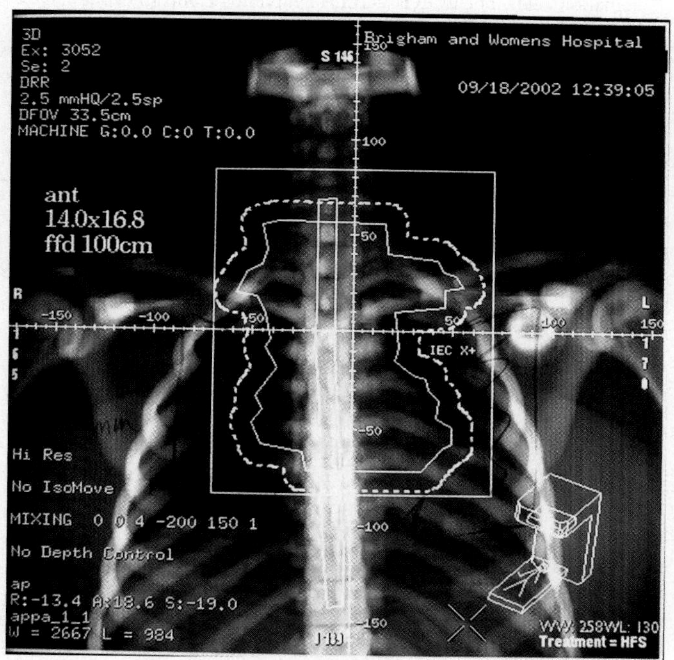

Figure 56-4 INVOLVED FIELD TO THE MEDIASTINUM.

FUTURE DIRECTIONS

Over the last several decades, tremendous advances have been made in the field of radiation oncology. The role of radiation therapy in the management of patients with hematologic malignancies has evolved, as systemic therapy options have improved, response assessment has become more reliable with functional imaging, and conformal radiation treatment planning and delivery have become more available. Future efforts include refining indications for radiation therapy in various settings, based on initial disease characteristics as well as response to treatment. In addition, optimal radiation doses and treatment fields need to be standardized. Finally, modern radiation therapy techniques including IMRT, image-guided therapy, four-dimensional radiation therapy, and dose painting may be applied to selected cases to further improve tumor targeting while sparing normal tissues.

REFERENCES

1. Paumier A, Ghalibafian M, Gilmore J, et al: Dosimetric benefits of intensity-modulated radiotherapy combined with the deep-inspiration breath-hold technique in patients with mediastinal Hodgkin's lymphoma. *Int J Radiat Oncol Biol Phys* 82:1522, 2012.
2. Wang H, Li YX, Wang WH, et al: Mild toxicity and favorable prognosis of high-dose and extended involved-field intensity-modulated radiotherapy for patients with early-stage nasal NK/T-cell lymphoma. *Int J Radiat Oncol Biol Phys* 82:1115, 2012.

3. Cella L, Liuzzi R, Magliulo M, et al: Radiotherapy of large target volumes in Hodgkin's lymphoma: Normal tissue sparing capability of forward IMRT versus conventional techniques. *Radiat Oncol* 5:33, 2011.
4. Weber DC, Peguret N, Dipasquale G, et al: Involved-node and involved-field volumetric modulated arc vs. fixed beam intensity-modulated radiotherapy for female patients with early-stage supra-diaphragmatic Hodgkin lymphoma: A comparative planning study. *Int J Radiat Oncol Biol Phys* 75:1578, 2009.
5. Chera BS, Rodriguez C, Morris CG, et al: Dosimetric comparison of three different involved nodal irradiation techniques for stage II Hodgkin's lymphoma patients: Conventional radiotherapy, intensity-modulated radiotherapy, and three-dimensional proton radiotherapy. *Int J Radiat Oncol Biol Phys* 75:1173, 2009.
6. Eich HT, Diehl V, Gorgen H, et al: Intensified chemotherapy and dose-reduced involved-field radiotherapy in patients with early unfavorable Hodgkin's lymphoma: Final analysis of the German Hodgkin Study Group HD11 trial. *J Clin Oncol* 28:4199, 2010.
7. Ferme C, Eghbali H, Meerwaldt JH, et al: Chemotherapy plus involved-field radiation in early-stage Hodgkin's disease. *N Engl J Med* 357:1916, 2007.
8. Herbst C, Rehan FA, Brillant C, et al: Combined modality treatment improves tumor control and overall survival in patients with early stage Hodgkin's lymphoma: A systematic review. *Haematologica* 95:494, 2010.
9. Picardi M, De Renzo A, Pane F, et al: Randomized comparison of consolidation radiation versus observation in bulky Hodgkin's lymphoma with post-chemotherapy negative positron emission tomography scans. *Leuk Lymphoma* 48:1721, 2007.
10. Miller TP, Dahlberg S, Cassady JR, et al: Chemotherapy alone compared with chemotherapy plus radiotherapy for localized intermediate- and high-grade non-Hodgkin's lymphoma. *N Engl J Med* 339:21, 1998.
11. Horning SJ, Weller E, Kim K, et al: Chemotherapy with or without radiotherapy in limited-stage diffuse aggressive non-Hodgkin's lymphoma: Eastern Cooperative Oncology Group study 1484. *J Clin Oncol* 22:3032, 2004.
12. Reyes F, Lepage E, Ganem G, et al: ACVBP versus CHOP plus radiotherapy for localized aggressive lymphoma. *N Engl J Med* 352:1197, 2005.
13. Bonnet C, Fillet G, Mounier N, et al: CHOP alone compared with CHOP plus radiotherapy for localized aggressive lymphoma in elderly patients: A study by the Groupe d'Etude des Lymphomes de l'Adulte. *J Clin Oncol* 25:787, 2007.
14. Phan J, Mazloom A, Jeffrey Medeiros L, et al: Benefit of consolidative radiation therapy in patients with diffuse large B-cell lymphoma treated with R-CHOP chemotherapy. *J Clin Oncol* 28:4170, 2010.
15. Gospodarowicz M, Lippuner T, Pintilie M, et al: Stage I and II follicular lymphoma: Long-term outcome and pattern of failure following treatment with radiation therapy alone. *Int J Radiat Oncol Biol Phys* 45:217a, 1999.
16. Vaughan Hudson B, Vaughan Hudson G, MacLennan K, et al: Clinical stage 1 non-Hodgkin's lymphoma: Long-term follow-up of patients treated by the British National Lymphoma Investigation with radiotherapy alone as initial therapy. *Br J Cancer* 69:1088, 1994.
17. Mac Manus M, Hoppe R: Is radiotherapy curative for stage I and II low-grade follicular lymphoma? Results of a long-term follow-up study of patients treated at Stanford University. *J Clin Oncol* 14:282, 1996.
18. Lawrence T, Urba W, Steinberg S, et al: Retrospective analysis of stage I and II indolent lymphomas at the National Cancer Institute. *Int J Radiat Oncol Biol Phys* 14:417, 1988.
19. Hayabuchi N, Jingu K, Masaki N, et al: Nodular histiocytic lymphoma, emphasizing results of stage I disease treated by radiotherapy. A report of the Japan Lymphoma Radiation Therapy Study Group (JLRTG). *Am J Clin Oncol* 13:501, 1990.
20. Soubeyran P, Eghbali H, Bonichon F, et al: Localized follicular lymphomas: Prognosis and survival of stages I and II in a retrospective series of 103 patients. *Radiother Oncol* 13:91, 1988.
21. Pendlebury S, el Awadi M, Ashley S, et al: Radiotherapy results in early stage low grade nodal non-Hodgkin's lymphoma. *Radiother Oncol* 36:167, 1995.
22. Kamath S, Marcus R, Lynch J, et al: The impact of radiotherapy dose and other treatment-related and clinical factors on in-field control in stage I and II non-Hodgkin's lymphoma. *Int J Radiat Oncol Biol Phys* 44:563, 1999.
23. Eich HT, Heimann M, Stutzer H, et al: Long-term outcome and prognostic factors in early-stage nodal low-grade non-Hodgkin's lymphomas treated with radiation therapy. *Strahlenther Onkol* 185:288, 2009.
24. Guadagnolo BA, Li S, Neuberg D, et al: Long-term outcome and mortality trends in early-stage, Grade 1-2 follicular lymphoma treated with radiation therapy. *Int J Radiat Oncol Biol Phys* 64:928, 2006.
25. Campbell BA, Voss N, Woods R, et al: Long-term outcomes for patients with limited stage follicular lymphoma: Involved regional radiotherapy versus involved node radiotherapy. *Cancer* 116:3797, 2010.
26. Tsai HK, Li S, Ng AK, et al: Role of radiation therapy in the treatment of stage I/II mucosa-associated lymphoid tissue lymphoma. *Ann Oncol* 18:672, 2007.
27. Goda JS, Gospodarowicz M, Pintilie M, et al: Long-term outcome in localized extranodal mucosa-associated lymphoid tissue lymphomas treated with radiotherapy. *Cancer* 116:3815, 2010.
28. Girinsky T, Specht L, Ghalibafian M, et al: The conundrum of Hodgkin lymphoma nodes: To be or not to be included in the involved node radiation fields. The EORTC-GELA lymphoma group guidelines. *Radiother Oncol* 88:202, 2008.
29. Eich HT, Muller RP, Engenhart-Cabillic R, et al: Involved-node radiotherapy in early-stage Hodgkin's lymphoma. Definition and guidelines of the German Hodgkin Study Group (GHSG). *Strahlenther Onkol* 184:406, 2008.
30. Campbell BA, Voss N, Pickles T, et al: Involved-nodal radiation therapy as a component of combination therapy for limited-stage Hodgkin's lymphoma: A question of field size. *J Clin Oncol* 26:5170, 2008.

CHAPTER 57

PATHOBIOLOGY OF ACUTE MYELOID LEUKEMIA

Michael Andreeff and Alfonso Quintás-Cardama

Human leukemias have posed unique clinical and conceptual challenges since their initial identification by Rudof Virchow 150 years ago. They continue to elicit fascination by those who study their biology, molecular genetics, and clinical presentation and have proven to be sensitive to chemotherapy, but are also incurable, depending on their cytogenetics and molecular genetics. This chapter summarizes our present, evolving knowledge of acute myeloid leukemia (AML) molecular pathophysiology.

Acute leukemias are clonal disorders that arise from hematopoietic progenitors developing either in the lymphoid or myeloid pathway or from primitive stem cells with multilineage potential. The genesis of human myeloid leukemia involves the deregulation of differentiation and maturation programs of the hematopoietic myeloid lineage that develops from primitive stem progenitor cells with multilineage potential. Myeloid leukemias have been linked to acquired somatic chromosomal translocations or inversions. These genomic rearrangements alter gene expression patterns that result in subversion of the programs regulating cell proliferation, differentiation, and survival. These changes are believed to determine the process of leukemic transformation,[1] a hypothesis has been supported by results obtained from gene manipulation studies in murine models.[2,3]

Chronic myeloid leukemia (CML) was the first cancer associated with a specific chromosomal abnormality. This aberrancy, first identified as a minute chromosome, is now known as the Philadelphia chromosome, which results from the t(9;22) balanced reciprocal translocation. The molecular consequence of the Philadelphia translocation is the generation of the oncogene *BCR-ABL1* that encodes the chimeric BCR-ABL protein with constitutive kinase activity. Extensive structural biology studies prompted the investigation of rationally designed small molecules that target the tyrosine kinase activity of the BCR-ABL kinase for the treatment of CML. The impressive results obtained with the first agent of this kind, imatinib mesylate, laid the foundation for the extensive development of targeted therapies of other leukemias and solid tumors. However, these initial results were partially offset by the realization that most patients receiving imatinib harbor residual disease[4] and that responses in patients with CML in accelerated phase (AP) or blastic phase (BP), when they occur, are generally short lived.[5] These shortcomings have propelled further studies to understand the mechanisms of resistance to tyrosine kinase inhibitor (TKI) therapy and the development of novel agents to override these limitations.

Acute myeloid leukemias are clinically characterized by accumulation of immature blastic cells that exhibit uncontrolled growth, lack normal differentiation, and exhibit much decreased apoptosis. The different AML phenotypes are classified, mostly by morphologic criteria, into subtypes according to the predominance of a particular myeloid lineage. The acquired somatic mutations that underlie the molecular pathogenesis of AML target an ample group of transcription factors and signaling pathways that result in the abrogation of orderly myeloid differentiation and cell death that all control population size. The current paradigm of AML pathogenesis implies a multistep process that involves at least two different types of genetic alterations. One type of alterations involves typically the deregulation of transcription factors that modulate hematopoietic development. Frequently, these arise from chromosomal translocations, and the resulting chimeric fusion proteins impair differentiation of a particular myeloid lineage, thus specifying the AML subtype. A second class of alterations affects intracellular signaling involved in cell survival and proliferation, such as protein receptors with tyrosine kinase activity.

Over 3 decades, investigation of clonal chromosomal abnormalities in leukemic cells obtained from patients with myeloid leukemia and the development of transgenic mouse models have been used to deconstruct the molecular pathways leading to leukemic transformation. These approaches have impacted our understanding of the molecular changes involved in the pathogenesis of these disorders and have uncovered potential therapeutic targets. This chapter describes the current state of knowledge of the molecular events involved in the pathogenesis of both myeloid leukemias.

PHILADELPHIA-CHROMOSOME LEUKEMIAS

Myeloid leukemias (both acute and chronic) result from the neoplastic transformation of a hematopoietic stem cell. The hallmark genetic abnormality driving the pathogenesis "Philadelphia chromosome" leukemias is the balanced translocation t(9;22)(q34;q11), which cytogenetically results in the Philadelphia chromosome[6,7] and molecularly gives rise to the *BCR-ABL1* hybrid gene.[8,9] The *BCR-ABL1* gene encodes a protein kinase, BCR-ABL, which is constitutively activated in CML. Classically, CML has been described as a disease that evolves in three phases. Most patients are diagnosed in the chronic phase (CP), characterized by overproduction of immature myeloid cells and mature granulocytes in the bone marrow (BM) and peripheral blood. Left untreated, most patients progress to blast phase, characterized by a peripheral blood or BM blast percentage of over 30%, usually preceded by an accelerated phase.[10] The estimated risk of transformation to BP is 5% to 10% per year during the first 2 years after diagnosis, but the annual progression rate increases to up to 20% to 25% thereafter.[10,11] CML in BP is characterized by remarkable resistance to chemotherapeutic drugs.

The BCR-ABL1 Oncogene

The *ABL1* gene is the human homologue of the v-*abl* oncogene carried by the Abelson murine leukemia virus (A-MuLV).[12] *ABL1* encodes the 145-kd nonreceptor tyrosine kinase ABL that localizes at several subcellular sites, including the nucleus, cytoplasm, mitochondria, the endoplasmic reticulum, and the cell cortex, where it interacts with a large variety of cellular proteins, including signaling adaptors, other kinases, phosphatases, transcription factors, and cytoskeletal proteins.[13] ABL is expressed in most tissues, and its structure is organized in functional domains.[14,15] In turn, *BCR* encodes a protein with serine-threonine kinase activity. The fusion of the BCR and ABL1 genes results in the activation of the c-*ABL1* protooncogene to its oncogenic form.[16,17] Several experimental models, such as *BCR-ABL1*–expressing CD34$^+$ cells in culture [18,19] or retrovirally transduced *BCR-ABL*-positive mouse cells,[20-22] have demonstrated that the *BCR-ABL1* is central to the pathogenesis of CML. Moreover, mice expressing a *BCR-ABL1* isoform with a point mutation in the adenosine triphosphate (ATP)–binding pocket of ABL, which results in inactivation of the kinase activity, do not develop leukemia even when the mutant transcript is expressed in long-term repopulating hematopoietic stem cells. These findings ultimately corroborate that ABL kinase activity is essential for *BCR-ABL1*-mediated leukemogenesis in vivo[15,22] and provide the rationale for the targeted use of TKIs for the treatment of CML. However, unlike other fusion oncogenes such as *MLL-ENL* or *MOZ-TIF2*, *BCR-ABL1* can transform hematopoietic stem cells but cannot transform committed progenitors lacking the capacity of self-renewal.[23] This has been shown in experiments in which flow-sorted populations of common myeloid progenitors and granulocyte-monocyte progenitors were transduced with either *MOZ-TIF2* or *BCR-ABL1*.[23] Unlike BCR-ABL1–transduced progenitors, those expressing MOZ-TIF2 could be serially replated in methylcellulose cultures and resulted in AML in vivo that could be serially transplanted.[23]

The breakpoints within the *ABL1* gene at 9q34 takes place within a large area that spans more than 300 kilobases (kb) at its 5′ end and can occur upstream of exon Ib; downstream of exon Ia; or, more frequently, between exons Ib and Ia.[24] In contrast, breakpoints within *BCR* map to three distinct areas known as *breakpoint cluster regions*. In most patients with CML, and in approximately one-third of those with Philadelphia chromosome–positive B-cell acute lymphoblastic leukemia (B-ALL), the break occurs within a 5.8-kb area spanning BCR exons e12-e16 (formerly called b1-b5), referred to as the *major breakpoint cluster region* (M-*bcr*). A fusion transcript with either b2a2 or b3a2 junctions is possible because of alternative splicing, thus giving rise to a 210-kd protein ($p210^{BCR\text{-}ABL1}$).[25] In two-thirds of patients with Philadelphia chromosome–positive B-ALL and in rare cases of CML, the *BCR* breakpoint localize to an area of 54.4 kb between exons e2′ and e2, termed the *minor breakpoint cluster region* (m-*bcr*), generating an e1a2 transcript that translates into a 190-kd protein ($p190^{BCR\text{-}ABL1}$). It has been suggested that patients with CML carrying $p190^{BCR\text{-}ABL1}$ may have a worse prognosis than those expressing the classical $p210^{BCR\text{-}ABL1}$ isoform.[26] A third breakpoint cluster region (μ-*bcr*), downstream of exon 19, has been occasionally identified in patients with CML, giving rise to a 230-kd fusion protein ($p230^{BCR\text{-}ABL1}$), which has been associated with a phenotype similar to that of chronic neutrophilic leukemia.[27] The leukemogenic potential of all three transcripts has been demonstrated in murine models. However, the tyrosine kinase activity of the different BCR-ABL variants differs significantly, with $p230^{BCR\text{-}ABL1}$ having the least activity and conferring only partial growth factor independence relative to the potent protein kinase $p190^{BCR\text{-}ABL1}$,[28,29] which may explain the more benign clinical course of patients with $p230^{BCR\text{-}ABL1}$.

Anatomy and Autoregulation of the BCR-ABL Protein

The N-terminus of BCR-ABL members consists of the "Cap" region, which is present in two different isoforms generated by alternative splicing of the first exon, termed 1a and 1b. ABL 1b contains a C_{14} myristoyl saturated fatty acid moiety covalently linked to the N-terminus and is expressed at higher levels than type 1a, which is not myristoylated. ABL also contains a tyrosine kinase domain that is preceded by a Src-homology-2 (SH2) and an SH3 domain. These three domains or motifs are highly conserved both in terms of sequence and spatial organization. Moreover, ABL has a long C-terminus extension, known as the last exon region, which contains protein–protein interaction sites responsible for the diverse subcellular localizations and functions of the protein.[13] The last exon region contains four proline-rich SH3 motifs that function as binding sites for the SH3 domains of adaptor proteins such as Crk, Grb2 (growth-factor-receptor-bound 2) and Nck,[30,31] a DNA-binding domain, an actin-binding domain, three nuclear localization signals, and one nuclear export signal, which allows c-Abl to shuttle between the nucleus and the cytoplasm in response to environmental stimuli.

BCR also exhibits a complex architectural modularity at the N-terminus highlighted by the presence of coiled-coil oligomerization domain, a serine/threonine kinase domain, a Dbl/CDC24 guanine-nucleotide exchange factor homology domain and a pleckstrin homology domain, a putative calcium-dependent lipid binding site, and a RAC guanosine triphosphatase-activating protein domain. Also in BCR, the tyrosine residue 177 (Y177) serves as docking site for growth factor receptor-bound protein 2 (GRB2), GRB10, 14-3-3, and the ABL proteins, through its SH2 domain.[15]

In simple terms, the Ph chromosome causes the replacement of the endogenous autoregulatory domain of ABL with erroneous coding sequences from BCR. In this novel protein, BCR-ABL, the tight temporal and spatial regulation of ABL is lost, resulting in constitutively high levels of tyrosine kinase activity. In *BCR-ABL1*–positive cells, both SH3 and SH2 domains in ABL function as an autoinhibitory structure that maintains the kinase domain in an off state.[32-34] Crystal structures of ABL have shown that the myristoyl modification at the extreme end of the N-terminal segment of ABL 1b engages with the C-terminal lobe of the ABL catalytic domain. This interaction induces conformational changes that facilitate the docking of the SH2 and SH3 domains onto the kinase domain[32,35] in a manner that closely resembles the inactive conformation of SRC.[13,36-38] Thus, binding of the myristoyl group to the pocket in the C-terminal lobe appears essential for adopting an autoinhibited conformation of ABL 1b, and forms of ABL 1b lacking the myristoyl group show constitutive tyrosine kinase activity.[13] The elements in ABL 1a that replace the function of the myristoyl group of ABL 1b have not been elucidated yet. In structures of inactive BCR-ABL, the SH2 and SH3 domains stabilize an inactive conformation of the kinase domain in which a prominent α-helix (helix αC) in the N-terminal lobe (N-lobe) of the kinase is displaced inwardly toward the active site, forming an ion pair between the conserved residues Lys271 and Glu286 residues[37] while the SH2 domain remains tightly bound to the C-lobe of the kinase. In this conformation, the rotation of the helix αC results in the displacement of important catalytic residues out of the active site, which precludes the access of ATP and the peptide substrate to the active site.[13] Of interest, several structural analyses have shown that the last exon region of ABL may be dispensable for SH3 domain–dependent autoinhibition in vitro.[34,39] In addition, ample evidence indicates that BCR is an important mediator of ABL deregulation. X-ray crystal structural analysis of the oligomerization domain of BCR-ABL (residues 1–72 or BCR_{1-72}), which includes the coiled-coil domain (BCR_{30-65}), has shown that two monomers associate in an antiparallel dimer that stacks to form a tetramer.[40] It is tempting to hypothesize that the fusion of BCR activates the activity of the ABL kinase via dimerization-mediated autophosphorylation of BCR-ABL molecules. Furthermore, the kinase activity, transformation, phosphorylation of tyrosine residues in the activation loop of the catalytic domain, and the leukemogenic potential of BCR-ABL are remarkably impaired by mutations of the coiled-coil domain secondary to impairment of oligomerization.[41] Accordingly, transformation by BCR-ABL devoid of the coiled-coil domain of BCR can be partially restored by deletion of the SH3 domain.[42]

Signaling Pathways Downstream of BCR-ABL

The leukemogenic activity of the BCR-ABL fusion tyrosine kinase relies upon its ability to promote gain-of-fitness changes that translate into abrogation of growth-factor/adhesion dependence, morphologic transformation, growth advantage, and enhanced proliferation.[20] These effects result from the activation of numerous downstream effector pathways by the BCR-ABL oncoprotein. The BCR autophosphorylation site Y177 is essential for *BCR-ABL1*–mediated leukemogenesis.[43,44] *BCR-ABL1* oncogenes in which Y177 is mutated to phenylalanine (Y177F) largely abolish GRB2 binding and abrogate BCR-ABL–induced RAS activation.[45] Therefore, despite preservation of the kinase activity of ABL, *BCR-ABL1-Y177F* impairs the transformation of primary BM cultures.[45] In a stem cell transplantation (SCT) model of CML, transfection of the mutant *BCR-ABL1-Y177F* results in a remarkably reduced ability to induce a myeloproliferative disorder (MPD) in mice.[45] The Y177 residue constitutes a high-affinity docking site for the SH2 domain of growth factor receptor–bound protein 2 (GRB2). GRB2, which in turn, recruits SOS (a guanine-nucleotide exchanger of *RAS*) that activates RAS,[15] and the scaffold adapter GRB2-associated binding protein 2 (GAB2) through its SH3 domain.[15] Tyrosine phosphorylation of GAB2 in *BCR-ABL1*–transformed cells requires Y177 of BCR-ABL and the GRB2 SH3 binding site in GAB2.[46] Therefore, BCR-ABL–induced GAB2 phosphorylation is mediated by a GRB2-GAB2 complex. This interaction is required for the full activation of the phosphatidylinositol 3-kinase (PI3K)–AKT and the RAS-ERK pathways as well as for the optimal proliferation and migration of Ba/F3 cells in response to BCR-ABL. As a consequence, BCR-ABL cannot transform primary myeloid cells from *GAB2*$^{(-/-)}$ mice.[46] The interaction of GRB2 and GAB2 is also critical for the activation of SHP2 (also known as PTPN11), which is required for the normal activation of the RAS extracellular signal-regulated kinase pathway that most receptor tyrosine kinases signal through.[15]

BCR-ABL also phosphorylates the SRC family kinases (SFKs) HCK, LYN, and FGR. Phosphorylation of HCK leads to recruitment of signal transducer and activation of transcription 5 (STAT5),[15,47] which results in dimerization and translocation of STAT5 molecules to the nucleus, where they modulate gene transcription through binding to cognate DNA sequences. However, the leukemogenic role of STAT5 in CML has been controversial. BCR-ABL–induced STAT5 phosphorylation and activation may occur either or indirectly through phosphorylation by Janus kinase 2 (JAK2) [48] or by SFKs.[49] In earlier experiments, retroviral transduction of *BCR-ABL1* into BM still induced a CML-like MPD in *STAT5a*$^{(-/-)}$*STAT5b*$^{(-/-)}$ mice.[50] The role of STAT5 has been recently revisited.[51,52] Inactivation of STAT5 with siRNA in human samples from patients with CML impairs Philadelphia chromosome–positive myeloid colony formation. Also, fetal liver hematopoietic progenitors from mice that have the entire *STAT5ab* locus deleted were incapable of generating leukemia in recipient mice after retroviral transduction with *BCR-ABL1*.[51] Additionally, BCL-X, which is repressed by the transcription factor interferon consensus sequence binding protein (ICSBP),[53] is transcriptionally activated by STAT5 in CML.[54] A series of knock-out mice studies have also shown the dispensability for *BCR-ABL1*–mediated leukemogenesis of several other factors such as CBL, interleukin-3 (IL-3), and granulocyte-macrophage colony-stimulating factor (GM-CSF).[55,56] Recently, it has been demonstrated that *BCR-ABL1* retrovirus-transduced BM from mice lacking the SFKs HCK, LYN, and FGR efficiently induced CML but not B-ALL, suggesting a prominent role these kinases in Philadelphia chromosome–positive lymphoid malignancies.[57] In keeping with these observations, ablation of LYN by siRNA in primary CML cells impaired leukemic cell viability and colony formation in primary cells from patients with Philadelphia chromosome–positive CML in lymphoid BP but had less effect on myeloid BP cells.[58] Interestingly, BCR-ABL–activated SFKs, which may be essential for transition to lymphoid BP, remain fully active in imatinib-treated mouse leukemic cells, suggesting an additional benefit of agents with potent anti-SFK activity (e.g., dasatinib) for patients with CML in lymphoid BP and Philadelphia chromosome–positive B-ALL.[59]

Although the individual contribution of some downstream elements activated by BCR-ABL may appear negligible when evaluated individually in knock-out systems, there is evidence supporting a cooperative role of some of these factors in the pathogenesis of CML. When *BCR-ABL1*–positive K562 cells were induced to express dominant negative forms of RAS, PI3K, or STAT5, marked apoptosis was observed in cells coexpressing two of the three dominant negative mutants in any combination.[60] These results suggest that a cooperative interplay among these factors is necessary for the full realization of the leukemogenic potential of BCR-ABL kinase.

It has been recently reported that mice deficient in the enzyme 12/15-lipoxygenase (12/15-LO) develop a MPD that progresses to transplantable leukemia independent from ABL dysregulation.[61] Cells isolated from chronic stage 12/15-LO-deficient mice *(Alox15)* exhibit increased activation of the PI3K–AKT pathway as well as hyperphosphorylation of the transcription factor interferon consensus sequence binding protein (ICSBP), translating into increased BCL-2 expression and leukemic cell survival.[61] ICSBP is a tumor suppressor and a negative regulator of granulocyte differentiation.[62] Forced expression of ICSBP inhibited the *BCR-ABL1*–induced CML-like disease in vivo.[63] Notably, all of the effects observed in *Alox15* mice were reversed upon treatment with a PI3K inhibitor. 12/15-LO expression suppressed the growth of a human CML-derived cell line, which in aggregate, suggests that 12/15-LO is an important suppressor of MPD by virtue of its PI3K-dependent regulation of ICSBP and their downstream target genes in vivo.[61]

JUNB is a component of the activator protein 1 family of transcription factors that has been shown to act as a tumor suppressor in myeloid cells,[64] antagonizing the RAS downstream target JUN, thus inhibiting cell proliferation and survival. Modifications of *JUNB* expression may have a role in the pathogenesis of CML. Transgenic mice specifically lacking *JUNB* in the myeloid lineage (*JunB*$^{-/-}$Ubi-*JunB* mice) developed an MPD that closely resembled human CML, beginning at 4 months of age, including progression to BP in 16% of mice.[65,66] Furthermore, only *JUNB*-deficient long-term self-renewing hematopoietic stem cells from diseased mice were able to induce CML-like disease in recipient mice after transplantation.[66]

Some of the elements involved in BCR-ABL signal transduction provide the rationale for the development of targeted therapies for patients with CML.

Transformation to Blast Phase or Acute Leukemia

Evolution of CML to BP is characterized by the development of a marked degree of resistance to treatment that is difficult to overcome by currently available therapies. The mechanisms responsible for the transition from the CP of CML to the BP remain poorly understood. This has been caused, at least in part, by the lack of adequate animal models of *BCR-ABL1*–induced leukemia with a long myeloproliferative phase necessary for assessing mechanisms of disease progression. Although little is known about the mechanisms involved in transformation to BP, continued expression or activity of BCR-ABL kinase and the acquisition of additional cytogenetic and molecular changes are observed in the majority of patients with CML during evolution to BP.[67] Approximately 80% of patients with CML develop additional nonrandom cytogenetic aberrancies in Philadelphia chromosome–positive metaphases. This phenomenon is known as *clonal evolution* and reflects the genetic instability frequently associated with advanced stages of the disease.[68]

Clonal evolution is believed to play a prime role in CML progression. The most frequent secondary cytogenetic abnormalities encountered in patients with clonal evolution are trisomy 8 (34%), isochromosome 17 (20%), and duplicate Ph chromosome (38%),[69] which have been linked to c-*Myc* overexpression, loss of 17p, and *BCR-ABL1* overexpression, respectively.[70-72] Other cytogenetic aberrancies, such as trisomy 19, trisomy 21, trisomy 17, and deletion 7, have been identified in fewer than 10% of cases of clonal evolution.[73] These genetic lesions are more frequently associated with myeloid than with lymphoid CML-BP. In addition, 10% to 15% of patients with CML present with deletions of the derivative chromosome 9, which may be a reflection of genomic instability leading to more rapid progression to BP than those lacking this abnormality.[74] The detrimental prognosis conferred by deletions of the derivative chromosome 9 appears to be offset by imatinib therapy.[75] Other cytogenetic abnormalities have been detected in Philadelphia chromosome–negative metaphases of patients with CML with an incidence ranging from 2% to 17% and have been occasionally linked to development of myelodysplasia or AML.[76,77]

Myeloid progenitors from patients with CML in AP or BP have increased β-catenin levels compared with levels in control participants. Self-renewal of hematopoietic stem cells in mice entails activation of the β-catenin pathway, which results in the translocation of β-catenin to the nucleus, where it interacts with lymphoid enhancer factor/T-cell factor (LEF/TCF) transcription factors and regulates the transcription of genes such as *MYC* and *cyclin D1*.[78] It has been shown that progression to BP is associated with expansion of the myeloid progenitor fraction, consisting mainly of granulocyte–macrophage progenitors, rather than expansion of the pool of hematopoietic stem cells. Of note, CML granulocyte–macrophage progenitors display *BCR-ABL1* amplification and activation of the β-catenin pathway, enhancing the self-renewal activity and leukemic potential of these cells.[79]

One of the most common gene mutations in CML-BP involves the *p53* gene, which is mutated in 25% to 30% of patients with myeloid BP, and the exon 2 of the *INK4A/ARF* locus, which is deleted in 50% of cases of lymphoid BP.[71] Deletion of exon 2 of the *INK4A/ARF* locus results in loss of *p16* and *p14/ARF* expression, which regulate cell cycle progression and the G_1/S checkpoint by inhibiting the G_1 phase cyclin D-Cdk4/Cdk6 and promoting p53 upregulation, respectively.[71] Based on the fact that ARF enhances p53 levels by interfering with the activity of MDM2, the principal negative regulator of p53,[80] homozygous deletion at the *p16/ARF* locus observed in lymphoid BP might represent a functional equivalent of *p53* mutation in myeloid BP.[71] Two other elements upregulated by BCR-ABL in CML-BP are the transcription factors encoded by *EVI-1* and *HOXA9,* which can cooperate with BCR-ABL in blocking myeloid differentiation and enhancing survival advantage.

Notably, BCR-ABL enhances SET expression during progression to BP.[81] SET is a nucleus/cytoplasm-localized phosphoprotein that potently inhibits the tumor suppressor protein phosphatase 2A (PP2A). In turn, PP2A is a phosphatase that regulates cell proliferation, survival, and differentiation.[82]

In summary, progression to CML-BP is characterized by a multitude of heterogenous cytogenetic and molecular alterations responsible for reduced apoptosis, enhanced proliferative potential, and differentiation arrest observed in CML-BP cells. A better understanding of these abnormalities, which will undoubtedly depend on the development of better animal models of advanced CML phase, is warranted to design rational therapies for patients in BP.

ACUTE MYELOID LEUKEMIA

Acute myeloid leukemia is a heterogeneous disease with regard to acquired genetic alterations, including cytogenetic aberrancies as well as gene mutations and changes in gene expression. Most cases of AML are sporadic and occur as a consequence of acquired somatic mutation in hematopoietic stem cells. Cytogenetic aberrations are detected in approximately 50% to 60% of patients with AML at the time of diagnosis and constitute the strongest predictor of clinical outcome.[83-86] However, there is significant variation in clinical outcome across different cytogenetic aberrations. In addition, there is enormous variability in prognosis within the same group of karyotypic alterations, indicating that other molecular events play a major role in the pathogenesis of AML. Identification of these abnormalities is needed to better understand AML, to improve the prognostic value of the cytogenetic analysis, and to better stratify patients with AML. In patients whose pretreatment karyotype is abnormal, cytogenetic analysis is customarily used to document complete remission after remission induction therapy. Multiple translocation breakpoints have been identified and cloned over the past decade from patients with AML. It is possible to classify these translocations based on the structure and function of the genes involved. Frequently, these balanced reciprocal translocations involve the fusion of two transcription factors important in normal hematopoiesis such as core binding factor (CBF), retinoic acid receptor alpha (RARa), homeobox (HOX) family members, and members of the ETS family of transcription factors. Of critical importance has been the discovery of mutations in several elements involved in survival, proliferation, and differentiation, such as the receptor tyrosine kinase receptors FMS-like tyrosine kinase 3 (FLT3), and KIT. The discovery of these mutations has added significant complexity to the pathogenesis of AML but also helped to better classify, stratify, and prognosticate different subsets of patients with AML. Moreover, this has unveiled novel targets that have spurred the development of experimental agents for this disease. Recent progress in deep-sequencing has facilitated genome-wide analysis of AML. Numerous new mutations have been reported that require further analysis regarding their roles as "driver" or "bystander" mutations.

Prognosis Based on Cytogenetic Analysis

Acquired structural chromosome aberrancies are detected at diagnosis in the BM of 50% to 60% of patients with AML .[83-85,87] Three distinct risk groups—favorable, intermediate, and adverse—can be established based on karyotypic findings. All large cytogenetic studies of AML concur that patients with t(15;17)(q22;q12-21) have an excellent prognosis and those with t(8;21)(q22;q22) or inv(16)(p13q22)/t(16;16)(p13;q22) have a relatively favorable prognosis. By contrast, patients with inv(3)(q21q26)/ t(3;3)(q21;q26), -7 or a complex karyotype (i.e., at least three chromosome aberrations) have a poor clinical outcome. The presence of the poor risk cytogenetic abnormalities -5, del(7q), -17/17p-, -18, or -20 is frequently associated with complex karyotypes.[87] Most large studies evaluating the prognosis of karyotypic abnormalities in AML have been undertaken in patients younger than 60 years of age.[83-85] The value of the pretreatment cytogenetic analysis has been recently corroborated in trials involving older patients with AML.[88,89] In these studies, the longest survival was observed in patients with CBF AML.[88,89] Patients with normal karyotype at diagnosis are classified in the intermediate prognostic category.[83-85] However, the prognosis within this subset of patients is highly variable, likely because of the presence of a heterogeneous group of molecular alterations undetectable by standard karyotypic analysis. A flurry of recent studies has highlighted the prognostic importance of different molecular markers in patients with normal karyotype (e.g., *NPM1, FLT3,* and *KIT* mutations). The complex interactions among these molecular abnormalities have not been elucidated yet.

Pathogenesis

In AML, the enormous complexity and diversity of genetic and molecular genotypes exceeds the number of recognizable clinical and morphologic phenotypes. A working formulation that rationally categorizes the wealth of available genetic and emerging molecular information is therefore necessary. A currently accepted notion of AML pathogenesis involves the cooperation of two different types of genetic abnormalities or mutations. The most frequently mutated genes in AML encode transcription factors, thus emphasizing the critical role of these "master" regulators in the control of hematopoietic cell development. Translocations that inappropriately activate transcription factor genes display specificity for hematopoietic cells blocked in defined stages of differentiation. A direct consequence of these mutations is the impairment of the processes of maturation and differentiation of cells of the myeloid lineage. A second type of mutations is those that confer a proliferative and survival advantage to cells (activating mutations).[90] An example of the former include the CBF translocations and RARα and MLL gene rearrangements. Examples of the latter include mutations in receptor tyrosine kinases such as KIT or the FLT3 genes.[90] Some of the mutations conferring proliferative and survival advantage correlate with karyotypic aberrations observed in patients with AML at diagnosis.

Mutations Interfering With Transcription in Acute Myeloid Leukemia

Two distinct groups of transcriptionally active proteins play a major role in the fate of hematopoietic progenitors. The first group consists of master regulatory transcription factors, which, similar to AML1, are implicated in the development of all the hematopoietic lineages. Disruption of the signaling stemming from this type of proteins results in complete failure of the hematopoietic program. A second category of transcription factors intervenes more specifically in the development and each hematopoietic lineage. Examples of this type of transcription factors are GATA-1, which skews the development of hematopoietic progenitors toward the erythroid lineage, and C/EBPα, which promotes granulocytic differentiation. The activity of some transcription factors depends on the cell type in which they are expressed. For instance, PU.1 induces B-lymphoid or myeloid differentiation (depending on its expression levels) when expressed in early hematopoietic progenitors, but it induces monocytic differentiation when expressed in committed myeloid precursors. Mutations and rearrangements of some transcription factors regulate the activity of different elements involved in signal transduction networks and of other transcription factors implicated in leukemogenesis. To identify the critical pathways responsible for AML pathogenesis, it is imperative to decipher with accuracy the cross-talk among the different classes of transcription factors and their mutated counterparts.

Core Binding Factor Rearrangements

Mutations involving CBF rearrangements are detectable in approximately 15% of patients with AML and are generally linked to a favorable prognosis. CBF is a heterodimeric transcription factor that consists of a DNA binding α-subunit, encoded by one of three members of the RUNX family (*RUNX1 or AML1, RUNX2,* and *RUNX3*), and a ß-subunit encoded by the *CBFβ* gene that increases DNA-binding affinity to the complex. CBF regulates the expression of an array of genes that modulate hematopoiesis, such as IL-3, GM-CSF, and the macrophage colony-stimulating factor (M-CSF) receptor. The CBFβ–RUNX3 complex is involved in B-cell maturation and the silencing of the *CD4* gene during T-cell maturation.[91] A *CBFα2* knock-out murine model renders a phenotype characterized by early embryonic death; central nervous system hemorrhage; and despite the presence of a normal yolk sac, absence of definitive hematopoiesis.[92,93] Rearrangements of *AML1* and *CBFβ* with other genes result in chimeric proteins that disrupt the CBF complex and represses transcription activation.[94] A variety of chromosomal translocations involving either *AML1* or *CBFβ* have been identified in AML. CBF AML include those expressing inv(16)/t(16;16), which gives rise to the fusion of *CBFβ* with the *smooth muscled myosin heavy chain* gene (MYH*11* or *SMMHC*), and t(8;21), which is associated with the fusion transcript composed of the *AML1* and the *eight-twenty-one (ETO)* genes. The AML1 gene has been found implicated in other fusion transcripts detected in AML, such as those involving the *ecotropic viral integration 1 (EVI1)* or *translocation ets leukemia (TEL)* genes in AML carrying the t(3;21) and t(12;21) translocations, respectively. Trisomy 13 has been shown to be strongly associated with AML1 mutations and FLT3 gene overexpression in AML.[95] Several types of *CBFβ-MYH11* transcripts have been described, depending on the fused exons of the *CBFβ* and *MYH11* genes, with almost 85% of cases presenting the transcript type A and 15% the transcripts D and E or other rarer isoforms.[96,97] In addition to the expression of these fusion oncoproteins, the normal unrearranged genes (e.g., *AML1*) continue to be expressed and both modulate the activity of each other. For instance, in AML expressing the CBF translocation *AML1-ETO,* this fusion oncogene acts as a dominant negative inhibitor of *AML1,* as evidenced in transcriptional activation assays[98] and knock-in murine models.[99] In fact, coexpression of *AML1-ETO* and *AML1* gives rise to an identical phenotype than that of embryos that completely lack *AML1*.[99] Similarly, the *CBFβ-MYH11* oncoprotein is a dominant negative inhibitor of CBF both in transactivation assays and during development.[100,101] Induction of *CBFβ-MYH11* expression or AML1-loss in BM does not appear to impair the maintenance of long-term hematopoietic stem cells. In knock-in *CBFβ-MYH11* chimeras, *CBFβ-MYH11* expression alters adult multilineage hematopoietic differentiation.[102] The multistep nature of leukemia progression in inv(16) AML expressing *CBFβ-MYH11* was also corroborated in these murine model in which gain of additional mutations induced by chemical or retroviral mutagens was necessary for the development of AML.[102,103] Interestingly, this phenotype was rescued in *CBFβ*$^{-/-}$ mice expressing *CBFβ* from the hematopoietic specific promoters *TIE2* or *GATA1,* further underscoring the key role of *CBFß* during hematopoietic differentiation.[104,105] *CBFß* also modulates the effect of *CBFβ-SMMHC* in adult hematopoiesis and leukemogenesis. In mice with a *CBFβ* knock-out allele and a conditional *CBFβ MYH11* knock-in allele, *CBFβ* modulated *CBFβ MYH11*–mediated leukemia development, suggesting that *CBFß* upregulation may efficiently counteract differentiation defects in human AML with inv(16).[106] In a conditional *CBFβ MYH11* knock-in mouse model, Cre-mediated induction of *CBFβ MYH11* in adult mice resulted in a drastic reduction in the numbers of B cells and platelets and the development of an abnormal myeloid progenitor population with deficient proliferation capacity in BM.[107] This study provides evidence in vivo that leukemia fusion proteins that affect hematopoietic differentiation may maintain normal number of hematopoietic stem cells with deficient repopulation function while creating preleukemic myeloid progenitors that can be targets for AML transformation.[107]

In summary, genetic rearrangements of CBF are frequent in patients with AML and usually occur through balanced reciprocal translocations, accounting for approximately 25% of cases of all cases of AML. Patients with CBF AML have a relatively favorable prognosis, which can be improved by postremission therapy with high-dose cytarabine.[108]

PML-RARα Rearrangements

Translocations involving the *retinoic acid receptor (RAR)* locus on chromosome 17, such as t(15;17)(q22;q11), are linked to the phenotype of acute promyelocytic leukemia (APL),[109-114] which comprises 10% to 15% of all cases of adult AML. The t(15;17)(q22;q11) gives rise to the *PML-RARα* transcript that encodes a fusion protein containing most of the functional domains of RARα (including the *RAR* binding domain and the DNA binding domain) and the majority of the *PML* gene. The breakpoints within the PML gene cluster locate to three different regions referred to as bcr1, bcr2, and bcr3.[115]

In addition to t(15;17)(q22;q11), there are at least two other variant translocations involving *RARα* associated with the APL phenotype. These include t(11;17)(q23;q21) and t(5;17)(q35;q21), which lead to the fusion of the *RARα* gene to the promyelocytic leukemia zinc finger *(PLZF)* and nucleophosmin *(NPM)* genes, respectively.[116] Other genes, such as *NuMA* and *STAT5,* have been found as much rarer *PML* translocation partners. The leukemogenic effect of *PML-RARα* has been demonstrated in transgenic models.[117,118] In these models, the development of APL occurred after a long preleukemic phase characterized by myeloproliferation, suggesting that additional genetic events are necessary for leukemogenesis. In fact, recurring, nonrandom cytogenetic abnormalities have been identified in PML-RARα transgenic mice that progress to APL.[119-121] Oncogenic *RAS* mutations have been identified in 10% to 15% of patients with AML,[122,123] suggesting a likely role as cooperating second hits in leukemogenesis. Oncogenic *N-RAS* and *K-RAS* mutations have been detected in 4% to 10% of patients with APL in two large studies.[123,124] It has been shown that conditional expression of oncogenic *K-RAS* from its endogenous promoter cooperates with *PML-RARα* in mice to induce a rapid-onset high-penetrance lethal APL-like disease.[125]

Transgenic mice expressing *PML-RARα, NPM/RARα,* or *PLZF/RARα* under the control of a human *cathepsin G* minigene have been recently generated.[126] In all three transgenic models, leukemia developed with variable penetrance after a variably long latency. Notably, distinct cytomorphologic features were induced by each fusion gene, with *hCG-NPM/RARα* leukemic cells resembling monoblasts, those expressing *hCG-PML/RARα* resembling promyelocytic blasts, and those expressing *hCG-PLZF/RARα* displaying a phenotype of terminally differentiated myeloid cells.[126] The PML-RARα oncoprotein disrupts the interaction of retinoic acid and *RARα*, which converts the latter into a transcription activator.[127] As a consequence, in APL, there is maturation arrest of hematopoietic progenitors at the promyelocyte stage. *PML-RARα* expression also disrupts the localization of native PML, causing it to relocalize from discrete nuclear structures, the PML nuclear bodies, into microspeckled aberrant structures.[128,129] Similar to CBF fusion proteins, the PML-RARα oncoprotein is considered to act as a dominant negative inhibitor of the PML protein, as well as the major heterodimeric partner of RARα, RXRα (retinoid X receptor).[128] PML-RARα recruits and complexes with several corepressors, including the nuclear corepressor (N-CoR). N-CoR inhibits transactivation from RARα target genes through the recruitment of the molecules sin3 and histone deacetylases, which in turn inhibit the binding of transcription factors and the binding of the transcriptional machinery to promoters, resulting in inhibition of gene expression for hematopoietic differentiation. Similarly, the PML moiety of the PML-RARα protein interacts with the DAXX corepressor. Mutations preventing DAXX recruitment, albeit allowing PML-RARα dimerization, abrogated the ability of PML-RARα to block hematopoietic differentiation and immortalize cells.[130]

All-trans retinoic acid (ATRA) is the mainstay of the treatment for patients with APL, inducing leukemic cell differentiation and remission in patients with t(15;17)/*PML-RARα* or t(5;17)/*NPM-RARα*.[131] Similarly, arsenic trioxide (As_2O_3) has been demonstrated to be effective in the treatment of de novo as well as of ATRA-resistant t(15;17)/*PML-RARα* APL.[132] Current evidence suggests that the combination of ATRA and As_2O_3 may represent an alternative to chemotherapy for the treatment of APL expressing *PML-RARα*.[133] Comparison of gene expression profiles set by *PML-RARα* and *PLZF-RARα* in the absence of ATRA therapy has demonstrated the inhibition of genes involved in DNA repair, repression of myeloid transcriptional regulators, and activation of the WNT–catenin and Jagged–NOTCH pathways, which promote self-renewal of leukemic cells.[134] Interestingly, patients with APL harboring t(15;17)(q22;q11)/*PLZF-RARα* fail to respond to ATRA. Paradoxically, both *PML-RARα* and *PLZF-RARα* contain identical *RAR* sequences and inhibit ATRA-induced gene transcription as well as cell differentiation. Both fusion proteins recruit the nuclear corepressor N-CoR–histone deacetylase complex through the *RARα* CoR box. Although ATRA can induce dissociation of N-CoR from PML-RARα, it does not affect its association with the PLZF-RARα fusion protein, thus resulting in persistent block in gene expression and hematopoietic differentiation.[135] This insensitivity is mediated by the N-terminal PLZF moiety of the chimera. Not surprisingly, histone deacetylase inhibitors antagonize the oncogenic activities of the PML-RARα fusion protein and partially relieve the transcriptional repression by PLZF and the inhibitory effect of PLZF-RARα on ATRA response.[117,135,136] Whereas conditional expression of the PML-RARα protein suppressed the expression of the transcription factor *PU.1,* treatment of APL cell lines and primary leukemic cells with ATRA restored the expression of the transcription factor *PU.1* and induced neutrophil differentiation.[137]

MLL Gene Rearrangements

Mixed-lineage leukemia (MLL), also known as ALL-1, HRX, or HTRX1, is the human homolog of Drosophila TRX and constitutes a maintenance factor for the homeobox (HOX) group of proteins, which are central to cell fate during development and hematopoiesis.[138] The N-terminus of *MLL,* which contains the AT-hook DNA-binding motif and a region homologous to DNA methyltransferase, is always retained in the fusion protein, but the C-terminus, which contains the activation and SET domains, is always replaced by the fusion partner.[139] The *MLL* AT hooks bind to the minor groove of DNA, which facilitates the binding and recruitment of transcription factors to enhancer and promoter elements.[140] This might explain the HOX gene upregulation and transformation detected in leukemia-associated MLL gene rearrangements.

MLL fusion genes can initiate both myeloid and lymphoid leukemogenic programs in primary human hematopoietic cells depending on the identity of the fusion partner, as well as by microenvironmental signals.[141] Most translocation junctions cluster within the 8.3-kb *breakpoint cluster region* (bcr) of the *MLL* gene at chromosome band 11q23.[142] Approximately 4% of patients with de novo AML have balanced translocations or insertions involving the *MLL* gene. *MLL* gene fusions are highly associated with previous therapy with topoisomerase II inhibitors such as etoposide and with the monocytic FAB-subtype M5a. The estimated incidence of this type of rearrangements in secondary treatment-related AML is 2% to 12%.

Similar to other genes involved in the pathogenesis of AML, *MLL* is critical both in embryonic development and in hematopoiesis. Mice lacking the *MLL* gene perish very early during embryonic development,[143,144] and *MLL*$^{(+/-)}$ mice display defects in hematopoiesis, including anemia. In AML, more than 65 different chromosomal regions have been thus far identified as *MLL* fusion partners.[145] All *MLL* rearrangements contain invariably a truncated MLL gene product expressed from its own promoter. For instance, the *MLL-AF9* fusion transcript gives rise to AML when knocked in to the *MLL* locus,[146,147] and *MLL-AF4* can transform primary hematopoietic cells.[148] In addition, some patients with AML present with rearrangements of *MLL* in which *MLL* is not fused with a partner gene but rather is elongated by means of an in-frame partial tandem duplication (*MLL*-PTD) of exons 11-5 or 12-5.[149] *MLL*-PTD occur chiefly in normal karyotype AML or in trisomy 11 and can be identified in 5% to 10% of all AML cases. Approximately 4% to 7% of patients with AML with normal cytogenetics carry *MLL*-PTD, which confers an especially poor prognosis.[150] It has been recently shown that *MLL*-PTD is associated with increased histone H3/H4 acetylation and methylation of H3 Lys4 at *cis*-regulatory *HOXA* sequences, indicating that *MLL* gene rearrangement can directly alter *HOXA* gene expression.[151] AML associated with *MLL* gene rearrangements portends an unfavorable prognosis.

Rearrangements Involving *HOX* Genes

HOX genes are frequently overexpressed in leukemia.[152] Expression of *HOX* genes is tightly regulated during hematopoietic ontogeny. *HOX* genes are expressed in early hematopoietic progenitors but are undetectable in terminally differentiated cells. Gene expression profiling analysis showed that the *HOXA4, HOXA9, HOXA10, PBX3,* and *MEIS1* homeobox genes are coexpressed across diverse cytogenetic groups, suggesting a coregulated pathway with pathogenetic relevance in a subgroup of AML.[153] Deregulation of *HOX* genes occurs in AML by different mechanisms. *HOX* genes are mainly disrupted via chromosomal translocation. For instance, *HOXA9* and *HOXD13* are deregulated through the t(7;11) and t(2;11) translocations, respectively,[154] giving rise to fusion proteins between the HOX protein and the nucleoporin 98 kDa (NUP98) nuclear protein. The NUP98 moiety of HOXA9-NUP98 has transactivating capacity and interacts with the transcriptional coactivator *creb binding protein (CBP)/p300.*[140] HOXA9-NUP98 is predominantly localized to the non-nucleolar portion of the nucleus rather than to the nuclear membrane, which seems to indicate that nucleoporin fusion genes might affect transport of mRNA through the nuclear membrane.[140] Other nucleoporing-containing fusion genes have identified *NUP98* and *NUP214* (also known as *CAN*) fused to *HOXA9, HOXD13, DEK,* and the putative RNA helicase *DDX10*.[140] Overexpression of *HOXA6, HOXA7, HOXA9,* and the HOX cofactor *myeloid ecotropic viral integration site 1 (MEIS1)* has also been correlated with chromosome 11q23 abnormalities involving the MLL protein, which directly regulates the expression of *HOX* genes.[155] The *caudal-type homeobox transcription factor 2 (CDX2),* a *HOX* gene involved in anteroposterior axis definition and intestinal epithelial cell differentiation,[156] is overexpressed in 90% of patients with AML despite its lack of expression in hematopoietic progenitors.[157] *CDX2* overexpression in primary murine hematopoietic progenitors resulted in transplantable AML in vivo, coinciding with a threefold upregulation in *HOXB6* expression,[157] a protein that is overexpressed in 40% of cases of AML with a normal karyotype.[158] This suggests the possibility that *CDX2*-mediated deregulation of *HOX* genes is a major pathway to leukemogenesis. Supporting this hypothesis is the fact that *CDX4* expression is deregulated in 25% of cases of AML.[159]

Mutations in the *C/EBPα* Gene

The *C/EBPα* gene, which encodes the CCAAT/enhancer-binding-protein-α, is a member of the family of leucine zipper (bZIP) transcription factors that couples lineage commitment to terminal differentiation and cell cycle arrest in the process of myeloid differentiation.[160] *C/EBPα* plays a crucial role in regulating the balance between cell proliferation and differentiation.[161,162] It initiates growth arrest through induction of *p21* and by disrupting the E2F transcriptional complexes during the G1 phase of the cell cycle.[163,164] Mutations in the *C/EBPα* gene occur in 15% to 19% of patients with AML and normal cytogenetics.[165-167] The latter consist of either in-frame C-terminal mutations in the bZIP domain that mediates DNA binding and homo- and heterodimerization with other CEBP proteins or N-terminal nonsense mutations that result in premature termination of the *C/EBPα* protein and lead to complete loss of *C/EPBα* function owing to the dominant negative inhibition of wild type *C/EBPα*–DNA binding and transactivation.[160] *C/EBPα* mutations increase the capacity of BM myeloid progenitors to proliferate and predispose mice to a granulocytic myeloproliferative disorder and transformation of the myeloid compartment of the BM.[165] It has been shown that *FLT3* mutations in human AML inhibit the function of *C/EBPα* by ERK1/2-mediated phosphorylation, which may explain the differentiation block of leukemic blasts.[168] Patients harboring *C/EBPα* mutations present with higher percentages of peripheral blood blasts, lower platelet counts, and less frequent extramedullary involvement and are less likely to carry the deleterious *FLT3* and *MLL-PTD* mutations.[166] In the absence of specific *C/EBPα* mutations, decreased expression may serve as an alternative mechanism that disrupts *C/EBPα* gene function. For example, *AML1-ETO* appears to indirectly suppress *C/EBPα* expression by inhibiting positive autoregulation of the *C/EBPα* promoter.[169] In fact, patients with AML and t(8;21) have up to sixfold less *C/EBPα* mRNA than patients with AML and a normal karyotype.[169] Conditional expression of *C/EBPα* in *AML1-ETO*-positive AML cell lines results in neutrophilic differentiation.[169] Importantly, *C/EBPα* mutations have been shown to be associated with a favorable prognosis in patients in the cytogenetic intermediate-risk category and may improve risk stratification in patients with normal cytogenetics.[166,167]

Mutations in the *PU.1* Gene

The transcription factor PU.1 encoded by the *Sfpi1* (spleen focus-forming virus proviral integration) gene is indispensable for myelomonocytic differentiation during normal hematopoiesis[170] and for regulating the commitment of multipotent hematopoietic progenitors.[171] Aberrant levels of expression of PU.1 are leukemogenic. Transcriptional control of *Sfpi1* gene expression is regulated by a distal upstream regulatory element (URE) that is highly conserved.[172] Knock-out of URE reduces expression of *PU.1* by 80% in the BM and leads to the development of AML in mice.[173] This suggests that reduced PU.1 levels are sufficient to support the survival of myeloid progenitors but not to sustain their differentiation, possibly because of deregulation of the expression of some cytokine receptors.[173] Interestingly, the course of AML in mice after knockdown of *PU.1* includes a preleukemic stage during which immature myelomonocytic precursors accumulate in the BM followed by a leukemic phase with elevated leukemic blasts in peripheral blood.[173] Repressed *PU.1* transcription has been reported in AML expressing *PML-RARα*[137] or internal tandem duplication *FLT3 (FLT3-ITD)* mutations,[174] and *AML1-ETO* functionally inactivates PU.1 by displacing its coactivator JUN. By means of genome-wide transcriptional analysis of hematopoietic stem cells isolated from mice in which *PU.1* was knocked down at the preleukemic stage, it has been shown that the transcription factors *c-JUN* and *JUNB* were among the top-downregulated targets.[175] Restoration of *c-JUN* expression in preleukemic cells rescued the *PU.1* knockdown-initiated myelomonocytic differentiation block, but restoration of *JUNB* led to loss of leukemic self-renewal capacity and abrogated the development of AML in NOD/SCID (nonobese nondiabetic/severe combined immune deficient) mice transplanted with leukemic *PU.1*-knockdown cells.[175] Despite of the evident leukemogenic potential of deregulated *PU.1*, mutations in this transcription factor have been rarely found in human AML.[176-178]

Mutations Altering Signal Transduction

Mutations of the Fms-Related Tyrosine Kinase 3 Gene

The *FLT3* gene locates to chromosome band 13q12 and encodes a membrane-bound structurally related to other class III tyrosine kinase receptors such as KIT, FMS, and platelet-derived growth factor receptor (PDGFR).[179] In the BM, FLT3 expression is restricted to CD34$^+$ cells and a subset of dendritic precursors, where it regulates proliferation, differentiation, and apoptosis of hematopoietic cell progenitors.[179] A series of models has investigated the role of FLT3 signaling in leukemogenesis. Retroviral transfection of primary murine BM cells with mutant *FLT3* fails to cause leukemia in mice but results in an oligoclonal fatal myeloproliferative disease after a latency period.[180,181] Internal tandem duplication (ITD) of the *FLT3* gene, occurring within the *FLT3* juxtamembrane domain (exons 14 and 15), is among the most prevalent mutations detected in patients with AML and normal karyotype, being detected in about 30% of cases.[182-184] Moreover, 7% of patients with AML harbor missense point mutations affecting the activation loop of the tyrosine kinase domain of FLT3 coded by exon 20.[182-184] A variety of kinase domain mutations have been reported. Most are point mutations such as substitution of aspartate residue 835 with a tyrosine (D835Y, which is the most frequent mutation), histidine, valine, or glutamate. Alternatively, other mutations include small deletions (Δ835, Δ836) and insertions. Evidence suggests that *FLT3* mutations occur in leukemic stem cells. In fact, 84% of patients with AML carrying *FLT3-ITD* mutations exhibit the same mutation at relapse.[185] Both *FLT3-ITD* and *FLT3* kinase domain mutations give rise to a constitutively active FLT3 protein that promotes ligand-independent proliferation and survival of leukemic cells.[184] Oncogenic activation of *FLT3-ITD* mutations activates aberrant signaling, including STAT5, and repression of myeloid transcription factors such as *PU.1* and *C/EBPα*.[186] In addition to STAT5, FLT3 signals through the PI3K/AKT and the mitogen-activated protein kinase (MAPK) pathways.[187] Interestingly, *FLT3-ITD* mutations collaborate with *AML1-ETO* in inducing acute leukemia in a murine BM transplantation model.[188] Patients carrying *FLT3* gene mutations have been largely associated with worse prognosis than those carrying wild type *FLT3*.[182,187,189,190] Small-molecule TKIs directed against the constitutively activated FLT3 protein such as PKC412,[191] lestaurtinib,[192] sorafenib,[193] or tandutinib[194] have shown encouraging results in early clinical trials, although complete responses have been rarely achieved. Further development of these agents must be pursued in combinatorial approaches including standard chemotherapy.

Mutations of the *KIT* Gene

The *KIT* gene, located at chromosome band 4q11-12, encodes a 145-kDa transmembrane receptor tyrosine kinase of the type III subgroup.[195] Structurally, the KIT protein is characterized by five immunoglobulin-like domains in the extracellular portion of the receptor, a transmembrane and juxtamembrane domains, and an intracellular kinase domain.[195] KIT is expressed in hematopoietic stem cells as well as in mast cells, germ cells, melanocytes, and interstitial cells of Cajal, among others.[195] Upon binding of the ligand stem cell factor (SCF) to the extracellular immunoglobulin-like domains, KIT undergoes homodimerization and autophosphorylation at the Y568 and Y570 tyrosine residues of the juxtamembrane domain, which activates downstream signaling pathways involved in proliferation, differentiation, and survival.[195] Gain-of-function point mutations in the kinase domain of KIT result in ligand-independent constitutive activation of KIT signaling, which leads to uncontrolled cell proliferation and resistance to apoptosis.[196] Activation of the KIT tyrosine kinase by somatic mutation has been documented in a variety of human malignancies, including CBF AML, systemic mastocytosis, and gastrointestinal stromal tumors.[197-199] In AML, most *KIT* mutations cluster within exon 17, which encodes the KIT activation loop (A-loop) in the kinase domain, and in exon 8,[197,200-203] which encodes a highly conserved region in the extracellular portion of the KIT receptor, which is believed to play a role in receptor dimerization.[204] Interestingly, *KIT* mutations at exon 17 in patients with inv(16) occur exclusively at codon D816,[197,201] but in patients with t(8;21), they map primarily to codons D816 or N822.[197] *KIT* mutations confer a higher risk of relapse in patients with CBF AML.[197] Akin to other mutations of genes encoding tyrosine kinases in AML, such as *FLT3 ITD*, gain-of-function *KIT* mutations may serve as a target for TKIs. Indeed, variable responses to imatinib administered both as single-agent or in combination with other chemotherapeutics have been reported in CBF AML with *KIT* mutations at exon 8, but patients with *KIT D816* mutations did not show any response.[205] In vitro studies have shown that *KIT D816* mutations can be effectively targeted with TKIs such as PKC412[206] or dasatinib.[207] The activity of these agents warrants further investigation in clinical trials of patients with CBF AML harboring *KIT* mutations.

Mutations of the *RAS* Gene

RAS oncogenes encode a family of membrane-associated proteins that regulate signal transduction by binding to a variety of membrane receptors. In so doing, RAS proteins play important roles in the regulatory processes of proliferation, differentiation, and apoptosis. Abnormalities in *RAS* genes have been implicated in the pathogenesis of AML.[208] Mutations in all *RAS* gene homologs, *NRAS, KRAS,* and *HRAS,* take place at codons 12, 13, and 61. All RAS proteins possess a consensus guanosine triphosphate (GTP) binding motif that critical for intracellular signaling.[209] The RAS proteins oscillate between a GTP- and a guanosine diphosphate (GDP)–bound state. GDP-bound RAS is incapable of activating signal transduction pathways.[209,210] *NRAS* mutations appear to be the most frequent *RAS* mutations in patients with AML, being detected in 10% to 30% of patients.[122,208,209,211] Mutated RAS proteins are constitutively activated, which is held in their GTP-bound status. *NRAS* rapidly and efficiently induced an AML-like disorder in a mouse BM transduction and transplantation model, indicating that mutated *NRAS* can function as an initiating oncogene in the induction of myeloid malignancies.[212] Despite the potential implication of *NRAS* mutations in AML pathogenesis, their prognostic impact in AML remains controversial, with some studies associating the presence of these mutations with a poor prognosis[213,214]; others suggesting a favorable prognosis[215]; and some others in which the prognostic impact of *NRAS* mutations was neutral for overall survival, event-free survival, or disease-free survival.[122,123,211]

RAS may represent a potential therapeutic target in AML. Farnesyl transferase inhibitors (FTIs) constitute a class of drugs that targets the farnesylation of RAS proteins (required for the attachment of this protein to the plasma membrane).[216] This posttranslational modification is critical for RAS-mediated cell transformation.[217] However, the nonpeptidomimetic FTI tipifarnib used in combination with standard idarubicin and cytarabine induction chemotherapy has not improved the results compared with historical control participants in a recently reported study.[218]

Other Genetic Events Implicated in the Pathogenesis of Acute Myeloid Leukemia

Mutations of the Nucleophosmin Gene

The *nucleophosmin member 1 (NPM1)* gene located at chromosome band 5q35, encodes a nucleus-cytoplasm shuttling protein implicated in preventing nucleolar protein aggregation, regulation of ribosomal protein assembly, initiation of centrosome duplication, and regulation of the oncosuppressors *p53* and *p19ARF* and their partners (i.e., HDM2/MDM2).[219,220] The mechanisms whereby *NPM1* is involved in leukemogenesis have not been elucidated yet. *NPM1* is involved in control of primitive hematopoiesis, and *NPM1* is haploinsufficient for the control of proper centrosome duplication, resulting in genomic instability that results in a syndrome reminiscent of human myelodysplasia. The NPM1 protein regulates the ARF-p53 tumor-suppressor pathway.[221] Translocations involving the *NPM* gene cause cytoplasmic dislocation of the NPM protein. Mutations of *NPM1* result in the shift of the NPM1 protein into the cytoplasm and constitute the most frequent genetic aberration found in AML with normal karyotype.[220,221] Given that NPM1 is thought to have a tumor-suppressor function, alterations in its subcellular localization from the nucleus to the cytoplasm may be crucial for malignant transformation.[221] *NPM1* mutations are found in approximately 35% of adult patients with primary AML (excluding PML) and have been linked to a higher complete remission rate after induction chemotherapy.[221] Most of the cases (60%-80%) carrying a mutant *NPM1* gene correspond to patients with AML and normal karyotype.[221] A polymorphism of nucleotide T deletion at position 1146 in the *NPM1* 3′-untranslated region has been reported in 60% to 70% of patients with AML and in healthy volunteers.[222,223] *NPM1* mutations are typically heterozygous, and except for anecdotal cases involving the splicing donor site of *NPM1* exon 9 and exon 11, most mutations are restricted to exon 12.[221,224,225] The most common *NPM1* mutation is a duplication of a TCTG tetranucleotide at position 956 to 959 and accounts for 75% to 80% of cases.[220,225] Interestingly, *FLT3-ITD* mutations were seen twice as often in patients with mutated *NPM1* as in cases with wild type *NPM1,* suggesting a possible mechanistic link between *FLT3* and *NPM1* mutations.[220-222] Because immunohistochemical detection of cytoplasmic *NPM1* is predictive of *NPM1* mutations in AML[226] and these are associated with a better prognosis, the detection of NPM1 mutations may represent a valuable tool both for outcome prediction as well as for monitoring of minimal residual disease. Although NPM1 represents an attractive therapeutic target, the pharmacologic inhibition of this protein might be difficult given the fact that *NPM1* can function both as an oncogene and a tumor-suppressor gene,[219] depending on gene dosage, expression levels, interacting partners, and compartmentalization. In fact, partial functional loss and aberrant overexpression of *NPM1* both lead, through separate mechanisms, to abnormal cell growth.[219,220] The development of adequate experimental animal models of *NPM1*-positive AML will be critical to further ascertain the role of *NPM1* in the pathogenesis of AML and to test the efficacy of novel agents targeting NPM1.

Overexpression of the *BAALC* and *ERG* Genes

High expression of the brain and acute leukemia, cytoplasmic *(BAALC)* gene can be found in some patients with AML. Overexpression of *BAALC* mRNA in peripheral blood blasts has been shown to portend an adverse clinical outcome in patients younger than 60 years of age.[227] These have been confirmed in several independent studies. In one study, 307 patients younger than 60 years of age with AML and normal karyotype were analyzed.[190] BAALC overexpression predicted for failure to achieve complete response, primary resistant disease, and a remarkably shorter overall survival.[190] Results of another study suggested that high *BAALC* expression may represent a prognostic marker that is particularly useful in AML with normal karyotype lacking *FLT3*-ITD and *C/EBPα* mutations.[167]

The v-ets erythroblastosis virus E26 oncogene homolog (avian) *(ERG)* gene maps to chromosome band 21q22 and is involved in regulating and promoting cell differentiation, proliferation, and tissue invasion.[228] In one study, 84 patients with AML and a normal karyotype were analyzed for *ERG* expression using real-time polymerase chain reaction.[229] Patients with the highest *ERG* expression levels had a worse cumulative incidence of relapse than those with low expression ($P < .001$). Whereas in patients with low *ERG* expression, the median survival had not been reached and the estimated 5-year survival was 51%, those with high *ERG* expression had an overall survival time of 1 to 2 years and an estimated 5-year rate survival of 19%. Interestingly, the adverse impact on overall survival conferred by high *ERG* expression was only observed in patients with low *BAALC* expression.[229]

In addition, mutations in IDH1 and IDH2,[230-232] ASXL1,[233] and DNMT 3A[234] have been reported.

Spliceosome Mutations

Alternatively spliced transcriptional isoforms are commonly found in the transcriptome of neoplastic cells, which often express specific transcripts that confer some survival advantage. But almost all genes are multi-exonic, and 95% of eukaryotic multi-exonic genes are alternatively spliced using the highly conserved splicing machinery that consists of small nuclear ribonucleoproteins (snRNPs) or associated protein factors. A spliceosome is a complex of snRNA and protein subunits that removes introns from a transcribed pre-mRNA (hnRNA) segment. Each spliceosome is composed of five small nuclear RNAs (snRNAs) and a range of associated protein factors. It catalyzes the removal of introns and the ligation of the flanking exons. Surprisingly, cancer-associated alternative splicing is not only the consequence of cis-acting DNA mutations in intron–exon boundary recognition sites, but recent next-generation sequencing projects have identified frequent somatic mutations in core splicing components in MDS[235,236] and secondary AML.[237] Eight different splicing component mutations have been identified (U2AF35, SF3B1, SRSF2, ZRSR2, SF3A1, PRP40B, SF1, and U2AF65); they are heterozygous and usually mutually exclusive.[235] Their overall frequency is 45% to 85%, and the most frequently abnormal gene, *SF3B1,* is mutated in up to 85% of refractory anemia with ring sideroblasts (RARS).[236] SRSF2 is mutated in 30% of CMML. Acquired mutations in these splicing factors are also found in chronic lymphocytic leukemia (9%-14%), myeloproliferative neoplasms, and de novo AML.[237,238] Interestingly, mutations in SF3B1 and DNMT3A, which encode a DNA methyltransferase, appear to co-associate.[238]

A recent report[239] of genome-wide analysis of alternative splicing in 81 AML and selected analysis in 193 AMLs found that alternative splicing is a common event involving many genes in any given patient. NOTCH2-Va (74 %), FLT3-Va (50 %), and CD13-Va (60 %) were the most frequently expressed variants in AML and NOTCH2-Va expression was negatively associated with overall survival ($P = .008$).

The molecular and biologic consequences of these mutations are not at all clear; early results are contradictory. Likewise, the potential of these splice variants as therapeutic targets has not yet been sufficiently explored.

FUTURE DIRECTIONS

Significant advances have been made over the past decades regarding the understanding of the mechanisms involved in the pathogenesis of myeloid leukemias. Most of this knowledge has been derived from the constant refinement of genetically engineered murine models of leukemia. These models have been particularly fruitful to demonstrate the multistep nature of the leukemogenic process based on the cooperation of a diversity of genetic abnormalities necessary for the development of human leukemias. A better understanding of the molecular underpinnings of myeloid leukemia has provided the opportunity to identify therapeutic targets. The development of targeted therapies against myeloid malignancies is epitomized by the remarkable success of the small-molecule kinase inhibitor imatinib mesylate in patients with CML. The main pathogenetic driver in CML can be ascribed to a single molecular defect, the BCR-ABL kinase. This has facilitated the development of a highly effective targeted agent such as imatinib, which constitutes the current standard for the treatment of CML. However, most patients receiving imatinib still harbor measurable amounts of residual leukemic cells, indicating that single-agent therapy with this TKI may not cure CML. It is likely that the complete eradication of leukemic cells in CML will be accomplished by using combinatorial approaches. In addition, a significant percentage of patients will develop mutations within the kinase domain of *ABL1* that will hinder the binding of imatinib and other small molecule inhibitors. Both nilotinib and dasatinib, second-generation ABL kinase inhibitors, have proven efficacious against most clinically relevant mutants, with the exception of T315I. Several agents, such as Aurora kinase inhibitors and JAK2, are currently under clinical development based on their in vitro activity against this mutation. Importantly, unlike patients with CML in CP, neither imatinib nor the potent second-generation TKIs nilotinib or dasatinib has proved effective in CML-BP, a condition that displays molecular features reminiscent of those of AML.

In AML, the discovery that mutation-induced deregulation of several tyrosine kinase receptors (e.g., KIT, FLT3) provides a survival and proliferative advantage to AML cells has opened the avenue of targeted therapies in this disease. The currently available agents directed against these kinases have produced short-lived responses. This is most likely because AML results from the alteration of multiple key elements in the homeostasis of the myeloid progenitors. A better understanding of the molecular pathways downstream of each of the oncogenes involved in the pathogenesis of AML will help extend the concept of targeted therapy of this disorder beyond the isolated paradigm that constitutes the success of ATRA therapy in patients with PML expressing *PML-RARα*. The efficacy of ATRA and arsenic trioxide in PML not only conveys the hope that therapy for other types of AML may diverge from the current practice of administration of cytotoxic agents but also underscores the therapeutic potential of targeting transcription factors for the treatment of AML. Translocation-generated oncogenic fusion proteins involving transcription factors are truly "tumor-specific" and as such provide novel targets for therapy. However, designing therapeutic modalities aimed at modulating transcription factors remains challenging. Several strategies deserve consideration, including (1) chimeric peptides that by binding both a transcription factor and a target DNA sequence can displace fusion oncoproteins away from proliferation-inducing genes,[240] (2) fusion proteins such as Tat-HoxB4 that allow entry of drugs into the cell nucleus to change the cellular phenotype,[241] and (3) reexpression of silenced genes by introducing large regulatory DNA sequences.[242] To further develop these strategies, it will be necessary to gain better insight of the early events of the leukemogenic process and into the biology of leukemia stem cells.

Finally, a mutagenic role of the very chemotherapy used to induce patients into remissions has been reported.[243] Hence, certain molecular changes observed at relapse may be induced by different antileukemic therapies, emphasizing the need for nongenotoxic therapies.[244,245]

SUGGESTED READINGS

Abelson HT, Rabstein LS: Lymphosarcoma: Virus-induced thymic-independent disease in mice. *Cancer Res* 30:2213, 1970.

Bartram CR, de Klein A, Hagemeijer A, et al: Translocation of c-abl oncogene correlates with the presence of a Philadelphia chromosome in chronic myelocytic leukaemia. *Nature* 306:277, 1983.

Bernards A, Rubin CM, Westbrook CA, et al: The first intron in the human c-abl gene is at least 200 kilobases long and is a target for translocations in chronic myelogenous leukemia. *Mol Cell Biol* 7:3231, 1987.

Daley GQ, Van Etten RA, Baltimore D: Induction of chronic myelogenous leukemia in mice by the P210bcr/abl gene of the Philadelphia chromosome. *Science* 247:824, 1990.

Druker BJ, Guilhot F, O'Brien SG, et al: Five-year follow-up of patients receiving imatinib for chronic myeloid leukemia. *N Engl J Med* 355:2408, 2006.

Druker BJ, Sawyers CL, Kantarjian H, et al: Activity of a specific inhibitor of the BCR-ABL tyrosine kinase in the blast crisis of chronic myeloid leukemia and acute lymphoblastic leukemia with the Philadelphia chromosome. *N Engl J Med* 344:1038, 2001.

Faderl S, Talpaz M, Estrov Z, et al: The biology of chronic myeloid leukemia. *N Engl J Med* 341:164, 1999.

Feller SM, Knudsen B, Hanafusa H: c-Abl kinase regulates the protein binding activity of c-Crk. *Embo J* 13:2341, 1994.

Groffen J, Stephenson JR, Heisterkamp N, et al: Philadelphia chromosomal breakpoints are clustered within a limited region, bcr, on chromosome 22. *Cell* 36:93, 1984.

Hantschel O, Superti-Furga G: Regulation of the c-Abl and Bcr-Abl tyrosine kinases. *Nat Rev Mol Cell Biol* 5:33, 2004.

Heisterkamp N, Jenster G, ten Hoeve J, et al: Acute leukaemia in bcr/abl transgenic mice. *Nature* 344:251, 1990.

Huntly BJ, Shigematsu H, Deguchi K, et al: MOZ-TIF2, but not BCR-ABL, confers properties of leukemic stem cells to committed murine hematopoietic progenitors. *Cancer Cell* 6:587, 2004.

Kelliher MA, McLaughlin J, Witte ON, et al: Induction of a chronic myelogenous leukemia-like syndrome in mice with v-abl and BCR/ABL. *Proc Natl Acad Sci U S A* 87:6649, 1990.

Laneuville P: Abl tyrosine protein kinase. *Semin Immunol* 7:255, 1995.

Look AT: Oncogenic transcription factors in the human acute leukemias. *Science* 278:1059, 1997.

Lugo TG, Pendergast AM, Muller AJ, et al: Tyrosine kinase activity and transformation potency of bcr-abl oncogene products. *Science* 247:1079, 1990.

McCormack E, Bruserud O, Gjertsen BT: Animal models of acute myelogenous leukaemia: Development, application and future perspectives. *Leukemia* 19:687, 2005.

Melo JV: The diversity of BCR-ABL fusion proteins and their relationship to leukemia phenotype. *Blood* 88:2375, 1996.

Nowell P, Hungerford DA: A minute chromosome in human chronic granulocytic leukemia. *Science* 132:1497, 1960.

Pane F, Frigeri F, Sindona M, et al: Neutrophilic-chronic myeloid leukemia: A distinct disease with a specific molecular marker (BCR/ABL with C3/A2 junction). *Blood* 88:2410, 1996.

Quackenbush RC, Reuther GW, Miller JP, et al: Analysis of the biologic properties of p230 Bcr-Abl reveals unique and overlapping properties with the oncogenic p185 and p210 Bcr-Abl tyrosine kinases. *Blood* 95:2913, 2000.

Ramaraj P, Singh H, Niu N, et al: Effect of mutational inactivation of tyrosine kinase activity on BCR/ABL-induced abnormalities in cell growth and adhesion in human hematopoietic progenitors. *Cancer Res* 64:5322, 2004.

Ravandi F, Cortes J, Albitar M, et al: Chronic myelogenous leukaemia with p185(BCR/ABL) expression: Characteristics and clinical significance. *Br J Haematol* 107:581, 1999.

Ren R: Mechanisms of BCR-ABL in the pathogenesis of chronic myelogenous leukaemia. *Nat Rev Cancer* 5:172, 2005.

Rowley JD: Letter: A new consistent chromosomal abnormality in chronic myelogenous leukaemia identified by quinacrine fluorescence and Giemsa staining. *Nature* 243:290, 1973.

Shivdasani RA, Orkin SH: The transcriptional control of hematopoiesis. *Blood* 87:4025, 1996.

Sokal JE, Baccarani M, Russo D, et al: Staging and prognosis in chronic myelogenous leukemia. *Semin Hematol* 25:49, 1988.

Sokal JE, Baccarani M, Tura S, et al: Prognostic discrimination among younger patients with chronic granulocytic leukemia: Relevance to bone marrow transplantation. *Blood* 66:1352, 1985.

Zhang X, Ren R: Bcr-Abl efficiently induces a myeloproliferative disease and production of excess interleukin-3 and granulocyte-macrophage colony-stimulating factor in mice: A novel model for chronic myelogenous leukemia. *Blood* 92:3829, 1998.

Zhao RC, Jiang Y, Verfaillie CM: A model of human p210(bcr/ABL)-mediated chronic myelogenous leukemia by transduction of primary normal human CD34(+) cells with a BCR/ABL-containing retroviral vector. *Blood* 97:2406, 2001.

For complete list of references log on to www.expertconsult.com.

CHAPTER 58

CLINICAL MANIFESTATIONS AND TREATMENT OF ACUTE MYELOID LEUKEMIA

Stefan Faderl and Hagop M. Kantarjian

Acute myeloid leukemia (AML) is a rare hematopoietic neoplasm of mainly older patients. About 12,000 persons are diagnosed with AML in the United States each year. Whereas the overall age-adjusted incidence rate is 3.4 per 100,000 persons, it is as low as less than 2 per 100,000 for people under 65 years to greater than 15 per 100,000 for those 65 years or older. About 9000 patients are expected to die each year with AML. Its high malignant potential, rapid progression, universally fatal outcome if left unattended to, and challenging clinical course continue to focus a high level of interest.

There has been a constant evolution of the understanding of many aspects of the biology of AML as it relates to blasts and their interactions with and interdependence on the microenvironment. Identification of molecular abnormalities has led to a reappraisal of the heterogeneity of AML.[1] That cytogenetic-molecular classifications have important practical implications and determine therapy is evident in the case of acute promyelocytic leukemia (APL), where differentiation therapy even in the absence of chemotherapy is highly effective. On the other hand, the so-called core binding factor (CBF) leukemias are exquisitely sensitive to cytarabine. Following identification of pathophysiologically relevant signaling pathways, numerous small molecules and other drugs are being developed for targeting these pathways. Despite recent progress, the essentials of AML therapy have not changed much in three decades and remain rooted in cytarabine/anthracycline combinations during induction followed by postremission therapy with either chemotherapy or stem cell transplant.[2] Challenges ahead include (1) identification of molecularly defined subgroups, (2) development of more powerful and specific targeted small-molecule inhibitors, (3) combination of new drugs with established treatments, and (4) definition of the best therapeutic approach for older patients.

PRESENTATION OF ACUTE MYELOID LEUKEMIA AT DIAGNOSIS

The signs and symptoms of AML mostly reflect the predominant cytopenias. With the exception of patients who have a history of an antecedent hematologic disorder such as a myelodysplastic syndrome (MDS), patients present with a short history (1 to 8 weeks) of constitutional complaints (fatigue, lack of energy, malaise, profuse sweats), manifestations of bleeding (such as from gums, bruising in the skin, epistaxis, menorrhagia), and fevers. Fevers should always be presumed to be secondary to infections even in the absence of an identifiable focus and lead to rapid institution of antibiotic therapy. "Tumor fever" is uncommon and remains a diagnosis of exclusion. Extramedullary infiltrations of leukemia cells in the gingiva, skin, lymph nodes, or other organs occur occasionally. Bone pains are infrequent even with excessive leukocytosis and should raise the suspicion of an acute lymphoblastic leukemia (ALL), especially in children. Likewise, signs and symptoms referable to central nervous system (CNS) involvement (cranial nerve defects and other focal neurologic abnormalities, mental status changes, seizure activity) are rare with the exception of AML with monocytic/monoblastic differentiation.

Given the nonspecific nature of the presenting symptoms, the physical examination elicits a variety of findings that in their aggregate can lead to a correct suspicion of the diagnosis of acute leukemia, but it is impossible to distinguish AML from ALL by the clinical presentation or examination findings alone. Patients may present with pallor, ecchymoses or petechiae, enlargement of lymph nodes, or rarely, hepatosplenomegaly. Examination of the lungs may reveal signs of symptoms of an infectious process. Some patients with AML will have no abnormal findings at physical examination.

The laboratory evaluation should include blood counts with evaluation of the blood smear, a standard chemistry panel (electrolytes, urea nitrogen, creatinine, total bilirubin, transaminases, uric acid, lactate dehydrogenase [LDH]), and coagulation studies, including prothrombin time (PT), partial thromboplastin time (PTT), and fibrinogen levels. Anemia and thrombocytopenia are universal. The white blood cell count (WBC) can vary from low to high but will range from 5000/μL to 100,000/μL in most patients. The highest WBC numbers are seen in myelomonocytic leukemias. A WBC exceeding 100,000/μL is considered an emergency, which requires immediate efforts to reduce the disease burden (e.g., leukapheresis, chemotherapy) because leukostasis may ensue in several vascular beds with potentially catastrophic consequences. However, there is not always a good correlation of the aggressiveness of the AML with the elevation of the WBC, and far lower WBC levels may elicit life-threatening symptoms. The WBC should therefore be assessed in the context of the patient's overall physical condition and other clinical and laboratory abnormalities (e.g., LDH, uric acid). Disseminated intravascular coagulation (DIC) is often seen in patients with myelomonocytic AML, APL, and any high-WBC AML in general. PT, PTT, and fibrinogen levels should be carefully followed. Subclinical DIC is common in other forms of AML as well. Abnormalities of renal and hepatic values may represent infiltration of these organs, even if subclinical.

Imaging studies are of little help in diagnosis but allow assessment of complications (pneumonia, cerebral bleed). At a minimum a chest x-ray examination is warranted. In view of findings of any neurologic deficit at presentation, the threshold for noncontrast computed tomography (CT) scan of the brain should be low. Further evaluations should be based on the clinical assessment of the patients.

CLASSIFICATION OF ACUTE MYELOID LEUKEMIA AND PROGNOSTIC FACTORS

The first systematic attempt to classify AML goes back to the French-American-British (FAB) group, which described subtypes mainly based on blast percentage, degree of differentiation, and on lineage involvement, which relied mainly on cytochemistry and then later on immunophenotype. The diagnostic algorithm now includes a morphologic assessment (including application of stains and cytochemical reactions), immunophenotyping by flow cytometry, and assessment of karyotype and molecular studies (Fig. 58-1).

Blast percentage is best determined on a 500-cell differential of the marrow aspirate. Three broad types of myeloblasts have been defined within the FAB classification and are essentially based on the granular content and nuclear features of the blasts (type 1: agranular basophilic cytoplasm, nucleus with fine chromatin and two to four distinct nucleoli; type 2: basophilic cytoplasm with 20 or fewer

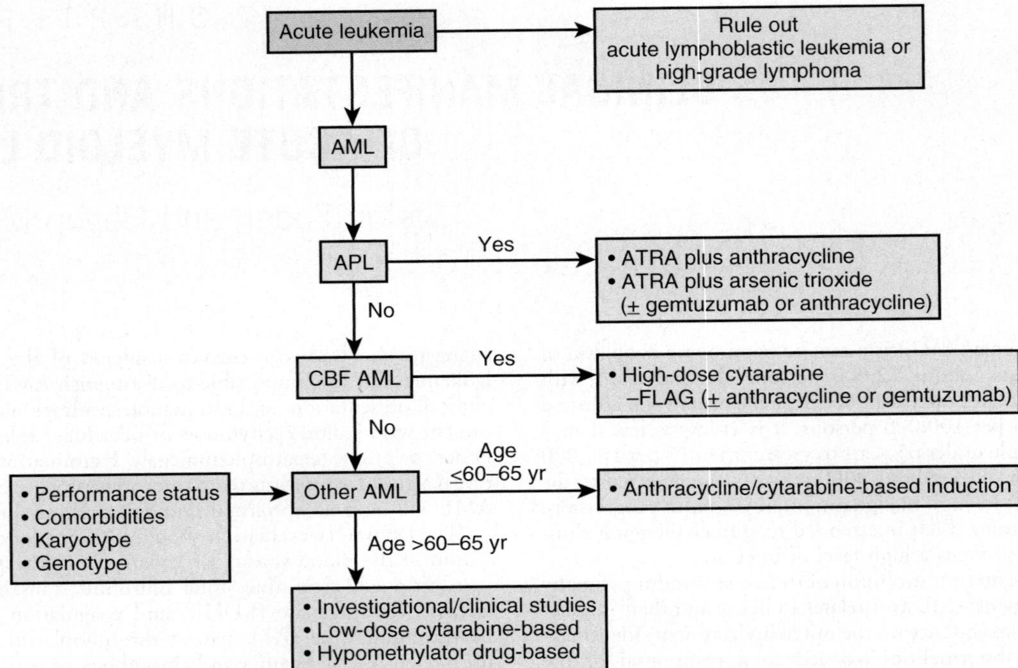

Figure 58-1 DIAGNOSTIC ALGORITHM OF ACUTE MYELOID LEUKEMIA (AML). The diagnostic workup consists of a morphologic assessment (including application of stains), immunophenotyping by flow cytometry, and assessment of the karyotype. Whereas morphologic assessment by itself is often not specific enough (including use of special stains), flow cytometry is nowadays always required to confirm the lineage assignment (myeloid versus lymphoid) and stage of differentiation. In more than 95% of cases, a lineage can thus be assigned to the blast phenotype. In only a few cases, no lineage-specific antigens are expressed (acute undifferentiated leukemia) or antigens of more than one lineage are present (mixed-phenotype acute leukemia). In the latter scenario, antigens of several lineages can be found on one blast population (biphenotypic) or several types of blasts, each expressing a more or less lineage-specific set of antigens (bilineal) can be detected. Karyotyping may add additional diagnostic information in some of those morphologically ambiguous situations but is far more useful prognostically in most other patients. The combined assessment applying the aforementioned methods, including information from the patient's prior history (exposure to previous chemotherapy agents and/or radiation therapy), forms the basis for the classification of AML, according to the World Health Organization system as per its most recent revision in 2008 (see Table 58-1). *MPO,* Myeloperoxidase; *WHO,* World Health Organization.

azurophilic granules and similar nuclear features as type 1 blasts; type 3: basophilic cytoplasm with more than 20 azurophilic granules), although the morphologic features of blasts are even more varied (Fig. 58-2). Promyelocytes have moderately basophilic cytoplasm with numerous azurophilic granules, and monoblasts and promonocytes usually exhibit folded/convoluted nuclei and may contain prominent acidophilic nucleoli. Promyelocytes, promonocytes, and atypical pronormoblasts may be considered as blast equivalents in some defined AML subgroups (APL, acute monoblastic leukemia, and acute erythroleukemia, pure erythroid type). Micromegakaryocytes and pronormoblasts are not considered blasts (see Fig. 58-2). Auer rods are rod-like filaments of aggregated primary granules that are found in 30% to 50% of newly diagnosed patients with AML and if present are one of the hallmark morphologic features to establish a diagnosis of AML (see Fig. 58-2, *C*) . AML marrows are typically hypercellular with decreased or absent megakaryocytes. Exceptions, however, exist. Samples of marrows of older patients or those with therapy-related AML may be hypocellular and include dysplastic changes of one or several blood lineages. Prominent dysplasia may suggest a previous diagnosis of MDS but can also be found in patients with de novo AML, where the prognostic significance of dysplastic changes is far less clear. Cases with extensive fibrosis may represent a preceding myeloproliferative disorder or acute megakaryocytic leukemia.

Several cytochemical reactions are in use to further highlight morphologic characteristics (myeloperoxidase [MPO], periodic acid–Schiff, Sudan black B, naphthol AS-D chloroacetate esterase [specific esterase], α-naphthyl acetate/butyrate esterases [nonspecific esterases], acid phosphatase) (Fig. 58-3). Among those, MPO is the most specific granulocytic marker, and the presence of MPO in at least 3% of the blasts is consistent with a diagnosis of AML. Absence of MPO staining does not rule out the possibility of AML because it is typically not present in AML with minimal differentiation, acute monoblastic leukemia, and acute megakaryocytic leukemia. Monoblastic leukemias are stained by nonspecific esterases. Whereas the MPO reaction is relatively uncomplicated and results are available quickly, this is not the case with most of the other cytochemical reactions, and their diagnostic utility is therefore often outdone by immunophenotyping by flow cytometry.

The limited scope of the FAB system became inadequate in view of rapidly growing information from cytogenetic-molecular abnormalities, their association with prognosis, and, in some cases, prediction of response to therapy. Although the hallmark of the diagnostic workup of AML remains a thorough assessment of Wright or Wright-Giemsa–stained blood and marrow smears, cytochemistry, and evaluation of the immunophenotype, cytogenetic-molecular markers are rapidly becoming the defining features of AML subtypes. The most recent World Health Organization (WHO) classification of AML primarily incorporates karyotype and genetic abnormalities together with morphologic descriptions related to dysplasia-related changes and remnants of the FAB system and information regarding exposure to prior chemotherapy and/or radiation therapy (Table 58-1).

The 2008 WHO classification divides AML into a number of broad categories. The first is AML with recurrent genetic abnormalities. This includes AML with relatively common genetic and cytogenetic changes: AML with t(8;21)(q22;q22), RUNX1-RUNX1T1 (Fig. 58-4); AML with inv(16)(p13.1q22) or t(16;16)(p13.1;q22),

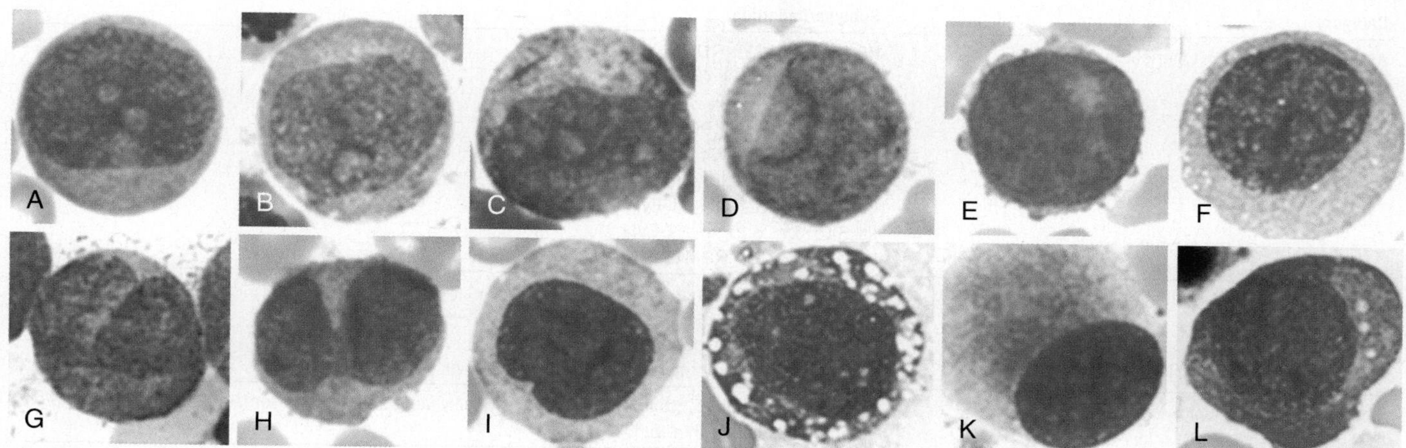

Figure 58-2 SPECTRUM OF BLASTS, BLAST EQUIVALENTS, AND OTHER CELLS. Blast cells in acute myeloid leukemia (AML) exhibit a wide spectrum of morphologic features. Initially, according to the French-American-British classification, there were three types of blasts depending on the granule content **(A** to **C).** However, blasts with nuclear invagination (frequently associated with NPM and/or Flt-3 mutations) **(D),** blasts with pseudopods (frequently shown to be megakaryoblasts) **(E),** and monoblasts **(F)** are also quite distinctive. Blast equivalents include granular or hypogranular promyelocytes **(G** and **H)** for acute promyelocytic leukemia, promonocytes **(I)** for AML with a monocytic component, and atypical pronormoblasts (frequently with cytoplasmic vacuoles) **(J)** for acute erythroleukemia of the pure erythroid type. Micromegakaryocytes **(K)** and pronormoblasts **(L)** are not considered blasts when considering AML.

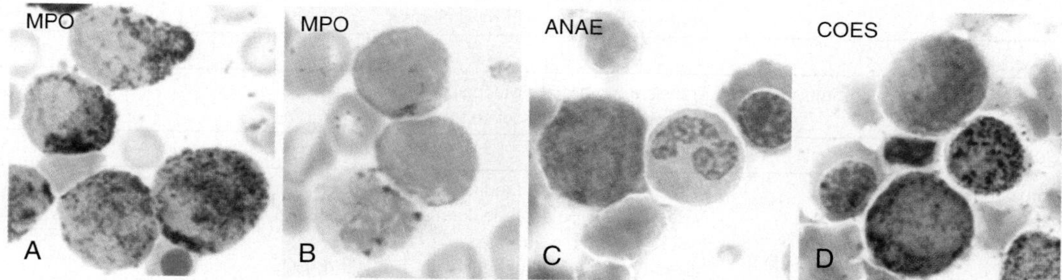

Figure 58-3 CYTOCHEMISTRIES: MYELOPEROXIDASE (MPO), α-NAPHTHYL ACETATE ESTERASE (ANAE), AND COMBINED ESTERASE (COES) REACTIONS. The MPO reaction is easily performed, can be done in less than a few minutes, and provides important initial information about the lineage of the blasts, particularly in cases in which morphologic assessment is difficult. In many laboratories it is routinely performed for all new acute leukemias. The MPO reaction should be interpreted in the blastic population and expressed as a percentage of blasts that are positive. **A,** The positive MPO reaction is strong. **B,** The reaction is weak and seen in only some blasts. A counterstain would have obscured the weak reaction product. A weak MPO reaction is not uncommon in cases of acute myeloid leukemia (AML) associated with myelodysplasia (as in **B**). The neutrophils in such cases are also only weakly positive (bottom cell, **B**). The ANAE reaction is a nonspecific esterase reaction positive in most monocytic cells (**C,** *orange-brown* cell on *left* compared to negative neutrophil, and erythroid cell, *middle* and *right*). The ANAE reaction is interpreted as positive cells as a percentage of nonerythroid elements. A significant monocytic component is usually defined as 20% or greater of the nonerythroid elements and is usually required for making a diagnosis of acute myelomonocytic leukemia. It is notable that in some cases of AML with inv(16) (i.e., AML with abnormal eosinophils), the monocytes are ANAE negative. A COES reaction uses another nonspecific esterase reaction for monocytes, α-naphthyl butyrate esterase, together with the specific esterase, chloroacetate esterase for granulocytes. The combination allows simultaneous evaluation of granulocytes (blue reaction product) and monocytes (orange-brown reaction product). **D,** Acute myelomonocytic leukemia. A monocyte *(top),* a granulocyte *(right),* and a myelomonocytic hybrid cell that exhibits both the orange-brown and blue reaction products *(bottom).*

CBFB-MYH11 (Fig. 58-5); AML with t(15;17)(q22;q12); PML-RARA (Fig. 58-6); and AML with t(9;11)(p22;q23), MLLT3-MLL (Fig. 58-7). However, this category now also includes cases with relatively uncommon genetic changes, and these are AML with t(6;9)(p23;q34), DEK-NUP214; AML with inv(3)(q21q26.2) or t(3;3)(q21;q26.2), RPN1-EVI1; and AML with t(1;22) (p13;q13), RBM15-MKL1 (Fig. 58-8). Provisional entities based on expression of exclusively molecular abnormalities have also been proposed, underlining the significance that molecular testing holds for the future, and these include AML with mutated nucleophosmin gene (NPM1; see Fig. 58-8, *G, H*), and AML with mutated CEBPA.. A second large category of AML is that of AML with myelodysplasia-related changes. These cases are defined in one of three ways: as AML in patients having a history of MDS, AML with multilineage dysplasia recognized morphologically (Fig. 58-9), or AML associated with a myelodysplastic-related cytogenetic abnormality. The next category in the classification is that of therapy-related AML. This category was retained from the 2001 WHO classification, although the distinctions between diseases associated with alkylating agents or radiation and those with topoisomerase II inhibitors were abandoned. Many patients receive complex therapeutic regimens including both types, making the initial distinction difficult. The next category of AML is a "wastebasket" of sorts for AML cases that do not fit the categories already described. These are considered "not otherwise specified" and for the most part are classified using the FAB classification (AML with minimal differentiation, AML without maturation, acute myelomonocytic leukemia, acute monocytic or monoblastic leukemia, acute erythroleukemia, acute megakaryoblastic leukemia,

Table 58-1 Classification of Acute Myeloid Leukemia According to the Revised World Health Organization Classification (2008)

Category	Subtype/Definition
AML with recurrent cytogenetic abnormalities	t(8;21)(q22;q22); RUNX1-RUNX1T1* inv(16)(p13.1q22); CBFB-MYH11* t(16;16)(p13.1q22); CBFB-MYH11* t(15;17)(q22;q12); PML-RARA* t(9;11)(p22;q23); MLLT3-MLL t(6;9)(p23;q34); DEK-Nup214 inv(3)(q21q26.2); RPN1-EVI1 t(3;3)(q21;q26.2); RPN1-EVI1 t(1;22)(p13q13); RBM15-MKL1
AML with MDS-related changes	Morphologic features of MDS, or Prior history of MDS or MDS/MPN, or MDS-related karyotype, and None of the recurrent genetic abnormalities above
Therapy-related myeloid neoplasms	Late complications of cytotoxic chemotherapy (alkylating agents, topoisomerase II inhibitors) and/or ionizing radiation therapy†
AML, not otherwise specified	AML with minimal differentiation AML without maturation AML with maturation Acute myelomonocytic leukemia Acute monoblastic/monocytic leukemia Acute erythroid leukemia Acute megakaryoblastic leukemia Acute basophilic leukemia Acute panmyelosis with myelofibrosis
Myeloid sarcoma	
Myeloid proliferations related to Down syndrome	Transient abnormal myelopoiesis Myeloid leukemia associated with Down syndrome
Blastic plasmacytoid dendritic cell neoplasm	
Acute leukemia of ambiguous lineage	Acute undifferentiated leukemia Mixed-phenotype acute leukemia with t(9;22)(q34;q11.2); BCR-ABL1 t(v;11q23); MLL rearranged Mixed-phenotype acute leukemia, B/myeloid, NOS Mixed-phenotype acute leukemia, T/myeloid, NOS
Provisional entities	AML with mutated NPM1 AML with mutated CEBPA NK-cell lymphoblastic leukemia/lymphoma

AML, Acute myeloid leukemia; *MDS,* myelodysplastic syndrome; *MPN,* myeloproliferative neoplasm; *NK,* natural killer.
*Diagnosis of AML regardless of percentage of blasts.
†Excluded are patients with AML who have transformed from MPN.

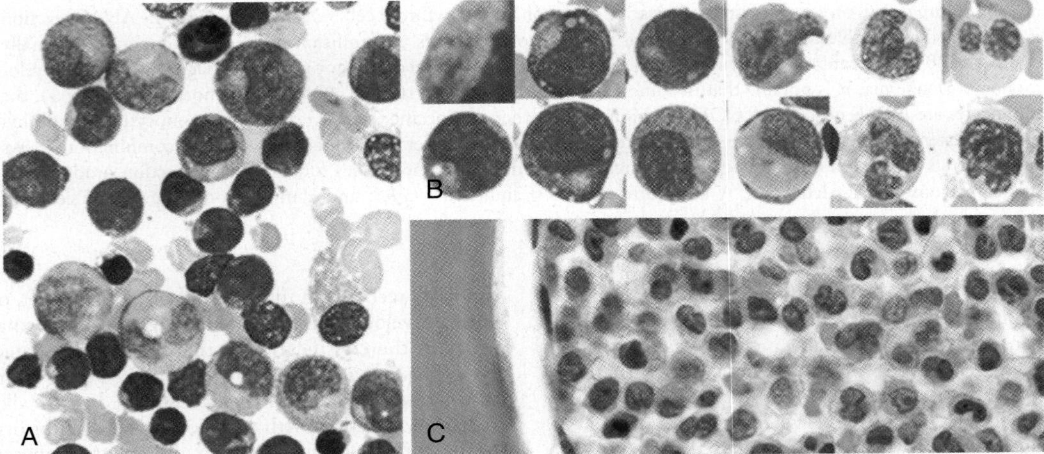

Figure 58-4 ACUTE MYELOID LEUKEMIA (AML) WITH t(8;21)(q22;q22), (RUNX1-RUNX1T1). **A,** Low-power, Wright-stained bone marrow aspirate smear showing increased blasts associated with differentiating myeloid cells. **B,** Details illustrating some of the features associated with this leukemia. They include blasts with long thin Auer rods *(top left),* immature cells with abnormal eosinophilic globules (*top* and *bottom, second from left*), abnormal salmon-colored granulation in the maturing cells, sometimes associated with a basophilic periphery (*top* and *bottom, fourth from left*), and slightly abnormal features in the mature neutrophils *(far right).* Pseudo–Chédiak-Higashi granules were not seen in this case. **C,** Biopsy specimen illustrates the significant degree of maturation that can sometimes be seen. In fact, in some cases the blast count can be less than 20%, but the diagnosis of AML can still be made with the cytogenetic finding of t(8;21).

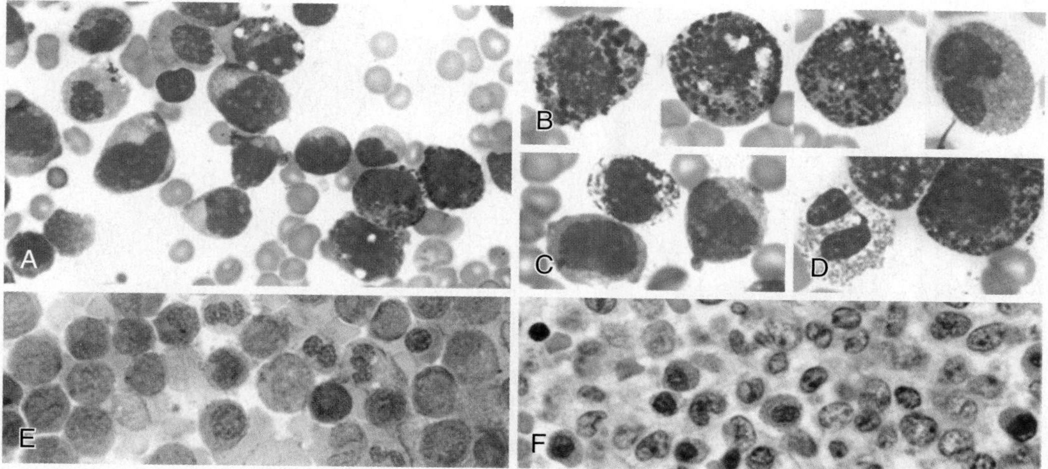

Figure 58-5 Acute myeloid leukemia (AML) with abnormal bone marrow eosinophils and inv(16)(p13.1;q22) or t(16;16)(p13.1;q22), (CBFB-MYH11). **A,** Low-power, Wright-stained bone marrow aspirate showing blasts, monocytic cells, granulocytic cells, and abnormal eosinophils. **B,** Features of the abnormal eosinophils in three abnormal eosinophils *(left three cells).* Note the abnormal basophilic granules in the eosinophilic myelocytes. These granules are large, tend to cluster or coalesce, and are interspersed among the large eosinophilic granules, which are more difficult to see. As the eosinophils mature, the abnormal basophilic granules are less prominent and sometimes disappear *(far right).* A common misconception is that the basophilic granules are the granules of basophils and that the abnormal eosinophils are "hybrid cells." This is not true. **C,** A basophil in the same case *(top cell)* for comparison. **D,** Some cells from a case of reactive eosinophilia, also for comparison. Immature eosinophils *(cell to the right)* do have primary blue granules. However, they are usually less prominent and less atypical than the basophilic granules of the abnormal eosinophils. It is notable that the monocytes in cases of AML with inv(16) or t(16;16) are sometimes α-naphthyl acetate esterase (ANAE)–reaction negative. **E,** Negative ANAE reaction. **F,** Abnormal eosinophils cannot be recognized in hematoxylin-eosin–stained sections of the biopsy.

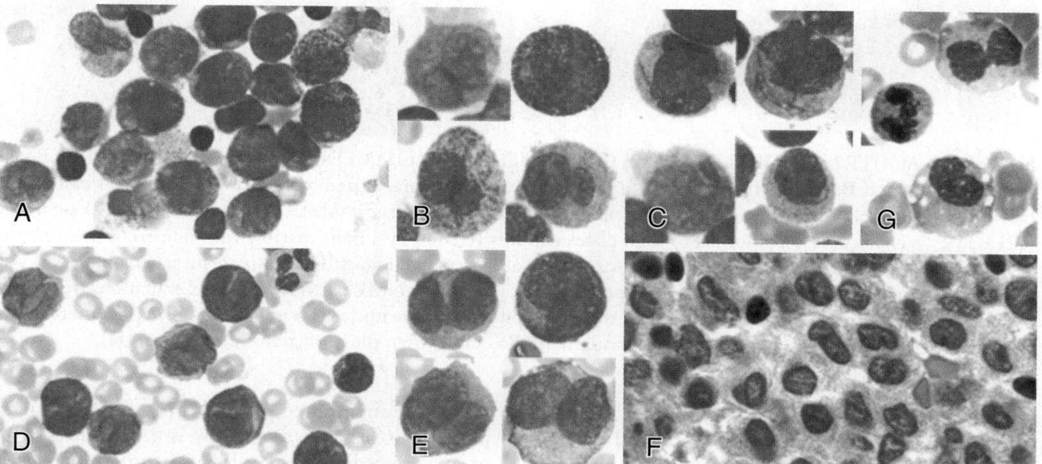

Figure 58-6 ACUTE PROMYELOCYTIC LEUKEMIA (APL), ACUTE MYELOID LEUKEMIA WITH t(15;17)(q22;q12)(PML-RARA). **A** to **C,** APL. **D** and **E,** Hypogranular or microgranular subtype. **F,** Bone marrow biopsy. **G,** APL cells maturing after all-trans retinoic acid (ATRA) therapy. In the typical granular type of APL **(A),** the abnormal promyelocytes can exhibit variable morphologic features. Even within the same case, the granules can range from coarse, dark, and dense to fine and dust-like **(B).** The nuclei in the abnormal promyelocytes frequently exhibit a bilobed, dumbbell, or reniform shape. This is a diagnostically important feature, which can sometimes be difficult to recognize beneath the granules **(B).** Auer rods can be single, multiple, coalesced into Auer bodies, and even present in maturing cells **(C).** The microgranular type usually presents with an elevated white blood cell count **(D).** Although granules cannot be readily appreciated at the light microscope **(E),** granules can be demonstrated by electron microscopy. The abnormal nuclear shapes (bilobed, dumbbell, and reniform) can be easily appreciated **(E).** Bone core biopsy sample typically shows sheets of cells with abundant granular cytoplasm **(F).** After ATRA therapy the abnormal promyelocytes mature to abnormal neutrophils (**G,** *top and bottom right,* compared to normal neutrophil, *left*). These can be seen for weeks after therapy and do not signify a failed response to the differentiating agent.

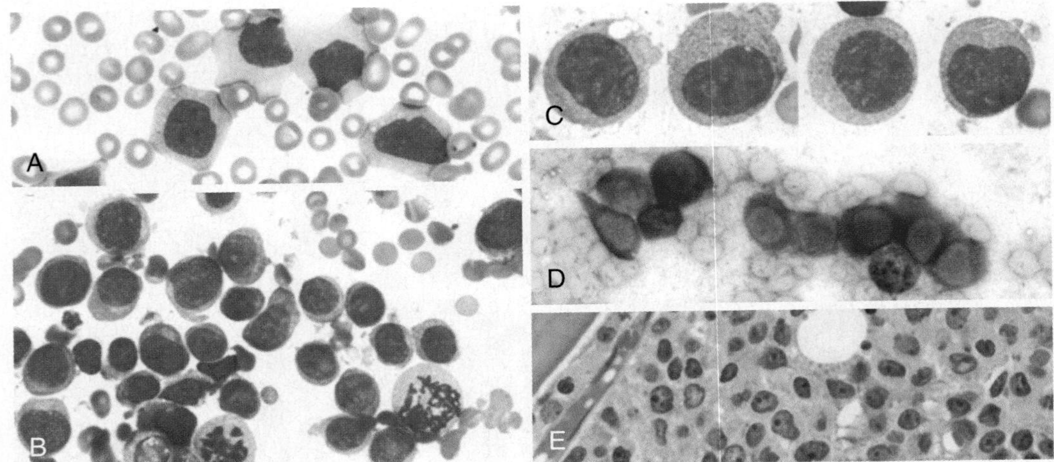

Figure 58-7 ACUTE MONOBLASTIC LEUKEMIA WITH t(9;11)(p22;q23), (MLLT3-MLL). Acute monoblastic leukemia with t(9;11). **A,** Such cases typically present with high counts because of circulating monoblasts. **B, C,** Bone marrow aspirate is packed with monoblasts and shows few granulocytic elements. **D,** Absence of a granulocytic component can be illustrated with the combined esterase reaction, in which most of the cells show the α-naphthyl butyrate reaction product *(orange-brown),* with only rare granulocytes with the blue reaction product from the chloroacetate esterase reaction. **E,** The biopsy sample is usually packed with sheets of monoblasts with fine nuclear chromatin and abundant pink cytoplasm.

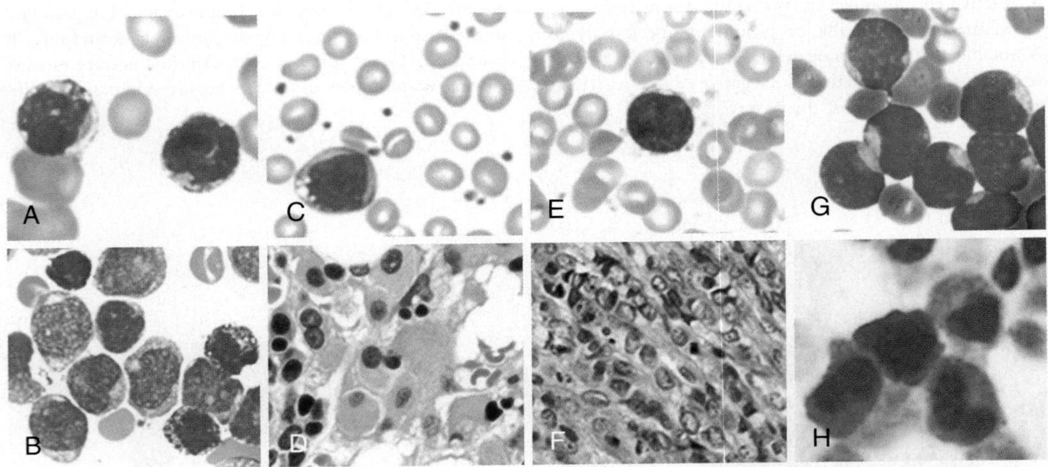

Figure 58-8 ACUTE MYELOID LEUKEMIA (AML) WITH LESS-COMMON CYTOGENETIC AND GENETIC CHANGES. **A** and **B,** AML with t(6;9)(p23;q34). These cases are characterized by marrow dysplasia and basophilia. However, the morphologic characteristics can be quite varied among cases. AML with inv(3)(q21q26.2) or t(3;3)(q21;q26.2) is characterized by normal or high platelet counts **(C)** and by a bone marrow with numerous micromegakaryocytes **(D).** AML with t(1;22)(p13;q13) is uncommon and occurs in infants. The blasts are megakaryoblasts **(E)** but in the bone marrow can have a sarcomatous appearance **(F).** AML with NMP or NPM and Flt-3 mutations frequently presents with high peripheral blasts counts, and the blasts sometimes have nuclear invaginations **(G).** NPM mutation is associated with the abnormal cytoplasmic localization of NPM rather than the normal nuclear staining **(H).**

AML with maturation, acute basophilic leukemia). The AML-like disease of acute panmyelosis with myelofibrosis is included in this group (Fig. 58-10). Lastly, the classification now includes myeloid sarcoma (Fig. 58-11), myeloid proliferations associated with Down syndrome (see Chapter 62), and the unusual blastic plasmacytoid dendritic cell neoplasm. The latter is an aggressive malignancy of plasmacytoid dendritic cells that frequently involves the blood and bone marrow (Fig. 58-12).

Prognostic factors are best divided into patient-related features that predict likelihood of surviving induction chemotherapy and disease-related factors that determine resistance to chemotherapy.[3] Among the former, age, performance status, and basic assessment of organ function (hepatic, renal, cardiac) have the greatest impact. Comorbidity scores such as the hematopoietic cell transplantation comorbidity index (HCTCI) have been applied to identify patients unfit for chemotherapy and may be particularly useful in older patients. Resistance to therapy is determined by presence or absence of an antecedent hematologic disorder such as MDS, exposure to previous chemotherapy and/or radiation therapy (therapy-related AML), and biologic features of the blasts themselves. Among the latter, karyotype continues to be the most important pretreatment prognostic feature dividing patients into those with favorable (CBF leukemias associated with t(8;21) and inv(16) or t(16;16); APL with t(15;17)), unfavorable (complex abnormalities, monosomies such as -5 and -7 among others), and intermediate prognosis (mainly diploid) (Fig. 58-13).[4] The prognostic power of karyotype is nowadays augmented by including molecular abnormalities. Genotype analysis adds most in patients with normal cytogenetics. Many molecular markers are being investigated (e.g., Flt-3, NPM1, CEBPA, Ras, KIT, IDH1 and IDH2, MLL, TET2). Testing for NPM1, CEBPA, and

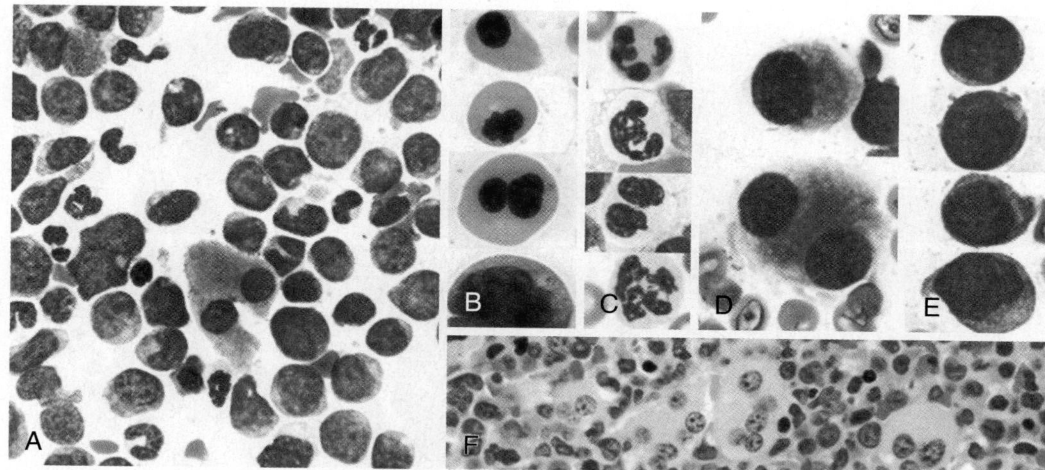

Figure 58-9 ACUTE MYELOID LEUKEMIA WITH MULTILINEAGE DYSPLASIA. **A,** Bone marrow aspirate shows increased blasts and maturing cells with dysplastic features. **B** to **D,** Details of the dysplasia. **B,** Maturing erythroid elements exhibit megaloblastoid change and bizarre nuclear abnormalities. **C,** Dysplastic granulocytes *(bottom three)* are compared to a rare normal granulocyte *(top)*. The dysplastic forms have pale cytoplasm and abnormal nuclear shapes with hypolobation, hypersegmentation, and prominent nuclear excrescences. **D,** Dysplastic micromegakaryocytes have single or double small nuclei but mature cytoplasm with platelet material within. **E,** Increased blasts. **F,** Dysplasia is difficult to appreciate on a biopsied section. This is true except for the megakaryocytes. Dysplastic megakaryocytes can be recognized on the biopsy specimen by their abnormally small nuclei, which are sometimes multiple and widely spaced.

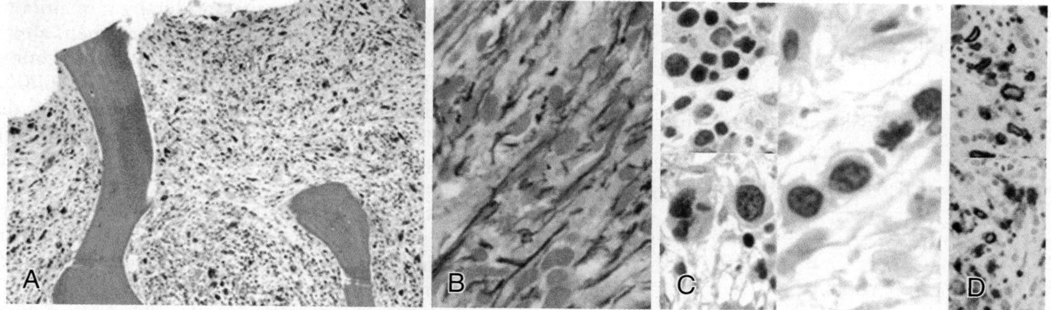

Figure 58-10 ACUTE PANMYELOSIS WITH MYELOFIBROSIS. **A,** Bone marrow biopsy specimen shows a loosely packed marrow with a swirling appearance to the cellular elements due to underlying fibrosis. **B,** The latter is illustrated on the reticulin stain. **C,** Proliferations of erythroid cells *(top left),* megakaryocytes *(bottom left),* and immature cells within the fibrotic areas *(right)*. **D,** Immunohistochemical staining shows increased megakaryocytes (*top,* CD61) and increased blasts (*bottom,* CD34).

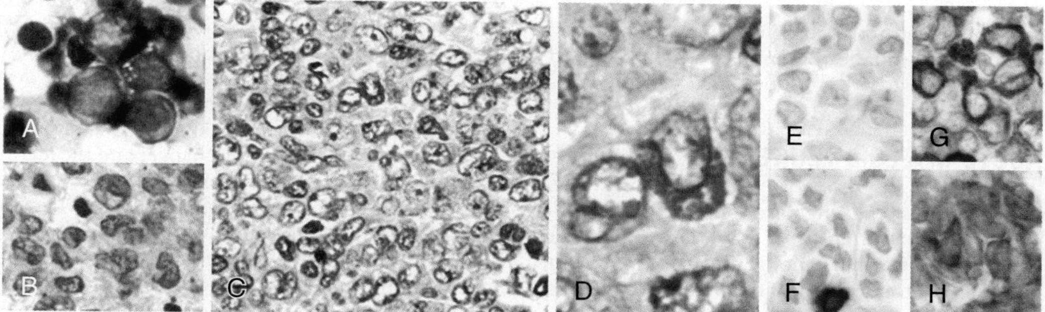

Figure 58-11 MYELOID SARCOMA. Myeloid sarcomas can sometimes present a diagnostic challenge. In this case the touch imprints **(A)** and frozen section preparation **(B)** from a mass lesion in the cecal area from a 44-year-old patient were thought to represent a high-grade lymphoma. However, initial immunohistochemical stains did not support the diagnosis, and on closer inspection of the tumor and with subsequent immunomarkers, a diagnosis could be reached. The tumor **(C)** is composed of sheets of noncohesive cells. A diagnostic clue to the origin was the presence of eosinophilic myelocytes **(D),** which indicate that some tumor cells have the capacity to differentiate to eosinophils. The granules of neutrophilic myelocytes cannot be recognized on tissue section. The immunohistochemical stains showed the cell to be CD45+ (not shown), B, and T marker negative **(E** and **F),** but myeloid marker (myeloperoxidase and CD33) positive **(G** and **H).** Cytogenetic analysis showed the case was inv(16)(p13.1;q22).

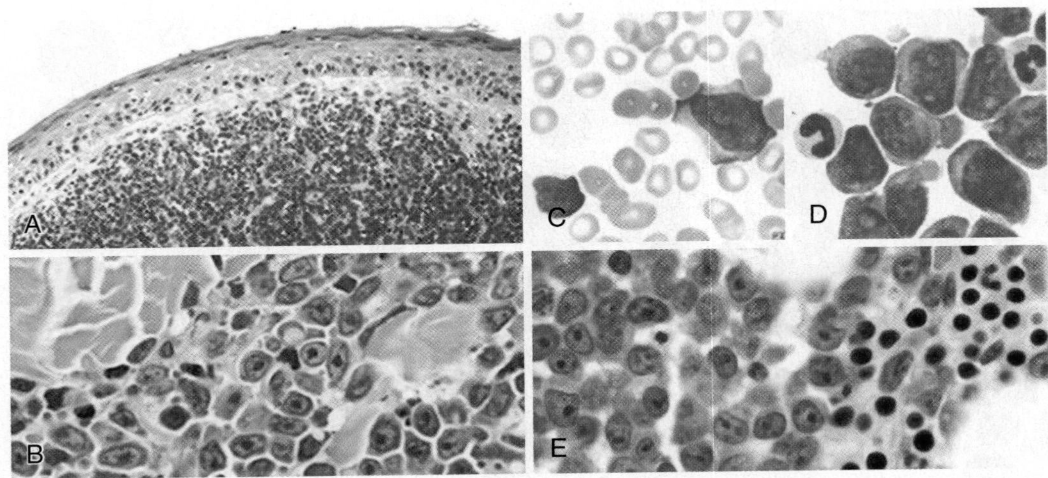

Figure 58-12 BLASTIC PLASMACYTOID DENDRITIC CELL NEOPLASM. The blastic plasmacytoid dendritic cell tumor is an unusually aggressive malignancy that was previously called *hematodermic* malignancy. It is now classified in the acute myeloid leukemia category of myeloid neoplasms. It frequently presents in the skin with a blastic proliferation of cells in the dermis **(A** and **B)**, which inevitably spreads to the blood **(C)**, and bone marrow **(D** and **E)**.

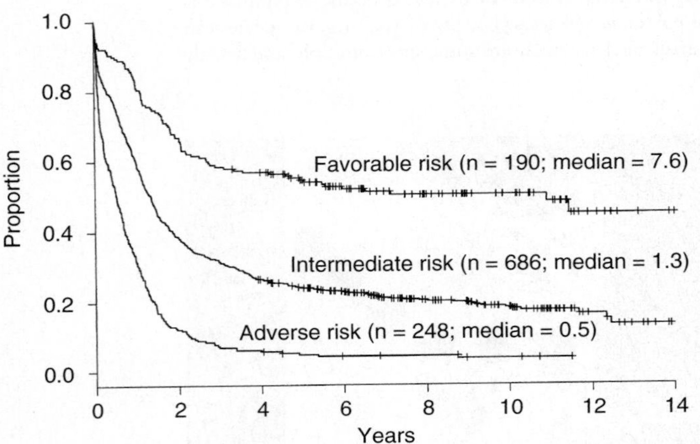

Figure 58-13 DISEASE-FREE SURVIVAL BY CYTOGENETIC RISK GROUP. *(Data from Byrd JC, Mrózek K, Dodge RK, et al: Pretreatment cytogenetic abnormalities are predictive of induction success, cumulative incidence of relapse, and overall survival in adult patients with de novo acute myeloid leukemia: Results from Cancer and Leukemia Group B (CALGB 8461),* Blood *100:4325, 2002.)*

Flt-3 mutations is recommended today in general practice. A panel on behalf of the European LeukemiaNet has proposed a standardized reporting for correlation of cytogenetic and molecular genetic data.[1]

THERAPY FOR ACUTE MYELOID LEUKEMIA

AML therapy is one of the most challenging of oncologic interventions (Fig. 58-14). Interventions often need to be fast, physicians need to deal with a multitude of complications (disease or treatment related), and any patient's condition can change rapidly. Given its complexity, treatment of patients with AML requires a multidisciplinary effort including oncologists, pharmacists, specifically educated nursing staff, and various consulting services (infectious disease, pulmonology, nephrology, cardiology). Supportive care is an essential part of AML therapy and plays an ever more important role, including transfusion services and symptom control measures.

The general approach to AML therapy depends on the AML subtype (APL, CBF leukemias, other) as well as age and performance status of the patient (high-intensity versus low-intensity therapy). Treatment of older patients (generally defined as older than 60 to 65 years) increasingly differs from that of younger patients, and hence this chapter follows this development by addressing the two age groups separately.

Treatment of AML consists of induction and postremission therapy. The goal of induction is to produce a complete remission (CR) and that of postremission therapy to maintain it by eliminating residual disease. CR is defined as achievement after chemotherapy of less than 5% marrow blasts, a neutrophil count of greater than 1000/μL, a platelet count of greater than 100,000/μL, independence of red blood cell transfusions, and resolution of all signs and symptoms referable to AML. CR defines a landmark point in time because patients who achieve CR on any given day after beginning therapy have longer survival subsequent to that day than patients who are resistant to therapy on the day in question. Lesser response criteria (CR without platelet recovery, CR with incomplete blood recovery including neutropenia, partial remission, morphologic leukemia-free state) may serve as useful end points in the context of investigational studies (phase I, II, or III), but they do not carry the same significance for survival as does CR. Postremission therapy consists of repeated cycles of chemotherapy or hematopoietic stem cell transplantation (HSCT) in its various forms (autologous, allogeneic, haploidentical, cord blood, reduced intensity). The role of HSCT for AML therapy will be the topic of a separate chapter of this book. The debate as to which patients should receive chemotherapy consolidation versus HSCT is most divisive for patients with intermediate-risk disease. In this population, characterization of the genotype has become most helpful in guiding that decision.

Leukemia has been at the forefront of the development of "targeted" therapy, mostly small-molecule drugs directed against defined intracellular proteins (e.g., kinases). Not surprisingly, given the increasing number of genetic changes and the identification of diverse signaling pathways of leukemic blasts, the specter of "personalized therapy" also looms high in AML therapy. Despite intense research activity, to date no "targeted" drug has been approved for this indication (with the exception of gemtuzumab ozogamicin [GO], an anti-CD33 monoclonal antibody–calicheamicin conjugate with activity in some subtypes of AML, but whose approval was recently revoked by the Food and Drug Administration [FDA]).

Therapy for Younger Adults

Standard Induction Therapy

Induction therapy is based on the combination of cytarabine and an anthracycline. Cytarabine, an analogue of a physiologic pyrimidine

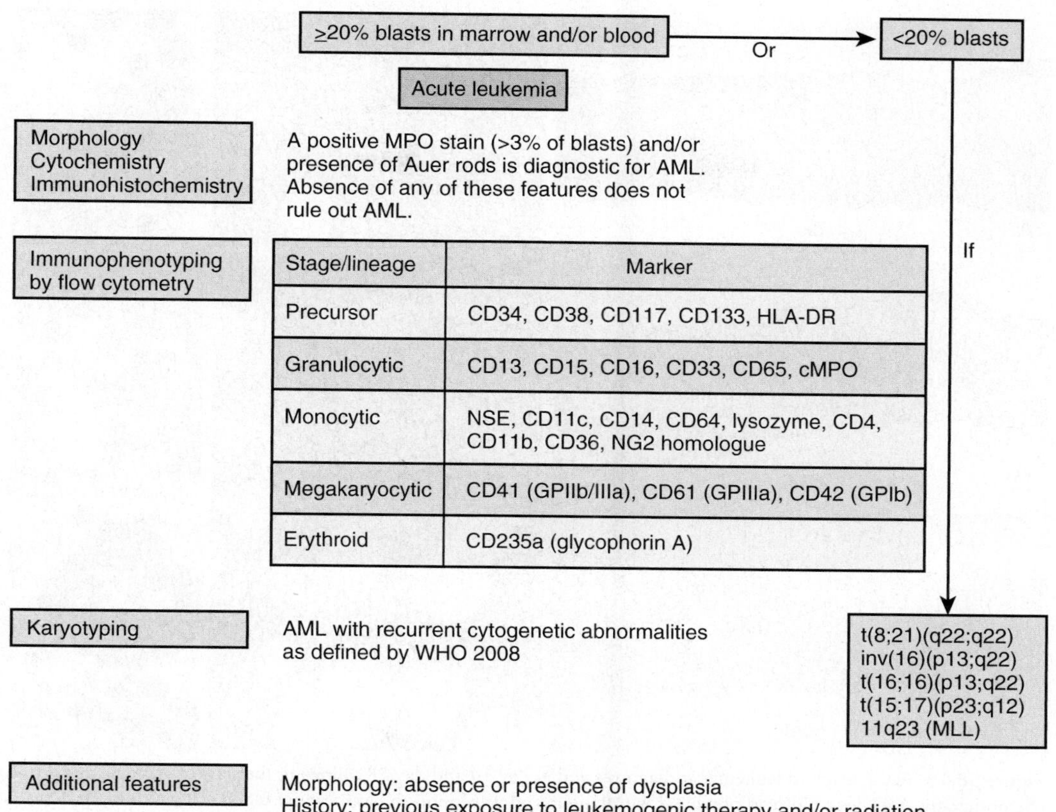

Figure 58-14 GENERAL DIAGNOSTIC APPROACH TO ACUTE MYELOID LEUKEMIA THERAPY. *AML,* Acute myeloid leukemia; *APL,* acute promyelocytic leukemia; *ATRA,* all-trans retinoic acid; *CBF,* core binding factor; *FLAG,* fludarabine, cytarabine (ara-C), and granulocyte colony-stimulating factor.

nucleoside, is an antimetabolite that requires intracellular conversion to its triphosphate compound, ara-CTP, and incorporation into deoxyribonucleic acid (DNA) to become active. When given by itself at standard doses of 100 to 200 mg/m^2 intravenously (IV) daily for 5 to 7 days, it produces CR rates of around 40%. Anthracyclines (daunorubicin, idarubicin, aclarubicin) act by stabilizing the normally occurring complex between DNA and the enzyme topoisomerase II, thereby leading to apoptotic cell death. Daunorubicin, the most frequently used anthracycline, achieves similar CR rates as with cytarabine alone. The combination of cytarabine at 100 to 200 mg/m^2 as a continuous IV infusion (its serum half-life is only 15 minutes) daily for 7 days and daunorubicin at 45 to 60 mg/m^2 IV daily for 3 days on days 1 to 3 has become known as the "3+7" regimen and, for more than 40 years, has been the standard induction combination for most patients with AML. Remission rates range from 60% to 80%, and long-term disease-free survival is about 35%.[5] Patients who fail to achieve remission may be divided into those who die during induction, mainly as a consequence of multisystem organ failure in the wake of infections, and those who survive induction therapy but whose blasts remain resistant to chemotherapy regardless of whether or not marrow hypoplasia was achieved during treatment. Whereas induction mortality is low among patients younger than 50 years, it can increase substantially in older patients.

In clinical practice, patients undergo a repeat marrow study between 14 and 21 days from the start of treatment (Fig. 58-15). If the marrow continues to show blasts and is cellular, a reinduction is usually given. The reinduction may be a repetition of the induction, be it attenuated (e.g., "2+5") or intensified as intermediate-dose cytarabine (IDAC) or high-dose cytarabine (HiDAC). If the day 14 or 21 marrow is hypoplastic, supportive care continues and marrow studies are repeated every 1 to 2 weeks until it becomes clear whether the patient is going into CR or not. If in CR, postremission therapy starts shortly thereafter, whereas in case of no response, treatment is often changed. Although reinductions lead to remissions, these are usually shorter lasting. The degree of neutrophil and platelet recovery at the time of remission has prognostic significance. Higher neutrophil and platelet counts at the time of remission are predictive of better relapse-free survival. In some cases a regenerating marrow may have an increased number of blasts, which may look like persistent leukemia. Further follow-up marrow studies will show reduction in blasts concomitant with a rise of neutrophils and platelets.

Many modifications to the 3+7 regimen have been tried to improve outcome. Giving 10 instead of 7 days of cytarabine (3+10), increasing the dose of cytarabine from 100 mg/m^2/day to 200 mg/m^2/day, adding a third drug (e.g., mitoxantrone, etoposide, thioguanine, topotecan, fludarabine) or modulators of drug resistance, and priming leukemic blasts with hematopoietic growth factors (granulocyte colony-stimulating factor [G-CSF], granulocyte-macrophage colony stimulating factor) are not any better and not recommended. Giving cytarabine as a continuous infusion rather than twice-daily, short IV infusions achieved slightly better response rates.

The choice of anthracycline has been the subject of an ongoing debate. Substitution of daunorubicin by doxorubicin produced more toxicity without added benefit. In three randomized trials of idarubicin versus daunorubicin, the combination of idarubicin with cytarabine produced higher response rates and a survival advantage in at least one study. However, most would nowadays agree that daunorubicin 45 mg/m^2 daily for 3 days is not appropriate and no longer standard of care in AML.[6] Recent studies analyzed the impact of higher doses of daunorubicin on AML induction outcome. A large study from Japan randomly assigned 1057 newly diagnosed patients with AML under 65 years to receive daunorubicin 50 mg/m^2 daily for 5 days or idarubicin 12 mg/m^2 daily for 3 days in combination with cytarabine 100 mg/m^2 by continuous IV infusion daily for 7 days. There were no differences in CR (77.5% versus 78.2%, P = .79), 5-year overall survival (48% in both groups, P = .54), or 5-year

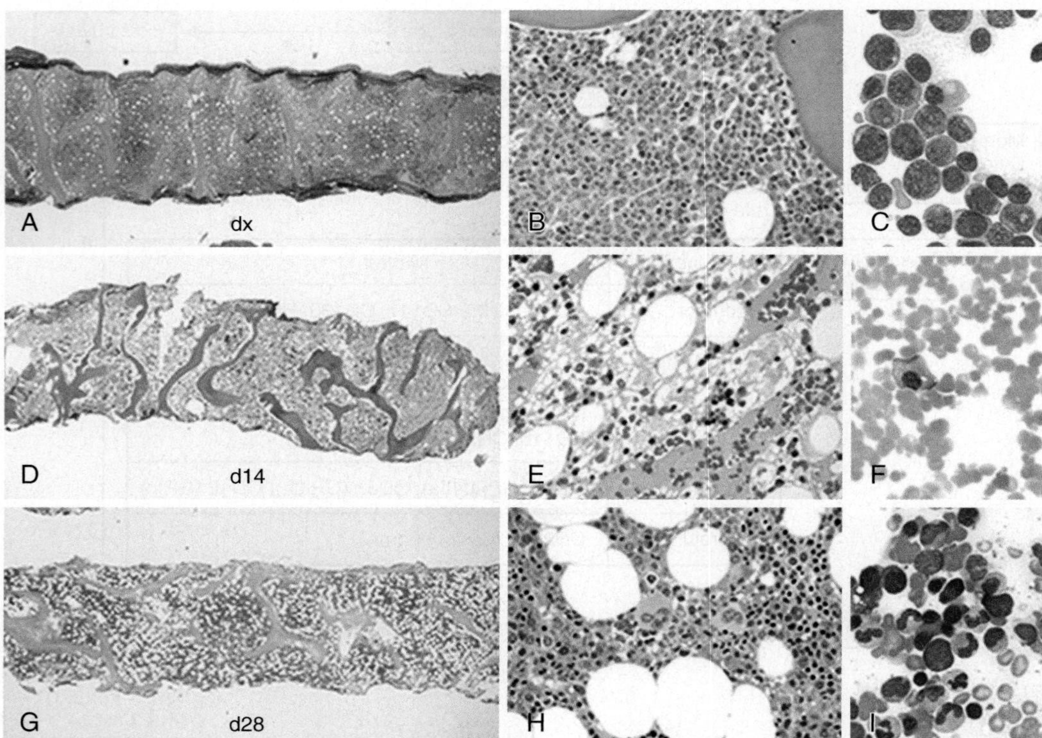

Figure 58-15 Acute myeloid leukemia at diagnosis and at day 14 and day 28 following the start of standard induction chemotherapy. A 43-year-old man presented with fatigue and was found to have a white blood cell count of 70,300/μL composed of mostly blasts. A bone marrow study **(A** to **C)** showed a hypercellular bone marrow (90% cellular) packed with blasts (80%). The blasts were myeloperoxidase positive and had the following phenotype: CD34+, HLA-DR+, CD117+, CD13+, CD33+ with partial CD15 and CD11b. Cytogenetic analysis demonstrated a normal male karyotype, and molecular studies showed wild-type Flt-3 and NPM1. The patient was treated with standard induction chemotherapy, and a day 14 bone marrow study **(D** to **F)** showed chemoablation effects with an empty marrow, stromal injury, dilated sinuses, and only scattered stromal cells and plasma cells with no obvious blasts. A bone marrow study performed at day 28 **(G** to **I)** showed regenerative changes with trilineage hematopoiesis.

relapse-free survival (41% in both groups, P = .97).[7] The French ALFA-9801 study randomized AML induction patients (age 50 to 70 years) to one of three anthracycline arms: daunorubicin 80 mg/m^2 daily for 3 days and idarubicin 12 mg/m^2 daily for 3 days and 4 days, respectively. Complete remission rates favored idarubicin (83%, 78%, and 70% for idarubicin × 4, idarubicin × 3, and daunorubicin, respectively, P = .04), and there was a trend for better survival.[8] A study by the Eastern Cooperative Oncology Group (ECOG) randomized patients between the ages of 17 and 60 years with untreated AML to receive the 3+7 combination with either standard-dose daunorubicin (45 mg/m^2 daily × 3) or high-dose daunorubicin (90 mg/m^2 daily × 3).[9] High-dose daunorubicin achieved higher rates of CR (70.6% versus 57.3%, P<.001) and improved median overall survival (23.7 months versus 15.7 months, P = .003), an improvement limited to patients younger than 50 years and with intermediate cytogenetics. High-dose daunorubicin did not lead to a higher incidence of adverse events (particularly cardiomyopathy and infectious complications). In conclusion, rather than the type of anthracycline, what matters most is to use an adequate dose.

HiDAC as part of the induction has been investigated in several randomized trials. A metaanalysis of trials encompassing 1691 patients arrived at the following conclusions: there were no differences between HiDAC and standard-dose cytarabine (SDAC) with respect to percent CR and rates of persisting leukemia and early death; 4-year overall and recurrence-free survival, on the other hand, were significantly better with HiDAC but at the cost of more toxicities (infections, nausea/vomiting, CNS).[10] HiDAC benefited mostly patients who already were more likely to achieve CR (i.e., patients with intermediate and favorable karyotype). The major drawback of HiDAC during induction is that it may make further consolidation therapy difficult. The Medical Research Council (MRC) AML 15 trial randomized 635 patients to receive fludarabine, cytarabine (ara-C), G-CSF, and idarubicin (FLAG-Ida; fludarabine 30 mg/m^2 on days 2 to 6, cytarabine 2 g/m^2 on days 2 to 6, idarubicin 10 mg/m^2 on days 4 to 6, and G-CSF on days 1 to 7) and 631 to receive cytarabine (ara-C), daunorubicin, and etoposide (ADE; daunorubicin 50 mg/m^2 on days 1, 3, 5; cytarabine 100 mg/m^2 on days 1 to 8; and etoposide 100 mg/m^2 on days 1 to 5), the latter representing the SDAC arm.[11] While there were no significant differences in response rate, fewer patients on FLAG-Ida relapsed. However, more myelosuppression and deaths in CR offset the survival benefit. A recent study by the Dutch-Belgian Cooperative Trial Group for Hemato-Oncology (HOVON) and the Swiss Group for Clinical Cancer Research (SAKK) Collaborative Group randomized patients with newly diagnosed AML (ages 18 to 60 years) to HiDAC (cytarabine 1 to 2 g/m^2) or IDAC (cytarabine 0.2 to 1 g/m^2).[12] HiDAC provided no advantage in any prognostic subgroup but resulted in more severe adverse events, prolonged hospitalizations, and delayed neutrophil and platelet recovery. HiDAC during induction remains investigational.

Standard Postremission Therapy

Once in a morphologic CR, there are still as many as 10^9 leukemia cells present below the threshold of detection by light microscopy (minimal residual disease). Further therapy is therefore necessary to reduce this number and minimize the chances of relapse. In a series of clinical studies in which patients did not receive postremission therapy, relapse was universal, and the median remission duration was about 4 months.

There is still debate about details of postremission therapy with regard to dose, number of cycles, or whether or not there is a role for maintenance. In a classic Cancer and Leukemia Group B (CALGB) study patients with newly diagnosed AML received the 3+7 combination and once in CR were randomized to SDAC (100 mg/m² continuous IV infusion daily × 5), IDAC (400 mg/m² continuous IV infusion daily × 5), or HiDAC (3 g/m² IV over 3 hours every 12 hours on days 1, 3, and 5) for a total of four cycles. This was followed by an additional four cycles of 2+5, a consolidation-maintenance omitted from all subsequent CALGB studies. The probability of remaining in continuous CR after 4 years was 24% for SDAC, 29% for IDAC, and 44% for HiDAC (P = .002). Among several randomizations in the AML MRC12 trial 1193 patients received induction therapy with either standard-dose daunorubicin, cytarabine (ara-C), and thioguanine (S-DAT) or double the standard dose of cytarabine (H-DAT).[13] In consolidation, patients then received either a total of four or five courses (including induction). There was no difference in outcome between the induction arms, and no difference for the addition of a fifth course. The Japan Adult Leukemia Study Group (JALSG) conducted a randomized study in 781 patients younger than 65 years in CR who received either three courses of HiDAC (2 g/m² IV twice daily for 5 days) or four courses of conventional standard-dose multiagent chemotherapy.[14] There was no difference between the groups with respect to 5-year disease-free survival (43% versus 39%, P = .724) or 5-year overall survival (58% versus 56%, P = .954). The study showed a beneficial effect of HiDAC only in the group of patients with favorable cytogenetics.

HiDAC in consolidation benefits mostly patients who are younger than 60 years and those with favorable cytogenetics, but to a far lesser extent those with intermediate and unfavorable karyotypes. Postremission therapy should be guided by the risk profile of the patient (based on cytogenetics and genotype; Table 58-2).

CBF leukemias are characterized by translocation t(8;21), inv(16), or t(16;16) and at the molecular level by a disruption of CBF transcription genes, which play a crucial role in hematopoietic differentiation. CBF AMLs occur in about 15% of patients with AML. CBF AMLs are very sensitive to cytarabine-based therapy. Remission rates are close to 90%, and long-term overall survival reaches 60%. Postremission therapy with HiDAC (e.g., 3 g/m² IV every 12 hours on days 1, 3, and 5) for three to four cycles is considered adequate. Some questions persist with regard to the optimal number of cycles, intensification, and addition of further drugs. One cycle (with a cumulative dose of up to 18 g/m² of cytarabine) is worse than three or four cycles (cumulative dose 54 mg/m² to 72 mg/m²). On the other hand, giving two cycles in combination with idarubicin, daunorubicin, or mitoxantrone is comparable to three or four cycles with HiDAC. According to the MRC AML10 trial, one consolidation cycle of IDAC (cumulative dose of 5 g/m²) was equivalent to three or four consolidation cycles as given in the CALGB studies. In recent studies, the addition of gemtuzumab (GO) to cytarabine-based conventional chemotherapy was shown to improve survival for patients with a favorable karyotype.[15] Given the excellent responsiveness to chemotherapy vis-à-vis the higher risk for treatment-related mortality and morbidity with stem cell transplant, there is no well-established role for transplant as consolidation for CBF AML. Some patients with CBF AML fare worse despite the apparent favorable karyotype. Long-established poor prognostic factors include older age, a high WBC at presentation, presentation with granulocytic sarcoma and t(8;21), and expression of CD56. An important factor associated with worse survival is the presence of KIT mutations. Mutations of KIT (more frequently of exon 17 than exon 8) occur in up to one-third of patients with inv(16) and about 20% of those with t(8;21). Although remission rates do not differ, relapse is more likely with mutated than wild-type KIT. Screening for KIT mutations should routinely follow cytogenetic analysis. Leukemic blasts with activated KIT could be targeted with novel tyrosine kinase inhibitors. Given the higher relapse rate, allogeneic stem cell transplant in this situation is also advocated by some.

Table 58-2 Postremission Therapy by Cytogenetic-Molecular Profile

Prognostic Group	Subgroups	Chemotherapy (HiDAC)	HSCT
Favorable		Yes	No
	KIT+ CBF	Yes	Yes
Intermediate		Yes	Yes
	Flt-3/ITD+	Yes	Yes
	Flt-3/D835+	Yes	No
	NPM1+*	Yes	No
	CEBPA+*	Yes	No
	NPM1-Flt-3/ITD+	Yes	Yes
Unfavorable		No	Yes

*Without concomitant expression of Flt-3/ITD or IDH1. In the case of CEBPA, only if the mutation is biallelic.
HiDAC, High-dose cytarabine; *HSCT,* hematopoietic stem cell transplant.

Patients with diploid cytogenetics and mutations of either NPM1 or biallelic mutations of CEBPA in the absence of Flt-3/ITD (fms-related tyrosine kinase 3 gene/internal tandem duplication) have a similarly favorable outcome to that of patients with CBF AML (without mutations of KIT) and are not referred for HSCT in first remission. There is also evidence that patients with mutations of Ras benefit from higher doses of cytarabine. Whether or not this obviates the need for a transplant in remission is not clear.

Patients with intermediate-risk AML are the largest group (about 60% of AML). These patients are induced with the 3+7 combination followed by up to four cycles of HiDAC (3 g/m² IV twice daily on days 1, 3, and 5) in consolidation. Because long-term disease-free survival remains suboptimal, there is an ongoing debate about how to approach these patients, and in particular the role of transplant.[16] Most randomized studies in the past demonstrated similar overall survival whether patients received intensive consolidation therapy, autologous, or allogeneic HSCT, where an improvement of relapse likelihood following transplant was offset by a higher transplant-related mortality. According to a more recent metaanalysis of 24 prospective trials including 6007 patients evaluating allogeneic HSCT versus nonallogeneic HSCT therapies for AML in first CR, both relapse-free survival and overall survival were significantly better for patients with intermediate- and poor-risk AML if they underwent allogeneic HSCT. The intermediate-risk group is heterogeneous, and the prognosis of patients with cytogenetically normal karyotype differs widely. Identification of gene mutations is helpful to gauge prognosis and, within a limited scope, to guide therapy. Although data are sparse, transplant can be deferred in patients with cytogenetically normal karyotype and favorable genotype (mutations of NPM1 or biallelic mutations of CEBPA without Flt-3/ITD). On the other hand, transplant in first CR should be considered in patients with unfavorable genotypes (e.g., Flt-3/ITD abnormalities). The presence of a Flt-3/ITD mutation may not matter as much as the mutated allele burden, so that quantification will likely play an increasing role. The picture is even less clear in most of the other mutations, for which data remain sparse and conflicting.

Outcome remains dismal for patients with adverse-risk cytogenetics. These patients have a low cure rate with standard chemotherapy and should be referred for transplant or clinical trials if available.

Therapy for Older Patients

Although arbitrary, *older* usually refers to patients who are 60 years and above. In an analysis of Surveillance, Epidemiology, and End Results (SEER) cancer registries and Medicare administrative claims, the estimated median survival of 2657 older patients with AML was 2 months with a 2-year survival rate of 6%.[17] However, only one-third of patients received treatment for AML, assuming that therapy was considered futile and palliation more appropriate. Older patients do worse for various reasons. Comorbidities are frequent, and they are more likely to have a poor performance status. Hence tolerance to intensive chemotherapy and its myelosuppressive and immunosuppressive consequences is diminished. There are also differences intrinsic to the biologic behavior of AML blasts in older and younger patients. Patients over age 60 are more likely to have secondary AML (following MDS), express unfavorable cytogenetics, and have reduced sensitivity to anthracyclines, and they more often express multidrug-resistant phenotypes. Nevertheless, older patients should not be precluded from therapy. As the SEER analysis also showed, patients who were treated lived on average 6 months longer. Other studies have also demonstrated the benefits of induction therapy over supportive care only, with respect to survival and quality of life.

Induction Therapy for Older Patients

Three options are conventional chemotherapy, clinical trials, and palliative care. Given the poor outcome with conventional therapy (median survival 10 months; induction mortality around 20%, which may exceed 50% in patients with a poor performance status), it can be argued that almost no one in this age-group should be treated with conventional therapy. Yet older patients are not a homogenous group, and outcome varies. Several prognostic models have been designed to identify patients who may do well with conventional therapy versus those who will not (Table 58-3). These models are based on easily accessible clinical information but are mainly derived from retrospective analyses and require validation in prospective clinical trials.

Among conventional therapy, low-intensity approaches can be distinguished from intensive (i.e., standard-dose cytarabine) therapy. Low intensity is indicated for patients who are "unfit" for chemotherapy, that is, who are older (e.g., older than 70 to 75 years), have a limited performance status, and at the same time do not display disease features (adverse karyotype, treatment-related AML) with a high likelihood of resistance. In the National Cancer Research Institute AML 14 Trial, 217 patients considered unfit for intensive chemotherapy were randomized to low-dose cytarabine at 20 mg subcutaneously twice daily for 10 days or hydroxyurea.[18] Both survival and remission rate (18% versus 1%; $P<.001$) were superior with low-dose cytarabine with the exception of patients with adverse cytogenetics, who did poorly on either treatment arm. Hypomethylating agents are widely used in the treatment of myeloid disorders such as MDS and increasingly in AML. Azacitidine 75 mg/m^2 subcutaneously daily for 7 days was compared to conventional care (best supportive care, low-dose cytarabine, or intensive chemotherapy) in a subset of 113 patients (median age 70 years) entered on a randomized MDS study but had 20% to 29% blasts.[19] Median overall survival was 24.5 months in the azacitidine group and 16 months in the conventional care group ($P = .005$). The median survival of 16 months in the control arm, compared with median survival of 4 to 7 months in the other AML studies of older patients suggests that this subset is not truly representative of older AML (e.g., based on exclusion of proliferative AML). In two single-arm trials, decitabine 20 mg/m^2 IV daily for 5 and 10 days achieved CR rates of 24% and 47%, respectively, and overall median survival times of 7.7 months and slightly longer than 1 year, respectively.[20,21] Notably, induction mortalities remained low, and responses also occurred in patients with unfavorable karyotypes, an important difference from low-dose cytarabine. Standard intensive therapy consists of 3 days of an anthracycline with 7 to 10 days of cytarabine 100 to 200 mg/m^2 per dose. Doses should not be attenuated based on age alone. As for younger patients, the choice of anthracycline does not matter as long as the particular agents are used at equitoxic doses. In a large randomized trial, daunorubicin 90 mg/m^2 daily × 3 was compared to daunorubicin 45 mg/m^2 daily × 3 in combination with standard-dose cytarabine. The high-dose daunorubicin arm achieved higher rates of CR, notably after only one course. A survival benefit was seen for patients ages 60 to 65 years.

Table 58-3 Prognostic Models in Older Patients With Acute Myeloid Leukemia

Model	Predicted Factor	Negative Prognostic Scores
Study Alliance Leukemia	Survival Disease-free survival	CD34 expression >10% WBC >20 ×10^9/L Age >65 yr LDH >700 units/L NPM1 status wild-type*
UK Medical Research Council (UKMRC)	Survival	Adverse cytogenetic group Elevated WBC† Poor performance status† Older age† Secondary AML
Acute Leukemia French Association (ALFA)	Survival	High-risk cytogenetics ± Age ≥75 yr Performance status ≥2 WBC ≥50 × 10^9/L
M.D. Anderson (MDACC)	Remission rate Induction mortality Survival	Age ≥75 yr Secondary AML‡ AHD duration ≥6‡ (12) mo Treatment outside LAFR Unfavorable cytogenetics WBC ≥25 × 10^9/L‡ Hemoglobin ≤8 g/dL‡ Creatinine >1.3 mg/dL Performance status >2 LDH >600 units/L§
Hematopoietic cell transplantation comorbidity index	Early mortality Survival	Dyspnea Coronary artery disease, CHF, MI, or EF <50% Chronic hepatitis, elevation of bilirubin and/or transaminases Cirrhosis Elevations of creatinine, dialysis, renal transplant Secondary AML Depression/anxiety requiring therapy Continued use of antimicrobial therapy after day 0 BMI >35 kg/m^2

AHD, Antecedent hematologic disorder; *AML*, acute myeloid leukemia; *BMI*, body mass index; *CHF*, congestive heart failure; *EF*, ejection fraction; *LAFR*, laminar air flow room (isolation floor); *LDH*, lactic dehydrogenase; *MI*, myocardial infarction; *WBC*, white blood cell count.
*Favorable and high-risk groups were defined solely by cytogenetic aberrations. Above factors served to further divide the intermediate-risk group into good intermediate versus adverse intermediate.
†As continuous variables.
‡Only significant for prediction of remission.
§Only significant for prediction of survival.

Investigational treatments are helpful where unfavorable prognostic factors predominate. *Investigational* does not a priori mean low intensity. Patients with an excellent performance status but high-risk disease because of an unfavorable karyotype, preceding MDS, or therapy-related AML may be appropriate candidates for high-intensity programs, whereas low-intensity protocols are indicated for patients with a poor performance status, comorbidities, or those who do not want to undergo intensive chemotherapy. Table 58-4 summarizes the experience with investigational regimens.

Table 58-4 Investigational Induction Therapies for Older Patients With Acute Myeloid Leukemia

Drug(s)	N	Median Age (yr) (range)	OR (%)	CR (%)	Median Survival (mo)	Early Mortality (%)
Clofarabine	112	71 (60-88)	46	38	9.8	9.8
Clofarabine + low-dose cytarabine	54	70 (60-82)	67*	63*	11.4	19
Tipifarnib + etoposide	84	77 (70-91)	40	25	5.3	11
Laromustine	85	72 (60-87)	32	23	3.2	14
Idarubicin/cytarabine + lomustine	508	70 (60-86)	68	68†	12.7†	16
High-dose lenalidomide	33	71 (60-88)	30	NA	4	24

CR, Complete remission; *OR,* overall response.
*Significantly higher than with clofarabine alone.
†Significantly higher than with idarubicin plus cytarabine alone.

Patients with a performance status of 3 or 4, severely abnormal organ function, or who are very old (older than 80 years) may be candidates for supportive care because their expected treatment-related mortality is high, and any gains will be minimal with currently available therapies. These decisions are very individual and need to be thoroughly discussed with patients and their families.

Postremission Therapy for Older Patients

To administer repetitive cycles of modest-dose consolidation therapy is a reasonable strategy for patients with good performance status and no adverse cytogenetics. Unlike in younger patients, HiDAC is less effective and, given its higher potential for toxicity in older patients is also less likely to be feasible. There are conflicting data as to the number of postremission cycles (four have been equal to one), the intensity of postremission therapy (one intensive consolidation cycle was better than 1 year of oral maintenance; in another study six cycles of outpatient consolidation were superior to one short but more intense course), and whether or not prolonged maintenance could be beneficial (as suggested in one study).[1] It is expected that the AML genotype will influence the choice of postremission therapy also in older patients, but data are preliminary and require confirmation from larger studies.

HSCT has been hampered by lack of suitable donors and high treatment-related mortality of standard transplant procedures. Reduced-intensity conditioning transplant has opened this treatment modality to a wider range of older patients as demonstrated by a recent analysis showing no significant impact of age on nonrelapse mortality, relapse, disease-free survival, and overall survival. Selection of patients for HSCT would presumably follow guidelines described in younger patients with the caveat that for older patients long-term disease control is more difficult to achieve.

Maintenance Therapy

Whereas most patients achieve CR following induction, only a third maintain it and do not relapse. Some patients will receive an allogeneic HSCT in first remission, but for most, therapy is terminated with completion of the consolidation, and a "watch and wait" strategy is pursued thereafter. To minimize the likelihood of relapse, postconsolidation maintenance therapy strategies have been tried. The graft-versus-leukemia effect following allogeneic HSCT plays a significant role in the reduction of the risk for relapse, and this effect is to a great part mediated by T-cell activation. Therefore nontransplant maintenance strategies have also been aimed at stimulating tumor-specific cytotoxic T lymphocytes and natural killer (NK) cells. Interleukin-2 (IL-2) is a potent effector-activating cytokine with evidence in preclinical models of antileukemic activity. Although at high doses IL-2 was able to induce responses in patients with active disease, the drug-related toxicities precluded these doses, and lower dose schedules have been evaluated instead in patients in CR.[8] None of these studies demonstrated an advantage of low-dose IL-2 maintenance immunotherapy with regard to disease-free and overall survival. An individual patient data metaanalysis from six randomized controlled trials has confirmed this observation. The only study with positive results supplemented IL-2 with histamine dihydrochloride to enhance the function of cytotoxic antileukemic lymphocytes.[22] In this phase III trial, 320 patients with AML and a median age of 57 years were randomly assigned to receive ten 21-day cycles of Il-2 plus histamine dihydrochloride or observation. The results revealed significantly improved 3-year leukemia-free survival (40% versus 26%; $P = .01$) for the treated patients. However, this benefit only included patients who were in their first CR, and overall survival was not affected in either group. Other concepts have been developed based on hypomethylating agents, which are well tolerated and can be administered over longer periods of time. Results are at best inconclusive, including when used after transplant. At this moment, there is no accepted role for maintenance therapy in AML.

Minimal Residual Disease

Minimal residual disease (MRD) remains below the threshold of detection by morphologic and immunohistochemical means. It is estimated that patients in morphologic CR still harbor up to 10^9 leukemic cells, which constitute an important reservoir for later recurrences. Although many of the biologic aspects of MRD remain unknown, the increasingly easy availability of highly sensitive laboratory assays has made the detection of MRD more practical and attractive. Measuring MRD has several advantages: (1) to improve the assessment of the quality of response, (2) to diagnose recurrence earlier, (3) to determine the intensity of postremission therapy, and (4) to prevent a full-blown clinical relapse while still at the level of a molecular relapse. It should be understood that these goals remain theoretical and especially with regard to points 3 and 4 are unproven (with APL as the only exception).

Two techniques are used for the detection of MRD: flow cytometry and reverse-transcriptase polymerase chain reaction (RT-PCR). Flow cytometry is applicable to almost all patients and is based on the identification of an aberrant leukemia immunophenotype. RT-PCR requires identifiable markers such as fusion transcripts (e.g., PML-RARA, RUNX1-RUNX1T1, CBFB-MYH11, DEK-CAN), overexpressed (WT1) or mutated (NPM1, Flt-3) genes. Both assays are comparable in sensitivity, but RT-PCR testing is less specific. Important issues are (1) the threshold of detection that is predictive for relapse; (2) when MRD testing should be done; and (3) if it is predictive for relapse, whether early intervention based on MRD levels is helpful. Different thresholds have been defined in clinical studies, but their validation is lacking. There is some evidence that high levels of MRD following induction are important but that levels at the end of consolidation matter most for overall survival. The only subtype of AML for which MRD measurements are integrated into clinical decision making in daily clinical practice is APL, which will be addressed in a separate section of this chapter. For all others, implications from MRD testing remain investigational and confined to clinical studies.

Acute Myeloid Leukemia Salvage Therapy

Most patients with AML will require salvage therapy either because they relapsed or because they did not respond to induction therapy (primary refractory). Most relapses occur within the first 2 years following achievement of remission. In an analysis of 1069 consecutive AML patients in first CR who were treated and followed at M.D. Anderson Cancer Center, the yearly risks for treatment failure were 69%, 38%, 17%, 8%, and 7% in the first to fourth year, respectively. With a probability of relapse-free survival of 84% at 6 years for patients who were alive and disease-free at 3 years, it is reasonable to consider patients cured once they have been in CR for at least 3 years. For patients older than 60 years with intermediate-risk cytogenetics, the relapse-free survival was only 56%, indicating that in older patients, a substantial risk for relapse remains even beyond 3 years in remission.

The prognosis for patients in relapse is likely to be guarded, but outcomes are more heterogeneous than the first impression may imply. The two most important predictors for prognosis are the duration of first remission and the number of previous salvage regimens. In a study of 243 patients with AML who have received first salvage therapy, the likelihood of CR was 60% if the duration of the first remission exceeded 1 year and only 19% for patients with shorter remissions. Treatment was not strongly associated with prognosis. Breems et al[23] presented a prognostic score based on a multivariate analysis of 667 patients who were in first relapse. They identified four clinical parameters (duration of first remission, cytogenetics at diagnosis, age at relapse, and previous HSCT or not) and identified three risk groups. In the favorable group, CR was achieved in 85% of patients and overall survival at 5 years was 46%. In the intermediate- and poor-risk groups the numbers for CR were 60% and 34% and for 5-year survival were 18% and 4%, respectively. Prognosis is worse for patients after second salvage, but even then survival expectations at 1 year vary between 2% and 24% depending on a set of clinical variables. In a study of patients with AML who were primary refractory to at least one cycle of HiDAC-based induction therapy, the subsequent CR rate was only 22% with a CR duration of around 9 months and median survival of only 3.8 months.[24]

The goal of salvage therapy is to provide sufficient disease control to allow for an HSCT. Although few patients will be successfully referred for transplantation, outcome is better than with chemotherapy, and 5-year survival expectations following HSCT may vary from 15% (in primary induction failure) to 40% (in secondary remission after first relapse).

There are no standardized salvage chemotherapy regimens. The choice is largely determined by the first remission duration, the patient age, and to a lesser degree the cytogenetics at presentation. Patients with remission durations exceeding 1 year may be successfully reinduced with a regimen similar to the induction. For most patients this means intermediate-dose (1 g/m^2 per dose) or higher-dose (2 to 3 g/m^2 per dose) cytarabine, which is commonly combined with other agents such as anthracyclines and/or fludarabine (e.g., fludarabine, cytarabine [ara-C], idarubicin [FAI]; fludarabine, cytarabine [ara-C], and G-CSF [FLAG]). Mitoxantrone and etoposide are sometimes used, but their efficacy is rather modest and the regimen is associated with severe mucositis. In a recent large international multicenter randomized trial of 326 patients with relapsed and refractory AML, patients received either intermediate-dose cytarabine (1 g/m^2 daily for 5 days) or cytarabine plus clofarabine, a second-generation deoxyadenosine analogue. Although response rates and event-free survival were superior in the combination arm, there was no difference in overall survival. Patients with short remission durations or refractory disease have poor response rates and even worse survival with conventional drugs and are therefore appropriate candidates to participate in clinical trials.

Investigational Therapies

The two most common scenarios in which investigational programs merit serious considerations are situations in which blasts are predictably resistant to therapy and in which patients are unfit for conventional therapy because of age and/or performance status.

Inhibitors of Flt-3

Mutations of the Flt-3 gene are among the most common abnormalities in patients with diploid cytogenetics. ITDs have been associated with high relapse likelihood and worse overall survival. Several inhibitors of Flt-3 have been tested in clinical trials, including lestaurtinib (CEP-701), midostaurin (PKC412), sorafenib (BAY 43-9006), tandutinib (MLN518), semaxanib (SU5416), sunitinib (SU11248), KW-2449, and quizartinib (AC220). Various factors influence the activity of these agents. Blasts with a low mutant allelic burden of Flt-3/ITD may be less dependent on Flt-3 signaling. Whether or not there is an association of the size of the ITD fragment with outcome is controversial. Secretion of Flt-3 ligand is another resistance mechanism under discussion. The spectrum of activity of most of the Flt-3 inhibitors extends to other kinases so that there are differences with regard to specificity between these agents. Also in clinical studies is the anti- Flt-3 monoclonal antibody IMC-EB10, which in preclinical studies showed antiproliferative activity against wild-type and mutant Flt-3 samples.

Single-agent activity for most of the Flt-3 inhibitors is modest, consisting of reductions of circulating or marrow blasts without reaching objective response criteria. The exception has been quizartinib, which achieved CR rates of up to 28% in patients with Flt-3/ITD mutations (13% without) and durable responses in some.[25] Combination therapy of Flt-3 inhibitors with chemotherapy is of larger interest. Although a randomized study of chemotherapy alone versus chemotherapy plus lestaurtinib involving 224 patients in first relapse showed no improvement of response rate or survival, several frontline studies have suggested improved responses in Flt-3/ITD-mutated patients.[26] Large randomized trials in newly diagnosed patients with Flt-3/ITD mutations are under way to validate the benefit of these drugs.

Other Inhibitors of Cellular Signaling Pathways

Cellular signaling pathways control maturation, differentiation, proliferation, apoptosis of marrow blasts, and other crucial cellular processes. Defects in one or several of the signaling cascades in the form of constitutive activation of kinases or dysfunction of adaptor proteins and transcription factors can trigger or propagate the leukemia phenotype. Conversely, many small-molecule targeted drugs are now in clinical trials that aim to abrogate abnormally activated kinases and other enzymes and reverse this process. Compared to the success of tyrosine kinase–inhibitor therapy in chronic myeloid leukemia, the clinical impact of this approach in AML is still limited.

Signaling through Ras/Raf/MEK is activated in many cancers and has been one of the first targets for small-molecule kinase inhibitors. In a phase I study of tipifarnib, a farnesyltransferase inhibitor, in adults with refractory acute leukemias, 29% of patients responded. Later studies proved disappointing with similar survival between tipifarnib and supportive care in older patients with untreated AML. However, a two-gene genetic signature has highlighted subgroups of patients with higher response to tipifarnib, and combination studies with agents such as etoposide appear more promising as well.

Inhibitors of MEK1/2 have demonstrated clinical activity in the salvage therapy for AML. Of 39 patients with relapsed or secondary AML, a third responded if the blasts had mutated KRAS or NRAS, compared with only 8% without mutations of Ras. The study highlights the importance of identifying particular cytogenetic-molecular signatures indicative of increased responsiveness to a specific group of drugs.

Other targets are BCL2 and other antiapoptotic proteins; multidrug resistance proteins; the ubiquitin-proteasome pathway; protein kinase C signaling; aurora kinases, which play an important role in the formation and organization of the mitotic spindle apparatus; the mammalian target of rapamycin (mTOR); and components of the microenvironment (e.g., proangiogenic proteins, cell adhesion molecules).

Epigenetic Therapy

Hypermethylation of CpG-rich islands of DNA together with changes in the conformation of histone proteins (e.g., deacetylation of histone proteins results in tighter packaging of chromosomal material and hence decreased transcriptional activity) lead to suppression of the expression of several genes, some of which function as tumor suppressor genes. In contrast to gene mutations, these epigenetic modifications are not permanent and can be reversed. Two drugs commonly used to affect this change are the DNA methyltransferase (DNMT) inhibitors azacitidine and decitabine ("hypomethylating agents"). Although FDA approved only for patients with MDS, they are widely used for adults with AML within and outside (off label) clinical studies. Because their use is predominantly for older patients with AML, some of the clinical experience has already been addressed.[19-21] Combination trials of DNMT inhibitors with histone deacetylase inhibitors and studies randomizing patients between hypomethylating agents and standard cytotoxic chemotherapy (e.g., decitabine versus low-dose cytarabine) are being conducted.

Gemtuzumab Ozogamicin

GO is a humanized anti-CD33 monoclonal antibody that is chemically linked to a cytotoxic moiety called calicheamicin. Upon binding to CD33, internalization, and dissolution of the link, calicheamicin is released intracellularly and inhibits DNA synthesis, resulting in apoptosis. Three phase II studies evaluated GO in patients with AML in first relapse and demonstrated a CR rate of 16% and a rate for CR without adequate platelet recovery of another 13%, culminating in an overall response rate of 29%. These studies provided the basis for the FDA approval of GO in 2000. Combinations of GO with cytotoxic chemotherapy resulted in hepatic toxicities, namely, venoocclusive disease (sinusoidal obstruction syndrome), that were not observed before. Although this problem was largely resolved by adjusting the GO doses to as low as 3 mg/m^2 in combinations, the expanded spectrum of toxicities plus the observation that GO failed to improve outcome of patients led the FDA to revoke the approval in 2010. However, one large multicenter trial by the MRC has since shown that GO in combination with cytotoxic chemotherapy improves survival in the frontline therapy for patients with favorable cytogenetics.[15] These results were mirrored in a smaller single-center trial in which the combination of FLAG with GO in patients with CBF leukemias resulted in superior event-free survival compared to historical controls of idarubicin plus cytarabine. A trend for better relapse-free survival with GO chemotherapy in patients with favorable cytogenetics was also seen in SWOG study S0106. GO has also been shown to be effective and safe for patients with APL. Identification of niche populations of patients who still derive benefit from GO has led to a resurgence of interest in the drug, which is currently available only through clinical studies.

Novel Cytotoxic Agents

Clofarabine is a second-generation deoxyadenosine nucleoside analogue with substantial structural similarity to its predecessors fludarabine and cladribine. The addition of two halogen molecules provides clofarabine with a more favorable pharmacokinetic profile and distinct spectrum of activity. Clofarabine has been used as single agent and in combination with standard cytotoxic agents (cytarabine, anthracyclines, cyclophosphamide) in patients with both untreated and relapsed/refractory AML. A multicenter study of 112 patients 60 years or older with untreated AML showed a CR rate of 38% with an overall response rate of 46%. Median survival of all patients regardless of response was 9.8 months, and early mortality was 9.8%. Combination studies, including those for younger patients with untreated disease, are under way. Other novel nucleoside analogues such as sapacitabine are in clinical trials.

Laromustine is a novel sulfonylhydrazine alkylating agent with unique properties compared to older alkylators such as BCNU. In an international phase II study laromustine was given as a single IV infusion to patients who were 60 years or older with untreated AML. The CR rate was 23% with an overall response rate of 32%. Early mortality was 14%. Although these patients were older with at least one predefined adverse characteristic at the time of diagnosis, the median overall survival was only 3.2 months. As for other novel cytotoxic drugs, their main use will be in combination treatments, which may require changes in dose and schedules, much of which remains unexplored at the present time.

ACUTE PROMYELOCYTIC LEUKEMIA

APL has unique clinical, pathophysiologic, and therapeutic features. The median age at diagnosis is about 40 years, and it is more frequent in Hispanics and the obese. Despite its rarity (approximately 10% of all AML diagnoses) it is important to promptly diagnose. If managed appropriately APL has the most favorable prognosis of all AMLs. On the other hand, coagulopathies in concert with thrombocytopenia can result in catastrophic bleeding events (especially inside the CNS) with a high early mortality. In 80% of the cases, APL cells are hypergranular with many Auer rods. A microgranular variant (M3v) is often associated with leukocytosis. APL cells are strongly positive MPO staining and lack expression of CD34 and HLA-DR.

APL is almost always the result of translocation t(15;17) that leads to fusion of the gene for retinoic acid receptor alpha (RARA) with the promyelocytic leukemia gene (PML). In very rare cases (<5%) translocation partners other than PML on chromosome 15 result in alternative fusion genes (e.g., PLZF-RARA, NPM-RARA, NuMA-RARA, STAT5-RARA) whose significance lies in possible resistance to all-trans retinoic acid (ATRA). PML-RARA is an abnormal retinoic acid (RA) receptor that represses transcription of a number of RA-activated target genes. It does so mainly by recruiting large protein complexes through the coiled-coil domain of PML, which in turn act as potent transcriptional corepressors. Pharmacologic doses of RA release the corepressors, allow recruitment of coactivators, and thus result in the transcription of previously silenced genes. This leads to a sudden arrest in proliferation and a differentiation response that can be seen in vitro and in vivo within a few days following administration of ATRA (Fig. 58-16). APL is the most dramatic example of the success of differentiating therapy, which has proved disappointing in other forms of AML.

The clinical activity of ATRA was first demonstrated in a study from China, where oral ATRA alone when given over 30 to 90 days achieved CR rates of 85%, an observation that was later confirmed by groups in North America and Europe. ATRA not only achieved high CR rates comparable to chemotherapy alone, but also improved the coagulopathy. ATRA therapy has also been associated in 10% to 25% of patients with the "retinoic acid syndrome" (nowadays referred to as *differentiation syndrome* because it is also seen with other differentiating agents). It occurs within a few days of start of therapy and presents with signs and symptoms resembling capillary leak and respiratory distress syndrome: fever, dyspnea, hypoxemia, pulmonary infiltrates, weight gain, peripheral edema, renal and hepatic dysfunction, and ascites. Differentiation syndrome carries a high mortality unless recognized and managed promptly. Therapy consists of holding the differentiating agent and instituting steroids (e.g., dexamethasone 10 mg for 3 to 5 days with a slow taper over 2 weeks). This intervention will rapidly reverse the manifestations of

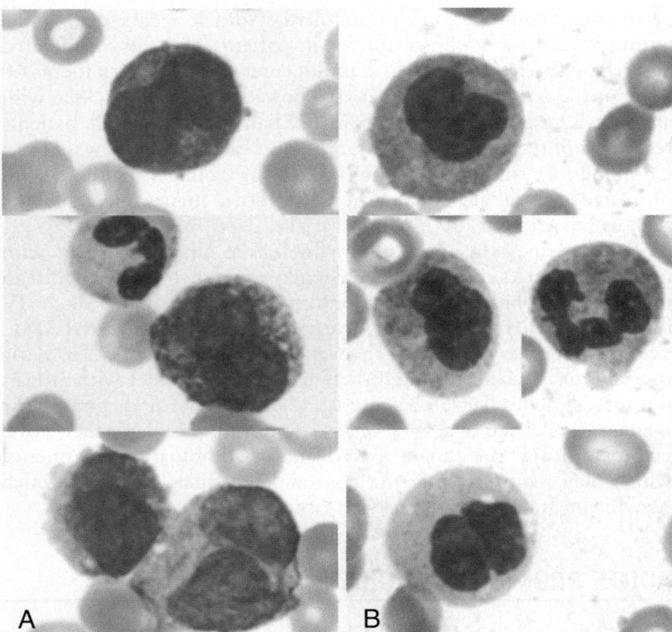

Figure 58-16 Effect of all-trans retinoic acid (ATRA) therapy on acute promyelocytic leukemia (APL) cells. ATRA therapy in APL causes the malignant promyelocytes **(A)** to differentiate, and the effects of differentiation can be seen within days of treatment **(B).** The differentiated APL cells are still somewhat atypical, frequently with bilobed nuclei (compare to normal neutrophil [**B,** *insert center right*]).

differentiation syndrome and has substantially reduced mortality to below 5%. Some investigators have proposed prophylactically using steroids in patients who present with WBC of greater than 10,000/μL.

ATRA alone is insufficient therapy because all patients will eventually relapse. Clinical studies confirmed significantly better disease-free survival for the combination of ATRA plus chemotherapy. In the French APL 93 trial concurrent administration of ATRA with chemotherapy achieved a lower relapse rate at 2 years (6%) compared to sequential administration (16%, $P = .04$) given identical CR rates of 92%. Optimal induction therapy for patients with APL therefore is the combination of ATRA with an anthracycline (daunorubicin or idarubicin). In two large trials from Italy (Italian Group for Haematological Diseases in Adults [GIMEMA]) and Spain (PETHEMA), CR rates were 95% and 89%, respectively, and 2-year disease-free survival was 79%.[27] Sanz et al[27] proposed a risk-stratification model based on WBC and platelet count. High-risk was defined as a WBC of greater than 10,000/μL at diagnosis with significant differences in relapse-free survival between patients with high-, intermediate-, and low-risk disease.

Monitoring response during induction consists of morphologic assessments of blood smears and marrow in addition to serial measurements of PML/RARalpha by RT-PCR assays. The differentiation response of the leukemic blasts may be delayed; therefore repeat marrow studies are not recommended before the blood counts recover at around 4 to 6 weeks of therapy. In some instances a repeat marrow assessment 1 to 2 weeks later may be necessary to establish the response. No early intervention or change of therapy should be undertaken during this time.[28] By the end of induction and with achievement of a morphologic remission, it is very likely that there has also been a complete cytogenetic response. However, molecular testing by RT-PCR is frequently still positive, which at this early point in therapy should not be interpreted as a sign of treatment resistance.

The role of cytarabine during induction and consolidation therapy remains controversial. In two randomized studies of ATRA/anthracycline ± cytarabine from the AML MRC15 trial and the European APL Group, rates for CR and induction failure were comparable, but in the European trial (using daunorubicin as opposed to idarubicin in the MRC trial) the risk for relapse was increased when cytarabine was omitted from the treatment regimen. On the other hand, in the MRC15 trial not only was there no difference in relapse rate, the cytarabine-treated patients experienced a small increase of deaths and higher use of medical resources. In a joint analysis of the European results with those of the PETHEMA group, the benefit of cytarabine was restricted to patients with higher-risk disease. Current recommendations provide an option of using cytarabine in younger patients with WBC of greater than 10,000/μL.

Arsenic trioxide (ATO) has potent antiapoptotic activity in APL cells. Whereas its precise mechanism of action is not well-defined and almost certainly depends on additional mechanisms, it is one of the most active drugs available against APL with high single-agent response rates in relapsed patients. In a study by M.D. Anderson Cancer Center ATRA and ATO were combined in newly diagnosed patients with APL.[29] High-risk patients also received GO. Of 82 patients, 74 achieved CR with an overall response rate of 92%. Among the low-risk group, the CR rate was 95% and no patient relapsed, with an estimated 3-year survival rate of 85% for the whole study group. The combination of ATRA and ATO is currently recommended for patients who are older and/or intolerant to therapy with anthracyclines. Single-agent ATO without ATRA may be particularly attractive where medical resources are scarce and access to cheaper therapies is an economic necessity. In two studies, one from India and one from Iran, single-agent ATO achieved CR rates of close to 85% with 3-year survival rates of 86% (India) and 5-year survival rates of 64% (Iran). Patients with higher-risk disease appeared to respond equally favorably. ATO can cause prolongation of the QTc interval, which may lead rarely to serious cardiac arrhythmias. It is recommended to check an electrocardiogram before each course of therapy and maintain electrolytes such as potassium and magnesium at high-normal levels throughout therapy.

Postremission therapy consists of consolidation and maintenance. Although there remains considerable debate about particular aspects of the consolidation (addition of ATRA, role of ATO, value of cytarabine), the general recommendation is to give another two or three anthracycline-based cycles, typically in conjunction with ATRA because the latter has been shown to reduce relapse risk. There is less agreement on the addition of cytarabine as has already been discussed. ATO in consolidation has been explored in a large randomized U.S. Intergroup study. Addition of ATO to a standard induction and consolidation therapy has significantly improved event-free and disease-free survival. The purpose of consolidation therapy is to convert a morphologic and cytogenetic remission into a durable molecular response. For patients who have achieved a molecular response, maintenance therapy for 1 to 2 years with ATRA ± mercaptopurine and methotrexate has been recommended. Later studies, in particular a large trial by the GIMEMA group, questioned the benefit of ATRA-based maintenance. There are ongoing randomized studies exploring the benefit of maintenance therapy, but it appears likely that the impact of maintenance on overall outcome has changed now that ATRA and ATO are being used earlier during treatment. Whereas maintenance may not be of much use for low-risk patients, it may be considered for high-risk patients who have become molecular responders after consolidation.

RT-PCR testing is essential in the follow-up of patients with APL. In no other leukemia, with the possible exception of chronic myeloid leukemia, does molecular testing play such a critical role and influence clinical decision-making processes. Patients who do not achieve a molecular response by the end of the consolidation (usually 3 months into CR) have a poorer prognosis with a higher likelihood of relapse. Furthermore, these patients have a better survival with early intervention rather than at the time of morphologic relapse. Whereas no further monitoring may be necessary for molecular responders with low-risk disease because of the very low relapse likelihood, monitoring should take place every 3 months for 2 years for patients with high-risk disease, those older than 60 years, and patients for whom treatment delays occurred during consolidation. Positive

PCR test results should be confirmed by a second PCR test within 1 to 4 weeks. If the repeat test results are negative, no further action is necessary; however, close prospective monitoring should be applied.

ATO is effective therapy for patients with relapsed APL, including those with persistent PCR-positive disease. Morphologic remissions are observed in up to 90% and molecular remission in 70% to 80% of patients, respectively.[30] Overall survival at 3 years is between 50% and 70%. Addition of ATRA to ATO may provide little further benefit if ATRA was already part of the induction/consolidation, which is the case most of the time. HSCT should follow achievement of a second remission. Autologous HSCT is recommended for patients who have again achieved a molecular response. For those whose PCR results remain positive despite ATO-based therapy, allogeneic HSCT is another option. CNS involvement at the time of relapse is rare, so that there is no commonly agreed-upon strategy of CNS prophylaxis. Whereas some groups such as the National Comprehensive Cancer Network advocate prophylactic intrathecal therapy for patients in second morphologic remission, the Spanish PETHEMA group showed that two independent risk factors for CNS disease are hyperleukocytosis (WBC >10,000/μL) and occurrence of CNS hemorrhage during induction. Whereas under those circumstances the incidence of CNS involvement has been as high as 5.5%, it was not higher than 1.2% at 5 years for the remainder of the patients.

ADDITIONAL ISSUES IN ACUTE MYELOID LEUKEMIA THERAPY

Hyperleukocytosis

Hyperleukocytosis is defined as a WBC of greater than 100,000/μL (Fig. 58-17). Presumably this should reflect an increase of blasts close to this level although this distinction is not always followed very closely in clinical practice. Myeloid blasts are less deformable than normal myeloid cells and adhere to vessel walls and extramedullary tissues due to a complex array of adhesion molecules, which distinguishes them from lymphoid blasts. Hyperleukocytosis is a medical emergency with a high mortality rate mainly due to pulmonary and CNS complications from bleeding (secondary to anatomic disruption of the endothelial lining of blood cells, DIC, or both) and direct tissue infiltration with inflammatory responses. It is therefore imperative that efforts be undertaken to reduce the blast burden as soon as possible. Because red blood cell transfusions increase the viscosity of blood flow, they should be used judiciously or if possible avoided as long as the WBC remains high. Leukapheresis is a fast and effective method for WBC reduction. Although it has an immediate effect in reducing early mortality, there has been no impact on survival. Leukapheresis does not affect cellular plugs that are already formed in a vascular territory, nor does it affect inflammatory reactions in tissues infiltrated by blasts. Rapid administration of cytotoxic chemotherapy with or without leukapheresis therefore plays an important role. The most effective drug is cytarabine. Hydroxyurea is an oral alternative that is well tolerated and easy to administer. However, hydroxyurea does not effectively infiltrate tissues and thus may not reach extravascular blast infiltrates. Care must be taken to avoid tumor lysis syndrome, using adequate hydration and uricosuric agents, and to meticulously follow electrolyte levels and renal function.

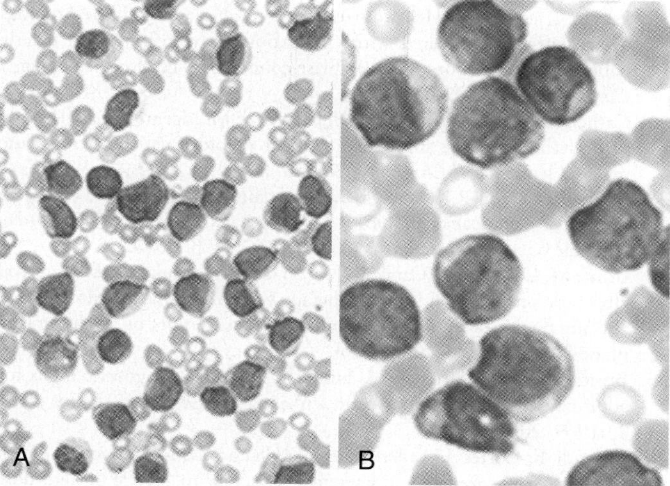

Figure 58-17 HYPERLEUKOCYTOSIS IN ACUTE MYELOID LEUKEMIA. The patient was a 23-year-old man who presented with several weeks of abdominal pain, weight loss, and fatigue. He was found to have a marked leukocytosis of 165,300/μL composed of mostly blasts (**A** and higher-power **B**), which were shown to be myeloblasts by flow immunophenotyping. The patient developed some shortness of breath and hypoxia and underwent two cycles of leukapheresis and hydroxyurea before induction. Molecular analysis revealed the leukemia to have an Flt-3-ITD mutation.

Myeloid Sarcoma

Myeloid sarcoma (granulocytic sarcoma, chloroma) is an extramedullary myeloid tumor composed of myeloid blasts. Myeloid sarcomas can occur in any tissue but most commonly present in the skin, lymph nodes, gastrointestinal tract, testes, CNS, soft tissue, and bones. They can easily be confused with lymphomas and soft tissue sarcomas. Myeloid sarcomas may be isolated; they may occur together with marrow involvement or precede it. In a few instances they may be the relapse manifestation of patients who have been treated for AML in the past. In the context of chronic myeloid malignancies (e.g., MDS, myeloproliferative neoplasms, chronic myeloid leukemia, chronic myelomonocytic leukemia) their appearance represents progression to a blast phase. Myeloid sarcoma even when isolated should be treated systemically with chemotherapy as for any other patient with AML. Radiation therapy may be of help in a few instances to optimize local control. However, in the absence of systemic therapy, subsequent development of systemic AML is very likely. There is controversy over whether patients with myeloid sarcoma do better or worse than those with AML. A recent retrospective comparison between patients with and without isolated myeloid sarcoma and a cohort of AML patients suggests no significant differences in survival and a possible survival benefit with HSCT for all groups.

Central Nervous System Disease

CNS involvement occurs in less than 5% of patients with AML and is therefore much rarer than in ALL. Consequently, there is no role for CNS prophylaxis. Before HiDAC, inv(16) AML was associated with a 30% incidence of CNS leukemia, particularly intracerebral masses. This particular problem has been virtually eliminated with the use of HiDAC but may still be noted in patients with inv(16) AML in whom HiDAC is not delivered. In the presence of symptoms suggestive of CNS disease, further workup should be pursued. Symptoms are due to raised intracranial pressure, mass effect, or infiltration of cranial nerves. Whereas CT scan is a convenient modality to rule out significant anatomic disruptions, it is not very sensitive to detect more subtle signs of leptomeningeal disease, and, if concerns persist, a magnetic resonance imaging scan of the brain (or any other CNS structure where disease is suspected) should be obtained. Lumbar puncture is a crucial component of the workup. Blasts in the cerebrospinal fluid may range from a few cells to several thousand. Treatment consists of intrathecal therapy with cytarabine and/or methotrexate via lumbar route or Ommaya reservoir. The dose of methotrexate should be reduced by 50% if administered into an Ommaya reservoir. A typical schedule includes twice-weekly intrathecal doses until the cerebrospinal fluid becomes clear. The frequency is then changed to weekly for 2 months, then every other week for 2 months, followed by monthly injections for up to 1 year. Radiation therapy can be a useful alternative, especially in the case of localized lesions such as isolated cranial nerve findings. Although high-dose cytarabine penetrates the blood-brain barrier and may have contributed to a lower rate of CNS involvement over the years, it by itself is not sufficient therapy once there is CNS disease. The risk for CNS involvement is higher in AML with any type of monoblastic differentiation and those cases with a high WBC (>100,000/μL) at presentation. Although some authorities have recommended routine screening for CNS disease in these patients, this is not common practice.

Pregnancy

AML diagnosis is a rare event during pregnancy. In a case-control study of 785 women with AML ages 15 to 50 years compared with 1576 age- and sex-matched controls, AML occurred at a rate of 1.3% in the pregnant group and 3.4% in the control group, resulting in an odds ratio of 0.44 in favor of the women who were pregnant. The response to treatment is not affected by pregnancy. AML therapy during the first trimester is problematic due to the toxic and teratogenic effects of chemotherapy on the fetus. Under those circumstances, termination of pregnancy before institution of induction therapy should be strongly considered. Pregnancy outcome during the second and third trimester is much more favorable, in which successful treatment of the AML and delivery of normal infants have been reported. Daunorubicin may be preferable over idarubicin because the latter is more lipophilic and has a higher DNA affinity, raising the specter of higher maternal-fetal transfer and toxicity to the fetus.[1] It is not advisable to delay therapy once the diagnosis of AML is made given the high risk for maternal death. In situations where the leukemia behaves indolently and women are close to delivery, a conservative approach can be chosen with supportive care and induction of labor as soon as possible. These decisions are based on clinical judgment and discussion with the patient.

FUTURE DIRECTIONS

The backbone of AML therapy has not changed substantially in the previous three decades and is heavily dependent on cytarabine in combination with other cytotoxic chemotherapy. Molecular signatures and identification of signaling pathways that are abnormally activated or regulated in AML blasts are contributing to a more complex picture of the biology of AML, provide more accurate prognostic information, and ultimately offer targets for drug development.

REFERENCES

1. Döhner H, Estey EH, Amadori S, et al: Diagnosis and management of acute myeloid leukemia in adults: Recommendations from an international expert panel, on behalf of the European LeukemiaNet. *Blood* 115:453, 2010.
2. Rowe JM, Tallman MS: How I treat acute myeloid leukemia. *Blood* 116:3147, 2010.
3. Foran JM: New prognostic markers in acute myeloid leukemia: Perspective from the clinic. *Hematology Am Soc Hematol Educ Program* 2010:47, 2010.
4. Byrd JC, Mrózek K, Dodge RK, et al: Pretreatment cytogenetic abnormalities are predictive of induction success, cumulative incidence of relapse, and overall survival in adult patients with de novo acute myeloid leukemia: Results from Cancer and Leukemia Group B (CALGB 8461). *Blood* 100:4325, 2002.
5. Burnett A, Wetzler M, Löwenberg B: Therapeutic advances in acute myeloid leukemia. *J Clin Oncol* 29:487, 2011.
6. Feldman EJ: Too much ara-C? Not enough daunorubicin? *Blood* 117:2299, 2011.
7. Ohtake S, Miyawaki S, Fujita H, et al: Randomized study of induction therapy comparing standard-dose idarubicin with high-dose daunorubicin in adult patients with previously untreated acute myeloid leukemia: The JALSG AML201 Study. *Blood* 117:2358, 2011.
8. Pautas C, Merabet F, Thomas X, et al: Randomized study of intensified anthracycline doses for induction and recombinant interleukin-2 for maintenance in patients with acute myeloid leukemia age 50 to 70 years: Results of the ALFA-9801 Study. *J Clin Oncol* 28:808, 2010.
9. Fernandez HF, Sun Z, Yao X, et al: Anthracycline dose intensification in acute myeloid leukemia. *N Engl J Med* 361:1249, 2009.
10. Kern W, Estey EH: High-dose cytosine arabinoside in the treatment of acute myeloid leukemia. *Cancer* 107:116, 2006.
11. Burnett AK, Hills R, Milligan D, et al: Attempts to optimize induction and consolidation chemotherapy in patients with acute myeloid leukaemia: Results of the MRC AML 15 Trial. *Blood* 114:200 (abstract 484), 2009.
12. Löwenberg B, Pabst T, Vellenga E, et al: Cytarabine dose for acute myeloid leukemia. *N Engl J Med* 364:1027, 2011.
13. Burnett AK, Hills RK, Milligan DW, et al: Attempts to optimize induction and consolidation treatment in acute myeloid leukemia: Results of the MRC AML 12 trial. *J Clin Oncol* 28:586, 2010.
14. Miyawaki S, Ohtake S, Fujisawa S, et al: A randomized comparison of 4 courses of standard-dose multiagent chemotherapy versus 3 courses of high-dose cytarabine alone in postremission therapy for acute myeloid leukemia in adults: The JALSG AML210 Study. *Blood* 117:2366, 2011.
15. Burnett AK, Hills RK, Milligan D, et al: Identification of patients with acute myeloblastic leukemia who benefit from the addition of gemtuzumab ozogamicin: Results of the MRC AML15 trial. *J Clin Oncol* 29:369, 2011.
16. Gupta V, Tallman MS, Weisdorf DJ: Allogeneic hematopoietic stem cell transplantation for adults with acute myeloid leukemia: Myths, controversies, and unknowns. *Blood* 117:2307, 2011.
17. Menzin J, Lang K, Earle CC, et al: The outcomes and costs of acute myeloid leukemia among the elderly. *Arch Intern Med* 162:1597, 2002.
18. Burnett AK, Milligan D, Prentice AG, et al: A comparison of low-dose cytarabine and hydroxyurea with or without all-trans retinoic acid for acute myeloid leukemia and high-risk myelodysplastic syndrome in patients not considered fit for intensive treatment. *Cancer* 109:1114, 2007.
19. Fenaux P, Mufti GJ, Hellström-Lindberg E, et al: Azacitidine prolongs overall survival compared with conventional care regimens in elderly patients with low bone marrow blast count acute myeloid leukemia. *J Clin Oncol* 28:562, 2010.
20. Cashen AF, Schiller GJ, O'Donnell MR, et al: Multicenter, phase II study of decitabine for the first-line treatment of older patients with acute myeloid leukemia. *J Clin Oncol* 28:556, 2010.
21. Blum W, Garzon R, Klisovic RB, et al: Clinical response and miR-29b predictive significance in older AML patients treated with a 10-day schedule of decitabine. *Proc N Acad Sci* 107:7473, 2010.
22. Brune M, Castaigne S, Catalano J, et al: Improved leukemia-free survival after postconsolidation immunotherapy with histamine dihydrochloride and interleukin-2 in acute myeloid leukemia: Results of a randomized phase 3 trial. *Blood* 108:88, 2006.
23. Breems DA, Van Putten WLJ, Huijgens PC, et al: Prognostic index for adult patients with acute myeloid leukemia in first relapse. *J Clin Oncol* 23:1969, 2005.
24. Ravandi F, Cortes J, Faderl S, et al: Characteristics and outcome of patients with acute myeloid leukemia refractory to 1 cycle of high-dose cytarabine-based induction chemotherapy. *Blood* 116:5818, 2010.
25. Cortes J, Foran J, Ghirdaladze D, et al: AC220, a potent, selective, second generation FLT3 receptor tyrosine kinase (RTK) inhibitor, in a first-in-human (FIH) phase 1 AML study. *Blood* 114:abstract 636, 2009.
26. Levis M, Ravandi F, Wang ES, et al: Results from a randomized trial of salvage chemotherapy followed by lestaurtinib for patients with FLT3 mutant AML in first relapse. *Blood* 117:3294, 2011.

27. Sanz MA, Martin G, Rayon C, et al: A modified AIDA protocol with anthracycline-based consolidation results in high antileukemic efficacy and reduced toxicity in newly diagnosed PML/RARalpha-positive acute promyelocytic leukemia. PETHEMA group. *Blood* 94:3015, 1999.
28. Sanz MA, Lo-Coco F: Modern approaches to treating acute promyelocytic leukemia. *J Clin Oncol* 29:495, 2011.
29. Ravandi F, Estey E, Jones D, et al: Effective treatment of acute promyelocytic leukemia with all-trans-retinoic acid, arsenic trioxide, and gemtuzumab ozogamicin. *J Clin Oncol* 27:504, 2009.
30. Shen ZX, Chen GQ, Ni JH, et al: Use of arsenic trioxide (As2O3) in the treatment of acute promyelocytic leukemia (APL): II. Clinical efficacy and pharmacokinetics in relapsed patients. *Blood* 89:3354, 1997.

CHAPTER 59

MYELODYSPLASTIC SYNDROMES: BIOLOGY AND TREATMENT

Daniel J. DeAngelo and Richard M. Stone

Over the past several decades, many terms have been used to describe the bone marrow (BM) failure syndromes, which often terminate in an overt acute leukemia. The terms include refractory anemia (RA), preleukemia, smoldering acute leukemia, oligoblastic leukemia, refractory dysmyelopoietic anemia, and myelodysplastic syndrome.[1-5] Patients typically present with varying degrees of anemia, leukopenia, and thrombocytopenia, rendering many transfusion dependent or susceptible to infection or hemorrhage. The term *myelodysplastic syndrome* (MDS) is the currently accepted norm that is used to describe this clinical entity. MDS may arise either de novo or secondary to ionizing radiation, toxins, or chemotherapeutic drug exposure.[6-11] The natural history of these syndromes ranges from an acute precipitous decline over several weeks to a chronic condition that lasts many years. The actual incidence of MDS is unknown. Unfortunately, the incidence rates of MDS were not reported to the National Cancer Institute's Surveillance Epidemiology and End Results (SEER) Program until 2001. Estimates in Europe range from 3 to 20 cases per 100,000, but in the United States, more than 10,000 new cases are diagnosed each year (median age, 76 years).[12-14] The incidence in men is significantly higher than in women (4.5 vs. 2.7 per 100,000). MDS is rarely seen in patients younger than age 50 years but rapidly increases with advancing age and may equal the incidence of acute myeloid leukemia (AML) by the eighth decade of life.[15-17] For example, the age-specific incidence rates of MDS are approximately 5 per 100,000 for ages 60 to 69 years, but increase to approximately 50 per 100,000 for ages 70 to 79 years.[18]

The various pathologic entities of MDS previously were classified by the French-American-British (FAB) Cooperative Group into five subtypes based on a set of criteria that included BM morphology and the percentage of myeloblasts,[19] with the presence of greater than 30% myeloblasts classified as AML. The FAB classification scheme, based largely on the histologic changes within the BM, has been extremely useful in assessing prognosis in patients with MDS, but the arbitrary division between MDS and AML based on the presence or absence of 30% myeloblasts is biologically inconsistent. In large studies, patients with refractory anemia with excess blasts in transformation (RAEB-T) and AML have similar outcomes. As a result, the World Health Organization (WHO) has adopted the definition of AML in a patient with 20% or greater myeloblasts and have removed the antiquated term RAEB-T.[20]

Most patients with MDS have progressive cytopenias, and a large fraction of patients eventually develop overt AML.[21] Patients with secondary AML from an underlying MDS typically are treated with multiagent chemotherapy in an attempt to delete the leukemic clone.[22] Nevertheless, the same problems exist as with MDS: advanced age, therapy-related toxicity, and resistant disease. Stem cell transplantation (SCT) remains the best chance for cure, but this strategy is not appropriate for the majority of patients because of their advanced age. Treatment of MDS ultimately is intended to extend overall survival by both improving the peripheral blood cytopenias and delaying the leukemic transformation. However, the more immediate goal of therapy is to relieve symptoms and improve the quality of life while minimizing side effects.

BIOLOGY

Pathogenesis

Myelodysplasia is the result of a transformation of a myeloid stem cell. A hematopoietic stem cell (HSC) is capable of self-renewal and can give rise to more differentiated progeny.[23-26] As the stem cell differentiates, it becomes lineage specific. An early pluripotent stem cell can give rise to both lymphoid and myeloid cells. However, the neoplastic transformation of the myeloid stem cell is the initial event that leads to myelodysplasia.[27] MDS rarely transforms into acute lymphocytic leukemia, thus suggesting that the MDS myeloid stem cell has lost its lymphopoietic potential.[28,29] A poorly defined transforming event(s) affects the pluripotent myeloid stem cell in MDS, thus conferring a growth advantage that eventually leads to development of monoclonal hematopoietic progeny. Many genetic mutations regulate this process, and these alterations determine both the biology and clinical aspects of the disease.[30]

The clinical hallmark of patients with myelodysplasia is the development of ineffective hematopoiesis (Fig. 59-1). Interestingly, cellular turnover within the BM often is increased in most patients with myelodysplasia.[31] Cell kinetic studies have revealed a dramatic increase in the rate of cell division. The peripheral cytopenias are thought to be secondary to an increase in apoptosis, or programmed cell death, resulting in a futile increase in cell cycling.[32,33] Impaired cellular function is another important clinical feature of myelodysplasia. Erythroid precursors have a decreased response to erythropoietin (EPO), which may contribute to subsequent anemia.[34] In addition, terminally differentiated cells in MDS have functional defects. Mature granulocytes have decreased myeloperoxidase activity,[35-37] and platelets may have impaired aggregation properties.[38] The oncogenic pathway is not a single-step process. Sequential genetic changes are required to change a transformed myelodysplastic stem cell into a true neoplasm that often leads to development of AML.[39]

Myelodysplastic syndrome is a clonal hematopoietic disorder.[40] BM cytogenetic analysis has been a great asset in the evaluation of the clonal nature of the MDS stem cell.[41-43] The clonal nature of MDS has been best elucidated by the use of X-inactivation studies.[44,45] These studies use restriction fragment length polymorphism (RFLP) analysis to study the differences between the methylation patterns of inactive versus active X chromosomes. RFLP analysis using the phosphoglycerate kinase and hypoxanthine phosphoribosyltransferase genes as well as the polymorphic genes of glucose-6-phosphate dehydrogenase all have demonstrated clonal hematopoiesis within the granulocyte, monocytic, erythroid, and megakaryocytic lineages in patients with MDS.

Apoptosis

Programmed cell death, referred to as apoptosis, is an important and active cellular process that regulates cell and lineage population.[46] The rate of apoptosis is finely regulated by the ratio of proapoptotic

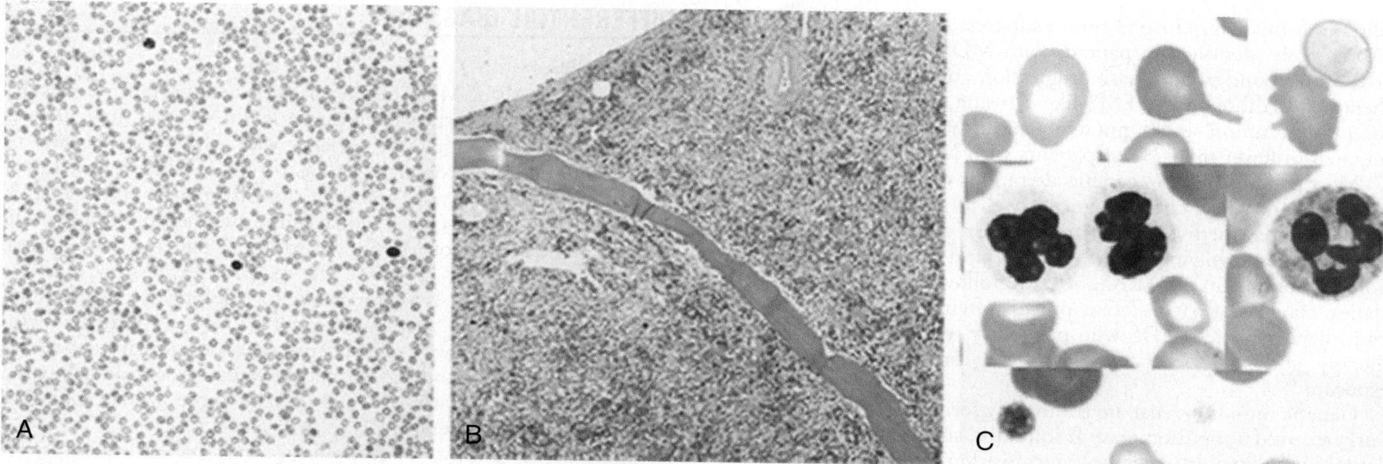

Figure 59-1 ELEMENTS OF MYELODYSPLASTIC SYNDROME. Myelodysplastic syndromes are generally characterized by cytopenias **(A)** caused by ineffective hematopoiesis **(B),** which is related to multilineage dysplasia **(C). A,** This patient presented with a white blood cell count of 1500/μL, hemoglobin 8.9 g/dL, and platelet count 47,000/μL. **B,** The bone marrow was hypercellular, indicating ineffective hematopoiesis. **C,** Evidence of trilineage dysplasia was apparent on the peripheral smear. Anisocytosis with macro-ovalocytes and poikilocytosis is seen in the red blood cells (**C,** *top*). The latter included the somewhat uncommon finding of Cabot ring forms *(right).* A large proportion of the granulocytes were severely hypogranular (**C,** *middle left*) compared to some normal forms still in the circulation *(right).* Platelets (**C,** *bottom*) were decreased in number, and many were severely hypogranular (*middle,* barely visible) compared with residual normal platelets *(left).*

proteins, such as c-Myc, p53, Bax, and Bad, to the antiapoptotic proteins, which include Bcl-2 and Bcl-XL.[47-50] Increased apoptosis has been documented within CD34+ BM cells in patients with MDS.[51] This increased apoptosis seems to be highest in patients with RA compared with those with RAEB and may account for the cytopenias that are the hallmark of early-stage MDS.[52-55] For example, the intracellular ratio of c-Myc to Bcl-2 is higher in CD34+ cells in patients with MDS compared with those from normal patients or patients with AML.[56] In addition, an increased level of apoptosis is associated with increased levels of inhibitory cytokines, such as tumor necrosis factor-α (TNF-α).[57] TNF-α is increased across all MDS subtypes and may inhibit the development and maturation of the hematopoietic precursors. TNF-α may increase the production and secretion of other proapoptotic cytokines, such as interleukin-8 (IL-6), transforming growth factor β, interferon-γ, and Fas ligand. Use of growth factors, such as erythropoiesis-stimulating agents (ESAs) and granulocyte colony-stimulating factor (G-CSF), has been shown to decrease the rate of apoptosis in some patients.[58-60] These findings suggest that increased levels of apoptosis is associated with early-stage MDS, but decreased levels of apoptosis may help propagate the transformation from MDS to AML.[52,54,61-63]

Hematopoiesis

The colony-forming capacities of the pluripotent HSCs and their progeny are low or absent in many patients with MDS.[64] The BM cells as well as peripheral T cells from patients with MDS seem to produce lower levels of granulocyte-macrophage colony-stimulating factor (GM-CSF), IL-3, macrophage colony-stimulating factor (M-CSF), and IL-6. The colony-forming unit granulocyte-macrophage (CFU-GM) is less responsive to both G-CSF and GM-CSF in patients with MDS.[65,66] These findings are more dramatic in patients with the higher grade MDS. In addition, the erythroid progenitor cell, burst-forming unit-erythroid (BFU-E), is less responsive to EPO in vitro.[64] There also seems to be a direct correlation between the size of the BFU-E and the EPO level in patients with MDS. These findings may help explain the peripheral blood cytopenias in patients with MDS and the observation that additional EPO is of limited clinical benefit.

Epigenetic

Epigenetics is the alteration of gene expression without altering the primary DNA sequence.[67-70] These modifications can occur at multiple levels, the most common involving DNA methylation. DNA methylation involves the addition of methyl groups to a cytosine residue.[71-73] Cytosine methylation typically occurs when a cytosine is followed by a guanine in the so-called CpG pair. CpG pairs are underrepresented within the human genome, but when they do occur, they occur clustered in so-called CpG islands. These CpG islands typically are located proximal to gene promoter regions and regulate gene expression.[74,75] For example, methylation of CpG islands is associated with gene silencing. The process of gene silencing may be physiologic in the case of both imprinted genes as well as regulating gene dosage of genes on the X chromosome in females.[67] Tumor suppressor genes are thought to undergo this aberrant gene silencing mechanism, leading to abnormal physiologic consequences.

Epigenetic changes in MDS and AML have become increasingly important. For example, the promoter methylation of the α-catenin gene *CTNNA1* may be an important underlying abnormality involving the loss of chromosome 5.[76] Other examples include promoter methylation of the p15INK4B gene.[72,77,78] This gene often is hypermethylated in patients with therapy-related MDS or therapy-related AML. In addition, methylation changes of this gene are seen more frequently in patients with loss of chromosome 7 and in patients who progress from RA to RAEB.[78]

Genetic Pathways Involved in Disease Progression

The genetic changes that occur in patients who transform from MDS to AML are numerous, complicated, and involve a multistep process characterized by activation of specific oncogenes as well as inactivation of tumor suppressor genes.[39] RAS mutations are frequently identified in patients with hematologic malignancies.[79-81] In patients with MDS, RAS was mutated in as many as one-third of the cases, with the highest frequency in patients with chronic myelomonocytic leukemia (CMML).[82] The FMS oncogene encodes for M-CSF and, similar to RAS, is most preferentially seen in patients with CMML.

Mutations involving the p53 tumor suppressor gene on chromosome 17p is rarely identified in patients with MDS, but when seen, they often correspond with disease progression and resistance to chemotherapy.[83,84] Although the FMS-like tyrosine receptor III (FLT-3) is the most common single mutated gene in patients with AML, it is mutated in fewer than 3% of patients with MDS.[85-88]

Most patients develop genetic alterations that include the gain or loss of part or whole chromosomes as well as specific gene mutations and promoter methylation changes.[89] For example, patients with abnormalities involving chromosome 5 and 7 often acquire additional mutations in p53, RAS, or both, followed by promoter methylation changes of p15.[87,90] This process often is involved in patients with therapy-related MDS who previously received alkylating agent therapy and typically occurs 3 to 5 years after chemotherapy exposure.[88]

Genetic mutations that are commonly seen in patients who previously received a topoisomerase II inhibitor, such as the anthracycline doxorubicin, involve the complex acquisition of chromosomal translocations often involving the mixed lineage leukemia (MLL) gene on 11q23.[91-101] More than 30 different translocations have been identified that involve 11q23, and they account for approximately 5% of all translocations that occur in acute leukemia. Reciprocal translocations involving the 11q23 gene have been described in patients with acute lymphoblastic leukemia (ALL), AML, acute biphenotypic leukemia, and MDS. Other chromosomal translocations that are seen less commonly after anthracycline exposure include the AML1 gene on 21q22 often leading to translocation of t(3;21),[91] the core-binding factor β (CBF-β) gene on chromosome 16 leading to inversion of chromosome 16 [inv(16)],[92] and the retinoic acid receptor α (RAR-α) gene on chromosome 17 characterized by translocation t(15;17) and development of acute promyelocytic leukemia.[93-95] In addition, mutations of the NUP98 gene on chromosome 11p15 have been associated with exposure to topoisomerase II inhibitors.[96,97] These cytogenetic changes characterized by specific chromosomal abnormalities, with the notable exception of NUP98 on 11p15, subsequently develop RAS, BRAF, c-KIT, or FLT-3 mutations followed by changes in the methylation pattern within the p15 promoter.[98,99]

Patients with a normal cytogenetic karyotype or other nonspecific chromosomal abnormalities often evolve from an MDS to an AML phenotype with a different and distinct process. These patients typically develop acquisition of a RAS mutation or another mutation involving a transcription factor,[100] which are known as class II mutations, or mutations involving tyrosine kinases, which are known as class I mutations. Examples of class I mutations include FLT-3, c-KIT, c-FMS, and JAK2.[101,102] Also included are genes further downstream within the RAS-BRAF-MEK-ERK pathway. They include N-RAS, K-RAS, BRAF, and PTPN11. This class of mutations results in the constitutive activation of the cell cycle leading to an increase in cell proliferation. For example, whereas mutations in RAS are commonly seen in monocytic subtypes of AML and in CMML, PTPN11 genes are commonly mutated in juvenile myelomonocytic leukemia.[103,104] The class I mutations are considered "late events" in the pathogenesis of leukemia but are thought to cooperate to a high degree with class II mutations. Examples of class II mutations that can be seen in patients who transform from MDS to AML include CCAAT enhancer-binding protein α (CEBPα), AML1, and rarely internal tandem duplications of MLL (MLL-PTD).[105-107]

As expected, patients with de novo and therapy-related MDS and AML have heterogeneous clinical presentations but often have similar cytogenetic abnormalities.[89,108,109] Although three distinct cytogenetic subgroups can be identified (chromosome 5/7, MLL gene on 11q23, and normal karyotype), many different genetic pathways have been outlined for patients with therapy-related MDS and therapy-related AML. Some of these changes are more consistent with the clinical presentation of MDS (e.g., −5/5q− or −7/7q−), but other abnormalities are more often related to the presentation of overt AML [e.g., translocations involving 11q23, inv(16), and t(15;17)]. However, the frequent association of both class I and II mutations argues strongly for their cooperative nature in the development of MDS and AML.[110]

DIFFERENTIAL DIAGNOSIS

Before a diagnosis of MDS can be made, it is important to consider alternative diagnoses, especially if the patient is younger than 50 years (Table 59-1). Although most patients with MDS have normal or hypercellular BM, approximately 10% to 15% of patients have hypocellular BM that may be difficult to distinguish from aplastic anemia.[111] The presence of a clonal chromosomal abnormality will confirm the diagnosis of MDS.[112] In addition, patients with aplastic anemia typically have greater TNF receptor expression than do patients with MDS.[113] It is important to rule out the diagnosis of paroxysmal nocturnal hemoglobinuria (PNH).[114] Patients with hypocellular MDS have a clinical presentation similar to patients with aplastic anemia and have a better overall prognosis compared with other patients with MDS, especially those who respond to immunosuppressive therapy.[115,116]

Similarly, the presence of myelofibrosis may make adequate assessment of the BM aspirate difficult.[117,118] Patients with significant fibrosis within the BM cavity often have an unaspiratable or aspicular aspirate specimen. Therefore, the ability to analyze the BM aspirate for dysplastic features is markedly limited. However, in some patients, the diagnosis of myelodysplasia can be easily made, and the BM biopsy shows an increased number of reticulin fibers.[119] Reticulin stain, typically by silver impregnation, is an important method for identifying underlying BM fibrosis but should be distinguished from marked collagen fibrosis, which is often seen in patients with chronic idiopathic myelofibrosis (agnogenic myeloid metaplasia with myelofibrosis). Extensive mature collagen fibrosis can be demonstrated by trichrome stain and is extremely uncommon in patients with MDS. Although BM fibrosis can be seen in all subtypes of MDS, it is more

Table 59-1 Predisposing Factors and Epidemiologic Associations of Patients With Myelodysplastic Syndrome

Heritable
CONSTITUTIONAL GENETIC DISORDERS
Trisomy 8 mosaicism
Familial monosomy 7
Down syndrome (trisomy 21)
Neurofibromatosis 1
Germ cell tumors [embryonal dysgenesis del(12p)]
CONGENITAL NEUTROPENIA
Kostmann syndrome
Shwachman-Diamond syndrome
DNA REPAIR DEFICIENCIES
Fanconi anemia
Ataxia telangiectasia
Bloom syndrome
Xeroderma pigmentosum
Pharmacogenomic polymorphisms (GSTq1-null)
Acquired
SENESCENCE
MUTAGEN EXPOSURE
Alkylator therapy (chlorambucil, cyclophosphamide, melphalan, N-mustards)
Topoisomerase II inhibitors (anthracyclines)
β-Emitters (^{32}P)
Autologous stem cell transplantation
Environmental or occupational (benzene)
Tobacco
Aplastic anemia
Paroxysmal nocturnal hemoglobinuria

frequent in CMML and therapy-related MDS.[120] Patients with MDS and fibrosis can be distinguished from patients with chronic idiopathic myelofibrosis.[121] The latter entity is associated with marked splenomegaly, an unusual feature in patients with MDS regardless of the degree of BM fibrosis. The absence of splenomegaly and an unusually rapid progressive clinical course helps distinguish patients between MDS and chronic idiopathic myelofibrosis, which usually is more indolent. Other disorders to consider in cases of extensive fibrosis include chronic myeloid leukemia (CML), especially accelerated phase disease, and acute megakaryocytic leukemia (FAB-M7).[122]

Variants of CML as well as atypical CML can be difficult to distinguish from CMML.[123] The WHO currently lists CMML in its own category; therefore, it is no longer considered part of the MDS.[20] Nevertheless, the differential is important. CML is distinguished by the presence or absence of a *BCR-ABL1* fusion gene.[124] The term *atypical CML* represents a diffuse group of disorders that are BCR negative.[125] Their clinical prognosis is somewhat worse than in patients with BCR-ABL given the inability to target a tyrosine kinase. Patients with atypical CML often have a short overall survival time and poor response to therapy. Clinically, they can be distinguished from patients with other forms of MDS by an increase in basophilia and progressive leukocytosis as well as organomegaly, specifically splenomegaly.[126] These patients typically have marked thrombocytopenia and eventually develop BM failure without transformation to AML. In a review of 76 BCR-negative patients from the MD Anderson Cancer Center, the median overall survival was 24 months, with AML transformation in 8 patients. Chromosomal abnormalities were seen in 30% of patients, with trisomy 8 the most common abnormality identified. Patients with atypical CML can be difficult to separate clinically and pathologically from patients with MDS or other myeloproliferative disorders.

Dysplastic hematopoiesis is a common finding accompanying human immunodeficiency virus (HIV) infection.[127,128] An HIV serologic test must be obtained to exclude HIV infection, especially in patients with high-risk lifestyles, as well as young patients. The typical BM aspirate and biopsy findings in patients with HIV infection include a hypercellular BM and evidence of trilineage dysplasia, which is most predominant within the erythroid lineage.[129,130] The erythroid hematopoiesis almost always is megaloblastic, and reticulated fibrosis is often seen in BM biopsies. Most patients have polyclonal plasma cell expansion, and lymphoid aggregates and granulomas are often seen. The differential diagnosis of erythrodysplasia in patients with HIV infection includes medications, opportunistic infections, or a direct effect of HIV on the hematopoietic progenitor cells. These findings reaffirm the need for serologic screening for HIV in patients with unexplained cytopenias.

A number of drugs can cause erythrodysplasia and complicate the evaluation and diagnosis of a patient with cytopenias. These medications include valproic acid,[131] mycophenolate mofetil,[132] ganciclovir,[132,133] alemtuzumab,[134] nucleoside analogues such as fludarabine and cytarabine, and the antimetabolites mercaptopurine and methotrexate. The BM changes associated with these medications include macrocytic anemia, reduced neutrophil lobation, and frank neutropenia and thrombocytopenia. In fact, some patients may have trilineage dysplasia, making an accurate diagnosis difficult.

Nutritional deficiencies must be excluded in any patients in whom the diagnosis of MDS is being entertained. These include vitamin B_{12} and folate deficiency[135] and copper deficiency.[136,137] Copper deficiency in adult patients is rare but can occur after gastrectomy, prolonged parenteral nutrition, or even enteral feeding if copper is not included in the formulation. Rarely, copper deficiency develops after ingestion of large amounts of zinc supplements because zinc excess results in concomitant copper deficiency. Clinically, patients with copper deficiency present with signs and symptoms of profound anemia. In addition, copper deficiency may cause a variety of neurologic complications, including central nervous system demyelination, peripheral neuropathy, myelopathy, and even optic neuritis. In patients with severe cooper deficiency, hemoglobin levels may fall as low as 3.5 g/dL. The mean corpuscular volume (MCV) often is normal or slightly increased, and the red blood cells (RBCs) on the peripheral smear are hypochromic and microcytic. Patients typically present with mild neutropenia with neutrophil counts of 1000/mL. BM examination will reveal a cellular BM with early erythroid vacuolization and moderate numbers of ringed sideroblasts.

A number of drugs may induce sideroblastic anemia, including isoniazid[138] and chloramphenicol.[139,140] Cycloserine and pyrazinamide also have been implicated in rare cases. With isoniazid, the anemia is modest, with hematocrits typically in the 26% range, low MCV, and dimorphic RBC morphology. Abundant ringed sideroblasts are present within the BM, and typically the anemia is rapidly reversed with discontinuation of the offending agent. However, administration of large doses of pyridoxine up to 200 mg/day may accelerate reversal of the anemia.

Although chloramphenicol typically produces a ringed sideroblastic anemia, an idiosyncratic BM failure syndrome associated with chronic administration also can be seen. When this occurs, a prominent feature within the BM is vacuolization, specifically of the early erythroid precursors. Patients often have marked reticulocytopenia and increased serum iron levels. In most cases, the anemia is reversed with discontinuation of the drug; however, some patients may have profound, long-lasting evidence of BM failure.

Sideroblastic anemia is associated with alcoholism with or without folate and vitamin B_{12} deficiency.[141] As many as one-third of patients who have chronic alcoholism may have sideroblastic changes within the BM, including dimorphic erythroid cells. Patients often have a markedly elevated MCV, which is impressively uniform. The ringed sideroblasts often disappear within days to weeks after discontinuation of alcohol intake.[142] However, concurrent vitamin deficiencies or liver disease may further affect the peripheral blood cytopenias and, importantly, the recovery phase.

CLINICAL FINDINGS IN PATIENTS WITH MYELODYSPLASTIC SYNDROMES

Erythroid Cells

The diagnosis of myelodysplasia in patients with anemia, neutropenia, thrombocytopenia, or a combination thereof depends on the demonstration of dysmorphic features within the BM (Table 59-2 and Fig. 59-2). Both a BM aspirate and a biopsy should be obtained. An aspirate usually can assess cellular morphology and quantitation of myeloblasts, but accurate assessment of BM cellularity and localization of immature precursors require a review of the biopsy sections. Occasionally, multiple sampling is required to make a definitive diagnosis because the affected BM is distributed unevenly or the patient develops progressive dysplastic features over time.

Almost all patients with MDS (>90%) present with fatigue and lethargy, which is associated with chronic anemia.[143] The anemia most often is macrocytic, with a significantly reduced reticulocyte index. The most recognized morphologic abnormality of the RBCs on examination of the peripheral blood smear consists of oval macrocytes; however, in rare cases, teardrop cells or dacrocytes, elliptocytes, and acanthocytes are seen.[144] It remains essential to exclude other causes of macrocytic anemia in this population, including vitamin B_{12} and folate deficiency.[145] The anemia in patients with MDS is a result of ineffective erythropoiesis. EPO levels usually are normal or elevated.[3,146] In addition, most patients have evidence of abnormal iron utilization. Other patients have evidence of increased fetal hemoglobin synthesis,[147] abnormal RBC antigens,[148] increased RBC fragility, and low levels of pyruvate kinase. The latter two abnormalities may result in an abnormal Ham test result secondary to increased hemolysis.[149]

It is important to exclude the diagnosis of PNH even in patients without a history of thromboembolic disorders. The most efficient test is the absence of polyinositol glycol–associated antigens by flow cytometric analysis because of the absence of the PIG-A gene. PNH

Table 59-2 Physical Examination, Medical History, and Laboratory Tests Aiding in the Diagnosis of Myelodysplastic Syndrome

MEDICAL HISTORY
Duration of symptoms
History of blood disease
History of exposure to occupational toxins or cytotoxic agents
Medication history
Alcohol intake
Comorbid conditions
PHYSICAL EXAMINATION
Pallor
Petechiae
Purpura
Bruising
Tachypnea
Signs of infection
Splenomegaly
LABORATORY TESTING
Complete blood count with a manual differential
Reticulocyte count
Vitamin B_{12} and folate levels
Consider methylmalonic acid and red blood cell folate levels
Iron, total iron-binding capacity, and ferritin level
Thyroid-stimulating hormone level
Lactate dehydrogenase
Antinuclear antibody
Coombs test and haptoglobin
Serum erythropoietin level
Human leukocyte antigen (histocompatibility antigens) typing in appropriate patients
Paroxysmal nocturnal hemoglobinuria screen
BONE MARROW TESTING
Hematopathology
Percentage of blasts on 200 cell aspirate differential
Presence or absence of Auer rods
Percentage of cellularity of bone marrow biopsy
Iron stain on aspirate (ringed sideroblasts)
Iron stain on biopsy (storage)
Dysplastic features (% and number of dysplastic lineages)
Cytogenetics (karyotype of 20 metaphase cells)
Fluorescent in situ hybridization
Flow cytometry (not useful for quantitation)

is diagnosed by the absence of CD55 and CD59 on RBCs and the absence of CD11b on monocytes.[150,151] Some patients have a small clone of PNH cells, but this finding is of unclear clinical significance.[152,153] Other possible features of MDS include disordered α- and β-globin chain synthesis[154,155] and hemoglobin H inclusions.[156]

Morphologic features within the BM aspirate include megaloblastic erythroid precursors, often with multiple nuclei or asynchronous maturation of the nucleus and cytoplasm. Occasionally, ringed sideroblasts, which are RBC precursors with iron-laden mitochondria, can be identified (see Fig. 59-2).[157] Ringed sideroblasts are defined by the presence of at least five Prussian blue—staining iron granules encircling more than one-third of the nucleus of an erythroblast. The presence of ringed sideroblasts without morphologic features of dysplasia also can be seen in unrelated congenital and malignant hematologic conditions. RA and refractory cytopenia with multilineage dysplasia (RCMD) typically are differentiated from refractory anemia with ringed sideroblasts (RARS) and refractory cytopenia with multilineage dysplasia and ringed sideroblasts (RCMD-S) by the presence of greater than 15% ringed sideroblasts.[158]

One unusual feature of the FAB or WHO classification scheme occurs when greater than 50% of the total cellularity is composed of erythroid precursors.[19] In this case, if greater than 30% of the nonerythroid cells are myeloblasts, a diagnosis of erythroleukemia is made (FAB-M6A,or WHO AML, NOS, acute erythroid leukemia, erythroid/myeloid type). This differs from the pure erythroleukemia described by Deguglielmo (FAB-M6B).

Myeloid Cells

A large proportion of patients, approximately 50%, with MDS either present with neutropenia or develop neutropenia as a result of disease progression.[159] Not only is MDS associated with a quantitative neutrophil defect but also with qualitative defects. Patients with MDS often have a reduced inflammatory response to infections. Patients with MDS have diminished production of many hematopoietic growth factors, and these likely account for the qualitative neutrophil defects and their reduced phagocytic properties. Despite this, recurrent infections occur in only 10% of patients,[160] but this is the cause of death in approximately one-fifth of the patients with MDS.[161]

The most common infections in patients with MDS are bacterial, usually from the lower respiratory tract, skin, or perineal area. Recurrent infections can occur even in the absence of severe neutropenia, likely from granulocyte functional impairment. In patients with CMML,[162,163] the monocytes are also derived from defective HSCs and similar qualitative defects in terms of cell adhesion and phagocytic and cell killing properties leading to an increased rate of infections.

Abnormalities of the myeloid series range from subtle to rather striking (Fig. 59-3).[19] They include a left shift toward more immature forms, even without an excess of myeloblasts. The myeloid precursors also may show asynchronous maturation of the nucleus and cytoplasm as manifested by a lack of granule formation. The nucleocytoplasmic dyssynchrony is most clearly represented in the early myeloid cells, or *abnormal promyelocytes*. Their granular cytoplasm, reticulated nucleus, and prominent Golgi apparatus characterize these dysplastic promyelocytes. The more mature granulocytes often are hypogranulated and may be hypolobated as well. Granulocytes with a bilobed nuclear structure are referred to as pseudo–Pelger-Huet cells.[164] There is a congenital abnormality in pediatric patients in which all of the neutrophils are bilobed or hyposegmented; this is termed the *Pelger-Huet anomaly*, which is a benign condition.

The most critical finding in patients with MDS is the presence and quantification of the myeloblasts. The absolute proportion of myeloblasts reflects the defect in the differentiation capacity of the abnormal HSC and represents the most important prognostic finding. The diagnosis of AML is established if there are more than 20% myeloblasts based on the WHO classification scheme or greater than 30% based on the older FAB criteria.[19,20] Quantification of myeloblasts should be performed on a cellular and spicular BM aspirate and not by flow cytometric analysis because the latter can be affected by peripheral blood dilution of the sample.

Megakaryocytes

Thrombocytopenia is present in approximately half of patients with MDS and may represent the only cytopenia in 5% of cases.[165] The finding of thrombocytosis is uncommon and typically associated with either the 5q syndrome[166] or a JAK2 mutation, as is the case in patients with refractory anemia with ringed sideroblasts and thrombocytosis (RARS-T).[167] As in the case with neutrophils, patients with MDS often have both a quantitative as well as a qualitative defect with their platelets.[38] The latter can be identified by careful examination of the peripheral blood smear, on which giant or agranular platelets often are identified. Upon examination of the BM, the megakaryocytes often are small or micromegakaryocytic and contain fewer nuclear lobes (hypolobated) than their normal counterparts (Fig. 59-4).[19,164,168] In patients with the 5q syndrome, the megakaryocytes are nonlobated and mononuclear.[166]

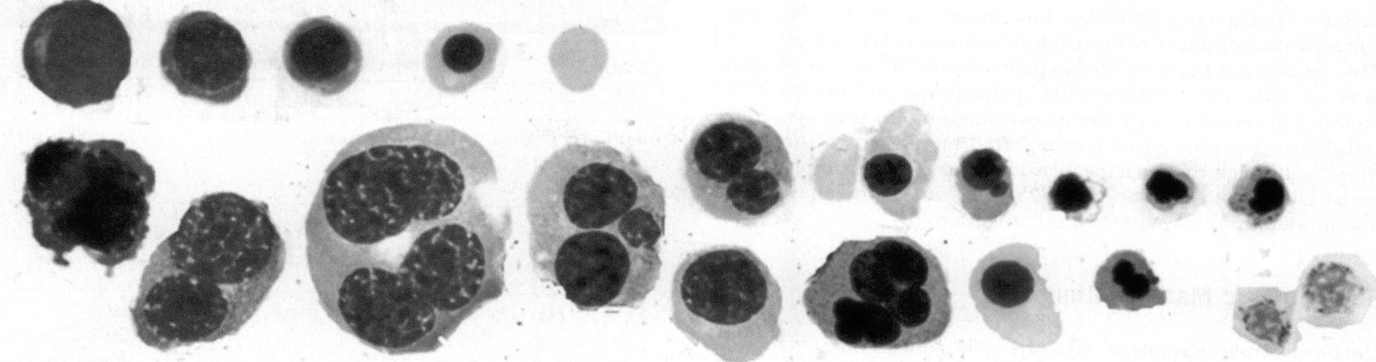

Figure 59-2 ERYTHROID DYSPLASIA. Examples of dysplastic erythroid precursors *(bottom)* compared to those with normal morphology in the sequence of erythroid maturation *(top)*. The dysplastic forms include (*left* to *right*) abnormal immature forms with multinucleation; maturing forms with multinucleation and nuclear-to-cytoplasmic dyssynchrony; and more mature forms with megaloblastoid change, nuclear budding, cloverleaf forms, cytoplasmic vacuolization, and cytoplasmic stippling. Ringed sideroblasts *(far right)* also are evidence of erythroid dysplasia. Photomicrographs are from patients with refractory cytopenia with multilineage dysplasia and ringed sideroblasts.

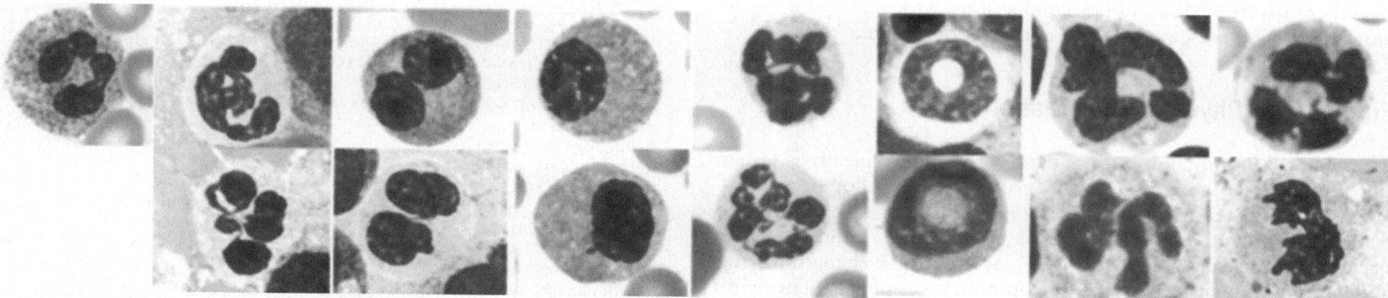

Figure 59-3 GRANULOCYTIC DYSPLASIA. Granulocytic dysplasia is most evident in mature neutrophils and can be contrasted to features of normal forms *(far left, top)*, which are usually still present as a subpopulation of the total cells in most cases. Granulocytic dysplasia is characterized by *(left to right, starting at second column)* reduced cytoplasmic granulation, nuclear hypolobation (resulting in the binuclear or single-lobed pseudo–Pelger-Huet forms), hypersegmentation, ringed forms ("rodent cells"), cells with nuclear twinning, and cells with excessive nuclear excrescences. Photomicrographs are from a number of cases of refractory cytopenia with multilineage dysplasia and refractory anemia with excess blasts.

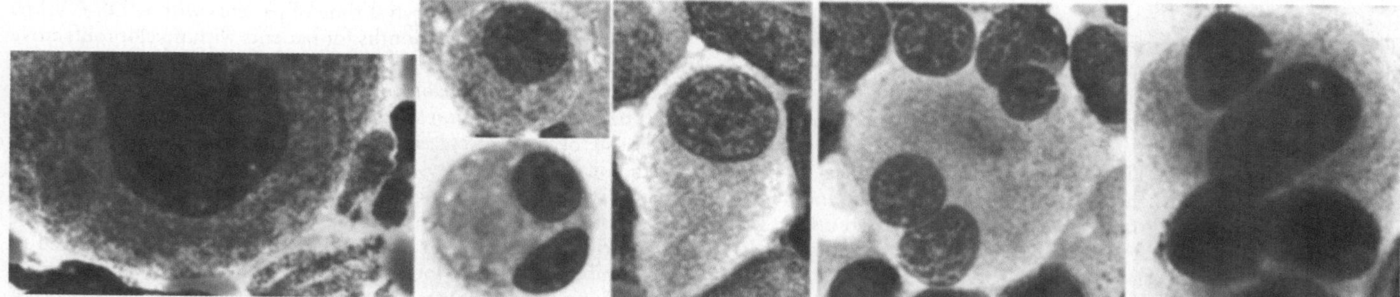

Figure 59-4 MEGAKARYOCYTIC DYSPLASIA. Dysmegakaryopoiesis is most obvious with the presence of micro-megakaryocytes and abnormal larger forms *(panels 2-5)*. These are compared with a normal megakaryocyte at same magnification *(panel 1, far left)*. Micro-megakaryocytes have single, two, or four small nuclei, which indicate a low-ploidy level. Normal low-ploidy megakaryocytes can be seen in the bone marrow, but these are immature forms and do not have mature granular cytoplasm with platelet material, as do the micro-megakaryocytes. Larger dysplastic megakaryocytes have multiple, small, widely spaced nuclei. Photomicrographs are from a number of cases of refractory anemia with excess blasts and refractory cytopenia with multilineage dysplasia.

Patients may have disproportionately prolonged bleeding times and abnormalities in platelet aggregation studies.[38,169-171] These may be present even in patients with normal platelet counts. The hallmark is an acquired Glanzmann defect, characterized by abnormal platelet glycoprotein IIb/IIIa. A falling platelet count often is a marker of disease progression. Patients with MDS are at risk for spontaneous bleeding and have increased risk for hemorrhage after surgery and trauma. Again, this is true even in patients without thrombocytopenia.

Autoimmune Manifestations

Immunologic and rheumatologic complications occur frequently in patients with MDS.[172-174] Patients can present with acute episodes of seronegative oligoarthritis or polyarthritis[175,176] as well as symptoms of cutaneous vasculitis, polymyositis, or peripheral neuropathies. Lupus-like symptoms have been reported at the time of the presentation of cytopenias in patients complaining of systemic features of fever, polyarthritis, polychondritis, pleuritis, pericarditis, or even hemolytic anemia. Presentations involving mucocutaneous ulcerations, iritis, polymyositis, peripheral neuropathy, inflammatory bowel disease, and RBC aplasia have been reported in patients with MDS.[177] In addition, cases of relapsing polychondritis, polymyalgia rheumatica,[172,178,179] Raynaud phenomenon, pyoderma gangrenosum, Sjögren syndrome, and glomerulonephritis have been reported, but their association is less clear.[180] Although these paraneoplastic processes may complicate the initial clinical presentation of MDS, they are often responsive to immunosuppressive agents such as corticosteroids.[181]

Dermatologic Manifestations

Cutaneous complications of MDS are rather uncommon.[182] Neutrophilic dermatosis (Sweet syndrome) is one exception. It is characterized by painful plaque-like lesions that often are associated with fever and arthralgias. These lesions can be present on the face, neck, or upper or lower extremities. Sweet syndrome usually responds to corticosteroid or dapsone therapy. It is often present in patients who are transforming to AML. Other dermatologic presentations include monocytic infiltrates, which are more common in patients with CMML[163,183,184]; chloroma or granulocytic sarcoma, which if present would constitute AML; and petechial lesions, which are common in any patient who presents with severe thrombocytopenia.

Findings on Physical Examination

The physical examination of a patient with MDS typically is rather unrevealing (see Table 59-2). Most patients have pallor because of anemia; petechiae is less commonly present as a result of thrombocytopenia.[185] Signs and symptoms of an infectious process, either bacterial or fungal, should be ruled out. Splenomegaly, hepatomegaly, and lymphadenopathy are rather uncommon except for patients with CMML.[163]

Table 59-3 French-American-British Classification Criteria*

Subtype	Abbreviation	Peripheral Blood	Bone Marrow
Refractory anemia	RA	Blasts <1%	Blasts <5%
Refractory anemia with ringed sideroblasts	RARS	Blasts <1%	Blasts <5%, and >15% ringed sideroblasts
Refractory anemia with excess blasts	RAEB	Blasts <5%	Blasts 5%-20%
Refractory anemia with excess blasts in transformation	RAEB-T	Blasts >5%	Blasts 20%-30% or Auer rods
Chronic myelomonocytic leukemia	CMML	Monocytes >1 × 10^9/L	Any of the above
Acute myelogenous leukemia	AML		Blasts >30%

*Description of syndromes from Bennett J, et al: Proposals for the classification of the myelodysplastic syndromes. *Blood* 51:189, 1982.
WHO 2008 classification:
Refractory anemia with unilineage dysplasia
Refractory anemia
Refractory neutropenia
Refractory thrombocytopenia
Refractory anemia with ring sideroblasts
Refractory cytopenia with multilineage dysplasia (with or without ringed sideroblasts)
Refractory anemia with excess of blasts-1
Refractory anemia with excess of blasts-2
Myelodysplastic syndrome, unclassifiable
Myelodysplastic syndrome with deletion 5q

CLASSIFICATION AND PROGNOSIS OF PATIENTS WITH MDS

Classification Systems

The MDS are a heterogeneous group of clonal hematologic disorders characterized by persistent peripheral blood cytopenias and proliferation of myeloblastic leukemia cells.[21] Since the early 1980s, several groups have developed classification schemes for patients with MDS that can be used for prediction of survival as well as rate of transformation to overt AML. The FAB consensus conference in 1982 described a classification scheme that includes both AML and myelodysplasia.[19] Five categories of MDS were described based on the BM morphology of BM aspirates, specifically requiring patients to have greater than 10% dysplasia within two or more cell lines. Patients were separated into five groups primarily based on the percentage of myeloblasts within the BM aspirate. These categories are RA, RARS, RAEB, RAEB-T, and CMML (Table 59-3). The diagnosis of acute leukemia required at least 30% myeloblasts within the BM or peripheral blood; patients with 30% or fewer myeloblasts were classified as having myelodysplasia.

With the exception of RARS and CMML, the subgroups of MDS are stratified by the percentage of blasts within the peripheral blood or BM. The first two categories, RA and RARS, have fewer than 5% myeloblasts in the BM. Patients with RA and RARS tend to have a longer median overall survival time and a lower rate of progression to acute leukemia than patients in the other categories. Patients with RAEB and RAEB-T have between 5% and 20% or between 21% and 30% myeloblasts within the BM, respectively. These patients often have more severe cytopenias, an increased risk of progression toward acute leukemia, and a shorter overall survival time. Patients with CMML represent a heterogeneous group.[162,163] Some patients have a more MDS-like picture, with significant pancytopenia and trilineage dysplasia within the BM. Other patients have more of a myeloproliferative-like picture, with elevated white blood cell (WBC) count, peripheral monocytosis, splenomegaly, and hypermetabolic symptoms. The median survival time of patients with MDS-CMML was 23 months versus 15 months for patients with myeloproliferative disorder (MPD)-CMML (P = .31), and both groups had nearly identical risk of progression to AML.[186,187]

The FAB classification scheme led to marked improvement in the diagnosis of myelodysplasia. It also served as a general prognostic predictor. However, there still exists considerable variation within the groups with respect to overall survival and clinical features. Several prognostic systems have been devised to better predict the outcome of individual patients. For example, prognosis is inversely related to the number of BM myeloblasts, and cytogenetics have an extremely important impact on overall survival.[188] The International Myelodysplastic Syndrome Risk Analysis Workshop (IMRAW) has developed an International Prognostic Scoring System (IPSS) based on an analysis of more than 800 patients (Table 59-4).[189] This analysis revealed that the most important variables for overall prognosis were specific cytogenetic abnormalities, percentage of myeloblasts within the BM, and number of the lineages involved in the cytopenia. Other adverse prognostic features include age older than 60 years and male sex. Isolated loss of the Y, 5q, or 20q chromosome or the presence of a normal karyotype is associated with a favorable prognosis. Adverse prognostic cytogenetic features included abnormalities of chromosome 7 or complex cytogenetic changes defined as having more than three cytogenetic anomalies. This scoring system divided patients into four categories: low, intermediate-1, intermediate-2, and high-risk groups. The overall median survival for these groups was 5.7, 3.5, 1.2, and 0.4 years, respectively.[189] There are several limitations of using the IPSS for individual patients. First, the IPSS is heavily

Table 59-4 International Prognostic Scoring System for Myelodysplastic Syndrome

Overall Score*	Median Survival (Years)	25% AML Evolution (Years)
Low (0)	5.7	9.4
Intermediate-1 (0.5-1.0)	3.5	3.3
Intermediate-2 (1.5-2.0)	1.2	1.1
High (≥2.5)	0.4	0.2

Data from Greenberg P, Cox C, LeBeau MM, et al: International scoring system for evaluating prognosis in myelodysplastic syndromes (published erratum appears in *Blood* 91:1100, 1998). *Blood* 89:2079, 1997.
AML, Acute myelogenous leukemia.
*The overall score is the sum of the scores from the percent of bone marrow myeloblasts, karyotype, and cytopenias.
The percent of myeloblasts are scored as follows: <5% = 0; 5%-10% = 0.5: 11%-20% = 1.5: 21%-30% = 2.0.
Cytogenetic features associated with good prognosis are scored as 0 and include normal karyotype, loss of Y, 5q–, or 20q–; those associated with a poor prognosis are scored as 1.0 and include abnormalities of chromosome 7 or three or more cytogenetic changes; all other cytogenetic abnormalities are scored as 0.5 and are of intermediate prognosis.
A score of 0 refers to a patient with either zero or one cell lineage cytopenia, and a score of 0.5 is assigned to two or more lineage cytopenias. Lineage cytopenias are defined as hemoglobin <10 g/dL, absolute neutrophil count <1800/mm^3, and platelet count <100,000/mm^3.

weighted on the percentage of blasts within the BM aspirate.[190] Second, only a limited number of cytogenetic abnormalities were described within the IPSS, and their prognostic importance is significantly underestimated. Finally, the various cytopenias not only have the same impact on the overall IPSS score but by themselves they are clinically meaningless.

A significant limitation of the FAB classification scheme derives from the arbitrary boundaries imposed within the continuum of disease categories. Patients with RAEB, RAEB-T, and AML likely represent a similar biologic process. Use of 30% myeloblasts within the BM as the division between myelodysplasia and acute leukemia is not biologically consistent and often leads to confusion in the recommendation of treatment options. The European Association of Hematopathologists and the Society for Hematopathology developed a new WHO classification scheme.[20] The WHO defines AML as having a myeloblast count of 20% or greater and drops the RAEB-T category (Table 59-5). Inclusion of CMML in MDS under the older FAB classification scheme was problematic, so within the new WHO classification scheme, CMML has been removed from the MDS category and placed within the myelodysplastic and myeloproliferative disorders (Table 59-6). This change seems more consistent with not only clinical presentation but also with the many treatment choices that are offered to patients with CMML. A new category, refractory cytopenia with multilineage dysplasia (RCMD), also was proposed. This category allows for the classification of patients with morphologic dysplasia within their BM aspirate but who present with isolated neutropenia or thrombocytopenia instead of the typical anemia.

In addition to the number of myeloblasts, the FAB and WHO classification scheme are based on the degree of hematopoietic dysplasia. The FAB classification required patients to have 10% or greater dysplasia in two or more hematopoietic lineages. The WHO modified this requirement, and unilineage erythrodysplasia now is classified as RA or RARS depending on the presence or absence of ringed sideroblasts. Importantly, the dysplasia must have been present for more than 6 months, and no other causes of erythrodysplasia could be present. The WHO introduced a new category of refractory cytopenia with multilineage dysplasia with or without ringed sideroblasts: RCMD and RCMD-S, respectively. Although often subtle, patients with multilineage dysplasia have a significantly poorer overall survival as well as leukemia-free survival compared with patients with unilineage dysplasia.

Table 59-5 World Health Organization Classifications of MDS

Refractory anemia with unilineage dysplasia
- Refractory anemia
- Refractory neutropenia
- Refractory thrombocytopenia

Refractory anemia with ring sideroblasts
Refractory cytopenia with multilineage dysplasia (with or without ring sideroblasts)
Refractory anemia with excess of blasts-1
Refractory anemia with excess of blasts-2
Myelodysplastic syndrome, unclassifiable
Myelodysplastic syndrome with deletion 5q

The World Health Organization has reclassified chronic myelomonocytic leukemia (CMML) within the myeloproliferative disorders (MPD) and RAEB-T to "AML with multilineage dysplasia." Acute myeloid leukemia (AML) is now classified as ≥20% myeloblasts.
The following are considered AML regardless of blast percentage: t(8;21)-AML1/ETO, t(15;17)-PML/RARA, inv(16) or t(16;16)-CBFβMYH11, and 11q23-MLL.

Table 59-6 World Health Organization Criteria for Diagnosis of Chronic Myelomonocytic Leukemia

Peripheral blood monocytosis >1000/mL.
No evidence of Philadelphia chromosome or *BCR-ABL1* gene
Less than 20% myeloblasts, monoblasts, and promonocytes within the peripheral blood or bone marrow
Dysplastic changes in one or more myeloid lineages. If myelodysplasia is absent or minimal, the diagnosis of CMML can be made if the above three criteria are met and:
Acquired clonal cytogenetic abnormality is present in bone marrow cells *or*
Persistent monocytosis for >3 months and all other causes of monocytosis have been excluded
CMML-1: Blasts <5% in peripheral blood and <10% in bone marrow
CMML-2: Blasts 5%-19% in peripheral blood or 10%-19% in bone marrow

From Vardiman JW, Harris NL, Brunning RD: The World Health Organization (WHO) classification of the myeloid neoplasms, *Blood* 100:2292, 2002.

The WHO classification system has been modified using prognostic scoring variables based on transfusion requirements as well as similar cytogenetic abnormalities within the IPSS.[191] The newer WHO classification-based scoring system (WPSS) is able to stratify patients into five risk groups (Table 59-7). Whereas the very-low-risk group has a survival of 11.3 years and 7% risk of transformation into AML at 10 years, the very-high-risk group has a survival of 0.7 years and 50% risk of transformation into AML at 8 months. Although this scoring system has been validated on a separate cohort of patients, use of the WPSS has not gained widespread popularity. What is clear from the WPSS is that the definition of RBC transfusion "dependency" requires further confirmation and prospective large cohort studies.

Other parameters for evaluating the prognosis of MDS have been assessed in a series of scoring systems that follow different clinical or cytogenetic features, which include WBC count, hemoglobin, platelet count, age, sex, lactate dehydrogenase, and immunophenotyping.[190,192-196] For example, the CD44 antigen, which is a transmembrane glycoprotein, is expressed on BM mononuclear precursor cells as well as peripheral granulocytes and erythrocytes.[193,197] Serum CD44 levels typically are increased in patients with MDS as well as AML and ALL. Increased expression of CD44-6v has been associated with shorter survival time in patients with AML. Flow cytometric analysis has been used to evaluate expression of CD44 on early myeloid cells that coexpress CD66. CD66 typically is expressed on monocytes as well as immature myeloid cells. Low CD44 coexpression on CD66

Table 59-7 World Health Organization–Based Prognostic Scoring System for Predicting Survival in Patients With Myelodysplastic Syndrome

	Points			
Variables	**0**	**1**	**2**	**3**
WHO subtype	RA, RARS, 5q−	RCMD, RCMD-RS	RAEB-1	RAEB-2
Transfusion requirement	None	Yes*	—	—
IPSS cytogenetic risk	Good	Intermediate	Poor	—

IPSS, International Prognostic Scoring System; *RA,* refractory anemia; *RAEB,* refractory anemia with excess blasts; *RAEB-1,* 5%-9% myeloblasts; *RAEB-2,* 10%-19% myeloblasts; *RCMD,* refractory cytopenias with multilineage dysplasia; *RS,* ringed sideroblasts; *WHO,* World Health Organization.

*Defined as 1 unit of red blood cells every 8 weeks over a 4-month period.

WPSS Risk Group	Score
Very low	0
Low	1
Intermediate	2
High	3-4
Very high	5-6

WPSS, World Health Organization classification-based scoring system.

Overall Score	Median Survival (Years)	Cumulative Acute Myelogenous Leukemia Evolution at 5 Years
Very low (0)	11.8	0.03
Intermediate (1)	5.5	0.14
Intermediate (2)	4.0	0.33
High (3-4)	2.2	0.54
Very high (5-6)	0.8	0.84

Adapted from Malcovati L, Porta MG, Pascutto C, et al: Prognostic factors and life expectancy in myelodysplastic syndromes classified according to WHO criteria: A basis for clinical decision making, *J Clin Oncol* 23:7594, 2005.

myeloid cells typically is seen in the early stages of MDS as opposed to increased CD44 expression on CD66-weak myeloid cells, which often is seen in the later stages of myelodysplasia, that is, in patients with increased number of blasts. A shift in CD44 expression therefore often has been associated with a trend toward immaturity or increased number of blasts in patients with MDS; therefore, CD44 expression profiling may be useful as a separate prognostic marker for patients with MDS. However, large prospective studies are warranted.

The angiogenic process is extremely important in the growth and metastasis of many solid tumors.[198,199] Its role in hematopoietic malignancies is less well characterized. Both vascular endothelial growth factor and basic fibroblast growth factor are expressed by myeloblasts. Furthermore, analysis of BM samples from patients with untreated AML showed increased microvessel density.[199,200] Vascular endothelial growth factor has been linked to the promotion of atypical localization of immature myeloid precursors, which is a poor prognostic marker in patients with MDS, especially for signaling out those patients who are at highest risk for disease progression.[119,201,202] Furthermore, microvessel density is markedly higher in patients with RAEB-T compared with the other MDS subtypes, suggesting a role between angiogenesis and transformation to acute leukemia in patients with MDS.

Red Blood Cell Transfusion Dependence

Red blood cell transfusion dependence is associated with a poorer overall survival in patients with MDS. In a retrospective study of 239 patients with low-risk MDS 19% were RBC transfusion dependent and had shorter survival than did patients who had not recently undergone transfusions.[203] A similar retrospective study of 467 patients by Malcovati et al[191] also demonstrated that RBC transfusion dependency in patients with MDS had a negative impact on both overall survival and leukemia-free survival. The negative effect was dependent on the number of transfusions per month and was an independent prognostic variable regardless of cytogenetic risk assessment.

The etiology for the shorter survival in patients with MDS who are RBC transfusion dependent is unclear. Some patients had secondary hemochromatosis as assayed by increased serum ferritin levels, and some patients developed cardiac dysfunction or arrhythmias.[203] Although iron overload is suggested to be a significant component in the increased mortality of transfusion-dependent patients with MDS, prospective studies are needed to accurately assess the effect of iron chelation on survival and subsequent prognosis in patients with MDS who are RBC transfusion dependent.

CYTOGENETIC AND MOLECULAR ABNORMALITIES

Careful examination of the BM aspirate to detect cytogenetic abnormalities is a critical part in establishing the diagnosis of MDS. Although approximately 60% of patients with MDS have a normal karyotype, the presence of characteristic cytogenetic abnormalities may establish the diagnosis in cases in which the dysplastic changes within the BM aspirate are subtle (see Table 59-4).[21] Furthermore, documentation of additional cytogenetic changes may imply an evolving clonal evolution and development of a neoplastic process.

Abnormal karyotypes are identified in about half of all cases of MDS and in more than 80% of therapy-related cases.[6,188] The most common abnormality is trisomy 8. Other common abnormalities include monosomy 5 or 7; loss of the Y chromosome; or deletions involving the long arms of chromosomes 5, 7, 11, 13, and 20. Complex karyotypes, defined as three or more abnormalities, are seen in approximately 15% of cases of MDS and portend an unfavorable prognosis. Chromosomal abnormalities are most often associated with the FAB subtypes RAEB and RAEB-T. The presence of a deletion of the long arm of chromosome 5 (5q−) as the sole abnormality is seen most often in patients with RA[145]; monosomy 7 is rarely seen in this MDS subgroup. Translocations involving platelet-derived growth factor receptor-β (PDGFR-β) have been identified in 5% to 10% of patients with CMML. The first case was identified in a patient with a translocation involving the transcription factor TEL on chromosome 12,[204] but many other fusion partners have now been described. The TEL–PDGFR-β receptor gene product produces a chronic myeloproliferative disorder in mice and is a potential target for tyrosine receptor kinase inhibition with imatinib therapy.

Therapy-related MDS is associated with specific chromosomal abnormalities.[108] Patients who develop MDS or AML after exposure to alkylator therapy often have either a partial loss or complete monosomy of chromosome 5 or 7.[6,7,109] Patients who were exposed to topoisomerase II inhibitors typically present with a monocytic acute leukemia and not MDS. These patients have a high frequency of chromosomal rearrangements involving the MLL gene on 11q23[91] or less commonly the AML1 gene on 21q21. Other chromosomal abnormalities associated with therapy-related MDS include 3p14-21, 6p21, 12p11-17, and 19p13. Mutations involving p53 on chromosome 17p have been described and are associated with a long latency period between toxin exposure and the diagnosis of MDS or AML.[205,206]

Several diagnostic tests have increased the ability to detect cryptic cytogenetic anomalies. Fluorescent in situ hybridization (FISH) uses specific DNA probes to identify each chromosome individually.[207] This method can screen hundreds of cells and does not depend on analysis of dividing cells during metaphase. Thus, the sensitivity can be dramatically increased, but use of FISH is limited to detection of standard cytogenetic abnormalities. Polymerase chain reaction analysis can detect specific gene translocations in either the BM or blood. This assay is rapid and can detect abnormalities present in fewer than 1 in 10,000 cells but also is limited to detection of standard cytogenetic abnormalities.

It is important to realize that a normal karyotype does not exclude the diagnosis of MDS. Normal karyotypes are see in about half of all cases of MDS. This is thought to be attributable to the limitations of standard G banding or the failure of the neoplastic clone to divide in culture. Spectral karyotype analysis or "chromosomal painting" can identify cryptic balanced and unbalanced translocations in most patients with MDS.

Cytogenetic Correlation With Prognosis

One of the limitations with the IPSS is the limited information that was available on cytogenetic data. Cytogenetic analysis since has been performed in more than 2000 patients with MDS and was successful in 97% of these patients.[208] Clonal cytogenetic abnormalities were seen in 52.3% of patients. These included numeric as well as structural chromosomal abnormalities. The limitation in terms of prognosis is the varying degree by which patients receive therapy; therefore, the impact of karyotypic abnormalities on the natural history of myelodysplasia was studied in 1286 patients treated with supportive care only (see Table 59-4). Therefore, how overall and leukemia-free survival are affected by therapeutic intervention is unclear.

In patients with a normal karyotype (n = 612), the median survival time was 53 months. This is compared with an 8.7-month survival time for patients with complex abnormalities. The most frequent abnormality involved deletion of chromosome 5q, which occurred in 30% of patients who had a cytogenetic abnormality or 58% of all patients with successful cytogenetic analysis. Isolated deletion of 5q was seen in 14% of patients with clonal abnormalities. Other frequent abnormalities included monosomy 7 or 7q deletion in 21% and trisomy 8 (+8) in 16% of patients with MDS. Less common abnormalities are listed in Table 59-8.

Favorable prognosis measured as a median survival of approximately 3 years was seen in patients with translocations involving chromosome 1q, translocation involving 7q, any chromosome 12 abnormality, translocation involving 17q with a noncomplex karyotype, monosomy 21, trisomy 21, as well as for loss of chromosome X. Median survivals had not been reached for patients with del9q, del12p, and del15q. The favorable survival for these patients was seen only if patients has no additional abnormalities. In addition, 21 other chromosomal aberrations were identified, but their rarity did not allow for prognostic relevance. Therefore, even though numerous cytogenetic abnormalities have been identified, the rarity of a few cytogenetic abnormalities makes prognostic impact limited.

Abnormalities with intermediate prognosis, defined as median survival between 1 and 3 years, was seen in patients with chromosome 3q rearrangements, translocations involving 11q23 as a noncomplex karyotype, and trisomy 19. In addition, regardless of the specific aberrations, an overall correlation was seen between prognosis and extent of abnormalities. Patients with three or more abnormalities had a median survival of 17 months, patients with four to six abnormalities had a median survival of 9 months, and patients with more than six abnormalities had a median survival of only 5 months. This analysis further demonstrates the cytogenetic impact of a complex karyotype on the prognosis of patients with MDS. Cytogenetic analysis remains an important factor in treatment selection as well as monitoring response to therapy. What is unclear from this type of analyses is the impact of pharmacologic therapy on the prognosis of patients with MDS based on their cytogenetic abnormalities.

Table 59-8 Frequency and Median Survival of Cytogenetic Prognostic Subgroups

Anomaly	Frequency (%)	Median Survival (Months)
Good-Prognosis Cytogenetics		
del(9q), NC	0.4	NR
del(15q), NC	0.4	NR
t(15q), NC	0.4	NR
del(12p), NC	0.8	108.0
+21, NC	1.1	100.8
–Y, +1	0.4	84.6
del(5q), isolated	8.2	80.0
+21, or +1	0.8	80.0
del(5q), NC	10.7	77.2
del(20q), isolated	1.9	71.0
del(20q), NC	2.2	71.0
–X, NC	0.5	56.4
No (normal karyotype)	49.5	53.4
del(5q), +1	2.5	47.0
+8, or +1	1.2	44.0
–Y, NC	2.7	39.0
–Y, sole	3.5	36.0
+1/+1q, NC	0.4	34.7
t(1q), NC	0.6	34.7
t(7q), NC	0.6	34.7
t(11q), NC	0.5	32.1
–21, NC	0.5	32.0
Intermediate-Prognosis Cytogenetics		
del(11q), NC	0.9	26.1
+8, NC	5.0	23.0
+8, isolated	3.8	22.0
t(11q23), NC	0.5	20.0
Rea 3q, NC	0.5	19.9
+19, NC	0.4	19.8
del(7q), isolated and NC	0.6	19.0
Any 3 abnormalities	2.8	17.1
del(11q), isolated	0.6	15.9
–7, +1	0.9	14.4
–5, NC	0.4	14.6
–7, sole	2.3	14.0
–7, NC	3.2	14.0
Poor-Prognosis Cytogenetics		
Complex, all	13.4	8.7
t(5q), NC	0.4	4/4
4-6 abnormalities	5.3	9.0
>6 abnormalities	3.9	5.0

From Haase D, Germing U, Schonz J, et al: New insights into the prognostic impact of the karyotype in MDS and correlation with subtypes: Evidence from a core dataset of 2124 patients. *Blood* 110:4385, 2007.
NC, Noncomplex karyotype (≤3 abnormalities); *NR,* not reached.

CLINICAL SYNDROMES

Patients with MDS often present with symptoms of ineffective hematopoiesis.[209] They usually seek medical attention complaining of recurrent infections, bleeding, easy bruising, progressive fatigue and lethargy, or dyspnea on exertion. Occasionally, patients present without symptoms but with abnormal peripheral counts, such as neutropenia, anemia, thrombocytopenia, or a combination of all three. It is important to realize that bleeding can also occur in nonthrombocytopenic patients because of dysfunctional platelets. Patients either die of progressive BM failure or progress to overt AML. A subgroup of patients with less than 5% myeloblasts, RA, or RARS may die of nonhematologic causes, which typifies this affected elderly patient population. In general, patients with MDS have a shorter overall survival time than age-matched control participants, suggesting that BM failure may be additive to other comorbid diseases.[21]

Myelodysplastic syndrome has been reported to coexist with other hematologic malignancies, the most frequent being multiple myeloma, even in previously untreated patients.[210,211] MDS also has been described in patients with hairy cell leukemia, chronic lymphocytic leukemia, non-Hodgkin lymphoma, and large granular lymphocytic leukemia.[212] The association of MDS with these other hematopoietic malignancies suggests a common myeloid or lymphoid stem cell as the transforming cell. However, the association may simply be a statistically random association or be therapy related in some cases. The coexistence of MDS with another hematologic malignancy significantly complicates the treatment options.

5q– Syndrome

Patients with myelodysplasia represent several unique clinical cohorts. Patients with an isolated loss of the short arm of chromosome 5 [del5(q31-q35), or 5q–] are characterized by a prolonged clinical course that progresses to acute leukemia in fewer than 25% of cases.[213,214] Interestingly, anemia seems to be the principal laboratory abnormality. Neutropenia, if present, typically is mild, and platelet counts often remain elevated. The striking pathologic feature is the presence of mononuclear micromegakaryocytes identified in the BM biopsy (Fig. 59-5, *A-C*).

Women account for a larger proportion of cases, up to 70%.[215,216] Patients with 5q– deletions must be distinguished from patients with additional cytogenetic abnormalities because these patients often have a more rapid progression to AML. The large arm of chromosome 5 is rich in genes encoding both cytokines and cytokine receptors.[217] Haploinsufficiency of the ribosomal protein encoding RPS14 gene has been shown to cause the phenotypic features of 5q– syndrome.[218] RNA interference (RNAi) screening technology confirmed the notion that 5q– syndrome is caused by a defect in ribosomal protein RPS14. In addition, a link has been established between acquired 5q– syndrome

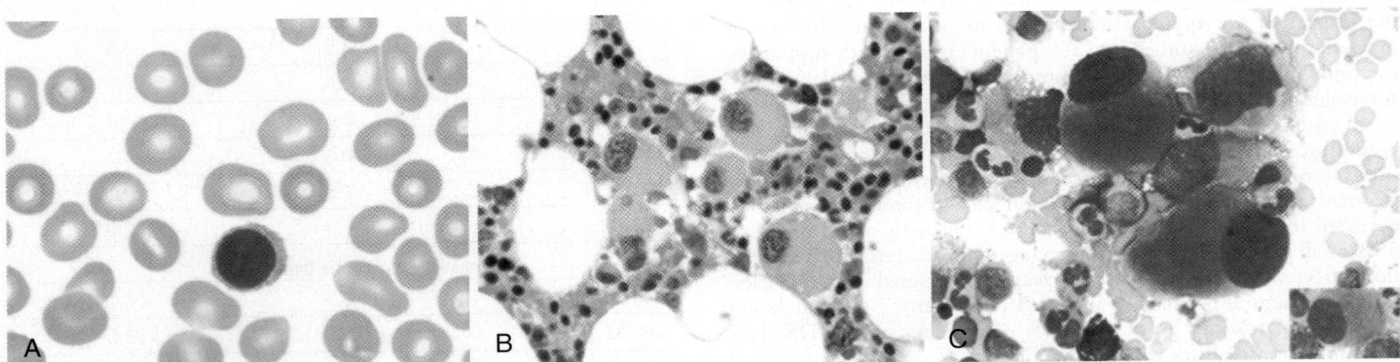

Figure 59-5 SPECIFIC MYELODYSPLASTIC SYNDROMES. The 5q– syndrome (**A** to **C**); hypocellular myelodysplastic syndrome (**D** and **E**), and myelodysplastic syndrome with fibrosis (**F** and **G**). The 5q– syndrome has specific morphologic correlates. There is a macrocytic anemia **(A)** and a cellular bone marrow characterized by increased small monolobated megakaryocytes (**B** and **C**). The megakaryocyte nuclei have little segmentation and are fairly round. Although some true micro-megakaryocytes may be present (**C,** *inset*, same magnification), the typical monolobated forms are not as tiny as the micro-megakaryocytes.

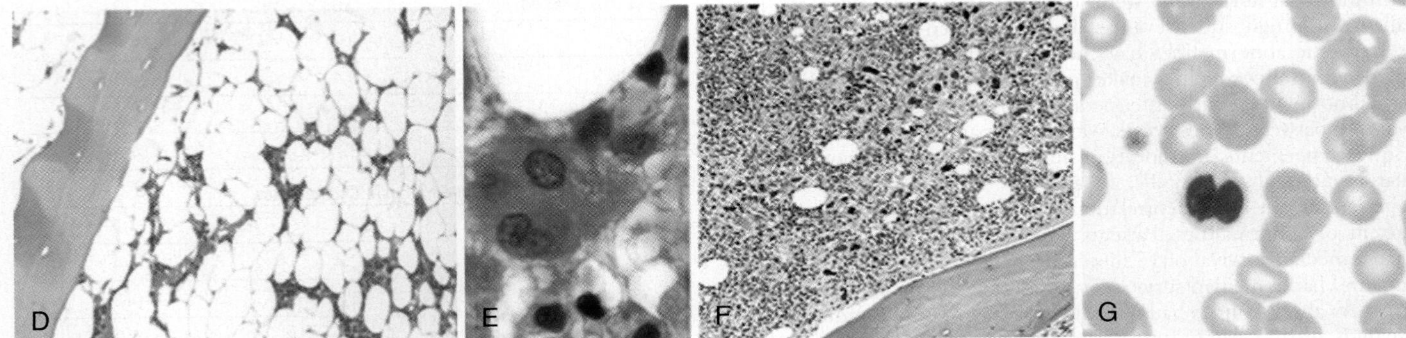

Figure 59-5, cont'd SPECIFIC MYELODYSPLASTIC SYNDROMES. Hypocellular myelodysplastic syndrome (**D** and **E**) can present a diagnostic problem and can be difficult to differentiate from aplastic anemia. Dysplasia may be difficult to evaluate if the smears are paucicellular. The finding of dysplastic megakaryocytes (note small widely separated nuclei, **E**) on the biopsy sample can be helpful. Myelodysplastic syndrome with fibrosis **(F)** can be difficult to differentiate from myeloproliferative neoplasms (MPN). However, the lack of large megakaryocytes, which typically are see in the MPNs along with presence of dysplasia in the circulating neutrophils **(G)** are useful clues to the correct diagnosis.

and congenital BM failure syndromes such as Diamond-Blackfan anemia. Because of the uniqueness of the 5q– syndrome, it often is considered separately from the other myelodysplastic disorders. Patients typically require RBC transfusion as their principal treatment, so careful attention must be paid to management of iron overload. Lenalidomide (Revimid) has been approved for patients with a chromosome 5q abnormality who are transfusion dependent, and its use is discussed in the treatment section.[219,220]

Hypocellular Myelodysplastic Syndromes

The majority of patients with myelodysplasia have hypercellular or normocellular BM. Hypocellular BM is found in a minority of patients (<15%) and is referred to as hypoplastic myelodysplasia (see Fig. 59-5, *D* and *E*).[221] In this subgroup of patients, the morphologic features of the BM may be difficult to differentiate from aplastic anemia, and the definitive diagnosis can sometimes be made from cytogenetic analysis. Cytogenetic abnormalities are rarely found in patients with aplastic anemia. The differential diagnosis of patients with a hypoplastic BM includes not only aplastic anemia but also drug toxicity, PNH, and T-cell large granular lymphocytic leukemia.[222,223] These entities usually can be excluded by flow cytometric analysis of the BM aspirate. The natural history of hypoplastic myelodysplasia is similar to that of the standard variants.

Myelodysplastic Syndrome With Myelofibrosis

Substantial reticulin fibrosis is rarely found in patients with myelodysplasia (see Fig. 59-5, *F* and *G*), although there is an increase incidence in patients with CMML. Myelodysplasia with myelofibrosis can be difficult to distinguish from chronic idiopathic myelofibrosis (agnogenic myeloid metaplasia with myelofibrosis).[121,224] The presence of trilineage dysplasia and the absence of hepatosplenomegaly support the diagnosis of myelodysplasia. However, some cases, may reflect an evolving transformation to a leukemic process, with profound BM fibrosis such as is often seen in acute megakaryocytic leukemia (FAB-M7). Myelofibrosis can occur in all MDS subtypes, and mild fibrosis is seen in more than two-thirds of cases. Marked fibrosis is much rarer and is thought to be present in only approximately 10% of cases.

Patients who develop MDS with myelofibrosis often have rapidly progressive cytopenias, usually without splenomegaly, and often have a poor prognosis.[117,118] Peripheral blood smear usually reveal the heralded "teardrop" cell, and the BM is markedly hypercellular with fibrosis and often dysplastic megakaryocytic proliferation with hypolobated megakaryocytes; many patients have an increased number of myeloblasts. The differential diagnosis is complicated and includes idiopathic or primary myelofibrosis, postpolycythemia vera myelofibrosis with myeloid metaplasia, post–essential thrombocythemic myelofibrosis with myeloid metaplasia, accelerated phase CML, acute leukemia (usually M7 or AML with dysplasia), and acute myelofibrosis.

Myelodysplastic Syndrome—Myeloproliferative Neoplasm Overlap Syndromes

CMML is the quintessential disorder having characteristic findings of both MDS and myeloproliferative neoplasm (MPN) (Fig. 59-6, *A*).[158,162,163] Because the majority of patients with CMML have evidence of trilineage dysplasia, the FAB cooperative group categorized CMML as a subtype of MDS. The FAB criteria for diagnosis included a peripheral monocyte count of 1000/mm^3, less than 5% blasts in the blood, less than 20% blasts in the BM, and absence of Auer rods. The new WHO classification system places CMML with juvenile myelomonocytic leukemia and atypical or BCR-negative CML into the new subgroup MDS–MPD (see Table 59-6).[21]

Many patients with CMML also present with splenomegaly, hepatomegaly, lymphadenopathy, tissue infiltration, or serous effusions.[162,186,187,225] Pleural, pericardial, synovial, and ascitic effusions all have been reported in patients with CMML and are associated with a high circulating monocyte count. Patients with CMML can have vastly different presentations. Certain patients with CMML present with profound cytopenias and marked dysplasia, but other patients have a predominately myeloproliferative form. Because of these two rather distinct clinical presentations, some clinicians separate CMML into two separate entities, with the proliferative form characterized by WBC count greater than 12,000/mm^3, presence of organomegaly, and constitutional symptoms. The nonproliferative form of CMML is characterized by a low WBC count with a relative monocytosis, and complications from cytopenias tend to dominate the clinical picture. The overall prognosis of both forms of CMML is similar, with median overall survival of 19 months, and the absolute number of BM blasts is the dominant prognostic feature.[187]

A subgroup of patients, usually with the proliferative form of CMML, is characterized by the balanced translocation t(5;12)(q33; p13).[204] The consequence of the t(5;12) translocation is fusion of the

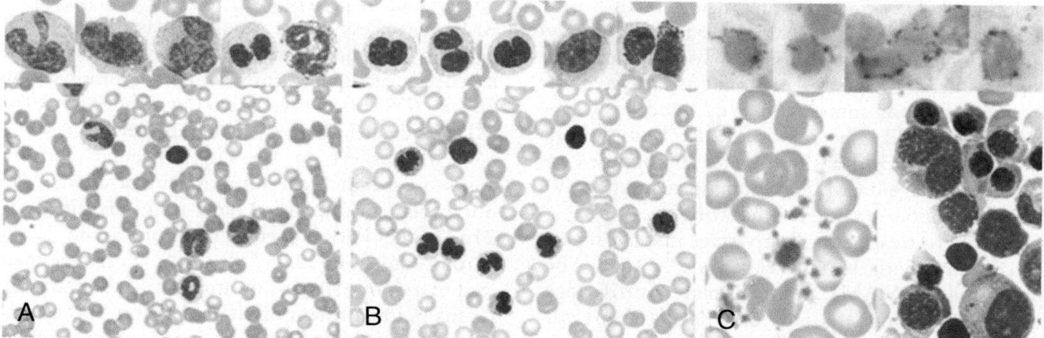

Figure 59-6 OVERLAP SYNDROMES. Chronic myelomonocytic leukemia **(A)**, "atypical chronic myelogenous leukemia," *BCR-ABL1*–negative **(B)**, and refractory anemia with ringed sideroblasts and thrombocytosis (RARS-T) **(C)**. In chromic myelomonocytic leukemia, there can be granulocytic dysplasia and cytopenias (e.g., anemia, thrombocytopenia), but the characteristic feature is the presence of an absolute monocytosis **(A)**. "Atypical chronic myelogenous leukemia" (*BCR-ABL1* negative) is essentially a "high-count" myelodysplastic syndrome. There typically is severe granulocytic dysplasia. The absence of an absolute monocytosis excludes chronic myelomonocytic leukemia from the diagnosis. The case shown is characterized by numerous pseudo–Pelger-Huet cells, immature hypogranular granulocytic precursors, and some basophils **(B)**. Refractory anemia with ringed sideroblasts and thrombocytosis is characterized by anemia and thrombocytosis in the blood (**C,** *left*), hypercellular marrow with erythroid proliferation (**C,** *right*), and ringed sideroblasts (**C,** *top*).

tyrosine kinase domain of PDGFR-β to a member of the *ETS* family of transcription factors TEL. Fusion of TEL to PDGFR-β constitutively activates the tyrosine kinase domain of PDGFR-β, leading to increased myeloid proliferation. PDGFR-β on chromosome 5q33 also is disrupted by t(5;7), t(5;14), and t(5;10) translocations, resulting in fusion of the tyrosine kinase domain of PDGFR-β to HIP1, CEV14, and H4/D10S170, respectively.[226] The understanding of these findings has led to novel therapeutic approaches using the tyrosine kinase inhibitor imatinib mesylate, with remarkable efficacy and durable responses.[183,227] Unfortunately, PDGFR-β is present in only a minority of cases of CMML.

Therapy-Related Myelodysplastic Syndromes

Therapy-related MDS is becoming more important given the increased dose density currently being administered to patients, for example, those with breast carcinoma.[228-231] Furthermore, the use of myeloid growth factors may inadvertently increase this risk.[232] Therapy-related MDS and AML remain one of the most serious long-term complications of current cancer therapy and often are induced by well-defined chemotherapeutic agents or radiation. The incidence of secondary or therapy-related MDS is increasing.[228] The term *secondary myelodysplasia* refers to the development of disease after either exposure to environmental or therapeutic toxins or from a previously diagnosed hematopoietic disorder. The term *therapy related* should be specifically attributed to the presentation of MDS or AML after the use of intensive chemotherapy or radiation therapy.

Many patients with therapy-related MDS/AML have common chromosomal aberrations or gene mutations. Most importantly, patients with therapy-related MDS behave in a more aggressive fashion regardless of FAB or WHO classification subtype. Patients with therapy-related MDS are not included in the IPSS schema; therefore, specific prognostic factors are limiting. The risk of secondary MDS is highest in patients who already have been exposed to alkylating agent therapy. The cytogenetic abnormalities of alkylating agent therapy–related MDS/AML are quite distinct.[6,10,109] They include either a total loss or a deletion of the long arm of either chromosome 5 or 7. A higher than normal risk for developing therapy-related MDS/AML has been described in long-term survivors of Hodgkin lymphoma, non-Hodgkin lymphoma, multiple myeloma, and gastrointestinal cancers, specifically those treated with semustine (methyl-CCNU).[233-236] The estimated actuarial risk in patients treated for Hodgkin lymphoma is between 6% and 9%. A 17% actuarial risk has been reported in patients treated for multiple myeloma.

The risk of developing MDS after adjuvant treatment of breast cancer, small cell lung cancer, testicular cancer, or ovarian cancer is low but increases with use of regional radiation therapy. Topoisomerase II inhibitors also can induce therapy-related AML[91] but typically involves a balanced translocation of chromosome band 11q23 and less commonly involves 3q26 and 21q22. The topoisomerase II inhibitors include the epipodophyllotoxins and anthracyclines. As opposed to prior exposure from alkylating agents, MDS seldom precedes therapy-related AML caused by the topoisomerase II inhibitors.

Use of adjuvant therapy for treatment of early-stage invasive breast carcinoma has been associated with therapy-related MDS/AML. The incidence of therapy-related MDS/AML after treatment of early-stage breast cancer with mastectomy alone is only 0.27%.[229,237,238] A case-control study of 82,700 women treated for early-stage breast cancer during the 1970s and 1980s reported that the typical cyclophosphamide, methotrexate, and fluorouracil (CMF) regimens with a low cumulative dose of cyclophosphamide is associated with an additional five cases of leukemia for every 10,000 women treated over 10 years.[239] However, with the current use of anthracycline-based adjuvant chemotherapy regimens (cyclophosphamide, epirubicin, fluorouracil [CEF]; or fluorouracil, Adriamycin [doxorubicin], cyclophosphamide [FAC]), the risk of therapy-related MDS/AML has increased compared with the classic CMF regimen. Rates of therapy-related MDS/AML now approach 1.5% after 5 to 10 years of follow-up. There is an even greater risk in women who received radiotherapy.[240,241] In patients who receive four cycles of standard anthracycline and cyclophosphamide therapy (cyclophosphamide 600 mg/m^2 and doxorubicin 60 mg/m^2 per cycle), the risk appears quite low. In one study, the incidence of therapy-related MDS/AML in patients who receive four full cycles of cyclophosphamide and anthracycline chemotherapy was only 0.1% with the median follow-up of 5 years. However, women seem to have a higher risk for therapy-related MDS/AML in the National Surgical Adjuvant Breast and Bowel Project (NSABP) protocols B-22 and B-25 in which a higher dose of cyclophosphamide as well as doxorubicin were used.[237] Of potential importance was the use of G-CSF in these regimens. In one retrospective study of patients with breast cancer, use of G-CSF was associated with doubling of the risk of therapy-related MDS/AML.[232]

A history of autologous BM transplantation (BMT) has been associated with a substantial risk of developing therapy-related MDS and AML.[240,242-249] The cumulative probability of developing therapy-related MDS/AML after autologous SCT ranges from 4% to 14%, depending on the series. A retrospective study by Friedberg et al[250] reported a 19.8% actuarial risk of developing MDS by 10 years. All of the 552 patients analyzed in this study were treated with cyclophosphamide and total body irradiation. The patients who developed MDS had on average a lower number of cells reinfused per kilogram at autologous BMT. The increased incidence of therapy-related MDS/AML has been associated with use of radiation therapy as part of the conditioning regimen, but other risk factors include advanced stage, number and type of prior courses of chemotherapy, and exposure to radiation therapy before transplantation. The prognosis of patients with therapy-related MDS or AML remains extremely poor.

Therapy-related MDS and AML are characterized by three distinct groups of cytogenetic abnormalities.[89,108] The first is an unbalanced aberration along chromosome 5 or 7. Patients typically have loss of the whole chromosome 5 or 7 or loss of various parts, specifically the long arm of chromosome 5 or 7. Another frequently observed abnormality is the gain of a whole chromosome 8 (trisomy 8).[39] Abnormalities of chromosomes 5, 7, and 8 are seen in 15% to 25% of cases in de novo MDS but comprise approximately 50% to 70% of cases with therapy-related MDS. Similarly, they occur in 15% to 25% of cases of de novo AML but in 40% to 50% of therapy-related AML. A second cytogenetic subgroup comprises recurrent balance translocations involving the MLL gene on chromosome 11q23.[251,252] Patients with this abnormality typically present with AML without a myelodysplastic prodrome. From 15% to 20% of patients with therapy-related AML have rearrangements of the MLL gene; this abnormality typically is not seen in patients with therapy-related MDS. In fact, the WHO has redefined patients with MLL gene rearrangements or patients with t(8;21) or t(16;16) or inv(16) as having AML regardless of the absolute blast count.[20,158] The final group of patients with therapy-related MDS consists of patients with a normal karyotype or other chromosomal aberrations. This group comprises 50% to 60% of de novo MDS but only 5% to 10% of therapy-related MDS and 10% to 15% of therapy-related AML.

With respect to specific molecular abnormalities, the most common specific gene mutation involves the MLL gene on 11q23, but other abnormalities have been identified, namely, AML1 on 21q22, the RARA locus on chromosome 17q21, and CBFB on chromosome 16q22.[93,94,97,105,107,252-254] Rearrangements of these genes lead to a dominant loss of function of the transcription factor, which results in impairment of differentiation. It is thought that by interfering with myeloid differentiation, leukemia will result. In addition, other abnormalities have been identified, including mutations of the nucleophosmin gene NPM1, which has been designated a class II mutation in leukemogenesis.[255] The critical genetic consequences of unbalanced chromosome aberrations in MDS and AML are unclear. Deletions of chromosome 17p13 or loss of whole chromosome 17 were thought to involve the p53 gene.[206,256-259] In addition, data have suggested that monosomy 5 or loss of the long arm of chromosome 5 is related to haploinsufficiency of the *EGR1* gene.[260] However, a study from the Look laboratory at the Dana Farber Cancer Institute has implicated haploinsufficiency and promoter methylation of

CTNNA1, the gene encoding α-catenin.[76] How either of these genetic defects relates to the haploinsufficiency of the ribosomal protein encoding RPS14 remains unclear.[218]

Refractory Anemia With Ringed Sideroblasts with Thrombocytosis

Some patients with MDS present with marked thrombocytosis. Most patients have RARS but with a markedly elevated platelet count and therefore have been reclassified as having RARS-T (see Fig. 59-6, *C*).[167,261-264] BM aspirate and biopsy show features consistent with a myeloproliferative and myelodysplastic overlap syndrome. Importantly, the megakaryocytes resemble those seen in essential thrombocythemia. Patients with RARS-T often have evolved from a low-grade MDS category, such as RA or RARS, but have acquired a Janus kinase 2 (JAK2) V617F mutation. This mutation is relatively uncommon in other patients with MDS; therefore, RARS-T represents another JAK2 mutation-associated chronic myeloproliferative disorder.[265-267]

According to the WHO, patients with RARS-T are classified under the provisional MDS/MPD category and listed as unclassifiable.[268] Given the rarity of this syndrome, definitive estimates of overall survival and time to leukemic transformation are unclear. However, a retrospective analysis of 23 patients with RARS-T revealed a 5-year survival of 86% compared with 62% in patients with RARS who did not have a JAK2 V617F mutation.

3q21-q26 Syndrome

Patients with MDS who contain a 3q21-q26 cytogenetic abnormality often have profound trilineage dysplasia, especially of the megakaryocytes.[269] Patients can present with either MDS or AML and typically have a normal or increased platelet count. Cytogenetic analysis at the time of diagnosis often reveals at t(1;3), inv(3), or t(3;3) abnormality. Patients with these cytogenetic abnormalities have an extremely poor response to chemotherapy and, as a result, a poor overall prognosis. The peripheral blood smear often reveals giant platelets or even circulating megakaryocytic fragments. In addition, hypogranular megakaryocytic forms and micromegakaryocytes may be present in the BM aspirate. These morphologic abnormalities involving the megakaryocytes are accompanied clinically with an increased risk of bleeding despite either a normal or increased absolute platelet count. Platelet aggregation studies show decreased platelet aggregation to collagen and epinephrine and may explain the increased risk of bleeding seen in these patients.[38,171]

TREATMENT

General Principles

Treatment of patients with MDS remains challenging for several reasons. First, patients with this disorder are likely to be elderly, so comorbid disease and performance status are critical components in deciding on specific therapy. Second, the disease is heterogeneous, making therapies for one type of MDS less optimal than those for others. Given the lack of precise pathophysiologic understanding of more than a few MDS subtypes, designing truly targeted therapies is impossible. We are left with agents that deal with abnormalities generally thought to play a role in MDS, such as underactive or overactive apoptosis, failure to express silenced genes required for hematopoietic cell differentiation, or overabundant angiogenic signaling. Finally, there is no widely accepted standard of care in that very few, if any, modalities have been definitively proven to change the natural history of this disease. Until recently,[270] response criteria for MDS were not standard, making for difficult interpretation of the multiple phase II trials that included trial-specific response criteria.

The primary goal of most therapeutic strategies in neoplastic diseases is improvement in overall survival. Although this remains the desired result for treatment of patients with MDS, less formidable achievements also might be useful. Such benefits might include a delay in time to transformation to leukemia, response rate (rigorously defined), decrease in transfusions, decreased infection, hematologic improvement, and improved quality of life. The only modality historically associated with an appreciable degree of long-term disease-free survival is allogeneic BMT.[270,271] This modality is resource intense, potentially highly toxic, and heretofore available only to a minority of patients with MDS because of age and performance status requirements. On the other hand, analysis of the role of the myriad other valuable medical therapies is complicated (see boxes on Management Guidelines for a Newly Diagnosed Patient With

Management Guidelines for a Newly Diagnosed Patient With Myelodysplasia

The only known curative modality for patients with MDS is SCT. Therefore, all appropriate candidates should be considered for SCT. They include patients younger than 70 years (age 75 years at some centers), with a reasonable performance status and no significant comorbidity. Retrospective data from the International Bone Marrow Transplant Registry suggest that patients with low-risk disease (IPSS low or intermediate-1) should undergo SCT only at the time of disease progression (see text and Table 59-10). Disease progression includes progressive, clinically significant cytopenias such as progressive RBC or platelet transfusion dependency or transformation to a high-risk disease. Transformation to high-risk MDS typically is manifested by an increase in the number of bone marrow blasts but also could represent accumulation of additional cytogenetic abnormalities.

Patients with low-risk disease should be carefully analyzed for the presence of a deletion of the long arm of chromosome 5. Patients with a deletion of 5q or those who have the 5q syndrome should start taking lenalidomide at the time they become RBC transfusion dependent. For patients with hypoplastic MDS who are younger than 6 years of age, have a low transfusion requirement, and have no increase in marrow myeloblasts, immunosuppressive therapy should be considered with ATG and a calcineurin inhibitor. In all other patients with low-risk MDS, the addition of an ESA should be considered, but only in patients with a serum EPO level less than 500 mU/mL. For patients who do not respond to initial ESAs, addition of a myeloid growth factor (GC-SF or GM-CSF) should be considered. In patients who do not respond or those with an elevated EPO level, aggressive supportive care should continue. The addition of a hypomethylating agent, such as azacytidine or decitabine, may improve the hematologic parameters, but the overall experience of hypomethylating agents in patients with low-risk MDS is limited. The addition of lenalidomide is another option for patients who have isolated anemia, but lenalidomide has no impact on the myeloid or megakaryocytic lineages in patients without the 5q abnormality. Although controversial, iron chelation therapy can be considered for patients with low-risk MDS and a serum ferritin level greater than 1000 mcq/L.

All patients with high-risk MDS classified by an IPSS score of intermediate-2 or higher or patients with more than 10% bone marrow blasts should be seen at a transplant center for consideration of SCT if they are appropriate candidates. For patients who are not eligible for transplantation, a hypomethylating agent should be initiated at the time of presentation. Hypomethylating agents such as azacytidine and decitabine are associated with a small but reproducible complete remission rate, and evidence from Europe has demonstrated that azacytidine may improve the median overall survival. In addition, regardless of the IPSS risk category, all patients should be considered for clinical trial participation. Hopefully, novel strategies will make an impact not only on patient quality of life but also improve the median survival of patients with MDS.

Role of Iron Chelation in the Management of Patients With Myelodysplasia

The development of secondary hemochromatosis is associated with significant morbidity in chronic hemoglobinopathies such as thalassemia major, Blackfan-Diamond syndrome, and sickle cell anemia. Iron chelation therapy has been shown to improve the outcome in patients with these disorders. However, the same cannot be said for patients with MDS. The majority of patients with MDS become RBC transfusion dependent because they are exposed to a significant amount of intravenous iron. Each unit of packed RBCs has approximately 200 to 250 mg of elemental iron. More than 75% of patients with MDS who receive chronic RBC transfusions will develop evidence of secondary hemochromatosis documented by a serum ferritin level of 1000 mg/mL or higher. This typically occurs after patients have received a total lifetime of 40 units of packed RBCs. Nevertheless, it remains difficult to document true organ failure as a result of iron overload in most patients with MDS. In patients with MDS, a serum ferritin level of 1000 mg/mL or higher is associated with a reduced median overall survival. What has not been demonstrated in a prospective fashion is whether the addition of iron chelation therapy can improve survival.

Patients with high-risk MDS have a shortened overall survival time as a result of progressive cytopenias resulting in infection, bleeding diatheses, or transformation to AML. In these patients, the role of iron chelation therapy is unlikely to improve the median survival. However, in patients with low-risk MDS, the natural history of the disease is markedly different. Many patients have an indolent course, with a median overall survival longer than 3 years. In addition, use of disease-modifying agents, such as lenalidomide, in patients with 5q syndrome may alter the natural history of the disease.

Two studies have demonstrated that iron chelation therapy is associated with an improved median survival in patients with low-risk MDS. Both studies have limitations. In the Canadian study, which was a retrospective analysis of 178 patients, only 18 patients received iron chelation therapy. The other study from the French MDS group was a nonrandomized prospective analysis of 165 patients of whom 46% received iron chelation therapy. In this latter study, various regimens of iron chelation were used, but no formal assessment of individual iron stores was made. Thus, the role of iron chelation therapy for patients with MDS is unclear. If it has a role, it should be reserved for patients with low-risk MDS because they are expected to have a prolonged median survival time, especially patients who are benefiting from their therapy.

Myelodysplasia, Role of Iron Chelation in the Management of Patients With Myelodysplasia, Myelodysplastic Syndromes in Young Patients, and Erythropoietin-Stimulating Agents in Patients With Myelodysplastic Syndromes).

Supportive Care

If there is standard therapy for patients with MDS (other than relatively rare young patients who may be BMT candidates), it is supportive care. Supportive care generally consists of administration of blood products and antibiotics when needed. Most also would consider use of iron chelation therapy and hematopoietic growth factors as reasonable supportive care adjuncts.

The development of hematopoietic growth factor therapy held both promise and peril as a therapeutic strategy in the treatment of patients with MDS. Certainly, if the platelet count, hematocrit, and neutrophil count are low, use of an agent that could stimulate growth of the appropriate precursor cell might prove beneficial in

Myelodysplastic Syndromes in Young Patients

Although MDS typically occurs in patients older than 60 years (median age, 70 years), younger individuals also can be affected. Data on the treatment of young patients with MDS who have an indolent or low-risk presentation are unclear. When the IPSS was developed, few patients were younger than 60 years, but it was clear that young patients within the low and intermediate-1 risk groups had significantly better survival than did older patients within the same IPSS risk group. Because the outcome from SCT is related to patient age, the best approach for young patients with MDS who have a low to intermediate-1 IPSS score remains debated.

Cutler et al[389] demonstrated a superior outcome when patients in low or intermediate-1 IPSS risk groups were transplanted at the time of disease progression as opposed to the time of their initial diagnosis. Furthermore, data from the German registry revealed that 86% of patients younger than 50 years with low-risk disease were alive at 20 years, and patients with an intermediate-1 IPSS score had a median survival of 176 months. Therefore, patients with low or intermediate-1 risk MDS who are younger than 50 years should be observed, and SCT should be delayed until disease progression. Disease progression includes the development of significant transfusion requirements, progressive cytopenias, or transformation to a higher IPSS subgroup.

ameliorating symptoms and complications associated with the given cytopenia. On the other hand, it was recognized early on that in most cases, the pathophysiology of MDS had nothing to do with the failure of growth factor availability. For example, levels of EPO, the renally elaborated protein that regulates RBC production,[272] usually are elevated in anemic patients with MDS[273]; however, the intrinsically diseased BM cannot respond. Moreover, it has been recognized for some time that leukemic cells, the neoplastic counterparts of normal BM stem cells, harbor growth factor receptors and can be induced to proliferate in vitro in response to these agents.[274] As such, it was feared that particularly the myeloid growth factors might be leukemogenic in patients with MDS. Although clinical studies have failed to confirm a major deleterious leukemogenic effect, they also have shown that these treatments do not prevent infection or prolong life expectancy. Nonetheless, when used selectively, hematopoietic growth factors may be useful in the management of certain patients with MDS.

Management of Red Blood Cell Transfusion Dependence

Because most patients with MDS are anemic, which is a major factor in fatigue and poor quality of life, the issue of primary management of this finding is critical. Transfusion of packed RBCs, generally when the patient is symptomatic or when the hemoglobin falls below 8 to 9 mg/dL, is the usual approach. RBCs should be irradiated to prevent transfusion-associated graft-versus-host disease (GVHD).[275] Whether routine depletion of WBCs to reduce alloimmunization is required is controversial.[276] Despite the caveat about high EPO levels in MDS patients, patients can respond meaningfully to this agent, perhaps because a blunted response curve[277] allows pharmacologic doses of recombinant EPO to stimulate erythropoiesis in MDS. The potential for exogenous EPO to raise the hematocrit, decrease transfusion requirements, and possibly improve the quality of life in patients with MDS spurred the generation of many phase II and III trials with various doses and schedules of EPO. Although the initial trials generally used three times per week dosing (based on the successful use of this drug in patients with renal failure),[278] the impracticability of this approach (based on third-party payment rules requiring patients receive drug administration in a doctor's office) have generated weekly dosing schedules. Moreover, the availability of long-acting EPO[279] has furthered the use of more intermittent schedules.

Erythropoietin-Stimulating Agents in Patients With Myelodysplastic Syndrome

The safety of ESAs, recombinant human erythropoietin (rh-EPO; Epogen or Procrit) and darbepoetin (Aranesp) has come into question, specifically in patients with chemotherapy-induced anemia and chronic renal failure. ESAs can increase hemoglobin and ameliorate the symptoms from anemia that develop in patients with cancer who are undergoing chemotherapy and those with chronic renal failure. However, treatment also increases the risk of thromboembolic complications. Increased risk of tumor recurrences also has been noted.

For patients with chronic renal failure, two trials have demonstrated that patients assigned to a high targeted hemoglobin experience significantly more adverse events, including death, chronic heart failure, myocardial infarction, and stroke than do patients assigned to lower targeted hemoglobin. Use of ESAs for treatment of anemia in patients with MDS has remained a standard approach used by most physicians. Interestingly, most physicians are unaware that this remains an off-label use because regulatory authorities have not approved ESAs for use in patients with MDS. The efficacy of ESAs in MDS has been difficult to tabulate given the changing definition of response. Now with most authors using the IWG criteria for response, we have a better appreciation for the low but reproducible responses seen with use of ESAs in patients with MDS. The hemoglobin response from an ESA in patients with MDS ranges from 20% to 40%. It is important to note that a major hemoglobin response includes the development of transfusion independence as well as an increase in hemoglobin of at least 2 g/dL from baseline measurements.

There have been many concerns regarding the safety of ESAs in patients with MDS. Importantly, no significant adverse events, including thromboembolic complications, have been noted in multiple studies. Mounting evidence indicates that a lower baseline serum EPO level is associated with a higher response rate; therefore, all patients should have a baseline EPO level measured before initiation of an ESA (see text and Table 59-9). Patients with serum EPO levels greater than 500 mU/mL have such a low response rate to ESAs that alternative strategies should be considered first. ESA treatment requires a long duration to see maximum benefit, and because of increased iron utilization, concurrent iron administration may be required to achieve a maximum response. In addition, use of ESAs did not appear to be associated with higher rates of progression to AML. More importantly, it appears that amelioration of chronic anemia in patients with MDS not only may improve their quality of life but also may change the natural history of the disease (see text).

Selected phase II trials[280-283] using recombinant human erythropoietin (rh-EPO) in patients with MDS report response rates in the 25% range. However, definitions of response are highly variable, most trials were conducted before common use of the International Working Group (IWG) criteria,[270] and the clinical benefit of such responses can be quite heterogeneous. For example, an increase in hemoglobin of 1 to 2 mg/dL could have biologic but very little clinical significance unless the patient becomes transfusion independent. Older patients with MDS who have clinical or subclinical impairment of renal function leading to a relatively lower level of serum EPO for a given degree of anemia might be good candidates for a therapeutic trial with this agent.

Although most patients with MDS have abundant supplies of iron because of prior transfusion or high gut absorption, a small subset of patients may be iron deficient. Therefore, it is important to review iron stores at the time of diagnostic BM examination and, if absent, to provide supplemental iron because EPO responsiveness requires an iron-replete state. Because response to EPO in MDS may be delayed, the drug should be continued for at least 8 weeks before therapeutic failure is declared. Although the drug is well tolerated, keeping severely anemic or heavily transfusion-dependent patients on EPO for long periods makes little sense and is costly. Several studies have suggested that adding the myeloid growth factor G-CSF at low doses to EPO can enhance the erythropoietic response.[284-286] Using the combination of EPO plus G-CSF initially or adding G-CSF after the effect of EPO is stable or waning may lead to response rates in the 40% range, which appear to be higher than with EPO alone. Nonetheless, the lack of a true prospective randomized trial of EPO with or without G-CSF has limited the wide acceptance of this strategy.

Table 59-9 Algorithm for Predicting Response to Erythropoietin and Granulocyte Colony-Stimulating Factor in Lower Risk Myelodysplastic Syndrome*

Parameter	Value of Parameter	Score
Serum erythropoietin	<100 mU/mL	+2
	100-500 mU/mL	+1
	>500 mU/mL	−3
RBC transfusions	<2 units/mo	+2
	≥2 units/mo	−2
Score	**Response**	
Score >+1	Good response = 74%	
Score −1 to +1	Intermediate response = 23%	
Score <−1	Poor response = 7%	

Adapted from Hellstrom-Lindberg E, Ahlgren T, Bequin Y, et al: Treatment of anemia in myelodysplastic syndromes with granulocyte colony-stimulating factor plus erythropoietin: Results from a randomized phase II study and long-term follow-up of 71 patients. *Blood* 92:68, 1998.
*Response definitions:
Complete = Stable hemoglobin >11.5 g/dL.
Partial = Increase in hemoglobin with >1.5 g/dL or cessation of red blood cell (RBC) transfusion.

For patients with low-risk MDS, rh-EPO remains the most commonly used initial therapeutic approach for treatment of patients with MDS who are transfusion dependent to RBCs. In patients with MDS, only 15% to 30% will experience an erythroid response to rh-EPO. There are good predictive features for an observed response. Predictors for response to EPO are unclear. A decision model was developed by Hellstrom-Lindberg[286] (Table 59-9). Patients with MDS who had an EPO level less than 500 mU/mL, low RBC transfusion requirements, and BM blasts less than 10% had a favorable chance of responding to rh-EPO. Interestingly, the presence of a deletion 5q with or without additional cytogenetic abnormalities did not affect the response rate but did shorten the response duration.[287] In addition, patients who do not have RARS[288,289] have a higher and more durable response. The Nordic MDS group suggested that patients with multilineage dysplasia have a poorer response to rh-EPO compared with patients with unilineage erythroid dysplasia (75% vs. 9%; P = .003).[290] However, this has not been uniformly observed. The addition of a granulocyte colony-stimulating factor (G-CSF or GM-CSF) to single-agent rh-EPO can increase response rates by 20% to 40%.[60,284,286,291-293] Darbepoetin, a hypersialated erythropoietin-stimulating agent (ESA), has a longer half-life than rh-EPO and has yielded similar response rates when administered at intervals of every 1 to 3 weeks.[293] Response durations to either ESA agent range from 1 to 2 years, with longer responses associated with lower blast percentage as well as a low to intermediate IPSS score.

Few data regarding the safety of ESA use in patients with MDS are available. Use of ESAs for treatment of chemotherapy-induced anemia and chronic renal insufficiency has been associated with increased morbidity and mortality in many but not all randomized trials. In patients with chronic renal insufficiency, a hemoglobin level of 10 to 12 g/dL was often targeted in a randomized trial in which patients assigned to a targeted hemoglobin of 13.5 g/dL experienced significantly more adverse events, including death, chronic heart failure, myocardial infarction, and stroke compared with patients assigned to a lower targeted hemoglobin.[294] These findings have been supported by a more recent meta-analysis of nine randomized studies comparing different hemoglobin targets, suggesting that patients with higher hemoglobin concentration display significantly higher rates of all-cause mortality, including complications from arteriovenous access thrombosis as well as from poorly controlled hypertension.[295]

As for patients with MDS, amelioration of anemia is thought to improve quality of life, specifically in responding patients. In addition, decreasing the need for transfusion support may have a dramatic impact on RBC supplies as well as decrease the risk of secondary hemochromatosis. More important is the observation that transfusion dependency has a negative impact on the natural history of patients with MDS.[191] A retrospective case-matched study of patients with MDS treated with supportive care compared with rh-EPO demonstrated that patients with a low RBC transfusion requirement (<2 units of RBCs per month) had a significant survival advantage with the addition of rh-EPO (hazard ratio, 0.56; $P = .015$).[296] Of major importance is the fact that administration of rh-EPO had no significant adverse effect on leukemic evolution. In fact, there was a suggestion that responding patients had a lower risk of AML progression compared with patients who did not respond. These findings were corroborated by another study of 419 patients with MDS who were treated with an ESA.[287] Patients were compared with case-matched control participants with MDS managed by supportive care without use of rh-EPO. Similarly, a survival advantage was observed in the responding patients. Finally, a phase III prospective cooperative group trial also demonstrated a survival advantage in patients with MDS treated with rh-EPO with or without use of the myeloid growth factor G-CSF.[291] This was compared with best supportive care. The median survival time in patients responding to treatment was 53 months compared with 23 months in nonresponding patients. These data importantly suggest that decreasing RBC transfusion requirements and resolution of severe anemia in patients with MDS may improve not only overall survival in low-risk patients but also decrease the risk for AML progression.

Management of Neutropenia

Because of the quantitative and qualitative defects in neutrophils, infections are common in patients with MDS and are a source of considerable morbidity and occasional mortality.[21] No data support the routine use of prophylactic granulocyte transfusions or antibiotics in MDS. When fears about the ability of the myeloid growth factors G-CSF and GM-CSF to stimulate clinically meaningful blast cell proliferation were diminished, studies conducted in the late 1980s and early 1990s documented the efficacy of these agents in routinely increasing the number of normal WBCs.[297-300] However, the few randomized studies performed did not demonstrate a decrease in the infection rate or an improvement in life expectancy despite achieving blood count improvement.[301] Such a discrepancy may reflect the maturation of dysfunctional or hypofunctional neutrophils that, although increased in number, cannot provide significant host defense benefit. Moreover, the mortality rate from infectious causes in MDS before conversion to AML probably is low. Although selected patients with recurrent suppurative infections might be candidates for myeloid growth factors, these agents should not be routinely used in MDS.

Management of Thrombocytopenia

Patients with MDS, particularly with more advanced subtypes, may have severe chronic thrombocytopenia with associated mucosal bleeding. Thrombocytopenia, defined as platelet count less than $100 \times 10^9/L$, occurs in 40% to 65% of patients with MDS. This problem may become life threatening if a significant bleed occurs in the brain or gastrointestinal tract. The reported incidence of hemorrhagic complications ranged from 3% to 53%, and the frequency of death as a result of hemorrhage was 14% to 24% of such cases.[165] Nonetheless, platelet transfusions should be used judiciously in MDS because overuse may result in alloimmunization and failure to respond to subsequent transfusions even if leuko-poor products are used.[276] As in the case of RBC transfusions, platelets should be irradiated before use.[275] Therefore, rather than giving transfusions below a certain threshold, as is routinely done after chemotherapeutic administration,[302] it makes more sense to use clinical bleeding as the trigger. Use of the antifibrinolytic agent ε-aminocaproic acid can be considered for the thrombocytopenic patient who is bleeding but is not responding to transfusional therapy.[303]

Levels of thrombopoietin, the homeostatic hormone responsible for maintaining normal platelet counts, are elevated in thrombocytopenic patients with MDS,[304] making response to pharmacologic doses of the recombinant protein unlikely. However, neither native thrombopoietin nor its pegylated derivative megakaryocyte growth and development factor (MGDF) has been tested in patients with MDS. MGDF underwent limited testing as a supportive agent in patients with AML after induction chemotherapy.[305,306] Not only was MGDF not associated with a decrease in bleeding or need for platelet transfusions in AML, but its development was discontinued because of development of antiplatelet antibodies and thrombocytopenia in normal volunteers. IL-11, a cytokine with pleiotropic effects, is approved for use as a supportive agent for prophylaxis against severe thrombocytopenia after myelointense chemotherapy for solid tumor patients.[307] Limited testing of this agent alone in MDS patients[308] or after myelosuppressive therapy with the antibody–toxin conjugate gemtuzumab ozogamicin demonstrated side effects (e.g., fluid retention) and limited efficacy.

AMG531 (romiplostim) is a thrombopoiesis-stimulating Fc-peptide fusion protein (peptibody) that is being investigated in patients with idiopathic thrombocytopenic purpura.[309] AMG531 binds and activates the thrombopoietin receptor myeloproliferative leukemia virus oncogene (c-Mpl). Phase II studies have demonstrated durable platelet responses in patients with idiopathic thrombocytopenic purpura and the ability of these patients to subsequently discontinue corticosteroid therapy. AMG531 also is being developed in patients with chemotherapy-induced thrombocytopenia as well as in patients with MDS. A phase I/II study of AMG531 in patients with low-risk MDS who also were thrombocytopenic has been completed. Durable platelet responses were seen in 54% of patients with a decreased need for transfusions and a lower number of severe hemorrhagic events in responding patients.[310] Future studies will further explore the response rates of AMG531 in patients with MDS-related thrombocytopenia as well as patients currently undergoing hypomethylating therapy who develop thrombocytopenia as a complication of therapy.

Eltrombopag (SB-497115) is an oral nonpeptide thrombopoietin receptor agonist that binds to the transmembrane domain of the Mpl receptor, thereby inducing proliferation and differentiation of megakaryocytes.[311] Eltrombopag increased platelet production in patients with thrombocytopenia secondary to hepatitis C virus infection and in adult patients with relapsed or refractory chronic idiopathic thrombocytopenic purpura. Its use in patients with MDS has not been reported.

Management of Iron Overload

In patients with MDS, particularly those with indolent histologic subtypes or good prognoses based on the IPSS schema, administration of well over 100 units of packed RBCs is not unusual. The high iron load associated with such transfusion requirements may be harmful to the liver, pancreas, heart, and central nervous system.[312] Chelation therapy with either deferoxamine by continuous subcutaneous administration or the oral agent deferasirox (ICL670) can be administered to such patients, usually after they have received at least 25 to 30 units of blood.[313,314] Side effects of deferoxamine include cataract formation and chronic skin irritation from the subcutaneous injections. Chronic administration of deferoxamine is cumbersome,[315] is not well tolerated, and chelates only approximately 25 mg/day of iron, which compares unfavorably with the 250 mg given in a single unit of blood. Although beneficial in children with thalassemia who receive frequent transfusions,[316] the role of desferoxamine is limited in patients with MDS.

Deferasirox initially is administered at a dose of 20 mg/kg once per day and escalated to 30 or 40 mg/kg/day depending on the response. Typical side effects include development of gastrointestinal toxicity principally manifested as abdominal pain, nausea, vomiting, and diarrhea. Unfortunately, these side effects make dose escalation difficult in some patients. Deferasirox typically is used in patients with low-risk MDS and has been associated with decreases in serum ferritin levels. Prospective randomized trials using this agent in patients with low-risk MDS are warranted before its use can be universally recommended.

The development of secondary iron overload is difficult to define.[209] Secondary iron overload often is defined in patients with serum ferritin level greater than 1000 mg/mL. Patients who have an elevated serum ferritin level greater than 1000 mg/mL have decreased overall survival.[191,317] Whether poorer clinical outcomes are related to increased number of transfusions, a consequence of iron overload, or are caused by progressive BM dysfunction and failure that results in lower hemoglobin levels is unclear. Although these data are provocative, further evaluation and independent validation are needed, especially because few patients live long enough to develop definitive complications of iron overload.

Agents With Limited Efficacy

In the past, virtually every patient with MDS was given pyridoxine (vitamin B6), probably because of its safety and the fact that rare children with congenital dysmyelopoiesis may respond.[318] However, reports of adults who actually benefit are rare. Androgen therapy, formerly a mainstay in the treatment of patients with BM failure caused by aplastic anemia or myelodysplasia, is rarely used today because of the lack of supporting data and its untoward side effects.[319] Danazol is a weak androgen and possibly has immunosuppressive properties. Although danazol therapy occasionally improves anemia and thrombocytopenia,[320] the rarity of such responses and the associated side effects have led to abandonment of its typical use.

Immunosuppressive Therapy

For many years, patients with MDS were treated with steroids. Response rates in the 20% range were noted, but the increased use of prednisone in patients with myelodysplasia clearly led to more complications than benefit.[321] Nonetheless, several pieces of evidence have caused resurgence in enthusiasm for immunosuppressive therapy for MDS. First, autoimmune phenomena, often polyarthritis,[174] can be associated with MDS. Treatment with steroids in such cases may ameliorate the autoimmune manifestations and improve blood counts.[181] Patients with MDS have aberrant autoimmune hematopoietic inhibitory activity. In a subset of patients, clonal amplification of T lymphocytes has been demonstrated. The implication of this T-cell repertoire is that it suppresses hematopoiesis through a $CD8^+$ cytotoxic T-lymphocyte–mediated pathway.

Hypoplastic MDS bears morphologic similarity to aplastic anemia. Some patients with aplastic anemia who initially respond to immunosuppressive therapy may progress to MDS,[322] which suggests that these two entities share a common pathophysiology, that of T-cell–mediated suppression of a primitive BM stem cell. Indeed, antithymocyte globulin (ATG), the mainstay of nontransplant therapy for aplastic anemia,[323] has a role in certain patients with MDS. A report from the National Cancer Institute suggests that patients with MDS who are young and have low platelet counts may benefit from a trial of ATG, with response rates as high as 50%.[324] The pretreatment variables associated with a higher response to immunosuppressive therapy include younger age (<60 years) and short duration of RBC transfusion dependency (<6 months). Interestingly, findings have shown the presence of a PNH clone or the presence of human leukocyte antigen (HLA) DR15 phenotype is another predictor for response to ATG in MDS.[325] It was originally thought that only those patients with hypoplastic MDS would respond, but now it seems clear that BM hypoplasia is not a requirement for response, that rabbit or horse ATG can be used, and that patients with excess blasts rarely respond.[326]

Although no randomized trials have confirmed a survival benefit in patients treated with immunosuppressive therapy, a comparison of more than 800 patients in the IMRAW managed for prognostic variables showed that immunosuppressive therapy was associated with an improved overall survival time (8.1 vs. 5.2 years; $P < .001$).[116] Immunosuppressive therapy also was associated with a decreased risk of leukemic transformation ($P = .001$). The benefit in overall survival caused by decreased leukemic transformation was seen in patients with low and intermediate-1 IPSS who were younger than 60 years of age. In addition, investigators from Prague have shown that approximately 40% of patients with indolent subtype MDS may respond to cyclosporine A.[327] Although a large randomized trial testing the usefulness of ATG in MDS is ongoing, young patients with MDS who do not have excess BM blasts should be considered for a trial of immunosuppression.

Manipulating the Microenvironment

The pathophysiology of MDS is complex. However, it is increasingly recognized that the BM microenvironment, including endothelial cells, fibroblasts, and other stromal cells, as well as immune effector cells and certain elaborated cytokines may have critical roles in maintenance of the neoplastic MDS clone. For example, microvessel density is increased in the BM of patients with AML and MDS,[199] and proangiogenic substances such as vascular endothelial growth factor may be required for growth of neoplastic stem cells.[200] Second, at least in the indolent MDS subtypes, peripheral cytopenias in the presence of hypercellular BM have suggested overabundant apoptosis, perhaps because of stromal cell secretion of proapoptotic substances such as TNF.[62] Attempts to modify TNF availability with use of phosphodiesterase inhibitors such as pentoxyphylline in combination with the steroids and ciprofloxacin (pentoxyphylline, ciprofloxacin, and dexamethasone [PCD] therapy)[328] or with the direct anti-TNF molecule etanercept (Enbrel),[329] as used in rheumatoid arthritis,[61] have led to transient and low-level responses in MDS. Amifostine, a thiol-containing compound approved for use as a chemoprotectant and radioprotectant,[330] alone[331] or in combination with PCD,[332] has limited biologic activity, with clinical responses that are too rare to justify the routine use of any of these strategies without an ability to predict which patients will respond.

The proangiogeneic and proapoptotic cytokine milieu of MDS may be counteracted by agents such as thalidomide, which has been effective in treatment of patients with refractory myeloma.[294] Studies suggest that thalidomide can lead to a significant improvement in the need for transfusions in approximately 20% of patients with low-grade MDS subtypes.[333,334] However, many in the typical older patient population are poorly tolerant of the constipation, somnolence, and neuropathy typically associated with thalidomide use. The potent and better tolerated thalidomide analogue lenalidomide (Revimid), which has activity in patients with advanced multiple myeloma,[219,220,335] may well be a real advance in "microenvironment-directed" therapy in MDS. Arsenic trioxide, which is approved for use in relapsed acute promyelocytic leukemia[336] and may modify the cytokine and angiogenic milieu in MDS, has shown only limited clinical activity.[337,338]

Lenalidomide

Lenalidomide is a thalidomide derivative (CC5013) that has more potent inhibition of TNF-α and other inflammatory cytokines compared with the parent compound. In addition, lenalidomide has greater capacity to promote T-cell activation and suppress angiogenesis. Importantly, lenalidomide lacks much of the neurotoxicity of thalidomide but still has myelosuppressive properties. A phase I study (MDS-001) was performed in patients with MDS who had symptomatic anemia and did not respond to treatment with ESAs.[220] Patients received doses of lenalidomide at 25 mg/day, 10 mg/day, or 10 mg/day for 21 days of a 28-day cycle, and 56% of patients experienced a durable erythroid response per the IWG. Twenty of 32 patients who previously were RBC transfusion dependent became independent of transfusion. Importantly, erythroid response rates were dependent on the presence of deletion of chromosome 5q, with 10 of 12 patients responding compared with 57% of patients with a normal karyotype and 12% of patients with abnormal karyotype. For patients with a 5q abnormality, responses were durable, with a median duration of major erythroid response exceeding 2 years. The dose-limiting toxicities were different than expected from thalidomide and predominantly included myelosuppression, specifically within the first month of therapy. In fact, grade 3 or greater neutropenia occurred in 58% of patients and grade 3 or greater thrombocytopenia in 50% of patients.

Two multicenter confirmatory trials were performed in patients with MDS and a low or intermediate-1 risk IPSS score. Patients were transfusion dependent and had not responded to an ESA. The MDS-002 study was performed in patients without a 5q abnormality, and lenalidomide was started at a dose of 10 mg/day or 10 mg/day on days 1 to 21 of a 28-day cycle.[339] The overall transfusion response rate was 43,% with 26% of patients achieving transfusion independence. The median duration of response was 41 weeks. Although only a minority of patients had clonal cytogenetic abnormalities 19% experienced a cytogenetic response. The principal toxicity remained myelosuppression, with 30% and 25% of patients developing grade 3 or greater neutropenia and thrombocytopenia, respectively.

A second phase II trial (MDS-003) was performed in transfusion-dependent patients with MDS who contained a deletion of chromosome 5q using a similar dosing regimen as in the MDS-002 study.[219] A total of 148 patients were enrolled, and erythroid responses were seen in 76% of patients, with an amazing 67% of patients achieving a transfusion-independent state. In addition, complete cytogenetic responses were seen in 73% of patients and partial cytogenetic responses in 45% of patients. Development of a cytogenetic response was associated with achievement of transfusion independence. Surprisingly, the presence of additional chromosomal abnormalities was not associated with a decreased erythroid or cytogenetic response rate. Myelosuppression was extremely common in patients with chromosome 5q abnormality, and grade 3 or greater neutropenia or thrombocytopenia was reported in 55% and 44% of patients, respectively. A retrospective analysis suggested that patients who experience a 50% reduction in platelet count or grade 3 myelosuppression during the first 8 weeks of therapy had a higher incidence of response compared to patients who did not have myelosuppression. Exogenous use of myeloid growth factors was effective in treatment-related neutropenia.

The long-term outcome of lenalidomide use for treatment of patients with MDS who harbinger a deletion of chromosome 5q has been analyzed.[340,341] The data confirm a long median duration of response of 2.2 years, with some patients responding for more than 5 years. Higher response rates were seen by multivariate analysis for patients with the "actual" 5q syndrome, RBC transfusions of fewer than 4 units per 8 weeks, low-risk IPSS score, and age younger than 70 years. Using Kaplan-Meier estimates, responders had a 10-year overall survival estimate of 78% compared with 4% for patients who failed to respond. Unfortunately, these data are retrospective but nevertheless suggest that lenalidomide may change the natural history of patients with MDS who concurrently have a chromosome 5 abnormality.

Differentiation Therapy

Can the putative block in normal hematopoietic differentiation in patients with MDS be reversed by pharmacologic agents? Many compounds, including the vitamin A analogue retinoic acid,[342] the protein kinase C inhibitors phorbol ester[343] and brysotatin,[344] polar-planar solvents such as phenylbutyrate[345] and hexamethylene bisacetamide,[346] and nucleoside analogues such as low-dose cytarabine (ara-C),[78] can promote maturation of leukemic cells in tissue culture. One of the first clinical efforts with one of these agents suggested that low-dose cytarabine produced responses in patients with MDS without causing aplasia.[347] Initial enthusiasm for low-dose cytarabine in MDS faded because of studies suggesting a low response rate in meta-analysis and that some of the responses really occurred because of hypoplasia, much as would be expected from standard chemotherapy.[348,349] A randomized trial conducted by the Medical Research Council demonstrated a superior overall survival compared with best supportive care in elderly patients with AML or high-risk MDS.[350]

A randomized trial of retinoic acid versus observation, one of the few such efforts in MDS, failed to show any discernible benefit for patients enrolled in the experimental arm.[351] Phase II clinical trials with phenylbutyrate[352] and hexamethylene bisacetamide[353] each produced a few impressive responses, but the low frequency of efficacy and the requirement for cumbersome prolonged infusions prevented major interest. Although not a differentiating agent, melphalan, an orally available alkylating agent, has produced complete remissions in limited testing in patients with MDS.[354]

The mechanism of retinoic acid's differentiation activity in acute promyelocytic leukemia is inhibition of histone deacetylase-mediated transcriptional repression engendered by the PML-RARA fusion protein consequent to the characteristic t(15;17) chromosomal abnormality.[355] Several compounds that, unlike retinoic acid, have direct histone deacetylase inhibitory capability are in development as potential therapeutic agents for MDS. Depsipeptide has undergone phase I testing in patients with AML.[356] The drug appears to be well tolerated and inhibits histone acetylation in vivo. Other histone deacetylase inhibitors, including phenylbutyrates, suberoylanilide hydroxamic acid (Vorinostat), valproic acid, MS-275, LAQ823, LBH589 (panobinostat), and MGCD0103, are undergoing phase I testing in patients with MDS and related disorders.[357,358] Not surprisingly, attempts have already been made to combine DNA hypomethylating agents with histone deacetylase inhibitors in the form of azacytidine plus phenylbutyrate[359] or decitabine plus valproic acid.[360] Such efforts require careful consideration of optimal scheduling and ample ancillary studies to determine if the presumed targets really are affected.

Hypomethylating Agents

Progress in the field of epigenetics,[361] including thoughts concerning promoting expression of transcriptionally silent genes that might be required for the differentiated phenotype, has rekindled interest in the use of small molecules to promote hematopoietic maturation in patients with MDS. Structural barriers to transcription result from either overmethylation of DNA[73] or underacetylation of the histone DNA coat.[362] Cells from patients with MDS typically display overmethylation of genes such as p15INK4B,[363] which argues in favor of the relevance of this mechanism.

The greatest recent therapeutic advance in the management of patients with MDS was highlighted by a phase III trial, albeit with early crossovers permitted, of the putative DNA hypomethylating agent azacytidine given subcutaneously daily for 7 days every 28 days versus observation in patients with MDS conducted by the Cancer and Leukemia Group B.[364] Randomization to azacytidine was associated with a response rate of 60% (mostly hematologic improvement), delay in transformation to AML, and improved quality of life measured by several validated instruments.[365] The benefit of azacytidine was apparent in patients with both high- and low-risk MDS; a trend toward improvement in overall survival in the azacytidine arm did not reach statistical significance. The side effect profile of the drug included mild nausea and vomiting and transient myelosuppression in some patients. Azacytidine, which now can be given intravenously, is metabolized in vivo to another hypomethylating agent decitabine.

Decitabine (5-aza-2′-deoxycytidine) has significant activity in patients with MDS based on a phase II trial performed in Europe[366] and a low-dose trial performed at the MD Anderson Cancer Center.[164] A phase III trial was performed in 170 patients with IPSS intermediate-1 or higher risk. Patients were randomized to receive either decitabine at a dose of 15 mg/m^2 given intravenously every 8 hours for 3 days or supportive care.[367] The overall response rate in patients treated with decitabine was 17%, including 9% complete remissions. Unfortunately, no effect was observed in terms of overall survival, but in a subgroup analysis, patients with intermediate-2 and high IPSS scores who received decitabine had a longer median time of progression to AML or death compared with patients who received supportive care alone (12.0 months vs. 6.8 months; $P = .03$). One of the difficult issues with this study is that 43 patients received only two cycles of therapy, yet more than two cycles or 3.3 months of therapy on average was required to demonstrate a clinical response. Both decitabine and azacytidine have been approved by the U.S. Food and Drug Administration and are being tested against supportive care in multi-institutional prospective phase III trials.

A randomized bayesian phase II trial of patients with MDS was conducted at the MD Anderson Cancer Center. Decitabine was administered in one of three schedules: 10 mg/m^2 intravenously for 10 days, 20 mg/m^2 intravenously for 5 days, or 20 mg/m^2 intravenously for 5 days.[368] All three groups of patients received the same total dose of decitabine, 100 mg/m^2. The 20 mg/m^2 intravenously for 5 days arm was preferentially enrolled, suggesting that this may be the superior regimen. The overall response rate was 48%, with 34% of patients entering a complete remission. Although these results seem to be superior to those achieved using the 3-day regimen, they must be confirmed in a multicenter trial.

Signal Transduction Inhibitors

In MDS subtypes associated with excess blasts, highly analogous to the situation in AML, the underlying biologic problem may include overproliferation or lack of apoptosis within the stem cell compartment. Insofar as there are patients with MDS whose disease behaves more like AML, one can think of the same therapies that are in use or in development for the more aggressive neoplasm. Moreover, older adults with AML in particular are generally presumed to have blasts that emanate from a primitive stem cell, similar to MDS.[97] As such, remission induction chemotherapy is a variable therapeutic alternative for some patients with MDS.

The constitutively activated tyrosine kinases BCR-ABL in CML[124] and FLT-3 in 30% of cases of AML[102] represent important drug targets. The development of imatinib for treatment of patients with CML[369] has revolutionized the treatment of patients with gastrointestinal stromal cell tumors based on the ability of imatinib to inhibit c-KIT,[370] idiopathic hypereosinophilic syndrome based on its ability to inhibit PDGFR-α.[371] Similarly, the rare patients with the MDS subtype CMML whose cells harbor a cytogenetic abnormality, such as t(5;12), a translocation that activates PDGFR-β,[226,227] also exhibit striking responses to imatinib.[183,227] Therefore, it is important to carefully scrutinize the cytogenetic results in patients with MDS, especially those with CMML, for any translocation involving the long arm of chromosome 5, for the potential of initiating imatinib therapy.

Several drugs that can inhibit the activated version of the FLT-3 tyrosine kinase are in development, particularly for use in AML.[372,373] However, rarely, and again probably more likely in CMML, patients with MDS may have one of two activating FLT-3 mutations, either a so-called *internal tandem duplication,* a copy of between 9 and 300 base pairs in the juxtamembrane region, or a mutation in the activation loop, usually a point mutation yielding a D835Y amino acid substitution.[102] As such, a few patients with primary MDS have been treated with PKC412, one of the FLT-3 inhibitors currently in clinical trials, and responses have been noted.[373] Identifying other tyrosine kinases that may be activated in MDS, and the drugs that inhibit them could yield future therapeutic advances.

Another cell-signaling therapeutic target in MDS is mutationally activated RAS, a 20-kd guanine nucleotide binding protein.[374] Because a mutation in a RAS family member occurs in approximately 20% to 40% of patients with MDS and most commonly in CMML, drugs that inhibit this enzyme are in development. The so-called *farnesyltransferase inhibitors* were developed because they inhibited an enzyme that catalyzed a key step in the posttranslational modification of RAS, preventing attachment of the farnesyl group required for movement to the cell membrane and enzyme activation.[375] Phase I and II trials with farnesyltransferase inhibitors have been completed in patients with MDS and AML.[376] One of the most important conclusions from these trials, in addition to the presence of only modest clinical activity, was that responses occurred exclusively in patients whose cells did not have RAS mutations, suggesting the likelihood of alternative targets, perhaps farnesylation of some of the many other proteins undergoing this posttranslational modification step, including lamin A or Ras homolog gene family B (RHOB).[377]

Induction Chemotherapy

Use of cytotoxic chemotherapy for treatment of patients with MDS was generally considered to be an unhelpful strategy based on the typically older age of these patients and their poor tolerance of chemotherapy. Moreover, the proximal nature of the stem cell defect in MDS suggests that patients would be resistant to chemotherapy, based on overexpression of proteins mediating pleiotropic drug resistance,[378] and would have limited normal stem reserve, making them prone to severe myelosuppression. However, Estey et al[379] demonstrated that patients with MDS can respond as well, or as poorly, to chemotherapy as those with AML if the key prognostic factors of age and cytogenetic status are controlled for. Complete response rates range from 40% to 50%. Unfortunately, these responses tend to be short lived, even with consolidation chemotherapy, which does support the intrinsic nature of chemotherapy resistance in MDS. Curative intensive consolidation regimens with high-dose ara-C is appropriate only for younger adults with de novo AML in first remission[380] and therefore has no role in the treatment of older patients with MDS, given that older adults with AML do not benefit from such an intensive approach.

The notion that selected patients with MDS might benefit from chemotherapy[379] was altered by the change in the definition of AML and MDS in the new WHO classification system. Patients with 20% or greater blasts, as opposed to 30% in the older FAB system, now are considered to have AML.[20] Second, patients with balanced chromosomal translocations associated with a favorable prognosis, such as inv(16), t(8;21), and t(15;17), are considered to have AML at any level of BM or peripheral blood leukemic cell involvement.[20] Applying the new definitions of MDS, relatively few patients are obvious chemotherapy candidates.

Induction chemotherapy may be useful in relatively younger patients with high-risk MDS, defined as greater than 10% blasts in the BM or with serious cytopenias. Such patients can be considered for nonmyeloablative or reduced-intensity conditioning allogeneic transplant.[381] Chemotherapy may be useful as a cytoreductive step before a reduced-intensity transplant, but prospective data are lacking. Although regimens containing topotecan alone or with ara-C[382] have activity in patients with MDS, this novel agent is no better than standard anthracycline and ara-C combination regimens[383] and should not be used routinely. Similarly, gemtuzumab ozogamicin, an antibody–toxin conjugate that is associated with a 30% remission rate in relapsed AML,[382] is expensive, myelosuppressive, and not particularly efficacious in patients with MDS.[384]

Stem Cell Transplantation

Recognition that the stem cell defect in MDS is proximal and pervasive suggested that allogeneic transplant would be required to eliminate the malignant clone, thereby making cure a possibility. Numerous studies suggested that up to 60% of selected patients with low-risk MDS and 20% to 40% of patients with high-risk disease can experience long-term disease-free survival after allogeneic transplantation from a matched donor.[270,271,385-387] Albeit in a relatively young and well population, no other modality, including chemotherapy[379] or autologous BMT,[388] is associated with a similarly high success rate. Despite concern that high-dose chemotherapy with autologous BM or peripheral blood stem cell rescue would be an unworthy approach given that neoplastic stem cells would be difficult to eliminate in MDS and would grow poorly as an autograft, European investigators reported appreciable disease-free survival when this modality is used as consolidation therapy in MDS patients achieving remission with chemotherapy.[388] However, because these patients likely would be more typical of an AML population, autologous BMT still is considered an experimental procedure for MDS.

An important treatment decision concerns the appropriate timing of transplantation, especially in low-risk disease. Upfront SCT potentially can take advantage of relatively healthier BM, with waiting until disease progression delaying transplant-related morbidity. Cutler et al[389] analyzed a national database registry of transplant patients with MDS and their outcomes to perform a decision analysis addressing this question. They found that for low and intermediate-1 IPSS groups, delayed SCT was associated with better overall survival (Table 59-10). In contrast, for intermediate-2 and high IPSS groups, SCT at diagnosis maximized overall survival. The analysis focused only on full ablative conditioning regimens. Nevertheless, all patients with MDS who are reasonable transplant candidates based on age and comorbidity should undergo a formal consultation with transplantation specialist.

One clear advantage of allogeneic transplant in MDS, beyond the obvious benefit provided by the proffering of normal stem cells, is the powerful graft-versus-leukemia effect.[383] Evidence that neoplastic MDS cells are targets for killing by the graft emanates from data demonstrating a lower relapse after allogeneic, compared with syngeneic, transplants, the higher relapse rate after T-cell–depleted grafts, and mildGVHD.[390] The apparent safety of unrelated matched transplants has improved recently because of the advent and routine use of molecular HLA typing.[391] Although allogeneic transplant seems an attractive option, a major problem remains the mortality associated with regimen-related toxicity and GVHD, especially given the older age of the typical MDS patient. Use of nonmyeloablative or reduced-intensity conditioning, seeking to maximize the graft-versus-leukemia to toxicity ratio, is being used with increasing frequency.[381,392,393] Although it appears that reduced-intensity conditioning allogeneic transplantation can be accomplished with an acceptable short-term

Table 59-10 Decision Analysis of Allogeneic Bone Marrow Transplantation for Myelodysplastic Syndrome

	Overall Survival (Years)		
International Prognostic Scoring System Category	***Immediate Transplant***	***Transplant in 2 Years***	***Transplant at Progression***
Low	6.51	6.86	7.21
Intermediate-1	4.61	4.47	5.16
Intermediate-2	4.93	3.21	2.84
High	3.20	2.75	2.75

From Cutler CS, Lee SJ, Greenberg P, et al: A decision analysis of allogeneic bone marrow transplantation for the myelodysplastic syndromes: Delayed transplantation for low-risk myelodysplasia is associated with improved outcome. *Blood* 104:579, 2004.

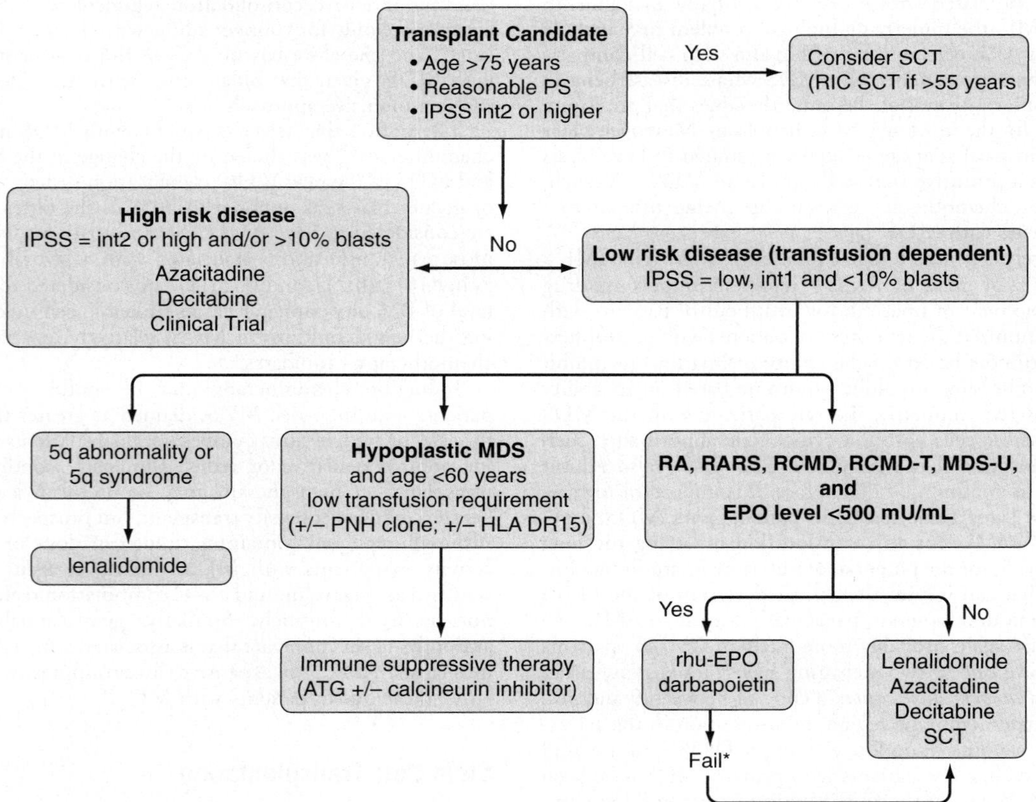

Figure 59-7 ALGORITHM FOR MANAGEMENT OF A PATIENT WITH MYELODYSPLASTIC SYNDROME. *PNH,* Paroxysmal nocturnal hemoglobinuria; *PS,* performance status; *RIC,* reduced-intensity conditioning regimen; *SCT,* stem cell transplant. *, consider adding G-CSF.

mortality rate in patients with MDS up to age 70 to 75 years, long-term data on efficacy are lacking.[394-396] Cord blood transplants could extend the availability of allogeneic transplantation to greater numbers of patients with MDS. This technique may prove feasible in older adults, especially if it is associated with an acceptable risk of GVHD.[397,398]

FUTURE DIRECTIONS

Despite recent advances in therapy for MDS, the need for improvement is great. Almost all patients with MDS should be referred for a clinical trial. Treatment recommendations involving available approaches and agents can be derived for a given patient but generally not without prolonged discussion between the physician and the patient and his or her family (Fig. 59-7). All patients younger than 70 years with high-risk disease according to the IPSS (intermediate-2 or high) and who have a related or unrelated matched donor should be considered for allogeneic BMT if feasible. Patients older than 55 years should consider reduced-intensity conditioning SCT, but the long-term efficacy data are lacking. Use of hypomethylating agents as a form of "cytoreduction" before SCT is being investigated. Patients with high-risk MDS who are not considered SCT candidates should initiate treatment with a hypomethylating agent such as azacytidine or decitabine. Patients with low-risk disease have many options. Patients with a chromosome 5q deletion or the 5q– syndrome who are RBC transfusion dependent should receive lenalidomide. Patients with low-risk disease who are RBC transfusion dependent and do not have a 5q abnormality have many options. If their serum EPO levels are less than 500 mU/mL, they should be started on an ESA, either rh-EPO or darbepoetin. If this treatment fails, then addition of a myeloid growth factor, such as G-CSF, should be considered. ATG should be considered for treatment of hypoplastic MDS in patients younger than 60 years who have modest transfusion requirements, a recent diagnosis, and a low blast count. Nonresponding patients with low-risk disease should consider lenalidomide if the goal is only an erythroid response, or a hypomethylating agent should be considered in patients with pancytopenia. Clinical trial participation should be considered for all patients because this is the only way that we can try to make strides in improving the survival of patients with MDS.

SUGGESTED READINGS

Barabe F, Kennedy JA, Hope KJ, et al: Modeling the initiation and progression of human acute leukemia in mice. *Science* 316:600, 2007.

Burnett AK, Milligan D, Prentice AG, et al: A comparison of low-dose cytarabine and hydroxyurea with or without all-trans retinoic acid for acute myeloid leukemia and high-risk myelodysplastic syndrome in patients not considered fit for intensive treatment. *Cancer* 109:1114, 2007.

Bussel JB, Cheng G, Saleh MN, et al: Eltrombopag for the treatment of chronic idiopathic thrombocytopenic purpura. *N Engl J Med* 357:2237, 2007.

DeAngelo DJ: Role of imatinib-sensitive tyrosine kinase in the pathogenesis of chronic myeloproliferative disorders. *Semin Hematol* 44:S17, 2007.

Girtovitis FI, Ntaios G, Papadopoulos A, et al: Defective platelet aggregation in myelodysplastic syndromes. *Acta Haematol* 118:117, 2007.

Haase D, Germing U, Schonz J, et al: New insights into the prognostic impact of the karyotype in MDS and correlation with subtypes: Evidence from a core dataset of 2124 patients. *Blood* 110:4385, 2007.

Hershman D, Neugut AI, Jacobson JS, et al: Acute myeloid leukemia or myelodysplastic syndrome following use of granulocyte colony-stimulating factors during breast cancer adjuvant chemotherapy. *J Natl Cancer Inst* 99:196, 2007.

Huff JD, Keung YK, Thakuri M, et al: Copper deficiency causes reversible myelodysplasia. *Am J Hematol* 82:625, 2007.

Jones PA, Baylin SB: The epigenomics of cancer. *Cell* 128:683, 2007.

Joslin JM, Fernald AA, Tennant TR, et al: Haploinsufficiency of EGR1, a candidate gene in the del(5q), leads to the development of myeloid disorders. *Blood* 110:719, 2007.

Kantarjian H, Fenaux P, Sekeres MA, et al: Phase 1/2 study of AMG 531 in thrombocytopenic patients with low-risk myelodysplastic syndrome: Update including extended treatment. *Blood* 110:250a, 2007.

Kantarjian H, Giles F, List A, et al: The incidence and impact of thrombocytopenia in myelodysplastic syndromes. *Cancer* 109:1705, 2007.

Kantarjian H, Oki Y, Garcia-Manero G, et al: Results of a randomized study of 3 schedules of low-dose decitabine in higher-risk myelodysplastic syndrome and chronic myelomonocytic leukemia. *Blood* 109:52, 2007.

Kouzarides T: Chromatin modifications and their function. *Cell* 128:693, 2007.

Kouzarides T: SnapShot: Histone-modifying enzymes. *Cell* 131:822, 2007.

Lancet JE, List AF, Moscinski LC: Treatment of deletion 5q acute myeloid leukemia with lenalidomide. *Leukemia* 21:586, 2007.

Liu TX, Becker MW, Jelinek J, et al: Chromosome 5q deletion and epigenetic suppression of the gene encoding alpha-catenin (CTNNA1) in myeloid cell transformation. *Nat Med* 13:78, 2007.

Ma X, Does M, Raza A, Mayne ST: Myelodysplastic syndromes: Incidence and survival in the United States. *Cancer* 109:1536, 2007.

Melchert M, Kale K, List A: The role of lenalidomide in the treatment of patients with chromosome 5q deletion and other myelodysplastic syndromes. *Curr Opin Hematol* 14:123, 2007.

Opel M, Lando D, Bonilla C, et al: Genome-wide studies of histone demethylation catalysed by the fission yeast homologues of mammalian LSD1. *PLoS ONE* 2:e386, 2007.

Phrommintikul A, Haas SJ, Elsik M, et al: Mortality and target haemoglobin concentrations in anaemic patients with chronic kidney disease treated with erythropoietin: A meta-analysis. *Lancet* 369:381, 2007.

For complete list of references log on to www.expertconsult.com.

CHAPTER 60

ALLOGENEIC HEMATOPOIETIC STEM CELL TRANSPLANTATION FOR ACUTE MYELOID LEUKEMIA AND MYELODYSPLASTIC SYNDROME IN ADULTS

John Koreth, Joseph H. Antin, and Corey Cutler

Recent advances in molecular diagnostics are shedding considerable light on genetic underpinnings of myelodysplastic syndrome (MDS) and acute myeloid leukemia (AML). However, with notable exceptions both diseases remain therapeutic challenges. Fortunately, our ability to provide more precise prognostic information has corresponded with advances in transplantation technology. We are increasingly able to apply transplantation to older people and those with comorbidities and to use alternative donors in patients without matched family members. By applying molecular prognostic criteria we can provide transplantation to patients with poor outcomes on conventional therapy and we can avoid transplant-related toxicity in those patients who are likely to do well with supportive care or nontransplant therapy.

Allogeneic hematopoietic stem cell transplantation (HSCT) is curative in MDS and AML due to a combination of the cytotoxicity of the preparative conditioning regimen and the donor-mediated immunologic graft-versus-leukemia (GVL) effect. Regimen intensity ranges from high-dose myeloablative conditioning (MAC) that induces profound and prolonged pancytopenia to reduced-intensity conditioning (RIC) that induces milder cytopenias and is more appropriate for older patients and those with comorbidities in whom MAC may be intolerable. The risk-benefit ratio of conditioning regimen intensity varies with factors like patient age, comorbidities, and relapse risk. In general, more intense regimens cause more treatment-related morbidity and mortality but are associated with a lower relapse rate. Conversely, there are more relapses in RIC HSCT, but the procedure is more tolerable.[1]

ACUTE MYELOID LEUKEMIA

AML displays considerable clinical heterogeneity with markedly variable survival, traditionally defined by prognostic factors of patient age, blast morphology, white blood cell count, prior MDS or cytotoxic therapy, remission status, and karyotype, but increasingly further refined by novel molecular markers. In addition to a burgeoning number of new prognostic indicators, there are now novel AML therapeutic agents in clinical trials, which also constitute an alternative to usual cytotoxic chemotherapy.

However, AML also constitutes the leading indication for HSCT worldwide, accounting for 7026 of 21,516 allogeneic HSCT (33%) in 2006.[2,3] Moreover, the use of molecular tissue typing in conjunction with better control of treatment-related complications has increased the use of alternative donors. Data from the Center for International Blood and Marrow Transplant Research (CIBMTR) indicate that 1286 of 1778 allogeneic HSCT (72%) undertaken for AML in 1998 involved related donors, compared to 1223 of 2557 allogeneic HSCT (48%) in 2008. In contrast, the number of unrelated donor HSCT for adult AML increased from 297 in 1998 to 1017 in 2008, while the number of umbilical cord blood (UCB) transplantations increased from 11 to 130 over the same time period.[4] It is likely that the ability to use donors that are not histocompatible will further increase the pool of patients in whom HSCT is an effective therapy.[5]

Matched Related Donor HSCT for Adult Acute Myeloid Leukemia in First Complete Remission

Cytogenetics is the most powerful prognostic indicator in AML, both at the time of diagnosis and at relapse, and can also direct choice of curative postremission therapy, especially for adult patients less than 60 years of age.[6,7] Adult AML patients can be stratified into good-risk, intermediate-risk, and poor-risk groups on the basis of numeric and/or structural chromosomal abnormalities and the presence of specific mutations (see Chapter 58).

Numerous groups prospectively evaluated the relative benefits of allogeneic HSCT versus nonallogeneic therapies (consolidation chemotherapy or autologous HSCT) in adult AML patients 18 to 60 years of age in first complete remission (CR1). Treatment allocation was by biologic assignment as a surrogate for true randomization, with allogeneic HSCT for patients with available human leukocyte antigen (HLA)–matched sibling donors (donor group) and nonallogeneic consolidation for those lacking matched sibling donors (no-donor group). Some of these studies further stratified postremission outcomes by cytogenetic risk. Individual studies, when analyzed on an intent-to-treat (ITT) donor versus no-donor basis, typically demonstrated that allogeneic HSCT was effective at improving disease-free survival, but overall survival benefit was hard to document because of graft-versus-host disease (GVHD) and other treatment-related mortality.

In an effort to overcome some of the limitations of individual trials, a recent meta-analysis of over 6000 patients in 24 biologic treatment assignment trials was undertaken. This study confirmed that overall survival was in fact better in allogeneic matched related donor transplantation in AML-CR1, with a hazard ratio (HR) of death at 0.90 (95% confidence interval [CI], 0.82 to 0.97).[8] Importantly, when stratified by cytogenetic risk, there was an overall survival benefit of allogeneic transplantation (Table 60-1) for both intermediate-risk (HR, 0.83; 95% CI, 0.74 to 0.93) and poor-risk (HR, 0.73; 95% CI, 0.59 to 0.90) cytogenetic groups, but not for good-risk AML-CR1 (HR, 1.07; 95% CI, 0.83 to 1.38) (Fig. 60-1). These findings were particularly relevant for patients with normal cytogenetic AML, who constitute the largest subgroup and for whom no consensus regarding optimal postremission treatment was previously available. These studies did not have the benefit of prognostic assignment based on FLT3, NPM1, or other molecular markers.

Prognostic Factors for Acute Myeloid Leukemia in First Complete Remission

Good-Risk Acute Myeloid Leukemia

In general, the 15% to 20% of AML patients with core binding factor (CBF) leukemia—t(8;21) (q22;q22) and inv(16)(p13.q22)—are considered to have good-risk disease, with a long-term disease-free survival of approximately 50% to 60% after consolidation chemotherapy. However, retrospective studies have identified activating

Table 60-1 Allogeneic Transplantation Guidelines for Adult Acute Myeloid Leukemia

AML Category	Prognostic Impact	Allogeneic Transplantation	Notes
AML-CR1: younger adults			
Good-risk disease			
APL	Favorable	No	APL is treatable by chemotherapy
CBF-AML without mKIT	Favorable	No	t(8;21) AML with high WBC count at diagnosis may have worse prognosis
CBF-AML with mKIT	Unfavorable	Possible: MRD, MUD Uncertain: MMUD, UCB, haplo	
Intermediate-risk disease			
CN-AML with CEBPA	Favorable	No	Benefit likely restricted to DM-CEBPA
CN-AML with NPM1 but not FLT-3-ITD	Favorable	No	
Other intermediate-risk disease	Unfavorable	Yes: MRD Likely acceptable*: MUD Possible†: MMUD, UCB, haplo	
Poor-risk disease			
Monosomal karyotype absent	Unfavorable	Yes: MRD, MUD Likely acceptable†: MMUD, UCB, haplo	
Monosomal karyotype present	Very unfavorable	Yes: MRD, MUD. Acceptable†: MMUD, UCB, haplo	
AML-CR1: older adults	Unfavorable	Yes: MRD, MUD Likely acceptable†: MMUD, UCB	
AML-CR1: t-AML, AML/MDS	Unfavorable	Yes: MRD, MUD Acceptable†: MMUD, UCB, haplo	
AML-CR2	Very unfavorable	Yes: MRD, MUD Acceptable†: MMUD, UCB, haplo	
AML not in remission	Very unfavorable	Yes: MRD, MUD Uncertain: MMUD, UCB, haplo	For selected patients: good performance status, little comorbidity, lower leukemic burden; CIBMTR risk score may be useful

AML, Acute myeloid leukemia; *APL,* acute promyelocytic leukemia; *CBF,* core binding factor; *CIBMTR,* Center for International Blood and Marrow Transplant Research; *CN,* cytogenetically normal; *CR1,* first complete remission; *CR2,* second complete remission; *haplo,* haploidentical; *MDS,* myelodysplastic syndrome; *MMUD,* mismatched unrelated donor; *MRD,* matched related donor; *MUD,* matched unrelated donor; *t-AML,* therapy-related AML; *UCB,* umbilical cord blood; *WBC,* white blood cell.
*If no sibling donor available.
†If no timely matched donor available.

mutations in C-KIT (mKIT)—a member of the type III receptor tyrosine kinase family—at exon 17 (mKIT 17) or exon 8 (mKIT 8) in approximately 30% of CBF AMLs that are associated with increased relapse incidence and likely poorer survival, though results from individual studies vary.[9,10] For instance, in an analysis of 61 patients with inv(16), mKIT was associated with 5-year relapse rate of 56% compared with 29% ($P = 0.05$) without mKIT mutations. This effect is especially prominent with mKIT17, where 80% relapsed compared with 29% without the mutation ($P = 0.002$). Similarly, in 49 patients with t(8;21), the 5-year relapse rate was 70% in the presence of mKIT mutations compared with 36% with wild-type mKIT ($P = 0.017$). These relapse rates are similar to that of poor-risk AML, suggesting a potential benefit of allogeneic HSCT in this subset.

Intermediate-Risk Acute Myeloid Leukemia

The intermediate-risk cytogenetic group is heterogeneous and includes cytogenetically normal disease as well as those with karyotypic abnormalities not meeting criteria for good- or poor-risk AML. It constitutes the largest risk category, accounting for approximately 40% to 50% of adult AML patients less than 60 years of age. Long-term disease-free survival of approximately 40% to 45% is anticipated after consolidation chemotherapy. However, identification of mutations with prognostic importance such as mutant FLT3 internal tandem duplication (ITD), NPM1, and CEBPA (CCAAT/enhancer binding protein-α) can help further individualize the decision regarding allogeneic transplantation.

Patients with FLT3-ITD have inferior survivals compared to those without FLT3-ITD.[11,12] The negative impact of FLT3-ITD appeared abrogated by allogeneic transplantation in CR1 when assessed on an ITT donor versus no-donor basis, although in this analysis the patients were not preferentially assigned transplantation on this basis. The finding of allogeneic transplantation benefit therefore remains to be prospectively validated. The nucleophosmin 1 (NPM1) and CEBPA mutations are associated with good outcomes independent of HSCT, and most investigators do not offer HSCT in first remission.[11,13-15] The favorable impact of NPM1 mutations appears to persist even in older patients.[16] There is a growing list of additional prognostic markers undergoing evaluation in AML. These include

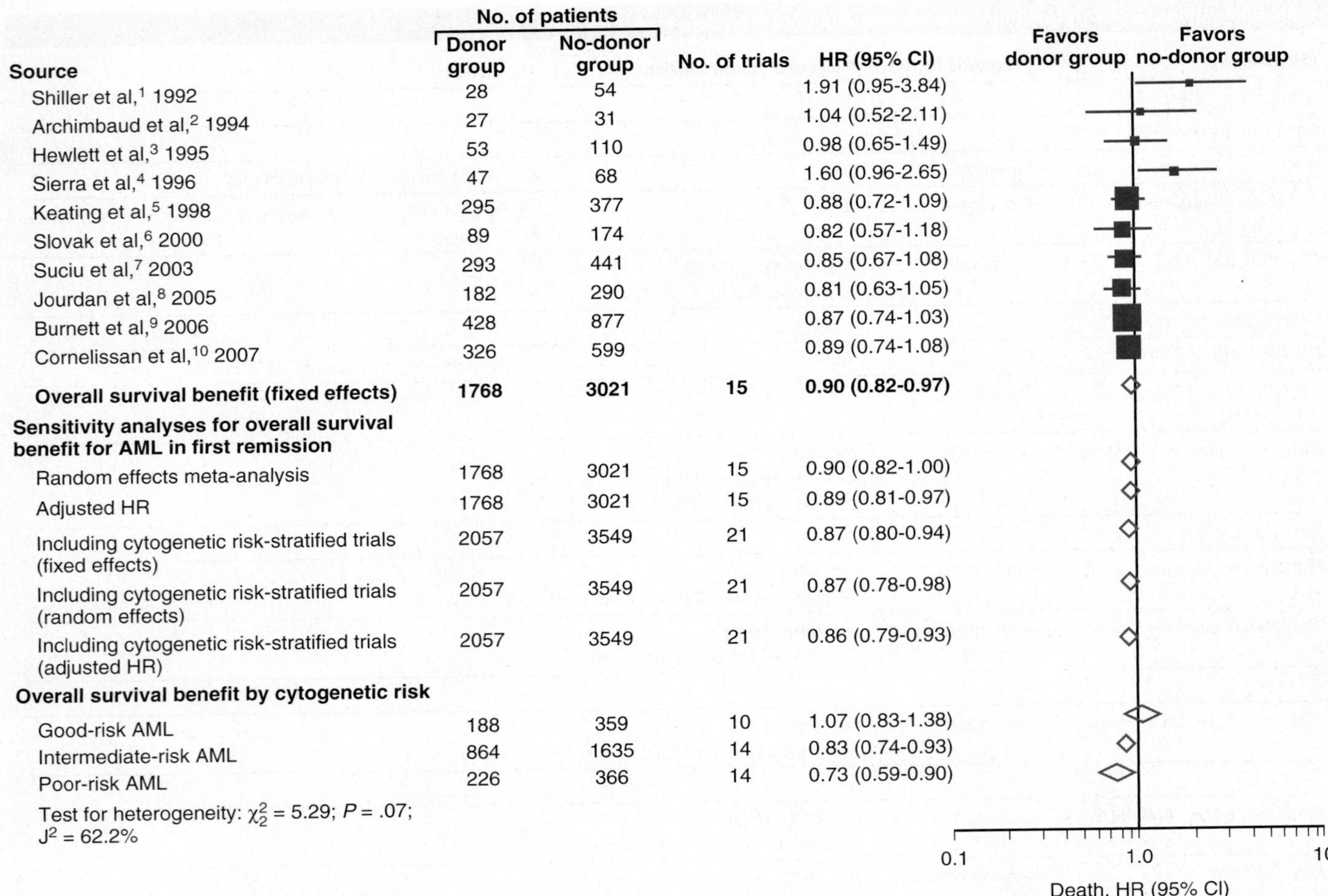

Figure 60-1 META-ANALYSIS OF OVERALL SURVIVAL BENEFIT IN FIRST COMPLETE REMISSION OF ACUTE MYELOID LEUKEMIA FOR YOUNGER ADULTS. *AML,* Acute myeloid leukemia; *CI,* confidence interval; *HR,* hazard ratio. *(Redrawn from Koreth J, Schlenk R, Kopecky KJ, et al: Allogeneic stem cell transplantation for acute myeloid leukemia in first complete remission: Systematic review and meta-analysis of prospective clinical trials,* JAMA 301:2349, 2009. *Sources cited within Fig. 60-1 can be found following the reference list online at expertconsult.com.)*

mutation analysis of RAS, WT1, RUNX1, MLL, TET2, IDH1/2, p53; expression levels of individual genes like EVI1, ERG, MN1, and BAALC; and gene expression and micro–ribonucleic acid (miRNA) profiling.[6,11,17] Many mutations appear to be linked with poorer outcomes (e.g., EVI1, MLL, IDH1/2, p53), although some (e.g., TET2, RAS) appear to not have a significant impact on survival. Low expression levels of BAALC, ERG, and possibly WT1 appear associated with better AML outcomes. It is important to integrate the gene mutation and expression markers to better assess their overall impact in AML clinical management. If validated, such analyses highlight the ability of carefully selected novel markers to further delineate prognosis within intermediate-risk AML. This suggests that this category of risk will gradually disappear as prognostic precision improves. Although the better-prognosis subgroup within intermediate-risk AML may not benefit from early allogeneic transplantation, it appears to be the preferred postremission therapy for intermediate-risk AML patients at higher risk for relapse, including those lacking favorable gene mutations like NPM1 without FLT3-ITD, or mutant CEBPA.

Poor-Risk Acute Myeloid Leukemia

In poor-risk AML relapse rates are high and survival rates are anticipated to be 15% or lower with conventional consolidation therapy. Allogeneic HSCT with a matched sibling or unrelated donor results in long-term survival of 30% to 40% and is considered the treatment of choice for younger adults aged less than 60 years of age with poor-risk AML. There is, however, a subgroup of poor-risk AML that may have particularly adverse prognosis, for whom additional novel therapeutic strategies may be necessary.

The monosomal karyotype (MK) is defined by the presence of a single autosomal monosomy, in association with at least one additional monosomy or non–good risk structural chromosomal abnormality (i.e., excluding CBF mutation AML).[18] In the original report, MK-positive AML patients had a long-term survival of only 3% to 4%, and these generally dismal chemotherapeutic outcomes have been confirmed by other investigators.[19] Allogeneic transplantation appears to only partly ameliorate the impact of MK-positive karyotype, which remained an adverse prognostic factor after HSCT, and was associated with a high relapse risk of 62% at 4 years.[20] Improving outcomes in MK-positive AML must be a high priority for improving AML survival.

Transplantation Regimen Intensity

Myeloablative HSCT remains the standard of care for younger adults with AML. However, treatment-related mortality after MAC remains appreciable, especially in older patients or those with comorbidities. Lower-intensity regimens offering less treatment-related toxicity are gaining in popularity. One report retrospectively compared RIC transplantation with chemotherapy in high-risk AML on a donor versus no-donor basis. They identified a leukemia-free survival benefit in the donor group (54% versus 30%, $P = 0.01$).[21] Several groups have compared MAC versus RIC transplantation, documenting similar overall and leukemia-free survival, with some reporting lower treatment-related mortality offset by increased relapse risk, especially for patients not in complete remission at time of HSCT. A recent CIBMTR study compared 3731 MAC, 1041 RIC, and 407 nonmyeloablative transplantations, reporting adjusted 5-year overall survivals of 34%, 33%, and 26%, respectively.[22] The authors concluded that, although nonmyeloablative transplantation had increased relapse and impaired survival, RIC and MAC regimens had similar overall and leukemia-free survival. A prospective randomized trial of MAC versus RIC transplantation in AML-CR1 patients greater than 40 years of age is underway in the Blood and Marrow Transplantation Clinical Trials Network to validate these findings. If confirmed, RIC transplantation might represent a new standard of care, especially in older or sicker AML-CR patients for whom the toxicity of MAC transplantation might be prejudicial. Conversely, patients with good performance status but high AML relapse risk might be preferentially selected for MAC.

Alternative Donor Transplantation

HSCT from an HLA-matched sibling donor has been the standard of care for prospective biologic treatment assignment studies evaluating postremission therapies. Patients lacking sibling donors could be considered for alternative donors: unrelated adult donors, UCB, or haploidentical donor transplantation.

Unrelated Adult Donors

Given the very poor outcomes after nonallogeneic therapy in poor-risk AML, and the documented benefit of HLA-matched sibling donor HSCT, clinical practice has been to undertake HLA-matched unrelated donor transplantation for younger adults with poor-risk AML in CR1 who lack sibling donors. A retrospective analysis of HLA-matched sibling compared with unrelated donor HSCT in poor-risk AML-CR1 documented comparable outcomes with HLA-matched siblings and HLA well-matched unrelated donors with 3-year overall survival of 45% compared with 53% ($P = 0.63$).[23] Outcomes were not as good for partially HLA-mismatched unrelated donors (one-locus HLA mismatch), with 3-year overall survival of 31% ($P = 0.026$). Smaller prospective studies have also shown equivalent results, confirming the suitability of well-matched unrelated donor HSCT in poor-risk AML.[24,25]

There is limited data comparing HLA-matched sibling with unrelated donors in intermediate-risk AML, although at least one study documented similar outcomes with either donor type.[26] Current practice is to offer HLA-matched unrelated donor HSCT to intermediate-risk AML patients in first remission, especially if there are adverse molecular lesions.

Umbilical Cord Blood

Another important issue is the use of UCB transplantation for AML in CR1. These data are harder to interpret because most studies have reported outcomes for "acute leukemia," rather than restricted to AML-CR1. A European registry study documented similar outcomes of UCB versus unrelated donor bone marrow (BM) transplantation in adults with acute leukemia, whereas a contemporaneous CIBMTR study showed better outcomes with HLA-matched unrelated donor BM transplantation, but similar outcomes of UCB and HLA-mismatched unrelated donor BM transplantation.[27,28] A recent large analysis of adult acute leukemia (including 880 AML patients) compared the outcomes of single-unit 4-6/6 HLA-matched (HLA-A, -B, -DRB1) UCB with 8/8 or 7/8 HLA-matched (HLA-A, -B, -C, DRB1) BM or peripheral blood stem cell (PBSC) transplantation and documented similar leukemia-free survival regardless of stem cell source or degree of HLA match. There was higher treatment-related mortality after UCB transplantation.[29] Transplantation in CR1 resulted in similar 2-year leukemia-free survivals of 44%, 50%, 52%, 39%, and 41% with UCB, 8/8 PBSC, 8/8 BM, 7/8 PBSC, and 7/8 BM transplantation, respectively. In contrast, a Japanese study evaluated outcomes of 484 AML patients receiving 4-6/6 UCB compared with 8/8 unrelated donor BM transplantation and documented a similar relapse risk with UCB transplantation, but higher treatment-related mortality and worse overall and leukemia-free survival.[30]

Double-unit UCB (DUCB) transplantation is commonly used for larger patients. Indeed, since 2005 the number of adults receiving DUCB has exceeded those receiving single-unit UCB products. Limited data suggest similar outcomes of myeloablative DUCB, HLA-matched unrelated, and sibling donor HSCT in hematologic malignancies.[31] However, only a subset of patients had AML. The role of DUCB in AML remains to be better demarcated. In general however, current clinical practice envisages use of UCB transplantation in younger adults with high-risk AML in CR1 who lack suitable HLA-matched donors.

Haploidentical Donors

There are no studies of haploidentical transplantation that allow a precise recommendation for patients with AML. Several strategies have been used in high-risk patients, and the outcomes are encouraging.[5,32-34] Haploidentical transplantation is particularly interesting given the potential enhancement of GVL activity by natural killer cells and allogeneic T cells responding to the HLA disparity.

Relapsed, Refractory, and Induction-Failure Acute Myeloid Leukemia

Outcomes are impaired for AML patients not in remission at the time of allogeneic HSCT, although the literature in this regard is limited, heterogeneous, and likely subject to patient selection and publication bias. A large analysis of MAC HSCT for acute leukemia in relapse or in primary induction failure (including 1673 AML patients) documented a 3-year overall survival of 19% in AML.[35] On multivariable analysis, risk factors at time of HSCT of poor-risk cytogenetic AML, CR1 duration of less than 6 months, circulating AML blasts, performance score of less than 90%, and lack of an HLA-matched sibling donor predicted for 3-year survivals ranging between 42% (zero risk factors) and 6% (three or more risk factors). The major cause of death remains AML relapse, and innovative strategies to reduce leukemic burden before transplantation and enhance GVL effect after transplantation are required to improve survival of this extremely high-risk patient population.[36] The ability to rapidly proceed to allogeneic transplantation may also be important given the dismal outcome of chemotherapy alone, suggesting a role for expeditious UCB and haploidentical BM transplantation in this setting, especially for patients achieving a remission.

Therapy-Related Acute Myeloid Leukemia

Therapy-related AML (t-AML) currently accounts for approximately 10% to 20% of newly diagnosed AML, and its incidence is likely to rise in the future, given increasing cancer survivorship. Postremission therapy using conventional chemotherapy is usually not curative with the rare exception of CBF-AML, specifically inv(16) and t(15;17). Allogeneic HSCT is less effective in t-AML and in AML arising from antecedent MDS. The poorer survival appears multifactorial, due to poor-risk cytogenetics, lower likelihood of entering remission, older patient age, and impaired organ function from prior cancer therapy; although some reports documented similar posttransplantation survival compared to de-novo AML when adjusted for risk factors like disease status and cytogenetics.[4,37] An observational analysis of 545 patients with t-AML identified four risk factors influencing HSCT outcomes: age greater than 35 years, poor-risk cytogenetics, AML not in remission, and lack of well-matched donors. A prognostic score could stratify outcomes from 5-year overall survivals of 50% (zero risk factors) to 4% (four risk factors).[38]

Acute Myeloid Leukemia in Older Adults

AML incidence rises with age, with a median age at diagnosis of 67 years (Surveillance, Epidemiology and End Results data: http://seer.cancer.gov/). For AML patients older than 60 years, consolidation chemotherapy is unlikely to be curative (Fig. 60-2). Even after adjusting for increased incidence of poor prognosis features like adverse cytogenetics, secondary AML, and poorer performance status, older age remains an independent predictor of poor survival with conventional chemotherapy. Although allogeneic HSCT is a curative therapy in the older age-group, there is considerable reluctance to refer these patients for transplantation, in contrast to younger adults with AML, in part due to outdated assumptions regarding the tolerability of allogeneic transplantation, but also due to lack of comparative data regarding outcomes.

Several reports have documented the feasibility of RIC transplantation with acceptable toxicity and reasonable survival in patients 60 years of age and above, including those with AML. Indeed, chronologic age alone does not appear to be a prognostic factor in RIC allogeneic transplantation for AML.[39,40] In a case-control study comparing RIC transplantation with chemotherapy for AML patients 60 to 70 years of age, allogeneic HSCT was associated with lower relapse risk (32% versus 81%, $P < 0.001$), greater treatment-related mortality (36% versus 4%; $P < 0.001$), and longer 3-year leukemia-free survival (32% versus 15%, $P = 0.001$), with a borderline 3-year overall survival benefit (37% versus 25%, $P = 0.08$).[41]

Overall, for physically fit older AML patients, especially those between 60 and 70 years of age, a donor search should be undertaken promptly at diagnosis, and they should be offered the option of potentially curative allogeneic transplantation upon entering complete remission.

Relapse After Transplantation

AML relapse after allogeneic transplantation is common, has a very poor prognosis, and remains a leading cause of death in this disease. The treatment recommendations for patients with disease relapse after HSCT include withdrawal of immune suppression, donor lymphocyte infusion (DLI), chemotherapy, second allogeneic transplantation, or supportive care.[42] Taper of immune suppression and DLI are used especially in patients without GVHD. DLI has limited efficacy, in the range of 15% to 30%, for patients with relapsed AML, and many responses are incomplete or temporary. Outcomes are better in patients who relapsed beyond 6 months after HSCT, those with lower leukemic burden (less than 35% bone marrow blasts), patients with good-risk cytogenetics, and those who achieved remission before DLI.[43] A second allogeneic HSCT has demonstrable but limited efficacy, and duration of remission of more than a year after initial HSCT is the major predictor of survival.[44]

TRANSPLANTATION FOR MYELODYSPLASTIC SYNDROME

The MDSs comprise a heterogeneous group of clonal hematologic stem cell disorders characterized by varying degree of cytopenias and risk for transformation into acute leukemia[45] (see Chapter 59). The incidence and prevalence of MDS has increased significantly over the last 20 years as a result of increasing longevity of the population and increasing physician awareness.[46-48] New therapeutic options such as hypomethylating agents, immunomodulatory drugs, and differentiation induction agents may improve hematologic parameters and reduce transfusion requirements,[49] and even prolong survival,[50] but allogeneic HSCT is the only known curative therapeutic option.

MDS is currently the third most common indication for allogeneic HSCT as reported to the CIBMTR.[3] MDS is a disease predominantly of older individuals, and with the increased use and acceptance of RIC into the eighth decade of life, it is anticipated that transplantation volume for MDS will continue to increase in the coming years.

Clinical Results in Myeloablative Transplantation

There are few reports of transplantation uniquely for patients with the myelodysplastic disorders, because most reports include both patients with AML and those with MDS. Those few analyses that do exist unfortunately often present biased results, because there is inherent patient selection in the reported studies. The bias in these analyses, although recognized by physicians and patients alike, is often overlooked, because patients who choose early HSCT often identify with those included in the analysis to justify their decision.

One of the largest reports of MAC HSCT for MDS is from the Seattle group. Using a targeted busulfan strategy in patients undergoing related or unrelated donor HSCT, results were presented stratified by pretransplant International Prognostic Scoring System (IPSS; see Chapter 59) risk score.[51,52] Patients were prospectively enrolled in the targeted busulfan treatment program; however, the decision to undergo transplantation was based upon physician and patient preference. Results in this study were correlated with IPSS stage, suggesting that outcomes were improved with HSCT at an earlier disease stage. This would be expected, because patients with earlier-stage disease have had less treatment for their disease (thus less comorbidity) and may also have more indolent disease biology. Among the patients in the lowest IPSS score group there were no relapses, whereas

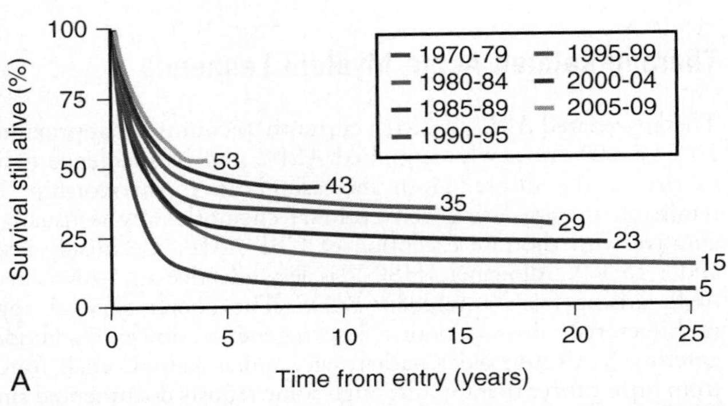

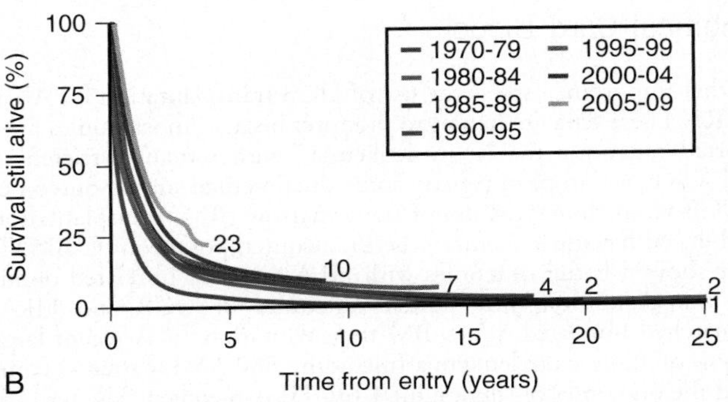

Figure 60-2 CHANGE IN ACUTE MYELOID LEUKEMIA OVERALL SURVIVAL WITH TIME. **A,** Age 15 to 59 years. **B,** Age 60 years or greater. *(Data from Burnett A, Wetzler M, Lowenberg B: Therapeutic advances in acute myeloid leukemia,* J Clin Oncol *29:487, 2011.)*

the relapse rate was 42% for patients in the highest IPSS category. As a consequence, 3-year survival was 80% in the lowest IPSS risk group but was under 30% for patients in the high IPSS category.

Similarly, de Witte et al[53] examined outcomes of HSCT for patients with earlier-stage MDS (refractory anemia or refractory anemia and ringed sideroblasts). This analysis studied 374 patients who underwent HSCT from either matched, sibling, or unrelated donors. Both standard MAC and RIC regimens were used. IPSS score could be calculated in fewer than half of the patients, and HSCTs were performed over a decade-long period, such that inherent differences in transplantation technology resulted in improved overall survival over time. Although factors such as conditioning intensity, stem cell source, and donor status did not affect outcome, recipient age and duration of identified MDS diagnosis were important predictors of overall survival. Earlier transplantation was associated with an absolute increase in overall survival of 10% at 4 years (57% versus 47%, $P = 0.02$) and was associated with improved relapse-free survival in multivariable analysis. Despite the finding of improved outcome with earlier HSCT, this should not be interpreted as a recommendation for early HSCT in individuals with low-risk MDS, because the authors did not compare outcomes to a cohort of patients treated with supportive care alone.

Clinical Results in Reduced-Intensity Conditioning Transplantation

It appears that late relapses after MAC HSCT are not common,[54] but high-intensity regimens are associated with higher treatment-related mortality.[55] Thus many groups have moved toward a reduction in conditioning intensity.

Previously HSCT was available to only a minority of patients with MDS, because 75% of patients are older than 60 years at diagnosis and are not candidates for MAC regimens. Because older patients have a poorer prognosis than their younger counterparts, there is a great impetus to develop strategies for older individuals. Within the RIC literature, there is great variability in the reported conditioning intensity; however, the commonality of these regimens is that they can be safely offered to patients previously deemed to be too old or to have too much comorbidity for high-dose therapy.

The City of Hope group has reported on their outcomes using a RIC regimen of fludarabine and melphalan in 43 patients with MDS or AML. Overall survival was 53% at 2 years, with a 16% relapse rate.[56] Treating over 90 patients with AML (n = 74) or AML (n = 22) using a targeted busulfan and fludarabine regimen, de Lima et al[57] reported 1-year treatment-related mortality of only 3%, without a compromise in antitumor activity. Using this more commonly applied RIC regimen of fludarabine with busulfan, albeit with different intensities (and including some patients with AML), other groups have demonstrated similar outcomes, with treatment-related mortality of 13% to 27%, relapse rates of 23% to 32%, disease-free survival of 38% to 68%, and overall survival of 39% to 79%.[58-61]

With the increased acceptance of RIC preparative regimens, and the resultant reduction in treatment-related mortality, determination of the optimal timing of HSCT will be critical.

Comparative Results: Myeloablative and Reduced-Intensity Regimens in Myelodysplastic Syndrome

Several analyses have compared RIC with conventional MAC transplantation, and the majority of them suggest similar outcomes. The premise behind all of these comparisons is that RIC should be associated with a reduction in early treatment-related mortality, whereas MAC approaches should be associated with a reduction in disease relapse. The net effect of these two opposing risks is no difference in outcomes. For example, at the Dana-Farber Cancer Institute, the outcomes of 136 patients with advanced MDS or acute myelogenous leukemia who underwent transplantation were compared when stratified by conditioning regimen intensity.[1] Overall survival at 2 years was the same following RIC as for MAC transplantation (28% versus 34%, $P = 0.89$); however, the causes of treatment failure were significantly different, with more relapse in the RIC group (61% versus 38%, $P = 0.02$), but higher treatment-related mortality in the MAC group (32% versus 15% at 100 days) as anticipated. Overall treatment-related mortality, however, was no different ($P = 0.28$). In this report, patients were treated according to patient and physician preference, whereas in a similar single-center analysis reported by Martino et al,[62] patients were prospectively assigned to RIC or $CD34^+$ selected MAC transplantation based on patient age. In this analysis, nonrelapse mortality and overall survival were no different between groups.

Similar to single-center studies, large retrospective database studies comparing RIC and high-intensity HSCT have been performed. A CIBMTR review of the outcomes of 550 patients 50 years of age or older who underwent matched sibling donor HSCT showed no difference in MAC and RIC outcomes.[3] In an even larger CIBMTR analysis that included both patients with MDS and those with AML, patients were stratified into MAC, RIC, and truly nonmyeloablative subgroups. Although results for MDS alone are not available, overall outcomes indicated less-favorable long-term results for nonmyeloablative regimens when compared with higher-intensity regimens.[22] In an analysis by the European Group for Blood and Marrow Transplantation (EBMT) of over 800 patients with MDS, the 3-year relapse rate was significantly higher after RIC (HR, 1.64; $P = .001$), but with less treatment-related mortality (HR, 0.61; $P = .015$), leading to similar 3-year overall survival (45% versus 41%, $P = 0.8$). When limited to individuals above 50 years of age, no difference in outcome stratified by conditioning intensity (32% versus 30%, $P = 0.73$) was noted.[63] Competing risk cumulative incidences for relapse and nonrelapse mortality are shown in Fig. 60-3.

It is important to consider that none of these retrospective studies adjusted for comorbidity, and it is almost certain that if reanalyzed, the RIC cohorts would contain a higher proportion of patients with more comorbid conditions. Because only a minority of studies have suggested that regimen intensity is important for long-term outcomes, some patients have now opted for earlier RIC transplantation, even without comorbidity, because treatment-related morbidity and mortality after this procedure is lower than after traditional MAC transplantation. In order to compare outcomes prospectively among patients eligible to undergo both MAC and RIC transplantation, the Bone Marrow Transplant Clinical Trials Network has embarked upon a randomized, controlled trial in patients 18 to 65 years of age.

Using Prognostic Models to Define the Role and Timing of Transplantation

Clinical, Laboratory, and Cytogenetic Prognostic Factors

Comparative registry analyses have documented the benefit of HSCT over conventional supportive and disease-modifying agents in MDS[64]; however, this should not be interpreted as an indication for HSCT in all patients. Despite the curative potential of HSCT, transplantation carries substantial risk for early morbidity and mortality, and careful consideration must be made regarding the appropriateness of each potential recipient and the timing at which transplantation is offered. Despite this, all patients who are potential candidates for HSCT should be referred to a transplantation center early in their disease course so that a discussion regarding the appropriateness of transplantation can occur and a donor search can be initiated, where appropriate. The correct timing of HSCT is therefore of paramount importance, and decisions regarding the timing of HSCT should be made on more than patient preference alone.

The most widely used clinical prognostic system is the IPSS. Not only does this combined clinical and laboratory scoring system predict nontransplantation outcomes, but the IPSS at the time of HSCT can predict MAC outcomes as well.[65,66] A Markov decision

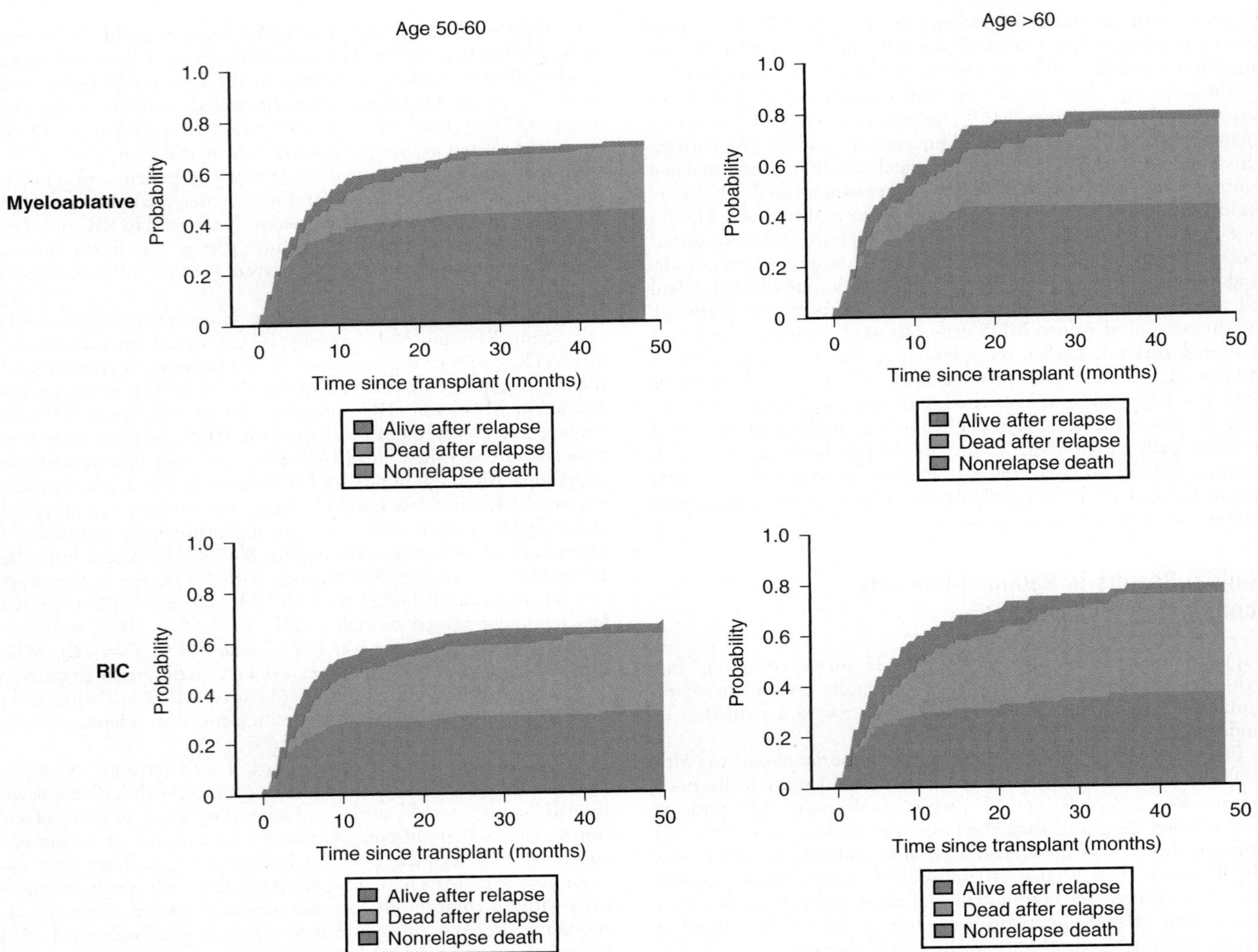

Figure 60-3 COMPETING RISK CUMULATIVE INCIDENCES FOR RELAPSE AND NONRELAPSE MORTALITY AMONG INDIVIDUALS ABOVE AGE 50 YEARS. *RIC,* Reduced-intensity conditioning. *(Data from Lim Z, Brand R, Martino R, et al: Allogeneic hematopoietic stem-cell transplantation for patients 50 years or older with myelodysplastic syndromes or secondary acute myeloid leukemia,* J Clin Oncol *28:405, 2010.)*

model can help determine if HSCT at the time of initial diagnosis, delayed a fixed number of years, or at the time of leukemic transformation is the optimal strategy when IPSS score at the time of diagnosis is considered. Data from several large, nonoverlapping databases demonstrated that the optimal treatment strategy for patients with low and intermediate-1 IPSS disease was to delay transplantation until the time of leukemic progression. Immediate transplantation was recommended for patients with intermediate-2 and high-risk IPSS scores, even when adjustment for quality of life was considered.[65]

A shortcoming of this analysis was the inability to provide treatment decision guidance at other clinically relevant times for patients not undergoing immediate HSCT, because other important clinical events, such as a new transfusion requirement, recurrent infection, or recurrent bleeding episodes certainly could be considered triggers to move on to transplantation. Thus it is useful to subdivide patients with lower-risk MDS into more-refined prognostic groups that may benefit from HSCT.

Transfusion frequency and resultant iron overload have both been demonstrated to be important prognostic factors in HSCT outcomes. Platzbecker et al[67] compared the effects of transfusion dependency at the time of HSCT. Even though the transfusion-dependent group had more low-risk features, overall survival was inferior, with a 3-year overall survival of 49% compared with 60% in the transfusion-independent group ($P = 0.1$). The Pavia group examined a cohort of patients stratified by IPSS to determine the relevance of the newer World Health Organization (WHO) histologic classification scheme and to determine if transfusion requirement influenced outcomes among different IPSS groups. For patients with low- and intermediate-1 risk IPSS scores, the WHO histologic classification scheme significantly differentiated survival among the different histologic subtypes within each IPSS range.[68] More importantly, the authors demonstrated a significant effect on survival based on the requirement for transfusion support. As would be expected, outcomes in patients with higher-grade myelodysplasia were affected less by transfusion requirement than were patients with less-advanced WHO histologic classifications. As a result, the impact of transfusion requirement was then incorporated into the WHO Prognostic Scoring System (WPSS).[69] In this system, the effect of regular transfusion requirement (defined as requiring at least one transfusion every 8 weeks in a 4-month period) was given the same regression weight as progressing between cytogenetic risk groups. In contrast to the initial IPSS publication, which carries prognostic information only at the time of initial MDS diagnosis, this model was time dependent, such that patients could be continually reevaluated by the scoring model and updated prognostic information could be generated at any time in the patient's treatment course. As such, the development of new cytogenetic changes or the development of a transfusion need adds useful information that helps guide treatment decisions, including the decision to proceed to HSCT as well as estimating transplantation outcomes.[70] Determining at which WPSS stage transplantation outcomes are superior to nontransplantation therapy has yet to be determined.

A limitation of both the IPSS and WPSS scoring systems is that they do not account for many important cytogenetic changes. An analysis of cytogenetics in over 2000 individuals with MDS identified several favorable karyotypes that were associated with median survivals that ranged from 32 to 108 months, as well as karyotypes associated with an intermediate prognosis.[71] Some have suggested that adverse cytogenetics be given the same weight as an elevated blast count in the IPSS modeling scheme.[72]

It is worth noting that the majority of the prognostic models discussed here relate largely to patients undergoing high-intensity conditioning HSCT, whereas this procedure is not recommended for the vast majority of patients with MDS because of the age distribution of this patient population. Therefore prognostic models developed specifically for older patients are required. In addition, the optimal timing of RIC transplantation needs to be addressed in a prospective clinical trial, or in the absence of the feasibility of this approach, with mathematical Markov modeling.

Molecular Prognostic Factors

Perhaps even more than in AML, mutation analysis undoubtedly led to a shift from rudimentary clinical prognostic models to molecularly defined models for prognosis and to guide therapy in MDS. As many as 75% of patients can be found to have one or more mutations.[73] Numerous individual genes and whole genome expression profiling have demonstrated significant associations with MDS outcome, although none of these molecular signatures have been tested yet to determine their impact on transplantation outcome. Nonetheless, these gene aberrations are useful in recommending HSCT in the face of an adverse clinical prognosis. The following presents some of the better-characterized lesions and their impact on MDS outcomes.

TET2: TET2 is the most commonly mutated gene in MDS, mutated in over 20% of MDS patients.[74] TET2 is involved in the conversion of 5-methylcytosine to 5-hydroxymethylcytosine and is thus important in the epigenetic modulation by deoxyribonucleic acid (DNA) methyltransferases.[75] Although prevalent, TET2 does not appear to offer prognostic information in MDS.[73,76]

ASXL1: Mutations in ASXL1, a member of the enhancer of trithorax and polycomb (ETP) family, are similar in frequency to mutations of TET2,[77] but they carry prognostic information. Thol et al[78] demonstrated a significantly shorter overall survival with a shortened time to leukemia progression among patients with frameshift mutations in this gene.

IDH1: The citric acid cycle gene IDH1 is mutated in a small proportion of patients with MDS. However, when mutated, it was associated with very poor outcome (14% versus 52% 2-year survival) in a large MDS cohort (n = 153).[79] This finding was not noted in a recent multigene analysis, where, in contrast, the homologue IDH2 had borderline prognostic significance.[73]

DNMT3A: Changes in DNA methylation have been extensively studied in MDS. Point mutations in one of two de novo methylation genes, DNMT3A, have been shown to be present in 8% of MDS patients.[80] These mutations are associated with an adverse prognosis.

EZH2: The protein encoded by EZH2 is a histone methyltransferase that influences stem cell renewal and likely acts as a tumor suppressor in myeloid malignancies.[81,82] In their multigene mutation analysis, Bejar et al[73] noted that mutations in this gene were associated with the highest adjusted hazard for death among 439 patients.

Other mutations: TP53, which is prognostic in many other tumor types appears to be prognostic in MDS.[73] Similarly, the DNA repair gene RUNX1 appears prognostic in MDS.[73] Other genes relevant in AML and other myeloid diseases, such as FLT3, NPM1, and JAK2 appear to have limited utility in prediction of MDS prognosis.[83,84]

In addition to individual gene mutations, the use of whole genome microarray gene expression profiling has been used to estimate prognosis in MDS. Mills et al[85] developed a hierarchic microarray-based risk score on 110 primary MDS samples and were able to stratify the risk for leukemic transformation and predict overall survival using their model.

As the number of patients with a defined molecular signature subtype of MDS that have undergone HSCT increases, the overall benefit (or lack thereof) for early HSCT can eventually be determined. Until then, and in the absence of specific effective therapeutics for each of the molecular adverse-risk subtypes, we can continue to recommend HSCT for patients who carry one or more of these high-risk molecular signatures.

Incorporating Comorbidity for Patient and Conditioning Intensity Selection Before Transplantation

With increased comorbidity comes an increase in the rate of adverse outcomes in hematologic malignancies, and, in particular, in the treatment of MDS.[86] Age alone cannot be used as a surrogate for comorbidity, as demonstrated by an analysis of over 500 individuals with MDS who underwent a first RIC transplantation.[87] Several comorbidity scores have been developed to help provide prognostic information in myeloid malignancies. In MDS, the Hematopoietic Cell Transplantation Comorbidity Index, developed by Sorror and colleagues,[88,89] has been shown to carry prognostic value, even in patients with MDS not undergoing transplantation.[90] The consideration of comorbidity before HSCT is even more relevant now that RIC has been shown to be effective in the treatment of MDS, and patients can elect to undergo RIC transplantation (see Comparative Results: Myeloablative and Reduced-Intensity Regimens in MDS). Patients were divided into four separate groups, with each group being defined on the basis of comorbidity and malignant disease risk. Within each of the four risk groups, patients who underwent MAC and RIC were compared with each other. As expected in each of the four groups, the RIC arm experienced higher relapse rates but lower treatment-related mortality rates when compared to the MAC arm. As a result, disease-free and overall survival was similar between conditioning arms in all four groups.[89]

The effects of elevated ferritin levels on HSCT until recently have been largely limited to patients undergoing MAC transplantation.[91] We previously reported that an elevated pre-HSCT serum ferritin level was strongly associated with lower overall and disease-free survival in patients with AML and MDS after transplantation, and this was largely attributable to increased treatment-related mortality.[91] Similarly, a prospective single-institution study of 190 adult patients undergoing MAC HSCT demonstrated that elevated pretransplantation serum ferritin level was associated with increased risk for 100-day mortality, acute GVHD, and bloodstream infections or death as a composite endpoint.[92] It has now been recognized that elevated ferritin level can predict inferior outcomes even after RIC transplantation.[63] As a laboratory prognostic factor, ferritin should be considered a marker of comorbidity, because ferritin is a marker of inflammation. As such, ferritin levels could influence the decision to pursue high-intensity or reduced-intensity HSCT. Optimally, if high-intensity HSCT is planned, proceeding before the accumulation of a critical amount of iron should be pursued, or, alternatively, chelation therapy before HSCT can be considered, although this latter approach has not yet been demonstrated to be effective in prospective clinical trials.

Pretransplantation Therapy

The role of cytoreductive chemotherapy before HSCT for MDS remains controversial. Many analyses have demonstrated that outcomes are improved with lower disease burden at the time of HSCT,[93] but previously only conventional chemotherapy was offered. The analyses that compare chemotherapy to no chemotherapy before HSCT are inherently biased, because patients who do poorly or expire with chemotherapy are not included in HSCT outcome data and might have had favorable outcomes if not exposed to cytotoxic agents. On the other hand, responsiveness to chemotherapy may indicate more favorable disease biology and this has been correlated with improved outcomes after HSCT.[94]

With the advent of DNA hypomethylating therapy, the use of conventional chemotherapy has diminished for MDS patients. The effect of DNA hypomethylating therapy on HSCT outcomes has recently been studied by several groups.[95-97] Compared retrospectively, it does not appear that pretransplantation hypomethylating therapy offers a survival advantage,[90] but these agents continue to be used widely to prevent disease progression and to reduce transfusion needs while donor selection is performed in patients destined to undergo transplantation. There may be some advantage to the use of these agents before HSCT, because DNA hypomethylating therapy has been shown to upregulate the expression of cancer-testis antigens,[98,99] killer immunoglobulin-like receptor (KIR) ligands,[100] HLA molecules,[101] and other minor antigens on tumor cells,[102] all of which may enhance graft-versus-MDS effects. Lack of response to DNA hypomethylating therapy is associated with a very poor prognosis [103] and should be an indication for transplantation referral. Finally, hypomethylating agents have been used after transplantation to reduce the risk for relapse,[104] but more studies will need to be undertaken before this type of therapy can be routinely recommended.

FUTURE DIRECTIONS

Despite the progress that has been made in conventional therapy for both AML and MDS, allogeneic HSCT has the best track record for curing the disease. Although HSCT has limitations, reductions in toxicity, improvements in donor availability, and new strategies to enhance GVL while limiting GVHD promise to further improve survival. Advances in mutation analysis provide insights into the pathophysiology of MDS and AML and suggest routes for targeted therapy. However, in many circumstances targeted therapy may not be feasible, and thus the utility of molecular prognostic indicators is to identify patients who will benefit from early transplantation.

SUGGESTED READINGS

Alessandrino EP, Della Porta MG, Bacigalupo A, et al: WHO classification and WPSS predict posttransplantation outcome in patients with myelodysplastic syndrome: A study from the Gruppo Italiano Trapianto di Midollo Osseo (GITMO). *Blood* 112:895, 2008.

Brunstein CG, Fuchs EJ, Carter SL, et al: Alternative donor transplantation: Results of parallel phase II trials using HLA-mismatched related bone marrow or unrelated umbilical cord blood grafts. *Blood* 118:282, 2011.

Burnett A, Wetzler M, Lowenberg B: Therapeutic advances in acute myeloid leukemia. *J Clin Oncol* 29:487, 2011.

Cutler CS, Lee SJ, Greenberg P, et al: A decision analysis of allogeneic bone marrow transplantation for the myelodysplastic syndromes: Delayed transplantation for low-risk myelodysplasia is associated with improved outcome. *Blood* 104:579, 2004.

Dohner H, Estey EH, Amadori S, et al: Diagnosis and management of acute myeloid leukemia in adults: Recommendations from an international expert panel, on behalf of the European LeukemiaNet. *Blood* 115:453, 2010.

Eapen M, Rocha V, Sanz G, et al: Effect of graft source on unrelated donor haemopoietic stem-cell transplantation in adults with acute leukaemia: A retrospective analysis. *Lancet Oncol* 11:653, 2010.

Farag SS, Maharry K, Zhang MJ, et al: Comparison of reduced-intensity hematopoietic cell transplantation with chemotherapy in patients aged 60-70 years with acute myelogenous leukemia in first remission. *Biol Blood Marrow Transplant* 2011.

Fenaux P, Mufti GJ, Hellstrom-Lindberg E, et al: Efficacy of azacitidine compared with that of conventional care regimens in the treatment of higher-risk myelodysplastic syndromes: A randomised, open-label, phase III study. *Lancet Oncol* 10:223, 2009.

Greenberg P, Cox C, LeBeau MM, et al: International scoring system for evaluating prognosis in myelodysplastic syndromes. *Blood* 89:2079, 1997.

Gupta V, Tallman MS, He W, et al: Comparable survival after HLA-well-matched unrelated or matched sibling donor transplantation for acute myeloid leukemia in first remission with unfavorable cytogenetics at diagnosis. *Blood* 116:1839, 2010.

Gupta V, Tallman MS, Weisdorf DJ: Allogeneic hematopoietic cell transplantation for adults with acute myeloid leukemia: Myths, controversies, and unknowns. *Blood* 117:2307, 2011.

Koreth J, Schlenk R, Kopecky KJ, et al: Allogeneic stem cell transplantation for acute myeloid leukemia in first complete remission: Systematic review and meta-analysis of prospective clinical trials. *JAMA* 301:2349, 2009.

Lee JH, Lim SN, Kim DY, et al: Allogeneic hematopoietic cell transplantation for myelodysplastic syndrome: Prognostic significance of pre-transplant IPSS score and comorbidity. *Bone Marrow Transplant* 45:450, 2010.

Lim Z, Brand R, Martino R, et al: Allogeneic Hematopoietic Stem-cell transplantation for patients 50 years or older with myelodysplastic syndromes or secondary acute myeloid leukemia. *J Clin Oncol* 28:405, 2010.

Litzow MR, Tarima S, Perez WS, et al: Allogeneic transplantation for therapy-related myelodysplastic syndrome and acute myeloid leukemia. *Blood* 115:1850, 2010.

Luger SM, Ringden O, Zhang MJ, et al: Similar outcomes using myeloablative vs reduced-intensity allogeneic transplant preparative regimens for AML or MDS. *Bone Marrow Transplant* 47:203, 2012.

Malcovati L, Germing U, Kuendgen A, et al: Time-dependent prognostic scoring system for predicting survival and leukemic evolution in myelodysplastic syndromes. *J Clin Oncol* 25:3503, 2007.

Malcovati L, Porta MG, Pascutto C, et al: Prognostic factors and life expectancy in myelodysplastic syndromes classified according to WHO criteria: A basis for clinical decision making. *J Clin Oncol* 23:7594, 2005.

McClune BL, Weisdorf DJ, Pedersen TL, et al: Effect of age on outcome of reduced-intensity hematopoietic cell transplantation for older patients with acute myeloid leukemia in first complete remission or with myelodysplastic syndrome. *J Clin Oncol* 28:1878, 2010.

Rockova V, Abbas S, Wouters BJ, et al: Risk stratification of intermediate-risk acute myeloid leukemia: Integrative analysis of a multitude of gene mutation and gene expression markers. *Blood* 118:1069, 2011.

Schanz J, Steidl C, Fonatsch C, et al: Coalesced multicentric analysis of 2,351 patients with myelodysplastic syndromes indicates an underestimation of poor-risk cytogenetics of myelodysplastic syndromes in the international prognostic scoring system. *J Clin Oncol* 29:1963, 2011.

Schlenk RF, Dohner K, Krauter J, et al: Mutations and treatment outcome in cytogenetically normal acute myeloid leukemia. *N Engl J Med* 358:1909, 2008.

Walter RB, Pagel JM, Gooley TA, et al: Comparison of matched unrelated and matched related donor myeloablative hematopoietic cell transplantation for adults with acute myeloid leukemia in first remission. *Leukemia* 24:1276, 2010.

For complete list of references log on to www.expertconsult.com.

CHAPTER 61

ACUTE MYELOID LEUKEMIA IN CHILDREN

Michael C. Wei, Gary V. Dahl, and Howard J. Weinstein

Pediatric acute myeloid leukemias (AMLs) represent a clinically and biologically heterogeneous group of diseases caused by the malignant transformation of a hematopoietic stem cell or myeloid progenitor cell. The proliferative advantage of the leukemic stem cell, coupled with impairments in differentiation and inhibition of apoptosis, is thought to arise from acquired genetic alterations that lead to accumulation of immature or blast cells in the bone marrow. The blasts eventually suppress normal hematopoiesis and infiltrate other organs and tissues. Conventionally, the French-American-British (FAB) cooperative group classified AML into eight subtypes (M0 to M7) based primarily on blast cell morphology and reactivity with histochemical stains. More recently, the World Health Organization (WHO) developed a new classification system that included cytogenetics and lowered the percentage of blasts in the marrow required to make a diagnosis of AML from 30% to 20%. AML accounts for approximately 20% of acute leukemias in children and 80% of those in adults. In contrast to cure rates for childhood acute lymphoblastic leukemia (ALL), cure rates for AML have improved only modestly over the past 2 decades. The use of intensive consolidation chemotherapy with allogeneic stem cell transplants in selective patient groups and better supportive care have resulted in overall survival (OS) rates approaching 70% in some clinical trials. Although some subgroups, such as patients with Down syndrome and acute megakaryoblastic leukemia (AMKL), acute promyelocytic leukemia (APL), and core binding factor leukemias with t(8;21) or inv(16), have excellent outcomes, others continue to have poor outcomes. Much has been learned about the prognostic impact of cytogenetic abnormalities, mutations in specific genes such as FLT3 and CEBPA, and response to therapy as measured by minimal residual disease (MRD). Current cooperative group trials incorporate these factors into risk-adapted therapy such as the recommendation for stem cell transplant for patients at highest risk for relapse. Challenges still remain in how to best identify those patients at risk for relapse and to tailor therapy based on this risk with therapy intensification or novel targeted therapy.

EPIDEMIOLOGY

Approximately 550 new cases of AML are diagnosed each year in children ages 0 to 19 years in the United States. In contrast to the early-age peak (3 to 4 years) for childhood ALL, the incidence of AML is quite constant from birth throughout the first 10 years, with a slight peak in late adolescence. AML also accounts for the majority of the very rare instances of congenital leukemia. The predominance of AML in this age group may in part be due to the inclusion of infants with the transient myeloproliferative disorder associated with Down syndrome (see discussion later in this chapter). There is no difference in incidence between males and females. There is no known relationship between race and the incidence of AML, although Hispanics experience the highest rate of leukemia per million population, from 1.3- to 1.7-fold higher than other racial/ethnic groups.

The incidence and subtypes of acute leukemia in children do not have significant geographic variation. In Japan, China, and among the Maori of New Zealand, however, the rates of AML are the highest. In India and Kuwait, the lowest rates are reported. Patterns of presentation also vary. For example, an unusually high percentage of children diagnosed with AML in Turkey and several African countries present with myeloblastomas or chloromas involving the orbital area. APL accounts for 5% to 8% of pediatric AML cases, and its frequency varies more widely geographically, with increased incidence in Italy and South and Central America. In addition, APL is uncommon in the first decade of life, and its incidence plateaus during early adulthood.

As in other forms of leukemia, the precise cause of AML is unknown. The vast majority of children with AML have no obvious predisposing factors. Known risk factors include several congenital/genetic disorders, ionizing radiation, and certain drug or toxin exposures (Table 61-1). For example, occupational exposure to benzene and treatment with alkylating agents or topoisomerase-II inhibitors (especially the epipodophyllotoxins etoposide or teniposide) are associated with an excess incidence of AML. The likelihood of developing secondary AML from epipodophyllotoxin therapy appears to be schedule- and cumulative dose–dependent. Increased risk has been noted with twice-weekly or weekly administration of etoposide/teniposide. In contrast to alkylating agent–induced AML, which generally causes chromosomal loss of 5q or 7q, the secondary leukemias observed after treatment with etoposide or teniposide are usually myelomonocytic or monocytic in morphology, have a shorter latency period (2 to 4 years), and usually have chromosomal translocations involving band 11q23 (MLL gene rearrangement). The MLL gene is also rearranged in 60% to 70% of cases of infant acute leukemia, and de novo AML, most frequently in AML with myelomonocytic or monocytic morphology. In utero exposure to naturally occurring topoisomerase II inhibitors such as dietary flavonoids has been hypothesized to increase the risk for MLL-rearranged infant AML. Children who were exposed to radiation from the atomic bombs in Japan had an increased incidence of leukemia, but no excess of leukemia was noted in Japanese children who were exposed prenatally to the atomic explosions. Several studies have addressed whether exposure to low-frequency, nonionizing radiation (e.g., electromagnetic fields) is leukemogenic but did not find an increased risk for acute leukemia in children exposed to residential magnetic fields.

Genetic factors predisposing to AML have been studied in twins and in children with certain genetic disorders. Unusual concordance of AML has been observed in monozygotic twins that approaches 100% for infant leukemias and a risk on the order of 1 in 10 for older twin pairs. These leukemias are the consequence of the transplacental passage of a single leukemic clone rather than a genetic predisposition in most cases. Patients with diseases associated with chromosome fragility and impaired deoxyribonucleic acid (DNA) repair mechanisms (e.g., Fanconi anemia and Bloom syndrome) are predisposed to develop AML. Children with congenital disorders of granulopoiesis and erythropoiesis, such as Kostmann syndrome and Diamond-Blackfan anemia, are also at increased risk for developing AML. The cumulative incidence of myelodysplastic syndrome or AML in patients with severe congenital neutropenia receiving long-term granulocyte colony-stimulating factor therapy is 21% after 10 years.

Children with trisomy 21 or Down syndrome have an approximately 10- to 20-fold increased risk for developing acute leukemia compared with children without Down syndrome. Although most

Table 61-1 Congenital Disorders or Acquired Factors Predisposing to Acute Myeloid Leukemia

GENETIC FACTORS
Down syndrome
Fanconi anemia
Bloom syndrome
Neurofibromatosis type 1
Klinefelter syndrome
Turner syndrome
CONGENITAL BONE MARROW FAILURE SYNDROMES
Kostmann syndrome
Diamond-Blackfan anemia
DRUGS
Benzene
Alkylating agents
Epipodophyllotoxins
Ionizing radiation

leukemia seen in children is lymphoid, in children with Down syndrome under the age of 4, more than 50% of cases are myeloid, and Down syndrome patients account for approximately 10% of all pediatric AML patients. From birth through 4 years of age, the incidence of AML (especially AMKL) is much greater than ALL in children with Down syndrome. In children with Down syndrome, the incidence of AMKL is up to 500-fold greater than in the general pediatric population. After 5 years of age, the ratio of ALL to AML reverts to that of the general pediatric population.

Children with neurofibromatosis 1 (NF1) are at increased risk for developing acute and chronic myeloid leukemias as well as certain benign and malignant tumors that primarily arise in cells derived from the embryonic neural crest. In patients with NF1 and leukemia, loss of both NF1 alleles in bone marrow blasts has been detected in some patients. These data are consistent with a tumor-suppressor function for the NF1 gene. Inactivation of NF1 may contribute to leukemogenesis by aberrantly activating the RAS signaling pathway.

PATHOBIOLOGY

Chromosomal Rearrangements

Chromosomal abnormalities are detected in blasts from 75% of children with AML and are important for diagnostic and prognostic purposes. The United Kingdom Medical Research Council (UK MRC) published the largest series of childhood AML cytogenetics, which defined 22 subgroups and showed that the distribution of chromosomal changes and the prognostic significance of these changes differed between adult and pediatric patients. Normal karyotype AML accounts for approximately 25% of pediatric patients, compared to 50% in adult AML. Most of the described chromosome changes are not unique to a specific age group, except for the 50% of 11q23 rearrangements seen in infants, the t(l;22)(pl3;ql3) in infants with AMKL, and the t(7;12)(q36;p13) translocation also seen in infants.

Many of the genes at the breakpoints of chromosomal translocations have been cloned and proven to be transcription factors involved in normal hematopoiesis and myeloid differentiation. The translocation t(8;21)(q22;q22) is the most frequently occurring translocation in AML at approximately 14% and is one of the core binding factor leukemias that has a favorable prognosis. Three-way rearrangements may occur. The t(8;21) is frequently associated with loss of a sex chromosome. The t(8;21) produces a fusion protein involving RUNX1/AML1 on chromosome 21 and RUNX1T1/ETO on chromosome 8. The RUNX1 gene encodes one of the DNA-binding α subunits of the heterodimeric core binding factor transcription factor complex. The chimeric fusion protein is thought to function as a transcriptional repressor and recruits corepressors that interfere with normal core binding factor–dependent transcription, thereby inhibiting differentiation and enhancing self-renewal. The RUNX1-RUNX1T1 fusion gene has been detected by molecular methods in patients with t(8;21) in long-term complete remission. In patients with t(8;21) AML, MRD quantitation by real-time reverse-transcriptase polymerase chain reaction (RT-PCR) allows for identification of patients with a higher risk for relapse.

Chromosomal abnormalities involving chromosome 16, inv(16)(p13;q22), or t(16;16)(p13;q22) constitute approximately 7% of AML, represent the second core binding factor leukemia, and are associated with a favorable prognosis and characteristic morphology. The morphology is characteristically myelomonocytic with the distinctive presence of dysplastic eosinophils containing a dense infiltration of large, violet-purple eosinophilic granules. CBFB, encoding the non–DNA binding β- subunit of the core binding factor heterodimer, is disrupted at the 16q22 breakpoint, and MYH11, encoding smooth muscle myosin heavy chain, is disrupted at the 16p13 breakpoint. The resultant fusion product, CBFβ–MYH11, exerts a dominant-negative effect on the core binding factor transcription factor complex, resulting in a block in myeloid differentiation. A high proportion of these leukemias have cooperating mutations thought to lead to increased cell proliferation.

Chromosome band 11q23 translocations are commonly seen in infants and toddlers with the myelomonocytic and monocytic morphology and secondary leukemias after epipodophyllotoxin therapy. Of the 75% of pediatric AML patients with an abnormal karyotype, 11q23 rearrangements were the largest subgroup at 16% of patients. The 11q23 translocation disrupts the MLL gene (mixed-lineage leukemia) that encodes a large protein with regions of homology to the Drosophila trithorax protein. In mammals the wild-type MLL protein functions as a histone methyltransferase involved in maintenance of homeobox (Hox) gene expression and plays a critical role in definitive hematopoiesis. MLL oncogenic rearrangements result in aberrant Hox gene expression and epigenetic chromatin changes. The most common 11q23 translocations observed in childhood AML are t(9;11)(p21;q23), t(11;19)(q23;p13.1), and t(10;11)(p12;q23), although more than 50 MLL translocation partners have been identified. The prognostic significance of the MLL translocation partner is controversial, with some groups reporting a favorable prognosis for t(9;11). MLL translocations are found in both ALL and AML, and the precise reasons for development of one or the other is likely related to the cell of origin and the biology of the specific MLL translocation.

The translocation t(15;17)(q22;q21) is associated with 95% of APL, including both the hypergranular and the hypogranular variants. This has a favorable prognosis because of molecularly targeted differentiation therapy. The cloning of the breakpoint revealed rearrangement of a retinoic acid receptor gene RARA fused to the PML gene. The PML-RARA hybrid gene is expressed in leukemic cells from most patients with APL, though rarely other fusion partners, such as PLZF-RARA t(11;17)(q23;q21) or NPM-RARA t(5;17)(q35;q21), have been reported. The PML-RARA fusion protein is an abnormal retinoic acid receptor with decreased sensitivity to retinoic acid, thereby antagonizing normal differentiation. This molecular marker (PML-RARA transcript) provides a convenient assay for diagnosing APL and determining the presence of MRD. Before the RARA gene was shown to be rearranged in t(15;17), observations were made that APL cells differentiated in response to retinoic acid both in vitro and in vivo. Now it is understood that the mechanism involves driving differentiation by saturating the retinoic acid receptor with pharmacologic levels of retinoic acid.

Cell of Origin and Biologic Properties of Leukemia Stem Cells

Cytogenetic studies and assays using X-linked polymorphisms suggested the clonal nature of AML. The chromosomal changes vary but predominantly involve balanced translocations, deletions, or inversions and are restricted to the leukemic cells. The bone marrow karyotype returns to normal when the disease is in complete remission. At relapse, often the original clone reappears (plus or minus additional genetic changes), suggesting that the leukemic clone was suppressed, but not eliminated, by treatment. Emerging evidence based on careful analysis of copy number alterations and whole-genome sequencing supports a clonal evolution model of leukemia, in which multiple, genetically distinct leukemic subclones are present at diagnosis. One clone may dominate at diagnosis and reemerge at relapse, or a related but distinct subclone may emerge at relapse.

There is evidence that the cell of origin in AML may be a primitive hematopoietic stem cell (HSC). Studies of human AML leukemic stem cells (LSCs) transplanted into immunodeficient mice indicated that the LSC closely resembles primitive HSC immunophenotypically. However, model systems of human AML using AML oncogenes introduced into phenotypically defined populations of mouse bone marrow cells have demonstrated that both primitive HSC and more differentiated granulocyte-macrophage precursors can be transformed and give rise to AML. Thus more committed progenitors have the potential to be transformed, but whether this occurs in human disease remains uncertain.

Although bulk leukemic blasts have limited capacity for self-renewal, the LSC hypothesis posits that LSCs have the ability to self-renew and generate precursors that give rise to the entire leukemic hierarchy when xenotransplanted into immunodeficient mice. Attempts have been made to define LSC immunophenotypically using cell surface markers such as CD34 and CD38; however, recent studies have shown a remarkable plasticity in the immunophenotype of leukemia-initiating cells. There may be many cells with stem cell–like properties that differ in their genetic profile and ability to initiate leukemia. The frequency of LSCs is thought to be quite rare, but that view is being challenged. Many AML LSCs are found in a quiescent state, which may explain why some patients relapse after treatment with agents that target rapidly dividing cells. Identification of LSCs and targeting therapy to these cells is a major goal of AML research.

Cooperating Mutations

Some oncogenic AML translocations can be generated in utero, indicating a long latency for the development of disease. Given this latency, additional secondary mutations are thought to be required for an initiated cell to progress to overt leukemia. A cooperativity model of leukemogenesis suggests that there are two types of mutations required, one conferring a proliferative or survival advantage and another that impairs hematopoietic differentiation. Although most chromosomal translocations act to impair differentiation, many cooperating mutations affect cellular proliferation. The most frequent known examples in pediatric AML include KIT, RAS, and FMS-like tyrosine kinase-3 (FLT3) mutations. A review of 170 pediatric AML samples showed that 40% harbored a mutation in one of these three genes. Mutations in RAS, a critical mediator of growth signal transduction mutated in many cancers, were found in 37 of 99 pediatric AML samples. Mutated RAS synergizes with nuclear fusion genes to accelerate leukemia latency in mouse models. FLT3 is a receptor tyrosine kinase important for cell proliferation and differentiation. Mutations, including the internal tandem duplication (ITD) or activating loop mutations, are thought to lead to constitutive activation of the receptor. FLT3-ITD expression induces a myeloproliferative disease (but not frank AML) in mice; however, FLT3-ITD increases the penetrance of APL in a PML-RARA model. Somatic FLT3 mutations are found in 10% to 20% of pediatric AML, and most studies have found a lower frequency than that in adult AML.

Analysis of copy number variations (genomic deletions and duplications) using single-nucleotide polymorphism (SNP) arrays indicates, in contrast to ALL, additional copy number variations in AML are rare. Instead, additional mutations are likely to be point mutations or structural changes below the detection level limit of SNP arrays. Many new somatic mutations in AML blasts are being

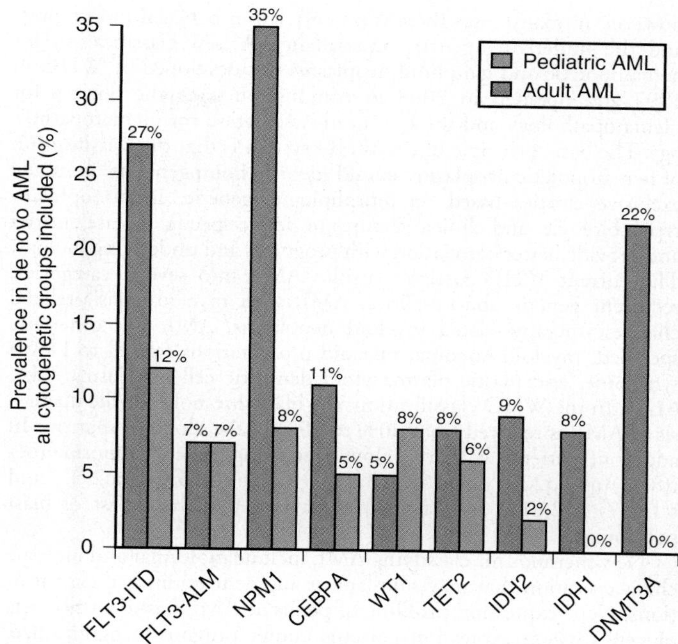

Figure 61-1 PREVALENCE OF GENETIC MUTATIONS IN ADULT VERSUS PEDIATRIC ACUTE MYELOID LEUKEMIA. *AML,* Acute myeloid leukemia. *(Modified from Ho PA, Kutny MA, Alonzo TA, et al: Leukemic mutations in the methylation-associated genes DNMT3A and IDH2 are rare events in pediatric AML: A report from the Children's Oncology Group.* Pediatr Blood Cancer *57:204, 2011.)*

uncovered by whole-genome sequencing. Whole-genome sequencing of adult AML samples revealed mutations in isocitrate dehydrogenase 1 (IDH1) and IDH2 and in DNA methyltransferase 3A (DNMT3A). These mutations were associated with aberrant DNA methylation patterns and found to be prognostically significant. Retrospective studies of pediatric AML samples indicate that these mutations are rare in pediatric AML and not prognostically significant in multivariate regression analysis. These studies highlight some of the molecular genetic differences in pediatric versus adult AML and also potentially reflect a difference in biology (Fig. 61-1). Whether new mutations discovered by sequencing represent driver or passenger mutations will require further study.

Besides altered proliferation and differentiation properties, AML cells, and particularly AML LSC, may also evade host immune surveillance systems by upregulating the CD47 antigen that functions as a "don't eat me" antiphagocytosis signal for the SIRPα receptor on macrophages. Antibodies that block CD47 make AML cells susceptible to macrophage phagocytosis in animal models and are being developed for human clinical trials.

CLASSIFICATION

Careful examination of both the blood smear and the bone marrow aspirate is required to establish the diagnosis of AML, because approximately 10% of patients with acute leukemia do not have circulating blasts at diagnosis. Various methods are available for characterizing the blast cell population in patients with acute leukemia. These include morphologic interpretation of Wright-Giemsa–stained specimens in conjunction with cytochemistry, chromosome analysis, immunophenotyping, and molecular genetic analysis. Precise diagnosis and classification are essential for successful treatment and biologic investigation of the childhood leukemias.

The FAB group recognizes eight subgroups of AML and also requires a minimum of 30% bone marrow blasts for the diagnosis of AML. The FAB system provides a useful morphologic classification;

however, in many cases there is no correlation between morphology and the underlying genetic abnormality. A new classification for hematopoietic and lymphoid neoplasms was developed by WHO in 1997 and updated in 2008 in conjunction with the Society for Hematopathology and the European Association for Hematopathology. The basic principle of the WHO system is that the classification of hematopoietic neoplasms should identify homogeneous, mutually exclusive entities based on morphologic, genetic, immunophenotypic, biologic, and clinical features to define specific disease entities and provide better correlation with prognosis and underlying biology. The current WHO system classifies AML into several categories: recurrent genetic abnormalities, AML with myelodysplasia-related changes, therapy-related myeloid neoplasms, AML not otherwise specified, myeloid sarcoma, myeloid proliferations related to Down syndrome, and blastic plasmacytoid dendritic cell neoplasm (Table 61-2). In the WHO classification, the blast threshold for the diagnosis of AML is reduced from 30% to 20% in the blood or marrow. In addition, patients with the clonal recurring genetic abnormalities t(8;21)(q22;q22), inv(16)(p13;q22) or t(16;16)(p13;q22), and t(15;17)(p22;q12) are classified as having AML regardless of blast percentage.

New methods for classifying AML include molecular and biologic characterization that may supplant or augment traditional classifications. Gene expression profiling of pediatric AML has identified sets of genes whose expression patterns confer prognostic significance. However, expression-based classifiers have to date not shown any advantage over cytogenetics. Another classification schema based on the pattern of basal and stimulated intracellular phosphoprotein phosphorylation measured by multiplex flow cytometry has described new subsets of AML and has promising prognostic utility. AML can also be classified based on differences in DNA methylation profiles, reflecting altered epigenetics in known AML subtypes and also defining new AML subtypes.

Table 61-2 2008 World Health Organization Classification of Acute Myeloid Leukemia

Acute myeloid leukemia with recurrent genetic abnormalities
Acute myeloid leukemia with t(8;21)(q22;q22); RUNX1-RUNX1T1 (formerly AML1-ETO)
Acute myeloid leukemia with inv(16)(p13.1q22) or t(16;16)(p13.1;q22); CBFB-MYH11
Acute promyelocytic leukemia with t(15;17)(q22;q12); PML-RARA
Acute myeloid leukemia with t(9;11)(p22;q23); MLLT3-MLL
Acute myeloid leukemia with t(6;9)(p23;q34); DEK-NUP214
Acute myeloid leukemia with inv(3)(q21q26.2) or t(3;3(q21;q26.2); RPN1-EVI1
Acute myeloid leukemia (megakaryoblastic) with t(1;22)(p13;q13); RBM15-MKL1
Acute myeloid leukemia with myelodysplasia-related changes
Therapy-related myeloid neoplasms
Acute myeloid leukemia, not otherwise specified
Classify as:
Acute myeloid leukemia, minimally differentiated
Acute myeloid leukemia without maturation
Acute myeloid leukemia with maturation
Acute myelomonocytic leukemia
Acute monoblastic/monocytic leukemia
Acute erythroid leukemia
Pure erythroid leukemia
Erythroleukemia, erythroid/myeloid
Acute megakaryoblastic leukemia
Acute basophilic leukemia
Acute panmyelosis with myelofibrosis
Myeloid sarcoma
Myeloid proliferations related to Down syndrome
Transient abnormal myelopoiesis
Myeloid leukemia associated with Down syndrome
Blastic plasmacytoid dendritic cell neoplasm

Modified from Vardiman JW, Thiele J, Arber DA, et al: The 2008 revision of the World Health Organization (WHO) classification of myeloid neoplasms and acute leukemia: Rationale and important changes, *Blood* 114:937, 2009.

CLINICAL MANIFESTATIONS

The initial signs and symptoms in the majority of children with AML include some degree of pallor, fatigue, skin or mucosal bleeding, or fever or infection that has not responded to appropriate antibiotic therapy. These signs and symptoms reflect the anemia, thrombocytopenia, and neutropenia secondary to diminished production of normal blood cells due to bone marrow infiltration with leukemic blasts. AML, in contrast to chronic myelogenous leukemia, is rarely diagnosed as an incidental finding on a routine complete blood cell count in an asymptomatic child. Bone pain and arthralgias are less common presenting symptoms in children with AML than those with ALL. Massive hepatosplenomegaly is uncommon except in infants with AML. Thrombocytopenia and/or disseminated intravascular coagulation (DIC) is the usual cause of hemorrhage in patients with AML. Bleeding is usually not observed until the platelet count falls below 20,000/μL unless there is an associated coagulopathy. Patients with APL are most at risk for DIC, but infants with myelomonocytic and monocytic AML are also at increased risk. Ocular pathology includes retinal hemorrhages due to coagulopathy, leukostasis, and leukemic infiltration, which may be asymptomatic.

Hyperleukocytosis can cause significant morbidity. Leukostasis refers to plugging of blasts in vessels with invasion of vessel walls, leading to hemorrhagic infarction of the brain, lung, or other organs. Children with AML who have leukocyte counts higher than 100,000/μL are much more susceptible to leukostasis than patients with ALL and comparable white blood cell (WBC) counts, because AML blasts are larger and less deformable. The most clinically relevant target organs for leukostasis are the brain and lung, with signs and symptoms including somnolence, seizures, stroke, tachypnea, and hypoxemia. Symptoms due to hyperleukocytosis require prompt treatment to quickly reduce the leukemic cell burden before the initiation of chemotherapy with leukapheresis, exchange transfusion in the case of infants, and oral hydroxyurea. Although extremely elevated WBC counts and leukostasis are rare in APL, leukapheresis should be avoided in these patients to prevent an exacerbation of DIC.

Congenital Leukemia

The clinical manifestations of leukemia diagnosed in the first 4 weeks of life differ in varying degrees from the typical findings in infants older than 6 months of age and older children with AML. Approximately one-half of newborns and infants younger than 2 months of age with AML have leukemia cutis. These babies have been described as looking like a "blueberry muffin" (Fig. 61-2). The skin lesions are described in the following section. It is important to note that these lesions may precede bone marrow manifestations of leukemia. Transient spontaneous remissions of leukemia cutis may occur but are usually followed within weeks by their reappearance in association with overt bone marrow involvement. In one review of 117 patients with congenital leukemia, there were 6 spontaneous remissions. Spontaneous remission of congenital AML has most often been observed with t(8;16)(p11;p13). Some experts suggest a period of observation only for the infant with leukemia cutis (MLL negative) as well as those with t(8;16), but overall it is recommended that chemotherapy be used for congenital leukemia.

Extramedullary Leukemia

The most common sites of extramedullary leukemia in children with AML include skin, gingiva, and central nervous system (CNS) and myeloblastomas in the head and neck area (Fig. 61-3).

Extramedullary involvement with AML is more common in infants than in older children. The skin lesions of leukemia cutis are often widespread, range in size from several millimeters to several centimeters, and are palpable as freely mobile, generally painless subcutaneous nodules. The color of the overlying skin may be salmon, red-brown, or bluish to slate gray (see box on Extramedullary AML: Myeloid Sarcoma and Leukemia Cutis). Testicular involvement is extraordinarily rare in children with AML and, like CNS leukemia, is commonly associated with the myelomonocytic and monocytic AML.

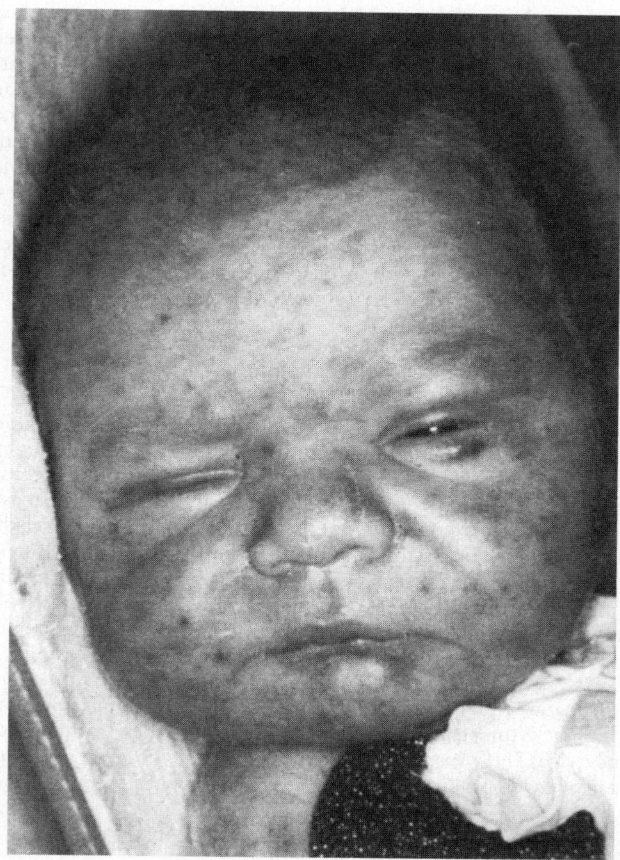

Figure 61-2 LEUKEMIA CUTIS AS COMMONLY SEEN IN CONGENITAL LEUKEMIA.

The most common pathologic finding of AML in the CNS is that of meningeal infiltration by blasts (Fig. 61-4), but epidural or brain parenchymal myeloblastomas have also been described. The incidence of meningeal leukemia at diagnosis in children with AML ranges from 5% to 15%, but most children are asymptomatic. The rare symptomatic patient with CNS leukemia may have headache, vomiting, papilledema, or a cranial nerve palsy (facial nerve is most common). In contrast, patients with cerebral leukostasis present with seizures, somnolence, or stroke secondary to areas of hemorrhage and infarction in brain tissue.

Fewer than 5% of newly diagnosed patients with AML have myeloblastomas, also known as granulocytic sarcomas or chloromas. These "solid tumors" of myeloid blasts may occur anywhere but are

Extramedullary Acute Myeloid Leukemia: Myeloid Sarcoma and Leukemia Cutis

The management of acute myeloid leukemia (AML) presenting with extramedullary disease, including myeloid sarcoma and leukemia cutis, is challenging. Diagnosis of myeloid sarcoma by biopsy is necessary if there are no other indications of leukemia. Diagnosis of leukemia cutis should always be through biopsy and not fine-needle aspiration, and samples need to be prepared for analysis by immunohistochemistry and cytogenetics/fluorescence in situ hybridization (FISH). Treatment should be with systemic chemotherapy based on risk stratification of the underlying disease cytogenetics and mutational profile. Radiation therapy as consolidation should be considered, especially if there is an incomplete response with chemotherapy alone and with careful evaluation of site and potential toxicities. Imaging of myeloid sarcoma sites by computed tomography (CT), positron emission tomography (PET), or magnetic resonance imaging (MRI) can be used to monitor response to treatment. There may be prognostic significance of extramedullary disease occurring at certain sites such as the orbit, but this should not influence choice of systemic therapy. The presence of leukemia cutis is a marker of aggressive disease. Isolated myeloid sarcoma or leukemia cutis relapse should be treated as a systemic relapse, because progression to systemic relapse is almost universal. Leukemia cutis as relapse after transplant is particularly difficult to treat. Total skin electron beam irradiation can be used and often achieves a transient response with cessation of new lesions and regression of old lesions, but recurrence or progression is typical. Caution must be used with concurrent chemotherapy that may induce a radiation recall reaction.

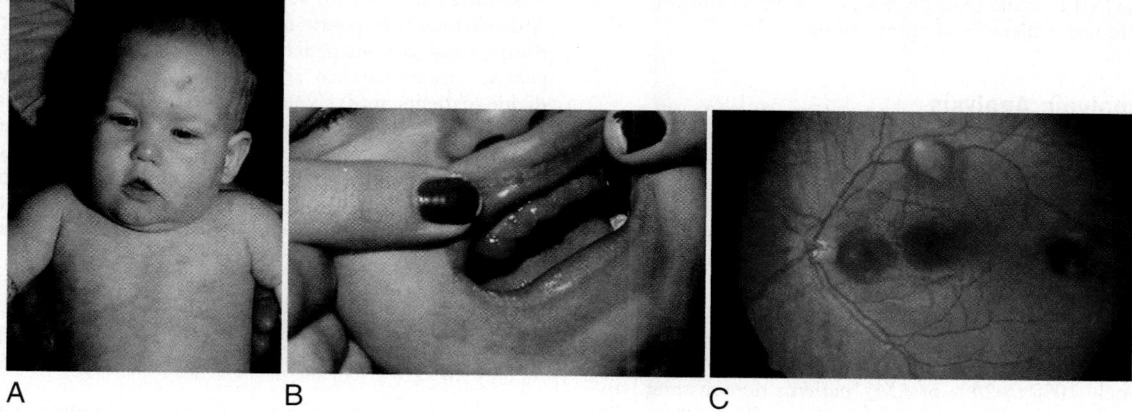

Figure 61-3 **A,** Monoblastic leukemia cutis at diagnosis; lesion on forehead preceded disseminated rash by 6 to 8 weeks. **B,** Gingival infiltration with M5a leukemia in a 21-month-old girl. **C,** Retinal infiltration at presentation of M4 disease in a 5-year-old boy.

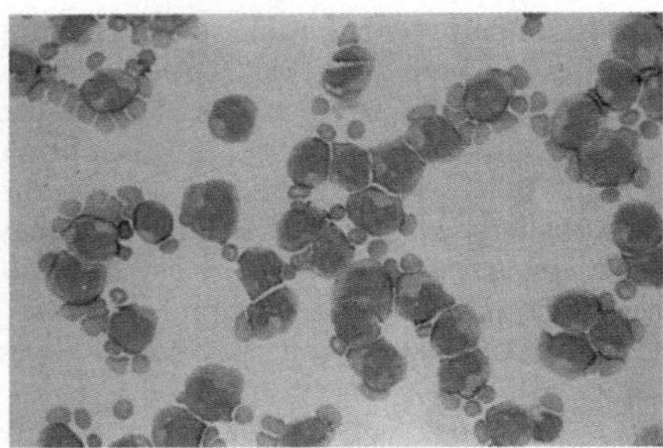

Figure 61-4 CEREBROSPINAL FLUID DOUBLE-CONCENTRATE CYTOCENTRIFUGE PREPARATION OF MONOCYTIC ACUTE MYELOID LEUKEMIA CELLS.

primarily detected in the bones and soft tissues of the head and neck (often orbits), and in intracranial or epidural locations. Myeloblastomas may herald overt bone marrow involvement with AML by weeks to months and are associated with t(8;21) and, in infants, with myelomonocytic and monocytic AML.

LABORATORY MANIFESTATIONS

The initial WBC count at presentation in children with AML is variable (1000/μL to 500,000/μL). Approximately 15% to 20% of children have WBC counts higher than 100,000/μL. Marked leukocytosis is associated with myelomonocytic and monocytic subtypes and congenital leukemia, whereas lower leukocyte counts are commonly seen in patients with APL. The leukocyte differential in most patients includes fewer than 1000 neutrophils per microliter and a variable percentage of blasts. In approximately 10% of patients, no peripheral blasts are detectable. Most patients with AML have a normocytic anemia, with occasional teardrop forms and nucleated red blood cells noted on the peripheral smear. The rare hemolytic anemia associated with AML is usually microangiopathic, secondary to DIC. Approximately 50% of children with AML present with platelet counts of fewer than 50,000/μL.

The definitive diagnosis of acute leukemia is made by examination of the bone marrow aspirate. In most patients, the bone marrow is hypercellular, with 20% to 90% blasts. The bone marrow biopsy may be hypocellular, especially in patients with a history of prior myelodysplastic syndrome (MDS), Fanconi anemia, or paroxysmal nocturnal hemoglobinuria. Dysplastic changes have recently been reported in patients with de novo AML and appear to have no prognostic significance. Conventional cytogenetic analysis of chromosome banding is usually sufficient to detect recurrent chromosomal rearrangements. Fluorescence in situ hybridization tests for specific chromosomal rearrangements and is often used for t(8;21) and 11q23 rearrangements (MLL break-apart probes); it can detect subtle abnormalities that are not evident in banding studies.

Immunophenotypic Analysis

Normal hematopoietic cells undergo changes in expression of cell surface markers as they mature from stem cells into cells of a committed lineage. Monoclonal antibodies have been developed that react with lineage-specific and stage-specific lymphoid and myeloid activation and differentiation antigens. By using a combination of monoclonal antibodies recognizing B-cell, T-cell, and myeloid antigens and flow cytometry, it is possible to confirm the diagnosis of AML and to differentiate AML from ALL if morphologic findings are inconclusive (<15% of cases).

Approximately 10% to 25% of AML patients demonstrate lymphoid antigen expression on myeloid blasts, and similarly 4% to 25% of ALL patients demonstrate expression of at least one myeloid antigen on the blast cell surface. The expression of lymphoid antigens in AML lacks prognostic significance. In most instances of hybrid or mixed-lineage acute leukemia, there is coexpression of lymphoid and myeloid markers on the same blast, but in rare cases there have been two distinct populations of blasts. The pathogenesis of these mixed-lineage leukemias remains poorly understood. They may represent a leukemic transformation in a primitive stem cell, or the aberrant expression of a lymphoid gene in a myeloid leukemia. Because few instances of true biphenotypic leukemia have been described, the prognosis is unclear. In a pediatric study, 14 of 16 patients with lymphoid antigen–positive AML expressed a T-cell marker. Interestingly, several of these patients had a poor response to AML induction therapy but subsequently responded to an ALL induction regimen. Despite this, children with AML whose blasts express lymphoid antigens should be treated initially on AML protocols.

Table 61-3 Risk Group Stratification in Children's Oncology Group Acute Myeloid Leukemia Trial COG AAML0531

Risk group
Low risk: core binding factor leukemia (inv[16]/t[16:16], t[8;21])
High risk: -7, -5, 5q-, FLT3-ITD high allelic ratio, >15% blasts at end of course 1
Intermediate risk: absence of low-risk or high-risk features

FLT3-ITD, FLT3 internal tandem duplication.

DIFFERENTIAL DIAGNOSIS

The diagnosis of AML is usually straightforward after an examination of the peripheral blood and bone marrow. Other diagnoses that can sometimes cause diagnostic difficulty include the myeloproliferative disorders (e.g., juvenile myelomonocytic leukemia), myelodysplastic (preleukemic) syndromes, and overwhelming bacterial infections that result in leukemoid reactions or neutropenia secondary to a bone marrow maturation arrest in granulocytic precursors. In the last situation, the bone marrow may be confused with APL, but with resolution of the infection, granulocytic maturation ensues. The differential diagnosis of congenital leukemia is somewhat more challenging, in part because of the leukoerythroblastic peripheral blood picture noted in neonates with hypoxia or sepsis. Congenital viral infections, including cytomegalovirus, herpes simplex, human immunodeficiency virus (HIV), and rubella, need to be ruled out as well as the transient myeloproliferative disorder associated with trisomy 21.

PROGNOSIS

Prognostic factors in AML depend on disease characteristics such as cytogenetics, FAB subtype, and associated mutations; host factors; and response to therapy. Favorable-risk patients with APL or Down syndrome patients with acute megakaryoblastic leukemia are treated with separate therapeutic regimens. Although many factors are prognostic, most current pediatric protocols use cytogenetics, additional genetic mutations such as FLT3-ITD, and response to therapy to divide patients into favorable, intermediate, and unfavorable risk groups that are assigned to risk-adapted regimens. There is no standard risk stratification among all of the worldwide cooperative groups. The current Children's Oncology Group (COG) risk stratification is summarized in Table 61-3 and will likely change in the future as new factors identifying better- and poor-risk features are identified.

Disease-Associated Risk Factors

Cytogenetics

Favorable-risk cytogenetics include the core binding factor leukemias with inv(16) or t(8;21) and APL with t(15;17). The St. Jude AML02 study reported 3-year event-free survival (EFS) greater than 84% and 3-year OS greater than 90% for both core binding factor leukemia groups. The Italian Pediatric Hematology and Oncology Group AIDA 0493 trial for APL reported a complete remission (CR) rate of 96%, 10-year EFS of 76%, and 10-year OS of 89%. Poor-risk cytogenetics include monosomy 7 and del(5q). UK MRC AML 10 and 12 trials reported 10-year OS of 32% and 27%, respectively. A novel finding from this study was the poor outcome with abnormalities of 12p with an OS of 35%. Monosomy 5, an adverse cytogenetic marker in adult AML, was not reported in this pediatric series. Abnormalities of 3q, an adverse prognostic factor in adults, had an OS of 57%. Complex karyotype (more than three independent abnormalities) was not an independent prognostic abnormality when adjusted for the presence of other prognostic cytogenetic changes. The 10-year EFS for t(6;9) was 10% with small numbers of patients. Intermediate-risk patients include all others not designated favorable or high risk. Of note, patients with 11q23/MLL rearrangements demonstrated no difference in outcome when compared to patients without MLL rearrangements, with a 10-year OS of 61% in the MRC data.

Non–Down Syndrome Acute Megakaryoblastic Leukemia

Whereas Down syndrome patients less than 4 years of age with AMKL have a favorable prognosis with reduced-intensity chemotherapy, non–Down syndrome patients have a poor prognosis with OS 14% in one single-institution review of 29 patients. Survival was higher in patients who underwent allogeneic stem cell transplant rather than chemotherapy alone. Predominantly seen in infants with non–Down syndrome AMKL, t(1;22)(p13;q13) accounts for one-third of patients with non–Down syndrome AMKL. The WHO recognizes t(1;22) as a distinct biologic entity, and the expression of the fusion gene RBM15-MKL1 can induce AMKL in mouse models. Patients with AMKL and t(1;22) have a better prognosis; in a series of 11 patients the 3-year EFS was 50%, and these patients may not need transplant compared to other patients with non–Down syndrome AMKL without t(1;22).

Leukocyte Count

A WBC count greater than 100,000/μL has been considered a poor prognostic factor. In the St. Jude AML02 trial, however, patients with WBC above or below 50,000/μL had similar outcomes. WBC count is prognostic in APL, and children with WBC greater than 10,000/μL have a higher risk for relapse. The presence of acute mixed-lineage or biphenotypic leukemia (AML with lymphoid-associated antigens) does not influence prognosis.

Genetic Mutations

Additional mutations or aberrant gene expression beyond the characteristic chromosomal translocations are found in AML blasts that have biologic and prognostic significance. As discussed earlier, patients with a somatic FLT3-ITD produce an abnormal protein that confers constitutive activation. FLT3-ITD mutations are found in approximately 12% of pediatric AML and have a poor prognosis regardless of subtype of usually less than 30%. FLT3 activating loop mutations do not appear to be prognostically significant. Because a proportion of patients with FLT3-ITD do well, the role of the wild-type allele has been studied, and the ratio of mutant FLT3-ITD allele to wild-type FLT-3 allele PCR products has been found to be prognostic in retrospective analyses. A mutant to wild-type allelic ratio of greater than 0.4 is being studied prospectively by the COG. The St. Jude collaborative group places patients with FLT3 mutation into a poor-risk category and is evaluating this risk stratification prospectively.

CEBPA encodes the CCAAT/enhancer binding protein-α protein that functions as a basic leucine zipper domain transcription factor that regulates proliferation and granulocytic differentiation. Mutations in CEBPA that cause a premature stop or disrupt the DNA-binding domain were found in adult patients with minimally differentiated AML, AML without maturation, and normal karyotype AML, and these mutations conferred a favorable prognosis. CEBPA mutations were found in 4.5% of a series of 847 pediatric patients and found to be an independent favorable prognostic factor.

The Wilms tumor suppressor gene WT1 is a zinc-finger protein transcription factor. WT1 mutations occur in the zinc-finger DNA-binding domain and are predicted to disrupt DNA binding, but the prognostic significance of WT1 mutations or overexpression has been controversial. Nucleophosmin (NPM1) is a nucleocytoplasmic shuttling protein that regulates the P53-ARF tumor suppressor pathway. Mutations in NPM1 have been found that alter its intracellular localization, and mutated NPM1 is associated with better response to induction and survival in adults. There have been conflicting reports on the prognostic significance of NPM1 mutations in pediatric AML. KIT receptor tyrosine kinase mutations were found in adult core binding factor AML and also pediatric AML but were not found to be prognostically significant. NRAS mutations had no clinical prognostic implication. There have been studies of gene expression levels (WT1, VLA-4, VEGFC, BRE) that divide patients into groups based on whether gene expression is above or below the median and then compare the outcome of the groups. Such studies are difficult to adapt moving forward given the continuous nature of the gene expression variable.

Host Factors

Host factors that influence prognosis include age, race, and body mass index (BMI). Age at diagnosis less than 2 years or greater than 10 years has been found to influence outcome in some studies. In AML02, age greater than 10 years was an adverse prognostic factor, but the recent COG AAML03P1 study of 305 patients did not show an adverse impact of age. Some racial disparities in outcome have been studied, with a trend toward inferior outcome in African American patients compared to white patients. Patients who are underweight (<10%) or overweight (>90%) based on BMI have had worse OS and increased treatment-related mortality.

Response to Treatment

Response to treatment is assessed by morphology and MRD. UK MRC AML 10 reported that primary induction failure with greater than 15% blasts after one course of induction was associated with an extremely poor outcome with survival of 22%. Patients with 5% to 15% blasts had similar survival as patients with complete remission with less than 5% blasts by morphology.

MRD analysis detects leukemic blasts at much higher sensitivity than traditional bone marrow morphologic analysis. MRD can be measured with flow immunophenotyping or PCR for specific translocations or genes associated with disease. Assays with RT-PCR for many of the common gene rearrangements in AML are now available for diagnostic purposes and for following minimal residual leukemia. Genetic markers suitable for RT-PCR studies are found in almost 50% of AML patients. One disadvantage is that leukemic cells may vary in the amount of transcript per cell for an individual chromosomal rearrangement or between patients, making precise quantitation challenging. Flow immunophenotyping can detect an aberrant leukemic phenotype in more than 85% of AML patients at 0.1% to 0.01% residual cells, and detection of more than 0.1% MRD after one round of induction or at end of consolidation was associated with a significantly worse risk for early relapse and OS. Importantly, immunophenotyping detected residual leukemia in 27% to 34% of cases in morphologic remission. In the St. Jude AML02 trial, MRD greater than 1% after induction 1 was an independent prognostic factor for survival. This effect was most pronounced in high-risk patients; MRD was not a significant predictor of relapse or induction

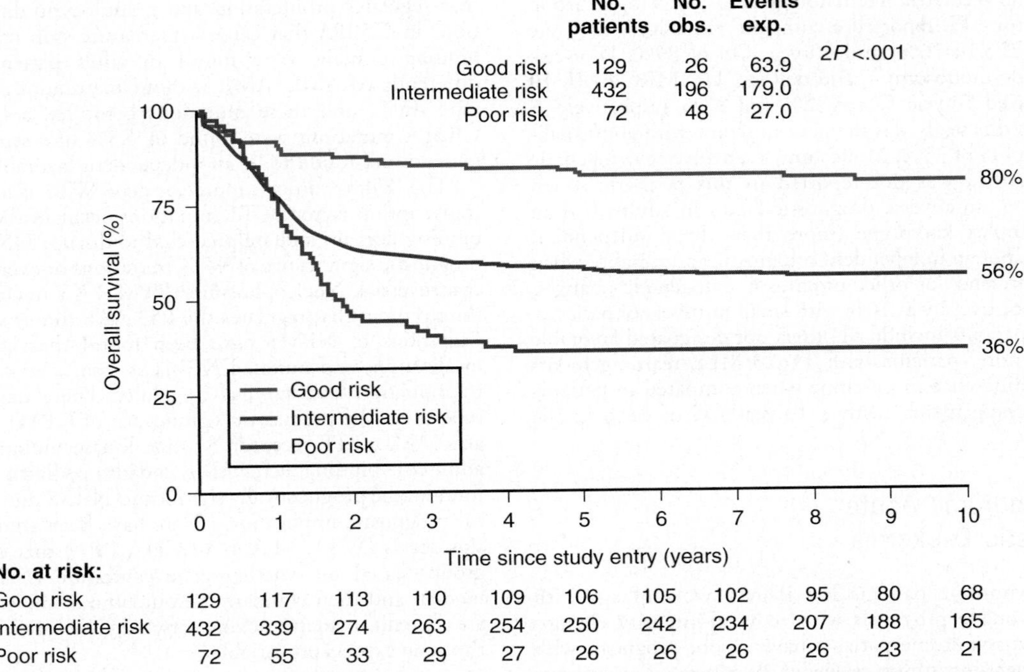

Figure 61-5 OVERALL SURVIVAL IN UNITED KINGDOM MEDICAL RESEARCH COUNCIL AML 10 AND 12 TRIALS BASED ON RISK STRATIFICATION. *Exp.,* Expected; *obs.,* observed. Good risk: t(8;21) and inv(16); poor risk: abn(12p), t(6;9), abn(5q), monosomy 7, t(9;22); intermediate risk: patients not included in the other two groups. *(From Harrison CJ, Hills RK, Moorman AV, et al: Cytogenetics of childhood acute myeloid leukemia: United Kingdom Medical Research Council treatment trials AML 10 and 12.* J Clin Oncol *28:2674, 2010.)*

failure among patients with low-risk or standard-risk disease. CCG-2961 studied MRD levels greater than 0.5% and found 13% of patients with responsive disease (<30% blasts) had occult leukemia, and the presence of occult leukemia was an independent risk factor for OS. Dutch Childhood Oncology Group and MRC results indicate that MRD after induction 1 is a significant independent prognostic factor. The Berlin-Frankfurt Muenster (BFM) group, however, has suggested that MRD is not more predictive of relapse than other traditional prognostic factors such as cytogenetics. Remission by MRD instead of morphology and whether MRD-positive patients benefit from intensified therapy is being studied.

Overall, the use of cytogenetics, MRD, and specific gene markers to predict patients with higher risk for relapse must be further studied prospectively. Current classification schemes predict prognosis for three broad risk categories (Fig. 61-5). There are differences in the prognostic utility of specific gene mutations in adult and pediatric AML. Eventually prospective studies may be used to stratify specific intermediate- or high-risk patients for more intensive or targeted therapy or hematopoietic stem cell transplantation (HSCT). Cooperative groups differ significantly in risk-assignment strategies (see Table 61-3). These classification schema still do not accurately predict specific patients who will ultimately relapse, and newer markers such as phospho-flow must be measured against these established prognostic factors.

THERAPY

The long-term survival (>5 years) rate for children with AML has increased from less than 10% to approximately 60% to 70% during the past 30 years (Table 61-4). This improved cure rate has resulted from more effective remission induction chemotherapy and better strategies to prevent relapse. Current regimens for treating pediatric AML consist of aggressive induction therapy based on a combination of cytarabine and anthracycline to achieve complete remission, followed by consolidation with high-dose cytarabine-based blocks of chemotherapy or stem cell transplant. The decision on transplant depends on risk for relapse, availability of a matched sibling or unrelated donor, and risk for transplant-related mortality. Unlike ALL, there is no extended maintenance therapy, except for APL. Intrathecal CNS treatment and prophylaxis is important, and most groups do not use CNS irradiation. Improvements in supportive care have also been important, making it safe and feasible to treat patients with myelosuppressive doses of chemotherapy. All children with AML should be referred to a pediatric oncology center for treatment and are usually enrolled on a cooperative group clinical trial.

Supportive Care

Excellent supportive care to facilitate children's surviving therapy without significant morbidity is of paramount importance. Before chemotherapy is started, the infant or child should be stabilized with regard to renal, metabolic, hematologic (anemia, bleeding, DIC, leukostasis), and infectious disease issues. A double-lumen indwelling central venous catheter should be placed early in the treatment course. The metabolic derangements associated with leukemic cell death (tumor lysis syndrome) include hyperuricemia, hyperkalemia, hyperphosphatemia, and hypocalcemia. The tumor lysis syndrome is seen more often in children with ALL (especially T cell and mature B cell) than in those with AML. Uric acid nephropathy is avoided by prompt attention to hydration, alkalinization of the urine, and administration of allopurinol. Alternatively, recombinant urate oxidase (rasburicase) converts uric acid to more soluble allantoin and is now used with outstanding efficacy in children expected to have tumor lysis syndrome.

Children with AML are at especially increased risk for bacterial and fungal infections during therapy- and leukemia-induced neutropenia. The most commonly encountered fungal infections are due to *Candida* and *Aspergillus* species. Given the high risk for fungal disease, it is reasonable to provide antifungal prophylaxis during AML therapy; however, there is no standard antifungal prophylactic

Table 61-4 Outcomes From Recent Cooperative Group Pediatric Acute Myeloid Leukemia Trials

	Years of Study	No. of Patients	Early Deaths (%)	Complete Remission Rate (%)	3- or 5-yr EFS	SE	3- or 5-yr OS	SE	First Author
NOPHO-AML 2004	2004-2009	151	1.3	92	57	5	69	5	Abrahamsson
COG AAML03P1	2003-2005	340	1.5	87	53	6	66	5	Cooper
SJCRH AML02	2002-2008	232	0.9	94	63	4	71	4	Rubnitz
JCACSG AML99	2000-2002	240	1.7	95	62	6	76	5	Tsukimoto
BFM-98	1998-2003	473	3.2	88	49	3	62	3	Creutzig
CCG-2961	1996-2002	901	6	88	42	3	52	4	Lange
UK MRC AML 12	1994-2002	445	4	92	56		66		Gibson

BFM, Berlin-Frankfurt Muenster; *CCG,* Children's Cancer Group; *COG,* Children's Oncology Group; *EFS,* event-free survival; *JCACSG,* Japanese Childhood AML Cooperative Study Group; *NOPHO,* Nordic Society for Pediatric Hematology and Oncology; *OS,* overall survival; *SE,* standard error; *SJCRH,* St. Jude Children's Research Hospital; *UK MRC,* United Kingdom Medical Research Council.

regimen. Fluconazole is effective against most *Candida* species but has no activity against *Aspergillus* species. Current commercially available agents with anti-*Aspergillus* activity that have been used in AML patients include the triazoles (itraconazole, voriconazole, and posaconazole), the echinocandins (caspofungin, micafungin, and anidulafungin), and amphotericin B deoxycholate or the lipid preparations of amphotericin. In patients with AML, septicemia due to α-hemolytic streptococcal organisms is associated with high-dose cytarabine, a component of most AML therapeutic protocols. The α-hemolytic streptococcal infections have a high rate of recurrence and associated toxicities during subsequent episodes of intensive chemotherapy. Physicians caring for these children must maintain a high index of suspicion and be prepared to institute appropriate antibiotic coverage in the event of fever or unexplained illness. Administration of prophylactic antibiotics (cefepime, vancomycin, ciprofloxacin) during periods of neutropenia are being studied to prevent septicemia. Prolonged periods of neutropenia have been treated with hematopoietic growth factors (granulocyte or granulocyte-macrophage colony-stimulating factor) during induction and after cycles of intensification chemotherapy, although not all protocols use them. Blood products should all be leuko-poor and irradiated to prevent transfusion-associated graft-versus-host disease. Platelet transfusions are recommended prophylactically if the platelet count is lower than 10,000/μL. The most disturbing gastrointestinal toxicity during therapy is an enterocolitis involving the distal ileum, cecum, and proximal colon. This syndrome is referred to as typhlitis or the right lower quadrant syndrome and is noted in approximately 10% of patients. The signs and symptoms of typhlitis develop approximately 10 to 14 days after the start of chemotherapy. Treatment recommendations include bowel rest and double-coverage broad-spectrum antibiotics for gram-negative organisms. Surgery is rarely needed and is reserved for intestinal perforation, abdominal wall fasciitis, or massive bleeding.

One percent to 2% of children with AML still die within the first several days to a week after diagnosis. These early deaths usually result from intracranial hemorrhage from either a coagulopathy or CNS leukostasis. If the leukocyte count is greater than 100,000/μL, it is important to initiate urgent measures to prevent leukostasis with leukapheresis, exchange transfusion, or hydroxyurea.

Remission Induction

Because of the narrow therapeutic index of the active agents in AML, all induction regimens (except for APL) are designed to produce rapid bone marrow hypoplasia, an apparent prerequisite for successful remission induction. The combination of cytarabine (7 days) and daunorubicin (3 days), known as the "7+3" regimen, has been the traditional backbone of induction chemotherapy. Approximately one-third of these patients require two courses of induction to achieve a remission. Protocols using intensified induction by timing or dose intensity (10 to 12 days of cytarabine or high-dose cytarabine) have demonstrated improved remission rates between 83% and 94% with superior OS (see Table 61-4). Children's Cancer Group CCG-2891 compared standard timing, allowing for hematologic recovery, with intensive timing during induction and found that remission rates were similar but EFS was improved with intensive timing. The addition of a third agent such as etoposide or thioguanine during induction is now widely used, and a randomization of DAT (daunorubicin, cytarabine [ara-C], thioguanine) versus ADE (cytarabine [ara-C], daunorubicin, etoposide) in MRC AML 10 showed no significant differences between the two induction regimens. Patients receiving intensified induction have had statistically significant increases in disease-free survival compared with those patients randomized to standard 7+3 induction. These data are consistent with the hypothesis that more effective early leukemic cell kill reduces the likelihood of a subsequent relapse in children and adults with AML. Lower remission rates are seen in patients with therapy-related AML, a history of a prior MDS, and certain cytogenetic findings or gene mutations (see Prognosis). Because of the requisite period of bone marrow hypoplasia and the greater impairment of bone marrow reserve in patients with AML, the remission induction phase of therapy is more toxic than for patients with ALL. A major concern is the appropriateness of current dose adjustments made in chemotherapy protocols for infants less than 1 year of age (generally based on milligram-per-kilogram arbitrary dose reductions of 25%). Prospectively controlled pediatric and adult cooperative group studies have shown that daunorubicin is preferable to doxorubicin because it is associated with less oral mucositis and gastrointestinal toxicity. Several adult and pediatric AML studies have explored the benefits of substituting either mitoxantrone or idarubicin for daunorubicin. Mitoxantrone is at least as effective as daunorubicin. Idarubicin is not superior to daunorubicin for remission induction and is associated with more marrow toxicity and greater number of days until neutrophil recovery. Gemtuzumab ozogamicin is a humanized monoclonal antibody against CD33 conjugated to the calicheamicin toxin. This antigen-directed therapy has been combined safely with standard induction and consolidation regimens. Hepatotoxicity, including venoocclusive disease, has been reported. Gemtuzumab ozogamicin was recently withdrawn from the United States due to lack of clear-cut benefit in improving overall outcome.

Acute Promyelocytic Leukemia

In the past, approximately 65% to 75% of patients with APL entered remission after a standard induction with daunorubicin and cytarabine. The remission induction period, however, was associated with significant early mortality secondary to hemorrhagic complications. Prompt all-trans retinoic acid (ATRA) therapy, without waiting for confirmation of molecular diagnosis, has reduced, but not eliminated, these hemorrhagic complications. ATRA appears to downregulate tissue factor expression and thereby reduces the severity and duration of DIC in APL patients. At present, all patients should be carefully followed with serial coagulation studies (partial thromboplastin time, prothrombin time, fibrinogen, and fibrin split products). The optimal management of coagulopathy is controversial.

European and American clinical trials have established the current standard front-line therapy, which combines ATRA with anthracycline-based chemotherapy for remission induction and consolidation chemotherapy and with ATRA continuing during 2 years of maintenance, resulting in complete remission rate greater than 90% and OS higher than 80%. The ATRA-induced remissions are associated with differentiation of the blasts/promyelocytes into mature granulocytes. Recent results support a potential role for the addition of cytarabine for patients at higher risk for relapse with initial WBC count greater than 10,000/μL. Unlike other AML subtypes, APL patients benefit from a maintenance course of ATRA-containing therapy for a duration of 2 years.

Arsenic trioxide (As_2O_3 or ATO) has impressive activity in relapse and de novo APL. ATO binds the PML moiety of the PML-RARA oncoprotein, leading to the recruitment of the small ubiquitin-like protein modifier (SUMO)-conjugating enzyme UBC9 and subsequent degradation of PML-RARA. The potential benefit of arsenic in consolidation remains controversial despite the results of the U.S. Intergroup study showing a significant benefit in EFS and OS for patients receiving two courses of arsenic given immediately after CR. The rare (1% of APL) variant PLZF-RARA t(11;17)(q23;q21) is insensitive to ATRA or ATO; other rare alternative rearrangements seen in APL may be treatable with ATRA.

ATRA is associated with several life-threatening complications, including severe respiratory distress and capillary leak syndrome and pseudotumor cerebri (more common in pediatric patients). The retinoic acid syndrome (respiratory distress and weight gain) has been successfully managed in most patients by temporary cessation of ATRA and administration of dexamethasone. The symptoms of pseudotumor cerebri disappear within days after withdrawal of ATRA, and the drug can usually be safely restarted at a reduced dose. This syndrome has also been seen in response to treatment with ATO and thus might better be termed the *differentiation syndrome.*

The ability to detect PML-RARA messenger RNA by RT-PCR is a useful method of monitoring the efficacy of therapy. When used at the 10^{-4} sensitivity level, persistent positive RT-PCR findings after the consolidation phase strongly predict hematologic relapse. Those patients in molecular relapse can be reinduced and treated with stem cell transplant. ATO can be used to achieve remissions in those patients who relapse after ATRA treatment.

Central Nervous System Leukemia

All pediatric AML studies include intrathecal chemotherapy, because isolated CNS relapse occurs in approximately 20% of children with AML who did not receive any CNS-directed therapy, and CNS relapse is associated with worse survival. Cytarabine alone or triple intrathecal therapy with cytarabine, methotrexate, and hydrocortisone are the most commonly used regimens worldwide. In contrast to ALL, the finding of blasts in the CSF at diagnosis in children with AML does not adversely affect prognosis. An accepted approach for the treatment of CNS leukemia is weekly intrathecal chemotherapy until the CSF is clear of blasts. In some protocols, this is followed by CNS irradiation at the end of systemic chemotherapy.

Treatment in Remission

Without further treatment after standard induction chemotherapy, more than 90% of patients relapse within 1 year, and the remainder relapse by 2 years. The intensity and duration of chemotherapy in remission, as well as the role of HSCT in first remission, have been areas of active investigation and controversy during the past decades. In the 1970s, pediatric AML studies tested whether modestly myelosuppressive combination chemotherapy given in remission would improve OS. These protocols led to a plateau in disease-free survival of 15% to 20% at 5 years. In an effort to improve upon these disappointing results, other approaches were explored, including early intensification or consolidation chemotherapy and HSCT. Allogeneic HSCT provided an opportunity for delivering very high doses of chemotherapy and/or irradiation and possibly stimulating a graft-versus-leukemia effect. Although the initial studies were not randomized, the results suggested a benefit for either the intensification of chemotherapy or HSCT early in first remission. Cytarabine, the single most active agent in AML, was the prototype drug for intensification, because laboratory and clinical studies indicated that a log increase in its dose could overcome certain mechanisms of resistance. Approximately 40% of patients with AML who are refractory to standard doses of cytarabine achieve a complete remission with high-dose cytarabine. The superiority of high-dose compared to standard-dose cytarabine has also been confirmed in a prospective randomized clinical trial in adults with AML. Most pediatric AML studies that were initiated in the 1980s and 1990s included several consolidation cycles of high-dose cytarabine. These protocols resulted in 5-year leukemia-free survival plateaus of 35% to 60%. Clinical studies in the most recent decade have evolved and indicate that timed sequential induction and therapies using repeated courses of intensive consolidation result in 5-year EFS rate of 50% to 60%. High-dose cytarabine is given alone or in combination with other agents such as mitoxantrone, asparaginase, or etoposide. The optimal number of consolidation chemotherapy cycles has not been determined but is usually two to three cycles. Maintenance chemotherapy with oral thioguanine and standard doses of cytarabine given after consolidation chemotherapy has not been shown to further increase the proportion of patients in long-term remission. Patients who receive maintenance have a poor salvage rate if relapsed because of clinical drug resistance.

Haploidentical natural killer cell transplant is a novel regimen to maintain remission after consolidation. In the St. Jude NKAML pilot study, 10 favorable- or standard-risk patients in remission received an immunosuppressive regimen followed by KIR-mismatched natural killer (NK) cell infusion. The 2-year EFS was 100% with minimal toxicity, and this approach is being studied further.

Hematopoietic Stem Cell Transplantation in First Remission

Allogeneic HSCT from a histocompatible family donor was first evaluated in children and young adults with AML in first remission in the mid-1970s. Published data from many pediatric AML bone marrow transplant series show 5-year EFS rates ranging from 56% to 74%. Many of the early transplant studies, however, were not prospectively designed and therefore were biased in their selection criteria, were not controlled for the timing of HSCT in first remission, and excluded patients who were eligible for a transplant but who relapsed before the procedure. In an effort to avoid these and other biases, it was suggested that the outcomes of studies comparing HSCT to chemotherapy be analyzed according to the intention-to-treat analysis, which includes all eligible patients (i.e., those having a matched family donor) and not just individuals who actually received the transplant. When the data are analyzed in this way, there is still a statistically significant OS advantage for allogeneic HSCT compared with chemotherapy in some studies. In the setting where no matched related donor was available, three randomized trials concluded that autologous stem cell transplant was not beneficial compared to intensive chemotherapy for consolidation (see box on Role of Hematopoietic Stem Cell Transplantation in Pediatric Acute Myeloid Leukemia).

Allogeneic HSCT early in first remission using an HLA-matched related donor results in a significantly better disease-free survival rate as compared with chemotherapy but is limited to approximately 20% of patients with a suitable donor. There is significant risk for acute (acute graft-versus-host disease, interstitial pneumonia, hepatic veno-occlusive disease) and chronic morbidity (growth problems, gonadal toxicity, secondary malignancy, and chronic graft-versus-host disease)

Role of Hematopoietic Stem Cell Transplantation in Pediatric Acute Myeloid Leukemia

Outcomes in pediatric acute myeloid leukemia (AML) show a benefit for allogeneic transplant in first remission for select patients, but the risk for treatment-related mortality with transplant must be weighed against the improved outcomes with chemotherapy alone because of sequential dose-intensive regimens. The choice of chemotherapy versus hematopoietic stem cell transplantation (HSCT) in first remission therefore depends on prognostic factors and the availability of a suitable donor. The authors recommend matched related or, if a sibling donor is unavailable, matched unrelated HSCT for patients with high-risk features, including monosomy 7, FLT3 internal tandem duplication mutation, and patients with refractory disease after two courses of induction. Allogeneic HSCT in first remission should also be considered for non–Down syndrome patients with French-American-British (FAB) M7 morphology given recent reports of poor outcomes with this subtype. Favorable-risk patients (i.e., Down syndrome M7, inv[16], t[15;17], t[8;21]) should be treated with chemotherapy alone. All other patients without high-risk features in first remission should be treated with consolidative chemotherapy alone, because multiple studies have shown equivalent outcomes compared to autologous or allogeneic transplant. For these patients without high-risk features, matched related or matched unrelated HSCT should be reserved for relapsed disease. An autologous transplant should be considered in second remission when there is no suitable allogeneic donor. Haploidentical transplants are still considered experimental but show promise as an alternative especially with a KIR mismatch.

FLT3

Patients with FLT3 internal tandem duplication (FLT3-ITD) mutation are at a higher risk for relapse, with estimates of overall survival at approximately 30%. The optimal management of these patients is still controversial, and there are several approaches by different cooperative groups. The Children's Oncology Group has identified subsets of patients who are at higher risk, based on the ratio of polymerase chain reaction amplification of wild-type versus FLT3-ITD alleles. The St. Jude collaborative group places patients with FLT3-ITD and minimal residual disease of 0.1% or more in the high-risk category. The United Kingdom Medical Research Council does not assign risk category based on FLT3-ITD status, but patients with FLT3-ITD are randomized to receive lestaurtinib. Kinase inhibitors such as lestaurtinib, sorafenib, and newer agents are being studied in combination with standard acute myeloid leukemia therapy, but their efficacy has not been proven, and they should be used in the context of a clinical trial. For consolidation most agree that hematopoietic stem cell transplantation (HSCT) with matched sibling donor is warranted for FLT3-ITD patients. There are not enough data to definitively recommend alternative donor transplantation in the absence of a matched sibling donor; however, it is not unreasonable to offer alternative donor HSCT given the poor prognosis of these patients.

and mortality with allogeneic transplant. Therefore an outstanding question is the identification of risk groups that benefit from matched related donor transplant. For those children with AML who have a relatively favorable prognosis after treatment with chemotherapy (e.g., t[15;17], t[8;21], inv[16], Down syndrome), it is reasonable to reserve HSCT for early relapse or second remission. Retrospective analysis of four cooperative group clinical trials by Horan et al showed no benefit for matched related donor transplant in the favorable-risk group patients.

In the same meta-analysis with intermediate-risk patients, there was a trend toward increase in 8-year OS in patients undergoing transplant versus chemotherapy alone (62% ± 7% versus 51% ± 5%, $P = 0.06$) due to decreased incidence of relapse. However, although AML99, NOPHO 93, MRC 10, and MRC 12 showed significant improvement in disease-free survival in patients with matched related donors, the OS difference was not significant. Many patients treated with chemotherapy alone in CR1 who relapsed could be salvaged. Therefore matched related donor transplant may be reserved for relapse in intermediate-risk patients, especially normal karyotype patients with wild-type FLT3 and CEBPA or NPM1 mutations that appear to confer favorable risk.

For poor-risk patients, outcomes for patients undergoing related HSCT was similar to chemotherapy alone. In AML02 high-risk patients with MRD greater than 1% after induction 1, HSCT showed a trend toward OS benefit (43% ± 12% versus 23% ± 10%, $P = 0.14$). Options for therapy intensification in poor-risk patients is limited, and most groups recommend transplant with matched related donor if available. Whether poor-risk patients benefit from alternative donor transplant (matched unrelated donor, cord blood) is not established. Recent advances have made the risk for toxicity with alternative donors approach that of matched related donors.

Although FLT3-ITD is a poor prognostic factor, whether to transplant based on the presence of FLT3-ITD alone is controversial. Data from MRC suggest that FLT3-ITD by itself is not a reason for transplant. In 683 adults comparing donor versus no-donor, the relapse risk was decreased if a donor was available and there was a trend toward benefit in OS, but this effect was seen in both FLT3-ITD and FLT3 wild-type AML. Data from COG showed that in individuals with a matched related donor, FLT3-ITD is no longer prognostic, suggesting that FLT3-ITD patients benefit from transplant. However, in this study by Meschinchi et al, 4-year OS comparison for FLT3-ITD patients in remission treated with HSCT versus chemotherapy alone was not significantly different (64% ± 29% versus 48% ± 17%, $P = 0.4$). It may be the case that FLT3-ITD patients benefit from allogeneic transplant, but larger studies of OS in pediatric patients with FLT3-ITD comparing transplant versus chemotherapy alone in intention-to-treat analysis and taking into account cytogenetic risk group are needed. Incorporation of other factors such as MRD may also help in identifying FLT3-ITD patients in need of transplant (see box on FLT3).

HSCT should be considered in first remission for children with high-risk features and be reserved for use in second remission or early relapse in all others. The decision to use HSCT for intermediate-risk patients in CR1 remains controversial. Up to 50% to 60% of patients with AML who achieve second remission and receive allogeneic transplantation appear to be long-term leukemia-free survivors. Patients with refractory disease or who relapse after intensive therapy within a year of diagnosis have a very poor prognosis with any form of therapy, including HSCT.

Myeloid Proliferations Related to Down Syndrome

Myeloid proliferations related to Down syndrome were recognized as a distinct category in the 2008 WHO classification of AML because of their unique genetic and clinical characteristics. These proliferations are seen as a transient abnormal myelopoiesis in neonates, and myeloid leukemia in young children. Some neonates with Down syndrome or trisomy 21 mosaicism may manifest a transient myeloproliferative disorder (TMD). This intriguing syndrome is diagnosed in 10% of neonates with Down syndrome, usually during the first week of life. TMD cannot be readily distinguished from congenital AML. The blasts have been shown to be clonal in origin, and there is complete clinical and hematologic recovery in approximately 80% of children with TMD within weeks to 3 months without therapy. Infants with TMD or transient leukemia may have very elevated

WBC counts with circulating blasts (megakaryoblasts or erythroblasts), hepatosplenomegaly, and an increased percentage of blasts in the bone marrow. There is a small subgroup of infants with TMD who die of liver failure and multiorgan system failure. In some of these patients, hepatic fibrosis is associated with megakaryoblast infiltration of the liver. Because the majority of infants with TMD never require any therapy in the first months of life, these neonates should be observed and given supportive care. However, for the small group of infants with liver failure or hydrops fetalis, a course of low-dose cytarabine may be helpful.

Data from retrospective surveys indicate that 30% of infants with TMD eventually develop AML (mostly AMKL) before 4 years of age. It is not known whether this is a recurrence of the original disease or the appearance of a new disease. Before the onset of AML, there is often a several-month prodrome characterized by thrombocytopenia and bone marrow myelofibrosis with dysplastic megakaryocytes. Mutations in the GATA-1 gene, an erythroid/megakaryoblastic transcription factor, are present in the blast cells from infants with TMD as well as patients with Down syndrome and AMKL.

An unexpected finding has been the high cure rate of AML in children with Down syndrome AMKL, including those who had TMD as neonates. This may in part be due to an increased in vitro sensitivity of Down syndrome myeloblasts to chemotherapy, especially cytarabine and daunorubicin. In in vitro studies with cytarabine, there is greater generation of ara-C triphosphate (ara-CTP) compared to myeloblasts from children without Down syndrome. Excellent results have been obtained with reduced-intensity therapy, with 91% OS in BFM trials, as compared to 56% survival in non–Down syndrome M7 AML. Reduced-intensity therapy is especially important because of increased susceptibility to anthracycline-induced cardiotoxicity in Down syndrome patients. Reducing chemotherapy is also advisable in Down syndrome AML patients because they appear to be more susceptible to treatment-related mortality, especially in intensive-timed regimens. Thus most cooperative groups treat Down syndrome AML on reduced-intensity regimens.

Therapy-Related AML

AML as a secondary malignancy after chemotherapy for another malignancy represents a difficult-to-treat subgroup of pediatric AML. Risk for therapy-related AML is primarily related to treatment with alkylating agents and epipodophyllotoxins. Common cytogenetic abnormalities include loss or deletions of chromosomes 5 and 7 and 11q23 MLL rearrangements. These patients are often heavily pretreated with ongoing morbidity from prior treatment. Complete remission rates in CCG-2951 were 50%, compared to 72% for de novo AML. OS in small series range from 14% to 26%. These patients should be treated with intensive induction therapy. There is little data comparing allogeneic stem cell transplant versus chemotherapy for consolidation, but in most reports survivors had undergone transplant.

Management of Relapse

The prognosis for children who do not enter remission with frontline chemotherapy or who suffer an on-therapy relapse is very poor. Intensive reinduction therapies and HSCT for second complete remission are associated with significant treatment-related morbidity and mortality. Chemotherapy options are sometimes limited due to cumulative anthracycline exposure. Many different chemotherapy regimens have been evaluated in children and adults with refractory or relapsed AML. Relapse regimens that have been investigated include high-dose cytarabine with L-asparaginase or mitoxantrone, etoposide (VP-16) and amsacrine with or without azacitidine, fludarabine and cytarabine, and 2-chlorodeoxyadenosine (2-CDA). Clofarabine is a nucleoside analogue that shows promise in relapsed leukemia as monotherapy or in combination with other agents. Other investigational agents include farnesyltransferase inhibitors, inhibitors of the mammalian target of rapamycin, kinase inhibitors, proteasome inhibitors, and epigenetic modifiers.

The best predictor of response to chemotherapy after relapse is the duration of the first remission. Children who relapse within 1 year after achieving remission have a substantially lower likelihood of achieving a second remission when compared with those patients who relapse later. The complete remission rate is 30% to 40% for the former group and 60% to 70% for the latter group. Fewer than 20% of the complete responders are projected to remain in remission for more than 2 years, unless they receive an HSCT.

The projected 5-year survival rate after an allogeneic or autologous HSCT in second remission is 40% to 60%. Because of the higher rate of relapse after an autologous compared to an allogeneic HSCT, there is growing experience with matched unrelated donor transplants using bone marrow or cord blood. In selected patients (short duration of first remission or early relapse), it is reasonable to undertake an HSCT without an attempt at inducing a second remission. This is feasible only if a transplant option is immediately available and the patient is clinically stable. A second transplant for multiply relapsed AML is feasible.

For relapsed patients without a matched related or unrelated donor, haploidentical transplants have become an option. Outcomes are typically worse compared to matched related transplants. However, mismatch at the KIR locus has been suggested to lead to improved outcomes in haploidentical transplants owing to NK cell alloreactivity. A subset of killer immunoglobulin-like receptors (KIRs) expressed on NK cells will inhibit NK cell function when engaged by specific major histocompatibility class I proteins. In HSCT, NK donor cells are thought to help eliminate recipient leukemia cells if the recipient cells do not express the cognate major histocompatibility epitope for the donor's inhibitory KIR. For matched unrelated transplants, the effect of KIR mismatch is not as clear.

Less than 5% of patients who achieve remission develop isolated CNS relapse. Risk factors for CNS relapse include age less than 2 years, hepatosplenomegaly, CNS disease at diagnosis, high WBC count, monocytic morphology, and chromosome 11q23 abnormalities. A COG study of 33 patients with isolated CNS relapse reported OS of 26%. Outcome following systemic versus local therapy was similar, suggesting that the rare patients with CNS relapse can be treated with local therapy alone, although this conclusion should be interpreted with caution because of the retrospective nature and small number of patients in this study.

FUTURE DIRECTIONS

The major challenge for the future is to continue improvement on all fronts for the care of patients with AML, including understanding the biology of the leukemic stem cell, disease classification, supportive care, development of more-effective therapies, and how to deliver the optimal combination of therapy for an individual patient. Although improved over past rates, the 5-year EFS rate is still only approximately 50% to 60%, and a substantial portion of children with AML continue to relapse and ultimately die of their disease. The primary cause of relapse is the development of drug resistance, and newer insights into the multiple mechanisms of drug resistance are beginning to be elucidated. Not to be overlooked is the importance of optimizing supportive care, because the treatment-related mortality with AML is still substantial.

Risk stratification and optimal treatment for different risk groups is a major issue. Current cytogenetics-based stratification schemes have identified good-risk patients (core binding factor leukemias, APL, and Down AMKL) but fare poorly in identifying intermediate-risk and high-risk patients who will ultimately relapse. Prospective incorporation of information on genetic mutations, MRD, gene expression, epigenetic profiles, and phospho-flow will better delineate at-risk patients. In most cases, these risk factors and their effect on prognosis will differ in pediatric versus adult AML.

Once patients are stratified, new therapies are needed that interfere with leukemia-related biologic processes. Lestaurtinib, a small-molecule inhibitor of FLT3, has selective toxicity against FLT3-ITD AML cell lines and in mouse models, but cells can develop resistance to FLT3 inhibition. Other FLT3 inhibitors are in various stages of development and clinical trials testing. Sorafenib is a Raf kinase inhibitor that also has activity against FLT3-ITD in vitro and in mouse models. The proteasome regulates the levels of many intracellular proteins, including NF- κB, and proteasome inhibition has been effective in myeloproliferative disorders. Bortezomib is a proteasome inhibitor that has in vitro activity and synergy with chemotherapeutic agents against primary AML cell lines. Regulation of epigenetic modifications with histone deacetylase and DNA methyltransferase inhibitors is also another promising area of research. Intriguing, novel efforts to screen libraries of small molecules based on their effect on gene expression signatures has yielded unexpected compounds active in promoting differentiation of AML. Antibodies targeting CD47-expressing leukemia stem cells are being developed. Many of these new agents are being tested up front in high-risk patients in a risk-adapted strategy and in the relapse setting. Eventually it may be possible to target the genetic lesions of leukemic cells in other AML subtypes, as exemplified by the use of ATRA in APL or imatinib in chronic myelogenous leukemia. In a completely different approach, the use of NK cells has been studied as a cell-based therapy outside of HSCT. NK cells from haploidentical donors, but mismatched at the KIR locus, can be isolated and infused into recipients and expanded in vivo using a combination of immunosuppressive agents and interleukin-2 to provide an antileukemia effect. This approach has been used to successfully maintain remission in low- and standard-risk patients treated with chemotherapy alone.

The improved ability to measure MRD by PCR, immunophenotyping, or specific genetic alterations should result in giving therapy when leukemic burden is smaller and selected intensification of therapy in the presence of residual leukemia. Through the development of new agents, improved monitoring, intelligent use of biologic response modifiers, and limiting the use of HSCT to high-risk patients, therapy can be closely tailored to improve outcome. For high-risk patients, the increasing availability of alternative sources of hematopoietic stem cells from unrelated bone marrow or cord blood donors will greatly expand the use of HSCT in all phases of therapy. Strategies based on preclinical models are also being developed that will hopefully achieve a more favorable balance of the graft-versus-host and graft-versus-leukemia reactions.

SUGGESTED READINGS

Abrahamsson J, Forestier E, Heldrup J, et al: Response-guided induction therapy in pediatric acute myeloid leukemia with excellent remission rate. *J Clin Oncol* 29:310, 2011 Jan. 20.

Barnard DR, Woods WG: Treatment-related myelodysplastic syndrome/acute myeloid leukemia in survivors of childhood cancer—an update. *Leuk Lymphoma* 46:651, 2005 May.

Cooper TM, Franklin J, Gerbing RB, et al: AAML03P1, a pilot study of the safety of gemtuzumab ozogamicin in combination with chemotherapy for newly diagnosed childhood acute myeloid leukemia. *Cancer* 118:761, 2012.

Creutzig U: Less toxicity by optimizing chemotherapy, but not by addition of granulocyte colony-stimulating factor in children and adolescents with acute myeloid leukemia: Results of AML-BFM 98. *J Clin Oncol* 24:4499, 2006 Aug. 22.

Figueroa ME, Lugthart S, Li Y, et al: DNA methylation signatures identify biologically distinct subtypes in acute myeloid leukemia. *Cancer Cell* 17:13, 2010 Feb. 10.

Gamis AS, Howells WB, DeSwarte-Wallace J, et al: Alpha hemolytic streptococcal infection during intensive treatment for acute myeloid leukemia: A report from the Children's Cancer Group study CCG-2891. *J Clin Oncol* 18:1845, 2000 May.

Gibson BE, Wheatley K, Hann IM, et al: Treatment strategy and long-term results in paediatric patients treated in consecutive UK AML trials. *Leukemia* 19:2130, 2005 Dec.

Harrison CJ, Hills RK, Moorman AV, et al: Cytogenetics of childhood acute myeloid leukemia: United Kingdom Medical Research Council Treatment trials AML 10 and 12. *J Clin Oncol* 28:2674, 2010 Jun. 1.

Ho PA, Alonzo TA, Gerbing RB, et al: Prevalence and prognostic implications of CEBPA mutations in pediatric acute myeloid leukemia (AML): A report from the Children's Oncology Group. *Blood* 113:6558, 2009 Jun. 25.

Ho PA, Kutny MA, Alonzo TA, et al: Leukemic mutations in the methylation-associated genes DNMT3A and IDH2 are rare events in pediatric AML: A report from the Children's Oncology Group. *Pediatr Blood Cancer* 57:204, 2011 Aug.

Johnston DL, Alonzo TA, Gerbing RB, et al: The presence of central nervous system disease at diagnosis in pediatric acute myeloid leukemia does not affect survival: A Children's Oncology Group study. *Pediatr Blood Cancer* 55:414, 2010 Sep.

Lange BJ, Smith FO, Feusner J, et al: Outcomes in CCG-2961, a Children's Oncology Group phase 3 trial for untreated pediatric acute myeloid leukemia: A report from the Children's Oncology Group. *Blood* 111:1044, 2007 Oct. 25.

Ley TJ, Mardis ER, Ding L, et al: DNA sequencing of a cytogenetically normal acute myeloid leukaemia genome. *Nature* 456:66, 2008 Nov. 6.

Majeti R, Chao MP, Alizadeh AA, et al: CD47 is an adverse prognostic factor and therapeutic antibody target on human acute myeloid leukemia stem cells. *Cell* 138:286, 2009 Jul. 23.

Massey GV, Zipursky A, Chang MN, et al: A prospective study of the natural history of transient leukemia (TL) in neonates with Down syndrome (DS): Children's Oncology Group (COG) study POG-9481. *Blood* 107:4606, 2006 Jun. 15.

Pui C-H, Howard SC: Current management and challenges of malignant disease in the CNS in paediatric leukaemia. *Lancet Oncol* 9:257, 2008 Mar.

Rubnitz JE, Inaba H, Dahl G, et al: Minimal residual disease-directed therapy for childhood acute myeloid leukaemia: Results of the AML02 multicentre trial. *Lancet Oncol* 11:543, 2010 Jun. 1.

Rubnitz JE, Inaba H, Ribeiro RC, et al: NKAML: A pilot study to determine the safety and feasibility of haploidentical natural killer cell transplantation in childhood acute myeloid leukemia. *J Clin Oncol* 28:955, 2010 Feb. 18.

Testi AM, Biondi A, Lo-Coco F, et al: GIMEMA-AIEOPAIDA protocol for the treatment of newly diagnosed acute promyelocytic leukemia (APL) in children. *Blood* 106:447, 2005 Jul. 15.

Tsukimoto I, Tawa A, Horibe K, et al: Risk-stratified therapy and the intensive use of cytarabine improves the outcome in childhood acute myeloid leukemia: The AML99 Trial from the Japanese Childhood AML Cooperative Study Group. *J Clin Oncol* 27:4007, 2009 Aug. 18.

Vardiman JW, Thiele J, Arber DA, et al: The 2008 revision of the World Health Organization (WHO) classification of myeloid neoplasms and acute leukemia: Rationale and important changes. *Blood* 114:937, 2009 Jul. 30.

Wells RJ, Woods WG, Buckley JD, et al: Treatment of newly diagnosed children and adolescents with acute myeloid leukemia: A Children's Cancer Group study. *J Clin Oncol* 12:2367, 1994 Nov.

Woods WG, Neudorf S, Gold S, et al: A comparison of allogeneic bone marrow transplantation, autologous bone marrow transplantation, and aggressive chemotherapy in children with acute myeloid leukemia in remission. *Blood* 97:56, 2001 Jan. 1.

CHAPTER 62

MYELODYSPLASTIC AND MYELOPROLIFERATIVE NEOPLASMS IN CHILDREN

Franklin O. Smith and Mignon L. Loh

The myelodysplastic (MDS) and myeloproliferative neoplasms (MPN) are a heterogeneous group of clonal stem cell disorders that result in ineffective hematopoiesis and an increased risk of developing acute myeloid leukemia (AML). In children, MDS and MPN are now classified into three main groups: MDS, juvenile myelomonocytic leukemia (JMML), and transient myeloproliferative disorder (TMD) in children with Down syndrome. Whereas in MDS, ineffective hematopoiesis results in progressive cytopenias, in MPN, at least initially, ineffective hematopoiesis leads to excessive proliferation frequently characterized by increased peripheral blood counts. MDS and MPN are rare in children. Chronic myeloid leukemia (CML), characterized by the Philadelphia chromosome (*BCR/ABL* positive) is seen in both children and adults, but other forms of MPN (polycythemia vera [PV], essential thrombocythemia [ET], primary myelofibrosis [PMF], chronic neutrophilic leukemia [CNL], chronic eosinophilic leukemia [CEL], chronic basophilic leukemia [CBL], chronic myelomonocytic leukemia [CMML], systemic mastocytosis [SM], and stem cell leukemia–lymphoma syndrome [SCLL]) are exceedingly rare in children. Readers interested in CML and disorders that are predominantly found in adults are referred to in Chapters 59 and 66 to 69. In contrast, two MPNs are uniquely pediatric: JMML and Down syndrome-associated TMD.

MYELODYSPLASTIC SYNDROMES

The MDS are a heterogeneous group of disorders characterized by ineffective hematopoiesis, impaired maturation of hematopoietic cells, progressive cytopenias, and dysplastic changes in the bone marrow (BM).

Epidemiology

Myelodysplastic syndrome is a common malignancy of adults with an incidence of 50 cases per million in people older than the age of 60 years.[1] In contrast, MDS accounts for only 3% to 7% of all hematologic malignancies in children, with an unknown true incidence. Several population-based studies have been performed with reported incidences of 4.0 cases per million in Denmark,[2] 3.1 per million in British Columbia,[3] and 1.35 per million in the United Kingdom.[4] The median age of presentation is 6.8 years with an equal sex distribution.[4-6]

Pathobiology

As in adults, MDS in children can be considered as primary (de novo) or secondary. In adults, two predominant patterns of primary, de novo MDS have been observed. In the first of these patterns, the disease is indolent in nature and is characterized by prolonged survival, little accumulated genetic damage, and a low probability of progression to AML. This group of diseases is best exemplified by the 5q-syndrome, an entity not seen in children. Far more common in adults is a disease characterized by the accumulation of genetic damage, progression to BM failure, and a high probability of developing AML. This form of the disease is characterized as a mutator phenotype.[7] The primary myelodysplastic syndromes seen in children appear to share this mutator phenotype.

As in adults, secondary MDS in children can also arise as sequelae from exposure to chemotherapy and radiation; however, MDS in children may also result from constitutional BM failure syndromes including Fanconi anemia, severe congenital neutropenia (SCN), Shwachman-Diamond syndrome, congenital amegakaryocytic thrombocytopenia, dyskeratosis congenital. and Diamond-Blackfan anemia.

Ongoing studies are now defining the molecular pathogenesis and interrelationships among MDS, myeloproliferative syndromes (MPS), and AML.[8-10] Accumulating data suggest that aberrant signal transduction resulting from acquired somatic mutations encoding proteins leading to hyperactivation of the Ras pathway may stimulate proliferation without concomitant differentiation.[9] This has been clearly demonstrated in CML *(BCR-ABL)*.[11,12] A number of other putative pathogenetic mutations have been identified in other myeloproliferative disorders, including *JAK*2V617F mutations in PV, ET, and PMF[13]; *KIT*D816V mutations in SM[14]; *FIPL1-PDGFRA* in CEL-SM[15]; *ZNF198-FG4FR1* mutations in SCLL[16]; *RAS/NF1/PTPN11* mutations in JMML[17-19]; and *GATA1* mutations in TMD (Fig. 62-1).[20]

AML is the result of cooperating mutations in genes that confer a proliferative and survival advantage without effecting differentiation (e.g., activating mutations in receptor tyrosine kinases [FLT3, c-kit]) and genes that impair differentiation and apoptosis (e.g., loss of function mutations in transcription factors [CBF, AML/ETO]) (Fig. 62-2). This multistep model for the pathogenesis of AML is supported by murine models,[21,22] the analysis of leukemia in twins,[23-26] and the analysis of patients with familial platelet disorder with a propensity to develop AML (FDP/AML syndrome).[27] Finally, several mutations have been described in adult MDS that do not appear at all or are only rarely found to be present in children with MDS, including *TP53, CSF1R (FMS)*,[28] *NRAS* and *KRAS2*.[29]

More recently, methylation studies in children with advanced MDS have demonstrated hypermethylation of the CDKN2B (p15) gene[30] or *CALCA* and *CDKN2B* genes.[31] Although the frequency of hypermethylation in children is similar to that seen in adults, the clinical significance of hypermethylation in children with MDS is not yet known. Finally, whole-genome sequencing of adult MDS samples revealed a high frequency of novel mutations in components of RNA spicing mechanisms.[32] The relevance of this unique finding to children with MDS is currently uncertain.

Classification

Until recently, MDS in children was poorly defined, characterized, classified, and reported. In fact, MDS was not included in the International Classification of Childhood Cancer until 2005.[33] Also contributing to this lack of information was the use of classification and prognostic systems designed for adults that have had limited applicability to children. A number of classification systems for children and adults have now been proposed. The most commonly used system is the French-American-British (FAB) system originally

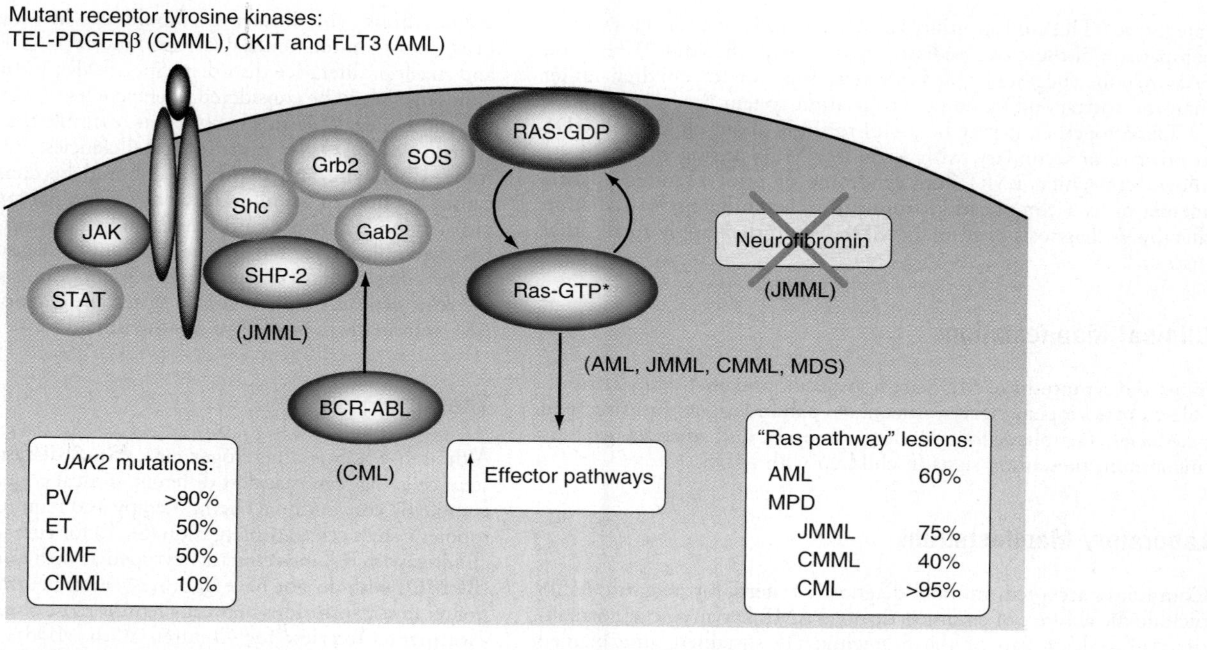

Figure 62-1 OVERVIEW OF RAS SIGNALING WITH MOLECULES HARBORING MUTATIONS IN PATIENTS WITH MYELOID MALIGNANCIES. *AML,* Acute myeloid leukemia; *CML,* chronic myeloid leukemia; *CMML,* chronic myelomonocytic leukemia; *ET,* essential thrombocythema; *GDP,* guanosine diphosphate; *GTP,* guanosine triphosphate; *JMML,* juvenile myelomonocytic leukemia; *MPD,* myeloproliferative disorder; *PV,* polycythemia vera.

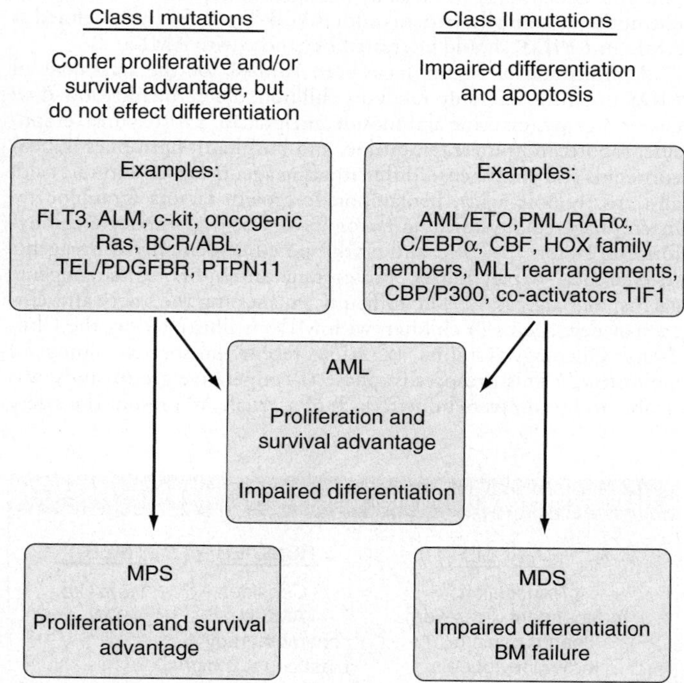

Figure 62-2 COOPERATING MUTATIONS IN ACUTE MYELOID LEUKEMIA (AML), MYELOPROLIFERATIVE SYNDROMES (MPS), AND MYELODYSPLASTIC SYNDROMES (MDS). *BM,* Bone marrow.

proposed in 1982.[34] This classification system recognized five forms of MDS in adults: refractory anemia (RA), refractory anemia with ringed sideroblasts (RARS), refractory anemia with excess of blasts (RAEB), refractory anemia with excess of blasts in transformation (RAEB-T), and CMML. Using this system, whereas RAEB, and RAEB-T were commonly reported in children, RA and RARS were thought to be rare in children. However, a population-based study in the United Kingdom showed 25% of childhood MDS cases to be RA

Table 62-1 Proposed Pediatric Myelodysplastic Syndrome Classification

I. COMBINED MYELOPROLIFERATIVE AND MYELODYSPLASTIC DISEASES
Juvenile myelomonocytic leukemia
Chronic myelomonocytic leukemia
BCR/ABC-negative chronic myeloid leukemia
II. DOWN SYNDROME DISEASE
Transient myeloproliferative disease
Myelodysplasia syndrome or acute myeloid leukemia
III. MYELODYSPLASTIC SYNDROME
Refractory cytopenias with multilineage dysplasia (RCMD)
RCMD-EB

or RARS4 suggesting inaccurate diagnosis or reporting of these subtypes in other pediatric studies. CMML has only rarely been reported in children.

Additional subtypes of MDS are now recognized that do not fit well into the FAB system, including hypoplastic MDS, therapy-related MDS, refractory cytopenias with trilineage dysplasia, MDS associated with myelofibrosis, and MDS associated with inherited disorders (congenital neutropenias, Shwachman-Diamond syndrome, Fanconi anemia), Down syndrome, neurofibromatosis type 1, and mitochondrial cytopathies.[35,36] Therefore, the World Health Organization (WHO) recently proposed changes to the FAB criteria to account for many of these subtypes.[37,38] Other significant changes included elimination of the RAEB-T subtype with reclassification of MDS with greater than 20% blasts as AML and reassignment of CMML and JMML to a new category of MDS/MPN.

Despite these improvements to the FAB system found in the WHO classification, there are still a number of limitations for children. Therefore, several pediatric-based classification systems for MDS and MPS have been proposed. Among these is a system to parallel the WHO classification (Table 62-1).[39] A second system based on category, cytology, and cytogenetics (CCC) allows for classification of individual patients into a very large number of categories.[40] The clinical utility of this system is unclear. However, a comparison of these two pediatric systems with the adult WHO and FAB systems suggested that both were superior for children rather than the corresponding adult classification system.[41]

Taken together, it may be useful to think about childhood MDS as primary or secondary, with secondary MDS arising either from a known congenital BM failure syndrome or prior acquired aplastic anemia or as a complication from prior chemotherapy or radiation therapy. A diagnosis of primary MDS would then apply to all other cases.

Clinical Manifestations

Signs and symptoms of MDS are nonspecific and are usually attributable to pancytopenia (fever, infections, pallor, fatigue, bruising, and petechiae). Lymphadenopathy, hepatomegaly, and splenomegaly are uncommon presenting signs in children with MDS.

Laboratory Manifestations

Commonly accepted minimal diagnostic criteria for pediatric MDS include the absence of common de novo AML karyotypic abnormalities and at least two of the following: (1) sustained, unexplained anemia; neutropenia or thrombocytopenia; dysplastic morphology in the erythroid; granulocytic or megakaryocytic lineages (at least bilineage) and (2) an acquired, sustained clonal cytogenetic abnormality and 5% or more blasts in the BM.[7,39] Almost half of all children with MDS in a series reported by Kardos et al[42] presented with refractory cytopenia, most notably neutropenia and thrombocytopenia.

Morphologically, the BM may be hypocellular, normocellular, or hypercellular. A diagnosis of MDS is made based on the presence of dysplastic changes in at least two cell lineages. The dysplastic changes in the granulocytes (hypogranulation, nuclear hyposegmentation, megaloblastoid maturation, and a left shift with an increased number of myeloblasts), megakaryocytes (micro-megakaryocytes, abnormal megakaryocyte nuclei), monocytes (increase in BM monocytes, abnormal granulation with persistence of azurophilic granules, hemophagocytosis, abnormal nuclei, and giant forms), or erythroid lineages (megaloblastoid maturation, nuclear budding and multinucleated forms, and ringed sideroblasts) can be multiple and varied. Similar dysplastic changes can occur in the peripheral blood for each of these lineages. Although dysplastic changes in the BM are a common feature of MDS, it is important to remember that dysplasia, unto itself, is not diagnostic of MDS because dysplastic features are associated with other conditions and can be found in normal BM donors.[43]

Although flow cytometric analysis can serve to quantitate the number of blasts based on aberrant cell surface antigen expression and detect populations of paroxysmal nocturnal hemoglobinuria (PNH)–like CD91 cells,[44] flow cytometric findings analysis is not generally diagnostic of MDS.

Cytogenetic abnormalities are seen in approximately half of children diagnosed with de novo MDS. Karyotypic abnormalities most commonly seen are –7, 7q–, and +8. Abnormalities in chromosomes 6, 9, 11, 12, and 13 are rare in children. Specific abnormalities seen in adults, including –5, 5q–, and –Y, are very rarely seen in children.

Differential Diagnosis

Although the history, physical examination, evaluation of the BM and peripheral blood, and cytogenetic analysis often make the diagnosis of MDS, other diseases should be considered. Congenital disorders such as Down syndrome, Fanconi anemia, Shwachman-Diamond syndrome, Diamond-Blackfan anemia, congenital dyserythropoietic anemias, and hereditary sideroblastic anemia should be considered. Hypoplastic MDS can be difficult to distinguish from severe aplastic anemia and may require prospective monitoring and serial BM examinations. The differential should also include AML with a low blast count, mitochondrial cytopathies such as Pearson syndrome, and myeloproliferative disorders. Specifically, PNH, although rare in children, should be considered. Deficiencies of vitamin B_{12} and folate can cause megaloblastic changes that resemble the dysplastic changes seen in MDS. Other nutritional deficiencies, including iron, thiamine, riboflavin, and pyridoxine, should be considered. Infections caused by human immunodeficiency virus, parvovirus, Epstein-Barr virus, cytomegalovirus, and human herpes virus 6 can cause changes that resemble MDS. Finally, the differential diagnosis should include toxins (insecticides, chemotherapy agents, and arsenic) as well as cytokine exposure and radiation. When the diagnosis is unclear, serial BM examinations may serve as a useful aid.

Therapy

Although MDS is a heterogeneous, clonal disease of hematopoietic stem cells that can manifest different clinical courses, it is not readily curable by conventional chemotherapy and requires allogeneic hematopoietic stem cell transplantation (SCT) for cure in most cases. Some children with RA and refractory cytopenias with multilineage dysplasia (RCMD) who do not have life-threatening neutropenia and who do not require transfusions may only require close observation (see box on Treatment Overview for Children With MDS). Although children with this disease may eventually develop progressive disease requiring SCT, they may have long periods when minimal treatment is required.[42] The use of AML-like chemotherapy for patients with RCMD with excess blasts (RCMD-EB) is controversial but may serve to "debulk" patients with a high percentage of blasts before SCT.[6,45,46] However, this potential benefit may be offset by toxicities associated with AML-like chemotherapy. Finally, patients with RAEB-T, which is now defined as AML, or t-MDS, should be treated like those with AML.

A multitude of agents have been studied for the treatment of MDS in adults but only rarely in children. These include low-dose chemotherapy (cytosine arabinoside, melphalan, hydroxyurea, etoposide, topotecan, 6-mercaptopurine, and busulfan), hormones (glucocorticoids and androgens), differentiating agents (13-*cis*-retinoic acid, all-trans retinoic acid), hematopoietic growth factors (granulocyte-macrophage colony-forming factor [GM-CSF], granulocyte colony-forming factor [G-CSF], and erythropoietin), demethylating agents (decitabine, 5-azacytidine), proteosome inhibitors, antiangiogenic agents, and arsenic.[47-62] The difficulty in assessing the safety and efficacy of new agents in children with MDS is illustrated by the Children's Oncology Group's (COG's) recent prospective study of amifostine.[63] This prospective phase II cooperative group study was unable to be completed due to lack of accrual. As a result, the safety

Treatment Overview for Children With MDS

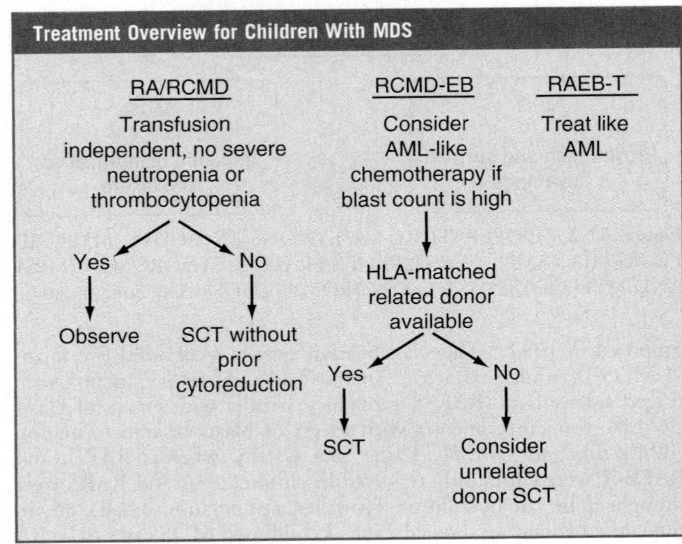

and efficacy of amifostine in children with MDS remains uncertain. Finally, although the potential to better control MDS in adults with azacitidine, decitabine, and arsenic is exciting, there are currently no safety or efficacy data to support the use of these agents in children with MDS.

Most children with MDS require allogeneic SCT for curative therapy. Although children have been included in published SCT studies for MDS that are largely focused on adult patients, several studies focus specifically on children.[64-69] Taken together, these studies suggest a probability of disease-free survival in about 50% of patients undergoing human leukocyte antigen (HLA)–matched related donor SCT. The Center for International Blood and Marrow Transplant (CIBMTR) recently published results for 118 children with MDS who underwent unrelated donor SCT.[68] Forty-six children had refractory cytopenia (RC), 55 with RAEB and 17 with RAEB-t. Relapse of disease was most likely in children with RAEB and RAEB-t with transplant-related mortality and highest in recipients of HLA-mismatched grafts. The 8-year probabilities of disease-free survival for children with RC, RAEB, and RAEB-t were 51%, 35%, and 29%, respectively (Fig. 62-3).

Prognosis

Although a number of methods have been developed to predict the outcome of adults with MDS, the system now most commonly used

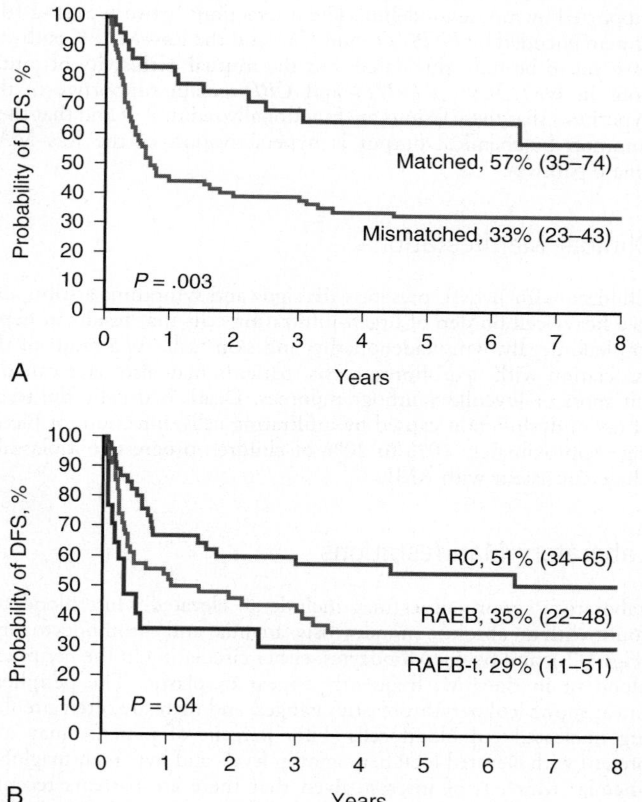

Figure 62-3 **A,** The 8-year probabilities of disease-free survival (DFS) after bone marrow transplantation (BMT): 57% for patients who received matched BMT (matched at human leukocyte antigen A, B, C, DRB1) and 33% for patients who received mismatched BMT. **B,** The 8-year probabilities of disease-free survival after BMT: 51% when transplantation was performed for RC, 35% when transplantation was performed for refractory anemia with excess of blasts (RAEB), and 29% when transplantation was performed for refractory anemia with excess of blasts in transformation (RAEB-T). *(Reproduced with permission from Woodard P, Carpenter PA, Davies SM, et al: Unrelated donor bone marrow transplantation for myelodysplastic syndrome in children.* Bio Blood Marrow Transplant *17: 723, 2011.*

in adults is the International Prognostic Scoring System.[70] This system uses percentage BM blasts, karyotype, and number of cytopenias to assign a score that is then used to predict outcome. Although it is an effective tool for adults, its value for children is very limited.[71]

Secondary Myelodysplastic Syndrome

Secondary MDS can develop in both children and adults after exposure to chemotherapy and radiation. Alkylating agents used to treat Hodgkin disease, non-Hodgkin lymphoma, and Ewing sarcoma are particularly concerning in children.[72-84] Interestingly, there is also evidence to suggest that the cardioprotectant dexrazoxane, a topoisomerase II inhibitor with a mechanism of action that is different from etoposide and doxorubicin, may have increased the incidence of secondary MDS and AML in children treated for Hodgkin disease.[85]

Treatment options for children with secondary MDS are limited. Although AML-like chemotherapy can induce a period of remission and reduction in BM blasts, it is not curative. Allogeneic SCT has curative potential, but outcomes remain poor, with only 20% to 30% of children surviving in reported series.[83,86,87] However, as noted earlier, recent data from the CIBMTR demonstrate that treatment failure with unrelated donor SCT is not higher compared with primary MDS.[68]

MYELOPROLIFERATIVE NEOPLASMS

Juvenile Myelomonocytic Leukemia

Juvenile myelomonocytic leukemia is classified by the WHO as an overlap MDS and MPN. It is an aggressive myeloid malignancy of young children with poor outcomes to conventional therapies. The diagnostic criteria are complex (Table 62-2), but recent advances in elucidating the molecular genetics of the disorder demonstrate that approximately 85% of children will harbor an alteration in one of five genes. Thus there is now international agreement on the diagnostic criteria[88] (see Table 62-2) with an emphasis on incorporating these molecular genetic criteria, and there is also recent progress toward defining common response criteria.

Table 62-2 Diagnostic Criteria for Juvenile Myelomonocytic Leukemia

CATEGORY 1 *All of the following:*	CATEGORY 2 *At least 1 of the following:*	CATEGORY 3 *At least 2 of the following:*
• Splenomegaly* • Absolute monocyte count (AMC) > 1000/μL • Blasts in PB/BM < 20% • Absence of the t(9;22) *BCR/ABL* fusion gene	• Somatic mutation in *RAS* or *PTPN11* • Clinical diagnosis of NF1 or *NF1* gene mutation • Homozygous mutation in *CBL* • Monosomy 7	• Circulating myeloid precursors • WBC > 10,000/μL • Increased fetal hemoglobin (Hgb F) for age • Clonal cytogenetic abnormality excluding monosomy 7 • GM-CSF hypersensitivity

From Chan RJ, Cooper T, Kratz CP, et al: Juvenile myelomonocytic leukemia: A report from the 2nd International JMML Symposium. *Leuk Res* 33:355, 2009.
The diagnosis of JMML is made if a patient meets all of the Category 1 criteria and one of the Category 2 criteria without needing to meet the Category 3 criteria. If there are no Category 2 criteria met, then the Category 3 criteria must be met.
*For the 7-10% of patients without splenomegaly, the diagnostic criteria must include all other features in Category 1 AND one of the parameters in Category 2 OR no features in Category 2 but two features in Category 3.

Epidemiology

The incidence of JMML in the United States has been estimated as 0.69 to 1.2 per million,[4,89] although its true incidence is currently not known, likely because of previous diagnostic imprecision. With the advent of molecular testing, the true incidence of this disease will be established in the coming years. There is a male predominance with a median age of diagnosis of 1.8 years.

Pathogenesis

Early clonality studies suggested that JMML arose at the level of at least an immature myeloid precursor cell.[88,90-94] More recent data suggest that JMML may arise in a pluripotent stem cell with involvement of the myeloid, erythroid, and megakaryocyte lineages as well as B lymphocytes and T lymphocytes.[88,95-97]

Several potential causative mutations in JMML cells have been identified, including loss of heterozygosity of NF1 in the context of patients with clinical neurofibromatosis 1 (15%),[98] activating RAS mutations (25%),[99,101] mutations in the *PTPN11* gene (see Fig. 62-1) (35%), and newly described mutations in *CBL* (10%–15%).[102-105] The identification of potential molecular mechanisms involved in the pathogenesis of JMML has been facilitated by two common human diseases (neurofibromatosis type 1 *[NF1]* and Noonan syndrome *[PTPN11]*) in which affected children are at a higher risk of developing JMML or a JMML-like MPN, and recent work demonstrates that children with germline CBL alterations also are at risk for developing JMML.

Approximately 10% to 15% of patients with JMML have clinically evident NFI,[88,98,106-108] and children with NF1 have a 500-fold increase in clonal malignant myeloid diseases, including JMML. The observation that individuals with NF1 are predisposed to JMML, the high incidence of *RAS* mutations in human cancers, and the identification of neurofibromin as a negative regulator that functions as a GTPase-activating protein that hydrolyzes Ras from its active GTP-bound state[88,109-111] led to the hypothesis that activation of the Ras–MAPK (mitogen-activated protein kinase) pathway plays a key role in the pathogenesis of this disease. Indeed, the demonstration of loss of heterozygosity of the wild-type *NF1* allele in leukemic cells from children with NF and JMML supports the observation that *NF1* functions as a tumor suppressor gene in myeloid malignancies. The mechanisms leading to loss of heterozygosity (LOH) of *NF1* in patients with JMML is unclear but is uniformly associated with the presence of acquired isodisomy of the mutant *NF1* allele.[112] In addition, accumulation of activated Ras proteins in these cells has provided evidence that the loss of *NF1* leads to excessive signaling downstream from Ras.[18,108,113,114] Abnormalities in *NF1* are also detected in an additional small percentage of JMML patients who do not display clinical manifestations of neurofibromatosis.[88,113] This finding is generally mutually exclusive of RAS mutations that occur in another 25% of patients, suggesting that both *NF1* and RAS mutations are sufficient to initiate JMML.[88,96,99,113,115,116-119] Indeed, accurate murine models of JMML have been engineered by several groups in which either the *NF1* gene has been homozygously deleted[120] or canonical *Nras* or *Kras*^{G12D} or *Ptpn11*^{E76K} alterations conditionally expressed.[121-123] The E76K knock-in mutation is embryonic lethal, but conditional expression of this allele results in a fatal MPN. One hallmark feature of human JMML is selective hypersensitivity of myeloid progenitors to low doses of GM-CSF in colony forming unit–granulocyte macrophage assays (CFU-GM), which is recapitulated in the mouse models and which is also associated with hyperactivation of the Ras–MAPK pathway as evidenced by increased levels of pERK. In 2001, Tartaglia et al[124] reported that constitutional mutations in *PTPN11* were causative of 50% of cases of Noonan syndrome (NS). NS is a common congenital disorder, with both acquired and sporadic forms. Patients affected by NS have cardiac defects (pulmonic stenosis of hypertrophic cardiomyopathy), variable levels of developmental delay, skeletal defects, and bleeding diatheses. Some children develop a JMML-like MPN in infancy that generally spontaneously recovers, although rare patients require chemotherapy or progress to frank JMML. Based on the knowledge that *PTPN11* encodes SHP-2, a nonreceptor protein tyrosine phosphatase that relays signals from activated growth factors to Ras, it was logical to hypothesize that somatic mutations in *PTPN11* might exist in the remaining cases of de novo JMML patients who did not have either clinical NF1 or harbor a RAS mutation. Indeed, 35% of patients with JMML were discovered to have mutations in *PTPN11* in residues altering the interaction between the N-SH2 and C-SH2 domains, leading to constitutive activity of the phosphatase.[17,102]

In 2009, Loh and colleagues[125] used single nucleotide polymorphism arrays to detect acquired isodisomy in a region of 11q in a subset of patients with JMML who did not have a known Ras pathway alteration. This led to the subsequent discovery of homozygous mutations in *CBL,* an E3 ubiquitin ligase that also serves as an important adaptor protein, as a fourth locus for genetic alterations in JMML.[103,105,125,126] Together with colleagues from the European Working Group on Childhood Myelodysplastic Syndromes, they then described that homozygous mutations in *CBL* first arise as germline events, with subsequent reduction to homozygosity in hematopoietic cells, in contrast to the lesions described in adults.[104] Specific germline features are found in the syndrome, although are not fully penetrant, and include cryptorchidism, hearing loss, and skeletal abnormalities. Analysis of family pedigrees indicate that transmission is autosomal dominant, although 50% of cases arise as spontaneous mutations. Others have confirmed these findings but in smaller series.[127,128]

Taken together, the early genetic data suggested that deregulated Ras–MAPK signaling is a common feature of JMML, which has been supported by mouse modeling. The interactions between SHP-2 (the protein encoded by *PTPN11*) and *CBL* and the Ras–MAPK pathway have yet to be fully elucidated, but the mutual exclusivity of mutations in *NF1,* RAS, *PTPN11* and *CBL* remain supportive of the hypothesis that these lesions are functionally redundant and that their common biochemical output is hyperactivation of the Ras–MAP kinase pathway.

Clinical Manifestations

Children with JMML present with signs and symptoms attributable to a heavy cell burden of organ-infiltrating cells that results in hepatosplenomegaly, lymphadenopathy, and skin rash. As a result of the association with neurofibromatosis, patients may also have café-au-lait spots or juvenile xanthogranulomas. Death is usually the result of organ dysfunction caused by infiltrating cells, infection, or bleeding. Approximately 10% to 20% of children progress to a blastlike phase consistent with AML.

Laboratory Manifestations

Laboratory abnormalities may include an elevated white blood cell count with an absolute monocytosis, anemia, and thrombocytopenia (Figs. 62-4 and 64-5). Monocytes, either circulating in the peripheral blood or in the BM, frequently appear dysplastic. The peripheral smear shows leukoerythroblastic changes, and there are often circulating nucleated red blood cells. Fifty percent of patients may also present with elevated fetal hemoglobin levels and hypergammaglobulinemia, which is of interest given that there are patients recently described with autoimmune lymphoproliferative syndromes who also harbor mutations in RAS, thus raising additional questions about other childhood BM disorders in which Ras–MAPK signaling is integral to pathogenesis. International criteria mandate that the BM has fewer than 20% blast cells at diagnosis. Other findings typical in the BM may include micro-megakaryocytes.

Differential Diagnosis

Traditionally, establishing a diagnosis of JMML was not easy because its clinical and laboratory presenting features can also be associated

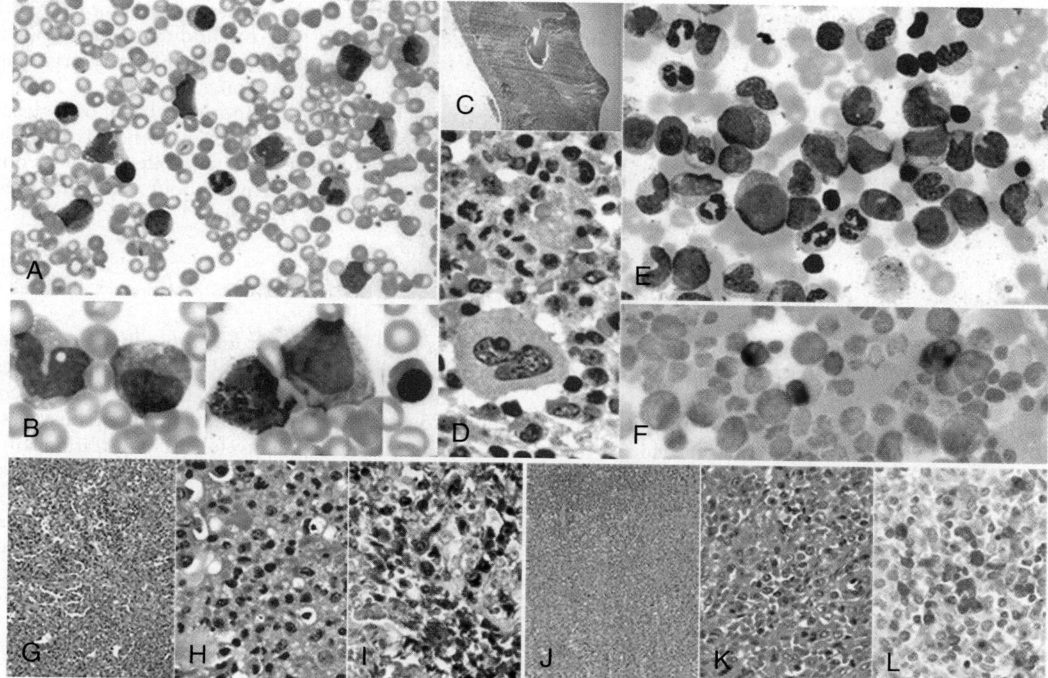

Figure 62-4 JUVENILE MYELOMONOCYTIC LEUKEMIA (JMML): BLOOD, BONE MARROW, LUNG, AND SPLEEN. The illustrations are from the case of a 3-year-old boy who was diagnosed with neurofibromatosis at birth. At 1 year of age, he presented with leukocytosis (58 K/μL). The peripheral blood (**A** and **B**) showed left-shifted granulocytes and increased monocytes (16%). A bone marrow biopsy (**C** and **D**) was hypercellular as a result of increased granulocytic and monocytic cells that could also be appreciated on the aspirate (**E**). Blasts accounted for only 4% of the bone marrow elements. A combined esterase reaction (**F**) illustrated the increased monocytes (α-naphthol butyrate esterase reaction positive; *orange/brown*) in the background of granulocytes (chloroacetate esterase reaction positive; *blue*). Cytogenetic analysis revealed monosomy 7. At age 2 years, the patient presented with respiratory distress, and a lung biopsy (**G** and **H**) demonstrated a monocyte infiltrate (lysozyme stain, **I**) consistent with involvement by JMML. This is not uncommon in such patients. At age 3 years, his blast count began to rise, and he underwent a splenectomy (which showed a marked infiltrate of immature and mature monocytes and granulocytic cells (**J** and **K**; lysozyme stain, **L**). After the splenectomy the patient underwent a successful stem cell transplant.

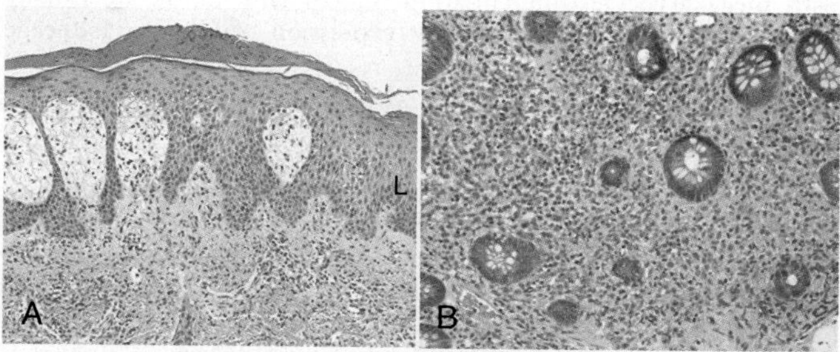

Figure 62-5 JUVENILE MYELOMONOCYTIC LEUKEMIA (JMML): SKIN AND GASTROINTESTINAL TRACT. Patients with JMML sometimes present with or develop skin nodules, which on biopsy show a myelomonocytic infiltrate in the upper and lower dermis **(A)**. Involvement can also be seen in the gastrointestinal tract **(B)**. *(The case was kindly provided by Dr. Elizabeth Hyjek, University of Chicago.)*

with other disorders, including infections (Epstein-Barr virus, cytomegalovirus, human herpes 6 virus, histoplasmosis, mycobacterium, and toxoplasmosis), class I Langerhans cell histiocytosis, hemophagocytic lymphohistiocytosis, Fanconi anemia, Kostmann syndrome, Shwachman syndrome, and Down syndrome. However, with a positive molecular mutation, patients who exhibit the category 1 features are now more easily diagnosed.

Therapy

Children with JMML can have a variable course, with rare patients having a spontaneous remission and long-term survival without treatment but others having a rapidly fatal course despite aggressive treatment.[129,130] Age, platelet count, and hemoglobin F level have been used to predict the clinical course of patients not undergoing SCT,[116] but biologic features that can reliably predict an individual patient's clinical courses are not currently known. Currently, the most adverse prognostic factor for outcome is older age at diagnosis.[131]

A wide variety of agents have been used to treat children with JMML, including AML-like chemotherapy,[46,107,132-136] low-dose chemotherapy,[137,138] interferon-α,[139] and 13-*cis*-retinoic acid.[110] Tipifarnib, a farnesyl transferase inhibitor, was tested in a phase II window by the COG. Although the evaluation of these treatment regimens has been complicated by a lack of consistent response criteria and assays to measure the burden of clonogenic JMML stem cells, the efficacy of chemotherapy appears to be limited. Allogeneic SCT offers the only known potential for cure, with about half of transplanted children surviving disease-free.[131,140] Rapid withdrawal of immunosuppression appears to be important in this disease, as mounting evidence supports a graft-versus-leukemia effect.[141] A number of issues related to SCT for JMML remain uncertain. Among these are the value of pretransplant splenectomy and the optimal conditioning regimen and graft-versus-host disease prophylaxis. In the absence of data to suggest superiority of radiation containing preparative regimens, most transplants now occur with chemotherapy-only preparative regimens. The most common cause of death after SCT is recurrent disease. A second SCT can be lifesaving for some children.[142,143] Donor leukocyte infusions are not often successful.[144]

Down Syndrome–Associated Transient Myeloproliferative Disorder

Epidemiology

Down syndrome is one of the most common congenital disorders, affecting approximately one in every 800 to 1000 live births. It has been demonstrated in a recent population-based study that children with Down syndrome have a 10- to 20-fold overall increased risk of developing leukemia,[145] a 150-fold increased risk of developing AML, and a 500-fold increased risk of acute megakaryocytic leukemia (AMKL). The median age of diagnosis of AMKL in individuals with Down syndrome is 2 years.[146] Transient myeloproliferative disorder, also known as transient abnormal myelopoiesis and transient leukemia, is thought to occur in at least 10% of children with Down syndrome, although it has been suggested that when cases of TMD that develop and resolve in utero or result in death before delivery are taken into account, the incidence may be as high as 20%.[147] Currently, it is estimated that approximately 20% to 30% of children with TMD subsequently develop AML, usually by 3 years of age. This estimate was validated in a recent prospective study conducted by the COG.[148] In this study, AML developed in 16% of Down syndrome children who had TMD at a median of 441 days (118-1085 days).

Pathobiology

The molecular pathogenesis of TMD and AMKL in children with Down syndrome is now providing valuable insights into myeloid leukemogenesis.[20] Recent studies have shown that virtually all patients with TMD and most patients with AMKL harbor mutations in the hematopoietic transcription factor *GATA1*.[149-153] *GATA1* is a double zinc finger DNA-binding transcription factor expressed primarily in hematopoietic cells. It is required for the development of red blood cells, megakaryocytes, mast cells, and eosinophils. A number of different mutations in *GATA1* have been identified, including insertions, deletions, missense mutations, nonsense mutations, and slice site mutations. All of these mutations lead to a block in the expression of the full-length 50-kd isoform of *GATA1* but allow for the expression of a smaller, 40-kd isoform *(GATA1s)*.[154] This smaller isoform lacks the N-terminal transactivation domain but retains both zinc fingers involved in DNA binding as well as interactions with its cofactor, friend of *GATA1* (FOG1).[149] Recent studies have shown that mutations that alter *GATA1–FOG1* binding in the N-terminal zinc finger or result in the expression of the *GATA1s* isoform uncouple megakaryocyte growth and differentiation.[155-157] Similar studies in cell lines derived from children with Down syndrome and AMKL have demonstrated that expression of *GATA1* led to erythroid differentiation whereas expression of *GATA1s* did not alter the characteristics of the cell line.[153] Taken together, current data suggest that the loss of *GATA1* and expression of *GATA1s* directly contribute to leukemogenesis. Although mutations in GATA1 may be sufficient to cause TMD, these mutations are not sufficient for the development of AMKL, as evidenced by the latency period between resolution of TMD and the development of AMKL as well as the observation that not all children with TMD and *GATA1* mutations will ultimately develop AMKL. Therefore, a multistep pathogenesis model is proposed in patients with Down syndrome in whom AMKL develops in clones with *GATA1* mutations and additional cooperating mutations. One potential "second-hit" mutation may occur in the JAK3 (Janus kinase 3) gene, a member of the JAK family of nonreceptor tyrosine kinases. Several gain-of-function mutations[158,159] and loss-of-function mutations in JAK3[160160] have been identified in both TMD and AMKL patient samples. Although mutations in *JAK3* might indeed represent a "second hit," the finding of mutations in TMD patients who have not progressed to AMKL may argue against *JAK3* as a second cooperating mutation.

Another particularly important area of investigation is the interaction between *GATA1* and chromosome 21. Identification of critical interactions between *GATA1* and relevant genes on chromosome 21 will serve to further inform us about the pathogenesis of leukemia in children with Down syndrome.

Clinical Manifestations

Patients with Down syndrome typically present with TMD within 3 months after birth, although TMD can be manifest at birth. Some of these children present with hydrops fetalis secondary to anemia and cardiac dysfunction. Although some patients may be asymptomatic, others can have myeloblast infiltration of the heart, liver, and spleen that can result in hepatosplenomegaly; hepatic fibrosis; pleural, pericardial, and peritoneal effusions; and disseminated intravascular coagulopathy. In some cases, organ dysfunction can be severe, with failure of the liver, heart, kidneys, and lungs. In the COG's recently published prospective study, death occurred in 21% of patients, although only 10% died as a result of TMD-associated problems.[148]

Laboratory Manifestations

The complete blood count in infants with TMD typically demonstrates an elevated white blood cell count with myeloblasts present (see Fig. 62-6). The percentage of circulating myeloblasts exceeds the percentage of BM myeloblasts. Rarely, a neonate without stigmata of Down syndrome will present with similar features—in these cases, workup for either trisomy 21 mosaicism or a PTPN11 mutation should be pursued. Flow cytometric analysis of the myeloblasts from TMD patients and AMKL associated with Down syndrome show many similarities between these disorders as well as patterns of cell surface antigen expression that is distinct from other types of AML in children.[161] Specifically, all TMD and AMKL blasts express CD45, CD38, and CD33, but the majority of cases express CD36 and CD34. CD41 and CD61 also are expressed, consistent with megakaryocyte differentiation. CD14 and CD64 are usually negative. Most cases have aberrant expression of CD7, a T-lineage antigen.

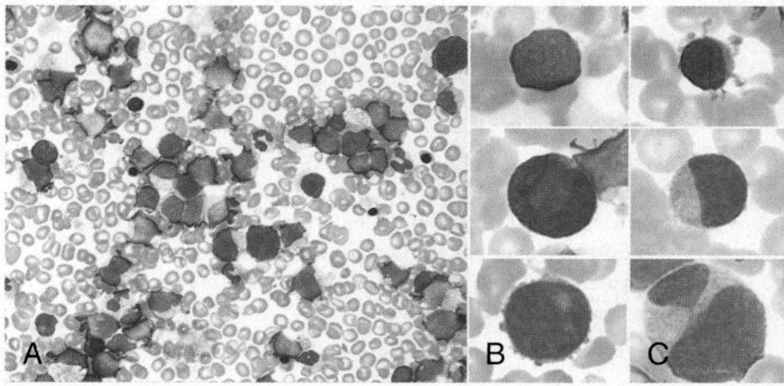

Figure 62-6 TRANSIENT MYELOPROLIFERATIVE DISORDER (TRANSIENT ABNORMAL MYELOPOIESIS AND TRANSIENT LEUKEMIA) OF DOWN SYNDROME. The patient was a premature newborn girl with trisomy 21 and a white blood cell count of 195,000/μL with 67% blasts **(A)**. The blasts were $CD34^+$, $CD33^+$ and $CD117^+$, and a portion exhibited CD41, a megakaryocyte marker. Morphologically, some of the blasts appeared to be megakaryoblasts **(B)**, sometimes with slight differentiation toward megakaryocytes **(C)**.

Therapy

The treatment of infants with TMD is generally supportive. Patients without significant organ dysfunction can be followed closely without medical intervention. In the COG's prospective study, peripheral blood blasts and TMD-associated symptoms resolved in 36 and 49 days, respectively, for observation patients.[148] In infants with significant organ impairment, a number of therapeutic approaches aimed at reducing the burden of myeloblasts are routinely used, including exchange transfusion, leukophoresis, and chemotherapy. According to reports using cytosine arabinoside in children with Down syndrome and AMKL,[162,163] cytosine arabinoside is the chemotherapeutic agent now most commonly used in infants with TMD. The efficacy of very low doses of cytosine arabinoside is being tested in prospective clinical trials. Several additional questions related to the treatment of infants with TMD are also the subject of ongoing clinical trials. Among these is the identification of high-, intermediate-, and low-risk populations with treatment stratified on the basis of risk group and a determination of whether treatment with very low dose cytosine arabinoside will prevent progression of TMD to AMKL and hepatic fibrosis.

Prognosis

Recent data from the COG reporting the results of the POG 9481 prospective clinical trial offer insights into the natural history of TMD and the identification of prognostic factors.[149] This study followed 48 children with TMD. Eighty-nine percent of infants achieved a spontaneous remission, 74% had a normalization of peripheral blood counts, and 64% maintained a clinical remission. Seventeen percent of infants had an early death. Factors associated with early death included a high white blood cell count ($P < .001$), increased bilirubin and liver function test values ($P < .005$), and a failure to normalize blood counts ($P < .001$). Nineteen percent of patients had a progression to AMKL at a median of 20 months. The greatest risk factor for progression to leukemia was the presence of karyotypic abnormalities in addition to trisomy 21 in blasts cells.

The COG's more recent A2971 study identified three groups of children with different outcomes based on the presence or absence of hepatomegaly and life-threatening symptoms.[148] Children with neither hepatomegaly nor life-threatening symptoms were at low risk of death (overall survival [OS], 92%); children with hepatomegaly alone had an intermediate risk of death (OS, 77%), and children with both hepatomegaly and life-threatening symptoms were at high risk of death (OS, 51%).

OTHER MYELOPROLIFERATIVE NEOPLASMS

Essential Thrombocythemia

Essential thrombocythemia has an estimated incidence of 1 to 1.25 cases per million in adults but is even rarer in children, with an estimated incidence of 0.09 cases per million.[165-169] Recent investigations in children and adults suggests that ET is a heterogeneous disease. Recently, mutations in *JAK2* have been reported in adults with *BCR-ABL*–negative MPNs, including ET, PV, and idiopathic myelofibrosis (IM). It has been proposed that ET consists of several subtypes, with some children and adults having monoclonal disease but others having polyclonal disease. Further investigation into the mutational status of V617F*JAK2* also demonstrates mutation-positive and -negative patients.[166,170] Studies suggest that a similar proportion of children and adults with somatic ET display polycythemia rubra vera-1 (PRV-1) RNA overexpression, V617FJAK2 mutations, and monoclonal disease.[171] Dominant activating mutations in c-MPL have been reported in rare cases of familial ET as opposed to JAK2 lesions.[171]

Patients with ET have thrombocythemia with an increased number of megakaryocytes in the BM. Platelet clumps on peripheral blood smears are common. Some patients have a concomitant increase in the number of peripheral blood granulocytes. The differential diagnosis includes familial ET (characterized by the dominant-positive activating mutation of *c-mpl*), other forms of MPS, and increased platelets as a reactive process.

Although the clinical course can be uncomplicated, patients can develop thromboembolic complications, including deep venous thrombosis, transient cerebral ischemia, and peripheral vascular ischemia. The clinical course for children is typically less aggressive than in adults, with fewer thrombotic episodes.[171,172] Adult patients have a median survival of at least 10 years, with most deaths caused by thrombosis.[173,174] Progression to AML has been reported in adult patients, usually those with a prior exposure to chemotherapy agents.

Asymptomatic children do not require treatment. A number of treatment approaches aimed at controlling thrombocytosis have been attempted for symptomatic patients, including hydroxyurea, interferon-α, and anagrelide.[175-177] The successful use of allogeneic BM transplantation has been reported for a small number of adult patients with ET.[178,179] Newer JAK2 inhibitors for patients harboring *JAK2* mutations are in the early phases of clinical development.

Idiopathic Myelofibrosis

Idiopathic myelofibrosis is rarely diagnosed in children[180] and should be differentiated from AMKL; metastatic neoplasms; and connective tissue, metabolic, and bone diseases. It is characterized by BM fibrosis, megakaryocytes with bizarre morphology, splenomegaly, anemia, and extramedullary hematopoiesis. IM is a clonal disorder with approximately half of adult patients having mutations in V617FJAK2.[181] Recent studies have suggested that angiogenic cytokines produced by megakaryocytes and monocytes and their receptors (platelet-derived growth factor receptors [PDGF-R], vascular endothelial growth factor receptor-2 [VEGF-R2] and fibroblast growth factor [FGF] receptor), may be involved in the pathogenesis of the myelofibrosis.[182]

Numerous treatment approaches have been attempted with variable degrees of success. These include splenectomy, splenic radiation, transfusions, androgens, corticosteroids, hydroxyurea, and interferon-α.[183-185] More recently, based on preliminary studies about the potential role of angiogenic cytokines and their receptors, new approaches have been tested, including the tyrosine kinase inhibitor imatinib[186,187] and the antiangiogenic agent thalidomide.[188,189] Selective JAK inhibitors have been successfully used in patients with IM with a dramatic improvement in the quality of life but without generalized reduction of the V617F JAK2 burden allele.[190] The U.S. Food and Drug Administration recently granted approval to the first of these agents, ruxolitinib, for adults with IM. However, the safety and efficacy of ruxolitinib in children is currently unknown. Finally, allogeneic transplantation has been used successfully, with resolution of BM fibrosis in donor-engrafted patients.[179,191,192] The survival in children is unknown with a median survival in adults of 4 years.

Polycythemia Vera

Polycythemia vera has an incidence of three cases per 100,000 in adults but is very rarely seen in children with fewer than 0.1% of PV patients diagnosed before 20 years of age.[193] PV in children is far more often the result of congenital or acquired causes of an increased red blood cell mass. These include primary familial polycythemia (characterized by specific mutations in the thrombopoietic gene [TPO], TPO receptor, or erythropoietic receptor gene) and secondary polycythemias caused by abnormal hemoglobins, cardiac and pulmonary disease, excessive erythropoietin, and a relative polycythemia that is the result of decreased plasma volume.

Polycythemia vera in children and adults is associated with clonal hematopoiesis,[194] V617F*JAK2* mutations,[171,195-199] overexpression of PVR-1 RNA,[200,201] and endogenous erythroid colony (EEC) growth.[202,203] However, in contrast to adults, children with PV are less likely to have V617F*JAK2* mutations and EEC growth.[171] Thus, although these biomarkers are useful diagnostic tools in adults, thereby necessitating a revision to the WHO's diagnostic criteria,[204] they may not be as helpful in the diagnosis of PV in children. Although the pathogenesis is currently unclear, patients also have abnormalities in tissue factor, endogenous anticoagulants mechanisms, hyperhomocysteinemia, and acquired von Willebrand syndrome.

Children with PV may present with signs and symptoms associated with an increased red blood cell mass such as headache, dizziness, fatigue, pruritus, night sweats, and a ruddy complexion. Hepatosplenomegaly may be present. As a result of hyperviscosity of the blood, elevated platelet counts, and coagulation abnormalities, patients can develop thromboses and central nervous system ischemia, although the incidence of thrombotic events may be lower than that reported in adults.[171]

Many different agents have been used to treat patients with PV, including chlorambucil,[205] melphalan,[206] 6-thioguanine,[207] uracil mustard,[208] busulfan,[209] carboquone,[210] anagrelide,[211] imatinib,[212] hydroxyurea,[213] radioactive phosphorous,[214] and interferon.[215] A total of seven randomized clinical trials have been conducted in adults using some of these agents.[216] Despite these efforts, the best approach to patients with PV remains unclear. Therefore, the British Committee for Standards in Haematology recently formulated recommendations for the initial management of PV.[217] Recommendations include phlebotomy to maintain a hematocrit level less than 45% aspirin unless contraindicated; and cytoreduction if there is poor tolerance to phlebotomy, symptomatic or progressive splenomegaly, evidence of disease progression, or thrombocytosis. For patients younger than 40 years of age, interferon was the recommendation for first-line cytoreduction with hydroxyurea and anagrelide as second-line. Currently, JAK inhibitors are in early phase clinical trials to determine maximally tolerated doses and have been well tolerated thus far. Finally, allogeneic transplantation has been successfully used to treat a limited number of adult patients.[178,179,218,219] Allogeneic transplantation is considered only for patients with significant thrombotic disease or progression to AML.

FUTURE DIRECTIONS

Although a clearer understanding of the biologic mechanisms underlying MDS in children is slow in coming, dramatic progress has been made in our understanding of the genetic and biologic mechanisms contributing to TMD, JMML, PV, ET, and IM. There exists a potential for targeted therapeutics for many of these disorders, with the first targeted agents now receiving approval for use in adults. However, the use of these agents in children remains investigational.

Progress for both MDS and MPN in children will require international cooperation. The rarity of these disorders and limitations in resources for pediatric cooperative cancer groups make clinical trials within each individual cooperative group increasingly difficult.

SUGGESTED READINGS

Bhatia S, Krailo MD, Chen Z, et al: Therapy-related myelodysplasia and acute myeloid leukemia after Ewing sarcoma and primitive neuroectodermal tumor of bone: A report from the Children's Oncology Group. *Blood* 109:46, 2007.

Crispino JD: GATA1 mutations in Down syndrome: Implications for biology and diagnosis of children with transient myeloproliferative disorder and acute megakaryoblastic leukemia. *Pediatric Blood Cancer* 44:40, 2005.

Gamis AS, Alonzo TA, Gerbing RB, et al: Natural history of transient myeloproliferative disorder clinically diagnosed in Down syndrome neonates: A report from the Children's Oncology Group Study A2971. *Blood* 118:6752, 2011.

Hasle H, Niemeyer CM: Advances in the prognostication and management of advanced MDS in children. *Br J Haematol* 154:185, 2011.

Hasle H, Baumann I, Bergstrasser E, et al: The International Prognostic Scoring System (IPSS) for childhood myelodysplastic syndrome (MDS) and juvenile myelomonocytic leukemia (JMML). *Leukemia* 18:2008, 2004.

Hasle H, Niemeyer CM, Chessells JM, et al: A pediatric approach to the WHO classification of myelodysplastic and myeloproliferative diseases. *Leukemia* 17:277, 2003.

Loh ML: Recent advances in the pathogenesis and treatment of juvenile myeolomonocytic leukemia. *Br J Haematol* 152:677, 2011.

Luna-Fineman S, Shannon KM, Atwater SK, et al: Myelodysplastic and myeloproliferative disorders of childhood: A study of 167 patients. *Blood* 93:459, 1999.

Niemeyer C, Kang M, Shin D, et al: Germline CBL mutations cause developmental abnormalities and predispose to juvenile myelomonocytic leukemia. *Nat Genet* 42:794, 2010.

Occhipinti E, Correa H, Yu L, et al: Comparison of two new classifications for pediatric myelodysplastic and myeloproliferative disorders. *Pediatr Blood Cancer* 44:240, 2005.

Shannon KM, O'Connell P, Martin GA, et al: Loss of the normal NF1 allele from the bone marrow of children with type 1 neurofibromatosis and malignant myeloid disorders [see comments]. *N Engl J Med* 330:597, 1994.

Strahm B, Nollke P, Zecca M, et al: Hematopoietic stem cell transplantation for advanced myelodysplastic syndrome in children: Results of the EWOG-MDS 98 study. *Leukemia.* 25:455, 2011.

Tefferi A, Gilliland DG: Oncogenes in myeloproliferative disorders. *Cell Cycle* 6:550, 2007.

Tefferi A, Thiele J, Orazi A, et al: Proposals and rationale for revision of the World Health Organization diagnostic criteria for polycythemia vera, essential thrombocythemia, and primary myelofibrosis: Recommendations from an ad hoc international expert panel. *Blood* 110:1092, 2007.

Tefferi A, Vainchanker W: Myeloproliferative neoplasms: Molecular pathophysiology, essential clinical understanding and treatment strategies, *J Clin Oncol* 29:573, 2011.

Vardiman JW, Thiele J, Arber DA, et al: The 2008 revision of the World Health Organization (WHO) classification of myeloid neoplasms and acute leukemia: Rationale and important changes. *Blood* 114:937, 2009.

Webb DK, Passmore SJ, Hann IM, et al: Results of treatment of children with refractory anaemia with excess blasts (RAEB) and RAEB in transformation (RAEBt) in Great Britain 1990-99. *Br J Haematol* 117:33, 2002.

Woodard P, Carpentaer PA, Davies SM, et al: Unrelated donor bone marrow transplantation for myelodysplastic syndrome in children. *Biol Blood Marrow Transplant* 17:723, 2011.

Woods WG, Barnard DR, Alonzo TA, et al: Prospective study of 90 children requiring treatment for juvenile myelomonocytic leukemia or myelodysplastic syndrome: A report from the Children's Cancer Group. *J Clin Oncol* 20:434, 2002.

For complete list of references log on to www.expertconsult.com.

CHAPTER 63

PATHOBIOLOGY OF ACUTE LYMPHOBLASTIC LEUKEMIA

Alejandro Gutierrez, Scott A. Armstrong, and A. Thomas Look

Normal lymphoid precursors undergo somatic recombination at their immunoglobulin *(Ig)* or T- cell receptor *(TCR)* gene loci,[1] and the successful completion of V(D)J recombination, with the resultant formation of a functional Ig or TCR, is required for the survival of lymphocyte precursors. Positive and negative selection steps ensure that only lymphocytes with Ig or TCRs that function appropriately within the context of an individual's immune microenvironment are allowed to proceed through the proliferation and differentiation steps required for the development of mature lymphocytes. This developmental process generates a repertoire of lymphocytes with unique variations in the antigen-recognition portions of the *Ig* or *TCR* genes, which form the foundation of a fully competent adaptive immune system that can recognize a countless variety of foreign antigens.

The acquisition of somatic genetic alterations involving oncogenes or tumor suppressors can lead to the dysregulated proliferation and clonal expansion of lymphoid precursors that are characteristic of acute lymphoblastic leukemia (ALL). Many genes that are critical to leukemogenesis have been identified through the cloning and characterization of genetic alterations induced by recurrent chromosomal translocations.[2-5] Additionally, a number of translocations have prognostic significance and are used in modern ALL treatment protocols to adjust the intensity of therapy. In many cases, the malignant transformation of lymphoid cells is the result of altered expression of transcription factors that play critical roles in normal B- and T-cell development, although it may also involve the aberrant expression of otherwise quiescent genes. More recent evidence has implicated members of signal transduction pathways in leukemogenesis.[6-8] Although the incidence of specific genetic alterations in ALL varies according to patient age, evidence is accumulating that the pathogenesis underlying malignant transformation in similar genetic alterations is similar across age groups.[9,10]

CLONAL ORIGIN OF LEUKEMIC LYMPHOID CELLS

Human ALL arises from a single progenitor cell that has acquired somatic genetic changes, which lead to dysregulated proliferation and differentiation arrest. The clonal origin of leukemia was first suggested by the identification of the Philadelphia chromosome in chronic myeloid leukemia (CML).[11] Subsequently, numerous lines of evidence have provided additional support for this theory, which is now generally accepted. Uniform structural and numerical chromosomal abnormalities are frequently demonstrated in all leukemic lymphoblasts from an individual patient. Identical rearrangements of *Ig* or *TCR* genes, which are somatic in origin, have been demonstrated in ALL cell populations.[2,12] Additionally, identical patterns of X-chromosome inactivation have been demonstrated within all cells of individual patients with ALL by allelic analysis of the glucose-6-phosphate dehydrogenase gene on the X chromosome.[13] Because X-inactivation occurs in early embryogenesis before somatically acquired mutations begin to promote the transformed phenotype, this is particularly strong evidence for the clonal origin of leukemia. In addition, the methylation patterns of restriction fragment length polymorphisms in X-linked genes, as detected by Southern blot analysis, have been used to show that even rare ALL cases with two completely different cytogenetic clones probably arise by clonal evolution from a single transformed progenitor.[14]

LINEAGE-SPECIFIC FEATURES OF LEUKEMIC LYMPHOBLASTS

An important advance in the understanding and treatment of ALL was the realization that malignant lymphoblasts share many of the features of normal lymphoid progenitors.[15-17] Thus, ALL cells rearrange their *Ig* and *TCR* genes and express components of antigen receptor molecules and other differentiation-linked cell-surface glycoproteins in ways that correspond to features of developing normal B and T lymphocytes. In many cases, leukemic cells appear to represent the clonal expansion of a lymphoid progenitor that has arrested its development at an early stage of B- or T-cell differentiation.[18] Furthermore, research continues with the goal of defining stem cell populations in lymphoblastic leukemia, such as those that have been identified in acute myeloid leukemia (AML).[19] However, with better understanding of the normal patterns of antigen-independent lymphoid cell development, it has become clear that leukemic lymphoblasts can show asynchronous gene expression with subtle variations in phenotype.[20] Hence, it should not be surprising that in some cases of ALL, the blast cell phenotypes differ from those of normal lymphocyte progenitors, which is likely a result of aberrant regulation of gene expression. Still, the general concept that leukemic cells should be classified according to their "normal" developmental stage remains an important one, providing a basis for the study of immunophenotype-specific genetic changes.

B-Cell Acute Lymphoblastic Leukemia

The diagnosis of mature B-cell ALL is based on the detection of surface Ig on leukemic blasts. This rare phenotype accounts for only 2% to 3% of ALL cases, and the lymphoblasts generally have distinctive morphology, with deeply basophilic cytoplasm containing prominent vacuoles; this morphologic pattern is designated L3 in the French-American-British (FAB) system.[21-23] Prominent clinical features include concomitant extramedullary lymphomatous masses in the abdomen or head and neck, frequent involvement of the central nervous system (CNS) and cranial nerves, and tumor lysis syndrome, often complicated by acute renal failure from uric acid nephropathy.

Acute B-cell leukemia appears to be a disseminated form of Burkitt lymphoma because these conditions share common cytogenetic, molecular genetic, immunologic, cytologic, and clinical features.[24] Acute B-cell leukemia does not respond well to chemotherapy traditionally used for childhood ALL. However, good outcomes have been obtained with treatments designed for Burkitt lymphoma, which involve relatively brief but intensive regimens that emphasize cyclophosphamide and the rapid rotation of antimetabolites in high dosages.[25-29] Thus, B-cell leukemia is the first form of ALL to be recognized as a distinct clinical entity based on immunophenotypic and cytogenetic features and the first to be treated by separate protocols designed specifically for the leukemia's unique features.

B-Precursor Acute Lymphoblastic Leukemia

Approximately 80% of ALL patients have lymphoblasts with phenotypes corresponding to those of B-cell progenitors.[23,30] These cases can be identified on the basis of cell surface expression of CD19 and at least one other recognized B lineage–associated antigen: CD20, CD24, CD22, CD21, or CD79[23,30]; most B-lineage ALL cases also express CD10 (common ALL antigen [CALLA]). The lymphoblasts may also express nuclear terminal deoxynucleotidyl transferase (TdT) or CD34. About one-fourth of B-progenitor ALL cases express cytoplasmic Ig μ heavy-chain proteins and are designated pre–B-cell ALL. Pre-B cases were originally shown to have a worse long-term response to therapy compared with early pre-B cases, an observation that was later attributed to the presence of the t(1;19) translocation that forms the *E2A–PBX1* fusion gene in about one-fourth of the pre-B cases.[31] However, with the introduction of more intensive, risk-adjusted treatment regimens, the prognosis for patients with t(1;19)+ ALL has improved significantly.[32,33]

DNA rearrangement of *Ig* genes occurs before heavy-chain gene expression in B-cell development, providing a genetic marker of B-lymphocyte ontogeny. Korsmeyer and coworkers[34,35] pioneered the use of heavy- and light-chain gene rearrangements to support an early B-lineage origin of most ALL blasts. This work was extended to establish synchrony between *Ig* gene rearrangements and the expression of B lineage–restricted cell surface antigens. However, *Ig* heavy-chain gene rearrangements have also been documented in about 15% of T-cell ALL cases and a similar percentage of AML cases.[36-38] Thus, caution must be exercised when assigning cell lineage on the basis of studies of *Ig* gene rearrangement.

The identification of specific immunophenotypic, genetic, and clinical features that predict response to therapy in patients with B-lineage ALL and the incorporation of these predictors into clinical decision making are now widespread in modern ALL treatment protocols. This ability to predict outcome in these patients has been closely tied to the remarkable improvements in therapy for children with this disease, which 50 years ago was universally fatal. However, many subgroups of pediatric and adult patients face a much poorer prognosis, and much progress remains to be made.

T-Cell Acute Lymphoblastic Leukemia

Leukemias of T-cell precursors can be identified and classified according to the sequence of expression of T-cell–associated surface antigens during normal thymocyte ontogeny.[39,40] In this tightly regulated process, the earliest T-cell precursors are characterized by the lack of expression of CD4 and CD8 surface markers. These double-negative (DN) thymocytes proceed through a series of differentiation stages (DN1-DN4 in mice; pro-T to pre-T in humans) during which the cells lose CD34 expression, gain CD1a expression, and the *TCR* genes *TCR-δ*, *TCR-γ*, and *TCR-β* become rearranged. The successful rearrangement of *TCR-β* drives the production of immature single-positive cells (ISPs) with a surface $CD4^+$, $CD8^-$, $sCD3^-$ phenotype ($CD4^-$ $CD8^+$ $sCD3^-$ in mice). These cells then differentiate into early double-positive ($CD4^+$, $CD8^+$) cells, at which point the *TCR-α* gene rearrangement occurs. Subsequently, these double-positive progenitors differentiate into late cortical thymocytes showing a loss of CD1 and a gain of surface CD3 expression. This thymic T-cell developmental process ends when mature $CD4^+$ or $CD8^+$ single-positive cells emerge from the thymus,[40,41] although further T-cell differentiation occurs in the periphery upon antigen presentation. Numerous investigators, using a battery of monoclonal antibodies specific for T-cell surface glycoproteins, have confirmed the close relationship between the recognizable patterns of surface antigen expression on leukemic T cells and the normal stages of thymocyte development.[42-45]

Lymphoblasts with a T-cell phenotype comprise approximately 15% of cases of ALL. These are often associated with distinctive clinical features that include high circulating leukocyte counts, a male predominance, CNS involvement, and a radiographically evident thymic mass in many cases at presentation. Historically, patients with T-cell ALL had an adverse prognosis compared with patients with B-lineage ALL, but this gap has narrowed with the intensification of therapy for these patients.[46-48] In marked contrast to B-precursor ALL, in which the availability of a wide range of clinical and genetic prognostic markers has allowed the development of treatment protocols tailored to an individual patient's risk of relapse, robust pretreatment prognostic markers had been lacking in T-ALL[49] until the recent identification of the early T-cell progenitor subtype of T-ALL.

Early T-Cell Progenitor Acute Lymphoblastic Leukemia

Recent work has identified a very high-risk subset of T-ALL cases characterized by differentiation arrest at the earliest identifiable stages of T-cell development, which are defined either by absence of biallelic TCRγ deletion (ABD), indicating differentiation arrest before TCR gene rearrangement, or by expression of a characteristic "early T-cell precursor" (ETP) phenotype.[50,51] These cases comprise 8% to 15% of pediatric T-ALL but appear to comprise a much higher fraction of T-ALL in adults,[52] thus providing one possible explanation for the significantly inferior outcomes of adults versus children with T-ALL. ABD/ETP T-ALL cases have recently been shown to harbor characteristic genetic alterations that include PTEN deletions and activating mutations of RAS, IL-7R, and FLT3, thus implicating these kinases, and the signal transduction pathways they regulate, as novel therapeutic targets in high-risk T-ALL.[50,52,53] Moreover, ETP T-ALL patients also harbor oncogenic alterations that are characteristic of AML or myelodysplastic syndrome (MDS), including *DNMT3A*, *IDH1/2*, and *EZH2* mutations,[52,53] suggesting that the cell of origin of ABD/ETP T-ALL may be a multipotent hematopoietic stem or progenitor cell rather than a committed T-cell progenitor. Indeed, approximately 20% of relapses in T-ALL patients with biallelic TCRγ rearrangements at diagnosis are characterized by absence of biallelic TCRγ deletion (ABD) at relapse.[50] It is implausible that a cell with a biallelic deletion of genomic DNA would reacquire the deleted sequences; thus, these data further support the hypothesis that, at least in some cases of high-risk T-ALL, the transformed leukemia-initiating clone is an immature progenitor characterized by differentiation arrest at an earlier stage than that of the bulk lymphoblast population at the time of T-ALL diagnosis.

Mixed-Lineage Leukemia

Acute mixed-lineage leukemias are defined by blast cells that coexpress markers of both the lymphoid and myeloid lineages. Two distinct forms of these leukemias are recognized: those with lymphoid morphology that coexpress myeloid-associated antigen[54,55] and those with myeloid morphology and reactivity to myeloperoxidase staining that coexpress cell-surface antigens normally restricted to lymphoid cells. The origin of mixed-lineage leukemias has not been established. One possibility is malignant transformation of pluripotent hematopoietic stem or progenitor cells that retain the ability to differentiate in both the myeloid and lymphoid lineages; another is immortalization of rare progenitor cells that normally coexpress features of both lineages; and a third is aberrant gene expression caused by specific genetic alterations.[56] There was initially considerable controversy over whether patients with lymphoid leukemia with expression of one or more myeloid cell surface antigens (e.g., CD13, CD33, or CD14) had an adverse prognosis. However, more recent data suggest that the coexpression of myeloid antigens in ALL does not carry an adverse prognosis in the setting of contemporary treatment regiments.[57-59] The expression of lymphoid markers in predominantly myeloid leukemias is relatively rare, and although some studies reported an adverse effect of T-lymphoid markers on outcomes,[60] more recent analyses did not demonstrate a significant prognostic value to lymphoid antigen expression in AML.[61]

GENETIC BASIS OF LYMPHOID LEUKEMIA

Multiple acquired genetic abnormalities are responsible for the aberrant proliferation and differentiation arrest characteristic of ALL. These include chromosomal rearrangements detectable by conventional cytogenetics, as well as lesions that are evident only by molecular analysis. The ability to identify these changes and the discovery that many of these can be used to predict response to therapy have led to risk-adapted therapy for patients with ALL. It is worth noting that the vast majority of patients with leukemia have normal constitutional karyotypes, indicating that the genetic abnormalities in ALL lymphoblasts are usually acquired somatically and thus are restricted to the malignant clone.

Chromosomal translocations are found in 75% of ALL patients (Fig. 63-1).[22,62] They can be broadly classified as recurrent lineage-restricted abnormalities, which account for approximately two-thirds of the translocations in ALL, or as "random" translocations, which

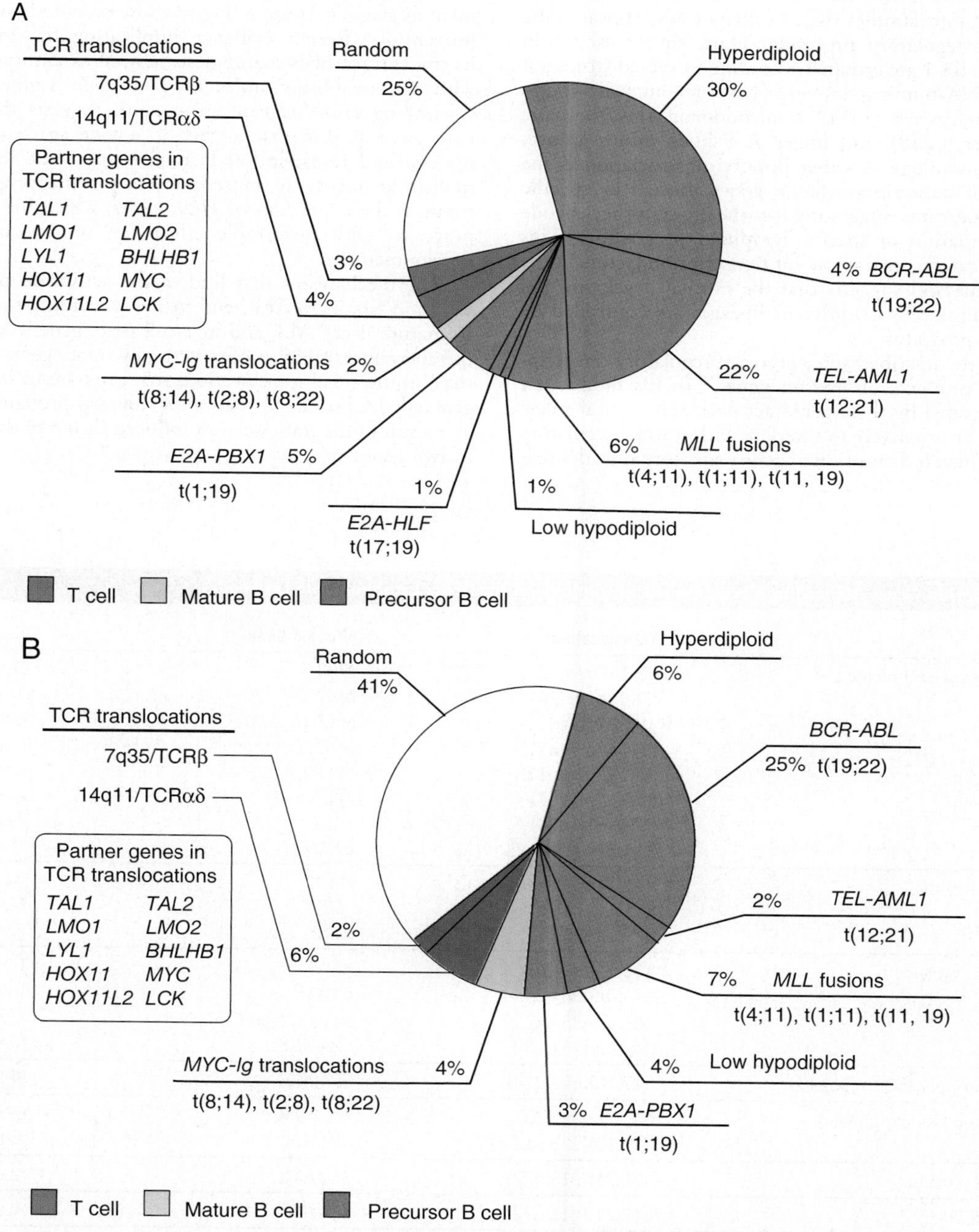

Figure 63-1 FREQUENCY OF THE MAJOR CHROMOSOMAL TRANSLOCATIONS IN PEDIATRIC (**A**) AND ADULT (**B**) ACUTE LYMPHOBLASTIC LEUKEMIA (ALL). The genes affected by chromosomal translocation are shown in *bold*. T-cell receptor (TCR) translocations in T-ALL can activate a number of different proto-oncogenes as shown in the *insert*, including *TAL1, LMO1/2, HOX11, HOX11L2,* and *MYC.*

have been identified only in single or very small numbers of cases. The characterization of genes that span the breakpoints of recurrent translocations has allowed the identification of genes that play critical roles in leukemogenesis.[3-5]

Central Role of Transcription Factors

Molecular studies on recurrent chromosomal translocations in ALL have demonstrated a central role for the aberrant expression of transcription factors in the pathobiology of leukemia (Table 63-1). The dysregulated expression of these transcription factors, which are often functionally normal, leads to abnormal proliferation and differentiation arrest of leukemic lymphoid and myeloid progenitors.[3-5] Conserved amino acid sequence motifs within the sequence-specific DNA binding domains of these nuclear trans-activating proteins allow them to be grouped into families that, in many cases, appear to be involved in similar regulatory processes. Thus, the transcription factor genes in Table 63-1 are grouped according to shared structural features of their DNA-binding domains: basic region helix–loop–helix (bHLH), cysteine-rich (LIM), homeodomain (HOX), basic region-leucine zipper (bZIP), zinc-finger, A-T hook minor groove, ETS-like, or runt homology. Another important association is the lineage restriction of transcription factor genes affected by specific chromosomal translocations, suggesting that the proteins they encode disrupt the differentiation of specific lymphoid progenitors. This interpretation implicates a central role for transcription factors in the initiation of leukemia and suggests that the normal developmental programs of progenitor cells of different lineages are controlled by different regulatory programs.

Rabbitts[63] has aptly described a key group of regulatory transcription factors as the products of "master genes." In his model, the nuclear proteins encoded by these genes act positively to upregulate critical target genes or negatively to interfere with normal regulatory pathways. The net effect is disruption of gene regulatory cascades that control and coordinate the expression of large numbers of proteins required for completion of lymphoid cell differentiation programs. Disruption of transcription factors in leukemic blasts occurs by at least two distinct mechanisms: the dysregulated expression of intact genes and the creation of chimeric transcription factors.

Developmental Biology of Oncogenic Transcription Factors

A surprising connection has emerged from studies of oncogenic transcription factors and the developmental proteins regulating segmentation in *Drosophila* because the DNA-binding domains of these proteins often show striking homology. The proteins participating in leukemogenesis interfere with a highly regulated network of hematopoietic transcription factors, leading to arrested cell development at stages corresponding to those of early lymphoid or myeloid progenitors. Recent evidence implicating the major *HOX* genes in the control of hematopoiesis as well as embryogenesis, together with the established roles of *Drosophila* segmentation genes in controlling *HOM-C* gene expression, suggests that the *HOX* loci may serve as proximal targets of a wide spectrum of hybrid and dysregulated transcription factors in the acute leukemias.[5] In this model, the oncogenic transcription factors inappropriately activate or suppress the expression of *HOX* genes, which in turn regulate gene programs with pleiotropic effects on normal hematopoietic cell development.

The mechanisms that lead to the activation of oncogenic transcription factors in ALL tend to vary according to the ALL subtype. In mature B-cell ALL and in T-cell ALL, genetic lesions that lead to the aberrant expression of structurally intact genes predominate, but the chromosomal translocations that often occur in B-precursor ALL generally lead to the formation of chimeric proteins, which produced as a result of the translocation-induced fusion of the coding sequence of two genes.

Table 63-1 Transcription Genes Affected by Chromosomal Breakpoints in the Acute Lymphoblastic Leukemias

Family*	Translocation	Affected Gene	Disease
Basic helix-loop-helix (bHLH) proteins	t(8;14)(q24;q32)	*MYC*	Burkitt lymphoma and
	t(2;8)(p12;q24)	*MYC*	B-cell ALL
	t(8;22)(q24;q11)	*MYC*	T-cell ALL
	t(8;14)(q24;q11)	*MYC*	T-cell ALL
	t(7;19)(q35;p13)	*LYL1*	T-cell ALL
	t(1;14)(p32;q11)	*TAL1*	T-cell ALL
	t(7;9)(q35;q34)	*TAL2*	T-cell ALL
	t(14;21)(q11.2;q22)	*BHLHB1*	
Cysteine-rich (LIM) proteins	t(11;14)(p15;q11)	*LMO1*	T-cell ALL
	t(11;14)(p13;q11)	*LMO2*	T-cell ALL
	t(7;11)(q35;p13)	*LMO2*	T-cell ALL
Homeodomain (HOX) proteins	t(10;14)(q24;q11)	*HOX11*	T-cell ALL
	t(7;10)(q35;q24)	*HOX11*	T-cell ALL
	t(5;14)(q35;q32.2)	*HOX11L2* and *BCL11B*	T-cell ALL
	t(1;19)(q23;p13)	*E2A-PBX1*	Pre-B-cell ALL
Basic-region/leucine-zipper (bZIP) proteins	t(17;19)(q22;p13)	*E2A-HLF*	EPB ALL
A-T hook minor groove binding proteins†	t(4;11)(q21;q23)	*MLL-AF4*	EPB ALL
	t(11;19)(q23;p13.3)	*MLL-ENL*	ALL or AML
ETS-like (TEL, ERG) proteins	t(12;21)(p13;q22)	*TEL-AML1*	ALL
Runt homology (AML1)	t(12;21)(p13;q22)	*TEL-AML1*	ALL

ALL, Acute lymphoblastic leukemia; *AML*, acute myeloid leukemia; *EPB*, early pre-B.
*Based on DNA-binding domain.
†Partial list of MLL fusions.

Dysregulated Expression of Structurally Intact Genes

Activation of *MYC* in B-Cell Acute Lymphoblastic Leukemia

The vast majority of cases of mature B-cell ALL and Burkitt lymphoma are characterized by a translocation that places one allele of *MYC* from chromosome 8 under the control of the regulatory elements of an *Ig* gene, either the heavy-chain gene on chromosome 14q32 or the κ or λ light-chain genes on chromosomes 2 and 22. This leads to the aberrant expression of *MYC,* a prototypical basic helix–loop–helix oncogenic transcription factor.[64-72] In the predominant t(8;14) translocation, the involved *MYC* locus is translocated into the heavy-chain gene on chromosome 14 adjacent to the coding sequences of the *Ig* constant region.[64-66] The coding sequences of the *Ig* variable region generally are reciprocally translocated to the distal tip of chromosome 8. In variant translocations, the *MYC* gene remains on chromosome 8, and portions of the respective light-chain genes are translocated to that chromosome downstream of the *MYC* locus.[67-71]

Although the *MYC* coding region is not structurally altered by translocation in most cases of B-cell ALL or Burkitt lymphoma, point mutations in the N-terminal phosphorylation domain of *MYC* commonly arise in these tumors at codons 58 or 62.[73-75] These codons are phosphorylation sites involved in the regulation of the activation and degradation of the protein,[76] and these mutations lead not only to the aberrant stabilization of MYC protein[77-79] but also inhibit the ability of *MYC* to activate the proapoptotic *BIM* gene while its ability to stimulate proliferation remains intact.[80]

The mechanisms by which *MYC* exerts its potent growth-promoting effects are complex and only partially understood. *MYC* is estimated to regulate the expression of 15% of the genome[81] and leads to the transcriptional activation of a large number of genes involved in cell division, growth, metabolism, adhesion, and motility.[82] It also leads to the transcriptional repression of many other genes, such as the cell cycle inhibitors p27 and p21. *MYC* exerts its transcriptional activity via the formation of heterodimers with its DNA-binding partner protein MAX–MYC–MAX heterodimers bind to canonical hexameric E-box DNA sequences (5′-CACGTG-3′) where they activate transcription.[83] MAX can also heterodimerize with other bHLHZip proteins, including MAD,[84] MXI-1 (MAD2),[85] and MNT.[86] Whereas transcriptional activation by MYC–MAX complexes promotes proliferation, binding by MAD–MAX and other MAX heterodimers produces opposite effects; for example, MAD inhibits MYC function both by competing with MYC for binding to MAX and by directly inhibiting transcription. Moreover, in addition to its well-established role as a transcriptional regulator, MYC is also an important regulator of microRNA expression and ribosome biogenesis,[87-90] thus implicating additional post-transcriptional regulation of protein expression through which MYC exerts its potent biologic effects.

BHLH, LIM, and *HOX* Genes in T-Cell Acute Lymphoblastic Leukemia

In leukemias with a T-cell phenotype, chromosomal breakpoints consistently involve the *TCR* enhancer (7q34) or the *TCRA/D* enhancer (14q11), both of which are highly active in committed T-cell progenitors and can cause dysregulated expression of transcription factor genes located at the breakpoint on the reciprocal chromosome involved in these phenotype-specific rearrangements.[91] The affected transcription factors include (2) genes encoding bHLH family members, such as *TAL1,*[92,93] *TAL2,*[94] *LYL1,*[95] *MYC,*[96-98] and BHLHB1[99]; (2) LIM-only domain *(LMO)* genes, such as *LMO1* and *LMO2*[100]; and (3) the orphan homeobox genes *HOX11* and *HOL11L1.*[37,101-106] The observation that T-ALL oncogenes act as master transcriptional regulators during the embryologic development of specific organ systems suggests that their aberrant expression in T-cell precursors may contribute to the onset of leukemia by disrupting the mechanisms that control cell proliferation, differentiation, and survival during the discrete steps of normal T-cell development. Gene expression profiling and mutational analyses have shown that cases of T-ALL can be separated into five subtypes based on the pattern of multistep genetic abnormalities that occur (Fig. 63-2).

The best characterized of the oncogenic transcription factors involved in T-ALL is *TAL1* (also known as *SCL*), which is altered by the t(1;14) or by site-specific deletions in approximately one-fourth of childhood T-ALL cases.[107-112] *TAL1* is aberrantly expressed in the leukemic cells of 60% of children and 45% of adults with T-ALL, and its expression is required for maintenance of the leukemic phenotype in human cell culture studies.[113] TAL1 acts as a master regulatory protein during early hematopoietic development and is required for the

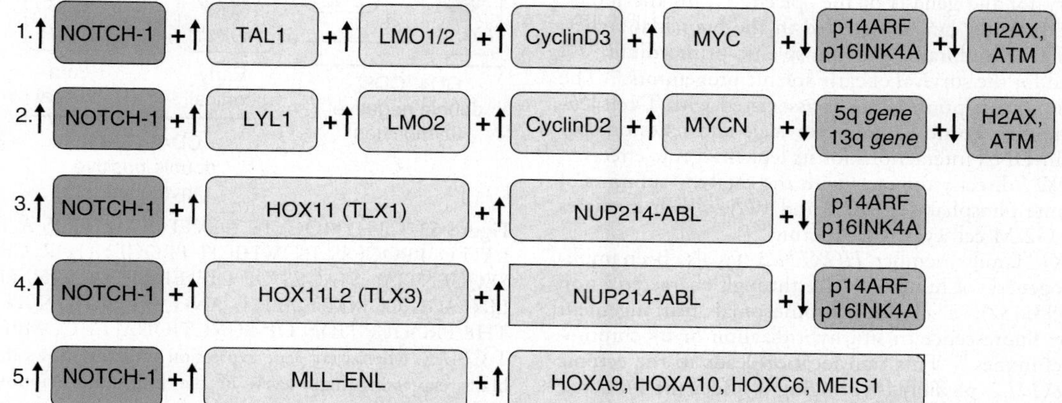

Figure 63-2 MULTISTEP ONCOGENIC PATHWAYS IN T-CELL ACUTE LYMPHOBLASTIC LEUKEMIA (ALL). Gene expression profiling and mutation analyses have revealed that five different multistep molecular pathways can lead to the malignant transformation of developing thymocytes. *NOTCH1* mutations are seen in samples from all five T-ALL subtypes. *HOX11, HOX11L2,* and *TAL1*-overexpressing cases show high levels of *MYC* expression and share the loss of the tumor suppressor genes *p16/INK4A* and *p14/ARF* on chromosome 9p. *HOX11* and *HOX11L2* are often associated with a novel *NUP214-ABL* episomal fusion gene, which may render these T-ALLs sensitive to imatinib. *LYL1*+ cases show high levels of expression of *N-MYC* and frequently have deletions affecting as yet unidentified loci on chromosomal arms 5q and 13q. Finally, *MLL–ENL*+ cases have a clearly distinct gene expression profile characterized by low expression of *MYC* and other genes involved in cell growth and proliferation but high expression of *HOXA9, HOXA10,* and *HOXC6* in concert with the *HOX* gene regulator *MEIS1. (Adapted from Armstrong SA, Look AT: Molecular genetics of acute lymphoblastic leukemia.* J Clin Oncol *23:6306, 2005, with permission.)*

generation of all blood cell lineages.[114,115] However, it does not seem to be required for the generation and function of hematopoietic stem cells (HSCs) during adult hematopoiesis.[116] This class II bHLH transcription factor binds to DNA by forming heterodimers with class I bHLH factors such as E2A.[117] Although TAL1 binding to promoter sites that are normally occupied by TAL1, E2A or HEB can lead to either repression or activation of transcription.[113] TAL1 appears to exert its leukemogenic effects largely via the inhibition of E2A activity.[118] The observation that loss of E2A function induces T-cell leukemias in mice[119,120] and that the DNA-binding domain of TAL1 is dispensable for transformation in transgenic mouse models[121] gives additional support to the notion that TAL1-mediated inhibition of E2A plays a central role in its pathogenesis in T-ALL.

The LIM-only domain genes, *LMO1/RBTN1/TTG1* and *LMO2/RBTN2/TTG2,*[100,122,123] encode proteins that possess duplicated cysteine-rich LIM domains involved in protein–protein interactions. LMO2 interacts with TAL1 in erythroid cells and in T-cell leukemias.[124-126] Moreover, homozygous disruption of *LMO2* in mice causes the same phenotype as described earlier for *TAL1* knock-outs, indicating that a multiprotein complex is required for normal hematopoietic development that involves LMO2, TAL1, and other proteins such as GATA1.[127-130] In addition, overexpression of *LMO1* or *LMO2* in thymocytes of transgenic mice leads to T-cell lymphomas, recapitulating human T-cell tumors,[131-135] and accelerates the onset of leukemias in *TAL1* transgenic mice lines.[126]

The homeodomain gene *HOX11* (also known as *TLX1*), located on chromosome 10, band 24, is one of the more interesting proteins activated by translocation into the vicinity of the *TCR* loci.[37,102,104-106] *HOX11* is the founding member of a family of *HOX* genes that includes *HOX11L1* and *HOX11L2*[106] and whose family members are characterized by the presence of a threonine in the third helix of the homeodomain, which confers specific DNA binding properties. *HOX11* was originally isolated from the recurrent t(10;14)(q24;q11) in T-ALL[37,102,104,105] and is aberrantly expressed in 5% of pediatric and up to 30% of adult T-ALL patients.[101,136,137] The relatively low frequency translocations involving the *HOX11* locus on 10q24, 2% to 5% in childhood T-ALL[105] and 14% in adult cases,[138] suggests that alternative mechanisms leading to *HOX11* overexpression account for the activation of this transcription factor oncogene in a significant fraction of T-ALL cases.

Similar to other *HOX* genes, *HOX11* plays an important role in embryonic development, and functions as a master transcriptional regulator necessary for the genesis of the spleen.[139,140] In the mouse embryo, *Hox11* expression can be detected in the branchial arches, restricted areas of the hindbrain, and the splenic primordium,[141,142] where it is required for the survival of early splenic progenitors.[140] The *HOX11* oncogenic transcription factor is associated with T-cell leukemogenesis at the early cortical thymocyte stage and relies on specific homeodomain-DNA interactions for its leukemogenic effects.[143] Additionally, *HOX11* directly interacts with the catalytic subunits of the serine–threonine phosphatases PP2A and PPA, which mediates disruption of the G2/M cell cycle checkpoint.[144]

A second *HOX11* family member, *HOX11L2,* has also been implicated in the pathogenesis of human T-ALL through characterization of the t(5;14)(q35;q32), a cryptic chromosomal rearrangement detectable only by fluorescence in situ hybridization or by chromosome painting techniques.[103] This translocation leads to the ectopic expression of *HOX11L2,* possibly by bringing it under the influence of regulatory elements in the *CTIP2/BCL11B* gene, which is highly expressed during T-lymphoid differentiation. In contrast to the predominance of *HOX11* expression in adult T-ALL cases, both the t(5;14) and expression of *HOX11L2* can be detected in 20% to 25% of children but in only 5% of adults with T-ALL.[101,137,145-147] The role of HOX11L2 as a master transcriptional regulator upstream of important pathways involved in cell fate determination is supported by its importance during embryonic development.[148] In mice, *Hox11l2* expression is essential for normal development of the ventral medullary respiratory center.[148] Mice deficient in this protein die soon after birth from respiratory failure that resembles congenital central hypoventilation syndrome in humans.

HOX11 and HOX11L2 are closely related in structure and have a high degree of homology at the amino acid level, especially in the homeobox domain, where their sequences differ by only three amino acids. The high level of structural homology in their DNA-binding domains supports the hypothesis that HOX11 and HOX11L2 may induce T-ALL through regulation of the same transcriptional targets. *HOX11* expression has recently been shown to induce T-ALL in mice and to disrupt the mitotic checkpoint via inhibition of *CHK1,* thus accounting for the association of *HOX11/HOX11L2* overexpression with aneuploidy, which is otherwise rare in human T-ALL.[149]

Recently, the analysis of gene expression profiling using oligonucleotide microarrays has shown that the expression of different transcription factor oncogenes such as *TAL1, LYL1, HOX11,* and *HOX11L2* is associated with distinct gene expression profiles. These unique signatures resemble those of thymocytes blocked at discrete stages of T-cell development (Fig. 63-3),[17] suggesting that transcription factor oncogenes contribute to the pathogenesis of T-ALL by interfering with critical regulatory networks that control cell proliferation, survival, and differentiation during T-cell development.[17] Based on the patterns of aberrant gene expression, human cases of T-ALL can be classified into five different subtypes (see Fig. 63-2).

HOXA Cluster Translocations in T-Cell Acute Lymphoblastic Leukemia

A recurrent inversion on chromosome 7 that places the *HOXA* cluster in the vicinity of the TCR β gene regulatory elements and that leads to activation of the entire *HOXA* cluster was recently discovered in approximately 5% of cases of T-ALL.[150,151] Many of these patients also carried cooperating oncogenic lesions consisting of *NOTCH1* gene mutations and deletions of 9p21.[152] This new translocation that directly activates *HOXA* gene expression provides additional evidence for the role of aberrant *HOXA* activation in leukemogenesis and in the pathogenesis of *MLL- and CALM-AF10*–rearranged leukemias.

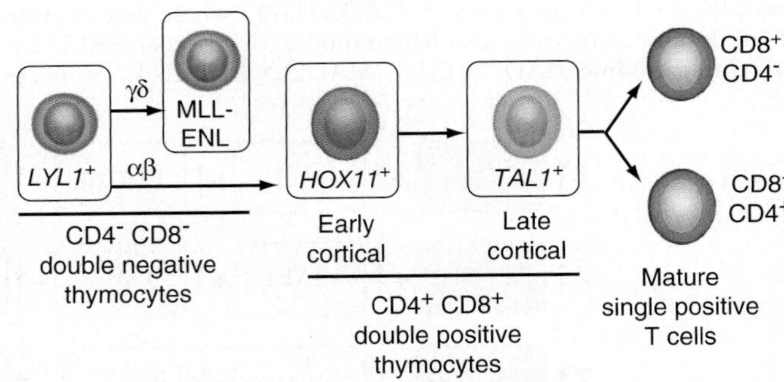

Figure 63-3 THYMOCYTE DEVELOPMENT IS A TIGHTLY REGULATED PROCESS IN WHICH PROGENITOR CELLS UNDERGO SEQUENTIAL STAGES OF DIFFERENTIATION, PROLIFERATION, LINEAGE COMMITMENT, AND SELECTION THAT RESULT IN THE PRODUCTION OF FUNCTIONALLY COMPETENT MATURE T CELLS. Microarray gene expression profiling shows that T-ALL lymphoblasts expressing high levels of the LYL1 transcription factor oncogene undergo an early arrest at the double-negative thymocyte ($CD4^-$, $CD8^-$) stage of development. In T-ALL cases with aberrant expression of HOX11, the leukemic cells show a developmental arrest at the double-positive ($CD4^+$, $CD8^+$) early cortical stage of thymocyte differentiation, but those with aberrant expression of TAL1 are arrested at the double positive late cortical stage. T-ALL cells with expression of the *MLL-ENL* fusion gene are characterized by an early arrest of differentiation with a gene expression signature that indicates commitment to the γ-delta lineage. *(Adapted from Ferrando AA, Neuberg DS, Staunton J, et al: Gene expression signatures define novel oncogenic pathways in T cell acute lymphoblastic leukemia.* Cancer Cell *1:75, 2002, and Ferrando AA, Look AT: Gene expression profiling in T-cell acute lymphoblastic leukemia.* Semin Hematol *40:274, 2003, with permission.)*

Other Genes Activated by Translocation

Transcription factors are not the only genes activated by translocation to the sites of the *Ig* or *TCR* genes. In cases of B-precursor ALL carrying the t(5;14), for example, the *IL-3* gene is activated by juxtaposition with the *Ig* heavy-chain locus.[153,154] Similarly, relocation to the *TCRB* locus activates expression of the *LCK* tyrosine kinase genes in T-ALL cases with the t(1;7).[155-157]

Chimeric Transcription Factor Genes

Formation of chimeric proteins whose functional domains come from two normally separate genes represents a second mechanism of aberrant transcription factor activation, which is more prevalent in B-precursor ALL. These chromosomal translocations result in the production of a chimeric protein by fusing the DNA-binding, dimerization, and trans-activation regions of discrete genes. This process is facilitated by the molecular structure of transcription factors in which discrete coding regions of each gene encode particular functional domains; this molecular structure likely arose for evolutionary reasons.

E2A-PBX1 Fusion Genes in Pre-B Cell Acute Lymphoblastic Leukemia

A well-known example of a chimeric transcription factor with oncogenic potential is the *E2A-PBX1* rearrangement, which results from the t(1;19)(q23;p13) chromosomal translocation present in about 5% of all B-lineage ALLs and in 25% of cases with a pre-B (cytoplasmic Ig-positive) phenotype.[32,91,158] This translocation fuses the transactivation domain of the *E2A* transcription factor on chromosome 19 to a homeobox gene *(PBX1)* on chromosome 1, leading to the expression of several forms of hybrid E2A-PBX1 oncoproteins.[159-161] *PBX1* is related to the *Drosophila exd* gene, a homeobox gene that plays a role in lymphocyte development.[162,163] The hybrid proteins resulting from the t(1;19) retain the amino-terminal trans-activation domains of E2A (AD1 and AD2) but not the bHLH DNA-binding/protein interaction domain.[160,161,164] The bHLH domain is replaced by the homeobox DNA-binding domain of PBX1, enabling the fusion protein to function as a chimeric transcription factor.[165-167]

The transforming potential of *E2A–PBX1* was first demonstrated by the rapid induction of AML in lethally irradiated mice repopulated with bone marrow stem cells that had been infected with recombinant retroviruses containing *E2A–PBX1* genes.[168] The fusion has also been shown to transform NIH-3T3 fibroblasts and induce T-cell lymphomas in transgenic mice.[169,170] Additional studies have shown that deletion of one of the E2A activation domains diminishes its transforming activity, but deletion of the PBX1 homeodomain has no effect.[170,171] However, the homeodomain and flanking sequences are required for interactions with other HOX proteins and for optimal binding of E2A–PBX1 to specific DNA sequences.[172-176] It thus appears that complex interactions between E2A–PBX1 and other HOX proteins target the fusion protein to specific target genes whose activation is critical to lymphoid cell transformation. The presence of the *E2A–PBX1* translocation was originally associated with a poor prognosis.[31] However, this translocation no longer imparts an adverse prognosis in the setting of modern risk-adjusted protocols for childhood ALL.[32,177-179]

E2A–HLF Fusion Genes in Early Pre-B Acute Lymphoblastic Leukemia

The t(17;19) is a rare recurrent chromosomal translocation that fuses the amino-terminal transactivation domains of E2A to the C-terminal DNA binding and dimerization domains of HLF,[180,181] which belongs to the PAR subfamily of bZIP transcription factors. Although E2A–HLF can bind DNA either as a homodimer or as a heterodimer with HLF and related proteins, no other PAR proteins are expressed in hematopoietic cells, and the E2A–HLF fusion binds DNA as a homodimer in cells harboring the t(17;19). Similar to E2A–PBX1, E2A–HLF can transform NIH–3T3 fibroblasts, a process that requires the HLF leucine zipper domain and the E2A transactivation domains.[182] E2A–HLF can also induce lymphoid tumors in transgenic mice.[183]

A major consequence of the activation of E2A–HLF in lymphoid precursors is dysregulation of the mechanisms that control programmed cell death in lymphoid progenitors. Expression of a dominant-negative form of E2A–HLF in t(17;19)-carrying cell lines blocks E2A–HLF function and results in apoptosis.[184] In normal pro-B lymphocytes, expression of E2A–HLF reversed IL-3-dependent and p53-induced apoptosis. HLF is the mammalian homologue of the nematode protein ces-2, which regulates the death of specific nerve cells in *Caenorhabditis elegans*.[184-186] Ces-2 is necessary for the death of the sister cells of a specific pair of serotonergic neurons during worm development. Ces-2 induces apoptosis by inhibiting the expression of *ces-1,* a prosurvival gene that normally inhibits programmed cell death by antagonizing the activity of the proapoptotic factor *egl-1*. This pathway, which is highly conserved through evolution, is disrupted by E2A–HLF fusion. Thus, in contrast to the proapoptotic role of ces-2 in the worm via repression of ces-1, E2A–HLF blocks apoptosis by inducing the expression of *SLUG,* a *ces-1* homologue normally responsible for protecting hematopoietic progenitors from DNA-damage–induced apoptosis.[187-190]

The t(17;19) is seen in fewer than 1% of ALL patients, typically occurs in adolescents, and is associated with disseminated intravascular coagulation and hypercalcemia at diagnosis. The t(17;19) seems to impart unfavorable prognosis because each of seven patients whose blasts expressed *E2A–HLF* died of leukemia despite aggressive therapy.[91] It seems likely that resistance to chemotherapy in these cases is mediated by the role of E2A–HLF in driving the expression of *SLUG* and inhibiting apoptosis.[190]

MLL Fusion Genes

Translocations involving chromosome 11 band q23 occur in approximately 80% of infant ALL cases, 5% of AML cases, and 85% of secondary AML cases that occur in patients treated with topoisomerase II inhibitors.[91] The gene bisected by 11q23 translocations is designated *MLL* (also known as *TRX1* or *ALL-1*), which is the human ortholog of the trithorax *Drosophila* gene.[191-194] The trithorax group family of proteins are positive regulators of homeobox gene expression and act antagonistically to the polycomb group of proteins.[195] Wild-type MLL positively regulates *HOX* gene expression and is required for both primitive and definitive hematopoiesis.[196-198] The MLL protein undergoes proteolytic processing by Taspase1, a specialized protease that cleaves the MLL protein into N-terminal (MLL^N) and C-terminal (MLL^C) fragments that remain associated through intramolecular protein–protein interaction domains.[199-201] MLL^N contains several DNA-binding domains, including AT-hook domains that nonspecifically bind the minor groove of DNA, a methyltransferase homology region (CxxC domain) that specifically binds unmethylated DNA, four plant homeodomain zinc fingers with an embedded bromodomain, and a transcriptional repression domain.[195] The C-terminal fragment MLL^C contains a transcriptional activation domain that recruits the histone acetyltransferase cAMP response element-binding protein (CBP) and a SET domain that is responsible for its histone 3 lysine 4 (H3K4) methyltransferase activity.[201] Recent studies have revealed that wild-type MLL is a member of a large multiprotein complex involved in chromatin modification and remodeling, together with histone deacetylases and members of the Swi/Snf chromatin-remodeling complex.[202]

MLL fusion oncogenes result from translocations whose breakpoints cluster between exons 5 and 11 of *MLL,* and the resultant fusion proteins retain the N-terminal region of *MLL,* including the AT-hook and CxxC domains that bind DNA in a sequence-nonspecific manner.[203] By contrast, the C-terminal domains that mediate the association of wild-type MLL with its endogenous chromatin modification–remodeling complex and its H3K4 methyltransferase activity are invariably lost from oncogenic MLL fusion proteins. Instead, the C-terminus of MLL fusion oncoproteins is provided by one of more than 60 different translocation partners, with common translocations such as the t(4;11), t(9;11), and t(11;19)(q23;p13.3) resulting in the in-frame fusion of *MLL* to *AF4, AF9,* and *ENL,* respectively. The unrelated t(11;19)(q23;p13.1) translocation results in fusion of MLL to ELL, the RNA polymerase II elongation factor.[204,205]

Formal proof that *MLL* fusions play a critical role in the development of leukemias has come from the generation of murine models of *MLL*-induced leukemias. Chimeric mice harboring a *MLL–AF9* fusion gene generated by homologous recombination developed leukemias with a latency of 4 to 12 months.[206] Retroviral transduction of *MLL–ENL, MLL–ELL,* and *MLL–CBP* fusion genes in hematopoietic precursors induces transformation upon transplantation into recipient mice.[207-209] Similar results were recently obtained with a model in which chromosomal translocations involving the *Mll* locus are induced by directed interchromosomal recombination in mice, a strategy that reproduces experimentally the initiating events in the pathogenesis of *MLL*-rearranged leukemias.[210] Interestingly, the introduction of MLL–AF9 into committed granulocyte-macrophage progenitors in the mouse leads to the reactivation of a subset of genes normally expressed only in HSCs and transforms these committed precursors into AML leukemic stem cells by imparting the properties of self-renewal,[211] suggesting that the leukemogenic lesion in MLL-rearranged leukemia might occur in a committed progenitor rather than in a pluripotent HSC.

The analysis of gene expression profiles in *MLL*-rearranged B-lineage leukemias has shown that these tumors have a characteristic gene expression signature that includes the upregulation of several *HOX* genes and the expression of numerous myeloid markers.[212-214] Both early B- and T-cell ALLs with MLL rearrangements showed a characteristic upregulation of specific *HOX* genes, including *HOXA9, HOXA10,* and *HOXC6* and the *HOX* gene regulator *MEIS1*.[212-214] These results, together with the demonstration that *HOXA9* plays important roles in the transformation of hematopoietic precursors by MLL fusion oncogenes in murine leukemia models,[215,216] emphasize the central role of *HOX* gene dysregulation in the pathogenesis of *MLL*-rearranged leukemias. Additionally, as discussed later in this chapter, overexpression or activating mutations of the FLT3 receptor tyrosine kinase are frequent in *MLL*-rearranged leukemias,[212,213,217,218] and a model of the multistep pathogenesis of *MLL*-rearranged ALL is depicted in Fig. 63-4.

Until recently, the precise mechanisms mediating the oncogenic activity of MLL fusion oncoproteins was unclear because MLL translocation partners have little sequence or functional similarity. However, recent work has shown that a number of distinct MLL translocation partners are functionally linked through their association in protein complexes that mediate transcriptional elongation.[219] Oncogenic MLL-fusion proteins associate with at least three such complexes, PAFc, DOT1L, and pTEFb (also known as SEC or AEP). PAFc, the polymerase-associated factor complex, regulates RNA polymerase II and associates with the amino-terminus of both wild-type MLL and MLL fusions.[220] The pTEFb complex (CDK9–cyclin T) phosphorylates RNA polymerase II; interacts with several MLL fusion partners, including ENL, ELL, AF4, and AF5; and co-purifies with several MLL fusion proteins.[221,222] The DOT1L complex consists of DOT1L; a histone H3 lysine 79 (H3K79) methyltransferase; and multiple MLL fusion partners, including AF9, ENL, and AF10.[223-228] Analysis of H3K79 methylation status has revealed increased methylation at genes overexpressed in MLL fusion-driven leukemias, including several direct targets of MLL fusions such as the 5′ HOXA cluster genes and MEIS1.[229-231] Interestingly, whereas the DOT1L methyltransferase is required for transformation of murine

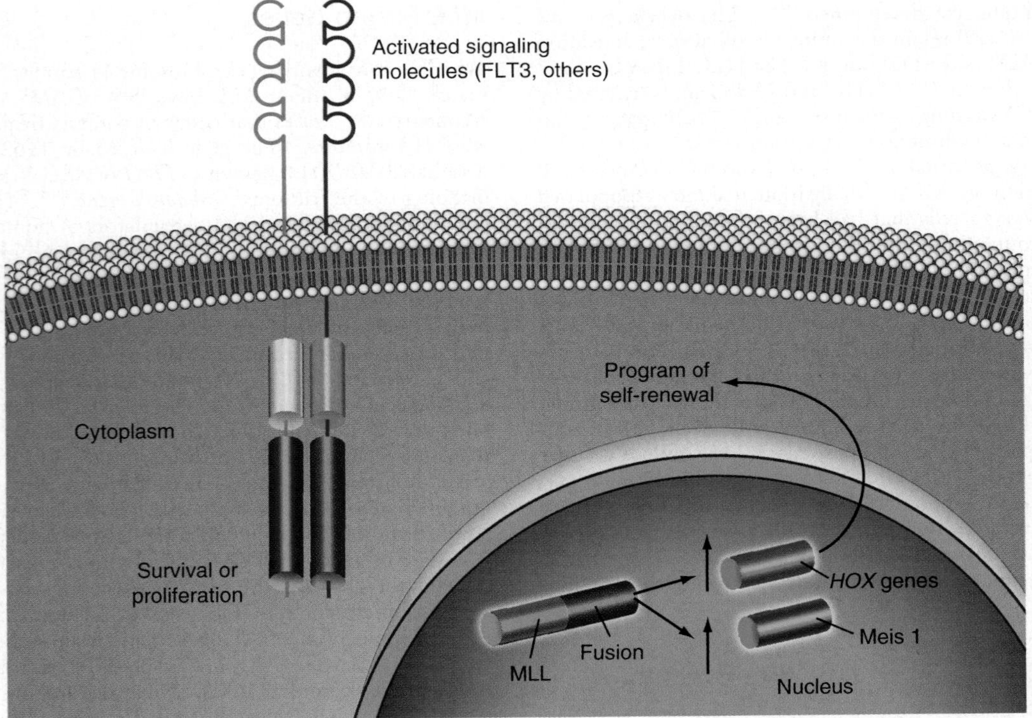

Figure 63-4 MULTISTEP PATHOGENESIS OF MLL-REARRANGED ACUTE LYMPHOBLASTIC LEUKEMIA (ALL). MLL translocations induce self-renewal in hematopoietic progenitors as a first step in leukemogenesis. The presence of FLT3 mutations in MLL-rearranged ALLs support activation of FLT3 or other kinases as cooperating events in this disease. Clinical trials designed to assess the efficacy of FLT3 inhibitors in MLL-rearranged ALL are being developed. *(Adapted from Armstrong SA, Look AT: Molecular genetics of acute lymphoblastic leukemia.* J Clin Oncol *23:6306, 2005, with permission.)*

bone marrow progenitors by MLL fusion oncoproteins, DOT1L plays a less prominent role in normal hematopoiesis, thus suggesting a therapeutic window for therapeutic targeting of DOT1L in MLL-driven leukemias.[227,232-235] Indeed, a small molecule inhibitor of DOT1L has recently been developed and demonstrates promising activity against MLL-positive leukemia cells in vitro and in vivo, with little toxicity in murine models.[236]

The presence of MLL rearrangements is associated with dismal outcomes despite aggressive chemotherapy in most cases of ALL.[23,237-239] Additionally, bone marrow transplantation (BMT) in first remission in these patients is not clearly beneficial and may actually be associated with a decrease in event-free and overall survival compared with chemotherapy alone.[239,240] However, the recent data implicating DOT1L as a promising therapeutic target in MLL-driven leukemias have generated considerable enthusiasm for the development of clinical DOT1L inhibitors for the treatment of MLL-rearranged leukemias.

CALM–AF10 Fusion Gene in T-Cell Acute Lymphoblastic Leukemia

The t(10;11)(p13;q14) detected in approximately 3% to 10% of T-ALL patients and in occasional AML patients and results in the fusion of *CALM,* encoding a protein with high homology to the murine clathrin assembly protein ap3, with *AF10,* a gene identified as an MLL partner in the MLL–AF10 fusion resulting from the t(10;11)(p13;q23).[241] Although the mechanism of action of CALM–AF10 remains incompletely understood, the expression of this fusion transcript has been associated with early arrest in T-cell development and to differentiation into the γ-δlineage in T-ALL.[242] Additionally, recent evidence suggests that aberrant upregulation of *HOX* gene expression appears to be involved in CALM–AF10-mediated leukemogenesis, at least in AML cells that carry this translocation.[243] Interestingly, analysis of a mouse model of CALM–AF10-induced AML suggests that the leukemia stem cell in this model has lymphoid characteristics, and cells from human patients with AML can be identified that have similar characteristics to the disease-propagating cell in this animal model.[244]

TEL–AML1 (ETV6-RUNX1) Fusion Gene in Early Pre-B Acute Lymphoblastic Leukemia

Although most t(12;21) translocations are not detectable by standard cytogenetic analysis, this translocation is detectable by molecular techniques in approximately 25% of childhood B-lineage ALL, which makes this the most common genetic lesion in pediatric ALL.[91] The *TEL–AML1* translocation often arises prenatally and is probably the initiating mutation in ALL, as evidenced by the identification of identical *TEL–AML1* translocations in identical twins with concordant ALL[245] and in retrospectively analyzed neonatal blood specimens of children diagnosed with ALL.[246] However, *TEL–AML1* is insufficient in causing leukemia because the incidence of detectable *TEL–AML1* fusions in the blood of normal newborns is about 100-fold greater than the incidence of leukemia.[247]

The molecular mechanisms mediating *TEL–AML1*-induced leukemogenesis remain poorly understood. This fusion gene encodes a chimeric protein that contains the helix–loop–helix (HLH) domain of TEL fused to nearly all of AML1 (also known as RUNX1 or CBFA2), including both the transactivation domain and the DNA- and protein-binding Runt homology domain. Both of these genes are found in other leukemia-related translocations, and both are essential for normal hematopoiesis. *TEL* was first identified in the t(5;12) in chronic myelomonocytic leukemia, where it is fused to the platelet derived growth factor receptor gene *(PDGFRB),* and is also fused to *ABL, MN1,* and *EVI1* in AML and to *JAK2* in T-ALL.[248] The role of TEL in hematopoiesis has been demonstrated with a conditional mouse model in which the absence of TEL in early development leads to the absence of fetal hematopoiesis. Interestingly, the inactivation of TEL in adult mice leads to the selective loss of HSCs from adult bone marrow, but hematopoiesis is sustained by committed precursors.[249] Most *TEL–AML1* leukemias show loss of the normal *TEL* allele, suggesting that the leukemogenic effect of TEL-AML1 may be mediated in part by loss of function of the *TEL* gene.[250-253]

AML1 is the DNA-binding component of the AML1–CBFß transcription factor complex disrupted by the t(8;21), t(3;21), and inv(16) in AML, making it the most common target of chromosomal translocations in leukemia. AML1 is a transcription factor that has been shown to be required for the expression of several hematopoietic genes involved in myeloid and lymphoid development, including *PU.1* and IL-3, although it can also act as a transcriptional repressor in some settings.[254] Homozygous disruption of the murine *AML1* gene or *CBFB* gene results in the lack of definitive hematopoiesis, indicating that genes regulated by AML1 are essential for normal hematopoietic development.[255,256] Additionally, rare familial mutations in the *AML1* DNA-binding domain lead to the familial platelet disorder and predisposition to myeloid malignancy syndrome.[257] However, the molecular pathways mediating *TEL–AML1*-induced leukemogenesis remain incompletely understood.

The presence of the *TEL–AML1* translocation is associated with an excellent prognosis, with event-free survival rates of approximately 90% in a variety of studies.[91,258,259] However, *TEL–AML1* may not represent an independent predictor of prognosis when age and white blood cell count at the time of diagnosis are taken into account in multivariate analysis.[259] Nevertheless, this translocation identifies a large subset of children with B-precursor ALL who appear to represent good candidates for less intensive therapy. The *TEL–AML1* translocation is associated with lower expression of the *MDR-1* multidrug resistance gene[260] and of genes involved in purine metabolism,[261] which might account for the particular efficacy of these cases to current combination chemotherapy regimens that rely heavily on methotrexate and mercaptopurine, agents that inhibit de novo purine synthesis.

Tyrosine Kinase Genes

BCR–ABL in B-Precursor Acute Lymphoblastic Leukemia

The $22q^-$ chromosomal marker, often called the Philadelphia (Ph) chromosome, which arises from the t(9;22)(q34;q11), was originally identified in patients with CML, although it is also found in about 4% of childhood cases and 25% of adult cases of ALL,[91] which are almost always of the B-precursor subtype. The t(9;22) generates a *BCR–ABL* fusion gene, consisting of 5′ (upstream) sequences from *BCR* and 3′ (downstream) sequences of ABL. The t(9;22) breakpoints on the distal tip of the long arm of chromosome 9 are scattered over a distance of nearly 200 kb within the first intron of the *ABL* proto-oncogene, upstream of the tyrosine kinase domain.[262-264] The breakpoints in the *BCR* gene on chromosome 22 cluster in two separate regions of that gene, known as the major breakpoint cluster region (M-bcr) or minor breakpoint cluster region (m-bcr). In two-thirds of cases of Ph-positive ALL, the breakpoint in the *BCR* gene occurs in the minor breakpoint cluster region (m-bcr), but in all cases of CML and about one third of cases of ALL, the breaks occur in the major breakpoint cluster region (M-bcr).[265] The fusion transcript more commonly present in ALL (m-bcr) encodes a 190-kd protein (p190), but the transcripts found in CML and some cases of ALL (M-bcr breakpoint) encodes a 210-kd hybrid protein (p210).[266-269] Both types of fusions generate chimeric oncoproteins that are activated as a tyrosine-specific protein kinase, similar to the v-abl protein.[270-272]

The ABL tyrosine kinase is localized both in the nucleus and in the cytoplasm of proliferating cells. It is normally activated by DNA damage downstream of ATM and appears to promote p53-mediated growth arrest.[273-276] Mice deficient in ABL develop a wasting syndrome and die soon after birth.[277,278] In contrast to the nuclear and cytoplasmic distribution of normal ABL, the BCR–ABL fusion oncoprotein has a cytoplasmic location and shows increased tyrosine kinase activity.[279,280] When expressed in murine hematopoietic precursors, both p190 and p210 transform hematopoietic cells in vitro and induce a syndrome similar to CML in mice.[281-284] Transformation by the BCR–ABL oncoprotein involves activation of the RAS–MAPK (mitogen-activated protein kinase) pathway, PI-3 and JUN kinases, c-CBL and CRKL, JAK–STAT, NFκB (nuclear factor kappa-B), Src, and cyclin D1.[285-292] Among these targets, the RAS, JUN–kinase, and PI-3 kinase pathways are involved in the induction of cell proliferation.[293] The BCR–ABL oncoprotein affects multiple aspects of cell homeostasis, including apoptosis, differentiation, and cell adhesion. An important cellular effect of BCR–ABL is the induction of cellular resistance to DNA damage agents such as cytostatic drugs and irradiation. After DNA damage, BCR–ABL extends the duration of the G2/M cell cycle checkpoint and facilitates DNA repair. It also upregulates the antiapoptotic *BCLXL* gene, contributing to the suppression of apoptotic cell death.[294]

The presence of the Philadelphia chromosome has historically been associated with an extremely poor prognosis in ALL patients despite treatment with intensified chemotherapeutic regimens.[295-297] However, these patients have been shown to have particularly good responses to allogeneic BMT in first remission, whether from matched sibling or from unrelated donors.[298-302] Moreover, the development of imatinib mesylate, a pharmacologic tyrosine kinase inhibitor targeting the BCR–ABL oncoprotein, has opened novel therapeutic opportunities for the management of Ph-positive ALL. The utility of imatinib as a single agent for BCR–ABL ALL is limited by the rapid development of drug resistance.[303,304] However, the combination of imatinib with conventional chemotherapy has led to remarkable improvements in outcome for patients with BCR–ABL ALL, with 3-year survival rates in children with this disease rivaling those obtained with BMT.[305]

Despite its activity, imatinib resistance remains a barrier to further therapeutic improvements in BCR–ABL ALL. Resistance most commonly emerges because of point mutations in the kinase domain of BCR–ABL, and a series of novel BCR–ABL1 kinase inhibitors have been developed that retain activity against many of these mutant oncoproteins.[306-308] Although not all BCR–ABL mutations that confer resistance can be overcome with newer agents, the potential of these newer BCR–ABL inhibitors with broader specificity to further improve outcomes is actively being investigated. Additionally, a novel pathway mediating resistance to BCR–ABL inhibition has recently been uncovered in BCR–ABL ALL lymphoblasts. Upon BCR–ABL inhibition, these cells markedly upregulate expression of the BCL6 transcription factor, a well-known oncogene that is often translocated in diffuse large B-cell lymphomas.[309] BCL6 then blocks activation of the p53 pathway via transcriptional repression of ARF and thus blocks the therapeutic efficacy of monotherapy with imatinib in BCR–ABL ALL cells. Importantly, inhibition of BCL6 activity generically or using a peptide inhibitor of BCL6 demonstrated marked activity in patient-derived BCR–ABL ALL cells grown in immunodeficient mice, highlighting the therapeutic relevance of these findings.[310]

NUP214–ABL1 in T-Cell Acute Lymphoblastic Leukemia

Although the *BCR–ABL1* translocation is rare in T-cell ALL, amplified episomes containing *NUP214–ABL1* fusion genes have recently been described in approximately 6% of children and adults with T-cell ALL.[311] These episomes appear to arise via a mechanism in which the genomic region of chromosome 9q34, which contains both the *NUP214* and *ABL1* genes, is circularized in a manner that leads to the fusion of these two genes. The breakpoint in the *ABL1* gene in all of these cases occurs in intron 1, which is the same breakpoint observed in Philadelphia-positive CML and B-precursor ALL, but the *NUP214* breakpoints are variable. The wild-type *NUP214* protein is a component of the nuclear pore complex and may contribute oligomerization motifs to the *NUP214–ABL1* fusion oncogene. The NUP214-ABL1 fusion protein has constitutively activated ABL1 tyrosine kinase activity, which is inhibited by the BCR–ABL kinase inhibitor imatinib.[311] The therapeutic potential of imatinib or second-generation tyrosine kinase inhibitors for *NUP214–ABL1*-positive T-cell ALL is of considerable interest.

FLT3 in *MLL*-Rearranged Acute Lymphoblastic Leukemia

FLT3 encodes a receptor tyrosine kinase that is highly expressed in early hematopoietic precursors, where it plays important functional roles.[312,313] Multiple studies have shown that activating mutations of *FLT3*, which lead to constitutive receptor tyrosine kinase activity even in the absence of ligand, are common in leukemic myeloblasts in patients with AML but are rare in adults with ALL.[314-316] However, gene expression studies demonstrated high expression of *FLT3* in most cases of ALL that involve MLL gene rearrangements or hyperdiploidy.[212,213,217] Additionally, activating mutations were identified in 18% of infants with MLL-rearranged ALL,[218] in 21% to 24% of hyperdiploid ALL cases,[7,218] and in all three cases of the prothymic CD117/KIT+ subtype of T-cell ALL in adults who were examined.[317]

In the absence of FLT3 ligand, wild-type FLT3 receptors are inactive because of autoinhibition mediated by the juxtamembrane domain of the receptor. Upon binding of FLT3 ligand, normal FLT3 receptors homodimerize, become activated by phosphorylation, and lead to the activation of signal transduction pathways that promote proliferation and cell survival.[318] Activating mutations of *FLT3* found in leukemias occur in two separate regions of the gene. In-frame tandem duplications in the juxtamembrane domain lead to loss of the autoinhibiton mediated by this domain, with subsequent dimerization and receptor activation in the absence of FLT3 ligand.[319] Alternatively, point mutations or insertions in the second tyrosine kinase domain of the FLT3 receptor lead to autophosphorylation and activation of downstream signaling in the absence of FLT3 ligand.[6,316,320] Small molecule inhibitors of the FLT3 kinase lead to apoptosis in AML cell lines in vitro and are currently undergoing phase I and II testing in adults with AML and MDS.[321] These small molecule inhibitors are also active against MLL-rearranged ALL cell lines[217,322] and hold promise as targeted therapies for cases of ALL that rely on aberrant activation of FLT3.

CRLF2 and *JAK2* Mutations in B-Precursor Acute Lymphoblastic Leukemia

The CRLF2 cytokine receptor binds its ligand, thymic stromal lymphopoietin (TSLP), as a heterodimeric complex with the IL-7 receptor subunit (IL-7R). TSLP–CRLF signaling plays physiologic roles during normal B-cell development and in inflammation. Genomic analyses of B-precursor ALL patient samples revealed recurrent deletions within the pseudoautosomal region of Xp22.3/Yp11.3 that result in overexpression of the entire coding region of CRLF2 under control of gene regulatory elements of P2RY8, a purinergic receptor that is expressed at high levels in ALL cells.[323-325] In some cases, such rearrangements are also accompanied by a Phe232Cys point mutation in CRLF2 that promotes constitutive dimerization and cytokine-independent growth.[324,325] CRLF2 rearrangements occur with especially high frequency in patients with Down syndrome[323-325] and have been found to portend a poor prognosis in adults.[324] Interestingly, aberrant CRLF2 expression very frequently co-occurs with JAK2 activating mutations, and these two genetic lesions collaborate to induce ligand-independent activation of downstream signal transduction pathways, suggesting that CRLF2 may act as a scaffold that is required for activation of oncogenic JAK-STAT signaling by JAK2 mutations in B-precursor ALL.[323-325] A number of JAK2 inhibitors have been developed for the treatment of myeloproliferative syndromes,[326] and these findings have thus generated considerable excitement to the application of such inhibitors to CRLF/JAK2-mutant B-precursor ALL.

Interleukin-7 Receptor Mutations in T-Cell Acute Lymphoblastic Leukemia

The IL-7R α is required for normal T-cell development, with inactivating IL7R mutations leading to severe combined immunodeficiency.[327] The IL-7R protein can heterodimerize with either IL2Rγ, resulting in the receptor for IL-7, or with CRLF2 to form the receptor for thymic stromal lymphopoietin.[328,329] Recently, point mutations in the IL-7R have been described in approximately 10% of T-ALL cases.[53,330,331] These point mutations often introduce a novel cysteine residue in the transmembrane domain of the protein that induces ligand-independent receptor dimerization and activation of downstream oncogenic signal transduction pathways, including JAK–STAT and PI3K–AKT. IL-7R mutations occur in approximately 10% of T-ALL cases and are enriched in the TLX3-rearranged and HOXA-overexpressing cases, thus suggesting the therapeutic utility of targeting this signal transduction pathway in T-ALL.

Mutated Genes

The activation of cellular proto-oncogenes by point mutation is difficult to detect because such lesions lack the cytogenetic abnormalities that signal other forms of transforming alterations. Genes of this type must first be identified in experimental systems so that investigators know in advance the types of activating point mutations that are likely to occur in human tumors. The prototypic genes of this class are NOTCH1 and members of the RAS family, with mutations that affect defined functional domains of the corresponding proteins.

NOTCH1 in T-Cell Acute Lymphoblastic Leukemia

The *NOTCH1* gene was discovered as a partner gene in a t(7;9) chromosomal translocation that is found in exceedingly rare cases of T-ALL in which *NOTCH1* is truncated and placed under the control of the TCR β locus.[332] *NOTCH1* plays several critical roles in promoting T-cell development[40,333-335] and is highly leukemogenic when expressed in murine T-cell precursors.[336] Despite the rarity of translocations involving this gene, a search for activating NOTCH1 mutations demonstrated that these are present in more than 50% of cases of T-ALL, and these occur in all molecular subtypes of T-ALL.[8] NOTCH1 is a transmembrane protein that is proteolytically processed during its transit to the cell surface, where it exists as a heterodimer consisting of extracellular and transmembrane subunits (Fig. 63-5). Upon ligand binding, the transmembrane subunit undergoes additional proteolytic cleavage within the plasma membrane, which leads to the release of its intracellular domain, known as ICN1 (intracellular domain of NOTCH1), into the cytosol. ICN1 subsequently translocates into the nucleus, where it is active as a transcription factor. Activating *NOTCH1* mutations in T-ALL can occur as either missense mutations in the heterodimerization domain, which allow constitutive proteolytic activation of the ICN1 domain,[8,337] or as frameshift mutations or stop codons that lead to truncation of the PEST domain.[8,338] PEST domains are protein sequences rich in proline (P), glutamate (E), serine (S), and threonine (T) that regulate the proteasomal degradation of proteins with short half-lives, thus these PEST-inactivating mutations impair the degradation of ICN1. Mutations in both regions are often found on the same allele in cases of T-ALL, and in experimental systems, mutations in both domains of the same gene indeed are synergistic.[8] Recent work has demonstrated that *MYC* is an important transcriptional target of *NOTCH1,* and it mediates many of the leukemogenic properties of *MYC* in human T-ALL cell lines.[339-341]

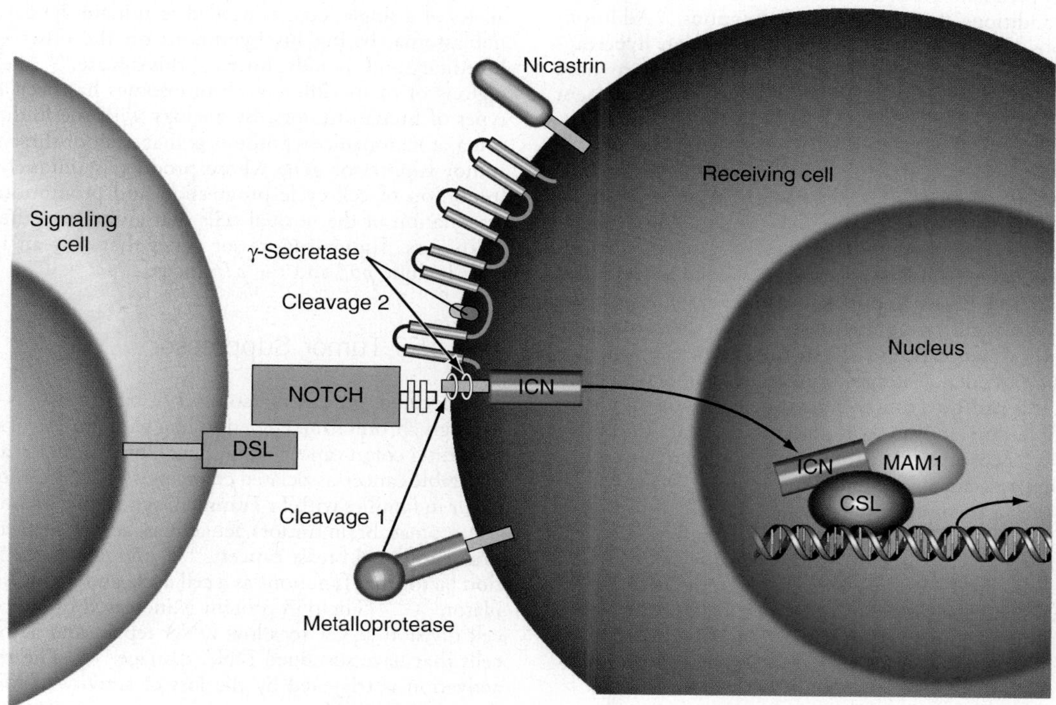

Figure 63-5 ACTIVATION OF NOTCH SIGNALING VIA EXTRACELLULAR AND INTRACELLULAR PROTEOLYTIC CLEAVAGE AND NUCLEAR TRANSLOCATION OF THE INTRACELLULAR NOTCH DOMAIN (ICN). Interaction with δ serrate ligand (DSL) stimulates proteolytic cleavage of NOTCH by metalloproteases and γ-secretase. This leads to the release of the intracellular ICN domain, which translocates to the nucleus, where it acts as a transcription factor to regulate gene expression. *(Adapted from Armstrong SA, Look AT: Molecular genetics of acute lymphoblastic leukemia.* J Clin Oncol *23:6306, 2005, with permission.)*

The proteolytic activation of the ICN domain of NOTCH1 upon ligand binding is mediated by γ-secretase, and γ-secretase inhibitors have previously been developed because of the role of this enzyme in the pathogenesis of Alzheimer disease. These inhibitors inhibit the growth of many T-ALL cell lines,[8,342] and trials of γ-secretase inhibitors in patients with T-ALL are currently underway.

RAS Gene Mutations

Human tumor DNAs were initially found to contain activated homologues of either *HRAS* or *KRAS*,[343,344] proto-oncogenes that were identified on the basis of their homology with viral oncogenes. Gene transfer methods identified an additional member of the RAS gene family, called *NRAS*,[345,346] that had not been observed as a component of a transforming retrovirus. Proto-oncogenes of the RAS family (*HRAS, KRAS,* and *NRAS*) encode 21-kDa proteins that are associated with the inner surface of the cytoplasmic membrane and are involved in growth factor receptor signaling.[347] The *RAS* proto-oncogenes are activated to the status of transforming oncogenes by somatic mutations that alter the amino acids specified by codons 12, 13, or 61. Mutated *RAS* genes lose their intrinsic GTPase activity and become insensitive to GAP proteins, thus accumulating in their active, GTP-bound conformation even in the absence of growth factor binding to surface receptors. Aberrant *RAS*-mediated signaling contributes to transformation through activation of the PI3K (phosphoinositide-3-kinase) and MAPK (mitogen-activated protein kinase) pathways.[347]

Activated *NRAS* genes appear to be preferentially involved in hematopoietic malignancies. They have been detected in myeloid cell lines,[348,349] in fresh leukemic cell samples from patients with AML or CML,[350-352] and in patients with MDS.[353] In ALL, mutations of codons 12, 13, or 61 of *NRAS* have been found in approximately 10% of patients, and *KRAS* mutations have been identified in 5% to 10% of patients.[354,355] *RAS* mutations are particularly common in cases of *MLL*-rearranged B-precursor ALL, in which 40% of cases have *KRAS* mutations and an additional 10% have *NRAS* mutations.[355] Additionally, *RAS* mutations have also been associated with high hyperdiploidy.[356] The presence of RAS mutations does not appear to have prognostic significance in the setting of contemporary treatment regimens.[354]

PTEN–PI3K–AKT Mutations in T-Cell Acute Lymphoblastic Leukemia

The PI3K–AKT signal transduction pathway, which is negatively regulated by the PTEN tumor suppressor, induces cellular growth and proliferation while inhibiting apoptosis and is aberrantly activated in a range of human cancers.[357-359] In T-ALL, recent work has identified a very high frequency of mutational activation of oncogenic signaling through this pathway, most often via deletions or truncating mutations of *PTEN,* but activating mutations of PI3K and AKT genes also occur.[360-363] Moreover, deletions of PTEN have been found to predict treatment resistance in clinical specimens,[53,360] and PTEN inactivation has been shown to induce resistance to inhibition of MYC and of NOTCH1 in zebrafish and murine models of T-ALL, further implicating PTEN loss in T-ALL treatment resistance.[362,364,365] Taken together, these findings thus suggest the potential clinical utility of PI3K-AKT pathway inhibitors in high-risk T-ALL, many of which are currently in human clinical trials.[366]

Gene Amplification

Gene amplification at the DNA level provides the cell a means to increase expression of critical genes whose products are ordinarily tightly controlled. Clinically important examples of proto-oncogene amplification have been documented in solid tumors of both adults and children. The *MYCN* gene, for example, is amplified from 10- to 300-fold in tumor cells from about one-third of cases of childhood neuroblastoma; such amplification has been linked to an advanced stage of disease and a poor prognosis.[367] However, the cytogenetic hallmarks of gene amplification—double-minute chromatin bodies and homogeneously staining regions—are rarely found in karyotypes of human leukemia cells, making it unlikely that high-level amplification of cellular proto-oncogenes is widespread in ALL. However, as noted earlier, the *NUP214–ABL1* fusion oncogene is amplified as a small, cytogenetically undetectable episome in T-ALL.

MYB Duplication in T-Cell Acute Lymphoblastic Leukemia

A duplication of the c-*MYB* gene was recently discovered in cases of T-ALL,[368-370a] and a chromosomal translocation that juxtaposes *c-MYB* to the TCR β gene regulatory elements was also identified in a small number of patients.[369] The discovery of this gene duplication involving a small region of the chromosome was made possible by recent technologic advances that now allow the high-resolution detection of small regions of focal amplifications and deletions. The *MYB* transcription factor is the cellular counterpart of the avian *v-MYB* avian myeloblastosis virus, which causes a rapidly fatal monoblastic leukemia in chickens and is essential for normal hematopoiesis, including T-cell development. The *MYB* duplication is mediated by homologous recombination between identical sequence regions that flank the gene,[370a] and its expression appears to be important in preventing T-lymphoblast differentiation because knock-down of *MYB* expression in T-ALL cell lines induces T-cell differentiation.[368]

Tumor Suppressor Genes

Much attention has been focused on tumor suppressors, whose loss of function via deletion or mutational inactivation leads to malignant transformation. Knudson first proposed that inactivation of both alleles of a single locus is needed to initiate the development of retinoblastoma, basing his hypothesis on the observed frequencies of hereditary and sporadic forms of this disease.[370b] Allelic loss of defined regions of many different chromosomes has been linked to specific types of human tumors. By analogy with the findings in retinoblastoma, a reasonable hypothesis is that each of these regions harbors a tumor suppressor gene whose product is uniquely involved in the inhibition of cell cycle progression and promotion of terminal differentiation of the normal cells that give rise to these different types of tumors. Tumor suppressor genes that play an important role in ALL include *p53* and the *p16* locus.

The *p53* Tumor Suppressor

p53, located on chromosome 17, band p13, is mutated or lost through chromosomal deletion in a wide variety of human tumors,[371] including colon cancer, lung cancer, breast cancer, and osteosarcoma. Heritable cancer-associated changes of the *p53* tumor suppressor gene occur in families with Li-Fraumeni syndrome, an unusual aggregation of sarcomas, brain tumors, leukemias, adrenocortical carcinomas, and premenopausal breast cancers.[372-375] *p53* encodes a 53-kDa transcription factor that functions as a cell cycle and apoptosis checkpoint regulator.[371,376-380] The p53 protein is increased by DNA damage, blocks cell division at G1 to allow DNA repair, and activates apoptosis in cells that have sustained DNA damage.[381-386] The mechanism of p53 activation is triggered by the loss of activity of MDM2 after DNA damage (via ATM) or oncogenic stress (via p14/ARF). As a negative regulator of p53, MDM2 induces the ubiqitination of p53 and its degradation by the proteasome. Hence, when MDM2 activity is abolished, p53 accumulates and certain cell cycle regulatory genes such as *p21*(*WAF1/CIP1/SDI1/CAP20*) and proapoptotic factor genes such as *BAX, PUMA,* and *NOXA* are transcriptionally activated.

p53 is also inactivated in a variety of hematopoietic malignancies, including B-cell ALL and Burkitt lymphoma, but is mutated or deleted in fewer than 3% of pediatric B-precursor or T-cell ALL cases at diagnosis.[387-389] It thus appears to play a limited role in the etiology of pediatric leukemia. However, *p53* mutations are seen in approximately 25% of relapsed T-cell ALL cases, suggesting a role for *p53* inactivation in the development of resistant disease.[387,388] In addition, *p53* mutations were detected in three of 10 ALL patients who failed on induction therapy or suffered early relapse, further supporting a role for *p53* inactivation in disease progression.[390,391]

The Cyclin-Dependent Kinase Inhibitors

The cyclin-dependent kinase (CDK) inhibitors, which include p15 (INK4B/MTS2), p16 (INK4A/MTS1/CDKN2), p18 (INK4C), p19 (INK4D), p21 (WAF1/CIP1/SDI1/CAP20), p27 (KIP1), and p57 (KIP2)m constitute a family of tumor suppressors that negatively regulate the cell cycle by inhibiting CDK phosphorylation of pRB.[392] The *INK4A* locus, located on the short arm of chromosome band 9q21, contains two different tumor suppressor genes, *p16INK4A* and *p14ARF* (*p19ARF* in mice),[393,394] each with a distinct promoter and first exon but common second and third exons. Despite this close relationship at the genomic level, p16 and p14 have totally unrelated amino acid sequences because they use different reading frames in their common second and third exons.[395] A third tumor suppressor gene, the CDK inhibitor *p15INK4B,* also resides in this region.[396,397] p16INK4A and p15INK4B directly inhibit cyclin D–CDK4/6 complexes and interfere with cell cycle progression. Cyclin D–CDK4/6 complexes promote entry into S phase through phosphorylation of the retinoblastoma protein, PRB, leading to the release of transcription factors, such as E2F, that promote entry into S phase. By contrast, p14ARF lacks a direct effect on the cell cycle machinery, acting instead to stabilize and upregulate p53 through the inhibition of MDM2.[396-400] The role of the *INK4a* locus in tumorigenesis was substantiated when mice with targeted disruption of exon 2 in *p16* developed tumors (primarily lymphomas and fibrosarcomas) whose induction was enhanced by the topical application of carcinogens and ultraviolet light.[401,402] The phenotype of the *p16/p19*$^{-/-}$ mice could be duplicated by selective mutation of the *p19ARF* gene (by targeting the first exon),[393] although mice deficient in *p16INK4A* with intact *p19ARF* also showed increased susceptibility to cancer.[401,402]

The short arm of chromosome 9 is the most frequent target of chromosomal alterations in human cancer. In particular, the human leukemias and lymphomas show a high frequency of 9p21 deletions involving both the *p16INK4A/p14ARF* and the *p15INK4B* loci. Epigenetic silencing of these tumor suppressor genes through hypermethylation of their promoter sequences represents an alternative mechanism of gene inactivation. Although *p16INK4A/p14ARF* and *p15INK4B* are homozygously deleted in 20% to 30% of B-precursor ALL cases and in 70% to 80% of T-cell ALL cases, epigenetic silencing of the p15INK4B promoter has been observed in 44% of primary B-lineage ALLs.[403-415]

FBW7 in T-Cell Acute Lymphoblastic Leukemia

FBW7 is an E3 ubiquitin ligase that targets the transcriptionally active intracellular form of NOTCH (ICN), MYC, and cyclin E for degradation, and this gene is inactivated by mutation or deletion in approximately 10% of T-ALL cases.[416] In T-ALL cell lines, *FBW7* mutation or homozygous deletion leads to resistance of NOTCH pathway inhibition by γ-secretase inhibitor therapy, likely because intracellular NOTCH protein levels remain high in the absence of FBW7-mediated degradation despite inhibition of γ-secretase activity. Additionally, tumor-derived FBW7 mutations maintain their ability to bind MYC but do not lead to its degradation, and these may act as dominant negative mutants that protect MYC from degradation.[416] More recent work has shown that FBW7 also targets the antiapoptotic protein MCL1 for proteasomal degradation in T-ALL, providing an additional oncogenic consequence resulting from inactivation of the FBW7 tumor suppressor.[417]

PAX5 and Other B-Cell Developmental Gene Alterations in B-Precursor Acute Lymphoblastic Leukemia

A recent high-resolution genome-wide analysis of B-precursor ALL cases using single nucleotide polymorphism arrays identified copy number alterations in a number of genes that play important roles in B-cell development.[418] Genes involved in B-cell development were found to be altered by deletion, amplification, mutation, or rearrangement in 40% of cases of B-precursor ALL. The most common abnormalities identified were deletions of *PAX5,* and, upon further analysis in other cases, other mechanisms that led to inactivation of *PAX5* were identified. These included a number of translocations that led to fusion proteins that maintained the ability to bind to PAX5 transcriptional targets but lost regulatory ability, thus having dominant negative activity, and inactivating point mutations that altered the transcriptional activity of *PAX5.* Deletions were also detected in the *TCF3, EBF1, LEF1, IKZF1,* and *IKZF3* genes, all of which play important roles in B-cell development.

Ikaros Mutations in High-Risk B-Precursor Acute Lymphoblastic Leukemia

Ikaros is a DNA-binding transcription factor that is required for the development of all lymphoid lineages, and expression of a dominant negative Ikaros mutation in mice was shown to lead to T-cell lymphomas.[419,420] However, the role of Ikaros in human leukemias was not appreciated until genomic analyses of B-precursor ALL patient samples revealed Ikaros (IKZF1) deletions in 29% of pediatric samples.[418] Ikaros deletions are strongly associated with BCR–ABL-positive ALL, and these are characteristically acquired at transformation of CML to ALL (lymphoid blast crisis).[421] Ikaros deletions predict a very high risk of treatment failure that appears to be independent of BCR–ABL, with patients with Ikaros-deleted, BCR–ABL negative ALL faring similarly poorly to those with BCR–ABL-positive ALL.[422] Interestingly, recent work has implicated mutational activation of CRLF2-JAK2 signaling in Ikaros-deleted, BCR–ABL-negative ALL.[423] Given the remarkable clinical activity of imatinib in high-risk BCR–ABL ALL, these findings thus suggest the need for clinical trials of small molecule inhibitors of JAK-STAT signaling in this high-risk subtype of B-precursor ALL.

Inactivation of LEF1 in T-Cell Acute Lymphoblastic Leukemia

The LEF1 transcription factor, a member of the LEF/TCF (lymphoid enhancer binding factor/T-cell specific transcription factor) family of DNA-binding transcription factors, is best known for its role as a positive mediator β-catenin transcriptional activity, a well-established oncogene.[424] Recent genomic analyses have identified mono- and biallelic deletions and truncating mutations of LEF1 in 18% of primary T-ALL patient samples, unexpectedly implicating LEF1 as a T-ALL tumor suppressor.[425] LEF1 inactivation is associated with a very young age at diagnosis, T-cell differentiation arrest at an early cortical stage of T-cell development, and activating NOTCH1 mutations. Moreover, T-ALL cases with LEF1 inactivation are characterized by the highest expression of MYC mRNA of any T-ALL subtype, a surprising finding given that LEF/TCF transcription factors transactivate MYC expression when bound to β-catenin.[426,427] In addition to their well-established functions as transcriptional activators, LEF/TCF transcription factors can also act as transcriptional repressors when bound to Groucho/TLE family members in the absence of β-catenin activation.[428] Although the precise mechanisms responsible for the pathogenic effect of LEF1 inactivation in T-ALL have not yet been established, these findings thus suggest the intriguing possibility that LEF1 may actively repress MYC in T-ALL cells lacking β-catenin activation, and that LEF1 inactivation in this context may promote maximal MYC overexpression downstream of other oncogenic lesions that drive MYC overexpression, such as NOTCH1 mutations.

BCL11B Inactivation in T-Cell Acute Lymphoblastic Leukemia

The BCL11B transcription factor is required for normal T-cell development. In murine T-cell progenitors, inactivation of BCL11B leads to developmental arrest at DN stages, acquisition of NK-like features, and aberrant self-renewal activity.[429-432] Monoallelic BCL11B deletions or point mutations have recently been identified in 9% to 16% of primary T-ALL patient samples.[149,433] The point mutations identified typically occur within the DNA-binding domains of BCL11B and are predicted to disrupt their ability to bind DNA. Moreover, previous work in murine models has shown that BCL11B suppresses T-lymphoblastic malignancies induced by p53 haploinsufficiency, radiation, or the BCR–ABL oncogene,[434,435] and BCL11B inactivation is a particularly common cooperating lesion in murine T-ALL induced by the TLX1 oncogene or by ATM deficiency.[149,436] In human T-ALL, recurrent cryptic t(5;14)(q35;q32) translocations juxtaposing BCL11B and TLX3 have been described, which result in BCL11B gene regulatory elements driving overexpression of TLX3.[103,437,438] These translocations were long thought to be pathogenic because of the resultant overexpression of the TLX3 oncogene. However, these recent findings indicate that both BCL11B inactivation and TLX oncogene overexpression are important pathogenic consequences of this translocation, thus representing two oncogenic events from a single genomic lesion.

PHF6 Mutations in T-Cell Acute Lymphoblastic Leukemia

T-ALL has a conspicuous male predominance, suggesting the potential involvement of tumor suppressors on the X-chromosome. Targeted mutational analysis of the X chromosome revealed one such candidate tumor suppressor, PHF6, which encodes a nucleolar protein of unknown function whose germline mutation leads to the Borjeson-Forssman-Lehmann syndrome (OMIM 301900), which is associated with severe mental retardation and facial dysmorphisms but is not known to be associated with T-ALL. Somatic PHF6 mutations were identified in 16% of pediatric and in 38% of adult T-ALL patient samples, were most often nonsense or frameshift mutations, and were associated with overexpression of the TLX1 or TLX3 oncogenic transcription factors.[439] The pathogenic consequences of PHF6 inactivation in T-ALL are presently unknown but are a matter of active investigation.

Abnormalities of Leukemia Cell Ploidy

Abnormalities of chromosome number, which generally occur in the absence of specific chromosomal translocations, have important prognostic implications in childhood ALL. Found in 25% to 30% of childhood ALL cases, hyperdiploidy of more than 50 chromosomes in the leukemic clone is one of the most powerful means of identifying patients with a very good prognosis.[91,258] In particular, trisomies of chromosomes 4, 10, and 17 impart a particularly good prognosis, and hyperdiploidy in the absence of these trisomies is less of a favorable prognostic factor.[440] As mentioned previously, activating mutations of *FLT3,* a receptor tyrosine kinase, are common in these patients. Patients with hyperdiploidy typically present with favorable prognostic indicators, such as age between 2 and 10 years, a low white blood cell count, and an early pre-B immunophenotype, and can expect cure rates that approach 90%.[441-443] The mechanism accounting for the favorable outcome of patients with hyperdiploid ALL remains elusive but may reflect an increased sensitivity to antimetabolite therapy[444] and a greater propensity to undergo apoptosis.[445] Conversely, hypodiploidy (<45 chromosomes) carries an extremely poor prognosis.[91,258,446] Overall, adults with ALL have significantly fewer numeric chromosomal abnormalities than do children; however, abnormalities of ploidy do also appear to have prognostic significance in adults because one large series demonstrated a favorable prognostic impact of hyperdiploidy, but adults with hypodiploidy had extremely poor outcomes.[33]

CHILDHOOD ACUTE LYMPHOBLASTIC LEUKEMIA: A MODEL FOR GENE-BASED RISK ASSESSMENT

Many of the chromosomal and molecular genetic abnormalities in the leukemic blasts of patients with B-precursor ALL are important predictors of response to currently available chemotherapy. Lymphoblasts from each new case of childhood ALL should be examined for molecular prognostic markers, including leukemia cell ploidy, *MLL* gene rearrangements, and the presence of *BCR–ABL* and *TEL–AML1* fusion transcripts. Additional clinical criteria that have prognostic significance, such as the age of the patient, the peripheral blood white blood cell count at diagnosis, and the presence of CNS involvement, are used by modern pediatric ALL treatment regimens to further adjust the intensity of therapy to an individual patient's risk of relapse. It is also worth noting that B-precursor ALL in patients younger than 1 year of age is associated with an extremely poor prognosis secondary to an exceedingly high rate of relapse, which is at least partly attributable to the very high frequency of MLL translocations in this population, and these patients are typically treated with unique treatment regimens designed specifically for infant ALL. In T-ALL, the paucity of clinically useful prognostic markers has greatly hindered progress toward personalized therapy, but the recent identification of differentiation arrest at the earliest stages of T-cell development as a marker of very poor prognosis,[50,51] together with the identification of mutations and gene expression signatures that closely resemble those of AML and HSCs,[52,53] has generated considerable excitement for the application of intensified, AML-like treatment regimens to this high-risk subset of T-ALL. Finally, response to treatment has independent prognostic significance. Induction failure, often defined in pediatric protocols as any morphologic evidence of leukemia at the end of the initial month of induction chemotherapy, represents a very poor prognostic factor and is an indication for BMT after remission is achieved in most centers. Additionally, sensitive flow cytometric and polymerase chain reaction–based methodologies for the detection of minimal residual disease (MRD) are now available, and the level of MRD after induction chemotherapy has recently been shown to provide an additional means of identifying patients at low or high risk of relapse.[447,448] With the availability of these prognostic indicators, there remains little justification for uniform treatment of newly diagnosed cases of ALL. Rather, modern trials emphasize risk-based therapy to reduce toxicity in patients likely to become long-term responders and to intensify therapy for those at high risk of relapse.

A risk classification scheme based on a patient's clinical features and on the genetic features of leukemic blasts has been proposed for patients with B-precursor or T-cell ALL who are 1 year of age or older (Table 63-2). Patients with *TEL–AML1* positivity or with simultaneous trisomies of chromosomes 4, 10, and 17 constitute the lower risk group and are candidates for reduced-intensity treatment regimens. The intermediate-risk group includes patients between the ages of 1 and 9 years with standard-risk age and leukocyte count, as defined by criteria of the National Cancer Institute, and whose leukemic lymphoblasts lack prognostically important genetic features. The high-risk group includes patients who meet any of the following criteria: age 10 years or older, high leukocyte counts at diagnosis, a T-cell immunophenotype, or a slow early response to therapy. Patients in the very high-risk group, defined by extreme hypodiploidy, *MLL* gene rearrangements, the *BCR–ABL* translocation, high MRD at the end of induction chemotherapy, or T-ALL blasts harboring the high-risk early T-cell progenitor (ETP) or absence of biallelic TCRγ deletion (ABD) markers are eligible for BMT in first remis-

Table 63-2 Clinical Risk Assignment in Childhood Acute Lymphoblastic Leukemia

Risk Group	Features	Recommended Therapy
Low risk	• Simultaneous trisomies of chromosomes 4, 10, 17 • *TEL–AML1* fusion	Less intensive antimetabolite-based chemotherapy
Intermediate risk	• Standard-risk age or leukocyte count without other genetic risk features	Intermediate antimetabolite-based chemotherapy
High risk	Presence of any of the following: • Age 10 years or older • T-cell immunophenotype • WBC count >50,000/mm^3 • CNS leukemia	Intensified multiagent chemotherapy with cranial radiation
Very high risk	• *BCR–ABL* translocation* • *MLL* translocations†‡ • Hypodiploidy <45 chromosomes • Induction failure or elevated MRD at the end of induction chemotherapy • T-ALLs with early T-cell progenitor (ETP) or absence of biallelic TCRγ deletion (ABD) markers	Allogeneic bone marrow transplantation in first remission

ALL, Acute lymphoblastic leukemia; *AML,* acute myeloid leukemia; *CNS,* central nervous system; *MRD,* minimal residual disease; *TCR,* T-cell receptor; *WBC,* white blood cell.
*Recent data also indicate excellent 3-year survival rates with the use of imatinib, a targeted BCR-ABL inhibitor, in combination with conventional chemotherapy.
†Current evidence suggests that bone marrow transplantation in first remission may not improve outcomes for children with MLL-rearranged ALL.
‡Although *MLL* translocations are almost always associated with very poor outcomes, patients with T-cell ALL who have the t(11;19) MLL-ENL translocation appear to have excellent outcomes with conventional chemotherapy.

sion. It is worth noting that the evidence supporting a benefit for BMT in first remission is especially strong in the presence of the *BCR–ABL* translocation, although its benefit in *MLL*-rearranged ALL remains unclear. Moreover, recent data in the setting of BCR–ABL ALL indicate that the combination of imatinib (a BCR–ABL inhibitor) with conventional chemotherapy leads to excellent short-term (3-year) survival rates, although longer follow-up will be required to ensure that long-term outcomes are comparable. Among several exceptions to this risk stratification criteria are T-ALL patients with the t(11;19) and expression of *MLL-ENL,* who have a favorable prognosis,[17,449] and infants younger than 1 year of age, in whom separate risk stratification criteria have been devised. The incorporation of highly predictive risk stratification methods into clinical trials, together with the development of novel molecularly tailored therapies, should eliminate the still significant risk of relapse in patients with newly diagnosed ALL, ensuring permanent cure without the hazard of acute or chronic complications.

FUTURE DIRECTIONS

The immediate applications of the emerging molecular information include a redefinition of risk classification schemes to emphasize the roles of somatically acquired genetic abnormalities that carry a defined prognosis and likelihood of therapeutic failure. Currently, patients are assigned to treatment according to their initial clinical features and, increasingly, the genetic and biologic properties of their leukemic cells. We are now in a position to view ALL as a group of heterogeneous diseases defined by discrete molecular lesions. As these lesions have been systematically analyzed in larger numbers of patients, it has been possible to devise new classification schemes for ALL that reflect prognosis with exquisite precision. The development of new drugs based on the molecular biology of ALL, whose promise is highlighted by the early success of imatinib in BCR–ABL–positive ALL, is clearly a priority for the future and will likely take the form of compounds developed to specifically interfere with oncoproteins expressed by each patient's leukemic blasts. Additionally, the discovery that several kinases play important roles in ALL pathogenesis has provided new opportunities for targeted drug development. The opportunity is now at hand to improve therapy through randomized trials coordinated on a nationwide or even worldwide scale that focus on key subsets of acute leukemia patients whose lymphoblasts harbor specific genetic abnormalities.

SUGGESTED READINGS

Comprehensive Reviews

Armstrong SA, Look AT: Molecular genetics of acute lymphoblastic leukemia. *J Clin Oncol* 23:6306, 2005.

Bernt KM, Armstrong SA: Targeting epigenetic programs in MLL-rearranged leukemias. *Hematology Am Soc Hematol Educ Program* 2011:354, 2011.

Pui CH, Robison LL, Look AT: Acute lymphoblastic leukaemia. *Lancet* 371:1030, 2008.

Specific Genetic Lesions in Acute Lymphoblastic Leukemia

Bernt KM, Zhu N, Sinha AU, et al: MLL-rearranged leukemia is dependent on aberrant H3K79 methylation by DOT1L. *Cancer Cell* 20:66, 2011.

De Keersmaecker K, Real PJ, Gatta GD, et al: The TLX1 oncogene drives aneuploidy in T cell transformation. *Nat Med* 16:1321, 2010.

Gutierrez A, Sanda T, Grebliunaite R, et al: High frequency of PTEN, PI3K, and AKT abnormalities in T-cell acute lymphoblastic leukemia. *Blood* 114:647, 2009.

Gutierrez A, Sanda T, Ma W, et al: Inactivation of LEF1 in T-cell acute lymphoblastic leukemia. *Blood* 115:2845, 2010.

Mullighan CG, Collins-Underwood JR, Phillips LA, et al: Rearrangement of CRLF2 in B-progenitor- and Down syndrome-associated acute lymphoblastic leukemia. *Nat Genet* 41:1243, 2009.

Mullighan CG, Goorha S, Radtke I, et al: Genome-wide analysis of genetic alterations in acute lymphoblastic leukaemia. *Nature* 446:758, 2007.

Weng AP, Ferrando AA, Lee W, et al: Activating mutations of NOTCH1 in human T cell acute lymphoblastic leukemia. *Science* 306:269, 2004.

Yoda A, Yoda Y, Chiaretti S, et al: Functional screening identifies CRLF2 in precursor B-cell acute lymphoblastic leukemia. *Proc Natl Acad Sci U S A* 107:252, 2010.

Zhang J, Ding L, Holmfeldt L, et al: The genetic basis of early T-cell precursor acute lymphoblastic leukaemia. *Nature* 481:157, 2012.

Clinical Implications of Acute Lymphoblastic Leukemia Genetics

Armstrong SA, Kung AL, Mabon ME, et al: Inhibition of FLT3 in MLL: Validation of a therapeutic target identified by gene expression based classification. *Cancer Cell* 3:173, 2003.

Coustan-Smith E, Mullighan CG, Onciu M, et al: Early T-cell precursor leukaemia: A subtype of very high-risk acute lymphoblastic leukaemia. *Lancet Oncol* 10:147, 2009.

Gutierrez A, Dahlberg SE, Neuberg DS, et al: Absence of biallelic TCRgamma deletion predicts early treatment failure in pediatric T-cell acute lymphoblastic leukemia. *J Clin Oncol* 28:3816, 2010.

Mullighan CG, Su X, Zhang J, et al: Deletion of IKZF1 and prognosis in acute lymphoblastic leukemia. *N Engl J Med* 360:470, 2009.

Schultz KR, Bowman WP, Aledo A, et al: Improved early event-free survival with imatinib in Philadelphia chromosome-positive acute lymphoblastic leukemia: A children's oncology group study. *J Clin Oncol* 27:5175, 2009.

For complete list of references log on to www.expertconsult.com.

CHAPTER 64

CLINICAL MANIFESTATIONS AND TREATMENT OF ACUTE LYMPHOBLASTIC LEUKEMIA IN CHILDREN

Sima Jeha and Ching-Hon Pui

Serial risk-directed clinical trials have optimized the combination of chemotherapeutic agents and, along with advances in supportive care, have led to current cure rates of childhood acute lymphoblastic leukemia (ALL) exceeding 85% compared with long-term survival less than 10% in the 1960s.[1] However, because ALL is the most common cancer in children, relapsed ALL remains the leading cause of death from a disease in this age group. Over the past decade, minimal residual disease (MRD) has become a major determinant in risk stratification, cranial irradiation has been successfully omitted from some frontline protocols, and the tyrosine kinase inhibitor (TKI) imatinib has revolutionized the treatment of patients with *BCR-ABL1* rearrangement. Our understanding of the immunology and molecular pathways involved in ALL is improving at a rapid pace, and several targeted therapies are showing promise in early clinical trials. The challenge is to successfully incorporate targeted therapy into personalized ALL regimens aiming at improving cure rates and reducing toxicity.[2]

EPIDEMIOLOGY

Acute lymphoblastic leukemia accounts for approximately 75% of all cases of childhood leukemia and is the most common pediatric cancer in developed countries, representing 23% of cancer diagnoses among children younger than 15 years of age. About 2400 children and adolescents are diagnosed with ALL each year in the United States, an annual rate of 30 to 40 per million. The peak incidence of ALL occurs around 4 years of age. This young age peak historically has appeared at different times in different countries and has been associated with major periods of industrialization, suggesting a causative role for environmental carcinogens. ALL occurs more frequently in boys than in girls at all ages.[3]

Acquired and inherited genetic factors play an essential role in ALL as supported by the demonstration of genetic abnormalities in leukemic cells of children with ALL as well as by clinical observations. Children with the constitutional chromosomal abnormality trisomy 21 (Down syndrome) are up to 15 times more likely to develop leukemia than children without Down syndrome. Genetic instability and DNA repair disorders (e.g., Bloom syndrome, ataxia telangiectasia, Fanconi anemia) are also associated with an increased risk of developing ALL.[4] Among identical twins, if one is diagnosed with ALL during the first year of life, the risk that the other twin will develop ALL is more than 70%, approaching 100% in twins with a single monochorionic placenta. Highest in infancy, this risk diminishes with increasing age at diagnosis in the first twin to about one in 10 in older children. If the first twin develops ALL by 5 to 7 years of age, the risk to the second twin is at least twice that in the general population, regardless of zygosity.[5] After the age of 7 years, the risk to the unaffected twin is similar to that for persons in the general population. The extraordinarily high concordance rate in monozygotic infants twins compared with dizygotic infant twins or nontwinned siblings results from the metastasis of leukemic cells from one twin to the other through shared placental circulation. The majority of infants with ALL have a chromosome translocation that results in the fusion of the *MLL* gene at 11q23 with a variety of partner genes but principally AF4. Identical twin infant pairs with concordant ALL share the same acquired *MLL* gene rearrangements.

The most common chromosome translocation in childhood ALL, t(12;21), results in ETV6(TEL)-RUNX1(AML1) fusion. In contrast to *MLL*-rearranged ALL, *ETV6-RUNX1* leukemias present after infancy and have a concordance rate of only 10% in identical twins. *ETV6-RUNX1* fusion can be found in as many as 1% of cord blood samples of normal newborn babies, a frequency 100 times higher than the prevalence of this subtype of leukemia, suggesting that additional postnatal mutations are necessary for malignant transformation. Analysis of Guthrie cards of 2- to 6-year old children with ALL showed that most did have detectable, clonotypic *ETV6-RUNX1* sequences at birth. In addition, identical *ETV6* and *RUNX1* breakpoints were present in each of twin pairs with a very asynchronous diagnosis, supporting the requirement for one or more additional postnatal events after in utero initiation. This interpretation suggests that *ETV6-RUNX1* initiates leukemogenesis but is insufficient for overt disease, and further genetic alterations are required. ETV6 deletions on chromosome 12p, the most frequent additional genetic abnormalities described in cases of ALL with *ETV6-RUNX1,* appear to be subclonal in fluorescence in situ hybridization (FISH) analysis of leukemic cells from nontwin patients. These findings indicate that *ETV6* deletion is a secondary or later event in leukemogenesis and suggest that leukemia might be initiated in utero but requires an essential second postnatal event (two hits).[6]

Several genetic, dietary, and environmental factors have been proposed to modify the risk of leukemia initiation. Children with various congenital immunodeficiency diseases, including Wiskott-Aldrich syndrome, congenital hypogammaglobulinemia, and ataxia telangiectasia, have an increased risk of developing lymphoid malignancies, as do patients under chronic treatment with immunosuppressive drugs. The loss of cellular immune surveillance capability for tumor antigens and the inability to self-regulate lymphoproliferative processes may contribute to malignant transformation in these patients. Absence of exposure to common infections in the first year of life is associated with a higher risk of developing *ETV6-RUNX1*–positive or hyperdiploid ALL in older children. A possible explanation is that in the absence of infection-driven modulation of the naive immune network in infants, subsequent infectious exposures could result in a highly dysregulated response to infections in older children, contributing to leukemogenesis. Exposure to ionizing radiation and certain toxic chemicals could also facilitate the development of acute leukemia. The high incidence of leukemia among survivors of atomic bomb explosions in Japan during World War II is well documented. Among survivors of the atomic bomb, there was no increase in the incidence of leukemia in children exposed to radiation in utero. This experience contrasts with other reports of an increased incidence of ALL in children exposed to medical diagnostic radiation both in utero and in childhood. Other evidence linking most environmental exposures to risk of childhood ALL has largely been inconsistent. Causation pathways are likely to be multifactorial, and it is probable that the risk of ALL from environmental exposure is influenced by genetic variation through the coinheritance of multiple low-risk variants.

PATHOBIOLOGY

Acute leukemias comprise a group of clonal disorders of maturation at an early phase of hematopoietic differentiation. ALL subtypes are a heterogeneous group of malignancies with distinctive immunophenotype and molecular pathogenesis that result in varying clinical characteristics and response to therapy. Accurate pathobiologic diagnosis is not only important for prognostic stratification but can also help define patient-specific therapeutic approaches.[7]

Lymphoblastic leukemias can arise from either B- or T-cell mutant hematopoietic cells capable of indefinite self-renewal. T-cell ALL can be classified into several distinct genetic subgroups that correspond to specific T-cell development stages and is frequently associated with translocations of T-cell receptor genes on chromosome 14q11 or 7q34 with other gene partners. Recent studies have identified a novel high-risk immature T-cell subtype termed *early T-cell precursor* (ETP) ALL with immunologic markers and gene expression reminiscent of double-negative 1 thymocyte that retains the ability to differentiate into both T-cell and myeloid, but not B-cell, lineages.[8] The discovery of its mutational spectrum recapitulated that of acute myeloid leukemia (AML) by whole-genome sequencing and a global transcription profile similar to that of normal hematopoietic stem cells (HSCs) and granulocyte macrophage precursors suggests that this subtype of leukemia is a stem cell leukemia. The prevalence of mutations in genes regulating cytokine receptor and Ras signaling, and histone modification further suggests that the addition of myeloid-directed therapy might improve the outcome of this subtype.[9] Most B-lineage leukemias are early precursor B cell, expressing CD19 and CD10 (or cALLa, the common acute leukemia antigen) but lacking surface or cytoplasmic immunoglobulin. The mature B-cell ALLs, or Burkitt-cell leukemia, are stratified separately and are not included in this chapter (see Chapters 81 and 83).

Recent advances in global genome analysis have enabled the identification of recurring alterations in genes and pathways with key roles in cell growth and tumorigenesis. Several observations suggest that multiple lesions are acquired subsequent to founding translocations to induce leukemogenesis. Single nucleotide polymorphism (SNP) array analysis demonstrated substantial differences in the frequency of copy number abnormality (CNA) among various ALL subtypes. *MLL*-rearranged cases had less than one CNA per case, suggesting that *MLL* is a potent oncogene that requires very few cooperating lesions to induce leukemia transformation, but *ETV6-RUNX1* and *BCR-ABL1* leukemias have more than six lesions per case.

Deletion or sequence mutation of the *IKZF1*, a gene that encodes the early lymphoid transcription factor IKAROS, is present in more than 80% of *BCR-ABL1*–positive ALL and in a novel high-risk subgroup of *BCR-ABL1*–negative ALL that has a gene expression profile significantly similar to that of *BCR-ABL1*-positive ALL.[10] The "*BCR-ABL1*-like" ALL occurs in as many as 7% to 9% of children with ALL. Approximately half of the *BCR-ABL1*–like cases have rearrangements of the lymphoid cytokine receptor gene *CRLF2,* with concomitant Janus kinases (JAKs) mutations in one-third of the *CRLF2*-rearranged cases.[11] This genotype is associated with high risk of relapse, independent of age, leukocyte count at diagnosis, cytogenetics, and levels of MRD after remission induction. A recent transcriptome sequencing study of 12 cases of *BCR-ABL1*–like cases (with whole-genome sequencing in two of them) identified structural alterations and mutations activating kinase and cytokine receptor signaling in all cases, including *EBF1-PDGFRB, NUP214-ABL1, RANBP2-ABL1, BCR-JAK2, STRN3-JAK2,* and activating mutations of *IL7R* or *FLT3.* Importantly, preclinical studies showed that primary leukemic cells harboring *PDGFRB* or *ABL1* fusion responded to ABL1 TKIs, and those harboring *BCR-JAK2* or mutated *IL7R* responded to JAK2 inhibitor, suggesting that these patients would benefit from the targeted therapy.[12] Another novel subtype of B-cell precursor ALL, characterized by *CRLF2* alterations (*PAR1* deletion and *IGH-CRLF2*), occurs in 5% to 7% of children with ALL and, remarkably, in approximately 50% of the cases with Down syndrome. These patients probably would require more intensive therapy because this genotype was associated with poor outcome in the reported series, albeit not independently significant in one.[13]

Experimental models have established that cooperative mutations are necessary to induce leukemia and contribute to the development of drug resistance. Association studies of ALL based on the candidate gene approach have evaluated a restricted number of polymorphisms in genes implicated in the metabolism of carcinogens, folate metabolism, protection of DNA from carcinogen-induced damage, and cell cycle regulation. Such studies highlight difficulties in conducting statistically and methodologically rigorous investigations into ALL risk. Genome-wide association studies of childhood ALL have recently demonstrated that common variation at four genetic loci [7p12.2 (*IKZF1*), 9p12 (*CDKN2A/CDKN2B*), 10q21.2 (*ARID5B*) and 14q11.2 (*CEBPE*)] confers a modest increase in risk, establishing a role for genetic susceptibility in the development of ALL. In addition to identifying common, low-penetrance susceptibility alleles, these data provide insights into disease causation by identifying risk variants and annotating genes involved in transcriptional regulation and differentiation of B-cell progenitors.

CLINICAL MANIFESTATIONS

Children with ALL present with nonspecific symptoms and signs reflecting the degree of disruption in bone marrow (BM) function and the extent of extramedullary infiltration. The most common presenting symptoms are fever, fatigue, pallor, petechiae, bruising, bleeding from mucosal surfaces, and pain (Table 64-1). Patients, especially young children, may present with bone pain, arthralgia, or refusal to walk because of leukemic infiltration of the bone or joint or because of expansion of the BM cavity by leukemic cells. The evolution of symptoms may proceed over a few days, weeks, or months. Less common presenting symptoms include headache, visual complaints, vomiting, respiratory distress, oliguria, and anuria. Occasionally, patients present with life-threatening infection or bleeding.

On physical examination, fever, pallor, petechiae, and ecchymoses may be present. The lymphoproliferative nature of the disease may

Table 64-1 Clinical Presentation of Acute Lymphoblastic Leukemia

Symptoms and Signs	Etiology	Management
Fever	Disease or infection	Always conduct fever workup and provide broad antimicrobial coverage until infectious etiology is ruled out
Fatigue, pallor	Anemia (ALL infiltrating BM)	RBC transfusion (slow if anemia is severe; avoid in hyperleukocytosis)
Petechiae, bruising, bleeding	Thrombocytopenia (ALL infiltrating BM)	Transfuse with platelets
Pain	Leukemia infiltrating bones or joints or expanding BM cavity	Establish diagnosis and start chemotherapy
Respiratory distress, superior vena cava syndrome	Mediastinal mass	Avoid sedation in the presence of tracheal compression; establish diagnosis as soon as possible and start chemotherapy

ALL, Acute lymphoblastic leukemia; *BM,* bone marrow; *RBC,* red blood cell.

be manifested as lymphadenopathy, splenomegaly, or less commonly hepatomegaly. Central nervous system (CNS) involvement is uncommon at presentation and in most instances is detected by screening lumbar puncture in high-risk patients who are asymptomatic at the time of the puncture (Fig. 64-1, *A* and *B*). Papilledema, retinal hemorrhages, and cranial nerve palsies should be ruled out on examination. CNS involvement usually is restricted to leptomeninges, and parenchymal mass lesions are uncommon. Epidural spinal cord compression is a rare but serious presenting finding and requires immediate chemotherapy and high-dose glucocorticoid therapy. Laminectomy or radiotherapy is generally not necessary because leukemias are very sensitive to chemotherapy at diagnosis. Overt testicular involvement occurs in only 2% of boys and usually presents as painless, asymmetric enlargement that can be distinguished from hydrocele by ultrasonography (Fig. 64-1, *C* and *D*). Less common presenting features include ocular involvement, subcutaneous nodules (leukemia cutis) (see Fig. 64-1, *E* and *F*) and enlarged salivary glands (Mikulicz syndrome). Approximately 55% of T-cell cases present with an anterior mediastinal mass. A bulky mediastinal mass can compresses the great vessels and trachea, resulting in superior vena cava syndrome and respiratory distress. Patients with a large mediastinal mass generally present with cough, dyspnea, orthopnea, dysphagia, stridor, cyanosis, facial edema, increased intracranial pressure, and sometimes syncope. When significant tracheal compression is present, general anesthesia should be avoided and procedures should be performed under local anesthesia. Immediate diagnosis and initiation of steroids and chemotherapy is essential to prevent respiratory failure.

Clinical laboratory data often reveal a broad spectrum of abnormal findings. Various degrees of anemia and thrombocytopenia are usually present at diagnosis. The presenting leukocyte counts range widely from 0.1 to 1500×10^9/L. Leukemic blasts may or may not be seen on peripheral smear. Approximately 45% of children have leukocyte counts less than 10×10^9/L, and 15% present with hyperleukocytosis (>100×10^9/L). Patients with hyperleukocytosis are at increased risk of CNS disease, tumor lysis syndrome, and leukostasis. Leukostasis may manifest as dyspnea, chest pain, alterations in mental status, cranial nerve palsies, or priapism. The majority of childhood ALL are B cell in derivation with approximately 12% to 15% of children with ALL having a T-cell immunophenotype. T-cell ALL usually occurs in patients older than 9 years of age with elevated leukocyte counts and is associated with CNS involvement. Coagulopathy, usually mild, can occur in T-cell ALL and is only rarely associated with severe bleeding. Elevated serum uric acid and lactate dehydrogenase levels are common in patients with a large leukemic cell burden. Patients with massive renal involvement can have increased levels of creatinine, urea nitrogen, uric acid, and phosphorus. Approximately 0.5% of patients have hypercalcemia at diagnosis, attributable to the release of parathyroid hormone-like protein from lymphoblasts and leukemic infiltration of bone; these patients tend to be in the older age group and present with low blast cell counts. This complication generally resolves rapidly with hydration and chemotherapy. Liver dysfunction caused by leukemic infiltration occurs in 10% to 20% of patients, is usually mild, and has no prognostic consequences. Because vincristine and daunorubicin are metabolized primarily through biliary excretion, modifications of the dosage of these agents are recommended if the direct bilirubin level is elevated.

Abnormalities of the bone, such as metaphyseal banding, periosteal reactions, osteolysis, osteosclerosis, or osteopenia, can be

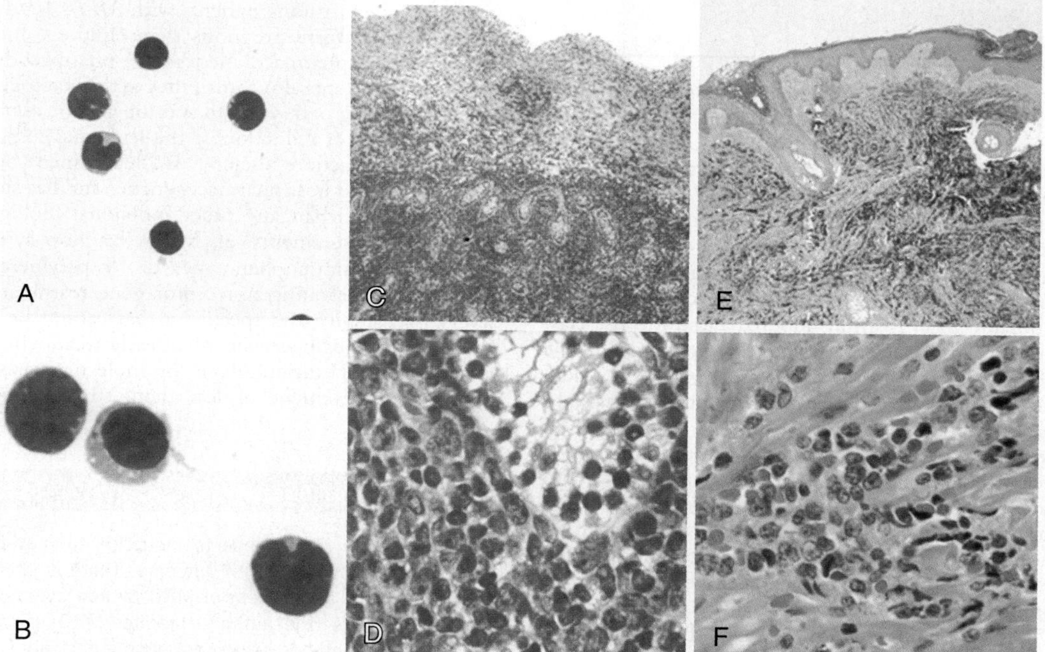

Figure 64-1 CENTRAL NERVOUS SYSTEM (CNS), TESTICULAR, AND SUBCUTANEOUS INVOLVEMENT IN CHILDHOOD ACUTE LYMPHOBLASTIC LEUKEMIA (ALL). CNS disease identified in the cerebrospinal fluid (CSF) by screening lumbar puncture at the time of diagnosis in a 12-year-old boy with high-risk precursor B-cell ALL. The total count of the CSF specimen was 6131/μL with 6076 white blood cells/μL and 98% blasts. **A** and **B,** The cytospin preparation shows mostly blasts, slightly altered morphologically by the preparation. In **B,** there is a small lymphocyte *(middle)* for comparison with the blasts. **C** and **D,** Testicular disease noted at relapse in a 13-year-old boy with precursor B-cell ALL. Note the infiltrate of blasts in the parenchyma of the testes, surrounding the seminiferous tubules. Immunostaining (not shown) demonstrated that the blasts were CD19+, CD10+, and TdT+. **E** and **F,** Cutaneous disease at diagnosis. The patient was an 8-year-old boy with a scalp lesion for 2 months that was initially treated with antibiotics. On biopsy, there was much crush artifact, but deep in the specimen, there was an infiltrate of blasts separating fibers **(F)** shown to be B-cell lineage. Interestingly, the patient had a normal complete blood count, but bone marrow was packed with blasts that had a precursor B-cell phenotype and a hyperdiploid karyotype.

demonstrated by radiographic studies in half of patients, especially those with low presenting leukocyte counts. Vertebral compression fracture can be detected in 2% of the cases, usually with low leukocyte count and hyperdiploidy (>50 chromosomes), and is not associated with adverse prognosis.

DIFFERENTIAL DIAGNOSIS

Children with ALL present with a variety of nonspecific symptoms that may mimic other conditions. Pancytopenia and fever are also presenting symptoms for aplastic anemia. Failure of a single cell line, as in transient erythroblastic anemia, idiopathic thrombocytopenic purpura, and congenital or acquired neutropenia, sometime produces a clinical picture that is difficult to distinguish from ALL. Routine BM aspiration is not necessary for patients with severe thrombocytopenia and no other hematologic or physical evidence of leukemia. However, BM aspiration should be performed to exclude leukemia in patients who require glucocorticoid treatment. Children with infectious mononucleosis or other acute viral illnesses may present with fever, adenopathy, splenomegaly, lymphocytosis, or pancytopenia. Fever, arthralgias, or a limp may frequently be confused with juvenile rheumatoid arthritis, which can also be associated with anemia, leukocytosis, and mild splenomegaly. Children with prominent bone pain frequently have nearly normal blood counts, a finding that can contribute to a delay in diagnosis. Immunostains and molecular studies help differentiate ALL from AML and other small blue cell malignancies that invade the BM, including neuroblastoma, rhabdomyosarcoma, Ewing sarcoma, and retinoblastoma. Infants may present with subcutaneous nodules (leukemia cutis) that look clinically like Langerhans cell histiocytosis.

PROGNOSIS

Contemporary regimens have abolished the prognostic impact of many clinical and biologic features, demonstrating that the single most important prognostic factor in childhood ALL is appropriate risk-directed therapy (Table 64-2). Accurate assessment of relapse hazard is an integral part of ALL therapy, so that only high-risk patients are treated aggressively, with less toxic therapy reserved for cases at lower risk of failure.

To facilitate comparison of treatment results among different clinical trials, participants in a 1993 workshop sponsored by the United States' National Cancer Institute adopted a uniform risk classification based on age and leukocyte count. Two-thirds of the patients who were 1 to 9 years old with precursor B-cell ALL and a leukocyte count less than 50 × 10^9/L were considered to be at standard risk of relapse; the other third was classified as high risk. This classification proved to be of limited prognostic value because up to one-third of patients designated as standard risk may relapse, and these criteria cannot be applied to T-cell ALL. Moreover, the prognostic impact of age and, to a lesser extent, leukocyte count is largely attributable to their association with specific genetic abnormalities. For example, the overall poor prognosis of infants younger than 12 months of age can be explained by the very high frequency of *MLL* rearrangements (70%–80%) in this age group,[14] and the overall favorable outcome of patients ages 1 to 9 years is related to the preponderance of cases (70%) with hyperdiploidy (>50 chromosomes) or *ETV6-RUNX1* (also known as *TEL-AML1*) fusion, which are both favorable genetic features. Thus a more reasonable strategy is to develop clinical prognostic risk categories based on their major immunophenotypic features and genetic characteristics.

Early pre-B ALL, lacking immunoglobulin synthesis, is the most common form of acute leukemia in children. The high-risk features previously ascribed to pre-B ALL (presence of cytoplasmic immunoglobulin M) are closely associated with the presence of the t(1;19) translocation and *E2A–PBX1* fusion. Prognostic distinctions among ALL immunophenotypes, including the negative prognostic impact once associated with T-cell ALL and pre-B ALL with *E2A-PBX1* fusion, have been abolished by recent improvements in risk-directed treatment. Aberrant expression of myeloid-associated antigens has been observed with certain genetic subtypes. CD15, CD33, and CD65 are expressed in ALL cases with a rearranged *MLL* gene, and CD13 and CD33 are expressed in cases with the *ETV6-RUNX1* fusion. Once associated with a poor outcome in some studies, myeloid-associated antigen expression has no prognostic impact in contemporary risk-directed treatment programs. The recently identified ETP ALL subtype is characterized by immature genetic and immunophenotypic features (CD1a negative, CD8 negative, and CD5 weak and the expression of stem cell or myeloid markers) and a dismal prognosis with conventional therapy.[9]

Acute lymphoblastic leukemia can be classified according to modal chromosomal number (ploidy) and specific genetic abnormalities of the leukemia stem line. Hyperdiploidy (>50 chromosomes per cell) is associated with an age of 1 to 10 years, a lower median leukocyte count, increased sensitivity to antimetabolite agents, and a favorable prognosis. A hypodiploid karyotype (<44 chromosomes per cell), by contrast, predicts a poor outcome. Molecular analysis can identify prognostically and therapeutically relevant subgroups that cannot be identified by karyotyping. *ETV6-RUNX1,* the most common specific genetic rearrangement in childhood ALL, has been associated with a good prognosis. With the exception of T-cell ALL with the t(11;19), the prognosis of cases with 11q23/*MLL* rearrangements is generally poor.

Genetic features do not entirely account for treatment outcome, and their prognostic impact also depends on the treatment efficacy. Although up to 15% of patients with hyperdiploidy greater than 50 chromosomes per cell or *ETV6–RUNX1* fusion have recurrences of their leukemia, a substantial proportion of the patients with the t(9;22) and *BCR-ABL1* fusion who are 1 to 9 years old and have low leukocyte counts at diagnosis may be cured with intensive chemotherapy alone.[15] Among patients with *MLL–AF4* fusion, infants and adults have a worse prognosis than children. Interindividual variability in the pharmacokinetics and pharmacodynamics of many antileukemic agents also contributes to the heterogeneity in treatment response among patients with specific genetic abnormalities.[16]

The degree of reduction of the leukemic cell clone early during remission induction therapy is determined by both leukemic cell genetics and host pharmacogenetics and has shown greater prognostic strength than any other individual biologic or host-related feature.[17] Measurements of MRD by flow-cytometric detection of aberrant immunophenotypes or by polymerase chain reaction (PCR) of clonal antigen–receptor gene rearrangements provides a level of sensitivity and specificity that cannot be attained by traditional morphologic assessment of early treatment response. Patients who achieve an immunologic or molecular remission, defined as leukemic involvement of less than 10^{-4} nucleated BM cells on

Minimal Residual Disease

The rapidity of response to induction therapy is an important independent predictor of outcome. There is strong concordance between the assessment of MRD by flow cytometry and by PCR methods. We (the authors) monitor MRD using primarily flow cytometry methods, which are simple and rapid, and we reserve PCR methods for the few patients (<5%) whose leukemic cells lack a suitable immunophenotype. About half of all patients show a disease reduction to 10^{-4} or lower after only 2 weeks of remission induction, and these patients appear to have an exceptionally good treatment outcome. Persistence of MRD of 10^{-4} or more at 4 months from diagnosis is associated with an especially dismal outcome. The adverse prognosis of high-risk slow early responders can be improved with intensification of induction and consolidation. Standard-risk cases may be spared the increased risk of early morbidity and mortality from intensive induction, provided that they receive postinduction intensification therapy.

Table 64-2 Prognostic Factors in Acute Lymphoblastic Leukemia

Factor	Prognosis	Clinical Application
Age		
<1 yr	MLL⁺ (70%–80% infants): Poor outcome MLL⁻ : Same outcome as for older children	MLL⁻: Do well on standard ALL therapy Potential role for FLT3 inhibitor for MLL+
1–9 yr	Standard risk	ALL biology may change risk
>9 yr	Higher risk	ALL biology may change risk
White Blood Cell Count		
$<50 \times 10^9$/L	Standard risk	ALL biology may change risk
$\geq 50 \times 10^9$/L	Higher risk	ALL biology may change risk
Central Nervous System		
CNS3	Higher risk	Therapy intensification
CNS2 Traumatic lumbar puncture with blasts	Higher risk of CNS relapse	CNS-directed therapy intensification
Testicular	Higher risk	Therapy intensification
Immunophenotype		
T cell	Higher risk	Poor outcome abolished with current therapy
Pre–B cell (cIgM+)	Higher risk	Poor outcome abolished with current therapy
Early pre–B cell	Standard risk	Genetics may change risk
ETP	Dismal prognosis	Ongoing studies exploring effective therapies
Ploidy		
>50 (DI >1.16)	Low risk	Good response to antimetabolites
<44	Higher risk	Therapy intensification
Genetic Alterations		
t(9;22)/*BCR-ABL1*	Higher risk	BCR-ABL inhibitors
t(4;11)/*MLL-AF4*	Higher risk	Potential role for FLT3 inhibitors and hypomethylating agents
t(1;19)/*E2A-PBX1*	Higher risk	Poor outcome cancelled on current therapy
t(12;21)/*ETV6-RUNX1*	Low risk	
IKZF1	Poor prognosis. Present in 80% BCR-ABL1+ and also in BCR-ABL1 like	Potential role for TKI, JAK inhibitors
NUP214-ABL1	High risk	Potential benefits from TKI
CRLF2	In 1/3 BCR-ABL1–like, associated with Hispanic or Latino ethnicity and poor outcome	Potential role for JAK inhibitors
CREBBP	Associated with drug resistance and relapse	Potential benefit from histone deacetylase inhibitors
Minimal Residual Disease		
Day 15 <0.01%	Excellent outcome	No benefit from second delayed intensification
Slow early responders	Higher MRD = Higher risk of relapse	Benefit from augmented delayed intensification
EOI >1%	Dismal prognosis	HSCT in first CR
4 mo >0.1%	Dismal outcome	HSCT in first CR

CNS, Central nervous system; *CR,* complete remission; *DI,* DNA index; *EOI,* end of induction; *HSCT,* hematopoietic stem cell transplantation; *MRD,* minimal residual disease; *JAK,* Janus kinase; *TKI,* tyrosine kinase inhibitor.

completion of remission induction, have a much more favorable prognosis than do those who do not achieve this status. Patients who are in morphologic remission but have a postinduction MRD level of 1% or more fare as poorly as those who do not achieve clinical remission by conventional criteria (≥5% blasts). About half of all patients show a disease reduction to 10^{-4} or lower after only 2 weeks of remission induction, and they appear to have an exceptionally good treatment outcome. The persistence of MRD (≥0.01%) beyond 4 months from diagnosis was associated with an estimated 70% cumulative risk of relapse. Patients with 0.1% MRD or more at 4 months had an especially dismal outcome. Most contemporary clinical trials have incorporated MRD detection into the risk classification system. Although MRD positivity is strongly associated with known presenting risk features, it has independent prognostic strength and is increasingly used in risk stratification of ALL in contemporary regimens.[18]

Currently, pediatric ALL patients are typically classified into three risk groups—low-, intermediate-, and high-risk (also referred to as standard-, high-, and very high-risk)—which are categories based on age, leukocyte count at diagnosis, blast cell immunophenotype, and genotype, as well as early treatment response. More recently, gene expression profiling of leukemic cells by the DNA microarray method has proved useful in identifying previously unrecognized genes whose expression may have prognostic significance. The predictive power of these newly identified expression signatures requires validation in prospective clinical trials.

THERAPY, INCLUDING STEM CELL TRANSPLANTATION

With the exception of patients with mature B-cell ALL, who are treated with short-term intensive chemotherapy, therapy for patients with ALL is administered over 2 to 3 years. Treatment starts with a 4- to 6-week remission-induction phase aimed at eradicating the initial leukemic cell burden and restoring normal hematopoiesis. The induction phase typically includes the administration of a glucocorticoid (prednisone or dexamethasone), vincristine, and at least a third drug (asparaginase, anthracycline, or both). A three-drug induction regimen appears sufficient for most standard-risk cases, provided they receive intensified postremission therapy. The benefit in long-term survival of using four or more drugs during induction is widely accepted in higher risk patients but less clear in lower risk patients. With this approach, 98% to 99% of patients can attain remission, as defined by fewer than 5% blasts in the BM and a return of neutrophil and platelet counts to near normal levels. Intrathecal chemotherapy is usually initiated at the start of treatment.

After remission induction, consolidation (or intensification) is given to eradicate drug-resistant residual leukemic cells. Therapy is tailored to the leukemia subtype and risk group. All patients benefit from a delayed intensification (or delayed reinduction), consisting of using drugs similar to those used in remission induction therapy after a 3-month period of a less intensive, interim maintenance chemotherapy. Double-delayed intensification with a second reinduction at week 32 of treatment improves outcome in patients with intermediate-risk leukemia but does not benefit patients with rapid early response. An augmented intensification regimen consisting of the administration of additional doses of vincristine and asparaginase during the myelosuppression period after delayed intensification and sequential escalating-dose parental methotrexate followed by asparaginase improved the outcome of high-risk patients whose disease had responded slowly to initial multiagent induction therapy.

After completion of induction and consolidation, patients receive a 2- to 2.5-year continuation (or maintenance) phase consisting of low-intensity metronomic chemotherapy designed to eradicate any residual leukemic cell burden. Weekly low-dose methotrexate and daily oral mercaptopurine form the backbone of most continuation regimens. Many groups add regular pulses of vincristine and corticosteroids to this regimen, although the benefit of these pulses and their optimal duration and frequency of administration in the context of contemporary therapy has not been established.[19] Adjusting chemotherapy doses to maintain a white cell count between 2 to 3×10^9/L and neutrophil counts between 0.5 and 1.5×10^9/L has been associated with a better clinical outcome. Overzealous use of mercaptopurine, to the extent that neutropenia necessitates chemotherapy interruption, reduces overall dose intensity and is counterproductive. The optimal duration of therapy remains unknown. Attempts to shorten therapy duration from 24 months to 12 or 18 months have resulted in a significant increase in relapses. Several studies showed no advantage to prolonging treatment beyond 3 years. A small number of patients with particularly poor prognostic features may undergo BM transplantation during first remission.

Radiation therapy was the first modality that was successfully used to prevent CNS relapse. The effectiveness of cranial radiation as preventive therapy was offset by substantial late effects in long-term survivors, including learning disabilities, multiple endocrinopathies, and an increased risk of second malignancies. Subsequent trials demonstrated that in the context of optimal systemic and intrathecal therapy, cranial irradiation can be reduced or even omitted altogether. Patients with high-risk genetic features, large leukemic cell burden, T-lineage ALL, and leukemic cells in the cerebrospinal fluid, even from iatrogenic introduction from a traumatic lumbar puncture at diagnosis, are at increased risk of CNS relapse and require more intense CNS-directed therapy.[20] Studies have successfully used triple intrathecal therapy with methotrexate, hydrocortisone, and cytarabine or intrathecal methotrexate alone. Systematically administered agents, including high-dose methotrexate, dexamethasone, and asparaginase, also contribute to prevention of extramedullary relapse.

Based on reports of more potent in vitro antileukemic activity and better CNS penetration, dexamethasone has replaced prednisone in many continuation regimens. Prednisone remains the preferred glucocorticoid during induction because of the relative increased toxicity associated with dexamethasone use.[21] Polyethylene glycol–conjugated asparaginase, a long-acting and less allergenic form, is progressively replacing the native *Escherichia coli* and is being increasingly administered intravenously instead of intramuscularly. Asparaginase derived from *Erwinia chrysanthemi* has a short half-life, and its use is currently limited to patients who are allergic to the *E. coli* formulations. The dose schedule for asparaginase should take into account the variability in the pharmacokinetic profile and potency among the different preparations.[22] Intensifying asparaginase therapy during the early phase of treatment benefits high-risk patients, particularly those with T-cell disease. Significant improvement was also reported in the outcome of patients receiving early intensification consisting of intermediate- or high-dose antimetabolite therapy.[23] The optimal dose of methotrexate depends on the leukemic cell genotype and phenotype, as well as host pharmacogenetic and pharmacokinetic parameters. Methotrexate at 2.5 g/m^2 is adequate for most patients with standard-risk B-cell precursor ALL, but a higher dose (5 g/m^2) may benefit those with T-cell or high-risk B-cell precursor ALL. This observation is consistent with the finding that T-lineage blast cells accumulate methotrexate polyglutamates less avidly than do B-lineage blast cells. The increased ability of hyperdiploid ALL blasts cells to accumulate methotrexate polyglutamate could partially explain the excellent outcome

Consolidation Therapy

The importance of a consolidation phase after remission induction is undisputed, but the treatment regimen and duration vary in the different childhood ALL studies. Commonly used strategies include high-dose methotrexate plus mercaptopurine, frequent pulses of vincristine and corticosteroid plus high-dose asparaginase for 20 to 30 weeks, and reinduction treatment with the same agents given during initial remission induction. Reinduction treatment has become an integral component of contemporary protocols. In one randomized study, double reinduction further improved treatment outcome in patients with intermediate-risk ALL, but additional pulses of vincristine and prednisone after a single reinduction course were not beneficial, suggesting that the increased dose intensity of other drugs, such as asparaginase, was responsible for the observed improvement. An "augmented" regimen including Capizzi methotrexate (escalating-dose intravenous methotrexate with no rescue followed by asparaginase) and additional doses of vincristine and asparaginase during periods of myelosuppression improved the outcome of patients with a slow early response to therapy.

High-Risk Central Nervous System Relapse

Patients with the following characteristics are at increased risk of CNS relapse and require more intense CNS-directed therapy:

1. Patients with high-risk genetic features
2. Large leukemic cell burden
3. T-lineage ALL
4. CNS-3 status (>5 WBC/μL CSF with presence of lymphoblasts on Cytospin)
5. CNS-2 status (<5 WBC/μL CSF with lymphoblasts)
6. Traumatic CSF with blasts

of children with hyperdiploid greater than 50 chromosomes per cell ALL treated on low-intensity antimetabolite-based regimens. Leucovorin rescue is necessary after treatment with high-dose methotrexate; however, overzealous rescue might counteract the antileukemic activity of methotrexate. Although the intensive asparaginase and high-dose methotrexate treatment has significantly improved the outcome for patients with T-cell ALL, the emergence of specific therapy such as the purine nucleoside analog nelarabine will likely increase the tendency to assign patients with T-cell ALL to a specific treatment protocol or strata.

It is generally recommended to give mercaptopurine at bedtime to patients with an empty stomach and to avoid taking it together with milk or milk products that contain xanthine oxidase, an enzyme that can degrade the drug. About 10% of the population inherit one wild-type gene encoding thiopurine methyltransferase (TPMT) and one nonfunctional variant allele, resulting in intermediate enzyme activity, but one in 300 people inherits two nonfunctional variant alleles and are completely deficient of this enzyme that catalyses the S-methylation of mercaptopurine to its inactive metabolite. Patients with heterozygous and especially homozygous deficiency of TPMT are at high risk of severe myelosuppression. Identification of these patients allows physicians to selectively guide reductions in mercaptopurine dosage without modifying the dose of methotrexate. Substituting thioguanine for mercaptopurine during continuation therapy was associated with a high incidence of profound thrombocytopenia and hepatic venoocclusive disease. Thioguanine use has therefore been limited to short pulses administered during consolidation therapy in some trials; mercaptopurine is selected for prolonged administration.

Because optimizing the administration of existing therapies is reaching its limit, further improvements in outcome will require the development of therapeutic approaches directed against rational therapeutic targets. An example is the significant improvement in the outcome of Philadelphia chromosome–positive (Ph+) ALL with the advent of TKIs targeting the constitutively active *BCR-ABL1* TKI in ALL subset. Ph+ ALL has historically had an extremely poor outcome, but recent studies have demonstrated dramatic improvements in treatment outcome with incorporation of *BCR-ABL1* inhibitors into Ph+ ALL treatment.[24] Recent identification of novel chimeric fusions involving kinases in ALL (e.g., NUP214–ABL1 and STRN3–JAK2) suggests that additional high-risk cases may benefit from targeted therapies directed at kinase signaling.

The expanded understanding of the biologic, immunologic, and genetic heterogeneity of ALL has enabled development of several novel therapeutic strategies.[25] Various monoclonal antibodies are showing promise in early clinical trials and may be incorporated into ALL regimens in the future.

Autologous transplantation has failed to improve outcome in ALL. Comparisons between allogeneic HSC transplantation (HSCT) and intensive chemotherapy have yielded inconsistent results because of the small numbers of patients studied and differences in case selection criteria. It is generally accepted that allogeneic HSCT is a treatment modality for patients with ALL who are predicted to respond poorly to intensive chemotherapy.[26] At present, patients with refractory leukemia (failure to enter morphologic remission after 4–6 weeks of induction therapy), high level of MRD (>1%) after remission induction, persistent MRD after consolidation treatment, and early hematologic relapse are candidates for allogeneic transplantation. It is crucial to reduce residual disease to, or close to, undetectable levels as outcome is superior if MRD is undetectable before HSCT and worsens with increasing MRD levels at the time of HSCT. Treatment approaches for adolescents and young adults with ALL have evolved considerably with the widespread adoption of pediatric-based protocols, which appears to have significantly improved survival and decreased the need for HSCT in this age group. The benefit of allogeneic HSCT in infants with t(4;11) ALL remains controversial and should be evaluated in the context of emerging molecular therapies such as FLT3 inhibitors and DNA methyltransferase inhibitors. Patients with the recently identified ETP ALL have a dismal prognosis (event-free survival of 22%), even though half of the patients received transplantation because of high MRD levels after remission induction. The therapeutic role of HSCT in this group of patients remains to be determined by studying a larger number of patients. Matched unrelated-donor or cord blood transplantation has yielded outcomes comparable to those obtained with matched related-donor HSCT and should be considered reasonable alternatives if a matched donor is not available. Many advances have been made in stem cell transplantation, such as prevention of graft-versus-host disease (GVHD), expansion of the pool of suitable unrelated or related donors, donor selection and tissue typing, acceleration of engraftment, enhancement of the graft-versus-leukemia effect, and supportive care. Because improvements in transplantation tend to parallel those in chemotherapy, the indications for transplantation in newly diagnosed and relapsed patients should be reevaluated periodically. For example, the presence of Philadelphia chromosome is no longer a clear indication for transplantation with the advent of TKIs.

Dose Schedule

The biologically equivalent doses among the different formulations of corticosteroids, thiopurines, and asparaginase are not clear. Trials comparing such agents should be cautiously interpreted, taking into account the dose schedule used and the effect of variability in the pharmacokinetic profile and potency among the agents involved. Simple modification of the dose or schedule may result in significant differences in efficacy and toxicity. Also, when comparing regimens containing high-dose intravenous methotrexate, the dose schedule of leucovorin rescue should not be ignored because it plays a crucial role in modulating the activity and toxicity of methotrexate.

ACUTE LYMPHOBLASTIC LEUKEMIA RELAPSE

Most relapses occur during treatment or within the first 2 years after its completion, although relapses have been reported as late as 10 years after initial ALL diagnosis. The most common site of relapse is the BM.[27] Relapse in extramedullary sites, such as the CNS and testes, has decreased to less than 5% and 2% respectively. Leukemia relapse occasionally occurs at other sites, including the eye, ovary, uterus, bone, muscle, tonsil, kidney, mediastinum, pleura, and paranasal sinus. Extramedullary relapse in children with ALL frequently presents as an isolated clinical finding. However, in studies that included MRD assays, many extramedullary recurrences were associated with MRD in the BM. A small fraction of patients experience a recurrence of acute leukemia with an immunophenotype different from that determined at diagnosis. Some of the cases represent relapse of original leukemic clones with a shift in immunophenotype, but others are secondary malignancies caused by the mutagenic effects of leukemia treatment, especially from epipodophyllotoxin. Patients with isolated BM relapse generally fare worse than those with isolated extramedullary relapse.[28] Factors indicating an especially poor prognosis are a short initial remission and a T-cell immunophenotype. Other adverse factors include t(9;22). The presence of MRD at the end of second remission induction is also a strong adverse prognostic indicator. Although chemotherapy may secure a prolonged second remission in children with ALL who experience late relapse (defined as >6 months after cessation of therapy), allogeneic HSCT is the treatment of choice for patients who experience hematologic relapse during therapy or shortly thereafter and for those with T-cell ALL. Patients with late-onset isolated CNS relapse who had not received cranial irradiation as initial CNS-directed therapy have a very high remission retrieval rate, with a long-term prognosis approaching that of newly diagnosed patients in those who had a long initial remission before the CNS event.

Genome-wide studies using matched diagnosis and relapse samples from the same patients are exploring the genetic basis of relapse.

Although 90% of the patients exhibit differential gaining or losing genetic lesions from diagnosis to relapse, most relapse samples are clonally related to diagnosis samples. Relapse clones could be present as minor populations at diagnosis and selected during treatment to emerge as the predominant clone at relapse displaying alterations of genes that have been implicated in treatment resistance. Almost 20% of relapsed cases have sequence or deletion mutations of *CREBBP,* which impair histone acetylation and transcriptional regulation of CREBBP targets, suggesting that the mutations may confer drug resistance and raising the possibility of using drugs to reverse the aberrant epigenetic programs, such as histone deacetylase inhibitors.[29] The next generation of deep sequencing technologies promises to unravel many more if not the full repertoire of genetic alterations in leukemia. Parallel gene expression studies, which have identified a proliferative gene signature that emerges at relapse and consistent upregulation of genes such as *survivin,* provide attractive targets for novel therapeutic intervention.

SUPPORTIVE CARE

Stringent supportive care significantly contributes to a favorable ALL outcome and should be initiated at diagnosis because remission induction is associated with an increased risk from cardiovascular, metabolic, and infectious complications. All febrile patients with or without documented infection should be given broad-spectrum intravenous antibiotics until an infectious disease can be excluded. Rapid turnover of leukemia cells before and immediately after the initiation of chemotherapy leads to metabolic disturbances, including hyperkalemia, hyperuricemia, hyperphosphatemia, and hypocalcemia. Patients with high levels of uric acid are at risk for the development of acute renal failure secondary to uric acid deposition in the kidneys. All patients require intravenous hydration to prevent or treat hyperuricemia and hyperphosphatemia. Allopurinol, a xanthine oxidase inhibitor, can prevent uric acid formation. Rasburicase, a recombinant urate oxidase that breaks down uric acid to allantoin (a readily excretable metabolite with five- to 10-fold higher solubility than uric acid), is more effective than allopurinol but is associated with methemoglobinemia or hemolytic anemia in patients with glucose-6-phosphate dehydrogenase deficiency because hydrogen peroxide is a byproduct of the uric acid breakdown.[30] Phosphate binders should also be used to prevent or treat hyperphosphatemia. Transfusions should be administered slowly in patients with severe anemia to prevent congestive heart failure. In patients with extreme hyperleukocytosis, packed red blood cell transfusion should be delayed until after leukocyte count is decreased to prevent complications of leukostasis. All blood products should be irradiated in patients who are receiving immunosuppressive therapy to prevent GVHD. Patients should avoid foods that may be contaminated with pathogens and reduce salt intake, which could induce hypertension and resultant seizure in patients receiving glucocorticoids during induction. Adolescents, obese individuals, and individuals with Down syndrome are at increased risk of hyperglycemia and other complications. Prophylactic use of trimethoprim–sulfamethoxazole (or pentamidine or atovaquone in patients with poor tolerance to trimethoprim–sulfamethoxazole) successfully prevents *Pneumocystis jiroveci* (formerly *carinii*) pneumonia. Dental evaluation at diagnosis and meticulous oral hygiene during chemotherapy minimize the oral complications of leukemia and its treatment. It is important to distinguish between herpes simplex viral infection and chemotherapy-induced oral mucositis. Occasionally, patients have nausea and substantial pain on swallowing caused by esophageal herpes simplex viral infection, candidiasis, or both. Oral candidiasis occurs frequently, especially in young children. Azole compounds (e.g., fluconazole, itraconazole, ketoconazole) are frequently used to treat fungal infections. It should be recognized that they can inhibit cytochrome P450 enzymes and increase the toxicities of various antileukemic agents, especially vincristine. On the other hand, concomitant administration of anticonvulsants that induce cytochrome P450 enzymes (e.g., phenytoin, phenobarbital, carbamazepine) increases the systemic clearance of several antileukemic agents and may adversely affect treatment outcome. Anticonvulsants that are less likely to induce the activity of cytochrome P450 enzymes (e.g., Keppra) are recommended in patients receiving chemotherapy. Photosensitive skin rash can occur during antimetabolite therapy. The rashes are erythematous, maculopapular, similar to atopic eczema, and most prominent on the face. Topical administration of simple emollients or a weak steroid preparation and avoidance of external exposure to sunlight should improve the skin condition. Patients with Down syndrome tolerate methotrexate poorly; appropriate dose adjustment is indicated. During each clinic visit, a thorough review of all drugs should be undertaken because of potential adverse interactions among them. In fact, chemotherapy can also interact with various food (e.g., grapefruit) and supplements (e.g., St. John's wort, folic acid).[31]

Drug Interactions

We have not yet reached a full understanding of the contribution of genetic polymorphisms to interindividual differences in drug effects to allow us to translate this new knowledge into clinical practice. However, by simply avoiding drug interactions, one can prevent increased toxicity or reduced efficacy of chemotherapy. Phenytoin and phenobarbital induce the activity of cytochrome P450 enzymes, significantly increasing the systemic clearance of several antileukemic agents that may adversely affect treatment outcome. We substitute these anticonvulsants with gabapentin or Keppra in patients receiving antileukemic therapy. On the other hand, azole compounds (e.g., fluconazole, itraconazole, ketoconazole) can inhibit cytochrome P450 enzymes and increase the toxicities of various antileukemic agents, especially vincristine.

LATE EFFECTS OF TREATMENT

The most problematic late effects of contemporary ALL therapy include neuropsychological impairments, bone morbidity, and obesity. Although neuropsychologic deficits are well-recognized side effects of cranial irradiation, intrathecal and systemic chemotherapy (especially methotrexate) can also cause brain atrophy and spinal cord dysfunction and contribute to the development of neurocognitive toxicities. Severe CNS toxicity has been attributed to cranial irradiation at doses of 2400 cGy or higher, but lower doses have also been associated with long-term neuropsychological impairments, especially in younger children. Obesity, which is most prevalent among female survivors of childhood ALL, may be related to cranial radiation and corticosteroids. Osteopenia, fractures, and osteonecrosis have been observed in up to 30% of survivors of childhood ALL. Osteonecrosis, which can lead to significant pain, loss of function, and total joint replacement, has been reported in approximately 8% of children with ALL, with the highest frequency observed in those diagnosed in adolescence. Ovarian and testicular function are relatively unaffected by most antileukemic therapy. Offspring of patients successfully treated for childhood ALL are expected to be as normal as the general population. Second malignant neoplasms, including malignant gliomas, meningiomas, and AML, occur with increased frequency in patients treated on regimens that include irradiation, epipodophyllotoxins, or alkylating agents.

FUTURE DIRECTIONS

As the cure rate approaches 90%, treatment response assessed by MRD measurements of submicroscopic leukemia has emerged as a powerful and independent prognostic indicator for gauging the intensity of ALL therapy. Children at high risk of relapse may now benefit from early intensification of therapy. The next goal is to reduce the intensity of therapy in children at very low risk of relapse, hence avoiding undue toxicity. The successful elimination of preventive cranial irradiation indicates that treatment reduction is feasible if done with caution and appropriate substitution with less toxic alternatives. Global genome analysis, in addition to refining leukemia classification, is helping identify potential molecular targets for therapy. Expanding the application of pharmacogenomics, a science that aims to define the genetic determinants of drug effects, will allow further personalized therapy in the future.

REFERENCES

1. Schrappe M, Nachman J, Hunger S, et al: Educational symposium on long-term results of large prospective clinical trials for childhood acute lymphoblastic leukemia (1985-2000). *Leukemia* 24:253, 2010.
2. Pui CH, Evans WE: Treatment of acute lymphoblastic leukemia. *N Engl J Med* 354:166, 2006.
3. Pui CH, Robison LL, Look AT: Acute lymphoblastic leukaemia. *Lancet* 371:1030, 2008.
4. Bienemann K, Burkhardt B, Modlich S, et al: Promising therapy results for lymphoid malignancies in children with chromosomal breakage syndromes (Ataxia teleangiectasia or Nijmegen-breakage syndrome): A retrospective survey1. *Br J Haematol* 155:468, 2011.
5. Schmiegelow K, Lausten TU, Baruchel A, et al: High concordance of subtypes of childhood acute lymphoblastic leukemia within families: Lessons from sibships with multiple cases of leukemia. *Leukemia* 26:675, 2011.
6. Zelent A, Greaves M, Enver T: Role of the TEL-AML1 fusion gene in the molecular pathogenesis of childhood acute lymphoblastic leukaemia. *Oncogene* 23:4275, 2004.
7. Pui CH, Carroll WL, Meshinchi S, et al: Biology, risk stratification, and therapy of pediatric acute leukemias: An update. *J Clin Oncol* 29:551, 2011.
8. Coustan-Smith E, Mullighan CG, Onciu M, et al: Early T-cell precursor leukaemia: A subtype of very high-risk acute lymphoblastic leukaemia1. *Lancet Oncol* 10:147, 2009.
9. Zhang J, Ding L, Holmfeldt L, et al: The genetic basis of early T-cell precursor acute lymphoblastic leukaemia. *Nature* 481:157, 2012.
10. Mullighan CG, Su X, Zhang J, et al: Deletion of IKZF1 and prognosis in acute lymphoblastic leukemia. *N Engl J Med* 360:470, 2009.
11. Harvey RC, Mullighan CG, Chen IM, et al: Rearrangement of CRLF2 is associated with mutation of JAK kinases, alteration of IKZF1, Hispanic/Latino ethnicity, and a poor outcome in pediatric B-progenitor acute lymphoblastic leukemia. *Blood* 115:5312, 2010.
12. Mullighan CG, Zhang J, Harvey RC, et al: JAK mutations in high-risk childhood acute lymphoblastic leukemia. *Proc Natl Acad Sci U S A* 106:9414, 2009.
13. Ensor HM, Schwab C, Russell LJ, et al: Demographic, clinical, and outcome features of children with acute lymphoblastic leukemia and CRLF2 deregulation: Results from the MRC ALL97 clinical trial. *Blood* 117:2129, 2011.
14. Kang H, Wilson CS, Harvey RC, et al: Gene expression profiles predictive of outcome and age in infant acute lymphoblastic leukemia: A Children's Oncology Group study. *Blood* 119:1872, 2011.
15. Arico M, Schrappe M, Hunger SP, et al: Clinical outcome of children with newly diagnosed Philadelphia chromosome-positive acute lymphoblastic leukemia treated between 1995 and 2005. *J Clin Oncol* 28:4755, 2010.
16. Evans WE, Relling MV: Moving towards individualized medicine with pharmacogenomics. *Nature* 429:464, 2004.
17. Stow P, Key L, Chen X, et al: Clinical significance of low levels of minimal residual disease at the end of remission induction therapy in childhood acute lymphoblastic leukemia. *Blood* 115:4657, 2010.
18. Schultz KR, Pullen DJ, Sather HN, et al: Risk- and response-based classification of childhood B-precursor acute lymphoblastic leukemia: A combined analysis of prognostic markers from the Pediatric Oncology Group (POG) and Children's Cancer Group (CCG). *Blood* 109:926, 2007.
19. Eden TO, Pieters R, Richards S: Systematic review of the addition of vincristine plus steroid pulses in maintenance treatment for childhood acute lymphoblastic leukaemia—an individual patient data meta-analysis involving 5,659 children1. *Br J Haematol* 149:722, 2010.
20. Pui CH, Howard SC: Current management and challenges of malignant disease in the CNS in paediatric leukaemia. *Lancet Oncol* 9:257, 2008.
21. Teuffel O, Kuster SP, Hunger SP, et al: Dexamethasone versus prednisone for induction therapy in childhood acute lymphoblastic leukemia: A systematic review and meta-analysis. *Leukemia* 25:1232, 2011.
22. van den BH: Asparaginase revisited. *Leuk Lymphoma* 52:168, 2011.
23. Matloub Y, Bostrom BC, Hunger SP, et al: Escalating intravenous methotrexate improves event-free survival in children with standard-risk acute lymphoblastic leukemia: A report from the Children's Oncology Group. *Blood* 118:243, 2011.
24. Schultz KR, Bowman WP, Aledo A, et al: Improved early event-free survival with imatinib in Philadelphia chromosome-positive acute lymphoblastic leukemia: A children's oncology group study. *J Clin Oncol* 27:5175, 2009.
25. Pui CH, Jeha S: New therapeutic strategies for the treatment of acute lymphoblastic leukaemia. *Nat Rev Drug Discov* 6:149, 2007.
26. Pulsipher MA, Peters C, Pui CH: High-risk pediatric acute lymphoblastic leukemia: To transplant or not to transplant? *Biol Blood Marrow Transplant* 17:S137, 2011.
27. Bailey LC, Lange BJ, Rheingold SR, et al: Bone-marrow relapse in paediatric acute lymphoblastic leukaemia1. *Lancet Oncol* 9:873, 2008.
28. Gaynon PS, Qu RP, Chappell RJ, et al: Survival after relapse in childhood acute lymphoblastic leukemia: Impact of site and time to first relapse–the Children's Cancer Group Experience1. *Cancer* 82:1387, 1998.
29. Mullighan CG, Zhang J, Kasper LH, et al: CREBBP mutations in relapsed acute lymphoblastic leukaemia. *Nature* 471:235, 2011.
30. Howard SC, Jones DP, Pui CH: The tumor lysis syndrome. *N Engl J Med* 364:1844, 2011.
31. Haidar C, Jeha S: Drug interactions in childhood cancer. *Lancet Oncol* 12:92, 2011.

CHAPTER 65

ACUTE LYMPHOBLASTIC LEUKEMIA IN ADULTS

Nitin Jain, Sandeep Gurbuxani, Charles Rhee, and Wendy Stock

Acute lymphoblastic leukemia (ALL) is a heterogeneous group of diseases characterized by clonal proliferation of lymphoid progenitors (lymphoblasts). Improved diagnostic tools permit accurate and prompt diagnosis and aid in evaluation of minimal residual disease (MRD). There have been significant advances in the past decade toward understanding disease pathogenesis, refinement of prognostic groups, and the development of novel therapies targeted toward specific disease subsets. These risk-adapted therapies are transforming the treatment strategies for adults with ALL and are beginning to result in significant improvements in survival.

EPIDEMIOLOGY

It is estimated that in the year 2012, 6050 men and women would be diagnosed with ALL in the United States. ALL is primarily a cancer of childhood; the peak incidence (7.7 in 100,000) occurs between the ages of 1 and 4 years, and approximately 60% of the patients are diagnosed before the age of 20 years. The incidence of ALL begins to decline with increasing age after the first decade of life. A second upward trend starts to emerge in the sixth decade of life, and a much smaller peak is seen in patients older than 85 years of age (1.8 in 100,000). Men have a slightly higher incidence of ALL than women (male-to-female ratio, 1.4 to 1). The overall age-adjusted rate of ALL has increased from 0.93 in 100,000 in the year 1975 to 1.47 in 100,000 in the year 2008. Similar increases in the incidence of ALL have also been reported in Scandinavia, the United Kingdom, and Italy. Although most investigators agree that this increase in the incidence is beyond what might be expected from better reporting, the actual cause(s) of this increased incidence remains largely speculative.

ETIOLOGY

A small minority of ALL cases (<5%) are associated with predisposing inherited syndromes such as Down syndrome, Bloom syndrome, ataxia telangiectasia, and Nijmegen breakage syndrome. However, the underlying etiology is not known in most cases. Although parental tobacco or alcohol use, exposure to pesticides or solvents, and cigarette smoking have all been implicated, only ionizing radiation has been significantly linked to increased risk of developing ALL. The vast majority of literature that attempts to identify causative agents for ALL is at best correlative; most of it borders on pure speculation and conjecture. Only recently has it been appreciated that the interaction between genetic predisposition and environmental factors involved in leukemogenesis is complex and may be different for different subtypes of ALL. Epidemiologic studies designed to identify environmental agents involved in leukemogenesis will therefore have to take into account the biologic subsets defined by morphology, immunophenotype, karyotype, and the molecular abnormalities and consider the possibility that for each of these subtypes, the causative agent may well be different. To adequately investigate these issues, future studies will require collaborative efforts studying large patient populations.

Despite the limitations described, it is relevant to review some of the recent advances in our understanding of the etiology of ALL. Greaves and colleagues have used DNA obtained from neonatal blood spots to demonstrate that ALL-associated chromosomal translocations (and hence a preleukemic clone) can be demonstrated in neonatal blood spots that are acquired in utero. Furthermore, these are present at 100-fold higher rate than the incidence of leukemia. These investigators hypothesize that overt leukemia evolves as a consequence of an abnormal lymphoid proliferation that occurs in response to exposure to an as yet unidentified infectious agent(s). Supporting this hypothesis are data that suggest that day care attendance associated with early exposure to common infectious agents is associated with a lower incidence of ALL. Similarly, industrialization associated with improved socioeconomic status and exposure to common infectious agents later in life has been postulated to result in abnormal and excessive lymphoid proliferation and leukemic transformation. Finally, an infectious etiology can also be evoked to explain leukemic clusters that occur when a previously unexposed community is exposed to infectious agents brought into the community by a large influx of residents as happens during urbanization of rural communities. However, it needs to be reiterated that all of these studies are at best correlative and not supported by direct experimental evidence. Furthermore, the infectious or environmental agent(s) responsible for this abnormal lymphoid proliferation remains elusive.

APPROACH TO DIAGNOSIS

While evaluation of morphology and immunophenotype are sufficient for making the diagnosis, current risk stratification relies on additional cytogenetic and molecular genetic information. Data from these tests is therefore an important adjunct to the initial diagnostic work up.

Initial laboratory evaluation starts with a complete blood count (CBC) and morphologic evaluation of a Giemsa-stained peripheral blood smear. An abnormality of at least one of the CBC parameters is detected in more than 90% of ALL patients at the time of diagnosis. Anemia and thrombocytopenia are common. The anemia is usually a normochromic, normocytic anemia accompanied by reticulocytopenia. The hemoglobin levels range from 30 to 174 g/L, and almost 50% of the patients have hemoglobin levels below 100 g/L. The median platelet count at presentation is approximately 55 to 60×10^9/L, and almost 60% to 70% of patients have platelet counts below 100×10^9/L. Although the total white blood cell (WBC) count may be low, normal or elevated, neutropenia is commonly present. In a Cancer and Leukemia Group B (CALGB) study, the median WBC count at presentation was 19.3×10^9/L. Almost one-third of the patients are likely to present with WBC count greater than 30×10^9/L. Blasts account for a variable proportion of the circulating WBCs, and the percent blast population can range from 0% to 100%. A leukoerythroblastic picture can sometimes be seen. In an extreme form, immature myeloid precursors and myeloblasts constitute the vast majority of cells in the peripheral blood. This should be kept in mind when attempting to make a diagnosis exclusively from peripheral blood. Eosinophilia as a presentation of ALL is extremely uncommon and is seen in association with specific chromosomal abnormalities, including t(5;14)(q31;q32) or, even less frequently, with 8p11-associated ALL. Eosinophilia associated with t(5;14) is reactive and due to overexpression of interleukin-3 (IL-3) on chromosome 5 driven by the IgH promoter on chromosome 14. The eosinophilia can be extremely pronounced and mask the blast population in this subset of patients.

Several metabolic abnormalities are present at the time of diagnosis and frequently reflect tumor burden. For example, lactate dehydrogenase (LDH) levels are frequently elevated, and almost 50% of the patients have levels between 300 and 1000 U/L. Elevated serum levels of calcium, potassium, and phosphorous have been noted. More importantly, elevated serum uric acid levels are frequently present and reflect tumor burden. Hyperuricemia needs to be carefully monitored and aggressively corrected to avoid renal failure, especially at the time of starting induction therapy.

MORPHOLOGY

Romanowsky-based stains such as Wright's Giemsa and Giemsa provide the greatest cytoplasmic detail for evaluation of cytomorphology of the cells in the peripheral blood smear, bone marrow (BM) aspirate smear, and touch imprints (Fig. 65-1). Most frequently, lymphoblasts are small to intermediate in size and have scant, agranular cytoplasm. B lymphoblasts are morphologically indistinguishable from T lymphoblasts, and this distinction relies on immunophenotyping. The nuclei are usually round, with uniformly dispersed "smudgy" chromatin and inconspicuous nucleoli (see Fig. 65-1, *C*). However, variations in morphology are common, and larger cells with abundant bluish gray cytoplasm, larger, somewhat irregular nuclei, and variably prominent nucleoli can be frequently seen (see Fig. 65-1, *D*). Even though the nuclear chromatin of these cells can be fine, it is never as finely dispersed as in a myeloblast. At the other end of morphologic spectrum are smaller cells with uniformly condensed, mature lymphocyte-like chromatin (see Fig. 65-1, *E*), and distinction from mature B-cell malignancies relies on immunophenotyping. Coarse azurophilic granules (see Fig. 65-1, *F*) can be seen in a subset of blasts in 5% to 8% of childhood ALLs and even more frequently in adult ALL patients. These have been reported in association with Philadelphia chromosome–positive (Ph$^+$) ALL and in ALL in Down syndrome patients. The granules are coarser than the granules seen in myeloblasts and are invariably myeloperoxidase negative (see later discussion of cytochemistry). Morphologic distinction between L1 and L2 category recommended in the French–American–British (FAB) classification has proven to be poorly reproducible and of little prognostic value. It has been abandoned in the current World Health Organization (WHO) classification.

Cytoplasmic vacuolation (see Fig. 65-1, *H*) can be seen in as many as 28% of childhood ALL patients. These lymphoblasts can be distinguished from leukemic presentation of Burkitt lymphoma (BL; see later discussion) based on other morphologic features such as a smaller cell size, lack of deep blue cytoplasm, and less coarse chromatin. However, when morphology is confounding, the distinction relies on immunophenotyping of the malignant cells. In contrast to BL cells, ALL blasts are precursor B cells that express terminal deoxynucleotidyl transferase (TdT) and lack surface immunoglobulin expression (see later discussion).

The trephine biopsy sections show hypercellular BM (Fig. 65-2). The sections are evaluated after staining with hematoxylin and eosin. The BM is usually packed with a relatively uniform population of

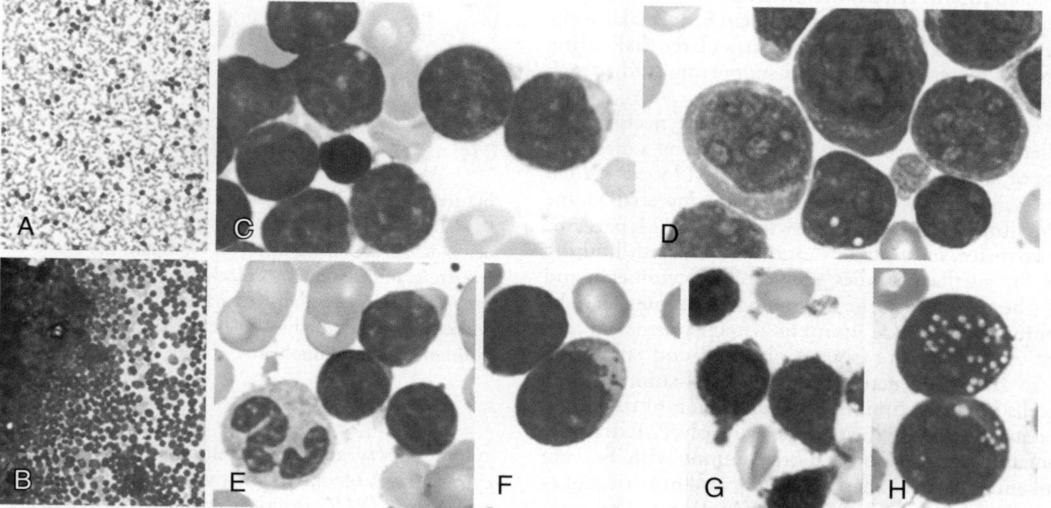

Figure 65-1 MORPHOLOGIC FEATURES OF ACUTE LYMPHOBLASTIC LEUKEMIA (ALL) IN THE BLOOD AND BONE MARROW (BM) ASPIRATE. In ALL, the peripheral blood count can be low, normal or high, although frequently it is high and composed of mostly blasts **(A)**. A similar range in cellularity is true regarding the BM **(B)**. Typically, lymphoblasts are small to intermediate in size and have round nuclei with dispersed chromatin and indistinct nucleoli. They have scant pale blue cytoplasm **(C)**. A small lymphocyte (**C**, *middle, left*) is useful for comparison. In many cases, the lymphoblasts are monotonous, but in some cases, the lymphoblast morphology is varied with some large cells, some cells with abundant cytoplasm, and other cells with prominent nucleoli **(D)**. In the older French–American–British (FAB) classification, these two patterns were referred to as ALL-L1 and ALL-L2, respectively, although they have been shown not to have any clinical significance. Other cytologic variants of lymphoblasts are shown in **E** to **H.** These include lymphocyte-like blasts **(E)**, blasts with azurophilic granules **(F)**, blasts with "hand-mirror" morphology **(G)**, and blasts with vacuoles **(H)**. The small lymphocyte-like blasts can be difficult to distinguish from chronic lymphocytic leukemia cells in the blood, making flow immunophenotyping important in the distinction. Lymphoblasts with granules can be misleading as they can be mistaken for myeloblast or monoblasts. The hand-mirror cells appear to be an artifact because they can be seen only focally on a smear. Vacuoles in the blasts can make the blasts difficult to distinguish from Burkitt cells (see also Fig. 65-7). However, flow cytometry can easily distinguish the immature ALL blasts from the mature B cells seen in a leukemic presentation of Burkitt lymphoma.

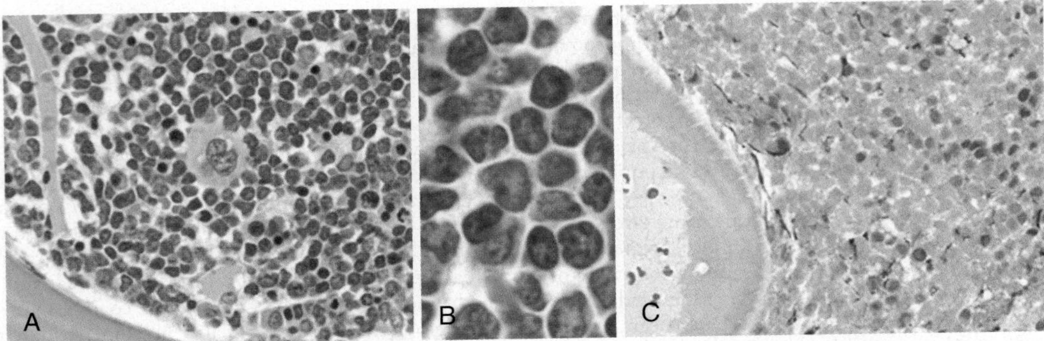

Figure 65-2 MORPHOLOGIC FEATURES OF ACUTE LYMPHOBLASTIC LEUKEMIA (ALL) IN THE BONE MARROW (BM) BIOPSY. The findings in the BM biopsy in ALL are varied, but frequently the biopsy is 100% cellular and packed with blasts **(A).** Sometimes there is some residual hematopoiesis with sparing of megakaryocytes as shown. A high power of the lymphoblasts is shown in **B** illustrating the fine, dispersed, and "blastic" chromatin pattern of the cells. Sometimes the BM can be hypocellular (not shown); however, the majority of the cells in such cases are blasts. Sometimes there is necrosis **(C).** The necrotic cells are referred to as "ghost" cells. They may retain some of their antigen expression as identified by immunostains; however, if the entire biopsy shows necrosis, a diagnosis should be made from the findings in the blood or a repeat BM may be necessary. Other tumors can present with BM necrosis.

small round blasts with round to oval nuclei. Less frequently, the blasts can be more pleomorphic with indented, convoluted, and variably sized nuclei. The chromatin is described as being finely dispersed or stippled and the nucleoli are usually not conspicuous. Brisk mitotic activity is almost always present. The effacement of the BM space is almost complete and uniform at the time of initial presentation. Minimal residual hematopoiesis is present; in most instances this is represented by a few megakaryocytes and some erythropoiesis. Normocellular or even hypocellular BMs at presentation have been described but are uncommon. Rarely, the initial presentation of ALL can be with an aplastic or markedly hypocellular BM. Making the diagnosis in this hypocellular context can be particularly challenging because of a paucity of material available for supporting studies such as cytogenetics and immunophenotyping.

Bone marrow biopsy can show partial or complete necrosis (see Fig. 65-2, *C*). When extensive necrosis is present, making a diagnosis can be challenging or almost impossible. A repeat BM biopsy should be attempted and will usually provide diagnostic material. Some increase in reticulin fibrosis is present in 60% to 70% of ALL patients. When fibrosis is extensive, an aspirate cannot be obtained, limiting material available for ancillary studies such as flow cytometry and cytogenetics. For these patients, the immunophenotyping can be performed by immunoperoxidase immunohistochemistry on the bone core biopsy. A second core can be obtained and submitted without fixation to the cytogenetic laboratory; evaluation can be performed from cells obtained from the disaggregation of the core.

Organs other than the BM can be frequently involved. Extramedullary or lymphomatous presentation is more common with T–acute lymphoblastic leukemia (T-ALL) than B–acute lymphoblastic leukemia (B-ALL) (described later in Clinical Manifestations). The cytomorphology of the malignant cells in extramedullary disease is similar to that described in the bone core biopsy. Lymph node involvement is usually diffuse but can be partial with sparing of the follicles.

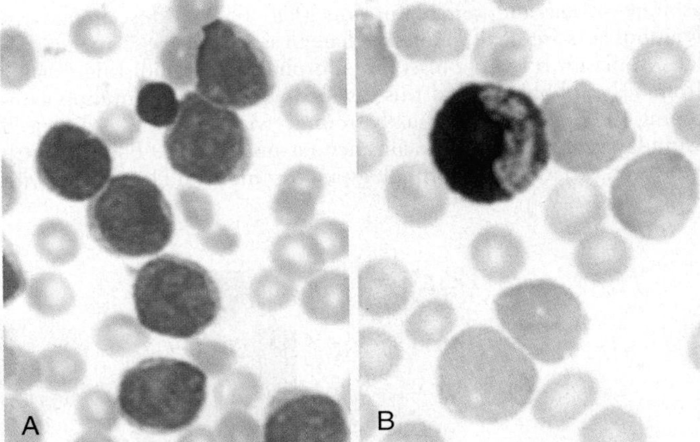

Figure 65-3 CYTOCHEMISTRY IN ACUTE LYMPHOBLASTIC LEUKEMIA. The blasts in acute lymphoblastic leukemia **(A)** are always myeloperoxidase reaction negative. **B,** Compare the blasts with a single positively reactive granulocyte with a black–blue reaction product. Evaluating for nonspecific esterase reactivity (α-naphthyl acetate esterase, or alpha naphthyl butyrate esterase) might also be performed when the blasts are difficult to distinguish from monoblasts.

CYTOCHEMISTRY

The use of cytochemistry to assign lineage has been largely replaced by flow cytometry evaluation of the leukemic blast immunophenotype. However, when available, the myeloperoxidase reaction (Fig. 65-3, *A* and *B*) permits a rapid distinction from acute myeloid leukemia (AML). The reaction detects the myeloperoxidase enzyme in the primary granules of myeloblasts and is specific for the myeloid lineage. An acute leukemia in which 3% or more of the cells are myeloperoxidase positive is considered myeloid. There is excellent concordance between the myeloperoxidase reaction detected by cytochemistry and the myeloperoxidase molecule detected by flow cytometry. A blocklike positivity has been described with the periodic acid-Schiff (PAS) reaction that detects glycogen in almost 50% of ALL cases.

IMMUNOPHENOTYPE

Based on large cooperative group studies in Europe and the United States, the incidence of B-ALL ranges from 75% to 80% and T-ALL from 15% to 25%. B lymphoblasts cannot be distinguished from T lymphoblasts by morphology. Extensive immunophenotypic characterization is therefore required for the appropriate classification of ALL and indeed distinction from certain subtypes of AML. When adequate material is available, immunophenotyping should be performed using multicolor flow cytometry so that multiple antigens can be detected simultaneously on the lymphoblasts (Fig. 65-4). When interpreting the immunophenotypic data, it is important to remember that no single antigen is specific for any given lineage and multiple

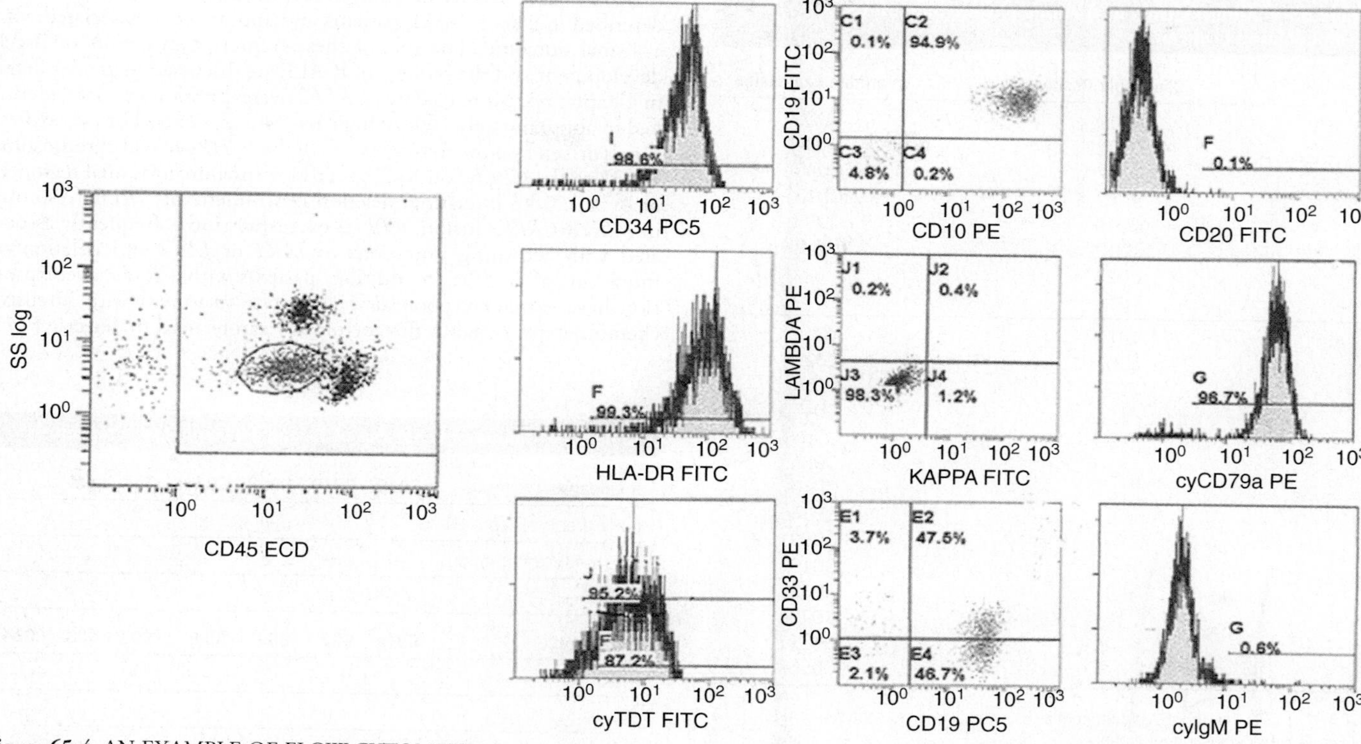

Figure 65-4 AN EXAMPLE OF FLOW CYTOMETRIC EVALUATION IN A CASE OF B–ACUTE LYMPHOBLASTIC LEUKEMIA (B-ALL). Selected histograms from a panel of markers used in the evaluation of ALL by flow cytometry are illustrated. The blasts are first identified by weak CD45 expression and low side scatter *(left histogram, circled population).* This is a useful gating strategy because it allows for an easy identification of the blast population and its separation from lymphocytes (with bright CD45) and nucleated red blood cells (with absent CD45 expression). Because no single antigen is specific for a lineage, multiple antigens are evaluated using multicolor flow cytometry. The phenotype illustrated is that of a common precursor B-ALL. In this case, the blasts are $CD34^+$, HLA-DR^+, TdT^+, $CD19^+$, $CD10^+$, $CD20^-$, $cyCD79a^+$, κ^-, λ^-, and $cyIgM^-$. There is weak and partial expression of the myeloid marker CD33.

antigens need to be evaluated to establish the correct diagnosis. The panel of antibodies used for flow cytometry of a new leukemia and the pattern of expression seen in B- and T-ALL are shown in Table 65-1. In addition, the combination of markers expressed on the B or T lymphoblasts can be reflective of the stage of development at which the transformation happened (Table 65-2). Of note, expression of myeloid antigens is seen frequently in B- and T-ALL, as is the expression of T-cell antigens in B-ALL and B-cell antigens in T-ALL. Expression of individual myeloid antigens should not be a deterrent to making the diagnosis of ALL. The criteria for diagnosis acute leukemias of ambiguous lineage, which would include mixed phenotype acute leukemia, have been extensively revised in the current WHO classification.

GENETICS

Chromosomal abnormalities can be detected in almost 80% of B-ALLs and 70% of T-ALLs. Cytogenetic classification remains the single most important prognostic factor in both pediatric and adult ALL. Numerical abnormalities as well as structural abnormalities that disrupt the function of transcription factors involved in hematopoietic development and differentiation are common. These genetic abnormalities define the biology of the disease and have an impact on treatment outcome. In addition, specific cytogenetic or molecular abnormalities are associated with unique phenotypic characteristics and are amenable to targeted therapy. Although Ph^+ ALL is the first subset of ALL to use a molecularly targeted tyrosine kinase inhibitor (TKI) therapy as frontline treatment, it is likely that more genetically defined entities will be targeted for specific therapy. This has been recognized in the 2008 WHO classification with a specific discussion on lymphoblastic leukemia/lymphoma with recurrent cytogenetic abnormalities (Table 65-3). Although the discussion in the current WHO classification is neither comprehensive nor complete, it does establish a framework for future discussion for appropriate classification of ALL. Association with distinct phenotypic properties or clinical behavior determines inclusion of specific entities in the 2008 classification.

Hyperdiploidy defined by the presence of more than 50 chromosomes is seen in almost 25% of pediatric patients and 4% to 5% of adult ALL patients. In addition to routine karyotyping or fluorescent in situ hybridization (FISH) analysis, hyperdiploid DNA content can be determined by flow cytometry using DNA binding fluorescent dyes and corresponds to a DNA content between 1.16 and 1.6. However, some studies have demonstrated that hyperdiploidy resulting from duplication of specific chromosomes (4, 10, and 17) is a better indicator of a favorable prognosis than the actual ploidy or the DNA content. In contrast, patients with a hypodiploid karyotype with a chromosome number below 46 is associated with an adverse prognosis. Another abnormality seen commonly in the pediatric age group but extremely rarely in the adult age group is a cryptic translocation, the t(12;21)(p13;q22)*(ETV6-RUNX1).* When present, it is associated with a favorable prognosis. Leukemias that harbor rearrangements of the *MLL* (mixed-lineage leukemia) gene at chromosome 11q23, most notably t(4;11)(q21;q23), present with high WBC counts and frequent central nervous system (CNS) involvement and are associated with poor clinical outcomes. Ph^+ ALL associated with t(9;22)(q34;q11.2) account for 25% of adult ALL. The presence of this translocation was invariably associated with a poor outcome before inclusion of TKIs into frontline treatment.

More recently, submicroscopic genomic alterations have been detected that have significant impact on the biology of ALL. These involve transcription factors such as *IKZF1* (Ikaros), *EBF,* and *PAX5.* Additionally, intrachromosomal amplification of chromosome 21

Table 65-1 Antigens Used for Immunophenotyping of Acute Lymphoblastic Leukemia*

	Commonly Positive	Variable Expression
B-ALL	CD19[†]	CD20
	cCD22[†]	CD34
	cCD79a[†]	CD45
	Pax5[‡]	CD13
	CD10	CD33
	sCD22	sIgM[§]
	CD24	
	TdT	
T-ALL	TdT	CD1a
	cCD3[‖]	CD2
	CD7	sCD3
		CD4[¶]
		CD5
		CD8[¶]
		CD10
		CD34
		CD99
		CD19
		CD33
		CD79a
		CD117
		CD56

B-ALL, B-acute lymphoblastic leukemia; *c,* cytoplasmic; *s,* surface; *T-ALL,* T-acute lymphoblastic leukemia.
*Antigens are listed approximately in order of frequency.
[†]Almost always positive.
[‡]Most specific for B lineage but can be positive in t(8;21) acute myeloid leukemia.
[§]Rarely present.
[‖]Only marker considered lineage specific.
[¶]Frequently coexpressed.

(iAMP21) that results in multiple copies of *RUNX1* has also been described in 2% of B-ALL patients and appears to be associated with a dismal outcome. The role of these transcription factors in B-cell development and the biology of B-ALL are discussed in greater detail in Chapter 63. More recently, *CRLF2* overexpression has been identified in approximately 14% of high-risk ALL patients. The overexpression is driven by either translocation of the *IGH2* gene on chromosome 14q32 to the *CRLF2* on Xp22.3/Yp11.3 (pseudoautosomal region 1) or by a 320-kb interstitial deletion centromeric of *CRLF2* resulting in *P2RY8-CRLF2* fusion. *CRLF2* overexpression is frequently associated with activating mutations of *JAK1* or *JAK2* and deletion or mutations of *IKZF1*. In addition, patients with *CRLF2* overexpression have extremely poor survival despite treatment with intensive chemotherapy. Notably, flow cytometry can be used to detect *CRLF2*

Table 65-2 Immunophenotypes of B- and T-Lymphocyte Progenitors

B Lineage	CD10	CD19	CD22	CD79a	TdT	IgM	
Early precursor (pro-B)	–	+	+	+	+	–	
Intermediate (common)	+	+	+	+	+	–	
Pre-B	+/–	+	+	+	+	C	
T Lineage	**CD1a**	**CD2**	**CD3**	**CD4**	**CD7**	**CD8**	**CD34**
Pro-T	–	–	C	–	+	–	+/–
Pre-T	–	+	C	–	+	–	+/–
Cortical T	+	+	C	+	+	+	–
Medullary T	–	+	C, S	*	+	*	–

C, Cytoplasmic; *Ig,* immunoglobulin; *S,* surface; *TdT,* terminal deoxynucleotidyl transferase.
*Medullary T lymphocytes are positive for either CD4 or CD8 but not both.

Table 65-3 Significant Features of B-Acute Lymphoblastic Leukemia With Recurrent Cytogenetic Abnormalities in the 2008 World Health Organization Classification

Cytogenetic Abnormality	Phenotype	Clinical Correlates	Incidence #
t(9;22)(q33;q11.2)	CD19⁺, CD10⁺, CD25⁺; frequent expression of myeloid antigens	Seen more frequently in adults; traditionally associated with extremely poor outcome; improved early event-free survival with targeted therapy	19% of all adult ALL patients; incidence increases with age
t(v;11q23) Common fusion partners include AF4 (4q21) and ENL (19p13)	CD19⁺, CD10⁻; aberrant expression of myeloid antigen CD15	Frequent presentation with high WBC count, CNS involvement	9% of Ph-negative adult ALL
t(12;21)(p13;q22) Cryptic translocation; requires FISH	CD19⁺CD10⁺; aberrant expression of myeloid antigen CD13	Sensitive disease with favorable outcome on standard therapy	2%-3% of Ph-negative adult ALL
Hyperdiploidy Chromosome number >50, <66 Extra copies of nonrandom chromosomes, most frequently 21,X,14, and 4	CD19⁺, CD10⁺; no distinctive phenotype	Sensitive disease with favorable outcome on standard therapy	10% of Ph-negative adult ALL
Hypodiploidy Chromosome number <46	CD19⁺, CD10⁺; no distinctive phenotype	Poor prognosis	4% of Ph-negative adult ALL
t(5;14)(q31;q32)	CD19⁺, CD10⁺; no distinctive phenotype	Reactive eosinophilia driven by IL-3 overexpression driven by the translocation; blasts may be <20% in the BM and undetectable in peripheral blood	Rare in adults
t(1;19)(q23;p13.3)	CD19⁺, CD10⁺; cytoplasmic μ⁺	No significant association with response to therapy on current protocols	3% of Ph-negative adult ALL

Data from Moorman AV, Harrison CJ, Buck GA, et al: Adult Leukaemia Working Party, Medical Research Council/National Cancer Research Institute. *Blood* 109:3189, 2007 and Pui CH, Relling MV, Downing JR: Acute lymphoblastic leukemia. *N Engl J Med* 350:1535, 2004.
ALL, Acute lymphoblastic leukemia; *BM,* bone marrow; *CNS,* central nervous system; *FISH,* fluorescent in situ hybridization; *IL-3,* interleukin-3; *WBC,* white blood cell.

overexpression in the clinical laboratory. As we acquire a better understanding of the effect of these genetic alterations on the biology of ALL, they are likely to have an impact on how we risk stratify ALL patients and indeed exploit these aberrations for targeted therapy.

Similar to B-ALL, translocations involving transcription factors are common in T-ALL. The most commonly involved genes include *HOX11* and *HOX11L2*. Other genes that have been described to be involved in T-ALL are *MYC, TAL1, LMO2*, and *LYL1*. Similar to t(12;21), translocations involving the *TAL1* gene are cryptic and require detection by molecular techniques. Activating mutations of the *NOTCH1* gene are detected in almost 50% of ALL patients. Although activating mutations of *NOTCH1* appear to be associated with disease pathogenesis, they do not appear to be associated with an adverse prognosis in the majority of studies; in fact, some pediatric studies suggest that NOTCH1-mutated T-ALL may have a relatively favorable response to current treatment regimens. Deletions of the *CDKN2A* gene on chromosome 9p are also particularly frequent as are mutations in the *FBXW7* gene, but neither has clear prognostic significance as single abnormalities. The significance of these mutations remains an area of active research.

CLINICAL MANIFESTATIONS

The clinical presentation of ALL encompasses a wide spectrum of symptoms that correlate with the degree of BM involvement and the resultant cytopenias, as well as the leukemic cell burden. Typical symptoms include fatigue, anorexia, night sweats, pallor, shortness of breath, bone pain, fever, and bleeding diathesis. Involvement of extramedullary sites may present with lymphadenopathy, hepatomegaly, or splenomegaly. Less commonly, ALL can involve the CNS, leading to headache, vomiting, lethargy, and cranial nerve palsies. Other extramedullary sites of involvement include the testis, tonsils, adenoids, breast, and gastrointestinal tract. Precursor T-cell ALL often presents with a large mediastinal mass with associated respiratory distress or possible signs of superior vena cava syndrome. Burkitt leukemia/lymphoma is frequently associated with CNS involvement and bulky adenopathy.

CLINICAL AND LABORATORY EVALUATION

The initial workup for patients with suspected ALL is detailed in Table 65-4. All patients should undergo a detailed history and physical examination. Family history should be ascertained. Laboratory evaluation should include CBC with differential; comprehensive metabolic panel, including liver function tests, LDH, and uric acid. Coagulation profile should also be obtained, although coagulation parameters are frequently normal at diagnosis. Human leukocyte antigen (HLA) testing should be obtained for patients who are potential candidates for allogeneic stem cell transplantation (aSCT).

All patients should undergo BM aspiration and biopsy for confirmation of diagnosis and for cytogenetic and molecular genetic evaluation. It is particularly important to send an aspirate (or peripheral blood if lymphoblasts are present) to the molecular oncology diagnostic laboratory to evaluate for the presence of the *BCR-ABL* fusion transcript using reverse transcriptase polymerase chain reaction (RT-PCR) because these patients will receive frontline therapy that includes a TKI.

A lumbar puncture should be performed at diagnosis to determine CNS involvement. In the event of increased risk of bleeding caused by severe thrombocytopenia or risk of cerebrospinal fluid contamination caused by high peripheral blood blasts, lumbar puncture should be performed by an experienced operator. It is prudent to administer intrathecal chemotherapy at the time of the diagnostic lumbar puncture after obtaining the necessary samples.

Table 65-4 Initial Evaluation of a Patient With Acute Lymphoblastic Leukemia

- Complete history (including family history)
- Physical examination
- CBC with differential
- Comprehensive metabolic profile, including LFTs
- LDH, uric acid
- Coagulation profile
- BM aspiration and biopsy (morphology, immunohistochemistry, flow cytometry, molecular and cytogenetic analysis)
- HLA typing of the patient (if a potential aSCT candidate)
- Lumbar puncture
- Chest radiography or CT imaging of the chest

aSCT, Allogeneic stem cell transplantation; *BM*, bone marrow; *CBC*, complete blood count; *CT*, computed tomography; *HLA*, human leukocyte antigen; *LDH*, lactate dehydrogenase; *LFT*, liver function test.

DIFFERENTIAL DIAGNOSIS

Acute lymphoblastic leukemia blasts can be easily distinguished from the reactive lymphocytes seen in viral infections because of the precursor phenotype of these cells. Low to weak expression of CD45 and expression of one or more precursor antigens such as TdT or CD34 is useful. In addition, precursor T-ALL cells express only cytoplasmic CD3 and no surface CD3, and B-ALLs frequently lack expression of CD20 while being CD19 positive. As previously mentioned, ALL cells can have some cytoplasmic vacuolation and need to be distinguished from leukemic presentation of BL. Unlike ALL, BL cells are mature B cells with bright surface immunoglobulin expression, very strong CD20 expression, and no expression of CD34. Diagnosis of BL is confirmed by the presence of an *MYC* translocation using FISH or cytogenetics. Other entities that require distinction from ALL depend on the age of presentation. In the pediatric age group, ALL blasts need to be distinguished from hematogones. Hematogones are normal B-cell precursors present within the BM. These are more abundant in childhood and decrease with increasing age. Hematogones may also be increased during hematopoietic regeneration, particularly after chemotherapy or BM engraftment after stem cell transplant. Hematogones possess a distinct pattern of antigen expression that recapitulates progressive B-cell maturation. This is reflected in progressive loss of antigens such as CD34, TdT, and CD10 and acquisition of CD20 and surface immunoglobulin expression (Fig. 65-5). Other diseases that need to be morphologically distinguished from ALL include small blue cell tumors, including Ewing sarcoma, neuroblastoma, and medulloblastoma. Ancillary studies, including immunophenotyping and cytogenetics, are helpful in making the distinction. In older adults, entities that can morphologically mimic ALL include blastoid mantle cell lymphoma, chronic lymphocytic leukemia, and prolymphocytic leukemia. These latter are all mature B-cell malignancies that can be distinguished from ALL based on the mature B-cell phenotype, including consistent expression of CD20 and surface immunoglobulins.

PROGNOSIS

Prognostication based on clinical and biologic risk factors has been useful in making informed decisions about postremission treatment options. Established risk factor for a poor prognosis with current chemotherapeutic approaches include age older than 60 years, elevated WBC count at diagnosis (>30,000/μL for B-cell ALL; >100,000/μL for T-cell ALL), pro–B cell or early T-cell immunophenotype, and cytogenetics (t(4;11)(q21;q23) and other *MLL* rearrangements, hypodiploidy, or a complex karyotype). The presence of the Philadelphia chromosome, t(9;22)(q34;q11.2) resulting in the *BCR-ABL* fusion gene was previously associated with very poor treatment outcomes. Recent addition of ABL kinase inhibitors

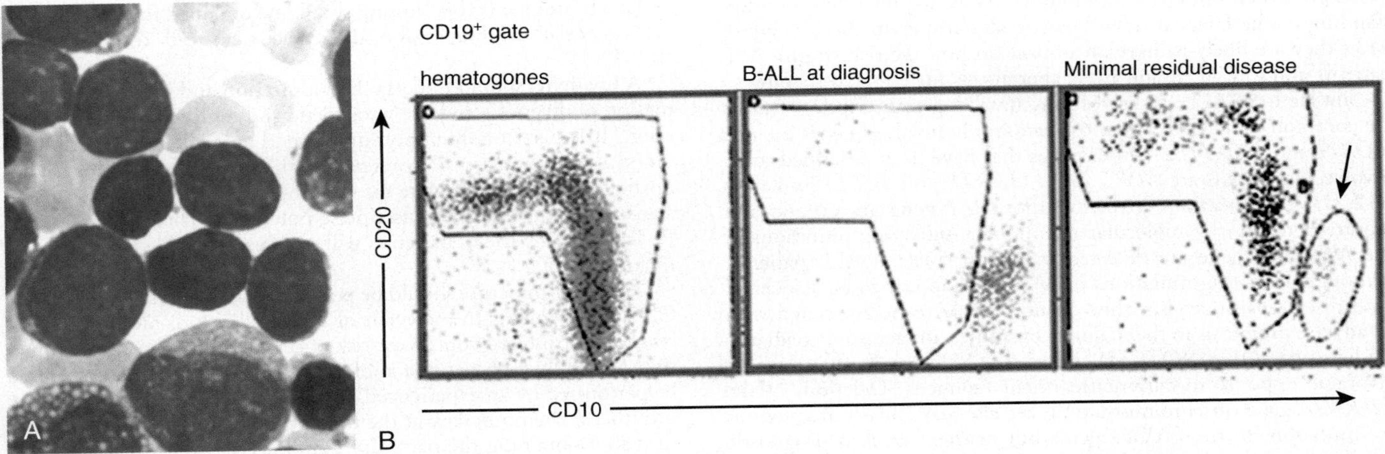

Figure 65-5 HEMATOGONES AND FLOW CYTOMETRIC EVALUATION OF MINIMAL RESIDUAL DISEASE (MRD). Hematogones are nonmalignant immature precursor B cells that are present in the bone marrow (BM). They are more commonly seen in pediatric patients but can be seen in adults during BM regeneration or associated with other conditions. **A,** They can be difficult to distinguish morphologically from malignant lymphoblasts because the cytologic features overlap significantly. **B,** Unlike malignant lymphoblasts, hematogones exhibit a spectrum of maturation that can be seen, for example, by analyzing CD10 and CD20 expression on $CD19^+$ cells *(left histogram)*. Hematogones are $CD10^+$, but as CD20 is expressed, CD10 is diminished. Lymphoblasts, on the other hand, frequently exhibit maturation arrest and over- or underexpression of markers. They can also exhibit aberrant markers. In the *middle histogram,* the B lymphoblasts from the initial diagnosis specimen can be seen *(red)*, and the CD10 and CD20 expression is outside the normal hematogone range with overexpression of CD10 and absence of CD20. This pattern can be used to identify MRD *(right histogram)* and distinguish regenerative hematogones *(black)* from residual or recurrent blasts *(red)* after therapy. Multiple markers and parameters are usually used to study posttherapy specimens in this way.

(molecularly targeted therapy), discussed in detail later, has improved the prognosis for these patients. Time to achievement of complete remission (CR) longer than 4 weeks has also been associated with a poor clinical outcome (Table 65-5).

Although different study groups have used slightly different variations of these risk factors, the presence of any one of the following is generally accepted as high risk (HR): high WBC count at diagnosis (>30,000/μL in B-cell ALL or >100,000/μL in T-cell ALL); cytogenetic abnormalities [hypodiploidy, t(4;11), t(9;22)]; age older than 60 years; pro–B cell phenotype; and time to remission longer than 4 weeks. All other patients are considered standard risk (SR).

Nevertheless, despite being labeled as SR, up to 40% to 50% of these adults eventually relapse. Thus, there is a need for refinement of prognostic markers for ALL patients. Recently, an early T-cell phenotype, the expression of $CD20^+$ and several recently described genetic mutations (*IKAROS, CRLF2,* and *JAK2;* and reviewed earlier in this chapter) have been identified as being associated with adverse outcomes from retrospective analyses.

Table 65-5 Markers for Poor Prognosis in Adult Acute Lymphoblastic Leukemia

Established Risk Factors	
Age	>60 years
Presenting WBC count	>30,000/μL (B-cell ALL); >100,000/μL (T-cell AL)
Immunophenotype	Pro–B cell; early T-cell
Cytogenetics	t(4;11)(q21;q23) and other *MLL* rearrangements t(9;22)(q34;q11.2) - Philadelphia chromosome Hypodiploidy (<44 chromosomes) Complex (>five abnormalities)
Therapy response	Time to complete remission >4 weeks
MRD	≥0.01% at 3-6 months after initiation of therapy*
Emerging Risk Factors	
Immunophenotype	CD20
Molecular	*BAALC* *IKAROS* *FUS* *ERG* *JAK* *CRLF2*

ALL, Acute lymphoblastic leukemia; *MRD,* minimal residual disease; *WBC,* white blood cell.
*Different studies have used different time points for MRD assessment.

MINIMAL RESIDUAL DISEASE

The identification and measurement of MRD (subclinical disease) using leukemia clone-specific quantitative PCR and flow cytometry is an independent prognostic that is now being used to guide postremission therapies in many pediatric and some adult ALL treatment studies. In general, these techniques have not yet been widely standardized; however, the majority of studies demonstrate that MRD detection during early postremission therapy is a reliable and independent predictor of relapse. The optimal time point for outcome prognostication based on MRD measurements varies from study to study; undoubtedly, some of this variability is the result of differences in the PCR technique used, the sensitivity of detection of MRD of the individual assay, and the treatment intensity and the population being studied. Nevertheless, the majority of studies indicate that MRD detection anywhere from 4 to 20 weeks from initiation of treatment is highly predictive of relapse. Thus current studies are using novel approaches to try to eradicate MRD during early remission or stratifying MRD-positive patients to early intensification with aSCT to try to improve survival for these patients at very high risk for relapse.

TREATMENT OF ACUTE LYMPHOBLASTIC LEUKEMIA

Combination chemotherapy is the cornerstone of ALL management. In the 1960s, investigators at the National Institutes of Health designed multidrug chemotherapy regimens given over many different courses for pediatric ALL patients. A similar approach was then introduced for adults with ALL. The Berlin-Frankfurt-Muenster (BFM) group in the 1980s conducted pioneering studies and showed that an intensive multidrug induction and consolidation chemotherapy followed by delayed intensification led to improvement in survival in the majority of children. These regimens combine drugs with varying mechanisms of action at different doses, often in complex schedules, which have largely evolved empirically. Only a few of these drugs have been tested individually in randomized clinical trials in adults with ALL; therefore, the relative contribution of each of the drugs in a multidrug regimen to the overall outcome is difficult to assess. Because there is an increased propensity for CNS involvement in ALL patients, all treatment regimens must also include CNS prophylaxis with intrathecal chemotherapy with or without cranial radiation.

The therapy for ALL is typically divided into three phases: (1) the remission induction phase, (2) remission consolidation or intensification, and (3) the maintenance (or continuation) phase. The remission induction and consolidation phases typically involve blocks of monthly treatment for 6 to 8 months followed by long-term maintenance, which is given for up to 3 years; thus, the treatment of ALL is long and challenging and requires tremendous attention to detail, compliance, and support. Because of these challenges and the relative rarity and biologic heterogeneity of the disease, it is recommended that patients are referred to larger academic centers for the evaluation and treatment to ensure the best possible survival rates. In the ensuing sections, the various components of treatment are reviewed. Special attention to the treatment of certain disease subsets are addressed because treatment of ALL is becoming increasingly based on its heterogeneity and the ability to adapt therapy to each of these subsets.

Effective chemotherapy regimens must be supplemented with adequate supportive care measures to obtain the best patient outcomes. Given the highly immunosuppressive nature of ALL treatment regimens, prophylaxis for *Pneumocystis carinii* with trimethoprim–sulfamethoxazole should be initiated early during treatment and continue throughout the consolidation and maintenance phases of chemotherapy. It is also reasonable to consider antifungal and antiviral prophylaxis during periods of neutropenia. Consideration may be given to antibacterial prophylaxis during periods of neutropenia. Fluoroquinolones such as levofloxacin are the preferred agent, although the optimal antibiotic choice should depend on local bacterial resistance patterns. Neutropenic fever in this group of patients must be treated as a medical emergency with immediate institution of intravenous (IV) antibiotics after obtaining the necessary cultures.

In an attempt to decrease the duration of neutropenia and improve remission rates, several groups have studied the role of granulocyte colony-stimulating factor (G-CSF) or granulocyte macrophage colony-stimulating factor (GM-CSF) during induction therapy. In the CALGB 9111 trial, 198 adults with untreated ALL were randomized to receive G-CSF (beginning 4 days after the start of induction until neutrophil recovery) versus placebo. The median time to neutrophil recovery (≥1000/μL for 2 days) significantly shortened to 16 days in the G-CSF arm compared with 22 days in the placebo arm. The duration of hospitalization was also significantly shorter in the G-CSF arm. There was a trend toward increased CR rate in the G-CSF arm. However, the infectious complications, disease-free survival (DFS), and overall survival (OS) were similar in the two arms. Thomas and colleagues randomized 236 ALL patients treated on the LALA-94 trial to receive G-CSF, GM-CSF, or no CSF. Use of G-CSF was associated with a significant decrease in time to neutrophil recovery, duration of hospitalization, and infections that were grade 3 or higher. Thus, use of G-CSF can allow for faster hematopoietic recovery, especially in elderly patients, and may decrease infectious complications; however, the prophylactic use of G-CSF has not been uniformly adopted, and many studies simply follow standard guidelines for use of growth factors in the setting of neutropenic fever.

All patients should be monitored carefully for tumor lysis syndromes especially those with risk factors such as elevated WBC counts, renal dysfunction, and elevated LDH at presentation. Patients must be provided adequate hydration and prophylaxis or treatment for hyperuricemia with allopurinol for the first week of induction. Rasburicase, a urate oxidase, can be considered for the treatment of hyperuricemia in cases with high proliferation rates.

REMISSION INDUCTION

The aim of induction therapy is to achieve maximal reduction of the leukemic burden to result in morphologic remission (<5% blasts with trilineage hematopoiesis) and normalization of the blood counts, with as little toxicity as possible. This is typically achieved using combination chemotherapy consisting of four or five systemically administered drugs and intrathecal chemotherapy over a period of approximately 3 to 4 weeks. Most current ALL induction regimens in adults are modeled after pediatric regimens and include a prolonged course of oral corticosteroid (prednisone or dexamethasone), weekly vincristine, and either weekly or pulsed anthracycline (doxorubicin, daunorubicin, or mitoxantrone). Many groups (CALGB, French GRAALL 2003, and BFM) have also used twice-weekly L-asparaginase as part of induction therapy and some have added cyclophosphamide (MD Anderson, GRAALL 2003, and GMALL 07/2003). With the current treatment regimens, very high CR rates in adults with ALL have been achieved in the range of 84% to 94% (Table 65-6). There have been few randomized comparisons between these different induction regimens; therefore, the choice of the regimen should depend on the treating physician's experience with a particular regimen. Most ALL regimens are designed to optimally deliver a variety of chemotherapeutic agents; thus, an entire treatment program should be selected at the time of diagnosis based on the patient's performance status and biologic risk factors. Whenever possible, these patients should be referred to centers that offer expertise in the treatment of ALL and where enrollment into clinical trials is available.

Traditionally, prednisone was the corticosteroid of choice during induction therapy for ALL trials. Studies in pediatric patients have shown lower relapse rates but higher toxicity (more sepsis, higher incidence of osteonecrosis) with dexamethasone. Dexamethasone penetrates the blood–brain barrier effectively and therefore may offer more direct CNS protection than prednisone. Comparative studies of prednisone versus dexamethasone have not been performed in adults, and some groups have incorporated prednisone (CALGB 10403, GRAALL-2003, and BFM); others have incorporated dexamethasone (CALGB 10102, MD Anderson, GMALL 07/2003) during the induction cycle. Anthracyclines form an important part of induction therapy. In an early trial from the CALGB (7612), patients were randomized to receive vincristine, prednisone, and L-asparaginase with or without daunorubicin. Significant improvements in CR rates and remission duration were noted with the addition of daunorubicin; anthracyclines have since become standard components of induction chemotherapy in adult and pediatric ALL. Different anthracyclines (doxorubicin, daunorubicin, and mitoxantrone) are thought to be clinically equivalent and, to date, dose intensification of anthracycline during induction has been tested in a variety of prospective clinical trials but has not been shown to definitely improve already high CR rates or to result in significant benefits in DFS. Addition of pulsed cyclophosphamide to induction chemotherapy has been studied with conflicting results. In the CALGB 8811 trial, addition of cyclophosphamide to the induction regimen was shown to lead to improved responses compared with historical control participants. However, in a prospective, randomized Italian GIMEMA 0288 study, the addition of cyclophosphamide did not influence CR rate or survival.

One of the regimens that is widely used in the United States and also results in high CR rates of approximately 90% is the hyper-CVAD (cyclophosphamide, vincristine, Adriamycin, and dexamethasone) regimen developed at the MD Anderson Cancer Center. The hyper-CVAD regimen differs from the pulsed weekly therapy developed by the pediatric groups and consists of four cycles of intensive infusional cyclophosphamide, vincristine, doxorubicin, and dexamethasone alternating with four cycles of high-dose methotrexate and high-dose cytarabine for a total of eight intensive treatment cycles.

Table 65-6 Clinical Trials With Various Chemotherapy Regimens for Adult Acute Lymphoblastic Leukemia

Trial	Patients *(n)*	Age in Years, Median (Range)	CR Rate (%)	Disease-Free Survival	Overall Survival	Comments
CALGB 8811[1]	197	32 (16-80)	85	46% at 3 years	36 months (median)	Five-drug induction regimen based on pediatric trials with earlier and more intensive L-asparaginase
CALGB 9111[2]	198	35 (16-83)	85	40% at 3 years	23 months (median)	Patients randomized to G-CSF vs. placebo; G-CSF significantly decreased time to neutrophil recovery and CR rate with no effect on DFS, OS, or toxicities
MDACC hyper-CVAD[3]	288	40 (15-92)	92	38% at 5 years	32 months (median)	Long-term follow-up results of hyper-CVAD regimen; regimen does not include asparaginase
GMALL 05/93[4]	1163	35 (15-65)	83		35% at 5 years	
GMALL 07/2003[5]	713	34 (15-55)	89		54% at 5 years	Risk-adapted SCT for HR and very HR groups
LALA 94[6]	922	33 (18-79)	84	30% at 5 years	23 months (median)	CR rate similar between IDA and DNR arms; significantly higher TRM with IDA; improved DFS for the IDA arm for patients receiving only chemotherapy; for SR patients, intensive consolidation did not affect outcomes
JALSG ALL-93[7]	263	31 (15-59)	78	30% at 6 years	33% at 6 years	Doxorubicin dose intensity did not improve outcomes; during maintenance phase, early sequential intensification compared with intermittent intensification did not affect DFS
JALSG ALL-97[8]	404	38 (15-64)	74	33% at 5 years	32% at 5 years	Induction and maintenance based on CALGB 8811; dose intensive doxorubicin during consolidation did not improve outcomes
GIMEMA 0288[9]	778	28 (12-60)	82	33% at 9 years	29% at 9 years	Addition of cyclophosphamide to induction did not influence CR rate or survival; responders to prednisone pretreatment had favorable outcomes
MRC UKALLXII/ECOG E2993[10]	1646 (Ph-)	(15-64)	90		43% at 5 years	Largest ALL trial to date; in a donor vs. no-donor analysis, those with a donor had improved OS and lower relapse rate; ASCT cannot replace consolidation or maintenance chemotherapy in any risk group
PETHEMA ALL-93[11]	222 high-risk ALL	27 (15-50)	82	35% at 5 years	34% at 5 years	Did not show beneficial effect of aSCT compared with ASCT or chemotherapy
GRAALL-2003[12]	225 Ph- ALL	31 (15-60)	94	59% at 3.5 years	60% at 3.5 years	Pediatric-inspired treatment regimen; in a historical comparison, significant increases in CR, EFS, and OS rates compared with LALA-94 trial; OS was improved for patients younger than 45 years only

ALL, Acute lymphoblastic leukemia; *aSCT,* allogeneic stem cell transplantation; *ASCT,* autologous stem cell transplantation; CALGB, Cancer And Leukemia Group B; *CR,* complete remission; *CVAD,* cyclophosphamide, vincristine, Adriamycin, and dexamethasone; *DFS,* disease-free survival; *DNR,* daunorubicin; *G-CSF,* granulocyte colony-stimulating factor; *HR,* high risk; *IDA,* idarubicin; *OS,* overall survival; *SCT,* stem cell transplantation; *SR,* standard risk; *TRM,* transplant-related mortality.

Some groups have also instituted a 5- to 7-day steroid prophase before starting the induction therapy. This results in gentle cytoreduction and reduces the risk of tumor lysis. The achievement of rapid cytoreduction during this steroid prophase has also been shown to be of prognostic value in several studies.

In summary, although all of the currently employed induction regimens in adults with ALL now routinely result in these very high CR rates of 80% to 90%, none of them has yet translated into the 80% to 85% DFS rates that are routinely achieved in pediatric ALL. In adult ALL, DFS generally has been reported to be at 40% to 45% at 3 years and 30% to 35% at 5 years (see Table 65-6). Thus, the main problem with the current treatment programs in adult ALL is disease relapse from the emergence of resistant disease and not in the failure to achieve CR.

POSTREMISSION THERAPY

As mentioned earlier, 80% to 90% of adults with previously untreated ALL achieve CR with induction chemotherapy. However, all patients relapse if no further chemotherapy is given. This underscores the need for effective postremission management strategies for these patients in first CR (CR1). As described earlier, adult patients with ALL have traditionally been stratified into SR or HR.

The type of postremission strategy is recommended to be based on the risk (risk-adapted approach), which implies more aggressive therapeutic approaches for HR groups compared with SR group. There have been three tested approaches for postremission therapies: (1) postremission chemotherapy modules followed by long-term maintenance chemotherapy; (2) allo-SCT; and least frequently, (3) autologous stem cell transplant (ASCT). Studies using these postremission strategies are reviewed below.

The optimal postremission strategy for SR adult patients is not clear. Conventionally, consolidation and maintenance chemotherapy has been the recommendation for this group of patients, given lower potential for toxicities and up to 40% to 60% survival at 5 years with this approach. Postremission chemotherapy typically consists of a variety of non–cross-resistant chemotherapeutic agents administered in treatment "modules" for a total of 6 to 8 months after achievement of remission. The postremission modules are typically 4 to 6 weeks in length and are modeled after successful pediatric regimens and often consist of consolidation module(s), interim maintenance modules that often focus on CNS prophylaxis (described in more detail below); and late intensification module(s), which is often quite similar to the induction chemotherapy course. The specific drugs and the sequence or combinations in which they used are different for each protocol but typically include cyclophosphamide, L-asparaginase (or pegasparaginase), methotrexate, cytarabine, 6-mercaptopurine, vincristine, and doxorubicin. Many of these protocols have evolved empirically with few randomized trials evaluating the impact of any of the modifications that have been developed (see Table 65-6).

A different approach to postremission therapy has been taken by the MD Anderson Cancer Center, which have reported long-term results of the hyper-CVAD regimen (also listed in Table 65-6). As described earlier in the induction section, patients received alternating cycles of hyperfractionated cyclophosphamide, vincristine, adriamycin, and dexamethasone hyper-CVAD (courses 1, 3, 5, and 7) alternating with high-dose methotrexate and cytarabine (courses 2, 4, 6, and 8) followed by maintenance therapy for 2 years with 6-mercaptopurine, methotrexate, vincristine, and prednisone (POMP). They identified the following factors to be independent poor prognostic factors for survival: older age, Ph^+ disease, leukocytosis, thrombocytopenia, poor performance status, and hepatomegaly. The 5-year OS for the good-risk (risk score, 0-1), intermediate risk (risk score, 2-3), and poor-risk groups (risk score, ≥4) were 62%, 34%, and 5%, respectively.

In summary, despite attempts to intensify postremission therapy with high doses of cytarabine and anthracycline, the OS rate of patients in all of the studies published in the past decade is approximately 30% to 50%, depending on risk factors and treatment approach. Notably, adults older than the age of 60 years have uniformly fared poorly with OS below 10%. Table 65-6 summarizes the major treatment questions, therapeutic approach and results of several of the recent large prospective cooperative group trials in the United States and Europe.

CENTRAL NERVOUS SYSTEM DISEASE: PROPHYLAXIS AND TREATMENT

Involvement of the CNS (Fig. 65-6) is uncommon at the time of diagnosis with most series reporting it at less than 10%. However, because many patients with CNS involvement may not be referred for clinical trial enrollment, this may be an underestimate of the true rate. In the MRC UKALL XII/ECOG E2993 trial, of the 1508 eligible patients, 77 (5%) had CNS involvement at diagnosis. Similarly, the French group reported a 7% (104 of 1493 patients) incidence of CNS disease at diagnosis. Risk factors for CNS disease at diagnosis have been varied in different studies. In the French trial (LALA-87 and LALA-94), risk factors included mediastinal mass associated with precursor T-cell immunophenotype, lymphadenopathy, higher hemoglobin level, and absence of the Philadelphia chromosome. In the MRC trial, the risk factors included a higher WBC count, precursor T-cell immunophenotype, and mediastinal mass. The presence of CNS disease at diagnosis has been shown not to affect the CR rate. The French group also reported no significant difference in the OS in patients with and without CNS disease at diagnosis. However, in the MRC trial, the OS at 5-year was lower in the CNS disease group (29% vs. 38%; $P = .03$), and they also reported that patients with CNS disease at diagnosis were twice more likely to relapse in the CNS. In the French study, younger age (<30 years), male gender, absence of the Ph chromosome, achievement of CR with one course, and use of transplant as postremission therapy had favorable impact on OS for patients presenting with CNS disease at diagnosis.

Induction therapy of ALL usually includes a lumbar puncture with introduction of intrathecal chemotherapy. For those presenting with CNS disease at diagnosis or in whom CNS disease develops later in the course of the treatment, immediate intensified CNS treatment is imperative. These patients should receive intrathecal chemotherapy (intrathecal methotrexate alone or together with cytarabine and steroid [triple intrathecal therapy]) twice-thrice weekly until clearing of cerebrospinal fluid along with initiation of systemic chemotherapy. Cranial irradiation (2400 cGy over 12 fractions) is considered necessary for the successful treatment of CNS disease with cranial nerve involvement.

Central nervous system prophylaxis is an essential component of therapy for all patients given the high incidence (30%-40%) of CNS relapse if the CNS prophylaxis is omitted. Now with the universal

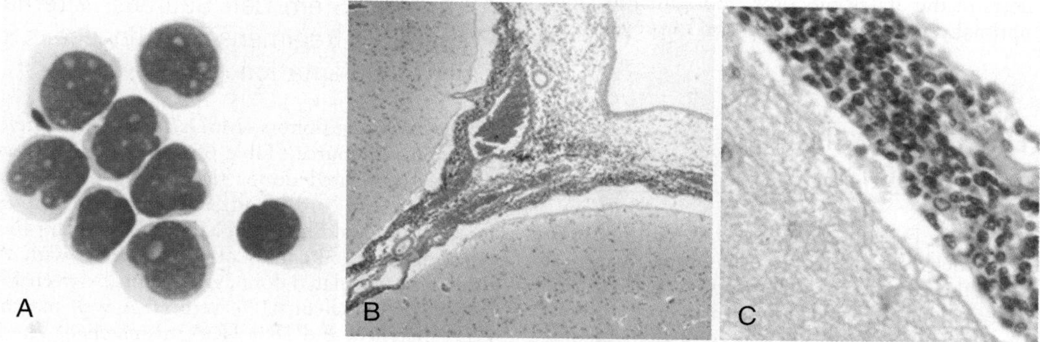

Figure 65-6 CEREBROSPINAL FLUID (CSF), AND CENTRAL NERVOUS SYSTEM DISEASE. Blasts in the CSF can be identified on a cytospin preparation. They have similar cytologic features as the blasts in the blood or bone marrow aspirate **(A)**. Histologic section of the brain is illustrated from a patient with ALL and leukemic meningitis. The sections show blasts within the leptomeninges (**B;** higher power, **C**).

adoption of CNS prophylaxis in the treatment regimens, the rates of CNS relapse have decreased substantially. CNS prophylaxis is typically administered by multiple rounds of intrathecal chemotherapy that are staggered over the entire treatment duration. In addition, the use of high-dose methotrexate and cytarabine also provides for CNS prophylaxis because both agents penetrate the blood–brain barrier. The intensive use of high-dose systemic methotrexate and frequent intrathecal therapy has often replaced the more traditional combination of CNS irradiation and intrathecal therapy that were the hallmarks of the earlier ALL regimens. This non–radiation-containing approach has resulted in effective CNS protection with rates of CNS relapse now routinely reported as occurring in fewer than 5% to 10% of cases. Adolescents and young adults (AYAs) treated on pediatric regimens with more intensive CNS prophylaxis have reported CNS relapse rates as low as 1%. The omission of cranial irradiation may prevent neurocognitive damage in adults. Although this has not been demonstrated in adult studies, definitive evidence from pediatric studies indicates that avoidance of cranial irradiation may prevent declines in cognitive function.

MAINTENANCE THERAPY

The goal of maintenance treatment is to prevent disease relapse by elimination of leukemia clones by long-term exposure to cytotoxic drugs. One of the commonly used regimens uses daily 6-mercaptopurine and weekly oral methotrexate with monthly vincristine and prednisone (POMP regimen). Some groups replaced prednisone with dexamethasone. The duration of maintenance treatment is generally 2 to 3 years (2 years for women and 3 years for men). Similar to the other components of adult ALL regimens, the adoption of long-term maintenance therapy derives from the benefit of maintenance therapy that has demonstrated in pediatric trials.

Although the benefit of maintenance therapy in adult trials has not been demonstrated in randomized trials, it has been shown that omission of maintenance treatment leads to worse clinical outcomes. In a CALGB study, 164 newly diagnosed ALL patients were randomized to receive daunorubicin or mitoxantrone during induction followed by 4 cycles of consolidation. No maintenance therapy was planned. There were significantly more relapses noted in this study with median remission duration of only 10 to 12 months. The study was stopped earlier than planned because remission duration was shorter than in historical control participants who had received maintenance therapy. Similar results were obtained by the Dutch-Belgian Haemato-Oncology Cooperative Group (HOVON), which treated 130 ALL patients with induction followed by 3 cycles of consolidation. No maintenance therapy was given. The estimated 5-year OS and DFS were only 22% and 28%, respectively. Pediatric regimens routinely incorporate CNS prophylaxis during the maintenance phase. Pediatric studies have also reported favorable impact on DFS of achieving adequate myelosuppression with the chemotherapy drugs during the maintenance phase. Thus, it appears that careful adjustment of the doses of the oral agents used during maintenance therapy to achieve optimal yet safe myelosuppression improves treatment outcomes.

ALLOGENEIC STEM CELL TRANSPLANT IN FIRST COMPLETE REMISSION

Despite attempts to improve DFS in adult ALL, OS with the standard chemotherapy regimens described above has been "fixed" at about 35% to 45% for the past decade. Thus, several groups have evaluated the role of treatment intensification with transplant (both aSCT and ASCT) as postremission therapy and compared the outcomes with the traditional chemotherapy approaches described previously. Conventionally, an aSCT has been reserved as the standard recommendation for only HR patients in CR1. In one of the earliest randomized trials to investigate the role of allogeneic transplant, the French LALA-87 study, patients in CR1 were assigned to donor group (if they had an HLA-matched related donor); the remaining patients (no-donor group) were randomized to ASCT versus chemotherapy. In this study, patients with HR ALL (defined as the presence of Philadelphia chromosome, or null leukemia [defined by a CD10- , CD20-immunophenotype], undifferentiated leukemia, or common leukemia with at least one adverse prognosis factor such as age older than 35 years, WBC count greater than 30,000/μL, or time to CR longer than 4 weeks) benefitted from aSCT. For the HR group, 5-year OS was 44% in the donor arm (n = 41), which was significantly better than the 20% in the no-donor arm (n = 55) (P = .03). The outcome of SR group was not improved with aSCT (5-year OS of 51% in the donor arm vs. 45% in the no-donor arm). Similar results were seen in a follow-up of LALA-94 trials with benefit of aSCT in HR group. In contrast, the Program Espa ol de Tratamiento en Hematologia (PETHEMA) ALL-93 trial failed to show benefit of aSCT in HR ALL patients.

In a recently published trial, the MRC UKALLXII/ECOG E2993 trial, all patients (younger than 50 years or 55 years or younger after 2003) in CR1, irrespective of risk status, were assigned to aSCT if they had an HLA-compatible sibling donor. All other patients were randomized to consolidation or maintenance therapy or to an ASCT. In this largest adult ALL trial to date, 1646 Ph-negative patients were enrolled; 1484 (90%) achieved CR1. After excluding patients who were older than 55 years old and those without available HLA typed siblings, 1031 CR1 patients (55% SR; 45% HR) were HLA typed. In a "genetic randomization" approach using donor (n = 443) versus no-donor (n = 588) analysis, OS benefit was seen for the donor arm when all patients were considered (5-year OS, 53% vs. 45%; P = .01). In a subgroup analysis, the survival benefit of transplant was restricted to patients who were younger than 35 years old. For patients older than 35 years of age or with adverse cytogenetics, OS was not better than with standard chemotherapy because of transplant-related toxicities, which resulted in early deaths.

In a report by the Dutch-Belgian HOVON group, patients younger than 50 to 55 years in CR1 were offered an aSCT. In a donor (n = 96) versus no-donor (n = 161) analysis for all patients, 5-year OS was 61% for the donor arm compared with 47% in the no-donor arm (P = .08). In subset analysis, the survival benefit of transplant was restricted to SR patients, which were those without any of the following HR features: presence of a high WBC count at diagnosis (>30,000/μL in B-ALL or >100,000/μL in T-ALL), cytogenetic abnormalities [t(4;11), t(1;19), t(9;22)], pro–B-cell immunophenotype, and CR achievement longer than 4 weeks from start of induction.

A meta-analysis of seven studies (with 1274 patients) that prospectively assessed OS using genetic randomization based on donor availability reported significantly better OS in the donor group versus the no-donor groups (hazard ratio; 1.29; P = .037), which was more pronounced in patients with HR features.

Alternative Stem Cell Sources; Alternative Preparative Regimens for Allogeneic Stem Cell Transplantation

Matched-sibling donors (MSDs) remain the preferred modality for the stem cell source (Table 65-7). For patients lacking an MSD, a matched unrelated donor (MUD) or an alternative donor source (e.g., umbilical cord blood [UCB]) should be pursued. In a Center for International Blood and Marrow Transplant Research (CIBMTR) registry study, outcomes of 169 patients with ALL in CR1 who underwent unrelated donor transplants between 1995 and 2004 were analyzed. A total of 41% were HLA well matched, 41% partially HLA matched, and 18% HLA mismatched. The majority (93%) of the patients had at least one HR feature. One-year transplant-related mortality (TRM) was high at 36%, and TRM at 5 years was 42%. The relapse rate at 5 years was 20% with 5-year DFS and OS of 38% and 39%, respectively. Factors associated with worse survival included

Table 65-7 Clinical Trials Evaluating Role of Myeloablative Allogeneic Stem Cell Transplant in Acute Lymphoblastic Leukemia

Trial	Patients (*n*)	Age in Years, Median (Range)	Conditioning Regimen/Donor	TRM	DFS/OS	Comments
GOELAL02[1]	41 (HR)	34 (15-52)	Etoposide/cyclophosphamide/TBI (12 Gy in 6 fractions) MSD	15%	DFS: 75% at 6 years; OS: 75% at 6 years	Showed improved survival with aSCT compared with ASCT
LALA 94[2]	100 (HR ALL excluding Ph+ ALL)	33 (15-55) for the entire study cohort of 922 patients	Cyclophosphamide/TBI (10 Gy as a single dose or 12 Gy in 6 fractions) MRD	18% at 3 years	3-year DFS: 47%	For high-risk ALL, aSCT was superior to an ASCT
PETHEMA-93[3]	222 HR patient underwent MSD (if available); if not, randomized to ASCT vs. chemotherapy	27 (15-50)	Cyclophosphamide/TBI (12 Gy in 6 fractions) MSD		5-year OS: 35%	No benefit of an MSD transplant for HR patients (compared with ASCT or chemotherapy only approach)
MRC UKALLXII/ ECOG E2993[4]	Patients assigned to aSCT if an MSD available (donor group); those without donors randomized to ASCT vs. chemotherapy	15-64	Etoposide/TBI (13.2 Gy in 6 fractions) MSD	NRM High risk (36% donor; 14% no-donor); Standard risk (20% donor; 7% no donor)	5-year OS: HR (41% donor, 35% no donor) SR (62% donor vs. 52% donor)	Beneficial effect of all-SCT limited to SR group only; relapse rate decreased with aSCT in both HR and SR groups
HOVON[5]	ALL in CR1 according to sibling donor vs. no-donor comparison HR: 46 donor; 73 no donor SR: 50 donor; 88 no donor	Donor 31 (16-55)	Cyclophosphamide/TBI (12 Gy in 6 fractions) MRD	HR: NRM at 5 years (15% donor vs. 4% no-donor) SR: NRN at 5 years (16% donor vs. 2% no-donor, $P = 0.01$)	HR: OS at 5 years (53% donor vs. 41% no donor) SR: OS at 5 years (69% donor vs. 49% no donor, $P = .05$)	Similar to the MRC UKALLXII/ ECOG E2993 trial, benefit of aSCT seems limited to SR patients

ALL, Acute lymphoblastic leukemia; *aSCT,* allogeneic stem cell transplantation; *ASCT,* autologous stem cell transplantation; *CR1,* first complete remission; *DFS,* disease-free survival; *HR,* high risk; *MRD,* minimal residual disease; *MSD,* matched-sibling donor; *OS,* overall survival; *SCT,* stem cell transplantation; *SR,* standard risk; *TBI,* total-body irradiation; *TRM,* transplant-related mortality.

WBC greater than 100 × 10^9/L, time to CR1 longer than 8 weeks, cytomegalovirus seropositivity, HLA mismatching, and T-cell depletion. The Minnesota group recently reported outcomes of myeloablative aSCT for ALL patients transplanted at their center and compared retrospectively the outcomes with respect to different donor sources. In an analysis restricted to 91 adult patients who received aSCT in CR1or CR2 from 1990 to 2005, there was no difference between the allogeneic donor sources (matched related donor vs. matched URD vs. UCB donor) for OS, DFS, or TRM.

Because the majority of older adults are not candidates for a myeloablative aSCT, reduced-intensity conditioning (RIC) approaches have been explored in this patient population (Table 65-8). The Seattle group recently reported outcomes of aSCT using nonmyeloablative conditioning in 51 patients with ALL (median age, 56 years), half of whom were Ph positive. For the Ph-negative group, the 3-year OS for those transplanted in CR1 was 52%. The incidence of chronic graft-versus-host disease, however, was high at 44%. A recent registry study examined the efficacy of RIC in 93 ALL patients and compared it with 1428 ALL patients receiving myeloablative conditioning for aSCT using either a sibling or unrelated donor in CR1/CR2. Interestingly, the TRM at 3 years was similar between the RIC and myeloablative regimens (32% vs. 33%, respectively). The relapse rate at 3 years was slightly higher in the RIC arm, although this was not statistically significant (35% vs. 26%; $P = .08$). The OS at 3 years was similar between the two groups (38% for RIC arm vs. 43% for myeloablative arm, $P = .39$). This was a retrospective registry study; however, it provides evidence that RIC regimens can lead to similar survival in adults with ALL as aSCT with a more intensive, myeloablative conditioning regimen. This is particularly compelling because the median age was significantly older for those receiving RIC (median age in RIC arm, 45 years vs. 28 years for myeloablative arm). The group from Minnesota has also reported encouraging results with the of UCB donor transplantation using a RIC regimen. Eighteen adults (median age, 49 years; range, 24-68 years) with high-risk ALL (majority Ph^+ ALL) received a with a cord blood transplant using a RIC conditioning regimen and reported 3-year OS, TRM, and relapse rates of 49%, 28%, and 33%, respectively. Notably, patients in CR1 had a TRM of only 8% with no events after 6 months. These results with UCB donor transplantation are promising and compare favorably to conventional aSCT with relatively low TRM in this high-risk population. Thus, RIC-based aSCT regimens with alternative donor sources should be considered for older adults in prospective clinical trials.

In summary, aSCT is a curative option for patients with ALL and can be considered the standard recommendation for patients with a good performance status but with adverse disease risk factors in CR1. There have been significant improvements in transplantation techniques (better supportive care, refinement of preparative regimens, uses of alternative donors as a source of stem cells) that are resulting in greater availability and improved transplant outcomes. At the same time, the TRM and mortality are significant, and aSCT has largely been offered only to patients younger than 60 years of age because of the poor tolerance of older adults to standard myeloablative transplant preparative regimens. Prospective incorporation of MRD evaluation may refine the ability to risk stratify patients who are at high risk of relapse and might benefit from aSCT in CR1. However, the benefit of a SCT for MRD-positive patients remains to be proven and has only been studied prospectively in a single study to date. Conversely, patients who were MRD negative in CR1 may best be treated by chemotherapy alone. Overall, the role of aSCT in CR1 merits further study, and it is important to refer these patients to clinical trials exploring such approaches.

Table 65-8 Clinical Trials Evaluating Role of Reduced-Intensity Conditioning Allogeneic Stem Cell Transplant in Acute Lymphoblastic Leukemia

Trial	Number of Patients	Age in Years, Median (Range)	Conditioning Regimen/Donor	Mortality	DFS/OS	Comments
Arnold[1]	22 (11 Ph^+)	38 (21-58)	Fludarabine/busulfan +/– ATG MSD or MUD	TRM: 45%	Median survival: 354 days	High TRM of the group; all patients with aGVHD had CR indicating toward GVL effect
Martino[2]	27 (11 Ph^+)	50 (18-63)	Fludarabine/melphalan (most cases) MSD or MUD	2-year TRM: 23%	2-year OS: 31%	100-day acute grade II-IV GVHD: 48%; cGVHD 72% (extensive in 39%)
Hamaki[3]	33 (14 Ph^+)	55 (17-68)	Different RIC regimens MSD or MUD	TRM: 27%	1-year OS: 39.6%	Grade II-IV aGVHD: 45%; cGVHD: 64%
Mohty[4]	97 (37 Ph^+)	38 (17-65)	Different RIC regimens MSD or MUD	NRM: 28% (for those transplanted in CR1: 18%)	2-year OS: 31% (for those transplanted in CR1: 52%)	Three factors associated with improved OS:CR1 at time of transplant, chronic GVHD, and woman donor
Stein[5]	24 (10 Ph^+)	47.5 (23-68)	Fludarabine/melphalan MSD or MUD	NRM at 2 years: 21.5%	OS at 2-years: 61.5%	75% aGVHD (62% grade II-IV aGVHD) 86% cGVHD (62% extensive)
Bachanova[6]	22 (14 Ph^+)	49 (24-68)	Fludarabine/cyclophosphamide/ TBI 200 cGy MRD ($n = 4$) or umbilical cord blood donor graft ($n = 18$)	TRM at 3 years: 27%	OS at 3 years: 50% (For CR1: 81%)	3-year OS for those in CR1 81% vs. 15% for those in CR2 or more ($P < .01$). For CR1: 8% TRM
Ram[7]	51 (25 Ph^+)	56 (8-69)	Fludarabine/TBI 200 cGy MSD or MUD	NRM at 3 years: 28%	OS at 3-years: 34%	Grade II-IV aGVHD: 53% Chronic extensive GVHD: 42%

aGVHD, Acute graft-versus-host disease; *ATG,* anti-thymocyte globulin; *CR1,* first complete remission; *CR2,* second complete remission; *DFS,* disease-free survival; *GVHD,* graft-versus-host disease; *GVL,* graft-versus-leukemia; *MSD,* matched-sibling donor; *MUD,* matched unrelated donor; *NRM,* non-relapse mortality; *OS,* overall survival; *RIC,* reduced-intensity conditioning; *TBI,* total-body irradiation; *TRM,* transplant-related mortality.

Autologous Stem Cell Transplantation

ASCT in CR1 has also been studied prospectively in several clinical trials. Dhedin and colleagues reviewed the data from the French LALA 85, 87, and 94 trials and compared the outcomes of patients in CR1 who were randomized to chemotherapy versus ASCT. There was no improvement in DFS or OS with the use of ASCT compared with postremission chemotherapy, but there was a lower incidence of relapse at 10 years (66% vs. 78%; $P = .05$). In the MRC UKALLXII/ECOG E2993 trial, 456 patients were randomized to chemotherapy versus ASCT in CR1. Patients randomized to chemotherapy had significantly better 5-year EFS (41% vs. 32%; $P = .02$); and OS (46% vs. 37%; $P = .03$). Thus, outside of a clinical trial, an ASCT cannot be recommended for ALL patients.

THERAPY FOR SPECIFIC DISEASE SUBSETS

Philadelphia Chromosome Positive Acute Lymphoblastic Leukemia

The Philadelphia chromosome [t(9;22)(q34;q11)], is the most common cytogenetic abnormality in adult ALL, and its incidence increases with age. Among patients older than 60 years old, 40% to 50% have the Philadelphia chromosome. Before the introduction of molecularly targeted therapy, Ph$^+$ ALL was associated with lower remission rates and a very poor prognosis with a median survival time of only approximately 9 months.

With the introduction of therapy using ABL-TKIs targeted to the aberrant BCR-ABL protein, the outcome of Ph$^+$ ALL has improved substantially and has been the major treatment advance for adults with ALL in the past 2 decades. Imatinib, the first targeted TKI developed for use in Ph$^+$ leukemias, has been combined with combination chemotherapy by various groups and this has substantially improved both CR rates and DFS (Table 65-9).

The MD Anderson was the first to report on the combination of imatinib with chemotherapy (hyper-CVAD). They used imatinib 600 mg/day on days 1 to 14 of induction, 600 mg continuously during courses 2 to 8 chemotherapy cycles, 800 mg during 2 years of maintenance therapy with monthly vincristine and prednisone, and then imatinib indefinitely. Thomas and colleagues recently reported long-term results of the Hyper-CVAD–Imatinib trial. The 3-year CR duration and OS rates were significantly superior in the hyper-CVAD–imatinib arm compared with historical control participants treated with hyper-CVAD alone (68% vs. 24% and 54% vs. 15%, respectively; $P < .001$). The Japanese have also reported impressive improvements compared to their control participants. In the JALSG ALL202 trial, imatinib, 600 mg/day, was added to standard induction followed by alternating cycles of high-dose methotrexate and high-dose cytarabine and imatinib 600 mg/day. Later maintenance therapy with imatinib 600 mg/day with monthly vincristine and prednisone was given. In a recent update, they reported results on 103 patients with Ph$^+$ ALL with a 97% CR rate and 3-year OS of 57%, both of which were significantly better than in historical control participants.

Older adults with Ph$^+$ ALL have also demonstrated improved survival with the addition of imatinib to chemotherapy regimens. Ottmann and colleagues reported for the German study group in which elderly (older than 55 years old) Ph$^+$ ALL patients were randomized to receive induction cycle with imatinib alone ($n = 28$) versus combination chemotherapy ($n = 27$). The CR rate was 96% in the imatinib arm, which was significantly better than the CR rate of 50% in the chemotherapy alone arm. This is the first prospective randomized controlled trial comparing imatinib with chemotherapy and clearly showed the superiority of the imatinib arm. There was no difference in the two arms with respect to DFS and OS, likely from the fact that all patients received imatinib-based consolidation or maintenance therapy. The Italian GIMEMA group treated 30 Ph$^+$ ALL patients (median age, 69 years; range, 61-83 years) with 7-day steroid pretreatment followed by induction treatment with only imatinib (800 mg/day) plus steroids. Impressively, all 29 evaluable patients achieved CR with 1-year DFS and OS of 48% and 74%.

There is general consensus that early TKI therapy is crucial, and most current treatment protocols include chemotherapy with continuous TKI therapy. In general, the TKI has been started with induction chemotherapy and continues throughout postremission therapy. However, Bassan and colleagues reported on 59 patients with Ph$^+$ ALL (NILG 09/00) in whom imatinib (600 mg/day) was added to each chemotherapy course for only 7 days, starting 3 days before chemotherapy, based on the hypothesis that imatinib would sensitize Ph$^+$ ALL cells to standard chemotherapy drugs. They reported a 92% CR rate with a 5-year OS of 38%.

Despite these significant advances in the treatment of Ph$^+$ ALL, relapses are still major challenges. Resistance to imatinib develops and most frequently results from the emergence of a resistant clone with ABL kinase domain mutations. These kinase domain mutations, including the frequently occurring T315I mutation, cause conformational changes in the ABL protein that prevent effective imatinib binding. Other potential mechanisms of resistance that have been described include reduced intracellular availability of imatinib and activation of alternative signaling pathways such as the Src-kinase pathways. Second-generation TKIs, dasatinib and nilotinib, are more potent kinase inhibitors and are also effective against many imatinib-resistant mutations (although not the T315I mutation). In addition, dasatinib has been shown to penetrate the CNS and thus may be particularly effective for ALL therapy.

Dasatinib has now been tested in several prospective trials for previously untreated Ph$^+$ ALL. MD Anderson investigators evaluated hyper-CVAD plus dasatinib in newly diagnosed Ph$^+$ ALL patients. Dasatinib, 100 mg/day, was given for the first 14 days of each of 8 cycles of alternating hyper-CVAD and high-dose cytarabine and methotrexate. Maintenance chemotherapy consisted of daily dasatinib 100 mg/day with monthly vincristine and prednisone for 2 years followed by dasatinib indefinitely. The median age of the 35 patients studied was 53 years (range, 21-79 years); 94% achieved CR. Of the patients who achieved CR, 61% patients achieved complete molecular remission, meaning that there was no detectable MRD using quantitative PCR for *BCR-ABL*. In a recent update to the hyper-CVAD and dasatinib study, the MD Anderson group reported that 24% patients underwent aSCT (16% in CR1; 8% CR2), and 3-year DFS and OS for the entire cohort were 49% and 62%, respectively. Foa and colleagues recently reported the results of the GIMEMA LAL1205 study in which dasatinib monotherapy (70 mg twice daily) with steroids was investigated for frontline treatment of 53 adult Ph$^+$ ALL patients (median age, 54 years). All patients achieved a complete hematologic response (CHR), and there were no induction deaths. BCR-ABL transcript levels decreased rapidly during induction therapy, and the percentage of patients achieving BCR-ABL levels below 0.001% increased from 23% at day 22 to 52% at day 85. Allo-SCT in CR1 was done in 18 (34%) patients. At 20 months, the OS was 69% and DFS was 51%. BCR-ABL levels of less than 0.001% at day 85 correlated with DFS. These results with dasatinib without any cytotoxic chemotherapy are encouraging but demonstrated that single-agent dasatinib is not sufficient to cure this disease.

Nilotinib is also a second-generation TKI that that has been evaluated in frontline therapy in a recently reported single-arm phase 2 study. Induction treatment consisted of vincristine, daunorubicin, oral prednisolone, and nilotinib (400 mg orallytwice daily). Patients in CR received either five courses of consolidation followed by 2-year maintenance therapy or an aSCT, depending on donor availability. Nilotinib was administered from day 8 of induction continuously until the end of maintenance or aSCT. Fifty consecutive patients were enrolled; 5 patients died during induction, and the remaining 45 (90%) patients achieved hematologic remission. More than 70% patients were able to receive aSCT. Estimated DFS and OS at 2 years were 71% and 66%, respectively, similar to rates observed with other

Table 65-9 Clinical Trials With Tyrosine Kinase Inhibitor Plus Chemotherapy for Adult Philadelphia Chromosome–Positive Acute Lymphoblastic Leukemia

Trial	Patients (*n*)	Age in Years, Median (Range)	CR Rate	Disease-Free Survival	Overall Survival	Comments
MDACC Hyper-CVAD Imatinib[1,2]	54	51 (17-84)	93%	68% at 3 years	In de novo patients 40 years of age or younger: 3-year OS was 90% with aSCT (n = 10) vs. 33% without aSCT (n = 6), P = .05.	First report of the combination of chemotherapy with a TKI Imatinib 600 mg/day on days 1-14 of induction; 600 mg continuously during courses 2-8; 800 mg during 2 years of maintenance therapy with monthly vincristine–prednisone; then imatinib indefinitely; allo-SCT in CR1 as feasible
JALSG ALL202[3-5]	103	45 (15-64)	97%	For those younger than age 55 years, 54 of 74 patients in CR1 who had aSCT, only 13% relapsed; among the 20/74 patients in CR1 who did not undergo SCT, 90% relapsed	57% at 3 years For patients younger than age 55 years, OS at 3 years was 75.0% for the transplanted group vs. 36.4% for the nontransplanted group	Standard induction plus imatinib 600 mg/day followed by alternating cycles of high-dose methotrexate and high-dose cytarabine and imatinib 600 mg/day; imatinib 600 mg/day with monthly vincristine–prednisone for maintenance
GRAAPH-2003[6,7]	45	45(16-59)	96%	43% at 4 years	52% at 4 years The 4-year OS in the aSCT, ASCT, and no SCT groups were 55%, 80%, and 25%, respectively	Imatinib was started with consolidation in good early responders (corticosensitive and chemosensitive ALL) or during the induction course in poor early responders
GMALL[8]	47 (alternating imatinib and chemotherapy)	46 (21-65)	NA because only CR patients were eligible	52% at 2 years	36% at 2 years	Coadministration of imatinib with induction cycle 2 led to CR rate of 95% and molecular CR rate of 52% of patients compared with 19% (significantly worse) in patients in the alternating treatment cohort
	45 (concurrent imatinib and chemotherapy starting after induction I)	41 (19-63)	95%	61% at 2 years	43% at 2 years	
GMALL[9]	28 (imatinib arm) 27 (chemotherapy arm)	66 (54-79) 68 (58-78)	96% 50% (significantly inferior to imatinib arm)	30% at 1.5 years 35% at 1.5 years	57% at 1.5 years 41% at 1.5 years	Patients older than age 55 years with de novo ALL and not eligible for aSCT; randomized to single-agent imatinib induction vs. multi-agent chemotherapy induction; subsequent consolidation or maintenance with imatinib plus chemotherapy for all patients
GIMEMA[10]	29	69 (61-83)	100%	48% at 1 year	74% at 1 year	7-day steroid pretreatment followed by induction treatment with imatinib (800 mg/day) plus steroids
NILG protocol 09/00[11]	59	45 (20-66)	92%	39% at 5 years	38% at 5 years	Imatinib (600 mg/day) was added to each chemotherapy course for 7 days starting 3 days before chemotherapy
UKALLXII/ ECOG2993[12]	175	Not reported	92%	54% at 3 years	42% at 3 years	Outcomes (CR, DFS, and OS) were significantly better compared with the historical pre-imatinib cohort; for the imatinib group, 3-year OS for patients who received aSCT was 59% vs. 28% for those who did not receive aSCT

ALL, Acute lymphoblastic leukemia; *aSCT*, allogenic stem cell transplantation; *ASCT*, autologous stem cell transplantation; *CR*, complete remission; *CR1*, first complete remission; *DFS*, disease-free survival; *NA*, not applicable; *OS*, overall survival; *SCT*, stem cell transplantation.

TKIs. Although these results are similar to other studies with dasatinib, most of the current trials in Ph⁺ ALL have incorporated dasatinib in the frontline therapy because of its potential advantage over nilotinib with respect to CNS penetration.

Role of Allogeneic Stem Cell Transplantation for Ph⁺ Acute Lymphoblastic Leukemia in the Era of Tyrosine Kinase Inhibitor–Based Therapy

Allo-SCT in CR1 has been the standard recommendation for Ph⁺ ALL in the pre-TKI era. Although the addition of TKI therapy has significantly improved the outcome of Ph⁺ ALL, many recent studies have also highlighted the continued role of aSCT for Ph⁺ ALL. In an update of the hyper-CVAD-imatinib protocol, the MD Anderson group reported that in a subgroup of patients younger than 40 years old, the 3-year OS was 90% with an aSCT compared with 33% without aSCT ($P = .05$). In the Japanese study, aSCT was performed in the CR1 in 54 of the 74 CR1 patients younger than 55 years of age. Relapse occurred in 13% (7 of 54) of the transplanted patients compared with 90% (18 of 20) in those who were not transplanted. Similarly, OS at 3 years was 75% for the transplanted group versus 36% for the nontransplanted group.

Similar results have been reported in preliminary form, by the MRC UKALLXII/ECOG E2993 trial group. In this study, 175 Ph⁺ ALL patients received imatinib plus chemotherapy (2003 onward). The authors reported that 44% of the patients were able to receive an aSCT per protocol, a number much higher than the 28% who were able to receive aSCT in the pre-imatinib era of this study (1993-2003). For the imatinib cohort, the 3-year OS for patients who received per protocol aSCT was 59% versus 28% for those who did not receive aSCT. In a recent update of the GMALL study, 219 of 335 (66%) Ph⁺ ALL patients treated with an imatinib-based chemotherapy regimen underwent aSCT in CR1. For the transplanted patients, the median OS was 57% after 3 years and 52% after 7 years compared with the dismal outcome of the nontransplanted group (3-year OS of only 14%). These studies provide a strong rationale for the continued recommendation for an aSCT in CR1 for Ph⁺ ALL patients.

The role and duration of TKI therapy after transplant is currently an area of active investigation. Wassmann and colleagues treated 27 Ph⁺ ALL patients with imatinib upon detection of MRD after SCT. Approximately 50% of patients achieved a molecular remission after a median of 1.5 months and these patients had a significantly longer time to progression (28.6 months vs. 3.6 months; $P < .001$) and OS (2-year OS, 80% vs. 23%; $P < .001$) compared with those who had persistent *BCR-ABL* transcript levels. The German group also reported results of a randomized study comparing prophylactic ($n = 26$) versus preemptive (after detection of bcr-abl transcripts, $n = 29$) imatinib after aSCT for Ph⁺ ALL. Imatinib was discontinued early in more than half the patients in both groups, mostly because of gastrointestinal toxicity. Prophylactic administration of imatinib significantly reduced the incidence of molecular relapse after the aSCT. The OS was similar in the two arms (5-year OS, 75%-80%). At the present time, it appears that continuing TKI therapy after transplant is an appropriate strategy. Studies evaluating MRD may provide guidance with the question of duration of posttransplant TKI therapy.

Newer TKIs such as ponatinib have shown promising activity in TKI-resistant Ph⁺ ALL and are discussed in the section Novel Therapies.

BURKITT LYMPHOMA/LEUKEMIA

Burkitt lymphoma is a mature B-cell lymphoma with an extremely short doubling time that often presents in extranodal sites or as acute leukemia. Thus, a brief description of the therapy is warranted in this chapter. Morphologically (Fig. 65-7), the malignant cells are intermediate in size, have round nuclei with small nucleoli, are intensely basophilic, and frequently have vacuolated cytoplasms. In BM biopsy and in tissue section, the tumor is classically described as having a "starry sky" appearance because of the presence of multiple tingible body macrophages with phagocytized cellular debris. Immunophenotypically, the tumor cells express moderate to strong levels of surface IgM with light chain restriction, indicating origin of the tumor from a mature B cell. The tumor cells also universally express the B-cell antigens CD19 and CD20 and germinal center associated markers such as CD10 and BCL6. Unlike B-ALL, BL cells do not express CD34 or TdT. The genetic basis of the disease is the underlying MYC translocation at band 8q24 to either the immunoglobulin heavy chain region on chromosome 14 or less commonly at the lambda (22q11) or kappa (2p12) loci.

Prompt diagnosis and recognition of this entity is essential because this is now highly curable leukemia (in the range of 65%-80% in recent trials); however, failure to institute appropriate therapy at diagnosis for Burkitt leukemia/lymphoma results in emergence of early resistance and dismal outcomes. Traditional CHOP (cyclophosphamide, hydroxydaunomycin, vincristine [Oncovin], and prednisone) chemotherapy is inadequate and should not be used. Treatment should be initiated quickly and consists of aggressive combination chemotherapy with CNS prophylaxis. These patients are at high risk for the development of tumor lysis syndrome; therefore, aggressive hydration and administration of allopurinol and/or rasburicase is important. All current regimens rely on short intensive courses of chemotherapy that incorporates fractionated doses of alkylating agents, high doses of methotrexate and cytarabine, and intensive

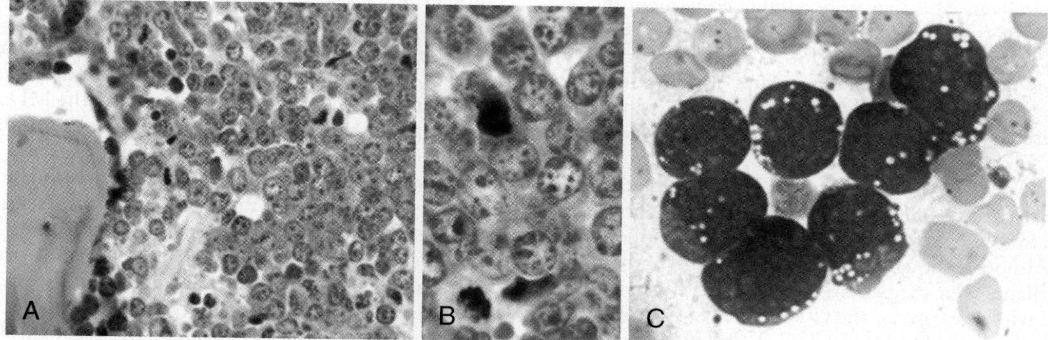

Figure 65-7 BURKITT LEUKEMIA/LYMPHOMA (**A** to **C**). Bone marrow biopsy and aspirate features of Burkitt leukemia/lymphoma are illustrated. The bone marrow (or lymph node) will show sheets of highly proliferating intermediate-sized neoplastic cells with a syncytial appearance. The cells are monotonous but have a stippled intermediate chromatin pattern with multiple small nucleoli. On the aspirate (**C**), the Burkitt cells have an intermediate size, a denser chromatin than lymphoblasts, and deeply blue cytoplasm with prominent vacuoles.

intrathecal prophylaxis. In the United States, commonly used regimens include CODOX-M/IVAC, CALGB 9251, and hyper-CVAD. With these regimens, approximately 80% achieve CR, and 2-year survival is around 60% to 70%. In the CALGB 9251 trial, 52% of the patients were alive and in continuous CR at a median follow-up of 5.1 years. Because Burkitt lymphoma/leukemia has a predisposition for CNS involvement, aggressive CNS-directed therapy is essential and typically consists of intrathecal administration of methotrexate, cytarabine, and hydrocortisone. Recurrence after the first 2 years rarely occurs; therefore, maintenance therapy has not been shown to be beneficial and is not recommended.

Because of the strong expression of CD20 in mature B-cell ALL, several groups have incorporated rituximab into the frontline chemotherapy regimen with impressive further improvements in survival. The hyper-CVAD–rituximab regimen was reported in 31 patients with newly diagnosed Burkitt lymphoma/leukemia with a CR rate of 86% and a 3-year survival rate of 89%. Similarly, the addition of rituximab to the treatment in both the GMALL and CALGB regimens has proven feasible with OS of 91% (3 years) and 79% (2 years), respectively. Based on these exciting improvements in survival, the addition of anti-CD20 targeting to frontline therapies for BL is now considered the standard of care.

ADOLESCENTS AND YOUNG ADULTS WITH ALL: THE INTERSECTION BETWEEN PEDIATRIC AND ADULT ONCOLOGY

Evaluation of the outcomes of young adult patients, here defined as patients between the ages of 15 and 21 years old, presents specific challenges. Because of community referral patterns, these patients may be treated by either pediatric or adult oncologists. As such, the treating physician may view a patient in this age group either as an older child or as a younger adult. The oncologist will choose a regimen most appropriate for the population usually seen by that particular physician. A number of comparisons of the clinical outcome of adolescents enrolled on adult and pediatric clinical trials (Table 65-10) have resulted in interesting observations about what that appropriate treatment regimen should be and have guided the design of a number of prospective clinical trials designed specifically for AYAs with ALL.

Retrospective Comparison of Pediatric and Adult Cooperative Group Trials in Adolescents and Young Adults

The retrospective comparisons summarized in Table 65-10 were performed by large cooperative groups throughout the world and examined the outcome of the AYA patients treated on pediatric or adult cooperative group trials in ALL that were conducted contemporaneously. The majority of these retrospective comparison studies demonstrated a significant survival advantage for AYA patients treated by the pediatric versus the adult cooperative group. The first of these trials to have been reported highlights many of the interesting questions posed by these comparisons and is reviewed briefly below. The CALGB and the Children's Cancer Group (CCG) examined the outcome of 321 AYA patients between 16 and 20 years of age treated on consecutive trials from 1988 to 2001. The two patient groups were well matched for biologic features, including immunophenotype and cytogenetics. Although the age range was the same in both groups examined, the median age of the patients in the CALGB studies was 19 years compared with 16 years for the CCG patients. CR rates were identical—90% for both CALGB and CCG AYAs. However, CCG AYAs had a 63% EFS at 7 years and 67% OS at 7 years in contrast to the CALGB AYAs, in which 7-year EFS was only 34%. A difference in pattern of relapse was also noted. The incidence of CNS relapses was significantly higher in CALGB AYAs (11%) compared with the CCG AYAs (1.4%) ($P < .001$).

Table 65-10 Retrospective Comparison of Trials Involving Adolescent and Young Adult Acute Lymphoblastic Leukemia Patients

Trial Comparison	AYA Patients/ Median Age (Years)	CR Rate (%)	Survival Rate
United States			(7-year OS)
CALGB (adult)	124/19	90	46%
CCG (pediatric)	197/16	90	67%
France			(5-year EFS)
LALA-94 (adult)	100/18	83	41%
FRALLE-93 (pediatric)	77/16	94	67%
The Netherlands			(5-year EFS)
HOVON (adult)	73/20	91	38%
DCOG (pediatric)	47/12	98	71%
Italy			(2-year OS)
GIMEMA (adult)	95/16	89	71%
AIEOP (pediatric)	150/15	94	80%
United Kingdom			(5-year OS)
UKALLXII/E2993 (adult)	67/15-17	94	56%
ALL97 (Pediatric)	61/NA	98	71%
Sweden			(5-year OS)
Adult ALL Group (adult)	99/18	90	39%
NOPHO-92 (pediatric)	36/16	99	74%
Finland			(5-year OS)
Finnish Leukemia (adult)	97/19	97	60%
NOPHO (pediatric)	128/13	96	67%

ALL, Acute lymphoblastic leukemia; *AYA*, adolescent and young adult; *CR*, complete remission; *EFS*, event-free survival; *NA*, not applicable; *OS*, overall survival.

Since the initial report of these findings in 2000, multiple national European cooperative groups have reported similar results with improvement in the outcome of AYAs treated on pediatric compared with adult protocols, and these are summarized in Table 65-10. Although the treatment approaches differ among countries, several treatment themes have emerged as being potentially important. Pediatric studies throughout the world use considerably more treatment with nonmyelosuppressive drugs, including glucocorticoids (both dexamethasone and prednisone), vincristine, and L-asparaginase. CNS prophylaxis is typically administered earlier, with a greater frequency and for a more prolonged period during pediatric group trials. Finally, long-term maintenance therapy was also continued for a longer period in pediatric cooperative group trials. Based on additional retrospective data from Finland and the MD Anderson Cancer Center, it appears that treating patients in a uniform fashion by an experienced group of physicians and nurses is also a very important component in the successful treatment of young adults with ALL.

To begin to address the many unanswered questions that have been raised by the retrospective comparison trials and to determine whether AYA patients treated by adult hematologists and oncologists can achieve similarly improved outcomes to the pediatricians for this age group, prospective cooperative group trials are being conducted in North America and in Europe. Early results from several of these trials have recently been reported. The PETHEMA Protocol ALL-96 addressed the toxicity and results of a pediatric-based protocol in 35 adolescent (ages 15-18 years) and 46 young adults (ages 19-30 years) with SR ALL. In this trial, patients received a standard five-drug, 5-week induction course followed by two cycles of early consolidation, maintenance with monthly reinforcement cycles for 1 year after remission, and standard maintenance chemotherapy for up to 2 years after CR. The AYAs were well-matched for pretreatment characteristics. The CR rate was 98%, and with median follow-up of 4.2 years, the 6-year EFS and OS were 61% and 69%, respectively. The only significant predictor of poor EFS for the entire group was a slow response to initial induction therapy (>10% blasts remaining in BM aspirate done on day 14 of induction therapy). Thus, the investigators concluded that a pediatric regimen was tolerable and efficacious in AYAs with ALL up to the age of 30 years.

Two pilot studies from French adult cooperative groups have also demonstrated the feasibility of using modified pediatric-inspired regimens in adults with ALL, but the age range of these studies extends well into the middle years of adult life. In the French Acute Lymphoblastic Leukemia Pediatric group (FRALLE) study, 28 Ph$^-$ adult ALL patients 16 to 57 years old were treated on the FRALLE 2000 protocol consisting of a prednisone prophase, four-drug induction including L-asparaginase, consolidation, delayed intensification, and maintenance chemotherapy. Four-year DFS was 90% versus 47% seen in matched historical control participants. In the Group for Research in Adult Acute Lymphoblastic Leukemia (GRAALL)- 2003 study, 225 patients with Ph$^-$ ALL 15 to 60 years old (median, 31 years) were treated between 2003 and 2005 with five-drug induction, dose-intense consolidation, delayed intensification, and 2-year maintenance therapy. Notably, aSCT for patients younger than 55 years was recommended in this trial and makes interpretation of this trial more problematic. The CR rate was 93.5%. Among the 139 CR patients, 71 actually underwent transplantation in CR1 and were censored at the time of transplant. At 42 months, EFS was 55% versus 41% when comparing patients from an earlier French trial, the LALA-94, and the OS was 61%, significantly better than 41% the OS in the LALA-94 ($P < .001$). The benefit of the GRAALL approach was not statistically significant in patients older than 45 years of age because of a significant increase in treatment-related mortality of 23% compared with 5% TRM for patients younger than 45 years old. The investigators concluded that the use of a pediatric inspired regimen in adults up to 45 years old was tolerable and markedly improved outcome for "younger" adults with ALL. This regimen included older adults up to the age of 60 years and used only a modified pediatric regimen that did not use the dose intensity of corticosteroids, asparaginase, and vincristine that are routinely used in current pediatric regimens. Another difference from the pediatric regimens is that all patients in these trials still received prophylactic cranial irradiation. Also, the majority of CR1 patients actually underwent aSCT, which is not the approach used by pediatric groups. Thus, any interpretation of the contribution of the "chemotherapy" intensification component of these trials to DFS is very difficult. The Dana-Farber Cancer Institute consortium has also extended its successful pediatric regimen to older patients 18 to 50 years old. The trial design here was a true pediatric approach with intensification of *Escherichia coli* L-asparaginase, glucocorticoids, and vincristine for patients up to 50 years old; aSCT was not routinely recommended. Early results from this completed phase II trial have recently been presented. Ninety-four patients were evaluable, with a median age of 28 years (range, 18-50). Seventy-nine patients (84%) achieved a CR after 1 month of intensive induction therapy. With a median follow-up time of 45 months, the group reports an estimated DFS rate for all patients of 66% and OS rate of 65%. For the 74 patients with Ph$^-$ ALL, DFS was 70%, and OS was 68%.

The largest prospective trial to evaluate the feasibility of using a pediatric regimen in AYA patients treated by adult medical hematologists and oncologists is ongoing in North America (CALGB-10403). The U.S. adult and pediatric cooperative groups are currently enrolling a total of 300 young adults 16 to 39 years old on a prospective phase II trial (CALGB-10403) that uses one treatment arm of a successful Children's Oncology Group (COG) protocol for adolescents (and HR children with ALL).

These prospective trials are demonstrating that it is possible to achieve significant improvements in outcome for AYAs with ALL, although many challenges remain to ensure access to care, to minimize treatment toxicity, and to develop and follow specific survivorship monitoring plans. The next generation of studies, linked to important biologic, psychosocial, and pharmacologic correlates, will result in further insights into optimizing the comprehensive approach to treatment and follow-up for this significant group of patients with ALL and may be the next step to achieving the high cure rate and successful transition back to "normal" life now routinely achieved in children with ALL. One of the other important issues that is beginning to be addressed in prospective trials is if these pediatric regimens can improve outcome for young adults, up to what age can this type of therapy be safely and successfully delivered?

OLDER ADULTS WITH ACUTE LYMPHOBLASTIC LEUKEMIA

Older adults (generally defined as older than 60 years old) constitute a challenging subset of ALL patients with worse prognosis reported in many studies compared with their younger counterparts. Most studies demonstrate that adults older than 60 years old have survival rates below 15%. Various factors contribute to the poor outcome of these patients, both patient related (e.g., the presence of comorbidities, less likely to be eligible for aSCT, poor tolerance of intensive chemotherapies) and disease related (more likely to have unfavorable disease characteristics such as the presence of Philadelphia chromosome). It is important to note that many large clinical trials have excluded patients older than 60 years of age; therefore, clinical outcome data for this group are sparse. Annino and colleagues reviewed results of 679 elderly patients (variably defined as older than 50 to older than 65 years of age, depending on the study) from 19 studies and reported a CR rate of 59% (range, 31%-85%) with an early mortality rate of 23% (range, 7.5%-50%) and 2-year OS of 15% to 19%, all of which are inferior to younger ALL patients. With hyper-CVAD regimens, the CR rate and 3-year survival for patients 60 years old or older ($n = 58$) were 88% and 29%, respectively. In a pooled analysis of six consecutive CALGB clinical trials, the CR rate and 3-year survival for patients 60 years old or older ($n = 197$) were 61% and 15%, respectively.

Sancho and colleagues reported results of the Spanish PETHEMA-ALL 96 trial looking specifically at the outcomes of Ph$^-$ ALL patients who were 55 years of age or older. They initially treated 10 patients with an induction regimen consisting of vincristine, daunorubicin, prednisone, asparaginase, and cyclophosphamide. However, 7 of the 10 patients died during induction. Asparaginase and cyclophosphamide were then omitted from the induction cycle, and 23 additional patients were treated with a CR rate of 70%; the induction death rate was reduced to 22%. The 2-year DFS and OS for the entire series were 46% and 39%, respectively.

Because most patients in this age group may not be eligible for conventional myeloablative aSCT, consideration should be given for RIC-based aSCT. Initial results with the use of RIC conditioning have been favorable, and long-term data are awaited (see earlier section on allogeneic stem cell transplant).

Many novel agents are being evaluated for this group of patients given poor prognosis with the currently available therapies. The GRAALL-SA1 randomized phase II trial compared the efficacy and toxicity of pegylated liposomal doxorubicin (Peg-Dox) versus continuous-infusion doxorubicin (CI-Dox) in patients 55 years of age and older with Ph$^-$ ALL patients. Use of Peg-Dox led to significant lower toxicities; however, there was a trend toward a lower CR rate, more refractory disease, and higher relapse rate in the Peg-Dox arm compared with CI-Dox arm. Other novel therapies are detailed in the Novel Therapies section later, and consideration should be given to incorporation of any promising agents into frontline therapies for older patients given the lack of progress with dose intensification of traditional agents. Management of elderly patients with Ph$^+$ ALL is discussed in the Ph$^+$ ALL section; the incorporation of TKIs into frontline therapy has already made significant improvements in DFS for these high-risk patients.

RELAPSED ACUTE LYMPHOBLASTIC LEUKEMIA

As described earlier, with standard therapies for ALL, long-term DFS is only around 30% to 40%. Thus, the majority patients with ALL relapse despite the administration of postremission treatment. Postrelapse therapies will lead to a second CR (CR2) in 30% to 40% of patients with a 5-year OS of only around 10%. An aSCT is the only chance for long-term cure in these patients and must be considered for all patients.

In the largest report of relapsed adult ALL patients to date, Fielding and colleagues analyzed the outcomes of relapsed adult ALL patients who were treated in the MRC UKALLXII/ECOG E2993 trial. Of the 1508 evaluable patients, 1372 (91%) achieved CR1, of whom 609 (44% of the CR1 patients) relapsed at a median of 11 months. The 5-year OS was only 7% for the relapsed patients, which was significantly worse compared with 38% for the newly diagnosed ALL patients in this study. The median OS for the relapsed patients was 5.5 months. The site of the relapses were BM alone (86%), CNS alone (4%), BM plus CNS (5%), and other extramedullary sites (4%). The majority of the relapses (81%) occurred within 2 years of diagnosis. In this series, none of the 55 patients who had CNS involvement at relapse were alive at 5 years. Receiving aSCT after relapse led to significant improved outcomes compared with chemotherapy alone (5-year OS, 23% for matched sibling SCT vs. 4% for the chemotherapy-alone arm).

Tavernier and colleagues reported outcomes of 421 ALL patients who experienced first relapse treated on the French LALA-94 trial. A CR2 was achieved in 44% patients with a median DFS of 5.2 months and median OS of 6.3 months. Factors associated with favorable outcome after relapse included transplant performed in CR2, CR1 of longer than 1 year's duration, and platelet count greater than 100,000/μL at relapse. The outcomes after relapse were not influenced by risk stratification at diagnosis or the treatment received during first CR. An aSCT was performed in 24% (n = 99) of the relapsing patients (in CR2 [n = 61] or with active disease at the time of SCT [n = 38], directly as a salvage therapy after relapse [n = 14], or after failure of salvage regimen [n = 24]). Median OS from an aSCT was 6.7 months with 5-year OS of 25% with a significantly higher OS at 3 years after aSCT in CR2 compared with those with active disease at the time of SCT.

Oriol and colleagues reported the outcomes of 263 ALL patients in first relapse treated in four consecutive PETHEMA trials. CR2 was achieved in 45% of patients, a rate similar to that in the French LALA trials. The median OS after relapse was 4.5 months with a 5-year OS of 10%. Factors associated with a favorable outcome after relapse included age younger than 30 years and CR1 duration of longer than 2 years. The best subgroup of patients was younger than 30 years old with CR1 longer than 2 years in which the 5-year DFS and OS were 53% and 38%, respectively.

Thus, patients with relapsed ALL continue to be a challenging subgroup of patients, and novel therapies (see later discussion) may improve outcomes by improving CR2 rates and increasing the percentage of patients who could be candidates for aSCT.

NOVEL THERAPIES

Many new agents are being investigated for patients with ALL, both in the relapsed and frontline setting. Clofarabine is a purine nucleoside analog that is currently approved by the United States FDA for the treatment of pediatric patients with relapsed or refractory ALL who have failed two prior regimens. The response rate CR, CR with incomplete recovery of platelets [CRp], and partial response [PR]) for this group of patients is approximately 30%. There are emerging data on the use of clofarabine in adults with relapsed or refractory ALL. Kantarjian and colleagues reported 17% response rate (CR, CRp, PR) with single-agent clofarabine in adults with relapsed or refractory ALL. Based on the modest single-agent activity, studies evaluating the role of the combination of clofarabine with cytarabine or cyclophosphamide are being conducted. The Southwest Oncology Group Study S0530 was a phase 2 trial of a combination of clofarabine and cytarabine for relapsed or refractory ALL patients (n = 37) and demonstrated a response rate of 17% (CR/CRp), which was not better than that reported as a single agent. Clofarabine has also been studied as a "bridge" to an aSCT in which the goal is to use clofarabine to provide adequate cytoreduction before an aSCT. The COG is now testing the addition of clofarabine to frontline therapy in an attempt to improve the outcomes for high-risk children and adolescents.

Nelarabine is a prodrug, which is demethylated by adenosine deaminase to the deoxyguanosine analog (ara-G). T lymphoblasts are sensitive to the cytotoxic effects of nelarabine, and this drug has been studied in T-cell ALL in the relapsed or refractory setting. DeAngelo and colleagues treated 26 patients with T-cell ALL and 13 patients with T-cell lymphoblastic lymphoma with nelarabine. The median age was 34 years (range, 16-66 years). The CR rate was 31% with a 1-year OS of 28%. Neurotoxicity was seen in many patients. Nelarabine is currently approved in the United States for both pediatric and adult patients with T-cell ALL and T-cell lymphoblastic lymphoma who have failed at least two chemotherapeutic regimens. The COG is currently testing the addition of nelarabine in frontline setting for T-ALL. The U.S. Intergroup and GMALL also have such trials in the planning stage.

Vincristine is an important component of ALL treatment. In preclinical models, encapsulation of vincristine into sphingomyelin liposomes or "sphingosomes" has been shown to lead to increased efficacy without increased neurotoxicity compared with conventional vincristine. A phase II trial of single-agent sphingosomal vincristine (2.0 mg/m^2 every 2 weeks) in 16 patients with relapsed or refractory ALL reported an overall response rate of 14%. A weekly schedule has also been evaluated in a phase I study in 36 relapsed or refractory ALL patients with a maximum tolerated dose of 2.25 mg/m^2/wk. Dexamethasone (40 mg) was given on days 1 to 4 and on days 11 to 14 of each 4-week cycle. The CR rate was 19% overall; it was 29% for those who underwent therapy as their first salvage treatment. Based on these results, an international phase III trial has been initiated to examine the benefit of the liposomal vincristine in frontline therapy of older adults with ALL.

L-asparaginase (asparaginase) is an important component of ALL therapy and has been incorporated into most ALL trials. ALL cells are unable to produce asparagine and are dependent on plasma levels of this amino acid for protein synthesis. Depletion of asparagine results in inhibition of protein synthesis and subsequent apoptotic leukemic cell death. Traditionally, native enzyme derived from *E. coli* has been used. However, this preparation can be immunogenic, leading to hypersensitive reactions and development of cross-reacting antibodies. Polyethylene glycosylated (PEG)–asparaginase, formed by covalently attaching polyethylene glycol to the native *E. coli* enzyme, has been developed and offers lower immunogenicity and a longer half-life. Douer and colleagues treated 25 newly diagnosed adult ALL patients (median age, 27 years; range, 17-55 years) with the adult ALL BFM protocol in which 14 injections of *E. coli* asparaginase were replaced by a single dose of pegaspargase (2000 IU/m^2 IV) on day 16 of induction therapy. After the single dose, asparagine deamination was complete in all patients after 2 hours and in 100%, 81%, and 44% on days 14, 21, and 28, respectively. No allergic reactions or pancreatitis was observed, and a CR was achieved in 24 of the 25 patients. The CALGB 9511 trial used pegaspargase (2000 IU/m^2 subcutaneously, two doses during induction and two during first intensification) as part of the five-drug induction regimen. Of the 85 evaluable patients, those with effective asparagine depletion (defined by enzyme levels >0.03 U/mL plasma for 14 consecutive days after pegaspargase administration) had improved DFS and OS compared with those without effective asparagine deletion. Thus, use of pegaspargase appears safe and effective in adults, and it may replace native L-asparaginase as the agent for asparagine deletion. To avoid systemic toxicities, a novel preparation of L-asparaginase in which L-asparaginase is encapsulated within red blood cells (GRASPA) has been developed and is in early phase testing in Europe.

TARGETED AGENTS

Given the established role of rituximab in many lymphoid malignancies, including BL (as described earlier), a similar approach has recently been tested in precursor B-cell ALL. Studies have shown that up to 20% to 40% pre-B ALL express CD20 (≥20% leukemia cells positive). In a retrospective analysis, the MD Anderson group reported the poor prognostic value of CD20 expression in adult precursor B-cell ALL. They subsequently incorporated rituximab into a modified hyper-CVAD regimen for patients with CD20 expression of 20% or greater. When analyzing the younger cohort of patients (younger than 60 years of age), incorporation of rituximab led to very significant improvement in 3-year OS of 75% compared with 47% in historical control participants ($P = .003$). In this study, the addition of rituximab did not improve the outcomes of patients older than 60 years old. The GMALL has substantiated these results.

CD22 is a commonly expressed antigen on the precursor B-cell lymphoblasts and therefore represents an attractive target. Epratuzumab, a humanized monoclonal antibody against CD22, has also activity in a subset of patients with ALL. In a COG pilot study, epratuzumab in combination with standard reinduction chemotherapy was evaluated in 15 pediatric patients with relapsed ALL. There was rapid clearing of surface CD22 antigen, and 9 of 15 patients achieved a CR. More recently, a conjugated anti-CD22 antibody has been introduced with promising results. Inotuzumab ozogamicin, a CD22 monoclonal antibody attached to immunotoxin calicheamicin, has shown activity in non-Hodgkin lymphoma and is currently being evaluated in ALL patients. In a preliminary report, 49 relapsed or refractory ALL patients were treated with inotuzumab IV on an every-3-week schedule. The drug was well tolerated with an overall response rate of 57% in patients with relapsed or refractory ALL. Additional phase I studies to determine the optimal dose and schedule of inotuzumab are underway. Moxetumomab pasudotox is a recombinant immunotoxin composed of the variable domain of anti-CD22 monoclonal antibody fused to a truncated form of *Pseudomonas* exotoxin A. In a phase I, dose-escalation study, 21 pediatric patients with relapsed or refractory ALL were enrolled. The drug was well tolerated. In this heavily pretreated patient population (median number of prior therapies, four), preliminary efficacy results are encouraging with hematologic improvement in 41% and CR in 24% of the patients.

Blinatumomab is a novel antibody (BiTE antibody) designed to engage the patient's T cells to CD19-expressing target B cells, resulting in a cytotoxic T-cell response. Preliminary results of an exploratory phase II trial of single-agent blinatumomab in adult patients with relapsed or refractory precursor-B ALL were recently reported. Blinatumomab was administered by continuous IV infusion for 28 days followed by a 14-day rest. Responding patients could proceed to an aSCT or receive up to total of 5 cycles of blinatumomab. Of the 18 evaluable patients, 12 achieved CR with a CR rate of 67%. All CR patients achieved MRD negativity by the second cycle. These data are particularly encouraging because a CR rate of 67% in the relapsed or refractory setting with a single-agent therapy is unprecedented, and responses appear to be durable. Incorporation of blinatumomab into the frontline therapy is planned by the U.S. Intergroup.

Because approximately 70% of all (both precursor B-cell and precursor T-cell) ALL patients express CD52, alemtuzumab, a humanized anti-CD52 monoclonal antibody, has been evaluated in ALL as an agent for eradication of MRD during postremission therapy. In a phase I/II study (CALGB 10102), dose escalation of alemtuzumab was tested in 24 CD52$^+$ ALL patients in CR1 in which it was given to a target dose of 30 mg administered subcutaneously three times a week for 4 weeks during postremission therapy. Serial assessment of MRD using clone-specific PCR was possible in 11 of 24 cases, and a median 1-log decrease in MRD was noted in the 20- and 30-mg cohorts. Alemtuzumab, as a single agent, has limited activity in relapsed or refractory pediatric and adult ALL. A combination of alemtuzumab and rituximab has recently been shown to lead to promising results in a NOD/SCID (nonobese nondiabetic/severe combined immune deficient) mouse model and should pave way for clinical trials exploring such an approach.

Ponatinib, an oral multiple TKI, is a potent pan–BCR-ABL inhibitor with activity against all tested imatinib-resistant mutants, including T315I. A dose-escalation phase I trial was recently reported, and 45 mg once daily was selected as a phase II dose. Preliminary results are very encouraging, especially in T315I mutant patients in whom all first- and second-generation TKIs are ineffective. Initial results from the pivotal phase 2 study of ponatinib (Ponatinib Ph+ ALL and CML Evaluation [PACE] trial) were recently reported. In the chronic myeloid leukemia blast phase/Ph$^+$ ALL cohort, 11 of the 30 (37%) patients who were resistant or intolerant to second-generation TKIs and 6 of the 22 (27%) patients with T315I mutations achieved a major hematologic remission. Other BCR-ABL kinase inhibitors such as bosutinib and INNO-406 and aurora kinase inhibitors such as MK-0457 have also been evaluated in Ph$^+$ ALL.

There has been an increasing understanding of the molecular biology of ALL, which may translate into newer therapeutic options. Mullighan and colleagues reported loss of the *IKZF1* gene on 7p12, which encodes the early lymphoid transcription factor Ikaros in 84% of BCR-ABL–positive ALL and in 28% of BCR-ABL–negative B-cell ALL. An *IKZF1* deletion was reported in 63% of 83 adult Ph$^+$ ALL patients treated in various GIMEMA trials. The presence of deletion of the *IKZF1* gene has been associated with poor prognosis with worse DFS and increased relapse risk. Patients with IKZF1 alteration have a gene expression profile similar to that of Ph$^+$ ALL, and one-third of such patients have rearrangements of the lymphoid cytokine receptor gene *CRLF2,* either alone or with mutations of the Janus kinase (JAK) genes *JAK1* and *JAK2*. This provides rationale to test JAK inhibitors as a targeted strategy for this group of patients.

NOTCH1 activation occurs in more than 50% of patients with precursor T-cell ALL and has been used as a therapeutic target. γ-Secretase is required for *NOTCH1* proteolytic activation, and small molecule γ-secretase inhibitors are being been tested in early phase clinical trials. Targeting the mTOR (mammalian target of rapamycin) pathway has also been studied both for patients with NOTCH1 activation and in other subsets of ALL patients.

AMD11070 is an orally available, small molecule inhibitor of CXCR4 and has been studied in ALL cell lines and mouse models as an agent to eradicate leukemic cells that are otherwise protected by stromal elements. Mice with murine Ph$^+$ ALL survived significantly longer when treated with a combination of nilotinib and AMD11070. Similarly, combination of vincristine and AMD11070 showed encouraging responses.

SURVIVORSHIP

Although fewer specific data are available on long-term complications of survivors of young adults with ALL, the long-term complications of successful treatment of children with ALL have been well described and include neurocognitive and neurologic dysfunction, endocrine and metabolic abnormalities (including obesity), bone toxicity (osteonecrosis), cardiac toxicity, and secondary malignancies. To guide the frequency and focus of medical visits and the ordering of appropriate surveillance tests, comprehensive guidelines have been published in many countries, including North America, where guidelines created by the COG, titled "Long-Term Follow-up Guidelines for Survivors of Childhood, Adolescent and Young Adult Cancers" are available at http://www.survivorshipguidelines.org and should be adopted by the adult oncology community.

FUTURE DIRECTIONS

Acute lymphoblastic leukemia is a heterogeneous group of diseases with varied clinical outcomes, depending on molecular, cytogenetic, and clinical characterization. There have been significant advances in our understanding of the molecular pathogenesis of this disease, which should translate into effective targeted therapies and better patient outcomes. Given the rarity of this disease, it is strongly recommended that patients are referred to centers of expertise, and it is crucial that patients be enrolled in clinical trials designed to evaluate subset-specific therapies to improve survival.

SUGGESTED READINGS

Bachanova V, Verneris MR, DeFor T, et al: Prolonged survival in adults with acute lymphoblastic leukemia after reduced-intensity conditioning with cord blood or sibling donor transplantation. *Blood* 113:2902, 2009.

Bassan R, Spinelli O, Oldani E, et al: Improved risk classification for risk-specific therapy based on the molecular study of minimal residual disease (MRD) in adult acute lymphoblastic leukemia (ALL). *Blood* 113:4153, 2009.

Borowitz MJ, Chan JKC: B-lymphoblastic leukaemia/lymphoma with recurrent genetic abnormalities. In Swerdlow SH, Camp E, Harris NL, et al, editors: *WHO classification of tumors of haematopoietic and lymphoid tissues*, Lyon, France, 2008, IARC, p 171.

Campana D: Minimal residual disease in acute lymphoblastic leukemia. *Hematology Am Soc Hematol Educ Program* 2010:7, 2010.

Cornelissen JJ, van der Holt B, Verhoef GE, et al: Myeloablative allogeneic versus autologous stem cell transplantation in adult patients with acute lymphoblastic leukemia in first remission: A prospective sibling donor versus no-donor comparison. *Blood* 113:1375, 2009.

DeAngelo DJ, Yu D, Johnson JL, et al: Nelarabine induces complete remissions in adults with relapsed or refractory T-lineage acute lymphoblastic leukemia or lymphoblastic lymphoma: Cancer and Leukemia Group B study 19801. *Blood* 109:5136, 2007.

Dhedin N, Dombret H, Thomas X, et al: Autologous stem cell transplantation in adults with acute lymphoblastic leukemia in first complete remission: Analysis of the LALA-85, -87 and -94 trials. *Leukemia* 20:336, 2006.

Fielding AK, Richards SM, Chopra R, et al: Outcome of 609 adults after relapse of acute lymphoblastic leukemia (ALL); an MRC UKALL12/ECOG 2993 study. *Blood* 109:944, 2007.

Foa R, Vitale A, Vignetti M, et al: Dasatinib as first-line treatment for adult patients with Philadelphia chromosome-positive acute lymphoblastic leukemia. *Blood* 118:6521, 2011.

Goldstone AH, Richards SM, Lazarus HM, et al: In adults with standard-risk acute lymphoblastic leukemia, the greatest benefit is achieved from a matched sibling allogeneic transplantation in first complete remission, and an autologous transplantation is less effective than conventional consolidation/maintenance chemotherapy in all patients: Final results of the International ALL Trial (MRC UKALL XII/ECOG E2993). *Blood* 111:1827, 2008.

Gale KB, Ford AM, Repp R, et al: Backtracking leukemia to birth: Identification of clonotypic gene fusion sequences in neonatal blood spots. *Proc Natl Acad Sci U S A* 94:13950, 1997.

Huguet F, Leguay T, Raffoux E, et al: Pediatric-inspired therapy in adults with Philadelphia chromosome-negative acute lymphoblastic leukemia: The GRAALL-2003 study. *J Clin Oncol* 27:911, 2009.

Kantarjian HM, O'Brien S, Smith TL, et al: Results of treatment with hyper-CVAD, a dose-intensive regimen, in adult acute lymphocytic leukemia. *J Clin Oncol* 18:547, 2000.

Kenkre VP, Stock W: Burkitt lymphoma/leukemia: Improving prognosis. *Clin Lymphoma Myeloma* 9:S231, 2009.

Larson RA, Dodge RK, Burns CP, et al: A five-drug remission induction regimen with intensive consolidation for adults with acute lymphoblastic leukemia: Cancer and leukemia group B study 8811. *Blood* 85:2025, 1995.

Lazarus HM, Richards SM, Chopra R, et al: Central nervous system involvement in adult acute lymphoblastic leukemia at diagnosis: Results from the international ALL trial MRC UKALL XII/ECOG E2993. *Blood* 108:465, 2006.

Marks DI, Wang T, Perez WS, et al: The outcome of full-intensity and reduced-intensity conditioning matched sibling or unrelated donor transplantation in adults with Philadelphia chromosome-negative acute lymphoblastic leukemia in first and second complete remission. *Blood* 116:366, 2010.

Mullighan CG, Su X, Zhang J, et al: Deletion of IKZF1 and prognosis in acute lymphoblastic leukemia. *N Engl J Med* 360:470, 2009.

O'Brien S, Thomas DA, Ohanian M, et al: Inotuzumab Ozogamycin (I0), a CD22 Monoclonal Antibody Conjugated to Calecheamicin, Is Active in Refractory-Relapse Acute Lymphocytic Leukemia (R-R ALL). *ASH Annual Meeting Abstracts* 118, 2011.

Pui CH, Robison LL, Look AT: Acute lymphoblastic leukaemia. *Lancet* 371:1030, 2008.

Ravandi F, O'Brien S, Thomas D, et al: First report of phase 2 study of dasatinib with hyper-CVAD for the frontline treatment of patients with Philadelphia chromosome-positive (Ph+) acute lymphoblastic leukemia. *Blood* 116:2070, 2010.

Rowe JM, Buck G, Burnett AK, et al: Induction therapy for adults with acute lymphoblastic leukemia: Results of more than 1500 patients from the international ALL trial: MRC UKALL XII/ECOG E2993. *Blood* 106:3760, 2005.

Stock W, La M, Sanford B, et al: What determines the outcomes for adolescents and young adults with acute lymphoblastic leukemia treated on cooperative group protocols? A comparison of Children's Cancer Group and Cancer and Leukemia Group B studies. *Blood* 112:1646, 2008.

Thomas DA, Faderl S, Cortes J, et al: Treatment of Philadelphia chromosome-positive acute lymphocytic leukemia with hyper-CVAD and imatinib mesylate. *Blood* 103:4396, 2004.

Thomas DA, O'Brien S, Faderl S, et al: Chemoimmunotherapy with a modified hyper-CVAD and rituximab regimen improves outcome in de novo Philadelphia chromosome-negative precursor B-lineage acute lymphoblastic leukemia. *J Clin Oncol* 28:3880, 2010.

Thomas X, Boiron JM, Huguet F, et al: Outcome of treatment in adults with acute lymphoblastic leukemia: Analysis of the LALA-94 trial. *J Clin Oncol* 22:4075, 2004.

Tomblyn MB, Arora M, Baker KS, et al: Myeloablative hematopoietic cell transplantation for acute lymphoblastic leukemia: Analysis of graft sources and long-term outcome. *J Clin Oncol* 27:3634, 2009.

Vignetti M, Fazi P, Cimino G, et al: Imatinib plus steroids induces complete remissions and prolonged survival in elderly Philadelphia chromosome-positive patients with acute lymphoblastic leukemia without additional chemotherapy: Results of the Gruppo Italiano Malattie Ematologiche dell'Adulto (GIMEMA) LAL0201-B protocol. *Blood* 109:3676, 2007.

Weng AP, Ferrando AA, Lee W, et al: Activating mutations of NOTCH1 in human T cell acute lymphoblastic leukemia. *Science* 306:269, 2004.

Wetzler M, Dodge RK, Mrozek K, et al: Prospective karyotype analysis in adult acute lymphoblastic leukemia: The cancer and leukemia Group B experience. *Blood* 93:3983, 1999.

Yanada M, Takeuchi J, Sugiura I, et al: High complete remission rate and promising outcome by combination of imatinib and chemotherapy for newly diagnosed BCR-ABL-positive acute lymphoblastic leukemia: A phase II study by the Japan Adult Leukemia Study Group. *J Clin Oncol* 24:460, 2006.

For complete list of references log on to www.expertconsult.com.

CHAPTER 66

CHRONIC MYELOID LEUKEMIA

Ravi Bhatia

Chronic myeloid leukemia (CML) is a hematopoietic malignancy originating from transformation of a primitive hematopoietic cell. Without treatment, CML progresses from an initial chronic phase (CP) characterized by marrow hyperplasia and increased numbers of circulating differentiated myeloid cells followed by advanced phases of disease (accelerated phase [AP] and blast crisis [BC]) marked by a block in differentiation, an accumulation of blasts, and a depletion of normal hematopoietic cells, especially white blood cells and platelets. CML was the first malignant disease found to be consistently associated with a specific cytogenetic abnormality, the Philadelphia chromosome (Ph), resulting in the formation of the BCR-ABL fusion oncogene. Study of BCR-ABL has led to sensitive methods to detect residual disease and predict outcome and to "targeted" therapy aimed at inhibiting abnormal tyrosine kinase activity resulting from the BCR-ABL fusion oncogene. In addition, CML was one of the first diseases demonstrated to be curable by hematopoietic cell transplantation (HCT). Thus CML has become the model for "tailored" therapy, in which various treatments can be escalated on the basis of molecular response.

ETIOLOGY/EPIDEMIOLOGY/GENETICS

Chronic myelogenous leukemia was recognized as a distinct entity, associated with massive splenomegaly and leukocytosis without other explanations, in the mid-1800s. The modern history of CML was initiated by Nowell and Hungerford in 1960. They used newly developed techniques to detect a small chromosome in metaphase preparations of marrow cells from CML patients. This abnormal chromosome was the first consistent chromosomal abnormality in human malignancies and was termed the *Philadelphia chromosome* after the city of its discovery. Rowley showed that the Philadelphia chromosome resulted from a translocation between chromosomes 9 and 22 [t(9;22)(q34;q11)] (Fig. 66-1). The genes involved in this translocation were cloned in the 1980s, and the t(9;22) translocation was shown to result from the fusion of the BCR (breakpoint cluster region) gene on chromosome 22 to the (Abelson leukemia virus) gene on chromosome 9, with formation of the BCR-ABL fusion oncogene. This oncogene codes for a constitutively active cytoplasmic tyrosine kinase, which is now believed to be the principal cause of the chronic phase of CML. Until the 1970s, CML was regarded as an incurable and inevitably lethal disorder. It was then recognized that selected patients can be cured, by allogeneic HCT. However, transplantation therapy for CML is limited by donor availability and the risk for life-threatening toxicity. More recently, imatinib mesylate and other tyrosine kinase inhibitors (TKIs) that specifically block the enzymatic action of the abnormal tyrosine kinase coded by the fusion oncogene have resulted in a high rate of remission and improved survival in CML patients.

Chronic myelogenous leukemia is the most common of the myeloproliferative diseases and represents 15% to 20% of all new leukemia cases. The annual incidence of CML is 1 to 1.5 cases per 100,000 population per year. The median age at diagnosis is 67 years and the incidence sharply rises with age. The disease occurs slightly more often in men than in women. Chronic myelogenous leukemia may occur in children, but only approximately 10% of cases occur in subjects between 5 and 20 years of age and represent only 3% of all childhood leukemias. Concordance of disease is not observed between identical twins. Radiation may play a role in some cases. Persons exposed to high-dose irradiation, including survivors of atomic bombing, have a significantly increased risk for leukemia. High-dose irradiation of myeloid cell lines in vitro induces the expression of BCR-ABL transcripts indistinguishable from those that characterize CML. The BCR-ABL gene can be detected at very low levels in a proportion of healthy individuals using a very sensitive PCR assay. These findings suggest that the fusion gene develops relatively frequently in hematopoietic cells, but only infrequently lead to leukemia development. The mechanism by which the Ph chromosome is first formed and the time required for progression to overt disease are unknown.

PATHOPHYSIOLOGY

CML is generally believed to develop from transformation of a primitive hematopoietic stem cell (HSC) by the BCR-ABL fusion gene. The progeny of transformed HSC have a proliferative advantage over normal hematopoietic cells, thus allowing the Ph-positive clone gradually to displace residual normal hematopoiesis. The translocation is found in cells of myeloid, erythroid, megakaryocytic and B-lymphoid origin, consistent with a hematopoietic stem cell origin of the disease. Hematopoietic expansion in patients with chronic-phase disease primarily involves an increase in myeloid cell mass, related to an expansion of mature cells, as well as increased numbers of precursor and progenitor cells. In chronic phase, the leukemic cells are minimally invasive and are primarily located in hematopoietic tissues including blood, bone marrow, spleen, and liver. The proliferative advantage of the malignant clone may be related to enhanced responsiveness to hematopoietic growth factors and/or reduced response to inhibitory factors. Chronic myelogenous leukemia progenitors also demonstrate defective adhesion to marrow stromal cells and extracellular matrix. Altered microenvironmental interactions may contribute to another feature of CML, which is abnormal progenitor trafficking with increased numbers of circulating progenitors and extramedullary hematopoiesis. Several observations indicate that although the Ph-positive clone displaces normal hematopoiesis, it does not destroy residual normal stem cells. For example, Ph-negative progenitors can be seen after cultures of CML cells in vitro can be selected on the basis of cell surface phenotype, and can be identified in the blood after high-dose chemotherapy. As described later in the Therapy section, treatment with agents such as interferon (IFN) or tyrosine kinase inhibitors can result in restoration of Ph-negative hematopoiesis in CML patients.

The BCR-ABL gene results from a chromosomal translocation that results in the fusion of the ABL gene on chromosome 9 and the BCR gene on chromosome 22 (Fig. 66-2). The translocation is related to a break in ABL upstream of exon a2 and in the major breakpoint cluster region of the BCR gene. This leads to juxtaposition of a 5′ portion of BCR and a 3′ portion of ABL on a shortened chromosome 22 (the derivative 22q-, or Ph). The resulting messenger RNA (mRNA) usually contains one of two BCR-ABL junctions, designated e13a2 (formerly b2a2) and e14a2 (or b3a2). Both

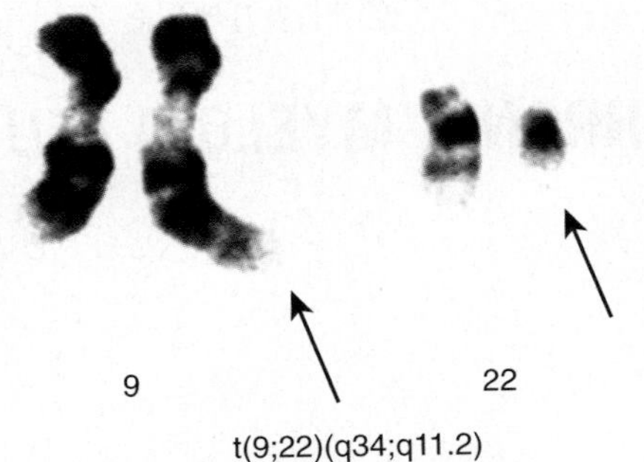

Figure 66-1 PARTIAL KARYOTYPE SHOWING THE t(9;22)(q34;q11). The Philadelphia chromosome is the derivative chromosome 22 *(right arrow)*.

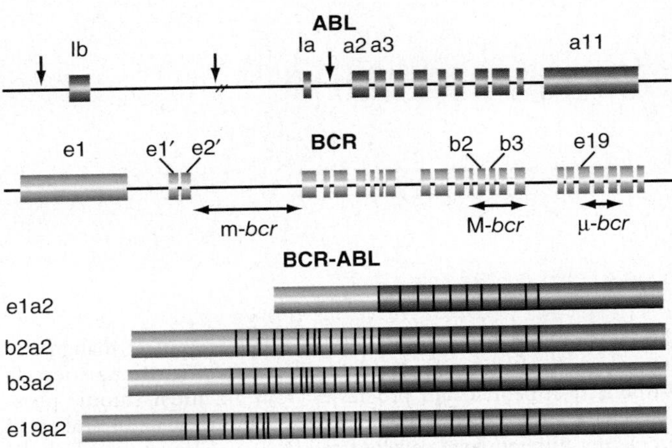

Figure 66-2 LOCATIONS OF THE BREAKPOINTS IN THE ABL AND BCR GENES AND STRUCTURE OF THE CHIMERIC mRNAs DERIVED FROM THE VARIOUS BREAKS. *(Modified from Deininger MW, Goldman JM, Melo JV, editors: The molecular biology of chronic myeloid leukemia,* Blood *96:3343, 2000.)*

BCR-ABL mRNA molecules are translated into a 210-kd fusion protein, referred to as *p210BCR-ABL*. Rarely, other variant breakpoints and fusions can give rise to full-length, functionally oncogenic BCR-ABL proteins, notably p190BCR-ABL (associated with an e1a2 mRNA junction) and p230BCR-ABL (associated with an e19a2 mRNA junction). Of patients with CML who have a normal-appearing karyotype, one-third have a cytogenetically occult BCR-ABL gene, usually located on a normal-appearing chromosome 22 but occasionally on chromosome 9. In the remaining patients with Ph-negative, BCR-ABL-negative disease, the molecular basis of leukemia is not known.

Some studies have suggested that pathogenesis of CML may be a multistep process, with development of clonal hematopoiesis preceding the t(9;22) translocation. However, there is substantial evidence to suggest that the generation of a classic BCR-ABL fusion gene in a hematopoietic stem cell is sufficient to initiate CML. Expression of BCR-ABL has been shown to transform mouse fibroblast cell lines, growth factor-dependent hematopoietic cell lines, and primary murine bone marrow cells. Expression of BCR-ABL in human CD34$^+$ cells also causes increased proliferation, reduced apoptosis, and altered adhesion and migration mimicking alterations seen in progenitor cells from CML patients. Transplantation of murine bone marrow cells made to ectopically express the BCR-ABL gene by retroviral transduction induces a myeloproliferative disorder (MPD) that closely resembles human CML with increased numbers of peripheral blood cells (with a predominance of granulocytes), splenomegaly, and extramedullary hematopoiesis, although the disease is much more fulminant than human CML. Initial development of transgenic and knock-in mouse models of CML was problematic. It appears to be crucial to express this oncogene in the proper cell type. Expression of BCR-ABL in B-cell lymphocytic and megakaryocytic precursors resulted in the development of B–acute lymphocytic leukemia (B-ALL) and megakaryocytic myeloproliferative syndrome. Specific expression of the oncogene in hematopoietic stem cells through a stem cell leukemia (SCL) enhancer to regulate expression induces development of a CML-like disease. Together, these studies indicate that BCR-ABL expression alone is sufficient to induce chronic-phase CML-like disease in mice.

The ABL gene encodes a nonreceptor tyrosine kinase that is expressed in most tissues (Fig. 66-3). Mice with homozygous disruption of the ABL gene demonstrate increased perinatal mortality, lymphopenia, and osteoporosis and are smaller, with abnormal head and eye development. The BCR gene also encodes a signaling protein that contains multiple modular domains (see Fig. 66-2). Although BCR-deficient mice develop normally, their neutrophils produce excess levels of oxygen metabolites following activation. The normally regulated tyrosine kinase activity of the ABL protein is constitutively activated by the juxtaposition of N-terminal BCR sequences. BCR acts by promoting protein dimerization, leading to phosphorylation of tyrosine residues in the kinase-activation loops and leading to constitutive activation of kinase activity. The fusion of BCR sequences to ABL also adds new regulatory domains/motifs to ABL, such as the growth factor receptor–bound protein 2 (GRB2) SH2-binding site. The uncontrolled kinase activity of BCR-ABL and enhanced interaction with a variety of effector proteins lead to deregulation of cell signaling mechanisms that regulate proliferation. The ABL protein is located in both the nucleus and the cytoplasm and shuttles between these two compartments, whereas the BCR-ABL is exclusively cytoplasmic and localizes to the cytoskeleton, where it appears to contribute to adhesion and migration abnormalities.

The structure of the BCR-ABL protein and the biochemical pathways affected have been extensively studied (see Fig. 66-3). However, most such interactions have been studied only in cell lines and conditions of forced overexpression. Their existence in primary leukemia cells and relevance to CML pathogenesis is not certain. The murine transduction-transplantation CML model has been helpful in studying the role of BCR-ABL domains and signaling interaction in primary hematopoietic cells. However, the murine CML model is not fully representative of human CML, and the role of different domains in development of disease in CML patients still needs to be confirmed. The ABL tyrosine kinase is crucial for oncogenic transformation. Mice that express a form of BCR-ABL with a point mutation in the ATP-binding site of ABL that inhibits its kinase activity do not develop leukemia. This suggests that the ABL kinase activity is essential for BCR-ABL leukemogenesis in vivo. The success of kinase inhibitor therapy for CML provides further proof of the importance of kinase activity in maintenance of human disease. Other important domains in BCR-ABL also regulate the kinase activity of ABL or connect to other downstream signaling pathways. The amino-terminal coiled-coil (CC) oligomerization domain of BCR is an important activator of ABL kinase activity, and also promotes the association of BCR-ABL with F-actin fibers. Phosphorylation of BCR at tyrosine 177 generates a GRB2-binding site, which is important for RAS activation. Mutation of the tyrosine-177 residue of BCR-ABL to phenylalanine (Y177F) largely abolishes its ability to bind GRB2, without affecting the kinase activity of ABL. The Y177F mutant has a greatly reduced ability to induce MPD in mice. A tyrosine phosphorylation site in the activation loop of the ABL kinase domain and the SH2 domain of ABL also contribute to RAS activation. Mutations in the SH2 domain of ABL and a Y1294F point mutation reduce the ability of BCR-ABL to induce a CML-like MPD in mice. The carboxy-terminal region of ABL is required for the proper function of normal ABL. However, deletion of the ABL actin-binding domain was reported to not affect the ability of BCR-ABL to induce CML-like MPD in mice, suggesting that this domain may be dispensable for BCR-ABL–mediated leukemogenesis. Certain BCR-ABL domains may have complementary or overlapping functions.

Many signaling proteins become phosphorylated in BCR-ABL–expressing cells and/or to interact with BCR-ABL through various

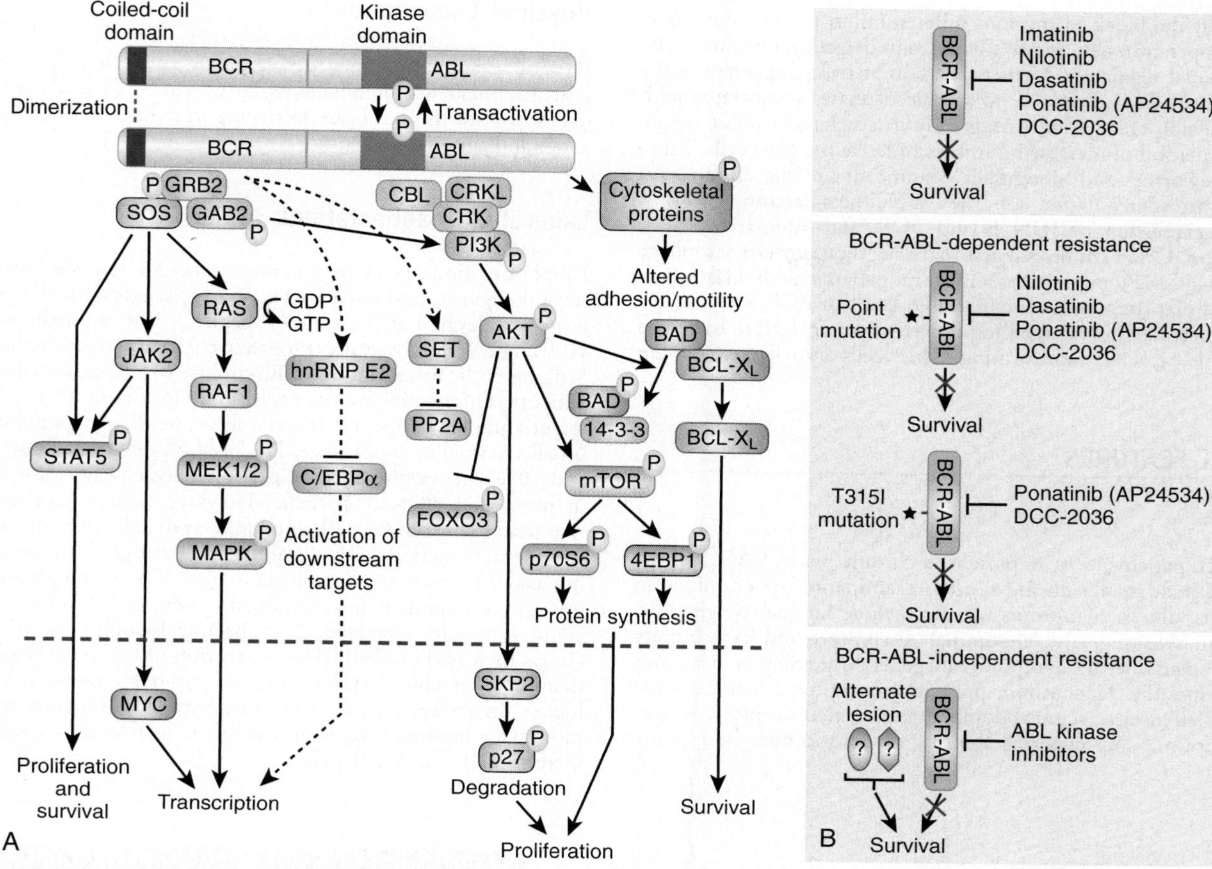

Figure 66-3 THE BCR-ABL SIGNALING NETWORK AND ABL KINASE INHIBITION. **A,** BCR-ABL signaling pathways activated in CML. Dimerization of BCR-ABL triggers autophosphorylation events that activate the kinase and generate docking sites for intermediary adapter proteins *(purple)* such as GRB2. BCR-ABL -dependent signaling facilitates activation of multiple downstream pathways that enforce enhanced survival, inhibition of apoptosis, and perturbation of cell adhesion and migration. A subset of these pathways and their constituent transcription factors *(blue)*, serine/threonine-specific kinases *(green)*, and apoptosisrelated proteins *(red)* are shown. A few pathways that were more recently implicated in CML stem cell maintenance and BCR-ABL -mediated disease transformation are shown *(orange)*. Of note, this is a simplified diagram and many more associations between BCR-ABL and signaling proteins have been reported. BCR-ABL is unstable upon disruption of primary CML cells; therefore, pharmacodynamic evaluation of BCR-ABL activity is performed by monitoring the tyrosine phosphorylation status of either CRKL or STAT5, with CRKL phosphorylation considered the most specific readout. **B,** Predicted effectiveness of ABL kinase inhibitors in three therapeutic scenarios: to inhibit native BCR-ABL *(top)*, to inhibit mutated BCR-ABL *(middle)*, and as a component in the control of CML involving a BCR-ABL -independent alternate lesion *(bottom)*. *(From O'Hare T, Deininger MWN, Eide CA, et al: Targeting the BCR-ABL signaling pathway in therapy-resistant Philadelphia chromosome-positive leukemia.* Clin Cancer Res *17:212, 2011.)*

functional domains. These interactions in turn activate signaling through mechanisms including RAS, PI3K, AKT, JNK, and SRC family kinases, protein phosphatase, STATs, nuclear factor-B, and MYC. BCR-ABL also induces expression of cytokines such as interleukin-3 (IL-3), granulocyte colony-stimulating factor (G-CSF), and granulocyte-macrophage colony-stimulating factor (GM-CSF). A CML-like MPD was still induced following expression of BCR-ABL in bone marrow cells from Stat5a$^{-/-}$Stat5b$^{-/-}$, Cbl$^{-/-}$, and Il-3$^{-/-}$GM-CSF$^{-/-}$ mice, indicating that these proteins may not be required for BCR-ABL-mediated leukemogenesis. BCR-ABL expression induced CML-like MPD but failed to induce B-ALL in mice that lacked the SRC family kinases LYN, HCK, and FGR, indicating the potential importance of the kinases in lymphoid blast crisis or ALL but not for MPD.

Progression to accelerated phase and blast crisis is associated with increase in immature blast cells that may be located within hematopoietic tissues or may infiltrate a number of extramedullary sites, including lymph nodes, skin, soft tissue, and the central nervous system. A number of molecular mechanisms, rather than a single gene defect, are likely to underlie the arrest of maturation, enhanced proliferation and survival, and increased tissue invasiveness that characterize blast crisis CML. Increased level of BCR-ABL expression is a common feature and appears to be a key factor in the development of features of blast crisis, through effects on cell signaling and on transcription and translation of important regulatory genes. Disease progression is related to susceptibility of the BCR-ABL-expressing clone to additional molecular changes. Additional cytogenetic and molecular changes are frequently seen during progression. Genetic instability in CML appears may be induced by several factors, including increased oxidative stress, reduced DNA repair, or reduced DNA damage checkpoint signaling response. Genetic changes observed in leukemic cells from blast-phase CML patients include nonrandom cytogenetic changes such as ++8, ++Ph, ++19, and I(17)q; point mutations in TP53, RB, and CDKN2A (p16^{INK4A}); and overexpression of EVI1 and MYC. Additional chromosome translocations are also observed, such as t(3;21)(q26;q22), which generates AML1-EVI1. Other CML-associated fusion genes include AML1-ETO, resulting from the t(8;21)(q22;q22) translocation; NUP98-HOXA9, resulting from the t(7;11)(p15;p15) translocation; and CBFβ-SMMHC, which results from inv(16)(p13;q22). These observations suggest that the block in myeloid differentiation in blast crisis may involve cooperation between BCR-ABL and defects in hematopoietic transcriptional regulators. Gene expression analyses suggest that the progression of CML from CP to advanced phase is associated with gene expression changes occurring early in accelerated phase before the accumulation of increased numbers of leukemia blast cells. Especially noteworthy and potentially significant in the progression program are deregulation of the WNT/beta-catenin pathway, decreased expression of JUN B and FOS, and alternative kinase deregulation. Other studies suggest that the granulocyte/macrophage progenitor (GMP) pool is expanded in patients with blast-phase CML, and that these cells have increased levels of BCR-ABL expression and increased WNT signaling activity that may lead to increased self-renewal capacity, transforming GMP cells into leukemic stem cells.[1,2]

CLINICAL FEATURES

History

Most CML patients (>90%) present in chronic phase. CML is often diagnosed incidentally during routine examination or examination for another illness. Symptoms usually include fatigue, weight loss, bone pain, sweating, and abdominal discomfort and early satiety related to splenomegaly. Symptoms are generally gradual in onset over weeks to months. Uncommon presenting symptoms include those related to leukostasis, acute abdominal pain related to splenic infraction, priapism, and hypermetabolism, hyperuricemia, and gouty arthritis.

Physical Examination

Physical examination may detect pallor and splenomegaly. In the past, the incidence of splenomegaly was often greater than 90% at diagnosis, but this has been decreasing in frequency since the disease is being diagnosed earlier.

Laboratory Manifestations

Laboratory findings at presentation generally include leukocytosis, thrombocytosis, and anemia (Fig. 66-4). The total leukocyte count is always elevated at the time of diagnosis and is usually over 25 × 10^9/L. The WBC count rises progressively if patients are left untreated. Striking cyclic variations in WBC counts have been described in rare patients. Differential counts reveal granulocytes at all stages of differentiation in peripheral blood cells. Circulating granulocytes are usually normal in appearance. The blast percentage is between 0.5% and 10%. Neutrophil alkaline phosphatase activity is low or absent in more than 90% of patients. However, activity can increase in response to infection, inflammation, and reduction of counts by treatment. Functional abnormalities of neutrophils are mild and are not associated with predisposition to infection. Although the proportion of eosinophils is usually not increased, the absolute eosinophil count is usually increased. The absolute basophil count is almost always increased in CML. The proportion of basophils is usually less than 15% in chronic-phase patients, although rarely, this may be higher. In contrast to mastocytosis, hyperhistaminemia is uncommon. The absolute lymphocyte count is increased as a result of an increase in T but not B cells.

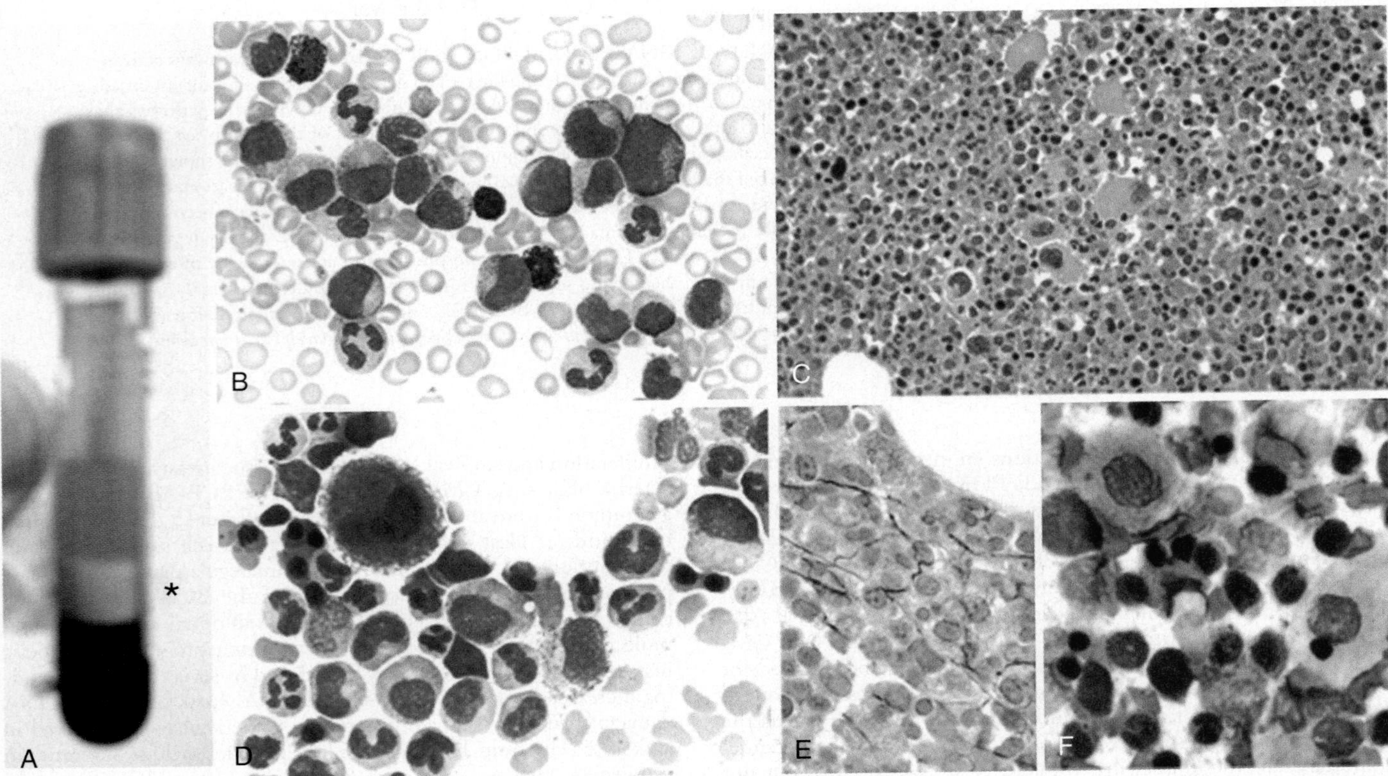

Figure 66-4 CHRONIC MYELOGENOUS LEUKEMIA, PERIPHERAL BLOOD TUBE, AND IMAGES OF BLOOD SMEAR AND BONE MARROW BIOPSY AND ASPIRATE IN CHRONIC PHASE. **A,** The spun tube of peripheral blood (EDTA collected) is from a patient with chronic phase CML who presented with a white blood cell count of about 600K/μL. Note the markedly expanded "buffy coat" layer *(asterisk)* due to the severe leukocytosis. **B,** Peripheral smear showing marked leukocytosis due to a granulocytic proliferation of all stages with particularly increased myelocytes and absolute basophilia. **C,** Bone core biopsy illustrating markedly hypercellular marrow due to granulocytic proliferation and increased small hypolobated megakaryocytes. **D,** Bone marrow aspirate showing the same granulocytic proliferation and small, "dwarf" megakaryocytes. Mild fibrosis as seen on reticulin stain **E,** and pseudo-Gaucher cells **(F).**

The platelet count is elevated in 50% of patients at the time of diagnosis. The platelet count may increase during the course of chronic phase. Platelet dysfunction may occur, but disorders of thrombosis and hemorrhage are rare. Thrombocytopenia is rare at diagnosis and usually is a sign of progression toward accelerated phase. A deficiency in the second wave of aggregation to epinephrine is the most common abnormality and is associated with deficiency of adenine nucleotides in the storage pool. The hematocrit is decreased in most patients at diagnosis. Red cells tend to show only mild alterations with increased variability of size and shape. Small numbers of nucleated red blood cells and mild reticulocytosis may be seen.

Chemical abnormalities seen in patients with untreated CML include hyperuricemia and hyperuricosuria. The formation of urate stones is common, and patients with underlying susceptibility may develop acute gouty arthritis or urate nephropathy. Patients have increased serum level of vitamin B_{12}–binding capacity related to release of transcobalamin I and II from mature neutrophils. The serum B_{12} level in CML is an average of 10-fold higher than normal. Serum LDH is elevated in CML. Pseudohyperkalemia may be seen related to release of potassium from WBC during clotting. Spurious hypoglycemia or hypoxemia may result from consumption by neutrophils after a sample is drawn.

Examination of the marrow usually reveals a very hypercellular marrow, with 75% to 90% marrow cellularity (see Fig. 66-4, *C-D*). The granulocytic-to-erythroid ratio is increased to 10:1 to 30:1, with increased granulopoiesis and reduced erythropoiesis. Eosinophils and basophils may be increased. Blasts usually represent less than 5% of cells. Presence of more than 10% blasts indicates transformation to accelerated phase. Megakaryocytes are typically smaller than usual and may have hypolobated nuclei. Megakaryocyte numbers may be normal or slightly decreased, but 40% to 50% of patients show moderate to extensive proliferation of megakaryocytes. Collagen type III detected by silver staining is typically increased (see Fig. 66-4, *E*). Approximately half of patients demonstrate increased reticulin fibrosis, which may be associated with increased megakaryocytes in marrow. Increased fibrosis may be associated with larger spleen size, anemia, and increased blasts in blood and marrow. Pseudo-Gaucher cells and sea blue histiocytes, secondary to increased marrow cell turnover, may be seen in 30% of specimens (see H5eC69, Fig. 66-4, *F*). The spleen shows enlargement related to infiltration of the cords of the red pulp with granulocytes at different stages of maturation. The liver may show infiltration with granulocytic cells in the portal areas and hepatic sinusoids.

Cytogenetic examination shows t(9;22)(q34;q11) and Ph chromosome in more than 90% of patients. Additional chromosomal abnormalities besides the Philadelphia chromosome are seen at diagnosis in 20% of patients including –Y and +8, and have not been shown to affect disease course. Variant Ph chromosomes are seen in 5% of patients, with complex rearrangement involving exchange of material with an additional chromosome besides chromosomes 9 and 22. In a small proportion of patients cryptic or complex translocations can be detected by fluorescence in situ hybridization (FISH) or polymerase chain reaction (PCR) assays. The methodology used for identifying BCR-ABL transcripts has evolved over the years. Initially it was possible only to identify the presence or absence of BCR-ABL transcripts by either single-step amplification or a two-step "nested" amplification with internal primers to increase the sensitivity. Real-time quantitative polymerase chain reaction (RQ-PCR) provides an accurate measure of the total leukemia cell mass, and the degree to which BCR-ABL transcripts are reduced by therapy correlates with progression-free survival. A consensus meeting at the National Institutes of Health (NIH) in October 2005 made suggestions for (a) harmonizing the different methodologies for measuring BCR-ABL transcripts in patients with CML undergoing treatment and using a conversion factor whereby individual laboratories can express BCR-ABL transcript levels on an internationally agreed scale; (b) using serial Q-PCR results rather than bone marrow cytogenetics or FISH for the BCR-ABL gene to monitor individual patients responding to treatment; and (c) detecting and reporting Ph-positive subpopulations bearing BCR-ABL kinase domain mutations. An international scale for comparison of BCR-ABL mRNA levels has been subsequently developed and implemented to facilitate common interpretation of data derived from individual laboratories and comparison of clinical studies, as well as to guide clinical decision. BCR-ABL values generated by different laboratories were aligned to the international scale such that major molecular response (MMR) was defined as BCR-ABL values of 0.1% or less. Alignment was achieved using laboratory-specific conversion factors calculated by comparisons of results of assays performed with patient samples against a reference method. A validation procedure was completed, and showed that there was good agreement between the overall MMR rates between different validated assays.[3]

In any new patient whose blood count suggests the diagnosis of a chronic myeloproliferative disorder, the detection of BCR-ABL transcripts in a blood specimen is probably the best way to confirm the diagnosis of CML. Current guidelines recommend that circulating BCR-ABL transcript numbers be measured and marrow cytogenetics be studied in every new patient with CML before initiation of treatment. Marrow cytogenetics is essential to identify any unusual translocations or additional cytogenetic abnormalities, and RQ-PCR for BCR-ABL at diagnosis will identify whether the commonly observed e13a2 (b2a2) or e14a2 (b3a2) transcripts are present or whether one of the less common fusion transcripts that are not amplified by the standard primer sets is present. This can prevent confusion if a patient on therapy has undetectable BCR-ABL transcripts because their transcripts were not amplified in the standard assay. If collection of marrow cells is not feasible, FISH performed on a blood specimen using dual probes for the BCR and ABL genes is an alternate method of confirming the diagnosis. FISH may also detect cytogenetically "silent" BCR-ABL rearrangements and deletions in the derivative 9q+, which have prognostic significance, and may therefore be performed in conjunction with marrow cytogenetics and RQ-PCR for BCR-ABL transcripts.

Natural History

The natural history of CML, determined more than 75 years ago, suggests a median survival from diagnosis of approximately 3 years. Without therapy, CML evolves from a chronic phase (CP) to an accelerated phase (AP) and eventually to blast crisis (BC). In approximately 25% of patients, there is no intervening AP between CP and BC (Table 66-1). Median survival times have been significantly prolonged with therapy (discussed later in the Therapy section). Following the introduction of imatinib treatment, a dramatic decrease in CML deaths was seen in age-adjusted death data from the U.S. Surveillance Epidemiology and End Results (SEER) (http://seer.cancer.gov/statistics/).[4] Long-term follow-up of CML patients who achieved complete cytogenetic response (CCR) 2 years after starting imatinib treatment, showed that CML-related deaths are uncommon and survival is not statistically significantly different from that of the general population.[5]

Accelerated Phase

In general, accelerated phase is characterized by symptoms of fever, night sweats, weight loss and bone pain, difficulty in controlling counts using conventional therapy, increased numbers of blasts and early myeloid cells in marrow and peripheral blood, and evidence of karyotypic evolution (Fig. 66-5). The World Health Organization (WHO) classification defines accelerated phase of CML as one or more of the following changes: (a) 10% to 19% myeloblasts in peripheral blood or bone marrow; (b) peripheral blood basophils higher than 20%; (c) persistent thrombocytopenia, less than 100×10^9/L; (d) persistent thrombocytosis, more than 1000×10^9/L unrelated to therapy; (e) increasing WBC count and increasing spleen size unresponsive to therapy; and/or (f) evidence of clonal evolution. The most common cytogenetic changes associated with disease evolution are an additional Ph chromosome, trisomy 8, isochrome I(17q), and trisomy 19.

Blast Crisis

The blast phase of CML resembles acute leukemia. Blast crisis is defined as having more than 20% blasts in the bone marrow or peripheral blood, the presence of large aggregates and clusters of blasts in the bone marrow biopsy, or the development of extramedullary blastic infiltrates. In approximately two-thirds of patients, the blasts have a myeloid or undifferentiated-like phenotype, whereas in the remaining third the blasts appear more lymphoid-like. Immunophenotypic analysis is recommended to characterize the nature of the blasts (Fig. 66-6). Extramedullary blast crisis most commonly affects the skin, lymph nodes, spleen, bone, or central nervous system, but it may occur elsewhere and may be of myeloid or lymphoid lineage.

Table 66-1 WHO Criteria for Accelerated and Blast Phases of CML

Accelerated phase	Diagnosis can be made if one or more of the following is present: Blasts 10% to 19% of peripheral blood white cells or bone marrow cells Peripheral blood basophils at least 20% Persistent thrombocytopenia (<100 × 10^9/L) unrelated to therapy, or persistent thrombocytosis (>1000 × 10^9/L) unresponsive to therapy Increasing spleen size and increasing WBC count unresponsive to therapy Cytogenetic evidence of clonal evolution (i.e., the appearance of an additional genetic abnormality that was not present in the initial specimen at the time of diagnosis of chronic phase CML) Megakaryocytic proliferation in sizable sheets and clusters, associated with marked reticulin or collagen fibrosis, and/or severe granulocytic dysplasia, should be considered as suggestive of CML-AP. (These findings have not yet been analyzed in large clinical studies; thus it is not clear whether they are independent criteria for accelerated phase. They often occur simultaneously with one or more of the other features listed.)
Blast crisis	Diagnosis can be made if one or more of following is present: Blasts 20% or more of peripheral blood white cells or bone marrow cells Extramedullary blast proliferation Large foci or clusters of blasts in bone marrow biopsy

PROGNOSIS

A number of prognostic scoring systems have been developed with the goal of predicting the length of chronic phase in individual patients. The best-known and widely used index was developed by Sokal and colleagues. An algorithm was identified, using spleen size, percentage of circulating blasts, platelet count, and age as prognostic factors for chronic-phase patients. However, the Sokal scale was based on therapies available at that time (busulfan, splenectomy), and newer systems for patients treated with IFN subsequently resulted in newer prognostic scoring systems. These scales, however, may have limited predictive value in the age of tyrosine kinase inhibitors.

Approximately 20% of patients with CML have deletions of chromosomal material of varying size on the derivative 9q+. These deletions presumably occur at the same time as the formation of the Ph chromosome, and are thus not considered to be additional clonal changes as would be suggestive of accelerated-phase disease. Patients with der 9q+ have a worse prognosis if they receive IFN therapy; it is unclear whether or not such deletions have a poor prognosis in patients receiving imatinib therapy.

Population-based studies investigating CML mortality in the imatinib era are now becoming available. They show that the pattern of mortality in CML patients related to high Sokal scores has became similar to those of intermediate scores induced by the use of imatinib in CP-CML patients.[4]

THERAPY

Definitions of Response to Treatment

Hematologic, cytogenetic, and molecular responses to treatment in CML have been defined (Table 66-2). A complete hematologic response is defined as the achievement of normal WBC and platelet counts and normal differential, along with the disappearance of all symptoms and signs of CML. A partial hematologic response is defined as a decrease in the WBC count to less than 50% of the pretreatment level or the normalization of the WBC count accompanied by persistent splenomegaly or immature cells in the peripheral blood. A complete cytogenetic response (CCR) is defined as the absence of Ph-positive metaphases in marrow cells, along with partial cytogenetic response as 1% to 34% Ph-positive metaphases. Major cytogenetic remission combines the percentages of complete and partial response. There is now increasing reliance on BCR-ABL mRNA levels for assessment of response. According to the international scale for comparison of BCR-ABL mRNA levels, a major molecular response (MMR) is defined as a value of 0.1% or less.[3] Lack of detection of BCR-ABL mRNA is referred to as a complete molecular response (CMR). Since the ability to detect BCR-ABL

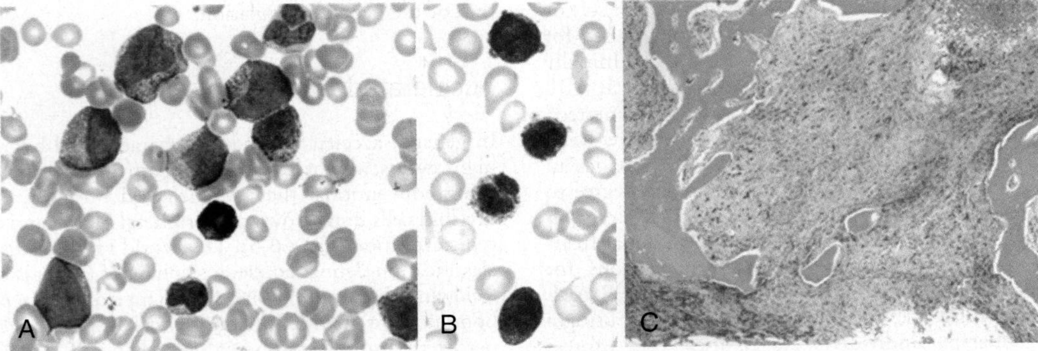

Figure 66-5 CHRONIC MYELOGENOUS LEUKEMIA, ACCELERATED PHASE. **A,** Peripheral smear showing increased immaturity in a case in which blasts were more than 10% of circulating leukocytes. **B,** Peripheral smear illustrating increased basophils, in a case in which basophils were more than 20% of circulating leukocytes. **C,** Bone core biopsy showing increased fibrosis and small dysplastic megakaryocyte. These findings are suggestive of accelerated phase.

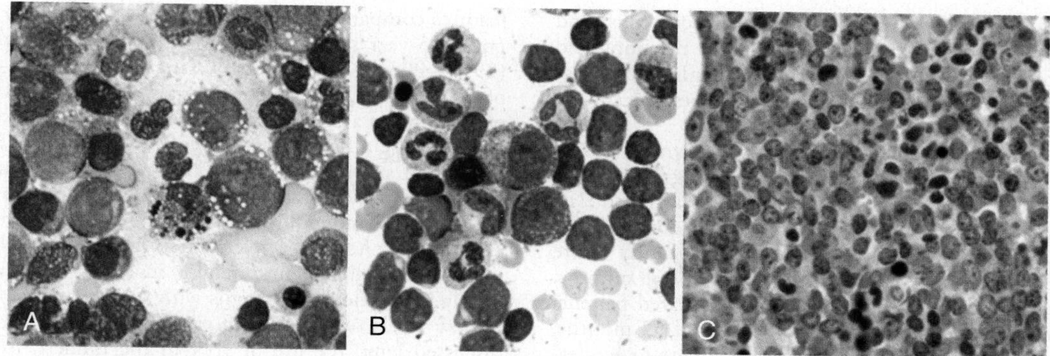

Figure 66-6 CHRONIC MYELOGENOUS LEUKEMIA, BLAST PHASE. **A,** Bone marrow aspirate showing myeloid blast phase associated with t(9;22) and inv(16). Note abnormal eosinophil *(center)*. **B,** Bone marrow aspirate showing lymphoid blast phase in the background of residual CML. **C,** Bone core biopsy illustrating focal blast phase.

Table 66-2 Response Definition and Monitoring

Hematologic Response	Cytogenetic Response	Molecular Response
Complete: Platelet count <450 × 10^9/L; WBC count <10 × 10^9/L; differential without immature granulocytes and with less than 5% basophils; nonpalpable spleen	Complete: Ph+ 0 Major: Ph+ 1%-35% Minor: Ph+ 36%-65 Minimal: Ph+ 66%-95% None: Ph+ <95%	Complete: BCR-ABL transcripts nonquantifiable and nondetectable* Major: ≤0.10%

BCR-ABL to control gene ratio according to the proposed international scale for measuring molecular response, with a standardized "baseline," as established in the IRIS trial, taken to represent 100% on the international scale, and a 3-log reduction from the standardized baseline (MMR) fixed at 0.10%.
*Qualified by the limit of sensitivity of the PCR assay employed.

mRNA depends on the sensitivity of the PCR assay, there is now consensus that CMR be defined based on assay sensitivity (e.g., $CMR^{4.0}$, where BCR-ABL mRNA levels are 0.01% or 4.0 log reduced).

Chemotherapy

Busulfan (BU) chemotherapy for CML was introduced in the 1950s. BU was administered in doses of 4 to 6 mg/day and then held when the WBC count fell to 30 × 10^9/L. The drug effect could persist for weeks, and the counts could fall further after therapy was discontinued. Busulfan therapy was associated with serious adverse effects, including prolonged aplasia, pulmonary fibrosis, and a syndrome simulating adrenal insufficiency.

Treatment with hydroxyurea (HU) was started as an alternative to busulfan. Hydroxyurea therapy is usually initiated at doses of 1 to 6 g/day in an attempt to lower counts. HU administered at doses of 1 to 2 g/day is then used to maintain blood counts in the normal range. Hydroxyurea is less toxic than busulfan. Its major adverse effect is reversible marrow suppression. In randomized trials, hydroxyurea was shown to prolong survival of patients with chronic-phase CML when compared with BU therapy. Median survival of hydroxyurea-treated patients was 5 years compared with 3.75-year median survival of busulfan-treated patients. Because neither drug results in significant selective suppression of the Ph-positive clone, the aim of therapy with these agents is to control disease and symptoms. Hydroxyurea is now commonly used to achieve control of counts simultaneous with, or prior to, initiation of treatment with imatinib or other disease-specific therapies.

Several other chemotherapeutic agents can be used to reduce the white cell counts in CML. Low-dose cytosine arabinoside can be used either as an intermittent bolus or as a daily infusion to control disease in cases where neither HU nor BU is proving useful. Cytosine arabinoside has also been used in combination with other agents, including IFN and imatinib in an attempt to enhance response.

Hyperuricemia and hyperuricosuria are frequently encountered problems in newly diagnosed and relapsed CML patients. Allopurinol, given at a dose of 300 mg daily and adequate hydration should be started before initiating treatment. Allopurinol should be discontinued after the WBC count has been controlled.

Interferon

Pioneering observational studies initiated in the 1980s by investigators at the MD Anderson Cancer Center provided evidence for efficacy of IFN in CML and indicated a 70% to 80% probability of complete hematologic remission in selected CML patients. Initial research involved the use of human leukocyte IFN, but subsequent clinical studies used recombinant human interferon-α (rIFN-α). Recombinant interferon-γ (rIFN-γ) has been shown to be relatively ineffective for CML. The potential mechanisms by which IFN works in CML are not understood but may include inhibition of increased proliferation, correction of the adhesion defect of the malignant progenitor in CML, or stimulating an immune response to CML. Rates for complete and partial cytogenetic remissions range from 0% to 38%. Evidence exists for a dose-response relationship, with IFN doses of 4 to 5 million units/m^2/day more likely to achieve remission (and toxicity) than lower doses. Durable remissions are more common in young patients, those treated soon after diagnosis, patients with less advanced stage disease, and those with favorable prognostic outlook. Hematologic remissions usually occur within 1 to 3 months after starting IFN. The median time to complete cytogenetic response is 9 to 18 months but may occur after 4 years of therapy. Durable cytogenetic responses, some lasting as long as 10 years, are more common in patients who achieve a complete cytogenetic response compared with partial cytogenetic remission.

Virtually all patients receiving IFN experience constitutional adverse effects, and discontinuation of treatment as a result of toxicity is necessary for 4% to 18% of patients compared with 1% of those receiving hydroxyurea. Acute adverse effects are generally mild to moderate and include flu-like symptoms such as fever, chills, and malaise. A constellation of other more severe acute reactions and chronic complications can occur. Overall, the mechanisms underlying the toxic effects are not well understood, but adverse effects 'are usually dose- and duration-dependent.

Randomized studies show an improvement in survival rates in patients receiving IFN compared with patients receiving busulfan or hydroxyurea. An Italian multicenter study randomly assigned 218 patients to receive IFN and 104 patients to receive HU or BU (the control group). Cytogenetic remissions were significantly more common in the IFN group. After a median follow-up of 68 months, the observed 6-year survival rate was 50% for IFN-treated patients and 29% for controls, with median survivals of 72 and 52 months, respectively. The time for progression from chronic phase to accelerated or blast phase was lengthened from 45 months to more than 72 months. In a German multicenter study, 622 patients were randomized to receive IFN, BU, or HU. The 5-year survival rate in the IFN group (59%) exceeded that of the BU group (32%) but was not significantly higher than that of the HU group (44%). Much of the discrepancy between the Italian and German findings can be explained by differences in case mix and treatment regimens. Two other randomized trials also showed benefit for IFN treatment compared with chemotherapy. The UK Medical Research Council randomly assigned 293 patients to receive IFN and 294 patients to receive HU or BU. The 5-year survival rate was 52% for the IFN group and 34% for the control group. A Japanese randomized control trial compared IFN (80 patients) with BU (79 patients). Hematologic and cytogenetic remission rates did not differ significantly. After a median follow-up of 50 months, the predicted 5-year survival rate was 54% for patients receiving IFN and 32% for those receiving BU.

The added value of combining IFN with cytosine arabinoside was shown in a French multicenter trial, wherein 360 patients were randomly assigned to receive IFN combined with cytosine arabinoside (20 mg/m^2/day for 10 days) and 361 patients to receive only IFN. After 3 years, the survival rate was 86% with IFN and cytosine arabinoside and 79% with IFN alone. The rate of hematologic response was higher in the IFN–cytosine arabinoside group than in the IFN group. Major cytogenetic responses were observed 12 months after randomization in 41% of patients treated with IFN-cytosine arabinoside and in 24% of patients treated with IFN only.

Thus accumulated evidence from randomized trials suggests that IFN improves survival in chronic-phase patients with favorable features compared with BU and HU. Metaanalysis suggests that the pooled 5-year survival rate is 57% (50%-59%) for IFN and 42% (29%-44%) for chemotherapy, which results from a delay in the onset of blast crisis. The controlled trials suggest that IFN increases life expectancy by a median of approximately 20 months compared with BU and HU. There is no direct evidence that IFN has a greater impact on survival than does HU for patients who are in the later stages of chronic phase (e.g., more than 1 year after diagnosis) or for those who are more ill (e.g., more than 10% to 30% blasts in peripheral blood). Adding cytosine arabinoside to IFN appears to add further survival benefit but also increases toxicity. Although IFN clearly is beneficial in patients with CML patients, benefit is limited by low levels of cytogenetic response and considerable toxicity. As discussed later, the use of IFN in the modern treatment of CML patients has been replaced by use of imatinib and other tyrosine kinase inhibitors.

Tyrosine Kinase Inhibitor Treatment

Because the tyrosine kinase activity of BCR-ABL plays a critical role in cellular transformation, it is an attractive target for inhibition. The introduction of TKIs into clinical practice has dramatically changed CML treatment. Tyrosine kinase inhibitor therapy, now the mainstay of treatment, is remarkably effective for chronic-phase CML, inducing remissions in most patients and leading to excellent survival. Tyrosine kinase inhibitor resistance can occur, especially in accelerated phase and blast crisis CML, usually as a result of tyrosine kinase domain point mutations. Resistance to imatinib can often be treated by "second generation" TKIs, dasatinib, or nilotinib, and there is evidence that these drugs may be even more effective than imatinib for front-line treatment of CML. Molecular endpoints that correlate with long-term outcomes have been developed and have been incorporated into guidelines to monitor response to tyrosine kinase inhibitors treatment (see box on Can Tyrosine Kinase Inhibitor Treatment Cure Chronic Myeloid Leukemia?).

Imatinib Mesylate

Imatinib mesylate is a small, 2-phenylaminopyrimidine molecule that inhibits the kinase activity of all proteins that contain ABL,

Can Tyrosine Kinase Inhibitor Treatment Cure Chronic Myeloid Leukemia?

An increasing proportion of CML patients treated with tyrosine kinase inhibitors may not have detectable levels of the BCR-ABL gene, even with sensitive PCR assays. This raises the question as to whether patients can actually be cured with tyrosine inhibitor treatment. Patients with negative PCR may still have significant numbers of residual malignant cells. The definition of a *cure* remains controversial. Although *cure* might theoretically require the total eradication of all leukemia cells, it can be argued that patients may be considered cured if low numbers of leukemia cells still persist but are not expected to be able to reestablish clinical disease. Such a situation may occur in CML after allogeneic transplantation in which a graft-versus-leukemia effect may help maintain remission. In AML associated with the t(8;21), many long-term survivors continue to demonstrate molecular evidence of this translocation. On the other hand, late relapses can be observed in patients with childhood ALL more than 10 years after remission, with molecular evidence that the relapse originated from the same clone that caused the disease originally.

Therefore it is important to consider whether BCR-ABL–expressing cells that escape elimination with imatinib include cells with leukemogenic potential. Mathematical modeling of the effect of imatinib on different hematopoietic cell compartments in CML suggests that leukemia stem cells are resistant to elimination by this drug. This is supported by evidence that BCR-ABL–positive stem and progenitor cells are retained in patients in CCR on imatinib treatment, including patients with sustained undetectable molecular evidence of disease by RT-PCR. In vitro treatment with tyrosine kinase inhibitors inhibits proliferation of CML primitive progenitors but only modestly increases apoptosis. Similarly, tyrosine kinase inhibitor treatment fails to eradicate primitive leukemia cells in a mouse model of CML. These observations suggest that TKI treatment does not eliminate primitive leukemogenic cells. On the other hand, some patients can maintain a BCR-ABL–negative status for more than 1 year following discontinuation of imatinib treatment. Although the long-term durability and frequency of such responses are not clear at present, these observations suggest that additional factors related to the frequency and leukemogenic potential of residual cells, or immune or microenvironmental factors determine the risk for relapse after discontinuation of tyrosine kinase inhibitor treatment.

In the future, a better understanding of these factors will allow for improved prediction of patients in whom treatment can be safely stopped. In addition, better understanding of the mechanisms underlying persistence of leukemogenic cells may allow development of improved strategies to enhance the number of CML patients in whom TKI treatment can be stopped and who are considered effectively "cured."

ABL-related gene (ARG) protein, or platelet-derived growth factor receptor, as well as the KIT receptor, at micromole concentrations.[6] Imatinib is a competitive inhibitor that acts at the ATP-binding site in the kinase domain to inhibit the normal binding of ATP and blocks the ability of BCR-ABL to phosphorylate tyrosine residues on its substrates (Fig. 66-7).

Initial phase 1 and phase 2 trials established that imatinib was well tolerated and induced hematologic as well as cytogenetic response in the majority of patients with chronic-phase CML in whom other treatments had failed.[7] In a phase II study, 532 chronic-phase patients who were refractory to or intolerant of IFN-α were treated with imatinib at a dose of 400 mg daily. A CHR was achieved in 95% of patients, major cytogenetic remission (MCR) in 60% of patients, and CCR in 41% of patients. With a median follow-up of 18 months, the estimated progression-free survival was 89%. Only 2% of patients discontinued therapy because of adverse events.

Subsequently the International Randomized Interferon and STI571 (IRIS) study compared imatinib at 400 mg daily with IFN-α plus cytosine arabinoside in 1106 newly diagnosed patients in first chronic phase. This study was closed with the conclusion that imatinib is the initial nontransplant treatment of choice for patients with newly diagnosed chronic-phase CML. This conclusion was based primarily on a higher rate of disease progression in the patient group receiving IFN plus cytosine arabinoside. In the initial report from this study, after a median follow-up of 19 months, the estimated rate of an MCR at 18 months was 87.1% (95% CI, 84.1-90.0) in the imatinib group and 34.7% (95% CI, 29.3-40.0) in the IFN plus cytosine arabinoside group (P <0.001).[8] The estimated rates of CCR were 76.2% (95% CI, 72.5-79.9) and 14.5% (95% CI, 10.5-18.5), respectively (P <0.001). At 18 months, the estimated rate of freedom from progression to accelerated-phase or blast-crisis CML was 96.7% in the imatinib group and 91.5% in the IFN group (P <0.001). Imatinib was better tolerated than combination therapy. In a subsequent 60-month follow-up report for this study, the estimated cumulative incidence rate of CHR, MCR, and CCR for patients on first-line imatinib was 98%, 92%, and 87% at 60 months (Fig. 66-8). Only 7% of patients progressed to advanced phase, and the estimated overall survival was 89%. Crossover between arms was permitted for treatment failure, and 382 (69%) of 553 patients originally allocated to the IFN/cytarabine arm crossed over to the imatinib arm at a median of 60 months from start of treatment. The main reason for crossover from IFN to imatinib was intolerance of treatment, but reasons also included disease progression and failure to achieve hematologic or cytogenetic response. During the sixth year of study treatment, there were no further reports of disease progression and the toxicity profile remained unchanged. Of all patients randomized to receive imatinib and still on study treatment, 63% showed CCR at last assessment. The estimated event-free survival at 6 years was 83%, and the estimated overall survival was 88%.[9]

A dose of 400 mg of imatinib daily is currently the standard dose for initiating therapy in newly diagnosed chronic-phase patients. Nonrandomized studies suggested that patients receiving initial therapy with 800 mg imatinib daily will achieve CCR more rapidly than patients receiving standard 400-mg daily doses. The Tyrosine Kinase Inhibitor Optimization and Selectivity (TOPS) study compared imatinib 800 mg/day (n = 319) to 400 mg/day (n = 157). Higher-dose imatinib provided faster response CCR rates at 6 months (57% versus 45%, respectively), but there was no significant difference between the arms at 12 months (70% versus 66%, respectively) or 24 months (76% in both groups). Similarly, no difference in EFS, progression-free survival (PFS), or overall survival was seen. However, a subset of patients who can tolerate higher doses of imatinib, without interruptions for side effects, can have a better response.[10]

Cumulative response estimates do not take into account patients who have left the study for a variety of reasons. It is also clear that the results of imatinib therapy in the community setting are less favorable. Thus only 55% of patients treated with first-line

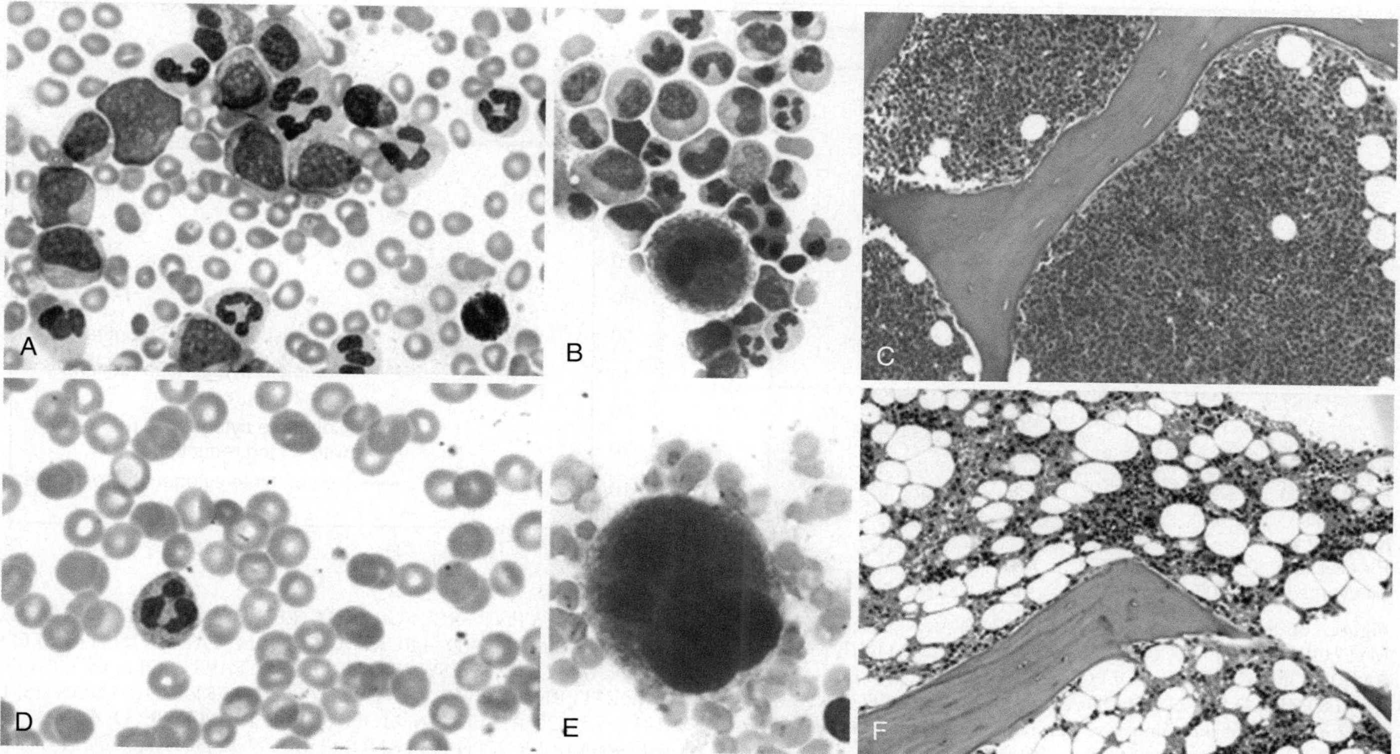

Figure 66-7 CHRONIC MYELOGENOUS LEUKEMIA, BEFORE AND 3 MONTHS AFTER IMATINIB THERAPY. Chronic-phase CML, as seen in the peripheral blood **(A)**, aspirate **(B)**, and biopsy **(C)**, and after 3 months of imatinib therapy (**D** to **F**). Note normalization of white cell count **(D)**, megakaryocyte size **(E)**, and marrow cellularity **(F)**.

imatinib in the IRIS study were still receiving imatinib at follow-up of 8 years, while the remainder had discontinued therapy as a result of inadequate therapeutic effect or toxicity. A report from the Hammersmith Hospital, which defined imatinib failure more broadly than the IRIS study as discontinuation of drug for any reason, including toxicity as well as a lack of major cytogenetic response, calculated 5 years EFS at only 63%.[11]

Comparison of health-related quality of life (QOL) of imatinib-treated patients and the general population indicated marked impairments of QOL in younger patients, especially between 18 and 39 years, related to physical and emotional problems. Women had worse QOL than men. The most frequently reported symptom was fatigue. Patients older than 60 years had QOL similar to that of the general population.[12]

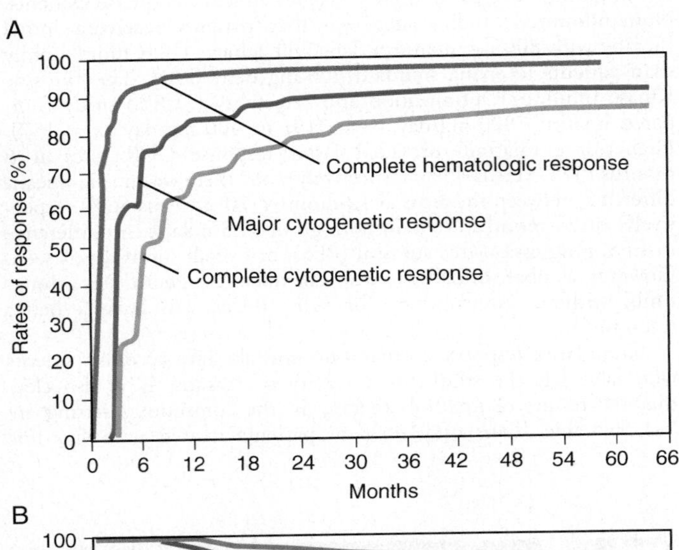

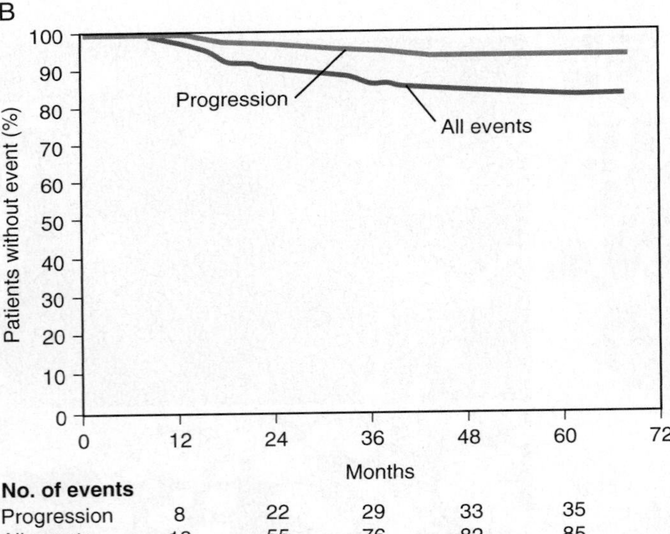

	12	24	36	48	60
No. of events					
Progression	8	22	29	33	35
All events	18	55	76	82	85
No. at risk					
Progression	513	461	431	409	280
All events	505	447	414	395	274

Figure 66-8 RESPONSE OF NEWLY DIAGNOSED CHRONIC MYELOID LEUKEMIA (CML) PATIENTS TO IMATINIB MESYLATE BASED ON 5 YEARS' FOLLOW-UP ON THE INTERNATIONAL RANDOMIZED INTERFERON AND STI571 (IRIS) STUDY. **A,** Kaplan-Meier estimates of the cumulative best response to initial imatinib therapy. **B,** Kaplan-Meier estimates of the rates of event-free survival and progression to the accelerated phase or blast crisis of CML for patients receiving imatinib. *(Data from Druker BJ, Guilhot F, O'Brien SG, et al: Five-year follow-up of patients receiving imatinib for chronic myeloid leukemia,* N Engl J Med *355:2408, 2006.)*

Prognostic Indicators

Pretreatment risk factors can predict the likelihood of achieving and maintaining response to imatinib. At 60 months, the estimated risk for disease progression was significantly higher for patients with a higher pretreatment Sokal score (estimated rates for high-risk, intermediate-risk, and low-risk groups of 17%, 8%, and 3%, respectively; $P<0.002$).

The achievement of certain milestones of response can also predict prognosis. For example, patients who do not experience a complete hematologic response by 3 months of treatment, any cytogenetic response by 6 months, or a major cytogenetic response by 12 months do poorly in comparison with patients achieving these milestones. Reduction of BCR-ABL levels observed with cytogenetic and quantitative PCR monitoring is also predictive of prognosis (Fig. 66-9). A landmark analysis indicated that at 60 months, 97% of the patients (95% CI, 94 to 99) who had achieved CCR at 12 months after the initiation of imatinib treatment (n = 350) had not progressed to accelerated phase or blast crisis (see Fig. 66-9). For patients who did not have an MCR within 12 months ($n = 73$), the estimate was 81% (95% CI, 70-92; P <0.001). Of interest, the Sokal score was not

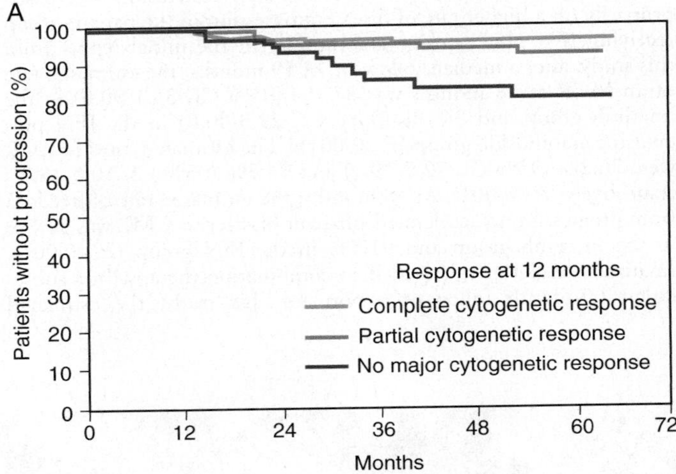

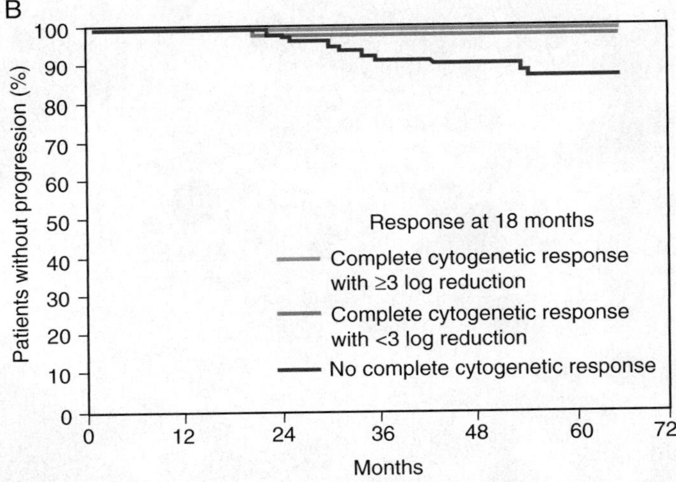

Figure 66-9 EVENT FREE SURVIVAL (EFS) OF NEWLY DIAGNOSED CHRONIC MYELOID LEUKEMIA (CML) PATIENTS TREATED WITH IMATINIB MESYLATE AFTER 7 YEARS' FOLLOW-UP ON THE INTERNATIONAL RANDOMIZED INTERFERON AND STI571 (IRIS) STUDY BASED ON MOLECULAR RESPONSE AT 6- **(A),** 12- **(B),** AND 18-MONTH **(C)** LANDMARKS. *(Data from Hughes TP, Hochhaus A, Branford S, et al: Long-term prognostic significance of early molecular response to imatinib in newly diagnosed chronic myeloid leukemia: An analysis from the International Randomized Study of Interferon and STI571 (IRIS),* Blood *116:3758, 2010.)*

predictive of risk for disease progression in patients who had a complete cytogenetic response (95%, 95%, and 99% in the high-risk, intermediate-risk, and low-risk groups, respectively; $P = 0.20$). The prognostic significance of molecular responses at 6-, 12-, and 18-month in predicting event-free survival (EFS) and time to progression to accelerated phase/blast crisis at 7 years was evaluated in the IRIS cohort. Patients with BCR-ABL mRNA levels >10% at 6 months and >1% at 12 months using the international scale had inferior EFS and higher rate of progression compared with all other molecular response groups. Conversely, patients who achieved major molecular response (BCR-ABL [IS] <0.1%) by 18 months enjoyed durable responses, with no progression, 95% EFS, and only 3% probability of loss of CCyR at 7 years.[13] An analysis from the Hammersmith group, patients with BCR-ABL mRNA levels >9.84% at 3 months had significantly lower 8-year probabilities of OS (56.9% versus 93.3%; $P < 0.001$), progression-free survival, cumulative incidence of CCyR, and complete molecular response than those with higher levels. Similarly, BCR-ABL mRNA levels >1.67% at 6 months and >0.53% at 12 months also identified patients at increased risk for progression.[14] These results indicate a strong association between the degree of reduction of BCR-ABL transcript numbers and long-term clinical outcome and have led to the adoption of time-dependent molecular response measurements in determining optimal response to therapy (Table 66-3).[15]

Lack of adherence to medication is a major underlying reason for failure of treatment. It has been reported, on multivariate analysis, that in CML patients treated with imatinib for some years, the adherence rate and failure to achieve a major molecular response were the only independent predictors for loss of CCR and discontinuation of imatinib, and poor adherence may be the predominant reason for inability to obtain adequate molecular responses.[16,17]

Results of Treatment in Accelerated Phase and Blast Crisis

A phase II study in accelerated-phase patients enrolled 235 patients. Some hematologic response was seen in 82% of patients, with 34% of patients achieving a CHR. A major cytogenetic response occurred in 24% of patients, with 17% complete responses. Estimated 12-month progression-free and overall survival rates were 59% and 74%, respectively.

A phase II study of 260 patients in myeloid blast crisis who were treated with imatinib showed an overall response rate of 52%, with sustained hematologic responses lasting at least 4 weeks in 31% of patients. Eight percent of patients achieved a complete remission with peripheral blood recovery. Another 4% of patients cleared their marrows to less than 5% blasts but did not meet the criteria for CR because of persistent cytopenias. Eighteen percent of patients either "returned" to chronic phase or had partial responses. Major cytogenetic responses were seen in 16% of patients, with 7% having complete cytogenetic responses. The median survival was 7 months. These results compare favorably with historical controls treated with chemotherapy for myeloid blast crisis in which the median survival is approximately 3 months. In patients with Ph-positive ALL, 29/48 (60%) responded to a single agent, imatinib. However, the duration of response was relatively short, with a median estimated time to disease progression of only 2 months.

Toxicity

Myelosuppression is particularly common in CML patients treated with imatinib and is more common in patients with advanced disease. In the phase III randomized trial of newly diagnosed patients in the chronic phase, grade 3 neutropenia (ANC <1000/mm^3) was experienced by 11% of patients, grade 4 neutropenia (ANC <500/mm^3) occurred in 2% of patients, grade 3 thrombocytopenia (platelets <50,000/mm^3) occurred in 6.9% of patients, and grade 4 thrombocytopenia (platelets <10,000/mm^3) occurred in less than 1% of patients. Myelosuppression can occur at any time during imatinib therapy, but it usually begins within the first 2 to 4 weeks of starting therapy for blast crisis, with a slightly later onset in patients in accelerated or chronic phase. Although grade 3 and 4 neutropenia is frequent, particularly in advanced phases, infectious complications are relatively rare, possibly related to the lack of mucous membrane

Table 66-3 Evaluation of Overall Response to Imatinib First-Line in Early Chronic Phase

	Response			
Evaluation Time (Months)	**Optimal**	**Suboptimal**	**Failure**	**Warnings**
Baseline	NA	NA	NA	High risk; CCA/Ph+*
3	CHR and at least minor CyR (Ph+ ≤65%)	No CyR (Ph+ >95%)	Less than CHR	NA
6	At least PCyR (Ph+ ≤35%)	Less than PCyR (Ph+ >35%)	No CyR (Ph+ >95%)	NA
12	CCR	PCyR (Ph+ 1%-35%)	Less than PCyR (Ph+ >35%)	Less than MMR†
18	MMR†	Less than MMR†	Less than CCR	NA
Any time during treatment	Stable or improving MMR†	Loss of MMR†; mutations‡	Loss of CHR; loss of CCR; mutations§; CCA/Ph+	Increase in transcript levels‖; CCA/Ph+

From Baccarani M, Cortes J, Pane F, et al: Chronic myeloid leukemia: An update of concepts and management recommendations of European LeukemiaNet, *J Clin Oncol* 27:6041, 2009.

CCA, clonal chromosome abnormalities; *CCR,* complete cytogenetic response; *CHR,* complete hematologic response; *CyR,* cytogenetic response; *MMR,* major molecular response; *NA,* Not applicable; *PCyR,* partial cytogenetic response; *Ph+,* Philadelphia chromosome positive.

*CCA/Ph+ is a warning factor at diagnosis, although its occurrence during treatment (i.e., clonal progression) is a marker of treatment failure. Two consecutive cytogenetic tests are required and must show the same CCA in at least two Ph+ cells.

†MMR indicates a ratio of BCR-ABL1 to ABL1 or other housekeeping genes of ≤0.1% on the international scale.

‡BCR-ABL1 kinase domain mutations still sensitive to imatinib.

§BCR-ABL1 kinase domain mutations poorly sensitive to imatinib.

‖The significance of the increase may vary by a factor of 2 to 10, depending on the laboratories.

Treatment recommendations:

- Optimal: Continue imatinib 400 mg/day.
- Suboptimal: Continue imatinib same dose; or test high-dose imatinib, dasatinib, or nilotinib.
- Failure: Dasatinib or nilotinib; third-generation agents or alloHSCT in patients who carry the T315I mutation; alloHSCT in patients who have experienced progression to AP/BP.

damage in patients on imatinib. Central nervous system and gastrointestinal hemorrhages may occur, most frequently in patients in blast crisis with platelet counts less than 20,000 and with uncontrolled leukemia. The primary goal in treating otherwise healthy patients in chronic phase is to avoid the risk for potentially dangerous neutropenia and platelet transfusion dependence. For patients with blast crisis or high-risk accelerated-phase disease (>15% blasts), a suggested approach is to balance risks and benefits, and support patients with a platelet count under 10,000/mm^3 or under 50,000/mm^3 with clinically evident bleeding with platelet transfusions. In the event of clinically significant bleeding, imatinib should be held immediately, until the bleeding is controlled. In patients whose absolute neutrophil count is less than 500/mm^3, imatinib should be continued if the marrow is hypercellular or if there are >30% blasts. In cases where the marrow is hypocellular and the ANC is <500/mm^3 for 2 to 4 weeks, imatinib may be held, the dose may be reduced, or myeloid growth factors can be used. Concurrent administration of growth factors and imatinib is well tolerated, and patients have not experienced a greater rate of relapse.[18]

The most common nonhematologic adverse events related to imatinib were nausea, muscle cramps, fluid retention, diarrhea, musculoskeletal pain, fatigue, and skin rashes. Only a minority of patients experienced grade 3 or 4 toxicity, and there was a low rate of discontinuance of therapy because of toxicity of 5%, 3%, and 2% in the phase II studies for blast crisis, accelerated phase, and chronic phase, respectively. The higher rate of severe toxicity in patients with advanced-phase disease may relate to the higher doses administered or to the poorer underlying health of patients. Most adverse effects can be managed successfully with supportive measures. Some toxicities (e.g., mild skin rashes, mild elevations of transaminases, bone pain, and arthralgias) may improve spontaneously despite continued therapy at the same dosage.

Imatinib Resistance

Both de novo and acquired resistance have been observed in imatinib-treated CML patients. The most commonly described mechanisms associated with resistance are point mutations in the BCR-ABL gene that prevent imatinib from inhibiting kinase activity and BCR-ABL gene amplification. BCR-ABL-independent mechanisms may also play a role in imatinib resistance in some patients. Activation of the SRC family kinases, LYN, has been demonstrated in cells from patients with acquired imatinib resistance. The Sawyers group, in an original study of nine patients who relapsed on imatinib treatment, detected BCR-ABL gene amplification in three patients and kinase domain mutations in six. Relapse was associated with reactivation of BCR-ABL kinase activity. Subsequent studies have shown that there are >90 different amino acid substitutions detected in imatinib-resistant patients ones (see Fig. 66-1), occurring with varying frequency.[19] The different mutations conferred varying degrees of imatinib resistance. In patients with stable chronic-phase disease, detection of mutations correlated with subsequent disease progression. Mutations have been found in some patients before the start of treatment, supporting a model in which preexisting BCR-ABL mutations that confer imatinib resistance acquire a selective clonal growth advantage during imatinib treatment.

Intensive efforts have been made to characterize the biologic and clinical significance of BCR-ABL kinase mutations and to develop kinase inhibitors with efficacy against the maximum number of mutants. The structure of the ABL kinase domain in complex with imatinib has been solved. This information sheds light on the mechanisms by which kinase domain mutations confer drug resistance. Mutations may affect residues that directly contact imatinib, such as a mutation resulting in substitution of isoleucine for threonine in the T315 position (T315I). Mutations in the P-loop of the ABL kinase prevent conformational changes required for imatinib binding. Imatinib captures and stabilizes the ABL kinase in its inactive conformation, but is sterically excluded from the active conformation. The M351T mutation and mutations in the activation loop result in the kinase remaining in the active conformation rather than the inactive conformation required for imatinib binding. Clinical experience with the second-generation TKIs dasatinib and nilotinib demonstrates that a much narrower spectrum of mutations retain insensitivity to these agents. These mutations are nonoverlapping, with the exception of the T315I mutation.

Knowledge of BCR-ABL mutation status is being integrated into therapeutic decision-making algorithms for patients. The European Leukemia Net guidelines for the use of mutation testing in management of CML patients recommends mutation testing in chronic-phase CML patients receiving first-line imatinib treatment only in case of failure or suboptimal response. Mutation analysis is recommended in imatinib-resistant patients receiving an alternative TKI in case of hematologic or cytogenetic failure.[19]

Second-Generation Tyrosine Kinase Inhibitors

Because the active conformations of ABL and SRC bear a high degree of structural similarity, compounds with SRC kinase inhibitory activity have been evaluated against native and mutant BCR-ABL. BMS-354825 (dasatinib, Sprycel) is a dual SRC-ABL kinase inhibitor that exhibits approximately 300-fold higher potency against native BCR-ABL. Dasatinib can effectively inhibit most clinically detected BCR-ABL kinase domain mutants at low nanomolar concentrations, with the notable exception of T315I. Another compound, AMN107 (nilotinib) was generated by rational modification of imatinib to enhance BCR-ABL kinase binding activity. Nilotinib binds ABL but with significantly increased avidity and can overcome resistance of most kinase domain mutants, with the exception of T315I. It is evident, however, that both agents have significant activity in imatinib-resistant CML. Of note, responses occurred in patients with and without BCR-ABL kinase domain mutations at trial entry, with the exception of patients with the T315I mutation. Responses in chronic phase and, to a lesser extent, in accelerated phase have been stable. In contrast, many patients with myeloid, and all patients with lymphoid, blast crisis, or Ph-positive ALL have relapsed. These data are similar to the results of the initial studies with imatinib and indicate that once the disease has progressed beyond the chronic phase, tyrosine kinase inhibitor-based monotherapy is not sufficient to induce lasting responses. Both dasatinib and nilotinib are approved for the treatment of patients with CML that is resistant to imatinib and those who are intolerant to the drug. Both agents are quite effective in resistant disease, yielding CCR in approximately 50% of chronic phase cases (for cases who discontinue imatinib because of drug intolerance, the CCR rates are >70%).

Because of this strong clinical activity, both drugs have been tried as first-line therapy in newly diagnosed chronic-phase CML. Two single-center trials of dasatinib and nilotinib have been performed at M.D. Anderson. At 18 to 24 months, both agents showed a similarly small, but consistent benefit in CCR over historical controls treated on imatinib trials. An Italian phase II study of nilotinib in newly diagnosed chronic phase cases showed a similarly high rate of CCR of >90% after 12 months of therapy. Dasatinib and nilotinib were compared with imatinib for frontline treatment of chronic phase CML. The Dasatinib Versus Imatinib Study in Treatment-Naïve CML (DASISION) study tested 100 mg dasatinib daily versus 400 mg imatinib daily.[20] The Evaluating Nilotinib Efficacy and Safety in Clinical Trials Newly Diagnosed Patients (ENESTnd) study compared two nilotinib doses (400 mg twice daily and 300 mg twice daily) with imatinib 400 mg daily.[21] Both studies found the experimental arms (dasatinib and nilotinib) to be superior to imatinib in achieving the primary endpoints (dasatinib: CCR by 12 months; nilotinib: MMR at 12 months). Patients treated with nilotinib had a significantly reduced risk for progression. Based on these results, both nilotinib and dasatinib were approved for frontline therapy of newly diagnosed chronic-phase CML patients in the United States in 2010.

The choice of TKI in newly diagnosed patients remains open to debate. Dasatinib and nilotinib are associated with faster and deeper reduction in leukemia burden. On the other hand, no differences in

OS have been observed yet, although follow-up is required and long-term data from the randomized clinical studies are needed to confirm the initial findings. Imatinib is less expensive, and there is longer experience with its use. A direct comparison between nilotinib and dasatinib has not been performed. Since their overall efficacy appears to be similar, the selection may be based primarily on side effect profile and convenience. Dasatinib treatment is associated with higher rates of myelosuppression and with pericardial and pleural effusion. In contrast, nilotinib can induce an increase in pancreatic enzymes, although radiographic/clinical pancreatitis is rarely noted. Hyperglycemia and hyperbilirubinemia are observed in some nilotinib-treated patients. Skin rash also is a prominent side effect of nilotinib therapy, but this is usually moderate and/or resolves spontaneously. Severe, uncontrolled diabetes and past pancreatitis may be considered as risk factors for nilotinib use, whereas patients with a history of hypertension, asthma, pneumonia, gastrointestinal bleeding, chronic obstructive pulmonary disease, congestive heart failure, autoimmune disorders, or concomitant aspirin use may be at increased risk for pleural and pericardial effusions, bleeding, and infection with dasatinib.

Drugs Targeting the T315I Mutation

The fact that the T315I mutant is not responsive to either dasatinib or nilotinib and that this mutant has been detected in some patients with acquired resistance to dasatinib and nilotinib underscores the need for drugs with T315I inhibitory activity.[22] Ponatinib is a multi-targeted kinase inhibitor active against all BCR-ABL mutants, including T315I. In a phase I study, more than 50% of patients in chronic phase, mostly patients in whom two or more TKIs had failed, attained CCR.[22,23] The CCR rate approached 100% in patients with the T315I mutation. Responses were less frequent and less stable in patients with advanced disease. The BCR-ABL switch pocket inhibitor DCC-2036 binds to an allosteric site in the enzyme and is also active against a broad spectrum of kinase domain mutants, including T315I.[24] This agent is undergoing clinical evaluation.

Residual Disease in Patients Treated With Tyrosine Kinase Inhibitors

Currently, the reverse-transcriptase polymerase chain reaction (RT-PCR) is the most sensitive method for detecting low numbers of BCR-ABL transcripts in a patient after apparently successful hematopoietic cell transplantation. Most patients who have been treated with imatinib and have responded well continue to demonstrate evidence of residual disease using sensitive PCR assays. Recent updates of clinical trials of imatinib in CP CML patients indicate that an increasing proportion of patients appear to enter a molecular remission over time, including some patients achieving a PCR-undetectable status. However, even patients with negative PCR (so-called complete molecular response) may still have significant numbers of residual malignant cells. Several groups have identified BCR-ABL–expressing leukemia stem cells in patients with sustained undetectable molecular residual remission. The French STIM (*St*op *IM*atinib) trial evaluated outcomes after imatinib discontinuation in patients with sustained undetectable MRD for more than 2 years. Approximately 40% of patients did not develop molecular recurrence after 1 year.[25] However, molecular relapse occurred in a substantial proportion of even this highly selected population. Patients with undetectable MRD after imatinib therapy continued to have BCR-ABL rearrangement detectable at the genomic level, indicating persistence of residual leukemic cells not detected by RT-PCR. It is important to note that residual leukemic cells with leukemia-initiating capacity have been shown to persist in CML patients in sustained molecular remission on imatinib.[26] Together, these data suggest that imatinib alone may not be capable of eradicating the leukemic cell clone, and at present, patients are recommended to continue medication indefinitely.

Allogeneic Hematopoietic Cell Transplantation

The Seattle team reported initial results of HLA-matched sibling donor hematopoietic cell transplants performed as therapy for 10 CML patients in 1982, and subsequently published a larger study on 167 patients transplanted from matched siblings through 1983. Long-term follow-up demonstrates that approximately 40% of patients transplanted in chronic phase nearly 20 years ago are surviving. Hematopoietic cell transplant became the first curative treatment in CML. Data from 4267 recipients of matched-sibling transplants reported to the IBMTR between 1994 and 1999 show a probability of survival of 69% ± 2% for 2876 patients transplanted within the first year from diagnosis, and 57% ± 3% for 1391 patients transplanted more than 1 year from diagnosis. Contemporary results from selected single institutions continue to demonstrate excellent outcomes with HCT, in part because of advances in preparative regimens, supportive care, and HLA typing for unrelated donors (Fig. 66-10). For example, the Seattle group has recently reported on their most recent trial using a preparative regimen of targeted busulfan plus cyclophosphamide (CY) in 131 consecutive chronic-phase CML patients. Survival 3 years posttransplant was 86%, and 87% of surviving patients were molecularly negative for BCR-ABL.

The outcome of allogeneic HCT in CML is influenced by many factors, the most important of which is the phase of disease. Other

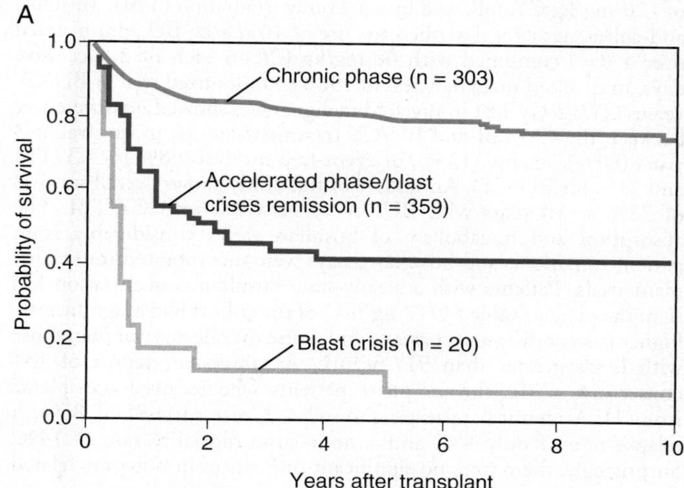

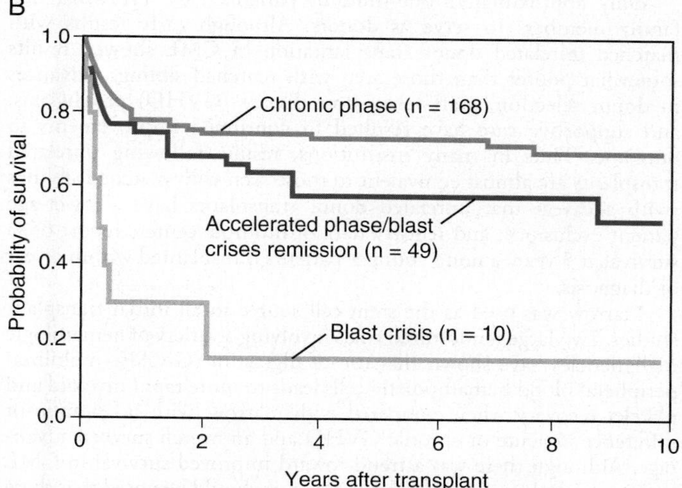

Figure 66-10 Probability of survival following **(A)** related donor transplantation and **(B)** unrelated donor transplantation for chronic myelogenous leukemia (CML), chronic phase (CP), accelerated phase (AP), and blast crisis (BC) performed after 1992, at the FHCRC, Seattle.

important variables include the type of donor used (related or unrelated), the source of the stem cell product (marrow or peripheral blood), and the age of the patient. Outcomes are superior for HCT in chronic phase compared with advanced phases of disease. In a Seattle analysis of 58 patients with accelerated-phase CML who received transplants from HLA-identical siblings, the 4-year probabilities of survival and event-free survival were 49 and 43%, and the probability of relapse was 12%. The outcome of transplantation for patients in blast crisis is uniformly poor, resulting in a high rate of disease recurrence and transplant-related deaths with event-free survivals of 43%, 18%, and 11% at 100 days, 1 year, and 3 years, respectively. Before the development of imatinib, only a small proportion of patients with blast-phase CML (generally, patients with lymphoid blast crisis) could achieve a hematologic remission with chemotherapy. Transplantation for patients with CML in remission after a previous blast phase results in cure rates somewhat worse than those seen in chronic-phase patients. Response rates of patients with CML in blast phase to imatinib are considerably higher than those seen with conventional chemotherapy. These responses tend to be short, particularly in the setting of lymphoid blast crisis. Limited data are available on the outcome of transplantation for patients with previous blast crisis who are once again in remission following treatment with imatinib, but these few patients seem to have a progression-free survival at 3 years of over 50%.

Preparative regimens have improved incrementally. The majority of patients treated in the early 1980s received a preparative regimen of 120 mg/kg CY, followed by total body irradiation (TBI). Tutschka and colleagues later described the use of 16 mg/kg BU administered over 4 days combined with 60 mg/kg CY on each of 2 successive days, in myeloid malignancies. In 1988 a randomized trial of BU/CY versus CY/12 Gy TBI in myeloid malignancies showed no differences between the CY/TBI and BU/CY treatment groups in survival at 3 years (80%), relapse (13%), or event-free survival (68% for CY/TBI and 71% for BU/CY). An update of this study shows overall survival of 78% at 10 years with BU/CY versus 64% with CY/TBI. The absorption and metabolism of busulfan varies considerably from patient to patient, and busulfan assays were incorporated into transplant trials. Patients with a steady-state busulfan concentration less than the median value (<917 ng/mL) of the cohort had a significantly higher risk for disease recurrence and worse overall survival than those with levels greater than 917 ng/mL. A subsequent report of 131 consecutive CML chronic-phase patients who received transplants from HLA-identical relatives showed a 3-year survival of 86%, a relapse rate of only 8%, and a nonrelapse mortality rate of 14%. Surprisingly, there were no significant differences in outcome related to patient age up to 65 years of age.

Only approximately one-third of patients have HLA-matched family members to serve as donors. Although early results with matched unrelated donor transplantation in CML showed results somewhat poorer than those seen with matched siblings, advances in donor selection, graft-versus-host disease (GVHD) prophylaxis, and supportive care have resulted in continued improvements in outcome. Thus in many institutions, results following unrelated transplants are almost equivalent to those seen with matched siblings (with a caveat that unrelated donor transplants have a lower-age patient exclusion), and registry data of multiple centers report 65% survival at 5 years among younger patients transplanted within a year of diagnosis.

Marrow was used as the stem cell source in all initial transplant studies. Two large randomized trials involving a variety of hematologic malignancies have shown that use of filgrastim (G-CSF)–mobilized peripheral blood hematopoietic cells leads to more rapid myeloid and platelet recovery when compared with marrow, with no significant difference in acute or chronic GVHD and an overall survival advantage. Although there was a trend toward improved survival in CML patients with the use of peripheral blood, it should be noted that these studies were not prospectively designed to address the role of peripheral blood versus marrow for individual disease states. Furthermore, the results of a randomized study of chronic-phase CML showed no statistically significant differences in outcome between the marrow and peripheral blood groups, though relapse rates were lower in the peripheral blood group and chronic GVHD occurrence was higher compared with patients transplanted with marrow.

Several studies have shown that an increased interval from diagnosis to transplant is associated with a worse transplant outcome, for patients treated in chronic phase. No single cause of failure is markedly increased with delay; rather there is a modest effect of delay on relapse rate and nonrelapse mortality. Thus the delay effect may be due in part to the advancing disease over time and/or the effect of the cumulative toxicity of prior therapy. An IBMTR report suggested that exposure to low-dose busulfan led to a worse outcome with subsequent transplantation. Reports have suggested that exposure to IFN might worsen the outcome of unrelated donor transplant, but data on the effect of IFN on matched-sibling transplantation were less clear. In a recent German report, the 5-year survival rate from transplant was 46% for the 50 patients who received IFN within the last 90 days before transplant and 71% for the 36 patients who did not. These observations suggest that IFN should be avoided, if possible, in the months immediately preceding allogeneic hematopoietic cell transplantation.

The form of GVHD prophylaxis used in the treatment regimens also influences the outcome of transplantation for CML, especially in chronic phase. Prevention of GHVD by removing T cells from the donor marrow was explored in a number of transplant studies in the 1980s. Although successful in reducing the incidence of GVHD, T-cell depletion in CML was associated with high rates of graft failure and relapse, leading to poorer disease-free and overall survival. These findings illustrated the critical role of the graft-versus-leukemia (GVL) effect in eradicating CML following allogeneic transplantation. Because of these observations, T-cell depletion was largely abandoned as a method to control GVHD in CML transplants. However, there has been renewed interest in the possibility of preventing GVHD without loss of a GVL effect by combining T-cell depletion with an intensified conditioning regimen and delayed reinfusion of viable donor lymphocytes.

Several studies have investigated the effect of prior imatinib and transplant outcomes. Early reports warned of an increase in regimen-related toxicity and mortality, especially from hepatic causes. Larger studies have failed to show a deleterious effect of pretransplant imatinib (Fig. 66-11). A study of only CML patients showed no difference in regimen-related mortality, survival, or relapse between 140 patients who received imatinib versus 200 historical controls. Curiously, in a few studies, the incidence of chronic GVHD has been significantly lower in patients receiving imatinib before transplant. However, an analysis from the CIBMTR of CML patients undergoing allogeneic transplantation showed that the cumulative incidence rates of acute and chronic GVHD and treatment related mortality (TRM) were not affected by prehematopoietic stem cell transplantation (SCT) IM exposure. On multivariate analysis conventional prognostic indicators remained the strongest determinants of transplant outcomes.[27] The biology underlying this effect is unknown. Allogeneic transplantation appears to be an effective treatment for T315I-mutated leukemias, providing acceptable survival rates with long-term control of the malignancy without detectable residual disease in some cases.[28]

In the period before the advent of tyrosine kinase inhibitors, allogeneic transplant was the front-line treatment of choice for CML, especially for younger patients. With the firm establishment of imatinib and other tyrosine kinase inhibitors as front-line therapy for CML with excellent outcomes on long-term follow-up, the number of patients undergoing allogeneic transplantation has declined dramatically. Currently, allogeneic transplantation is recommended for those patients in whom a second-generation TKI has failed, patients with TKI-resistant mutations such as T315I, and patients in accelerated phase or blast phase. The MD Anderson group reported outcomes of imatinib-resistant CML patients (chronic phase, $n = 34$; accelerated phase, $n = 9$; and blast crisis, $n = 4$) who underwent allogeneic transplantation. Nineteen patients (40%) had BCR-ABL mutations, 15 of whom had advanced disease. Thirty-two patients (68%) had a major molecular response after transplantation, with a

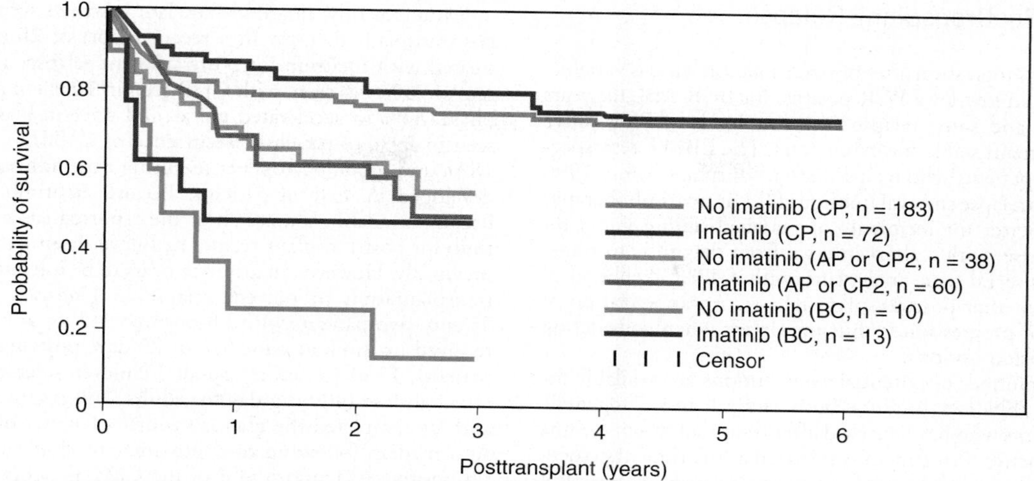

Figure 66-11 EFFECT OF PRIOR TREATMENT WITH IMATINIB ON OVERALL SURVIVAL AFTER TRANSPLANTATION. *CP2,* A return to chronic phase after treatment for accelerated phase or blast crisis disease. *(Data from Oehler VG, Gooley T, Snyder DS, et al: The effects of imatinib mesylate treatment before allogeneic transplantation for chronic myeloid leukemia,* Blood *109:1782, 2007.)*

2-year EFS of 36% and 58% for the mutant and nonmutant groups and a 2-year OS of 44% and 76%, respectively. These results confirm the effectiveness of transplantation as salvage treatment for TKI-resistant patients.[29] Since patients with mutations are more likely to develop advanced disease and have worse outcomes after transplantation, this procedure should be considered early for patients with poor response to a second-generation TKI.

Graft Versus Leukemia Effect in Chronic Myeloid Leukemia

Although evidence for a GVL effect can be found in many settings, nowhere is it as strong as in the setting of allogeneic HCT therapy for CML. Evidence in support of such an effect includes the following: the higher rates of relapse following syngeneic and T cell–depleted transplants compared with unmodified allogeneic transplants; the close association between the development of acute and chronic GVHD and freedom from relapse following non–T cell–depleted transplants; and the high response rate to donor lymphocyte infusions to treat posttransplant relapse (range from 50% to 100%), which is higher than in any other malignancy. The markedly increased relapse rates seen with T-cell depletion indicate a role for T cells in GVL. T cell targets might include minor histocompatibility antigens shared by most cells in the body, thus accounting for the association of GVL with GVHD. Alternatively, there may be polymorphic minor histocompatibility antigens, with expression limited to hematopoietic tissue. A third possible category of targets for the GVL effect in CML is the overexpression of protein targets in CML cells. Understanding the cells and their targets responsible for the potent GVL effect seen in CML will be critical to the development of more effective, less toxic transplant-based therapies in the future.

Reduced-Intensity Conditioning

Reduced-intensity conditioning (RIC) or nonablative transplant approaches have been introduced with the aim of avoiding the toxicities of high-dose preparative regimens while retaining GVL effects. These approaches are of particular relevance for patients with CML because their median age at diagnosis is 67 years. Using a preparative regimen consisting only of 200-cGy TBI, and GVHD prophylaxis using cyclosporine (CSP) and mycophenolate mofetil (MMF), McSweeney and colleagues reported complete molecular responses in five of nine patients transplanted for CML in chronic phase ($n = 6$) or accelerated phase ($n = 3$). The other four patients rejected their grafts. By adding 30 mg/m^2 fludarabine pretransplant, graft rejection has been eliminated as a problem following matched-sibling transplantation. Or and colleagues recently reported similar encouraging results using a preparative regimen of fludarabine, low-dose busulfan, and antithymocyte globulin. The MD Anderson group reported outcomes of 64 CML patients with advanced-phase disease (80% beyond first chronic phase), not eligible for myeloablative preparative regimens because of older age or comorbid conditions, who received transplants with fludarabine-based reduced intensity conditioning regimens (matched related, $n = 30$; one antigen-mismatched related, $n = 4$; matched unrelated, $n = 30$).[30] At 5 years, the overall survival (OS) and PFS were 33% and 20%, and TRM was 48%. In multivariate analysis, only disease stage at time of HSCT was significantly predictive for survival. These results indicate that reduced intensity transplantation may offer a safe and effective way to treat CML in the chronic phase, but alternative treatment strategies need to be explored in patients with advanced disease.

Residual Disease Posttransplantation

The detection of BCR-ABL transcripts posttransplant is a strong predictor of relapse following transplantation. In a study of 346 patients after transplantation, 40% of patients were positive for BCR-ABL residual disease at 3 months posttransplant, but this finding was not predictive of outcome, suggesting that eradication of the CML clone posttransplant takes an extended period of time. In contrast, at 6 or 12 months posttransplant, 27% of patients were BCR-ABL–positive and at this time the assay was a powerful predictor of outcome, as only 3% of PCR-negative patients eventually relapsed compared with 42% of PCR-positive patients. The predictive power of PCR detection of BCR-ABL among longer-term survivors is somewhat weaker. At 18 months posttransplant, 1% of 289 BCR-ABL-negative patients subsequently relapsed compared with 14% of 90 BCR-ABL-positive patients. The advent of reliable quantitative PCR testing further refined risk prediction of BCR-ABL detection. Olavarria and colleagues studied 138 transplant patients at 3 to 5 months posttransplant and were able to define patients as having a low risk for relapse (16%), an intermediate risk (43%), or a high risk (86%) based on BCR-ABL quantification. Further studies have confirmed the importance of quantitative BCR-ABL monitoring of minimal residual disease after transplantation for CML, which offers an obvious opportunity for early intervention for patients with residual or recurring disease.

Treatment of Posttransplant Relapse

The pace of disease progression after posttransplant relapse is variable; some patients remain low-level PCR-positive for BCR-ABL for years without relapsing, and some relapse with low levels of Ph-positive metaphases and remain stable for many years. The EBMT retrospectively studied 130 patients who relapsed after transplant before 1990 and noted that postrelapse survival (without DLI or imatinib therapy) was significantly better for recipients of matched-sibling grafts for chronic-phase disease, with a short interval from diagnosis to transplant but a long interval from transplant, with a 42% likelihood of being alive 10 years after posttransplant relapse. An appreciation of the likely tempo of progression is thus important when considering treatment intervention options.

An increasing number of potential interventions are available for relapsing disease. IFN can produce both clinical and cytogenetic remissions in patients who have relapsed after transplantation. Results with IFN appear better if treatment is initiated at the time of cytogenetic relapse instead of waiting until hematologic relapse, because IFN induces molecular remissions in some individuals treated early. A large number of studies now demonstrate cytogenetic complete response rates of 50% to 100% in patients treated with DLI for clinically relapsed chronic-phase CML. Response rates tend to be higher for patients treated earlier at the time of cytogenetic relapse and lower for patients in accelerated phase. The two major complications of DLI are transient marrow failure and the development of GVHD. Marrow failure only occurs in patients treated in hematologic relapse and likely reflects clearance of host hematopoiesis before donor hematopoiesis recovers; this is of particular concern for patients in full-blown hematologic relapse with no evidence of residual donor hematopoiesis. Treatment earlier in the course of relapse can avoid this complication. The overall incidence of GVHD following DLI is approximately 50% in most series. Most early studies of DLI involved a single infusion of a relatively large number of donor T cells. It has since been reported that large numbers of T cells are tolerated with less GVHD if administered in a fractionated fashion rather than as a single bulk dose. A recent report from the EBMT provides further support for starting at lower doses of lymphocytes and escalating dosage as required.

More recently, imatinib mesylate has been shown to be active as posttransplant therapy. In a recent report of 28 patients who were treated with imatinib for posttransplant relapse, an overall response rate of 79% was seen, with CHR seen in 100% of patients in chronic phase, 83% in accelerated phase, and 43% in blast crisis. CCR was seen in 29% of patients. Recurrence of GVHD disease was seen in 18%, and granulocytopenia requiring dose adjustments of imatinib developed in 43% of patients. Because imatinib has only recently become available, almost all of the reported cases treated with imatinib for posttransplant relapse had never been treated with the drug previously. However, imatinib appears to be tolerated given early after transplantation to prevent relapse in high-risk Ph-positive cases. Twenty-two patients with Ph-positive ALL or advanced-phase CML received imatinib at a median of 28 days postengraftment. Of these patients, 17 of 19 adults and all 3 children tolerated imatinib at the targeted dose (400 mg/day for adults, 260 mg/m^2/day for children), and 19 completed the planned course of 1 year of imatinib therapy. At a median follow-up of approximately 1½ years, 12 of 15 of the Ph-positive ALL and 5 of 7 of the CML patients were in molecular remission.

Autologous Transplantation

The rationale for autologous transplantation in CML has been provided by the experimental and clinical evidence for persistence of polyclonal Ph-negative progenitors capable of reconstituting hematopoiesis in CML patients. This is most dramatically demonstrated by the high rate of cytogenetic and molecular response in CML patients treated with tyrosine kinase inhibitors. Furthermore, it was shown that transplantation of autologous cells may allow restoration of Ph hematopoiesis. Initial studies carried out using unmanipulated autologous marrow or blood cells indicated that autologous transplantation could reestablish CP in patients with advanced disease and induce cytogenetic responses in a small proportion of CML CP patients. Subsequent studies indicated that depletion of Ph-positive progenitors by ex vivo graft manipulation was associated with cytogenetic remission posttransplant. Another approach to depleting

Management of the Newly Diagnosed Chronic Myeloid Leukemia Patient

What should be the initial management for CML patients? After years of clinical research, we know (a) imatinib is remarkably effective for patients treated in chronic phase, because greater than 85% of patients obtain a complete cytogenetic response and approximately 70% of cases remain in CCR at 5 years of follow-up; (b) second-generation tyrosine kinase inhibitors, dasatinib and nilotinib, used as first-line treatment for chronic phase CML may be even more effective, resulting in faster and more profound reduction in BCR-ABL levels; (c) allogeneic transplantation is generally associated with 10-year survival rates of 70% or better for younger patients in early chronic phase; and (d) outcome for patients receiving TKI treatment can be effectively monitored by sensitive RT-PCR assays.

Imatinib has become the initial treatment of choice for patients with CML. For patients diagnosed during chronic phase, imatinib is a reasonable first choice of therapy. However, in view of the association between cytogenetic and molecular responses on imatinib and survival, it is reasonable to suggest that the faster and deeper reduction in disease burden using the second-generation agents may reduce the risk for progression when compared with imatinib. The tolerability of the newer agents appears to be comparable to imatinib, although follow-up is shorter and the long-term effects of treatment are not known. It is notable that differences in overall survival have not been observed as yet. In addition, low-risk chronic-phase patients demonstrate excellent survival with imatinib. In addition, imatinib is considerably less expensive than the newer agents and a generic form will soon be available, reducing costs further. Careful monitoring of imatinib response could potentially identify the subset of patients who will benefit from second-generation tyrosine kinase inhibitor treatment. Longer-term follow-up of patients from the front-line studies and better prognostication measures for response to individual agents will be required to resolve these issues. Until then, the choice of first-line TKI is dependent on individual preference based on risk group, toxicity profile, dosing schedule, and economic factors.

For patients with chronic-phase disease, tyrosine kinase treatment can be initiated with simultaneous workup of family donors and unrelated donors. Criteria for failure or suboptimal response have been developed. Certainly, the failure of imatinib treatment to achieve a complete hematologic response at 3 months of treatment, lack of any cytogenetic response by 6 months, or lack of a major cytogenetic response by 12 months is an indication to switch therapy. By a conservative approach, patients should achieve a complete cytogenetic response by 18 months of therapy. Similarly, BCR-ABL mRNA levels greater than 10% at 6 months and greater than 1% at 12 months (using the international scale) are indicators to switch treatment. Patients who relapse after a CCR, especially those with ABL point mutations, should consider alternative therapy, including transplant. For patients diagnosed in accelerated phase or in blast crisis, initial treatment with dasatinib results in better responses than those seen with imatinib, but in general, these responses tend to be short-lived; thus advanced-phase patients should consider transplantation as soon as possible.

malignant cells from the graft was to treat patients before harvesting marrow or peripheral blood for transplantation, also called *in vivo purging*. However, remissions following autologous transplantation were usually of short duration. In addition, the procedure was often associated with significant toxicity and delayed recovery. Although the compiled results of 200 autologous transplants at eight different centers in Europe and North America indicated a possibility of improved survival, it is not possible to make any definite conclusions in the absence of controlled clinical trials. A meta-analysis of six trials in which patients were randomly allocated to receive autologous HCT or an IFN-based regimen did not show an advantage for HCT.

Autologous HCT has now fallen out of favor in view of the excellent results of tyrosine kinase inhibitor treatment in CML patients. Pilot studies to collect PBSC from patients who have received imatinib and achieved CCR, for use for autologous HCT in case of later progression, have been reported. The PBSC collection process is well tolerated and Ph-negative collections are more consistently achieved than with previous strategies. Although the target numbers of $CD34^+$ cells is usually attained, a subset of patients are unable to reach this target. Furthermore, many patients mobilize suboptimally and require multiple collections, possibly as a result of the effects of imatinib on normal hematopoiesis and the mobilization process. Collections are usually Ph-negative, but molecular evidence of disease is usually found. Collection of PBSC from patients responsive to tyrosine kinase inhibitors may form the framework of any future attempts to perform autologous transplantation in CML; however, additional strategies are needed to further deplete leukemia cells from PBSC collections and to improve therapy for residual disease posttransplant. At this point, autologous HCT for CML should be limited to investigational trials for patients who lack allogeneic donors and for those in whom tyrosine kinase inhibitors have failed (see box on Management of the Newly Diagnosed Chronic Myeloid Leukemia Patient).

REFERENCES

1. Perrotti D, Jamieson C, Goldman J, et al: Chronic myeloid leukemia: Mechanisms of blastic transformation. *J Clin Invest* 120:2254, 2010.
2. Goldman JM, Melo JV: Chronic myeloid leukemia—Advances in biology and new approaches to treatment. *N Engl J Med* 349:1451, 2003.
3. Branford S, Fletcher L, Cross NC, et al: Desirable performance characteristics for BCR-ABL measurement on an international reporting scale to allow consistent interpretation of individual patient response and comparison of response rates between clinical trials. *Blood* 112:3330, 2008.
4. Corm S, Roche L, Micol JB, et al: Changes in the dynamics of the excess mortality rate in chronic phase-chronic myeloid leukemia over 1990–2007: A population study. *Blood* 118:4331, 2011.
5. Gambacorti-Passerini C, Antolini L, Mahon FX, et al: Multicenter independent assessment of outcomes in chronic myeloid leukemia patients treated with imatinib. *J Natl Cancer Inst* 103:553, 2011.
6. Druker B, Tamura S, Buchdunger E, et al: Effects of a selective inhibitor of the Abl tyrosine kinase on the growth of Bcr-Abl positive cells. *Nature Medicine* 2:561, 1996.
7. Druker BJ, Talpaz M, Resta DJ, et al: Efficacy and safety of a specific inhibitor of the BCR-ABL tyrosine kinase in chronic myeloid leukemia. *N Engl J Med* 344:1031, 2001.
8. O'Brien SG, Guilhot F, Larson RA, et al: Imatinib compared with interferon and low-dose cytarabine for newly diagnosed chronic-phase chronic myeloid leukemia. *N Engl J Med* 348:994, 2003.
9. Hochhaus A, O'Brien SG, Guilhot F, et al: Six-year follow-up of patients receiving imatinib for the first-line treatment of chronic myeloid leukemia. *Leukemia* 23:1054, 2009.
10. Cortes JE, Baccarani M, Guilhot F, et al: Phase III, randomized, open-label study of daily imatinib mesylate 400 mg versus 800 mg in patients with newly diagnosed, previously untreated chronic myeloid leukemia in chronic phase using molecular end points: Tyrosine kinase inhibitor optimization and selectivity study. *J Clin Oncol* 28:424, 2010.
11. de Lavallade H, Apperley JF, Khorashad JS, et al: Imatinib for newly diagnosed patients with chronic myeloid leukemia: Incidence of sustained responses in an intention-to-treat analysis. *J Clin Oncol* 26:3358, 2008.
12. Efficace F, Baccarani M, Breccia M, et al: Health-related quality of life in chronic myeloid leukemia patients receiving long-term therapy with imatinib compared with the general population. *Blood* 118:4554, 2011.
13. Hughes TP, Hochhaus A, Branford S, et al: Long-term prognostic significance of early molecular response to imatinib in newly diagnosed chronic myeloid leukemia: An analysis from the International Randomized Study of Interferon and STI571 (IRIS). *Blood* 116:3758, 2010.
14. Marin D, Ibrahim AR, Lucas C, et al: Assessment of BCR-ABL1 Transcript levels at 3 months is the only requirement for predicting outcome for patients with chronic myeloid leukemia treated with tyrosine kinase inhibitors. *J Clin Oncol* 30:232, 2012.
15. Baccarani M, Cortes J, Pane F, et al: Chronic myeloid leukemia: An update of concepts and management recommendations of European LeukemiaNet. *J Clin Oncol* 27:6041, 2009.
16. Ibrahim AR, Eliasson L, Apperley JF, et al: Poor adherence is the main reason for loss of CCyR and imatinib failure for chronic myeloid leukemia patients on long-term therapy. *Blood* 117:3733, 2011.
17. Marin D, Bazeos A, Mahon FX, et al: Adherence is the critical factor for achieving molecular responses in patients with chronic myeloid leukemia who achieve complete cytogenetic responses on imatinib. *J Clin Oncol* 28:2381, 2011.
18. Deininger MW, O'Brien SG, Ford JM, et al: Practical management of patients with chronic myeloid leukemia receiving imatinib. *J Clin Oncol* 21:1637, 2003.
19. Soverini S, Hochhaus A, Nicolini FE, et al: BCR-ABL kinase domain mutation analysis in chronic myeloid leukemia patients treated with tyrosine kinase inhibitors: Recommendations from an expert panel on behalf of European LeukemiaNet. *Blood*118:1208, 2011.
20. Kantarjian H, Shah NP, Hochhaus A, et al: Dasatinib versus imatinib in newly diagnosed chronic-phase chronic myeloid leukemia. *N Engl J Med* 362:2260, 2010.
21. Saglio G, Kim DW, Issaragrisil S, et al: Nilotinib versus imatinib for newly diagnosed chronic myeloid leukemia. *N Engl J Med* 362:2251, 2010.
22. Santos FP, Quintas-Cardama A: New drugs for chronic myelogenous leukemia. *Curr Hematol Malig Rep* 6:96, 2011.
23. O'Hare T, Shakespeare WC, Zhu X, et al: AP24534, a pan-BCR-ABL inhibitor for chronic myeloid leukemia, potently inhibits the T315I mutant and overcomes mutation-based resistance. *Cancer Cell* 16:401, 2009.
24. Chan WW, Wise SC, Kaufman MD, et al: Conformational control inhibition of the BCR-ABL1 tyrosine kinase, including the gatekeeper T315I mutant, by the switch-control inhibitor DCC-2036. *Cancer Cell* 19:556, 2011.
25. Mahon FX, Rea D, Guilhot J, et al: Discontinuation of imatinib in patients with chronic myeloid leukaemia who have maintained complete molecular remission for at least 2 years: The prospective, multicentre Stop Imatinib (STIM) trial. *Lancet Oncol* 11:1029, 2010.
26. Chu S, McDonald T, Lin A, et al: Persistence of leukemia stem cells in chronic myelogenous leukemia patients in prolonged remission with imatinib treatment. *Blood* 118:5565, 2011.
27. Khoury HJ, Kukreja M, Goldman JM, et al: Prognostic factors for outcomes in allogeneic transplantation for CML in the imatinib era: A CIBMTR analysis. *Bone Marrow Transplant* 2011.
28. Basak G, Torosian T, Snarski E, et al: Hematopoietic stem cell transplantation for T315I-mutated chronic myelogenous leukemia. *Ann Transplant* 15:68, 2010.
29. Jabbour E, Cortes J, Santos FP, et al: Results of allogeneic hematopoietic stem cell transplantation for chronic myelogenous leukemia patients who failed tyrosine kinase inhibitors after developing BCR-ABL1 kinase domain mutations. *Blood* 117:3641, 2011.
30. Kebriaei P, Detry MA, Giralt S, et al: Long-term follow-up of allogeneic hematopoietic stem-cell transplantation with reduced-intensity conditioning for patients with chronic myeloid leukemia. *Blood* 110:3456, 2007.

CHAPTER 67

THE POLYCYTHEMIAS

Marina Kremyanskaya, Vesna Najfeld, John Mascarenhas, and Ronald Hoffman

Under normal conditions, the red blood cell (RBC) mass in humans is tightly controlled and remains relatively constant in a given individual. The numbers of senescent RBCs lost daily are replaced by newly formed ones by a carefully controlled network of growth factors and progenitor cells. Erythropoiesis can be augmented by a variety of stimuli that increase the delivery of oxygen to tissues. This delicate balance can be disturbed by various pathologic conditions and can result in either reduced numbers of RBCs (anemia) or excessive numbers of RBCs (polycythemia). Hematocrit values over 52% in males and over 48% in females are abnormal and require further evaluation to determine if the patient has an absolute increase in the RBC mass and investigation of its cause. The RBC mass is defined as being increased if it is greater than 125% above that expected for sex and body mass. The measurement of the RBC mass is a diagnostic study that is now available at a dwindling number of tertiary care centers, making other diagnostic studies pivotal in evaluating patients with elevated hematocrit levels. Polycythemic states can be caused by a variety of disorders that can be attributed to several pathophysiologic mechanisms. Determination of the etiology of an individual's polycythemia is a critical step in defining the patient's appropriate prognosis and treatment plan. Primary polycythemias are the result of innate abnormalities involving hematopoietic progenitors and stem cells that lead to constitutive overproduction of RBCs, which are accompanied by low erythropoietin (EPO) levels. By contrast, secondary polycythemias are the consequence of a number of conditions that lead to increased EPO production, which acts on normal progenitors to overproduce RBCs. In a small number of patients, the cause of erythrocytosis cannot be determined; these patients are classified as having idiopathic erythrocytosis (IE). Approximately one-third of these patients have low EPO levels; the remainder have inappropriately normal or elevated EPO levels. This latter group presumably has a secondary form of erythrocytosis, although a mechanism leading to the absolute erythrocytosis is frequently not defined.

ERYTHROPOIESIS

Red blood cell production can be influenced by numerous factors, including nutrients, growth factors, numbers and function of bone marrow (BM) progenitor and precursor cells, and cellular receptors and transcription factors. The hematopoietic growth factor EPO is considered to be the physiologic regulator of the terminal phases of erythropoiesis. Alterations in its production are followed by adjustments in the rate of formation of RBCs. In humans, EPO production is controlled by the relative supply of oxygen to the kidneys, the major site of EPO. In states of severe hypoxia, EPO production can be increased up to 1000-fold. A large body of information is available addressing EPO physiology in patients with erythrocytosis. After phlebotomy of a healthy person, EPO excretion increases, and an inverse logarithmic relationship between hematocrit and EPO excretion rates is observed. Patients with secondary erythrocytosis caused by chronic hypoxia have either normal or increased basal values, but they also have increased values after reduction of the hematocrit to normal levels by phlebotomy. By contrast, EPO excretion is invariably subnormal in patients with polycythemia vera (PV), which demonstrates that this disorder is not a result of excessive EPO production.

Different levels of EPO are required at the erythroid precursor and progenitor cell levels. In addition, multipotent myeloid progenitors and primitive erythroid progenitors (burst-forming units–erythroid [BFU-E]), both of which ultimately contribute to erythropoiesis, require additional growth factors such as stem cell factor (SCF), interleukin-3 (IL-3), granulocyte macrophage-colony stimulating factor (GM-CSF), or thrombopoietin (TPO) to promote their proliferation and maturation. In addition, erythroid cell proliferation is also controlled by nuclear receptors such as the glucocorticoid receptor. Glucocorticoids have been shown to maintain erythroblasts in a proliferative state, blocking their terminal maturation in response to EPO and stem cell factor.

ERYTHROPOIETIN, OXYGEN SENSING, AND HYPOXIA-INDUCIBLE FACTOR

Under normal conditions, EPO production is mediated by the decreased oxygen content of hemoglobin within RBCs, termed *hypoxemia,* which leads to decreased oxygen delivery to tissues. Regulation of oxygen homeostasis is critical to survival. In humans, oxygen sensing occurs at many levels, leading to both acute and chronic adaptation. The acute reduction of the availability of oxygen leads to the initiation of a cascade of adaptive events that sets in place compensatory events to correct the lack of oxygen supply. Low oxygen levels, or hypoxia (60 mm Hg), in humans cause oxygen-sensing chemosensory cells to undergo rapid membrane depolarization within seconds, leading to the production of action potentials, influx of calcium ions, and release of the neurotransmitters that result in stimulation of the brain stem that controls the respiratory and cardiovascular systems.[1] These chemosensory cells are found within the glomus cells of the carotid body located at the bifurcation of the internal and external carotid arteries. The released neurotransmitters activate the nerve endings of the carotid body sensory nerve to convey to the central nervous system signals that command ventilation to fight hypoxia, resulting in an increase of the lung ventilation rate and restoration of normal oxygen tension to vital organs. In addition, there are changes in blood pressure and heart rate to maximize oxygen delivery. The carotid body is the organ with the greatest blood flow within the body. Activation of the carotid body results in the sensation of breathlessness experienced by individuals at high altitudes. During chronic hypoxia when the carotid body is permanently active, there is marked enlargement of the carotid body because of an increase in capillaries and a marked reduction in the mean distance from the capillaries to the edge of the chemoreceptor cells.

In response to chronic hypoxia, multiple compensatory mechanisms come into play over several days in the kidneys, the major site of EPO production. Hypoxic stimulation results in production of hypoxia-inducible factor-1 (HIF-1), the major factor responsible for transcriptional activation of the EPO gene. Analysis of proteins that bind to the EPO enhancer under hypoxic conditions led to the identification of HIF. The HIF transcriptional system is a master

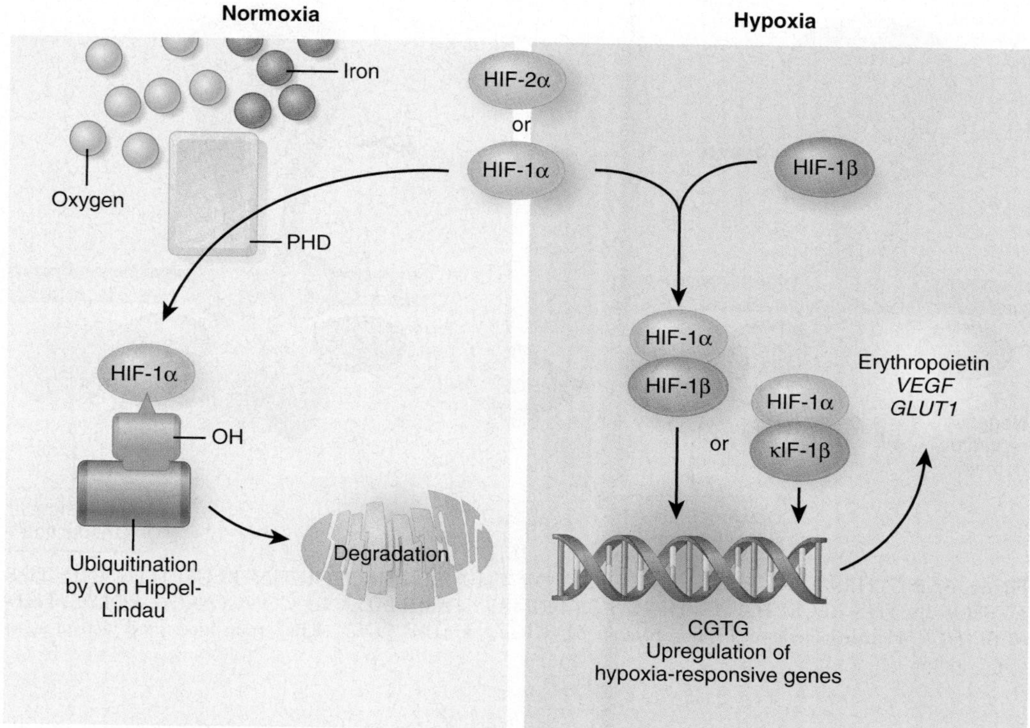

Figure 67-1 SCHEMATIC REPRESENTATION OF THE RELATIONSHIP BETWEEN HYPOXIA SENSING AND ERYTHROPOIETIN PRODUCTION. *GLUT,* Glucose transporter 1; *HIF,* hypoxia-inducible factor; *PHD,* proline hydroxylase; *VEGF,* vascular endothelial growth factor.

regulator of the hypoxic response controlling a large number of genes in multiple cell types. HIF-1 is a heterodimeric protein consisting of HIF-1α and HIF-1β, which is required for normal development of the heart, blood vessels, and blood cells.[2] The levels of HIF-1α increase exponentially as the oxygen concentration declines. As the key mediator of cellular oxygen maintenance, HIF-1 facilitates body oxygen delivery and responses to oxygen deprivation by regulating the expression of gene products that are involved in cellular energy metabolism and glucose transport, angiogenesis, erythropoiesis and iron metabolism, pH regulation, apoptosis, cell proliferation, and cell–cell and cell–matrix interactions. Classic HIF target genes include phosphoglycerate kinase, glucose transporter-1, vascular endothelial growth factor (VEGF), and EPO. The HIF proteins are members of the Per–ARNT–Sim family of heterodimeric basic helix–loop–helix transcription factors (Fig. 67-1).

In contrast to the constitutively expressed, HIF-1β subunits, HIF-1α is an oxygen-labile protein that becomes stabilized in response to hypoxia. HIF-1α mRNA and protein levels are induced by hypoxia, and HIF-1α protein levels decay rapidly with return to normoxia. The posttranslational regulation of HIF-1α protein accounts for the majority of the regulation of this gene. Normoxia-induced, ubiquitin-mediated degradation of the HIF-1α protein is the major regulator of HIF-1α levels, thereby reducing the stimulus for additional EPO production. The targeting and subsequent polyubiquitination of HIF-1α require the von Hippel-Lindau (VHL) protein, oxygen, and three different iron-requiring proline hydroxylase enzymes (PHD) (see Fig. 67-1). The PHD proteins exist in three isoforms, PHD1, PHD2, and PHD3. HIF-1α is hydroxylated by all three isoforms but primarily by PHD2.The prolyl hydroxylation of HIF-1α is necessary for the binding of HIF-1α to VHL, which is the substrate-recognition subunit of an E3 ubiquitin-protein ligase. Different parts of the HIF-1α chains have different functions. The amino terminus part of HIF-1α is involved in DNA binding and dimerization, and the carboxy terminus portion has regulatory functions. One domain at the carboxy terminus influences transcriptional activity without affecting HIF-1α protein levels, and the other region, termed the oxygen-dependent degradation domain (ODD), affects protein abundance. The ODD is divided into an amino terminus and a carboxy terminus subdomain. The VHL protein physically interacts with the ODD of HIF-1α, targeting it for ubiquitination and destruction by the proteasome. Iron-chelating drugs can also block the interaction of HIF-1α with the VHL protein, suggesting a role for iron in the degradation of HIF-1α.

Under normoxic conditions, hydroxylation of HIF-1α is essential for HIF proteolytic degradation by promoting interaction with the VHL tumor-suppressor protein through hydrogen bonding to the hydroxy proline-binding pocket in the VHL-β domain. As oxygen levels decrease, hydroxylation of HIF decreases, and HIF-1α then no longer binds VHL. As a result, it becomes stabilized, dimerizes with HIF-1β, and activates transcription of target genes. The activity of PHDs depends on the availability of molecular oxygen, which qualifies these enzymes as oxygen sensors. In addition, these dioxygenases require 2-oxoglutarate as a cosubstrate and vitamin C to keep their central nonheme iron in the ferrous state. Although PHD-2 appears to be the hydroxylase that is essential for HIF-1α degradation under normoxic conditions, PHD-3 is important for hydroxylation of HIF-1α during reoxygenation. Different effects of individual PHDs on HIF-1α and HIF-2α hydroxylation indicate that the stability of individual HIF-1α subunits and their target gene expression might be affected by tissue- and cell-type differences in PHD expression and activity levels. The activity of PHDs can be modulated by mitochondrial reactive oxygen species, implicating mitochondria in oxygen sensing. Another protein termed HIF-2α has been identified that under hypoxic conditions dimerizes with HIF-1β and activates the transcription of a set of target genes that overlap with the target genes regulated by HIF-1α /HIF-1β heterodimers. HIF-1α is expressed by all nucleated cells, but HIF-2α is expressed by specific cell types, including vascular endothelial cells, renal interstitial cells, hepatocytes, cardiomyocytes, and astrocytes. HIF-2α appears to play a critical role in regulating EPO production in adult mammals, and HIF-1α is also important during yolk sac erythropoiesis. HIF-1 also controls the absorption and delivery of iron to the BM through its repression of hepcidin and activation of genes encoding transferrin and the transferrin receptor.

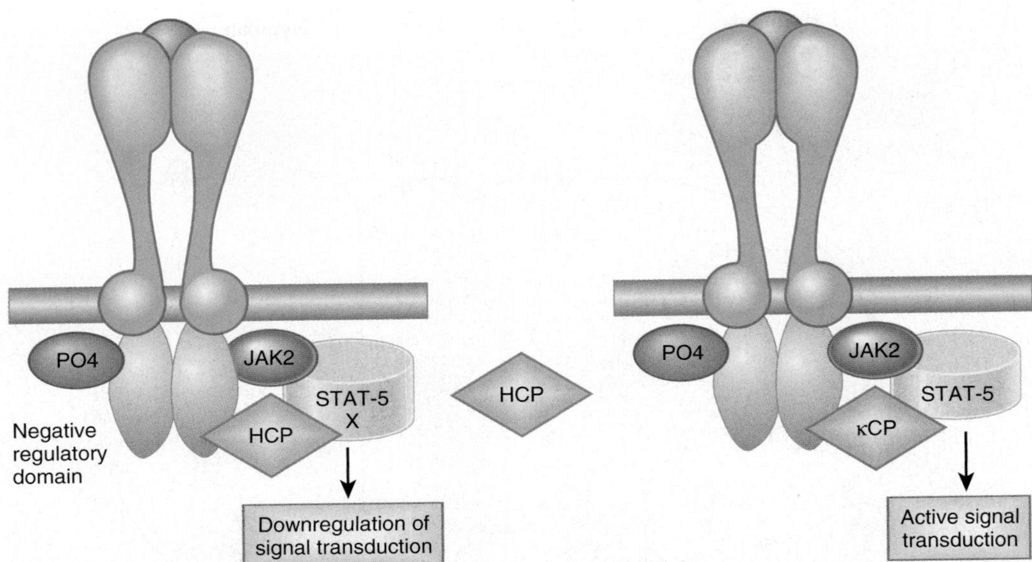

Figure 67-2 SCHEMATIC REPRESENTATION OF THE ERYTHROPOIETIN RECEPTOR AND THE DEFECT IN THE RECEPTOR UNDERLYING PRIMARY FAMILIAL AND CONGENITAL POLYCYTHEMIA. *HCP,* Hematopoietic cell phosphatase; *JAK,* Janus kinase; *STAT,* signal transducer and activator of transcription.

von Hippel-Lindau syndrome is a hereditary cancer syndrome that is associated with exaggerated responses to hypoxia caused by posttranslational abnormalities in HIF.[3] VHL syndrome is characterized by a propensity for developing clear cell renal carcinomas, retinal hemangioblastomas, cerebellar and spinal hemangiomas, pancreatic and renal cysts, islet cell tumors of the pancreas, and pheochromocytomas. The tumors result from somatic mutations that cause a loss of heterozygosity (LOH) of the *VHL* gene. VHL disease affects approximately one in 35,000 individuals and is transmitted in an autosomal dominant manner. Individuals with VHL disease carry one wild-type VHL allele and one inactivated VHL allele. This inactivation can occur by somatic mutation or hypermethylation. Tumor or cyst development is linked to somatic inactivation or loss of the remaining wild-type VHL allele. Approximately 20% to 37% of VHL patients have large or partial germline deletions, 23% to 27% have nonsense or frame-shift mutations, and 30% to 35% have missense mutations. More than 150 different VHL mutations linked to VHL disease have been reported. The tumors linked to VHL inactivation are often highly vascular and can produce angiogenic factors such as VEGF. In addition, renal cell carcinoma, cerebellar hemangioblastomas, and pheochromocytomas have been associated with paraneoplastic erythrocytosis caused by overproduction of EPO. Overproduction of HIF-inducible mRNAs is the hallmark of VHL protein defective cells. Genotype–phenotype correlates in VHL disease suggest that VHL has functions independent of HIF regulation that might play a role in tumor formation. VHL protein has other binding partners, including atypical protein kinase C and a family of deubiquitinating enzymes named VHL-interacting deubiquitinating enzymes 1 and 2. In addition, pVHL has been involved in numerous cellular processes, including regulation of extracellular matrix, cytoskeleton stability, cell cycle control, and differentiation. VHL disease is not associated with erythrocytosis.

THE ERYTHROPOIETIN RECEPTOR

Interaction of EPO with the EPO receptor (EPOR) present on the erythroid progenitor and precursor cells leads to its homodimerization, resulting in (1) stimulation of cell division, (2) differentiation by induction of erythroid-specific gene expression, and (3) prevention of erythroid progenitor and precursor cell apoptosis. The cytoplasmic portion of the EPOR contains a positive regulatory domain that interacts with Janus kinase 2 (JAK2) (Fig. 67-2). Immediately after EPO binding, JAK2 phosphorylates itself, the EPOR, and other proteins such as STAT5 (signal transducer and activator of transcription 5). This JAK2–STAT5 signaling plays an essential role in EPO/EPOR-mediated regulation of erythropoiesis. Consistent with their essential roles in erythropoiesis EPO, EPOR- and JAK2-deficient mice die embryonically from severe anemia.

The C-terminal cytoplasmic portion of the EPOR also possesses a negative regulatory domain. Hematopoietic cell phosphatase (HCP, also known as SHP-1 or PTP N6) interacts with this portion of the EPOR and downregulates signal transduction by promoting dephosphorylation (see Fig. 67-2). Inactivation of the HCP-binding site leads to prolonged phosphorylation of JAK2–STAT5. Another negative regulator of erythropoiesis, suppressor of cytokine signaling-3 (SOCS-3), binds to the cytoplasmic portion of the EPOR and suppresses EPO-dependent JAK2–STAT5 signaling. Thus deletion of the distal C-terminal cytoplasmic portion of the EPOR abolishes negative regulatory elements and results in increased proliferation of erythroid progenitor cells. Mutations in the *EPOR* gene have been observed in some patients with primary familial and congenital polycythemia (PFCP) and are occasionally found in erythroleukemia (see Fig. 67-2). Such secondary growth factors as insulin-like growth factor-1 (IGF-1) and the components of the renin–angiotensin system (RAS) may also influence the production of RBCs.

THE RENIN–ANGIOTENSIN SYSTEM AND HEMATOPOIESIS

The RAS regulates fluid and electrolyte homeostasis and blood pressure and has been hypothesized to also play a role in the regulation of erythropoiesis. The primary function of angiotensin during development is the regulation of tissue growth and differentiation. Angiotensin II (AngII) is a ligand for two distinct receptors, type 1 and type 2 (AT1 and AT2). AT1 appears to play a major role in the regulation of cell proliferation.

The RAS was first postulated to influence erythropoiesis in the 1980s after the use of angiotensin-converting enzyme (ACE) inhibitors to treat hypertension was shown to result in anemia. In animals, increased blood levels of renin (a major regulator of AngII synthesis) were found to result in elevated serum EPO levels and erythrocytosis. In humans, the infusion of AngII also increases serum EPO levels.

The pathway underlying AngII-driven EPO secretion is unknown. However, some investigators have suggested that AngII modulates renal EPO production through changes in renal perfusion and sodium reabsorption. This hypothesis is based on the presumption that reduced oxygen pressure in the kidneys triggers HIF-1α to induce release of EPO. AngII also directly stimulates proliferation of hematopoietic progenitors in vitro, and inhibition of this effect with ACE inhibitors induces apoptosis of erythroid progenitors in renal transplantation patients. ACE-1 knockout mice develop a normocytic anemia that can be fully reversed by infusion of AngII. ACE-related anemia is most pronounced in patients with renal insufficiency or end-stage renal disease and in patients who have received a renal allograft. The pathogenesis of this anemia is not clear, but reduced levels of circulating EPO are not solely responsible, suggesting that there might be other contributing factors. The AT1 receptor is present on erythroid progenitors, and its ligand, AngII, augments EPO stimulation of erythropoiesis. The involvement of JAK2 kinase in AngII signaling suggests that this signal transduction pathway mediated by EPO and AngII might overlap. Postrenal transplant erythrocytosis likely can be accounted for by activation of the RAS.

DEFINITION AND CLASSIFICATION OF POLYCYTHEMIA

The term *polycythemia* is a literal translation from Greek, meaning "too many cells in the blood," and refers to an increase in the RBC mass; it is frequently used interchangeably with the term *erythrocytosis*. Polycythemia may be due to a myriad of causes (Table 67-1). The polycythemias can be classified as relative and absolute. Relative polycythemia is a disorder in which the patient characteristically has a modest elevation of the hematocrit level without an elevated RBC mass but rather because of contraction of the plasma volume. The absolute polycythemias are accompanied by an actual increase in the circulating RBC mass. Polycythemias can also be classified according to the responsiveness of their erythroid progenitor cells to growth factors or the circulating levels of such growth factors. Primary polycythemias are characterized by increased sensitivity of the erythroid progenitors to regulatory growth factors as a result of acquired somatic or inherited germline mutations expressed by hematopoietic progenitor cells (HPCs). In contrast, secondary polycythemias are characterized by an increase in regulatory growth factors, primarily EPO, and normal responsiveness of their erythroid progenitors to these growth factors. These conditions can usually be distinguished by in vitro assays of erythroid progenitor cells, quantitation of serum EPO levels, and detection of somatic JAK2 mutations. In a small number of patients, the cause of erythrocytosis cannot be determined; these patients are classified as having IE.

Table 67-1 Differential Diagnosis of the Polycythemias

Relative or Spurious Polycythemia

1. Decreased plasma volume—reduced fluid intake, marked loss of body fluids (diaphoresis, vomiting, diarrhea, "third spacing")
2. Gaisböck syndrome
3. Overfilling of blood in collection vacuum tubes

Absolute Polycythemia

1. Secondary polycythemia
   A. Acquired
      Hypoxia
      - Pulmonary disease
      - Cyanotic congenital heart disease
      - Hypoventilation syndromes: sleep apnea, Pickwickian syndrome
      - High altitude
      - Smokers' polycythemia, hookah polycythemia, carbon monoxide intoxication caused by industrial exposure

      Postrenal transplantation erythrocytosis
      Aberrant erythropoietin production
      - Tumors: renal cell carcinoma, Wilms tumor, hepatic carcinoma, uterine leiomyomata, virilizing ovarian tumors, vascular cerebellar tumors
      - Miscellaneous renal and hepatic disorders: solitary renal cysts, polycystic kidney disease, renal artery stenosis hydronephrosis, viral hepatitis

      Endocrine disorders: Cushing syndrome, primary aldosteronism
      Androgen use
      Erythropoietin use
   B. Congenital Polycythemias
      - Abnormal high-affinity hemoglobin variants
      - Bisphosphoglycerate deficiency
      - Congenital methemoglobinemia
      - Chuvash polycythemia (von Hippel Lindau mutations)
      - Prolyl hydroxylase mutations
      - Hypoxia-inducible factor gene mutations
2. Primary polycythemias
   - Primary congenital and familial polycythemia
   - Polycythemia vera

RELATIVE POLYCYTHEMIA

Individuals with a modestly increased venous hematocrit level that is not accompanied by an increased RBC mass are frequently thought to be polycythemic by imprecise yet widely accepted medical practice. Frequently, these individuals are thought to be polycythemic owing to the lack of appreciation by a clinician of what constitutes the upper limit of normal values for a hematocrit (52% in males and 48% in females). Such individuals frequently prove not to have an absolute polycythemia as defined by an actual increase in the measured RBC mass. *Relative* or *spurious polycythemia* is a term used to describe an elevation of the hematocrit level either caused by an acute transient state of hemoconcentration associated with intravascular fluid depletion or a chronic sustained relative polycythemia caused by contraction of the plasma volume (see Table 67-1).

Transient polycythemias may be a result of acute depletion of the plasma volume from a variety of disorders, including protracted vomiting or diarrhea, plasma loss from external burns, sudden cold exposure or protracted exercise, insensible fluid loss from fever, sepsis, diabetic ketoacidosis, or acute ethanol intoxication. These elevations of hematocrit can be easily corrected by appropriate replacement of intravascular fluids.

Gaisböck syndrome, first described in 1905, is a benign condition observed mainly in obese, hypertensive, middle-aged, male smokers. Alcohol, diuretics, obesity, hypoxia, psychological stress, and excess catecholamine secretion have been identified as possible causes of relative polycythemia. Such individuals can have a chronic modest to moderate elevation of the hematocrit level associated with a normal RBC mass and low plasma volume, which has been attributed to reduced venous compliance, or they can have a high normal RBC mass with either a normal or slightly decreased plasma volume. The primary significance of the identification of a patient with relative polycythemia is the recognition of the increased risk of developing thrombotic vascular events likely caused by excessive smoking, hypertension, and obesity associated with this disease. The optimal therapy is unknown, but treatment is generally directed at correction of the patient's underlying cardiovascular risk factors.

It is also important to emphasize that overfilling of blood collection vacuum tubes can result in pseudopolycythemia, pseudothrombocytopenia, and pseudoleukopenia as a result of inadequate sample mixing. Careful attention to such a seemingly trivial detail can help avoid expensive, unnecessary diagnostic workups.

ABSOLUTE POLYCYTHEMIAS

Primary Familial and Congenital Polycythemia

This is an autosomal dominant disorder. Although PFCP is uncommon, it is more prevalent than polycythemia caused by high-oxygen-affinity hemoglobin mutants or a 2,3-biphosphoglycerate deficiency. Unlike patients with PV, patients with PFCP lack splenomegaly and do not progress to acute leukemia. It is not unusual for these patients to present with headaches, dizziness, epistaxis, and exertional dyspnea that resolve with normalization of the hematocrit level.[4] An increased incidence of cardiovascular events and premature morbidity and mortality has been reported in some affected members, but many appear to have a benign clinical course. Although clinical symptoms are relieved by phlebotomy, the increased risk of cardiovascular morbidity is not corrected by maintaining a normal hematocrit. Characteristic laboratory findings are (1) an increased hematocrit and RBC mass without an increased leukocyte or platelet count, (2) no activating mutation of JAK2, (3) a normal hemoglobin–oxygen dissociation curve, (4) low serum EPO levels, and (5) in vitro hypersensitivity of erythroid progenitors to EPO. Even though PFCP is present at birth, many affected patients are incidentally diagnosed later in life after the performance of routine blood counts or when evaluated in the context of multiple family members having polycythemia. It is of interest that one individual so affected was an accomplished cross-country skier who had won medals at the Olympic Games. To date, 16 mutations of the EPOR associated with PFCP have been described, leading to a loss in the negative regulatory domain of the EPOR.

The physiologic basis for EPO-mediated activation of erythropoiesis is as follows: EPO activates its receptor by conformational changes of its dimers, leading to initiation of an erythroid-specific cascade of events. The first signal is initiated by the binding of a tyrosine kinase to the EPOR and its phosphorylation and activation of a transcription factor, STAT5, which regulates erythroid-specific genes. This "on" signal is negated by dephosphorylation of the EPOR by HCP, that is, the "off" signal. Truncation of the EPOR leads to a loss in the negative regulatory domain of the EPOR, a binding site for HCP, leading to a gain-of-function mutation of the EPOR (see Fig. 67-2). In addition the negative regulation of erythropoiesis by SOCS-3, CIS and SHIP1 is presumed to contribute to the underlying cause of PFCP.

Recently, alternative explanations for the increased sensitivity of erythroid progenitors to EPO of patients with PFCP have been provided. EPOR downregulation provides another mechanism by which EPO desensitization can occur. EPOR downregulation is a complex process that involves EPOR-induced internalization or ubiquitination and degradation by proteasomes. EPO-induced receptor internalization is an efficient means of rapidly reducing EPO responsiveness. All of the truncated mutants associated with PFCP are associated with failure to internalize the EPOR, contributing to prolonged signaling through the EPOR. The EPOR degradation process removes all of the phosphorylated tyrosine residues in the intracellular domain of the receptor, thereby preventing further signal transduction. The remaining part of the EPO–EPOR complex is then internalized and degraded by lysosymes. The E3 ligase B-transducin repeat containing protein-1 (B-Trcp-1) is responsible for EPOR ubiquitination and degradation. Mutations of the B-Trcp abolish EPOR ubiquitination and degradation, making BaF3 cells expressing the EPORs hypersensitive to EPO. Each of the PFCP mutations involving the EPOR results in the loss of the binding site for B-Trcp-1. These findings suggest that the EPO hypersensitivity in PFCP might not only be attributable to a failure to recruit negative regulators such as phosphatases to inactivate JAK2 but that these mutant receptors are defective in EPO-induced receptor downregulation.

The effect of a truncated EPOR is not always predictable. Some patients who inherit an EPOR mutation are not polycythemic. This observation suggests that undefined environmental or genetic factors may mask the development of polycythemia. Also, the heterogeneity of the polycythemic phenotype observed in a PFCP animal model appears to be strain dependent. This indicates that gene modifiers or epigenetic factors may mask the development of the full PFCP phenotype.

Mutations of genes encoding proteins other than the EPOR account for most cases of PFCP. Mutations of the EPOR have been found in only 10% to 20% of subjects with PFCP. Additional disease-causing genes and their mutations have yet to be identified. In patients with erythrocytosis who are JAK2V617F negative and do not have a JAK2 exon 12 mutation and who have lifelong erythrocytosis associated with a low serum EPO level, a mutational analysis of the EPOR should be pursued.

SECONDARY POLYCYTHEMIAS

Secondary polycythemias can be either congenital or acquired (see Table 67-1). Conditions leading to hypoxia, such as high altitude, cyanotic heart disease, or chronic lung disease, may result in physiologic polycythemia mediated by increased levels of EPO. There are marked variations in EPO levels and the subsequent erythroid response in the face of chronic hypoxia, suggesting that some of these factors may be genetically determined. The same degree of renal tissue hypoxia may induce substantially different levels of EPO production in response to high altitude. It is likely that these individual variations are a function of genetic differences in hypoxia sensing and the hypoxia response pathways; the exact mechanism has been the subject of recent investigations. For purposes of simplicity and clinical diagnostic usefulness, the secondary polycythemic disorders are divided into those that are acquired and those that are congenital. It should be kept in mind that this division, although useful for differential diagnosis, is artificial. Patients with inherited germline mutations, for instance, can develop an EPO-secreting pheochromocytoma or renal cell cancer, and a patient with PV can smoke and have chronic obstructive pulmonary disease (COPD). In other instances, polycythemia caused by a germline mutation can be masked by an acquired environmental factor or another gene-modifying mutation.

Acquired Secondary Polycythemias

Polycythemias of Cyanotic Heart Disease and Pulmonary Disease

Patients with cyanotic heart disease and pulmonary disease frequently have arterial hypoxemia, leading to increased production of EPO and polycythemia. Excessive EPO production occurs when the Pa_{O_2} is sustained below 67 mm Hg as a result of severely impaired pulmonary mechanics. Because patients with severe pulmonary disease and secondary erythrocytosis frequently have elevated plasma volumes, the degree of elevation of the hematocrit level may be modest. Hematocrit levels as high as 65% or rarely 75% have, however, been reported. Moderate elevations of the hematocrit have been estimated to occur in 20% of patients with COPD. Polycythemia in this setting can contribute to pulmonary hypertension, pulmonary endothelial cell dysfunction, reduced cerebral blood flow, hyperuricemia, gout, and an increased risk of venous thromboembolic disease.

Why some patients with pulmonary disease and congenital heart disease develop polycythemia but others do not is not clear. Increased oxygen-carrying capacity may improve oxygen delivery; however, it is not obvious at what hematocrit level the resultant elevation in blood viscosity impairs blood flow to the tissues, leading to a reduction in oxygen uptake. In addition, oxygen uptake to the tissues is markedly influenced by whole blood volume. Thus, whereas the optimal hematocrit level for oxygen delivery is about 45% in normovolemic subjects, it rises to over 60% in hypervolemic states, likely as a result of engorgement of the vascular bed and a decrease in peripheral resistance. Furthermore, chronic exposure to hypoxia leads to respiratory alkalosis that in turn promotes the synthesis of 2,3-bisphosphoglycerate (2,3-BPG), facilitating increased oxygen delivery to tissues.

The practical relevance of an elevated hematocrit level in this clinical situation is whether and at what level it is harmful or beneficial.[5] An extremely elevated hematocrit level may be detrimental to optimal oxygen delivery. Extreme but not moderate polycythemia caused by chronic hypoxia may affect systemic vascular function by altering blood viscosity, vessel wall shear stress, reduced endothelial cell–derived nitric oxide release, and increasing the secretion of endothelin. Although it is widely accepted that erythrocytotic pediatric patients with cyanotic heart disease are at an increased risk for developing cerebrovascular accidents, the literature provides conflicting data as relates to the prevalence of such events among adults. A 10% to 13.6% prevalence of stroke and transient ischemic attacks (TIAs) has been reported in a cohort of adult patients with cyanotic heart disease, but others have claimed that such events are rare.

Iron deficiency occurs in more than 30% because of the total depletion of iron stores to support erythropoiesis. Microcytic iron-deficient RBCs are rarely found, and despite the iron deficiency, these patients frequently have normal mean corpuscular volumes but high mean corpuscular hemoglobin concentrations, which might maximize the amount of hemoglobin within an individual RBC, thereby maximizing oxygen delivery. In the past, compensatory erythrocytosis was thought to lead to an increased plasma viscosity, leading to a compromised microcirculation, resulting in such symptoms as headache, sluggish mentation, dizziness, blurry vision, muscle weakness, or paresthesias. In reality, such symptoms are rare in patients with chronic compensated secondary erythrocytosis, and the secondary erythrocytosis is viewed as a physiological desirable response to chronic hypoxia. The symptoms delineated above are likely attributable to decreased tissue oxygen delivery rather than hyperviscosity.

The treatment of hyperviscosity secondary to erythrocytosis in cyanotic heart disease with prophylactic phlebotomy was once a core therapeutic strategy but today is rarely used. In fact, phlebotomy has been reported to have harmful rather than beneficial effects in adults with cyanotic congenital heart disease. Many question if the beneficial effects attributed to phlebotomy represented a placebo effect. Because almost one-third of these patients are iron deficient even though their RBC indices do not reflect this, routine assessment of the patient's iron status is suggested with gradual supplementation with sufficient iron to attain appropriate compensatory levels of erythropoiesis but avoiding excessive sudden increases in the degree of erythrocytosis. The present evidence indicates that prophylactic phlebotomy promotes the development of iron deficiency, decreases exercise tolerance, and increases the number of cerebrovascular events. Currently, experts in this field recommend that phlebotomy should be restricted to individuals with symptoms with extreme erythrocytosis (hematocrit >65%) and preoperatively to improve hemostasis. Clinical data to justify these recommendations are lacking. Phlebotomy must be followed by the infusion of an equal volume of fluids to maintain intravascular volume and blood flow as well as to provide a dilutional effect to reduce the hematocrit level. A 1:1 replacement with 0.9% normal saline has been recommended, but others have suggested replacing the volume of blood removed with 1:1 fresh-frozen plasma infused over 30 to 60 minutes. Hydroxyurea therapy has been used occasionally to reduce erythropoiesis in this situation to reduce the need for phlebotomy, but little evidence exists for this approach. The superiority of hydroxyurea therapy versus phlebotomy therapy has not been documented. Hydroxyurea might act not only by suppressing RBC production but also by promoting macrocytic RBC formation, thereby increasing RBC deformability and decreasing RBC adhesiveness.

Chronic oxygen therapy in patients with severe COPD has resulted in relief of hypoxia and a modest reduction in hematocrit levels. Pharmacologic interventions, including theophylline, inhaled nitric oxidesildenafil, or antagonism of the renin–angiotensin pathway with losartin, may also reduce the degree of pulmonary hypertension or secondary erythrocytosis.

Obstructive Sleep Apnea–Induced Polycythemia

Obstructive sleep apnea syndrome is characterized by repetitive episodes of partial or complete obstruction of airflow during sleep. Common symptoms include loud snoring and breathing pauses observed by a bed partner, feelings of nonrefreshing sleep, and excess daytime sleeping. Although the evidence is largely anecdotal, secondary polycythemia is a widely recognized complication of long-standing sleep apnea, being found in 5% to 10% of those with nocturnal apnea and hypopnea. Similarly, 25% of those with unexplained polycythemia are subsequently found to have sleep apnea. The mechanism by which sleep apnea causes polycythemia is unclear. Differences in EPO levels between normoxic and hypoxemic patients referred for suspected sleep apnea have not been documented. Obstructive sleep apnea is also associated with an increased risk of developing cardiovascular diseases, including systemic hypertension, pulmonary hypertension, cardiac arrhythmias, atherosclerosis, ischemic heart disease, and stroke. Intermittent hypoxia is thought to be a major cause of cardiovascular complications. These patients undergo repeated episodes of hypoxia and normoxia. The hypoxia leads to ischemia, and the reoxygenation causes a sudden increase of oxygen. This reoxygenation phase results in the production of reactive oxygen species and the promotion of oxidative stress, leading to an inflammatory response and the development of vascular complications.

Conversely, PV may induce central sleep apnea by decreasing cerebral blood flow to diencephalic respiratory centers, and patients so affected can have complete resolution of their sleep disorder with normalization of their blood counts.

Pickwickian Syndrome and Polycythemia

Pickwickian syndrome or obesity–hypoventilation syndrome, seen in morbidly obese individuals, is characterized by chronic hypoxemia and hypercapnia caused by alveolar hypoventilation, with a resultant increase in EPO production, polycythemia, and cor pulmonale. The three principal causes are the high cost of the work of respiration in morbidly obese individuals, dysfunction of the respiratory centers, and repeated episodes of nocturnal obstructive apnea. Effective treatments include surgically induced weight loss, nasal continuous positive airway pressure ventilation, and the respiratory stimulant medroxyprogesterone acetate.

Polycythemia Caused by High Altitude

Polycythemia caused by the hypoxic conditions encountered by high-altitude dwellers would appear at first glance to represent a universal adaptive process to altitude. High altitude results in hyperventilation, alkalosis, and shifting of the O_2 dissociation curve to the left, leading to the impaired release of O_2 from hemoglobin and ultimately tissue hypoxia. This tissue hypoxia results in markedly increased EPO production, leading to increased plasma iron turnover, reticulocytosis, and a rising hematocrit level. Residents of the Andes Mountains who live 4200 m above sea level frequently have 30% higher hematocrit levels than individuals living at sea level.

People native to high altitudes (highlanders) live in a hypobaric hypoxic environment characterized by a low ambient partial pressure of oxygen. In response to this environment, they develop alveolar hypoxia, hypoxemia, and polycythemia. Healthy highlanders develop pulmonary hypertension, right ventricular hypertrophy, and an increased amount of smooth muscle cells in the distal pulmonary arterial branches, which leads to increased pulmonary vascular resistance and pulmonary artery pressure as compared with individuals living at sea level. The importance of these structural changes in the pulmonary vasculature in highlanders is confirmed by the slow decline of pulmonary artery pressure, which is normalized after living for 2 years at sea level. Despite these adaptive changes, healthy highlanders are able to perform physical activities similar to or often even more strenuous than those living at sea level. In fact, there are differences in ventilation rates between athletes performing at sea level and those at high altitudes. Ventilation rates of athletes increase normally during exercise at sea level, but relative hypoventilation occurs in highlanders. This relative hypoventilation is characteristic of Andean natives and has been ascribed to desensitization of the carotid bodies to the hypoxic stimulus. The erythrocytosis observed in individuals who reside at high altitudes for relatively short periods of time (days) can also be attributed in part to excessive water loss and contraction of the plasma volume. Total acclimatization of an individual who moves from sea level to a high altitude may actually require years. Individuals who reside at sea level and are acutely exposed to high altitudes are at increased risks of developing deep venous thrombosis, pulmonary infarction, retinal hemorrhage, and ischemic digits because of increased blood viscosity. High-altitude climbers frequently combat these problems by intravenous administration of isotonic saline, with considerable success.

The chronic responses of various ethnic and racial groups to high altitudes are quite variable. Andean natives, known as the Quechua and Ayamara Indians, experience a gradual increase in their hemoglobin levels with age. In addition, hemoglobin values are almost 10% higher in those living at 5500 m above sea level than in those living at 4355 m above sea level. Curiously, their Tibetan and Ethiopian counterparts living at similar altitudes do not respond to the resultant chronic hypoxia by increasing their hematocrits.[6] It has been suggested that high levels of nitrous oxide in the exhaled breath of Tibetans may improve oxygen delivery by inducing vasodilatation and increasing blood flow to tissues, thus making the compensatory increased RBC volume unnecessary. Interestingly, Tibetans and Ethiopians have lived much longer as mountain dwellers than the Quechua or Ayamara Indians, suggesting that extreme elevation of the RBC mass is a maladaptation that Tibetans and Ethiopians have avoided by adopting more physiologic compensatory mechanisms. Many residents of the Tibetan plateau reside at elevations exceeding 4000 m and experience oxygen concentrations that are about 40% lower than experienced at sea level. Human adaptation to a high-altitude environment has been believed to be the result of advantageous genetic mutations and selective pressure.[7] These genetic adaptations are shared by common ancestors within East Asian but not Central and South Asian populations and confer characteristics including adaptation to hypoxia, the absence of CMS, and high offspring survival rates. Polymorphisms in the *EPAS1* gene that encodes HIF-2α, and the *EGLN1* gene, which encodes PHD2, have been positively selected and have been shown to be associated with the key adaptive features in Tibetans. The putative advantageous haplotypes of *EGLN1* and *EPAS1* have revealed negative correlations with hemoglobin levels in Tibetans compared with lowlander Han Chinese. These Tibetans apparently are able to maintain sufficient oxygenation of tissues at high altitudes without increasing RBC numbers. Variations in *ELGN1* and *EPAS1* have also been linked to susceptibility to developing high altitude pulmonary edema. Other factors can contribute to the development of erythrocytosis in high-altitude dwellers. Many inhabitants of the mining community of Cerro de Pasco (altitude, 4280 m) with excessive erythrocytosis (mean hematocrit, 76%; range 66%–91%) have been shown to have toxic serum cobalt levels, suggesting that other EPO-promoting factors such as cobalt might augment the hypoxia-inducing effect on EPO, causing the extreme polycythemias.

This individual variability of elevation of serum EPO levels in high-altitude dwellers and the resultant increase in RBC mass appears widespread. For example, acclimatization to moderately high altitudes when combined with low-altitude training (so-called living high, training low) improves sea-level performance in endurance athletes, in part because of the erythropoietic effects of altitude exposure. This substantial individual variability in response to all forms of altitude training correlates with improved athletic performance and with elevation of EPO levels. A large component of this individual variability appears to be related to differences in the peak and rate of decay of the increase in EPO in response to altitude exposure. These observations suggest that genetically determined variables account for individual responses to hypoxia.

Chronic mountain sickness (CMS) is a pathological loss of adaptation to altitude by highlanders. CMS is a clinical syndrome that occurs in native or lifelong residents living above 2500 m. Anecdotal reports of families or people being particularly susceptible to CMS are frequently cited as evidence that certain individuals have an innate susceptibility to develop CMS. It is characterized by excessive erythrocytosis (females, Hb >19 g/dL; males, Hb >21 g/dL); severe hypoxemia; and in some cases, moderate or severe pulmonary hypertension that may lead to the development of cor pulmonale and congestive heart failure. The clinical picture of CMS gradually disappears after descending to lower altitudes and reappears after returning to high altitudes. The prevalence of CMS is higher in men than women and increases with altitude, aging, associated lung disease, history of smoking, and air pollution. CMS is a public health problem in populations of mountainous regions of the world living above 2500 m. In China alone, 80 million people live above that altitude, but in South America, 35 million people live above 2500 m. CMS is a common problem in these areas. Bolivian investigators have reported a prevalence of CMS in 6% to 8% of males in La Paz (3600 m) and a hospital frequency of 28%. Chinese investigators have reported an overall prevalence of 5.6% in Chinese Han immigrants and 1.2% in Tibetan natives living in the Qinghai Tibetan plateau. The major mechanism underlying the development of CMS is relative alveolar hypoventilation. Healthy highlanders characteristically hyperventilate. A gradual decline in the rate of alveolar ventilation in these individuals leads to progressive loss of adaptation to chronic hypoxia and the development of CMS. The main components of this syndrome include (1) alveolar hypoventilation leading to relative hypercapnia and increasing hypoxemia; (2) excessive polycythemia leading to increased blood viscosity and expansion of the total lung blood volume; (3) pulmonary hypertension and right ventricular hypertrophy that may evolve to hypoxic cor pulmonale and heart failure; and (4) neuropsychiatric symptoms, including sleep disorders, headache, dizziness, and mental fatigue. Physical examination reveals cyanosis of the nail beds, ears, and lips in contrast to the ruddy color that is characteristic of a healthy highlander. In some cases, the face is almost black, and the mucosa and conjunctiva are dark red. The fingers are frequently clubbed, and auscultation of the heart reveals an increased pulmonary second sound. The patients are frequently hypertensive and have evidence of heart failure. Chest radiographic and electrocardiographic findings are characteristic of right atrial and right ventricular hypertrophy. The cardiac hemodynamic values of patients with CMS and healthy highlanders and those living at sea level are shown in Table 67-2. Criteria for the diagnosis of CMS have been recently published and are useful in identifying CMS patients as well as monitoring their response to treatment.

The definitive treatment for CMS is descent to lower altitudes or sea level. The degree of polycythemia decreases after a few weeks or months, and eventually the hematocrit level returns to sea-level values. Pulmonary hypertension and right ventricular hypertrophy gradually resolve and disappear after 1 to 2 years of living at sea level. Phlebotomy or isovolemic hemodilution can reduce the excessive erythrocytosis and hyperviscosity. A variety of drugs has also been evaluated for the treatment of patients with CMS. Ten weeks of the respiratory stimulant medroxyprogesterone acetate at doses of 60 mg/day led to a reduction of the hematocrit level from 60% to 52% and an increase in arterial oxygen saturation from 84% to 90% in 17 highlanders with excess erythrocytes. Medroxyprogesterone use, however, was associated with a loss of libido in men and therefore is infrequently used in this population. Therapy with almitrine, a respiratory stimulant, or enalapril, an ACE inhibitor (10 mg/day for 30 days), has resulted in even more modest reductions of hematocrit levels. Acetazolamide therapy has been evaluated in a small double-blind, placebo-controlled, randomized clinical trial of patients with CMS. Acetazolamide is an inhibitor of carbonic anhydrase and stimulates ventilation by promoting the development of metabolic acidosis. Furthermore, acetazolamide reduces renal EPO production. Patients with CMS were randomized to receive placebo or acetazolamide therapy at a dose of 250 or 500 mg/day for 21 days. Drug therapy at both doses of acetazolamide resulted in reduction of hematocrit levels by 7% ($P < .001$) and serum EPO levels by 50% to 67% ($P < .1$), with an increase in nocturnal oxygen saturation levels of 5% ($P < .01$). According to this small study, 250 mg of acetazolamide daily appears to be an inexpensive, nontoxic, effective therapy for CMS. Whether this conclusion can be validated by larger clinical trials and can be implemented successfully in large populations of patients with CMS has yet to be determined.

Table 67-2 Frequency of JAK2V617F Mutations in Polycythemia Vera, Essential Thrombocytosis, and Primary Myelofibrosis

	JAK2V617F Detection Method	PV: JAK2V617F (Homozygous)	ET: JAK2V617F (Homozygous)	PMF: JAK2V617F (Homozygous)
James et al	Sequencing	89 (30)	43	43
Levine et al	Sequencing	74 (25)	32 (3)	35 (9)
Kralovics et al	Sequencing	65 (27)	23 (3)	57 (22)
Baxter et al	Sequencing	97 (26)	57 (0)	50 (19)
Jones et al	ARMS/pyrosequencing	81 (33)	41 (7)	43 (29)
Levine et al	Allele specific/Taqman	99	72	39

Data from Levine RL, Wernig G: Role of JAK-STAT signaling in the pathogenesis of myeloproliferative disorders. *Hematology Am Soc Hematol Educ Program* 233, 2006.
ET, Essential thrombocytosis; *PMF,* primary myelofibrosis; polycythemia vera.

Smokers' Polycythemia or Carbon Monoxide–Induced Polycythemia

Smoking is the most common cause of secondary polycythemia. Those affected have a carboxyhemoglobin-induced increase in RBC mass or decrease in plasma volume, either of which is reversible with smoking cessation. Excessive carbon monoxide exposure can also be attributed to exposure to industrial emissions and automobile exhaust. Carbon monoxide binds to hemoglobin with a more than 200 times greater affinity than oxygen, resulting in not only occupation of one of the heme groups of hemoglobin but also an increase in the O_2 affinity by the remaining heme group. Individuals smoking even one pack of cigarettes a day frequently have elevated hematocrit levels. These patients characteristically have normal blood gases and elevation of carboxyhemoglobin levels, resulting in a reduction in $P_{50}o_2$. The elevation of the hematocrit level is reversed with the interruption of the smoking behavior. Increased hematocrit levels have been observed in 3% to 5% of heavy smokers. Although these patients are not immune to thrombotic complications, the number of thromboembolic events is lower than in patients with PV. A retrospective review of patients with either PV or smokers' polycythemia found that 60% of those with PV had thromboses, but only 41% of those with smokers' polycythemia were so affected (P <.05). Recently, polycythemia has also been reported to be associated with hookah use. A hookah is an oriental pipe containing tobacco often mixed with molasses and fruit flavors connected by a long flexible tube that draws the smoke to the bowl of water. Hookah use exposes the user to generous amounts of carbon monoxide, resulting in erythrocytosis.

Postrenal Transplantation Erythrocytosis

Postrenal transplantation erythrocytosis (PTE) is defined as a persistently elevated hematocrit level greater than 51% after renal transplantation without an elevation of the WBC (WBC) count or platelet count. PTE is a potentially dangerous condition found in approximately 10% to 15% of renal allograft recipients. PTE usually develops within 8 to 24 months after a successful renal transplantation and resolves spontaneously within 2 years in about 25% of patients despite persistently good renal allograft function. PTE is more common in males and may recur in the same patient after a second successful renal transplantation. Factors that increase the likelihood of its development are a lack of EPO therapy before transplantation, a history of smoking, diabetes mellitus, transplant-related renal artery stenosis, retention of the native kidney, low serum ferritin levels, and normal or high pretransplantation EPO levels. PTE is also more frequent in patients who do not experience rejection. At higher hematocrit levels (usually >60%), thrombotic events may complicate the clinical course of patients with PTE.

Approximately 60% of patients with PTE experience malaise, headache, plethora, lethargy, and dizziness. In addition, from 10% to 20% develop thromboembolic complications involving either arteries or veins. Retention of the native kidney is essential for the development of PTE in most cases. Although the transplanted kidney produces EPO under normal regulatory mechanisms, the native kidney overproduces EPO despite the development of erythrocytosis. Frequently, the PTE resolves with removal of the native kidney. Plasma EPO levels are higher (10-fold) in patients with PTE than in nonerythrocytotic renal transplant recipients. In addition, erythroid progenitor cells isolated from patients with PTE are hypersensitive to EPO.

The molecular basis of PTE remains unclear; AngII is believed, however, to play an important role in its pathogenesis by sustaining the secretion of EPO. Growing evidence indicates that increased AT1R expression makes erythroid progenitor cells hypersensitive to AngII. Furthermore, AngII can modulate release of erythropoietic stimulatory factors, including EPO and IGF-1. Because men comprise almost all of the transplant recipients who develop PTE, androgens are thought to play a role in the development of the syndrome. Androgens can directly affect erythroid progenitor cells or stimulate EPO production or actually the RAS. Treatment of patients with PTE includes intermittent phlebotomy or administration of drugs. The ACE inhibitor enalapril suppresses the renin–angiotensin pathway and virtually eliminates the need for therapeutic phlebotomy in these patients. Maximal reduction of hemoglobin levels is evident 6 months after starting therapy with either ACE inhibitor or angiotensin receptor blockers. Some patients are exquisitely sensitive to these medications and may become severely anemic. The AT1R antagonist losartan has been shown to be as effective in treating PTE as are ACE inhibitors. Therapy is usually begun at hematocrit levels above 55% with the hope of maintaining hematocrit levels below 50% to reduce the risk of thrombosis. Furthermore, the ACE inhibitor fosinopril in an open-label crossover trial with theophylline was shown to produce a dramatic reduction in hematocrits in patients with PTE (51.3%–43.7%; P <.005). Low doses of ramipril, another ACE inhibitor, normalized the hematocrit level in 26 of 27 patients with PTE after a mean of 127 days of therapy.

Polycythemia Accompanying Kidney and Liver Diseases and Neoplastic Disorders

Polycythemia has been reported in association with kidney diseases such as renal cell carcinoma, renal artery stenosis, hydronephrosis, Wilms tumor, and polycystic kidney disease, paragangliomas, and pituitary adenomas. Renal tumors account for approximately one-third of cases of tumor-associated polycythemias. The tumor tissue has been demonstrated to produce excessive amounts of EPO, and the erythrocytosis resolves with surgical resections of the tumor. The mechanisms underlying the activation of the EPO gene have been related to somatic mutation of the VHL gene in clear cell renal carcinomas. Clear cell carcinoma is associated with erythrocytosis and high serum EPO levels caused by increased expression of EPO mRNA, HIF-1α, and HIF-2α.[8] These abnormalities were related to a point mutation in the VHL gene that impaired the bindings of HIF-1α to VHL, leading to its accumulation and increased production of EPO. Polycythemia is also a well-described paraneoplastic manifestation of hepatocellular carcinoma in 2.5% to 10% of patients and is again caused by the production of EPO by the tumor. Polycythemia in hepatoma patients is strongly related to tumor burden and elevated α-fetoprotein levels. Polycythemia has also been associated with cerebellar hemangioblastomas and very large uterine fibromas. In tumor-associated erythrocytosis, EPO production has been shown to be autonomous of hypoxic stimuli. Paragangliomas are tumors arising from extra-adrenal paragangliar neural crest cells. Most paragangliomas arise retroperitoneally or within the peritoneal cavity and are associated with high EPO levels and erythrocytosis. After tumor resection, reduction of the EPO levels and erythrocytosis occurs. Germ line mutations involving two Krebs cycle enzymes, fumarate hydratase and succinate dehydrogenase, have been implicated in the hereditary paraganglioma–pheochromocytoma syndrome. In tumors deficient in these enzymes, fumarate and succinate accumulate, which inhibits PHD, leading to accumulation of HIF-1α and eventually resulting in erythrocytosis. In another patient with a paraganglioma who did not have the inherited syndrome but had extreme erythrocytosis, a mutation in PHD2 was demonstrated in germ line cells. In this patient's tumor, tumor analysis showed LOH with the mutant allele predominating, which was associated with a loss of function. The degradation of both HIF-1α and HIF-2α was increased. These data indicate that PHD2 can act as a tumor suppressor gene. The tumor suppressor activity of PHD2 has also been reported in sporadic endometrial, breast, and pancreatic cancers with inactivating mutations ultimately leading to the increased production of growth factors that contribute to tumor growth.

Polycythemia in Endocrine Disorders

Polycythemia is also associated with Cushing syndrome, acromegaly, and primary aldosteronism. Secondary polycythemia can also be seen in 24% of older hypogonadal men receiving long-term androgen replacement therapy and a significant number of competitive athletes taking anabolic steroids. For instance, in a small study of professional bodybuilders, 67% of those examined had hematocrit levels above 50%. The effectiveness of drug screening in athletic competitions is demonstrated by the very low rate of positive test results for androgens (<2% of 170,000 tests) on random testing at the Olympic Games and other international events. Despite previous assertions regarding increased EPO excretion after androgen therapy, none of the athletes examined had elevated levels of EPO. Recombinant human EPO has also been abused by athletes competing in endurance sports and can be detected by analyzing the individual's hematocrit level, reticulocyte count, percentage of macrocytic RBCs, serum EPO level, serum transferrin receptor level, and electrophoretic mobility of the EPO molecule (recombinant EPO is less negatively charged than endogenous EPO).

Congenital Secondary Polycythemias

High-Oxygen-Affinity Hemoglobins and Bisphosphoglycerate Deficiency

More than 100 mutations of hemoglobin lead to increased oxygen affinity and thus decreased oxygen delivery and compensatory polycythemia (see Chapter 41). These mutations involve either the α- or β-chain globin chains. Such polycythemias are usually well tolerated in young patients but may lead to thrombotic complications in older patients. High-oxygen-affinity hemoglobin variants are transmitted as autosomal dominants. Phlebotomy therapy of such patients has been reported to be of no beneficial value and has been shown to decrease exercise tolerance and anaerobic threshold. The best test to detect a high-oxygen-affinity hemoglobin relies on the determination of hemoglobin dissociation kinetics and P50 (partial pressure of O_2 at which hemoglobin is 50% oxygenated). If cooximetry is not available, the P50 can be mathematically estimated from a venous blood gas measurement by using a computer algorithm, which is available online.

Whereas a $P_{50}O_2$ below 17 mm Hg is indicative of a mutant hemoglobin with high oxygen affinity, a level above 35 mm Hg is strongly suggestive of a mutant hemoglobin with a low oxygen affinity. Hemoglobin electrophoresis is not a reliable screen to rule out hemoglobin mutations because only about half of these mutants are electrophoretically distinguishable. A hemoglobin electrophoresis will reveal the presence of an abnormal hemoglobin only if the mutation leads to a change in electrical charge. In 30 hemoglobin variants, such a charge differential was not present, and high-performance liquid chromatography or mass spectrometry followed by polymerase chain reaction (PCR)–directed sequencing was required to make the diagnosis.

A rare cause of congenital polycythemia is 2,3-BPG (previously known as 2,3-DPG) deficiency (see Chapter 42). 2,3-BPG is synthesized in RBCs and binds to hemoglobin, thereby reducing its affinity for oxygen. An absence of 2,3-BPG therefore leads to increased affinity of hemoglobin for oxygen, resulting in a lifelong hypoxic stimulus and erythrocytosis.

Congenital methemoglobinemias, whether caused by cytochrome b5 reductase mutations or globin mutations, may be associated with mild polycythemia (see Chapter 41). When hemoglobin is oxidized to methemoglobin, all of the four subunits of the tetramer may be affected, eliminating the oxygen transport capacity of hemoglobin.

Hypoxia Inducible Factor Pathway Mutations Leading to Erythrocytosis

Alterations of a number of proteins in the HIF pathway have been shown to lead to increased EPO production and erythrocytosis (see Fig. 67-1).[9] Chuvash polycythemia (CP) is an autosomal recessive disorder associated with germline mutations of VHL and erythrocytosis. CP was first described in the mid-1970s and is endemic in the Chuvash population of the Russian republic. The serum EPO concentration in affected individuals is elevated compared with healthy first-degree family members, although some patients may have normal serum EPO levels. They also have elevated levels of VEGF and plasminogen activator inhibitor-1. The erythroid progenitors of patients with CP are also hypersensitive to EPO; thus CP has characteristics of both primary and secondary polycythemias. A homozygous missense mutation in the VHL gene, VHL598C→T mutation, has been identified in CP patients. The disorder is characterized by high hemoglobin levels (usually >20 g/L), increased plasma EPO levels, varicose veins, vertebral hemangiomas, low blood pressure, and an elevated concentration of VEGF. The defective VHL gene product is not capable of promoting the ubiquitin-mediated degradation of HIF-1α and HIF-2α, thereby leading to increased levels of both of these proteins and increased elaboration of EPO. Inheritance occurs as an autosomal recessive, and the frequency of the allele has been estimated to be at 0.057 in the Chuvash population. Several other similar types of mutations in VHL have been described that have been observed in a variety of other ethnic groups. A number of heterozygotes with erythrocytosis have been reported, which can likely be accounted for by an as yet undiscovered additional defect. CP is associated with a high mortality rate from thrombotic and hemorrhagic vascular complications. Cerebrovascular events are especially common causes of death. The median age of death from cerebrovascular events is 42 years. Estimated survival to age 65 years is 29% for individuals with CP and 64% for age-matched community members. There is a perfect genotype–phenotypic correlation, with all patients with CP being homozygotes for the mutation. Interestingly, heterozygous carriers do not develop erythrocytosis but do have lower blood pressures and do not seem to be at increased risk for tumors, which contrasts with patients with VHL syndrome. Patients with CP also have larger livers, spleens, and kidneys than control patients, which has been attributed to enhanced cellular proliferation caused by HIF-2α suppression of p21Cip1.

Germline mutations of VHL alleles have been reported in several patients with apparent congenital polycythemia that had no evidence of developing a tumor; some of these subjects had germline mutations of both VHL alleles. Other subjects with congenital polycythemia of various ethnicities, including Pakistanis, Punjabis, African Americans, and whites, harboring homozygosity for the CP VHL mutation or double heterozygosity for CP and other VHL mutations, have been found. The VHL598C→T mutation has been shown to originate in a single haplotype in the Chuvash patients, as well as in whites, Asian Indians, and one African American individual. Homozygosity of this mutation appears to be the most common genetic defect leading to congenital polycythemia. The mutation originated from a single founder 12,000 to 51,000 years ago. This suggests that such wide dissemination from the original founder may be associated with some survival advantage for heterozygotes carrying this mutation. Such an advantage might be related to a subtle improvement of iron metabolism, erythropoiesis, embryonic development, energy metabolism, or some other yet unknown effect.

von Hippel-Lindau mutations are likely the most common cause of congenital polycythemias, greatly exceeding the number of patients with hemoglobin chain mutations. In point of fact, in one study of more than 200 unrelated subjects with apparently congenital polycythemia, none had a 2,3-BPG deficiency, two had a globin mutation (Hgb Vanderbilt, and Hemoglobin San Diego), and 12 had EPOR mutations to account for their polycythemia. By contrast, when 50 patients were examined for the VHL mutation, 22 had VHL mutations, most of them being the CP VHL mutation, occurring either homozygously or in combination with another VHL mutation. The failure of patients with CP to develop VHL syndrome tumors is consistent with the concept that deregulation of H1F-1α and VEGF are not sufficient to cause tumors. A cluster of patients with clinical features identical to patients with CP has been documented on the island of Ischia in the Bay of Naples, Italy. All of these patients also had the VHL598C→T mutation. Twelve of the 14 patients were homozygotes, and two were heterozygotes. The homozygotes had symptoms identical to patients in Chuvashia with this mutation. Unlike heterozygotes in Chuvashia, the heterozygotes from Ischia developed erythrocytosis associated with high EPO levels, which raises the possibility that genetic alterations of additional components of the oxygen-sensing pathway other than VHL may contribute to the development of erythrocytosis in the Italian patients. The disorder in Ischia has a gene frequency even higher than that in Chuvashia, with 14% of the population estimated to be heterozygotes, which has led to the suggestion that heterozygotes have a survival advantage, perhaps caused by heterozygosity conferring protection from developing anemia.

The Chuvash mutation has also been shown to have a profound effect on the cardiopulmonary system. Patients with CP have significant abnormalities of cardiopulmonary physiology, including elevated basal ventilation rates and increased pulmonary vascular tone, with extremely high ventilatory rates and heightened pulmonary vasoconstriction and heart rates in response to acute hypoxia. These observations indicate that the VHL–HIF pathway might also play a central role in calibrating the pulmonary system to hypoxic challenges. Such undesirable exaggerated hypoxic responses and the resulting elevated pulmonary vascular hypertension may contribute to the morbidity and mortality associated with CP. Increased expression of endothelin-1 has been documented in patients with CP. Endothelin-1 has been associated with the development of hypoxia-related pulmonary hypertension. Endothelin-1 receptor inhibitors might therefore be useful in reversing the associated pulmonary hypertension in these patients. Treatment strategies for patients with CP have included phlebotomy, aspirin, and occasionally chemotherapy. It is unknown whether such therapeutic strategies alter the natural history of this disorder. A variety of HIF-1 inhibitors being currently evaluated for the treatment of tumor patients might potentially also be useful for the treatment of patients with CP.

Recently, the CP-VHL mutants have been shown to affect EPO signaling in erythroid progenitor cells of patients with CP. JAK2 phosphorylation of STAT5 triggers not only erythroid progenitor development but also a negative feedback mechanism by transactivating the expression of SOCS family members which bind and inhibit activated JAKs by promoting their ubiquination and protosomal degradation. The CP mutation causes conformational changes leading to a tight CP–VHL–SOCS1 association, thereby slowing phosphorylated JAK2 degradation. These events lead to hyperactivation of the JAK2–STAT pathway in erythroid progenitor cells causing their hypersensitivity to EPO, which likely contributes to the excessive erythrocytosis characteristic of CP.

Additional genetic abnormalities of oxygen sensing have been reported that lead to familial polycythemia. A heterozygous C-to-G change at base 950 of the coding sequence of PHD2 (P317R mutation) was first detected in all three affected family members with this syndrome. Hydroxylation of HIF-1 by PHD2 facilitates its interaction with VHL, thereby favoring its ubiquitination and degradation by the proteosome.[10] The failure of PHD2 P317R to bind the HIF-1 and HIF-2α and promote HIF hydroxylase activity ultimately leads to increased HIF-l and EPO levels, resulting in the development of erythrocytosis. The PHD2 P317R mutation is inherited as an autosomal dominant trait in contrast to the CP defect, which is an autosomal recessive disorder. Polycythemic patients with PHD2 P317R do not have any evidence of tumors characteristic of the VHL syndrome. Additional mutations in PHD2 have been reported that lead to erythrocytosis. All of these mutations are germline and heterozygous encoding predicted mutant full-length PHD2 proteins. Two of these patients with PHD mutations also have an exon 12 JAK2 mutation that is associated with PV. The interaction between these two defects requires further study.

A series of HIF-2α gain of function mutations have also been reported to lead to familial erythrocytosis.[9] These mutations lead to weakened bonds between PHD2 and HIF-1α, resulting in less hydroxylation of HIF-1α and subsequent recognition of HIF-1α by VHL. Many of these patients present in their twenties, although patients have also been diagnosed in their fifties with erythrocytosis associated with high EPO levels. All patients have heterozygous mutations, suggesting that one allele is sufficient to cause erythrocytosis. It is not unusual for patients to have a clinical history of thrombotic disorders, but there does not appear to be an increased incidence of cancer.

Neonatal Polycythemia

Because of the high oxygen affinity of fetal hemoglobin, many neonates have markedly elevated hematocrit levels. Babies with hematocrit levels over 65% have more neurologic and functional impairments and are more likely to be born to diabetic mothers. Although phlebotomy has been recommended, there is little evidence that it has been beneficial for these babies.

Drug-Induced Erythrocytosis

The administration of EPO, corticosteroids, or androgens to an excessive degree has each been associated with reversible erythrocytosis. Androgens have been shown to simulate EPO production and to directly affect erythroid progenitor cells. Approximately 5% of patients receiving long-term testosterone therapy for testosterone deficiency syndrome develop erythrocytosis. Androgens activate HIF-1 and HIF-1-regulated gene expression, leading to increased expression of VEGF and presumably EPO. Rarely, erythrocytosis can be the presenting manifestation of Cushing syndrome. Blood doping refers to the use of EPO to increase the RBC mass and enhance oxygen delivery with the hope of increasing endurance performance in athletes. A monitoring of an athlete's hematologic profile longitudinally provides some insight into the likelihood of blood doping playing a role in the development of erythrocytosis

The development of paradoxical polycythemia in three patients with VHL syndrome and central nervous system or retinal hemangioblastomas treated with the VEGF receptor inhibitor SU5416 is surprising but has been reported. The cause of these phenomena remains unknown. In addition, reversible erythrocytosis has been reported with the use of the tyrosine kinase inhibitors sunitinib and sorafenib in over 20% of patients with a variety of metastatic malignancies including renal cell carcinoma, hepatomas, and melanomas. The erythrocytosis associated with these drugs is not associated with further elevation of EPO levels but has been suggested to be a consequence of sensitization of erythroid cells to EPO.

POLYCYTHEMIA VERA

Polycythemia vera is a clonal, chronic, progressive myeloproliferative neoplasm (MPN) often of insidious onset characterized by an absolute increase in RBC mass and also usually by leukocytosis, thrombocytosis, and splenomegaly. PV leads to excessive proliferation of erythroid, myeloid, and megakaryocytic elements within the BM. Vaquez first described this clinical entity in 1892, noting the characteristic physical findings. At the turn of this century, Cabot and Osler independently associated the name PV with this clinical disorder.

Polycythemia vera differs from many other hematologic malignancies in that prolonged survival is enjoyed by most patients if the excessive production of RBCs and platelets can be controlled. This prolonged survival, however, can be punctuated by the development of other syndromes, such as myelofibrosis (MF), termed post-PV MF, and acute leukemia (Fig. 67-3). Frequently, patients present asymptomatically to a physician only to find that they have splenomegaly, isolated erythrocytosis, or thrombocytosis. Left untreated, these patients will become symptomatic, owing to the excessive production of RBCs, platelets, or both, leading to arterial or venous thromboses, aquagenic pruritus, and symptoms caused by increasing splenomegaly. After a number of years, the erythrocytotic phase of the disease frequently becomes inactive, and the patient may no longer have the sequelae of excessive RBC production. Subsequently, these patients can develop post-PV MF, which is frequently indistinguishable from another MPN, primary MF (PMF). Finally, a significant proportion of these patients will go on to develop acute myeloid leukemia (AML). Only a limited number of patients undergo this orderly transition; many patients transition from the polycythemic phase directly into an acute leukemia or a myelodysplastic disorder.

The transition from one phase of this MPN to another is not necessarily unidirectional. A number of cases of presumed PMF have been described in which chemotherapy treatment has resulted in a striking decrease in BM fibrosis associated with the development of erythrocytosis and a syndrome that is virtually indistinguishable from de novo PV. The constantly changing clinical picture of this malignant hematologic disorder requires careful observation and treatment to deal with the numerous problems that can be encountered.

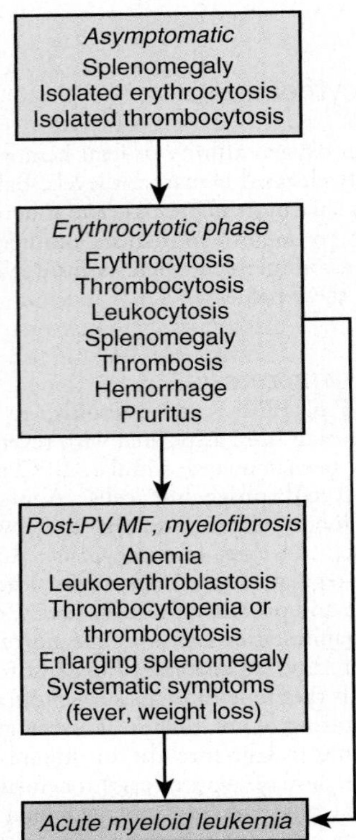

Figure 67-3 EVOLUTION OF POLYCYTHEMIA VERA (PV). *MF,* Myelofibrosis.

EPIDEMIOLOGY

Polycythemia vera is the most common primary polycythemia. Reported incidence rates are around 2.8 per 100,000 persons per year. It is important to emphasize that no or very few population-based estimates of the prevalence of this disorder are presently available. Actual determination of its prevalence has been a difficult process because of the need in the past to pursue an extensive diagnostic evaluation to differentiate this disorder from other causes of spurious or absolute erythrocytosis. The diagnosis of PV has been simplified by the identification of PV-associated mutations (JAK2V617F and JAK2 exon 12 mutations), permitting for the first time molecular epidemiologic studies. The prevalence of the JAK2V617F mutation in a normal population in Denmark was recently determined to be 0.2%, with 63% of these individuals not having a previously detected hematological malignancy.[11] The presence of the mutation was associated with increasing age, male sex, and a lower cumulative survival. Several groups have reported that 50% of patients with a splanchnic vein thrombosis without an overt MPN are JAK2V617F positive and that more than 50% of these individuals subsequently develop an MPN. However, the incidence of the mutation with unprovoked thromboembolism in the more usual sites (deep venous thrombosis involving the leg veins or pulmonary embolism) ranges between 0.2 and 1.0%. Such data have led to the conclusion that systematic screening for JAK2V617 in such a patient population is not warranted.

The prevalence of PV has been reported by several investigators to be higher among American Jews and lower among African Americans. The reported lower incidence in African Americans might reflect a referral bias characteristic of centers with research interest in MPN because the authors, when practicing in several large urban areas, have observed a considerable number of African Americans with MPNs, including PV. The incidence of the disorder is greater among Ashkenazi Jews, who originate from eastern and central Europe, than among Arabs and Sephardic Jews. Interestingly, extremely low occurrence rates have been reported from Japan. These findings suggest that important genetic factors might be involved in the biogenesis of this disorder. The importance of genetic factors in the origin of this disease is further emphasized by reports of multiple cases of JAK2V617F or JAK2 exon 12 mutation–positive and –negative MPN, including PV, within multiple generations of a number of families. These forms of familial PV must be distinguished from PFCP, CP, and polycythemia associated with mutations in the HIF pathway. The reports of families in which multiple members have PV first raised the possibility that a genetic predisposition to acquire such mutations exists in these families that is inherited in an autosomal dominant pattern with decreased penetrance. Clinical analyses of affected family members confirmed that they have clonal hematopoiesis and that their clinical manifestations are identical to patients with sporadic PV. In a large population study recently reported from Sweden, the relatives of MPN patients were shown to have a significantly increased risk of developing a Philadelphia chromosome–negative MPN and possibly chronic myeloid leukemia.[12] It was estimated that first-degree relatives of MPN patients have a five- to sevenfold greater risk of developing an MPN, again supporting the hypothesis that common strong susceptibility genes predispose one to develop PV, essential thrombocytosis (ET), PMF, and possibly CML.

One notable exception to the low prevalence of PV in Japan has been the higher incidence observed among populations exposed to atomic bomb explosions. The possibility that radiation exposure is an etiologic factor in the generation of PV was also raised by the observation in the United States of four cases of PV 10 to 20 years after a nuclear explosion in which 3000 military observers were exposed. An epidemiologic investigation that focused on occupational exposure among petroleum refinery and chemical plant workers has revealed an increased incidence of PV relative to the general population. In this study, the increased incidence of PV was linked to similar increases in the frequency of multiple myeloma and non-Hodgkin lymphoma, suggesting involvement of a putative environmental toxin that may have broad hematopoietic toxicity. The possibility of environmental factors contributing to the development of PV was recently raised by the identification of a cluster of patients with JAK2V617F-positive PV in an area of Eastern Pennsylvania that contained numerous sources of hazardous materials including, waste coal power plants and U.S. Environmental Protection Agency Superfund sites. What possible environmental factors might contribute to this fourfold increase in the number of PV cases is currently the subject of intense investigation.

Slightly more men than women develop PV, the male-to-female ratio being approximately 1.2 to 1. The average age at diagnosis is 60 years, but the disease is observed not infrequently in female patients younger than 30 years of age. In several large studies, 5% of patients with PV were younger than 40 years of age, 1% were younger than 25 years at diagnosis, and 0.1% were younger than 20 years. Small numbers of patients with PV have been reported who presented during childhood. More importantly, in several of these children, hepatic vein thrombosis (Budd-Chiari syndrome) was the initial manifestation of the disease. In fact, a 7-month-old infant with PV and an acquired somatic JAK2V617F mutation that likely occurred in utero has been reported.

Pathobiology

Considerable speculation has centered on the pathobiology of the erythrocytosis that characterizes PV. The expanded RBC mass in PV patients is due to a two- to threefold increase in the production of RBCs by a hyperplastic BM and is not attributable to prolongation of the RBC lifespan. Granulocyte and platelet production is also increased in this disorder. This overly exuberant production of all cellular elements of the blood suggests that the basic defect resides at the level of the hematopoietic cellular hierarchy from which each of these cells originates, the pluripotent hematopoietic stem cell (HSC).

A variety of studies have documented serum EPO levels in patients with PV, secondary erythrocytosis, and relative polycythemia in normal adults. Serum EPO levels have been shown to be subnormal in patients with PV, elevated in many but not all cases of secondary erythrocytosis, and normal in patients with relative polycythemia, indicating that PV cannot be an abnormality of EPO production.

In 1951, Dameshek postulated that chronic myeloid leukemia, PV, essential thrombocythemia, and PMF were related disorders, which he called MPD, but are now termed MPNs because of the evidence that these disorders are hematologic malignancies.

Since the mid-1970s, data have accumulated that conclusively demonstrate PV to be the result of a neoplastic proliferation of hematopoietic cells. The cellular origin of the disorder was first established by the analysis of glucose-6-phosphate dehydrogenase (G6PD) isoenzymes in African American women who were heterozygous for this X-linked gene. This approach was based on the random irreversible inactivation of one X chromosome in each female somatic cell during embryogenesis. Inactivation of the same X chromosome occurs in the progeny of these cells. A normal African American female heterozygous for G6PD will therefore have approximately equal populations of BM cells with a different G6PD isoenzyme. The G6PD isoenzymes can be readily distinguished by electrophoretic methods.

This approach was exploited in a seminal study by Adamson and coworkers in an effort to determine the cellular origin of PV. They presumed that cells composing a tumor that arises from a single cell in a G6PD heterozygote would express a single isoenzyme type, but a neoplasm originating from multiple cells would express both isoenzyme types. These investigators found that circulating RBCs, granulocytes, and platelets obtained from African American female patients who were G6PD heterozygotes express the same isoenzyme, but skin and cultured BM fibroblasts obtained from these same patients demonstrate both isoenzymes. They concluded that PV represented a clonal proliferation of neoplastic HSCs and was not multicellular in origin or the consequence of excessive proliferation of normal HSCs.

The clonality of blood cell production in PV has subsequently been confirmed using restriction fragment length polymorphisms of the active X chromosome. A monoclonal pattern of X chromosome inactivation has been defined in RBCs, granulocytes, monocytes, and platelets in female patients with PV.

On the basis of the knowledge that RBC production in PV is not associated with excessive EPO production, numerous investigators hypothesized that the erythroid progenitor cell in this disorder is no longer subject to physiologic regulators. PV BM can form substantial numbers of erythroid colonies in vitro in the absence of exogenous EPO, but normal human BM is incapable of forming such colonies without the addition of EPO. These erythroid colonies were termed *endogenous colonies*. When erythroid PV and normal BM were subsequently assayed in the presence of EPO, PV BM was characterized by a higher cloning efficiency. Additional observations suggested that the altered response to cytokines was not restricted to EPO but included a variety of other cytokines and that this cytokine hypersensitivity was characteristic of progenitor cells committed to a variety of other lineages.

In addition, BM cells cloned from African American female G6PD heterozygotes with PV in the presence and absence of exogenous EPO revealed that the erythroid colonies that formed in the absence of exogenous EPO contained the same G6PD isoenzyme type as that expressed by peripheral blood elements. Thus the so-called endogenous erythroid colonies arose from the abnormal clone that was responsible for supplying RBCs, granulocytes, and platelets to the peripheral blood. When exogenous EPO was added, increasing numbers of colonies were formed containing cellular elements expressing the other G6PD isoenzymes; presumably, these colonies originated from cells not involved in the malignant process. Similarly, small numbers of granulocyte–macrophage colonies not originating from the PV clone were also observed in these assays. These data collectively indicate the existence of malignant and nonmalignant populations of HPCs in PV BM. The relative frequency of the neoplastic clone in relation to normal progenitor cells was further examined by Adamson and coworkers, who, by monitoring the proportion of neoplastic erythroid clones and their numeric relationship to normal clones over a period of several years, showed disease progression to be associated with a significant decline in the frequency of normal progenitor cells and increasing proportion of the neoplastic clone. Erythroid progenitor cells from PV patients are, in fact, abnormally sensitive to the actions of this EPO. This increased responsiveness allows these cells to form colonies in the presence of small amounts of EPO. Most PV patients possess two distinct populations of erythroid progenitor cells: a normally EPO-responsive population and a population of cells similar in proliferative and maturational behavior in vitro but requiring little or no EPO. These investigators suggested that the proliferation of the normal progenitor cells in vivo was at a disadvantage.

A number of investigators have demonstrated that the increased responsiveness of these BM progenitor populations extends to their responses to other cytokines, including SCF, IL-3, GM-CSF, and IGF-1. These studies also demonstrated that BM fractions enriched for granulocyte–macrophage progenitors as well as megakaryocyte progenitors from the patients had a heightened responsiveness to IL-3 and GM-CSF. The dogma that the hyperresponsivity of PV progenitor cells to a variety of growth factors (EPO, IL-3, GM-CSF, steel factor) is the underlying defect that leads to PV has been universally accepted.

Many investigators have examined the possibility that the hematopoietic defect in PV could be accounted for by genetic alteration of cytokine receptors expressed by affected hematopoietic cells. In PV, the EPOR is structurally similar to the normal EPOR, and mutations in the EPOR are not directly involved in the pathobiology of PV. Furthermore, no significant differences in the number, dissociation constant, or internalization rate of receptors for steel factor have been detected in the erythroid progenitor cells of PV patients.

Identification of JAK2V617F Mutation in PV

For more than 2 decades, a number of research groups have been searching for the genetic defect underlying PV. Most groups predicted that this defect involved the signaling pathways downstream of the EPOR. These pathways include the tyrosine kinase JAK2 and the transcriptional signal transducers and activators of transcription STAT3 and STAT5. The initial discovery of a mutation was predicated on a somewhat simplistic yet revealing set of experiments performed by Vainchenker and colleagues in France and reported in 2005.[13] They observed that the inhibition of JAK2 by a small molecule (AG490) or by small interfering RNA (siRNA) reduced EPO-independent colony formation by PV BM mononuclear cells. This observation prompted them to directly sequence JAK2 in the hematopoietic cells of PV patients and to discover a single recurrent point mutation. A guanine-to-thymine mutation was observed that resulted in a substitution of valine to phenylalanine at codon 617 within the pseudokinase domain (JH2) of JAK2 (JAK2V617F) (Fig. 67-4). These findings were quickly confirmed by several different groups. Kralovics et al[14] had previously identified a region of LOH on chromosome 9p in PV and identified a 6·2-Mbp region common to all PV patients screened. Because this region contained JAK2, with its known role in erythropoiesis, it was screened for mutations and the same JAK2V617F mutation identified. Three other groups targeted JAK2 as part of a global sequencing screen of tyrosine kinases and phosphatases in MPDs. Analysis of germline DNA demonstrated that JAK2V617F is an acquired somatic mutation present exclusively in hematopoietic cells. All patients with PV have a population of erythroid progenitor cells that are homozygous for the mutation. Using quantitative PCR, patients can be divided into those with a low allele

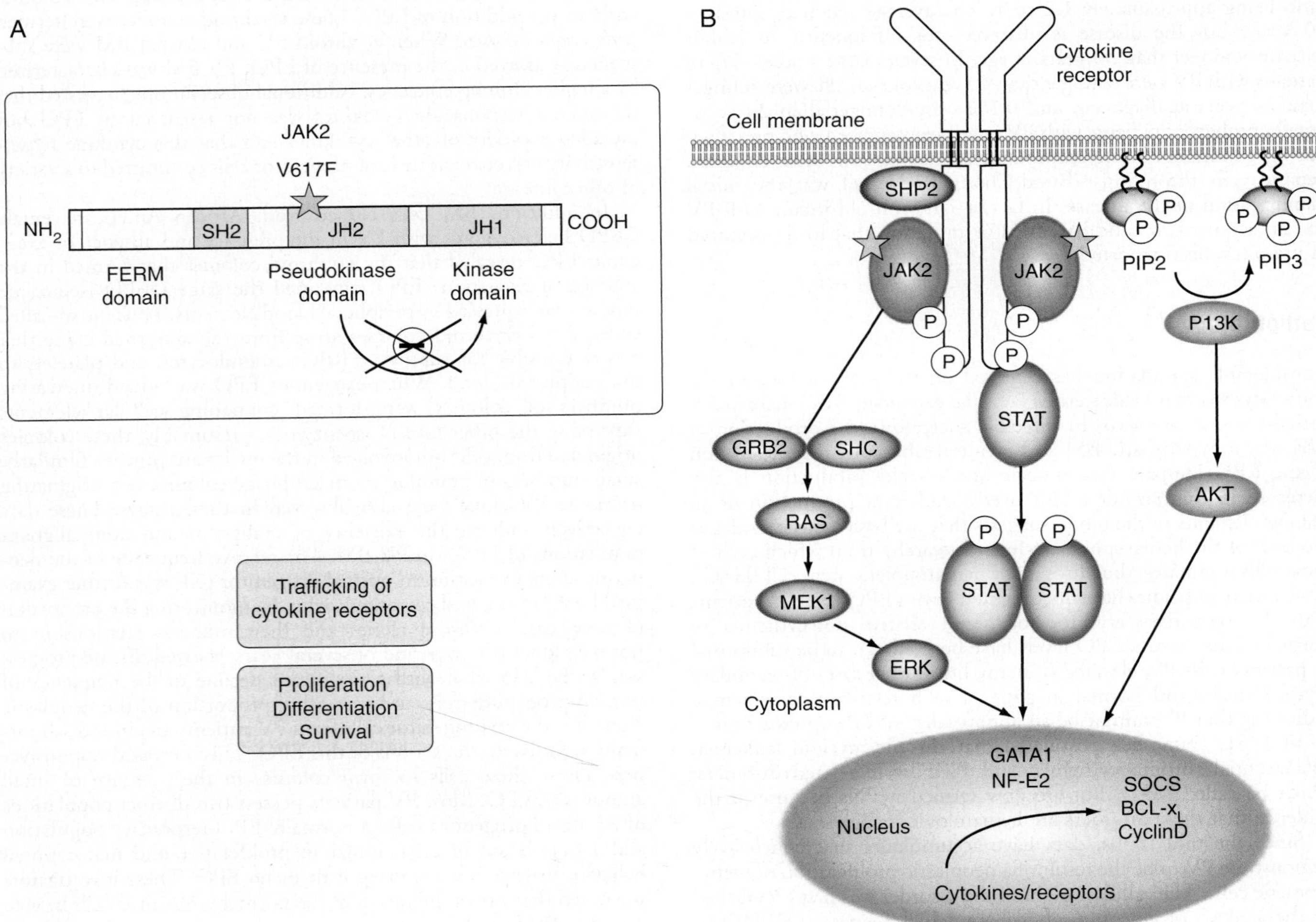

Figure 67-4 JAK2V617F SIGNALING IN MYELOPROLIFERATIVE DISORDERS. **A,** Structure of JAK2V617F: the mutation is located in pseudokinase Janus kinase (JAK) homology domain 2 (JH2) and disrupts the autoinhibition of this regulatory domain. Consequently, the tyrosine kinase corresponding to the JH1 domain is constitutively activated. **B,** In the presence of a homodimeric cytokine receptor (e.g., erythropoietin receptor [EPOR]), the two JAK2V617F proteins bound to the intracellular domain of the receptor transphosphorylate its tyrosine residues. In turn, STAT5 (signal transducer and activator of transcription 5), phosphatidylinositol 3-kinase (PI3K), and renin–angiotensin system (RAS) signaling pathways are activated, leading to the downstream modulation of transcription and protein levels for cell cycle, proliferation, and apoptosis-related factors. *Bcl-X_L,* B cell lymphoma-extra large; *ERK,* extracellular signal-related kinase; *GATA,* GATA-binding factor; *GRB,* growth factor receptor-bound protein; *MEK1,* dual specificity mitogen-activated protein kinase kinase 1; *NF,* nuclear factor; *P,* Phosphate; PIP2 and PIP3, phosphatidyl inositol bi- and triphosphate; *SH2,* src homology 2; *SOCS,* suppressor of cytokine signaling. *(From Delhommeau F, Pisani DF, James C, et al: Oncogenic mechanisms in myeloproliferative disorders.* Cell Mol Life Sci *6363:2939, 2006.)*

burden of JAK2V617F in granulocytes ha (<50%) and patients with a higher burden of JAK2V617F (>50%). A subset of patients with PV are homozygous for JAK2V617F, which was demonstrated to be the result of mitotic recombination and duplication of the mutant allele (Fig. 67-5). The occurrence of this mitotic recombination event has been observed during the clinical course of individual patients, leading to JAK2V617F heterozygote patients becoming homozygotes over time. The concept of the conversion of JAK2V617F low burden to high burden is further supported by the observation that the median duration of disease at the time of evaluation was 48 months in high-burden PV patients as compared with 23 months in low-burden PV. These observations are consistent with a multistep pathogenesis of PV. The first step consists of the acquisition of JAK2V617F, which results in a low allele burden of JAK2V617F, followed by a second step, homologous recombination, that leads to JAK2V617F homozygous progenitor cells and eventually granulocytes with a high burden of JAK2V617F. It remains unknown at present if a lesion occurring before acquisition of the JAK2V617F mutation predisposes an individual to acquire JAK2V617F.

A number of groups have reported the frequency of JAK2V617F in patients with MPNs (see Table 67-2). The mutational frequency of JAKV617F in PV is greater than 95% of cases. Approximately 50% to 60% of patients with ET and PMF are also *JAK2V617F* positive. ET is distinguished from PV by being associated with a low allele burden. In the overwhelming majority of cases, PV is characterized by a population of JAK2V617F homozygous colonies with some heterozygous and wild-type colonies. By contrast in ET, there are few homozygous colonies, with the majority being heterozygous or wild type. The majority of ET and PMF patients who are negative for *JAK2V617F* have clonal hematopoiesis, which indicates that these JAK2V617F diseases likely are the consequences of other genetic events, several of which have recently been described and are discussed in Chapter 69. The *JAK2V617F* allele has also been observed in a limited number of patients with chronic myelomonocytic leukemia, myelodysplastic syndromes (MDS), refractory anemia with ringed sideroblasts and thrombocytosis, and AML, although most *JAK2V617F* mutations in AML occur in patients with a preceding diagnosis of PV, ET, or PMF. JAK2V617F is an acquired somatic mutation, does not appear in nonhematopoietic cells, and has not been detected in patients with secondary erythrocytosis. Moreover, JAK2V617F has not been observed in lymphoid malignancies, although other mutations in *JAK2* have been identified in 10% of patients with pediatric high-risk ALL.

Other JAK2 Mutations in Polycythemia Vera

Other mutations of JAK2 associated with erythrocytosis, however, can also constitutively activate JAK2 kinase activity. Several gain-of-function mutations affecting JAK2 exon 12 within an area immediately adjacent to pseudokinase domain of JAK2V617F-negative patients have been identified in 2.5% to 3.4% of PV patients and approximately 30% of JAK2V617F-negative PV. To date, 17 different such mutations have been identified.[14] Two-thirds of patients with a JAK2 exon 12 mutation presented with an isolated erythrocytosis and distinctive BM morphology and had reduced serum EPO levels, but the remainder of patients have erythrocytosis plus leukocytosis, thrombocytosis, or both. These exon 12 mutations perturb the autoinhibitory domain of JAK2. JAK2 exon 12 mutations have not been reported in patients with ET or PMF but have been occasionally observed in patients with refractory anemia and ringed sideroblasts associated with thrombocytosis. Erythroid colonies cloned from their blood samples in the absence of exogenous EPO were most frequently heterozygous for the mutation, with homozygous colonies only rarely occurring, but colonies homozygous for the mutation occur in most PV patients with JAK2V617F, suggesting that a JAK2 exon 12 mutation results in a stronger activation of the JAK2-mediated intracellular signaling pathways. Patients with exon 12 mutations can develop

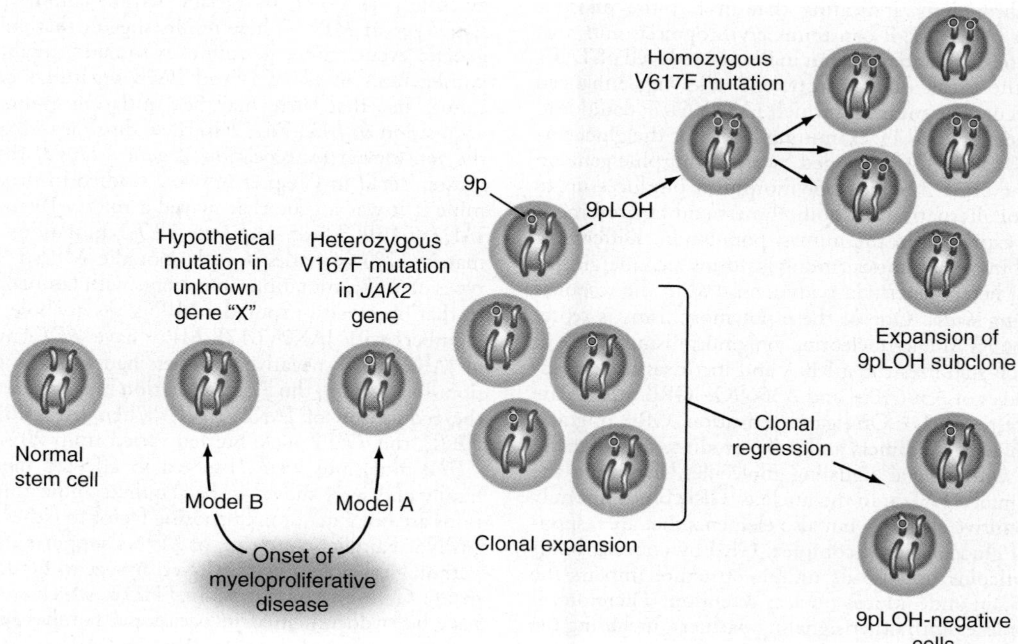

Figure 67-5 POSSIBLE ROLE OF JAK2V617F IN THE BIOLOGY OF MYELOPROLIFERATIVE DISORDERS. The chromosome 9 with the wild-type *JAK2* sequence (G) is depicted in *white,* and the chromosome 9 with the G-T transversion (T) is shown in *red. Circles* symbolize the nuclei of the cells. Deletion of the telomeric part of wild-type chromosome 9p as a potential mechanism for 9pLOH is shown on the *left.* Alternatively, mitotic recombination could also result in 9pLOH, shown on the *right.* The events during mitosis and the resulting cell progeny after mitotic recombination of chromosome 9p are also shown. *(Adapted from Kralovics R, Passamonti F, Buser AS, et al: A gain-of-function mutation of JAK2 in myeloproliferative disorders.* N Engl J Med *352:1779, 2005.)*

thrombotic episodes and can evolve into post-PVMF or acute leukemia. BaF3 cells expressing the murine EPOR and carrying exon 12 mutations can proliferate without added IL-3. They also exhibited increased phosphorylation of JAK2 and extracellular signal-related kinase (ERKs) as compared with cells transduced by wild-type JAK2 or JAK2V617F. This mutation resulted in a myeloproliferative disorder phenotype, including erythrocytosis, in retroviral murine BM transplantation model. JAK2 exon 12 mutations, therefore, might define a distinctive MPN that affects patients who had previously been carrying a diagnosis of IE. In several series, approximately 2.7% of patients with a clinical syndrome that resembles PV have been observed who have a wild-type JAK2. The existence of such patients may be the result of several factors, including limited sensitivity of the assay used for genotyping; prior treatment with interferon (INF), which might eliminate the JAK2 mutations; or lack of efforts to exclude inherited genetic disorders associated with erythrocytosis that have been described in this chapter. Alternatively, additional acquired genetic lesions that have yet to be described may be responsible for the disease phenotype.

JAK2V617F Is Likely Not the Disease-Initiating Event in Polycythemia Vera

Despite data generated using a variety of mouse models suggesting that JAK2V617F might be sufficient for the development of PV, increasing evidence shows that PV is not solely initiated by JAK2V617F. The fact that JAK2V617F has been identified in patients with three phenotypically related but clinically distinct MPN suggests that additional genetic or epigenetic events likely contribute to the phenotypic divergence of these disorders. These differing disease phenotypes have been hypothesized to be caused by striking differences in the degree to which the mutation activates the JAK–STAT pathway. Mutant JAK2 activates multiple cytokine receptor associated pathways, including STAT1 and STAT5, which can have competing consequences. STAT1 appears to be activated in association with JAK2V617F ET but not PV. Inhibition of STAT1 in ET progenitor cells enhances erythropoiesis, indicating that in ET, the phospo-STAT1 response to JAK2V617F constrains erythropoiesis and promotes megakaryocytic differentiation, but in PV, the reduced pSTAT1 response removes the break on erythropoiesis, allowing enhanced erythropoiesis to occur. The means by which JAK2V617F could lead to MPNs was further explored by examining SNPs for the glucocorticoid receptor (GR). The GR is encoded by a polymorphic gene on human chromosome 5q31-32. This polymorphism produces up to 256 combinations of alternative GR homodimers and heterodimers, which are variably expressed in the human population. Differences in ligand or DNA-binding affinities among isoforms are emerging as the leading cause of heterogeneity in body mass and in the response to GR ligands during stress. One of these polymorphisms is represented by the A3669G single-nucleotide polymorphism (SNP) in exon 9 of GR, which stabilizes the mRNA and increases the expression of GRβ (half-lives of A3669G+ and A3669G− GRβ mRNA are >6 and <6 hours, respectively). On ligand activation, GRα migrates to the nucleus both as homodimers and as heterodimeric tetrameric protein complexes with several signaling molecules, including the phosphorylated form of STAT-5. In the nucleus, GRα binds not only glucocorticoid-responsive elements but also elements that are responsive to each type of glucocorticoid complex. GRβ by contrast binds poorly to glucocorticoids because its unique structure impairs the ligand-binding domain and induces nuclear retention. Therefore, it does not form complexes with other signaling partners, including the phosphorylated form of STAT-5, and by forming heterodimers with GRα, it impairs ligand binding of this isoform and acts as a dominant negative regulator of GR function within the cells. The A3669G polymorphism, which stabilizes GRβ mRNA, had greater frequency in PV and MF patients than in normal control participants or patients with essential thrombocythemia. It has been suggested that JAK2V617F may be responsible for activation of alternative GR splicing in MPN EBs. After the alternative splicing is activated, the presence of the A3669G polymorphism, by stabilizing GRβ mRNA, may favor its translation, generating amounts of protein adequate for GRα neutralization, resulting in expansion of the erythroid precursor pool and delaying terminal differentiation, thereby contributing to the development of erythrocytosis in PV.

The role of JAK2V617F in the underlying pathogenesis of PV has been extensively explored using either restricted fragment length polymorphism analysis or the presence of marker cytogenetic abnormalities in patients with MPNs. It was demonstrated that the percentage of granulocytes and platelets that are JAK2V617F positive is often lower than the percentage of granulocytes belonging to the malignant clone. In addition, these marker cytogenetic abnormalities may occur before or after the acquisition of JAK2V617F. Furthermore JAK2V617F-negative erythroid colonies have been cloned in vitro in the absence of the addition of EPO, a hallmark of PV, indicating the presence of an undefined molecular lesion that precedes the JAK2V617 mutation.[15] These findings suggest that the acquisition of JAK2V617F is a relatively late event that is preceded by another genetic event that leads to clonal hematopoiesis. The acquisition of the JAK2V617F apparently occurs in this background of clonal hematopoiesis. Additional information that indicates that JAK2V617f is a relatively late event in the multistep pathogenesis of PV is the observation that the blasts cells from patients with JAK2V617F AML are negative for this mutation in 50% of instances, suggesting that the leukemia originates in residual normal stem cells or in the preJAK2 V617F clone. This observation is discussed in greater detail in Chapter 69.

Several investigators have reported families in which multiple members have an MPN and have analyzed the JAK2V617F status of family members. The members of 72 families with multiple members with MPN were analyzed for *JAK2V617F* mutational status. Somatic *JAK2V617F* mutations were identified in some, but not all, family members with MPNs. Interestingly, in some families, both *JAK2V617F*-positive and -negative members with MPN were observed. A small number of relatives who were JAJ2V617F negative and did not have a diagnosis of PV, ET, or PMF had hematopoietic cells that formed endogenous erythroid colonies in vitro. Disease evolution can be highly variable within families presenting with the same type of MPN. These results suggest that an as yet unidentified genetic event, either germline or somatic, might contribute to the pathogenesis of PV, ET, and PMF, regardless of *JAK2* mutational status, and that there may be "initiating events" that precede the acquisition of *JAK2V617F* in these disorders. Acquired mutations of the ten–eleven translocation 2 gene *(TET2)* that are discussed in greater detail in Chapter 69 were studied in these families to determine if it was a gene that played a role in PV before acquisition of JAK2V617F. These acquired *TET2* mutations occur in approximately 12% of patients with sporadic MPNs. The frequency and types of *TET2* mutations in patients with familial MPNs were similar to that observed in sporadic MPNs. As a whole, 20% of the family members with JAK2V617F MPN have *TET2* mutations, and 17% of JAK2V617F-negative members had a MPN with a *TET2* mutation. In addition, the *TET2* mutation may occur either before or after the acquisition of JAK2V617F. When JAK2V617F coexisted with *TET2,* the *TET2* allele burden varied from 20% to 60%. Different *TET2* mutations were observed in affected members of the same family and were shown to be acquired, indicating that *TET2* mutations are not a major predisposing factor to either sporadic or familial MPNS. Familial clustering of MPNs supports the evidence that the pathological phenotype is driven by yet to be defined susceptibility genes. Germline mutations in PHD2, which were discussed earlier, have been documented in occasional families with multiple family members affected by JAK2V617F MPNs. Mutated PDH2 has been proposed to be capable of acting as a tumor suppressor gene, but whether it plays any role in predisposing to familial MPNs will require further study. The germline constitutive JAK2 haplotype, called GGCC or 46/1, has been shown to be a susceptibility factor for the development of JAK2V617F-positive PV and PV characterized by exon 12 mutations.[16] How this JAK2 SNP promotes the development of typical MPNs remains the subject of great speculation, but two hypotheses have been proposed: (1) hypermutability of the chromosome region facilitates the acquisition of somatic mutation, or (2) the JAK2 SNP confers a selective proliferative advantage, the so-called fertile ground hypothesis.

The JAK2V617F Mutation Is Present in Hematopoietic Stem Cells in Polycythemia Vera

Previous studies had demonstrated that the majority of patients with PV had clonal involvement of multiple lineages, including myeloid, erythroid, and lymphoid cells. These results suggested that PV originates in hematopoietic progenitors with the ability to differentiate into multiple lineages. In addition, LOH at 9p24, now known to correspond to homozygous JAK2V617F mutations, can be identified in both myeloid and lymphoid cells in some patients with PV, further suggesting that the underlying mutations occur in progenitor cells with the ability to differentiate into multiple hematopoietic lineages.

The JAK2V617F mutation has been detected in hematopoietic colony-forming cells and more mature progeny, such as neutrophils and platelets. Populations of cells enriched for HSCs, common myeloid progenitors (CMPs), granulocyte–macrophage progenitors (GMPs), and megakaryocytic–erythroid progenitors (MEPs) from patients with PV have been analyzed for the presence of the *JAK2V617F* mutation. *JAK2V617F* was detected in HSCs, CMPs, GMPs, and MEPs from patients with PV, supporting that PV is a disorder that arises in HSCs and involves the myeloid, erythroid, and megakaryocytic lineages. These data indicate that the *JAK2V617F* mutation in PV originates in lymphomyeloid progenitor cells.[17] The functional effects of the *JAK2V617F* mutation on HSC or precursor cells has been the subject of conflicting data originating from several laboratories with some investigators indicating that JAK2V617F is associated with an expansion of the HSC with skewing of the differentiation program toward the erythroid and megakaryocytic differentiation program and others indicating that JAK2V617F leads to expansion of more differentiated erythroid and megakaryocytic precursor cells but not stem cells. The expansion of JAK2V617F-positive cells has been attributed to responses to tumor necrosis factor-α (TNF-α). MPNs are characterized by increased levels of TNF-α, and JAk2V617F-positive HPCs compared with HPCs with wild-type JAK2, have been shown to be resistant to the inhibitory effects of this cytokine, thereby selecting for the malignant clone and facilitating its expansion.

Structural and Functional Aspects of JAK2V617F-Mediated Transformation

The *JAK2V617F* mutation occurs within the JH2 domain of JAK2, which has significant homology to the kinase domain of JAK2 (JH1) but lacks catalytic activity (see Fig. 67-4). The JH2 domain exerts an inhibitory effect on JAK2 kinase activity, and the V617F mutation is predicted to disrupt this inhibition. In vitro kinase assays with JAK2V617F and wild-type JAK2 have revealed that JAK2V617F has greatly increased kinase activity, as assessed by autophosphorylation and by substrate phosphorylation. Ectopic expression of JAK2V617F in either epithelial or hemopoietic cell lines results in autophosphorylation of mutant JAK2, but not the wild-type (WT) JAK2, and activation of downstream signaling events. BAF3 or FDCP cell lines expressing the EPOR and engineered to stably express JAK2V617F are largely independent of the addition of exogenous growth factors and are hypersensitive to EPO. Coexpression of JAK2 V617F and a homodimeric type 1 cytokine receptor (EPOR, TPOR, or G-CSFR) facilitates the transformation of cells to growth factor independence, suggesting that the mutant JAK2 requires a receptor scaffold to be active. This contrasts with the effects of the *TEL–JAK2* fusion gene, which can readily transform cells on its own, presumably because of the strong homodimerization effects of the TEL moiety. Ectopic expression of JAK2V617F can also sensitize cells to the effects of IGF1, a characteristic feature of PV progenitors.

Expression of JAK2V617F in hematopoietic cells activates intracellular signaling pathways downstream of the EPOR, including STAT5, STAT3, the MAP kinase pathway, and the phosphatidylinositol 3-kinase (PI3K)–Akt pathway.[18] STAT5 is normally phosphorylated by the cytokine receptor–JAK2 complex, and phosphorylated STAT5 then translocates to the nucleus and activates the transcription of target genes. The target genes of STAT5 include Bcl-X_L, an important antiapoptotic protein known to be expressed in increased levels in PV proerythroblasts. The possibility that STAT5-mediated activation of Bcl-X_L is important in the pathogenesis of PV was suggested by observations that expression of either constitutively active STAT-5 or Bcl-X_L resulted in spontaneous erythroid colony formation. In normal cells, DNA damage increases the activity of an amiloride-sensitive sodium hydrogen exchange isoform 1, which raises the intracellular pH, which in turn causes nonenzymatic deamidation of Bcl-xL. The deamidation pathway has been shown to be inhibited in a variety of MPNs, including PV, leading to less apoptosis. Interestingly, this defect in deamidation was reversed by treatment with a JAK2 inhibitor, suggesting that this defect might be a consequence of mutated JAK2. Furthermore, the degree of apoptosis can also be altered by p53 levels. JAk2V617F appears to functionally inactivate p53 by upregulating MDM2, an E3 ubiquitin ligase, thereby decreasing the degree of apoptosis. In addition, cells expressing JAK2V617F display constitutive activation of the MAP kinase pathway (as assessed by phosphorylation of ERK), and of the PI3K pathway (as assessed by phosphorylation of AKT). Furthermore, JAK2 has been shown to play a role in cellular myeloproliferative leukemia virus oncogene (MPL) trafficking. JAK2V617F might also lead to the decreased expression of mpl by platelets observed in PV patients. Furthermore, JAK2V617F and activated STAT5 have been shown to increase the expression of 6 phosphofructokinase/fructose-2,6 bisphosphatase 3 (PFKFB3), which controls glycolytic flux through 6-6-phosphofructo-1-kinase. PFKB3 is required for JAK2V617F-dependent lactate production, oxidative metabolic activity, and glucose activity, thereby promoting cell proliferation. It is important to note that many other oncogenic tyrosine kinases activate the same signal transduction pathways, and the role and requirement for each of these signaling pathways in the transformation of hematopoietic cells by JAK2V617F remain unknown. Although once thought to reside strictly in the cytoplasm of cells, a growing body of evidence indicates that both JAK1 and JAK2 are present in the nucleus of certain cells under conditions associated with high rates of cell proliferation. Nuclear JAKs have been reported to affect gene expression by activating other transcription factors besides STATs and influencing epigenetic events by phosphorylating H3 and activating global gene expression. JAK2V617F may alter chromatin structure by selectively phosphorylating the arginine methyltransferase PRMT5, impairing PRMT5 methyltransferase activity by negatively affecting its association with methylsome protein 50. Reduced PRMT5 activity increases HPC proliferation and promotes erythroid differentiation.

Many PV patients have a low burden of *JAK2V617F* as assessed by DNA sequencing, suggesting that there is either a subpopulation of cells that are homozygous for *JAK2V617F* mixed with wild-type cells or a clonal population of cells with one wild-type copy of *JAK2* and one mutant copy of *JAK2*. In PV, data from clonality or quantitative *JAK2V617F* assessment and from colony assays suggest that most PV patients have a subpopulation of cells homozygous for *JAK2V617F*, but in ET, clonal progenitor cells are heterozygous for *JAK2V617F*. It is therefore important to determine whether the wild-type allele can interfere with the ability of JAK2V617F to constitutively signal in the heterozygous state and whether there is an effect of gene dosage on the activation of signal transduction pathways. Transient coexpression of wild-type JAK2 does not interfere with the ability of JAK2V617F to autophosphorylate even when wild-type JAK2 is expressed at higher levels than the mutant kinase. This suggests that JAK2V617F kinase activity is unaffected by coexpression of wild-type JAK2. In contrast, when JAK2V617F and wild-type JAK2 were coexpressed in Ba/F3 cells, cytokine-independent growth was attenuated, suggesting in this cellular context that wild-type JAK2 is able to interfere with JAK2V617F-mediated transformation. SOCS proteins bind to the JH1 catalytic loop and target JAK2 for degradation.[19] SOCS1 and SOCS3 bind to the catalytic groove belonging to JAK2 and inhibit its catalytic activity. SOCS3 binds to the EPOR and JAK2 to inhibit EPOR signaling. SOCS proteins inhibit JAK2 by functioning as E3 ubiquitin ligases. Although SOCS1, SOCS2, and SOCS3 inhibit phosphorylation of wild-type JAK2, they are incapable of blocking phosphorylation of JAK2V617F. On the basis of their findings, SOCS3 appears to be unable to inactivate JAK2V617, and SOCS3 itself is not degraded but accumulates and actually promotes the further phosphorylation of JAK2V617F. Such dysregulation likely enhances JAK2V617F-induced cell proliferation and prolongs signaling. These data have been suggested as an explanation for why JAK2V617F hematopoiesis predominates in PV heterozygotes. Low levels of JAK2V617F signaling in JAK2V617F heterozygotes likely induce SOCS3, which would downregulate JAK2 wild-type signaling and enhance signaling by JAK2V617F, permitting the malignant clone to predominate.

Additional Mutations Associated With Polycythemia Vera

After the application of whole-genome assays (comparative genomic hybridization and SNPs) as well as whole-genome sequencing, an increasing number of mutations have been observed in the patients with Philadelphia chromosome–negative MPNs. These mutations are not unique to any of the MPNs and are associated with AML and MDS.[18] Four of these genes—*EZH2, ASXL, DNMT3a,* and *TET2*—participate in the epigenetic control of transcription and are discussed in greater detail in Chapter 69. *EZH2* mutations occur in 3% of PV patients, 7% to 16% of PV patients have *TET2* mutations, and 5% to 7% have mutations of *DNMT3a; ASXL* mutations are rare in PV (<7%). Each of these mutations may precede JAK2V617F, but the converse may also occur. Each of these mutations are far less frequent in PV and ET than PMF, supporting that these events may combine to generate a more accelerated phase of the classic MPN that phenotypically presents as MF. In addition, several other mutations, including IDH1/2, IKZF deletions, NRAS/KRAS, p53 mutations, and RUNX1 mutations, rarely occur in PV but are all associated with transformation of an underlying MPN such as PV to acute leukemia.

The Hypercoagulable State That Characterizes Polycythemia Vera

Thrombosis is a major cause of morbidity and mortality in PV patients. These thrombotic events are most frequently microcirculatory and arterial, but venous thromboses are also of important clinical significance. The increased risk for thrombosis can be attributed to abnormalities in the vessel wall, blood cell components, and the dynamics of blood flow.

In the European Collaboration on Low-Dose Aspirin in Polycythemia Vera (ECLAP) study, the incidence of cardiovascular complications was higher in patients older than 65 years (5.0% of patients per year; hazard ratio [HR], 2.0; confidence interval [CI], 1.22-3.29; $P<.006$) or with a history of thrombosis (4.93% of patients per year; HR, 1.96; 95% CI, 1.29-2.97; $P = .0017$). Patients both with a history of thrombosis and older than 65 years had the highest risk of developing additional cardiovascular events (10.9% of patients per year; HR, 4.35; 95% CI, 2.95-6.41; $P<.0001$).[20] These data confirm previous findings that increasing age and history of thrombosis are the two most important prognostic factors for the development of vascular complications.

This information does not negate the increased incidence of thrombotic incidents also observed in younger patients with this disorder. In a series of 58 PV patients younger than 40 years of age, a disturbingly high incidence of life-threatening thrombotic events was observed. In fact, seven of the 10 patients in this series who died during the period of observation died from thrombotic events—four from Budd-Chiari syndrome, one from a pulmonary embolism, and two from cerebral thrombosis. Therefore, although a significant factor, preexisting atherosclerotic disease is not the sole etiologic factor in the genesis of thrombosis in PV. Some have suggested an important role for smoking as a secondary factor leading to the increased incidence of thrombotic events in this patient population.

The principal hemorrheologic abnormality in PV is an elevated whole blood viscosity. The blood viscosity in PV is higher than that of normal control participants at all shear rates. In a retrospective analysis of PV patients with histories of vascular thrombosis, a strong correlation in univariate analysis between hematocrit level and the development of thrombotic episodes, including many cerebrovascular occlusions, was demonstrated. Cerebral blood flow is reduced in patients with PV in whom the hematocrit level is 53% to 62%. These abnormalities were observed even in patients with hematocrits at the lower levels of normal, that is, 46% to 52%. Reductions in cerebral blood flow are correctable with phlebotomy. Reduction of the hematocrit by relatively small amounts frequently led to substantial improvements in whole blood viscosity and cerebral blood flow. Some PV patients apparently still maintain a higher than normal whole blood viscosity despite the normalization of the hematocrit, suggesting that an increase in hematocrit may not be the only factor responsible for increased blood viscosity. There appear to be important gender differences as related to the location of thromboses in PV patients. Women appear to have a higher incidence of thromboses within the abdominal cavity involving the portal, mesenteric, or hepatic vessels but a comparable rate of other vascular complications. Several groups have reported that patients with splanchnic vein thromboses frequently have endothelial cells that are affected by JAK2V617F, suggesting that in such individuals, their MPN might originate not at the level of the HSC but rather at the level of a hemangioblast, from which myeloid and endothelial cells originate. Such JAK2V61F-positive endothelial cells have been shown to exhibit a high efficiency of adhering to normal mononuclear cells, thereby likely leading to an increased risk of thrombosis.

A number of possible explanations have been suggested for the observed relationship between hematocrit level and the development of thrombotic events in PV patients. Platelet adhesion and thrombus formation on the vascular subendothelium are determined in part by the rate at which platelets are transported to the vascular surface. In a polycythemic condition in which increased numbers of RBCs are present, a greater number of intercellular collisions between RBCs and platelets occurs. These collisions could lead to increased platelet movement in a direction perpendicular to blood flow. This facilitation of platelet transport to the vessel wall may be an important factor in the development of thrombosis. An alternative explanation for the association between hematocrit level and the risk of thrombosis is based on the knowledge that blood viscosity is particularly sensitive to hematocrit levels. Increased hematocrits lead to increased blood viscosity, in turn leading to increased peripheral vascular resistance and an actual reduction in blood flow to a variety of organs, predisposing them to the development of thrombosis. The issue of hematocrits and thrombosis in PV has been prospectively investigated in a recent analysis of 1638 patients enrolled in the ECLAP study. In this prospective study, despite recommendations of maintaining hematocrit levels fewer than 45%, only 50% of patients achieved this target during the follow-up, and 10% had hematocrit levels above 50%. These different hematocrit values were not associated with different thrombotic outcomes as assessed using univariate and multivariable analysis. The clinical significance of this finding appears to be relevant for the construction of future therapeutic guidelines and is being validated in prospective randomized clinical trials. Additional factors have been implicated in the development of thrombosis in PV patients. Almost all patients with PV are iron deficient. Decreased RBC deformability has been said to accompany iron deficiency, leading to increased blood viscosity and a decreased ability of RBCs to pass through small-bore polycarbonate filters. This increased membrane stiffness, however, might be counterbalanced by the effect of a reduced RBC size on the adherence of blood platelets to arteriolar subendothelium. RBC size is a major determinant of platelet adherence, with larger RBCs leading to increased platelet adherence and smaller RBCs to decreased platelet adherence. Whether the increased membrane stiffness associated with iron deficiency is counterbalanced by the decreased platelet adherence associated with smaller RBCs is yet to be determined.

Thrombocytosis and qualitative platelet abnormalities occur frequently and are likely to be important contributory factors to the development of thrombosis.[21] Some investigators have implicated uncontrolled thrombocytosis as a cause of thrombosis in these patients, but this relationship has not been confirmed by others. Increased plasma and urinary thromboxane production has been linked to increased platelet activation in these patients. A low-dose aspirin regimen selective for inhibition of platelet cyclooxygenase has been found to suppress increased thromboxane production in vivo and to clinically benefit patients with PV. Furthermore, elevated levels of serum VEGF and plasma TPO have been observed in patients with PV. These growth factors have been shown to lead to platelet activation.

Despite conflicting data, no clear clinical relationship between platelet number or function and the incidence of hemorrhage or thrombosis in PV patients has been delineated. An argument in favor of a role of elevated platelet numbers in the genesis of thrombosis in PV and ET is the observation in patients with ET that a reduction of excessive platelet numbers with the use of hydroxyurea is associated with a reduction in the risk of developing thrombotic events. However, this should not be taken as evidence that the reduction in developing additional vascular events was caused by platelet count normalization alone; very likely, it may be related to the suppression by hydroxyurea of each of three myeloid lineages. In line with this interpretation are the results of a randomized study performed by the Medical Research Council in the United Kingdom (PT-01) in which patients with ET were randomized to receive either hydroxyurea or anagrelide therapy. This study showed that hydroxyurea therapy rather than anagrelide, a selective platelet number–reducing drug, was associated with a reduction in the number of arterial thrombotic events, especially in JAK2V617F patients. In a recently reported analysis of the ECLAP study, the rate of thrombosis in PV patients during follow-up did not vary according to different platelet numbers. Select patients with PV have, however, been afforded prompt resolution of vascular complications such as erythromelalgia or TIAs after institution of platelet antiaggregating agents or cytoreduction. It is important to emphasize that erythromelalgia does not resolve in PV patients with phlebotomy alone or with anticoagulation but requires the use of platelet antiaggregating agents or reduction of platelet numbers. What distinguishes the clinical courses of these patients from those of others is unknown. These reports coupled with the knowledge of abnormal thromboxane metabolism of platelets in PV provide substance to the belief that platelets contribute to the generation of the thrombotic and hemorrhagic tendencies observed in PV. Although a number of clinical assessments of platelet function have been used to identify patients who are potentially at a high risk of developing a life-threatening hemorrhagic or thrombotic event, the results of these studies to date have been very disappointing. It appears that the etiology of thrombosis and hemorrhage in PV is multifactorial and that the available tools are inadequate to identify patients at highest risk.

An elevation of WBC number occurs in 50% to 60% of PV patients, which may also have a detrimental effect on the rheology of the microcirculation in PV. An analysis of the ECLAP database showed that a baseline WBC count above $15{,}000 \times 10^6\ L^{-1}$ was associated with the development of major arterial events, mainly myocardial infarction. Similar results were shown in two additional studies in patients with ET. Activated leukocytes may release proteases and oxygen radicals that alter endothelial cells and platelets so as to favor the development of a prothrombotic state. A series of markers of leukocyte activation, including expression of membrane CD11b and leukocyte alkaline phosphatase antigen, cellular elastase content, plasma elastase levels, and myeloperoxidase levels, are elevated in patients with PV. Limited and conflicting data are available as to whether or not there is a correlation between the presence of platelet–leukocyte interactions and thrombotic events. Moreover, the association between these functional abnormalities and the presence of JAK2V617F is unclear. Increased expression of leukocyte adhesion molecules increases the adhesion of leukocytes to platelets and the endothelium. These cell to cell interactions stimulate the activation of endothelial cells and platelets and induce the release from activated leukocytes reactive oxygen species as well as proteases that are capable of impairing a number of hemostatic processes. Platelet–leukocyte aggregates are increased in number in PV and are associated with an increased propensity to thrombose. In addition, the prothrombotic state in PV has been attributed to an acquired resistance to the naturally occurring anticoagulant, protein C, which is associated with reduced levels of protein S. The loss of protein S in PV patients is especially profound in those with a high JAK2V617F allele burden, but its cause remains unknown, although some have speculated that it is the consequence of the degradation of protein S by the increased levels of neutrophil elastase. PV patients with a high allele burden may represent a subpopulation with a particular high risk of developing a thromboembolic event.

Polycythemia Vera and the Risk of Hemorrhage

Patients with PV are also at an increased risk of developing life-threatening hemorrhagic complications. Abnormalities in platelet function and number have been implicated as the cause of this hemorrhagic tendency. Qualitative platelet abnormalities frequently found in these patients include platelet hypofunction as demonstrated by defective in vitro platelet aggregation, acquired storage pool disease, platelet membrane defects, increased platelet reactivity as demonstrated by enhanced platelet aggregation, increased plasma β-thromboglobulin levels, and shortened platelet survival. With platelet counts greater than $1000 \times 10^9\ L^{-1}$, the development of acquired von Willebrand syndrome has been reported and is associated with life-threatening hemorrhagic episodes.

Post–Polycythemia Vera Myelofibrosis and Acute Myeloid Leukemia

A major cause of morbidity and mortality in PV results from the transition from the polycythemic phase of the disease to post-PV MF and to acute leukemia. Post-PV MF is characterized by cytopenias, MF, and extramedullary hematopoiesis. In a variety of MPNs, the fibroblastic component of the BM has been shown not to be directly involved in the malignant process but to be a reactive event to the neoplastic clone. Several investigators have suggested that the release of growth factors, particularly platelet-derived growth factor (PDGF), fibroblast growth factor, and transforming growth factor-β from megakaryocytes or platelets, which are present in abundance in patients with MPNs, might be responsible for this fibroblastic proliferation. Whether the use of any particular therapeutic agents for treatment of PV accelerates the development of PV related MF remains hotly debated, although it is well established that the use of alkylating agents such as piprobroman or chlorambucil increases the risk of developing acute leukemia. It remains a source of debate if treatment with hydroxyurea increases the risk of developing MF or AML. The bulk of evidence does not support a clear leukemogenic role for this drug that is the standard of care for high-risk PV patients. Nevertheless, as a cautionary principle, it is wise to consider carefully the use of this agent in very young subjects and in those carrying cytogenetic abnormalities and to avoid it in pregnant women and in patients previously exposed to alkylating agents. In a recent report in which patients were treated exclusively with hydroxyurea with an average follow-up of 16.3 years, the cumulative incidence of AML/MDS in the patients treated with hydroxyurea alone was 7.3%, 10.7%, and 16.6% at 10, 15, and 20 years, respectively, and was significantly lower than in patients treated with the alkylating agent piprobroman.[22] However, patients treated with hydroxyurea had a greater chance of developing MF (at 20 years, 31.6% vs. 21.3%). Whether hydroxyurea really is leukemogenic is difficult to say from this study because such long-term follow-up of patients not receiving any chemotherapeutic agents is not available; the possibility therefore exists that these rates of evolution merely reflect the natural history of the disease. In 50% of cases of JAK2V617F MPNs, the blast cells that represent the progeny of the leukemia-initiating clone are JAK2V617F negative, suggesting that the leukemia originates from a clone distinct from the JAK2V617F-positive clone. This coexistent JAK2V617F-negative clone appears to have a higher propensity to undergo leukemic transformation. JAK2V617F therefore does not appear to be a prerequisite for leukemic transformation of MPNs, suggesting that additional genetic events are required for full transformation to occur. SNP–array analysis has shown that genomic alterations occur at an increased frequency during the period of blastic transformation and that no single gene or molecular pathway is sufficient to cause transformation. A surprising correlation has been observed between the phenotype of the preceding MPN and the JAK2 mutational status of the leukemic blasts after transformation. In contrast to JAK2 wild-type AML in this setting, evolution to JAK2V617F-positive leukemias is invariably preceded by a myelofibrotic transformation of ET/PV or JAK2V617F-positive PMF. Because of these observations, myelofibrotic transformation of ET or PV is thought by many to represent an accelerated phase of the initial MPN preceded by genetic changes that result in evolution to MF and eventually leukemia. JAK2 wild-type leukemia, by contrast, usually arises in patients with chronic phase PV or ET that do not undergo evolution to MF. Some have suggested that these leukemias are therapy related. The reversion from JAK2V617F to wild-type JAK2 in these leukemias has been shown not to be caused by homologous recombination. Two models have been proposed to account for the clonal relationship between JAK2 wild-type AML and its preceding MPN: (1) both the chronic MPN and the AML arise from a shared pre-JAK2V617F founder clone and (2) the chronic MPN and the AML arise from two independent stem cells (Fig. 67-6).It remains possible that each model is viable and operates in different individual patients.

CLINICAL MANIFESTATIONS

The principal clinical manifestations of PV can largely be attributed to the excessive production of cells belonging to each of the myeloid lineages affected by the malignant process, including RBCs, platelets, and WBCs. With the implementation of laboratory tests during annual physical examinations, increasing numbers of people are being diagnosed with PV before the symptoms related to this neoplastic process become apparent. Symptomatic patients with PV may present to a physician with a myriad of nonspecific complaints, including headaches, weakness, pruritus, dizziness, excessive sweating, visual disturbances, paresthesias, joint symptoms, abdominal distress, a

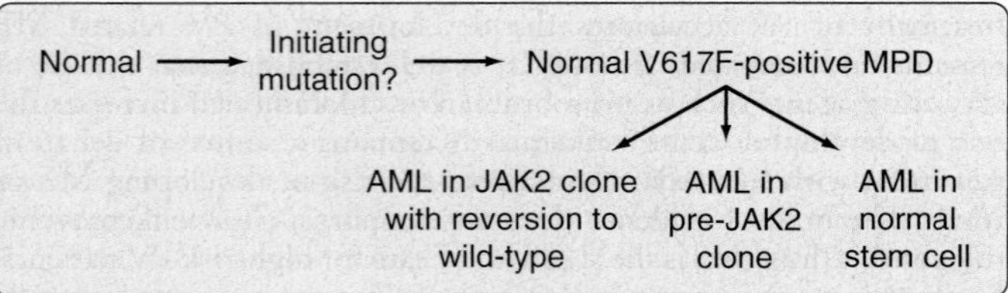

Figure 67-6 MODELS FOR THE DEVELOPMENT OF JAK2V617F-NEGATIVE ACUTE MYELOID LEUKEMIA (AML) FROM JAK2V617F-POSITIVE MYELOPROLIFERATIVE DISORDER (MPD). Three possible models are shown, in which V617F$^-$ AML could develop from (1) a V617F$^+$ cell that subsequently reverts to V617F$^-$, (2) a cell that had some other initiating mutation before *JAK2*, or (3) a normal stem cell. *JAK*, Janus kinase. *(From Campbell PJ, Baxter EJ, Beer PA, et al: Mutation of JAK2 in the myeloproliferative disorders: Timing, clonality studies, cytogenetic associations, and role in leukemic transformation.* Blood *108:3548, 2006.)*

thrombotic or hemorrhagic episode, and weight loss. Thrombosis is a frequent presenting event. Two-thirds of such thrombotic events occur either at presentation or before diagnosis and the remainder most often during the first 10 years of follow-up. At diagnosis, one-third of patients have already lost 10% of their body weight, presumably secondary to the hypermetabolism associated with this disorder, and complaints of fatigue are common. Arthropathies are frequently observed and are largely caused by the clinical manifestations of gout. The hyperproliferative BM state characteristic of PV and the increased nucleoprotein degradation are contributory factors in the development of hyperuricemia.

The principal findings on physical examination of a patient with PV include ruddy cyanosis, conjunctival plethora, hepatomegaly, splenomegaly, and hypertension.

Untreated patients are at particularly high risk for thrombotic and hemorrhagic events. In several large series of patients with PV, thrombosis was the cause of death in 30% to 40% of patients. Arterial thrombotic events account for two-thirds of such events, with venous thrombotic events representing the remainder. Ischemic stroke, myocardial infarction, and TIAs are the most common arterial thrombotic events. Patients may also present with deep venous thrombosis in the lower extremities, pulmonary embolism, or peripheral vascular occlusions. The cumulative rate of thrombosis ranges from 2.5% to 5% per patient per year. The prevalence of thrombosis at diagnosis ranges from 34% to 39%. It is not unusual for patients with PV to develop thromboses at unusual anatomic sites; in particular, thromboses are relatively frequent in the splanchnic veins, including the splenic, hepatic, portal, and mesenteric vessels or cerebral sinus veins, thrombosis of the vena cava, and intraventricular thrombosis. A particularly serious thrombotic event associated with PV is Budd-Chiari syndrome, which results from hepatic venous or inferior vena caval thrombosis and obstruction. These events lead to hepatic venous outflow obstruction, increased hepatic sinusoidal pressure, and portal hypertension. Portal venous perfusion of the liver is frequently reduced, leading to portal venous thrombosis and hypoxic damage of liver parenchymal cells. This cascade of events results in centrilobular hepatic necrosis, centrilobular fibrosis, and nodular regenerative fibrosis, which culminates in the development of cirrhosis of the liver. The cause of Budd-Chiari syndrome can be identified in 75% of cases, including hereditary and acquired prothrombotic disorders, trauma, and infection. PV account for 10% to 40% of all cases of Budd-Chiari syndrome. Paroxysmal nocturnal hemoglobinuria is also a frequent cause of Budd-Chiari syndrome. Because BM cells from 87% of patients with idiopathic Budd-Chiari syndrome form erythroid colonies in the absence of EPO, such patients were in the past believed to have a forme fruste of an MPN. The identification of these latent MPNs, without elevated blood counts, has been facilitated by screening for JAK2V617F. These patients tend to be younger and female and to have normal blood counts caused by hemodilution and hypersplenism, which mask an elevated RBC mass.[23] Many of these patients (37%) also have another predisposing factor for thrombosis such as exposure to oral contraceptives, antiphospholipid antibodies, factor V Leiden, or protein C deficiency. The JAK2V617F mutation has been reported in 32.7% patients of 831 patients with an idiopathic splanchnic vein thrombosis. The mutation was present in 49% of patients at diagnosis of the idiopathic form of splanchnic vein thrombosis of which 60% were diagnosed as having a coexisting MPN; more than 52% of the remaining patients went on to develop an MPN after a median of 49 months. JAK2V617F was detected in 45% of patients with Budd-Chiari syndrome, and at least in one series, neither exon 12 JAK2 mutations nor MPL mutations were observed. Furthermore, additional patients (6.9%) have idiopathic splanchnic vein thrombosis who have a BM histopathologic picture diagnostic of an MPN but are JAK2V617F negative. The diagnostic value of low serum EPO level in Budd-Chiari syndrome has been questioned because elevated levels have been attributed in JAK2V617F-positive patients to necrotic liver tissue.

There are fulminant, acute, subacute, and chronic forms of Budd-Chiari syndrome. These clinical manifestations depend on the extent and rapidity of hepatic vein occlusion and the development of venous collaterals to decompress the venous sinusoids. One should always consider a diagnosis of Budd-Chiari syndrome in any patient with an MPN with ascites, upper abdominal pain, and liver function abnormalities. This syndrome is characterized by hepatosplenomegaly, ascites, edema of the peripheral extremities, and distention of superficial abdominal veins caused by resultant portal hypertension. Routine biochemical determinations of hepatocellular function and injury are frequently of little diagnostic value in patients with suspected Budd-Chiari syndrome. Doppler ultrasonography is the best tool for screening patients for Budd-Chiari syndrome. This test has a sensitivity and specificity of 85%. Characteristic findings include an absence of flow in the hepatic veins or nonvisualization of the hepatic vein. Contrast-enhanced computed tomography (CT) scanning and magnetic resonance imaging (MRI) are useful in better defining the hepatic venous anatomy. Hepatic venous and inferior vena caval catheterization is a key diagnostic procedure indicating the sites of venous obstruction. The diagnosis can be definitively made by a spider web pattern on hepatic venography. Transjugular liver biopsy specimens usually reveal intense congestion and cellular atrophy.

It has been emphasized that patients with PV can present with portal or hepatic vein thrombosis with normal hemoglobin or hematocrit values. Such patients have leukocytosis, thrombocytosis, or splenomegaly. Screening for the JAK2 mutation should be systematically carried out in such situations and may substitute for BM examinations in individuals who are JAK2V617F positive. In patients with an idiopathic form of splanchnic vein thrombosis but who are JAK2V617F negative, a BM aspirate and biopsy are recommended to exclude the possibility of a JAK2V617F-negative MPN. Gastrointestinal bleeding or an increase in plasma volume that is a consequence of splenomegaly often accounts for the normal blood counts in such patients with Budd-Chiari syndrome. The factors operational in the PV patient that lead to the development of hepatic vein thrombosis are believed to be multiple. Whereas splenomegaly causes increased portal blood flow, extramedullary hematopoiesis within the hepatic sinusoids frequently obstructs hepatic blood flow, and JAK2V617F-positive endothelial cells might affect adhesion to monocytes, leading to aggregation of blood elements. These processes are surely important contributory factors in addition to the other previously discussed risk factors that lead to the development of thrombosis in this patient population.

Neurologic abnormalities occur in almost 60% to 80% of untreated or poorly controlled PV patients and include TIAs, cerebral infarction, cerebral hemorrhage, fluctuating dementia, confusional states, and choreic syndromes. In addition, complaints of dizziness, paresthesias, visual disturbances, tinnitus, and headaches have been attributed to the increased blood viscosity and reduced cerebral blood flow caused by erythrocytosis. The transient neurologic symptoms can also be the consequence of small infarcts in the region of the basal ganglia, which can be detected by CT. These small infarcts are known as lacunae and result from the occlusion of small penetrating arteries, which are particularly susceptible to thrombosis. Cerebrovascular thrombosis occurs more often in PV patients than in the general population. Symptoms caused by intermittent carotid or vertebral basilar artery insufficiency (or both) occur so frequently in PV that it is suggested that every patient with focal cerebrovascular insufficiency should at least have a complete blood count test to exclude the diagnosis of an underlying MPN.

Thrombosis of the dural sinus or cerebral veins (CVT) is an uncommon form of stroke, usually affecting young individuals. CVT represents about 0.5% to 1% of all strokes. Headache, generally indicative of an increase in intracranial pressure, is the most common symptom in CVT. Clinical manifestations of CVT may also depend on the location of the thrombosis. The superior sagittal sinus is most commonly involved, which may lead to headache, increased intracranial pressure, and papilledema. A motor deficit, sometimes with seizures, can also occur. Scalp edema and dilated scalp veins may be seen on examination. For lateral sinus thromboses, symptoms related to an underlying condition (middle ear infection) may be noted, including constitutional symptoms, fever, and ear discharge. Pain in the ear or mastoid region and headache are typical. Hemianopia, contralateral weakness, and aphasia may sometimes be seen owing to cortical involvement. Approximately 16% of patients with CVT have thrombosis of the deep cerebral venous system (internal cerebral vein, vein of Galen, and straight sinus), which can lead to thalamic or basal ganglial infarction. Cavernous sinus thrombosis is usually associated with a primary infectious etiology involving a focus in the face, throat, mouth, ear, or sinuses. Aseptic cavernous sinus thrombosis is an extremely rare phenomenon that has been reported in patients with PV. These patients present with monocular blindness and the characteristic features of ipsilateral cavernous sinus thrombosis, and only retrospectively is the diagnosis of PV made. Therefore, patients found to have this symptom complex who have no known infectious predisposing causes should be carefully evaluated to rule out this diagnosis. The most sensitive diagnostic technique is MRI in combination with magnetic resonance venography.

Thrombosis of large-caliber arteries is a relatively rare event in PV patients, but there have been case reports of thromboses within the chambers of the heart, leading to refractory congestive heart failure and acute aortic occlusion. Such catastrophic thrombotic events in the heart or large vessels would suggest that cardiac catheterization be performed with some caution.

Polycythemia vera frequently manifests with symptoms caused by peripheral vascular disease. In these cases, patients may first be seen by surgeons or dermatologists. Intense redness or cyanosis of the digits with or without burning, classic erythromelalgia, digital ischemia with palpable pulses, or thrombophlebitis without another known cause may be the presenting symptoms.

Erythromelalgia is characterized by burning pain in the digits, an objective sensation of increased temperature, and relief by cooling. PV is the most common cause of erythromelalgia and is one of the few disorders in which digital ischemia with or without ulceration may exist in the presence of palpable pulses. Other disorders that can lead to this abnormality include embolism, trauma, cutaneous infarction, neuritis, infection, and various types of arteritis. Painful and ulcerating toes and fingers have frequently been observed to be presenting symptoms in patients with PV. The likelihood that arterial insufficiency is the cause of such ulceration is quite small in patients who have a palpable dorsalis pedis and posterior tibialis pulses; in this situation, the possibility of an underlying hematologic disorder such as PV should be entertained. Foot pain at rest is a distressing but not widely recognized symptom of PV. In patients with this complaint, peripheral pulses are of normal character, and cutaneous circulation appears to be adequate. The pain is most severe at night, is dull in nature, and occurs primarily in the feet or legs. These symptoms have been shown to be the results of platelet activation and aggregation in vivo, which preferentially occur in arterioles. If untreated, erythromelalgia can progress to ischemic acrocyanosis or gangrene. Phlebotomy alone in PV does not improve erythromelalgia. These symptoms can be abolished by reducing the platelet counts to normal levels and can be rapidly reversed after the institution of antiplatelet aggregation therapy. Therefore, the cause of erythromelalgia appears to be closely linked to abnormal arachidonic acid metabolism that occurs within platelets in this disorder.

Retrospective reviews have revealed a higher than expected number of patients with PV and pulmonary hypertension. Proposed etiologies include direct obstruction of pulmonary arteries by circulating megakaryocytes, extramedullary hematopoiesis in the pulmonary parenchyma, smooth muscle hyperplasia induced by release of PDGF from activated platelets, chronic disseminated intravascular coagulation, and unrecognized recurrent thrombotic events. ET-1 has been associated with development of hypoxia-related pulmonary hypertension and VEGF with protection from this complication. The diagnosis of pulmonary hypertension is made, on average, 9.5 years after the diagnosis of the underlying MPN and is associated with a poor prognosis, with death usually occurring as a result of congestive heart failure or pneumonia. Although anecdotal reports have claimed improvements in patients' pulmonary artery pressure with control of the underlying disease, others have not found any change in serial measurements of 11 patients' pulmonary arterial pressures despite good disease control.

As many as 30% to 40% of patients with PV experience some sort of hemorrhagic event, which can be relatively trivial, such as epistaxis or gingival hemorrhage, or can be life-threatening, such as gastrointestinal hemorrhage or hematomas involving vital organs. The gastrointestinal tract is a frequent site of hemorrhagic complications because patients with PV are predisposed to portal vein thrombosis and resultant variceal bleeding and peptic ulcer disease. Gastroduodenal erosions and ulcers and *Helicobacter pylori* infection are all significantly more common in PV patients than in control patients with dyspepsia. This may be partly attributable to altered mucosal blood flow as a result of increased plasma viscosity or increased histamine release caused by peripheral blood basophilia. Cerebral hemorrhage is a common cause of morbidity and mortality. Bleeding events frequently occur with the use of aspirin or other drugs that impair platelet function; an association between the hemorrhage and the use of high doses of these platelet-paralyzing drugs has been made in almost one-third of such instances. Low-dose aspirin therapy has, however, been reported not to lead to an increased incidence of life-threatening hemorrhagic events. Spontaneous bleeding in patients with PV is relatively rare, although spontaneous retropharyngeal hematomas leading to acute upper airway obstruction or hematomas in the groin have been reported.

Patients with PV who undergo surgical procedures are at a very high risk of developing postoperative complications. In one series of 62 major operations on 54 patients with PV, postoperative complications occurred in 49% of patients; 52% of complications were from hemorrhage, 18% from thrombosis, and 14% from hemorrhage and thrombosis. The postoperative mortality rate in this patient population was 18%. In another series of 15 patients five had serious complications secondary to thrombosis and hemorrhage. A study by an Italian group evaluated retrospectively 311 surgical interventions in 105 patients with PV and 150 with ET: 24 arterial or venous thrombosis (7.7%), 23 major hemorrhages (7.3%), and five surgery-related deaths (1.6%) were observed within 3 months of the procedure. PV patients with uncontrolled erythrocytosis before surgery have been shown to have the highest complication rate. Patients with inadequately controlled disease had a 79% incidence of complications, but in those with adequate hematologic control before surgery, the rate of perioperative and postoperative complications was reduced to 28%. In addition, the duration of disease control was an important factor in decreasing surgical risk; a prolonged period of effective disease control before surgery reduced the complication rate to 5%. Complication rates after surgery can therefore be dramatically reduced by appropriate therapeutic interventions with normalization of blood counts. The chief deterrent to such an approach has been the failure by physicians to recognize the risk associated with PV in the surgical setting.

Generalized pruritus occurs in approximately 40% of cases of PV. Water contact, such as during showers or bathing, induces attacks of intolerable pruritus. There appears to be no clear relationship between the degree of the pruritus and severity of the disease, and 20% of patients continue to experience itching despite reduction of their hematocrits to normal levels. Aquagenic pruritus is significantly more common among JAK2V617F homozygous patients than heterozygotes. The degree of pruritus is so severe in some patients that they are unable to tolerate bathing at all and find it necessary to substitute gentle skin swabbing or to simply not bathe. The etiology of the pruritus in PV remains uncertain. Several groups have attempted to implicate elevated blood and urine histamine levels in its pathobiology. A strong correlation between skin mast cell numbers and the severity of itching has been demonstrated, and mast cells in PV have been shown to be JAK2V617F positive. However, the failure of the pruritus to respond to antihistamine therapy in many patients suggests that abnormally high histamine levels probably do not constitute the sole factor in its development.

Iron deficiency has also been implicated as a factor contributing to pruritus in PV patients who are almost invariably iron deficient. Iron substitution therapy has resulted in symptomatic improvement, but this approach is less than optimal because it frequently results in uncontrollable erythrocytosis.

The development of post-PV MF was increased with prolonged duration of disease and is directly related to the duration of long-term follow-up, but the influence of the modality used to treat the initial PV phase of the disease on the rate of transformation to this more accelerated form of the disease remains uncertain. Post-PV MF should be considered the natural evolution of PV. Criteria for the diagnosis of post-PV MF have recently been proposed (Table 67-3) and can be used as a guide for documenting this transition in disease phenotype, which in reality represents a point in the continuum of PV. For patients with disease duration greater than 10 years, the hazard ratio was 15.24 (95% CI, 4.22-55.06; $P<.0001$). The median interval between the diagnosis of PV and the development of post-PV MF is 13 years. Post-PV MF is characterized by (1) increasing splenomegaly, (2) teardrop RBC morphology, (3) extensive BM fibrosis, (4) a leukoerythroblastic blood picture, and (5) a normal or decreasing RBC mass. The patients may be entirely asymptomatic but often complain of fatigue, dizziness, weight loss, and anorexia. Splenomegaly can lead to abdominal pain caused by repeated splenic infarcts and to early satiety caused by mechanical obstruction of the upper gastrointestinal tract. Patients with post-PV MF are virtually all JAK2V617F positive and characteristically have high JAK2V617F allele burdens (see Chapter 69).

The anemia that characterizes post-PV MF is primarily a result of splenic pooling, ineffective erythropoiesis, and extramedullary production of RBCs with a shortened RBC survival. Patients positive for JAK2V617F are less likely to require blood transfusions but have a poorer survival. Occasionally, the anemia is exacerbated by folate or iron deficiency. Before assuming that a patient has entered post-PV MF, it is prudent to assess BM iron stores. Replacement therapy with iron may lead to the resurgence of erythropoiesis and prevent the faulty categorization of disease progression.

Bleeding abnormalities caused by thrombocytopenia or qualitative platelet abnormalities are especially common during this phase of the disease. Frequent instances of epistaxis or ecchymoses occur, and gastrointestinal hemorrhage caused by esophageal varices arising from portal hypertension is a recurrent problem. The majority of hemorrhagic events are minor in nature. Frequently, patients have generalized wasting characterized by progressive asthenia and weight loss. Severe hyperuricemia, leading to secondary gout or uric acid nephropathy, may also complicate the clinical course.

The median survival for patients with post-PV MF is 5.7 years. Patients with post-PV MF are at a high risk for the development of

Table 67-3 International Working Group for Myelofibrosis Research and Recommended Treatment Criteria for Post-PV MF

Required Criteria:

1. Documentation of a previous diagnosis of polycythemia vera as defined by the WHO criteria
2. Bone marrow fibrosis grade 2–3 (on 0–3 scale) or grade 3–4 (on 0–4 scale)

Additional Criteria (Two Are Required):

1. Anemia or sustained loss of requirement of either phlebotomy (in the absence of cytoreductive therapy) or cytoreductive treatment for erythrocytosis
2. A leukoerythroblastic peripheral blood picture
3. Increasing splenomegaly defined as either an increase in palpable splenomegaly of ≥5cm (distance of the tip of the spleen from the left costal margin) or the appearance of a newly palpable splenomegaly
4. Development of ≥1 of three constitutional symptoms: >10% weight loss in 6 months, night sweats, unexplained fever (>37.5°C)

Adapted from Proposed criteria for the diagnosis of post-polycythemia vera and post-essential thrombocythemia myelofibrosis: A consensus statement from the international working group for myelofibrosis research and treatment. *Leukemia* 22:437, 2008.
WHO, World Health Organization.

acute leukemia. Of patients who develop post-PV MF, approximately 18% will undergo leukemic transformation after 3 years and likely a greater number with longer follow-up. Patients with post-PV MF with a hemoglobin less than 10 g/dL, platelet count less than 100 × 10^9 and WBC counts that exceed 30 × 10^9/L have a poorer prognosis than individuals with fewer of these prognostic variables.

The leukemic transformation of PV has been extensively described. The possibility that a relationship exists between the therapeutic modality used during the erythrocytotic phase and the frequency of development of acute leukemia has been a point of heated discussion. Some of the controversy surrounding this question was formerly caused by a lack of understanding of the basic origins of PV. Clinical hematologists in the 1950s and 1960s frequently thought of PV as a benign hematologic abnormality and believed that therapeutic interventions either with alkylating agents or radiotherapy were solely responsible for the development of acute leukemia. That concept has proved erroneous, and PV, similar to the other MPNs, has been shown to be a clonal malignant hematologic disorder. The evolution to acute leukemia can therefore be thought of as a natural consequence of this malignant disorder, which can be accentuated by the therapeutic interventions already discussed. In fact, 25% of patients who develop MPNs have never been exposed to any form of cytotoxic therapy.

Further insight into the relationship between acute leukemia and PV has been best provided by the results of the PV Study Group (PVSG), which described a randomized trial comparing the use of phlebotomy, chlorambucil, and ^{32}P for the treatment of this disorder. The incidence of acute leukemia was approximately 1.5% in patients treated with phlebotomy alone, 17.5% in patients treated with chlorambucil, and 10.9% in patients treated with ^{32}P after over 15 years of follow-up. The incidence of acute leukemia in the patients treated with phlebotomy alone is therefore much higher than that expected in a normal age-matched control group, again indicating that leukemia is a natural evolutionary event in the clinical course of an individual with PV. The incidence of acute leukemia can be increased, however, by the institution of therapy with either alkylating agents or ^{32}P. The time course for the development of acute leukemia appears to be dependent on the treatment used to control the polycythemia. The development of acute leukemia in patients treated with phlebotomy in the PVSG trial was limited to the first 5 years of treatment, suggesting that the development of acute leukemia is not solely attributable to the prolongation of survival. In contrast, analysis of the hazard function was virtually flat for patients treated with chlorambucil from years 2 to 7 after randomization; however, the risk for acute leukemia became alarmingly high after 10 years of study, suggesting that the risk of acute leukemia increases with time even after the drug has been stopped. One half of the cases of acute leukemia in the chlorambucil arm occurred in the first 5 years, with the remainder equally split between the second and third 5-year periods. In contrast, 60% of the cases of acute leukemia in the group treated with radioactive phosphorus occurred 6 to 10 years after randomization. Of particular concern is the high incidence of leukemia recently reported in patients who were initially treated with radioactive phosphorous or busulphan and then switched to maintenance therapy with hydroxyurea, previously believed to be a nonleukemogenic agent. These findings suggest that a combination of radiotherapy (^{32}P) or an alkylating agent, busulphan, and another chemotherapeutic agent (hydroxyurea) may particularly increase the risk of leukemia. Approximately 30% to 50% of patients with PV who develop acute leukemia have previously entered the post-PV MF phase. In contrast, approximately 50% of patients progress directly from the erythrocytotic phase to acute leukemia. The phenotype of the leukemia cells that characterize the leukemic phase is overwhelmingly myeloid, although rare cases of lymphoblastic and biphenotypic leukemias have been reported. Patients with JAK2V617F-positive MPN are also at a higher risk of developing both additional hematologic malignancies and solid tumors. In addition, low-grade lymphoproliferative disorders such as chronic lymphocytic leukemia have been shown to coexist in patients with a variety of MPNs, including PV, and not to have an adverse effect on prognosis.

The development of leukemia sometimes can be abrupt, however. In some instances, a preleukemic phase characterized by refractory anemia with excess blasts has been described. In fact, half of such cases of acute leukemia in one series were preceded by a myelodysplastic disorder.

A surprising finding that provides some insight into the origins of acute leukemia occurring in PV patients has been provided from studies of the JAK2V617F status of the leukemia blast cells of such patients. Surprisingly, in about 50% of these patients, the leukemic cells were JAK2V617F negative even though in excess of 90% of the PV patients are JAK2V617F positive. Patients with JAK2V617F-positive MPN who developed JAK2V617F-negative leukemias had a shorter time between the diagnosis of the original MPN and the leukemic transformation (3 + 2 vs. 10 + 7 years, respectively) than patients with JAK2V617F-positive leukemias. The possible origins of JAK2V617F-negative leukemias from JAK2V617F-positive MPNs are diagrammatically presented in Fig. 67-6. The AML could potentially originate in the normal stem cell pool that persists in MPD patients, or it could originate in a malignant clone that has not acquired the JAK2V617F mutation. The other possibility remains that the chronic MPN and the AML represent two subclones originating from a common ancestor and that the leukemic transformation results in loss of JAK2V617F.

LABORATORY MANIFESTATIONS

Laboratory evaluation of patients with erythrocytosis involves the careful use of a broad range of diagnostic studies. These studies must be used in a rational manner or the evaluation can become extremely costly. Because PV is a panmyelosis, the overwhelming number of patients has elevated hematocrits, WBC counts, and platelet counts. The diagnosis of PV has been greatly simplified by the discovery of the JAK2V617F mutation, which is present in more than 90% of PV patients. Hematocrit values greater than 52% in males and greater than 48% in females are abnormal and require further evaluation. Documentation of the absolute increase in RBC mass is rarely required and is a test that is available at smaller and smaller numbers of institutions. A hematocrit value greater than 60% in men or greater than 55% in women is almost always associated with an absolute erythrocytosis. In men suspected of polycythemia with a hematocrit level below 60% and women with a hematocrit level below 55%, blood volume measurement is suggested, if available, for determining whether the elevated hematocrit level is actually attributable to an expanded RBC mass. Occasionally, an elevated RBC mass can actually be present in the face of a normal hematocrit value. In cases of splenomegaly caused by portal hypertension, an expanded plasma volume may mask an elevated RBC mass. In addition, iron deficiency can also lead to a normalization of the hematocrit in PV, making the diagnosis difficult. PV is associated with a 20% to 30% frequency of peptic ulcers and gastritis, which can be associated with blood loss. In this situation, thrombocytosis may be exacerbated as a consequence of the iron deficiency. Iron supplementation is not necessary to make a diagnosis of an MPN because of the availability of molecular diagnostic studies. Administration of iron to such patients must be performed carefully to avoid a rapid increase in RBC mass, which can be associated with a high risk of thrombosis. If the patient is JAK2V617F positive and has microcytosis and iron studies indicative of iron deficiency, one can be certain that the patient has an MPN, which is likely PV. The true type of MPN will become apparent with continued follow-up.

The criteria for establishing an RBC mass has previously been based on values expressed as milliliters per kilogram of total body weight. Because adipose tissue is considerably less vascular than lean tissue, it may not contribute equally to the RBC mass. Therefore, RBC mass measurements based solely on body weight can be misleading. RBC mass measurements more closely correlate with lean body mass than total body weight. Measured RBC mass values in obese subjects are regularly lower when expressed as milliliters per kilogram of total body weight than those observed in lean individuals. To overcome this difficulty, the International Council for Standardization in Haematology has presented formulas to calculate normal RBC mass values based on lean body mass, surface area, height, and weight. An elevated RBC mass is now defined as being 25% greater than the mean predicted value of an RBC mass for that individual rather than basing evaluations on the volume per kilogram of total body weight.

Leukocytosis is present in approximately two-thirds of cases and seems to be proportional to the burden of JAK2V617F. Thrombocytosis is observed in 50% of cases. Abnormalities of RBC, WBC, and platelet morphology are frequently observed. The morphologic RBC changes observed during the erythrocytotic phases are characteristic of iron deficiency and include microcytosis, hypochromia, and frequently polychromatophilia. Some anisocytosis and poikilocytosis can be seen as well. Fetal hemoglobin levels and the number of RBCs containing fetal hemoglobin, known as F cells, may be increased. The WBCs are characterized by normal morphology, although the numbers of basophils, eosinophils, and immature myeloid forms can be increased. Platelet morphology is also quite striking in PV. Frequently, megathrombocytes (platelets the sizes of RBCs) are seen on the peripheral blood smear. Patients frequently have platelet counts of less than 1×10^6 mm^{-3}, but it is not unusual to observe a patient with a platelet count higher than this value. PV-related MF is characterized by a leukoerythroblastic blood picture, with the appearance in the peripheral blood of dacryocytes or teardrop RBCs, myelocytes, metamyelocytes, and (rarely) blasts and promyelocytes in addition to nucleated RBCs in the peripheral blood.

Platelet aggregation studies do not correlate frequently with the risk of bleeding episodes. The most common abnormalities are decreased primary and secondary aggregation to either or both epinephrine and adenosine diphosphate and decreased response to collagen with generally a normal response to arachidonic acid. An abnormal platelet storage pool disease is a characteristic feature and is caused by abnormal platelet activation. Prothrombin times (PT) and partial thromboplastin times (aPTT), as well as fibrinogen levels, are usually normal. Profound abnormalities of the PT and aPTT, however, are frequently reported. This is largely a laboratory artifact caused by the extreme erythrocytosis, which results in a relatively smaller volume of plasma being present in the whole blood sample. Coagulation assays are performed on blood anticoagulated with sodium citrate, and the citrate concentration in the anticoagulant is calibrated to chelate the plasma calcium and inhibit coagulation reactions. All coagulation assays include the addition of calcium chloride to neutralize the excess citrate and provide free calcium to mediate coagulation reactions. In patients with extreme erythrocytosis, the ratio of citrate in the collection tube to the volume of plasma is too high; therefore, excess citrate is present, and the standard amount of calcium chloride added during the performance of the PT and aPTT is insufficient to neutralize the excessive citrate, and the coagulation assays are frequently and factually prolonged. To avoid this problem, the clinician should calculate the relative amount of plasma compared with the normal amount and remove the corresponding volume of sodium citrate from the blood collection tube. Normal values can then be confidently anticipated in patients with erythrocytosis. A shortened fibrinogen half-life has been detected in some patients with PV and a significantly increased fractional catabolic rate of the plasma fibrinogen pool per day. In addition, elevated platelet β-thromboglobulin and plasma β-thromboglobulin levels are observed. The constellation of findings is indicative of increased platelet turnover. Prothrombin fragments F1 and 2, thrombin–antithrombin complex, and D-dimer levels are frequently elevated in PV patients. These are enzyme–inhibitor complexes or byproducts of active thrombosis that serve as a biochemical signature of the hypercoagulable state that characterizes PV.

An acquired von Willebrand syndrome occurs frequently in patients with PV and ET who have extreme elevations of platelet numbers. This syndrome is characterized by a normal or prolonged bleeding time, normal factor VIII level, and normal von Willebrand factor (vWF) antigen level, but abnormal vWF ristocetin cofactor actively associated with a decrease or absence of large vWF multimers. This acquired defect resembles type II vWF disease. Because the molecular size of vWF is a major determinant of its adhesive function and the larger multimers are most active in achieving hemostasis, the deficiency of large vWF multimers is associated with a bleeding tendency. The decrease in the frequency of large vWF multimers occurs in patients with platelet counts over 1000×10^9 L^{-1}. This abnormality has been reported not only with patients with severe thrombocytosis caused by MPN but also in patients with reactive thrombocytosis. An inverse correlation between the proportion of large vWF multimers and platelet numbers has been observed. In addition, normalization of the platelet count is accompanied by restoration of a normal vWF multimer pattern. These findings suggest that thrombocytosis of any etiology may favor the adsorption of larger forms of vWF multimers onto platelet membranes, resulting in their removal from the circulation and subsequent degradation by platelet-associated proteases. Although patients with MPN frequently have bleeding tendencies, this is not the case in secondary thrombocytosis, possibly because of the limited periods of extreme thrombocytosis observed in such patients. Patients with PV with clinical courses punctuated by hemorrhagic events, extreme thrombocytosis, and acquired von Willebrand syndrome should not receive aspirin therapy if they are having a thrombotic episode but should be phlebotomized, and platelet reduction therapy should be initiated. Patients with PV and acquired von Willebrand syndrome have recurrent bleeding from mucous membranes and the digestive tract and easy bruisability. These symptoms frequently resolve with normalization of the platelet count.

Deficiencies of one or more natural anticoagulants as well as antiphospholipid antibody syndrome have been observed in patients with PV and thrombosis. These studies indicate that either familial or acquired antithrombin III deficiency, protein C or S deficiency, factor V Leiden mutation, or the prothrombin G gene mutation may contribute to the hypercoagulable state observed in PV. Of note, although hyperhomocysteinemia caused by deficiency of cobalamin or folate can be found in 32% to 56% of PV patients, there is no agreement as to its role in the genesis of thrombotic episodes. Such inherited disorders associated with the erythrocytosis of PV provide a scenario that frequently favors thrombosis in affected individuals. In attempting to determine if a patient with PV and an active thrombosis has such an inherited predisposition, it is important to be aware that proteins C and S as well as antithrombin III levels can be low in patients with an ongoing acute thrombosis or liver cirrhosis. Normal prothrombin and factor VII levels in such patients eliminate liver cirrhosis as a cause of the reduction of these circulating anticoagulants. Individuals with inherited prethrombotic conditions frequently have levels of specific proteins below 10% to 20% of normal during periods of active thrombosis.

The leukocyte alkaline phosphatase activity level is elevated in 70% of patients. Moreover, recent data indicate an increase of neutrophil elastase levels in granulocytes and in plasma that correlates with JAK2 mutational status. Whereas serum vitamin B_{12} concentrations have been found to be elevated in 40% of patients, serum vitamin B_{12}–binding proteins are elevated in 70% of patients. Hyperuricemia occurs in an overwhelming number of patients, and elevated histamine levels are also frequently observed. BM aspirates and biopsies obtained at the time of diagnosis of patients with PV are hypercellular and display characteristic erythroid, granulocytic, and megakaryocytic hyperplasia. The cellular elements (Fig. 67-7) are frequently morphologically normal. Iron stores are almost uniformly absent in pretreatment biopsy specimens. Significant increases in BM reticulin may be present in biopsies obtained early in the course but also may develop during the erythrocytotic phase and may be present for long periods before the onset of the post-PV MF. It is important to emphasize that individuals may have considerable BM fibrosis, which occurs as a consequence of the underlying MPN. The presence of minimal BM fibrosis should not be considered a harbinger of the development of post-PV MF. In patients with post-PV MF, a moderate to marked increase in reticulin fiber is observed, either simultaneously with or within 1 year of this clinical transformation.

Several investigators have attempted to use BM biopsy morphology as a differential diagnostic tool to differentiate between PV and

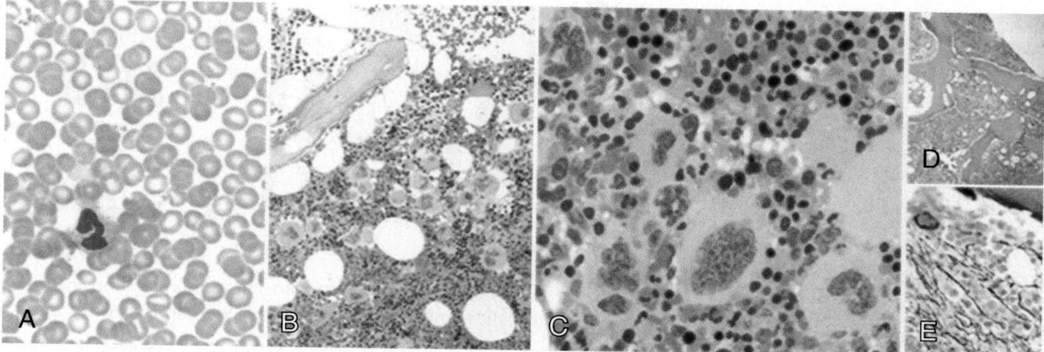

Figure 67-7 PHOTOMICROGRAPH OF BONE MARROW BIOPSY OBTAINED FROM A PATIENT WITH POLYCYTHEMIA VERA IN MYELOFIBROTIC PHASE DEMONSTRATING HYPERCELLULARITY AND INCREASED NUMBER OF MEGAKARYOCYTES (×160).

secondary forms of erythrocytosis. The marked hypercellularity and megakaryocytic hyperplasia that are the hallmarks of MPNs are useful parameters for identifying such individuals (see Fig. 67-7). It is imperative to use the BM biopsy rather than the aspirate specimens for this purpose. It has been suggested that those PV patients with minor BM fibrosis are at an increased risk to develop a thrombotic episode or to evolve into post-PV MF but not acute leukemia during the course of their disease.

The pathologic appearance of the spleen in PV depends on the stage of the disease at which the organ is examined. Spleens from patients in the erythrocytotic phase of the disease are characterized by striking congestion with mature erythrocytes. Small numbers of hematopoietic precursor cells are frequently present. By contrast, spleens examined during the PV-related MF phase are characterized by prominent numbers of foci of extramedullary hematopoiesis, with representation of all BM precursor elements.

The proliferative capacity of PV HPCs has been shown to be a useful laboratory adjunctive study. PV HPC form endogenous erythroid colonies in vitro, which is a tool that can be used to study patients with features of PV who are JAK2V617F negative or who do not have an exon 12 mutation of JAK2. It is important to emphasize that although the presence of endogenous colonies in the blood is indicative of PV, the inability to detect these colonies does not entirely eliminate the diagnosis. Assays of BM cells are indicated when endogenous colonies are not detectable in the peripheral blood. Because of the lack of quality assurance in the performance of such clonal erythroid progenitor cell assays in some laboratories, some reservations concerning their widespread use as diagnostic tools have been expressed.

Allele-specific PCR methods can be used to detect the JAK2V617 or an JAK2 exon 12 mutation in approximately 95% of patients with PV. The very high frequency of JAK2V617F in PV has dramatically improved our ability to diagnose this disease. Patients with isolated erythrocytosis associated with normal neutrophil and platelet counts but low serum EPO levels and the formation of erythroid colonies by peripheral blood mononuclear cells in the absence of EPO in vitro are the characteristic phenotype of patients with the exon 12 mutation. BM biopsies from these patients were slightly hypercellular with isolated erythroid hyperplasia. Megakaryocytes were morphologically normal and not clustered. The exon 12 mutations were frequently present at low levels in granulocyte DNA but were readily identifiable in endogenous erythroid colonies generated in vitro. Because granulocyte involvement with JAK2 exon 12 mutations is low, it is important to sequence DNA from BM cells or from endogenous erythroid colonies generated in vitro to make this diagnosis. At diagnosis, serum EPO levels in PV are either reduced or at the lower limits of normal. Even after normalization of the hematocrit, the serum EPO level in PV remains low in two thirds of patients.

Arterial blood gas measurements are frequently performed to rule out hypoxia as a cause of erythrocytosis. In PV with extreme thrombocytosis, such routine measurements can prove to be misleading. Spurious hypoxemia can frequently be attributed to either significant

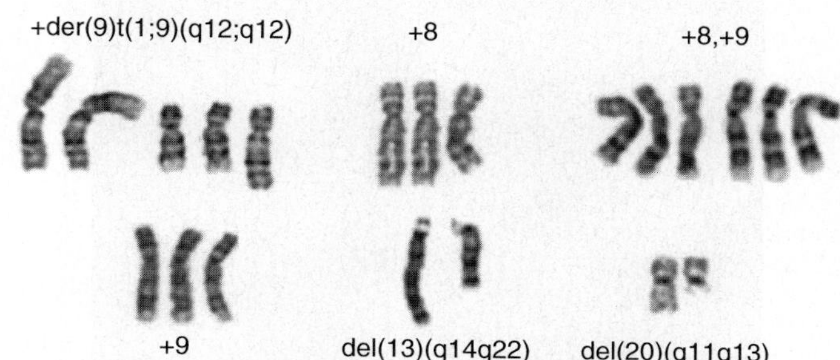

Figure 67-8 Most frequent chromosomal abnormalities associated with polycythemia vera at diagnosis include *(top row)* a gain of derivative(9)t(1;9), resulting in three copies of the long arms of chromosome 1 and three copies of the long arms of chromosome 9, including Janus kinase 2 (JAK2); gain of chromosome 8 and simultaneous gain of both chromosomes 8 and 9 *(bottom row)*; gain of chromosome 9 alone; interstitial deletion of chromosome 13, c; and interstitial deletion of chromosome 20.

leukocytosis or thrombocytosis caused by in vitro consumption of oxygen, the so-called platelet and leukocyte larceny. In this situation, pulse oximetry can be a useful tool for establishing the patient's true oxygenation status.

CYTOGENETIC ABNORMALITIES

The occurrence of nonrandom cytogenetic abnormalities in PV is anticipated because this is a feature of most hematologic malignancies. Such abnormalities have been observed without a single characteristic abnormality defined; the most frequent abnormalities are the gain of chromosome 9 as well as 9p, deletion of chromosome 20q, gain of the long arms of chromosome 1, trisomy 8, and deletion of chromosome 13 (Fig. 67-8). Balanced translocations are rarely observed in PV. At diagnosis, approximately 28% of patients have a recurrent clonal chromosome marker. Interphase fluorescence in situ hybridization (FISH) testing with eight probes for loci most frequently associated with PV and other Ph-negative MPNs occasionally identifies cryptic +9p, del(20q) or del(13q) abnormalities and thus may increase the frequency of detecting a chromosomal rearrangement at diagnosis to 29% to 30%.[24] However, interphase FISH (I-FISH) does not appear to significantly increase the detection rate in untreated patients. Among 387 patients with PV cytogenetically studied at the authors' institution between 1984 and April 2011, 28% had cytogenetic abnormalities at diagnosis. I-FISH studies alone (without cytogenetic examination) using an MPN panel of 12 probes revealed that 29% of patients had genomic changes (Fig. 67-9). The frequency of detection of cytogenetic abnormalities in PV increases over time, with 35% to 55% of patients having clonal cytogenetic abnormalities after extended follow-up and more than 80% of those patients in whom acute leukemia eventually develops. The detection

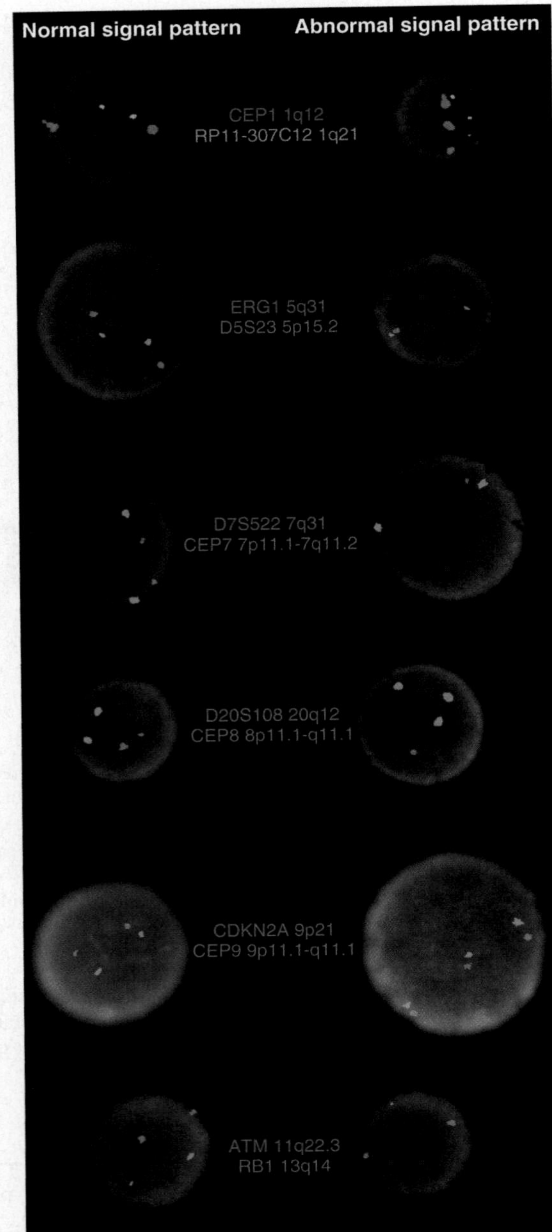

Figure 67-9 Myeloproliferative neoplasm fluorescence in situ hybridization (FISH) panel includes 12 loci on eight different chromosomes for detection of the most frequent chromosomal rearrangements when cytogenetics are either not available or in conjunction with conventional cytogenetics for detection of cryptic abnormalities. Discrepancy in frequency of abnormality detected by interphase FISH and conventional cytogenetics are present and often suggest a proliferative advantage of the abnormal clone.

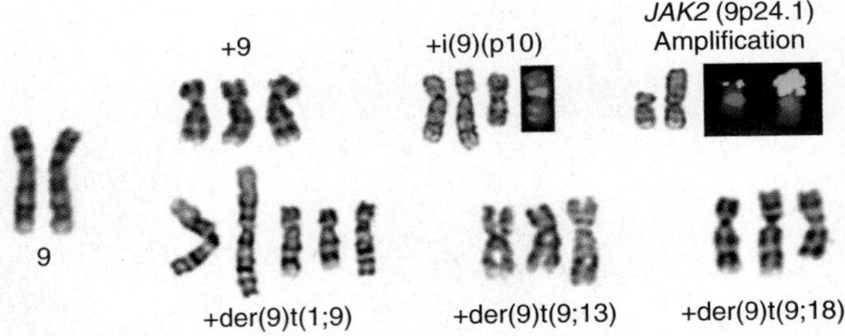

Figure 67-10 Numerous chromosomal abnormalities resulting in trisomy, tetrasomy, or amplification of the short arms of chromosome 9.

of these abnormalities during the disease progression is higher with I-FISH because del(20q) or +9p may be associated with a proliferative advantage. Therefore, progression from a normal to abnormal karyotype is an important adverse prognostic parameter.

Trisomy of the long arms of chromosome 1 is a recurrent abnormality present in about 4% to 6% of patients with PV and an abnormal karyotype. This abnormality has also been described in PMF and other myeloid malignancies. Specifically, 70% of patients with post-PV MF develop trisomy 1q as a result of unbalanced translocations. There are three types of chromosome 1q abnormalities identified in PV: (1) unbalanced translocations such as der(1)t(1q; other chromosome); (2) duplication of the long arms, most frequently q21, q31-32 chromosomal regions; and (3) jumping 1q translocations. Trisomy 1q rarely occurs alone and is most frequently found translocated to another chromosome creating a balanced +1q translocation. The recipient chromosome most frequently involved is chromosome 6 followed by chromosome 9. Jumping translocations are rare cytogenetic phenomenon whereby a part of one chromosome is translocated to several recipient chromosomes, creating multiple related clones within a single patient. Jumping 1q in MPN occurs in 4.2% of cytogenetically abnormal MPN; 86% of such patients progress to AML after an average of 8 months. After it is acquired, the prognosis tends to depend on a copy number of 1q, suggesting that 1q jumping translocations are associated with both disease progression and poor prognosis.

Gain of chromosome 8 is a recurrent abnormality not only in Ph-negative MPN, but it is also one of the three most frequent abnormalities in MDS and is present in 10% of patients with malignant hematopoietic disorders of both myeloid and lymphoid lineages. The prognostic significance in PV is unknown. Some patients with PV with trisomy 8 do not acquire other abnormalities after 20 years. The simultaneous presence of both +8 and +9 is PV specific and is observed in 3% to 4% of PV cases; it is rarely seen in other hematologic malignancies. In PV, trisomy 8 has been demonstrated in myeloid cells but not in lymphoid cells. The genetic consequences of trisomy 8 are unclear, although recent studies suggested a role for microRNAs that are localized on chromosome 8. MicroRNAs are small noncoding RNAs (≈19-25 nucleotides in length) that act as regulators of gene expression by inducing translational inhibition and cleavage of target mRNAs.

Trisomy 9 and gain of the short arms of chromosome 9 is most frequently and almost exclusively observed in PV. There are three types of 9p abnormalities in PV: (1) about 30% of patients have uniparental disomy of 9p region; (2) numerical gain, such as different chromosomal rearrangements that contribute to trisomy, tetrasomy, or amplification of 9p; and (3) unbalanced translocations, of which the most frequent, +der(9)t(1;9), results in a trisomy of both 9p and 1q and appears to be relatively specific abnormality in PV patients (Fig. 67-10). This rearrangement provides an extra copy of mutated *JAK2*. Another recurrent and rare chromosome abnormality resulting in trisomy 9p and three copies of mutated *JAK2* is der(18)t(9;18)(p13;p11)/der(9;18)(p10;q10). I-FISH has been used to detect cryptic chromosome 9 rearrangements. FISH uncovered chromosome 9 rearrangements in 53% of patients with abnormal FISH patterns, indicating that a gain of 9p is the most frequent genomic alteration in PV. The association between the trisomy of 9p and PV was one of the keys to the identification of the JAK2V617F mutation. Cytogenetic studies of 9p and LOH do not indicate any terminal losses or deletions along the entire short arm of chromosome 9, indicating that the LOH is attributable to mitotic recombination. The prognostic significance of +9/+9p is still unknown.

Interstitial deletions of the long arms of chromosome 13 are not specific for PV and are more frequently observed in PMF than in PV. About 1% to 13% of cytogenetically abnormal patients with PV have del(13q). Among patients with del(13q), about 91% have breakpoints in 13q12-14 to q21-22 regions. Fine FISH mapping has defined the commonly deleted region to 13q13.3-q14.3

encompassing Rb1 and two microsatellite loci, D13S319 and D13S25. Cryptic del(13q) occurs and is easily identified with the FISH method. Deletions are heterogenous and may involve one, two, or all three loci, including Rb1. However, structural rearrangements of Rb1 have not been reported in patients with PV. Balanced translocations of 13q14 have rarely been reported in PV, and several studies have shown that submicroscopic deletions involving the same commonly deleted region as defined by del(13q) are present in those apparently balanced translocations.

Del(20)(q11q13), an interstitial deletion of the long arm of chromosome 20, is the second most common cytogenetic abnormality in PV (Fig. 67-11). Del(20)(q11q13) is not diagnostic of PV because it also occurs in PMF and ET as well as in MDS and AML. Heterogeneity of the breakpoints is suggested by the observation that two minimally deleted regions (MDRs) characterize different disorders. A 2.7-Mb spanning D20S10-8 (proximal) and D20S481 (distal) is identified in Ph-negative MPN, and a 2.6-Mb region spanning R52161 (proximal) and Wi-12515 (distal) region is found in other malignancies. Two commonly deleted regions (CDR), CDR1 spanning 2.4 Mb between bands 20q11.23 and 20q12 and CDR2 encompassing 1.8 Mb within 20q13.12, have been identified. The commonly retained region 1(CRR1) spans 1.9 Mb within 20q11.21 and CRR2 encompasses 2.5 Mb within 20q13.33.[25] High-resolution genotyping did not reveal any somatic copy neutral LOH within these regions. Because deletion of chromosomal material may result in the loss of one or several tumor suppressor genes, investigations to date of candidate genes within the deleted segments have failed to identify any mutations within deleted segments. In contrast, haploinsufficiency of the *L3MBTL1* gene, the human homolog of the *Drosophila* L(3)MBT polycomb group tumor suppressor gene located on the 20q12 within a region commonly deleted in several myeloid malignancies, may play a role in erythropoiesis in PV. Downregulation of the L3MBTL1 expression in primary hematopoietic stem progenitor cells (HSPCs), causes an enhanced commitment to and acceleration of erythroid differentiation. Moreover, overexpression of L3MBTL1 in primary hematopoietic $CD34^+$ cells as well as in 20q-cell lines limits erythroid differentiation. Knock-out of L3MBTL1 enhances the sensitivity of HSPCs to EPO, with increased EPO-induced phosphorylation of STAT5, AKT, and mitogen-activated protein kinase (MAPK) as well as detectable phosphorylation in the absence of EPO. Therefore, haploinsufficiency of L3MBTL1 may contribute to erythroid differentiation in PV. It has also been demonstrated that L3MBTL1 is important for the normal progression of cells through mitosis because both overexpression and loss of activity can affect cell division. There is evidence that 20q deletions may impair the release of granulocytes into the peripheral blood. Some patients with PV and 20q deletion in BM cells have cytogenetically normal peripheral blood granulocytes, which has been attributed to del(20q) cells being preferentially retained or destroyed in the BM. I-FISH and SNP-A greatly enhance detection of del(20q) not identified with metaphase cytogenetics. The significance of this abnormality remains unknown because it may be dormant for many years before cells with del(20q) gain proliferative advantage. It is important to emphasize, however, that patients with del(20q) have been observed without further karyotypic instability for more than 10 years.

Other rare recurrent chromosomal abnormalities may occur at the onset of the disease or are associated with disease progression. Most notable are interstitial deletions of the long arms of chromosomes 5 and 7; both have been reported at diagnosis and are associated with disease progression. Loss of P53 as a result of del(17p) or other chromosomal rearrangements is a rare finding in PV and appears to be related to disease progression. Deletion (17p) is not PV specific because it is found in many other myeloid malignancies.

One can conclude that chromosome abnormalities such as +8, +9, and del(20)(q11q13) might be related to the biogenesis of the disease rather than occurring as a consequence of the chemotherapy used to treat the patients. However, it appears that in some patients, an abnormal clone (abnormalities of chromosome 5, 7, or 17) develops as a consequence of therapy with chemotherapeutic agents. Some investigators have suggested that patients with cytogenetic abnormalities at diagnosis have a statistically significant poorer survival rate than those in whom a normal karyotype is observed. This influence of cytogenetic abnormalities on prognosis has, however, not been verified.

Genomic aberrations detected by high-resolution SNP microarray demonstrated that indeed many patients are genetically normal at diagnosis except for, as already mentioned, uniparental 9p disomy, which is detected in about 30% of PV patients. However, disease progression is characterized by an increased number of genomic changes, some of which may not be cytogenetically detectable.

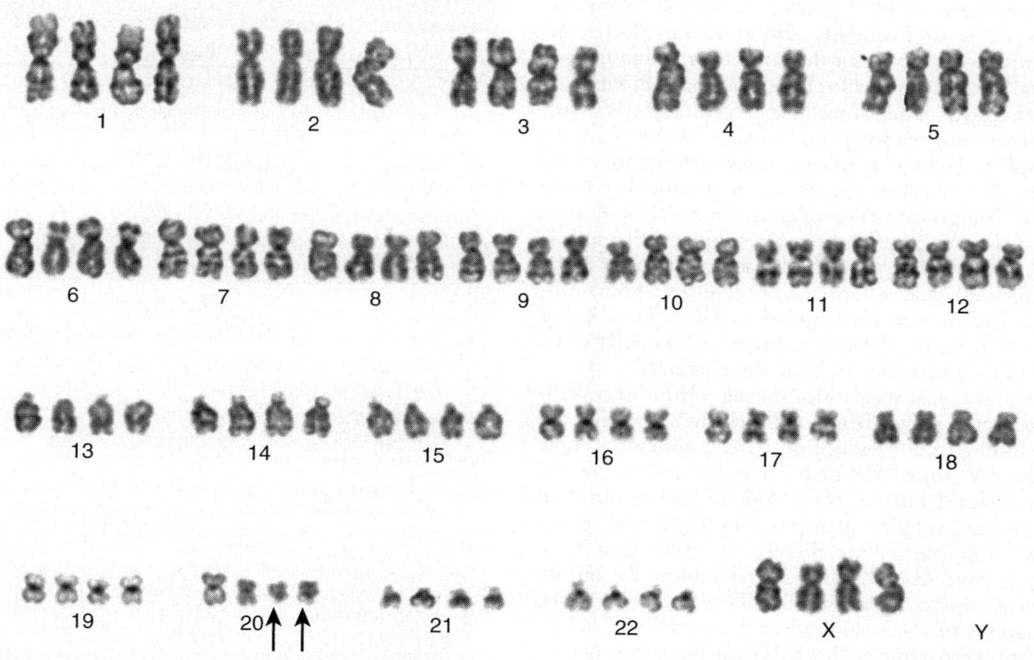

Figure 67-11 A karyotype from a dividing megakaryocyte showing (*arrows*) two copies of deleted 20q in a cell with 92 chromosomes.

Moreover, in a limited number of patients tested, abnormal methylation pattern does not seem to play a crucial role in the pathogenesis of JAK2V617F mutation–positive PV.

DIFFERENTIAL DIAGNOSIS

In most patients, establishing the cause leading to erythrocytosis is not difficult. Initially, it is critical to be certain that one is dealing with a patient with an absolute erythrocytosis. A hematocrit level greater than 60% on several occasions in men or greater than 55% in women, however, is associated with an elevated RBC mass in virtually every case. Testing for JAK2V617F and JAK2 exon 12 mutations can be extremely useful in diagnosing PV and is now common practice to make a diagnosis in any patient who is suspected of having PV. The presence of splenomegaly is an important finding on clinical examination, and adjunctive laboratory findings include normal arterial oxygen saturation, elevated leukocyte alkaline phosphatase activity, and JAK2V617F assays. Splenic sizing by ultrasonography can be useful in documenting splenic enlargement when the spleen is not palpable by physical examination.

It is initially important to differentiate PV from the large number of other causes of secondary erythrocytosis. Characteristically, the patient with PV will present with erythrocytosis, leukocytosis, thrombocytosis, and splenomegaly and is positive for JAK2V617F. The BM biopsy shows hypercellularity with trilineage hyperplasia. In individuals with less pronounced disease, it is important to determine the SaO_2 using an arterial blood gas, the carboxyhemoglobin level, and the $P_{50}O_2$ in patients with other family members with erythrocytosis to exclude obvious causes of secondary erythrocytosis. Because smokers' polycythemia is the most frequent cause of erythrocytosis, it is wise to measure carboxyhemoglobin levels early on in the investigation. In addition, a PaO_2 greater than 67 mm Hg or an O_2 saturation greater than 95% as quantitated on an arterial blood gas is helpful in ruling out hypoxic conditions that lead to erythrocytosis. In patients with intermittent hypoxia, such as sleep apnea syndrome or alveolar hypoventilation caused by obesity, such blood gas determinations can be normal. A low $P_{50}O_2$ is indicative of a hemoglobin mutant with high O_2 affinity, leading to tissue hypoxia and erythrocytosis. These patients often have multiple family members with erythrocytosis. Tests that can be especially useful for this purpose are the serum EPO level, the ability of BM cells to form erythroid colonies in the absence of exogenous EPO, and a JAK2V617F determination. Patients with PV most frequently exhibit serum EPO levels below the 95% confidence intervals for the range observed in normal control participants. It is not unusual to have a normal EPO level in some patients with hypoxic causes of secondary erythrocytosis unless the hypoxia exists over an extended period of time. A normal EPO level cannot be used to exclude a hypoxic cause of erythrocytosis. EPO measurements do, however, remain an important diagnostic tool. Elevation of EPO levels in the face of erythrocytosis is indicative of a hypoxic cause of secondary erythrocytosis, but extremely low levels of EPO (<4 mIU/mL) are virtually diagnostic of PV. It is the patient with erythrocytosis and a normal EPO level in whom additional adjunctive diagnostic tests are required to define the cause of erythrocytosis. The availability of genetic markers such as JAK2V617 or JAK2 exon 12 mutations clearly expedite the diagnosis.

Incorporating a mutational screen into the algorithm for investigating a case of suspected polycythemia will help to streamline the diagnosis of PV, although the presence of a JAK2 mutation alone does not distinguish PV from PMF or ET. Clinical criteria for the diagnosis of PV have been defined by the World Health Organization (WHO), which serves as a uniform platform with which to diagnose PV. It is important, however, for the clinician to realize that some patients undoubtedly have an MPN disorder resembling PV but do not fulfill all the diagnostic criteria of the PVSG or the WHO. The criteria for the diagnosis of PV including the use of the JAK2V617 assay and histopathologic parameters have recently been provided by the WHO (Table 67-4). These criteria are the consensus of many experts working in this field and represent an advance in this field. There will always be unusual cases with clinical characteristics that cannot be pigeonholed into a particular diagnostic category. If asymptomatic; these patients should be followed carefully until the disorder evolves into a more recognizable entity. This would appear prudent to avoid unnecessary therapeutic interventions. If these patients have serious symptoms, the individual physician must make treatment decisions on the basis of the risk-to-benefit ratio for that patient.

A particularly difficult dilemma occurs when evaluating patients with isolated pure erythrocytosis. These patients have elevated RBC masses, normal WBC counts, normal platelet counts, no evidence of splenomegaly, and no evidence of any recognizable cause of secondary erythrocytosis. Clearly, some of these patients have JAK2V617F-positive PV or mutations of exon 12 JAK2 leading to isolated erythrocytosis. The familial congenital form of polycythemia caused by truncation of the EPOR, characterized by increased sensitivity of erythroid progenitor cells to EPO, can be easily distinguished from PV. These patients frequently present in childhood, and this disorder is characterized by isolated erythrocytosis that is associated with an increased risk of thrombotic events. There is a strong family history of polycythemia. In contrast to PV, the BM progenitor cells are hypersensitive to EPO, yet no colonies form in the absence of EPO. The patient with profound erythrocytosis but who is negative for JAK2V617F as well as exon 12 JAK2 mutations and does not have erythrocytosis caused by smoking, cyanotic heart disease, an EPO-secreting tumor, residing at a high altitude, or sleep apnea remains a diagnostic dilemma. All patients should have a good family and drug history obtained, an arterial oxygen saturation study and a carboxyhemoglobin measurement, and measurement or calculation of a p50 and quantitation of a 2,3BPG level and a serum EPO level. If these studies are unrewarding, these patients should then be investigated for mutations in the hypoxia-responsive element of the human EPO gene,HIF-2α and HIF-1α, VHL, PHD1,2,3, STAT5, LNK, and TET2. Some of these tests can be performed by commercial labs, but often one will have to contact an academic reference lab to complete such an extensive investigative effort.

Polycythemia vera must also be differentiated from the other MPNs, such as CML, ET, and PMF. Such classification has major prognostic implications and influences important therapeutic decisions, including the use of tyrosine kinase inhibitors such as imatinib,

Table 67-4 Proposed Revised World Health Organization Criteria for Polycythemia Vera

Diagnosis
Requires the presence of both major criteria and one minor criterion *or* the presence of the first major criterion together with two minor criteria.
Major Criteria
1. Hemoglobin >18.5 g/dL in men and 16.5 g/dL in women *or* another evidence of increased RBC volume*
2. Presence of *JAK2V*617F or other functionally similar mutation such as *JAK2* exon 12 mutation
Minor Criteria
1. Bone marrow biopsy showing hypercellularity with trilineage hyperplasia (panmyelosis) with prominent erythroid, granulocytic, and megakaryocytic proliferation
2. Low serum erythropoietin level
3. Endogenous erythroid colony formation in vitro

Data from Tefferi, Thiele J, Orazi A, et al: Proposals for revision of the World Health Organization diagnostic criteria for polycythemia vera, essential thrombocythemia, and primary myelofibrosis: From an ad hoc international expert panel. *Blood* 110:1092, 2007.

*Hemoglobin or hematocrit >99th percentile of method-specific reference range for age, sex, altitude of residence, *or* hemoglobin >17 g/dL in men and 15 g/dL in women if associated with a documented and sustained increase of at least 2 g/dL from an individual's baseline value that cannot be attributed to correction of iron deficiency, *or* elevated red blood cell mass >25% above mean normal predicted value.

dasatinib, and nilotinib. With the distinctive cytogenetic abnormalities and molecular genetic abnormalities that are unique to CML (Philadelphia chromosome, *BCR-ABL* gene fusion), these two disorders should not be difficult to differentiate. Occasional patients with an MPN have been shown to have both JAK2V617F as well as *BCR-ABL;* whether this unusual occurrence takes place in two different clones and thereby represents two independent MPNs or a single clone and is caused by the predisposition of such patients to acquire mutations in their hematopoietic cells is a subject of speculation. This association has been reported in about 2% of CML patients with the CML disease phenotype predominating in most.

Patients with PMF can present with abnormalities that are virtually indistinguishable from those of patients with PV-related MF. Almost 50% of PMF are JAK2V617F positive, but more than 90% of patients with post-PV MF are JAK2V617F positive. The survival of patients with the latter disorder is much shorter than that of patients with the former condition. Some patients with presumed PMF may actually develop PV after the institution of chemotherapy.

A preceding history of PV permits differentiation between these two situations. ET and PV with marked thrombocytosis can easily be confused. When the RBC mass is used as a definitive diagnostic test, a distinction between ET and the erythrocytotic phase of PV is usually readily apparent. This measurement, however, can be normal or actually low in patients with PV who are iron deficient because of bleeding or excessive phlebotomy. Campbell and coworkers[25] have recently used sensitive PCR-based methods to assess the JAK2 mutational states in 806 patients with ET. The mutation was present in more than 50% of patients with ET. JAK2V617F-positive ET patients were characterized by multiple features that resembled those of patients with PV, including higher hemoglobin levels, higher WBC counts, more prominent BM erythroid and granulocytic hyperplasia, a higher incidence of venous but not arterial thrombosis, low serum EPO levels, and lower serum ferritin levels. Surprisingly, JAK2V617F-negative patients had higher platelet counts. Furthermore, JAK2V617F-positive ET patients had a higher probability of developing PV with longer follow-up. Acquisition of homozygosity for the JAK2V617 caused by homologous recombination is likely the critical event in the development of PV in JAK2V617F ET patients. Homozygosity for JAK2V617F occurs in at least 30% of patients with PV but is extremely rare in ET.

PROGNOSIS

The prognosis of a patient with PV depends on the nature and severity of the complications that occur during the clinical course of that particular patient's disorder. In addition, an individual patient's prognosis depends on the duration of the erythrocytotic phase or the time to transition to post-PV MF or acute leukemia. Survival is also influenced by whether appropriate treatment is instituted during the erythrocytotic phase of the illness. Patients who have uncontrolled erythrocytosis are at an extremely high risk for the development of thromboses. The median survival time from the onset of symptoms has been reported in a study that is over 4 decades old to be as short as 1.5 years in untreated patients, but this number seems excessive because of the relatively large number of patients who are diagnosed during routine examinations and are asymptomatic for prolonged periods of time. Determination of the optimal management of patients with PV has been a difficult task because the disease, when treated, is associated with a survival period of approximately 17 years. Studies of new potential therapeutic interventions therefore require prospective studies with prolonged follow-up times before meaningful results can be generated determining their ability to improve upon overall survival.

Increasing age and history of vascular events have consistently proven to be independent predictors of developing additional thromboses in patients with PV. In the ECLAP trial, the incidence of cardiovascular complications was higher in patients older than 69 years of age, patients with a history of thrombosis, and patients with WBC counts higher than 15,000 × 109 L^{-1}. Conventional cardiovascular risk factors, including hypertension, hyperlipidemia, diabetes, and smoking, are assumed to be associated with the same relative risk of developing thrombosis in PV patients as that observed in the general population. Although practicing hematologists are frequently concerned about elevated platelet counts in PV patients, several reports have failed to show any association between platelet count and thrombotic events, suggesting that therapies in PV targeting reduction of platelet numbers are ill conceived.

Table 67-5 Risk Stratification in Polycythemia Vera Based on Thrombotic Risk

Risk Category	Age >60 Years or History of Thrombosis	Cardiovascular Risk Factors*
Low	No	No
Intermediate	No	Yes
High	Yes	

Data from Finazzi G, Barbui T: How I treat patients with polycythemia vera. *Blood* 109:5104, 2007.
*Hypertension, hypercholesterolemia, diabetes, and smoking (see text). Extreme thrombocytosis (platelet count >1500 × 10^9 L^{-1}) is a risk factor for bleeding. Its role as a risk factor for thrombosis is uncertain. An increasing leukocyte count has been identified as a novel risk factor for thrombosis, but confirmation is required.

These data have led to stratification of therapy in patients with PV based on clearly identifiable risk factors (Table 67-5) of developing additional thrombotic events. The development of acute leukemia was a relatively rare event in PV, occurring in 22 of 1638 patients in the ECLAP observational study after a median of 8.4 years from the time of diagnosis. Older age as well as treatment with P^{32}, busulphan, and pipobroman was associated with a four- to eightfold increased risk of developing AML of an MDS compared with patients treated with phlebotomy alone, hydroxyurea, or INF. For reasons not presently understood, patients presenting with PV and low blood cholesterol levels are at an especially high risk for developing acute leukemia.

Recently, the effect of JAK2V617F allele frequency on the prognosis of PV patients has been examined. More than 95% of patients with PV are JAK2V617F positive, and their mutational load can be determined by allele-specific PCR. Approximately 30% of PV patients have a high JAK2V617F burden (>50%), and the remainder have a lower burden (<50%), with the small numbers being wild type. Some investigators, but not all, have reported that high burdens of JAK2V617F in PV patients are associated with larger splenic volumes, more frequent aquagenic pruritus, a higher incidence of thrombotic events, and a higher rate of evolution into MF and acute leukemia.

High leukocyte counts (>15,000 × 10^9/L) at the time of diagnosis has been identified as another independent predictor of developing a major thrombosis in PV patients. In addition, others have suggested that this parameter is predictive of evolution to MF and an overall inferior survival time.

The choice of therapeutic agents used to treat the erythrocytotic phase of disease clearly influences patient outcomes. The use of alkylating agents and radioactive phosphorous is associated with an established risk for leukemic transformation or evolution to MDS. Clearly, this risk is also associated with increased duration of the disease. The effect of hydroxyurea on leukemic transformation rates is an area of controversy. In addition, the influence of long-term INF therapy on disease outcomes is not at present clearly defined.

THERAPY

A cumulative duration of survival for PV patients treated with modern strategies of between 15 and 17 years has been reported. Despite the implementation of standard therapeutic strategies, the mortality rate of PV patients is increased by 1.84 compared with age- and sex-matched populations. At present, the goals of therapy are directed toward normalization of blood counts in an attempt to avoid additional thrombotic events. Therapy is also stratified based on the presumed risk of an individual patient to develop additional thrombotic episodes, with low-risk patients being treated with phlebotomy therapy alone plus a therapy directed toward paralysis of platelet function and high-risk patients receiving not only phlebotomy plus antiplatelet therapy but also some form of myelosuppressive therapy (hydroxyurea, INF, anagrelide, busulfan). At present, the therapeutic goals are to reduce the risk of thrombosis by normalizing the hematocrit levels to 45% or lower in males and 42% or lower in females, but the relationship between maintaining hematocrit levels under target values and clinically relevant outcomes remains the subject of much spirited speculation rather than being based on a firm foundation of evidence. In a retrospective analysis, Spanish investigators reported that maintaining the hematocrit below 45% was not associated with a decreased thrombotic risk. These data should not be interpreted to mean that phlebotomy therapy for excessive erythrocytosis should be abandoned, but rather that the need to maintain patients below hematocrits of 45% likely does not provide any advantage. Previous studies have indicated a lack of a relationship between thrombocytosis at diagnosis or during the period of follow-up with thrombotic complications, yet in the Spanish study, there was an association between lack of reduction of platelet numbers below 400×10^9/L and an increased risk of thrombosis, and that persistence of leukocytosis was associated with a greater risk of hematologic transformation and shorter survival time but not a reduced incidence of thrombosis. Whether therapy should be directed at normalization of platelet or leukocyte numbers is unclear. Phlebotomy therapy alone is the standard of care for low-risk PV patients. Several investigators have, however, suggested that patients have serious nonhematologic symptoms secondary to the iron deficiency that inevitably accompanies repeated phlebotomies. A careful evaluation of symptoms fails to provide convincing evidence that undue fatigue occurs as a result of iron deficiency in PV patients with normal or elevated hematocrit values. Phebotomized PV patients do not experience dysphagia or the esophageal changes associated with chronic iron deficiency. The two symptoms that have been observed to occur regularly are picophagia, a pica consisting of compulsive ice eating, and restless leg syndrome. These symptoms can be resolved with ingestion of extremely small amounts of oral iron, which might increase the need for phlebotomy therapy (see box on General Principles of Therapy).

A series of studies, although completed more than 30 years ago, by the Polycythemia Vera Study Group has answered several very important questions regarding the efficacy and associated complications of particular therapeutic modalities. These investigations have aided in the identification of optimal therapy for individual patients, which must be selected on the basis of age and comorbid disease status to minimize treatment-related complications.

The first PVSG randomized trial (01 trial) evaluated three treatment strategies: (1) phlebotomy alone to maintain the hematocrit level at less than 45%; (2) intravenous ^{32}P, 2.3 mCi/m^2 repeated every 12 weeks, if needed (maximum, 5 mCi per dose) supplemented by phlebotomy to maintain the hematocrit level at less than 45%; and (3) myelosuppression with chlorambucil 10 mg/day orally for 6 weeks and then daily on alternate months with necessary dose reductions and supplemental phlebotomy. More than 400 patients were randomly assigned to this protocol. The median survival duration from entry into the study until death was 9.1 years for patients treated with chlorambucil, 10.9 years for those treated with ^{32}P, and 12.6 years for the phlebotomy group. Long-term survival was inferior for patients treated with chlorambucil compared with those treated with ^{32}P or phlebotomy. An early finding was the appearance during the first 5 years of a significant excess of deaths from acute leukemia in the chlorambucil arm, which reached 17% after 15 years of follow-up. As a result, the chlorambucil arm was discontinued, and patients were assigned randomly to one of the other two arms. Even though no statistical difference in overall survival between ^{32}P and phlebotomy alone was apparent through the first 10 years, the morbidity and mortality associated with each type of therapy were attributable to distinctly different causes. Thrombosis as a cause of death was much more frequent in the phlebotomy-only group during the first 5 to 7 years of follow-up. Analyses of factors associated with thrombosis revealed that the performance of phlebotomy, the rate of phlebotomy, advancing age, and history of previous thrombosis were statistically significant factors predictive of this outcome. In contrast, the use of ^{32}P led to a lower rate of thrombosis during the first 5 years, but the incidences of leukemias, lymphomas, and nonhematologic malignancies increased during the next 5 years to nearly 10%. After a 15-year period of observation, the incidences of leukemia and lymphoma in the chlorambucil group had risen to 17%. A statistically significant increase in skin and gastrointestinal cancers occurred in the ^{32}P- and chlorambucil-treated cohorts compared with the group treated with phlebotomy alone (see box on Algorithm for Management of Patients With Polycythemia Vera).

General Principles of Therapy

1. The etiology of erythrocytosis must be correctly categorized to be certain the patient has PV. This will avoid inappropriate exposure of patients with nonmalignant disorders to potential leukemogenic agents. To this end, a major contribution is played by incorporating a JAK2V617F and exon 12 JAK2 mutational determinations in the diagnostic workup, and in this way, early phases of PV can be recognized as well. In individuals with erythrocytosis without a JAK2 mutation, search for mutations in VHL, PHD2, HIF-1 and HIF-2 should be considered.
2. Therapy should be individualized.
3. Initially, the hematocrit should be reduced to 45% as soon as possible. The speed of phlebotomy will depend on patients' general medical conditions (250-500 mL every other day). Elderly patients with compromised cardiovascular or pulmonary systems should be more carefully phlebotomized (twice a week), or smaller volumes of blood should be removed.
4. Hematocrit levels should be maintained at 45%.
5. The use of chemotherapeutic agents should be avoided in low-risk PV patients, and treatment with hydroxyurea or INF should be reserved for high-risk patients. Be on the look-out for toxicities from each of these agents.
6. Hyperuricemia is treated with allopurinol (100-300 mg/day).
7. Pruritus is treated empirically with cyproheptadine 4 to 16 mg/day or, if unsuccessful, INF-α therapy 3.0×10^6 units subcutaneously three times a week. A role of selective serotonin uptake inhibitors (paroxetine 20 mg/day or fluoxetine 10 mg/day) or with phototherapy has been proposed. Dramatic relief occurs with the institution of JAK2 inhibitors, and these agents should be used as a component of an experimental trial or if the patients have features that justify the diagnosis of post-PV MF syndrome.
8. Elective surgery or dental procedures should be delayed until hematocrit and platelet counts have been normalized for more than 2 months. Aspirin should be withdrawn at least 1 week before surgery. If emergency surgery is contemplated, phlebotomy and cytapheresis should be pursued.
9. Women and men who are contemplating having children should be treated by phlebotomy plus low-dose aspirin therapy (81 mg/day or with INF-α) to avoid teratogenic effects of chemotherapy. Such avoidance will also prevent deleterious effects on fertility. During pregnancy, therapy is frequently not necessary; if it is, phlebotomy plus low-dose aspirin should be exclusively used. If phlebotomy control is inadequate, treatment with INF-α should be pursued.

Algorithm for Management of Patients With Polycythemia Vera

Low-risk young patients (age <60 years) and no history of thrombosis, platelet count <1.5 × 10⁶ mm⁻³

Phlebotomy + low-dose aspirin (81 mg/day) to maintain hematocrit lower than 45% in males and lower than 42% in females. Aspirin should not be used in patients with histories of a hemorrhagic episode or with extreme thrombocytosis (>1.5 × 10^6 mm^{-3}) or acquired von Willebrand syndrome.

↓

Thrombosis or hemorrhage
Systemic symptoms
Severe pruritus refractory to histamine antagonists
Painful splenomegaly

↓

Hydroxyurea 15-20 mg/kg (unless younger than 40 years, pregnant, intolerant to hydroxyurea; consider pegylated INF)

↓

Pegylated INF 45 to 180 μg/wk or INF - (3 × 10^6 units three times a week; alter dose depending on response and toxicity). Consider the use of pegylated INF, which can be administered once weekly.

↓

If platelet control is inadequate or patient cannot tolerate interferon, one option is the use of anagrelide. However, the use of this drug is controversial. In this case, supplemental phlebotomy is required to maintain hematocrit lower than 45% in males and lower than 42% in females, and the use of hydroxyurea should be considered, especially if patient continues to have thrombotic episodes.

↓

If the patient has increasing splenomegaly, systemic symptoms, or repeated thromboses despite adequate dose of hydroxyurea (2-3 g/day), start busulphan, 4 to 6 mg/day orally for 4 to 8 weeks. It should be mentioned that the sequential use of hydroxyurea and busulphan may be associated with an increased risk of leukemia. Supplemental phlebotomy may be required.

Painful splenomegaly

↓

Splenectomy + continued systemic therapy

↓

High-risk patients (age >60 years), previous thrombosis, platelet count >1.5 × 10⁶ mm⁻³

Phlebotomy to hematocrit of 42% in females and 45% in males

Aspirin (81 mg/day) to be given only in patients with platelet counts <1.5 × 10^6 mm^{-2}

Myelosuppressive therapy with hydroxyurea 30 mg/kg orally for 1 week

Then 15 to 20 mg/kg

↓

If patient continues to have thrombotic episodes and has extreme thrombocytosis or cannot tolerate hydroxyurea

Consider pegylated INF 45 to 180 μg/wk or add busulphan 4-6 mg/d orally for 4 to 8 weeks.

If on bisulphan, stop when blood counts are normalized or platelet count is lower than 300,000 mm^{-3}.

Occasional supplemental phlebotomy if hematocrit is >42% in females and greater than 45% in males; when patient relapses (patient is symptomatic), initiate busulphan therapy again at same dose.

Patient age >70 years

Phlebotomy + low-dose aspirin + hydroxyurea

↓

No response or poor compliance

Busulphan 4 to 6 mg/day orally for 4 to 8 weeks. Stop when blood counts are normalized or platelet count is lower than 300,000 mm^{-3}.

Given the paradox of equal 10-year survivals but demise because of distinct causes in comparable populations of patients treated by phlebotomy alone or by phlebotomy plus ^{32}P, the PVSG pursued strategies to reduce the thrombotic risk in the phlebotomy-only group. One study attempted reduction of the thrombotic risk by combination antiplatelet therapy. It appeared possible that therapy directed toward altering platelet function might reduce the frequency of thrombosis. Therefore, a randomized trial was performed in which phlebotomy, supplemented with the platelet antiaggregating agents aspirin and dipyridamole, was compared with ^{32}P (PVSG trial 05). The outcome for the group treated with phlebotomy, aspirin, and dipyridamole was disappointingly inferior to the ^{32}P results. In fact, more thromboses occurred in the former than in the latter group, but surprisingly, there was also a significantly greater incidence of severe gastrointestinal hemorrhages.

Renewed impetus for the use of nonchemotherapeutic agents for the treatment of PV was provided by an extensive natural history study of 1213 patients reported by the Gruppo Italiano Studio Policitemia. They showed that the age- and gender-standardized mortality rate of patients with PV was 1.7 times greater than the mortality rate of control participants in the general Italian population. In addition, four times as many patients who had previously received ^{32}P, alkylating agents, or hydroxyurea died of cancer compared with patients treated with phlebotomy alone. When this group combined the total number of deaths and the number of nonfatal myocardial infarctions and strokes, they found an unsatisfactory risk-to-benefit profile in patients treated with chemotherapeutic agents and suggested that antithrombotic strategies, such as low-dose aspirin, be carefully evaluated for use in the care of patients with PV.

In light of more recent knowledge of the dose requirements for selective antiplatelet therapy with aspirin, it appears that the PVSG study of platelet antiaggregating agents might have failed because of the use of excessive aspirin dosages (900 mg/day). Such aspirin doses appear to diminish vascular endothelial production of the platelet antiaggregatory factor, prostacyclin I_2 (PGI_2).

Polycythemia vera platelets are known to have a generalized abnormality of arachidonate metabolism that is characterized by enhanced synthesis of thromboxane A_2, which likely reflects stimuli to platelet activation. The exact mechanism responsible for enhanced platelet synthesis of thromboxane A_2 in PV remains unknown and requires further investigation. A low-dose aspirin regimen (50 mg/day for 7-14 days) has been shown to suppress more than 80% of the excretion of the metabolites of thromboxane A_2. A pilot study was performed in which the toxicity of low-dose aspirin therapy in PV patients was evaluated. A very-low-dose aspirin regimen (40 mg/day) was chosen to prevent thrombosis yet minimize the risk of bleeding. After follow-up of the low-dose aspirin treatment group and control group, low-dose therapy was shown not to be associated with an increased incidence of bleeding complications. Aspirin therapy was well tolerated and was associated with complete inhibition of platelet cyclooxygenase activity. A large, randomized, placebo-controlled clinical trial testing the risk-to-benefit ratio of low-dose aspirin therapy in preventing thrombotic episodes in PV has been completed. Treatment with low-dose aspirin (100 mg/day) compared with placebo reduced the risk of the combined end points of nonfatal myocardial infarction, nonfatal stroke, pulmonary embolism, major venous thrombosis, or death from cardiovascular courses. Overall mortality and cardiovascular mortality, however, was not reduced significantly by aspirin therapy. Importantly, the incidence of major bleeding episodes was not significantly increased in the aspirin group. It is important to emphasize that patients require aggressive phlebotomy therapy to the appropriate target hematocrit levels as well as the appropriate use of myelosuppressive agents as primary therapy, with the addition of aspirin serving as an adjunct to this strategy. The conclusions of this study have been questioned by several investigators. In addition, a retrospective analysis performed by independent investigators of the 630 patients treated by the ECLAP group has concluded that low-dose aspirin therapy in PV patients was associated with a statistically nonsignificant reduction in the risk of fatal thrombotic episodes without an increased risk of bleeding.[26] This meta-analysis is surely not a ringing endorsement of the widespread use of aspirin therapy, which is a strategy that has been indiscriminately used worldwide to treat such patients. Because it is unlikely that the value of aspirin therapy will be examined in a properly powered randomized trial, it is suggested that since aspirin therapy is a relatively innocuous therapy it should be used in high-risk patients judiciously. However, it should be avoided in patients with extremely high platelet counts who are at risk for hemorrhage. There is no evidence at present to indicate the necessity of its use in patients with low-risk disease.

It is interesting to compare the results of the PVSG study with those of a randomized trial of ^{32}P versus busulphan for the treatment of PV conducted by the European Organization for Research and Treatment of Cancer (EORTC). The two studies were comparable in size, design, and duration of follow-up. In the EORTC trial, induction courses of busulphan 4 to 6 mg/day for 4 to 8 weeks were compared with ^{32}P treatment. Patients treated with busulphan had a survival advantage over ^{32}P-treated patients. This difference was due primarily to a threefold greater incidence of fatal thrombotic events in the ^{32}P group. Interestingly, the incidence of leukemia in both groups was very low (<2%), with an overall malignancy rate of less than 10% (involving mostly solid tumors).

It is reasonable to conclude from this trial that busulphan is a myelosuppressive agent with limited leukemogenic potential when used on an intermittent schedule. A retrospective study of patients in England treated with phlebotomy and intermittent busulphan supports these same conclusions.

After the disappointing results experienced with the alkylating agent chlorambucil, the PVSG began a nonrandomized phase II investigation of hydroxyurea, an S-phase–specific ribonucleotide reductase inhibitor. The hope was that this agent would be nonleukemogenic. Of 53 patients with PV treated with hydroxyurea who had never received other forms of myelosuppression, after follow-up for a median period of 8.6 years and a maximum follow-up of 795 weeks, 5.4% developed acute leukemia compared with 1.5% of patients treated with phlebotomy alone on the original PVSG randomized study.

In a comparable trial from Israel 71 patients were treated with hydroxyurea for a mean duration of 7.3 years. Remarkably, the incidence of thrombosis was only 6%, indicating the impressive potential of hydroxyurea to lower the incidence of thrombosis in patients with PV, confirming an observation previously made by another group. The incidence of leukemia in the Israeli trial was 5.6%. In another retrospective series, the incidence of acute leukemia and myelodysplasia in patients with PV treatment of hydroxyurea alone was 6.9%. In patients treated first with busulphan and then hydroxyurea, the rate of acute leukemia and myelodysplasia was 13.8%. Twenty-two patients developed AML and MDS in the ECLAP study that enrolled 1638 patients. AML and MDS were diagnosed after a median of 8.4 years from the diagnosis of PV; the variable associated with progression was older age, but overall disease duration (>10 years) failed to reach statistical significance. Exposure to P^{32}, busulphan, and pipobroman but not hydroxyurea alone had an independent role in producing an excess risk for progression to AML and MDS compared with treatment with phlebotomy or INF. The potential leukemia-promoting potential of hydroxyurea has been readdressed in two recent studies. Kiladjian and coworkers[22] reported the results of a randomized trial of hydroxyurea versus piprobroman that was initiated in 1980; the overall survival was 20.3 years in the hydroxyurea-treated group compared with 15.4 years for the patients treated with piprobroman. The incidence of AML and MDs in the piprobroman group was dramatically higher, which is not unexpected because pipribroman is an alkylating agent. This trial was designed with a cross-over option, but 93 patients only received piprobroman. The incidence of AML and MDS in the patient group that only received hydroxyurea was 7.3%, 10.7%, and 16.6% at 10, 15, and 20 years, respectively. Such high rates of transformation have not been previously reported, and because there was not a control arm treated with phlebotomy alone, one cannot determine if this represents the natural history of PV or a potential leukemogenic effect of hydroxyurea. Interestingly, no difference in the incidence of vascular events was seen between the two arms. This same question was again addressed in a nested case control study performed in Sweden.[27] The most important observation was that 25% of patients with various MPNS (68% had PV) who evolved to AML and MDS had not been exposed to any chemotherapeutic agent, indicating that the risk of leukemic evolution was higher than had been previously appreciated. The use of radioactive phosphorous and alkylating agents, but not hydroxyurea, was associated with a higher rate of AML and MDS. These reports indicate that nontreatment-related factors play a major role in the development of AML and MDS, and the contribution of hydroxyurea based on the best available evidence is at best minimal, but likely not totally without risk. However, the documented ability of hydroxyurea to lower the incidence of thrombotic events and its very limited leukemogenic potential makes this drug a very useful chemotherapeutic agent in older, high-risk patients with disease that cannot be controlled with phlebotomy alone. Excessive myelosuppression, macrocytosis, hypersegmentation of polymorphonuclear leukocytes, cutaneous actinic keratosis, squamous cell carcinoma of the skin, hyperpigmentation, stomatitis, painful leg ulcers, creatinine elevations, and jaundice have been attributed to the use of hydroxyurea. Aphthous and leg ulcers occur in 9% of patients, usually after approximately 10 months of therapy (see Fig. 67-12).[28] Rarely, cycling of platelet and leukocyte counts but not RBCs occurs while patients are being treated with hydroxyurea. In this situation, the authors have maintained patients on a fixed dose of hydroxyurea rather than chasing cycling platelet counts. In addition, the use of hydroxyurea requires patient compliance and careful monitoring of blood counts to avoid the sequelae of excessive myelosuppression.

Some clinical investigators have suggested that a program of phlebotomy alone would be the most appropriate for younger patients, who have not experienced a cerebrovascular or cardiovascular event. Strong consideration should be given to the use of phlebotomy therapy in conjunction with low-dose aspirin therapy in addition to the use of such apparently nonleukemogenic drugs as INF-α in this younger patient population.

Anagrelide, a selective inhibitor of platelet production, has been used to treat thrombocytosis in PV patients with thrombotic or hemorrhagic complications. This agent appears to be nonleukemogenic and acts by impairing megakaryocyte maturation. Its use leads to a selective reduction in platelet numbers, and it has been effective in patients refractory to hydroxyurea and INF. This drug does not effectively control the erythrocytosis and leukocytosis or systemic symptoms associated with PV and therefore was suggested to be used as a supplement to phlebotomy therapy. The time to complete response generally ranges between 17 and 25 days. The dose of anagrelide required to control thrombocytosis remains constant over time in most patients. When anagrelide is discontinued, platelet counts returned to pretreatment levels within 5 to 7 days. The simultaneous administration of anagrelide and low-dose aspirin has been

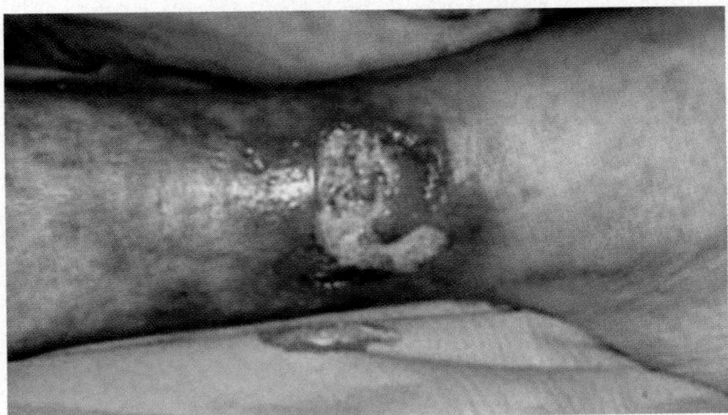

Figure 67-12 EXAMPLE OF A HYDROXYUREA-INDUCED LEG ULCER. *(From Soutou B, Aractingi S: Myeloproliferative disorder therapy: Assessment and management of adverse events: A dermatologist's perspective.* Hematol Oncol *27:11, 2009.)*

reported to lead to a significant increase of bleeding manifestations. Clinicians presume that the effects of anagrelide observed in ET patients will be relevant to patients with PV. This assumption has not been tested in a randomized clinical trial. Anagrelide therapy should be reserved for patients with recent thromboses (e.g., myocardial infarction, stroke, migraines, erythromelalgia) and with thrombocytosis that cannot be controlled with INF or hydroxyurea therapy alone. It can also be used in combination with hydroxyurea to minimize adverse events that accompany the use of each drug alone. Anagrelide should not be used in pregnant patients because it can easily cross the placenta, leading to adverse effects on the platelet count of the fetus.

Approximately 15% to 20% of patients treated with anagrelide discontinue the medication because of nonmyelosuppressive side effects. The spectrum of adverse effects involved neurologic (headaches and dizziness), cardiac (vasodilatation, fluid retention, congestive heart failure, palpitations, and tachycardia), and gastrointestinal (nausea) toxicities. These toxicities reflect the novel mechanism of action of anagrelide as a cyclic nucleotide phosphodiesterase inhibitor. Anagrelide should be used with caution in patients with known or suspected cardiac disease because of its ability to promote fluid retention. Because many patients with PV are elderly, careful attention to fluid status should be maintained to avoid slipping into congestive heart failure after the initiation of anagrelide.

Interferon-α therapy has been explored for several decades for the treatment of PV patients, but its positive effects have been more greatly appreciated during the past 5 to 7 years.[29] Its effects on myeloid malignancies are likely the consequence of its broad range of biologic activities, including direct effects on malignant cells, enhancement of antitumor immune responses, induction of proapoptotic genes, inhibition of angiogenesis, and promotion of the cycling of dormant malignant stem cells. Because of the recent development of "targeted" therapies, the use of IFN has been dramatically reduced over the past decade. The increasing awareness of the multistep pathogenesis of many malignancies has suggested, however, that such an approach using target-specific agents is not universally effective. This awareness provided the rationale for the use of an agent such as INF-α that might be especially useful for the treatment of a disease in which multiple genetic, epigenetic and environmental factors contribute to its origin and progression. INF-α promotes apoptosis of a variety of tumor cell types. The induction of apoptosis by INF-α involves the activation of a number of INF-stimulated genes that mediate this response. Gene expression studies have identified more than 15 INF stimulated genes with proapoptotic functions. Although these INF-stimulated genes alone are probably not sufficient to induce apoptosis, their cumulative effects likely result in apoptosis. These mediators of apoptosis include caspase 4, caspase 8, TNF-related apoptosis-inducing ligand (TRAIL), Fas/CD95, the X-linked inhibitor of apoptosis (XIAP), death-activating protein kinases, INF regulatory factors, dsRNA-activated protein kinase, and *PML* (acute promyelocytic leukemia gene). The induction of caspase 8 and caspase 4 by INF may sensitize tumor cells to death receptor (TRAIL and Fas L)–mediated apoptosis. The ability of INF to induce apoptosis is independent of cell-cycle arrest, the presence of wild-type p53, or expression of Bcl-2 family members but appears to always involve the FAS-associated death domain (FADD)/caspase 8 signaling, activation of the caspase cascade, which leads to disruption of mitochondrial potential and eventual DNA fragmentation. Conflicting evidence exists as to the role that STAT1 and STAT2 play in INF-induced apoptosis. It appears most likely that the PI3K and JAK–STAT pathways act independently of each other in mediating INF-α–induced apoptosis and that the particular pathway operating is dependent on the target cell type. Several of these pathways may actually act together to contribute to IFN-α–induced apoptosis of tumor cells. Type 1 IFNs suppress the ability of normal human HPCs to proliferate in vitro in the presence of cytokine combinations. IFN-α acts directly against HPCs; this inhibitory activity has been documented using $CD34^+$ cell populations. This inhibitory role of IFN-α has been shown to synergize with the inhibitory activities of IFN-γ, which is likely produced by BM auxiliary cells in response to IFN-α. PV $CD34^+$ cells are more sensitive to the inhibitory effects of IFN-α than normal HPCs. The myelosuppressive effects of IFN-α can also be partly attributed to the inhibition of the paracrine production of several stimulatory hematopoietic growth factors, including GM-CSF and IL-11, and inhibition of the production of IL-1 receptor antagonist by BM stromal cells. INF-α therapy of hepatitis patients is frequently complicated by dose-limiting thrombocytopenia. This has led to a more careful examination of the effects of INF-α on normal megakaryocyte development. This cytokine directly inhibits megakaryocyte HPC proliferation and differentiation by blunting the JAK–STAT signaling responses that occur in response to TPO and impairs TPO-induced intracellular signaling by upregulating SOCS-1 expression. INF-α reduces TPO-induced activation of MPL, as well as phosphorylation of JAK2, JAK3, and STAT5. Furthermore, INF-α directly inhibits cytoplasmic maturation and platelet production by megakaryocytes but not the proliferation of megakaryocyte progenitor cells or endomitosis of human megakaryocytes.

The ability of type 1 INFs to inhibit HPC proliferation and maturation has been documented to occur independently of the STAT pathway. Type 1 INFs activate the p38 MAPK, a proline-directed serine/threonine kinase that is required for INF-stimulated gene transcription through interferon sensitive response element (IRSE). The pharmacologic blockade of p38 in IFN-treated PV HPCs reverses the inhibitory effects of INF-α. The inhibitory activities of type 1 INF against normal and malignant HPCs involve several additional downstream signaling pathways, including the Crkl adaptor protein, the MAPK-interacting kinase 1 (Mnk), a MAPK-regulated kinase that phosphorylates the eukaryotic initiation factor 4e, and the Schlafen family of proteins that includes several members that regulate cell-cycle progression and growth arrest. The relative contribution of each of these pathways to the antiproliferative effects of INF-α on HPCs requires further investigation. P38 MAP kinase activation by INF-α has been reported to promote apoptosis of PV $CD34^+$ cells. Activation of p38 MAP kinase results in mitochondrial translocation of the proapoptotic protein Bax, leading to the induction of apoptosis.

Interferon has also been shown to be able to affect HSC behavior. High levels of INF-α induce murine HSCs to exit from a normally quiescent state and to transiently proliferate. In these studies, the HSC proliferative response was not observed in HSCs that lacked the INF receptor or STAT1. However, HSCs that lacked the INF receptor did respond to INF-α if they were mixed with wild-type cells, suggesting that other cytokines such as INF-γ that are elaborated by BM auxiliary cells may be responsible for this biologic activity. In support of this hypothesis is the recent report that IFN-γ is also capable of inducing HSC cycling. The effect of IFNs on HSC cycling appears to occur by a pathway that is distinct from the pathway which mediates their antiproliferative effect on HPC. STAT1 is required for the IFN-α–mediated exit of HSC from dormancy, suggesting that this effect is mediated by canonical type 1 IFN signaling. It remains uncertain whether human HSCs respond in a similar fashion to IFN-α, and clonal stem cells from MPN patients cycle at a higher rate than the small reservoir of normal HSCs that persist in such patients.

In the United States, the pioneering study of Silver[30] in 1988 documented the clinical effectiveness of IFN-α in controlling erythrocytosis as well as pruritus and other constitutional symptoms in PV patients, and Austrian and French groups reported during the same period evidence that IFN-α was also effective in reducing thrombocytosis in ET patients. A number of clinical trials have been performed subsequently using several different commercial preparations of IFN. Recent reviews of the literature found more than 400 PV and ET patients who participated in clinical trials. A meta-analysis of these studies has proven problematic. First, various forms of IFN were used, and one cannot exclude the possibility that each of these preparations of IFN might have different effects that might influence response rates or disease evolution. Furthermore, heterogeneous response criteria were used to evaluate efficacy. The recently proposed response criteria for use in MPNs clinical trials provided by the European LeukemiaNet might be helpful to avoid such a dilemma in the future. In almost all PV and ET trials, IFN-α therapy rapidly normalized platelet numbers and corrected the degree of leukocytosis and erythrocytosis, allowing reduction in the requirement for phlebotomies within a few months. In both diseases, an objective hematologic response was observed in about 80% of patients, including complete freedom from phlebotomies in PV in 60% of patients. In addition, IFN-α was also able to reduce PV-associated pruritus in a significant number of patients and appears to be an effective drug for this purpose. However, toxicity associated with IFN-α therapy was not trivial, leading to the discontinuation of treatment in almost 25% of patients. A pegylated form of INF has been used with increasing frequency to treat patients with a variety of MPNs with great success. This form of INF can be administered once weekly, and its use is associated with a more favorable toxicity profile. Several phase 2 studies using peg-IFNα-2a in PV and ET showed similarly impressive hematologic response rates compared with standard IFN-α but with less associated toxicity (<10% of patients discontinued therapy during the first year of therapy). In addition, these studies showed for the first time evidence of significant molecular responses as documented by a clear reduction in the JAK2V617F allele burden after IFN-α treatment.[30] A specific effect of IFN-α against the MPN clone had previously been suggested by occasional studies showing reversion from monoclonal to polyclonal patterns of hematopoiesis (based on X chromosome inactivation pattern studies) or disappearance of a marker chromosomal abnormality present before treatment. The discovery of the JAK2V617F mutation provides a tool with which to measure molecular response to a variety of therapeutic approaches in MPN, an end point not available before the discovery of this mutation in 2005. Overall, the two clinical trials with peg-IFNα-2a showed a meaningful and progressive reduction in the JAK2V617F allele burden in about 70% of PV and 40% of ET patients. Importantly, the JAK2V617F mutation became undetectable (with 1% sensitivity PCR assays) in 24% of PV patients in the French "PVN-1" study after about 3 years' median follow-up, and in 14% and 6% of PV and ET patients, respectively, in the U.S. study after about 2 years' median follow-up. Combining both studies, 12 of 64 (19%) PV patients achieved a molecular complete response (MCR). Of note, each of these MCRs occurred after the 12th month of treatment, but hematologic responses occurred within a few weeks. Prolonged exposure (>12 months) to peg-IFNα-2a seems to be an important factor in achieving MCR. The reduction in the JAK2V617F allele burden was not influenced by the cumulative dose of peg-IFNα-2a in the PVN-1 study, but toxicity was clearly dose dependent in the U.S. study. Taken together, these results indicate that peg-IFNα-2a therapy is best initiated at very low doses that are gradually increased until hematologic response is achieved; this strategy avoids cessation of therapy and allows sufficient exposure to the drug to allow for the achievement of a molecular response. These results are in agreement with studies from Denmark, showing major molecular responses in PV after long-term treatment with IFNα-2b that could persist after IFN-α was discontinued. Finally, five of seven patients who achieved MCR in the PVN-1 study have maintained this response after peg-IFNα-2a was discontinued (≤30 months after discontinuation), with none experiencing hematologic relapse. Such long-term clinical and molecular responses after the discontinuation of treatment have previously been reported after IFN-α therapy in MPN patients, an effect that has not been reported with other currently available therapies. It is important to emphasize that the elimination of JAK2V617F in this setting is not necessarily indicative of cure of the MPN and that clinical implications of these molecular responses remain uncertain and require validation. It has been shown that molecular relapse can rapidly occur after IFN-α discontinuation in some cases. In one patient with a biclonal JAK2V617F/TET2-mutated PV, peg-IFNα-2a treatment did not affect the TET2-mutated cells, but the JAK2V617F clone was eradicated. Nevertheless, prolonged periods of time (≤40 months, personal unpublished data) during which the patient remained in complete hematologic remission without any cytoreductive therapy after peg-IFNα-2a withdrawal was observed in several patients of the PVN-1 study even though low levels of the JAK2V617F allele (≈5%) were still detected. Such results suggests that despite the disease not being eradicated, long-term exposure to peg-IFNα-2a was sufficient to modify the clinical expression of the MPN for a sustained period of time.

In addition to clinical, hematologic, and MCRs achieved in a significant proportion of PV and ET patients, IFN-α therapy has also been shown recently to reverse BM histopathologic abnormalities in selected cases of both PV and PMF. Thus IFN-α seems to be the uniquely available drug able to induce complete resolution of all clinical, biologic, and morphologic abnormalities in selected MPN patients, raising the hope that a curative outcome might be possible in a subset of such patients. These observations lead one to question the validity of the current therapeutic strategies for PV and ET patients in which myelosuppressive therapy is exclusively used in subpopulations of patients at high risk for developing additional thrombotic events. If IFN-α is shown in a large prospective trial to eliminate clinical, histologic, cytogenetic, and molecular evidence of disease with acceptable toxicity, one might also consider early treatment of low-risk patients when the tumor burden is still low.

Intolerance to therapy with INF-α leads to drug withdrawal in 14% of patients. INF is not a leukemogenic drug but it is not an innocuous agent, necessitating careful follow-up of patients receiving such treatment. Initially, all patients experience flulike symptoms, which are controllable with acetaminophen or aspirin. Such symptoms usually resolve spontaneously after several months of therapy. More serious side effects, including excessive suppression of blood counts, irritability, high fevers, severe asthenia, reversible lower extremity bilateral neuritis, retinopathy, hypothyroidism, depression, sarcoidosis and left-sided heart failure, may require cessation of INF-α therapy. Exacerbation of the depression is a serious side effect of INF and should be considered as a rationale for denying patients this treatment option unless unusual circumstances exist. The role of pegylated INF therapy versus hydroxyurea therapy will be defined only after the performance of a randomized phase III trial in newly diagnosed high-risk ET and PV patients.

The use of small molecule inhibitors of JAK2 for the treatment of advanced forms of MF has recently received approval by regulatory agencies in the United States and likely will in the near future in Europe. The use of ruxolitinib or other JAK2 inhibitors in PV patients has been exclusively explored in patients who are resistant or intolerant to hydroxyurea. These agents appear capable of reducing hematocrit levels, reducing the need for phlebotomy, and reducing the degree of splenomegaly, but have not been associated with dramatic changes in histopathologic abnormalities, platelet numbers, WBC numbers, JAK2V617 allele burden, or elimination of cytogenetic abnormalities. These drugs both in PV and PMF have a remarkable effect on reducing the severity of intractable pruritus that not infrequently affects PV patients. Indiscriminate use of such JAK2 inhibitors in PV patients is discouraged. Patients considering such options should be entered on clinical trials that are constructed to assess their role in the treatment of PV. Symptomatic management of the PV patient may be complicated by the occurrence of intractable pruritus. Normally, the pruritus occurs on exposure to sudden body cooling, especially after a warm bath, and is experienced by as many as 40% to 60% of patients treated with phlebotomy. Aquagenic pruritus is not unique to PV, and in one series of patients presenting to a dermatology clinic, 31% had PV, but in the remainder, an underlying hematologic malignancy could not be detected. Aquagenic pruritus in MPN patients and in patients without an associated malignancy was associated with lactose intolerance. In some instances, multiple family members are affected, suggesting that genetic factors might predispose individuals to this symptom. In some studies, basophils and mast cells have been shown to be involved by JAK2V617F in patients with aquagenic pruritus and PV, likely leading to the elaboration of mediators that lead to itching. The frequency of pruritus appears to be somewhat lower in patients treated with myelosuppressive agents. This observation is related to the probable relation between pruritus and degranulation of tissue mast cells and circulating basophils. Some uncontrolled studies have attributed pruritus to hyperhistaminemia or severe iron deficiency, with relief associated with the use of histamine antagonists or ferrous sulfate. Iron replacement is frequently not possible because it can lead to dangerous elevations of the RBC mass. In a number of instances, however, iron replacement has been possible with disease control with INF-α. The association between pruritus and tissue infiltration by mast cells would appear to explain the response of occasional patients to photochemotherapy with psoralens and ultraviolet irradiation. At present, INF therapy for pruritus appears to be extremely useful. In addition, 80% of patients with pruritus have been reported to respond to paroxetine or fluoxetine, selective serotonin uptake inhibitors. Other effective options include anticonvulsant drugs such as pregabalin. As mentioned, the JAK2 inhibitors are extremely effective in relieving the pruritus associated with PV, but in occasional patients, this effect, unfortunately, is not sustained.

Budd-Chiari syndrome is a catastrophic illness that can lead to significant morbidity and mortality in a patient with PV. Patients with MPN are at a high risk of developing this syndrome. Independently, the use of oral contraceptive pills and congenital and acquired thrombophilic factors are involved in its development. A number of cases of hepatic vein thrombosis have been reported in nonpolycythemic women taking oral contraceptives. Although no data are available, one must be concerned about the use of oral contraceptives in women with PV.

The optimal approach to the problem of Budd-Chiari syndrome is obviously preventive and involves maintenance of normal blood values in the patient with PV. When the Budd-Chiari syndrome develops, the prognosis without treatment is dismal. The goals of therapy are to prevent further propagation of thrombus, relieve the intense hepatic congestion, and manage the severe ascites that often plague these patients. If untreated, these patients often have a slowly progressive course, with deterioration and death occurring within 3.5 years. Spontaneous resolution of the hepatic vein occlusion rarely occurs. Diuretics may be of value in the treatment of the ascites but do not affect the long-term outcome. Thrombolytic therapy within 24 hours of onset of diagnosis with urokinase (240,000 units/hr for 2 hours followed by 60,000 units/hr) or tissue plasminogen activator (0.5-1.0 mg/hr) directly infused into the thrombosed hepatic vein for 24 hours results occasionally in success. Even if therapy is delayed for 2 to 3 weeks, a favorable outcome can be achieved in some instances with thrombolytic therapy. Such therapy is not innocuous because bleeding can complicate the course of therapy. Angioplasty of localized segments of the hepatic vein can result in the relief of symptoms in the majority of patients, but the risk of restenosis is high. Anticoagulant therapy with Coumadin may have a role in the prevention of further clot formation, but there has been no definitive evidence that such therapy promotes resolution of established thromboses. Several newer anticoagulants that act by direct thrombin or factor Xa inhibition have no natural antidote and are being increasingly used for various prophylactic and therapeutic indications. As such, these new anticoagulants will inevitably pose major challenges in the treatment of MPN patients who are at high risk of bleeding. Indiscriminate use of such anticoagulants before considering the downsides of their lack of reversibility in a group of patients at such a high risk of hemorrhage is likely not prudent and will require further careful study.

The clinical deterioration of patients with Budd-Chiari syndrome results from damage to the hepatocytes from necrosis associated with marked elevation in sinusoidal pressure coupled with ischemia from reduced hepatic arteriole perfusion. The only rational therapeutic intervention, therefore, involves some sort of portal vein decompression to achieve an effective reduction of sinusoidal pressure. A variety of surgical procedures resulting in portal-splenic decompression have been shown to be of value in patients with Budd-Chiari syndrome. Transjugular intrahepatic portosystemic shunt (TIPS) placement has been used as a bridge to liver transplantation. Recent technical advances in the procedure and the introduction of specially coated stents have greatly improved the frequency of shunt patency, sometimes avoiding the need for liver transplantation. The indications for TIPS include recurrent variceal bleeding and refractory ascites. Surgical portosystemic shunts may reverse hepatic necrosis and prevent cirrhosis. The 5-year survival rate after surgical shunts ranges from 75% to 94%. Liver transplantation is a potential option for treatment of those patients with continued hepatic decompensation. The indications for liver transplantation are cirrhosis, fulminant hepatic failure, and failure of a portosystemic shunt. The overall actuarial survival at 1 year was 76% and was 68% at 10 years. Because PV is a slowly progressive disease, transplantation should not be withheld from these patients. Pretransplant predictors of mortality based on a multivariable analysis were impaired renal function and a history of a shunt. The hematologic consequences of polycythemia must be aggressively treated in the posttransplantation setting; the hepatic vein occlusion may reoccur in the transplanted liver.

Therapy of cerebral vein thrombosis and sinuses includes anticoagulation with heparin to arrest the thrombotic process and to prevent pulmonary embolism. Low-molecular-weight heparin (LMWH) should be started as soon as the diagnosis is confirmed even in the presence of hemorrhagic infarcts. After the acute phase, oral anticoagulants are given for 6 months after a first episode or longer if the MPN is not well controlled. There is currently no available evidence from randomized clinical trials regarding the efficacy or safety of thrombolytic therapy.

The performance of any surgical procedures on patients with PV is, as previously discussed, accompanied by excessively high morbidity and mortality. Elective surgery should not be contemplated unless the patient's hematologic values have been normalized for several months. The longer the hematologic control has been in effect, the lower the incidence of postoperative complications. If emergency surgery is required, the patient should be phlebotomized rapidly until a normal hematocrit is reached, and platelets should be available in case excessive perioperative or postoperative bleeding occurs. After emergency or elective surgery, the patient should be mobilized as soon as possible, and strong consideration should be given to anticoagulation with LMWH unless the patient has some contraindication. Dental extractions can also result in excessive hemorrhage and should not be performed unless the patient is under strict hematologic control.

Perhaps the most difficult and frustrating period encountered during the clinical course of a patient with PV is the development of post-PV MF. The origins, manifestations, and management options are discussed in detail in Chapter 69.

Limited information is available concerning the treatment of patients who develop acute leukemia after PV. The overwhelming majority of such cases involve myeloid leukemias. The leukemia is frequently preceded by post-PV MF but not always. Patients with post-PV MF and acute leukemia frequently have greater than 20% blasts in the peripheral blood but far fewer blast cells in the BM, which has led to a hypothesis that the leukemia is originating from an extramedullary site, particularly the spleen. These cases tend to have a more indolent course, but patients with a greater degree of BM infiltration have a more highly proliferative form of leukemia that is associated with an even more aggressive course. The optimal treatment of such patients is unknown. In elderly adults with significant comorbidities, the choice not to institute chemotherapy is a reasonable option. These patients are frequently elderly, and poor results with standard regimens have been reported. Patients rarely achieve a complete remission but rather return to a clinical condition that resembles their original MPN for limited periods of time. In a retrospective analysis on 23 patients with leukemic transformation of PV, the median patient age was 68 years, and leukemia developed a median of 12.8 years from the diagnosis of PV. Twelve of the 14 patients in whom cytogenetic analyses were performed had complex cytogenetic abnormalities associated with high-risk leukemias. Fifteen patients were treated with palliative measures and had a median survival of 2.5 months. Of the eight patients treated with standard induction therapy, one obtained a complete remission, and seven died without obtaining a response. The median survival time of these chemotherapy-treated patients was 5.6 months. The median survival time of the entire cohort of 23 patients was 2.9 months. This poor outcome is likely the result of clinical and biologic features of the acute leukemia, advanced patient age, unfavorable cytogenetics, and patient comorbidities associated with advanced age. Selected patients are likely to tolerate and to have a favorable outcome with allogeneic stem cell transplantation and reduced intensity conditioning. In fact, the only long-term survival with post-PV leukemia has been observed in patients receiving allogeneic stem cell transplantation. Whether the patients should receive some form of induction chemotherapy before receiving conditioning therapy for preparation of the transplant or proceed directly to transplant is a decision that varies from patient to patient and from center to center. Most patients with PV-related acute leukemia should be considered candidates for experimental therapeutic strategies. Recently, promising results with the use of DNA hypomethylating agents such as decitabine or azacitidine have been reported with 50% to 60% of patients achieving clinically significant responses persisting for 6 to 24 months in the majority of cases. These chemotherapeutic regimens can frequently be administered as an outpatient but require treatment for at least six monthly cycles before clinical responses can be evaluated. Although many of these patients do not achieve true complete remissions (CRs), their prolonged survival and quality of life, at least based upon single-institutional studies, appears to be superior to that achieved with standard induction chemotherapy. Rare clinical responses have also been reported with the use of the oral JAK2 inhibitor bruxolitinib. The use of hypomethylating agents, JAK2 inhibitors, or both is now being explored as bridging therapies before patients receive allogeneic transplants.

Polycythemia vera occurs frequently during the childbearing years. A discussion of contraception options is imperative because the use of oral contraceptive pills may be associated with an increased risk of deep venous thrombosis as well as splanchnic vein thrombosis. It seems prudent to entertain alternative forms of contraception with such individuals. Discontinuation of hydroxyurea in both men and women desiring to have a child are recommended. Hydroxyurea is capable of inducing azoospermia in men, frequently limiting their ability to father a child. Pregnancy is itself a prothrombotic condition. PV in a pregnant individual has been reported to lead to an increased incidence of fetal wastage, with 30% of pregnancies in PV patients terminating in spontaneous abortions. In addition, preeclampsia occurs more frequently in these women. A team approach requiring close communication between an obstetrician skilled in providing care for high-risk pregnancies and the responsible hematologist provides the optimal integration of care to the mother and the child. Pregnancy in PV patients is frequently associated with a gradual normalization of blood values, and it is not unusual for a woman who has required extensive therapy for control of her disease to no longer require phlebotomies during pregnancy. Delivery appears not to be complicated by excessive hemorrhage, but the postpartum period carries an increased risk of venous thrombosis. Although some degree of hematocrit level normalization can be explained by expansion of the plasma volume or by nutritional deficiencies that occur during pregnancy, it is unlikely that these factors can be solely responsible. It seems more reasonable to assume that the high estrogen levels characteristic of pregnancy suppress erythropoiesis. After completion of the pregnancies, the patients' hematologic values slowly drift back to their previously elevated values in parallel with the return to normal estrogen levels. Because pregnancy is usually associated with spontaneous control of the polycythemic state, no specific therapy is required except for careful observation. If needed, therapy should be limited to phlebotomy and low-dose aspirin therapy because of the mutagenic effects of chemotherapeutic agents. Aggressive treatment of hypertension is imperative, as well as attention to the risk of developing preeclampsia and toxemia, which should be treated in a standard fashion. In individuals with a history of repeated spontaneous abortions associated with placental infarction, consideration should be given to low-dose aspirin with LMWH therapy, making sure that these agents are discontinued at the time of delivery to avoid the risk of excessive hemorrhage. If this approach is not successful, INF therapy is suggested because it is not known to be leukemogenic or teratogenic and does not cross the placenta. In the puerperium, thromboprophylaxis with 6 weeks of LMWH therapy is recommended. Aggressive intervention with hematocrit levels maintained below 45% and aspirin therapy with LMWH is associated with a positive outcome for the pregnancy. Breastfeeding is recommended if the mother is receiving therapy with heparin or Coumadin as long as the baby receives adequate supplementation with vitamin K. Rapid mobilization of the mother after delivery is of great importance.

Because PV is ultimately a stem cell disorder, it should be possible to achieve a cure with stem cell transplantation. Thus far, the majority of patients undergoing allogeneic stem cell transplantation have been relatively young (<50 years of age) and have been transplanted after evolution to MF, MDS, or acute leukemia. Transplantation during the polycythemia phase of the disease is rarely appropriate.

FUTURE DIRECTIONS

The discovery of JAK2V617F mutations has led to a more comprehensive understanding of the pathophysiology of the MPNs, including PV. There is no question that the diagnostic tests for JAK2V617F and exon 12 mutations of JAK2, as well as mutations in HIF-1, HIF-2, the EPO receptor, and PHD have revolutionized the diagnostic approach to patients with erythrocytosis. Continued efforts are clearly needed to identify the so-called pre-JAK2V617 mutation and to assess its effects on stem cells. PV is a stem cell disease that will ultimately require curative therapies at a minimum to reduce the numbers or at best to eliminate malignant stem cells if curative small molecule therapies are to become a reality. Before the JAK2V617F allele burden is used as a biomarker for outcomes of novel therapeutic approaches to treat patients with PV, studies are needed to determine the extent of reduction of allele burden that would be predictive of altering the natural history of PV and eliminating complications from thrombotic episodes or evolution to MF or acute leukemia. The use of drugs affecting only JAK2 are unlikely to be curative because multiple genetic and epigenetic events likely contribute to the origins and progression of PV. Randomized clinical trials of combinations of drugs, rather than single drugs, and comparing these outcomes with the standard of care are more likely to lead to significant advances in improving the natural history of PV patients.

REFERENCES

1. Gonzalez C, Agapito MT, Rocher A, et al: A revisit to O2 sensing and transduction in the carotid body chemoreceptors in the context of reactive oxygen species biology. *Respir Physiol Neurobiol* 174:317, 2010.
2. Lee FS, Percy MJ: The HIF pathway and erythrocytosis. *Annu Rev Pathol* 6:165, 2011.
3. McMullin MF: HIF pathway mutations and erythrocytosis. *Expert Rev Hematol* 3:93, 2010.
4. Huang LJ, Shen YM, Bulut GB: Advances in understanding the pathogenesis of primary familial and congenital polycythaemia. *Br J Haematol* 148:844, 2010.
5. Spence MS, Balaratnam MS, Gatzoulis MA: Clinical update: Cyanotic adult congenital heart disease. *Lancet* 370:1530, 2007.
6. Wang B, Zhang YB, Zhang F, et al: On the origin of Tibetans and their genetic basis in adapting high-altitude environments. *PLoS One* 6:e17002, 2011.
7. van Patot MC, Gassmann M: Hypoxia: Adapting to high altitude by mutating EPAS-1, the gene encoding HIF-2alpha. *High Alt Med Biol* 12:157, 2011.
8. Wiesener MS, Seyfarth M, Warnecke C, et al: Paraneoplastic erythrocytosis associated with an inactivating point mutation of the von Hippel-Lindau gene in a renal cell carcinoma. *Blood* 99:3562, 2002.
9. Lee FS: Genetic causes of erythrocytosis and the oxygen-sensing pathway. *Blood Rev* 22:321, 2008.
10. Albiero E, Ruggeri M, Fortuna S, et al: Isolated erythrocytosis: Study of 67 patients and identification of three novel germ-line mutations in the prolyl hydroxylase domain protein 2 (PHD2) gene. *Haematologica* 97:123, 2012.
11. Nielsen C, Birgens HS, Nordestgaard BG, et al: The JAK2 V617F somatic mutation, mortality and cancer risk in the general population. *Haematologica* 96:450, 2011.

12. Landgren O, Goldin LR, Kristinsson SY, et al: Increased risks of polycythemia vera, essential thrombocythemia, and myelofibrosis among 24,577 first-degree relatives of 11,039 patients with myeloproliferative neoplasms in Sweden. *Blood* 112:2199, 2008.
13. James C, Ugo V, Le Couédic JP, et al: A unique clonal JAK2 mutation leading to constitutive signalling causes polycythaemia vera. *Nature* 434:1144, 2005.
14. Kralovics R, Passamonti F, Buser AS, et al: A gain-of-function mutation of JAK2 in myeloproliferative disorders. *N Engl J Med* 352:1779, 2005.
15. Nussenzveig RH, Swierczek SI, Jelinek J, et al: Polycythemia vera is not initiated by JAK2V617F mutation. *Exp Hematol* 35:32, 2007.
16. Jones AV, Chase A, Silver RT, et al: JAK2 haplotype is a major risk factor for the development of myeloproliferative neoplasms. *Nat Genet* 41:446, 2009.
17. Jamieson CH, Gotlib J, Durocher JA, et al: The JAK2 V617F mutation occurs in hematopoietic stem cells in polycythemia vera and predisposes toward erythroid differentiation. *Proc Natl Acad Sci U S A* 103:6224, 2006.
18. Vainchenker W, Delhommeau F, Constantinescu SN, et al: New mutations and pathogenesis of myeloproliferative neoplasms. *Blood* 118:1723, 2011.
19. Kota J, Caceres N, Constantinescu SN: Aberrant signal transduction pathways in myeloproliferative neoplasms. *Leukemia* 22:1828, 2008.
20. Landolfi R, Marchioli R, Kutti J, et al: Efficacy and safety of low-dose aspirin in polycythemia vera. *N Engl J Med* 350:114, 2004.
21. Landolfi R, Di Gennaro L, Falanga A: Thrombosis in myeloproliferative disorders: Pathogenetic facts and speculation. *Leukemia* 22:2020, 2008.
22. Kiladjian JJ, Chevret S, Dosquet C, et al: Treatment of polycythemia vera with hydroxyurea and pipobroman: Final results of a randomized trial initiated in 1980. *J Clin Oncol* 29:3907, 2011.
23. Kiladjian JJ, Cervantes F, Leebeek FW, et al: The impact of JAK2 and MPL mutations on diagnosis and prognosis of splanchnic vein thrombosis: A report on 241 cases. *Blood* 111:4922, 2008.
24. Najfeld V, Montella L, Scalise A, et al: Exploring polycythaemia vera with fluorescence in situ hybridization: Additional cryptic 9p is the most frequent abnormality detected. *Br J Haematol* 119:558, 2002.
25. Campbell PJ, Scott LM, Buck G, for the United Kingdom Myeloproliferative Disorders Study Group, Medical Research Council Adult Leukaemia Working Party, and the Australasian Leukaemia and Lymphoma Group, et al: Definition of subtypes of essential thrombocythaemia and relation to polycythaemia vera based on JAK2 V617F mutation status: A prospective study. *Lancet* 366:1945, 2005.
26. Squizzato A, Romualdi E, Middeldorp S: Antiplatelet drugs for polycythaemia vera and essential thrombocythaemia. *Cochrane Database Syst Rev* CD006503, 2008.
27. Björkholm M, Derolf AR, Hultcrantz M, et al: Treatment-related risk factors for transformation to acute myeloid leukemia and myelodysplastic syndromes in myeloproliferative neoplasms. *J Clin Oncol* 29:2410, 2011.
28. Soutou B, Aractingi S: Myeloproliferative disorder therapy: Assessment and management of adverse events: A dermatologist's perspective. *Hematol Oncol* 27:11, 2009.
29. Kiladjian JJ, Mesa RA, Hoffman R: The renaissance of interferon therapy for the treatment of myeloid malignancies. *Blood* 117:4706, 2011.
30. Silver RT: Recombinant interferon-alpha for treatment of Polycythemia Vera. *Lancet* 1:403, 1988.

CHAPTER 68

ESSENTIAL THROMBOCYTHEMIA

Ronald Hoffman, Marina Kremyanskaya, Vesna Najfeld, and John Mascarenhas

Essential thrombocythemia (ET) is a chronic myeloproliferative neoplasm (MPN) characterized by platelet counts in excess of 450 × 109/L, profound bone marrow (BM) megakaryocyte hyperplasia, leukocytosis, splenomegaly, a clinical course punctuated by hemorrhagic or thrombotic episodes, and possible evolution to myelofibrosis (MF) and acute leukemia. ET is a clinically heterogeneous disorder with more than half of patients meeting the criteria for diagnosis being asymptomatic at presentation. ET was first described in 1934 by Epstein and Goedel, who described a patient with an elevated platelet count who had repeated hemorrhagic episodes.

Originally, many clinical investigators questioned whether ET represented a distinct clinical entity. However, extensive descriptions of larger numbers of patients have provided information to dispute this initial skepticism. In 1951, Dameshek speculated that ET might represent one of the myeloproliferative disorders that are now recognized to be hematologic malignancies. Recent investigations have confirmed this concept and clearly demonstrated that the disorder is typically a clonal hematologic malignancy. Many patients, however, meet the criteria for the diagnosis of ET but have polyclonal hematopoiesis.

In 2005, a breakthrough in our understanding of the pathogenesis and management of ET was made with the discovery of the *JAK2V617F* mutation in the majority of patients with chronic MPN. This finding has had a major impact on the classification of and diagnostic approaches to the MPNs as well as creating drug development strategies based on our increasing understanding of their molecular pathogenesis.

EPIDEMIOLOGY

The true incidence of ET is unknown because extensive epidemiologic studies are not available. Although many investigators have indicated that this disorder is very rare, information from several institutions suggests that it occurs considerably more frequently than originally believed. After the incorporation of a platelet channel in automated complete blood cell counts, extreme thrombocytosis has been shown to be a relatively common occurrence in a general hospital setting. The incidence of ET has been reported to be approximately 1.5 to 2.4 patients per 100,000 population annually. Interestingly, a significant increase in the annual incidence rate of ET from 0.69 to 4.35 patients per 100,000 inhabitants through the years 1983 to 1999 was observed in the city of Goteborg, Sweden. This trend was not observed for polycythemia vera (PV) and was most likely attributable to the standard use of automated blood cell counters over the past few decades and likely will in the future be further accentuated by the recent use of a lower threshold platelet count for diagnosis, the availability of *JAK2V617F* testing, and the implementation of World Health Organization's diagnostic criteria. ET and PV have been reported to have an approximately 1 : 1 relative incidence, although a recent epidemiologic study in Sweden indicated that PV was more than twice as common as ET. The Swedish study also indicated that first-degree relatives of patients with an MPN, including ET, had a five- to sevenfold increased risk of developing an MPN, supporting the concept that there are common, strong, shared susceptibility genes that predispose individuals to develop one of the MPNs.[1] The Janus kinase 2 *(JAK2)* mutation has been shown not to be acquired randomly but instead to arise preferentially on a specific *JAK2* haplotype (46/1). The *JAK2* 46/1 haplotype has been shown not only to predispose to *JAK2V617F* positive ET but also to cases of ET with mutations of the thrombopoietin receptor and, surprisingly, to ET not associated with such acquired mutations, again indicating genetic factors playing a role in the susceptibility to developing ET. Recently, the risk of developing ET was shown to be higher in carriers of constitutional *CHEK2* gene mutations.[2] *CHEK2* is a tumor suppressor gene that protects cells from excessive proliferation by regulating cell division. Germline *CHEK2* mutations have been also associated with Li-Fraumeni syndrome, some lymphoid and solid tumors malignancies, and myeloid malignancies. The manner by which germline *CHEK2* mutations might contribute to the development of ET remains the subject of speculation, but it is most closely associated with onset at a young age.

Based on population studies, the disorder appears to occur in individuals with a median age of 67 to 73 years, but in single-institution studies, the median age at diagnosis has been reported to be lower (50-57 years). In most series, there appears to be no gender predilection; although in several reports, a higher prevalence in women has been noted. This discrepancy might be due to an equal frequency in older patients of both sexes but to a second peak frequency at around 30 years of age for women.

Cases of ET have been reported in patients in the pediatric age group, but this is an unusual occurrence. A review of the literature cannot accurately determine the risk of thrombosis or bleeding of ET in childhood, but the clinical course is not entirely benign. The incidence of ET in childhood has been reported to be approximately 1 per 10^7 population, which is 60 times lower than that in adults. Approximately 30% of children with this disorder experience thrombotic or hemorrhagic complications at diagnosis or later in their course, and 50% have splenomegaly. Interestingly, in a recent study, only 20% of pediatric patients with ET, compared with 45% of adult ET patients, had clonal hematopoiesis, and 20% were *JAK2V617F* positive compared with 60% of adult patients.

Several families with multiple members having ET have been described. The prevalence of the *JAK2V617F* mutation in familial cases of MPN has been analyzed in 72 families, including 174 patients (68 with ET). The *JAK2* mutation was found in half of patients with ET, a similar proportion as observed in sporadic, nonfamilial cases. Among 46 families with at least two cases of PV, ET, or primary MF (PMF), the *JAK2* mutation was absent in six families, heterogeneously distributed in 18, and present in all patients with MPN in 22. Thus the *JAK2* mutation does not seem to be required for the development of ET or other MPNs, and this familial clustering cannot be accounted for by the prevalence of *JAK2* 46/1 haplotype.

PATHOBIOLOGY

Greater insights into the mechanisms leading to thrombocytosis in ET have been gained. Patients with ET have normal or near-normal platelet survival. The thrombocytosis is due to increased platelet production by megakaryocytes. Effective platelet production is increased as much as 10-fold and is associated with an increase in megakaryocyte clustering, volume, nuclear lobe number, and nuclear ploidy.

ET is typically a clonal hematopoietic disorder originating at the level of the pluripotent hematopoietic stem cell. Subsequent analyses have revealed, however, that a significant proportion of nonclonally derived leukocytes exist in addition to the clonally derived population of leukocytes in patients with ET. In one study of 42 patients with ET, 31 patients exhibited clonality of at least one hematopoietic lineage, but the remaining 11 patients had polyclonal origin of all lineages studied. The biogenesis of polyclonal ET remains ill defined.[3] It is possible that small numbers of normal hematopoietic stem cells persist to account for this admixture of nonclonal populations. It has been reported by several groups that ET patients with polyclonal hematopoiesis have fewer thrombotic complications. Interestingly, in some patients, monoclonality of hematopoiesis is restricted to platelets despite the polyclonal origin of the other lineages. Other studies, however, have indicated a common origin of granulocytes, platelets, and B lymphocytes in this disorder. Such studies raise the possibility that the malignant transformation leading to ET occurs at a number of cellular stages along the hematopoietic cellular hierarchy.

The biologic behavior of megakaryocyte progenitor cells present either in the BM or in the peripheral blood of patients with ET has been extensively studied. In each of these studies, the use of serum-containing culture systems has led to the detection of increased numbers of assayable progenitors. These data support the concept that the principal abnormality is an expansion of the progenitor cell pool. In addition, colonies were noted to appear in the absence of exogenous cytokines. A second subpopulation of colony-forming unit–megakaryocyte (CFU-MK) assayed from patients with ET was also shown to remain responsive to the addition of cytokines, suggesting the presence of both an MPN clone not requiring exogenous cytokines.

Several laboratories have demonstrated that megakaryocyte progenitor cells isolated from ET patients are characterized by increased sensitivity to the action of several cytokines, including interleukin-3 (IL-3), IL-6, and thrombopoietin. Investigators have explored the possibility that the defect in ET might actually be due to resistance to inhibitors of megakaryocytopoiesis; ET CFU-MK are significantly less sensitive to the inhibitory effects of transforming growth factor-β (TGFβ) and have a limited response to the inhibitory effects of high concentrations of autologous platelet lysates. TGFβ was shown to be primarily responsible for the inhibitory activity present in such platelet lysates. Some combination of increased sensitivity to growth factors that promotes platelet production and disrupted sensitivity to negative regulators of thrombopoiesis at the level of the megakaryocyte progenitor cell or megakaryoblast likely accounts for the thrombocytosis in patients with ET.

Erythroid progenitor cells in ET can also proliferate in response to the small amounts of cytokines. Erythroid colony formation in the absence of exogenous erythropoietin is a hallmark of the proliferative defect that characterizes PV. Burst-forming unit–erythroid can be assayed from both BM and peripheral blood of patients with ET and form erythroid colonies in the absence of exogenous erythropoietin. Such an abnormality in these nonpolycythemic patients probably indicates an underlying intracellular defect shared by progenitor cells in many MPNs. Thrombopoietin is the primary physiologic regulator of thrombopoiesis. This growth factor acts by binding to its cell surface receptor, MPL. The thrombopoietin receptor is expressed by $CD34^+$ hematopoietic progenitor cells, megakaryocytes, and platelets. Normal or slightly elevated thrombopoietin levels have been observed in patients with ET. This is in contrast to erythropoietin levels in PV and ET, which are uniformly decreased. Furthermore, expression of the thrombopoietin receptor and its mRNA have been shown to be dramatically reduced in the platelets of patients with ET. A possible explanation for the diminished expression of platelet MPL and the associated thrombocytosis has been provided by the study of several animal models, which has confirmed that decreased expression of MPL in late-stage megakaryocytes and platelets concurrent with persistent expression of MPL on early megakaryocytes and progenitor cells results in thrombocytosis. Thrombopoietin serum levels are controlled by platelet mass through MPL-mediated thrombopoietin uptake and degradation. The reduced platelet MPL expression occurs not only in ET but also in PV and PMF and has been shown to be a downstream event of *JAK2V617F* and likely results in the decreased capacity of platelets to absorb thrombopoietin, resulting ultimately in an increased megakaryocyte mass and thrombocytosis.

Whereas the *JAK2V617F* mutation is present in 40% to 60% of patients with ET, gain-of-function mutations involving the thrombopoietin receptor, *MPLW515L* and *MPL515K*, are present in approximately 1% to 3% of patients with ET.[4] About 60% of patients with *MPL* mutations have the *W515L* mutation and 40% the *W515K* mutation. The mutant allele burden is greater than 50% in 50% of *W515K* patients as compared with 17% of *W515L* patients. More than 50% of patients with MPL mutant alleles are also *JAK2V617F* positive. In ET, both *JAK2V617F* and MPL mutations arise preferentially on a specific constitutional *JAK2* 46/1 haplotype. Two hypotheses have been proposed to account for this predilection: 46/1 is inherently genetically more unstable (hypermutability hypothesis) or 46/1 confers a growth advantage that favors the predominance of *JAK2V617F* hematopoiesis (fertile ground hypothesis). The association of MPL mutations with the *JAK2* 46/1 haplotype strongly favors the hypermutability hypothesis rather than the fertile ground hypothesis.

JAK2 is a cytoplasmic tyrosine kinase that plays a key role in mediating intracellular signaling from a variety of growth factors, including IL-3, erythropoietin, granulocyte macrophage colony-stimulating factor (GM-CSF), granulocyte colony-stimulating factor (G-CSF), and thrombopoietin. Coexpression of *JAK2V617F* with a homodimeric type 1 cytokine receptor (including erythropoietin, thrombopoietin, or G-CSF) is necessary for hormone activation of JAK-STAT (signal transducer and activator of transcription) signaling pathways and for hematopoietic cell proliferation to become growth factor independent. The *JAK2V617F* mutation is present in ET patients with both clonal and polyclonal hematopoiesis. Patients with clonal hematopoiesis have a higher *JAK2V617F* allele burden (26%) than patients with polyclonal hematopoiesis (16%). The relative size of the *JAK2V617F* clone is often small and remains stable over time in patients with both clonal and polyclonal hematopoiesis. Although an allele burden higher than 50% indicating the presence of granulocytes homozygous for *JAK2V617F* has been found in 70% of PV patients, it has been observed less frequently in ET patients. All PV patients have assayable erythroid colonies that are homozygous for *JAK2V617F*, even in PV patients with a low burden of *JAK2V617F*. By contrast hematopoietic colonies cloned from ET patients are occasionally *JAK2V617F* homozygous. The transition from *JAK2* heterozygous to homozygous progenitors is a consequence of homologous recombination. These studies suggest that such an event is characteristic of PV but rarely occurs in ET. If such an event occurred in ET, it would likely lead to a transition from an ET phenotype to a PV phenotype. Some investigators, but not all, have reported a higher allelic burden of *JAK2V617F* in platelets compared with granulocytes in patients with ET, and that the allelic burden in PV and PMF is higher in granulocytes than platelets. *JAK2V617F* is observed only in platelets in rare patients with ET. *JAK2V617F* can be detected not only in granulocytes and platelets of ET patients but also erythroblasts. Recently, Lambert and coworkers,[3] using single-nucleotide polymorphism (SNP) genotyping of the *JAK2V617F* mutant alleles reported that there were at least two *JAK2V617F* mutational events occurring in 10 of 11 cases, suggesting that multiple independent abnormal clones were involved in the origination of ET. Others have, however, reported that the true prevalence of biallelic *JAK2* mutations is approximately 5% to 10%. These findings are in contrast to the results obtained in PV patients in whom only a single SNP is associated with the mutated *JAK2*. These data have led some investigators to question if such biallelic *JAK2V617F* forms of ET truly represent a malignant disease but are rather a benign stem cell clonal disease.

One of the ongoing mysteries of the biology of *JAK2V617F* has been the lack of insight of how this mutation can participate molecularly in such phenotypically diverse MPNs. Increased basal signaling in both early and later stages of myeloid differentiation appears to be common to all MPN. In PV, *JAK2V617F* produces an increased phosphorylation of STAT. In PV, uniformly increased phosphorylated STAT3 and STAT5 in BM cells has been observed, but in ET, normal or increased phosphorylated STAT3 but reduced phosphorylated STAT5 has been noted. STAT3 is a pivotal regulator of megakaryocytopoiesis that might provide an explanation for its exclusive upregulation in ET. To further examine the differences between hematopoiesis in *JAK2V617F* ET and PV, the gene expression changes in *JAK2V617F* heterozygous erythroid colonies have been examined. Erythroblasts from ET patients were characterized by enhanced expression of genes associated with interferon (INF) signaling and phosho-STAT1 compared with PV erythroblasts.[5] STAT1 is essential for INF-γ signaling. Increased STAT1 in normal $CD34^+$ cells has been shown to favor megakaryocytic but reduce erythroid differentiation, creating a differentiation pattern that resembles ET. Furthermore, inhibition of STAT1 signaling in ET hematopoietic progenitor cells led to enhanced erythropoiesis and reduced megakaryocytopoiesis. These studies suggest that in ET, *JAK2V617F* induces simultaneous activation of STAT5 and STAT1 pathways, but in PV, the relative reduced levels of phosphol-STAT1 reduces a brake favoring more profound erythropoiesis. The MPL mutations occurring in ET patients trigger conformational changes in the receptor, bringing in close proximity two molecules of bound *JAK2* for transphosphorylation and activation of the signaling cascade.

The methodology used to detect *JAK2V617F* can influence the proportion of ET patients documented to be positive for the mutation. The frequency of *JAK2V617F*-positive ET ranges from 40% to 60% of cases. This still leaves a subset that does not possess MPL mutations and that is *JAK2V617F* negative. ET patients without mutated *JAK2* are characterized by a lower expression pattern of JAK/STAT target genes and lower levels of STAT3 phosphorylation, indicating that alternative signaling pathways are likely responsible for the ET phenotype in these patients. This hypothesis has been verified by the description of a patient with *JAK2V617F*-negative ET who also lacked an MPL mutation but was characterized by an acquired t(5;9) chromosomal translocation that resulted in the fusion of *KANK1* and platelet-derived growth factor receptor β (PDGFRβ).[6] In this patient, the *KANK1* gene is disrupted. *KANK1* is a putative tumor suppressor gene present at 9p24, a region that is deleted in a variety of cancers. *KANK1* expression has been shown to be diminished in patients with *JAK2V617F* PV and ET. *KANK1* inhibits cell migration and actin polymerization through the modulation of Rho GTPases, which play a role in the terminal phases of platelet generation. *KANK1*–PDGFRβ activates STAT5 transcription factors but does not require JAKs, indicating that other signaling pathways result in the thrombocytosis observed in such patients.

The clinical phenotype of patients with *JAK2V617F*-positive and -negative ET appears to differ. At diagnosis, patients with the mutation tend to be older and to have a higher hemoglobin level and a higher neutrophil count but a lower platelet count than patients with *JAK2V617F*-negative ET. Patients with *JAK2V617F*-positive ET have a BM that is more hypercellular and is characterized by greater degrees of erythroid and granulocytic hyperplasia. Serum erythropoietin levels are lower in *JAK2V617F*-positive patients, and they have lower serum ferritin levels. In addition, the rate of thrombosis has been suggested by some, but not all, investigators to be higher in *JAK2V617F*-positive ET patients. Furthermore, a greater number of ET patients who have the mutation eventually go on to develop PV. *JAK2V617F*-positive patients have been reported to require smaller doses of hydroxyurea to lower their platelet counts. Campbell et al have hypothesized that because *JAK2V617F*-positive ET shares many phenotypic similarities with PV, these two disorders should be considered as a continuum rather than being categorized as two separate diseases. The presence of the *MPLW515K* mutations in ET patients has been reported to be associated with lower hemoglobin levels and higher platelet counts as well as preferential expansion of the numbers of megakaryocytes at the expense of erythroid precursors as observed in BM biopsy specimens.

Discordance between the percentage of clonal granulocytes and the percent of *JAK2V617F*-positive granulocytes has led some investigators to speculate that the development of a clonal form of ET may precede the acquisition of the *JAK2V617F* mutation or that other mutations might be playing a role in the origins of ET. In mouse models, the inhibitory adaptor protein Lnk has been shown to be associated with downmodulation of erythropoietin and thrombopoietin signaling. Lnk can bind to wild-type *JAK2*, *JAK2V617F*, wild-type MPL, and *MPLW515L*. Lnk levels are upregulated and correlate with an increase in the *JAK2V617F* allele burden in MPN patients. In *JAK2V617F*-positive ET, Lnk mRNA expression is upregulated and serves to modulate *JAK2V617F*-mediated cell regulation. Thrombopoietin-mediated signaling regulates Lnk expression at both the mRNA and protein levels. Furthermore, acquired Lnk mutations have been observed in 1% to 5% of ET patients without *JAK2V617F*. The inactivating Lnk mutations in ET patients result in JAK/STAT activation, leading to high levels of STAT3 and STAT5 activation, leading to either ET or PMF.[7]

An additional gene that is mutated in ET is *TET2* (the ten–eleven translocation gene, which encodes for a hydroxylase that is able to hydroxylate methylated cytosine). These mutations result in loss of function, leading to increased DNA methylation and a reduction in hydroxymethyl cytosine. *TET2* mutations occur in 11% of ET patients but are not specific to ET because they can also occur in a variety of other myeloid malignancies. Mutations in *TET2* can occur either before or after mutations of *JA2V617F* or *MPL*. Mutations in the gene for isocitrate dehydrogenase (IDH) occur in 0.9% of ET patients and can functionally lead to similar effects as *TET2* mutations on DNA methylation. Furthermore, disrupting mutations of ASXL, which occur in 36% of PMF patients, are infrequent in ET as are mutations of *CBL* or *EZH2*.

Furthermore, the transcription factor NF-E2 has been shown to be overexpressed in the cells of patients with MPNs independent of the presence or absence of *JAK2V617F*. NF-E2 acts as an epigenetic transcriptional regulator and chromatin modifier. Genetically engineered mice that overexpress NF-E2 have been created and are characterized by extreme thrombocytosis and leukocytosis, normal hemoglobin levels, and BM hypercellularity, a clinical picture similar to that observed in ET patients.[8] These animals die of gastrointestinal hemorrhagic events, and 15% evolve to a form of acute myeloid leukemia (AML). The upregulation of NF-E2 can be corrected by treatment with inhibitors of histone deacetylases, suggesting that downregulation of NF-E2 using similar agents in ET patients should be explored, especially because the use of histone deacetylase inhibitors is frequently associated with dose-limiting thrombocytopenia.

The cause of the increased risk of developing hemorrhagic and thrombotic events associated with ET remains the subject of investigation. Thrombotic complications occur most frequently in patients older than age 60 years; patients with a history of a thrombotic event; and individuals with cardiovascular risk factors, including tobacco use, hypertension, or diabetes mellitus, but hemorrhagic events occur almost exclusively in individuals with extremely high platelet counts ($>1000 \times 10^9$/L).[9] In addition, leukocytosis (>11,0000/L) and *JAK2V617F* positivity have been associated with the development of arterial thromboses. Platelet counts in excess of 1000×10^9 are associated with a lower risk of developing arterial thromboses. The incidence of thrombotic events in ET patients ranges from 1.5 to 6.6 percent per patient-year. The thrombotic events in ET are largely arterial, but venous thromboses also occur not infrequently.[10] *JAK2V617F*-positive patients compared with patients without the mutation have a higher risk of developing thrombotic events, but a dose-dependent correlation between allele burden and the development of clinical symptoms has not been demonstrated. A subset of young patients who are asymptomatic and remarkably free of such complications has also been described. Unfortunately, catastrophic thrombotic complications can be seen in both young and elderly patients. The age-related differences in the frequency of these events have been attributed to the coexistence of vascular disease in older patients.

Some progress has been made in defining the relationship between platelet numbers and the risks for thrombotic and hemorrhagic events in ET. In a randomized trial of patients at a high risk of developing

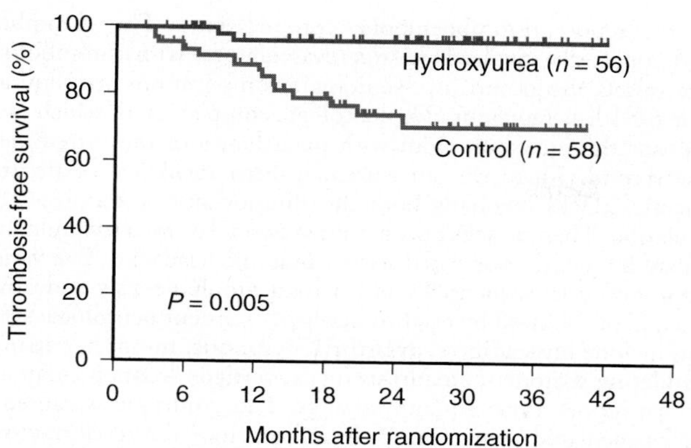

Figure 68-1 PROBABILITY OF THROMBOSIS-FREE SURVIVAL IN 114 PATIENTS WITH ESSENTIAL THROMBOCYTHEMIA TREATED WITH HYDROXYUREA OR LEFT UNTREATED. *(From Cortelazzo S, Finazzi G, Ruggeri M, et al: Hydroxyurea for patients with essential thrombocythemia and a high risk of thrombosis.* N Engl J Med *332:1132, 1995.)*

a thrombotic event (older than 60 years of age, a history of a thrombotic episode, or both), the reduction of platelet numbers was highly effective in preventing additional thrombotic events (Fig. 68-1). Furthermore, the incidence of thrombotic events has been shown to be closely correlated with the duration of thrombocytosis.

Several groups have now confirmed that the degree and duration of bleeding in ET patients is correlated with platelet numbers. Bleeding events appear to occur exclusively when the platelet counts are excessively high and are reduced in number when the platelet count returns to normal. The clinical spectrum of bleeding in ET patients closely resembles that observed in von Willebrand disease. Several groups have now shown that high platelet counts (>1000 × 10^9/L) are associated with an acquired form of von Willebrand syndrome and that reduction of platelet numbers is associated with correction of the von Willebrand syndrome–like abnormalities and cessation of bleeding episodes.[11] The mean platelet count in patients with ET and acquired von Willebrand disease is 2050 ± 1107 × 10^9/L. An increase in the number of circulating platelets appears to favor the adsorption of larger von Willebrand multimers onto platelet membranes, resulting in their removal from the circulation and their subsequent degradation.

Platelets in patients with ET have been known for a considerable time to be qualitatively abnormal. Although both increased and decreased platelet reactivity has been described, these findings have not been definitively associated with thrombohemorrhagic complications with two noteworthy exceptions—erythromelalgia, in which the prompt relief of symptoms by cyclooxygenase inhibitors provides direct evidence that prostaglandins play a role in the development of vascular occlusion, and acquired von Willebrand syndrome, which is a major cause of bleeding in patients with ET. Recently, both ET and PV platelets have been shown to contain a large proportion of immature platelets that have been recently released from the BM. Such immature platelets have increased hemostatic activity as demonstrated by a heightened response to thrombin and greater expression of P-selectin. Hydroxyurea has been shown to be capable of reducing the number of immature platelets in ET, which might partly be responsible for the reduced thrombotic risk associated with its use.

Abnormal platelet aggregation has been reported in 35% to 100% of patients with ET. The majority of such studies have used conventional platelet aggregation studies performed on platelet-rich plasma. The simultaneous measurement of platelet aggregation and adenosine triphosphate–dense granule release by whole-blood platelet lumiaggregometry has been used to study platelet function in ET patients with the hope of identifying patients at a risk of developing thrombosis. A prospective analysis of large cohorts of patients has not been performed to confirm the utility of such assays.

Abnormal aggregation studies have not been successful in predicting the incidence of episodes of hemorrhage or thrombosis. In ET, platelet aggregation is classically defective in response to epinephrine, adenosine diphosphate (ADP), and collagen but is usually normal with arachidonic acid and ristocetin. Characteristically, in ET, the first wave of aggregation is diminished, and the second wave of aggregation is absent in response to epinephrine. Interestingly, preincubation of ET platelets with thrombopoietin partly corrects the impaired aggregation in response to epinephrine, ADP, and collagen. An acquired form of platelet storage pool disease occurs frequently in ET. Platelet α-granule content and the release of the content of granules are abnormal, resulting in elevated plasma levels of platelet factor-4 and β-thromboglobulin.

Because the content of α-granule constituents has been reported to be normal in ET megakaryocytes, the synthesis of these molecules is not believed to be abnormal; rather, the release of α-granule constituents is believed to be a consequence of platelet activation. The finding of an acquired storage pool defect again does not correlate with platelet numbers or with the occurrence of clinical symptoms. Numerous individual functional platelet abnormalities have been demonstrated. A defect in the metabolism of arachidonic acid by lipoxygenase has been documented, as have decreased numbers of platelet receptors for prostaglandin D_2 and adrenergic receptors for epinephrine. Platelets from patients with thrombotic episodes have been found to be capable of increased generation of thromboxanes and to have an increased affinity for fibrinogen. Elevations in β-thromboglobulin and serum thromboxane levels in ET patients are validated indices of enhanced in vivo platelet activation and possibly thrombin generation. Such abnormalities are not present in patients with secondary thrombocytosis and may provide some explanation for the high incidence of thrombosis associated with ET. The antithrombotic activity of aspirin has been attributed to its ability to permanently and selectively inactivate platelet cyclooxygenase-1 (COX-1), thereby blocking thromboxane biosynthesis. This action has served as the rationale for the widespread use of aspirin in ET patients for thrombosis prophylaxis in the absence of valid controlled clinical trials. Recently, however, COX-2 has been shown to be overexpressed by the megakaryocytes and platelets of ET patients; COX-2 can also contribute to the enhanced biosynthesis of thromboxanes in ET.[12] Low-dose aspirin can only partially correct this enhanced thromboxane synthesis, likely because of the increased COX-2 activity associated with the increased rate of platelet generation associated with ET, providing the rationale for the use of more aggressive aspirin scheduling or the addition of thromboxane receptor A_2 antagonists to reduce the incidence of thrombotic events.

The platelet activation observed in ET has also been linked to Src, which is a nonreceptor tyrosine kinase particularly abundant in platelets. In thrombin-stimulated platelets, Src kinase is required for platelet aggregation. In normal resting platelets, Src is silent, but its catalytic activity is activated in response to specific stimuli. In ET platelets, Src kinase is dephosphorylated into its potentially active form as a consequence of its interaction with the tyrosine phosphatase, Src-homology 2 (SHP-2). ET platelets are therefore primed for stimulation by low concentrations of thrombin for faster Src signaling, which ultimately leads to platelet cytoskeleton rearrangement and aggregation. In ET, Src dephosphorylation may be triggered in vivo by a variety of stimuli, including a high platelet count, high shear stress, high concentrations of thrombopoietin, and procoagulant activities. This preactivation of Src that is characteristic of ET and the related platelet hyperactivity is likely to account for the hypercoagulable state that is emblematic of ET.

Microvascular thrombosis causing digital or central nervous system ischemia leads to a variety of clinical syndromes closely associated with ET. The survival of platelets in ET patients with erythromelalgia and thrombosis has been shown to be reduced to 4.2 ± 0.2 days compared with normal platelet survival in asymptomatic ET patients (6.6 ± 0.3 days) and patients with reactive thrombocytosis (8.0 ± 0.4 days). Thrombosis in this setting is associated with an increased platelet turnover, which can be quantitated flow cytometrically by measuring the number of platelets most recently released into the circulation (reticulated platelets). Treatment of erythromelalgia with aspirin increased mean platelet survival from 4.0 ± 0.3 days to

6.9 ± 0.4 days and was associated with a significant elevation of platelet numbers. These findings suggest that erythromelalgia results from platelet-mediated thrombosis of the arterial microvasculature of the extremities. Complete correction of this ischemic circulatory defect is associated with the use of platelet cyclooxygenase inhibitors, such as aspirin and indomethacin. Agents that do not inhibit platelet cyclooxygenase, such as coumadin, sodium salicylate, dipyridamole, sulfinpyrazone, and ticlopidine, are not active in the treatment of this disorder. Dazoxiben is capable of inhibiting platelet malondialdehyde and thromboxane B_2 synthesis but does not correct the symptoms of erythromelalgia. These findings suggest that prostaglandin endoperoxides play a role in the generation of platelet-associated thrombosis in ET.

One intriguing explanation for the increased risk of thrombosis in patients with ET has been the observation that the total amount of thrombin generated on the platelet surfaces of patients with ET is markedly greater than that generated on the platelet surfaces of normal control participants or patients with reactive thrombocytosis. The molecular basis of this abnormality has not been defined, but it remains possible that an abnormal membrane structure of ET platelets may account for the enhanced thrombin potential that may lead to a relatively high thrombotic risk. Increased numbers of platelet microparticles, as well as increased platelet–neutrophil and platelet–monocyte complexes have been observed in patients with ET. Platelet microparticles support thrombin generation and leukocyte activation. Increased numbers of platelet microparticles have been associated with the development of vascular thrombosis.

Recently, in vivo leukocyte activation has been shown to occur in ET and to be associated with signs of activation of both the coagulation cascade and endothelial cells. Such platelet and leukocyte activation may play a role in the generation of the prethrombotic state that characterizes ET. Interestingly, the presence of the *JAK2* mutation is associated with a greater degree of platelet and leukocyte activation in these patients. Activated neutrophils are able to bind platelets, which triggers the expression of tissue factor as well as endothelial cell activation and damage. From a clinical point of view, several studies have demonstrated that an increased leukocyte count (>11,000 × 10^9) in patients with ET is an independent risk factor for developing arterial thrombosis, especially myocardial infarction, and is associated with an inferior survival rate.[13] Therefore, an important role for leukocytes in the pathogenesis of thrombosis in ET is becoming more evident. Presumably, the leukocytosis in ET patients leads to thrombosis by damaging the vascular endothelium because of the release of reactive oxygen species, intracellular proteases, or both. In addition, a high percentage of leukocytes from ET patients has been shown to have platelets present in phagocytic vacuoles, presumably leading to enhanced platelet clearance. This leukocyte-mediated clearance of platelets has been shown to be diminished in individuals with prior thrombotic episodes.

Direct involvement of endothelial cells of MPN patients by *JAK2V617F* has been recently reported by several groups, which might lead to endothelial dysfunction in subsets of MPN patients, further enhancing the thrombotic predisposition to the development of splanchnic vein thromboses.

CLINICAL MANIFESTATIONS

The presenting symptoms of patients with ET are quite variable. Many patients (12%–67%) reach medical attention fortuitously as a result of the extreme degree of thrombocytosis detected when obtaining a routine blood cell count. In two series, in fact, 76% to 84% of cases were asymptomatic, and the diagnosis was made incidentally. Most patients present with symptoms related to small- or large-vessel thrombosis or minor bleeding. The thrombotic events at diagnosis and during follow-up occurred at rates of 10% to 29% and 8% to 31%, respectively. In general, arterial events predominate over venous events. Presentation with a major bleeding episode is unusual. After thrombocytosis has been detected, 13% to 37% of patients relate symptoms resulting from hemorrhagic events, and 22% to 84% of patients report thromboembolic complications. The thrombotic events primarily involved the microvasculature, with thrombosis of large vessels also occurring. Neurologic complications are common. Table 68-1 lists representative neurologic complaints, of which headache was the most common, with paresthesias of the extremities a close second. There was an extremely high incidence of transient ischemic attacks involving both the anterior and posterior cerebral circulation. These attacks have a sudden onset, last for a few moments, and are frequently associated with a pulsatile headache. The various symptoms occur sequentially rather than simultaneously and can be preceded or followed by erythromelalgia. Transient neurologic symptoms include unsteadiness, dysarthria, dysphoria, motor hemiparesis, scintillating scotomas, amaurosis fugax, vertigo, dizziness, migraine-like symptoms, syncope, and seizures. The syndrome is caused by platelet-mediated ischemia and thrombosis in end-arterial microvasculature. It is not unusual for these symptoms to eventually progress to definitive cerebral infarcts.

Microvascular circulatory insufficiency involving the toes and fingers is frequent. Such events can lead to digital pain, enhanced by warmth; distal extremity gangrene, and classic erythromelalgia. The term *erythromelalgia* refers to a syndrome of redness and burning pain in the extremities. Erythromelalgia, which is characterized by a burning pain and a dusky congestion of swollen extremities, is usually preceded by paresthesias. Cold provides relief to these symptoms, and heat intensifies the symptoms. Patients prefer to wear shoes or slippers without socks and elevate their feet. These symptoms may progress in intensity and lead to peeling of the skin in affected appendages or affected toes or fingers, which then may become cold and ischemic with a dark purplish tinge. Erythromelalgia symptoms

Table 68-1 Frequency of Neurologic Complaints Associated With Essential Thrombocythemia

Manifestations	Patients (*n*)
Headache	13
Paresthesias	10
Posterior cerebral circulatory ischemia	9
Anterior cerebral circulatory ischemia	6
Visual disturbances	6
Epileptic seizures	2
Total number of patients	33

Data from Jabaily J, Iland HJ, Laszlo J, et al: Neurologic manifestations of essential thrombocythemia. *Ann Intern Med* 99:513, 1983.

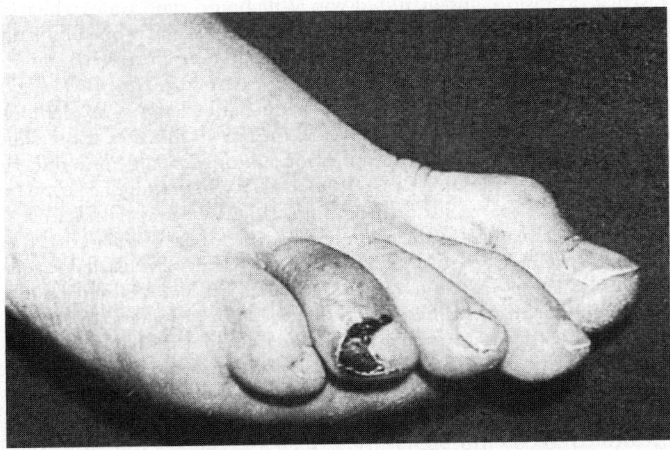

Figure 68-2 GANGRENE OF THE TOE IN A PATIENT WITH ESSENTIAL THROMBOCYTHEMIA.

are asymmetric in the majority of cases. Symptoms related to coronary artery disease or transient ischemic attacks may precede or accompany the onset of erythromelalgia. Occasionally, hemorrhagic episodes may occur in patients experiencing erythromelalgia. Platelet counts in patients with erythromelalgia are frequently below 1000 × 10^9/L, except in patients with concomitant occurrence of erythromelalgia and hemorrhage. The relief of such pain for several days after a single dose of aspirin is diagnostic of erythromelalgia. The specific microvascular syndrome of erythromelalgia is readily explained by platelet-mediated arteriolar inflammation and occlusive thrombosis leading to acrocyanosis and even gangrene.[14] Skin biopsies from affected sites reveal arteriolar lesions without involvement of venules, capillaries, or nerves. The arteriolar endothelial cells are swollen and the vessel walls thickened by cellular swelling and deposition of intracellular material. Compared with atherosclerotic circulatory obstruction, arterial pulses in patients with erythromelalgia remain normal. Other patients develop platelet-mediated acral inflammation and arterial thrombosis, which can progress to ischemic acrocyanosis or necrosis of fingers, toes, and, rarely, the tip of the nose (Fig. 68-2).[15]

Although thrombosis of the microvasculature is generally more frequent, thrombosis of large veins and arteries in patients with ET still occurs commonly.[16] Patient symptoms frequently occur related to large-vessel thrombosis, mostly in the arteries of the legs, the coronary arteries, and the renal arteries. Involvement of the carotid, mesenteric, and subclavian arteries is frequent, and patients characteristically have venous thromboses involving the splenic vein, hepatic veins, or veins of the legs and pelvis. Unexplained thrombosis of the hepatic veins leads to Budd-Chiari syndrome, and thrombosis of the renal vein can result in the development of the nephrotic syndrome.[17] Splanchnic vein thromboses occur predominantly in young women with ET. Patients with this complication are at a high risk of having a poor survival because of hepatic failure or transformation to MF or acute leukemia. It is worth noting that a fraction of patients with idiopathic splanchnic vein thrombosis may present with normal or near-normal blood counts but have an occult MPN based on genetic or histopathologic abnormalities. In a recent review of more than 800 patients with splanchnic vein thrombosis without a diagnosis of an MPN, a mean of 32.7% of patients were *JAK2V617F* positive. More than 50% of these patients subsequently were diagnosed with an MPN. In addition, 2.6% of patients with a cerebral sinus and vein thrombosis were also shown to be *JAK2V617F* positive. These studies suggest that all cases of splanchnic vein thrombosis and likely cerebral sinus and vein thrombosis should be tested for *JAK2V617F* to identify patients with an occult MPN. This high prevalence of *JAK2V617F* positivity has not been observed in individuals with more common kinds of thrombotic events. Priapism is a rare complication of ET, presumably caused by platelet sludging in the corpus cavernosum. In addition, myocardial ischemia and infarction associated with normal coronary angiograms has been reported in patients with ET as has a high incidence of anginal symptoms. A high incidence of aortic and mitral valvular lesions has been reported in patients with MPN, including ET. These valvular lesions resemble previous descriptions of nonbacterial thrombotic endocarditis and may occasionally be the origin of the peripheral arterial emboli observed in these patients. In addition, acute renal failure has been observed after thrombosis of renal arteries and veins in patients with ET. Pulmonary hypertension secondary to alveolar capillary plugging by platelets and megakaryocytes has also been reported in patients with ET.

Hemorrhagic events occur in 3% to 11% of patients with ET; the primary site of bleeding is the gastrointestinal tract.[11] Other sites of bleeding may be the skin, eyes, urinary tract, gums, tooth sockets (after extraction), joints, or brain. Bleeding most often is not severe but occasionally may require red blood cell (RBC) transfusion support. The postoperative period appears to be an extremely precarious time, with a high incidence of bleeding episodes during the immediate postoperative period. This hemorrhagic tendency is likely caused by postsurgical thrombocytosis and the development of acquired von Willebrand syndrome or the use of antithrombotic prophylaxis therapy. Bleeding is closely correlated with a significant increase in platelet counts in excess of 1500 × 10^9/L and is associated with pseudohyperkalemia. It is important to emphasize that individual patients can experience both thrombotic and hemorrhagic episodes and that patients are not necessarily consistent "bleeders" or "clotters."

Appreciation of the risk of developing thrombohemorrhagic events in asymptomatic patients with ET who are younger than 40 years of age is imprecise at best. Such patients are thought to be at a low risk of developing thrombotic episodes unless they have experienced a prior thrombotic episode or have associated cardiovascular risk factors. With their anticipated long survival, such patients are, however, at a considerable risk of eventually developing symptomatic MF several decades after the initial diagnosis of their MPN. The most common thrombotic complications include migraine headaches in 20% and erythromelalgia in 5% of the patients. Life-threatening hemorrhagic episodes are rare. The degree of leukocytosis has been suggested by some investigators to be useful in discriminating between young patients with a low or high risk to develop a thrombotic episode.

A meta-analysis has revealed that the JAK2V617 mutation is associated with a twofold higher risk of developing either a venous or arterial thrombosis but does not influence the risk of suffering from a hemorrhagic event. Regardless, it is conceivable that the significantly more advanced age and elevated hematocrit and leukocyte levels in mutation-positive patients might contribute to the apparent association between *JAK2V617F* and thrombosis reported in some studies. Vannucchi et al[4] have reported that rare ET patients with a high *JAK2V617F* allele burden are at a particularly higher risk of developing cardiovascular events.

Patients with ET who are older than 60 years of age who have had a prior thrombotic event have a greater risk of developing additional thrombotic events (Table 68-2). By contrast, the incidence of thrombotic and hemorrhagic complications in asymptomatic patients with ET who are younger than 60 years of age who have platelet counts of less than 1500 × 10^9/L has been shown to be comparable to a normal control population. Gender, hypertension, diabetes mellitus, hypercholesterolemia, and smoking have been shown to be independent risk factors for developing arterial thrombotic complications in ET (see Table 68-2). Investigators continue to search for other acquired or congenital defects of hemostatic mechanisms, such as the factor V Leiden mutation, prothrombin G20210A gene mutation, and so on, to better understand why many patients remain asymptomatic but others experience a serious thrombosis. Screening of patients for such thrombophilic states may identify patients at an even higher risk for both arterial and venous thrombotic events.

Pregnancy is not contraindicated in patients with ET. The outcome of pregnancy in patients with ET has recently been the subject of intense investigation. The rate of having a successful pregnancy is 61% compared with an 85% to 90% rate in normal women. The rate of spontaneous abortions ranges from 39% to 44% compared

Table 68-2 Risk Stratification in Essential Thrombocythemia Based on Thrombotic Risk*

Risk Category	Age >60 Years or History of Thrombosis	Cardiovascular Risk Factors
Low	No	No
Intermediate	No	Yes
High	Yes	Yes

Data from Finazzi G, Barbui T: Risk-adapted therapy in essential thrombocythemia and polycythemia vera. *Blood Rev* 19:243, 2005.
*Cardiovascular risk factors: hypertension, hypercholesterolemia, diabetes, smoking, and congestive heart failure. Extreme thrombocytosis (platelet count >1500 × 10^9/L) is a risk factor for bleeding. Its role as a risk factor for thrombosis in essential thrombocythemia is uncertain.

with the miscarriage rate of 10% to 15% in normal pregnancies. Loss of the fetus late in the pregnancy is also more common in women with ET than in those without ET (5%–9.6% versus 0.5%). Placental infarction is often responsible for intrauterine fetal growth retardation (5%). Abruptio placenta has been reported in 3.6% of cases, a rate that is higher than that observed in the general population (1%). Major thrombotic episodes occur in 3% of these pregnancies while major bleeding episodes occur in 2% of cases. These rates are higher than that observed in the overall population of pregnant women.[18] The average platelet count at the beginning of pregnancy in patients with successful pregnancies was 1010×10^9/L, and it was 977×10^9/L among those with an unsuccessful outcome; thus the baseline platelet count is not predictive of pregnancy outcome. ET patients with the *JAK2V617F* mutation have been reported to be at a higher risk of developing complications with pregnancy. During the second trimester, a spontaneous decline in platelet counts was reported, reaching a nadir of 599×10^9/L. This decrease in platelet numbers seems larger than the reduction observed in normal pregnancies, which has been attributed to an increase in plasma volume. The mechanism for this reduction in platelet numbers is not known but could involve placental or fetal production of a factor that downregulates platelet production. In the postpartum period, the platelet counts return to their earlier levels, and rebound thrombocytosis may occur in some patients. This is thought to increase the probability of vascular complications during this period to a level similar to that observed in other conditions of thrombophilia.

In the large majority of cases, the fetal losses in pregnant ET women occur during the first trimester. In one series, 65% of the miscarriages occurred in 17% of women. Thus a previous history of spontaneous abortion may be the greatest risk factor for the development of subsequent spontaneous abortions.

Physical examination findings are relatively unremarkable in patients with ET. Most patients are not severely ill at diagnosis, with a median Karnofsky score of 90% being reported in one series. Splenomegaly is detectable in 40% to 50% of patients, and approximately 20% have hepatomegaly. During the course of the disorder, a further increase in the degree of hepatosplenomegaly may be observed in patients who are developing post-ET MF. Recently, skin manifestations of the MPN have been reported to be relatively common, ranging from paraneoplastic lesions, including vascular, neutrophilic plaques, and unexplained dermatoses. Rarely, vascular changes result in microcirculatory flow abnormalities, leading to a vasculities resulting in classic purpura that may progress to skin necrosis. This should be distinguished from leg ulcers that occur in patients being treated with hydroxyurea. Occasionally, patients also develop pyoderma gangrenosum or Sweet syndrome.

LABORATORY MANIFESTATIONS

The hallmark of ET is a sustained and unexplained elevation of the platelet count (≥450 × 109/L). The level of thrombocytosis required for the diagnosis is arbitrarily determined, the range being 450 to greater than 1000 × 109/L.[3] Accompanying leukocytosis is a common finding. A leukoerythroblastic blood picture, as well as teardrop-shaped RBCs are not features of ET but are suggestive of an early form of MF. Mild eosinophilia (>400/mm^3) and basophilia (>100/mm^3) have been reported in more than one-third of patients.

The most common morphologic abnormalities are variations in RBC size and shape and the presence of megathrombocytes (Fig. 68-3). The BM is usually normocellular or slightly hypercellular without a significant increase in granulopoiesis or erythropoiesis. Increased numbers of enlarged megakaryocytes with hyperlobulated or deeply folded nuclei that cluster in small groups along sinuses are the hallmarks of ET (see Fig. 68-3). Reticulin fibrosis is not significantly evident. A great deal of controversy currently surrounds distinguishing "true ET" from an early prefibrotic form of MF in which the BM is characteristically hypercellular with pronounced proliferation of granulocytes and reduced erythroid precursors. The megakaryocytes are increased in number but are loosely clustered or located along the endosteal bone surface. The megakaryocytes contain hyperchromatic, hypolobulated bulbous, or irregularly folded nuclei with an abnormal nuclear-to-cytoplasmic ratio. The histopathologic criteria for this form of PMF have been combined with clinical criteria (minor criteria) by the World Health Organization (WHO).[19] Two minor criteria are required to make a diagnosis of early PMF, including a leukoerythroblastic blood picture, increased serum LDH, anemia, and splenomegaly (Table 68-3). These minor criteria are important because the diagnosis of early PMF cannot be made without their fulfillment according to WHO criteria. Based on the 2008 WHO Diagnostic Criteria, the presence of modest BM reticulin fibrosis excludes the diagnosis of ET but is supportive rather of a diagnosis of an early form of MF. By contrast, the diagnostic criteria for ET defined by the British Committee for Standards in Hematology still classifies patients with grade 2 reticulin fibrosis on a scale of 0 to 4 as having ET. These two sets of diagnostic criteria are provided in Table 68-3 and are of importance because their implementation determines who one classifies as having "true" ET or an early form of MF. Although select hematopathologists can reproducibly distinguish ET from the early prefibrotic form of MF, it remains uncertain whether this distinction is broadly applicable. In fact, in one study of six European hematopathologists analyzing BM biopsies from 102 nonfibrotic patients with sustained thrombocytosis, in more than 50% of cases the classification of individual cases was not

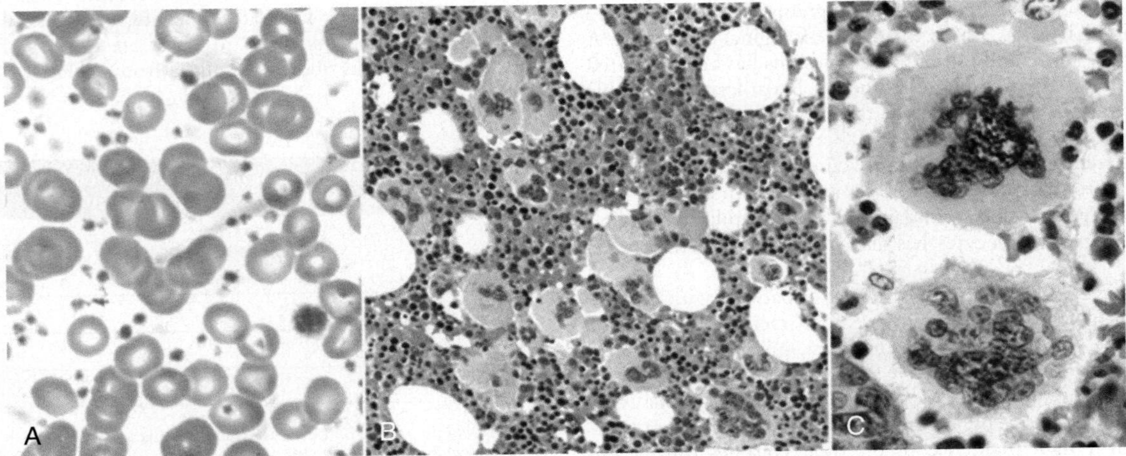

Figure 68-3 ESSENTIAL THROMBOCYTHEMIA (ET): PERIPHERAL BLOOD SMEAR AND BONE MARROW BIOPSY. The peripheral blood smear in ET shows a marked thrombocytosis with anisocytosis (varying sizes) of the platelets **(A)**. The bone marrow **(B)** is hypercellular and exhibits a marked proliferation of large and giant megakaryocytes in loose clusters with other hematopoietic elements in the background. The large megakaryocytes **(C)** tend to be extensively lobulated.

Table 68-3 Proposed Revised World Health Organization Criteria for the Diagnosis of Primary Myelofibrosis and Essential Thrombocythemia and British Committee for Standards in Hematology Criteria for Diagnosis of Essential Thrombocythemia

Proposed Revised WHO Criteria for Primary Myelofibrosis

Major Criteria

1. Presence of megakaryocyte proliferation and atypia,* usually accompanied by either reticulin or collagen fibrosis or in the absence of significant reticulin fibrosis, the megakaryocyte changes must be accompanied by an increased BM cellularity characterized by granulocytic proliferation and often decreased erythropoiesis (i.e., prefibrotic cellular phase disease)
2. Not meeting WHO criteria for PV,† CML,‡ MDS,§ or other myeloid neoplasm
3. Demonstration of JAK2617V->F or other clonal marker (e.g., MPL515W->L/K) or in the absence of a clonal marker, no evidence of BM fibrosis caused by underlying inflammatory or other neoplastic diseases‖

Minor Criteria

1. Leukoerythroblastosis¶
2. Increase in serum LDH level¶
3. Anemia¶
4. Palpable splenomegaly¶

Diagnosis requires meeting all three major criteria and two minor criteria.

BM, Bone marrow; *CML,* chronic myeloid leukemia; *LDH,* lactate dehydrogenase; *MDS,* myelodysplastic syndrome; *PV,* polycythemia vera; *WHO,* World Health Organization.
*Small to large megakaryocytes with an aberrant nuclear-to-cytoplasmic ratio and hyperchromatic, bulbous, or irregularly folded nuclei and sense clustering.
†Requires the failure of iron replacement therapy to increase hemoglobin level to the PV range in the presence of decreased serum ferritin. Exclusion of PV is based on hemoglobin and hematocrit levels, and RBC mass measurement is not required.
‡Requires the absence of *BCR-ABL.*
§Requires absence of dyserythropoiesis and dysgranulopoiesis.
(ParaMarks)Secondary to infection, autoimmune disorder or other chronic inflammatory condition, hairy cell leukemia or other lymphoid neoplasm, metastatic malignancy, or toxic (chronic) myelopathies. It should be noted that patients with conditions associated with reactive myelofibrosis are not immune to primary myelofibrosis, and the diagnosis should be considered in such cases if other criteria are met.
¶Degree of abnormality could be borderline or marked.

Proposed Revised World Health Organization Criteria for Essential Thrombocythemia

1. Sustained platelet count ≥450 × 10^9/L*
2. BM biopsy specimen showing proliferation mainly of the megakaryocytic lineage with increased numbers of enlarged, mature megakaryocytes; no significant increase or left shift of neutrophil granulopoiesis or erythropoiesis
3. Not meeting WHO criteria for PV,† PMF,‡ CML,§ MDS,‖ or other myeloid neoplasm
4. Demonstration of *JAK2V617F* or other clonal marker or in the absence of a clonal marker, no evidence for reactive thrombocytosis¶

Diagnosis requires meeting all four criteria.

From Tefferi A, Thiele J, Orazi A, et al: Proposals and rationale for revision of the World Health Organization diagnostic criteria for polycythemia vera, essential thrombocythemia, and primary myelofibrosis: Recommendations from an ad hoc international expert panel. *Blood* 110:1092, 2007.
BM, Bone marrow; *CML,* chronic myeloid leukemia; *MDS,* myelodysplastic syndrome; *PV,* polycythemia vera; *WHO,* World Health Organization.
*During the workup period.
†Requires the failure of iron replacement therapy to increase hemoglobin level to the PV range in the presence of decreased serum ferritin. Exclusion of PV is based on hemoglobin and hematocrit levels, and red blood cell mass measurement is not required.
‡Requires the absence of relevant reticulin fibrosis, collagen fibrosis, peripheral blood leukoerythroblastosis, or markedly hypercellular BM for age accompanied by megakaryocyte morphology that is typical for PMF—small to large with an aberrant nuclear-to-cytoplasmic ratio and hyperchromatic, bulbous, or irregularly folded nuclei and dense clustering.
§Requires the absence of *BCR-ABL.*
‖ Requires absence of dyserythropoiesis and dysgranulopoiesis.
¶Causes of reactive thrombocytosis include iron deficiency, splenectomy, surgery, infection, inflammation, connective tissue disease, metastatic cancer, and lymphoproliferative disorders. However, the presence of a condition associated with reactive thrombocytosis does not exclude the possibility of ET if the first three criteria are met.

British Committee for Standards in Hematology Criteria for Diagnosis of Essential Thrombocythemia

Requires A1-A3 or A1+A3-A5
A1: Sustained platelet count >450 × 10^9/L
A2: Presence of an acquired pathogenetic mutation (e.g., in *JAK2* or MPL)
A3: No other myeloid malignancy, especially PV, PMF, CML, or MDS
A4: No reactive cause for thrombocytosis and normal iron stores
A5: BM aspirate and trephine biopsy showing increased megakaryocyte numbers displaying a spectrum of morphology with predominant large megakaryocytes with hyperlobated nuclei and abundant cytoplasm

From Harrison et al: Br. J Haemotol 149:352, 2010.
BM, Bone marrow; *CML,* chronic myeloid leukemia; *JAK2,* Janus kinase 2; *MDS,* myelodysplastic syndrome; *MPL,* thrombopoietin receptor; *PMF,* primary myelofibrosis; *PV,* polycythemia vera.

reproducible or fell into the category of unclassifiable MPN.[20] In 70% to 80% of ET patients, iron stores were present in the BM, albeit at reduced levels. Almost all patients have normal serum ferritin levels. The absence of iron stores in 30% of patients may merely be an epiphenomenon of a chronic MPN and not truly reflective of an iron deficiency state. Platelet aggregation study results are frequently abnormal, most often demonstrating an impaired aggregation response to epinephrine, ADP, and collagen but not to arachidonic acid and ristocetin. Spontaneous platelet aggregation has been reported to occur frequently in such patients, but this has not been a universal finding.

Approximately 25% of patients with ET have been reported to have elevated uric acid levels at diagnosis. The average value of the serum potassium at diagnosis is usually within the normal range, although 23% of patients have been reported to have pseudohyperkalemia, and caused by the degranulation of platelets when in vitro clotting releases potassium. Both excessive numbers of RBCs and leukocytes can also be associated with these phenomena. The pseudohyperkalemia can be documented by measuring plasma instead of serum potassium levels and the lack of electrocardiographic findings associated with true hyperkalemia. Pseudohypoxemia has also been observed in ET patients with extreme degrees of thrombocytosis. Acquired von Willebrand syndrome is associated almost uniformly with a platelet count greater than 1500×10^9/L, a prolonged bleeding time, a normal factor VIII coagulant activity, and a von Willebrand antigen level but a decreased von Willebrand factor–ristocetin cofactor activity and collagen binding activity, as well as a decrease or absence of large von Willebrand factor multimers simulating a type II von Willebrand disorder. The enhanced thrombotic risk of ET patients has been associated with a reduction in the concentration of one of the natural anticoagulants, including protein S, antithrombin III protein C, and resistance to activated protein C. These studies indicate that such a genetic deficiency of one of the natural anticoagulants might further contribute to the thrombotic tendency of patients with ET. The serum vitamin B_{12} level can be increased in 25% of cases.

In ET, BM karyotypes are characteristically normal. The absence of the Philadelphia chromosome and the *BCR/ABL* rearrangement excludes the diagnosis of chronic myeloid leukemia (CML). The Philadelphia chromosome or the *BCR/ABL* rearrangement that is seen in patients with CML must be searched for in patients who present with a high platelet count because of the observation that thrombocytosis may be the initial laboratory abnormality in patients with CML. Rare patients share two molecular markers of MPNs (*JAK2V617F* and *BCR/ABL*). Because the prognosis and management for ET and CML are very different, it is important to rule out CML as the cause of the elevation in platelet numbers. Aneuploidy is seen in the minority of cases at diagnosis. In fact, ET is associated with a definite chromosomal abnormality in only 7.8% of cases, but with disease progression, there is an increased risk of aneuploidy. Specific chromosome abnormalities associated with ET have not been described, but abnormalities observed in PV and PMF as well as in myelodysplastic syndrome (MDS) such as trisomy 1q, deletions of 5q, 13q and 20q, trisomy 8 as well as monosomal karyotypes have been reported. Many nonspecific chromosomal rearrangements have also been observed such as a complex karyotype, presence of a marker chromosome, and unusual translocations. Molecular cytogenetic studies in ET have not been performed extensively. In one reported study, addition of fluorescence in situ hybridization (FISH) increased detection of chromosomally abnormal clones by 15%. But in 21 patients studied with oligoarray comparative genomic hybridization, one additional patient with deletion 13q was identified compared with conventional cytogenetics. In 12 pediatric ET patients, chromosomal abnormalities were not detected. Leukemic transformation of ET is characterized by development of an abnormal karyotype in 60% to 100% of patients. Consistent chromosomal abnormalities associated with ET progression in *JAK2V617F*-positive patients are der(1)t(1;9) and der(1;7)(q10;p10). Of the eight reported ET patients with der(1;7), five received previous chemotherapy (chlorambucil, hydroxyurea, pipobroman, melphalan, cytosine arabinoside, anthracycline), and six transformed to acute leukemia. Although der(1)t(1;9) is a consistent nonrandom rearrangement associated with de novo PV and with PV progression, four ET patients had der(1)t(1;9) with different breakpoints (p13;p13) and (q10;p10). In ET, similar to PV, PMF, and other myeloid disorders, formation of trisomy 1q alone or subsequent formation of jumping +1q translocations should be considered a clonal marker associated with disease progression or transformation to AML. As has been previously mentioned, approximately 50% of ET patients are *JAK2V617F* positive with only 4% having a high allele burden. Approximately 3% to 5% of patients have activating MPL mutations.

DIFFERENTIAL DIAGNOSIS

Thrombocytosis is a common finding. There are numerous causes of primary, secondary, and spurious forms of thrombocytosis. A listing of the conditions that can lead to thrombocytosis is provided in Table 68-4. Primary thrombocytosis includes both acquired and hereditary forms. In acquired forms of primary thrombocytosis, the genetic abnormalities are present exclusively in hematopoietic cells, but in the hereditary forms, these underlying defects can be detected in both somatic and germ line cells and are inherited. The discovery of *JAK2* and MPL mutations has provided definitive diagnostic tools with which to diagnose the MPNs, including ET. These mutations, however, can be found only in about half of ET patients. Hence, it is reasonable to consider *JAK2V617F* analysis and a search for a mutation in MPL when evaluating patients with otherwise unexplained thrombocytosis. A positive test result indicates an underlying MPN. However, further investigations, including a BM biopsy (see Table 68-3) as well as a cytogenetic analysis, are still required to differentiate ET from the other chronic MPNs as well as from myelodysplastic disorders presenting with thrombocytosis, such as the 5q− syndrome and refractory anemia with ringed sideroblasts associated with thrombocytosis (RARS-T) (see Table 68-4) and early forms of PMF.

For those patients who present with thrombocytosis who are *JAK2* negative, the first step in determining the cause of thrombocytosis is to exclude reactive forms of thrombocytosis.[21] The causes of secondary or reactive forms of thrombocytosis are numerous, but the most common causes are infection, inflammation, hemolysis, severe exercise, malignancy, hyposplenism, and other causes of an acute phase response (see Table 68-4). In a hospital population, patients with extreme thrombocytosis ($>1000 \times 10^9$/L) are not particularly rare in adult or pediatric patient populations. Examination of the blood smear is important to avoid confusion with so-called pseudothrombocytosis. This occurs in a number of conditions in which platelet-sized particles of red or white blood cell fragments (CLL, TTP, hemoglobin H disease), schistocytes, microspherocytosis, and cryoglobulinemia are erroneously enumerated as platelets by automatic particle counters. Confirmation of increased numbers of platelets by examination of the peripheral smear will avoid misdiagnosis and unnecessary clinical evaluation.

Table 68-4 Conditions Associated With Thrombocytosis

Conditions
Primary Thrombocytosis
Malignancies
Essential thrombocythemia
Polycythemia vera
Primary myelofibrosis
Chronic myeloid leukemia
Refractory anemia with ringed sideroblasts and thrombocytosis
Chronic myelomonocytic leukemia
MDS/MPN overlap
Familial thrombocythemia (inherited mutations in thrombopoietin or thrombopoietin receptor)
Secondary (Reactive) Thrombocytosis
Blood loss or iron deficiency
Infection
Inflammation
Disseminated malignancy
Hemolysis
Drug therapy
Hyposplenism
Cytokine administration
Spurious Thrombocytosis
Schistocytes
Cytoplasmic fragmentation of neoplastic cells
Cryoglobulinemia
Bacteria

MDS, Myelodysplastic syndrome; *MPN*, myeloproliferative neoplasm.

Whereas reactive thrombocytosis accounts for more than 88% to 97% of cases, thrombocytosis caused by an MPN accounts for only a minority of cases. Reactive thrombocytosis is more common in all age groups except those in the eighth decade and older. A significant number of patients with reactive thrombocytosis have platelet counts greater than $1000 \times 10^9/L$. It is therefore impossible to distinguish between reactive thrombocytosis and thrombocytosis caused by an MPN based solely on the degree of thrombocytosis. Thrombotic and hemorrhagic events infrequently occur in patients with reactive thrombocytosis. These findings are in contrast to the enhanced risk of these two complications in patients with ET. This relatively high frequency of extreme thrombocytosis in an acute care hospital emphasizes the need for caution in making a diagnosis of ET (Table 68-5). A number of groups have shown that reactive thrombocytosis may be a consequence of the elaboration of known cytokines in response to the underlying inflammatory or neoplastic disorder and are accompanied by an elevated erythrocyte sedimentation rate or a high C-reactive protein (CRP). Elevated levels of IL-1, IL-6, GM-CSF, G-CSF, and thrombopoietin have been detected in such patient populations and frequently in individuals with thrombocytosis caused by an underlying MPN. Elevation of thrombopoietin levels has not only been found in patients with reactive thrombocytosis but also in patients with ET. IL-6–induced thrombocytosis is mediated in part by secondary thrombopoietin production by the liver in inflammatory disorders and malignant diseases. Thus as opposed to erythropoietin levels being helpful in differentiating primary from secondary causes of erythrocytosis, the level of thrombopoietin cannot be used to differentiate ET from secondary causes of thrombocytosis. CRP is an acute phase reactant, the hepatic synthesis of which is mediated by IL-6. CRP levels are high in patients with high levels of IL-6. In one series, whereas 81% of patients with reactive thrombocytosis had elevated IL-6 or CRP levels, patients with uncomplicated thrombocytosis secondary to an MPN had undetectable IL-6 levels. Low levels of both IL-6 and CRP are strongly indicative of the thrombocytosis being the consequence of an underlying MPN.

Both familial forms of thrombocytosis and thrombocytosis that accompanies hematologic malignancies are examples of primary thrombocytoses. The MPNs are characterized by clonal hematopoiesis, but in the familial forms of thrombocytosis, hematopoiesis is polyclonal. An abnormality of thrombopoietin production or of the thrombopoietin receptor has been documented to be the basis of these inherited disorders leading to thrombocytosis.

Four different mutations have been reported in which excessive thrombocytosis has been attributed to increased thrombopoietin production. A Dutch family with 11 family members and a Japanese family with eight family members were reported with a hereditary form of thrombocytosis that was inherited as an autosomal dominant. The thrombopoietin receptor in the Dutch family was normal, yet there was a G-to-C transversion in the splice donor site of intron 3 of the thrombopoietin gene. All of the affected members of the Dutch family were shown to have elevated thrombopoietin levels. In this family, a point mutation in the thrombopoietin gene was believed to lead to systemic overproduction of thrombopoietin, leading to a familial form of thrombocytosis. This was the first example of a human disease caused by increased efficiency of mRNA production. Actually, the translation of full-length thrombopoietin is almost completely inhibited by the presence in the 5′ untranslated region of seven AUG codons, which create seven upstream reading frames (uORFs). These uORFs are potent inhibitors of translation, and mutations in this area cause thrombocytosis by eliminating the normal physiological inhibition of thrombopoietin mRNA translation. Three additional families with thrombocytosis caused by a similar genetic mechanism have been identified.

Another form of familial thrombocytosis has been attributed to germ line mutations of MPL (MPL-S505N, MPL-K39N, and MPL-P106L). MPL-S505N was first described in a Japanese pedigree of familial thrombocytosis that is inherited in an autosomal dominant fashion. This disorder has been attributed to a dominant-positive activating mutation of the cellular receptor of MPL. Eight additional Italian families with thrombocytosis and MPL-S505N have been identified.

A polymorphism of the thrombopoietin receptor (MPL Baltimore, MPL-K39N) that is accompanied by thrombocytosis has also been described. This polymorphism is caused by a single nucleotide substitution that results in a lysine to asparagine (K39N) substitution in the ligand-binding domain of MPL. The polymorphism occurs exclusively in African Americans and appears to have an autosomal dominant pattern of inheritance with incomplete penetrance because some heterozygotes have normal platelet counts but others have thrombocytosis. Approximately 7% of African Americans are heterozygous for MPLK39N. The mutation in the homozygous state is associated with extreme thrombocytosis with a reduced expression of platelet MPL, which has been proposed to affect the receptor's ability to bind thrombopoietin, resulting in its reduced clearance and increased stimulation of megakaryocytopoiesis. MPL-P106L is another mutation associated with familial thrombocytosis that has been found in 6% of Arabs.

Subjects with familial forms of thrombocytosis are characteristically diagnosed at earlier ages than patients with ET. These disorders were initially considered to be associated with a benign clinical course, but follow-up of such families for longer periods of time has corrected this misperception. Overall, 23 members of a Dutch and a Polish family with a form of thrombocytosis attributed to excessive thrombopoietin production were shown to have similar thrombotic and hemorrhagic complications as individuals with ET. Also, these family members experienced vasomotor symptoms, including erythromelalgia and Raynaud phenomena, that responded to aspirin therapy but not hydroxyurea therapy. Furthermore, many of these patients developed splenomegaly as well as BM histopathologic findings that resemble an MPN, including BM hypercellularity, clustering of megakaryocytes, and a mild increase of BM fibrosis. Surprisingly, more prolonged follow-up of members of the Dutch family have revealed progression to symptomatic MF in one individual and progression to acute leukemia in a second family member. The patient with acute leukemia had not received any chemotherapeutic agents, and evaluation of the strength of the relationship between this high thrombopoietin condition and the development of acute leukemia requires further investigation of these families. Similarly, patients with the activating mutation of MPL, MPL-S505N also have a high incidence of major thrombotic events, including stroke, myocardial infarction, and Budd-Chiari syndrome. In adult patients, overt BM reticulin and collagen fibrosis associated with mild reductions in hemoglobin levels have been observed, but no differences in platelet counts, incidence in thrombotic episodes, or splenomegaly have been

Table 68-5 Clinical and Laboratory Features Helpful in Distinguishing Essential Thrombocythemia from Reactive Thrombocytosis* (Revised)

Feature	ET	RT
Chronic platelet increase	+	–
Known causes of RT	–	+
Thrombosis or hemorrhage	+	–
Splenomegaly	+	–
BM reticulin fibrosis	+	–
BM megakaryocyte clusters	+	–
Abnormal cytogenetics	+	–
Increased acute phase reactants	–	+
Spontaneous colony formation†	+	–
JAK2V617F mutation	+	–

Modified from Tefferi A, Hoagland HC: Issues in the diagnosis and management of primary thrombocythemia. *Mayo Clin Proc* 69:651, 1994.
BM, bone marrow; *ET,* essential thrombocythemia; *RT,* reactive thrombocytosis.
*Acute phase reactants include C-reactive protein and fibrinogen.
†Erythroid colonies.

observed when one compares these individuals with ET patients. In women with MPL-S505N, hematopoiesis is polyclonal, and the mutation is observed not only in hematopoietic tissues but also other somatic tissues. Family members who are affected by this mutation appear to have a significantly shorter survival time than nonaffected family members who did not have thrombocytosis, with affected individuals dying most frequently of thrombotic events or complications of MF. By contrast, individuals with either MPL-K39N or MPL-P106L, which both involve the extracellular domain of MPL affecting its ability to bind thrombopoietin, do not have an increased risk for thrombosis, splenomegaly, or BM fibrosis. Because the median age of diagnosis of patients with these familial forms of thrombocytosis is 17 years, these disorders should be carefully considered in all *JAK2V617F-*, *MPLW515L-*, and *MPL515K*-negative children with multiple family members with thrombocytosis.

Table 68-3 outlines the recently updated WHO and British Committee for Standards in Hematology criteria for the diagnosis of ET that incorporates JAK2V7617F and MPL mutational analyses. RBC mass and plasma volume studies, if available, are sometimes helpful in differentiating between *JAK2V617F*-positive ET with borderline elevated hematocrits from patients with PV, but such patients likely represent a continuum of evolution of a *JAK2V617F*-positive hematologic malignancy. BM karyotypic analysis or studies for the *BCR-ABL* fusion gene are imperative in every patient to exclude the diagnosis of CML or to detect another clonal hematologic malignancy. This step is necessary because the natural history of these disorders is very different, and early therapeutic intervention with specific medical therapy for CML, such as with imatinib, dasatinib, or nilotinib, is essential.

Occasionally, ET might be distinguished from refractory anemia with ring sideroblasts and thrombocytosis (RARS-T), which has been recognized by the WHO classification of hematologic malignancies. These patients present with thrombocytosis that is associated with a moderate to severe anemia and frequently splenomegaly. Their BMs are characterized by the morphologic features of ET and the presence of more than 15% ringed sideroblasts. This entity likely represents a heterogeneous, poorly defined disorder that includes a spectrum of conditions sharing features of an MPN and a myelodysplastic disorder. This entity is associated with *JAK2V617F* in 58% of reported patients and a MPLW515 mutation in 7% of reported patients. Occasional patients with thrombocytosis and increased ringed sideroblasts but without anemia have also been described. Patients with RARRS-T have a similar prognosis as ET patients. RARS-T has been recently shown to be associated with somatic mutations of *SF3B1,* a gene encoding a core component of the RNA splicing machinery.[22] In RARS-T, the allele burden of mutant *SF3B1* ranges from 17% to 62%. The *SF3B1* mutations are associated with expanded but ineffective erythropoiesis. RARS-T therefore likely results from a combination of *SF3B1* and *JAK2* or *MPL* mutations.[23] About 25% of patients with RARS-T have wild-type *SF3B1,* suggesting that other molecular defects can be associated with RARS-T.

Because patients with early forms of MF frequently present with thrombocytosis, this form of PMF can frequently be difficult to distinguish from ET. This early form of PMF was previously referred to as a prefibrotic form of PMF. In the prefibrotic phase of PMF, nucleated RBCs, teardrop-shaped RBCs, immature myeloid cells, and megathrombocytes are observed in the peripheral blood. In the BM biopsy, the megakaryocytes are markedly abnormal, a morphologic finding that is helpful in distinguishing this entity from ET. In prefibrotic PMF, the megakaryocytes often appear in clusters adjacent to the sinusoids; deviations in the nuclear cytoplasmic ratio in the megakaryocytes are observed with abnormal patterns of chromatin clumping, and plump clouds similar to a balloon-shaped lobulation of the nuclei are observed associated with minimal fibrosis or even absent reticulin fibrosis during this stage of PMF.

The presence of clonal hematopoiesis, at least in one lineage, quickly establishes the diagnosis of ET. Unfortunately, techniques to study clonality are currently not widely available and are restricted to the evaluation of female patients. Such studies may be particularly useful in young female patients with thrombocytosis. Probes for a variety of genes on the X chromosome can be informative for clonal analysis of blood cell production in more than 72% of female Americans. In such patients, analysis of restriction fragment length polymorphisms can be used to establish a pattern of clonal hematopoiesis, which is indicative of a hematologic malignancy and establishes the diagnosis of ET in a young female patient with thrombocytosis who is *JAK2V617F* negative. Polyclonal hematopoiesis is found in all cases of reactive and familial thrombocytosis. Polyclonal hematopoiesis, however, does not exclude the diagnosis of ET because in several series, almost one-third of patients who met the clinical criteria for ET had polyclonal hematopoiesis in all studied lineages. The biogenesis of this polyclonal form of ET is poorly understood. Initial studies, however, have suggested that women with polyclonal hematopoiesis may have fewer thrombotic complications than those with clonal hematopoiesis.

A number of diagnostic tests, including splenic volume estimates using ultrasound evaluations and assays of BM progenitor cells (erythroid or megakaryocyte), have been suggested as useful means of differentiating reactive thrombocytosis from ET (see Table 68-5). Insufficient numbers of patients, as well as a lack of long-term follow-up, make it impossible to assess the clinical value of such tests. As outlined earlier, the most important step in improving the diagnosis of ET has been the identification of the *JAK2V617F* mutation in about 50% of patients with ET. The current availability of this relatively simple molecular test makes it easier to establish the diagnosis of ET, although the utility of the test is limited by suboptimal negative predictive value and lack of diagnostic specificity.

At times, it is impossible to define the cause of an individual patient's thrombocytosis. In an asymptomatic patient, the resolution of this problem is easy: one should simply provide follow-up and determine whether the degree of thrombocytosis increases. If additional clues to the cause of the thrombocytosis are subsequently revealed, a diagnosis will become apparent. In a patient with thrombohemorrhagic difficulties, one must make a presumptive diagnosis of the cause of the thrombocytosis and then, after weighing the benefits versus the risks of various treatment plans, determine whether reduction of platelet numbers or simple observation is indicated. Some reassurance is provided by reports of larger cohorts of patients, each with platelet counts of greater than 1000×10^9/L, have been followed for years. Virtually none of the patients with reactive thrombocytosis developed a cerebrovascular accident, thrombophlebitis, or a peripheral arterial thrombosis.

PROGNOSIS

The probability that a patient with ET will survive 10 years ranges from 64% to 80%. In a large study from Spain with extensive follow-up, there was no substantial difference between the probability of survival of patients with ET and that of a control population. However, a study of 322 consecutive patients seen at the Mayo Clinic and followed for a median follow-up of 13.6 years showed a different pattern. Survival of patients with ET was similar to that of the control population during the first decade of disease, but the survival became significantly worse thereafter. Multivariable analysis identified an age at diagnosis of 60 years or older, leukocytosis, tobacco use, and diabetes mellitus as independent predictors of poor survival. The risk of developing leukemia or MF was low in the first 10 years (1.4% and 3.8%, respectively) but increased substantially in the second (8.1% and 19.9%, respectively) and third (24.0% and 28.9%, respectively) decades of the disease. The presence of the *JAK2V617F* mutation did not influence either survival or the rate of leukemic transformation. The rate of leukemic transformation was, however, higher in patients with platelet counts above 1000×10^9/L and abnormal hemoglobin levels. The development of MF was heralded by the appearance of immature myeloid precursors and dacryocytes in the blood smear and increased serum lactate dehydrogenase levels followed by a reduction in platelet numbers and progressive splenomegaly. This does not represent an instance of misdiagnosis but rather the natural evolution of the underlying hematologic malignancy. In addition, some patients, especially women who are iron deficient, may have their erythrocytosis masked and thus may truly have PV, although with the finding of an elevated platelet count, a diagnosis of ET may have been made or patients with *JAK2V617F* positive are known not infrequently to evolve to a picture that resembles PV as has been previously discussed.

A major determinant of the prognosis of a patient with a presumptive diagnosis of ET depends on the discrimination of whether such patients actually have true ET or an early form of MF based on histopathologic and clinical criteria adopted by the WHO (see Table 68-3).[24] Although some investigators believe that these histopathologic criteria cannot be widely implemented because of interobserver differences, the recent examination of large numbers of cases in a blinded fashion has shed some light on the clinical significance of the implementation of the WHO criteria. In a group of 891 patients with a prior diagnosis of ET with BM biopsies evaluated retrospectively histopathologically, 16% were reclassified as having an early or prefibrotic form of MF. Thrombosis rates and *JAK2V617F* positivity were similar in the two groups. However, patients with an early form of MF had higher leukocyte counts, lower hemoglobin levels, higher platelet counts, higher lactic dehydrogenase levels, greater numbers of circulating $CD34^+$, cells and a greater incidence of palpable splenomegaly than patients with true ET. Survival was reported to be significantly inferior for those patients with the early form of PMF compared with patients with histopathologically validated ET (Fig. 68-4). In one series with a median follow-up of approximately 7 years, the median survival of patients with ET ranged from 16 to 21 years, and the survival of the patients with the early form of MF ranged from 10.8 to 14.4 years with the majority of deaths being attributed to progression to overt PMF and acute leukemia. Although the patients with ET enjoyed a more favorable outcome, the 15-year cumulative incidences of overt MF and acute leukemia were still 9.3% and 2.1%, respectively, emphasizing the seriousness of this diagnosis, especially in younger patients.

Death of ET patients predominantly results from thrombotic complications, but transformation to AML is an important cause of mortality. The phenotype of the blast cell can be myeloid, myelomonocytic, megakaryocytic, of mixed lineage, or even lymphoblastic. According to the data mentioned earlier, the risk of patients with ET transforming into acute leukemia is greater than that of normal individuals. This is a phenomenon shared with the other MPN. The risk of developing acute leukemia after treatment with hydroxyurea alone increases only slightly (3%–4%), but the sequential use of hydroxyurea with other cytotoxic agents, such as busulfan or pipobroman, significantly increases the risk of developing a secondary leukemia.

The development of acute leukemia is associated with a deletion of the short arm of chromosome 17, which is most frequently deleted in hydroxyurea-treated patients, but a trisomy of the long-arm of chromosome 1 and monosomy 7q has been observed in patients treated with pipobroman. These cytogenetic abnormalities are believed to be induced by the use of these chemotherapeutic agents. The median survival after the development of myelodysplasia or leukemic transformation is 4 months. Acute leukemia, which develops after ET, is frequently refractory to standard induction chemotherapy but has been recently reported to be responsive to hypomethylating agents, including 5-azacytidine and decitabine. Because allogeneic stem cell transplantation can be curative, rapid referral to a transplant center is recommended if the patient has an appropriate performance status and an allogeneic stem cell donor is available.

THERAPY

The goal in treating patients with ET is to prevent additional thrombotic and hemorrhagic events without increasing the risk of transformation to post-ET MF or AML. Both age (>60 years of age) and a history of a prior thrombosis are predictors of a patient developing additional thrombotic events during follow-up (Table 68-6). Other predictors of cardiovascular morbidity include a history of smoking, hypertension, diabetes mellitus, and congestive heart failure and a white blood cell count greater than 11 × 109/L. Ironically, patients with platelet counts greater than 1000 × 109 /L have a lower risk of

Table 68-6 Risk Factors for Thrombosis in 100 Patients With Essential Thrombocythemia

Risk Factor	Incidence of Thrombosis (% Patient-Yr)	Relative Risk (95% CI)	P
Age (yr)			
<40	1.7	1.0*	
40–60	6.3	3.9 (0.7–21.5)	NS
>60	15.1	10.3 (2.1–51.5)	<.001
Previous Thrombosis			
No	3.4	1.0*	<.0005
Yes	31.4	13.0 (4.1–1.5)	

Data from: Finazzi G, Barbui T: Risk-adapted therapy in essential thrombocythemia and polycythemia vera. *Blood Rev* 19:243, 2005.
CI, Confidence interval; *NS*, not significant.
*Reference category.

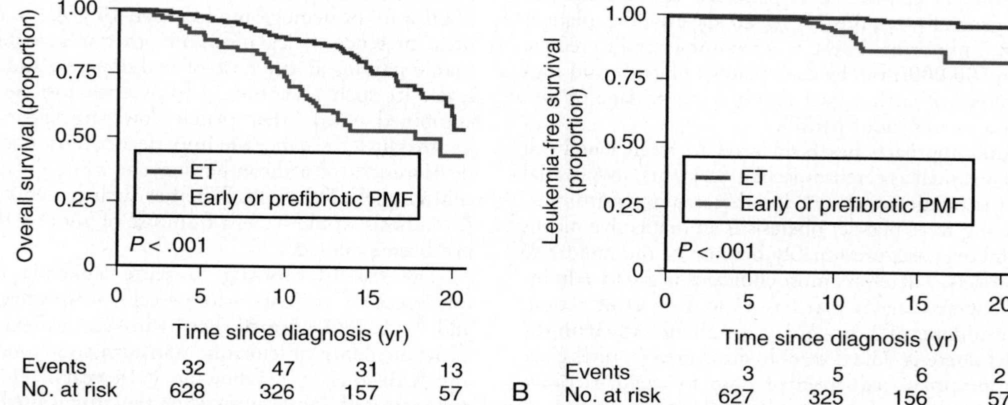

Figure 68-4 Overall **(A)** and leukemia-free **(B)** survival of patients with true essential thrombocythemia (ET) versus early or prefibrotic primary myelofibrosis (PMF). *(Data from Barbui T, Thiele J, Passamonti F, et al: Survival and disease progression in essential thrombocythemia are significantly influenced by accurate morphologic diagnosis: An international study.* J Clin Oncol *29:3179, 2011.)*

developing an arterial thrombosis. These parameters have been widely used by clinicians to stratify ET patients according to their risk for developing additional thrombotic events. Such stratification strategies have been used to make decisions on the need to use agents that are capable of reducing platelet counts. It is important to emphasize that such risk factors have been identified based on retrospective analyses of registries of ET patients that have largely not been created using modern molecular and histopathologic diagnostic tools. Using such patient stratification strategies, patients have been placed into high-, intermediate-, or low-risk groups based on their predicted risk of developing an additional life-threatening thrombotic event. This strategy is uniformly implemented throughout Europe and North America. The benefit of this strategy is based on a single clinical trial that indicated that the reduction of platelet numbers to less than 600 × 109/L with hydroxyurea therapy was associated with a reduction of developing additional thrombotic events compared with a control group (see Fig. 68-1). This study involved a total of 114 patients, and the median follow-up period was only 27 months.[25] Greater degrees of platelet suppression have not been shown to be associated with further reduction in the possibility of developing a thrombotic episode, which in hydroxyurea-treated high risk patients has been reported to be 1.66% patients per year. Although the implementation of such a strategy is widely accepted, it is important to be aware that this approach is not based on robust data that one associates with modern day evidence-based medicine. In fact, in several studies, an elevated leukocyte count of above 11 × 109/L has been more closely associated with the risk of developing additional thromboses than the degree of elevation of the platelet count. These conflicting reports in the literature among experts in this field makes it increasingly more difficult to be dogmatic about who to treat with platelet-lowering agents. The risk stratification of patients should not be ignored, and patients with a life-threatening thrombosis or disabling symptoms because of microcirculatory problems should receive drugs that lower the platelet count, but it seems somewhat robotic to treat every individual with ET older than 60 years of age with a similar strategy unless they have serious cardiovascular comorbidities. Obviously, if a patient of any age has excessive thrombocytosis and a thrombotic or hemorrhagic event, that patient must be treated, but for asymptomatic ET patients in so-called high-risk categories, the decision to embark upon a strategy including platelet-lowering agents is in reality a murky one that is more based on personal treatment decisions than volumes of data.

The treatment of asymptomatic low-risk patients with ET is controversial and remains largely problematic, yet greater insight into the management of such patients has recently been gained. Management of ET patients with life-threatening hemorrhagic or thrombotic episodes is more straightforward. Life-threatening thrombotic events require platelet pheresis in combination with the institution of myelosuppressive therapy. In this situation, immediate physical removal of large numbers of platelets is preferred because chemotherapeutic agents generally require 18 to 20 days before platelet counts can be reduced to normal levels. It is recommended to reduce the platelet count to 500,000/mm^3 by each platelet pheresis and suggested that achievement of such a goal requires the passage of two blood volumes over a 3- to 4-hour period.

Such a therapeutic approach has been used to treat acutely ill patients with problems, such as cerebrovascular accidents, myocardial infarction, transient ischemic attacks, or life-threatening gastrointestinal hemorrhage. Long-term platelet pheresis is an ineffective means of controlling thrombocytosis, presumably because of the rapid rate of production of platelets. Therefore, most clinicians begin by administering a chemotherapeutic agent that has a rapid onset of action, such as hydroxyurea at doses of 2 to 4 g/day, simultaneously with the institution of platelet pheresis. The dose of hydroxyurea requires close monitoring with appropriate reduction of dose to avoid excessive myelosuppression.

In patients found to have ET and who are clearly symptomatic and fall into the high-risk group, little controversy exists as to the need for lowering platelet numbers. The large number of thrombotic complications that occur in patients with ET who smoke points to the urgent need for these patients to stop smoking immediately. Most investigators try to normalize the platelet count or to reach a platelet count at which the symptoms of the high-risk patient resolve. Although major bleeding episodes requiring hospitalizations are rare, patients with extreme thrombocytosis (>1500 × 10^9/L), acquired von Willebrand syndrome, and history of hemorrhagic episode are clearly at risk for developing additional bleeding complications. These patients require reduction of the increased platelet numbers to the normal range with use of a variety of agents, including hydroxyurea, anagrelide, or INF-α. According to some authors, such patients should avoid exposure to aspirin even if they have hemorrhagic complications and thrombotic episodes simultaneously.

Another situation that requires treatment is discomfort caused by erythromelalgia or progression of erythromelalgia to frank gangrene. Such patients respond within days to low-dose aspirin therapy or platelet reduction therapy.

During the 1980s and 1990s, hydroxyurea became the drug of choice for the treatment of ET. The impetus for this practice was based on the knowledge that agents such as ^{32}P and alkylating agents such as melphalan and busulfan were leukemogenic. The popularity of the ribonucleoside reductase inhibitor, hydroxyurea, for the management of ET was due to the belief in the early 1970s that it was nonleukemogenic. Hydroxyurea can be administered at a dose of 15 mg/kg initially with adjustment of the dose to maintain a platelet count (at the least) below 600 × 10^9/L without inducing significant neutropenia. After the agent is started, frequent monitoring of blood counts is mandatory to avoid the development of neutropenia until the maintenance dose is determined. The use of this drug in a high-risk group of patients with reduction of platelet numbers to less than 600 × 10^9/L has resulted in reduction of thrombotic events compared with a control population. The reduction of platelet numbers to this level did not entirely eliminate the occurrence of additional thrombotic episodes.

Hydroxyurea use is associated with some toxicity, including dose-related neutropenia, nausea, stomatitis, hair loss, nail discoloration, and lower extremity and oral ulcerations as well as squamous cell carcinoma of the skin. Many of these problems resolve with withdrawal of the drug or dose reduction, but leg ulcers can be persistent, sometimes requiring skin grafting. These ulcers typically heal within 1 to 9 months of cessation of therapy. Such leg ulcers have been reported to occur in 9% of patients treated with hydroxyurea and are an indication for immediate discontinuation of therapy and elimination of any rechallenge with the drug. Hydroxyurea is also not universally successful in controlling the thrombocytosis; resistance to hydroxyurea has been reported in 11% to 17% of cases. The criteria for defining resistance or intolerance to hydroxyurea have been established by an International Working Group. They include a platelet count greater than 600 × 10^9/L after 3 months of at least 2 g/day of hydroxyurea (2.5 g/day in patients with a body weight >80 kg); platelet count greater than 400 × 10^9/L and WBC less than 2500/mm^3 or hemoglobin less than 10 g/dL at any dose of hydroxyurea; presence of leg ulcers or other unacceptable mucocutaneous manifestations at any dose of hydroxyurea; and hydroxyurea-related fever. In such situations, hydroxyurea can be substituted for (or combined with) other platelet-lowering agents. These criteria for hydroxyurea resistance are imperfect because they do not include the development of a thrombotic event while on therapy, which is the central goal of therapy. Whether such patients who develop a new thrombosis would benefit from use of another therapeutic agent has not been explored.

The risk of evolving to acute leukemia is extremely low in untreated ET patients. More recent prospective studies both in ET and PV have confirmed that hydroxyurea therapy is associated with a low incidence of leukemic transformation when used alone (<5%) and with long-term follow-up (≤14 years). However, the leukemic risk increased significantly when the drug is used before or after treatment with alkylating agents, particularly busulfan. One can conclude from these studies that hydroxyurea therapy alone is less leukemogenic than alkylating agents or P^{32} alone, but a small increased risk for the development of leukemia secondary to its use can not be completely excluded. Of concern is the observation that a high proportion of the AMLs and myelodysplastic disorders occurring in ET patients treated with hydroxyurea alone have morphologic, cytogenetic, and molecular characteristics of the 17p deletion syndrome. These patients are reported to have a typical form of dysgranulopoiesis characterized by hypolobulated polymorphonuclear leukocytes with small vacuoles in neutrophils and p53 mutations.

An alternative to hydroxyurea is therapy with anagrelide. Data on the use of anagrelide in ET suggest that it is nonleukemogenic when used in patients with ET. When considering the risk-to-benefit ratio, one can conclude that hydroxyurea therapy is first-line therapy for ET patients at a high risk of developing an additional thrombosis, including those older than 60 years of age or with a history of a thrombotic episode or with significant other cardiovascular risk factors. Such nonleukemogenic drugs as INF-α, anagrelide, or pegylated INF appear to be good choices in symptomatic patients younger than 40 years of age.

Anagrelide is a member of the imidazo (2,1-b)quinazolin-2-1 series of compounds. When studied in humans, it was noted that anagrelide in small doses produced thrombocytopenia. The drug acts primarily by reducing megakaryocyte size and ploidy and decreasing megakaryocyte proliferation. Anagrelide therefore appears to lower platelet counts primarily by interfering with the development of megakaryocytes. Anagrelide suppresses megakaryocytopoiesis by selectively reducing the expression levels of GATA-1,FLI-1,NFE-2, and FOG-1 in cells belonging to the megakaryocytic lineage.[26] The effects of anagrelide do not involve thrombopoietin-mediated signal transduction events. GATA-1 and FOG-1 play critical roles in megakaryocytic differentiation. Anagrelide in low doses is effective in lowering the platelet count in 93% of patients. Most importantly, it is effective despite resistance to prior therapies. Resistance to anagrelide therapy has not been documented, but occasionally patients have been observed to require extraordinarily high doses to control the excessive thrombocytosis. The recommended initial dose is 0.5 mg orally two to four times a day. The dose should be increased by 0.5 mg/wk to control thrombocythemia. The dose of anagrelide should not exceed 10 mg/day or 2 mg/dose. Excessive use will result in predictable thrombocytopenia and increase the likelihood of side effects. The median maintenance dose in patients with ET is 2 mg/day administered in divided doses. Data on more than 3000 patients with a variety of MPNs complicated by extreme thrombocytosis are available. In addition, follow-up of more than 500 patients for more than 5 years had been reported. Anagrelide has been shown to be an effective drug in the treatment of ET, resulting in a median time to response of 2.5 to 4 weeks. An effect on platelet numbers is usually noted in 6 to 10 days. Anagrelide leads to a reduction in hematocrit in 36% of patients, but it has no effect on white blood cell numbers, systemic symptoms, or the degree of splenomegaly. In a long-term study of 35 young patients (17-48 years) followed for a median of 10.8 years (range, 7-15.5 years), more than 3-g/dL decreases in hemoglobin level were reported in eight cases (24%). Most important, the reduction in platelet numbers attributed to anagrelide use has been reported to be associated with a decrease in symptoms attributable to the thrombocythemia. Anagrelide use in 1700 patients reduced the incidence of thrombohemorrhagic episodes related to thrombocytosis associated with MPNs from 0.66 symptoms per patient before therapy to 0.07 symptoms per patient after 28 to 30 months of therapy.

The most common side effects of anagrelide resulted from its vasodilatory and positive inotropic actions. These effects resulted in complaints of headache, dizziness, fluid retention, palpitations, and high-output cardiac failure. The vasodilatory effect leads to reduced renal blood flow, resulting in fluid retention. In addition, gastrointestinal complications, such as nausea, abdominal pain, and diarrhea, are prominent. These side effects usually develop within 2 weeks of initiation of therapy and frequently diminish in severity or resolve within 2 weeks of continued therapy. Because of its ability to promote fluid retention and the development of tachyarrhythmias, anagrelide therapy should be used with caution in patients with cardiac disease and should be administered carefully to elderly patients. If congestive heart failure or arrhythmias other than tachycardia develop, anagrelide therapy should be discontinued. Prolonged anagrelide therapy may be associated with a potentially irreversible drug-induced cardiomyopathy that is reminiscent of tachycardia-induced cardiomyopathy. Dose reduction can be used to lessen the degree of tachycardia or fluid retention. Before the institution of anagrelide, it is recommended that a basic cardiac evaluation be performed, including an assessment of cardiac risk factors, a careful cardiac history, and an electrocardiogram, which can be used as a baseline if the patient develops rhythm disturbances. Patients should avoid caffeine if feasible because it might trigger palpitations. Acetaminophen may be useful for treatment of the headaches. The carrier for the anagrelide is lactose, and patients who develop nausea, diarrhea, and abdominal pain with anagrelide therapy are frequently lactase deficient, and the use of LactAid results in resolution of such symptoms. Although most adverse effects are mild or moderate, in one series, therapy was discontinued in 16% of patients because of intolerable side effects, especially headache, nausea, fluid retention, and, rarely, frank congestive heart failure. Anagrelide has no mutagenic activity, but its use is not currently advised during pregnancy. Because of its small molecular weight, it is believed to be capable of crossing the placenta and thus may lead to fetal thrombocytopenia. Anagrelide does not appear to be leukemogenic. Anagrelide therefore appears to be a suitable drug for the treatment of young, symptomatic patients with ET and for those who are resistant or refractory to front-line treatment with hydroxyurea.

The approval of anagrelide for ET patients was based on the completion of phase 2 trials, and its superiority to the standard of care was never validated by the performance of a randomized phase 3 trial until recently. Hydroxyurea and anagrelide have now been compared head to head in a large randomized trial of 809 high-risk patients with ET, all treated also with low-dose aspirin (75 mg/day).[27] Overall, patients randomized to anagrelide (and aspirin) were more likely to reach the composite primary end point of major thrombosis (arterial or venous), major hemorrhage, or death from vascular causes (P = .03) (Fig. 68-5). When individual end points were assessed, arterial thrombosis, major hemorrhage, and the development of MF were all significantly more frequent in patients treated with anagrelide (P = .004, .008, and .01, respectively). Anagrelide and aspirin seemed to offer at least partial protection from thrombosis because the prevalence of thrombotic events (8% at 2 years) was significantly less than

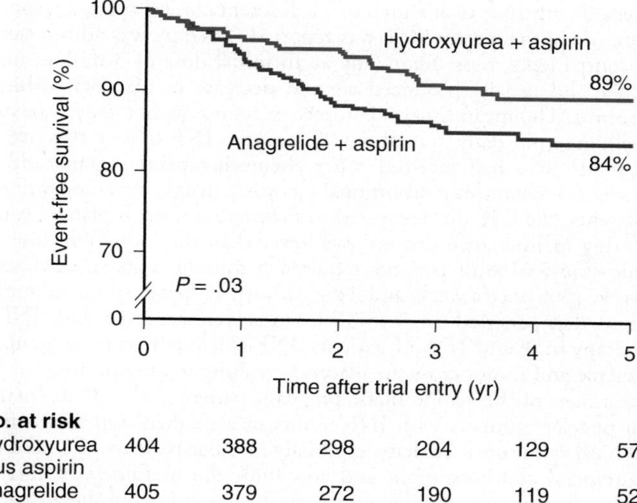

No. at risk						
Hydroxyurea plus aspirin	404	388	298	204	129	57
Anagrelide plus aspirin	405	379	272	190	119	52

Figure 68-5 EVENT-FREE SURVIVAL IN A HYDROXYUREA-TREATED GROUP COMPARED WITH AN ANAGRELIDE-TREATED GROUP. Primary end points were arterial or venous thrombosis, serious hemorrhage, or death from any of these causes. *(From Harrison CN, Campbell PJ, Buck G, et al: Hydroxyurea compared with anagrelide in high-risk essential thrombocythemia.* N Engl J Med *353:33, 2005.)*

Table 68-7 Choice of Drugs for Treatment of Patients With High-Risk Essential Thrombocythemia

Age (yr)	Treatment of Choice	Second Line
<50	Interferon	Anagrelide Hydroxyurea
50–75	Hydroxyurea	Interferon Anagrelide
>75	Hydroxyurea	Anagrelide Busulfan

that observed in the control arm of a previous study (28%). Intriguingly, the number of venous thromboses was less frequent in patients treated with anagrelide (P = .006). In addition patients with *JAK2V617F*-positive ET were more sensitive to therapy with hydroxyurea but not anagrelide. Also, the incidence of discontinuation of anagrelide therapy because of drug-related adverse events was significantly greater than that observed with patients receiving hydroxyurea. Based on this large randomized study, hydroxyurea is presently considered first-line therapy for patients with high-risk ET (Table 68-7). Although equivalent control of the platelet count was achieved with both agents, hydroxyurea proved superior, perhaps because of its ability to reduce not only platelet numbers but also leukocyte numbers, which have been associated with thrombosis in ET patients. In addition, the combination of anagrelide and low-dose aspirin was associated with a higher incidence of bleeding episodes, suggesting that aspirin therapy might be best avoided in patients being treated with anagrelide.

Interferon-α has been used to treat the thrombocytosis associated with MPN with increasing frequency since the 1990s. INF-α acts by directly inhibiting megakaryocyte colony formation and secondarily by inhibiting the expression of thrombopoietic-stimulating cytokines, such as GM-CSF, G-CSF, IL-3, and IL-11 and by stimulating the production of negative regulators of megakaryocytopoiesis, such as IL-1ra (receptor agonist) and macrophage inflammatory protein 1 (MIP-1a). INF-α inhibits thrombopoiesis by suppressing thrombopoietin-induced phosphorylation of the *JAK2* substrates, MPL and STAT5. Furthermore, INF-α also induces the production of suppressor of cytokine signalling-1 (SOCS-1), which inhibits thrombopoietin-mediated cell proliferation. In a total of 212 patients treated with INF-α in a total of 11 different clinical trials, a response rate of approximately 90% was reported. Therapy was administered to outpatients, most frequently at an initial dose of 3 million units daily, and usually produced a rapid decrease in platelets within 2 months. The mean time to complete response with a daily dose of 3 million units daily was about 3 months. INF-α was effective in patients who had received other chemotherapeutic agents and in patients resistant to conventional cytotoxic drugs. In the majority of patients, the INF dose required to maintain a normal platelet count during maintenance therapy was lower than the induction dose. In one study, 61% of patients required 3 million units three times a week, 15% once a week, and 24% daily. In addition, sustained remissions that persisted for 3 to 36 months were achieved with INF-α therapy in 9% to 16% of patients. INF-α is reported to be nonmutagenic and to not cross the placenta, making it a useful drug for the treatment of the symptomatic pregnant patient with ET. Reduction in platelet numbers with INF results in a marked improvement in clinical symptoms. Toxicity, especially in older patients, the need for parenteral administration, and cost limit the usefulness of INF-α. Side effects include flulike symptoms during induction therapy, such as fever, bone and muscle pain, fatigue, lethargy, and depression. Symptoms are frequently controlled with acetaminophen. Long-term administration of INF-α can result in mild weight loss; alopecia; retinal abnormalities; rarely, a reversible form of sarcoidosis and a reversible form of left-sided heart failure; and the development of autoimmune conditions, including thyroiditis leading to hypothyroidism and autoimmune hemolytic anemia. Patients may develop neutralizing antibodies to recombinant INF, leading to a concomitant rise in platelet numbers. In such a situation, use of leukocyte INF-α results in an excellent response. In one review, it was reported that 25% of 273 patients failed to continue to receive INF therapy either because of poor compliance or side effects.

A semisynthetic protein polymer conjugate of INF-α 2b, pegylated INF (PEG-IFNa2b), was anticipated to be superior to unmodified INF as related to its adverse event profile and efficacy when used to treat ET patients. This formulation of INF provides prolonged activity that permits once-weekly dosing. Normalization of blood counts occurred after a median time of 2 to 3 months; 12% of patients discontinued therapy because of inability to tolerate the drug, and 17% did not achieve normalization of their platelet counts. The majority of side effects were WHO grade 1 or 2, although some encountered grade 3 toxicity, primarily fatigue and flulike symptoms. More importantly, no thromboembolic or hemorrhagic complications occurred during the period of treatment, although 12 thrombotic events occurred in 42 patients (24%) in the 24 months before the institution of therapy. This form of INF, however, appears to lead to a similar frequency and severity of side effects during long-term use as experienced with conventional INFs. Interestingly, the use of another pegylated form of INF (peg-IFNα-2a) in patients with PV was able to decrease the percentage of mutated *JAK2* allele in 24 of 27 treated patients from a mean of 49% to a mean of 27%. The use of this form of INF appeared to be associated with fewer side effects than standard forms of INF or peg-IFNa-2b. This form of pegylated IFN has been used to treat approximately 40 patients with ET with more than 75% of patients achieving a complete hematologic remission.[28] Almost 40% of patients with *JAK2V617F*-positive ET had a reduction in their *JAK2V617F* allele burden with occasional patients no longer having detectable *JAK2V617F*, leading to their being classified as having achieved a complete molecular remission. Although hematologic remissions were frequently achieved after 3 months of therapy, the effects on *JAK2V617F* were observed after 6 months of treatment. Most patients were successfully treated with 45 to 90 μg/weekly, and 22% of patients ceased therapy because of toxicity. Surprisingly, the hematologic and molecular responses persist for a number of months after discontinuation of therapy, suggesting that intermittent therapy may be an acceptable means of chronically administering this drug. No data indicating whether IFN therapy delays or prevents the evolution to MF are available. To gain a more comprehensive assessment of the clinical usefulness of INF-α, a prospective clinical trial comparing INF-α with hydroxyurea in patients with ET is underway at numerous sites in North America and Europe. Until the results of this trial are available, INF-α or anagrelide should be considered as reasonable alternatives to hydroxyurea in a patient younger than 40 years of age who has had a previous thrombotic episode (see Table 68-7), but which drug is the standard of care in so-called high-risk patients will require data emanating from the randomized trial. Although many clinicians have presumed that IFN will prove to be the superior agent, this conclusion is clearly premature and is based on small phase 2 trials. One should keep in mind that at the initiation of the randomized trial comparing hydroxyurea with anagrelide, most participants presumed that anagrelide would be the optimal therapy, which was disproven. The present randomized trial comparing IFN with hydroxyurea is therefore of utmost importance to provide the evidence for what the standard of care should be. A number of small molecule inhibitors of *JAK2* have been evaluated for the treatment of ET patients. These agents reproducibly lower platelet counts, but the definition of the appropriate role of such agents in the treatment of ET patients will require their careful evaluation in well-controlled clinical trials.

The use of platelet antiaggregating agents remains an important area of investigation. Patients with ET have an increased predisposition to hemorrhage, which is likely potentiated by the use of drugs that affect platelet function. Transient ischemic attacks and erythromelalgia associated with ET respond rapidly to aspirin alone. In erythromelalgia, symptoms disappear for 2 to 4 days after administration of a single dose of aspirin. Although these agents surely have a role in the treatment of these specific complications, their use should be pursued with extreme caution because of the increased risk of hemorrhage. Kessler et al have determined that 32% of bleeding episodes in patients with extreme thrombocytosis and MPN occurred concurrently with the use of antiinflammatory agents.

Low-dose aspirin therapy has been uniformly recommended for virtually all patients with ET independent of their risk of developing a thrombotic event.[29] These recommendations are somewhat surprising because they are based on 2 clinical trials of the effects of low-dose aspirin therapy in PV patients, and such a trial with aspirin has never been performed with a population of ET patients. Furthermore, an independent analysis of the data from these two trials by the Cochrane Collaboration indicated that the use of low-dose aspirin therapy was associated with a statistically nonsignificant reduction in the risk of fatal thrombotic events and was not associated with an increased risk of bleeding episodes. Furthermore, after a retrospective study of 198 patients with low-risk ET, Alvarez-Larrán et al[30] concluded that antiplatelet therapy did not reduce the incidence of thrombotic events and might increase the bleeding risk if platelet counts are greater than 1000×10^9/L or aspirin is used in patients with a bleeding history (Table 68-8). Aspirin should be used with caution in patients with peptic ulcer disease. Such patients who require aspirin benefit from the concurrent use of a proton pump inhibitor such as omeprazole rather than switching them to clopidogrel. This more critical evaluation of the evidence supporting the indiscriminate use of aspirin therapy in ET patients requires serious reconsideration of this practice. In patients who absolutely require aspirin therapy, one should avoid the simultaneous administration of aspirin with a nonsteroidal antiinflammatory drug (NSAID) such as ibuprofen or naproxen because such NSAIDs are known to compete with aspirin for a common binding site on COX-1 that prevents aspirin from gaining access to and acetylating its target serine. This antagonism can be overcome by separating the time of administration of these two agents. The judicious use of aspirin in patients with a history of a thrombotic episode seems reasonable, but low-dose aspirin therapy must be restricted to patients with platelet counts of less than 1500 $\times 10^9$/L and not be used in patients receiving anagrelide therapy unless they have experienced an arterial thrombotic event. The diagnosis of acquired von Willebrand syndrome should be excluded before aspirin use and considered a contraindication to the use of aspirin. Whether all patients with low-risk ET should be uniformly treated with aspirin remains speculative because prospective randomized clinical trials including appropriate numbers of patients so as to assure the resolution of this dilemma have not been completed to date.

A continuing clinical controversy revolves around the question of whether any treatment is indicated in patients with ET in whom the platelet count elevation is initially detected fortuitously and who remain largely asymptomatic. Such a decision is particularly important because the use of most chemotherapeutic agents is associated with an increased risk of the development of leukemia, and the use of platelet antiaggregating agents is not without risk. The need for such treatment can be questioned because in several studies, a relationship between the frequency of thrombotic episodes and degree of platelet elevation has not been established. One should not lapse into a false sense of security in deferring therapy, however, because the course of ET can include infrequent but dangerous thromboembolic complications, and patients may function normally for long periods of time without experiencing a life-threatening event. In a retrospective study of 99 consecutive low-risk ET patients (age younger than 60 years) who presented with extreme thrombocytosis (platelet count $>1000 \times 10^9$/L) but without a previous history of thrombohemorrhagic complications, the incidence of major thrombosis and hemorrhagic events was shown to be similar during follow-up to those who were treated with prophylactic cytoreductive therapy and those who did not receive such therapy. If the clinician feels compelled to use some therapeutic intervention in young, asymptomatic patients, low-dose aspirin (81 mg/day) appears to be effective in the treatment of microvascular complications, and its use is associated with limited toxicity. Still, it seems reasonable to withhold therapy in younger, asymptomatic patients until the development of a clinically significant thrombotic or hemorrhagic event. Patients older than 60 years of age with other significant risk factors for cardiovascular complications are probably best served by immediate institution of therapy.

The management of pregnant patients with ET remains problematic.[18] The major goal of any therapeutic intervention in pregnant patients with ET should be the prevention of the vasoocclusive events that lead to placental infarction; intrauterine fetal growth retardation; and, in some cases, fetal death. Patients with *JAK2V617F*-positive ET are at a higher risk of developing such complications. In one large series, there was no significant relationship between the fetal outcome and the degree of maternal thrombocytosis or the presence of disease complications. In this series, there were no instances of excessive bleeding or other related complications during delivery. This group did not recommend the use of therapeutic platelet pheresis and, in fact, claimed that specific therapy (aspirin, heparin, or platelet pheresis) did not alter the clinical course. However, of the many patients reported in the literature who did not receive any therapy, a significant number experienced either spontaneous abortion or intrauterine deaths. Low-dose aspirin (81 mg/day), because of its profound effect on events involving the microcirculation, such as erythromelalgia and transient ischemic events, has been used with increasing frequency in pregnant patients during the first and second trimesters. Low-dose aspirin therapy is safe in pregnant women. It is recommended that aspirin be discontinued at least 1 week before delivery to avoid bleeding complications such as an epidural hematoma during delivery or during the postpartum period. Because of the high risk of bleeding in patients with platelet counts greater than 1000×10^9/L with acquired von Willebrand syndrome, aspirin therapy is contraindicated. There is limited experience reported in the literature with aspirin therapy alone, and although the results are promising, the sample size is too small to confirm a beneficial effect. The observed true birth rate, however, was 75% in those receiving aspirin compared with 43% in the group in the literature who received no therapy. Aspirin therapy has, however, recently been found to be ineffective in preventing complications in *JAK2V617F*-positive pregnant ET patients. Chemotherapeutic drugs should be avoided during the period of conception and especially during the first trimester. Both

Table 68-8 Outcome in Patients With Low-Risk Essential Thrombocythemia Followed With Careful Observation or Treated With Antiplatelet Therapy

	Observation (848 Person-Years)		Antiplatelet therapy (802 Person-Years)		
	Events (*n*)	Incidence Rate (95% CI)	Events (*n*)	Incidence Rate (95% CI)	*P*
Thrombosis (arterial and venous)	15	17.7 (107–29.3)	17	21.2 (13.2–34.1)	.6
Arterial thrombosis	8	9.4 (4.7–18.9)	13	16.2 (9.4–27.9)	.2
Venous thrombosis	7	8.2 (3.9–17.3)	4	4.9 (1.9–13.3)	.4
Bleeding	5	6.0 (2.5–14.5)	10	12.6 (6.8–23.4)	.09

From Alvarez-Larrán A, Cervantes F, Pereira A, et al: Observation versus antiplatelet therapy as primary prophylaxis for thrombosis in low-risk essential thrombocythemia. *Blood* 116:1205, 2010.

hydroxyurea and busulfan are known teratogens in animal models. In addition, busulfan and hydroxyurea reduce fertility in men. Because the greatest risk of thrombosis is postpartum, thrombosis prophylaxis should be initiated in the form of low-molecular-weight heparin and low-dose aspirin after delivery unless the patient is hemorrhaging. These measures should be continued for 6 weeks. Mothers receiving INF, anagrelide, or hydroxyurea should refrain from breastfeeding.

With the availability of INF to treat ET, it is difficult to justify the use of chemotherapeutic agents during the time of conception or during the first two trimesters of gestation. INF-α therapy is not known to be leukemogenic or teratogenic, and because it does not cross the placenta, its use may be considered during pregnancy. The manufacturers of INF-α still advise that INF-α not be used during pregnancy because adverse effects on the fetus cannot be ruled out. The effect of INF-α on male fertility remains uncertain. Anagrelide therapy should be avoided in pregnant patients because of its potential to lead to fetal thrombocytopenia.

Because none of the strategies described earlier has been tested in large clinical trials, one must develop a therapeutic strategy for an individual pregnant patient. In a patient who lacks a history of spontaneous abortions and who is totally asymptomatic but is found to be pregnant, no therapy is presently indicated, although low-dose aspirin therapy (81 mg/day) can be initiated without appreciable risk and can be continued throughout the pregnancy. Its use should be discontinued 1 week before delivery. Aspirin therapy is contraindicated in patients with platelet counts greater than $1500 \times 10^9/L$ and patients with acquired von Willebrand syndrome. If a patient has experienced a thrombohemorrhagic episode or if the platelet count is rising to levels above $1500 \times 10^9/L$, therapy with a platelet-reducing agent is indicated. Platelet pheresis therapy can be attempted in selected patients, but if incomplete control is obtained, INF-α therapy is, at this point, the best option. Several successful pregnancies have been observed in patients receiving INF-α therapy. Patients with a history of a previous spontaneous abortion appear to be at a particularly high risk of developing subsequent spontaneous abortions if left untreated. At the minimum, low-dose aspirin therapy in this patient population is a reasonable therapeutic approach.

Hormone replacement therapy including oral contraceptives and estrogen replacement hormone therapy remains controversial in patients with ET. Each of these agents in the normal population is associated with an increased incidence of arterial and venous thrombosis. Intuitively, it would seem wise to avoid such agents in patients with ET who are already at an increased risk of developing thrombosis. Gangat et al retrospectively reviewed the consequences of such hormonal interventions in 305 women. Oral contraceptive therapy was associated with a high incidence of venous thrombosis occurring within the abdominal cavity, but estrogen replacement hormone therapy in menopausal women did not appear to be associated with an increased incidence of thrombosis. This observation is surprising and might be a consequence of the limited numbers of patients included within this study.

If a patient with ET develops a thrombotic episode, anticoagulation with low-molecular-weight heparin and then transition to an oral anticoagulant is recommended. The thrombotic episode places a patient into a high-risk group in which myelosuppressive therapy is clearly indicated. Whether patients should have lifelong anticoagulation or should receive only 6 to 12 months of anticoagulation after they are in a complete hematologic remission has not been investigated in a systematic fashion. Because the data necessary to make this decision are not available, this decision can only be made at the discretion of the treating physician. In one small series of patients with an MPN and Budd-Chiari syndrome from a single center, long-term anticoagulation was successfully avoided by treating these patients without oral anticoagulants but with chronic hydroxyurea and aspirin therapy. Whether such an approach is really optimal requires a more systematic randomized clinical trial. Antiplatelet therapy has been shown to reduce the risks of deep venous thrombosis and of pulmonary embolism in a variety of high-risk groups. In patients who have a new thrombosis while they are in complete hematologic remission and are optimally anticoagulated, some consideration should be given to adding low-dose aspirin if the risk of hemorrhage is not excessive.

FUTURE DIRECTIONS

Essential thrombocythemia is a hematologic malignancy with its own distinct clinical manifestations and associated complications. Better means of identifying patients at risk for developing fatal thrombotic or hemorrhagic complications are necessary to provide the basis with which to develop the optimal care of such patients. The ability to reduce the incidence of thrombohemorrhagic episodes with cytoreductive therapy in high-risk patients is well established.

Multi-institutional studies comparing the efficacy of such promising agents as INF-α or pegylated INF for the treatment of high-risk patients compared with hydroxyurea are currently being pursued. The use of low-dose aspirin therapy to reduce the number of episodes of erythromelalgia and transient ischemic attacks is widely practiced, but whether aspirin therapy should be indiscriminately used remains a subject of dispute that will only be resolved with the completion of appropriately powered clinical trials. Another pressing question that requires resolution is the degree of reduction of platelet or leukocyte numbers required for optimal management of ET patients.

Finally, the discovery of the *JAK2V617F* and MPL mutations have already had a major impact on disease classification during routine clinical practice. Diagnostic strategies have now incorporated screening for the *JAK2* and MPL mutations, although their prognostic significance remains to be clearly established. This new understanding of the molecular pathogenesis of MPN has led to the development of novel targeted therapies. The use of specific *JAK2* inhibitors for ET patients should be carefully studied in well-controlled clinical trials in which significant end points such as incidence of thrombosis, hemorrhage, and transformation to MF and acute leukemia are incorporated as end points. This is critical because the degree of reduction of platelet numbers has not served as a suitable biomarker for the development of these complications. The treatment of ET presently depends on the opinions of a small group of experts who develop treatment paradigms without the execution of randomized trials that are required for decisions to be made based on evidence. If this field is to progress, greater efforts toward the completion of well-powered clinical trials will be clearly necessary (see box on Personal Approach to Therapy of Essential Thrombocythemia).

Personal Approach to Therapy of Essential Thrombocythemia

The optimal therapy for patients with ET remains uncertain. Therapy is geared toward interventions to reduce the potential for developing thrombotic episodes. Patients with the greatest risk of developing a thrombus have a number of characteristics, including age 60 years or older, history of a thrombotic event, leukocytosis (WBC ≥11,000 × $10^9/L$), and cardiovascular risk factors (hypertension, hypercholesterolemia, diabetes mellitus, obesity). Patients with ET or prefibrotic form of MF can frequently present with elevated platelet counts and are treated in a similar fashion by us. No known therapy is available that is capable of reversing the BM fibrosis in such patients or delaying or eliminating evolution to MF. Certain concepts, however, apply to all patients. All patients with ET should stop smoking to minimize the risk factors associated with atherosclerotic disease. Indiscriminant use of high doses of NSAIDs should be avoided because this

Personal Approach to Therapy of Essential Thrombocythemia—cont'd

practice can lead to an increased risk of hemorrhage. Use of such agents is particularly frequent in elderly patients in whom ET is common. In patients with a life-threatening thrombotic or hemorrhagic episode, plateletpheresis should be initiated in addition to starting them on hydroxyurea therapy.

In high-risk patients, cytoreductive therapy has been shown to lessen the chance of developing additional thrombotic events with the reduction of extreme thrombocytosis to platelet counts below 600,000 × 10^9/L. High-risk patients include patients older than 60 years of age and patients with a history of a previous thrombotic episode, including erythromelalgia, transient ischemic attacks, or large vessel thrombosis. Even though this treatment philosophy has been considered common practice, the recommendation to treat patients older that the age of 60 years who have not experienced a thrombotic episode with cytoreductive therapy is not based on robust data from multiple randomized trials. Asymptomatic high-risk patients without cardiovascular risk factors may not necessarily benefit from this treatment, and the decision on how to treat them should be based on individual assessment.

At present, no therapy is indicated in asymptomatic patients younger than 60 years of age. If a patient has a platelet count greater than or equal to 1500 × 10^9/L and acquired von Willebrand syndrome with bleeding symptoms, platelet reduction therapy is indicated to avoid the high risk of hemorrhage. In totally asymptomatic patients with platelet counts greater than 1500 × 10^9/L, we frequently observe the patients and do not feel compelled to treat them. Patients with acquired von Willebrand syndrome should clearly avoid the use of aspirin.

In patients requiring platelet reduction therapy, the choice among the use of anagrelide, INF-α, pegylated INF, or hydroxyurea therapy is based on patient age, ease of administration, and drug-related toxicity. Randomized trials comparing these treatments in high-risk patients are ongoing. Until the results are available, we use the following strategy. In patients older than 50 years, hydroxyurea therapy is the treatment of choice, but in younger patients, we prefer to initiate therapy with INF-α. INF therapy should be avoided in patients with a history of depression, autoimmune disorders, or retinitis. If the patient cannot tolerate INF-α or it is not available, we feel comfortable treating symptomatic patients younger than 50 years of age with anagrelide or hydroxyurea. Although we remain concerned about the leukemogenic potential of hydroxyurea, the risk appears to be low if not associated with the prior use of an alkylating agent. The development of malleolar ulcers is a frequent complication of hydroxyurea treatment and is a signal for the elimination of hydroxyurea as a therapeutic agent for that particular patient.

Patients who initially receive hydroxyurea and no longer respond to this agent or experience toxicity and require another agent should not receive an alkylating agent. This sequence of administration is associated with an extremely high risk of leukemic transformation. Patients who have had a trial of hydroxyurea and require further treatment should receive either anagrelide, INF-α, or pegylated INF. Doses of each of these agents required for disease control will, of course, be dependent on the target platelet level that one hopes to achieve. Strict control to a platelet count of lower than 600 × 10^9/L does not appear to be necessary. In these patients, the addition of low-dose aspirin (81 mg/day) should be considered; it is less clear to us if patients who achieve better platelet control with cytoreductive therapy should also be so treated. However, in studies from Europe addressing this question in PV, the approach of combining aspirin with cytoreduction therapy appears to minimize thrombotic complications. The use of anagrelide and aspirin in combination should be avoided because of the high risk of a hemorrhage. In patients with thrombotic episodes, especially episodes involving the microcirculation or large vessels, we administer low-dose aspirin (81 mg/day). This dose of aspirin does increase the number of bleeding episodes to a modest degree but is effective in the treatment of thrombotic events. This low-dose aspirin therapy is given in addition to an agent, which reduces platelet numbers.

Hydroxyurea can be started at a dose of 1 g/day and then adjusted to achieve the target platelet count (≤600 × 10^9/L) without developing leukopenia. Anagrelide is initiated at 0.5 mg twice daily and increased by 0.5 mg/day every 5 to 7 days if platelet counts do not begin to drop. The usual dose to achieve platelet number control is 2.0 to 2.5 mg/day. Alternatively, combination therapy with anagrelide and hydroxyurea may be considered. Some patients do not tolerate either hydroxyurea or anagrelide. In this patient group, INF-α therapy is initiated at 3 million units three times per week subcutaneously or consideration to therapy with a pegylated form of interferon (peg-IFNα-2a) should be given. Another choice is busulfan at 4 mg/day for 2-week courses every time the platelet count rises above the normal range. Busulfan therapy is reserved for patients older than 70 years.

Complications even in young, otherwise healthy patients with platelet counts greater than 2000 × 10^9/L are unusual. However, these marked elevations of platelet numbers can be anxiety-provoking situations for the patient and the clinician.

In certain situations, in young, low-risk patients, treatment should be instituted. Surgery can increase the risk of thrombosis, and the use of antiinflammatory agents can increase the risk of bleeding postoperatively. Under these circumstances, the platelet count should be lowered to the normal range. In pregnant patients with ET, low-dose aspirin therapy is the first treatment option. If the patient develops symptoms as a result of thrombosis, platelet reduction therapy is necessary, and INF-α therapy is the treatment of choice.

In a patient with ET and a serious acute hemorrhagic event, the site of bleeding should be determined immediately, and any antiplatelet aggregating agents should be stopped. Although the platelet count may be high, these platelets should be considered to be qualitatively abnormal, leading to defective hemostasis. The patient may have acquired von Willebrand syndrome. In patients with acquired von Willebrand syndrome, DDAVP (desmopressin) or factor VIII concentrates containing von Willebrand factor can be used immediately at the same time chemotherapy is being administered. If acquired von Willebrand syndrome is not present, the transfusion of normal platelets is suggested. In patients with persistent hemorrhage, immediate reduction of the platelet count can be achieved by platelet pheresis. If this approach fails, some consideration to the use of activated factor VIIa should be given. Hydroxyurea at 2 to 4 g/day for 3 to 5 days should be administered immediately and then reduced to 1 g/day. All patients receiving hydroxyurea should be monitored for the onset of granulocytopenia or thrombocytopenia. Reduction of platelet counts is usually observed within 3 to 5 days of hydroxyurea treatment.

In contrast, patients with acute arterial thrombosis require immediate institution of platelet antiaggregating agents. Aspirin at a dose of 81 mg/day is suggested. Patients with erythromelalgia or transient ischemic attacks will have a rapid cessation of symptoms after the use of low-dose aspirin. In a patient with a life-threatening arterial thrombosis, the platelet count should be lowered with either a combination of apheresis and hydroxyurea or with hydroxyurea alone, depending on the severity of the event. If the arterial thrombosis involves the microcirculation and is not life threatening (transient ischemic attacks or erythromelalgia), immediate low-dose aspirin therapy is indicated, and platelet reduction therapy (hydroxyurea, anagrelide, or INF-α) can be initiated using a standard dose and schedule.

REFERENCES

1. Landgren O, Goldin LR, Kristinsson SY, et al: Increased risks of polycythemia vera, essential thrombocythemia, and myelofibrosis among 24,577 first-degree relatives of 11,039 patients with myeloproliferative neoplasms in Sweden. *Blood* 112:2199, 2008.
2. Janiszewska H, Bak A, Pilarska M, et al: A risk of essential thrombocythemia in carriers of constitutional *CHEK2* gene mutations. *Haematologica* 97:366, 2012.
3. Lambert JR, Everington T, Linch DC, et al: In essential thrombocythemia, multiple *JAK2*-V617F clones are present in most mutant-positive patients: A new disease paradigm. *Blood* 114:3018, 2009.
4. Vannucchi AM, Antonioli E, Guglielmelli P, et al: Characteristics and clinical correlates of MPL 515W>L/K mutation in essential thrombocythemia. *Blood* 112:844, 2008.
5. Chen E, Beer PA, Godfrey AL, et al: Distinct clinical phenotypes associated with *JAK2V617F* reflect differential STAT1 signaling. *Cancer Cell* 18:524, 2010.
6. Medves S, Noël LA, Montano-Almendras CP, et al: Multiple oligomerization domains of *KANK1*-PDGFRbeta are required for *JAK2*-independent hematopoietic cell proliferation and signaling via STAT5 and ERK. *Haematologica* 96:1406, 2011.
7. Vainchenker W, Delhommeau F, Constantinescu SN, et al: New mutations and pathogenesis of myeloproliferative neoplasms. *Blood* 118:1723, 2011.
8. Kaufmann KB, Gründer A, Hadlich T, et al: A novel murine model of myeloproliferative disorders generated by overexpression of the transcription factor NF-E2. *J Exp Med* 209:35, 2012.
9. Carobbio A, Thiele J, Passamonti F, et al: Risk factors for arterial and venous thrombosis in WHO-defined essential thrombocythemia: An international study of 891 patients. *Blood* 117:5857, 2011.
10. Vannucchi AM: Insights into the pathogenesis and management of thrombosis in polycythemia vera and essential thrombocythemia. *Intern Emerg Med* 5:177, 2010.
11. Palandri F, Polverelli N, Catani L, et al: Bleeding in essential thrombocythaemia: A retrospective analysis on 565 patients. *Br J Haematol* 156:281, 2012.
12. Dragani A, Pascale S, Recchiuti A, et al: The contribution of cyclooxygenase-1 and -2 to persistent thromboxane biosynthesis in aspirin-treated essential thrombocythemia: Implications for antiplatelet therapy. *Blood* 115:1054, 2010.
13. Barbui T, Carobbio A, Rambaldi A, et al: Perspectives on thrombosis in essential thrombocythemia and polycythemia vera: Is leukocytosis a causative factor? *Blood* 114:759, 2009.
14. Michiels JJ, ten Kate FJ: Erythromelalgia caused by platelet-mediated arteriolar inflammation and thrombosis in thrombocythemia. *Ann Intern Med* 102:466, 1985.
15. Hanoun M, Röth A, Dührsen U, et al: Acral ischemia as a presenting manifestation of essential thrombocythemia. *Int J Hematol* 94:219, 2011.
16. Reikvam, H, Tiu RV: Venous thromboembolism in patients with essential thrombocythemia and polycythemia vera. *Leukemia* 26:563, 2011.
17. Kiladjian JJ, Cervantes F, Leebeek FW, et al: The impact of *JAK2* and MPL mutations on diagnosis and prognosis of splanchnic vein thrombosis: A report on 241 cases. *Blood* 111:4922, 2008.
18. Valera MC, Parant O, Vayssiere C, et al: Essential thrombocythemia and pregnancy. *Eur J Obstet Gynecol Reprod Biol* 158:141, 2011.
19. Tefferi A, Thiele J, Orazi A, et al: Proposals and rationale for revision of the World Health Organization diagnostic criteria for polycythemia vera, essential thrombocythemia, and primary myelofibrosis: Recommendations from an ad hoc international expert panel. *Blood* 110:1092, 2007.
20. Wilkins BS, Erber WN, Bareford D, et al: Bone marrow pathology in essential thrombocythemia: Interobserver reliability and utility for identifying disease subtypes. *Blood* 111:60, 2008.
21. Harrison CN, Bareford D, Butt N, et al: British Committee for Standards in Haematology. Guideline for investigation and management of adults and children presenting with a thrombocytosis. *Br J Haematol* 149:352, 2010.
22. Malcovati L, Papaemmanuil E, Bowen DT, et al: Chronic Myeloid Disorders Working Group of the International Cancer Genome Consortium and of the Associazione Italiana per la Ricerca sul Cancro Gruppo Italiano Malattie Mieloproliferative. Clinical significance of SF3B1 mutations in myelodysplastic syndromes and myelodysplastic/myeloproliferative neoplasms. *Blood* 118:6239, 2011.
23. Hellstrom-Lindberg, E, Cazzola M: The role of *JAK2* mutations in RARS and other MDS. *Hematology Am Soc Hematol Educ Program* 52, 2008.
24. Thiele J, Kvasnicka HM, Müllauer L, et al: Essential thrombocythemia versus early primary myelofibrosis: A multicenter study to validate the WHO classification. *Blood* 117:5710, 2011.
25. Cortelazzo S, Finazzi G, Ruggeri M, et al: Hydroxyurea for patients with essential thrombocythemia and a high risk of thrombosis. *N Engl J Med* 332:1132, 1995.
26. Ahluwalia M, Donovan H, Singh N, et al: Anagrelide represses GATA-1 and FOG-1 expression without interfering with thrombopoietin receptor signal transduction. *J Thromb Haemost* 8:2252, 2010.
27. Harrison CN, Campbell PJ, Buck G, et al: United Kingdom Medical Research Council Primary Thrombocythemia 1 Study. Hydroxyurea compared with anagrelide in high-risk essential thrombocythemia. *N Engl J Med* 353:33, 2005.
28. Quintás-Cardama A, Kantarjian H, Manshouri T, et al: Pegylated interferon alfa-2a yields high rates of hematologic and molecular response in patients with advanced essential thrombocythemia and polycythemia vera. *J Clin Oncol* 27:5418, 2009.
29. Harrison, C, Barbui T: Aspirin in low-risk essential thrombocythemia, not so simple after all? *Leuk Res* 35:286, 2011.
30. Alvarez-Larrán A, Cervantes F, Pereira A, et al: Observation versus antiplatelet therapy as primary prophylaxis for thrombosis in low-risk essential thrombocythemia. *Blood* 116:1205, 2010, quiz 1387.

CHAPTER 69

PRIMARY MYELOFIBROSIS

John Mascarenhas, Vesna Najfeld, Marina Kremyanskaya, and Ronald Hoffman

Primary myelofibrosis (PMF) is a chronic, malignant hematologic disorder characterized by splenomegaly, leukoerythroblastosis, teardrop poikilocytosis (i.e., dacryocytes), some degree of bone marrow (BM) fibrosis, increased BM microvessel density, and extramedullary hematopoiesis (EMH). In PMF, there is a profound hyperplasia of morphologically abnormal megakaryocytes and clonal populations of monocytes that may be responsible for the BM fibrosis due to the local release of fibrogenic growth factors. This disorder was first described in 1879 by Heuck. Fibrosis of the BM is not unique to PMF and may accompany many other disorders (Table 69-1). The designation PMF rather than idiopathic myelofibrosis was chosen by an international group of hematologists and hematopathologists to reflect our greater understanding of the origins of this disorder. Furthermore, this same group created the terms post–polycythemia vera (PV) myelofibrosis (post-PV MF) and post–essential thrombocythemia (ET) myelofibrosis (post-ET MF) to identify MF that is preceded by a history of PV or ET. In PMF, the BM fibrosis is believed to occur in response to the progeny of a clonal proliferation of hematopoietic stem cells (HSCs). This syndrome frequently leads to progressive BM failure. In 1951, Dameshek included PMF among the myeloproliferative disorders (MPDs). This hypothesis was largely based on clinical observations of patients with PV, chronic myeloid leukemia (CML), and ET who developed BM fibrosis and a clinical picture resembling PMF. Dameshek also noticed that each of these myeloproliferative neoplasms (MPNs) frequently terminates in a leukemic phase. In 2008, the World Health Organization (WHO) modified the terminology of myeloproliferative disorders to MPNs to correctly reflect the malignant nature of these related hematologic cancers.[1]

EPIDEMIOLOGY

Few epidemiologic studies are available to estimate the incidence of PMF. Because the chronic MPNs have not been considered in the past to be malignancies, case registries have limited data on the incidence of such chronic MPN as PMF. Review of previously published reports indicated an annual incidence rate in European, Australian, and North American localities ranging from 0.5 to 1.3 cases per 100,000 persons. The annual incidence rate of PMF in Olmstead County, Minnesota, was determined to be 1.33 cases per 100,000 persons, and in southeast England, the annual incidence has recently been reported to be 0.37 per 100,000 persons. In Japan, PMF is considered a rare disorder. The incidence of MF among survivors who were 10,000 m or less from the hypocenter of the atomic bomb explosion at Hiroshima, however, was 18 times the incidence reported from the remainder of Japan. These patients became symptomatic an average of 6 years after the bomb blast. Such data indicate a strong link between excessive radiation exposure and development of PMF, which is further substantiated by the high incidence of MF in patients who have received the contrast material Thorotrast (which contains 232Th, a radioactive element with a half-life of 1.41 × 1010 years). Thorotrast is taken up and retained indefinitely by cells of the reticuloendothelial system, which results in continuous irradiation of the liver, spleen, lymph nodes, and BM. Chronic exposure to several industrial solvents, including benzene and toluene, has also been associated with development of PMF. Unlike PV, where clusters of patients have been identified in Eastern Pennsylvania, raising the concern for possible environmental effects of waste-coal and Superfund sites, there are no definitive epidemiologic studies supporting environmental exposures in PMF. PMF has been reported as a complication of chronic benzene poisoning since the chemical was first used in the leather and shoe industries during the 1930s and 1940s. The average age at diagnosis of PMF is approximately 65 years, and most patients are diagnosed between 50 and 69 years of age. In several series, men have been affected more frequently than women, but others have failed to confirm this male predominance. Rarely, PMF has been reported in the pediatric age group. Evidence of genetic transmission exists: a higher incidence has been reported in Ashkenazi Jews than in Arabs who both live in Northern Israel.

PATHOBIOLOGY

The cellular origins of PMF were first explored in an African American female PMF patient who was heterozygous for isoenzymes of glucose-6-phosphate dehydrogenase (G6PD).These studies showed that the circulating hematopoietic cells were derived from a common HSC and that the BM fibroblasts were nonclonal in origin. Using X chromosome gene probes, the clonal origin of hematopoiesis in PMF was confirmed. The cytogenetic composition of BM fibroblasts of a PMF patient who had a clonal cytogenetic abnormality present in hematopoietic cells was shown to be absent in the BM fibroblasts, indicating that the fibroblasts were not involved by the malignant process. The development of extensive fibrosis of the BM in PMF is frequently preceded by a hypercellular phase of variable duration. The diagnosis depends on the demonstration of atypical megakaryocytes, BM hypercellularity, and minimal BM fibrosis within BM biopsies and the exclusion of other MPNs. An analysis of X-linked restriction fragment length polymorphisms of blood cells of patients at various stages of PMF demonstrated clonal hematopoiesis in advanced stages of PMF and in the prefibrotic phase. An *NRAS* mutation present in the hematopoietic cells of a PMF patient indicated that T and B cells were also involved in the malignant process in some patients, perhaps providing some explanation for the immunologic abnormalities associated with PMF. Similarly, fluorescence in situ hybridization (FISH) techniques have been used to detect clonal cytogenetic abnormalities in myeloid and in purified B- and T-cell lymphocytes in patients with PMF. These studies indicate that PMF is a clonal hematologic malignancy originating in primitive hematopoietic cells capable of producing lymphoid and myeloid cells and that the BM fibrosis represents a secondary reaction of BM stromal cells not involved by the process. If BM fibrosis is truly an epiphenomenon of the neoplastic hematopoietic cell proliferation, it may be expected to disappear if this cell population is eradicated. Reversal of MF has been observed after allogeneic stem cell transplantation (SCT) and infrequently seen after long-term administration of chemotherapy or interferon (INF). Such findings indicate that the BM fibrosis in PMF is not irreversible and is clearly a secondary consequence of the neoplastic cellular proliferation.

When PMF mononuclear cells are cloned in semisolid media, erythroid and megakaryocyte colony formation occurs in the absence

Table 69-1 Conditions Associated With Myelofibrosis

NONMALIGNANT CONDITIONS
Infections: tuberculosis, histoplasmosis
Renal osteodystrophy
Vitamin D deficiency
Hypoparathyroidism
Hyperparathyroidism
Gray platelet syndrome
Systemic lupus erythematosus
Scleroderma
Radiation exposure
Osteopetrosis
Paget disease
Benzene exposure
Thorotrast exposure
Gaucher disease
Primary autoimmune myelofibrosis
MALIGNANT DISORDERS
Primary myelofibrosis
Other chronic myeloproliferative disorders: polycythemia vera, chronic myeloid leukemia, essential thrombocythemia
Acute myelofibrosis
Acute myeloid leukemia
Acute lymphocytic leukemia
Hairy cell leukemia
Hodgkin lymphoma
Myelodysplasia with myelofibrosis
Multiple myeloma
Systemic mastocytosis
Non-Hodgkin lymphoma
Carcinomas: breast, lung, prostate, stomach

of added exogenous cytokines, a finding common to other MPNs. These findings suggest that possible genetic mutations activating several intracellular signaling pathways responsible for normal hematopoiesis might account for this autonomous in vitro hematopoiesis. In addition to a population of autonomous proliferating megakaryocyte progenitor cells, a second and more common population remains dependent on the addition of exogenous growth factors. The hypothesis that BM fibrosis in PMF is a secondary process has been explored by many groups who uniformly found that fibroblasts derived from BM explants obtained from PMF patients displayed the same physical and proliferative characteristics as normal BM fibroblasts. PMF and normal BM fibroblasts exhibited anchorage and serum dependence, contact inhibition of growth, and similar production of hematopoietic colony stimulating activities. These data suggest that BM fibroblasts and their precursor cells in PMF patients do not differ from those of normal subjects.

Many of the peripheral blood abnormalities associated with PMF may be attributed to the EMH that is characteristic of this disorder. EMH has been previously attributed to the reactivation of quiescent HSCs, which are retained at sites of prior embryonic hematopoiesis, especially in the spleen. This hypothesis has been questioned because of the observation that the spleen is not a prominent site of fetal hematopoiesis in humans and by the observation that EMH occurs in a wide variety of sites in PMF that cannot be accounted for by the fetal reversion hypothesis. CD34$^+$ cells in PMF exit from the BM; because of abnormal trafficking patterns, they are filtered out by the spleen, accumulate progressively, and continue to proliferate. Ultimately, there is an unequal distribution of CD34$^+$ cells, with a twofold greater number being present in the spleen than the BM. The EMH within the spleen is characterized by disturbances of splenic architecture, including an increased presence of megakaryocytes and their progenitor cells. Intravascular hematopoiesis within the sinusoids of the BM is a conspicuous finding in PMF. The characteristic changes of the BM vascular architecture consist of increased quantities of collagen type IV deposits associated with increased BM microvessel density, resulting in increased blood flow. The excessively dilated BM sinusoids in PMF contain prominent intraluminal foci of hematopoiesis. Evolution of the fibroosteosclerotic changes in PMF is accompanied by a striking accumulation of collagen IV and a marked luminal expansion and irregularity. The formation of a network of blood vessels has been shown to be triggered by a broad variety of tumor cells as a consequence of the production and release of angiogenic factors and is therefore not specific to PMF. This increase in BM microvessel density in PMF has been confirmed using immunohistochemical methods and has been shown to correlate with increased spleen size and to be an independent risk factor for overall survival. Vessels from patients with PMF are frequently markedly abnormal and appear as localized vascular nests consisting of numerous short vessels that are highly branched and tortuous. The increased BM microvessel density in PMF is probably mediated by megakaryocyte α-granule constituents. Transforming growth factor beta (TGF-β) and vascular endothelial growth factor (VEGF), for instance, have a profound effect on angiogenesis. The evolution of the fibroosteosclerotic process in PMF appears to be a coordinated process closely related to the vascular proliferation and also modulated by growth factors present within abnormal megakaryocytes.

Osteosclerosis is a prominent clinical feature of many patients with PMF frequently manifesting itself as bone pain. The osteosclerosis is a consequence of cytokines produced by the malignant BM cells or stroma conditioned and activated by an interaction with PMF cells. PMF-associated osteosclerosis can be reversed after allogeneic SCT with the establishment of normal hematopoiesis. Studies of both PMF patients and animal models of PMF indicate that both TGF-β and stromal cell–derived osteoprotegerin, a member of the TNF receptor family, play pivotal roles in the development of osteosclerosis. Osteoprotegerin is a decoy receptor for the receptor activator of the nuclear factor kappa-B ligand (RANKL). RANKL is a transmembrane protein expressed on the cell surface of osteoblasts that can be cleaved into a soluble form by proteases. Both soluble and membrane bound RANKL attach to RANK, a cell receptor expressed by osteoclast precursors to stimulate osteoclastogenesis. RANKL and osteoprotegerin are positive and negative regulators of osteoclast differentiation, respectively. Osteoprotegerin can reduce the production of osteoclasts by inhibiting the differentiation of osteoclast progenitor cells into mature osteoclasts, leading to the development of osteosclerosis. TGF-β is also a negative regulator of osteoclastogenesis through direct stimulation of transcriptional secretion of osteoprotegerin and downregulation of RANKL. In patients with PMF, it remains unknown if the degree of osteosclerosis is corrected with increased levels of osteoprotegerin.

A number of angiogenic growth factors, including basic fibroblast growth factor (bFGF) and VEGF, have been implicated as causative factors of the increased BM microvessel density observed in the BMs of PMF patients. Elevated serum VEGF levels have been reported in PMF, and increased expression of bFGF has been reported in PMF megakaryocytes and platelets. These angiogenic cytokines are the products of the abnormal megakaryocytes present in PMF BM, and the increased BM microvessel density observed is ultimately a consequence of a cytokine release characteristic of PMF megakaryocytes. The role of megakaryocytes in the development of fibrosis in PMF is further supported by the megakaryocytic hyperplasia with dysplastic or necrotic megakaryocytes that characterizes this disorder; by the increased circulating megakaryocytes and megakaryocyte progenitors that are present in PMF; by the association of BM fibrosis and acute megakaryocytic leukemia; and by the presence of MF in gray platelet syndrome, an inherited disorder of platelet α-granules. Ineffective megakaryocytopoiesis in PMF has been hypothesized to lead to the liberation of excessive amounts of such growth factors, leading to BM fibroblast proliferation and collagen synthesis. The platelet-derived growth factor (PDGF) content of platelets from PMF patients is decreased, indicating that a release or leakage of such growth factors by BM megakaryocytes may occur. PMF platelet PDGF and TGF-β levels have been found to be 2.0- to 3.0-fold and 1.5- to 3.0-fold higher, respectively, in PMF than in normal control participants, but

EGF levels in PMF were similar to those of control platelets. The roles of PDGF and TGF-β in the biogenesis of PMF probably are not restricted to promoting fibroblastic proliferation but are also related to the effect of these two growth factors on synthesis, secretion, and degradation of extracellular matrix components.

TGF-β enhances fibronectin and collagens types I, III, and IV as well as chondroitin or dermatan sulphate and proteoglycan gene expression. TGF-β decreases the synthesis of various collagenase-like enzymes that degrade extracellular matrices while at the same time stimulating the synthesis of protease inhibitors such as plasminogen activator inhibitor 1. The net effect of these complex interactions is the accumulation of extracellular matrix, which probably contributes to further progression of fibrosis. Additional growth factors probably are involved in the development of progressive fibrosis in PMF. Circulating megakaryocytic cells and platelets from PMF patients have been shown to possess high levels of bFGF. Because bFGF is devoid of a secretion peptide signal, bFGF is not present in media conditioned by megakaryocytic cells from PMF patients. bFGF is a potent angiogenic factor and is a mitogen for human BM stromal cells. Elevated platelet, megakaryocyte, and serum bFGF levels have been reported in PMF patients with progressive fibrosis. BFGF may be released or leaked from dysplastic and necrotic PMF megakaryocytes or platelets. These findings suggest that bFGF may also contribute to the progressive fibrosis and pronounced angiogenesis frequently observed in PMF. The mechanism by which the pathologic release of growth factors from megakaryocytes occurs in PMF remains unknown. Some have suggested that impaired megakaryocyte emperipolesis might lead to this liberation of fibrogenic cytokines. *Emperipolesis* is defined as the random entry of hematopoietic cells into the cytoplasm of megakaryocytes. This group documented increased emperipolesis of neutrophils and eosinophils in PMF and the liberation of myeloperoxidase-positive granules by the engulfed neutrophils. They correlated the degree of emperipolesis in PMF BM biopsies with the degree of BM fibrosis. They suggested the abnormal P-selectin distribution in megakaryocytes accounted for the selective sequestration of granulocytes by PMF megakaryocytes.[2]

In a number of reports, elevated thrombopoietin levels have been reported in patients with PMF. This unanticipated elevation of plasma thrombopoietin levels was not caused by enhanced production of thrombopoietin mRNA by BM fibroblasts or BM cells but was probably caused by the reduced expression of the thrombopoietin receptor by the platelets and megakaryocytes of PMF patients, leading to decreased clearance of thrombopoietin. Activated Janus kinase 2 (JAK2) has been shown to strongly promote cell surface localization and enhance protein levels of myeloproliferative leukemia virus (MPL). This effect has been shown to be caused by stabilization of the mature endoglycosidase H-resistant form of the receptor. In ET and PMF, platelets and megakaryocytes are characterized by lower MPL protein levels and most of receptors are immature Endo-H sensitive. These data suggest that a defect in JAK2 or an associated protein may be involved in the reduction of the mature MPL observed in MPN patients.

Vannucchi and colleagues studied mutant mice with reduced expression of the transcription factor GATA1 to further define the role of megakaryocytes and the development of BM fibrosis. These mice frequently develop anemia and die during gestation or after birth. The few animals that survive to adulthood recover from the anemia but remain thrombocytopenic throughout life because of a block in megakaryocyte maturation into proplatelets that results in megakaryocyte hyperplasia in the BM and the spleen and increased production of TGF-β. These animals develop a clinical picture after 15 months that closely resembles that of PMF, including anemia, teardrop red blood cells (RBCs), fibrosis of the BM and spleen, EMH in the liver, and progenitor cell mobilization into the peripheral blood. Unlike PMF in humans, the MF in the GATA1-low mice is not the consequence of a clonal disorder and does not progress to acute leukemia. Mutations in the GATA1 functional pathway in human PMF have not been described. However, at the protein level, a large number of the megakaryocytes in the BM of PMF patients are GATA1 negative, suggesting that whatever the genetic defect leading to PMF is, it involves the pathway that affects the posttranscriptional or posttranslational regulation of GATA1 in megakaryocytes. Given the central role played by GATA1 in megakaryopoiesis, it is not surprising that megakaryocytes with low GATA1 content are characterized by common morphologic abnormalities. These abnormalities include a lack of proper organization of the α-granules; abnormal P-selectin localization on the demarcation membrane system; increased emperipolesis of neutrophils through the demarcation membrane system; and increased levels of para-apoptosis, a TUNEL-negative process of cell death mediated by neutrophils and macrophages. It is conceivable that at least some of these megakaryocytes alterations may play a central role in the pathobiology of PMF. In addition, Garimella and coworkers have provided evidence that the osteosclerosis observed in GATA1-low mice is caused by the elaboration of bone morphogenetic proteins by megakaryocytes. Bone morphogenetic proteins cause abnormal stimulation of BM osteoprogenitor cells, resulting in overgrowth of cancellous bone and osteosclerosis.

Megakaryocytes are not the only cells capable of releasing cytokines that promote BM fibrosis. Levels of macrophage colony stimulating factor, a cytokine that regulates macrophage development and proliferation, are elevated in the serum of PMF patients. Monocytes and macrophages from patients with PMF can produce greater quantities of TGF-β and interleukin-1 (IL-1) than those from normal control participants. IL-1 and TGF-β are fibroblast mitogens that induce extracellular matrix protein production. Monocyte adhesion to extracellular matrix proteins has been shown to lead to the overproduction of IL-1 and TGF-β by PMF monocytes. Monocyte adhesion molecule through the adhesion molecule, CD44, appears to be involved in the induction of fibrogenic cytokines by mediating the interaction between monocytes and accumulated extracellular matrix protein deposits. The proinflammatory transcriptional factor nuclear factor kappa-B (NFκB) plays a pivotal role in the elaboration of IL-1 and TGF-β in the activation of NFκB monocytes and that of PMF patients. These investigators suggest that NFκB stimulates TGF-β production by influencing intracellular IL-1 levels and may serve as another potential therapeutic target for the treatment of PMF. An alternative means by which NFκB might be activated was recently described. MicroRNA (MiRNA) 146a functions to downregulate TNF receptor associated factor 6 (TRAF6) and IL-1 receptor associated kinase-1 (IRAK1), two of the signal transducers of NFκB. MiRNA-146a therefore serves to dampen the effects of NFκB activation by terminating an inflammatory response via a negative feedback loop with deletion of miRNA 146a, resulting in NFκB activation. These investigators have shown that miRNA-146a leads to a syndrome in mice that closely resembles human PMF (BM fibrosis, splenomegaly, anemia, thrombocytopenia, EMH), which is accompanied by cells within the spleen and BM having increased transcription of NFκB regulated genes. Whether such a defect in miRNAs influencing NFκB occurs in human PMF has yet to be explored. Abnormal cytokine expression in PMF is thought to represent an inflammatory response to the disease phenotype that contributes not only to the development of BM fibrosis, osteosclerosis, and increased BM microvessel density, but also PMF associated constitutional symptoms including weight loss, anorexia, pruritus, bone pain, and night sweats. Elevated levels of IL-8 and IL-2R have been closely correlated with the presence of constitutional symptoms, the requirement for RBC transfusions, and leukocytosis as well as inferior overall survival and leukemia-free survival. These observations raise the possibility that mutational events leading to the malignant transformation of hematopoietic cells in PMF may also lead to activation of transcriptional programs that promote hematopoietic cell survival and disease progression. The elevation of a variety of cytokines may therefore not only be responsible for the numerous epiphenomenon that occur as a consequence of the presence of these malignant cells but also act on the malignant clone affecting the proliferation and differentiation in differing microenvironments characteristic of the BM and various extramedullary sites, including the spleen. Ultimately, this may increase the risk of disease progression or leukemic transformation.

In 2005, greater insight into the molecular origins of the MPN was gained after the discovery of a gain-of-function mutation of an autoinhibitory domain of the JAK family of protein tyrosine kinases, which is involved in cytokine receptor signalling.[3] The JAK2V617F mutation results from a valine to phenylalanine mutation at amino acid JAK2V617F, which leads to ongoing phosphorylation activity, which then can bind to a cytokine receptor and promote signal transducer and activator of transcription (STAT) recruitment. This mutation is the likely cause of the hypersensitivity to cytokines that characterizes hematopoietic progenitors from each of the MPN. In a mouse BM transplant model, BM cells transduced with JAK2V617F results in a clinical phenotype that closely resembles PV including erythrocytosis, EMH, and BM fibrosis. Although 90% of patients with PV are JAK2V617F positive, approximately 50% of PMF patients harbor this mutation. The JAK2V617F mutation is homozygous in 13% of patients with PMF but in 30% of patients with PV. Homozygosity has been attributed to homologous recombination. Homozygosity of JAK2V617F in PMF patients is associated with a more frequent occurrence of unfavorable cytogenetic abnormalities. There is conflicting data as to whether the clinical course of patients with JAK2V617F-positive and JAK2V617F-negative PMF differ. Additional somatic mutations have been identified in patients with PMF that likely play a role in the biogenesis of PMF. A mutation in the transmembrane domain of the thrombopoietin receptor (cMPL) has been documented in 9% of patients with JAK2V617F-negative PMF (MPLW515L or MPLW515K).[4] Pardanani and coworkers have provided data to support the coexistence of MPL515L, MPL515K, and MPL wild-type (WT) alleles in the same patient. Furthermore, 30% of PMF patients with mutations of cMPL also have the JAK2V617F mutation. By studying archival material, the burden of MPL515L, MPK515K, and JAK2V617 in PMF patients has been shown to remain constant throughout the clinical course of patients with PMF. In a murine BM transplant assay, expression of MPLW515L but not WT MPL resulted in a rapidly progressive, fully penetrable, lethal MPN (18 days) characterized by marked thrombocytosis, leukocytosis, splenomegaly, hepatomegaly, BM megakaryocytic hyperplasia, and BM fibrosis but not erythrocytosis. These data have suggested that the MPL mutation favors the development of thrombocytosis but the JAK2V617F mutation favors the development of erythrocytosis. PMF patients with MPL515L/K mutations as compared with MPL WT PMF are older, present with more severe anemia, and are more likely to require transfusional support. Although 50% of patients with PMF have clonal hematopoiesis and lack mutations of either JAK2 or cMPL, they have a similar clinical phenotype to patients with the recently identified somatic mutations. It is therefore difficult to attribute to either of these mutations as the sole cause of PMF. It appears, however, that the genetic origins of PMF represent the culmination of multiple genetic and possibly epigenetic events. Additional genetic events which might play a role in this process have been defined by the efforts of a number of laboratories. Comparative genomic hybridization has shown that gains of cytogenetic material occur in more than 50% of PMF patients and most commonly involve gains of 9p, 2q, 3p, chromosome 4, 12q, and 13q. These chromosomal sites may harbor additional genes that play a role in the origins of PMF.

Further insight into the phenotypic heterogeneity of JAK2V617F-positive and -negative MPNs has recently been provided. Immunohistochemical analyses of BM have shown that PV is characterized by increased expression of phosphorylated STAT3 and STAT5 protein, but PMF is characterized by reduced expression of STAT3 and STAT5. This expression pattern was independent of JAK2V617F status. Such observations suggest that additional or alternative molecular events occur in PMF and PV that might play a role in the development of their distinctive clinical phenotypes.

A growing list of additional mutations have been identified in PMF over the past several years, providing further insight into the complex molecular pathology of this disease.[5] Many of these mutations impact the epigenome and can coexist in PMF CD34$^+$ cells. None of the genetic or epigenetic lesions identified thus far are specific to PMF, clearly aid in prognostication, or appear to be disease-initiating events. Table 69-2 lists the molecular lesions that have been characterized in patients with PMF.

Translocation ten-eleven oncogene family member 2 (TET2) located on chromosome 4q24 has been noted in many myeloid malignancies at a frequency of approximately 15%. Acquired somatic mutations throughout the 11 exons of this gene result in compromised catalytic activity of an α-ketoglutarate dependent enzyme responsible for oxidation of 5-methylcytosine (5mC) to 5-hydroxymethylcytosine (5hmC) in DNA. Low levels of 5hmC result in a hypermethylation phenotype at CpG sites in various DNA promoter regions. TET2 mRNA has been found to be highly expressed in Lin$^-$, Sca-1$^+$, c-Kit^{hi} multipotent progenitors cells isolated from the BM and thymus of C57BL/6 mice. This expression pattern was maintained in myeloid progenitor cells but low in mature granulocytes. Moreover, in patient samples when compared with normal control sample, low 5hmC levels correlated with a significant decrease in DNA hypermethylation supporting a role of TET2 loss of function leading to DNA hypermethylation. It is currently believed that TET2 mutations result in loss of function and lead to the accumulation of 5hmC in DNA promoting DNA hypermethylation that may inhibit cells from differentiating beyond a HSC-like state. In vitro studies reveal that TET2 deficiency restrains hematopoietic cells from normal differentiation patterns and skews in favor of the monocyte/macrophage lineage with transgenic animals with knockout of TET2 having a phenotype resembling chronic myelomonocytic leukemia. Alterations in TET2 include base substitutions, out-of-frame insertions or deletions, and splice site mutations have been shown to occur in 15% to 20% of patients and that these mutations were more common in older patients. In families with multiple family members having an MPN, all TET2 mutations were almost universally acquired, and their incidence was similar to that of patients with sporadic PMF. Clonal analysis studies in MPN patient samples failed to define a consistent temporal sequence of acquisition of TET2 mutations with respect to JAK2 mutations and can occur late in the progression of MPNs. These two genetic events appear to occur independently. The clinical correlation of TET2 mutation status in PMF patients does not appear to provide a new prognostic marker. TET2 mutations can be found in PMF patients with and without

Table 69-2 Acquired Genetic Lesions Identified in Patients With Primary Myelofibrosis

Gene	Location	Mutation	Frequency
Janus kinase 2 (JAK2)	9p24 exon 14 9p24 exon 12	JAK2V617F	65% Infrequent
Ten-eleven translocation 2 (TET2)	4q24		17%
Enhancer of zeste homolog 2 (EZH2)	7q36.1		13%
Myeloproliferative leukemia virus (MPL)	1p34 exon 10	MPLW515L/K	5%-10%
Casitas B-lineage lymphoma (CBL)	11q23.3	Exons 8 and 9	6%
Isocitrate dehydrogenase (IDH 1 and 2)	2q33.3/15q26.1		4%
Ikaros family zinc finger 1 (IKZF1)	7p12		Infrequent
Additional sex Combs-like 1 (ASXL1)	20q11.1		Infrequent

the JAK2V617F mutation and did not influence rate of thrombosis, leukemic transformation or overall survival. It was noted in multivariate analysis that the presence of TET2 mutation did correlate with anemia (hemoglobin <10 g/dL) in PMF.

Isocitrate dehydrogenase 1 and 2 *(IDH 1/2)* located on chromosome 2q33.3 and 15q26.1, respectively, encode NADP$^+$ dependent enzymes that catalyze the oxidative decarboxylation of isocitrate to α-ketoglutarate. Mutant IDH forms preferentially transform α-ketoglutarate to 2-hydroxyglutarate and appear to promote tumorigenesis by inducing hypoxia-inducible factor 1α (HIF-1α). *IDH 1/2* mutations are found at a frequency of approximately 4% in PMF and can coexist with mutations in JAK2, MPL, and TET2. The specific IDH mutant variants seen in MPNs (IDH1R132C, IDH1R132S, IDH2R140Q) all affect arginine residues. IDH 1/2 mutations do not appear to predict for survival in PMF but do have prognostic significance in multivariate analysis in blast phase disease (PMF-BP). It is not yet clear if different IDH mutation variants carry different biologic or prognostic consequences in PMF. A significant association between IDH 1/2 mutation and non-46/1 haplotype has been observed and supports a theory that PMF patients that are nullizygous for the 46/1 haplotype are more susceptible to acquiring additional molecular lesions that contribute to a poor prognosis.

Additional sex combs-like 1 *(ASXL1)* gene is located on chromosome 20q11.1 and is responsible for encoding an enhancer of the trithorax group (trxG) and polycomb group (PcG) proteins (ETP) chromatin modifier complex. The PcG proteins (repress) and trxG proteins (activate) serve to regulate gene expression of homeotic genes, such as *Hox* genes via histone methylation. ASXL mutations have been identified in various myeloid malignancies and in highest frequency in myelodysplastic syndrome (MDS) and CMML. In a study of 64 MPN cases, ASXL1 mutations were found in five MPN patients (three with PMF), all of whom were negative for the JAK2 mutation. ASXL1 mutations can be found in the MPN HSC, suggesting acquisition early in the pathogenesis of MPNs, but the clinical significance of this mutation in PMF is not yet clear.

The Casitas B-lineage lymphoma *(CBL)* proto-oncogene is located on chromosome 11q23.3 and is believed to play a role in the maintenance of the hematopoietic pluripotent stem cell pool. CBL has the capacity to downregulate and upregulate tyrosine kinase activity by either serving as an adaptor protein and recruiting downstream targets of the pathway or by activation of E3ubiquitin-protein ligase activity and the subsequent recycling of the receptor through internalization of the receptor/ligand complex or lysosomal-directed destruction. CBL mutations were first appreciated in MPNs in the setting of mutational screening of acquired uniparental disomy of chromosome 11q with a total of 27 CBL variants identified in MPNs. Within a cohort of 579 MPN patients screened, three patients with PMF were identified with CBL mutations at an overall frequency of 6%. The majority of the CBL mutations identified were located in the RING or linker domains, resulting in impaired ubiquitin ligase activity. Additionally, the oncogenic activity of selected CBL mutant variants was tested in vitro in the ability to confer growth factor independence to IL-3 dependent cell line 32D and demonstrated enhanced proliferation in transformed cells overexpressing WT FLT3.

Ikaros is a Kruppel-like zinc finger transcription factor that has pleiotrophic function important in the development of normal hematopoiesis and is encoded by the Ikaros family zinc finger 1 *(IKZF1)* gene located at 7p.12. Mutations involving IKZF1 have been identified as a molecular event leading to transformation of chronic phase MPNs to blast phase disease and appearing to occur after the acquisition of JAK2V617F. The mutational frequency in chronic phase MPN is very low at 0.2% in contrast to 21% of blast phase MPN patients and is highly associated with del7p. The effect of *IKZF1* mutation was studied in mouse primary progenitor cells with shRNA-mediated IKZF1 deficiency and is associated cytokine hypersensitivity and increased p-STAT5 expression.

Enhancer of zeste homolog 2 *(EZH2)* gene located on chromosome 7q36.1 encodes the catalytic subunit of the histone methyltransferase polycomb repressor complex 2 (PRC2), and mutations in this gene have also been described in MPN patients. PRC2 is a multiprotein enzyme complex (EZH2, SUz12, EED and YY1) responsible for the trimethylation of lysine 27 on histone H3 (H3K27me3). Additionally, PRC2 can recruit other polycomb complexes, DNMTs and HDACs to the gene site, resulting in chromatin compaction and additional repressive activity. Upregulation of *EZH2* gene expression has been documented in MPNs, most frequently in PMF patients, suggesting a potential role of tumor suppressor gene silencing as a mechanism in disease progression. In a study of 614 patients with myeloid malignancies, 42 cases were found to have a total of 49 *EZH2* mutations. Thirty PMF patients were analyzed in this cohort, and 13% were found to have an EZH2 mutation. Microarray and single-nucleotide polymorphism (SNP) analysis did not show association with copy number alterations or uniparental disomy. Because of small patient numbers and short follow-up, it was not possible to gauge the true prognostic significance of mutated EZH2 in PMF. Retrospective studies using archived MPN BM samples to assess for EZH2 mutations have also not shown to hold prognostic significance in PMF.

A number of investigators have shown that myeloid cells in PMF (RBCs, white blood cells [WBCs], and megakaryocytes and platelets) are clonal and that they harbor the JAK2V617F or MPL515L/K mutations. Furthermore B, T, and natural killer cells isolated from PMF patients in selected cases are JAK2V617F or MPL515 L/K positive. These studies indicate that JAK2V617F and MPL mutational events originate in a cell capable of generating both myeloid and lymphoid cells such as the pluripotent HSC. The ability of primitive human hematopoietic cells to engraft sublethally irradiated immunodeficient mice is the standard surrogate in vivo assay for human HSCs. PMF CD34$^+$ cells are capable of engrafting NOD/SCID (nonobese nondiabetic/severe combined immune deficient) mice and generating myeloid and B cells that are clonal, JAK2V617F positive, and carry a patient-specific marker chromosomal abnormality.[6] The differentiation program of PMF CD34$^+$ cells after transplant into NOD/SCID mice was also remarkably different from that of normal CD34$^+$ cells, producing greater numbers of CD34$^+$, CD33$^+$, and CD41$^+$ cells but fewer CD19$^+$ cells. This predisposition to produce greater numbers of megakaryocytes has been further explored by incubating PMF, PV, and CD34$^+$ cells in vitro in the presence of stem cell factor and thrombopoietin. PMF CD34$^+$ cells displayed a far greater proliferative capacity and produced greater numbers of megakaryocytes that were characterized by a resistance to undergo apoptosis in vitro caused by overexpression of the antiapoptotic factor Bcl-XL. The megakaryocyte hyperplasia in PMF, therefore, could be accounted for by two factors, an increased ability of CD34$^+$ cells to generate megakaryocytes and the accumulation of megakaryocytes caused by Bcl-xL overexpression. Although Bcl-xL overexpression has been linked to JAK2V617F, PMF megakaryocyte Bcl-xL overexpression also occurred to a similar degree in megakaryocytes generated from CD34$^+$ cells isolated from individuals with both JAK2V617F-positive and -negative disease.

Bone marrow megakaryocytes PMF have been reported to produce greater amounts of TGF-β than MKs generated in vitro from normal volunteers or patients with PV.[7] An immunophilin FK506 binding protein 51 (FKB51) is overexpressed in PMF megakaryocytes, and that FKB51 overexpression leads to activation of NFκB in PMF MKs. Cells with activated NFκB produce greater amounts of TGF-β. This effect of NFκB is likely indirect because NFκB cannot directly increase transcription of TGF-β because its promoter does not have NFκB binding sites. These studies suggest that NFκB or TGF-β inhibitors might be useful in preventing the progression of BM fibrosis in PMF.

The number of unilineage and multilineage hematopoietic progenitor cells constitutively mobilized into the blood of PMF patients is dramatically increased. The number of CD34$^+$ cells present in the peripheral blood in PMF is 360 times greater than in normal control participants and 18 to 30 times higher than in patients with PV or ET. These findings are so striking that some investigators have suggested that the quantitation of CD34$^+$ cells in the peripheral blood might serve as a means of discriminating PMF from other MPNs. A level of 15 × 10^6/L of CD34$^+$ cells in peripheral blood allows differentiation of PMF from PV and ET. The numbers of circulating CD34+ cells tend to increase as the disease progresses and that there is a close correlation between patients presenting with more than 300 × 10^6 CD34+ cells/L of peripheral blood and imminent evolution to leukemia. These findings suggest that PMF CD34+ cell trafficking abnormality is caused by the inability of these cells to be retained within the BM or their premature release into the peripheral blood.

Primary myelofibrosis is characterized not only by the constitutive mobilization of CD34+ hematopoietic cells but also endothelial progenitor cells into the peripheral blood. Endothelial progenitor cell mobilization predominates during the prefibrotic phase of PMF while hematopoietic stem/progenitor cell mobilization occurs characteristically in more clinically advanced phases of the disease. This dysregulation of stem cell trafficking likely ultimately leads to the seeding of extramedullary sites with primitive hematopoietic and endothelial cells, which results in production of EMH within the liver and spleen as well as a variety of other organs. Several proteolytic pathways have been documented to play a role in cytokine-mediated stem cell mobilization. Proteins released by activated neutrophils cleave vascular adhesion molecule-1 (VCAM-1) expressed by stromal cells, leading to the disruption of a key adhesive interaction between VCAM-1 and very late antigen-4 (VLA-4) expressed by HSCs and progenitor cells. The interaction between stromal cell–, endothelial cell–, and osteoblast-derived stromal cell–derived factor-1 (SDF-1) and the CXC chemokine receptor-4 (CXCR-4) expressed by HSCs and progenitor cells is also believed to determine patterns of stem cell trafficking. Proteases, including neutrophil elastase, soluble matrix metalloproteinase-9 (MMP-9), and cell-bound MMP-9, have been shown to play a role in the constitutive mobilization of CD34+ cells that occurs in PMF patients. The concentrations of soluble VCAM-1, a degradation product of VCAM-1, is elevated in the plasma of PMF patients, and these levels correlate with the absolute numbers of CD34+ cells in the peripheral blood. In addition, these elevated levels of proteases have been shown to be responsible for degradation of the chemokine SDF-1, which plays a role in retention of CD34+ cells within the BM because the degradations products lack the ability to attract CD34+ cells, thereby favoring their mobilization. Furthermore, CXCR-4 expression by PMF CD34+ cells is downregulated, which may account for altered SDF-1–CXCR-4 interactions participating in CD34+ cell mobilization. This downregulation of CXCR4 expression can be reversed in vitro by treatment with chromatin modifying agents, suggesting that this eve2nt might be attributable to epigenetic events. Furthermore, the expression levels of CXCR4 were significantly lower in patients with a high burden of JAK2V617F (allele frequency, 75%) compared with patients with low-burden JAK2V617F, suggesting the dependence of gene expression on the frequency of the mutated allele. Similar degrees of CD34+ cell mobilization are observed in post-ET and post-PV MF as occurs in PMF. In PV patients, Passamonti and coworkers have demonstrated a relationship between JAK2V617F gene dosage and the degree of constitutive mobilization of CD34+ cells, suggesting that such mobilization may be a consequence of the transition from JAK2V617F heterozygosity to homozygosity that is accompanied by granulocyte activation. Drugs that target the proteases responsible for constitutive CD34+ cell mobilization may present an intriguing strategy to prevent the establishment of extramedullary sites of hematopoiesis in patients with PMF.

The kinetics of engraftment of normal stem cells after allogeneic SCT in PMF patients and the slow regression of fibrosis after transplant lead one to question if the distorted BM architecture associated with fibrosis in PMF actually disrupts the functions of the BM microenvironment. In PMF patients, normal stem cells engraft after transplant and hematopoietic cell recovery occurs before the BM fibrosis has resolved. These observations raise some questions concerning the prospects for success with strategies for the treatment of patients with PMF that are directed solely toward reversing the BM fibrosis rather than eliminating the malignant clone and its progeny. Furthermore, in mouse models of MF, inhibition of TGF-β1 was capable of preventing the development of BM fibrosis but did not rescue animals from a fatal MPN.

CLINICAL MANIFESTATIONS

Table 69-3 lists the symptoms and physical findings of patients with PMF at presentation.

Approximately 25% of patients are entirely asymptomatic and come to medical attention because of an enlarged spleen detected during routine physical examination or because of an abnormal blood cell count or peripheral blood smear. The most common symptom in PMF is fatigue, which in the majority of patients affects the quality of daily life and social activities. Fatigue may be the result of anemia, which leads to the associated complaints of weakness, dyspnea on exertion, and palpitations. But when patients were questioned with the aid of specific questionnaires, fatigue was found to be a significant burden even in patients who were not anemic. The presence of anemia, splenomegaly, and other features associated with advanced disease favored the development of higher levels of fatigue. Other nonspecific constitutional symptoms, including fever, night sweats, pruritus, bone pain, and weight loss, are present at diagnosis in 20% to 50% of patients with PMF and are more frequent in older patients.

With enlargement of the spleen, various syndromes characterized by abdominal discomfort emerge. Pressure of the spleen on the stomach may lead to delayed gastric emptying and early satiety. Patients may merely complain of a dull, heavy sensation in the left upper quadrant. Pain of extreme severity, simulating an acute abdominal emergency, is produced by splenic infarction. Pressure of the spleen on the colon or small bowel may be responsible of severe, disabling diarrhea.

Thrombotic episodes may rarely be the presenting feature of the disease or may occur during its course with a probability of 9.6% at 5 years, a rate higher than in the control general population. Thrombosis may be venous (cerebral venous sinus thrombosis, splanchnic vein thrombosis, deep venous thrombosis, pulmonary thromboembolism) or arterial (stroke, transient ischemic attacks, retinal artery occlusion, myocardial infarction, angina pectoris, and peripheral arterial disease). The cellular phase of PMF with thrombocytosis and presence of cardiovascular risk factors such as hypertension, smoking, hypercholesterolemia, and diabetes are the independent predictors of thrombosis.[8] After splenectomy, the rate of thrombosis increases and is associated with the development of thrombocytosis after the procedure. A systematic review of PMF patients with the *JAK2V617F*

Table 69-3 Summary of Symptoms and Physical Findings of Patients With Primary Myelofibrosis Detected at Diagnosis

Symptom or Finding	Incidence (%)
Asymptomatic	16-30
Fatigue	47-71
Fever	5-15
Weight loss	7-39
Night sweats	6-21
Symptoms due to enlarged spleen	11-48
Bleeding	5-20
Gout or renal stones	6-13
Pallor	60
Petechiae or ecchymoses	15-20
Splenomegaly	89-99
Hepatomegaly	39-70
Peripheral edema	13
Evidence of portal hypertension	2-6
Lymphadenopathy	1-10
Jaundice	0-4

mutation failed to clearly define a statistically significant increased risk of thrombosis in this population, and further studies with larger numbers of PMF patients need to be conducted.

Bleeding problems may complicate the clinical course of PMF patients. Bleeding may be trivial, as manifested by petechiae and ecchymoses, or it may be life-threatening as a result of uncontrollable esophageal bleeding. It may result from thrombocytopenia or poor platelet function. Bleeding may be only initially encountered during a surgical procedure such as splenectomy; in this case, the bleeding diathesis may result from inapparent disseminated intravascular coagulopathy (DIC) and has the potential for catastrophic consequences.

Occurrence of isolated sites of ectopic sites of myeloid metaplasia has been reported, particularly in the pulmonary, gastrointestinal, central nervous, and genitourinary systems. EMH can rarely occur in the skin, manifesting as nontender, occasionally pruritic red, pink, or violaceous plaques, papules, or hemangioma-like nodules. These dermal infiltrates, when biopsied, are composed of combinations of myeloid, erythroid, and megakaryocytic cells. Patients with nonsplenic ectopic myeloid metaplasia present with cough and "large lung tumors," headache, or paralysis resulting from "brain tumors or spinal cord tumors," small bowel obstruction, or intractable ascites from ectopic implants of hematopoietic tissue in the gut or peritoneum. Myeloid metaplasia of the renal pelvis, ureters, and bladder and renal parenchymal infiltration have been observed. Expansion of hematopoietic tissue at the urethral meatus may be confused with a urethral carbuncle. Such strategically localized sites of EMH may lead to renal failure or obstruction of both kidneys and bladder dysfunction. Ascites occurring in a patient with PMF may result from peritoneal or mesenteric implants of extramedullary hematopoietic tissue or from portal hypertension. If the ascites result from peritoneal implants, the fluid is always exudative and sterile and frequently contains myeloid, erythroid, and megakaryocytic elements. Such cytologic studies should routinely be performed on ascitic or pleural fluid obtained from patients with PMF. Unusual sites of EMH have been reported in the gallbladder and lacrimal fossae.

Table 69-3 lists the prominent physical findings in patients with PMF.[9] Splenomegaly serves as the hallmark of the disease. Its extent may vary, but massive splenomegaly, with the organ occupying the entire left side of the abdomen and extending into the pelvis, may occur in 35% of patients. Hepatomegaly occurs in almost 70% of cases, and lymphadenopathy is observed in 10% to 20%, but the degree of nodal enlargement is frequently only moderate. Other important physical findings include pallor, peripheral edema, jaundice, and bony tenderness. Acute monoarticular inflammation caused by secondary gout is seen in 6% of patients.

Portal hypertension may occur and is a result of massive increases in hepatic blood flow and intrahepatic obstruction. Clinical features of portal hypertension, such as ascites or esophageal varices, occur in 9% to 18% of patients with PMF. Occasionally, cirrhosis or evidence of thrombosis of the portal or hepatic veins has been reported. In patients with portal hypertension, thrombotic lesions in small- or medium-sized portal veins and in extrahepatic portal veins were observed. Nodular regenerative liver hyperplasia occurred in 14.6% of cases and correlated closely with the presence of portal vein lesions. They concluded that thrombosis is the most likely cause of portal venous obliteration and portal hypertension in PMF and that clinically significant thrombosis confined to small intrahepatic veins or large hepatic veins should be considered in any patient with PMF. In this autopsy series, portal and hepatic venous disease occurred even in the absence of signs of portal hypertension. Such a finding is consistent with subclinical thrombosis with recanalization occurring fairly commonly in this patient group.

Rarely, the development of PMF can be preceded by the appearance of multiple cutaneous edematous plaques and nodules characteristic of the Sweet syndrome, a cutaneous process occurring in response to a number of hematologic malignancies. Pyoderma gangrenosum has been reported to be associated with PMF, and atypical pyoderma gangrenosum is reported to be a complication at splenectomy incision.

Primary myelofibrosis may be associated with the development of pulmonary hypertension. These patients present with progressive dyspnea, signs of biventricular heart failure, and rapidly increasing hepatosplenomegaly. An elevation in pulmonary artery pressure can be documented by transthoracic Doppler echocardiography and right heart catheterization. Many of these patients succumb to cardiopulmonary complications within 18 months of the documentation of pulmonary artery hypertension. The development of pulmonary artery hypertension can be attributed to thromboembolic disease, EMH diffusely involving the lung, or pulmonary fibrosis due to the elaboration of fibrogenic cytokines from dysfunctional circulating megakaryocytes and platelets. BM fibrosis also occurs in patients with primary pulmonary hypertension and can be associated with anemia and thrombocytopenia. These patients can be distinguished from patients with PMF by their lack of high levels of circulating $CD34^+$ cells, teardrop RBCs, hematopoietic cell clonality, and JAK2V617F negativity.

The nephrotic syndrome can occasionally be associated with PMF. Renal EMH is a constant finding in these cases, but renal biopsy may reveal also a picture of mesangioproliferative glomerulopathy or membranous glomerulonephritis. Immunocomplexes deposition with subepithelial electron dense deposits caused by immunodysfunction of PMF has been proposed as the pathogenetic explanation for this association.

Primary myelofibrosis may be associated with a preexisting or simultaneously appearing autoimmune disease, such as systemic lupus erythematosus (SLE), scleroderma, primary biliary cirrhosis, ulcerative colitis, polyarteritis nodosa, or juvenile rheumatoid arthritis. In addition, autoimmune forms of MF have been described distinct from PMF and are most commonly associated with SLE. These patients characteristically have cytopenia and BM fibrosis but have a limited degree of splenomegaly and only mild numbers of teardrop RBC and immature myeloid cells in the peripheral blood. Patients with autoimmune MF frequently have a positive direct antiglobulin test result and antinuclear antibodies (ANAs) but are JAK2V617F negative.

LABORATORY MANIFESTATIONS

Careful examination of the peripheral blood smear and BM (Fig. 69-1) permits ready diagnosis of PMF. Leukoerythroblastosis with teardrop RBCs strongly suggests this diagnosis. The leukoerythroblastic condition is characterized by the presence of nucleated RBCs and immature myeloid elements in 96% of cases. Megathrombocytes and megakaryocytic fragments are frequent findings. The number of teardrop erythrocytes (i.e., dacryocytes) decreases after splenectomy or institution of chemotherapy, which has led some to suggest that splenic fibrosis causes the development of these RBC changes. In approximately 60% of patients, hemoglobin levels drop to less than 10 g/dL. The degree of anemia is not infrequently difficult to estimate by hemoglobin or hematocrit determinations because individuals with large spleens often have expanded plasma volumes and apparent anemia, which is largely dilutional in nature. Most patients have normochromic normocytic RBC indices. The anemia may be caused by decreased production because of erythroid hypoplasia or ineffective RBC production and shortened RBC survival. The cause of the hemolytic anemia is usually multifactorial, with contributions from hypersplenism, a defect in RBCs resembling paroxysmal nocturnal hemoglobinuria, and antierythrocyte autoantibodies.

Hypochromic microcytic anemia resulting from iron deficiency secondary to blood loss may develop in 5% of PMF patients. Blood loss may be caused by leaking esophageal varices, duodenal ulceration, gastritis, or intravascular hemolysis. Occasionally, a patient with PMF may develop an occult malignancy or a site of EMH within the gastrointestinal tract, which may serve as a bleeding source. Unexplained microcytosis (mean corpuscular volume >80 fL) has been reported as a laboratory feature in PMF and in general has not been shown to have prognostic relevance. Macrocytic anemia may complicate PMF. Folic acid absorption is normal in these patients, and the folic acid deficiency probably results from increased use.

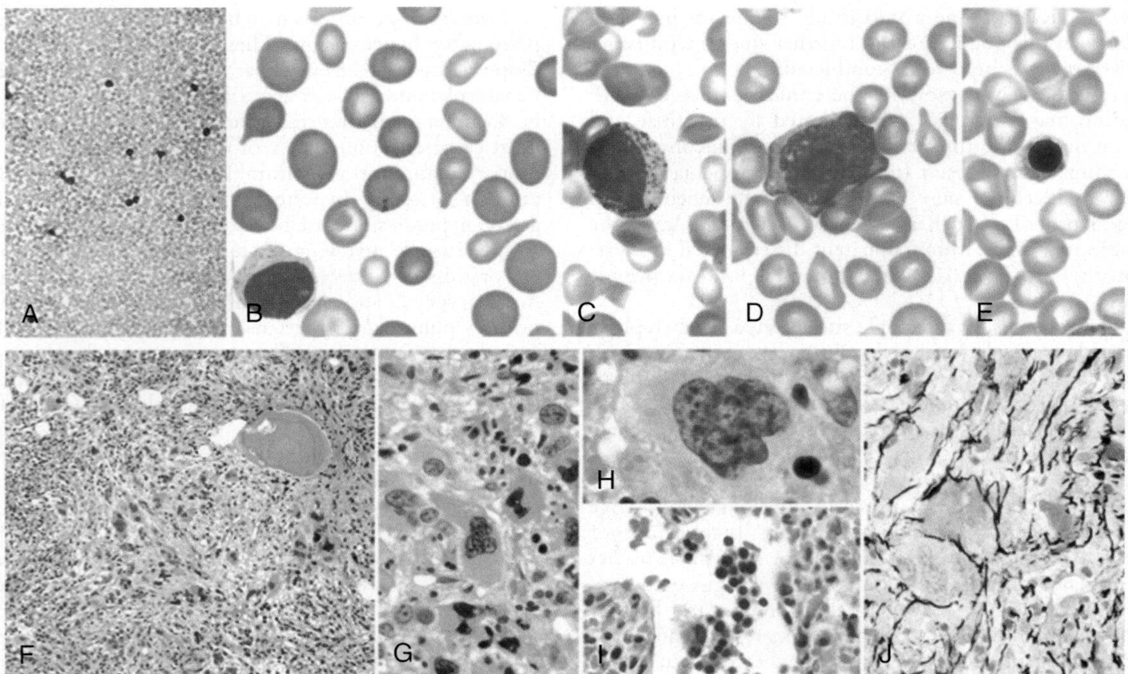

Figure 69-1 PRIMARY MYELOFIBROSIS (PMF). Peripheral blood and bone marrow (BM) biopsy. The leukocyte count can vary in PMF from leukopenia to marked leukocytosis. In the case illustrated, the count was normal **(A)**. However, the smear showed numerous dacryocytes, or teardrop forms **(B)**, and a leukoerythroblastic picture (**C** to **E**), that is the presence leukoblasts, or immature granulocytic precursors **(C)**, including myeloblasts **(D)**, and circulating nucleated red blood cells or erythroblasts **(E)**. The BM biopsy is frequently hypercellular **(F)** and comprised of an atypical megakaryocytic and granulocytic proliferation **(G)** in which some of the megakaryocytes have atypical and pyknotic nuclei. Other megakaryocytes **(H)** are considered to have nuclei that are "cloudlike." The BM biopsy frequently shows sinusoidal hematopoiesis **(I)** and significant fibrosis as illustrated by a reticulin stain **(J)**.

Leukopenia can occur in 13% to 25% of patients, and leukocytosis is seen in one-third. Occasional blast cells and granulocytes with the pseudo–Pelger-Huët anomaly are frequent findings. The leukocyte alkaline phosphatase score is high in more than half of patients but low in about one-third. Platelet counts of less than 100,000/mm^3 are observed in 31% of patients, and platelet counts of more than 800,000/mm^3 have been observed in 12%. In the prefibrotic phase of the disease, almost 90% of patients had platelet counts greater than 500,000/mm^3. Defective platelet aggregation is common, and platelets frequently do not respond to collagen or epinephrine. A variety of qualitative platelet anomalies have been documented by abnormal in vitro aggregation patterns. In 15% of patients, abnormalities suggestive of ongoing DIC are found, including decreased platelet numbers, decreased levels of factor V and VIII, and increased fibrin-split products. Usually, when DIC occurs in PMF, it produces no symptoms and unfortunately may only become clinically apparent after surgical intervention. Associated liver dysfunction may also be a contributory factor to prolongation of the prothrombin time.

Additional laboratory abnormalities are quite common. In one series, lactic acid levels were elevated in 95% of patients, bilirubin levels in 40%, uric acid in 60%, and alkaline phosphate and serum glutamic oxaloacetic transaminase levels in 50%. Patients with PMF have decreased levels of total cholesterol. The ratio of high-density lipoprotein cholesterol to low-density lipoprotein cholesterol is diminished.

A variety of immunologic abnormalities have been reported in PMF, including the presence of ANAs, elevated rheumatoid factor titers, direct Coombs test positivity, lupus-type circulating anticoagulants, hypocomplementemia, BM lymphoid nodules, and increased circulating immune complexes. In one series of 50 patients with PMF, increased quantities of circulating immune complexes were detected in 39% and found to be associated with increased disease activity as manifested by increased transfusion requirements, bone pain, and fever. Some investigators have suggested that abnormalities of the complement system may be important in the disease progression of PMF, and others have hypothesized that low levels of C3 may predispose these patients to develop serious bacterial infections. A remarkably high incidence of monoclonal gammopathies has been reported in PMF, with such benign gammopathies occurring in 8% to 10% of patients in some series. A number of cases of the simultaneous occurrence of a plasma cell dyscrasia and PMF have been reported.

Successful BM aspiration is unusual, accomplished in only six of 48 cases in one series, with the tap completely dry in 50% of cases. A BM biopsy is necessary in all cases for the diagnosis and monitoring of the disease. The amount of residual hematopoietic cellular tissue and the degree of BM fibrosis are the key elements that should be assessed. Some caution should be taken in using repeated BM biopsy specimens to diagnose PMF. A BM biopsy performed at the site of a previous bone injury during the healing process frequently results in confusion because of primary callus formation at that site. Most BM biopsies in PMF are hypercellular and are remarkable for increased numbers of megakaryocytes. BM fibrosis and osteosclerosis were seen in 67% and 54% of cases, respectively. The characteristic morphologic features include patchiness of the hematopoietic cellularity and the reticulin fibrosis, some microscopic fields being cellular and others depleted of hematopoietic cells. The amount of reticulin may vary from field to field. The megakaryocytes are increased in numbers and often are arranged around and within the sinuses and not always clustered in groups. They are large with irregular, roundish, cloudlike nuclei and distended BM sinusoids frequently containing intravascular hematopoiesis. The BM biopsies reveal a substantial increase in vascularity. The BM microvessels are more tortuous and branched than observed in normal control participants. The increased microvessel density is correlated with increased VEGF expression by megakaryocytes. A rare histologic variant of PMF is the so-called MF with fatty BM in which the BM is characterized by myeloid hypoplasia associated with fairly complete fatty substitution, mimicking the BM of aplastic anemia. These patients frequently have areas of clusters of densely aggregated hematopoietic elements exhibiting the histopathologic characteristics of PMF and large numbers of hematopoietic progenitors circulating in their peripheral blood. This variant of PMF is likely caused by the abnormal trafficking of hematopoietic cells from the BM to extramedullary sites, consistent with the osteosclerosis observed in patients with PMF, increased thickness of some bone units with new lamellae and focal areas of woven bone. There is a net decrease in osteoclast number and conversion of trabecular pillars into plates.

Progressive fibrosis is frequently observed in patients who did not have maximal MF at the time of the initial biopsy. Thiele and colleagues presented data to indicate an early prefibrotic subtype of PMF with no or minimal BM reticulin and another phase with conspicuous fibrosis and osteosclerotic changes of the BM.[10] Based on a careful histomorphometric evaluation of the BM, they concluded that in a subset of patients there was a progressive fibroosteosclerotic process during the evolution of the disease that was paralleled by an increase in numbers of small megakaryocytes with irregular perimeters and megakaryocytes with naked nuclei. The clinical and morphologic findings of patients with the prefibrotic stage of PMF have been further characterized. Although a steady progression to BM fibrosis has been demonstrated in patients with the prefibrotic phase, fibrosis may remain static or diminish in the more advanced stages of PMF.

Different scoring systems for pathologically grading the BM cellularity and fibrosis have been used with the aim of staging and documenting progression of the disease. In a recent European consensus conference, the importance of age-dependent decrease in cellularity was recognized (Table 69-4). Grading of MF was simplified by using four easily reproducible categories, including differentiation between reticulin and collagen. A consensus was reached that the density of fibers must be assessed in relation to the hematopoietic tissue. This feature is especially important to avoid a false impression of a reduced fiber content in fatty or edematous BM samples after treatment. The progression of BM fibrosis in PMF is accompanied by expression of subsets of collagenases that is independent of the JAK2V617F status.

Morphologic examination of the spleen reveals foci of EMH in the sinusoids of the red pulp, where megakaryocytes, myeloid elements, and nucleated erythroid elements are seen. Follicular atrophy in the white pulp frequently occurs. The extramedullary hematopoietic cells belonging to each of the myeloid lineages can be distributed in the spleen diffusely or be limited to macronodules. The

Table 69-4 Grading of Myelofibrosis According to the European Consensus Criteria

Grading	Description*
MF-0	Scattered linear reticulin with no intersections (cross-overs) corresponding to normal bone marrow
MF-1	Loose network of reticulin with many intersections, especially in perivascular areas
MF-2	Diffuse and dense increase in reticulin with extensive intersections, occasionally with focal bundles of collagen, focal osteosclerosis, or both
MF-3	Diffuse and dense increase in reticulin with extensive intersections and coarse bundles of collagen, often associated with osteosclerosis

Data from Thiele J, Kvasnicka HM, Facchetti F, et al: European consensus on grading bone marrow fibrosis and assessment of cellularity. *Haematologica* 90:1128, 2005.

*The quality of the reticulin stain should be assessed by detection of normal staining in vessel walls as internal control. The degree of myelofibrosis should be assessed by disregarding lymphoid nodules and vessels and disregarding fibers framing adipocytes. Areas of prominent scleredema or scarring should be included in the overall grading of myelofibrosis. Fiber density should be assessed in hematopoietic areas.

predominance of immature granulocytic forms is associated with an especially poor prognosis. Pathologic examination of the liver reveals hematopoietic cellular elements within the sinusoids. Sinusoidal dilatation is a common finding, as well as prominent intrahepatocyte and Kupffer cell hemosiderin deposition. A marked increase in the hepatic reticulin network has also been observed.

Approximately 30% to 50% of patients with PMF have karyotypic abnormalities at diagnosis. It is important to perform cytogenetic analysis on this patient population to exclude rare cases of chronic myelogenous leukemia with associated BM fibrosis. Detection of a Philadelphia chromosome or *BCR-ABL1* fusion gene is diagnostic of CML and excludes the diagnosis of PMF. In cases that are Philadelphia chromosome negative, it is prudent to perform FISH or polymerase chain reaction analysis for *BCR-ABL1*.

Because of BM fibrosis, it is often difficult to obtain optimal numbers of metaphase cells for cytogenetic analysis. In the past, a substantial percentage of patients with PMF had a "dry tap" or were uninformative, thereby making cytogenetic analysis challenging. Although cytogenetic analysis of PMF remains time consuming and laborious, cytogenetic studies are now informative in about 99% of patients from unstimulated peripheral blood specimens. This success is due to the presence of large numbers of immature hematopoietic cells (including CD34-positive cells) present in the peripheral blood combined with the use of an MPN interphase FISH panel that allows for essentially all PMF patients to be examined for the most frequent cytogenomic changes (see Figure 67-3). There is a high concordance rate (92%) between conventional cytogenetics and interphase FISH for the 12 most frequent chromosomal abnormalities detected in PMF. Although detection of clonal chromosomal abnormalities in a small proportion of metaphase, but not interphase cells, is a rare observation (≈2% of all patients), it demonstrates the importance of applying both technologies when evaluating PMF patients at diagnosis.

Among the Philadelphia chromosome-negative MPNs, PMF has the highest rate of chromosomal abnormalities at diagnosis. Deletions of the long arms of chromosomes 13 and 20, trisomy 8 and abnormalities of chromosomes 1, 7, and 9 constitute more than 80% of all chromosomal changes detected in PMF (Fig. 69-2). None of these lesions are specific for PMF because they are also detected in PV, ET, MDS, and other myeloid malignancies. Deletion of the long arm of chromosome 13 is substantially more frequent in PMF than in PV. Fine FISH mapping has defined the commonly deleted region to 13q13.3-q14.3 encompassing *RB1, D13S319,* and *D13S25* loci. As mentioned in Chapter 67, del(20q) and +9/+9p are more frequent in PV than in PMF. Multiple copies of 9p result in trisomy/tetrasomy or amplification of *JAK2* and each of these abnormalities has been reported in PMF. A 2.7-Mb region on chromosome 20, spanning D20S108 (proximal) and D20S481 (distal) is deleted in all Philadelphia chromosome–negative MPNs. A different region is deleted in other myeloid malignancies, but a common 1.6 kb region may constitute the major site responsible for loss of heterozygosity. High resolution SNP array karyotyping recently identified a novel 20p13 amplification in 55% of 20 patients at the time of PMF diagnosis. Within this band, *SIRPB1* gene locus is present in four copies. Currently, the role of *SIRPB1* gene in PMF remains unknown.

With disease progression from PV/ET to MF, the frequency of cytogenetic abnormalities increases to 70% to 90%. The types of chromosomal abnormalities observed in these cases are similar to those seen at diagnosis of PV/ET or PMF, but through subclonal evolution, they may become very complex. The number of genomic alterations are more than two or three times greater in the blast phase as in the chronic phase. Specific regions on 12p *(ETV6),* 17p *(P53),* and on 21q *(RUNX1)* are frequently altered and associated with disease progression.

Investigation of PMF by a comparative genomic hybridization technique suggests that genomic aberrations are much more common than has been previously indicated by conventional cytogenetic analysis and occur in the majority of cases. Gains of 9p were the most frequent finding, occurring in 50% of patients, suggesting that genes on 9p may play a crucial role in the pathogenesis of PMF. This

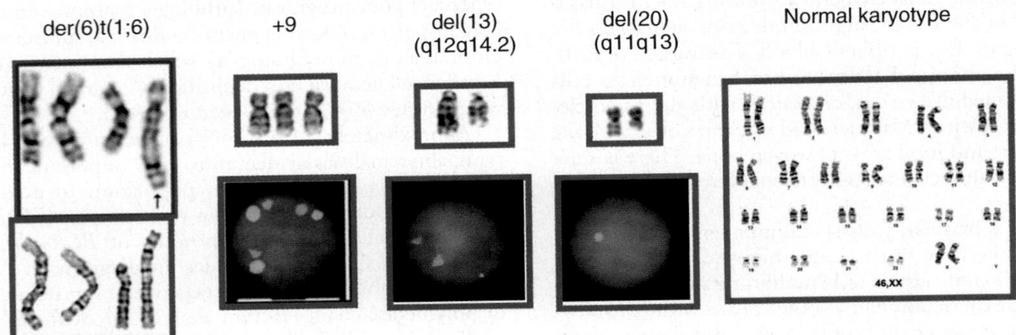

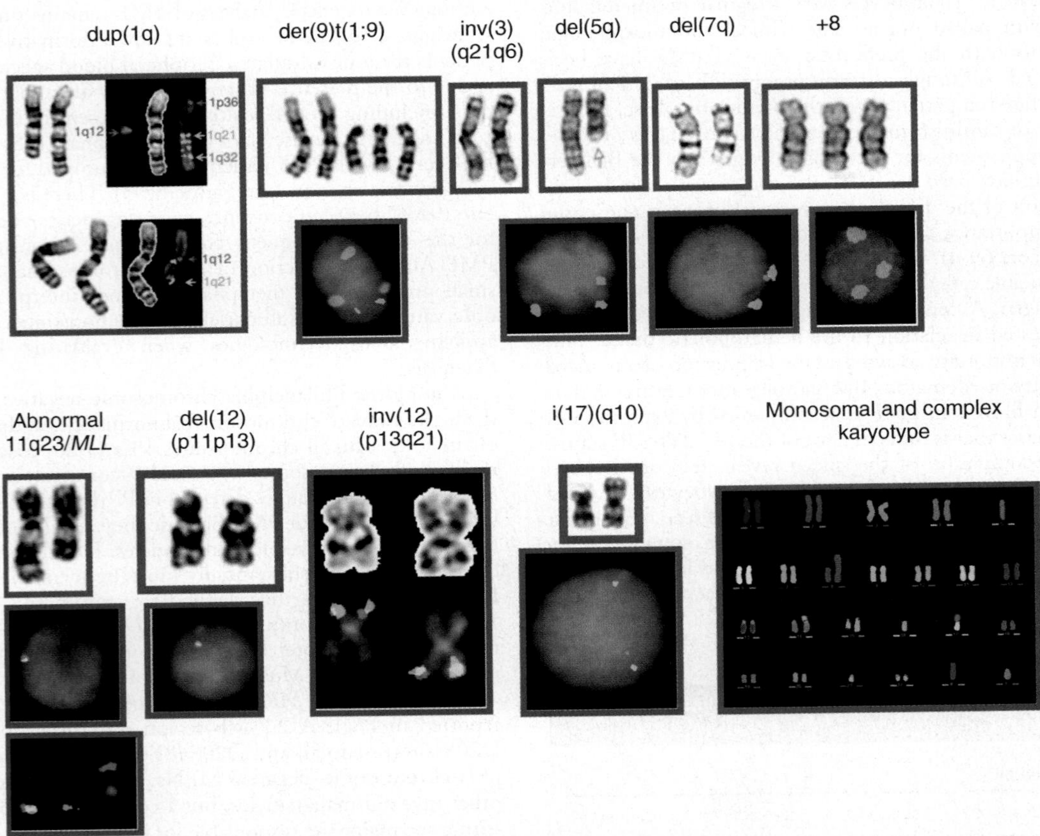

Figure 69-2 CYTOGENETIC FINDINGS IN PRIMARY MYELOFIBROSIS (PMF). The *top row* shows chromosomal abnormalities and corresponding interphase fluorescence in situ hybridization (FISH) findings associated with a favorable prognosis. They include unbalanced translocations between chromosomes 1 and 6 (both the short and long arms of chromosome 6) resulting in a gain of 1q, sole abnormality of chromosomes 9, 13, and 20 as well as the normal karyotype. Abnormalities include a gain of chromosome 9 and interstitial deletions of the long arm of chromosome 13 and 20. The *bottom row* shows chromosomal abnormalities and corresponding interphase nuclei after FISH studies associated with an unfavorable prognosis. They include duplication and trisomy 1q. The most frequent abnormality associated with polycythemia vera–related PMF is der (9)t(1;9), resulting in a gain of 1q *(red)* and 9p. Inversion of chromosome 3, -5/del(5q) *(red)* and -7/del(7q) *(red)* are rare in PMF as are rearrangement of 11q23 and deletion of the short arms of chromosome 12. Sole trisomy 8 is a frequent abnormality associated with PMF, and rearrangements of 12q are almost exclusively identified in PMF. The chromosomal abnormalities associated with the most dismal prognosis are heterozygous 17p loss *(red)* and monosomal or complex karyotype.

observation, together with the observation that loss of heterozygosity at 9p was a frequent stem cell defect in PV, served as a foundation for the discovery of the JAK2*V617F* mutation in MPN.

In PMF, the proportion of patients with the JAK2*V617F* mutation in granulocytes has been reported to range from 35% to 95%. The detection rate for JAK2V617F is much higher for patients with post-PV MF (91%) than PMF (45%) or post-ET MF (39%). In PV, a high burden of JAK2V617F allele has been associated with an increased rate of evolution to MF. Such wide differences in the mutational frequencies can be attributed to the different sensitivity of the techniques used to detect the mutation and to differences in the case mix of the reported series (i.e., proportion of primary and secondary PMF cases). The JAK2V617F mutation in PMF is associated with an older patient age at diagnosis and a history of thrombosis or pruritus. The clinical utility of performing mutational studies in patients with PMF has been well defined in making a definitive diagnosis of PMF. More recently, a common JAK2 germline haplotype (46/1) that is identified by the rs12343867 SNP was found to affect disease susceptibility in PMF regardless of JAK2 mutational status. In a study of 130 PMF patients, the 46/1 haplotype was found in both JAK2V617F-positive and -negative cases at a frequency of 50% and 36%, respectively. Nullizygosity for the JAK2 46/1 haplotype (rs12343867 TT genotype) was found to be associated with a shortened survival in PMF, and this was independent of other clinical parameters or karyotype. This has led the authors to propose that the non-46/1 haplotypes may be associated with a more biologically and thus clinically aggressive form of PMF.

Gain-of-function mutations of the thrombopoietin receptor, MPLW515L and MPLW515K, are present in patients with PMF at a frequency of approximately 5%, 1% of patients with ET but not patients with PV. MPL mutations may occur concurrently with the normal V617F mutation, suggesting that these alleles may have functional complementation in MPN. In all cases, the MPLW515K/L mutant allele is present in excess of the JAK2V617F allele. In contrast to acute myeloid leukemia (AML), mutations in the receptor tyrosine kinases KIT, FMS, and FLT3 have not been documented in PMF.

The number of circulating cells expressing the CD34 antigen, a phenotypic marker of hematopoietic stem and progenitor cells, in patients with PMF has been reported to be more than 300 times higher than in normal volunteers and 18 to 30 times higher than in patients with PV or ET. The clinical utility of the cytofluorimetric measurement of $CD34^+$ cells as a diagnostic marker of PMF is hampered by the fact that a small number of subjects with PMF exhibit a normal number of $CD34^+$ cells in the peripheral blood. Cases with a very mild disease phenotype or absent or slight reticulin BM fibrosis account for the majority of these patients. High values of $CD34^+$ cells ($>200 \times 10^6$/L) have been proposed as an indicator of an accelerated phase of the disease.

On radiographic examination, the characteristic features of PMF are a diffuse increase in bone density and increased prominence of the bony trabeculae. This increased bone density may be patchy and can produce a mottled appearance. Such abnormalities have been reported in 25% to 66% of patients with PMF.

Noninvasive imaging of BM is a promising means of evaluating the BM cellularity and distribution in PMF. Magnetic resonance imaging (MRI) can portray the conversion or reconversion of fatty to cellular BM. Fibrotic BM is easily distinguished from cellular BM by its strikingly low signal intensity with all pulse signals. The BM patterns in the proximal femurs of PMF patients have been reported to be correlated with the clinical severity of the disease. BM MRI has been used to differentiate PMF from ET, where the BM adipose tissue is preserved, but in PMF, the adiposity of the BM is reduced.

DIFFERENTIAL DIAGNOSIS

A patient with hepatosplenomegaly, peripheral cytopenias, teardrop poikilocytosis, leukoerythroblastosis, and BM fibrosis probably has PMF, but other disorders may also lead to this clinical picture (see Table 69-3 and Fig. 69-3). The WHO diagnostic criteria were revised,

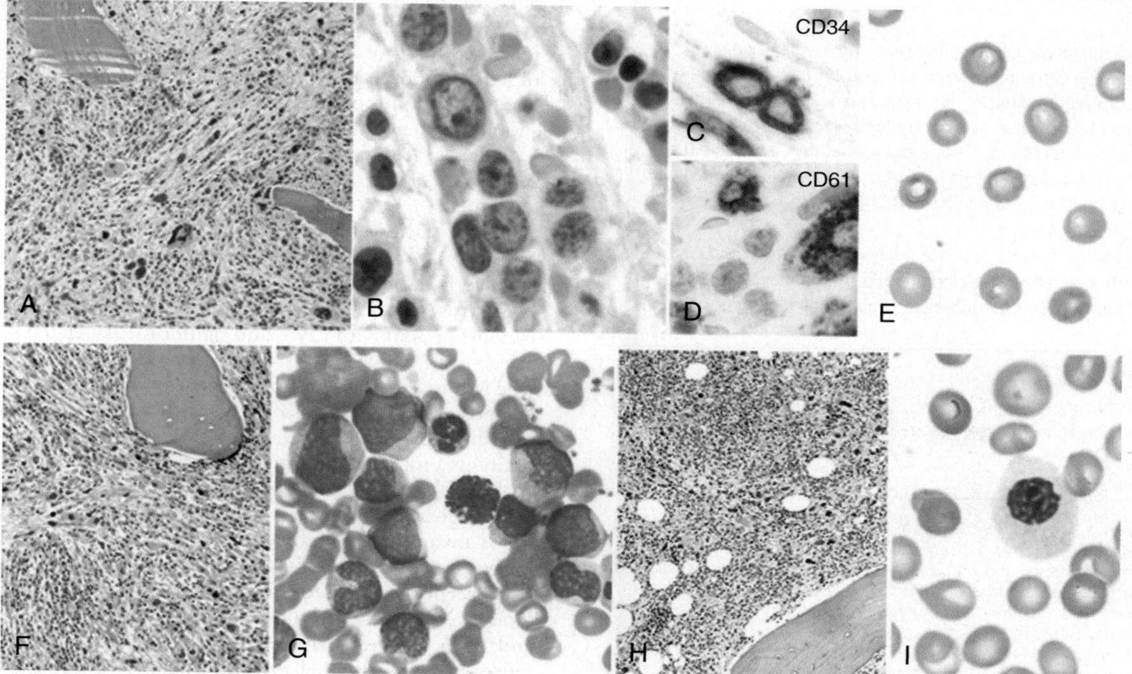

Figure 69-3 DIFFERENTIAL DIAGNOSTIC CONSIDERATIONS IN PRIMARY MYELOFIBROSIS (PMF). **A** to **E,** Acute panmyelosis with myelofibrosis (APMF). **F** and **G,** Chronic myelogenous leukemia (CML) in an advance phase with fibrosis. **H** and **I,** Myelodysplastic syndrome (MDS) with fibrosis. The bone marrow (BM) biopsy of APMF, CML in advanced phase with fibrosis, and MDS with fibrosis can all look similar to PMF at low power (**A,** **F,** and **H**). In APMF, the distinction from PMF is made in part by seeing increased immature cells on the biopsy (**B**) interspersed with other hematopoietic precursors. These are usually $CD34^+$ (**C**) but in contrast to acute megakaryoblastic leukemia are usually CD61 negative (**D**). Also, the peripheral blood usually shows pancytopenia with neither teardrop red blood cells nor a leukoerythroblastosis (**E**). Although the biopsy of CML presenting in an advanced phase can resemble PMF (**F**), the peripheral blood usually shows a classic granulocytosis with left shift and basophilia (**G**). In the case illustrated, the 30-year-old female patient had fibrotic BM (**F**) but presented with a white blood cell count of 148,000/L showing a full spectrum of granulocytes, increased blasts (22%), and basophilia. P210 *BCR/ABL1* was demonstrated. The bone marrow biopsy in MDS with fibrosis has small megakaryocytes (**H**), but dysplasia is otherwise difficult to evaluate in the absence of an aspirate, and one must rely on the peripheral blood to identify dysplasia, as in the severely dysplastic neutrophil (**F**).

incorporating testing for JAK2V617F and activating MPL mutations as well as greater emphasis on histomorphologic criteria which allow one to distinguish early phases of PMF from ET (Table 69-5). The WHO criteria are based on the recognition of a prefibrotic form of PMF without reticulin fibrosis and that the primary diagnostic features of PMF are increased megakaryocyte numbers, megakaryocyte morphology, and abnormalities of granulocyte mutation. Secondary MF frequently occurs in patients with lymphoma or metastatic carcinoma of the stomach, prostate, lung, or breast. The clinician should be extremely careful in making the diagnosis of PMF in a patient who has a history of a primary neoplasm. Demonstration of carcinoma cells in the BM establishes that metastatic carcinoma is the cause of the BM fibrosis. Careful breast examination and mammography are indicated in all women suspected of having PMF to exclude the possibility of metastatic breast cancer. The finding of blastic or lytic bone lesions in patients with MF suggests the presence of an underlying carcinoma. Disseminated tuberculosis and histoplasmosis have been associated with the development of secondary MF. Caseating or noncaseating granulomas observed on BM biopsy suggest the presence of these infectious disorders. Identification of the causative organisms by culture techniques should be pursued.

A number of other primary hematologic disorders can also be accompanied by BM fibrosis. A variety of overlap syndromes that share features of both PMF and MDS have been reported and are seen frequently in clinical practice. These so-called overlap syndromes have pathological and clinical features of both MPN and MDS and are characterized by BM hypercellularity, dysplasia of various myeloid lineages, and proliferative features yet also ineffective hematopoiesis, modest hepatosplenomegaly, and some degree of BM fibrosis. These patients are occasionally JAK2V617F positive and frequently have TET2 mutations. Such patients frequently present with cytopenias and are at a high risk of developing acute leukemia. These cases indicate the limitations of adhering to strict disease classifications and underscore that a continuum exists between MPNs and MDS. The peripheral blood and BM findings that allow differentiation of these disorders and can be enhanced by JAK2V617F and MPLW515L/K mutational analysis. Patients with the variant MDS with MF frequently present with cytopenias and have dysplastic cellular abnormalities indistinguishable from those of other patients with myelodysplasia. Their BMs, however, are characterized by the presence of BM fibrosis and a striking megakaryocytic hyperplasia, with a predominance of small hypolobulated forms, in some cases surrounding fibrosis. Reticulocytopenia is characteristic of these patients, as are teardrop RBCs and a clinical picture of leukoerythroblastosis. Unlike patients with PMF, patients with myelodysplasia and BM fibrosis do not have hepatic or splenic enlargement extending more than 3 cm below the costal margin. The overall survival time of patients with this variant of myelodysplasia has been reported to be 30 months, with death resulting from the effects of cytopenias or transformation to acute leukemia. Additional studies have indicated that the presence of MF in patients with myelodysplasia was associated with a particularly short survival time (9.6 months) compared with patients with myelodysplasia without fibrosis (17.4 months).

Hairy cell leukemia can also be confused with PMF. In one study, five of 61 patients who had originally been diagnosed as having PMF were shown retrospectively to have had hairy cell leukemia. Hairy cell leukemia can present as pancytopenia with splenomegaly and is associated with a dry BM tap. In one series, BM reticulin content was increased in 26 of 29 patients with hairy cell leukemia. The presence of hairy mononuclear cells possessing tartrate-resistant acid phosphatase or the appropriate phenotype in the peripheral blood or BM should facilitate differentiation of PMF from hairy cell leukemia (see Chapter 77). This exercise is important because of the different modalities of treatment that can be successfully used for hairy cell leukemia.

Bone marrow fibrosis can occur in patients with other MPNs, especially PV and CML, and less frequently with ET. In CML, progressive BM fibrosis may herald the onset of accelerated disease or blast crisis. MF in CML occurs in two distinct patterns, one in which patients present with CML and significant associated BM fibrosis and a second in which the MF develops late in the course of the CML. The MF in the latter group appears at a mean of 36 months after the diagnosis of CML, is associated with a mean survival time of 4.9 months from the detection of MF, and therefore represents an ominous prognostic sign.

Post-PV MF occurs in 5% to 15% of patients with PV. This transition occurs, on average, 10 years after the initial diagnosis of PV is made, but in individual cases, it may appear after shorter or longer intervals. PMF is clinically indistinguishable from post-PV MF except for the previous history of erythrocytosis in the latter group. Of patients with post-PV MF, 25% to 50% develop leukemia, and 70% are dead within 3 years of this transition. Post-PV MF represents a transitional myeloproliferative syndrome with relatively grave prognostic implications. MF has also been reported after ET. These investigators claimed that these patients did not represent individuals with prefibrotic stages of PMF but rather evolution of patients with true ET. They estimated the probability of developing such a complication to be 3% 5 years after diagnosis, 8% at 10 years, and 15% at 15 years, and considered this evolution to BM fibrosis a major long-term complication of ET. This evolution of ET was reported not to be associated with or prevented by the use of cytotoxic agents. Others have, however, suggested that most individuals with a presumptive diagnosis of ET whose disease evolved into post-ET MF had prefibrotic PMF if strict diagnostic criteria were used. They have conjectured that a considerable number of patients who carry a

Table 69-5 Proposed Revised World Health Organization Criteria for Primary Myelofibrosis*

MAJOR CRITERIA

1. Presence of megakaryocyte proliferation and atypia,[†] usually accompanied by either reticulin or collagen fibrosis, or, in the absence of significant reticulin fibrosis, the megakaryocyte changes must be accompanied by an increased bone marrow cellularity characterized by granulocytic proliferation and often decreased erythropoiesis (i.e., prefibrotic cellular-phase disease)
2. Not meeting WHO criteria for PV,[‡] CML,[§] MDS,[‖] or other myeloid neoplasm
3. Demonstration of *JAK2*617V >F or other clonal marker (e.g., *MPL*515W >L/K) or in the absence of a clonal marker, no evidence of bone marrow fibrosis caused by underlying inflammatory or other neoplastic diseases[¶]

MINOR CRITERIA

1. Leukoerythroblastosis**
2. Increase in serum lactate dehydrogenase level**
3. Anemia**
4. Palpable splenomegaly**

Data from Tefferi A, Thiele J, Orazi A, et al: Proposals and rationale for revision of the World Health Organization diagnostic criteria for polycythemia vera, essential thrombocythemia, and primary myelofibrosis: Recommendations from an ad hoc international expert panel, *Blood* 110:1092, 2007.

CML, Chronic myeloid leukemia; *MDS,* myelodysplastic syndrome; *PV,* polycythemia vera; *WHO,* World Health Organization.

*Diagnosis requires meeting all three major criteria and two minor criteria.

[†]Small to large megakaryocytes with an aberrant nuclear-to-cytoplasmic ratio and hyperchromatic, bulbous, or irregularly folded nuclei and dense clustering.

[‡]Requires the failure of iron replacement therapy to increase hemoglobin level to the polycythemia vera range in the presence of decreased serum ferritin. Exclusion of polycythemia vera is based on hemoglobin and hematocrit levels. Red blood cell mass measurement is not required.

[§]Requires the absence of *BCR-ABL.*

[‖]Requires the absence of dyserythropoiesis and dysgranulopoiesis.

[¶]Secondary to infection, autoimmune disorder or other chronic inflammatory condition, hairy cell leukemia or other lymphoid neoplasm, metastatic malignancy, or toxic (chronic) myelopathies. It should be noted that patients with conditions associated with reactive myelofibrosis are not immune to primary myelofibrosis, and the diagnosis should be considered in such cases if other criteria are met.

**Degree of abnormality could be borderline or marked.

diagnosis of ET already are actually in a prefibrotic phase of PMF. Careful prospective natural history studies using strict histopathologic criteria are still required to resolve this controversy.

Acute panmyelosis with myelofibrosis (APMF) represents a clinical entity distinct from PMF. This disorder has also been termed acute MF, acute myelosclerosis, acute megakaryocytic MF, and acute myelodysplasia with MF. APMF is exceedingly rare and corresponds to fewer than 1% of the cases of AML. Patients characteristically present with pancytopenia, fever, absence of clinically significant splenomegaly, minimal or absent teardrop poikilocytosis, and fibrotic BM. The BM is characterized by the appearance of immature myeloid cells and the blast cells, which frequently express megakaryocytic phenotypic properties. Survival ranges from 1 to 9 months after diagnosis. Its distinction from PMF is important because aggressive chemotherapy and possibly SCT are the treatments of choice. Even though some authors consider APMF a form of acute megakaryoblastic leukemia (AMKL), the WHO criteria for diagnosing APMF are somewhat distinct from those for AMKL. The main requirement for the diagnosis of AMKL is a minimum of 20% BM blasts, a percentage that is significantly higher than observed in APMF. In addition, the blasts in all cases of AMKL stain strongly for CD61 and CD41 and are negative for myeloperoxidase. In contrast, APMF is characterized by a lower percentage of blasts within a polymorphic cellular background, which includes erythroblasts, megakaryocytes, and maturing myeloid elements with variability in their relative proportions from case to case. The blasts in APMF did not express significant reactivity to megakaryocytic phenotypic markers but are identifiable by their strong reactivity with CD34 and occasional reactivity with myeloperoxidase. These results emphasized the panmyelotic nature of APMF. In PMF, the peculiar cytologic characteristics of the megakaryocytes, which include anisocytosis with a predominance of large size forms arranged into tight cellular clusters, the abnormal chromatin clumping with hyperchromatic nuclei and clumped (cloud shape) nuclear lobulation as well as the characteristic stromal changes that include the presence of intrasinusoidal hematopoiesis, allow for a distinction from these more acute disorders.

Up to 12% of patients who present with MF have been reported to have an underlying autoimmune disorder such as SLE, although in the authors' clinical practice, this is an extraordinary rare event. Primary autoimmune MF (primary AIMF) likely represents a distinct clinicopathologic syndrome unrelated to other well-defined autoimmune disorders. Eight diagnostic criteria for AIMF, including grade 3 or 4 reticulin fibrosis in the BM, lack of clustered or atypical megakaryocytes, lack of dysplasia or eosinophilia or basophilia, lymphoid infiltration of the BM, lack of osteosclerosis, absent or mild splenomegaly, presence of autoantibodies, and absence of disorders associated with MF, have been outlined. The appearance of the BM in AIMF is indistinguishable from that of PMF. Autoimmune MF occurs predominantly in females with a broad clinical spectrum. Patients may present with MF in the setting of established SLE or in patients with minimal manifestations of an autoimmune disorder as in primary AIMF. The presence of teardrop erythrocytes or leukoerythroblastosis in a patient with lupus suggests autoimmune MF. Such patients universally have a positive ANA test result or an elevated anti-DNA titer. Because the physical manifestations of an autoimmune disease may not be evident, all patients with MF should have an ANA test to exclude an autoimmune etiology. Moreover, a diagnosis of AIMF is important because the cytopenias and BM fibrosis in this disorder may partially resolve with steroid or methotrexate therapy. However, it must be pointed out that the place of primary AIMF in the classification of fibrotic disorders needs a more precise definition requiring the absence of mutations that include JAK2V617F, MPLW515L, and MPLW515K.

PROGNOSIS

The median overall survival period from the time of diagnosis of PMF varies from series to series but is approximately 5 years (Fig. 69-4). Individual survival times have been reported to range from 1 year to more than 30 years. The primary causes of death include infection, leukemic transformation, heart failure, bleeding, hepatic failure caused by EMH of the liver, portal hypertension, renal failure, pulmonary embolism, and posttransplantation. The incidence of acute leukemia as a terminal event ranges from 5% to 22%, depending on the series cited (Fig. 69-5). Approximately half of the patients who develop acute leukemia have not received previous treatment

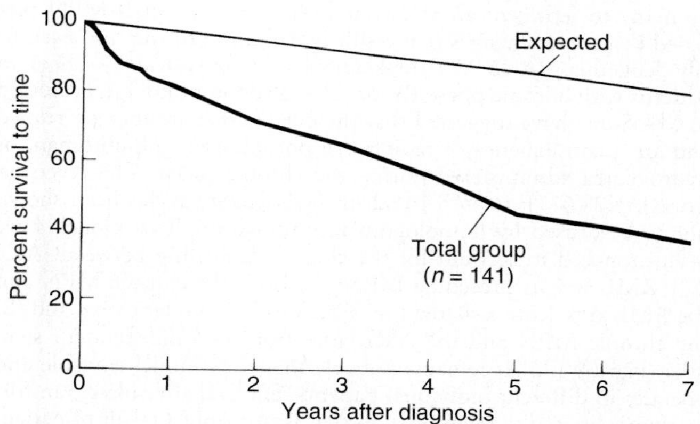

Figure 69-4 OVERALL SURVIVAL FROM THE TIME OF DIAGNOSIS OF 141 PATIENTS WITH PRIMARY MYELOFIBROSIS. *(Data from Silverstein MN:* Agnogenic myeloid metaplasia, *Acton, MA, 1975, Publishing Sciences Group, p 197.)*

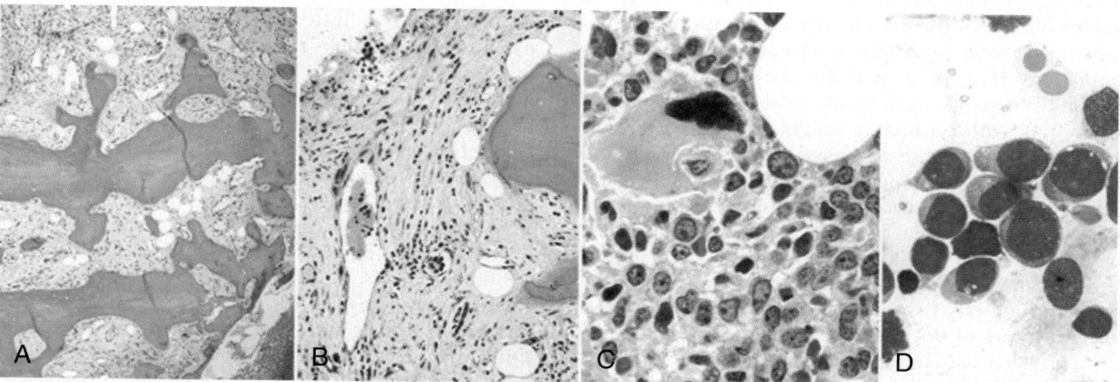

Figure 69-5 DISEASE PROGRESSION IN PRIMARY MYELOFIBROSIS (PMF). Marked osteosclerosis (**A** and **B**) and acute leukemia (**C** and **D**). In some patients, PMF progresses to severe osteosclerosis in which there is markedly thickened and irregular bone formation **(A)** and a bone marrow space that is fibrotic and nearly depleted of hematopoietic elements **(B).** A terminal transformation to acute leukemia (**C** and **D**) occurs in 5% to 22% of cases.

with alkylating agents or radiotherapy, suggesting that the evolution into acute leukemia may be part of the natural history of PMF. The actuarial cumulative risk of death from leukemic transformation at 1 and 5 years after diagnosis has been reported to be 2% and 16%, respectively. Immunologic and morphologic characterization of the blast phenotypes comprising these leukemias reveals that a typical myeloid phenotype is most commonly detected; other cell lineages, such as megakaryocytic, erythroid, lymphoid, and even stem cell phenotype, may also be involved, leading to the existence of mixed myeloid and hybrid transformations. Megakaryoblastic transformations have been detected in one-third of cases in one series, an incidence higher than that found in de novo AML. In 50% of cases of JAK2V617F MPNs, the blast cells that represent the progeny of the leukemia initiating clone are JAK2V617F negative suggesting that the leukemia originates from a clone distinct from the JAK2V617F-positive clone. This coexistent JAK2V617F-negative clone appears to have a higher propensity to undergo leukemic transformation. JAK2V617F therefore does not appear to be a prerequisite for leukemic transformation of MPNs, suggesting that additional genetic events are required for full transformation to occur. SNP array analysis has shown that genomic alterations occur at an increased frequency during the period of blastic transformation and that no single gene or molecular pathway is sufficient to cause transformation. A surprising correlation has been observed between the phenotype of the preceding MPN and the JAK2 mutational status of the leukemic blasts after transformation. In contrast to JAK2 WT AML in this setting, evolution to JAK2V617F leukemias is invariably preceded by a myelofibrotic transformation of ET or PV or PMF. Because of these observations, myelofibrotic transformation of ET or PV are thought by many to represent an accelerated phase of the initial MPN preceded by genetic changes that result in evolution to MF and eventually leukemia. JAK2 WT leukemia by contrast usually arises in patients with chronic phase PV or ET that do not undergo evolution to MF. Some have suggested that these leukemias are therapy related and are a consequence of radioactive phosphorous, pipobroman, or hydroxyurea administered during the chronic phase. The reversion from JAK2V617F to WT JAK2 in these leukemias has been shown not to be caused by homologous recombination. Two models have been proposed to account for the clonal relationship between JAK2 WT AML and its preceding MPN: (1) Both the chronic MPN and the AML arise from a shared pre-JAK2V617F founder clone, and (2) the chronic MPN and the AML arise from two independent stem cells (Fig. 69-6).[11] It remains possible that each model is viable and operates in different individual patients. Survival after blast transformation is limited, a phenomenon that is probably a result of patient age and the aggressive biology of these leukemias. Leukemic transformation of PMF has been reported to be fatal in 98% after a median of 2.6 months. Successful leukemia remission induction therapy in these patients is an extremely rare event. Patients should therefore be sent for stem cell transplant before leukemic transformation.

Several clinical and biologic parameters that are characteristic of patients at diagnosis have been used to identify subgroups of patients with different outcomes. Some investigators have suggested that there are two subpopulations of patients in PMF: short-lived and long-lived subpopulations of patients. Such efforts at developing prognostic parameters have met with conflicting results, with the exception that anemia at presentation is consistently associated with short survival. Dupriez and associates developed an extremely simple scoring system, the Lille scoring system, based on two adverse prognostic factors—hemoglobin level less than 10 g/dL and WBC count less than 4000/mm^3 or more than 30,000/mm^3 and were able to stratify patients into three groups The low-risk (zero factors), intermediate-risk (one factor), and high-risk (two factors) groups were associated with median survival times of 93, 26, and 13 months, respectively. Other scoring systems that use simple clinical hematologic parameters have been subsequently proposed. In another study, the presence of a hemoglobin level of 10 g/dL or higher, a platelet count of at least 100 × 10^9/L, and less than 3% circulating blasts predicted a median survival of approximately 15 years compared with less than 5 years in the remaining patients.

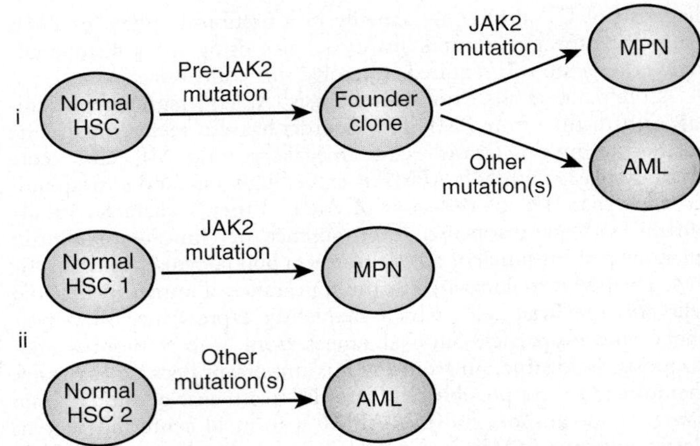

Figure 69-6 MODELS TO EXPLAIN PROGRESSION FROM A JANUS KINASE 2 (JAK2) MUTANT MYELOPROLIFERATIVE NEOPLASM TO A JAK2 WILD-TYPE LEUKEMIA. In model 1 (i), the two phases of disease are phylogenetically related, having arisen from a shared (pre-JAK2) founder clone, but in model 2 (ii), the two phases of disease are clonally unrelated, reflecting transformation of independent stem cells. *AML,* acute myeloid leukemia; *HSC,* hematopoietic stem cell. *(From Beer PA, Delhommeau F, LeCouédic JP, et al: Two routes to leukemic transformation after a JAK2 mutation-positive myeloproliferative neoplasm.* Blood *115:2891, 2010.)*

The International Working Group for Myelofibrosis Research and Treatment (IWG-MRT) developed an international prognostic scoring system (IPSS) based on 1054 patients diagnosed with PMF.[12] (Table 69-6 and 69-7) compare four validated prognostic scoring systems for patients with PMF. The overall median survival for this group was 69 months, and multivariate analysis identified age older than 65 years, presence of constitutional symptoms, hemoglobin below 10 g/dL, leukocyte count above 25 × 10^9/L, and peripheral blood blasts 1% or greater as significant risk factors. The sum of the risk factors allows for allocation into discrete risk groups. Four risk groups can be discerned with non-overlapping survival curves based on this model with median survivals of 135, 95, 48, and 27 months for low (0), intermediate-1 (1), intermediate-2 (2), and high-risk (3-5) groups, respectively. Although the presence of JAK2V617F was associated with age older than 65 years, it did not influence survival in this study. The presence of cytogenetic abnormalities exerted an influence on the intermediate risk groups only. A cohort of 525 PMF patients was followed over time to assess the prognostic influence of the five IPSS clinical variables acquired during the course of disease rather than at presentation. The IPSS variables were analyzed as time-dependent covariates in a multivariate Cox proportional hazard model. Anemia was found to have the most significant hazard ratio for survival. The advantage of this dynamic IPSS (DIPSS) is the ability to assess real-time prognosis as a patient acquires each clinical feature. An age-adjusted DIPSS (aaDIPSS) was also proposed for patients younger than the age of 65 years and may be particularly useful when applied to young patients in the context of risk assessment for SCT. Most recently, an attempt to further refine the DIPSS based on the incorporation of unfavorable karyotype, platelet count below 100 × 10^9/L and transfusional status within the scoring system was reported. Additionally, in this review of 793 PMF patients, a poorer, leukemia-free survival was predicted by the presence of thrombocytopenia or unfavorable karyotype with a 10-year risk of 31% (hazards ratio [HR], 3.3; 95% confidence interval [CI], 1.9-5.6).

Although cytogenetic studies are an integral part of a variety of prognostic scoring systems for many hematologic malignancies, for similar purpose in PMF, this has not been as well developed. However, substantial progress has been made during the past few years to allow for the use of cytogenetics as a prognostic indicator. Initially, a group from MD Anderson performed a retrospective analysis of 256 patients (36% had an abnormal karyotype) and determined that baseline cytogenetic status was useful in predicting survival. Sole deletions of

Table 69-6 Prognostic Scoring Systems for Primary Myelofibrosis

Risk Factor	Lille	IPSS	DIPSS	DIPSS Plus
Anemia (hemoglobin)	X (<10 g/dL)	X (<10 g/dL)	X (<10 g/dL)	X (<10 g/dL)
Leukocytosis (white blood cell count)	X (<4 or >30 x 10^9/L)	X (>25 x 10^9/L)	X (>25 x 10^9/L)	X (>25 x 10^9/L)
Peripheral blood blasts		X (≥1%)	X (≥1%)	X (≥1%)
Constitutional symptoms		X	X	X
Age (years)		X (>65)	X (adjusted for age)	X
Karyotype				X (unfavorable*)
Platelet				X (<100 x10^9/L)
Transfusion status				X

DIPSS, Dynamic international prognostic scoring system; *IPSS*, international prognostic scoring system.
*Unfavorable karyotype includes complex or sole or two abnormalities that include +8, -7/7q-, i7/7q-, i(17q), -5/5q-, 12p-, inv(3), or 11q23 rearrangements.

Table 69-7 Median Survival of Each Risk Group in Four Prognostic Scoring Systems for Primary Myelofibrosis

Risk Group	Lille	IPSS	DIPSS	DIPSS Plus
Low	93 months	135 months	Not reached	185 months
Intermediate-1	26 months	95 months	170 months	78 months
Intermediate-2		48 months	48 months	35 months
High	13 months	27 months	18 months	16 months

DIPSS, Dynamic international prognostic scoring system; *IPSS*, international prognostic scoring system.

chromosomes 13 and 20 or trisomy 9 alone or in the presence of other abnormalities were associated with a median survival time similar to those with a normal karyotype (63 and 46 months, respectively). By contrast, abnormalities of chromosomes 5 or 7 or three or more abnormalities were associated with a median survival time of 15 months. In the more expanded Mayo Clinic study of 433 patients, a two-tier cytogenetic risk stratification after a median follow-up of 4 years was established.[13] Because cytogenetic analysis is not yet incorporated in the IPSS, the following cytogenetic current schema should be carefully considered.[14] Patients with favorable karyotype include sole chromosome 1 translocations or duplication, del(13q), del(20q), trisomy 9, other sole abnormalities, two abnormalities excluding unfavorable type, and a normal karyotype. A 5-year survival rate was 51% with a median survival of 5.2 years was observed (see Fig. 69-5). The 5-year survival for patients with an unfavorable karyotype, including a sole trisomy 8, sole abnormalities of chromosomes 5 or 7, inversion of chromosome 3, isochromosome 17q, deletion 12p or 11q23 rearrangement as well as two abnormalities including the unfavorable type and a complex karyotype was 8% with a median survival of 2 years. Moreover, multivariable analysis demonstrated that karyotype ($P = .001$) and platelet count ($100 < \times 10^9$/L [$P = .04$]) but not IPSS ($P = .27$) predicted leukemia-free survival: the 5-year leukemic transformation rates for unfavorable versus favorable karyotype were 46% and 7%, respectively ($P < .0001$). The implementation of these recommendations observations needs confirmation from multiple institutions. Specifically, gain of chromosome 1q, occurring in 22% of PMF, is believed to be associated with disease progression, and jumping 1q translocations was reported to be associated with imminent transformation to AML in a majority of patients. In PMF, the region on chromosome 1 that is most frequently duplicated or occurring in trisomy is between 1q21-32 and 1q32-44 band regions (see Fig. 69-3). This 1q region has been reported in unbalanced translocations with many chromosomes, although more specific PMF translocation involves der(6)t(1;6) (q21-23;p21-23 or q27). In contrast, in patients with PV-related MF, the most frequent recurrent 1q abnormality involves der(9)t(1;9) (q21;q12), resulting also in trisomy 9p. A new cytogenetic risk category, monosomal karyotype (MK), also defines an unfavorable risk category. An MK is defined as having two or more autosomal monosomies or a single autosomal monosomy associated with at least one structural abnormality. This is a rare cytogenetic change associated with median survival of 6 months and a 2-year leukemic transformation rate of 29.4%. At diagnosis of PMF, detection of MK is associated with extremely poor overall and leukemia-free survival.

Patients who have normal diploid karyotype at baseline that remains unchanged during the period of observation have a similar median survival to those with favorable abnormalities (36 vs. 31 months, respectively). The most unfavorable cytogenetic abnormalities include i(17q), which results in the loss of 17p, and heterozygous loss of P53, inversion of chromosome 3 and MK.

Most studies have indicated that the overall survival of patients with JAK2V617F-positive and -negative PMF are similar; however, patients with JAK2V617F-positive disease and a low allele burden (<25%) have been shown to have a shorter survival time. In addition, mutations in MPL or TET2 do not appear to influence overall or leukemia-free survival. A number of investigators have attempted to correlate the presence of a variety of more recently identified mutations with disease outcomes of patients with PMF. EZH2 mutations have been identified in 6% of patients with PMF, 3% of PV patients, 3% of patients with post-PV MF, and 9.4% of patients with post-ET MF. More than 40% of the patients with EZH2 mutations were JAK2V617F, 6% have a TET2 mutation, and, 22% harbored an ASXL mutation. Concurrent EZH2 mutations and MPL mutations have not been observed. EZH2 mutations are usually present at the diagnosis of the chronic MPN and are maintained universally in the leukemic blasts at the time of transformation to AML. EZH2 mutated patients are characterized by more profound leukocytosis and larger spleens and have a higher percentage of blasts. The survival of patients with EZH2 mutations was clearly inferior because they clustered in patients with IPSS scores associated with high-risk disease. In addition, IDH mutations, albeit rare in PMF patients, have been associated with an inferior survival in JAK2V617F-positive patients, raising the possibility of the cooperation between IDH mutations and JAK2V617F in leukemic transformation.

Therapy

The optimal forms of treatment for PMF have not yet been defined, but reports of successful nonmyeloablative allogeneic SCT provide hope for cure of a subpopulation of these patients, and the recent approval of small molecule JAK2 inhibitors that are effective in reducing the degree of splenomegaly and alleviating systemic symptoms is an important therapeutic advance. A conservative approach to management is generally accepted, with observation of asymptomatic patients and therapeutic intervention reserved for patients with symptoms.[15] Hydroxyurea appears to be a useful agent for the treatment of PMF. Its use has been associated with significantly reduced platelet numbers and a reduction of megakaryocytic abnormalities, as well as a significant reduction of MF. Some investigators have hypothesized that hydroxyurea-induced suppression of megakaryocytopoiesis causes a reduction in the levels of platelet-derived fibrogenic cytokines, resulting in reduced fibroblast proliferation and deposition of reticulin. Moderate doses (20-30 mg/kg) of hydroxyurea given twice or three times weekly are effective and safe in PMF patients requiring treatment. Similar reports have appeared after the use of daily busulfan with responding patients achieving hematologic remission and some reversal of BM fibrosis. Not only did hematologic parameters, including the hemoglobin and hematocrit levels, improve, but a reduction of the number of teardrop erythrocytes and the degree of leukoerythroblastosis has been reported in occasional patients. Most importantly, the quality of life of these individuals improved. Judicious use of busulfan is recommended in this setting, however, because of its potential for producing delayed BM suppression. Melphalan administered at low doses (2.5 mg given three times a week) has also been reported to be well tolerated and capable of producing less hematologic toxicity than busulfan. Among patients with severe anemia requiring transfusion therapy, 38% became transfusion independent, and 20% experienced a 50% reduction in their transfusion requirement. Approximately 54% of patients with symptomatic splenomegaly experienced a clinically significant reduction in spleen size. The median duration of the response to melphalan therapy was somewhat longer than 2 years. The disease of more than 20% of the patients receiving melphalan evolved into the leukemic phase. It is impossible to determine whether melphalan therapy played a role in this evolution or if this rate of blastic transformation was a consequence of the advanced stage of the disease at the time of treatment. The use of this agent was associated with acceptable toxicity, with only 13% of patients stopping their therapy because of the development of cytopenias and 17% requiring a dose reduction because of hematologic toxicity.

Interferon-α therapy has been reported to have activity in some patients with PMF. It can be useful in suppressing thrombocytosis and inhibiting the activity of PDGF, which stimulates the proliferation of fibroblasts.[16] A combination of INF, granulocyte-macrophage colony-stimulating factor (GM-CSF), and erythropoietin (EPO) in seven patients with an early form of PMF was investigated. Six of seven patients enjoyed marked reductions in spleen size. Each of these patients had an increase of 1 g/dL or more in the hemoglobin concentration. In one patient, the degree of BM fibrosis was diminished. These investigators suggested that INF might decrease the rate of fibrosis if administered chronically during the early course of this disease. Others have not reported similar effects in patients with more advanced phases of the disease. In one series, only four of 11 patients were able to complete 1 year of therapy; the other seven patients discontinued the drug because of unacceptable toxicity or the development of severe cytopenias. No clinically significant improvement was observed in any of these patients. INF therapy did not appear to alter the degree of BM fibrosis, osteosclerosis, or angiogenesis. A small phase II pilot study in PMF patients demonstrated responses in patients with prefibrotic hypercellular PMF treated with low doses of IFN-α-2b over an extended period (median duration, 3 years). Four patients with JAK2V617F-positive PMF were followed over time, and although all had clinical responses, only one had a significant reduction in mutant allele burden. The drug was generally well tolerated at doses between 1 and 2 million units weekly, and responses in the BM included reduction in reticulin fibrosis and abnormal cellular morphology. Eleven patients with PMF were treated with a pegylated form of INF-α-2b (PEG-IFNα-2b) at starting dose between 2 and 3 μg/kg/week; only a single patient with PMF responded. Although the pegylated form of this drug allows for weekly injections, the toxicity profile was found to be similar to the standard formulation and for many patients limits the duration of therapy. The most common grade 3/4 toxicity was fatigue and thrombocytopenia. Because of the recent encouraging results reported with PEG-IFN-α-2a (Pegasys) in PV patients, this form of INF-α has also been tested in MF patients. The French Groupe d'Etudes des Myelofibrosis (GEM) and France Intergroupe des Syndromes Myeloproliferatifs conducted a study of 18 patients with PMF and post-ET/PV MF treated with Pegasys.[17] Of the four PMF patients included in this study, one had a CR, two had a minor response, and one had no response by EUMNET criteria. Responses were associated with improvement in the degree of anemia, leukocytosis, and thrombocytosis but not splenomegaly and appeared to be irrespective of JAK2 status. Comprehensive reviews of the literature suggest that modest benefits may be derived from INF-α therapy for PMF after patients have entered the more advanced phases of the disease. Further large randomized studies are warranted in patients with the prefibrotic phase of PMF to determine the effects of this modality of treatment on disease-free survival, overall survival, quality of life, and progression to more advanced phases of PMF or evolution to acute leukemia. Before such trials are completed, INF therapy at any phase of PMF should be considered an experimental form of therapy and not embarked upon unless the patient is participating in a clinical trial.

Therapy is indicated for PMF patients with the following conditions: symptoms attributable to anemia, pressure symptoms related to splenomegaly, bleeding problems, life-threatening thrombocytopenia, significant hyperuricemia bone pain, systemic symptoms (fevers, night sweats and weight loss), and portal hypertension and life-threatening gastrointestinal bleeding. Hyperuricemia should be aggressively treated in all patients with PMF. Hydration and chronic administration of allopurinol (300 mg/day) are suggested.

Anemia is a common problem in patients with PMF. It is usually multifactorial in origin; contributing factors are folate deficiency, iron deficiency, ineffective erythropoiesis, erythroid hypoplasia, and hemolysis. Patients with documented nutritional deficiencies should receive folate, iron supplementation, or both. Transfusion therapy with packed RBCs is clearly indicated in patients who are symptomatic from their anemia. Chronic transfusion therapy is frequently required, and the clinician should try to attain a hemoglobin level at which symptoms resolve. Long-term transfusion therapy potentially may lead to the development of iron overload syndrome. Thus serious consideration should be given to early institution of iron chelation therapy. For a handful of patients, transfusion requirements have been reported to be reduced after desferrioxamine or deferasirox therapy. Because an oral effective iron chelator, deferasirox, is now available, therapy should be initiated early in the course of the disease when repeated cell transfusion therapy is required. The remainder of approaches to anemic patients deals with therapeutic interventions designed to avoid or diminish the number of transfusions administered.

Low-dose dexamethasone has been reported to be useful in the treatment of patients with transfusion-dependent PMF. Whether these cases represent steroid responses of autoimmune-induced MF and not classic PMF remains unknown. Low-dose melphalan therapy has been successfully used to reduce the transfusion requirements of a reasonable number of PMF patients. Corticosteroids (e.g., prednisone 1 mg/kg/day taken orally) have also been successfully used for treatment of the hemolytic anemia associated with PMF. A 2-g increase in hemoglobin in 29% of men and 52% of women receiving steroid therapy for PMF-associated hemolytic anemia. Folate should be simultaneously administered to all such patients. Even more encouraging results have been reported with simultaneous administration of busulfan and corticosteroids, with clinical responses lasting 6 to 12 months. After patients have reached a peak response, tapering of prednisone should be initiated to determine an acceptable maintenance dose. The hemolytic process frequently recurs after such tapering. It is important to be aware that the hemolytic anemia in patients with PMF may also be a consequence of a coexisting secondary form of paroxysmal nocturnal hemoglobinuria. Paroxysmal cold hemoglobinuria associated with a Donath-Landsteiner antibody should also be excluded as a cause of hemolytic anemia. Furthermore, patients with PMF who receive multiple transfusions are candidates for developing delayed hemolytic transfusion reactions that occasionally may be severe and persistent. The direct antiglobulin test result is usually positive in this setting. It is generally believed that additional transfusions in these patients with delayed hemolytic transfusion reactions should be avoided if possible. Other therapeutic options for PMF-associated hemolytic anemia include therapy with intravenous immunoglobulins and recombinant human erythropoietin-α (rHuEPO).

Anemia caused by erythroid cell hypoplasia as well as ineffective erythropoiesis in PMF may respond to anabolic steroids. A number of preparations have been suggested, including testosterone enanthate (600 mg/wk intramuscularly), stanozolol (12 mg/day taken orally), nandrolone (3 mg/kg/week intramuscularly), fluoxymesterone (10 mg taken orally three times daily), and oxymetholone (50 mg taken orally four times daily). A good response, as defined by a decrease or total avoidance of transfusion therapy, occurs in about 50% of patients. A course of 3 to 6 months of androgen therapy is indicated to identify responsive patients, but the development of hepatic dysfunction or virilizing side effects may limit long-term androgen administration. Patients with associated chromosomal abnormalities have been reported to be less likely to respond to androgen therapy. Danazol, a synthetic attenuated androgen, has also been useful in reducing the requirement for RBC transfusion support and correction of thrombocytopenia. Danazol appears to be a potentially effective therapy for PMF, which is mainly characterized by BM failure. Thirty-three patients with PMF who were either transfusion dependent or had hemoglobin levels below 10 g/dL were reported to be treated with an initial dose of 600 mg/day of danazol.[18] Of the 30 evaluable patients, a favorable response was seen in 11 (37%), with 27% having a complete response. The median time to response was 5 months (range, 1-9 months). Variables associated with response were lack of transfusion requirement and higher hemoglobin levels. In eight of 30 patients (27%), a moderate increase of liver enzyme levels was reported. It is unknown whether any of the anabolic steroids preparations are superior to the others or whether they are superior to danazol in improving anemia of PMF.

The experience with the use of rHuEPO in PMF has been recently reviewed by Cervantes and colleagues in a total of 51 patients, documenting that 28 (55%) of these patients responded to rHuEPO treatment, including 16 complete and 12 partial responses. Endogenous serum EPO levels inappropriately low for the degree of anemia is predictive of a favorable response to rHuEPO. Serum EPO levels below 125 U/L were found to be associated with a favorable response to rHuEPO therapy. Responses can be associated with a limited enlargement of the spleen.

The use of darbepoetin, a novel hyperglycosylated erythropoiesis-stimulating protein, has been reported in 20 PMF patients. With an initial weekly dose of 150 μg, increased to 300 μg, when no response was observed after 4 to 8 weeks, eight patients (40%) responded to treatment, including six complete and two partial responses, and five maintained their response after a median follow-up of 12 months (range, 4-22 months). The median time to response was 2 months. Univariate analysis indicated that older age was the only factor associated with a favorable response to treatment (P <.006). None of the patients with elevated serum EPO levels responded. Treatment was usually well tolerated, and patients can be successfully switched from rHuEPO to darbepoetin.

Multiple trials have explored the use of thalidomide in the treatment of anemia in PMF based on the drug's antiangiogenic, immunomodulatory, and antiinflammatory actions. A pooled analysis of five small phase II studies published from 2000 to 2002 have indicated that 29% of patients with moderate to severe anemia experience an increase in hemoglobin or reduction or elimination of blood transfusion requirements with thalidomide therapy at a standard dose of 200 to 800 mg/day. Nevertheless, most of the patients treated with these doses had adverse effects that resulted in an attrition rate of greater than 50% after 3 months. Moreover, increases of WBC numbers or platelet counts were frequently reported to be associated with such serious adverse events as pericardial effusions secondary to myeloid metaplasia. Using a dose-escalation design and starting with a low dose of thalidomide (50 mg/day), 31% of patients with transfusion-dependent anemia were reported to experience a response after treatment. A combination of low-dose thalidomide (50 mg/day) with prednisone has been reported to be a better tolerated regimen and equally or more effective than standard-dose treatment. Although the size of the patient population was limited, with this regimen, 40% of patients with an RBC transfusion requirement became transfusion independent, and 95% of the patients were able to complete the 3-month course of therapy with acceptable toxicity. The median hemoglobin level was reported to increase by 1.8 g/dL after low-dose thalidomide and prednisone therapy. This regimen also had a significant effect on the degree of thrombocytopenia and resulted in a reduction in the degree of splenomegaly in almost 10% of the patients. These responses were frequently maintained after therapy was halted. More recent reports provided further evidence that higher doses of thalidomide were not more effective than lower doses. A prospective phase II B, randomized, double-blind, multicenter trial compared therapy with 200 to 400 mg of thalidomide with placebo and documented that in the thalidomide group, only 10 of 26 patients completed 6 months of treatment and that no difference was observed between the thalidomide and placebo groups as regards improvement of hemoglobin levels or reduction of the number of RBC transfusion required. In addition, experience with thalidomide therapy in a two-stage phase II dose-escalation trial in 44 patients with advanced PMF has been reported. Starting at 200 mg/day and increasing to 800 mg as tolerated, the median tolerated dose was 400 mg for a median duration of 3 months; and 20% of the patients experienced improvement in their degree of anemia (21% became transfusion independent). Recently, a more potent thalidomide analog, lenalidomide, has been evaluated in 68 symptomatic patients with PMF at two institutions. Oral lenalidomide was administered at a dose of 10 mg/day if the platelet count was greater than 100,000/mm^3 or at a dose of 5 mg/day if the platelet count was less than 100,000/mm^3 for 3 to 4 months. The overall response rates were 22% for patients with anemia, 33% for patients with splenomegaly, and 50% for thrombocytopenia. Several patients normalized their hemoglobin levels or became RBC transfusion independent. The most common associated toxicities were grade 3 and 4 neutropenia and thrombocytopenia, which occurred in approximately 30% of patients but resolved with discontinuation of therapy. In several patients with del(5)(q31)-associated PMF or post-PV MF, lenalidomide therapy was associated with reduction of the numbers of cells with a marker chromosome as assayed by FISH and reduction of the JAK2V617F burden. Lenalidomide therapy in combination with prednisone therapy in PMF has been evaluated in a phase 2 trial within the Eastern Cooperative Oncology Group and appears to be modestly active and myelosuppressive.[19] Forty-two MF patients with anemia were treated with lenalidomide at 10 mg/day in combination with a 3-month prednisone taper. Grade 3 and higher myelotoxicity was noted in 88% of patients, and a response rate of 23% by IWG-MRT was obtained (19% clinical improvement in anemia or 10% clinical improvement in spleen size). In a single institution, thalidomide therapy and lenalidomide therapy for PMF was compared by retrospectively analyzing the results of three phase 2 trials performed that included 125 patients at this single center. They concluded that lenalidomide plus prednisone therapy was more effective than single-agent thalidomide or lenalidomide therapy. These results are of limited value because lenalidomide therapy plus prednisone therapy was never compared with that achieved with low-dose thalidomide and prednisone, which is associated with less myelosuppression. In this report, low-dose lenalidomide plus prednisone was not associated with an increased incidence of thrombotic events in the absence of any thromboprophylaxis. Some patients who failed to respond to thalidomide or lost their response to thalidomide did achieve significant responses with lenalidomide therapy. Whether either of these immunomodulatory drugs (IMiDs) is superior to the other is the subject of speculation, which would require a large randomized clinical trial. The mechanism by which these agents achieve these clinical responses also remains larger speculation.

Because IMiDs as a class have shown activity in MF and their use is often undermined by neurotoxicity or myelosuppression, recent interest in the structurally related but more potent pomalidomide in the treatment of MF-associated anemia has led to the completion of several early phase studies and an ongoing randomized phase 3 study. The first study to evaluate the response of pomalidomide in MF was a phase 2 randomized, double-blind, placebo-controlled adaptive design study with four treatment arms. This study reported an overall response in anemia of 24% (10 patients), and 15 of these patients achieved transfusion independence that was durable at 7.5 months. Pomalidomide at 0.5 mg/day with or without a prednisone taper was found to have better responses in anemia with less toxicity compared with pomalidomide at 2 mg/day with or without prednisone. Grade 3/4 myelosuppression and neurotoxicity were not frequent adverse events. A single-center phase 2 study of low-dose pomalidomide was conducted at Mayo Clinic.[20] A cohort of 58 patients were treated with pomalidomide at 0.5 mg/day. Of the 42 transfusion-dependent JAK2V617F-positive MF patients, 10 had significant responses in anemia with nine patients achieving transfusion independence. Although there were no spleen responses, a 58% response in thrombocytopenia for those with baseline platelets below 100×10^9 cells/L was noted. The anemia response was predicted by peripheral blood basophilia within the first month of therapy and the absence of massive splenomegaly and was restricted to MF patients who were JAK2V617F positive. Pomalidomide was also evaluated in a dose escalation phase 1/2 setting with the purpose of determining if higher doses of pomalidomide were more effective in reversing the anemia associated with MF. Doses of 3 mg/day given for 21 of 28 consecutive days were found to be the maximum tolerated dose, and myelosuppression the dose-limiting toxicity without any added response in anemia. The randomized, placebo-controlled, phase 3 RESUME trial is currently ongoing and will provide a definitive answer to the benefit of this IMiD in the treatment of anemia in MF.

Pressure symptoms caused by splenic enlargement can be treated initially with cytotoxic chemotherapy. Busulfan, melphalan, and hydroxyurea have each been used for this purpose. A significant reduction in spleen size with relief of pressure symptoms occurs in 70% of patients receiving chemotherapy.[3] Responses are unfortunately short lived, lasting a median of only 4.5 months. Only 16% of patients with long-term maintenance therapy enjoy sustained relief of symptoms. Hematologic toxicity often necessitates cessation of therapy. Inhibition of the activated JAK–STAT pathway is an attractive therapeutic target in PMF and during the past 5 years has been the focus of both industry and academia in the development of oral small molecule inhibitors. Ruxolitinib, a selective JAK1 and JAK2 tyrosine kinase inhibitor, has recently been approved for the treatment of patients with PMF; this is the first drug approved by the U.S. Food and Drug Administration (FDA) where the indication for use is intermediate- or high-risk MF. The phase 1/2 study determined the optimal starting dose of 15 mg twice daily and that thrombocytopenia and worsening anemia were dose-limiting toxicities.[21] A dose-dependent suppression of phospho-STAT3 was seen in both WT and mutated JAK2 patients treated with ruxolitinib, demonstrating that the drug does not discriminate between mutated and WT JAK2 in its inhibitory activity. Fifty-two percent of treated patients achieved a greater than 50% reduction in splenomegaly for greater than 12 months that was irrespective of their JAK2 mutational status. The debilitating symptoms associated with MF were dramatically improved, and this was correlated with reduction in inflammatory cytokines believed to be mediated through inhibition of JAK1 signaling. This compound was then evaluated in two randomized phase 3 trials, COMFORT 1 (United States, Canada, and Australia) in which ruxolitinib therapy was compared with a placebo control and COMFORT 2 trial (Europe) in which ruxolitinib therapy was compared with the best available therapy.[22,23] The results of each of these trials are remarkably similar, and each trial was adequately powered. Patients with intermediate-2 or high-risk MF as assessed using the IPSS were eligible regardless of JAK2 mutational status. All patients had platelet counts over 100×10^9/L and had a spleen palpated at least 5 cm below the left costal margin. In COMFORT 1, the primary endpoint of 35% or greater reduction in spleen volume was met at 24 weeks in 41.9% of the ruxolitinib-treated cohort and only 0.7% in the placebo group. This response was maintained 48 weeks or more in 67% of treated patients. Fig. 69-7 shows the percent change in spleen volume from baseline at week 24 for individual patients on both arms of this trial and depicts the contrast of spleen reduction in ruxolitinib-treated patients compared with the majority of patients in the placebo arm who had an increase in spleen volume. There were 13 deaths in the ruxolitinib arm and 24 deaths in the placebo arm, revealing a survival benefit for MF patients treated with ruxolitinib with an HR of 0.50 (CI, 0.25, 0.98; $P = .33$). Although grade 3/4 anemia and thrombocytopenia were frequent in the ruxolitinib arm (45.2% and 12.9%, respectively), discontinuation for these events was extremely rare. The primary endpoint in the COMFORT 2 trial was met at 48 weeks with 28% of patients in the ruxolitinib arm and 0% in the BAT arm achieving at least a 35% reduction in spleen volume. The mean length of palpable spleen decreased by 56% at 48 weeks compared with an increase of 4% in the BAT arm. Sophisticated disease-specific quality of life tools were used to evaluate the effects of ruxolitinib therapy on the systemic symptoms that have been presumed to be a consequence of the increased elaboration of inflammatory cytokines modulated by JAK1 signaling. The effects of ruxolitinib were, however, limited in that reversal of histomorphologic abnormalities, including BM fibrosis or osteosclerosis, significant reduction in the JAK2V617F allele burden, and loss of marker cytogenetic abnormalities indicating that the underlying malignant potential of PMF is not affected by this therapy. In addition, abrupt discontinuation of ruxolitinib therapy was associated with rapid return to baseline levels of splenomegaly and severity of the systemic symptoms that at times can be disabling. More gradual tapering of this agent or the use of a short steroid taper is recommended to avoid this complication. Ruxolitinib is an important new agent for the palliation of symptomatic splenomegaly and the debilitating symptoms seen in patients with PMF. The survival data from the COMFORT 1 trial, although modest, are intriguing and suggest that even if an appreciable impact on abnormal BM histopathology or molecular or cytogenetic responses is not seen with ruxolitinib, suppression of the JAK pathway decreases the risk of death, perhaps simply by improving the overall performance status of an individual. The use of ruxolitinib in patients with platelet counts below 100×10^9/L remains experimental, thereby limiting the number of patients who can be treated with this agent. The need to treat patients who are asymptomatic with limited splenomegaly is not apparent since treatment does not appear to affect the underlying

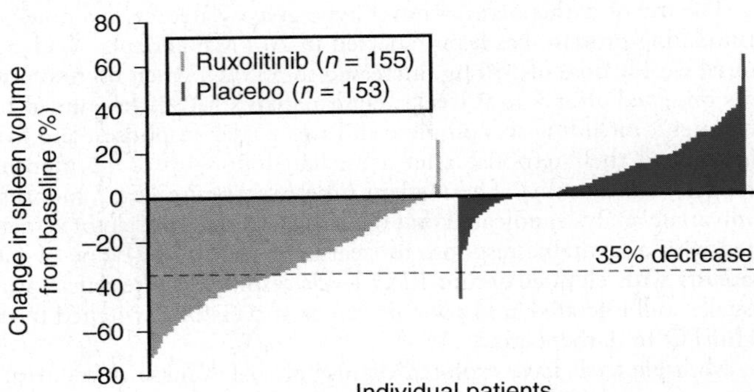

Figure 69-7 REDUCTION IN SPLENIC VOLUME WITH RUXOLITINIB THERAPY IN THE COMFORT 2 TRIAL. The waterfall plot shows the percent change from baseline in spleen volume at week 24 (in 139 patients in the ruxolitinib group and 106 in the placebo group) or at the last evaluation before week 24 (in 16 patients in the ruxolitinib group and 47 in the placebo group). Data for one patient with a missing baseline value are not included on the graph. Most patients in the ruxolitinib group (150 of 155) had a reduction in spleen volume, but most patients in the placebo group had either an increase in spleen volume (102 of 153 patients) or no change (15 of 153 patients). *(Data from Verstovsek S, Mesa RA, Gotlib J, et al: A double-blind, placebo-controlled trial of ruxolitinib for myelofibrosis.* N Engl J Med *366:799, 2012.)*

malignant disorder. A number of other small molecule inhibitors of JAK2 are under various phases of clinical development. These agents have different specificities or toxicity profiles and require evaluation in clinical trials to determine their utility in comparison with ruxolitinib.

Splenic irradiation frequently has been used for treatment of the painful, large spleen syndrome. Irradiation in fractions of 0.15 to 1 Gy administered daily or by an intermittent fractionation schedule (i.e., two or three times a week) to a total dose per treatment course of 2.5 to 6.5 Gy may be effective. Responses are transient, lasting an average of 3.5 months, and hematopoietic toxicity is frequently significant. Splenic irradiation is especially useful for treatment of splenic pain of sudden onset and for treatment of ascites caused by implants of hematopoietic tissue. Radiation therapy should be considered as a temporary measure to be used in patients who are too ill to tolerate splenectomy or chemotherapy. In one series, the median duration of response to irradiation was 6 months, and the median survival after irradiation was 20 months. Splenic irradiation is limited by myelosuppression with significant prolonged cytopenias, which is not predictable and is not correlated with the doses of radiation administered. Splenectomy after irradiation can be associated with increased complications, and irradiation should probably be administered only to patients who are not candidates for surgery.

Radiotherapy offers a viable treatment option and sometimes may be the therapy of choice for the treatment of patients with symptomatic hepatomegaly, peritoneal and pleural implants or pulmonary infiltration leading to ascites or pleural effusions, and EMH in vital organs leading to organ dysfunction. Because of the inherent sensitivity of myeloid tissue to radiation and profound BM suppression that may occur after irradiation, therapy is usually initiated at low doses (20-25 cGy/day), with modification of the dose as the clinical situation dictates. An alternative approach using intraperitoneal administration of cytosine arabinoside has been used to treat ascites in PMF. Therapy is initiated at 0.77 mg/kg/day to achieve a concentration of 30 mg per 2 L of peritoneal fluid. The dosage is advanced so that the patient eventually receives 1 g or 13.5 mg/kg/day. Abdominal pain is the most common adverse effect associated with this approach. Low-dose, single-fraction, whole-lung radiotherapy has also been useful in treating pulmonary artery hypertension associated with PMF.

Splenectomy remains a viable option even in the face of the recent availability of JAK2 inhibitors in patients with hemolysis, thrombocytopenia, painful splenomegaly, recurrent splenic infarction, and portal hypertension refractory to other therapeutic modalities or in individuals with leukopenia or thrombocytopenia that prevents one from resorting to therapy with chemotherapeutic agents or a JAK2 inhibitor. Splenectomy in patients with PMF is associated with a postoperative morbidity rate of 15% to 30% and a mortality rate of almost 10%. These events largely result from episodes of bleeding, infection, and thrombosis.[24] After splenectomy, 77%, 50%, 40%, and 30% of patients, respectively, have been reported to experience long-term improvement in symptomatic splenomegaly, anemia, portal hypertension, and severe thrombocytopenia. Bleeding and thrombotic complications, however, complicate the course of 25% of patients with PMF, and 6.7% of patients die during the perioperative period. Postoperatively, the major long-term complications include leukocytosis, thrombocytosis, and accelerated hepatic enlargement. Such adverse events can frequently be controlled with the immediate institution of hydroxyurea therapy during the postoperative period or if treatment with 2-chlorodeoxyadenosine therapy is unsuccessful. The appropriate implementation of splenectomy can result in the improved quality of life of PMF patients who frequently do not have other therapeutic options available. Because splenectomy is associated with significant morbidity and mortality, the physician should only resort to this strategy if thrombocytopenia, anemia, or symptomatic splenomegaly is unresponsive to less invasive approaches. Patients should only be considered for this procedure if their performance status allows one to anticipate a favorable surgical outcome with some certainty. Excessive delay of the decision to undergo splenectomy may result in a missed window of opportunity because the patient may become increasingly debilitated, no longer making him or her a viable surgical candidate. Histopathologic and cytogenetic features of the patient's BM did not predict the likelihood of response for the cytopenias to splenectomy. Progressive hepatomegaly and marked thrombocytosis occurred, respectively, in 16% and 22% of patients after splenectomy. The latter was associated with increased risk of thrombosis and decreased postoperative survival duration. An extraordinarily high rate of leukemic transformation has been observed after splenectomy. Whether this was a function of the absence of the spleen or more likely the consequence of the natural history of the disease is unknown. It has been suggested that splenectomy is an independent risk factor for leukemic transformation, stemming from a disruption of the host–tumor relationship, but others argue that patients with late-stage PMF who required splenectomy might be undergoing leukemic transformation in areas of splenic EMH without overt BM transformation. This population may be destined to develop leukemic transformation, and the need for splenectomy may only serve to identify this group of patients before such an event. 2-Chlorodeoxyadenosine therapy can be a particularly useful agent for patients with increased hepatomegaly, rapidly rising white blast cell counts, an extreme degree of thrombocytosis after splenectomy or for patients with these same clinical features who have not undergone splenectomy. The drug can be administered every 4 weeks according to one of two dosing schedules (0.1 mg/kg/day intravenously by continuous infusion for 7 days, or 5 mg/m^2/day for 2 hours intravenously for 5 consecutive days). Responses occur usually by the second cycle, and the medium duration of response is 6 months. 2-Chlorodeoxyadenosine can be extremely useful in controlling the excessive myeloproliferation in patients awaiting an allogeneic stem cell transplant.

Excessive bleeding in patients with PMF can be a result of thrombocytopenia, qualitative platelet defects, or DIC. Based on clinical observations, it is recommended that splenectomy be avoided in patients with DIC. Actively bleeding patients with consumption coagulopathy should receive platelet and plasma replacement therapy. Low-dose heparinization has resulted in improvement in some patients.[3] Platelet transfusions are suggested in bleeding patients who are thrombocytopenic or have normal platelet counts but who are known to have qualitative platelet abnormalities. Factor VII infusions should be considered in patients with bleeding refractory to platelet transfusion.

Allogeneic SCT is a potentially curative option in patients with PMF who have an appropriate donor available. Successful transplantation is associated with gradual resolution of BM fibrosis and normalization of hematopoiesis (see box on Algorithm for Selection of Appropriate Patients for Stem Cell Transplantation Stratified According to Risk Status).

Most of the knowledge of allogeneic SCT with conventional conditioning regimens comes from two series of transplants with more than 50 patients each. In the two cohorts of 55 and 56 PMF patients, the median age of transplanted patients was 42 and 43 years; treatment-related mortality (TRM) was 27% and 33%; and 5-year survival was 47% and 58%, respectively. The 5-year probability of treatment failure caused by relapse or persistent disease after transplantation was 36%, and the failure of sustained engraftment was 10.7% and occurred solely in patients receiving transplants from alternative donors. A hemoglobin level of 10 g/dL or less and osteomyelosclerosis before transplantation adversely affected the outcome. The probability of grade III or IV acute graft-versus-host disease (GVHD) was 33%, with 16 of 45 patients developing extensive chronic GVHD. Multivariate analyses demonstrated the influence of age on 5-year survival (14% for patients 45 years or older compared with 62% for those younger than 45 years). In an update from the Seattle group, the experience with 95 PMF patients who received busulfan, a total-body irradiation conditioning reagent, was provided. The 7-year actual survival rate was 61%, although 10% of patients died of recurrent or a persistent disease and the non–relapse-related mortality at 5 years was 34%. An even higher 1-year cumulative nonrelapse mortality of 48% was reported from two Canadian centers in 25 patients. These reports of myeloablative allo-HSCT in PMF provide evidence that engraftment can be achieved and that a complete and durable remission of the disease can occur in approximately 50% of patients. However, owing to the poor transplant outcomes in older patients, enrollment to this procedure represents a major therapeutic dilemma in PMF patients who are primarily diagnosed at ages in excess of 60 years.

The advent of nonmyeloablative, reduced-intensity conditioning (RIC) regimens for allogeneic SCT has expanded the use of the procedure to older patients. As a result of diminished transplantation-related toxicity, it has been possible to investigate the usefulness of allo-SCT in patients with PMF previously believed to be unsuitable candidates because of advanced age. The use of RIC regimens in older patients with PMF has resulted in lower TRM and achievement of histohematologic responses.

Rondelli and coworkers reported retrospectively the outcome of 21 PMF patients with a median age of 54 years and a range from 27 to 68 years who were transplanted at various centers using RIC regimens. All patients had an intermediate or high disease, taking into account hemoglobin and WBC count values. However, no patient had undergone leukemic transformation. Different conditioning regimens, most of which contained fludarabine, resulted in a TRM of 10% and 2-year overall survival rates of 87%. Eighteen patients were alive 12 to 122 months (median, 31 months) after transplant, and 17 were in remission (1 after a second transplant), with a relapse rate of 14%. Thirty-three percent of the patients developed acute GVHD grades II to IV, and 72% developed chronic GVHD. Posttransplant chimerism analysis showed more than 95% donor cells in 18 patients, and two patients achieved complete donor chimerism after donor lymphocyte infusion (DLI). The European Group for Blood and BM Transplantation has performed a prospective study of RIC conditioning for allogeneic SCT.[25] This study was performed at multiple sites and included 103 patients who received a RIC conditioning regimen of busulfan and fludarabine followed by an allogeneic stem cell graft from related ($n = 33$) or unrelated donors ($n = 70$). The estimated 5-year event-free survival and overall survival was 51% and 67%, respectively . As can be seen in Fig. 69-8, human leukocyte antigen (HLA) mismatching and advanced disease remain poor prognostic parameters, but even in this high-risk group, the overall survival was approximately 40%. Of course, older patients had a less favorable outcome than younger patients, but individuals older than 55 years of age have an overall survival of 48%. Remarkably, patients younger than 55 years of age had a 5-year overall survival rate of 82%. Elimination of JAK2V617F after transplant was associated with a reduced incidence of relapse. The Seattle group has reported their single-center experience that included 100 patients using modern conditioning regimens and reported a day 100 mortality rate of 13%, a relapse rate of 11%, and a 7-year actuarial survival of 61% for HLA-matched related and unrelated transplants. In a retrospective study of allogeneic SCT of 30 PMF patients between the ages of 60 and 78 years transplanted at four different centers, 3-year overall survival and progression-free survival rates of 45% and 40% were reported, respectively. One of the limitations of widely applying allogeneic SCT to more patients with PMF is the lack of access to appropriate donors. Recently, Takagi and coworkers from Japan reported surprisingly positive results with cord blood grafts for RIC allogeneic transplantation in adults (median age, 57.5 years) with various hematologic disorders associated with extensive BM fibrosis (PMF, post-MPN AML, and MDS-related AML). The estimated probability of survival at 4 years for this group was 28.6%, which is modest but considerably superior to that which would be anticipated with presently available chemotherapy regimens for such high-risk disease. This study provides the rationale for the further evaluation of RIC allogeneic transplant for eligible PMF patients lacking an HLA-matched sibling or unrelated donor with the use of alternative sources of grafts such as cord blood units or possibly haploidentical donors. Occasionally, patients with PMF after allogeneic transplant can experience relapse of their underlying disease, failure of engraftment, or graft failure. Relapse can frequently be treated with donor lymphocyte infusions. Second RIC allogeneic transplants should be considered for individuals who do not respond to donor lymphocyte infusions or experience difficulty with engraftment or late graft failure.

The feasibility of viewing allogeneic SCT as the preferable therapeutic option for intermediate- and high-risk PMF continues to be an area of great debate. Not all patients are candidates for allogeneic transplantation because of comorbidities or a poor performance status because of the systemic effects of the underlying PMF. Although the JAK2 inhibitors are largely palliative, they do reduce the degree of splenomegaly and often improve the performance status of such

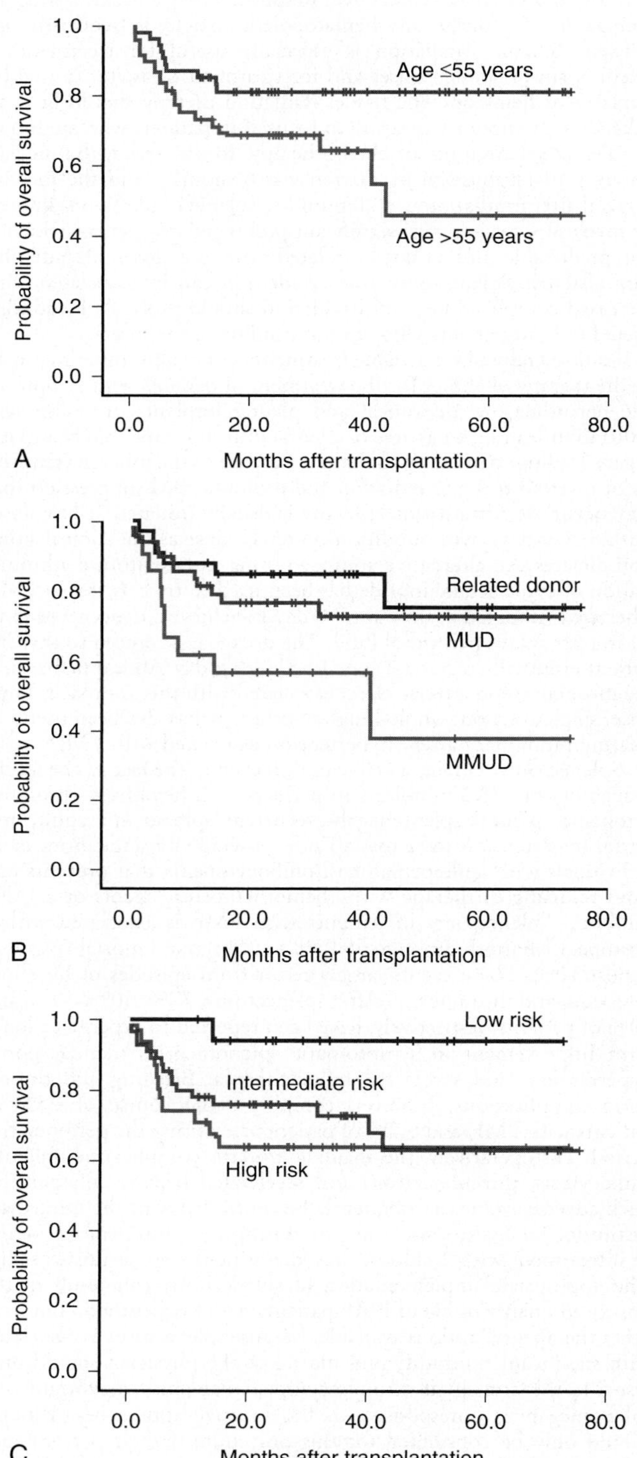

Figure 69-8 Survival of patients with myelofibrosis after reduced-intensity allogeneic stem cell transplantation according to age **(A)**, donor **(B)**, and Lille risk profile **(C)**.

Algorithm for Selection of Appropriate Patients for Stem Cell Transplantation Stratified According to Risk Status

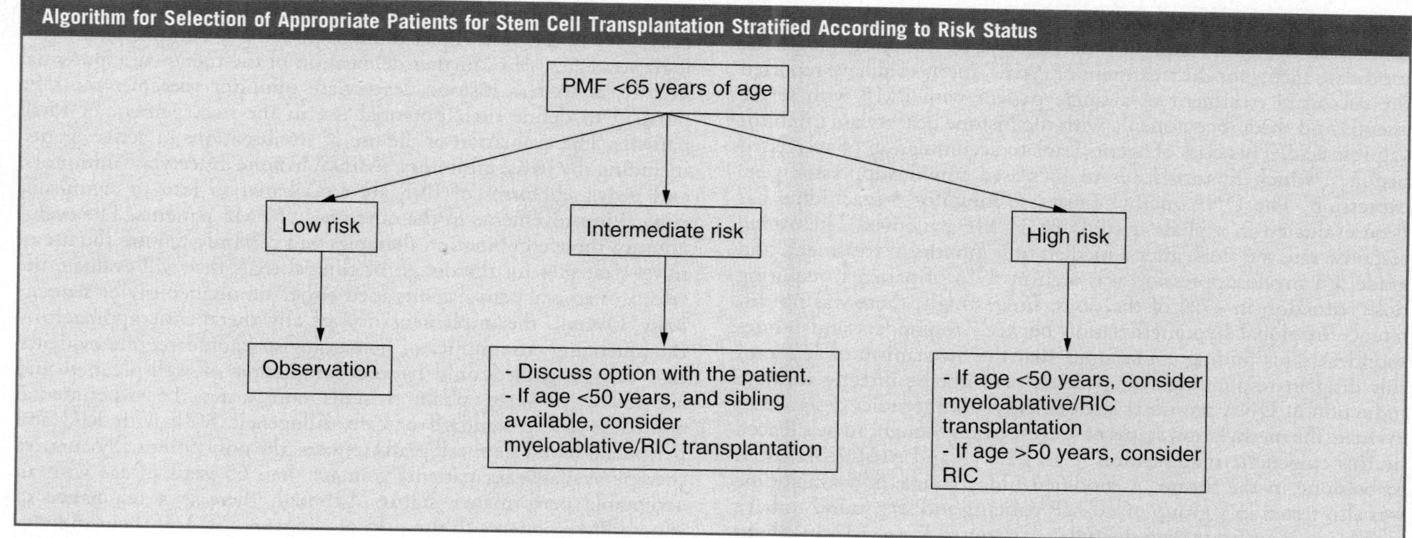
PMF <65 years of age
Low risk
Intermediate risk
High risk
Observation
- Discuss option with the patient.
- If age <50 years, and sibling available, consider myeloablative/RIC transplantation
- If age <50 years, consider myeloablative/RIC transplantation
- If age >50 years, consider RIC

patients, frequently resulting in weight gain, and improve their candidacy for transplant. The reported outcomes with JAK2 inhibitor therapy, albeit limited in regard to overall survival, might actually increase the number of patients who will ultimately be eligible for transplant because of the improvements in performance status. This approach is currently being evaluated within the MPD-RC.

The fact that allogeneic RIC transplant is curative in appropriate patients is undeniable, and the improvements in the design of conditioning regimens and supportive therapy make this a viable first-line approach for individuals with HLA-matched donors and advanced disease. Whether such an approach should also be implemented in patients with earlier phases of the disease is a point of contention that requires further careful investigation. This decision is especially important in young patients with early forms of PMF because their disease is likely to eventually progress, and the best results with allogeneic transplant have been reported in such low-risk patients. The flaw in the argument to proceed with immediate transplant in young patients with early PMF is the exposure to significant mortality and morbidity in a patient population that frequently can anticipate a decade or more of a good quality life with no or minimal therapeutic interventions. Although longer term follow-up data and larger studies are desirable, nonmyeloablative transplantation appears to be a promising therapeutic option in older patients with PMF before leukemic transformation.

Many unresolved issues remain to be clarified concerning the optimal strategy for allo-SCT in PMF. The need for splenectomy before allo-SCT remains a major issue. Splenectomy before allo-HSCT in PMF results in faster hematopoietic recovery. The role of splenectomy before HSCT should be evaluated in prospective studies. Our initial observations in patients who were prepared with fludarabine and melphalan and then received an allogeneic HSCT suggest that even extensive splenomegaly (>30 cm longitudinal size by computed tomography scan) does not prolong hematologic reconstitution after transplant, thereby avoiding delays of going to transplant caused by prolonged postoperative recovery times after splenectomy.[26]

The establishment of valid complete remission criteria of PMF after allogeneic SCT remains a major issue because the conventional criteria for response after allo-SCT are often influenced by GVHD, infections, or poor graft function and cannot be used. Conversely, normal blood counts and disappearance of disease-related symptoms do not exclude residual disease. Molecular markers of minimal residual disease monitoring have been evaluated as a biomarker for long-term disease-free survival. A highly sensitive method to monitor and quantify V617F-positive cells in mutation-positive patients with PMF after SCT allowed detecting minimal residual disease. This method has proven useful as a parameter for complete remission assessment and as a guide for instituting adoptive immunotherapy.

Autologous transplantation has also been investigated based on the premise that BM fibrosis and EMH are related to the bulk of the neoplastic clone and therefore successful debulking using high-dose chemotherapy may interrupt the disease process and improve the disease manifestations at least until the reestablishment of the abnormal clone in the BM by the "contaminated" autologous graft is achieved. This hypothesis was tested in a study in 21 patients with PMF. The median patient age was 59 years. The conditioning regimen consisted of oral busulfan (16 mg/kg). The median times to neutrophil and platelet recovery were 21 days and 21 days, respectively. Five patients required backup stem cell infusions because of delayed engraftment. The 2-year actuarial survival rate was 61%. Six patients died of non–relapse-related causes ($n = 3$) or disease progression ($n = 3$). Transfusion independence was achieved in 10 of 17 anemic patients and four patients with platelet counts of less than 100×10^9/L responded with durable counts of more than 100×10^9/L. Although this study clearly demonstrates the feasibility of this procedure, the role of autologous transplantation in PMF remains uncertain.

With increased understanding of the biology of PMF, a number of phase I and II studies have examined more rational therapy for PMF. NFκB has been shown to be upregulated in megakaryocytes and CD34$^+$ HSC in patients with PMF and is believed to contribute to the elaboration of TGF-β from megakaryocytes and monocytes. In a TPO^{high} murine model, deregulation of MPL signaling results in a phenotype that mimics PMF. Treatment of these mice with bortezomib resulted in decreased expression of TGF-β1 and osteoprotegerin with improvement in myeloproliferation and reduction in retuclin fibrosis and osteosclerosis. Bortezomib, a proteosome inhibitor with the ability to downregulate NFκB, appears to be an effective strategy in MF. A multicenter pilot phase 2 study of nine MF patients treated with bortezomib was conducted. Seven of the patients experienced at least grade 3 toxicity of which the majority were nonhematologic. No appreciable clinical responses were seen in this study. The MPD-RC also conducted a phase I/II trial of single-agent bortezomib in 12 MF patients in the phase I portion of the study and found the MTD to be 1.3 mg/m^2 given on days 1, 4, 8, and 11 of a 28-day cycle with a dose-limiting toxicity of thrombocytopenia. There were no cases of clinical improvement in the 16 evaluable phase 2 MF patients, and there was no statistically significant reduction in TGF-β from baseline. Interestingly, although bortezomib did not reduce VEGF levels from baseline, it did induce significant reduction in median vessel density within the BM and exerted a detrimental effect of downregulating CXCR4 expression in CD34$^+$ MF cells.

The identification of various epigenetic defects in PMF has also provided novel therapeutic targets, and preclinical studies are actively being translated into early phase clinical trials. Shi et al presented data suggesting that chromatin-modifying agents such as DNA methyltransferase inhibitors and histone deacetylase inhibitors might be candidate agents for the treatment of PMF.[27] Inoue et al have reported the successful treatment of a single patient with PMF with severe anemia and thrombocytopenia with the histone deacetylase inhibitor valproic acid. This class of agents leads to accumulation of acetylated histones, which in turn leads to increased tumor suppressor gene expression. The DNA methyltransferase inhibitor 5-azacitidine has been evaluated in a phase 2 study in 34 MF patients.[28] The overall response rate was 24% after a median of 5 months of treatment, and grade 3/4 myelosuppression was seen in 29% of patients, requiring dose reduction in 47% of the cases. Interestingly, there was no difference in global hypomethylation between responders and nonresponders. This finding could argue that the mechanism of action of this drug in responding MF patients may not be directly through induction of DNA promoter site demethylation. Studies designed to evaluate the methylation status of specific genes thought to be silenced by this epigenetic modification (e.g., $p15^{INK4b}$ and p16INK4a) need to be done in the future. A modified 5-day course of 5-azacitidine was also tested in a group of 10 MF patients and was found to have even less response rate than the full 7-day course. Case series highlight the potential role of decitabine in the treatment of MF in blast phase, and initial reports of subcutaneous low-dose decitabine in advanced MF also appears to hold promise and is currently being evaluated in larger studies. LBH589 (panobinostat) is a potent pan-deacetylase inhibitor that has also been evaluated in PMF patients in two separate trials with thrombocytopenia as the dose-limiting toxicity and the demonstration of a signal of clinical activity that is associated with enhanced histone acetylation. A report of the results of long-term administration of low-dose panobinostat in MF patients demonstrated the potential to alleviate constitutional symptoms, reduce splenomegaly, improve anemia, eliminate peripheral blood leukoerythroblastosis, reduce BM reticulin and collagen fibrosis, and restore normal BM morphology in a small number of patients. A phase II study of panobinostat at a dose of 25 mg orally TIW weekly is currently ongoing, and studies combining this agent with ruxolitinib are ongoing, and the results are highly anticipated. The therapeutic potential for the use of chromatin-modifying agents for the treatment of PMF patients is an exciting approach and requires further careful evaluation in well-designed clinical studies.

FUTURE DIRECTIONS

More rational therapies for PMF should evolve from further enhancement of the understanding of the cellular and molecular biologic abnormalities underlying PMF. Studies defining the relative contributions of acquired genetic mutations, epigenetic events, as well as the influence of the BM and splenic microenvironment on the origins of PMF, disease progression, and events leading to leukemic transformation are required. Because PMF originates at the level of the HSC, the identification of novel drugs that eliminate such malignant stem cells is likely the most direct route to potentially curative pharmacologic strategies. Also, further delineation of the therapeutic potential of INF as well as histone deacetylase inhibitor therapies must be pursued to define their potential use in the management of PMF patients. The evaluation of the use of combinations of active agents, including the JAK2 inhibitors, IMiDS, histone deacetylase inhibitors, and pegylated forms of INF are anticipated to lead to significant clinical improvements in the outcomes of PMF patients. The evaluation of these combination therapies will certainly require the use of novel strategies for the design of clinical trials that will evaluate the effects of several active agents used either simultaneously or sequentially. Overall, the implementation of any therapeutic approach by the practicing community of hematologists should require evidence that can be gained only by the completion of well-planned and adequately powered phase 3 trials comparing the experimental approach to the standard of care. Allogeneic SCT with RIC and peripheral blood stem cell grafts remains the only potentially curative therapy available for patients younger than 65 years of age with an acceptable performance status. Although there is a reluctance to expose PMF patients to the risks of allogeneic SCT, if their underlying disorder is associated with a poor prognosis, this risk appears to be warranted. Because early forms of PMF are associated with survival of well over a decade, many individuals have been even more reluctant to expose such patients to experimental therapeutic agents or allogeneic transplant. Unfortunately, progression to more advanced forms of MF is anticipated in younger patients. Exploration of therapeutic agents that can delay or even prevent disease progression or identification of the appropriate role of allogeneic stem cell transplantation in this low-risk group will require additional study. The decision to proceed to transplant requires a detailed discussion of the risks and benefits of such a high-risk but potentially curative procedure. The establishment of multi-institutional cooperative groups to evaluate such novel therapies and treatment strategies for PMF patients remains a continuing critical need. No single institution has sufficient numbers of patients to perform this ever-growing number of required investigative efforts. Only with the completion of such rigorous evaluations of individual therapeutic strategies will one be able to determine the value of a continuously growing number of potentially active agents used alone or in combination. Each new therapy will likely be evaluated using not only a number of clinical endpoints but also surrogate biomarkers and consideration of the immediate and long-term toxicities associated with their use documented. The European Myelofibrosis Network and the IWG for Myelofibrosis Research and Treatment have independently developed objective criteria by which responses to experimental therapeutic agents can be judged.[29,30] Furthermore, quality of life tools have become more widely used in the evaluation of such experimental therapeutic agents. The presently available instruments used for this purpose are clearly imperfect and will require modification to be more effective in evaluating the impact of a particular treatment strategy. Because it is likely that a large

Case Vignettes

How should PMF patients with thrombocytopenia be treated?

Platelet count 50 to 100 × 10^9/L:

It is important to ensure that vitamin B_{12} or folate deficiency is not contributing to the low platelet count as well as suppression from prior chemotherapeutic agents. Chemotherapeutic agents such as hydroxyurea can be used in patients with marked splenomegaly because initially this can result in an improvement in platelet count as the spleen is reduced in volume. Patients can also be treated with thalidomide or lenalidomide in combination with prednisone. These first-generation IMiDs can sometimes improve cytopenias and reduce splenomegaly in PMF patients, and in some cases, this response can persist even after drug discontinuation. Lenalidomide can induce cytopenias to a greater extent than thalidomide, and this needs to be taken into consideration before the use of this agent in this setting. In a phase II trial, pomalidomide was reported to have a response rate of 58% in increasing the baseline platelet count by greater than 50% in patients with baseline platelets above 50 × 10^9/L. This second-generation IMiD will need to be evaluated in patients with platelet counts below 50 × 10^9/L. The use of JAK2 inhibitors in patients with reduced platelets counts remains a subject of research because these agents are associated with thrombocytopenia. For patients with symptoms related to splenomegaly and constitutional symptoms, a recently FDA-approved JAK1/2 inhibitor, ruxolitinib, is being evaluated in a clinical trial in MF patients with this platelet

Case Vignettes—cont'd

range. Patients can also be enrolled in other JAK2 inhibitor clinical trials in which reduced platelet counts are acceptable or in clinical trials with other agents in development. If thrombocytopenia worsens with the current treatment plan, then proceed with the strategy outlined below.

Platelet count 20 to 50 × 10^9/L:

Thalidomide or lenalidomide in combination with prednisone can be attempted to correct anemia in these PMF patients but rarely improve the platelet count in a clinically meaningful way. Most clinical trials involving a variety of therapeutic agents including JAK2 inhibitors will require baseline platelets above 50 × 10^9/L. In patients who are experiencing life-threatening bleeding, in addition to aggressive immediate platelet transfusions, splenectomy is a reasonable therapeutic option.

Platelet count below 20 × 10^9/L

The treatment choices are truly limited for these patients. Intervention is also dependent on the clinical picture with emphasis on addressing bleeding. Supportive therapy with frequent platelet transfusions is a possibility, but it is likely not sustainable in the long term. It is our practice to transfuse if platelets are below 10 × 10^9/L unless there is no evidence of mucosal bleeding or life-threatening hemorrhage. Occasionally, patients may have an improvement in the degree of thrombocytopenia with steroids; however, this has not been systematically evaluated. About 20% to 30% of patients with severe thrombocytopenia will have significant improvement in platelet counts after a splenectomy. Aggressive platelet transfusional support is necessary before, during, and after splenectomy in many cases. However, splenectomy in patients with PMF is associated with a postoperative morbidity rate of 15% to 30% and mortality rate of close to 10%. These numbers, however, are highly dependent on the institutional experience and the operating surgeon. Splenectomy can also result in EMH in the liver, causing hepatomegaly, which may require the administration of judicious amount of chemotherapeutic agents (hydroxyurea, busulfan, cladribine). Severe thrombocytopenia is an adverse prognostic feature. Such patients who are eligible for stem cell transplant and have available donors should be considered for transplantation. TPO mimetics have been associated with increased BM fibrosis when used for the treatment of ITP and have not been evaluated in the setting of PMF-associated thrombocytopenia. Additionally, patients with extreme thrombocytopenia and signs of leukemic transformation can be considered for therapy with decitabine or azacytidine with aggressive platelet transfusional support and then should proceed on to allogeneic SCT if a donor is available and the patient's performance status is appropriate.

Which patients should be considered for allogeneic stem cell transplantation?

Allogeneic SCT is the only potential curative treatment option for PMF. Patients with poor risk features and decreased probability for survival should be considered for SCT because of the not insignificant risk of transplant related morbidity and mortality. All patients younger than 70 years of age and their siblings should be HLA typed at the time of diagnosis to determine if there is a potential match. Patients between the ages of 65 and 70 years with available related donors should be evaluated based on their performance status and comorbid conditions. Patients younger than 65 years with good performance status and available donors (either related or fully matched unrelated) should be encouraged to undergo evaluation for SCT soon after the diagnosis and preferably within a clinical trial. Patients with high- or intermediate-risk disease with available donors should consider transplantation before developing debilitating symptoms or significant worsening in their performance status. Patients with low-risk disease should be closely monitored without intervention but should proceed to transplantation with evidence of disease progression. For patients with available donors but poor performance status because of symptoms of MF, a course of treatment with ruxolitinib can be considered with a goal of improvement in performance status associated with reduction of splenomegaly and constitutional symptoms. These patients may become more viable transplant candidates with this pretransplant treatment approach. Splenectomy before transplant is not essential to ensure adequate engraftment. Currently, SCT using RCI regimens, haploidentical donors, and cord blood grafts are being evaluated.

Which PMF patients are appropriate for JAK2 inhibitor therapy???

Not all patients require treatment with JAK2 inhibitor therapy. Patients with symptomatic splenomegaly or debilitating MF-related symptoms are potential candidates for treatment with ruxolitinib. Inhibition of JAK1/2 is associated with myelosuppression and could further compromise existing cytopenias. In patients with splenomegaly and constitutional symptoms with adequate blood counts, a course of hydroxyurea should be considered. If the patient fails hydroxyurea or has debilitating symptoms, then ruxolitinib would be the appropriate agent. Ruxolitinib is currently approved for patients with intermediate- and high-risk MF and has yet to be explored in cases of symptomatic patients with low-risk disease. Additionally, this drug has not yet been fully evaluated in MF patients with platelet counts below 100 × 10^9/L. Ruxolitinib could also be used in patients with poor performance status before allogeneic SCT as a means to improve their performance status and promote weight gain in an attempt to optimize them for SCT. Although the COMFORT 1 trial reported a modest improvement in survival at a median of 51 weeks of treatment with ruxolitinib, the exact mechanism that would provide for this survival benefit is not yet understood, and this agent should not be given with the primary goal of disease process modification and increased survival. Patients started on ruxolitinib need to have frequent monitoring of blood counts, and if discontinued, the dose should be either tapered or a pulse of steroid therapy considered to avoid the rapid reappearance of systemic symptoms and splenomegaly.

number of such agents will be evaluated in patients with PMF in the future, it is recommended that a uniform standard be adopted so that the relative efficacy of any new therapeutic approach can be more easily judged. The integration of these new classes of agents can also be incorporated into the conditioning regimens that are used before allogeneic SCT; this approach will also likely contribute to significant improvements in outcomes in PMF patients undergoing allogeneic stem cell transplant.

REFERENCES

1. Swerdlow SH, Campo E, Harris NL, et al: *WHO classification of tumours of haematopoietic and lymphoid tissues,* ed 4, 2008.
2. Schmitt A, Jouault H, Guichard J, et al: Pathologic interaction between megakaryocytes and polymorphonuclear leukocytes in myelofibrosis. *Blood* 96:1342, 2000.
3. James C, Ugo V, Le Couédic JP, et al: A unique clonal JAK2 mutation leading to constitutive signalling causes polycythaemia vera. *Nature* 434:1144, 2005.
4. Pardanani AD, Levine RL, Lasho T, et al: MPL515 mutations in myeloproliferative and other myeloid disorders: A study of 1182 patients. *Blood* 108:3472, 2006.
5. Tefferi A: Novel mutations and their functional and clinical relevance in myeloproliferative neoplasms: JAK2, MPL, TET2, ASXL1, CBL, IDH and IKZF1. *Leukemia* 24:1128, 2010.
6. Xu M, Bruno E, Chao J, et al: MPD Research Consortium: Constitutive mobilization of CD34+ cells into the peripheral blood in idiopathic

myelofibrosis may be due to the action of a number of proteases. *Blood* 105:4508, 2005.

7. Ciurea SO, Merchant D, Mahmud N, et al: Pivotal contributions of megakaryocytes to the biology of idiopathic myelofibrosis. *Blood* 110:986, 2007.
8. Cervantes F, Alvarez-Larrán A, Arellano-Rodrigo E, et al: Frequency and risk factors for thrombosis in idiopathic myelofibrosis: Analysis in a series of 155 patients from a single institution. *Leukemia* 20:55, 2006.
9. Silverstein MN, Gomes MR, ReMine WH, et al: Agnogenic myeloid metaplasia. Natural history and treatment. *Arch Intern Med* 120:546, 1967.
10. Thiele J, Kvasnicka HM, Werden C, et al: Idiopathic primary osteomyelofibrosis: A clinico-pathological study on 208 patients with special emphasis on evolution of disease features, differentiation from essential thrombocythemia and variables of prognostic impact. *Leuk Lymphoma* 22:303, 1996.
11. Beer PA, Delhommeau F, LeCouédic JP, et al: Two routes to leukemic transformation after a JAK2 mutation-positive myeloproliferative neoplasm. *Blood* 115:2891, 2010.
12. Cervantes F, Dupriez B, Pereira A, et al: New prognostic scoring system for primary myelofibrosis based on a study of the International Working Group for Myelofibrosis Research and Treatment. *Blood* 113:2895, 2009.
13. Tefferi A, Jimma T, Gangat N, et al: Predictors of greater than 80% 2-year mortality in primary myelofibrosis: A Mayo Clinic study of 884 karyotypically annotated patients. *Blood* 118:4595, 2011.
14. Hussein K, Pardanani AD, Van Dyke DL, et al: International Prognostic Scoring System-independent cytogenetic risk categorization in primary myelofibrosis. *Blood* 115:496, 2010.
15. Tefferi A: How I treat myelofibrosis. *Blood* 117:3494, 2011.
16. Kiladjian JJ, Mesa RA, Hoffman R: The renaissance of interferon therapy for the treatment of myeloid malignancies. *Blood* 117:4706, 2011.
17. Ianotto JC, Kiladjian JJ, Demory JL, et al: PEG-IFN-alpha-2a therapy in patients with myelofibrosis: A study of the French Groupe d'Etudes des Myelofibroses (GEM) and France Intergroupe des syndromes Myeloproliferatifs (FIM). *Br J Haematol* 146:223, 2009.
18. Cervantes F, Alvarez-Larrán A, Domingo A, et al: Efficacy and tolerability of danazol as a treatment for the anaemia of myelofibrosis with myeloid metaplasia: Long-term results in 30 patients. *Br J Haematol* 129:771, 2005.
19. Mesa RA, Yao X, Cripe LD, et al: Lenalidomide and prednisone for myelofibrosis: Eastern Cooperative Oncology Group (ECOG) phase 2 trial E4903. *Blood* 116:4436, 2010.
20. Begna KH, Mesa RA, Pardanani A, et al: A phase-2 trial of low-dose pomalidomide in myelofibrosis. *Leukemia* 25:301, 2011.
21. Verstovsek S, Kantarjian H, Mesa RA, et al: Safety and efficacy of INCB018424, a JAK1 and JAK2 inhibitor, in myelofibrosis. *N Engl J Med* 363:1117, 2010.
22. Verstovsek S, Mesa RA, Gotlib J, et al: A double-blind, placebo-controlled trial of ruxolitinib for myelofibrosis. *N Engl J Med* 366:799, 2012.
23. Harrison C, Kiladjian JJ, Al-Ali HK, et al: JAK inhibition with ruxolitinib versus best available therapy for myelofibrosis. *N Engl J Med* 366:787, 2012.
24. Tefferi A, Mesa RA, Nagorney DM, et al: Splenectomy in myelofibrosis with myeloid metaplasia: A single-institution experience with 223 patients. *Blood* 95:2226, 2000.
25. Kröger N, Holler E, Kobbe G, et al: Allogeneic stem cell transplantation after reduced-intensity conditioning in patients with myelofibrosis: A prospective, multicenter study of the Chronic Leukemia Working Party of the European Group for Blood and Marrow Transplantation. *Blood* 114:5264, 2009.
26. Ciurea SO, Sadegi B, Wilbur A, et al: Effects of extensive splenomegaly in patients with myelofibrosis undergoing a reduced intensity allogeneic stem cell transplantation. *Br J Haematol* 141:80, 2008.
27. Shi J, Zhao Y, Ishii T, et al: Effects of chromatin-modifying agents on CD34+ cells from patients with idiopathic myelofibrosis. *Cancer Res* 67:6417, 2007.
28. Quintás-Cardama A, Tong W, Kantarjian H, et al: A phase II study of 5-azacitidine for patients with primary and post-essential thrombocythemia/polycythemia vera myelofibrosis. *Leukemia* 22:965, 2008.
29. Barosi G, Bordessoule D, Briere J, et al: European Myelofibrosis Network: Response criteria for myelofibrosis with myeloid metaplasia: Results of an initiative of the European Myelofibrosis Network (EUMNET). *Blood* 106:2849, 2005.
30. Tefferi A, Barosi G, Mesa RA, et al: IWG for Myelofibrosis Research and Treatment (IWG-MRT): International Working Group (IWG) consensus criteria for treatment response in myelofibrosis with myeloid metaplasia, for the IWG for Myelofibrosis Research and Treatment (IWG-MRT). *Blood* 108:1497, 2006.

CHAPTER 70

EOSINOPHILIA, EOSINOPHIL-ASSOCIATED DISEASES, CHRONIC EOSINOPHIL LEUKEMIA, AND THE HYPEREOSINOPHILIC SYNDROMES

Marina Kremyanskaya, Steven J. Ackerman, Joseph H. Butterfield, John Mascarenhas, and Ronald Hoffman

Since the initial identification of the eosinophilic granulocyte (Fig. 70-1) by Paul Ehrlich in 1879, an extensive number of diseases and conditions characterized by blood and/or tissue eosinophilia (Table 70-1) have been identified. Researchers have also gained a better understanding of the unique cellular characteristics of activated tissue and peripheral blood eosinophils; their preformed granule protein constituents and inducible lipid, oxidative, and cytokine products; and the eosinophil's proinflammatory and cytotoxic potential in the pathogenesis of allergic, parasitic, neoplastic, and a variety of other idiopathic disease processes. Recognition of the eosinophil as a proinflammatory effector cell has fueled a surge of interest in this granulocyte's role in a growing number of disorders.

Studies of the biochemistry, biologic activities, and in particular, the localization in tissues of the distinctive enzymatic and nonenzymatic cationic protein constituents of the eosinophil's secondary or specific granules have provided convincing evidence for its role in the pathogenesis of inflammation and tissue damage in eosinophil-associated diseases. In addition, identification of specific granule constituents in tissues has supplied additional evidence for the participation of eosinophils in diseases not normally associated with tissue or blood eosinophilia. Investigations of the biochemistry, functions, and localization in tissues of these unique enzymatic and nonenzymatic cationic proteins have now provided compelling evidence supporting a pathologic effector role for the eosinophil in directly inducing tissue damage. These five distinctive cationic granule protein constituents include the two major basic proteins (MBP-1, MBP-2), eosinophil peroxidase (EPX), and the two ribonucleases eosinophil cationic protein (ECP) and eosinophil-derived neurotoxin (EDN). Eosinophils also have the capacity to express toxic oxidative intermediates, eicosanoid and other lipid mediators of inflammation, and cytokines that are integral to their normal and pathologic role in disease. This chapter provides an overview of current knowledge and understanding of eosinophil biology, focusing principally on clinical disorders associated with hypereosinophilia—in particular, hypereosinophilic syndrome (HES).

Eosinophilia is defined as the presence of greater than 450 to 500 eosinophils/microliter of blood as normally measured by sampling peripheral blood.[1] The process of determining the cause of eosinophilia is often a frustrating experience for both physician and patient, one that may still result in a significant number of patients being classified as having hypereosinophilia of unknown etiology. HES is a group of disorders marked by sustained overproduction of eosinophils and tissue infiltration. In addition to the striking and sometimes profound eosinophilia associated with the syndrome, HES is characterized by a predilection for end-organ damage most commonly involving the heart, with the development of eosinophilic endomyocardial fibrosis and related cardiac pathologies. Heart disease can, however, also develop with eosinophilias due to other causes, for example, tropical eosinophilia and certain cancers. The initial defined criteria for HES were originally provided by Chusid and colleagues and served to distinguish HES patients from those with identifiable (reactive) causes of eosinophilia. Of interest, the more recent identification of subgroups of patients who have profound idiopathic eosinophilia (IE) characteristic of HES but do not go on to develop end-organ damage characteristic of HES (e.g., patients with episodic angioedema with eosinophilia) complicates the diagnosis, treatment, and management of patients with profound eosinophilia of unknown etiology. HES remains a useful term, but with increasing understanding of the variants of the syndrome, it is likely more accurate to use the term as a diagnostic feature rather than to define a primary hematologic disease. Myeloproliferative neoplasm (MPN) associated with eosinophilia can occur in patients who may or may not present with organ damage. Furthermore, 10% to 15% of patients with HES have been shown not to have a myeloid malignancy; rather, their eosinophilia is driven by an abnormal clonal $CD3^-CD4^+$ T-cell population producing interleukin-5 (IL-5). This variant is referred to as *lymphocytic variant hypereosinophilia*. Furthermore, a small number of patients with a clinical picture of HES have been shown to have myeloid malignancies associated with fusion proteins involving platelet-derived growth factor receptor (PDGFRA or PDGFRB) or the fibroblast growth factor receptor (FGFR). These disorders are categorized by the World Health Organization (WHO) as myeloid and lymphoid malignancies associated with eosinophilia and genetic abnormalities. Chronic eosinophilic leukemia (CEL) is considered an MPN and is referred to as *CEL not otherwise specified (CEL-NOS)*. These patients have peripheral blood eosinophilia (>30%), lack mutations in PDGFR, KIT, or FGFR, and have less than 20% blasts or features of acute myeloid leukemia, including inversion of chromosome 16, but they have other cytogenetic or molecular markers indicative of clonal hematologic malignancies and a blast cell count greater than 2% in the peripheral blood and 5% in the bone marrow. Acute eosinophilic leukemia (AEL), by contrast, is a variant of acute myeloid leukemia (AML) characterized by greater than 30% of nucleated marrow cells being eosinophils and greater than 20% being myeloblasts. The wide variety of these categories indicates the heterogeneity of what was previously termed *HES* and emphasizes the importance of incorporating histomorphologic criteria, as well as molecular and genetic criteria, when evaluating such patients. Those patients in whom reactive and clonal eosinophilia have been excluded are classified as having idiopathic eosinophilia. Some of these IE patients have end-organ damage associated with eosinophilia and suffer from the clinical syndrome of HES.

EPIDEMIOLOGY

No population-based data are available to indicate the incidence or prevalence of the heterogeneous syndromes referred to as *HES*. An attempt to estimate these data has been made by using the Surveillance, Epidemiology and End Results (SEER) database sponsored by the National Cancer Institute. A crude incidence of 0.035 cases per 100,000 person years was obtained, and the male-to-female ratio was 1.47. The average age at diagnosis was 52.5 years, and the peak incidence was in individuals 65 to 74 years of age. Infrequent cases

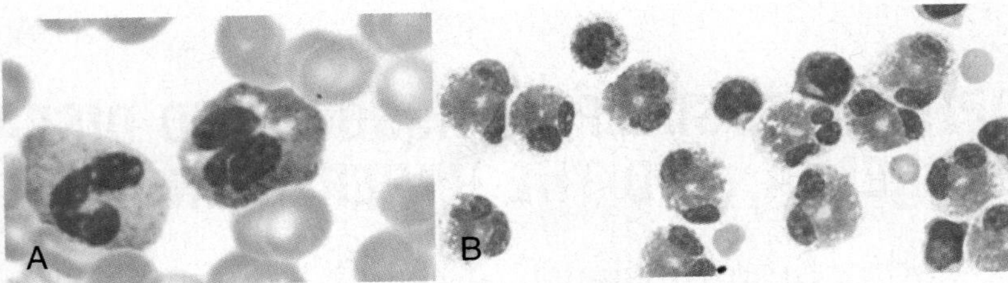

Figure 70-1 EOSINOPHIL AND EOSINOPHILIA. **A,** Eosinophil in a standard peripheral blood smear *(center)* compared with a neutrophilic granulocyte *(left)*. The eosinophil usually has a bilobed nucleus and heavily condensed chromatin usually with two lobes. The granules are considerably larger than those of a neutrophil and are spherical *red-orange* and refractile. They fill the cytoplasm and frequently overlie the nucleus. **B,** An eosinophilia is illustrated in a CSF specimen from a patient with hydrocephalus and a V-P shunt; apparently the eosinophilia is due to an allergic response.

have been described in infants and children.[2] These data have serious limitations and emphasize the need for more comprehensive epidemiologic data using currently available diagnostic criteria. Of interest, the overwhelming number of patients with FIP1L1-PDGFRA variants of hypereosinophilia are males.

PATHOPHYSIOLOGY

Eosinophil Morphology

Eosinophils contain three distinct membrane-bound granule populations that are produced during their differentiation from hematopoietic progenitor cells (Fig. 70-2). These include (a) round, uniformly electron-dense primary granules, present mainly at the eosinophilic promyelocyte/myelocyte stages; (b) specific or secondary granules, containing an electron-dense crystalloid core surrounded by a less dense granular matrix (>95% of granules in mature eosinophils and the morphologic hallmark of this granulocyte); and (c) less well-characterized small granules, which may contain catalase and may be functionally analogous to lysosomes and peroxisomes of other cells and which serve as sites for hydrolytic enzymes such as acid phosphatase and arylsulfatase.[3] The large, specific granule is the major repository for the eosinophil's cytotoxic and proinflammatory cationic proteins, which also confer its tinctorial (eosinophilic) properties. Eosinophils also contain lipid bodies, non–membrane-bound lipid-rich organelles often confused with granules, and present in many types of leukocytes and other cells. Normal eosinophils contain greater numbers of lipid bodies than neutrophils, and the numbers of lipid bodies increase during eosinophil activation in vitro and engagement in inflammatory reactions in vivo. Although the functions of lipid bodies are incompletely understood, they incorporate fatty acids such as arachidonate and likely serve as intracellular depots for its storage and metabolism, as suggested by the lipid body localization of all the principal eosinophil eicosanoide-forming enzymes, including 5-lipoxygenase, leukotriene C4 synthase, and cyclooxygenase. These four organelles, along with vesiculotubular structures and small vesicles involved in transport and secretion in the activated cell, serve as the major subcellular sites for the eosinophil's armamentarium of preformed cytotoxic and inflammatory mediators.

EOSINOPHIL DEVELOPMENT, RECRUITMENT, AND ACTIVATION

Eosinophilopoiesis

Eosinophils are derived from marrow $CD34^+$ cells in response to a number of T cell–derived eosinophilopoietic cytokines and growth factors, including IL-3, GM-CSF, and IL-5. Although eosinophils and basophils are thought to share a common bipotential progenitor, there is no evidence for a similar progenitor that gives rise only to eosinophils and mast cells. Eosinophil-committed hematopoietic progenitors (EoP) are identified within the $CD34^+$ progenitor population as IL-5Rα^+CD34$^+$CD38$^+$IL-3Rα^+CD45RA$^-$ cells and are distinct from the common myeloid progenitor (CMP) population that gives rise to the other myeloid lineages. Eosinophil development is controlled by the transcription factors GATA-1, GATA-2, C/EBPα, and C/EBPε. IL-3, GM-CSF, and IL-5 affect the eosinophil lineage at three different levels: (a) commitment, proliferation, and differentiation of hematopoietic progenitors in the bone marrow; (b) priming, activation, and survival in the blood and tissues; and (c) recruitment and tissue localization. Although activated T cells are likely the primary source of cytokines responsible for eosinophil differentiation and the development of reactive eosinophilia in disease, other cell types, including mast cells, macrophages, natural killer cells, endothelial cells, and stromal cells such as fibroblasts, are also producers of GM-CSF. IL-5, produced primarily by activated T_{H2}-type helper T cells and mast cells, stimulates the proliferation and differentiation of murine-activated B cells and regulates the production of eosinophils in vitro and in vivo. Both IL-3 and GM-CSF affect other hematopoietic cell lineages, whereas IL-5 is more eosinophil-specific and plays a crucial role in regulating the terminal differentiation and postmitotic activation of eosinophils. IL-5 is therefore a late-acting cytokine that demonstrates maximum activity on an eosinophil progenitor pool that is first expanded by the earlier-acting cytokines such as IL-3 or GM-CSF.[4] Although IL-3 and GM-CSF participate in the proliferation of progenitors to the eosinophil lineage, IL-5 is both necessary and sufficient for eosinophil development to proceed in vivo. In humans, IL-5 does not appear to have any effect on B cells or other lymphoid lineages, and its activity, high-affinity receptor, and functions are restricted to eosinophils and basophils. The expression of the high-affinity receptor for IL-5 is an important prerequisite and very early lineage-specific event in the hematopoietic differentiation program for both of these granulocytes. Overexpression of IL-5 is observed in many eosinophil-associated diseases and IL-5 transgenic mice develop profound eosinophilia, indicating that IL-5 plays an important role in promoting the production and function of eosinophils in vivo. These observations have been confirmed and expanded in studies of IL-5 knock-out mice, which produce basal levels of normal eosinophils in the bone marrow but do not develop blood and tissue eosinophilia, airway hyper-reactivity, or lung damage in the murine ovalbumin allergic asthma model or eosinophilic responses to helminth parasites. For these reasons, IL-5 and its receptor have proven to be excellent targets for therapeutic intervention in eosinophil-associated inflammatory diseases.

Mobilization and Migration of Eosinophils to Sites of Inflammation

In a normal individual, eosinophils produced in the bone marrow reside only briefly in the peripheral circulation in transit to

Table 70-1 Diseases, Syndromes, and Conditions Commonly Associated With Peripheral Blood Eosinophilia and/or Tissue Eosinophilia

INFECTIOUS AGENTS

Parasitic Infections

Tropical eosinophilia
Visceral larval migrans (VLM, toxocariasis)
Helminth infections
Filariasis *(Wuchereria bancrofti, Brugia malay)*
Onchocerciasis
Schistosomiasis
Fascioliasis
Paragonimiasis
Strongyloidiasis
Trichinosis
Hookworm
Ascariasis
Echinococcosis/hydatid disease

Fungal Infections

Coccidioidomycosis
Cryptococcosis (CSF eosinophilia) in HIV

ALLERGIC DISEASES

Asthma (atopic and intrinsic, nasal polyps, aspirin intolerance syndromes)
Bronchopulmonary aspergillosis
Allergic rhinitis
Urticarias (acute allergic and chronic idiopathic)
Atopic dermatitis
Acute drug (hypersensitivity) reactions (interstitial nephritis, cholestatic hepatitis, exfoliative dermatitis)

RESPIRATORY TRACT DISORDERS

Hypersensitivity pneumonitis (rare)
Allergic bronchopulmonary aspergillosis
Eosinophilic pneumonia
Transient pulmonary infiltrates (Löeffler syndrome)
Prolonged pulmonary infiltrates with eosinophilia (PIE syndrome)
Tropical pulmonary eosinophilia (TPE)
Bronchiectasis
Cystic fibrosis

ENDOCRINOLOGIC DISORDERS

Addison disease

GASTROINTESTINAL DISEASES

Inflammatory bowel disease (IBD)
Eosinophilic gastroenteritis, eosinophilic esophagitis (EE)
Allergic gastroenteritis (young children)
Celiac disease (when associated with EE)

TOXIC REACTIONS TO INGESTED AGENTS

Eosinophil myalgia syndrome (L-tryptophan)
Toxic oil syndrome

REACTIONS TO CYTOKINE THERAPIES

IL-2 and IL-2 plus lymphokine activated killer (LAK) cells
GM-CSF therapy

CUTANEOUS DISORDERS

Atopic dermatitis
Immunologic skin diseases
Scabies
Myiasis
Chlamydial pneumonia of infancy
Scarlet fever and pneumococcal pneumonia (convalescent phase)
Cat scratch disease
Eosinophilic cellulitis (Wells syndrome)
Episodic angioedema with eosinophilia
Chronic idiopathic urticaria
Bullous pemphigoid
Herpes gestationis
Angioblastic lymphoid hyperplasia (Kimura disease)

IMMUNODEFICIENCY SYNDROMES

Wiskott-Aldrich syndrome
Selective IgA deficiency with atopy
Hyper-IgE recurrent infection syndrome (Job syndrome)
Swiss-type and sex-linked combined immunodeficiency
Nezelof syndrome
Graft-versus-host-disease (GVHD)

CONNECTIVE TISSUE DISEASES

Vasculitis/Collagen Vascular Disorders

Hypersensitivity vasculitis
Allergic granulomatosis with angiitis (Churg-Strauss syndrome)
Serum sickness
Eosinophilic fasciitis
Sjögren syndrome
Rheumatoid arthritis (severe)

NEOPLASTIC, MYELOPROLIFERATIVE, AND LYMPHOPROLIFERATIVE NEOPLASMS AND SYNDROMES

Neoplastic
Ovarian carcinoma
Solid tumors (mucin-secreting, epithelial cell origin)
Chronic eosinophil leukemia
Idiopathic hypereosinophilic syndromes (HES)
Systemic mastocytosis
Myeloproliferative
Chronic myelogenous leukemia (CML) acute myelogenous leukemia (AML) and myelodysplastic syndrome (MDS)
Myelomonocytic leukemia with bone marrow eosinophilia (M4Eo, inversion 16)
Lymphoproliferative
T Cell lymphocytic leukemia
Lymphomas (T Cell, Hodgkin disease)
Angioimmunoblastic lymphadenopathy

RARE CAUSES

Chronic active hepatitis
Chronic dialysis
Acute pancreatitis
Postirradiation
Hypopituitarism

Modified and updated from Mahanty S, Nutman, TB: Eosinophilia and eosinophil-related disorders. In Middleton EJ, Reed CE, Ellis EF, et al, editors: *Allergy: Principles and practice*, ed 4, St Louis, 1993, Mosby-Year Book, pp 1077.

extravascular sites. They tend to localize preferentially in certain tissues and organs exposed to the external environment, principally in the submucosal membrane and loose connective tissue of the skin, gastrointestinal tract, genital tract, and lungs. In contrast, the acute and chronic inflammatory recruitment of eosinophils into tissues occurs primarily in response to the early- and late-phase components of immediate hypersensitivity reactions, but also in association with a variety of immunologic reactions, diseases, and idiopathic syndromes.[5] In addition, diurnal variations in the eosinophil intravascular compartment are well documented, with minimum numbers of blood eosinophils appearing early in the morning and the greatest numbers appearing late at night, mirroring circadian rhythms in circulating adrenal corticosteroids. Likewise, diurnal variations have also been documented to occur in the mobilization, recruitment, and activation of eosinophils in tissues, for example, in diseases such as nocturnal asthma.

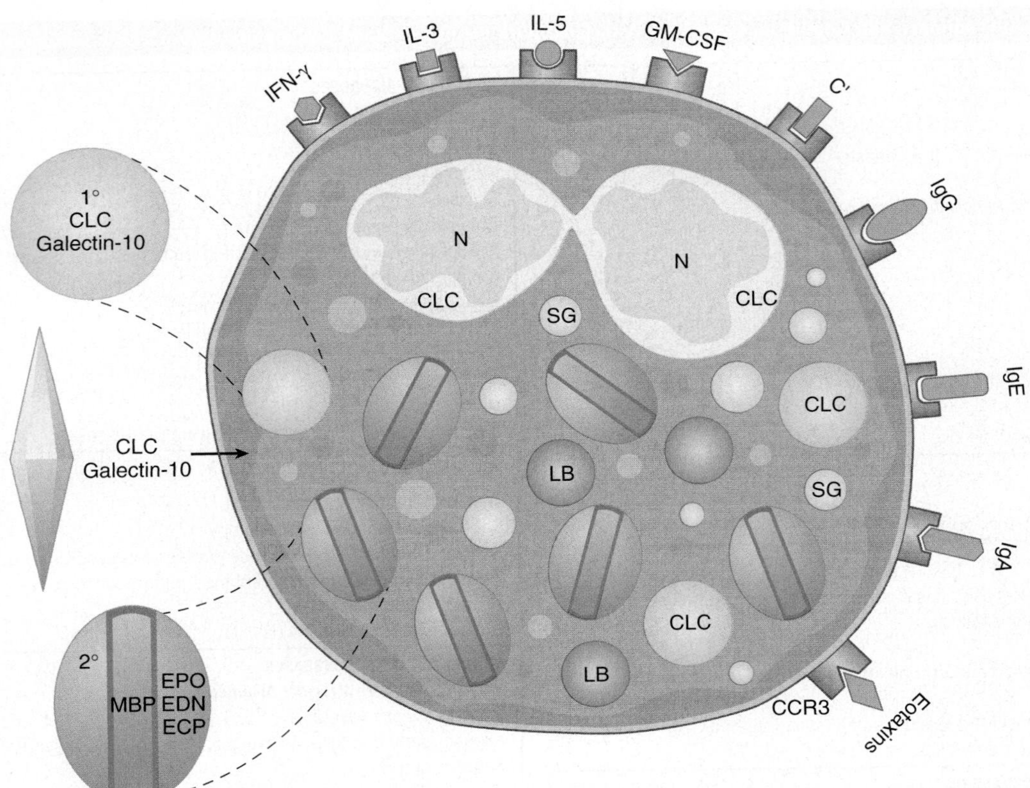

Figure 70-2 SCHEMATIC STRUCTURE OF THE MATURE HUMAN EOSINOPHIL. Primary (1°) and secondary (2°) granules, small granules (SG), and non–membrane-bound lipid bodies (LB) are shown, as are the major cell surface cytokine, chemokine, immunoglobulin, and complement receptors. Also indicated are the subcellular localizations of the eosinophil granule cationic proteins, major basic protein (MBP), eosinophil peroxidase (EPX), eosinophil cationic protein (ECP), and eosinophil-derived neurotoxin (EDN) in the secondary granule and the Charcot-Leyden crystal (CLC) protein (galectin-10) in the coreless primary granule, and the nucleus and cytosolic space beneath the plasma membrane. *(Redrawn from Gleich GJ, Adolphson CR, Leiferman KM: The biology of the eosinophilic leukocyte.* Annu Rev Med *44:85, 1993.)*

Although eosinophils may represent only a component of an inflammatory infiltrate composed of neutrophils, monocytes, and/or lymphocytes, the mechanisms by which they are selectively recruited in large numbers in certain situations remains the subject of investigation. The mobilization of eosinophils from the vasculature involves their rolling and adherence to vascular endothelium via L-selectin, followed by interactions with intercellular adhesion molecule-1 (ICAM1) through CD18/CD11a,b–dependent mechanisms and migration in response to specific cytokines or chemoattractants. Adherence via CD18-independent mechanisms involves binding to cytokine-activated endothelial cells using either E-selectin, also known as *endothelial leukocyte adhesion molecule 1 (ELAM1)* or *vascular cell adhesion molecule 1 (VCAM1)*. Selective recruitment of eosinophils likely involves adhesion to VCAM via the β_1 integrin very late activation antigen-4 (VLA-4), which is expressed by eosinophils but not by neutrophils. Because no single chemokine identified thus far is uniquely specific for eosinophils, including the eotaxins (see later), selective eosinophil recruitment likely involves the complex interaction of multiple adhesion pathways and chemotactic gradients of the eotaxins. The inflammatory mediators identified to function as potent eosinophil chemoattractants include the complement fragment C5a and platelet-activating factor (PAF), along with a number of the eosinophil-active cytokines, including IL-3, IL-5, and GM-CSF, which also prime eosinophils for enhanced migratory responses to agents such as PAF, fMLP, LTB_4, and IL-8. Other potent eosinophil chemoattractants identified thus far are approximately 1000-fold more active than PAF and C5a and include IL-2, as well as the $CD8^+$ T cell–derived lymphocyte chemoattractant factor (LCF) that utilizes CD4 expressed on the activated eosinophil as its receptor. The chemokine regulated on activation, normal T Cell expressed and secreted (RANTES), which is a chemoattractant for certain T-cell subsets and monocytes but not for neutrophils, is likewise a potent stimulus for eosinophil migration; its production by the $CD4^+$ T-cell component of cutaneous and pulmonary allergen-induced late-phase reactions may contribute to the eosinophil infiltration characteristic of these responses. The most potent and eosinophil-selective chemoattractants identified are the eotaxins (eotaxin-1, -2, -3), chemokines that bind and signal through the CCR3 receptor expressed by eosinophils. The selective signals that regulate eosinophil accumulation in tissues in eosinophil-associated diseases have been characterized. Two interrelated mechanisms for the tissue accumulation of eosinophils have been identified and shown to be linked to pathophysiology of the eosinophilic disorders. Interleukin-5 has been shown to play a critical role in the expansion and terminal differentiation of eosinophil progenitor cells in response to allergenic or other stimuli in peripheral tissues. T_{H2} T cell–derived cytokines such as IL-4 and IL-13 operate within tissues to regulate the transmigration of eosinophils from the vascular bed, a process that exclusively promotes tissue accumulation of eosinophils over other leukocytes, probably by activating eosinophil-specific adhesion pathways on endothelial cells and by regulating the production of IL-5 and eotaxin expression in the target tissue compartment. IL-5 and eotaxin likely cooperate locally to selectively and synergistically promote eosinophilia, the former working both systemically and within tissues to promote the local eosinophil chemotactic signals provided by the latter. The regulation of IL-5 and eotaxin levels within tissues by cytokines, including IL-4 and IL-13, allows T_{H2} cells to coordinate both tissue and peripheral blood eosinophilia. These observations highlight the importance of targeting both IL-5 and eotaxin/CCR3 signaling pathways to block eosinophil-associated inflammation and tissue injury.

Mast cells, which normally reside in mucosal tissues and at interfaces with allergens, play an especially important role in eosinophilopoiesis. Mast cells provide the immediate stimuli upon activation to initiate the allergic inflammatory cascade, resulting in eosinophil recruitment during the later phases following an allergen encounter.[6] Mast cells and eosinophils are increased in numbers in nonallergic inflammatory and neoplastic conditions. Both mast cells and eosinophils express CCR3 and respond to eotaxins and RANTES (CCL5), leading to recruitment of both cell types to tissues. Mast cell–derived heparin can bind and stabilize eotaxins. Mast cells and eosinophils can interact with each other through soluble mediators or by direct cell-to-cell contact. Mast cells can also be induced to produce IL-3 and IL-5. Mast cell proteases appear to have a dual action on eosinophil functions. Mast cell–derived chymase suppresses eosinophil apoptosis and induces the release of IL-6, CXCL8, CCL2, and CXCL1 from eosinophils. Beta-tryptase, on the other hand, can cleave eotaxin and RANTES and can potentially limit eosinophil chemotaxis. Eosinophils in turn produce stem cell factor (SCF), which can attract more mast cells into the tissue and protect them from apoptosis. Simultaneous downregulation of eosinophil and mast cell activation can be achieved by inhibitory surface molecules, such as CD300a and the so-called sialic acid binding immunoglobulin-like lectins (SIGLECs), which are expressed by human eosinophils, basophils, and mast cells. Mature forms of both mast cells and eosinophils express SIGLEC8, a cell surface marker with lectin activity. SIGLEC8 induces eosinophil apoptosis and inhibits IgE-mediated mast cell activation, thereby providing a common mechanism to limit inflammation caused by the coexistence of both cell types.[7] SIGLEC8-induced eosinophil death is surprisingly augmented by the presence of GM-CSF and IL-5. SIGLECs apparently act as a failsafe mechanism that counteracts the effects of antiapoptotic cytokines that promote eosinophil survival at sites of inflammation. The SIGLECs provide a potential therapeutic target for the treatment of diseases mediated by eosinophils. For instance, Churg-Strauss syndrome and chronic urticaria, both characterized by increased tissue eosinophilia, have been successfully treated with intravenous immunoglobulins that contain SIGLEC8 autoantibodies. These autoantibodies are agonistic and promote eosinophil cell death.

Eosinophil Activation in Disease: Eosinophil Heterogeneity

Eosinophils secrete their preformed granule constituents and newly synthesized lipid, cytokine, and peptide mediators of inflammation upon stimulation (Fig. 70-3). Peripheral blood eosinophils from patients with eosinophilia and eosinophils from an inflammatory environment within tissues are heterogeneous with regard to their capacity for stimulation and secretion of the described mediators. Eosinophils from blood and tissues of patients with eosinophilia differ from their normal counterparts by a variety of morphologic, biochemical, and functional characteristics, some of which appear to be linked to a significant decrease in cell density. A distinction is made between the populations of "normodense" (normal-density) and "hypodense" (light-density) eosinophils isolated from the peripheral blood and tissues. The blood of normal individuals contains less than 10% of eosinophils with densities less than 1.082 g/mL, whereas patients with eosinophilia can have markedly increased numbers of hypodense cells. Hypodense eosinophils possess a variety of properties consistent with their being primed and/or activated in vivo. Activated hypodense eosinophils are morphologically characterized by increased vacuolization, decreased granule size and content of granule cationic proteins such as MBP, and increased numbers of cytoplasmic lipid bodies. The numbers of surface receptors for a variety of eosinophil-active agonists, including complement cleavage fragments of C3 (CR1 and CR3), immunoglobulins (IgE, IgA), cytokines, and PAF, are expressed to a greater degree by hypodense eosinophils, as are a number of membrane surface antigens such as CD4. Functionally, hypodense eosinophils show increased metabolic activity, oxygen consumption, and generation of superoxide anion, as well as an increased capacity for the synthesis and secretion of LTC_4 and certain cytokines, enhanced chemotaxis, and augmented cytotoxicity for antibody-coated targets.

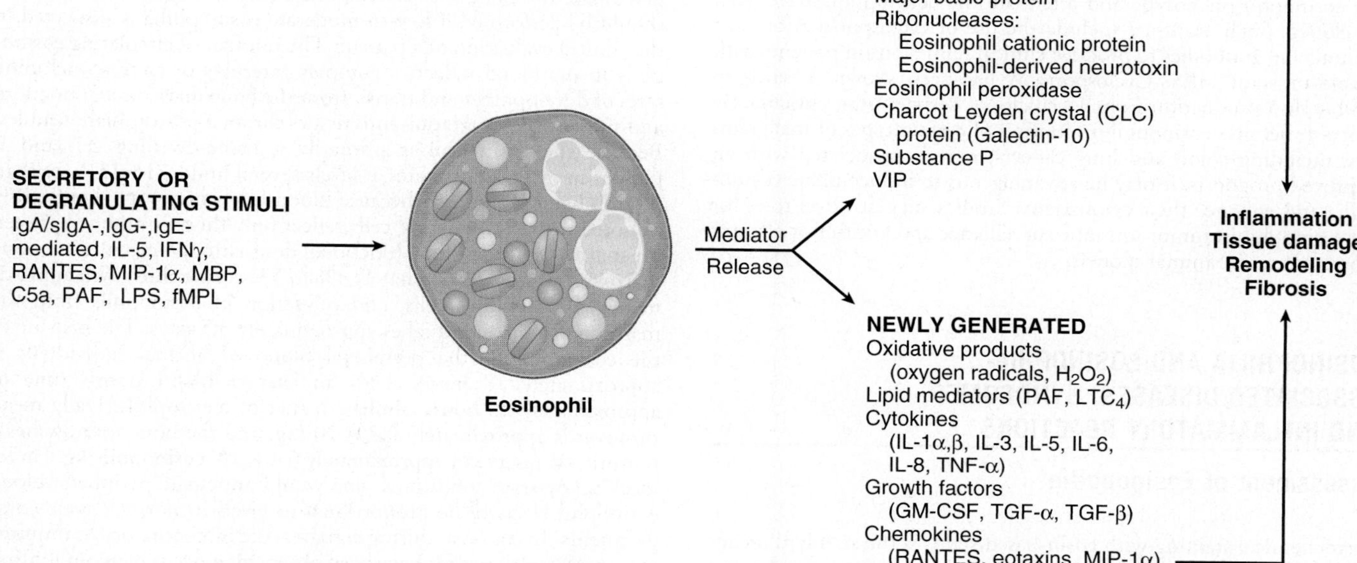

Figure 70-3 EOSINOPHIL SECRETORY/DEGRANULATING STIMULI AND EOSINOPHIL-DERIVED INFLAMMATORY MEDIATORS. The listed factors have been shown to stimulate the secretion of inflammatory mediators from the eosinophil. These mediators may be either preformed, such as the eosinophil granule-derived cationic proteins, or newly generated mediators such as oxidative products, lipid mediators (e.g., LTC_4), inflammatory or hematopoietic cytokines, chemokines, and growth factors. Release of these mediators leads to tissue inflammation, damage, remodeling, and fibrosis. *(Redrawn from Furuta GT, Ackerman SJ, Wershil BK: The role of the eosinophil in gastrointestinal diseases.* Curr Opin Gastroenterol *11:541, 1995.)*

The mechanism by which eosinophils are activated in vivo has been largely defined through the in vitro analysis of factors capable of prolonging eosinophil survival and inducing the development of the hypodense phenotype. The incubation of normal peripheral blood eosinophils with GM-CSF, IL-3, IL-5, and interferons (IFN-α and IFN-γ), either alone or in co-culture with endothelial cells or fibroblasts, induces the development of the hypodense activated phenotype characteristic of eosinophils isolated from patients with hypereosinophilic disorders. In addition, the eosinophilopoietic cytokines (IL-3, IL-5, and GM-CSF) prolong the survival of mature normodense and hypodense eosinophils in vitro (and possibly in vivo in tissues, likely by preventing apoptosis). The exposure of eosinophils to the previously discussed factors in vitro does not precisely recapitulate all the functional characteristics of the in vivo activated, tissue-derived cell, suggesting a requirement for additional, as yet undefined, factors that may include interaction of adhesion receptors with their ligands during eosinophil recruitment and migration into the tissue or stromal cell–derived factors.

Precise relationships between the percentage of hypodense eosinophils and the clinical nature of an eosinophilic disorder have not been clearly defined. Rough correlations have been reported between disease severity and numbers of circulating hypodense eosinophils for particular hypersensitivity disorders such as allergic asthma and allergic rhinitis. However, a significant overlap exists in the percentage of hypodense peripheral blood eosinophils in hypereosinophilic disorders of varying severity, such as bronchial asthma, HES, and certain helminth infections. Because eosinophils reside primarily within tissues for the majority of their lifespan, it is not surprising that their heterogeneity in the peripheral circulation is at best a crude reflection of disease severity. In vitro models of eosinophil heterogeneity suggest a number of pathways for the development of eosinophil subpopulations, including acute exposure to mediators generated in immediate-type hypersensitivity reactions (e.g., PAF, eosinophil-active cytokines such as GM-CSF, IL-3, IL-5, IFN, or TNF) or more chronic exposure to eosinophil-active cytokines in combination with as-yet-undefined factors in tissues as discussed earlier. Regardless of the specific mechanisms or mediators underlying eosinophil priming or activation, the development of eosinophil heterogeneity as a reflection of the functional, proinflammatory capacity of the cell in vivo indicates that these processes can be manipulated therapeutically. For example, in disorders such as HES, in which excessive levels of IL-5 have been demonstrated therapies aimed at modulating IL-5 levels to normalize the eosinophil phenotype and attenuate the eosinophilia have been developed. Such examples include the use of cyclosporin A or IL-5 neutralizing antibodies to produce clinical remissions in patients with steroid-resistant HES. Cyclosporin A has been shown in vitro to inhibit IL-5 production from T-cell clones derived from patients. By contrast, because eosinophil infiltration of certain types of malignancies, including colon and lung cancers, may be associated with an improved prognosis, it may be advantageous to induce tissue eosinophilia and enhance their cytotoxicity. Studies suggest novel roles for the eosinophil in tumor immune surveillance and antitumor effector cell responses in animal models.

EOSINOPHILIA AND EOSINOPHIL-ASSOCIATED DISEASES, SYNDROMES, AND INFLAMMATORY REACTIONS

Assessment of Eosinophilia

Histochemical staining with eosin-based stains is the standard means of identifying eosinophils in both blood and tissues (hematoxylin and eosin) (see Fig. 70-1). Other histochemical dyes such as chromotrope 2R are more definitive in tissues, and Fast Green or Luxol Fast Blue can be used in blood smears or cytocentrifuge preparations to specifically distinguish the mature eosinophil from polymorphonuclear leukocytes and basophils. The chemical characteristics of the fluid or tissue in which the eosinophil is analyzed, and most important, the eosinophil's degree of maturity, activation, secretion, and/or degranulation can induce significant variability in histochemical characteristics using Romanovsky-type metachromatic stains. For example, eosinophils in urine, as found in eosinophilic cystitis or interstitial nephritis, are best detected with a Hansel stain. As a result, it is now appreciated that the definitive identification of the eosinophil's participation in a particular inflammatory response or disease may require immunochemical localization using specific monoclonal or polyclonal antibodies to eosinophil-specific granule proteins such as MBP, eosinophil peroxidase, or ECP, all of which have been used to identify eosinophil infiltration and secretion or degranulation in tissues where they have been missed by more classic histochemical techniques. For peripheral blood, manually performing absolute eosinophil counts or using automated counting systems will provide a much more reliable estimation of eosinophil numbers than will microscopic differential counting of blood smears combined with total leukocyte counts, especially in situations in which there is an absolute leukocytosis or leukopenia for another lymphoid or myeloid lineage. Circulating eosinophils are generally present in low numbers in normal healthy individuals with consensus absolute counts ranging from 35 to 350 eosinophils/mm^3 (mean 125 for adults; 225 for children under 12 years). The broad range of variability in normal blood eosinophil levels reflects the multiple sources of both subtle and more obvious physiologic effects due to diurnal variation in endogenous glucocorticoid levels, degree of atopy in the general population, and other factors that can include exercise, emotional stress, and hormonal influences of the menstrual cycle.

Clinical Assessment of Eosinophilia: Peripheral Blood Versus Tissue Eosinophils

The low numbers of eosinophils in the blood compared with neutrophils and lymphocytes, coupled with their primary localization in tissues, makes accurate quantitation and interpretation of blood eosinophil counts difficult. As noted earlier, a cell differential count fraught with sampling error when eosinophils constitute less than 3% to 5% of total peripheral blood leukocytes. Furthermore, automated cell counters may not accurately enumerate eosinophils unless they are present in sufficiently high numbers, and they can miss eosinophil peroxidase-deficient cells. A manual differential or absolute cell count should be performed if low-to-moderate eosinophilia is suspected in the clinical evaluation of a patient. The number of circulating eosinophils in the blood reflects a complex interplay of factors, including rates of development and transit from the bone marrow, margination, and subsequent emigration into tissues through postcapillary venules. Because the eosinophil is primarily a tissue-dwelling cell and is present in extravascular sites at levels several hundred-fold more than in peripheral blood, and because blood levels may vary significantly as noted earlier, circulating cells reflect only those in transit between the marrow and their final functional destination. Normal adult bone marrow contains approximately 3% to 5% eosinophils, with approximately 40% mature cells, and migration of eosinophils from the marrow into the blood takes approximately 3.5 days. The half-life of the eosinophil in the peripheral blood of normal individuals is approximately 18 hours, with an average blood transit time of approximately 26 hours, similar to that of neutrophils. Daily mean turnover is approximately 0.2×10^9/kg, and the bone marrow has a postmitotic reserve of approximately 0.1×10^9 eosinophils/kg. Under ideal steady-state conditions, one would anticipate peripheral blood eosinophil levels to be proportional to levels in normal tissue compartments. In contrast, during certain acute inflammatory or immune responses, temporal lags have been observed to occur between infiltration into reactive tissue sites and the induction of eosinophil development and emigration from the marrow, resulting in the development of eosinopenia or delayed blood eosinophilia, or both. Moreover, in more chronic eosinophil-associated inflammatory conditions, tissue eosinophilia may be prominent in the absence of any peripheral blood eosinophilia, for example, in certain skin diseases. Thus the clinical assessment of peripheral blood eosinophilia, although diagnostically important, must be interpreted with these caveats in mind.

The list of diseases, syndromes, and inflammatory processes associated with peripheral blood (>450-500 eosinophils/mm^3) or tissue eosinophilia, or both, is quite extensive (see Table 70-1). Of course, the most common causes are infections with parasitic helminths and allergic diseases and their related inflammatory reactions. Effective clinical assessment of patients with eosinophilia requires taking a careful and detailed history, including travel information (e.g., where the patient has lived; drug use, including intravenous drugs, L-tryptophan, vitamin supplements, and other over-the-counter medications; diet; allergic symptomatology).[8] Hypoadrenalism is associated with eosinophilia because of the reduced levels of glucocorticoids. In addition, the systemic nature of many of the nonallergic/noninfectious conditions involving eosinophilia dictates that a careful history of fever, weight loss, myalgias, arthralgias, arthritis, rashes, and lymphadenopathy be obtained as well. Symptomatic or asymptomatic eosinophilia in patients taking drugs associated with known eosinophil-related drug reactions strongly dictates that their use be discontinued, in which case follow-up evaluation should be done to confirm that the eosinophilia and related symptoms have resolved. Patients with eosinophilia who have resided in or visited areas endemic for helminths or other parasites should be examined for intestinal and blood-borne infections, with additional serologic evaluation as necessary to identify the causative agent. It is important to be aware that the degree of eosinophilia associated with parasitic infections is determined by the development, migration, and distribution of the specific parasite and the host's immune response. Eosinophilia is most pronounced in infections such as trichinosis, strongyloides, ascaris, schistosomiasis, filariasis, and gnathostmiasis, which have a phase that involves migration through tissues. Once the more common and obvious causes of eosinophilia have been excluded, the differential diagnosis of eosinophilia becomes more difficult because of the complexity and number of potential organ systems and conditions involved (see Table 70-1).

Monitoring of Eosinophil Activity

Monitoring of eosinophil activity in situ has become more routine. Reasons for this include an increased appreciation for the importance of the greater numbers of tissue eosinophils compared with the number in circulating and their activated status, due to cytokine exposure in the tissue microenvironment. Tissue biopsies have become more routinely used for the clinical evaluation of eosinophil function in diseases involving the skin, lungs, lymph nodes, heart, and other tissues. The difficulties inherent in accurately determining the numbers of eosinophils make routine clinical evaluation of tissue eosinophils somewhat impractical. Alternative approaches such as analysis of tissue secretions from affected organs (e.g., bronchoalveolar lavage of the lung) have been used with success in evaluating eosinophil function in asthma. In addition to the more routine histochemical identification and enumeration of eosinophils and the immunochemical localization of secreted eosinophil granule cationic proteins in tissue biopsies, two other methods have been extensively used to monitor eosinophil activation, secretion, and involvement in disease pathogenesis: (1) the identification of activated eosinophils by staining with a monoclonal anti-ECP antibody EG2 that recognizes a secreted, deglycosylated form of the protein and (2) measurement of the eosinophil granule cationic proteins such as MBP, ECP, and EDN by radioimmunoassay or enzyme-linked immunosorbent assay (ELISA) in various body fluids including serum, plasma, urine, sputum, nasal lavage, and BAL fluid. Under controlled sampling conditions, measurements of these eosinophil granule products have served as excellent biomarkers of eosinophil secretory activity in vivo and eosinophil involvement in a variety of allergic, parasitic, and certain inflammatory and skin diseases not normally associated with blood or tissue eosinophilia. Examples include assays of MBP and ECP in bronchoalveolar lavage and nasal lavage in asthma and allergic rhinitis, in serum and plasma in lymphatic filariasis, and in skin diseases such as chronic idiopathic urticaria. Such measurements likely reflect in vivo secretion in tissues and/or secretory activity of eosinophils in the fluid sampled and have provided compelling evidence for relationships between eosinophil secretory activity and disease severity.

PATHOGENESIS OF EOSINOPHIL-ASSOCIATED END-ORGAN DAMAGE IN HYPEREOSINOPHILIC SYNDROME

Sustained eosinophilia, regardless of origin (whether reactive, clonal, or idiopathic), has the capacity to lead to end-organ damage. The multiple manifestations of such eosinophil-associated end-organ damage are considerable (Table 70-2). However, not all cases of sustained hypereosinophilia necessarily lead to end-organ damage. For example, patients with syndromes such as eosinophilic pneumonia and episodic angioedema with eosinophilia characteristically fail to develop the cardiac damage characteristic of HES patients. Experimentally, IL-5 transgenic mice, which develop extremely high numbers of peripheral blood eosinophils, do not develop significant end-organ damage, suggesting that other factors in addition to IL-5 are likely necessary for eosinophil tissue damage. Because of rather limited experience, it is not currently known whether true myeloproliferative eosinophilic disorders of clonal origin have the capacity to

Table 70-2 Major Organ Involvement and Prominent Clinical Features of Patients With the Hypereosinophilic Syndrome*

PRIMARY ORGAN INVOLVEMENT†
Hematologic‡[100]
Cardiovascular[58]
Cutaneous[56]
Neurologic[54]
Pulmonary[49]
Splenic[43]
Hepatic[30]
Ocular[23]
Gastrointestinal[23]
CLINICAL MANIFESTATIONS§
Eosinophilic endomyocardial disease
Skin lesions (e.g., angioedema, urticaria)
Anorexia and weight loss
Thromboembolic disease
Lymph node and/or spleen enlargement
Ophthalmologic complications
Fever, excessive sweating
Gastrointestinal involvement, including diarrhea
Central nervous system disease
Pulmonary involvement
Psychiatric disturbances
Myalgia
Arrhythmias
Renal impairment
Splenic infarction
Diarrhea alone
Arthralgia
Pericarditis

*Listed in order of frequency.
†Average percentage of 105 patients from American, French, and English studies combined.
‡Reproduced from Spry CJ: The hypereosinophilic syndrome: Clinical features, laboratory findings and treatment. *Allergy* 37:539, 1982.
§Reproduced from Weller PF, Bubley GJ: The idiopathic hypereosinophilic syndrome. *Blood* 83:2759, 1994.

lead to end-organ damage. Of note, HES patients in the National Institutes of Health (NIH) series who ultimately developed cardiac disease exhibited features suggestive of a diagnosis of a myeloproliferative neoplasm, including splenomegaly, thrombocytopenia, anemia, elevated B_{12} levels, cytogenetic abnormalities, and circulating myeloid precursors and myeloid dysplasia. As noted earlier, eosinophils express a number of granule cationic protein mediators capable of inducing thrombotic events, endothelial and endocardial damage, and neurotoxicity (the ribonucleases EDN and ECP). Eosinophil granule MBP and ECP are potent cellular toxins capable of damaging normal host cells and tissues in a manner reminiscent of end-organ damage associated with tissue eosinophilia. In addition, the eosinophil has the capacity to undergo a potent respiratory burst on activation, generating reactive oxidative species that can directly, or in association with eosinophil peroxidase, induce oxidant-mediated tissue damage. However, the mechanisms by which eosinophils induce thrombosis and thromboembolic events associated with hypereosinophilic diseases remain unclear, especially because consistent systemic alterations in coagulation and fibrinolytic pathways in these patients have not been identified. The eosinophil granule cationic proteins do, however, appear to have the capacity to alter thrombomodulin activity, suggesting one possible mechanism for thromboembolism in hypereosinophilic heart disease.[9]

HYPEREOSINOPHILIC SYNDROME

Hypereosinophilic syndrome (HES) is a group of disorders that are marked by a sustained overproduction of eosinophils.[10] The cause of HES can be attributed to several well-defined entities. Approximately 10% to 15% of patients with HES do not have a myeloid malignancy but rather an abnormal clonal $CD3^-CD4^+$ T-cell population that has been shown to produce interleukin-5 (IL-5) in vitro. This variant is referred to as *lymphocytic variant hypereosinophilia.* Furthermore, a small number of patients with a clinical picture of HES have been shown to have myeloid malignancies associated with mutations involving platelet-derived growth factor receptor (PDGFRA or PDGFRB) or the fibroblast growth factor receptor (FGFR). These disorders are categorized by the World Health Organization (WHO) as myeloid and lymphoid malignancies associated with eosinophilia and genetic abnormalities. Those patients with HES in whom a specific etiology cannot be identified are classified as having idiopathic eosinophilia. Some of these IE patients have end-organ damage associated with their eosinophilia and suffer from the clinical syndrome of HES.

HES is characterized by a predilection for end-organ damage, most commonly involving the heart, with the development of eosinophilic endomyocardial fibrosis and related cardiac pathology. The currently defined criteria for HES (Table 70-3) include (a) persistent eosinophilia of greater than 1500 eosinophils/mm^3 for more than 6 months; (b) exclusion of other potential etiologies for the eosinophilia, including parasitic, allergic, or other causes; and (c) signs and symptoms of organ system dysfunction or involvement that appear related to the eosinophilia or are of unknown cause in the clinical presentation. Total leukocyte counts are often less than 25,000/mm^3 with 30% to 70% eosinophils. However, extremely high leukocyte counts (>90,000/mm^3) may be associated with a poor prognosis in some patients. These three primary features of the syndrome, including sustained eosinophilia of unknown etiology or disease association, along with evidence of organ involvement (see Table 70-3), are the defining characteristics of HES. The clinical manifestations of HES, as well as their frequency at presentation, are summarized in Table 70-2. The most commonly encountered features in approximately 50% to 75% of patients include the cardiovascular manifestations, especially endomyocardial disease and its associated thromboembolic complications, the major causes of morbidity (and mortality) in HES.

Table 70-3 Criteria for the Diagnosis of the Idiopathic Hypereosinophilic Syndrome

Eosinophils >1500/mm^3 for at least 6 months
Reactive causes of eosinophilia excluded
Known eosinophilic disease entities excluded
Evidence of eosinophilic end-organ damage
Clonal eosinophilic disorders excluded
FACTORS FAVORING A DIAGNOSIS OF HES
Elevated serum immunoglobulins
Elevated levels of tumor necrosis factor or interleukins (IL-5)
Elevated serum IgE levels
Good therapeutic response to corticosteroids

Reproduced with permission from Brito-Babapulle F: Clonal eosinophilic disorders and the hypereosinophilic syndrome. *Blood Rev* 11:129, 1997.

Differential Diagnosis of Hypereosinophilic Syndrome

As shown in Table 70-1, a large number of diseases have been identified that are associated with reactive, secondary eosinophilia and hypereosinophilia. Their clinical presentations vary significantly and must be clearly distinguished from HES. In particular, a number of eosinophilic diseases and syndromes of questionable or unknown etiology must be differentiated from HES, according to clinical and pathologic parameters. A number of these eosinophilic syndromes have pathologies that are generally restricted to specific organs (e.g., eosinophilic gastroenteritis and eosinophilic pneumonia) and lack the multiplicity of end-organ damage generally seen in HES. In disorders such as eosinophilic gastroenteritis, eosinophilic esophagitis, and eosinophilic cystitis, localized tissue eosinophilia may not be accompanied by eosinophilia in the peripheral blood. For reasons that remain unclear, these syndromes lack the propensity to develop toward secondary eosinophil-mediated cardiac disease. The major eosinophil-associated vasculitis is Churg-Strauss syndrome, which is characterized by a history of blood eosinophilia greater than 10%, asthma, pulmonary infiltrates (nonfixed), abnormalities in the paranasal sinuses, gastrointestinal and cardiac manifestations, mononeuropathy or polyneuropathy, extravascular eosinophilic infiltrates in blood vessels, renal insufficiency, and proteinuria.[11] Necrotizing vasculitis of small arteries and veins and extravascular granulomas are characteristic findings in biopsies from most, but not all Churg-Strauss patients. Asthma, peak eosinophil counts of greater than 1500/mm^3, and systemic vasculitis involving two or more extrapulmonary organs are the identifying characteristics of these patients. Although neurologic, pulmonary, and possibly paranasal findings may accompany HES, asthma is characteristically absent. Nevertheless, it may be difficult to make a clear-cut distinction between HES and Churg-Strauss syndrome in some patients, especially since responses to high-dose corticosteroids would be identical for both at the outset. T cells are critical in the development of Churg-Strauss syndrome and are thought to secrete increased levels of IL-5, IL-4, and IL-13, which promote mobilization and activation of eosinophils. Inhaled allergens, infections, vaccinations, drugs, and the use of leukotriene receptor antagonist therapy for asthma have each been associated with the development of Churg-Strauss syndrome. Autoantibodies to antineutrophil cytoplasmic antigens are detectable in 30% to 40% of cases, which suggests a role for B cells in its pathogenesis, leading to the use of rituximab as a therapeutic agent.

Eosinophilic syndromes with cutaneous involvement can generally be distinguished from HES by the histopathology of biopsied skin lesions. These syndromes include Kimura disease (angiolymphoid hyperplasia with eosinophilia), Wells syndrome (eosinophilic cellulitis), eosinophilic fasciitis, and eosinophilic pustular folliculitis. The syndrome of episodic angioedema with eosinophilia, characterized by a clinical course of periodic recurring episodes of angioedema, urticaria, fever, and marked blood eosinophilia, is not associated with end-organ cardiac damage and has thus been distinguished from HES. The eosinophil myalgia syndrome, induced by ingestion of "tainted" L-tryptophan, is relegated to mainly historic interest, since there have not been any new cases following removal of the tainted L-tryptophan from the market.

A differential diagnosis of HES requires the exclusion of all identifiable eosinophilias of reactive, secondary etiologies (see Table 70-1). These especially include eosinophilias due to parasitic infections caused predominantly by helminthic parasites, but also by two enteric protozoans, *Dientamoeba fragilis* and *Isospora belli.* In adults, filarial infections and strongyloidiasis are most likely to elicit pronounced and prolonged eosinophilias, in contrast to *Trichinella spiralis* infections, which cause an acute eosinophilia that does not persist without reinfection. Infections with *Strongyloides stercoralis,* which have the capacity to induce marked hypereosinophilia that mimics HES, are particularly important to exclude, especially because HES has been misdiagnosed in patients with unsuspected strongyloidiasis, and treatment of these patients with immunosuppressive glucocorticoids can lead to disseminated, often fatal disease. Serial stool examinations and, in particular, assays for *Strongyloides* infection should be performed (e.g., strongyloides agar plate culture) since serologic ELISA assays may cross-react with other helminth infections such as filariasis, ascaris lumbricoides, and schistosomiasis. Parasitic helminth infections not amenable to or detectable by routine stool examinations, including tissue or blood-dwelling helminths causing filariasis, trichinosis, or visceral larval migrans (*Toxocara canis* infections in children), should be evaluated by diagnostic examinations of blood, tissue biopsies, or specific serologic tests (ELISAs) that are currently available.

CLINICAL MANIFESTATIONS OF HES

Hematologic Findings

The definitive hematologic manifestation of HES is sustained eosinophilia of 30% to 70%, with total leukocyte counts ranging from 10,000/mm^3 to 30,000/mm^3 (Fig. 70-4). However, extremely high leukocyte counts of greater than 90,000/mm^3 are not uncommon in some patients with HES, although they are often associated with a poorer prognosis. Blood smears from patients with HES generally show more or less normal, mature eosinophil morphology, including typical bilobed nuclei and granule-rich cytoplasm. However, eosinophilic myeloid precursors may also be noted, though less commonly, and eosinophils may also exhibit morphologic abnormalities including nuclear hypersegmentation, decreased size and/or numbers of secondary granules, and cytoplasmic vacuolization. The presence of myeloblasts and/or dysplastic findings in the peripheral blood may suggest an alternative, clonal etiology such as AML or a myelodysplastic syndrome. Ultrastructurally, HES eosinophils may show a selective loss of secondary granule components (crystalloid MBP-containing core or granular matrix, or both), decreased numbers and/or size of granules, and increased numbers of cytoplasmic lipid bodies and tubulovesicular structures that may be involved in eosinophil secretion of secondary granule contents during the process of piecemeal degranulation.

In addition to the hypereosinophilia, patients with HES may also present with an absolute neutrophilia, further contributing to their overall increased leukocyte counts. This may include band forms, less mature precursors, and alterations in neutrophil nuclear segmentation and cytoplasmic granules. Basophilia, when seen in some HES patients, is usually minimal. Levels of leukocyte alkaline phosphatase may be abnormally elevated or decreased in HES patients, and serum vitamin B_{12} and B_{12}-binding proteins can be normal or elevated. Platelet counts are decreased or increased in 31% and 16% of patients, respectively. Approximately 50% of HES patients may be anemic, with nucleated erythrocytes being present in the peripheral blood. The bone marrow in these patients is hypercellular with significant increases in the percentage of eosinophils (generally from 25% to 75% of marrow elements) and a clear left shift in eosinophil maturation. Myeloblasts are generally normal in number, and marrow fibrosis is rare. Splenomegaly has been reported in approximately 43% of HES patients (see Table 70-2). Hypersplenism in these individuals may contribute to the development of both thrombocytopenia and anemia. Splenic pain induced by capsular distention or infarction is a frequent complication of splenic involvement. The progressive leukocytosis with hypereosinophilia in these patients, along with the hypercellular bone marrow and lack of increased numbers of myeloblasts, can make it difficult to distinguish HES from other myeloproliferative neoplasms.

Cardiovascular Findings

Cardiac manifestations occur in approximately 50% to 60% of patients and are a major cause of morbidity with an associated 5-year mortality of 30% (Table 70-4; also see Table 70-2). Prior to the advent of early diagnosis, improved management, and newer therapies, cardiac disease was the leading cause of morbidity and mortality in HES patients. The cardiac and thromboembolic manifestations of HES are likely eosinophil-mediated. However, the risks for developing cardiac disease are not necessarily related to the extent or duration of the eosinophilia, as patients who ultimately develop cardiac involvement are more likely to be males with an HLA-Bw44

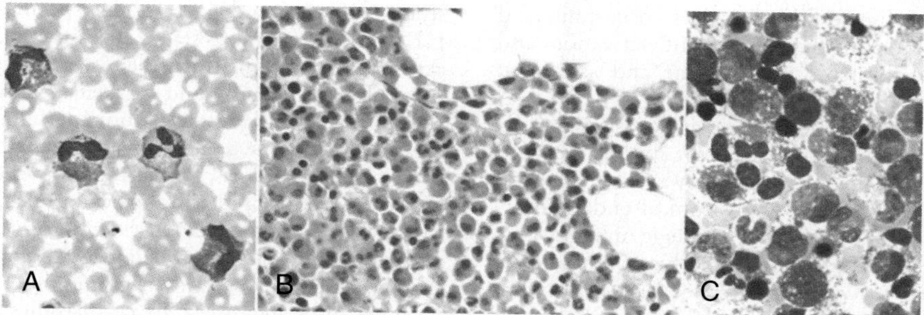

Figure 70-4 HYPEREOSINOPHILIC SYNDROME. This illustration is from the case of a 38-year-old woman who was found to have a marked eosinophilia when she presented with headaches, nausea, and vomiting. Her WBC was 16,900/μL, with 36% eosinophils (**A**). Her bone marrow was hypercellular and showed sheets of eosinophils (**B**). On the aspirated material (**C**), eosinophils and eosinophilic precursors accounted for more than 70% of the cells. The patient had no obvious infectious process and no allergies. There was no malignancy associated with eosinophilia such as T-cell lymphoma, Hodgkin lymphoma, or other myeloid disease. Peripheral blood lymphocyte phenotyping showed no abnormal T-cell subset. Cytogenetic analysis showed a normal female karyocyte, and FISH analysis for del 4q12 showed no deletion of CHIC2.

Table 70-4 End-Organ Damage Produced by Hypereosinophilia

ORGAN/SYSTEM	
Cardiac	***Pulmonary***
Constrictive pericarditis	Pulmonary infiltrates
Endomyocardial fibrosis	Fibrosis
Myocarditis	Pleural effusions
Intramural thrombi	Pulmonary emboli
Valve regurgitation	***Ocular***
Cardiomyopathy	Microthrombi
Coronary artery spasm	Vasculitis
Neurologic	Retinal arteritis
Thromboemboli	***Connective tissue***
Peripheral neuropathy	Arthralgias
Central nervous system dysfunction	Effusions
Epilepsy	Polyarthritis
Dementia	Raynaud phenomenon
Eosinophilic meningitis	Digital necrosis
Dermatologic	***Gastrointestinal***
Angioedema	Ascites
Urticaria	Diarrhea
Papulonodular lesions	Gastritis
Mucosal ulcers	Colitis
Vesicobullous lesions	Pancreatitis
Microthrombi	Cholangitis
	Budd-Chiari syndrome

Reproduced from Brito-Babapulle F: Clonal eosinophilic disorders and the hypereosinophilic syndrome. *Blood Rev* 11:129, 1997.

phenotype, develop splenomegaly and thrombocytopenia, have elevated vitamin B_{12} levels, and have abnormal hypogranular and vacuolated blood eosinophils and circulating early myeloid progenitors. In contrast, those HES patients who do not develop heart disease tend to be females with angioedema, hypergammaglobulinemia, and increased serum IgE levels and immune complexes. The cardiac damage seen in HES, progressing from early necrotic changes through thrombosis and fibrosis, is identical to that seen in patients with hypereosinophilias of diverse etiologies, including tropical eosinophilias caused by loiasis; filarial infections; parasitic infections such as trichinosis and visceral larval migrans, drug reactions or administration of GM-CSF; eosinophil leukemia; eosinophilia due to various solid tumors or lymphomas; and Churg-Strauss syndrome. Because identical forms of cardiac pathology can develop in patients with hypereosinophilias of diverse etiologies, and because some patients never go on to develop cardiac involvement, the pathogenesis of eosinophil-associated cardiac disease likely involves eosinophils and as-yet-undefined factors required for the recruitment, activation, and secretion of eosinophilic constituents in the heart and associated cardiovascular tissues.

The pathology of eosinophilic endomyocardial fibrosis is similar to that of tropical endomyocardial fibrosis, except for the frequent absence of eosinophilia in the latter disorder. However, the general absence of hypereosinophilia in patients with tropical endomyocardial fibrosis is thought to be a function of the late stage of helminthic disease in which the heart disease develops. The histopathology of cardiac involvement in HES is well characterized and can evolve through three sequentially defined stages for which eosinophils and secretion of eosinophil-derived mediators may be directly involved. These include (a) an initial acute necrotic stage of short duration (5 weeks) involving active endomyocarditis, (b) a later thrombotic stage (10 months) with mural thrombus formation over endocardial lesions, and (c) a late fibrotic stage (after approximately 2 years of illness) with development of endomyocardial fibrosis. The early necrotic stage with damage to the endocardium involves marked eosinophil and lymphocyte infiltration of the myocardium with myocardial necrosis, formation of eosinophilic microabscesses, and eosinophil degranulation. However, this early necrotic stage of cardiac disease is usually not recognized clinically. Echocardiography and angiography may fail to detect abnormalities at this early stage of the disease because ventricular thickening has not yet occurred and endomyocardial biopsies, generally from the right ventricle, are required to make the diagnosis of cardiac involvement. Treatment of HES patients with corticosteroids during this acute necrotic stage may avert or control the subsequent development of myocardial fibrosis. However, patients often present at the later stages of the cardiac involvement. In the second stage, thrombi form over the damaged endocardium in either of the ventricles or the atrium, generally with sparing of the aortic and pulmonary valves. Progressive scarring at sites of mural thrombus formation ultimately leads to the late fibrotic stage, with endomyocardial fibrosis resulting in a restrictive cardiomyopathy and mitral or tricuspid valve regurgitation, or both. The more common clinical manifestations in the later progressive stages of endomyocardial fibrosis include dyspnea, chest pain, signs of left or right ventricular congestive heart failure, or both, murmurs from mitral valve regurgitation, cardiomegaly, and T-wave inversions. Most patients who progress to this stage of HES cardiomyopathy will benefit from standard medical therapies for congestive heart failure or, where hemodynamically indicated, mitral valve replacement. Two-dimensional echocardiography is a sensitive method for detecting cardiac abnormalities in these patients, with visualization of mural thrombi and the various manifestations of fibrosis, including thickening of the mitral valve and its supporting structures. Approximately 80% of HES patients have echocardiographic abnormalities, with thickening of the left ventricular free wall the most common finding (68% of patients). Cardiac catheterization may also be useful for demonstrating elevated right and left ventricular end diastolic pressures, and angiography may be used to visualize valvular incompetence. Although electrocardiographic changes in these patients are common, they are not specific to HES. Recently, intractable coronary artery spasm has been reported as the sole cardiovascular manifestation of HES. Cardiac magnetic resonance imaging with late enhancement with gadolinium may be helpful in detecting myocardial fibrosis and signs of inflammation as well as being of use in monitoring the patient's clinical course. Although each of these imaging procedures may be useful diagnostically or in following the clinical course of an individual patient, endomyocardial biopsy from the right or left ventricle remains the gold standard diagnostic procedure.

Histopathologic evaluation of the heart of HES patients generally shows four dominant features: (a) endocardial fibrosis and thickening, including involvement of mitral valve and supporting structures; (b) mural thrombus and granulation tissue on the endocardium with extensive infiltration by eosinophils; (c) thrombotic and fibrotic involvement of small intramural coronary vessels, including inflammatory cells and eosinophils; and (d) eosinophilic infiltration of the endocardium and, in some cases, of the myocardium. In a multicenter study of biopsy and postmortem specimens of cardiac tissue from HES patients at various stages of eosinophilic endomyocardial disease, activated eosinophils (identified by staining with the EG2 anti-ECP monoclonal antibody) and marked intracardiac extracellular deposition of eosinophil granule cationic proteins were identified mainly in areas of acute tissue damage on and beneath the endocardium in areas of myocardial necrosis, and in the walls of small vessels. The presence of activated eosinophils and toxic granule proteins in the lesions early in this disease suggests an active role for eosinophils and their products in inducing endocardial damage and myofibrillar injury, although the mechanisms involved in eosinophil recruitment into the heart have yet to be identified. In vitro studies have shown that secretion products of activated eosinophils can damage heart cell plasma membranes in rats. In addition, eosinophil peroxidase in the presence of hydrogen peroxide and bromide or thiocyanate ion can damage the endothelium of an isolated rat heart, and eosinophil granule proteins can impair thrombomodulin activity, findings that support a role for these eosinophil products in the development of endocardial injury and subsequent thrombotic events in HES. The in vitro findings that eosinophil secretion products such as EDN can induce fibroblast proliferation, that ECP alters fibroblast proteoglycan synthesis, and that MBP can augment IL-1 or TGF-β–induced production of inflammatory cytokines (IL-6 and IL-11) by fibroblasts, confirm that eosinophils play a pivotal role in the development of endocardial fibrosis in later stages of the disease. Treatment involves medical interventions to prevent heart failure as well as to prevent symptoms. Prophylactic anticoagulation is warranted to avoid thrombotic complications. Unless the patient has an FIP1L1-PDGFRA fusion gene in which imatinib is the therapy of choice, corticosteroids are the mainstay of therapy. Occasionally, surgical resection of ventricular masses or heart valve replacement is indicated.

Pulmonary Findings

Approximately 50% of HES patients have pulmonary involvement, with the most common symptom being a chronic and persistent (usually nonproductive) cough. Although the physiologic basis for pulmonary involvement in HES is not known, it may be secondary to congestive heart failure or numerous other factors, including infiltration and sequestration of eosinophils in lung tissues or pulmonary emboli originating from ventricular thrombi. Although bronchospasm has been noted in some patients, asthma is quite rare in HES. Transudative pleural effusions are the most common abnormality in patients with frank congestive heart failure. In contrast to chronic eosinophilic pneumonia, the pulmonary infiltrates seen in 14% to 28% of HES patients were either diffuse or focal, without any preference for particular regions of the lung. Pulmonary infiltrates in HES may or may not clear with prednisone treatment, and pulmonary fibrosis can develop in patients with endomyocardial fibrosis.

Neurologic Manifestations

As noted in Tables 70-2 and 70-4, neurologic involvement is quite common in HES (approximately 50% of patients), including three different types of manifestations. The first form of neurologic involvement is caused by thromboemboli, which may originate from intracardiac thrombi in the left ventricle. These thromboembolic episodes may occur even before overt cardiac disease is visible by echocardiography. Patients with thrombotic complications may experience embolic strokes or transient ischemic attacks that may be multiple and recurrent, and these episodes may occur even though the patient is adequately anticoagulated. The second type of neurologic manifestation involves primary diffuse central nervous system (CNS) dysfunction of unknown etiology. HES patients may variably exhibit changes in behavior, confusion, ataxia, and loss of memory. The third neurologic abnormality noted in HES is the development of peripheral neuropathy, which can occur in approximately 50% of HES patients exhibiting neurologic involvement. This includes symmetric or asymmetric sensory polyneuropathies, including sensory deficits, painful paresthesias, or mixed sensory and motor defects. These neuropathies may improve with steroid administration or other treatments, may be stable or continue to progress despite therapy, or may improve or resolve with time. The histopathology of the involved nerves usually shows varying degrees of axonal loss, without evidence of vasculitis or direct or peripheral eosinophil infiltration. The presence in eosinophils of two granule cationic proteins, EDN and eosinophil cationic protein, both equally potent in inducing a neurotoxic and paralytic syndrome known as the Gordon phenomenon when injected (intrathecally) into rabbits, has led to the hypothesis that these proteins might be responsible for inducing the various neuropathies commonly seen in HES. The histopathology of the cerebrocerebellar dysfunction in the brains of experimental rabbits undergoing the Gordon phenomenon includes a spongiform degeneration of white matter and loss of Purkinje cells, changes not comparable to the peripheral axonal nerve damage seen in HES. Both EDN and ECP (related, approximately 16-kDa cationic proteins with 70% amino acid sequence homology) are members of the ribonuclease gene family and possess potent ribonuclease activity and cellular toxicities in vitro. However, no direct evidence shows that these ribonucleases and cellular toxins have the capacity to mediate the types of neurologic damage seen in HES, nor have these proteins been visualized by immunochemical means at sites of HES neuropathology. Marked elevations in CSF levels of IL-5, MBP, and EDN have been documented in children with raccoon roundworm infections, progressive neurologic deterioration, and deep white matter changes on magnetic resonance images of the brain. Thus the pathogenesis of the encephalopathic, CNS, and peripheral manifestations of HES-associated neuropathy remains poorly defined.

Cutaneous Manifestations

The skin is frequently involved in HES pathology, with cutaneous manifestations present in greater than 50% of patients (see Table 70-2). The skin lesions associated with HES most commonly fall into three categories: (a) angioedematous and urticarial lesions; (b) erythematous, pruritic papules and nodules; and (c) mucosal ulcerations (see Table 70-4).[12] Patients with angioedema and urticaria are more likely to have a benign disease course that is responsive to corticosteroids, without the development of cardiac or neuropathic complications. A subgroup of HES patients with cyclical angioedema and eosinophilia are now considered to have a syndrome (episodic angioedema with eosinophilia) that is distinct from classic HES. These patients have a disorder with recurrent attacks of angioedema, urticaria, fever, and bodyweight gain that can be quite pronounced. These clinical manifestations are associated with marked leukocytosis and eosinophilia during the episodes. In HES patients who develop papular or nodular lesions (Fig. 70-5), the lesions usually improve

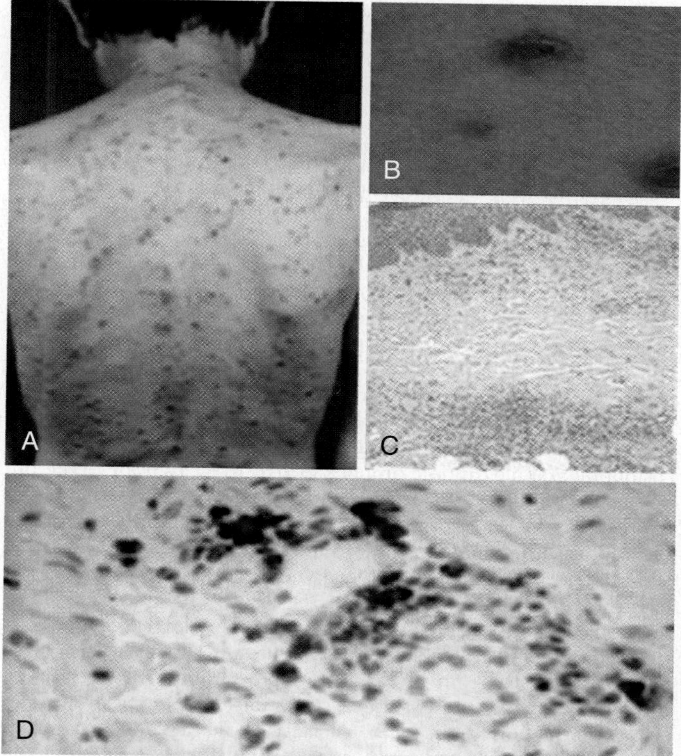

Figure 70-5 DERMATOLOGIC MANIFESTATIONS OF HES. Erythematous pruritic papules and nodules (**A**). Partially centrally ulcerated (**B**) hematoxylin-eosin-stained biopsy tissues demonstrating inflammatory cell infiltrates largely consisting of eosinophils and lymphocytes (**C**). Larger magnification of perivascular infiltrate with numerous eosinophils (**D**). *(From Plötz, S.G., Hüttig B, Aigner B, et al: Clinical overview of cutaneous features in hypereosinophilic syndrome.* Curr Allergy Asthma Rep *12:85, 2012.)*

concomitantly with positive responses to systemic therapy. Dermal biopsies in these patients generally show mixed cellular infiltrates, including eosinophils, without signs of vasculitis. Perivascular eosinophilic infiltrates are also found in these lesions. The aquagenic erythematous pruritic eruptions and indurated papules and nodules in some HES patients respond to psoralen and ultraviolet light A therapy (PUVA); in some cases, this treatment is accompanied by a return of eosinophil counts to normal. PUVA therapy may also be effective for the cutaneous manifestations of HES associated with HIV infection (exfoliative erythroderma, linear flagellate plaques). HES-associated pruritus and nodular lesions have also been controlled with Dapsone (75-150 mg/day) and prednisone therapy. Oral sodium cromoglycate (cromolyn sodium) given before meals has also been reported to be efficacious, though neither of these agents had any effect on peripheral eosinophilia. Severe and sometimes incapacitating mucocutaneous ulcerations may be a prodrome to HES and indicate a subset of HES patients with a poor prognosis. These lesions can appear at multiple sites, including the mouth, nose, pharynx, penis, esophagus, stomach, and anus; lesions can flare up independently of other clinical manifestations of HES. Biopsies of the ulcerative lesions usually show mixed cellular infiltrates, without a predominance of eosinophils or any evidence of vasculitis or microthrombi. These ulcers have generally been resistant to treatment with topical or systemic corticosteroids, colchicine, and hydroxyurea, but they have recently been shown to respond to IFN-α with complete and durable remissions.

Eosinophils are present in many skin diseases and, in certain conditions, may constitute part of the diagnostic histopathology. Although eosinophils in general may not be prominent in many cutaneous diseases, ample evidence now shows that they may nevertheless participate in the pathogenesis of cutaneous inflammation and contribute to edematous reactions in atopic dermatitis, syndromes associated with acute and chronic urticarias, IgE-mediated late-phase reactions, chronic dermatitis associated with parasitic infections (such as onchocerciasis, episodic angioedema with eosinophilia, eosinophilic cellulitis), and skin lesions associated with rIL-2 administration for advanced malignancies. Indirect evidence includes the ability of the eosinophil to elaborate its granule cationic proteins (some of which are capable of inducing release of vasoactive amines from basophils and mast cells and inducing cutaneous wheal-and-flare reactions following direct injection into human skin) and production of lipid mediators such as LTC_4 and PAF, both potent inducers of vascular permeability in vivo. In addition, levels of eosinophil-active IL-5 are elevated in patients who have episodic angioedema with eosinophilia and those who have eosinophil-associated toxicity due to IL-2 administration, as well as in the acute inflammatory response (Mazzotti reaction) in human patients with onchocerciasis treated with diethylcarbamazine.

By far, the most conclusive evidence for eosinophil participation in the etiology of the skin diseases remains the immunochemical analysis of skin biopsies showing prominent extracellular deposits of eosinophil granule cationic proteins such as MBP, ECP, or EDN, but not neutrophil products (neutrophil elastase), in affected but not unaffected skin, and in the absence of prominent numbers of intact eosinophils in lesional infiltrates. One example is the IgE-mediated late-phase reaction that follows the wheal-and-flare response characteristic of type I, IgE-mediated hypersensitivity. This classic late-phase reaction, which is characterized clinically by erythema, edema, pruritus, and tenderness peaking 6 to 12 hours after intradermal antigen or anti-IgE challenge, involves infiltration by mononuclear cells, neutrophils, basophils, and eosinophils presumably in response to mast cell degranulation, along with extensive extracellular deposition of eosinophil MBP and neutrophil granule products. The secretion and extracellular deposition of eosinophil granule constituents, shown to possess potent cytotoxic and proinflammatory activities in edematous and eczematous lesions, clearly suggests that eosinophils may contribute to the pathogenesis of both acute and chronic skin diseases, including the cutaneous lesions associated with HES. However, studies elucidating the mechanisms that regulate eosinophil recruitment, activation, and secretion in the skin are still needed to more clearly understand the dynamics of eosinophil participation in these cutaneous disorders and to identify potential therapeutic approaches to selectively block their influx and function.

NEW DEFINITIONS OF HYPEREOSINOPHILIC SYNDROME

HES is not a monolithic diagnosis but a clinical syndrome that can be attributed to a variety of distinct pathologic mechanisms (see box on Diagnosis and Workup of Hypereosinophilic Syndrome). At least two pathogenetic forms of HES—myeloproliferative and lymphocytic variants—have been defined. The MPN form of HES is characterized by hepatosplenomegaly, circulating myeloid precursors, increased serum tryptase levels, anemia, thrombocytopenia, marrow fibrosis, immature myeloid marrow precursor cells, and genetic and cytogenetic abnormalities associated with myeloid neoplasms. These disorders can be accompanied by mutations in PDGFRA, PDGFRB, or FGFR in as few as 10% to 20% of patients with HES. The discovery of these genetic lesions was prompted by reports indicating that some patients with HES or CEL respond to imatinib mesylate with complete hematologic and cytogenetic remissions—in most patients, remission was achieved at fourfold lower doses than those typically used to treat chronic myelogenous leukemia (CML) (100 mg/day versus 400 mg/day). These data suggested that these BCR-ABL–negative patients might possess abnormal gene fusion products or activating mutations that generate novel tyrosine kinase targets of imatinib. These findings sparked a "reverse" bedside-to-bench translational research effort by several research laboratories to rapidly identify the constitutively active tyrosine kinase targets of imatinib in these HES patients. Possible targets included the known activated kinases such as ABL, PDGFR, or c-KIT, all of which had been shown to be inhibited by imatinib mesylate. These efforts led to the successful identification of an activated tyrosine kinase gene fusion on chromosome 4q12, which is produced by a novel interstitial chromosomal deletion of the CHIC2 domain, fusing an uncharacterized human gene known as FIP1-like-1 (FIP1L1) to the platelet-derived growth factor receptor-α gene (PDGFRα). These findings have significantly changed the current paradigm for the diagnosis and treatment of patients with HES and CEL.[13] Of importance, not all HES and CEL patients respond to imatinib, and the majority of patients who do respond with hematologic remissions have been male and not female. It is also important to note that approximately 40% of the patients who do respond to imatinib lack the FIP1L1-PDGFRA gene fusion, suggesting genetic heterogeneity in HES/CEL, which led to the discovery of activating mutations in PDGFRA and PDGFRB that generate imatinib-sensitive constitutively active tyrosine kinases. The FIP1L1-PDGFRA can be detected by fluorescence in situ hybridization (FISH) or by nested polymerase chain reaction (PCR) but not by classical cytogenetics. Eosinophilia is the hallmark of this disorder; it is a multisystem disorder with manifestations secondary to infiltration of tissues with eosinophils and release of proinflammatory mediators and toxic granules. Endomyocardial fibrosis and restrictive cardiomyopathy are the most life-threatening consequences of F1PL1-PDGFRA–positive MPN. PDGFRB fusion partners remain uncommon causes of clonal eosinophilia, which occurs more commonly in men in their late 40s. The disorders associated with these abnormalities are also responsive to imatinib.

The mechanism of action by which the FIP1L1-PDGFRA gene fusion leads to the proliferation and differentiation of the eosinophil lineage over other myeloid lineages in these patients is unclear. Initial investigations suggested that STAT5 may be one of the downstream targets of FIP1L1-PDFGRA tyrosine kinase activity. Studies have demonstrated that retroviral transduction-mediated overexpression of STAT5a in umbilical cord blood–derived $CD34^+$ human stem/progenitor cells selectively amplifies their commitment, proliferation, and terminal differentiation to the eosinophil lineage in vitro in the presence of IL-5 and that STAT5 activation by tyrosine kinases such as BCR-ABL can contribute to the transformation of leukemic cells. A murine transgenic model revealed that the FIP1L1-PDGFRA

Diagnosis and Workup of Hypereosinophilic Syndrome

Patients presenting with eosinophilia of unknown etiology should undergo a thorough clinical and laboratory evaluation consisting of the following:

- Complete/detailed history and physical examination
- Review of all medications (including herbal medications and nutritional supplements); withdrawal of all noncritical medications
- Complete blood count with total eosinophil count and review of peripheral blood smear
- Hepatic and renal function tests, urine analysis
- Vitamin B_{12} level
- Serologic assays: erythrocyte sedimentation rate, rheumatoid factor, human immunodeficiency virus (HIV)
- Serum tryptase level
- Quantitation of total IgE level
- Cardiac troponin level
- Stool for ova, parasites ×3
- Serologic assays for *Strongyloides, Trichinella, Toxocara, Entamoeba histolytica, Echinococcus,* filariasis, and schistosomiasis
- Bone marrow aspirate and biopsy
- Cytogenetics, FISH, and molecular analyses (PDGFRA, PDGFRB, FGFR1 fusion genes, BCR-ABL, JAK2 V617F, KIT D816V, clonal TCR gene rearrangement)
- T-cell phenotyping by flow cytometry
- Chest radiograph; computed tomographic scan of chest, abdomen, and pelvis
- Electrocardiogram and echocardiogram
- Pulmonary function tests

Diagnostic Criteria for HES/CEL

1. Persistent eosinophilia of greater than 1500 eosinophils/mm^3 for more than 6 months
2. Exclusion of other potential "reactive" etiologies for the eosinophilia including parasitic, allergic, or other causes, *and*
3. Presumptive signs and symptoms of organ system dysfunction or involvement that appears related to the eosinophilia or is of unknown cause in the clinical presentation

fusion gene itself is not sufficient to induce an HES/CEL–like disease independently; rather, it requires a second event, that is, overexpression of IL-5.

Eosinophilic disorders due to fusions of FGFR1 are rare but affect patients of all ages with a slight male predominance. This disorder is defined by the rearrangement of the FGFR1 at the chromosome 8p11-12 locus resulting in the creation of fusion proteins with constitutive activation of FGFR1 tyrosine kinase. The most common translocations include t(8;13)(p11;q12); t(6;8)(q27;p11); t(8,9)(p12;q33). The clinical pictures associated with these fusion proteins are quite diverse. Patients with t(8;13)(p11q12) often present with leukocytosis and basophilia rather than eosinophilia and develop lymphadenopathy and T-cell lymphoma, whereas patients with t(6;8) develop disease associated with hypereosinophilia and tonsillar involvement and monocytosis. These disorders are extremely rare and are associated with a poor prognosis with an overall survival of 16 months. These disorders do not respond to imatinib and the few long-term survivors have received allogeneic stem cell transplants. The characteristic genetic abnormalities are best detected using FISH or PCR rather than classical cytogenetics.

CEL-NOS is an MPN defined by a high degree of eosinophilia associated with HES but absence of PDGFRA, PDGFRB, and FGFR1 rearrangements and greater than 2% blasts in the peripheral blood or greater than 5% but less than 20% blasts in the marrow and/or evidence of clonality due to the presence of cytogenetic abnormalities. CEL-NOS is a rare disorder that has been observed in 12.5% of patients with MDS and is associated with a poorer prognosis than other forms of MDS. Progression to blastic transformation (>20% blast cells) in patients with stable disease has been documented. Idiopathic HES is diagnosed in those patients with profound eosinophilia and accompanying tissue damage but no evidence of reactive hypereosinophilia or clonal eosinophilopoiesis. These patients account for 65% to 80% of patients with HES.

Other Genetic Abnormalities Associated With HES

Other TK fusion genes, for example, involving ABL or JAK2, have also been reported in diverse eosinophilia-associated myeloid neoplasms. Disorders with FGFR1 and JAK2 fusion genes are resistant to imatinib and other clinically available tyrosine kinase inhibitors. Fusion genes involving FLT3 are uncommon. An ETV6-FLT3 fusion has been identified in several patients with an eosinophilia-associated MPN who achieved rapid complete hematologic response and complete cytogenetic response after 3 months of taking sunitinib. A secondary blast phase caused by clonal evolution was diagnosed after 6 months, and a second complete hematologic response after taking sorafenib occurred but the patient relapsed 2 months later. A second heavily-pretreated patient with an initial diagnosis of T-lymphoblastic lymphoma and died from sunitinib-induced pancytopenia. Patients with systemic mastocytosis (SM) carry the D816V KIT mutation. Even though these patients often present with features similar to patients with hypereosinophilia, the FIP1L1-PDGFR1 fusion and D816V KIT mutation appear to be mutually exclusive oncogenic lesions. The presence of KIT mutation places these patients into the SM diagnostic category.

Lymphomas and Hypereosinophilia

A number of lymphomas may be associated with the development of eosinophilia, including Hodgkin lymphoma, T-cell lymphoblastic lymphoma, and adult T-cell leukemia/lymphoma, but the eosinophilia is generally much more modest than that seen in HES.[14] In contrast, there are several reports of patients presenting with classic clinical and hematologic features of HES who have gone on to develop acute lymphoblastic leukemia or T-cell lymphoma. In a number of T-cell lymphoma cases, the accompanying eosinophilias were shown to be associated with the production of eosinophilopoietic cytokines (GM-CSF, IL-3, or IL-5) by the lymphoma cells. Most T-cell malignancies associated with eosinophilias have acquired the ability to produce cytokines capable of promoting eosinophilopoiesis. A significant number of patients with peripheral T-cell lymphomas, including Sezary syndrome and mycosis fungoides, develop reactive blood eosinophilia above 700/microliter, which serves as a poor prognostic factor. Eosinophil-mediated end-organ damage is rare in this situation. Eosinophilia is an uncommon finding in patients with B-cell lymphomas, with the exception of Hodgkin lymphoma. Mild peripheral blood eosinophilia has been observed in about 15% of patients with Hodgkin lymphoma with the Reed-Sternberg cells being responsible for excessive IL-5 production. An extreme reactive form of eosinophilia can be associated with rare cases of B-cell acute lymphoblastic leukemia. In 10% of such cases, a t(5;14) translocation is associated with high levels of IL-3. These patients have extreme eosinophilia and can develop eosinophil-mediated end-organ damage. Congestive heart failure occurs in 30% of patients at diagnosis and can be rapidly reversed with the administration of steroids. Effective treatment of this B-cell ALL results in disappearance of the hypereosinophilia, which reappears if relapse occurs.

The Lymphocytic Variant of HES

The lymphocytic variant of HES (L-HES) represents a distinct clinical entity characterized by the overproduction of cytokines capable of promoting eosinophilopoiesis, primarily IL-5, by an aberrant T-cell phenotype ($CD3^-CD4^+$), and the presence of clonal rearrangements of the T-cell receptor in some, but not all, patients.[15] This syndrome can precede the development of overt T-cell lymphoma. Involvement of the skin is the most common presenting symptom. Serum elevation of IgE and the chemokine TARC is common. The variant occurs equally in males and females and is characterized by skin involvement, gastrointestinal symptoms, obstructive lung disease, and rarely, endomyocardial fibrosis. This variant accounts for 10% to 15% of HES patients. Rare patients have cyclical angioedema and eosinophilia accompanied by cyclical increases of IL-4, suggesting that this is a variant of L-HES. These patients characteristically respond to steroids and not imatinib.

Eosinophil Leukemia

True acute eosinophilic leukemias have several distinguishing characteristics such as a marked increase in the numbers of immature blood and/or bone marrow eosinophils, greater than 20% blast forms in the bone marrow, tissue infiltration with immature eosinophilic cells, and a clinical course and findings that tend to resemble other acute leukemias, including anemia, thrombocytopenia, and increased susceptibility to infections. However, the cardiac and neurologic manifestations of HES can also develop in eosinophil leukemia.

In contrast, CNS infiltration by eosinophils and the tendency to produce bone myeloblastomas are features more frequently associated with acute eosinophil leukemia. Chromosomal abnormalities may occur with both HES and CES-NOS, but eosinophil leukemia is more frequently associated with chromosomal anomalies characteristic of other acute myeloid leukemias including 8:21 and 10p+11q− translocations and trisomy 1. In addition, eosinophil leukemia has been reported as a variant of the M4Eo phenotype of acute myelomonocytic leukemia with eosinophilia, linked to inversion of chromosome 16.

Familial Eosinophilia

Familial clustering of HES is extremely rare but has been observed with Churg-Strauss syndrome and eosinophilic esophagitis. In one family, multiple family members had marked eosinophilia from birth, but only a minority of family members developed symptomatic HES with cardiac involvement.

THERAPY AND PROGNOSIS FOR HYPEREOSINOPHILIC SYNDROME

The earlier literature on HES is filled with reports of poor to dismal patient prognosis. For example, a 1975 review indicated an average survival time of 9 months, with a 3-year survival of only 12%. The high morbidity and mortality likely reflect the fact that most HES patients tended to present late with more advanced disease, in particular, significant cardiovascular problems. Deaths in these patients were generally the result of congestive heart failure and secondary complications of endomyocardial disease, including bacterial endocarditis, progressive valvular incompetence, and the thromboembolic sequelae. However, earlier diagnosis of HES, improved clinical and echocardiographic methods for monitoring, and the use of cardiac medications and cardiothoracic surgical procedures not previously available have resulted in more successful prevention and management of cardiac disease in these patients, considerably improving clinical outcomes and survival. A report in 1989 of 40 HES patients reported 80% survival after 5 years and 42% survival at 10 and 15 years. Thus for many patients, prevention and management of HES end-organ damage, in particular the cardiac sequelae, result in prolonged survival persisting over decades. Supportive therapies for managing the cardiovascular complications of HES, along with therapies aimed at controlling the eosinophilia to prevent end-organ damage, are the mainstay of HES treatment regimens. Treatment should focus on controlling end-organ damage, not just on suppressing or eradicating the eosinophilia, especially as the severity of cardiovascular complications of HES does not necessarily correlate with the duration or level of eosinophilia. Although more aggressive treatment (e.g., cytotoxic chemotherapy or bone marrow transplant) may be indicated in selected patients, the current goal is chronic maintenance therapy. Clearly, all causes of reversible eosinophilia, such as parasite infections, should be treated after careful documentation of the infectious agent. The most prudent approach to treating patients with Churg-Strauss syndrome is to have biopsy-proven disease before embarking on a regimen of high-dose corticosteroids and cyclophosphamide. After achievement of a clinical response or remission, a low dose of prednisone is suggested as maintenance therapy. If unacceptably high doses of prednisone are required for disease control, methotrexate as a maintenance agent is recommended. Interferon alpha or the anti-IL-5 neutralizing antibody mepolizumab also permit the reduction of steroids to more acceptable levels.

Initial Therapeutic Options

It is difficult to predict the duration and severity of eosinophilia that predispose individual patients to end-organ damage. Generally, patients meeting the diagnostic criteria for HES (see Table 70-3), without any overt evidence of organ dysfunction or severe symptoms and with eosinophil counts less than 1500 to 2000 eosinophils/mm^3, can be monitored closely and periodically without treatment for at least 6 months and possibly indefinitely, as long as their complete blood counts are stable, their echocardiograms normal, and no new clinical signs or symptoms of end-organ involvement appear. Periodic reinvestigation of the etiology of the eosinophilia is highly appropriate and recommended every 3 to 6 months to reconfirm the diagnosis of HES. Given the poor prognosis for patients with HES, those patients who have PDGFRA/B abnormalities should be treated with imatinib even in the absence of end-organ dysfunction since this treatment is so effective[16] (see box [flowchart] on Treatment Algorithm for Patients With Severe Eosinophilia). The hematologic benefit of imatinib in FIP1L1-PDGFRA–positive HES has been confirmed in multiple studies. The optimal treatment and dosing strategy for imatinib is not fully defined, and a number of different studies have been performed with imatinib dosing ranging from 100 mg to 400 mg daily. A daily dose of 100 mg appears to be sufficient to induce complete hematologic and molecular remission in most patients, although some patients require doses of up to 400 mg daily. Maintenance doses of 100 to 200 mg weekly may be effective in achieving molecular remission in some patients.[17] The efficacy of imatinib in patients with FIP1L1-PDGFRA HES was evaluated in a multicenter prospective study in an Italian prospective cohort of 27 patients with a median follow-up period of 25 months.[18] Complete hematologic remission was achieved in all patients within 1 month, and all patients achieved complete molecular remission after a median of 3 months of treatment. Patients on imatinib remained PCR-negative during a median follow-up of 19 months. Despite the durable molecular remissions observed in these patients, discontinuation of the drug leads to relapse of the disease.[19] Molecular remissions can be achieved again upon reintroduction of imatinib. Second-generation tyrosine kinase inhibitors such as nilotinib or dasatinib are effective in patients intolerant of imatinib. Frequently, patients resistant to imatinib experience a response with interferon α, but they should be considered candidates for allogeneic stem cell transplantation.

Overall, imatinib is well tolerated at the low dose of 100 mg daily with minimal hematologic and nonhematologic toxicities. However, in a few cases, development of severe left ventricular dysfunction has been reported soon after treatment initiation. Close monitoring of patients is recommended during this time period. Currently, prophylactic use of steroids during the first 7 to 10 days of imatinib treatment is recommended for patients with known cardiac disease. Unlike the experience of patients with CML, only rare cases of imatinib resistance have been described in the 10 years of treating

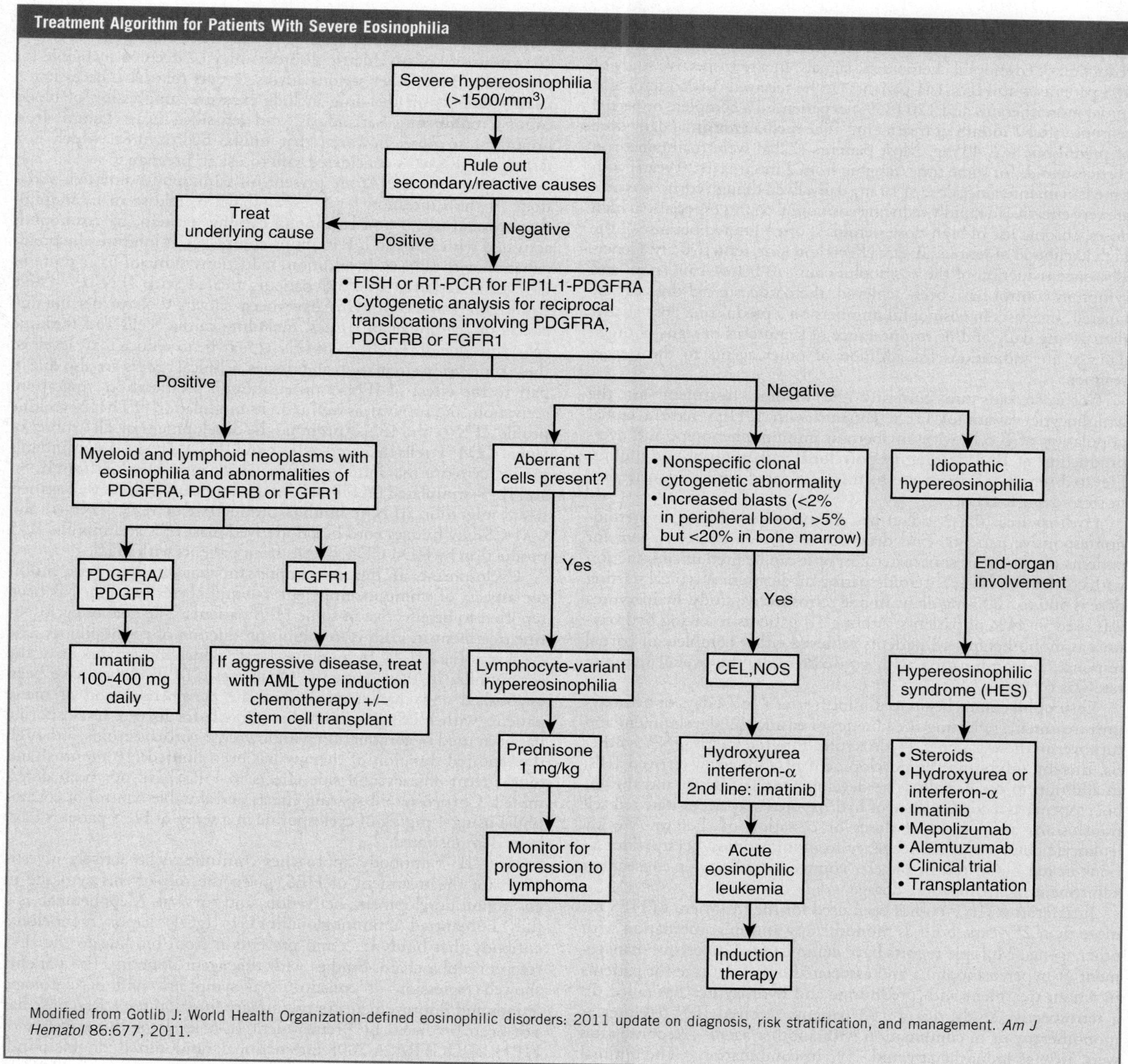

Modified from Gotlib J: World Health Organization-defined eosinophilic disorders: 2011 update on diagnosis, risk stratification, and management. *Am J Hematol* 86:677, 2011.

FIP1L1-PDGFR positive disease. Most of the mutations are the T674I mutation within the ATP-binding domain of PDGFRα and occur during the blast phase of the disease. This mutation is analogous to the T315I BCR-ABL mutation in CML, which renders it resistant to imatinib, nilotinib, and dasatinib.

In patients with rearrangement variants other than FIP1L1-PDGFRA, literature (consisting of case reports and small case series) indicates that treatment with imatinib at 400 mg daily can result in durable hematologic and cytogenetic remissions.[20] In patients with FGFR1 mutations, imatinib is not an effective treatment option and thus is not recommended. In many of these patients, the disease follows an aggressive course, often culminating in AML in 1 to 2 years. Therefore intensive chemotherapy followed by allogeneic stem cell transplantation is recommended. Imatinib at doses of 400 to 500 mg/day may also be considered for FIP1L1-PDGFRA mutation–negative patients with myeloproliferative features of disease such as elevated serum tryptase. Only 23% of such patients who receive imatinib experience complete or partial response. Occasionally sorafenib and other second-generation tyrosine kinase inhibitors have been used successfully to treat imatinib resistance. No reports of cure with imatinib have been reported. Patients may remain in remission for some months after discontinuation of therapy; however, eventual relapse is inevitable. Molecular monitoring for detection of minimal residual disease in patients on a constant dose of imatinib is recommended in order to detect early relapse, which should prompt an immediate increase in imatinib dose.

For the majority of hypereosinophilic patients with strictly an idiopathic form of HES (including the absence of abnormalities of PDGFRA, PDGFRB, and FGFR1) corticosteroids (usually prednisone at 1 mg/kg) is considered frontline therapy and is usually effective in achieving rapid reductions in the eosinophil count. Steroids act through the glucocorticoid receptors that are present in the cytoplasm of eosinophils. The mechanisms of action by which corticosteroids induce eosinopenia are multiple and not completely understood. Possible mechanisms include disruption of eosinophilopoiesis, induction of apoptosis, eosinophil sequestration into the spleen or lymph nodes and reduction of eosinophil chemotactic signals. In a retrospective study of 188 patients with HES, 141 patients (75%) received corticosteroids as initial monotherapy, and 120 (85%) experienced a complete or partial response after 1 month of treatment.[21] The median maximal daily dose of prednisone was 40 mg. Most patients (72%) were maintained on corticosteroids for some time, ranging from 2 months to 20 years, with a median maintenance dose of 10 mg daily. Even though corticosteroids are very effective in rapidly reducing eosinophil counts especially at high doses, chronic use of high-dose steroids is often limited because of the high likelihood of serious adverse effects and long-term toxicity. Generally, once reduction of the eosinophil count to below 1500/mm^3 and symptom control have been achieved, the corticosteroid dose can be tapered. Increases in eosinophil numbers on a prednisone dose greater than 10 mg daily and/or reappearance of symptoms or signs of organ damage are indications for addition of other agents to the steroid regimen.

Corticosteroids are currently the firstline treatment for the lymphocytic variant of HES. Patients with L-HES have a clonal population of T cells with an aberrant immunophenotype and overproduction of IL-5, leading to polyclonal expansion of eosinophils. Elevated serum IgE levels are further associated with responsiveness to steroids in L-HES.

Hydroxyurea (0.5-2 g/day) has demonstrated efficacy in steroid-nonresponsive patients. This drug can also be an effective agent for patients intolerant of corticosteroids, or it can be used in conjunction with corticosteroids as a steroid-sparing medication. A typical starting dose is 500 to 1000 mg daily. In one retrospective study, hydroxyurea was used in 34% of patients. Among 18 patients receiving hydroxyurea as monotherapy, 13 patients achieved either complete or partial response. In combination with corticosteroids, the overall response rate was 69%.[21]

Eosinophil counts begin to diminish after 7 to 14 days of hydroxyurea treatment, reflecting the kinetics of eosinophil development and turnover in these patients. Hydroxyurea interferes with DNA synthesis, thereby inhibiting the development of all marrow-derived cells, in addition to eosinophils. The development of anemia and thrombocytopenia as a consequence of hydroxyurea may necessitate red cell transfusions and decreased doses or cessation of therapy. Weekly leukocyte counts may be necessary to monitor idiosyncratic fluctuations in red blood cell or platelet counts, as well as for consequent adjustment of hydroxyurea dosage.

Interferon-α (INF-α) has been used for the treatment of HES for more than 25 years, both as monotherapy and in combination with other agents. Multiple reports have demonstrated successful management of hypereosinophilia and associated organ damage for patients in whom treatment with prednisone and hydroxyurea has failed. In a retrospective study, 46 of 188 patients received IFN-α either as monotherapy or in combination with another agent—response rates were 50% as monotherapy and 75% in combination.[21] The optimal starting dose of INF-α has not been defined, but the initial dose required to induce normalization of eosinophil count is often higher than the dose required to maintain remission. Usually, therapy is initiated at 1 million units three times weekly by subcutaneous injection, and the dose is titrated up to 3 to 4 million units three times weekly as needed for individual patients to achieve control of the eosinophil count. Improvements in the eosinophil count have been associated with improvement in splenomegaly and hepatomegaly, as well as reductions in cardiac and thromboembolic complications, mucosal ulcers, and skin manifestations. Treatment with pegylated IFN-α-2b on a weekly schedule has also been effective in the treatment of HES.[22] INF-α treatment has been reported to result in cytogenetic remissions in patients with cytogenetic abnormalities. Side effects of short- and long-acting formulations of IFN-α are often dose dependent and include fatigue and flu-like symptoms that often improve with long-term administration and can be easily controlled with acetaminophen. Exacerbation of autoimmune disorders, such as autoimmune thyroiditis, psoriasis, ulcerative colitis, and others have been reported. Exacerbation of depression, including development of suicidal ideation and development of psychosis, is a serious side effect that needs to be carefully assessed at each visit; thus patients with a known history of psychiatric disorders may be deemed ineligible for this medication. Other serious adverse events that have necessitated taking patients off the drug include excessive suppression of blood counts, retinopathy, sarcoidosis, and left-sided heart failure. It is important to note, however, that unlike hydroxyurea, which is a teratogen, IFN-α is considered safe to use in pregnancy.

Receptors for IFN-α are present on eosinophils, although variations in the expression levels exist. In vitro, release of eosinophil-derived neurotoxin and eosinophil cationic protein, by eosinophils activated with IgA and IgE immune complexes, is inhibited by preincubation with IFN-α. In addition, reductions in major basic proteins have been reported in HES patients treated with IFN-α.[23] These eosinophil granule proteins have been shown to have detrimental effects on a number of tissues, including cardiac cells and Purkinje cells; thus one of the effects of IFN-α may be to reduce toxic levels of these proteins in circulation and tissues. Clinical results are also due in part to the effect of IFN-α on eosinophil proliferation, migration, activation, and survival, as well as on its modulation of Th1/2 cytokine profile. IFN-α and IFN-γ promote the development of Th1 subset of clonal CD4$^+$ T cells that secrete IL-2 and IFN-γ. IFN-γ is a proinflammatory cytokine that inhibits differentiation of eosinophils from IL-3– and IL-5–stimulated umbilical cord mononuclear cells, as well as their tissue migration. IFN-α inhibits production of IL-5, TNF-α, and GM-CSF by human cord blood–derived mast cells and inhibits IL-5 production by CD3$^-$CD4$^+$ T cells from patients with HES.

Cyclosporine, an immunosuppressant that interferes with multiple aspects of immunocompetent T-lymphocyte function, has been reported to be effective in some HES patients. The goal of cyclosporine treatment in HES is to inhibit production of eosinophilopoietic cytokines (i.e., IL-5) by putative T-cell clones thought to drive the eosinophilia in these patients. Of interest, T-cell clones have been established and characterized from the peripheral blood of many patients with HES, providing the rationale for its use. Cyclosporine has been used in conjunction with low-dose corticosteroids, although the reported duration of therapy has been limited (10 months) and longer-term efficacy and side effects in HES have not been determined. Corticosteroid-sparing effects and durable control of eosinophilia using 4 mg/kg of cyclosporine in a series of HES patients have been demonstrated.

Anti–IL-5 antibody approaches continue to be actively investigated for the treatment of HES, given the role of this cytokine in eosinophil development, activation, and survival. Mepolizumab is a fully humanized immunoglobulin G1 (IgG1) kappa monoclonal antibody that binds IL-5 and prevents it from binding to the IL-5 receptor alpha chain. Studies with this agent done in HES patients showed regression of constitutional symptoms and dermatologic lesions and improvements in pulmonary function tests. Response has not been predicted by pretreatment IL-5 levels or the presence of FIP1L1-PDGFRA. A 2008 international, randomized, double-blind, placebo-controlled trial of mepolizumab in patients with FIP1L1-PDGFRA–negative HES demonstrated a corticosteroid-sparing effect of mepolizumab.[24] In patients requiring 20 to 60 mg of prednisone per day to maintain eosinophil count less than 1000 per microliter and stable clinical status, 84% of patients in the mepolizumab group (compared with 43% of patients in the placebo group) achieved the primary end point of reduction of the prednisone dose to 10 mg or less for 8 or more consecutive weeks. Rates of adverse events were similar in treated and placebo groups. Mepolizumab is not yet FDA-approved for the treatment of HES but may be available through compassionate use protocol for patients with life-threatening, treatment-resistant disease.

Reslizumab is a humanized IgG4 anti–IL-5 monoclonal antibody that is currently in clinical trials for eosinophilic esophagitis and in pediatric patients for eosinophilic asthma, but it has not yet been evaluated extensively for patients with HES. Early studies showed improvements in eosinophil counts and clinical symptoms in 75% of patients. More studies are needed to evaluate the treatment potential of this antibody.[25]

Alemtuzumab is anti-CD52 monoclonal antibody being evaluated for the treatment of HES based on the rationale that eosinophils express CD52 antigen. It has been used for the treatment of therapy-resistant eosinophilic disorders with variable results.[26] In 10 of 11 patients, alemtuzamab induced hematologic remission; however, this response was not sustained off-therapy.

Historically, a number of cytotoxic agents have been used to treat HES, refractory to steroids and hydroxyurea. The use of these agents is now limited, given the availability of other, more effective and less toxic treatments. Vinca alkaloids are effective in HES, and vincristine (1.0-1.5 mg/m^2 at biweekly intervals), which produces a permanent mitotic arrest by disrupting spindle microtubules, has been shown to be beneficial in some patients. However, the use of vincristine can lead to liver failure and is limited by neurologic complications that may be indistinguishable from the peripheral neuropathies associated with HES. Because vincristine decreases blood eosinophil counts in 1 to 3 days, it may be particularly useful for acute treatment of patients with marked hypereosinophilia (>100,000 eosinophils/mm^3). Other chemotherapeutic agents that have been used with some success in a limited number of patients include etoposide (VP-16) and alkylating agents such as chlorambucil. In particular, etoposide, a podophyllotoxin derivative and topoisomerase II inhibitor that induces DNA damage, has been used successfully in a number of patients to date. Administration of oral followed by parenteral etoposide after cessation of hydroxyurea treatment has been reported to control symptoms and eosinophil counts for prolonged period of 18 months, but its use was ultimately withdrawn because of marrow suppression. Use of oral pulses of chlorambucil has been reported at doses ranging from 4 to 10 mg/m^2 daily for 4 consecutive days approximately every second month for 2 years with some efficacy in patients refractory to steroids and intolerant of hydroxyurea.

Leukapheresis

Plasma and leukapheresis have no defined role in the long-term management of HES. The use of leukapheresis has generally been restricted to emergency situations for patients developing profoundly high eosinophil counts. However, cell counts rebound rapidly to pretreatment levels within 1 day of the procedure. Even multiple repeated sessions of leukapheresis are usually not sufficient to induce more than a transient decrease in blood eosinophil levels. Five repeated plasma and leukapheresis sessions over a period of 2 weeks were reported to significantly decrease blood eosinophilia; however, continued sessions were insufficient by themselves to lower blood eosinophil counts to acceptable levels. The mechanism by which plasmapheresis transiently decreases eosinophil levels is entirely speculative but has been suggested to involve a temporary removal or decrease in the levels of circulating eosinophilopoietic factors.

Anticoagulation and Antiplatelet Agents

Because thrombotic and thromboembolic events are frequently serious complications of HES, anticoagulants have often been used, especially in those patients with clear evidence of thromboemboli, neurologic symptoms, and cardiac involvement. Commonly used agents include warfarin, antiplatelet agents, and heparin. However, the efficacy of anticoagulation or antiplatelet agents has not been clearly established in HES disease, and many patients treated with these agents have continued to have thrombotic events, despite their adequate use.

Splenectomy

As previously noted, splenomegaly has been used in HES patients, and hypersplenism in these individuals may contribute to thrombocytopenia, anemia, and splenic infarction. Splenic pain induced by capsular distention or infarction is a known complication of HES. In HES, splenectomy has the capacity to ameliorate platelet sequestration from hypersplenism and to relieve the pain associated with splenic distention and infarction.

Stem Cell Transplantation

Experience reported with stem cell transplantation for the treatment of HES is quite limited; however, it has been attempted for aggressive and treatment-resistant disease.[27] Reports of stem cell transplantation for refractory HES include several successes with patients apparently in complete remission with the clinical course complicated in some by the development of graft-versus-host-disease (GVHD) requiring cyclosporin-A therapy. In another report, the patient relapsed 40 months after transplantation but survived for more than 44 months. Only in HES cases with an extremely aggressive course unresponsive to standard therapies or in young patients with a refractory course of disease and clinical features suggestive of a myeloproliferative neoplasm (e.g., chromosomal abnormalities) should allogeneic stem cell transplantation be considered a treatment option. Without greater understanding of the underlying mechanisms responsible for the overproduction of eosinophils and the aggressive development of end-organ damage in some of these patients, the risks associated with stem cell transplantation may outweigh its more routine use in treatment of this disorder.

Cardiac Surgery

Treatment of the cardiovascular sequelae of HES continues to be a therapeutic challenge. Surgical intervention in eosinophilic heart disease does not appear to carry any risk for disease recurrence at the operative sites. For patients who develop significant compromise of valvular function, endomyocardial thrombosis, or fibrosis, cardiac surgery has the capacity to provide substantial clinical and quality-of-life improvements. Mitral valve and/or tricuspid valve repair or replacements have been reported in more than 50 eosinophilic patients. Endomyocardectomy and thrombectomy, as performed for advanced-stage Löeffler endomyocardial fibrosis, have also been used effectively in some HES patients, and ventricular decortication may be performed in combination with valve replacement. For mitral valve replacements, mechanical valves have proven problematic because of recurring thrombotic episodes despite adequate anticoagulation, suggesting the use of porcine valves whenever possible. HES patients who have received valve replacements have generally experienced long-term improvement in cardiac function, provided the eosinophilia remains controlled.

FUTURE DIRECTIONS

The heterogeneous nature of HES, ranging from patients with clear features of myeloproliferative disorders (including cytogenetic abnormalities) to patients with more benign clinical courses (such as episodic angioedema with eosinophilia), suggests that multiple disease processes are likely at play. Current research aimed at defining the cause of HES and mechanisms regulating the development of eosinophil-mediated end-organ damage in eosinophil-associated diseases in general should ultimately lead to more selective and improved therapies. The therapeutic targets for these efforts are likely to include (a) IL-5 and its high-affinity receptor; (b) underlying T-cell clones (either immunocompetent or occult T-lymphoid malignancies) that elaborate IL-5 or GM-CSF tissue- or organ-specific dysfunctional elaboration of eosinophil-active chemoattractant factors such as eosinophil-selective chemokines (the eotaxins); (c) vascular endothelial adhesion molecules (VCAM/VLA-4); and (d) undefined mechanisms that induce the overproduction of eosinophils and/or serve to recruit and activate eosinophils selectively in certain tissues and organs.[28] The essential absence of end-organ damage in some syndromes of hypereosinophilia contrasts starkly with the morbidity (and mortality) associated with the development of endomyocardial fibrosis in HES and certain other eosinophilias. Because HES patients are clearly a heterogeneous group, clinical management based on current knowledge must be specifically tailored to the individual, with the overall goal of controlling the eosinophilia and, in particular, the eosinophil-mediated end-organ damage. The clinical and surgical management of patients with IE and HES has evolved significantly. Current treatment options facilitate the control or eradication of eosinophilia and end-organ damage in most HES patients. The efficacy of imatinib mesylate in patients with HES has led to the identification of the FIP1L1-PDGFRA gene fusion, which encodes a pathogenetically relevant and constitutively active tyrosine kinase. This seminal finding had led to a reclassification of hypereosinophilias into several well-defined clinical entities and has stimulated research that may ultimately translate into improved clinical characterization and therapeutic options. For patients with imatinib-resistant forms of CEL or those with classic HES that does not respond to conventional therapies such as glucocorticoids, hydroxyurea, and IFN-α, treatment options such as stem cell transplantation may hold promise for durable disease remissions. Treatment with IFN-α should be considered as an initial firstline option for the management of imatinib-nonresponsive HES, either alone or in combination with other therapies. Finally, humanized anti–IL-5 antibody (mepolizumab) is available through compassionate use protocols at several institutions. The clinical data with this agent look highly promising for the treatment of a wide range of patients with *FIP1L1-PDGFRA*-negative HES and possibly other eosinophilias—for example, eosinophilic gastrointestinal syndromes such as eosinophilic esophagitis.

Future research on HES and CEL will likely focus on the molecular basis of imatinib responsiveness in both FIP1L1-PDGFRA–positive and –negative patients, specifically addressing how the constitutively activated FIP1L1-PDGFRA or other fusion- or mutant-activated kinases selectively lead to chronic hypereosinophilia and end-organ damage. Studies of the effects of imatinib on the proliferation and terminal differentiation of bone marrow–derived eosinophil progenitors, as well as the survival and intracellular signaling pathways in eosinophils from imatinib-responsive patients, may be particularly revealing in terms of the downstream targets of these novel kinases. Clearly, more carefully controlled clinical trials are required to define evidence-based information with which to treat this patient population.

REFERENCES

1. Valent P, Horny HP, Bochner BS, et al: Controversies and open questions in the definitions and classification of the hypereosinophilic syndromes and eosinophilic leukemias. *Semin Hematol* 49:171, 2012.
2. Schwartz LB, Sheikh J, Singh A: Current strategies in the management of hypereosinophilic syndrome, including mepolizumab. *Curr Med Res Opin* 26:1933, 2010.
3. Valent P, Gleich GJ, Reiter A, et al: Pathogenesis and classification of eosinophil disorders: A review of recent developments in the field. *Expert Rev Hematol* 5:157, 2012.
4. Gauvreau GM, Ellis AK, Denburg JA: Haemopoietic processes in allergic disease: Eosinophil/basophil development. *Clin Exp Allergy* 39:1297, 2009.
5. Kita H: Eosinophils: Multifaceted biological properties and roles in health and disease. *Immunol Rev* 242:161, 2011.
6. Gotlib J, Akin C: Mast cells and eosinophils in mastocytosis, chronic eosinophilic leukemia, and non-clonal disorders. *Semin Hematol* 49:128, 2012.
7. Nutku-Bilir E, Hudson SA, Bochner BS: Interleukin-5 priming of human eosinophils alters siglec-8 mediated apoptosis pathways. *Am J Respir Cell Mol Biol* 38:121, 2008.
8. Mejia R, Nutman TB: Evaluation and differential diagnosis of marked, persistent eosinophilia. *Semin Hematol* 49:149, 2012.
9. Wang JG, Mahmud SA, Thomas JA, et al: The principal eosinophil peroxidase product, HOSCN, is a uniquely potent phagocyte oxidant inducer of endothelial cell tissue factor activity: A potential mechanism for thrombosis in eosinophilic inflammatory states. *Blood* 107:558, 2006.
10. Gotlib J: World Health Organization-defined eosinophilic disorders: 2011 update on diagnosis, risk stratification, and management. *Am J Hematol* 86:677, 2011.
11. Vaglio A, Moosig F, Zwerina J: Churg-Strauss syndrome: Update on pathophysiology and treatment. *Curr Opin Rheumatol* 24:24, 2012.
12. Plötz SG, Hüttig B, Aigner B, et al: Clinical overview of cutaneous features in hypereosinophilic syndrome. *Curr Allergy Asthma Rep* 12:85, 2012.
13. Apperley JF, Gardembas M, Melo J, et al: Response to imatinib mesylate in patients with chronic myeloproliferative diseases with rearrangements of the platelet-derived growth factor receptor beta. *N Engl J Med* 347:481, 2002.
14. Roufosse F, Garaud S, de Leval L: Lymphoproliferative disorders associated with hypereosinophilia. *Semin Hematol* 49:138, 2012.
15. Simon HU, Plötz SG, Dummer R, et al: Abnormal clones of T cells producing interleukin-5 in idiopathic eosinophilia. *N Engl J Med* 341:1112, 1999.
16. Jovanovic JV, Score J, Waghorn K, et al: Low-dose imatinib mesylate leads to rapid induction of major molecular responses and achievement of complete molecular remission in FIP1L1-PDGFRA-positive chronic eosinophilic leukemia. *Blood* 109:4635, 2007.
17. Helbig G, Stella-Holowiecka B, Majewski M, et al: A single weekly dose of imatinib is sufficient to induce and maintain remission of chronic eosinophilic leukaemia in FIP1L1-PDGFRA-expressing patients. *Br J Haematol* 141:200, 2008.
18. Baccarani M, Ciloni D, Rondoni M, et al: The efficacy of imatinib mesylate in patients with FIP1L1-PDGFRalpha-positive hypereosinophilic syndrome. Results of a multicenter prospective study. *Haematologica* 92:1173, 2007.
19. Klion AD, Robyn J, Maric I, et al: Relapse following discontinuation of imatinib mesylate therapy for FIP1L1/PDGFRA-positive chronic eosinophilic leukemia: Implications for optimal dosing. *Blood* 110:3552, 2007.
20. Gotlib J, Cools J: Five years since the discovery of FIP1L1-PDGFRA: What we have learned about the fusion and other molecularly defined eosinophilias. *Leukemia* 22:1999, 2008.
21. Ogbogu PU, Bochner BS, Butterfield JH, et al: Hypereosinophilic syndrome: A multicenter, retrospective analysis of clinical characteristics and response to therapy. *J Allergy Clin Immunol* 124:1319, 2009.
22. Butterfield JH: Treatment of hypereosinophilic syndromes with prednisone, hydroxyurea, and interferon. *Immunol Allergy Clin North Am* 27:493, 2007.
23. Butterfield JH, Weiler CR: Treatment of hypereosinophilic syndromes–the first 100 years. *Semin Hematol* 49:182, 2012.
24. Rothenberg ME, Klion AD, Roufosse FE, et al: Treatment of patients with the hypereosinophilic syndrome with mepolizumab. *N Engl J Med* 358:1215, 2008.
25. Walsh GM: Reslizumab, a humanized anti-IL-5 mAb for the treatment of eosinophil-mediated inflammatory conditions. *Curr Opin Mol Ther* 11:329, 2009.
26. Verstovsek S, Tefferi A, Kantarjian H, et al: Alemtuzumab therapy for hypereosinophilic syndrome and chronic eosinophilic leukemia. *Clin Cancer Res* 15:368, 2009.
27. Ueno NT, Anagnostopoulos A, Rondon G, et al: Successful non-myeloablative allogeneic transplantation for treatment of idiopathic hypereosinophilic syndrome. *Br J Haematol* 119:131, 2002.
28. Menzies-Gow A, Ying S, Sabroe I, et al: Eotaxin (CCL11) and eotaxin-2 (CCL24) induce recruitment of eosinophils, basophils, neutrophils, and macrophages as well as features of early- and late-phase allergic reactions following cutaneous injection in human atopic and nonatopic volunteers. *J Immunol* 169:2712, 2002.

CHAPTER 71

MAST CELLS AND SYSTEMIC MASTOCYTOSIS

John Mascarenhas, Animesh Pardanani, Marina Kremyanskaya, and Ronald Hoffman

MAST CELLS

Discovery

The discovery of mast cells is credited to Paul Ehrlich, who first described a subgroup of cells ("Mastzellen") localized to a large extent around blood vessels within a number of tissues; these cells were thought to be larger than white blood cells and to contain "protoplasmic deposits" (granules) that reacted in a characteristic manner with aniline dyes. Ehrlich stressed that the identification of mast cells was based primarily on a specific histochemical reaction that rendered the cellular granules metachromatic, not simply on the morphologic appearance of these cells. Several years later, Ehrlich also discovered a peripheral blood basophilic granulocyte in patients with myeloid leukemia and suggested that this cell (blood mast cell, basophil, or mast leukocyte) had its origin in the bone marrow with subsequent residence in the peripheral blood. Mast cell nuclei are typically round to oval, whereas basophils have lobulated nuclei similar to granulocytes.

Origin

Normal mast cells originate from a $CD34^+$ cell population in the bone marrow.[1] Mast cells are released into the circulation in a primitive state and undergo terminal maturation/differentiation after migrating into tissues, where they ultimately reside. Mouse models were first used to investigate the origin and development of mast cells. In a C57BL/6-bg^j/bg^j, beige Chediak-Higashi–syndrome mouse model, the giant mast cell granules were used as a morphologic marker for donor-derived cells. Here, cells from the bone marrow, peripheral blood, liver, thymus, or lymph nodes of beige mice were transplanted into irradiated, congenic C57BL/6 +/+ mice, or alternatively, the beige mouse was parabiosed with a congenic +/+ mouse, dominant white-spotting (W)– or steel (Sl)–locus mutant mice (vide infra) that are profoundly deficient in mast cells. The mast cells in skin and other organs in the adult W/W^v mouse could be restored to normal levels after transplantation with bone marrow cells from congenic +/+ mice.

The relationship between human mast cells and cells belonging to other leukocyte lineages remains unclear. Although mast cells share several features with basophils, namely presence of cytoplasmic basophilic granules, expression of high-affinity IgE receptors (FcεRI), and release of histamine upon stimulation, the two cell types are considered to be distinct. Unlike mast cells, basophils circulate in the blood as mature cells and are thought to be incapable of proliferation; basophils undergo apoptosis after their recruitment and activation in the tissues. Studies of developmental pathways in murine models have not been conclusive as to how mast cell–committed progenitors are generated. It remains uncertain as to whether there is a shared bipotent progenitor for mast cells and basophils or whether mast cells are derived directly from multipotent progenitor cells. Eosinophils and basophils, by contrast, share a common bipotent progenitor cell. However, molecular studies in patients who have received cells from patients with systemic mastocytosis (SM) have revealed that a pathogenetically relevant mutation, Kit Asp816Val (D816V), is found primarily in mast cells and not basophils, thus suggesting that the two cells do not arise from a common progenitor cell. Furthermore, it has been proposed that mast cells and basophils, both of which contain metachromatic granules, can be distinguished on the basis of cellular immunophenotype, gene expression profile, or growth factor responsiveness. The primary cytokine for mast cell growth and differentiation is stem cell factor (SCF)/C-KIT ligand. Other cytokines (including IL-3, IL-4, IL-5, IL-6, and IL-9), however, do not independently promote the generation of mast cells but may enhance the activity of SCF. Mast cells resemble monocytes based on several characteristics, including their responsiveness to IL-4, the expression of mast cell tryptase in human monocytic cell lines, and the ability of murine mast cells to adopt monocytic features in vitro.

Growth, Proliferation, Survival

The interaction between SCF and its cognate receptor C-KIT plays a key role in regulating mast cell growth and differentiation. Kit is expressed on hematopoietic progenitors and is downregulated upon differentiation into mature cells belonging to all lineages, except mast cells, which retain high levels of C-KIT expression. Insight into the biologic function of Kit and SCF has been derived from observations of mice carrying specific mutations at the dominant white-spotting or steel loci, respectively. A double dose of mutant alleles at either locus produces common pleiotropic effects, including a profound decrease in mast cell number, coat color abnormalities/white-spotting (piebaldism), macrocytic anemia, reduced fertility, and abnormalities in intestinal pacemaker activity. Despite the shared phenotype between W- and Sl-mutant mice, the mechanism underlying the defect in hematopoiesis is quite different. In W/W^v mice, for instance, transplantation of bone marrow cells from congenic +/+ mice corrected both the anemia and mast cell deficiency, which indicated the defect was an intrinsic stem cell disorder. Many independent mutations of the W locus have been described; the alleles are semidominant and vary in their phenotypic effect on hematopoiesis, pigmentation, and fertility in the homozygous and heterozygous state. By contrast, the defect is cell-extrinsic in Sl/Sl^d mice; when skin from either W/W^v or Sl/Sl^d mice was grafted onto the back of congenic +/+ mice, mast cells were found to populate the grafted skin from W/W^v mice but not in skin from Sl/Sl^d mice. Furthermore, the hematologic defects in Sl/Sl^d mice were not corrected by transplantation of bone marrow cells from a congenic +/+ host, indicating that the disorder is microenvironmental in nature.

Activation and Function

Mast cells are ubiquitous and are found in virtually all tissues, but they are most numerous at anatomic sites that are in contact with the environment, such as the mucosa of airways and gut, as well as in the skin. Although mast cells have been long identified as key cellular mediators of the allergic inflammatory response, they have a myriad of other physiologic functions, including a key role in innate immunity. The study of mast cell function in humans has been difficult for several reasons. First, these cells are relatively inaccessible; in general, primary culture of mast cells (including those derived from cord blood or peripheral blood–derived progenitor cells) is cumbersome, the yield of cells is quite limited, and it is presently unclear whether fully mature mast cells can be obtained by this approach. Second, there appears to be significant variation in the functional properties of mast cells depending on the anatomic location from which they are isolated (e.g., skin versus intestinal mucosa). Third, mast cells display considerable phenotypic plasticity, with many autocrine, paracrine, or systemic factors influencing various aspects of cell phenotype. Consequently, investigators have often relied on transformed mast cell leukemia cell lines (e.g., HMC-1, LAD-1, LAD-2) or murine animal models for experimental studies of mast cell function. Mouse strains that exhibit a profound mast cell deficiency include (a) C-KIT/W mutant mice (e.g., W/W^v mice; vide infra) also display non–mast cell phenotypic abnormalities including sterility, which entails complex breeding strategies, and (b) W^{sh}/W^{sh} mice, which carry an inversion mutation upstream of the C-KIT coding region, display abnormal pigmentation and reduced mast cell number but have relatively preserved hematopoiesis and fertility. The aforementioned mice can be selectively reconstituted with mast cells by systemic (intravenous) or local (e.g., intradermal, intraperitoneal) transfer; this adoptive transfer of genetically compatible, in vitro cultured mast cells (e.g., from bone marrow cells) provides a useful model (i.e., "mast cell knock-in mice") for the study of mast cell function in vivo. It remains unclear, however, whether observations generated using cell lines or mouse experiments can be extrapolated to humans, given that neoplastic transformation significantly alters normal cellular function and the marked interspecies differences in mast cell biology. Mast cells undergo activation, classically following cross-linking of FcεRI-bound IgE by multivalent allergens in sensitized individuals. The tissue mast cell burden is dynamic and has been noted to increase in chronic allergic inflammatory states. Non-IgE triggers for mast cell mediator release include anaphylatoxins of the complement system (C3a and C5a), neuropeptides (e.g., vasoactive peptides, somatostatin, substance P), proteoglycans (heparin), prostaglandins, lipopolysaccharides, chemokines (e.g., CCL3, MIP1α), Toll-like receptors, proteases (tryptase, chymase, carboxypeptidase) and cytokines (TNF). Other non-IgE triggers for mast cell activation include specific cytokines, such as SCF, and to some extent IL-4 (in cooperation with SCF) as well as IL-3. Upon activation by either IgE-dependent or IgE-independent mechanisms, these mediators are released. Mast cells are primed for multiple cycles of degranulation-mediator release, and display distinct patterns of mediator release depending upon the strength and type of stimulus that is provided. Mast cells display a wide spectrum of "activation levels" in vivo; however, the mechanisms regulating the secretory phenotype of mast cells in a given individual is not completely understood. The key mast cell mediators include (a) vasoactive amines, particularly histamine; (b) several distinct tryptases (α, β, and γ) that comprise the principal protein component of mast cells; (c) anionic proteoglycans (e.g., heparin, chondroitin sulphate) that confer metachromasia upon staining with toluidine blue; (d) various lipid mediators; these arachidonic acid-derived eicosanoids, which include leukotriene C_4, leukotriene B_4, and prostaglandin D_2, mediate vasodilation, vasopermeability, smooth muscle constriction, mucus secretion, as well as other proinflammatory processes; (e) other proteases (e.g., chymase, carboxypeptidase A); and (f) specific cytokines. The secreted cytokines, which recruit and activate specific cells, include IL-3 (basophils), IL-5 (eosinophils), tumor necrosis factor-α/IL-8 (neutrophils), and IL-4/IL-13 (T and B lymphocytes). Mast cells mediate not only early-phase (e.g., anaphylaxis, acute asthma) but also late-phase allergic responses, as well as non–type I hypersensitivity reactions through the aforementioned mediators. Furthermore, mast cells mediate upregulation of T_H2-responses and allergen-specific IgE biosynthesis, which contribute to host defenses against parasitic infections. Mast cells have also been implicated in other nonallergic diseases, including viral and bacterial infections, autoimmune disorders, as well as in angiogenesis related to cancer, although their role(s) in these conditions has not yet been precisely delineated.

Role of C-KIT and Stem Cell Factor in Mast Cell Biology

C-KIT is the cellular homolog of the V-KIT oncogene of the Hardy-Zuckerman 4 feline sarcoma virus and encodes for Kit, which belongs to the type III subfamily of receptor tyrosine kinases. Members of this receptor tyrosine kinase subfamily share both sequence similarity and a common overall structure, with an extracellular domain containing five immunoglobulin-like motifs that bind SCF, a short transmembrane (TM) domain that anchors Kit to the cell membrane, a cytoplasmic tyrosine kinase (TK) domain that is split by an insert sequence into ATP-binding and phosphotransferase regions, and a juxtamembrane (JM) domain that lies between the TM and TK domains. C-KIT is located on human chromosome 4, in a region (4q11-q12) homologous to a region of mouse chromosome 5, that includes the W gene locus. Additional studies sought to determine whether the W locus was linked to murine C-KIT.[2] Using interspecific backcross analyses, the two were shown to be tightly linked, and C-KIT was subsequently found to be disrupted in two spontaneous mutant W alleles, W^x, and W, confirming that Kit was encoded by the W locus. Specific mutations at the W locus, such as W (78, amino acid TM/JM deletion), W^{37} (JM missense mutation), or W^v, W^{41}, and W^{42} (TK missense mutations), result in a loss-of-function phenotype and point to the critical role of individual domains/regions in Kit function. The common phenotypic denominator of mutations at the W locus is reduced Kit tyrosine kinase activity, whether by expression of decreased numbers of Kit receptors with normal kinase activity (W^{44}, W^{57}, and W^x alleles) or expression of normal numbers of kinase-defective Kit (W^{37}, W^{42}, W^{41}, W^v, W^{55} alleles).

SCF was initially isolated from medium conditioned by Buffalo rat liver cells and exhibited ex vivo growth factor activity toward primitive hematopoietic progenitors, as well as mast cells. The subsequent purification, cloning, and mapping of SCF revealed it to be syntenic with the Sl locus on mouse chromosome 10, and SCF sequences were found to be deleted in a number of mutant Sl alleles such as Sl^d and Sl^{12H}. SCF was shown to be a ligand for Kit by cross-linking of ^{125}I-labeled SCF to Kit-expressing cells, and the administration of recombinant SCF in vivo rescued both the macrocytic anemia and the mast cell deficiency exhibited by Sl/Sl^d mice. The steel-Dickie (Sl^d) mutation is a 4.0-kb deletion within the gene SCF, which renders Sl^d capable only of encoding a soluble truncated growth factor that lacks both transmembrane and cytoplasmic domains. SCF is synthesized by a variety of mesenchymal cells, including fibroblasts, that express the cytokine as a transmembrane protein that may be proteolytically cleaved to generate a soluble form; two distinct isoforms with differential susceptibility to proteolysis are synthesized. Soluble SCF exists as a homodimer in plasma and can crosslink two Kit receptors on the cell surface, thereby leading to activation of Kit, as well as downstream signal transduction. SCF promotes mast cell development, survival of mature mast cells, as well as adhesion of mast cells to extracellular matrix proteins. SCF also regulates mediator release from human mast cells, potentially by both IgE-dependent and IgE-independent mechanisms.

Mast cells and eosinophils frequently are each present in atopic disorders such as allergic disorders, atopic dermatitis, and asthma. Mast cells provide the intermediate stimuli upon activation that leads to eosinophil recruitment. Both mast cells and eosinophils express CCR3 and respond to eotaxins and CCL5 (RANTES), leading to localization of both cell types to inflamed tissues. Eosinophils can produce SCF, which can attract more mast cells and delay their apoptosis. This cross-talk between eosinophils and mast cells plays a key role in the activation and eventual downregulation of inflammation.

SYSTEMIC MASTOCYTOSIS

SM is a clonal hematologic malignancy that has been included as a myeloproliferative neoplasm and is characterized by the excessive growth and accumulation of immunophenotypically abnormal mast cells in one or more tissues. The bone marrow is involved in almost all cases. The clinical features and course of SM vary widely from an indolent form associated with a normal life expectancy to a highly aggressive form associated with organ failure and a short survival. In contrast to normal mast cells, neoplastic mast cells are more variable in appearance, ranging from round to fusiform variants, with long, polar cytoplasmic processes; they additionally display cytoplasmic hypogranularity with uneven distribution of fine granules, as well as atypical nuclei with monocytoid appearance.[3] Immunophenotypic evaluation of mast cells reveals frequent expression of aberrant markers in SM patients.

Epidemiology

Epidemiologic data on SM are scarce. The true incidence of this rare group of heterogeneous disorders is unknown, and SM is considered an orphan disease in the United States that affects all ethnic groups equally. CM is more common in children than in adults, and it is usually transient and self-limited. A slight male predominance has been observed, and the median age at time of SM diagnosis was 55. The median survival of this cohort of SM patients was 63 months, which is inferior to the age- and sex-matched U.S. population with the exception of ISM, which carries a normal life expectancy. The excess of deaths occurs in the first 3 years from time of diagnosis.

Pathobiology

Current evidence points to an important role for gain-of-function mutations in C-KIT, particularly Kit D816V, in the pathogenesis of mastocytosis. It remains to be determined whether additional genetic events are necessary for neoplastic transformation of mast cells and for full expression of the mastocytosis phenotype. Other specific mutations, such as FIP1L1-PDGFRA and Kit F522C, although rare, exhibit specific genotype-phenotype associations in mastocytosis patients and hence deserve specific mention in this section.

Kit D816V

Furitsu and colleagues showed that Kit expressed on HMC-1 cells, an immature mast cell line, was constitutively phosphorylated and activated in the absence of SCF.[4] Sequencing of C-KIT in these cells revealed two point mutations, one in the juxtamembrane region at codon 560 and nucleotides 1699-1701 (V560G; GTT → GGT) and the other in the tyrosine kinase at codon 816 and nycleotides 2467-2469 (D816V; GAC → GTC) domain. Two rodent cell lines, P815 (mouse mastocytoma) and RBL-2H3 (rat mast cell leukemia), were subsequently found to possess mutations corresponding to human D816V (i.e., D814Y and D817Y, respectively). These mutations, in human, mouse, and rat Kit, were shown to be constitutively activating when expressed in the human embryonic kidney cell line 293T. Soon after this came the first report of the detection of the Kit D816V mutation in blood mononuclear cells from patients with SM and associated non–mast cell myeloid neoplasms but not in patients with indolent or aggressive SM, solitary mastocytomas, or chronic myelomonocytic leukemia.[5] Point mutations of the Kit are the most common genetic abnormality in SM and result in a substitution of valine for aspartate at codon 816 of exon 17 termed *Asp816Val* or *D816V*. More than 95% of patients with SM have this mutation. Additional Kit mutations, involving D816 or an adjacent amino acid residue (e.g., D816Y, D816F, D816H, I817V or VI815–816, and D820G) or other domains (extracellular, transmembrane, or juxtamembrane) have also been identified in mastocytosis. The juxtamembrane mutations include V560G, K509I, and V559A; some are rare alleles detected in germline DNA in cohorts with familial forms of mastocytosis. Of interest, several kindreds with combined familial gastrointestinal stromal cell tumors and SM, both of which are associated with gain-of-function Kit mutations, have also now been described.

Kit signaling is believed to regulate multiple transcriptional targets through downstream targets, which include PI3K-Akt, the Src family of kinases, Ras/ERK, phospholipase Cγ, MAPK, and JAK-STAT.[6] Both PI3-kinase and Src-kinase signaling pathways converge to activate JNK and RAC1 and bone marrow–derived mast cell proliferation but not apoptosis and require an intact JNK/RAC1 pathway for Kit ligand–induced proliferation of mast cells. Because of the many complex signaling pathways that are activated downstream from Kit, diverse biologic functions such as chemotaxis, differentiation, proliferation, and survival of clonal mast cells are likely influenced by Kit-activating mutations.

Although activating Kit mutations are clearly associated with human mastocytosis, they do not occur universally, and whether individual mutations are necessary and sufficient to cause mast cell transformation remains currently unresolved. Introduction of human Kit D816V (or its murine homologs) into IL-3-dependent cell lines—Ba/F3 (pro–B-lymphocyte), IC-2 (mast cell), or FDC-P1 (myeloid)—results in their cytokine-independent growth. Furthermore, subcutaneous injection of mutant Kit V559G– or Kit D814V–bearing Ba/F3 cells into nude mice led to the appearance of large mastocytomas, with all the mice subsequently dying of mast cell leukemia. These experiments do not, however, provide direct confirmation of the neoplastic transformation potential of activating Kit mutations since the IL-3–dependent cell lines are immortalized and have acquired a priori the capacity to self-renew. Investigators have introduced activated Kit (V559G or D814V) by using retroviral vectors into murine bone marrow cells and injected these cells into mast cell–deficient irradiated W/W^v mice. In vitro colony assays revealed that Kit D814V, and to some extent Kit V559G, resulted in cytokine-independent growth of both mast cell and non–mast cell myeloid colonies. Furthermore, a proportion of the transplanted mice developed acute leukemia, likely of B-lymphoid origin; in addition, a subset of transgenic mice expressing Kit D814V developed acute leukemia/lymphoma of immature B-cell origin at 10 to 80 weeks of age. In another study, human Kit D816V was introduced into murine fetal liver cells, with induction of megakaryocytic differentiation, in the absence of cytokines. In the presence of SCF, Kit D816V–expressing cells showed increased mast cell differentiation, as did Kit–wild-type (WT)–expressing cells. The Kit D816V–expressing cells, however, were not transformed, as assessed by colony assays, regardless of the absence or presence of SCF. Furthermore, introduction of Kit D816V induced both myeloid and mastocytic differentiation patterns of Ba/F3 cells but did not enhance their growth. Thus experimental data from mouse studies conflict as to whether activating Kit mutations are sufficient to cause oncogenic transformation. Similarly, Kit D816V mutation alone may not be sufficient to cause oncogenic transformation in humans. This is consistent with the observation that most mastocytosis patients with this mutation alone have indolent disease. In addition, B cells and monocytes carrying mutated C-KIT display a nonmalignant behavior pattern, despite being derived from the same precursor that gives rise to mast cells within the lesions present in mastocytosis patients. Thus it is possible that Kit D816V may affect the differentiation and apoptosis potential of human mast cells rather than providing a potent proliferative signal. In support of this theory, Kit D816V positive human bone marrow mast cells, but not normal mast cells, survive in vitro in the absence of SCF. Moreover, enhanced expression of the antiapoptotic protein BCL-XL was found in lesional mast cells in patient bone marrow biopsies. D816V KIT suppression of the pro-apoptotic BH3-only death regulator BIM was observed in neoplastic mast cells. Bim has been shown to act as a tumor suppressor in a variety of myeloid neoplasms. Evidence to support mutant Kit signaling as a mechanism driving malignant mast cell proliferation is supported by the finding of high expression levels of microphthalmia-associated transcription factor (MITF).[7] Investigators have shown that MITF expression is upregulated by Kit signaling in primary SM cells and cell lines through downregulation of repressive miRNAs (miR-539 and miR-381). The critical gene targets of MITF responsible for mast cell proliferation remain unclear. Of interest, high MITF levels are not found in all cases of mastocytosis, suggesting that there are likely other cooperative factors inducing abnormal mast cell proliferation. It is also possible that Kit D816V affects mast cell function; for instance, it has been shown that hematopoietic progenitors and mast cells carrying Kit D816V migrate to SCF to a greater extent.

In a large prospective cohort study of adult patients with SM, disease phenotype and Kit genotype were correlated with age of disease onset. This study of 142 patients with histologically confirmed mastocytosis showed that although genotypic differences were observed, clinical features of adult patients with mastocytosis were the same regardless of whether their disease began in childhood or adulthood. The demonstration of KitD816V in 40% of adult patients with childhood-onset SM would suggest that pediatric patients with Kit mutations have a higher probability of the disease persisting into adulthood.

The bone marrow microenvironment in SM is often altered with increased angiogenesis, osteosclerosis, and variable amounts of fibrosis being observed. Neoplastic mast cells express oncostatin M (OSM), a fibrogenic and angiogenic modulator that appears to be mediated by Kit D816.[8] Ba/F3 cells induced to express Kit D816V produce enhanced levels of OSM mRNA as well as protein product, and HMC-1.2 cells with mutated Kit expressed significantly greater amounts of OSM than did wild-type Kit HMC-1.2 cells. Furthermore, STAT5 knockdown results in inhibition of OSM production in this cell line. Neoplastic mast cells have been shown to express elevated levels of cytoplasmic and nuclear p-STAT5, which has been attributed to Kit D816V.

FIP1L1-PDGFRA

SM patients frequently exhibit eosinophilia (SM-eo), and in at least some cases the eosinophils appear to be derived from the neoplastic clone. A subset of cases with eosinophilia harbor the FIP1L1-PDGFRA oncogene, which results from an interstitial deletion in chromosome 4q12 that removes a segment of DNA involving CHIC2 gene, leading to constitutive activation of the platelet-derived growth factor receptor A. PDGFRA tyrosine kinase activity is uniquely sensitive to inhibition by imatinib mesylate. FIP1L1-PDGFRA cannot be detected with classic cytogenetic methods and its detection requires either the use of fluorescence in situ hybridization or reverse transcriptase polymerase chain reaction. In these patients, FIP1L1-PDGFRA involves mast cells and eosinophils in addition to lymphocytes, suggesting that this disorder originates in a multipotent hematopoietic progenitor cell. The bone marrow mast cell infiltration pattern in these patients is similar to that in the typical SM patients with Kit D816V, in that the mast cells are diffusely distributed, with fewer pathonomonic mast cell clusters. The patients harboring FIP1L1-PDGFRA can be classified as having chronic eosinophilic leukemia (CEL), although at least some cases fulfill the criteria for both systemic mastocytosis and CEL, leading in the past to their classification as systemic mastocytosis, subtype SM-CEL. In the 2008 World Health Organization (WHO) classification of myeloid neoplasms, however, FIP1L1-PDGFRA disease was not considered a type of SM but rather was included in a major new category designated as myeloid and lymphoid neoplasms with eosinophilia and abnormalities of PDGFRA, PDGFRB, and FGFR1. The FIP1L1-PDGFRA fusion and the D816V Kit mutation appear to be mutually exclusive oncogenic events. Gain-of-function Kit and PDGFRA mutations have also been identified in gastrointestinal stromal cell tumors. Intriguingly, in both gastrointestinal stromal cell tumors and mastocytosis patients, Kit and PDGFRA mutations appear to be alternative and mutually exclusive genetic events.

In a murine model of chronic eosinophilic leukemia in which FIP1L1/PDGFRA is expressed in hematopoietic stem cells and IL-5 is over-expressed by T cells, mast cell infiltration of the bone marrow and other organs was increased when compared with control mice transplanted with cells overexpressing IL-5. Intestinal mast cell infiltration in the mouse was diminished by administration of neutralizing C-KIT antibody, suggesting synergy between SCF-activated Kit signaling with FIP1LI/PDGFRA–induced mastocytosis. Additionally, in vitro studies show that bone marrow–derived mast cells that are forced to express FIP1L1/PDGFRA proliferate and differentiate in the absence of cytokines and that SCF can induce greater migration than control bone marrow mast cells lacking this gene fusion product.

Other Mutations/Polymorphisms

The presence of Kit D816V alone does not explain the remarkable clinical heterogeneity of human mastocytosis. Kit mutations are not consistently detected in some patients, such as those with children who have cutaneous mastocytosis. Also, other mutations, polymorphisms, and/or karyotypic abnormalities have been detected in mastocytosis, which likely influence the disease phenotype regardless of whether these lesions coexist with Kit D816V. Of note, loss-of-function mutations have also been detected in mastocytosis; the dominant-negative Kit E839K mutation and the IL-4 receptor alpha chain polymorphism Q576R, which are thought to limit mast cell growth and differentiation, are both associated with relatively limited forms of mastocytosis.

Recently, a growing number of overlapping novel mutations have been identified in MPNs. Although the clinical significance of these individual mutations remains unclear, they reveal a complex molecular pathogenesis underlying MPN disorders. Fourteen different mutations involving the TET2 (TET oncogene family member 2) gene located on chromosome 4q24 have been documented in 29% of bone marrow samples from SM patients. Of interest, none of the FIP1L1-PDGFRA–associated SM cases were found to have TET2 mutations. A statistically significant association between the presence of TET2 mutations and monocytosis and female sex was seen. The presence of TET2 mutations did segregate with Kit-D816V, was found in all SM subgroups, and did not influence survival in nonindolent SM.

RAS proteins are membrane-associated GTPases integral for intracellular signaling mediating cell proliferation, differentiation, and survival. Recently, activating NRAS mutations have been identified in 2 of 8 patients tested with advanced mastocytosis but not found in patients with indolent disease.[9] Some data suggest that the acquisition of NRAS mutations preceded Kit mutations.

The interleukin-13 (IL-13) promoter gene polymorphism 1112c/T has also been associated with SM and not cutaneous mastocytosis (CM) and is correlated with elevated serum levels of tryptase and adult onset of SM. Higher levels of IL-13 have been documented in SM patients, and neoplastic MC cells have been shown to express the IL-13 receptor and to proliferate to a greater degree in the presence of IL-13.

Fusion of the lymphoma-related oncoprotein nucleophosmin (NPM) with anaplastic lymphoma kinase (ALK) results in the NPM-ALK fusion gene. This gene, when expressed in a murine transplant model in lethally irradiated IL-9 transgenic mice, results not only in the formation of lymphoma, but in an SM-like disease with atypical multifocal dense MC-infiltrates in visceral organs. Neither IL-9 expression nor NPM-ALK alone was sufficient to produce the histopathologic findings of SM in these mice; both were required to act in concert to cause a mastocytosis-like disease. It is possible that the downstream signaling pathways that are activated by NPM-ALK tyrosine kinase are shared with Kit, serving to regulate growth and survival of neoplastic MCs.

Classification

The classification of disorders characterized by SM has evolved over the years; the first recognition of cutaneous mast cell disease came from Unna's observation in 1887 that the lesions characteristic of urticaria pigmentosa (UP) lesions were histologically composed of mast cell infiltrates. Although the systemic nature of mastocytosis had been alluded to by Sézary and others in the early 1900s, systemic mast cell infiltrates were first histologically demonstrated by Ellis in

1949. Subsequently, a dichotomous view prevailed, wherein benign mastocytosis was separated from malignant mastocytosis, based on the presence or absence of several clinical features, including UP and organomegaly, particular cytologic and cytochemical features of bone marrow mast cells, as well as the clinical course. Based on the recognition that not all patients classified as having benign mastocytosis have a favorable outcome, and that malignant mastocytosis was composed of relatively distinct clinicopathologic entities, updated classifications have been proposed, generally with four or five subgroups. Updated diagnostic criteria and consensus classification for mastocytosis were proposed and adopted by WHO in 2008.[10] This classification system incorporates advances in our understanding of mastocytosis, including the role of C-KIT mutations, aberrant expression of cell surface immunophenotypic markers on neoplastic mast cells, and mast cell mediators as surrogate measures of mast cell number and/or function.

The current WHO classification identifies seven mastocytosis variants (Table 71-1): cutaneous mastocytosis (CM), indolent systemic mastocytosis (ISM), systemic mastocytosis with an associated clonal hematologic non–mast cell lineage disease (SM-AHNMD), aggressive systemic mastocytosis (ASM), mast cell leukemia (MCL), mast cell sarcoma (MCS), and extracutaneous mastocytoma (EM). ISM can also be further subdivided into two subvariants, isolated bone marrow mastocytosis (BMM) and smoldering systemic mastocytosis (SSM). In addition, two relatively rare variants of mastocytosis with characteristic clinicopathologic features have also been described: well-differentiated systemic mastocytosis (WDSM) and systemic mastocytosis without skin involvement associated with recurrent anaphylaxis (SM-ana). The WHO classification of mastocytosis mandates a number of investigations to define the exact subtype of disease. Identification of B findings (Table 71-2) alone, such as more than 30% mast cells in the bone marrow or serum tryptase greater than 200 ng/mL, is indicative of a high systemic mast cell burden (e.g., smoldering SM), whereas the additional presence of C findings (Table 71-3), such as cytopenias, pathologic fractures, hypersplenism, and so on, indicates impaired organ function directly attributable to mast cell infiltration and the presence of aggressive disease (e.g., ASM). A large retrospective study of 342 individuals with SM seen at the Mayo Clinic observed over approximately 30 years determined the distribution of the incidence of ISM, SM-AHNMD, ASM, and MCL as 46%, 40%, 12%, and 1%, respectively.

Table 71-1 World Health Organization Variants of Mastocytosis

1. Cutaneous mastocytosis (CM)
   a. Maculopapular CM
   b. Diffuse CM
   c. Mastocytoma of skin
2. Indolent systemic mastocytosis (ISM)
   a. Smoldering systemic mastocytosis (SSM)
   b. Isolated bone marrow mastocytosis
3. Systemic mastocytosis with an associated clonal hematologic non–mast cell lineage disease (SM-AHNMD)
   a. SM-MDS
   b. SM-MPD
   c. SM-CEL
   d. SM-CMML
   e. SM-NHL
4. Aggressive systemic mastocytosis (ASM)
   With eosinophilia (SM-eo)
5. Mast cell leukemia (MCL)
   Aleukemic MCL
6. Mast cell sarcoma (MCS)
7. Extracutaneous mastocytoma (EM)

CEL, Chronic eosinophilic leukemia; *CMML*, chronic myelomonocytic leukemia; *MDS*, myelodysplastic syndrome; *MPD*, myeloproliferative disorder; *NHL*, non–Hodgkin lymphoma.

Clinical Manifestations

The clinical manifestations of SM reflect the consequences of either mediator release from mast cells or infiltration of mast cells into virtually any tissue. Mast cell disease has a varied clinical presentation with symptoms that may be broadly grouped as follows:

Skin Rash

Three major forms of cutaneous mastocytosis are recognized by the WHO. The most common is urticaria pigmentosa (also referred to as *maculopapular cutaneous mastocytosis [MPCM]*); the others are diffuse cutaneous mastocytosis and solitary mastocytoma of the skin. The skin lesions are typically yellowish tan to reddish brown macules and may less frequently present as nodules or plaques (Fig. 71-1). The lesions generally involve the extremities, trunk, and abdomen, but spare sun-exposed areas, including the palms, soles, and scalp. The lesions commonly exhibit an urticarial response to mechanical stimulation such as stroking or scratching (Darier sign or dermographic urticaria). Darier sign has been reported rarely in leukemia cutis and cutaneous T-cell lymphomas but is considered pathognomonic for CM. Biopsies of UP/MPCM lesions demonstrate multifocal MC aggregates mainly around blood vessels and around skin appendages in the papillary dermis (Fig. 71-2). An increase in dermal MC, in the absence of typical UP lesions, is not considered diagnostic of CM, given the relatively nonspecific nature of such a finding. Children account for nearly two-thirds of all reported cases of cutaneous mastocytosis, with a majority of cases arising before the age of 2 years. In contrast, most adult MCD patients with UP/MPCM present with systemic disease (often indolent) that is most commonly revealed by a bone marrow biopsy done as part of the diagnostic workup. CM is often associated with systemic symptoms related to the release of mast cell mediators. Flushing, itching, blistering, diarrhea, abdominal pain, vomiting, hypotension, headache, and bone pain are frequent accompanying symptoms. The course of pediatric mast cell disease is usually benign and transient. Skin lesions have a tendency to undergo partial or complete remission during puberty in the majority of children.

Table 71-2 "B" Findings: Indication of High Mast Cell Burden

1. Infiltration grade (mast cells) greater than 30% in bone marrow in histology and serum total tryptase levels greater than 200 ng/mL
2. Hypercellular marrow with loss of fat cells, discrete signs of dysmyelopoiesis without substantial cytopenias, or WHO criteria for an MDS or MPD
3. Organomegaly: palpable hepatomegaly, splenomegaly, or lymphadenopathy (on CT or ultrasound) greater than 2 cm without impaired organ function

MDS, myelodysplastic syndrome; *MPD*, myeloproliferative disorder; *WHO*, World Health Organization.

Table 71-3 "C" Findings: Indication of Impaired Organ Function Attributable to Mast Cell Infiltration

1. Cytopenia(s): Absolute neutrophil count <1000/μL or hemoglobin <10 g/dL or platelets <100,000/μL
2. Hepatomegaly with ascites and impaired liver function
3. Palpable splenomegaly with hypersplenism
4. Malabsorption with hypoalbuminemia and weight loss
5. Skeletal lesions: large-sized osteolysis or severe osteoporosis causing pathologic fractures
6. Life-threatening organopathy in other organ systems that is definitively caused by an infiltration of the tissue by neoplastic mast cells

Symptoms Related to Mast Cell Degranulation

Most adult patients in this category have a low systemic mast cell burden, commonly exhibit CM lesions, and generally have indolent disease. Presenting symptoms include pruritus, urticaria, angioedema, flushing, bronchoconstriction, neuropsychiatric manifestations, and hypotension.[11] Aggregation of high affinity receptors for IgE on mast cell surfaces elicits the release of preformed granule-associated inflammatory mediators that lead to mediator-related symptoms. Gastrointestinal features such as nausea, vomiting, abdominal pain, diarrhea, and malabsorption may be prominent in some patients. GI symptoms occur in 60% to 80% of patients. Histamine receptor stimulation increases gastric acid production, which may cause peptic ulcer disease with potential morbidity from a bleeding peptic ulcer and/or perforation. Peptic ulcer disease has been reported in about 25% of cases. Presyncope, episodic vascular collapse, and sudden death represent the more dramatic clinical presentations of mast cell mediator release.

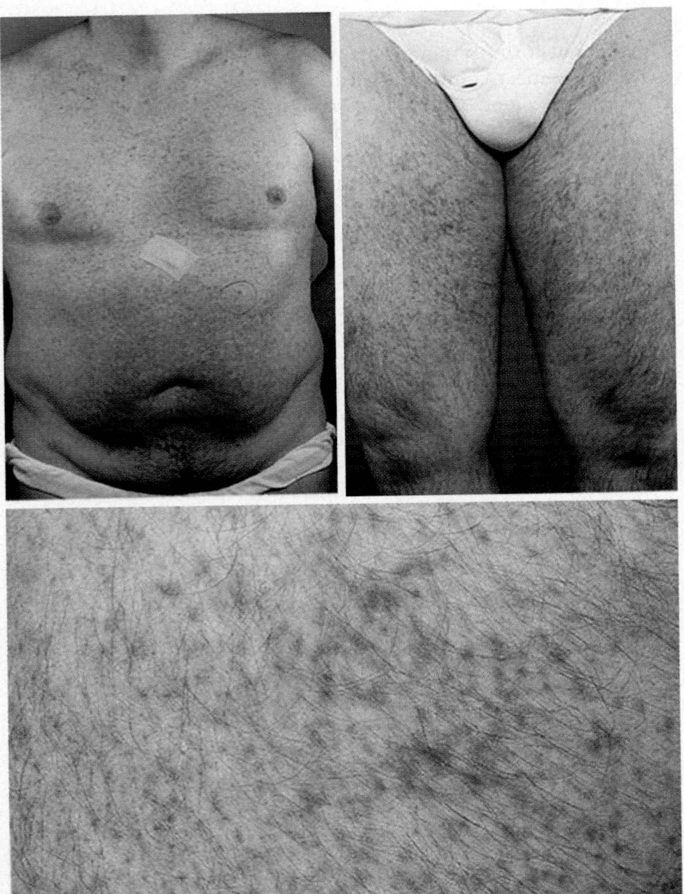

Figure 71-1 URTICARIA PIGMENTOSA LESIONS IN A PATIENT WITH CUTANEOUS MASTOCYTOSIS.

Headaches are known to be a significant contributor to SM-related disability and include migraine and tension-type headaches. Primary headache syndromes usually parallel mast cell activation and concurrent mast cell degranulation symptoms (i.e., pruritus and rhinorrhea).[12] Mast cells have been identified in the dura mater, in association with connective tissue, neural, and vascular components in patients with SM. Primary cough headaches and migraines with a high incidence of auras appear to be particularly common associated neurologic manifestations of SM.

Severe life-threatening anaphylaxis can be triggered by the release of MC-derived vasoactive mediators. The actual trigger or provoker of MC degranulation is not always readily identifiable. In approximately 3% of cases of mastocytosis, severe life-threatening anaphylaxis can occur.[13] Prolonged hypotension following anaphylaxis and cerebral hypoxia have been identified as the major causes for disability and death in these cases. Neither the subtype of mast cell disease nor the degree of mast cell burden appears to correlate with the severity or frequency of severe anaphylaxis. Severe life-threatening or disabling anaphylaxis to Hymenoptera venom is associated with SM. A primary cause of disability is cerebral hypoxia following anaphylactic shock, which is frequently seen after bee or wasp stings in patients with a high burden of mast cells. Anaphylactic symptoms are more common in males who have mastocytosis with elevated IgE levels.

Musculoskeletal Symptoms

Patients may have indolent or aggressive disease and present with poorly localized bone pain, diffuse osteoporosis or osteopenia, myalgias, arthralgias, pathologic fractures, skeletal deformities, and/or compression radiculopathies. In the absence of typical cutaneous lesions (i.e., UP/MPCM) or mast cell–mediator–release symptoms, the diagnosis of SM may prove challenging, and diagnosis is frequently delayed in this setting. In such cases, SM must be distinguished from other disorders, including osteoporosis, metastatic cancer, Paget disease, and multiple myeloma. Vertebral osteoporosis

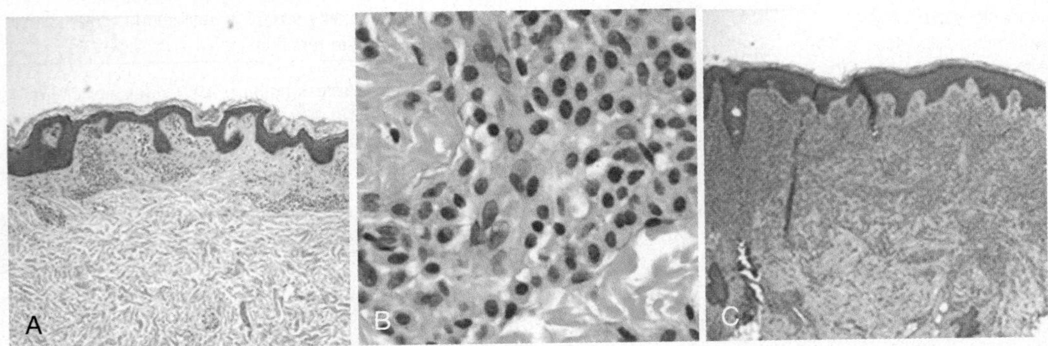

Figure 71-2 CUTANEOUS MASTOCYTOSIS. A skin biopsy of urticaria pigmentosa or maculopapular mastocytosis shows multiple focal aggregates of mast cells around blood vessels or skin appendages in the papillary dermis (**A**). The mast cells are plump with abundant cytoplasm and typically accumulate around vessels (**B,** *center*). In solitary mastocytoma of the skin or in diffuse cutaneous mastocytosis, the mast cell infiltrate is more extensive as it infiltrates the papillary and reticular dermis and may even extend into the subcutaneous tissues. The mast cells are bland and without cytologic atypia. In these disorders, there should be no evidence of systemic involvement. Evidence of systemic disease would indicate systemic mastocytosis.

and fractures are frequently seen in ISM; thus spine radiographs and bone densitometric assays should routinely be performed in this patient population.

Symptoms Related to Organomegaly/Organopathy

SM patients in this category are generally older, do not have CM lesions, frequently exhibit organomegaly and mast cell atypia (i.e., high-grade morphology), and commonly experience an aggressive disease course. Organ infiltration by neoplastic mast cells may lead to hepatomegaly (with or without liver dysfunction and ascites), splenomegaly (with or without hypersplenism), lymphadenopathy, large osteolytic lesions (with or without pathologic fractures), and infiltration of the small intestine with malabsorption, hypoalbuminemia, and weight loss. Extensive marrow involvement may result in anemia and eventually leads to pancytopenia.

Laboratory Manifestations

The diagnosis of SM is based on the identification of abnormal mast cells by morphologic, immunophenotypic, and/or genetic (molecular) criteria in various organs.

Bone Marrow Histology

The mast cell burden in normal bone marrow is very low (<0.1%) and increases significantly in SM patients. Increased numbers of tissue mast cells can appear in the marrow or in a variety of other organs in response to a variety of allergic reactions, autoimmune disorders, or non–mast cell cancers. Mast cells can be increased in such diverse disorders as eosinophilic gastritis, chronic gastrointestinal neoplasms, parasitic infections, inflammatory bowel disease, atopic dermatitis, asthma, and allergic rhinitis. Hodgkin disease, for instance, is frequently associated with mast cell infiltration that correlates directly with disease severity; yet the mechanisms underlying this relationship remain unclear. In Hodgkin disease, mast cells promote the growth of tumors by modifying the tumor microenvironment. The microenvironments of many other tumors, which are composed of stromal cells such as endothelial cells, fibroblasts, and immune cells, provide a supportive niche that promotes the growth and invasion of tumors. Mast cells accumulate in the microenvironment of these tumors, leading to significant organ involvement, and their presence is associated with poor prognosis. These reactive forms of mastocytosis must be distinguished from the various forms of SM. Reactive mast cells are small with round, centrally located nuclei. The diagnosis of SM is most frequently established by histologic and immunohistochemical examination of bone marrow aspirate and biopsy specimens. The bone marrow is virtually always involved in adults and shows characteristic histologic features; in contrast, histologic criteria for organ involvement beyond the marrow have not been clearly defined or widely accepted to date. Furthermore, a bone marrow examination allows determination of whether an associated clonal non–mast cell lineage hematologic disorder is present. The pathognomonic lesion is characterized by the presence of multifocal, dense mast cell aggregates, frequently in perivascular and/or paratrabecular locations (Fig. 71-3). These aggregates may be relatively monomorphic (composed mainly of fusiform mast cells) or polymorphic, with mast cells admixed with lymphocytes, eosinophils, neutrophils, histiocytes, endothelial cells, and fibroblasts. Eosinophils are commonly observed at the periphery of mast cell aggregates (often focally), but increased numbers of eosinophils may also be seen in areas not involved by mast cells. Although irregular trabecular thickening is commonly noted, particularly when mast cell aggregates abut

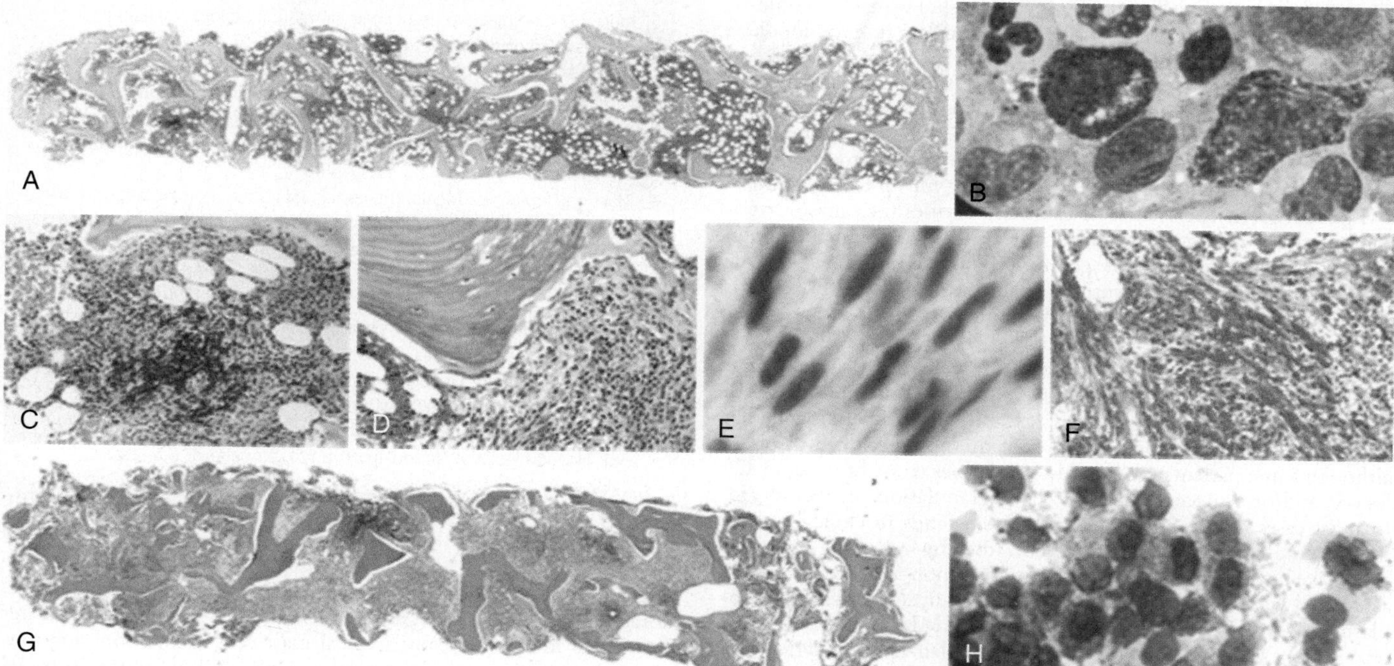

Figure 71-3 SYSTEMIC MASTOCYTOSIS. Bone marrow biopsy (**A**) shows multiple small foci of involvement by systemic mast cell disease. The aspirate (**B**) contained only scattered mast cells (mast cells do not aspirate well). The involved areas on the biopsy include nodules of mast cells (**C**, and *far left bottom* in **A**) with central accumulations of lymphocytes resulting in the so-called bull's eye pattern, and paratrabecular foci (**D**, and *far right bottom* in **A**) along thickened bone. The latter can easily mimic lymphoma in the bone marrow, which can also exhibit a paratrabecular pattern of infiltration. High power of the mast cell involvement (**E**) illustrates the typical fusiform or spindled appearance of the mast cells. A mast cell tryptase immunohistochemical stain (**F**) is quite useful diagnostically. CD117 and CD25 were also positive. A second case (**G**) illustrates extensive involvement by an aggressive systemic mastocytosis. Note the extensive replacement of the marrow space and the marked osteosclerosis. Numerous mast cells are seen on the aspirate (**H**).

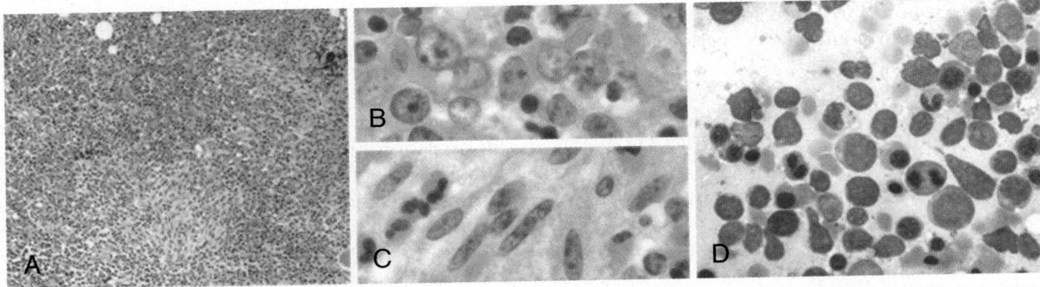

Figure 71-4 SYSTEMIC MASTOCYTOSIS WITH AN ASSOCIATED CLONAL HEMATOLOGIC NON–MAST CELL DISORDER. Low-power depiction of bone marrow (**A**) from a 57-year-old female with systemic mastocytosis associated with acute myeloid leukemia. A focus of mast cells is present (**A**, *bottom center*) in the hypercellular marrow. High-power depictions of the same area (**B**) demonstrate increased immature cells, including blasts, and the mast cell focus (**C**) composed of fusiform mast cells associated with eosinophils. The mast cells were shown to be mast cell tryptase–positive, $CD25^+$ and $CD117^+$. The marrow aspirate (**D**) illustrates increased myeloblasts associated with multilineage dysplasia.

the trabeculae, other cases may be characterized by a marked thinning of bone marrow trabeculae and osteopenia. Mast cell infiltrates are commonly associated with a dense network of reticulin fibers; in cases with diffuse marrow infiltration by monomorphous, spindled mast cells that resemble fibroblasts, a diagnosis of primary myelofibrosis may be erroneously made, especially when accompanied with a decrease in normal hematopoietic elements.

Three distinct patterns of bone marrow mast cell infiltration have been described in SM.[14] The most common, type I pattern, is frequently associated with UP and indolent disease; the mast cells are focally increased (generally 10% to 30% of marrow cellularity), with normal distribution of fat and other hematopoietic elements in the uninvolved marrow space. A spectrum of atypical morphologic features, including cell spindling, cytoplasmic hypogranulation or uneven granule distribution, cytoplasmic processes, and nuclear abnormalities, is seen in mast cells from these patients. Much less commonly, the mast cells may appear relatively normal. In contrast, the type II pattern consists of a significant increase in granulopoiesis in areas not involved by mast cells, as may be seen in ASM patients; some of these cases meet WHO criteria for diagnosis of a clonal non–mast cell lineage hematologic disorder associated with mastocytosis (SM-AHNMD) (Fig. 71-4). The latter (i.e., SM-AHNMD) is the second most common mastocytosis category (more common than ASM) and may account for up to one-third of SM patients. The coexistence of these two entities (i.e., mastocytosis and non–mast cell neoplasm) likely reflects their origin in a common multipotent hematopoietic progenitor cell, although in rare cases the two may develop independently. The diagnosis of SM-AHNMD is established by WHO criteria, for both the mastocytosis and non–mast cell neoplasm components (Table 71-4). In most SM-AHNMD cases, a diagnosis of mastocytosis is made incidentally, usually after an examination of bone marrow for evaluation of the non–mast cell hematologic disorder. In such cases, it is difficult to ascertain whether mastocytosis existed before the onset of the non–mast cell disorder, although some patients provide historical clues (time of onset of UP lesions and/or symptoms of mast cell degranulation) in this regard. In most cases, the non–mast cell neoplasm tends to clinically overshadow the mastocytosis component, thereby reflecting its more aggressive biologic nature. The most frequent non–mast cell disorders associated with mastocytosis are the chronic myeloproliferative neoplasms (except BCR-ABL–positive CML), AML, and MDS.[15] The recognition that chronic myelomonocytic leukemia (CMML), a hybrid myeloproliferative–myelodysplastic disorder, is commonly associated with mastocytosis supports the contention that dysmyelopoiesis is a prominent feature of SM. In some cases, the bone marrow mast cell involvement may be obscured by the non–mast cell neoplasm if only conventional stains are employed (vide infra). In this regard, mast cell infiltrates are more easily identified within sheets of monotonous blasts in AML than within the polymorphic infiltrates seen in myeloproliferative or myelodysplastic disorders. Patient characteristics associated with type II pattern include older age, absence of UP lesions, organomegaly, anemia, eosinophilia, greater than 10% morphologically atypical mast cells in the bone marrow, elevated serum tryptase level, and a rapid clinical course. Type III pattern is characterized by diffuse marrow infiltration with atypical mast cells of high-grade morphology, frequently with circulating mast cells. MCL (Fig. 71-5) is characterized by increased numbers of mast cells in bone marrow (>20% in aspirate smear) and peripheral blood (>10%), with associated bone marrow failure manifested as peripheral cytopenias. The mast cells are immature, sometimes blastic, and often have sparse metachromatic granules, and hence may be missed

Table 71-4 World Health Organization Diagnostic Criteria for Variants for Systemic Mastocytosis

1. Indolent systemic mastocytosis (ISM): Meets criteria for SM. No "B" or "C" findings. No evidence of associated clonal hematologic malignancy/disorder. In this variant, the mast cell burden is low; skin lesions are almost invariably present.
    - *Bone marrow mastocytosis:* As above, with bone marrow involvement, but no skin lesions.
    - *Smoldering systemic mastocytosis:* As above, but with two or more "B" findings and no "C" findings.
2. Systemic mastocytosis with associated clonal hematologic non–mast cell lineage disease (SM-AHNMD): Meets criteria for SM and criteria for an associated, clonal hematologic non–mast cell lineage disease (MDS, CMPD, AML, lymphoma, or other hematologic neoplasm that meets the criteria for a distinct entity in the WHO classification).
3. Aggressive systemic mastocytosis (ASM): Meets criteria for SM. One or more "C" findings. No associated clonal hematologic malignancy/disorder. No evidence of mast cell leukemia.
    - *Lymphadenopathic mastocytosis with eosinophilia:* Progressive lymphadenopathy with peripheral blood eosinophilia, often with extensive bony involvement, and hepatosplenomegaly, but usually without skin lesions. Cases with rearrangement of PDGFRA are excluded.
4. Mast cell leukemia: Meets criteria for SM. Bone marrow biopsy shows diffuse infiltration, usually interstitial pattern, by atypical, immature mast cells. Bone marrow aspirate smears show 20% or more mast cells. Mast cells account for 10% or more of peripheral blood white cells.
    - *Aleukaemic mast cell leukemia: A rare variant.* As above, but <10% of WBCs are mast cells. Usually without skin lesions.
5. Mast cell sarcoma: Unifocal mast cell tumor. No evidence of SM. No skin lesions. Destructive growth pattern. High-grade cytology.
6. Extracutaneous mastocytoma: Unifocal mast cell tumor. No evidence of SM. No skin lesions. Nondestructive growth pattern. Low-grade cytology.

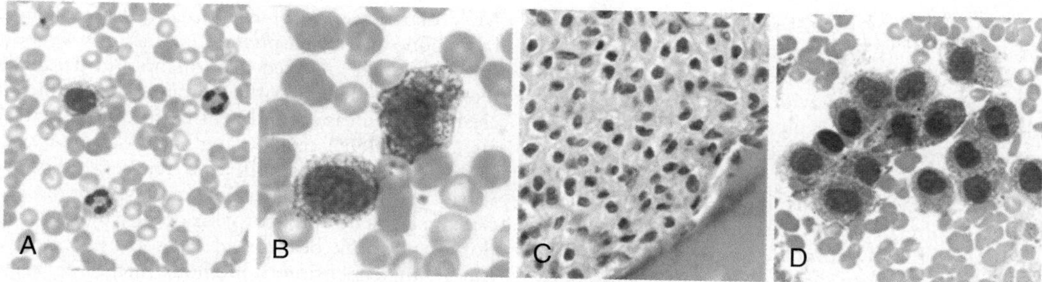

Figure 71-5 MAST CELL LEUKEMIA. Low-power depiction of peripheral blood (**A**), showing two granulocytes and a single immature mast cell with sparse metachromatic granules. Two additional circulating mast cells are also illustrated (**B**). The marrow biopsy was packed with mast cells (**C**). Note the cells are held apart from one another because of their abundant cytoplasm. A similar pattern of infiltration is seen in hairy cell leukemia and in acute promyelocytic leukemia. The aspirate (**D**) shows sheets of immature and hypogranular mast cells.

on routine staining unless tryptase and/or immunophenotyping studies are performed. Rare aleukemic variants of MCL have also been described. Rarely, patients may present with increased numbers of metachromatically granulated, primitive, blast-like cells. In such cases, differentiating MCL from tryptase-positive and/or Kit D816V–positive AML or acute basophilic leukemia is a diagnostic challenge in the absence of well-defined criteria. The aforementioned histologic patterns appear to be relevant for assessing patient prognosis. In one study, mastocytosis patients with a type I pattern (ISM) had an actuarial 5-year survival rate of 75%, compared with 17% and 0% for patients with type II (ASM or SM-AHNMD) and type III (MCL) patterns, respectively. Although mast cell cytologic atypia (large, irregularly shaped nuclei, increased mitotic activity, decreased numbers of metachromatic granules, etc.) has been historically proposed by some authors as criteria for aggressive mastocytosis, such proposals have not been broadly accepted or implemented in routine practice.

In general, mast cells may not be readily recognized by standard staining procedures such as Giemsa, toluidine blue, or naphthol AS-D chloroacetate esterase (Leder stain), particularly when associated with significant hypogranulation or with abnormal nuclear morphology, and may be confused with a variety of other cells that include fibroblasts, histiocytes, hairy cells, and monocytes, particularly in polymorphic bone marrow mast cell aggregates. Furthermore, the metachromatic staining properties of mast cells may be significantly diminished or lost with conventional tissue processing, particularly decalcification with acidic solutions that is necessary for sectioning of paraffin-embedded bone marrow tissue. Among the immunohistochemical markers, staining for tryptase is considered the most sensitive, being able to detect even small-sized mast cell infiltrates (i.e., composed of 10 to 15 cells) (see Fig. 71-3).[16] Given that virtually all mast cells (regardless of their stage of maturation, activation status, or tissue site) express tryptase, staining for this marker detects even those infiltrates that are primarily composed of immature, poorly granulated mast cells. Tryptase immunostaining is particularly useful for assessing the diffuse pattern of mast cell infiltration, particularly when the cells are loosely distributed, in contrast to discrete mast cell aggregates. It must be emphasized that neither tryptase nor other immunohistochemical markers such as chymase, Kit/CD117, or CD68 can distinguish between normal and neoplastic mast cells. Also, abnormal basophils seen in some cases of acute and chronic basophilic leukemia, as well as in chronic myeloid leukemia, and blasts in some AML cases may be tryptase positive and may prove difficult to distinguish from mast cells. In contrast, immunohistochemical detection of aberrant CD25 expression by bone marrow mast cells appears to also be a reliable diagnostic tool in SM, given its ability to detect abnormal mast cells in all subtypes of mastocytosis, including the rare cases with loosely scattered, interstitial mast cells.[17] A unilateral bone marrow biopsy may not be sufficient to exclude low levels (early stages) of mast cell involvement. In a retrospective analysis of 23 mastocytosis patients who underwent bilateral bone marrow biopsies, 4 cases (17%) had unilateral involvement only. Three of the four patients had low serum tryptase levels (<25 ng/mL); hence the diagnosis of SM may not have been established without bilateral biopsies.

Mast Cell Immunophenotyping

As mentioned previously, the qualitative and semiquantitative profiling of cell surface antigens by multiparametric flow cytometry can be extremely useful in distinguishing normal bone marrow mast cells from their pathologic counterparts in SM.[18] Normal mast cells typically express Kit/CD117 and FcεRI, and their typical profile is $CD117^{++}/Fc\varepsilon RI^{+}/CD34^{-}/CD38^{-}/CD33^{+}/CD45^{+}/CD11c^{+}/CD71^{+}$. These cells do not express certain myeloid markers (CD14 and CD15) or lymphoid lineage markers, except CD22. Neoplastic mast cells typically express CD25 and/or CD2, and the abnormal expression of at least one of these two antigens is considered a minor criterion toward the diagnosis of SM, according to the WHO. Overexpression of CD63, CD69, CD58, CD33, and CD11c by neoplastic mast cell is also observed. In general, the detection of CD25 on mast cells, by either flow cytometry or immunohistochemistry, appears to be the more reliable marker (relative to CD2), although some authors have noted significant variation in the percentage of CD2-positive cases by flow cytometry depending on the specific antibody-fluorochrome conjugate used. Consistent with flow cytometry data, it has been reported that screening for CD2 expression by immunohistochemistry may have relatively low diagnostic value because a significant proportion of cases stain negative, and CD2 expression on bone marrow mast cells is generally weak in the cases that are positive. In a large study conducted by REMA (Spanish network on mastocytosis), the sensitivity and specificity of CD2 versus CD25 expression in the diagnosis of SM was evaluated in 886 bone marrow and 153 non–bone marrow extracutaneous tissue samples.[19] The inclusion of CD2 did not improve the sensitivity and decreased the specificity of this test when compared with evaluating CD25 expression alone (sensitivity 100%, specificity 99.2%). This group proposes future modification of the WHO diagnostic criteria to replace the minor criterion of CD2 and/or CD25 by bone marrow, peripheral blood, or other extracutaneous tissue mast cells to a major criterion of exclusive CD25 expression.

Interval monitoring of CD25 expression on bone marrow mast cells may represent one approach for assessing presence of residual disease in patients undergoing mast cell–cytoreductive therapy, generally for the aggressive forms of mastocytosis. Other aberrant immunophenotypic features of neoplastic mast cells include abnormally high expression of complement-related markers such as CD11c, CD35, CD59, and CD88, as well as increased expression of the CD69 early-activation antigen, and the CD63 lysosomal-associated protein. Three distinct immunophenotypic patterns were determined by flow cytometry analysis in 123 SM patients: an immature immunophenotype present in ASM (CD25$^+$/CD2-/CD63$^+$/CD69$^+$) and MCL (CD25$^+$/CD2$^-$/CD63$^-$/CD69$^-$) and a mature activated or resting phenotype (CD25$^-$/CD2$^-$). Each pattern was associated with distinct genetic markers and clinical behavior.

Peripheral blood CD34$^-$ cells, which express C-KIT when isolated and cultured, give rise to mature mast cells, indicating that this population represents a mast cell precursor. The number of peripheral blood CD34$^-$ C-KIT$^+$ cells in SM patients is significantly higher than that in normal donors and correlates with the severity of mastocytosis (higher in ASM and SM-AHNMD compared with ISM) and has been used to determine disease severity, detect early relapse, and assess treatment response.[20]

Serum Tryptase Measurements

The measurement of tryptase (a mast cell enzyme with trypsin-like enzymatic activity) levels in biologic fluids (serum) has proven to be a useful disease-related marker in SM and is included as a minor criterion for diagnosing the condition according to WHO guidelines, provided that certain conditions are satisfied.[10] There are two major forms of mast cell tryptase: alpha (subtypes α_1 and α_2) and beta (subtypes β_1, β_2, and β_3). Mature β_2-tryptase is stored in mast cell secretory granules as an enzymatically active tetramer complexed with proteoglycans and is released only during granule exocytosis, thereby largely reflecting mast cell activation.[21] In contrast, the precursor forms of both α-tryptase and β-tryptase are constitutively secreted by mast cells, and the combined total serum levels (including precursor and mature tryptase forms) are thought to correlate with systemic mast cell number, albeit with effects related to tryptase haplotype and gender. The commercially available fluoroimmunoenzymatic assay measures total tryptase levels; in healthy individuals, levels range from 1 to 15 ng/mL, whereas in most patients with SM, total serum tryptase levels exceed 20 ng/mL. In cases of suspected mastocytosis, it is important that serum tryptase levels be interpreted in the appropriate context. Elevated levels of serum tryptase have been documented in patients with non–mast cell myeloid malignancies, including acute myeloid leukemia (AML), myelodysplastic syndrome (MDS), and chronic myeloid leukemia (CML), which mandates exclusion of such non–mast cell myeloid disorders before reaching a diagnosis of SM. Furthermore, levels of serum tryptase, particularly mature β-tryptase, are frequently elevated in association with anaphylaxis or a severe allergic reaction. Total tryptase levels may also be useful for monitoring treatment response in mastocytosis patients; interpretation of levels, however, must take into account other clinical/laboratory data, given the potential inherent variability of tryptase levels, as well as other possible confounding effects, such as administration of radiocontrast agents or narcotics, that may lead to mast cell degranulation.

Recently, REMA created a simple clinical score based on age, sex, serum baseline tryptase level, the presence of presyncope/syncope, and the presence of pruritus, hives, or angioedema to predict bone marrow mast cell clonality. In a prospective study, the clinical utility of the REMA score was validated in 158 patients with MCAS in the absence of MIS to predict not only bone marrow mast cell clonality but also the diagnosis of SM by WHO criteria (before a bone marrow study).[22] The REMA score was found to be more sensitive than the serum baseline tryptase level of >20 ng/L alone in predicting a diagnosis of SM.

Molecular Studies

In patients with mastocytosis, molecular studies are clearly important diagnostically; moreover, these studies are becoming increasingly important from a therapeutic standpoint as well. Recent studies underscore the high prevalence of the Kit D816V gain-of-function mutation in mastocytosis patients, with high correlation between mutation detection and the proportion of lesional/clonal cells in the sample, as well as the sensitivity of the screening method employed. Molecular detection of Kit mutations are preferably performed on fresh bone marrow aspirate, clot sections, or bone marrow biopsy specimens that are fixed in formalin and decalcified in EDTA. The likelihood of detecting the mutation in peripheral blood mononuclear cells in a case of indolent mastocytosis (with low probability of circulating clonal cells), using a low-sensitivity screening test (e.g., DNA sequencing), is quite low. The sensitivity of detection may be enhanced by enriching lesional mast cells or other clonal cell populations (e.g., neutrophils or eosinophils) by laser-capture microdissection or magnetic bead-based cell sorting, respectively. Furthermore, use of higher-sensitivity methods, including allele-specific PCR or PCR with peptide nucleic acid (PNA) probes, to clamp the wild-type allele combined with mutant allele detection with hybridization probes dramatically enhances the probability of mutation detection in bulk cells (sensitivity $=10^{-3}$). Using a higher sensitivity method, the D816V mutation has been detected in virtually all patients with ISM or ASM (93%), but less frequently in patients with WDSM (vide infra) (29%). Kit mutations other than D816V (e.g., I817V, VI815-816) were rarely detected (<3%). Notably, most mastocytosis patients with poor prognosis harbored Kit D816V in two or more bone marrow myeloid cell populations (81%), in contrast to patients with indolent mastocytosis (27%).

WDSM may represent a distinct, albeit genetically heterogeneous, subtype of SM. A subset of WDSM cases carries the F522C germline mutation located in the Kit transmembrane domain. In contrast to other SM subtypes, mast cells in WDSM do not (aberrantly) express either CD2 or CD25 antigens and are mature in appearance.

The FIP1L1-PDGFRA mutation can be detected by either fluorescence in situ hybridization (FISH) or PCR-based assays. Some investigators have suggested that PCR (particularly, nested PCR) is a more reliable screening test for FIP1L1-PDGFRA (relative to FISH) in primary eosinophilia, given the low sensitivity of FISH in some cases. Limitations of PCR-based assays include the possibility of an unusual FIP1L1-PDGFRA transcript, given the heterogeneity of breakpoints with the FIP1L1 locus and other mechanisms (e.g., cryptic splice sites), which may lead to a false-negative test result. Finally, although real-time quantitative PCR assays for monitoring FIP1L1-PDGFRA transcript levels have been described, its precise utility in assessing either depth of response with therapy (i.e., detection of minimal residual disease) or for molecular relapse remains unclear at this time.

Biochemical markers can also be used to predict bone marrow involvement in SM. Serum tryptase and urine N-methylhistamine and N-methylimidazole acetic acid have been shown in a study to have high pretest accuracy in predicting the probability of ISM in a given individual with SM-related symptoms.

Differential Diagnosis

The WHO diagnostic criteria for SM are provided in Table 71-5, and the diagnostic criteria for the diagnosis of the SM variants (including ISM, SM-AHNMD, ASM, MCL, MCS, and EM) are presented in Table 71-4. Because mast cells can be seen in other conditions and the treatment approach to ASM/MCL would differ from that of ISM, it is important that a rigorous clinical and laboratory evaluation be performed on an individual with suspected mast cell disease.

The presence of mast cells in a bone marrow aspirate smear or histologic sections prompts a pathologist to a differential diagnosis that includes not only SM but also acute basophilic leukemia, mast cell hyperplasia, myeloid neoplasms with eosinophilia and PDGFR abnormalities, myelomastocytic leukemia, and tryptase-positive AML. Appreciating mast cell cytology (normal, atypical type I, atypical type II, metachromatic blasts) and the pattern of mast cell infiltration (interstitial, diffuse dense, focal dense, tryptase-positive compact round cell infiltrate of the bone marrow) allows for discrimination among these disease entities, and confirmation of D816V Kit further supports the diagnosis of SM.

Table 71-5 World Health Organization Criteria for Diagnosis* of Systemic Mastocytosis

MAJOR
Multifocal dense infiltrates of mast cells in bone marrow or other extracutaneous organ sections (>15 mast cells aggregating)
MINOR
a. >25% mast cells in tissue sections or bone marrow aspirate smears that are spindle-shaped, immature or have atypical morphology
b. C-KIT point mutation at codon 816V detected in bone marrow, blood, or another extracutaneous organ
c. Expression of CD2 and/or CD25 in neoplastic mast cells
d. Baseline serum tryptase persistently >20 ng/mL (not valid in presence of another non–mast cell clonal disorder)

*Diagnosis of systemic mastocytosis requires three minor criteria *or* the sole major plus minor criteria.

SM should be distinguished from mast cell hyperplasia states or mast cell activation syndromes (MCAS) with or without the morphologic and/or molecular abnormalities that characterize a neoplastic proliferation. MCAS is a heterogeneous group of mast cell–related diseases characterized by episodic symptoms that are attributed to mast cell degranulation, including flushing, lightheadedness, dermatographism, crampy abdominal pain, diarrhea, life-threatening hypotension, and neuropsychiatric symptoms (headache, poor concentration, and memory loss). Heat and consumption of alcohol are known to stimulate mast cell mediator release. This includes signs and symptoms involving the dermis, gastrointestinal track, pulmonary system, musculoskeletal system, cardiovascular system, and nervous system. MCAS identifies a group of patients with unexplained or recurrent anaphylaxis without skin lesions or with diseases that do not meet criteria for the diagnosis of SM. Consideration of this diagnosis requires the elimination of a variety of disorders that can mimic the characteristic symptoms. These disorders include carcinoid syndrome pheochromocytoma, medullary thyroid carcinoma, estrogen or testosterone deficiency, inflammatory bowel syndrome, reactions to environmental stimuli, and allergic reactions. The existence of mast cell activation disorders causing sudden and sometimes life-threatening symptoms has been recognized for many decades, but these cases fail to meet the full diagnostic criteria of a mast cell proliferative disorder such as SM. These patients appear to have a hyperresponsive/hypersensitive mast cell population rather than an expanded mast cell population, and long-term follow-up is indicated. Because of the absence of definitive diagnostic criteria for these types of mast cell diseases, proposed diagnostic criteria have been developed.[23] Table 71-6 shows the proposed criteria for MCAS, which require the ruling out of other primary and secondary causes, documentation of urinary or serum markers of mast cell activation, a decrease in frequency or severity of symptoms with antimediator therapy, and the presence of episodic symptoms consistent with mast cell mediator release that affect two or more organ symptoms. This classification scheme will require validation in prospective multicentered clinical trials. A classification has been proposed that distinguishes secondary MC disorders (allergic diseases, physical urticarias, chronic autoimmune urticaria, or associated chronic inflammatory or neoplastic disorders), primary MC disorders (hypotension with mastocytosis or monoclonal mast cell activation syndrome [MMAS]), and idiopathic MC disorders (anaphylaxis, angioedema, urticaria, MCAS). Monoclonal MCAS is characterized by the demonstration of multifocal mast cell clusters of atypical morphology (spindle-shaped and hypogranulated), mast cell CD25 expression, and/or the presence of C-KIT D816V point mutation.[23] Patients who do not meet these criteria are considered to have an idiopathic MCAS. A useful way to distinguish among SM, MMAS, MCAS, and idiopathic anaphylaxis (IA) is provided in Table 71-7.

A set of clinical and laboratory features that is helpful in distinguishing patients with Kit D816V–positive SM with eosinophilia

Table 71-6 Proposed Criteria for the Diagnosis of MCAS0*

1. Episodic symptoms consistent with mast cell mediator release affecting two or more organ systems, evidenced as follows: a. Skin: urticaria, angioedema, flushing b. Gastrointestinal: nausea, vomiting, diarrhea, abdominal cramping c. Cardiovascular: hypotensive syncope or near syncope, tachycardia d. Respiratory: wheezing e. Naso-ocular: conjunctival injection, pruritus, nasal stuffiness
2. A decrease in the frequency or severity or a resolution of symptoms with antimediator therapy: H_1- and H_2-histamine receptor inverse agonists, antileukotriene medications (cysteinyl leukotriene receptor blockers or 5-lipoxygenase inhibitor), or mast cell stabilizers (cromolyn sodium).
3. Evidence of an increase in a validated urinary or serum marker of mast cell activation: Documentation of an increase of the marker to greater than the patient's baseline value during a symptomatic period on two or more occasions or, if baseline tryptase levels are persistently >15 ng/mL, documentation of an increase of the tryptase level above baseline value on one occasion. Total serum tryptase level is recommended as the marker of choice; less specific (also from basophils) are 24-hour urine histamine metabolites or PGD_2 or its metabolite 11-β-prostaglandin F_2.
4. Rule out primary and secondary causes of mast cell activation and well-defined clinical idiopathic entities.

PGD_2, Prostaglandin D_2.
*MCAS remains, for now, an idiopathic disorder; however, in some cases it could be an early reflection of a monoclonal population of mast cells, in which case it could, with time, meet the criteria for MMAS as one or two minor criteria for mastocytosis are fulfilled.

from individuals with the FIP1L1-PDGFRA–positive myeloid neoplasms with eosinophilia has been created. In the D816V Kit–positive group, gastrointestinal symptoms, urticaria pigmentosa, thrombocytosis, median serum tryptase value, and the presence of dense mast cell aggregates in the bone marrow are more frequently observed as compared with FIP1L1-PDGFRA–positive patients. By contrast, male sex, cardiac and pulmonary symptoms, median peak absolute eosinophil count, the eosinophil-to-tryptase ratio, and elevated serum B_{12} levels were higher or more common in the FIP1L1-PDGFRA–positive group. A scoring system incorporating these clinical and laboratory parameters has been created, which can be helpful in predicting whether patients with peripheral eosinophilia and increased marrow mast cell burden carry the D816V Kit mutation or the FIP1L1-PDGFRA, which is important for developing treatment decisions (Table 71-8).

Prognosis

In a retrospective study of 342 adult patients with SM (46% ISM, 12% ASM, 40% SM-AHNMD, 1% MCL) seen at Mayo Clinic, Kit D816V was detected in 68% of patients (78% ISM, 82% ASM, and 60% SM-AHNMD).[24] Survival was superior in the ISM group and was similar to the age- and sex-matched control population, with leukemic transformation occurring as a rare event. Median survival for SM-AHNMD, ASM, and MCL cases was approximately 2 years, 3.5 years, and 2 months, respectively. Median survival for ISM was more than 16 years and was not reached for the BMM subvariant (Fig. 71-6). Advanced age, weight loss, anemia, thrombocytopenia, hypoalbuminemia, and excess bone marrow blasts were identified by multivariable analysis as independent adverse prognostic factors for survival. This large study validates the prognostic significance of WHO diagnostic categories and further justifies therapeutic intervention with a goal to reduce systemic mast cell burden in patients with ASM, MCL, and ISM with severe anaphylaxis. ISM has a low rate of disease progression, and most patients will enjoy a normal life expectancy.[25] The presence of Kit mutations in mast cells, myeloid and lymphoid cells, and an elevated serum β_2-microglobulin has been

Table 71-7 Comparison of Clinical and Diagnostic Features for SM, MMAS, MCAS, and IA

Features	SM	MMAS	MCAS	IA
Baseline tryptase	>20	Normal or mildly increased	Normal or mildly increased	Normal
C-KIT D816V	+	+	–	–
Multifocal mast cell aggregates	+	–	–	–
Aberrant CD25	+	+	–	–
UP	+/–	–	–	–
Mediator-release symptoms	+	+	+	+
Hypotensive episodes	+/–	+/–	+/–	+/–
Urine N-MH or PGD_2	Increased at baseline	Increased during symptoms	Increased during symptoms	Increased during symptoms
Response to antimediator therapy	+	+	+	+/–

Modified from, Akin C, Valent P, Metcalfe DD: Mast cell activation syndrome: Proposed diagnostic criteria. *J Allergy Clin Immunol* 126:1099, 2010.
IA, Idiopathic anaphylaxis; *N-MH,* N-methylhistamine; *PGD_2,* prostaglandin D_2; *MCAS,* mast cell activation syndrome; *MMAS,* monoclonal mast cell activation syndrome; *SM,* systemic mastocytosis.

Table 71-8 Clinicopathologic Features of Eosinophilia-Associated FIP1L1-PDGFRA–Rearranged Myeloid Neoplasms Versus D816V Kit–Positive Systemic Mastocytosis

Features	FIP1L1-PDGFRA–Rearranged	D816V KIT–Positive
Gender	Overwhelmingly male	Less gender skewing
Bone marrow mast cell aggregates	Loose clusters/ interstitial	Dense aggregates
AEC/tryptase ratio	>100	≤100
Treatment	Imatinib-sensitive	Imatinib-resistant; second-generation TKIs (e.g., midostaurin)
Symptom profile	Cardiac/pulmonary	Gastrointestinal/urticaria pigmentosa/vascular
Vitamin B_{12} level	Elevated	Normal

Modified from Gotlib J, Akin C: Mast cells and eosinophils in mastocytosis, chronic eosinophilic leukemia, and non-clonal disorders. *Semin Hematol* 49:128, 2012.
AEC, Absolute eosinophil count; *TKIs,* tyrosine kinase inhibitors.

shown to be predictive of transformation to more aggressive disease. In a prospective study of patients with ISM, age above 60 years and the development of SM-AHNMD were associated with a poor survival, with a probability of death of 2.2% (+/– 1.3%) and 11% (+/– 5.9%) at 5 and 25 years, respectively.

Treatment

Adults with SM generally seek treatment for one or more of the following disease manifestations: skin rash (e.g., UP), symptoms of mast cell degranulation, and/or symptoms related to skeletal involvement or organomegaly/organopathy from mast cell infiltration. Although the treatment of SM has largely been empirically derived, recent advances in our understanding of the molecular pathogenesis of this condition allows for the identification of specific disease subtypes that are uniquely sensitive (or resistant) to specific therapies. Consequently, in this era of increasingly greater access to molecular testing, it is important that SM patients be molecularly profiled for presence or absence of relevant pathogenetic mutations, to enable optimal therapeutic decisions to be possible. The relative rarity of mastocytosis, its biologic heterogeneity, and (historically) the lack of simple, widely accepted treatment response criteria have hitherto served as barriers to development of

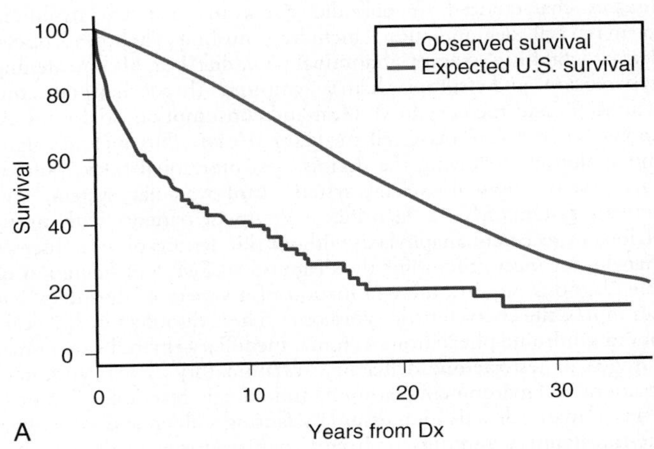

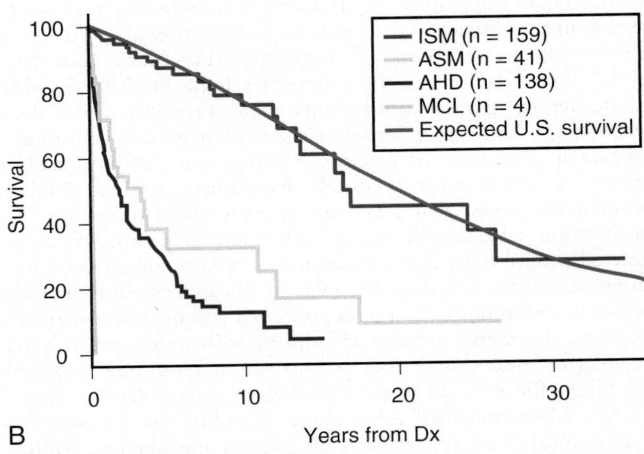

Figure 71-6 SURVIVAL OF SYSTEMIC MASTOCYTOSIS PATIENTS. **A,** The observed Kaplan-Meier survival for systemic mastocytosis patients *(red)* compared with the expected survival of the age- and sex-matched U.S. population *(blue)*. **B,** The observed Kaplan-Meier survival for patients with systemic mastocytosis, classified by disease subtypes ISM *(red)*, ASM *(green)*, AHNMD *(yellow)*, and MCL *(purple)* compared with the expected survival of the age- and sex-matched U.S. population *(blue)*.

Investigational Therapies for Patients With Systemic Mastocytosis

Response Criteria

In order to standardize evaluation of therapies in systemic mastocytosis (SM), it is essential to have uniform response criteria to compare novel therapeutic approaches. For a comprehensive review of the consensus statements on diagnostics, treatment recommendations, and response criteria in mastocytosis by leading world experts in this field, refer to the published results of the Working Conference on Mastocytosis in 2005 (as reported in the European Journal of Clinical Investigation[28]).

Proposed response criteria for cutaneous mastocytosis (CM) or "mastocytosis in the skin (MIS)" include complete regression, or CR (complete disappearance of affected skin lesions); major regression, or MR (reduction in lesions by >50%); partial regression, or PR (reduction in lesions by 10% to 50%); and no regression, or NR (<10% reduction in cutaneous lesions).

Since tryptase levels tend to reflect the mast cell burden in SM, tryptase can be used as a surrogate marker for measuring response to cytoreductive agents. The added value of using soluble-Kit, soluble-CD25 and histamine as markers of disease response is not known. Proposed response criteria for SM include complete resolution, or CR; major response, or MR (>50% reduction in severity and/or significant decrease in frequency, B → A or C → B); partial response, or PR (10% to 50% reduction in severity, no major decrease in frequency); no response, or NR (<10% reduction, no decrease in frequency); and continuous CR, or CCR (symptom-free interval of at least 2 years following initiation of therapy).

The use of consensus response criteria will better enable a uniformed and agreed-upon standard for comparing the clinical response of various agents with differing mechanisms of action.

Tyrosine Kinase Inhibitors

Dasatinib (BMS354825) is an orally bioavailable thiazolecarboxamide that is structurally unrelated to imatinib. It is a dual Src/ABL kinase inhibitor that is more potent than imatinib, and it demonstrates inhibitory activity against a number of BCR-ABL mutations linked to imatinib resistance in CML, but not T315I. Dasatinib inhibits cell lines harboring Kit WT or Kit D816V at nanomolar concentrations. In contrast to imatinib, dasatinib binds to the ABL and Kit ATP-binding sites regardless of the activation-loop conformation. In a large phase II study with 33 SM patients (28 Kit-D816V–positive) were treated with dasatinib at 70 mg twice daily or 140 mg once daily.[29] The ORR was 33%, 2 Kit wild-type patients achieved a CR for up to 15 months in one case, and 9 patients (including Kit D816V–positive SM) had improvements in disease-related symptoms, including rash, diarrhea, bone pain, headaches, itching, fatigue, shortness of breath, indigestion, and decrease or elimination of anaphylactic reactions. Treatment-related adverse events were similar to those seen in previous studies in Ph+ MPNs. It would appear that despite in vitro Kit-D816V inhibitory activity, dasatinib does not exhibit disease-modifying activity in patients with Kit D816V–positive SM, and it is not clear which subgroup of SM may have the best response to this therapy.

Nilotinib (AMN107) is a more potent small-molecule kinase inhibitor with activity against a number of BCR-ABL mutations linked to imatinib resistance in CML, but not T315I. Nilotinib also has in vitro inhibitory activity against cell lines harboring Kit WT or Kit V560G (juxtamembrane mutant) but has limited activity against Kit D816V (IC_{50} in micromolar range). These data suggest that nilotinib may be a less-than-ideal candidate for treatment of patients with systemic mastocytosis, of whom a majority carry the Kit D816V mutation.

Masitinib (AB1010) is a potent oral multityrosine kinase inhibitor selective for C-KIT and PDGFRα/β, as well as for Lyn and Fyn, which are important regulators of IgE-mediated mast cell degranulation. The drug was not effective in inhibiting Kit D816V–driven mast cell proliferation in vitro. This agent was studied in a proof-of-concept, multicentered, nonrandomized, phase IIa study of 25 patients with indolent SM or CM suffering from disease-related symptoms (pruritus, flushing, depression, and reduced quality of life [QOL]) at dose levels of 3 or 6 mg/kg/day over a 12-week core study period.[20,30] Patients were entered into this study if they were refractory to at least one previous treatment and had involvement of at least one organ, with absent Kit D816V. During the 12-week treatment period masitinib significantly reduced SM-associated symptoms and improved QOL. The authors postulated that the clinical response of masitinib in patients with the D816V mutation may be explained in part to the inhibition of Lyn and Fyn, leading to reduced mast cell degranulation. Drug-related adverse events (edema 44%, nausea 44%, muscle spasms 28%, rash 28%) were observed in 84% of patients and were mostly mild to moderate, occurring within the first 12 weeks, and manageable with symptomatic treatments. A single patient experienced reversible agranulocytosis. Depression has been associated with SM and estimated at a prevalence of approximately 64%; masitinib has been shown to improve depression in 67% of cases in a study of 35 patients with indolent SM. Recently, a single patient with MCL was found to have a previously unidentified mutation in Kit (dup[501-502]) and was successfully treated with masitinib, inducing complete resolution of circulating mast cells, decrease in serum histamine and tryptase, and clinical improvement.

Midostaurin (PKC412) is an N-benzoyl-staurosporine, with inhibitory activity against protein kinase C (PKC), FLT3 (FMS-like tyrosine kinase-3), Kit mutants (D816Yand D816V), vascular endothelial growth factor receptor-2 (VEGFR-2), PDGFR, and fibroblast growth factor receptor (FGFR) tyrosine kinases. PKC412 potently inhibits growth of cell lines harboring Kit D816V, and early data suggest activity in patients with advanced SM. In a phase II study, midostaurin administered to 26 patients with SM (4 ASM, 14 SM-CMML, 3 SM-MDS, 1 SM-MDS/MPN, 4 MCL) at a dose of 100 mg twice daily achieved a major response rate of 38%, which included normalization of hypoalbuminemia, improvement in anemia/thrombocytopenia, resolution of transaminitis, improvement in pleural effusions and ascites, and restoration of weight. A patient with MCL had a near complete response. The most common side effects noted were nausea, vomiting, diarrhea, and fatigue. A phase III trial of midostaurin is currently being pursued; the results of this trial are eagerly awaited to determine the true potential of this drug in treating SM patients.

Based on in vitro studies demonstrating that midostaurin could inhibit D816V Kit–transformed Ba/F3 cell growth, a single patient with MCL and an associated myelodysplastic syndrome (MDS)/myeloproliferative neoplasm [MPN]) was treated with midostaurin and obtained a partial response. The patient had resolution of liver function abnormalities, reduction in peripheral blood mast cell percentage, serum histamine level, and decrease in Kit phosphorylation and D816V Kit–mutation frequency; however, the patient died after 3 months of therapy as a result of leukemic transformation.

Additional small-molecule Kit inhibitors in various stages of preclinical and clinical development for the treatment of patients with mastocytosis include **MLN518,** a quinazoline-based tyrosine kinase inhibitor, which inhibits cell lines harboring Kit D816V, as well as juxtamembrane mutant-Kit; **AP23464/AP23848,** ATP-based inhibitors that have low-nanomolar inhibitory activity against Kit D816V; and **EXEL-0862,** a novel multi–tyrosine kinase inhibitor (FGFR, VEGF, PDGFR, and FLT3) that has been shown to have greater inhibitory activity against the HMC-1.2 cell line, which harbors both Kit D816V and Kit V560G, as compared with HMC-1.1, which harbors the juxtamembrane Kit V560G mutation alone.

Thus far, treatment with small-molecule kinase inhibitors has been mostly disappointing and to date has not resulted in improvement in survival. Other than rare cases of SM with specific Kit mutations involving the transmembrane domain (F522C

Continued

Investigational Therapies for Patients With Systemic Mastocytosis—cont'd

and K5091) that are exquisitely responsive to imatinib therapy, therapeutic intervention is largely palliative, aimed at alleviating skin manifestations (urticaria, pruritus) and gastrointestinal complaints (nausea, vomiting, diarrhea, abdominal pain) and avoiding severe anaphylactic reactions.

Non–Tyrosine Kinase Inhibitors

17-AAG (17-[Allylamino]-17-demethoxygeldanamycin) is a geldanamycin derivative that binds to heat shock protein 90 (Hsp90), thus enhancing the proteasomal degradation of several Hsp90 client kinases, including mutant Kit. In one report, a dose-dependent decrease in phosphorylation of Kit, AKT, and STAT3 was observed in both HMC-1.1 and HMC-1.2 cells. Furthermore, 17-AAG inhibited patient-derived neoplastic mast cells ex vivo, relative to mononuclear cells. 17-AAG is currently in phase II clinical trials for the treatment of mastocytosis. STA-9090 is another novel Hsp90 inhibitor that has shown preclinical activity in growth inhibition, caspase 3/7-dependent apoptosis, and downregulation of phosphorylated Kit in malignant mast cell lines and in primary malignant mast cells expressing wild-type or D816V Kit.

IMD-0354 is an NF-κB inhibitor that has been shown to suppress neoplastic mast cell proliferation preferentially over that of normal mast cells. Cyclin D3 expression was shown to be depressed after HMC-1 cells were exposed to IMD-0354, suggesting that constitutive activation of Kit by D816V mutation promotes NF-κB activity and the downstream upregulation of cyclin D3, leading to cell cycle progression.

Polo-like kinase-1 (PLK1) is a serine/threonine kinase that plays an essential role in mitosis and has recently been shown to be active in primary neoplastic mast cells and MCL cell lines. **BI2536** is a small-molecule inhibitor of PLK1 that has been evaluated in preclinical studies and demonstrated antiproliferative activity in SM cell lines and primary neoplastic mast cells (with associated mitotic arrest and apoptosis), but not in normal mast cells. This drug acted in synergy with midostaurin in inhibiting in vitro growth of neoplastic cells.

Obatoclax (GX015-070) inhibits BCL-2/BCL-XL and MCL 1, which has been shown to be expressed in SM. In vitro studies have shown antiproliferative effects in both SM primary cells and cell lines; these effects were augmented when obatoclax was combined with bortezomib, a proteasome inhibitor that promotes the expression of Bim.

SMA-ZnPP and **PEG-ZnPP** are Hsp32 inhibitors that target Kit-inducible heme oxygenase-1 (HO-1) in neoplastic mast cells and inhibit proliferation of SM cell lines in vitro. Hsp32 inhibitors cooperate with midostaurin in suppressing proliferation and inducing apoptosis in mast cells. Hsp32 appears to be an important survival factor in SM and serves as a novel drug target in future clinical trials.

RAD001 (everolimus) is a novel oral mammalian target of rapamycin (mTOR) inhibitor that was tested in an open-label phase II study in 10 patients with SM. Since constitutive Kit signaling leads to activation of the mTOR pathway, preclinical rationale was established for the use of this oral agent in SM. Although four patients experienced a subjective improvement in symptoms for a median duration of 3 months, no objective clinical responses were seen.

Homoharringtonine is a protein synthesis inhibitor that has been shown to inhibit the in vitro growth of imatinib-sensitive HMC-1.1 cells harboring the Kit V560G mutation and imatinib-resistant HMC-1.2 cells harboring the Kit V560G and D816V mutations. Additionally, in a murine MCL model with imatinib-resistant Kit D814Y mast cells, antitumor activity with homoharringtonine was observed, and mice had prolonged survival. The antiproliferative and proapoptotic activity was associated with inhibition of Kit-dependent phosphorylation of downstream signaling molecules such as AKT, STAT3/STAT5, and ERK1/2. Evaluation of homoharringtonine in clinical trial is warranted.

Since CD25 is almost universally and aberrantly expressed on the surface of neoplastic mast cells in patients with SM, it may serve as a novel therapeutic target. **Denileukin diftitox (Ontak)** is a DNA-derived cytotoxic protein composed of the amino acid sequences of diphtheria toxin fragments A and B and IL-2 amino acid sequences, which directs the agent to the IL-2 receptor (of which CD25 is a subunit). A pilot study conducted in eight symptomatic treatment–naive and refractory SM patients failed to show any clinical activity or any reduction in marrow mast cell burden or tryptase level with denileukin diftitox treatment. It is thought that the disappointing results of this trial are due to the finding that coexpression of the other IL-2 receptor subunits is lacking in malignant mast cells and is required for optimal binding of this agent.

Since mast cells are known to be a rich source of inflammatory cytokines (such as TNF-α and IL-6) and these cytokines may play a role in the pathogenesis of SM, a pilot study was conducted of two patients with SM-AHNMD myeloma who were treated with **lenalidomide (Revlimid),** an immunomodulating drug with potent activity in patients with myelodysplastic syndrome and 5q minus syndrome and active in the treatment of multiple myeloma. At a daily dose of 10 mg, lenalidomide did not improve SM features such as bone marrow mast cell burden, serum tryptase levels, or SM-related symptoms. In vitro studies also failed to show a signal of activity of lenalidomide in primary mast cells from the patients with aggressive or indolent SM or in HMC-1 cell lines. It is unlikely that larger clinical trials with lenalidomide in SM will be pursued.

evidence-based therapies for this disorder. Although the therapy of SM patients needs to be individualized, the general approaches to therapy are described in the following treatment sections. When appropriate, clinical trial options should be considered for SM patients requiring therapy (see box on Investigational Therapies for Patients With Systemic Mastocytosis). We refer the reader to specialized dermatology texts for the treatment of cutaneous mastocytosis.

Treatment of Mast Cell Degranulation Symptoms

Although mast cell cytoreductive agents (e.g., interferon, chemotherapy) can often effectively ameliorate symptoms of mast cell degranulation, these agents may have significant adverse effects; hence the initial approach to these patients emphasizes measures to prevent mast cell degranulation, as well as use of medications for symptom relief. In all cases, avoidance of triggers for mast cell degranulation (e.g., animal venoms, extremes of temperature, mechanical irritation, alcohol, emotional and physical stress) remains the cornerstone of therapy. Some patients cannot tolerate certain drugs or chemicals such as opioid analgesics, alcohol, aspirin or other nonsteroidal antiinflammatory medications and contrast dyes; the patient history often provides useful clues in this regard. A detailed workup to provide allergen avoidance guidelines is recommended in patients with mastocytosis. Skin testing can be done safely, and the results correlate with the symptoms of allergy- and antigen-specific IgEs. Lifelong venom immunotherapy should be considered in patients with IgE-mediated Hymenoptera venom allergy. Furthermore, appropriate precautionary measures during anesthesia and surgery are recommended in these patients.

Noncytoreductive therapy of mast cell degranulation symptoms includes the use of oral H_1- (e.g., hydroxyzine, diphenhydramine, fexofenadine, cetirizine, cyproheptadine, chlorpheniramine) and H_2- (e.g., ranitidine, famotidine) antihistamines for pruritus and peptic ulcer symptoms, respectively, and orally administered cromolyn sodium for nausea, abdominal pain, and diarrhea. Use of the latter is supported by Level I evidence. In a double-blind crossover study, cromolyn sodium was found to be therapeutically equivalent to a combination of cimetidine and chlorpheniramine for the treatment of mastocytosis-related symptoms. Corticosteroids are occasionally used for treating recurrent hypotensive episodes, ascites, and diarrhea with malabsorption. Patients with a propensity toward vasodilatory shock should wear a medical alert bracelet and carry an EpiPen injector for self-administration of subcutaneous epinephrine. In the rare case of a patient with severe and/or recurrent life-threatening degranulation-related events that are refractory to the aforementioned agents, cautious consideration may be given to the use of cytostatic or cytoreductive agents (such as 2-CdA); however, the potential adverse effects, including potentially mutagenic effects, of such agents must always be kept in mind and their use should be preceded by a full discussion of the potential risks and benefits with the patient.

Treatment of Organomegaly/Organopathy Symptoms

Cytoreductive therapy, especially chemotherapy, is generally reserved for patients with progressive symptomatic disease and for organopathy (C findings) that is directly related to tissue mast cell infiltration. In certain patients, however, it can be difficult to distinguish whether the organopathy relates to mast cell infiltration or whether it represents an immunologic response to the disease or an associated non–mast cell neoplasm (SM-AHNMD). Currently used first- and second-line therapeutic agents include the following:

Interferon-Alpha (IFN-α)

Interferon-alpha (IFN-α) is often considered the first-line therapy for progressive symptomatic disease, including in the presence of a concurrent non–mast cell myeloproliferative disorder (e.g., CMML). IFN-α is generally started at the dose of 1 million units (MU) subcutaneously three times per week, followed by gradual escalation to 3 to 5 MU three to five times per week, if tolerated. IFN-α (with or without concomitant corticosteroids for synergistic effect) has been reported to improve symptoms of mast cell degranulation, decrease bone marrow mast cell infiltration, and ameliorate mastocytosis-related ascites/hepatosplenomegaly, cytopenias, skin findings, and osteoporosis. Overall response rates to IFN-α therapy are approximately 20% to 60% (depending on the subtype), but they are extremely difficult to estimate, given the heterogeneous presentation of patients with mastocytosis, use of variable treatment dosages, generally short follow-up, and use of nonuniform treatment response criteria in published studies. The optimal dose and duration of IFN-α therapy for systemic mastocytosis remains uncertain. In a prospective multicenter study, all four patients receiving the highest IFN-α dose (i.e., >3 MU/m^2/day) responded to treatment. The time to best response may be up to 12 months or longer and delayed responses to therapy have been described. The addition of prednisone at doses of 20 to 60 mg/day with a slow taper over weeks to months did not appear to improve the response rates, but it can improve tolerability of IFN-α. A significant proportion of patients may experience clinical and/or biochemical relapse within several months of IFN-α treatment being discontinued, highlighting the largely cytostatic effect of IFN-α on neoplastic mast cells. IFN-α is associated with a variable, but significant, incidence (up to 50%) of dose-limiting toxicity, including flu-like symptoms, bone pain, fever, worsening cytopenias (particularly in patients with baseline organomegaly/cytopenias), depression, retinitis, and hypothyroidism. Anaphylaxis, as a response to IFN-α injections, has been described. Consequently, the dropout rate with IFN-α treatment due to adverse events is not trivial, and whether the addition of corticosteroids to IFN-α improves either treatment tolerance or efficacy remains to be proven in a randomized setting.

2-Chlorodeoxyadenosine/Cladribine

Single-agent 2-chlorodeoxyadenosine/cladribine (2-CdA) is effective in treating all subgroups of IFN-α refractory/intolerant SM patients; variable treatment schedules have been used in this setting. In SSM, 2-CdA can effectively reduce mast cell burden and improve symptoms, but in rapidly progressive ASM and MCL, this agent alone may not be effective in inducing durable responses. In a prospective multicenter pilot study of 10 patients, 2-CdA (0.1 to 0.13 mg/kg by a 2-hour IV infusion on days 1 through 5 every 4 to 8 weeks for 6 cycles) was found to be therapeutically active in all mastocytosis subsets. Although all patients had a clinical response, and bone marrow mast cell cytoreduction was also noted in 9 of 10 patients, no complete remissions were observed. Also, in a preliminary report of 33 SM patients treated with 2-CdA (0.15 mg/kg by a 2-hour IV infusion or subcutaneously for 5 days every 4 to 12 weeks for 1 to 6 cycles), major, partial, or no responses were seen in 24, 2, and 7 patients, respectively. Twenty six patients (first- and second-line therapy) were treated with 2-CdA at doses of 5 mg/m^2 or 0.13 to 0.17 mg/kg/day for 5 days as a 2-hour intravenous infusion. At a median of 3 cycles (range 1-9), an objective response rate (ORR) of 55% was observed and was essentially uniform in response throughout subcategories. Myelosuppression was the major adverse effect seen in approximately one-third of cases in each study. In a French study, 44 SM patients that had either failed symptomatic therapy and/or IFN therapy were treated with 2-CdA at 0.15 mg/kg/day for 5 days every 1 to 2 months for a median of 4 cycles. The median time to response was 20 months, and ORRs were 89%, 58%, 67%, 100% in ISM, ASM, CM, SSM, respectively.[26] Responses were seen in individual symptoms, normalization of eosinophil counts, and improved tryptase levels.

Imatinib Mesylate (Gleevec)

Imatinib mesylate (Gleevec) is an orally bioavailable small-molecule inhibitor of Kit, ABL, Arg, and PDGFR tyrosine kinases. The identification of gain-of-function mutations involving Kit and PDGFRA genes (known imatinib targets) in the pathogenesis of systemic mastocytosis has obvious therapeutic implications in this regard. Consistent with predictions from in vitro data, the clinical experience to date suggests that the vast majority of mastocytosis patients (who harbor Kit D816V) are likely to be refractory to imatinib therapy. In contrast, clinically meaningful responses have been observed for patients with wild-type Kit–associated mastocytosis and rare patients with Kit juxtamembrane mutations (e.g., F522C, K509I), suggesting that this subgroup of patients has imatinib-responsive disease. Imatinib has largely had disappointing results in clinical trials of patients with mastocytosis, and this is in large part due to the high frequency of D816V expression in patients, which is predictive for nonresponse. Overall response rates have ranged from 18% to 36% and include improvements in symptoms, UP, and organomegaly, as well as reduction in MC bone marrow burden and other biomarkers (e.g., serum tryptase). A response rate of 36% in Kit D816V–positive patients has been reported in one study,[27] whereas in another study, no patients with Kit D816V responded. In a Mayo Clinic study, the highest response rate was seen in SM-AHNMD. The drug has been used at a starting dose of 400 mg daily (+/− initial low-dose steroids) with a taper to 200 mg daily in responding patients that continue to receive maintenance therapy.

Patients with bone marrow involvement by abnormal mast cells who harbor FIP1L1-PDGFRA also uniformly achieve complete clinical, histologic, and molecular/cytogenetic responses with low-dose imatinib therapy, in the absence of mutations that confer imatinib resistance (PDGFRAT764I), which may be acquired with clonal evolution. Finally, imatinib is predicted to be effective in SM with specific mutations such as V560G and del419, although clinical proof of this supposition is lacking to date. The remarkable efficacy of imatinib in treating mastocytosis patients harboring specific mutations provides proof of principle for the development of molecularly targeted therapies for this disease, as well as a treatment-relevant molecular classification. It is currently recommended that patients with primary eosinophilia, particularly in the presence of increased bone marrow mast cells or increased serum tryptase level (i.e., SM-CEL), be screened for the presence of FIP1L1-PDGFRA by either FISH or reverse transcriptase–polymerase chain reaction (RT-PCR). Imatinib mesylate, generally at the 100-mg daily dose level, is considered to be first-line therapy for this group of patients. Initiation of imatinib therapy in patients with clonal eosinophilia harboring FIP1L1-PDGFRA can rarely lead to cardiogenic shock, resulting from rapid onset of eosinophil lysis/degranulation in the endomyocardium. Consequently, consideration may be given to starting imatinib concurrently with corticosteroids, particularly in the presence of either an abnormal echocardiogram or an elevated serum troponin level before treatment. In contrast to its effectiveness with FIP1L1-PDGFRA, most studies show that imatinib is not therapeutically beneficial for patients carrying Kit D816V, who make up the majority of SM patients. This mutation maps to the Kit enzymatic site and disrupts the imatinib-binding site. For patients harboring D816V or those without detectable imatinib-sensitive mutations, IFN-α may represent an attractive initial treatment option. Although a modest clinical benefit may be observed with imatinib at 400 mg daily in some patients without either Kit D816V or FIP1L1-PDGFRA, the use of imatinib in this setting remains investigational. Currently, imatinib is the only FDA-approved drug for the treatment of SM and is specifically indicated in the treatment of adult patients with ASM who do not have Kit D816V or who have an unknown mutation status.

In patients in whom symptomatic therapy is not sufficient and cytoreductive therapy is not effective, hematopoietic stem cell transplantation (HSCT) can be considered. Only limited reports exist of HSCT with myeloablative conditioning. A pilot study of three SM patients treated with a nonmyeloablative HSCT using an HLA-identical sibling has been reported. A highly immunosuppressive conditioning regimen was used to reduce transplant-related mortality (TRM) while allowing for engraftment and the induction of a graft-versus-mast-cell (GVMC) effect. Although TRM was not an issue, mast cell degranulation events complicated the treatment in two of the three cases. The three patients experienced progressive disease, and the longest duration of response was 39 months. Optimal cytoreduction with cladribine or interferon prior to HSCT may improve the ability of nonmyeloablative HSCT to effectively exploit the GVMC effect and lead to durable remissions and possibly cure in cases of aggressive SM. Currently, HSCT remains experimental in the treatment of SM.

FUTURE DIRECTIONS

The approach to a patient with systemic mastocytosis continues to be challenging, with many unanswered questions relating to aspects of (a) diagnosis, (b) pathogenesis, (c) clinical presentation, and (d) treatment of this heterogeneous disorder. At the diagnostic interface, a uniform approach to molecular testing is lacking at present; consensus is needed regarding the specific molecular assay(s) as well as biologic material(s) that are considered optimal for mutation analysis in mastocytosis patients. Advances in the understanding of SM pathogenesis have identified a number of potential drug targets in addition to Kit. Although effective control of MC mediator-related symptoms is obtained in most cases, effective control of mast cell burden is not uniformly controlled with current therapeutic strategies, and an unmet need for improved treatment approaches continues to exist. Ongoing and future clinical trials need to combine tyrosine kinase inhibitors, chemotherapeutics, and other novel agents that target Kit-independent oncogenic pathways in synergistic antiproliferative activity directed against the neoplastic mast cell. Optimally, what is needed are innovative, well-designed clinical trials combining agents directed against relevant molecular and biologic targets in the neoplastic mast cells that are conducted in cooperative multiinstitutional settings.

REFERENCES

1. Kirshenbaum AS, Kessler SW, Goff JP, et al: Demonstration of the origin of human mast cells from CD34+ bone marrow progenitor cells. *J Immunol* 146:1410, 1991.
2. d'Auriol L, Mattei MG, Andre C, et al: Localization of the human c-kit protooncogene on the q11-q12 region of chromosome 4. *Hum Genet* 78:374, 1988.
3. Stevens EC, Rosenthal NS: Bone marrow mast cell morphologic features and hematopoietic dyspoiesis in systemic mast cell disease. *Am J Clin Pathol* 116:177, 2001.
4. Furitsu T, Tsujimura T, Tono T, et al: Identification of mutations in the coding sequence of the proto-oncogene c-kit in a human mast cell leukemia cell line causing ligand-independent activation of c-kit product. *J Clin Invest* 92:1736, 1993.
5. Nagata H, Worobec AS, Oh CK, et al: Identification of a point mutation in the catalytic domain of the protooncogene c-kit in peripheral blood mononuclear cells of patients who have mastocytosis with an associated hematologic disorder. *Proc Natl Acad Sci U S A* 92:10560, 1995.
6. Ronnstrand L: Signal transduction via the stem cell factor receptor/c-Kit. *Cell Mol Life Sci* 61:2535, 2004.
7. Lee YN, Brandal S, Noel P, et al: KIT signaling regulates MITF expression through miRNAs in normal and malignant mast cell proliferation. *Blood* 117:3629, 2011.
8. Hoermann G, Cerny-Reiterer S, Perné A, et al: Identification of oncostatin M as a STAT5-dependent mediator of bone marrow remodeling in KIT D816V-positive systemic mastocytosis. *Am J Pathol* 178:2344, 2011.
9. Wilson TM, Maric I, Simakova O, et al: Clonal analysis of NRAS activating mutations in KIT-D816V systemic mastocytosis. *Haematologica* 96:459, 2011.
10. Arock M, Valent P: Pathogenesis, classification and treatment of mastocytosis: State of the art in 2010 and future perspectives. *Expert Rev Hematol* 3:497, 2010.
11. Castells M, Austen KF: Mastocytosis: Mediator-related signs and symptoms. *Int Arch Allergy Immunol* 127:147, 2002.
12. Smith JH, Butterfield JH, Cutrer FM: Primary headache syndromes in systemic mastocytosis. *Cephalalgia* 31:1522, 2011.
13. Wimazal F, Geissler P, Shnawa P, et al: Severe life-threatening or disabling anaphylaxis in patients with systemic mastocytosis: A single-center experience. *Int Arch Allergy Immunol* 157:399, 2012.
14. Horny HP, Parwaresch MR, Lennert K: Bone marrow findings in systemic mastocytosis. *Hum Pathol* 16:808, 1985.
15. Travis WD, Li CY, Yam LT, et al: Significance of systemic mast cell disease with associated hematologic disorders. *Cancer* 62:965, 1988.
16. Horny HP, Valent P: Histopathological and immunohistochemical aspects of mastocytosis. *Int Arch Allergy Immunol* 127:115, 2002.
17. Sotlar K, Horny H-P, Simonitsch I, et al: CD25 indicates the neoplastic phenotype of mast cells: A novel immunohistochemical marker for the diagnosis of systemic mastocytosis (SM) in routinely processed bone marrow biopsy specimens. *Am J Surg Pathol* 28:1319, 2004.
18. Escribano L, Garcia Montero AC, Nunez R, et al: Flow cytometric analysis of normal and neoplastic mast cells: Role in diagnosis and follow-up of mast cell disease. *Immunol Allergy Clin North Am* 26:535, 2006.
19. Morgado JM, Sánchez-Muñoz L, Teodosio CG, et al: Immunophenotyping in systemic mastocytosis diagnosis: 'CD25 positive' alone is more informative than the 'CD25 and/or CD2' WHO criterion. *Mod Pathol* 25:516, 2012.
20. Georgin-Lavialle, S, Lhermitte L, Baude C, et al: Blood CD34-c-Kit+ cell rate correlates with aggressive forms of systemic mastocytosis and behaves like a mast cell precursor. *Blood* 118:5246, 2011.
21. Schwartz LB: Diagnostic value of tryptase in anaphylaxis and mastocytosis. *Immunol Allergy Clin North Am* 26:451, 2006.
22. Alvarez-Twose I, González-de-Olano D, Sánchez-Muñoz L, et al: Validation of the REMA score for predicting mast cell clonality and systemic mastocytosis in patients with systemic mast cell activation symptoms. *Int Arch Allergy Immunol* 157:275, 2011.
23. Akin C, Valent P, Metcalfe DD: Mast cell activation syndrome: Proposed diagnostic criteria. *J Allergy Clin Immunol* 126:1099, 2010.
24. Lim KH, Tefferi A, Lasho TL, et al: Systemic mastocytosis in 342 consecutive adults: Survival studies and prognostic factors. *Blood* 113:5727, 2009.

25. Escribano L., Alvarez-Twose I, Sánchez-Muñoz L, et al: Prognosis in adult indolent systemic mastocytosis: A long-term study of the Spanish Network on Mastocytosis in a series of 145 patients. *J Allergy Clin Immunol* 124:514, 2009.
26. Hermine O, Hirsh I, Damaj G, et al: Long Term Efficacy and Safety of Cladribine In Adult Systemic mastocytosis: A French Multicenter Study of 44 Patients. *ASH Annual Meeting Abstracts* 116:1982.
27. Droogendijk HJ, Kluin-Nelemans HJ, van Doormaal JJ, et al: Imatinib mesylate in the treatment of systemic mastocytosis: A phase II trial. *Cancer* 107:345, 2006.
28. Valent P, Akin C, Escribano L, et al: Standards and standardization in mastocytosis: Consensus statements on diagnostics, treatment recommendations and response criteria. *Eur J Clin Invest* 37:435, 2007.
29. Verstovsek S, Tefferi A, Cortes J, et al: Phase II study of dasatinib in Philadelphia chromosome-negative acute and chronic myeloid diseases, including systemic mastocytosis. *Clin Cancer Res* 14:3906, 2008.
30. Paul C, Sans B, Suarez F, et al: Masitinib for the treatment of systemic and cutaneous mastocytosis with handicap: A phase 2a study. *Am J Hematol* 85:921, 2010.

CHAPTER 72

PATHOLOGIC BASIS FOR THE CLASSIFICATION OF NON-HODGKIN AND HODGKIN LYMPHOMAS

Elaine S. Jaffe, Stefania Pittaluga, and John Anastasi

The classification of malignant lymphomas has undergone significant changes over the past 50 years. The current approach is based on the integration of morphologic, phenotypic, genetic, and clinical features that allows the identification of distinct disease entities (see box on Principles of the Classification of Lymphomas Based on the REAL/WHO Classifications). This practical approach to lymphoma categorization was initially proposed by the International Lymphoma Study Group in 1994 and formed the basis of the Revised European-American Classification of Lymphoid Neoplasm (REAL). It was then adopted by the World Health Organization (WHO) classification of neoplasms of the hematopoietic and lymphoid tissues, published in 2001 and updated in 2008 (Table 72-1). The WHO classification represents a significant achievement in terms of cooperation, communication, and consensus among pathologists, hematologists, and oncologists. Furthermore, it recognizes that any classification system, in order to be viable and applicable, should evolve and incorporate new data resulting from emerging technologies in the field of hematopathology as shown by the inclusion of gene expression profiling (GEP) data in the more recent edition. These studies have led to the identifications of new prognostic and diagnostic categories. Major improvements in sequencing technologies now provide a great opportunity to examine the cancer genome for large-scale identification of genomic alterations in a more comprehensive manner, and by combining analysis of genome, transcriptome, and exome sequences, new insights will be gained into pathogenetic mechanisms and implementation of more targeted and personalized therapies.

Principles of the Classification of Lymphomas Based on the Revised European-American Classification of Lymphoid Neoplasm/World Health Organization Classifications

- Each disease is defined as a distinct entity based on a constellation of morphologic, clinical, and biologic features.
- The cell of origin is the starting point of disease definition.
- Some lymphoid neoplasms can be identified by routine morphologic approaches. However, for most diseases, knowledge of the immunophenotype and molecular genetics or cytogenetics plays an important role in differential diagnosis.
- A disease-based approach to classification facilitates discovery of molecular pathogenesis.
- The sites of presentation and involvement are important clues to underlying biologic distinctions. Extranodal lymphomas differ in many respects from their nodal counterparts.
- Many lymphoma entities display a range in cytologic grade and clinical aggressiveness, making it difficult to stratify lymphomas according to clinical behavior. A number of prognostic factors influence clinical outcome, including stage, international prognostic index, cytologic grade, gene expression profile, secondary genetic events, and the host environment.

This chapter focuses on the classification of neoplasms derived from mature B cells, T cells, and natural killer (NK) cells with emphasis on malignant lymphoma. The chapter provides a framework for the subsequent chapters on Hodgkin lymphoma and non-Hodgkin lymphoma (NHL) in reviewing the major entities according to the WHO classification.

PRECURSOR B-CELL AND T-CELL NEOPLASMS

B-Lymphoblastic Leukemia and Lymphoma

Most B-lymphoblastic leukemias and lymphomas (B-LBL) present as leukemia; lymphomatous presentations occur in approximately 5% to 10% of cases. Frequent sites of involvement include the lymph nodes, skin, soft tissue, and bone. Skin lesions in children frequently present in the head and neck region, including the scalp. Progression to leukemia occurs in the vast majority of cases if a complete remission is not obtained. The disease is most common in children and young adults.

Cytologically, B-LBL is composed of lymphoblasts that are usually somewhat larger than small lymphocytes but smaller than the cells of diffuse large cell lymphoma (Fig. 72-1). The cells have finely stippled chromatin with sparse cytoplasm and inconspicuous nucleoli. The nuclei may be round or convoluted. Mitotic figures are common, in keeping with the high-grade nature of the neoplasm. The differential diagnosis of B-LBL includes blastic plasmacytoid dendritic cell neoplasm, which can occur in children, and shows a marked predilection for skin. Extensive immunophenotypic studies are required for the differential diagnosis.

The lymphoblasts of B-LBL usually express markers of B-cell lineage such as CD19, PAX-5, and cytoplasmic CD22. They often lack CD20, which is usually expressed at later stages of B-cell differentiation after light chain gene rearrangement has occurred. PAX-5, a B-cell transcription factor, is a useful diagnostic marker in this instance. However, it should be noted that PAX-5 is not restricted to the B-cell lineage and may be expressed in some neuroendocrine carcinomas, particularly Merkel cell carcinoma, which is often in the differential diagnosis of small blue round cell tumors involving the skin.

In the 2008 WHO classification, B-LBL is further subdivided into distinct subsets characterized by recurrent genetic abnormalities. These are associated with distinctive clinical or phenotypic features and have important prognostic implications.

The impact of new technologies in the classification of lymphoblastic leukemia and lymphoma and targeted therapy are addressed in Chapters 63 and 64.

T-Lymphoblastic Lymphoma and Leukemia

Most lymphoblastic lymphomas and leukemias (T-LBLs) are cytologically indistinguishable from their B-cell counterparts. The blasts have finely distributed chromatin, inconspicuous nucleoli, and sparse pale cytoplasm. Nuclear irregularity is variable. This is a disease of adolescents and young adults, with an increased male-to-female ratio.

Table 72-1 World Health Organization Classification of Tumors of Hematopoietic and Lymphoid Tissues (2008)*

B-cell lymphoblastic leukemia/lymphoma
  Multiple variants listed based on cytogenetic findings
B-cell lymphoblastic leukemia/lymphoma

MATURE B-CELL NEOPLASMS

Chronic lymphocytic leukemia/small lymphocytic lymphoma
B-cell prolymphocytic leukemia
Splenic marginal zone lymphoma
Hairy cell leukemia
Splenic B-cell lymphoma/leukemia, unclassifiable
  Splenic diffuse red pulp small B-cell lymphoma
  Hairy cell leukemia—variant
Lymphoplasmacytic lymphoma
  Waldenström macroglobulinemia
Heavy chain diseases
  α-Heavy chain disease
  γ-Heavy chain disease
  μ-Heavy chain disease
Plasma cell myeloma
Solitary plasmacytoma of bone
Extraosseous plasmacytoma
Extranodal marginal zone lymphoma of mucosa-associated lymphoid tissue (MALT lymphoma)
Nodal marginal zone lymphoma
  Pediatric nodal marginal zone lymphoma
Follicular lymphoma
  Pediatric follicular lymphoma
Primary cutaneous follicle center lymphoma
Mantle cell lymphoma
Diffuse large B-cell lymphoma (DLBCL), not otherwise specified
  T-cell/histiocyte rich large B-cell lymphoma
  Primary DLBCL of the central nervous system
  Primary cutaneous DLBCL, leg type
  EBV positive DLBCL of the elderly
DLBCL associated with chronic inflammation
Lymphomatoid granulomatosis
Primary mediastinal (thymic) large B-cell lymphoma
Intravascular large B-cell lymphoma
ALK-positive large B-cell lymphoma
Plasmablastic lymphoma
Large B-cell lymphoma arising in human herpesvirus 8–associated multicentric Castleman disease
Primary effusion lymphoma
Burkitt lymphoma
B-cell lymphoma unclassifiable, with features intermediate between diffuse large B-cell lymphoma and Burkitt lymphoma
B-cell lymphoma unclassifiable, with features intermediate between diffuse large B-cell lymphoma and classical Hodgkin lymphoma

MATURE T-CELL AND NATURAL KILLER (NK) CELL NEOPLASMS

T-cell prolymphocytic leukemia
T-cell large granular lymphocytic leukemia
Chronic lymphoproliferative disorder of NK cells
Aggressive NK cell leukemia
Systemic EBV positive T-cell lymphoproliferative disease of childhood
Hydroa vacciniforme-like lymphoma
Adult T-cell leukemia/lymphoma
Extranodal NK cell/T-cell lymphoma, nasal type
Enteropathy-associated T-cell lymphoma
Hepatosplenic T-cell lymphoma
Subcutaneous panniculitis-like T-cell lymphoma
Mycosis fungoides
Sézary syndrome
Primary cutaneous CD30-positive T-cell lymphoproliferative disorders
  Lymphoid papulosis
  Primary cutaneous anaplastic large cell lymphoma
Primary cutaneous γ-δ T-cell lymphoma
Primary cutaneous CD8-positive aggressive epidermotropic cytotoxic T-cell lymphoma
Primary cutaneous CD4-positive small/medium T-cell lymphoma
Peripheral T-cell lymphoma, not otherwise specified
Angioimmunoblastic T-cell lymphoma
Anaplastic large cell lymphoma, ALK positive
Anaplastic large cell lymphoma, ALK negative

HODGKIN LYMPHOMA

Nodular lymphocyte predominant Hodgkin lymphoma
Classical Hodgkin lymphoma
Nodular sclerosis Hodgkin lymphoma
Lymphocyte-rich classical Hodgkin lymphoma
Mixed cellularity classical Hodgkin lymphoma
Lymphocyte-depleted classical Hodgkin lymphoma

*Provisional entities are shown in *italics*.

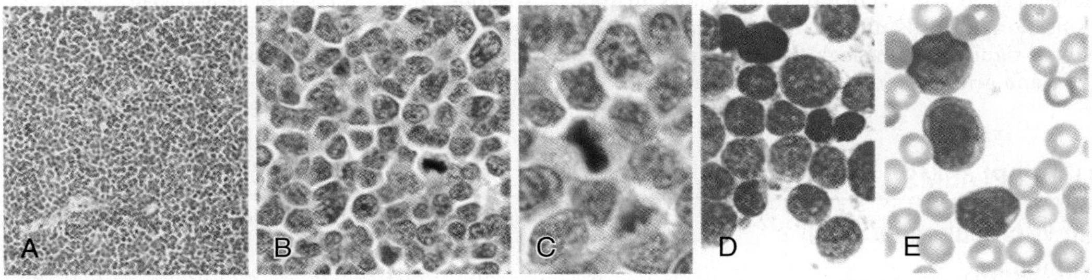

Figure 72-1 LYMPHOBLASTIC LYMPHOMA. Low-power **(A)** and higher power **(B)** views showing a diffuse infiltrate of intermediate-sized cells with high mitotic rate and finely dispersed "blastic" nuclear chromatin **(C).** Touch imprints performed at the time of the biopsy **(D)** illustrate the fact that the lymphoma cells are nearly identical to circulating lymphoblasts seen in acute lymphoblastic leukemia **(E).** The precursor B type cannot be easily distinguished from the precursor T-cell type without immunophenotyping.

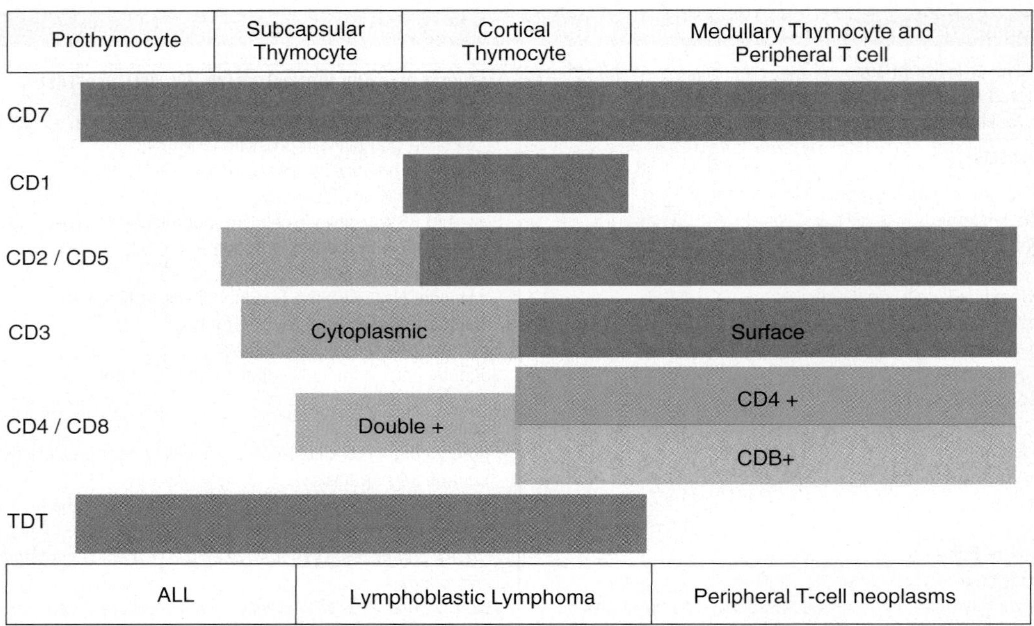

Figure 72-2 T-CELL NEOPLASMS RELATED TO STAGES OF T-CELL DIFFERENTIATION. *ALL,* Acute lymphoblastic leukemia.

About 50% to 80% of patients present with an anterior mediastinal mass, usually with involvement of the thymus gland. This is a high-grade lymphoma; the rapidly growing mass may be associated with airway obstruction. Bone marrow (BM) involvement is common, and progression to a leukemic picture occurs in the absence of effective therapy.

In lymph nodes, T-LBL has a diffuse pattern of infiltration. There is little stromal reaction, and the blasts infiltrate the nodal parenchyma with streaming of cells around vascular structures and spilling over the capsule. Mitotic figures are frequent with a starry-sky pattern seen in approximately one-third of cases.

By immunophenotypic studies, the blasts have an immature T-cell phenotype that correlates with different stages of intrathymic maturation based on the expression of numerous transcription factors. The blasts also express terminal deoxynucleotidyl transferase (TdT) (Fig. 72-2). The earliest T cell–associated antigen with some lineage specificity is CD7. However, it is also expressed in rare cases of acute myeloid leukemia as evidence of lineage infidelity, often present in primitive hematopoietic malignancies. CD3, linked to the T-cell antigen receptor, is detectable in the cytoplasm before its surface expression and thus may be negative when examined on fresh cells or by routine flow cytometry unless permeabilization techniques are used to detect cytoplasmic antigens. It should be noted that the normal thymocytes encountered in a lymphocyte-rich thymoma are phenotypically similar to the cells detected in T-LBL. The differential diagnosis can be quite challenging, especially on needle core biopsies and immunohistochemical analysis, and molecular studies may be necessary. The classification of B-LBL and T-LBL has attained greater accuracy and prognostic significance through the application of GEP, copy number analysis, and genome-wide profiling of structural DNA alterations.[1]

MATURE B-CELL NEOPLASMS

Chronic Lymphocytic Leukemia/Small Lymphocytic Lymphoma

Chronic lymphocytic leukemia/small lymphocytic lymphoma (CLL/SLL) usually presents in adults with generalized lymphadenopathy, frequent BM and peripheral blood involvement, and often hepatosplenomegaly. Presentation as leukemia, that is, CLL, is more common than as lymphoma, SLL. Even in patients with a lymphomatous presentation, careful examination of the blood may reveal a circulating monoclonal B-cell component. Nevertheless, some patients present with generalized adenopathy, and although progression to CLL is frequent, it does not necessarily occur in all cases.

The increased sensitivity of immunophenotypic and molecular methodologies has resulted in the detection of clonal lymphoid proliferations with a CLL phenotype in the general population even in the absence of clinical lymphocytosis, a condition now designated monoclonal B-cell lymphocytosis (MBL) (see box on Early Events in Lymphoid Neoplasia). The International Workshop on CLL proposed new diagnostic criteria that were then included in the WHO classification of 2008. Recent studies have indeed shown that the absolute count of monoclonal B cells greater than 5.0×10^9/L is clinically more relevant than the absolute lymphocyte count in predicting outcome.[2] Similar to peripheral blood, small clonal populations with a CLL phenotype can be detected in lymph nodes as an incidental finding and appear to represent a tissue counterpart of MBL.[3] At a recent workshop of the European Association for Haematopathology and the Society of Hematopathology (Uppsala, September 2010), the term *lymph node involvement by monoclonal CLL-type B cells of unknown clinical significance* was suggested for such lesions, borrowing from terminology of plasma cell neoplasms.

Histologically, the lymph node involved by CLL/SLL shows diffuse architectural effacement (Fig. 72-3), although occasional residual naked germinal centers can be observed. The predominant cell type is a small lymphocyte with clumped chromatin, but a spectrum of nuclear morphology is usually seen. Pseudofollicular growth centers or proliferation centers are present in the majority of cases and contain a spectrum of cells ranging from small lymphocytes to prolymphocytes and paraimmunoblasts. The prolymphocytes and paraimmunoblasts have more dispersed chromatin and more prominent nucleoli usually centrally placed. The presence of proliferation centers is also a helpful criterion in the differential diagnosis with mantle cell lymphoma (MCL), which may show otherwise some overlapping features with CLL. If needed, immunophenotypic studies can be helpful in this differential diagnosis.

CLL/SLL is characterized by $CD5^+$, $CD23^+$, B cells expressing dim CD20, and usually dim surface immunoglobulin (sIg). The lack of staining for Cyclin D1 can help rule out MCL. CLL has been shown

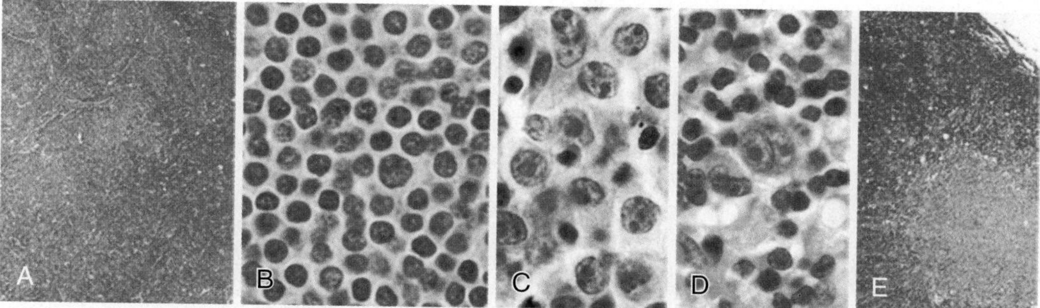

Figure 72-3 SMALL LYMPHOCYTIC LYMPHOMA (SLL). Low-power view **(A)** illustrates a diffuse effacement of the lymph node. A monotonous population of small lymphocytes is seen at higher power **(B)**. These have fairly round nuclear contours, condensed nuclear chromatin, and inconspicuous or absent nucleoli. Only rare larger cells are present. SLL can transform to large cell lymphoma **(C)** and occasionally to Hodgkin lymphoma **(D)**. Patients can also develop worsening lymphadenopathy from viral infections such as herpes simplex virus, in which the node typically shows focal necrosis **(E)**.

Early Events in Lymphoid Neoplasia

- In recent years, there has been a greater appreciation of early events in lymphoid neoplasia.
- These early lesions can in some ways be considered equivalent to benign neoplasms in the epithelial system.
- These are clonal proliferations of B cells or T cells that carry genetic aberrations associated with specific forms of lymphoid neoplasia, including CLL, multiple myeloma, follicular lymphoma, and mantle cell lymphoma.
- Examples include monoclonal gammopathy of undetermined significance, MBL, follicular lymphoma in situ, mantle cell lymphoma in situ, lymphomatoid papulosis, patch stage of mycosis fungoides, and primary cutaneous $CD4^+$ small/medium T-cell lymphoma.
- Early lesions appear to lack the secondary and tertiary "hits" seen in lymphoid neoplasms that are clinically significant, and most patients have a very low risk of clinical progression.
- Challenges for the future are:
  - To define the precise genetic features that distinguish early lesions from lymphoma.
  - To assess the risk of clinical progression.
  - To determine how these patients should be managed clinically.

to have a greater degree of heterogeneity biologically, and different subgroups have been identified based on immunoglobulin heavy chain mutational status, cytogenetics, ZAP-70 expression, and CD38 expression.[4] The latter two have been used as partial surrogate markers for the mutational status. ZAP-70 expression correlates with an unmutated status and a poorer prognosis. In fact, ZAP-70 expression has been suggested to be more clinically relevant than mutation status when the two markers are discordant. The use of CD38 as a surrogate marker for mutational status is less useful, but its high expression is also associated with a poor prognosis. Recently, additional new recurrent somatic mutations have been identified in CLL using whole-genome and -exome sequencing techniques, and some of them have been associated with clinical outcome.[5]

Histologic transformation over time may occur in CLL, a phenomenon known as Richter syndrome. Short of progression to diffuse large B-cell lymphoma (DLBCL), lymph nodes may show an increased number of prolymphocytes and paraimmunoblasts, recently proposed as "accelerated phase."[6] A Hodgkin-like transformation has also been described in CLL/SLL. This transformation can take one of two forms. In some cases, Reed-Sternberg (RS) cells and mononuclear variants are seen in a background of small round B lymphocytes, consistent with CLL. The process lacks the rich inflammatory background characteristic of Hodgkin lymphoma, such as eosinophils, plasma cells, and histiocytes. However, patients with this type of Hodgkin transformation appear to progress to a process that is more typical of Hodgkin lymphoma, with loss of the B-cell small lymphocytic component. In other instances, classical Hodgkin lymphoma (CHL) of the mixed cellularity or nodular sclerosis subtype may be seen in patients with a history of CLL. Studies have implicated Epstein-Barr virus (EBV) in the Hodgkin type of Richter transformation. The RS cells and variants are EBV positive and in some cases have been shown to be derived from the CLL clone. In other instances, diverse clonal origins are shown.

Lymphoplasmacytic Lymphoma

The term lymphoplasmacytic lymphoma (LPL) should be limited to cases that do not fulfill the criteria for any other type of B-cell neoplasm with plasmacytic differentiation. Also, the definition of Waldenström macroglobulinemia (WM) and its relationship to LPL have been complex. The WHO classification (2008) adopted the approach advocated at the second international workshop on WM, which defined WM as the presence of an IgM monoclonal gammopathy of any concentration associated with BM involvement by LPL.[7] Hence, LPL and WM are not synonymous, with WM defying a subset of LPL.

This is a disease of adult life that usually presents with BM involvement and sometimes with nodal and splenic involvement (splenomegaly), vague constitutional symptoms, and anemia (see Chapter 86). The tumor consists of a diffuse proliferation of small lymphocytes, plasmacytoid lymphocytes, and plasma cells, with or without Dutcher bodies (see Fig. 72-4). The growth pattern is often interfollicular with sparing of the sinuses. The cells have surface and cytoplasmic Ig, usually of IgM type, usually lack IgD, and express B cell–associated antigens (CD19, 20, 22, 79a). They are usually negative for CD5 and CD10. CD25 or CD11c may be weakly expressed in some cases. The lack of CD5 and the presence of strong cytoplasmic Ig are useful in distinction from CLL. The postulated normal counterpart is thought to be a postfollicular medullary cord B cell based in part on the presence of somatic mutations in the Ig heavy- and light-chain variable region genes.

Deletion of 6q21–22.1 occurs in about half of cases but is not a specific finding.[8a] LPL shows morphological and immunophenotypic overlap with some cases of marginal zone lymphoma with plasmacytic differentiation. Recent studies have identified recurrent mutations of *MYD88* in LPL but not in marginal zone lymphomas, confirming these are distinct entities, and providing a genetic test for diagnosis.[8b]

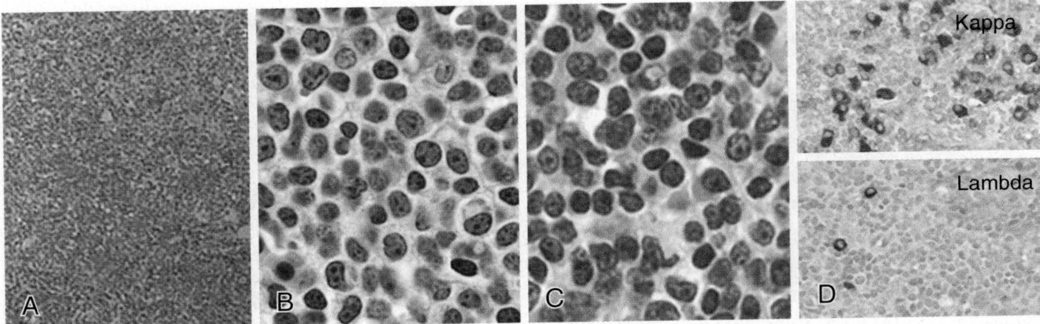

Figure 72-4 LYMPHOPLASMACYTIC LYMPHOMA (LPL). LPL and Waldenström macroglobulinemia have nearly identical morphology. There is a diffuse infiltrate **(A)** of small lymphocytes that have plasmacytoid features or interspersed plasma cells (**B,** bone marrow; **C,** lymph node). Intranuclear inclusions can sometimes be seen. Evaluation for κ and λ by immunohistochemical stains can demonstrate clonality in the plasma cells and plasmacytoid lymphocytes **(D).**

Mantle Cell Lymphoma

Mantle cell lymphoma is a distinct entity that has been more precisely defined in recent years through the integration of immunophenotypic, molecular genetic, and clinicopathologic studies. The molecular hallmark of MCL is the t(11;14)(q13;q32) involving cyclin D1 *(CCND1)* and the IGH@ gene. Cyclin D1 overexpression is believed to be essential in the pathogenesis of MCL. However, rare variants negative for cyclin D1 with similar immunomorphology and gene expression signature have been identified. Cyclin D1–negative forms usually express either cyclin D2 or cyclin D3, which may functionally substitute for cyclin D1. Sox11 is overexpressed in most cyclin D1–positive and –negative cases.[9]

The postulated normal counterpart is the CD5$^+$ "naive" B cell, sIgM$^+$ and sIgD$^+$, which can be found in the peripheral blood and in the mantle of reactive germinal centers. Mutational analysis of the rearranged immunoglobulin variable region genes shows few or no somatic mutations; however, similarly to CLL, a subset of MCL has mutated *IG* genes.

Recently, because of the widespread use of immunohistochemistry, early involvement of lymph node by cells carrying t(11;14) translocation with subsequent overexpression of cyclin D1 has been documented in several cases, so-called "in situ MCL." Most often these represent an incidental finding, but some cases eventually progress to overt MCL.[10] In some cases, in situ MCL is detected in a lymph node involved by another lymphoma type, such as follicular lymphoma (FL). The risk of progression of in situ MCL is difficult to ascertain because the number of reported cases is few. In a recent multicenter retrospective study, it was noted that the expression of SOX-11 was more frequently associated with progression to MCL because the majority of in situ cases lacked SOX-11 expression.[10] Also similar to FL in situ, a distinction should be made between partial involvement by MCL with a mantle zone pattern and in situ MCL. The latter refers to a reactive lymph node with cyclin D1–positive cells limited to an otherwise normally appearing follicle mantle; these cases tend not to progress, and they should not be labeled as lymphomas.

Another newly identified variant is an indolent form of MCL characterized by a leukemic phase without nodal disease but often with long-standing splenomegaly. These patients have an indolent clinical course and do not appear to require aggressive chemotherapy.[11] These cases carry t(11;14) with few additional chromosomal abnormalities and lack expression of SOX11 in contrast to conventional MCL.

Mantle cell lymphoma occurs in adults (median age, 62 years), with a high male-to-female ratio. Most patients present with advanced stage at diagnosis. Common sites of involvement include the lymph nodes, spleen, BM, and lymphoid tissue of Waldeyer ring. Gastrointestinal tract involvement is frequent and is associated with the picture of lymphomatous polyposis.

The hallmark of MCL is a very monotonous cellular composition. In the typical case, the cells are slightly larger than a normal lymphocyte with finely clumped chromatin, scant cytoplasm, and inconspicuous nucleoli (Fig. 72-5). The nuclear contour is usually irregular or cleaved. Some cytologic variants, blastoid (blastic) and pleomorphic, tend to be associated with a more aggressive course and adverse biologic features, such as tetraploidy or p53 mutation or deletion. The proliferation rate was previously identified as prognostically important based on scoring of Ki67-positive cells. More recently, GEP, using genes involved in cell cycle progression and DNA synthesis, has identified a proliferation signature that delineates cohorts with varied prognosis. These correlate to some extent with cytologic subtype.[12] For example, the blastoid variant has a high proliferation rate using both Ki67 and GEP.

Follicular Lymphoma

Follicular lymphoma is the most common subtype of NHL within the United States and accounts for approximately 45% of all newly diagnosed cases. It has a peak incidence in the fifth and sixth decades of life and is rare before the age of 20 years. Men and women are equally affected. FL is less common in black and Asian populations. Most patients have stage 3 or 4 disease at diagnosis, with generalized lymphadenopathy. Staging evaluation usually detects BM involvement. Approximately 10% of patients have circulating malignant cells. However, careful immunophenotypic or molecular analyses may disclose peripheral blood involvement in a higher proportion of patients. A more accurate prognostic index than the IPI, the FLIPI, has been proposed for FL and has been widely adopted.

The natural history of the disease is associated with histologic progression in both pattern and cell type (Fig. 72-6). A heterogeneous cytologic composition is one of the hallmarks of FL. Usually, all of the follicle center cells are represented but in varying proportions. It should be stressed that the variation in cytologic grade is a continuum, and therefore precise morphologic criteria for subclassification are difficult to establish.

According to the WHO classification, all low-grade FLs are combined into a single category, grade 1 to 2, all containing overall a predominance of centrocytes with fewer than 15 centroblasts per high-power field (hpf). FL grade 3 (with >15 centroblasts/hpf) is further subdivided into grades 3A and 3B based on the presence or absence of centrocytes in the background. Other factors that may influence outcome in FL include the tumor microenvironment, highlighted initially by GEP.[13]

The vast majority of FL (≈85%) are associated with a t(14;18) involving rearrangement of the *BCL2* gene. This translocation appears to result in constitutive expression of Bcl-2 protein, which is capable of inhibiting apoptosis in lymphoid cells. The cells of FL accumulate and are at risk to acquire secondary mutations, which may be

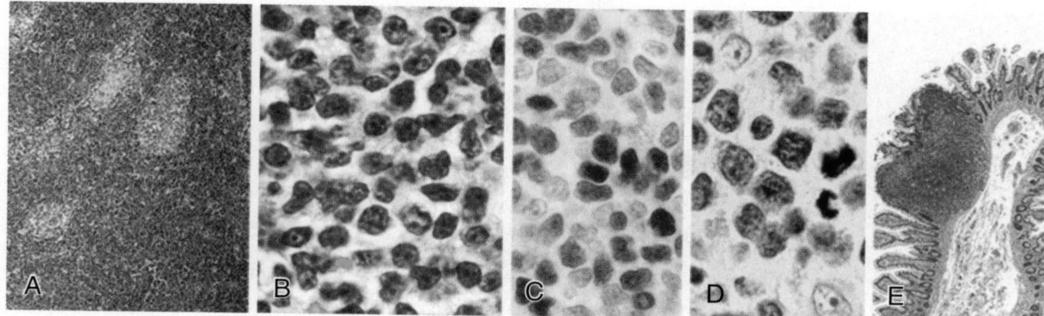

Figure 72-5 MANTLE CELL LYMPHOMA (MCL). At low power, MCL can show a diffuse, vaguely nodular, or mantle zone pattern. In the latter, the neoplastic mantle zones are expanded and can become confluent leaving "naked" germinal centers **(A).** At higher power, the lymphoma cells are small or slightly enlarged **(B).** They have irregular nuclear contours, especially compared with small lymphocytic lymphoma, and they have a dense chromatin. Typically, cases are positive for cyclin D1 expression **(C),** which is related to the t(11;14) involving IgH and *CCND1*. Some cases can develop a "blastoid" transformation **(D),** although some cases can present as a "blastoid" variant. Such cases are characterized by cells with an intermediate size, a high mitotic rate, and finely dispersed "blastic" chromatin. Sometimes when the "blastoid" cases develop a leukemic phase, they can be difficult to distinguish morphologically from acute lymphoblastic leukemia. In such cases, flow immunophenotyping is needed to resolve the differential diagnosis. MCL can also present with gastrointestinal involvement **(E)** as in lymphomatoid papulosis.

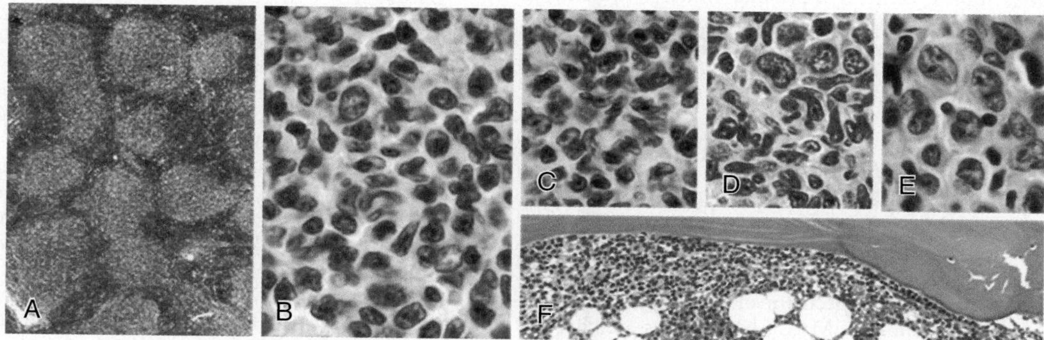

Figure 72-6 FOLLICULAR LYMPHOMA (FL). FL shows effacement of the normal lymph node architecture because of an accumulation of neoplastic lymphoid follicles that lack the features of reactive follicles **(A).** They are crowded, show back-to-back localization, lack distinct mantle zones, and show no polarity. The lymphoma cells are highly irregular **(B)** with elongated, twisted, or clefted nuclear contours and dense chromatin. FL is typically graded into grade 1 or 2 (1/2; **C, D**), or 3 **(E),** depending on the number of large cells seen at higher power (see text). FL typically involves the bone marrow with lymphoma cells spreading along the bone **(F).** This localization is termed "paratrabecular."

associated with histologic progression. It has been postulated that the *BCL2/IGH@* translocation occurs during immunoglobulin gene rearrangement in the BM at the pre–B cell stage of development. This fact might contribute to the difficulty in eradicating the neoplastic clone with chemotherapy.

Biologically, the pathogenesis of most cases of FL grade 3B differs from that of FL grade 1 and 2 in lacking the BCL2/IGH@ but also differs from DLBCL in having a low incidence of BCL6 aberrations.[14] These data provide a biologic explanation for the greater curability of grade 3 FL with aggressive therapy, although some studies have not found support for this hypothesis. Differences in diagnostic criteria might account for this apparent discrepancy, and the correlation between grade 3A versus 3B and molecular alterations is imprecise. In light of these data, cytologic grading is assuming less importance in clinical trials and clinical practice. Evolution toward a molecularly defined classification of FL is a possibility for the future.

The phenomenon of localization of FL cells to isolated germinal centers within a lymph node has been termed in situ FL.[15] This pattern may be seen with FL at other sites of disease or may be the only manifestation of disease in some patients. The risk for progression in this latter group is not fully established, but if no other evidence of FL is seen at initial clinical evaluation, the likelihood of evolution to clinically significant FL is low. Indeed, this translocation can be found in the peripheral blood and lymphoid organs of healthy individuals and suggests that the *BCL2/IGH@* translocation is necessary but not sufficient for the development of FL.[16] "In situ FL" (also termed intrafollicular neoplasia) is a distinctive lesion and should be distinguished from partial involvement by FL.[15] In the true "in situ" lesion, clusters of B cells strongly positive for CD10 and BCL2 are localized to germinal centers in an otherwise reactive lymph node. It often represents an incidental finding in a lymph node biopsied for other reasons. The term "FL-like B-cells of unknown significance" was recently proposed for this lesion.[17]

The 2008 WHO classification recognizes other lymphomas of follicle center derivation that may resemble nodal FL but exhibit significant differences either clinically or biologically. These include pediatric FL, primary intestinal FL, and cutaneous lymphomas of follicle center cell derivation. Intestinal FL, most often presenting in the duodenum, is associated with the BCL2/IGH@ translocation but usually presents as isolated mucosal polyps with a low risk of dissemination.[18] Conversely, pediatric FL is often extranodal at presentation, usually grade 3B, and not associated with translocations of BCL2. At least some cases have been shown to have a different molecular pathogenesis.[19,20] These tumors are usually associated with a good prognosis, and in some patients, complete remissions may be

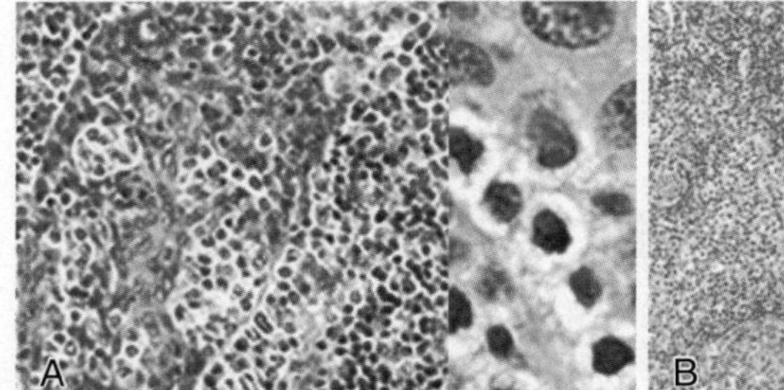

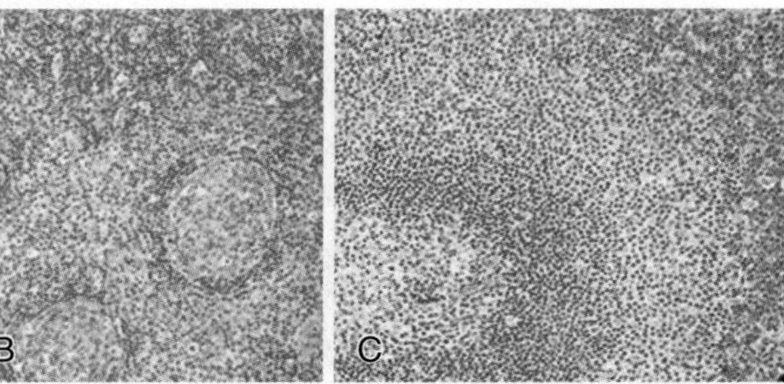

Figure 72-7 MARGINAL ZONE LYMPHOMA. Marginal zone lymphomas commonly occur at extranodal sites arising from mucosa-associated lymphoid tissue (MALT). MALT lymphomas typically infiltrate or invade into epithelial structures, resulting in "lymphoepithelial lesions" **(A).** They are composed of small- to intermediate-sized cells with abundant clear cytoplasms (**A,** *detail*). The normal lymph node does not have a marginal zone, but primary nodal marginal zone lymphomas (NMZL) can occur. They infiltrate the node in what would be a marginal zone pattern with an expansion of cells peripheral to mantle zone **(B).** The spleen does have a normal marginal zone, and this can give rise to a splenic marginal zone lymphoma (SMZL). Early on, these show expansion of the marginal zone areas **(C)** but later can become more diffuse, infiltrating the red pulp. In the case illustrated, the spleen weighed 1700 g.

obtained with either surgical excision or local radiation therapy. The pediatric variant of FL is more common in males than females.

Primary cutaneous follicle center lymphoma, which frequently lacks the *BCL2* translocation and BCL2 expression, is now considered by the WHO classification as a separate entity.[17] However, when BCL2 expression is detected, the possibility that this may represent a secondary site of involvement should be considered.

Extranodal Marginal Zone Lymphoma of Mucosa-Associated Lymphoid Tissue Type

Most lymphomas of marginal-zone derivation present in extranodal sites and have the histopathologic and clinical features identified by Isaacson and Wright as part of the spectrum of mucosa-associated lymphoid tissue (MALT) lymphomas. MALT lymphomas are characterized by a heterogeneous cellular composition that includes marginal-zone or centrocyte-like cells, monocytoid B cells, small lymphocytes, and plasma cells (Fig. 72-7, *A*). In most cases, large transformed cells are infrequent. Reactive germinal centers are nearly always present. When follicular colonization occurs, the process may simulate FL. Clonality is confirmed by molecular and or immunohistochemical studies.

MALT lymphomas have been described in nearly every anatomic site but are most frequent in the stomach, lung, thyroid, salivary gland, and lacrimal gland. Other less common sites of involvement include the orbit, breast, conjunctiva, bladder and kidney, and thymus gland. Widespread nodal involvement is infrequent, as is BM involvement. The clinical course is usually quite indolent, and many patients are asymptomatic. MALT lymphomas tend to relapse in other MALT-associated sites.

MALT lymphomas of the salivary gland and thyroid are usually associated with a history of autoimmune diseases. Helicobacter gastritis is frequent in most patients with gastric MALT lymphomas. Other infectious agents have been described in MALT lymphomas involving the skin *(Borrelia burgdorferi),* ocular adnexae *(Chlamydia psittaci),* and small intestine *(Campylobacter jejuni);* however, in this latter group, a causal relationship has not yet been demonstrated. Chronic antigen stimulation is critical to both the development of a MALT lymphoma and the maintenance of the neoplastic state. Indeed, in some cases, antibiotic therapy and the eradication of *Helicobacter pylori* have led to the spontaneous remission of gastric MALT lymphoma in cases lacking genetic aberrations.

By immunophenotype, MALT lymphomas are positive for B cell–associated antigens CD19, CD20, and CD22 but are negative for CD5 and CD10. The absence of cyclin D1 is useful in ruling out MCL, especially in intestinal disease. Rare cases of MALT lymphoma have been reported to be CD5 positive, and in some but not all instances, this has been associated with more aggressive disease.

MALT lymphomas also have several recurring cytogenetic abnormalities, including t(11;18)(q21;q21), t(1;14)(p22;q32), t(14;18)(q32;q21), t(3;14)(q27;q32), and t(3;14)(p14.1;q32), which are observed with variable frequency, often depending on the anatomic site. Although several genes are involved in these translocations, at least three of them—(t(11;18), t(1;14) and t(14;18)—share a common pathway, which leads to the activation of nuclear factor kappa-B (NFκB) and its downstream targets. By genome-wide DNA profiling integrated with GEP, differences were detected among the three different main types of marginal zone lymphomas, lending support to the current WHO classification, which separates these three entities.[21]

The WHO Clinical Advisory Committee recommended that the term *high-grade MALT* not be used for extranodal large cell lymphomas in a "MALT" site and in fact stated that this term should be avoided because of its ambiguity. The clinical significance of increased transformed cells is still uncertain. The putative cell of origin of MALT lymphoma is a post-germinal center B-cell.

Nodal Marginal Zone Lymphoma

Nodal marginal zone lymphoma (NMZL) is a primary nodal disease, which resembles other marginal zone lymphomas, extranodal or splenic types. These patients often present with BM involvement and tend to have a more aggressive clinical course than those with extranodal MALT. The neoplastic proliferation is polymorphous and composed of monocytoid B cells and plasmacytoid cells with interspersed large blastlike cells. There is an expansion of the marginal zone area, often with preservation of the nodal architecture (Fig. 72-7, *B*). The mantle zone may be intact, attenuated, or effaced. The immunophenotype is similar to other MZL, that is, CD20 positive, CD10 negative, and CD5 negative, with variable expression of IgD (weak to negative). Because there are no precise immunophenotypic or genotypic markers of NMZL, the diagnosis is sometimes one of exclusion. The differential diagnosis with LPL may be problematic. A variant of nodal MZL occurs in children; these cases shows a striking male predominance, present with localized disease, and can be managed with local therapies.[22]

Splenic Marginal Zone Lymphoma

Splenic marginal zone lymphomas (SMZLs) present in adults and are slightly more frequent in women than men. The clinical presentation is splenomegaly, usually without peripheral lymphadenopathy. The

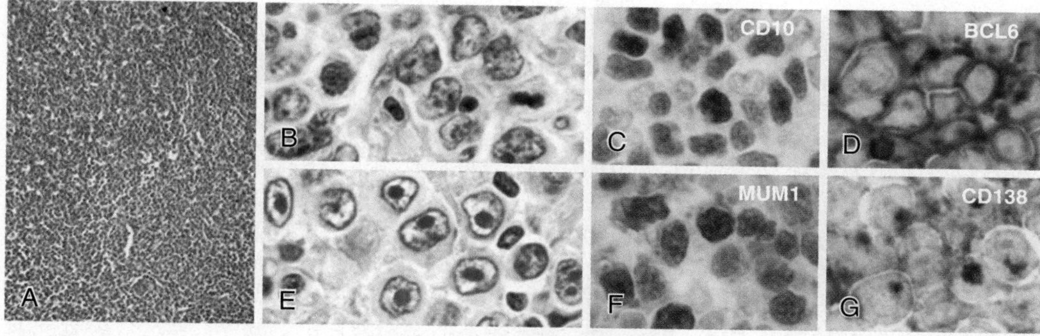

Figure 72-8 DIFFUSE LARGE B-CELL LYMPHOMA (DLBCL). The low power illustration demonstrates the diffuse nature of the process **(A).** At high power **(B),** there are sheets of large cells. Those with a vesicular nuclear chromatin and variable numbers of nucleoli along the nuclear membrane are referred to as centroblasts. These typically have a germinal center gene expression profile and a germinal center immunophenotype with expression of BCL6 and CD10 (**C** and **D**). Those cases composed of large cells with a single prominent nucleolus **(E)** are called immunoblastic and commonly have an activated B-cell (ABC) gene expression profile and an ABC phenotype with expression of Mum-1, CD138 (**F** and **G**), and IFR-4. The correlation of morphology and immunophenotype is not always exact.

majority of patients have BM involvement, but there is usually only a modest lymphocytosis, with elevations in the lymphocyte count usually less than that seen in CLL. Some evidence of plasmacytoid differentiation may be seen, and patients may have a small M component. The abundant pale cytoplasm evident in tissue sections may also be seen in blood smears. The course is indolent, and splenectomy may be followed by a prolonged remission.

Histologically, the spleen shows expansion of the white pulp but usually some infiltration of the red pulp is present as well (see Fig. 72-7, *C*). A characteristic biphasic pattern in the neoplastic white pulp has been described, with the neoplastic cells surrounding regressed follicles. The immunophenotype of these cells resembles that of other marginal-zone B-cell lymphomas; however, IgD expression is more frequently observed. Progression to DLBCL can be seen.

Although the molecular pathogenesis of SMZL has not been delineated, a frequent cytogenetic alteration involving deletions of the region 7q(22-32) has been reported.[23] Studies of the Ig variable genes have also revealed the presence of mutations suggesting a postfollicular origin, but variations in this profile have been observed. The differential diagnosis of SMZL includes other unspecified B-cell lymphomas of the spleen, including splenic lymphoma with villous lymphocytes (SLVL), and hairy cell variant. The latter have been grouped together under splenic B-cell lymphoma/leukemia unclassifiable, and the interrelationship among these disorders is not fully resolved.

> **Varied Basis for the Recognition of Diverse Entities Among Aggressive B-Cell Neoplasms**
>
> **Cell of Origin, in Part as Determined by Gene Expression Profiling**
> - Activated B cell versus germinal center B cell
> - Thymic B cell of PMBL
>
> **Clinical Factors**
> - Anatomic site (e.g., CNS, mediastinum, intravascular)
> - Advanced age, background of chronic inflammation
>
> **Etiologic Factors**
> - EBV, HHV-8
>
> **Molecular Pathogenesis**
> - *BCL6, C-MYC, ALK, BCL2, MYD88* (translocations, amplification, mutation)
>
> *ABC,* Activated B cell; *CNS,* central nervous system *GCB,* germinal center B cells; *PMBL,* primary mediastinal large B-cell lymphoma.

Diffuse Large B-Cell Lymphoma, Not Otherwise Specified

Diffuse large B-cell lymphoma is one of the more common subtypes of NHL, representing up to 40% of cases. It has an aggressive natural history but responds well to chemotherapy. The complete remission rate with modern regimens is 75% to 80%, with long-term disease-free survival approaching 50% or more in most series. This lymphoma may present in lymph nodes or in extranodal sites. Frequent extranodal sites of involvement include bone, skin, thyroid, gastrointestinal tract, and lung.

Diffuse large B-cell lymphoma represents one of the most heterogeneous categories in the WHO classification, and attempts to identify prognostic groups based on morphology and phenotype have shown limited usefulness and reproducibility (see box on Varied Basis for the Recognition of Diverse Entities Among Aggressive B-Cell Neoplasms). To address these issues, DLBCLs were among the first cases to be analyzed by cDNA array technology and more recently also by genome-wide analysis.[24] By GEP, three groups were identified based on the differential expression of a large set of genes, namely germinal center–like group (GCB), activated B cell–like group (ABC), and primary mediastinal (thymic) large B-cell lymphoma (PMBL). The expression profile reflects a corresponding non-neoplastic counterpart, which shares similarity with germinal center B cells (GCB), and postgerminal center B cells (ABC). A unique signature was identified by GEP in PMBL, which shared similarities with CHL cell lines, including constitutive activation of the NFκB and recurrent gains and amplification of c-Rel. More recently, frequent genetic defects have been identified in the BCR-signaling and NFkB pathways in the ABC subtype providing new insight in the pathogenesis of DLBCL and new potential therapeutic targets.[25,26a] Recurrent mutations in the GCB type of DLBCL appear to target histone-modifying genes.[24,26b] Somatic mutations in *EZH2* also have been identified in FL, another tumor of germinal center derivation.

Diffuse large B-cell lymphomas are composed of large, transformed lymphoid cells with nuclei at least twice the size of a small lymphocyte (Fig. 72-8). The nuclei generally have vesicular chromatin, prominent nucleoli, and basophilic cytoplasm, resembling the centroblasts of the normal germinal center. The immunoblastic variant is characterized by cells with prominent central nucleoli and abundant deeply staining cytoplasm. Although there is no absolute correlation between morphology and GEP, the majority of centroblastic DLBCL falls into the GCB group and the majority of immunoblastic into the ABC group.

Algorithms based on immunophenotype have been proposed as surrogates for cDNA microarray using CD10/BCL-6 positivity for GCB and Mum-1/IRF-4 for ABC with the addition of BCL-2 in

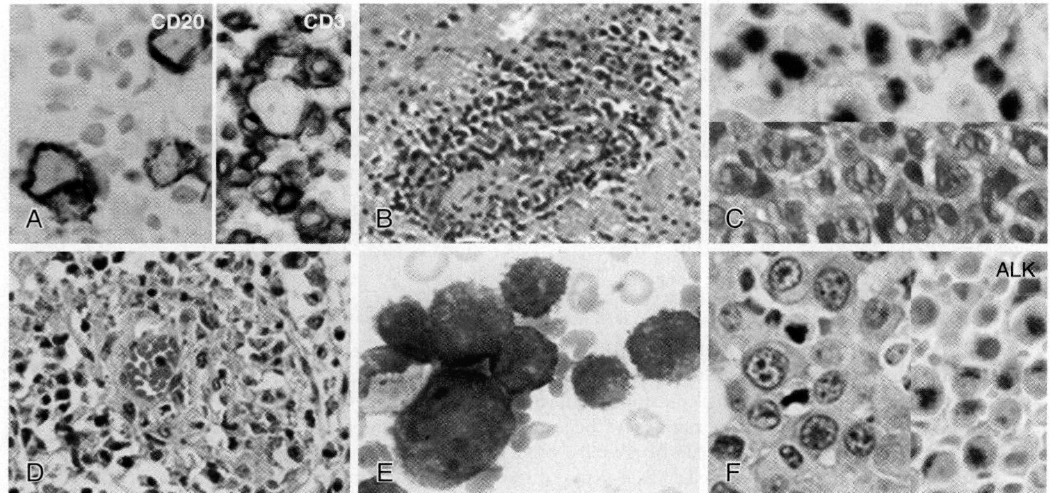

Figure 72-9 DIFFUSE LARGE B-CELL LYMPHOMA (DLBCL) VARIANTS AND SUBTYPES. T-cell/histiocyte-rich large B-cell lymphoma is illustrated in **A,** where a CD20 immunostain *(right)* identifies scattered large B cells, which are associated with a prominent background of small reactive T cells (CD3; *left*). Sometimes there are numerous histiocytes in the background or an admixture of reactive T cells and histiocytes. Primary DLBCL of the central nervous system usually shows a perivascular distribution (**B**). Epstein-Barr virus (EBV)–positive DLBCL of the elderly can have variable morphologic features sometimes with a polymorphic mixture of large cells and small lymphocytes and plasma cells. Sometimes they can be monomorphic and composed of large cells, which are positive for EBV-encoded RNA (EBER) (**C,** *bottom* and *top*). Lymphomatoid granulomatosis (**D**) also has a perivascular distribution and is composed of a mix of malignant large EBV-positive B cells and reactive T cells. Primary effusion lymphoma usually is diagnosed from cytologic preparations (**E**) and by flow cytometric and molecular techniques. Although the tumor cells do not generally form masses, recent reports have identified a solid variant. Plasmablastic B-cell lymphoma is quite rare and can show ALK positivity as a consequence of a translocation of *ALK* (**F**).

combination with IPI and may improve the stratification of DLBCL. However, there is as yet no consensus for the best model to address the heterogeneity of DLBCL, and the correlation with GEP has been questioned.[17]

Diffuse Large B-Cell Lymphomas: Other Variants and Subtypes

The spectrum of aggressive B-cell lymphomas has broadened in recent years, incorporating new entities based on unique clinical features such as age or anatomic site, viral pathogenesis (EBV, human herpesvirus 8 [HHV-8]), or distinctive pathological features.[27]

T-cell or histiocyte-rich large B-cell lymphoma (THRLBCL) is now considered a distinct clinical pathologic entity rather than a morphologic variant of DLBCL (see Fig. 72-9, *A*). It has been associated with aggressive clinical behavior and often presents in younger patients than typical DLBCL with advanced stage and BM involvement. The relevance of the microenvironment and recruitment mechanism of the inflammatory cells, which are the main histological component, has been the focus of recent studies.[28]

The WHO classification recognizes that some lymphomas arising in certain anatomic sites may have distinctive features both clinically and biologically. Among these are *primary DLBCL of the central nervous system (CNS)* and *primary cutaneous DLBCL, leg type.* Primary DLBCL of the CNS (see Fig. 72-9, *B*) has some distinctive features based on GEP and shares some similarities with DLBCL arising in other immune privileged sites such as the testis.[17] Primary cutaneous DLBCL, leg type, has a GEP resembling the ABC type of DLBCL, presents most often in elderly women, and generally has an aggressive clinical course. As with nodal DLBCL, Bcl-2 expression is an adverse prognostic factor.

There are several EBV-positive B-cell lymphoproliferations that are often grouped with DLBCL. *EBV-positive DLBCL of the elderly* is a provisional entity in the 2008 WHO classification.[29] It appears to develop as a consequence of decreased immune surveillance. The morphological spectrum is broad and includes polymorphous and more monomorphic tumors (see Fig. 72-9, *C*). Most cases have an aggressive clinical course and should be distinguished from atypical hyperplasia associated with EBV and lesions with a self-limited course, such as EBV-positive mucocutaneous ulcer.

Lymphomatoid granulomatosis is an EBV-positive B-cell lymphoproliferative disorder (LPD) associated with an inflammatory background rich in T cells (Fig. 72-9, *D*). The lung is nearly always involved, with the skin, kidney, liver, and brain being frequently affected as well. *DLBCL associated with chronic inflammation* was first described in association with chronic pyothorax but now has been associated with EBV-driven large B-cell proliferations in diverse clinical settings, usually associated with a confined anatomic space and a background of chronic inflammation. These cases appear to have a good prognosis if successfully resected.

Several LPDs are associated with HHV-8/Kaposi sarcoma–associated herpesvirus. These include *primary effusion lymphoma (PEL)* and *multicentric Castleman disease (MCD),* as well as lymphomas arising in the context of MCD. The cells of PEL are usually coinfected with EBV, and the disease is most often diagnosed in the setting of HIV infection and immunosuppression. Although pleural or peritoneal effusions are most common (Fig. 72-9, *E*), extracavitary PEL can present as a tumor mass, usually in extranodal sites. PEL has a phenotype resembling that of terminally differentiated B cells (i.e., plasmablastic).

Two other lymphomas with a plasmablastic phenotype include *plasmablastic lymphoma (PBL)* and *ALK-positive large B-cell lymphoma.* PBL is usually positive for EBV, most often extranodal, and associated with immunosuppression from either HIV infection or advanced age. Recent studies have identified a high incidence of MYC translocations in PBL.[30] ALK-positive large B-cell lymphomas show overexpression of ALK (Fig. 72-9, *F*), usually as a consequence of translocation involving the ALK gene. They mainly affect older individuals but can occur at any age. Interestingly, IgA is most often expressed.

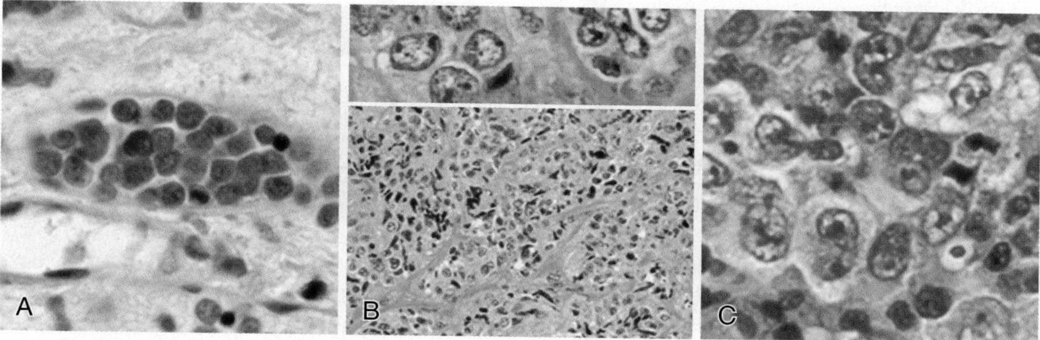

Figure 72-10 DIFFUSE LARGE B-CELL LYMPHOMA (DLBCL) VARIANTS (INTRAVASCULAR, MEDIASTINAL, UNCLASSIFIABLE). In intravascular lymphoma, also known as angiotropic lymphoma, the large B cells are confined to the inside of vessels **(A)**. Paradoxically, they do not spread to the blood. Primary mediastinal (thymic) large B-cell lymphoma typically shows sclerosis and large B cells immeshed in the fibrosis (**B,** *top* and *bottom*). An unclassifiable type of lymphoma has features intermediate between large B-cell lymphoma and Hodgkin lymphoma. In the case illustrated **(C)**, the male patient presented with a mediastinal mass. The cells were $CD30^+$ and only variably positive for CD45 as in Hodgkin lymphoma, but they were strongly and uniformly positive for CD20 and PAX5. They also strongly expressed the B-cell transcription factors OCT2 and BOB1.

Intravascular Large B-Cell Lymphoma

Intravascular large B-cell lymphoma is a rare form of DLBCL characterized by the presence of lymphoma cells only in the lumens of small vessels, particularly capillaries (Fig. 72-10, *A*). These cells are nearly always of B-cell phenotype, often with aberrant expression of CD5. The tumor cells are large, with vesicular nuclei and prominent nucleoli, resembling centroblasts or immunoblasts. Lymph node involvement is rare, and the tumor presents in extranodal sites, most readily diagnosed in the skin. Neurologic symptoms associated with plugging of small vessels in the CNS are common. The disease is often not diagnosed until autopsy because of the lack of definitive radiologic or clinical evidence of disease and diverse symptomatology.

Primary Mediastinal (Thymic) Large B-Cell Lymphoma

Primary mediastinal large B-cell lymphoma has emerged in recent years as a distinct clinicopathologic entity, typically arising in young women, with a peak incidence in the fourth decade of life. Patients present with a mediastinal mass with frequent superior vena caval syndrome. Regional lymph nodes may be involved, but spread to distant nodal sites is uncommon. Frequent extranodal sites of involvement, particularly at relapse, include the liver, kidneys, adrenal glands, ovaries, gastrointestinal tract, and CNS.

Histologically, PMBL is characterized by fine compartmentalizing sclerosis, and large lymphoid cells with abundant pale cytoplasms (Fig. 72-10, *B*). An origin from medullary thymic B cells has been proposed. The cells express CD20 and CD79a but do not express surface Ig. Recently, expression of the MAL gene has been detected in PMBL and not in other DLBCLs.[31] PMBL usually lacks rearrangement for BCL2, BCL6; however, *REL* amplification is a common feature. A common cytogenetic abnormality seen in approximately 50% of cases includes gains in 9p, which may be associated with amplification of Janus kinase 2 *(JAK2)*. Recently, GEP studies have found that PMBL bears a distinct molecular signature that differs from that of other DLBCLs and shares features of CHL.

B-Cell Lymphoma, Unclassifiable, With Features Intermediate Between Diffuse Large B-Cell Lymphoma and Classical Hodgkin Lymphoma

A new aspect of the 2008 WHO classification is the inclusion of borderline categories, one of which manifests features intermediate between DLBCL, especially PMBL, and CHL (see Fig. 72-10, *C*). These tumors are sometimes referred to as *gray zone lymphomas*. A close relationship between PMBL and CHL was supported by GEP.[31] TRAF1 expression and *c-REL* amplification also were seen in both types of neoplasms and could be detected with suitable immunohistochemical studies.

Gray zone lymphomas are more common in males than females, present with bulky mediastinal masses, and appear to have a more aggressive clinical course than PMBL or CHL. A recent study using methylation profiling identified gray zone lymphomas as having a signature distinct from both CHL and PMBL. However, by fluorescence in situ hybridization, gray zone lymphomas, PBMCL, and CHL share a number of common cytogenetic aberrations, including gains at 2p16.1 (*REL/BCL11A* locus), 9p24.1 *(JAK2/PDL2)* and rearrangements of 16p13.13 (*CIITA)*. It is not clear how these patients should be approached therapeutically, but they appear to benefit from combine modality therapy (systemic chemotherapy and radiation).

Burkitt Lymphoma

Burkitt lymphoma (BL) is most common in children and accounts for up to one-third of all pediatric lymphomas in the United States. It is the most rapidly growing of all lymphomas, with 100% of the cells in cell cycle at any time. It usually presents in extranodal sites. In non-endemic regions, such as the United States, frequent sites of presentation are the ileocecal region, ovaries, kidneys, or breasts. Jaw presentations, as well as involvement of other facial bones, are common in African or endemic cases and are seen occasionally in nonendemic regions. BM involvement is a poor prognostic sign.

Burkitt lymphoma is one of the more common tumors associated with human immunodeficiency virus (HIV). It can present at any time during the clinical course. In some patients with HIV infection, BL may be the initial acquired immunodeficiency syndrome (AIDS)–defining illness.

The pathogenesis of BL is related to the translocations involving the *MYC* oncogene, which are seen in virtually 100% of cases and often constitute the sole karyotypic abnormality. Most cases involve the *IGH@* gene on chromosome 14 and less frequently the light-chain genes on chromosomes 2 and 22.

African BL occurs in regions endemic for malaria, and it has been postulated that the pathogenesis appears similar to that seen with HIV infection; recent GEP data also support a common pathogenetic mechanism.[32]

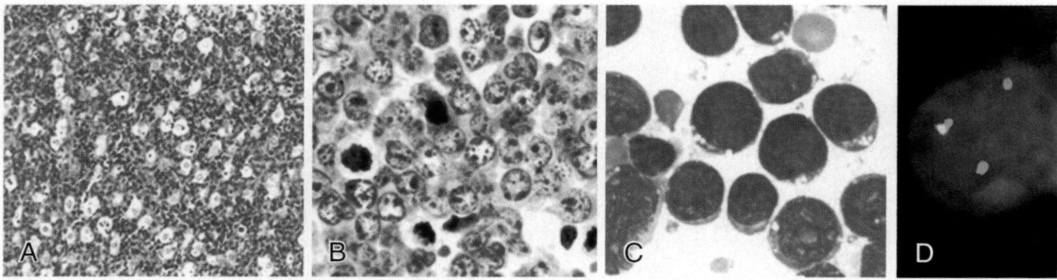

Figure 72-11 BURKITT LYMPHOMA (BL). At low power, BL gives a classic "starry sky" appearance because of numerous histiocytes or tingible body macrophages with clear cytoplasm *(stars),* in a background of darkly stained tumor cells **(A).** At high power, the cells exhibit a very high mitotic rate and are intermediate in size with an almost stippled nuclear chromatin **(B).** On a Wright-stained touch preparation or in the blood or bone marrow aspirate, the cells also have a characteristic appearance with deep blue cytoplasm typically with vacuoles **(C).** Fluorescence in situ hybridization with a probe that spans *MYC* will show a break-apart signal **(D)** indicating that the *MYC* has translocated to a partner chromosome.

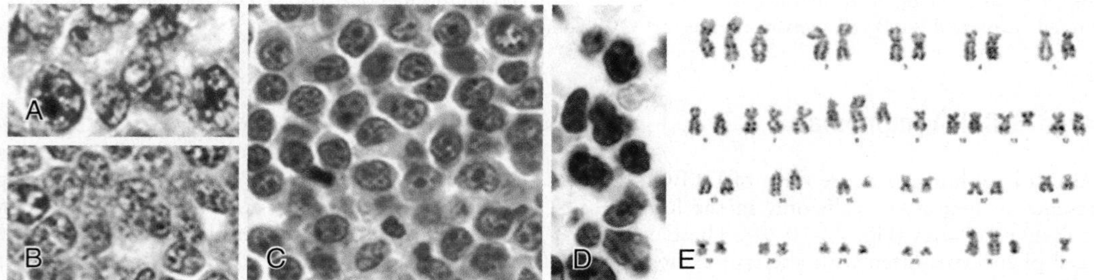

Figure 72-12 B-CELL LYMPHOMA, UNCLASSIFIABLE WITH FEATURES INTERMEDIATE BETWEEN DIFFUSE LARGE B-CELL LYMPHOMA (DLBCL) AND BURKITT LYMPHOMA (BL). Examples of DLBCL **(A)** and BL **(B)** are for comparison. In **C,** the lymphoma cells are intermediate in size and not as large as the DLBCL but without the typical characteristics of BL cells. The cells had a high Ki67 rate **(D)** and a B-cell phenotype with CD10 and BCL2 expression (not shown). The karyotype had a t(14;18) as in follicular lymphoma but was complex and involved the *MYC* gene in multiple translocations **(E).** The karyotype was as follows: 51,XY,+X,+1,dup(1)(q32q44),der(1) del(1)(p21p36.3)dup(1)(q32q44),t(6;8)(p21.1;q24.1),+7,+del(?8) (p11.2p23),der(8)i(8)(q10)t(8;11)(q24.1;q13),-9,der(11)t(8;11)(q24.1;q13), t(14;15)(q32;q15), t(14;18)(q32;q21.3),+21,+mar[13]/46,XY[1]. *(The karyotype was kindly provided by Dr. Yanming Zhan of Northwestern University).*

Epstein-Barr virus is closely linked to BL in endemic regions but is less frequently seen (15%-20%) in sporadic cases. In other regions characterized by low socioeconomic status and EBV infection at an early age, BL is often EBV positive in the range of 50% to 70%. These data support the concept that the EBV is a cofactor for the development of BL. Cytologically, BL is monomorphic (Fig. 72-11). The cells are medium in size with round nuclei, moderately clumped chromatin, and multiple (two to five) basophilic nucleoli. The cytoplasm is deeply basophilic and moderately abundant. These cells contain cytoplasmic lipid vacuoles, which are probably a manifestation of the high rate of proliferation and high rate of spontaneous cell death. The starry sky pattern characteristic of BL is a manifestation of the numerous benign macrophages that have ingested karyorrhectic or apoptotic tumor cells.

Burkitt lymphoma has a mature B-cell phenotype. The cells express CD19, CD20, CD22, CD79a, and monoclonal surface Ig, nearly always IgM. CD10 is positive in nearly all cases, and CD5, CD23, and BCL-2 are consistently negative.

B-Cell Lymphoma, Unclassifiable, With Features Intermediate Between Diffuse Large B-Cell Lymphoma and Burkitt Lymphoma

Historically, it has been difficult for pathologists to distinguish some DLBCL with a very high growth fraction from BL with atypical cytology. In addition, there are cases that have a molecular GEP of BL but carry additional cytogenetic abnormalities, most often involving *BCL2* or *BCL6*. These double- and triple-hit lymphomas have a very aggressive clinical course. To recognize and delineate these cases, this borderline category was created in the 2008 WHO classification (Fig. 72-12). However, it should not be used for otherwise typical DLBCL with a *MYC* translocation. The clinical impact of MYC overexpression in DLBCL has not been fully resolved; in some series, has been associated with a more aggressive clinical course, but in most such cases in adults, C-*MYC* translocation occurs in the setting of multiple genetic aberrations.[27] This unclassified category also should not be used for cases of BL with atypical cytologic features, which are retained under the heading of BL and have a better prognosis when treated appropriately.

T-CELL AND NATURAL KILLER CELL LYMPHOMAS

Overview of the Classification of T-Cell Neoplasms

Although the definition of precursor T-cell or lymphoblastic neoplasms is straightforward, the classification of peripheral T-cell lymphomas has been controversial. These are uncommon, representing fewer than 15% cases of NHL. Most previously published classification schemes for the malignant lymphomas in the United States or Europe have been based on B-cell malignancies because these are far more common than their T-cell counterparts. T-cell and NK cell lymphomas show significant variation in incidence in different geographic regions and racial populations.

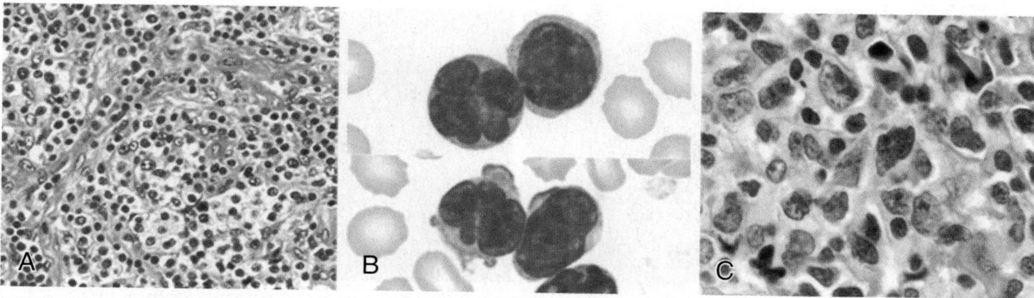

Figure 72-13 T-CELL LYMPHOMA. In angioimmunoblastic T-cell lymphoma (AILT), the lymph node shows effacement because of a vascular proliferation of post-capillary venules and clustered large cells with clear cytoplasms in the background of plasma cells, immunoblasts, and small lymphocytes **(A).** The peripheral blood in adult T-cell leukemia/lymphoma (ATLL) has classic "flower-cells" **(B).** Peripheral T-cell lymphoma (PTCL) is heterogeneous, but typically there is a mixture of small and large neoplastic T cells **(C).**

Natural Killer Cell and T-Cell Subsets and the Classification of Peripheral T-Cell and Natural Killer Cell Neoplasms

Innate Immune System	*Adaptive Immune System*
Does not require antigen sensitization	Characterized by specificity and memory
NK cells, NK/T cells, γ-δ T cells	Effector and memory T cells
Cell-mediated cytotoxicity	Act principally through cytokines and chemokines
Mainly cutaneous and other extranodal sites	Mainly nodal lymphomas
Children and adults	More often in adults

The classification of T-cell and NK cell neoplasms proposed by the WHO emphasizes a multiparameter approach, integrating morphologic, immunophenotypic, genetic, and clinical features. Clinical features play particular importance in the subclassification of these tumors, partly because of the lack of specificity of other parameters (see box on Natural Killer and T-Cell Subsets and the Classification of Peripheral T-Cell and Natural Killer Cell Neoplasms).

In contrast to B-cell lymphomas, specific immunophenotypic profiles are not associated with most T-cell lymphoma subtypes. Although certain antigens are commonly associated with specific disease entities, these associations are not entirely disease specific. Presently, specific genetic features have not been identified for many of the T-cell and NK cell neoplasms, although there are few exceptions.

Angioimmunoblastic T-Cell Lymphoma

Angioimmunoblastic T-cell lymphoma (AILT) was initially proposed as an abnormal immune reaction or form of atypical lymphoid hyperplasia with a high risk of progression to malignant lymphoma. Because the majority of cases show clonal rearrangements of T-cell receptor genes, it is now regarded as a variant of T-cell lymphoma. The median survival is generally less than 5 years.

Angioimmunoblastic T-cell lymphoma presents in adults; most patients have generalized lymphadenopathy, hepatosplenomegaly, skin rash, and prominent constitutional symptoms. They also usually have polyclonal hypergammaglobulinemia and other hematologic abnormalities such as Coombs-positive hemolytic anemia. Rituximab has been used in some recent clinical trials in an attempt to control some of the effects of B-cell hyperactivity in this disease. Patients may also show evidence of immunodeficiency with recurrent opportunistic infections that may ultimately lead to their demise.

The nodal architecture is generally effaced, but peripheral sinuses are often open and even dilated. At low power, there is usually a striking proliferation of high endothelial venules (HEV) with prominent arborization (see Fig. 72-13, *A*). Follicles are typically regressed, but there is a proliferation of dendritic cells around HEV. The atypical T cells have clear cytoplasms and are associated with small lymphocytes, immunoblasts, plasma cells, and histiocytes. The abnormal cells are usually positive for CD3, CD4, CD10, and CD279 (PD-1), a phenotype characteristic of follicular T-helper cells. This relationship is also confirmed by recent GEP data. CXCL13, a chemokine involved in B-cell trafficking into the germinal centers, is also expressed in AILT.

Epstein-Barr virus–positive large B-cell blasts are nearly always present in the background, and progression to EBV-positive DLBCL has been reported in rare cases. Atypical B-cell proliferations that are negative for EBV also occur, presumably related to the T-helper follicular function of the neoplastic cells in promoting the activation and migration of bystander B cells. However, the exact role of EBV in AILT remains uncertain.

Adult T-Cell Leukemia/Lymphoma

Adult T-cell leukemia/lymphoma (ATLL) is a distinct clinicopathologic entity associated with the retrovirus HTLV-I, which is found clonally integrated in the T cells. HTLV-1 infection is endemic in Southwestern Japan and in the Caribbean basin. The disease has a long latency, and affected individuals usually are exposed to the virus very early in life. The virus may be transmitted in breast milk and through exposure to blood and blood products. The cumulative incidence of ATLL is estimated to be 2.5% among HTLV-1 carriers.

The median age of affected individuals is 45 years. Patients may present with leukemia or generalized lymphadenopathy. Other clinical findings include lymphadenopathy, hepatosplenomegaly, lytic bone lesions, and hypercalcemia. Cutaneous involvement is seen in the majority of patients. The acute form of the disease is associated with a poor prognosis and a median survival of less than 2 years. Complete remissions may be obtained, but the relapse rate is nearly 100%.

Chronic and smoldering forms of the disease are seen less commonly and are associated with minimal lymphadenopathy. The predominant clinical manifestation is skin rash, with only small numbers of atypical cells in the peripheral blood.

The cytologic spectrum of ATLL is extremely diverse (Fig. 72-13, *B*). The cells are often markedly polylobated and have been referred to as flower cells. Peripheral blood involvement is very common but often in the absence of BM disease. Immunophenotypically, the neoplastic cells are positive for mature T-cell antigens, such as CD2, CD3, and CD5; they are typically CD4/CD25 positive, a phenotype that resembles regulatory T (Tregs) cells. Some cases express FoxP3 but usually in a minority of tumor cells. The function of the tumor cells as Treg cells may correlate with the associated immunodeficiency.

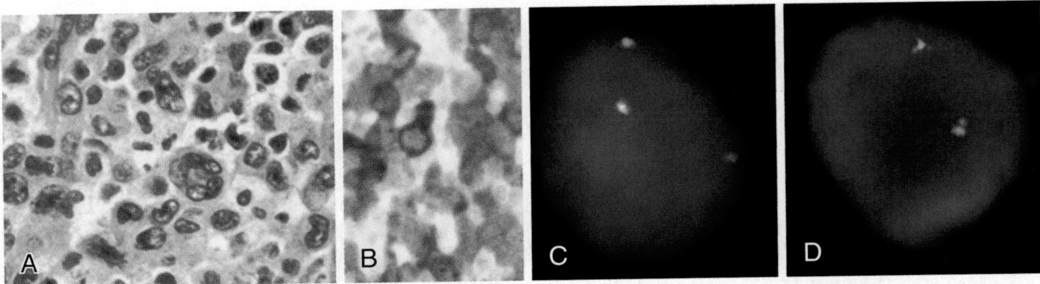

Figure 72-14 T-CELL LYMPHOMA: ANAPLASTIC LARGE CELL LYMPHOMA (ALCL). ATCL is characterized by a mix of pleomorphic malignant large T cells **(A),** which include "wreath cells" *(center)* and "hallmark cells" *(bottom right).* **B,** The presence of ALK staining with nuclear and cytoplasmic localization *(right)* is associated with the t(2;5). A translocation of ALK can be identified with a break-apart probe that spans *ALK* but is split when *ALK* is translocated to one of a number of partners. A cell with a translocated *ALK* is pictured in **C** and a normal cell in **D**.

Peripheral T-Cell Lymphomas, Not Otherwise Specified

Peripheral T-cell lymphomas, not otherwise specified (PTCL, NOS) is a diagnosis of exclusion and is admittedly a heterogeneous category with most cases being nodal in origin. Therefore, not unexpectedly, the cytologic spectrum is very broad[33] (Fig. 72-13, *C*). An inflammatory background is frequent, consisting of eosinophils, plasma cells, and histiocytes. If the epithelioid histiocytes are numerous and clustered, the neoplasm fulfils the criteria for the lymphoepithelioid cell variant of PTCL. The T-zone variant is composed of small- to medium-sized cells that preferentially involve the paracortical regions of the lymph node.

There is also a rare follicular variant composed of TFH cells that are restricted to the lymphoid follicles.

Clinically, PTCL, NOS most often presents in adults with generalized lymphadenopathy, hepatosplenomegaly, and frequent BM involvement. Constitutional symptoms, including fever and night sweats, are common, as is pruritus. The clinical course is aggressive, although complete remissions may be obtained with combination chemotherapy. However, the relapse rate is higher than in aggressive B-cell lymphomas, including DLBCL.

PTCL, NOS, as defined in the WHO classification, remains heterogeneous. It is likely that individual clinicopathologic entities will be delineated in the future from this broad group of malignancies. Thus far, immunophenotypic criteria have not been helpful in delineating subtypes. Most cases have a mature T-cell phenotype and express one of the major subset antigens: CD4 > CD8. These are not clonal markers, and antigen expression can change over time. Loss of one of the pan T-cell antigens (CD3, CD5, CD2, or CD7) is seen in 75% of cases, with CD7 most frequently being absent. GEP studies have shown some cases with a profile resembling AILT. Cases with a high proliferation signature appear to have a more aggressive clinical course, but GEP has not led to the delineation of distinctive subtypes as independent entities.

Anaplastic Large Cell Lymphoma, ALK Positive

Anaplastic large cell lymphoma (ALCL) is characterized by pleomorphic or monomorphic cells, which have a propensity to invade lymphoid sinuses (Fig. 72-14). Because of the sinusoidal location of the tumor cells and their lobulated nuclear appearance, this disease when first observed was suspected to be of histiocytic origin. A consistent feature is the strong expression of CD30 antigen, a diagnostic hallmark. However, CD30 expression is not specific for ALCL and can be seen in a variety of conditions, of course, including CHL. Systemic ALCL is associated with a characteristic chromosomal translocation, t(2;5)(p23;q35), involving *NPM/ALK* genes, respectively. A number of variant translocations have been identified that involve partners other than *NPM*. All lead to overexpression of ALK, although the cellular distribution of *ALK* varies according to the gene partner.

The cells of classical ALCL have large, often lobulated nuclei with small basophilic nucleoli, so-called hallmark cells. The cytoplasm is usually abundant and amphophilic, and there are distinct cytoplasmic borders. A prominent Golgi region is generally visible. Small cell and lymphohistiocytic variants constitute part of the entity and appear to be associated with a more aggressive clinical course.[34]

The cells exhibit an aberrant phenotype with loss of many of the T cell–associated antigens. Both CD3 and CD5 are negative in more than 50% of cases. CD2 and CD4 are positive in the majority of cases. CD8 is usually negative. ALCL cells, despite the CD4-positive/CD8-negative phenotype, exhibit positivity for the cytotoxic-associated antigens TIA-1, granzyme B, and perforin. In addition, clusterin is generally present in ALCL and represents another useful diagnostic marker. By molecular studies, in most of the cases, a T-cell receptor rearrangement is found, confirming a T-cell origin.

Anaplastic large cell lymphoma is most common in children and young adults, and a marked male predominance is noted. Although most patients present with nodal disease, a high incidence of extranodal involvement has been reported (involving skin, bone, and soft tissue). Approximately 75% of cases present with advanced stage and systemic symptoms. Although these lymphomas have an aggressive natural clinical history, they respond well to chemotherapy. Overall survival and disease-free survival are significantly better among ALK-positive than ALK-negative cases. Both ALK-positive and -negative ALCL have better prognoses than other PTCLs, with a plateau in the survival curve seen in both groups.[35]

Anaplastic Large Cell Lymphoma, ALK Negative (Provisional Entity)

It has been controversial whether ALCL negative for ALK is a separate entity or part of the spectrum of PTCL, NOS. Part of the controversy relates to the lack of absolute criteria to recognize these cases. They should be morphologically and phenotypically similar to ALK-positive ALCL, with strong CD30 expression and a cytotoxic phenotype. They occur in an older age group than the ALK positive, and as already noted, appear to have a better prognosis than other PTCL, NOS.

Primary Cutaneous Anaplastic Large Cell Lymphoma

The primary cutaneous form of ALCL is closely related to lymphomatoid papulosis and differs clinically, immunophenotypically, and at the molecular level from the systemic form. Lymphomatoid papulosis and cutaneous ALCL are part of the spectrum of CD30-positive cutaneous T-cell lymphoproliferative diseases. Small lesions are likely to regress. Patients with large tumor masses may develop disseminated disease with lymph node involvement. However,

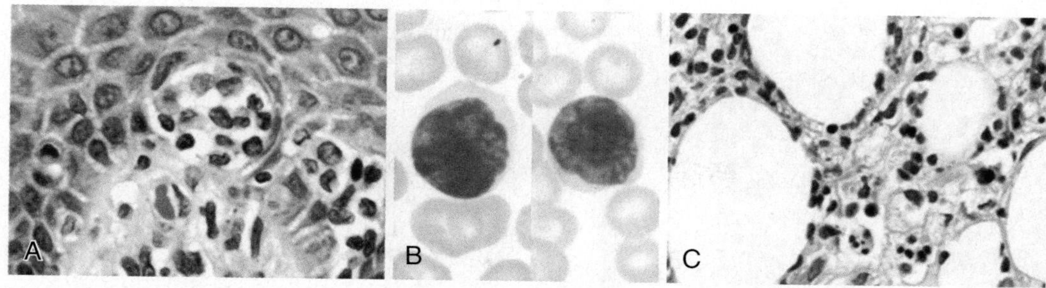

Figure 72-15 T-CELL LYMPHOMA: MYCOSIS FUNGOIDES/SÉZARY SYNDROME AND SUBCUTANEOUS PANNICULITIS-LIKE T-CELL LYMPHOMA (SPTCL). In mycosis fungoides, there is a dermal infiltrate with some malignant T cells infiltrating into the epithelium (Pautrier microabscesses) **(A).** Sézary cells with convoluted nuclear folding are seen in **B**. The peripheral nuclear outline is fairly rounded, but the internal nuclear detail shows complex nuclear folding giving rise to a convoluted and cerebriform look. A case of SPTCL is illustrated and shows an abnormal lymphoid infiltrate in the subcutaneous fat **(C).** This is associated with hemophagocytosis *(bottom center)* and necrosis.

primary cutaneous ALCL is a more indolent disease than other T-cell lymphomas of the skin. Because the skin nodules may show spontaneous regression, usually a period of observation is warranted before the institution of any chemotherapy. Cutaneous ALCL is CD30 positive but ALK negative, lacking translocations involving the *ALK* gene. However, recent studies have identified translocations of the *IRF4* gene in cutaneous ALCL.[36]

Mycosis Fungoides and Sézary Syndrome

Mycosis fungoides and Sézary syndrome are now regarded as separate diseases but are closely related and often considered together from a clinical and biologic standpoint.[37] Both are primary cutaneous T-cell malignancies derived from mature $CD4^+$ skin-homing T cells. Skin involvement may be manifested as multiple cutaneous plaques or nodules (Fig. 72-15, *A*). Sézary syndrome is characterized by erythroderma and a leukemic phase.[38] Lymphadenopathy is usually not present at presentation and, when identified, is associated with a poor prognosis. In early stages, enlarged lymph nodes may only show dermatopathic changes (category I). If malignant cells are present in significant numbers and are associated with architectural effacement (category II or III), the prognosis is significantly worse.

Cytologically, the small cells of mycosis fungoides demonstrate cerebriform nuclei with clumped chromatin, inconspicuous nucleoli, and sparse cytoplasm. Epidermotropism is usually a prominent feature. Sézary syndrome presents with exfoliative erythroderma and circulating cerebriform lymphocytes known as Sézary cells (Fig. 72-15, *B*). The typical phenotype is $CD2^+$, $CD3^+$, $CD5^+$, $CD4^+$, and $CD8^-$. However, CD8-positive variants of mycosis fungoides have been described and are more common in children. The absence of CD7 is a constant feature but may also be seen in reactive conditions and therefore is of limited diagnostic value. Aberrant expression of other T-cell antigens may be seen but mainly occurs in the advanced (tumor) stages. Inactivation of p16 *(CDKN2A)* and *PTEN* has been identified in some cases and may be associated with disease progression.

Subcutaneous Panniculitis-Like T-Cell Lymphoma

Subcutaneous panniculitis-like T-cell lymphoma (SPTCL) usually presents with subcutaneous nodules, primarily affecting the extremities and trunk. The nodules range in size from 0.5 cm to several centimeters in diameter. In its early stages, the infiltrate may appear deceptively benign, and lesions are often misdiagnosed as panniculitis. However, histologic progression usually occurs, and subsequent biopsies show more pronounced cytologic atypia, permitting the diagnosis of malignant lymphoma.

Atypical lymphoid cells rim individual fat cells. Admixed reactive histiocytes are frequently present, particularly in areas of fat infiltration and destruction. Vascular invasion may be seen in some cases, and necrosis and karyorrhexis are common (see Fig. 72-15, *C*).

The neoplastic cells are CD8-positive T α-β cells, with tumors composed of γ-δ T cells now included under primary cutaneous γ-δ T-cell lymphomas.[39] The cells display an activated cytotoxic immunophenotype (positive for TIA-1, granzyme B, and perforin). These proteins may be responsible for the cellular destruction seen in these tumors.

A hemophagocytic syndrome is less often seen in SPTCL than in panniculitis-like tumors of γ-δ T-cell derivation, but whenever seen, is associated with an adverse prognosis.[40] Patients present with fever, pancytopenia, and hepatosplenomegaly. The cause of the hemophagocytic syndrome appears related to cytokine production by the malignant cells.

Primary Cutaneous γ-δ T-Cell Lymphoma

Primary cutaneous γ-δ T-cell lymphoma is considered a distinct entity, which can involve the subcutis, the dermis, or with epidermal infiltration. These are clinically aggressive tumors. The cells have a cytotoxic phenotype, and similar to normal γ-δ T cells, lack CD5 and express cytotoxic molecules. They may be CD8 positive, or more often, double negative for CD4 and CD8. Although the skin is the most common presenting site, similar lymphomas of γ-δ T-cell origin can present in other extranodal sites, most often the gastrointestinal tract.[41] The cells are invariably EBV negative and show clonal rearrangement of T-cell receptor genes.

Primary Cutaneous CD8-Positive Aggressive Epidermotropic Cytotoxic T-Cell Lymphoma and Primary Cutaneous CD4-Positive Small/Medium T-Cell Lymphoma

These are provisional entities listed in the 2008 WHO classification. *Primary cutaneous CD8-positive aggressive epidermotropic cytotoxic T-cell lymphoma* is an aggressive cutaneous neoplasm that shares many clinical features with primary cutaneous γ-δ T-cell lymphomas but is derived from cytotoxic α-β T cells. As the term implies, the neoplastic cells show prominent epidermotropism.

Primary cutaneous CD4-positive small/medium T-cell lymphoma most often presents with localized skin lesions. It is associated with an excellent prognosis and requires only limited localized therapy unless multiple skin lesions are present. Some authors have questioned whether this lymphoid proliferation should be considered a form of "pseudolymphoma," often containing T-cell clones but

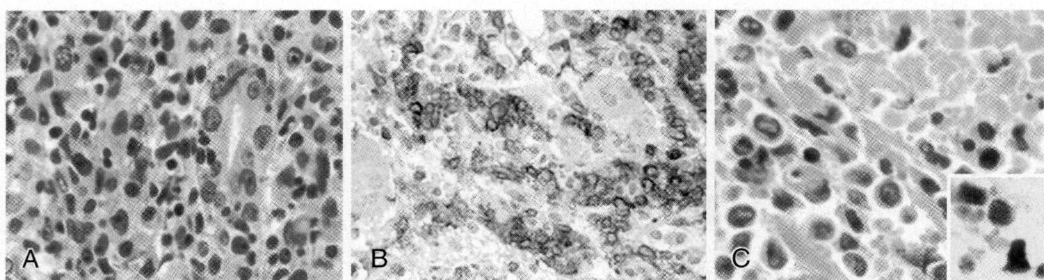

Figure 72-16 T-CELL LYMPHOMA. In enteropathy-associated T-cell lymphoma (EATL) **(A),** there is an abnormal T-lymphoid proliferation with infiltration into the gastrointestinal glandular elements *(center right).* Bone marrow involvement of hepatosplenic gamma δ T-cell lymphoma (HSTCL) is illustrated with a CD2 stain showing the characteristic sinusoidal distribution of the lymphoma **(B).** Extra nodal natural killer cell/T-cell lymphoma typically has marked necrosis **(C).** The malignant cells are Epstein-Barr virus (EBV) positive by in situ hybridization for EBV encoded RNA *(insert).*

having limited potential for progression.[42] The lesions are rich in B cells, and the proliferating T cells have a T_{FH} phenotype.

Enteropathy-Associated T-Cell Lymphoma

Two variants of enteropathy-associated T-cell lymphoma (EATL) are recognized in the WHO 2008, EATL types I and II. EATL type I is associated with either overt or clinically silent gluten-sensitive enteropathy and is largely seen in patients of European extraction; the type II form has a more worldwide distribution. Patients usually present with abdominal symptoms, including pain, small bowel perforation, and associated peritonitis. The clinical course is aggressive, and most patients have multifocal intestinal disease.[43]

In EATL type I, the cytologic composition is somewhat varied; the neoplastic cells show prominent invasion of the mucosa and are cytotoxic T cells most often of α-β origin. The cells also express the homing receptor CD 103 (HML-1) (Fig. 72-16, *A*). Cells with anaplastic features positive for CD30 may be present. In EATL type I, the adjacent small bowel usually shows villous atrophy associated with celiac disease. In EATL type II, the infiltrate is monomorphic composed of medium-sized cells with clear cytoplasm showing prominent epitheliotropism. They are CD56 positive, CD8 positive, and most often of γ-δ T-cell derivation. An association with celiac disease is only seen sporadically, and this form of the disease is relatively common in Asia. Other PTCLs can present with intestinal disease and should be distinguished from EATL. These include the EBV-positive extranodal T-cell/NK cell lymphomas and γ-δ T-cell lymphomas. Both EATL types I and II share some genetic aberrations, including chromosomal gains on 9q33-34.

Hepatosplenic T-Cell Lymphoma

Hepatosplenic T-cell lymphoma (HSTCL) presents with marked hepatosplenomegaly in the absence of lymphadenopathy. The great majority of cases are of γ-δ T-cell origin. Most patients are male, with a peak incidence in young adults. Although patients may respond initially to chemotherapy, relapse has been seen in the vast majority of cases, and the median survival is less than 3 years. Rare long-term survival has been seen after allogeneic hematopoietic cell transplantation.

The cells of HSTCL are usually moderate in size, with a rim of pale cytoplasm. The nuclear chromatin is loosely condensed, with small inconspicuous nucleoli. The pattern of infiltration mimics the homing pattern of γ-δ T cells with marked sinusoidal infiltration in liver and spleen. Abnormal cells are usually present in the sinusoids of the BM but may be difficult to identify without immunohistochemical stains (see Fig. 72-16, *B*). The neoplastic cells also have a phenotype that resembles that of normal resting γ-δ T cells. They are often negative for both CD4 and CD8, although CD8 may be expressed in some cases. CD56 is typically positive. The neoplastic cells express markers associated with cytotoxic T cells, such as TIA-1. However, perforin and granzyme B are usually negative, suggesting that these cells are not activated. Isochromosome 7q is a consistent cytogenetic abnormality and is often seen in association with trisomy 8.

Extranodal Natural Killer Cell/T-Cell Lymphoma, Nasal Type

Extranodal NK cell/T-cell lymphoma, nasal type, is a distinct clinicopathologic entity highly associated with EBV. It is much more common in Asians than in Europeans.[44] Clusters of the disease also have been reported in Central and South America in individuals of Native American heritage, suggesting that ethnic background (i.e., genetic risk factors) may play a role in the pathogenesis of these lymphomas. It affects adults (median age, 50 years), and the most common clinical presentation is a destructive nasal or midline facial lesion. Palatal destruction, orbital swelling, and edema may be prominent. NK cell/T-cell lymphomas have been reported in other extranodal sites, including skin, soft tissue, testis, upper respiratory tract, and gastrointestinal tract. The clinical course is usually aggressive, with a slightly improved median survival in patients with localized disease, in which local radiation therapy may be useful.[44] A hemophagocytic syndrome is a common clinical complication and adversely affects survival.

Extranodal NK cell/T-cell lymphoma, nasal type, is characterized by a broad cytologic spectrum (see Fig. 72-16, *C*). Although the cells express some T cell-associated antigens, most commonly CD2, other T-cell markers, such as surface CD3, are usually absent. The cells express cytoplasmic CD3 but lack T-cell receptor gene rearrangement. In support of an NK cell origin, the cells are usually CD56 positive but do not express CD57 or CD16. EBV is positive in 100% of cases by in situ hybridization.

Aggressive NK cell leukemia is a closely related entity. It presents at a younger age than extranodal NK cell/T-cell lymphoma and is associated with systemic disease and a fulminant clinical course. It has a similar phenotype, EBV association, and epidemiology.

There are other EBV-positive T-cell and NK cell proliferations that are seen mainly in children. These include *systemic EBV-positive T-cell lymphoproliferative disease, hydroa vacciniforme-like lymphoma,* and *mosquito bite allergy,* the latter usually being derived from NK cells. All are seen most often in Asian children but also are reported in Central and South America in individuals of Native American origin. Whereas the latter two conditions affect mainly the skin and have a more indolent clinical course, the systemic disease has a very aggressive clinical course with survival measured in weeks. Systemic

EBV-positive T-cell LPD may arise in a background of chronic active EBV infection.

Hodgkin Lymphomas

Hodgkin lymphoma and NHL have long been regarded as distinct disease entities based on their differences in pathology, phenotype, clinical features, and response to therapy. It is now accepted that the malignant cell of Hodgkin lymphoma is an altered B cell. Therefore, it is not surprising that both biologic and clinical overlaps should occur between these two lymphoma groups, as also shown by GEP in PMBL and cell lines derived from CHL. Although we have become aware of this closer relationship from the histogenetic point of view (hence the name Hodgkin lymphoma), these disorders are still treated with different modalities.

The diagnosis of CHL depends on the identification of Hodgkin/Reed-Sternberg (HRS) cells in an appropriate inflammatory background composed of small T lymphocytes, plasma cells, histiocytes, and granulocytes (often eosinophils).[45] All cases of CHL share certain immunophenotypic and genotypic features. Neoplastic cells are $CD30^+$, $CD15^{+/-}$, $CD45^-$, and EMA^-. Expression of B cell–associated antigens is seen in up to 75% of cases. However, when present, CD20 staining is weaker than that seen in normal B cells with variable in intensity among individual tumor cells. CD79a is usually negative. Ig and T-cell receptor genes are usually germline because of the paucity of tumor cells in the inflammatory background, but using microdissection and polymerase chain reaction amplification for clonal rearrangement of the Ig genes can generally be shown. In addition, the presence of somatic mutations indicates transit through the germinal center.

Sufficient evidence has emerged in recent years to warrant the recognition of nodular lymphocyte-predominant Hodgkin lymphoma (NLPHL) as a distinct entity. Although it resembles other types of Hodgkin lymphoma in having a minority of putative neoplastic cells on a background of benign inflammatory cells, it differs morphologically, immunophenotypically, and clinically from classic Hodgkin lymphoma. The preferred term of Hodgkin lymphoma over Hodgkin disease reflects current knowledge concerning the nature of the neoplastic cell as a lymphocyte.

Nodular Lymphocyte-Predominant Hodgkin Lymphoma

Nodular lymphocyte-predominant Hodgkin lymphoma (NLPHL) usually has a nodular growth pattern (Fig. 72-17) with or without diffuse areas; it is rarely purely diffuse. Nodularity may be more easily recognized using immunohistologic stains with anti–B-cell or antifollicular dendritic cell (FDC) antibodies. Progressively transformed germinal centers are often seen in partially involved lymph nodes or other lymph node sites. The atypical cells have vesicular, polylobated nuclei and small nucleoli. These had been called lymphocytic or histiocytic (L&H) cells, or "popcorn" cells, but the term *LP cell* is now preferred.[17] Although these cells may be very numerous, usually no diagnostic HRS cells are found. The background is predominantly lymphocytes with or without epithelioid histiocyte clusters. Plasma cells are infrequent, and eosinophils and neutrophils are rarely seen. Occasionally, sclerosis may cause lesions to resemble nodular sclerosis.

The atypical cells are $CD45^+$-expressing B cell–associated antigens (CD19, 20, 22, 79a), $CDw75^+$, $EMA^{+/-}$ $CD15^-$, $CD30^{-/+}$, and usually SIg^- by routine techniques, although one study reported light-chain restriction. Neoplastic cells positive for IgD are more often found in male patients, median age 21 years.[46] J chain has been demonstrated in many cases. Small lymphocytes in the nodules are predominantly B cells with a mantle zone phenotype. However, numerous T cells are present, with T cells positive for CD57 and PD-1 (CD279) surrounding the LP cells. The proportion of T cells tends to increase over time in sequential biopsies. A prominent meshwork of FDC is present within the nodules. LP cells, when isolated by microdissection, have clonally rearranged Ig genes with evidence of somatic hypermutation.

NLPHL occurs at all ages, in adults more commonly than in children, and in men more than in women. It usually involves peripheral lymph nodes with sparing of the mediastinum. It is usually localized at diagnosis but rarely may be disseminated. Survival is long, with or without treatment, for localized cases. However, when disseminated, the prognosis is often poor. Patients with advanced stage disease may benefit from treatment regimens used for aggressive B-cell lymphomas. Late relapses have been reported to be more common than in other types of Hodgkin lymphoma; it may be associated with or progress to large B-cell lymphoma. Progression to a process resembling T-cell/histiocyte rich large B-cell lymphoma may also been seen.

Classic Hodgkin Lymphoma, Nodular Sclerosis

This variant is most common in adolescents and young adults, but can occur at any age; female cases equal or exceed those in males. The mediastinum is commonly involved; stage and bulk of disease have prognostic importance. Classic Hodgkin lymphoma, nodular sclerosis (NSCHL), is often curable; however, in long-term survivors the risk of secondary malignancies is increased, especially in those receiving both radiation and chemotherapy. NSCHL of the mediastinum

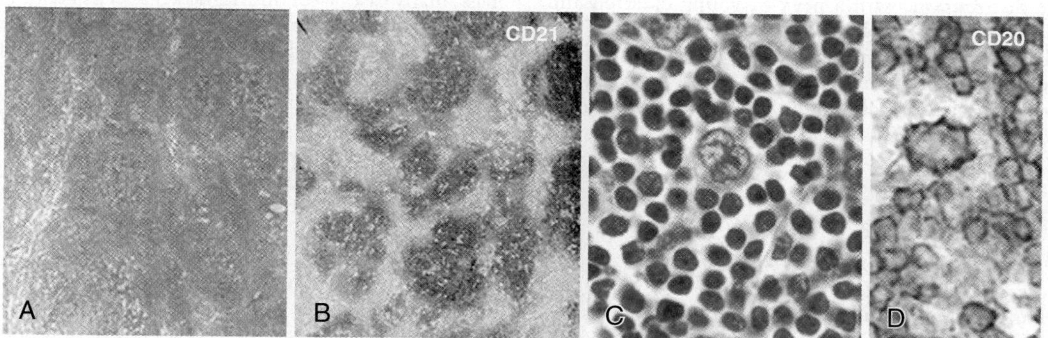

Figure 72-17 NODULAR LYMPHOCYTE PREDOMINANT HODGKIN LYMPHOMA (NLPHLP). Low-power illustration shows vague expansile nodules that efface the lymph node architecture **(A)**. The nodules can be accentuated with a stain for germinal center dendritic cells, CD21 **(B)**. This indicates that the nodules are germinal center derived. The neoplastic components are the so-called "LP" cells (previously called "L&H" cells or "popcorn" cells) **(C)**. Unlike the neoplastic cells of classical Hodgkin lymphoma, these LP cells stain brightly for CD20 **(D)** and are typically $CD45^+$, $CD30^-$, and $CD15^-$.

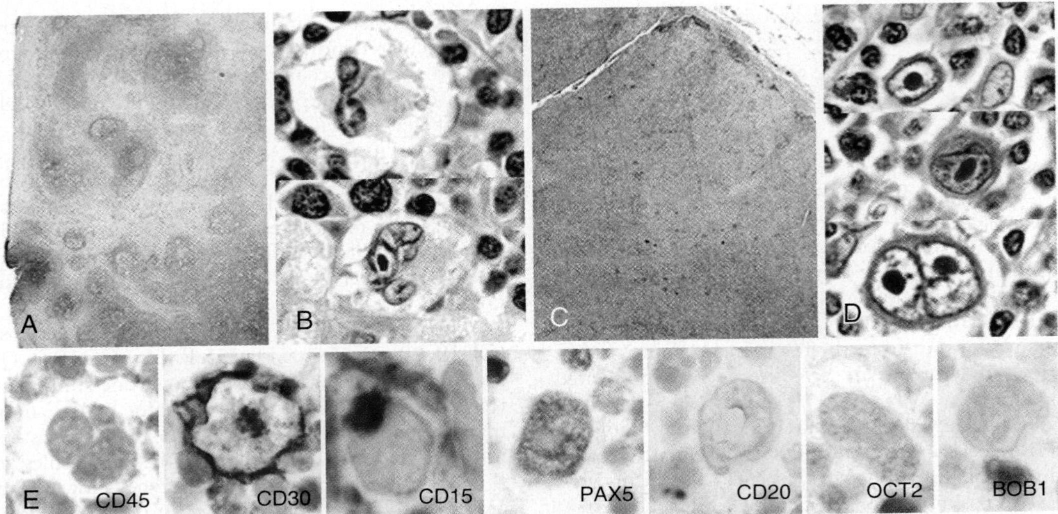

Figure 72-18 CLASSICAL HODGKIN LYMPHOMA, NODULAR SCLEROSING TYPE AND MIXED CELLULARITY TYPE. In nodular sclerosing Hodgkin Lymphoma, broad bands of sclerosis typically divide the lymph node into cellular nodules **(A).** The nodules contain a mixed cellular infiltrate and scattered neoplastic cells with lobular nuclei and retracted cytoplasm **(B).** In mixed cellularity Hodgkin lymphoma, the lymph node is usually diffusely effaced and is without fibrosis **(C).** Classic mononuclear and bi- and multinuclear Hodgkin (H) and Reed-Sternberg (RS) cells are present **(D).** Both the lacunar and HRS cell are typically $CD45^-$, $CD30^+$, $CD15^+$, weak $PAX5^+$, and $CD20^-$. The B-cell transcription factors OCT2 and BOB1 are variable but usually not both or uniformly positive **(E).**

is thought to be closely related to PMBL, and both types of tumors can be seen in the same patient, either as composite malignancy, or sequentially.[47]

The tumor has at least a partially nodular pattern with fibrous bands separating the nodules in most cases (see Fig. 72-18, *A* and *B*). Diffuse areas may be present, as is necrosis. The characteristic cell is the lacunar-type RS cell, which may be very numerous. Diagnostic RS cells are usually also present. The background contains lymphocytes, histiocytes, plasma cells, eosinophils, and neutrophils. It can be graded according to the proportion of the tumor cells and the presence of necrosis (grades I and II). However, grading is considered optional. The immunophenotype and genotype are characteristic of CHL. However, EBV is infrequently positive (<15% of cases).

Classic Hodgkin Lymphoma, Mixed Cellularity

Patients are usually adults; men outnumber women, and the stage is often advanced. The course is moderately aggressive but is often curable. Classic Hodgkin lymphoma, mixed cellularity (CHLMC) has a bimodal age distribution, with a peak in young children and again in older adults. It is often EBV positive, seen in up to 75% of cases. Both CHLMC and the lymphocyte depleted form can be associated with underlying HIV infection. The infiltrate is diffuse without band-forming sclerosis, although fine interstitial fibrosis may be present (Fig. 72-18, *C* and *D*). HRS cells are of the classic type.

Classic Hodgkin Lymphoma, Lymphocyte Depletion

Classic Hodgkin lymphoma, lymphocyte depletion (CHLLD) is the least common variant of CHL and is most common in older people, in HIV-positive individuals, and in non-industrialized countries. It frequently presents with abdominal lymphadenopathy, spleen, liver, and BM involvement without peripheral adenopathy. The stage is usually advanced at diagnosis. It shares many features with CHLMC and appears to represent a continuum with this variant, associated with more frequent neoplastic cells and fewer normal T cells.[45]

The infiltrate is diffuse and often appears hypocellular owing to the presence of diffuse fibrosis and necrosis. Relative to the number of normal lymphocytes, there are large numbers of HRS cells and occasional bizarre "sarcomatous" variants with a paucity of other inflammatory cells. The immunophenotype is characteristic of CHL. Because the histologic differential diagnosis often includes large B- or T-cell lymphoma or ALCL, immunohistochemistry should be performed in most cases. EBV is positive in the majority of cases.

Classic Hodgkin Lymphoma, Lymphocyte Rich

Classic Hodgkin lymphoma, lymphocyte rich (CHLLR) may be nodular or diffuse and contains relatively infrequent HRS cells, which are of the classic type, rather than the LP variants seen in NLPHL. There are infrequent eosinophils or plasma cells. In the nodular form, the HRS cells are seen at the periphery of B cell–rich nodules, mainly in the marginal zone. The neoplastic cells have the immunophenotype of classic HRS cells but morphologically may be difficult to distinguish from LP cells in some cases. Thus, in the past, many cases were misdiagnosed as NLPHL.[48] The genetic features are similar to those of the other variants of CHL. Patients usually present with localized disease and tend to be older than patients with NLPHL.

SUGGESTED READINGS

Campo E, Swerdlow SH, Harris NL, et al: The 2008 WHO classification of lymphoid neoplasms and beyond: Evolving concepts and practical applications. *Blood* 117:5019, 2011.

Carvajal A, Sua L, Silva N, et al: "In Situ" Mantle Cell Lymphoma (MCL), an incidental finding with an indolent clinical course. *Lab Invest* 91:1228, 2011.

Dave SS, Wright G, Tan B, et al: Prediction of survival in follicular lymphoma based on molecular features of tumor-infiltrating immune cells. *N Engl J Med* 351:2159, 2004.

Dojcinov SD, Venkataraman G, Pittaluga S, et al: Age-related EBV-associated lymphoproliferative disorders in the Western population: A spectrum of reactive lymphoid hyperplasia and lymphoma. *Blood* 117:4726, 2011.

Fernandez V, Salamero O, Espinet B, et al: Genomic and gene expression profiling defines indolent forms of mantle cell lymphoma. *Cancer Res* 70:1408, 2010.

Gibson SE, Swerdlow SH, Ferry JA, et al: Reassessment of small lymphocytic lymphoma in the era of monoclonal B-cell lymphocytosis. *Haematologica* 96:1144, 2011.

Gine E, Martinez A, Villamor N, et al: Expanded and highly active proliferation centers identify a histological subtype of chronic lymphocytic leukemia ("accelerated" chronic lymphocytic leukemia) with aggressive clinical behavior. *Haematologica* 95:1526, 2010.

Horn H, Schmelter C, Leich E, et al: Follicular lymphoma grade 3B is a distinct neoplasm according to cytogenetic and immunohistochemical profiles. *Haematologica* 96:1327, 2011.

Jaffe ES, Harris NL, Stein H, et al: Classification of lymphoid neoplasms: The microscope as a tool for disease discovery. *Blood* 112:4384, Dec 1 2008.

Jaffe ES, Pittaluga S: Aggressive B-cell lymphomas: A review of new and old entities in the WHO classification. *Hematology Am Soc Hematol Educ Program* 506, 2011.

Jegalian AG, Eberle FC, Pack SD, et al: Follicular lymphoma in situ: Clinical implications and comparisons with partial involvement by follicular lymphoma. *Blood* 118:2976, 2011.

Malavasi F, Deaglio S, Damle R, et al: CD38 and chronic lymphocytic leukemia: A decade later. *Blood* 118:3470, 2011.

Morin RD, Mendez-Lago M, Mungall AJ, et al: Frequent mutation of histone-modifying genes in non-Hodgkin lymphoma. *Nature* 476:298, 2011.

Mozos A, Royo C, Hartmann E, et al: SOX11 expression is highly specific for mantle cell lymphoma and identifies the cyclin D1-negative subtype. *Haematologica* 94:1555, 2009.

Mullighan CG: New strategies in acute lymphoblastic leukemia: Translating advances in genomics into clinical practice. *Clin Cancer Res* 17:396, 2011.

Ngo VN, Young RM, Schmitz R, et al: Oncogenically active MYD88 mutations in human lymphoma. *Nature* 470:115, 2011.

Oschlies I, Salaverria I, Mahn F, et al: Pediatric follicular lymphoma–a clinico-pathological study of a population-based series of patients treated within the Non-Hodgkin's Lymphoma–Berlin-Frankfurt-Munster (NHL-BFM) multicenter trials. *Haematologica* 95:253, Feb 2010.

Owen RG, Treon SP, Al-Katib A, et al: Clinicopathological definition of Waldenström's macroglobulinemia: Consensus panel recommendations from the Second International Workshop on Waldenstrom's Macroglobulinemia. *Semin Oncol* 30:110, 2003.

Pasqualucci L, Dominguez-Sola D, Chiarenza A, et al: Inactivating mutations of acetyltransferase genes in B-cell lymphoma. *Nature* 471:189, 2011.

Puente XS, Pinyol M, Quesada V, et al: Whole-genome sequencing identifies recurrent mutations in chronic lymphocytic leukaemia. *Nature* 475:101, 2011.

Rinaldi A, Mian M, Chigrinova E, et al: Genome-wide DNA profiling of marginal zone lymphomas identifies subtype-specific lesions with an impact on the clinical outcome. *Blood* 117:1595, 2011.

Rosenwald A, Wright G, Wiestner A, et al: The proliferation gene expression signature is a quantitative integrator of oncogenic events that predicts survival in mantle cell lymphoma. *Cancer Cell* 3:185, 2003.

Roulland S, Faroudi M, Mamessier E, et al: Early steps of follicular lymphoma pathogenesis. *Adv Immunol* 111:1, 2011.

Salaverria I, Philipp C, Oschlies I, et al: Translocations activating IRF4 identify a subtype of germinal center-derived B-cell lymphoma affecting predominantly children and young adults. *Blood* 118:139, 2011.

Schmatz AI, Streubel B, Kretschmer-Chott E, et al: Primary follicular lymphoma of the duodenum is a distinct mucosal/submucosal variant of follicular lymphoma: A retrospective study of 63 cases. *J Clin Oncol* 29:1445, 2011.

Shanafelt TD, Ghia P, Lanasa MC, et al: Monoclonal B-cell lymphocytosis: Biology, natural history and clinical management. *Leukemia* 24:512, 2010.

Valera A, Balague O, Colomo L, et al: IG/MYC rearrangements are the main cytogenetic alteration in plasmablastic lymphomas. *Am J Surg Pathol* 34:1686, 2010.

Van Loo P, Tousseyn T, Vanhentenrijk V, et al: T-cell/histiocyte-rich large B-cell lymphoma shows transcriptional features suggestive of a tolerogenic host immune response. *Haematologica* 95:440, 2010.

Vitolo U, Ferreri AJ, Montoto S: Lymphoplasmacytic lymphoma-Waldenstrom's macroglobulinemia. *Crit Rev Oncol Hematol* 67:172, 2008.

Watkins AJ, Huang Y, Ye H, et al: Splenic marginal zone lymphoma: Characterization of 7q deletion and its value in diagnosis. *J Pathol* 220:461, 2010.

For complete list of references log on to www.expertconsult.com.

CHAPTER 73

ORIGIN OF HODGKIN LYMPHOMA

Ralf Küppers

More than 150 years ago, Thomas Hodgkin described several cases of a lymphoproliferative disease, which was later named Hodgkin disease. This malignancy, which is now called Hodgkin lymphoma (HL), has been one of the most enigmatic forms of lymphomas for a long time. This is due to several key features of the disease: First, the pathognomonic and suspected tumor cells of HL, the mononuclear Hodgkin and the bi- or multinucleated large Reed-Sternberg cells, are very rare in the tumor tissue, often accounting for only about 1% of the cells. Thus the molecular analysis of these cells was very much hampered until methods became available to isolate these cells by microdissection from tissue sections. Second, the Hodgkin and Reed-Sternberg (HRS) cells have a very unusual immunophenotype, which does not resemble any normal cell in the hematopoietic system. Therefore immunophenotyping, which was very informative in revealing the cellular derivation of most other lymphoid malignancies, did not help to uncover the cellular origin of HRS cells. Third, only a few cell lines could be established from HL patients, these lines were rather heterogeneous, and for hardly any of these lines was the derivation from the HRS cells in the patient unequivocally shown. Hence it was initially difficult to draw firm conclusions from the study of such lines. Although HL still harbors many secrets, exciting novel insights into the cellular origin of the HRS cells and the pathogenetic processes in their generation have been obtained in the last years, which will be discussed in this chapter.

CLASSIFICATION OF HODGKIN LYMPHOMA

HL is subdivided into classical HL, which accounts for about 95% of cases, and nodular lymphocyte predominant HL (NLPHL). The tumor cells are called *HRS cells* in classical HL and *lymphocyte predominant (LP) cells* in NLPHL (until recently, the tumor cells in NLPHL were called lymphocytic and histiocytic [L&H] cells). Classical HL and NLPHL differ in the histologic picture, the morphology and immunophenotype of the tumor cells, and multiple clinical features. Classical HL is further subdivided into four subforms: nodular sclerosis, mixed cellularity, lymphocyte-rich classical, and lymphocyte depletion HL. Again, differences in the histologic picture and HRS cell morphology are the basis for this subtyping (see Chapter 72 for a detailed description).

B-cell Development and Differentiation

Because we now know that HRS and LP cells are derived from B cells (see later), a brief outline of B-cell development and differentiation is given first. B cells are generated in the bone marrow from hematopoietic stem cells in a multistep developmental process. The key determinant for B-cell development is the generation of a functional B-cell receptor (BCR), which is composed of two identical immunoglobulin (Ig) heavy chains and two identical light chains, the latter of which can be of the κ or λ type. B-cell development is initiated when common lymphoid progenitors undergo gene rearrangements at the Ig gene heavy chain locus. The variable part of the antibody heavy chain is composed of three gene segments: variable (V), diversity (D) and joining (J). First, a randomly selected D_H gene segment is rearranged to one J_H gene segment. In the next step, a V_H gene segment is rearranged to a D_H-J_H joint. If the rearrangement is in-frame and productive, a heavy chain can be expressed and the developmental stage of a pre-B cell is reached. In the next step, V_κ to J_κ rearrangements occur to generate a κ light chain. If this is not successful, V gene rearrangement processes take place at the λ light chain locus. B cells expressing a functional (and nonautoreactive) BCR are released into the periphery and express their BCR as IgM and IgD receptors—that is, two different classes of the heavy chain constant region. The first D_H-J_H rearrangements are not completely specific for B-lineage cells, but $V_HD_HJ_H$ rearrangements and light chain gene rearrangements are highly specific for B cells. Thus their detection in a cell unequivocally defines that cell as a B cell. Moreover, because of the availability of multiple V, D, and J gene segments and additional diversity generated at the joining sites of the rearranging gene segments, a V(D)J rearrangement (in particular for the heavy chain locus) is unique for each B cell and thus can be used as a clonal marker for B cells deriving from the same mature B cell.

If B cells are activated through binding of antigen to their BCR and through cognate help from T-helper cells, the cells undergo a T-dependent immune response in specific histologic structures, the germinal centers (GC), in lymph nodes or other secondary lymphoid organs. In these follicles, activated B cells undergo massive clonal expansion and further diversify their BCR through two processes: somatic hypermutation and class switching. The process of somatic hypermutation introduces point mutations and some deletions and duplications at a very high rate into the Ig heavy and light chain V region genes. This randomly modifies amino acids in the V regions, and in a selection process involving follicular dendritic cells and follicular T-helper cells, B cells expressing mutated BCR with increased affinity to the stimulating antigen are positively selected, whereas B cells acquiring unfavorable mutations undergo apoptosis within the GC microenvironment (Fig. 73-1). Unfavorable mutations include clearly destructive mutations, such as nonsense mutations and deletions or duplications causing reading frame–shifts that prevent expression of a BCR as such. Other disadvantageous replacement mutations still allow BCR expression but reduce the affinity to the antigen. After multiple rounds of proliferation, mutation, and selection, positively selected B cells expressing a high-affinity BCR differentiate into long-lived memory B cells or plasma cells and exit the GC. Many GC B cells also undergo class switching before they are selected into the memory or plasma cell pool. In class switching, the originally expressed Cμ and Cδ heavy chain constant region genes (encoding IgM and IgD, respectively) are replaced by downstream-located Cγ, Cα, or Cε genes, encoding IgG, IgA, and IgE heavy chains, respectively, so that antibodies with altered effector functions are generated. At all stages of their development, B lineage cells are selected for expression of the appropriate BCR, and cells failing this selection are eliminated.

Cellular Origin of Lymphocyte Predominant Cells in Nodular Lymphocyte Predominant Hodgkin Lymphoma

LP cells in NLPHL express multiple typical B cell markers, such as the surface molecules CD20 and CD79 and the transcription factors PAX5, OCT-2, and BOB1 (Table 73-1).[1] LP cells mostly lack

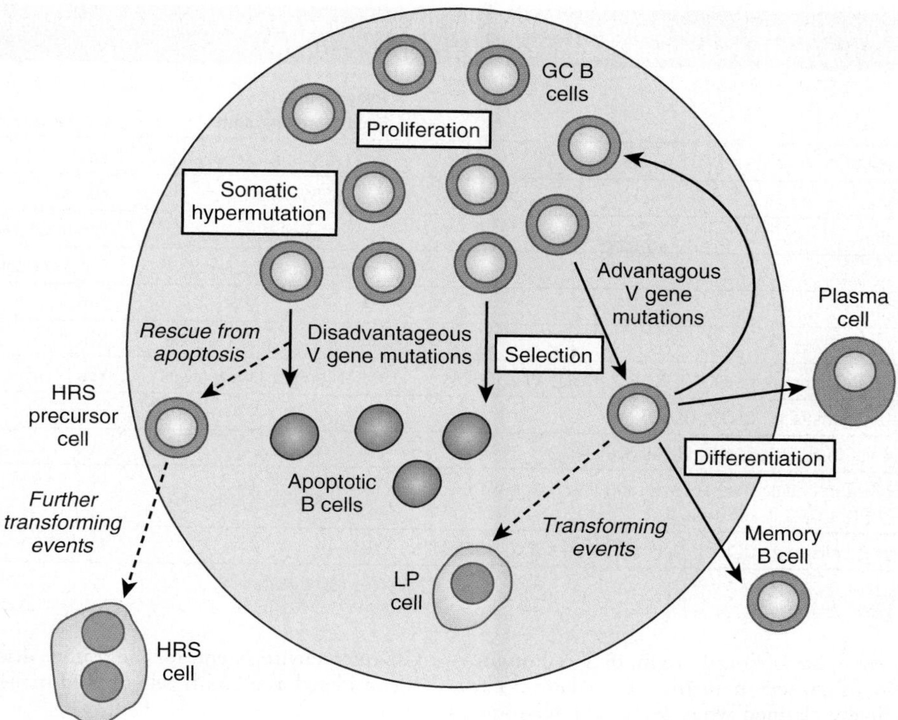

Figure 73-1 THE GERMINAL CENTER REACTION AND A SCENARIO FOR HODGKIN AND REED-STERNBERG AND LYMPHOCYTE PREDOMINANT CELL DERIVATION. Antigen-activated B cells that receive costimulatory signals from T-helper cells establish germinal center (GC) reactions in T-dependent humoral immune responses. In the GC, the activated B cells undergo massive clonal expansion in the dark zone. The proliferating GC B cells are called *centroblasts.* In the centroblasts, the process of somatic hypermutation is activated, which introduces somatic mutations at a very high rate into rearranged Ig V genes. Centroblasts migrate into the light zone and become resting centrocytes. Centrocytes are then selected based on their BCR. Most Ig V gene mutations will be disadvantageous (e.g., when they cause premature stop codons or lead to aminoacid changes that reduce the affinity of the BCR to the immunizing antigen) and will cause apoptotic death of the respective B cells. GC B cells acquiring affinity-increasing mutations will be positively selected by interaction with T-helper cells and follicular dendritic cells (not shown). Positively selected centrocytes may either return to the dark zone for further rounds of proliferation, mutation, and selection, or they differentiate into memory B cells or plasma cells and exit the GC. LP cells of NLPHL express functional Ig V genes and proliferate in a follicular microenvironment resembling GC. Thus these cells are likely derived from selected GC B cells. HRS cells in classical HL often carry destructive Ig V gene mutations, indicating that they derive from GC B cells that normally would have undergone apoptosis (i.e., pre-apoptotic GC B cells). Initial transforming events in HRS cell pathogenesis might have occurred already at a pre–GC B cell differentiation stage, or they might happen in the GC. In EBV-positive cases, EBV is a good candidate for a factor that allows GC B cells with destructive Ig V gene mutations to escape from apoptosis.

expression of markers of other hematopoietic cell lineages. Thus their immunophenotype suggests a B-cell origin. Moreover, LP cells are located in follicular structures in close association with follicular dendritic cells and GC-type T-helper cells, suggesting a close relationship with GC B cells. Indeed, LP cells express the transcription factor BCL6, the main regulator of the GC B cell differentiation program. They also express activation-induced cytidine deaminase (AID), an enzyme that regulates somatic hypermutation and class switching in GC B cells. Thus all of these phenotypic features point to a GC B cell origin of LP cells (see Table 73-1). This was further corroborated at the genetic level when clonally rearranged and productive Ig V region genes were amplified from isolated LP cells. These rearrangements were always somatically mutated. In some cases, intraclonal diversity of V region genes was observed, indicating ongoing somatic hypermutation during clonal expansion. Therefore the Ig V gene analysis further strongly supported a GC B cell origin of LP cells (Fig. 73-1). The detection of the same V gene rearrangements in all LP cells of a given NLPHL case was also important, because this firmly established for the first time the monoclonality of the LP cells, a hallmark for tumor cells. A recent gene expression profiling study of primary LP cells indicated that LP cells have partly downregulated a fraction of typical B cell genes and that their gene expression pattern indicates a relationship to late GC B cells on the way to becoming post-GC memory B cells.[2]

Cellular Origin of Hodgkin and Reed-Sternberg Cells in Classical Hodgkin Lymphoma

As mentioned earlier, HRS cells show a very peculiar immunophenotype that does not resemble any normal hematopoietic cell type. HRS cells express markers of different cell lineages in a fraction or even most cases, including B cell genes (e.g., PAX5, IRF4), T cell genes (e.g. Notch-1, GATA3), natural killer cell genes (ID2), myeloid genes (e.g., CD15, CSF1R), and dendritic cell markers (e.g., CCL13, fascin, restin) (Table 73-1).[2-4] Therefore immunohistochemical studies could not resolve the cellular origin of HRS cells. In addition, the first cell lines established from HL patients and presumed to be

Table 73-1 Comparison of Phenotypic and Genetic Features of Hodgkin and Reed-Sternberg Cells of Classical Hodgkin Lymphoma and Lymphocyte Predominant Cells of Nodular Lymphocyte Predominant Hodgkin Lymphoma

Feature	Hodgkin and Reed-Sternberg cells	Lymphocyte Predominant cells
Somatically mutated Ig V genes	Yes (very rare exceptions)	Yes
Crippling Ig V gene mutations	Yes (>25% of cases)	No
Ongoing somatic hypermutation	No	Yes (moderately)
Presumed cellular origin	Pre-apoptotic GC B cells	Positively selected, mutating GC B cells
Rare cases with a T-cell origin	Yes (<5%)	No
B-cell receptor expression	No	Yes
Expression of B-cell transcription factors (e.g., OCT2, BOB.1, PU.1, PAX5, E2A)	Rarely and/or at low levels	Yes
Expression of B-cell surface antigens (e.g., CD19, CD20)	No or rarely	Yes
Expression of GC B cell markers (e.g., BCL6, AID, HGAL, GCET)	No or rarely	Yes
Expression of molecules involved in antigen presentation and interaction with T-helper cells (e.g., CD40, CD80, CD86, MHC class II)	Yes	Yes
Expression of markers of non-B cells (e.g., CCL13, Notch1, GATA3, ID2, CSFR1)	Yes	No
EBV infection of tumor cells	Yes (30%-40%)	No

derived from HRS cells were either of B-cell origin, of T-cell origin, or of nonlymphoid origin (discussed in further detail later). The origin of HRS cells was finally clarified when HRS cells microdissected from tissue sections were analyzed for rearranged Ig V region genes. These studies revealed that HRS cells in nearly all cases carry clonal Ig heavy and light chain gene rearrangements.[5] This established their B-cell nature, because such rearrangements are highly specific for B cells. Moreover, with rare exceptions, the rearranged V region genes were highly mutated, pointing to a derivation from GC or post-GC B cells.[5] Intraclonal V gene diversity was not observed, showing that the process of somatic hypermutation is no longer active in these cells. There is also indication that many HRS cell clones underwent class-switch recombination, a further antigen-driven and B cell–specific process. Thus these genetic features of the rearranged Ig genes unequivocally demonstrate that the HRS cells are derived from mature B cells that had been activated by antigen. Although some initial studies reported polyclonality of HRS cells, these results could not be verified, and additional analyses firmly established the monoclonality of the HRS cells in a given case.

Surprisingly, in about a quarter of the cases of classical HL, the Ig V gene rearrangements carried clearly destructive mutations that rendered originally functional V region genes nonfunctional.[5] Such "crippling" mutations included deletions and insertions causing loss of the correct reading frame, as well as nonsense mutations. As discussed earlier, destructive mutations regularly happen in mutating GC B cells, but this normally results very efficiently in the removal of the cells by apoptosis. Thus it is highly likely that the GC B cells that acquired the destructive mutations already carried some transforming events that allowed them to escape apoptosis (Fig. 73-1). Of note, most disadvantageous mutations that cause apoptosis of normal GC B cells are likely replacement mutations that reduce affinity to the antigen or that interfere with the proper folding and/or pairing of the Ig heavy and light chains. These mutations cannot be easily recognized by looking at the V gene sequences. Thus the clearly crippling mutations likely represent only the "tip of the iceberg," and we have speculated that HRS cells, as a rule, derive from the pool of pre-apoptotic GC B cells (Fig. 73-1).[5] Rare cases of classical HL with unmutated V region genes have also been described. In such cases, the HRS cells may stem from pre-GC B cells. However, because GC B cells acquire their apoptosis proneness upon entering the GC even before starting to undergo hypermutation, it is also conceivable that such cases may originate from GC founder cells.

Decisive steps in HL pathogenesis, therefore, become effective or take place in GC B cells. Thus although some final transforming events may well occur when HRS precursor cells have already left the GC microenvironment, for the reasons discussed earlier, classical HL is considered as a GC B cell–derived malignancy.

T Cell–Derived Classical Hodgkin Lymphoma

The observation that in a fraction of cases the HRS cells express several T cell markers (e.g., CD3, granzyme B, perforin, T cell intracellular antigen 1) prompted studies aimed to clarify whether in such cases the HRS cells might derive from T cells. Analysis of HRS cells from several cases with T cell marker expression showed that most of these cases nevertheless are B cell–derived. However, several cases were identified that lacked Ig V gene rearrangements and that showed clonal T-cell receptor gene rearrangements.[6,7] Thus these cases have a T cell origin. Because the cellular origin of a lymphoma clone is a key factor for current lymphoma classification, it is a matter of debate whether lymphomas with HRS cells of T cell origin should be called *HL* or whether they should be considered a rare, separate type of T-cell lymphoma. However, because these cases are very rare (likely accounting for less than 5% of classical HL), because it is so far not possible to identify them by immunohistochemistry, and because it is unclear whether such cases differ in their clinical behavior from B cell–derived classical HL, there is currently no easy way to resolve this issue. Notably, in gene expression studies of HL cell lines, HDLM2 (a T cell–derived HL cell line) clustered more closely to B cell–derived HL cell lines than to other T-cell lymphoma lines, suggesting that B cell– and T cell–derived HRS cells have a similar gene expression pattern.

Hodgkin Lymphoma Cell Lines

Tumor cell lines are very valuable tools for detailed genetic, biochemical, and functional studies of a malignancy. Thus there have been many attempts to establish such lines from HL patients. However, this has proved to be a very difficult task, and less than 10 HL cell lines exist. A main reason for the difficulty in growing HRS or LP cells in culture is most likely their dependence on survival signals from the cellular microenvironment in the disease-affected lymph nodes. Of note, all of the existing HL lines are derived from end-stage patients and were not established from lymph nodes, but rather from peripheral blood, bone marrow, or pleural effusions. This suggests that only when the HRS cells have become independent from the lymph node microenvironment in the patient do they also have a chance to survive in suspension culture. The existing HL lines are

Table 73-2 Characteristics of Hodgkin Lymphoma Cell Lines*

Cell Line	Hodgkin Lymphoma Subtype	Cellular Origin	Known Genetic Lesions in Oncogenes or Tumor Suppressor Genes	Remarks
L428	Classical	B cell	NFKBIA, NFKBIE, SOCS1, TP53	
L540	Classical	T cell		
L591	Classical	B cell		Only EBV-positive line
L1236	Classical	B cell	TNFAIP3, CD95, SOCS1, TP53	Only line with proven origin from HRS cells in patient
KMH2	Classical	B cell	NFKBIA, TNFAIP3, CYLD	
HDLM2	Classical	T cell	TNFAIP3, SOCS1, TP53	
UHO-1	Classical	B cell	TNFAIP3, TRAF3	
SUP-HD1	Classical	B cell		
DEV	NLPHL	B cell	BCL6 (translocation)	

*A few additional lines have been published (HO, ZO, HD-70, HKB-1), but these have not been used in published studies in recent years, so it is unclear to the author whether they still exist, and very little is known about their phenotypic, functional, and genetic features.

L428, L540, L591, L1236, KMH2, HDLM2, UHO-1, SUP-HD1 and DEV (Table 73-2). Most lines are of B-cell origin, but HDLM2 and L540 are T cell–derived. L591 is the only HL line that is Epstein-Barr virus (EBV)–positive. Among primary cases of classical HL, about 30% to 40% show an infection of the HRS cells by EBV (see further details later). Notably, L591 cells do not have the typical EBV gene expression pattern of primary EBV-infected HRS cells, which should be kept in mind when using this line for gene expression or functional studies. The DEV line was originally reported as being derived from a case of classical HL, but subsequent more-detailed phenotypic and gene expression studies indicated that this is indeed the only existing cell line from a patient with NLPHL. Although the phenotype and genotype of these lines fits well with their presumed origin from HRS cells (or LP cells in the case of DEV), L1236 is the only cell line for which the derivation from the HRS cell clone of the patient from which it was established was unequivocally proven. In 1998 a line from a pediatric HL patient was established (HKB-1), but no further studies with this line were reported. Originally, the CO line was also published as an HL cell line. However, later studies showed that this line represents a cell culture contamination. Also the HD-Myz line was for a long time considered to be a classical HL cell line. However, it was later discovered that the phenotype of the line differs in key aspects from the phenotype of the primary HRS cells of the respective patient. Even more important, HD-Myz lacks Ig- and T-cell receptor gene rearrangements and is presumably of myeloid origin. Considering the fact that all informative HL cases that have been studied in detail for a lymphoid origin have turned out to be B cell–derived, or in rare cases T cell–derived, the nonlymphoid origin of HD-Myz argues against its derivation from HRS cells; thus this line should no longer be used as a model for HL.

Relationship Between Hodgkin Cells and Reed-Sternberg Cells

The population of HRS cells is always composed of a mixture of mononuclear Hodgkin cells and bi- or multinucleated Reed-Sternberg cells. It is thus an intriguing question how these two types of cells are related to each other. It was proposed that cell fusion might be involved in the generation of Reed-Sternberg cells from Hodgkin cells. However, in HL cell line models, fusions of Hodgkin cells resulting in the generation of Reed-Sternberg cells were rendered unlikely. Indeed, there is now firm evidence from studies of HL cell lines that Reed-Sternberg cells develop from mononuclear Hodgkin cells through a process of endomitosis, that is, nuclear division without cellular division. It was also discussed whether the whole HRS cell clone could derive from a cell fusion (e.g., a fusion of a B cell with a non-B cell). Such a scenario was attractive because it might have provided an explanation for the mixed immunophenotype and the usually aneuploid karyotype of the HRS cells. However, generation of the HRS cell clone through fusion was excluded by molecular studies.

Potential Hodgkin and Reed-Sternberg Precursor or Stem Cells

Another interesting question is whether the rare CD30$^+$ HRS cells represent the whole tumor cell clone in the HL tissue or whether further tumor clone members are present among the smaller, CD30$^-$ cells in the microenvironment. A fluorescence in situ hybridization study combined with CD30 immunostaining for cells with numeric chromosomal aberrations argued in favor of the existence of tumor cells among CD30-negative cells.[8] However, only two cases were studied, and numeric chromosomal aberrations (i.e., trisomies) are not stringent clonal markers. In a single-cell Ig V gene analysis of EBV-positive HRS cells and EBV-infected CD30-negative cells, it was found that the HRS cells and the small CD30$^-$ EBV-infected B cells carried distinct V gene rearrangements in nearly all instances.[9] Because EBV infection of HRS cells is a clonal event, so that in EBV$^+$ HL cases all members of the tumor clone should carry the virus, this finding was taken as an argument that the HRS cell clone does not have additional members among CD30-negative lymphocytes.

In several types of tumors, cancer stem cells were identified. These cells are defined as rare cells that have a particular proliferative potential and that sustain the tumor clone, whereas the bulk of the tumor clone lacks the potential to regrow to a full tumor. One study described the existence of HRS precursor cells in HL that fulfill at least some key features of cancer stem cells. In that work, it was reported that CD20$^+$BCR$^+$CD30$^-$ cells belonging to the HRS cell clone exist in the peripheral blood of HL patients and that these cells express the stem cell marker aldehyde dehydrogenase.[10] However, this finding was criticized because the markers for a clonal relationship between the HRS and non-HRS cells were unreliable and even argued, in part, against a relationship of the cells.[11] Moreover, a previous highly sensitive study that searched for HRS clone members in the peripheral blood failed to identify such cells.[12] Thus there is currently no convincing evidence for the existence of CD20$^+$BCR$^+$ HRS stem cells. In any case, it needs to be considered that HRS cells carry clonal and somatically mutated Ig V gene rearrangements; thus if HRS stem cells exist, they must be mature GC-derived B cells that carry the same Ig gene rearrangements and mutation pattern as the HRS cells.

The issue of potential subpopulations among the HRS cell clone with specific features in terms of proliferative potential and chemotherapy resistance was also addressed by searching for *side population cells,* which are defined as cells that extrude the Hoechst dye 33342, usually because they express drug transporters of the ABC family, such as the multidrug resistance 1 gene. In several types of tumors, side population cells were shown to share features with cancer stem cells (e.g., increased proliferative potential and chemotherapy resistance). Side population cells were indeed detected at low frequency (about 0.5% of cells) in some HL cell lines, and these cells showed increased resistance to chemotherapeutic drugs.[13,14] The side population cells had the phenotype of small Hodgkin cells and they were positive for CD30 and negative for CD19 and CD20. Hence these cells are different from the cells identified earlier as potential HRS stem cells. Notably, side population cells were able to reestablish the full HRS cell clone upon subcloning. However, not all HL cell lines showed side population cells, arguing against a general role of these cells in the maintenance of the HRS cell clone. Moreover, although side population cells were also identified in cell suspensions of HL lymph nodes, it remains to be clarified whether these cells belong to the HRS cell clone. Thus, there are exciting developments regarding the potential existence of subpopulations among the HRS cell clones with specific biologic features, but additional studies are needed to characterize these cells and reveal their relevance for the HRS clone in vivo.

Lessons From Composite Lymphomas

Composite lymphomas are very rare lymphomas in which an HL and a non-Hodgkin lymphoma (NHL) occur in the same patient. In a strict definition of composite lymphoma, this happens concurrently, but there are also cases where an HL may occur either before or after an NHL in the same patient. There are a few cases where the two lymphomas are not related to each other and hence represent the chance occurrence of two unrelated malignancies developing in parallel in a patient. However, in most composite lymphomas that have been molecularly studied for their clonal relationship, it was found that the lymphomas share a common origin.[15,16] The detailed study of the rearranged Ig V genes of such cases revealed that although, in many cases, the clonally related V region genes of the lymphomas share a number of somatic mutations, there are often additional mutations that were present only in the HRS cells and others only in the NHL B cells.[15,16] This showed that the two lymphomas have a common precursor, most likely a mutating GC B cell, and that the two lymphomas most likely developed from two distinct members of the GC B cell clone (Fig. 73-2). Thus these composite lymphomas usually do not represent the transformation of one lymphoma into the other but, rather, the parallel development of the two malignant clones from a common, premalignant precursor cell. It is likely that some transforming events were already present in the common precursor, but distinct daughter cells of this GC B cell later acquired different mutations, leading to the generation of the two distinct B-cell malignancies (Fig. 73-2). Therefore composite lymphomas are intriguing models to study the multistep transformation process in lymphomagenesis. In an initial study of several composite lymphomas for shared and distinct transforming events, examples for such genetic lesions were indeed identified.[17]

A further important aspect of the molecular studies of composite lymphomas is that they provide further evidence for the derivation of HRS cells in classical HL from GC B cells, because the clonal relationship with shared and distinct somatic Ig V gene mutations of an HRS cell clone and a typical GC B cell–derived lymphoma (e.g., follicular lymphoma or diffuse large B-cell lymphoma) strongly supports a common GC B-cell origin of both malignancies.

The Role of Epstein-Barr Virus in Classical Hodgkin Lymphoma

In about 40% of cases of classical HL in the Western world, and in about 90% of childhood HL cases in Central and Southern America, HRS cells are infected by EBV. Molecular analyses of EBV$^+$ cases showed that EBV infection of HRS cells is a clonal event (i.e., EBV

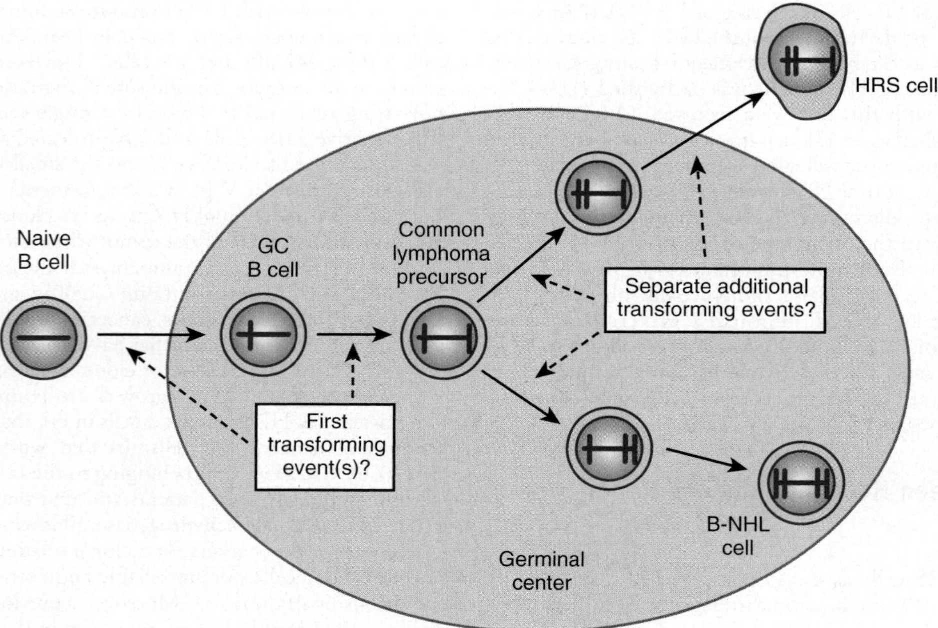

Figure 73-2 SCENARIO FOR THE GENERATION OF COMPOSITE LYMPHOMAS. Composite lymphomas are very rare combinations of a classical HL and an NHL. Detailed molecular analysis of rearranged Ig V genes in several such cases revealed that, in most instances, the two lymphomas are clonally related. Notably, the pattern of both shared and distinct V gene mutations in the majority of these cases revealed that the two lymphomas share a common precursor, but developed separately from this precursor. The direct clonal relationship of HRS cells with typical GC B cell–derived NHL is a further strong argument for a GC derivation of HRS cells. The horizontal line within the cells indicates an Ig V region gene; the vertical lines indicate somatic Ig V gene mutations. *(Modified from Bräuninger A, Hansmann ML, Strickler JG, et al.: Identification of common germinal center B-cell precursors in two patients with both Hodgkin's disease and non-Hodgkin's lymphoma,* New Engl J Med *340:1239, 1999.)*

infected or was already present in the founder cell of the HRS cell clone. EBV-positive HRS cells typically show a latency II gene expression pattern, which is characterized by expression of the EBV nuclear antigen 1 (EBNA1) and the two latent membrane proteins 1 and 2a (LMP1 and LMP2a, respectively). EBNA1 is essential for the replication of the EBV episome in proliferating cells. LMP1 is an oncogene, and one of its main functions is to cause constitutive NF-κB activation by mimicking an activated CD40 receptor. LMP2a has a cytoplasmic motif that resembles the signaling motif of the BCR. LMP2a can, on the one hand, diminish BCR signaling by recruiting BCR signaling components away from the BCR, but on the other hand, it mimics a tonic BCR signal. Strikingly, all HRS cell clones with clearly destructive Ig V gene mutations that prevent the expression of a BCR at all were found to be EBV-positive.[18] Hence it appears that in GC B cell precursors of HRS cells that acquired BCR-destructive mutations, EBV is essential to rescue these cells from apoptosis upon loss of BCR expression. This scenario is supported by studies showing that EBV can rescue BCR-deficient GC B cells from apoptosis, and that LMP2a has an important role in this process.[19] Whether the BCR-mimicking function is still important in the established HRS cell clone is unclear. The downregulation of most components of BCR signaling in HRS cells indicates that LMP2a does not have this role in the established HRS cell clone.

Genetic Lesions in Hodgkin and Reed-Sternberg and Lymphocyte Predominant Cells

The molecular analysis of HRS and LP cells for genetic lesions is hampered by the rarity of these cells. Nevertheless, we are now aware of a number of transforming events, especially for HRS cells. The recognition of constitutive activity of the NF-κB transcription factor, which is normally only transiently activated in lymphocytes, prompted studies of whether gene mutations might cause this deregulated activity. Inactivating mutations in the gene NFKBIA, which encodes the main inhibitor of NF-κB (i.e., IκBα) were detected in 10% to 20% of cases of classical HL (Fig. 73-3).[1] Also mutations in the NFKBIE gene were found. Genomic gains of the REL gene, encoding one of

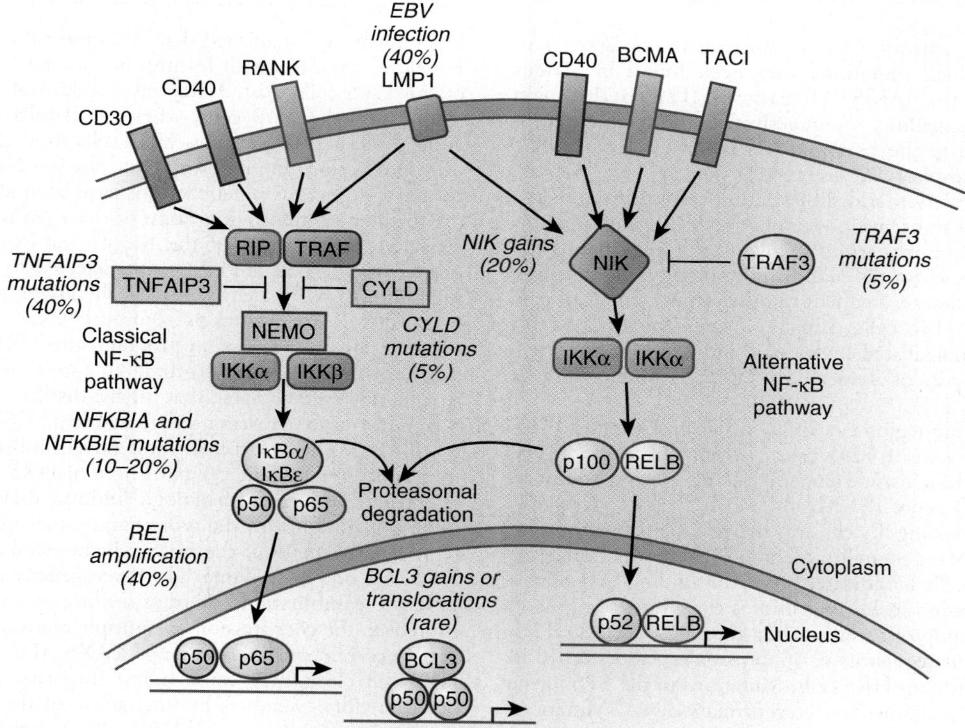

Figure 73-3 MECHANISM OF NF-κB ACTIVATION IN HODGKIN AND REED-STERNBERG CELLS. A classical and an alternative NF-κB signaling pathway are distinguished. In the classical NF-κB pathway, stimulation of numerous receptors (e.g., RANK, CD30, and CD40) leads via TNF receptor–associated factors (TRAFs) and other associated factors, such as the receptor-interacting protein (RIP), to activation of the IKK complex. The IKK complex is composed of IKKα, IKKβ, and NEMO. The activated IKK complex phosphorylates the NF-κB inhibitors IκBα and IκBε, which are encoded by the NFKBIA and NFKBIE genes, respectively. The phosphorylation marks the IκB factors for ubiquitinylation and subsequent proteasomal degradation. Thus the NF-κB transcription factors (e.g., p50/p65 or p50/REL heterodimers) are no longer retained in the cytoplasm and translocate into the nucleus, where they activate multiple genes. The signal transduction from TRAFs/RIP to the IKK complex can be inhibited by A20/TNFAIP3, which removes activating ubiquitins from RIP and TRAFs and additionally links ubiquitins to these molecules to mark them for proteasomal degradation. In the alternative NF-κB pathway, activation of receptors such as BCMA, CD40, and TACI causes stimulation of the kinase NIK, which then activates an IKKα complex. Activated IKKα processes p100 precursors to p52 molecules, which translocate as active p52/RELB NF-κB heterodimers into the nucleus. HRS cells show constitutive activity of the classical and alternative NF-κB signaling pathways. This activity is mediated by diverse mechanisms, including receptor signaling through CD40, RANK, BCMA, and TACI; genomic REL and NIK amplifications; destructive mutations in the TNFAIP3, NFKBIA, and NFKBIE genes; and signaling through the EBV-encoded latent membrane protein 1. HRS cells may also harbor nuclear BCL3/$(p50)_2$ complexes, and in a few cases the strong BCL3 expression appears to be mediated by genomic gains or chromosomal translocations of this gene. In rare instances, inactivating mutations in the inhibitory factors TRAF3 and CYLD have been found. *(Modified and updated from Küppers R: The biology of Hodgkin's lymphoma,* Nature Rev Cancer *9:15, 2009.)*

the NF-κB factors, are present in about 40% of classical HL. More recently, inactivating mutations in TNFAIP3, a further negative regulator of NF-κB, were detected in 40% of HRS cell clones.[20,21] Of interest, most cases with TNFAIP3 mutations were EBV-negative, suggesting that EBV infection and TNFAIP3 mutations are alternative mechanisms in HL pathogenesis. Reestablishing wild-type TNFAIP3 in HL cell lines reduced NF-κB activity and survival, establishing that TNFAIP3 functions as a tumor suppressor gene in this lymphoma.[21] For CYLD, another tumor suppressor gene and negative regulator of NF-κB, inactivating mutations were found in one HL cell line, but not in several primary cases of HL studied, indicating that mutations in this gene also occur in HRS cells, albeit at a low frequency. Rare mutations were recently also found in TRAF3, a negative regulator of the noncanonical NF-κB pathway. Finally, the NIK kinase gene, encoding a major activating factor for the noncanonical NF-κB pathway, shows gains in 20% of classical HL.[22]

Although LP cells of NLPHL also show constitutive NF-κB activity,[2] no destructive mutations were found in TNFAIP3 and NFKBIA in these cells.[23] Because there are also no indications for REL gains in LP cells, and because these cells are not infected by EBV, the mechanisms causing NF-κB activation in HRS and LP cells are strikingly different.

A second signaling pathway that shows constitutive activity in HRS cells and for which mutations have been found in various pathway members is the JAK/STAT pathway. This is the main pathway for cytokine signaling. Upon activation of cytokine receptors, JAK kinases bind to the receptors and become activated. The activated JAKs then phosphorylate and thereby activate STAT factors, which upon phosphorylation and dimerization translocate into the nucleus and function as transcription factors. Frequent genomic gains of JAK2 and also rare translocations involving this gene have been detected in HRS cells. However, activating point mutations in the JAK2 gene, although they are frequent in other types of hematologic diseases, are absent in HRS cells. SOCS1, a main inhibitor of this signaling pathway, is inactivated by somatic mutations in the HRS cells in about 40% of cases of classical HL.[24] SOCS1 mutations were also found in LP cells.[25]

Notably, the genomic region on 9p24, which harbors the JAK2 gene and which shows gains in HRS cells, also encompasses the gene JMJD2C, which encodes a histone demethylase, and the programmed death 1 (PD-1) ligand genes PD-L1 and PD-L2.[26,27] PD-1 ligands can inhibit PD-1–expressing T cells and thereby may contribute to the immunosuppressive microenvironment in HL.[26] A functional role of JMJD2C in HRS cells is indicated from the finding that down-regulation of its expression in HL cell lines is toxic for these cells.[27]

Because disturbed apoptosis seems to be a key aspect of classical HL pathogenesis, numerous regulators of apoptosis were also studied in HL cell lines and/or primary HRS cells. Mutations in the TP53 gene were found in three HL cell lines and a few primary cases.[28] Mutations in the CD95 gene were found in less than 10% of cases, and no mutations were found in the CD95 signaling components CASP8, CASP10, and FADD.[28] Moreover, no mutations were detected in the proapoptotic gene BAD; mutations in ATM are also very rare.[28]

Chromosomal translocations, usually involving one of the Ig loci and an oncogene, are a hallmark of most B cell lymphomas. Also in classical HL, chromosomal breaks involving the Ig loci were detected by fluorescence in situ hybridization in about 20% of cases. However, the translocation partners are in most cases unknown. In a few instances, BCL2, BCL3, BCL6, or MYC were identified as partners of the translocations. This also includes composite lymphomas in which the clonally related classical HL and the B cell NHL were found to carry the identical translocation—for example, a BCL2-IgH translocation in a composite classical HL/follicular lymphoma.[17] Notably, Ig locus–associated translocations usually function by causing deregulated expression of the translocated oncogene that has been brought under the control of the Ig regulatory elements, which are active in normal B cells and B cell NHL. Because the Ig loci are largely silenced in HRS cells, it is still unclear whether the partner genes of Ig locus–associated translocations in HRS cells are still active and pathogenetically relevant. Perhaps the translocations were important during early stages of HRS cell pathogenesis, when the lymphoma precursor cells still had a B-cell gene expression program, but became less important during later stages of the multistep transformation process. Alternatively, it should also be considered that translocations might function by mechanisms other than Ig enhancer–driven oncogene overexpression (e.g., promoter replacement or tumor suppressor gene inactivation).

Recently, recurrent translocations involving the MHC class II transactivator gene CIITA were found in about 15% of classical HL.[29] These translocations involved heterogeneous partner genes and seemed to function by impairing CIITA function and hence dampening MHC class II expression.

For LP cells of NLPHL, few genetic lesions are known. Besides the SOCS1 mutations mentioned earlier, translocations involving the BCL6 gene are frequently found.[30] BCL6 encodes a transcription factor that orchestrates the GC B-cell differentiation program and that has an oncogenic function when constitutively expressed in B cells.

FUTURE DIRECTIONS

It is now firmly established that HRS and LP cells stem from mature B cells. A few cases with features of classical HL and a T-cell origin of the HRS cells exist. HRS cells in classical HL appear to derive from crippled GC B cells, whereas LP cells likely originate from antigen-selected GC B cells. HRS cells show deregulated activation of multiple signaling pathways, and for the NF-κB and JAK/STAT pathway, numerous genetic lesions have been identified that contribute to the deregulated activation of these pathways. HRS cells show a nearly complete loss of the B-cell gene expression program.[4] As normal GC B cells are stringently selected to express a functional, high affinity BCR, the lost B-cell phenotype may be related to the origin of HRS cells from pre-apoptotic GC B cells: by losing the B cell–typical gene expression program, the HRS cell precursors may escape from the pressure to undergo apoptosis as "failed B cells." It should, however, be noted that further distinct subpopulations of GC B cells are currently being recognized (e.g., $CD30^+$ GC B cells), and it will be important to take these novel findings into consideration for a refinement of the cellular origin of HRS and LP cells.

The recent molecular biologic findings about HRS cells also offer some explanations for the typical and rather unique immunophenotypic heterogeneity of the HRS cells between cases and also among HRS cells of a given clone. The heterogeneity is likely due in part to different combinations of transforming events between HL cases. Moreover, the coexpression of multiple master regulators of different hematopoietic cell lineages (e.g., PAX5, ID2, Notch1) within one HRS cell clone may cause major fluctuations in gene expression between clone members by fluctuation of the competing transcription factors. Finally, because HRS cells are intimately interacting with multiple types of cells in their microenvironment, both by cellular interactions and through cytokines and chemokines, variations in the direct surrounding of HRS cells may cause differences in gene expression in these cells.

Further work is needed to fully understand the transforming events that lead to the generation of malignant HRS and LP cell clones, but with the availability of new methods, such as massively parallel sequencing of tumor genomes, it can be expected that major progresses will be made in the near future.

REFERENCES

1. Küppers R: The biology of Hodgkin's lymphoma. *Nat Rev Cancer* 9:15, 2009.
2. Brune V, Tiacci E, Pfeil I, et al: Origin and pathogenesis of nodular lymphocyte-predominant Hodgkin lymphoma as revealed by global gene expression analysis. *J Exp Med* 205:2251, 2008.
3. Lamprecht B, Walter K, Kreher S, et al: Derepression of an endogenous long terminal repeat activates the CSF1R proto-oncogene in human lymphoma. *Nat Med* 16:571, 2010.

4. Schwering I, Bräuninger A, Klein U, et al: Loss of the B-lineage-specific gene expression program in Hodgkin and Reed-Sternberg cells of Hodgkin lymphoma. *Blood* 101:1505, 2003.
5. Kanzler H, Küppers R, Hansmann ML, Rajewsky K: Hodgkin and Reed-Sternberg cells in Hodgkin's disease represent the outgrowth of a dominant tumor clone derived from (crippled) germinal center B cells. *J Exp Med* 184:1495, 1996.
6. Müschen M, Rajewsky K, Bräuninger A, et al: Rare occurrence of classical Hodgkin's disease as a T cell lymphoma. *J Exp Med* 191:387, 2000.
7. Seitz V, Hummel M, Marafioti T, et al: Detection of clonal T-cell receptor gamma-chain gene rearrangements in Reed-Sternberg cells of classic Hodgkin disease. *Blood* 95:3020, 2000.
8. Jansen MP, Hopman AH, Bot FJ, et al: Morphologically normal, CD30-negative B-lymphocytes with chromosome aberrations in classical Hodgkin's disease: The progenitor cell of the malignant clone? *J Pathol* 189: 527, 1999.
9. Spieker T, Kurth J, Küppers R, et al: Molecular single-cell analysis of the clonal relationship of small Epstein-Barr virus-infected cells and Epstein-Barr virus–harboring Hodgkin and Reed/Sternberg cells in Hodgkin disease. *Blood* 96:3133, 2000.
10. Jones RJ, Gocke CD, Kasamon YL, et al: Circulating clonotypic B cells in classic Hodgkin lymphoma. *Blood* 113:5920, 2009.
11. Küppers R: Clonogenic B cells in classic Hodgkin lymphoma. *Blood* 114:3970, 2009.
12. Vockerodt M, Soares M, Kanzler H, et al: Detection of clonal Hodgkin and Reed-Sternberg cells with identical somatically mutated and rearranged VH genes in different biopsies in relapsed Hodgkin's disease. *Blood* 92:2899, 1998.
13. Nakashima M, Ishii Y, Watanabe M, et al: The side population, as a precursor of Hodgkin and Reed-Sternberg cells and a target for nuclear factor-κB inhibitors in Hodgkin's lymphoma. *Cancer Sci* 101:2490, 2010.
14. Shafer JA, Cruz CR, Leen AM, et al: Antigen-specific cytotoxic T lymphocytes can target chemoresistant side-population tumor cells in Hodgkin lymphoma. *Leuk Lymphoma* 51:870, 2010.
15. Bräuninger A, Hansmann ML, Strickler JG, et al: Identification of common germinal-center B-cell precursors in two patients with both Hodgkin's disease and Non-Hodgkin's lymphoma. *N Engl J Med* 340:1239, 1999.
16. Marafioti T, Hummel M, Anagnostopoulos I, et al: Classical Hodgkin's disease and follicular lymphoma originating from the same germinal center B cell. *J Clin Oncol* 17:3804, 1999.
17. Schmitz R, Renné C, Rosenquist R, et al: Insight into the multistep transformation process of lymphomas: IgH-associated translocations and tumor suppressor gene mutations in clonally related composite Hodgkin's and non-Hodgkin's lymphomas. *Leukemia* 19:1452, 2005.
18. Bräuninger A, Schmitz R, Bechtel D, et al: Molecular biology of Hodgkin and Reed/Sternberg cells in Hodgkin's lymphoma. *Int J Cancer* 118:1853, 2006.
19. Mancao C, Hammerschmidt W: Epstein-Barr virus latent membrane protein 2A is a B-cell receptor mimic and essential for B-cell survival. *Blood* 110:3715, 2007.
20. Kato M, Sanada M, Kato I, et al: Frequent inactivation of A20 in B-cell lymphomas. *Nature* 459:712, 2009.
21. Schmitz R, Hansmann ML, Bohle V, et al: TNFAIP3 (A20) is a tumor suppressor gene in Hodgkin lymphoma and primary mediastinal B cell lymphoma. *J Exp Med* 206:981, 2009.
22. Steidl C, Telenius A, Shah SP, et al: Genome-wide copy number analysis of Hodgkin Reed-Sternberg cells identifies recurrent imbalances with correlations to treatment outcome. *Blood* 116:418, 2010.
23. Schumacher MA, Schmitz R, Brune V, et al: Mutations in the genes coding for the NF-κB regulating factors IκBα and A20 are uncommon in nodular lymphocyte–predominant Hodgkin's lymphoma. *Haematologica* 95:153, 2010.
24. Weniger MA, Melzner I, Menz CK, et al: Mutations of the tumor suppressor gene SOCS-1 in classical Hodgkin lymphoma are frequent and associated with nuclear phospho-STAT5 accumulation. *Oncogene* 25: 2679, 2006.
25. Mottok A, Renné C, Willenbrock K, et al: Somatic hypermutation of SOCS1 in lymphocyte-predominant Hodgkin lymphoma is accompanied by high JAK2 expression and activation of STAT6. *Blood* 110:3387, 2007.
26. Green MR, Monti S, Rodig SJ, et al: Integrative analysis reveals selective 9p24.1 amplification, increased PD-1 ligand expression, and further induction via JAK2 in nodular sclerosing Hodgkin lymphoma and primary mediastinal large B-cell lymphoma. *Blood* 116:3268, 2010.
27. Rui L, Emre NC, Kruhlak MJ, et al: Cooperative epigenetic modulation by cancer amplicon genes. *Cancer Cell* 18:590, 2010.
28. Schmitz R, Stanelle J, Hansmann M-L, et al: Pathogenesis of classical and lymphocyte-predominant Hodgkin lymphoma. *Annu Rev Pathol* 4:151, 2009.
29. Steidl C, Shah SP, Woolcock BW, et al: MHC class II transactivator CIITA is a recurrent gene fusion partner in lymphoid cancers. *Nature* 471:377, 2011.
30. Wlodarska I, Nooyen P, Maes B, et al: Frequent occurrence of BCL6 rearrangements in nodular lymphocyte predominance Hodgkin lymphoma but not in classical Hodgkin lymphoma. *Blood* 101:706, 2003.

CHAPTER 74

HODGKIN LYMPHOMA: CLINICAL MANIFESTATIONS, STAGING, AND THERAPY

Dennis A. Eichenauer, Andreas Engert, and Volker Diehl

In his historic 1832 paper, "On Some Morbid Appearances of the Absorbent Glands and Spleen," Thomas Hodgkin presented the clinical history and postmortem findings of the massive enlargement of lymph nodes and spleens of seven patients. Hodgkin assumed that rather than an inflammatory condition or an infectious disease such as syphilis or tuberculosis, these pathologic findings more resembled an autonomous lymphatic process that started in the lymph nodes located along the major vessels in the neck, chest, or abdomen.

In 1865, Sir Samuel Wilks for the first time linked Thomas Hodgkin's name to the disease that he described as "Cases of the Enlargement of the Lymphatic Glands and Spleen (or Hodgkin's Disease)." He was also the first to describe Hodgkin lymphoma (HL)–associated B symptoms such as weight loss and fever. In 1878, Greenfield was the first to publish drawings of the pathognomonic giant cells, which later were named after Carl Sternberg (1898) and Dorothy Reed (1902), who contributed the first definitive microscopic descriptions of HL.

Because HL was frequently clinically associated with tuberculosis, for a long time it was considered to be a peculiar form of a granulomatous disease such as tuberculosis. Despite the very strong evidence for the malignant nature of HL over the past century, it has been only recently shown that Hodgkin and Reed-Sternberg (HRS) cells are definitely clonally expanding, pre-apoptotic, germinal center–derived B lymphocytes that resemble true malignant cells.[1-2] (See Chapter 73.)

The management of HL has undergone a paradigm shift as a result of the availability of effective first-line regimens inducing high remission rates, the use of combined chemoradiotherapy and the introduction of effective salvage chemotherapy followed by autologous stem cell transplantation (ASCT) in relapsed HL, and a more sensitive realization of the magnitude of treatment-related late effects. Future developments will be based on a better understanding of biologic prognostic factors and the implementation of PET imaging to allow a more individualized treatment approach. In addition, novel drugs used in combination with classical chemotherapy protocols may increase efficacy and decrease toxicity of HL treatment.

ETIOLOGY, EPIDEMIOLOGY, AND GENETICS

Incidence and Age of Onset

HL is a rare disease with an annual incidence of 2 to 3 cases per 100,000 persons in Europe and the United States. In industrialized countries, the onset of HL has a bimodal distribution, with a first peak occurring in the third decade and a second peak occurring after the age of 50 years. Because of more refined molecular, cytologic, and immunohistologic techniques offering sensitive discrimination between HL subtypes and non-Hodgkin lymphoma (NHL), the second peak seems to have disappeared, mainly because the lymphocyte-depleted subtype of HL was recognized more frequently as large B-cell lymphoma. Slightly more men than women (1.4 : 1) develop HL. Among the group of young adults, the most common subtype is nodular sclerosing HL (NSHL) (Fig. 74-1). The frequency of the mixed-cellularity HL (MCHL) subtype increases with age, whereas the incidence of the NSHL subtypes reaches a plateau in the group of young adults older than 30 years so that MCHL is the subtype most often observed in older patients. According to the World Health Organization (WHO) classification, the subtypes of lymphocyte-rich classic HL (LRCHL), nodular lymphocyte-predominant HL (NLPHL) and lymphocyte-depleted HL (LDHL) are less commonly diagnosed, with a frequency of 3% to 5% (LPHL and LRCHL, respectively) and less than 1% (LDHL) in Western countries (Table 74-1). Incidence of this disease varies greatly between developing and industrialized countries. In developing countries, the disorder occurs predominantly during childhood, and its incidence decreases with age, whereas in industrialized countries, young children are much less commonly diagnosed with HL compared with adolescents or young adults. In industrialized countries, there are associations for early birth order, low number of siblings and playmates, high level of maternal education, single-family dwellings during childhood, and occurrence of HL in younger patients.

Role of Epstein-Barr Virus in the Pathogenesis of Hodgkin Lymphoma

Several studies have suggested that the Epstein-Barr virus (EBV) might be a transforming agent in HL. Mueller and colleagues analyzed EBV titers in predisease sera and found enhanced EBV activation before the onset of HL. Patients with a history of EBV-related infectious mononucleosis had a twofold to threefold increased risk for the development of HL. Another study confirmed that patients with a serologically diagnosed infectious mononucleosis had a fourfold increased relative risk for EBV-positive but not EBV-negative HL. The estimated median incubation time from mononucleosis to EBV-positive HL was 4.1 years, making a causal association between mononucleosis-related EBV infection and the EBV-positive subgroup of HL likely in young adults.[3]

To substantiate the role of EBV in HL, a number of researchers investigated EBV in HRS cells using novel molecular techniques and found that EBV-DNA is more often present in the tumor cells of HL patients in developing than in industrialized countries. In Western countries, about 50% of all cases of classic HL are EBV-positive (i.e., carry the virus within the tumor cells) (Fig. 74-2), with 15% to 30% of NSHL cases being positive and up to 70% of MCHL subtypes harboring EBV-DNA. In comparison, 90% or more of HRS cells are positive for EBV in developing countries. It was also shown that an impaired immune status may contribute to the development of EBV-positive HL in older patients.

HRS cells in EBV-positive patients show an expression pattern of EBV-encoded genes resembling that found in endemic nasopharyngeal carcinoma or in a subset of T-cell lymphomas, called *type 2 latency*. This pattern includes expression of the EBV-latent genes LMP1, LMP2, and EBNA1. Recently, it was shown by three independent studies that EBV can rescue B-cell receptor (BCR)–deficient germinal center B cells from apoptosis, adding evidence that EBV plays a role in the malignant transformation in HL.

Because EBV is present in only half of the tumor cells in HL patients from the Western world, investigators were prompted to

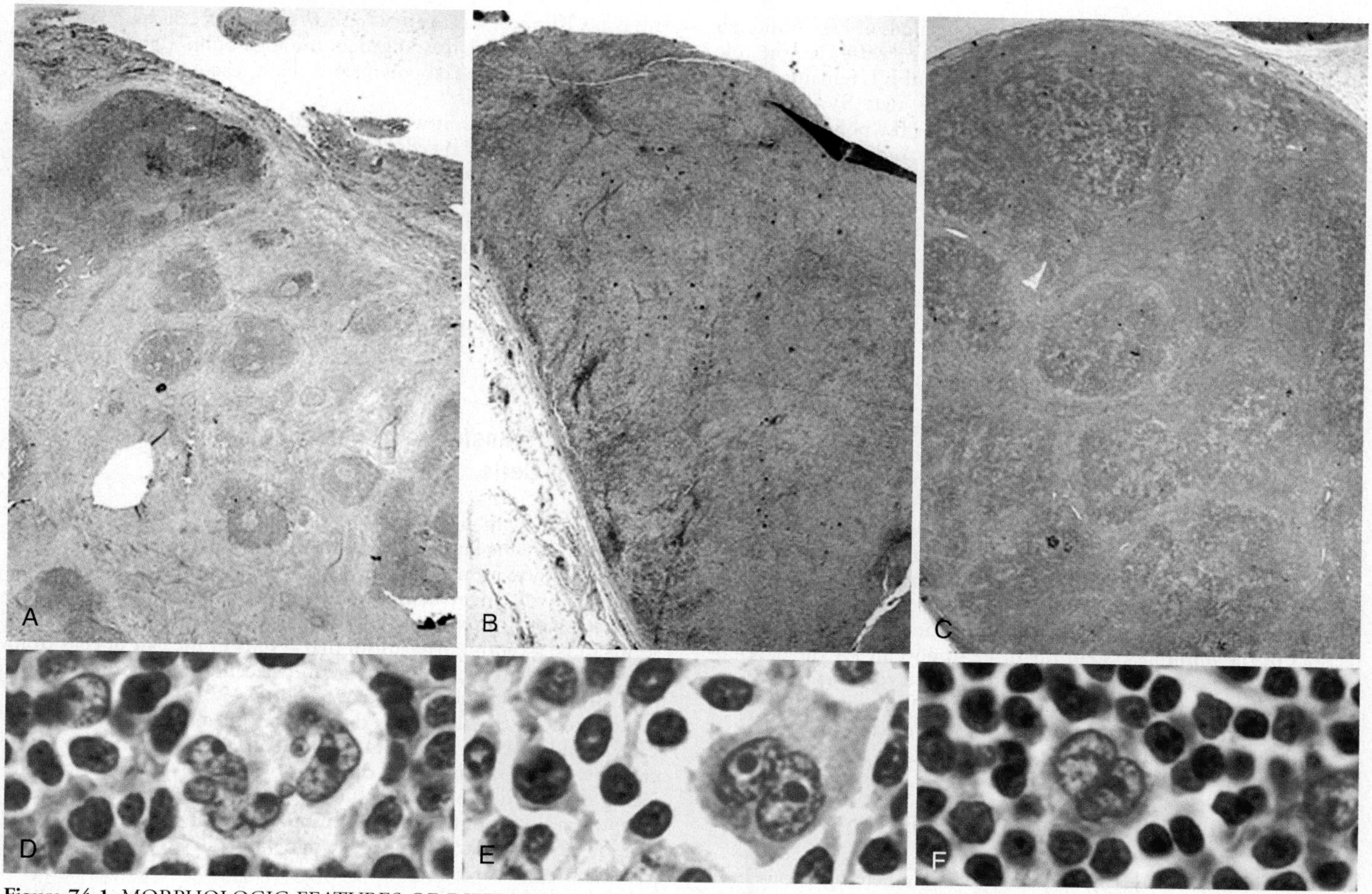

Figure 74-1 MORPHOLOGIC FEATURES OF DIFFERENT SUBTYPES OF HODGKIN LYMPHOMA. A low-power view of nodular sclerosing HL **(A)**, showing dense bands of fibrosis *(pink material)* dividing the node into cellular nodules. A similar low-power view of mixed cellular type **(B)** illustrating diffuse and patchy effacement of the normal lymph node architecture. In nodular lymphocyte predominance type **(C),** the node shows multiple vague expansile nodules. Sometimes these compress adjacent tissue and normal vasculature, giving the appearance of thin sclerotic bands, but this is not sclerosis as in the nodular sclerosing type. High-power illustrations of the associated neoplastic cells in these three variants. Lacunar cell variants **(D)** are the most prominent neoplastic cells in the nodular sclerosing type. These cells have lobulated nuclei and a clear space around the nucleus due to contraction of the cytoplasm in formalin-fixed tissue. More typical Reed-Sternberg cells can also be seen. In the mixed cellular type, classic mononuclear Hodgkin cells and binuclear Reed-Sternberg cells **(E)** are usually readily identified. In the nodular lymphocyte predominance type, the neoplastic cells are referred to as *LP cells* or *L&H (lymphocyte/histiocyte) cells* or *popcorn cells* because of their appearance **(F)**. In all types there are various numbers of reactive lymphocytes, plasma cells, histiocytes, eosinophils, and other acute inflammatory cells in the background.

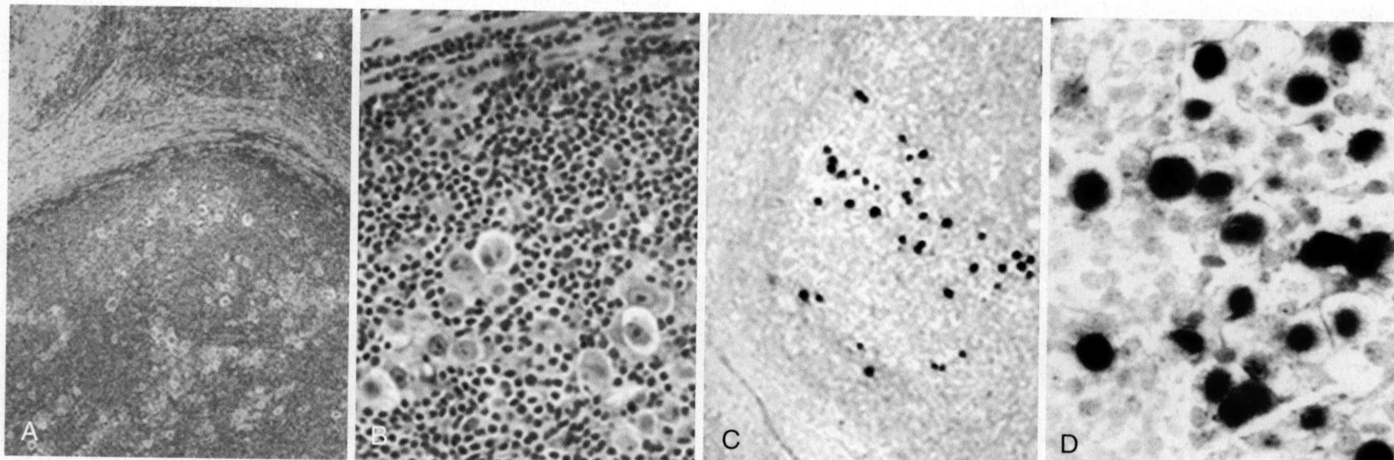

Figure 74-2 EBV DEMONSTRATED IN A CASE OF CLASSIC HODGKIN LYMPHOMA. Histologic sections **(A** and **B)** showing nodular sclerosing Hodgkin lymphoma with sclerotic bands, cellular nodules, and the HRS variant, lacunar cells. Epstein-Barr virus demonstrated by in situ hybridization by EBER (EBV-encoded RNA) identified by a black/blue reaction product, at low and high power **(C** and **D)**.

search for other viruses involved in the pathogenesis of HL. Although measles virus has been discussed to be associated with HL, the role of viruses other than EBV in the pathogenesis of HL remains uncertain. More specifically, despite initial reports that SV40 virus is present in a variety of lymphomas including HL, polyoma viruses were not detected in HL samples in follow-up studies.

Taken together, these data suggest that EBV is involved in the transformation process in EBV-positive HL cases. In EBV-negative cases, a "hit and run" mechanism was hypothesized, but evidence of EBV as a transforming agent in negative cases is scant.

Inheritance Pattern

In general, a family history of hematopoietic malignancy is associated with an approximately twofold increased risk to develop HL. More specifically, the risks of family members of patients affected by HL for developing the same disease are three to nine times those of the expected values. These observations led to the hypothesis that at least a portion of cases occur as an inherited disorder. Mack and colleagues found that of 179 monozygotic twin pairs with HL, both twins developed HL in 10 pairs, strongly supporting the idea of a genetic component in a subset of HL. Recent linkage studies correlated family or personal history of autoimmune or chronic inflammatory disease with the development of HL, suggesting that certain characteristics of the immune system might be important for the development of HL. However, familial HL is estimated to constitute only a minority of cases. No consistent mechanism of inheritance has been identified, and evidence for a genetic translocation unique to all cases of familial HL is lacking.

Hodgkin and Reed-Sternberg Cells and Their Origins

The affected tissue in HL is characterized by a heterogeneous infiltrate with typical mononucleated and multinucleated giant cells in an inflammatory background composed of stroma, lymphocytes, histiocytes, eosinophils, and monocytes. In classic HL (cHL), the giant cells are called *HRS cells,* and in NLPHL, they are called *lymphocyte predominant (LP) cells* (see Fig. 74-1). Typically, HRS cells represent only 0.1% to 1% of the affected tissue.

Because immunophenotyping did not lead to the identification of the origin of the HRS cells, molecular approaches were used to resolve this issue. Küppers was the first to show that HRS cells harbor somatically mutated clonal rearranged immunoglobulin (Ig) heavy chain genes by using single-cell polymerase chain reaction (PCR) methods on primary HRS cells.[2]

From these results, it was concluded that HRS cells were derived from germinal center B cells (Fig. 74-3). Amplification of identically rearranged and mutated Ig genes from different HRS cells showed they were clonal in origin—a key criterion of malignancy. HRS cells expand clonally within one affected lymph node, clonally disseminate in advanced-stage disease, and recur even after clinical complete remission (CR). Some studies indicate that in a small subset of HL, the HRS cells are probably of T-cell origin. In contrast, LP cells in NLPHL harbor ongoing mutations in their rearranged Ig genes and therefore seem to be malignant B cells at a different stage of maturation.

Table 74-1 Hodgkin Lymphoma Subtypes According to the WHO Classification

Nodular-sclerosing classic Hodgkin lymphoma
Mixed-cellularity classic Hodgkin lymphoma
Lymphocyte-rich classic Hodgkin lymphoma
Lymphocyte-depleted classic Hodgkin lymphoma
Unclassifiable classic Hodgkin lymphoma
Nodular lymphocyte–predominant Hodgkin lymphoma

Malignant Transformation of Hodgkin and Reed-Sternberg Cells

Despite significant progress in understanding the cellular origin of HRS cells, little is known about the mechanisms responsible for the initial transformation event. EBV has been identified as a virus with potential involvement in the transformation of a subpopulation of HL cases. Constitutive activation of nuclear factor–kappa B (NF-κB) seems to be a central mechanism that results in the exit of cells from the hostile environment of the germinal center and contributes to their proliferation and resistance to apoptosis.

Infected HRS cells express the EBV-encoded latent genes LMP1, LMP2, and EBNA1. Products of the latent genes have transforming capacity. LMP1, for instance, can transform primary B cells by mimicking the function of constitutively active CD40, a transmembrane receptor molecule of the TNF receptor family. Physiologically, CD40 ligation results in activation of a signaling cascade terminating in activation of the transcription factor NF-κB. NF-κB itself initiates transcription of proinflammatory and antiapoptotic genes. Constitutively, activation of NF-κB has been demonstrated to be a characteristic feature of HRS cells. Abrogation of constitutive NF-κB activation results in massive, spontaneous apoptosis of HRS cells by downregulation of an antiapoptotic signaling network, thereby providing evidence for its central role in the transformation and acquisition of the apoptosis-resistant phenotype.

SUMMARY OF MECHANISMS UNDERLYING MALIGNANT TRANSFORMATION

Although much has been learned about the derivation of the HRS cells, little is known about the basic mechanisms underlying malignant transformation of HL. The HRS cells in HL are derived from pre-apoptotic germinal center B cells in most cases, but in some cases, they are of T-cell origin. The expression of EBV-latent genes in EBV-positive cases (50%) may play a role in cellular transformation by upregulating the transcription factor NF-κB. The events underlying

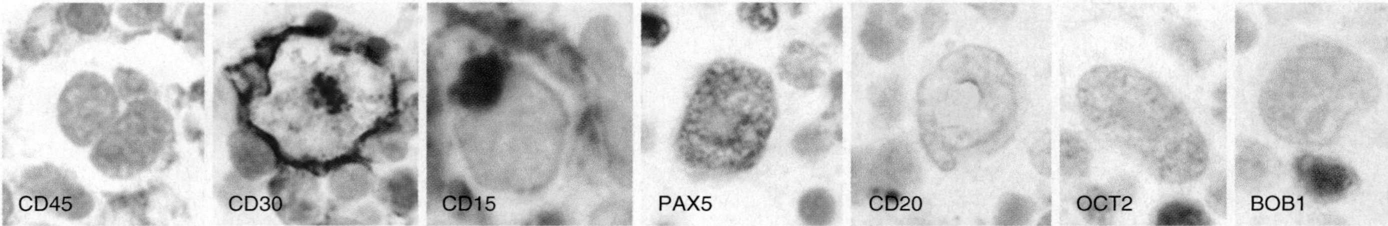

Figure 74-3 THE IMMUNOPHENOTYPE OF THE NEOPLASTIC CELLS IN CLASSIC HODGKIN LYMPHOMA. The cells typically are CD45-negative, CD30-positive, and CD15-positive with membranous and Golgi staining. The cells show nuclear staining for PAX5, a B-cell transcription factor, but the staining is usually weak compared with normal B cells. Typically, the cells are CD20-negative, but some cases can show partial or weak CD20. Last, the cells from classic Hodgkin lymphoma can weakly express one of the two other B-cell transcription factors: OCT2 and BOB1. They usually do not express both.

the transformation process in the EBV-negative cases, however, are still not understood. Several studies have focused on the apoptosis-resistant phenotype of HRS cells, and some data suggest that constitutively expressed FLICE-inhibitory protein (FLIP), a protein that inhibits FAS-mediated apoptosis, contributes to apoptosis resistance in HL. Genetic instability is a typical feature of HRS cells, and studies point to distinct genetic imbalances rather than subtile genetic alterations such as point mutations or microsatellite instability. Besides NF-κB, other transcription factors are deregulated in HRS cells, contributing to the lost B-cell identity of malignant cells in HL. The discovery that the HRS cells themselves contribute to the ineffective immune response by expressing immunosuppressive cytokines or by expressing chemokines that predominantly attract Th2 lymphocytes that are incapable of cell killing has widened our understanding of the environmental cross talk of these peculiar cells.

DIAGNOSIS AND STAGING

From the beginning, it was postulated that HL spread from one lymph node area by contiguity to adjacent lymph node chains. Only in the middle of the 20th century was this knowledge used by investigators such as Peters, Kaplan, Tubiana, and Musshoff for the development of strategies for the treatment of this disorder.

The applicability of new radiologic techniques and the information derived from routine exploratory staging laparotomies have provided important insights into the presentation and evolution of HL. Although there is strong evidence that HL starts in a single group of lymph nodes and then spreads by the lymphatic route, mounting data suggest that the gradually more aggressive tumor cells tend to disseminate through the bloodstream rather early and disseminate to organs such as bone marrow, liver, and lung. For the initial diagnosis of HL, an excisional biopsy of a suspicious lymph node should be performed. Assessment of the bone marrow is important for staging and for an evaluation of the normal bone marrow cells before therapy. Bone marrow involvement occurs in less than 5% of patients.

The extent of HL can be classified using the four-stage Ann Arbor classification. The absence (A) or presence (B) of systemic symptoms (e.g., fever, night sweats, and weight loss) further characterizes the severity of disease. The Cotswolds classification is a modification of the Ann Arbor classification, using information from staging and treatment gathered over the past 20 years. This classification was proposed in 1989 during a meeting held in the Cotswolds, England. Information about prognostic factors such as size of the mediastinal mass, the presence of bulky nodal disease, and the extent of subdiaphragmatic disease is included in this classification.

The staging procedures recommended for determining the extent of disease have become less invasive in recent years. Staging laparotomy and splenectomy are no longer used. Computed tomography (CT) of neck, chest, abdomen, and pelvis is routinely performed in the diagnostic evaluation of a patient with HL.

Two thirds of patients with newly diagnosed HL have radiographic evidence of intrathoracic involvement. A *large mediastinal mass* has been arbitrarily defined as a mass in which the ratio is greater than one third for the largest transverse diameter of the mediastinal mass over the transverse diameter of the thorax at the diaphragm on a standing posteroanterior chest radiograph. Alternatively, others have defined extensive mediastinal disease as greater than 35% of the thoracic diameter at T5-6 or wider than 5 or 10 cm.

Gallium 67 scintigraphy, previously used in evaluating the mediastinum or in the evaluation of residual masses in HL patients after treatment, has been replaced by FDG-PET. According to the international harmonization project, FDG-PET can be used to improve staging techniques at initial diagnosis by detecting lesions not detected by CT, to assess tumor response while on treatment, and to evaluate residual tumor masses at the end of treatment, allowing discrimination between active lymphoma and fibronecrotic tissue.[4]

When FDG-PET is used in addition to conventional imaging techniques for the initial workup of patients, approximately 10% of HL patients are up-staged and another 10% down-staged but it remains unclear whether patients would benefit from a subsequent change of the treatment plan. Therefore the value of FDG-PET for initial staging of HL patients is limited. When assessing early tumor response rates in HL patients after two or three cycles of chemotherapy, Hutchings and Gallamini found a significant correlation between the PET results and the clinical outcome of patients in terms of progression-free survival (PFS) and overall survival (OS).[5] Whether such an early PET response will be useful to tailor therapies more individually in the future needs to be clarified by prospective trials currently ongoing worldwide.

If PET is used at the end of treatment, it shows an excellent negative predictive value. In the HD15 trial from the German Hodgkin Study Group (GHSG), patients with advanced HL who had residual lesions larger than 2.5 cm after chemotherapy underwent PET examination. Patients with a positive PET received additional localized radiation, whereas those patients with a negative PET did not receive further treatment. The negative prognostic value (defined as the proportion of PET-negative patients without progression, relapse, or the need for radiation within 12 months) was 94.6%. Thus PET-guided radiation in patients with advanced HL was adopted as standard within the GHSG.

CLINICAL FEATURES

Patients with NSHL or MCHL have a central pattern of lymph node involvement (e.g., cervical, mediastinal, paraaortic). In most patients with cHL, primary lymphadenopathy occurs in the left cervical or supraclavicular region or in the mediastinum. NSHL patients more often have a supradiaphragmatic onset of disease. MCHL patients present with smaller disseminated nodes and predominantly subdiaphragmatic nodes or organ involvement. In contrast, certain nodal chains (e.g., mesenteric, hypogastric, presacral, popliteal) are seldom involved. Patients with NLPHL typically present with involved peripheral nodes in the cervical, submandibular, axillary, or inguinal region. NLPHL is mostly diagnosed in early stages. B symptoms and involvement of the spleen or other organs rarely occur. The spleen is involved more frequently in patients with adenopathy below the diaphragm, systemic symptoms and MCHL histology. Involvement of the liver is rare and mainly occurs with concomitant splenic involvement. Infiltration of the bone marrow at diagnosis is uncommon, usually focal, and almost always associated with extensive disease, systemic symptoms, and unfavorable histology.

Bulky lymph node involvement or a contiguous collection of smaller lymph nodes (>10 cm in diameter) may result in regional complications such as vascular, tracheal, bronchial, or gastrointestinal compression or obstruction. Invasion of adjacent anatomic regions such as the lung, pericardium, pleura, chest wall, or bone can occur in patients with HL. Effusions of the pericardium, pleural cavity or peritoneal cavity are often associated with extranodal involvement and invasive growth into neighboring structures. Despite a large mediastinal mass, superior vena cava syndrome is seldom observed; if it occurs, it is often associated with venous thrombosis.

Compared with NHL, bulky infradiaphragmatic lesions with obstructive symptoms are rare in HL. Spleen involvement is often subclinical and sometimes hard to diagnose with modern imaging techniques. Tumor involvement is not necessarily associated with splenic enlargement; a small spleen can have diffuse HL involvement.

Hematopoietic spread to organs is mainly seen in the lung, liver, bone marrow, and bone, and it must be distinguished from disease invasion into adjacent organs by an extranodal tumor that penetrates the capsule of a lymph node. Skin involvement is seen very rarely and can appear as small, opaque, or red papules or as ulcerating lesions. Involvement of the central nervous system can occur by extension from nodes within the paraaortic region through the intervertebral foramina, manifesting as neurologic symptoms and pain.

A considerable number of undiagnosed patients with HL present with systemic symptoms before the discovery of enlarged lymph nodes. Typical symptoms include fever, drenching night sweats, and weight loss (i.e., B symptoms). The characteristic HL-associated fever (i.e., Pel-Ebstein type) occurs intermittently and recurs at variable intervals over several days or weeks. Fever and drenching night sweats are identified in 25% of all patients at the time of initial presentation, increasing to 50% of patients with more advanced disease. Other nonspecific symptoms include pruritus, fatigue, and the development of pain shortly after drinking alcohol. This pain is usually transient at the site of nodal involvement and may be severe. Pruritus, although not a defined B symptom, may be an important systemic symptom of disease, although it affects less than 20% of patients. It often occurs months or even a year before the diagnosis of HL. The underlying pathophysiologic mechanisms leading to pruritus are unknown, but possible causes include an intrinsic production of cytokines such as growth factors by the HRS cells and an autoimmune reaction in which a number of cytokines are activated by tumor lysis.

CHOICE OF TREATMENT

Prognostic Factors and Treatment Groups

Prognostic factors define the likely outcome of the disease of an individual patient at diagnosis allowing selection of appropriate treatment strategies. Despite an enormous effort to define clinically relevant and generally acceptable prognostic factors, there are still two major methods for dividing HL patients according to a risk- or prognosis-adapted therapeutic approach: stage and systemic symptoms. A third factor meets general transatlantic acceptance: massive local tumor burden (i.e., bulky disease >10 cm in diameter). Prognostic factors are rarely the subject of specific clinical studies but are recognized and evaluated using data from large cohorts of uniformly treated, well-documented, and reliably followed patients, usually from large clinical trials.

In the United States, some centers still treat HL patients according to the traditional separation of early stages (stage I-IIA), representing about 45% of newly diagnosed patients, and advanced stages (III-IV, A and B, or any stage with bulky disease >10 cm in diameter or B symptoms), representing about 55% of newly diagnosed patients. Patients with early-stage disease are treated with combined-modality strategies. Patients with advanced-stage disease are assigned to intensive chemotherapy protocols, sometimes followed by adjuvant radiotherapy.

The European Organization for Research and Treatment of Cancer (EORTC), in the H1 and H2 trials, identified additional prognostic factors that are now used to assign clinical stage I or II patients to a more unfavorable-prognosis group. The EORTC has, since 1982, defined clinical stage I or II (supradiaphragmatic only) patients as having an early unfavorable prognosis HL if any of the following factors is present: age older than 50 years, asymptomatic with an ESR higher than 50 mm/h, B symptoms with an ESR higher than 30 mm/h, and a large mediastinal mass (Table 74-2). In previous trials, stage II disease with MCHL or LDHL histology and number of involved regions had also been counted as adverse factors.

The GHSG has, since 1988, assigned clinical stage I or II patients to an intermediate group if they have any of the following adverse factors: large mediastinal mass (>⅓ of maximum thoracic diameter), three or more involved nodal areas, elevated ESR, and localized extranodal infiltration (Table 74-2). It can be difficult to distinguish consistently between extranodal lesions and stage IV disease, so various assessments of the prognostic value of this feature have been obtained by different investigators.

Currently, the following general treatment strategies are widely used in the United States and in Europe:

1. Early stages, favorable: combined-modality approaches (2-4 cycles of chemotherapy plus involved-field radiation)
2. Early stages, unfavorable (intermediate): combined-modality approaches (4-6 cycles of chemotherapy plus involved-field radiation)

Table 74-2 Allocation of Hodgkin Lymphoma Patients to Treatment Groups

Treatment Group	EORTC/GELA	GHSG
Limited-stage patients	CS I-II without risk factors (supradiaphragmatic)	CS I-II without risk factors
Intermediate-stage patients	CS I-II with ≥1 risk factors (supradiaphragmatic)	CS I, CS IIA with ≥1 risk factors CS IIB with risk factors C/D, but not A/B
Advanced-stage patients	CS III-IV	CS IIB with risk factors A/B, CS III/IV
Risk factors	(A) Large mediastinal mass (B) Age ≥50 years (C) Elevated ESR (D) ≥4 nodal areas	(A) Large mediastinal mass (B) Extranodal disease (C) Elevated ESR (D) ≥3 nodal areas

3. Advanced stages: extensive chemotherapy (6-8 cycles) with or without consolidating localized radiation

An attempt has also been made to identify very good risk and very poor risk subgroups. The EORTC has investigated the use of localized radiotherapy in a “very favorable subgroup” of early-stage patients. Inclusion criteria were stage IA disease for female patients younger than 40 years and NSHL or NLPHL histology without an elevated ESR or large mediastinal mass. However, the failure rate was 29% at 6-year follow-up, and this policy was abandoned. Similarly, advanced-stage patients at particularly high risk for failure were treated with early high-dose chemotherapy (HDCT) with autologous stem cell transplantation (ASCT). Currently, only patients who relapse after first-line treatment receive HDCT followed by ASCT. HDCT/ASCT is not included in standard treatment strategies for initially diagnosed HL.

The EORTC includes in its advanced-stage cohort stage III and IV patients only, without regard to other factors, as did the U.S. National Cancer Institute and several U.S. cooperative groups. Certain other trial groups also include stage I-II patients in the advanced-stage group, if they have B symptoms or bulky disease. The GHSG includes both stage III-IV patients and patients with stage IIB disease and a large mediastinal mass and/or E-lesions in the advanced-stage cohort (Table 74-2). The gradual shift towards more intensive therapy is based on the incorporation of prognostic factors into treatment algorithms.

Prognostic Factors for Advanced-Stage Hodgkin Lymphoma

International consensus about longer and better-controlled follow-up periods with the observation of a greater frequency of treatment failure events has permitted the identification of more conclusive and generally applicable prognostic factor analyses for advanced-stage disease. The International Prognostic Factor Project produced an International Prognostic Score (IPS), which, although not necessarily completely comprehensive, is widely accepted.

All of the factors included in the IPS were shown to be highly significant in a multivariate analysis of data from 5141 patients, and their prognostic power was confirmed in an independent sample. All seven factors were associated with similar relative risks of between 1.26 and 1.49. It was recommended that these factors should be combined into a single score by counting the number of adverse factors resulting in an integer prognostic score between 0 and 7. However, even patients with five or more factors (7% of cases) had a 5-year failure-free rate of more than 40%. The best failure-free rate was close to 80% for patients with at most one adverse factor (29%

of cases), suggesting that a group of advanced-stage patients with a relatively favorable prognosis could be recognized (1618 patients included in the final analysis for freedom from treatment failure according to whether the prognostic score was 0 to 2 or 3 or higher).[6]

A number of other factors have been shown to correlate with prognosis in advanced stages, but their independent importance has not been proven because of conflicting results or lack of validation in a large independent data set. These include pathologic grade in NSHL, the amount of tissue eosinophilia, inguinal involvement, serum lactic dehydrogenase concentration, and beta-2 microglobulin level.

In conclusion, the three-level scheme of division into early favorable, early unfavorable (intermediate), and advanced-stage cases remains a suitable instrument to tailor therapy. Because clinical and biologic factors do not discriminate the 10% to 15% of advanced-stage patients who will progress or experience an early relapse (<12 months), biologic molecular parameters are urgently needed to save most patients from overtreatment or intensify treatment for patients resistant to the best modern treatment modalities. There is hope that current approaches using on-treatment imaging techniques such as PET, gene expression profiles of primary tumor material, individual drug metabolism, or cytokine profiles of serum samples will detect patterns that distinguish low-risk from standard-risk and poor-risk patients.

EARLY-STAGE HODGKIN LYMPHOMA

Early Favorable Disease

The treatment of early-stage HL is changing. In the 1990s, extended-field irradiation was considered standard treatment. However, because of the high relapse rate and the increased frequency of long-term effects, the use of extended-field radiotherapy has been abandoned by most study groups. Instead, a brief chemotherapy combined with involved-field irradiation is the current standard of care for early favorable HL.

Extended-field radiotherapy alone produces CR in 90% to 98% of patients with early favorable HL. Unfortunately, 30% to 40% of those patients relapse, but salvage chemotherapy or combined-modality treatment yields remissions in most of these cases. As a result, approximately 75% to 85% of patients with early favorable disease who receive extended-field radiotherapy as first-line treatment are alive after 10 years.[7]

Combined-Modality Treatment With Extended-Field Irradiation Versus Extended-Field Radiotherapy Alone

To reduce the high relapse rates observed with radiotherapy alone, combined-modality therapies were introduced and compared with radiotherapy alone in patients with early favorable HL. The HD7 trial (1994-1998) of the GHSG randomized 650 patients with early favorable HL to extended-field radiation alone or to two courses of ABVD (i.e., doxorubicin [Adriamycin], bleomycin, vinblastine, and dacarbazine) (Table 74-3) and extended-field radiation therapy. The final analysis after a median follow-up of 87 months showed an advantage in freedom from treatment failure (FFTF) in the patients receiving ABVD (88%) compared with those treated with irradiation alone (67%, P <0.0001) (Fig. 74-4). Probably because of effective salvage therapy, overall survival (94% and 92%) did not differ between the two treatment arms.[7]

Results were similar in an American Intergroup phase III trial comparing three cycles of doxorubicin (Adriamycin) and vinblastine (AV) plus subtotal lymphoid irradiation with subtotal lymphoid irradiation alone in clinical stage IA-IIA patients with supradiaphragmatic disease that did not undergo staging laparotomy. The trial had to be closed after the second interim analysis because of a significantly superior failure-free survival rate for patients in the combined-modality arm (94% versus 81%, respectively, at a median follow-up of 3.3 years). However, the two previously described studies used extended-field radiotherapy and did not address the issue of whether radiation therapy could be reduced safely when coadministering chemotherapy.

Table 74-3 The ABVD Regimen

Drug	Dose	Route	Schedule
Doxorubicin	25 mg/m²	IV	Days 1 + 15
Bleomycin	10 mg/m²	IV	Days 1 + 15
Vinblastine	6 mg/m²	IV	Days 1 + 15
Dacarbazine	375 mg/m²	IV	Days 1 + 15

Recycle day 29

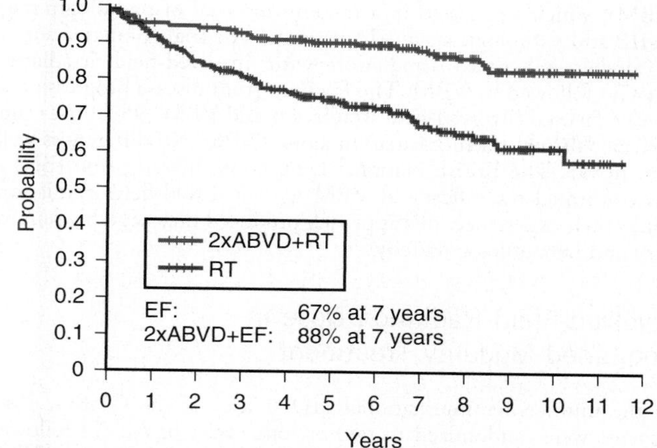

Figure 74-4 FREEDOM FROM TREATMENT FAILURE AMONG PATIENTS TREATED WITHIN THE GHSG HD7 TRIAL FOR EARLY FAVORABLE HODGKIN LYMPHOMA. *Blue,* Combined-modality treatment (2 cycles of ABVD plus extended-field radiotherapy). *Purple,* Radiotherapy alone (extended-field radiotherapy). *(Engert A, Franklin J, Eich HT, et al: Two cycles of doxorubicin, bleomycin, vinblastine, and dacarbazine plus extended-field radiotherapy is superior to radiotherapy alone in early favorable Hodgkin's lymphoma: Final results of the GHSG HD7 trial,* J Clin Oncol *25:3495, 2007.)*

Combined-Modality Treatment With Involved-Field Radiotherapy Versus Extended-Field Radiotherapy Alone

Randomized trials of combined-modality therapy have been based on the premise that this approach results in a very high freedom from recurrence rate and that this high degree of efficacy can even be maintained when using less toxic chemotherapy and radiation approaches. In the EORTC H7F trial (333 favorable patients), six cycles of the EBVP regimen (i.e., epirubicin, bleomycin, vinblastine, and prednisone) plus involved-field irradiation were compared with mantle and para-aortic-splenic nodal irradiation for favorable-prognosis clinical stage IA-IIA patients. At 10 years, the event-free survival rate was significantly better for patients on the combined-modality arm compared with those receiving radiation alone (88% versus 78%, P = 0.01). Survival rates were similar (92%). Because the H7U trial showed that EBVP is less efficient than a hybrid of MOPP (mechlorethamine, vincristine [Oncovin], procarbazine and prednisone) and ABVD, the latter regimen was used in subsequent studies.

The EORTC H8F trial (1993-1998) compared three cycles of MOPP/ABV and involved-field irradiation against mantle and para-aortic-splenic irradiation for favorable-prognosis clinical stage IA-IIA patients. Because relapse-free survival differed significantly between the two treatment arms (98% versus 74%; P <0.001), it was concluded that combined-modality treatment was the new gold standard of therapy. Taken together, this EORTC trial was the first to demonstrate that subtotal nodal irradiation could be safely replaced by a combined-modality regimen, because reduced radiotherapy (involved-field radiotherapy) in combination with chemotherapy was shown to be superior to subtotal nodal irradiation.[8]

With the objective of reducing acute toxicity and chronic morbidity, Horning and colleagues developed a presumably less toxic chemotherapy regimen of vinblastine, bleomycin, and methotrexate (VBM), which was tested in a randomized trial of pathologic stage IA-IIB and pathologic stage IIIA patients. The trial compared subtotal nodal/total nodal irradiation with involved-field irradiation (44 Gy) followed by VBM. The freedom from disease progression at 5 years favored involved-field irradiation and VBM (95%) over subtotal nodal/total nodal irradiation alone (70%). No differences were seen in OS. The British National Lymphoma Investigation (BNLI) has confirmed the efficacy of VBM with involved-field irradiation, but in their experience, this approach produced unacceptable pulmonary and hematologic toxicity.

Involved-Field Radiation Dose in Combined-Modality Treatment

In the multicenter international HD10 trial of the GHSG, 1370 patients were randomized to two or four cycles of ABVD followed by 20 or 30 Gy of involved-field radiation therapy. At 5 years, FFTF and OS rates were very similar in all treatment arms; thus the least-toxic approach (two cycles of ABVD followed by 20 Gy of IF-RT) was adopted as the novel standard for early favorable HL.[9]

The GHSG follow-up trial for patients with early favorable HL, HD13, was designed to determine whether the rather toxic components of the ABVD regimen of bleomycin (lung) and dacarbazine (gastrointestinal) can safely be eliminated in combined-modality treatment schedules. The data safety monitoring committee closed the AV and the ABV arm prematurely in 2005 and 2006 due to a fourfold increase in HL-related events compared with ABVD and AVD. Randomization into the other arms was continued as planned until 2009. Thus final results of the trial are pending.

Two randomized trials tested chemotherapy-only approaches for early-stage patients. The EORTC/GELA H9F trial (n = 783) evaluated doses of 36 Gy, 20 Gy, or no radiation to involved sites in patients who have achieved complete remission after six cycles of EBVP (n = 591). The final analysis with arm comparison showed higher relapse rates than expected in the chemotherapy-only arm, which had to be closed early. The event-free survival at 4 years was 87%, 84%, and 70% for 36 Gy, 20 Gy, and no radiation therapy, respectively (P <0.001) showing that involved-field radiation could not be skipped when combined with a mild chemotherapy regimen. Although data are not yet mature, it was postulated that a dosage of 20 Gy is equally efficient as 36 Gy in these patients.

Meyer and colleagues published results of a trial conducted by the National Cancer Institute of Canada Clinical Trials Group and the Eastern Cooperative Group. Patients with stage I-IIA were allocated to a favorable and an unfavorable cohort (inclusion criteria: age >40 years, ESR >50 mm/h, mixed-cellularity or lymphocyte-depleted histology, and >4 sites of involvement) before random assignment to ABVD as single modality or a radiotherapy-containing treatment. Patients in the chemotherapy-only group received up to six cycles of ABVD. Patients in the radiotherapy group were treated with subtotal nodal irradiation only or two cycles of ABVD and subtotal nodal irradiation, if allocated to the favorable or the unfavorable cohort, respectively. There was a statistically significant difference in terms of freedom from progression in favor of the radiation-containing regimen (93% versus 87%), but rates for event-free survival and OS did not reach statistical significance at a median follow-up time of 4.2 years. It might be speculated that the reduced freedom from progression rate for the chemotherapy-only arm will be outweighed by a reduced rate of long-term toxicities and secondary malignancies. This needs to be confirmed in a longer follow-up.

Recommendations and Future Directions for Early Favorable Hodgkin Lymphoma

Current clinical trials are evaluating the use of alternative chemotherapy combinations, shortened courses of chemotherapy, chemotherapy with smaller radiation fields or lower radiation doses, and chemotherapy without radiation therapy. Fortunately, HL-related death of patients with early favorable disease is unusual, and OS is not a useful parameter to evaluate midterm results in early-stage HL. Current trials should be judged by freedom from first recurrence rates and acute morbidity. On the basis of the available data, it can be concluded that patients with early favorable HL benefit from a short course of ABVD chemotherapy in combination with involved-field radiotherapy. Although there is some evidence that radiotherapy might not be necessary for those patients that achieve a CR after two courses of ABVD chemotherapy, it is still advisable to treat all patients with early favorable HL with a combined-modality regimen since long-term results on patients treated with chemotherapy only are pending. Ongoing studies using PET after two courses of ABVD and giving involved-field radiotherapy only to PET-positive patients (e.g., the GHSG HD16 trial) will demonstrate whether consolidative radiotherapy is necessary in case a metabolic CR is achieved after two cycles of ABVD.

Early Unfavorable Disease

It is generally accepted that early unfavorable HL should be treated with a combination of chemotherapy and radiotherapy. However, the prognostic impact of a single risk factor, the optimal chemotherapy regimen, the number of chemotherapy cycles, the field sizes, and the dosage of radiation within these fields are subjects of debate.

Trials to Identify the Best Chemotherapy Regimen

Based mainly on trial results from advanced HL, ABVD has also become the standard regimen for clinical stage I-II patients. In clinical trials, ABVD was thus compared with more intense regimens. The GHSG HD11 trial compared four cycles of ABVD with four cycles of BEACOPP (i.e., bleomycin, etoposide, doxorubicin (Adriamycin), cyclophosphamide, vincristine (Oncovin), procarbazine, and prednisone) in baseline dosage followed by involved-field radiotherapy at a dose of 20 or 30 Gy. The final results of the HD11 trial were published in 2010. FFTF after $BEACOPP_{baseline}$ was superior compared with that observed after ABVD when chemotherapy was followed by 20 Gy of involved-field radiotherapy. In contrast, no significant outcome differences between both chemotherapy protocols were detected in patients who received a 30 Gy radiation dose. Treatment-related toxicity was more frequently observed with $BEACOPP_{baseline}$. As a direct consequence, $BEACOPP_{baseline}$ was not adopted as new standard chemotherapy for early unfavorable HL.

Interim results of the EORTC H9U trial were similar. In this study, patients were randomized into three treatment arms consisting of four cycles of ABVD, six cycles of ABVD, or four cycles of $BEACOPP_{baseline}$, each followed by 30 Gy of involved-field radiotherapy. An interim analysis at a median follow-up of 4 years showed no significant differences regarding event-free survival and OS between the treatment arms while increased toxicity was observed with $BEACOPP_{baseline}$.

Significant outcome improvements in patients with early unfavorable HL were seen after the introduction of the $BEACOPP_{escalated}$ protocol (Table 74-4) in the treatment of these patients within the

Table 74-4 The BEACOPP$_{escalated}$ Regimen

Drug	Dose	Route	Schedule
Bleomycin	10 mg/m^2	IV	Day 8
Etoposide	200 mg/m^2	IV	Day 1-3
Doxorubicin	35 mg/m^2	IV	Day 1
Cyclophosphamide	1250 mg/m^2	IV	Day 1
Vincristine	1,4 mg/m^2 max. 2 mg	IV	Day 8
Procarbazine	100 mg/m^2	PO	Day 1-7
Prednisone	40 mg/m^2	PO	Day 1-14
G-CSF		Subcutaneous	From Day 8

Recycle day 22

GHSG HD14 trial. Patients were randomized to either four cycles of ABVD followed by 30 Gy of involved-field radiotherapy or a more intensified treatment protocol consisting of two cycles of BEACOPP$_{escalated}$ followed by two cycles of ABVD ("2+2") and the same radiotherapy. A preplanned interim analysis including 1010 patients at a median observation of 3 years revealed a significant superiority in FFTF for the 2+2 arm so that randomization for the trial was closed prematurely. The final analysis of HD14 including 1623 patients confirmed these results. At 5 years, the FFTF rate among patients who received the intensified 2+2 chemotherapy was significantly superior to that among patients who received four cycles of ABVD (94.7% versus 89.3%).

Radiation Field and Dose

In preceding studies, the GHSG randomized responding patients with early unfavorable disease to dosage of 40 Gy of extended-field irradiation or 20 Gy of extended-field irradiation plus 20 Gy of involved-field radiotherapy (HD1 trial) with no outcome difference. In the follow-up trial (HD5), patients received 30 Gy of extended-field irradiation plus 10 Gy to sites of bulky disease. These trials demonstrated that radiation dose in the extended field can safely be reduced to at least 30 Gy (with 10 Gy delivered to bulky tumors) when given after two cycles of alternating ABVD and COPP (i.e., cyclophosphamide, vincristine [Oncovin], procarbazine and prednisone). Similarly, other groups have aimed at improving combined-modality treatment for HL patients with early unfavorable disease. The cooperative study reported by Zittoun and colleagues compared six cycles of MOPP sandwiched around 40 Gy of radiotherapy applied in an involved-field or extended-field technique. No differences in terms of disease-free survival and OS were observed.

An Italian study headed by the Milan group enrolled patients in a randomized study comparing subtotal nodal irradiation with involved-field irradiation after four cycles of ABVD. At a median follow-up of 12 years, treatment outcomes were very similar in both arms (freedom from progression rates of 94% and 93%; survival rates of 96% and 94%, respectively).

In their H8U trial, the EORTC compared six cycles of MOPP/ABV plus 36 Gy of involved-field irradiation, four cycles MOPP/ABV plus 36 Gy of involved-field irradiation, and four cycles of MOPP/ABV plus subtotal lymphoid irradiation. At a median follow-up of 92 months, there were no differences among the three arms in terms of response rates, failure-free survival, and OS, leading to the conclusion that four cycles of chemotherapy followed by involved-field radiation should be the standard of care for patients with early unfavorable HL.[8]

The question of whether radiation fields can be reduced to the involved field after adequate chemotherapy was also the subject of the GHSG HD8 trial. This trial compared 30 Gy of extended-field irradiation plus 10 Gy to sites of bulky disease (>5 cm in diameter) with 30 Gy of involved-field radiotherapy plus 10 Gy to bulky disease sites after two alternating cycles of COPP/ABVD. Between 1993 and 1998, 1204 patients were randomized. The median observation time was 54 months. The OS rate for all eligible patients was 91%, and the FFTF rate was 83%. Comparisons of both arms showed similar rates for freedom from treatment failure (86% and 84%) and OS at 5 years (91% and 92%). No significant differences were found between the two arms in terms of complete remission, progressive disease, relapse, death, and secondary neoplasias. In contrast, acute side effects (including leukopenia, thrombocytopenia, nausea, and gastrointestinal and pharyngeal toxicity) occurred more frequently in the extended-field arm, so four cycles of chemotherapy plus 30 Gy of involved-field radiotherapy was adopted as standard of care within the GHSG.

Recommendations and Future Directions of Early Unfavorable Hodgkin Lymphoma

The outcome of treatment for patients with early unfavorable HL has improved dramatically in the past three decades. This results primarily from the use of combined-modality therapy, because radiation therapy alone or chemotherapy alone historically was associated with recurrence rates of approximately 50%. Four cycles of chemotherapy followed by 30 Gy of involved-field radiotherapy is a new standard for patients with unfavorable-prognosis early-stage HL. Most clinical trials are exploring new combinations of more effective chemotherapy and reduced radiation doses to determine optimal treatment, with the aim of decreasing late morbidity and mortality while maintaining a high probability of freedom from recurrence. Whether four to six cycles of chemotherapy without irradiation—at least in patients with complete metabolic response after chemotherapy as assessed by FDG-PET—can produce long-lasting remissions has not been determined. Trials such as the ongoing HD17 trial are addressing this issue.

ADVANCED-STAGE HODGKIN LYMPHOMA

Treatment Strategies

MOPP: Pioneer Combination Therapy

Until the middle of the 20th century, patients with advanced stages of HL were considered incurable. With the advent of more effective drugs, DeVita and colleagues at the National Cancer Institute were the pioneers who paved the way for the incredible success of modern chemotherapy in oncology by achieving a CR rate of 80% and cure in more than 50% among advanced-stage HL patients with the drug combination MOPP.

Despite the promising initial results with MOPP therapy, many investigators used alternative regimens to improve the efficacy or/and reduce toxicity. The omission of single drugs, such as the alkylating agents nitrogen mustard or procarbazine, from the MOPP regimen was associated with inferior CR rates, as shown by the Cancer and Leukemia Group B (CALGB). Therefore, at that time, the four-drug principle was considered the standard with which any other drug combination had to be compared.

ABVD: Second Combination Regimen

Despite great accomplishments with MOPP and MOPP-like regimens, there were major drawbacks. Between 15% and 30% of the patients did not obtain CR, and only about 50% of patients could be cured. The use of MOPP was associated with significant acute toxicity and with an increased risk for sterility and acute leukemia because of the alkylating agents included in this schema.

In 1975, Bonadonna and colleagues introduced the ABVD regimen for the treatment of patients who had failed MOPP therapy. Vinblastine had demonstrated high activity as a single agent and lacked cross-resistance with vincristine. Doxorubicin and bleomycin were also very active drugs and produced objective responses in about 50% of patients. Dacarbazine was added because it was active as a single agent and showed synergism with doxorubicin.

The Milan group compared MOPP and ABVD, using three cycles of each drug combination, followed by extended-field irradiation and three additional cycles of the same chemotherapy regimen. The comparison demonstrated a significant superiority for ABVD, with freedom from progression rates of 63% for MOPP compared with 81% for ABVD.

The pivotal CALGB trial of treatment for advanced HL, which compared MOPP, ABVD, and alternating MOPP/ABVD without additive radiotherapy, revealed equal therapeutic results for ABVD and MOPP/ABVD as far as progression-free survival and OS rates were concerned. Both regimens were superior to MOPP. ABVD had less germ cell and hematopoietic stem cell toxicities. Long-term follow-up of this study demonstrated a 45% to 50% progression-free survival rate and a 65% OS rate for ABVD and MOPP/ABVD.[10]

Treatment Duration

Many groups have compared different lengths of treatment and numbers of cycles. From these studies, although the optimal duration or total dose of drugs is not known precisely, it becomes evident that at least six, but maximally eight, cycles of an anthracycline-containing drug combination appear to be sufficient.

Newer Chemotherapy Regimens

The comparable efficacy of ABVD and combinations containing alkylating agents at higher doses in recent trials indicates that cure of advanced-stage HL patients is possible without alkylating agents. However, the pulmonary toxicity of bleomycin, which is especially pronounced in children and in combination with mediastinal irradiation, remains a major problem associated with ABVD. A number of drugs showing significant responses in relapsed HL have become candidates for use in first-line therapy. The topoisomerase II inhibitor etoposide has been of special interest since promising response rates have been reported after single-agent use in refractory HL. Based on these considerations, several etoposide-containing drug regimens have been developed.

Stanford V is a seven-drug regimen, consisting of doxorubicin, vinblastine, nitrogen mustard, bleomycin, vincristine, etoposide, and prednisone. The program is applied weekly over a total of 12 weeks. Sophisticated consolidation radiotherapy to sites of initial bulky disease has been employed. In a phase II trial, 126 patients were recruited. The estimated 5-year freedom from progression rate was 89%, and the OS rate was 96% at a median observation time of 5.4 years. However, results were not reproducible and were clearly inferior in a randomized comparison with ABVD and MOPPEB-VCAD (mechlorethamine, vincristine [Oncovin], procarbazine, prednisone, epidoxirubicin, bleomycin, vinblastine, lomustine [CeeNu], melphalan, and vindesine), which in part may be explained by the use of smaller consolidating radiation fields in the randomized setting.

Dose Density and Dose Intensity

Experiences with treating several tumors in animal models have demonstrated a clear relationship between chemotherapy dose and tumor response. Retrospective analyses of drug delivery with MOPP chemotherapy showed that patients with HL who received less than the intended doses had inferior outcomes. Such dose-response relationships also were observed independently with nitrogen mustard, procarbazine, and vincristine.

Until recently, no prospective, randomized trials that analyzed the role of dose intensity in the treatment of advanced-stage HL had been conducted. In 1992, the GHSG initiated a series of clinical trials to address the role of dose intensity in advanced HL in a comprehensive way. Starting with a mathematical model of tumor growth and chemotherapy effects, the data from 705 patients with advanced-stage disease who were treated in previous GHSG studies were reassessed. The investigators predicted that moderate dose escalation would increase tumor control by 10% at 5 years. Thus the BEACOPP regimen was devised. After establishing excellent tolerability and efficacy of the regimen in a pilot trial, a second regimen of escalated BEACOPP was developed in which the doxorubicin dose was increased to a fixed level and doses of cyclophosphamide and etoposide were increased in a stepwise fashion with G-CSF support. Maximum tolerated doses were determined in a multicenter pilot study as 190% of the standard dose for cyclophosphamide and 200% for etoposide.

The GHSG then designed a three-arm study, the HD9 trial, comparing COPP/ABVD, standard BEACOPP, and escalated BEACOPP in patients with advanced HL. Radiotherapy was administered to bulky disease at diagnosis or residual disease after eight cycles of chemotherapy. About two-thirds of patients received consolidation radiotherapy. In September 1996, at the time of a planned interim analysis, the COPP/ABVD arm of this trial was closed to accrual because of superior outcomes in the BEACOPP arms. In the final analysis in June 2001, 1201 patients were evaluated. Superiority over the COPP/ABVD arm for freedom from treatment failure was observed, with 87% for escalated BEACOPP, 76% for baseline BEACOPP, and 69% for COPP/ABVD after a median of 5 years, a highly significant result. A major difference was observed in the rate of primary progressive disease during initial therapy, which was significantly lower with escalated BEACOPP (2%) than with baseline BEACOPP (8%) or COPP/ABVD (10%) (P <0.001). The OS rates were 83% for COPP/ABVD, 88% for baseline BEACOPP and 91% for escalated BEACOPP. The survival differences were highly significant (P <0.002), and the survival difference between the COPP/ABVD and the $\text{BEACOPP}_{\text{escalated}}$ regimen reached an impressive degree of significance (P <0.002). These results were confirmed and became even more significant in a 10-year update analysis of the trial published in 2009 (Fig. 74-5).[11]

As expected, escalated BEACOPP was associated with a greater degree of hematologic toxicity, including the need for a greater number of red blood cell and platelet transfusions. Second malignancies, including AML possibly related to etoposide, were reported: with escalated BEACOPP, 9 cases of AML/MDS; with baseline BEACOPP, 4 cases of AML/MDS; and with COPP/ABVD, 1 case of AML/MDS. However, the total rate of secondary neoplasias was highest in the COPP/ABVD arm, with 4.2% compared with 3.4% in the $\text{BEACOPP}_{\text{escalated}}$ arm. The death rate at 5 years, including all

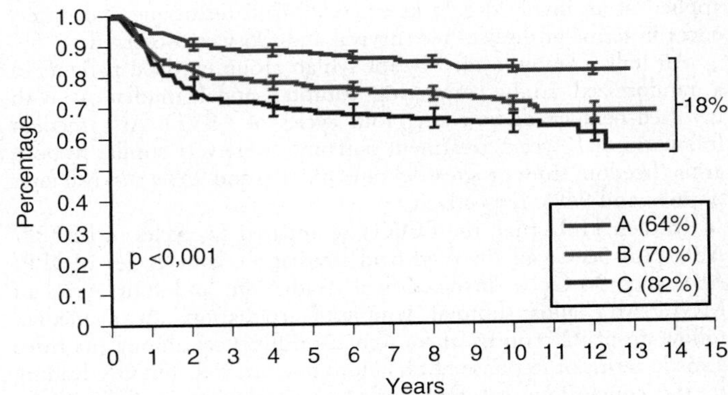

Figure 74-5 FREEDOM FROM TREATMENT FAILURE AT 10 YEARS AMONG PATIENTS TREATED WITHIN THE GHSG HD9 TRIAL FOR ADVANCED HODGKIN LYMPHOMA. **A,** COPP/ABVD. **B,** $\text{BEACOPP}_{\text{baseline}}$. **C,** $\text{BEACOPP}_{\text{escalated}}$. *From Engert A, Diehl V, Franklin J, et al: Escalated-dose BEACOPP in the treatment of patients with advanced-stage Hodgkin's lymphoma: 10 years of follow-up of the GHSG HD9 study.* J Clin Oncol *27:4548, 2009.*

acute and late causes of deaths, was 18.8% (49 of 260 patients) for the COPP/ABVD arm, 13% (61 of 469 patients) for baseline BEACOPP, and 8.6% (40 of 460 patients) for escalated BEACOPP.

Dosage, dose intensity, and total dose are decisive factors when comparing similar drug regimens. It is difficult to predict the relative efficacy of regimens that use different drugs. As mentioned above, Hasenclever proposed a theoretical framework as a first step to accomplish that task. Different drug doses in a regimen are assumed to be roughly additive in an efficacy scale when appropriately weighted. If the drug weights are known, a total chemotherapy dose can be derived. This total dose must be further corrected for different treatment durations, assuming a typical regrowth kinetic for each lymphoma entity. The resulting quantity, the effective dose, is a reasonable first-order predictor of relative treatment efficacy. Hasenclever derived drug weight estimates from a model-based metaanalysis of all randomized chemotherapy comparing trials of treatment for HL and provided an estimate of the slope of the effective dose-cure rate relationship.

Applying the effective dose model and using the weights estimated from trials up to 1998, MOPP/ABVD, MOPP/ABV, and baseline BEACOPP were predicted not to be notably different from ABVD in cure rates (all within ±5%) because their effective doses are similar. However, Stanford V was predicted to be of reduced efficacy when given with less additional radiotherapy while escalated BEACOPP was predicted to be of increased efficacy when compared with ABVD. These predictions were confirmed by the randomized trials mentioned above.

The 14-Day Variant of the BEACOPP-21 Regimen: BEACOPP-14

Increased dose intensity can be achieved by two means: increasing the dosage in the same timeframe or shortening the intervals between the treatment courses and shortening the time scale in which drugs are applied. The experiences with the highly effective but toxic $\text{BEACOPP}_{\text{escalated}}$ regimen (given in 21-day intervals) led the GHSG to consider a BEACOPP variant, in which the drug dosage and time architecture were altered according to the effective dose model of Hasenclever, with the hope of accomplishing the same efficacy but with a reduced toxicity.

The result was the development of a time-intensified $\text{BEACOPP}_{\text{baseline}}$ regimen, which was given in 14-day intervals and administered with G-CSF support for advanced-stage HL (BEACOPP-14). In a multicenter pilot study, the GHSG tested the feasibility, toxicity, and efficacy of the regimen in 99 patients in stage IIB with large mediastinal masses or extranodal disease (23%) or stage III-IV disease (77%) from July 1997 until March 2000. The final analysis with 94 evaluable patients was performed in August 2002. Ninety-one percent of patients received eight cycles of therapy; 77% were given within 16 days, and 94% were given within 22 days. Seventy percent of patients received consolidation radiotherapy. Seven patients with initial bulky disease were not irradiated. Eighty-eight patients (94%) achieved a CR, and only four patients had progressive disease. With a median follow-up of 34 months, five patients relapsed, only one developed a high-grade NHL, and three patients died, one of toxicity and two of progressive disease. The estimated rate for FFTF was 90%, and the OS rate was 97%.

Acute hematotoxicity was moderate, ranging between that of the escalated and the baseline BEACOPP regimen, with 75% of patients experiencing WHO grade 3 or 4 leukopenia. Twenty-three percent of patients experienced thrombocytopenia, and 65% had anemia, in a few cases necessitating the use of erythropoietin or blood transfusions. Since treatment results with the BEACOPP-14 regimen were promising, the regimen was thus included in the randomized HD15 trial as one comparator. Final results of this trial comparing the standard treatment consisting of eight cycles of escalated BEACOPP with six cycles of escalated BEACOPP and eight cycles of BEACOPP-14 will be available soon.

Role of Radiotherapy in Advanced-Stage Hodgkin Lymphoma

Several reports have indicated that patients treated with chemotherapy alone failed to respond or progressed, primarily in previously involved nodal sites. However, the benefits of consolidating radiotherapy must be balanced with the risk for serious side effects, particularly a second malignancy in the irradiated field.

To overcome the insufficient power of randomized studies with too few patients to detect a relevant difference, Loeffler and colleagues performed a metaanalysis of 14 studies involving more than 1700 patients. Two study designs were compared; in the additional design, irradiation was added to the same chemotherapy regimen, and in the parallel design, more cycles of chemotherapy were substituted for irradiation. In the additional design, radiotherapy reduced the hazard rate by about 40%. The benefit of irradiation was most pronounced among patients with mediastinal involvement and provided no reduction in relapse among patients with stage IV disease. There was no survival benefit detected for radiotherapy in any subgroup analyzed. In the parallel design, there was no significant difference in disease-free survival. However, OS was significantly higher among patients treated with chemotherapy alone. In the combined-modality group, there were more deaths from causes other than HL.

An important issue is determining the added efficacy of radiotherapy as adjuvant treatment to modern anthracycline-containing chemotherapy and the added late toxicity of this combined-modality treatment. Prospective, randomized trials, such as the comparison of MOPP/ABV hybrid plus or without consolidation radiotherapy by the EORTC, are needed to address these questions. In this trial, patients in complete remission after MOPP/ABV received two further chemotherapy cycles followed by randomization to involved-field radiotherapy or observation. This important study recruited patients for more than 10 years and completed the accrual with 739 patients in 2000. The final analysis published in 2003 showed that involved-field irradiation did not improve relapse-free survival or OS in patients who already achieved a CR with MOPP/ABV. Remarkably, those who reached a partial remission and were treated with additional involved-field irradiation had comparable overall outcomes compared with those who reached a CR. The added late toxicity associated with irradiation was not evaluated in this report because of the short observation time of 79 months.[12]

In the GHSG HD15 trial, patients with residual lymphoma of less than 2.5 cm after chemotherapy were not irradiated. Patients with residual lymphoma of more than 2.5 cm after chemotherapy underwent FDG-PET. Patients who were still PET-positive received consolidating localized irradiation; patients who were PET-negative were not irradiated. The negative prognostic value (NPV) of the PET examination in this situation was 94.6% so that PET-guided consolidating after adequate chemotherapy appears to be possible without an increased frequency of relapses.

Recommendations and Future Directions in Advanced Hodgkin Lymphoma

Advanced Hodgkin lymphoma has become a curable disease for the majority of patients. First-line treatment with six to eight cycles of ABVD is the widely accepted standard. However, the more aggressive $\text{BEACOPP}_{\text{escalated}}$ regimen induces a clinically relevant superior progression-free survival that translates into an improved OS in indirect comparisons. Ongoing well-designed prospectively randomized studies are currently evaluating these two approaches, and valid results will be available in the near future. In the meantime, some speculate that the early PET response-adapted design of the latest study generation will render this question redundant. Scientific interest is currently focused on these questions: (1) whether two cycles of the less-toxic ABVD regimen should be escalated to the more aggressive BEACOPP in case of PET-2 positivity, or (2) whether, after an aggressive induction therapy with two cycles of BEACOPP, further treatment can be deescalated. Both approaches aim at finding the best balance between toxicity and efficacy for the benefit of each individual patient. Unfortunately, both approaches are not tested against each other within a single randomized trial; therefore the current debate on the standard treatment of advanced-stage Hodgkin lymphoma will very likely continue. Maybe, the future question will not be: ABVD or BEACOPP; but: do we start with BEACOPP or ABVD and switch according to the findings of an early interim PET.

PRIMARY PROGRESSIVE AND RELAPSED HODGKIN LYMPHOMA

Depending on stage and risk factor profile, up to 95% of patients with HL achieve complete remission after first-line treatment. Depending on their initial treatment, patients who relapse have different treatment options, including radiotherapy for localized disease in previously nonirradiated areas, conventional salvage chemotherapy, or HDCT followed by ASCT. Conventional chemotherapy is the treatment of choice for patients relapsing after initial radiotherapy for early-stage HL. The survival of these patients is at least equal compared with patients who initially present with advanced disease and receive chemotherapy. In contrast, patients with relapsed HL after primary chemotherapy generally have a poorer prognosis. These patients are mostly treated with HDCT with ASCT.

Newer approaches such as sequential HDCT or allogeneic SCT (aSCT) have been investigated in cases of relapsed HL. Because more aggressive approaches are associated with increased toxicity, an accurate pretreatment prognostic assessment of patients is required to help select the most appropriate therapeutic regimen.

Prognostic Factors for Patients Relapsing After Primary Radiotherapy

The relapse rate after primary radiation therapy is 30% to 35%, and most relapses occur within 3 years after completion of radiotherapy, although late relapses after 4 years have been observed in 5% to 7% of patients. This small fraction of late disease recurrence is noteworthy because this is generally a more favorable prognostic group when treated with systemic therapy. Their OS rate is not different from that of patients who never relapse.

Most patients who relapse after radiotherapy are treated with systemic combination chemotherapy, often with the inclusion of involved-field radiotherapy if an affected nodal site was previously nonirradiated. The long-term survival of patients varies significantly according to the pattern of relapse. Four major prognostic factors for response to second-line therapy include age (> 40 or 50 years), stage at relapse, duration of CR (<12 months versus >12 months) and the type of therapy used for the treatment of relapse (i.e., chemotherapy alone or chemotherapy and radiation). In some series, mixed-cellularity or lymphocyte-depleted histology were also adverse prognostic factors.

Prognostic Factors for Patients Relapsing After Primary Chemotherapy

It was first noticed in 1979 that the length of remission to first-line chemotherapy had a marked effect on the ability of patients to respond to subsequent salvage treatment. In 1992, the National Cancer Institute updated its experience with the long-term follow-up of patients who relapsed after combination-chemotherapy regimens. Derived primarily from investigations involving failures after MOPP and MOPP variants, the conclusions are relevant to other chemotherapy programs. On this basis, chemotherapy failures can be divided into three subgroups:

1. Primary progressive HL (approximately 10% of all cases) (i.e., patients who never achieved a CR or relapse less than 3 months after completion of treatment)
2. Early relapses within 12 months of complete remission (approximately 15% of all cases)
3. Late relapses after complete remission lasting longer than 12 months (approximately 15% of all cases)

Prognostic Factors for Patients With Primary Progressive Hodgkin Lymphoma

Patients with primary progressive disease, defined as progression during induction treatment or within 90 days after the end of treatment, have a poor prognosis particularly when treated with conventional salvage regimens. The 8-year overall survival rate is between 0% and 8%.

The GHSG retrospectively analyzed 206 patients with primary progressive disease to determine the outcome after salvage therapy. Rates for the 5-year freedom from second failure and OS for all patients were 17% and 26%, respectively. As reported from a number of transplantation centers, the 5-year freedom from second failure and OS rates for patients treated with HDCT were 42% and 48%, respectively, but only 33% of all patients were able to receive HDCT.

Insufficient stem cell harvests, poor performance status and older age contribute to an ineligibility to undergo HDCT. In a multivariate analysis, Karnofsky performance score at the time to progression ($P < 0.0001$), age ($P = 0.019$), and attainment of a temporary remission to first-line chemotherapy ($P = 0.0003$) were significant prognostic factors for survival. Patients with none of these risk factors had a 5-year OS rate of 55%, compared with an OS rate of 0% for patients with all three of these unfavorable prognostic factors.[13]

HDCT is an effective treatment for a proportion of patients with primary progressive HL. Because of the poor outcomes of HL patients with progressive disease, future trials must aim at identifying patients at very high risk for induction failure and modifying primary treatment in this group to avoid progressive disease.

Prognostic Factors for Early and Late Relapsed Hodgkin Lymphoma

Many prognostic factors have been described for patients relapsing after first-line chemotherapy. These include age, gender, histology, relapse sites, stage at relapse, B symptoms, performance status and extranodal relapse. The impact of these variables is difficult to assess because of a variety of confounding factors, small numbers of patients and inclusion of patients with primary progressive HL into analyses. Multivariate analyses were not performed systematically.

Lohri and colleagues observed favorable outcomes for patients with risk factors such as an initial stage of less than stage IV at diagnosis, an absence of B symptoms at relapse, and an initial remission duration of more than 12 months. The 5-year failure-free survival rate was 82% for patients lacking all three parameters and 17% for those with one or more risk factors. Reece and associates reported an analysis of 58 patients treated with HDCT and ASCT at the same institution. Three prognostic subgroups were identified according to the presence of the following parameters at relapse: B symptoms, extranodal disease, and initial remission duration of less than 12 months. Patients with no risk factors had a 3-year progression-free survival of 100%, compared with 81% in patients with one factor, 41% in those with two factors, and 0% in patients with all three adverse risk factors. The GHSG performed the largest retrospective analysis on prognostic factors in relapsed HL published to date ($n = 422$). After testing several variables, the most relevant factors were combined into a prognostic score. This score was calculated on the basis of duration of first remission, stage at relapse, and presence of anemia at relapse. Early recurrence within 3 to 12 months after the completion of primary treatment, relapse with stage III or IV disease, and reduced hemoglobin levels at relapse (<10.5 g/dL for female patients, <12 g/dL for male patients) were counted in a score with possible values of 0, 1, 2, and 3, in order of worsening prognosis. This prognostic score allows the examiner to distinguish patients with different rates of freedom from second failure and OS. The actuarial 4-year rates for freedom from second failure and OS for patients relapsing after chemotherapy with three unfavorable factors were 17% and 27%, respectively. In contrast, patients with none of the unfavorable factors had rates of freedom from second failure and OS at 4 years of 48% and 83%, respectively.

Treatment of Primary Progressive and Relapsed Hodgkin Lymphoma

Patients who relapse after achieving an initial CR can achieve a second CR with salvage treatment, including radiotherapy for localized relapse in previously nonirradiated areas, conventional salvage chemotherapy or HDCT followed by ASCT. Salvage radiotherapy alone offers an effective treatment option for a selected subset of patients with relapsed HL. This applies to patients with localized relapses in previously nonirradiated areas. In a retrospective analysis from the GHSG database including 624 relapsed or refractory HL patients, 100 patients were eligible to receive salvage radiotherapy alone: the 5-year freedom from second failure (FF2F) and OS rates were 28% and 51%, respectively. Prognostic factors for OS were B symptoms and stage at relapse, whereas performance status and duration of first remission were significant for FFTF. The survival of patients treated with conventional chemotherapy after relapse of early-stage disease is only marginally worse than that of patients with newly diagnosed advanced-stage disease. Rates of disease-free survival and OS are 52% and 67%, respectively.

The optimal treatment for recurrence after primary chemotherapy is HDCT followed by ASCT in all patients who are eligible for this treatment modality. HDCT followed by ASCT has been shown to produce long-term disease-free survival rates of 30% to 65% in patients with refractory or relapsed HL. The reduction of early transplantation-related mortality from rates of 10% to 25% reported in earlier studies to less than 5% in later studies has led to the widespread acceptance of HDCT and ASCT.

Two randomized clinical trials independently showed the superiority of HDCT followed by ASCT when compared with conventional salvage treatment. In a British trial, patients with relapsed or refractory HL were treated with a combination of BCNU (carmustine), etoposide, cytosine arabinoside, and melphalan at a conventional-dose level (mini-BEAM) or a high-dose level followed by ASCT. The actuarial 3-year rate for event-free survival was significantly better for patients who received HDCT (53% versus 10%).[14]

The largest randomized, multicenter trial including patients with refractory or relapsed HL was performed by the GHSG/EBMT. Patients were randomly assigned to four cycles of DexaBEAM (i.e., dexamethasone, BCNU, etoposide, cytosine arabinoside, and melphalan) or two cycles of DexaBEAM followed by HDCT (BEAM) and ABMT/ASCT. The final analysis of 144 evaluable patients revealed that among 117 patients with partial remission or CR after two cycles of chemotherapy, the FFTF rate for the HDCT group was 55% compared with 34% for the patients receiving additional two cycles of standard chemotherapy. OS did not significantly differ.[15]

Sequential High-Dose Chemotherapy

Sequential HDCT has increasingly been used in the treatment of solid tumors and hematologic and lymphoproliferative disorders. Initial results from phase I and II studies indicate that this kind of therapy offers safe and effective treatment. In accordance with the Norton-Simon hypothesis, non–cross-resistant agents are administered at short intervals after initial cytoreduction. In general, the transplantation of peripheral blood stem cells (PBSCs) and the use of growth factors allow the application of the most effective drugs at the highest possible doses at intervals of 1 to 3 weeks. Sequential HDCT enables the highest possible dosing over a minimum period of time (i.e., dose intensification).

In 1997, a multicenter phase II trial with a sequential high-dose chemotherapy program and a final myeloablative course was started to evaluate the feasibility and efficacy of this novel regimen in patients with relapsed HL. Patients between the ages of 18 and 60 years with histologically proven primary progressive HL or with first or higher grade of relapse with no prior HDCT and an ECOG performance status 0 to 1 were eligible for this study.

Treatment consisted of two cycles of DHAP (i.e., dexamethasone, cytosine arabinoside, and cisplatin [Platinol]) in the first phase to reduce tumor burden before HDCT. Patients with partial or complete remissions after DHAP received sequential HDCT consisting of cyclophosphamide (4 g/m^2), methotrexate (8 g/m^2), vincristine (1.4 mg/m^2), and etoposide (2 g/m^2). The final myeloablative course was BEAM followed by ASCT with at least 2×10^6 CD34$^+$ cells/kg.

At final analysis, 102 patients were available for the evaluation. Of those, 12 patients had experienced multiple relapses, 17 had progressive disease, 29 had early relapses, and 44 had late relapses. After a median follow-up of 30 months, results were as follows: the response rate after DHAP was 80% (72% CR, 8% partial remissions). Toxicity was tolerable, two treatment-related deaths were observed. FFTF and OS rates were 62% and 81% for patients with early relapse, 65% and 81% for patients with late relapse, 41% and 48% for patients with progressive disease, and 39% and 48%, respectively, for patients with multiple relapses.

Based on these results, the GHSG, EORTC, and EBMT initiated a prospective, randomized study to compare the effectiveness of a standard HDCT (BEAM) with a sequential HDCT after initial cytoreduction with two cycles of DHAP. Initially, 284 patients who had histologically confirmed early or late relapsed HL or who were in second relapse with no prior HDCT received two cycles of DHAP. Then 241 of these patients who had no change, partial remission, or CR after the two cycles of DHAP were centrally randomized to receive BEAM followed by ASCT or high-dose cyclophosphamide plus high-dose methotrexate/vincristine plus high-dose etoposide followed by a final myeloablative course with BEAM and ASCT. The final results of this trial were published in 2010. No significant differences in terms of treatment outcome were observed, but toxicity was increased in patients who received sequential HDCT (Fig. 74-6). Thus sequential HDCT was not adopted as standard of care in patients with relapsed HL eligible for HDCT.[16]

The Role of Nonmyeloablative Allogeneic Stem Cell Transplantation in Hodgkin Lymphoma

Given the high nonrelapse mortality of myeloablative aSCT in HL, the use of reduced intensity nonmyeloablative conditioning regimens represents a possible alternative. The goal of this strategy is to reduce the treatment-related toxicity while providing sufficient immunosuppression to facilitate donor engraftment with a subsequent graft-versus-lymphoma effect. Several published regimens exist, ranging from the truly nonmyeloablative single fraction total body irradiation with a dose of 2 Gy to moderately myelosuppressive chemotherapy-based regimens that often combine fludarabine with an alkylating agent such as melphalan or busulfan. The marked reduction of upfront toxicity with these regimens theoretically extended the applicability of aSCT to older patients, patients with comorbidities, and particularly those for whom ASCT had previously failed.

In recent years, several groups reported on the outcome of patients with relapsed HL treated with reduced-intensity conditioning and aSCT. However, these reports are often difficult to interpret because of differences in patient populations and conditioning regimens used. In general, transplant-related mortality was lower as compared with classical myeloablative conditioning regimens. A reduction in transplant-related mortality was shown by the Lymphoma Working Party of the EBMT, retrospectively comparing patients who had

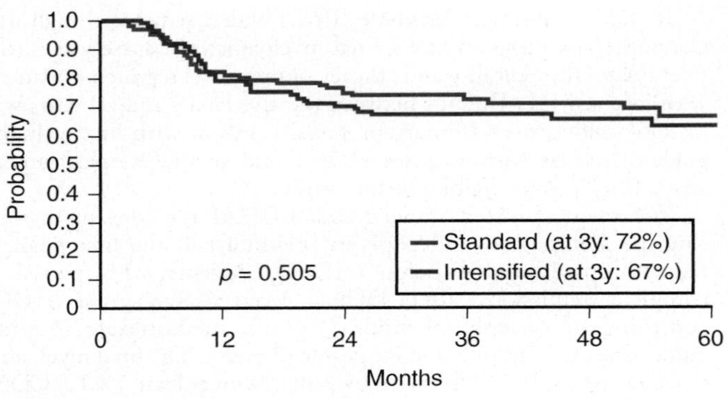

Pts. at risk						
Standard	119	92	75	55	35	22
Intensified	122	90	75	53	34	22

Figure 74-6 PROGRESSION-FREE SURVIVAL AMONG PATIENTS TREATED WITHIN THE HD-R2 TRIAL FOR RELAPSED HODGKIN LYMPHOMA. *Standard,* Two cycles of DHAP plus HD-BEAM plus ASCT. *Intensified,* Two cycles of DHAP plus HD-cyclophosphamide plus HD-methotrexate/vincristine plus HD-etoposide plus HD-BEAM plus ASCT. *(Josting A, Muller H, Borchmann P, et al: Dose intensity of chemotherapy in patients with relapsed Hodgkin's lymphoma,* J Clin Oncol *28:5074, 2010.)*

standard myeloablative conditioning with patients who received reduced-intensity regimens. Transplant-related mortality at 1 year was 46% in the myeloablative group and 23% in the reduced-intensity group ($p = 0.003$).[17]

There is mounting evidence that successful aSCT in HL needs a combination of an effective salvage chemotherapy and a moderately intensive pretransplant conditioning regimen to keep the disease under control and to allow the withdrawal of immunosuppression and/or the use of donor lymphocyte infusions to achieve an effective graft-versus-lymphoma response.

Another retrospective analysis by the EBMT included a total of 285 patients with relapsed or refractory HL treated with reduced intensity aSCT. The aim of the study was to identify prognostic factors predicting long-term outcome. Sixty patients died from nonrelapse mortality at a median of 91 days (ranging from 1 day to 20 months) following transplantation. The cumulative incidence estimates of nonrelapse mortality at 100 days, 1 year, and 3 years after aSCT were 10.9%, 19.5%, and 21.1%, respectively. In multivariate analysis, nonrelapse mortality was associated with poor performance status, chemorefractory disease, age of more than 45 years, and transplantation before 2002. With a median follow-up of 26 months (range 3 to 94 months), 126 patients were alive and 159 had died. The Kaplan-Meier estimates of overall and progression-free survival at 1, 2, and 3 years were 67% and 52%, 43% and 39%, and 29% and 25%, respectively. Refractory disease and poor performance status were identified as risk factors for poor overall and progression-free survival. Patients with none of these risk factors had a 3-year progression-free and overall survival of 42% and 56% compared with 8% and 25% for patients presenting with one or two risk factors. In an analysis restricted to patients who had relapsed after a prior ASCT, relapse within the first 6 months after transplant was associated with a significantly worse disease progression rate (RR = 1.9 [1.2-3.1] $p = 0.01$) and reduced progression-free survival (RR = 1.9 [1.2-2.9] $p = 0.003$) after reduced-intensity aSCT. In summary, reduced-intensity aSCT may be an effective salvage strategy for selected patients with good risk features who relapse after ASCT. The major limit of this approach, however, is the poor tumor control reported after reduced-intensity conditioning with relapse rates of 59% at 3 years. Further optimization of an aSCT approach in HL, particularly related to the optimal re-induction regimen and a better selection of patients who might benefit, is warranted.

SPECIAL CONSIDERATIONS

Nodular Lymphocyte-Predominant Hodgkin Lymphoma

NLPHL is a rare HL subtype accounting for about 5 % of all cases. Immunophenotype and the clinical course of NLPHL differ substantially from cHL. However, current standard treatment of NLPHL is not different from cHL standard treatment for most stages, a fact that can be explained by the rarity of the disease and, consequentially, a lack of clinical trials evaluating novel treatment approaches in NLPHL.

Clinical Presentation

Because of the rarity of this disease, distinct clinical features were not recognized in detail until the European Task Force on Lymphoma (ETFL) conducted an analysis comprising 219 patients with histologically confirmed NLPHL. Another analysis, in which characteristics of 394 NLPHL patients were compared with characteristics of 7904 cHL patients, was performed by the GHSG. Both analyses revealed that NLPHL was more often diagnosed in early stages. B symptoms, bulky and extranodal disease, elevation of the erythrocyte sedimentation rate and of the lactic dehydrogenase, and involvement of three or more nodal areas were less frequently found than in cHL.[18]

Treatment Results

In the GHSG analysis, FFTF (88% versus 82%) and OS (96% versus 92%) rates in NLPHL patients were superior when compared with cHL.[18] This might be due in part to the increased rate of NLPHL patients diagnosed in early stages. Patients with early favorable NLPHL in clinical stage IA have an excellent OS that is close to 100%. Different approaches can be applied in these patients. Those include watch-and-wait, radiotherapy, combined-modality strategies, and treatment with anti-CD20 antibodies.

Treatment of Early Favorable Stages

The major goal of NLPHL treatment in early stages is to induce as little acute and late toxicity as possible. Particularly in children with NLPHL, treatment strategies focus on avoiding long-term side effects such as secondary malignancies, infertility, growth retardation, hypothyroidism, and damage of heart and lung. In an attempt to postpone treatment, watch-and-wait strategies after diagnostic lymphadenectomy were evaluated in smaller series of patients. In one study including 27 pediatric patients, 13 underwent lymphadenectomy only, 10 were treated with combined-modality treatment, 1 had involved-field radiotherapy, and 3 received chemotherapy only. At a median follow-up of 70 months, OS for all 27 patients was 100% with an event-free survival rate of 69%. The event-free survival rate in the watch-and-wait group was 42% compared with 90% in those patients who had additional treatment. Patients with residual lymphoma after the diagnostic operation clearly had an inferior event-free survival when receiving no further treatment. Thus watch-and-wait must be regarded as an experimental strategy and cannot be routinely recommended in clinical practice.

For most NLPHL patients in early favorable stages, radiotherapy is the mainstay of treatment. In a smaller series including 36 stage I/IIA patients that were either treated with involved-field radiotherapy or a modified localized radiation, event-free survival and OS rates were 95% and 100%, respectively, after 5 years. A larger Australian series analyzed 202 stage I/II patients treated with radiotherapy in mantle field technique or reverted Y field. In this group of patients, the progression-free survival was 82% with an OS of 83% at a median follow-up of 15 years. In GHSG studies, a total of 131 patients with stage IA NLHPL were treated with different treatment modalities, including extended-field radiotherapy (45 patients), involved-field radiotherapy (45 patients), and combined-modality treatment (41 patients). Median follow-up was 78 months for the extended-field radiotherapy-treated group, 17 months for those patients treated with involved-field radiotherapy, and 40 months for those who received combined-modality treatment. Overall, 99% of patients achieved a CR. There was no difference in terms of FFTF among the treatment modalities applied. Similar results were seen in a recently published large single institution retrospective study by Chen and colleagues including 113 patients with stage I or II NLPHL. In this study, outcome of patients treated with involved-field radiotherapy, extended-field radiotherapy, or combined-modality treatment was also comparable with a shorter follow-up for patients receiving involved-field radiotherapy only.[19] Although longer follow-up is required for a more comprehensive picture, the efficacy and tolerability of involved-field radiotherapy has resulted in the recommendation of this treatment modality by the GHSG for patients with stage IA NLPHL without risk factors. The EORTC has also adopted involved-field radiotherapy as standard of care for stage IA NLPHL. Similarly, the guidelines panel of the U.S. National Cancer Center Network (NCCN) recommends small-field radiotherapy as the treatment of choice for stage IA NLPHL.

In a phase II study conducted by the GHSG, 28 NLPHL patients with clinical stage IA without risk factors received four weekly doses of rituximab. The recently published final analysis showed an overall response rate of 100%. However, at a median follow-up of 43 months, 25% of patients had relapsed so that rituximab alone appears to be less effective than radiotherapy.

A North American Group conducted a trial including both patients with first diagnosis of NLPHL and relapsed disease. Patients received either four weekly doses of rituximab without further treatment (limited treatment) or four weekly doses of rituximab followed by repeated rituximab administrations every 6 months (extended treatment). Preliminary results indicate that extended administration of rituximab might prolong freedom from progression. After a median follow-up of 30 months, the median freedom from disease progression was not reached in the extended treatment group and 24 months in the limited treatment group.

Treatment of Early Unfavorable and Advanced Stages

The treatment of early unfavorable and advanced NLPHL is usually identical to the treatment of cHL. This is based on larger analyses performed by several groups that revealed similar treatment results of NLPHL and cHL patients when treated with protocols widely accepted in the treatment of HL. The GHSG analysis reported that 86% of patients in early unfavorable and 77% of patients in advanced stages reached CR. This compares with rates of 83% and 78%, respectively, in cHL patients. Only 0.3% of NLPHL patients experienced progressive disease compared with a rate of 3.9% in cHL patients. Although the overall relapse rate was very similar (NLPHL 8.1% versus 8.0% in cHL), early relapses were more frequent in patients with cHL (3.2% versus 0.8% in NLPHL), whereas late relapses were more frequent in NLPHL patients (7.4% versus 4.7% in cHL). With a median follow-up of 50 months, no significant differences between NLPHL and cHL were observed in terms of OS rates (96% in NLPHL versus 92% in cHL).[18] Similar data were reported by the ETFL. Here, at a median follow-up of 8 years, OS rate was 89% in both NLPHL and cHL.

Treatment of Relapsed NLPHL

If possible, NLPHL patients with suspected relapse should undergo a renewed biopsy since transformation into aggressive non-Hodgkin lymphoma must be excluded. In the ETFL analysis, 14% of NLPHL relapses were identified as cHL and 10% as NHL. However, patients with NLPHL showed a tendency to more favorable survival after relapse as compared with cHL patients ($p = 0.05$), but this finding must be handled with care: more NLPHL patients had been diagnosed in early stages at primary diagnosis and were treated with less intensive first-line treatment than most cHL patients.

With the advent of the anti-CD20 monoclonal antibody rituximab in the treatment of CD20-positive lymphomas, some phase II studies using this antibody were initiated in patients with relapsed or refractory NLPHL. This was based on the fact that in NLPHL not only the reactive background usually stains strongly for CD20—more important, the malignant LP cells are CD20-positive. In a study conducted by the GHSG, 14 patients were treated with weekly rituximab at a dose of 375 mg/m^2 for 4 consecutive weeks. Overall response rate was 86%. Eight patients achieved CR, and four patients partial remission. At a short median follow-up of 12 months, nine patients were in remission. An update analysis on this study including 15 patients who had reconfirmed NLPHL reported an overall response rate of 94%. With a median follow-up of 63 months, the median time to progression was 33 months; the median OS was not reached.[20] Similar results were reported from Stanford on 22 less intensively or previously untreated NLPHL patients who received rituximab. Here, response rate was 100%, but nine patients relapsed. However, with excellent response rates even in heavily pretreated patients, anti-CD20 antibodies such as rituximab and novel follow-up products might become an inherent part in future strategies for the treatment of NLPHL, possibly in combination with classical chemotherapy protocols such as ABVD or others.

Transformation into Non-Hodgkin Lymphoma

The possibility of transformation from NLPHL into aggressive non-Hodgkin lymphoma is well documented. Two recent analyses independently indicated higher transformation rates than previously reported. In one analysis including 164 patients initially diagnosed with NLPHL, the 10-year cumulative transformation rate was 12%. Another analysis including 95 NLPHL patients reported an actuarial risk for transformation to aggressive lymphoma of 7% at 10 years and of 30% at 20 years.[21]

Hodgkin Lymphoma in the Older Adult Patient

Clinical experience and data from large trials indicate that patients older than 60 years have a higher risk for treatment failure and experience more treatment-related toxicity than younger patients.[22] Regarding the incidence of HL in older adult patients, the most accurate assessments were derived from population-based studies. Two Swedish studies covering the years from 1979 to 1988 and 1973 to 1994 showed a proportion of 31% and 26% of HL patients older than 60 years, respectively. The Scotland and Newcastle Lymphoma Group (SNLG) data demonstrated that from 1979 to 2003, 624 (20%) of 3373 patients registered in the population registry were over 60 years.

The patient's physical and mental condition, disease history, and the presence of concurrent disorders influence the treatment strategy. Age in general is no contraindication against aggressive treatment, but compared with younger patients fewer older adult patients receive the intended chemotherapy dose. The survival analysis of one large comprehensive analysis performed by the GHSG showed a significantly poorer treatment outcome for older adult patients in terms of 5-year OS (65% versus 90%) and FFTF (60% versus 80%).[22] However, biologically young patients in good physical and mental condition should be treated in a stage-adapted manner.

ABVD is regarded as standard chemotherapy for most older adult HL patients. In early favorable and unfavorable stages, two to six cycles of ABVD followed by IF-RT represent a widely accepted standard of care. In advanced stages, six to eight cycles of ABVD are usually being given. However, ABVD is associated with an increased toxicity and mortality in older adult patients, so a relevant proportion of these patients might not be eligible for this regimen.

More aggressive regimens should be avoided in elderly patients since they were shown to cause unacceptable toxicity. The GHSG HD9 elderly trial was designed for patients ages 66 to 75 years in stages IIB to IV. Patients were randomized between eight cycles of COPP/ABVD (26 patients) and eight cycles of $BEACOPP_{baseline}$ (42 patients). Eighteen patients with bulky or residual disease after chemotherapy received consolidating radiotherapy. The full number of planned treatment cycles was given to 18 patients (69%) in the COPP/ABVD group and to 23 patients (55%) in the $BEACOPP_{baseline}$ group. The CR rate was the same in both treatment arms (76%), and no difference occurred regarding the number of patients with progressive disease (8% for COPP/ABVD and 7% for BEACOPP baseline). The disease-specific FFTF at 5 years was better for the more aggressive $BEACOPP_{baseline}$ regimen than for COPP/ABVD (74% versus 55%, $p = 0.13$). This did not translate into a superior OS at 5 years owing to more treatment-related fatal events in the $BEACOPP_{baseline}$ arm (21% versus 8% for COPP/ABVD).

Since etoposide was thought to contribute to the poorer tolerability of BEACOPP in older adult patients, the GHSG then developed a new BEACOPP variant especially for this patient cohort. This new schedule, BACOPP, contained no etoposide, whereas the dose of doxorubicin was increased (from 25 mg/m^2 to 50 mg/m^2). Sixty patients (92%) were eligible for the final analysis of the phase II trial evaluating the regimen. In total, 51 patients showed CR (85%), two had partial remissions (3%), and four had primary progression of disease (7%). WHO grade III to IV toxicities were documented in 52 patients (87%). With a median observation of 33 months, 18 deaths (30%) have been observed, including seven therapy-associated fatal outcomes. Thus with a therapy-associated death rate beyond 10%, this regimen also requires modification and is not recommended for routine use.

Another phase II study by the GHSG investigated the incorporation of gemcitabine into the first-line treatment of older patients. Bleomycin and dacarbazine were replaced from the ABVD backbone by gemcitabine and prednisone, resulting in the PVAG regimen. The recently performed final analysis included 59 patients with early unfavorable and advanced HL. Of these, 78% achieved a CR/CRu (complete remission unconfirmed). Three-year estimates for OS and progression-free survival were 66% and 58%.

Since HDCT followed by ASCT is not possible in most older adult patients, second-line treatment is generally of palliative nature. Several single-agents including gemcitabine and trofosphamide were described to be active in a relevant portion of patients. In addition, it may be possible to treat relapsed older adult HL patients with a second polychemotherapy—for instance, with a regimen that has been developed years ago and used by the Scottish and Newcastle Lymphoma Group (SNLG) as palliative therapy over a prolonged period. The regimen is a well-tolerated all-oral schedule consisting of prednisolone, etoposide, chlorambucil, and CCNU (PECC). Recently, an update on the use of the protocol in relapsed HL from the SNLG database demonstrated a CR rate of 58% in the 12 included patients who were older than 60 years. This finding suggests that PECC might have a useful role in the treatment of relapsed HL in older adult patients.[23] Treatment for patients with impairment of lung, liver, heart, or kidney should be adapted individually. Single drugs with organ-specific toxicities (e.g., bleomycin and doxorubicin) may be omitted, replaced, or modified in dose. Involved-field radiotherapy or the use of less aggressive drugs, such as gemcitabine and vinorelbine with or without dexamethasone are possible treatment alternatives in case standard treatment is impossible. Of note, a concomitant application of bleomycin and gemcitabine should be avoided since a high incidence of pulmonary toxicity was observed in one trial.

Hodgkin Lymphoma During Pregnancy

The peak incidence of HL occurs at female reproductive age. Therefore the association with pregnancy is not uncommon. HL is the fourth most common cancer occurring during pregnancy. One case of HL occurs per 1.000 to 6.000 deliveries. Several studies have shown that pregnancy is not associated with a worse clinical course and that the 20-year survival rate of pregnant women with HL is not different from that of nonpregnant women.

The clinical presentation of HL is not influenced by pregnancy. However, there are significant limitations regarding staging and treatment of pregnant patients. CT and PET scans should be avoided since limiting radiation exposure to the fetus is essential especially during early stages of gestation. Ultrasound is helpful for assessing the fetal status and detecting tumor lesions in the abdomen of the mother. Magnetic resonance imaging can complete the radiologic staging because it does not seem to be associated with risk to the fetus. Decisions about the need for a chest radiograph should be made on the basis of clinical examination.

In case HL is diagnosed during the first trimester, and disease requires immediate therapeutic intervention, most experts agree that a therapeutic abortion should be encouraged since the risk is high for negative effects on the development of the fetus if antineoplastic drugs are applied during that period. If an immediate start of therapy is indicated and the mother does not want to have an abortion, low-dose supradiaphragmatic irradiation or application of vinblastine monotherapy may be considered. In cases with no need for an immediate therapeutic intervention, the start of treatment should be deferred.[24]

In the second or third trimester, patients with stage I or II disease may be closely observed, and treatment can be postponed until an early delivery is achieved. If there is any sign of accelerated disease progression, especially supradiaphragmatic lymphadenopathy, radiotherapy alone is recommended. Most studies recommend doses of 10 to 36 Gy applied as mantle field or involved-field irradiation with abdominal shielding. At this time of fetal development, the risk for adverse sequelae for the child from supradiaphragmatic irradiation is low. Pregnant HL patients in the second or third trimester who present with infradiaphragmatic lymphadenopathy or advanced disease should receive combination chemotherapy. Because most chemotherapeutic agents freely cross the placenta and enter the fetal circulation, the patient and the fetus should be monitored closely. Application of cytotoxic drugs shortly before birth may be particularly hazardous because the placenta is also the primary means of drug elimination, and metabolism and excretion are delayed in the neonate. The current concept is that antimetabolites, especially methotrexate must not be given since they carry a high risk for teratogenesis, whereas doxorubicin, bleomycin, etoposide, and the vinca alkaloids appear acceptable. Thus the ABVD regimen may be used when chemotherapy is indicated beyond the first trimester. Because chemotherapeutic agents accumulate in the milk, mothers are best advised not to breast-feed during treatment.

Hodgkin Lymphoma in HIV-Positive Patients

Epidemiology and Clinical Presentation

In patients with HIV infection, HL is diagnosed more frequently than in the general population. Given the background incidence of HL in the population groups at high risk for HIV infection, researchers conducting epidemiologic studies during the first years of the HIV epidemic in North America and Europe had difficulties including HL in the spectrum of HIV-associated cancers. However, with the spread of the epidemic and longer survival of infected people, the impact of HL in HIV-positive patients could be better recognized. All studies available to date strongly support the evidence that persons infected with HIV have about a 10-fold higher risk for developing HL than do HIV-negative persons. Such an excess risk is more pronounced in HIV-infected individuals with moderate immune suppression as found in patients undergoing antiretroviral therapy. In contrast to HIV-negative patients with HL, the mixed-cellularity subtype is also more frequently found in HIV-positive HL patients and almost all cases are EBV-associated, a fact that also contrasts to what is observed in HIV-negative HL patients.

Treatment of Hodgkin Lymphoma in HIV-Positive Patients

The optimal therapy for HL in HIV-positive patients has not been defined yet. Because most patients present with advanced stages, treatment consists mainly of combination chemotherapy regimens, but the complete remission rates achieved with these regimens remain lower than in patients without HIV infection and OS is only about 1.5 years. Because of the low overall incidence of HIV-related HL, no randomized controlled trials have been conducted in this setting. After results with rather mild treatment protocols were disappointing, the widespread introduction of antiretroviral therapy allowed the use of more aggressive chemotherapeutic regimens such as Stanford V or BEACOPP. From 1997 to 2001, 59 consecutive patients were treated with Stanford V in a prospective phase II study. Treatment was well tolerated, and 69% of the patients completed therapy with no dose reduction or delay in chemotherapy administration. The most important dose-limiting side effects were bone marrow toxicity and neurotoxicity. Eighty-one percent of the patients achieved CR, and at a median follow-up of 17 months, 56% of patients were alive and disease-free. The estimated 5-year OS was 59%. Within the German group, treatment with BEACOPP in baseline dosage showed promising results in terms of CR, toxicity, and median survival. In contrast, the use of escalated BEACOPP cannot be recommended for HIV-positive patients.[25] Recently, the results of a large prospective phase II study with ABVD have been published. Within a cooperative network in Spain, 62 HIV-positive patients with HL received standard ABVD plus antiretroviral therapy. The scheduled six to eight ABVD cycles were completed in 82% of cases. Of the 62 patients, 6 died during induction, 54 (87%) achieved CR, and 2 were resistant. The 5-year overall and event-free survival probabilities were 76% and 71%, respectively. The immunologic response to antiretroviral therapy had a positive impact on overall ($p = 0.002$) and event-free survival ($p = 0.001$).

Because a large portion of HIV-positive patients with HL have progress or relapse, the use of HDCT and ASCT in this setting has been evaluated by several groups and the data published so far have demonstrated the feasibility of this approach; thus it can be considered the standard of care in progressive or relapsed patients.

SEQUELAE OF TREATMENT

Cardiac Complications

Chemotherapy-Associated Cardiac Complications

The most relevant cardiotoxic drugs used in the treatment of HL are anthracyclines. Anthracycline-associated toxicity may occur at different intervals after therapy. Cardiotoxicity often presents as electrocardiographic changes, arrhythmias, or cardiomyopathy leading to congestive heart failure. Anthracycline-associated cardiotoxicity is caused by direct damage of the myoepithelium and is strongly related to the cumulative dose applied. Doses less than 500 mg/m^2 are usually well tolerated. The total dose of anthracyclines used in the first-line therapy of HL is relatively low compared with treatment regimens used in the treatment of breast cancer or pediatric malignancies. The cumulative dose of eight cycles is 400 mg/m^2 for ABVD and 280 mg/m^2 for escalated BEACOPP. However, most patients are treated with less than eight cycles of anthracycline-containing chemotherapy.

Whether cardiac toxicity observed after chemotherapy and radiotherapy is additive or synergistic remains unclear. However, several clinical studies showed that anthracycline-containing therapy may increase the radiation-related risk for congestive heart failure and valvular disorders by two- to three-fold compared with radiotherapy alone.[26]

Radiotherapy-Associated Cardiac Complications

Radiation-associated heart disease in cancer survivors includes a wide spectrum of cardiac pathologies such as coronary artery disease, myocardial dysfunction, valvular heart disease, pericardial disease, and electrical conduction abnormalities. Radiation-associated heart diseases, except for pericarditis, usually present 10 to 15 years after exposure, although nonsymptomatic abnormalities may develop much earlier. The long delay before expression of serious damage probably explains why radiation sensitivity of the heart has previously been underestimated.

Radiation causes both increased mortality and increased morbidity. Epidemiologic studies on HL survivors show relative risk estimates for cardiac deaths in the range of two- to sevenfold higher than the general population, depending on the patient's age. An increased risk was observed for patients irradiated at young age, depending on the radiation technique used and the duration of follow-up. In a Dutch study on HL patients treated before the age of 41, standardized incidence ratios for the development of various heart diseases were three- to fivefold higher when compared with the general population, even after a follow-up of more than 20 years.[26] The persistence of an increased risk over prolonged follow-up is a major concern because this implies increasing absolute excess risks over time, based on the rising incidence of cardiovascular diseases with age.

The heart volume included in the radiation field influences the risk for cardiotoxicity, although there are still many uncertainties regarding dose- and volume-effect relationship. A reduction regarding the risk for death from cardiovascular diseases other than myocardial infarction has been reported in HL patients treated after partial shielding of the heart and restriction of the total, fractionated, mediastinal dose to less than 30 Gy. Therefore the number of radiotherapy-associated cardiac long-term sequelae might decrease in the upcoming years.

Secondary Neoplasia

Radiotherapy and certain chemotherapeutic agents such as nitrogen mustard, procarbazine, cyclophosphamide, and etoposide are well known to have the potential to induce the development of secondary malignancies.

The highest incidence of acute leukemia usually spikes within the first 10 years after initial treatment. Several analyses on incidence and outcome of secondary leukemia were performed. The largest report, which came from the GHSG, retrospectively assessed 5411 patients with HL treated within the group's studies conducted between 1981 and 1998. After a median observation time of 55 months, incidence of secondary AML/MDS was 1%. Most patients were treated with COPP/ABVD, COPP/ABVD-like combinations or BEACOPP. With a median observation of 24 months, only one patient had not died from secondary AML/MDS.[27] The classical form of a treatment-related leukemia is characterized by a latency period of 3 to 5 years, a preceding myelodysplastic phase with trilineage bone marrow dysplasia, and abnormalities of chromosome 5 and/or 7. Topoisomerase II inhibitors, especially the epipodophyllotoxins, have been implicated in the development of a clinically and cytogenetically distinct form of secondary AML. When compared with classical secondary AML induced by alkylating agents, etoposide-related AML typically occurs sooner after exposure, generally lacks a preceding myelodysplastic phase, and is characterized by balanced translocations involving chromosome bands 11q23 and 21q22.

Secondary NHL occurring after HL include intermediate- or high-grade lymphomas and present similar to lymphomas seen in patients with chronic suppression of the immune system. There is a cumulative risk of about 1.5% at 15 years for the development of these lymphomas. In general, outcome of patients with secondary NHL is worse than that of patients with primary NHL. However, some patients with secondary NHL achieve durable remission after adequate chemotherapy.

The incidence of solid tumors after HL treatment increases with time and does not reach a plateau, even in the second decade after treatment. The causative role of radiotherapy and chemotherapy is debated, but most epidemiologists tend to place greatest blame on intensive irradiation with large fields and high doses. The organs at major risk appear to be lung and breast, especially among women who were irradiated at a young age during development of the breast. A retrospective analysis by the GHSG with a median follow-up of 72 months revealed an overall cumulative risk to develop a solid secondary malignancy of 2% with relative risk estimates for secondary malignancies of lung, colon, and breast at 3.8%, 3.2%, and 1.9%, respectively. Other secondary cancers observed after successful treatment for HL include sarcomas, melanomas, and bone tumors. As indicated by registry-based reports, the portion of patients with secondary solid tumors among HL survivors will further increase with longer follow-up since radiotherapy-related secondary malignancies, in particular, have a latency of decades from exposure to the carcinogenic noxa to the diagnosis of the secondary cancer.

Gonadal Dysfunction

Of total male patients in advanced stages of HL, 78% have inadequate pretreatment semen quality as a result of the lymphoma itself. The mechanisms involved are still unknown; however, possible factors include damage of the germinal epithelium, disturbances in the hypothalamic-hypophyseal axis, immunologic processes associated with cancer that impair spermatogenesis, and the dysregulated release of cytokines. In a recent study by the GHSG, male fertility was assessed in a total of 202 patients. In pretreatment semen analyses, only 20% of patients had normal sperms. Azoospermia was observed in 11%, and other dysspermia was reported in 69% of patients.

Intensive alkylating agent–based combinations such as BEACOPP are highly gonadotoxic in males. In a recent study, posttreatment sperm analyses performed at a median of 17.4 months after completion of therapy revealed azoospermia in 64% of patients, other forms of dysspermia in 30%, and normal sperm analysis results in only 6% of cases. No statistically significant difference was found in the posttreatment status between a group of patients treated with eight cycles of $BEACOPP_{baseline}$ (with a cumulative cyclophosphamide dose of 5200 mg/m^2) and a group treated with eight cycles of $BEACOPP_{escalated}$ (with a cumulative cyclophosphamide dose of 10.000 mg/m^2). In contrast, ABVD, probably the most widely used regimen in the treatment of HL, is less gonadotoxic, with gonadal damage that might be only transient. However, because of the gonadotoxic effects of many drugs used in the current treatment of HL, cryoconservation should be offered to every young male before starting with chemotherapy.

Gonadal complications affect female patients as well. As with males, alkylating agents are most commonly involved in treatment-associated gonadal damage in female patients. In a retrospective analysis by the GHSG, the menstrual status after HL treatment of 405 female patients younger than 40 years was analyzed. With a median follow-up of 3.2 years, 51.4% of women who had received eight cycles of escalated BEACOPP had continuous amenorrhea. Amenorrhea was significantly less common in women treated with two cycles of ABVD (3.9%), two cycles of alternating COPP/ABVD (6.9%), four cycles of alternating COPP/ABVD (37.5%), or eight cycles of BEACOPP baseline (22.6%). In a multivariate analysis, amenorrhea was most pronounced in women with advanced-stage HL, women older than 30 years of age at treatment, and women who did not take oral contraceptives during chemotherapy.[28] After ABVD alone, chemotherapy-induced ovarian failure is less likely, especially when women are younger than 30 years at the time of treatment. Older women have a significantly lower likelihood of ovarian recovery than those of younger age. In the GHSG analysis, 40% of women younger than 30 years of age experienced amenorrhea after treatment with eight cycles of escalated BEACOPP, compared with 70% of women aged 30 or older.

Quality of Life

A review of most randomized clinical trials in HL reveals that quality of life (QOL) has been neglected as primary or even secondary outcome measure in the past. However, the number of clinical trials evaluating health-related QOL (HRQOL) is increasing. It has become widely accepted that the multidimensional approach of HRQOL assessment reflects the patient's situation and reveals important information for the process of treatment evaluation. With the constantly growing cohort of long-term survivors indicating the progress of cancer therapy, new approaches in HRQOL assessment are needed in order to deal with the particular problems of these long-term survivors. Several studies have highlighted the difficulties that survivors may experience long after treatment ends, such as general fatigue, health fragility, and social and financial problems. These findings have been demonstrated in studies in which an HRQOL approach has been used. Since most of these studies used a cross-sectional design, the need exists for new approaches to describe patient situations more precisely, to detect reasons for maladaptation, and to identify patients at high risk for developing problems.

Combined comprehensive approaches could help to overcome the difficulties in assessing HRQOL in long-term survivors. Furthermore, this approach can be used with few modifications in the assessment of normal control persons. It seems plausible that many years after treatment, daily living circumstances have a stronger impact on a patient's HRQOL. Therefore it is essential to also have reference data from age- and gender-matched healthy persons for the interpretation of HRQOL results. In addition, a more comprehensive approach that accounts for each patient's life situation is necessary to represent the complexity of HRQOL. Results from studies by the EORTC/GELA and the GHSG within the next few years should reveal whether this approach is successful. Quality-of-life assessment should benefit patients by defining relevant issues, even long after initial treatment. Well-designed prospective studies must evaluate disease- and therapy-independent predisposing factors for long-term HRQOL functions as well as those factors associated with the applied therapy or the lymphoma itself.

NEW DRUGS IN HODGKIN LYMPHOMA

Despite the excellent cure rates achieved with current first-line protocols, treatment of relapsed or refractory HL has remained a field o f unmet medical need. Relapse after HDCT and ASCT, in particular, is associated with poor prognosis and a median OS of less than 3 years. This section provides a brief introduction to some of the new drugs being used in HL treatment, including monoclonal antibodies, immunotoxins, radioimmunoconjugates, and small molecules.

Anti-CD30 Antibody-Based Approaches

Because it is selectively overexpressed on HRS cells, CD30 is considered a privileged target antigen for antibody-based immunotherapy of cHL. However, despite encouraging preclinical data, results of phase I/II clinical trials with naked first-generation anti-CD30 antibodies were disappointing. Both first-generation antibodies applied in HL patients, MDX-060 and SGN-30, showed only modest clinical activity when given as single agent. In a phase I/II trial, a total of 72 patients with CD30-positive malignancies, including 63 patients with multiple relapsed HL, were treated with MDX-060, but only 6 patients achieved an objective response and only 25 had stable disease. In another phase II trial using a different monoclonal antibody (SGN-30), none of the 38 HL patients responded. Several possible reasons may explain this lack of activity, including poor binding properties in vivo and a neutralization of the antibodies by the soluble form of CD30 shed from the target cells.

The most advanced and promising anti-CD30 construct so far is the antibody-drug conjugate SGN-35 (brentuximab vedotin) consisting of the antibody cAC10 and the synthetic antimitotic agent monomethylauristatin. In a phase 1 trial, 42 patients with relapsed HL, 2 patients with systemic anaplastic large cell lymphoma, and 1 patient with angioimmunoblastic T-cell lymphoma were included. With a median of three prior lines of treatment, 86% of patients showed reductions in target lesion size. Side effects were mainly mild and manageable.[29] A pivotal phase II trial including 102 HL patients with relapse after HDCT and ASCT finished recruitment at the end of 2009.

Antibody-Based Strategies Targeting Other Antigens

CD25 (interleukin-2 receptor) is expressed on a few normal cells and can consistently be found on malignant cells in a number of lymphoma entities, including HL. Therefore a rationale follows to target CD25 with antibodies and antibody-based constructs. Efficacy and safety of a radioimmunoconjugate consisting of an anti-CD25 antibody (daclizumab) and radioactive yttrium-90 (daclizumab-90Y) were evaluated in a phase II trial including 30 heavily pretreated HL patients (1 to 8 prior lines of treatment). Response rate was promising, with 19 patients achieving either partial (7 patients) or complete (12 patients) remission. Only six patients showed disease progression. However, because the drug also exhibited relevant toxicity, with seven patients showing an insufficient platelet count recovery and three patients developing MDS, the future role for this treatment approach is unclear despite its clearly proven antilymphoma activity.

Small Molecules

An increasing number of small molecules have become available in recent years. As examples of this group of drug, the immunomodulatory drug lenalidomide, the histone deacetylase inhibitor panobinostat, and the mTOR inhibitor everolimus will be described in this section.

The efficacy of the thalidomide-derivate lenalidomide has been independently reported by different groups as a single-agent treatment in HL patients who had relapsed after ASCT. In an individual patient program conducted by the GHSG, 12 patients with a median of six prior therapies received lenalidomide at doses of 25 mg/day for 21 days of each 28-day cycle. Of these patients, 50% responded to treatment. Hematologic and nonhematologic side effects were mostly mild and manageable and did not prevent continuation of treatment at the initial dose level.[30]

An interim analysis of a phase II trial using the same treatment schedule reported the outcome of 15 patients with relapsed disease, 13 of whom had not responded to their prior treatment. Partial remission or CR was achieved by 33% of evaluable patients, and another 25% had stable disease lasting 6 months or longer. In this trial, treatment was also well tolerated; thus lenalidomide appears to be active in a relevant portion of heavily pretreated patients without excessive or treatment-limiting toxicity. Therefore lenalidomide can also be considered as a possible part of combination therapies with other small molecules, antibodies, or conventional chemotherapy.

Histone deacetylases are a family of enzymes involved in diverse activities, including cell proliferation, survival, angiogenesis, and immunity. In recent years, several histone deacetylase inhibitors were developed for clinical use, including vorinostat, MGCD0103, and panobinostat. Larger trials have already finished recruitment, but no final analyses are available to date.

The PI3K/Akt/mTOR pathway is aberrantly activated in many cancer entities. This pathway was also shown to be dysregulated in HRS cells by several mechanisms, including activation of CD30 and CD40; thus it is considered a possible target pathway for novel treatment approaches. Safety and activity of the mTOR inhibitor everolimus were proven in a phase II study including 19 patients who continuously received 10 mg of the drug. Of these patients, 47% responded to treatment, with eight patients achieving partial remission and one achieving a complete remission. No excessive toxicity was observed. Thus the drug is currently undergoing further clinical studies.

REFERENCES

1. Stein H, Hummel M: Cellular origin and clonality of classic Hodgkin's lymphoma: Immunophenotypic and molecular studies. *Semin Hematol* 36:233, 1999.
2. Kuppers R, Rajewsky K, Zhao M, et al: Hodgkin disease: Hodgkin and Reed-Sternberg cells picked from histological sections show clonal immunoglobulin gene rearrangements and appear to be derived from B cells at various stages of development. *Proc Natl Acad Sci USA* 91:10962, 1994.
3. Hjalgrim H, Askling J, Rostgaard K, et al: Characteristics of Hodgkin's lymphoma after infectious mononucleosis. *N Engl J Med* 349:1324, 2003.
4. Cheson BD, Pfistner B, Juweid ME, et al: Revised response criteria for malignant lymphoma. *J Clin Oncol* 25:579, 2007.
5. Gallamini A, Hutchings M, Rigacci L, et al: Early interim 2-[18F]fluoro-2-deoxy-D-glucose positron emission tomography is prognostically superior to international prognostic score in advanced-stage Hodgkin's lymphoma: A report from a joint Italian-Danish study. *J Clin Oncol* 25:3746, 2007.
6. Hasenclever D, Diehl V: A prognostic score for advanced Hodgkin's disease. International Prognostic Factors Project on Advanced Hodgkin's Disease. *N Engl J Med* 339:1506, 1998.
7. Engert A, Franklin J, Eich HT, et al: Two cycles of doxorubicin, bleomycin, vinblastine, and dacarbazine plus extended-field radiotherapy is superior to radiotherapy alone in early favorable Hodgkin's lymphoma: Final results of the GHSG HD7 trial. *J Clin Oncol* 25:3495, 2007.
8. Ferme C, Eghbali H, Meerwaldt JH, et al: Chemotherapy plus involved-field radiation in early-stage Hodgkin's disease. *N Engl J Med* 357:1916, 2007.
9. Engert A, Plutschow A, Eich HT, et al: Reduced treatment intensity in patients with early-stage Hodgkin's lymphoma. *N Engl J Med* 363:640, 2010.
10. Canellos GP, Anderson JR, Propert KJ, et al: Chemotherapy of advanced Hodgkin's disease with MOPP, ABVD, or MOPP alternating with ABVD. *N Engl J Med* 327:1478, 1992.
11. Engert A, Diehl V, Franklin J, et al: Escalated-dose BEACOPP in the treatment of patients with advanced-stage Hodgkin's lymphoma: 10 years of follow-up of the GHSG HD9 study. *J Clin Oncol* 27:4548, 2009.
12. Aleman BM, Raemaekers JM, Tirelli U, et al: Involved-field radiotherapy for advanced Hodgkin's lymphoma. *N Engl J Med* 348:2396, 2003.
13. Josting A, Rueffer U, Franklin J, et al: Prognostic factors and treatment outcome in primary progressive Hodgkin lymphoma: A report from the German Hodgkin Lymphoma Study Group. *Blood* 96:1280, 2000.
14. Linch DC, Winfield D, Goldstone AH, et al: Dose intensification with autologous bone-marrow transplantation in relapsed and resistant Hodgkin's disease: Results of a BNLI randomised trial. *Lancet* 341:1051, 1993.
15. Schmitz N, Pfistner B, Sextro M, et al: Aggressive conventional chemotherapy compared with high-dose chemotherapy with autologous haemopoietic stem-cell transplantation for relapsed chemosensitive Hodgkin's disease: A randomised trial. *Lancet* 359:2065, 2002.
16. Josting A, Muller H, Borchmann P, et al: Dose intensity of chemotherapy in patients with relapsed Hodgkin's lymphoma. *J Clin Oncol* 28:5074, 2010.
17. Sureda A, Robinson S, Canals C, et al: Reduced-intensity conditioning compared with conventional allogeneic stem-cell transplantation in relapsed or refractory Hodgkin's lymphoma: An analysis from the Lymphoma Working Party of the European Group for Blood and Marrow Transplantation. *J Clin Oncol* 26:455, 2008.
18. Nogova L, Reineke T, Brillant C, et al: Lymphocyte-predominant and classical Hodgkin's lymphoma: A comprehensive analysis from the German Hodgkin Study Group. *J Clin Oncol* 26:434, 2008.

19. Chen RC, Chin MS, Ng AK, et al: Early-stage, lymphocyte-predominant Hodgkin's lymphoma: Patient outcomes from a large, single-institution series with long follow-up. *J Clin Oncol* 28:136, 2010.
20. Schulz H, Rehwald U, Morschhauser F, et al: Rituximab in relapsed lymphocyte-predominant Hodgkin lymphoma: Long-term results of a phase 2 trial by the German Hodgkin Lymphoma Study Group (GHSG). *Blood* 111:109, 2008.
21. Al-Mansour M, Connors JM, Gascoyne RD, et al: Transformation to aggressive lymphoma in nodular lymphocyte-predominant Hodgkin's lymphoma. *J Clin Oncol* 28:793, 2010.
22. Engert A, Ballova V, Haverkamp H, et al: Hodgkin's lymphoma in elderly patients: A comprehensive retrospective analysis from the German Hodgkin's Study Group. *J Clin Oncol* 23:5052, 2005.
23. Proctor SJ, Lennard AL, Jackson GH, et al: The role of an all-oral chemotherapy containing lomustine (CCNU) in advanced,fs progressive Hodgkin lymphoma: A patient-friendly palliative option which can result in long-term disease control. *Ann Oncol* 21:426, 2010.
24. Pereg D, Koren G, Lishner M: The treatment of Hodgkin's and non-Hodgkin's lymphoma in pregnancy. *Haematologica* 92:1230, 2007.
25. Hartmann P, Rehwald U, Salzberger B, et al: BEACOPP therapeutic regimen for patients with Hodgkin's disease and HIV infection. *Ann Oncol* 14:1562, 2003.
26. Aleman BM, van den Belt-Dusebout AW, De Bruin ML, et al: Late cardiotoxicity after treatment for Hodgkin lymphoma. *Blood* 109:1878, 2007.
27. Josting A, Wiedenmann S, Franklin J, et al: Secondary myeloid leukemia and myelodysplastic syndromes in patients treated for Hodgkin's disease: A report from the German Hodgkin's Lymphoma Study Group. *J Clin Oncol* 21:3440, 2003.
28. Behringer K, Breuer K, Reineke T, et al: Secondary amenorrhea after Hodgkin's lymphoma is influenced by age at treatment, stage of disease, chemotherapy regimen, and the use of oral contraceptives during therapy: A report from the German Hodgkin's Lymphoma Study Group. *J Clin Oncol* 23:7555, 2005.
29. Younes A, Bartlett NL, Leonard JP, et al: Brentuximab vedotin (SGN-35) for relapsed CD30-positive lymphomas. *N Engl J Med* 363:1812, 2010.
30. Boll B, Borchmann P, Topp MS, et al: Lenalidomide in patients with refractory or multiple relapsed Hodgkin lymphoma. *Br J Haematol* 148:480, 2010.

CHAPTER 75

ORIGIN OF NON-HODGKIN LYMPHOMA

Matthew S. McKinney and Sandeep S. Dave

Over the past 2 decades, discoveries in basic immunology and the pathogenesis of malignancies have significantly advanced our understanding of the origin of lymphoid neoplasms. These diseases have been reexamined and grouped based on recurrent chromosomal rearrangements, histologic patterns, and gene expression profiles. The multiple revisions to the World Health Organization's classification schemes for lymphomas reflect this progress. As with other cancers, acquisition of sequential mutations and recurrent chromosomal rearrangements involving oncogenic pathways as transformation events characterize B-cell lymphomas. Many of these derangements occur as a result of disordered genetic recombination and somatic hypermutation events intended to support adaptive immunity.

An evolving understanding of the steps involved in normal B-cell development has provided further insights into the development of this diverse group of malignancies because most non-Hodgkin lymphomas (NHLs) reflect stages of B-cell development. The application of gene expression profiling (GEP) and massively parallel high-throughput sequencing, as well as a better appreciation of the contribution of microRNAs (miRNAs) and epigenetic alterations to lymphoma pathogenesis, have shed new light on the mechanisms underlying lymphomagenesis. Correlation of these findings with the clinical outcomes has further refined prediction of outcome and has suggested targets for novel therapies.

This chapter reviews the most common B-cell NHLs with regard to classification using prevailing views regarding genetic or genomic classification of these disorders. Additionally, insights regarding pathogenesis, prognosis, and possible therapeutic targets gleaned from genomic approaches are discussed.

OVERVIEW OF B-CELL LYMPHOMAS

B-cell lymphomas often represent immortalized, "frozen" stages of B-cell development. The goal of early B-cell development is to produce mature B cells expressing surface immunoglobulin M (IgM) that can efficiently recognize cognate antigen. After this is accomplished, B cells develop along pathways involving germinal center (GC), mantle, and marginal zones in lymphoid organs where they encounter antigen in association with activated antigen-presenting cells (APCs). Differentiation of mature B cells into plasma cells after somatic hypermutation is the final step in B-cell development and is critical to the development of effective humoral immunity. Antibody diversity is accomplished through the process of somatic V(D)J recombination at the pro–B cell stage via recombinase activating genes (*RAG1* and *RAG2*) followed by trafficking to GCs, where they proliferate rapidly with dividing times of 6 to 8 hours. High-affinity B-cell clones produced in part via activation-induced cytidine deaminase (AID) expression and somatic hypermutation (SHM) are favored because of protection from apoptosis. Through this mechanism, protective antibodies are produced at the risk of exposing antigen-stimulated B cells to genetic lesions caused by the molecular machinery utilized to create V(D)J recombination and SHM. Many NHLs exhibit translocations of driver oncogenes to highly active Ig loci, implying that recombination events intended to produce high-affinity antibodies are misdirected and instead produce immortalized B cells representing stages of B-cell development. Furthermore, mutations in oncogenes or tumor suppressors frequently occur in a pattern consistent with SHM at these loci. When considered together with the recurrent chromosomal rearrangements noted in NHL, this confirms the notion that these neoplasms stem from mature B cells that have entered (or are poised to enter) GCs.

Subsets of NHL recapitulate this pattern of normal B-cell differentiation at the histologic, molecular, and genomic levels and serve as a template for the classification of these diseases. This template can be applied to the entire spectrum of B-cell neoplasms as outlined in Fig. 75-1, suggesting that NHLs form as a result of genetic alterations developed along this process. B-cell differentiation must be carefully choreographed at the molecular and genomic level because the expression of the *RAG* genes and AID cause DNA strand breaks and put the nascent lymphocyte at risk of oncogene overexpression and tumor suppressor deletion. Moreover, a coordinated regulation of gene expression is required to allow such genomic revision without triggering reflexive, protective apoptotic pathways and to allow appropriate B-cell differentiation. GC B cells highly express BCL6, and its functions are critically important to regulation of cell survival and differentiation. Targets of BCL6 also include cell cycle regulators (p21, p27) and TP53, which may overall work to facilitate cell cycle progression in the face of ongoing AID-mediated DNA strand breaks. BCL6 also represses *PRDM1*/Blimp1 and serves to prevent plasmacytic differentiation. Plasma cell differentiation is mediated by upregulation of IRF4 and nuclear factor kappa-B (NFκB), which establish characteristic regulatory programs.

Genetic lesions altering these pathways are found recurrently in NHL. *BCL6* rearrangements occur in diffuse large B-cell lymphoma (DLBCL) and other lymphomas, and constitutively active NFκB signaling is associated specifically with aggressive phenotypes of DLBCL. Translocations of *BCL2,* which is expressed at very low levels in GCs, occur in almost all follicular lymphomas (FLs) and illustrate the dangers of aberrant recombination events in the GCs because *BCL2* translocation appears to be a primary event in the formation of these tumors.

Recent work has also suggested a role for miRNAs in B-cell development. Multiple miRNAs are required at various steps across B-cell development, and patterns of miRNA expression can be correlated to individual stages of B-cell maturation. In particular, miR-150 and mi17~92 clusters downregulate pre–B cell development, and miR-155 has been implicated in disordered humoral immunity and the development of NHL. Interestingly, mi17~92 appears to drive oncogenic mTOR (mammalian target of rapamycin) signaling in GC origin DLBCLs as well. Important regulators of germinal center B (GCB) transition, including LMO2 and Blimp1, appear to be regulated by miRNAs, and maintenance of this phenotype may play a role in NHL formation. Interestingly, miRNA profiles in NHL also reflect their cell of origin, highlighting their importance in maintaining the B-cell phenotype.

Antigen stimulation of the B-cell receptor (BCR) is important in both B-cell maturation and the development of NHL. The BCR consists of a multimeric signaling complex, including CD79A and CD79B, which acts through the immunoreceptor tyrosine activation motif on CD79B and leads to a cascade of molecular events involving SYK and BTK signaling. The end-result of this cascade is an increase in cellular proliferation through activation of NFκB target genes and

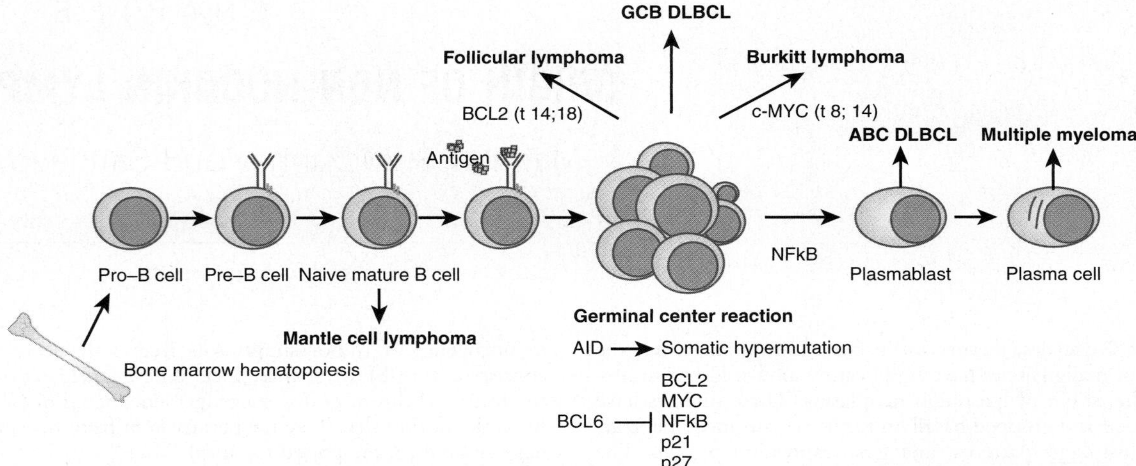

Figure 75-1 CLASSIFICATION OF COMMON NON-HODGKIN LYMPHOMAS (NHLs) IN RELATION TO B-CELL DEVELOPMENT IN GERMINAL CENTERS (GCs). Hematopoiesis results in B-cell precursors that ultimately produce immunoglobulin M (IgM) that recognize cognate antigen via activation of recombinase activating genes (*RAG1* and *RAG2*) and a GC reaction occurs. A regulatory program relying on BCL6 regulation of cell proliferation and apoptosis occurs at this point, and rearrangements presumed to occur along this course result in post-GC lymphomas, including follicular lymphoma, Burkitt lymphoma, and diffuse large B-cell lymphoma (DLBCL). The underlying molecular biology of NHL subsets (and other lymphoid neoplasms) reflects the GC step and other stages of B-cell development. For example, gene profiling of DLBCL reveals that whereas activated B cell–like (ABC) DLBCL reflects the plasmablast stage along normal B-cell development, multiple myeloma expressesion profiles more consistent with differentiated plasma cell origin.

other cellular machinery. Almost all NHLs express surface Ig, suggesting that functional BCR signaling is important at some point in the process of lymphoma formation. Analysis of Ig SHM patterns in lymphoma samples further suggests that antigen-induced selective pressure is important in the pathogenesis of NHL. The antigen(s) involved in this process are unknown, and it is also unclear whether ongoing antigen stimulation is important in subsets of NHL.

Epidemiologic studies have bolstered the argument that chronic immune activation and inflammation are connected with NHL development; these data also suggest that immune surveillance plays a role in the origin of NHL. DLBCL and Burkitt lymphoma (BL) occur more frequently in immunocompromised hosts and are often Epstein-Barr virus (EBV) positive. HIV/AIDS is a significant risk factor for post-GC neoplasms, and this risk is attenuated with the use of highly active antiretroviral therapy. For example, the risk of central nervous system lymphomas is increased more than 1000-fold in patients with AIDS. NHL also occurs more frequently in acquired or inherited immunodeficiencies such as common variable immunodeficiency and severe combined immunodeficiency and with solid organ and hemopoietic transplantation. Situations in which chronic infection or inflammation occurs have also been linked to NHL. Gastric MALT *(Helicobacter pylori),* hepatosplenic T-cell lymphoma (associated with infliximab use), and thyroid NHL (Hashimoto thyroiditis) are specific instances in which the development of lymphoid malignancy can be traced to chronic inflammation, either of microbial or autoimmune etiology. A critical association with EBV has been noted for NHL and is most frequently seen in posttransplant lymphoproliferative disorder, a disease that occurs in the setting of organ transplantation and immunosuppression targeting cellular immunity.

Beyond these factors, the contributions of modifiable risk factors and heredity appear to play only a small role in NHL development. Any increased risk contributed by inherited genetic factors appears to be almost negligible. Furthermore, several environmental factors (pesticides, Agent Orange, radiation exposure) have been implicated in NHL, but the associations between these agents and lymphomagenesis are difficult to prove. Pesticide exposure does appear to have a dose-effect relationship with regard to NHL pathogenesis and has been linked to recurrent t(14;18) cytogenetic rearrangements that are noted in DLBCL and FL.

Together, these observations reinforce the notion that NHLs originate from disordered lymphoid development. Factors related to immune surveillance, lymphoid proliferation, or Ig gene rearrangement appear to be the most important factors for the development of NHL.

DIFFUSE LARGE B-CELL LYMPHOMA

Diffuse large B-cell lymphoma is the most common subtype of NHL (≈25% of all NHL) and is responsible for more patient deaths than any other form of lymphoma. This entity often presents at an advanced stage, and around 50% of all patients fail to respond long-term to standard chemotherapy programs; the vast majority of those patients will eventually succumb to their disease. Even prior to the availability of gene expression profiling technology. It was clear clinically (based on tumor morphology, immunohistochemical staining, and patient outcomes) that DLBCL is a heterogeneous disease. Advances in molecular biology and genomic technologies have clarified the basis for some of this observed heterogeneity, and it has become clear that DLBCL comprises a diverse group of lymphomas that have distinct cellular origins, recurrent gene mutations, and chromosomal rearrangements that dictate their behavior. It is also clear that the stromal environment appears to play a key role in the development and progression of DLBCL, as with other cancers.

GENE EXPRESSION PROFILES DEFINE DIFFUSE LARGE B-CELL LYMPHOMA SUBTYPES (Table 75-1)

Gene expression profiling has identified GCB and activated B cell–like (ABC) DLBCL subsets that express gene signatures that mimic GCs and activated B cells (Figs. 75-2 and 75-3). Roughly 30% of DLBCLs cannot be classified using this system and have been deemed unclassified DLBCL. There are thousands of genes that differ between these subtypes at the GEP level, which is a magnitude similar to that seen between acute myeloid and lymphoblastic leukemias, which have profoundly different mechanisms of origin and natural histories.

Germinal center B DLBCLs express a characteristic spectrum of genes and have ongoing AID-mediated somatic hypermutation as

Table 75-1 Frequency of Recurrent Genetic Aberrations in Diffuse Large B-Cell Lymphoma Subtypes

Rearrangement, Amplification, or Deletion	ABC DLBCL	GCB DLBCL	PMBL	Notes
BCL2 translocation t(14;18)	0%	40%-50%	20%	Alternatively translocated to light chain loci 5%-10% of time
BCL2 amplification	34%	10%	16%	
BCL6 translocation t(3;V)(q27;V)	25%	10%	20%	Variable translocation partners (14q32, 2p11, 22q11, 4p11, 6p21, 11q23)
3q amplification	25%	0%	<5%	
9q24 amplification	5%	0%	45%	
PRDM1/PRDM1 deletion/mutation	25%	0%	Unknown	
REL amplification	0	15%	25%	
MYC rearrangement t(8;14)(q24;q32)	5%-10% of all DLBCLs			25%-30% occur with t(14;18)(q32;q21)
TP53 deletion	Mutations, deletions, or both in 20% of DLBCLs			

Compiled from Iqbal J: Distinctive patterns of BCL6 molecular alterations and their functional consequences in different subgroups of diffuse large B-cell lymphoma. *Leukemia* 21:2332, 2007; Iqbal J, Neppalli VT, Wright G, et al: BCL2 expression is a prognostic marker for the activated B-cell-like type of diffuse large B-cell lymphoma. *J Clin Oncol* 24:961, 2006; Iqbal J, Weisenburger DD, Greiner TC, et al: Molecular signatures to improve diagnosis in peripheral T-cell lymphoma and prognostication in angioimmunoblastic T-cell lymphoma. *Blood* 115:1026, 2010; Pasqualucci L. Inactivation of the *PRDM1*/BLIMP1 gene in diffuse large B cell lymphoma. *J Exp Med* 203:311, 2006; and Tam W: Mutational analysis of *PRDM1* indicates a tumor-suppressor role in diffuse large B-cell lymphomas. *Blood* 107:4090, 2006.
DLCBL, Diffuse large B-cell lymphoma.

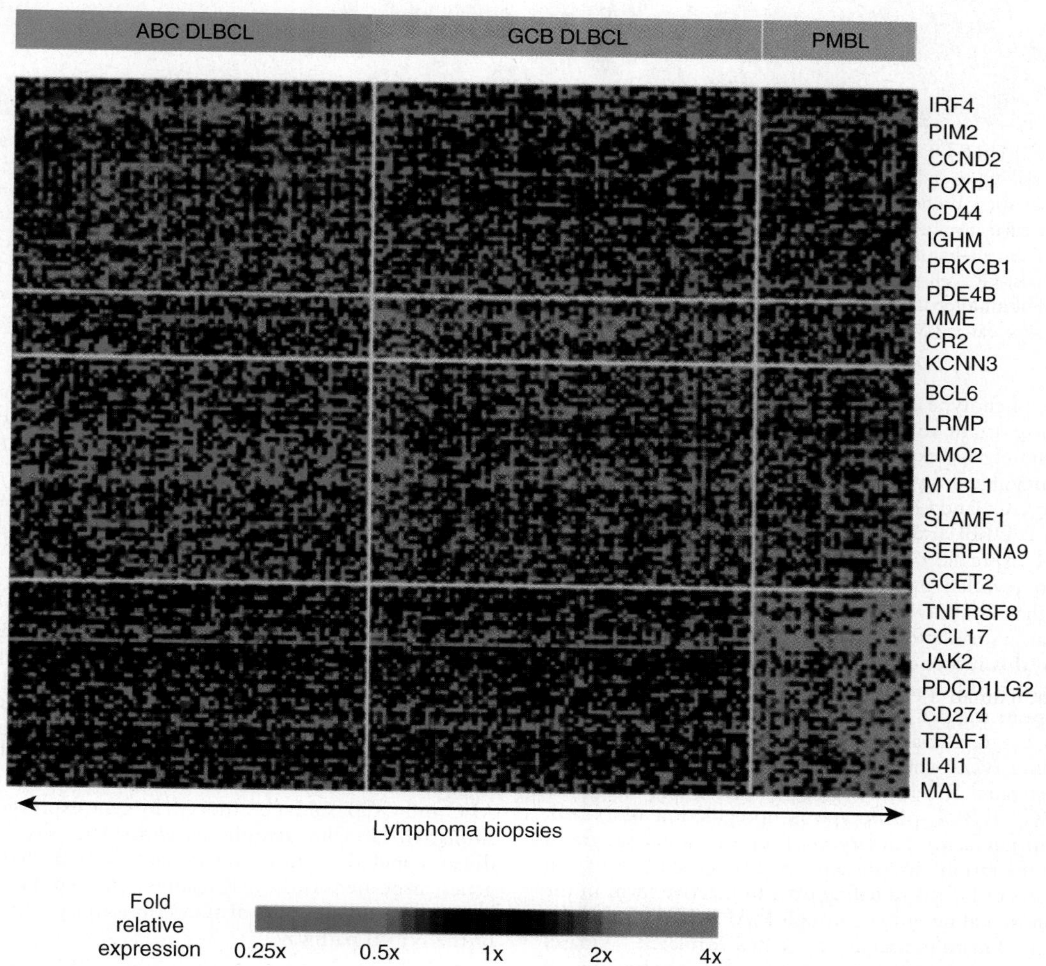

Figure 75-2 GENES CHARACTERISTICALLY EXPRESSED BY SUBGROUPS OF DIFFUSE LARGE B-CELL LYMPHOMA (DLBCL). Activated B-cell–like (ABC) DLBCL, germinal center B cell–like (GCB) DLBCL, and primary mediastinal B-cell lymphoma (PMBL). Each column represents gene expression data from a single DLBCL biopsy sample, and each row represents expression of a single gene. Relative gene expression is indicated according to the color scale shown. *(See Alizadeh, AA: Distinct types of diffuse large B-cell lymphoma identified by gene expression profiling.* Nature *403:503, 2000.)*

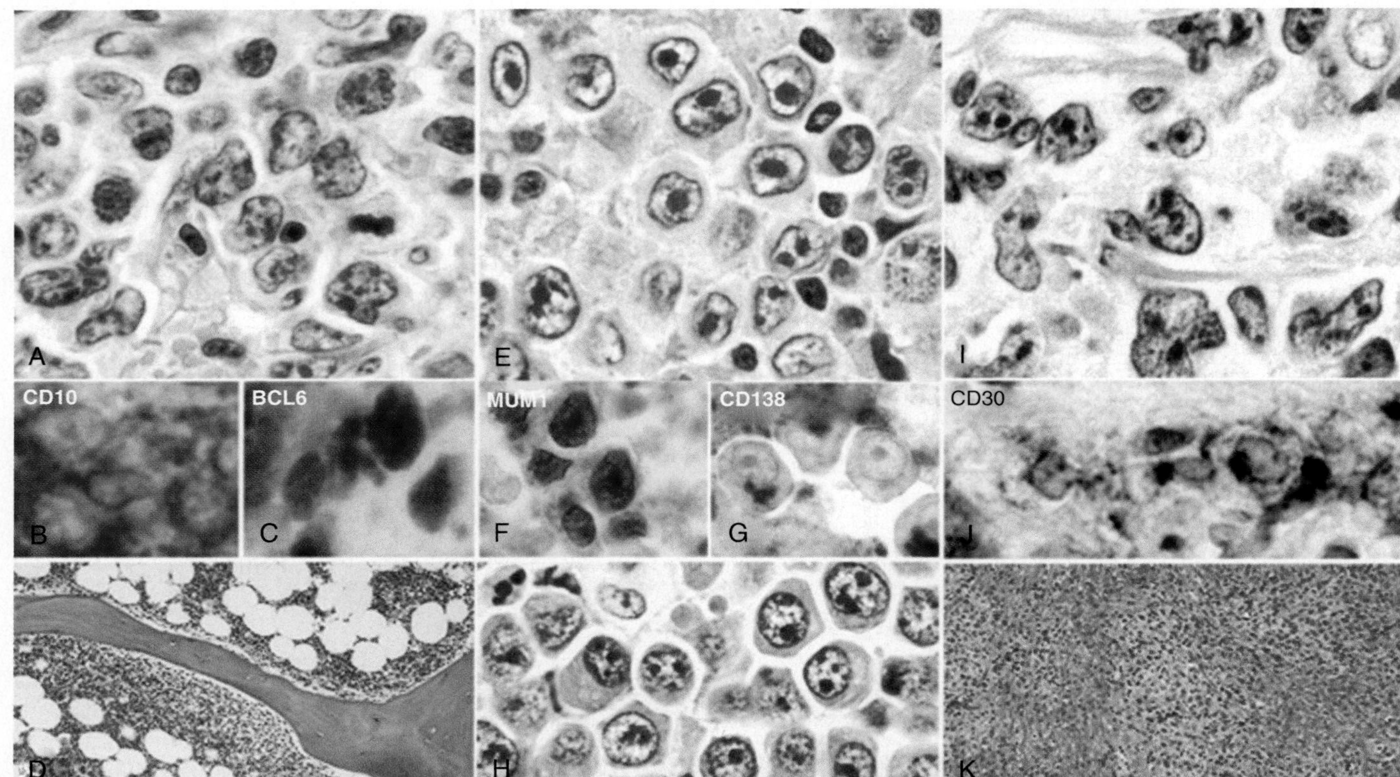

Figure 75-3 THREE TYPES OF DIFFUSE LARGE B-CELL LYMPHOMA DELINEATED BY HISTOLOGIC PATTERNS. Germinal center B cell–like (GCB), activated B-cell–type, and primary mediastinal B-cell lymphoma (PMBCL) type. GCB, or germinal center (GC)–derived large B-cell lymphomas usually have a centroblastic morphology **(A),** are CD20$^+$, and express the GC markers CD10 **(B)** and BCL6 **(C).** In this case, the patient's staging bone marrow **(D)** showed paratrabecular involvement by small cleaved cells (centrocytes), indicating that the large B-cell lymphoma likely arose from a lower grade follicular lymphoma. Activated B cell–like large B-cell lymphoma can sometime have an immunoblastic morphology **(E)** and can typically express MUM1 **(F)** and CD138 **(G).** These post-GC cell types of lymphomas can also have a plasmablastic morphology **(H),** as sometimes seen in HIV-related cases. PMBCLs are frequently composed of multilobated centroblasts **(I).** They are typically CD45$^+$, CD20$^+$, and usually CD30$^+$ **(J)** but CD15 negative. Surface immunoglobulin may be negative on such cases. PMBL is commonly associated with fibrosis, which is present in broad bands **(K)** or surrounding individual cells (as in **I**).

well as a histologic phenotype consistent with GC origin. BCL6 and LMO2 are both important to the transcriptional program of GCs and are commensurately overexpressed in GCB DLBCLs. Conversely, *PRDM1* is downregulated by BCL6, which results in decreased *PRDM1* activity in GCs, and GCB DLBCLs display a similar pattern. Histologically, GCB DLBCLs are characterized by CD10 expression and lack of IRF4 expression. Evaluation of Ig loci within GCB DLBCLs has also revealed evidence of ongoing SHM, which is further evidence that GCB DLBCLs reflect the biology of normal GC B cells and that dysregulation of pathways involved in GC formation might lead to this subset of DLBCL.

Alternatively, the ABC subtype of DLBCL expresses a post-GC phenotype but appears trapped just before differentiation into plasma cells. ABC DLBCLs are characterized by downregulation of many GC genes, including *BCL6* and *LMO2,* and by expression of genes associated with activated B cells and plasma cells. One of the hallmarks of the ABC DLBCL phenotype is upregulation of NFκB. NFκB is a transcription factor that targets a number of gene programs governing cell proliferation, immortality, and angiogenesis within NHLs. The effectors of NFκB signaling exist in inactive form in the cytosol and require signaling either through MAPK/ERK (mitogen-activated protein kinase/extracellular signal-regulated kinase) signaling (the canonical NFκB pathway) or through ligation of CD40–LTbR–BAFF-R (B-cell activating factor receptor), which results in phosphorylation of the inactive complex and translocation of either the p50–RelA or p52–Rel B complexes to the nucleus and subsequent transcription of target genes. In ABC DLBCL cell lines, a signaling complex involving CARD11, BCL10, and MALT1 (the CBM complex) constitutively activates NFκB signaling and selective knock-down of any of the components of this complex using RNAi or small molecule inhibitors and is lethal to ABC cell lines. Interestingly, a few GCB cell lines also demonstrate activation of NFκB and mutations in the NFκB pathway, which might confer sensitivity to inhibition of this pathway in those tumors. The mechanisms by which DLBCLs acquire and maintain constitutive NFκB activity are still being elucidated and may provide insights into the origin and into possible treatments for this entity.

Primary mediastinal B-cell lymphoma (PMBL) represents a distinct subset of patients that have sometimes been classified as DLBCL. PMBL was originally identified based on the clinical characteristics of the disease. Patients with PMBL are generally young (third or fourth decades of life), predominantly women, and present with a large mediastinal mass; outcomes with chemoimmunotherapy for PMBL are generally superior to those with other subtypes of DLBCL. GEP studies revealed that PMBL could be clearly delineated from ABC and GCB, subtypes. Indeed, by gene expression, PMBL appears similar to Hodgkin lymphoma with many shared features in both diseases, including the expression of CD30. Both diseases also express genes associated with JAK (Janus-activated kinase)–STAT (signal transducer and activator of transcription) signaling as well as targets of the NFκB pathway.

Molecular Pathogenesis of Diffuse Large B-Cell Lymphoma

Investigation of the molecular landscape of DLBCL has revealed a set of recurrent cytogenetic and molecular abnormalities associated with pathogenesis. Chromosomal translocations involving *BCL6*, *BCL2*, and *MYC* (v-*myc* myelocytomatosis viral oncogene homolog) occur frequently in DLBCL, and these translocations appear to reflect cell-of-origin phenotype. 3q27 rearrangement with Ig gene partners is the most common rearrangement seen in DLBCL and occurs in about 30% of both the ABC and GCB subtypes. This genetic rearrangement upregulates the *BCL6* gene, resulting in an oncogenic phenotype. Additional mutations in the transcriptional regulatory program of *BCL6* may also occur with alternative translocation. Notably, *BCL6* translocations appear to not be sufficient for lymphoma formation as evidenced by mice bearing t(3;14) translocations that develop NHL at a low rate. *BCL2* translocations occur in a minority of GCB DLBCLs but are not seen in the ABC phenotype; this mirrors the situation in FL, in which *BCL2* overexpression results in disordered GC transit. *MYC* rearrangements additionally occur in DLBCL (≈5% of cases), sometimes with rearrangements of *BCL2*, *BCL6*, or both. These tumors, sometimes termed *double-hit lymphomas*, display an aggressive phenotype seemingly intermediate between BL and DLBCL.

Oncogenic mutations and areas of chromosomal amplification or deletion also appear important in the pathogenesis of DLBCL. Upregulation of c-REL occurs in about 20% of GCB tumors through amplification of the 2p locus. Amplification of *MYC* and *BCL2* may also occur through this mechanism. *TP53* mutations and SHM of other loci, including *PIM1*, *BCL6*, and *MYC*, also appear to contribute to lymphoma formation and progression. Mutations in *CARD11* causing constitutive NFκB activation have been described in a subset of both ABC and GCB DLBCLs and appear to drive oncogenesis in these tumors. Overall, the patterns of gene mutation and recurrent cytogenetic abnormalities add further complexity to the classification of DLBCLs.

Recurrent mutations of genes involved in DLBCL pathogenesis have also been reported. Inactivating mutations of *PRDM1* and mutation in genes regulating NFκB signaling *(TNFAIP3, MYD88, CARD11)* have been noted in ABC DLBCL subtypes. *CD79B* and *BCL2* have also been found to harbor mutations in DLBCL and other NHLs. Most recently, several groups have reported analyses of whole-genome, exome, or transcriptome data from the application of massively parallel sequencing in DLBCLs. These studies identified novel mutations in genes that play roles in histone modification as well as a number of other processes in DLBCLs. A series that performed RNA sequencing on 127 NHL samples (including 83 DLBCL tumors) found 651 coding single nucleotide variants (cSNVs), many of which were not previously documented in malignancies. Truncating deletions in tumor suppression genes *(TP53, TNFRSF14, CREBBP)* were among the most significantly mutated genes and other heavily mutated genes not previously known to be involved in DLBCL pathogenesis (including *MLL2, BTG1,* and *GNA13*). *MLL2* contained cSNVs in 26% of tumors and most often occurred as a heterozygous defect, and sometimes multiple mutations occurred in trans MLL2 functions as a H3K4-specific methyltransferase responsible for regulation of transcription of developmental genes. Ostensibly, MLL2 might serve to deregulate genes involved in differentiation or development and act in conjunction with other oncogenes to facilitate NHL. Other groups have confirmed mutations in *MLL2* and other genes *(CREBBP/EP300)* that coordinate chromatin acetylation, leading to the hypothesis that mutations in histone-modifying genes lead to DLBCL and other NHLs. Further work is needed to understand how these genetic lesions may be targeted for DLBCL treatment.

The Tumor Microenvironment and Diffuse Large B-Cell Lymphoma

The complexities of antigen presentation and recognition and regulation of B-cell proliferation that occur in GCs suggest that the microenvironment may play a role in the origin and progression of DLBCL. Tumor-infiltrating T cells have been correlated to longer survival in patients with DLBCL, and failure of immune editing is likely responsible for the increase in NHL in HIV-positive and immunosuppressed persons. GEP has been used to define stromal elements related to DLBCL progression. In one series, hierarchical clustering was used to define three groups among DLBCL samples by GEP. Clusters identifying gene signature termed *oxidative phosphorylation*, *BCR proliferation*, and *host response* were identified; notably, the host response group exhibited gene expression profiles associated with T and natural killer cells, dendritic cells, and macrophages. This work illustrates that patterns of stromal involvement in DLBCL could play a key role in pathogenesis. In another series involving biopsy specimens from 414 patients treated with chemotherapy and immunochemotherapy, two gene signatures characterizing patterns of tumor stroma best predicted survival (Figs. 75-4 and 75-5). Improved survival was noted with a pattern that included genes associated with the extracellular matrix and histiocytic infiltration. The converse was true for gene profiles correlating to angiogenesis because these were associated with far worse overall survival.

Although it is not known what roles distinct lymph node subsets play in the pathogenesis of lymphoma, it is clear from these studies that the tumor microenvironment plays a role in the origin of NHL.

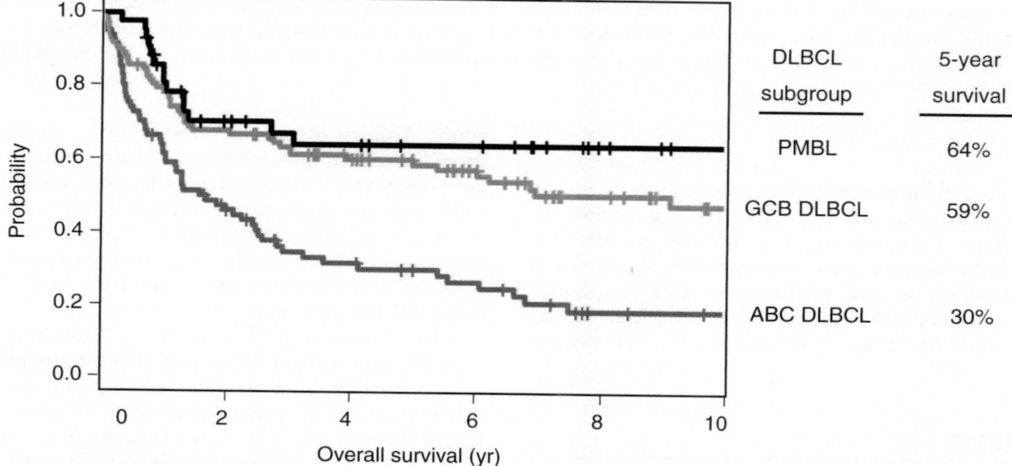

Figure 75-4 KAPLAN-MEIER PLOT OF OVERALL SURVIVAL FOR DIFFERENT DIFFUSE LARGE B-CELL LYMPHOMA SUBGROUPS TREATED WITH ANTHRACYCLINE-CONTAINING CHEMOTHERAPEUTIC REGIMENS. *(From Rosenwald, A: The use of molecular profiling to predict survival after chemotherapy for diffuse large-B-cell lymphoma.* N Engl J Med *346:1937, 2002.)*

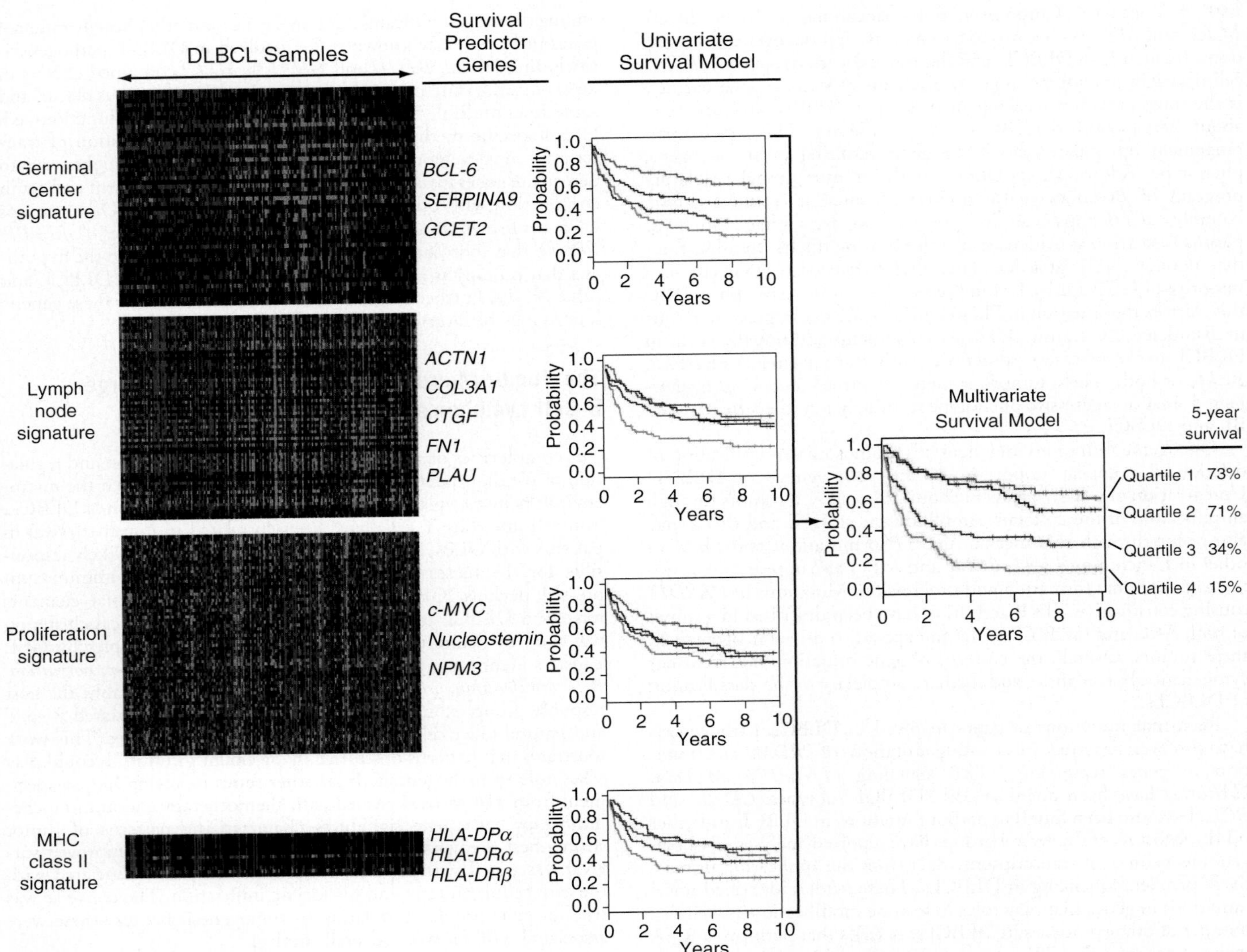

Figure 75-5 GENE EXPRESSION–BASED MODEL OF SURVIVAL AFTER CHEMOTHERAPY FOR DIFFUSE LARGE B-CELL LYMPHOMA (DLBCL). The *left panel* shows the expression of the four gene expression signatures used to create the survival model in DLBCL. Whereas expression of the germinal center, lymph node, and major histocompatibility class II signatures is associated with favorable prognosis, expression of the proliferation signature is associated with inferior survival. Representative genes from each signature used to create the survival model are shown. For each signature, patients were divided into four equal quartiles based on the expression of the signature in their biopsy samples. The four Kaplan-Meier plots in the middle depict the survival of patients in each signature quartile. These four signatures were combined into a multivariate model of survival, and patients were divided into four quartile groups based on this model. The Kaplan-Meier plot at the *right* depicts the survival of each quartile group of the multivariate model. *HLA,* Human leukocyte antigen. *(From Rosenwald, A: The use of molecular profiling to predict survival after chemotherapy for diffuse large-B-cell lymphoma.* N Engl J Med *346:1937, 2002.)*

Conclusions

Diffuse large B-cell lymphoma represents a heterogeneous group of B-cell neoplasms with a distinct underlying biology, prognosis, and response to therapy. Recent genomic approaches to studying DLBCL have identified a number of interesting potential targets for better prognostic stratification and treatment of this lymphoma entity. More work is needed to this end and to better understand the origin of DLBCL and the role of stromal factors in disease progression.

BURKITT LYMPHOMA

Burkitt lymphoma (BL) is a highly aggressive lymphoma entity characterized by a high mitotic rate, extranodal spread, and early death, but it is frequently curable with high-intensity multi-agent chemotherapy. It was first described more than 50 years ago as a disease in young Africans in association with EBV infection. Since then, the sporadic and immunodeficiency-related forms of the disease have been described. Subsequent work has shown that translocation of the *MYC* gene on chromosome 8q24 to the Ig locus occurs in virtually all cases of BL (Figs. 75-6 and 75-7 for an overview of BL). Given the high prevalence of *MYC* rearrangements and the high cure rates observed with chemotherapy, many have studied BL as a model for other B-cell lymphomas.

Overexpression of MYC occurs in association with a GC phenotype. BL tumors typically display the immunophenotypic characteristics of GC B cells, and genetic and genomic studies have reinforced this notion of GC origin. In virtually all cases, rearrangements are found between the MYC locus and one of the Ig genes, most commonly with the IgH locus at 14q32.33 in more than 80% of cases. Alternative rearrangements involving MYC and the κ or λ light chain regions are also noted in the minority of cases. Two different patterns of rearrangement and somatic hypermutation have been noted among the three types of BL. In endemic BL, chromosome 14 breakpoints

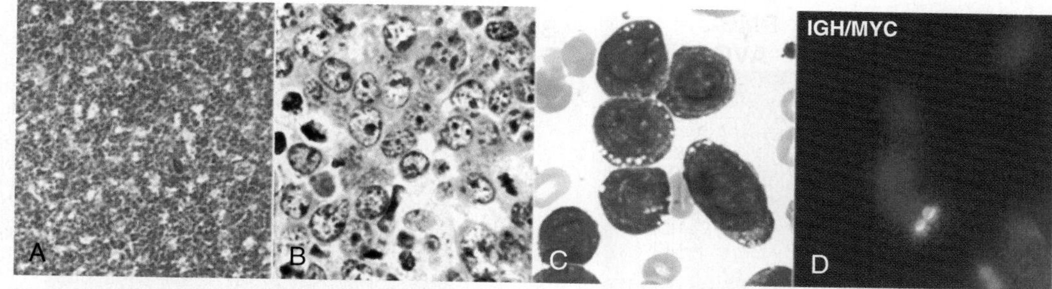

Figure 75-6 BURKITT LYMPHOMA (BL). **A,** A case of BL illustrated at low power showing the "starry sky" appearance. This appearance is attributable to the dense proliferating cells producing the "dark sky," and the scattered lighter staining tingible body macrophages ("stars") phagocytizing dying cells. **B,** Higher magnification image illustrating the syncytia of intermediate-sized cells with coarse chromatin and multiple nucleoli. Note the tingible body macrophage with abundant light cytoplasm and ingested debris *(center bottom).* **C,** Burkitt cells as seen on a Wright-stained bone marrow aspirate in a patient with BL. Notice deep blue cytoplasm with numerous vacuoles. **D,** Fluorescence in situ hybridization with probes to MYC and immunoglobulin h (IgH) illustrate the IgH–MYC fusion. *(Courtesy Dr. Yanming Zhang, University of Chicago.)*

can be mapped to J_H regions, indicating *RAG1-* or *RAG2*-mediated rearrangement occurring at the pro–B cell stage. In contrast, sporadic and immunodeficiency-related BL often demonstrate somatic hypermutation and rearrangement at chromosome 14 breakpoints related in Ig switch regions; this is consistent with GC or memory B-cell origin.

Translocations placing MYC downstream of Ig genes result in massive gene upregulation and oncogenesis by dysregulation of multiple pathways. In normal B cells, MYC regulates B-cell proliferation and differentiation and is tightly regulated by multiple mechanisms, including posttranslational modifications and transcriptional autoregulation and by other factors, including a careful balance of interactions with regulatory proteins. Under normal circumstances, MYC also induces a number of proapoptotic cellular mechanisms, which are then perturbed when MYC is overexpressed by the robust Ig gene promoters existing GC B cells. Constitutive induction of MYC expression in GCs via upstream Ig gene promoter then confers a neoplastic phenotype. Highlighting the complexities of MYC in this setting, even brief reversal of MYC overexpression may induce a reversion of tumors to a benign phenotype; this implies that c-*MYC*–Ig rearrangements might serve as the "switch" that drives BL formation in the context of GCs.

Recently, GEP has further examined the role of MYC in BL and revealed insights into the similarities and differences between BL and other GCB-origin NHLs. This work has further defined the differences between BL and DLBCLs carrying MYC rearrangements because these entities can be difficult to distinguish on histopathologic grounds alone. Although BL is characterized by gene expression profiles consistent with GC origin, a group of genes found in GCB DLBCL, including *LMO2, BCL2, CD80,* and *CD86,* are expressed only weakly in BL. BLs also express low amounts of NFκB and major histocompatibility class I molecules compared with DLBCL. These data also serve to allow the diagnostic distinction of BLs on molecular grounds. In two large studies, a fraction of DLBCLs were classified as BL in instances when there was DLBCL–BL overlap, causing disagreement among pathologists. The outcome with CHOP-like chemotherapy in these instances was associated with poorer survival. Furthermore, classic MYC t(8;14) rearrangements and intermediate molecular phenotypes were also associated with worse overall survival.

The development of a molecular diagnosis for BL aids in distinguishing BL from DLBCL and further illustrates the complexity of *MYC* rearrangements in NHL. Lymphoma entities containing MYC rearrangement in addition to rearrangements in *BCL2* or *BCL6* have been historically termed "double-hit" lymphomas. This subtype frequently has a clinical behavior distant from BL and is often associated with progressive disease, a high International Prognostic Index score, and poor response to intensive chemotherapy regimens. More work regarding this subtype of NHL is needed to understand its pathogenesis.

Aside from gene expression patterns related to GC origin, further genomic alterations may contribute to BL pathogenesis. TP53 is frequently mutated or deleted in a subset of BL tumors. EBV infection is also thought to play a role in the development of BL because virtually 100% of cases of endemic BL and 30% to 50% of all other BLs are associated with EBV positivity. The exact role of EBV in BL is unclear. Endemic BL is frequently associated with endemic malaria, which further suggests a complex interaction of the host immune response with microorganisms and other factors. Other host factors or genomic changes may further contribute to the development of BL.

Further work is needed to define what other genomic changes and host–environmental interactions contribute to the pathogenesis of BL. Ongoing studies seeking to define the entire spectrum of molecular, immunologic, genomic, and epigenetic changes associated with BL pathogenesis may further elucidate this process.

FOLLICULAR LYMPHOMA

Follicular lymphoma is a low-grade B-cell neoplasm that is also characterized by recurrent chromosomal rearrangements involving the IgH locus. It is the most common indolent NHL with more than 16,000 adults diagnosed yearly in the United States. It is characterized by significant heterogeneity with regards to histologic grade and overall survival, with more than 10% of patients surviving at least 15 years after diagnosis. A spectrum of histologic grading based on the density of centroblasts is also characteristic of this disorder, with higher FL grades resembling DLBCL. There is no clear association between grade and clinical outcome in the disease. Some patients with FL experience an aggressive clinical course and transformation to aggressive lymphomas, but others may experience disease progression only after many years with the disease. This review focuses on the classic rearrangements of *BCL2* and the additional molecular changes associated with FL development and with histologic transformation of FL to more aggressive subtypes (Figs. 75-8 and 75-9 for a schematic overview of FL).

BCL2 Rearrangements and Other Genomic Alterations in Follicular Lymphoma

Follicular lymphoma arises from GC B cells that have been immortalized at this stage of B-cell differentiation. Cytogenetic studies performed in the early 1970s defined a recurrent translocation involving the long arms of chromosomes 14 and 18 in more than 90% of FL cases. Further investigation revealed that this places the gene encoding the important antiapoptotic gene *BCL2* downstream of the Ig heavy chain transcriptional regulators. The BCL2 protein inhibits the

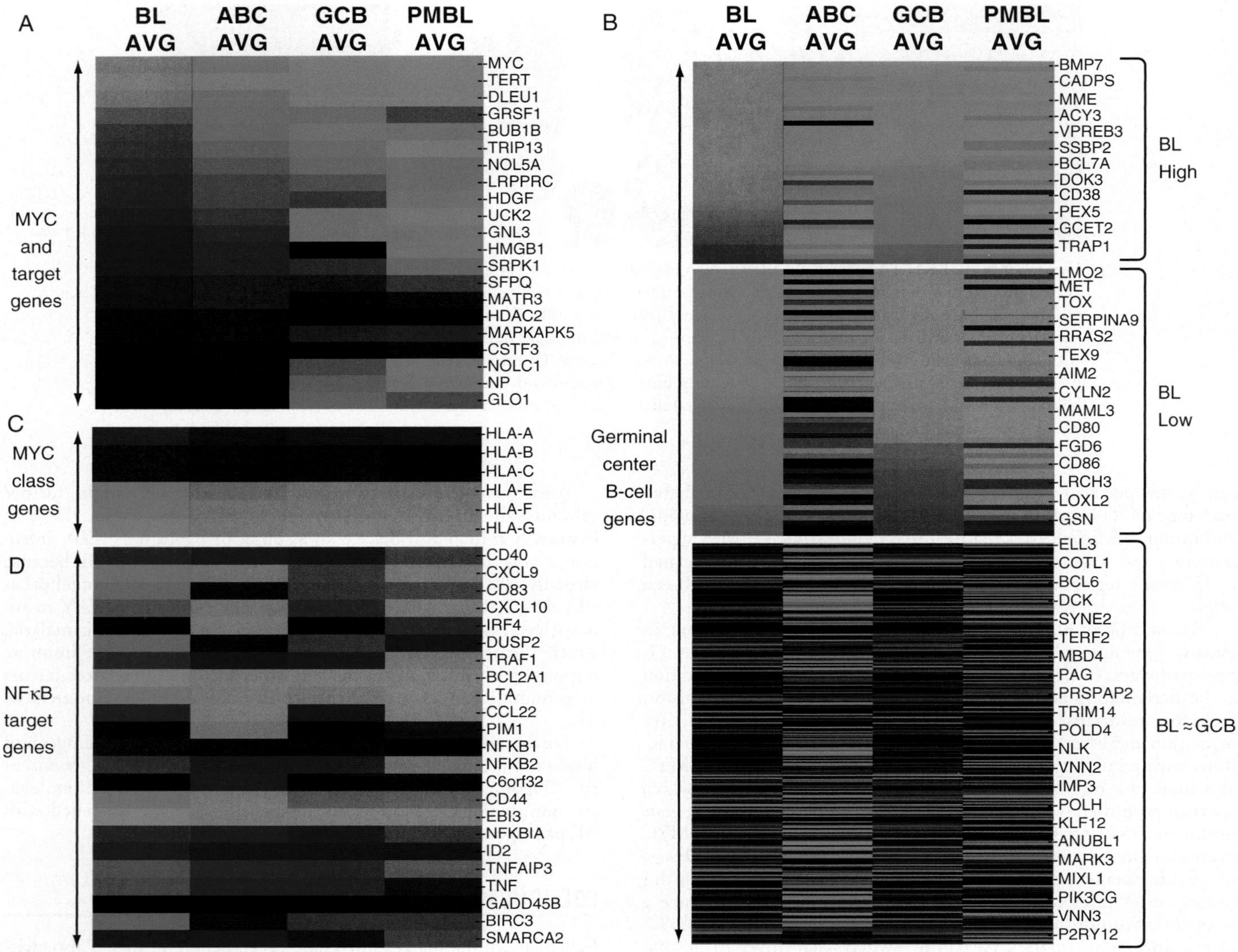

Figure 75-7 Relative expression of genes that distinguish Burkitt lymphoma (BL) from subgroups of diffuse large B-cell lymphoma (DLBCL)—activated B cell–like (ABC) DLBCL, germinal center B (GCB) DLBCL, and primary mediastinal B-cell lymphoma (PMBL)—is categorized into gene expression signatures: c-myc and its target genes **(A)**; genes that are expressed in normal germinal center (GC) B cells **(B)** and are expressed more highly (BL-high), less highly (BL-low), or equivalently (BL~GCB) in BL than in GCB DLBCL; major histocompatibility class I genes **(C)**; and genes targeted by the nuclear factor kappa-B (NFκB) signaling pathway **(D).** GC B-cell signature genes are those that were overexpressed in normal GC B cells, compared with blood B cells. The "BL-high" genes were expressed at levels twice as high in BL as in GCB DLBCL (P <.001). The "BL-low" genes were expressed at levels twice as high in GCB DLBCL as in BL (P <.001). The expression levels of the "BL~GCB" genes did not differ significantly between the two lymphoma subtypes. *(From Dave SS, Fu K, Wright GW, et al: Lymphoma/Leukemia Molecular Profiling Project: Molecular diagnosis of Burkitt's lymphoma.* N Engl J Med *354:2431, 2006.)*

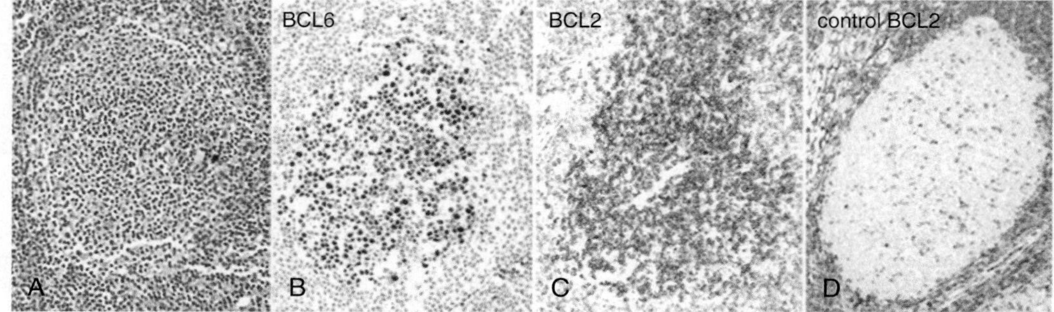

Figure 75-8 FOLLICULAR LYMPHOMA (FL). Details from a case of FL, grade 1 of 3 associated with t(14;18)(q32;q21). Malignant follicle **(A)** with immunohistochemical stains for the germinal center marker, BCL6 **(B),** and BCL2 **(C).** Note the overexpression of BCL2 compared with a reactive follicle **(D).**

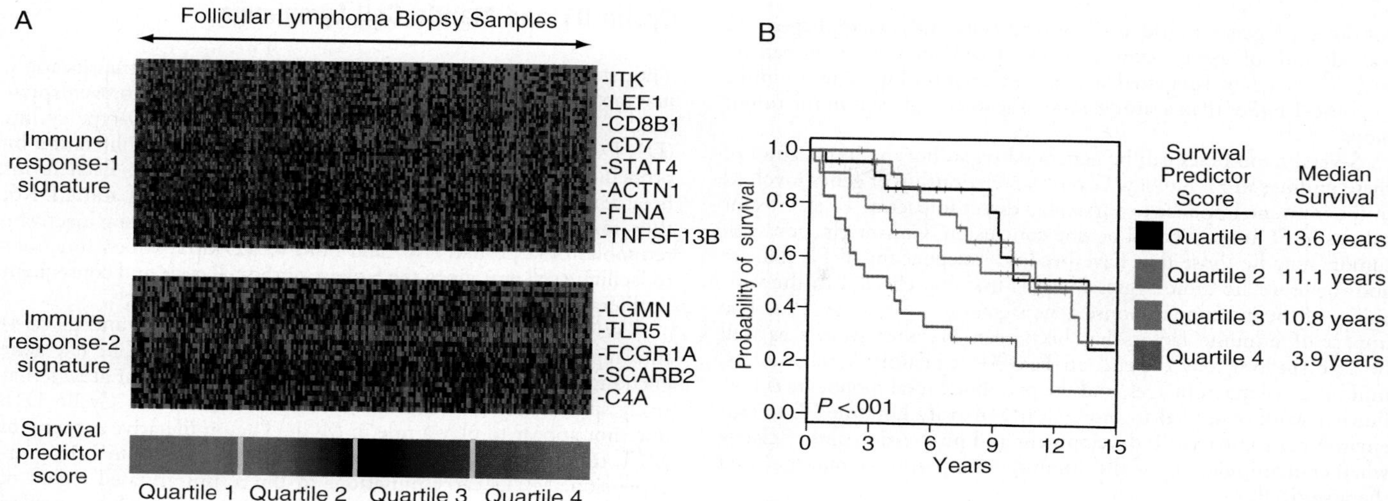

Figure 75-9 SURVIVAL IN FOLLICULAR LYMPHOMA (FL) CAN BE PREDICTED USING FEATURES OF THE TUMOR MICROENVIRONMENT. **A,** Two sets of coordinately expressed genes, termed the *immune response-1* and *immune response-2 signatures,* are associated with survival in FL. The expression pattern of each gene in these two signatures is shown for FL biopsy samples. Expression of the immune response-1 signature is associated with favorable survival after diagnosis, and expression of the immune response-2 signature is associated with adverse survival. These signatures are combined into a multivariate model of survival that generates a survival predictor score for each patient. Patients are ranked according to this survival predictor and divided into four equal quartiles as shown. **B,** Kaplan-Meier plot of overall survival of patients in the four quartiles of the survival predictor. *(**A,** see Dave SS, Wright G, Tan B, et al: Prediction of survival in follicular lymphoma based on molecular features of tumor-infiltrating immune cells. N Engl J Med 351:2159, 2004.)*

release of cytochrome c from mitoch in the process of apoptosis. In normal GCs, *BCL2* is essentially absent because selection of B-cell clones via apoptosis is an important step in the production of high-affinity Ig idiotypes. The t(14;18)(q32.3;q21.3) appears to be mediated by *RAG1/RAG2* in pre-GC B cells because *BCL2* is most often found juxtaposed to J chain exons. Isolated t(14;18) is not sufficient to induce FL because transgenic mice bearing this translocation develop lymphoid hyperplasia but require other genetic lesions to develop FL. Additionally, B cells with t(14;18) can be isolated from apparently normal individuals who never develop lymphoma, and *in situ* follicular hyperplasia with BCL2 overexpression has been noted on examination of otherwise normal lymph nodes. This suggests that other lesions must be acquired for development of FL; a preponderance of evidence suggests this occurs in GCs. Histologically, FL is characterized by an abnormal follicular architecture containing neoplastic cells. The follicles loosely resemble GCs but usually lack an appreciable mantle zone but generally occur in close proximity to follicular T-helper cells expressing CD3, CD4, CD57, PD1, and CXCL13. FL usually exhibits a CD10+BCL6+IRF8+ GC-like phenotype in association with ongoing somatic hypermutation, confirming GC or post-GC origin. One obvious hypothesis is that BCL2 overexpression dysregulates apoptosis such that GC transition and SHM result in further genomic and epigenomic changes that result in FL. This framework might need to be reexamined in the small proportion of FL cases that do not express BCL2.

Although BCL2 is thought to have a critical role in development of FL, nearly 30% of grade 3A and a majority of grade 3B FLs are t(14;18) negative. Alternative rearrangements involving the κ or λ light chains and *BCL2* may occur, but many t(14;18) FLs do not express BCL2. These entities express a post-GC CD10-IRF4-phenotype with 3q27/*BCL6* rearrangements and are associated with lower chemotherapy response rates as well as worse overall survival compared with t(14;18)-positive FLs. It is not clear how this subset of FL evolves from normal B cells, but this immunophenotype suggests a late- or post-GC origin. GEP and analysis of miRNA profiles of FL confirm this association. Leich et al analyzed gene expression profiles of 184 grade I-3A FLs, of which 17 were t(14;18) negative (six of these rearrangement-negative FLs still overexpressed BCL2). Analysis of this data showed enrichment of signatures associated with activated B cells, including NFκB signaling, and those associated with cell cycle, proliferation, and the tumor microenvironment. A study involving a similar cohort showed that a pattern of 17 miRNAs was differentially expressed between translocation positive and negative phenotypes. A group of five miRNAs was found to be downregulated in the t(14;18) group, and this correlated to overexpression of genes related to proliferation, apoptosis, and differentiation. Thus evidence for a post-GCB origin of t(14;18) translocation–negative FLs exists at the gene expression level. Further work is needed to fully understand how BCL2-negative FL develops.

Similar work with BCL2-positive FL has revealed the additional steps required for FL development after t(14;18). Further genomic changes and host factors have also been delineated for DLBCL arising from FL. Conventional cytogenetic studies in FL reveal recurrent duplications of 1p36 and 6q and gains of chromosomes 2, 8, 17, 21, and X. Additionally, SHM appears to affect glycosylation status of surface Ig, implicating BCR signaling in FL pathogenesis. Histologic transformation is associated with further mutations or deletions in *TP53* and *p16* and appears to occur by distinct mechanisms involving either clonal evolution or by transformation of a putative progenitor FL stem cell. Acquired rearrangement of the MYC oncogene can also occur and has been associated with an aggressive plasmablastic phenotype. Stromal factors with FL tumors also likely play a key role in FL propagation and have been studied as having prognostic consequence in FL as well.

Tumor Microenvironment and Survival in Follicular Lymphoma

Just as the lymphoid microenvironment is integral to the formation and function of GCs and immune factors predict survival in DLBCL, FL development appears to depend on stromal factors and the host immune response. In the largest study examining this relationship Dave et al performed gene expression analysis using whole-genome microarrays on 191 FL specimens with the goal of determining genomic predictors of survival. Genes identified were stratified into two groups based on correlation of expression with patient outcome (gene sets associated with good prognosis or poor prognosis). Hierarchical clustering then identified five survival gene sets within each of these groups; analysis revealed that a combination of two gene sets (immune response-1 and immune response-2) formed the best model for prediction of survival. Interestingly, immune response-1 consists of genes *(CD7, CD8B1, ITK, LEF1, STAT4)* associated with specific T-cell populations and macrophages. Conversely, immune response-2 consisted of genes found in dendritic cells and macrophages and was devoid of genes expressed by T-cell subsets. Comparison with T-cell genes suggested a complex relationship with immune response-1 rather than a simple preponderance of T cells in the tumor biopsy.

Several hypotheses can be generated regarding the implication of these findings in FL biology. Given the relationship of genes involved in the immune response to survival, a direct impact of T-cell effector subsets in FL tumors could be one conclusion. Conversely, poor-risk tumors may be those that have become independent of FL follicles and therefore are more aggressive; this may be reflected in the variability of the immune response gene signatures seen across FLs. The impact of immune factors has been seen in other studies as well because survival may depend on FoxP3+ regulatory T-cell subsets, infiltration of macrophages, and the peripheral total monocyte count. Further work is needed to more clearly identify how the FL microenvironment impacts FL development and progression and to clarify whether manipulation of the immune compartment may be used therapeutically.

MANTLE CELL LYMPHOMA

Mantle cell lymphoma (MCL) is characterized by the chromosomal translocation t(11;14)q13;q32, which places cyclin D1 under the transcriptional control of the IgH promoter. MCL is predominantly a disease of elderly men and is characterized by a rather short median survival of 5 to 7 years. Histologic evaluation divides MCL into classic and blastoid variants, with the blastoid subtype having worse survival. Subgroups can also be defined on the basis of somatic mutations in the IgH loci because Ig-mutated tumors tend to have a more indolent disease as is the case with chronic lymphocytic leukemia (CLL), another CD5+ neoplasm. This suggests two disparate origins for MCL with one subtype arising from pre-GC B lymphocytes and another stemming from cells that have encountered antigen and consequently have undergone SHM (see Fig. 75-10). Genomic approaches have also identified molecular profiles delineating MCL from histologically similar neoplasms and identified factors associated with survival. Notably, a minority of patients with MCL are cyclin D1 negative, and GEP has been useful in identifying this entity; further work in this area has identified numerous genomic lesions and molecular pathways involved in MCL. Herein the pathogenesis of MCL is reviewed focusing on the genomic and molecular basis of this disease.

Cyclin D1 and Mantle Cell Lymphoma

The genetic hallmark of MCL, the t(11;14) (q13; q32) translocation, juxtaposes the *CCND1* gene to the IgH locus, leading to overexpression of the cell cycle regulator cyclin D1. The three D-type cyclins (D1, D2, and D3) play an important role in cellular proliferation by propelling cells from G_1 to S phase of the cell cycle. Each forms heterodimers with the cyclin-dependent kinases CDK4 and CDK6, thus forming active kinase complexes. These complexes inactivate retinoblastoma protein (Rb) and bind to p27kip1, which functions to facilitate cell entry into the S phase of the cell cycle and consequent proliferation.

Cyclin D1 is not expressed in normal lymphocytes, and t(11;14) thus represents a pathogenic event in the origin of MCL. The gene encoding cyclin D1 *(CCND1)* consists of five exons that are alternatively spliced into two isoforms, cyclin D1a and D1b. Cyclin D1b does not appear to play a role in MCL. The proliferative capacity of MCL tumors appears closely tied to the degree of cyclin D1a overexpression. MCLs carry mutations in the 3′ untranslated region of *CCND1* that serve to stabilize cyclinD1a transcripts by removing miRNA (miR15/16) binding sites and deleting mRNA destabilizing elements. These sequences usually result in cyclin D1a being an unstable entity, with a half-life of less than 1 hour, but in MCL, these deletions or mutations result in cyclin D1a accumulation and increased cellular proliferation. Additional mutations in the translated regions of cyclinD1 result in protein stabilization through the blockade of GSK3β-mediated nuclear export of cyclin D1.

A minority of patients with MCL are cyclin D1 negative and are alternatively characterized by overexpression of cyclin D2 or D3 and cyclin D2. These derangements serve to deregulate the G_1–S transition in a manner similar to t(11;14) and highlight the theme that MCL is a disease created by cyclin complex–mediated cell cycle progression aided by upregulation of several molecular pathways associated with cellular proliferation and genomic instability.

Secondary Genomic Alterations in Mantle Cell Lymphoma

Beyond t(11;14), MCL is characterized by extensive genomic instability relative to other NHLs, and a variety of genetic lesions appears to drive proliferation of these tumors. Recurrent chromosomal losses, gains, and amplifications are seen in MCL, and many of these affect a large proportion of cases. Secondary genetic instability may occur

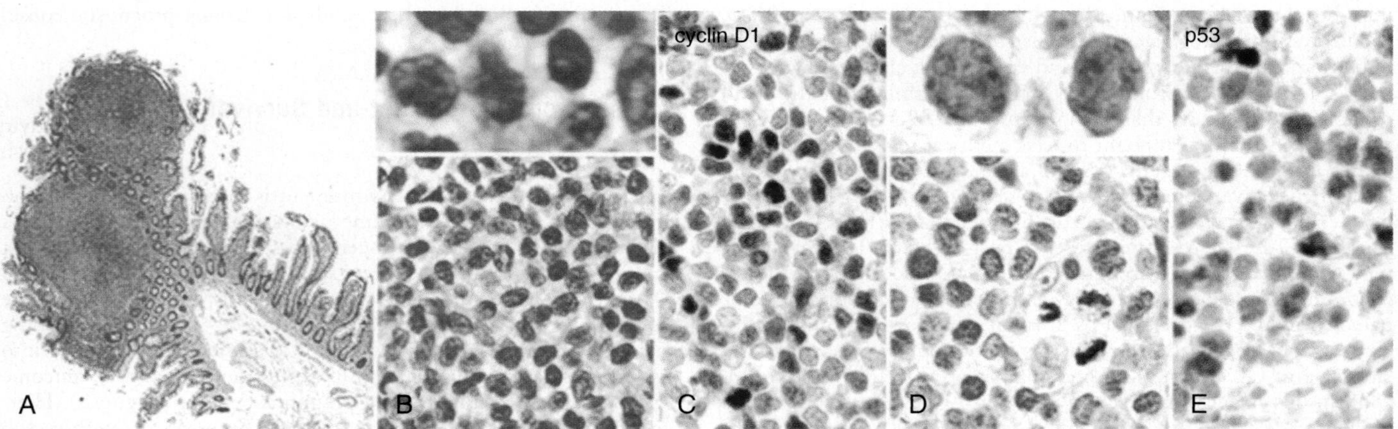

Figure 75-10 MANTLE CELL LYMPHOMA (MCL). **A,** A case of MCL presenting as lymphomatoid polyposis. **B,** The lymphoma cells are small to intermediate in size and have irregular nuclear contours and condensed nuclear chromatin. The cells were $CD19^+$, monoclonal B cells with λ light chain restriction, coexpression of CD5, FMC-7, and lack of CD23. **C,** The cells showed cyclin D1 expression by immunohistochemical staining. The t(11;14)(q13;q32) was detected by conventional cytogenetic analysis. **D,** In comparison, the blastoid variant of MCL has larger cells with a high mitotic rate and fine chromatin. **E,** These cases frequently overexpress p53 and are associated with a complex karyotype, including t(11;14).

as a result of aberrant DNA replication in the setting of deregulated S phase transition mediated by cyclinD1–CD4-complexes. Acquired lesions in genes mediating cellular response to DNA damage and microtubule dynamics may contribute to the accumulation of these alterations as well.

Many (30%–50%) of MCL cases are characterized by mutations or deletions in the DNA damage response pathway mediated by ATM and TP53 or modifiers of this pathway such as MDM2 and p14/ARF. *ATM* is often mutated with loss of the other chromosomal allele. TP53 may also be downregulated in these tumors via similar mechanisms, and overexpression of TP53-negative regulators MDM2 and MDM4 also occurs via copy number amplification. These overall serve to deregulate important cellular machinery involved in DNA damage repair, apoptosis, and cell cycle arrest, leading to increased cell cycle progression and proliferation in MCL. Further deletions at 9p21 occur frequently in MCL and serve to enhance cell cycle progression and block apoptosis. The 9p21 locus encodes p16(INK4a) and p14(ARF), which function as tumor suppressors. p16(INK4a) inhibits CDK 4/6 complex binding to cyclin D1, which results in decreased cell cycle progression. Deletion of p16(INK4a) in the setting of t(11;14) enhances proliferation in MCL and has been associated with worse overall survival. The function of p14(ARF) in MCL pathogenesis is less clear, but p14(ARF) blocks MDM2-mediated TP53 ubiquitination; p14(ARF) has other effects on cellular proliferation that usually work in a homeostatic pattern. Interestingly, cyclin D1 levels and INK4a/ARF deletions both correlate to a MCL proliferation signature created using GEP. Using a similar strategy, cyclin D1 expression levels and the presence of INK4a/ARF deletion have been used to create a predictor of overall survival using a cohort of MCL patients. Survival among groups stratified by this approach varies widely (from 6-7 years to <10 months), which confirms the importance of involvement of genes involved with the cell cycle and proliferation in MCL. This parallels the experience noted with histologic markers of tumor proliferation because Ki-67 (a marker of actively dividing cells) and the presence of blastoid features have previously been shown to correlate with worse outcomes.

When considered together, the recurrent deletions and mutations noted in MCL illustrate the importance of unchecked cell cycle progression in this disorder. DNA instability is another hallmark of MCL that appears to result from the blockade of cell cycle checkpoints in the setting of ongoing DNA damage. These factors are intertwined in a complicated fashion in MCL and further work to upregulate several diverse molecular pathways involved in cellular proliferation and survival.

Molecular Pathways and Profiles in Mantle Cell Lymphoma

A variety of molecular pathways have recently been described as being active in MCL. These include signaling pathways facilitating cellular proliferation, avoidance of apoptosis, evasion of immune editing, and cellular microenvironment interactions. As in other NHLs, GEP has been used to define a molecular diagnosis of MCL and identify genes and molecular pathways involved in its pathogenesis (Fig. 75-11).

Genomic approaches identify a subset of MCL that is cyclin D1 negative and has features similar to other CD5+ B-cell neoplasms such as CLL. Although such cases are indistinguishable by histologic analysis, GEP demonstrates that these tumors express gene signatures that are otherwise nearly identical to cyclin D1+ MCL but lack the classic t(11;14) rearrangement. Overexpression of other D cyclins (cyclin D2 or D3) via rearrangement, amplification, or other mechanisms is found in many of these cases; this is consistent with the underlying theme that MCL is a disease of disordered cell cycle progression. Using a similar approach, *SOX11* has been identified as a sensitive and specific marker of MCL regardless of cyclinD1 expression status. *SOX11* encodes an HMG-box transcription factor that regulates embryogenesis and is important in neural development. Because greater than 90% of MCL specimens overexpress *SOX11* and this finding is rare in histologically similar NHLs, *SOX11* is a potentially useful marker for improving the diagnosis of MCL. *SOX11* has also been incorporated into prognostic models of MCL using histologic, clinical, and GEP data. Reports regarding the clinical significance of *SOX11* have been conflicting. Thus further work is needed to understand the molecular mechanisms underlying *SOX11* expression in MCL and the implications in this disease.

Mantle cell lymphoma has also been characterized by expression of several molecular pathways that enhance cellular proliferation and metabolism and are tightly intertwined with abnormalities in cell cycle regulation. *Wnt 3* is a consistently overexpressed gene in MCL, and abnormal Wnt signaling may be one way in which MCLs bypass negative feedback loops controlling differentiation. Proliferation in MCLs may also depend on Wnt–Β-catenin signaling, but the impact of this pathway on patient survival or as a therapeutic target in MCL is unknown. Similar to ABC DLBCLs, the NFκB pathway is also active in MCL, and crosstalk between proliferation signaling between this pathway PI3K/AKT/mTOR and cell cycle signaling also appears to be important. Importantly, phosphatase and tensin homologue (PTEN), a molecule that has important roles in providing negative feedback to the mTOR pathway is also commonly deleted or acquires loss of function mutations in MCL. Taken together, these facts reinforce the fact that abnormalities in several diverse signaling pathways are required beyond t(11;14) for MCL to form. Further work is needed to define how to use these findings to build better prognostic models in this disease, and studies investigating the therapeutic utility of targeting these pathways are beginning.

OTHER NON-HODGKIN LYMPHOMAS

Gene expression profiling and high-throughput sequencing have been applied to other lymphomas in manners similar to the subtypes already described. Important discoveries regarding other NHLs such as marginal zone lymphomas, lymphoplasmacytic lymphoma, and peripheral T-cell lymphomas (PTCLs) have refined our understanding of how these diseases develop. Recurrent mutations in genes and involvement of molecular pathways governing control of apoptosis, cellular proliferation, and metabolism are recurrent themes in these NHL subtypes as well as those described earlier. In addition to being found in DLBCLs, *MYD88* L265P mutations have been reported in virtually all cases of lymphoplasmacytic lymphoma (Waldenstrom macroglobulinemia) and may serve as a marker to differentiate this disease from other indolent lymphomas. *NOTCH2* mutations have been noted in a subset of marginal zone lymphomas and have been found in DLBCLs and other NHLs. Gene clusters have also been developed for T-cell lymphomas and identify angioimmunoblastic T-cell lymphoma (AITL) as an entity distinct from other PTCLs; this work also has shown upregulation of genes involved in NFκB signaling in AITL. A subset of PTCL is characterized by t(2;5) (p23;q35), which joins the anaplastic lymphoma kinase-1 gene *(ALK)* next to *NPM-1* at 5q35. This creates an aberrant tyrosine kinase that appears to have a number of downstream transforming effects. ALK positivity is generally associated with response to cytotoxic chemotherapy in PTCL; however, better molecular predictors of response are needed. Whereas NFκB gene signature expression also correlates to improved survival in PTCL, tumors that exhibit increased markers of proliferation are associated with poor outcomes, as in other NHLs. Given that rarity of these tumors, it is difficult to make further associations between molecular markers and outcomes.

FUTURE DIRECTIONS

Non-Hodgkin lymphoma represents a complex group of related neoplasms that have quite disparate molecular characteristics. Given the lack of modifiable risk factors and varied prognosis with standard treatment (chemoimmunotherapy), a better understanding of the processes driving NHL is needed. Advances in technology have recently allowed whole-genomic surveys to identify the role of altered

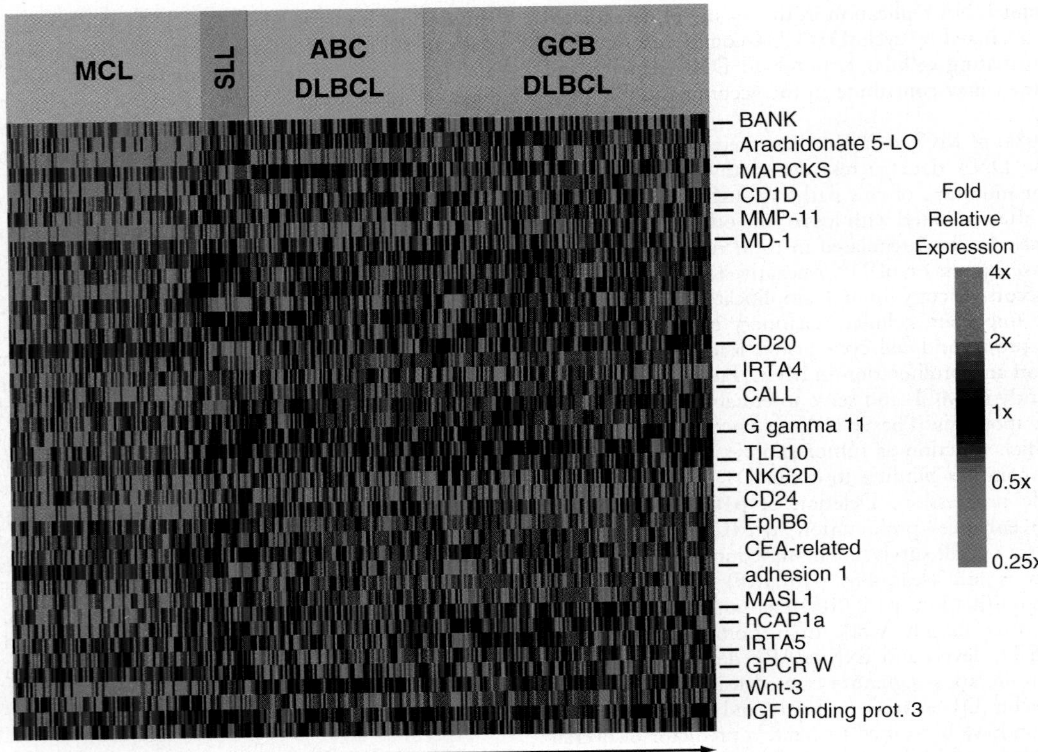

Figure 75-11 HIERARCHICAL CLUSTERING OF EXPRESSION MEASUREMENTS FROM 42 MANTLE CELL LYMPHOMA (MCL) SIGNATURE GENES THAT ARE MORE HIGHLY EXPRESSED IN MCL SAMPLES COMPARED WITH SMALL LYMPHOCYTIC LYMPHOMA (SLL), ACTIVATED B CELL–LIKE (ABC) DIFFUSE LARGE B-CELL LYMPHOMA (DLBCL), AND GERMINAL CENTER B (GCB) DLBCL SAMPLES. Each column represents a single lymphoma specimen, and each row represents expression of a single gene. *Red squares* indicate increased expression, and *green squares* indicate decreased expression relative to the median expression level according to the color scale shown. *(From Fu K, Weisenburger DD, Greiner TC, et al: Lymphoma/Leukemia Molecular Profiling Project: Cyclin D1-negative mantle cell lymphoma: A clinicopathologic study based on gene expression profiling.* Blood *106:4315, 2005 and Rosenwald A, Wright G, Wiestner A, et al: The proliferation gene expression signature is a quantitative integrator of oncogenic events that predicts survival in mantle cell lymphoma.* Cancer Cell *3:185, 2003.)*

genetics, transcription, and epigenetic regulation as contributors to the observed lymphoma phenotypes. This work will serve as the starting point for the unraveling of new diagnostic and prognostic markers, as well as therapeutic targets in a group of diseases in which such options are urgently needed.

SUGGESTED READINGS

Alizadeh AA: Distinct types of diffuse large B-cell lymphoma identified by gene expression profiling. *Nature* 403:503, 2000.

Bakhshi A, Jensen JP, Goldman P, et al: Cloning the chromosomal breakpoint of t(14;18) human lymphomas: Clustering around JH on chromosome 14 and near a transcriptional unit on 18. *Cell* 41:899, 1985.

Bea S, Zettl A, Wright G, et al: Lymphoma/Leukemia Molecular Profiling Project: Diffuse large B-cell lymphoma subgroups have distinct genetic profiles that influence tumor biology and improve gene-expression-based survival prediction. *Blood* 106:3183, 2005.

Dave SS, Fu K, Wright GW, et al: Lymphoma/Leukemia Molecular Profiling Project: Molecular diagnosis of Burkitt's lymphoma. *N Engl J Med* 354:2431, 2006.

Dave SS, Wright G, Tan B, et al: Prediction of survival in follicular lymphoma based on molecular features of tumor-infiltrating immune cells. *N Engl J Med* 351:2159, 2004.

de Boer CJ, van Krieken JH, Kluin-Nelemans HC, et al: Cyclin D1 messenger RNA overexpression as a marker for mantle cell lymphoma. *Oncogene* 10:1833, 1995.

Dolken G, Illerhaus G, Hirt C, et al: BCL2/JH rearrangements in circulating B cells of healthy blood donors and patients with nonmalignant diseases. *J Clin Oncol* 14:1333, 1996.

Fisher SG, Fisher RI: The epidemiology of non-Hodgkin's lymphoma. *Oncogene* 23:6524, 2004.

Fu K, Weisenburger DD, Greiner TC, et al: Lymphoma/Leukemia Molecular Profiling Project: Cyclin D1-negative mantle cell lymphoma: A clinicopathologic study based on gene expression profiling. *Blood* 106:4315, 2005.

Gracias DT, Katsikis PD: MicroRNAs: Key components of immune regulation. *Adv Exp Med Biol* 780:15, 2011.

Iqbal J: Distinctive patterns of BCL6 molecular alterations and their functional consequences in different subgroups of diffuse large B-cell lymphoma. *Leukemia* 21:2332, 2007.

Iqbal J, Neppalli VT, Wright G, et al: BCL2 expression is a prognostic marker for the activated B-cell-like type of diffuse large B-cell lymphoma. *J Clin Oncol* 24:961, 2006.

Iqbal J, Weisenburger DD, Greiner TC, et al: International Peripheral T-Cell Lymphoma Project: Molecular signatures to improve diagnosis in peripheral T-cell lymphoma and prognostication in angioimmunoblastic T-cell lymphoma. *Blood* 115:1026, 2010.

Jardin F, Gaulard P, Buchonnet G, et al: Follicular lymphoma without t(14;18) and with BCL6 rearrangement: A lymphoma subtype with distinct pathological, molecular and clinical characteristics. *Leukemia* 16:2309, 2002.

Jost PJ, Ruland J: Aberrant NF-kappaB signaling in lymphoma: Mechanisms, consequences, and therapeutic implications. *Blood* 109:2700, 2007.

Leich E, Zamo A, Horn H et al: MicroRNA profiles of t(14;18)-negative follicular lymphoma support a late germinal center B-cell phenotype. *Blood* 118:5550, 2011.

Lenz G, Nagel I, Siebert R, et al: Aberrant immunoglobulin class switch recombination and switch translocations in activated B cell-like diffuse large B cell lymphoma. *J Exp Med* 204:633, 2007.

Lenz G, Wright G, Dave SS, et al: Lymphoma/Leukemia Molecular Profiling Project: Stromal gene signatures in large-B-cell lymphomas. *N Engl J Med* 359:2313, 2008.

Magrath I: Epidemiology: Clues to the pathogenesis of Burkitt lymphoma. *Br J Haematol* 156:744, 2012.

McHeyzer-Williams M, Okitsu S, Wang N, et al: Molecular programming of B cell memory. *Nat Rev Immunol* 12:24, 2011.

Morin RD, Mendez-Lago M, Mungall AJ, et al: Frequent mutation of histone-modifying genes in non-Hodgkin lymphoma. *Nature* 476:298, 2011.

Pasqualucci L: Inactivation of the PRDM1/BLIMP1 gene in diffuse large B cell lymphoma. *J Exp Med* 203:311, 2006.

Rosebeck S, Rehman AO, Lucas PC, et al: From MALT lymphoma to the CBM signalosome: Three decades of discovery. *Cell Cycle* 10:2485, 2011.

Rosenwald A: The use of molecular profiling to predict survival after chemotherapy for diffuse large-B-cell lymphoma. *N Engl J Med* 346:1937, 2002.

Rosenwald A, Wright G, Leroy K, et al: Molecular diagnosis of primary mediastinal B cell lymphoma identifies a clinically favorable subgroup of diffuse large B cell lymphoma related to Hodgkin lymphoma. *J Exp Med* 198:851, 2003.

Rosenwald A, Wright G, Wiestner A, et al: The proliferation gene expression signature is a quantitative integrator of oncogenic events that predicts survival in mantle cell lymphoma. *Cancer Cell* 3:185, 2003.

Schaffner C, Idler I, Stilgenbauer S, et al: Mantle cell lymphoma is characterized by inactivation of the ATM gene. *Proc Natl Acad Sci U S A* 97:2773, 2000.

Tam W: Mutational analysis of PRDM1 indicates a tumor-suppressor role in diffuse large B-cell lymphomas. *Blood* 107:4090, 2006.

Volpe G, Vitolo U, Carbone A, et al: Molecular heterogeneity of B-lineage diffuse large cell lymphoma. *Genes Chromosomes Cancer* 16:21, 1996.

Wang LD, Clark MR: B-cell antigen-receptor signalling in lymphocyte development. *Immunology* 110:411, 2003.

CHAPTER 76

CHRONIC LYMPHOCYTIC LEUKEMIA

Thomas S. Lin, Farrukh T. Awan, and John C. Byrd

Over the past several decades, major advances have come in understanding both the biology that ultimately has translated to both helpful diagnostic tests and improved therapy for chronic lymphocytic leukemia (CLL). The plethora of information about CLL has increased dramatically and made management of what was a relatively straightforward disease quite complex. The authors herein provide a reference source focused on critical issues in clinical management of CLL that will hopefully help.

EPIDEMIOLOGY

Chronic lymphocytic leukemia is one of the most common types of leukemia in the Western Hemisphere. SEER estimates for 2010 indicated that approximately 14,570 patients (8520 men and 6050 women) would be diagnosed in the United States and that 4380 patients would die from CLL in 2010. The median age at diagnosis for CLL was 72 years from 2000 to 2005, according to the SEER database. The incidence of CLL increases proportionately by decade, as shown in Fig. 76-1. This figure illustrates that CLL is a very uncommon diagnosis before 45 years of age and infrequent (30% of total patients diagnosed) in patients before 65 years of age. The age-adjusted incidence rate was 4.2 per 100,000 men and women per year; 0.46% of men and women born in 2008 are expected to be diagnosed with CLL during their lifetime. The extended time of survival after diagnosis at 5 years is 80.8%, which explains the estimated prevalence of 105,643 patients living with CLL in the United States currently. Similar to other types of leukemia, the risk of dying from disease-specific causes increases proportionately with increasing age. Another analysis of the SEER database comparing outcome of elderly patients with CLL with age- and sex-matched healthy control participants demonstrated that CLL has the greatest impact on survival in the most elderly group of patients. However, even for patients diagnosed with CLL before the age of 50 years, Montserrat and colleagues demonstrated that the median expected life span is only 12.3 years compared with 31.2 years in age-matched control participants. Thus CLL is a significant health problem affecting all ages of patients with this disease.

Chronic lymphocytic leukemia is more common in men than women. Women diagnosed with CLL have 5- and 10-year overall survival (OS) rates that exceed those of men. CLL is most common in whites and decreases in frequency in a descending order among blacks, Hispanics, American Indians and Native Alaskans, and Asians and Pacific Islanders. The rarity of CLL among Asians and Pacific Islanders persists even in immigrants from these areas who have migrated to the Western Hemisphere. This implicates a possible genetic predisposition to the development of CLL. The relationship of environmental factors such as exposure to benzene and other chemicals to the development of CLL is not clearly defined. However, CLL is recognized as a service-connected illness among Vietnam War veterans who were exposed to Agent Orange. For patients in the theatre of the Vietnam conflict, it is important to identify this because additional compensation from the U.S. Veterans Administration is possible. Occupational or environmental exposure to radiation does not appear to predispose patients to a higher risk of developing CLL. For example, although the frequency of acute myeloid leukemia (AML), chronic myeloid leukemia (CML), and acute lymphoblastic leukemia (ALL) were increased among survivors of the atomic bomb at Hiroshima, no increase in CLL was appreciated. Recent studies of leukemia rates in inhabitants around the Chernobyl nuclear reactor accident site have supported this notion, where essentially all other types of leukemia were increased with the exception of CLL.

FAMILIAL CHRONIC LYMPHOCYTIC LEUKEMIA

Up to 10% of CLL patients have a first- or second-degree relative with CLL, making CLL one of the most common types of malignancy with familial predisposition. Newer studies identifying an even higher frequency of monoclonal B-cell lymphocytosis (MBL) in these families provides further evidence of inheritance in a subset of patients. Unlike other types of familial cancer, it is very uncommon for CLL patients to have large pedigrees with many affected distant relatives throughout an extensive family tree. Rather, the more common finding is for most patients to have one or two first- or second-degree relatives with this diagnosis. Large case-control studies concluded that the risk ratio (RR) for first-degree relatives of CLL probands to also have CLL was higher than that for most other cancers. Although the average RR for all cancers in a U.S. study was approximately 2.1, CLL showed an RR of 5.0, the fourth highest of all cancers. Relatives of patients with CLL also appear to have a higher frequency of other lymphoproliferative disorders and autoimmune diseases. Unlike a variety of other cancers that have known predisposing genes, identification of divergent genes in CLL has been generally elusive. To date, only a single germline mutation of death-associated protein kinase (DAPK) and LEU7 has been convincingly linked to familial predisposition in a single CLL family but not identified by others in additional families. Most other studies have been limited by weak evidence for linkage, and the occurrence at many loci was different between the studies. Two loci at chromosome bands 11p11 and 13q21 were backed by statistically significant evidence, but no genes at these sites have been implicated in familial CLL. This brings forth a common theme of divergent pathogenesis in familial predisposition of CLL. In a very small number of isolated families, there are likely driver mutations with a dominant pattern of inheritance such as the DAPK1 and LEU7 family. In conjunction with this, there are many collaborating, low phenotype associated genes in the majority of families in which familial disease is present, thereby explaining the failure of linkage studies to identify specific abnormalities. It is likely that significant advances will come over the next decade in identifying these collaborating genes with the ability to do whole-genome sequencing in large cohorts of patients. The role of anticipation in identifying other family members has been reported by several groups; patients with such a family history are generally diagnosed a median of 10 years earlier than other patients. However, other clinical features of CLL at diagnosis do not appear to be different. Thus patients with familial CLL do not appear to be genetically or clinically different from individuals with sporadic CLL.

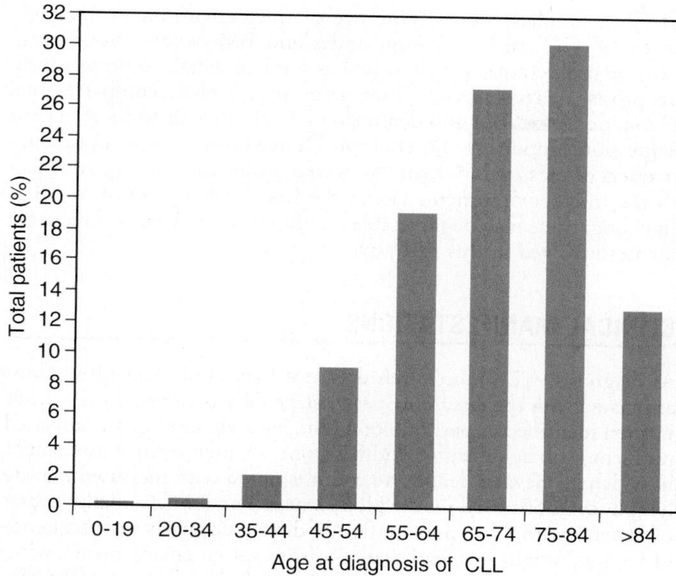

Figure 76-1 GRAPH SHOWING THAT CHRONIC LYMPHOCYTIC LEUKEMIA (CLL) IS A VERY UNCOMMON DIAGNOSIS BEFORE AGE 45 YEARS AND INFREQUENT (30% OF TOTAL PATIENTS DIAGNOSED) BEFORE AGE 65 YEARS.

PATHOBIOLOGY

The complexity of the biology of CLL has become increasingly apparent as the knowledge of the basic science of this disease has expanded. Despite these advances, many questions remain unsolved, including (1) the cell of origin from which CLL is derived, (2) the existence of a CLL stem cell as occurs in other leukemias, (3) the biological etiology of the divergent natural histories of IgV_H-mutated versus unmutated CLL, and (4) the existence and identification of infectious or other naturally occurring antigens that may drive the B-cell clone in this disease. Nonetheless, significant advances in our understanding of the roles of cytogenetics, immunology, and other relevant biological markers in predicting the natural history of disease progression and response to therapy in CLL make an understanding of the basic biology of CLL increasingly relevant and important to clinicians caring for CLL patients.

For many years, CLL was believed to represent a single disease that had a varied natural history. Basic research focused on understanding (1) the normal cell of origin from which CLL is derived, (2) the function of the B-cell receptor (BCR) in CLL, (3) the maturational point in B-cell development at which CLL occurs, and (4) the relevance and contribution of a self- or acquired antigen to driving the disease. The normal counterpart to the cell of origin of transformed CLL remains unknown. For many years, it was believed that CLL was not derived from a clonal stem cell, based on the inability of the leukemia cells to engraft and recapitulate the disease when tumor cells are inoculated or transplanted into immunocompromised mice. However, a recent seminal paper demonstrated that CD34-positive hematopoietic stem cells from CLL patients have a higher number of cells with B-lymphoid progenitor phenotype and develop clonal B cells characteristic of CLL when engrafted into immunocompromised mice. Notably, the CLL cells developing in these mice did not have the genetic features of the patient's CLL, suggesting that additional transforming event(s) in the clonal CLL cells occur(s). In addition, several whole exon and genome sequencing projects in CLL have identified genes, such as *NOTCH1* and *SF3B1*, that clearly have clinical relevance in CLL and point to new biologic areas that will be pursued moving forward. All of these observations are important scientific areas of active, ongoing study, and readers are referred to several recent definitive reviews for further information on the basic biology of CLL. The biology and genetics covered within this chapter focus predominately on areas relevant to clinicians who care for patients with CLL.

IgV_H Mutational Status

Two seminal manuscripts in 1999 demonstrated that the IgV_H gene had undergone somatic mutation, indicating that the patient's CLL arose after this point in B-cell maturation, in 60% of CLL patients at diagnosis. In an attempt to identify surrogate genes associated with IgV_H-unmutated disease, ZAP-70 overexpression was identified. The majority of IgV_H-unmutated CLL cells have ZAP-70 expression and demonstrate evidence of syk activation and other essential BCR downstream activation signals after ligation of surface IgM (sIgM) that is related to overexpression of this protein. In contrast, virtually all IgV_H-mutated patients lack significant ZAP-70 expression and do not signal after ligation by sIgM, but can often weakly signal through other alternative BCRs. Thus, although gene expression profiling demonstrates all CLL cells to be most closely related to memory B cells, IgV_H-unmutated and -mutated CLL cells differ significantly with respect to their ability to transduce intracellular signals after sIgM ligation. A common repertoire of mutational changes among CLL patients has also been documented that differs significantly from that found in the normal adult B-cell repertoire. These studies have prompted the hypothesis that CLL may represent an antigen-driven disease. Targeting BBCR signaling based on this represents an attractive pharmacologic option that is being actively pursued in preclinical and clinical studies of several therapeutic agents directed against signaling pathways downstream of the BCR.

Defective Apoptosis

Since its initial description and early characterization, CLL has been considered a disease of slow accumulation of tumor cells caused by disrupted or defective apoptosis. Multiple studies have demonstrated that CLL cells overexpress several antiapoptotic proteins, including bcl-2, mcl-1, bak, and X-linked inactivator of apoptosis protein (XIAP), and have diminished expression of compensatory proapoptotic proteins such as bax. Overexpression of bcl-2 and mcl-1 and an increase of the ratio of these proteins to bax have correlated not only with disrupted apoptosis but also shortened OS and poor response to therapy. Why are these antiapoptotic genes overexpressed in vivo? Studies have demonstrated that CLL cells have constitutive activation of several anti-apoptotic transcription factors, including nuclear factor kappa-B (NFκB), nuclear factor of activated T cells (NFAT), and signal transducer and activator of transcription 3 (STAT3). Each of these transcription factors can influence one or more of the antiapoptotic proteins that promote survival in vivo. The source of activation of these different transcription factors is not completely defined but may be partly attributable to autocrine and paracrine networks involving B-cell activation factor (BAFF), a proliferation inducing ligand (APRIL) vascular endothelial growth factor (VEGF), interleukin-4 (IL-4), and CD40. CLL cells are also maintained through contact with stromal cells (bone marrow [BM] and dendritic) and nurse similar cells through a complex interface of adhesion molecules and stromal survival factors such as stromal cell–derived factor (SDF). The importance of the in vivo environment to CLL survival is supported by the increase in apoptosis when CLL cells are cultured in vitro.

Genetic Abnormalities

Much of the advances in understanding the biology of acute leukemia have come from studying repetitively occurring cytogenetic abnormalities. Such detailed study of the genetics of CLL has been hindered by the inability to effectively induce proliferation of tumor cells for standard metaphase cytogenetic analysis and the poor response of CLL cells to B-cell mitogens. Nonetheless, several cytogenetic studies identified a variety of deletions, including del(11q22.3), del(17p13.1), del(13q14), and del(6q21-q23), as well as trisomy 12, as common abnormalities in CLL. The frequency of these abnormalities has been further refined through the use of interphase cells using fluorescence in situ hybridization (FISH), which does not require isolation of dividing cells. These studies have demonstrated that del(13q14) is by far the most common cytogenetic abnormality in CLL followed by trisomy 12, del(11q22.3), del(17p13.1), and del(6q22.3). Stimulation studies with CpG oligonucleotides plus IL-4 or CD40 confirmed the prevalence of these abnormalities and identified unbalanced translocations not generally observed with traditional metaphase cytogenetics. The prognostic implications of these unbalanced translocations appear to be significant. Similarly, complexity of karyotype, as already appreciated in acute leukemia, appears to be a driving poor prognostic factor in CLL. Interestingly, balanced translocations, which are more frequently observed in ALL and AML, are generally not observed in CLL.

The presence of recurrent deletions in CLL suggests the possibility of unique tumor suppressor genes in these different regions. Extensive pursuit of such genes within the 13q14 region failed to identify a viable tumor suppressor gene candidate for many years. However, in 2002, Croce and colleagues identified miR15 and miR16, two noncoding microRNAs, in the deleted region of 13q14. Noncoding RNAs range in size from 21 to 25 nucleotides and represent a newly recognized class of gene products whose function is to silence genes through binding to the 3′-untranslated region of specific genes to inhibit translation. This same group later showed that mir16 regulates expression of bcl-2, which is overexpressed in CLL and other B-cell lymphoproliferative disorders. Multiple different studies have associated specific miR expression with rapid disease progression, fludarabine resistance, and poor prognosis. In addition, miR34a has been directly related to the adverse outcome associated with p53 dysfunction. Further study of miRs in CLL is under way to elucidate their full role in the pathogenesis and progression of CLL.

Recurring Mutations in Chronic Lymphocytic Leukemia

Until the advent of whole-exon and whole-genomic sequencing, CLL was not typically associated with recurring mutations early in the pathogenesis of the disease. Probably best characterized are p53 mutations, which occur in only 3% to 5% of patients at diagnosis, often in conjunction with deletion of the alternative allele (at 17p13.1 loci) that is associated with rapid disease progression and poor survival. With treatment and subsequent relapse, the frequency of p53 mutations continues to increase proportionately and is most common in patients with Richter transformation. Thus p53 mutations are considered by most to be a secondary abnormality in CLL associated with progression. Nonetheless, p53 mutations or deletions have significant impact on consideration of treatment of CLL, and the 2008 International Workshop on CLL (IWCLL) criteria recommended that patients with p53 mutations with deletions be treated in a different manner than other CLL patients. Although detailed studies of ATM mutations have followed by several groups, the impact of this abnormality is less well defined, in particular as it relates to treatment response. Other recurring mutations in CLL, including SF3B1, NOTCH1, MYD88, XPO1, and ERK1, have been described with recent whole-exon and -genome sequencing efforts. The impact of these new different mutations in the pathogenesis of CLL is under active investigation.

Immune and Microenvironmental Features

The importance of progressive immune suppression with progression of CLL has become appreciated in both human CLL and murine models of this disease. The absolute number of T cells and natural killer (NK) cells in CLL patients at diagnosis has been shown to predict OS. In particular, expansion of suppressive T-regulatory cells has been documented as patients come closer to the time of requiring therapy. The immunosuppressive effects observed in CLL lie predominately with the CLL clone, as recently demonstrated in very elegant work by the Gribben laboratory in human and mouse models of CLL. Similarly, the importance of microenvironment compartments of CLL such as lymph nodes and BM, where stromal cells provide proliferative signals as well as survival signals to protect from apoptosis, are recognized. Wiestner's group examined compartmental blood, node, and BM and demonstrated definitive differences in gene expression supporting this concept. Derived from this work are biomarkers of measurable chemokines responsible for T-cell recruitment to the microenvironment. Given the link of these stimuli to BCR signaling, these may be targetable by inhibitory molecules directed at kinases involved in this pathway.

CLINICAL MANIFESTATIONS

At diagnosis, CLL most often does not have clinical manifestations associated with the disease. For early stage CLL patients, the diagnosis is often identified as part of blood tests for evaluation of an unrelated problem such as infection, kidney stone, or preoperative assessment in which an elevated leukocyte count is noted with increased mature lymphocytes observed on the blood smear. For a much smaller subset of patients with CLL, presentation of disease occurs as a consequence of fatigue, weight loss, early satiety (from spleen enlargement), petechiae (from low platelets), or new palpable lymph nodes. Patients with symptomatic CLL at diagnosis represent only 15% of those seen, corresponding to the more indolent nature of this disease at diagnosis. With additional follow-up, the majority of CLL patients will eventually manifest symptoms of the disease that ultimately lead to the need for treatment. The most common symptoms with progression include increasing fatigue (as a consequence of anemia and cytokines from disease), lymph node and spleen size, worsening hematologic parameters (anemia and thrombocytopenia), and rarely infiltration of other organs (kidney, lung, pleural space, skin) that necessitates initiation of treatment to palliate symptoms. Unusual symptoms generally not associated with CLL progression are night sweats, fevers, and weight loss. These are generally suggestive of Richter transformation.

Separate from direct CLL progression, the disease is also immunosuppressive, and with more advanced disease, an increase in infections is generally observed. This represents a major morbidity of CLL and is a leading contribution to mortality associated with this disease. Other manifestations of immune suppression, including higher rate of secondary malignancies and autoimmune complications, are also increased in CLL (see box on Initial Evaluation of Young Patients With Chronic Lymphocytic Leukemia).

DIAGNOSIS AND LABORATORY MANIFESTATIONS

The diagnosis of CLL, as defined by the IWCLL 2008 criteria, requires an absolute malignant B-cell lymphocyte count of greater than 5000/μL. This differs from the previous NCI criteria that required a total lymphocyte count of 5000/μL and emphasizes the need to quantify the malignant B-cell clone in the new diagnostic criteria. Morphologically, the lymphocytes must appear mature with fewer than 55% prolymphocytes (Fig. 76-2, *A–E*). The BM aspirate smear must show greater than 30% of all nucleated cells to be lymphoid, or the BM core biopsy must show lymphoid infiltrates consistent with CLL (Fig. 76-2, *F* and *G*). The overall cellularity must be normocellular or hypercellular. Immunophenotyping must reveal a predominant B-cell monoclonal population coexpressing the B-cell markers CD19, CD20, and CD23 and the T-cell antigen CD5 in the absence of other pan-T cell markers (see later section).

Patients may present with tumor cells immunophenotypically consistent with CLL but have predominately lymph node disease without a peripheral B-cell lymphocyte count of 5000/μL despite BM involvement. Although these patients are considered to have small lymphocytic lymphoma (SLL) and not true CLL by the NCI criteria, the most recent World Health Organization (WHO) classification considers such SLL patients to have CLL, given the similar immunophenotypic features, genetic findings, natural history, and complications of these two diseases. The clinical management of SLL

Initial Evaluation of Young Patients With Chronic Lymphocytic Leukemia

Only 10% of patients diagnosed with CLL are younger than 50 years of age, and these patients often present a diagnostic and therapeutic dilemma to hematologists initially evaluating them. The great majority of patients diagnosed before the age of 50 years will have early-stage CLL with a slightly higher predisposition to a prior first-generation relative with this disease. Additionally, these patients are generally of a higher economic status or have chronic fatigue or medical illnesses for which they have been undergoing routine blood testing, leading to diagnosis of CLL. When the diagnosis of CLL is made, these younger patients have a more challenging time understanding how the disease will impact them. For patients with no symptoms referable to CLL, we generally discuss complications of the disease during the first visit and have a detailed discussion regarding assessment of genetic risk factors predisposing to early disease progression, including select interphase chromosomal abnormalities [del(17p13.1) and del(11q22.3)] and IgV_H mutational status (unmutated). During this time, it is important to counsel patients that identification of high-risk genomic features can actually increase anxiety because no treatment intervention is indicated in the absence of symptoms, regardless of genomic profile, outside of a clinical trial. In our experience, the great majority of patients desire this testing. Despite the potential benefit of allogeneic SCT in younger patients with CLL, we generally mention this only as one treatment option used in this disease and do not pursue consultation or tissue typing of patients or siblings until patients are truly symptomatic from their disease. We provide considerable discussion about the promising new kinase inhibitors coming forward in the treatment of CLL, analogous to how imatinib impacted treatment of CML. During the second visit 4 to 6 weeks later, we review the results of these prognostic factors and answer additional questions that have arisen. Ultimately, the majority of patients have low-risk disease, and knowing this allows patients to take partial control of their disease and move on with their lives. Serial assessment of the psychological well-being of patients with CLL during this first year is incredibly important. At no place during the evaluation do we refer to CLL as being a good or favorable leukemia. In our experience, the most common reason for dissatisfaction toward the initial hematology evaluation is lack of explanation of the disease process or the minimization of CLL as a "good leukemia to have."

For young patients presenting with other chronic medical problems who are asymptomatic from their CLL, we follow the approach outlined above. More commonly, these patients have fatigue, mild anemia, or other symptoms that could be referable to the CLL. Additionally, this group is more commonly overweight or obese. In either setting, it is important to first think like an internist and pursue other causes for symptoms potentially referable to CLL. In particular, encouragement of both weight loss and a fixed exercise plan should be encouraged for fatigue and often improve quality of life and in other medical comorbidities. It is very important to note that younger patients with CLL can often go a decade or more without therapy, and early treatment of this patient group in the absence of symptoms still offers no proven long-term advantage. For this reason, our group remains very conservative on starting therapy for young patients with CLL.

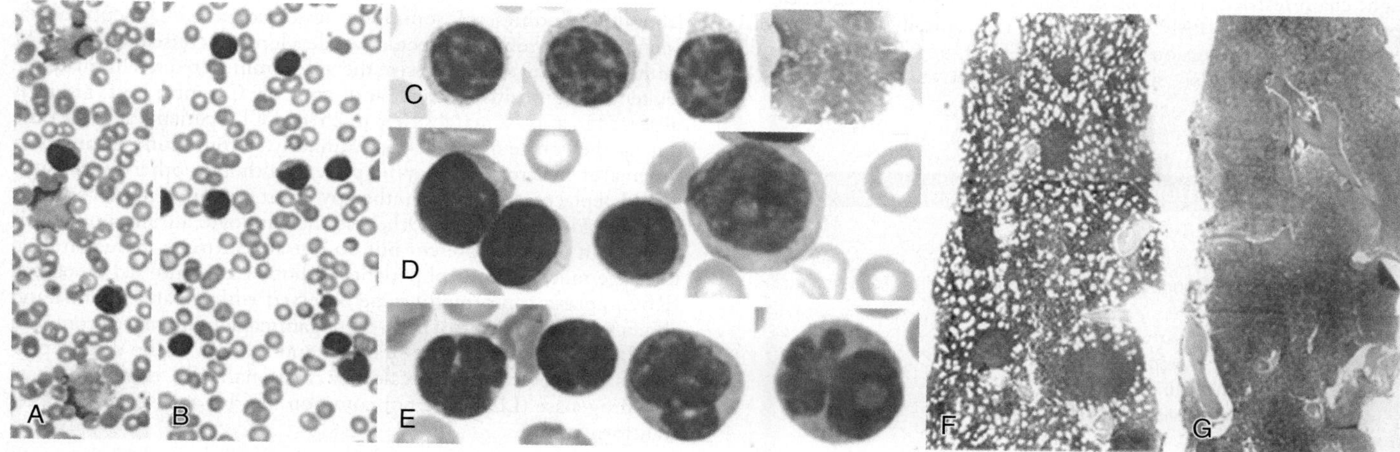

Figure 76-2 CHRONIC LYMPHOCYTIC LEUKEMIA (CLL). The peripheral blood smear **(A)** typically shows lymphocytosis and increased smudge cells as a result of the fragility of the CLL cells (see also smudge cell in **C,** *right side*). These can be avoided by making a preparation of blood and bovine serum albumin (22%) at a ratio of 11 drops of blood and 1 drop of albumin before preparing the slide **(B)**. Cytologic features of CLL cells differ. Classic cells have a small nucleus with a "soccer ball" chromatin pattern **(C)**. Some cases have increased large cells, or prolymphocytes, with more open chromatin and prominent "punched-out" nucleoli (**D;** prolymphocyte, *right side*). Other cases, sometimes referred to as "atypical," have clefted cells and large cells **(E)**. The bone marrow can show nodular infiltrates of CLL cells **(F)**, an interstitial infiltrate, or a diffuse infiltrate **(G)**.

patients should be similar to CLL with respect to diagnostic testing and treatment. However, SLL patients may not be eligible for some clinical studies in CLL if those trials follow IWCLL 2008 criteria and mandate a peripheral malignant B-cell lymphocyte count of 5000/μL for study entry.

The recent increase in diagnostic blood testing for other B-cell lymphoid cancers has led to recognition of a precursor to CLL called monoclonal B-cell lymphocytosis (MBL). Patients with MBL have circulating peripheral B cells immunophenotypically consistent with CLL but do not have enlarged lymph nodes, a malignant lymphocyte count greater than 5000/μL, or cytopenias. The frequency of MBL increases with age; 0.3% of patients younger than the age of 40 years have MBL compared with 2.1% of 40- to 60-year-old patients and 5.2% of 60- to 90-year-old patients. The frequency of MBL in family members of patients with a first-degree relative with CLL is significantly higher in both young and older patients. With the new IWCLL 2008 definition of CLL requiring 5000/μL malignant B lymphocytes, more cases of MBL exist than in the past with many patients being downstaged from early CLL to MBL. This bears significant clinical relevance because it may allow patients to obtain health and life insurance easier. Similar to the relationship of monoclonal gammopathy of undetermined significance and multiple myeloma, it appears that only a small proportion of patients with MBL develop overt CLL over time. Whereas genetic features such as IgV_H mutational status and cytogenetic abnormalities may predict for progression of CLL, it is unclear if these tests bear any relevance to predicting MBL progression. For this reason, we generally do not examine these tests in MBL patients.

LABORATORY MANIFESTATIONS

For many years, the diagnosis of CLL was made based on morphologic examination of the peripheral blood smear, which demonstrated mature lymphocytes with an abundance of smudge cells. Despite rigorous morphology, many diseases can mimic CLL in both appearance and clinical presentation, as summarized in Table 76-1, resulting in incorrect diagnoses. With the advent of new, more effective targeted therapies in CLL and other related diseases listed in Table 76-1, determining the correct diagnosis is of great importance. Flow cytometry, or immunophenotyping, has become a widely used diagnostic test that is currently performed in most reference pathology laboratories, and the use of flow cytometry is now the standard approach to establish the diagnosis of CLL (Fig. 76-3, for example). The diagnosis of CLL relies on immunophenotypic confirmation, and flow cytometry should therefore be performed on all CLL patients at diagnosis. CLL cells have a relatively consistent immunophenotype, which differentiates CLL from mantle cell lymphoma, hairy cell leukemia, follicular center cell lymphoma, splenic lymphoma with villous lymphocytes, and other indolent B-cell malignancies. Specifically, CLL cells express a variety of B-cell markers, including dim sIg, CD19, dim CD20 and CD23, as well as the pan T-cell marker CD5. κ or λ restriction is always present, establishing the presence of a clonal B-cell population, although sIg expression may be so dim that light chain restriction may be difficult to determine. In contrast, the presence of CD10, FMC7, or CD79b (all typically absent on CLL cells) or bright expression of CD11c, CD20, or CD25 (all typically dim on CLL cells) suggests an alternative low-grade B-cell lymphoproliferative malignancy. Expression of CD5 without CD23 suggests mantle cell lymphoma, and FISH for t(11;14) should be performed to exclude mantle cell lymphoma. Some genetic subsets of CLL are predisposed to variant antigen expression, particularly patients with trisomy 12. Repeating immunophenotyping after the initial diagnosis is not required unless there is a suspicion of transformation to a more aggressive histology or there is a need to assess BM response or antigen expression for an antibody directed therapeutic agent. Transformation of CLL (Fig. 76-4, *A* to *C*) to either prolymphocytic leukemia (PLL) or large cell lymphoma (Richter transformation) is often associated with immunophenotypic drift, where CD5 is lost and FMC7 expression is acquired. Additionally, expression of CD20 and surface immunoglobulin typically becomes brighter in PLL or Richter transformation. Although the morphologic appearance of prolymphocytes or large lymphoid cells in blood, BM or lymph nodes is typically adequate to make the diagnosis of transformation, flow cytometry may be useful in cases when morphologic findings are less clear.

Table 76-1 Diseases That Can Mimic Chronic Lymphocytic Leukemia

Follicular lymphoma
Mantle cell lymphoma
Monocytoid B-cell lymphoma or splenic lymphoma with villous lymphocytes
Hairy cell leukemia
Acute lymphoblastic leukemia
T-cell prolymphocytic leukemia
Large granular natural killer or T-cell leukemia

Patients with CLL often present with no symptoms, with the diagnosis being made as a consequence of asymptomatic enlarged lymph nodes or splenomegaly detected on physical examination or routine blood work done for another cause. Other patients present with symptoms of BM replacement (fatigue, dyspnea, or petechiae secondary to anemia and thrombocytopenia), symptomatic lymphadenopathy or hepatosplenomegaly, autoimmune complications (hemolytic anemia or idiopathic thrombocytopenic purpura), or B symptoms (fevers, night sweats, and weight loss). A small proportion of CLL patients will have pulmonary infiltrates at diagnosis that are representative of CLL involvement in some cases and active infection in others. Clearly, a wide spectrum of presentations exists for patients with CLL (see box on When Do I Consider a Transplant Evaluation in Chronic Lymphocytic Leukemia?).

In addition to blood and BM lymphocytosis, a few abnormal laboratory findings are commonly observed in CLL. Neutropenia, anemia, and thrombocytopenia can develop as a consequence of BM infiltration or myelosuppressive therapy administered to eliminate the leukemia. A positive direct antibody, or Coombs, test result is observed in approximately 10% to 25% of CLL patients at some time during the course of the disease. Similarly, autoimmune thrombocytopenia or neutropenia may be present, although other causes such as BM replacement or chemotherapy effect are much more common and should be excluded. Other nonhematologic autoimmune antibodies can rarely be present but do not appear to be more common than age-matched control patients without CLL. Pure red blood cell (RBC) aplasia can sometimes be observed with isolated anemia and absence of RBC precursor cells. Hypogammaglobulinemia is common in CLL and becomes more frequent and marked as the disease progresses. In contrast, hypercalcemia and markedly elevated lactate dehydrogenase (LDH) are not common in CLL and suggest Richter transformation.

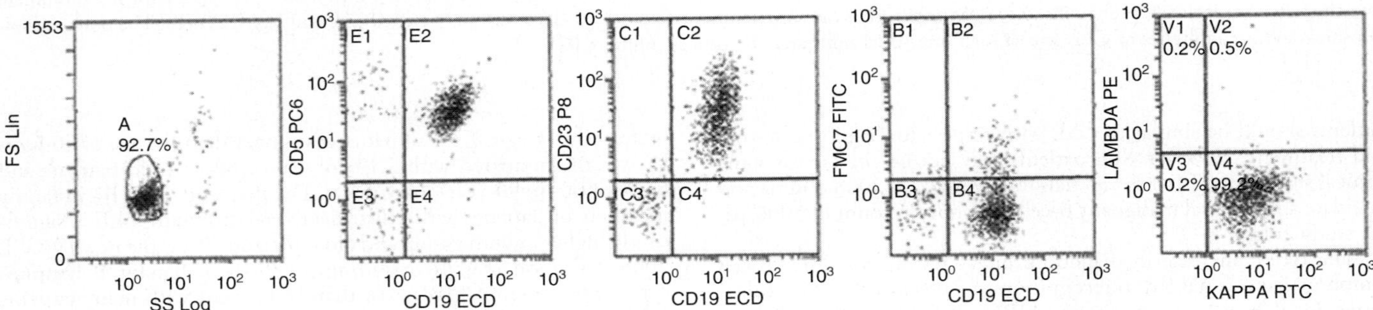

Figure 76-3 FLOW IMMUNOPHENOTYPING IN CHRONIC LYMPHOCYTIC LEUKEMIA (CLL). Flow data in a typical case of CLL. The phenotype is CD19⁺ clonal B cells with κ light chain restriction (weak to moderately intense), with coexpression of CD5 and CD23, but lack of FMC-7. The cells were CD38 negative.

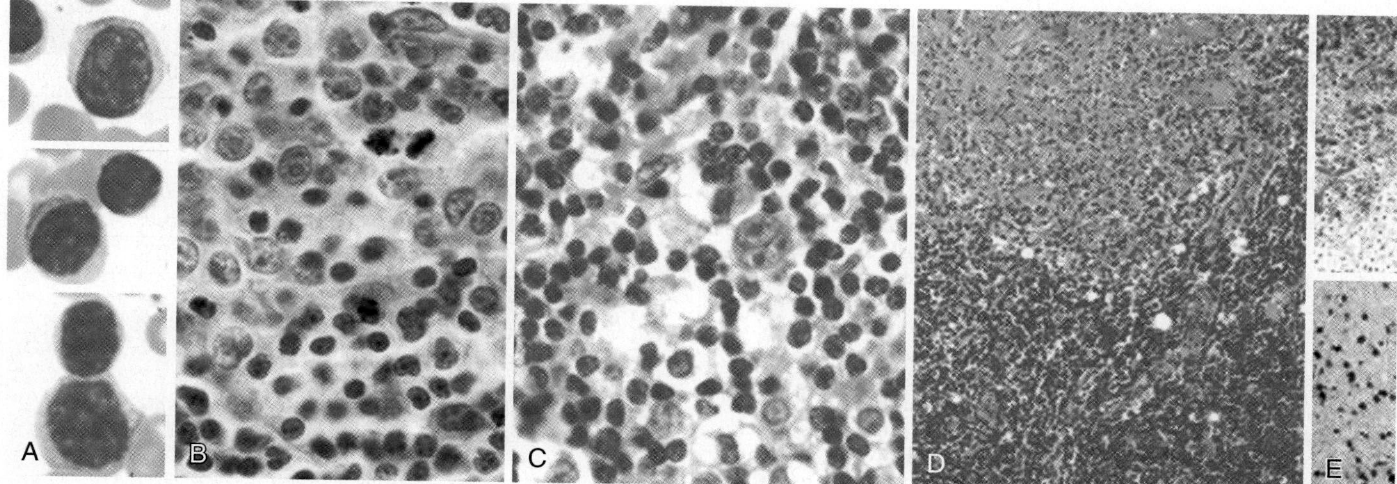

Figure 76-4 TRANSFORMATION IN CHRONIC LYMPHOCYTIC LEUKEMIA (CLL). Some patients of CLL develop increasing numbers of prolymphocytes (**A**) and a "prolymphocytic transformation." A Richter transformation is to a large-cell lymphoma (**B**; large cells, *upper left,* residual CLL, *lower right*). Occasionally, cases can transform to Hodgkin lymphoma (i.e., the Hodgkin variant of Richter syndrome) (**C**). With the use of fludarabine and other immunosuppressants, patient can also develop Epstein-Barr virus–related lymphadenopathies or lymphadenopathies with large areas of necrosis caused by herpes simplex virus (HSV). The case illustrated in **D** and **E** had both (**E;** *upper panel* shows an immunostain of HSV-1/2, and lower is EBER in situ hybridization).

When Do We Consider a Transplant Evaluation in Chronic Lymphocytic Leukemia?

With the introduction of nonmyeloablative stem cell transplantation, the morbidity and mortality associated with this therapy in CLL has decreased, and this option thereby has been extended to young and older patients alike. Additionally, extended follow-up in several transplant series has suggested that prolonged remissions can occur with this treatment approach, potentially providing the only curative therapeutic option for this disease. In general, we do not consider detailed discussion of transplant or referral for asymptomatic patients. When patients become symptomatic and require therapy for their CLL, we also consider if they would qualify for transplant. Approximately 50% of patients with CLL are 75 years of age or younger, have acceptable end-organ function, and lack comorbidities when symptomatic disease develops. It is this CLL patient group who may benefit from an allogeneic transplant consultation. Autologous transplant in CLL offers no opportunity for cure and is associated with treatment-related MDS/AML. For patients without del(17p13.1) attaining a complete remission to initial combination chemotherapy, we would never consider a consolidative SCT. However, for patients having only a partial response to combination therapy and who are likely to have only a short remission duration, consolidation transplant in the first partial remission should be strongly considered. Consolidation transplant after induction is generally pursued for patients with del(17p13.1) given the extreme poor outcome associated with this genetic group. For all patients relapsing after first therapy, we strongly recommend transplant evaluation and pursuit of this option after second treatment unless a complete remission is obtained again. For patients attaining a complete remission both to initial therapy and therapy at first relapse, remission duration can be prolonged and the allogeneic transplant can be delayed, particularly in the absence of high-risk genomic features. At the time of writing this chapter, introduction of kinase inhibitors appears to be altering the natural history of relapsed CLL similar to how imatinib influenced decisions of pursuing transplantation of CML in the 1990s. It is possible that the indication(s) for transplantation in CLL will change dramatically if these kinase inhibitors are eventually approved and alter long-term outcomes in CLL.

Table 76-2 Rai Staging System

Rai Stage at Diagnosis	Percent of Patients Never Requiring Chronic Lymphocytic Leukemia Therapy	Expected Survival in Months From Initial Diagnosis
0. Lymphocytosis $>5 \times 10^9$/L only	59	150
1. Lymph node enlargement	21	101
2. Spleen or liver enlargement	23	71
3. Anemia with hemoglobin <11 g/dL	5	19
4. Thrombocytopenia $<100 \times 10^{12}$/L	0	19

Adapted from Rai KR, Sawitsky A, Cronkite EP, et al. Clinical staging of chronic lymphocytic leukemia, *Blood* 46:219, 1975.

PROGNOSIS

Until recently, patients with CLL have been staged using either the Rai or Binet system. Both of these discriminate CLL by the sites of disease and degree of cytopenias induced by leukemia BM replacement. Patients can be categorized into three groups on the basis of these features. According to the modified Rai criteria, patients in the low-risk group (stage 0) have lymphocytosis without any other abnormality; patients in the intermediate-risk group (stages I and II) have, in addition to their lymphocytosis, enlarged lymph nodes, spleen, or liver; and patients in the high-risk group (stages III and IV) have anemia (hemoglobin <11.0 g/dL) or thrombocytopenia (platelets $<100 \times 10^9$/L). The median survival times for the Rai low-, intermediate-, and high-risk groups are similar to those of Binet stages A, B, and C: 12+, 8, and 2 years (Table 76-2). For early-stage patients with CLL (Rai low and intermediate stage and Binet stages A and B), a significant range of time to developing symptoms of CLL exists. The lack of survival advantage with early treatment, the observation that a subset of CLL patients will never require therapy, and the varied natural history of the disease have driven research efforts in CLL to identify specific biologic or clinical prognostic factors that predict time to progression.

Although lymphadenopathy is a common clinical feature of CLL and is incorporated into both major clinical staging systems, computed tomography (CT) scans are not commonly used to determine staging or to evaluate response to therapy outside of clinical trials. However, several studies have examined whether the incorporation of CT scans in initial staging or response evaluation may affect the ability to predict disease progression at diagnosis and assessment of clinical response to therapy. Although a few studies have suggested that these may help predict disease progression diagnosis, studies done serially at the time of treatment and for response show that CT scans generally do not impact assessment of response, progression-free survival (PFS), or OS. Additionally, CT scan identification of new nodal areas did not impact decisions for retreatment. Thus the use of CT scans in staging and response evaluation in CLL needs further study by well-designed, prospective clinical trials. However, CT scans should not be routinely incorporated in standard clinical use until their significance is evaluated within the context of such trials. Although CT scans have been the focus of greatest debate, the use of positron emission tomography (PET) should also be briefly discussed. Specifically, PET scans may be useful in detecting Richter transformation. In a single-institution study of 37 patients, PET scans identified 10 of 11 patients who had documented Richter transformation by tissue biopsy. However, nine patients had false-positive scans. Thus PET scans appear to be sensitive for Richter transformation, with a high negative predictive value, but specificity is poor. We generally use these studies to identify patients who warrant biopsy for Richter transformation and to localize where to biopsy.

With recent advances in the molecular biology of CLL, some prognostic factors such as BM infiltration pattern, which requires an invasive procedure at diagnosis, have not maintained their usefulness in predicting disease progression. Prognostic features outside of the traditional staging systems outlined above relative to daily practice are summarized below (Table 76-3).

Table 76-3 Evaluation of Chronic Lymphocytic Leukemia Patients at Diagnosis

History
B-symptom and fatigue assessment
Infectious history assessment
Occupational assessment for chemical exposure
Familial history of CLL and lymphoproliferative disorders
Preventive interventions for infections and secondary cancers
Physical Examination
LABORATORY ASSESSMENT
CBC with differential
Morphology assessment of lymphocytes
Chemistry, LFT enzymes, LDH
Flow cytometry assessment to confirm immunophenotype of CLL
Serum immunoglobulins
Serum β_2M levels
Interphase cytogenetics for del(17p13.1), del(11q22.3), del(13q14), del(6q21), and trisomy 12
IgV_H mutational analysis
Stimulated metaphase karyotype (if available)
Selected Tests Under Certain Circumstances
DAT, haptoglobin, reticulocyte count if anemia present
CT scan if unexplained abdominal pain or enlargement present
PET scan or biopsy (or both) if large nodal mass present
BM aspirate and biopsy if cytopenias present
Familial counseling if first-degree relative with CLL
Teaching
Varicella zoster identification instruction
Skin cancer identification
Disease education (Leukemia and Lymphoma Society, CLL Topics)

BM, Bone marrow; *CBC*, complete blood count; *CLL*, chronic lymphocytic leukemia; *CT*, computed tomography; *DAT*, direct antiglobulin test; *LDH*, lactate dehydrogenase; *LFT*, liver function test; *PET*, positron emission tomography.

Thymidine Kinase Activity and β_2-Microglobulin

Thymidine kinase is an enzyme involved in the salvage pathway of DNA synthesis and correlates with proliferative activity. Elevated thymidine kinase activity (TKA) has been observed to be predictive of early progression in a subgroup of untreated patients with smoldering CLL. β_2-Microglobulin (β_2M) is an extracellular protein component of the human leukocyte antigen (HLA) class I complex. β_2M has been shown to have significant prognostic relevance in lymphoma and multiple myeloma and correlates with disease burden in CLL. Hallek and colleagues examined 113 CLL and immunocytoma patients for β_2M levels and TKA and demonstrated that elevated TKA and β_2M both were independent predictors of shortened PFS. Keating et al confirmed the prognostic value of β_2M in 622 CLL patients, reporting that an elevated level was associated with a significantly shorter survival time for both untreated and previously treated patients. In this study, elevated β_2M was observed in patients with high tumor burden and extensive BM infiltration. In addition to disease progression, both β_2M and TKA have been associated with short duration of remission and inferior survival after treatment.

IgV_H Mutational Status

Although the malignant cell of CLL morphologically resembles a mature lymphocyte, genetic, immunologic, and phenotypic studies suggest that this cell is better designated as either a pregerminal or postgerminal B cell. Somatic mutations in the first and second complementarity-determining regions (CDR1 and CDR2) of the IgV_H genes are thought to occur in the germinal centers. Examination of IgV_H genes in patient cells suggests that there may be two subsets of CLL: leukemias whose cell of origin has successfully traversed the germinal center, resulting in the mutated IgV_H phenotype, and leukemias that are derived from naive B cells with the unmutated (germline) IgV_H sequence. Whereas approximately 60% of CLL patients have cells with mutated IgV_H genes (<98% identity to germline), the remaining patients have cells exhibiting unmutated IgV_H (≥98% sequence identity with germline), typical of pregerminal B cells. The prognostic significance of the absence of IgV_H gene mutations is substantial, with studies uniformly noting an inferior survival and high predisposition to requiring early treatment in this patient subset. A CLL Research Consortium study examined the impact of IgV_H mutation in 307 untreated CLL patients enrolled in a prospective tissue collection study. A total of 53% of these patients exhibited unmutated IgV_H genes, and this population had a significantly shorter median time to initial therapy (3.5 years) than those with mutated IgV_H (9.2 years; P <.001).

Because of the difficulties in determining IgV_H gene mutational status, researchers have sought surrogate markers for this parameter. Correlation between the absence of IgV_H gene mutations and elevated expression of the cell surface molecule CD38 on CLL cells was noted in one such report. In another work, ZAP-70 expression was shown to correlate with IgV_H gene mutational status. ZAP-70 is a T-cell receptor–associated tyrosine kinase that is aberrantly expressed in CLL cells, and ZAP-70 expression is generally found in patients with unmutated IgV_H but not in patients with mutated IgV_H. These two associated biomarkers appear to be linked directly to the difference in the behavior between these two genetic subtypes of CLL and are discussed independently. Other surrogate markers for the mutational status of the IgV_H gene have been reported, including methylation and subsequent silencing of TWIST2, a transcription factor that negatively regulates p53. TWIST2 methylation and silencing are preferentially observed in IgV_H-mutated CLL cases. Elevated levels of lipoprotein lipase and related genes have been noted in patients with IgV_H-unmutated disease. Additionally, it has been reported that IgV_H-mutated CLL cells have long telomeres with low telomerase activity, but IgV_H-unmutated patients have short telomeres with high telomerase activity. The extreme shortening of telomeres and elevated telomerase activity are associated with both genetic instability and disrupted apoptosis in other diseases, suggesting that a similar process occurs in IgV_H-unmutated CLL cells. Finally, distinct gene and microRNA (miRNA) expression profiles have also been correlated with IgV_H gene mutational status.

CD38 Expression

Retrospective studies have shown that CD38 is an independent prognostic marker in CLL, demonstrating that high CD38 expression is associated with both a shorter time from diagnosis to treatment and inferior survival. CD38 functional studies using CD31 and plexin B1 transfected fibroblasts have provided a biologic explanation for this observation. CD38 interaction with its ligand, CD31, in the presence of IL-2 results in upregulation of the survival receptor CD100 exclusively on proliferating CLL cells. This occurs with concomitant downmodulation of CD72, a negative regulator of immune response. The interaction between CD38 and CD100 on CLL cells and CD31 and plexin B1, respectively, on transfected fibroblasts results in enhanced survival and growth of CLL cells. Furthermore, the presence of nurse-like cells in CLL patients expressing high levels of CD31 and plexin B1 corroborates the interplay of CD38 and CD31 and provides further evidence of activation of circulating CD38-positive CLL cells by the microenvironment. This finding also may explain the aggressive nature of these CLL clones.

ZAP-70

ZAP-70 expression was identified as another surrogate marker for IgV_H gene mutational status by a cDNA microarray analysis of untreated CLL patients. Functional studies in ZAP-70–positive cases have shown that BCR ligation leads to increased phosphorylation of cytosolic proteins (Syk, BLNK, PLCγ), calcium mobilization, degradation of IκB, and ultimately NFκB target gene activation. Despite clear data showing that ZAP-70 is a prognostic factor, the reproducibility of this assay across laboratories has been problematic. Inconsistent measurement of ZAP-70 may be the cause because ZAP-70 is a labile protein, and laboratories have used different methods and reagents. Given the challenges of measuring ZAP-70 protein accurately, others have attempted to identify alternative markers or more stable readouts of ZAP-70 expression. For example, methylation of select regions in the proximal 5′ region of the ZAP-70 gene has been shown to correlate closely with expression of ZAP-70 and influence treatment outcome. Overall, despite the apparent usefulness of ZAP-70 in research laboratories for discriminating CLL patients at high risk for progression, this test currently is not useful for clinical practice.

Chromosomal Aberrations

Conventional metaphase cytogenetics can identify chromosomal aberrations in only 20% to 50% of CLL cases because of the low in vitro mitotic activity of CLL cells. Abnormalities noted in descending frequency of occurrence include trisomy 12; deletions at 13q14; structural aberrations of 14q32; and deletions of 11q, 17p, and 6q. In addition, a complex karyotype (three or more abnormalities) occurs in approximately 15% of patients and predicts for rapid disease progression, Richter transformation, and inferior survival. A recent study showed that the use of CD40L or the combination of IL-2 and CpG stimulation revealed translocations in 33 of 96 patients (34%). These translocations were both balanced and unbalanced, occurring in 13q14, 11(q21q25), 14q32, or regions also seen in lymphomas such as 1(p32p36), 1(q21q25), 2(p11p13), 6(p11p12), 6(p21p25), and 18q21. These data define a new prognostic subgroup of patients with significantly shorter median time from diagnosis to requiring therapy (24 vs. 106 months) and OS (94 vs. 346 months) compared with those without translocations. The frequency of these translocations in untreated patients was less common, suggesting that these accumulate with disease progression. Although of interest, these findings require additional prospective validation before being used as a standard prognostic tool for CLL patients.

Given the limitation of standard or stimulated karyotype analysis, interphase FISH has become the state-of-the-art technique for accurately distinguishing genetic subtypes of CLL. The largest study of interphase FISH resulted in improved sensitivity to detect partial trisomies (12q12, 3q27, 8q24), deletions (13q14, 11q22-23, 6q21, 6q27, 17p13), and translocations (band 14q32) in more than 80% of all cases. In a large study of 325 patients by Dohner and colleagues, a hierarchical model consisting of five genetic subgroups was constructed on the basis of regression analysis of CLL patients with chromosomal aberrations. Patients with a 17p deletion had the shortest median survival time (32 months) and the shortest treatment-free interval (TFI, months); patients with an 11q deletion followed closely with 79 months and 13 months, respectively. Whereas the favorable 13q14 deletion group had a long TFI of 92 months and a median survival of 133 months, the group without detectable chromosomal anomalies and those with trisomy 12 fell into the intermediate group with median survival of 111 and 114 months, respectively, and TFI of 33 and 49 months, respectively. According to this pivotal study, CLL patients are prioritized in a hierarchical order (deletion 17p13 > deletion 11q22-q23 > trisomy 12 > no aberration > deletion 13q14). The hierarchical model of cytogenetic abnormalities in predicting disease progression by FISH has been further confirmed by other studies. Of interest, patients with high-risk interphase cytogenetic abnormalities or other complex abnormalities are almost always found to have IgVH-unmutated CLL. The impact of high-risk interphase cytogenetics relative to disease progression, outside of its association with IgVH-unmutated CLL, in at least one study had less impact on outcome.

Preliminary Prospective Validation of New Biomarkers From the German Chronic Lymphocytic Leukemia Study Group

The CLL-1 Study of the German CLL Study Group (GCLLSG) is a randomized phase III study of early treatment with fludarabine versus observation in newly diagnosed CLL patients. Risk of progression is determined on the basis of lymphocyte-doubling time, thymidine kinase, and diffuse BM pattern. Differing from other early-intervention studies, patients with disease that meet one or more of the NCI 96 criteria (i.e., lymphocyte-doubling times <1 year) may enroll. Accompanying this study is the plan to assess interphase FISH, IgV_H mutations, and β_2M level to determine their independent prognostic significance compared with other variables. If shown to be of prospective importance relative to predicting early treatment progression, these laboratory tests would be incorporated into subsequent risk stratification criteria. IgV_H-unmutated disease represented 41% of patients at diagnosis. Patients with IgV_H-unmutated disease assigned to observation had a median time to symptomatic disease of only 2 years. High-risk karyotypes were present in 15% of cases, with the great majority being IgV_H unmutated. A preliminary analysis of the first 340 patients randomized to observation suggested that IgV_H-unmutated disease, high-risk interphase FISH, thymidine kinase, and lymphocyte-doubling time correlated with time to first treatment. Publication of these large prospective new prognostic factors will be important to determining the risk of CLL progression (see box on How Should Staging and Biomarkers Be Used for Treatment Decisions in Chronic Lymphocytic Leukemia Patients?).

How Should Staging and Biomarkers Be Used for Treatment Decisions in Chronic Lymphocytic Leukemia Patients?

Our understanding of the biology of CLL has improved dramatically, and many relevant biomarkers are now becoming useful for predicting when CLL will clinically progress. However, no study to date has demonstrated that earlier treatment will alter the natural history of the patient in even the higher risk groups with high progression rates. Therefore, at the present time, the use of staging and predictive biomarkers should be used only to provide patients with information relative to the expected course of their disease. Outside of a clinical trial, these results should never be used to initiate therapy in patients with asymptomatic disease and no indication for treatment. Before performing predictive tests, a detailed discussion of how these tests will be used with the patient should occur and the option of not performing them should be provided. In a subset of patients, significant anxiety can be produced by identifying high-risk features for which observation, without therapeutic intervention, remains the standard of care. Table 76-3 provides an example of the initial evaluation provided by our group when seeing a newly diagnosed patient. Because lymphocyte-doubling time is a prognostic feature in the progression of CLL, our approach is to follow patients every 3 months during the first year; if little change in clinical or laboratory parameters occurs at this point, we extend this time period to every 6 months in the absence of new complaints.

TREATMENT

Initiation of Treatment of Newly Diagnosed or Previously Untreated Patients

Many patients are incidentally diagnosed with CLL on routine complete blood count examination and are asymptomatic with a normal hemoglobin and platelet count at time of initial diagnosis. Expectant observation without therapy is the standard practice for such asymptomatic patients, and patients receive treatment only when their disease progresses. This practice is based on several studies that failed to show an improvement in OS when early therapeutic intervention with chlorambucil therapy was administered to asymptomatic patients. A meta-analysis of 2048 patients in six trials demonstrated no difference in death rate between patients who were randomized to early therapy (42.6%) and those with treatment deferred (41.6%). Thus patients with asymptomatic or early-stage disease derive no therapeutic benefit from early alkylating agent therapy. However, in these studies, chlorambucil was administered as initial therapy, and chlorambucil achieves complete response (CR) in few patients. The past decade has seen the development of more effective treatment regimens combining monoclonal antibody therapy with purine analogs (chemoimmunotherapy), which are able to achieve CR in a majority of previously untreated patients, and the increasing use of new molecular markers to risk stratify newly diagnosed CLL patients. Furthermore, it is now well established that CLL undergoes genetic clonal evolution over time with greater frequency in IgV_H-unmutated CLL, resulting in increasing resistance to therapy in this patient population. Thus the issue of early treatment needs to be reconsidered, particularly in patients with high-risk biological or molecular markers predicting a poor long-term prognosis, such as IgV_H-unmutated disease. Ongoing efforts within the GCLLSG will hopefully determine whether early intervention with chemoimmunotherapy regimens will improve long-term survival in patients with high-risk CLL.

To establish uniform clinical practice standards and ensure reproducible eligibility criteria for entrance into clinical studies, the IWCLL established guidelines for initiation of treatment. Indications to begin therapy included non-autoimmune cytopenias (Rai stage III and IV), bulky or symptomatic lymphadenopathy or hepatosplenomegaly, disease-related B symptoms or fatigue, extreme lymphocytosis (>300 × 109/L) or a rapid lymphocyte-doubling time, and autoimmune hemolytic anemia (AIHA) or thrombocytopenia not controlled with steroids. It is imperative to determine if a patient's symptoms are attributable to CLL or a comorbid medical condition because constitutional symptoms such as fatigue are nonspecific and can be caused by many etiologies in elderly patients with comorbid illnesses. In addition to the official IWCLL 2008 criteria for therapy, an increasing frequency of infections and slowly progressive anemia are other indications that can aid the practicing physician in deciding when to initiate therapy in patients with CLL. A summary of the IWCLL 2008 guidelines for treatment is provided in Table 76-4 with some minimal modifications used by our group.

Table 76-4 Modified Indications for Treatment of Chronic Lymphocytic Leukemia

Grade 2 or greater fatigue limiting life activities
B symptoms persisting for ≥2 weeks
Lymph nodes >10 cm or progressively enlarging lymph nodes causing symptoms
Spleen or liver with progressive enlargement or causing symptoms
Anemia (hemoglobin <11 g/dL) referable to CLL
Thrombocytopenia (platelets <100 × 10^{12}/L) referable to CLL or ITP poorly responsive to traditional therapy
WBC count >300 × 10^9/L on two occasions 2 weeks apart if no alternative comorbid diseases increase morbidity of treatment
Severe paraneoplastic (e.g., insect hypersensitivity, vasculitis, myositis) process related to CLL not responsive to traditional therapies

AIHA, Autoimmune hemolytic anemia; *CLL*, chronic lymphocytic leukemia; *ITP*, idiopathic thrombocytopenic purpura; *WBC*, white blood cell.

A useful paradigm for clinical practice is to institute treatment in CLL only for cytopenias or directly referable symptoms. When treatment is necessary, a variety of agents have been examined in clinical trials (outlined below). Previously identified biomarkers are used in selecting the initial treatment for CLL, and the utility of more recently identified biomarkers currently are under study by several groups. In general, patients with del(17p13.1) do not respond well to traditional therapy and should be considered for more aggressive interventions such as allogeneic stem cell transplantation (SCT) as part of initial therapy. Patients with del(11q22.3) appear to have improved outcome with hyperfractionated cyclophosphamide as part of the FCR (fludarabine–cyclophosphamide–rituximab) regimen. Additionally, several studies have shown that CLL patients older than 70 years of age or who have multiple comorbid illnesses do not benefit from fludarabine-containing regimens, and this needs to be factored into treatment algorithms. Below, we summarize the findings of clinical studies of different treatments for CLL; where such data exist, we integrate genomic biomarkers as well as clinical features, including age and comorbid illnesses. Different therapies are outlined below with attention to details related to their initial use in previously untreated CLL. Because many of these regimens were also developed in relapsed CLL, these data are also reviewed and later referred to in the section Treatment of Patients With Relapsed Chronic Lymphocytic Leukemia.

Cytotoxic Chemotherapy

Alkylating Agents

Chlorambucil and other alkylating agents have served as first-line therapy for CLL for many decades, and chlorambucil is still given as first-line therapy for some patients, particularly older patients and patients who cannot tolerate purine analog therapy. Chlorambucil is generally administered as a single pulse dose 40 mg/m^2 orally (PO) every 28 days with or without concomitant steroid therapy, although alternative dosing schedules are used, particularly in Europe. Chlorambucil is typically given without steroid therapy because the addition of steroids to alkylating agent therapy has not been shown to improve survival. Although a high-dose continuous dosing schedule of 15 mg/day PO has been evaluated in several large European studies and led to results superior to those of pulse therapy, high-dose therapy is associated with greater myelosuppression and frequently requires dose reduction, particularly in older or more fragile patients in whom chlorambucil is typically considered. Although high-dose therapy may be more effective if maximal cytoreduction is desired, the less intensive pulse dosing schedule should generally be used outside the setting of a clinical study. Because most studies of alkylating agent therapy predated widespread use of cytogenetic and biological risk factors, data on the effect of biomarkers on response to chlorambucil are limited. However, the existing data indicate that patients with del(11q22.3) or del(17p13.1) have a lower response rate and a shorter remission duration to chlorambucil compared with patients without these abnormalities. The primary advantages of chlorambucil are its well-established toxicity profile and its low cost; its primary disadvantages are its low CR rate, even in previously untreated patients, and the small possibility of developing myelodysplasia with extended therapy. Although not typically given as a single agent to younger patients, its use should be considered in older patients and other patients who may not tolerate fludarabine therapy. Given the benefit of the chimeric monoclonal anti-CD20 antibody rituximab as part of chemoimmunotherapy regimens with fludarabine, several pilot studies have been performed combining chlorambucil with rituximab. These have shown promising results and favorable toxicity profile, prompting an ongoing phase III study of this combination, compared with single-agent chlorambucil, by the GCLLSG. This phase III study also includes an experimental arm combining chlorambucil with the novel type II monoclonal anti-CD20 antibody obinutuzumab (GA-101). A similar phase III study comparing the combination of chlorambucil and the fully human anti-CD20 antibody ofatumumab has completed accrual. (Both obinutuzumab and ofatumumab are discussed later in this chapter.)

Bendamustine

Although typically classified as a bifunctional alkylator, bendamustine has an uncertain mechanism of action. Although the drug predominately promotes cytotoxicity by inducing DNA damage and reactive oxygen species, in NCI60 cell line studies, bendamustine displayed a distinct pattern of activity unrelated to other DNA-alkylating agents but closest to melphalan. Unlike other alkylating agents, bendamustine activates a base excision DNA repair pathway rather than an alkyltransferase DNA repair mechanism. Studies of bendamustine in a variety of solid tumors, non-Hodgkin lymphoma (NHL), multiple myeloma, Hodgkin disease, and CLL have shown single agent activity. Bendamustine has been widely used in Eastern Germany and several European countries for decades and was approved by the U.S. Food and Drug Administration (FDA) for treatment of CLL in 2008. This was based on a well-controlled, randomized phase III study comparing bendamustine 100 mg/m^2 intravenous (IV) on days 1 and 2 with chlorambucil 0.8 mg/kg PO on days 1 and 15 every 4 weeks for 6 cycles. A total of 319 patients were enrolled with an overall response rate (ORR) of 68% and 31% CR with bendamustine versus 31% ORR and 2% CR with chlorambucil treatment (P <.0001). The median PFS was significantly better (P <.0001) with bendamustine (21.6 vs. 8.3 months) than chlorambucil. Grade 3/4 hematologic toxicity and severe infections (grades 3-4) occurred more commonly with bendamustine. Overall, this study and others that have followed showed that bendamustine is well tolerated in young and old CLL patients. This agent has been effectively combined with rituximab and is currently being pursued as a phase III study by the GCLLSG.

Combination Chemotherapy With Alkylating Agents

A variety of trials combining alkylating agents and other cytotoxic agents have been performed. A phase III Eastern Cooperative Oncology Group (ECOG) study of chlorambucil and prednisone (CP) with or without vincristine (CVP) demonstrated no benefit in PFS for the CVP arm. The French CLL group showed that a modified CHOP (cyclophosphamide, Adriamycin, vincristine, prednisone) regimen was superior to CVP and achieved similar results as fludarabine monotherapy. A meta-analysis compared alkylating agent-based combination regimens with a single-agent regimen based on an alkylating agent and demonstrated no survival benefit. Given that alkylating agent–based combination regimens are associated with more toxicity and show no benefit over fludarabine-based therapy, our approach is to use the latter for most patients. Only in rare cases of de novo CLL do we consider alkylating agent–based combination therapy (i.e., a young patient without comorbid illnesses who has fludarabine toxicity that prohibits further use or a patient with renal failure who cannot receive fludarabine). In the relapse setting, although salvage lymphoma regimens such as CHOP-R, RICE, and ESHAP-R are used to treat CLL, clinical studies of these regimens in CLL are lacking, and the utility of these regimens is undefined.

Purine Analogs

The introduction of purine analogs in the 1980s by Grever and later Keating revolutionized CLL therapy, and fludarabine has demonstrated significant clinical efficacy in both relapsed and previously untreated CLL. Pentostatin was the first nucleoside analog that demonstrated clinical activity in CLL and related B-cell lymphoproliferative disorders; however, subsequent phase II studies showed modest activity, limiting further trials of this agent. Given its more favorable myelosuppression profile compared with other nucleoside analogs, pentostatin has been combined with other agents and shown favorable clinical activity and toxicity in selected populations. Two other nucleoside analogs, fludarabine and cladribine, were subsequently found to be clinically active in CLL. Phase II to III studies of cladribine monotherapy achieved similar clinical responses as alkylating agent–based treatment but were associated with more cytopenias and immune suppression. The FDA approved fludarabine for the treatment of CLL, and thus most studies of purine analog–based therapy in CLL have focused on fludarabine. The remainder of this section focuses predominately on clinical trials of fludarabine.

Fludarabine was initially approved by the FDA for alkylating agent–resistant CLL in 1991 based on two phase II studies demonstrating a high response rate to fludarabine in this patient subset, prompting several additional trials of fludarabine as monotherapy in relapsed and previously untreated CLL. After the observation of high response rates and a 33% CR rate in previously untreated CLL by Keating and colleagues, several large prospective randomized studies in previously untreated CLL patients compared alkylating agent–based regimens with fludarabine. These studies collectively established fludarabine as an accepted standard first-line therapy for CLL based on improved response rates and PFS. These studies are summarized in Table 76-4. A multicenter European study randomized 196 evaluable patients to fludarabine or cyclophosphamide, doxorubicin, and prednisone (CAP). The ORR favored fludarabine (60% vs. 44%), and this benefit was observed in both relapsed (n = 96; 48% vs. 27%) and previously untreated (n = 100; 71% vs. 60%) patients, although the difference was not statistically significant in the untreated group. Fludarabine achieved a longer median duration of response than did CAP, with a tendency toward longer OS in previously untreated patients. A randomized, multicenter American study confirmed these findings in 509 previously untreated CLL patients. Patients were randomized to receive fludarabine 25 mg/m^2 IV daily for 5 days every 28 days, chlorambucil 40 mg/m^2 PO every 28 days, or fludarabine 20 mg/m^2 daily for 5 days and chlorambucil 20 mg/m^2 PO every 28 days, for up to 12 cycles. Patients who failed to respond or relapsed were allowed to cross over to the other arm. The combination arm was closed because of excessive toxicity. Fludarabine achieved a superior CR rate, ORR, median duration of remission, and median duration of PFS (20%, 63%, 25 months, 20 months, respectively) than did chlorambucil (4%, 37%, 14 months, 14 months, respectively). However, there was no statistically significant difference in OS even at 10 years of follow-up (66 vs. 56 months), possibly because of the crossover design. A multicenter French study randomized 938 patients with previously untreated Binet stage B and C CLL to fludarabine, CHOP, or CAP. Although fludarabine achieved better response rates than CAP, OS (67-70 months) was identical in all three treatment groups. Thus single-agent fludarabine achieves superior response rates and duration of PFS to alkylating agent–based regimens. The impact of prognostic factors on response rates and duration of PFS to fludarabine was recently examined; patients with high-risk cytogenetic abnormalities, including del(11q22.3) and del(17p13.1), have significantly shorter PFS in response to fludarabine-based therapy than patients with other cytogenetic abnormalities.

However, the benefit of fludarabine does not apply to patients older than the age of 65 years. A phase III trial by the GCLLSG randomized 193 previously untreated CLL patients older than 65 years to fludarabine 25 mg/m^2 IV for 5 days every 28 days for 6 cycles or chlorambucil 0.4 to 0.8 mg/kg PO every 15 days for 12 months. Fludarabine achieved higher OR (72% vs. 51%) and CR rates (7% vs. 0%) and longer time to treatment failure (19 vs. 18 months). However, PFS was similar in both arms (19 months vs. 18 months), and OS was 46 months for fludarabine compared with 64 months for chlorambucil arm ($P = .15$). Thus the results achieved in younger patients do not necessarily apply to older patients with comorbid diseases or who otherwise cannot tolerate more aggressive therapies.

Combining Fludarabine With Alkylating Agent Therapy

Fludarabine was combined with cyclophosphamide (Flu/Cy) in three randomized phase III studies, based on two promising pilot studies in previously untreated CLL patients, with the goal of improving response rates and hopefully long-term survival. The GCLLSG randomized 375 previously untreated patients (age younger than 65 years) to standard fludarabine or Flu/Cy (fludarabine 30 mg/m^2 IV and cyclophosphamide 250 mg/m^2 IV daily for 3 days) every 28 days for 6 cycles. The ORR (94% vs. 83%), CR rate (24% vs. 7%), median PFS (48 vs. 20 months), and duration of treatment-free survival (37 vs. 25 months) all favored Flu/Cy, although there were more patients with cytopenias in the combination arm. Furthermore, no difference in OS was observed. EGOG randomized 278 patients to single-agent fludarabine or fludarabine 25 mg/m^2 on days 1 to 5, cyclophosphamide 600 mg/m^2 on day 1, and granulocyte colony-stimulating factor (G-CSF) support every 28 days for 6 cycles. Flu/Cy therapy achieved a superior ORR (74% vs. 59%), rates of CR (23% vs. 5%), and duration of PFS (32 vs. 19 months), although no OS advantage was observed. Most recently, the United Kingdom LRF CLL4 study randomized 777 patients to oral chlorambucil, fludarabine, or Flu/Cy. Patients randomized to Flu/Cy enjoyed superior ORR, CR rates, and 5-year PFS rates (94%, 39%, and 33%, respectively) to patients who received chlorambucil (72%, 7%, and 9%, respectively) or fludarabine (80%, 15%, and 14%, respectively).

Thus three large, prospective, randomized, multicenter studies in the United States and Europe have clearly demonstrated that Flu/Cy therapy is associated with better response rates and duration of PFS than single-agent fludarabine. However, no OS advantage for upfront Flu/Cy has been observed to date. Although toxicity has generally been manageable, greater hematologic toxicity has been observed with Flu/Cy. Additionally, patients older than 65 or 70 years, who make up the majority of CLL patients receiving initial therapy in clinical practice, have either been excluded or minimally represented in these trials. Further studies are needed to determine if Flu/Cy is as well tolerated and active in older patients as it is in younger patients. Finally, of these patients, long-term follow-up is required to determine the duration of remission, OS, and the incidence of potential late complications such as therapy-related myeloid neoplasia (tr-MN) to fully assess the utility of the Flu/Cy regimen. Indeed, the US Intergroup study of FC versus F suggested an increased risk of tr-MN in the FC arm. Examination of outcome by cytogenetic risk groups showed that patients with high-risk cytogenetic abnormalities, including del(11q22.3) and del(17p13.1), had a significantly shorter remission than patients in the groups with good- or intermediate-risk cytogenetic findings. Thus the addition of alkylating agents to fludarabine does not appear to alter the poor prognosis associated with high-risk cytogenetic abnormalities.

Rituximab

Rituximab is a chimeric murine monoclonal antibody that targets the CD20 antigen on the surface of normal and malignant B lymphocytes, and is the best studied and most widely used monoclonal antibody for the treatment of CLL and B-NHL. CD20, a calcium channel that interacts with the BCR complex, is an ideal target, because CD20 is expressed in 90% to 100% of CLL and B-NHL and is only minimally internalized or shed. Rituximab induces antibody-dependent cellular cytotoxicity (ADCC) and complement-dependent cytotoxicity (CDC), activates caspase 3, and induces apoptosis in CLL and B-NHL cells. Thus multiple mechanisms of action likely contribute to rituximab's effectiveness in CLL.

In phase I clinical studies in indolent B-NHL rituximab, 375 mg/m^2 IV was administered weekly for four doses, although the dose and length of treatment were empirically determined. The pivotal phase II trial of rituximab was pursued in 166 patients with relapsed or refractory indolent B-NHL, including SLL. Although an ORR of 60% was achieved in indolent follicle center B-NHL, only four of 30 patients (13%) with SLL/CLL responded. Similarly, disappointing results were obtained in several other small studies. Responses in each of these studies were predominately in the blood and nodal compartment with little improvement in BM disease. In contrast, two trials in which higher doses of rituximab weekly (≤2250 mg/m^2 per dose) or in which rituximab was administered thrice weekly (at 375 mg/m^2) to relapsed CLL patients showed improved response rate with response duration approaching that achieved in follicular B-NHL in prior trials. These studies established a role for single-agent rituximab in patients with relapsed CLL and lead to combination with other agents.

In contrast to studies in relapsed CLL, weekly single-agent rituximab demonstrated greater clinical efficacy when given to patients with previously untreated SLL/CLL. Forty-four previously untreated patients with SLL/CLL received 4-weekly doses of rituximab 375 mg/m^2; the ORR after the first course of rituximab was 51% (CR 4%). Twenty-eight patients with stable or responsive disease received additional 4-week courses of rituximab every 6 months for up to 4 cycles. However, there was only a modest increase in ORR (58%) and CR rates (9%), and the median duration of PFS of 19 months was shorter than the 36- to 40-month median duration of PFS reported by the same investigators using the same regimen in previously untreated patients with follicle center B-NHL. Nonetheless, this response duration compared favorably with the response duration achieved with fludarabine in the upfront setting, suggesting that rituximab is active and may have a role in the upfront therapy of SLL/CLL.

Rituximab is selective for the B-cell antigen CD20 and therefore has a relatively favorable toxicity profile. Toxicity associated with infusion of this agent commonly occurs with the first infusion of rituximab and may be greater in patients with CLL compared with patients with NHL. These symptoms generally include fever, rigors, transient hypoxemia, dyspnea, and hypotension, which are partly caused by an inflammatory cytokine release syndrome. Although poorly understood, CLL patients with platelet counts less than 50 × 1012/L may experience transient, severe thrombocytopenia associated with this infusional toxicity and may require platelet transfusions with the first one or two doses of rituximab. Patients with preexisting thrombocytopenia should therefore have a posttherapy platelet count after the first one or two doses of rituximab. Another uncommon but potentially severe toxicity is a tumor lysis syndrome, which is generally observed in patients with a high circulating peripheral lymphocyte count with CLL variants. Such patients should receive prophylactic allopurinol, hydration, and careful observation, and inpatient monitoring and administration of rituximab can be considered for the highest risk patients. Patients who develop tumor lysis syndrome after the first dose of rituximab can safely receive subsequent doses, especially after the number of circulating CLL cells is reduced. Other rare toxicities with rituximab therapy include delayed neutropenia, hepatitis B reactivation, skin toxicity, interstitial pneumonitis, serum sickness, and progressive multifocal encephalopathy. Patients with prior hepatitis B exposure, as indicated by positive serologies, should receive rituximab only if viral load testing indicates no active disease. Such patients should undergo regular viral load monitoring during and after completion of rituximab therapy, and prophylactic antiviral therapy may be considered to reduce the likelihood of viral reactivation. Patients who develop profound neutropenia, pulmonary, or skin toxicity with rituximab should not be challenged with repeated dosing. In general, rituximab is a very well-tolerated therapy, making it ideal for use in combination with other agents in patients with CLL.

Phase II Studies of Rituximab Chemoimmunotherapy

Given its activity and toxicity profile, rituximab has been combined with cytotoxic chemotherapy in the treatment of CLL, and clinical trials have examined several such chemoimmunotherapy regimens. Studies of chemoimmunotherapy in CLL have focused primarily on fludarabine-based combinations because of the established role of fludarabine therapy in this disease. The approval of bendamustine and potentially an alternative mechanism compared with alkylator agents and fludarabine has led to combination therapy of bendamustine with rituximab. Finally, given the recent recognition that elderly patients do not benefit from fludarabine-containing regimens, several trials have also combined rituximab with chlorambucil with promising results. Alternative regimens including FCR–mitoxantrone (FCR-M) and pentostatin, rituximab, and cyclophosphamide (PCR) have been published and used in CLL but are unlikely to be building blocks for improvement in CLL therapy in the future and are therefore not described below.

Fludarabine and Rituximab

The CALGB 9712 study randomized 104 previously untreated CLL patients to sequential or concurrent fludarabine and rituximab (FR) therapy. Patients received standard fludarabine 25 mg/m^2 days 1 to 5 every 4 weeks for 6 cycles with or without concurrent rituximab 375 mg/m^2 on day 1 of each cycle with an additional dose on day 4 of cycle 1. Patients in both arms received rituximab 375 mg/m^2 weekly for four doses beginning 2 months after completion of fludarabine; thus patients in the concurrent arm received 11 total doses of rituximab compared with four in the sequential arm. Patients receiving concurrent FR therapy enjoyed a superior CR rate (47% vs. 28%) and ORR (90% vs. 77%) to patients in the sequential arm. Retrospective comparison to a fludarabine only–containing treatment study performed previously by CALGB demonstrated improved PFS and OS compared with fludarabine treatment. Analysis of prognostic cytogenetic abnormalities demonstrated that patients with del(11q22.3) and del(17p13.1) have a shorter duration of response to this regimen. A recent update of this study with a median follow-up of 117 months showed that the median OS was 85 months with 71% of patients alive at 5 years. The median PFS was 42 months with 27% progression free at 5 years. Importantly, an estimated 13% of patients remained free of progression at almost 10 years of follow-up. IgV$_H$-mutated disease status was favorably associated with extended PFS and OS, but not having high-risk cytogenetics was associated with a favorable OS. Notably, there were no cases of treatment-related myeloid neoplasms occurring before relapse contrasting with prior studies with fludarabine- and alkylator-containing regimens.

Fludarabine, Cyclophosphamide, and Rituximab

The most active phase II results with chemoimmunotherapy have been achieved by the MD Anderson group with a combination FCR regimen in both previously treated and untreated CLL. A total of 177 evaluable patients with previously treated CLL received fludarabine 25 mg/m^2 and cyclophosphamide 250 mg/m^2 on days 2 to 4 of cycle 1 and on days 1 to 3 of cycles 2 to 6 in addition to rituximab 375 mg/m^2 on day 1 of cycle 1 and 500 mg/m^2 on day 1 of cycles 2 to 6. An ORR of 73% with a 25% CR rate and 16% nodular PR rate was reported, and 12 of 37 patients (32%) in CR achieved molecular remission. The same authors administered FCR to 300 previously untreated CLL patients; the ORR was 95%, with 72% of patients attaining a CR. Six-year PFS was 51%, and OS was 77%. Features associated with poor response included high β_2M, del(17p13.1), age older than 70 years, and elevated white blood cell count above 150 × 10^9/L. Late infections or other complications were uncommon except for treatment-related myeloid neoplasias (tr-MN), which occurred in 3% of patients. The outcome of patients with tr-MN was poor irrespective of treatment. In a multivariate analysis of patients receiving fludarabine-based therapy at MD Anderson, FCR therapy was significantly associated with improved survival, thereby validating the experience with FR, suggesting that rituximab therapy was improving OS.

The benefit of adding rituximab to FC was confirmed by the GCLLSG, which randomized 817 physically fit, previously untreated CLL patients, ages 30 to 81 years, to fludarabine 25 mg/m^2 on days 1 to 3 and cyclophosphamide 250 mg/m^2 IV on days 1 to 3, with or without rituximab 375 mg/m^2 day 0 of cycle 1 and 500 mg/m^2 day 1 of cycles 2 to 6 every 28 days for 6 cycles. A total of 761 patients were evaluable for response. FCR induced higher OR (95 vs. 88%) and CR rates (44 vs. 22%) than FC. Median PFS was 32.8 months for FC and 51.8 months for FCR, and the largest benefit for FCR was observed in Binet stage A and B patients. The OS rate at 37.7 months favored FCR over FC (84% vs. 79%; $P = .01$). FCR resulted in more grade 3 and 4 neutropenia (34% vs. 21%) and leukopenia (24% vs. 12%), but there was no difference in severe infections or treatment-related deaths between the two arms. As with other chemoimmunotherapy trials in CLL, neutropenia was more common with FCR than FC. Emerging from this study were numerous biologic correlative studies showing the most predictive test of long term PFS and OS was attainment of minimal residual disease (MRD)–negative disease by high-sensitivity flow cytometry. In addition, patients with unmutated IgV$_H$ disease had a shorter PFS and OS with both FCR and FC, although rituximab appeared to benefit both treatment groups. All genetic groups benefited from rituximab with the exception of the del(17p13.1) and normal karyotype patients, who had similar outcomes to FC or FCR treatment. Further long-term follow up of this study is ongoing for late complications and assessment of newer prognostic factors identified since initiation of this study. Thus the benefit of chemoimmunotherapy in the frontline treatment of CLL has been clearly demonstrated by studies of both FR and FCR.

Bendamustine and Rituximab

Based on promising single agent activity of bendamustine in previously treated CLL and in vitro studies demonstrating synergy between bendamustine and rituximab, the GCLLSG examined the feasibility and safety of this combination in a phase II study in 78 relapsed CLL patients. Bendamustine was administered at a dose of 70 mg/m^2 days 1 and 2 and rituximab at 375 mg/m^2 on day 0 of cycle 1 and 500 mg/m^2 on day 1 of cycles 2 to 6. Using an intent-to-treat analysis, the ORR was 59% with a CR of 9%. The median PFS was 14.7 months. Response was poor (7%) in the del(17p) patients. Severe infections occurred in 13% of patients. Grade 3 or 4 neutropenia, thrombocytopenia, and anemia were documented in 23%, 28%, and 17% of patients, respectively.

A follow-up study (CLL2M) included a total of 117 symptomatic, previously untreated CLL patients who were treated with bendamustine (90 mg/m^2 on days 1 and 2) and rituximab (375 mg/m^2 in cycle 1 and 500 mg/m^2 in cycle 2 to 6). Treatment was administered every 28 days for up to 6 cycles. Demographics of the patients included a median age of 64 years with 48% having Binet C disease. The ORR was 91%, and the CR was 33%. After 18 months, 76% of patients were still in remission, and median PFS had not been reached at the time of the report. The treatment was well tolerated with cytopenias and infections being most problematic. Treatment-related mortality (TRM) was 2.6%. Patients with all genomic groups except for del(17p13.1) responded favorably. Based on these encouraging phase II data, the GCLLSG initiated a phase III study comparing BR with FCR (CLL10) in previously untreated, physically fit CLL patients that is ongoing at this time.

Chlorambucil and Rituximab

Based on the success of chemoimmunotherapy and the potential absence of benefit of nucleoside analogs in elderly CLL patients, Hillmen and colleagues initiated a study in 100 elderly, previously untreated CLL patients combining rituximab (day 1; 375 mg/m^2 IV cycle 1, 500 mg/m^2 cycles 2-6) and chlorambucil (days 1-7; 10 mg/m^2/day PO) every 28 days for 6 cycles. Patients were permitted to receive 6 additional cycles of chlorambucil if they had evidence of continuing clinical response at 6 cycles. The median age was 70 years. OR rate on an intent-to-treat analysis was 82%, with nine patients achieving CR, 58 patients showing partial response (PR), 15 patients showing nodular PR (nPR), and 11 patients with stable disease (SD). Median PFS to date is 23.5 months. The response in this study was significantly higher in patients receiving chlorambucil alone in the CLL4 study, suggesting a benefit to rituximab. A second Italian phase II study using a similar combination regimen of chlorambucil and rituximab together demonstrated similar favorable response data. Based on these phase II data, a randomized phase III study comparing chlorambucil versus chlorambucil with either rituximab or obinutuzumab is currently ongoing by the GCLLSG, and a similar study is studying ofatumumab and chlorambucil versus single-agent chlorambucil in previously untreated elderly or unfit CLL patients (see box on What Is the Role of Rituximab in Chronic Lymphocytic Leukemia?).

What Is the Role of Rituximab in Chronic Lymphocytic Leukemia?

Studies of rituximab to this point have demonstrated modest single-agent clinical activity in both previously untreated CLL patients using the weekly dosing schedule and in the relapsed state using more intensive dosing regimens. Rituximab does not have activity against CLL with del(17p13.1). For this reason, rituximab monotherapy is generally used in either of these settings only if more definitive therapy cannot be administered because of other comorbid conditions. Rituximab's greatest contribution is to combination therapy both in symptomatic, previously untreated CLL patients and relapsed patients receiving the FR or FCR regimen, particularly in younger patients. Phase III studies have demonstrated the clear benefit of chemoimmunotherapy over traditional chemotherapy alone and, combined with multiple retrospective analyses, established chemoimmunotherapy as the standard of care in CLL. Several phase II studies have combined rituximab with other therapies such as bendamustine, chlorambucil, and pentostatin–cyclophosphamide that might be more tolerable to the more common older patients. Phase III studies with several of these agents are ongoing at this time. Inclusion of rituximab in alternative chemoimmunotherapy regimens for patients not appropriate for fludarabine-containing regimens is reasonable and our current practice approach. Although several phase II studies of maintenance rituximab have been published after completion of chemoimmunotherapy, the benefit of this is uncertain. Until ongoing phase III results are available justifying maintenance rituximab in CLL, it should not be used outside of the context of a clinical trial.

Alemtuzumab

Alemtuzumab is a humanized monoclonal antibody against CD52, a cell-surface glycopeptide expressed on virtually all human lymphocytes, monocytes, and macrophages, a small subset of granulocytes, but not erythrocytes, platelets, or hematopoietic stem cells. CD52 is expressed on all CLL cells and indolent B-NHL cells. The physiological function remains unknown, but crosslinking of CD52 on B-cell and T-cell lymphoma cell lines inhibits their cell proliferation. Alemtuzumab has been demonstrated to mediate apoptosis, CDC, and ADCC of CLL cells in vitro. CD52 is not shed, internalized, or modulated and is therefore an ideal antigen for targeted immunotherapy. However, the ubiquitous expression of CD52 on normal lymphocytes and monocytes is predictive of the increased neutropenia, lymphopenia, and infectious complications observed with alemtuzumab therapy.

Phase I studies of alemtuzumab have established a dose of 30 mg IV three times per week for 4 to 12 weeks. Alemtuzumab induced significantly more infusion-related toxicity than rituximab, but stepped-up dosing diminished initial infusion-related toxicity and made administration of the antibody tolerable and feasible. Three milligrams is given on the first day, 10 mg on day 2, and 30 mg on day 3; after dose escalation, patients receive 30 mg thrice weekly. Several clinical studies have established a role for alemtuzumab in CLL. In a multicenter European phase II study, alemtuzumab was administered at 30 mg thrice weekly for up to 12 weeks to 29 recurrent and refractory CLL patients. The ORR was 42%, but only one patient (4%) achieved a CR. Alemtuzumab cleared CLL cells from the peripheral blood in 97% of patients but was less effective at eliminating BM (36%) or nodal disease (7%).

The pivotal CAM211 trial administered the same regimen of alemtuzumab therapy to 93 heavily pretreated, fludarabine-refractory CLL patients. The ORR was 33%, but only 2% of patients achieved a CR. Median time to progression for responders was 9.5 months, with a median OS of 16 months for all patients and 32 months for responders. The median peripheral blood CLL count decreased by more than 99.9%, but the antibody was less effective against nodal disease, particularly in patients with bulky lymph nodes larger than 5 cm in diameter. Although 90% of patients with lymph nodes measuring less than or equal to 2 cm responded, with 64% achieving resolution of adenopathy, only 12% of patients with lymph nodes greater than 5 cm responded with no patients attaining resolution of their adenopathy. All patients were placed on prophylactic antibiotics and antiviral agents, and treatment-related toxicity was manageable. Patients with a poor performance status did markedly worse than patients with no or minimal symptoms from their disease, likely owing to their reduced ability to tolerate the hematologic and infectious side effects of alemtuzumab, and no patients with ECOG performance status greater than 1 responded to therapy. The activity of alemtuzumab was later confirmed by a multi-institutional, compassionate use study in 136 patients with fludarabine-refractory CLL.

The GCLLSG explored the use of subcutaneous (SC) alemtuzumab for patients with relapsed CLL in an attempt to diminish infusion-related toxicity associated with this regimen. This study administered alemtuzumab 3, 10, and 30 mg IV during week 1 followed by 30 mg SC thrice weekly for 4 to 12 weeks. A total of 109 heavily treated patients were treated. The ORR (34%), CR rate (4%), median duration of PFS (7.7 months), and median OS (19.1 months) were virtually identical to the results achieved with IV alemtuzumab in the CAM211 study. Additionally, the response rate was similar in patients with high-risk cytogenetic abnormalities with del(11q22.3) and del(17p13.1). Infusional toxicity with this treatment was minimal, and inflammation at the sites of injection was mild. Toxicity included grade 3/4 neutropenia (56%), thrombocytopenia (57%), and anemia. Grade 3/4 infections (29%) and cytomegalovirus (CMV) infections (8%) were also observed. In this study, long-term survival was best predicted by subsequent allogeneic SCT indicating the poor prognosis of this refractory patient group.

Based on promising data in relapsed disease, a phase II clinical trial of alemtuzumab administered at a dose of 30 mg SC three times per week for up to 18 weeks to 41 previously untreated patients with CLL was performed. Except for transient grade 1 to 2 fever, adverse reactions after the first were minimal. The ORR was 81% on an intent-to-treat basis, and 87% of the 38 patients who received at least 2 weeks of treatment responded. Alemtuzumab was more active in this setting with an ORR of 87% and CR of 29%. Some patients who achieved a CR in the BM required the full 18 weeks of therapy to do so, suggesting that prolonged administration was necessary to clear CLL cells from the BM. On the basis of these promising results in the upfront setting, the CAM307 study prospectively randomized 297 previously untreated CLL patients to oral chlorambucil 40 mg/m^2 every 4 weeks for 12 cycles or alemtuzumab 30 mg IV three times per week for up to 12 weeks. All patients on the alemtuzumab arm received prophylaxis for *Pneumocystis carinii* and varicella zoster. Alemtuzumab achieved a superior ORR (83% vs. 55%), CR rate (22% vs. 2%), and duration of PFS (23.3 vs. 14.7 months). Response in del(11q22.3) and del(17p13.1) patients was improved over chlorambucil, but the median PFS was less than 1 year, indicating a very modest benefit of this treatment. Non–infusion-related toxicity between the two treatment arms was similar except for more nausea with the chlorambucil and increased CMV viremia (52.4% vs. 7.5%) with alemtuzumab. This registration study had no late analysis for survival outcome or late toxicity associated with this treatment.

Owing to the ubiquitous expression of CD52 on lymphocytes and monocytes, immunosuppression and infectious complications constitute the most concerning toxicity of alemtuzumab. Although alemtuzumab also depletes B cells, CD8$^+$ T cells, NK cells, and monocytes, the antibody's most profound effect is its ablation of CD4$^+$ T lymphocytes. This delayed recovery of CD4$^+$ T-lymphocytes has been observed by multiple investigators. The absolute CD4$^+$ T-cell count reached a nadir of 2/μL by week 4 and increased only to 84/μL by week 12 in the CAM211 trial. Furthermore, alemtuzumab depleted CD52$^+$ myeloid peripheral blood dendritic cells, inhibiting the ability of peripheral blood mononuclear cells (PBMCs) to present antigen to purified CD4$^+$ T lymphocytes.

Given this prolonged immunosuppression, alemtuzumab should be administered carefully, particularly when the antibody is given in combination with other immunosuppressive agents such as fludarabine. Patients receiving alemtuzumab are at an increased risk for bacterial, fungal, viral, and other opportunistic infections as demonstrated by multiple clinical trials. For instance, 55% of patients in the CAM211 study developed infections (27% grade 3-4), and 13% experienced septicemia. Patients receiving alemtuzumab must therefore be placed on appropriate prophylaxis for *P. carinii* pneumonia and varicella zoster infection/reactivation. Additionally, CMV infection monitoring by PCR or hybrid capture assays should be performed regularly during and for at least 2 to 3 months after therapy with alemtuzumab. Alternatively, the MD Anderson group has demonstrated in a small randomized trial that valganciclovir prophylaxis during alemtuzumab treatment eliminates the risk of CMV reactivation. If prophylactic therapy is not used, patients who reactivate CMV should be treated appropriately. With these prophylactic measures, alemtuzumab can be administered safely and with acceptable infection-related morbidity in most patients. The approach of CMV monitoring and treatment of increasing CMV viremia is the approach that our group takes when administering alemtuzumab, caused by the cytopenias associated with valganciclovir and cost of this therapy that is prohibitive to most patients. Other toxicities with alemtuzumab, including infusion events (more common with IV administration) and cytopenias, are treated with traditional support provided to patients with leukemia. Although alemtuzumab received full marketing approval for initial and relapse therapy of CLL, this agent is very uncommonly used in CLL as monotherapy at this time because of the serious toxicity and modest benefit it offers to these patients.

Chemoimmunotherapy With Alemtuzumab

Several groups have pursued adding alemtuzumab, similar to rituximab, either concurrently or sequentially with several chemotherapeutic agents for the treatment of previously treated or symptomatic untreated CLL patients. Results of these studies have not yet translated to a standard therapy used for the treatment of patients with CLL. In virtually all of the studies, increased toxicity has been observed compared with standard regimens. Additionally, in two studies adding alemtuzumab to FCR, the MD Anderson group was unable to demonstrate added benefit in high-risk CLL patients. Because these approaches will likely not be applied in future treatment regimens for CLL, they are not summarized further.

Alemtuzumab as Consolidation Therapy After Chemotherapy

Given the ability of alemtuzumab to clear BM of CLL cells and to eliminate MRD, several investigators have examined the use of alemtuzumab as consolidation therapy after initial induction therapy with fludarabine. In one report, alemtuzumab was administered at a dose of 10 or 30 mg IV thrice weekly for 4 weeks to 58 patients who had responded to their most recent therapy but still had residual disease. The ORR was 53%, and the response rate was dose dependent; 65% of patients who received 30 mg responded compared with 39% of patients who received 10 mg. Eleven of 29 patients (38%) achieved MRD-negative BM, and the TTP was not reached after a median follow-up of 24 months. In addition, the TTP was significantly longer in patients who had no BM MRD after alemtuzumab consolidation. Similar findings were reported by the GCLLSG, which randomized 21 eligible patients, who had responded to fludarabine or Flu/Cy induction therapy but still had persistent disease, to observation ($n = 10$) or alemtuzumab 30 mg IV thrice weekly for up to 12 weeks ($n = 11$). The study was discontinued early as a result of increased toxicity in the alemtuzumab arm; six of 11 patients experienced grade 4 hematologic toxicity, and seven of 11 patients developed grade 3 or 4 infectious complications, including four patients with CMV. However, five of six evaluable patients had no MRD in the BM with alemtuzumab consolidation. After a median follow-up of 48 months, the median PFS favored the alemtuzumab arm (not reached vs. 20.6 months) with only three of 11 patients who received alemtuzumab relapsing. On the basis of these promising results, the GCLLSG FLL2i study is currently evaluating the optimal dose and schedule of alemtuzumab consolidation after initial fludarabine-based therapy.

The administration of alemtuzumab SC has also been examined in the consolidation setting in two additional trials. The CALGB 19901 study administered fludarabine 25 mg/m^2 IV daily for 5 days every 28 days for 6 cycles followed by alemtuzumab 30 mg either IV or SC thrice weekly for 6 weeks with previously untreated CLL. Of the 85 evaluable patients enrolled, four (5%) attained a CR, and 43 (51%) attained a partial response after fludarabine induction for an ORR of 55%. Thirty-nine patients received IV alemtuzumab for consolidation with improvement in CR to 27% and ORR to 73%. Twenty patients received SC alemtuzumab consolidation with improvement in CR to 17% and ORR to 69%. Toxicity from IV alemtuzumab included infusion-related reactions and infection. Mild local inflammation was common from SC alemtuzumab. Nine of 59 (15%) patients had CMV infections with one death. Given the lack of intensity of induction therapy with fludarabine, CALGB planned a second study with more intensive induction as part of CALGB 10101. Patients received fludarabine and rituximab (FR) similar to that administered in CALGB 9712 for 6 cycles. Three months after completion of FR, patients with stable disease or better response received SC alemtuzumab using stepped-up dosing week 1 followed by 30 mg three times per week for 5 weeks. The ORR was 90% and CR rate was 29%. Of 102 patients enrolled, 58 received alemtuzumab; 28 (61%) of 46 patients achieving PR after FR attained CR after alemtuzumab. By intent to treat for all patients at completion of therapy, the ORR was 90% and CR rate was 57%. With median follow-up of 36 months, the median PFS was 36 months, 2-year PFS was 72%, and 2-year OS was 86%. In patients achieving CR after FR, alemtuzumab was associated with five deaths resulting from infection (viral and *Listeria* meningitis and *Legionella,* CMV, and *Pneumocystis* pneumonias), which occurred up to 7 months after the last therapy. Most importantly, alemtuzumab in this study did not abrogate the adverse outcome associated with high-risk genetic features, including del(17p13.1), del(11q22.3), and IgV_H-unmutated CLL. Additionally, PFS and OS in this study did not appear better than the FR regimen previously reported by CALGB. Future efforts with this approach are not being pursued by the US Intergroup.

What Is Alemtuzumab's Role in Chronic Lymphocytic Leukemia?

As a result of the ubiquitous expression of CD52 on lymphocytes and monocytes, alemtuzumab causes significantly more hematologic and immune toxicity than does rituximab, and careful monitoring of and prophylaxis for potential infections is required for any administration of alemtuzumab. Although the different toxicities of alemtuzumab are manageable, its integration into CLL therapy has been somewhat challenging based on the difficulty of administering it with other myelosuppressive or immunosuppressive therapies used for CLL either concurrently or as consolidation therapy. Additionally, although it is effective in all high-risk groups based on genetic abnormalities, including those with del(17p13.1), it does not work well for patients with bulky lymph nodes. These numerous limitations have greatly impaired the use of alemtuzumab in the treatment of CLL. Furthermore, the advent of newer therapeutic agents with activity against del(17p13.1) may offer clinicians safer yet effective treatments for this high-risk population. Although several such agents have shown activity against genetically high-risk CLL, none of these agents has yet shown the ability to achieve CR in the BM and eradicate MRD to the same degree as alemtuzumab.

TREATMENT OF PATIENTS WITH RELAPSED CHRONIC LYMPHOCYTIC LEUKEMIA

The approach to reinitiating therapy for CLL patients who have relapsed after initial therapy is similar to that applied for initial therapy assessment. Patients need not receive therapy at the first sign of relapse. Rather, patients should have an indication for treatment, as discussed earlier. Patients should have repeat interphase FISH analysis of the peripheral blood or BM aspirate because patients may acquire additional cytogenetic abnormalities, most notably del(17p13.1), as their CLL becomes more advanced. The incidence of del(17p13.1) increases from 5% of patients at initial diagnosis to nearly half of heavily treated patients with advanced CLL, and acquisition of this abnormality has profound implications on treatment, as will be discussed later. IgV_H mutational analysis does not need to be performed if such information has been obtained previously because a patient's IgV_H mutational status does not change with time. A BM should be performed if cytopenias are present to confirm that CLL is the cause and to exclude other potential causes of cytopenias such as transformed lymphoma, prolonged BM toxicity from prior therapy, or development of treatment-related myelodysplasia. Patients should be treated according to the indications outlined in Table 76-4. An algorithm to our treatment approach to first relapsed CLL is summarized in Fig. 76-2. In general, for patients younger than the age of 70 years who have experienced a good remission with initial therapy for longer than 24 months, an FCR or BR regimen, preferably in combination with an investigational agent, is suggested. If a complete remission is obtained in the absence of del(17p13.1), our approach at this point is to observe. If a del(17p13.1) is present or a complete response to therapy is not obtained, we generally will consider a nonmyeloablative allogenetic SCT. For patients relapsing who are 70 years or older, retreatment with the same therapy, BR or an alternative antibody or investigational agent can be considered. In general, we do not administer FCR to this patient population owing to concerns of increasing toxicity.

Ofatumumab in Relapsed Chronic Lymphocytic Leukemia

Ofatumumab

Ofatumumab is a fully human type I anti-CD20 monoclonal antibody that was initially approved for the treatment of CLL in late 2009. In vitro, it has improved CDC, ADC, and direct killing (with cross-linking), compared with rituximab. Ofatumumab has a different binding epitope of CD20 than rituximab, binding to both the small and large extracellular loops of CD20, and a slower off rate as well. Ofatumumab is able to kill rituximab-resistant CLL cells because of greater induction of CDC and its ability to kill cells with low CD20 expression, which may be relevant given the low CD20 expression on CLL cells. Based on these promising data, a phase I/II study of ofatumumab, given at doses of 500 to 2000 weekly for four doses in 33 relapsed or refractory CLL patients, demonstrated that it is generally well tolerated even at higher doses. Ofatumumab was active, with an ORR of 50% in the highest cohort treated at 2000 mg. Infusion-related adverse events were similar to those reported with rituximab and decreased after the first infusion. Infections were fairly common, occurring in 51% of patients, including one fatal infection. These results prompted a pivotal, single-arm study of ofatumumab administered as 8 weekly infusions of ofatumumab followed by 4 monthly infusions. Patients received 300 mg as the first dose to minimize infusion-related reactions, and the dose was increased to 2000 mg for all subsequent infusions. Patients included in this study were required to be fludarabine refractory and to also be alemtuzumab-refractory (FA-refractory group; n = 95) or to have bulky lymphadenopathy larger than 5 cm (BF-refractory group; n = 111). The ORR, as assessed by an independent review committee, was 51% for the FA-refractory group and 44% for the BR-refractory group, with two CRs observed in the BF-refractory group. All other responses were partial. The median duration of response was 5.7 months in the FA-refractory group and 6.0 months in the BF-refractory group with most patients progressing during treatment. The median PFS was 5.5 months in both the FA-refractory and BF-refractory groups. Median OS was 14.2 months and 17.4 months, respectively. For rituximab-treated (n = 117), rituximab-refractory (n = 98), and rituximab-naive (n = 89) patients, the OR rates were 43%, 44%, and 53%, respectively; median PFS was 5.3, 5.5, and 5.6 months, respectively; and median OS was 15.5, 15.5, and 20.2 months, respectively. Thus prior exposure to rituximab did not affect the response to ofatumumab.

The presence of del(17p13.1) was associated with a lower response rate and shorter median PFS in both patient groups (37% vs. 56% and 3.3 months vs. 5.5 months in FA-refractory group; 22% vs. 49% and 3.8 vs. 5.6 months in BF-refractory group). Thus, in contrast to rituximab, ofatumumab is active as a single agent in del(17p13.1) CLL but has inferior activity compared with alemtuzumab. Toxicity included infusion-related reactions, infections, and cytopenias. This trial led to accelerated approval of ofatumumab for the treatment of patients with fludarabine- and alemtuzumab-refractory CLL, and a phase III study of ofatumumab versus physician's choice of therapy in bulky, fludarabine-refractory CLL is ongoing. Determination of the clinical superiority of ofatumumab over rituximab will require randomized trials comparing equivalent doses. Currently, several phase III studies of ofatumumab in combination with chlorambucil (initial treatment), FC (salvage), or as single agent maintenance therapy in CLL are ongoing.

Stem Cell Transplantation

For many years, autologous and allogeneic SCTs were generally used for treatment of CLL late in the course of the disease. However, trials of SCTs have indicated that patients with multiply relapsed and chemotherapy-resistant disease are at highest risk for both relapse and TRM. Additionally, many patients with heavily treated CLL cannot be adequately cytoreduced or disease control cannot be maintained for a sufficient period of time to obtain insurance approval and find a suitable allogeneic donor, producing a selection bias that often excludes patients with the most refractory or aggressive disease from actually receiving SCT. The recognition that patients with poor prognostic features such as del(11q22.3) and del(17p13.1) and patients who fail to achieve CR after receiving regimens such as FCR have a short remission duration to initial therapy has prompted many transplant centers to consider earlier application of allogenic SCT as therapy for CLL, including its use as consolidation treatment after induction therapy for the highest risk patients. Referral of high-risk CLL patients at the time of initial treatment to an experienced transplant center for evaluation, potential tissue typing of the patient and his or her siblings, and initiation of an unrelated donor search (if needed) should be considered. Although autologous SCT has been used historically as a treatment for CLL and has been reviewed elsewhere, nonmyeloablative allogeneic SCT is the preferred modality for most patients requiring a transplant unless a suitable allogeneic donor is not available. Autologous SCT is no longer utilized in CLL because of a lack of a survival advantage, only modest benefit in PFS, and a high risk of tr-MN with this modality. Therefore, autologous SCT is not reviewed in this chapter.

Myeloablative Allogeneic Stem Cell Transplantation

Allogeneic SCT offers several theoretical advantages over autologous SCT in CLL. The use of an allogeneic donor provides an immunologic graft-versus-leukemia (GVL) effect for patients with CLL. Limited data suggest that TBI-containing conditioning regimens are superior to chemotherapy-only regimens in CLL transplant patients. A small study of 25 patients demonstrated a 100-day TRM of 57% in patients who received busulfan and cyclophosphamide (Bu/Cy; $n = 7$), compared to 17% for patients who received a TBI regimen ($n = 18$). Five-year actuarial survival was 56% for 14 patients transplanted with TBI regimens during 1992-1999. A study of Cy/TBI in 28 CLL patients observed a 100-day TRM of 11%. Five-year PFS and OS were 78% and 78% for chemosensitive patients compared with 26% and 31% for refractory patients.

A retrospective EBMT study of 135 patients showed 54% 3-year OS and 40% 100-day TRM. The IBMTR reported similar findings, with 45% 3-year OS and 30% 100-day TRM in 242 patients. The high TRM may be explained in part by the late stage of the disease in many of these patients. Median time from diagnosis to SCT was 41 and 46 months in these two studies, and 37% of patients in the EBMT study were chemorefractory before transplant. In a Canadian study of allogeneic SCT in 30 CLL patients, the 5-year EFS and OS were both 39%, with 48% OS for patients with sibling donors. The role of unrelated donor allogeneic SCT was examined by a multicenter study in 38 patients, 92% of whom received TBI. Five-year FFS and OS were 30% and 33%, and TRM was 38%. Although there are no prospective randomized studies, a retrospective comparison showed a 3-year DFS of 57% for allogeneic SCT versus 24% for purged autologous SCT. Finally, allogeneic SCT appears to overcome the adverse prognosis associated with an unmutated IgV_H; an analysis of 34 CLL patients who underwent SCT found that only two of 14 patients who received allogeneic SCT relapsed, compared with 13 of 20 patients who underwent autologous SCT.

Thus myeloablative allogeneic SCT may provide superior DFS to patients with CLL compared with autologous SCT. Although the 3-year DFS after allogeneic SCT is approximately 50%, longer follow-up is needed to determine if the disease remissions are durable. However, this DFS advantage is offset by significantly higher TRM, thus limiting the use of allogeneic SCT in CLL. Limited data indicate that Bu/Cy may be particularly toxic in this population; by contrast, TBI regimens have acceptable TRM. To preserve the immunologic GVL effect while reducing TRM, the focus of clinical SCT research in CLL has turned to nonmyeloablative, or reduced-intensity, allogeneic SCT.

Nonmyeloablative Allogeneic Stem Cell Therapy

Ideally, the goal is to harness the GVL effect of allogeneic SCT for patients with CLL while reducing TRM from acute graft-versus-host-disease (GVHD), acute infection, and organ toxicity associated with myeloablative conditioning. Fludarabine, busulfan, and ATG were administered to 30 German CLL patients; the stem cell source was a matched related ($n = 15$) or unrelated ($n = 15$) donor. Grade 2 to 4 acute GVHD was observed in 56% of patients, and 75% developed chronic GVHD. Responses were seen in 93% of patients, with 40% achieving CR. Of note, it took up to 2 years for patients to achieve CR, suggesting a GVL effect. All patients achieved a molecular CR by PCR, but only six patients were in continued molecular CR after a median follow-up of 2 years. Two-year TRM, PFS, and OS were 15%, 67%, and 72%, respectively.

The EBMT retrospectively examined 77 CLL patients who received a variety of nonmyeloablative conditioning regimens, followed by allogeneic SCT. The 1-year TRM was 18%, and the 2-year probability of relapse was 31%. Two-year DFS and OS were 56% and 72%, respectively. Nineteen patients received donor lymphocyte infusions (DLIs) for relapse or incomplete donor chimerism, but only seven responded to DLI (37%). Unfortunately, this study was complicated by the heterogeneity of conditioning regimens and the use of ATG or Campath-1H for T-cell depletion of the grafts in 40% of patients. A retrospective analysis of 73 CLL patients who underwent nonmyeloablative SCT and 82 patients who underwent myeloablative allogeneic SCT showed that the TRM was significantly reduced in the former group, with a hazard ratio of 0.4; however, there was no difference in EFS or OS between the two groups.

Sixty-four patients received 200 cGy of TBI, with ($n = 53$) or without ($n = 11$) fludarabine followed by an allogeneic SCT from a related ($n = 44$) or unrelated ($n = 20$) donor. The 2-year DFS and OS were 52% and 60%, respectively, and the 2-year TRM was 22%. The incidence of relapse at 2 years was 26%, and the mortality due to relapse was 18%. Finally, a British study of 41 CLL patients who received fludarabine, melphalan, and alemtuzumab followed by an allogeneic SCT from a related ($n = 24$) or unrelated ($n = 17$) donor observed a 2-year OS and TRM of 51% and 26%. Eleven patients (27%) relapsed and received escalated donor lymphocyte infusions, but only three patients had a sustained response to DLI. Five patients (12%) have died of relapse.

Nonmyeloablative allogeneic SCT may be superior to autologous SCT in obtaining clinical and molecular remissions in high-risk CLL patients with unmutated IgV_H because of a GVL effect. Seven of nine patients (78%) in a German study became negative by PCR for allele-specific IgVH after d100 post-SCT; attainment of molecular CR occurred after DLI or development of chronic GVHD. In contrast, only six of 26 control CLL patients (23%) achieved a PCR-negative state after autologous SCT. Similar findings were reported by a Spanish study of nonmyeloablative SCT in 30 CLL patients. The 6-year EFS and OS were 92% and 90% for patients with unmutated IgV_H or del(11q). Several other studies from MD Anderson, Germany, and the University of Washington transplant groups have confirmed these findings. Thus an immunologic GVL effect appears to be important in CLL and may confer a long-term survival advantage for allogeneic SCT, given sufficient time.

Investigational Agents Currently in Phase II–III Testing for Relapsed CLL

Although numerous therapeutic agents are currently being tested in CLL, many of these agents will ultimately fail to gain an indication for CLL or are many years away from approval. Attention is therefore directed toward agents that are currently in phase III registration studies based on preliminary efficacy in relapsed CLL.

Lenalidomide

Lenalidomide, or 3-(4-amino-1,3-dihydro-1-oxo-2*H*-isoindol-2-yl)-2,6-piperidinedione (Revlimid), is an immunomodulatory drug (IMiD) that is a more potent analog of thalidomide. Lenalidomide is approved for marketing in multiple myeloma and transfusion-dependent myelodysplasia. Lenalidomide has clinical activity in a variety of other malignancies, including CLL. Two initial studies examining either an intermittent 25 mg PO daily for 21 days and 5 mg with dose escalation to 10 mg PO as tolerated given as continuous therapy were pursued initially in relapsed CLL. The higher dose, intermittent schedule was active with an ORR of 47% and 9% CR. Major side effects of this therapy were cytopenias, rash, and tumor flare, which in some cases can be life threatening. The continuous, low-dose regimen had a 32% intent-to-treat ORR with a 7% CR rate. Toxicity was less with this schedule but still included cytopenias in most. On the basis of these promising phase II clinical studies, a large, multicenter trial randomizing patients to low-dose (10 mg) or high-dose (25 mg) lenalidomide was undertaken, which was halted early because of life-threatening adverse events in patients receiving the higher dose of therapy. Subsequent studies have shown that lower doses of lenalidomide administered as continuous treatment in patients with relapsed CLL are feasible. These have prompted several single agent studies in symptomatic, previously untreated CLL in which the clinical activity has ranged from an ORR of 56% to 65% with up to 10% CR. Most provocative from these studies was the observation that lenalidomide reversed the hypogammaglobulinemia observed in CLL patients. PFS with this treatment is approximately 2 years. Toxicity, including tumor flare, cytopenias, rash, and infection, has been noted but is manageable.

In an attempt to understand both the pathogenesis of tumor flare and immunoglobulin recovery, laboratory work by our group and others has demonstrated that lenalidomide activates CLL cells to promote expression of CD154, CD80, and CD86 that makes them more immunogenic, visible to the immune system, and potentially proliferative in node and BM sanctuaries. These activated CLL cells also can serve as a second signal with T cells to promote normal B cells to produce antibody, thus possibly explaining why hypogammaglobulinemia is reversed in many of these patients. Other studies have shown lenalidomide enhances T-cell and NK cell response to CLL cells.

Moving forward, efforts with lenalidomide have focused in part on combining it with other agents, most notably anti-CD20 antibodies such as rituximab and ofatumumab, or as consolidation therapy after purine analog or bendamustine-based induction therapy. Preliminary reports have suggested diminished tumor flare when administered with therapeutic antibodies but increased cytopenias and adverse events when combined with chemoimmunotherapy regimens. Similarly, lenalidomide has been given as consolidation maintenance as part of several phase II chemoimmunotherapy trials. In one such study with PCR-based treatment, consolidation therapy with lenalidomide appeared to potentially extend PFS over that previously seen with PCR alone. Based on the clinical activity observed with lenalidomide, two phase III registration studies are currently underway examining lenalidomide versus chlorambucil for elderly CLL and as a consolidation therapy after second treatment for this disease. The recent recognition of the profound immunologic effects of lenalidomide on CLL suggest that it might also serve as an effective agent earlier in the course of the disease or as an adjuvant to vaccine-based approaches. These are currently being pursued at this time as well by several different groups. Because of the relative modest activity in heavily pretreated patients, other alternatives in first-line therapy, and potential for life-threatening tumor flair and other toxicity with lenalidomide, this agent should only be considered as part of a well-designed clinical trial despite its FDA approval for other indications (MDS and multiple myeloma).

Agents Targeting B-Cell Receptor Signaling Pathways

B-cell receptor signaling and microenvironmental signals are now known to be important in both proliferation and protection of CLL cells in BM and nodal sites. These findings have prompted the introduction of several novel, orally available kinase inhibitors. In particular, agents targeting the δ isoform of PI3-kinase and Bruton tyrosine kinase (Btk) have shown very promising clinical activity and, more importantly, durability of remission over time in refractory CLL patients. The results of these studies are summarized below.

Fostamatinib disodium is a multitargeted kinase inhibitor whose primary target is syk. An early phase I/II study of fostamatinib in NHL and CLL was undertaken based on preclinical data showing a potential for therapeutic benefit. This phase II study noted modest activity in NHL patients, but six of 11 (55%) CLL/SLL patients responded with rapid reduction of nodal disease and transient lymphocytosis suggestive of CLL cell compartmental mobilization. Because of off-target effects of this drug, tolerability was not optimal with many patients noting diarrhea, fatigue, cytopenias, hypertension, and nausea. Although this agent did not move forward for development in CLL, it served as the first hint that targeting syk and other BCR signaling pathways may be worthwhile.

GS1101 (formerly CAL-101) is an orally bioavailable, isoform specific, PI3-kinase-δ inhibitor that, at therapeutic levels obtained in patients, does not inhibit other isoforms of PI3-kinase. Genetic mouse models knocking out PI3-kinase delta demonstrate predominantly a B-cell defect, absent B1 lymphocytes, and disrupted BCR signaling. Preclinical studies by our group and later confirmed by others demonstrated that GS1101 promotes the apoptosis of CLL cells via a PI3-kinase-δ pathway and inhibits signals from the microenvironment that protects CLL cells from apoptosis. Based in part on these data, a phase I study in healthy volunteers showed this agent to be well tolerated, and subsequently a large phase I study in NHL, CLL, multiple myeloma, and AML was undertaken. GS1101 was active at all dose levels tested, with the dose-limiting toxicity being reversible transaminitis that generally occurs during the first 2 months of therapy in approximately 5% to 20% of patients, depending on histology. Although patients with NHL experienced a higher incidence of transaminitis, perhaps caused by occult liver involvement by tumor, the incidence of transaminitis was less than 5% in CLL patients. In the phase I study, 57 relapsed CLL patients have been treated with a median of 5 prior regimens. Notable with this treatment was that 90% had a 50% or greater nodal response but with 26% also having class specific lymphocytosis. However, 14 of 54 CLL patients (26%) achieved durable remissions that exceeded 1 year. Responses were noted across all genetic groups of CLL. Toxicity with this treatment included pneumonia and liver function abnormalities but not myelosuppression. Subsequent studies have been undertaken with GS1101 combining it with rituximab, ofatumumab, and bendamustine/rituximab, showing that combination therapy with GS1101 is feasible and does not result in increased liver toxicity. Given the high rate of response and durable remissions observed with GS-1101, registration studies with this agent in CLL are now being undertaken.

PCI32765 is a potent, irreversible inhibitor of Btk. Btk is a tyrosine kinase in the Tec family of tyrosine kinases and is an essential element of the BCR signaling pathway. Genetic knock-out or inactivation of Btk in mice produces predominantly a B-cell defect with absent B1 lymphocytes, diminished B cells, and disrupted BCR signaling. Mutations in Btk in humans result in a more profound humoral immune defect with absent B-cells, immunoglobulin, and infections. Preclinical work with PCI32765 demonstrated disruption of BCR signaling and in vivo activity in spontaneous canine lymphoma models with documented targeted inhibition of Btk. Preclinical trials demonstrated that PCI32765 promotes apoptosis of CLL cells, inhibits activation of PI3-kinase, ERK1, and NFκB by external microenvironment signals, and also prevents CLL proliferation. Collectively, these preclinical studies prompted phase I/II studies with PCI32765 in NHL and CLL. The phase I study of PCI32765 was completed after two dose levels above where Btk inhibition occurred without obtaining a maximum tolerated dose. At the highest dose, toxicity was quite mild, including grade 1/2 nausea, diarrhea, infections, rash, and fatigue. Activity was seen at all doses, including in nine of 16 CLL/SLL patients. A phase IB/II study in CLL patients was undertaken in which 61 patients with relapsed disease were treated daily at a dose of 420 mg ($n = 27$) or 840 mg ($n = 34$). The patients' median age was 60 years, and the median number of prior therapies was four. Median follow-up for the 420 mg and 840 mg cohorts was 12.6 months and 9.3 months, respectively. As with GS1101, the clinical response was characterized by early lymphocytosis accompanied by rapid reduction in the size of lymph nodes, later followed by reduction of lymphocytosis in the majority of patients. Response by IWCLL 2008 criteria was similar (67% and 68%) by dose, with 22% and 24% additional patients having 50% nodal reduction but incomplete resolution of lymphocytosis (nodal response). PFS was estimated to be 86% at 1 year. Of note, only three of 61 patients have gone off study because of progressive disease. Additionally, response has been noted independent of associated genetic abnormalities del(17p13.1). Subsequent studies have been undertaken with PCI3276 combining it with ofatumumab and bendamustine–rituximab, showing that these combinations are feasible. Based on these promising results, registration studies in CLL are now being undertaken with PCI32765.

At the time of writing this chapter, it is apparent that these new inhibitors of BCR signaling will have great impact on the treatment of CLL, particularly given the well-tolerated and durable remissions that are being achieved in relapsed patients. At select CLL centers that also focus on allogeneic SCT, a decline in the number of transplants is being observed based in part on the durable remissions induced in patients considering transplant who have elected to delay this option.

Chimeric Antigen Receptor T-Cell Therapy

To date, efforts at reverting T-cell immune suppression toward the tumor cells have been relatively limited. A major development has been preclinical and early phase I studies demonstrating that ex vivo transfected T-cells with chimeric T-cell receptors bearing both CD3 and also a B cell–specific antigen (most often CD19) have great potential to eradicate established B-cell tumors after administration into both xenograft models and, recently, patients with refractory CLL. Significant development and optimization with chimeric antigen receptor T-cell therapy (CAR-T) cells remains, however, before this can be readily administered widely.

Other Agents in Late Clinical Trials for Chronic Lymphocytic Leukemia

Several other promising therapeutics are in late phase II/III clinical trials for CLL. Those with documented activity in this disease that have potential to be approved for use in CLL are describe d here.

The cyclin-dependent kinase inhibitor flavopiridol is a first-generation molecule with approximately a 50% response rate in highly refractory CLL with the dose-limiting side effect of tumor lysis syndrome but producing durable remissions in a subset of CLL patients, including those with del(17p13.1). Off-target effects of flavopiridol promoting diarrhea and fatigue prompted transition to a second-generation CDK inhibitor dinaciclib, which has a more favorable therapeutic index. This agent has completed phase I studies in CLL with similar efficacy of flavopiridol, including dose-limiting toxicity of hyperacute tumor lysis syndrome but absent many of the off-target effects of flavopiridol. Dinaciclib will be entering a phase III licensing study for therapy of relapsed CLL.

The bcl-2 antiapoptotic protein is overexpressed in CLL and has been shown to disrupt apoptosis in this disease. Although the bcl-2 antisense molecule genasense did not meet the bar for regulatory approval in CLL, attempts to target bcl-2 with small molecule inhibitors have proceeded. The most potent inhibitor of bcl-2, Navitoclax (formerly ABT263), has demonstrated single agent activity in relapsed CLL with a target specific (BCL-XL) dose-limiting toxicity of profound thrombocytopenia. A second-generation inhibitor (ABT199) that lacks off-target effect on BCL-XL is now entering phase I studies.

GA101 is a type II human CD20 directed antibody that is also glycoengineered to have enhanced NK-cell mediated ADCC. As a type II CD20 antibody, GA-101 has the ability to induce direct apoptosis of CLL and NHL tumor cells but lacks CDC activity. GA101 has completed phase I studies in NHL and CLL where clinical activity was shown in a dose-dependent fashion. GA101 is now being tested in a phase III registration study in combination with chlorambucil versus chlorambucil alone. In addition, it is being tested as both a single agent in previously untreated CLL and also in combination with FC.

Therapeutic antibodies or small modular immune pharmaceuticals (SMIP) targeting surface antigens, including CD19 (Xm5574), CD37 (TRU-016, IMGN529 and MAb 37.1), and BAFF-R (VAY736), are under development. Additionally, therapeutic agents targeting signal transduction pathways (HSP-90 inhibitors, AKT inhibitors, ILK inhibitors, NFκB inhibitors, and PP2A activating agents) are in early clinical development. Finally, agents targeting epigenetic events or innate immune activation (CpG oligonucleotides or IL-21) have promising data to support their ongoing early clinical investigation.

Management of Chronic Lymphocytic Leukemia in Specialized Centers

Given the recent advent of prognostic markers and treatment options in CLL, a recent study that examined the impact of physician expertise on patient outcomes in CLL has shown that disease-specific expertise made significant differences in outcomes across all aspects of patient care from prognostic evaluation to choice of therapy. These findings suggest that the expertise of the physician caring for the patient with CLL/SLL is an independent prognostic variable that may not be related to the number of patients he or she manages. We therefore recommend that all patients with newly diagnosed CLL/SLL should be managed in consultation with a CLL expert at a tertiary care center with access to the most recent molecular diagnostic tools.

SPECIAL CLINICAL SCENARIOS IN CHRONIC LYMPHOCYTIC LEUKEMIA

Young Patients (Younger Than 50 Years of Age) With Chronic Lymphocytic Leukemia

As mentioned previously, CLL is a disease of elderly adults, with only 10% of patients being younger than the age of 50 years at diagnosis. Although CLL patients live for a prolonged period of time, young patients without comorbid illnesses have a great potential to have their lives significantly shortened by the disease, irrespective of their cytogenetic abnormalities. Additionally, stress associated with job performance, insurance coverage maintenance, and disease-related symptoms are most significant in this age group. Special attention to psychosocial issues related to CLL should occur early in the course of the disease to allow patients to maintain or resume their normal lifestyles as soon as possible. In the absence of impending need for therapy, our approach is generally not to empirically pursue HLA typing or examine transplant options before the development of symptomatic disease. When therapy is initiated for this group of patients, consideration of aggressive intervention to promote prolonged remission duration is always a top priority. SCT is generally considered for patients in this age group with CLL with high-risk cytogenetic abnormalities in first remission and for all patients who relapse after initial therapy unless high-risk cytogenetic abnormalities are not present and a complete response is attained.

Patients With Fludarabine-Refractory Chronic Lymphocytic Leukemia

Fludarabine-refractory CLL is generally considered to exist if a patient has not responded to a fludarabine-based therapy or relapses within 6 months of completing such a regimen. Several retrospective studies have documented a short survival time (9-12 months) and a particularly high frequency of both bacterial and opportunistic infections in this patient population. With the introduction of chemoimmunotherapy as initial therapy, another poor prognostic group includes patients relapsing within 2 years of FCR- or FR-based therapy. These patients have a significantly shorter PFS with subsequent therapies. New therapeutic agents such as bendamustine, ofatumumab, and alemtuzumab have been evaluated in this setting and have modest activity and produce relatively short remissions. New investigational agents (CAL-101, PCI-32765, CDK inhibitors, bcl-2 antagonists) have been evaluated in this patient population and demonstrated clinical activity. Consideration of allogeneic SCT in this setting is essential. The complexities of complications, poor therapeutic options, and acute features of this advanced CLL can put great strain on the patient, family members, and general hematologist alike. Referral of such patients to tertiary CLL centers for access to clinical trials and treatment of these specialized needs should be considered for patients with fludarabine-refractory or short remission chemoimmunotherapy CLL.

Richter Syndrome

Richter syndrome (RS), the development of high-grade lymphoma in patients with CLL, was described by Maurice Richter in 1928. Over the years, the classification of RS has expanded to include lymphoid malignancies such as Hodgkin disease, lymphoblastic lymphoma, PLL, and hairy cell leukemia (see Fig. 76-4, *A* to *C*). Incidence estimates range from 2.8% to 10.7%. Recent studies have suggested that the development of RS may be related to the evolution of an abnormal clone unrelated to the underlying CLL clone. Clearly identifiable risk factors for the development of RS are lacking, and its development has been shown to be independent of disease stage, duration of disease, type of therapy, or response to therapy. However, the presence of diffuse lymphomatous involvement, advanced Rai stage, IgV_H-unmutated disease, ZAP-70 expression, high LDH, del(17p13.1), high serum β_2M levels, and recently NOTCH1 mutations may predict the development of RS. RS is characterized by sudden onset of B symptoms (fever, night sweats, weight loss) and rapidly progressive lymphadenopathy at any anatomic site. Rarely, the lymphomatous clone may arise from the bone or an extranodal site. Laboratory abnormalities including anemia, neutropenia, and thrombocytopenia may be due to large-cell transformation in the BM. A rapid increase in the serum LDH is seen in the majority of patients. The diagnosis is generally made after examining the histology of a rapidly enlarging lymph node, which typically reveals large-cell lymphoma. PET scans can be helpful in these patients to localize the most hypermetabolic node for biopsy. Historically, RS has been treated with regimens similar to those used for the treatment of large-cell lymphomas involving multiple agents such as methotrexate, doxorubicin, cyclophosphamide, vincristine, prednisone, bleomycin, dexamethasone, cytarabine, and cisplatin (e.g., MACOP-B, CHOP-B, DHAP, and VAD). Recently, regimens incorporating oxaliplatin (OFAR) have been reported, although their benefit in RS is uncertain over traditional lymphoma regimens. Our institution prefers dose-adjusted infusional therapy (R-EPOCH) for the initial treatment of these patients. The duration of response and the OS rates are dismal, with most patients likely to die within 6 months of their diagnosis despite aggressive therapy. Long-term remissions and survival have been reported in a few patients after allogeneic SCT, but this approach is associated with a high TRM. When Richter transformation occurs, consolidation with allogeneic SCT is the preferred treatment.

Similar to RS, prolymphocytic transformation (PT) occurs in fewer than 10% of patients with CLL. PT is characterized by the appearance of large, immature prolymphocytes in the peripheral blood, which make up 10% to 50% of the peripheral circulating malignant lymphoid cells. These patients may be older with advanced disease and have more pronounced lymphadenopathy and splenomegaly. PT is associated with a poor outcome, with limited survival beyond 1 year. These patients often have del(17p13.1) but do appear to respond to many of the newer therapies coming forward for treatment of CLL. Allogeneic SCT may also be used as a potentially curative therapeutic option.

Secondary Malignancies in Chronic Lymphocytic Leukemia

Chronic lymphocytic leukemia is associated with an increased risk of secondary malignancies. These include not only hematologic malignancies such as MDS and AML associated with the use of chemotherapeutic agents but also solid tumors such as Kaposi sarcoma, malignant melanoma, and laryngeal and lung cancers. The increased incidence of secondary malignancies may be attributable to multiple reasons, including the immune dysfunction associated with CLL, the frequent infectious complications, the carcinogenic side effects of the various chemotherapeutic agents, and the increased and close medical surveillance that patients with CLL receive from trained oncologists.

Hypersensitivity in Chronic Lymphocytic Leukemia to Mosquitoes and Insect Bites and Treatment

Patients with chronic lymphocytic leukemia commonly exhibit an exaggerated cutaneous response to insect bites. This was first reported in 1965 by Robert Weed, who documented a hypersensitivity reaction to insect bites in eight of 97 patients with CLL over a 13-year period. The reaction is characterized histologically by the presence of a dermal infiltrate composed of a mixed population of T and B cells, eosinophils, and eosinophilic granule protein. The extent of eosinophilic degranulation may also correlate with the severity of symptoms. Clinically, these patients present with recurrent, painful, bullous eruptions that may be traced to an insect bite in some instances. In limited cases, we have also observed that CLL patients have hypersensitivity to bed bugs, and this should be considered in the differential diagnosis. Identification and avoidance of known triggers may be useful in some cases, but most patients are unable to identify the inciting exposure. Treatment with a short course of steroids is usually effective, but these patients frequently relapse and may require multiple courses of therapy. Dapsone and chlorambucil may also be useful in severe, recurrent cases.

Other cutaneous conditions are also common in CLL patients, with up to 45% reporting some form of skin involvement. These include petechial, purpural, or ecchymotic lesions related to thrombocytopenia; infectious eruptions such as herpes simplex and zoster; and direct leukemic involvement in fewer than 10% of all patients with advanced disease.

INFECTIONS IN PATIENTS WITH CHRONIC LYMPHOCYTIC LEUKEMIA

Infectious complications remain the leading cause of morbidity and mortality in patients with CLL. The incidence of infectious complications has been estimated to be as high as 80% with a mortality rate of approximately 60%. Various factors contribute to the increased incidence of infectious complications in CLL, the most important being progressive disease affecting host immunity through an impaired antibody response and hypogammaglobulinemia; weakened host cellular immune responses, including impaired macrophage function; a decrease in T-regulatory cells; and, finally, the acquired defects after immunosuppressive chemotherapy.

Recent studies have examined predictors of severe infections in patients with CLL. In their retrospective analysis of infection-related mortality in 280 patients, advanced age, clinical stage B or C disease, unmutated IgV_H, and positive CD38 status have been identified as independent predictors of both shorter time to first infection and infection-related mortality. Other risk factors that may also have an impact on development of infections include type of initial therapy and development of renal insufficiency.

Historically, sinopulmonary infections from encapsulated bacteria such as *Streptococcus pneumoniae* and *Haemophilus influenzae* have been the most common cause of infectious complications in patients with CLL. With the recent use of more potent cytotoxic chemotherapy and the resultant profound myelosuppression, an increased frequency of severe pulmonary infections, bacteremia, and gram-negative infections has been reported. Infections caused by atypical organisms such as *Listeria monocytogenes, Nocardia* spp., *Mycobacterium* spp., and *Neisseria meningitidis* are relatively infrequent in patients who receive conventional chemotherapy. Treatment for presumed infection should be initiated empirically in CLL patients who develop fever because fever in CLL patients usually indicates an active infection. Therapy should be tailored to the particular organ involved and the sensitivity of the organism. Prophylactic antibiotics can be initiated for debilitated patients with high-risk disease and significant immune dysfunction.

Viral infections are also commonly encountered in CLL patients (see Fig. 76-3, *D* and *E*). Herpesvirus infections are especially common in patients treated with nucleoside analogs and alemtuzumab. Chronic, indolent oropharyngeal and circumoral herpes simplex virus (HSV) outbreaks are more frequent than aggressive, disseminated visceral disease. Reactivation of Epstein-Barr virus (EBV) has been implicated in some cases of Richter transformation. Other viruses may cause severe systemic disease in patients with CLL. Varicella zoster virus (VZV) can cause herpes zoster, herpetic neuralgia, and rarely meningoencephalitis, parvovirus B19 can cause severe polyarthritis and pure RBC aplasia, and JC polyoma virus has been implicated in the development of progressive multifocal leukoencephalopathy. Management of these infections depends on early recognition of disseminated viral disease, timely initiation of antiviral therapy in cases of HSV and EBV, and a low threshold for the introduction of prophylactic acyclovir and supportive therapy. All patients should be provided instruction to identify the signs and symptoms of herpes virus infection at the time of diagnosis of CLL.

Fungal infections are not typically observed in CLL in the absence of treatment with corticosteroids or other immunosuppressive therapy for autoimmune complications arising from CLL. Cryptococcal meningitis, pneumonia, and fungemia are well-recognized events in patients with CLL and are associated with significant morbidity and mortality. More cases of *P. carinii* pneumonia, systemic candidiasis, and aspergillosis have been reported since the advent of combination nucleoside analog therapy with steroids. Treatment of the infection is dictated by the identification of the particular organism. Trimethoprim–sulfamethoxazole is routinely used as effective prophylaxis against *P. carinii* infections, especially during and immediately after the use of nucleoside analogs or alemtuzumab. Fungal prophylaxis with posaconazole may also be used during protracted therapy with high-dose steroids to avoid invasive aspergillosis.

Prophylactic Strategies for Infections

Routine use of prophylactic antibiotics is generally not used for CLL despite the higher frequency of infections observed in patients with this disease. Early recognition of signs and symptoms of infection and prompt initiation of empiric broad-spectrum antibiotics is probably a more feasible and cost-effective approach. When chemoimmunotherapy is used that includes a nucleoside analog or alemtuzumab therapy, prophylaxis for herpes simplex and varicella zoster should be used, particularly in older patients. Trimethoprim–sulfamethoxazole (or other alternative *P. carinii* pneumonia prophylaxis) should also be administered in this setting.

Hypogammaglobulinemia is virtually always present in advanced CLL, and several studies have examined whether intravenous immunoglobulin (IVIG) replacement therapy can reduce the incidence and severity of infectious complications. Patients receiving IVIG in a double-blind, placebo-controlled trial experienced significantly fewer bacterial infections than the placebo group. The therapy was well tolerated with few adverse reactions, but there was no observed benefit in terms of preventing viral or fungal infections. However, other studies have shown an almost 50% reduction in the number of serious infections per year with IVIG infusions. Limited data support the use of IVIG at a higher dose of 600 mg/kg every 4 weeks to reduce the number and severity of respiratory infections. However, the prohibitive cost of IVIG therapy and the fact that it has not been shown to prolong survival argues against its empiric use in all patients. IVIG should be used judiciously and reserved for patients with advanced disease and recurrent infections. The usual dose used is 200 to 400 mg/kg every 4 to 6 weeks as needed, with the aim of keeping the trough serum IgG concentration greater than 500 mg/dL. This is something our group routinely does for refractory patients or those who have more than two infections requiring hospitalization during 1 year.

Among the strategies for preventing infections in this patient population is immunization. CLL patients, however, typically respond poorly to pneumococcal and influenza vaccines. Advanced age, advanced disease stage, hypogammaglobulinemia, and low levels of soluble CD23 influence the rate of responses to immunizations. Soluble CD23, a degradation product of membrane-bound CD23, is involved in several aspects of B-cell activation and proliferation and has a synergistic effect on histamine release. Histamine has a direct inhibitory effect on immunoglobulin production by B cells in vitro via histamine type-2 (H2) receptors and acts as an immune regulatory factor that can be modulated by H2 receptor antagonists. Thus responses to vaccines may be further enhanced by adjuvant treatment with H2 blockers. Studies have shown that response to protein-conjugated vaccines may be enhanced by ranitidine in CLL patients to as much as 90% compared with 43% in the control group. Unfortunately, this response is not seen with polysaccharide vaccines. Recent studies have indicated that protein-conjugated vaccines may be more immunogenic, as shown by a more significant immune response to *Haemophilus influenzae* type b conjugate vaccine than to plain polysaccharide antigen. In light of the paucity of data on an appropriate immunization schedule, we suggest a modified immunization plan based on the recommendations of the Advisory Committee on Immunization Practices. This includes use of Prevnar 13 for pneumococcal prophylaxis and avoiding live vaccines, including the varicella zoster virus.

Growth factors such as G-CSF or granulocyte macrophage colony-stimulating factor (GM-CSF) can be used prophylactically in high-risk, severely neutropenic patients to shorten the duration and severity of neutropenia.

AUTOIMMUNE COMPLICATIONS OF CHRONIC LYMPHOCYTIC LEUKEMIA

Patients with CLL have a greater predisposition to develop autoimmune hematologic complications, including AIHA, idiopathic thrombocytopenia purpura (ITP), and pure RBC aplasia. AIHA occurs in up to 37% of CLL patients at some time during the course of their disease. A small proportion (10%-15%) of patients may present with AIHA at diagnosis. AIHA can have a varied presentation, with patients developing signs of anemia, including weakness, lethargy, dyspnea on exertion, and dizziness over a period of months.

Examination may reveal pallor, jaundice, hepatosplenomegaly and lymphadenopathy. Hemolysis can cause mild to moderate indirect hyperbilirubinemia, elevated LDH levels, and hemoglobinuria. The direct antiglobulin Coombs test result is positive in up to 74% of patients with CLL, but not all patients develop hemolysis. Most of the antibodies produced are warm reactive, but patients can occasionally present with cold agglutination syndrome. The antibodies are mostly polyclonal and usually a product of normal B cells rather than the leukemic clone.

In contrast to the high frequency of AIHA in CLL, ITP or ITP and AIHA, or Evans syndrome, occurs less frequently in CLL. These events can occur throughout the entire course of CLL and are much more difficult to diagnose because of the absence of multiple implicating laboratory features as seen with autoimmune hemolytic anemia.

Given the small number of patients with AIHA, there are no data from controlled trials to guide the management of AIHA. Glucocorticoids have been used since the 1940s and are considered the first line of therapy. Most patients will respond to prednisone at a dose of 1 mg/kg for 10 to 14 days followed by a slow taper over 2 to 3 months, depending on the extent of hemolysis. ORRs of up to 90%, with 65% CRs, have been reported with the use of steroids. Unfortunately, approximately 60% of patients relapse when steroid therapy is stopped. Rituximab 375 mg/m^2 weekly for four weeks is often effective for steroid-resistant AIHA or ITP and if steroid withdrawal is not possible. Because of the long-term morbidity of prolonged steroid administration in CLL and data demonstrating benefit to concurrent steroids and rituximab for rapid withdrawal of corticosteroids in ITP, our group recently has begun giving these two concurrently at diagnosis of ITP or AIHA unless contraindicated (e.g., hepatitis B). IVIG, the next line of treatment, induces responses in 40% of patients for both AIHA and ITP. Thrombopoietin agonists are effective for refractory ITP in CLL and could also be considered at this time. Cyclosporine A (CSA) has been used for refractory AIHA and ITP of CLL at 5 mg/kg/day given in divided doses twice daily. The dose should be adjusted to maintain a serum level of around 100 to 150 μg/dL. Other treatment modalities include splenectomy or splenic irradiation, alkylating agents, or therapy (FCR or FR directed at the disease if active). Treatment of the underlying CLL is generally required for long-term control of autoimmune cytopenias. However, our practice is to first control the autoimmune process with steroids or other therapies before considering treatment of the underlying CLL. Supportive therapy with periodic RBC transfusions is also important in the management of AIHA.

There are limited data on the routine use of erythropoiesis-stimulating agents (ESAs) in patients with Coombs-negative anemia. These agents are most effective in patients with low levels of endogenous erythropoietin and may improve the quality of life and reduce the frequency of transfusions in this subset of patients. However, given the recent data on the increased risk of thromboembolic events and higher sudden death rates in patients treated with these agents, judicious use is recommended. ESAs are never recommended when rapid correction of hemoglobin is required.

Pure RBC aplasia (PRCA) is a relatively rare T cell–dependent complication associated with CLL, but an incidence as high as 6% has been reported. PRCA was first described by Dameshek and colleagues in 1967. It is characterized by a hypoproliferative anemia that can be detected even in early-stage CLL and is thought to be caused by cytotoxic effects of suppressor T cells on erythroid progenitor cells. Higher numbers of these CD3, CD8, and CD57 coexpressing cells have been shown to gradually accumulate in the BM of patients with PRCA. Abeloff and Waterbury described the first remission of PRCA to cyclophosphamide therapy in 1974, and Chikkappa and colleagues described the first case of response to CSA. Subsequent larger studies have shown a response rate as high as 63% with 300 mg/day of oral CSA. Mild reversible nephrotoxicity may warrant dose adjustment in some patients. Most patients exhibit a response by having reticulocytosis within the first 10 to 14 days, but maximal response may occur an average of 10 weeks after the start of therapy. However, steroid therapy at a dose of 1 mg/kg/day of prednisone remains the first line of treatment. If a response is not obtained in 4 weeks, CSA should be added to the regimen. Other agents that have shown promising activity in treating PRCA include rituximab, IVIG, alemtuzumab, and antithymocyte globulin. Packed RBC transfusions are usually indicated in patients who are clinically symptomatic from severe anemia.

A number of other complications, most of which are autoimmune in nature, have been reported in patients with CLL. These complications include paraneoplastic pemphigus, angioedema caused by acquired C1-inhibitor deficiency, and nephrotic syndrome. As a result of autoimmune involvement of various organs, patients with CLL may have abnormal serum chemistry profiles and liver function tests.

FUTURE DIRECTIONS

Advances in the molecular biology of CLL over the past 2 decades have translated into new diagnostic tests that allow better assessment of initial prognosis and also to assign treatment. Additionally, multiple new therapies have come forward, and progress is being made to extend remission duration and improve the quality of life of CLL patients. Additionally, medications and interventions to support complications that arise from CLL have also been introduced. Overall, the future for patients with CLL remains brighter based on these past efforts and likely will improve further with continued laboratory and clinical research ongoing in this disease. In particular, the BCR kinase inhibitors have potential to transform treatment and outcome of patients with CLL.

FINANCIAL SUPPORT

This work was supported by the National Cancer Institute P01 CA95426, R01 CA095241, the American Cancer Society, the Leukemia and Lymphoma Society, and the D. Warren Brown Foundation.

SUGGESTED READINGS

Badoux XC, Keating MJ, Wang X, et al: Fludarabine, cyclophosphamide, and rituximab chemoimmunotherapy is highly effective treatment for relapsed patients with CLL. *Blood* 117:3016, 2011.

Badoux XC, Keating MJ, Wen S, et al: Lenalidomide as initial therapy of elderly patients with chronic lymphocytic leukemia. *Blood* 118:3489, 2011.

Chen CI, Bergsagel PL, Paul H, et al: Single-agent lenalidomide in the treatment of previously untreated chronic lymphocytic leukemia. *J Clin Oncol* 29:1175, 2011.

Crowther-Swanepoel D, Corre T, Lloyd A, et al: Inherited genetic susceptibility to monoclonal B-cell lymphocytosis. *Blood* 116:5957, 2010.

Dreger P, Döhner H, Ritgen M, et al: German CLL Study Group: Allogeneic stem cell transplantation provides durable disease control in poor-risk chronic lymphocytic leukemia: Long-term clinical and MRD results of the German CLL Study Group CLL3X trial. *Blood* 116:2438, 2010.

Eichhorst BF, Busch R, Stilgenbauer S, et al: German CLL Study Group (GCLLSG): First-line therapy with fludarabine compared with chlorambucil does not result in a major benefit for elderly patients with advanced chronic lymphocytic leukemia. *Blood* 114:3382, 2009.

Eichhorst BF, Fischer K, Fink AM, et al: German CLL Study Group (GCLLSG): Limited clinical relevance of imaging techniques in the follow-up of patients with advanced chronic lymphocytic leukemia: Results of a meta-analysis. *Blood* 117:1817, 2011.

Fabbri M, Bottoni A, Shimizu M, et al: Association of a microRNA/TP53 feedback circuitry with pathogenesis and outcome of B-cell chronic lymphocytic leukemia. *JAMA* 305:59, 2011

Fischer K, Cramer P, Busch R, et al: Bendamustine combined with rituximab in patients with relapsed and/or refractory chronic lymphocytic leukemia: A multicenter phase II trial of the German Chronic Lymphocytic Leukemia Study Group. *J Clin Oncol* 29:3559, 2011.

Hallek M, Cheson BD, Catovsky D, et al: International Workshop on Chronic Lymphocytic Leukemia: Guidelines for the diagnosis and treatment of chronic lymphocytic leukemia: A report from the International Workshop on Chronic Lymphocytic Leukemia updating the National Cancer Institute-Working Group 1996 guidelines. *Blood* 111:5446, 2008.

Hallek M, Fischer K, Fingerle-Rowson G, et al: International Group of Investigators; German Chronic Lymphocytic Leukaemia Study Group: Addition of rituximab to fludarabine and cyclophosphamide in patients with chronic lymphocytic leukaemia: A randomised, open-label, phase 3 trial. *Lancet* 376:1164, 2010

Herishanu Y, Pérez-Galán P, Liu D, et al: The lymph node microenvironment promotes B-cell receptor signaling, NF-kappaB activation, and tumor proliferation in chronic lymphocytic leukemia. *Blood* 117:563, 2011.

Jaglowski SM, Alinari L, Lapalombella R, et al: The clinical application of monoclonal antibodies in chronic lymphocytic leukemia. *Blood* 116:3705, 2010.

Kikushige Y, Ishikawa F, Miyamoto T, et al: Self-renewing hematopoietic stem cell is the primary target in pathogenesis of human chronic lymphocytic leukemia. *Cancer Cell* 20:246, 2011.

Knauf WU, Lissichkov T, Aldaoud A, et al: Phase III randomized study of bendamustine compared with chlorambucil in previously untreated patients with chronic lymphocytic leukemia. *J Clin Oncol* 27:4378, 2009.

Puente XS, Pinyol M, Quesada V, et al: Whole-genome sequencing identifies recurrent mutations in chronic lymphocytic leukaemia. *Nature* 475:101, 2011.

Robak T, Dmoszynska A, Solal-Céligny P, et al: Rituximab plus fludarabine and cyclophosphamide prolongs progression-free survival compared with fludarabine and cyclophosphamide alone in previously treated chronic lymphocytic leukemia. *J Clin Oncol* 28:1756, 2010.

Rossignol J, Michallet AS, Oberic L, et al: Rituximab-cyclophosphamide-dexamethasone combination in the management of autoimmune cytopenias associated with chronic lymphocytic leukemia. *Leukemia* 25:473, 2011.

Shanafelt TD, Drake MT, Maurer MJ, et al: Vitamin D insufficiency and prognosis in chronic lymphocytic leukemia. *Blood* 117:1492, 2011.

Sorror ML, Storer BE, Sandmaier BM, et al: Five-year follow-up of patients with advanced chronic lymphocytic leukemia treated with allogeneic hematopoietic cell transplantation after nonmyeloablative conditioning. *J Clin Oncol* 26:4912, 2008.

Stilgenbauer S, Zenz T, Winkler D, et al: German Chronic Lymphocytic Leukemia Study; Subcutaneous alemtuzumab in fludarabine-refractory chronic lymphocytic leukemia: Clinical results and prognostic marker analyses from the CLL2H study of the German Chronic Lymphocytic Leukemia Study Group. *J Clin Oncol* 27:3994, 2009.

Tam CS, Keating MJ: Chemoimmunotherapy of chronic lymphocytic leukemia. *Nat Rev Clin Oncol* 7:521, 2010.

Tam CS, O'Brien S, Wierda W, et al: Long-term results of the fludarabine, cyclophosphamide, and rituximab regimen as initial therapy of chronic lymphocytic leukemia *Blood* 112:975, 2008.

Wierda WG, Kipps TJ, Mayer J, et al: Hx-CD20-406 Study Investigators: Ofatumumab as single-agent CD20 immunotherapy in fludarabine-refractory chronic lymphocytic leukemia. *J Clin Oncol* 28:1749, 2010.

Wierda WG, O'Brien S, Wang X, et al: Multivariable model for time to first treatment in patients with chronic lymphocytic leukemia. *J Clin Oncol* 29:4088, 2011.

Woyach JA, Ruppert AS, Heerema NA, et al: Chemoimmunotherapy with fludarabine and rituximab produces extended overall survival and progression-free survival in chronic lymphocytic leukemia: Long-term follow-up of CALGB study 9712. *J Clin Oncol* 29:1349, 2011.

Zenz T, Eichhorst B, Busch R, et al: TP53 mutation and survival in chronic lymphocytic leukemia. *J Clin Oncol* 28:4473, 2010.

Zenz T, Mertens D, Küppers R, et al: From pathogenesis to treatment of chronic lymphocytic leukaemia. *Nat Rev Cancer* 10:37, 2010.

CHAPTER 77

HAIRY CELL LEUKEMIA

Farhad Ravandi

The most recent revision of the World Health Organization (WHO) classification of hematopoietic neoplasms is intended to provide a disease specific classification for the diagnosis and potential treatment of these disorders and has continued to further incorporate modern cytogenetics and molecular data to better define disease subsets that may be amenable to different treatment strategies. Hairy cell leukemia (HCL) is one of the diseases exemplifying the importance of the application of appropriate diagnostic techniques and treatment strategies in order to obtain the best results in the individual patient.[1] The disease was first described by Bouroncle and colleagues in 1958. The term *hairy cell leukemia* was first used to describe the disorder by Schreck and Donnelly in 1966 and is derived from the observation of hair-like projections from mononuclear cells giving rise to a frayed cell surface appearance.

The evolution of therapeutic strategies in patients with HCL over the past 25 years has led to a significant change in the natural history of the disease. Using the currently available drugs, the majority of patients with this disease achieve complete remission (CR), and the published survival curves from several large series are similar to those for appropriate age-matched individuals without the disease. At the same time, recent research efforts have led to a better understanding of the molecular mechanisms responsible for the disease pathogenesis. Several studies, using modern techniques, have demonstrated the persistence of minimal residual disease (MRD) after therapy with nucleoside analogs in the majority of patients without consensus on the significance of such MRD. The role of monoclonal antibodies, naked or conjugated with toxins, in the management of HCL, as well as their ability to eradicate MRD, is under investigation. The possibility of such strategies of chemoimmunotherapy leading to further improvements in the outcome of patients with HCL needs to be further investigated.

EPIDEMIOLOGY

HCL is an uncommon lymphoid malignancy, accounting for only 2% of lymphoid leukemias, with approximately 600 to 800 new patients diagnosed each year in the United States.[1] The disease is more common in whites and occurs more frequently in men than women by a ratio of 4 to 1.[1] The median age at diagnosis is reported by most studies to be in the 50s. However, it is possible that the disease is underreported in the older population. The Swedish Cancer Registry has maintained records on the incidence of the disease for several decades and has shown a stable incidence since the 1980s. It reports the median age at diagnosis of 62 years, suggesting less rigid diagnostic efforts in older patients.

HCL has been diagnosed in patients in their 20s and 30s but is exceptionally rare in children. Using data from the 17 population-based cancer registry areas in the United States, the National Cancer Institute's Surveillance Epidemiology and End Results (SEER) program reported that the incidence of the disease was stable in the decades between 1978 and 2004 with a rapid rise in age-specific incidence ratios until approximately 40 years and then at a slower pace beyond that age.

ETIOLOGY AND CELL OF ORIGIN

Several reports have suggested an association between development of HCL and exposure to several compounds, including benzene, organophosphorus insecticides, and other solvents. However, such association has not been confirmed by other reports. Exposure to radiation, wood dust, or agricultural chemicals, and a previous history of infectious mononucleosis have also been suggested as predisposing factors, but a direct, causal association has not been established with any of these or other factors.

Morphologically and phenotypically, the cells in HCL have no resemblance to any of the normal stages of B-cell development and maturation; past studies have debated their cell of origin. Initially, because of morphologic and functional similarities between hairy cells and cells of the monocyte/macrophage system, HCL tumor cells were thought to be derived from a cell transformed from the reticuloendothelium. Korsmeyer demonstrated the rearrangement of the B-cell receptor (BCR) immunoglobulin genes in HCL, demonstrating for the first time the B-cell origin of the disease. Recently, several studies have increased our understanding of the cell of origin in HCL allowing for a better description of pathogenic mechanisms responsible for its development.[2]

In lymphoid cells, the analysis of the immunoglobulin variable region genes provides a tool for the delineation of the clonal history of cells at which lymphoid neoplasms originate, identifying whether antigen encountered by a normal mature B cell has resulted in somatic mutation (Fig. 77-1). This process occurs within the germinal centers (GC) of lymph tissues and may be associated with isotype switching. The enzyme activation–induced cytidine deaminase (AICD) is critical for both processes. Tumor cells from various B-cell malignancies are arrested at a number of stages along normal B-cell differentiation, conserving the immunogenetic characteristics of the stage-specific cell. The analysis of immunoglobulin variable gene regions can provide information about whether the cell of origin has undergone somatic mutation and isotype switching. Several reports have clearly demonstrated that in more than 85% of patients with HCL the tumor cells express switched immunoglobulin isotypes, and their rearranged variable region genes have undergone somatic mutations.[3] Furthermore, HCL cells express AICD, the enzyme that is critical for both processes.[3] This suggests that the cell of origin in the majority of HCL cases has transited through the GCs of peripheral lymphoid tissue having undergone the GC reaction.[2] Of interest, in about 40% of cases of HCL, the leukemia cells express multiple immunoglobulin heavy chain isotypes, with dominance of IgG3 but only a single light chain, suggesting that clonally related multiple isotypes coexist in single hairy cells. Therefore this subset of the disease may be arrested at a point after isotype switching and before exit from the GC. However, other lines of evidence suggest a post-GC origin.[2]

Another study by Arons and colleagues provided evidence that in the majority of patients with classic HCL (83% of 102 cases), the cell of origin is post-GC with mutated immunoglobulin heavy chain variable region.[4] This contrasted with historic data for patients with CLL, in which case about half of cell origins are unmutated. They also reported higher usage of certain immunoglobulin gene families and a difference in mutational frequency among these genes.[4] Furthermore, by demonstrating that the mutations fulfilled

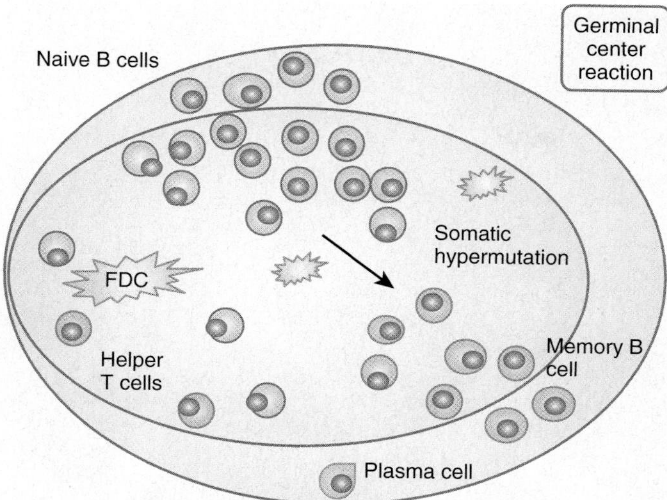

Figure 77-1 GERMINAL CENTER REACTION. The process of somatic hypermutation and isotypic switch in the germinal center.

predefined characteristics of a canonical and nonrandom event, Arons and colleagues provided further evidence suggestive of an antigen-driven process.

The post-GC origin of HCL is supported by gene expression profiling studies comparing HCL cells with cells from other lymphoid neoplasms, as well as with naive and memory B cells.[5] Samples from various HCL patients displayed a homogeneous pattern of gene expression that was clearly distinct from other B-cell lymphomas and was related to post-GC memory B cells.[5] Other investigators have reported this remarkably stable genome in HCL. Furthermore, when compared with memory B cells, HCL cells had a remarkable conservation of proliferation, apoptosis, and DNA metabolism programs but differed significantly in the expression of genes controlling cell adhesion and response to chemokines.[5] Against the hypothesis of a memory B-cell origin is the lack of expression by hairy cells of the memory B-cell marker, CD27. However, CD27-negative memory B cells have been described in humans, and hairy cells may lose this marker as a result of the neoplastic transformation.

As lymph node involvement in HCL is uncommon, the post-GC cell of origin is likely to originate from the spleen or the bone marrow, sites involved by the disease almost invariably. A number of reports have suggested that HCL may originate from the B cells of the splenic marginal zone (SMZ). Normal SMZ B cells are mainly memory B cells. Vanhentenrijk and colleagues, using comparative expressed sequence hybridization (CESH) studies, demonstrated that hairy cells had an expression profile consistent with a splenic expression signature that most likely reflected the expression profile of spleen-specific components, such as the sinusoidal lining cells from the red pulp and the marginal zone B cells from the white pulp.

Recently, Tiacci and colleagues reported the presence of *BRAF* V600E mutations in each of 47 patients with HCL and no mutations in the cells from patients with 195 peripheral B-cell lymphomas or leukemias, which were also evaluated.[6] Using whole-genome sequencing they identified, in an index patient, five missense somatic clonal mutations, including a heterozygous mutation in *BRAF* that resulted in a BRAF V600E variant protein.[6] Since *BRAF* V600F is known to be oncogenic in other tumors, Tiacci and colleagues focused on this mutation and analyzed the subsequent 46 cases as well as the patients with other lymphomas. They also demonstrated expression of phosphorylated MEK and ERK, showing constitutive activation of the RAF-MEK-ERK mitogen-activated protein kinase (MAPK) pathway in HCL.[6] This discovery has potential significance in the understanding of the pathogenic mechanisms of HCL; its applications in diagnosis and treatment of this disease are likely to increase with further research.

Table 77-1 Initial Work Up of a Patient With Suspected Hairy Cell Leukemia

History and physical examination
Complete blood count with differential counts
Review of peripheral blood smear
Serum chemistries
Bone marrow aspirate and biopsy with immunostains
Immunophenotyping by flow cytometry of peripheral blood and bone marrow
? Serum soluble markers such as CD25 and CD22
? Immune status analysis with CD4/CD8 lymphocyte subsets
Appropriate imaging, if febrile, to rule out infections

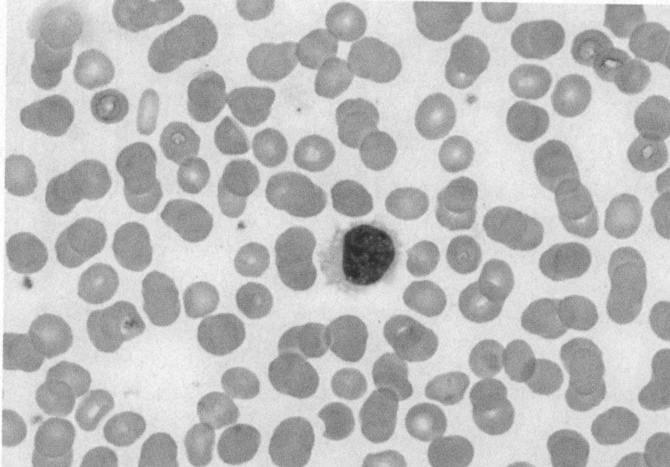

Figure 77-2 PHOTOMICROGRAPH OF A HAIRY CELL IN THE PERIPHERAL BLOOD. *(Provided by Jeffrey Jorgensen, Department of Hematopathology, UTMDACC.)*

CLINICAL PRESENTATION AND DIAGNOSIS

Typically, the majority of patients present with pancytopenia and splenomegaly with the associated fatigue, left upper quadrant abdominal pain, fever and infections, and/or bleeding problems (Table 77-1). Common presenting features include significant anemia, seen in up to 85% of patients, thrombocytopenia in about 60% to 80%, and leukopenia in 60% of patients; these cytopenias can be severe and life-threatening and are likely multifactorial, with hypersplenism and marrow infiltration being the more important contributors. Monocytopenia is a characteristic finding. Circulating hairy cells are typically scant in most patients and frequently absent. Hairy cells are small- and medium-sized lymphoid cells with an oval or indented (bean-shaped) nucleus with homogeneous chromatin that is less clumped than normal B cells (Fig. 77-2).[1] Nucleoli are typically absent or inconspicuous and the cytoplasm abundant and pale blue in color with circumferential "hairy" projections. Electron micrographs of hairy cells clearly demonstrate their distinctive and complex surface features with multiple surface folds and clusters of short microvilli, creating an appearance unique to hairy cells (Fig. 77-3).

Bone marrow involvement can be interstitial or patchy with the infiltrate characterized by widely spaced nuclei due to the abundant cytoplasm, giving rise to the commonly described "fried egg" appearance (Fig. 77-4).[1] Occasionally, an increase in the bone marrow reticulin fibrosis, as well as significant loss of the hematopoietic elements, leads to a "dry tap." Bone marrow fibrosis is caused by the production and assembly of a fibronectin matrix by hairy cells and the deposition of fine reticulin fibers (mainly composed of type III collagen fibrils) by fibroblasts.[2] Hairy cells express isoenzyme 5 of acid phosphatase, which imparts resistance to treatment with tartaric acid, with virtually all cases being positive for tartrate-resistant acid phosphatase (TRAP)

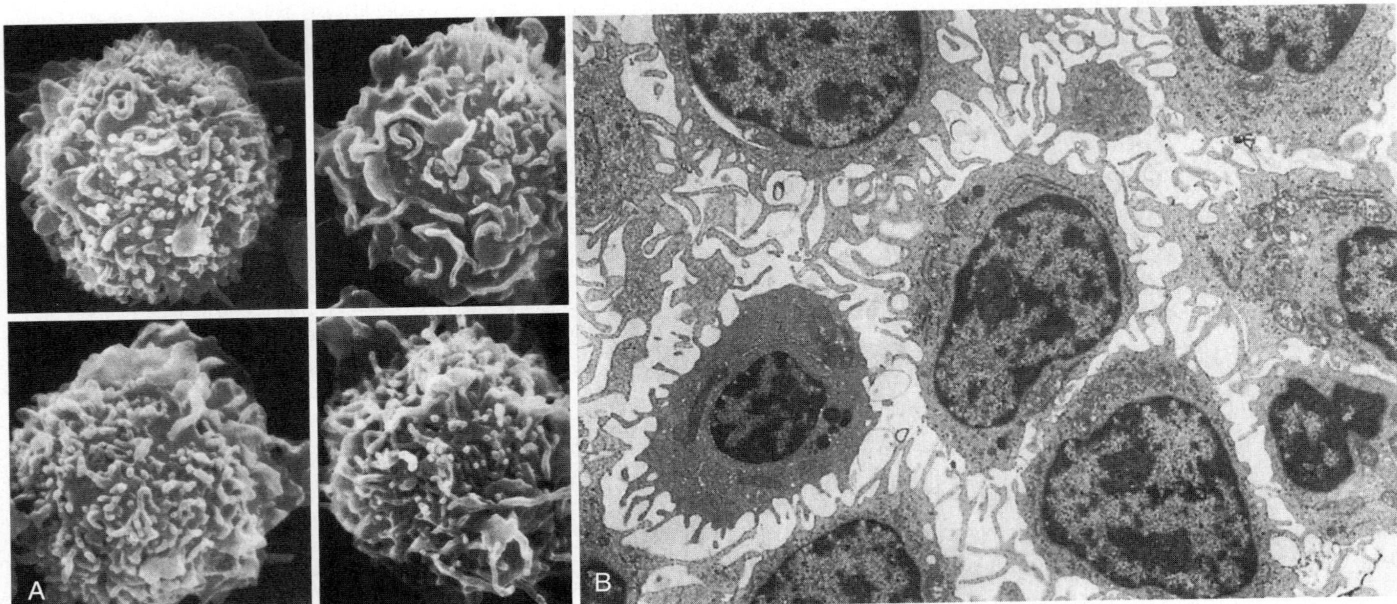

Figure 77-3 ELECTRON MICROGRAPH OF HAIRY CELLS. **A,** Ruffles and folds on the surface. **B,** Hair-like projections from the cytoplasm. *(Used with permission from Aaron Polliack, Emeritus Professor of Hematology, Hadassah University Hospital, Hebrew University Medical School, Jerusalem, Israel.)*

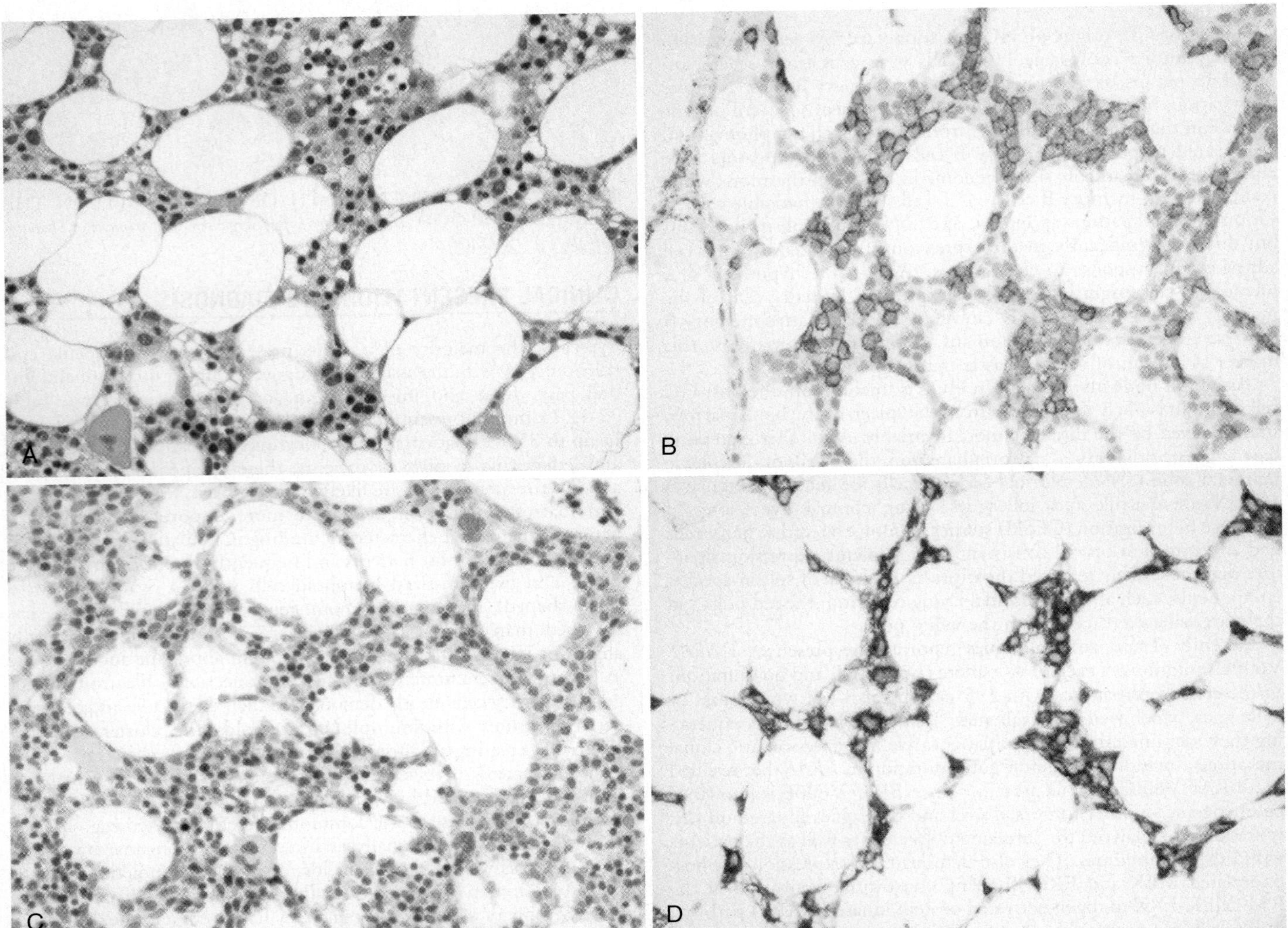

Figure 77-4 BONE MARROW FINDINGS IN HAIRY CELL LEUKEMIA. **A,** Bone marrow biopsy (H&E stain ×400). **B,** Bone marrow biopsy (CD20 stain ×400). **C,** Bone marrow biopsy (Annexin A1 stain ×400). **D,** Bone marrow biopsy (CD11c stain ×400). *(Provided by Jeffrey Jorgensen, Department of Hematopathology, UTMDACC.)*

(Fig. 77-5). Combined expression of DBA44 and TRAP by immunohistochemical analysis is highly specific and useful for arriving at the diagnosis. More recently, immunostaining for annexin A1 (ANAX1) has been reported to be very specific for HCL.[7] ANAX1 can be used to distinguish HCL from its variant form and from other lymphoid neoplasms such as splenic marginal zone lymphoma (SMZL).[1,7] Cyclin D1 (encoded by *CCND1* gene) is frequently expressed, but this is not secondary to translocation involving *CCNDI,* unlike mantle cell lymphoma. In a proportion of patients, the bone marrow is hypocellular with the loss of hematopoietic elements, which can result in an erroneous diagnosis of aplastic anemia. Immunostaining for antigens such as CD20 may be helpful to detect the abnormal B-cell infiltrate, hence prompting more specific stains for HCL.[1]

HCL cells have a characteristic immunophenotype with flow cytometry being an important element of diagnostic evaluation in this disease (Table 77-1). Hairy cells strongly express CD45 and gate within the monocytic region when analyzed by CD45 versus side scatter, which is typically devoid of monocytes. They exhibit a mature B-cell phenotype and commonly express one or more heavy chains and monotypic light chains (κ and λ light chains in equal numbers of patients). They express B-cell associated antigens CD19, CD20, CD22, FMC7, and CD79b but typically lack CD5, CD10 (positive in about 10%), and CD23 (positive in about 20%) expression. No single marker is specific for distinguishing HCL from other B-cell neoplasms; however, the antigens CD11c, CD103, CD123, as well as the interleukin (IL)-2 receptor α-subunit (CD25), are typically expressed in HCL. Bright expression of CD22 and CD20 is also seen, which can be important therapeutically. Among the patients evaluated in one study, CD52 was also universally expressed.

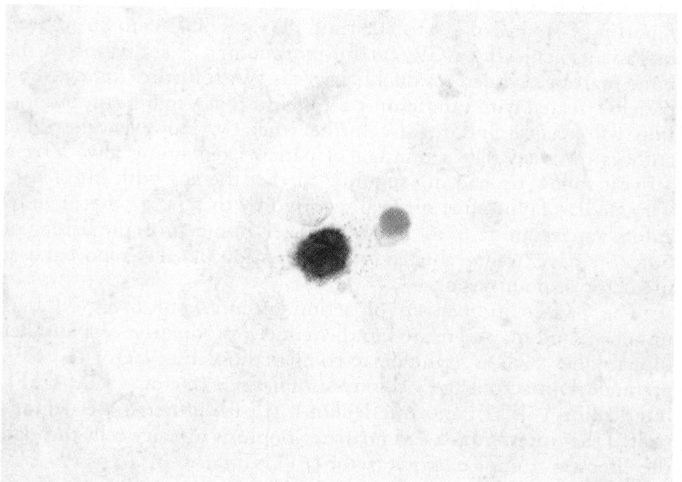

Figure 77-5 BONE MARROW ASPIRATE SMEAR (TRAP STAIN ×1000). *(Provided by Jeffrey Jorgensen, Department of Hematopathology, UTMDACC.)*

Splenic enlargement is present in the majority of patients and can be massive in about 20%. Splenic involvement is characterized by diffuse infiltration of the red pulp cords and sinuses, with atrophy and replacement of white pulp. Blood-filled sinuses lined by hairy cells (often referred to as *pseudosinuses* or *red blood lakes*) are often a prominent but not pathognomonic finding (Fig. 77-6).[1] Significant lymphadenopathy is uncommon and present only in the advanced stages of the disease. When involved, the lymph node enlargement is largely confined to the abdominal and retroperitoneal nodes. The infiltrates are distributed in the interfollicular and paracortical areas of the nodes and may extend through the capsule to the surrounding adipose tissue. Hepatomegaly is much less frequent, occurring in up to a third of patients. However, the liver is almost always involved with a mononuclear cell infiltrate in the sinusoids, portal areas or both. Unusual sites of disease involvement have been reported, including mediastinal and paravertebral masses, skeletal lytic lesions, pleural effusions and ascites, as well as involvement of skin, eye, the central nervous system, and the gastrointestinal tract. Other notable clinical features include a predisposition to infections and an uncommon association with autoimmune disorders such as polyarteritis nodosa, vasculitis, and rheumatoid arthritis.

Several cytogenetic abnormalities have been reported in HCL but no single abnormality is present consistently. Few cytogenetic studies have been reported because of the rarity of the disease, difficulty in obtaining marrow samples, and low responsiveness of hairy cells to common mitogens. In the reported series, chromosomes 1, 2, 5, 6, 11, 14, 19, and 20 are most frequently involved, with chromosome 5 and 14 abnormalities predominating. Deletions and mutations of p53, as well as overexpression of cyclin-D1, have been reported. Lack of reciprocal chromosomal translocations in HCL is consistent with a memory B-cell origin of the disease, because these translocations are thought to arise from mistakes in the immunoglobulin remodeling mechanisms, which are believed to be turned off in memory B cells.[2]

DIFFERENTIAL DIAGNOSIS

HCL must be distinguished from other indolent lymphoid neoplasms, such as B-prolymphocytic leukemia and SMZL, and most notably, from HCLv, the variant form of the disease. HCLv is a rare disorder accounting for approximately 10% of cases and occurring

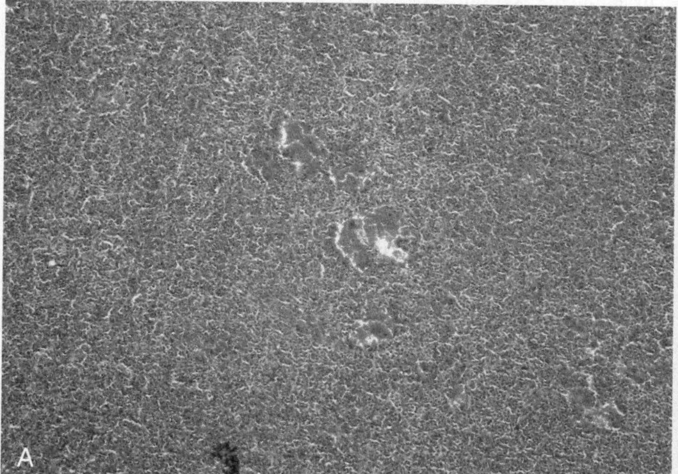

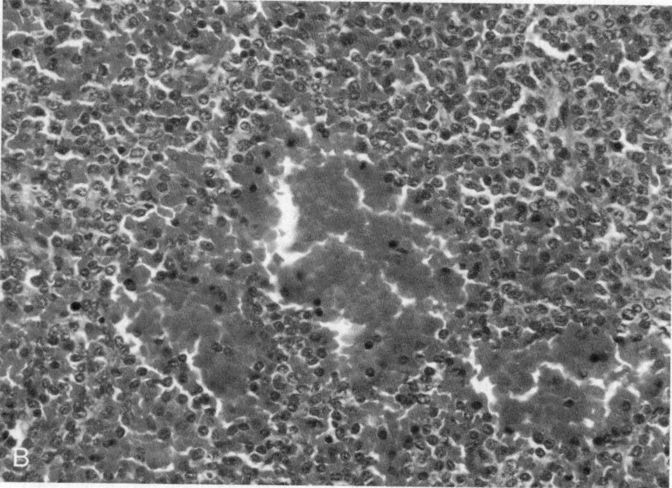

Figure 77-6 PATHOLOGIC FINDINGS IN THE SPLEEN. **A,** H&E stain (×100). **B,** H&E stain (×400). *(Provided by Roberto Miranda, Department of Hematopathology, UTMDACC.)*

Table 77-2 Immunophenotype of Hairy Cell Leukemia and Other Indolent Lymphoid Neoplasms

Disease	sIg	CD5	CD10	CD11c	CD20	CD22	CD23	CD25	CD103
HCL	+/–	–/+	–	++	+	+	–/+	+	++
CLL	+/–	++	–	–/+	+/–	–/+	++	–/+	–
B-PLL	++	+	–	–/+	+/–	+	+/–	–	–
HCLv	+/–	–	–	++	+	+	–	–	–/+
MCL	+	++	–	–	+	+	–/+	–	–
SMZL	+	–/+	–/+	+	+	+/–	–/+	–	–
FL	+	–	+	–	++	+	–/+	–	–

in the older population, with the median age being 71 years.[8] There are no reports of an association with exposure to carcinogens, radiation, or viral infections, and no specific underlying cause has been described. Patients often have an elevated WBC count (>10 × 10^9/L) including atypical hairy cells with prolymphocytic features and lack monocytopenia. Splenomegaly and cytopenias are present in the majority of patients, and the pattern of bone marrow and splenic involvement is similar to HCL and different from prolymphocytic leukemia and SMZL. The immunophenotypic expression of various lymphoid markers is also different in these disorders, with HCLv lacking CD25 expression, further assisting diagnosis (Table 77-2). Another aid in distinguishing HCL from HCLv is CD123 expression, which is positive in the former and negative in the latter. A number of chromosomal abnormalities, including translocations, have been reported in a few cases. Although HCLv has some similarities to HCL, the two conditions differ in a number of features, most notably being HCLv's lack of responsiveness to classic HCL therapies. As such, it is important to distinguish the two and consider them as separate diseases. HCL and HCLv have different immunoglobulin heavy (IGH) chain gene repertoires and somatic hypermutation patterns.[4] A recent report also suggested that high expression levels of AICD can distinguish HCL from HCLv, as well as from SMZL. However, the same group was unable to find distinct cytogenetic events to distinguish HCL from its variant, using high-resolution genomic profiling. Most recently, *BRAF* V600F mutations have been shown to occur exclusively in HCL samples and not in those from patients with HCLv and SMZL.

SMZL (previously referred to as *splenic lymphoma with villous lymphocytes [SLVL]*) exhibits some of the clinical and morphologic features of HCL but typically has a more prominent peripheral blood involvement, lacks TRAP expression, and has a different immunophenotype, including absence of expression of CD25 and CD103. HCL should be distinguished from other indolent lymphoid neoplasms such as chronic lymphocytic leukemia, prolymphocytic leukemia, and follicular lymphomas, but this distinction is typically easily made using the characteristic morphologic and immunotypic findings characteristic of these disorders (Table 77-2). Other disorders that should be included in the differential diagnosis include aplastic anemia, primary myelofibrosis, and systemic mast cell disorders.

TREATMENT

Indications for Therapy

HCL has an indolent course, with some patients surviving many years without receiving therapy and others not requiring further therapy despite persistence of residual morphologic evidence of the disease after the initial treatment.[9] Therefore a watch-and-wait strategy may be appropriate in the initial management of patients with limited or no manifestations of the disease. Disease progression that necessitates therapy is commonly evident by the development of progressive cytopenias and their associated complications, such as infections, bleeding, and progressive fatigue. No specific criteria for therapy have been established, but generally treatment is indicated when the patient has significant cytopenias, symptomatic organomegaly or adenopathy, infections, or constitutional symptoms such as fever, night sweats, or fatigue. Typical blood counts warranting therapy include an absolute neutrophil count < 1.0 x 10^9/L, a platelet count < 100 X 10^9/L, and/or a hemoglobin < 12.0 g/dL.

Historic Aspects of Therapy

Progress in the treatment of patients with HCL over the last 25 years has been significant, with survival curves now approaching those of age-matched cohorts without the disease. Before the introduction of interferon-α, splenectomy was used effectively to treat patients with HCL. Although splenectomy does not result in morphologic remissions in the bone marrow, the peripheral blood counts are normalized in up to 70% of patients. Progression of disease can be expected in about 45% within 5 years. Furthermore, there is an associated morbidity and mortality with the procedure. As such, splenectomy is no longer performed in this disease except in rare, selected patients.

The first report of effective treatment of HCL with interferon-α described several patients with progressive disease who received daily doses of 3 million units. Three patients achieved complete response (CR) with the other four having partial responses (PR). The activity of interferon-α in HCL was further confirmed by several large trials reporting CR rates of 4% to 30% and PR rates of 43% to 86%. Even in patients achieving a CR, careful morphologic examination of the bone marrow revealed residual hairy cells. With further follow-up of patients treated with interferon-α, it is clear that a significant proportion will relapse and require further therapy. However, the same authors reported that a number of patients remaining alive after a 10-year follow-up had not required further therapy with interferon. The median failure-free survival reported by these and other investigators ranges from 6 to 25 months. A number of predictors of outcome have been evaluated, with expression of CD5 reported as a predictor of poor response.

The precise mechanism of action of interferon-α in HCL is unknown and may be related to the reduced production of a number of cytokines such as granulocyte colony-stimulating factor (GCSF), granulocyte-macrophage colony-stimulating factor (GM-CSF), interleukin-3 (IL-3), and interleukin-6 (IL-6). Others have demonstrated that interferon-α can mediate apoptosis of hairy cells through the effects of tumor necrosis factor-α (TNF-α).

Treatment with interferon-α is associated with significant toxicity including flu-like symptoms, anorexia, fatigue, nausea and vomiting, diarrhea, skin rash, peripheral neuropathy, and central nervous system dysfunction (such as depression and memory loss). This and the introduction of nucleoside analogs that are generally more effective in achieving responses has led to the use of interferon being limited to rare cases and special circumstances.

Purine Nucleoside Analogs

Although there are no specific guidelines for the treatment of HCL, monotherapy with cladribine or pentostatin is the current established standard. Furthermore, despite the lack of a comparative study, a substantial number of data suggest that both drugs are equally effective in terms of response rate and durability.[10] The use of nucleoside analogs in treating lymphoid neoplasms can be traced back to the observation that children with the deficiency of the enzyme adenine deaminase (ADA) developed severe combined immunodeficiency (SCID). The accumulation of the triphosphorylated form of deoxyadenosine (dependent on the action of the enzyme deoxycitidine kinase [DCK]) is thought to be responsible for the lack of lymphocyte development. Similarly, after treatment with purine nucleoside analogs, the accumulation of deoxyadenosine triphosphate results in DNA strand breaks, inhibition of DNA repair, and apoptosis preferentially in lymphoid cells, rich in DCK and low in 5′ nucleotidase (the enzyme responsible for degrading deoxyadenosine monophosphate).

Table 77-3 Selected Published Reports of Cladribine Therapy for Hairy Cell Leukemia

Reference	Evaluable Patients (n)	CR (%)	PR (%)	OR (%)
INTRAVENOUS DAILY ADMINISTRATION (CONTINUOUS OR PULSED)				
Saven[15]	349	91	7	98
Goodman[16]	207	95	5	100
Tallman	50	80	18	98
Chadha[17]	85	79	21	100
Hoffman	49	76	24	100
Seymore[30]	46	78	11	89
Dearden	45	84	16	100
Juliusson	16	75	0	75
Zinzani*	21	81	19	100
Jehn	44	98	2	100
Robak[†13]	132	76	19	95
INTRAVENOUS WEEKLY ADMINISTRATION				
Lauria	30	73	27	100
Zinzani*	16	81	19	100
Robak[†13]	57	72	19	91
SUBCUTANEOUS ADMINISTRATION				
Juliusson[14]	73	81	13	94
Forconi[20]	58	72	19	91

CR, Complete response; *OR*, overall response; *PR*, partial response.
*Reports from the same publication.
†Numbers reported for the two arms of a randomized study.

Table 77-4 Alternative Dose and Schedules of Cladribine Therapy Reported in the Literature

Study	Dosing	Route of Administration	Responses
Saven[15]	0.1 mg/kg/day × 7 days	Continuous IV infusion	CR: 91%; PR: 7%
Juliusson[14]	3.4 mg/m²/day × 7 days	Subcutaneous injection	CR: 75% after 1 cycle, 85% after 2 cycles
Robak[13]	0.12 mg/kg/day × 5 days	2-hour IV bolus	CR: 76%; PR: 19%
Robak[13]	0.12 mg/kg/week × 6 weeks	2 hour IV bolus	CR: 72%; PR: 19%
Chacko	0.15 mg/kg/week × 6 weeks	3 hour IV infusion	CR: 100%
Lauria[12]	0.15 mg/kg/week × 6 weeks	2 hour IV bolus	CR: 76%; PR: 24%
Von Rohr	0.14 mg/kg/day × 5 days	Subcutaneous injection	CR: 76%; PR: 21%

Cladribine is a purine nucleoside analog resistant to deamination by ADA. It accumulates in lymphocytes rich in DCK and inhibits ribonucleotide reductase, impairing DNA synthesis and repair. Cladribine has been very effective for the initial therapy of HCL, with overall response rates ranging from 75% to 100% after a single course of the drug (Table 77-3). Piro and colleagues first reported 12 patients with HCL who received cladribine 0.1 mg/kg per day by intravenous continuous infusion for 7 days.[11] Eleven patients achieved CR, and one had PR.[11] Since then, other dose, routes of administration, and schedules of the drug have been used effectively (Tables 77-3 and 77-4). Weekly administration was evaluated in severely neutropenic patients in a pilot study in an effort to produce a less toxic strategy.[12] The authors reported a 73% CR rate, with an overall response rate of 100%. However, only 16% developed severe neutropenia and 8% infections.[12] In a more recent report, 132 patients with untreated HCL were randomized to receive cladribine either on 5 consecutive days or a novel schedule of 6 weekly doses.[13] The response rates, overall response rates, progression free, overall survival, and incidence of grade 3 and 4 infections were the same in the two arms.[13] The subcutaneous route was also evaluated after the initial demonstration that similar plasma levels to those seen with the intravenous route can be achieved subcutaneously. Juliusson and colleagues treated 73 patients with cladribine administered as a subcutaneous daily injection for 7 days and reported a CR rate of 81% after 1 (75%) or 2 courses.[14]

Despite the very high response rate to cladribine, responses are not universal and a significant proportion of patients relapse. Saven and colleagues reported the long-term outcome of 358 patients with HCL who were followed for a median of 52 months.[15] Of these patients, 26% relapsed after a median of 29 months.[15] The same group reported on 209 patients treated with cladribine with a follow-up period of at least 7 years.[16] Although the overall response rate was 100%, 76 (37%) patients relapsed after their first course of cladribine with a median time to relapse of 42 months.[16] Notably, the time to treatment failure curve did not show a plateau, indicating that the treatment is probably not "curative."[16] Outcome of patients achieving CR with their initial therapy is better than those achieving PR (Fig. 77-7). More recent publications have confirmed the high response rate of patients with HCL treated with cladribine and have provided long-term follow-up data.[17] Jehn and colleagues described a 12-year follow-up of 44 patients (including 11 with prior therapy before receiving cladribine) who received cladribine at the originally reported dose and schedule. The CR rate was 98%, and with a median follow-up of 8.5 years (range 0.1 to 12.2), 17 patients had relapsed. Eight of nine patients retreated with cladribine responded again. The overall survival at 12 years was 79%. Zinzani and colleagues reported the long-term outcome of 37 patients treated with one of two regimens of cladribine. Twenty-one patients received cladribine by a 2-hour infusion for 5 days, whereas 16 patients were treated with a once-weekly schedule for 5 weeks. A CR rate of 81% with an overall response rate of 100% was reported, with no difference between the two schedules. After a median follow-up of 122 months (range 54 to 156), the overall relapse rate was about 30% for both groups. The projected 13-year overall and relapse-free survival rates were 96% and 52%, respectively. Investigators at Northwestern University treated 86 consecutive patients with cladribine and reported a CR rate of 79%, as well as a PR rate of 21%.[17] The progression-free survival after 12 years was 54%. After a median follow-up of 9.7 years (range 0.3 to 13.8), 31 patients (36%) relapsed.[17] Of these, 23 were treated with a second course of cladribine; 12 (52%) achieved CR, and 7 (30%) achieved PR. The overall survival after 12 years was 87%.[17] The authors suggested that the lower CR rate in this study was due to their more stringent criteria for response, which included a requirement for resolution of splenomegaly and lymphadenopathy by CT scan as criteria for CR.[17]

Similar excellent responses have been achieved using pentostatin (Table 77-5). Overall CR rates of 44% to 89% have been reported with pentostatin administered intravenously at a dose of 2 to 4 mg/m² every 2 weeks. Spiers and colleagues were the first to report that a nucleoside analog (pentostatin) was capable of producing CRs in patients with HCL. The activity of pentostatin in HCL was confirmed in a number of larger studies by several investigators. Grever and colleagues conducted a large, randomized clinical trial comparing pentostatin with interferon-α in patients with previously untreated HCL.[18] Patients were randomized to receive either IFN-α 3 million

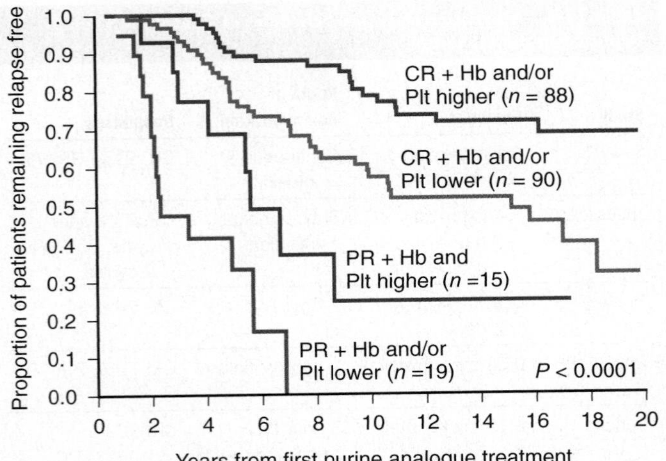

Figure 77-7 LONG-TERM FOLLOW-UP OF PATIENTS TREATED WITH NUCLEOSIDE ANALOG MONOTHERAPY. Excellent outcome for the majority, and significantly better relapse-free survival for patients achieving CR versus PR with initial therapy. *(Else M, Dearden CE, Matutes E, et al: Long-term follow-up of 233 patients with hairy cell leukaemia, treated initially with pentostatin or cladribine, at a median of 16 years from diagnosis.* Br J Haematol *145:733, 2009.)*

units subcutaneously three times per week or pentostatin 4 mg/m^2 intravenously every 2 weeks.[18] Patients who did not respond to initial treatment were crossed over. Confirmed complete and overall response rates were reported for 76% and 79% of patients treated with pentostatin, respectively, as compared with 11% and 38% of those treated with interferon-α.[18] Response rates were significantly higher (P <0.0001), and relapse-free survival was significantly longer with pentostatin than with interferon (P<0.0001).[18] Furthermore, patients who were initially assigned to receive interferon were frequently crossed over to pentostatin therapy, achieving a CR rate of 66%. In a follow-up report, Flinn and colleagues described the long-term outcome of 241 patients who were treated with pentostatin either as initial therapy or after failure of IFN-α.[19] The 5- and 10-year event-free survival rates were 85% and 67% respectively (Fig. 77-8). Other investigators have reported long-term follow-up data on patients treated with pentostatin. Maloisel and colleagues reported outcome of 230 evaluable patients with HCL treated with pentostatin, including 84 with pentostatin as the initial agent. They reported a CR rate of 79%, with an overall response rate of 96%. With a median follow-up of 63.5 months, 34 (15%) of 220 responding patients had relapsed. The estimated 5- and 10-year disease-free survival was 88% and 69%, respectively, and the estimated 5-year overall survival was 89%.

There are no prospective trials comparing the efficacy and durability of response between cladribine and pentostatin. Dearden and colleagues examined the outcome of the patients with the two agents at their institution and reported that 82% of 165 patients treated with pentostatin achieved a CR compared with 84% of 45 patients treated with cladribine. Relapse rates were 24% with pentostatin and 29% with cladribine after median follow-up of 71 and 45 months, respectively. They suggested a longer remission duration with pentostatin. However, with further follow-up, there appears to be no difference between the two agents with regard to disease-free survival (Fig. 77-9, *A*). Further follow-up data of these cohorts of patients have been reported.[10] With a median follow-up of 16 years, there was no significant difference in the outcome of the patients treated with the 2 drugs. After relapse or nonresponse, patients could be successfully retreated with pentostatin or cladribine but achieved lower response rates, with a decline in the proportion of patients achieving CR with second- and third-line therapy (Fig. 77-9, *A*).[10] However, CRs were equally durable after first, second, or third line of treatment. Complete responders and those with pretreatment hemoglobin >10.0 g/dL and platelet count >100 × 10^9/L had the longest

Table 77-5 Selected Published Reports of Pentostatin Therapy for Hairy Cell Leukemia

Reference	Evaluable Patients (n)	CR (%)	PR (%)	OR (%)
Kraut	23	87	4	91
Johnston	28	89	11	100
Dearden	165	82	15	97
Catovsky	148	74	22	96
Grever[18]	154	76	3	79
Rafel	78	72	16	88
Ribeiro	49	44	52	96
Maloisel	230	79	17	96

CR, Complete response; *PR,* partial response; *OR,* overall response.

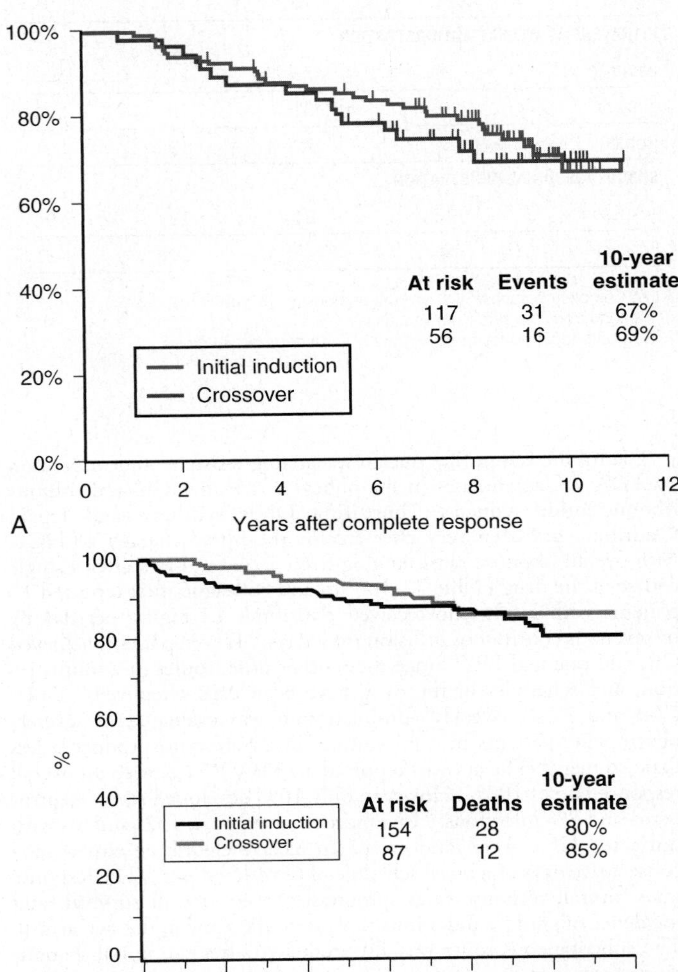

Figure 77-8 LONG-TERM FOLLOW-UP OF PATIENTS TREATED WITH PENTOSTATIN FOR THEIR INITIAL THERAPY OR FOLLOWING FAILURE OF INTERFERON-A AS A PART OF THE RANDOMIZED INTERGROUP STUDY. **A,** Relapse-free survival by phase of treatment. **B,** Overall survival by phase of treatment. *(Flinn IW, Kopecky KJ, Foucar MK, et al: Long-term follow-up of remission duration, mortality, and second malignancies in hairy cell leukemia patients treated with pentostatin.* Blood *96:2981, 2000.)*

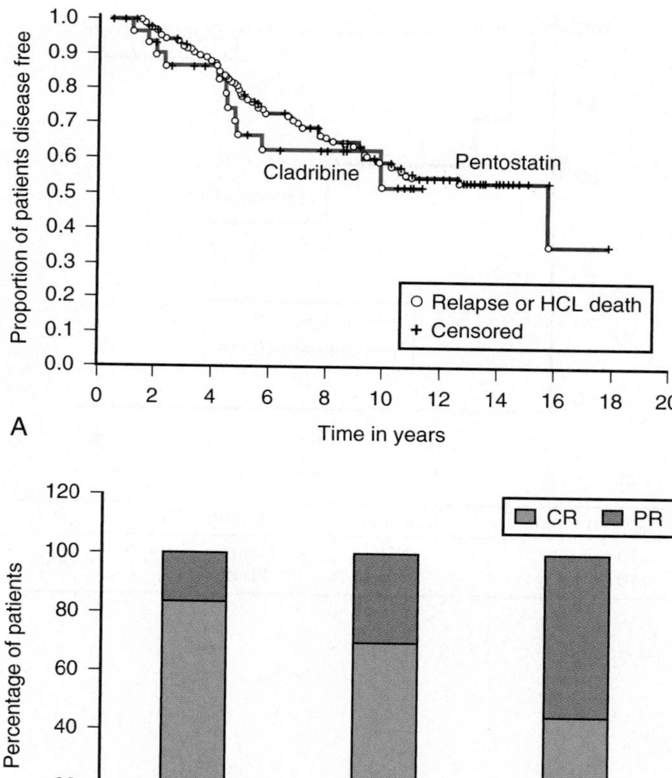

Figure 77-9 LONG-TERM FOLLOW-UP OF PATIENTS TREATED AT THE ROYAL MARSDEN HOSPITAL. **A,** Patients who received either cladribine or pentostatin as their initial therapy. **B,** Proportion of patients achieving CR and PR with first-, second-, and third-line therapy. *(Else MA, Ruchlemer R, Osuji N, et al: Long remissions in hairy cell leukemia with purine analogs.* Cancer *104:2442, 2005.)*

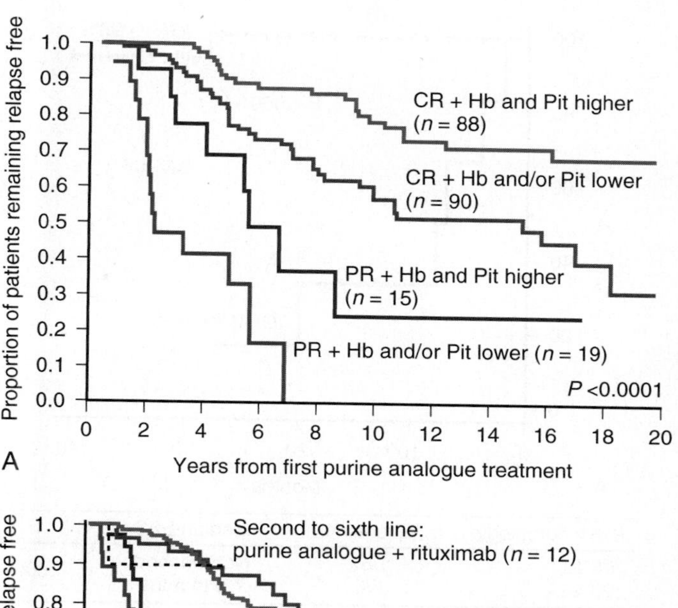

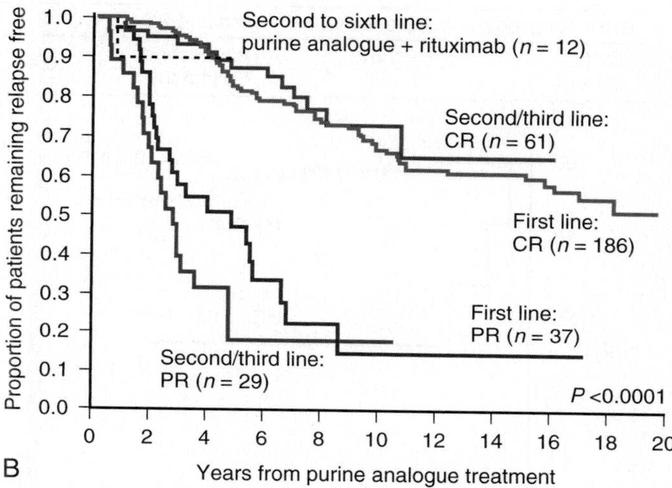

Figure 77-10 A, Relapse-free survival after initial therapy with nucleoside analogs by initial response and blood counts. **B,** Relapse-free survival analyzed by line of therapy and response to treatment. Complete responses were equally durable, whether achieved at first-, second-, or third-line single-agent treatment. *(Else MA, Ruchlemer R, Osuji N, et al: Long remissions in hairy cell leukemia with purine analogs.* Cancer *104:2442, 2005; and Else M, Dearden CE, Matutes E, et al: Long-term follow-up of 233 patients with hairy cell leukaemia, treated initially with pentostatin or cladribine, at a median of 16 years from diagnosis.* Br J Haematol *145:733, 2009).*

relapse-free survival (p <0.0001) (Fig. 77-10).[10] Patients who were in CR after 5 years had only a 25% risk for relapsing by 15 years.[10] These data suggest that both pentostatin and cladribine are highly effective in treating patients with HCL but not curative in all patients. Few predictors of response and long-term outcome have been reported, but the recent demonstration by two groups that patients with unmutated immunoglobulin heavy chain variable *(IGHV)* region gene were less likely to respond to cladribine suggests that further insight into the biology of the disease may potentially clarify mechanisms of resistance (Fig. 77-11).[20-21]

Monoclonal Antibodies

Several therapeutic options are now available for patients with relapsed HCL. The efficacy of the monoclonal antibody rituximab in treating these patients has been suggested by a number of studies (Table 77-6). Rituximab is a monoclonal antibody directed against the pan–B cell antigen (CD20), which is heavily expressed on the surface of hairy cells. Nieva and colleagues reported their experience with 4 weekly doses of rituximab in 24 patients with HCL who had failed prior treatment with cladribine. The overall response rate was 26%, with 13% CR and 13% PR. No unusual toxicity was reported. Lauria and colleagues treated 10 patients with relapsed/progressed HCL with 4 weekly doses of rituximab and reported 1 CR and 4 PR (overall response rate of 50%). Hagberg and colleagues treated 11

Table 77-6 Selected Published Reports of Rituximab Therapy for Hairy Cell Leukemia

Reference	Patients (n)	No Prior Therapy (n)	CR (%) (Untreated)	PR (%)	OR (%)
Lauria	10	0	10	40	50
Hagberg	11	3	55 (33)	10	65
Nieva	24	0	13	13	26
Thomas[22]	15	0	66	13	80
Zenhausern	25	0	32	48	80

CR, Complete response; *OR,* overall response; *PR,* partial response.

patients with HCL (including 3 previously untreated patients) with the same regimen of rituximab for 4 weeks. The response rate was 64%, with 6 CRs and 1 PR (including 1 CR in an untreated patient). The Swiss Group for Clinical Cancer Research reported their study of 4 weekly doses of rituximab in 26 patients with relapsed/progressed HCL, showing an 80% response rate, with 32% achieving CR.

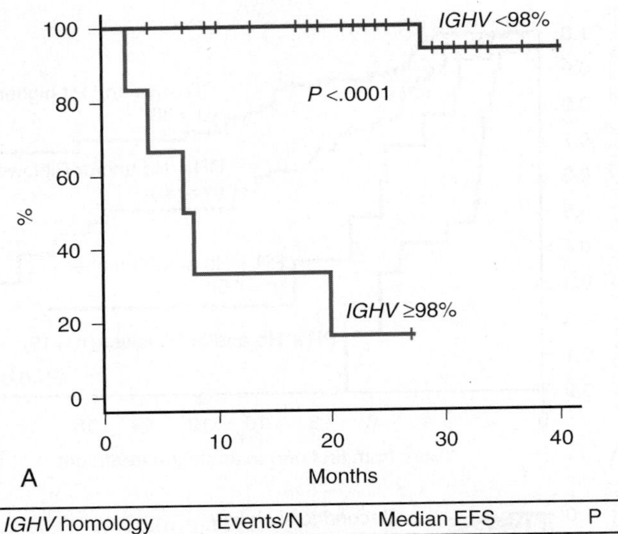

IGHV homology	Events/N	Median EFS	P
<98%	1/52	Not reached	<.0001
≥98%	5/6	7.5 months	

B

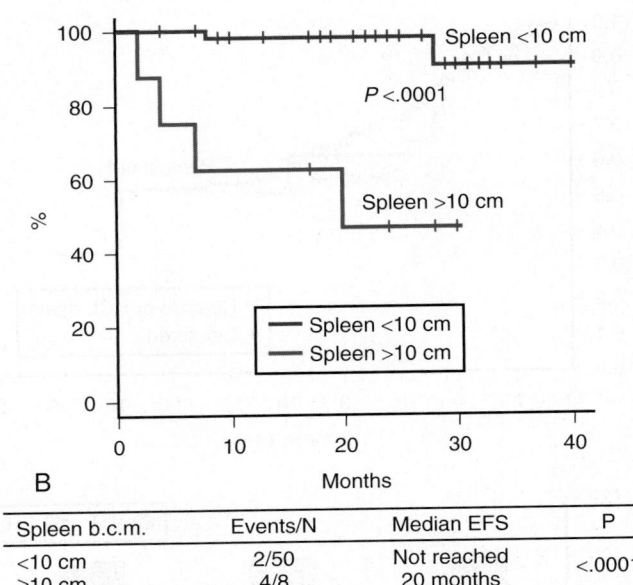

Spleen b.c.m.	Events/N	Median EFS	P
<10 cm	2/50	Not reached	<.0001
≥10 cm	4/8	20 months	

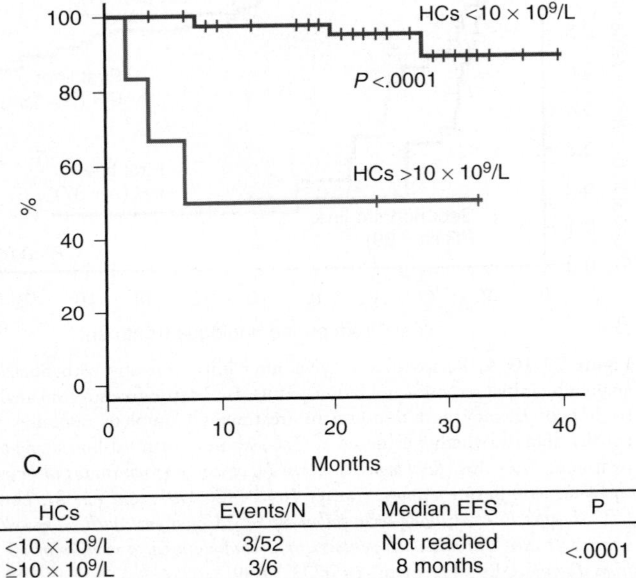

HCs	Events/N	Median EFS	P
$<10 \times 10^9/L$	3/52	Not reached	<.0001
$\geq 10 \times 10^9/L$	3/6	8 months	

Figure 77-11 PREDICTING RESPONSE AND OUTCOME OF THERAPY WITH CLADRIBINE BY ASSESSING *IGHV* MUTATIONAL STATUS (AS WELL AS BY SPLENOMEGALY AND LEUKOCYTOSIS). *(Forconi F, Sozzi E, Cencini E, et al: Hairy cell leukemias with unmutated IGHV genes define the minor subset refractory to single-agent cladribine and with more aggressive behavior.* Blood *114:4696, 2009.)*

Thomas and colleagues used an extended regimen of rituximab 375 mg/m^2 weekly for 8 doses to treat 15 patients with relapsed/refractory HCL and reported a response rate of 80%, including 8 (52%) CR, 2 (13%) CR with residual marrow disease, and 2 (13%) PR.[22]

Rituximab has been evaluated in a sequential strategy to improve responses in patients with HCL after treatment with cladribine.[23] Rituximab has also been used concomitantly to treat patients with refractory disease with reported excellent responses suggesting a possible synergy. The investigators from the Royal Marsden NHS Trust treated 18 patients with either pentostatin (n = 12) or cladribine (n = 6) in combination with rituximab after a median of 2 (range, 1 to 6) prior treatments and reported a CR rate of 89%. Toxicity with the combination was minimal, and with a median follow-up of 36 months, all 16 patients who had achieved CR remained in CR.

Other monoclonal antibody–based therapies have developed and are under investigation. BL22 is a recombinant immunotoxin containing the variable domains of the anti-CD22 monoclonal antibody RFB4 fused to a truncated pseudomonas endotoxin A.[24] In a dose-escalation study, 16 patients who were resistant to cladribine were treated with BL22 by intravenous infusion every other day for a total of 3 doses.[24] Response included 11 CR and 2 PR. The 3 nonresponders either had preexisting neutralizing antibodies or received low doses of the immunotoxin.[24] Toxicity included a cytokine-release syndrome and development of a reversible hemolytic-uremic syndrome in 2 patients.[24] In a larger phase I follow-up study of 46 patients with previously treated CD22+ lymphoid malignancies, including 31 with HCL, 61% achieved a CR and 19% experienced a PR, further demonstrating the activity of this agent in HCL. Neutralizing antibodies occurred in 11 (24%) of 46 patients (all HCL), and a reversible hemolytic uremic syndrome requiring plasmapheresis was observed in 1 patient with NHL during cycle 1 and in 4 patients with HCL during cycle 2 or 3. The median duration for CR was 36 months (range, 5 to 66 months). The maximum tolerated dose (MTD) was established at 40 μg/kg every other day ×3 doses. More recently, the results of a phase 2 study of the same drug in 36 patients with relapsed or refractory HCL was published.[25] Patients received BL22 at the MTD on cycle 1. Those achieving hematologic remission were observed while the others were retreated at 30 μg/kg every other day for three doses every 4 weeks beginning at least 8 weeks after cycle 1. The response after one cycle (CR, 25%; PR, 25%) improved when 56% were retreated (CR, 47%; PR, 25%).[25] A modified version of this agent, moxetumomab pasudotox (or HA22), has a superior affinity for CD22 and is under clinical development.

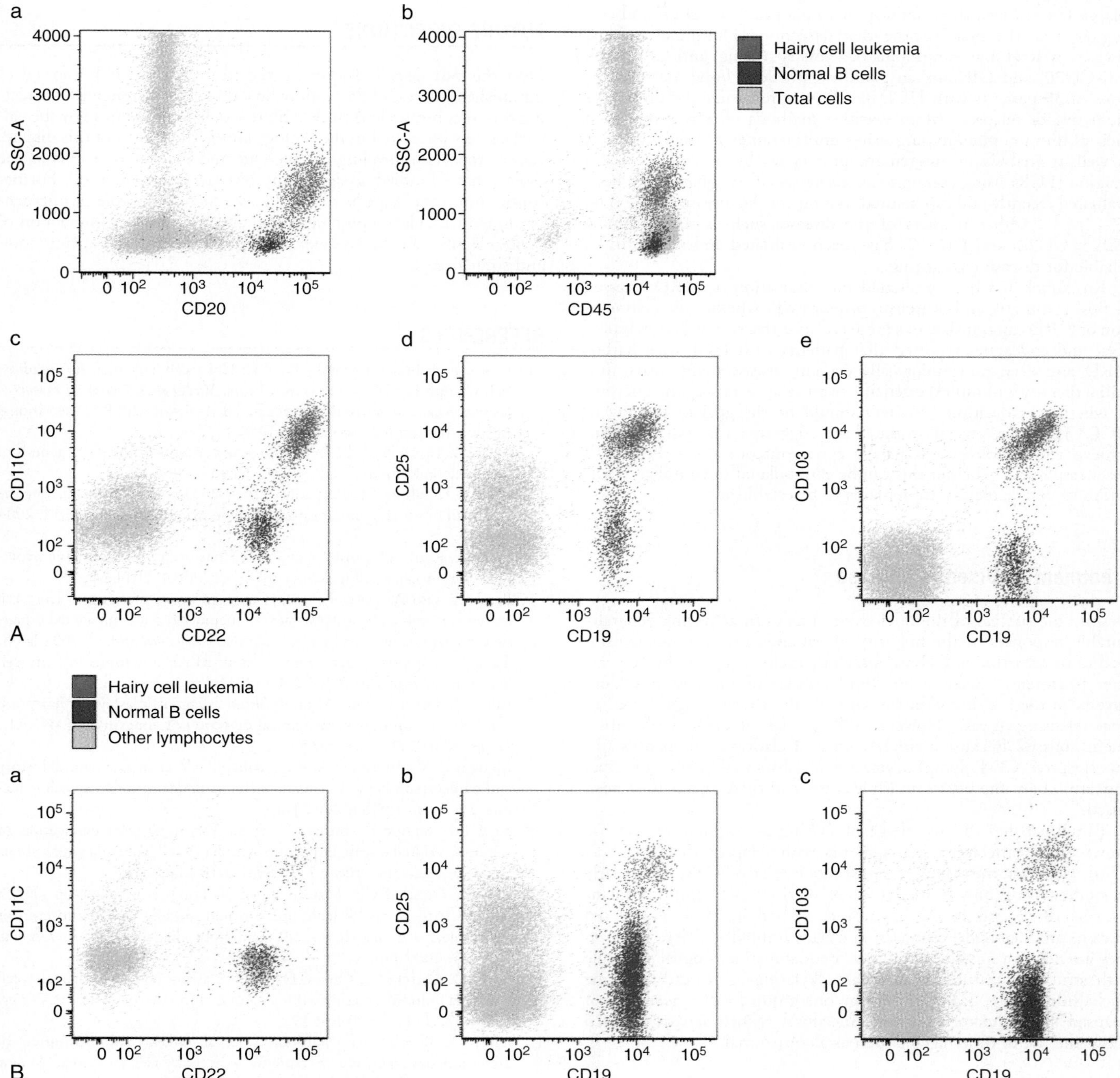

Figure 77-12 MONITORING MINIMAL RESIDUAL DISEASE IN HAIRY CELL LEUKEMIA. **A,** Total nucleated cells in a hemodilute bone marrow aspirate (*a* and *b*); total lymphocytes (*c* to *e*). Hairy cells (*red,* about 6% of total cellularity and 12% of lymphocytes) show increased side scatter (SSC) because of their high cytoplasmic complexity, compared with normal B cells *(blue).* Hairy cells often show increased expression of CD20 *(a).* On CD45 versus SSC gating plots *(b),* they may be mistaken for monocytes. Hairy cells usually show bright expression of CD11c and CD22 *(c)* and CD25 *(d)* and are positive for CD103 *(e).* **B,** Total lymphocytes from a posttherapy bone marrow aspirate, positive for minimal residual hairy cell leukemia, accounting for about 0.6% of total cellularity. Hairy cells *(red)* can be easily distinguished from normal B cells *(blue),* particularly on the basis of their bright expression of CD11c *(a)* and CD25 *(b)* and positivity for CD103 *(c).* In *a,* 30,000 total cells were collected; in *b* and *c,* 100,000. *(Courtesy Jeffrey Jorgensen, Department of Hematopathology, UTMDACC.)*

CD52 is also expressed on the surface of hairy cells, and an anecdotal report of a response to alemtuzumab has recently been published.

Minimal Residual Disease and Its Significance

Despite excellent responses, there is a definite relapse rate associated with therapy of HCL with both cladribine and pentostatin, and the relapse-free survival does not appear to plateau.[10] Wheaton and colleagues were the first to note that detection of minimal residual disease (MRD) by immunohistochemistry (using anti-CD45RO, anti-CD20, and DBA.44) in paraffin-embedded bone marrow sections of 39 patients with HCL in CR after receiving cladribine was predictive of relapse.[26] More sensitive methods of MRD detection such as immunophenotyping using multiparameter flow cytometry, as well as analysis of antigen receptor genes by polymerase chain reaction (PCR) using consensus or clone-specific primers, have been evaluated recently and can be used to monitor the disease course (Fig. 77-12).[23,27,28] Other markers of the disease, such as serum-soluble CD25, CD22, and CD307, have been evaluated and shown to be reliable for disease monitoring.[29]

Rituximab has been evaluated for eradication of MRD assessed by flow cytometry and consensus primer PCR; whether such elimination of MRD can translate to a longer relapse-free survival is unclear.[9,23] Sigal and colleagues reported that patients with HCL may harbor MRD and even morphologically evident disease many years after initial therapy without experiencing overt relapse, raising the question of whether eradication of MRD should be the goal of therapy in HCL.[9] However, several studies have suggested that patients who achieve a morphologic CR have a better outcome than those with lesser responses. Whether this can be extrapolated to complete eradication of detectable disease remains to be established.

Treatment of Disease Relapse

Despite the success of the nucleoside analogs in achieving generally durable responses in the majority of patients, they are not considered to be curative, with about 40% of patients relapsing by 10 years after treatment.[10] Second and third courses of nucleoside analogs have been used, either with the same or the alternate agent used to treat relapsing disease. However, CRs are less frequent with subsequent courses. Because a single course of cladribine or pentostatin can suppress $CD4^+$ lymphocytes for a substantial period of time, concerns about the use of multiple courses of these agents have been raised.[30]

Rituximab has the advantage of sparing T-lymphocytes and has shown significant activity in patients with relapsed disease (Table 77-6). However, the overall response rate is relatively low, particularly in studies using only 4 weekly doses of rituximab. Immunotoxins such as BL22 and HA22 have been studied in cases of relapsed disease, produce high responses, and have limited toxicity; however, they are not, as yet, widely available. Bendamustine, a novel molecule with structural features of both an alkylating agent and a purine nucleoside analog, has been used by one group for the treatment of relapsed and refractory disease. Anecdotal reports have circulated about the use of other agents such as alemtuzumab.

Incidence of Second Malignancies

Early studies suggested an association between HCL and development of second malignancies, but this link is controversial and has been refuted by other reports. The reported second cancers include melanoma, prostate cancer, gastrointestinal cancers, and non-Hodgkin lymphomas. Whether these second malignancies are related to the primary disease itself or to its treatment has also been debated. A number of long-term studies of patients treated with pentostatin or cladribine have not shown a statistically significant increased risk for second malignancies. It remains unclear whether the immunosuppressive effects of nucleoside analogs play a role in such susceptibility to developing a second malignancy or whether disease-related factors or perhaps increased monitoring of these patients are important.

FUTURE DIRECTIONS

Over the past decade, success in the treatment of HCL had led to diminished interest in developing new therapeutic strategies for treating this uncommon leukemia, with research confined to a few specialized centers interested in the biology and pathogenesis of this disease. Recent reports unraveling the biologic and molecular aspects of the disease have kindled a significant resurgence of interest.[2] Further studies into other aspects of the disease, such as the role of microenvironment, B-cell receptor signaling, and the complex interaction of various signaling pathways will likely provide better therapeutic tools and strategies.[2]

REFERENCES

1. Foucar K, Falini B, Catovsky D, et al: Hairy cell leukemia. In Swerdlow SH, Campo E, Harris NL, et al, editors: *WHO classification of tumors of haematopoietic and lymphoid tissues*, ed 4, Lyon, 2008, International Agency for Research on Cancer (IARC).
2. Tiacci E, Liso A, Piris M, et al: Evolving concepts in the pathogenesis of hairy-cell leukaemia. *Nat Rev Cancer* 6:437, 2006 Jun.
3. Forconi F, Sahota SS, Raspadori D, et al: Hairy cell leukemia: At the crossroad of somatic mutation and isotype switch. *Blood* 104:3312, 2004 Nov 15.
4. Arons E, Roth L, Sapolsky J, et al: Evidence of canonical somatic hypermutation in hairy cell leukemia. *Blood* 117:4844, 2011 May 5.
5. Basso K, Liso A, Tiacci E, et al: Gene expression profiling of hairy cell leukemia reveals a phenotype related to memory B cells with altered expression of chemokine and adhesion receptors. *J Exp Med* 199:59, 2004 Jan 5.
6. Tiacci E, Trifonov V, Schiavoni G, et al: BRAF mutations in hairy-cell leukemia. *N Engl J Med* 364:2305, 2011 Jun 16.
7. Falini B, Tiacci E, Liso A, et al: Simple diagnostic assay for hairy cell leukaemia by immunocytochemical detection of annexin A1 (ANXA1). *Lancet* 363:1869, 2004 Jun 5.
8. Matutes E, Wotherspoon A, Brito-Babapulle V, et al: The natural history and clinico-pathological features of the variant form of hairy cell leukemia. *Leukemia* 15:184, 2001 Jan.
9. Sigal DS, Sharpe R, Burian C, et al: Very long-term eradication of minimal residual disease in patients with hairy cell leukemia after a single course of cladribine. *Blood* 115:1893, 2010 Mar 11.
10. Else M, Dearden CE, Matutes E, et al: Long-term follow-up of 233 patients with hairy cell leukaemia, treated initially with pentostatin or cladribine, at a median of 16 years from diagnosis. *Br J Haematol* 145:733, 2009 Jun.
11. Piro LD, Carrera CJ, Carson DA, et al: Lasting remissions in hairy-cell leukemia induced by a single infusion of 2-chlorodeoxyadenosine. *N Engl J Med* 322:1117, 1990 Apr 19.
12. Lauria F, Bocchia M, Marotta G, et al: Weekly administration of 2-chlorodeoxyadenosine in patients with hairy-cell leukemia: A new treatment schedule effective and safer in preventing infectious complications. *Blood* 89:1838, 1997 Mar 1.
13. Robak T, Jamroziak K, Gora-Tybor J, et al: Cladribine in a weekly versus daily schedule for untreated active hairy cell leukemia: Final report from the Polish Adult Leukemia Group (PALG) of a prospective, randomized, multicenter trial. *Blood* 109:3672, 2007 May 1.
14. Juliusson G, Heldal D, Hippe E, et al: Subcutaneous injections of 2-chlorodeoxyadenosine for symptomatic hairy cell leukemia. *J Clin Oncol* 13:989, 1995 Apr.

15. Saven A, Burian C, Koziol JA, et al: Long-term follow-up of patients with hairy cell leukemia after cladribine treatment. *Blood* 92:1918, 1998 Sep 15.
16. Goodman GR, Burian C, Koziol JA, et al: Extended follow-up of patients with hairy cell leukemia after treatment with cladribine. *J Clin Oncol* 21:891, 2003 Mar 1.
17. Chadha P, Rademaker AW, Mendiratta P, et al: Treatment of hairy cell leukemia with 2-chlorodeoxyadenosine (2-CdA): Long-term follow-up of the Northwestern University experience. *Blood* 106:241, 2005 Jul 1.
18. Grever M, Kopecky K, Foucar MK, et al: Randomized comparison of pentostatin versus interferon alfa-2a in previously untreated patients with hairy cell leukemia: An intergroup study. *J Clin Oncol* 13:974, 1995 Apr.
19. Flinn IW, Kopecky KJ, Foucar MK, et al: Long-term follow-up of remission duration, mortality, and second malignancies in hairy cell leukemia patients treated with pentostatin. *Blood* 96:2981, 2000 Nov 1.
20. Forconi F, Sozzi E, Cencini E, et al: Hairy cell leukemias with unmutated IGHV genes define the minor subset refractory to single-agent cladribine and with more aggressive behavior. *Blood* 114:4696, 2009 Nov 19.
21. Arons E, Suntum T, Stetler-Stevenson M, et al: VH4-34+ hairy cell leukemia, a new variant with poor prognosis despite standard therapy. *Blood* 114:4687, 2009 Nov 19.
22. Thomas DA, O'Brien S, Bueso-Ramos C, et al: Rituximab in relapsed or refractory hairy cell leukemia. *Blood* 102:3906, 2003 Dec 1.
23. Ravandi F, Jorgensen JL, O'Brien SM, et al: Eradication of minimal residual disease in hairy cell leukemia. *Blood* 107:4658, 2006 Jun 15.
24. Kreitman RJ, Wilson WH, Bergeron K, et al: Efficacy of the anti-CD22 recombinant immunotoxin BL22 in chemotherapy-resistant hairy-cell leukemia. *N Engl J Med* 345:241, 2001 Jul 26.
25. Kreitman RJ, Stetler-Stevenson M, Margulies I, et al: Phase II trial of recombinant immunotoxin RFB4(dsFv)-PE38 (BL22) in patients with hairy cell leukemia. *J Clin Oncol* 27:2983, 2009 Jun 20.
26. Wheaton S, Tallman MS, Hakimian D, et al: Minimal residual disease may predict bone marrow relapse in patients with hairy cell leukemia treated with 2-chlorodeoxyadenosine. *Blood* 87:1556, 1996 Feb 15.
27. Sausville JE, Salloum RG, Sorbara L, et al: Minimal residual disease detection in hairy cell leukemia: Comparison of flow cytometric immunophenotyping with clonal analysis using consensus primer polymerase chain reaction for the heavy chain gene. *Am J Clin Pathol* 119:213, 2003 Feb.
28. Arons E, Margulies I, Sorbara L, et al: Minimal residual disease in hairy cell leukemia patients assessed by clone-specific polymerase chain reaction. *Clin Cancer Res* 12:2804, 2006 May 1.
29. Ravandi F, O'Brien S, Jorgensen J, et al: Phase II study of cladribine followed by rituximab in patients with hairy cell leukemia. *Blood* Aug 5 2011.
30. Seymour JF, Kurzrock R, Freireich EJ, et al: 2-chlorodeoxyadenosine induces durable remissions and prolonged suppression of CD4+ lymphocyte counts in patients with hairy cell leukemia. *Blood* 83:2906, 1994 May 15.

CHAPTER 78

CLINICAL MANIFESTATIONS AND TREATMENT OF MARGINAL ZONE LYMPHOMAS (EXTRANODAL/MALT, SPLENIC, AND NODAL)

Carlos A. Ramos

The term *marginal zone* refers to a histologic compartment located at the periphery of lymphoid follicles immediately outside their mantle zone.[1] The marginal zone is especially evident in the spleen, although identical areas have been observed in other lymphoid structures, including mesenteric lymph nodes and mucosa-associated lymphoid tissue (MALT) (Fig. 78-1).[2] Ordinarily, it is composed predominantly of B cells that are slightly larger than mantle zone lymphocytes and strongly positive for surface IgM, but weakly positive for IgD (in contrast to mantle zone cells, which are strongly positive for IgD).[3] Marginal zone B lymphocytes are thought to be involved in fast protective responses against pathogenic encapsulated bacteria that do not trigger classical T cell–dependent humoral immunity.[4] They are also assumed to be the physiologic counterpart of a group of non-Hodgkin lymphomas (NHL) that are currently referred to as *marginal zone lymphomas (MZLs)*.

Although MZLs share a common denomination, arising from histologic similarities, new genetic findings and longer follow-up studies have established that the currently recognized subtypes of MZLs, initially described in the Revised European-American Lymphoma (REAL) classification, are different diseases.[5] In the most recent WHO classification of tumors of the hematopoietic and lymphoid tissues,[6] these disorders comprise three distinct entities: extranodal MZL of MALT type (ENMZL), splenic MZL (SMZL) and nodal MZL (NMZL). Immunoproliferative small intestinal disease (IPSID), formerly known as alpha heavy chain (or Seligmann) disease, has been recently recognized as a variant of ENMZL.[7] In aggregate, MZLs represent approximately 10% of all NHL.[8] Clinically, they behave indolently and have a prolonged course. Therefore, management strategies share similarity with other low-grade lymphomas,[9] although specific biologic characteristics and particular pathophysiologic mechanisms determine unique therapeutic approaches in some of the subtypes. This chapter will summarize the clinical characteristics and current management strategies for the different types of MZL.

INITIAL EVALUATION OF MARGINAL ZONE LYMPHOMA

As for other lymphomas, biopsy of an adequate amount of tissue with review by a hematopathologist with expertise in the field is essential to establish the diagnosis. Excisional or incisional biopsies of a lymph node or suspicious mass, obtained by endoscopic or conventional means, are preferred. In patients without easily accessible nodes or masses, computed tomography (CT) or ultrasound-guided core needle biopsy is usually well tolerated and may be adequate for diagnosis. Fine-needle aspiration is not appropriate for diagnosis; sufficient material must be obtained for proper histologic examination and required immunophenotypic and genetic studies.

Physical examination with special attention to peripheral lymph nodes and the abdomen should be performed. Initial laboratory evaluation should include a complete blood count (cytopenias may be evidence of marrow infiltration or of autoimmunity) with evaluation of a peripheral blood smear (to exclude leukemic involvement) and basic biochemical studies, including lactate dehydrogenase (LDH) level, which is an important prognostic factor and a potential indicator of transformation from indolent to aggressive lymphoma. Serum protein electrophoresis and immunofixation may demonstrate a monoclonal immunoglobulin. β_2-microglobulin levels may have prognostic value[10] as in other indolent lymphomas.

Depending on the primary site of disease, specific procedures may be indicated. Gastrointestinal MZLs may require repeat staging endoscopies, during which an adequate number of biopsies should be obtained. For gastric ENMZL, the European Gastro-Intestinal Lymphoma Study (EGILS) group recommends a mapping procedure with a minimum of 10 biopsies taken from visible lesions and additional ones from macroscopically normal mucosa; the same procedure should be repeated to assess treatment response.[11] Since endoscopic biopsies are not transmural, endoscopic ultrasound (EUS) is a useful way to assess the depth of involvement, which has prognostic implications.[12-17] For head primaries, such as ocular adnexal ENMZL, appropriate directed examination and imaging studies (CT or magnetic resonance) are indicated.

STAGING OF MARGINAL ZONE LYMPHOMA

Imaging studies of the chest, abdomen, and pelvis, usually CT scans, should be obtained to adequately stage the disease. PET scan has been increasingly used for staging and evaluation of response to therapy in NHL, but it may be less useful in MZL because up to 60% of these lymphomas may be PET-negative, especially in early-stage gastric ENZML.[18] Some MZL series, however, document a PET-positivity rate of up to 80%.[19-23] Also for staging and, occasionally, for diagnostic purposes, bone marrow biopsy and aspirate are usually advocated, even in cases in which the likelihood of systemic disease is low, because any positive result has important implications for therapy.

Staging of MZL is similar to that of other lymphomas; the Ann Arbor system, or an adapted version,[24] is used most frequently (Table 78-1). Nonetheless, specific staging systems have been adopted for particular sites. Gastrointestinal MZL is often staged according to a modified Ann Arbor scheme, commonly known as the Lugano staging system,[25] which incorporates indices corresponding to depth of mucosal invasion and proximity of affected lymph nodes to the primary lesion (Table 78-1). Of note, stage IIE in the Lugano system may refer to lesions that extend by contiguity to adjacent organs and not necessarily to secondary involvement of lymph nodes. Recently, arguing that the dissemination patterns of extranodal lymphomas are essentially different from those of primary nodal lymphomas, the EGILS group has proposed a new staging system (the Paris staging system)[26] that is based on the TNM scheme used for solid tumors (Table 78-1). The International Society for Cutaneous Lymphomas (ISCL) and the cutaneous lymphoma task force of the European Organization of Research and Treatment of Cancer (EORTC) have also recently suggested a new, TNM-based staging system for cutaneous lymphomas other than mycosis fungoides and Sézary syndrome,[27] which may be used for the cutaneous forms of ENMZL (Table 78-2).

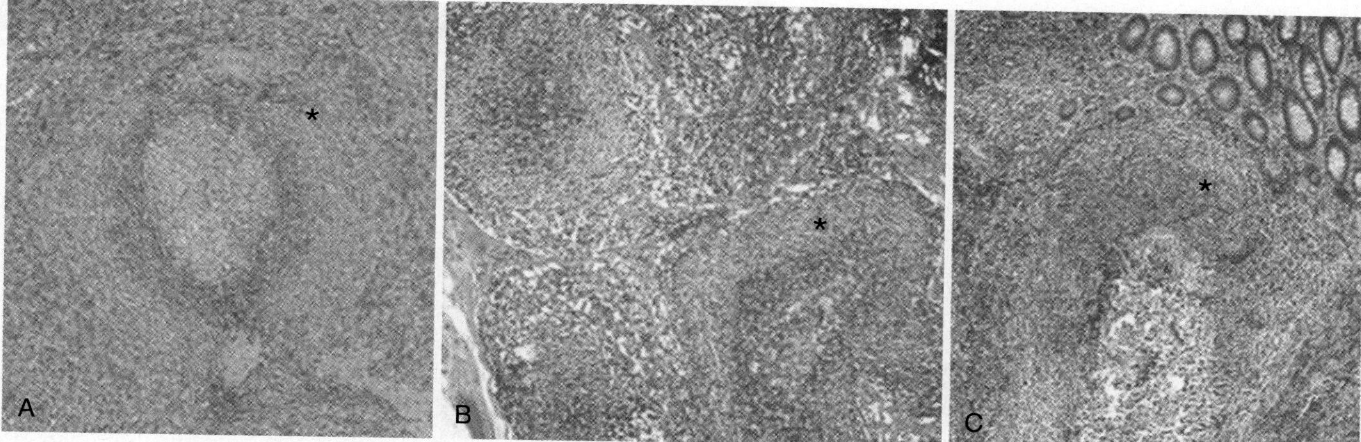

Figure 78-1 NORMAL MARGINAL ZONE CELLS. **A,** Marginal zone cells are seen most readily in sections from the normal spleen. The splenic white pulp typically has three distinctive layers: the germinal center, the mantle zone, and external to this, the marginal zone (see *asterisk*). **B,** Marginal zone cells are not usually seen in lymph nodes, but for some reason are sometimes present in mesenteric lymph nodes (see *asterisk*). They have a similar appearance to those in the spleen. **C,** In the gastrointestinal tract, the lymphoid tissue in Peyer's patches is believed to have a marginal zone equivalent (see *asterisk*). The cells are again external to the mantle zone and are believed to traffic between the epithelium and the lymphoid follicle.

Table 78-1 Staging Systems for Gastrointestinal Lymphomas

Adapted Ann Arbor System[24]	Lugano System[25]	Paris System[26]	Areas Involved*
IE1	I_1	T1 N0 M0	Mucosa to submucosa
IE2	I_2	T2 N0 M0	To muscularis propria or subserosa
		T3 N0 M0	To serosa
	IIE	T4 N0 M0	To adjacent organs
IIE1	II_1	T1-4 N1 M0	Regional lymph nodes†
IIE2	II_2	T1-4 N2 M0	Non-regional abdominal lymph nodes
IIIE	IV	T1-4 N3 M0	Extra-abdominal lymph nodes
IV		T1-4 N0-3 M1	Distant organs
		B1	Bone marrow

*In case of more than one visible lesion synchronously originating in the gastrointestinal tract, select the characteristics of the more advanced lesion.
†Anatomic designation of lymph nodes as *regional* according to site:
(a) stomach: perigastric nodes and those located along the ramifications of the celiac artery (i.e., left gastric artery, common hepatic artery, splenic artery);
(b) duodenum: pancreaticoduodenal, pyloric, hepatic, and superior mesenteric nodes; (c) jejunum/ileum: mesenteric nodes and, for the terminal ileum only, the ileocolic as well as the posterior cecal nodes; (d) colorectum: pericolic and perirectal nodes and those located along the ileocolic, right, middle, and left colic, inferior mesenteric, superior rectal, and internal iliac arteries.

EXTRANODAL MARGINAL ZONE LYMPHOMA OF MALT TYPE

Epidemiology and Manifestations

ENMZL is the most frequent of the MZL subtypes, accounting for approximately 8% of all NHL.[8] The median age of presentation is around 60, with a wide range spanning from the third to the ninth decades, and there is a slight female predominance (55%).[28] In contrast to most other indolent lymphomas, ENMZL frequently presents at a localized stage (≈40% stage I and ≈30% stage II), and the risk for systemic dissemination is low (albeit variable depending on primary location), which has important implications for the choice of therapy.

The most commonly affected primary site is the mucosa of the gastrointestinal tract, in particular the stomach (approximately 44% of all ENMZL cases) followed by the small intestine (≈7%). Ocular structures are also frequently involved (≈12%), namely, the orbit (≈40% of all ocular adnexal ENMZL), the conjunctiva (35%-40%), the lacrimal glands (10%-15%) and the eyelids (≈10%).[29] Other commonly affected sites include the bronchial mucosa (≈11% of all ENMZL cases), the skin (≈9%), the salivary glands (≈6%), and the thyroid gland (≈6%). More rarely reported sites are Waldeyer pharyngeal lymphoid ring, breast, liver, pancreas, urogenital tract, and central nervous system.[30-33] Findings at presentation depend on the specific organ affected. Gastric ENMZL may lead to dyspepsia, epigastric pain, nausea, anorexia, and manifestations of gastrointestinal bleeding.[34] Conjunctival ENMZL often forms a painless nodule or plaque that has a "salmon-pink patch" appearance and can be associated with erythema, chemosis, and foreign-body sensation.[35] Primary cutaneous ENMZL frequently presents as multiple red to violaceous papules, plaques, or nodules, most often on the trunk or extremities, in particular the arms, which very uncommonly ulcerate.[36] Salivary and lacrimal gland ENMZL is often preceded by sicca syndrome, with xerostomia or xerophthalmia. B symptoms are uncommon (≈15% of cases).[30]

IPSID usually affects young adults, with no gender predominance, and is seen most commonly in the Middle East and Northern Africa, usually in low socioeconomic status populations.[37] The disease affects the proximal small bowel diffusely and generally presents with a malabsorption syndrome, with steatorrhea, hypocalcemia, weight loss, abdominal pain, and fever. Cases involving the stomach, the colon, and very rarely, the respiratory tract have been described.[7]

Pathobiology and Differential Diagnosis

Etiology

ENMZL is strongly associated with chronic antigenic stimulation, including that deriving from chronic bacterial infections[15,17,38-56] or autoimmune disorders[57-61] (Table 78-3), although the strength of this correlation for some primary sites of disease is discordant among studies, suggesting a possible geographic variation. The common assumption about this association is that continual immune stimulation by bacterial or self-antigens leads to expansion of lymphoid

Table 78-2 ISCL/EORTC Staging System for Cutaneous Lymphomas Other Than Mycosis Fungoides and Sézary Syndrome[27]

Parameter*		Description
T		
T1		Solitary skin involvement
	T1a	Lesion <5 cm diameter
	T1b	Lesion >5 cm diameter
T2		Regional skin involvement: multiple lesions limited to 1 body region or 2 contiguous body regions†
	T2a	All-disease-encompassing in a <15-cm–diameter circular area
	T2b	All-disease-encompassing in a >15- and <30-cm–diameter circular area
	T2c	All-disease-encompassing in a >30-cm–diameter circular area
T3		Generalized skin involvement
	T3a	Multiple lesions involving 2 noncontiguous body regions
	T3b	Multiple lesions involving ≥3 body regions
N		
N0		No clinical or pathologic lymph node involvement
N1		Involvement of 1 peripheral lymph node region that drains an area of current or prior skin involvement
N2		Involvement of 2 or more peripheral lymph node regions or involvement of any lymph node region‡ that does not drain an area of current or prior skin involvement
N3		Involvement of central lymph nodes
M		
M0		No evidence of extracutaneous nonlymph node disease
M1		Extracutaneous nonlymph node disease present

*The ISCL/EORTC proposes to defer any stage groupings of the TNM classification until further information is available to validate specific stage grouping strategies.
†Definition of body regions: Head and neck: inferior border—superior border of clavicles, T1 spinous process. Chest: superior border—superior border of clavicles; inferior border—inferior margin of rib cage; lateral borders—midaxillary lines, glenohumeral joints (inclusive of axillae). Abdomen/genital: superior border—inferior margin of rib cage; inferior border—inguinal folds, anterior perineum; lateral borders—midaxillary lines. Upper back: superior border—T1 spinous process; inferior border—inferior margin of rib cage; lateral borders—midaxillary lines. Lower back/buttocks: superior border—inferior margin of rib cage; inferior border—inferior gluteal fold, anterior perineum (inclusive of perineum); lateral borders—midaxillary lines. Each upper arm: superior borders—glenohumeral joints (exclusive of axillae); inferior borders—ulnar/radial-humeral (elbow) joint. Each lower arm/hand: superior borders—ulnar/radial-humeral (elbow) joint. Each upper leg (thigh): superior borders—inguinal folds, inferior gluteal folds; inferior borders—mid-patellae, midpopliteal fossae. Each lower leg/foot: superior borders—mid-patellae, midpopliteal fossae.
‡Definition of lymph node regions: Peripheral sites: antecubital, cervical, supraclavicular, axillary, inguinal-femoral, and popliteal. Central sites: mediastinal, pulmonary hilar, paraortic, iliac.

Table 78-3 Chronic Antigenic Stimulation and Extranodal Marginal Zone Lymphoma

BACTERIAL INFECTIONS		
Organism	**Site**	**Prevalence (%)**
Helicobacter pylori[15,17,39-41]	Stomach	72-100
Campylobacter jejuni[42]	Intestine (IPSID)	≈70
Chlamydophila psittaci[43-52]	Conjunctiva	0-80
Borrelia burgdoferi[53-56]	Skin	0-42
AUTOIMMUNE DISORDERS		
Disease	**Site**	**Relative Risk**
Hashimoto thyroiditis*[58,59]	Thyroid	67-80
Sjögren syndrome[57,60,61]	Salivary and lacrimal glands	6.6-30.6

*Estimated by assuming cases of thyroid histiocytic lymphoma were ENMZL because these were published before the REAL classification.

elements in the connective tissue adjacent to the epithelium involved, initially leading to a process of reactive lymphoid hyperplasia. Persistent lymphocytic activation and proliferation predisposes to the accumulation of genetic errors that ultimately may result in antigen-independent growth and, consequently, lymphoma emergence.[62,63] The histologic distinction between the reactive inflammatory process associated with chronic infection (or autoimmunity) and lymphoma proper may be difficult, in which case demonstration of immunoglobulin gene monoclonality by molecular studies may aid in establishing the diagnosis of lymphoma.[64]

Histology

ENMZL is composed predominantly of morphologically heterogenous small B cells.[64] These resemble a spectrum spanning from small lymphocytes with scant cytoplasm to slightly larger cells with nuclei similar to those of centrocytes and having relatively abundant pale cytoplasm (leading possibly to a monocytoid appearance). These cells are located in the outer zone of reactive lymphoid follicles, extend into the interfollicular region and may sometimes colonize the germinal centers. Larger, immunoblast- or centroblast-like cells may be present in small numbers, but an abundance of these should raise suspicion for diffuse large B-cell lymphoma (DLBCL), which requires different management. According to the new WHO classification, the term *high-grade MALT lymphoma*, denoting the presence of sheets of transformed cells, should not be used and instead these tumors should be diagnosed as DLBCL.

Often there are lymphoid infiltrates invading and destroying glandular structures, with eosinophilic degeneration of epithelial cells (so-called lymphoepithelioid lesions), which are strongly suggestive of progression to lymphoma in cases where the differential diagnosis

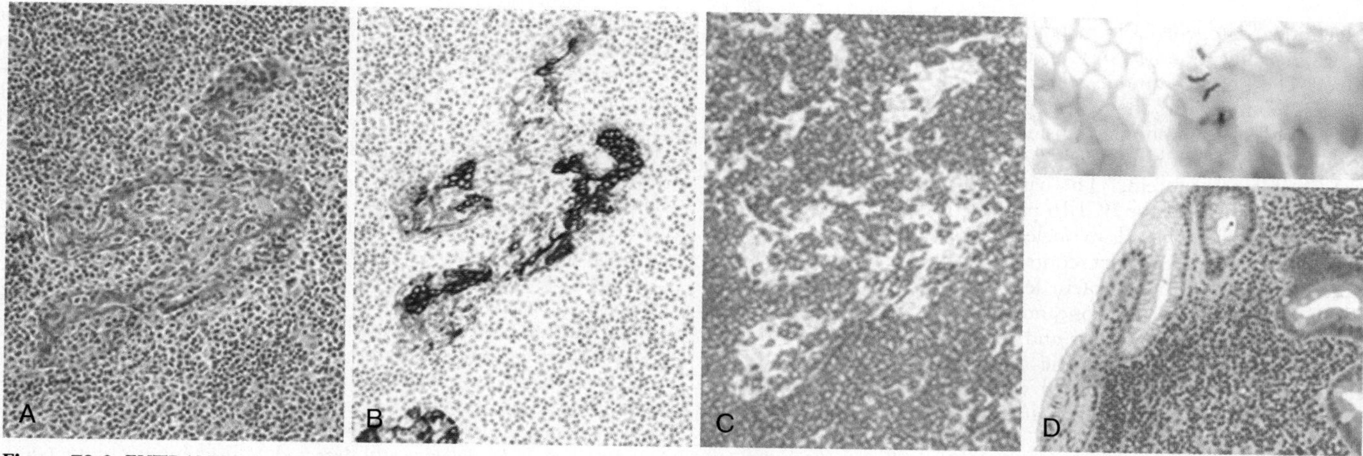

Figure 78-2 EXTRANODAL MARGINAL ZONE LYMPHOMAS OF MUCOSA-ASSOCIATED LYMPHOID TISSUE (MALT LYMPHOMAS). **A** to **C,** An example of a MALT lymphoma in the parotid gland is illustrated with various stains. The glandular tissue is overrun by lymphoid cells, which disrupt and destroy the gland. The resulting structure is referred to as a *lymphoepithelial lesion* **(A)**. These can be more clearly identified with a keratin stain **(B)** and with a B-cell stain such as CD20 **(C)**, which illustrate the glandular remnant and the B-cell proliferation. **D,** MALT lymphoma of the stomach is commonly associated with *H. pylori* infection, which can be identified by special stains *(top)*.

Table 78-4 Frequency of Common Genetic Aberrations in Extranodal Marginal Zone Lymphoma According to Primary Site of Disease

	Genetic Abnormality[31,32] *Genes Involved*[76]					
	t(11;18)(q21;q21)	t(14;18)(q32;q21)	t(1;14)(p22;q32)	t(3;14)(p14.1;q32)	+3*	+18*
Primary site	*API2/MALT1*	*IGH@/MALT1*	*IGH@/BCL10*	*IGH@/FOXP1*	*NFKBIZ, BCL6, FOXP1, ...*	*BCL2, NFATC1, ...*
Lung	36-53	6-10	2-7	0	20	7
Intestine (non-IPSID)	13-56	0	0-13	0	75	25
Stomach	6-26	1-5	0	0	11	6
Ocular adnexa	3-10	0-25	0	0-20	38	14
Salivary glands	0-5	0-16	0-2	0	55	19
Skin	0-4	0-14	0	0-10	20	4
Thyroid	0-17	0	0	0-50	17	0

All values expressed as percentages of cases.
*Mostly partial trisomies. Data summarized based on references noted.

with reactive lymphoid hyperplasia is in doubt (Fig. 78-2). Plasmacytic differentiation is frequent, especially in association with cutaneous, thyroid, and intestinal (IPSID) ENMZL and may pose differential diagnosis problems with lymphoplasmacytic lymphoma. These plasmacytoid cells often contain periodic acid–Schiff (PAS)–positive inclusions, known as Dutcher or Russell bodies, depending on whether they are located over the nucleus or in the cytoplasm, respectively.[65]

In gastric ENMZL, histology also plays an important role in establishing the diagnosis of *Helicobacter pylori* infection. All biopsy samples should have sections appropriately stained for its detection (see Fig. 78-2, *D*). Because proton pump inhibitors (PPIs) may decrease the sensitivity of detection, patients should stop taking these medications for at least 2 weeks before biopsies are obtained.[66,67]

Immunophenotype

ENMZL cells display common pan B-cell markers, such as CD19 and CD20. They are also usually positive for the complement receptors CD21 and CD35, antigens that are shared with follicular dendritic cells, and also for CD79a. Plasmacytoid cells can be CD138-positive. Helpful in the differential diagnosis with other indolent lymphomas, ENMZL are usually CD5-negative (in contrast to chronic lymphocytic leukemia/small lymphocytic lymphoma [CLL/SLL] and mantle cell lymphoma [MCL]), CD23-negative (in contrast to CLL/SLL), CD10-negative (in contrast to follicular lymphoma [FL]), and cyclin D1-negative (in contrast to MCL). They are also negative for BCL6, which may be helpful to exclude transformation to DLBCL. Except for IPSID, in which tumor cells express a truncated alpha heavy chain without any light chain, most ENMZL are typically positive for IgM or, less commonly, IgA or IgG, with light chain restriction. IgD expression is usually negative or very weak. These immunoglobulins may be secreted, especially when there is significant plasmacytic differentiation, and can give rise to a monoclonal band in the serum protein electrophoresis. The truncated heavy chains of IPSID usually do not appear as a monoclonal band because they co-migrate with other serum proteins but can be detected with anti-alpha heavy chain antibodies on immunofixation.

Genetics

Specific chromosomal aberrations have been associated with ENMZL, the frequency of which depends strongly on the primary site of disease (Table 78-4).[31,32] These abnormalities can be detected by conventional cytogenetics in metaphase plates or through fluorescent in situ hybridization (FISH) of interphase nuclei using specific probes. The most commonly observed abnormality is the t(11;18)(q21;q21), which fuses the API2 (apoptosis inhibitor-2 protein) and MALT1 (MALT lymphoma translocation-1 protein) genes in chromosomes 11 and 18, respectively, leading to expression of an API2-MALT1 chimeric protein.[68] The native MALT1 is part of a protein complex that includes the BCL10 protein (B-cell lymphoma protein 10) and that indirectly leads to nuclear factor kappa-B (NFκB) activation, a process under strict control by several upstream factors. Expression of the fusion protein leads to constitutive activation of NFκB via canonical[69] and noncanonical[70] pathways, which in turn leads to resistance to apoptosis and uncontrolled proliferation. The t(11;18) has a special prognostic significance in gastric ENMZL, because its presence is associated with worse response to antibiotherapy,[71] which is at least partly due to its higher prevalence in *H. pylori*–negative gastric ENMZL.[72]

Another, less frequently observed, abnormality is the t(14;18)(q32;q21). This translocation is different from that observed in follicular lymphoma, which involves the BCL2 gene, and instead brings the MALT1 gene under the influence of the immunoglobulin heavy chain gene promoter (IGH@), leading to overexpression of MALT1 and, through mechanisms akin to those of t(11;18), constitutive activation of NFκB. The t(1;14)(p22;q32) is seen even more rarely and causes overexpression of the BCL10 gene, which is placed under control of the IGH@ promoter, and, in turn, activation of the same pathways affected by MALT1. A fourth translocation, t(3;14)(p14.1;q32), described mostly in ocular, cutaneous, and thyroid ENMZL, involves the FOXP1 (forkhead box protein P1) transcription factor and the heavy chain promoter.[73] Although FOXP1 is overexpressed in these tumors, its exact significance in their biology is unknown.

Apart from the translocations described, all believed to be mutually exclusive, ENMZL has also been associated with gains of genetic material, in particular partial trisomies of chromosomes 3 (including regions affecting FOXP1, NFKBIZ [NFκB inhibitor zeta], and BCL6) and 18 (affecting NFATC1 [nuclear factor of activated T cells, cytoplasmic, calcineurin-dependent 1], and BCL2). Gains at 6p25 and losses at 6q (affecting TNFAIP3 [tumor necrosis factor, α-induced protein 3])[74,75] and 1p have also been reported.[76]

Consistent with a postgerminal center B-cell origin, ENMZL have rearranged immunoglobulin genes that display somatic hypermutation of their variable regions.[77] In the case of IPSID, there are deletions of the alpha heavy chain gene in the VH and CH1 regions, which result in the production of an abnormal heavy chain that cannot bind light chains to form a complete immunoglobulin molecule.[78]

Therapy for Early-Stage (I/II) Disease

Given its rarity, there are no randomized controlled trials defining the optimal treatment for ENMZL. Most recommendations arise from consensus panels based on data from retrospective or uncontrolled prospective trials. The most extensive body of data has been gathered on gastric ENMZL.

Gastric Extranodal Marginal Zone Lymphoma

This form of ENMZL has a strong association with active *H. pylori* infection. If histologic analysis of the gastric biopsies obtained during staging endoscopy fails to demonstrate *H. pylori*, noninvasive methods, such as breath tests, stool antigen test, or serology, should be used to exclude the infection. Although not necessarily a marker of active infection, the presence of antibodies against *H. pylori* in an individual not previously treated for this bacterium implicates it in the pathogenesis of the lymphoma.

The focus of therapy for *H. pylori*–positive disease is on eradication of the infection with one of the currently recommended regimens for this purpose. These commonly combine a PPI and clarithromycin with a second antibiotic, usually amoxicillin or metronidazole (triple therapy), but this is an issue in flux as resistance to clarithromycin is increasing in several regions.[79] Alternatively, quadruple therapy with a PPI, bismuth, tetracycline, and metronidazole can be used. Most authors recommend 10 to 14 days of treatment because of data suggesting better results than with 7-day courses. According to some authorities, eradication of *H. pylori* should be confirmed with an appropriate test, such as the urea breath test, at least 4 weeks after finishing antibiotherapy and 2 weeks after discontinuing PPI.[79] Pooled data from several prospective and retrospective studies suggest more than 90% eradication rates after initial antibiotherapy.[80] Persistent infection should be treated with a different course of antibiotics, preferably guided by sensitivity tests, because the same data suggests an eradication rate close to 100% after second- or third-line treatments. Repeat endoscopy with biopsies should be obtained 3 months after completion of antibacterial therapy in order to assess tumor response and also to allow histologic confirmation of *H. pylori* eradication. If *H. pylori* is still detected, a different antibiotic combination should be tried and the patient reassessed as above.[9,11]

Responses to therapy are classified according to biopsy findings on endoscopy. Complete histologic response (complete remission [CR]) should be confirmed by a second endoscopy 3 months later and is managed by observation and regular follow-up thereafter as clinically indicated. The presence of small residual lymphoid aggregates early after *H. pylori* eradication, corresponding to a category of *probable minimal residual disease* in the French Study Group of Adult Lymphomas (GELA) grading system for posttreatment evaluation, should also be managed as CR.[81] In some cases, these lymphoid aggregates have been shown to harbor cells with the same monoclonal rearrangements of the original tumor.[82] Nevertheless, these patients do not seem to have an increased risk for relapse and most will have evidence of complete response in a subsequent evaluation.[83]

Patients with overt residual (partial remission [PR]) or stable disease, as long as asymptomatic, can also be managed conservatively, with observation or antibiotherapy as appropriate, for several months. Of interest, responses may occur as late as more than 18 months after completion of antibiotic therapy.[41,83] Progressive or symptomatic disease should be managed with local therapy, with radiotherapy being preferred. Despite its established efficacy in disease control, gastrectomy, because of its immediate morbidity and long-term metabolic complications, is currently reserved for management of rare complications such as perforation or bleeding that cannot be controlled endoscopically.[9,11]

A recent metaanalysis of 1436 patients with early stage (IE-IIE1) *H. pylori*–positive disease on prospective or retrospective studies estimates an overall CR rate of 78% after eradication of *H. pylori*,[84] but with individual study remission rates anywhere from 47 to 100%.[15,17,39-41,82,85-109] On univariate analysis of available data from the same studies, adverse risk factors for achieving remission included the presence of t(11;18), stage greater than IE1, proximal (body or fundus) location of lesions, and Western (versus Asian) residence. No good evidence is available to support adjuvant chemotherapy after anti–*H. pylori* treatment as a means to prevent recurrence in localized gastric MALT lymphomas, although this has only been formally addressed with an additional single agent (chlorambucil).[110]

The management of early-stage *H. pylori*–negative disease is controversial, with some groups suggesting involved field radiation therapy or, if radiation therapy is contraindicated, systemic therapy with rituximab as initial treatment,[9] whereas others propose a trial of anti-*Helicobacter* therapy.[11] The rationale for the latter derives from anecdotal reports of CR in *H. pylori*–negative gastric ENMZL patients that were treated exclusively with antibacterials,[111] with a metaanalysis suggesting a response rate of up to 19%.[112] These patients are assumed to have been infected with *H. pylori* that was missed by diagnostic tests or with a different species of *Helicobacter*, several of which have been recently recognized.[113,114]

Responses to radiation therapy are excellent, with some series reporting CR rates of up to 100% with total doses as low as 30 Gy.[115,116] Recurrence rate is very low in these patients, but follow-up is limited for most series reported.

The optimal follow-up schedule is unknown, although most recommend periodic endoscopies every 3-6 months for the first 5 years and yearly thereafter.[9,11] Long-term follow-up data in patients with complete remission after *H. pylori* eradication document a 7.2% relapse rate overall (2.2% per year).[84] Some of these relapses were associated with *H. pylori* recurrence, and responses to retreatment for *H. pylori* were seen. Whether most complete remissions equate to cures is a question that will require longer follow-up studies. An additional argument in favor of periodic endoscopies is that *H. pylori* may be associated with an increased risk for gastric adenocarcinoma.[117]

Molecular studies should not be done routinely in follow-up biopsy samples, outside of a research protocol. Several studies have shown that molecular disease, defined by the presence of residual t(11;18) or monoclonal immunoglobulin as evidenced by PCR methods, may still be detected even with complete pathologic remissions.[93,118,119] However, this finding is not associated with an increased relapse rate and thus is not helpful for clinical management.

Ocular Extranodal Marginal Zone Lymphoma

The most frequently used treatment modality for all localized forms of ocular adnexal ENMZL is radiation therapy, with treatment specifics dependent on the exact location of the tumor in the orbit. Reported responses are very good, with CR rates of 83% to 100%.[120-128] Local recurrence rates vary between 0% and 17%, and distant recurrences can occur up to 25% over 10 years, although disease-specific survival approaches 100% in most series. The exact site of presentation correlates with the risk for systemic recurrence, the lowest being for conjunctival and the highest for eyelid primaries.[29] Long-term complications, such as cataract formation and xerophthalmia, occur in approximately half the patients.[129]

Based on the success of antibiotherapy for *H. pylori*–associated ENMZL and reports of the presence of *Chlamydophila psittaci* (by PCR, immunofluorescence, or electron microscopy) in ocular tissues of patients affected by ocular adnexal ENMZL, some authors have evaluated a course of an antichlamydial antibiotic in the management of these patients.[43-52] A few studies have reported PR or CR in a significant fraction of these patients. However, the recommendation to treat with a tetracycline at initial diagnosis is still controversial because the reported rates of association with *C. psittaci* are highly variable—some studies suggest prevalences as high as 80%, whereas others are not able to detect the organism in any of the patients. Additionally, a metaanalysis has suggested that the benefit of antibiotherapy may be restricted to specific geographic areas and, even then, is likely to be limited.[130]

Cutaneous Extranodal Marginal Zone Lymphoma

Results for both surgical excision and radiation therapy for limited disease are comparable, with CR rates approaching 100%. Both approaches have a relapse rate (usually limited to the skin) of around 45%. Encouraging results have also been obtained with intralesional injection of rituximab or α-interferon.[36]

Studies from Europe have suggested an association between *Borrelia burgdoferi* infection and ENMZL of the skin, although this has not been reproduced in Asian and American studies.[53-56] In view of this, similar to ocular lymphoma, it has been suggested that a course of a tetracycline may be a reasonable first approach, especially in locations where the association has been documented or when infection by *B. burgdoferi* is detected.

IPSID

Antibiotherapy (varying from single-agent tetracycline to triple-antibiotic therapy with ampicillin, metronidazole, and tetracycline, or an *H. pylori* regimen)[131-134] has long been recognized as being able to induce CR in early-stage disease. Recently, IPSID has been associated with chronic infection with *Campylobacter jejuni*.[42] Therefore treatment of early disease is directed at bacterial eradication. Historic rates of remission vary between 30% and 70%, depending on the study. Maximal responses may take more than 5 months of therapy, and relapses occur in a fraction of patients.

Other Extranodal Marginal Zone Lymphoma

Early-stage ENMZL in other primary sites is managed in a similar way to ocular adnexal or cutaneous forms. When feasible, surgery can be potentially curative and often may be done with primary diagnostic intent. If full resection is achieved, these patients may be observed. Otherwise, for sites not amenable to surgery or if there is residual disease after surgical excision (i.e., positive margins), radiation therapy is the usual preferred approach. If radiation is contraindicated and the patient is asymptomatic, observation is an option. Otherwise, systemic therapy as for advanced stage, preferably one with minimal toxicity, is appropriate.[9,135]

Therapy for Advanced-Stage (III/IV) Disease

The data regarding management of advanced-stage disease are also limited, because most large treatment series with long-term follow-up aggregate all indolent lymphomas and include only a small fraction of patients with MZL among other more frequent histologies. Thus most treatment approaches have been modeled after those for FL (see Chapter 79), and indeed the most common recommendation is that advanced ENMZL be managed as advanced FL.[9] In any case, there is some suggestion that responses may be better, possibly because of a usually lower burden of disease. Eligible patients should be included whenever possible in clinical trials.

As in other indolent lymphomas, extensive disease is likely incurable with current approaches, which together with a generally slow pace of progression means that systemic treatment is not always indicated. Since no benefit in survival has been demonstrated with early systemic treatment of asymptomatic disease, unless a treatable etiology has been identified, initial management of asymptomatic patients with expectant observation is acceptable. While on this watch-and-wait approach, patients should be reassessed approximately every 3 months with history, physical examination, complete blood counts, basic chemistry, and LDH. Any new symptoms or findings suggestive of transformation should be investigated with a repeat biopsy to rule it out. Routine repeat imaging studies are controversial but often used.

Indications for initiating systemic treatment include symptomatic disease due to mass effect or effusion, risk for local compressive disease, bulky lymphadenopathy, symptomatic splenomegaly, B symptoms, cytopenias due to bone marrow involvement, or rapid disease progression. Although unlikely to contribute to regression of established advanced disease, treatment of an underlying infection associated with the lymphoma (such as *H. pylori* for primary gastric ENMZL and *C. jejuni* for IPSID) is advisable in order to remove any inciting factor. Otherwise, as already mentioned, the same treatment approaches used for FL (see Chapter 79) are usually followed for ENMZL. Nonetheless, a few studies specifically addressing MZL are worth reviewing here.

Rituximab

Given its low toxicity, single-agent immunotherapy with rituximab has generated a lot of interest in the management of advanced disease. Two series of approximately 30 patients each, pooling early- and advanced-stage ENMZL, have reported overall response rates of around 75%,[136,137] with up to 48% CR in patients without previous therapy. In one of the series, median time to treatment failure was

22 versus 12 months in chemotherapy-naive versus non-naive patients, respectively.[136] Rituximab has activity in t(11;18)–positive disease.[137]

Alkylating Agents

Single-agent alkylators have also been used in this setting. A study of 24 patients with gastric ENMZL (stages IE or IV) treated with daily oral chlorambucil or cyclophosphamide for 12 to 24 months showed a CR rate of 75%, with the remaining patients achieving PR.[138] Remissions were durable in approximately half of the patients after a median follow-up time of 45 months. Another study of 21 patients (stages I to IV) treated with continuous alkylating drugs documented a CR rate of 42% and 89% in t(11;18)–positive and t(11;18)–negative disease, respectively.[139] After a median follow-up of 7.5 years, CR was sustained in all patients with translocation-negative disease, but in only one patient otherwise.

The combination of rituximab and chlorambucil has produced an impressive 100% CR rate in 13 patients with t(11;18)–positive gastric ENMZL (stages I to IV).[140] No relapses were observed after a median follow-up of 24 months, but long-term data are not available.

Purine Analogues

The purine analogue cladribine has also been used as single-agent therapy in a series of 25 patients (stages I to IV), and CR was obtained in 84% of them. After a median follow-up time of 80 months, seven patients experienced disease relapse.[141] Of note, one of the patients treated developed a myelodysplastic syndrome immediately after the third infusion of the drug.[142] Another purine analogue, fludarabine, has been used in combination with rituximab to treat a series of 22 patients (stages I to IV).[143] At the end of treatment (three cycles, with some patients requiring six), 90% of patients achieved a CR. The progression-free survival rate at 2 years in patients with gastric and extragastric ENMZL was 100% and 89%, respectively. Both purine analogues seem to have activity in t(11;18)–positive gastric ENMZL.

Other Single Agents

Other single chemotherapeutic agents whose use has been reported in ENMZL include oxaliplatin, bendamustine, bortezomib, and vorinostat. In a study of 16 patients (stages I to IV) treated with oxaliplatin, a CR rate of 56% with a median time to response of 4 months was observed.[144] Responses to bendamustine have been documented in patients with relapsed/refractory indolent lymphomas, a small fraction of which were ENMZL: in one series, three cases with CR and three PRs were seen in seven ENMZL patients[145]; in another, four CRs and one PR were observed in six patients.[146] Other studies of patients with relapsed, multiply treated indolent lymphomas report encouraging responses to bortezomib (two cases with PR out of two patients)[147] and vorinostat (one CR and one PR out of nine patients).[148] Long-term follow-up is not available; therefore, the role of these agents as first-line therapy has not been established.

Combination Chemotherapy

Combination chemotherapy regimens reported in ENMZL patients include CVP (cyclophosphamide, vincristine, and prednisone) followed by radiation therapy,[149] FM (fludarabine and mitoxantrone),[150] CHOP (cyclophosphamide, hydroxydaunomycin, vincristine [Oncovin], and prednisone) followed by CVP,[151] MCP (mitoxantrone, chlorambucil, and prednisone),[152] R-CHOP (rituximab, cyclophosphamide, hydroxydaunomycin, vincristine [Oncovin], and prednisone) and R-CNOP (rituximab, cyclophosphamide, mitoxantrone [Novantrone], vincristine [Oncovin], and prednisone).[153] These regimens have mostly been used in patients who were believed to have more aggressive disease. CR rates vary from 61% to 100%, with relapse rates reaching up to 36% on long-term follow-up. Advanced/transformed IPSID has usually been treated with combination chemotherapy, such as CHOP.[7,154]

Radioimmunotherapy

Radioisotope-conjugated forms of anti-CD20 antibodies (ibritumomab and tositumomab) have also been used both as first-line[155] therapy (eight CRs and one PR in nine patients with ocular adnexal ENMZL) and for relapsed disease[156,157] (three CRs and three PRs in six patients with ocular adnexal ENMZL; four CRs and one PR in six patients with a variety of primary sites). The combination of conventional radiation therapy and rituximab is currently being studied for early-stage follicular lymphoma.[158] There are no published studies of its use on ENMZL.

Therapy for Relapsed Disease

Limited relapses can be retreated, if feasible, with local therapy. Otherwise, treatment considerations are similar to those described for advanced disease. Symptomatic, relapsed extensive disease will usually require an alternative regimen to those previously used.

The role of hematopoietic stem cell transplantation is controversial because most series do not directly address ENMZL and thus most recommendations are again extrapolated from studies of FL.[159-163] Given that most young patients with relapsed systemic ENMZL are likely to succumb to complications of their disease, considering them for allogeneic stem cell transplantation is reasonable, although this should preferably take place on a clinical trial. Encouraging results have also recently been reported with high-dose therapy and autologous stem cell transplantation specifically for MZL.[164]

Prognosis

Overall, prognosis of limited stage ENMZL is excellent, as mentioned in each of the treatment subsections. Even for advanced disease, the expected overall survival at 5 years is greater than 90%, with some series showing survivals similar to those of early disease. As in other indolent lymphomas, transformation to aggressive forms (DLBCL) can occur, but this is thought to be a rare event (less than 10% of cases) associated with acquisition of additional genetic abnormalities.[33] Regardless, even patients in CR after first-line therapy can develop DLBCL. For instance, 0.05% of individuals with gastric ENMZL who underwent successful antibiotic treatment had evidence of DLBCL between 6 months to 2 years after achieving remission.[84] On the other hand, untreated IPSID tends to evolve to large-cell transformation.[7,154]

As for other lymphomas, the International Prognostic Index (IPI)[165] (see Chapter 81) predicts outcomes, with reported 5-year overall survivals of >90%, 70% to 80%, and 40% to 50% for patients with low, low-intermediate/high-intermediate, and high-risk scores, respectively.[28] Nonetheless, the utility of the IPI in ENMZL has been disputed.[166] One of the main criticisms to its use in patients with indolent lymphomas is that prognostic subgroups do not have a good discriminating power, because most patients are assigned to the favorable outcome groups and only very few patients are allocated to the adverse prognostic groups.[167] To circumvent this issue, modifications of the original IPI have been proposed in some cases,[168] but none has been universally adopted.

The recent explosion of genomic analysis of these neoplasms has also led to a plethora of findings that have been shown to have prognostic significance in ENMZL. For instance, the expression of FOXP1 in tumors predicts poor prognosis and transformation to diffuse large B-cell lymphoma.[169] Although these findings are not yet incorporated into clinical practice, as they become more widely available, they may be useful for risk stratification and therapeutic decisions (see box on Suggested Treatment Approach to Extranodal Marginal Zone Lymphoma).

SPLENIC MARGINAL ZONE LYMPHOMA

Epidemiology and Manifestations

SMZL (Fig. 78-3) is a rare disease, corresponding to <1% of all non-Hodgkin lymphomas.[8] The median age at diagnosis is around 65, but as with ENMZL, the age range is wide and there may be a slight female predominance. The vast majority of patients present with advanced-stage disease involving the spleen (with splenomegaly in more than 80% of patients), abdominal (mainly splenic hilar) lymph nodes, and in 83% to 94% of patients, the bone marrow.[170-173] Peripheral lymphadenopathy is, however, uncommon. Liver involvement is seen in up to one-fourth of patients, and rarely other nonhematopoietic sites can also be involved. B symptoms occur in approximately 25% to 60% of patients, depending on the series.[171,172]

Circulating villous lymphocytes (with short polar villi) can be seen in approximately two-thirds of patients (see Fig. 78-3, *B*) and frank lymphocytosis in up to one-half. This has led to a prior designation of *splenic lymphoma with villous lymphocytes* being given to a specific presentation of this disorder and explains why the disease was called *SMZL with or without villous lymphocytes* in a previous version of the WHO classification. Anemia is seen in about one-half to two-thirds and thrombocytopenia in one-fifth of cases, which can be the result of bone marrow involvement or an autoimmune process (seen in approximately 15% of patients). Between 25% and 40% of patients have a low-level circulating monoclonal immunoglobulin (mostly IgM),[172] and in a few patients, especially in those with active hepatitis C virus (HCV) infection, mixed cryoglobulins can be demonstrated, which can be associated with vasculitis.[174,175]

Pathobiology and Differential Diagnosis

Etiology

Approximately 10% to 20% of SMZL patients from European series have evidence of HCV infection,[170,173] and a significant fraction of these patients can achieve CR after successful treatment of the infection.[174,176] This raises the possibility that, like ENMZL, this disease is associated with chronic antigenic stimulation. However, no other infections have been described in clear connection to SMZL, despite a suggested association with *Plasmodium*,[177] and thus the etiology of most cases is unknown.

Histology

The classic histology of SMZL includes a population of small lymphocytes that surrounds or replaces the germinal centers of the lymphoid follicles of the white pulp, effacing their mantle zone, and progressively merging peripherally with larger, marginal zone–like cells.[178] These cells expand to the interfollicular zones and invariably invade the red pulp (see Fig. 78-3, *A*). A few scattered lymphoblasts are usually present, and as in ENMZL, plasmacytic differentiation can occur. Bone marrow involvement usually gives rise to nodular interstitial lymphoid infiltrates that resemble the histology of the spleen, although the cell types are usually admixed, without distinct zones. Peripheral blood involvement is typically associated with lymphocytes that have short polar villi (Fig. 78-3, *B*), as mentioned above, although the villi may be absent.

Suggested Treatment Approach to Extranodal Marginal Zone Lymphoma

Stage I/II

Gastric* H. pylori*–positive

- Antibiotic therapy
- Repeat endoscopy in 3-6 months
- If still *H. Pylori*–positive and no progression, alternative antibiotic therapy
- Repeat endoscopy in 3 months

Nongastric, gastric* H. pylori*–negative or not responding to antibiotic therapy

- Antibiotic trial for stage I gastric, ocular, or cutaneous?
- Involved field radiation therapy (30 Gy)

Stage III/IV or Relapsed after Antibiotic and Radiation Therapy

- Expectant observation until indication to treat
- Rituximab ± single-agent alkylator/purine analogue or combination chemotherapy (CVP/FND)

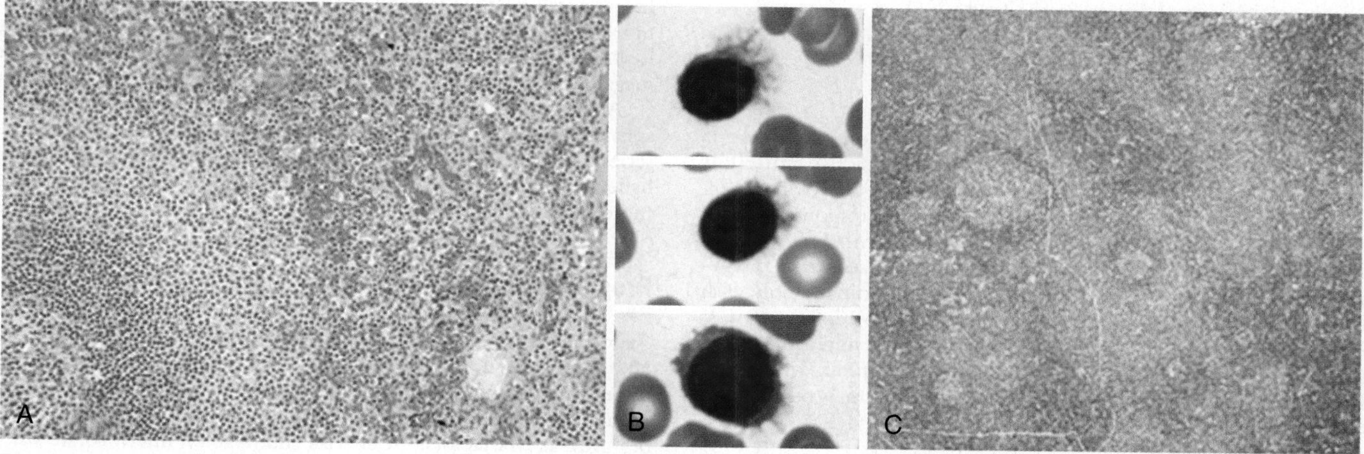

Figure 78-3 SPELINC MARGINAL ZONE LYMPHOMA, VILLOUS LYMPHOCYTES, AND PRIMARY NODAL MARGINAL ZONE LYMPHOMA. **A,** Splenic marginal zone lymphoma is characterized by an expansion of the marginal zone cells *(left)* and their spilling into the red pulp *(right)*. **B,** These cells can also become leukemic and can be recognized on the peripheral blood smear. Note the polar distribution of the cytoplasmic projections. **C,** Primary nodal marginal zone lymphoma is rare, and involvement of a node by extranodal disease must always be ruled out. NMZL is histologically characterized by an expansion of marginal zone cells (formerly referred to as monocytoid B cells) in between reactive germinal centers.

Immunophenotype

The phenotype of SMZL is similar to that of ENMZL (see earlier), but in contrast to the latter, SMZL is usually IgD-positive. The same differential diagnosis considerations apply; additionally, because this disease behaves as a chronic B-cell leukemia, it is of interest that SMZL is negative for annexin A1 and CD25 and usually negative for CD103 (in contrast to hairy cell leukemia).[178] Rare cases may be CD5-positive.[179]

Genetics

A substantial amount of genetic data on SMZL has been accumulated during the last decade. A recent review of 330 patients with SMZL documented del(7q) (affecting different loci in regions q21 to q36) as the most frequent cytogenetic abnormality (≈40% of patients).[173] Gains of genetic material from chromosomes 3 (≈25%), 8 (≈10%), and 12 (≈8%) were also seen frequently. Translocations involving 14q32, different from those seen in ENMZL, occurred in 12% of patients. The translocation t(11;18) was not seen in SMZL. More than 50% of cases had three or more cytogenetic aberrations. Deletions of 8p and 17p (TP53) have been seen in approximately 15% of cases analyzed with DNA microarrays.[76] The biologic significance of these chromosomal abnormalities is unclear at this point, although there are ongoing efforts at clarifying it.[180]

Approximately 50% to 60% of SMZL have evidence of somatic hypermutation of the immunoglobulin genes,[173,180-182] and there is some evidence that, similar to CLL, these cases may have better overall prognosis.[181] Both mutated and unmutated tumors display bias in variable region usage, with predominance of VH1-2 family genes. Intraclonal variation has also been described, which suggests the presence of ongoing mutational events in these lymphomas.[183]

Therapy

Since SMZL behaves indolently, in asymptomatic patients without significant or progressive cytopenias, expectant observation is a reasonable approach. The 5-year overall survival rate of 32 patients with asymptomatic SMZL who never received treatment was 86% in one published series.[184] In another series, 10 out of 14 untreated patients were alive between 1 and 6 years after diagnosis.[185]

Indications for lymphoma treatment are similar to those for advanced-stage ENMZL, including symptomatic splenomegaly. As for other forms of MZL, there are no data from randomized trials guiding selection of therapy, and most recommendations come from consensus opinions of experts in the field.[9]

Anti-HCV Therapy

In patients with evidence of active HCV infection, interferon-α (IFNα) with or without ribavirin (or possibly other active anti-HCV therapy) is recommended. A study of the effects of IFNα in SMZL showed eight complete and one partial hematologic responses in nine HCV-positive patients after clearance of HCV (with two of them requiring addition of ribavirin), versus no responses in six HCV-negative individuals.[176] One patient in CR treated initially only with IFNα had a relapse of the lymphoma with detectable levels of HCV RNA; treatment with interferon-α and ribavirin resulted in second complete virologic and hematologic responses. Of note, evidence of monoclonal immunoglobulin gene rearrangement may persist after successful treatment of HCV and SMZL.[174]

Splenectomy

In general, in symptomatic HCV-negative patients or in those whose disease does not respond to anti-HCV treatment, the most frequently used first-line therapy is splenectomy. A benefit of this procedure, which may often be done for diagnostic purposes in patients with localized disease, is the usual improvement of cytopenias occurring as a result of hypersplenism. Precise response rates to splenectomy are difficult to ascertain. All of 25 patients in a series treated with splenectomy alone had responses, including 2 CRs.[10] Most responses were durable: only 8 of these 25 patients experienced disease progression on long-term follow-up, with a median time to progression of 32 months (with a range of 4 to 137 months).[186] Moreover, all of 16 patients treated with first-line splenectomy in an earlier series had good responses, most likely partial (complete responses could not be assessed because of a lack of bone marrow assessment after treatment); 2 patients progressed subsequently.[185] Finally, another series of 28 patients documented a 5-year overall survival of 71% after splenectomy; no CRs were reported.[184]

Rituximab

For patients who progress after splenectomy or who have contraindications to surgery and require treatment, systemic therapy is appropriate. Rituximab has been used as single agent or in combination with chemotherapeutic drugs. The response rate to single-agent rituximab in a retrospective subseries of 25 patients with splenic and nonsplenic MZL was 88%, which compared favorably with that of 11 patients who received chemotherapy alone (55%).[187] In another retrospective study, rituximab was found to be an effective therapy in 10 of 11 patients with SMZL, with reduction in splenomegaly and improvement in blood counts.[188]

Chemotherapy

Single alkylating agents (chlorambucil or cyclophosphamide) have also been used for treatment of SMZL. Most series are very small, but all report a significant fraction of responses, albeit mostly partial. Fludarabine has produced encouraging results also,[189,190] but the efficacy of cladribine is controversial.[191,192] The use of combination chemotherapy (including CVP and CHOP) has also been reported, but differences between CHOP (or CHOP-like) therapy and other less-intensive regimens could not be demonstrated.[172] In a subseries of 19 patients treated with chemotherapy alone, the 5-year overall survival rate was 64%.[184]

Radiation Therapy

In patients ineligible for any of the aforementioned therapies, radiation therapy to the spleen can be used for symptomatic control. Even low-dose radiation (around 4 Gy) can result in resolution of splenomegaly and correction of cytopenias,[193] at least temporarily.

Although it is tempting to compare the results of observation, splenectomy and systemic therapy, this is not prudent. All published series have considerable selection bias, because patients who are believed to have more aggressive disease have been usually offered more-intensive therapies.

Prognosis

Reported 5-year overall survival rates vary from 65% to 78%,[172,184] with a median survival of 10.4 years.[10] The Italian Lymphoma Intergroup (ILI) has proposed a prognostic model using hemoglobin less than 12 g/dL, LDH higher than normal, and albumin less than 3.5 g/dL as risk factors.[170] Low-risk (no factors), intermediate-risk (1 factor), and high-risk (2 or more factors) patients have 5-year overall survivals of 83%, 72%, and 56%, respectively. Shorter survival has been associated with CD38 expression, unmutated variable region immunoglobulin genes, and expression of a specific set of NF-κB pathway genes (by gene expression array).[180] The presence of both

Suggested Treatment Approach to Splenic Marginal Zone Lymphoma

HCV-Positive
- Interferon-α and ribavirin (or other anti-HCV therapy)

HCV-Negative (or Not Responding to Anti-HCV Therapy) or Relapsed
- Expectant observation until indication to treat
- Splenectomy
- Rituximab ± single-agent alkylator/purine analogue or combination chemotherapy (CVP/FND)
- If contraindication to splenectomy and systemic therapy, low-dose splenic irradiation

del(8p) and del(17p) involving TP53 is associated with worse prognosis, although isolated deletion 17p is not.[76] Transformation to aggressive lymphoma may occur in around 10% of cases[10] (see box on Suggested Treatment Approach to SMZL).

NODAL MARGINAL ZONE LYMPHOMA

Epidemiology and Manifestations

NMZL represents between 1% and 2% of all non-Hodgkin lymphomas. The diagnosis requires the absence of extranodal or splenic disease, the presence of which makes ENMZL and SMZL more likely. The median age at presentation is around 60, and in most series there is a slight female predominance. Most patients present with asymptomatic lymphadenopathy. The most recent series report the presence of B symptoms in less than 20% of patients.[30,171,194-198] Except in three of the published series,[195-197] the majority of patients present with stage III or IV disease (approximately 70% to 80% of cases), with bone marrow involvement detected in up to two-thirds of cases. Anemia and thrombocytopenia have been described in up to 30% and 10% of cases, respectively. A monoclonal IgM is seen in approximately 10% of patients. A pediatric form, with excellent prognosis, has been recently recognized.[199]

Pathobiology and Differential Diagnosis

Etiology

As with SMZL, some series have reported an association with HCV in up to one-fourth of NMZL cases, but with a strong geographic variation.[194,195,197,198] No other clear association has been described.

Histology and Immunophenotype

The histology and immunophenotype of NMZL resembles that of ENMZL or SMZL (see Fig. 78-3, *C*).[200] The frequent presence of monocytoid B cells explains why this disease has been previously called *monocytoid B-cell lymphoma*[201] and *NMZL with or without monocytoid B cells*. A primary ENMZL should always be ruled out with appropriate studies (such as endoscopy) because 30% to 40% of cases presenting as NMZL may in fact represent nodal dissemination of an ENMZL of MALT type.[202,203]

Genetics

The genetic abnormalities most frequently associated with NMZL are partial trisomies of chromosomes 3 and 18, affecting the same regions as in ENMZL. None of the characteristic translocations of ENMZL are seen in NMZL, however.[76] Furthermore, del(7q) is also not observed. More than 75% of cases have mutated immunoglobulin genes.[195,204] Of interest, different VH immunoglobulin gene segments are predominantly involved in HCV-positive and HCV-negative patients, raising the possibility that distinct antigens drive different underlying chronic immune stimulation processes.[205]

Therapy

Few data are available to guide treatment of NMZL, and most recommendations are extrapolated from the management of FL.[9] As in other indolent lymphomas, expectant observation is appropriate for asymptomatic patients. Radiation therapy may be curative for early disease. Symptomatic advanced disease can be managed with the same general approach described for advanced ENMZL, although there is usually a tendency to use combination chemoimmunotherapy identical to that for FL as first-line treatment because of the generally worse outcomes with NMZL as compared with ENMZL.

Prognosis

Most series report worse prognosis for NMZL when compared with the other forms of MZL.[30] Overall survival rates at 5 years vary from 55% to 70% in most series, except for those containing a greater proportion of early-stage disease, which report 5-year survivals of up to 80%. Five-year progression-free survival is around 30%. Relapse in extranodal sites is rare. As in other lymphomas, the IPI correlates with outcomes, as does the Follicular Lymphoma International Prognostic Index (FLIPI)[206] (see Chapter 79). In a series of 47 patients, those with low-, intermediate-, and poor-risk FLIPI scores had a 5-year overall survival of approximately 90%, 70% and 35%, respectively.[194]

SUGGESTED READINGS

Al-Saleem T, Al-Mondhiry H: Immunoproliferative small intestinal disease (IPSID): A model for mature B-cell neoplasms. *Blood* 105:2274, 2005.

Armitage JO, Weisenburger DD: New approach to classifying non-Hodgkin's lymphomas: Clinical features of the major histologic subtypes. Non-Hodgkin's Lymphoma Classification Project. *J Clin Oncol* 16:2780, 1998.

Berger F, Felman P, Thieblemont C, et al: Non-MALT marginal zone B-cell lymphomas: A description of clinical presentation and outcome in 124 patients. *Blood* 95:1950, 2000.

Chacon JI, Mollejo M, Munoz E, et al: Splenic marginal zone lymphoma: Clinical characteristics and prognostic factors in a series of 60 patients. *Blood* 100:1648, 2002.

Craig VJ, Arnold I, Gerke C, et al: Gastric MALT lymphoma B cells express polyreactive, somatically mutated immunoglobulins. *Blood* 115:581, 2010.

Escalon MP, Champlin RE, Saliba RM, et al: Nonmyeloablative allogeneic hematopoietic transplantation: A promising salvage therapy for patients with non-Hodgkin's lymphoma whose disease has failed a prior autologous transplantation. *J Clin Oncol* 22:2419, 2004.

Fine KD, Stone MJ: Alpha-heavy chain disease, Mediterranean lymphoma, and immunoproliferative small intestinal disease: A review of clinicopathological features, pathogenesis, and differential diagnosis. *Am J Gastroenterol* 94:1139, 1999.

Fischbach W, Goebeler ME, Ruskone-Fourmestraux A, et al: Most patients with minimal histological residuals of gastric MALT lymphoma after successful eradication of *Helicobacter pylori* can be managed safely by a watch and wait strategy: Experience from a large international series. *Gut* 56:1685, 2007.

Hancock BW, Qian W, Linch D, et al: Chlorambucil versus observation after anti-*Helicobacter* therapy in gastric MALT lymphomas: Results of the international randomised LY03 trial. *Br J Haematol* 144:367, 2009.

Hermine O, Lefrere F, Bronowicki JP, et al: Regression of splenic lymphoma with villous lymphocytes after treatment of hepatitis C virus infection. *N Engl J Med* 347:89, 2002.

Ho L, Davis RE, Conne B, et al: MALT1 and the API2-MALT1 fusion act between CD40 and IKK and confer NF-κ B-dependent proliferative advantage and resistance against FAS-induced cell death in B cells. *Blood* 105:2891, 2005.

Husain A, Roberts D, Pro B, et al: Meta-analyses of the association between *Chlamydia psittaci* and ocular adnexal lymphoma and the response of ocular adnexal lymphoma to antibiotics. *Cancer* 110:809, 2007.

Lecuit M, Abachin E, Martin A, et al: Immunoproliferative small intestinal disease associated with *Campylobacter jejuni*. *N Engl J Med* 350:239, 2004.

Liu H, Ruskon-Fourmestraux A, Lavergne-Slove A, et al: Resistance of t(11;18) positive gastric mucosa-associated lymphoid tissue lymphoma to *Helicobacter pylori* eradication therapy. *Lancet* 357:39, 2001.

Malfertheiner P, Megraud F, O'Morain C, et al: Current concepts in the management of *Helicobacter pylori* infection: The Maastricht III Consensus Report. *Gut* 56:772, 2007.

Nathwani BN, Anderson JR, Armitage JO, et al: Marginal zone B-cell lymphoma: A clinical comparison of nodal and mucosa-associated lymphoid tissue types. Non-Hodgkin's Lymphoma Classification Project. *J Clin Oncol* 17:2486, 1999.

Rinaldi A, Mian M, Chigrinova E, et al: Genome-wide DNA profiling of marginal zone lymphomas identifies subtype-specific lesions with an impact on the clinical outcome. *Blood* 117:1595, 2011.

Rosebeck S, Madden L, Jin X, et al: Cleavage of NIK by the API2-MALT1 fusion oncoprotein leads to noncanonical NF-κB activation. *Science* 331:468, 2011.

Ruskone-Fourmestraux A, Fischbach W, Aleman BM, et al: EGILS consensus report. Gastric extranodal marginal zone B-cell lymphoma of MALT. *Gut* 60:747, 2011.

Salido M, Baro C, Oscier D, et al: Cytogenetic aberrations and their prognostic value in a series of 330 splenic marginal zone B-cell lymphomas: A multicenter study of the Splenic B-Cell Lymphoma Group. *Blood* 116:1479, 2010.

Schechter NR, Portlock CS, Yahalom J: Treatment of mucosa-associated lymphoid tissue lymphoma of the stomach with radiation alone. *J Clin Oncol* 16:1916, 1998.

Seligmann M, Danon F, Hurez D, et al: Alpha-chain disease: A new immunoglobulin abnormality. *Science* 162:1396, 1968.

Senff NJ, Noordijk EM, Kim YH, et al: European Organization for Research and Treatment of Cancer and International Society for Cutaneous Lymphoma consensus recommendations for the management of cutaneous B-cell lymphomas. *Blood* 112:1600, 2008.

Smedby KE, Vajdic CM, Falster M, et al: Autoimmune disorders and risk of non-Hodgkin lymphoma subtypes: A pooled analysis within the InterLymph Consortium. *Blood* 111:4029, 2008.

Stefanovic A, Lossos IS: Extranodal marginal zone lymphoma of the ocular adnexa. *Blood* 114:501, 2009.

Swerdlow SH, Campo E, Harris NL, et al, editors: *WHO classification of tumours of haematopoietic and lymphoid tissues*, Lyon, 2008, International Agency for Research on Cancer.

Weill JC, Weller S, Reynaud CA: Human marginal zone B cells. *Annu Rev Immunol* 27:267, 2009.

Zelenetz AD, Abramson JS, Advani RH, et al: NCCN Clinical Practice Guidelines in Oncology: Non-Hodgkin's lymphomas. *J Natl Compr Canc Netw* 8:288, 2010.

Zucca E, Bertoni F, Roggero E, et al: Molecular analysis of the progression from *Helicobacter pylori*-associated chronic gastritis to mucosa-associated lymphoid-tissue lymphoma of the stomach. *N Engl J Med* 338:804, 1998.

Zullo A, Hassan C, Cristofari F, et al: Effects of *Helicobacter pylori* eradication on early stage gastric mucosa-associated lymphoid tissue lymphoma. *Clin Gastroenterol Hepatol* 8:105, 2010.

For complete list of references log on to www.expertconsult.com.

CHAPTER 79

CLINICAL MANIFESTATIONS, STAGING, AND TREATMENT OF FOLLICULAR LYMPHOMA

John G. Gribben

Non-Hodgkin lymphoma (NHL) refers to all malignancies of the lymphoid system with the exception of Hodgkin disease. Development of the lymphoid system is a highly regulated process, characterized by differential expression of a number of cell-surface and intracytoplasmic proteins and antigen receptor gene rearrangements, somatic hypermutation, and class switching. Dysregulation of this orderly process can result in humoral deficiency, autoimmunity, or malignancy. The indolent B-cell lymphomas are mature peripheral B-cell neoplasms, excluding those diseases associated with an aggressive clinical course. Despite differences in cell of origin, molecular biology, clinical presentation, and clinical course, the indolent lymphomas share common features, including frequent localization to the principal lymphoid organs, a propensity for bone marrow infiltration and leukemic presentation, and generally, an indolent clinical course. The classification of NHLs has been a challenge for pathologists, as well as for practicing physicians. A number of classifications have been proposed over the years, leading to considerable confusion and difficulty in comparison of outcomes of clinical trials performed using different pathologic classifications. The World Health Organization (WHO) lymphoma classification lists nearly 100 different types of lymphoid neoplasms.[1] This classification uses all available information—morphology, cytochemistry, immunophenotype, and molecular genetics, as well as clinical features. The WHO classification does not include the terminology *indolent lymphoma*. This is a clinical rather than a pathologic term and applies to those lymphomas that tend to grow and spread slowly and produce few symptoms. Indolent lymphomas represent 35% to 40% of NHLs, and follicular lymphoma (FL) is the most common of the indolent lymphomas.

EPIDEMIOLOGY

It was estimated that in 2011 more than 66,000 cases of NHL would be diagnosed in the United States and that almost 20,000 patients would die of their disease (http://seer.cancer.gov/statfacts/html/nhl.html). NHL is extremely heterogeneous in its molecular pathophysiology, histology, and clinical course, and there are major differences in the incidence of subtypes in different geographic locations and among different racial and ethnic populations. This difference in geographic distribution is particularly striking for FL. In the Western world, FL is the second most common lymphoma, accounting for approximately 20% of all non-Hodgkin lymphomas. For example, the incidence of FL in Europe is approximately 2.18 cases per 100,000 persons per year.[2] Incidence rates of indolent lymphomas by gender are shown in Table 79-1. Although most cases are sporadic studies, there is an increased incidence in family members of affected individuals, with a relative risk of 2.3 for siblings of patients.[3] Differentiation of complex environmental factors from true inherited factors remains difficult. The complexity of the epidemiology of NHL mirrors the complexity of the disease and the complexity of the immune system. Since lymphomas do not constitute a single disease, it should come as no surprise that there is no single etiologic factor. The influence on immune dysregulation of viruses, chemicals, radiation, diet, and aging remains unclear. Immune suppression leads to increased incidence of aggressive lymphomas, but not usually indolent lymphomas. FL typically presents in middle age and in older adults, and the median age at diagnosis is 60 years. There is a slight female preponderance.[2]

PATHOGENESIS

FL (Fig. 79-1) is derived from germinal center B cells and maintains the gene expression profile of this stage of differentiation.[4] FL cells express CD19, CD20, CD22, and surface immunoglobulin, and 60% express CD10. A hallmark of the disease is the chromosomal translocation t(14.18) contributing to overexpression of the antiapoptotic protein BCL2. Morphologically, the disease is composed of a mixture of centrocytes and centroblasts. The third edition of the WHO classification of pathology recommended the use of grades 1, 2, and 3, applied according to the number of centroblasts (0-5, 6-15, and >15 per high-power field, respectively). Grade 3 was further subdivided into 3A (centrocytes still present) and 3B (sheets of centroblasts)—an increased percentage of centroblasts is predictive of poor outcome. A problem with this classification is that it was poorly reproducible among pathologists. Also problematic is the fact that there were no major biologic or clinical differences between grades 1 and 2, whereas grade 3B FL was biologically distinct from grades 1 through 3A, with features suggesting a close relationship to diffuse large B-cell lymphoma (DLBCL).[5] These considerations led to the recommendation to group together FL grades 1 through 3A as FL and to create a new category called FL3B. However, the gene signature in FL3B is closer to FL than to DLBCL.[6] The final classification combined FL grades 1 and 2 into a single category (FL1-2 of 3) and made the distinction between FL3A and FL3B optional rather than mandatory.[7] The fourth edition of the WHO classification recognizes some distinctive clinical and genetic subtypes of FL, including primary duodenal FL and the pediatric type of FL that lacks t(14:18) and usually presents with localized disease. Several variants of FL that lack t(14;18) have some distinctive features—for instance, predominantly diffuse FL with deletions of 1p36 that presents with localized bulky disease in the inguinal region. The gene expression profiles of FL cases with and without t(14;18) show some differences, with t(14;18)–negative FL resembling activated late-stage germinal center B cells.[8]

Although 85% of patients with FL have t(14;18), the pathogenesis of FL remains poorly understood. Recent studies have demonstrated frequent mutations, particularly inactivating mutations of the MLL2 gene, which occurred in 89% of FL cases examined.[9] The major mutations seen in FL are shown in Table 79-2. A notable feature of these findings is that many of the mutated genes are involved in transcriptional regulation. It is likely that posttranscriptional modification of histones is of key importance in germinal center B cells and that the deregulated histone modification due to these mutations is likely to result in reduced acetylation and enhanced methylation, which will act as as driving event in the development of FL. Attention has also been paid recently to the complex interaction among the malignant B cell, the host,[10] and the tumor microenvironment.[4,11,12]

Table 79-1 Incidence Rates of Indolent Lymphomas (Per 100,000 Population)

Type of Indolent Lymphoma	All	Male	Female
Follicular lymphoma	2.186	2.1	2.6
Small B lymphocytic lymphoma/ chronic lymphocytic leukemia	4.92	5.87	4.01
Lymphoplasmacytic lymphoma	0.83	1.0	0.6
Mantle cell lymphoma	0.45	0.64	0.27
Marginal zone lymphoma	0.42	0.4	0.45

From Sant M, Allemani C, Tereanu C, et al: Incidence of hematologic malignancies in Europe by morphologic subtype: Results of the HAEMACARE project. *Blood* 116:3724, 2010.

Table 79-2 Mutations in Follicular Lymphoma

Gene Name	Abbreviation	Location	Frequency at Diagnosis
Myeloid/lymphoid or mixed-lineage leukemia 2	MLL2	12q	89%
CREB-binding protein	CREBBP	16p	33%
Tumor necrosis factor receptor superfamily member 14	TNFRSF14	1p	25%
E1A-binding protein p300	EP300	22q	15%
Myocyte enhancer factor 2B	MEF2B	19p	13%
Enhancer of zeste homolog 2	EZH2	7q	11%

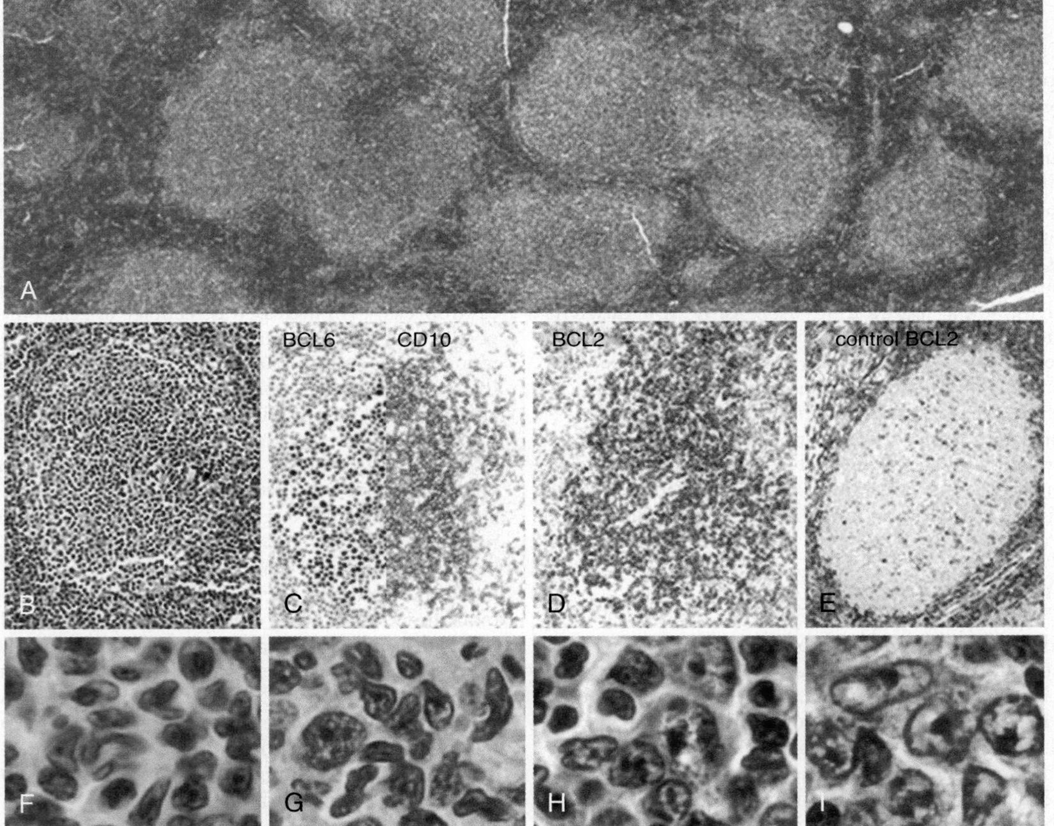

Figure 79-1 FOLLICULAR LYMPHOMA: MORPHOLOGIC AND IMMUNOPHENOTYPIC FINDINGS. **A,** A low-power photomicrograph illustrates a lymph node involved by follicular lymphoma. The lymphoma cells grow in nodules or follicles that resemble the normal lymphoid follicles of a reactive lymph node. However, in the lymphomatous growth, the follicles are crowded, show back-to-back localization, and lack many of the features of their reactive counterparts. At higher power **(B),** the neoplastic follicles lack mantle zones and the normal polarization of small and large germinal center cells (centrocytes and centroblasts, respectively), which occurs due to the cellular response to antigenic stimulation as it sweeps thorough the follicle. The neoplastic follicles stain for the germinal center marker, BCL6 and CD10 **(C);** however, they overexpress BCL2 **(D)** as a result of the associated translocation t(14;18), involving the IgH gene and BCL2. BCL2 is not much expressed in normal germinal center B cells (**E,** control for comparison). Follicular lymphoma is graded by the number of large neoplastic cells (centroblasts) present among the smaller neoplastic cells (centrocytes) (**F** to **I**). The grading system is not entirely accurate, but it provides some framework for subclassifying cases morphologically. Grade 1 is 0 to 5 centroblasts per average 40x field **(F);** between 6 and 15 is grade 2 **(G);** and more than 15 is grade 3A **(H).** Grades 1 and 2 are now considered together. When most of the cells in the neoplastic follicles are centroblasts without centrocytes, the case is considered grade 3B **(I)** (see text for further explanation of grading).

CLINICAL PRESENTATION

The majority of patients with FL present with lymphadenopathy in one or more sites. FL patients often present with a long history of having noticed painless increased lymph nodes over a number of years before presentation. Lymphadenopathy may wax and wane, and spontaneous remissions can occur, albeit rarely.[13] Disease transformation to a more aggressive histologic type is a common terminal event.[14]

Extranodal disease is relatively common and can affect any organ. The most common sites of extranodal disease include the bone marrow, skin, GI tract, and bone. Symptoms may be nonspecific or related to the site of disease involvement. Many patients are asymptomatic, but some, particularly those with bulky disease, may present with B symptoms defined as fever, drenching sweats, or weight loss of more than 10% of body weight. Patients may present with evidence of bowel obstruction from intraabdominal lymphadenopathy and retroperitoneal disease may manifest as obstructive uropathy. Inguinal disease may cause compression of the venous system with deep venous thrombosis. CNS involvement can occur, but this is uncommon in FL.

DIAGNOSIS OF INDOLENT LYMPHOMAS

Suggested guidelines for the diagnosis of indolent lymphomas have been outlined by the National Comprehensive Cancer Network (http://www.nccn.org/) and by the European Society for Medical Oncology.[15] In all cases, possible diagnosis should be confirmed by excisional biopsy of an accessible lymph node (LN) with review by an expert hematopathologist with expertise in lymphoma diagnosis. Fine-needle aspiration is not appropriate for diagnosis in these conditions, and sufficient material must be obtained for immunophenotyping and genetic studies as required for diagnosis and assay for prognostic markers. In patients without easily accessible peripheral nodes, computed tomography (CT) or ultrasound guided biopsy are typically well tolerated. Where possible, consent should be obtained for the procurement and storage of use of excess tissue from LN biopsies at the time of presentation and at each subsequent relapse of disease for research purposes to investigate the molecular biology of these diseases. Bone marrow biopsy provides essential information and should be performed routinely. The yield of bilateral bone marrow biopsy is moderately higher (15%) than that of unilateral biopsy.

Initial investigations are listed in Table 79-3. Physical examination should include careful examination of all peripheral lymph node groups, including the cervical, supraclavicular, axillary, and inguinal chains and examination of Waldeyer ring. Abdominal examination should focus on evaluation of any intraabdominal masses, with particular attention paid to detection of enlargement of the liver or spleen. The skin should be carefully examined. Patients may present with pleural or pericardial effusions, although this is less common than in the aggressive lymphomas.

Laboratory investigations should include a complete blood count to evaluate for cytopenias, which may be evidence of bone marrow infiltration or of autoimmunity. A white blood count with differential and examination of the peripheral blood smear may elucidate leukemic involvement with disease. Baseline electrolytes (including calcium and phosphate), creatinine levels, and liver function tests are important to determine organ dysfunction that may be related to direct infiltration by lymphoma. Elevation of lactate dehydrogenase (LDH) is an important prognostic factor and may be a useful indicator of transformation from indolent to aggressive lymphoma.

Initial staging workup also includes a CT scan of the chest, abdomen, and pelvis. Particular attention should be paid to sites of bulk disease and to the number of involved sites. Liver biopsy may be indicated based on abnormal imaging or laboratory testing.

Table 79-3 Initial Evaluation of Follicular Lymphoma

Physical examination with attention to peripheral nodes, abdomen
Complete blood count; evaluation of peripheral blood
Liver function tests; LDH; beta-2-microglobulin
CT scans of chest, abdomen, pelvis (PET scan if indicated)
Lymph node biopsy with review by an expert lymphoma histopathologist
Bone marrow biopsy/aspirate
Other studies as indicated

STAGING

The staging of NHL uses the Ann Arbor Classification (Table 79-4). CT scans have replaced lymphangiography. The impact of newer technologies such as positron emission tomography (PET), which are included in the revised guidelines for aggressive lymphomas,[16] has been much less studied in the indolent lymphomas. Considerable heterogeneity exists in uptake of fluorine-18 fluorodeoxyglucose based on histology, but PET demonstrates 94% sensitivity and 100% specificity for staging in FL.[17] Although data are still insufficient to recommend PET scans routinely in patients with FL, these scans can be useful to direct biopsy in cases in which transformation is suspected.

NATURAL HISTORY

Until recently, there was little evidence that the natural history of FL had changed over the last 30 years from the median survival of 10 years from diagnosis.[18] The overall probability of survival of FL patients treated at St. Bartholomew's Hospital is presented in Fig. 79-2. Evidence now shows that the introduction of monoclonal antibodies in combination with chemotherapy has finally led to an improvement in survival, with the result that the median survival is now 12 to 14 years.[19,20] The clinical course is extremely variable, with some patients having an extremely aggressive course and death within 1 year, whereas others may live for more than 20 years and never require therapy. Therefore prognostic markers are needed to help identify those patients who will have a good or poor prognosis. The Follicular Lymphoma International Prognostic Index (FLIPI), a five-factor prognostic index based on the clinical characteristics of age, stage, number of nodal sites, hemoglobin level, and LDH level (Table 79-5), defines three prognostic risk groups of almost equal numbers of patients.[21] This tool is useful in assessing the likely need for early treatment of patients and their potential outcome, as well as in comparing the outcomes of different clinical trials. A revised FLIPI2 (incorporating β_2 microglobulin, diameter of largest lymph node, bone marrow involvement, and hemoglobin level) may better discriminate the outcome for patients requiring treatment (Table 79-6).[22]

Table 79-4 Ann Arbor Staging

Stage	Criteria
I	Involvement of 1 lymph node (I) or 1 extralymphatic organ or site (IE)
II	Involvement of 2 or more lymph nodes on same side of diaphragm (II) or localized extralymphatic organ or site and 1 or more involved lymph node on same side of diaphragm (IIE)
III	Involvement of lymph nodes on both sides of diaphragm (III) or same side with localized involvement of extralymphatic site (IIIE), spleen (IIIS), or both (IIIS+E)
IV	Diffuse or disseminated involvement of extralymphatic organ or tissues with or without lymph node enlargement

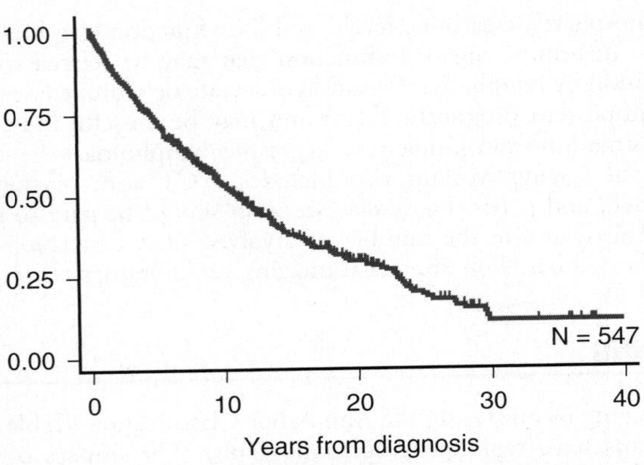

Figure 79-2 OVERALL PROBABILITY OF SURVIVAL OF PATIENTS WITH FOLLICULAR LYMPHOMA TREATED AT ST. BARTHOLOMEW'S HOSPITAL.

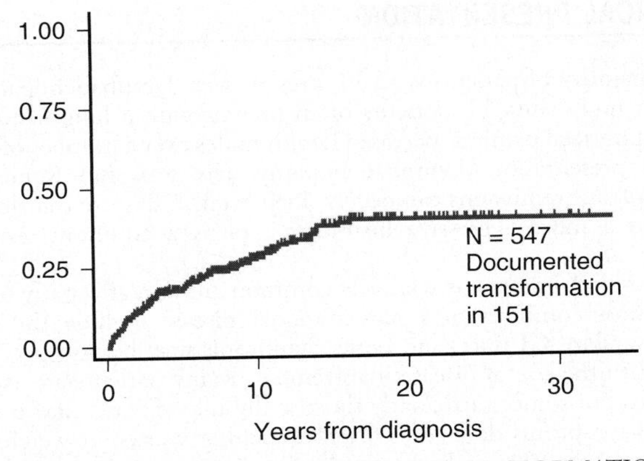

Figure 79-3 PROBABILITY OF RISK FOR TRANSFORMATION OF PATIENTS WITH FOLLICULAR LYMPHOMA.

Table 79-5 Factors Having Prognostic Significance in the FLIPI* and FLIPI2†

Parameter	Adverse Factor	HR
FLIPI1		
Age	≥60 years	2.38
Ann Arbor stage	III-IV	2.00
Hemoglobin level	<120 g/L	1.55
Serum LDH level	>ULN	1.50
Number of nodal sites	>4	1.39
FLIPI2		
Parameter	**Adverse Factor**	**HR (in Final Model)**
β_2 microbulin	>ULN	1.5
Bone marrow involvement	+	1.59
Hemoglobin level	<120 g/L	1.51
Largest diameter of LN	>6 cm	1.66
Age	>60 years	1.38

FLIP, Follicular lymphoma international prognostic index; *HR,* hazard ratio; *LDH,* lactate dehydrogenase, *ULN,* upper limit of normal.
*From Solal-Celigny P, Roy P, Colombat P, et al: Follicular lymphoma international prognostic index. *Blood* 104:1258, 2004.
†From Federico M, Bellei M, Marcheselli L, et al: Follicular lymphoma international prognostic index 2: A new prognostic index for follicular lymphoma developed by the international follicular lymphoma prognostic factor project. *J Clin Oncol* 27:4555, 2009.

Table 79-6 Outcome by FLIPI2

Risk Factor Level		% of Patients Alive at 5-year	PFS	OS
Low risk	0	18%	76%	96%
Intermediate risk	1-2	62%	46%	80%
High risk	3-5	20%	29%	59%

Data from Federico M, Bellei M, Marcheselli L, et al: Follicular lymphoma international prognostic index 2: A new prognostic index for follicular lymphoma developed by the international follicular lymphoma prognostic factor project. *J Clin Oncol* 27:4555, 2009.

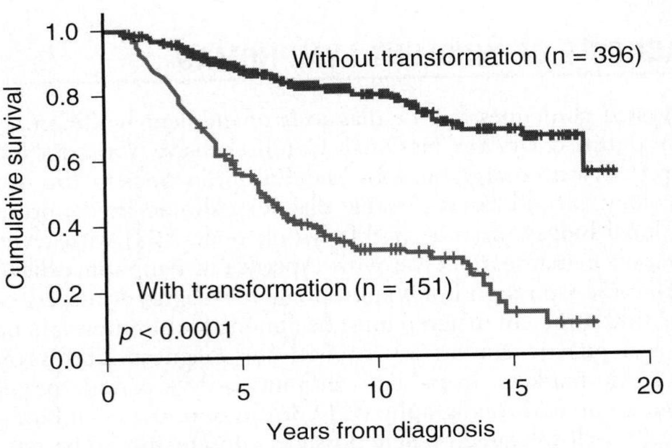

Figure 79-4 OVERALL PROBABILITY OF SURVIVAL OF PATIENTS WITH FOLLICULAR LYMPHOMA WHO HAVE AND HAVE NOT UNDERGONE HISTOLOGIC TRANSFORMATION.

An important factor for the prognosis of FL is histologic transformation of the disease.[14] This factor was evaluated in the database of patients treated for FL at St. Bartholomew's Hospital. Fig. 79-3 shows the actuarial risk for these patients undergoing histologic transformation; the survival of patients with and without transformation is illustrated in Fig. 79-4. Despite a considerable body of information on the pathologic and molecular events associated with HT, the pathogenesis of transformation remains elusive and the molecular events that have been identified have not been translated into changes in clinical practice. A major focus of research is the attempt to identify patients at high risk for transformation early in their clinical course, but this is not yet possible. The outcome of patients who undergo transformation after already having received multiple lines of therapy remains poor, but for those patients who undergo transformation and then receive their first therapy for the transformed disease, the use of chemoimmunotherapy has led to a significant improvement in prognosis.

TREATMENT OF FOLLICULAR LYMPHOMA

For most cases of FL, the goal of therapy has been to maintain the best quality of life and to treat patients only when they develop symptoms. Any alteration to this approach requires demonstration of improved survival with early institution of therapy or identification of criteria that define patients sufficiently "high risk" to merit early

Table 79-7 Treatment Strategies for Indolent Lymphomas

LOCALIZED DISEASE
Radiotherapy
"Watch and wait"
ADVANCED-STAGE DISEASE
"Watchful waiting"
Chemotherapy
Alkylating agents
Bendamustine
Purine analogues
Combination chemotherapy
Monoclonal antibodies
Unconjugated
Conjugated—radioimmunoconjugates and immunotoxins
Chemotherapy + monoclonal antibodies (chemoimmunotherapy)
High-dose chemotherapy plus autologous/allogeneic stem cell transplantation
Reduced-intensity conditioning allogeneic transplantation
Palliative radiotherapy

therapy. There are many available therapies but no consensus on an optimal first-line or relapse treatment. Despite the lack of data demonstrating any benefit for early therapy, patients are being treated earlier in their disease course. There is no clear-cut treatment pathway for patients with FL, and although we have a good evidence base to decide on a particular treatment, little or no data exist regarding the optimal sequencing of treatment approaches in this disease. In the absence of such data, treatment choices remain empiric and should always involve discussion regarding patient choice and the goal of therapy. These choices will likely become even more complicated by the many new treatment agents currently being investigated in preclinical and clinical studies—in particular, the novel monoclonal antibodies and agents that alter the antiapoptotic pathways and B-cell receptor signaling pathways. The impact of these new agents on practice will depend on the results of ongoing clinical trials.

Multiple treatment approaches exist for advanced stage low-grade lymphomas, and these patients are best treated in the setting of clinical trials. Options range from a watch-and-wait expectant management approach, to single-agent chemotherapy or monoclonal antibody therapy with rituximab, to combination chemoimmunotherapy with use of autologous or allogeneic stem cell transplantation (SCT) (Table 79-7). Patients remaining on an expectant course should be followed every 3 months with history, physical examination, and blood counts including LDH. Special attention should be paid to any change in symptoms that might be suggestive of transformation, which is an indication for repeat biopsy to examine for histologic evidence to confirm transformation. Repeat scanning is not routinely performed unless indicated by symptoms or signs.

Since there is no clearly defined treatment algorithm for most patients with indolent lymphomas, eligible patients should be included in clinical trials whenever possible. This ensures delivery of optimal care for patients and helps inform the design of subsequent trials, hopefully leading to cure. Information on available clinical trials can be found at the Clinical Trials registry and database (www.clinicaltrials.gov) (see box on Management of Follicular Lymphoma).

WHEN TO INSTITUTE THERAPY

Stage I-II (Limited Stage Disease)

Radiation therapy is the preferred treatment for the approximately 10% of patients who present with limited stage, nonbulky disease. This treatment option is offered with curative potential[23] but must be weighed against the potential toxicity of the radiation therapy to other tissues. In patients with large tumor burden or other adverse risk factors, systemic therapy is indicated. There is no proven role of radiation consolidation therapy.

Expectant management is the treatment of choice for asymptomatic patients with low-bulk disease until clear indications for initiation of treatment are seen, except for those patients enrolled in a clinical trial assessing the impact of early therapy. This approach is based on the demonstration of no survival advantage for institution of immediate treatment compared with deferred treatment until time of progression.[24] Three randomized trials, performed in the prerituximab era, confirmed no survival benefit for early therapy.[25-27] In a National Cancer Institute (NCI) study of 104 newly diagnosed patients with FL, deferred treatment was compared with immediate treatment with the ProMACE-MOPP regimen (see table 79-10) followed by total nodal irradiation. An updated analysis of these data is long overdue, but no difference in overall survival (OS) was found between the two arms of the study at the time of the last analysis.[25] The Groupe Pour l'Etude de Lymphome Folliculaire (GELF) used defined criteria for patients in whom immediate therapy was not believed to be indicated (Table 79-8) and randomized 193 patients to receive deferred treatment or to receive prednimustine 200 mg/m^2/day for 5 days per month for 18 months or IFN-α 5 MU/day for 3 months followed by 5 MU three times per week for 15 months.[26] The median OS time was not reached and the OS was the same in all three arms of the study. The British National Lymphoma Investigation (BNLI)[27] compared treatment in 309 patients with asymptomatic advanced-stage, indolent lymphoma—158 of these patients were randomized to receive immediate therapy with oral chlorambucil 10 mg per day continuously, and 151 patients were randomized to deferred treatment until disease progression (see Table 79-8). In both arms, local radiotherapy to symptomatic nodes was allowed. At a median follow up in the study of 16 years, no difference was seen in OS or cause-specific survival between the two groups.

A major clinical trial question is whether identification of clinical or molecular risk factors can help determine which patients are candidates for early therapy. A survival predictor score has been developed from gene expression profiling studies.[4] The results from this study suggest that the molecular determinants of biologic heterogeneity are already present in the diagnostic LN biopsies rather than by the later acquisition of secondary genetic changes. A major

Management of Follicular Lymphoma

Patients most often present with asymptomatic lymphadenopathy. The diagnosis should be made by excisional biopsy and review by an expert hematopathologist. In the absence of symptoms requiring treatment, an expectant "watch and wait" approach is the treatment of choice. While in this phase of treatment, patients should be followed every 3 to 6 months for history, physical examination, and laboratory results with radiologic restaging as clinically indicated. Once a decision to treat has been made, no clear treatment algorithm exists, and a number of treatment options are available. The treatment goal, whether palliative or potentially with curative intent, is dependent on the age and performance status of patients. Enrollment in a clinical trial should be the treatment of choice. For younger patients in whom high-dose therapy may be indicated later in their disease course, it is best to avoid profoundly myelotoxic regimens. The role of maintenance therapy in first remission using interferon-α remains controversial, and the use of rituximab maintenance therapy in first remission remains the focus of ongoing clinical trials. The choice of therapy after first relapse depends again on the goal of therapy; however, it is also dependent on the previous therapy, response, and duration of response. Autologous or allogeneic stem cell transplantation has a role to play in selected younger patients with this disease.

Table 79-8 Criteria for Delaying Treatment of Follicular Lymphoma

GELF*

All of the following:
- Maximum diameter of disease <7 cm
- Fewer than 3 nodal sites
- Absence of systemic symptoms
- Spleen <16 cm on CT
- No significant effusions
- No risk for local compressive symptoms
- No circulating lymphoma cells or marrow compromise (Hb < 10 g/dL, WBC < 1.5 or platelets <100,000/dL)

BNLI†

Absence of all of the following:
- B symptoms or pruritus
- Rapid generalized disease progression
- Marrow compromise (Hb ≤ 10 g/dL, WBC < 3.0 or platelets <100,000/dL)
- Life-threatening organ involvement
- Renal infiltration
- Bone lesions

*From Brice P, Bastion Y, Lepage E, et al: Comparison in low-tumor-burden follicular lymphomas between an initial no-treatment policy, prednimustine, or interferon alfa: A randomized study from the Groupe d'Etude des Lymphomes Folliculaires. Groupe d'Etude des Lymphomes de l'Adulte. *J Clin Oncol* 15:1110, 1997.
†From Ardeshna KM, Smith P, Norton A, et al: Long-term effect of a watch and wait policy versus immediate systemic treatment for asymptomatic advanced-stage non-Hodgkin lymphoma: A randomised controlled trial. *Lancet* 362:516, 2003.

Table 79-9 National LymphoCare Study Survey of Current Practice for Follicular Lymphoma in the United States, 2004 to 2007

ADVANCED-STAGE FL	
Treatment Strategy	% of Patients
"Watch and Wait"	17.7%
Rituximab monotherapy	13.9%
Chemotherapy plus rituximab	51.9%
R-CHOP	55%
R-CVP	23%
R-fludarabine-based	15%
R-other	6%
Chemotherapy alone	4%
LIMITED-STAGE FL	
"Watch and wait"	29%
Rituximab monotherapy	13%
Chemotherapy plus rituximab	30.4%
Radiation alone	23%

Data from Friedberg JW, Taylor MD, Cerhan JR, et al: Follicular lymphoma in the United States: First report of the national LymphoCare study. *J Clin Oncol* 27:1202, 2009.

component of the gene expression prognostic signature is related to immune cells in the tumor microenvironment.[11,12,28] Future guidelines for treatment will likely be based on clinical staging systems, genetic profiles, and immune response signatures, but these factors do not yet provide guidance in terms of who should have immediate therapy.

Little evidence is available to suggest that we should change our practice of "watch and wait" for the asymptomatic patient with low-bulk disease; regardless, data demonstrate that this practice is becoming much less common in the United States.[29] The National LymphoCare Study is a prospective observational survey designed to assess presentation, prognosis, treatment, and clinical outcomes in patients newly diagnosed with FL. The treating physician determines management according to clinical judgment with no prescribed treatment regimen; data are then recorded regarding histology, stage, therapy, response, relapse, and death. The first treatments offered are listed in Table 79-9. Among 2708 patients enrolled at 265 centers, only 17.7% of patients were initially observed; of these, 22% received active therapy within 1 year and 31% within 2 years. This observation is in stark contrast to the data from the BLNI study, demonstrating that censored for nonlymphoma death, 19% of patients and 40% for those older than 70 years who were randomized to expectant management still did not require therapy at 10 years.[27]

TREATMENT APPROACHES

Treatment is indicated in patients with symptomatic disease, bulky lymphadenopathy and/or splenomegaly, risk for local compressive disease, marrow compromise, or rapid disease progression. Once indicated, numerous treatment approaches are available (Table 79-10). Newly diagnosed patients (and their physicians) may be quite confused by the choice of vastly different treatment approaches—for instance, a "do nothing" approach versus a treatment associated with considerable morbidity and mortality, such as stem cell transplantation (SCT). Thus considerable consultation time is required to review available treatment approaches. Staging of response in indolent lymphomas is by the revised response criteria.[16] Depending on the treatment approach used, restaging after two to three cycles of therapy can be useful to ensure responsiveness, and the patient is then fully restaged after completion of therapy. Although curative approaches are being sought for aggressive lymphomas, the failure to achieve complete remission or complete eradication of disease does not have the same implication in indolent lymphomas as in aggressive lymphomas, and a PR may be a sufficient response to therapy to alleviate symptoms. The more commonly used regimens in indolent lymphoma cases are shown in Table 79-10.

In the absence of a clear standard of care with curative potential, optimal first-line treatment remains enrollment in randomized clinical trials wherever possible. In the National LymphoCare Study,[30] academic sites are more likely than community sites to treat patients in clinical trials (12% versus 4% of patients), but it is lamentable that only 6% of patients were enrolled in clinical trials. For patients who are not eligible for clinical trials or who refuse entry, data demonstrate higher response rates, longer duration of responses, and perhaps, improved survival with chemoimmunotherapy. Many investigators favor alkylator over fludarabine-based regimens for FL, based on concerns regarding the ability to obtain stem cells for later use for autologous SCT in patients who were treated with fludarabine.[31] It is suggested that more aggressive first-line therapy be offered to patients who progress within 1 year of presentation, because these patients have a worse outcome.[26] Older adult patients or those with poor performance status remain candidates for single-agent chlorambucil. Single-agent monoclonal antibody therapy is appropriate for patients who choose to avoid chemotherapy; this is a reasonable treatment choice based on the results of clinical trials of prolonged or maintenance therapy with rituximab. Although data suggest a survival advantage with the use of interferon (IFN)-α in combination with chemotherapy, this approach is associated with a significant side effect profile and is rarely used in the United States. Optimal results are seen when radioimmunoconjugates are used earlier in the disease course. There is no indication for the use of high-dose therapy and SCT in first remission in FL, unless as part of a clinical trial.

Data from the National LymphoCare Study[29] demonstrate that chemoimmunotherapy is now the treatment of choice of physicians in the United States (see Table 79-9). No randomized trials demonstrate a benefit for the addition of anthracyclines, but the

Table 79-10 Chemotherapy Regimens in Indolent Lymphomas

CVP (EVERY 21 DAYS)

- cyclophosphamide 750 mg/m^2 IV on day 1
- vincristine 1.4 mg/m^2, up to a maximal dose of 2 mg IV, on day 1
- prednisone 40 mg/m^2 daily PO on days 1 to 5

Patients being treated with R-CVP also received 375 mg/m^2 of rituximab IV on day 1 of each therapy cycle.[72]

CHOP (EVERY 21 DAYS)

- cyclophosphamide 750 mg/m^2 IV on day 1
- hydroxydaunomycin 50 mg/m^2 IV on day 1
- vincristine (Oncovin) 1.4 mg/m^2, up to a maximal dose of 2 mg IV, on day 1
- prednisone 100 mg daily orally on days 1 to 5

Patients being treated with R-CHOP also received 375 mg/m^2 of rituximab IV on day 1 of each therapy cycle[73] or by alternate schedule.[70]

CNOP (EVERY 21 DAYS)

- cyclophosphamide 750 mg/m^2 IV on day 1
- mitoxantrone (Novantrone) 10 mg/m^2 IV on day 1
- vincristine (Oncovin) 1.4 mg/m^2, up to a maximal dose of 2 mg IV, on day 1
- prednisone 50 mg/m^2 daily orally on days 1 to 5

CHVP-IFN (EVERY 28 DAYS FOR 6 MONTHS, THEN EVERY 2 MONTHS FOR 6 MONTHS)[88]

- cyclophosphamide 600 mg/m^2
- hydroxydaunomycin 25 mg/m^2
- etoposide (Vepesid) 100 mg/m^2 on day 1 (replaces original teniposide 60 mg/m^2 on day 1)
- prednisolone 40 mg/m^2 on days 1 to 5
- interferon-α-5, 3 times a week

Patients being treated with R-CHVP also received 375 mg/m^2 of rituximab IV on day 1 of each therapy cycle for six cycles.

FMD (EVERY 28 DAYS)

- fludarabine 25 mg/m^2 IV on days 1-3
- mitoxantrone 10 mg/m^2 IV on day 1
- dexamethasone 20 mg /day PO days 1 to 5

Patients being treated with R-FMD also received 375 mg/m^2 of rituximab IV on day 1 of each therapy cycle.

PROMACE-MOPP

Cycles repeated every 28 days

Day 1

- cyclophosphamide 650 mg/m^2 IV
- doxorubicin 25 mg/m^2 IV
- etoposide 120 mg/m^2 IV
- prednisone 60 mg/m^2 orally daily days 1-14

Day 8

- mechlorethamine 6 mg/m^2 IV
- vincristine 1.4 mg/m^2 (maximum 2 mg) IV on day 8
- procarbazine 100 mg/m^2 orally daily days 8-14

Day 15

- methotrexate 500 mg/m^2 IV on day 15
- leucovorin 50 mg/m^2 orally every 6 hours for four doses beginning 24 hours after methotrexate

R-HYPER-CVAD (EVERY 21 DAYS)*

Cycles I, 3, 5, and 7

- rituxumab 375 mg/m^2 IV on day 1
- cyclophosphamide (with mesna) 300 mg/m^2 IV over 3 hours every 12 hours on days 2-4 (total six doses)
- vincristine 1.4 mg/m^2 (maximum 2 mg) IV on days 5 and 12
- doxorubicin (Adriamycin) 16.6 mg/m^2 IV by continuous infusion on days 5-7
- dexamethasone 40 mg/day PO/IV on days 2-5 and days 12-15

Cycles 2,4, 6, and 8

- rituxumab 375 mg/m^2 IV on day 1
- methotrexate 200 mg/m^2 IV over 2 hours, followed by 800 mg/m^2 IV continuous infusion over 22 hours on day 2
- leucovorin 50 mg PO starting 12 hours after completion of methotrexate infusion, followed by 15 mg PO every 6 hours for 8 dosed until the methotrexate level is less than 0.1 μM/L
- cytarabine 3000 mg/m^2 IV over 2 hours every 12 hours on days 3 and 4 (4 doses total)

*From Romaguera JE, Fayad L, Rodriguez MA, et al: High rate of durable remissions after treatment of newly diagnosed aggressive mantle-cell lymphoma with rituximab plus hyper-CVAD alternating with rituximab plus high-dose methotrexate and cytarabine. *J Clin Oncol* 23:7013, 2005.

combination of rituximab, cyclophosphamide, hydroxydaunomycin, vincristine (Oncovin), and prednisone (R-CHOP) is heavily favored over rituximab, cyclophosphamide, vincristine, and prednisone (R-CVP) or fludarabine-based regimens. Choice to initiate therapy was associated with FLIPI, stage, and grade; however, FLIPI was not associated with the decision to use any specific treatment approach. Significant regional and center differences were observed, strongly suggesting that physician preference is the predominant factor that drives initial therapy. For example, initial "watch and wait" was used in 31% of cases in the Northeast but only in 13% in the Southeast; fludarabine-based chemoimmunotherapy was used in 18% of patients in Southwest but only in 3% in the Northeast.

Alkylating Agents

The alkylating agents chlorambucil and cyclophosphamide, with or without prednisone and CVP or CHOP, and other alkylator-based combination chemotherapy regimens have been the standard of therapy for FL decades. Single-agent alkylators at different doses and schedules produce overall response (OR) rates of 50% to 75% in FL.[32,33] Comparable response rates, but higher complete remission (CR) rates with longer progression-free survival (PFS), are seen with CVP compared with chlorambucil, but with no survival advantage.[34,35] The addition of anthracyclines has not improved the response rate or duration of the response,[36,37] but its use may be associated with a lower risk for histologic transformation.[25,38] This finding needs to be confirmed, particularly in the era of chemoimmunotherapy.

Bendamustine

Bendamustine is a potent alkylating agent that has been demonstrated to have substantial efficacy in NHL patients, including those with FL. Bendamustine is highly effective in rituximab-refractory FL and in patients whose disease is refractory to other alkylating agents. It has also demonstrated considerable efficacy in previously untreated FL, both alone and in combination with rituximab or other chemotherapeutic agents.[47,48] Increased understanding of the mechanisms of action of bendamustine and its efficacy in combination with rituximab in newly diagnosed or relapsed/refractory FL has led to investigation of other combinations. Ongoing studies are examining bendamustine with bortezomib, lenalidomide, temsirolimus, ofatumumab, GA101, and other novel agents.

Purine Analogues

The purine analogues have been studied extensively in various types of indolent lymphoma. Fludarabine monotherapy produces response rates of 65% to 84%, with 37% to 47% CR in previously untreated FL patients.[39] In a randomized trial of 381 previously untreated patients with indolent lymphoma, CR rates were higher with fludarabine than with CVP.[40] Fludarabine combinations result in increased response rates, with an 89% CR rate in an Eastern Cooperative Oncology Group (ECOG) trial combining fludarabine and cyclophosphamide (FC),[41] whereas fludarabine and mitoxantrone (FM) produced a 91% OR, 43% CR, and 2-year DFS of 63%.[42] A higher CR rare was seen with FM (68%) compared with CHOP (42%) in a randomized trial.[43] The use of alkylator-based regimens or purine analogue–based regimens appears to vary geographically, suggesting personal preference for the use of regimens in which the clinician has experience, rather than alterations of practice based on the results of the published studies. In CLL/SLL, fludarabine is associated with a higher response rate and longer duration of response than chlorambucil,[44] but with no OS advantage. The use of fludarabine in combination with cyclophosphamide is associated with a higher response rate and longer duration of response compared with fludarabine alone in randomized trials.[45] The highest response rates have been with fludarabine, cyclophosphamide, and rituximab (FCR).[46]

Biologic Therapy

Based on improved survival in clinical trials[21,49,50] and metaanalysis of phase III trial data,[51] IFN-α has been approved by the Food and Drug Administration (FDA) for the treatment of advanced-stage FL in combination with anthracycline-based chemotherapy. IFN-α has been widely used in Europe, but not in the United States, where it is believed that its toxicity profile outweighs any potential benefit. In the Southwest Oncology Group (SWOG) study,[52] 571 patients with stage III and IV indolent lymphoma were treated with ProMACE-MOPP, and 279 responding patients were randomized to 24 months of observation versus treatment with IFN-α. No statistically significant difference was seen in PFS or OS between the observation group and the IFN-α group at 4 years.

Monoclonal Antibody Therapy

Monoclonal antibodies are the most exciting agents to emerge in the treatment of indolent lymphomas. The most widely used monoclonal antibody is rituximab, a chimeric unconjugated antibody against the CD20 antigen. Rituximab is licensed by the FDA and the European Agency for the Evaluation of Medicinal Products (EMEA) for (1) the treatment of patients with relapsed or refractory, CD20-positive low-grade FL, (2) the first-line treatment of CD20-positive FL in combination with CVP chemotherapy, and (3) the treatment of CD20-positive low-grade NHL in patients with stable disease or patients who achieve a PR or CR following first-line treatment with CVP chemotherapy. The use of this agent has had a profound effect in improvement in survival in patients with FL.[19,20,53]

Following phase I studies,[54] rituximab at a dose of 375 mg/m^2 weekly for 4 weeks was selected for the pivotal phase II trial,[55] and although this remains the standard dose, the optimal dose and schedule of rituximab are still unknown. In relapsed FL patients, OR to rituximab monotherapy was 60% with a median PFS for responders of 13 months. Factors associated with lower response rates include chemoresistant disease,[55] bulky disease,[56] and treatment late in the disease course.[57] OR was 73% in previously untreated patients with low-bulk disease[58]; some of these patients have needed no further treatment and have no evidence of polymerase chain reaction (PCR)–detectable minimal residual disease (MRD) after 7 years.[59] Extended use with 8 weeks of treatment (instead of 4 weeks) is associated with improvement in OR and duration of response.[60] Comparable or even longer durations of response have been observed with retreatment.[61]

Table 79-11 Studies of Rituximab Maintenance Therapy in Indolent Lymphomas

Trial	Disease Setting	Diseases Included	Previous Therapy
ECOG[62]	First-line	Follicular Small lymphocytic	CVP
SAKK[63]	First-line Relapsed/refractory	Follicular Mantle cell	Rituximab
EORTC[64]	Relapsed/refractory	Follicular	CHOP vs. R-CHOP
GLSG[65]	Relapsed/refractory	Follicular Mantle cell	FCM vs. R-FCM
LYM-5[66]	Relapsed/refractory	Follicular Small lymphocytic	Rituximab

A number of trials in front-line and in relapsed/refractory patients have investigated the potential benefits of extended or maintenance rituximab treatment,[62-68] and all of these trials demonstrated prolonged time to progression in patients receiving maintenance rituximab (Table 79-11). Results from the E1496 randomized trial from ECOG and from the Cancer and Leukemia Group B (CALGB) comparing CVP alone with CVP followed by rituximab in patients with advanced-stage FL demonstrated that addition of rituximab maintenance significantly improved OS[62] and led to FDA approval for rituximab therapy in patients responding to CVP chemotherapy. The results of the PRIMA (primary rituximab and maintenance) study demonstrated an advantage in PFS for maintenance rituximab therapy offered after initial chemoimmunotherapy.[68] It is too soon to determine whether this will have an impact on OS, and questions remain as to whether this should become standard of care.[69]

Chemoimmunotherapy

In a phase II study, 40 patients with indolent lymphoma were treated with six infusions of rituximab (375 mg/m^2 per dose) in combination with six doses of CHOP chemotherapy (R-CHOP)[70]; OR was 95%, with 55% CR. In a phase II study of 40 patients with indolent lymphomas, rituximab in combination with fludarabine produced OR of 90%, with 80% CR, with similar response rates in treatment-naive and previously treated patients.[71]

A number of randomized trials show a benefit for the use of rituximab with chemotherapy compared with chemotherapy alone (Table 79-12).[64,72-75] Each study showed an improvement in time to treatment failure (TTF), and more recent follow-up data suggest improved OS in patients treated with chemoimmunotherapy compared with chemotherapy alone. A metaanalysis of these trials demonstrates that OS, OR, and disease control are significantly better with chemoimmunotherapy compared with chemotherapy for FL and mantle cell lymphoma.[76] Data from the German Low-Grade Study Group (GLSG) suggest that it is the addition of rituximab that has led to the recent improvement in survival of patients with FL.[20] An independently assessed analysis of the clinical benefits provided by rituximab in relation to cost concluded that it is a highly cost-effective treatment.[77]

The largest FL trial ever reported is the PRIMA study.[68] This study enrolled 1217 patients to receive initial chemoimmunotherapy. Treatment was from three possible regimens, but it is important to note that 75% of patients received R-CHOP. All patients had fulfilled the criteria for treatment, and 80% had FLIPI intermediate- or high-risk features. Responding patients were randomized to receive no further therapy or to receive 12 doses (every 8 weeks) for 2 years.

Table 79-12 Randomized Trials of Chemotherapy Versus Chemoimmunotherapy

Study	Treatment, Number of Patients	Median FU (months)	OR (%)	CR (%)	Median TTF (months)	OS (%)
M39021[72]	CVP, 159 R-CVP, 162	53	57 81	10 41	15 34 $p < 0.0001$	77 83 $p = 0.0290$
GLSG[73]	CHOP, 205 R-CHOP, 223	18	90 96	17 20	29 NR $p < 0.001$	90 95 $p = 0.016$
M39023[74]	MCP, 96 R-MCP, 105	47	75 92	25 50	26 NR $p < 0.0001$	74 87 $p = 0.0096$
FL2000[75]	CHVP-IFN, 183 R-CHVP-IFN 175	42	73 84	63 79	46% 67% $p < 0.0001$	84 91 $p = 0.029$

CR, Complete remission; *FU*, follow-up; *OR*, overall response.

Patients who received rituximab maintenance therapy had significantly better rates of 3-year PFS than did those who received observation (75% versus 58%), and the benefit to maintenance was observed in all FLIPI groups. Time to next treatment was also longer in the maintenance group than in the observation group. Increased toxicities were seen in the maintenance group, most being infections, but these were largely self-limiting.

Conjugated Radiolabeled Monoclonal Antibody Therapy

Complexing a radioisotope to a monoclonal antibody (radioimmunoconjugate) might be expected to improve efficacy over antibody therapy alone. Tositumomab complexes ^{131}I (radioactive iodine) to the anti-B1 antibody and has been studied extensively in the treatment of heavily pretreated patients[78] and untreated patients,[79] as well as for retreatment of indolent lymphomas.[80] Best responses are seen in previously untreated FL patients—95% OR, 75% CR, and 80% of assessable patients achieving eradication of PCR-detectable MRD patients treated with a single treatment course with tositumomab.[79] Median PFS was 6.1 years, with 40 patients remaining in remission for 4.3 to 7.7 years and no cases of myelodysplastic syndrome observed. A SWOG study investigated chemoimmunotherapy with six cycles of CHOP chemotherapy followed 4 to 8 weeks later by tositumomab in 90 patients with previously untreated, advanced-stage FL.[81] The OR was 91%, including 69% CR; at median follow-up time of 5.1 years, the estimated 5-year OS was 87% and PFS was 67%, which 23% better than CHOP alone on previous SWOG protocols. Ibritumomab tiuxetan is a ^{88}Y-labeled anti-CD20 antibody that produced an OR of 74% and 15% CR in 57 FL patients refractory to rituximab.[82] Toxicity is primarily hematologic, with nadir counts occurring at 7 to 9 weeks and lasting approximately 1 to 4 weeks. The risk for hematologic toxicity increased with dose delivered and with degree of baseline bone marrow lymphoma involvement.[83] An acceptable safety profile was observed in relapsed patients with less than 25% lymphoma marrow involvement, adequate marrow reserve, platelets greater than 100,000 cells/μL, and neutrophils greater than 1500 cells/μL.

High-Dose Therapy as Consolidation of First Remission

The role of high-dose therapy (HDT) and autologous SCT (ASCT) in FL patients during first remission has been explored in phase II trials[84,85] and in three phase III randomized trials.[86-88] The GLSG trial[86] recruited 307 previously untreated patients up to 60 years of age; patients who responded after induction chemotherapy with two cycles of CHOP or MCP (mitoxantrone, chlorambucil, and prednisone) were randomized to receive ASCT or IFN-α maintenance. Among 240 evaluable patients, the 5-year PFS was 64.7% for ASCT, and 33.3% in the IFN-α arm ($P < 0.0001$). Acute toxicity was higher in the ASCT group, but early mortality was below 2.5% in both study arms. Longer follow-up is necessary to determine the effect of ASCT on OS. In the Groupe Ouest Est des Leucemies Aigues et des Maladies du Sang (GOELAMS) study, 172 newly diagnosed advanced-stage FL patients were randomized either to CHVP (cyclophosphamide, hydroxydaunomycin, teniposide [Vumon], and prednisone) and IFN-α or to HDT followed by purged ASCT.[87] Patients treated with high-dose therapy had a higher response rate than those who received chemotherapy and IFN-α (81% versus 69%, $p = 0.045$) and a longer median PFS (not reached versus 45 months); however, because of an excess of secondary malignancies after transplantation, this did not translate into a better OS. A subgroup of patients with a significantly higher event-free survival rate after ASCT could be identified using the FLIPI. The GELF94 study enrolled 401 previously untreated advanced-stage FL patients who were randomized to receive CHVP plus IFN-α compared with four courses of CHOP followed by HDT with total body irradiation (TBI) and ASCT; OR rates were similar in both groups (79% and 78%, respectively), and 87% of eligible patients underwent ASCT. Intent-to-treat analysis after a median follow-up of 7.5 years showed no difference between the two arms for OS ($p = 0.53$) or PFS ($p = 0.11$). Long-term follow-up demonstrated no statistically significant benefit in favor of first-line ASCT in patients with FL, which the investigators conclude should be reserved for relapsed patients. A metaanalysis concluded that that HDT and ASCT does not improve overall survival in FL.[89] In view of these results, ASCT should be used in first remission only in the setting of clinical trials.

TREATMENT OF RELAPSED INDOLENT LYMPHOMA

The treatment options after relapse remain the same as for first-line therapy (see Table 79-5), and ideally, relapsed patients should be treated in clinical trials. Relapsed asymptomatic disease is not necessarily an indication for treatment, and patients can again be managed expectantly. A number of factors must be taken into account in planning therapy; it is not possible to define treatment at relapse without considering the goal of therapy (palliative versus potentially curative), performance status, previous therapy, response, and duration of response. Single-agent rituximab is approved for relapsed lymphoma and is widely used in this setting. A multicenter randomized trial in relapsed patients has demonstrated a survival advantage for chemoimmunotherapy with R-CHOP or with CHOP followed by rituximab compared with CHOP alone, as well as a further benefit for rituximab maintenance therapy.[64] For younger patients who are suitable candidates for either HDT and ASCT or reduced-intensity conditioning (RIC) allogeneic transplantation, referral to a transplant center should be considered early to discuss the potential role and timing of transplantation. Best results are seen when transplantation is considered early in the course of disease, before patients become chemorefractory, and HDT and ASCT remain an effective treatment approach for younger patients with chemoresponsive-relapsed disease. SCT approaches must be considered in the context of the improving results that are being seen with salvage therapy alone.

The Role of Transplant in Relapsed Indolent Lymphomas

Unlike its use with aggressive lymphomas, the use of high-dose chemotherapy with autologous SCT in the treatment of indolent lymphomas has not yet been fully established. The rationale for considering transplantation is that the disease is incurable using standard approaches; young patients with indolent lymphomas will die of their disease, and promising results have been observed in a number of phase II studies.[90-92] Detection of MRD has been a useful surrogate marker for tracking long-term PFS in patients examining the autologous stem cells or serial samples after transplantation.[92-96] A major concern relates to the risk for development of secondary myelodysplasia/acute myeloid leukemia.[97] The European Bone Marrow Transplant Registry (EBMTR)–sponsored CUP study (conventional chemotherapy, unpurged, purged autograft) is the only prospective randomized trial to assess the role of autologous SCT in patients with relapsed FL.[98] The results of the study suggest a PFS and OS advantage of ASCT over conventional chemotherapy, with 4-year OS of 46% for the chemotherapy arm, versus 71% for the unpurged and 77% for the purged ASCT arms. The study was closed early because of slow accrual with 140 of the planned 250 patients accrued and only 89 randomized.

Novel Agents

A large number of novel approaches are being studied in FL patients. These include monoclonal antibodies, idiotype vaccines, immunomodulatory agents, and novel kinase inhibitors. Combinations of monoclonal antibodies are being explored, such as combining anti-CD20 with anti-CD22 antibodies.[99] Several new anti-CD20 monoclonal antibodies are being evaluated in FL patients refractory to rituximab. These include several humanized antibodies designed to have less infusion toxicity and improved effector function.[100,101] GA101 is the first type II, glycoengineered, and humanized monoclonal anti-CD20 antibody[102] to enhance the activity of rituximab. Kinases involved in the B-cell receptor–signaling pathway are logical targets for therapy in FL. Clinical trial data have been presented for three kinase inhibitors, which target PI3 kinase p110d,[103] BTK,[104] and SYK,[105] respectively. These agents are now being examined in combination with monoclonal antibodies and chemotherapy. Since a hallmark of FL is overexpression of BCL2, this protein is also a logical target for small molecule inhibitors that can diminish the antiapoptotic activity of BCL2. Clinical responses have been observed in a phase I study examining the efficacy of navitoclax in lymphoid malignancies,[106] and this agent and similar compounds are currently also being evaluated in ongoing clinical trials alone and in combinations.

Allogeneic BMT

There is a trend toward the increasing use of allogeneic SCT (aSCT) in the management of indolent lymphomas. In a report of the International Bone Marrow Transplant Registry (IBMTR), results after SCT are described for 904 patients with FL.[107] Among these patients, 176 underwent aSCT, 131 underwent ASCT using purged stem cells, and 597 had ASCT using purged autologous stem cells. The transplant-related mortality (TRM) in these three groups was 30%, 14%, and 8%, respectively; disease recurrence occurred in 21%, 43%, and 58%, respectively; and 5-year overall survival was 51%, 62%, and 55%, respectively. The use of regimens involving TBI was associated with increased TRM but decreased risk for relapse. The use of aSCT was associated with increased TRM but significantly lower risk for disease recurrence, in keeping with a graft-versus-lymphoma effect in this disease. Trends suggest that outcomes are improving; this is highly likely to continue with the increased use of RIC regimens that have become increasingly common since the time these IBMTR data were collated. Long-term PFS has been observed after aSCT, even in patients with refractory FL.[108] In 29 FL patients, 11 of whom had refractory disease, the nonrelapse mortality rate was 24% and there was a 23% incidence of relapse. The 5-year OS was 58% with 53% event-free survival. Patients who have relapsed after previous autologous SCT have very poor outcomes. The outcome following myeloablative allogeneic SCT of 114 such patients has been reported from the IBMTR.[109] The treatment-related mortality was 22%, and the probability of disease progression was 52% at 3 years.

The use of TBI conditioning regimens and achievement of CR at the time of allogeneic SCT were associated with improved outcome. The use of RIC regimens appears to be associated with improved outcome. In 20 such patients, only one treatment-related mortality occurred (due to fungal infection), and the 3-year PFS was excellent, at 95%.[110] The outcome following RIC transplant regimen incorporating alemtuzumab immunosuppressive therapy has been reported for patients with 81 patients with lymphoma, including 41 with low-grade FL, 37 with high- or intermediate-grade FL, and 10 patients with MCL, 31 of whom had relapsed following previous autologous SCT.[111] Patients received a conditioning regimen consisting of alemtuzumab, fludarabine and melphalan; they also received short-course cyclosporine as prophylaxis for graft-versus-host disease (GVHD). The use of this conditioning regimen was associated with a low incidence of GVHD, and the treatment-related mortality was decreased in patients with low-grade compared with higher-grade histology. The 3-year PFS was 65% for patients with low-grade lymphoma, 50% for patients with MCL, and 34% for higher-grade lymphoma ($p = 0.002$). Donor lymphocyte infusion (DLI) was given to 36 patients, 21 for relapsed or persistent disease and 15 for persistence of mixed chimerism. The use of DLI to treat relapse after allogeneic SCT is solely dependent on the existence of a graft-versus-lymphoma effect. In seven patients with FL and SLL who had relapsed after prior allogeneic SCT, six patients responded; in four of these patients, the CRs were maintained for 43 to 89 months. The effectiveness of DLI to treat relapse after allogeneic SCT provides very strong evidence for a graft-versus-lymphoma effect that can be exploited in indolent lymphomas.[111,112] The role of RIC allogeneic SCT has been evaluated by the Cancer and Leukemia Group B in a phase II study to evaluate the safety and efficacy in patients with recurrent low-grade B cell malignancies, including 16 patients with FL.[113] The 3-year TRM was 9%, and the 3-year OS was 81%. The incidence of grade II-IV acute GVHD was 29%, and the extensive chronic GVHD was 18%.

SUGGESTED READINGS

Al Khabori M, de Almeida JR, Guyatt GH, et al: Autologous stem cell transplantation in follicular lymphoma: A systematic review and meta-analysis. *J Natl Cancer Inst* 104:18, 2012.

Campo E, Swerdlow SH, Harris NL, et al: The 2008 WHO classification of lymphoid neoplasms and beyond: Evolving concepts and practical applications. *Blood* 117:5019, 2011.

Cerhan JR, Wang S, Maurer MJ, et al: Prognostic significance of host immune gene polymorphisms in follicular lymphoma survival. *Blood* 109:5439, 2007.

Dave SS, Wright G, Tan B, et al: Prediction of survival in follicular lymphoma based on molecular features of tumor-infiltrating immune cells. *N Engl J Med* 351:2159, 2004.

Deconinck E, Foussard C, Milpied N, et al: High-dose therapy followed by autologous purged stem-cell transplantation and doxorubicin-based chemotherapy in patients with advanced follicular lymphoma: A randomized multicenter study by GOELAMS. *Blood* 105:3817, 2005.

Farinha P, Masoudi H, Skinnider BF, et al: Analysis of multiple biomarkers shows that lymphoma-associated macrophage (LAM) content is an independent predictor of survival in follicular lymphoma (FL). *Blood* 106:2169, 2005.

Federico M, Bellei M, Marcheselli L, et al: Follicular lymphoma international prognostic index 2: A new prognostic index for follicular lymphoma developed by the international follicular lymphoma prognostic factor project. *J Clin Oncol* 27:4555, 2009.

Fisher RI, LeBlanc M, Press OW, et al: New treatment options have changed the survival of patients with follicular lymphoma. *J Clin Oncol* 23:8447, 2005.

Horning SJ, Rosenberg SA: The natural history of initially untreated low-grade non-Hodgkin's lymphomas. *N Engl J Med* 311:1471, 1984.

Kaminski MS, Tuck M, Estes J, et al: 131I-tositumomab therapy as initial treatment for follicular lymphoma. *N Engl J Med* 352:441, 2005.

Lenz G, Dreyling M, Schiegnitz E, et al: Myeloablative radiochemotherapy followed by autologous stem cell transplantation in first remission prolongs progression-free survival in follicular lymphoma: Results of a prospective, randomized trial of the German Low-Grade Lymphoma Study Group. *Blood* 104:2667, 2004.

Montoto S, Fitzgibbon J: Transformation of indolent B-cell lymphomas. *J Clin Oncol* 29:1827, 2011.

Morin RD, Mendez-Lago M, Mungall AJ, et al: Frequent mutation of histone-modifying genes in non-Hodgkin lymphoma. *Nature* 476:298, 2011.

Press OW, Unger JM, Braziel RM, et al: Phase II trial of CHOP chemotherapy followed by tositumomab/iodine I-131 tositumomab for previously untreated follicular non-Hodgkin's lymphoma: Five-year follow-up of Southwest Oncology Group Protocol S9911. *J Clin Oncol* 24:4143, 2006.

Salles G, Seymour JF, Offner F, et al: Rituximab maintenance for 2 years in patients with high tumour burden follicular lymphoma responding to rituximab plus chemotherapy (PRIMA): A phase 3, randomised controlled trial. *Lancet* 377:42, 2011.

Solal-Celigny P, Roy P, Colombat P, et al: Follicular lymphoma international prognostic index. *Blood* 104:1258, 2004.

Swerdlow SH, Campo E, Harris NL, et al: *WHO classification of tumours of haematopoietic and lymphoid tissues*, ed 4, Lyon, 2008, IARC Press.

For complete list of references log on to www.expertconsult.com.

CHAPTER 80

MANTLE CELL LYMPHOMA

Michael Wang, Liang Zhang, Zhishuo Ou, Madhav V. Desai, Ken H. Young, Richard E. Champlin, Larry W. Kwak, and Jorge E. Romaguera

Mantle cell lymphoma (MCL) is a well-defined pathologic and clinical entity with an extremely variable clinical course. It is incurable using current approaches and has a poor prognosis after conventional chemotherapy when compared with other types of B-cell lymphomas. The major genetic feature of MCL is the presence of a t(11;14) translocation that results in the overexpression of cyclin D1 (CCDN1) in the tumor cells of virtually all patients. No standard treatment has been established to date; however, progress made towards elucidating the pathogenesis of MCL has led to novel approaches to therapy that have greatly improved patient outcomes.

DEFINITION AND HISTORY

Mantle cell lymphoma is classified as a subtype of B-cell lymphoma derived from CD5-positive antigen-naive pregerminal center B cells within the mantle zone that surrounds the normal germinal center follicles. Previously named *intermediate lymphocytic lymphoma, centrocytic lymphoma, lymphocytic lymphoma with intermediate differentiation,* and *marginal zone lymphoma,* MCL is now recognized as a distinct entity with a unique biology and aggressive clinical behavior.

EPIDEMIOLOGY

MCL represents approximately 6% (3% to 10%) of all non-Hodgkin lymphomas (NHLs) and accounts for 3000 to 4000 cases of lymphoma per year in the United States, with current median survival duration of up to 5 years. The median age at diagnosis is 68 years (range, 29 to 85 years), and the overall incidence of MCL is estimated to be 0.55 per 100,000 in the United States,[1] which increases with age. Given the relatively short median overall survival (OS), its prevalence is low, at 15,000 cases. Currently, there are no known etiologic agents for MCL.

CLINICAL FEATURES

The ratio of men to women diagnosed with MCL is about 4:1. The early symptoms usually include fever, heavy night sweats, unexplained weight loss, swelling of the lymph nodes, and splenomegaly. The typical presentation is that of a 64-year-old man with advanced disease who is asymptomatic (Table 80-1).[2] The spleen can be enlarged in 40% of patients, and 50% of patients can present with blood involvement, sometimes with an overt leukemic phase but more often with subclinical involvement, as detected by flow cytometry. Symptomatic gastrointestinal involvement occurs in 25% of MCL cases; at its most extreme, this is known as lymphomatous polyposis. Overall, gastrointestinal involvement can be detected in 90% of cases; half of these can be diagnosed only by panendoscopy and microscopic evaluation of random biopsies. Most cases are detected using colonoscopy.[3,4]

LABORATORY FEATURES

Morphologic Features

Histologically, MCL presents most frequently as a diffuse effacement of the lymph nodes, less frequently as nodules, and rarely as a mantle zone pattern, defined as >90% of the follicles presenting with preservation of the germinal center (Fig. 80-1).[5]

There are four cytologic variants of MCL. (1) Classic MCL is characterized by a monotonous population of small to intermediately sized lymphoid cells with slightly irregular nuclei, scant cytoplasm, and finely condensed chromatin. In some cases, the residual normal germinal center may be disrupted. (2) The small-cell variant is composed of small, round lymphocytes (which resemble chronic lymphocytic leukemia) and finely clumped chromatin. (3) The blastoid-cell variant is the most common and is characterized by large blastoid lymphocytes, appreciable nucleoli, and more abundant cytoplasm. (4) The pleomorphic variant is characterized by medium to large cells and prominent nuclei. The blastoid and pleomorphic variants are associated with a more aggressive clinical course. A rare monocytoid variant with features resembling marginal-zone B-cell lymphoma has also been reported.

Immunophenotypic Features

Immunophenotyping of MCL has revealed the positive expression of the B cell–associated antigens CD19, CD20, CD22, and CD79a; the aberrant expression of the T cell–associated antigens CD5 and CD43; and negative staining for CD7, CD8, and CD23. MCL stains are strongly positive for the antiapoptotic molecule BCL2 and negative for the germinal center markers CD10 and BCL6.[5] The diagnostic marker for MCL that is not encountered in other malignant lymphomas is the overexpression of cyclin D1, which is revealed most accurately in stains of formalin-fixed, paraffin-embedded lymph nodes or soft tissue.

Cytogenetic Features

The t(11;14)(q13;q32) translocation, which is characteristic of MCL and the central and primary event of lymphomagenesis, occurs in bone marrow at the pre–B-cell stage of differentiation when the B cell is initiating IG gene rearrangement with the recombination of the V(D)J segments.[6] The reciprocal chromosomal translocation involves the cyclin D1 (CCND1) gene on chromosome 11 and the IGH gene locus on chromosome 14. This results in increased expression of cyclin D1. A cell-cycle protein not normally expressed in lymphoid and myeloid cells, cyclin D1 promotes the transition from the G1 to the S phase of the cell cycle. In the rare cases of MCL in which cyclin D1 is not overexpressed, cyclin D2 or cyclin D3 is usually overexpressed,[7] suggesting that deregulation of other members of the highly conserved cyclin family may be an alternative

Table 80-1 Patient Characteristics at Presentation (304 Cases)

Characteristic	*n*
AGE (YEARS)	
<60	123
>60	178
SEX	
Male	230
Female	71
STAGE	
I-II	23
III-IV	267
STATUS (WHO)	
0–1	233
≥2	43
DH	
Elevated	6
Normal	140
IPI	
0-1	15
≥2	75
BONE MARROW INVOLVEMENT	
Yes	207
No	81
B SYMPTOMS	
Yes	107
No	155
EXTRANODAL INVOLVEMENT	
Yes	161
No	16

LDH, Lactate dehydrogenase; *IPI,* International Prognostic Index.

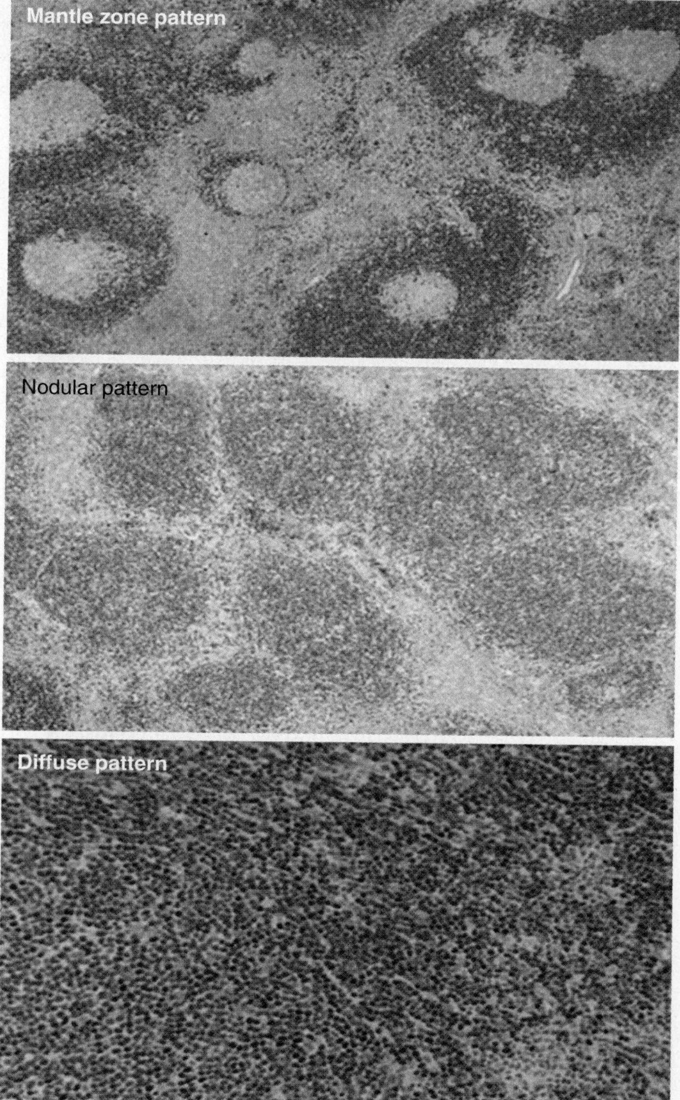

Figure 80-1 HISTOPATHOLOGY OF MANTLE CELL LYMPHOMA.

mechanism to cyclin D1 overexpression in MCL tumorigenesis. The transcription factor SOX-11 is highly expressed in these cyclin D1–negative MCL cases but absent in other types of mature B-cell lymphoma and thereby serves as a valuable biomarker for the differential diagnosis of MCL in these cases.

Although most cases of MCL have the conventional t(11;14)(q13;q32) chromosomal translocation, additional genetic events contributing to the progression of MCL have been clinically observed. In addition, low numbers of cells carrying the t(11;14) translocation have been found in the blood of 1% to 2% of healthy individuals without any evidence of disease.[8] Cytogenetic studies have revealed secondary genetic alterations (Table 80-2) that may be involved in the pathogenesis and progression of MCL and have shown that MCL has one of the highest levels of genomic instability among the malignant lymphoid neoplasms.[9] The analysis of primary MCL cells with relatively low-resolution conventional comparative genomic hybridization, high-resolution comparative genomic hybridization array, and single nucleotide polymorphism microarray combined with microarray gene-expression profiling studies has revealed that MCL has a characteristic profile of genomic alterations. In addition, the delineation of minimally altered regions has facilitated the identification of potential target genes (Table 80-2).[10-14]

Dysregulation occurs not only in the cell cycle, but also in the DNA damage–response and cell-survival pathways. The blastoid variant is associated with most of these genetic alterations. In addition, TP53 mutations, uniparental disomy involving TP53, INK4a/ARF homozygous deletions, and BMI1 amplifications are all known to contribute to MCL cell proliferation. Abnormalities in chromosome 17p have been observed in up to 26% of MCL cases[15] and have been associated with p53 mutations, which correlate with poor prognosis,[16] most likely owing to the impairment of the DNA damage–response pathway.

Biologic Pathways and Potential Therapeutic Targets

Comprehensive abnormalities identified in cell survival, DNA damage, cell-cycle regulation, and apoptosis pathways provide the biologic mechanisms responsible for the aggressive clinical behavior of MCL, its rapid relapse, and its short response to therapy. Its proliferation activity, which reflects these biologic mechanisms, is therefore believed to be the most valuable pathologic parameter for predicting the biologic behavior of MCL tumors.

A proposed model of MCL progression is depicted in Fig. 80-2.[6] Overall, CCND1 translocation is the primary or initial genetic event, followed by alterations in two major signaling pathways, INK4a/CDK4/RB1 and MDM2/TP53/P27. Studies indicate that secondary genetic alterations may reinforce the two major signaling pathways' effects, which include further enhancing cell proliferation, facilitating evasion of apoptosis, reducing immune control, and promoting interactions with the tumor microenvironment through constitutive activation of the Wnt, hedgehog, PI3K/AKT/mammalian target of rapamycin (mTOR), B-cell antigen receptor (BCR), and nuclear factor kappa-B (NF-κB) signaling pathways, as well as TP53 mutation and BMI1 amplification (Fig. 80-3).[17] These altered molecular pathways in MCL—including the often constitutively activated PI3K/AKT/mTOR, Wnt, hedgehog, BCR, and NF-κB pathways—provide insight into its pathogenesis. The overexpressed cyclin D1 complexes with CDK4, and this has at least two important downstream effects. The cyclin D1-CDK4 (or CDK6) complex leads to phosphorylation of the retinoblastoma gene RB1, with the net result (through the release of elongation factor 2 [EF2] transcription factors) being the progression of the lymphoma cells into S phase. The cyclin D1-CDK4 complex may also neutralize the ability of the CDK inhibitor p27 to induce G1 cell-cycle arrest.

Table 80-2 Main Genetic Anomalies, Including Losses and Gains, in Mantle Cell Lymphoma

	Main Genetic Losses	Main Genetic Gains
Low-resolution conventional comparative genomic hybridization (CGH)	1p13-p31, 2q13, 3p13-p14, 6q21-q26, 8p21, 9p21, 10p14-p15, 11q22-q23(ATM), 13q11-q13, 13q33-q34, 17p13(TP53)	3q25-qt28, 4p12-13, 7p11-22, 8p24(MYC), 8q21, 9q22, 10p12-p13(BMI1), 12q13-q14(CDK4), 13q31-q32, 15q22-q24,18q21-q22(BCL2)
High-resolution CGH-array and single nucleotide polymorphism microarray combined with microarray gene expression profiling	1p21.1,1p22.2-p22.3(CDKN2C), 1p32.3, 1q32(PROX1), 2q37.1(SP100), 6q23.3(TNFAIP3), 6q25(LATS1), 8p21.3, 9p21.2, 9p21.3(CDKN2A), 9q22.2-q22.31, 10p13, 11q22.3(ATM), 13q12.3-q13.1, 13q14.2(RB1), 13q33.2-q33.3, 17p13(TP53),19p13.1, 21q11.2	3q26.1-q26.32, 7p22.1-p22.3, 8q24.21(MYC), 10p12.2-p12.31 (BMI1), 11q13.3-q21, 12q14(MDM2), 13q231.3, 15q23, 18q21.33(BCL2)

Terms in parentheses are potential target genes.

One of these secondary alterations is the mutation of the ataxia-telangiectasia mutant (ATM) gene, which is seen in about 40% of MCL cases. ATM inactivation facilitates genomic instability in lymphoma cells by impairing their response to DNA damage. Also, PI3K, which is encoded by ATM, is a key kinase in this pathway. Notably, the PI3K-AKT pathway is upstream of mTOR, which is in turn upstream of cyclin D1, p27, and other regulatory proteins.[18,19]

Other genetic alterations affect two major signaling pathways: the Wnt canonical pathway (WCP) via β-catenin, which is important for normal cell growth and development, and an alternative pathway leading to JNK activation. Activation of β-catenin is a relatively frequent aberration in MCL, and several Wnt members are consistently overexpressed in MCL.[20]

The hedgehog signaling pathway can also be altered in MCL. This pathway is one of the key regulators of animal development, and sonic hedgehog (SHH) is the well-known ligand of the vertebrate pathway. SHH-GLI signaling molecules such as PTCH, SMO, GLI1, and GLI2 are expressed in human MCL cell lines and in primary MCL cells from patients. Downregulation of GLI transcription factors has been shown to significantly decrease the proliferation of MCL cells and increase the susceptibility of MCL cells to chemotherapy.[21]

Another pathway involved in the pathogenesis of MCL is the ubiquitin-proteasome pathway, the major nonlysosomal pathway through which intracellular proteins are degraded. By stabilizing the promoters of cyclins and repressors of CDK, proteasome inhibition leads to cell-cycle arrest and the induction of apoptosis.[22] This pathway plays an essential role in the activation of NF-κB by degrading its inhibitory protein, I-κB.[23] The NF-κB signaling regulates transcription factors that activate numerous genes involved in cell survival, apoptosis, and cell migration. Its persistent activity is associated with tumor formation, tumor growth, metastasis, and drug resistance in many cancer types, including B-cell lymphoma. Current therapeutic efforts to inhibit this central "switch" include using small molecules to block selected targets in the pathway.[24] Studies show that

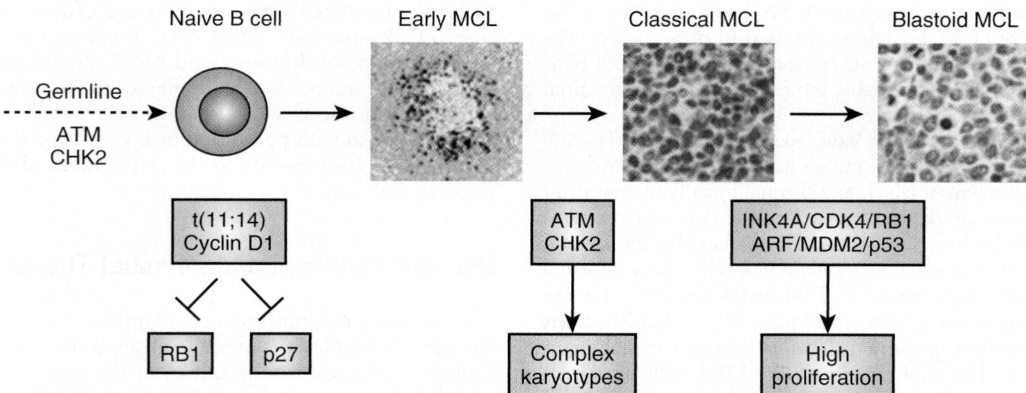

Figure 80-2 PROPOSED MODEL OF MOLECULAR PATHOGENESIS IN THE DEVELOPMENT AND PROGRESSION OF MANTLE CELL LYMPHOMA. The presence of ataxia-telangiectasia–mutated (ATM) or cell cycle checkpoint kinase 2 (CHK2) inactivating mutations in the germline of some patients suggests that they may facilitate the development of the tumor. The t(11;14) translocation occurs in an immature B cell and leads to the constitutive deregulation of cyclin D1 and early expansion of tumor B cells in the mantle zone areas of lymphoid follicles. Acquired inactivation of DNA damage response pathways may facilitate additional genetic alterations and the development of classical mantle cell lymphoma. Further genetic alterations may target genes of the cell cycle and senescence regulatory pathways, leading to more proliferative and aggressive variants of MCL.

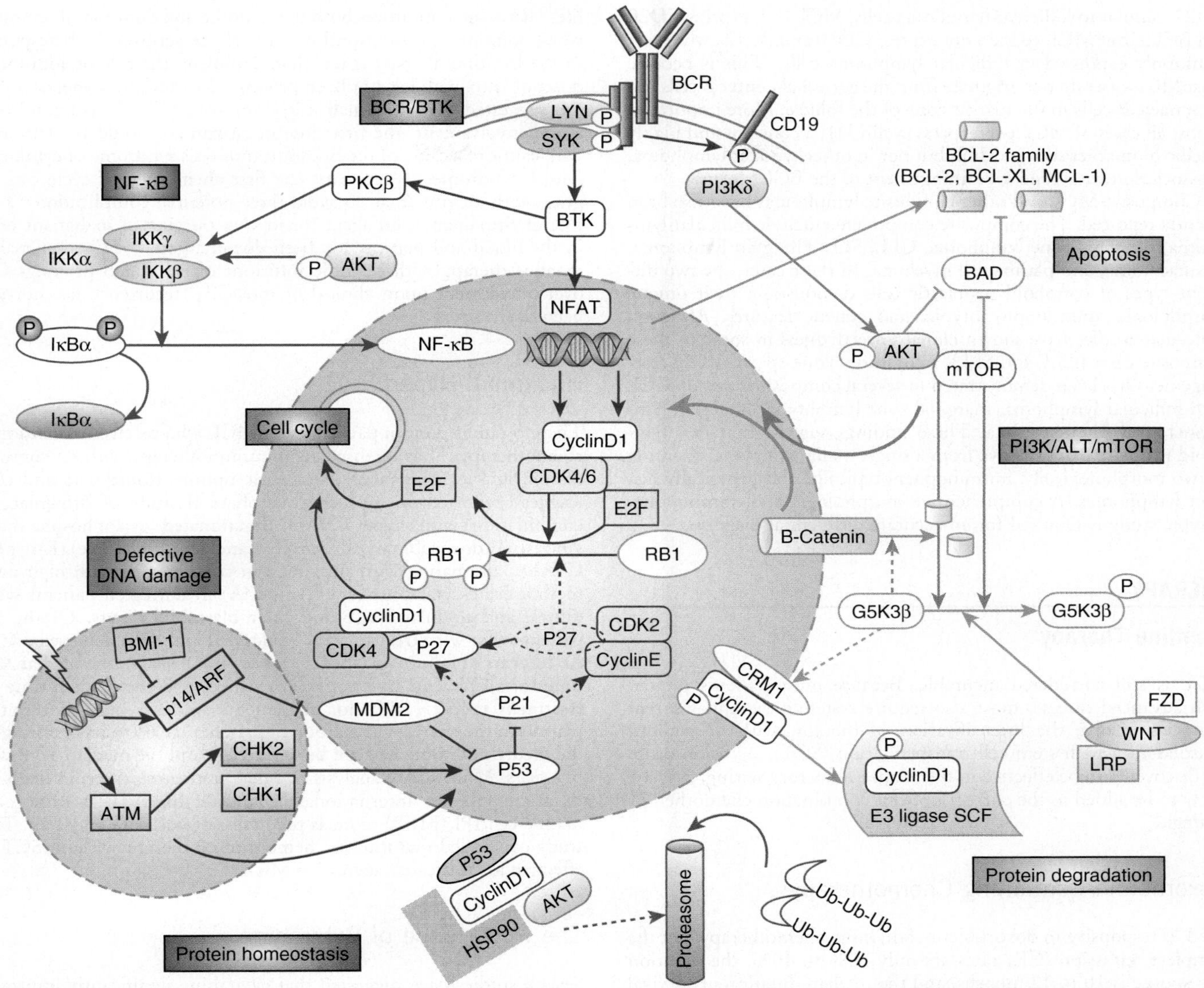

Figure 80-3 THE SIGNALING PATHWAYS CONTRIBUTING TO MANTLE CELL LYMPHOMA PATHOGENESIS. CCND1 translocation is the main primary or initial oncogenic event, which is followed by alterations in two major signaling pathways, the RB1 and P27 pathways. The secondary alterations may target genes functioning in these two major signaling pathways to further enhance MCL cell proliferation, which may be involved in the constitutive activation of BCR, Wnt, PI3K/AKT/mTOR, NF-κB, NFAT, HSP90, ATM, and other genes.

proteasome inhibitors, such as bortezomib (first generation) and carfilzomib (second generation), can be a novel approach for patients with relapsed/refractory MCL.[25,26]

Recent studies have reported constitutive activation of BCR signal transduction in MCL.[27] The lymphomagenesis of MCL is inseparable from B-cell development, because MCL is a type of B-cell lymphoma. Although the different subtypes of MCL have their own characteristics, BCR is associated with the pathogenesis of various subtypes of MCL, in most cases because BCR plays a key role in the process of B-cell differentiation and development. Many clinical studies have targeted BCR-associated kinases, including spleen tyrosine kinase (Syk), Bruton tyrosine kinase (Btk), and protein kinase C-beta (PKC-β). Intriguingly, Btk, a member of the Tec family of nonreceptor protein tyrosine kinases, has a well-defined role in the constitutively activated BCR signaling pathway in MCL. Clinical observations imply that Btk inhibition is a novel therapeutic approach in MCL. It is noteworthy that a recent phase I study of the novel small molecule PCI-32765, an irreversible Btk inhibitor, blocked B-cell activation and had antitumor activity in B-cell malignancies, including MCL, with favorable safety data.[28]

Recent molecular and genetic studies have revealed a subset of approximately 20% of MCL cases that have a relatively indolent clinical course. Prognosis in these patients is not affected by delaying initial therapy. These patients are clinically asymptomatic, their cases pathologically mimic low-grade B-cell lymphomas, and they usually present with leukemic phase or non-nodal involvement. Biologic mechanisms to explain this different clinical presentation have not yet been elucidated in this subset of cases.

DIFFERENTIAL DIAGNOSIS

The immunophenotype of MCL has some similarities to that of chronic lymphocytic leukemia (CLL) or small lymphocytic lymphoma (SLL) in that the lymphoma cells strongly express surface immunoglobulins M and D (IgM and IgD) and B cell–associated antigens CD19 and CD20 and aberrantly express the T-cell antigen CD5. Staining for B-cell antigens and Ig is stronger in intensity and more frequent in MCL than in CLL or SLL. In contrast to CLL or SLL cells, MCL cells express FMC7 and typically do not express

CD23. Similar to follicular lymphoma cells, MCL cells express CD20 and BCL2, but MCL cells do not express CD10 and BCL6, which are commonly expressed in follicular lymphoma cells.[5] This is because most MCL cases do not originate from the germinal-center B cells but from naive B cells in the mantle zone of the follicle. More important, almost all cases of MCL overexpress cyclin D1, a constant and highly specific biomarker seen in MCL but not in other types of lymphoma, in association with genetic rearrangement of the BCL1 locus.

Composite MCL and other composite lymphomas have also been recently reported. The composite components include follicular lymphoma, marginal zone lymphoma, CLL, SLL, Hodgkin lymphoma, plasmacytoma, and plasma cell myeloma. In these cases, the two different types of lymphoid neoplastic cells demonstrate their unique morphologic, immunophenotypic, and genetic features. Although molecular studies have shown clonal unrelatedness in some of these composite cases (CLL and SLL), a common clone-specific IGH rearrangement has been demonstrated in several composite cases of MCL with follicular lymphoma, marginal zone lymphoma, Hodgkin lymphoma, and plasmacytoma. These findings suggest that two lymphoid neoplasms may evolve from a single malignant clone, resulting in two morphologically, immunophenotypically, and genetically distinct lymphomas. A comprehensive morphologic and immunophenotypic study is required for an accurate differential diagnosis.

THERAPY

Frontline Therapy

MCL is still considered incurable. Because most patients present with advanced disease, most also require systemic therapy. Current strategies involve the intensification of therapy, with or without consolidation with stem cell transplantation (SCT). As novel drugs are discovered to be effective in the relapse/refractory setting, they are likely to be added to the current upfront combination chemotherapy strategies.

Doxorubicin-Containing Chemotherapy

MCL is responsive to doxorubicin-containing chemotherapy, but the complete remission (CR) rates are only 30% to 40%, the duration of response is 10 to 12 months, and the median duration of survival is 3 to 4 years, all of which are lower than these endpoints reported in other lymphomas.[29]

Fludarabine Alone or in Combination

Fludarabine is a purine analog that inhibits DNA synthesis by interfering with ribonucleotide reductase and DNA polymerase. In patients with previously untreated MCL, it yielded an overall response (OR) rate of 41% and a CR rate of 29%.[30] The median OS in that study was 2 years. However, fludarabine therapy is fraught with concerns regarding the ability to subsequently collect autologous stem cells, if needed. It has been reported that previous fludarabine therapy interferes with the quality of stem cells harvested and increases the risk for myelodysplastic syndrome/acute myeloid leukemia after autologous SCT.[31]

Importance of Rituximab

The anti-CD20 monoclonal antibody rituximab is the most important addition to the frontline treatment of lymphomas, including MCL. Rituximab alone produces a 38% response rate in patients with untreated MCL, results in a median response duration of 1.2 years, has very little hematologic or nonhematologic toxicity, and can be used in selected patients who would otherwise not tolerate cytotoxic therapy, thus prolonging and improving their quality of life.[32] Rituximab improves both the response and duration of response when combined in the frontline and relapse settings.[33-36] If response to the frontline therapy is less than complete, the role of additional doses of rituximab has not been proven.[37] In addition, a metaanalysis has suggested that rituximab might improve OS.[36] In patients with blood involvement, the first dose of rituximab should be delivered with caution because of the risk for tumor lysis syndrome or cytokine-release syndrome. If necessary, the first chemotherapy cycle can be given without rituximab to avoid these potential complications. The role of rituximab as an agent for in vivo purging of malignant cells in the blood and marrow has been documented.[38,39] Whether maintenance therapy with periodic infusions of rituximab prolongs OS over retreatment upon clinical or molecular recurrence has not yet been determined.

Rituximab-HyperCVAD

The OS rate is poor in patients with MCL who receive conventional chemotherapy. Thus intense chemoimmunotherapy without consolidation SCT is a potential therapeutic option. Romaguera and colleagues[40] reported on a prospective phase II study of rituximab in combination with hyper-CVAD (fractionated cyclophosphamide, vincristine, doxorubicin [Adriamycin], and dexamethasone) (R-hyper-CVAD), alternating with rituximab in combination with high-dose methotrexate-cytarabine (ara-C) (R-MA) in untreated patients with diffuse and nodular MCL and their blastoid variants. Of the 97 patients who were treated, 97% responded and 87% achieved a CR. At 10 years of follow-up (median follow-up, 8 years), the median OS time for all patients had not been reached, and the median time to treatment failure (TTF) for all patients was 4.6 years, without a plateau in the curves. For a group of patients age 65 years or younger, the median OS time had not been reached, and the median TTF was 5.9 years. Multivariate analysis revealed pretreatment serum levels of β_2 microglobulin, International Prognostic Index (IPI) score, and mantle cell IPI (MIPI) score as predictive of both OS and TTF. The study concluded that intense chemoimmunotherapy without SCT is effective for untreated aggressive MCL.[40]

The Importance of Cytarabine

Several studies have suggested that cytarabine significantly improves response to chemotherapy. These include, among others, a study in which a regimen consisting of dexamethasone, high-dose cytarabine (ara-C), and cisplatin (Platinol) (DHAP) further cytoreduced tumors that were not responding to cyclophosphamide, hydroxydaunomycin, vincristine (Oncovin), and prednisone (CHOP)[41] before autoSCT. Results of a more recent trial[42] showed that high doses of cytarabine significantly improved the results of an autoSCT-containing regimen when compared with identical prior historical data without cytarabine. In the latter study, rituximab was also added to the frontline therapy, but rituximab alone cannot likely account for the impressive results. Thus high doses of cytarabine are also an important component of intense non-SCT regimens.[43]

Intense Chemotherapy With or Without Stem Cell Transplantation

Several studies have intensified conventional therapy and/or incorporated consolidation high-dose chemotherapy followed by SCT as part of the frontline therapy. As seen in Table 80-3, more intense chemotherapy combinations have produced better rates of CR and longer durations of response.[44-46] Whether consolidation with SCT is needed as part of the frontline therapy is not clear, because intense chemoimmunotherapy regimens without consolidation SCT have produced similar results.[46]

Among conventional chemotherapeutic options, reported regimens include nucleoside analogues, particularly the R-FCM

Table 80-3 Therapy Results for Untreated Mantle Cell Lymphoma in More Than 20 Patients

Study	Regimen	Age (years)	No. of Patients	CR/CRu (%)	Outcome	Median Follow-Up (months)
Howard et al[37]	CHOP-R	31-69	40	48	Median PFS, 16.5 months	25
Lenz et al[33]*	CHOP-R	37-78	62	34	Median TTF, 21 months	18
Neelapu et al[44]	EPOCH-R	22-73	26	92	Median EFS, 22 months	46
Kahl et al[45]	Modified R-hyper-CVAD†	40-81	22	64	50% 3-year PFS	37
Fayad et al[46]	Hyper-CVAD-R + methotrexate-cytarabine-R	41-65	65	89	60% 5-year FFS	58
Magni et al[38]	R-HDS–autoSCT	23-65	28	100	10-year EFS of 57% for low-risk, 34% for high-risk MIPI	NA
Khouri et al[47]	Hyper-CVAD–autoSCT	38-66	33	100	43% 5-year DFS	49
Vandenberghe et al[48]	Chemo–autoSCT	24-70	195‡	67	33% 5-year PFS	44
Geisler et al[42§]	Maxi-CHOP–cytarabine autoSCT	38-65	160	90	56% 6-year EFS	41
Lefrere et al[41]	CHOP/DHAP–autoSCT	33-64	28	89	Median EFS 51 months	NA
Dreyling et al[49,50]	CHOP/interferon	35-65	122	28	25% 3-year PFS	25
	CHOP/autoSCT			81	54% 3-year PFS	
Evens et al[51]	CTAP/VMAC/autoSCT	39-63	25	76	54% 5-year EFS	66
Vigouroux et al[52]	CHOP/DHAP/autoSCT	40-63	30	87	40% 5-year PFS	55
Thieblemont et al[53]	Doxorubicin-containing + rituximab + DHAP/autoSCT	29-65	29	71	Median FFS 42 months	31
van't Veer et al[54]	R-CHOP + cytarabine/autoSCT	32-66	87	64	36% 4-year FFS	42
de Guibert et al[55]	R-DHAP/ autoSCT	47-74	24	92	65% 3-year FFS	28

DFS, Disease-free survival; *EFS*, event-free survival; *EPOCH*, etoposide, prednisone, vincristine (Oncavin), cyclophosphamide, and hydroxydaunomycin; *FFS*, failure-free survival; *R-CHOP*, rituximab, cyclophosphamide, hydroxydaunomycin, vincristine (Oncovin), and prednisone; *R-HDS*, rituximab with high-dose sequential therapy; *TTF*, time to treatment failure.
*Prospective randomized and statistically superior to CHOP without rituximab.
†Maintenance rituximab given every 6 months × 2 years.
‡15% underwent transplantation at relapse.
§Patients with molecular recurrence treated with rituximab and not counted as events.

(rituximab, fludarabine, cyclophosphamide, and mitoxantrone) regimen.[34] Of note is the bifunctional alkylating agent bendamustine, which, in combination with rituximab, has moved quickly to the frontline setting and shown similar efficacy as R-CHOP (rituximab, cyclophosphamide, hydroxydaunomycin, vincristine [Oncovin], and prednisone), with less toxicity, in a multiinstitutional prospective randomized trial.[56]

Risk for Central Nervous System Disease

There is no consensus on the risk for central nervous system disease in patients with MCL or the need for prophylaxis. Studies have reported a 4% incidence of central nervous system disease in patients with MCL and a 5-year actuarial risk of 26%.[57-59] Possible risk factors mentioned in these studies include the presence of blastoid cytology and an elevated proliferation rate.

Minimal Residual Disease

Current molecular techniques allow for the detection of 1 in 10^4 to 1 in 10^6 MCL cells, although the methodology used is currently not uniform among researchers. A recent report suggested a correlation between molecular recurrence and clinical recurrence,[39] a relationship used in a recent trial as a basis for preemptive treatment with rituximab before any clinical evidence of recurrence was detected.[42] However, other researchers have not seen this correlation, because the sensitivity of their molecular tests differed.[60]

THERAPY FOR RECURRENT AND REFRACTORY DISEASE

The inherent resistance of MCL to conventional chemotherapy is evident at relapse. Table 80-4 shows a summary of most reported single-agent and combination chemotherapy trials in MCL. Among the studies of salvage therapies, several successful ones have recently exploited their biologic insights.

Proteasome Inhibitors

Bortezomib, a first-in-class reversible proteasome inhibitor, has been shown to produce a 31% to 50% response rate as a single-agent therapy and has been approved by the U.S. Food and Drug Administration (FDA).[81,82] Salinosporamide A, a second-generation proteasome inhibitor, is a natural product that has significant effects on the proteasome and provides more potent and durable proteasome inhibition than does bortezomib.[83] Carfilzomib, another second-generation proteasome inhibitor, selectively and irreversibly disables the chymotrypsin-like activity of the proteasome.[84] Both salinosporamide A and carfilzomib hold promise for relapsed or refractory MCL. In addition, carfilzomib has been shown to be effective in multiple myeloma.

Zhang and colleagues[85] investigated the therapeutic efficacy of carfilzomib in MCL in vitro and in vivo and showed that carfilzomib inhibited the growth of not only the MCL cell lines but also freshly isolated MCL cells from patients in a dose-dependent manner. Of note, carfilzomib also inhibited the proliferation of PMA/ionomycin-activated or anti-CD3/anti-CD28 monoclonal antibody–activated

Table 80-4 Published Response Rates Due to Different Salvage Therapies for Relapsed/Refractory Mantle Cell Lymphoma

Study	Regimen	No. Patients	CR/CRu %	PR %	ORR %
Foran et al[32]	Rituximab	35	14	23	37
Gressin et al[61]	VAD ± chlorambucil	30	43	30	73
Foran et al[30]	Fludarabine	17	29	12	41
Kaufmann et al[62]	Rituximab, thalidomide	16	31	50	81
Dang et al[63]	Ontak	8	12.5	25	37.5
Cohen et al[64]	Cyclophosphamide, fludarabine	30	30	33	63
Goy et al[65]	Bortezomib	29	21	21	42
O'Connor et al[66]	Bortezomib	11	9	36	45
McLaughlin et al[67]	Fludarabine, mitoxantrone, dexamethasone	5	20	80	100
Seymour et al[68]	Fludarabine, cisplatin, cytarabine	8			88
Forstpointner et al[34]	Fludarabine, cyclophosphamide, mitoxantrone	24	0	46	46
Forstpointner et al[34]	Fludarabine, cyclophosphamide, mitoxantrone, rituximab	24	29	29	58
Rummel et al[56]	Bendamustine, rituximab	16	50	25	75
Fisher et al[25]	Bortezomib	141	8	25	33
Robak et al[69]	2-CdA, rituximab or rituximab/cyclophosphamide	9	22	45	67
O'Connor et al[70]	Epothilone, ixabepilone	15	0	1	7
Robinson et al[71]	Bendamustine, rituximab	12	59	33	92
Wiernik et al[72]	Lenalidomide	15	13	40	53
Witzig et al[73]	Temsirolimus	34	3	35	38
Ansell et al[74]	Low-dose temsirolimus	27	4	37	41
Inwards et al[75]	Cladribine	24	21	25	46
Coleman et al[76]	PEP-C (prednisone, cyclophosphamide, etoposide, procarbazine)	22	46	36	82
Rodriguez et al[77]	Gemcitabine, oxaliplatin, rituximab	14	64	14	78
Weide et al[78]	Bendamustine, mitoxantrone, rituximab	57	35	54	87
Lin et al[79]	Flavopiridol	10	0	0	0
Kouroukis et al[80]	Flavopiridol	28	0	11	11

cells but not resting peripheral blood mononuclear cells (PBMCs) from healthy donors. Flow cytometry using fluorescence-labeled annexin V and propidium iodide showed that carfilzomib induced apoptosis in both the cell lines and primary MCL cells in a time- and dose-dependent manner. Notably, carfilzomib did not induce apoptosis of normal PBMCs.

Carfilzomib was effective and therapeutic in an MCL mouse model established in severe combined immunodeficient (SCID) mice. Tumor growth was significantly inhibited after carfilzomib treatment compared with vehicle control, and the survival time of tumor-bearing mice was significantly prolonged in the treatment group. Western blot analysis showed that apoptosis of MCL cells was induced via the activation of caspase cascades and the PARP pathway. Pretreatment of cells with a pan-caspase inhibitor (z-VAD) but neither a caspase-8 inhibitor (z-IETD) nor a caspase-9 inhibitor (z-LEHD) alone completely blocked carfilzomib-induced apoptosis. The authors concluded that carfilzomib inhibited MCL cell growth and induced apoptosis via a caspase-dependent signaling pathway both in vitro and in vivo.[85]

Btk Inhibitor

Activation of the BCR signaling pathway contributes to the initiation and maintenance of B-cell malignancies. The Btk inhibitor PCI-32765 blocks B-cell activation and has antitumor activity in B-cell malignancies, including MCL, with favorable safety data.[86] PCI-32765, similar to other Btk inhibitors, was designed to inhibit Btk activation by selectively interacting with an ATP-binding site in the tyrosine kinase domain, preventing Btk phosphorylation and activation. PCI-32765, an orally bioavailable, selective, and irreversible inhibitor, was shown to block signaling downstream of Btk and completely and irreversibly inhibit B-cell activation.[87] Findings from a novel study imply that PCI-32765 inhibits MCL cell proliferation and chemokine secretion and interferes with MCL cell actin polymerization, highlighting the importance of BCR signaling and Btk in MCL and explaining the effect of the Btk inhibitor PCI-32765 on patients with MCL.[88] In that study, PCI-32765 effectively inhibited phospho-Btk, leading to reduced MCL cell growth. PCI-32765 also induced MCL cell apoptosis in a dose- and time-dependent manner in both MCL cell lines and primary cells.

A recent phase I study in patients with relapsed/refractory B-cell malignancies showed that the Btk inhibitor PCI-32765 is highly active and well tolerated. No cumulative toxicity was noted with a treatment duration of more than 6 months.[28] More recently, preliminary results of an ongoing phase II study of single-agent PCI-32765 in relapsed or refractory MCL have become available. In that study, PCI-32765 was administered orally at 560 mg daily (in continuous 28-day cycles) until disease progression. Bortezomib-naive and bortezomib-exposed cohorts were evaluated separately. Tumor response was evaluated every two cycles and classified by 2007 NHL International Workshop Group (IWG) criteria. A total of 48 (29 bortezomib-naive, 19 bortezomib-exposed) patients were enrolled and initiated treatment on study PCYC-1104 between February 16,

2011, and July 20, 2011. The median age is 67 years (62-72), and the median number of prior treatment regimens is two (range, one to five). Of the total patients, 24 (12 bortezomib-naive, 12 bortezomib-exposed) have undergone at least one follow-up tumor assessment and are evaluable for efficacy. Treatment has been well tolerated. No patients have discontinued treatment because of adverse events. The objective response rate (ORR) by IWG criteria is 67% (16/24); in the bortezomib-naive cohort, the ORR is 58% (7/12) and 75% (9/12) in the bortezomib-exposed cohort. To date, 35/39 patients remain on PCI-32765. Preliminary data from this phase II trial suggests that the potent Btk inhibitor PCI-32765 is well tolerated and induces a high rate of objective responses in patients with relapsed or refractory MCL. A phase III trial entitled "Safety and Efficacy of PCI-32765 in Subjects With Relapsed/Refractory MCL" is ongoing.[89] These preliminary results suggest that Btk inhibition is a novel therapeutic approach in MCL.

New Class of mTOR Inhibitors

mTOR is a key element of the PI3K/AKT pathway. Temsirolimus is a promising mTOR inhibitor that has been shown to produce a 38% OR rate.[73] Everolimus, an oral derivative of rapamycin, was shown to yield a 32% OR rate in patients with relapsed or refractory MCL.[90]

Flavopiridol: Cyclin D Kinase Inhibitor

Single-agent therapy with the cycline D kinase (CDK) inhibitor flavopiridol has not been effective, probably because of its schedule dependency. Recent research using flavopiridol in combination chemotherapy with a specific schedule suggests this is a promising approach.[56]

Immunomodulatory Drugs

Lenalidomide is an oral, antiangiogenic, antiproliferative immunomodulatory agent, and phase II studies of single-agent lenalidomide in lymphoma have yielded promising results, with 13% to 20% CR rates in relapsed or refractory MCL.[91,92] A phase I study demonstrated that when combined with rituximab, the combination therapy is well tolerated. Among 46 patients in a phase II trial, the ORR was 56.5%, the CR rate was 34.8%, and the PR rate was 21.7%. The median response duration was 18.9 months. The median progression-free survival was 12.4 months, and the median overall survival was 24.3 months. Oral lenalidomide plus rituximab is well tolerated and highly effective in patients with relapsed/refractory MCL.[93,94]

Stem Cell Transplantation

Since second and later remissions are predictably brief, SCT deserves consideration after cytoreduction with salvage chemotherapy. Unfortunately, relapsed or refractory MCL recurs after high-dose chemotherapy followed by rescue of autologous stem cells.[48,49,51-55] The current consensus is that the best result with the longest duration of disease control in the relapse setting is consolidation of a response, preferably a CR, with allogeneic SCT, based on evidence of graft-versus-lymphoma activity in MCL. A reduced-intensity allograft has been shown to produce progression-free survival (PFS)/event-free survival (EFS) rates of 40% to 80% and OS rates of 55% to 86% after a median follow-up of 2 to 3 years, with a 5% to 30% rate of acute graft-versus-host disease and up to a 24% treatment-related mortality rate.[95-99]

In addition, cure fractions may be emerging in patients who had received rituximab-containing autologous SCT in first remission and in patients who had received nonmyeloablative SCTs for relapsed or refractory MCL. After analysis of the results of long-term transplantation experience in patients with MCL, rituximab has been found to improve the outcome of patients undergoing autologous SCT and facilitated the effectiveness and durability of disease control in patients undergoing nonmyeloablative SCTs.[100]

Radioimmunotherapy Plus Chemotherapy

MCL is very sensitive to radiotherapy. Because the disease is advanced at presentation in a great majority of patients, radioimmunotherapy is an option worth exploring. The use of iodine I^{131}tositumomab as part of frontline therapy before any chemotherapy has been reported.[101] In 25 patients, the OR rate was 88%, the CR rate was 50%, and the molecular remission rate was 46%, all after just one dose of the radioimmunoisotope and before the start of CHOP chemotherapy. The median EFS duration was 21.6 months.

In the relapsed/refractory setting, single-agent ibritumomab tiuxetan-^{90}yttrium has resulted in a 41% OR rate and a 29% CR/CR, unconfirmed (CRu) rate but with a short time to progression of 5 months.[102] In another study in the relapsed/refractory setting, Gopal and colleagues[103] showed that radioimmunotherapy cytoreduced the tumor and was consolidated with high doses of cyclophosphamide and etoposide, followed by myloablative doses of iodine I^{131}tositumomab, resulting in a 100% OR rate, a 91% CR rate, and a 61% 3-year PFS rate.[103] Other researchers explored the use of standard doses of ibritumomab tiuxetan-^{90}yttrium as part of the preparative regimen for autoSCT in 41 patients with relapsed MCL and reported a 2-year OS rate of 90% and a 2-year PFS rate of 70% after a median follow-up of 18.4 months.[104]

Wang and colleagues[105] conducted a phase II trial to evaluate the safety and efficacy of ibritumomab tiuxetan-^{90}yttrium in patients with relapsed/refractory MCL. Thirty-four patients with a median age of 68 years (range, 52 to 79 years) received the therapeutic dose. The patients had received a median of three prior treatment regimens (range, one to six treatment regimens), including those that contained rituximab ($n = 32$) and bortezomib ($n = 7$). Of the 32 patients with measurable disease, 10 (31%) achieved CR or partial remission (PR). After a median follow-up of 22 months (range, 2 to 72+ months), an intent-to-treat analysis revealed a median EFS duration of 6 months and an OS duration of 21 months. The median EFS duration was 28 months for those who achieved PR or CR and 3 months for those whose disease did not respond (P <0.0001); the median EFS duration was 9 months for patients whose tumor measured less than 5 cm in the largest diameter before treatment and 3 months for those whose tumor measured 5 cm or more ($P = 0.015$). The single-agent activity of ibritumomab tiuxetan-^{90}yttrium and its favorable safety profile warrant its further development for the treatment of MCL.[105]

Lenalidomide Plus Rituximab

Rituximab, a chimeric anti-CD20 antibody, is associated with direct induction of apoptosis and antibody-dependent cell-mediated cytotoxicity with clinical efficacy in MCL. Lenalidomide, a novel immunomodulatory agent, sensitizes tumor cells and enhances antibody-dependent cell-mediated cytotoxicity. In a preclinical study, Zhang and colleagues[106] attempted to elucidate the mechanism of the lenalidomide-enhanced rituximab-mediated cytotoxicity of MCL cells. They found that lenalidomide and rituximab induced growth inhibition of both cultured and fresh primary MCL cells. Lenalidomide enhanced rituximab-induced apoptosis by upregulating phosphorylation of JNK, BCL2, and BAD; increasing the release of cytochrome-c; and enhancing activation of caspase-3, -8, and -9 and cleavage of PARP. In addition, lenalidomide activated natural killer (NK) cells and increased CD16 expression in $CD56^{low}CD16^{+}$ NK cells. Lenalidomide augmented the rituximab-dependent cytotoxicity of whole PBMCs but not NK cell-depleted PBMCs by 30%. Daily treatment with lenalidomide increased the number of NK cells by 10-fold in SCID mice, and the lenalidomide-rituximab combination decreased tumor burden and prolonged survival of the MCL-bearing

SCID mice. Taken together, these findings demonstrate that lenalidomide and rituximab have a synergistically therapeutic effect on MCL cells by enhancing apoptosis and rituximab-dependent NK cell–mediated cytotoxicity and may be an optimal combination in a clinical trial of relapsed/refractory MCL.[106]

Wang and colleagues[93] attempted to determine the maximum tolerated dose of lenalidomide plus rituximab in a phase I clinical trial and to evaluate the efficacy and safety of this combination in a phase II trial in patients with relapsed/refractory MCL. Four patient cohorts received escalating doses of oral lenalidomide daily on days 1 to 21 of each 28-day cycle. Intravenous rituximab was administered once a week for 4 weeks during the first cycle only. Patients were treated until disease progression or severe toxicity. Fifty-two patients were enrolled: 14 in phase I and 46 (including eight patients from the phase I portion) in phase II. Two patients experienced dose-limiting toxic events with lenalidomide at 25 mg daily. The maximum tolerated dose was 20 mg lenalidomide given daily on days 1 to 21 of each 28-day cycle, plus intravenous rituximab at 375 mg/m^2 for 4 weekly doses during the first cycle. In the phase II study, grade 3 to 4 toxicities included neutropenia (17% of cycles), lymphopenia (7% of cycles), and thrombocytopenia (5% of cycles). Only two episodes of febrile neutropenia occurred. In the phase II trial, the OR rate was 56.5%, the CR rate was 34.8%, and the PR rate was 21.7%. The median response duration was 18.9 months. The median PFS duration was 12.4 months, and the median OS duration was 24.3 months. All 13 patients who had received bortezomib therapy before enrollment achieved stable disease or better. These results demonstrate that oral lenalidomide plus rituximab is well tolerated and highly effective for patients with relapsed/refractory MCL.[93]

FUTURE DIRECTIONS

Prospects for patients with this incurable lymphoma have improved over the past decade as a result of current therapy and improvement in diagnostic tools and supportive therapy. In addition, newer therapies have been made available that might alter the OS of patients with disease recurrence. A recent study reported an improvement in OS duration from 2.7 years between 1975 and 1986 to 5.8 years between 1996 and 2004.[107] In that study, the authors concluded that the addition of doxorubicin and stem cell transplantation with rituximab, as well as improved patient care, most likely accounted for the longer survival. Another retrospective study of patients treated without intense initial chemotherapy and with watchful waiting for those with stable or indolent MCL reported a median OS duration of 5 years.[108] Determining whether intense therapy or a conservative approach will result in a longer OS duration will require additional studies. More important, it will require the accurate identification of subgroups of patients with MCL who will have better or worse prognoses. Only then can studies be compared more rationally and significant advances made in the management of MCL.

Most of the reported prognostic variables and models are retrospective and were devised with patients who received therapy in the form of a doxorubicin-containing regimen with or without rituximab. Molecular profiling has revealed a group of genes associated with proliferation that can identify patient subsets that differ by more than 5 years in median survival.[109] An immunohistochemical test for the proliferation antigen Ki-67 has also been shown to have prognostic value in a retrospective study of patients with MCL treated with a variety of regimens, most of which contained doxorubicin.[110] More recently, a five-gene model for predicting survival in MCL using frozen or formalin-fixed, paraffin-embedded tissue has been developed.[111] Other variables reported to be of prognostic importance are the pretreatment serum levels of β_2 microglobulin and lactate dehydrogenase, blastoid cytology, age, Ann Arbor stage, extranodal presentation, and constitutional symptoms.[2,43] The recently introduced MIPI uses four independent prognostic factors: age, performance status, lactate dehydrogenase level, and leukocyte count.[112] Fig. 80-4 shows survival curves using this model for the accurate stratification of patients with MCLs. Patients were classified according to the MIPI into low-risk (44% of patients, median OS not reached), intermediate-risk (35% of patients, 51 months OS duration), and high-risk (21% of patients, 29 months OS duration) groups. Retrospective applications of this model have shown some correlation with prognosis.[38,113]

With new therapies based on the knowledge of MCL biology and new prognostic models that can be used to tailor therapy and compare studies, the future of patients with MCL looks brighter.

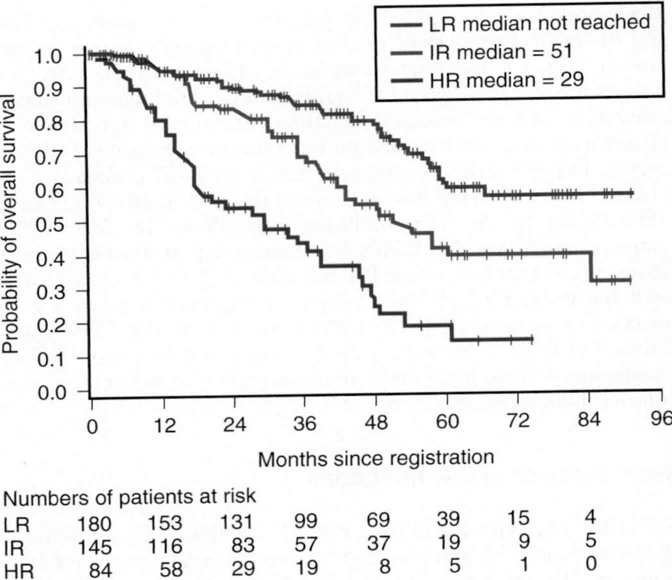

Numbers of patients at risk

LR	180	153	131	99	69	39	15	4
IR	145	116	83	57	37	19	9	5
HR	84	58	29	19	8	5	1	0

Figure 80-4 PROGNOSTIC GROUPS STRATIFIED ACCORDING TO THE MANTLE CELL INTERNATIONAL PROGNOSTIC INDEX.

SUGGESTED READINGS

Bea S, Salaverria I, Armengol L, et al: Uniparental disomies, homozygous deletions, amplifications, and target genes in mantle cell lymphoma revealed by integrative high-resolution whole-genome profiling. *Blood* 113:3059, 2009.

Cecconi D, Zamo A, Bianchi E, et al: Signal transduction pathways of mantle cell lymphoma: A phosphoproteome-based study. *Proteomics* 8:4495, 2008.

Dal Col J, Zancai P, Terrin L, et al: Distinct functional significance of Akt and mTOR constitutive activation in mantle cell lymphoma. *Blood* 111:5142, 2008.

Fisher RI, Bernstein SH, Kahl BS, et al: Multicenter phase II study of bortezomib in patients with relapsed or refractory mantle cell lymphoma. *J Clin Oncol* 24:4867, 2006.

Forstpointner R, Dreyling M, Repp R, et al: The addition of rituximab to a combination of fludarabine, cyclophosphamide, mitoxantrone (FCM) significantly increases the response rate and prolongs survival as compared with FCM alone in patients with relapsed and refractory follicular and mantle cell lymphomas: Results of a prospective randomized study of the German Low-Grade Lymphoma Study Group. *Blood* 104:3064, 2004.

Fu K, Weisenburger DD, Greiner TC, et al: Cyclin D1-negative mantle cell lymphoma: A clinicopathologic study based on gene expression profiling. *Blood* 106:4315, 2005.

Geisler CH, Kolstad A, Laurell A, et al: Long-term progression-free survival of mantle cell lymphoma after intensive front-line immunochemotherapy with in vivo-purged stem cell rescue: A nonrandomized phase 2 multicenter study by the Nordic Lymphoma Group. *Blood* 112:2687, 2008.

Gelebart P, Anand M, Armanious H, et al: Constitutive activation of the Wnt canonical pathway in mantle cell lymphoma. *Blood* 112:5171, 2008.

Greiner TC, Moynihan MJ, Chan WC, et al: p53 mutations in mantle cell lymphoma are associated with variant cytology and predict a poor prognosis. *Blood* 87:4302, 1996.

Hartmann E, Fernandez V, Moreno V, et al: Five-gene model to predict survival in mantle-cell lymphoma using frozen or formalin-fixed, paraffin-embedded tissue. *J Clin Oncol* 26:4966, 2008.

Hoster E, Dreyling M, Klapper W, et al: A new prognostic index (MIPI) for patients with advanced-stage mantle cell lymphoma. *Blood* 111:558, 2008.

Jares P, Colomer D, Campo E: Genetic and molecular pathogenesis of mantle cell lymphoma: Perspectives for new targeted therapeutics. *Nat Rev Cancer* 7:750, 2007.

Kahl BS: Frontline therapy in mantle cell lymphoma: The role of high-dose therapy and integration of new agents. *Curr Hematol Malig Rep* 4:213, 2009.

Kane RC, Dagher R, Farrell A, et al: Bortezomib for the treatment of mantle cell lymphoma. *Clin Cancer Res* 13:5291, 2007.

Khouri IF, Lee MS, Saliba RM, et al: Nonablative allogeneic stem-cell transplantation for advanced/recurrent mantle-cell lymphoma. *J Clin Oncol* 21:4407, 2003.

Lefrere F, Delmer A, Levy V, et al: Sequential chemotherapy regimens followed by high-dose therapy with stem cell transplantation in mantle cell lymphoma: An update of a prospective study. *Haematologica* 89:1275, 2004.

Lenz G, Dreyling M, Hoster E, et al: Immunochemotherapy with rituximab and cyclophosphamide, doxorubicin, vincristine, and prednisone significantly improves response and time to treatment failure, but not long-term outcome in patients with previously untreated mantle cell lymphoma: Results of a prospective randomized trial of the German Low Grade Lymphoma Study Group (GLSG). *J Clin Oncol* 23:1984, 2005.

Magni M, Di Nicola M, Carlo-Stella C, et al: High-dose sequential chemotherapy and in vivo rituximab-purged stem cell autografting in mantle cell lymphoma: A 10-year update of the R-HDS regimen. *Bone Marrow Transplant* 43:509, 2009.

Martin P, Chadburn A, Christos P, et al: Outcome of deferred initial therapy in mantle-cell lymphoma. *J Clin Oncol* 27:1209, 2009.

Perez-Galan P, Dreyling M, Wiestner A: Mantle cell lymphoma: Biology, pathogenesis, and the molecular basis of treatment in the genomic era. *Blood* 117:26, 2011.

Robinson KS, Williams ME, van der Jagt RH, et al: Phase II multicenter study of bendamustine plus rituximab in patients with relapsed indolent B-cell and mantle cell non-Hodgkin's lymphoma. *J Clin Oncol* 26:4473, 2008.

Romaguera JE, Fayad LE, Feng L, et al: Ten-year follow-up after intense chemoimmunotherapy with Rituximab-hyper-CVAD alternating with Rituximab-high dose methotrexate/cytarabine (R-MA) and without stem cell transplantation in patients with untreated aggressive mantle cell lymphoma. *Br J Haematol* 150:200, 2010.

Romaguera JE, Fayad L, Rodriguez MA, et al: High rate of durable remissions after treatment of newly diagnosed aggressive mantle-cell lymphoma with rituximab plus hyper-CVAD alternating with rituximab plus high-dose methotrexate and cytarabine. *J Clin Oncol* 23:7013, 2005.

Schulz H, Bohlius JF, Trelle S, et al: Immunochemotherapy with rituximab and overall survival in patients with indolent or mantle cell lymphoma: A systematic review and meta-analysis. *J Natl Cancer Inst* 99:706, 2007.

Tam CS, Bassett R, Ledesma C, et al: Mature results of the M. D. Anderson Cancer Center risk-adapted transplantation strategy in mantle cell lymphoma. *Blood* 113:4144, 2009.

Wang M, Fayad L, Wagner-Bartak N, et al: Oral Lenalidomide Plus 4 Doses of Rituximab Induces Prolonged Remissions in Relapsed/Refractory Mantle Cell Lymphoma: A Phase I/II Clinical Trial. *J Clin Oncol* 2011 In press.

Weisenburger DD, Armitage JO: Mantle cell lymphoma–an entity comes of age. *Blood* 87:4483, 1996.

Zhou Y, Wang H, Fang W, et al: Incidence trends of mantle cell lymphoma in the United States between 1992 and 2004. *Cancer* 113:791, 2008.

For complete list of references log on to www.expertconsult.com.

CHAPTER 81

DIAGNOSIS AND TREATMENT OF DIFFUSE LARGE B-CELL LYMPHOMA AND BURKITT LYMPHOMA

Kieron Dunleavy and Wyndham H. Wilson

Diffuse large B-cell lymphoma (DLBCL) and Burkitt lymphoma (BL) are the most common types of aggressive B-cell lymphoma. Although they share many clinical and biological features, the approach to their management is different; therefore, an accurate histologic diagnosis is of utmost importance. There have been several recent therapeutic advances in the management of these diseases, and both DLBCL and BL have high cure rates with current treatment approaches. Therefore, it is imperative to promptly evaluate patients with these diseases and expeditiously institute appropriate therapy.

DIFFUSE LARGE B-CELL LYMPHOMA

Epidemiology

Diffuse large B-cell lymphoma is the most prevalent histologic subtype of non-Hodgkin lymphoma (NHL) (of which there were more than 65,000 new cases in the United States in 2010) and comprises 30% to 40% of these diseases.[1,2] Although the median age at diagnosis is in the seventh decade of life, DLBCL affects children and adults of all ages, and it is slightly more common in males than females. Although the etiology of DLBCL is unknown in most cases, it can arise from transformation of an indolent lymphoma. A history of immunodeficiency is a significant risk factor, and individuals who are HIV positive have a 100 times higher incidence of developing DLBCL over those who do not have HIV.

Pathobiology

The pathobiology of DLBCL is very diverse, and within DLBCL, there are several morphologic variants that include centroblastic, immunoblastic, T-cell rich or histioctye-rich, and anaplastic subtypes, and progress in molecular profiling is further advancing this taxonomy. There are also several clinical-pathologic variants of DLBCL. Primary mediastinal B-cell lymphoma (PMBL), for example, commonly presents in young women and usually remains localized to the mediastinum (Fig. 81-1). Primary central nervous system lymphoma (PCNSL) is another rare subtype of DLBCL that rarely disseminates to extraneural sites and is much more commonly observed in HIV-positive individuals. It is important to recognize that DLBCL can also arise as a result of histologic transformation from an indolent lymphoma. Although this differentiation may not affect treatment choice initially, it will affect prognosis and natural history and therefore needs to be recognized at diagnosis.

The neoplastic cells of DLBCL express pan B-cell markers, including CD20, and surface or cytoplasmic immunoglobulin is often demonstrated. CD10, BCL6, and IRF4/MUM1 are variably expressed, and the proliferation index as measured by Ki67 staining is typically high. Approximately 30% of cases show abnormalities involving the *BCL6* gene, and translocation of the *BCL2* gene—a hallmark of follicular lymphoma—is present in 20% to 30% of cases. Approximately 10% of cases of DLBCL harbor a t(8:14) MYC translocation, and recently, several groups have demonstrated that this confers a much worse prognosis compared with MYC-negative cases when CHOP-type (cyclophosphamide, doxorubicin [Novantrone], vincristine [Oncovin], and prednisone) regimens are used.

Recently, gene expression profiling has defined a new molecular taxonomy for DLBCL. Morphologically indistinguishable tumors can show marked heterogeneity in gene expression, and these patterns of expression may be classified into signatures that correspond to the cellular origin of the lymphoma according to its stage of B-cell differentiation; on the basis of these signatures, DLBCL can be divided into at least three different subtypes: germinal center B-cell (GCB)–like, activated B-cell (ABC)–like, and primary mediastinal B-cell lymphoma (PMBL). Patients with GCB DLBCL have a significantly better survival than patients with ABC DLBCL after immunochemotherapy.

Clinical Features

The clinical presentation of DLBCL is variable and depends on a number of factors, including histology, patient age, and immune status. The disease typically presents with lymphadenopathy that can range from relatively asymptomatic to causing pain (Fig. 81-2), causing organ compromise such as ureteral obstruction or spinal cord compression. The involvement of bone marrow (BM) is much less frequent than with indolent lymphomas and is present in approximately 20% of cases.

Patients may have constitutional manifestations from the production of inflammatory molecules and a variety of other cytokines and chemokines produced by the lymphoma cells or host tissues. Such manifestations include weight loss, malaise, fevers, night sweats, and loss of appetite. Of these, unexplained weight loss of more than 10% of body weight and temperature higher than 38° C as well as drenching night sweats are referred to as "B" symptoms.

Investigation

History and Physical Examination

Patients should be questioned about systemic symptoms, and their performance status should be assessed (Table 81-1). It is important to determine if there is a history of potential causative factors such as prior malignancy, chemotherapy or radiation treatment, or autoimmune or immunodeficiency diseases. A history of infection with or exposure to various pathogens, including HIV and hepatitis B and C, should be excluded. A detailed physical examination should be performed with particular attention to lymph node (LN) regions. Skin involvement by DLBCL is rare (Fig. 81-3).

An accurate histologic diagnosis is imperative to determine the patient's prognosis and treatment; therefore, the single most important diagnostic test is a properly evaluated and technically adequate excisional tissue biopsy. With few exceptions, fine-needle aspiration is inadequate for diagnosis. Aggressive lymphoma should be diagnosed by an experienced hematopathologist familiar with the nuances and pitfalls of lymphoma diagnosis.

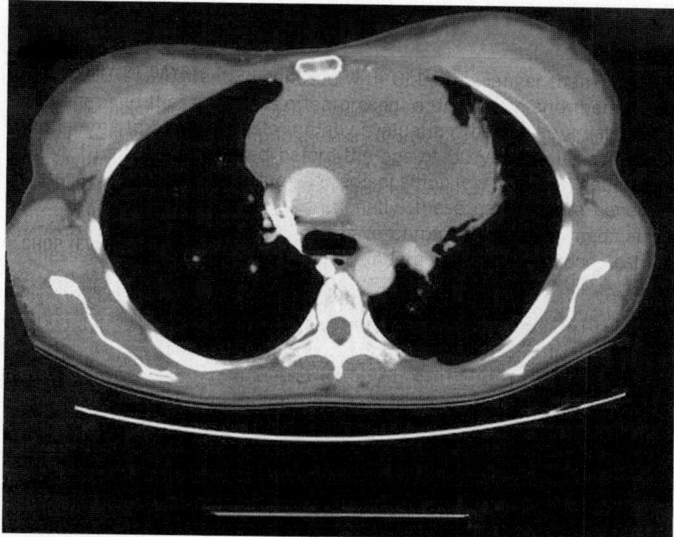

Figure 81-1 COMPUTED TOMOGRAPHY SCAN OF THE CHEST SHOWING A LARGE 17-CM ANTERIOR MEDIASTINAL MASS. A biopsy was consistent with primary mediastinal B-cell lymphoma.

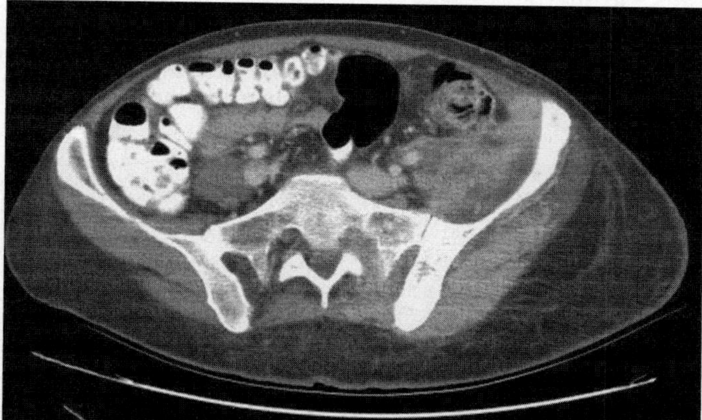

Figure 81-2 COMPUTED TOMOGRAPHY SCAN OF THE ABDOMEN SHOWING A LARGE LEFT-SIDED PSOAS MASS. A biopsy was consistent with diffuse large B-cell lymphoma.

Table 81-1 Eastern Co-operative Group Performance Scale

Performance Status	Definition
0	Asymptomatic
1	Symptomatic but fully ambulatory
2	Symptomatic and in bed <50% of the day
3	Symptomatic and in bed >50% of the day
4	Bedridden

Laboratory Investigations

Laboratory tests should include a complete blood count; serum chemistry, including lactate dehydrogenase (LDH); and human immunodeficiency virus (HIV) and hepatitis serology tests (Table 81-2). The latter should be included because it is important to identify patients with active hepatitis and a history of hepatitis B because they will likely require treatment with antivirals, monitoring, or both (see box on Hepatitis B Prophylaxis and Therapy During Lymphoma Treatment). Epstein-Barr virus (EBV) viral loads may also be useful

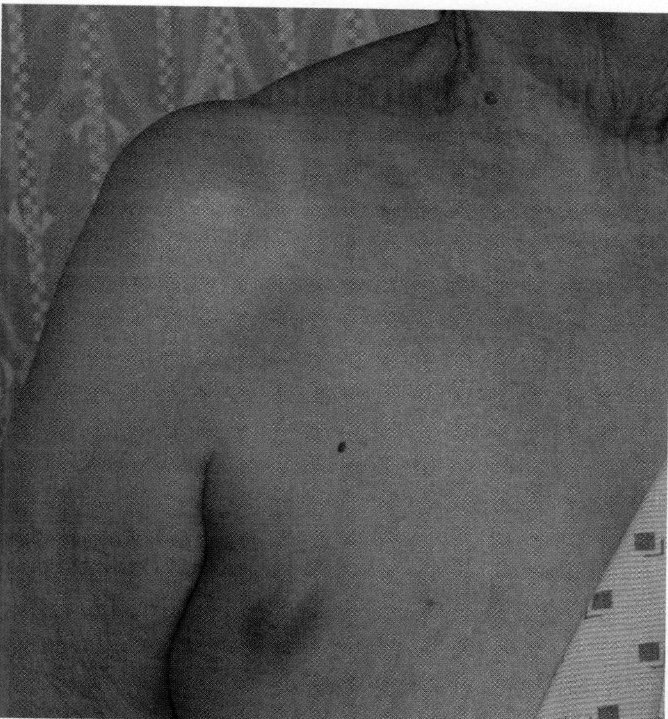

Figure 81-3 INFILTRATION OF THE RIGHT LOWER ANTERIOR CHEST WALL WITH DIFFUSE LARGE B-CELL LYMPHOMA.

Table 81-2 Staging Evaluation for Diffuse Large B-Cell Lymphoma

All Patients	As Clinically Indicated
History and physical examination	Other viral studies
CBC and chemistry (including LDH)	CT or MRI of the head
HIV and hepatitis B and C serology	Body PET scan
Chest radiograph	Additional imaging
CT scan of the chest, abdomen, and pelvis	CSF evaluation by cytology or flow cytometry
BM aspirate and biopsy	Other tests indicated by results of staging

BM, Bone marrow; *CBC,* complete blood count; *CSF,* cerebrospinal fluid; *CT,* computed tomography; *LDH,* lactate dehydrogenase; *MRI,* magnetic resonance imaging; *PET,* positron emission tomography.

Hepatitis B Prophylaxis and Therapy During Lymphoma Treatment

There is a risk of hepatitis B reactivation both from chemotherapy and rituximab, and this is a potentially fatal complication. We check hepatitis serology (hepatitis B surface antigen [HBsAg], hepatitis B surface antibody [anti-HBs], and hepatitis B core antibody [anti-HBc]) in all patients at diagnosis. Patients with active hepatitis B receive antiviral medication and LFTs, and hepatitis B viral loads are monitored closely. Patients with a history of hepatitis B infection should either receive antiviral prophylaxis or have the hepatitis B viral load monitored very closely (ideally on each cycle) with a low threshold to commence antiviral medications.

in specific lymphomas such as posttransplant lymphoproliferative disorders (PTLDs) and EBV-positive DLBCL of elderly adults. An elevated LDH level has adverse prognostic implications for patients with DLBCL.

Imaging and Staging

It is important to determine sites of disease involvement; therefore, imaging studies should include computed tomography (CT) scanning of the chest, abdomen, and pelvis. The need for additional imaging studies such as magnetic resonance imaging (MRI) and fludeoxyglucose positron emission tomography (FDG-PET) scanning depends on the clinical presentation and sites of disease. For example, if central nervous system (CNS) involvement is highly suspected, evaluation of the head by CT or MRI may be indicated. Involvement of the bone is best evaluated by MRI and PET scans. Although PET scanning is widely used for lymphoma imaging, it does not have a validated role in the initial staging of aggressive NHL.[3] However, it may be a useful adjunct to CT for staging in certain clinical scenarios.

Because involvement of the BM may impact management, it should be assessed in all patients with DLBCL. Patients at increased risk of CNS involvement should undergo lumbar puncture with evaluation of the cerebrospinal fluid (CSF) by cytology and flow cytometry.[4] Specifically, clinical presentations with several extranodal sites and elevated LDH level as well as particular sites such as the testis and BM are associated with an increased risk of CNS disease, and intrathecal prophylaxis should be considered (see box on Intrathecal Prophylaxis in Diffuse Large B-Cell Lymphoma).[5]

DLBCL is staged according to the Ann Arbor staging system (Table 81-3), which was originally developed for Hodgkin lymphoma (HL). However, because of the heterogeneity and hematogenous pattern of dissemination in NHL, in contrast to contiguous LN spread with HL, the staging system has more limited value. At the same time, important modifications to the Ann Arbor staging system made at the Cotswold Conference have made it more applicable to NHL.[6]

Table 81-3 Ann Arbor Staging System for Lymphomas

Stage*	Cotswold Modification of Arbor Classification
I	Involvement of a single LN region or lymphoid structure
II	Involvement of two or more LN regions on the same side of the diaphragm (the mediastinum is considered a single site, but the hilar LNs are considered bilaterally); the number of atomic sites should be indicated by a subscript (e.g., II_3)
III	Involvement of LN regions on both sides of the diaphragm: III_1 (with or without involvement of splenic hilar, celiac, or portal nodes) and III_2 (with involvement of paraaortic, iliac, and mesenteric nodes
IV	Involvement of one or more extranodal sites in addition to a site for which the designation E has been used

LN, Lymph node.
*All cases are subclassified to indicate the absence (A) or presence (B) of the systemic symptoms of significant fever (>38.0° C [100.4° F]), night sweats, and unexplained weight loss exceeding 10% of normal body weight within the previous 6 months. The clinical stage (CS) denotes the stage as determined by all diagnostic examinations and a single diagnostic biopsy only. In the Ann Arbor classification, the term *pathologic stage* (PS) is used if a second biopsy of any kind has been obtained, whether the result was negative or positive. In the Cotswold modification, the PS is determined by laparotomy; X designates bulky disease (widening of the mediastinum by more than one-third or the presence of a nodal mass >10 cm), and E designates involvement of a single extranodal site that is contiguous or proximal to the known nodal site.

Prognosis

To identify prognostic factors in NHL, an international project to correlate clinical variables and outcome in 2031 patients with untreated aggressive lymphoma was undertaken.[7] The following parameters were associated with inferior outcome: age older than 60 years, Ann Arbor stage III or IV disease, serum LDH level above normal range, Eastern Co-operative Oncology Group (ECOG) performance status of 2 or higher, and involvement of two or more extranodal sites. A clinical prognostic model, termed the International Prognostic Index (IPI), was developed using these five factors. In this model, 1 point was allocated for each feature and nicely stratified patients into four groups with 5-year survivals of 73%, 51%, 43%, and 26% for zero or one, two, three, and four or five risk factors, respectively, with CHOP-based treatment.[7] Based on this model, the IPI has become the standard in DLBCL for assessing clinical prognosis and treatment stratification within and comparison between clinical trials. Although it has yet to be fully revalidated in the rituximab era in prospective studies, a revised prognostic model for R-CHOP, termed Revised-IPI, was recently published based on a limited retrospective series (Table 81-4).[8]

Although not yet routinely performed in aggressive NHL, gene expression profiling is emerging as an important prognostic tool.[9-12] In DLBCL, overall survival is different in each group and superior in patients with the GCB compared with the ABC subtype. Using gene expression profiling, a molecular prognostic model of survival, independent of the IPI, has been developed for R-CHOP–treated DLBCL.[10] Although gene expression profiling is not routinely performed at diagnosis, several immunohistochemical models have been developed to predict GCB or non-GCB origin of the DLBCL.[13,14]

Intrathecal Prophylaxis in Diffuse Large B-Cell Lymphoma

In DLBCL, the role of intrathecal prophylaxis to prevent CNS recurrence is controversial and poorly studied, and there are several different approaches. Our approach is as follows. All patients at risk for CNS disease undergo a lumbar puncture at diagnosis, and CSF is checked by cytology and flow cytometry; if the results are positive, patients receive active treatment of the CNS. We administer intrathecal prophylaxis to all patients who fulfill either of the following criteria:

1. Two or more extranodal sites of disease involvement and an elevated LDH level
2. Certain extranodal sites of involvement that have been associated with an increased risk of CNS spread such as BM and testis

We use intrathecal methotrexate at a dose of 12 mg. We commence prophylaxis on cycle 3 day 1 and administer it on days 1 and 5 of cycles 3 through 6.

Table 81-4 Revised International Prognostic Index (R-IPI)*

No. of IPI Factors	IPI Score	Outcome	Overall Survival (%)
0	0	Very Good	94
1–2	1–2	Good	79
3, 4, or 5	3–5	Poor	55

From Sehn LH, Berry B, Chhanabhai M, et al: The revised International Prognostic Index is a better predictor of outcome than the standard IPI for patients with diffuse large B-cell lymphoma treated with R-CHOP. *Blood* 109:1857, 2007.
ECOG, Eastern Cooperative Oncology Group; *IPI,* International Prognostic Index; *LDH,* lactate dehydrogenase
*One point is given for the presence of each of the following characteristics: age older than 60 years, elevated serum LDH level, ECOG performance status ≥2, Ann Arbor stage III or IV, and more than two extranodal sites.

Although molecular profiling remains an experimental technique that is not widely available, it will likely help to improve pathologic diagnostic accuracy, predict outcome with greater precision, and help elucidate pathways of lymphomagenesis. This should lead to the identification of novel cellular targets, paving the way for more personalized therapy. The current integration of immunostaining and gene expression profiling into large prospective clinical trials is imperative to facilitate the investigation and development of new and useful prognostic models that may ultimately guide therapeutic choices.

Treatment

The mainstay of treatment for DLBCL is systemic chemotherapy; radiation treatment alone is inadequate and associated with high recurrence rates.[15] For early stage disease, whether or not radiation treatment adds benefit to chemotherapy has been controversial. Based on a randomized study that showed a survival advantage of limited course CHOP plus involved field radiation compared with full course CHOP in early stage (I/II) aggressive lymphoma, combined modality therapy became the standard.[16] However, longer patient follow-up showed a convergence of the overall survival curves because of late systemic relapses in the combined modality arm, thus reopening the debate on radiation.[16,17] In this regard, a prospective Groupe d'Etude des Lymphomes de l'Adulte (GELA) study randomized 576 elderly patients with favorable early stage aggressive lymphoma to receive CHOP alone (4 cycles) or CHOP plus radiation and found that combined modality therapy was not superior to chemotherapy alone.[18] Given these results and the improved outcome of R-CHOP, it is difficult to justify the routine use of radiation in early stage disease.

A possible exception to the omission of radiation, however, is in the treatment of primary mediastinal DLBCL (PMBL), depending on the chemotherapy regimen. In a study of 50 untreated patients with PMBL who received MACOP-B (methotrexate, ARA-C [Cytarabine], cyclophosphamide, Oncovin, prednisone, and bleomycin) followed by radiation, 66% had persistently positive gallium scans after chemotherapy, suggesting active disease. After consolidation radiotherapy, however, only 19% of patients had a positive gallium scan, and 80% were event free at 39 months of median follow-up.[19] This important study suggested that radiotherapy was necessary after chemotherapy in PMBL. Furthermore, historical evidence indicates that dose-intense regimens such as MACOP-B or VACOP-B (etoposide, doxorubicin, cyclophosphamide, vincristine, prednisone, and bleomycin) are superior to CHOP for PMBL, raising yet another question about the optimal chemotherapy for this disease.[20-22] Although the addition of rituximab to CHOP has improved the outcome for patients with DLBCL, there remains a high proportion of patients who do not achieve remission with R-CHOP, and in two recent studies, most of them received mediastinal radiation.[23,24] Recent results with the pharmacodynamically dose-adjusted regimen of doxorubicin, vincristine, and etoposide infused over 96 hours with bolus intravenous cyclophosphamide, rituximab and oral prednisone (DA-EPOCH-R) may be challenging the need for radiation in PMBL.[25-27] In a phase II study of DA-EPOCH-R in 40 patients with PMBL, 100% and 95% are alive and event free at a median 4-year follow-up, respectively, and only two patients required radiation treatment (see box on Treatment of Primary Mediastinal B-Cell Lymphoma).[27] These results suggest that DA-EPOCH-R obviates the need for radiation in almost all patients with PMBL, thus eliminating the risk of long-term toxicities such as secondary malignancies and heart disease. This is particularly important given that patients with PMBL are typically young and often women and are at increased risk of breast and other cancers as well as late-term toxicities.[28]

Systemic treatment is required for advanced stage DLBCL (Table 81-5). The CHOP regimen was developed some 30 years ago and was established as the standard by a randomized trial showing that CHOP was as effective as three other common albeit more complex or toxic regimens.[29] The fact that only 44% of patients achieved complete remissions (CRs) with CHOP, however, left significant room for improvement and spawned multiple studies aimed at improving treatment outcome.[29,30] Many of these studies focused on modifications to the CHOP platform. A GELA study compared doxorubicin; cyclophosphamide, vindesine, bleomycin, and prednisone (ACVBP) with CHOP in elderly patients with aggressive lymphoma and showed a superior 5-year event-free survival rate (EFS) of 39% and OS of 46% compared with 29% and 38% for CHOP, respectively.[31] Much of the benefit in the ACVBP arm, however, was due to a lower incidence of CNS progression, which could be attributed to the use of CNS prophylaxis with ACVBP. Furthermore, a previous study of ACVBP in low-IPI patients showed no benefit over m-BACOD, which was shown to be equivalent to CHOP.[32]

Treatment of Primary Mediastinal B-Cell Lymphoma

Patients with a diagnosis of PMBL undergo routine CT staging of chest, abdomen, and pelvis. We administer 6 cycles of DA-EPOCH-R. After 4 cycles of therapy, we repeat CT staging, and after 6 cycles, we perform CTs and an FDG-PET scan. If patients have responded and the posttherapy PET scan result is negative, we repeat CT scans every few months. If the FDG-PET result is positive, we attempt to perform a biopsy, and if there is residual disease, patients undergo mediastinal radiation treatment. If the FDG-PET result is suspicious (low SUV values), we repeat it in 4 to 6 weeks. If at this time, the result becomes negative, patients go into routine follow-up, and if it remains abnormal, we perform a biopsy and administer radiation if the biopsy confirms residual disease.

In aggressive lymphomas, high tumor proliferation determined by Ki-67 or MIB-1 immunohistochemistry has been shown to be an adverse prognostic finding with CHOP chemotherapy, suggesting that "kinetic" failure is a problem.[10,33] One strategy to overcome "kinetic" failure is to increase the dose density through frequent chemotherapy administration. The Deutsche Studiengruppe für Hochmaligne Non-Hodgkin Lymphome (DSHNHL) group evaluated the effect of dose density and etoposide in two four-arm studies of CHOP administered every 14 or 21 days with or without etoposide (CHOEP) in patients older than 60 years of age and low-risk patients 60 years of age or younger.[34,35] In the younger patients, CHOEP-21 demonstrated the best overall results with a CR rate of 88% versus 79% and EFS of 69% versus 58% at 5 years compared with standard CHOP-21, respectively.[35] In older patients, however, dose-dense CHOP-14 showed the best outcome with a CR rate of 76% versus 60% and EFS of 44% versus 33% at 5 years compared with standard CHOP-21.[34] Although these studies provided the best evidence that outcome could be improved through specific changes to the CHOP chemotherapy platform, it remains unclear why the optimal treatment differed in the studies given the continuum in disease biology across age.[10] The question of whether dose intensity can improve outcome has been and is being addressed in various other studies.[36,37]

An alternative strategy to dose density is to increase the fractional cell kill or efficacy of chemotherapy, thereby reducing the number of tumor cells that can survive and proliferate between cycles. Longer drug exposure may take advantage of the increased sensitivity of cycling cells, and in vitro studies have shown that prolonged low concentration exposure to vincristine and doxorubicin, compared with brief higher concentration exposure, can increase cytotoxicity by up to 1 log.[38] This approach was translated into the pharmacodynamically dose-adjusted DA-EPOCH regimen, which showed a promising progression-free survival (PFS) and OS of 70% and 73%, respectively, at 5-year median follow-up in newly diagnosed DLBCL.[25] Interestingly, high tumor proliferation was not found to be an adverse biomarker in this study.[25]

The development of rituximab has made the single greatest impact on the treatment of patients with DLBCL since CHOP was first introduced more than 30 years ago. The first study to show the benefit of rituximab was performed by GELA, in which patients older

Table 81-5 Treatment Regimens for Diffuse Large B-Cell Lymphoma

Study	Therapy	Patient group	Event-free Survival	Overall Survival	Reference
Phase III R-CHOP V CHOP	R-CHOP GELA	Age ≥60 yr All IPI	EFS: 47% at 5 yr	58% at 5 yr	39,40
Phase III R-CHOP V CHOP	R-CHOP U.S. Intergroup	Age ≥60 yr All IPI	FFS: 53% at 3 yr	NA	42
Phase III R-CHOP-like V CHOP	R-CHOP-like* MInT	Age ≤60 yr Low IPI	EFS: 79% at 3 yr	93% at 3 yr	44
Phase III ACVBP V CHOP	ACVBP GELA	Age ≥60 yr ≤1 IPI factor	EFS: 39% at 5 yr	46% at 5 yr	31
Single arm Phase II	DA-EPOCH-R NCI/CALGB	Age ≥18 yr All IPI	PFS: 81% at 62 mos	84% at 62 months	49
Phase III: four arms CHOP-14, CHOP-21, CHOEP-14, CHOEP-21	CHOEP-21 DSHNHL	Age 18–60 yr Good prognosis disease	EFS: 69.2% at 5 yr	NA	35
Phase III: four arms CHOP-14, CHOP-21, CHOEP-14, CHOEP-21	CHOP-14 DSHNHL	Age 61–75 yr All IPI	EFS: 43.8% at 5 yr	53.3% at 5 yr	34
Phase III: four arms R-CHOP-14 × 8, R-CHOP-14 × 6, R-CHOP-21 × 8, R-CHOP-21 × 6	R-CHOP-14 (X6) DSHNHL	Age ≥60 yr All IPI	EFS: 66% at 3 yr	78% at 3 yr	43
Phase III: two arms R-ACVBP V R-CHOP	R-ACVBP	Age 18–59 yr Only one adverse IPI prognostic factor	EFS: 81% at 3 yr	92% at 3 yr	46

ACVBP, Doxorubicin, cyclophosphamide, vindesine, bleomycin, and prednisone; *CHOEP,* cyclophosphamide, doxorubicin, vincristine, etoposide, and prednisone; *DA-EPOCH-R,* dose-adjusted etoposide, prednisone, vincristine, cyclophosphamide, and doxorubicin; *DSHNHL,* Deutsche Studiengruppe für Hochmaligne Non-Hodgkin'Lymphome; *GELA,* Groupe d'Etude Lymphomes d'Adultes; *IPI,* International Prognostic Index; *MACOP-B,* methotrexate, doxorubicin, cyclophosphamide, vincristine, prednisone, and bleomycin; *MInT,* MabThera International Trial; *NCI,* National Cancer Institute; *PmitCEBO,* prednisone, mitozantrone, cyclophosphamide, etoposide, bleomycin, and vincristine; *R-CHOP,* rituximab, cyclophosphamide, doxorubicin, vincristine, and prednisone.
*CHOP-like regimens included CHOP, CHOEP, MACOP-B, and PmitCEBO.

than 60 years were randomized to receive CHOP or R-CHOP.[39] In this study, the CR (76% vs. 63%) and 5-year EFS (47% vs. 29%) were higher with R-CHOP than CHOP, respectively, making R-CHOP the "de facto" standard in DLBCL.[39,40] Recently, long-term follow-up of this study was presented, and the benefit of R-CHOP remains significant.[41] The benefit of rituximab has also been confirmed by the U.S. Intergroup study in a similar patient population.[42]

With the benefit of rituximab established, investigators have gone on to explore its use in a variety of clinical settings and treatment strategies. The DSHNHL group explored the question of whether there was a difference in outcome between 6 or 8 cycles of treatment in a randomized study of 6 versus 8 cycles of CHOP-14, with or without rituximab, in elderly patients with DLBCL. In that study, termed the RECOVER-60 trial, they found no difference in outcome with 6 versus 8 cycles of treatment.[43] Although they showed an excellent 3-year EFS of 66% with R-CHOP-14 over 6 cycles, which is somewhat better than the GELA and U.S. Intergroup study results, one cannot conclude that R-CHOP-14 is superior to standard R-CHOP-21, given all the caveats of inter-study comparisons. The MabThera International Trial (MInT) studied the benefit of rituximab with CHOP-based treatment in younger patients (60 years of age and younger) with favorable characteristics defined as low-IPI risk; furthermore, nearly half of patients received involved field radiotherapy.[44] Similar to the other randomized rituximab studies, patients who received rituximab fared significantly better with a 3-year EFS of 79%. As an interesting aside, the MInT study also showed that rituximab obviated the benefit of CHOEP in younger patients.[44] The additive role of rituximab in the context of dose intensity has also been evaluated, and in a recent update of the largest study that compared R-CHOP-14 with R-CHOP-21, there was no difference in overall survival between the two arms.[45] Recently, the GELA group compared R-CHOP-21 with R-ACVBP in younger patients (age 18–59 years) and at a median follow-up of 44 months demonstrated a significantly improved overall and PFS in patients who received R-ACVBP.[46]

Rituximab has also been tested in combination with the DA-EPOCH regimen.[47-49] In a recent report of 69 patients treated in a multicenter study, 81% and 84% of patients were progression free and alive, respectively, at the median follow-up of 62 months.[49] Furthermore, PFS was 87%, 92% and 54% for patients with low/low-intermediate, high-intermediate and high-IPI risk groups. PFS and EFS were 100% and 94%, respectively, for patients with germinal center tumors and 67% and 58%, respectively, for patients with nongerminal center tumors. Evaluation of DA-EPOCH-R versus R-CHOP in untreated DLBCL is currently ongoing in the Cancer and Leukemia Group B (CALGB) cooperative group in conjunction with microarray analysis.

Although it is clear that rituximab has significantly improved the overall outcome of patients with DLBCL, several studies suggest its benefit is limited by tumor pathobiology.[50-52] Two studies found that rituximab benefit was primarily in Bcl-2 positive DLBCL, and another study showed that benefit was limited to Bcl-6 negative DLBCL.[50-52] These biomarkers are likely related to the new molecular taxonomy of DLBCL defined by gene profiling and suggest that rituximab may primarily benefit tumors derived from a nongerminal center B cell.[10,11,53] Recently, studies have suggested that molecular subtypes of DLBCL can be differentially targeted, and ongoing randomized studies are looking at the role of bortezomib when added to R-CHOP in nongerminal center DLBCL.[54,55]

Over the past few decades, there have been significant improvements in the outcome of patients with HIV-associated DLBCL, and these can be attributed to the widespread availability of combination antiretroviral therapy (CART) as well as advances in the therapeutics of these diseases.[56-58] Recently, the AIDS Malignancy Consortium in the United States reported excellent results with the DA-EPOCH-R regimen that were similar to survival outcomes in HIV-negative DLBCL.[59]

The role of high-dose chemotherapy and autologous stem cell transplantation (ASCT) in the initial treatment of patients with DLBCL remains controversial.[60,61] Although some studies have suggested benefit—recently, the GELA group reported promising results in high-risk DLBCL patients who received R-ACVBP followed by ASCT—this approach has not been compared with standard approaches.[62,63] ASCT is also associated with late toxicities, including leukemia and secondary myelodysplasia, which must be considered in the risk benefit of treatment.[64]

PRIMARY CENTRAL NERVOUS SYSTEM LYMPHOMA

Primary central nervous system lymphoma is a rare and highly aggressive lymphoma confined to the CNS and is usually of diffuse large B-cell histology. Its unique radiographic findings present challenges in evaluation, which have been recently addressed in a report of an international workshop to standardize criteria for baseline evaluation and response.[65] The incidence of PCNSL is particularly high in the setting of HIV infection, in which it often presents with multifocal disease and is virtually always associated with EBV. In contrast, PCNSL in HIV-negative patients often presents with solitary intracranial masses and is rarely associated with EBV (Fig. 81-4).

Treatment of PCNSL differs from systemic DLBCL because many chemotherapy agents do not adequately penetrate the blood–brain barrier. Radiotherapy has been a mainstay of treatment because it is effective and sidestepped the limitations of chemotherapy, but responses are usually short-lived, and virtually all patients relapse. High-dose methotrexate (HD-MTX), on the other hand, is a cytotoxic agent with good CNS penetration, but when used alone, PFS is a relatively short 7 months.[66] A logical step was to administer HD-MTX followed by whole-brain radiotherapy, and this resulted in an impressive 82% to 88% CR and median PFS rates of 32 to 40 months.[66-68] Unfortunately, such combined modality treatment is associated with severe long-term neurotoxicity.[66,69] For this reason, there has been much interest in developing regimens that obviate or defer the need for radiation until relapse. Most promising in this regard are combinations of HD-MTX with systemic agents that cross the blood–brain barrier, such as cytarabine, vincristine, and ifosfamide, particularly in patients younger than 60 years of age.[70] The Bonn group and others have adopted such an approach and have reported promising results with chemotherapy and deferred radiation in younger patients.[70,71] These results require further validation in trials. Studies are also addressing the role of immunochemotherapy with rituximab and other novel agents, which promise to further improve the outcome of patients with PCNSL.[72,73]

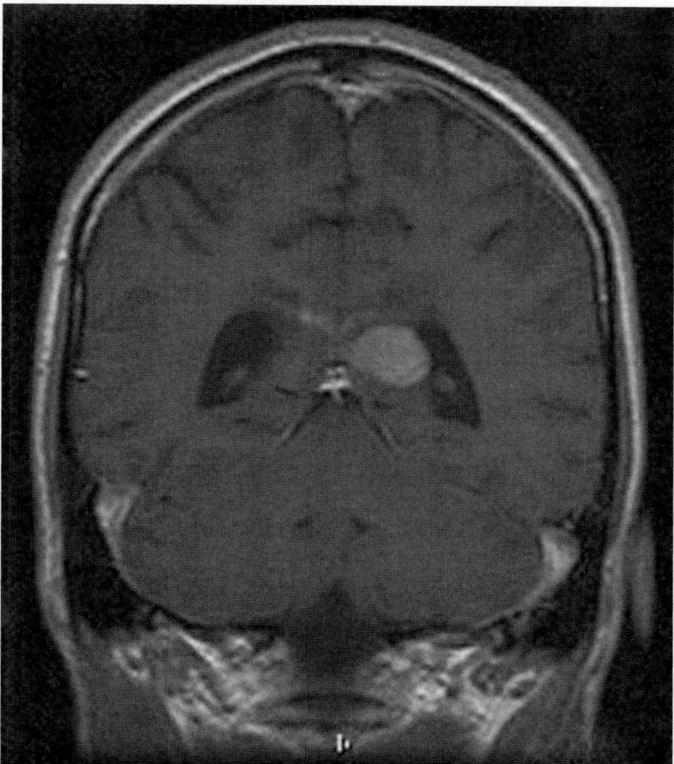

Figure 81-4 THIS GADOLINIUM-ENHANCED MAGNETIC RESONANCE IMAGING SCAN OF THE BRAIN SHOWS AN ENHANCING INFILTRATIVE MASS IN THE MAJOR FORCEPS OF THE CORPUS CALLOSUM. A biopsy was consistent with primary central nervous system lymphoma.

BURKITT LYMPHOMA

Epidemiology

Burkitt lymphoma mostly occurs in the first 2 decades of life, is more common in males, and accounts for some 2% of all lymphomas. There are three recognized clinical variants, and they vary in who they effect and how they present, and they also have morphologic and biological differences. Endemic BL occurs in equatorial Africa and Papua New Guinea, peaks in incidence in 4- to 7-year–old children, and is predominantly a male disease. Sporadic BL presents worldwide and is the most common variant in the Western world. It typically affects children and young adults and is more commonly observed in boys. Immunodeficiency-associated BL occurs in association with HIV infection and is approximately 1000 times more common in HIV-infected individuals.

Pathobiology

Burkitt lymphoma is highly aggressive and characterized by an extremely high proliferation fraction and a high fraction of apoptosis, and this accounts for its "starry sky" appearance. Although a leukemic phase of BL can occur in patients with advanced disease, it is very rare for BL to present purely as acute leukemia. Biologically, BL is derived from a germinal center B cell as indicated by its CD20+, CD10+, and TdT-negative immunohistochemical profile and gene expression profiling.[74] The neoplastic cells are usually negative or weakly positive for BCL2. Although EBV is virtually always detected in endemic BL, it is only present in 25% to 40% of sporadic and immunodeficiency-associated cases.

Although virtually all cases of BL have MYC translocations, usually at 8q24 to the IG heavy chain region, MYC translocations are not specific for BL and can be found in other aggressive B-cell lymphomas (Fig. 81-5). BL has a unique gene expression signature that is molecularly distinct from that of DLBCL. Studies have demonstrated that some cases of DLBCL by histology have gene expression profiles consistent with BL.[74-76] Given that BL does not respond well to CHOP-based treatments, this distinction by molecular profiling is important, and gene expression profiling may be useful in rare cases that would otherwise be diagnosed as DLBCL. Additionally, there are cases with a profile intermediate between that of DLBCL and BL; these cases typically harbor MYC and have a poor outcome with CHOP-based regimens.

Clinical Features

The clinical presentation of BL is variable and depends on the epidemiological subtype as well as other factors. In endemic BL, it is common for patients to present with jaw and other facial disease, and other extranodal sites of involvement include the ileocecum, gonads, kidneys, and breasts. The ileocecal area is the most common site of disease involvement in sporadic BL (Fig. 81-6), and jaw involvement is very rare. In immunodeficiency-associated BL, involvement of the ileocecum, LNs, and BM is commonly observed. Patients often present with advanced stage and bulky disease caused by the short doubling time of the tumor, and it is common for patients to develop tumor lysis syndrome (TLS) after the institution of therapy.

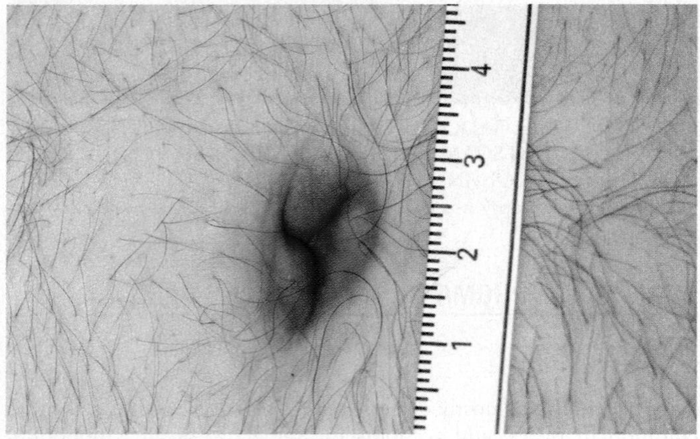

Figure 81-5 BURKITT LYMPHOMA (BL) INVOLVING THE UMBILICUS. This is an 18-year old man who presented with a history of abdominal pain. Computed tomography scan demonstrated a large intraabdominal mass extending up to the umbilicus, and a biopsy revealed it to be BL.

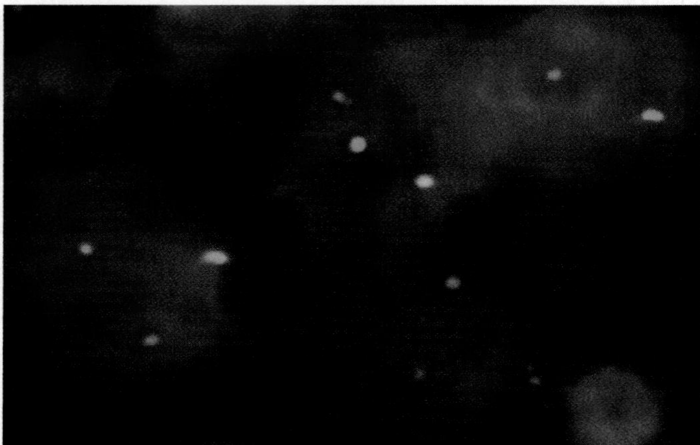

Figure 81-6 FLUORESCENT IN SITU HYBRIDIZATION SHOWING AN MYC TRANSLOCATION IN A PATIENT WITH DIFFUSE LARGE B-CELL LYMPHOMA.

Investigation

History and Physical Examination and Laboratory Investigations

Similar to patients with DLBCL, a detailed history and physical examination is required, and the diagnosis of BL should be made by an experienced hematopathologist. Given its association with HIV infection, it is imperative to perform an HIV test at diagnosis and to check hepatitis serologies.

Imaging and Staging

As with DLBCL, imaging studies should include chest radiography and CT scanning of the chest, abdomen, and pelvis. The need for additional imaging studies depends on the clinical presentation. A BM aspirate and biopsy should be performed in all patients, and all patients should undergo lumbar puncture with evaluation of the CSF by cytology and flow cytometry.[4] Although BL in adults is staged according to the Ann Arbor staging system, the Murphy staging system is often used in children.

Prognosis

Age, large tumor volume, and CNS involvement have been associated with a poor prognosis in the past. Although early studies demonstrated that HIV-positive patients with BL had a worse outcome, this has not been the case with newer treatment approaches.

Treatment

Burkitt lymphoma is a systemic disease and requires chemotherapy for all disease stages. Importantly, locoregional radiation does not improve survival and should be avoided. Although older studies demonstrated that surgical resection of abdominal disease improved outcome, indicating the importance of tumor volume, more effective and risk-adapted treatments have made surgical resection unnecessary except for specific complications such as obstruction, perforation, fistula, or bleeding.

Early treatment strategies for BL were modeled on acute lymphoblastic leukemia (ALL) regimens that used dose-intense and prolonged treatment with induction, consolidation, and maintenance phases. These approaches stand in contrast to the significantly less dose-intense regimens used in adults with "intermediate-grade" lymphoma, such as CHOP and CHOP-based regimens, that only produced a 50% to 60% EFS. Although dose intensity and dose density are important treatment components for BL, later studies indicated that shorter treatment durations were equally effective. Furthermore, the recognition that tumor volume is an important prognostic feature led to the use of risk adaptive approaches and a further reduction in treatment for patients with early stage disease. Several biological characteristics of BL have helped guide treatment strategies, including its high proliferative fraction. It has been recognized for years that BL is sensitive to multiple chemotherapy classes, and in endemic BL, cures were occasionally achieved with single-agent cyclophosphamide. Despite initial sensitivity, however, patients frequently relapsed, particularly those with higher volume disease. This apparent dichotomy can potentially be explained by the high tumor proliferation rate, resulting in "kinetic" failure. One strategy to overcome "kinetic" failure is to increase the dose density through frequent chemotherapy administration, a strategy used in most current BL regimens. Another strategy is to increase the fractional cell kill or efficacy of chemotherapy, thereby reducing the number of tumor cells that can survive and proliferate between cycles. Hence, BL regimens commonly use multiple chemotherapy agents in high doses and alternating cycles. They typically include anthracylines, epipodophyllotoxins, vinca alkaloids, and alkylators, as well as methotrexate and cytarabine, which are cell cycle active agents and take advantage of the high tumor proliferation. These agents, however, are administered in a variety of combinations and schedule, indicating the empiric nature of the actual combinations.

The risks of TLS and propensity for CNS dissemination in BL also have important treatment implications. All patients should receive TLS prophylaxis during the first cycle and undergo close monitoring of their electrolytes. The high risk of CNS involvement has prompted the use in the past of relatively high-dose intravenous methotrexate and cytarabine—both of which have CNS penetration—and intrathecal administration of these drugs. An important advance has been to reduce intrathecal treatment and eliminate whole-brain radiation for prophylaxis, which has significantly reduced CNS toxicity. A recently published FAB/LMB study demonstrated that patients with early stage BL had a high cure rate and very low rate of CNS relapse without the use of intrathecal chemotherapy.[77]

There are multiple highly effective regimens for BL; however, because of the rarity of the disease—there are only 1200 new cases in the United States each year—there are no good comparative studies of different therapies in BL. A variety of dose-intense short-duration regimens have achieved durable CRs in 47% to 84% of patients.[78-81] Included in these are the French LMB and German Berlin-Frankfurt-Munster (BFM) protocols and the National Cancer Institute CODOX-M/IVAC (cyclophosphamide, vincristine, doxorubicin, and HD-MTX alternating with ifosfamide, etoposide, and high-dose cytarabine; intrathecal methotrexate and cytarabine are also administered) regimen. These regimens are similar in their drug composition, short cycle length, and CNS prophylaxis. Although most BL occurs in children, Magrath and colleagues[82] demonstrated that adults have a similar disease outcome when treated with the same regimen and reported cure rates approaching 90%. Other groups have confirmed the efficacy of this regimen albeit with lower survival rates. In the United Kingdom, Mead et al[83] reported an overall EFS of 65% at 2 years. The hyper-CVAD regimen has also been tested in BL with good results (recently with the addition of rituximab).

Toxicity is an important clinical limitation of these regimens in adults, particularly in older patients and in patients who are immunosuppressed, in whom severe morbidity and even mortality occur. Therefore, one of the major therapeutic challenges in BL is to develop therapies that are as effective in achieving high cure rates as "standard" regimens but that also improve the therapeutic index and reduce toxicity complications. This approach has been investigated in a study using DA-EPOCH-R in BL. Based on the efficacy of the regimen in a DLBCL study—which suggested that DA-EPOCH overcomes the adverse effect of high proliferation, likely because of its infusional schedule—a study was undertaken in BL. A recent update reported an EFS of 97% in 29 patients at a median follow-up time of 57 months.[84] There were very low rates of TLS and other toxicities compared with conventional BL regimens. Many different approaches have been tested in patients who have HIV-associated BL. As with older patients, treatment-related toxicity can be an important consideration in this population, and regimens such as DA-EPOCH-R are well tolerated and effective.[84]

SALVAGE THERAPY

The salvage treatment of relapsed DLBCL should be approached in an individual manner because the choice of treatment is influenced by the time to recurrence, prior therapy, medical condition, and the potential for cure. Although most relapsed aggressive lymphomas require combination chemotherapy for adequate disease control, it is important to recognize that patients with local disease may be salvaged with radiation therapy. Examples include primary mediastinal DLBCL, which can remain local even at relapse, and PTLDs, which may have an isolated resistant EBV clone after chemotherapy.[85]

A variety of active salvage chemotherapy regimens are available for relapsed or refractory DLBCL.[86-92] Platinum-containing regimens, such as ESHAP (etoposide, methylprednisolone, cytosine arabinoside, and platinum) and ICE, are currently among the most widely used salvage treatment.[88,90,93] It is a commonly held notion that salvage treatment should include different agents from past treatment to avoid drug resistance. Recent evidence indicates, however, that sensitivity to apoptosis is a central cause of drug resistance and that drug-specific mechanisms are less important.[10,94] Hence, salvage regimens developed around the most active upfront agents should show high activity.[95] The addition of rituximab appears to enhance the activity of salvage regimens as demonstrated by results with R-ICE (rituximab, ifosfamid, carboplatin, and etoposide) and ICE (ifosfamid, carboplatin, and etoposide), which showed CRs of 53% and 27%, respectively.[88,93]

Patients with chemotherapy-sensitive disease have the best outcome with ASCT, and this is recommended at initial relapse; in the pre-rituximab era, this approach yielded OS and EFS rates in the range of 40% to 50% and 30% to 40%, respectively.[88,96] However, the improvement in upfront curability of DLBCL because of immunochemotherapy has diminished the efficacy of ASCT at relapse, which was recently demonstrated in the CORAL study, in which the 3-year EFS of patients who had initially received rituximab was merely 21% after ASCT.[97] Of course, patients with chemotherapy-resistant disease do poorly with ASCT and should be considered for experimental treatments such as allogeneic SCT.

The outcome for patients with BL who relapse after or progress during initial therapy is extremely poor, and there are no standard approaches that have been associated with good outcomes; therefore, experimental approaches such as allogeneic SCT (if it is feasible) should be considered.

Late Complications of Treatment and Follow-up

It is important to recognize that successful treatment may be associated with late complications that may not appear for decades. Among the major late-term complications are secondary malignancies, ischemic heart disease, anthracycline-related cardiotoxicity, and radiation- or bleomycin-induced pulmonary toxicity.[98] The risk of developing myelodysplastic disorders and acute myeloid leukemia is related to alkylator and topoisomerase inhibitor use and is enhanced by radiation. Radiation therapy increases the risk of malignancy in the treatment region, particularly breast cancer in women and lung cancer in smokers. Indeed, it is imperative to consider late-term toxicity when selecting treatment.

A general guideline for follow-up after initial therapy involves visits every 3 months for 2 years, every 6 months for 3 years, and annually thereafter. During these visits, examination of the LN areas, abdomen, thyroid, and skin is important. CT scans are recommended in routine follow-up. It is important to note that CT scans are associated with a relatively high radiation exposure and projected risks and should not be used unnecessarily.[99] PET scans are not recommended for routine follow-up because the high rate of false-positive scans is unlikely to offset the value of early detection. Indeed, the role of PET scans in the overall treatment of lymphomas needs to be prospectively studied.[100] Routine laboratory studies with blood counts, liver function tests, and LD should be performed. Patients with disease in the chest area can be followed with chest radiographs. Thyroid-stimulating hormone levels should be monitored annually in patients who received neck radiotherapy. Mammography for women should begin 10 years from the diagnosis of lymphoma or at age 40 years, whichever comes first.

FUTURE DIRECTIONS

Over recent years, we have made significant advances in elucidating the molecular biology of DLBCL and BL, and this has led to an era of enhanced and exciting drug discovery. In DLBCL in particular, many critical pathways and novel targets have been identified, and many small molecule inhibitors are being investigated and in development as a result of these advances. For example, in the ABC subtype of DLBCL, constitutive activation of nuclear factor kappa B (NF-κB) has been shown to be an important inhibitor of apoptosis, and this may lead to chemotherapy resistance. Therefore, bortezomib, an inhibitor of NF-κB, was tested in DLBCL, and outcomes according to molecular subtype suggested that it enhances the activity of chemotherapy in ABC but not GCB DLBCL.[54,55] Recent work has identified that chronic active B-cell receptor signaling is an important mechanism of ABC tumor cell survival; to test this clinically, studies in patients with ABC DLBCL are in progress targeting specific components of this pathway (Bruton tyrosine kinase [BTK] by PCI-32765).[101-104] In BL, cure rates are very high with conventional approaches, and the challenge for the future is to further develop strategies that maintain the efficacy of "standard" treatment but with much less toxicity. To advance the therapeutics of these diseases, it is critical to wisely choose which drugs should be developed and incorporated into upfront clinical trials and to pair drug development with understanding of tumor biology.

SUGGESTED READINGS

Alizadeh AA, Eisen MB, Davis RE, et al: Distinct types of diffuse large B-cell lymphoma identified by gene expression profiling. *Nature* 403:503, 2000.

Choi WW, Weisenburger DD, Greiner TC, et al: A new immunostain algorithm classifies diffuse large B-cell lymphoma into molecular subtypes with high accuracy. *Clin Cancer Res* 15:5494, 2009.

Coiffier B, Lepage E, Briere J, et al: CHOP chemotherapy plus rituximab compared with CHOP alone in elderly patients with diffuse large-B-cell lymphoma. *N Engl J Med* 346:235, 2002.

Coiffier B, Thieblemont C, Van Den Neste E, et al: Long-term outcome of patients in the LNH-98.5 trial, the first randomized study comparing rituximab-CHOP to standard CHOP chemotherapy in DLBCL patients: A study by the Groupe d'Etudes des Lymphomes de l'Adulte. *Blood* 116:2040, 2010.

Dave SS, Fu K, Wright GW, et al: Molecular diagnosis of Burkitt's lymphoma. *N Engl J Med* 354:2431, 2006.

Davis RE, Ngo VN, Lenz G, et al: Chronic active B-cell-receptor signalling in diffuse large B-cell lymphoma. *Nature* 463:88, 2010.

Dunleavy K, Little RF, Pittaluga S, et al: The role of tumor histogenesis, FDG-PET, and short-course EPOCH with dose-dense rituximab (SC-EPOCH-RR) in HIV-associated diffuse large B-cell lymphoma. *Blood* 115:3017, 2010.

Dunleavy K, Pittaluga S, Czuczman MS, et al: Differential efficacy of bortezomib plus chemotherapy within molecular subtypes of diffuse large B-cell lymphoma. *Blood* 113:6069, 2009.

Gisselbrecht C, Glass B, Mounier N, et al: Salvage regimens with autologous transplantation for relapsed large B-cell lymphoma in the rituximab era. *J Clin Oncol* 28:4184, 2010.

Hegde U, Filie A, Little RF, et al: High incidence of occult leptomeningeal disease detected by flow cytometry in newly diagnosed aggressive B-cell lymphomas at risk for central nervous system involvement: The role of flow cytometry versus cytology. *Blood* 105:496, 2005.

Hummel M, Bentink S, Berger H, et al: A biologic definition of Burkitt's lymphoma from transcriptional and genomic profiling. *N Engl J Med* 354:2419, 2006.

Lenz G, Davis RE, Ngo VN, et al: Oncogenic CARD11 mutations in human diffuse large B cell lymphoma. *Science* 319:1676, 2008.

Lenz G, Staudt LM: Aggressive lymphomas. *N Engl J Med* 362:1417, 2010.

Magrath I, Adde M, Shad A, et al: Adults and children with small non-cleaved-cell lymphoma have a similar excellent outcome when treated with the same chemotherapy regimen. *J Clin Oncol* 14:925, 1996.

Mead GM, Sydes MR, Walewski J, et al: An international evaluation of CODOX-M and CODOX-M alternating with IVAC in adult Burkitt's lymphoma: Results of United Kingdom Lymphoma Group LY06 study. *Ann Oncol* 13:1264, 2002.

Pels H, Schmidt-Wolf IG, Glasmacher A, et al: Primary central nervous system lymphoma: Results of a pilot and phase II study of systemic and intraventricular chemotherapy with deferred radiotherapy. *J Clin Oncol* 21:4489, 2003.

Pfreundschuh M, Trumper L, Kloess M, et al: Two-weekly or 3-weekly CHOP chemotherapy with or without etoposide for the treatment of elderly patients with aggressive lymphomas: Results of the NHL-B2 trial of the DSHNHL. *Blood* 104:634, 2004.

Pfreundschuh M, Trumper L, Kloess M, et al: Two-weekly or 3-weekly CHOP chemotherapy with or without etoposide for the treatment of young patients with good-prognosis (normal LDH) aggressive lymphomas: Results of the NHL-B1 trial of the DSHNHL. *Blood* 104:626, 2004.

Pfreundschuh M, Trumper L, Osterborg A, et al: CHOP-like chemotherapy plus rituximab versus CHOP-like chemotherapy alone in young patients with good-prognosis diffuse large-B-cell lymphoma: A randomised controlled trial by the MabThera International Trial (MInT) Group. *Lancet Oncol* 7:379, 2006.

Ruan J, Martin P, Furman RR, et al: Bortezomib plus CHOP-rituximab for previously untreated diffuse large B-cell lymphoma and mantle cell lymphoma. *J Clin Oncol* 29:690, 2011.

Sehn LH, Berry B, Chhanabhai M, et al: The revised International Prognostic Index (R-IPI) is a better predictor of outcome than the standard IPI for patients with diffuse large B-cell lymphoma treated with R-CHOP. *Blood* 109:1857, 2007.

Sparano JA, Lee JY, Kaplan LD, et al: Rituximab plus concurrent infusional EPOCH chemotherapy is highly effective in HIV-associated B-cell non-Hodgkin lymphoma. *Blood* 115:3008, 2010.

Swerdlow SH, Campo E, Harris NL, et al: *WHO classification of tumours of haematopoietic and lymphoid tissues,* Lyon, 2008, IARC.

van Besien K, Ha CS, Murphy S, et al: Risk factors, treatment, and outcome of central nervous system recurrence in adults with intermediate-grade and immunoblastic lymphoma. *Blood* 91:1178, 1998.

Wilson W, Jung SH, Porcu P, et al: A cancer and leukemia group B multi-center study of DA-EPOCH-rituximab in untreated diffuse large B-cell lymphoma with analysis of outcome by molecular subtype. *Haematologica* 2011.

Zinzani PL, Martelli M, Magagnoli M, et al: Treatment and clinical management of primary mediastinal large B-cell lymphoma with sclerosis: MACOP-B regimen and mediastinal radiotherapy monitored by (67) Gallium scan in 50 patients. *Blood* 94:3289, 1999.

For complete list of references log on to www.expertconsult.com.

CHAPTER 82

VIRUS-ASSOCIATED LYMPHOMA

Jennifer A. Kanakry and Richard F. Ambinder

There are five well-characterized human viruses that are generally accepted as important in lymphomagenesis (Table 82-1). These viruses may infect tumor cells (or their progenitors) or may act at a distance. The genomes of Epstein-Barr virus (EBV), Kaposi sarcoma–associated herpesvirus (KSHV, also known as *human herpesvirus 8* [HHV-8]), and human T-lymphotropic virus-1 (HTLV-1) are present in tumor cells. The viral genes expressed in tumor cells modulate cellular metabolism, proliferation, and cell death. In contrast, the human immunodeficiency virus (HIV) genome is generally not detected in tumor cells. Whether hepatitis C virus (HCV) genomes are present in lymphoma cells remains a subject of controversy.

Although viral infection plays a role in the pathogenesis of some lymphomas, lymphomagenesis is unusual. Only a small subset of infected people develops lymphoma. Furthermore, although primary viral infection may be followed by lymphomagenesis within days or weeks in exceptional circumstances, most lymphomas arise years or decades after primary infection. Indeed the term *adult* in adult T-cell leukemia/lymphoma (ATL) reflects the time lag between HTLV-1 infection in infancy and the evolution to malignancy. Geography and associated environmental exposures, host genetic factors, and immune status all modify risk.

Aspects of the biology and epidemiology of each of these viruses and their relationship with lymphomagenesis are reviewed. In addition, clinically important and distinctive features of diagnosis and treatment of the associated lymphomas are presented.

EPSTEIN-BARR VIRUS

Viral Biology

EBV is a gammaherpesvirus transmitted mainly through saliva.[1,2] After primary infection, some of the infected cells are driven to proliferate and thereby spread infection throughout the B-cell compartment. Ultimately, in the normal host, there is an immune response that controls infection and eradicates virus-infected proliferating cells. Thereafter the viral genome is harbored mainly in resting memory B lymphocytes that persist for life. These B cells that harbor virus elude immune surveillance in part because of their very restricted viral gene expression such that few viral antigens are presented. Occasionally there is activation of viral lytic gene expression (at least in some instances this occurs in concert with plasma cell differentiation) leading to production of infectious virions that may infect other B cells. T cell–mediated immune function keeps such proliferation in check.[3]

In vitro EBV immortalizes B cells such that they grow indefinitely as lymphoblastoid cell lines (LCLs) (Fig. 82-1). LCLs are tumorigenic in immunodeficient mice. In LCL, viral genomes are present as circular double-stranded deoxyribonucleic acid (DNA) episomes within the nucleus. The viral proteins required for immortalization include Epstein-Barr virus nuclear antigen-1 (EBNA1), a sequence-specific DNA-binding protein important in the maintenance of the viral episome; EBNA2, a transcription factor that has many effects similar to those of activated Notch receptors; and latent membrane protein-1 (LMP1), a constitutively activated member of the tumor necrosis factor (TNF) receptor superfamily, which most closely resembles CD40.[4] LMP1 activates the nuclear factor kappa-B (NFκB) pathway, which modulates cell proliferation and apoptosis.[5] Several other EBV proteins are also required for immortalization. Although EBV immortalization of B cells in vitro may offer some insights into tumorigenesis, some caution is required in using LCL as a tumor model. Most EBV tumors, including tumors of B-lineage cells, do not express many of the viral genes required for lymphocyte immortalization. The only tumors that express the full complement of viral proteins required for immortalization are those that arise in the most profoundly immunocompromised patients (organ or hematopoietic transplant recipients, patients with congenital immunodeficiency, or patients with far advanced acquired immunodeficiency syndrome [AIDS]). Thus in posttransplantation lymphoproliferative disorder (PTLD), tumor cells may resemble LCL in expressing many viral latency genes in association with normal karyotype (and few mutations of the cellular genome). It has been suggested that there is an inverse relationship between cellular mutations and viral gene expression in tumors.[6]

EBV gene expression may directly drive proliferation or inhibit apoptotic pathways as illustrated by lymphocyte immortalization. However, viral gene expression may also perturb normal lymphocyte biology. Thus LMP1 expression upregulates activation induced (cytidine) deaminase expression, which facilitates somatic hypermutation and immunoglobulin class switching.[7] LMP1 expression may also be important in the conversion of naive B-cells to post-germinal center memory B-cells. LMP2A allows B-cells that lack normal immunoglobulin expression to escape regulatory checkpoints and survive.[8]

Epidemiology of Viral Infection

EBV infection is ubiquitous. The vast majority of adults are infected worldwide. Primary infection is most often asymptomatic, especially when it occurs in childhood.[9] Primary infection may be associated with the syndrome of infectious mononucleosis. Symptomatic primary infection occurs more frequently in older children and in adults than in younger children. Other possible determinants of symptomatic primary infection include genetic factors and possibly the size of the viral inoculum.

Strain differences in EBV are well recognized.[10] However, the importance of these strain differences with regard to lymphomagenesis remains poorly understood. There is general agreement that the Type 1 strain EBV is most common worldwide and in tumors. The Type 2 strain virus has been identified in some African Burkitt lymphoma (BL) and in some AIDS-associated lymphoma. A-strain virus is more efficient at lymphocyte immortalization in vitro and lymphomagenesis in mouse models. The two strains of virus differ mainly in the EBNA2 gene, but differences are recognized in some other viral proteins as well.[11] Variations in the regulatory regions or coding regions of a variety of other genes including EBNA1, LMP1, and ZTA have been recognized and suggested to play a role in lymphomagenesis.

A simple classification of latent viral gene expression recognizes three patterns as shown in the Table 82-2.

Table 82-1 Viruses and Lymphomagenesis

Virus	Viral Genome in Tumor Cell	Lymphoma Type
EBV	Episomal	B, T, NK
KSHV	Episomal	B
HTLV-1	Integrated	T
HIV-1	Absent	B
HCV	Uncertain	B

EBV, Epstein-Barr virus; *HCV,* hepatitis C virus; *HIV-1,* human immunodeficiency virus type 1; *HTLV-1,* human T-lymphotropic virus-1; *KSHV,* Kaposi sarcoma–associated herpesvirus; NK, natural killer.

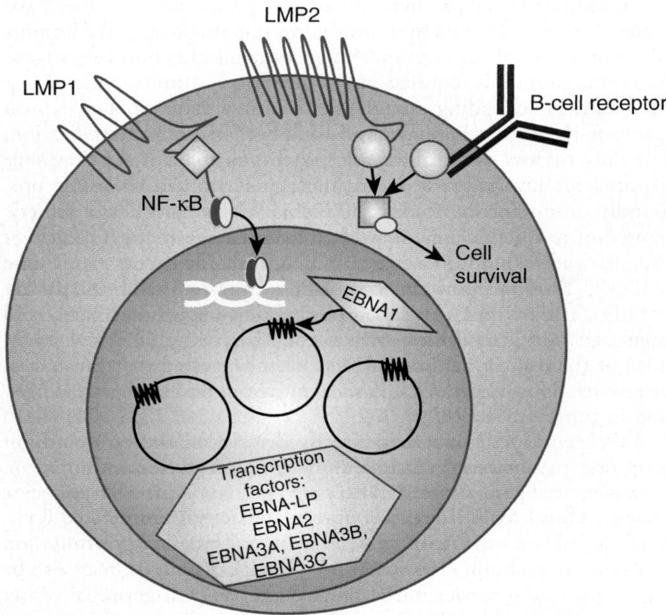

Figure 82-1 EPSTEIN-BARR VIRUS (EBV)–IMMORTALIZED B CELL. Normal B cells are readily immortalized in vitro with EBV. These cells express EBV nuclear and membrane proteins. The nuclear proteins include a protein expressed in all EBV-associated tumors, Epstein-Barr virus nuclear antigen 1 (EBNA1). This protein is required for episomal maintenance. Other viral nuclear proteins expressed are transcription factors. These include EBNA-LP, EBNA2, EBNA3A, EBNA3B, and EBNA3C. Two membrane proteins are expressed: latent membrane protein 1 (LMP1), which activates NFκB pathways, and LMP2A, which mimics B-cell receptor (immunoglobulin) signaling.

Epstein-Barr Virus Detection in Clinical Specimens

The sensitivity of polymerase chain reaction (PCR) makes detection of viral DNA straightforward, but the ubiquity of EBV infection, and the persistence of B cells that harbor EBV in all seropositive individuals, means that EBV DNA is readily detected in many specimens that include normal lymphocytes. Thus diagnosis of the EBV association in general requires viral detection specifically in tumor cells. Techniques for viral DNA detection by fluorescence in situ hybridization or related techniques, although greatly improved in recent years, remain the purview of research laboratories and are generally not readily applicable to clinical specimens. This reflects the relatively low copy number of the viral genome in tumor cells, typically 1 to 200 copies per cell. In contrast, in situ hybridization for the Epstein-Barr encoded ribonucleic acids (RNAs) has emerged as a laboratory standard.[12] These RNAs are polymerase 3 transcripts that are expressed at very high copy number (perhaps millions of copies per cell) in latently infected cells. The function(s) of these RNAs is disputed, but their use for the detection of virus in a variety of surgical specimens is generally accepted.

Table 82-2 Patterns of Epstein-Barr Virus Gene Expression in Latency

Latency	EBNA1	EBNA2, EBNA3A, EBNA3B, EBNA3C	LMP1	LMP2A
I	+			
II	+		+	+
III	+	+	+	+

EBNA1, Epstein-Barr virus nuclear antigen 1; *EBV,* Epstein-Barr virus; *LMP1,* latent membrane protein 1.

Viral antigens are detected by immunohistochemistry. In clinical laboratories, immunohistochemistry for LMP1 is commonly employed and is sensitive for the detection of EBV in Hodgkin lymphoma (HL). In a variety of other EBV-associated B- and T-cell malignancies, expression is variable. Thus failure to detect LMP1 expression does not exclude the presence of EBV except perhaps in HL. In principle, detection of EBNA1 should be universally applicable, although the low level of antigen expression and the cross-reactivity of available monoclonal antibodies have prevented immunohistochemistry for this antigen from emerging as a standard tool.

Association With Particular Types of Lymphoma

Some lymphoma types are nearly 100% EBV associated, including endemic BL, extranodal natural killer (NK)/T-cell lymphoma of the nasal type, early PTLD, lymphomatoid granulomatosis, diffuse large B-cell lymphoma (DLBCL) associated with chronic inflammation, EBV-positive DLBCL of older adults, and AIDS primary central nervous system (CNS) lymphoma (PCNSL).[13-16] Other lymphoma types are variably EBV associated. These include classic HL, PTLDs occurring many months or years after transplantation, and systemic AIDS-related lymphoma. Some lymphoma types appear never or almost never to be EBV associated, including follicular lymphoma, nodular lymphocyte-predominant HL, and mantle cell lymphoma. Table 82-3 lists the lymphomas that have been associated with EBV, associated cofactors, viral antigen expression, and an estimate of the percentage of tumors within each lymphoma subtype that harbor viral genomes.

Posttransplantation Lymphoproliferative Disorder

PTLD is a group of lymphoproliferative disorders ranging from polyclonal lymphoid hyperplasia to lymphomas that arise in patients after solid organ or hematopoietic stem cell transplantation (HSCT).[17] PTLD, especially in the first few months after transplantation, is highly associated with EBV (Fig. 82-2, *A, B*). EBV gene expression in PTLD corresponds to latencies 2 and 3.[18] Broad expression of viral proteins is seen only in immunosuppressed hosts, perhaps reflecting that many of these proteins are commonly targeted by cytotoxic T cells.

B cells that harbor EBV are able to proliferate in the setting of posttransplantation immunosuppression at least in part due to decreased T-cell surveillance.[19] HSCT patients that receive grafts that have been T-cell depleted develop EBV-associated PTLD at very high rates. Treatment of rejection in solid organ transplant recipients with agents such as the monoclonal antibody OKT3, which targets $CD3^+$ cells, is associated with markedly increased risk for PTLD.[20] Treatment strategies such as the use of rituximab and infusion of EBV-specific cytotoxic T cells have been quite effective in treating or preventing PTLD (see box on Epstein-Barr Virus-Associated Positive Posttransplant Lymphoproliferative Disorder).

Table 82-3 Epstein-Barr Virus-Associated Lymphoma

Type	Cofactors	Viral Gene Expression	Approximate % EBV Associated	Comment
PTLD	Immunosuppression, allograft	Latency II or III	50-95	Early days/months after transplantation are more commonly associated with EBV
Sporadic BL		Latency I	20 in the United States	Higher in Latin America
Endemic BL	Malaria	Latency I	>95	
AIDS BL	HIV	Latency I	30	
HL		Latency II	30 in the United States	Higher % in mixed cellularity, in males, in Hispanics
AIDS PCNSL	HIV	Latency II or III	>95	
Nasal-type NK cell	More common in Asia	Latency II	>95	
AIDS PEL	HIV and KSHV	Latency I	>75	

AIDS, Acquired immunodeficiency syndrome; *BL,* Burkitt lymphoma; *EBV,* Epstein-Barr virus; *HIV,* human immunodeficiency virus; *HL,* Hodgkin lymphoma; *KSHV,* Kaposi sarcoma–associated herpesvirus; *NK,* natural killer; *PCNSL,* primary central nervous system lymphoma; *PEL,* primary effusion lymphoma; *PTLD,* posttransplantation lymphoproliferative disorder.

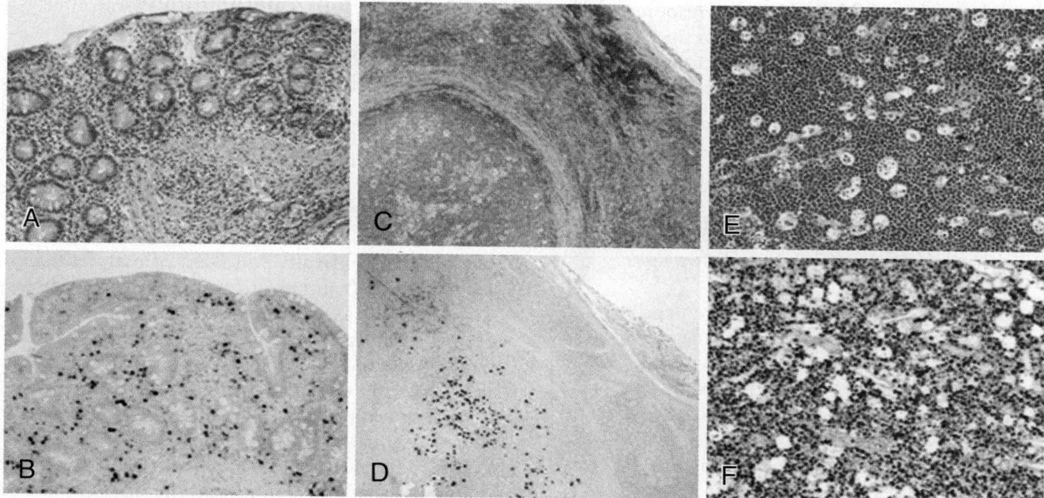

Figure 82-2 EXAMPLES OF EPSTEIN-BARR VIRUS (EBV)–RELATED LYMPHOMAS. Posttransplantation lymphoproliferative disorder (PTLD), polymorphic type, EBV+ occurring in the gastrointestinal tract of a 15-month-old girl following an orthotopic liver transplant (**A** and **B**). There was a mildly atypical lymphocytic infiltrate in the duodenal mucosa composed of small lymphocytes, plasma cells, and occasional large cells (**A**). The infiltrate was EBV+ as demonstrated by in situ hybridization for Epstein-Barr–encoded RNA (EBER) (**B**). Hodgkin lymphoma, nodular sclerosing type, EBV+ (**C** and **D**). The hematoxylin-eosin section shows a portion of a lymph node from a cervical lymph node biopsy of an 8-year-old girl. There are bands of sclerosis forming a cellular nodule, and within the nodule there is a mixed inflammatory infiltrate and scattered large cells with contracted cytoplasm consistent with lacunar cells (**C**). The immunophenotype of these cells was that of classic Hodgkin lymphoma, and the cells were EBER+ (**D**). EBV is seen more frequently in mixed cellularity Hodgkin lymphoma but can be seen in 10% to 40% of cases of nodular sclerosing type. It is even more frequent in cases associated with human immunodeficiency virus (HIV; see text) and in resource-poor regions. Burkitt lymphoma, sporadic type, EBV+ (**E** and **F**). A section of the cervical lymph node biopsy of a 9-year-old girl with a rapidly enlarging neck mass is shown. The section illustrates the classic morphologic features of Burkitt lymphoma with a "starry sky" appearance, sheets of intermediate-sized cells with multiple small nucleoli and high mitotic rate. The cells were virtually all EBER+ (**F**). EBV can be seen in about 20% to 30% of cases of sporadic Burkitt lymphoma and is essentially always positive in endemic cases.

Hodgkin Lymphoma

Approximately 30% of HL tumors in the United States and Europe are EBV associated (Fig. 82-2, *C, D*).[21,22] Epidemiologic studies in Denmark and Sweden suggest that individuals with a history of symptomatic infectious mononucleosis are at increased risk for EBV-associated HL, but not for EBV-negative HL or other lymphomas.[23] The period of risk peaks at about 2 years but continues to be elevated for at least 10 years after symptomatic mononucleosis.

Higher EBV associations are seen in Latin America, Africa, and parts of Asia. Factors associated with EBV tumor positivity include mixed cellularity and lymphocyte-depleted classic HL histologic subtypes, male gender, low socioeconomic background, history of symptomatic infectious mononucleosis, and Hispanic ethnicity.[21,24,25] Organ and hematopoietic stem cell transplant recipients and HIV-positive patients are more likely to develop HL than the general population, and approximately 90% of the tumors are EBV associated.[26]

The EBV gene expression pattern in HL is latency II even when HL occurs in immunocompromised populations.[27] LMP1 and LMP2A may mimic signaling of B-cell receptors and thus protect B cells lacking functional immunoglobulin expression from apoptotic signaling. Approximately 20% of HL lack productive immunoglobulin gene rearrangements. These tumors appear to be exclusively EBV associated.

The EBV association of HL appears not to have prognostic import in young adult patients but is associated with poorer survival in older patients in several reports.[22] Treatment strategies involving adoptive therapy with EBV-specific T cells expanded in vitro are under study.[28]

Burkitt Lymphoma

Endemic BL is nearly 100% associated with EBV, whereas sporadic and HIV-associated BL are much more variably EBV associated (see Table 82-3 and Fig. 82-2, *E, F*).[29] Viral expression is latency I (i.e., EBNA1 is the only viral protein consistently expressed). The defining feature of BL is a translocation between c-Myc on chromosome 8 and one of the immunoglobulin genes on chromosomes 2, 14, or 22. It has been generally presumed that falciparum malaria is a cofactor in endemic BL, and the distribution of BL in Africa corresponds to the distribution of holoendemic malaria. However, little is understood of the pathogenesis or interaction between these infectious cofactors. The characteristic presentation of BL is different in the endemic versus sporadic settings, but there is no evidence to link these presentations specifically with the virus. The virus-tumor association does not guide diagnosis, therapy, or estimation of prognosis at present.

Epstein-Barr Virus-Associated Positive Posttransplant Lymphoproliferative Disorder

A 55-year-old renal transplant patient presents with acute renal failure 5 months after transplant. She is found on imaging to have an obstructing mass in the transplanted kidney. She undergoes kidney biopsy, and Epstein-Barr virus (EBV)–positive posttransplant lymphoproliferative disorder (PTLD) involving the transplanted organ is diagnosed. Treatment options include rituximab; decreasing immunosuppression (acknowledging the associated risk for organ rejection); changing immunosuppressive agents—switching a calcineurin inhibitor for a mammalian target of rapamycin (mTOR) inhibitor; combination chemotherapy; or, in the case of renal transplant, removal of the transplanted organ and withdrawal of immunosuppression.

Diffuse Large B-cell Lymphoma Associated With Chronic Inflammation

EBV-associated lymphomas sometimes arise in the setting of long-standing chronic inflammation.[15] This was first described in Japanese patients with a remote history of pulmonary tuberculosis treated with thoracoplasty with resulting chronic pyothorax, although many more cases have since been reported. These patients developed EBV-associated DLBCL of the pleural lining and associated lung tissue decades after thoracoplasty. Similar cases of aggressive, EBV-associated B-cell lymphomas have been reported to arise in patients at the sites of chronic inflammation associated with various implants, surgical mesh, or in the lung after chronic empyema.

KAPOSI SARCOMA–ASSOCIATED HERPESVIRUS

Virus and Tumor Epidemiology

KSHV (HHV-8) is a gammaherpesvirus that, unlike EBV, has a low prevalence worldwide.[30] The virus is endemic in certain areas, such as in sub-Saharan Africa and the Middle East, and has an intermediate prevalence in Mediterranean countries. Transmission is believed to be predominately through saliva. Similar to EBV, KSHV latently infects B cells; viral genes that promote cell survival are implicated in lymphomagenesis.

KSHV was discovered in Kaposi sarcoma but is also present in two lymphoproliferative diseases: primary effusion lymphoma (PEL) (Fig. 82-3, *A, B*) and multicentric Castleman disease (MCD).[16,31] PEL occurs almost exclusively in HIV-positive patients, particularly in men who have sex with men, and typically when CD4 counts are less than 100/mm^3. PELs are usually dually infected with KSHV and EBV, but KSHV is always present. KSHV-associated MCD, although much more common in HIV-infected populations, also occurs in the general population.

MCD is a KSHV-associated, immunoglobulin M (IgM) λ–producing nonclonal lymphoproliferative disorder typically involving the mantle zone of lymph nodes and the spleen. The KSHV-positive cells in MCD are always EBV negative. These cells express a broad range of KSHV lytic antigens, and high KSHV copy numbers are reported in plasma. Evolution into or coassociation with an aggressive lymphoma, often of plasmablastic phenotype, is not uncommon.

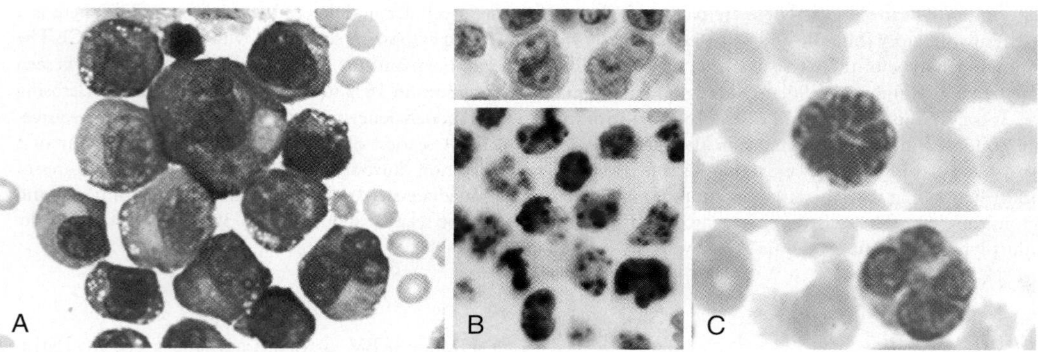

Figure 82-3 EXAMPLES OF KSHV- AND HTLV-1-ASSOCIATED LYMPHOPROLIFERATIVE DISEASE. Primary effusion lymphoma (**A** and **B**). **A,** The pleural tap had a high cell count, and the cytospin preparation revealed a markedly pleomorphic cell population with large and giant cells with deep-blue cytoplasm. **B,** A cell block was prepared *(top)* so that in situ hybridization studies could be performed. These studies showed the cells to be KSHV+ by immunohistochemistry for latency associated nuclear antigen-1 (LANA-1) *(bottom)* and EBV+ by EBER in situ hybridization (not shown). **C,** Adult T-cell leukemia/lymphoma in a patient who was HTLV-1+. The peripheral smear showed the classic "flower" cells. *EBER,* Epstein-Barr–encoded RNA; *HTLV-1,* human T-lymphotropic virus-1; *KSHV,* Kaposi sarcoma–associated herpesvirus. *(**A** and **B** courtesy Dr. Elizabeth Hyjek, University of Chicago.)*

Within the HIV population, nearly all cases of MCD are KSHV associated; this viral association is not as strong among HIV-negative MCD patients. High expression of viral interleukin-6 (vIL-6) is thought to contribute to the systemic inflammation seen in this disorder.[32] The KSHV-associated lymphomas that arise in association with MCD are not nodal equivalents of PEL; rather these plasmablastic lymphomas are uniformly EBV negative and express IgM λ.[16]

Diagnostic and Therapeutic Considerations

The requisite finding in PEL is a lymphomatous effusion, which can be pleural, pericardial, or peritoneal, without associated lymphadenopathy or masses, arising in the setting of immunocompromise. Often, patients with HIV/AIDS will present with PEL in addition to other KSHV-associated diseases, such as Kaposi sarcoma and MCD, so thorough evaluation and staging should be undertaken at diagnosis. On cytologic examination, the PEL tumor cells are large with prominent nucleoli. The effusion cells are clonal B cells with CD45 positivity but typically lack other specific B-cell lineage markers, although CD30 and CD38 positivity can be seen. BCL6 mutations are frequently detected. Tumor cells always harbor KSHV as demonstrated by staining for KSHV-associated latency-associated nuclear antigen-1 (LANA-1). In MCD there is characteristically λ light chain restriction.[33] This does not reflect clonality as assessed by study of Ig DNA rearrangements. Rather it reflects a tendency for the virus to selectively infect cells expressing λ or to selectively drive such cells to proliferate.

Treatment of PEL is most commonly combination chemotherapy. Outcomes remain quite poor. Treatment of MCD with targeted therapies has been more successful, including the use of rituximab and IL-6 inhibition.[34,35] Antivirals such as ganciclovir and valganciclovir have shown clinical activity in MCD, because viral lytic replication is a feature of this disease.[36]

HUMAN T-LYMPHOTROPIC VIRUS-1

Viral Biology

HTLV-1 is a retrovirus with a single-stranded RNA genome.[37,38] Following infection there is reverse transcription and integration of proviral DNA into the host genome. HTLV-1 infects a variety of cell types but persists in CD4⁺ T lymphocytes. Viral infection within the host is spread from cell to cell through direct cell-to-cell contact. As with EBV, the proliferation of HTLV-1–infected lymphocytes plays a central role in ensuring viral persistence.

The HTLV-1 protein Tax plays a central role in T-lymphocyte immortalization and transformation (Fig. 82-4).[37,39] Tax affects NFκB and the serine/threonine kinase AKT pathways with diverse proliferative and antiapoptotic effects. As with some of the immunodominant EBV antigens expressed in proliferating lymphocytes, Tax expression is targeted by cytotoxic T cells. Another viral protein, Hbz, suppresses Tax expression, allowing transformed T cells to elude immune surveillance.[40] Tax interferes with various DNA repair pathways and induces reactive oxygen species, facilitating the development of aneuploidy.[37,39] Tax leads to functional inactivation of p53 and may interfere with the spindle assembly checkpoint that normally operates in mitosis to preserve euploidy.

Epidemiology of Viral Infection and Adult T-Cell Leukemia/Lymphoma

HTLV-1 is endemic in particular regions of Japan, Africa, South America, and some Caribbean islands.[40,41] As assessed by seroprevalence, rates up to 37% are found on the southwestern Japanese islands of Shikoku, Kyushu, and Okinawa, whereas most other areas of Japan have an intermediate prevalence of 1% to 5%. In the United States

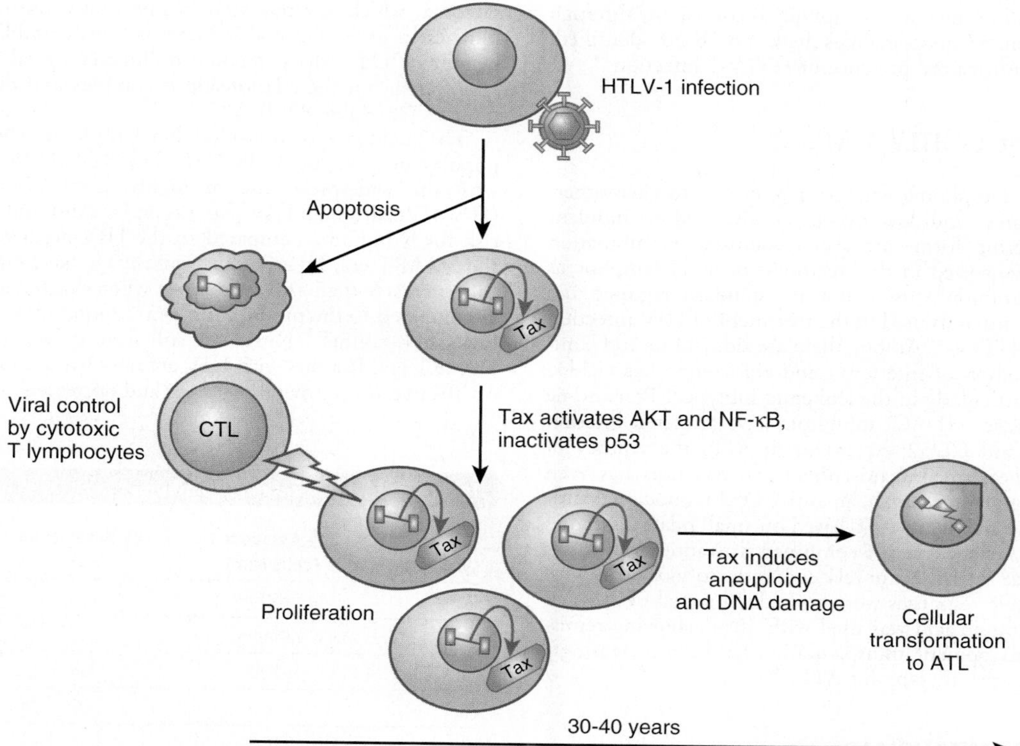

Figure 82-4 HTLV-1 AND THE EVOLUTION OF ADULT T-CELL LEUKEMIA/LYMPHOMA. Following HTLV-1 infection, many cells undergo apoptosis, but some infected CD4⁺ T cells are driven to proliferate by the effects of Tax on the nuclear factor kappa-B (NFκB) pathway and on the AKT pathway. Tax is also suggested to result in inactivation of p53, aneuploidy, and deoxyribonucleic acid (DNA) damage. Over many decades malignancy evolves. *HTLV-1,* Human T-lymphotropic virus-1.

the incidence in blood donors is 0.025%. It has been estimated that about 20 million individuals are infected worldwide. The major mode of transmission in endemic areas is from mother to child in breast milk, although infection is also transmitted through sexual intercourse, transfusion of cellular blood products, and the sharing of needles and syringes. Evidence has been presented that HTLV-1 infection persists in association with certain human leukocyte antigen (HLA) types and may be more readily transmitted from mother to child when these HLA types are shared.

ATL is more common in men than in women and typically presents in the fourth or fifth decade of life. Perhaps as a function of the long latency period, cases of ATL following blood transfusion or needle sharing are vanishingly rare. The lifetime risk for ATL has been estimated to be in excess of 6% in men who are HTLV-1 carriers in an endemic region of Japan, although in other settings the risk may be much lower.[42] As with EBV, the subset of the infected population that develops lymphoma is quite small.

Adult T-Cell Leukemia/Lymphoma Diagnostic Considerations

There is a spectrum of HTLV-1–associated leukemia/lymphoma.[38] Twenty percent of ATL cases present with a lymphomatous subtype dominated by lymphadenopathy and hepatosplenomegaly. Cutaneous infiltration, lytic bone lesions, malignant effusions, and involvement of the CNS and other extranodal sites are not uncommon.[40] Hypercalcemia is common, particularly in leukemic forms. Presentations reflecting immune dysfunction such as strongyloidiasis with dissemination, *Pneumocystis jiroveci* pneumonia (PJP), mycobacterium, or cryptococcal infection are common. In the leukemic subtype of ATL, the classic findings on peripheral blood smear are lymphocytes with flower-shaped nuclei (Fig. 82-3, *C*).

Histologically ATL shows lymph node effacement by large, atypical T cells usually expressing CD4$^+$, CD25$^+$, and CD52$^+$, with variable CD30 and CD15 expression. Aneuploidy is consistent, although characteristic cytogenetic abnormalities have not been identified. Serologic analysis confirms the presence of HTLV-1 infection.[38]

Therapies Specific to HTLV-1 ATL

ATL is an aggressive lymphoma with poor responses to chemotherapy, high relapse rates, and low overall survival. More indolent chronic and smoldering forms are also recognized. Combination chemotherapy regimens used in the treatment of other lymphomas or leukemias are commonly used, but no standard regimen has emerged.[38,43] Several antivirals used in the treatment of HIV infection have activity against HTLV-1. Among them are zidovudine and lamivudine. The combination of interferon and zidovudine has yielded promising results, particularly in the leukemic subtype.[38] Proteasome and histone deacetylase (HDAC) inhibitors have attracted interest. Given high CD25 and CD52 expression in ATL, the efficacy of monoclonal antibodies aimed against these two receptors has been investigated. Thus far alemtuzumab, an anti-CD52 monoclonal antibody, may have some activity in ATL based on small phase II studies and case reports.[44,45] Arsenic trioxide combined with interferon-α has been shown to induce remissions in relapsed, refractory patients with ATL, although durable responses were limited. In a trial of 20 ATL patients, all-trans retinoic acid was used with 40% achieving remission. Allogeneic hematopoietic transplantation has been increasingly recognized as an effective therapy for ATL.[46,47]

HIV-ASSOCIATED LYMPHOMAS

Viral Biology and Pathogenesis

HIV-1 is a retrovirus that infects CD4$^+$ T cells and monocytes.[48,49] It appears to establish a lifelong reservoir in CD4$^+$ T cells.[50] Viral infection may lead to cell death or establishment of latency in resting cells. HIV infection is spread either through new rounds of virion production with cellular infection or cell-cell fusion. There is no evidence to suggest that infected cells are driven to proliferate. This is in contrast to HTLV-1 and EBV, where proliferation of infected cells appears to play a key role in establishing the long-term viral reservoir and perhaps in mediating lymphomagenesis. The lymphomas that are increased in HIV-infected patients (Table 82-4) are of B-cell lineage, and there is no substantial evidence that HIV infection of B cells is important in the pathogenesis of these lymphomas. Rather it appears that the HIV infection compromises cellular immunity, decreasing immune surveillance of EBV- and KSHV-infected B cells. In addition, HIV infection stimulates proliferation of B lymphocytes and perhaps genetic aberrations in the proliferating cells.[51] Many possible mechanisms have been invoked, including (1) direct stimulation of B cells by HIV antigens or antigens associated with opportunistic infection; (2) stimulation of B cells by cellular proteins (CD40 ligand) incorporated into the HIV virion leading to expression of activation-induced deaminase, an enzyme that mediates double-strand DNA breaks; and (3) dysregulation of B cells as a consequence of T-cell dysfunction.[16,51,52]

There is also some evidence that host biology may contribute to lymphomagenesis. In particular, there are a variety of genetic polymorphisms that influence susceptibility to HIV-1 infection, such as CCR5-Δ32.[53,54] Individuals who are homozygous for this polymorphism are much less likely to be infected by HIV than others. Some evidence has emerged to suggest that in heterozygotes who are infected, HIV progression is slowed and there is less likelihood of lymphomagenesis. Many of these lymphomas are associated with EBV, KSHV, or both (see Table 82-4).

Epidemiology

Lymphoma is increased in all HIV risk groups, in contrast to Kaposi sarcoma, which is rarely seen in injection drug users (or in hemophiliacs in an earlier era).[55] There is a well-established relationship between CD4$^+$ cells per cubic millimeter overall and the risk for lymphoma, but the relationship is complex and differs among lymphomas (see Table 82-4).

The incidence of non-Hodgkin lymphoma (NHL) in the HIV population, particularly PCNSL (Fig. 82-5, *A* to *C*), has decreased with the widespread use of highly active antiretroviral therapy (HAART), although HIV patients on HAART still carry an increased risk for lymphoma compared to the HIV-negative population.[55] In the HAART era, HIV patients on average have higher CD4$^+$ counts (often greater than 100 cells/mm^3) when diagnosed with lymphoma as compared to the pre-HAART era. Among HIV patients with very low CD4$^+$ counts,[56] NHLs are still seen at rates similar to the pre-HAART era. Patients with HIV are now living much longer because of effective antiretroviral regimens and decreased rates of opportunis-

Table 82-4 HIV-Associated Lymphoma

Lymphoma	CD4 Association (cells/mm^3)	EBV Association (%)	Other Cofactors
PCNSL	<50	>95	
DLBCL	Variable	40	
BL	>100	30	
HL	>100	90	
PEL	<100	>75	KSHV

BL, Burkitt lymphoma; *DLBCL*, diffuse large B-cell lymphoma; *EBV*, Epstein-Barr virus; *HIV*, human immunodeficiency virus; *HL*, Hodgkin lymphoma; *KSHV*, Kaposi sarcoma–associated herpesvirus; *PCNSL*, primary central nervous system lymphoma; *PEL*, primary effusion lymphoma.

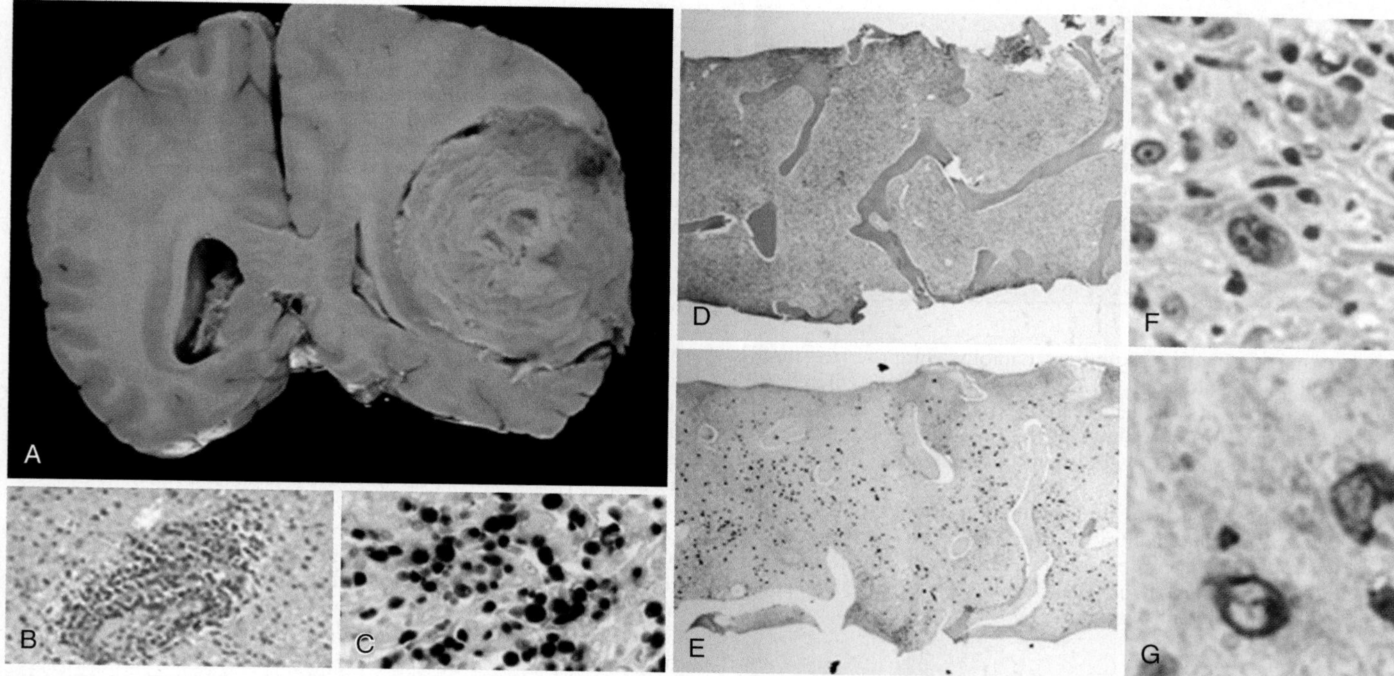

Figure 82-5 EXAMPLES OF HUMAN IMMUNODEFICIENCY VIRUS (HIV)–RELATED LYMPHOMAS. Primary central nervous system (CNS) lymphoma in HIV+ patients (**A** to **C**). Gross appearance (coronal section) of the brain from an autopsy of a 24-year-old HIV+ female patient with temporo-parietal mass due to a primary CNS lymphoma (**A**). The patient died from uncal and cingulate herniation. Biopsy section from another patient showing a perivascular infiltrate of large lymphoma cells. This is the typical pattern of involvement by CNS lymphoma (**B**). The cells were shown to be $CD20^+$ B cells and were EBER+ (**C**). A diagnosis can be made without biopsy when magnetic resonance imaging studies show characteristic features and EBV is demonstrated in the cerebrospinal fluid by polymerase chain reaction (see box on AIDS Primary Central Nervous System Lymphoma). Hodgkin lymphoma extensively involving the bone marrow in an HIV+ patient with stage IVB disease (**D** to **G**). The bone marrow biopsy was entirely replaced with Hodgkin lymphoma associated with dense sclerosis (**D**). An EBER study shows scattered positive cells throughout the marrow (**E**), corresponding to the Hodgkin and Reed-Sternberg cells (**F**), which were $CD30^+$ as illustrated (**G**). Hodgkin lymphoma infrequently involves the bone marrow in HIV-negative cases but some HIV+ patients can first present with extensive bone marrow disease (see box on HIV Hodgkin Lymphoma). *(**A** courtesy Dr. Peter Pytel, University of Chicago.)*

HIV Hodgkin Lymphoma

A 42-year-old human immunodeficiency virus (HIV)–positive patient, on highly active antiretroviral therapy (HAART) with a CD4 count of 324 cells/mm^3 and undetectable viral load, presents with fever, weight loss, and a palpable axillary lymph node. Hodgkin lymphoma (HL) is diagnosed on excisional biopsy, and Epstein-Barr virus (EBV) positivity is demonstrated by Epstein-Barr–encoded RNA (EBER) in the Reed-Sternberg tumor cells. Although he lacks additional lymphadenopathy, a bone marrow biopsy is performed, and it shows involvement by HL. He has stage IVB disease. *Pneumocystis jiroveci* pneumonia prophylaxis is started despite adequate CD4 count in anticipation of chemotherapy. His HAART regimen is reviewed for potential antiviral-chemotherapy drug interactions. He receives six cycles of full-dose, first-line chemotherapy and achieves a complete remission.

tic infection. As a result, malignancy has emerged as the major cause of mortality in HIV populations with access to antiretroviral therapy.[57,58]

With the widespread use of HAART, the incidence of HL in HIV-seropositive patients has not declined; patients with $CD4^+$ counts between 150 and 199 cells/mm^3 actually have higher risk for HIV-associated HL than patients with $CD4^+$ counts of less than 50 cells/mm^3.[3,59]

Diagnostic Considerations Specific to Lymphoma in Patients With HIV

Lymphomas in HIV-infected patients are more likely to present with B symptoms such as fever and night sweats, and advanced stage, including bone marrow, extranodal, and CNS involvement. Thus the approach to diagnosis is somewhat different than the approach in the HIV-negative patient.

Unexplained fever and sweats in an HIV-seropositive patient, even in the absence of lymphadenopathy, are sufficient to warrant consideration of HL. Patterns of disease involvement also differ in HIV-infected patients. Contiguous spread so characteristic of classic HL in other settings is less common in HIV HL. Bone marrow–only presentations of HL are not uncommon (Fig. 82-5, *D* to *G*), and the possibility of HL should be in the differential diagnosis even in the absence of lymphadenopathy.

Patients with HIV-associated NHL have higher rates of extranodal involvement, including bone marrow and CNS disease, as well as higher stage disease and more aggressive tumors on average.[72] Therefore it is recommended that all HIV-seropositive patients with aggressive NHL undergo a diagnostic lumbar puncture. The routine use of CNS intrathecal chemotherapy prophylaxis in all HIV-seropositive NHL patients is controversial but reasonable and typically done in particularly high-risk patients, such as those with BL, marrow or testicular involvement, or extranodal disease.

Imaging is often more difficult to interpret in HIV patients than in other settings. Lymphadenopathy associated with HIV infection or opportunistic infection is common, and the presumption that enlarged lymph nodes reflect the presence of lymphoma in patients with known lymphoma or history of lymphoma is not as safe as in

> **AIDS Primary Central Nervous System Lymphoma**
>
> In acquired immunodeficiency syndrome (AIDS) primary central nervous system lymphoma (PCNSL), Epstein-Barr virus (EBV) polymerase chain reaction of the cerebrospinal fluid is positive approximately 90% of the time and rarely positive in patients with AIDS but without PCNSL. When EBV is detected in the cerebrospinal fluid of an AIDS patient, coupled with characteristic magnetic resonance imaging findings, this is sufficient to diagnose AIDS PCNSL without a confirmatory brain biopsy.

other settings. Positron emission tomography–computerized tomography (PET-CT), although useful, must also be interpreted with caution insofar as HIV infection itself, opportunistic infection, and immune reconstitution following the initiation of antiretroviral therapy are all associated with signal on metabolic imaging with fluorodeoxyglucose.

$CD4^+$ counts can help to guide evaluation insofar as $CD4^+$ counts of greater than 300 cells/mm^3 are typically associated with BL or HL,[60] whereas these diagnoses would be unlikely in patients with very low $CD4^+$ counts of less than 50 cells/mm^3 (see box on AIDS Primary Central Nervous System Lymphoma).[61]

Treatment

Aggressive chemotherapy for HIV-associated lymphoma was initially associated with morbidity and mortality related to immunocompromise. A phase III randomized study identified a reduced-dose regimen as preferable to standard dose.[63] Lower doses were not associated with higher lymphoma cure rates but were associated with less chemotherapy-related morbidity and mortality. However, with the evolution of supportive care, including PJP prophylaxis and neutrophil growth factors, tolerance of chemotherapy improved. With effective antiretroviral therapy, long-term outcomes improved as well.[64,65] And with full-dose therapies, some evidence emerged to suggest that stage-for-stage outcomes might be as good or better in patients with HIV-associated lymphoma compared to those without HIV.[66] At the outset of therapy a series of questions must be addressed.

Regimen

Rituximab, cyclophosphamide, hydroxydaunomycin, vincristine, and prednisone (R-CHOP); and rituximab, infusional etoposide, prednisone, vincristine, cyclophosphamide, and hydroxydaunomycin (R-EPOCH) have emerged as standard regimens.[67,68] As in the treatment of DLBCL in patients without HIV infection, the value of infusional chemotherapy remains controversial. A recent pooled retrospective analysis favored the infusional regimen.[69] However, insofar as the trials were conducted sequentially (R-CHOP between 1998 and 2002, and R-EPOCH between 2002 and 2006), it is difficult to exclude other factors such as the availability of better antiretroviral agents, improvements in supportive care, or changes in the population studied. However, there is general agreement that rituximab improves outcome, at least in patients with $CD4^+$ counts of greater than 50 cells/mm^3.

BL typically requires more intensive treatment regimens than those used for DLBCL.[70] Thus there has been concern about using these regimens in the HIV-seropositive population. A small retrospective study of cyclophosphamide, vincristine (Oncovin), doxorubicin, and methotrexate (CODOX-M)/ifosfamide, etoposide, and cytarabine (IVAC) for BL that included 14 patients with HIV showed HIV-seropositive patients to have similar progression-free survival, overall survival, and complete response rates as compared to the HIV-negative BL patients. In a prospective Spanish study, HIV-seropositive and HIV-seronegative BL patients were treated with six cycles of intensive chemotherapy and rituximab and were found to have comparable outcomes regardless of HIV status.[71] In this study all HIV-seropositive patients were required to be on HAART to enroll, and the majority had $CD4^+$ counts of greater than 200 cells/mm^3. Granulocyte colony-stimulating factor support was used throughout chemotherapy cycles, as well as PJP and other antimicrobial prophylaxis. Differences in induction-related mortality, duration of neutropenia, progression-free survival, or overall survival were not detected, although HIV-seropositive patients did have significantly more severe mucositis and infectious complications.

Dose

Most would agree that dose reduction is appropriate in patients with low $CD4^+$ count (<100 cells/mm^3), history of ongoing opportunistic infection, performance status below 75%, or compromised organ function. Some regimens begin with a 50% dose reduction in cyclophosphamide dose for $CD4^+$ count of less than 100 cells/mm^3 with a built-in dose escalation for the next cycle if well tolerated.[64,68]

Chemotherapy regimens of varying intensity depending on $CD4^+$ count, performance status, and International Prognostic Index score have been studied, including a comparison of low-dose CHOP to standard-dose CHOP, with no differences found in overall survival based on the intensity of the chemotherapy regimen.[66] In patients with very low $CD4^+$ counts, low-dose chemotherapy is a reasonable treatment option, while maintaining the possibility of long-term disease-free survival in some.

Antiretroviral Therapy

A few key special issues in considering concurrent antiretroviral and lymphoma therapy include concerns about shared toxicities, drug-drug interactions, and risk for inability to comply with consistent antiretroviral dosing. Zidovudine is myelosuppressive and can exacerbate pancytopenia associated with lymphoma therapy. If patients are already on a zidovudine-containing regimen, it is generally possible to substitute an alternative regimen before the initiation of lymphoma therapy. Many antiretroviral agents alter the metabolism of drugs used in lymphoma treatment. This has been a particular concern when infusional chemotherapy regimens are used, and some investigators have chosen to stop chemotherapy before initiation of such regimens.[64] However, in trials involving infusional chemotherapy that allowed patients already on a stable antiretroviral regimen to remain on that regimen during lymphoma treatment, major problems were not noted.[68] Nausea and vomiting associated with chemotherapy regimens may interfere with regular antiviral dosing. Intermittent antiretroviral therapy raises concerns about the development of a resistant strain of HIV. Because of the concern that initiation of antiretroviral therapy with cytotoxic chemotherapy might result in such resistance, many recommend delaying initiation of antiretroviral therapy until an appropriate regimen to control nausea and vomiting is established. Stopping antiretroviral therapy also carries with it some risks. When antiretroviral therapy includes drugs with different half-lives, stopping treatment may result in the longest-lived agent being present in the absence of other antiretroviral agents. This is particularly an issue for long-lived nonnucleoside reverse transcriptase inhibitors. Even a single dose of such agents in the absence of other antiretroviral agents may lead to resistance to that class of agents. Thus when an interruption of antiretroviral therapy is planned, specific strategies have been advocated, including a "staggered stop" or a change to a regimen with components that have similar half-lives.[62]

For patients already on antiretroviral treatment at the time of lymphoma diagnosis, the particulars of the regimen should be considered during the pretreatment evaluation. Atazanavir and indinavir are associated with hyperbilirubinemia as a result of UGT1A1 inhibition.[62] This is an unconjugated hyperbilirubinemia similar to that occurring with Gilbert syndrome. Elevated total bilirubin in such patients is not indicative of hepatic involvement or other serious hepatic dysfunction and should not guide decisions about chemotherapy dose adjustments. Ritonavir inhibits the clearance of midazolam, phenytoin, and voriconazole and other agents metabolized by the cytochrome P-450 CYP3A4 pathway.

Supportive Care

Although PJP prophylaxis is recommended only when the CD4+ count is less than 200 cells/mm³ for HIV patients not receiving cytotoxic chemotherapy, prophylaxis is universally recommended for HIV patients receiving cytotoxic chemotherapy. The following are also commonly used: fungal prophylaxis with fluconazole; herpes simplex and varicella prophylaxis with acyclovir, valacyclovir, or famciclovir; quinolone prophylaxis when neutrophil counts fall below 1000 cells/mm³; and granulocyte growth factors.

Bone Marrow Transplantation in HIV Patients

Autologous bone marrow transplant has been successful in HIV-seropositive NHL patients, with these patients having adequate stem cell mobilization, nonrelapse mortality rates comparable to those for HIV-negative patients, count recovery within 2 weeks of stem cell rescue, and maintained control of HIV viral loads and CD4+ counts after high-dose chemotherapy.[73,74] There have also been successful reduced-intensity allogeneic bone marrow transplants in HIV-seropositive patients, making the possibilities for treating HIV patients with NHL even more vast, even in those patients with chemotherapy-resistant disease (see box on Autologous Bone Marrow Transplant in an HIV-Seropositive Hodgkin Lymphoma Patient).[75]

HEPATITIS C VIRUS

Viral Biology and B-Lymphocyte Proliferation

HCV is an enveloped positive-strand RNA virus.[76,77] Infection involves interactions between E2, a viral structural protein with two hypervariable regions, and a cellular protein CD81 present on hepatocytes and B lymphocytes. A polyprotein is translated from viral RNA and is cleaved by cellular and viral proteases, including NS3, to yield proteins required for viral replication. The RNA-dependent RNA polymerase that replicates the viral genome lacks proofreading capacity, thus generating genetic heterogeneity among viral progeny. Viral replication occurs predominantly in the liver, but some evidence suggests that B cells may also be infected.

Chronic infection can be associated with mixed cryoglobulinemia, a systemic vasculitis that results from clonal expansion of B cells producing an IgM autoantibody against IgG, leading to deposition of immune complexes on endothelial surfaces, resulting in inflammation.[78] Several hypotheses have been advanced with regard to how HCV might drive B-cell proliferation. There is controversy as to whether infection of B cells plays any role in this process. A lymphoma cell line that produces infectious HCV has been reported. Even in the absence of infection of B cells, interaction of the HCV E2 protein with CD81 on B cells may drive B-cell proliferation or lower the threshold for other B-cell stimuli to drive proliferation. Ig signaling may be activated by Ig-virus complexes, and Toll-like receptor 7 signaling may be activated by viral RNA. Finally, it is noted that E2 binding triggers expression of activation-induced deaminase, an enzyme that is important in generating somatic hypermutation and that has also been implicated in mediating mutations thought to play a role in DLBCL lymphomagenesis.[77]

Autologous Bone Marrow Transplant in an HIV-Seropositive Hodgkin Lymphoma Patient

A 38-year-old human immunodeficiency virus (HIV)–positive patient with CD4+ count of 485 cells/mm³ is diagnosed with classic Hodgkin lymphoma (HL) and treated with doxorubicin (Adriamycin), bleomycin, vinblastine, and dacarbazine (ABVD), achieving a complete remission. Two years later he presents with retroperitoneal lymphadenopathy and is found on biopsy to have relapsed HL. He is treated with salvage chemotherapy with complete response, as well as good performance status and no active infections. His HIV remains well controlled on antiretroviral therapy. He is deemed an excellent candidate for high-dose therapy and undergoes consolidation with autologous bone marrow transplant.

Epidemiology of Viral Infection and Associated Lymphoma

The association between HCV and lymphoma was first recognized in patients with HCV-associated type II mixed cryoglobulinemia, an autoimmune extrahepatic manifestation of HCV infection.[79] There followed demonstration of an increased risk for certain subtypes of B-cell lymphoma (marginal zone lymphoma [MZL], lymphoplasmacytic lymphoma and to a lesser extent DLBCL in HCV-infected patients).[80-83] For example, in Taiwan the rate of chronic HCV infection in patients with NHL was 11%, 10-fold higher than in the general Taiwanese population.[84] Among HCV-infected patients with lymphoma, nodal and splenic MZL, but not mucosa-associated lymphoid tissue (MALT) lymphomas, were increased. The HCV-lymphoma association is more apparent in some countries than others, with the association being established most clearly in Italy and Japan. A multitude of studies in regions or countries where HCV infection is less prevalent have failed to identify any association with lymphoma.[85-87]

Further evidence in support of an etiologic relationship comes from studies in which successful treatment of HCV was followed by lymphoma regression.[88] The most dramatic illustration comes from patients with splenic lymphoma with villous lymphocytes treated with ribavirin and interferon.

Certain HCV genotypes may confer increased risk for NHL, with genotypes 2a/III and 2b/IV seen more frequently in the HCV-seropositive patients that develop NHL.

Diagnostic Considerations

In contrast to EBV-, KSHV-, or HTLV-1–associated tumors, there is no established role for studies demonstrating HCV nucleic acid or protein in tumor cells. Thus serologic study and measurement of HCV copy number are the only tools available for inferring an association. We recommend checking HCV serologic characteristics in all patients with B-cell lymphomas most commonly associated with chronic HCV infection.[89] In addition, screening patients with chronic HCV for a monoclonal gammopathy and cryoglobulinemia may be of benefit to identify patients at highest risk for malignant transformation. Elevated serum γ-globulin levels have been found to be a predictor of NHL among patients with type II mixed cryoglobulinemia.[90] In patients who are HCV seropositive, we evaluate HCV RNA in plasma.

Therapy

In patients with indolent lymphomas and untreated HCV infection, antiviral treatment may obviate the need for cytotoxic chemotherapy and should be considered as an initial therapeutic strategy. The studies showing that antiviral therapy may lead to regression of HCV-associated lymphomas involved treatment with ribavirin and interferon. In the last year new antiviral agents have become available, notably protease inhibitors specific for the HCV protease. Likelihood of response to older therapy is a function of viral genotype, host genetics (IL28R polymorphisms play a critical role in response to protease inhibitors) and other factors. The field is rapidly evolving, and colleagues with specific expertise in appropriate antiviral approaches should be consulted.[76]

Rituximab has posed an interesting dilemma for the treatment of patients with HCV and lymphoma. It has been reported that HCV plasma RNA increases following rituximab treatment, and there is certainly the possibility that elimination of B cells for 3 to 18 months following treatment may compromise humoral responses to the evolution of HCV quasispecies. However, in studies to date overall survival is not inferior.[91] Similarly, combination chemotherapy is safe in patients with HCV infection.[92] Rituximab is specifically recommended for the treatment of HCV-associated cryoglobulinemia (although as in the treatment of Waldenström macroglobulinemia, it must be appreciated that the initial response to rituximab may be an increase in the IgM paraprotein level, necessitating plasmapheresis).

Aspects of Therapy

With regards to the use of rituximab to treat B-cell lymphomas in patients with HCV, overall survival is not inferior, although there do appear to be increased rates of hepatotoxicity and rises in HCV viral load during therapy. Similarly, combination chemotherapy is safe in patients with HCV infection, although HCV RNA levels can rise during treatment. Interestingly, patients with HCV and splenic MZL have had regression of their tumors with treatment for HCV infection with interferon-α and ribavirin, an effect not seen in HCV-negative patients with splenic MZL treated with the same regimen.

FUTURE DIRECTIONS

In this chapter a variety of virus-associated lymphomas and lymphoproliferative diseases have been reviewed. For most of these lymphomas, standard antiviral drugs do not have a role in treatment. There are, however, several exceptions, and these are worth highlighting. Antiviral therapy for HCV-associated splenic lymphoma with villous lymphocytes is accepted as a standard approach and likely has a role in the treatment of other HCV-associated indolent lymphomas. Similarly, ganciclovir or valganciclovir appears to have a role in the management of MCD associated with KSHV in HIV patients. And of course there is an established role for antiretroviral therapy in the treatment of HIV patients with malignancy. There are virus-targeted therapies that are broadly accepted as standard, including adoptive immunotherapy with EBV-specific T cells for PTLD. The use of targeted T cells also has promise in other settings, including EBV-associated HL. Other virus-targeted therapies are being developed. Some involve vaccination; others involve induction of viral genes in tumor cells, rendering them more susceptible to pharmacologic treatment. Finally, it may ultimately be possible to prevent some kinds of lymphoma by preventing viral infection or altering the host response to viral infection.

SUGGESTED READINGS

Balsalobre P, Diez-Martin JL, Re A, et al: Autologous stem-cell transplantation in patients with HIV-related lymphoma. *J Clin Oncol* 27:2192, 2009.

Barta SK, Lee JY, Kaplan LD, et al: Pooled analysis of AIDS malignancy consortium trials evaluating rituximab plus CHOP or infusional EPOCH chemotherapy in HIV-associated non-Hodgkin lymphoma. *Cancer* doi: 10.1002/cncr.26723. [Epub ahead of print], 2011.

Bazarbachi A, Suarez F, Fields P, et al: How I treat adult T-cell leukemia/lymphoma. *Blood* 118:1736, 2011.

Bower M, Newsom-Davis T, Naresh K, et al: Clinical features and outcome in HIV-associated multicentric Castleman's disease. *J Clin Oncol* 29:2481, 2011.

Carbone A, Cesarman E, Spina M, et al: HIV-associated lymphomas and gamma-herpesviruses. *Blood* 113:1213, 2009.

Choi I, Tanosaki R, Uike N, et al: Long-term outcomes after hematopoietic SCT for adult T-cell leukemia/lymphoma: Results of prospective trials. *Bone Marrow Transplant* 46:116, 2011.

Chuang SS, Liao YL, Chang ST, et al: Hepatitis C virus infection is significantly associated with malignant lymphoma in Taiwan, particularly with nodal and splenic marginal zone lymphomas. *J Clin Pathol* 63:595, 2010.

Engels EA, Pfeiffer RM, Landgren O, et al: Immunologic and virologic predictors of AIDS-related non-Hodgkin lymphoma in the highly active antiretroviral therapy era. *J Acquir Immune Defic Syndr* 54:78, 2010.

Epeldegui M, Hung YP, McQuay A, et al: Infection of human B cells with Epstein-Barr virus results in the expression of somatic hypermutation-inducing molecules and in the accrual of oncogene mutations. *Mol Immunol* 44:934, 2007.

Evens AM, Roy R, Sterrenberg D, et al: Post-transplantation lymphoproliferative disorders: Diagnosis, prognosis, and current approaches to therapy. *Curr Oncol Rep* 12:383, 2010.

Giordano TP, Henderson L, Landgren O, et al: Risk of non-Hodgkin lymphoma and lymphoproliferative precursor diseases in US veterans with hepatitis C virus. *JAMA* 297:2010, 2007.

Guech-Ongey M, Simard EP, Anderson WF, et al: AIDS-related Burkitt lymphoma in the United States: What do age and CD4 lymphocyte patterns tell us about etiology and/or biology? *Blood* 116:5600, 2010.

Heslop HE, Slobod KS, Pule MA, et al: Long-term outcome of EBV-specific T-cell infusions to prevent or treat EBV-related lymphoproliferative disease in transplant recipients. *Blood* 115:925, 2010.

Hishizawa M, Kanda J, Utsunomiya A, et al: Transplantation of allogeneic hematopoietic stem cells for adult T-cell leukemia: A nationwide retrospective study. *Blood* 116:1369, 2010.

Ito M, Kusunoki H, Mochida K, et al: HCV infection and B-cell lymphomagenesis. *Adv Hematol* 2011:835314, 2011.

Jaffe ES, Campo E, Swerdlow SH, et al: The 2008 WHO classification of lymphoid neoplasms and beyond: Evolving concepts and practical applications. *Blood* 117:5019, 2011.

Keegan TH, Glaser SL, Clarke CA, et al: Epstein-Barr virus as a marker of survival after Hodgkin's lymphoma: A population-based study. *J Clin Oncol* 23:7604, 2005.

Kelly GL, Rickinson AB: Burkitt lymphoma: Revisiting the pathogenesis of a virus-associated malignancy. *Hematology Am Soc Hematol Educ Program* 2007:277, 2007.

Kitahata MM, Achenbach CJ, Saag MS: Age at cancer diagnosis among persons with AIDS. *Ann Int Med* 154:642; author reply 643, 2011.

Levine AM: HIV-associated lymphoma. *Blood* 115:2986, 2010.

Libra M, Polesel J, Russo AE, et al: Extrahepatic disorders of HCV infection: A distinct entity of B-cell neoplasia? *Int J Oncol* 36:1331, 2010.

Matsuoka M, Jeang KT: Human T-cell leukaemia virus type 1 (HTLV-1) infectivity and cellular transformation. *Nat Rev Cancer* 7:270, 2007.

Matsuoka M, Jeang KT: Human T-cell leukemia virus type 1 (HTLV-1) and leukemic transformation: Viral infectivity, Tax, HBZ and therapy. *Oncogene* 30:1379, 2011.

Moore PS, Chang Y: KSHV: Forgotten but not gone. *Blood* 117:6973, 2011.

Ratner L, Harrington W, Feng X, et al: Human T cell leukemia virus reactivation with progression of adult T-cell leukemia-lymphoma. *PLoS One* 4:e4420, 2009.

Rudek MA, Flexner C, Ambinder RF: Use of antineoplastic agents in patients with cancer who have HIV/AIDS. *Lancet Oncol* 12:905, 2011.

Savoldo B, Goss JA, Hammer MM, et al: Treatment of solid organ transplant recipients with autologous Epstein Barr virus-specific cytotoxic T lymphocytes (CTLs). *Blood* 108:2942, 2006.

Sparano JA, Lee JY, Kaplan LD, et al: Rituximab plus concurrent infusional EPOCH chemotherapy is highly effective in HIV-associated B-cell non-Hodgkin lymphoma. *Blood* 115:3008, 2010.

Uldrick TS, Polizzotto MN, Aleman K, et al: High-dose zidovudine plus valganciclovir for Kaposi sarcoma herpesvirus-associated multicentric Castleman disease: A pilot study of virus-activated cytotoxic therapy. *Blood* 117:6977, 2011.

Vereide DT, Sugden B: Lymphomas differ in their dependence on Epstein-Barr virus. *Blood* 117:1977, 2011.

For complete list of references log on to www.expertconsult.com.

CHAPTER 83

MALIGNANT LYMPHOMAS IN CHILDHOOD

Kala Y. Kamdar, John T. Sandlund, Jr., and Catherine M. Bollard

Malignant lymphomas are the third most common malignancy among children and adolescents.[1-3] Among children under 15 years of age, non-Hodgkin lymphoma (NHL) is more frequent; however, in patients up to 18 years of age, Hodgkin disease is predominant. NHLs in children are usually extranodal diffuse high-grade tumors, whereas low- and intermediate-grade nodal lymphomas predominate in adults. These differences are speculated to reflect maturational changes in the function and composition of the immune system.[2] The different histologies explain in part the differing clinical features, disease course, and treatment strategies used in adults and children.

The differences in treatment approach and disease subtypes are less striking in adults and children with Hodgkin disease. However, there are significant challenges in the management of children with Hodgkin disease because of the sequelae of therapy, such as radiation-induced bone growth abnormalities, endocrine dysfunction, and chemotherapy-related sterility. Of greater concern are the radiation- and chemotherapy-related second malignancies and late cardiac deaths. Current trials are examining ways to reduce the toxicity of therapy without compromising the excellent outcome generally achieved.

EPIDEMIOLOGY

The incidence of NHL increases steadily throughout life, in contrast to Hodgkin disease, which has a bimodal age distribution peaking in early and late adulthood.[2] Although NHLs may occur at any age in childhood, they are infrequent among children younger than 3 years of age—the median age at presentation is approximately 10 years. NHL is two to three times more frequent in boys than in girls and is almost twice as common in whites as in African Americans; the reasons for these differences have yet to be determined.[4]

Specific populations at risk for the development of NHL include those with either congenital or acquired immunodeficiency conditions.[5] Inherited immunodeficiency syndromes include Wiskott-Aldrich syndrome, X-linked lymphoproliferative syndrome (XLP), and ataxia-telangiectasia (AT). The recognition of these syndromes in children with newly diagnosed NHL is important for appropriate therapeutic design. For example, involved field irradiation and radiomimetics should be avoided in children with AT. Additionally, children with AT are at increased risk for the development of cyclophosphamide-induced hemorrhagic cystitis; therefore they should receive vigorous hydration and uroprotectants (e.g., MESNA) when receiving any dose of cyclophosphamide. XLP should be considered in any male with a high-grade B-cell lymphoma who either develops a late recurrence (second occurrence) of a high-grade B-cell lymphoma or has a brother with either a high-grade B-cell lymphoma or fatal infectious mononucleosis. Children with acquired immunodeficiency conditions predisposing to the development of NHL include those who have received posttransplant immunosuppressive therapy and those with acquired immunodeficiency syndrome (AIDS).

Differences exist in both the incidence and proportion of histologic subtypes in different parts of the world. For example, the NHLs are very rare in Japan but occur quite frequently in equatorial Africa. Burkitt lymphoma, which accounts for about half of all childhood cancers in equatorial Africa, is the predominant NHL histologic subtype in both equatorial Africa and northeast Brazil.[6] There are also geographic differences in both the clinical and biologic features of certain NHL subtypes.[7,8]

CLASSIFICATION

After Thomas Hodgkin described the disease bearing his name in 1832, various schemes emerged to classify the tumors now collectively referred to as the *NHLs*. Several classification schemes were developed based on histopathologic features and the putative cell of origin. In an attempt to reduce the confusion of multiple classification schemes, the National Cancer Institute (NCI) sponsored a workshop to design a single classification scheme for clinical usage. This scheme, published in 1982 and referred to as the *NCI Working Formulation,* was widely accepted for almost 2 decades. In the Working Formulation, the NHLs of childhood are predominantly diffuse high-grade tumors and can be divided among three major subgroups: lymphoblastic, small noncleaved cell, and large cell lymphomas.

In the past decade, additional classification schemes were designed to improve on the NCI Working Formulation. Because of the problems associated with attempts to classify lymphoid neoplasms into categories based on presumed normal cell counterparts, the International Lymphoma Study Group proposed a classification system for lymphoid neoplasms[9] predicated on a practical approach to categorizing these diseases using available immunologic and molecular genetic techniques in addition to the standard morphologic criteria. This Revised European-American Classification of Lymphoid Neoplasms (REAL Classification) has been endorsed by many of the world's leading lymphoma pathologists, and it has served as the basis for the World Health Organization (WHO) classification of hematopoietic and lymphoid tumors.[10] Both the REAL and WHO classification systems include related lymphoid leukemias and recognize that NHL and acute lymphoblastic leukemia (ALL) represent different stages of evolution within specific morphologically and immunologically defined disease categories—an observation recognized by clinicians caring for children with lymphoid neoplasms and reflected in current clinical practice, which prescribes similar therapies for lymphomas and leukemias of related phenotype.

In the REAL and WHO classification systems, non-Hodgkin lymphomas are classified on the basis of phenotype (B lineage versus T lineage versus NK cell lineage) and differentiation (precursor versus mature). Hence NHLs that occur commonly in children appear in three major categories: lymphoblastic lymphoma (precursor B-cell lymphoma and precursor T-cell lymphoma), mature B-cell NHL (Burkitt and Burkitt-like lymphoma and diffuse large B-cell lymphoma), and anaplastic large cell lymphoma (mature T-cell or null-cell types).

The clinical and biologic characteristics of NHL in children are summarized in Table 83-1 and illustrated in Fig. 83-1, *A-C.*

Lymphoblastic Lymphoma

Lymphoblastic lymphoma (LBL) and acute lymphoblastic leukemia (ALL) are often considered two clinical presentations of the same disease. Patients with a mass and fewer than 25% bone marrow lymphoblasts are designated as having LBL, whereas patients with at least 25% bone marrow involvement have ALL. In contrast to ALL, more than 75% of LBL cases demonstrate a precursor T-cell immunophenotype (T-LBL), with the remainder showing a precursor B-cell immunophenotype (pB-LBL).[11-13]

Epidemiology

LBL constitutes 22% to 28% of childhood NHL. There is a 2 : 1 male predominance for LBL, but the incidence of lymphoblastic lymphoma remains constant across the pediatric age group for both boys and girls.[14]

Table 83-1 Characteristics of Non-Hodgkin Lymphoma in Children

Subtype	Proportion of Cases in BFM Studies (%)[11]	Phenotype	Primary Site	Translocation	Affected Genes
Lymphoblastic	26	T cell B cell	Mediastinum or head and neck	t(1;14)(p32;q11) t(11;14)(p13;q11) t(11;14)(p15;q11) t(10;14)(q24;q11) t(7;19)(q35;p13) t(8;14)(q24;q11) t(1;7)(p34;q34)	*TCRαδ-TAL1* *TCRαδ-RHOMB2* *TCRαδ-RHOMB1* *TCRαδ-HOX11* *TCRβ-LYL1* *TCRαδ-MYC* *TCRβ-LCK*
Burkitt	49	B cell	Abdomen or head and neck	t(8;14)(q24;q32) t(2;8)(p11;q24) t(8;22)(q24;q11)	*IgH-cMYC* *Ig6-cMYC* *Ig8-cMYC*
DLBCL	13	B cell	Mediastinum, abdomen, head and neck	t(8;14)(q24;q32) t(14;18)(q32;q21)	*IgH-cMYC* *IgH-BCL2*
ALCL	13	T-cell indeterminate	Mediastinum, abdomen, head and neck, bone, soft tissue or skin	t(2;5)(p23;q35)	*NPM-ALK*

ALCL, Anaplastic large cell lymphoma; *BFM,* Berlin-Frankfurt-Münster; *DLBCL,* Diffuse large B-cell lymphoma; *Ig,* immunoglobulin; *TCR,* T-cell receptor.

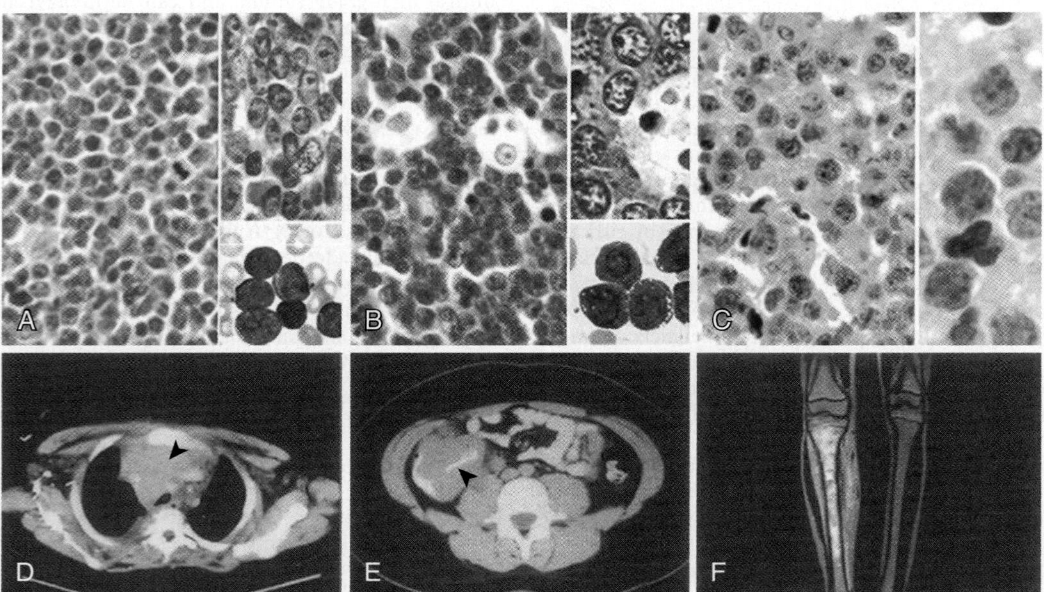

Figure 83-1 HISTOLOGIC AND CLINICAL FEATURES OF THE NON-HODGKIN LYMPHOMAS OF CHILDHOOD. The upper panels (**A** to **C**) demonstrate the appearance in hematoxylin and eosin sections of lymphoblastic lymphoma (**A**); Burkitt lymphoma/leukemia (**B**); and large B cell lymphoma, centroblastic with multilobulated nuclei (**C**). The inserts in **A** and **B** demonstrate the appearance of Wright-stained specimens of the lymphoblasts and the neoplastic cells of Burkitt leukemia/lymphoma, respectively. The lower panels (**D** to **F**) show clinical presentations of the three histologic subtypes of lymphoma: airway compression by lymphoblastic lymphoma of the anterior mediastinum on computed tomography of the chest (**D**), encasement of the bowel lumen by Burkitt lymphoma on abdominal computed tomography (**E**), and tibial bone disease in primary lymphoma of the bone (**F**). *(Reproduced, in part, with permission from Sandlund JT, Downing JR, Crist WM: Non-Hodgkin's lymphoma in childhood,* N Engl J Med *334:1238, 1996.)*

Pathobiology

LBL arises from precursor T or B lymphoblasts at varying stages of differentiation. Morphology is similar to that of ALL, with lymphoblasts of small or medium size and with scant cytoplasm, round or convoluted nuclei, fine chromatin, and indistinct or small nucleoli (see Fig. 83-1, *A*). Stains show positivity for periodic acid-Schiff, variable positivity for Sudan black B and nonspecific esterase, and negativity for myeloperoxidase. Immunophenotyping shows TdT positivity. T-LBL is usually positive for CD7 and surface or cytoplasmic CD3, with variable expression of CD2, CD5, CD1a, CD4, and CD8. CD10 expression is more frequent in T-LBL (40%) than T-ALL (less than 10%), possibly related to maturational stage, with T-ALL more frequently demonstrating an immature phenotype.[13,15,16] B-lineage markers are positive in pB-LBL. Unlike ALL, there are no known cytogenetic prognostic factors for LBL. Recurrent cytogenetic anomalies are seen in about half of childhood T-ALL but have not been well defined in T-LBL. Literature is scarce regarding typical chromosomal aberrations for T-LBL, with most published aberrations reported for T-ALL. The most common chromosomal translocations for both T-LBL and T-ALL involve the T-cell receptor (TCR) gene loci at chromosome 14q11 or 7q34, resulting in the juxtaposition of an oncogenic partner gene with the regulatory region of one of the TCR gene loci and subsequent deregulation of the reciprocal partner gene. Common partner genes seen in T-ALL and T-LBL include *TAL1, MYC, HOXA* gene cluster, and *MYB*. Other chromosomal abnormalities described for T-LBL and T-ALL include *NOTCH1* mutations, alterations of chromosome 9p containing *CDKN2A/CDKN2B* loci, and deletions in chromosome 6p.[17-19]

Clinical Manifestations

The clinical features at presentation vary with primary site and extent of disease spread. Patients with T-LBL frequently present with an anterior mediastinal mass (75%), which may cause respiratory symptoms, airway compromise, dysphagia, or superior vena cava syndrome (see Fig. 83-1, *D*). Pleural effusions are common when a mediastinal mass is present, and lymphadenopathy above the diaphragm is frequent. Bone, skin, bone marrow, central nervous system (CNS), abdominal organs, other lymph nodes, and occasionally testes may also be involved. Children with pB-LBL are less likely to present with a mediastinal mass, but a higher frequency of cutaneous involvement occurs with pB-LBL.[20-23] Bone lesions are also common in pB-LBL.[22,24] CNS involvement at diagnosis is seen in 4% to 5% of patients with LBL.[22,25]

Differential Diagnosis

LBL is distinguished from ALL by having less than 25% bone marrow involvement and from myeloid malignancies being positive for TdT and negative for myeloperoxidase. T-LBL and pB-LBL are differentiated by flow cytometry.

Prognosis (Staging)

After obtaining tissue diagnosis, staging is performed with imaging (computed tomography of neck, chest, abdomen, and pelvis), bilateral bone marrow evaluation, and lumbar puncture. Bone scans are only done if clinically indicated. Childhood NHL, including LBL, is most commonly staged using the Murphy classification (Table 83-2).[26]

With current therapies based on ALL protocols, LBL has a long-term survival greater than 90% in low-stage disease and greater than 80% in advanced-stage disease[27] (Table 83-3). Children with CNS disease have the worst outcome, but CNS disease is less common in T-LBL than in T-ALL. The Children's Oncology Group (COG) demonstrated that minimal disseminated disease at diagnosis has prognostic value, as indicated by flow cytometric evidence of tumor cells in bone marrow. In 99 children with T-LBL treated on the A5971 study, 2-year EFS was 68.1% ± 11.1% for patients with ≥1% T-LL cells in bone marrow by flow cytometry methods, as compared with 90.7% ± 4.4% for patients with lower degree of marrow involvement.[28] Minimal disseminated disease at diagnosis was associated with an increased likelihood of bone marrow or distant recurrence but not local recurrence. On NHL-BFM trials, adolescent females with T-LBL had poorer outcomes than adolescent males despite similar presenting characteristics. In 45 adolescents with T-LBL, the 5-year EFS was 57% for females and 92% for males ($p = 0.004$). This gender difference was not observed in children younger than 15 years old on NHL-BFM trials.[29] One adult study for T-cell ALL has demonstrated poorer outcomes in females than in males,[30] but a prognostic impact of gender has not been found in other pediatric or adult studies for LBL. Although adolescent age itself has not been established as a poor prognostic factor as it has for ALL, adult outcomes for LBL are inferior to pediatric outcomes.[31]

Table 83-2 Murphy Staging of Non-Hodgkin Lymphoma

STAGE I
Single tumor (extranodal) or involvement of a single anatomic area (nodal), with the exception of the mediastinum and abdomen.
STAGE II
Single tumor (extranodal) with regional node involvement.
Two or more nodal areas on the same side of the diaphragm.
Two single (extranodal) tumors, with or without regional node involvement, on the same side of the diaphragm.
Primary gastrointestinal tract tumor (frequently in the ileocecal area), with or without involvement of associated mesenteric nodes; completely resected.
STAGE III
Two single tumors (extranodal) on opposite sides of the diaphragm.
Two or more nodal areas on opposite sides of the diaphragm.
Primary intrathoracic tumor (mediastinal, pleural, or thymic).
Extensive primary intraabdominal disease.
Paraspinal or epidural tumor, regardless of other sites of involvement.
STAGE IV
Any of the above with initial involvement of the central nervous system and/or bone marrow.

Modified from the classification proposed by Murphy (Murphy SB, Fairclough DL, Hutchison RE, et al: Non-Hodgkin's lymphomas of childhood: An analysis of the histology, staging, and response to treatment of 338 cases at a single institution, *J Clin Oncol* 7:186, 1989.)

Therapy

Two potentially life-threatening situations requiring urgent intervention must be considered in children with LBL: (1) mediastinal tumor with airway obstruction or superior vena cava syndrome and (2) tumor lysis syndrome. Because of the cardiac and respiratory risks associated with anesthesia or sedation in children with a large mediastinal mass, the least-invasive procedure for obtaining a tissue sample should be chosen. In children with peripheral lymphadenopathy, lymph node biopsy under local anesthesia may be possible. In children who cannot tolerate a procedure, pretreatment with steroids or radiation may be necessary to stabilize the patient. Since pretreatment may diminish the ability to accurately diagnose a patient, a tissue biopsy should be obtained as soon as it is possible to do so safely. Tumor lysis syndrome is characterized by metabolic consequences of the breakdown of lymphoma cells causing renal failure if severe. Hyperuricemia, hyperkalemia, and hyperphosphatemia must be

Table 83-3 Outcomes for Lymphoblastic Lymphoma

Protocol	n =	Stage	Regimen	EFS
CCG 551[33]	164	I-IV	LSA_2L_2 (multidrug, cyclic chemotherapy, ± XRT)	64% (5-year)
POG 8314 and 8719[141]	46	I-II	CHOP + maintenance	63% (5-year)
NHL-BFM 86 and 90				
T-LBL[27]	105	I-IV	ALL-type (protocols I, M, ± II, maintenance, ± CRT)	90% (5-year)
pB-LBL[142]	27	I-IV	ALL-type (Protocols I, M, ± II, maintenance, ± CRT)	73% (10-year)
NHL-BFM 95[37]	156	III-IV, CNS-neg	ALL-type (Protocols I, M, ± II, no pCRT)	82% (5-year)
EORTC 58881[143]	119	I-IV, CNS-neg or -pos	ALL-type (BFM-based), no CRT	78% (6-year)
St. Jude NHL13[36]	41	III-IV, CNS-neg	ALL-type, intensive TIT, no pCRT	83% (5-year)

ALL, Acute lymphoblastic leukemia; *BFM*, Berlin-Frankfurt-Münster; *CCG*, Children's Cancer Group; *CHOP*, cyclophosphamide, hydroxydaunomycin, vincristine (Oncovin), prednisone; *CRT*, cranial radiation therapy; *EFS*, event-free survival; *LBL*, T-cell lymphoblastic lymphoma; *NHL*, Non-Hodgkin lymphoma; *pB-LBL*, precursor B-cell lymphoblastic lymphoma; *POG*, Pediatric Oncology Group; *TIT*, triple intrathecal therapy; *T-LBL*, T-cell lymphoblastic lymphoma; *XRT*, radiation therapy.

aggressively managed by hyperhydration, rasburicase and/or allopurinol, and close monitoring. Children with NHL can also present with epidural masses and associated neurologic deficits caused by spinal cord compression. If the diagnosis is known, chemotherapy should be started as soon as possible. If the diagnosis is not known, or if there is a sluggish response to chemotherapy, emergent steroids or low-dose radiation therapy may be considered in consultation with a radiation oncologist.

For stage I and II disease, cooperative group studies have shown that short, pulsed chemotherapy regimens are effective for some pediatric NHL such as Burkitt lymphoma (90% OS) but are inferior for treatment of LBL (60% OS).[32,33] However, the Berlin-Frankfurt-Münster (BFM) group showed excellent outcomes for LBL with extended combination chemotherapy based on ALL treatment with induction, consolidation, and maintenance phases lasting a total of 24 months (90% 5-year EFS).[27] Even patients with stage III and IV LBL had good outcomes on ALL-type therapy.[34,35] This ALL-like therapy has now become standard for LBL (see Table 83-3). The Children's Oncology Group is currently risk-stratifying patients with T-LBL based on the presence of minimal disease in the bone marrow at presentation and on radiologic response to induction therapy, with high-risk patients eligible for randomization to additional therapy. CNS prophylaxis is needed for LBL, but chemotherapy prophylaxis has not proven inferior to prophylactic cranial irradiation in CNS-negative patients, even with advanced-stage disease.[22,36,37] Additionally, the Pediatric Oncology Group did not demonstrate a survival advantage of high-dose methotrexate for T-LBL, although its utility in T-ALL is still being evaluated.[35]

Burkitt Lymphoma

Burkitt lymphoma (BL) was first described by Dennis Burkitt in the 1950s in Uganda.[38] First thought to be endemic to equatorial Africa, it was subsequently observed in Europe and North America. The WHO classification recognizes three variants: (1) sporadic BL, occurring throughout the world and more common in children, adolescents, and young adults; (2) endemic BL, occurring primarily in sub-Saharan Africa and New Guinea, with some unique clinical features but morphologically identical to sporadic BL; and (3) immunodeficiency-associated BL, observed primarily in patients with HIV and less commonly in the setting of other immunodeficiencies. The WHO and REAL classifications also recognize the controversial entity of Burkitt-like lymphoma, with features intermediate between BL and diffuse large B-cell lymphoma (DLBCL). Burkitt-like lymphoma is rare in children, and the clinical value of this classification is unclear. When there is greater than 25% bone marrow involvement, it is designated Burkitt leukemia (FAB L3 subtype of ALL) but is treated similarly to Burkitt lymphoma.[10,39]

Epidemiology

Sporadic BL constitutes approximately 35% to 50% of childhood NHL and is much more common in boys than in girls (4:1 ratio), with a peak incidence between 5 and 14 years of age.[11,14] Endemic BL associated with Epstein-Barr virus (EBV) in more than 85% of cases accounts for approximately half of all childhood cancers in equatorial Africa. In contrast, sporadic BL is most common in the United States and Europe and is associated with EBV in only 15% of cases.[40]

Pathobiology

BL is composed of monomorphic, small, noncleaved cells with round nuclei, clumped chromatin, and basophilic cytoplasm (see Fig. 83-1, *B*). A high uniform proliferation index is seen, with the Ki-67 positivity approaching 100%. The classic "starry sky" appearance of BL seen under low-power microscopy is caused by tingible body macrophages scattered among malignant cells. Burkitt-like lymphoma has a gene expression signature that is similar to Burkitt lymphoma but has more variation in nuclear size and shape, with larger cells and larger nucleoli similar to DLBCL.[41-43] BL cells show mature B-cell features and usually express surface immunoglobulins. B-cell markers such as CD19, CD20, and CD22 are usually present, and the majority express CD10 (CALLA). BL is negative for TdT and BCL-2. CD21, the EBV receptor, is more commonly seen in endemic BL than in sporadic BL.

Characteristic chromosomal translocations suggest that BL develops from genetic aberrations during immunoglobulin gene rearrangement or attempted immunoglobulin class switching in a B-cell precursor. These translocations, usually t(8;14) or infrequently t(8;22) or t(2;8), juxtapose the *c-Myc* gene (involved in cellular proliferation) with immunoglobulin locus regulatory elements, resulting in c-Myc overexpression. In sporadic cases, the predominant chromosome 8 breakpoints usually occur within the *c-Myc* gene, whereas they are upstream of the gene in endemic cases. Other cytogenetic abnormalities, such as gain of 7q and deletion of 13q, are uncommon.[44,45]

Clinical Manifestations

BL is an extremely fast-growing malignancy. The most common primary sites of sporadic BL are the abdomen and the lymph nodes of the head and neck.[46,47] Abdominal disease presentation, which is often associated with nausea, vomiting, and abdominal pain, carries a risk for intestinal perforation, obstruction, and gastrointestinal bleeding. Abdominal lymphoma often arises from the distal ileum causing intestinal obstruction secondary to intussusception or compression by an expanding mass encasing the bowel (see Fig. 83-1, *E*). BL can involve testes, bone, skin, bone marrow, and CNS. CNS involvement at diagnosis, occurring in about 9% of patients, is associated with a worse outcome.[25] Endemic BL frequently involves the abdomen, jaw, paraspinal region, orbit, and CNS.

Differential Diagnosis

In DLBCL, another mature B-cell lymphoma, the cells are usually larger and additional cytogenetic abnormalities, such as BCL-6 gene rearrangements or t(14;18), may be seen, although these abnormalities are more common in adult DLBCL. Ki-67 staining in less than 95% of the cells or positivity for BCL-2 is helpful in excluding a diagnosis of BL. Burkitt-like lymphoma is a controversial diagnosis with some morphologic features more similar to DLBCL, including larger cells, but commonly with *c-Myc* translocations and a clinical behavior similar to classic BL.[41,48] TdT negativity is helpful in distinguishing BL from pB-LBL.

Prognosis (Staging)

The risk group classification developed by the French Society of Pediatric Oncology (SFOP) is widely used on current protocols incorporating risk-adapted therapy (Table 83-4). This system takes into account whether localized disease has been resected and the adverse prognosis associated with CNS or bone marrow involvement. Localized or CNS-negative advanced-stage cases of BL have greater than 90% long-term survival with current therapies, with approximately 79% event-free survival (EFS) for CNS-positive BL.[49] Cytogenetic abnormalities such as gain of 7q, deletion of 13q, and partial duplication of 1q carry a poor prognosis. Suboptimal response to initial cytoreduction is also associated with worse prognosis, and poor responders are often stratified to more intensive chemotherapy on current regimens. High levels of lactate dehydrogenase (LDH) at diagnosis also carries a worse prognosis and is frequently incorporated in risk-classification schemes. Age greater than 15 years has a worse outcome for mature B-cell malignancies, but this may be primarily due to DLBCL rather than BL.

Therapy

Tumor lysis syndrome must be anticipated as a major risk in newly diagnosed Burkitt lymphoma. To help prevent this complication, children at risk should be vigorously hydrated (3 to 4 L/m^2/day with D_5 ¼ NaCl and 40 mEq/L $NaHCO_3$; there should be no added potassium) and started on allopurinol, a xanthine oxidase inhibitor. The urine pH should be maintained at about 7.0; at a more alkaline pH, phosphorus is less soluble, and at a more acidic pH, uric acid is less soluble. In some cases, mannitol followed by furosemide is required to maintain urine output. Uricolytic agents, which have been used for many years in Europe, directly cleave the uric acid molecule and result in a precipitous drop in serum uric acid levels within a few hours. The use of uricolytic agents (e.g., urate oxidase, uricase, rasburicase) has proven to be superior to allopurinol to reduce rapidly the level of serum uric acid and improve renal function. Rasburicase has significantly reduced the need for hemodialysis consequent to tumor lysis syndrome. Recent protocols incorporate a prophase of reduced intensity to decrease the risk for severe tumor lysis syndrome.[50] In the setting of abdominal BL, intestinal perforation, obstruction, or gastrointestinal bleeding may not occur until after the initiation of chemotherapy as the lymphoma begins to regress.

A multinational cooperative study demonstrated that localized resected mature B-cell NHL (including both BL and DLBCL) could be cured without significant toxicity by two courses of COPAD (cyclophosphamide, vincristine, prednisolone, and doxorubicin) without intrathecal chemotherapy. Four-year OS was 99.2%.[51] Advanced-stage BL requires aggressive combination chemotherapy with CNS prophylaxis (Table 83-5). Cyclophosphamide, methotrexate, and cytarabine at high doses have been used most recently, with or without anthracyclines and epipodophyllotoxins. Therapy should be started as quickly as possible upon presentation, because this tumor grows very rapidly, and subsequent cycles should be administered in an intensive fashion as soon as recovery occurs from the last cycle. CNS prophylaxis is needed—without it, approximately 30% to 50% of patients will relapse in the CNS,[52] whereas only 6% to 11% develop CNS relapse if adequate prophylaxis is given.[25] CNS prophylaxis includes high-dose methotrexate (and cytarabine in high-risk patients) to penetrate the CNS, together with intensive intrathecal chemotherapy. Risk-adapted therapy used in the SFOP LMB-89 study conferred an excellent 5-year EFS of 91% in advanced-stage patients without bone marrow or CNS involvement and approximately 79% to 84% with bone marrow or CNS disease. Treatment intensity was escalated based on tumor burden and response to therapy. These are the best published outcomes to date, but these regimens have significant hematologic toxicity; thus growth factor and blood product support is needed.[49] The French-American-British

Table 83-4 SFOP Risk Group Classification of Mature B-Cell Lymphomas

Group	Extent of Disease
Group A	Completely resected stage I Completely resected abdominal stage II
Group B	Nonresected stage I and stage II Any stage III CNS-negative stage IV with BM involvement, 5%-25%
Group C	CNS-positive stage IV Stage IV with BM involvement ≥25% (mature B-cell ALL)

ALL, Acute lymphoblastic leukemia; *BM*, bone marrow; *CNS*, central nervous system; *SFOP*, French Society of Pediatric Oncology.

Table 83-5 Outcomes for Burkitt Lymphoma

Protocol	*n* =	Stage	Regimen	EFS
CCG 503	279	I-III	COMP	61% (10-year)
POG 8314 and 8719[141] 8617[144]	171	I-II IV	CHOP Total B (multiagent, high-dose)	89% (5-year) 79% (4-year)
LMB 89[49]	459	Stage I-IV		92% (5-year)
		Group A	COPAD	98% (5-year)
		Group B	COP, COPADM, CYM, M1	92% (5-year)
		Group C	COP, COPADM, CYVE, M1-M4	84% (5-year)
NHL-BFM 90[34]	413	I-IV	Multiagent, risk-adapted	89% (6-year)

CCG, Children's Cancer Group; *CHOP*, cyclophosphamide, hydroxydaunomycin, vincristine (Oncovin), prednisone; *COMP*, cyclophosphamide, vincristine (Oncovin), methotrexate, prednisone; *COPAD*, cyclophosphamide, vincristine (Oncovin), prednisone, and doxorubicin; *COPADM*, COPAD plus methotrexate; *CYM*, cytarabine, methotrexate; *CYVE*, cytarabine, etoposide (Vepesid); *EFS*, Event-free survival; *LMB*, Lymphome Malins de Burkitt; *M*, maintenance; *NHL-BFM*, non-Hodgkin lymphoma Berlin-Frankfurt-Münster; *POG*, Pediatric Oncology Group;.

(FAB)/LMB-96 study successfully reduced therapy for intermediate-risk (Group B) patients without a compromise in survival. In this study, a reduction in the cumulative dose of cyclophosphamide and omission of a multi-agent maintenance cycle for Group B patients resulted in a reduction in toxicity while maintaining the effectiveness seen on LMB-89.[50] However, intensity of therapy could not be safely reduced for Group C patients.

Rituximab is a mouse/human chimeric monoclonal antibody against CD20, highly expressed in BL and DLBCL. In adults, the addition of rituximab to CHOP chemotherapy is beneficial for DLBCL[53,54] and has been given safely in combination with intensive BL therapy.[55] In children, single-agent rituximab showed activity for BL in a phase II window study for newly diagnosed patients.[56] The Children's Oncology Group is evaluating the safety and efficacy of adding rituximab to the LMB backbone for the treatment of BL.

Local radiation therapy has no role in BL because it is chemosensitive and often diffuse. CNS radiation has been used in the past for CNS involvement at diagnosis but did not show an impact on outcome in this group. Surgery is no longer routinely used for Burkitt lymphoma. However, patients with localized disease resected at diagnosis are eligible for reduced chemotherapy, as noted earlier.

Diffuse Large B-Cell Lymphoma

DLBCL includes a heterogeneous group of neoplasms of transformed B cells, accounting for 10% to 13% of pediatric NHL.[11] Primary mediastinal disease, termed *primary mediastinal B-cell lymphoma (PMBCL),* occurs in 20% of childhood DLBCL cases. DLBCL has some distinctive biologic and clinical features, described in more detail in the following sections.[57]

Epidemiology

The incidence of DLBCL increases with age, being more common in the second decade of life.[14,58] It is rare in children younger than 4 years of age. Although DLBCL is more common in boys than girls (in a 2.1 : 1 ratio), the gender difference is less notable than in BL. PMBCL occurs more frequently in adolescents, with no gender difference.[57]

Pathobiology

Most pediatric DLBCL cases have a germinal-center or postgerminal-center mature B-cell phenotype.[58] Nuclei are usually more than twice the size of normal lymphocytes (see Fig. 83-1, *C*). They express pan-B cell antigens, including CD19, CD20, CD22, and CD79a, with or without surface immunoglobulin. Most express CD10 and BCL6, and approximately 40% express BCL2. However, breaks or translocations in *BCL2* and *BCL6* are rare in pediatric DLBCL. Unlike adult DLBCL, pediatric cases rarely demonstrate the t(14;18) translocation.[57,58] Gene profiling has led to subclassification of adult cases into germinal center B cell–like, activated B cell–like, and type 3 (those not belonging to the first two groups) phenotypes. The great majority of children have the germinal center B cell–like phenotype.[51,58] Of note, this phenotype has a better prognosis in adults, and childhood DLBCL outcomes are better than adult outcomes. Morphologic variants of DLBCL include centroblastic, immunoblastic, anaplastic, and T cell/histiocyte—rich variants.[59] Although DLBCL is clearly heterogeneous, the clinical value of these distinctions is unclear in children.

PMBCL is thought to originate from medullary thymic B cells. B-lineage antigens and CD30 are often positive, but surface immunoglobulin and HLA class I and II molecules are absent or incompletely expressed.[57] *MYC, BCL2,* and *BCL6* genes are not rearranged. PMBCL is associated with gains in chromosome 9p (involving JAK2) and 2p (involving c-rel). They commonly demonstrate inactivation of SOCS1.[60,61] Variable degrees of sclerosis occur in PMBCL,[62] as well as occasional lymphocytes, eosinophils, and Reed-Sternberg–like cells, sometimes leading to confusion with Hodgkin lymphoma.

Clinical Manifestations

DLBCL is often more localized than BL and is less likely to involve the bone marrow or CNS.[25] Nodal disease is more commonly seen in DLBCL than in BL, but extranodal disease is frequent. Common sites of involvement include the abdomen, mediastinum, bone (see Fig. 83-1, *F*), and head and neck, particularly Waldeyer ring. PMBCL is locally invasive and frequently associated with SVC syndrome or airway compression. Pleural or pericardial effusions are present in approximately 40% of PMBCL cases,[62] and kidney metastases are frequent.[57]

Differential Diagnosis

The differential diagnosis of DLBCL encompasses BL, pB-LBL, and nodular lymphocyte predominant Hodgkin lymphoma. BL is distinguished from DLBCL by morphology, although atypical BL shows more pleomorphism than typical BL. BCL2 negativity, high cell proliferation, and translocations involving *c-Myc* may suggest BL but are not definitive. DLBCL, with its mature phenotype, differs from pB-LBL by a lack of TdT expression. DLBCL and nodular lymphocyte predominant Hodgkin lymphoma share some similar features and derive from a common B-cell clone. DLBCL may represent the clonal progression of nodular lymphocyte predominant Hodgkin lymphoma. PMBCL can also be confused with Hodgkin lymphoma and an adequate biopsy is essential for diagnosis. PMBCL and other DLBCL are distinguished clinically—PBMCLs typically reside within the thymic area, whereas mediastinal DLBCLs usually involve mediastinal lymph nodes.

Prognosis (Staging)

Murphy classification is used to stage DLBCL.[63] No difference in outcomes exists between Burkitt lymphoma and DLBCL based on histology, and the treatment is identical in children.[57] The outcome for DLBCL is better for children than adults, with 5-year OS of 90% for children using current therapies. Prognosis is poorer for children who have DLBCL with *c-Myc* rearrangements and for those with PMBCL (5-year EFS of 65% to 70%).[44,62] Adolescent females fared worse than adolescent males with DLBCL on NHL-BFM protocols.[29] In the setting of PMBCL, an LDH level of 500 units/L or more carries a worse prognosis.[62] BCL2 expression is not an unfavorable prognostic factor in children with DLBCL, in contrast to adults with DLBCL.[58]

Therapy

In children, all mature B-cell lymphomas are usually treated similarly with good results. Despite biologic and clinical differences, BL therapy is effective in DLBCL (Table 83-6).[57] Risk-adapted therapy with LMB (SFOP study) or B-NHL (BFM study) backbones consists of short, dose-intense courses of chemotherapy, including steroids, vincristine, high-dose methotrexate, cyclophosphamide, doxorubicin, cytarabine, etoposide, and intrathecal chemotherapy.[34,49,50,64] As described for BL, risk-adapted therapy based on LMB-89 and LMB-96 are also the current standard of care for childhood DLBCL.[49,50] Rituximab can improve adult outcomes for DLBCL when added to CHOP or CHOP-like therapy, but the benefit has not been proven in children.[53,54,65] Adult data suggest that rituximab may allow diminished use of agents with serious acute or late toxicities, warranting further study.[54] Children with localized primary DLBCL of the bone have excellent outcomes in Pediatric Oncology Group studies using

Table 83-6 Outcomes for Diffuse Large B-Cell Lymphoma

Protocol	*n* =	Stage	Regimen	EFS
POG studies				
8314 and 8719[141]	72	I-II	CHOP	88% (5-year)
9315[60]	73	III-IV	APO + antimetabolite	64% (4-year)
LMB 89[49]	63	I-IV	Multiagent, risk-stratified	89% (5-year)
NHL-BFM 90[34]	56	I-IV	Multiagent, risk-adapted	95% (6-year)

APO, doxorubicin (Adriamycin), prednisone, vincristine (Oncovin); *CHOP*, cyclophosphamide, doxorubicin, vincristine (Oncovin), prednisone; *EFS*, Event-free survival; *LMB*, Lymphome Malins de Burkitt; *NHL-BFM*, non-Hodgkin lymphoma Berlin-Frankfurt-Münster; *POG*, Pediatric Oncology Group;.

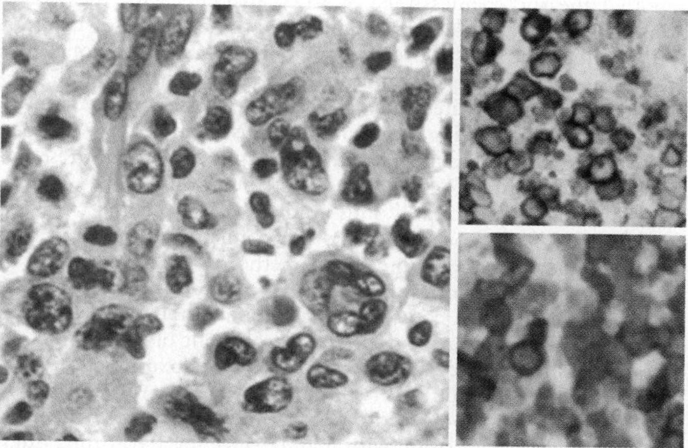

Figure 83-2 HISTOLOGIC AND IMMUNOPHENOTYPIC FEATURES OF ANAPLASTIC LARGE CELL LYMPHOMA. The section shows anaplastic cells including a "wreath cell" and a staining pattern with bright CD30 (Ki-1)-positivity *(top right)* and ALK-positivity *(bottom right)*. The nuclear and cytoplasmic staining by ALK would predict that the case has the t(2;5).

modified CHOP therapy without radiation for a total duration of 9 weeks.[66] Having evolved from BL regimens, DLBCL treatment has traditionally included intrathecal chemotherapy for CNS prophylaxis. Since the risk for CNS involvement is lower for DLBCL than for BL, it is unclear if CNS-directed therapy should be as intensive.[25,57] Local radiation has no role in frontline DLBCL therapy.[57]

Anaplastic Large Cell Lymphoma

Most childhood NHLs previously classified as large cell lymphomas fall into the category of anaplastic large cell lymphomas (ALCLs) in the REAL and WHO classification. This entity was first described in 1985 as a clinicopathologic variant of large cell lymphoma with a predilection for young patients.[67]

Pathobiology

ALCLs are characterized by the proliferation of large, pleomorphic cells with one or more prominent nucleoli (Fig. 83-2). The cells preferentially involve lymph node sinuses and extranodal sites (notably skin, bone, and soft tissue), where they grow in a cohesive pattern. The cells express epithelial membrane antigen (EMA) and CD30 (Ki-1) antigen—a 120-kd membrane-bound molecule and a member of the tumor necrosis factor (TNF) receptor superfamily—previously found in association with Hodgkin disease. A soluble (88-kd) form of the CD30 molecule is found in high levels in the serum of nearly all patients with ALCL.[68] Marked elevation of soluble CD30 levels in patients with ALCL correlates with higher risk for relapse, and soluble CD30 levels correlate with clinical disease status, returning to normal with attainment of complete remission and increasing with disease recurrence.

The anaplastic large cell lymphomas are associated with chromosomal rearrangements involving the long arm of chromosome 5 at position q35.[69] In most cases, this translocation includes material from chromosome 2p23 [t(2;5)(p23;q35)], resulting in the fusion of the NPM nucleolar phosphoprotein gene on chromosome 5q35 to anaplastic lymphoma kinase (ALK), a tyrosine kinase gene on chromosome 2p23. The hybrid protein produced from the translocation links the amino terminus of nucleophosmin (NPM) with the catalytic domain of ALK.[70] Deregulated expression of the truncated ALK may contribute to malignant transformation. The chimeric NPM-ALK protein is clearly oncogenic, perhaps through triggering of antiapoptotic signals via phosphatidylinositol 3-kinase/AKT, although secondary molecular events may be required for lymphomagenesis.

Immunologic and molecular biologic studies reveal that most cases of Ki-1$^+$ anaplastic large cell lymphomas are derived from activated T cells, although cases of non-T cell, non-B cell (null cell), and more rarely, B cell occur.[71] Based on extended testing for T-cell antigens and examination of the configuration of T-cell receptor genes, many null cell cases are, in fact, T-lineage neoplasms, although a minority may be derived from natural killer (NK) cells.[72] The diagnosis of ALCL can be difficult, and many cases are initially misdiagnosed as Hodgkin disease. In many cases, the diagnosis of ALCL can be confirmed by molecular techniques (RT-PCR) to detect the fusion gene resulting from t(2;5). Variant translocations in which ALK is involved with other partner genes on other chromosomes limit the application of RT-PCR for diagnosis. However, the t(2;5) results in the expression of the NPM-ALK fusion protein, whereas the variant translocations result in upregulation of ALK. The ALK1 monoclonal antibody recognizing the formalin-resistant epitope of both the NPM-ALK chimeric protein and normal ALK thus serves as a useful diagnostic reagent for identifying cases of ALCL. It should be noted that the distribution of ALK staining varies depending on the translocation. Further, ALK expression is a feature of inflammatory myofibroblastic tumors (IMT); however, confusion with ALCL can be minimized by testing for other hematopoietic markers, and the distinction is not usually difficult for experienced pathologists.

Clinical Manifestations

ALCL is rare, accounting for approximately 8% to 13% of childhood NHLs and roughly 30% to 40% of the pediatric large cell lymphomas. Approximately one-third of the cases present with localized disease, whereas the majority have advanced disease at presentation, although bone marrow and central nervous system involvement is uncommon.[73] A rare leukemic presentation of ALCL possibly associated with the small cell variant of ALCL has been described. Systemic symptoms (fevers, weight loss) are frequently present in advanced-stage disease. Cutaneous (spontaneously regressing) lesions sometimes accompany disease at other sites, but skin involvement is not universal.[67] A variety of presenting sites—both nodal and extranodal—can occur, including the mediastinum, gastrointestinal tract, and bone. Further, tumors may invade adjacent structures and be associated with ascites and other intraabdominal sites of disease, including kidney, liver, and lymph nodes. The outcome of children with ALCL in most series has been good (with survival rates ranging from 70% to 85%), albeit inferior to that of children with Burkitt and diffuse large B cell lymphomas (Table 83-7).

Diagnosis and Differential Diagnosis

Immunophenotyping and immunohistochemistry is critical for the definitive diagnosis of ALCL. The typical ALCL immunophenotype

Table 83-7 Outcomes for Anaplastic Large Cell Lymphoma

Protocol	n =	Stage	Regimen	EFS
POG 8314 and 8719[79]	72	I-II (resected)	CHOP ± maintenance	88% (5-year)*
CCG 5941[76]	86	Nonlocalized	Multiagent, + maintenance	68% (5-year)
NHL-BFM 90[80]	9	I-II (resected)	Multiagent, risk-adapted (short-pulse B-NHL–type therapy)	100% (5-year)
	65	II (nonresected)-III		73% (5-year)
	14	IV and multifocal bone involvement		79% (5-year)
ALCL-99[75]	225	I-IV	Multiagent, risk-adapted, 3-6 cycles chemotherapy	81% (5-year)

ALCL, anaplastic large cell lymphoma; *BFM*, Berlin-Frankfurt-Münster; *CCG*, Children's Cancer Group; *CHOP*, cyclophosphamide, hydroxydaunomycin, vincristine (Oncovin), prednisone; *EFS*, Event-free survival; *NHL*, non-Hodgkin lymphoma; *POG*, Pediatric Oncology Group.
*ALCL and DLBCL combined.

is CD30⁺, CD15⁻, CD45⁺, in contrast to Hodgkin lymphoma, which is typically CD30⁺ and CD15⁺. More than 60% of cases of ALCL express one or more T-cell antigens (CD3⁺, CD43, or CD45RO) and ALK protein is detected in most cases (over 60%).

Prognosis (Staging)

The disease stage of ALCL is determined according to the staging system described by Murphy (see Table 83-2).[26] As for other types of childhood NHL, stages I and II are considered limited-stage disease, whereas stage III represents advanced-stage disease. Stage IV is reserved for children with bone marrow or central nervous system involvement. For older adult patients with cutaneous CD30⁺ ALCL, the 5-year disease-free survival appears to be determined by the extent of limb involvement; however, this has not been shown in children, possibly because primary cutaneous ALCL is rare in the pediatric population.[74]

For systemic ALCL, studies have suggested that the stage of disease may be more important than the expression of the ALK protein. The European Intergroup for Childhood Non-Hodgkin Lymphoma (EICNHL) defined three factors (mediastinal involvement, visceral involvement, and skin lesions) associated with poorer prognosis in childhood ALCL.[75] This group conducted a multivariate analysis (merging preexisting databases from BFM, SFOP, and the United Kingdom Children's Cancer Study Group [UKCCSG] studies) and identified poor prognosis (one or more risk factors) and standard risk groups with 5-year PFS of 61% and 89% respectively. However, it is important to note that this study was not done as a prospective collaborative study. In contrast, the Children's Cancer Group (CCG) Study 5941 (CCG-5941) reported that only bone marrow involvement significantly changed the 5-year survival rate.[76]

The presence of ALK autoantibodies appears to be associated with decreased clinical risk factors and lower clinical stage, resulting in a lower cumulative incidence of relapses.[77] No correlation exists between outcome and the ALK translocation type. However, recently, the SFOP group have shown that for patients with ALK-positive ALCL, the presence of a small cell or lymphohistiocytic component is associated with a worse prognosis.[78]

Therapy

The optimal treatment approach for patients with ALCL has yet to be determined, as evidenced by a wide range of successful treatment strategies. In the United States, children with advanced stage CD30⁺ ALCL are generally treated with non-ALCL large cell lymphoma regimens, with long-term event-free survival rates ranging from 60% to 75%[75,76,79,80] (see Table 83-7). In a randomized trial performed by the POG, addition of intermediate-dose methotrexate and high-dose cytarabine did not improve on the 70% 4-year event-free survival achieved with APO alone.[81] The BFM reported 3-year EFS of approximately 80% using a Burkitt lymphoma–based strategy.[80] Regimens designed specifically for children with CD30⁺ ALCL have been developed by the French (SFOP) and German groups.[82] The SFOP also reported the successful salvage of ALCL patients with the weekly administration of single-agent vinblastine.[83] The impact of incorporating vinblastine into two different frontline treatments for ALCL (the BFM B-cell approach [multinational European trial] and APO [COG trial in the United States]) was then studied in randomized fashion. Patients receiving the vinblastine plus chemotherapy regimen had a better EFS in the first year after therapy (91%) than those not receiving vinblastine (74%); however, at the 2-year follow-up, EFS was 73% for both groups.[84] This study also showed that infusing methotrexate 1 g/m^2 over 24 hours was comparable to 3 g/m^2 over 3-hour infusions without intrathecal methotrexate.[85] However, 3 g/m^2 of methotrexate had less toxicity.

Other studies have come to no firm conclusions. For example, (1) the POG-9317 trial demonstrated no benefit of adding methotrexate and high-dose cytarabine to 52 weeks of doxorubicin (Adriamycin), prednisone, and vincristine (Oncovin), or APO, regimen[81] and (2) the CCG-5941 study, which evaluated a more intensive induction and consolidation with maintenance for 1 year total duration of therapy, had similar outcomes but with significant hematologic toxicity.[76]

Relapsed Non-Hodgkin Lymphoma Management

There is no standard treatment for relapsed NHL. Treatment usually consists of intensive chemotherapy to induce a complete or partial response, followed by autologous or allogeneic stem cell transplant. Recent studies suggest that allogeneic transplant may be more effective than autologous transplant for relapsed NHL, particularly for lymphoblastic lymphoma.[86] Outcomes are significantly better for patients with a complete remission before transplant. Radiation may be useful before transplant in selected patients with an incomplete response to chemotherapy.

Outcomes vary by histologic subtype. Relapsed BL and DLBCL is often chemoresistant, and survival is only 10% to 20%. The Children's Oncology Group used rituximab, ifosfamide, carboplatin, and etoposide (R-ICE) for salvage therapy in this population, achieving a 60% response rate (complete and partial).[87] Patients who achieve a complete remission should proceed to stem cell transplant. Relapsed LBL is also frequently chemoresistant, and reported survival is 10% to 40%.[88-90] Salvage regimens used for ALL may be employed for LBL, and nelarabine has demonstrated a 40% response rate in this setting for T-ALL and T-LBL in a phase II COG study.[91] Survival for relapsed ALCL is better than for other non-Hodgkin lymphomas, reaching 40% to 60%.[29,88,92] Vinblastine monotherapy as salvage therapy resulted in a complete remission rate of 83% in one study.[93] Brentuximab vedotin, an antibody against CD30, has been used successfully in adults with relapsed ALCL but has not been well studied in children yet.[94] Crizotinib, an ALK inhibitor, has also shown promise in adults in early clinical trials for relapsed ALCL patients and is undergoing phase I evaluation in children.[95] Autologous transplant has been used successfully for some patients, but allogeneic transplant may have better outcomes and is preferred for patients with bone marrow or CNS involvement, early relapse, and CD3-positive ALCL.[29,86,96]

Posttransplant Lymphoproliferative Disorder

The biology of posttransplant lymphoproliferative disorder (PTLD) is discussed in Chapter 52. Therefore this section merely serves to summarize the issues specific for pediatric patients with this diagnosis. The pediatric populations where PTLD is most frequently seen include patients with congenital immune deficiencies and patients after bone marrow or solid organ transplant. A particularly high risk is seen in stem cell transplant recipients with underlying immunodeficiencies such as Wiskott-Aldrich syndrome.[97] Patients with primary, congenital immunodeficiencies such as X-linked agammaglobulinemia and ataxia telangiectasia have an incidence of EBV-associated lymphoproliferative disease (LPD) ranging from 0.7% to 15%.[98] The incidence of PTLD after solid organ transplant is higher in children than in the adult population. The disease is heterogeneous but in children it is most frequently of B-cell origin and associated with EBV. In the United States, approximately 150 new cases are diagnosed in children each year.

Numerous therapeutic approaches to PTLD have been explored in children but generally there has been a paucity of multicenter collaborative studies for this disease. Withdrawal or reduction of immunosuppression is often considered as firstline therapy for PTLD, but the success of this maneuver depends on whether the patient can recover sufficient immune system function to eradicate EBV-infected B cells. For the pediatric HSCT patient, strategies have included reduction in immune suppression, rituximab,[99] donor lymphocyte infusions,[100] and EBV-specific T cell–directly therapy.[101] The advantages of T cell–based therapies over antibody therapy is that EBV-specific T cell–immune reconstitution is restored, thus reducing the risk for disease recurrence. Responses to donor-derived EBV-specific T-cell therapies developed at multiple centers for pediatric patients range from 70% to 85%.[101,102] Immune-based therapies are generally preferred in this population since the use of chemotherapy in patients with LPD after HSCT is associated with high mortality rates secondary to increased infectious complications.[103] However, hydroxyurea and immune-based therapies may be an option for patients with CNS disease.[104] After solid organ transplant (SOT), modalities such as radiotherapy or surgical resection for localized LPD can result in complete remissions. One study evaluated the efficacy of low-dose cyclophosphamide and prednisone for pediatric patients with PTLD after SOT. All patients had progressed despite reduction of immune suppression and received six cycles of chemotherapy. The 2-year event-free and overall survival rates were 67% and 73%, respectively.[105] More recently, in a phase II study (COG-ANHL0221), the Children's Oncology Group evaluated the addition of the CD20 monoclonal antibody to the previously reported regimen of low-dose cyclophosphamide and prednisone, but the results are still pending (http://clinicaltrials.gov/show/NCT00066469). Finally, for patients refractory to these low-dose regimens or patients with definitive features of malignancy, standard lymphoma chemotherapy regimens are used depending on histologic subtype (e.g., BL versus DLBCL versus HL-directed therapy).

Hodgkin Lymphoma

Epidemiology

Hodgkin lymphoma (HL) accounts for 10% of all lymphomas and approximately 10% of pediatric cancers[2] and has a bimodal incidence, with one peak at 15 to 34 years of age and a second peak in the sixth decade. In children, the highest peak is among 15- to 19-year-olds (29 per million per year) and is least frequent in children under 5 years. There is an age-dependent sex predominance, with a male predominance in children under 5 years (male-to-female ratio of 5.3 : 1) and a slight female predominance in children ages 15 to 19 years (male-to-female ratio of 0.8 : 1). HL (especially the nodular sclerosing subtype) is classically associated with higher socioeconomic status, increased incidence in single-family homes, smaller family sizes, and a higher level of maternal education. In contrast, mixed-cellularity HL is inversely related to socioeconomic status. It is commonly postulated that delayed exposure to an environmental antigen may trigger development of HL, and higher rates of certain childhood infections (e.g., varicella, measles, mumps, rubella) are negatively associated with HL development.[106]

HL has been shown to have a genetic predisposition, although this is incompletely understood. Siblings of HL patients have a two- to ninefold increased risk for developing HL. There is also an increased risk among parent-child pairs, though not between spouses, supporting a genetic rather than a uniquely environmental predisposition. Environmental factors are nevertheless involved in HL. Approximately 40% of all HL cases in economically developed countries harbor EBV in the Hodgkin and Reed-Sternberg (HRS) cells. EBV positivity of the malignant HRS populations is more common in children under 10 years of age and is highly associated with childhood HL with mixed cellularity subtype (approximately 80% of cases) characteristically seen in developing countries. The EBV latent membrane protein 1 (LMP1) may be the key in the oncogenic process, since it can elicit B lymphocyte transformation in vitro.[107]

A relationship also exists between the development of Hodgkin lymphoma and cell-mediated immune deficiency with an increased incidence in patients with HIV and CVID. It remains unclear whether the underlying immune deficiency commonly seen in Hodgkin lymphoma is primary, secondary, or both.[107]

Pathobiology

Hodgkin lymphoma is generally considered to be slow growing with a tendency to spread to contiguous lymph nodes. Only in advanced stages is there evidence of blood vessel invasion and spreading to more distant organs.[108] Over the past 30 years, advances in the treatment of pediatric HL have been significant—over 85% of children are now cured with chemotherapy and/or radiation even with stage III/IV disease.

HL is notable for the characteristic B cell–derived HRS cells found in a background of an inflammatory microenvironment usually comprising Tregs, Th2 T cells, macrophages, and eosinophils. The REAL/WHO classification identifies two main subtypes: classical HL and lymphocyte predominant HL. Classical Hodgkin lymphoma accounts for the majority of cases in adolescents and young adults and is characterized by HRS cells, which are usually $CD15^+$ and $CD30^+$. HRS cells do not express B-cell markers such as CD19 and CD79A, although CD20 is expressed in approximately 5% to 10% of cases. Mixed-cellularity HL accounts for approximately one-third of cases diagnosed in children younger than 10 years. The histopathology shows frequent HRS cells on a background of normal reactive immune cells, including T lymphocytes, plasma cells, eosinophils, macrophages, and histiocytes. Lymphocyte-predominant HL and lymphocyte-rich classical HL may both have nodular appearances, but the former is more commonly CD15 negative and usually has strong CD20 and CD45 positivity, thus distinguishing it from classical Hodgkin lymphoma.[109]

Clinical Manifestations

The majority of pediatric patients with HL present with painless, firm, "rubbery" lymphadenopathy, most commonly in the cervical/supraclavicular regions. Over 70% of adolescents and young adults present with mediastinal disease, which can be asymptomatic. This presentation is less frequent in younger children and may be related to a lower incidence of nodular sclerosis HL and a greater frequency of mixed-cellularity or lymphocyte-predominant HL in this group. Approximately one-quarter of patients present with systemic "B" symptoms including fevers, weight loss, and night sweats. The majority of pediatric patients presenting with HL have stage I, II, or III disease (involvement of lymph nodes and/or the spleen only) with a minority (approximately 15%) presenting with stage IV disease (noncontiguous extranodal involvement such as bone marrow, lung, liver, and/or bone).

Staging

Pediatric Hodgkin lymphoma is staged using the Ann Arbor staging system (with subsets A and B used for the absence or presence of B symptoms, respectively).[110] Briefly, stage I involves a single lymph node region. Stage II involves two or more lymph node regions on the same side of the diaphragm. Stage III involves lymph node regions above and below the diaphragm. For stages I to III, if extension to an adjacent extralymphatic region/organ is present, the designation E is added (e.g., stage IIE). Thus stage III HL with splenic involvement is designated stage IIIE. Finally, stage IV disease refers to multifocal, noncontiguous involvement of one or more extralymphatic organs or tissues, with or without involvement of associated lymph nodes. Isolated extralymphatic organ involvement with distant nodal involvement is also considered stage IV.

Treatment

Despite the excellent outcomes for children with HL, there is still no ideal therapeutic approach. Generally, combination chemotherapy with low-dose involved-field radiation is used with varying intensities and duration, usually depending on disease stage and prognostic factors such as disease bulk and B symptoms. However, studies of late effects in these patients[111] has fueled cooperative groups in particular to explore regimens with decreased radiation and/or chemotherapy doses, especially for children with low-risk disease. The general consensus, however, is that chemotherapy should be given to all HL patients, with or without radiation. The exception to this approach is patients with stage I, completely resected, nodular lymphocyte-predominant HL, who can achieve cure with surgery alone.[112]

Chemotherapeutic agents used for the initial treatment of pediatric HL are similar to those used for adults and include alkylating agents, steroids, vinca alkaloids, antimetabolites, doxorubicin, bleomycin, dacarbazine, and etoposide. However, doxorubicin (Adriamycin) is associated with cardiac toxicity, and bleomycin can lead to pulmonary fibrosis. Therefore many cooperative group studies have developed hybrid regimens using lower cumulative doses of alkylators, doxorubicin, and bleomycin especially for low-risk (stages I to IIA; no bulk; no B symptoms) and intermediate-risk (all stage I and II patients not classified as early stage; stage IIIA; stage IVA) disease. As shown in Table 83-8, the COPP/ABV (cyclophosphamide, vincristine (Oncovin), procarbazine, prednisone alternating with doxorubicin (Adriamycin), bleomycin, and vinblastine) regimen is one such example.[113] To preserve male fertility, etoposide has been substituted for procarbazine in the OEPA (vincristine [Oncovin], etoposide, prednisone, doxorubicin [Adriamycin]) studies developed by the German pediatric Hodgkin lymphoma group and dacarbazine for procarbazine in subsequent courses, resulting in an excellent EFS rate with no difference in outcome between boys and girls.[114] DBVE (doxorubicin, bleomycin, vincristine, and etoposide) and ABVE-PC (doxorubicin [Adriamycin], bleomycin, vincristine, and etoposide plus prednisone and cyclophosphamide) have been used in POG studies and, more recently, in COG trials.[115,116] Despite the inclusion of etoposide, the secondary leukemia rate appears very low in patients treated with DBVE or ABVE-PC without dexrazoxane.[115,116] Further, investigators from Stanford University Medical Center, Dana-Farber Cancer Institute, Massachusetts General Hospital, Barbara Bush Children's Hospital at Maine Medical Center, and St. Jude Children's Research Hospital have excellent results with low-risk disease with the VAMP regimen (vincristine, doxorubicin [Adriamycin], methotrexate, and prednisone)[117] (see Table 83-8).

Published clinical trial outcomes for low- and intermediate-risk pediatric HL patients (summarized in Table 83-8) have achieved 5-year EFS rates of 92% and 85%, respectively. For patients with high-risk disease (e.g., stages IIIB, IVB) POG used a risk-adapted approach with ABVE-PC plus low-dose involved field radiation therapy (LD-IFRT). Rapid early responders (RERs), defined by response on CT scanning after three ABVE-PC cycles, received 21 Gy involved-field radiation. Slow early responders (SERs) received two additional ABVE-PC cycles before radiation. For RERs the 5-year EFS was 86%, and for SERs, 83% ($P = 0.85$).[116] The Children's Cancer Group used intensive chemotherapy with cytarabine/etoposide, COPP/ABV or CHOP (2 cycles of either), plus or minus LD-IFRT. The 5-year EFS for stage IV patients was 90% for those who received RT and 80% for those who did not, leading to the

Table 83-8 Treatment Outcome for Low/Intermediate-Risk Pediatric Hodgkin Lymphoma

Study	*n* =	"Early Stage"	Prescribed Treatment	Cycles	Radiation	EFS
SFOP MDH-90[145]	171	IAB-IIAB	VBVP	4 cycles	20, IF	91% (5-year)
Stanford, St. Jude, et al (5 centers)[117]	110	IAB-IIAB	VAMP	4 cycles	15-25, IF	93% (5-year)
CCG5942[113]	215	IAB-IIAB (no mediastinal or bulky disease)	COPP-ABV	4 cycles	21, IF None	97% (3-year) 91% (3-year)
GPOH[114]	394	IAB-IIA	OEPA (males) OPPA (females)	2 cycles	20-35, IF None	94% (5-year) 97% (5-year)
POG9226[115]	46	IA, IIA, IIIA (no bulk)	DBVE	4 cycles	25, IF	91% (5-year)
POG8625[146]	159	IA, IIA, IIIA (no bulk)	MOPP-ABVD MOPP-ABVD	3 cycles 2 cycles	None 25, IF	83% (8-year) 91% (8-year)
POG9425[116]	262	IB, IIB, IIIB, IVA	ABVE-PC	3 cycles (±) 2 cycles based on response	21, IF	84% (5-year)

ABVE-PC, Doxorubicin (Adriamycin), bleomycin, vincristine, etoposide, prednisone, cyclophosphamide; *CCG,* Children's Cancer Study Group; *COPP-ABV,* cyclophosphamide, vincristine (Oncovin), procarbazine, prednisone, doxorubicin (Adriamycin), bleomycin, vinblastine; *DBVE,* doxorubicin, bleomycin, vincristine, etoposide; *GPOH,* Society for Pediatric Hematology/Oncology; *IF,* involved field; *MOPP-ABVD,* mechlorethamine, vincristine (Oncovin), procarbazine, prednisone, doxorubicin (Adriamycin), bleomycin, vinblastine, dacarbazine; *OEPA,* vincristine (Oncovin), etoposide, prednisone, doxorubicin (Adriamycin); *OPPA,* vincristine (Oncovin), prednisone, procarbazine, doxorubicin (Adriamycin); *POG,* Pediatric Oncology Group; *SFOP,* French Pediatric Oncology Society; *VAMP,* vinblastine, doxorubicin (Adriamycin), methotrexate, prednisone; *VBVP,* vinblastine, bleomycin, etoposide (Vepesid), prednisone.

conclusion that RT should be given for these patients when used with this chemotherapy combination.[113] Finally, in the German GPOH-HD 95 trial, patients with stages IIEB, IIIEA, IIIB, or IV received six cycles OPPA (vincristine [Oncovin], prednisone, procarbazine, doxorubicin [Adriamycin]) for girls and six cycles OEPA for boys. Patients achieving complete remission (defined by CT scan) after chemotherapy were not irradiated, and all others received involved-field radiotherapy. In the high-risk groups however, the DFS was significantly worse for nonirradiated patients compared with patients who received RT (79% versus 91%), again confirming that with this regimen, radiation was needed for high-risk disease.[114]

Management of Relapsed Hodgkin Lymphoma

For patients who relapse, response depends on whether or not they had favorable disease at diagnosis and whether the relapse is confined to an area of initial involvement after chemotherapy and no radiation. These patients can generally be salvaged with chemotherapy and involved-field radiation therapy, and even without hematopoietic stem cell transplant, results are very acceptable. For all other patients, treatment of refractory, progressive, or relapsed disease includes induction chemotherapy with multiple chemotherapeutic agents not generally used in the initial therapy (e.g., gemcitabine, vinorelbine, carboplatin/cisplatin, ifosfamide, and more recently, brentuximab), followed by high-dose chemotherapy and autologous stem cell rescue. Conditioning regimens are generally alkylator based,[118] and the frequently reported regimens are CBV (cyclophosphamide, carmustine [BiCNU], and etoposide [VP-16]), BEAM (carmustine [BiCNU], etoposide, cytarabine [ara-C], and melphalan), and BEAC (carmustine [BiCNU], etoposide, cytarabine [ara-C], and cyclophosphamide).[119-121] None of these conditioning regimens produces a superior outcome in pediatric patients, and CVB and BEAM remain the most widely used. The role of local radiation therapy either before or after HSCT is still unclear, although TBI is now generally not used.[122,123] Although an overall DFS of approximately 50% is consistently reported with this approach, the reported range is 20% to 60% because outcomes are related to prognostic factors such as disease burden and chemosensitivity.[119,120,124,125]

The role of allogeneic HSCT has also been investigated for patients with relapsed/refractory HL, although never in a prospective, randomized manner.[126] The use of submyeloablative regimens (generally fludarabine based) may reduce transplant-related mortality rates while still achieving a graft-versus-lymphoma (GVL) effect in patients receiving allografts; this warrants further investigation in the pediatric population.[127,128] Finally, investigational therapies such as targeted T-cell therapies are being explored for pediatric HL patients with relapsed disease, either as adjuvant therapy after transplant or for relapsed disease.[129]

In summary, most children with HL are initially treated with risk-adapted chemotherapy alone or in combination with low-dose involved-field radiotherapy involving carefully designed radiation fields to achieve local disease control while minimizing bystander organ toxicity. Especially for low-risk patients, some studies suggest that the overall survival for patients receiving chemotherapy alone may be similar to that for patients receiving chemotherapy plus radiotherapy, despite possible differences in EFS. This is due to the fact that it is usually possible to salvage relapse after initial therapy.[114] If salvage therapy for such patients can be targeted and relatively nontoxic (e.g., using novel agents such as brentuximab),[130] then using a less-intense initial regimen may be appropriate. Currently, however, salvage therapy for the majority of patients is typically more toxic and can lead to an unacceptable incidence of late events such as cardiac toxicities and secondary malignancies.[131] Therefore strategies using a less-intense upfront regimen should be investigated only within the context of a clinical trial. Future clinical studies should attempt to address this important issue by evaluating the prognostic significance of achieving PET-negative disease after one or two cycles of chemotherapy and the use of upfront brentuximab to replace more toxic modalities such as bleomycin and radiation therapy.

Rare Subtypes of Lymphoma

Other subtypes that are observed rarely in children deserve mention, but the rarity of these neoplasms in children makes generalizations and therapeutic recommendations difficult. Follicular lymphomas (characterized by the arrangement of malignant cells in aggregates separated by normal cells), which account for approximately 30% of adult NHLs, are extremely rare in children. Children with follicular lymphomas tend to present with early-stage disease and cervical lymph node involvement (although primary tumors of the testis have been reported[132]) and have an excellent prognosis.[133] Unlike most cases of follicular lymphoma in adults, in which aberrant expression of BCL2, usually as a result of the t(14;18) translocation, is thought to play an important role in lymphomagenesis, the majority of cases of follicular lymphomas in children demonstrate neither the t(14;18) nor BCL2 expression. BCL2 expression appears to occur more frequently in older children and is associated with advanced-stage disease at presentation and a more aggressive clinical course.[133]

Marginal zone B cell lymphomas arising in mucosa-associated lymphoid tissue (MALT) can arise in extranodal sites. They tend to present with localized disease and infrequently disseminate. Natural killer cell lymphoma and NK-like T-cell lymphomas usually involve the upper aerodigestive tract (midline lethal granuloma, angiocentric T-cell lymphoma), but these can present in the skin as well. Such cases are rare in children and follow a very aggressive clinical course; these lymphomas are often fatal but may respond to high-dose chemotherapy with stem cell transplantation.[134] Peripheral T-cell lymphomas include a variety of neoplasms that have not yet been further specified. Although these lymphomas are rare in children, they generally present at advanced stage, often in association with systemic symptoms and hemophagocytic syndrome, and an aggressive course of treatment is the rule.

FUTURE DIRECTIONS

Although there have been dramatic improvements in the treatment of children with NHL and HL over the past 25 years, approximately 25% of children with these tumors still relapse or fail to respond to initial therapy. Additionally, late effects such as anthracycline-related cardiomyopathy, secondary malignancies such as epipodophyllotoxin-related acute myeloid leukemia, and endocrine abnormalities such as cyclophosphamide-related azoospermia remain a concern.[131,135] Thus a major task is to develop treatment strategies that provide a cure for the remaining 25% while also reducing treatment-related morbidity. Several approaches appear promising.

The identification of both clinical and biologic features at the time of diagnosis that predict treatment failure will enable investigators to refine existing risk-adapted therapeutic approaches. Strategies to be considered for children at high risk for treatment failure include the intensification of existing regimens and the incorporation of new active or novel agents. More-intensive therapy may require either autologous or allogeneic hematopoietic stem cell support. The administration of colony-stimulating factors may be necessary in some cases, although their role in therapy remains controversial. Novel approaches include the incorporation of immunotherapeutic agents into multiagent chemotherapy regimens. For example, there is increasing experience with the anti-CD20 antibody (rituximab) in pediatric patients with B-cell lymphomas.[56] A radiolabeled form of this product (yttrium-90 Zevalin) has also yielded promising preliminary results in children.[136] $CD30^+$ lymphomas, such as ALCL, mediastinal B-large cell lymphoma, and Hodgkin disease, are also candidates for CD30 antibody therapy. Novel immunotherapeutic approaches include the use of surface protein–specific cytotoxic T lymphocytes; this approach is effective in the prevention and treatment of EBV-related posttransplant lymphoproliferative disease, NHL and HL.[101,129] Agents targeting specific molecular lesions (e.g., the ALK inhibitor for ALCL) are promising and are already in phase I studies in children and the implementation of anti-idiotype and antisense strategies are also being studied.

The continued investigation of molecular abnormalities and pathogenic mechanisms of malignant transformation associated with childhood lymphomas is essential. Microchip gene arrays have already identified clinically relevant subtypes of large B-cell lymphomas in adults.[137] Gene array analyses of Burkitt lymphoma, anaplastic large cell lymphoma, and T-lymphoblastic disease have also been reported.[138] Similar studies are ongoing for childhood lymphomas and preliminary results for T-lymphoblastic leukemia/lymphoma have been published.[139] Comprehensive molecular characterization of childhood lymphomas may help to further refine disease classification, provide a means of detecting minimal residual disease (MRD) during clinical remission and enhance our assessment of early response.[140] Monitoring is facilitated by the finding that the level of MRD in the peripheral blood is comparable to that in the bone marrow in children presenting with advanced-stage lymphomas. Additionally, a more complete understanding of the molecular pathogenesis of pediatric HL and NHLs will provide clues to new and better treatments directed toward tumor-specific molecular lesions.

SUGGESTED READINGS

Asselin BL, Devidas M, Wang C, et al: Effectiveness of high-dose methotrexate in T-cell lymphoblastic leukemia and advanced-stage lymphoblastic lymphoma: A randomized study by the Children's Oncology Group (POG 9404). *Blood* 118:874, 2011.

Bradley MB, Cairo MS: Stem cell transplantation for pediatric lymphoma: Past, present and future. *Bone Marrow Transplant* 41:149, 2008.

Burkhardt B, Oschlies I, Klapper W, et al: Non-Hodgkin's lymphoma in adolescents: Experiences in 378 adolescent NHL patients treated according to pediatric NHL-BFM protocols. *Leukemia* 25:153, 2011.

Campo E, Swerdlow SH, Harris NL, et al: The 2008 WHO classification of lymphoid neoplasms and beyond: Evolving concepts and practical applications. *Blood* 117:5019, 2011.

Castellino SM, Geiger AM, Mertens AC, et al: Morbidity and mortality in long-term survivors of Hodgkin lymphoma: A report from the Childhood Cancer Survivor Study. *Blood* 117:1806, 2011.

Cooney-Qualter E, Krailo M, Angiolillo A, et al: A phase I study of ^{90}yttrium-ibritumomab-tiuxetan in children and adolescents with relapsed/refractory CD20-positive non-Hodgkin's lymphoma: A Children's Oncology Group study. *Clin Cancer Res* 13:5652s, 2007.

Dave BJ, Nelson M, Sanger WG: Lymphoma cytogenetics. *Clin Lab Med* 31:725, 2011.

Dave SS, Fu K, Wright GW, et al: Molecular diagnosis of Burkitt's lymphoma. *N Engl J Med* 354:2431, 2006.

Donaldson SS, Link MP, Weinstein HJ, et al: Final results of a prospective clinical trial with VAMP and low-dose involved-field radiation for children with low-risk Hodgkin's disease. *J Clin Oncol* 25:332, 2007.

Ducassou S, Ferlay C, Bergeron C, et al: Clinical presentation, evolution, and prognosis of precursor B-cell lymphoblastic lymphoma in trials LMT96, EORTC 58881, and EORTC 58951. *Br J Haematol* 152:441, 2011.

Haddy TB, Adde MA, McCalla J, et al: Late effects in long-term survivors of high-grade non-Hodgkin's lymphomas. *J Clin Oncol* 16:2070, 1998.

Jaglowski SM, Linden E, Termuhlen AM, et al: Lymphoma in adolescents and young adults. *Semin Oncol* 36:381, 2009.

Le Deley MC, Reiter A, Williams D, et al: Prognostic factors in childhood anaplastic large cell lymphoma: Results of a large European intergroup study. *Blood* 111:1560, 2008.

Le Deley MC, Rosolen A, Williams DM, et al: Vinblastine in children and adolescents with high-risk anaplastic large-cell lymphoma: Results of the randomized ALCL99-vinblastine trial. *J Clin Oncol* 28:3987, 2010.

Link MP, Donaldson SS, Berard CW, et al: Results of treatment of childhood localized non-Hodgkin's lymphoma with combination chemotherapy with or without radiotherapy. *N Engl J Med* 322:1169, 1990.

Link MP, Shuster JJ, Donaldson SS, et al: Treatment of children and young adults with early-stage non-Hodgkin's lymphoma. *N Engl J Med* 337:1259, 1997.

Lorsbach RB, Shay-Seymore D, Moore J, et al: Clinicopathologic analysis of follicular lymphoma occurring in children. *Blood* 99:1959, 2002.

Magrath IT: African Burkitt's lymphoma. History, biology, clinical features, and treatment. *Am J Pediatr Hematol Oncol* 13:222, 1991.

Mauz-Korholz C, Gorde-Grosjean S, Hasenclever D, et al: Resection alone in 58 children with limited stage, lymphocyte-predominant Hodgkin lymphoma-experience from the European network group on pediatric Hodgkin lymphoma. *Cancer* 110:179, 2007.

Murphy SB: Pediatric lymphomas: Recent advances and commentary on Ki-1–positive anaplastic large-cell lymphomas of childhood. *Ann Oncol* 5:31, 1994.

Murphy SB: Classification, staging and end results of treatment of childhood non-Hodgkin's lymphomas: Dissimilarities from lymphomas in adults. *Semin Oncol* 7:332, 1980.

Murphy SB, Fairclough DL, Hutchison RE, et al: Non-Hodgkin's lymphomas of childhood: An analysis of the histology, staging, and response to treatment of 338 cases at a single institution. *J Clin Oncol* 7:186, 1989.

Nachman JB, Sposto R, Herzog P, et al: Randomized comparison of low-dose involved-field radiotherapy and no radiotherapy for children with Hodgkin's disease who achieve a complete response to chemotherapy. *J Clin Oncol* 20:3765, 2002.

Patte C, Auperin A, Gerrard M, et al: Results of the randomized international FAB/LMB96 trial for intermediate risk B-cell non-Hodgkin lymphoma in children and adolescents: It is possible to reduce treatment for the early responding patients. *Blood* 109:2773, 2007.

Salzburg J, Burkhardt B, Zimmermann M, et al: Prevalence, clinical pattern, and outcome of CNS involvement in childhood and adolescent non-Hodgkin's lymphoma differ by non-Hodgkin's lymphoma subtype: A Berlin-Frankfurt-Münster Group Report. *J Clin Oncol* 25:3915, 2007.

Sandlund JT, Downing JR, Crist WM: Non-Hodgkin's lymphoma in childhood. *N Engl J Med* 334:1238, 1996.

Schwartz CL, Constine LS, Villaluna D, et al: A risk-adapted, response-based approach using ABVE-PC for children and adolescents with intermediate- and high-risk Hodgkin lymphoma: The results of P9425. *Blood* 114:2051, 2009.

Stein H, Foss HD, Durkop H, et al: CD30(+) anaplastic large cell lymphoma: A review of its histopathologic, genetic, and clinical features. *Blood* 96:3681, 2000.

Reiter A, Klapper W: Recent advances in the understanding and management of diffuse large B-cell lymphoma in children. *Br J Haematol* 142:329, 2008.

Uckun FM, Sensel MG, Sun L, et al: Biology and treatment of childhood T-lineage acute lymphoblastic leukemia. *Blood* 91:735, 1998.

For complete list of references log on to www.expertconsult.com.

CHAPTER 84

T-CELL LYMPHOMAS

Owen A. O'Connor, Enrica Marchi, Govind Bhagat, Paolo Corradini, Joan Guitart, Steven T. Rosen, and Timothy M. Kuzel

The T-cell lymphomas are a heterogeneous group of diseases. They can be divided into those diseases that predominantly arise within the skin, and are thus referred to as the *cutaneous T-cell lymphomas* (CTCLs), and those that do not primarily arise in the skin, namely, the mature or peripheral T-cell lymphomas (PTCLs). Like the B-cell malignancies, each of these subcategories of T-cell lymphoma can be divided into indolent and aggressive diseases, each associated with its own treatment principles. Although CTCL is considered a mature T-cell lymphoma, these diseases are for the most part indolent in nature. They are characterized by a variety of clinical entities, each with its own unique biology and presentation. The mature or peripheral T-cell lymphomas typically arise in lymph nodes, extranodal sites, or as leukemic disease and are for the most part very aggressive diseases. The separation of the T-cell lymphomas into cutaneous or noncutaneous is largely intended to highlight some of the general differences in behavior, though clearly there is overlap. Some forms of CTCL can involve nodal and extranodal sites, and some forms of PTCL can involve the skin. Given the marked differences in biology, clinical behavior, and treatment of these two categories of T-cell lymphoma, this chapter has organized them into their own sections.

THE PERIPHERAL T-CELL LYMPHOMAS (NONCUTANEOUS)

The mature or peripheral T-cell lymphomas are a heterogeneous group of diseases. Similar to the B-cell neoplasms, there are some entities that are known to be relatively indolent, such as the CTCLs and CD30-positive anaplastic large cell lymphomas (ALCLs) of the skin. Most PTCL entities are, however, considered highly aggressive diseases that respond poorly to conventional chemotherapy. Among the most common subtypes are PTCL not otherwise specified (NOS), angioimmunoblastic lymphoma, angioimmunoblastic T-cell lymphoma (AITL), and the ALCLs. Although these diseases are considered to carry an unfavorable prognosis compared to their B-cell counterparts, select molecular entities, such as ALK-positive ALCL, are associated with a favorable prognosis, comparable to that seen with diffuse large B-cell lymphoma (DLBCL).

It is estimated that there were approximately 66,360 cases of non-Hodgkin lymphoma (NHL) in the United States in 2011, of which the T-cell lymphomas account for approximately 5% to 10% of all cases.[1] The median age at diagnosis is 59 years, which is slightly less than the median age of 66 for patients with NHL in general. Like other forms of lymphoma, the T-cell lymphomas are diseases of older adults, with approximately 40% of cases occurring between the ages of 55 and 74, and only about 5% of cases occurring after the age of 85. Between 2004 and 2008, Surveillance Epidemiology and End Results (SEER) reported the age-adjusted incidence rate of T-cell lymphoma as approximately 1.8 per 100,000 men and women. The incidence rates among all races in males and females is approximately 2.3 and 1.4 per 100,000 individuals, respectively, in contrast to 24 and 16.5 cases per 100,000 males and females for NHL. The disease is almost twice as frequent in males as females.[1] In general, the disease is far more common in Asia. For example, the International Peripheral T-Cell and Natural Killer/T-Cell Lymphoma Study noted that T-cell lymphomas accounted for only 5% to 10% of all NHL cases in Western countries and about 10% to 20% in Asian countries.[2] Rudiger et al[3] have reported that the frequency of PTCL in Vancouver, for example, was roughly 1.6%, compared to the 18.3% frequency in Hong Kong.

Although rare in the West, subtypes of PTCL are not uncommon in the Eastern hemisphere and in Central and South America. Geographic and ethnic variability have been cited as reasons for the differences in the prevalence of some types of PTCL. Exposure to certain infectious or environmental agents is thought to account for some of the geographic variation, especially with regard to human T-lymphotropic virus-1 (HTLV-1) infection and occurrence of adult T-cell leukemia/lymphoma (ATL), as well as Epstein-Barr virus (EBV) infection and the development of natural killer (NK)/T-cell lymphoma (NKTCL) in Asia, the Caribbean, and Central and South America. Globally the three most common subtypes of PTCL are PTCL-NOS (25.9%), AITL (18.5%), and ALCL (12%).[2] PTCL-NOS is recognized as being slightly more common in North America, with a lower incidence in Europe and Asia, whereas AITL is more common in Europe as compared to Asia or North America. Enteropathy-associated T-cell lymphoma (EATL) is associated with celiac disease (which itself is associated with leukocyte antigen DQ), which is more common in European populations.[4] Similarly, EBV-associated lymphomas are primarily seen in Japan, Korea, and northern China, as well as immigrant populations from South America in North America. These data suggest that there may be a variety of both genetic and environmental factors that may predispose to T-cell lymphomas, many of which are only now being identified in larger epidemiologic studies.

Classification

The classification of the PTCLs has evolved substantially over the past several decades. Older classification schemes failed to incorporate all the necessary immunophenotypic, cytogenetic, morphologic, and clinical data to subclassify these diseases, as now presented in the context of the World Health Organization (WHO) classification system. The most recent WHO classification published in 2008 recognizes more than 22 different subtypes of T-cell lymphoma distributed among four different subcategories. As shown in Table 84-1 and Fig. 84-1, these subcategories are divided into nodal, extranodal, cutaneous, and leukemic, each based on the predominant clinical behavior of that disease entity.

The nodal group consists of PTCL-NOS, which is the most common subtype of PTCL, accounting for roughly one-quarter of all PTCL cases. Other subtypes included ALCL and AITL. In ALCL there is a significant impact of specific cytogenetic features on prognosis. The ALK-positive forms of ALCL, which are characterized by the nucleophosmin (NPM)-ALK translocation [t(2;5)] have a highly favorable prognosis, whereas those variants that are ALK negative carry a relatively poor prognosis. Other than the presence of the ALK translocation as determined by fluorescence in situ hybridization (FISH), there is no way to differentiate these diseases on strictly morphologic or immunophenotypic grounds. As such, the appropriate therapeutic recommendations for these two diseases obligatorily involve an understanding of this specific cytogenetic feature. Each of

Table 84-1 WHO Classification of the Mature T-Cell Lymphomas

Leukemic	T-cell prolymphocytic leukemia T-cell large granular lymphocytic leukemia Aggressive NK-cell leukemia Indolent large granular NK-cell lymphoproliferative disorder (provisional) Adult T-cell leukemia (HTLV-1, ATL)
Extranodal	Extranodal NK/T-cell lymphoma, nasal type Enteropathy-associated T-cell lymphoma Hepatosplenic T-cell lymphoma Subcutaneous panniculitis-like T-cell lymphoma (αβ T-cell lineage only) Primary cutaneous γδ-T-cell lymphoma
Nodal	ALCL, systemic or cutaneous ALCL:ALK positive [t(2;5)] ALCL:ALK negative (provisional) PTCL-NOS
Cutaneous	Mycosis fungoides/Sézary syndrome Primary cutaneous CD30⁺ T-cell LPD LYP and primary cutaneous ALCL Primary cutaneous CD4⁺ small/medium T-cell lymphoma (provisional) Primary cutaneous CD8⁺ aggressive epidermotropic cytoxic T-cell lymphoma (provisional)
Other	Systemic EBV-positive T-cell LPD of childhood Hydroa vacciniforme–like lymphoma

ALCL, Anaplastic large cell lymphoma; *ATL,* adult T-cell leukemia/lymphoma; *EBV,* Epstein-Barr virus; *HTLV-1,* human T-lymphotropic virus-1; LPD, lymphoproliferative disease; *LYP,* lymphomatoid papulosis; *NK,* natural killer; *NOS,* not otherwise specified; *PTCL,* peripheral T-cell lymphoma; *WHO,* World Health Organization.

these ALCL variants accounts for about 5% to 6% of all cases of PTCL. Similarly, it is often a significant diagnostic challenge to discriminate ALK-negative ALCL from PTCL-NOS. AITL is the second most common subtype of PTCL, accounting for about 18% to 19% of all cases of PTCL. It, uniquely, can also be associated with an EBV-infected clonal B-cell population.

The extranodal subtypes of PTCL are associated with their own unique clinical behavior. This subcategory can include very rare and aggressive diseases like hepatosplenic γδ-T-cell lymphoma. The γδ designation refers to the composition of dimeric protein that makes up the T-cell receptor (TCR). Approximately 95% of all PTCLs possess TCRs that carry the αβ-heterodimer, whereas the γδ-T-cell lymphomas, like hepatosplenic T-cell lymphoma, possess a TCR composed of the γδ-chains. The disease is thought to be derived from a highly primitive γδ-T-cell that has a penchant for infiltrating the liver and spleen. EATL accounts for less than 5% of all PTCL cases. EATL is highly associated with celiac disease, which itself is far more prevalent in Europe. As a result, EATL accounts for only about 6% of all PTCL cases in North America, about 10% in Europe, and less than 2% in Asia, where celiac disease is very uncommon. Panniculitis-like T-cell lymphoma is another subtype of extranodal PTCL. It accounts for less than 1% of all cases of PTCL and is associated with a very aggressive course and resistance to chemotherapy. The immunophenotype of the disease is usually CD3 and CD8 positive and CD4 negative. In addition, the disease can exhibit rearrangements in the TCR of the αβ or γδ variety. This rare form of lymphoma is often misdiagnosed, frequently being confused with the panniculitic-like lesions seen in lupus. It usually presents with subcutaneous nodules that may be necrotic, making rebiopsy the only avenue to diagnosis.

The leukemia subtypes of T-cell lymphoma largely consist of ATL, which is commonly associated with the HTLV-1 retrovirus. The immunophenotype is typically CD3 and CD5 positive, CD7 negative, with positivity for CD4 and CD25 in the majority of cases. ATL is associated with HTLV-1 infection in the clonal T-cell in 100% of cases. Typically the interval between viral infection and onset of lymphoma is long, on the order of 10 to 40 years, with usually less than 5% of infected individuals actually developing ATL. The disease is typically very aggressive, often involving the bone marrow and lymph nodes, though smoldering and chronic forms of ATL do exist and are often managed differently.

Pathobiology

The PTCLs comprise many rare subsets of NHLs that arise from postthymic T cells or NK cells, which can occur at nodal or extranodal sites. Over recent years there has been some progress in disease characterization and classification. Unlike B-NHLs, the pathogenesis of PTCL is poorly understood, and the cell of origin of many PTCL entities is unknown at present. Progress in understanding the etiology of PTCL and the associated pathogenetic molecular alterations is hampered by the rarity and heterogenous nature of this disease.

Anaplastic Large Cell Lymphoma

ALK-positive ALCL is one of the best characterized types of PTCL (Fig. 84-2). The chromosomal translocation t(2;5)(p23;q35) generates an NPM-ALK fusion protein leading to the constitutive activation of the ALK tyrosine kinase, which can be detected in 55% to 85% of systemic ALCL, with higher frequencies seen in children and young adults.[5,6] Alterations in multiple different signaling pathways have been described as a consequence of ALK translocations, which include the Janus-activated kinase 3 (JAK3)/signal transducer and activator of transcription (STAT3), phosphatidylinositol 3-kinase (PI3-kinase)/protein kinase (AKT)/mammalian target of rapamycin (mTOR), and the phospholipase C-γ (PLC-γ)–mediated Ras–extracellular signal-regulated kinase (ERK) pathways. In addition, abnormalities of CD30 signaling, MYC, and growth factor receptor–bound protein 2 (Grb2) (an adaptor protein) have also been reported.[5] A role for active Notch1 signaling has been proposed in ALK-positive ALCL, similar to that proposed in classic Hodgkin lymphoma (HL).[7] The cell of origin of ALK-positive ALCL has been debated. A cytotoxic T-cell origin has been proposed; however, there is speculation that the "null cell" phenotype could reflect a common end point for lymphomas arising from different T-cell subsets. Expression of Th17-associated molecules leading to the activation of a Th17 differentiation program has recently been reported for ALK-positive ALCL.[8]

Variant translocations involving ALK and other partner genes have been documented in a minority of cases.[5] Immunohistochemical staining for ALK can influence one's suspicion for such translocations, because an altered pattern of staining (cytoplasmic, membranous, or nucleolar instead of the nuclear and cytoplasmic) is observed depending on the ALK fusion partner (see Fig. 84-2). Pathologic consequences of the variant translocations are not adequately understood at present. The genetic basis for differences in the histopathologic subtypes of ALK-positive ALCL is similarly unclear. Differences in gene expression profiles between certain morphologic subtypes have been reported.[9] It is possible that these reflect differences in the tumor composition with regard to the admixture of nonneoplastic cells. Although molecular alterations associated with the different subtypes have not been well characterized, comparative genomic hybridization (CGH) array studies of NPM-ALK and variant ALK translocation–associated ALCL have reported similar recurrent secondary genetic abnormalities.[10] The genetic basis of aggressive disease in some patients with ALK-positive ALCL also remains to be elucidated. Of interest, secondary MYC translocations have been reported in some cases with adverse outcomes.[11,12]

ALK-negative ALCL shows morphologic and phenotypic similarity with ALK-positive ALCL; however, its histogenesis is not known at present. Array CGH analysis of ALK-positive and ALK-negative ALCL highlighted differences in secondary aberrations between the

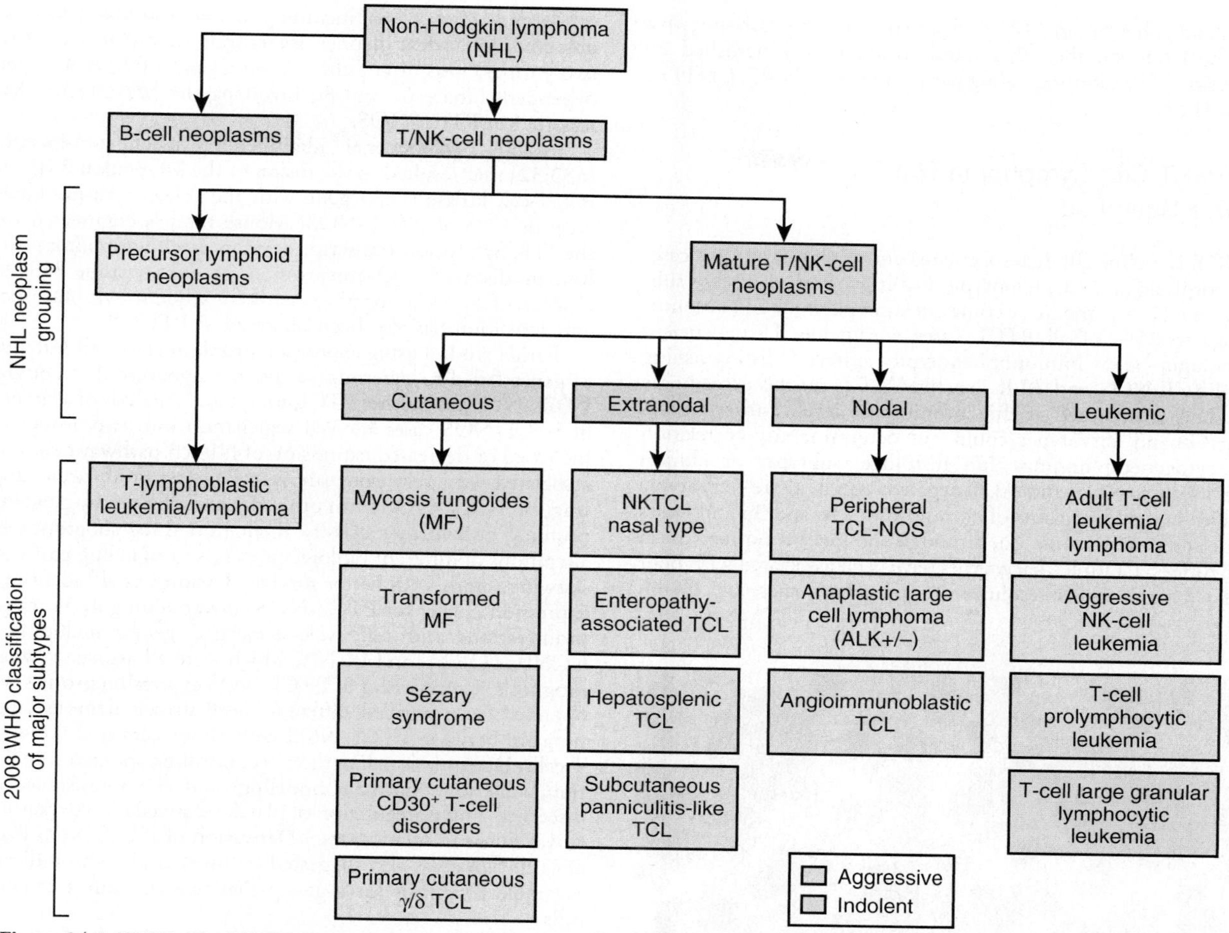

Non-Hodgkin lymphoma (NHL)

- B-cell neoplasms
- T/NK-cell neoplasms
  - Precursor lymphoid neoplasms
    - T-lymphoblastic leukemia/lymphoma
  - Mature T/NK-cell neoplasms
    - Cutaneous
      - Mycosis fungoides (MF)
      - Transformed MF
      - Sézary syndrome
      - Primary cutaneous CD30⁺ T-cell disorders
      - Primary cutaneous γ/δ TCL
    - Extranodal
      - NKTCL nasal type
      - Enteropathy-associated TCL
      - Hepatosplenic TCL
      - Subcutaneous panniculitis-like TCL
    - Nodal
      - Peripheral TCL-NOS
      - Anaplastic large cell lymphoma (ALK+/–)
      - Angioimmunoblastic TCL
    - Leukemic
      - Adult T-cell leukemia/lymphoma
      - Aggressive NK-cell leukemia
      - T-cell prolymphocytic leukemia
      - T-cell large granular lymphocytic leukemia

NHL neoplasm grouping

2008 WHO classification of major subtypes

Aggressive

Indolent

Figure 84-1 WHO CLASSIFICATION OF THE MATURE T-CELL NEOPLASMS. *NK,* Natural killer; *NOS,* not otherwise specified; *TCL,* T-cell lymphoma.

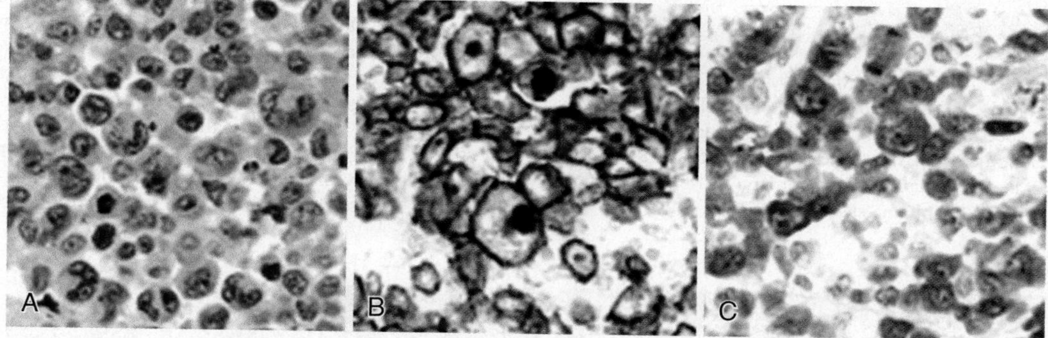

Figure 84-2 ANAPLASTIC LARGE CELL LYMPHOMA. Anaplastic large cell lymphoma has variable morphologic features but is typically composed of large, highly irregular "anaplastic" cells, which include giant cells sometimes with a wreath-like or horseshoe-shape nuclei, and "hallmark" cells, which are cells with a folded-up nucleus with an embryo shape **(A).** The cells are typically brightly CD30 positive **(B).** ALK1 staining with cytoplasmic and nuclear localization **(C)** is associated with the t(2;5)(p23;q35) translocation, whereas other patterns are associated with the variant translocations **(C).** Whether ALK1-negative cases should be considered as a separate group or classified together with peripheral T-cell lymphoma not otherwise specified is somewhat debatable (see text).

two subtypes.[10] Early analyses of gene expression profiles of ALK-positive and ALK-negative ALCL indicated deregulation of certain common kinase-signaling cascades and regulators of apoptosis.[13] ALK-positive and ALK-negative ALCL were shown to differ with regard to alterations in cell cycle regulators based on unsupervised analysis of expression profiles (overexpression of cyclin D3 in ALK-positive ALCL and underexpression of p19INK4D in ALK-negative ALCL). ALK-positive ALCL is associated with overexpressed genes encoding signal transduction molecules (Syk, Lyn, and Cdc37) and showed lower expression of transcription factors (HoxC6 or HoxA3) in comparison with ALK-negative ALCL.[13] Lamant et al,[9] using supervised analysis, described overexpression of BCL6, PTPN12, CEBPB, and SERPINA1, genes implicated in immune or inflammatory responses, regulation of the NF-κB signaling, and leukocyte migration and adhesion, in ALK-positive compared to ALK-negative ALCL. The latter, on the other hand, could be distinguished by overexpression of cytokine-signaling pathway genes (CCR7, CNTFR, IL22, and IL21).

Peripheral T-Cell Lymphoma Not Otherwise Specified

PTCL-NOS is a clinically heterogeneous entity that comprises cases lacking morphologic and phenotypic features of other disease subtypes (Fig. 84-3). It is the most common subtype of PTCL, accounting for up to 25% of all PTCL cases worldwide. Using current histopathologic and immunophenotypic criteria distinguishing between PTCL-NOS and ALK-negative ALCL can be exceedingly difficult. This is mirrored at the chromosome level. Earlier studies analyzing G-band karyotypes could not determine any correlation between cytogenetic findings and histologic subtypes or clinical outcome.[14] PTCL-NOS and ALK-negative ALCL share karyotypic abnormalities, including gains of chromosomes 1q and 3p and losses of material on chromosome 6q, although the loci on 6q have been shown to differ.[15] Complex karyotypes have been associated with poor prognosis. Using higher-resolution approaches, such as CGH, overlapping aberrations, including 6q and 13q losses, have also been observed, but a few distinct aberrations were detected between the two entities.[16] Recurrent chromosome gains of 7q that target cyclin-dependent kinase 6[17] and 8q involving the MYC locus[18] have been reported in PTCL-NOS.

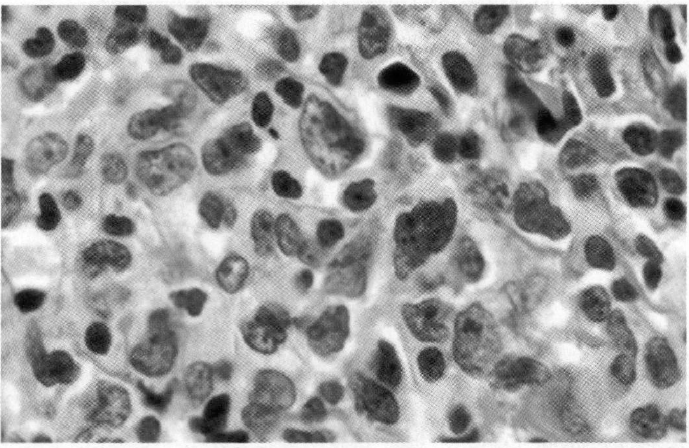

Figure 84-3 PERIPHERAL T-CELL LYMPHOMA NOT OTHERWISE SPECIFIED (PTCL-NOS). PTCL-NOS is morphologically heterogeneous. Typically, cases have a spectrum of small to large lymphoma cells, frequently with irregular nuclear borders and sometimes with clear cytoplasm. Other cases can have more of a predominance of small or large cells. Features of the other defined types of T-cell lymphoma should be lacking.

In 2006, Streubel et al[19] identified a recurrent translocation t(5;9)(q33;32) that resulted in the fusion of the interleukin 2 (IL-2) inducible T-cell kinase (ITK) gene with the spleen tyrosine kinase (Syk) gene in 17% of PTCL-NOS. Mouse models engineered to express the ITK-Syk fusion transcript develop T-cell lymphomas mimicking human disease.[20,21] Overexpression of Syk tyrosine kinase in the absence of Syk translocations with consequent Syk phosphorylation and activation has also been observed in PTCL.[22]

Earlier studies using expression profile analysis of limited numbers of genes failed to determine a distinct signature that could separate PTCL-NOS from other PTCL subtypes.[23] Analysis of a larger number of PTCL-NOS cases allowed segregation into two groups based on increased or decreased expression of NF-κB pathway genes, the latter associated with very poor survival. Ballester et al[24] were able to distinguish PTCL-NOS from other disease subtypes by gene expression profiling and further classify them into three subgroups based on alterations of different biologic processes or signaling pathways, some showing trends with better survival. Cuadros et al[25] identified a gene expression cluster for PTCL-NOS corresponding to 55 transcripts of proliferation- and cell cycle–associated genes, including CCNA, CCNB, TOP2A, and PCNA, which were all associated with a poor prognosis. Comparison of PTCL-NOS expression profiles with those obtained from purified different T-cell subsets demonstrated a relationship between PTCL-NOS with either activated $CD4^+$ or $CD8^+$ T cells. Deregulation of pathways controlling apoptosis, cell proliferation, adhesion, matrix remodeling, and chemoresistance could be discerned, and upregulation of platelet-derived growth factor receptor α was noted in many cases.[26] Derivation of PTCL-NOS from different cell types was also suggested by Iqbal et al,[8] who indicated a less favorable prognosis for a group that had signatures of cytotoxic T cells.

Angioimmunoblastic T-Cell Lymphoma

AITL was originally referred to as "angioimmunoblastic lymphadenopathy (AILD) with dysproteinemia" because it was considered to represent a state of deregulated immune response. Its categorization as a lymphoma was based on the detection of clonal TCR gene rearrangements (Fig. 84-4). Gains of chromosomes 3q, 5q, and 21 have been described as recurrent alterations, although the genes affected by these changes are not known.[15] Recent reports have described similarities between gene expression profiles of AITL and T-follicular helper (TFH) cells, with AITL overexpressing genes characteristic of

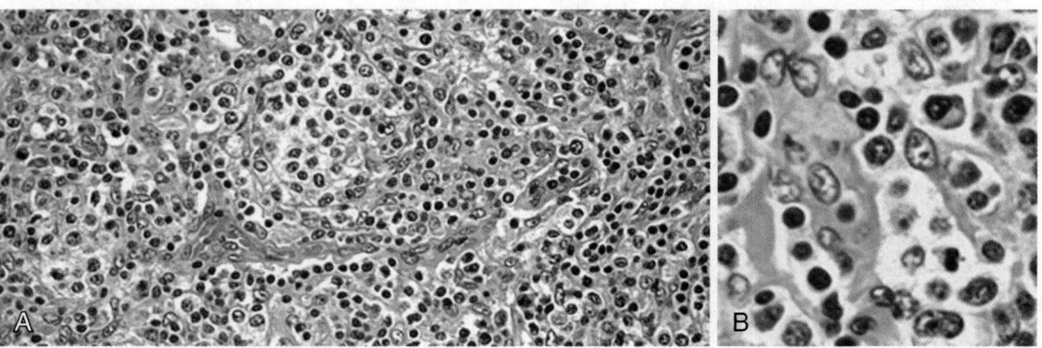

Figure 84-4 ANGIOIMMUNOBLASTIC T-CELL LYMPHOMA (AITL). A prominent feature of AITL is the prominent vasculature in the background. The vessels usually show branching and prominent endothelial cells **(A).** The cellular component is made up of a mix of plasma cells, immunoblasts, and small lymphocytes; the lymphoma cells can be of intermediate or large size and they tend to cluster and exhibit clear cytoplasm **(A, B).** Some cases can develop a superimposed Epstein-Barr virus–driven large B-cell lymphoma.

normal TFH cells (CXCL13, BCL6, PDCD1, CD40L, and NFATC1).[27] Numerous studies have confirmed the phenotypic profile of AITL to be similar to TFH cells.[28] A role for the tumor microenvironment has also been proposed in AITL pathogenesis.[8] Although vascular endothelial growth factor (VEGF) transcripts detected in AITL were originally thought to be derived from the vascular stroma of these neoplasms, expression of VEGF and its receptor (KDR) by the tumor cells was also demonstrated by Piccaluga et al.[29] It should be mentioned that recent immunophenotypic studies have also uncovered other types of PTCL with a TFH phenotype, including subsets of PTCL-NOS.[30] This might be one of the explanations for the inability of gene expression profiling to segregate AITL from subsets of PTCL-NOS in some instances.[29] Whether this indicates an origin of such PTCL from a TFH precursor or acquisition of a TFH phenotype due to derangement of transcriptional circuits remains to be seen. Genome-sequencing studies underway might establish developmental or mechanistic links between different PTCL subtypes. Such studies have already begun to provide insights into similarities and differences among PTCL subtypes. Quivoron et al[31] discovered an increase in T-cell progenitors and genesis of T-cell lymphomas in mice engineered to disrupt the function of the TET2 gene. On sequencing human lymphoma specimens, they found heterozygous insertions and deletions leading to TET2 frameshift and nonsense mutations in 33% of AITL and a smaller subset of other T-cell lymphomas. Other mutations, including those affecting the second allele, occurred later in lymphomagenesis. The same group then analyzed a large series of PTCL, including PTCL-NOS and AITL, and detected DNMT3A mutations in 73% of cases that had TET2 mutations (including both disease subtypes), suggesting possible oncogenic cooperation between TET2 and DNMT3A mutations and deregulation of cytosine methylation and demethylation processes in T-cell lymphomas.[32a] On screening a variety of PTCL subtypes for IDH1 and IDH2 mutations, Cairns et al[32b] detected heterozygous IDH2 mutations only in AITL (20% in a discovery set and 45% in a validation set), which resulted in an R172 substitution in the majority of cases. Unlike other neoplasms associated with IDH mutations, no IDH1 mutations were detected. The prognostic implications of this mutation, if any, are unclear at present. It also remains to be seen whether this mutation is specific for AITL or other subtypes of PTCL derived from TFH cells.

Natural Killer/T-Cell Lymphoma

NKTCL is associated with EBV infection, and episomal and/or viral integration into the deoxyribonucleic acid (DNA) of neoplastic T or NK cells can be detected (Fig. 84-5). However, other as yet–uncharacterized cooperating genetic and environmental agents likely also play roles in disease pathogenesis. Recurrent deletions of 6q21-25 were described in NKTCL by Wong et al.[33] Array CGH analysis of aggressive NK-cell leukemias and extranodal NKTCL, nasal type, has highlighted genomic differences between the two entities, with gains of 1q and losses of 7p15.1-p22.3 and 17p13.1 being detected more frequently in aggressive NK-cell leukemias, and gains of 2q and losses of 6q16.1-q27 and 11q22.3-q23.3, among others, being more commonly observed in NKTCL, nasal type.[34] A recent study incorporating gene expression analysis with array CGH mapped a novel tumor suppressor gene, HACE1, to the 6q21 region, but the role of this gene in disease pathogenesis remains to be defined.[35] These authors also reported overexpression of granzyme H and overexpression of PDGFRA in NKTCL similar to what has been described in PTCL-NOS. Amplifications of the C-REL gene have been detected in subsets of NKTCL.[36] More recently, deletions of two 6q21 regions detected in 36% of analyzed cases were further characterized by oligonucleotide array CGH and functional studies, which led to the identification of PRDM1 (BLIMP1) and FOX03 as novel tumor suppressors in NKTCL.[37] Rare PRDM1 mutations were also found. Küçük et al[38] confirmed a tumor suppressor role for PRDM1 and described monoallelic deletions and promoter hypermethylation of this gene in a significant percentage of NKTCT.

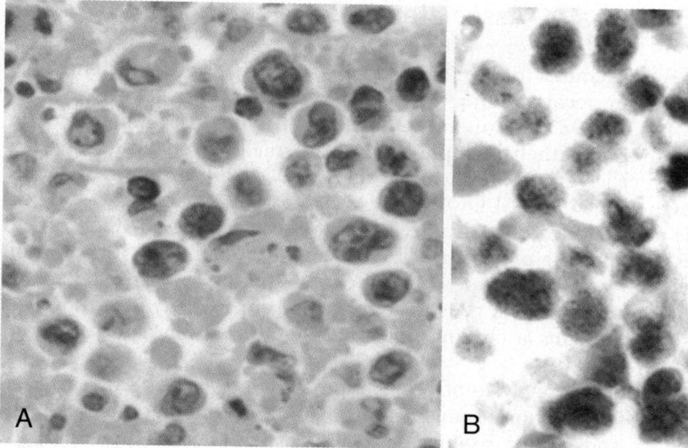

Figure 84-5 NATURAL KILLER (NK)/T-CELL LYMPHOMA, NASAL TYPE. The nasal type of NK/T-cell lymphoma **(A, B)** is usually associated with marked necrosis and karyorrhectic material indicating high cell turnover. The lymphoma cells are variable from case to case, but they invariably are Epstein-Barr virus (EBV) positive as demonstrated by in situ hybridization for EBV-encoded ribonucleic acid (RNA; **B**).

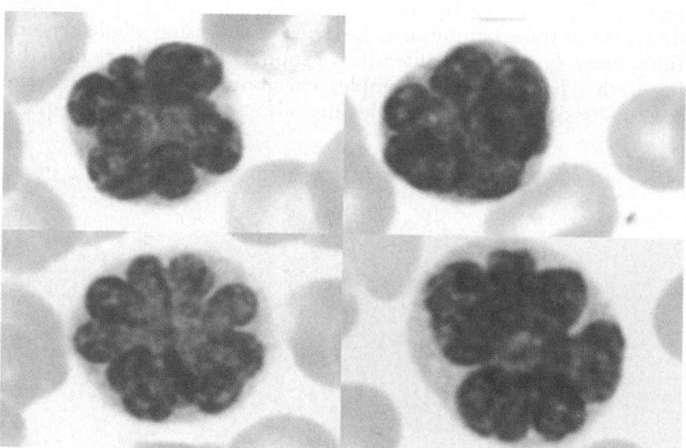

Figure 84-6 HUMAN T-LYMPHOTROPIC VIRUS-1–ASSOCIATED LEUKEMIA/LYMPHOMA. The leukemic process (adult T-cell leukemia/lymphoma) is characterized by circulating neoplastic T cells with a "flower-like" form. In some cases this cytologic feature is more prominent than in others.

Human T-lymphotropic Virus-1–Associated Acute T-Cell Leukemia/Lymphoma

HTLV-1 is a retrovirus that is transmitted via infected T cells present in body fluids, especially breast milk and semen, and blood of carriers of the HTLV-1 provirus. Clinicopathologic subsets of HTLV-1–associated lymphomas include acute ATL, smoldering ATL, lymphomatous ATL, and chronic ATL (Fig. 84-6). ATL is characterized by infection and clonal expansion of $CD4^+$ T cells in the vast majority of cases. Disease pathogenesis involves viral and host factors. A variety of viral proteins with transforming activity have been described, but the Tax protein is the best characterized. The NF-κB transcription factor is one of its targets.[39] Array CGH has highlighted differences in chromosomal alterations between subtypes and could provide hints regarding genes targeted by these alterations.[40] C-REL and IRF-4 expression has been associated with resistance of ATL to antiviral agents.[41]

Enteropathy-Associated T-Cell Lymphoma

EATL accounts for less than 5% of PTCL (Fig. 84-7). Currently, two types are recognized, EATL type 1 ($CD8^-$ and usually $CD56^-$) and type 2 ($CD8^+$ and often $CD56^+$). EATL type 1 is thought to arise from intraepithelial lymphocytes of the small bowel and is associated with celiac disease, occurring in individuals who carry human leukocyte antigen (HLA) DQ2 or DQ8 haplotypes, whereas EATL type 2 is unrelated to celiac disease. Refractory celiac disease (RCD) type II is considered a precursor of EATL, and approximately 50% of individuals with RCD type II develop EATL within 5 years.[42] There are little data regarding genetic abnormalities in RCD type II; however, recurrent gains at chromosome 1q22-q44 have been reported in one study.[43]

Genomic analyses of EATL type 1 have revealed recurrent gains and losses of chromosomal regions that might contain potential oncogenes and tumor suppressor genes. Using microsatellite markers, Baumgartner et al[44] detected frequent amplifications of 9q34 (40%) and slightly less frequent recurrent gains at 5q33.3-34 and 7q31 in EATL. Analysis of these patterns suggested two different disease types, one characterized by gains of 9q34 and another exhibiting allelic imbalances at 3q27.[44] A role for amplification of Notch1 and ABL1 genes, located on chromosome 9q, has been proposed as possible pathogenetic aberrations in EATL.[44,45a] Using CGH, Zettl et al[45b] confirmed the high frequency of 9q gains in EATL (58%) and further refined the minimal region of aberration as 9q33-q34. Recurrent gains at 7q, 5q, and 1q and losses of 8p, 9p, and 13q have been described in these lymphomas. Deleeuw et al,[46] using whole genome tiling array–based CGH, identified genomic abnormalities underlying both types of EATL. Complex chromosomal gains of 9q were seen in 70% of cases and virtually mutually exclusive losses of 16q21.1 in 30% of cases. Of note, gains of 1q and 5q were more frequently observed in EATL type 1, while gains of the MYC locus (8q24) were detected more often in EATL type 2. Segmental amplifications of the 9q31.3-qter chromosomal region or deletions in 16q12.1 were seen in both types of EATL. Recent array CGH analysis of Asian EATL type 2 also detected a high frequency of 9q33-q34.1 gains (80% of cases), suggesting similarities with cases occurring in the West, and documented other recurrent alterations, including gains of 6p21.1-21.31 and 19q, and losses of 3p12.1-p12.2 and 3q26.31.[47] Gene expression analysis of these lymphomas has not yet been performed to determine alterations of any particular signaling, survival, or metabolic pathway.

Hepatosplenic T-Cell Lymphoma

Hepatosplenic TCL is a rare PTCL, which has been associated with underlying immune dysfunction (Fig. 84-8). It is most commonly of γδ-T-cell lineage; however, lymphomas bearing the αβ-TCR have been described, as have occasional cases lacking surface TCR. Isochromosome 7q [i(7)(q10)] is reported to be a frequent recurrent chromosomal aberration, but specific abnormalities of particular genes have not been defined.[48] Of interest, i(7)(q10) has been detected in hepatosplenic T-cell lymphoma irrespective of the phenotype (γδ or αβ). Moreover, an increase in the number of 7q signals was detected in some cases that had features of cytologic progression, suggesting a tendency of the neoplastic cells to increase the dosage of the i(7)(q10) as the disease evolves.[49] Miyazaki et al,[50] using unsupervised analysis of gene expression profiles, were able to classify hepatosplenic γδ-TCL as a distinct cluster but were not able to discriminate between other types of γδ-TCL and αβ-TCL. This could

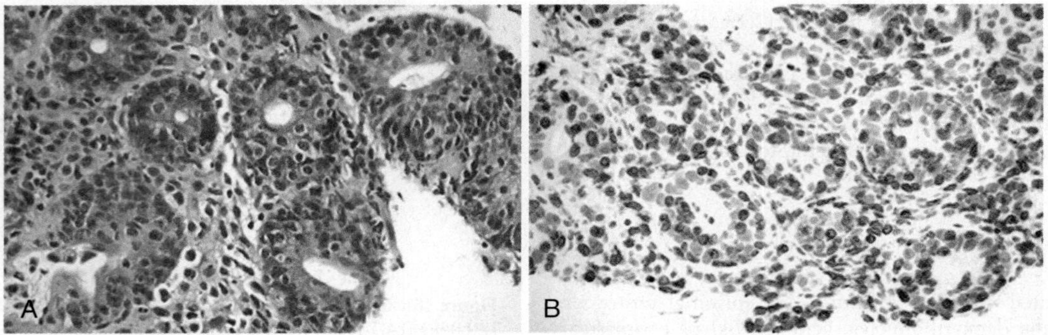

Figure 84-7 ENTEROPATHY-ASSOCIATED T-CELL LYMPHOMA. In enteropathy-associated T-cell lymphoma there is prominent infiltration of gastrointestinal glandular elements by neoplastic T cells **(A).** These are typically $CD3^+$ **(B)** and almost always $CD5^-$ and $CD4^-$ negative, and CD8, and CD56 variable, depending on the type.

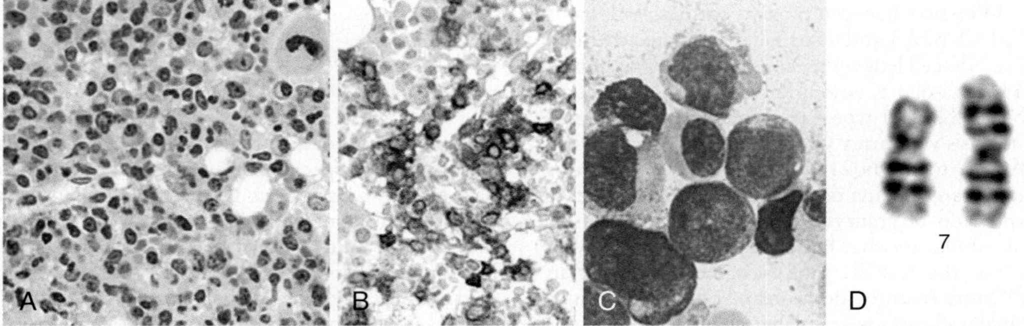

Figure 84-8 HEPATOSPLENIC T-CELL LYMPHOMA. Hepatosplenic γδ-T-cell lymphoma is commonly diagnosed from a bone marrow biopsy specimen in a patient being evaluated for hepatosplenomegaly. The bone marrow typically shows a subtle lymphoid infiltrate **(A),** which becomes more evident with a T-cell stain such as CD3 **(B).** This highlights the classic sinusoidal distribution of the lymphoma. Lymphoma cells may be seen in the circulation or in the marrow aspirate and can resemble monocytes or blasts **(C).** The lymphoma is typically associated with isochromosome 7q, as illustrated in the partial karyotype **(D).**

be due to part of the signature being derived from splenic tissue. Of interest, the authors were able to discern overexpression of NK cell–associated transcripts, such as killer-cell immunoglobulin (Ig)-like receptor (KIR) genes and killer lectin-like receptors.

Clinical Manifestations

PTCLs, with the exclusion of CTCL, recapitulate the general presentation of aggressive NHL, which can vary depending on histologic features, patient age, and immune status. PTCL generally presents with lymphadenopathy, and patients can range from being asymptomatic to presenting with serious organ compromise. PTCL can present as nodal, extranodal, leukemic, and cutaneous disease, which are discussed separately. An extranodal presentation is common in PTCL and often contributes to a delay in the diagnosis. When compared to aggressive B-cell lymphomas, patients with PTCL tend to present with more advanced disease, a poorer performance status, and frequently B symptoms. Patients may have constitutional manifestations because of the production of inflammatory molecules and a variety of other cytokines and chemokines produced by the lymphoma cells and host tissues. Paraneoplastic features, including eosinophilia, hemophagocytic syndrome, and autoimmune phenomena, have been well described in different PTCL subtypes. For example, the AITL is often characterized by systemic symptoms, skin rash, organomegaly, hypergammaglobulinemia, and hemolytic anemia. It affects older adults, and patients frequently present with peripheral lymphadenopathy, hepatosplenomegaly, skin rash, and constitutional symptoms. By contrast, hepatosplenic T-cell lymphoma, which often occurs in young adults, is characterized by marked hepatosplenomegaly and bone marrow involvement.

Laboratory Manifestations

Laboratory tests should include a complete blood count, serum chemistry determination (including lactate dehydrogenase [LDH]), human immunodeficiency virus status, and other viral studies, including HTLV-1 status and EBV in appropriate cases. The level of β_2-microglobulin is usually normal compared to that found with the B-cell lymphomas.

Differential Diagnosis

Accuracy in diagnosis of the PTCLs more often than not requires the consensus of hematopathologists with a specific expertise in this field. Diagnosis is based on examination of peripheral blood or tissue biopsy specimen for histologic features supplemented by detailed immunohistochemistry, flow cytometry, cytogenetics, and molecular genetics. Expert hematopathologic review is essential for the correct classification of the different subtypes, given the often poor concordance among hematopathologists in matching the diagnosis. Detailed clinical information is obviously important in making the correct diagnosis. For example, in patients from Japan, information regarding HTLV-1 status is essential to aiding the pathologist in distinguishing between lymph node involvement due to PTCL-NOS and ATL. Because this disease also occurs in the West, HTLV-1 status should be evaluated in patients at high risk for the disease or from endemic areas. Other diagnoses such as AITL and EATL are often clarified by the clinical information. For cases in which it is difficult to distinguish between different entities, gene expression profiling may become helpful in the future for confirming the correct diagnosis.

Prognostic Factors

The majority of PTCLs are associated with a very poor prognosis as compared to their B-cell counterparts[2] (Fig. 84-9). Treatment outcomes for PTCL patients are substantially inferior to those for their B-cell lymphoma counterparts. Lymphomas derived from the T-cell lineage have been shown to be an independent negative prognostic factor.[51] The International Peripheral T-Cell and Natural Killer/T-Cell Lymphoma study reported that the overall survival (OS) and failure-free survival (FFS) at 10 to 15 years was only 10%. The International Prognostic Index (IPI), which is based on age, performance status, LDH level, stage, and extranodal involvement, appears to be useful in determining the prognosis for certain PTCL subtypes. However, even patients in the best risk categories (IPI 0 or 1) do not have a favorable outcome, and patients in the high-risk categories have a very short survival. When compared to the IPI curves seen for patients with B-cell lymphoma, the curves seen for patients with T-cell lymphoma essentially identify two risk categories, those with IPI 0 or 1 having a relatively more favorable outcome and those with IPI 2 or higher with an unfavorable outcome. In contrast to what is seen in patients with B-cell lymphoma, there is limited separation of the curves. When analyzed as a function of the histopathologic subset, the 5-year OS for patients with PTCL-NOS and AITL with IPI 0 or 1 was only 56% and 50%, respectively, whereas for those patients with IPI 4 or 5 it was 11% and 25%, respectively. Among patients with ALCL, the 5-year survival for IPI 0 or 1 is roughly 90% and 74% for the ALK-positive and ALK-negative patients, respectively. Patients with IPI 2 or higher have a poor outcome, with 5-year survivals of only 33% and 13% in the ALK-positive and ALK-negative populations, respectively. These observations confirm that IPI is an important predictor even in ALK-positive ALCL. The IPI has been less useful in stratifying patients with other subtypes of PTCL, including those with ATL, EATL, hepatosplenic T-cell lymphoma, or extranasal NKTCL.

Other prognostic models have been developed specifically for patients with PTCL. The Prognostic Index for PTCL (PIT) was developed based on risk factors that include age, LDH level, performance status, and bone marrow involvement. When applied to a PTCL-NOS population, the PIT stratified patients into more distinct prognostic groups compared to the IPI. Of 322 patients studied, 20% had no adverse features, 34% had one, and 20% had three or more. The 5-year OS for the most favorable subgroup with no adverse prognostic features was 62% compared to 18% for patients with three or four prognostic factors.[52] Despite improved stratification, the so-called favorable-risk population of patients with PTCL still had a strikingly poor outcome.

Efforts to improve on the more traditional clinically-based scoring systems have been proposed. The Bologna scoring system[53] was developed integrating both patient-specific and tumor-specific characteristics (age >60 years, performance status, LDH level, and Ki-67 protein ≥80%), stratifying patients into low-risk (score 1), intermediate-risk (score 2), and high-risk disease (score 3), with median overall survivals of 37, 23, and 6 months, respectively. Although the scores seem to be able to stratify the patient population, it is clear that there is no really favorable population of patients. The prognostic capability of the Bologna score was validated by Briones et al.[54]

Recently the International Peripheral Lymphoma Study (IPLS) showed that the 5-year OS of 340 patients with PTCL-NOS was only 32% (after 3 years' follow-up), whereas the 5-year FFS was only 20%[55,56] (Fig. 84-10). In this analysis, each of the prognostic factors in the IPI was a highly significant predictor of OS and FFS ($P < .001$; Fig. 84-11). The overall IPI was predictive of both OS and FFS, whereas the PIT was predictive of only survival. Bone marrow involvement was not a robust predictor of OS ($P = .03$) or FFS ($P = .06$) (Fig. 84-12). The PIT did not prove to be superior to the IPI in predicting the survival of patients with PTCL-NOS. Only one group with relatively good FFS was identified using both models. The IPLS evaluated other potential predictive factors by univariate analysis, establishing that the following factors were adverse prognostic factors of OS and FFS, respectively: B symptoms ($P = .004$; $P = .014$), bulky disease greater than or equal to 10 cm ($P = .005$; $P = .004$), elevated serum C-reactive protein level ($P = .018$; $P = .008$), circulating tumor cells ($P < .001$; $P < .001$), and a platelet count of less than 150×10^9/L ($P < .001$; $P < .001$). For unclear reasons, hypergammaglobulinemia fell out as a favorable prognostic

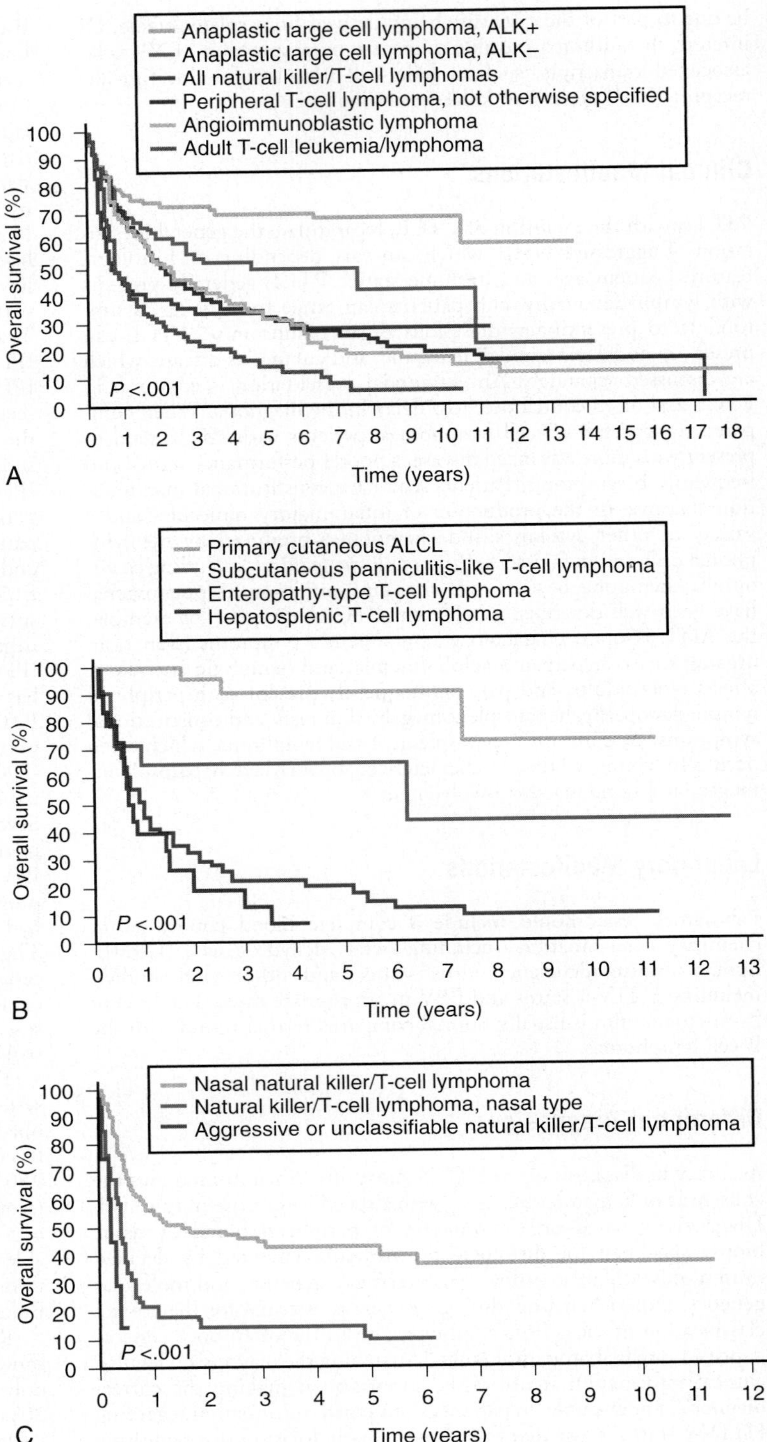

Figure 84-9 A, Overall survival of patients with the common subtypes of peripheral T-cell lymphoma (PTCL). **B,** Overall survival of patients with less-common subtypes of PTCL. **C,** Overall survival of patients with natural killer/T-cell lymphoma. *(Data from Vose J, Armitage J, Weisenburger D: International peripheral T-cell and natural killer/T-cell lymphoma study: Pathology findings and clinical outcomes.* J Clin Oncol 26:4124, 2008.)

factor for OS and FFS ($P = .04$; $P = .03$). When the data were analyzed in a multivariate analysis, after controlling for IPI, only bulky disease greater than or equal to 10 cm was still predictive of survival with a hazard ratio (HR) of 2.1 for OS ($P = .019$) and 2.5 for FFS ($P = .003$), whereas a platelet count of less than 150×10^9/L was predictive of FFS (HR = 1.6, $P = .016$).

The IPLS also explored the impact of several pathologic features that were associated with inferior OS and FFS, including the following: Ki-67 index more than 25%, the presence of transformed tumor cells more than 70%, significant numbers of EBV-positive B cells (Epstein-Barr encoded ribonucleic acid [EBER] 3-4$^+$), and CD56 and CD30 expression by more than 20% on tumor cells. EBV positivity was predictive of an adverse survival only in patients younger than 60 years and was independent of a history of immunosuppressive therapy or autoimmune disorders. Factors that appeared to be favorably associated with improved OS and FFS included lymphoepithelioid (Lennert) variant and background CD8$^+$ T cells constituting more than 10% of the population. Several clinicopathologic factors were identified to be of prognostic significance by univariate analysis, but only bulky disease (>10 cm) and thrombocytopenia (<150×10^9 cells/L) were predictive of OS.

Probably the most important prognostic factor for any subtype of PTCL is the presence or absence of ALK in ALCL. The OS of ALK-positive ALCL is substantially better than that seen for ALK-negative

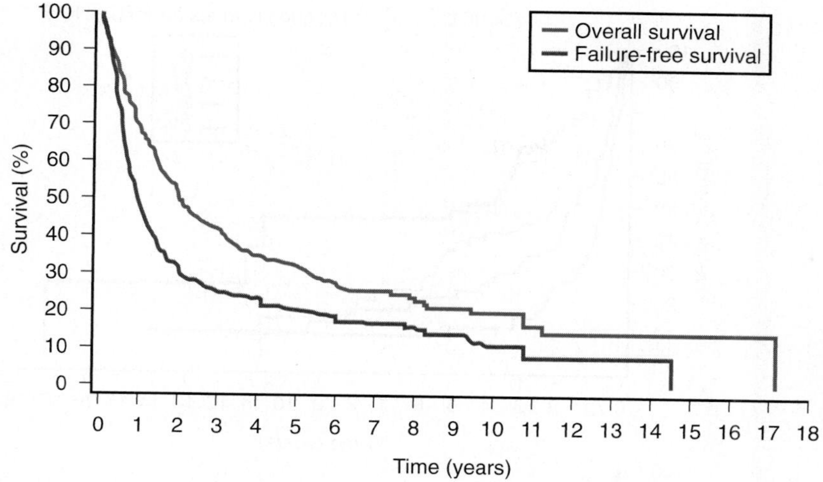

Figure 84-10 OVERALL SURVIVAL AND FAILURE-FREE SURVIVAL OF 340 PATIENTS WITH PERIPHERAL T-CELL LYMPHOMA NOT OTHERWISE SPECIFIED. *(Data from Weisenburger DD, Savage KJ, Harris NL, et al: Peripheral T-cell lymphoma, not otherwise specified: A report of 340 cases from the International Peripheral T-cell Lymphoma Project.* Blood *117:3402, 2011.)*

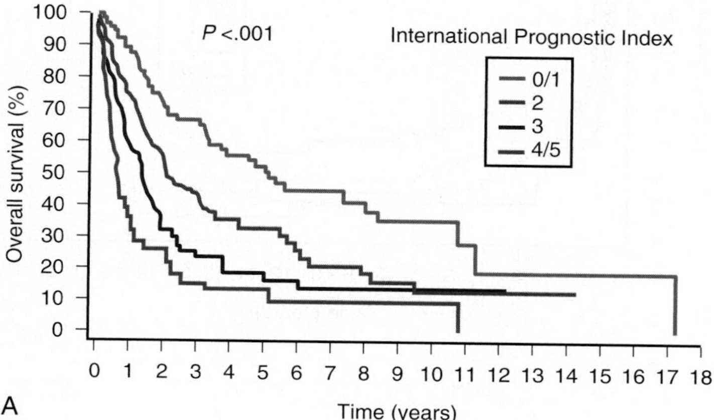

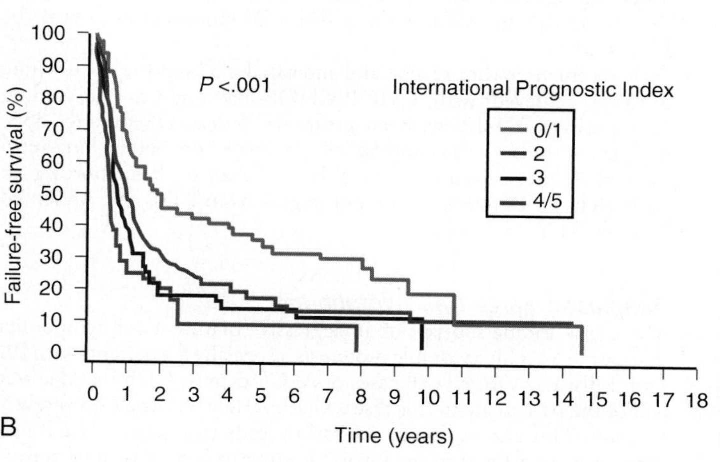

Figure 84-11 OVERALL SURVIVAL **(A)** AND FAILURE-FREE SURVIVAL **(B)** OF 315 PATIENTS WITH PTCL-NOS ACCORDING TO THE INTERNATIONAL PROGNOSTIC INDEX. *(Data from Weisenburger DD, Savage KJ, Harris NL, et al: Peripheral T-cell lymphoma, not otherwise specified: A report of 340 cases from the International Peripheral T-cell Lymphoma Project.* Blood *117:3402, 2011.)*

ALCL (71% ± 6% versus 15% ± 11%, respectively). However, within the good prognostic category of ALK-positive ALCL, survival was 94% ± 5% for the low/low-intermediate risk group (age-adjusted IPI 0 to 1) and 41% ± 12% for the high/high-intermediate risk group (age-adjusted IPI ≥2). Multivariate analysis identified ALK expression and the IPI as independent variables that were able to predict survival among T/null primary, systemic ALCL.[56]

More recently, recognizing the biologic and clinical heterogeneity of PTCL, investigators have begun to develop subtype-specific prognostic models. Although potentially interesting, these models still need to be validated in large studies.

Therapy

Standard of Care

CHOP-Like Therapy in Mature T-Cell Lymphomas

The treatment for the PTCLs has largely mirrored the strategies employed for the treatment of DLBCL. Consequently, CHOP (cyclophosphamide, hydroxydaunomycin, vincristine [Oncovin], and prednisone) has emerged as the "standard of care" despite disappointing outcomes. The milestone SWOG trial that compared CHOP

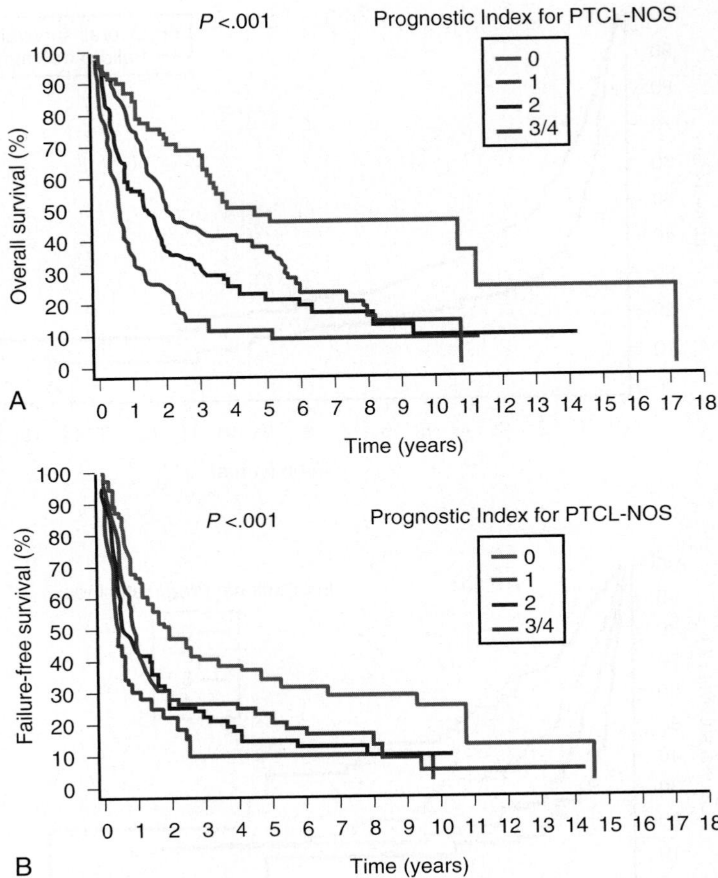

Figure 84-12 OVERALL SURVIVAL **(A)** AND FAILURE-FREE SURVIVAL **(B)** OF 315 PATIENTS WITH PTCL-NOS ACCORDING TO THE PROGNOSTIC INDEX. *PTCL-NOS,* Peripheral T-cell lymphoma not otherwise specified. *(Data from Weisenburger DD, Savage KJ, Harris NL, et al: Peripheral T-cell lymphoma, not otherwise specified: A report of 340 cases from the International Peripheral T-cell Lymphoma Project.* Blood *117:3402, 2011.)*

with the second- and third-generation dose-intensive regimens in aggressive lymphoma established that CHOP exhibited the same efficacy and less toxicity than the other regimens.[57] This landmark trial was based on the use of a histopathologic classification system when immunophenotyping was not yet routinely applied to all cases. Unfortunately, there are no large randomized prospective studies that compare the benefit of anthracycline-based therapies to other combination regimens in PTCL.

Conventional chemotherapy such as CHOP has led to disappointing results in patients with T-cell lymphomas. When the main subgroups of T-cell lymphomas were analyzed, only ALCL with the t(2;5) translocation (NPM-ALK fusion protein) had an equivalent or superior prognosis compared to patients with DLBCL.[51,56] The LNH87 study conducted by the Groupe d'Etudes des Lymphomes de l'Adulte showed that the use of anthracycline-containing chemotherapy regimens in T- and B-cell lymphomas were able to induce the complete remission (CR) in 54% versus 63% of the patients, with an OS of 41% and 53% and an event-free survival (EFS) of 33% and 42%, respectively.[51] The same group published the results of the LNH84 study, in which they employed a dose-intense consolidation. Again, although there was no difference in the response rate, patients with T-cell lymphomas relapsed more frequently and earlier as compared to patients with B-cell lymphoma.[58] More recently the CHOEP regimen (cyclophosphamide, hydroxydaunomycin, vincristine [Oncovin], etoposide, and prednisone) was retrospectively studied by the German High-Grade Non-Hodgkin Lymphoma Study Group in 343 patients with T-cell lymphoma, including PTCL-NOS, ALCL, and AITL, who had been included in seven German high-grade phase 2 or phase 3 aggressive NHL treatment studies. The main purpose was to determine whether the addition of etoposide or shortening of the interval of chemotherapy from 3 weeks to 2 weeks affected survival.[59] In older adult patients, neither shortening the interval nor the addition of etoposide improved the EFS and OS.

A recent literature review and metaanalysis[60] reported a CR rate of 52% achieved with CHOP/CHOP-like regimens (excluding ALK-positive ALCL), with an estimated 5-year OS of only 35% in PTCL. This is in contrast to the 65% or better long-term survival frequently reported in DLBCL. Select studies reporting on the activity of various combination regimens in PTCL are presented in Table 84-2.

Anaplastic Large Cell Lymphoma

ALCL is a unique subtype of an aggressive mature T-cell lymphoma that carries a highly favorable prognosis, especially for patients with IPI 1 or 2 disease. Virtually all cases of ALCL express CD30, and about half of the patients with this disease harbor the t(2;5)(p21;q35) translocation. This chromosomal aberration leads to fusion of the NPM gene with the ALK tyrosine kinase, leading to its constitutive activation. As discussed earlier, the presence of the ALK translocation confers a highly favorable prognosis, and determination of the ALK status by FISH is imperative in all cases of ALCL, especially those in which the differential diagnosis also includes PTCL-NOS. The National Comprehensive Cancer Network guidelines recommend standard CHOP-based chemotherapy for these patients, sometimes combined with radiation for bulky disease, leading to remission rates close to 80%. Patients who experience relapse of their disease typically exhibit the same poor prognosis as patients with other subtypes of PTCL. Patients with ALK-negative ALCL carry the same poor prognosis as other subtypes of mature T-cell lymphoma and may be suitable candidates for clinical trials in both the up-front and relapsed settings.

Table 84-2 Summary of Retrospective Up-Front Studies in Peripheral T-Cell Lymphoma

Regimen	PTCL Subtypes	n	CR (%)	OS	Reference
Anthracycline-based	NK/T nasal	24	66.7	Not Reported	Kwong et al, 1997, *Br Jr Haematol*
Anthracycline-based	PTCL-NOS	24	69.6	2 yr 63%	Cheung et al, 1998, *J Clin Oncol*
	NK/T nasal	51	56.0	2 yr 43%	
Anthracycline-based	PTCL-combined	174	49.0	4 yr 38%	Lopez-Guillermo et al, 1998, *Annals of Oncol*
	PTCL-NOS	95	47.0	4 yr 32%	
	ALCL	30	69.0		
	AITL	22	37.0		
	NK/T nasal	14	46.0		
	EATL	12	27.0		
CHOP-like	AITL	33	60.6	5 yr 36%	Pautier et al, 1999, *Leuk and Lymph*
CHOP-type ± RT	NK/T nasal	7	28.6		Ribrag et al, 2001, *Leuk*
CMT	NK/T nasal	61	65.6	5 yr 41%	Cheung et al, 2002, *Int J of Rad Oncol Bio*
CHOP ± RT	PTCL-combined	78	52.6	5 yr 36%	Kim et al, 2002, Eur j of Cancer
	ALCL	13	69.2		
	PTCL-NOS	31	51.6		
	AITL	5	40.0		
	NK/T nasal	25	52.0		
Anthracycline-based	PTCL-combined	66	62.0	5 yr 55%	Reiser et al, 2002, *Leuk and Lymph*
	ALCL	19	79.0		
	PTCL-NOS	28	60.7		
	AITL	7	28.6		
Adriamycin-based	Non-ALCL PTCL	96		5 yr 26%	Rudiger et al, 2002, *Ann Oncol*
Anthracycline-based + RT	NK/T nasal	47	65.9		Chim et al, 2004, *Blood*
CHOP-based	NK/T nasal local	18	50.0	5 yr 15%	Li et al, 2004, *Cancer*
CHOP-based + RT	NK/T nasal local	27	74.1	5 yr 59%	
CHOP-based	NK/T nasal systemic	10	60.0	5 yr 30%	
CHOP-based + RT	NK/T nasal systemic	10	30.0	5 yr 20%	
CHOP-type	PTCL-Nos	117	64.1	5 yr 35%	Savage et al, 2004, *Annals of Oncol*
	ALCL	33	55.0	5 yr 43%	
	AITL	10	70.0	5 yr 36%	
	NK/T nasal	17	73.0	5 yr 24%	
	EATL	9	33.0	5 yr 22%	
CT + RT	NK/T nasal	16		5 yr 42%	You et al, 2004, *Annals of Oncol*
CT	NK/T nasal	15		5 yr 20%	
CHOP	Non-ALCL PTCL	24	58.0	3 yr 43%	Escalón et al, 2005, *Cancer*
CHOP intensive	Non-ALCL PTCL	52	59.0	3 yr 49%	
CHOP/COPBLAM-V + RT	NK/T nasal	16	37.5	5 yr 59%	Kim et al, 2005, *Jap J of Clin Oncol*
RT	NK/T nasal	33	52.0	5 yr 76%	
CHOP-type	PTCL-combined	125	53.0	5 yr 43%	Sonnen et al, 2005, *Br J of Haem*
	ALCL	21	71.0	5 yr 61%	
	PTCL-NOS	70	55.0	5 yr 45%	
	AITL	34	36.0	5 yr 28%	
CHOP-based + RT	NK/T nasal	71	84.5	5 yr 76%	Li YX et al, 2006, *J Clin Oncol*
CHOP alone	NK/T nasal	3	33.3		
Anthracycline-based	PTCL-NOS	340		5 yr 32%	Vose et al, 2008, *Oncology*
	ALK-negative	72		5 yr 49%	
	ALCL	243		5 yr 32%	
	AITL	136		5 yr 42%	
	NK/T nasal	62		3 yr 20%	
	EATL				

AITL, Angioimmunoblastic T-cell lymphoma; *ALCL*, anaplastic large cell lymphoma; *CHOP*, cyclophosphamide, hydroxydaunomycin, vincristine (Oncovin), and prednisone; *CMT*, combined modality therapy; *COPBLAM-V*, cyclophosphamide, vincristine (Oncovin), prednisone, bleomycin, doxorubicin (Adriamycin), and procarbazine; *CR*, complete remission; *CT*, chemotherapy; *EATL*, enteropathy associated T-cell lymphoma; *NK*, natural killer; *NOS*, not otherwise specified; *OS*, overall survival, *PTCL*, peripheral T-cell lymphoma; *RT*, radiotherapy.

Nasal NKTCL—Combined-Modality Versus Single-Modality Approaches

Radiotherapy is considered the most active treatment for early-stage nasal NKTCL.[61] For patients with limited stage IE or stage IE disease without any adverse factors, radiotherapy alone should be pursued with curative intent.[62] For patients with extensive stage I and II disease, radiotherapy followed by consolidation with chemotherapy is commonly used. Because of the intrinsic drug resistance frequently seen in this disease, chemotherapy is not recommended as primary treatment in early-stage nasal NKTCL. Extranodal NKTCL is generally refractory to CHOP-based chemotherapy and is often associated with the expression of the multidrug resistance genes.[61]

Despite the benefit of radiotherapy in this disease, a uniformly accepted standard of care has yet to be identified. Recently a phase I/II study using concurrent chemotherapy and radiotherapy was reported.[63] Patients were treated concurrently with radiotherapy and chemotherapy, which included carboplatin, etoposide, ifosfamide, and dexamethasone. Among the 26 patients reported, the objective response rate (ORR) was 81% with 77% CR. The most common grade 3 nonhematologic toxicity was mucositis (30% of patients), which was related to the radiotherapy. With a median follow-up of 32 months, the study reported a 2-year OS of 78%, which compares very favorably with the historical control group, which received radiotherapy alone (45%). Increasingly, many physicians are considering combined-modality therapy as the best up-front treatment for this disease, despite the potentially significant associated toxicity.

Newer approaches for patients with advanced NKTCLs have explored integrating L-asparaginase into a dexamethasone (steroid), methotrexate, ifosfamide, and etoposide–based backbone (SMILE). Yong et al[64] treated 18 patients that were refractory to CHOP with L-asparaginase, vincristine, dexamethasone, and involved field radiotherapy. The ORR was 83.3%, with 10 (55.6%) of the patients achieving CR, and five (27.8%) achieving partial response (PR). The 5-year overall survival rate was 55.6%. Results of the preliminary clinical study indicated that the L-asparaginase-based salvage regimens significantly improved the response rate and 5-year survival rate. A prospective phase II trial has been reported with the SMILE regimen in patients with newly diagnosed stage IV or relapsed refractory NKTCLs.[65] Among the 39 patients treated, 29 (74%) completed the planned treatment. The responses included 15 patients in CR and 14 in PR, with early deaths due to infection in 4 patients. Infection was the most commonly observed toxicity, seen in 41% of the patients. Based on these studies, we conclude that L-asparaginase may have a role, either in the up-front setting or for patients with relapsed or refractory disease.

Adult T-Cell Leukemia/Lymphoma—Role of Antiviral Agents

In patients with ATL the results of chemotherapy have been uniformly poor, leading to a consensus recommendation to enroll patients when possible in a clinical trial in either the up-front or relapsed or refractory setting. Although there is again no standard of care for these patients, the general sentiment is that CHOP-based chemotherapy regimens are insufficient. Owing to the comparatively higher incidence of ATL in Japan, many studies regarding the management of ATL come from Asia. The Japanese evaluated a complex combination regimen of VCAP (vincristine, cyclophosphamide, doxorubicin [Adriamycin], and prednisone), AMP (doxorubicin [Adriamycin], ranimustine [MCNU], and prednisone), and VECP (vindesine, etoposide, carboplatin, and prednisone) against CHOP-14 in ATL.[66] A total of 118 patients were enrolled in the trial and treated with either six courses of VCAP-AMP-VECP every 4 weeks or eight courses of biweekly CHOP. The CR rate was higher in the VCAP-AMP-VECP arm than in the CHOP-14 arm (40% versus 25%, respectively), and the progression-free survival (PFS) at 1 year was 28% in the VCAP-AMP-VECP arm compared to 16% in the CHOP arm. The OS at 3 years was 24% in the VCAP-AMP-VECP arm and 13% in the CHOP arm. Overall, the toxicity in the VCAP-AMP-VECP arm was higher than in the CHOP-14 arm, with substantially more grade 3 or 4 cytopenias in the VCAP-AMP-VECP arm, which included three toxic deaths. Because most patients with ATL do not have curable disease when treated with these chemotherapy regimens, it is reasonable to consider allogeneic stem cell transplantation (SCT) in patients who show responses to chemotherapy. Although this experience is very limited, there is some suggestion that there may be benefit in some patients.[67]

Infection with HTLV-1 can cause ATL. Nineteen patients with acute or lymphomatous forms of ATL were treated with oral zidovudine (200 mg five times daily) and interferon-α (Intron A; 5 to 10 million units subcutaneously each day). Seven of these patients either relapsed or were refractory to combination chemotherapy. Major responses were achieved in 58% of the patients (11 of 19), including complete remission in 26% (5 of 19). Four patients in whom prior cytotoxic therapy had failed experienced major responses, two of which were complete remissions. Six patients have survived for more than 12 months, with the longest remission since the discontinuation of treatment lasting more than 59 months.[68] A recent metaanalysis evaluated 116 patients with acute ATL, 18 patients with chronic ATL, 11 patients with smoldering ATL, and 100 patients with ATL lymphoma.[69] The 5-year OS rates were 46% for 75 patients who received first-line antiviral therapy ($P = .004$), 20% for the 77 patients who received first-line chemotherapy, and 12% for the 55 patients who received first-line chemotherapy followed by antiviral therapy. The metaanalysis suggested that patients with acute, chronic, and smoldering ATL significantly benefited from first-line antiviral therapy, whereas patients with ATL lymphoma experienced a better outcome with chemotherapy. In acute ATL, 82% of patients were alive at 5 years with antiviral therapy, and 100% of patients with chronic and smoldering ATL were alive at 5 years. Multivariate analysis showed that first-line antiviral therapy significantly improved OS (HR = 0.47; 95% confidence interval [CI], 0.27 to 0.83; $P = .021$). Prospective studies are warranted to better define the role of antiviral therapy in treatment of ATL.

Angioimmunoblastic T-Cell Lymphoma—The Role of Cyclosporin and Rituximab

AITL is one of the most common forms of PTCL with peculiar clinical and pathologic features. Although the normal counterpart has been recently identified as the TFH) cell, the nonneoplastic cells typically represent the quantitatively major component of AITL. Clinically the manifestations of the disease reflect a dysregulated immune and/or inflammatory response rather than being the direct complication of tumor growth,[70] supporting the concept of a paraneoplastic immunologic dysfunction. Despite the use of different intensive anthracycline-based chemotherapies, AITL is an aggressive disease compared to other PTCLs, for which the optimal therapeutic strategy is still not defined. Given the considerable immune dysregulation present in AITL, the possible role of cyclosporine A (CsA) has been investigated.[71] Twelve patients were treated with CsA; 10 out of 12 patients had failed prior therapy with either chemotherapy and/or steroids (one to two prior regimens). Two patients were untreated because of age or comorbid conditions. Three patients achieved CR and five a PR for an overall response rate of 67%, suggesting a possible role for CsA in this setting. In AITL, symptoms linked to B-lymphocyte activation are common, and variable numbers of CD20$^+$ large B-blasts, often infected by EBV virus, are found in the neoplastic tissues. It has recently been investigated that the disruption of putative B- and T-cell interactions and/or depletion of the EBV reservoir by anti-CD20 monoclonal antibody (rituximab) might improve clinical outcome observed with conventional chemotherapy. Twenty-five newly diagnosed patients were treated in a phase II study with eight cycles of rituximab plus chemotherapy (R-CHOP21). The complete response rate was 44%, the 2-year PFS rate was 42%, and OS was 62%. This trial showed no clear benefit of adding rituximab to conventional chemotherapy[72] (see box on Treatment of Peripheral T-Cell Lymphoma).

Treatment of Peripheral T-Cell Lymphoma

Given that the mature T-cell lymphomas are relatively rare diseases, there is a lack of large randomized clinical trials comparing the "standard" CHOP and CHOP-like regimens to other more-intensified chemotherapy strategies, or even other novel drug platforms. Our approach involves tailoring the treatment to the specific histologic subtype and age of the patient. From the outset, we send HLA typing for possible allogeneic stem cell transplant, assuming the patient is eligible, and request immunohistochemical staining of the primary tissue for CD30. Where possible, we preferentially try to put all patients on a clinical trial. For the majority of peripheral T-cell lymphomas, our standard initial approach is to use an etoposide-based regimen (CHOEP or EPOCH), especially for young patients or older adult patients with an excellent performance status. As alluded to earlier, there are some data to suggest a reduced failure-free interval and higher complete response rate. For patients with a poor performance status or older adult patients, standard CHOP administered on an every-21-day basis for six to eight cycles would be our preferred recommendation. In select cases, where an older adult patient is not a candidate for combination chemotherapy and requires palliative care, we have successfully used single-agent gemcitabine to obtain disease control and improve performance status. Those patients who attain a complete remission are usually referred for an autologous stem cell transplant. Those patients who do not attain a complete remission with standard frontline chemotherapy are typically referred for treatment with one of the drugs recently approved by the FDA for patients with relapsed or refractory disease, including pralatrexate, romidepsin, or brentuximab vedotin (if $CD30^+$ positive). For patients who relapse or are refractory to frontline and beyond therapy, we typically consider allogeneic stem cell transplant, assuming they are transplant eligible and have an appropriate HLA match.

CHOEP, Cyclophosphamide, hydroxydaunomycin, vincristine (Oncovin), etoposide, and prednisone; *CHOP,* cyclophosphamide, hydroxydaunomycin, vincristine (Oncovin), and prednisone; *EPOCH,* etoposide, prednisone, vincristine (Oncovin), cyclophosphamide, and hydroxydaunomycin; *FDA,* Food and Drug Administration; *HLA,* human leukocyte antigen.

Role of Stem Cell Transplantation in Treatment

Because of the poor results often seen with conventional chemotherapy in patients with PTCL, many investigators have begun to explore intensive treatments, including high-dose chemotherapy followed by autologous or allogeneic SCT in both a frontline therapy and in patients who have relapsed. Despite the growing number of reports, one must keep in mind a series of limitations: (1) most of the studies are retrospective; (2) randomized trials between standard chemotherapy and SCT have not been published so far; (3) many prospective studies of autologous SCT (ASCT) include both first-line and relapsed patients with diverse subtypes of T-cell lymphoma, making the results very heterogeneous and difficult to interpret.

High-Dose Chemotherapy and Autologous Stem Cell Transplantation

High-dose chemotherapy followed by ASCT is currently accepted as the treatment of choice for patients with relapsed aggressive B-cell lymphoma, resulting in 40% to 50% long-term disease-free survival, as demonstrated by the pivotal PARMA study.[73] The role of ASCT in TCL is less clear, and the burning issue is whether or not autografting during first or subsequent remissions may be of clinical benefit.

The Spanish Lymphoma/Autologous Bone Marrow Transplant Study Group (GELTAMO) reported the results of 123 patients with high-risk PTCL who received an ASCT in the salvage setting: the 5-year OS and PFS were 45% and 34%, respectively. In this analysis, having more than one factor of the adjusted-IPI or a high β_2-microglobulin level at transplant was identified as adverse prognostic factors.[74] Moreover, PFS and OS of patients in second or subsequent CR at transplant (35% and 57%, respectively) were superior as compared to those in more than a second PR (23% and 33%) or with refractory disease (10% and 9%). Other groups have underscored the importance of being in CR at the time of transplant to achieve a long-term survival.[75] This is not surprising and is a recurring theme in many transplant studies.

Some studies have focused on the different results between PTCL-NOS and ALCL, emphasizing that the histologic subtype can influence the outcome after ASCT.[76-79] The Toronto group compared relapsed and refractory PTCL patients with those affected by DLBCL, who were transplanted for the same indications over the same period. The 3-year OS and EFS were 48% and 37%, respectively, for PTCL, compared to 53% and 42% for DLBCL.[76,77] Nevertheless, a significantly different outcome has been demonstrated when the major subtypes of PTCL were analyzed separately. Patients with PTCL-NOS had an inferior EFS (3-year EFS, 23%) when compared to patients with DLBCL. In contrast, patients with ALCL exhibited a similar outcome to patients with DLBCL. These results are consistent with the data from a retrospective study of the Memorial Sloan-Kettering Cancer Center that reported a 5-year PFS of 24% for relapsed or refractory ALK-negative ALCL.[77] The more favorable prognosis of ALCL after ASCT was confirmed also by studies from Northern Europe investigators.[78,79]

Overall the prognosis of ALK-negative PTCL seems poor when ASCT is used for relapsed disease, where long-term remissions have been observed in less than one-third of the patients. Those who benefited the most are the patients with ALK-positive ALCL in CR at the time of transplant or those with a low IPI. Based upon the poor results of both front-line standard chemotherapy and ASCT in the salvage setting, high-dose chemotherapy has been investigated as first-line treatment.[80-84,85b] Although there are no randomized prospective trials comparing frontline ASCT with standard chemotherapy, the results of some retrospective and prospective phase II studies are suggesting a role for this approach (Table 84-3). In a retrospective analysis, the Japan registry demonstrated that the long-term outcome of PTCL was better in patients transplanted in first CR or PR than those not in remission (5-year OS, 72.9% versus 45.8%; PFS, 73.1% versus 42.2%).[80] The British Society of Bone Marrow Transplantation (BSBMT) and Stanford University reported similar data. The 2-year OS and PFS were 62% and 59%, respectively, for patients receiving ASCT as consolidation during first CR.[81,86] The Spanish group published a retrospective analysis of 74 patients undergoing SCT after the achievement of CR with first-line anthracycline-based induction chemotherapy.[82] After a median follow-up of 67 months, 5-year OS and PFS were 68% and 63%, respectively, and the main cause of death was disease progression. In multivariate analysis only the PIT score was significantly associated with OS and PFS. Although data about ALK expression were lacking, patients affected by ALCL had a significantly better outcome as compared to other PTCL subtypes. The same authors published the results of a prospective study in 26 high-risk nodal PTCL patients, excluding those with ALK-positive ALCL.[87] The patients who were positron emission tomography–positive after three cycles of dose-escalated CHOP (MegaCHOP) received salvage chemotherapy followed by autologous transplant. At a median follow-up of 35 months, 3-year OS and PFS of the entire cohort of patients were 73% and 56%, respectively, whereas those patients who were rescued by high-dose chemotherapy achieved a 2-year disease-free survival of 63%.

An Italian multicenter prospective study employed high-dose sequential chemotherapy followed by ASCT as first-line treatment in 62 patients with high-risk PTCL (stage III-IV and/or age-adjusted IPI >1) including 19 ALK-positive ALCL patients.[83] On an intent-to-treat analysis, only 46 of 62 patients (74%) completed the whole

Table 84-3 Prospective Studies of Up-Front High-Dose Chemotherapy and Autologous Stem Cell Transplantation in T-Cell Lymphomas

Reference	No. of Patients, Age (% Autografted)	Disease	Induction and Conditioning	CR After ASCT* (%)	TRM	Survival	Median Follow-Up (mo)
87	26, 44 yr (73%)	11 PTCL-NOS 8 ALCL 7 AITL	MegaCHOP BEAM	65%	4%	3-yr OS 73% PFS 56%	35
83	62, 43 yr (74%)	28 PTCL-NOS 19 ALCL-ALK positive 10 AITL 5 others	HDS-CT MitoMel or BEAM	66%	5%	12-yr OS 34% DFS 55%	76
84	83, 47 yr (66%)	32 PTCL-NOS 13 ALK negative ALCL 27 AITL 11 others	CHOP TBI/CY	56%	4%	3-yr OS 48% PFS 36%	33
85a	160, 57 yr (70%)	62 PTCL-NOS 31 ALK negative ALCL 30 AITL 37 others	CHOEP/IFE BEAM	79%	10%	3-yr OS 50% PFS 43%	45
85b	41, 47 yr (41%)	20 PTCL-NOS 12 AITL 9 others	CHOP/ESHAP BEAM or BEAC	NA	7%	4-yr OS 39% PFS 30%	38

AITL, Angioimmunoblastic T-cell lymphoma; *ALCL,* anaplastic large cell lymphoma; *ASCT,* autologous stem cell transplantation; *BEAC,* carmustine (BCNU), cytarabine (ara-C), etoposide, cyclophosphamide; *BEAM,* carmustine (BCNU), etoposide, cytarabine (ara-C), and melphalan; *CHOEP,* cyclophosphamide, hydroxydaunomycin, vincristine [Oncovin], etoposide, and prednisone; *CHOP,* cyclophosphamide, hydroxydaunomycin, vincristine (Oncovin), and prednisone; *CR;* complete remission; *CY,* cyclophosphamide; *DFS,* disease-free survival; *ESHAP,* etoposide, methylprednisolone (Solu-Medrol), cytarabine (ara-C), cisplatin; *HDS-CT,* high-dose sequential chemotherapy; *IFE,* ifosfamide, etoposide; *MegaCHOP,* dose-escalated CHOP; *MitoMel,* mitoxantrone, melphalan; *mo,* months; *NA,* not available; *OS,* overall survival; *PFS,* progression-free survival; *PTCL-NOS,* peripheral T-cell lymphoma unspecified; *TBI,* total body irradiation; *TRM,* transplant-related mortality; *yr,* years.
*Percentage refers to the whole population on study.

program. Progressive disease during the induction phase was the main obstacle for proceeding to ASCT and the main reason for treatment failure. The high progression rate led to disappointing 12-year OS and EFS curves (34% and 30%, respectively). However, in the cohort of patients who underwent ASCT, the response rate was high: 89% of these patients achieved CR. As in the Spanish study, patients with ALCL had the most favorable OS and EFS (62% and 54%, respectively, compared to 21% and 18% of non-ALCL). On the other hand, when patients with PTCL-NOS were in CR at the time of transplant, the EFS was 62% versus 10% for those not in CR. The CR status remained a significant predictor of long-term outcome in the multivariate analysis.

More recently the German group published the results of a prospective multicenter study employing myeloablative doses of cyclophosphamide and total body irradiation as the conditioning regimen for 83 ALK-negative ALCL patients who were at least in partial remission after six CHOP cycles.[84] Similar to the Italian data, 34% of the patients did not complete the study protocol because of progressive disease. The estimated 3-year OS was 71% for patients who underwent ASCT compared to 11% for those who did not.

To increase the number of patients undergoing ASCT in complete or at least partial remission, some recent trials were designed that focused on a more intense pretransplant phase. The Nordic Lymphoma Group included a dose-dense induction phase for 160 PTCL patients. After six cycles of CHOEP every 2 weeks, 85% of the patients achieved CR and 70% could undergo ASCT at the last follow-up. Five-year OS and PFS were 50% and 43%, respectively. A Spanish group used alternating CHOP and ESHAP (etoposide, methylprednisolone [Solu-Medrol], cytarabine [ara-C], cisplatin) in the induction phase of 41 ALK-negative patients: 58% of the patients were in CR or PR after the induction phase, but only 41% of them underwent ASCT.[85b]

From the studies reported above, two important messages emerge clearly: (1) one of the reasons for treatment failure is disease progression before ASCT, therefore the intent-to-treat analyses give unsatisfactory PFS and OS curves; (2) for the two-thirds of the patients who are able to undergo the ASCT as frontline therapy, the results, especially for patients in CR before transplant, appear better as compared to those observed with patients receiving an ASCT after relapse.

Although most of the published data include different histologic subtypes of T-cell NHL, during recent years some efforts have been made to define the role of ASCT in specific subtypes. AITL patients have a median survival of 18 months after conventional chemotherapy, with less than 50% of the patients achieving CR. A retrospective analysis of the European Group for Blood and Marrow Transplantation in 146 AITL patients demonstrated an OS and PFS of 59% and 42%, respectively, at 4 years.[88] The PFS was greater in patients who received ASCT in CR, 56% at 4 years, compared to 23% in the case of patients with chemotherapy-refractory disease. EATL is another very poor-prognosis PTCL, commonly associated with celiac disease. Because of its rarity, very few data on EATL treatment are available. In a prospective observational study using ASCT as first-line treatment, 5-year OS was 60% versus 22% for patients treated with standard chemotherapy.[89]

In conclusion, the role of ASCT in T-cell NHL may be summarized as follows: (1) ALK-positive ALCLs have a favorable outcome after ASCT, but they also do well with conventional chemotherapy, allowing this strategy to be possibly delayed to the salvage setting; (2) patients affected by PTCL seem to have an advantage when transplanted in first CR; (3) in order to validate the results in larger cohorts of patients and with longer follow-up, all PTCL patients should be enrolled in prospective trials including ASCT as first-line treatment; (4) clinical protocols should be designed with an innovative pretransplant phase in order to achieve the best disease response before transplant and increase the number of patients who are able to get an ASCT. Novel agents might be useful to induce a response in patients having refractory disease before SCT.

Even in the absence of randomized trials, the current standard of care is the use of ASCT for young patients frontline.

Allogeneic Stem Cell Transplantation

Allogeneic SCT has been generally used in T-cell lymphomas with progressive or refractory disease after several lines of chemotherapy or in case of relapse after an autologous transplant. This strategy can provide the infusion of lymphoma-free graft and the potentially active graft-versus-lymphoma effect. The survival after myeloablative allogeneic SCT has been heavily influenced by the high nonrelapse mortality (NRM), mainly related to graft-versus-host disease, infections, and acute organ toxicities. Retrospective comparative analyses of autologous versus allogeneic SCT in aggressive lymphomas presented some selection bias because patients receiving allogeneic SCT usually had more advanced disease, more prior therapies, and/or bone marrow involvement.[90] However, these studies demonstrated that allogeneic SCT induced a lower relapse risk compared to ASCT, but the high NRM offset any survival benefit. The results of some studies using allogeneic SCT as therapeutic strategy are listed in Table 84-4.

A small retrospective comparative study by the GELTAMO group evaluated the outcome of patients receiving autologous (n = 29) or allogeneic SCT (n = 7) for PTCL. The 3-year OS was 39% and 29% for autologous and allogeneic SCT, respectively. However, the majority of patients in the group receiving allogeneic grafts in CR died because of transplant-related complications.[91] In 2006 a Japanese group published the first large analysis on the outcome of T-cell NHL after myeloablative allogeneic SCT from matched related and unrelated donors.[92] Fifty-one patients were retrospectively described, and, in univariate analysis, OS was better for PTCL compared to B-cell NHL or other T-cell NHL.

During the last 15 years, reduced-intensity conditioning (RIC) regimens have been increasingly used in relapsed lymphomas in order to reduce the NRM, thus making this strategy feasible in older adult or heavily pretreated patients.[93] In 2004 one of the first papers of RIC allogeneic SCT reported 56% of patients alive and in complete remission after 1.4 years.[94] The first prospective study evaluated the outcome of 17 relapsed PTCL patients after a fludarabine-based RIC regimen: 14 of 17 enrolled patients were alive (12 in CR) after a median follow-up of 28 months with an estimated 3-year NRM, OS, and PFS of 6%, 81%, and 64%, respectively.[95] In this study, there were some data suggesting the existence of a graft-versus-T-cell lymphoma effect, based on the following observations: (1) the achievement of durable responses with allogeneic SCT in patients who had already failed a previous ASCT and (2) the demonstration of clinical responses to donor lymphocyte infusions. These preliminary results were then supported by a larger Italian multicenter retrospective study with a longer follow-up. In this study, the 5-year outcome showed an NRM, OS, and PFS of 12%, 50%, and 40%, respectively, and a plateau in the survival curves after 36 months, suggesting that these patients have been cured by allogeneic SCT.[96] Following multivariate analyses, age over 45 years and refractory disease were independent prognostic factors, highlighting that the timing of allogeneic SCT can significantly influence the final clinical outcome. Similarly, in a French retrospective study of 77 PTCL patients receiving allogeneic SCT with both RIC or myeloablative regimens, those patients with chemosensitive disease or with less than two prior lines of chemotherapy experienced a better outcome.[97] In both the Italian and French studies, the survival was not significantly different among the

Table 84-4 Studies of Allogeneic Stem Cell Transplantation in T-Cell Non-Hodgkin Lymphoma

Reference	No. of Patients (age)	Disease	Conditioning	Previous ASCT (%)	TRM	Survival	Median Follow-Up (mo)
RETROSPECTIVE DATA							
97	77 (36 yr)	27 PTCL-NOS 27 ALCL 11 AITL 12 others	MA: 74% RIC: 26%	25	33%	5-yr OS 57% EFS 53%	43
Dodero (2011)	52 (47 yr)	23 PTCL-NOS 9 ALK-positive ALCL 11 AITL 9 others	RIC: Thio/Flu/CY	52	12% (5 yr)	5-yr OS 50% PFS 40%	67
98	45 (48 yr)	45 AITL	MA: 56% RIC: 44%	33	25% (1 yr)	3-yr OS 64% PFS 53%	29
100	52 (46 yr)	20 PTCL-NOS 6 ALCL 5 AITL 12 others	MA: 60% RIC: 40%		27% (3 yr)	3-yr OS 41% PFS 30%	49
PROSPECTIVE DATA							
95	17 (41 yr)	9 PTCL-NOS 4 ALK-negative ALCL 4 AITL	RIC: Thio/Flu/CY	47	6% (2 yr)	3-yr OS 81% PFS 64%	28
99	10 (45 yr)	4 PTCL-NOS 2 AITL 3 ALCL 1 other	RIC: Flu/Bu/CY	20	30%	7-month 7 alive 6 in CR	7
Shustov (2011)	17 (57 yr)	7 PTCL-NOS 4 AITL 1 ALCL 6 others	RIC: Flu/TBI	41	19% (3 yr)	3-yr OS 59% PFS 53%	40

AITL, Angioimmunoblastic T-cell lymphoma; *ALCL,* anaplastic large cell lymphoma; *CR,* complete remission; *EFS,* event-free survival; *MA,* myeloablative conditioning; *OS,* overall survival; *PFS,* progression-free survival; *PTCL-NOS,* peripheral T-cell lymphoma unspecified; *RIC,* reduced-intensity conditioning; *TBI,* total body irradiation; *Thio/Flu/Cy,* thiotepa, fludarabine, cyclophosphamide; *TRM,* transplant-related mortality; *yr,* years.

histologic subtypes of T-cell lymphoma (of note, the majority of ALCLs had an unknown ALK mutational status), although AITL did slightly better. In support of this finding, a European Group for Blood and Marrow Transplantation retrospective analysis on 45 AITL patients undergoing an allogeneic SCT between 1998 and 2005 showed a relapse risk of 20% at 3 years with a PFS of 53% and an OS of 64%.[98]

In the last few years a growing number of retrospective and prospective studies have demonstrated the feasibility and efficacy of allogeneic SCT in relapsed and refractory T-cell NHL, including the extranodal subtypes.[99-102]

In conclusion, allogeneic SCT can be offered in relapsed and refractory T-cell NHL based on the following observations: (1) in all studies the survival curves seem to reach a plateau after 24 to 36 months, suggesting the potential curability of the disease; (2) delaying allogeneic SCT too long from diagnosis may significantly impair the results, thus allogeneic SCT should be performed during a chemosensitive relapse; (3) RIC regimens have increased the feasibility of allogeneic SCT by reducing the NRM and may be used, at least in older and heavily pretreated patients. The future will hopefully see the combination of new agents with allogeneic SCT to improve the results in the significant proportion of refractory patients.

Emerging New Drugs for PTCL

There is little question that one of the most promising new areas in PTCL research is new drug development. Over the past several years, three new drugs, all with relatively unique mechanisms of action, have been approved for the treatment of patients with relapsed or refractory disease. These drugs, which all now have substantial data demonstrating their marked single-agent activity in these diseases, have created a unique opportunity to build non–CHOP-based platforms for treatment. In addition to the three drugs already approved, many new drugs are in various stages of clinical development, with very promising signals (Table 84-5). We will discuss some of these new agents and how they are beginning to change the treatment paradigms for PTCL.

Pralatrexate

Pralatrexate is a novel antifolate with very high affinity for the reduced folate carrier. The reduced folate carrier is an oncofetal protein expressed at relatively high levels on the surface of malignant cells.[103] The carrier is responsible for transporting into the cell natural folate required for DNA biosynthesis. Pralatrexate, designed to have a high affinity for the folate receptors, is rapidly internalized into the cell, where it undergoes efficient polyglutamylation by the folylpolyglutamate synthase, which enhances the affinity of the drug for dihydrofolate reductase and increases its intracellular retention.[104]

A phase "II-I-II" study of pralatrexate in patients with relapsed or refractory NHL established the maximum tolerated dose as 30 mg/m^2 weekly for 6 of 7 consecutive weeks of treatment.[105] The dose-limiting toxicity was determined to be mucositis, which was largely controlled with the addition of folic acid and vitamin B_{12}. These data revealed an ORR of 31% among the entire population of patients with both B- and T-cell lymphoma (n = 48 evaluable), of which 8 patients obtained a CR. Among the 20 evaluable patients with B-cell lymphoma, the ORR was 5%, of which there were no CRs. Among the 26 evaluable patients with T-cell lymphoma, the ORR was 54%, of which there were 8 CRs.[105] All the complete remissions, many of which were very durable and included patients who had responded to prior methotrexate, were seen exclusively in patients with PTCL.

These data gave rise to a pivotal study of pralatrexate in patients with most subtypes of relapsed or refractory PTCL. The Pralatrexate in Patients With Relapsed or Refractory Peripheral T-Cell Lymphoma (PROPEL) study was an international, open-label, single-arm trial in which pralatrexate was administered at a dose of 30 mg/m^2 weekly for 6 of 7 consecutive weeks. At the time, it was the largest study ever conducted in this patient population. Of 115 patients enrolled, 111 were treated with pralatrexate.[106] Overall, the patient population was very heavily pretreated, with the median number of prior therapies being 3, with a range of 1 to 12. Twenty percent of patients in PROPEL had received more than five lines of prior chemotherapy. The response rate among the 109 evaluable patients was 29%, which included 12 CRs (11%), with a median duration of response of 10.1 months. The most common grade 3 or 4 toxicities included

Table 84-5 Recent FDA-Approved and Emerging New Drugs in Peripheral T-Cell Lymphoma

Drug	Disease/No. of Patients	Overall Response Rate	Complete Response Rate	PFS/DOR	Reference
Pralatrexate (Accelerated approval 2009)	Relapsed/refractory PTCL N = 111	29%	11%	Median DOR = 10.1 mo	106
Romidepsin (Accelerated approval 2011)	Relapsed/refractory PTCL N = 130	25%	15%	Median DOR = 17 mo	117
Brentuximab vedotin (Accelerated approval 2011)	CD30$^+$ anaplastic large cell lymphoma N = 58	86%	57%	Median DOR = 12.6 mo	Advani et al, 2011
KW-0761	HTLV-1 ATL N = 27	13 of 26 (50%)	8 of 13 (61%)	PFS = 5.2 mo	124
Bortezomib	Relapsed/refractory CTCL and PTCL N = 12	8 of 12 (67%) (2 patients with PTCL)	2 of 12 (17%) (1 of 2 patients with PTCL)	Not reported	129
Lenalidomide	Relapsed/refractory PTCL				
	N = 10 (Zinzani)	30%	3 of 10	Not reported	132
	N = 24 (Dueck)	30%	0 of 7	Median PFS 96 days	131
Alisertib	Relapsed/refractory PTCL N = 8	4 of 8 (50%)	2 of 4	Not reported	133

ATL, Adult T-cell leukemia/lymphoma; *CTCL*, cutaneous T-cell lymphoma; *DOR*, duration of response; *FDA*, Food and Drug Administration; *HTLV-1*, human T-lymphotropic virus-1; *PFS*, progression-free survival; *PTCL*, peripheral T-cell lymphoma.

thrombocytopenia and mucositis. These data led to pralatrexate becoming the first drug ever approved by the U.S. Food and Drug Administration (FDA) for PTCL, receiving accelerated approval in late 2009.

More recently, pralatrexate has been reported to potently synergize with gemcitabine,[107] bortezomib,[108] and the histone deacetylase (HDAC) inhibitor depsipeptide.[109] These data have now led to a number of phase I clinical trials exploring the merits of these drug combinations.

Histone Deacetylase Inhibitors

The HDAC inhibitors (HDACI) appear to exhibit a consistent pattern of activity in T-cell neoplasms, with little to no activity in B-cell lymphoid malignancies. HDACs play a crucial role in modulating the balance between open and closed chromatin, which in turn modulates transcriptional activation. Histone acetyltransferases acetylate the ε-amino moieties of lysine residues found both in histone and nonhistone protein. Acetylation of histone proteins facilitates an open chromatin structure, leading to access by transcription factors and thus transcriptional activation. Conversely, HDACs facilitate deacetylation of chromatin, which leads to a closed chromatin structure and transcriptional silencing. Although the modulation of chromatin structure has been long postulated as one of the key mechanisms for HDACI activity, it is now widely recognized that these drugs are more appropriately recognized as more general protein deacetylase inhibitors. In this capacity, it is also recognized that HDACI may functionally affect tumor cell growth and survival by modulating the posttranslational state of different proteins, which leads to activation or inactivation of various tumor suppressor genes or oncogenes. For example, it is known that acetylation controls Notch function.[110] This example provides additional clues into how these drugs might affect the balance between growth and survival pathways of tumor cells. Other studies have highlighted that the relative proportion of different HDACs in tumor cells might lead to dysregulated growth. For example, PTCL tissue is known to be characterized by overexpression of HDAC1, HDAC2, and HDAC6 as well as acetylated histone 4 (H4).[111,112] Although it is not known precisely what genes are affected by the dysregulation of these HDACs, it clearly provides additional insight into the mechanism by which this class of drugs might be able to affect a unique set of intracellular pathways in PTCL.

The first HDAC inhibitor approved for the treatment of cancer was vorinostat, or SAHA.[113] Vorinostat is a hydroxamic acid derivative known to be a potent class 1-2 inhibitor of HDAC. Early developmental clinical studies performed with both intravenous and oral vorinostat demonstrated that the drug could inhibit HDACs, leading to accumulation of acetylated H3/H4.[114,115] These studies also demonstrated that the drug was well tolerated for extended periods of time, with dose-limiting toxicities of fatigue, diarrhea, and anorexia for the oral formulations, and myelosuppression for the intravenous formulations. Expanded phase II experiences with vorinostat confirmed single-agent activity in Hodgkin disease–transformed lymphomas and CTCL. These data gave rise to pivotal studies in CTCL leading to FDA approval in 2006.

Another HDAC inhibitor has been shown to be more active in PTCL, depsipeptide, also known as *romidepsin.* Romidepsin is a potent macrolide HDAC inhibitor isolated from *Chromobacterium violaceum.* An early phase I-II trial demonstrated that romidepsin exhibited marked single-agent activity in patients with relapsed or refractory CTCL and PTCL.[116] In fact, among 47 patients with relapsed or refractory PTCL, excluding patients with transformed mycosis fungoides (MF) and HTLV-1 ATL, which were included in the PROPEL study, an ORR of 38% was noted, including 8 patients who attained a CR. The most common toxicities were very similar to those reported for vorinostat and included nausea, fatigue, and transient thrombocytopenia. The median duration of response was roughly 8.9 months, and responses were seen in most of the PTCL subtypes studied. These data gave rise to an international, open-label, pivotal phase II study of romidepsin in patients with relapsed or refractory PTCL who had received at least one line of prior therapy. Of the 131 patients enrolled, 130 had histologically confirmed PTCL. The median number of prior therapies was two, with a range of one to eight. The ORR was 25%, which included 19 (15%) CRs, and the median duration of response was 17 months.[117] These data led to a conditional approval of romidepsin in patients with relapsed or refractory PTCL by the FDA in June of 2011.

More recent data have now suggested that pralatrexate and romidepsin appear to display synergistic activity in models of T-cell lymphoma.[109] These data are now being used as a rationale to support a multicenter phase I study that will define the maximum tolerated dose of this regimen, and then the tolerability and activity in a subpopulation of patients with PTCL.

Brentuximab Vedotin

Monoclonal antibodies have emerged as potentially important new therapeutic tools in the treatment of many subtypes of NHL. Monoclonal antibodies are now being developed against a host of other cell surface proteins, including the chemokine receptor CCR4, and other surface proteins like CD4 and more recently CD30. CD30 (also known as TNFRSF8) is a 120-kD transmembrane protein of the tumor necrosis factor family and a known tumor marker found on many kinds of lymphoma.[118,119] The receptor is found on the surface of only activated T cells, and some B cells. CD30 is found on virtually all cases of ALCL, and the majority of cases of HL, where it is seen on the surface of the Reed-Sternberg cell. It is also expressed by several nonlymphoid malignancies, including embryonal carcinoma and some cases of non–small cell lung cancer. Clinical trials with the chimeric anti-CD30 monoclonal antibody were uniformly disappointing in patients with ALCL and HL.[120,121] For example, among 38 patients with HL and 41 patients with ALCL treated with SGN-30, no responses were seen in patients with HL, whereas 2 patients with ALCL achieved a CR.[120] Similar results have been reported with other anti-CD30 monoclonal antibodies.

Conjugation of small molecules to highly targeted monoclonal antibodies to create an antibody drug conjugate offers a promising way to deliver highly toxic drugs to select populations of cells. The conjugation of a highly potent antimicrotubule agent, monomethyl auristatin E to the anti-CD30 monoclonal antibody creates a novel antibody drug conjugate called SGN-35, or brentuximab vedotin. Clinical trials of this drug in patients with HL and ALCL have demonstrated remarkable activity in these CD30-expressing diseases. A pivotal trial of brentuximab vedotin in patients with relapsed or refractory ALCL produced an ORR of 86%, with a CR rate of 57%.[71] These remissions were found to be very durable, with a median response duration of 12.6 months and a median duration of response among patients in CR of 13.2 months. The majority of patients enrolled in the study exhibited poor prognostic features: 72% of patients had ALK-negative ALCL, 63% of patients were refractory to front-line therapy, and 22% of patients had never responded to any prior therapy. These results recently led the FDA to grant accelerated approval to brentuximab vedotin in patients with ALCL. Ongoing studies are now exploring the benefits of this drug in combination with standard up-front chemotherapy regimens like CHOP.

KW-0761

Another novel cell surface protein for which there is now a targeted drug is the CCR4 chemokine receptor, which is encoded by the CCR4 gene. CCR4 has also recently been designated CD194.[122,123] The CCR4 protein belongs to the G protein–coupled receptor family and is a receptor for many different cytokines that influence the behavior of leukocytes. CCR4 is known to be expressed on T-helper type 2 (Th2) cells and regulatory T cells (Tregs). Several studies have demonstrated that CCR4 is expressed at relatively high levels on select T-cell neoplasms, including HTLV-1 ATLL. KW-0761 is a defucosylated humanized IgG1 anti-CCR4 monoclonal antibody that enhances antibody-dependent cellular cytotoxicity and has been evaluated in multicenter phase I and II studies in patients with relapsed, aggressive CCR4-positive ATL.[124,125]

Patients received intravenous infusions of KW-0761 once a week for 8 weeks at a dose of 1.0 mg/kg. The phase II study of KW-0761 was conducted in 28 patients with relapsed or refractory ATL. The overall response rate was 50%, including eight complete responses, and the median PFS and OS were 5.2 and 13.7 months, respectively.[124] The most common adverse events were infusion reactions (89%) and skin rashes (63%), which were manageable and reversible in all cases. Albeit relatively early, this study demonstrated clinically meaningful antitumor activity in patients with relapsed aggressive ATL, with an acceptable toxicity profile. Further investigation of KW-0761 for treatment of ATL and other T-cell neoplasms are now warranted.

Miscellaneous Agents

The drugs mentioned above all represent agents that have been studied in a reasonable number of patients with T-cell lymphoma. In addition to these there are select other agents with very early and potentially promising signals of activity in PTCL. The proteasome inhibitors, including bortezomib and carfilzomib, have marked activity in multiple myeloma and mantle cell lymphoma.[126-128] Although the experience in PTCL is modest, 10 patients with CTCL and 2 with PTCL were treated with bortezomib at a dose of 1.3 mg/m^2 on a day 1, 4, 8, and 11 schedule. Although the ORR was reported to be 67%, dramatic responses were seen in patients with advanced CTCL, and one of the two patients with PTCL experienced a complete remission.[129] Emerging data have now demonstrated that the proteasome inhibitors potently synergize with the HDACI[130] and pralatrexate, which is leading now to combination studies in patients with PTCL.[108]

Another novel class of drugs with a signal of activity in the T-cell lymphomas includes the immunomodulatory drug lenalidomide. This class of drugs is thought to increase the immunologic synapse by increasing NK cell activity against the lymphoma cells. In one report, lenalidomide was administered orally for 21 days on a 28-day cycle at a dose of 25 mg daily in 24 patients with relapsed or refractory PTCL with an ORR of 30% being reported (7 responses among 23 evaluable patients), with no CR.[131] Responses were seen in patients with ALCL, AITL, and PTCL-NOS. The median PFS was 96 days. Similar results were reported among 10 patients with relapsed and refractory PTCL-NOS, where 3 CRs were reported.[132]

Preliminary reports from a phase II study of a novel Aurora-A kinase inhibitor, MLN8237/alisertib, in patients with aggressive NHL have recently demonstrated activity in patients with PTCL. Although the ORR was 32%, four of eight patients with relapsed or refractory PTCL experienced a response, including some complete remissions.[133] These data have now prompted a large international randomized study of alisertib in patients with relapsed or refractory PTCL, in which patients will be randomized to either the Aurora-A kinase inhibitor or a drug selected at the investigator's discretion (pralatrexate, romidepsin, or gemcitabine).

Future Directions

Over the past several years there has been a remarkable increase in our understanding of the diversity within the PTCLs. The appreciation that the mature T-cell lymphomas represent a vast spectrum of both indolent and aggressive subtypes, commonly associated with diverse clinical pictures with substantial global variation, has shaped how we now classify and think about these diseases. Even prognosticating the outcomes of patients with these diseases has become remarkably complicated, because each subtype of PTCL is now widely recognized as possessing its own unique clinical behavior and thus its own unique response to different therapeutic approaches. Eventually these prognostic models will be used to better risk stratify patients at diagnosis, allowing physicians to institute the optimal treatment plan earlier, which may include ASCT for select patients and allogeneic SCT for those with relapsed or refractory disease. Unquestionably, however, the increase in the number of new drugs available for the treatment of this group of diseases has begun to reshape our options when considering the management of patients with relapsed and refractory disease. As these new drugs are used with increasing frequency, each having significant single-agent activity in these traditionally chemotherapy-resistant diseases, the emergence of novel non–CHOP-based drug combinations will likely emerge, with the intent of tailoring the use of these combinations of drugs to patients with specific disease subtypes based upon an assessment of an individual patient's risk due to his or her specific disease subtype.

CUTANEOUS T-CELL LYMPHOMAS

The T-cell NHLs include a wide variety of clinical disorders with different prognoses. The WHO classification of hematopoietic malignancies suggests that more than 10 discrete clinicopathologic entities can be considered part of this family. This portion of the chapter focuses on the disorders that would be encompassed by the diagnosis *cutaneous T-cell lymphoma* (Table 84-6). The most common subtypes of CTCLs are the epidermotropic variants MF and the related leukemic variant, Sézary syndrome (SS).

Epidemiology

CTCLs account for 71% of the 3844 cutaneous lymphomas diagnosed in the United States between 2001 and 2010. MF and SS are the most common CTCL subtypes worldwide, constituting 54% of the CTCLs and an annual incidence of approximately four cases per million people.[135,136] MF and SS are the most common primary lymphomas involving the skin.[137,138] Data collected from the SEER program showed a rapidly increasing incidence from 0.2 cases per 100,000 people in 1973 to 0.4 cases per 100,000 people in 1984. This corresponds to approximately 1000 new cases each year in the United States. Whether this represented a true increase in incidence or was attributable to a better awareness and therefore more frequent recognition of this disease has not been resolved. Since that time the incidence rate of CTCL has stabilized at 0.36 cases per 100,000 persons, and the mortality rate has declined. The incidence of MF/SS increases with advancing age, as does the incidence of NHLs in general. The average age at presentation is approximately 50 years. Although cases in very young patients have been reported, most patients are at least 30 years of age.[139,141] MF/SS is seen in all racial groups. There is a 1.6 : 1 ratio of African Americans to whites and a 2.2 : 1 ratio of men to women with this disorder. MF is less common in the Asian population. Clusters of cases of MF/SS within families have been reported. An association with histocompatibility antigens AW31, AW32, B8, BW35, and DR5 has been described.[142] However, a solid genetic predisposition or inherited genetic defect has not been demonstrated.

Pathobiology

The T lymphocyte is central to the body's ability to mount an immune response and is the precursor of neoplastic cells in MF/SS. Sézary cells respond to phytohemagglutinin and perform T-cell immunoregulatory functions similar to normal lymphocytes.[143,144] The clonal nature of CTCL has been demonstrated by Southern blotting or polymerase chain reaction methods for analysis of the TCR.

The development of monoclonal antibodies directed against different T-cell antigens has allowed for more precise identification of surface markers on the malignant T cells.[145] Most cases of MF and SS are composed of the helper memory or effector T cells with a CD4$^+$CD45RO$^+$ phenotype. In most instances, the cells express the

Table 84-6 Comparison of EORTC and WHO Classifications of Primary Cutaneous Lymphoma

EORTC Classification	WHO Classification
CUTANEOUS T-CELL LYMPHOMA	
Indolent clinical behavior	Mycosis fungoides
Mycosis fungoides variants	Mycosis fungoides variants
Follicular mycosis fungoides	Follicular mycosis fungoides
Pagetoid reticulosis	Pagetoid reticulosis
CTCL, large cell, CD30+	Primary cutaneous CD30+ ALCL (CD30+ lymphoproliferative disease, including lymphomatoid papulosis)
Lymphomatoid papulosis	
Aggressive clinical behavior	Sézary syndrome
Sézary syndrome	Peripheral T-cell lymphoma, unspecified (most); extranodal NK/T-cell lymphoma, nasal type
CTCL, large cell, CD30−	
PROVISIONAL ENTITIES	
CTCL, pleomorphic, small/medium sized	
Subcutaneous panniculitis-like T-cell lymphoma	Subcutaneous panniculitis-like T-cell lymphoma
CUTANEOUS B-CELL LYMPHOMA	
Indolent clinical behavior	Extranodal marginal zone B-cell lymphoma
Primary cutaneous immunocytoma (marginal zone B-cell lymphoma)	
Follicle center cell lymphoma (any grade)	
Intermediate clinical behavior	
Primary cutaneous large B-cell lymphoma of the leg	
PROVISIONAL ENTITIES	
Primary cutaneous plasmacytoma	Plasmacytoma
Intravascular large B-cell lymphoma	Diffuse large B-cell lymphoma (intravascular)

ALCL, Anaplastic large cell lymphoma; *CTCL*, cutaneous T-cell lymphoma; *EORTC*, European Organization for Research and Treatment of Cancer; *NK*, natural killer; *WHO*, World Health Organization.

pan–T cell antigens CD2 (the sheep erythrocyte receptor), CD3, and CD5. CD7 is a T-cell marker expressed in early differentiation, but usually absent in T cells homing to the skin. Although benign conditions may show some downregulation of CD7, marked deletion of CD7 is commonly used by the pathologist as an ancillary confirmatory test for CTCL. Flow cytometry provides a sensitive method for detecting early peripheral blood involvement in patients by detection of $CD4^+$, $CD26^-$ T-cell populations. A small subset of MF is characterized by the expression of CD8, a marker that is essentially never expressed in SS. Low expression of the α-chain component of the IL-2 receptor (CD25) is detected with heterogeneous expression by the malignant cells in less than half of the patients. The implication of this finding is of uncertain significance, because both activated T cells and immunoregulatory T cells can express CD25. Key signaling pathway alterations that affect MF and SS include Notch overexpression, Fas underexpression, and the association of PKC inhibition with apoptosis.[146-148]

Cytogenetic analyses have demonstrated numeric and structural chromosomal abnormalities in MF/SS,[149] although usually in advanced-stage disease. Hyperdiploidy and complex karyotypes are common. Nonrandom deletions of chromosomes 1, 6, 8, 10, and 17 have been reported with gains in chromosome 17q and 4p occurring in more than 25% of cases. Regions of the genome that include genes encoding the TCR do not appear to be involved, suggesting that the genetic basis for malignant transformation in MF/SS appears to be different from that involved in other T-cell malignant disorders.

Modest data exist on the aberrant expression of oncogenes and suppressor genes in MF/SS. Loss of heterozygosity is identified in 30% to 60% of patients, commonly at 9p, 10q, 1p, and 17p. Loss of heterozygosity in early stages of disease is associated with a threefold increase in mortality.[150] Various mutations involving the Fas pathway are commonly seen from the early stages of lymphomagenesis, reflecting an initial accumulation of abnormal lymphocytes secondary to abnormal proapoptotic pathways. Mutant forms of the P53 tumor suppressor gene are observed rarely, usually in tumor stage and large cell transformation of MF.[151] LYT-10, a member of the NF-κB family of transcription factors associated with translocations in lymphoid malignancies, is rearranged in a small proportion of cases.[152] However, BCL2, a gene whose rearrangement is characteristic of follicular B-cell lymphomas and which slows programmed cell death, is overexpressed in MF. Constitutive phosphorylation of STAT3 (a member of the transcription factor family that contributes to the diversity of cytokine responses) has been reported and suggests that these malignant T cells are activated.[145,153] Altered expression or release of select cytokines or their receptors, including IL-1, IL-2R, IL-4, IL-5, IL-6, IL-7, IL-8, IL-12, and TGF-β receptor II, has been noted.[154] IL-7 and IL-15 have been identified as growth factors for MF/SS and shown to regulate expression of the BCL2 and MYB oncogenes and stimulate DNA binding of STAT proteins.[155,156] There is recent evidence suggesting that SS and MF may follow different molecular pathways with dysregulation of genes encoding c-Myc and c-Myc regulatory proteins commonly associated with SS but not with MF.

The cause of MF/SS remains unknown. It is considered to be a sporadic disease without compelling evidence of transmissibility. Several viruses have been implicated in the pathogenesis of MF/SS, including HTLV-1 and HTLV-2, herpes simplex virus, human herpesvirus 6, and EBV. However, a viral cause of MF/SS has not been proven, and no epidemiologic evidence supports these hypotheses.

Investigators have suggested that prolonged antigenic stimulation via exposure to contact allergens or superantigen stimulation associated with infections may lead to enhanced immune responses with subsequent mutations in apoptotic pathway leading directly or indirectly to the development of MF/SS. Sézary cells respond in vitro to superantigenic exotoxins, and colonization by *Staphylococcus aureus* may influence disease activity.[157] Several reports suggested that exposure to metals or their salts, pesticides or herbicides, and organic solvents (halogenated or aromatic hydrocarbons) could be related to the development of MF/SS.[158] However, two well-designed case-control studies have failed to support these observations.[159,160]

Various theories have been advanced to explain the epidermotropism of malignant T cells in MF/SS. Organ-specific affinity to skin and other organs has been recognized in subsets of normal T cells. Homing of CTCL cells to the skin is probably mediated by more than one adhesion receptor mechanism. CTCL cells express cutaneous lymphocyte antigen, a skin homing receptor that interacts with E-selectin expressed by dermal venules.[145,161,162] Furthermore, the cutaneous lymphocyte antigen T lymphocytes also typically express the CCR4 chemokine receptor, which binds to chemokines produced by the skin, such as the CC-chemokine ligands 17 and 22. Peripheral blood mononuclear cells bind to cultured keratinocytes exposed to interferon-γ. The major histocompatibility complex class II proteins, along with intercellular adhesion molecule 1 present on keratinocytes, attract and bind lymphocytes. Additional chemokine receptors, such as CXC chemokine receptors 3 and 4, as well as unique integrins, have been shown to have corresponding ligands or integrin receptors on dermal Langerhans cells, suggesting a relationship between the malignant T cells and host immune cells. The chemokine receptor CCR4 is expressed by a spectrum of CTCL cells, and an anti-CCR4 monoclonal antibody has significant activity against these diseases.[163]

An additional feature of MF/SS cells is the production of a cytokine profile consistent with Th2 cells.[164] The Th2 cells produce IL-4, IL-5, and IL-6, and they are inhibited by interferon-γ. The expression of immunomodulatory molecule IL-17 is also increased in MF and SS.[165] The Th2 cells are critical for stimulating antibody- and eosinophil-mediated responses. Hypergammaglobulinemia and eosinophilia are often seen in advanced cases of MF/SS and are consistent with a Th2 profile. Stimulation of Th2 cells inhibits the Th1 subpopulation of lymphocytes involved in cell-mediated immunity. Progression of MF/SS is associated with immune suppression as a result of depletion of this T-cell subset. The Th2 cytokine profile may explain the decrease in tumor-infiltrating lymphocytes during tumor progression. In addition to the effect of cytokines secreted by the neoplastic cells, the malignant $CD4^+$ cells express antigens (e.g., Fas ligand) that may directly mediate elimination of the $CD8^+$-infiltrating lymphocytes by induction of apoptosis.[166] $CD4^+$ T cells from MF skin lesions have an effector memory phenotype, whereas T cells from SS skin lesions display central memory characteristics[167] with the expression of the lymph node chemoattractant CCR7, which is not expressed in MF.

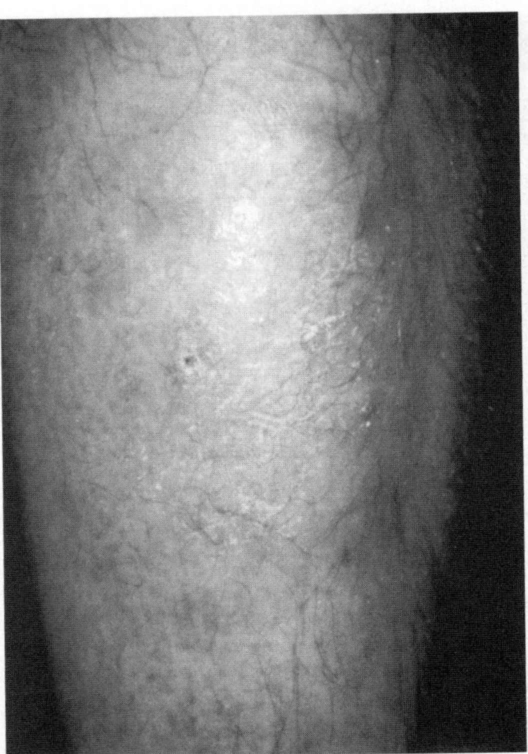

Figure 84-13 ERYTHEMATOUS AND SCALY PATCH LESION OF MYCOSIS FUNGOIDES.

Clinical Presentation

Alibert[168] reported the first case of MF in 1806. His patient developed a skin eruption that progressed into mushroom-like tumors, prompting the term *mycosis fungoides.* Later in the 19th century, Bazin[169] defined the three classic cutaneous phases (patch, plaque, and tumor stage) of the disease. The recognition of the clinical triad of intensely pruritic erythroderma, lymphadenopathy, and abnormal hyperconvoluted cells in the peripheral blood led to the description of SS.[170]

MF is the prototype of CTCL observed in over 50% of CTCL cases. The initial course of patients with MF is usually indolent. Most patients give a history of antecedent skin lesions, usually nonspecific erythematous patches that can mimic eczema or psoriasis. In many cases, there is an orderly progression from limited patches to more generalized patches, plaques, tumors, and nodal or visceral involvement. However, some patients may present with extensive skin involvement and tumor lesions, whereas other patients have limited patch disease that remains unaltered for the patient's entire life. The characteristic patch lesion is typically poorly demarcated, lightly erythematous, and scaly, with a predilection for sun-protected areas, such as the lower abdomen or buttocks (Fig. 84-13). The texture can vary from poikilodermatous atrophic cases to serpiginous annular lesions or markedly keratotic patches. Plaque lesions are more indurated, have well-demarcated margins, and some scaling (Fig. 84-14). Plaques can arise from patch lesions or previously uninvolved areas of skin. The distinction between a patch and a plaque is often subjective, with a low rate of interpersonal agreement among experts. Tumor lesions tend to appear in advanced cases, frequently associated with previous patches or plaques, and are commonly associated with histologic evidence and large cell transformation. They can be located on any part of the body. Ulceration of these lesions is common, and secondary infection is a major cause of morbidity (Fig. 84-15). Tumors may be the initial presentation in a small percentage of patients (d'emblée presentation, Vidal and Brocq, 1889).

SS patients present with generalized desquamative erythroderma, pruritus, and circulating malignant cells. Peripheral blood usually shows a significant number or percentage of hyperconvoluted atypical lymphocytes (Fig. 84-16). Approximately 5% to 10% of all newly reported cases of CTCL are SS. In its most advanced form, patients with SS suffer from alopecia, ectropion, leonine facies, hyperkeratosis, nail dystrophy, fissuring of the palms and soles, and severe

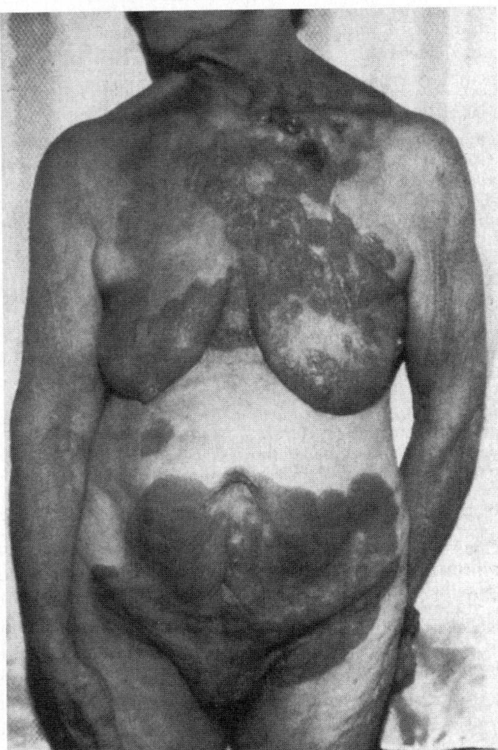

Figure 84-14 PLAQUE LESION OF CUTANEOUS T-CELL LYMPHOMA.

pruritus and cutaneous pain. Many other entities can clinically mimic this disease, including drug eruptions, atopic dermatitis, contact dermatitis, and erythrodermic psoriasis. A number of variant presentations of CTCL are described in the following sections.

Clonal Dermatitis

Clonal dermatitis is a term introduced by Wood et al[180] that included a variety of lymphocyte-rich dermatoses, often characterized by clonal T-lymphocyte proliferations. Clinically they exhibit a myriad of cutaneous presentations from poikiloderma (atrophic patches) to hyperpigmented areas resembling pigmented purpuric dermatosis.

Large Plaque Parapsoriasis

Large plaque parapsoriasis is the classic premalignant lesion of MF. It most commonly consists of a few scattered, erythematous to brown plaques that are usually larger than 6 cm.[172] There is a predilection for the buttocks and intertriginous areas. Histologic examination shows a superficial lymphocytic infiltrate with minimal nuclear atypia. Epidermotropism is scant or absent, and dermal fibrosis correlates with the chronicity of the process. Plaques can persist for decades before a frank evolution to MF occurs. Approximately 10% to 30% of patients ultimately develop an overt malignant transformation. Large plaque parapsoriasis is more likely to evolve into MF than small plaque lesions.

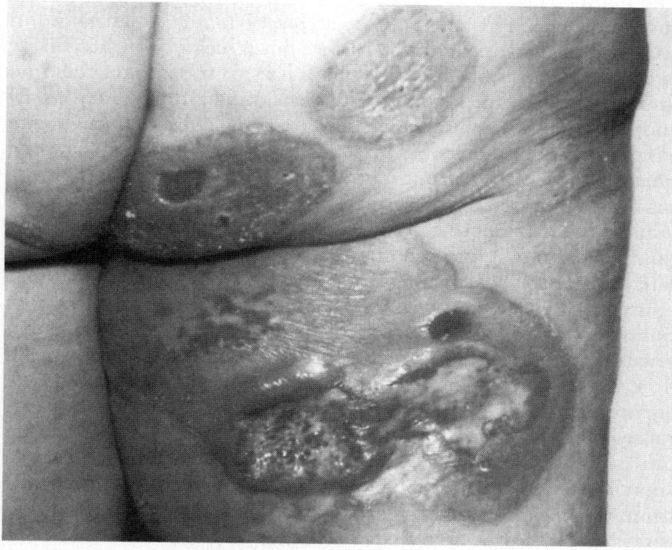

Figure 84-15 ULCERATED TUMORS ARISING FROM MYCOSIS FUNGOIDES PLAQUES.

Follicular Mucinosis

Follicular mucinosis manifests with grouped erythematous follicular papules or boggy or indurated nodular plaques, notably devoid of hair (Fig. 84-17).[173] There is a predilection for the head and neck area, especially the forehead, which has the highest density of pilosebaceous units. Histopathologic evaluation reveals cells in sebaceous glands often associated with destruction of hair follicle structures due to infiltration by a T-lymphocytic process. This condition may be idiopathic or associated with MF. Even idiopathic cases can be associated with clonal T-lymphocytic infiltration.[174] In general, patients older than 40 with a more generalized cutaneous involvement and a chronic course are more likely to develop associated MF. No cases of MF have been reported in children with alopecia mucinosa, although a few reports of Hodgkin disease have been reported in children with follicular mucinosis.[175] Patients with folliculotropic MF and follicular mucinosis are reported to have a worse prognosis, stage for stage, which may be caused by inability of topical treatment to penetrate to the deeper layers of the process.[176]

Lymphomatoid Papulosis

Lymphomatoid papulosis is characterized by recurrent crops of self-healing, red-brown, centrally necrotic, asymptomatic papules and nodules (Fig. 84-18).[177] This entity represents 10% to 15% of all CTCL cases. Patients may have a few lesions or more than 100 at a time. Histologic evaluation reveals an atypical $CD4^+$ lymphocytic infiltrate with a variable mixed inflammatory infiltrate (Fig. 84-19). These may be primarily small cerebriform cells similar to those seen in MF (type B), but most often there are larger $CD30^+$ cells with prominent nucleoli resembling Reed-Sternberg cells (type A). A third variety of lymphomatoid papulosis (type C) with sheets of anaplastic large cells resembling $CD30^+$ large cell lymphoma ($CD30^+$ LCL) has also been reported.[178] TCR gene rearrangement studies demonstrate a clonal origin. Although the typical course is usually indolent, spanning decades, approximately 15% of patients develop MF, HL, or NHL during their lifetime.[179] A direct link between lymphomatoid papulosis, CTCL, and Hodgkin disease was demonstrated in a patient with the three lymphoproliferative disorders arising from a common T-cell clone as shown by TCR gene studies.[180]

Pagetoid Reticulosis

Pagetoid reticulosis (i.e., Woringer-Kolopp disease) is a rare condition affecting young adults. It typically manifests with a solitary, hyperkeratotic, often verrucous plaque on the lower limb.[181] Biopsy results show atypical cerebriform lymphocytes with a perinuclear halo almost exclusively localized within the intraepidermal compartment.[182] Extracutaneous dissemination is exceedingly rare. Most cases have a $CD8^+$ phenotype, although $CD4^+$ cases or double-negative ($CD4^+$/CD8) cases have been reported. Frequently the tumor cells express CD30, but TCR gene rearrangement study results are often

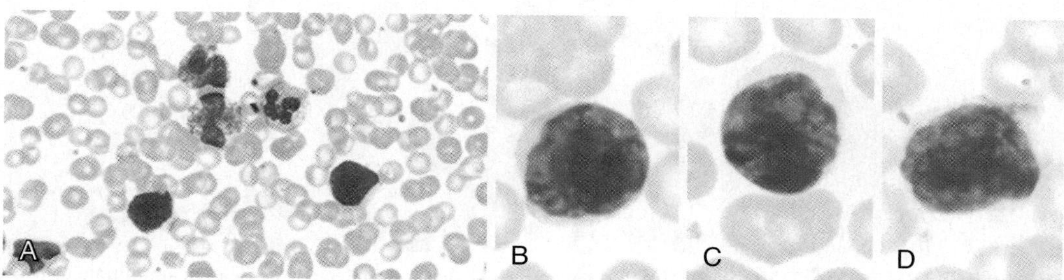

Figure 84-16 SÉZARY CELLS. Peripheral smear **(A)** with Sézary cells associated with eosinophilia. Note the cerebriform nuclei with fine chromatin **(B** to **D)**. The hyperconvoluted nature of the nuclei is evident as complex nuclear folds seen through the chromatin.

negative. Whether pagetoid reticulosis should be considered a localized form of MF or a reactive pseudomalignant process is debatable. Although most cases have an indolent protracted course, generalized and sometimes aggressive variants have been reported.[183] Cases presenting with a solitary lesion are extremely indolent and could be considered a reactive or pseudolymphomatous process. At the opposite end of the spectrum there are patients with extensive ulcerative plaques formerly known as *generalized pagetoid reticulosis* or *Ketron-Goodman disease* that now are diagnosed as the $CD8^+$ aggressive intraepidermal T-cell lymphoma.

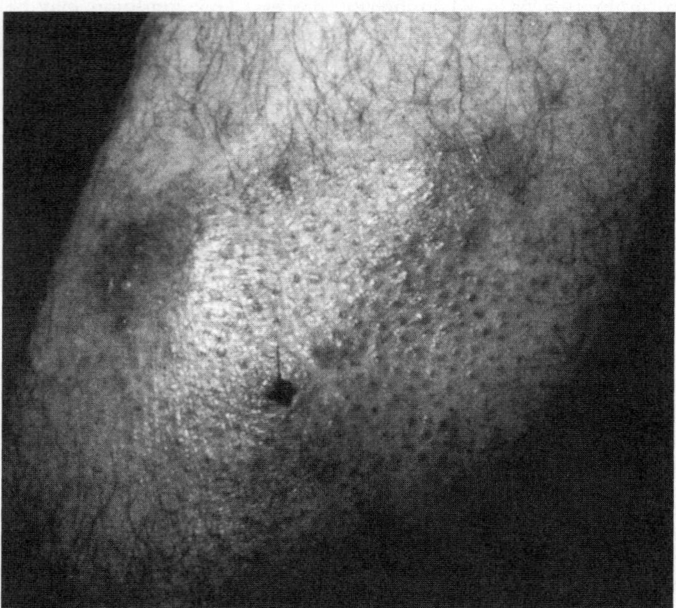

Figure 84-17 FOLLICULAR MUCINOSIS SHOWING A PATCH OF ALOPECIA WITH FOLLICULAR PROMINENCE.

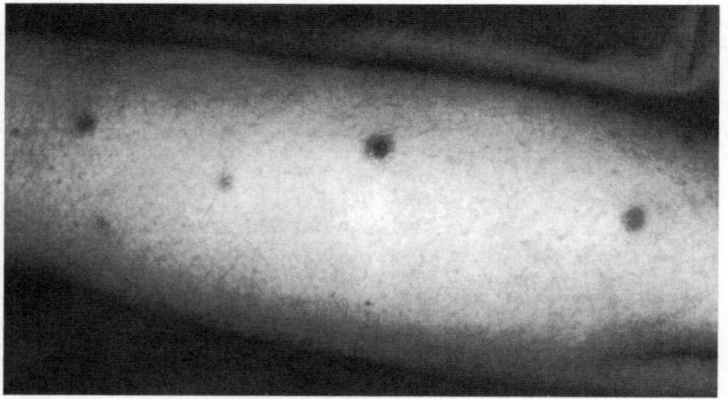

Figure 84-18 LESIONS OF LYMPHOMATOID PAPULOSIS APPEAR IN CROPS AND CONSIST OF ULCERATED PAPULES AND SCARS.

Granulomatous Slack Skin

In granulomatous slack skin syndrome, an extremely rare disorder, clonal $CD4^+$ T cells elicit a reactive granulomatous response that destroys the elastic fibers, rendering skin slack, fibrotic, and inelastic (Fig. 84-20).[184] Changes characteristic of MF are often found within the epidermis and papillary dermis, and the reticular dermis contains numerous histiocytes with multinucleated giant cells and elastophagocytosis. Some patients with granulomatous MF do not have destruction of the elastic fibers with slack skin changes. The differential diagnosis includes sarcoidosis and tuberculoid leprosy. An increased incidence of HL has been reported in this patient population.

Laboratory Manifestations

The gold standard in the diagnosis of MF/SS is light microscopic examination of a skin biopsy specimen. Characteristic findings include a band-like infiltrate involving the papillary dermis containing small, medium-sized, and occasionally large mononuclear cells with hyperchromatic, hyperconvoluted (cerebriform) nuclei and variable numbers of admixed inflammatory cells often expanding into adnexal structures (hair follicles and sweat glands).[154,185] Epidermal exocytosis of single or small clusters of neoplastic cells is a characteristic finding (Fig. 84-21, *A, C, D*). The presence of Pautrier microabscesses, defined as four or more atypical lymphocytes arranged in an aggregate in the epidermis, is classic but is seen in only a minority of cases. Reticular fibroplasia of the papillary dermis is also a common finding. Tumor-stage lesions demonstrate a more diffuse, superficial and deep, dermal infiltrate with fewer reactive cells and an absence of epidermotropism (Fig. 84-21, *B, E, F*). The malignant T-cell clone often evolves into large cell morphology during tumor progression, although rare cases show large cell morphology from the early patch lesions.[186] The presence of large cells in a skin lesion should be distinguished from "large cell transformation," which displays rapid skin, node, and visceral progression, is refractory to treatment, and is associated with poor survival. The histologic features in SS may be similar to those of MF. However, the cellular infiltrates in SS are more often monotonous, and epidermotropism may be absent.

Lymph node involvement initially involves the paracortical regions. Progression is associated with small to large clusters of atypical cells with preserved nodal architecture, followed by partial or total effacement of the node by neoplastic cells. Visceral involvement is a late clinical feature. Variable peripheral blood involvement can be demonstrated in all stages of skin disease, although it is most prevalent in patients with tumor or erythrodermic presentations. Patients with SS present with high circulating neoplastic cells, typically more

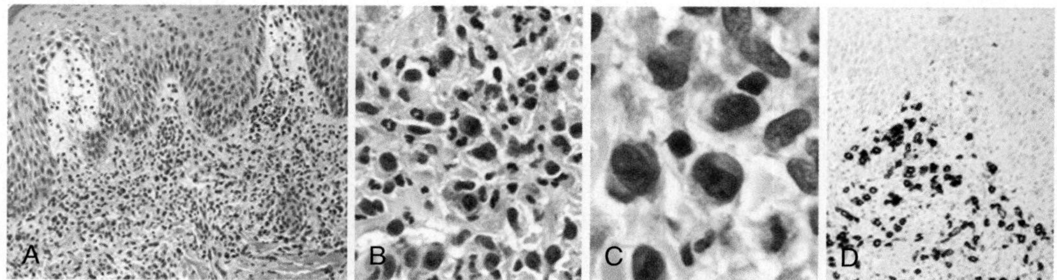

Figure 84-19 LYMPHOMATOID PAPULOSIS. Low power **(A)** shows a moderately dense dermal infiltrate of lymphoid cells admixed with inflammatory cells, including neutrophils and eosinophils **(B).** The lymphoid cells are varied but include atypical large forms **(C),** which are brightly positive for CD30 **(D).** *(Courtesy Drs. Vesna Petrovic-Rosic and Mark Racz, University of Chicago.)*

than 1000 cells/mL (B2), but a lower count may be noted initially (B1). Bone marrow biopsy results are typically negative. However, some involvement may be detected by flow cytometry in many cases of SS or advanced MF but rarely influences management outside an investigational setting. A staging bone marrow aspirate and biopsy is not recommended, unless unexplained cytopenias are seen.

The malignant cells are typically CD3$^+$, CD4$^+$, CD45RO$^+$, CD8$^+$, and CD30$^+$ by immunohistochemical analysis. CD7 is not expressed by cells from the early disease stages. More aggressive variants and advanced forms of CTCL may have cells with multiple pan–T cell antigen deletions, especially CD2, CD5, and even CD4. TCR genes are clonally rearranged and can be documented in most cases by Southern blotting or polymerase chain reaction assays when a sufficient malignant infiltrate exists.

Analysis of peripheral blood may reveal an elevated LDH level, mostly in patients with high-blood-burden SS and bulky advanced MF. Eosinophilia and hypergammaglobulinemia are not uncommon is SS patients. A limited number of patients have an associated monoclonal gammopathy. Elevated serum β_2-microglobulin and IL-2 receptor levels have also been observed in advanced cases.

Imaging studies for classic MF/SS are generally of modest utility. Computed tomographic scans of the chest, abdomen, or pelvis should be reserved for patients with SS, nodal involvement, or CTCL variants. In an investigational setting, electron microscopy, cytogenetics, and molecular analyses have shown that a higher percentage of patients have occult involvement of internal organs.

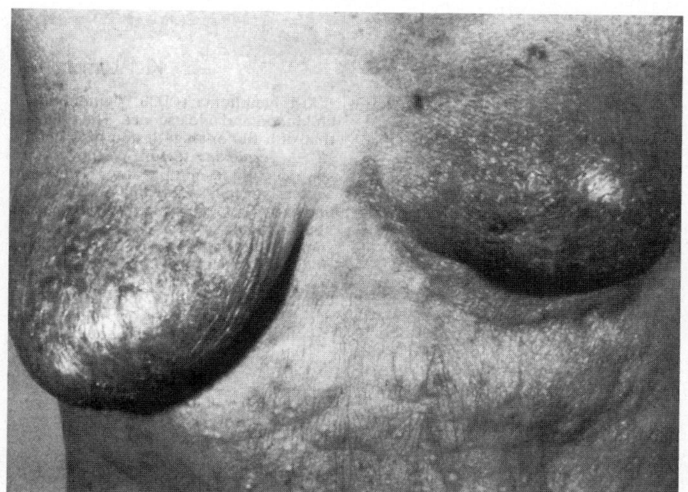

Figure 84-20 LESIONS OF GRANULOMATOUS SLACK SKIN WITH DESTRUCTION OF THE DERMAL ELASTICITY.

Differential Diagnosis

Primary CTCL represents a heterogeneous group of disorders with considerable variability in histologic characteristics, phenotype, and prognosis. The Kiel Classification, the Working Formulation, and the Revised European-American Lymphoma (REAL) classification system were developed for NHLs and were not designed to provide an adequate characterization of the spectrum of CTCL. To address the deficiencies of the previously proposed systems, a more clinically useful classification was developed by the European Organization for Research and Treatment of Cancer (EORTC).[3] WHO has proposed a classification with nearly 90% concordance with the EORTC classification (see Table 84-6). A number of other disorders in which malignant T cells infiltrate the skin should be distinguished from MF/SS. These disorders are discussed in the following sections.

CD30 Lymphoproliferative Disorders

CD30 lymphoproliferative disorders include lymphomatoid papulosis, primary cutaneous ALCL, and a spectrum of borderline cases. By definition ALCL presents with single or multiple tumors measuring more than 2 cm and with a tendency for ulceration and steady growth. Borderline lesions are smaller but also tend to have a prolonged course, often with spontaneous resolution.

Lymphomatoid Papulosis

Lymphomatoid papulosis is characterized by recurrent crops of self-healing, red-brown, centrally necrotic, asymptomatic papules and

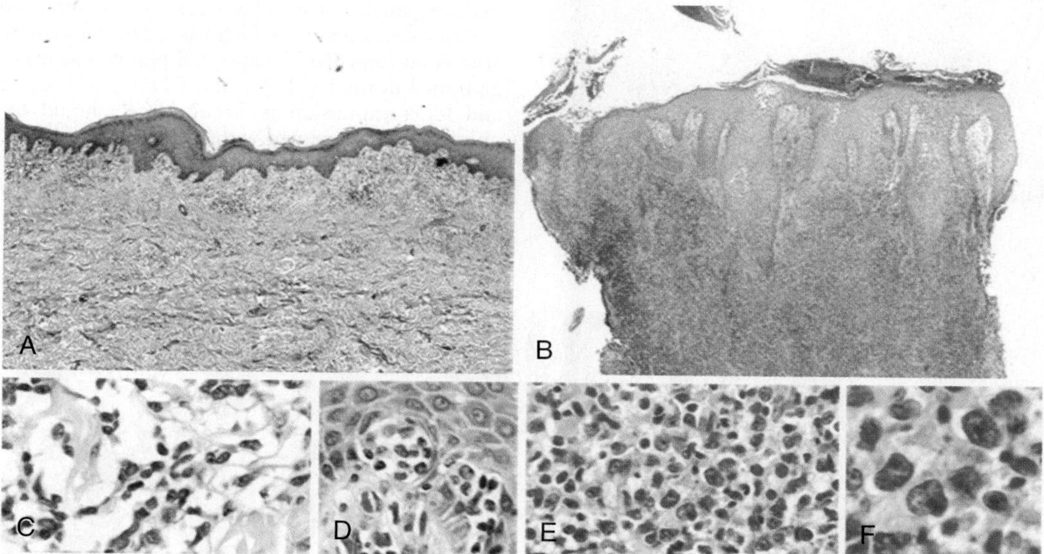

Figure 84-21 MYCOSIS FUNGOIDES, PLAQUE STAGE AND TRANSFORMED TUMOR STAGE. Plaque stage (**A, C,** and **D**) demonstrates a band-like infiltrate (**A** and **C**) with some epidermotropism in the form of Pautrier microabscesses **(D).** In the tumor stage (**B, E,** and **F**) there is a deep and dense infiltrate without significant epidermotropism. The cells are mostly large and atypical (**E** and **F**) and CD30$^+$ (not shown). *(Courtesy Drs. Vesna Petrovic-Rosic and Mark Racz, University of Chicago.)*

nodules. This entity represents 10% to 15% of all CTCL cases. Patients may have a few lesions or more than 100 at a time. Histologic evaluation reveals an atypical $CD4^+$ lymphocytic infiltrate with a variable mixed inflammatory infiltrate. These may be primarily small cerebriform cells similar to those seen in MF (type B), but most often there are larger $CD30^+$ cells with prominent nucleoli resembling Reed-Sternberg cells (type A). A third variety of lymphomatoid papulosis (type C), also considered borderline ALCL, presents with sheets of large cells resembling $CD30^+$ large cells. TCR gene rearrangement studies demonstrate a clonal origin. Although the typical course is usually indolent, spanning decades, approximately 15% of patients develop MF, cutaneous ALCL, and very rarely HL or NHL during their lifetime. A direct link between lymphomatoid papulosis, CTCL, and Hodgkin disease was demonstrated in a patient with the three lymphoproliferative disorders arising from a common T-cell clone as shown by TCR gene studies.

CD30-Positive Cutaneous T-Cell Lymphoma

Primary cutaneous $CD30^+$ LCL typically occurs in adults presenting with solitary or localized (ulcerating) nodules or tumors (Fig. 84-22).[187] Regional lymph node involvement is seen in 25% of patients at presentation. These primary cutaneous $CD30^+$ LCLs are probably closely related to lymphomatoid papulosis, regressing atypical histiocytosis, and primary cutaneous Hodgkin disease. The tumor has a favorable prognosis, and often complete or partial spontaneous regression occurs. This is in contrast to primary noncutaneous $CD30^+$ LCL, which can be seen in children or adults and which carries a poor prognosis.[188] These primary cutaneous lesions, in contrast to nodal or pediatric cases, have been shown to rarely have the chromosomal translocation t(2;5) associated with overexpression of the anaplastic lymphoma kinase (ALK negative). Histopathology consists of diffuse nonepidermotropic infiltrates with cohesive sheets of large $CD30^+$ tumor cells (Fig. 84-23). In most instances, the tumor cells have anaplastic morphologic characteristics, showing round, oval, or irregularly shaped nuclei; prominent (eosinophilic) nucleoli; and abundant cytoplasm. Less commonly, the neoplastic cells have a pleomorphic or immunoblastic appearance. Reactive lymphocytes are often present, but infiltrating eosinophils are often less conspicuous. The immunophenotype of this disorder is characteristically $CD4^+$, with more than 75% of neoplastic cells expressing CD30. In contrast to the poor outcome of MF that has transformed to a $CD30^+$ large cell variant, primary cutaneous $CD30^+$ LCLs are associated with an excellent prognosis. Radiotherapy is the preferred treatment for solitary or localized disease, with combination chemotherapy reserved for patients with generalized skin lesions or extracutaneous dissemination. Surgical excision may be adequate in many cases. In advanced cases, 5-year survival exceeds 30%.

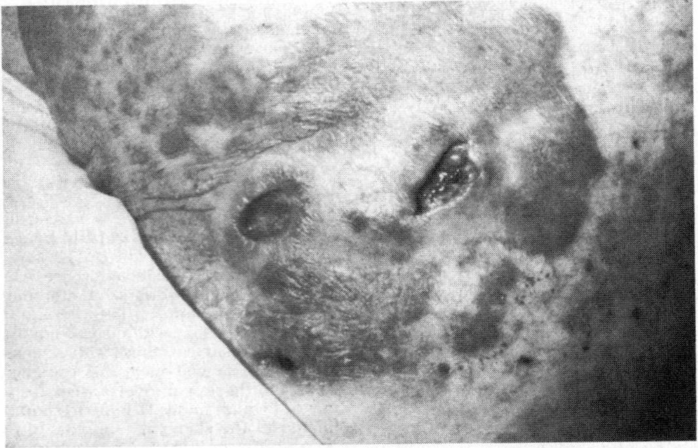

Figure 84-22 LESIONS OF $CD30^+$ LARGE CELL LYMPHOMA WITH ULCERATION.

CD30-Negative Cutaneous T-Cell Lymphoma

These rare presentations often classified as CTCL, NOS, or d'emblée presentation, tend to have an aggressive clinical course. Patients present with localized or generalized plaques, nodules, or tumors.[189] Histopathologic evaluation demonstrates that infiltrates are nonepidermotropic with variable numbers of medium-sized to large pleomorphic T cells with or without cerebriform nuclei and immunoblasts. The tumor cells are $CD4^+$ with $CD30^-$ or expression restricted to a few scattered tumor cells. The infiltrate is often accompanied by a mixed infiltrate with reactive B cells and granulomatous or histiocytic component. Multiagent chemotherapy is used in most instances, with radiation therapy reserved for patients with localized disease. The 5-year survival rate is less than 20%.

Pleomorphic Small or Medium-Sized Cutaneous T-Cell Lymphoma

Pleomorphic small or medium-sized cutaneous T-cell lymphoma is a rare entity. Patients typically present with a single red-purplish nodule or tumor involving the head and neck regions. Rarely are multiple nodules noted. The neoplastic cells are accompanied by many reactive B cells and histiocytes, which has led to the hypothesis that they may arise from follicular T-helper cell population expressing BCL6, programmed death-1 (PD-1), and CD10. Typically, CD30 is negative, and CD4 expression is strong. TCR should be positive. In our opinion, cases presented with a single lesion should not be diagnosed as lymphomas because, despite its clonal nature, the prognosis is invariably benign. Recent publications have confirmed that these lesions were called *pseudolymphomas* in the past without significant

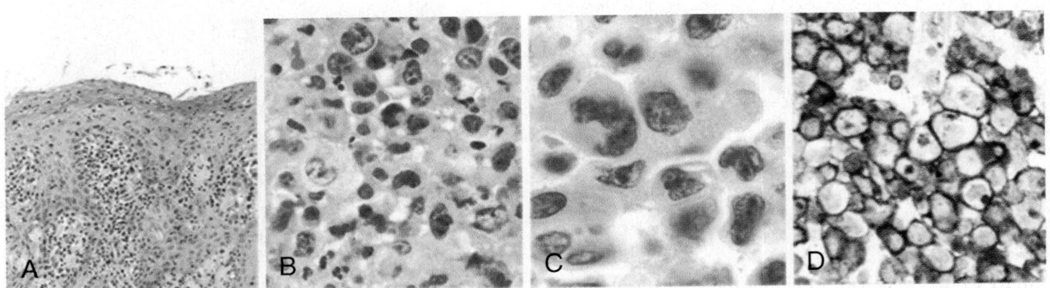

Figure 84-23 CUTANEOUS ANAPLASTIC LARGE CELL LYMPHOMA. Sheets of tumor cells are present in the dermis **(A)** and are associated with marked pseudoepitheliomatous hyperplasia. The cells are quite varied and bizarre **(B)** and frequently show abnormal "embryoid" shapes **(C)** constituting the "hallmark" cells. There is bright staining with CD30 **(D)**. ALK staining (not shown) is typically negative.

consequences. However, patients presenting with multiple lesions are part of the d'emblée presentation and should be approached with caution, including full staging and systemic therapy. Patients with more generalized disease have been treated with regimens used for indolent NHLs. Five-year survival rates are 100% in unilesional cases and exceed 60% in patients with more extensive disease.

Subcutaneous Panniculitis-Like T-Cell Lymphoma

Subcutaneous panniculitis-like T-cell lymphoma is a rare entity. Patients, typically younger and female, present with asymptomatic deep subcutaneous nonulcerated nodules and plaques involving the legs.[191,192] Systemic symptoms are common, including fevers, fatigue, and anorexia. Overlapping or preceding signs of lupus erythematosus or other autoimmune conditions are commonly observed. Histopathologic examination reveals a subcutaneous infiltrate with pleomorphic medium-sized T cells mixed with a reactive lymphoid infiltrate and some histiocytes. Tumor cell necrosis, karyorrhexis, and erythrophagocytosis are common findings. Differential diagnosis includes the frequently fatal but nonneoplastic cytophagic histiocytic panniculitis. Neoplastic infiltration of deep blood vessels can be noted in some cases.[193] Immunophenotyping reveals postthymic T-cell markers with $CD8^+$ phenotype and expression of cytotoxic markers like TIA-1 and granzyme B. By definition the tumor cells are negative for EBV markers and lack expression of the γδ heterodimer. However, T-cell clonality including the γ- or β-gene is commonly identified. The prognosis is fairly good with a 5-year survival rate over 80% with the exception of patients with a concurrent hemophagocytic syndrome (fevers, cytopenias). Cases in which the panniculitic findings coexist with lupus erythematosus may behave in a clinically indolent fashion.

Primary Cutaneous γδ-T-Cell Lymphoma

Cutaneous γδ-T-cell lymphoma is a rare condition that tends to present with extensive panniculitis-like plaques on the extremities with a tendency to ulcerate during the course of the disease.[192,193] A subset of patients present with single lesions resembling an infection process or with extensive chronic erythematous and scaly patches resembling MF. Several of our patients had comorbidities associated with immune suppression, including autoimmune conditions or other lymphoproliferative conditions or malignancies. Chronic antigen stimulation has been hypothesized to play a role in the pathogenesis of cutaneous γδ-T-cell lymphoma. Patients often present with a high level of LDH and constitutional symptoms and succumb to the disease, often associated with hemophagocytic syndrome. For the most part, all therapies have shown modest effectiveness. Sustained remissions have not resulted from radiation, immune therapy, or multiagent chemotherapy. However, a case with complete remission for 23 months following ASCT has been observed. Cytotoxic features like necrosis, hemorrhage, and vasculitis are commonly encountered. The immunophenotype is characterized by CD4/CD8 double negativity (with some $CD8^+$ cases), lack of CD5 expression, and expression of cytotoxic granules.

Primary Cutaneous Aggressive Epidermotropic $CD8^+$ T-Cell Lymphoma

This extremely rare condition, formerly known as generalized pagetoid reticulosis or Ketron-Goodman syndrome, constitutes less than 1% of all cutaneous lymphomas.[194] The term *Berti lymphoma* is often used to refer to this condition. Men are affected more commonly, and patients present with extensive erosive patches with frequent mucosal involvement. Occasionally the lesions are exophytic and hemorrhagic, resembling pyogenic granuloma. The course is invariable and rapidly fatal with exceptional cases reported surviving following ASCT. Histologically the infiltrate is markedly epidermotropic and adnexotropic, infiltrating into hair follicles and sweat glands, eventually becoming hemorrhagic and ulcerated. The cells are also of intermediate size, always expressing CD8 as well as other T-cell markers such as CD7 and CD45RO.

Extranasal Natural Killer/T-Cell Lymphoma

EBV-induced extranasal NKTCLs rarely appear in the skin as the initial site of presentation.[195] This condition is mostly reported in Asia and Latin America with rare cases seen in the United States. Although occasional cases remain localized in the skin, most of these lymphomas eventually involve other sites commonly affected in cytotoxic lymphomas such as the testes or the gastrointestinal tract. A careful ear, nose, and throat evaluation to rule out nasopharyngeal involvement is important. The lesions are mostly large ulcerated tumor lesions with hemorrhagic and necrotic appearance. Histologically the tumor is composed of a deep infiltrate with intermediate-sized lymphocytes with cytotoxic changes, hemorrhage, and necrotic debris. A histologic landmark is the presence of angiocentric and angiodestructive features. The immunophenotype is characterized by the expression of CD3ε in the cytoplasmic membrane, as well as CD56. Cytotoxic cytoplasmic granules are always identified, and EBV in the tumor cells can be demonstrated by the expression of EBER or LMP1. A lymphoproliferative disorder resembling hydroa vacciniforme has been reported almost exclusively in Latin America, especially in the Andes region, where the combination of high altitude with intense ultraviolet rays triggers this process, which is mostly seen in vulnerable indigenous patients. The patients present with facial edema, hepatosplenomegaly, and necrotizing hemorrhagic lesions triggered by sun exposure or arthropod bite reactions. These conditions are all very aggressive, and patients often succumb to hemophagocytic syndrome. Multiagent chemotherapy has not been effective, and perhaps the only hope for these individuals is an allogeneic SCT.

Lymphomatoid Granulomatosis

Lymphomatoid granulomatosis is a rare multiorgan disease of the lungs, nasopharynx, joints, and peripheral and central nervous systems.[196] Cutaneous involvement occurs in 25% to 50% of patients. Though nodules are most common, some patients have nonspecific macules, papules, or ulceration. Histologic evaluation reveals an angiocentric, polymorphous infiltrate of atypical lymphocytes and histiocytes surrounding and invading blood vessels within the dermis. Molecular and immunologic studies suggest a mature clonal helper T-cell process. However, reports have suggested a massive reactive T-cell infiltrate driven by a small number of clonal B cells.[195]

EBV DNA sequences are frequently present, and their role in the pathogenesis of this disorder remains poorly defined. Though the clinical course is variable, the prognosis for patients with diffuse pulmonary involvement or evolution to high-grade lymphoma is poor, with a median survival of less than 2 years. Treatment that depends on histologic findings and extent and location of disease may include corticosteroids, radiotherapy, and chemotherapy. Interferon has shown significant activity against this disease.[196] Related conditions include the recently reported EBV-induced mucocutaneous ulcer seen in immunosuppressed patients and B-cell lymphomas of older adults.

Adult T-Cell Leukemia

ATLL is in most instances a rapidly progressive T-cell neoplasm expressing a helper phenotype that is described earlier in this chapter.[197,198] It is endemic in southern Japan and the Caribbean islands and is associated with the retrovirus HTLV-1. However, most HTLV-l–infected patients remain asymptomatic, and only 2% to 4% develop ATL. The clinical presentation is polymorphous and can resemble MF or SS. Cutaneous lesions are variable, ranging from a rash simulating a viral exanthem, to annular lesions resembling erythema multiforme, to large tumors and plaques similar to MF (Fig. 84-24). Advanced stages of the disease, which affects a younger population than seen with MF, are characterized by visceral involvement, immunodeficiency, elevated LDH level, and hypercalcemia. Malignant lymphocytes often have convoluted or multilobed nuclei and can be detected in the peripheral blood in 75% of patients. The neoplastic T cells express high levels of the IL-2 receptor (CD25). For purposes of treatment and prognosis, it is wise to view ATL as a spectrum with two subgroups, acute and all others, with treatment, though inadequate, reserved for those with acute ATL. Therapeutic options include multiagent chemotherapy and antibody or recombinant toxins directed against the IL-2 receptor. Patients with acute ATL have poor survival rates, with a median duration of 4 to 6 months. Patients with disease that is not "acute" are considered to have "smoldering" disease and have lesions that may wax and wane in size and shape despite treatment.

Prognosis

The goals of treatment in MF are the relief of symptoms with improved quality of life, generally through prevention or delay in development of advanced skin disease and improvement in cosmetics. Despite some uncontrolled clinical trial results that have been reported to suggest "cures" in this disease, the general perception remains that this disease is not curable with standard therapies available today. The disease behaves similarly to other low-grade lymphomas, with periods of remission gradually becoming shorter with subsequent therapeutic interventions. Unlike B-cell low-grade lymphomas, however, advanced-stage MF is associated with a relatively short median life expectancy. Patients with significant nodal involvement (LN3 or LN4) or extensive skin involvement (T4) have median life expectancies of 30 to 55 months[199,200] (Table 84-7)]. A driving force in the development of treatments for this disease is the goal of altering the natural history for this group of poor-prognosis patients.

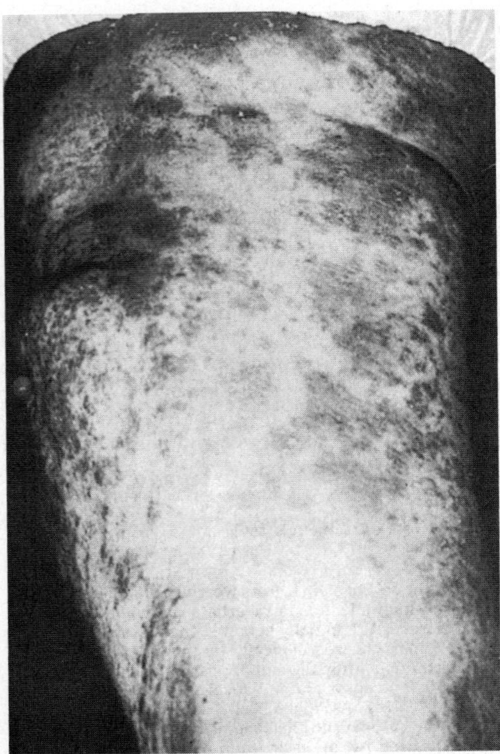

Figure 84-24 SKIN LESIONS IN ADULT T-CELL LYMPHOMA/LEUKEMIA.

No clinical trial has determined that aggressive early therapy is better than sequential palliative approaches or investigational approaches,[201] and new treatments continue to be developed and tested for these patients.

In 1979 the staging committee at an international workshop on MF proposed a staging system based on the international tumor-node-metastasis (TNM) system (see Table 84-7).[202] This classification was based on the evaluation of 347 patients and a multivariate analysis of potential prognostic factors. This group identified several independent prognostic factors: extent of skin disease at diagnosis (T), type of lymph node (N) involvement, presence or absence of peripheral blood (PB) involvement, and presence or absence of visceral (M) involvement. The group also translated this staging into a recommended clinical staging system (see Table 84-7). Investigators at the National Cancer Institute retrospectively analyzed 152 patients who

Table 84-7 TNM Staging System for Cutaneous T-Cell Lymphomas

Classification	Description
T	Skin
T0	Clinically or histopathologically suspicious lesions
T1	Limited plaques, papules, or eczematous patches covering 10% of the skin surface
T2	Generalized plaques, papules, or erythematous patches covering 10% of the skin surface
T3	Tumors (one or more)
T4	Generalized erythroderma Pathology of T1 to 4 is diagnostic of a cutaneous T-cell lymphoma. When more than one T stage exists, both are recorded and highest is used for staging. Record other features if appropriate (e.g., ulcers, poikiloderma, scale)
N	Lymph nodes
N0	No clinically abnormal peripheral lymph nodes
N1	Clinically abnormal peripheral lymph nodes (record number of sites)
NP0	Biopsy performed, not CTCL
NP1	Biopsy performed, CTCL
PB	Peripheral blood
PB0	Atypical circulating cells not present (≤5%)
PB1	Atypical circulating cells not present (>5%), record total white blood cell count, total lymphocyte count, and percentage of abnormal cells
M	Visceral organs
M0	No visceral organ involvement
M1	Visceral involvement (must have pathologic confirmation), record organ involved
Staging	
Stage IA	T1, N0 NP0, M0
Stage IB	T2, N0 NP0, M0
Stage IIA	T1-2, N1 NP0, M0
Stage IIB	T3, N0 NP0, M0
Stage III	T4, N0 NP0, M0
Stage IVA	T1-4, N0,1 NP1, M0
Stage IVB	T1-4, N0,1 NP0,1, M1

CTCL, Cutaneous T-cell lymphoma; *TNM,* tumor-node-metastasis.

underwent uniform pathologic staging.[203] They were able to identify three distinct prognostic groups. Good-risk patients had plaque-only skin disease without lymph node, blood, or visceral involvement, and a median survival of more than 12 years. Less than 10% of patients with stage 1A (limited patch) and less than 30% with stage 1B (extensive patch or plaque) progress to more advanced disease. Intermediate-risk patients had skin tumors, erythroderma, or plaque disease with lymph node or blood involvement (but no visceral disease) and a median survival of 5 years. Poor-risk patients had visceral disease or complete effacement of lymph nodes by lymphoma, and a median survival of 2.5 years.

In addition to the classic TNM staging, implementation of techniques such as flow cytometry, cytogenetic analysis, and determination of nuclear contour indices may also improve diagnostic and prognostic specificity. Flow cytometry and cytogenetic analysis are complementary techniques. Flow cytometry allows the detection of cell populations with a normal (diploid) number of chromosomes versus abnormal (aneuploid) numbers, and cytogenetic analysis precisely identifies the individual chromosomal structure and number. Bunn et al[204] demonstrated that in MF/SS the presence of aneuploidy during the clinical course was associated with more aggressive disease. Hyperdiploid cell clones were demonstrated in patients with large-cell histology, aggressive disease, and shortened survival time. Specific chromosomal deletions also influenced prognosis.[205]

The nuclear contour index has been used by several groups in an effort to separate "benign" cutaneous lymphocytic disorders, such as lymphomatoid papulosis and pityriasis lichenoides, from MF/SS.[206,207] Electron microscopy allows the calculation of a value based on the degree of nuclear folding; this nuclear contour index is significantly greater in patients with MF than in other benign conditions.

The density of epidermal Langerhans cells in biopsy samples, as determined by immunoperoxidase stains, has been identified as a prognostic feature.[208] Epidermal Langerhans cells are necessary for antigen recognition and processing in the normal immune response. Patients with Langerhans cell densities greater than 90 cells/mm^2 had a significantly reduced risk for death from MF/SS as compared with those with lower densities. There was no prognostic significance identified for the presence or absence of CD30-positive cells. It has been noted that the presence of cytotoxic CD8$^+$ T lymphocytes in the skin infiltrate is associated with a more favorable prognosis.[209]

Occasionally patients may develop a more clinically aggressive lymphoma concurrent with a change in the histologic appearance of the neoplastic cells and the pace of their disease. This progression from typical small, convoluted lymphocytes to larger lymphocytes, such as those associated with large cell lymphoma, has been documented.[210,211] Whether this conversion is secondary to prior therapeutic modalities used remains uncertain.

The gold standard for the diagnosis of MF is still routine histopathologic evaluation with adequate clinical correlation. Early lesions of MF are frequently accompanied by heavy infiltrates of benign reactive T cells, hampering the detection of abnormal T-cell clones by any laboratory method. Hence most adjuvant laboratory methods are not helpful at the precise time when they are most needed.

Therapy

Therapy can be conveniently divided into two approaches: topical (skin directed), such as psoralen plus ultraviolet A (PUVA), topical chemotherapy application (nitrogen mustard or carmustine), external beam radiotherapy, and total-skin electron beam radiotherapy, and systemic (skin and viscera directed), such as interferons, oral or parenteral chemotherapy, photopheresis, oral retinoids, and investigational new compounds (Table 84-8). No studies have demonstrated that one topical therapy is more effective than another, and patient and investigator preference remains the most important discriminating factor governing choice. However, as the biology of the neoplastic cell has become better understood,[202] it is clear that some therapies may actually have topical and systemic effects through alterations in the body's cytokine milieu and ability to mount a host response against the neoplastic cell.[203] Furthermore, knowledge regarding signaling pathways in the neoplastic cells in MF/SS offers hope that future development of targeted treatment approaches will soon be available. Investigational approaches combining therapies also remains an active research strategy (see box on Algorithm for Care of Patients With Mycosis Fungoides or Sézary Syndrome).

Table 84-8 Therapeutic Options for Mycosis Fungoides

TOPICAL THERAPY
Ultraviolet A with psoralen
Ultraviolet B
External beam radiation therapy
Total-skin electron beam radiation
Topical chemotherapy
Topical retinoids
SYSTEMIC THERAPY
Photophoresis
Interferon-α
Oral retinoids
Targeted therapies
Single-agent chemotherapy
Combination chemotherapy
Stem cell transplantation
Investigational agents

Phototherapy

8-Methoxypsoralen (8-MOP) is a member of a family of photoactivated compounds (furocoumarin derivatives), which may inhibit DNA and ribonucleic acid (RNA) synthesis through formation of monofunctional or bifunctional thymine adducts, gene mutations, or sister chromatid exchanges.[212,213] The cross-strand formed between DNA strands results in a halt in cell division, as well as oxidative damage to cytoplasmic organelles and cell membranes. These drugs are active only if the tissue containing the psoralen compound is exposed to ultraviolet A (UVA). The mechanism of cell cytotoxicity for many cancer therapies involves the induction of apoptosis. Yoo et al[217] demonstrated that peripheral blood mononuclear cells from SS patients and controls exposed in vitro to PUVA undergo apoptosis. Unfortunately, normal and neoplastic lymphocytes were equally sensitive to the apoptosis induced by PUVA (as opposed to with psoralen alone). However, macrophages appeared to be resistant to apoptosis induction and phagocytized apoptotic lymphocytes (but not nonapoptotic lymphocytes). Apoptosis induction may be the ultimate end point yielding benefit, but an immunologic effect due to monocyte phagocytosis and antigen presentation resulting from effector cells may also be present.

Photochemotherapy units with UVA lamps emit a continuous spectrum of long UVA in the range of 320 to 400 nm with peak emission between 350 and 380 nm. Initial exposure times of patients to high-output UVA are based on the degree of pigmentation before therapy, history of ability to tan, and the output of the photochemotherapy units. Exposure times are increased with each treatment depending on the patient's response and evidence of erythema. The initial UVA dose is between 0.5 and 2.0 J/cm^2 and can be increased by approximately 0.5 J/cm^2 per treatment as tolerated. The psoralen compound is ingested 2 hours before the UVA exposure. Topical psoralen protocols are also available. UV-blocking glasses should be worn for 24 hours after administration of 8-MOP. Therapy is typically given three times weekly until complete clearing occurs. The frequency of treatments can then be reduced, but some maintenance therapy (once every 2 to 4 weeks) may prolong the duration of remission. As data have emerged regarding the long-term risks of second skin malignancies after PUVA, the advisability of this maintenance therapy has been questioned.

Algorithm for Care of Patients With Mycosis Fungoides or Sézary Syndrome

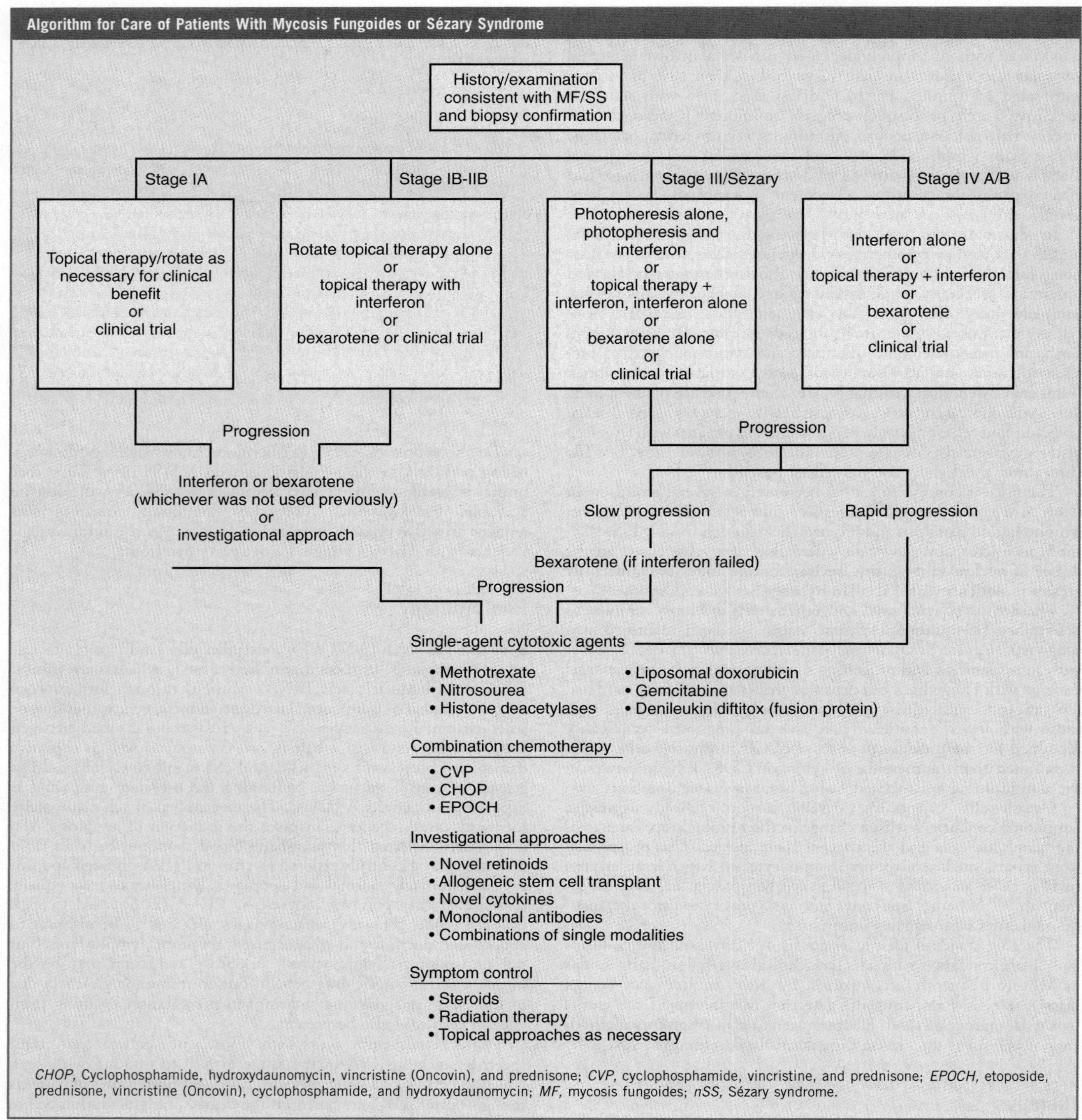

CHOP, Cyclophosphamide, hydroxydaunomycin, vincristine (Oncovin), and prednisone; *CVP*, cyclophosphamide, vincristine, and prednisone; *EPOCH*, etoposide, prednisone, vincristine (Oncovin), cyclophosphamide, and hydroxydaunomycin; *MF*, mycosis fungoides; *nSS*, Sézary syndrome.

Initial trials using PUVA benefited psoriasis patients.[215] Clinical trials with PUVA for patients with MF soon followed.[216] These studies all demonstrated high rates of remission in the early stage (patch or plaque stage of disease). The Scandinavian study group reported a 58% CR rate for these patients within 4 to 12 months of initiation of therapy.[217] Maintenance therapy was associated with a remission duration of up to 53 months. In these early studies, the same group also reported a surprisingly high rate of objective remissions in tumor-stage patients of 83%.[218] In a large series, 82 patients were followed for a median of 43 months.[219] An ORR was observed in 95% of patients, with a 65% complete clearance rate. Ninety percent of these patients had early-stage disease (stage IA-IIA). A single patient with tumor-stage disease attained a short remission with PUVA alone. Two of six patients with generalized erythroderma cleared completely (no evidence of circulating neoplastic lymphocytes). Given the difficulty in treating advanced-stage patients with PUVA alone, we usually restrict PUVA therapy to patients with stage IA-IIA disease (see Table 84-7), monitoring patients with tumor disease closely for progression.

Side effects associated with PUVA are quite tolerable. Nausea or vomiting due to psoralen ingestion is observed occasionally, and erythema, pruritus, and chronic dry skin are effects of the UVA damage. Long-term PUVA exposure has been associated with a number of delayed effects. These include dry skin, lichenification, keratosis, and rarely amyloid deposition in the skin.[220] Most important is the late development of iatrogenic (basal and squamous) carcinomas,[221] secondary malignant melanomas of the skin,[222] and rarely cataract formation. Because the cumulative dose of PUVA is correlated with the risk for developing a second skin cancer, routine use of maintenance therapy may be less desirable, especially for patients with an excellent prognosis (stage IA). Despite these problems, the long remissions induced, the ease of administration, and the lack of interactions with other therapeutic modalities make PUVA an attractive early intervention.

Narrow-band UVB (wavelength of 311 nm) is emerging as a valid alternative to PUVA for patients with limited patch or plaque disease. Although probably not as effective as PUVA, initial studies reported response rates near 70%.[223] The advantages of narrow-band UVB are that oral psoralen is not required and there may be less of a photocarcinogenic effect. The role for maintenance therapy has not been established.

UVA-1 is a modality of phototherapy that uses high-energy UVA1 (340 to 400 nm) output, which penetrates deep into the dermis. Resolution of tumor lesions has even been reported using this therapeutic approach.[224] However, the reduction in circulating $CD4^+$ cells raises the possibility that chronic use of this modality could be immunosuppressive.

Radiation Therapy

The CTCLs have been shown to be radiosensitive.[225] External-beam radiation adequately controls local areas of otherwise resistant MF or provides palliation in cases of bulky tumor lesions.[226,227] Unfortunately, the cumulative dosage that can be given to patients over time is limited due to organ toxicity. Side effects consisting of leukopenia, thrombocytopenia, and radiation-induced dermatitis may prevent long-term therapy with other agents. Newer techniques involving total nodal irradiation, fractionated total body irradiation, and limited fraction lesional irradiation all may have a role to play in the development of multimodality approaches to this disease. There has been little comparative research into methodology for external beam radiation that provides guidance to clinicians.

We recently reviewed our outcomes with a single fraction of external beam radiation, which was hypothesized to optimize convenience and minimize expense to patients.[228] Two hundred seventy individual lesions in 58 patients were primarily treated with more than 700 cGy (97%). With a mean follow-up of 41 months, 94.4% of lesions completely responded, and 3.7% partially responded. Predictors of poor response included lower extremity lesion, tumors, and lesions exhibiting large cell transformation. Lesions treated with electrons had a higher complete remission rate than those treated with photons. Cost estimates suggested multifractionated radiation was 200% more expensive than the single fraction.

The limitations of external beam radiation led to increasing use of electron beam radiotherapy for cases of MF confined to the skin. Linear accelerator–generated electron beams are scattered by a penetrable plate placed at the collimator site. The energy of the electrons is reduced to 4 to 7 MeV and allows adequate field distribution. Because of this low energy level, the beam only penetrates the surface several millimeters to 1 cm into the dermis. Patients may be treated using six-field or rotational treatments.[229,230] The total skin surface can be treated without significant internal organ toxicity. Most patients are able to tolerate total doses of approximately 3000 to 3600 cGy over an 8- to 10-week period.[230]

An excellent review compared results of external beam therapy at Stanford University with those achieved in Hamilton, Ontario.[231] The results cited in this paper reflect the extensive expertise of both centers in the delivery of this therapy and may not be applicable to centers where this approach is less frequently used. For patients with stage IA-IIA disease (see Table 84-7), almost 65% to 95% of patients achieved a complete remission. Treatment delivered without adjuvant therapies is associated with a relatively high rate of relapse in patients of all stages except stage IA. Ten-year relapse-free survival rates at the two centers ranged from 33% to 52% for this good-prognosis group. However, for stage IB and more advanced disease, 10-year unmaintained remission rates were only 16% or less. Higher-risk patients may be "induced" with external beam radiation and then placed on topical chemotherapy or systemic treatments such as extracorporeal photopheresis for "maintenance." Still the benefits of therapy may extend beyond crude estimates of relapse rates or survival. Patients with tumor lesions, generalized erythroderma, peripheral blood or nodal involvement, and even visceral spread can be successfully palliated with electron beam radiation therapy as well. Side effects, however, can be occasionally extreme, including scaling, dryness of skin, erythema, edematous extremities, telangiectasia formation, skin ulceration, and hair or sweat gland loss (usually transient but occasionally permanent). Careful radiation dosimetric techniques are required to ensure adequate skin treatment without excessive organ toxicity.[230] We do not use electron beam radiotherapy early in the course of the disease because other topical therapies have been developed that yield similar response rates with less potential toxicity. The long duration of remissions observed in patients with stage IA disease does not equate with cure, because their life expectancy is essentially the same as age-matched controls, and these patients may simply have indolent biology. One group has reported our experience with multiple courses of therapy.[232] They re-treated 15 patients with relapsed MF a mean of 41 months after the initial course of electron beam therapy. All patients had received intervening therapies for disease control. Eleven of the 15 had a CR with their first cycle of radiation. The second course achieved six CRs and nine partial remissions. The median duration of the initial CR was 11 months. The median duration of CR to the second course of therapy was only 3 months, suggesting radioresistance had developed between the first and second cycles in many patients. In general, toxicity was thought to be tolerable.

Topical Drug Therapy

The initial therapies for MF focused on treatment of the skin disease. Patients have long been known to benefit from the application of topical steroids. Zackheim et al[236] reported a 63% complete response rate with twice-daily applications in stage T1 patients but only a 25% complete response rate in stage T2 patients. Novel approaches by dermatologists to apply chemotherapy topically to avoid systemic therapy complications have also been devised. Mechlorethamine hydrochloride was the first topical agent evaluated to demonstrate efficacy in MF.[234] The solution used for topical application contains 10 to 20 mg of mechlorethamine dissolved in 50 to 100 mL of tap water (no vesicant activity at this low concentration). Although several methods may be used for administration, self-administration at home to the entire skin surface is preferred. The concentration may need to be varied depending on patient tolerance and sensitivity.[235] The time to initial response is usually short, approximately 1 to 2 weeks, but long-term application is usually required to obtain the maximum response.

Several large studies have been completed demonstrating the benefit of mechlorethamine, especially in early-stage disease.[236,238] One by Vonderheid et al[237] reported their experience with topical mechlorethamine and found that it compared favorably with results achieved with electron beam treatment. CRs were seen in 80%, 68%, and 61% of patients with limited plaque, extensive plaque, and tumor lesions, respectively. The corresponding median duration of remissions was in excess of 15, 5, and 12 months, respectively. It is difficult to draw definite conclusions from these data, because many patients included in the analysis also received intravenous mechlorethamine or methotrexate, and some may have received radiation therapy. Several patients have relapsed as long as 8 years after the completion of therapy, suggesting that follow-up times must be long to compare various topical therapies for early-stage disease. Hoppe et al[97,232] confirmed these findings using an ointment-based

(Aquaphor or polyethylene glycol) topical mechlorethamine, which may be associated with a lower incidence of cutaneous sensitivity. Formal testing of polyethylene glycol formulations for the treatment of early-stage disease has been completed, and an assessment of relative benefit compared to standard formulations is awaited.

For early-stage disease, topical mechlorethamine offers an efficient, convenient (outpatient treatment), and relatively inexpensive treatment option. Side effects consist of delayed hypersensitivity in approximately 35% of patients, although ointment-based solutions appeared to offer a reduced risk for allergic contact dermatitis. Once hypersensitivity develops, patients can be desensitized by injecting minute daily doses of mechlorethamine over a period of several weeks.[238] This should be done only in a medical setting with appropriate anaphylaxis precautions observed. Other investigators had difficulty replicating the results using this risky procedure, and topical desensitization has become much more common. Constantine et al[242] propose that therapy should be transiently discontinued until clearance of the allergic dermatitis is achieved (using topical steroids if necessary). Then 0.01 to 0.1 mg per 100 mL of the drug should be applied daily for 1 week. If this dilution is tolerated, the dosage is doubled weekly until the dose achieved is often identical to the initial concentration that induced the hypersensitivity.

Some clinicians, however, believe that a mild hypersensitivity reaction may have beneficial antitumor effects. Ratner et al[243] previously demonstrated that plaque lesions of MF cleared when exposed to topical doses of 2,4-dinitrochlorobenzene, a known universal inducer of delayed hypersensitivity responses. Anergic individuals failed to improve. Other known sensitizing agents yielded similar but less dramatic responses. Some hypersensitivity may be beneficial; the generalized erythroderma and pruritus are usually poorly tolerated when severe, however, and some alteration in therapy is required.

An increased risk for secondary skin cancers in patients receiving long-term mechlorethamine has been observed. Some physicians have expressed concern regarding the safety of family members or health care workers secondarily exposed to the topical solutions. Home treatment with topical mechlorethamine has been shown to result in aerosolized drug levels, which may result in mucous membrane or ocular irritation.[241] However, we are unaware of any documented adverse outcomes and believe this to be a theoretical concern rather than a practical one.

Several other topical agents have been tested and shown to be of benefit in the treatment of MF, including cytarabine, dianhydrogalactitol, dacarbazine, guanazole, teniposide, hydroxyurea, thiotepa, and methotrexate.[242] However, topical carmustine is the only agent that has demonstrated clinical use.[243] A stock solution is created with 300 mg carmustine in 150 mL of 95% ethanol (sufficient for 30 days of treatment). The patient then adds 5 mL of the 0.2% stock solution to 60 mL of room-temperature tap water. This solution can then be applied to the general body surface, with the exception of the head, genitals, palms, soles, and intertriginous zones, unless involved by disease. Applications are planned to occur daily for 2 to 6 months, if necessary. Brief exposures to double-dose solution can be used for resistant disease. Results in 188 patients with patch or plaque disease demonstrate efficacy similar to that of topical mechlorethamine.[243] For limited patch disease, there was a failure-free rate of 90% at 3 years. For more extensive patch-stage disease the freedom from treatment failure rate at 3 years was 62%. Some patients have been managed for as long as 10 years with topical carmustine. Side effects of contact dermatitis are less frequent with this agent, but systemic side effects, mainly leukopenia, are more common. This drug may be helpful for the treatment of patients who do not tolerate topical mechlorethamine, because there is no cross-sensitivity.

Hamminga et al[247] performed one of the few prospective trials comparing total-skin electron beam radiation to topical mechlorethamine. A total of 42 patients with MF localized to the skin (no documented nodal or visceral involvement) were treated. Patients were not randomized to their treatment; rather, the physician based the decision on patient health, availability of the linear accelerator, and the distance the patient lived from the clinic. In patients with minimal skin disease, no difference in outcome was observed. In more advanced skin disease, a trend toward superior initial response was seen with electron beam therapy, but there was a high relapse rate in those patients, necessitating subsequent therapy.

Systemic Chemotherapy

Currently systemic chemotherapy is reserved for those patients with relapsed or refractory disease after topical interventions or for those patients with advanced nodal or visceral disease at presentation. Many of the patients treated with chemotherapy have also previously been treated with cytokine-based or other nontraditional chemotherapeutic agents before systemic chemotherapy is considered. With that in mind, a number of trials have been published reporting results using agents developed many years ago for other indications but still in use for the treatment of MF/SS today. Recently, novel agents are being increasingly studied for efficacy in MF/SS based upon a rationale developed with molecular or proteomic data. An example of such agents is the HDACI. Vorinostat (SAHA) has been approved by the FDA for the treatment of the cutaneous manifestations of CTCL in patients in whom bexarotene therapy (see Retinoids) has failed,[113,245-247] and a related HDAC inhibitor, romidepsin (depsipeptide or FR901228), was more recently approved for the treatment of CTCL and PTCL. The mechanism of action of these drugs has been described previously in this chapter.

Approved Chemotherapy Agents for CTCL

Vorinostat 400 mg daily orally was tested in an open-label trial of 74 patients who had progressed on at least two prior systemic therapies. The ORR (skin only) was 29.5%, with 1 CR and 18 PRs. Common adverse events included diarrhea (49%) and fatigue (46%). Grade 3 events were less common but included fatigue (5%), deep venous thromboses/pulmonary emboli (5%), and thrombocytopenia (4%).

Reports from the National Cancer Institute with romidepsin have provided confirmatory results of the use of this class of agent for the treatment of patients with T-cell lymphomas, including some with MF/SS.[248,249] In these reports of several phase I and phase II trials, 10 of 20 patients with MF/SS appeared to have had a PR. Since these studies were published, two clinical trials have been reported demonstrating activity in CTCL. In a large multicenter open-label phase II trial of romidepsin, 96 patients with relapsed stage IB to IVA MF/SS (71% had stage IIB or higher) received standard dosing of 14 mg/m^2, on days 1, 8, and 15 every 28 days.[250] Importantly in these trials, total disease burden, not just skin involvement, was assessed to determine the response rates. The overall response rates was 34%, with 7% of patients achieving a CR. The median response duration was 15 months. Common adverse events included nausea/vomiting in over 56% of patients, asthenia in 44%, and diarrhea in 14%, but again grade 3 toxicities were much less frequent, but also included fatigue in 6%. The HDACI have been linked to cardiac abnormalities and especially arrhythmias. However, in this large trial, events such as cardiac failure, atrioventricular block, and ventricular tachycardia were rare, occurring typically in less than 1% of patients. Avoiding other drugs that may also cause cardiac arrhythmias seems prudent in patients treated with HDACI. The second confirmatory trial was led by investigators at the National Cancer Institute.[251] Seventy-one patients (87% with stage IIB or higher) with heavily pretreated MF/SS (median four prior treatments) were treated with romidepsin at the same dose as described earlier. Again the overall response rate was 34% with 6% CR. Although GI disturbances and fatigue were common in this trial in over 40% of patients, myelosuppression was seen more frequently, with 5% to 10% of patients experiencing grade 3 granulocytopenia and thrombocytopenia. Cardiac arrhythmias were again uncommon, but T-wave/ST changes were seen in the majority of patients, and grade 1 QTc prolongation was seen in 10% of patients.

In general then, toxicity to romidepsin and vorinostat has included alterations in the cardiac conduction that could potentially predispose to arrhythmias, and treatment of patients has required ongoing telemetry monitoring in some trials, but no evidence for acute or chronic impairment in cardiac function has been noted. Vorinostat demonstrated drug-related grade 1 electrocardiographic changes in five patients and grade 2 in one patient. Therefore it appears safe to use these agents in the outpatient setting with a periodic assessment of cardiac rhythm and QTc interval with an electrocardiogram based on the judgment of the practitioner.

Unfortunately, romidepsin has been shown to be a substrate for the multidrug resistance (MDR) protein (a *p*-glycoprotein) and upregulates the expression of MDR1. Preliminary molecular analyses confirmed the upregulation of MDR1. These data suggest that when resistance to this agent develops, other chemotherapeutic drugs handled by MDR1 may be rendered ineffective. Several patients demonstrated increased surface expression of the CD25 component of the high-affinity IL-2 receptor after treatment. This protein is a target for denileukin diftitox (DD), discussed elsewhere in this chapter as a therapy for MF, suggesting that strategies for combination therapy approaches could be devised to enhance responses to both agents.

Approved Chemotherapy Agents for Cancer But Not for CTCL

Older agents studied previously include alkylating agents like chlorambucil or cisplatin, the microtubule inhibitors etoposide, vincristine, and vinblastine, or the antitumor antibiotics, like bleomycin and doxorubicin.[252-255] In general, the response rates are modest, and duration of response is typically less than 6 months.

McDonald and Bertino[259] reported particularly good results with the antimetabolite methotrexate administered intravenously followed by oral citrovorum factor. Patients received 1 to 5 mg/kg of intravenous methotrexate every 5 days. If a patient tolerated the lowest dose, each subsequent dose was escalated. After five intravenous doses, patients were switched to oral methotrexate (25 to 50 mg) with oral citrovorum as weekly maintenance. All 11 patients achieved "good" or better clearing (>60%) for a median duration of 24 months. Mucositis and skin ulcerations were the most significant toxicity witnessed. Myelosuppression was mild in general. The related compound, trimetrexate has also been reported to be effective in treating CTCL.[257]

As discussed previously, a newer folate analogue, pralatrexate, has also been shown to have substantial activity against PTCL. In early-phase trials several patients with CTCL were felt to benefit, and therefore a trial was designed specifically for MF/SS patients to identify an effective and tolerable dose.[258] Starting with dose de-escalation design at 30 mg/m^2/wk intravenously for 3 of 4 weeks, ultimately 15 mg/m^2/wk was identified as the recommended dosage for further exploration. Twenty-nine patients received this dose for a median of four cycles, and the ORR was 45% (1 CR unconfirmed [CRu]/12 PR). No median response duration had been identified at the time of publication but ranged from 1 day to 372 days. Mucositis (17% grade 3), skin toxicity (7% grade 3), and fatigue (3% grade 3) were common with the use of this agent at the recommended dose. To date no comparison trials of pralatrexate to methotrexate have been performed to assess the relative cost and benefit differences.

Subsequently the benefits of adding 5-fluorouracil to the methotrexate-based regimen, exploiting the synergy between these agents, were evaluated.[259] The methotrexate was administered as a 24-hour continuous infusion at 60 mg/m^2. Immediately after this infusion, 5-flourouracil (20 mg/kg each 24 hours) was continuously infused for 36 to 48 hours. Oral citrovorum factor (10 mg/m^2) was administered intravenously 6 hours after cessation of the methotrexate infusion and then orally for five additional doses. The methotrexate dose was escalated to a maximum of 120 mg/m^2, as allowed by toxicity and response. Ten patients were treated for an average duration of 33 months (range, 3 to 78 months). The number of cycles administered ranged from 5 to 45. All patients achieved a partial remission. Initial cycles were given every 5 to 8 days. Once a good response was achieved, cycles were administered every 3 months as maintenance. Other groups anecdotally reported success with low doses of oral methotrexate. In general these regimens appear to be fairly well tolerated.

The purine antimetabolites have been shown to be active in the treatment of MF/SS. These compounds do not have a single mechanism of action, but all ultimately interfere with intracellular regulation of deoxyribonucleotide pools and this imbalance partially explains the cytotoxicity. This family of drugs includes 2′-deoxycoformycin (DCF), fludarabine phosphate, and 2-chlorodeoxyadenosine (2-CdA).[260]

DCF is a transition-state inhibitor of adenosine deaminase. Inhibition of this enzyme, necessary for the conversion of adenosine to inosine, results in accumulation of 2-deoxy-ATP and subsequent inhibition of the enzyme ribonucleotide diphosphate reductase necessary for DNA synthesis in dividing cells. DCF is also effective against cells in the resting state, where ribonucleotide diphosphate reductase levels are barely detectable. It has been shown that deoxy-ATP accumulation in resting lymphocytes results in increased DNA strand breaks over time; this results in the activation of Ca^{2+}/Mg^{2+}-dependent endonuclease that produces double-stranded DNA strand breaks at internucleosomal regions and also activation of a poly–adenosine diphosphate (ADP)–ribose polymerase that consumes nicotinamide adenine dinucleotide and adenosine triphosphate (ATP). These perturbations lead to apoptotic cell death.

Fludarabine phosphate represents the fluorinated derivative of adenine arabinoside (ara-A). This compound was known to retain cytotoxic action against leukemias and was resistant to degradation by adenosine deaminase. Solubility was poor, however, unless the 5′-monophosphate derivative was used; hence fludarabine monophosphate is the 5′-monophosphate form of F-ara-A. Similar to the mechanism of action of cytarabine or ara-A, fludarabine phosphate requires phosphorylation by deoxycytidine kinase to the active triphosphate metabolite F-ara-ATP. Again, this triphosphate derivative inhibits ribonucleotide reductase, resulting in nucleotide pool imbalances, which prevent DNA repair and ultimately cause apoptosis.

2-CdA represents another chemical modification of deoxyadenosine, which renders the drug resistant to adenosine deaminase. After activation by deoxycytidine kinase, the triphosphate derivative similarly inhibits ribonucleotide reductase and accumulates intracellularly, perturbing the deoxyribonucleotide pool balance, resulting in DNA damage and cell death.

Enzymes such as cytoplasmic 5′-nucleotidase catalyze the degradation of the active triphosphate derivatives discussed earlier. Cells with relatively greater levels of the activation enzymes versus degradation enzymes were identified as likely clinical targets. Lymphoid disorders make good targets for these agents because they contain high levels of deoxycytidine kinase and low levels of 5′-nucleotidase and depend on polymerase-α for DNA repair. Because it was known that T-lymphoblastoid cell lines were most sensitive to these drugs, it was thought that T-lymphocyte disorders would be sensitive in vivo to these agents.

A number of studies treating patients with MF/SS have been performed with these drugs. Table 84-9 shows the results in these studies. Four studies used DCF as a single agent at doses ranging from 3.75 to 10 mg/m^2 daily for three doses every 21 to 28 days.[261-264] Twenty-five patients with MF/SS were included in these studies[261-263]; overall, 3 CRs (12%) and 12 PRs (48%) were documented. The fourth study represents the largest phase II experience reported for the treatment of MF/SS and other CTCLs.[264] Twenty-seven eligible patients were treated for 3 consecutive days at 3.75 mg/m^2/day. Essentially, 80% of the doses in the trial were delivered at 3.75 or 5.0 mg/m^2/day. Twenty-one of 24 response-evaluable patients had SS (14 patients), tumor-stage MF (6 patients), or large cell transformation of MF (1 patient). Patients had failed a median of three prior treatments before enrollment. The overall response rate for patients with MF/SS was 66% (five CRs and nine PRs). Most responses were short-lived because the median duration of response in patients with tumor-stage disease was 2 months (range, 1 to 2 months) and the median duration of response in erythrodermic disease was 3.5 months (no range given, but two patients had responses of at least 17 months).

Table 84-9 Response Rates Observed in Clinical Trials With Purine Antimetabolite Agents

Drug	Overall Response Rate (%)	Reference
DCF	66	119
DCF	100	120
DCF	54	121
DCF	66	122
Fludarabine	18	123
2-CdA	28	124
2-CdA	38	125
2-CdA	18	126
2-CdA	100	127

DCF, 2′-Deoxycoformycin; *2-CdA*, 2-chlorodeoxyadenosine.

The use of fludarabine for the treatment of MF/SS has also been assessed in a single, large phase II trial by Von Hoff et al.[268] They treated 33 patients who were good-risk disease (i.e., no prior systemic therapy) or poor-risk disease (i.e., prior systemic therapy) with fludarabine alone at doses of 25 and 18 mg/m^2 for the two groups, respectively. One complete response and five partial responses were obtained for an overall response rate of 18%.

2-CdA has been evaluated as a single agent for the treatment of MF/SS in 21 patients who had failed at least one prior therapy.[266] There were three CRs and three PRs (overall response rate of 29%). The median duration of response in this heavily pretreated group, however, was only 4 months. Three other groups have also reported results in small numbers of MF patients.[267-269] A total of 21 patients were reported when the studies are pooled. Seven patients achieved responses, giving an overall ORR of 33%, remarkably similar to results from the prior large, single-institution study.

The similarity in mechanism of action of these compounds would suggest that toxicity associated with the various compounds would be similar. This has definitely not been the case, however. There are distinct differences in the spectrum of acute and chronic toxicities with these agents. DCF and fludarabine are associated with higher rates of nausea or vomiting and alopecia than commonly associated with 2-CdA. The most significant toxicities with DCF and fludarabine, however, are neurotoxicity and immunosuppression. Approximately 15% of patients developed sepsis, and 10% developed an opportunistic infection, such as disseminated toxoplasmosis, cytomegalovirus infection, *Pneumocystis carinii* pneumonia, atypical mycobacterial infection, and fungemia in studies. Another 15% developed severe neurotoxicity in the form of confusion, motor weakness, paresthesias, and central nervous system demyelination. Treatment with 2-CdA is extremely well tolerated acutely but may result in somewhat greater myelosuppression than the other agents. This myelosuppression may even be more significant when the agent is used to treat T-lymphocyte disorders as compared to B-cell diseases. In the study by Betticher et al,[270] significant decrements in neutrophils and lymphocyte populations occurred in 46% and 41% of patients, respectively. In a study of 2-CdA, we reduced the days of therapy delivered by continuous infusion to 5 days from the usual 7 because of a perception that the toxicity, primarily prolonged thrombocytopenia, was unacceptable. These results suggest that patients treated with these agents should be carefully evaluated for infectious complications, especially opportunistic infections, and that prophylactic antibiotic therapy should be considered during and after therapy if significant immunosuppression is documented. In addition, one should carefully consider the value of continuing to administer cycles of therapy if there is no evidence of further improvement in clinical response, because of the risk for suddenly developing prolonged cytopenias that may limit future therapeutic approaches. In general it is not apparent that one purine antimetabolite is dramatically superior from these studies, although DCF has a slightly higher overall response rate. It has been observed repeatedly in these studies that occasional patients with SS may have striking and durable responses to treatment, but ideally other agents emerging may allow for higher response rates with less toxicity in this population.

A relatively new class of antineoplastic agents, the proteasome inhibitors, also have activity in CTCL. In vitro activity of bortezomib against CTCL cell lines has been demonstrated, thought to be due to a decrease in NF-κB expression observed, and this reduction resulted in marked increase in spontaneous apoptosis.[270] These data formed the rationale for performing a clinical trial. Zinzani et al[129] reported a small phase II trial of 10 evaluable patients with stage IV or greater MF. In this limited sample, there was one CR and six PR observed, with a range of response durations of 7 to 14 months at the time of the report. Toxicity was as expected, with nearly 20% of patients experiencing grade 3 neutropenia and thrombocytopenia. Additional studies are ongoing with this agent in combination with other agents for histologically aggressive T-cell lymphomas.

Combination chemotherapy has often been employed for MF/SS patients with advanced disease at presentation or with progression. Usually alkylating agents are used, in combination with doxorubicin or vinca alkaloids.[271,272] Response rates of 80% to 100% have been achieved, with longer durations of remission than observed with single-agent therapy. There have been no trials comparing different aggressive combination regimens. High response rates with perhaps less toxicity have been observed in treating other NHLs using infusional combination regimens such as etoposide, prednisone, vincristine (Oncovin), cyclophosphamide, and hydroxydaunomycin (EPOCH). A trial in CTCL suggested comparable activity to a bolus schedule, with greater risk for febrile neutropenia and bacteremia associated with indwelling catheters required for the infusion.[273]

It is our philosophy that this disease behaves similarly to other low-grade lymphomas (e.g., B-cell type), with periods of remission becoming shorter with subsequent therapeutic interventions. However, as noted, advanced-stage MF is associated with a relatively short median life expectancy. Patients with significant nodal involvement or extensive skin disease (T4 in particular) have median life expectancies of 30 to 55 months.[200] A driving force in the development of treatments for this disease is the goal of altering the natural history for this group of poor-prognosis patients, or for delaying the development of poor-prognosis disease. There is no clinical trial of any modality that has demonstrated a survival benefit as compared with a control group. Kaye et al[204] demonstrated more than a decade ago that combination chemotherapy (and total-skin electron beam radiation therapy) did not provide a more favorable survival or even clinically significant delays in time to recurrence for patients, compared with standard palliative, less-aggressive therapies. New drugs or approaches are still being developed with the goal of altering the disease state in poor-prognosis patients.

Because of the pressing need to identify new strategies to provide more durable remissions or even curative therapy for advanced CTCL, new drugs continue to be tested. On the basis of the clinical evidence of possible activity in early-phase testing, several drugs have been evaluated. In a phase II trial of 44 patients with relapsed MF or PTCL (unspecified), a dose of gemcitabine was administered at 1200 mg/m^2 over 30 minutes for 3 weeks every 28 days.[274] There were 5 (11%) CRs and 26 (59%) PRs (overall response rate 70.5%). The median duration of response ranged from 15 months for CRs to 10 months for those patients with PR. There appeared to be no difference in response type between patients with MF and PTCL. In a second trial at the MD Anderson Cancer Center with gemcitabine administered similarly but at a dose of 1000 mg/m^2, investigators documented a 68% overall response rate (17/25), with two patients developing a CR.[275] Toxicity included myelosuppression in the majority of patients and development of a hemolytic uremic syndrome in two older adult patients. Most recently gemcitabine was studied as a first-line systemic treatment in 27 patients with stage T3 or T4 MF/SS.[276] The overall response rate was 70% (19/27), with six CRs. The median time to progression was 10 months. Toxicity was generally mild.

The camptothecins are a family of compounds that inhibit topoisomerase I, an enzyme required for unwinding strands of DNA for transcription and replication. In early-phase studies it was recognized that the administration of 9-aminocamptothecin (9-AC) by continuous infusion to maintain a drug concentration above a threshold level coupled with duration of exposure was important to ensure adequate inhibition of the target enzyme. In these studies at appropriate concentrations, activity was identified in NHLs,[277] and it was therefore appropriate to study in MF/SS. We undertook a trial of intravenous 9-AC in patients with MF/SS.[278] The trial was prematurely closed after 12 patients received 30 cycles. There were 2 PRs (17%) in a heavily pretreated population of patients; however, 6 of the 12 patients (50%) developed indwelling catheter infections, and 3 patients died 4 to 8 weeks after the last dose of 9-AC. The toxicity was deemed too excessive to justify this dose, route, and schedule of administration. This study nicely demonstrates the hazards of chemotherapy in this patient population, including the underlying risk for infection and the relative contraindication to indwelling catheters (hence a bias toward agents administered as short infusions through peripheral catheters, or oral agents, and the importance of prophylactic antibiotics if excessive invasive procedures are anticipated).

Another drug empirically tested for the treatment of MF/SS is pegylated doxorubicin based on the historic activity of doxorubicin against NHLs. The process of encapsulating the doxorubicin in pegylated liposomes creates stable, long circulating carriers of the drug that result in greater tumor cell uptake versus normal cell uptake. This may reduce normal cardiotoxicity and myelosuppression. The drug is approved for use against Kaposi sarcoma but has been evaluated in a small group of patients with MF in Europe. Six patients in this pilot study received pegylated liposomal doxorubicin at 20 mg/m^2 every 4 weeks.[279] Four patients achieved a CR and one other patient achieved a partial remission. The overall response rate was 83%. The median duration of response was not reported. Grade 3 adverse events were few and included one patient with lymphopenia and two with anemia. No other severe adverse effects were noted. A larger retrospective multicenter report of this agent administered intravenously at 20 to 40 mg/m^2 every 2 to 3 weeks in 34 patients has also been conducted.[280] Overall, 15 patients achieved a CR and 15 achieved a PR (response rate of 88%), with EFS of 12 months. Toxicity was similarly manageable.

The ability to biopsy skin lesions for studies of tumor cells in MF/SS has resulted in this disease being a favorable setting for the evaluation of candidate therapeutic agents and exploration of rational therapeutic development. The knowledge gained regarding the human genome and the new studies of proteomics are increasingly allowing investigators to test new drugs at appropriate dosages, by correct schedule of administration, and to generate, prove, or refute hypotheses regarding mechanism of action or resistance. A number of studies of such agents have recently been completed and may lead to further drug testing in search of enhanced therapeutic activity in MF or perhaps achieve cure of MF.

An example of such an achievement has been the work with temozolomide for the treatment of MF/SS. This agent is an oral imidazotetrazine that has shown activity in solid tumors, such as brain tumors and melanoma. It has been determined that mechanisms of resistance to this agent include expression of high levels of the scavenger protein O^6-alkylguanine-DNA alkyltransferase (AGT) in tumor cells. This protein is implicated in the recognition and repair of alkylator-induced DNA damage introduced by chloroethylnitrosourea (e.g., bis-chloroethylnitrosourea or BCNU) or methylating agents (temozolomide).[281] The presence of the AGT protein imparts resistance by removing toxic lesions formed at the O^6 position of guanine. Chloroethylnitrosourea cross-links are prevented from forming by the removal of the chloroethyl lesion from the O^6 position before rearrangement or by the reaction with the intermediate, 1,O^6-ethanoguanine, to form a cross-link between DNA and the repair protein. The AGT protein is inactivated in the process.[282] Studies evaluating AGT levels in patients with brain tumors receiving BCNU therapy support the role of AGT in resistance to chloroethylating and methylating agents. Retrospective and prospective human studies have demonstrated a correlation between AGT concentration and clinical outcome after treatment with BCNU.[283]

Because of the unique sensitivity of MF to topical BCNU, we were interested in exploring levels of AGT in a variety of patients with various stages of MF/SS. Patients with patch or plaque lesions expressed low levels of the AGT protein compared with a number of controls with reactive dermatitis, and the level of AGT increased correlating with the stage of MF/SS (i.e., patients with malignant lymphocytes harvested from peripheral blood or involved lymph nodes had higher levels of AGT than those with patch or plaque lesions).[284] Given this data, we initiated a prospective trial of temozolomide in relapsed patients with MF/SS, correlating response to levels of AGT and other known resistance proteins (such as the family DNA mismatch repair proteins).

Twenty-six patients with relapsed heavily pretreated stage IB-IVB disease were evaluated.[285] The overall response rate was 27% with two complete responders. Median disease-free survival was 4 months. We hypothesized that the optimal phenotype that would predict for good response to therapy would be low levels of AGT combined with normal levels of several DNA mismatch repair proteins. Interestingly, hypermethylation of these DNA repair proteins has been reported to result in silencing of the genes and to correlate with lack of the proteins as assessed by immunohistochemical techniques in patients with MF.[286] This hypermethylation may be more prevalent in more advanced tumor lesions and suggests that a propensity for mutations may precede clinical progression. It also suggests that patients might benefit from treatment with a demethylating agent in combination with temozolomide. Unfortunately, in the trial above, pretreatment levels of O^6-methylguanine-DNA methyltransferase (MGMT) and the mismatch repair genes mutL homolog 1 (MLH1)/mutS homolog 2 (MSH2) were not predictive of response to the temozolomide.

Role of Stem Cell Transplantation

The natural evolution of the use of chemotherapy for this disease has been to use dose-intensified approaches with hematopoietic reconstitution with autologous[287] or allogeneic bone marrow or stem cells.[288] There are few reports in the literature of such treatment programs in well-designed prospective clinical trials.

Given the propensity of Sézary cells to be detectable despite a lack of clinical evidence even in early-stage disease if sophisticated molecular techniques are used, it is likely that reinfusion of neoplastic cells may occur with autologous bone marrow transplantation. The lack of dramatic benefit in low-grade B-cell lymphomas for autologous bone marrow transplantation similarly suggests that this approach will not benefit patients. We had a very limited experience with autologous bone marrow and SCT at our center and abandoned it, because of rapid progression of disease, in favor of allogeneic SCT.

Allogeneic SCT has been presumed to be curative in small percentages of patients with low-grade B-cell lymphomas, and this approach has now been investigated in the small subset of young MF/SS patients with HLA-identical siblings or HLA-matched unrelated donors who have poor-prognosis disease and have demonstrated relapse or resistance to interferons, chemotherapy, and topical therapies. In an early study, a single patient treated with cyclophosphamide and total body irradiation was reported to achieve complete remission after allogeneic SCT, but relapse occurred by day 70, necessitating additional therapy.[289] The patient remained in complete remission and was alive at least 6 years after the transplantation. In light of this, we and others have begun to explore this approach in patients with MF/SS who are young and have matched donors available.[290] We have used marrow-derived stem cells enriched with peripheral blood–derived stem cells or peripheral blood stem cells only. We believe that in appropriate patients this approach should continue to be explored; older patients may benefit from strategies involving the use of RIC regimens that involve less myeloablative preparative regimens and rely on the effects of the donor marrow to create a graft-versus-lymphoma effect for disease control. Molina et al[294] reported promising data using allogeneic SCT for patients with refractory MF/SS. Each of the seven patients treated had failed a median of seven therapies. Although one patient received a myeloablative conditioning regimen, five received a reduced-intensity regimen consisting of fludarabine and melphalan. Each of the patients achieved a clinical remission and resolution of molecular and cytogenetic evidence of the disease. After a median follow-up of 56 months, six of the eight patients were alive and free of evidence of lymphoma. The other two patients died of transplant-related complications. This small study provided the impetus to further develop allogeneic SCT strategies for the treatment of advanced CTCL refractory to standard therapies at many centers.

A metaanalysis from reports before 2008 of 20 allogeneic and 19 ASCTs was reported by Wu et al[295]and includes some of the patients described here. The majority of patients in both groups received myeloablative chemotherapy and total-skin electron beam as preparative regimens, with the remainder in the allogeneic SCT group receiving RIC regimens. In the ASCT group event-free survival was only 20% at 1 year and 0% at 5 years, statistically significantly less the 65% and 60%, respectively, in the allogeneic SCT group. Overall survival was also significantly better in the allogeneic SCT group, confirming our impressions regarding the limitations of ASCT for this disease.

Since this metaanalysis was published, two larger single-institution or multiinstitution reports have been published. A European group reported the outcomes on 60 patients with MF/SS (36/24) who received either a matched related donor (mRD) or matched unrelated donor (mUD) (45/15) allogeneic SCT.[293] Survival at 3 years was 54%. A multivariate analysis suggested that recipients of mRD SCT had better progression-free and overall survival than patients receiving mUD SCT transplants, and reduced-intensity transplants had less nonrelapse mortality without increased relapse of disease.

A single-institution trial in the United States reported the outcome of 19 patients treated with total-skin electron beam and nonmyeloablative allogeneic SCT in advanced MF/SS.[294] The complete response rate was 58%. Relapse was sometimes treated with reduced immunosuppression or donor lymphocyte infusions. With a median follow-up of 19 months, the median overall survival had not been reached.

Other Established Treatments for CTCL

Extracorporeal Photopheresis

An adaptation of the use of psoralen with UVA called extracorporeal photopheresis has been described by Edelson et al.[298] Patients ingest 0.6 mg/kg of oral 8-methoxypsoralen before a treatment. The treatment consists of routine leukapheresis with isolation of the mononuclear cell fraction. The cells are then exposed to UVA ex vivo within a special chamber inside the pheresis device. In the initial report, Edelson et al documented an 88.5% loss of lymphocyte viability compared with control patients treated with the drug alone. Overall, 64% of patients responded to therapy, with the best results in those with generalized erythroderma and, presumably, higher circulating Sézary cell levels. The mechanism is not thought to be directly cytotoxic, but rather to induce a host immune response to the reinfused altered Sézary cells, possibly through activation of circulating dendritic cells.[296] This theory would explain the findings of some investigators that patients without leukemic involvement do poorly with such therapy. This treatment modality has resulted in the best results in SS patients with erythroderma of short duration and with adequate $CD8^+$ blood counts.

Several other groups have reported their experiences with photopheresis.[297,298] When the data are analyzed on an intent-to-treat basis, overall response rates of 36% to 52% were observed. Only 12% to 18% achieved CR. These investigators attempted to wean patients from therapy as clearing of lesions was documented. Ultimately, most responders developed recurrent disease. Many trials are under way combining extracorporeal photopheresis with other active modalities.

Toxicity is mild and includes occasional nausea, erythematous flares, and temperature elevations. Patients may develop hypotension during leukapheresis, which usually responds to saline infusions.

Interferons

Interferon-α is an active agent for the treatment of MF.[299-303] Dosages and routes of administration have differed among studies. Initially, high-dose interferon was used, with maximum doses of 36 to 50 million International Units. Bunn et al[302,303] and Olsen et al[300] independently demonstrated complete response rates of 10% to 27% in heavily pretreated patients. The duration of response was only 5.5 months. Later trials of untreated patients with doses of 3 to 18 million International Units given subcutaneously daily have demonstrated response rates of 80% to 92%. From all these studies, it appears that a reasonable and tolerable single-agent dose is 12 million International Units/m^2 administered subcutaneously daily. We recommend starting at 3 million International Units and gradually increasing as treatment is tolerated by the patient.

In a single trial, the results of treatment of 16 refractory CTCL patients with interferon-γ were reported.[304] Five patients experienced PRs (response rate 31%) with a median duration of 10 months (range, 3 to 32+ months).

Side effects of all interferons are dose dependent. Most common adverse effects are constitutional symptoms, consisting of fever, chills, myalgias, malaise, and anorexia. Rarely, cytopenias, elevations of liver function test results, renal dysfunction, cardiac dysfunction, or changes in mental status can be seen. Patients need to be monitored closely while on interferon.

Retinoids

Vitamin A and its natural and synthetic analogues are known as retinoids. These compounds have diverse biologic effects, influencing differentiation and proliferation of a number of structures during development.[305] In addition, some compounds have been shown to influence immune function.[306,307] Clinically, a number of approved formulations have demonstrated efficacy in MF and SS.

Many of the trials of retinoids for MF/SS were performed decades ago with limited patient numbers. Treatment with isotretinoin (13-cis-retinoic acid), a nonaromatic retinoid, has been associated with clinical benefit in a number of trials. Overall objective responses have been described in 33 of 56 patients treated in three clinical trials.[308-310] A monoaromatic retinoid compound, etretinate, did not achieve similar results when tested as monotherapy for MF in several trials[311-317] but did show efficacy in a trial for the treatment of parapsoriasis en plaques.[315] A polyaromatic retinoid demonstrated efficacy in a small trial. Objective responses were observed in three of six patients (one CR and two PRs).

Vitamin A Derivatives Not Approved for CTCL

There has been a resurgence of interest in retinoids for the treatment of hematologic malignancies with the approval of all-trans retinoic acid (ATRA) for acute promyelocytic leukemia. The mechanism of biologic effect for retinoids is better understood given the advances in basic sciences over the past decades. ATRA has been studied in 33 patients with relapsed MF who had not had prior exposure to oral retinoids.[313] Patients received 45 mg/m^2 daily in two divided doses for up to 2 years. In 29 evaluable patients, 5 responses were observed (1 CR, 4 PRs) for an ORR of 17% with a median duration of response of 4.5 months. Another seven patients (24%) had stable disease. The most common toxicities included headache (37%) and mucous membrane dryness (80%). Only one patient experienced severe elevation of lipid levels. ATRA works through binding to specific retinoic acid receptors (RAR family α, β, and γ), which then bind to retinoic acid response elements located upstream of gene promoters, providing transcriptional control of proteins.

Approved Vitamin A Derivatives for CTCL

A second family of receptors, the retinoid X family of receptors (RXR), has been identified.[312,313] Bexarotene is a synthetic retinoid that selectively binds this family of receptors. Unfortunately, as is the case with the retinoids that bind the RAR family of receptors, it is not known ultimately the expression of which genes is altered to achieve the clinical benefits observed. This compound has been tested in separate trials of early- and advanced-stage patients. At the 300 mg/m^2 dosage daily (dose recommended by the FDA), 54% of the 94 advanced-stage patients in an open-label phase II study responded to therapy (2% CRs).[313] The median duration of response was 299 days. The early disease trial showed similar response rates. The toxicity spectrum is somewhat different from the RAR-specific retinoids, including more frequent severe elevations of lipid levels (although rarely associated with pancreatitis), hypothyroidism, and less frequent headaches and dry mucous membranes. The compound can also be used topically. A phase I/II trial of the topical bexarotene demonstrated a 63% response rate (21% clinical CRs) in primarily early-stage patients with lesional application.[312] Toxicity was mostly local irritation with erythema.

The favorable toxicity profile has led to a number of combination-modality trials using retinoids. Some of these small trials have combined retinoids with interferon-α and have reported response rates of 40% to 50%. Combinations of retinoids with PUVA have been suggested to result in clinical benefit in less time with less exposure to ultraviolet radiation. These experiences have been generally limited and often uncontrolled, making definitive conclusions impossible. Larger randomized trials would be needed to determine if routine use of such combinations should be undertaken off of an investigational trial except in rare cases.

Monoclonal Antibodies

Targeted therapy has become a reality for the treatment of many types of cancer, including MF/SS. Although the most common approach has been with the use of antibodies that target antigens expressed by the tumor cells (e.g., rituximab), another class of compounds known as recombinant fusion proteins has been developed, the prototype being DD, for the treatment of CTCL.

Approved Monoclonal Antibodies for Cutaneous T-Cell Lymphoma

DD is a single-chain protein in which the receptor-binding domain of native diphtheria toxin is replaced by the sequences encoding the IL-2 gene (CD25).[316] Once this molecule binds to the high-affinity IL-2 receptor, the fusion toxin is internalized by receptor-mediated endocytosis and is proteolytically cleaved within endosomes to liberate the free ADP-ribosyl transferase activity of diphtheria toxin into the cytosol, where it then inhibits protein synthesis.[314,318]

In early phase I studies with DD, the response rate of CTCL patients who demonstrated at least 20% expression of the IL-2 receptor was 30%.[319] A phase III study comparing various dose levels of DD demonstrated a similar response rate, but there was significant toxicity that led to a high drop-out rate (constitutional symptoms, infusional reactions such as hypotension, chest pain or dyspnea, and a vascular leak syndrome).[320] Based on this trial the drug was approved for the treatment of relapsed/refractory CD25-expressing CTCL.

Recently two dose levels of DD were compared to placebo in patients with stage IA to III disease.[321] This clinical trial is one of the larger studies conducted in MF/SS to date and provides interesting information because it is one of the few to include a placebo control arm. Overall 144 patients were enrolled, all with 20% or higher expression of CD25 on a skin biopsy specimen and randomized in a 1:1:1 fashion to either 18 mcg/kg DD, 9 mcg/kg DD, or the placebo with the primary end point being overall response rate. The response rates were 49.1%, 37.85%, and 15.9%, respectively, and both DD dose arms were statistically superior to the placebo. PFS (median >2 years) in the DD arms was also superior compared with placebo (median 4 months). Moderately severe and severe adverse events were both greater in the DD arms than placebo, but there was no dose effect with regard to safety.

Because of the toxicity spectrum of DD, we limit the use of this agent to patients who have failed several systemic agents (often bexarotene and interferon) previously and have more threatening disease such as the presence of skin tumors or nodal involvement. It is important to note that the pivotal trials did not allow concomitant use of corticosteroids to prevent nausea and infusional reactions. Subsequently a retrospective case review of patients pretreated with corticosteroids suggested a more favorable toxicity profile and a response rate of nearly 60%.[322] The nature of the trial limits the conclusions to be drawn but suggests that aggressive pretreatment with steroids can make this drug a useful addition to treat patients with advanced relapsed MF.

Approved Targeted Agents for Cancer But Not for Cutaneous T-Cell Lymphoma

Targeted therapies against unique tumor antigens continue to be tested, such as the monoclonal antibody alemtuzumab. This antibody is directed against CD52 and presumably works through antibody-dependent cellular cytotoxicity and activation of complement-dependent cytolysis[323-326] but may also induce apoptosis without complement activation. A number of trials of this agent in various stages of MF/SS have been reported. The initial phase II study using alemtuzumab in 50 patients with low-grade NHL, including 8 patients with MF, demonstrated a 50% response rate in MF (4 of 8 patients, 2 CR).[327] In a phase II multicenter study of 22 patients with advanced MF (n = 15) and SS (n = 7) refractory to PUVA, radiotherapy, or systemic chemotherapy, intravenous treatment with 30 mg alemtuzumab three times a week for 12 weeks resulted in an ORR of 55%, with 32% of patients in CR and 23% in PR.[328] Higher response rates were demonstrated in patients with erythroderma and those with fewer previous treatment regimens. Both patients with tumor-stage disease had progressive disease on alemtuzumab. Kennedy et al[332] studied the efficacy of alemtuzumab in CTCL patients (stage IIB to IV) and demonstrated a PR in three (38%) with infectious complications in seven of eight patients. Two of the responders had SS, and these findings support our perspective that alemtuzumab may be most helpful in patients with erythrodermic MF and SS. Therefore we conducted a trial in 19 heavily pretreated patients with erythrodermic MF or frank SS. In this trial the patients received a variety of subcutaneous, intravenous, or both routes of administration. The overall response rate was 84% (47% CR and 37% PR). Median PFS was 6 months, but median overall survival was 41 months despite the advanced-stage disease and extensive prior therapy. We did not experience the dramatic infectious or cardiac events some investigators have reported, likely because of the routine inclusion of prophylactic antiviral, antifungal, and antipneumocystis agents.[330]

Another target of therapy for MF/SS is CD30. As noted earlier, this antigen is expressed in a variety of malignancies, including advanced HL, ALCL, and often the lesions of tumor-stage or transformed MF. As previously discussed, brentuximab vedotin (SGN-35), is an antibody to CD30 conjugated to a derivative of auristatin E (monomethyl auristatin E), which inhibits microtubules and induces apoptosis in target cells. It has been approved for the treatment of relapsed HL and systemic ALCL that express CD30. There are now efforts under way to determine its efficacy in primary cutaneous ALCL and MF. Several studies have been reported in a preliminary fashion. Recently, investigators at Stanford led a trial of this molecule in MF/SS with all levels of expression of CD30.[331] At the time of the preliminary report, 15 patients with MF/SS (13 stage IIB to IV MF/SS, 9 with large cell transformation) were included. Seven of the patients had less than 10% CD30 expression, 7 had 10% to 50% expression, and 1 had more than 50% expression by immunohistochemical analysis. An objective response was observed in 60% of the patients and in all cohorts by expression level of CD30. Toxicity was generally mild, including fatigue, peripheral neuropathy, rash, and infusion reactions. Two patients with pretreatment expression of CD30 developed antigen loss during treatment. Definitive trials to determine its efficacy in MF/SS and cutaneous ALCL are planned.

Investigational Approaches

Because of the chronic relapsing nature of MF, new therapies with different mechanisms of action are needed to circumvent tumor resistance. A variety of such approaches are under investigation. These include the use of existing or newly developed retinoid compounds or combinations of retinoids with other agents.[332] Other combination modalities under study include retinoids, interferons, and chemotherapy or radiation therapy[333] and total-skin electron beam radiotherapy followed by photopheresis or chemotherapy.[334] Given the lack of benefits of combination chemotherapy and radiotherapy previously, the role of such approaches should remain investigational. Another less toxic combination approach has been the simultaneous administration of interferon and phototherapy.[335] An overall response rate of 92% has been observed with this combination in all stages of patients, many of whom had been previously treated with other therapies.

Another approach to the therapy of this disease has involved new drugs to exploit the biologic characteristics of these neoplastic cells. For example, Notch signaling has been shown to be dysregulated in a variety of T-lymphocyte neoplasms. It has also been shown that Notch1 is expressed in tumor cells in many advanced-stage patients with MF/SS.[146] There are specific inhibitors of Notch signaling that induce apoptosis in MF/SS cell lines, and this is an elegant example of how these molecular breakthroughs could be exploited to develop new approaches to the treatment of this disease.

Knowledge of the unique cytokine milieu associated with these neoplastic T cells has led to trials testing cytokines that may inhibit the growth of these cells, such as IL-12[335] or IL-2.[336] Vaccine approaches may be practical.

Significant amounts of basic and practical research have been performed in an attempt to control this disease, and future treatment approaches will likely depend on further understanding of the molecular and genetic bases of these disorders. We hope that one of the strategies under development or study will lead to treatments that can control the disease and symptomatic effects or even cure this neoplasm in the majority of afflicted patients.

SUGGESTED READINGS

Beljaards RC, Kaudewitz P, Berti E, et al: Primary cutaneous CD30-positive large cell lymphoma: Definition of a new type cutaneous lymphoma with a favorable prognosis. A European multicenter study on 47 cases. *Cancer* 71:2097, 1993.

Duvic M, Talpur R, Ni X, et al: Phase 2 trial of oral vorinostat (suberoylanilide hydroxamic acid, SAHA) for refractory cutaneous T-cell lymphoma (CTCL). *Blood* 109:31, 2007.

Duvic M, Talpur R, Wen S, et al: Phase II evaluation of gemcitabine monotherapy for cutaneous T-cell lymphoma. *Clin Lymphoma Myeloma* 7:51, 2006.

Kuzel TM, Roenigk HH, Jr, Samuelson E, et al: Effectiveness of interferon alfa-2a combined with phototherapy for mycosis fungoides and the Sézary syndrome. *J Clin Oncol* 13:257, 1995.

Molina A, Zain J, Arber DA, et al: Durable clinical, cytogenetic, and molecular remissions after allogeneic hematopoietic cell transplantation for refractory Sézary syndrome and mycosis fungoides. *J Clin Oncol* 23:6163, 2005.

Olsen E, Duvic M, Frankel A, et al: Pivotal phase III trial of two doses of DAB389IL2 (Ontak) for the treatment of cutaneous T-cell lymphoma. *J Clin Oncol* 19:376, 2001.

Rook AH, Gottlieb SL, Wolfe JT, et al: Pathogenesis of cutaneous T-cell lymphoma: Implications for the use of recombinant cytokines and photopheresis. *Clin Exp Immunol* 107:16, 1997.

Siegel R, Pandolfino T, Guitart J, et al: Cutaneous T-cell lymphoma: Review and current concepts. *J Clin Oncol* 18:2908, 2000.

Van Doorn R, van Haselen CW, van voorst Vader PC, et al: Mycosis fungoides: Disease evolution and prognosis of 309 patients. *Arch Dermatol* 136:504, 2000.

Vowels BR, Cassin M, Vonderheid EC, et al: Aberrant cytokine production by Sézary syndrome patients: Cytokine secretion pattern resembles murine TH2 cells. *J Invest Dermatol* 99:90, 1992.

Willemze R, Kerl H, Sterry W, et al: EORTC classification for primary cutaneous lymphomas: A proposal from the Cutaneous Lymphoma Study Group of the European Organization for Research and Treatment of Cancer. *Blood* 90:354, 1997.

Wood GS, Bahler DW, Hoppe RT, et al: Transformation of mycosis fungoides: T-cell receptor beta gene analysis demonstrates a common clonal origin for plaque-type mycosis fungoides and CD30+ large-cell lymphoma. *J Invest Dermatol* 101:296, 1993.

For complete list of references log on to www.expertconsult.com.

CHAPTER 85

PLASMA CELL NEOPLASMS

Nikhil C. Munshi and Sundar Jagannath

Multiple myeloma (MM) is a malignancy involving terminally differentiated plasma cells. It includes a spectrum of plasma cell disorders ranging from monoclonal gammopathy of unknown significance (MGUS), a relatively benign condition, to smoldering MM (SMM), the symptomatic malignant disorder MM and its more aggressive form, plasma cell leukemia with circulating myeloma cells in the blood. Various other plasma cell disorders belong to the same group of conditions, including Castleman disease, α heavy-chain disease, and Waldenström macroglobulinemia. MM is characterized by the presence of clonal plasma cells, and production in the majority of cases of a monoclonal immunoglobulin or its fragment with subsequent involvement or effects on organ function. There are five classes of immunoglobulins, and the dysfunctional plasma cells can produce any one of the five immunoglobulin subtypes, including immunoglobulin G (IgG), IgA, IgM, IgD, and IgE. Infrequently, heavy-chain components of the immunoglobulin are not produced by the myeloma cells, and the disease manifests as production and secretion of light chain only, which would either be κ or λ type. Very rarely, myeloma fails to produce any significant amount of protein and manifests as a nonsecretory MM. With more recently available free high-sensitivity, free light-chain testing, the frequency of true nonsecretory MM has significantly decreased.

EPIDEMIOLOGY

Multiple myeloma accounts for 1% of all malignancies and is the second most common hematologic malignancy with prevalence of around 10%. The prevalence of MM was around 64,615 in 2008, and it is estimated that 20,520 men and women (11,400 men and 9120 women) will be diagnosed with and 10,610 men and women will die of myeloma in 2011. It is a disease involving a relatively older population with a median age at diagnosis of 69 years and median age at death of 74 years (Fig. 85-1, *A*). Fewer than 5% of patients at diagnosis are younger than age 40 years. Myeloma is more frequent in men than women and in African Americans as opposed to whites in the United States (Fig. 85-1, *B*). The incidence of MM in black men is approximately 14.5 per 100,000 per year compared with 10.2 per 100,000 per year in black women. The corresponding incidence is 7.2 and 4.6 per 100,000 in white men and women, respectively. Although the Asian population has a lower incidence of myeloma compared with their white counterparts, ethnic groups, including Hawaiians, female Hispanics, female American Indians from New Mexico, and Alaskan natives, experience higher incidence rates than those of the U.S. white population from the same geographic regions. Although there has been some increase in the incidence of MM, it is primarily attributed to better detection and surveillance for the disease as well as overall aging of the population worldwide. Moreover, there has been improvement in overall survival (OS) times for patients with MM from 3 to 7 years and longer.

HISTORICAL ASPECTS

The first published clinical description of a patient with myeloma was made by Dr. Henry Bence Jones in 1850 describing a patient, Thomas Alexander McBean, who presented with symptoms of fatigue, diffuse bone pain, and urinary frequency. Urinalysis showed a urinary protein with a peculiar heat property (now called *Bence Jones proteins*). The disease was, however, given the name MM by Rustizky in 1873 after his observation of multiple bone lesions in a similar patient. A larger review of this disease by Kahler in 1889 also led to it being called Kahler disease, especially in Europe. Subsequently, investigative advances defined the disease further with descriptions of plasma cell and radiographic abnormalities in 1900 by Wright, bone marrow (BM) aspiration in 1929, electrophoresis in 1937, and immunoelectrophoresis identifying the heavy and light chains in 1953, confirming the monoclonality of immunoglobulins in this disease. In recent years, recurrent chromosomal translocations have defined subgroups of myeloma patients, and gene expression profiling and proteomic studies are providing a greater molecular understanding of the disease. Similarly, the influence of the BM microenvironment on myeloma cell growth and survival has been explored and led to the identification of novel therapeutic targets. The first randomized study in myeloma compared urethane with placebo and indicated that the survival of patients receiving urethane was inferior to that observed with a placebo.

Progress in myeloma therapy started with the first successful use of a chemotherapeutic agent in myeloma with racemic mixture of D- and L-phenylalanine mustards (Sarcolysine) in 1958 by Blokhin and colleagues; use of melphalan in 1962 by Bergsagel and colleagues; use of high doses of glucocorticoids in 1967; and subsequent use of melphalan in combination with prednisone, which is used even today. With the use of high-dose therapy (HDT) with melphalan by McElwain and Powles in 1983, complete remissions (CRs) were achieved in a proportion of patients, and the identification of novel agents such as thalidomide and its immunomodulatory analogue lenalidomide and the proteasome inhibitor bortezomib during the past 10 years targeting both myeloma cells as well as the BM microenvironment have further improved responses and OS.

PATHOBIOLOGY

Multiple myeloma, as with a number of other malignancies, remains a disease that is initiated and sustained by genomic changes that provide uncontrolled proliferative advantages to the tumor cells. Myeloma represents the classic multistep transformation process with an initial premalignant stage, MGUS, demonstrating a number of recurrent cytogenetic abnormalities as well as gene expression changes (Table 85-1). It has been now well documented that all MM develops from MGUS, suggesting that the initial event required for transformation to MGUS provides the first step in a multistep process.[1]

Cytogenetics

Multiple myeloma is characterized by a significant molecular and genomic heterogeneity affecting tumor clones. Karyotypes in MM are usually complex, with both number and structural abnormalities in chromosome observed (Fig. 85-2).[2] Although chromosomal abnormalities using conventional cytogenetics in newly-diagnosed patients

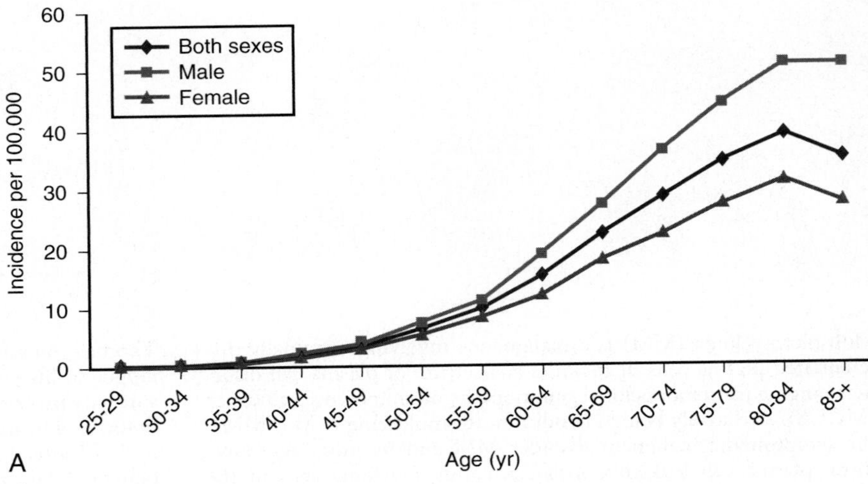

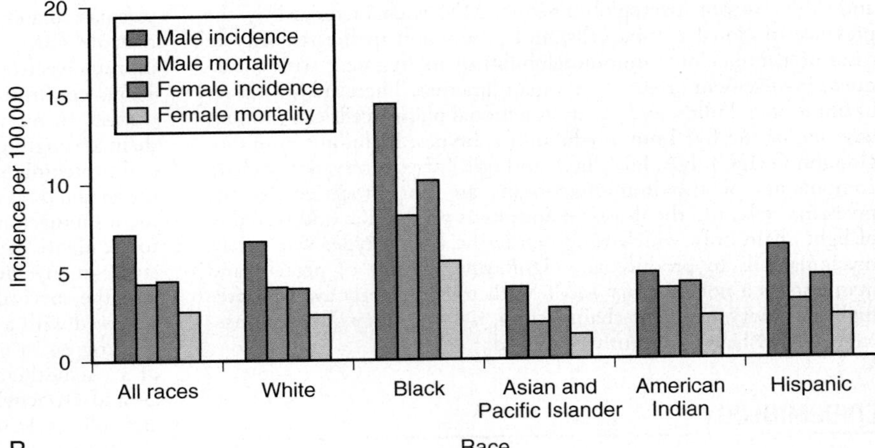

Figure 85-1 A, Multiple myeloma (MM) average annual age- and gender-specific incidence per 100,000 population in the United States in 2009. **B,** MM average annual race-specific incidence per 100,000 population in the United States in 2009. An increase in incidence is noted with advancing age, men are affected more than women, and a higher incidence is observed in blacks than whites.

Table 85-1 Recurrent Cytogenetic Changes in Myeloma

Chromosomal Abnormality	Frequency (% patients)	Genes Involved
Common Cytogenetic Alterations		
Hyperdiploidy	50-60	Unclear
Hypodiploid	20	Unclear
Pseudodiploid	15	Unclear
del(17p)	8	p53
t(4:14):	15	FGFR3, MMSET
t(11;14):	20	cyclin D1
t(14;16):	3	c-maf
t(14;20)	1	maf-b
t(6p25 or 6p21;14)	1	IRF-4 or CCND3
t(8;14)	5	c-myc
t(9;14)	<1	PAX-5
del(13) or (13q)	50	unclear
Recently Identified Alterations		
1q+:		35%
1p-:		30%
5q+:		50%
12p-:		10%

are detected in only 30-50% of patients due to the low proliferative activity of MM cells, in advanced stages when cells usually have a higher proliferative index, a greater number of abnormalities are identified. Importantly, using fluorescent in situ hybridization (FISH) as well as flow cytometry–based DNA aneuploidy analysis, genomic alterations are observed in more than 90% of the patients with MM. These results suggest that the normal cytogenetics observed in the majority of the patients is derived from normal cellular components of the BM and not from the cells belonging to the myeloma clone. Although detection of karyotypic changes in MGUS and SMM is extremely low, again because of the very low frequency of proliferating cells in these indolent conditions, using FISH shows that up to 50% of the patients with MGUS and SMM have genomic alterations.

In a study of 542 patients, gain, loss, or translocations involving the p or q arm of every single chromosome has been described in MM. Despite this complexity, several recurrent changes are observed. The most prominent amongst them is hyperdiploidy, which commonly involves gains of the whole chromosome 3, 5, 7, 9, 11, 15, 19, or 21. Additional recurrent abnormalities include loss of chromosome 13, t(4;14)(p16;q32), t(11;14)(q13;q32), or t(14;16)(q23;q32). The common chromosomal region involved in these translocations is 14q32 region, which contains the IgH gene, suggesting that this abnormality may be an early important event in the development of plasma cell disorders. This has been confirmed using FISH analysis of interphase cells showing its involvement in approximately 47% of MGUS patients and more than 70% of patients with MM. In other patients, translocation partners involve the λ light-chain region on chromosome 22. This abnormality is observed in 17% of patients

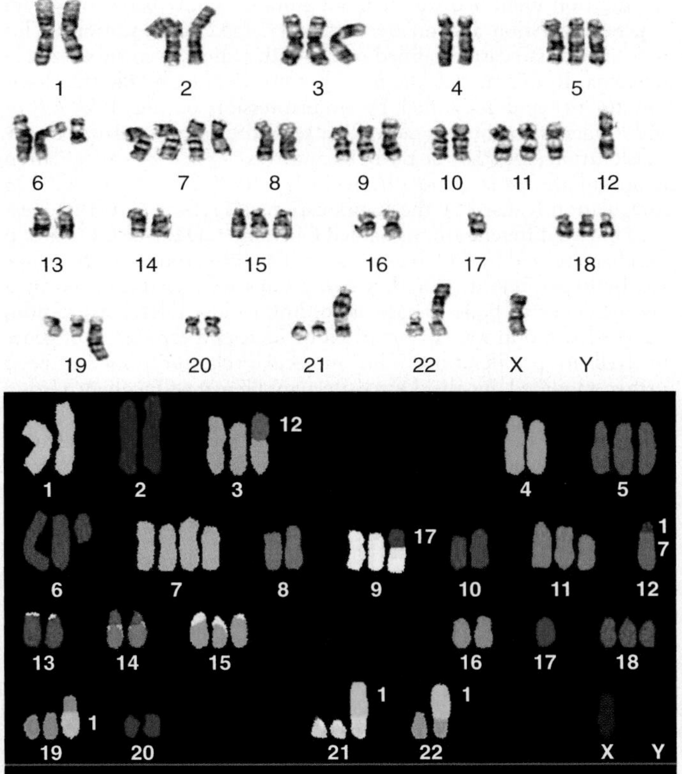

Figure 85-2 A SPECTRAL KARYOTYPE SHOWING SIGNIFICANT KARYOTYPIC ABNORMALITIES IN A PATIENT WITH MYELOMA. *(Courtesy J.R. Sawyer.)*

with MM. Translocations involving the κ light-chain genes on chromosome 2 are rare. The frequency of various common translocations in MM is provided in Table 85-1.

Hyperdiploidy

Almost half of MM patients have a hyperdiploid karyotype (>46 chromosomes), and fewer than one-quarter of the patients have a hypodiploid karyotype (<46 chromosomes). Hyperdiploid MM is a relatively homogeneous group with median quartile of 54 chromosomes involving nonrandom gains. Interestingly, trisomies mostly involve odd-numbered chromosomes, 3, 5, 7, 9, 11, 15, 19, and 21. The structural abnormalities observed in MM are not exclusive for nonhyperdiploid MM because they are also observed in hyperdiploid patients along with the hyperdiploid changes. Of note, most (if not all) of the human myeloma cell lines are derived from patients with the nonhyperdiploid genomic changes, which may reflect the difference in proliferative potential between these two categories. Hyperdiploidy has been reported to be associated with a better prognosis based on retrospective analyses. This has been confirmed more recently using interphase FISH approach to define ploidy. However, a study by the International Myeloma Foundation (IFM) showed that hyperdiploidy was not an independent prognostic factor but was associated with a lower incidence of other independent poor risk features such as del(13), t(4;14), and del(17p).[3]

Translocations Involving 14q32

Chromosomal region 14q32 has been identified as a recurrent site of translocations in myeloma. Unlike mantle cell lymphoma, in which the IgH breakpoint is near the site targeted by VDJ recombination, the breakpoint on14q32 in MM is located within the IgH or the switch region. This suggests that the translocations are caused by either somatic hypermutation or switch recombination. In all, more than 25 different chromosomal regions have been involved in translocations involving 14q32 region; the major translocation partners involving this IgH gene location are 4p16, 6p21, 11q13, and 16q23. The t(11;14)(q13;q32) translocation is present in approximately 20% of myeloma patients and involves the cyclin D1 gene.[4] Although this translocation leads to upregulation of cyclin D1, its role in oncogenesis is unknown. Despite known molecular functions of cyclin D1 in cell cycle and proliferation, the t(11;14) myelomas have a low proliferative index, appearing morphologically as small mature plasma cells or lymphoplasmacytic cells expressing CD20. Initial studies suggested a better survival outcome in patients with this translocation; however, larger studies have failed to confirm this observation.

The t(4;14)(p16;q32) is a cryptic translocation not easily detectable by conventional karyotyping. It leads to a unique dysregulation of two genes located at 4p16 region, the gene for the fibroblast growth factors 3 (FGFR3) located on the telomeric side of the breakpoint and MM SET domain (MMSET) located on the centromeric side. The translocation leads to the molecular activation of FGFR3 gene transcription. FGFR3 is one of the four high-affinity tyrosine kinase receptors for FGF. FGFR-mediated signaling results in signal transducer and activator of transcription 3 (STAT3) phosphorylation and activation of the mitogen-activated protein kinase (MAPK) pathway. It is not expressed in normal plasma cells and is shown to have oncogenic potential both in vitro and in vivo studies. Interestingly, about one-third of the patients with t(4;14) do not overexpress FGFR3. The translocation also generates a novel chimeric IGH–MMSET gene by disrupting the MMSET gene within its first intron. MMSET plays a crucial role in chromatin remodeling as well as transformation in MM.

Several studies have confirmed that a poor prognosis is associated with the t(4;14); however, some of the newer therapies such as bortezomib are able to overcome the poor outcomes associated with t(4;14). It is interesting to note that genetic studies using FISH have identified the presence of del(13) in at least 85% of the patients with t(4;14). The reasons for this strong association are so far unknown. Both FGFR3 and MMSET are potential therapeutic targets, and several tyrosine kinase inhibitors are currently being tested to inhibit FGFR3 function.

The t(14;16)(q32;q23) involves the *c-maf* gene located at the 16q23 breakpoint. c-*maf* is a basic zipper transcription factor that positively regulates cyclin D2 and ITGB7. Although this translocation is reported in only 5% of MM patients, it is observed in 25% of MM cell lines, suggesting its role in cell proliferation as well as association with aggressive behavior of the disease. t(14;16) is considered to be associated with a poor prognosis. The other translocation partner of 14q32 is 20q11, observed in fewer than 5% of patients, and it dysregulates *MAFB* expression, another basic transcription factor belonging to the MAF family, with as yet unclear molecular consequences. It is also considered to be associated with a poor outcome; however, studies have been very small because of its infrequent occurrence.

Although c-myc is increasingly considered to play a role in myeloma pathobiology, t(8;14) translocations involving c-myc are rarely reported in myeloma, unlike Burkitt lymphoma, in which it is considered a classic feature. Almost 20% of patients with 14q32 translocation have other partners with unclear clinical or molecular significance.

Deletion 17p

Loss of the short arm of chromosome 17, (del(17p)) has been described in about 10% of patients with early stage MM. The deletion involves the major part of the short arm of chromosome 17 with consequent loss of number of genes. The most prominent gene in this region is TP53, which has been the focus of most investigations. However, p53 abnormalities represent an important late event associated with progression to an aggressive form of the disease. A study of p53 gene mutations in 52 patients with myeloma showed that seven of 52 patients had p53 abnormalities, all with advanced clinically aggressive acute or leukemic stage of MM. Because p53 is involved in cell death induced by most therapeutic agents, its inactivation may lead to the chemoresistance and consequent poor prognosis observed in patients with del(17p). However, this hypothesis has yet to be confirmed. In contrast to translocations involving the 14q32 region, del(17p) is considered as a secondary event mostly acquired during evolution. Patients presenting with a del(17p) have a poor prognosis despite the use of novel agent combinations or HDT and transplant. Mutations of the *TP53* gene are a rare event in myeloma, especially at diagnosis.[3]

Deletion 13q14

Deletion of chromosome 13 or part of its long arm is detected in approximately 15% to 20% of the patients by conventional cytogenetics and by interphase FISH in 50% of the patients. Interestingly, del(13q) is also detected in 50% of patients with MGUS by FISH, predominantly in a small subpopulation of cells, indicating that it is a secondary genetic event occurring after initial clonal expansion. Although the retinoblastoma gene is present in the deleted region, the exact molecular consequence of del(13q) has not yet been ascertained. A number of studies, especially with conventional agents as well as HDT, have identified del(13q) to be a poor prognostic feature in myeloma; however, recent studies have identified that there is an association between del(13q) and t(4;14) and in the absence of t(4;14), del(13q) by itself is not associated with a poor prognosis, especially with the use of novel agents.[3] However, del(13q) detected by conventional cytogenetics is still considered a poor prognostic feature. Interestingly, del(13q) is also common in chronic lymphocytic leukemia but does not confer an adverse prognosis.

Abnormalities of the 1q Region

Recent studies have reported the biological role and prognostic implications of a gain of 1q. In fact, this is one of the frequently reported cytogenetic abnormalities in MM, being described in about one-third of the patients. This abnormality has also been reported in a number of other hematologic and solid tumors. A gain of 1q21 chromosomal region or overexpression of the *CKS1B* gene located in this region is associated with a poor outcome; however, further studies are required to ascertain the clear prognostic impact of 1q gains. A number of important genes in addition to CKS1B are located in this region, including the interleukin-6 (IL-6) receptor.[3]

GENOMICS

Expression Profiling

Several investigators have performed high-throughput expression profiling to better understand the pathobiology of myeloma, develop prognostic models, identify new targets for drug development and develop personalized medicine approaches. In these studies, RNA is extracted from purified CD138$^+$ myeloma cells and hybridized on high-density arrays to evaluate expression of genes from the whole transcribed genome. One of the first such analyses using unsupervised clustering identified sequential genetic changes from normal plasma cells to plasma cells from patients with MGUS and MM and provided clues to the molecular basis for malignant transformation and potential therapeutic targets.

Expression profiling in combination with cytogenetic changes has been used to classify myeloma into phenotypic and molecular subgroups as well as for prognosis. The molecular classification compared profiles from MM cells with those from MGUS representing an initial indolent form of the disease and MM cell lines representing cells with a more aggressive phenotype. A later, more detailed classification identified different subgroups, mainly based on cyclin D gene expression and on the different 14q32 translocations. This molecular classification refined in 2006 identified seven subclasses of myeloma. In this model, the first class was defined by the translocation t(4;14) and identified by overexpression of the *MMSET* or *FGFR3* genes (or both genes). The second class was related to the translocations t(14;16) or t(14;20) and was defined by upregulation of one of the *MAF* genes. Individuals with CCND1 or CCND3 upregulation (caused by the translocations t(11;14) or t(6;14)) clustered in two different groups named CD1 and CD2. The CD2 group was characterized by CD20 expression. The fifth group was characterized by hyperdiploidy. The last two groups were characterized by a low incidence of bone disease, according to low DKK1 expression, and the last group was characterized by increased expression of genes involved in proliferation. This molecular classification has been further modified by the Dutch-Belgian Hemato-Oncology Group (HOVON). This analysis did not confirm the "low bone disease" group, but three other subgroups were identified: one group characterized by overexpression of cancer testis antigen genes, another group defined by overexpression of positive regulators of the nuclear factor kappa-B (NFκB) pathway, and a third subgroup enriched for "myeloid" genes (unclear significance).[5]

Copy Number Alteration

DNA-based high-throughput techniques such as array comparative genomic hybridization (array-CGH) and high-density single nucleotide polymorphism (SNP) arrays have identified recurrent copy number alterations. These studies have identified significant molecular heterogeneity (Fig. 85-3).[6] Copy number alterations (CAN) have been observed in 98% of evaluated 192 newly diagnosed patients with MM. Two distinct groups were observed in these patients: One group of patients shows a hyperdiploid phenotype with gains of chromosomes 3, 5, 7, 9, 11, 15, 18, 19, and 21 or loss of chromosomes 13, 22, and X (in female cases). The second group is characterized by gain or loss of subchromosomal region. This includes deletion of 1p, 6q, 8p, 12p, 14q, 16p, 16q, and 20p, as well as amplification of 1q and 6p. The genomic heterogeneity observed within the hyperdiploid group is driven by the presence of gain of copies of chromosome 1q or chromosome 11, chromosome 13 loss, or chromosome 5 gain. Subclasses of hyperdiploid MM patients and their correlation with gene expression profiles provide a basis for identifying therapeutically targetable genes. The molecular basis of this genomic heterogeneity may stem from uncontrolled recombination activity, which may drive continued acquisition of genomic changes.

To identify genetic events underlying the genesis and progression of MM, a high-resolution analysis of recurrent copy number alterations using array comparative genomic hybridization (aCGH) and expression profiles were prepared from a collection of MM cell lines and outcome-annotated clinical specimens.[7] Attesting to the molecular heterogeneity of MM, distinct genomic subtypes along with 87 discrete minimal common regions (MCRs) within recurrent and highly focal CNAs were identified. The genes residing in these regions provide a genomic framework to understand the biology of MM as well as identify potential therapeutic targets.

Transcriptome Modifiers

Alternate splicing is an important posttranslational modification that allows production of multiple protein isoforms, and more than 90% of human genes undergo alternative splicing. The spliced isoform frequency varies between tissues, and these protein isoforms may have related, distinct, or even opposing functions. Changes in alternative splicing has been reported in myeloma cells compared with normal plasma cells, and these changes have been correlated with an effect on overall clinical outcome.

MicroRNAs are a class of small noncoding RNAs that cleave specific targeted transcripts, inhibiting translational of specific genes.

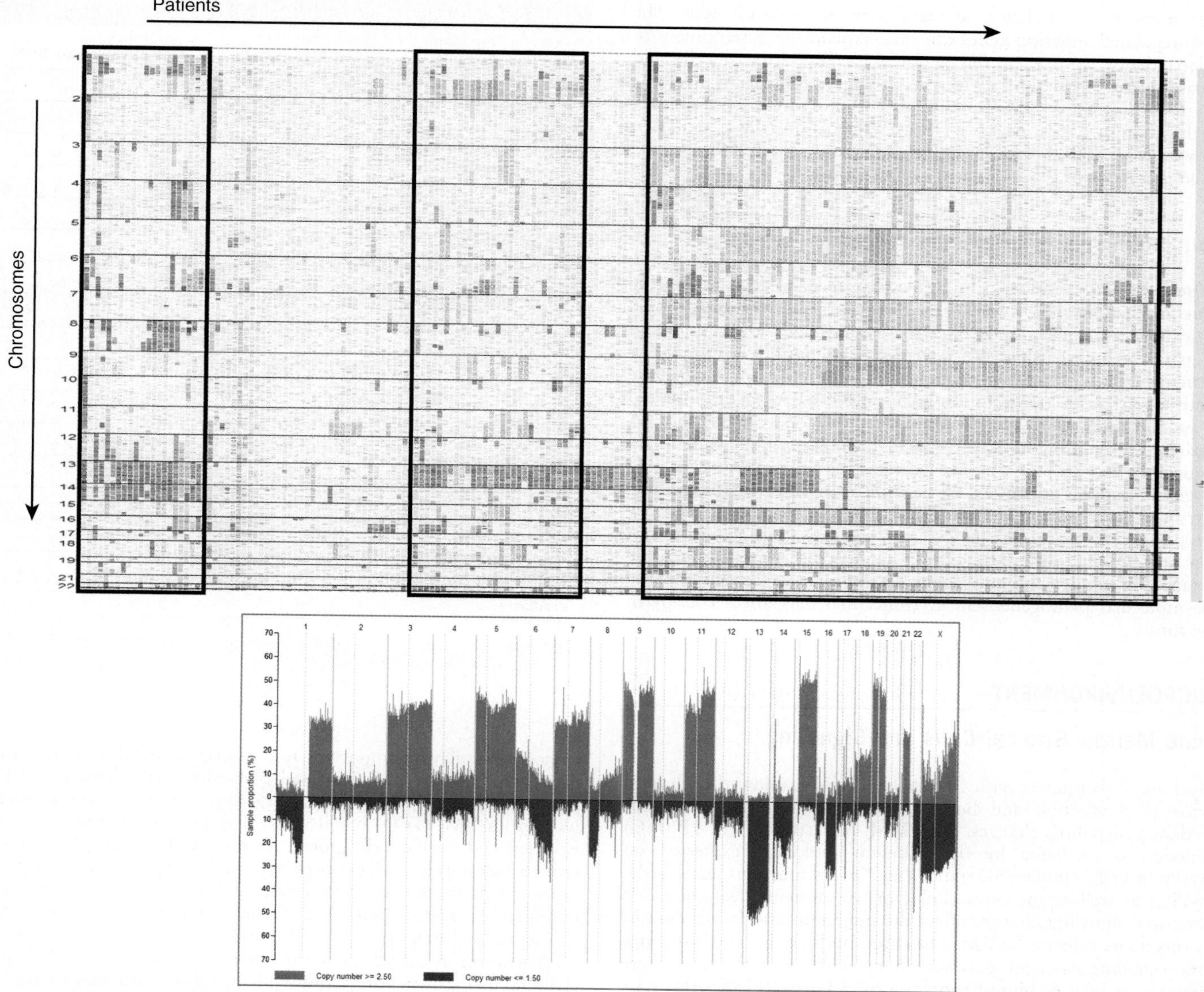

Figure 85-3 UNSUPERVISED HIERARCHICAL CLUSTERING OF SINGLE NUCLEOTIDE POLYMORPHISM (SNP) ARRAY–BASED DATA IN 192 PATIENT SAMPLES. Each column represents a patient and SNPs are arranged from 1p(tel) to Xq(tel) from top to bottom, so copy number changes are depicted from top to bottom for each chromosome. *Red* suggests gain, and *blue* suggests loss of copy number *(upper)*. Recurrence of copy-number abnormalities (CNAs) across 192 MM patients in chromosomal order. *Red* or *blue bars* denote gain or loss of chromosome material *(lower)*. The figure identifies recurrent areas of gains and losses in MM with identification of genomic subgroups and potential therapeutic targets. *(Adapted from Avet-Loiseau H, Li C, Magrangeas F, et al: Prognostic significance of copy-number alterations in multiple myeloma.* J Clin Oncol *27:4585, 2009.)*

Differences in expression patterns of microRNAs have been observed between MM and MGUS. For example, miRs -32, and -17-92 are overexpressed only in MM, but MiRs-21, -106b-25, and -181a/b show a similar expression pattern in both MM and MGUS but are highly expressed compared with normal plasma cells, providing a possible clue to events underlying progression from MGUS to MM. MiRs 15a/-16, are present on chromosome 13, and their downregulation is described in a subset of myeloma. Although this does not strictly correlate with chromosome 13 deletion, which is observed in almost half of MM patients, a potential effect of these MiRs on MM cell proliferation has been described. A similar attempt at correlating observed cytogenetic changes and their effects on MiR expression has identified overexpression of miR-let 7e, -125-5p, and -99b in patients with t(4;14) translocation and miRs -1 and -133a in patients with t(14;16) MM. A causal relationship between changes in these MiR expressions and their effects on target genes and eventual phenotypic changes in myeloma still needs to be established.[8] As in gene expression profiling, microRNA expression profile also identifies subgroups with different clinical outcomes, highlighting a significant role of microRNAs in MM biology and possibly as a therapeutic target. An integrated analysis of mRNA and miR profiling has now begun to identify regulatory networks that combine microRNA–mRNA pairs that may drive the eventually behavior of tumor cells. One such network combines p53/MDM2 expression with the downregulation of miRs -192, -194, and -215 in subset of MM. Such analysis will help explain some of the genomic changes observed in myelomagenesis and its progression.

A genome-wide methylation profile has identified hypomethylation, a characteristic that differentiates nonmalignant from malignant plasma cells.[9] Different methylation patterns have been observed between MGUS and MM cells, explaining their effect of gene expression patterns and the behavior of myeloma cells. Similarly, differential or downregulated expression of genes involved in cell–cell signaling and cell adhesion in plasma cell leukemia cells can be explained by the observed remethylation of these genes in leukemic cells. The downregulated adhesion genes can then explain the development of independence from their interaction with BM stromal cells and release in the circulation. Epigenetic changes modulating myeloma cell growth and survival genes have also been reported. For example, methylation of p16, a negative cell cycle regulator, is reported as an early event in MGUS. However, p16 methylation has not been shown to be predictive of OS in a larger cohort study.

Sequencing

Gene sequencing studies in myeloma have to date failed to identify a predominant mutation driving the disease process. A whole-genome or -exome sequencing study of 39 patients (22 whole genomes and 17 whole exomes) using 30X coverage has identified a number of recurrent unique but low-frequency mutations involving histone methyltransferases, transcription factor IRF4, BRAF, genes involved in protein translation, and genes involved in blood coagulation.[10] A separate study using massively parallel whole-genome paired end sequencing on paired samples collected 6 months apart in two myeloma patients identified 29 somatic rearrangements, including three that were present only in the second sample, suggesting both the presence of genomic changes early on as well as acquisition of new changes over time. These initial sequencing efforts confirm the potential of whole-genome sequencing to provide a true insight into the molecular pathogenesis in myeloma that may affect therapy in the future.

Table 85-2 Phenotypic Characterization of Plasma Cells

Adhesion Molecule	Normal Plasma Cells	Multiple Myeloma Cells
CD138	+	+
CD19	+	–
CD28	–	–
CD38	+	+
CD40	+	+
CD45	+	–*
CD27	–	+
CD11a	+	–
CD11b	–	–
CD44	+	+
CD54	+	+
CD56	–	+
CD58	–	+
LFA-1	–	–/+
RHAMM	–	+
VLA-4	+	+
VLA-5	+	+

RHAMM, Hyaluronan-mediated motility receptor; *VLA,* very late antigen.
*CD45 on immature myeloma cells.

MICROENVIRONMENT

Bone Marrow Stromal Cells and Signaling

Myeloma cells interact with BM stromal cells, leading to both local cytokine production and both cytokine-mediated and adhesion-mediated signaling changes. The MM–BM stromal cell (BMSC) adhesion is mediated by the adhesion molecules expressed on myeloma cells (Table 85-2) and their interacting partners on the BMSCs as well as the extracellular matrix proteins. Adhesion and associated signaling changes affect the migration and localization of the myeloma cells in the BM. Moreover, proliferative and antiapoptotic signaling cascades activated in myeloma as a result of these interactions include phosphatidylinositol-3 kinase (PI3K)/Akt, Ras/Raf/mitogen-activated protein kinase (MAPK) kinase (MEKK)/extracellular signal-related kinase (ERK), Janus kinase (JAK) 2/signal transducers and activators of transcription 3 (STAT 3), and NFκB pathways. These pathways lead to MM cell growth, survival, antiapoptosis, and development of drug resistance (Fig. 85-4).[11]

For example, syndecan-1, a cell surface transmembrane heparan sulfate proteoglycan present on MM cells, interacts with type I collagen and regulates the growth of MM cells; it also mediates increased osteoclast activity. Elevated levels of syndecan-1 shed into serum correlate with increased tumor mass, decreased matrix metalloproteinase-9 activity in serum, and a poor prognosis.

Various cellular components constitute the BM milieu, including osteoclasts, osteoblasts, endothelial cells, and immune cells, each contributing differently and distinctly to the overall effect of the microenvironment. For example, the cross-talk between tumor cells and components of the BM composed of osteoclasts and osteoblasts helps propagate not only the development of osteolytic lesions but also consequent survival and proliferation of MM cells. Several cytokines and signaling pathways have been identified as important mediators in the disruption of the osteoclast–osteoblast axis.[12] Impaired osteoblastogenesis is caused by the release of WNT inhibitors such as DKK1 have been studied, and neutralizing DKK1 antibody suppresses tumor-induced bone resorption and MM growth in vivo. Restoring normal bone homeostasis by disrupting this cross-talk thus represents a potential strategy to create a hostile niche for tumor growth. Similarly, endothelial cell proliferation and increased angiogenesis play an important role in plasma cell disorders. Compared with normal BM, increased BM microvessel density (MVD) has been observed in MGUS and MM. There is a stage-related increase in BM MVD that is also correlated with prognosis. Both vascular endothelial cell growth factor (VEGF) and hepatocyte growth factor (HGF) have been reported to be angiogenic factors expressed in myeloma. These results also suggest angiogenesis as a potential therapeutic target in myeloma and explains in part the efficacy of thalidomide and lenalidomide.

Activation of NFκB has been observed in myeloma cells, especially following their interaction with BMSCs. A number of abnormalities contributing to the dysregulation of NFκB and constitutive activation of the noncanonical NFκB pathway have been described,[11] In two separate studies, it has been shown that the NFκB pathway can be activated, either by deletions of NFκB inhibitors (e.g., TRAF3 or CYLD) or by activation of NFκB activators (e.g., NIK or CD40). Inactivating mutations of TRAF3 and elevated expression of NIK by genomic alterations or protein stabilization have been described and may explain the mechanism whereby MM cells achieve autonomy from the BM microenvironment.

Cytokines

Myeloma cell growth, survival, antiapoptosis, and drug resistance are in part mediated by a number of cytokines produced by MM cells as well as BMSCs. In fact, the production of cytokines is significantly modulated by MM–BMSC interactions and includes IL-6, insulin-like growth factor-1 (IGF-1), VEGF, tumor necrosis factor-α (TNF-α), transforming growth factor-β (TGFβ), IL-17, IL-21, CXC-chemokine ligand 12 (CXCL12), and others.[11]

Interleukin-6

Interleukin-6 is one of the most important cytokines, mediating both growth and survival of MM cells. IL-6 plays an important role in the

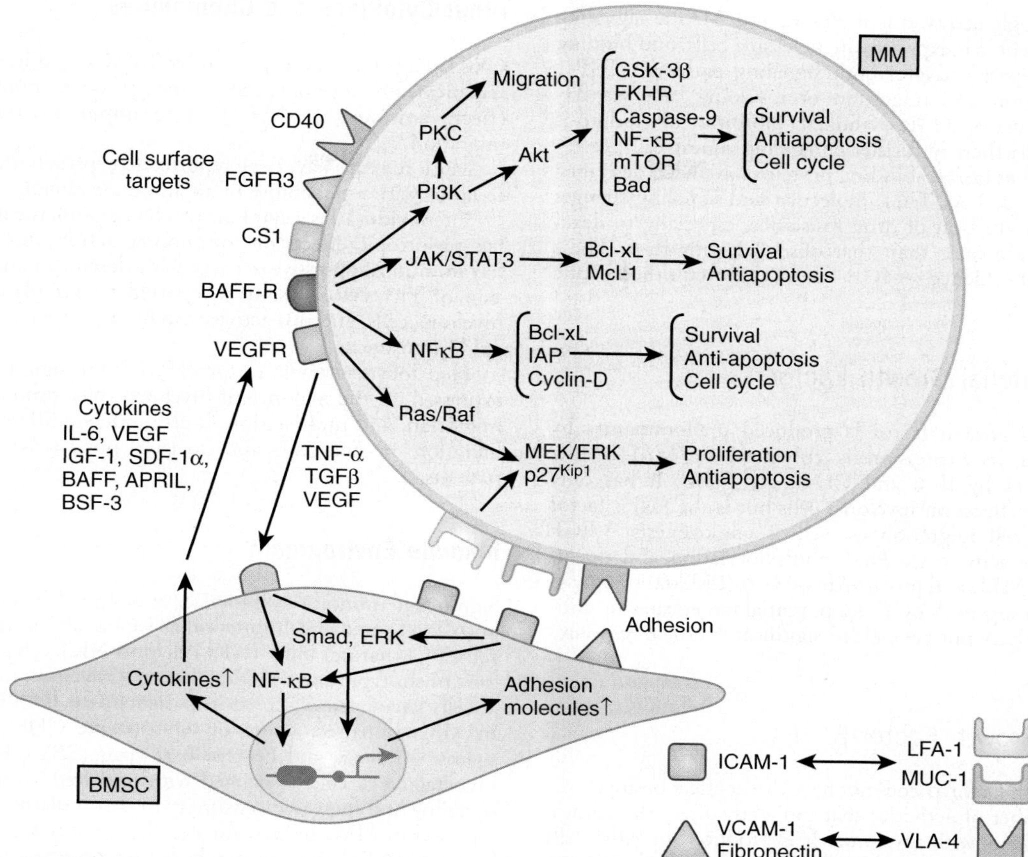

Figure 85-4 GROWTH OF THE MULTIPLE MYELOMA (MM) CELL IN THE BONE MARROW (BM) MICROENVIRONMENT. The interaction and adhesion of MM cells to the BM stromal cells (BMSCs) lead to adhesion- and cytokine-mediated signaling. MM cells binding to BMSCs induce the activation of p42/44 mitogen-activated protein kinase (MAPK) and nuclear factor kappa-B (NFκB) in BMSCs. The activation of NFκB upregulates adhesion molecules on BMSCs. Cytokines secreted through this interaction include interleukin-6 (IL-6) secretion, tumor-necrosis factor-α (TNF-α), and vascular endothelial growth factor (VEGF) to activate the main signaling pathways (p42/44 mitogen-activated protein kinase [MAPK], Janus kinase [JAK]/signal transducer and activator of transcription 3 [STAT3], or phosphatidylinositol 3-kinase [PI3K]/AKT) and their downstream targets, which triggers MM cell growth, survival, and migration. The RAS/RAF/MAPK kinase (MEK)/MAPK pathway mediates proliferation of MM cells. JAK/STAT3 along with upregulation of BCL-X_L and MCL1 mediates survival. PI3K/AKT through downstream activation of BAD and NFκB or inactivation of caspase-9 mediates antiapoptosis. NFκB and forkhead in rhabdomyosarcoma (FKHR) modulate cyclin D and KIP1, thereby regulating cell cycle progression. Signaling through PI3K induces downstream protein kinase C (PKC) activity and MM cell migration. *APRIL,* A proliferation-inducing ligand; *BAFF,* B-cell activating factor; *BSF-3,* B-cell stimulating factor; *ERK,* extracellular signal-related kinase; *FGFR3,* fibroblast growth factor receptor 3; *ICAM1,* intercellular adhesion molecule 1; *IGF1,* insulinlike growth factor-1; *IL,* interleukin; *LFA1,* lymphocyte function–associated antigen 1; *MEK,* MAPK/ERK kinase; *mTOR,* mammalian target of rapamycin; *muc1,* mucin 1; *SDF-1α,* stromal cell–derived factor-1α; *VCAM1,* vascular cell adhesion molecule 1; *VLA4,* very-late antigen 4. *(Adapted from Hideshima T, Mitsiades C, Tonon G, et al: Understanding MM pathogenesis in the bone marrow to identify new therapeutic targets.* Nat Rev Cancer *7:585, 2007.)*

terminal differentiation and the proliferation of normal plasmablasts. The IL-6 receptor that is composed of an α chain (gp80) and a signal-transducing β chain (gp130) is expressed by myeloma cells. IL-6 binding to its receptor activates Ras/RAF/MEK/ERK, JAK/STAT, and PI3K/AKT signaling pathways, mediating growth, survival, and drug resistance, respectively. The major source of IL-6 production is the BM stroma with myeloma cells contributing to a smaller extent. IL-6 production is induced by MM-BMSC interactions as well as by other cytokines, including TNF-α and VEGF in the BM milieu. IL-6 mediates mainly in a paracrine fashion but also has, to some extent, autocrine activity. IL-6 has a number of other activities, including being responsible for the number of symptoms observed in patients, inducing anemia and thrombocytosis, inducing T regulatory as well as Th17 cells with associated immunosuppression, and mediating enhanced bone resorption by osteoclasts. Additionally, IL-6 promotes coagulation without affecting fibrinolysis and induces a prothrombotic state by increasing expression of fibrinogen, factor VIII, and von Willebrand factor and by increasing production of platelets as well as activation of endothelial cells, overall inducing a prothrombogenic state. Importantly, it confers resistance to antitumor agents, especially dexamethasone. Myeloma cells shed IL-6Rα and soluble IL-6R, which can transduce the response of myeloma cells to IL-6. High serum levels of IL-6 as well as IL-6R are considered to predict poor prognosis. Both IL-6 and IL-6R are thus therapeutic targets, and antibodies targeting them are in advanced stages of clinical development.

Insulinlike Growth Factor-1

Insulinlike growth factor-1, similar to IL-6, is a mitogenic factor secreted by myeloma cells and mediates growth and survival of myeloma cells through activation of PI-3K and MAPK signaling pathways. IGF-1 receptor is expressed by myeloma cells, and binding of IGF-1 to its receptor activates both signaling pathways. IGF-1 also mediates adhesion and migration of myeloma cells via β1-integrin and upregulates FLIP, X-linked inhibitor of apoptosis (XIAP), and A1/Bfl1, thereby further enhancing tumor cell growth and survival. A number of IGF-binding proteins have been described that modulate IGF-1 activity. These molecular and signaling changes collectively lead to induction of drug resistance, especially to dexamethasone, which is greater than that observed with IL-6. These results have provided evidence for IGF-1 as an important therapeutic target.

Vascular Endothelial Growth Factor

Vascular endothelial growth factor is produced predominantly by myeloma cells, and its expression is enhanced by MM–BMSC interaction as well as by IL-6 and CD40 activation. It has only modest proliferative effects on myeloma cells but is the major factor affecting myeloma cell migration as well as angiogenesis. VEGF mediates part of its activity via Flt-1 phosphorylation and downstream activation of MEK and protein kinase C-α (PKC-α) signaling. Although these data suggest VEGF as a potential target, specific anti-VEGF therapeutics have not yet yielded significant clinical responses in myeloma.

Transforming Growth Factor-β

Transforming growth factor-β does not have direct effect on myeloma cells but has a number of activities that indirectly affect the clinical presentation of patients with myeloma. It is produced by MM cells and induces secretion of IL-6 by BMSCs. Importantly, it induces immunosuppression characteristic of myeloma and may also affect normal plasma cell development and function, thereby contributing to suppressed uninvolved immunoglobulin production in myeloma. It is also a major cytokine that affects T-helper cell development, especially T regulatory cells and Th17 cells.

Interleukin-17 and Proinflammatory Cytokines

Elevated levels of Th17 cells along with increased levels of serum IL-17 and associated proinflammatory cytokines, IL-21, IL-22, and IL-23, are observed in patients with myeloma. IL-17 has multiple effects in myeloma, including induction of myeloma cell growth; suppression of immune function, especially in association with IL-22; and induction of bone disease by inducing osteoclast number and function. IL-17 also induces IL-6 production by BMSCs, thereby augmenting its myeloma growth–inducing effects. IL-17 triggers phosphorylation of JAK1, STAT3, and ERK1/2. TNF-α upregulates expression of both IL-21 and of IL-21 receptor (IL-21R), and IL-21 induces proliferation and inhibits apoptosis of myeloma cells independent of IL-6 signaling.

Tumor Necrosis Factor-α

Tumor necrosis factor-α is primarily a mediator of inflammation. It is produced by myeloma cells and has no significant direct effect on myeloma cells. However, it mediates part of its activity through induction of IL-6 production by BMSCs. It induces activation of NFκB and adhesion molecules with a resultant increase in binding of myeloma cells to BMSC and mediates cell adhesion–mediated drug resistance. Antibodies specifically targeting TNF-α have not shown clinical activity. However, novel agents such as bortezomib and the immunomodulatory agents thalidomide and lenalidomide have potent anti–TNF-α activity and can overcome drug-resistance by eliminating TNF-α–induced NFκB activation.

Other Cytokines and Chemokines

CXCL-12 (SDF-1) is expressed by BMSCs, and its receptor CXCR4 is expressed by myeloma cells. It induces only a minimal proliferative effect; however, it plays a more important role in mediating migration.

Myeloma cells have been reported to express both IL-15 and IL-15 receptor with a possibility of an autocrine circuit.

Interleukin-10 is a cytokine produced primarily by monocytes and has pleiotropic effects on immunoregulation and inflammation. It has immunosuppressive activity with downregulation of the expression of Th1 cytokines. It is reported to stimulate proliferation of myeloma cells, and this activity can be abrogated by antibodies to the gpl30 transducer.

Hepatocyte growth factor (HGF), through its receptor c-met expressed on the majority of myeloma cells, promotes cell invasion, migration, and proliferation. It also induces differentiation and proliferation of osteoclasts and increases bone resorption in myeloma patients.

Immune Environment

Significant immune dysfunction is observed in myeloma involving both T cells and B-cell function as well as abnormalities in dendritic cell (DC), natural killer (NK) cell, and NKT-cell activity.[13-15] Significant phenotypic and functional aberrations in both $CD4^+$ and $CD8^+$ T cells have been observed in patients with both MGUS and MM. In MM, impaired action of viral-specific $CD8^+$ cells, particularly against influenza and Epstein-Barr virus (EBV), has been reported. Hyperactive T cells associated with impaired T-cell receptor (TCR) signaling and increased sensitivity to costimulatory signals have been reported in MM. In fact, further abnormalities of the TCR variable β-chain (TCR-Vβ) repertoire have been observed after chemotherapy in MM patients. A reduction in $CD4^+$ T-cell numbers and $CD4^+$:$CD8^+$ T-cell ratio is observed in the peripheral blood of MM patients. Persistent proliferative activity of both $CD4^+$ and $CD8^+$ T cells has been observed in both MGUS and MM, which plays a possible role in controlling tumor cell growth and survival. Overall hyperactivity, clonal expansion, and homeostatic proliferation of T-cell activity are observed. Moreover, $CD4^+$ and $CD8^+$ T cells from the BM of patients with MGUS are able to mount a strong immune response against autologous MGUS plasma cells; however, similar responses are not observed with T cells from the BM of MM patients, suggesting the role of the immune system in controlling plasma cell growth in MGUS and loss of immune surveillance in MM. Although in MM, T cells are dysfunctional in the BM, these cells can be stimulated in vitro leading to restored function. Regulatory T cells (Tregs): The $CD4^+$/$CD25^+$ T-helper cells specifically express forkhead box protein (Foxp) 3 and actively suppress inappropriate immune responses maintaining immune homeostasis. In MM, Tregs are lower in number and are dysfunctional. This may be mediated by elevated IL-6, sIL-6R and TGFβ levels. Another report suggests that after short exposure to IL-2, purified Tregs from MM patients are able to induce suppressive activity in vivo and in vitro. Therapy such as lenalidomide, granulocyte colony-stimulating factor (G-CSF), and allogeneic stem cell transplantation (SCT) may directly or indirectly affect Treg and may account for some of the observed variations in Treg number and function in MM. T-helper 17 (Th17) specifically express retinoic acid–related orphan receptor-γt (ROR-γt) and produce IL-17, which provides protection against certain bacterial, fungal, and viral infections. Development of Th17 cells is also determined by TGFβ and IL-6, which are upregulated in MM. In myeloma, an increased number of Th17 cells are reported with an associated increase in serum levels of IL-17 and other proinflammatory cytokines such as IL-21, IL-22, and IL-23. IL-17 has been reported to support myeloma cell growth, suppress immune function, and induce osteoclastogenesis, supporting bone disease in MM. These effects make Th17 cells an important therapeutic target in MM. γδ T cells possess a distinct TCR and represent a small subset of T cells involved in generating an antimyeloma response. γδ T cells are considered a bridge between innate and adaptive immunity and are able to kill major histocompatibility (MHC) class I chain-related protein A (MICA)–positive MM cells via the NKG2D (a NK-cell triggering receptor) pathway. Interestingly, MICA expression is significantly higher in plasma cells from MGUS patients. Bisphosphonates have been shown to activate γδ T cells, which may in part explain their weak antimyeloma activity.

Significant B-cell and plasma cell dysfunction is observed in MM as represented by suppressed uninvolved immunoglobulins. For example, in patients with IgA myeloma, there is suppression of serum IgG and IgM levels. This is not considered to be mediated by high levels of monoclonal paraprotein because suppressed immunoglobulins have also been observed in patients with nonsecretory disease. An explanation for this observation remains elusive; however, suppressed uninvolved immunoglobulins predispose patients to infectious complications because they reduce the patient's ability to generate a specific humoral immune response to infections or vaccinations. For example, a study evaluating the serologic responses to vaccinations against influenza, streptococcus pneumoniae, and *Haemophilus influenzae* in 52 MM patients reported that only 19% developed protective antibody titer levels against influenza, 39% against streptococcus pneumoniae, and 41% against *H. influenzae* type b. These observations suggest the necessity to define suitable immunization protocols for patients with MM and the need to study the humoral and cellular responses after vaccination in terms of clinical efficacy, magnitude, and duration of response. Both B- and T-cell immune function is also affected by the therapeutic agents themselves with further increase in the risk of infectious complications (e.g., the increased risk of herpes zoster after bortezomib treatment or bacterial infections after dexamethasone use in MM). Recovery of uninvolved immunoglobulins to normal levels after effective therapy has been associated with both improved survival and protection from infectious complications.

Alterations in NK cell number have been observed in MM and are correlated with disease burden (e.g., high numbers of NK cells have been observed in patients with a low tumor burden). NK cells are considered to have a potential therapeutic role, and the immunomodulatory drugs (thalidomide, lenalidomide, and pomalidomide) enhance NK cell–mediated cytotoxicity against MM cells. Invariant natural killer T cells (iNKTs), which constitute an innate lymphocyte lineage with potential for a potent antitumor immune response through the production of Th1 cytokines, are functionally defective in MM; however, these cells can be cultured in vitro with restored function, suggesting the possibility of their adoptive transfer as a potential therapeutic strategy in MM.

Dendritic cells are important antigen-presenting cells (APCs) that generate effective immune responses, including antitumor responses. DC dysfunction partly mediated by cytokines such as VEGF, IL-10, and TGFβ is reported in MM. However, it is possible to improve the defective DC function by in vitro generation. A number of studies have used DC-based vaccination strategies, including vaccinations with DCs pulsed with the idiotype protein. DCs pulsed with MM antigen-directed peptides or MM cell lysate and fusion of MM cells with DCs have been reported to lead to an antimyeloma immune response after vaccination.

CLINICAL MANIFESTATIONS

Patients with MM present with a number of signs and symptoms that are either related to BM infiltration by plasma cells or caused by manifestations of end-organ damage involving renal dysfunction, bone lesions, or immunoparesis. However, in up to 20% of the patients, MM may present entirely as an asymptomatic disease diagnosed on routine blood work. The symptoms may also be related to deposition of paraproteins in various organs as either light-chain deposition or amyloid deposits or caused by cytokines such as IL-6 or VEGF produced by the myeloma cells or the BM stromal cells. Because of improvement in routine blood work and the availability of sensitive tests, the clinical presentation in myeloma has changed over the past 25 years (Table 85-3). Overall, patients are more frequently being diagnosed with asymptomatic disease than presenting with symptoms. For example, patients are presenting less often with bone pain, pathological fractures, and renal failure as well as hyperviscosity. Various clinical features of myeloma are summarized in Table 85-4.

Bone Disease

Almost two-thirds of patients with MM present with bone pain as their main symptom. The mechanism of bone involvement is

Table 85-3 Changing Clinical Presentation of Patients With Myeloma

	Kyle (%)	Riccardi (%)
Symptoms related to MM	90	66
Bone pain	68	37
Pathologic fracture	60	34
Hypercalcemia	30	18
Renal failure (Cr >2.0 mg/dL)	29	10
Anemia (high <12 g/dL)	62	39
Hyperviscosity (>1.8 cp)	89	55

Cr, Creatinine; *MM,* multiple myeloma.

Table 85-4 Clinical Features of Multiple Myeloma

Bone Destruction
Pain
Fractures
Spinal cord compression
Radicular pain
Hypercalcemia
Polyuria, polydipsia
Nausea, vomiting
Renal Failure
Nausea, vomiting
Malaise, weakness
Amyloidosis
Peripheral neuropathy
Dependant edema
Organomegaly
Bone Marrow Infiltration
Anemia
Bleeding tendency
Reduced Globulins
Recurrent infections
Pneumonia
Cryoglobulins
Raynaud phenomenon
Acrocyanosis
Hyperviscosity
Shortness of breath
Transient ischemic attacks
Deep venous thrombosis
Retinal hemorrhage
Epistaxis

multifactorial, including direct bone destruction by the unbalanced hyperactivity of osteoclasts and suppression of osteoblastic activity. This is further accentuated by the cytokine milieu generated in the BM microenvironment by interaction between myeloma cells and BMSCs; this includes IL-6, IL-1β, TNF-α, and MIP1α.[12] A member of the TNF family, RANKL (receptor activator of nuclear factor κ-B ligand), also plays an important role in osteoclast growth and differentiation via its receptor located on osteoclasts. RANKL is secreted by stromal cells and osteoblasts, and induces differentiation and maturation of osteoclast progenitors. Osteoprotegerin (OPG) acts as a decoy receptor for RANKL and plays a significant role in development of bone disease in myeloma. In myeloma, the soluble syndecan produced by myeloma cells occupies and sequesters OPG, leading to excess RANKL activity that induces osteoclast differentiation and proliferation with the development of consequent lytic bone lesions. Importantly, myeloma cells also secrete Dick Kopf–related protein 1 (DKK-1), which has significant osteoblast inhibitory activity, leading to suppression of new bone formation, further contributing to bone disease in myeloma.[16] Thus DKK-1 has become an important therapeutic target to improve bone anabolic effects in myeloma. These factors together lead to osteoporosis and lytic bone lesions. Additionally, direct infiltration of bone by myeloma cells also causes bone destruction. Overall, one observes pain that is aggravated on movement and also collapse of vertebrae, leading to a decrease in height as well as symptoms of nerve compression. Besides pain, involvement of the extremities or spine leads to lack of mobility and associated problems, including predisposition to thrombotic events.

Hypercalcemia

Hypercalcemia is observed in approximately 25% to 30% of patients with myeloma and is usually a manifestation of higher burden of the disease. Its occurrence is related to bone involvement as well as production of various cytokines that lead to increased bone resorption and calcium release. Hypercalcemia manifests as mental status changes, lethargy, nausea and vomiting, and constipation. In extreme cases, one can also develop seizure activity. A normal serum calcium level in the presence of high paraprotein or low albumen level may require calculation or measurement of ionized calcium levels to assess true and effective serum calcium levels. Hypercalcemia can also induce renal failure caused by dehydration and it is to be considered a hematologic emergency, meriting prompt intervention.

Renal Failure

Renal insufficiency is one of the frequent and serious complications of myeloma with a multifactorial etiology.[17] The most common and reversible cause of renal failure is light-chain tubular cast deposition or light-chain deposition disease (commonly associated with κ light chains). Similarly, proteins can be deposited as amyloid, predominantly involving λ light chain (specifically λ light-chain subtype 6) with development of kidney failure. Amyloidosis is quite often associated with nephrotic (syndrome) range proteinuria. The proteinuria observed in patients with amyloid is more nonspecific, which differs from conditions with light-chain cast nephropathy with predominantly excess of light-chain excretion in the urine. Another common cause is hypercalcemia leading to osmotic diuresis and prerenal dysfunction associated with volume depletion. Additional mechanisms of renal failure in myeloma include renal calcium deposition with interstitial nephritis, use of nonsteroidal antiinflammatory drugs for pain control, hyperuricemia, intravenous contrast dye use for imaging purposes, chemotherapy-induced nephrotoxicity, and use of bisphosphonates. The development of light-chain cast nephropathy has been reported to be associated with Tom-Horsfall protein, which promotes heterotypic aggregation of light chains with deposition in the distal tubules of the kidney. Patients with renal failure are often asymptomatic. However, when symptoms are present, they are predominately malaise, weakness, nausea, or vomiting.

Anemia

Anemia is one of the common presenting symptoms in myeloma and is symptomatically associated with fatigue and shortness of breath. Anemia usually is normochromic normocytic and has a number of etiologic factors associated, including inadequate erythropoietin production caused by renal dysfunction, erythropoietin unresponsiveness predominately caused by various cytokines produced in myeloma, dilution caused by significantly increased immunoglobulin levels, and BM infiltrative processes.[18] Part of the development of anemia may also be related to high IL-6 levels. In patients who have had a number of treatments, quite often anemia is related to repeated rounds of chemotherapy. Erythropoietin administration therefore is an important supportive measure for the symptomatic treatment of anemia in myeloma. In one study, improvement in hemoglobin was observed in 60% of treated patients, and responses were observed in those with low erythropoietin levels compared with normal or high level (72% vs. 20%).

Neurologic Symptoms

Patients with MM present with a number of neurologic symptoms related either to direct involvement of the nervous system or the impact of cytokine or paraproteins on the nervous system. The most common abnormality is compression of the spinal cord or nerve roots, giving rise to pain as well as various degrees of neurologic dysfunction, including, in several cases, paraplegia with loss of bladder and bowel control. Cord compression is considered a neurologic emergency requiring prompt intervention, which in fact might allow complete recovery of function as well as resolution of a majority of the symptoms. In this setting, an urgent magnetic resonance imaging (MRI) followed by radiotherapeutic or surgical intervention is immediately warranted. Peripheral neuropathy is another common manifestation observed in almost one-third of the newly diagnosed patients, if analyzed using sophisticated and sensitive methods. Peripheral neuropathy also can develop because of a therapeutic intervention, especially agents such as thalidomide, bortezomib, and vincristine. Moreover, a constellation of symptoms associated with POEMS syndrome (polyneuropathy, organomegaly, endocrinopathy, monoclonal gammopathy, and skin changes) includes prominent sensory neuropathy associated with sclerotic myeloma. Paraneoplastic central nervous system (CNS) manifestations have been occasionally reported in myeloma and are considered to be related to clonal immunoglobulin targeting various CNS cells or structure. Furthermore, the polyneuropathy in myeloma is caused by multiple other factors, including amyloid deposits, infiltrative processes with other protein deposits, metabolic causes related to hypercalcemia or hyperviscosity, immune processes, or cytokine effects. IgM-related neuropathy is well described in which case a myelin-associated globulin (MAG) has been described in 50% of the patients. The presence of MAG provides diagnostic clues as well as a parameter to follow therapy. Traditionally, meningeal involvement has been described very rarely in myeloma; however, with prolonged survival with novel agents, it is being seen more frequently. This type of complication is usually observed with high-risk disease. Finally, intracranial plasmacytomas involving brain parenchyma, either from the skull or from the skull base, has been reported in advanced cases.

Hyperviscosity

Hyperviscosity is less frequent in myeloma compared with Waldenström macroglobulinemia, in which higher molecular weight IgM molecules frequently cause an increase in viscosity. In general, hyperviscosity in IgG myeloma is extremely uncommon. For hyperviscosity to develop, generally an IgG greater than 10 g/dL, IgA greater than 7 g/dL, and IgM greater than 5 g/dL is required to cause symptomatology. Occasionally, certain physicochemical characteristics of immunoglobulin may lead to self-aggregating properties and induce viscosity even at a lower level. This has been reported with IgG3, which is more frequently associated with hyperviscosity among various IgG myelomas. The commonly observed symptoms are related to circulatory decline involving vital organs, leading to complaints of headache, visual symptoms, shortness of breath, bleeding complications such as nosebleeds, and eventually mental status changes. The confirmation of viscosity can be obtained by measuring viscosity, which may exceed 4.0 cp units; however, symptoms at lower levels of viscosity have been observed. Therapy is instituted more on the basis of symptomatology than absolute measured levels of viscosity and requires prompt institution of plasmapheresis with quick resolution of symptoms.

Infections

Infections are some of the most important causes of morbidity and a common cause of mortality in myeloma. Because of compromised T- and B-cell functions, myeloma patients are at a significant high risk of developing recurrent bacterial as well as viral and fungal infections. As described earlier, various factors lead to an inability of myeloma patients to mount a humoral immune response to antigens or an infectious challenge.[19] The patients are susceptible to polysaccharide-encapsulated organisms as well as enteric gram-negative bacilli. Further susceptibility to infections also stems from therapeutic intervention, especially with corticosteroids. For example, fungal infections, most commonly, oral thrush, are observed after high-dose dexamethasone-based therapy, and herpes zoster is observed frequently after bortezomib-based therapy. In both cases, prophylactic antibiotics or antivirals are indicated. A number of cases of therapy-induced activation of mycobacterium tuberculosis in developing countries have been reported. The risk of infection is highest during the first 2 months of initiation of therapy when both myeloma-related immunosuppression as well as therapy-related immunosuppression increase the predisposition to infectious complication. Prompt diagnosis of infectious complications and quick institution of therapy or preferably initial prophylactic measures prevent major complications.

Coagulation Disorders

Both BM suppression with cytopenias and coagulation abnormalities are observed in myeloma. Myeloma might be associated with both bleeding-related problems as well as thrombotic events. The coagulation abnormalities are related to high levels of paraprotein that interfere with normal coagulation pathways as well as platelet dysfunction caused by either decreased number or function. The coagulation abnormalities include conditions similar to acquired deficiency of factor VIII. The hypercoagulable state is observed in 15% of patients with IgG myeloma and one-third of patients with IgA myeloma and is related to hyperviscosity, acquired activated protein C resistance, lupus-like anticoagulants with thromboembolic complications, acquired deficiency of protein S, and a therapy-related hypercoagulable state specifically with immunomodulatory agents such as thalidomide and lenalidomide. In the absence of prophylactics measure, these agents have been reported to cause deep venous thrombosis (DVT) in 10% to 20% of these patients, in whom the thrombotic risk increases with associated use of dexamethasone, other chemotherapeutic agents, or a previous history of DVT or immobility.

Thrombocytosis is more frequently associated with myeloma than thrombocytopenia, mainly driven by the high level of IL-6, which drives growth and maturation of megakaryocytes. Rarely, extensive BM infiltration by myeloma cells, and more commonly, extensive chemotherapeutic intervention with BM compromise leads to thrombocytopenia in the advanced stages of the disease.

Amyloidosis

The monoclonal protein, specifically the light chain, can get deposited in various organs as an insoluble fibrillar protein, amyloid, affecting organ dysfunction. Around 20% of patients with primary amyloidosis (AL) also have a concurrent diagnosis of MM, and all patients with AL-amyloid have clonal light chain production. Although clinically overt amyloidosis is observed less frequently in myeloma, intense investigation to identify amyloid deposits using fat pad biopsies, concurrent staining of BM with Sudan black, and obtaining rectal biopsy can identify some level of amyloid deposit in almost one-third of the patients. Patients with amyloid deposits can present with a number of features primarily related to their organ damage, including renal and cardiac dysfunction and symptoms suggesting carpal tunnel syndrome. Classic presentations of advance amyloid include cutaneous fragility around the eyelids with raccoon eyes and macroglossia. Patients with advanced amyloid with myeloma have a poor overall outcome; however, therapeutic intervention currently remains the same as in patients with myeloma with amyloidosis.

LABORATORY MANIFESTATIONS

Investigations to Detect Clonality

Protein Electrophoresis

A serum protein electrophoresis is performed to quantitate the monoclonal proteins present in myeloma.[20] In 70% of the patients, the monoclonal protein is IgG; in 20%, it is IgA; and in 5% to 10% of patients, it is light chains only. Fewer than 1% of patients have monoclonal protein, which is IgD, IgE, or IgM, or truly nonsecretory myeloma. The identification of the exact type of paraproteins in both serum and urine requires immunofixation (Fig. 85-5). This should be performed at the time of initial diagnosis and needs to be repeated to confirm achievement of complete response. Patients who produce intact immunoglobulins can also produce excess light chain, leading to a diagnosis that has both heavy and light chains (e.g., patients can have IgG κ and κ light-chain myeloma). Associated with the presence of a monoclonal protein, the uninvolved immunoglobulins are suppressed in MM. For example, patients with IgG myeloma have suppressed IgA and IgM. In a setting where all three immunoglobulins are suppressed, one should suspect either light chain–only disease or the possibility of IgD or IgE MM. Very rarely, a biclonal or triclonal pattern of immunoglobulins is observed, more often with the same light chain but rarely with different heterotypic light chains. This may suggest truly separate clones, especially with separate light chains. Quantitation of Bence Jones proteins in urine is still important both for the diagnosis of myeloma as well as for follow-up. It is important to note that free light-chain measurement in urine is not informative. Those patients with only monoclonal protein in the urine require frequent 24-hour Bence Jones proteins measurements for follow-up. Therapeutically, patients with all the various types of immunoglobulins are treated with a similar approach; however, a patient with IgA myeloma appears to have an inferior survival. The immunoglobulin isotype remains constant in a given patient over the natural history of the disease; however, occasionally, a patient producing one immunoglobulin at the time of diagnosis, at relapse, or with advanced disease may present with only the same light chain as initially observed with the original immunoglobulin (light-chain escape) or occasionally may become nonsecretory. Both the changes are reflective of the change in plasma cells to a more aggressive or undifferentiated form. Because of the observed light-chain escape, patients without initial Bence Jones proteins detection in urine will require periodic 24-hour urine Bence Jones proteins measurements on follow-up.

The unique sequences that are observed with the idiotype protein (CDR3) have been used as a marker that specifically identifies tumor cell clone and has been applied to polymerase chain reaction–based methodology to detect minimal residual disease (MRD) with high sensitivity. Early studies using such molecular methods for detecting MRD have identified patients who achieve molecular CRs that are associated with improved overall outcome.

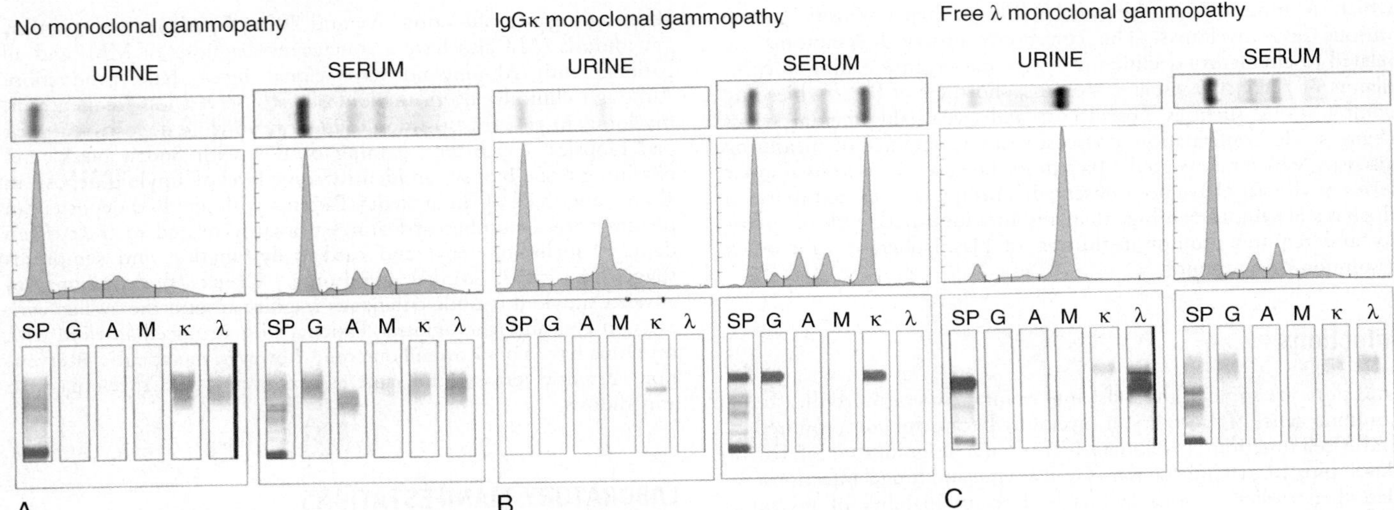

Figure 85-5 REPRESENTATIVE PATTERNS OF SERUM ELECTROPHORESIS AND IMMUNOFIXATION. In each figure, the *lower panels* represent immunofixation patterns, *middle panels* are the densitometric tracing of the gel, and *upper panels* are agarose gel of urine sample *(left)* and serum *(right)*. **A,** The normal pattern of serum and urine protein on electrophoresis. Because there are many different immunoglobulins in the serum, their differing mobilities in an electric field produce a broad peak. **B,** In monoclonal gammopathies, the predominance of a product of a single cell produces a sharp peak. The immunofixation identifies the type of immunoglobulin (e.g., κ light chain in urine and IgG κ in serum). **C,** In patients with light chain–only disease, a clonal band is observed only in urine with no clear peak in serum (e.g., γ light chain in urine with no distinct immunofixation positivity in serum). *(Courtesy Dr. Neal I Lindeman, with permission.)*

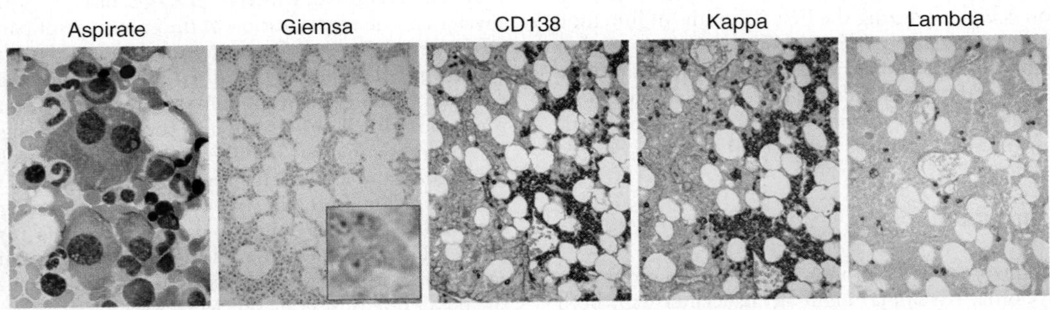

Figure 85-6 BONE MARROW EXAMINATION FROM A PATIENT WITH IMMUNOGLOBULIN G (IgG) κ MYELOMA SHOWING NEOPLASTIC PLASMA CELLS AT VARIOUS STAGES OF DIFFERENTIATION. The cells are CD138$^+$ and κ light-chain positive but λ negative. *(Courtesy Dr. Ruben Carrasco, MD, with permission.)*

Serum-Free Light Chain

This test measures light chain that is not associated with heavy chain that forms the intact immunoglobulin molecule. The presence of serum-free light chains provides an additional marker and measurement of plasma cell proliferation, and its quantitation has allowed us to determine protein levels in a number of patients who were previously considered oligo or nonsecretory. For example, 80% of patients with previously diagnosed nonsecretory myeloma have measurable serum-free light chains. Routine use of serum-free light chain measurements is indicated for diagnosis, response evaluation, and prognosis. As shown later, in patients with MGUS and SMM, the serum-free light-chain ratio allows for identification of patients with an increased likelihood of progression to symptomatic myeloma. As initially hoped, measurement of serum-free light chain does not replace the measurement of Bence Jones proteins in 24-hour urine collection.

Bone Marrow Examination

Except for patients with solitary plasmacytoma, the presence of clonal plasma cells (>5%) is usually observed in all plasma cell disorders.[21] Ten or greater percentage of clonal plasma cells in the BM aspirate or biopsy (whichever is higher if both done) is required to differentiate MGUS from SMM and for diagnosis of MM. The quantitation of plasma cells should be performed with at least a 200 cell count, and confirmation of clonality is essential for diagnosis, which can be done either by immunostaining using κ/λ staining or by flow cytometry (Figs. 85-6 and 85-7). In absence of clear BM involvement, a biopsy-proven soft tissue or bony plasmacytoma is also adequate for diagnosis (Fig. 85-8). Cytogenetics and FISH studies should be performed on BM samples at the time of diagnosis and if initially confirmed as low-risk disease, then should be repeated on BM performed at the time of relapse. Although important for prognostication, cytogenetic or FISH-identified abnormalities are not adequate for diagnosing MM from MGUS or SMM. A seven-color flow cytometry panel is also now used on BM samples to detect MRD.

Investigation to Detection of End-Organ Damage

The diagnosis of a plasma cell disorder is based on the presence of a monoclonal protein and clonal plasma cells. However, the diagnosis of MGUS/SMM that currently does not require therapeutic

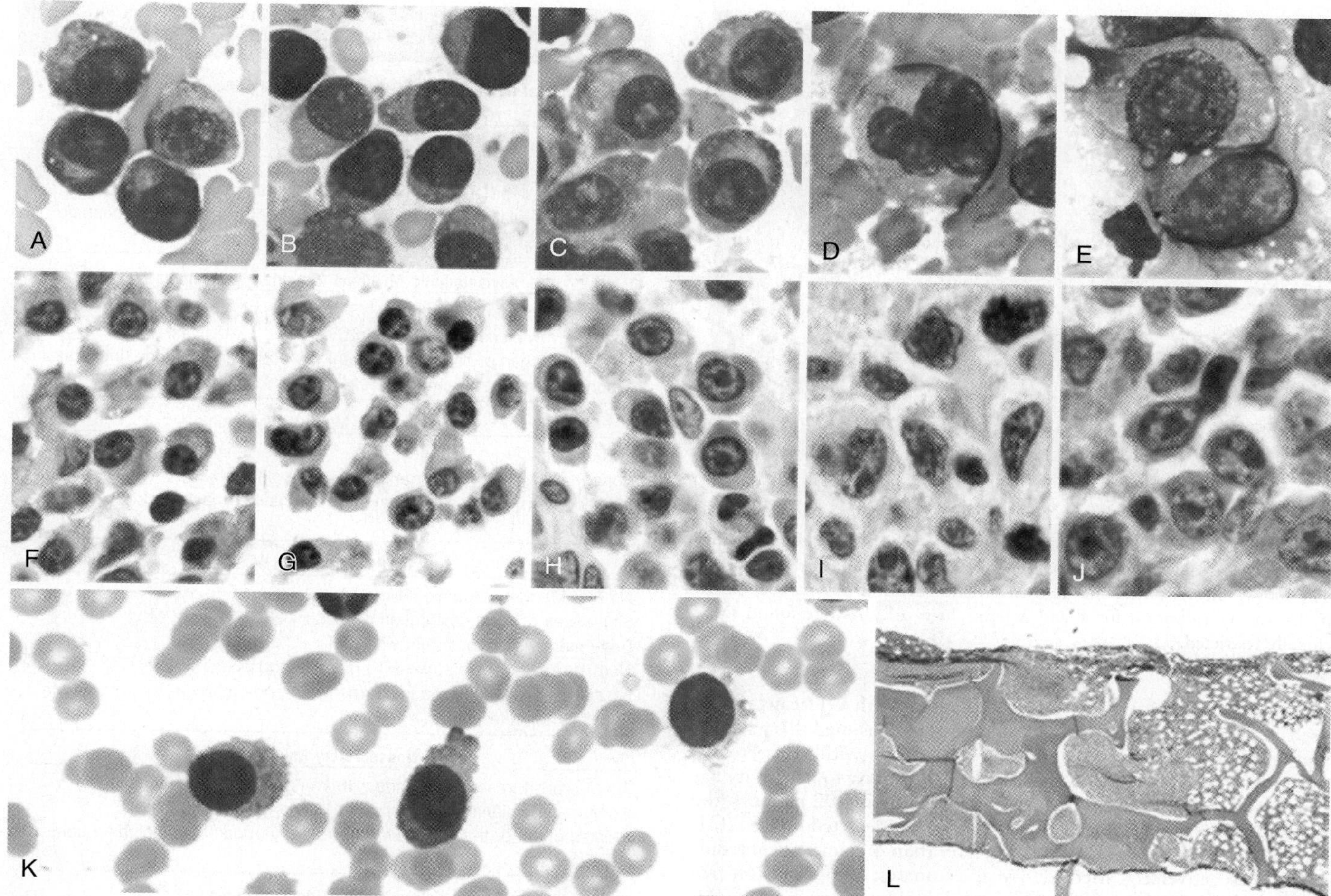

Figure 85-7 MORPHOLOGIC SPECTRUM OF NEOPLASTIC PLASMA CELLS IN MULTIPLE MYELOMA. There is significant morphologic heterogeneity in the plasma cells as seen on the bone marrow aspirate (**A** to **E**) and biopsy (**F** to **J**). The plasma cells can sometimes be fairly normal appearing (**A** and **F**); they can be "lymphocyte-like" and difficult to distinguish from lymphoplasmacytic lymphoma (**B** and **G**); they frequently can exhibit cytologic atypia with prominent nucleoli and nuclear to cytoplasmic dyssynchrony (**C** and **H**); they can exhibit anaplastic features (**D** and **I**), and they can show "blastic" features (**E** and **J**). Myeloma can also have a leukemic phase **(K)** and can be associated with osteosclerosis **(L),** as sometime seen in association with POEMS syndrome (polyneuropathy, organomegaly, endocrinopathy, monoclonal gammopathy, and skin changes).

intervention and active symptomatic MM that needs treatment is based on the detection of end-organ damage, which includes bone lesions, anemia, renal dysfunction, and hypercalcemia. The details of the diagnostic criteria are listed in Table 85-5.[21]

Radiographic Evaluation

The standard evaluation of bone lesions in myeloma is by a skeletal survey that includes plain radiographs of the entire skeleton. The presence of characteristic lytic lesions is considered diagnostic for myeloma (Fig. 85-9). Rarely, in POEMS syndrome, bone lesions are osteosclerotic. The bone lesions do not always resolve after effective therapy. Because of the absence or suppression of osteoblastic activity, the bone scan is diagnostically not a useful investigative tool in myeloma. Almost all patients with myeloma have osteoporosis caused by unbalanced osteoclastic activity. Bone mineral density (BMD) measurement by dual-energy x-ray absorptiometry helps identify osteoporosis and is considered a useful investigation. However, it is not uniformly used because all patients receive bisphosphonates, making the measurement of BMD irrelevant in therapeutic decision making. Details of various imaging modalities and their roles in myeloma diagnostics are described in Table 85-6.

Magnetic resonance imaging, computed tomography (CT), and positron emission tomography (PET) are increasingly used in MM patients. MRI allows assessment of the degree of BM involvement and judges involvement of the spinal cord. One-third of the patients have generalized hyperintensity on MRI of the skeleton, another third predominantly have focal lesions in the background of low level of BM involvement, and the another third have a mixed picture with focal lesions in the background of generalized involvement of the BM. MRI is indicated in all patients with a suspected diagnosis of solitary plasmacytoma and is indicated in SMM to identify any focal BM involvement. Identification of multiple lesions not observed on a skeletal survey allows prediction of progression and early intervention.

In symptomatic myeloma, MRI can be considered as routine evaluation to detect unsuspected focal lesions; assess the extent of involvement of the BM, especially in the spine and pelvis; and explore the possibility of cord compression. MRI is an important investigation in patients with nonsecretory myeloma and becomes a critical investigation to evaluate response. Normalization of MRI findings after achieving CR is a good prognostic feature and is being considered as one of the features to better define CR.

Computed tomography scans have been used to evaluate focal lesions and obtain fine-needle biopsy for cytologic analysis. CT scans provide a better picture of the bone component and can also be used

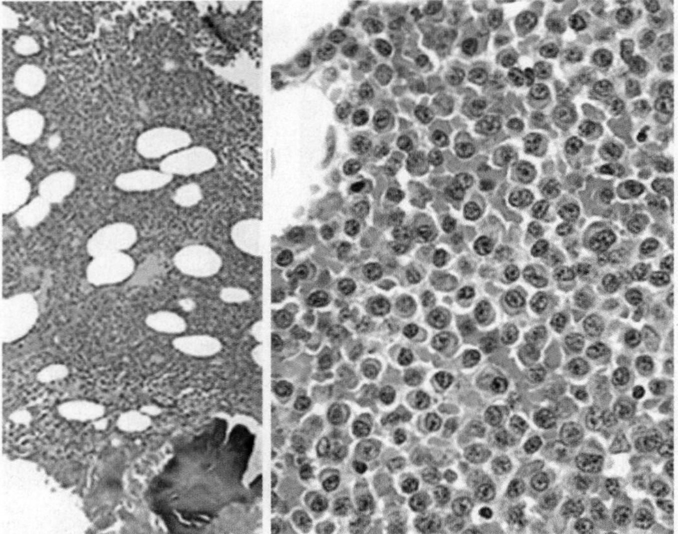

Figure 85-8 SOLITARY PLASMACYTOMA OF BONE. Bone biopsy from a 50-year-old male patient with a solitary bone lesion in the humerus. The biopsy shows some bone destruction and sheets of plasma cells which by in situ hybridization for κ and λ light-chain mRNA were found to be clonally restricted.

to judge the integrity of the bone. PET along with CT scans can be used to define the extramedullary disease as well as medullary lesions and complements MRI for follow-up of patients with nonsecretory myeloma (Fig. 85-10). Conversion of PET positivity to negativity has prognostic significance. In one prospective study in 192 patients, the presence at baseline of at least three focal lesions detected by PET/CT, a standardized uptake value (SUV) greater than 4.2, and extramedullary disease adversely affected 4-year estimates of progression-free survival (PFS; ≥3 FLs: 50%; SUV >4.2: 43%; presence of EMD: 28%) and SUV greater than 4.2 and EMD also correlated with shorter OS (4-year OS rates: 77% and 66%, respectively). In this study, post-therapy persistence of PET positivity predicted for poor outcome as compared with those with negative PET/CT (PFS, 66%; OS, 89%).

Renal Function

A serum creatinine greater than 173 mmol/L is considered to represent end-organ damage. Because absolute creatinine values do not incorporate the patient's age it may underrepresent the extent of renal dysfunction. There has been consideration of using the creatinine clearance as a more optimal diagnostic criteria. Because myeloma patients are older and have other comorbidities such as diabetes and hypertension that by themselves also affect renal function, it is necessary to establish the relationship between renal dysfunction and the plasma cell disorder (e.g., the presence of Bence Jones proteinuria may be required to support such a relationship). In the absence of Bence Jones proteinuria, a renal biopsy may be necessary. This may be even more critical in patients who otherwise fit the criteria for MGUS or SMM but have renal dysfunction. It is important to note that a renal biopsy is not required for everyone but only when the physician is uncertain as to the cause of the renal dysfunction. A biopsy is not currently required for light-chain cast nephropathy if Bence Jones protein is present as the predominant urinary protein. Other causes of renal dysfunction should be considered before attributing renal dysfunction to myeloma.

Hemogram and Serum Calcium

A standard hemogram is performed to detect anemia. The level of anemia considered to be diagnostic for myeloma is hemoglobin

Table 85-5 Diagnostic Criteria for Multiple Myeloma, Myeloma Variants, and Monoclonal Gammopathy of Unknown Significance

Monoclonal Gammopathy of Undetermined Significance or Monoclonal Gammopathy, Unattributed/Unassociated
M protein in serum <30 g/L
Bone marrow clonal plasma cells <10%
No evidence of other B-cell proliferative disorders
No myeloma related organ or tissue impairment (no end-organ damage, including bone lesions)
Asymptomatic Myeloma (Smoldering Myeloma)
M protein in serum >30 g/L *or*
Bone marrow clonal plasma cell ≥10%
No related organ or tissue impairment (no end-organ damage, including bone lesions) or symptoms
Symptomatic Multiple Myeloma
M protein in serum or urine*
Bone marrow (clonal) plasma cells* or plasmacytoma
Related organ or tissue impairment (end-organ damage, including bone lesions)
Solitary Plasmacytoma of Bone
No M protein in serum or urine†
Single area of bone destruction caused by clonal plasma cells
Bone marrow not consistent with MM
Normal skeletal survey (and MRI of spine and pelvis if done)
No related organ or tissue impairment (no end-organ damage other than solitary bone lesion)†
Nonsecretory Myeloma
No M protein in serum or urine with immunofixation
Bone marrow clonal plasmacytosis ≥10% or plasmacytoma
Related organ or tissue impairment (end-organ damage, including bone lesions)
Extramedullary Plasmacytoma
No M protein in serum or urine†
Extramedullary tumor of clonal plasma cells
Normal bone marrow
Normal skeletal survey
No related organ or tissue impairment (end organ-damage including bone lesions)
Multiple Solitary Plasmacytomas (± Recurrent)
No M protein in serum or urine†
More than one localized area of bone destruction or extramedullary tumor of clonal plasma cells, which may be recurrent
Normal bone marrow
Normal skeletal survey and MRI of spine and pelvis if done
No related organ or tissue impairment (no end-organ damage other than the localized bone lesions)
Myeloma-Related Organ or Tissue Impairment (End-Organ Damage)
Calcium levels increased: serum calcium >0-25 mmol/L above the upper limit of normal or >2-75 mmol/L
Renal insufficiency: creatinine >173 mmol/L
Anemia: hemoglobin 2 g/dL below the lower limit of normal or hemoglobin <10 g/dL
Bone lesions: lytic lesions or osteoporosis with compression fractures (MRI or CT may clarify)
Other: symptomatic hyperviscosity, amyloidosis, recurrent bacterial infections (more than two episodes in 12 months)

CT, Computed tomography; *MM,* multiple myeloma; *MRI,* magnetic resonance imaging.
*If flow cytometry is performed, most plasma cells (>90%) will show a neoplastic phenotype.
†A small M component may sometimes be present.

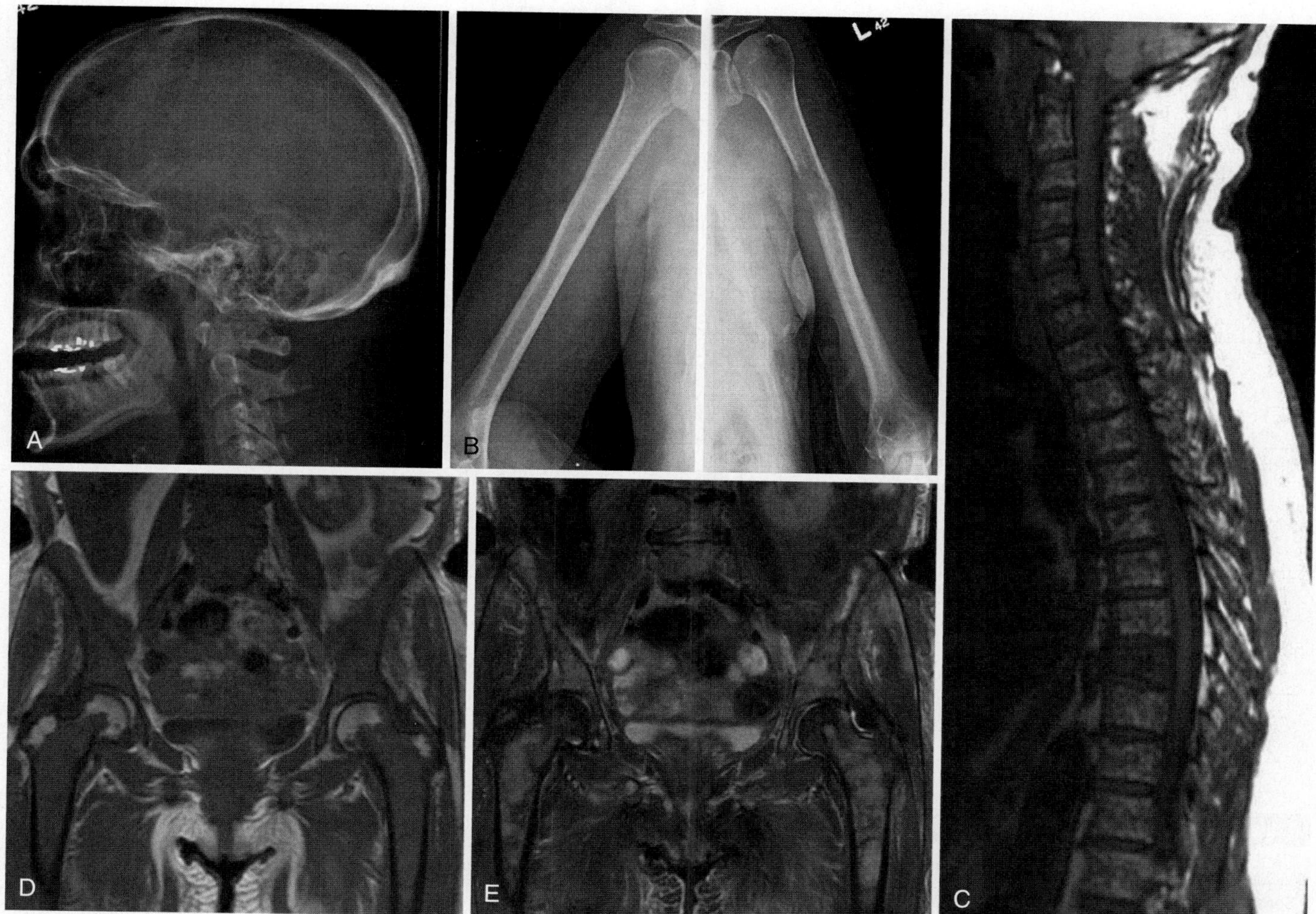

Figure 85-9 **A** and **B,** Typical skeletal changes on radiography. Example of "punched-out" lytic lesions in the skull and humerus. **C** to **E,** Magnetic resonance imaging pattern in multiple myeloma in the spine and pelvis showing diffuse involvement with focal lesions. *(Courtesy Dr. Nikhil Ramaiya, MD.)*

2 g/dL below the lower limit of normal or the patient's baseline or hemoglobin below 10 g/dL. It is necessary to exclude other causes of anemia. Circulating plasma cells are frequently observed in patients with MM. Serum calcium is measured and corrected for albumin, or in occasional cases ionized calcium is considered.

PROGNOSIS

Myeloma is a heterogeneous disease with 20% of patients having a survival time of less than 2 years, but more than 15% of patients have more than a 10-year survival time. Therefore, it is critically important to identify disease features that may allow identification of low- versus high-risk disease to better tailor therapeutic intervention. Moreover, such risk stratification permits the physician to predict life expectancy and allows development of strategies to evaluate the results of clinical trials. Various prognostic variables have been identified, including tumor burden–related factors such as β_2-microglobulin, more than three lytic bone lesions, hypercalcemia, and soluble IL-6 receptor; tumor biology–related factors such as cytogenetic or FISH-identified abnormalities, genomic changes, plasma cell–labeling index, IgA myeloma, C-reactive protein (CRP) and lactate dehydrogenase (LDH); tumor microenvironment–related factors such as BM microvessel density, serum soluble syndecan-1 levels, soluble CD16, and BM plasmacytoid DC number; patient-related factors such as age, renal failure, albumin, and performance status; and finally, treatment-related factors such as achieving CR or a very good partial response and the performance of tandem autologous transplants.

Among these features, the international staging system using serum albumin and β_2-microglobulin levels; cytogenetic or FISH changes, and newer genomic correlates of outcome have been validated in a number of studies and are considered the standard of care as predictive markers in myeloma. A short list of investigations to be performed for risk stratification of MM patients is detailed in Table 85-7.[22]

International Staging System

The International Staging System (ISS) described in Table 85-8 uses simple chemical tests (serum albumin and β_2-microglobulin) to predict outcome.[23] ISS staging is able to predict both event-free survival (EFS) and OS (Fig. 85-11) and is valid irrespective of age, geographic region, study site, standard or HDT, method of albumin measurement, and use of novel agents. Although it is universally applicable, it does not include the genetic makeup of the myeloma cells and thus lacks an important consideration that drives the disease process.

Cytogenetics and Fluorescent in Situ Hybridization

By conventional cytogenetics, detection of any abnormality is considered to predict an adverse outcome. Of course, the recurrent chromosomal changes, t(4;14), t(14;16), as well as loss of 13q34 and 17p13 identified using traditional cytogenetic methods carry a poor

Table 85-6 Imaging Modalities for Disease Assessment in Myeloma

	Use	Sensitivity and Specificity	False-Negative Test Results	False-Positive Test Results
Bone scan	Not useful as a screening tool	Vary	Pure osteolytic lesions	Trauma Inflammation Benign tumor Healing
Radiography	Skeletal survey is used for standard work up of myeloma Assesses risk of fracture Useful to detect progression but not useful to determine tumor response	Low sensitivity	Low disease burden Osteopenia	Trauma Inflammation Benign tumor Healing
CT	For anatomic detail in axial skeleton Possible follow-up of tumor response especially in extramedullary disease	High sensitivity	Low disease burden	Trauma Inflammation Benign tumor Healing
MRI	Detection of spinal cord compression Can help distinguish benign from malignant vertebral compression fracture Useful to assess response and progression, especially in non-secretory myeloma	High sensitivity and specificity	Diffuse marrow infiltration	Edema
PET/CT	Useful for extramedullary disease Possible follow-up of tumor response	High specificity	Low disease burden in marrow only	After chemotherapy
Bone density	Measures osteoporosis Response to bisphosphonates	High specificity and sensitivity		Age-related osteoporosis

CT, Computed tomography; *MM*, multiple myeloma; *MRI*, magnetic resonance imaging; *PET*, positron emission tomography.

Table 85-7 Risk Stratification in Multiple Myeloma

Investigation Recommended for Risk Stratification
Serum albumin and β_2-microglobulin to determine ISS stage
BM examination for t(4;14); t(14;16) and del(17p) on identified PC by FISH
LDH
Immunoglobulin type: IgA
Histology: plasmablastic disease or plasma cell leukemia
Additional Investigation for Risk Stratification
Cytogenetics
Gene expression profiling
Labeling index
MRI or PET
DNA copy number alteration by CGH/SNP array

BM, Bone marrow; *CGH*, comparative genomic hydridization; *FISH*, fluorescent in situ hybridization; *ISS*, International Staging System; *MRI*, magnetic resonance imaging; *PC*, plasma cells; *PET*, spositron emission tomography; *SNP*, single nucleotide polymorphism.

Table 85-8 International Staging System of Multiple Myeloma Patients

Stage	Criteria	Median Survival (mo)
I	Serum β_2 microglobulin <3.5 mg/L	62
	Serum albumin ≥3.5 g/dL	
II*	Not stage I or III	44
III	Serum β_2 microglobulin ≥5.5 mg/L	29

Data from Greipp PR, San Miguel J, Durie BG, et al: International staging system for multiple myeloma. *J Clin Oncol* 23:3412, 2005.
*There are two categories for stage II: serum β_2 microglobulin <3.5 mg/L but serum albumin <3.5 g/dL; or serum β_2-microglobulin 3.5 to <5.5 mg/L irrespective of the serum albumin level.

prognosis. Hyperdiploidy and t(11;14) translocations detected by cytogenetics have been reported in some studies to predict a favorable outcome.

As described earlier, because of a low proliferative index, cytogenetic abnormalities are only detected in a small number of patients, and interphase FISH is used to detect specific genetic aberrations. Among these abnormalities, patients with t(4;14) (15% of the patients) have a poor prognosis. In some early studies, use of bortezomib and lenalidomide has been shown to at least partly overcome poor risk associated with this abnormality. The del(17p) observed in 8% to 10% of the patients remains a poor risk feature not overcome by novel agent–based therapies.[3] Although the p53 gene resides in this region of deletion, a clear biological confirmation of its role is lacking. p53 mutations have only been detected in very small number of patients. In patients without t(4;14) or del(17p), the presence of del13 is not considered to predict a poor outcome (Fig. 85-12). Moreover, the presence of del13 observed in patients with MGUS and SMM without clear correlation with clinical outcome also raises questions about the role of del13 in myeloma progression and prognosis. As shown in Table 85-1, newer additional chromosomal changes are being identified with clinical correlation; gains of chromosome 1q, and loss of 1p are two such regions which are considered to predict a poor outcome. Additional studies are needed to confirm their significance.

High-Throughput Genomic Studies

Further analysis of genomic changes that drive the disease process has been performed using the high-throughput microarrays profiling techniques. Copy number alterations (CNAs) have been studied using either SNP[6] or CGH[7] arrays, and expression of genes has been evaluated using the expression profile arrays covering the whole expressed genome. These studies have correlated with clinical outcomes in myeloma.

The IFM-DFCI collaborative group has evaluated CNAs and correlated with survival outcomes in 192 newly diagnosed patients with

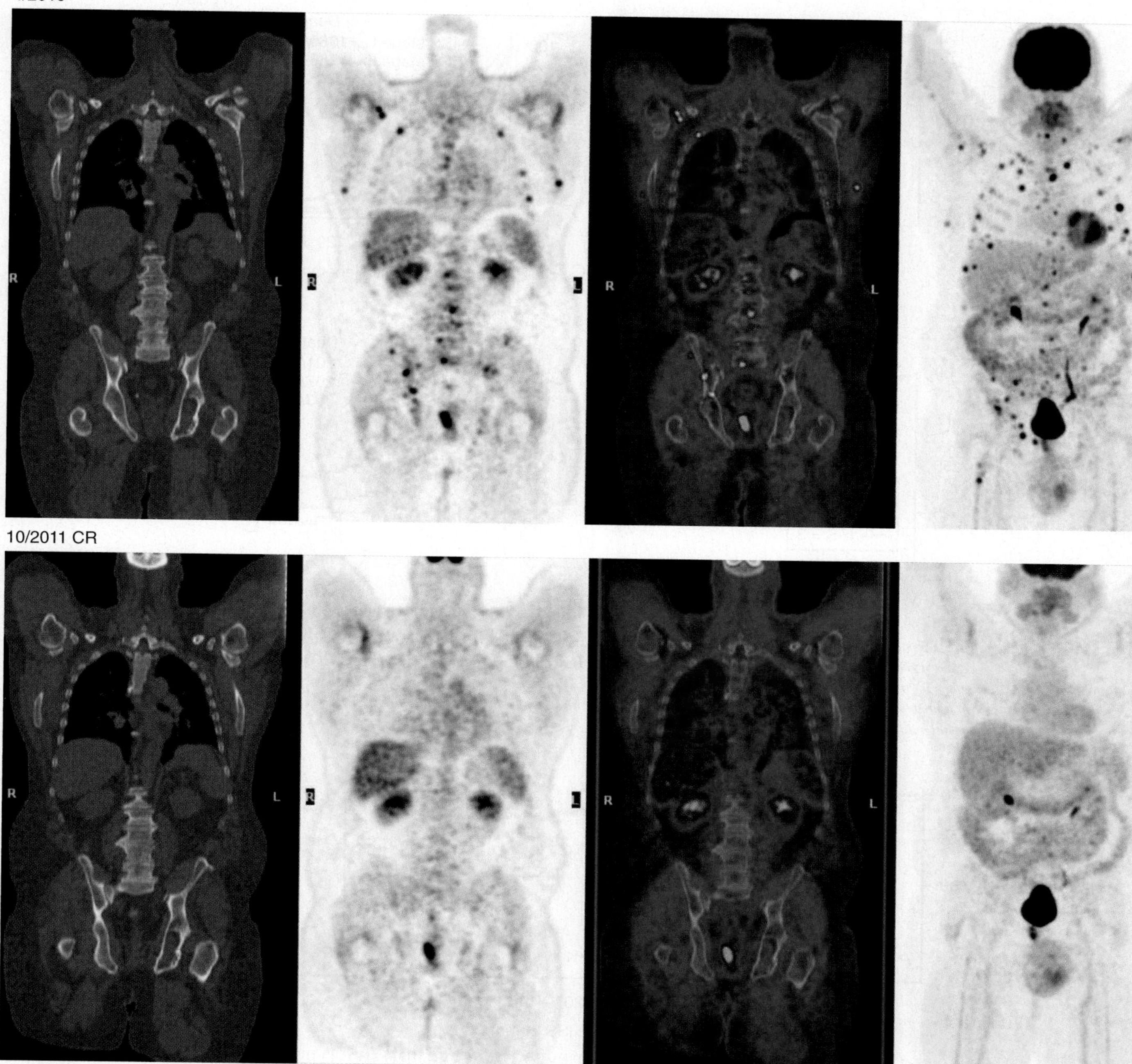

Figure 85-10 POSITRON EMISSION TOMOGRAPHY/COMPUTED TOMOGRAPHY SCAN SHOWING MULTIPLE FDG-AVID LESIONS IN THE SKELETON *(UPPER PANEL)* WITH THEIR RESOLUTION ON ACHIEVING COMPLETE REMISSION (CR) *(LOWER PANEL)*. The images are CT in the *first row,* PET rear view in the *second row,* fusion of CT and PET in the *third row,* and PET front view in the *last row.*

MM who were uniformly treated. A univariate analysis identified amplifications of 1q and deletions of 1p, 12p, 14q, 16q, and 22q to be associated with a poor prognosis, but amplifications of chromosomes 5, 9, 11, 15, and 19 conferred a superior outcome. A multivariate analysis identified amp(1q23.3), amp(5q31.3), and del(12p13.31) as the most significant independent adverse markers (*P* <.0001). This model has been further validated in an independent cohort of 273 patients, confirming the utility of SNP profiling for prognostication.[6]

Using gene expression profiling, a 70-gene model has been proposed by the UAMS group.[24] This signature for survival identifies three groups of patients with high-, intermediate-, and low-risk disease and has been applied across various groups. Similarly, a 15-gene model is proposed by the IFM group classifying patients into two risk groups.[25] Interestingly, there is no common gene between the two models. This can be explained by differences in the treatment in different patient groups, differences in the platform used and is more likely caused by the redundancy and overlapping functions of the genes regulating various pathways. Both of the models have been better at identifying poor-risk patients. A larger scale study incorporating various genomic correlates in the future will be required to identify and validate signatures that can identify risk categories and hopefully response to therapies.

DIFFERENTIAL DIAGNOSIS

The diagnosis of MM is essentially based on laboratory results. No single or group of symptoms is pathognomonic of MM. A significant

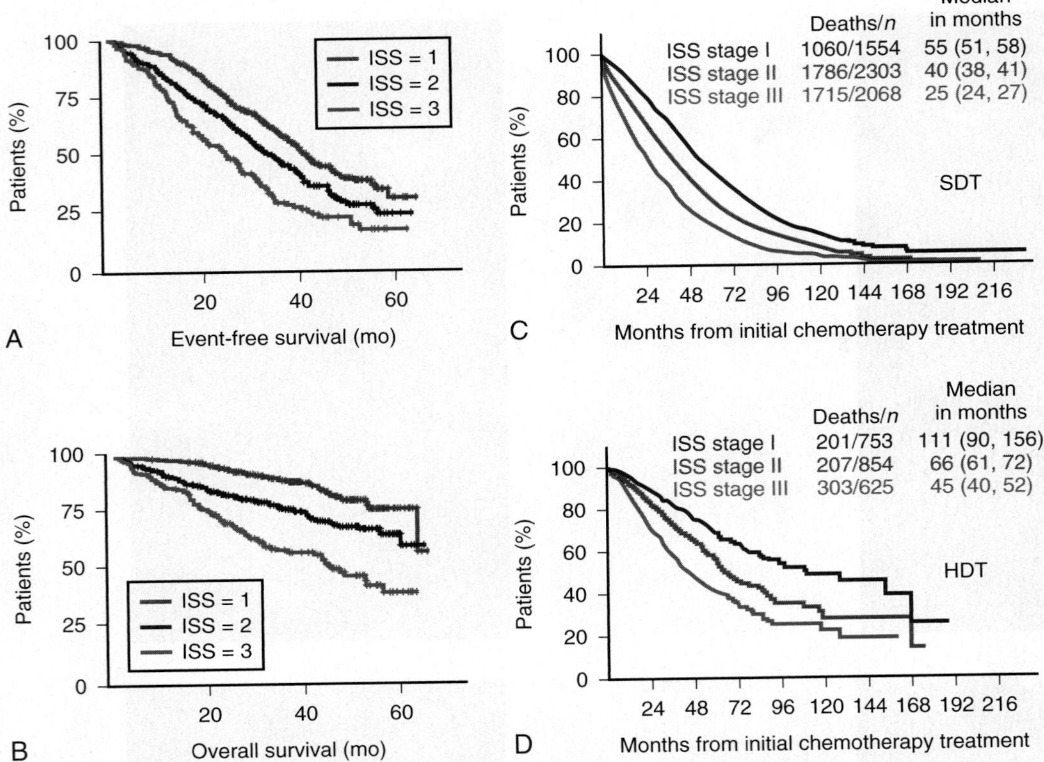

Figure 85-11 International Staging System (ISS) predicts both event-free survival **(A)** and overall survival **(B)** and overall survival with both standard-dose therapy (SDT) **(C)** and high-dose therapy (HDT) **(D)**. *(A and B from Avet-Loiseau H, Attal M, Moreau P, et al: Genetic abnormalities and survival in multiple myeloma: The experience of the Intergroupe Francophone du Myélome.* Blood *109:3489, 2007; C and D from Greipp PR, San Miguel J, Durie BG, et al: International staging system for multiple myeloma.* J Clin Oncol *23:3412, 2005.)*

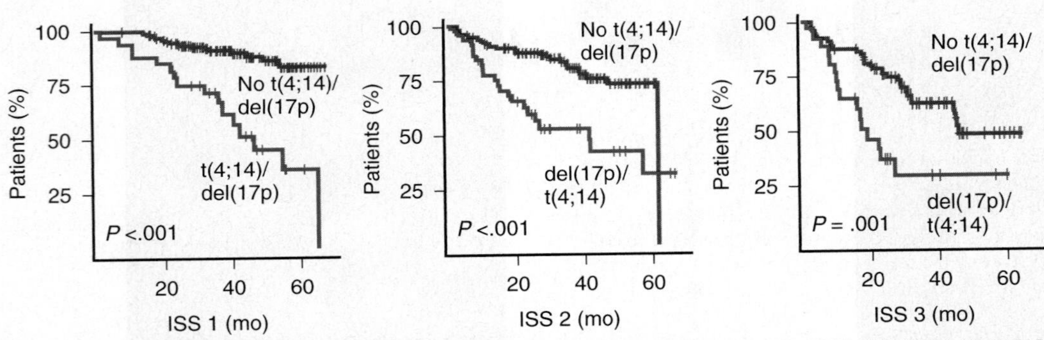

Figure 85-12 KAPLAN-MEIER ESTIMATES OF SURVIVAL ACCORDING TO THE INTERNATIONAL STAGING SYSTEM (ISS) STAGES AND t(4;14) OR del(17p). Overall survival (in months). *Blue lines* indicate patients presenting t(4;14) or del(17p); *red lines* indicate those lacking the aberrations. *(From Avet-Loiseau H, Attal M, Moreau P, et al: Genetic abnormalities and survival in multiple myeloma: The experience of the Intergroupe Francophone du Myélome.* Blood *109:3489, 2007.)*

number of patients remain asymptomatic, and the diagnosis is usually delayed. Most frequently, in a relatively asymptomatic patient, the investigation is carried out because of increased total protein levels, proteinuria, renal dysfunction, or bone pain. An older patient with any of these features or unexplained back pain, anemia, or recurrent infection should be screened for myeloma. Unexplained and marked elevation of an erythrocyte sedimentation rate also warrants an investigation for a diagnosis of plasma cell disorder. The diagnosis is based on two steps: first, the detection of a monoclonal protein and monoclonal plasma cells, and second, identification of end-organ damage. This is essential to differentiate early stage plasma cell disorders such as MGUS or SMM from active symptomatic myeloma. When a diagnosis of MM is suspected, investigations are carried out as detailed in Table 85-9. Evaluation for a monoclonal protein includes electrophoresis of serum proteins as well as 24-hour urine collection and serum-free light-chain measurements. Both serum protein electrophoresis and quantitative immunoglobulins are required to quantitate, and an immunofixation is important at the time of diagnosis to identify the type of paraprotein present. The BM is examined for the presence of clonal plasma cell mainly by histology but also importantly by immunostaining or flow cytometry using κ/λ staining. Determination and quantitation of clonal plasma cells is required to differentiate SMM from MGUS. Detailed investigation to look for organ damage is then undertaken to look for bony lesions, renal dysfunction, anemia, and hypercalcemia. In patients in whom hyperviscosity is suspected, in addition to measuring serum viscosity, a funduscopic examination is useful. Detailed diagnostic criteria are summarized in Table 85-5.[21]

Table 85-9 Evaluation of Multiple Myeloma Patients

Evaluation for Diagnosis Evaluation for Monoclonal Protein
Serum protein electrophoresis, immunofixation
Quantitative immunoglobulin by nephelometric method
24-hour urine collection for electrophoresis and Bence Jones protein assessment and immunofixation
Serum-free light chain and ratio
Evaluation for Clonal Plasma Cells
BM aspirate and biopsy for
Histology
Clonality by immunostaining or flow cytometry by κ/λ staining
Fine-needle aspiration of plasmacytoma if indicated
Evaluation for end-organ damage
Hemogram to detect anemia
Chemistry panel for renal function and calcium
Radiologic evaluation: skeletal survey
MRI as indicated for confirmation
Evaluation for risk stratification
β_2-microglobulin and serum albumin for ISS stage
Cytogenetics and FISH on BM sample
LDH
CRP
Other Investigations for Selected Patients
Abdominal fat pad or rectal biopsy for amyloid
Solitary lytic lesion biopsy
Serum viscosity if IgM component or high IgA levels or serum M-component >7 g/dL
Immunofixation for IgD or IgE in select cases

BM, Bone marrow; *CRP,* C-reactive protein; *FISH,* fluorescent in situ hybridization; *Ig,* immunoglobulin; *ISS,* International Staging System; *LDH,* lactate dehydrogenase; *MRI,* magnetic resonance imaging.

TREATMENT

Treatment of underlying plasma cell dyscrasias is warranted when organ or tissue function is compromised. The damage to the organ or functional impairment could be caused by the underlying plasma cell clone or related to the monoclonal protein. The acronym CRAB (hypercalcemia, renal impairment, anemia, and bone disease) is helpful in this regard. Symptomatic hyperviscosity, amyloidosis, monoclonal immunoglobulin deposition disease, recurrent bacterial infections (more than two major infections), and progressive peripheral neuropathy are also indications for initiation of treatment. The constellation of polyneuropathy, organomegaly, endocrinopathy, monoclonal gammopathy and the skin changes in the setting of osteosclerotic myeloma (POEMS syndrome) may present a challenging diagnosis but is always an indication for treatment.

Monoclonal Gammopathy of Unknown Significance and Smoldering Multiple Myeloma

MGUS is characterized by serum paraprotein below 3 g/dL and BM plasmacytosis below 10% and absence of amyloidosis, a solitary plasmacytoma, Waldenström macroglobulinemia, or a B-cell lymphoproliferative disorder. The diagnosis of MGUS is often incidental when a serum or urine protein electrophoresis and immunofixation are ordered as a part of a battery of tests. The test may have been ordered for evaluation of elevated globulin in the serum, proteinuria, peripheral neuropathy, osteoporosis, immune disorders, or hypogammaglobulinemia.[26,27] The rate of progression of MGUS to MM is 1% per year. These patients can be further risk stratified based on serum M spike level less than 1.5 g/dL, IgG isotype and a normal serum free light-chain ratio (Fig. 85-13). The presence of all of these factors would be low risk with only a 2% chance for progression at 20 years

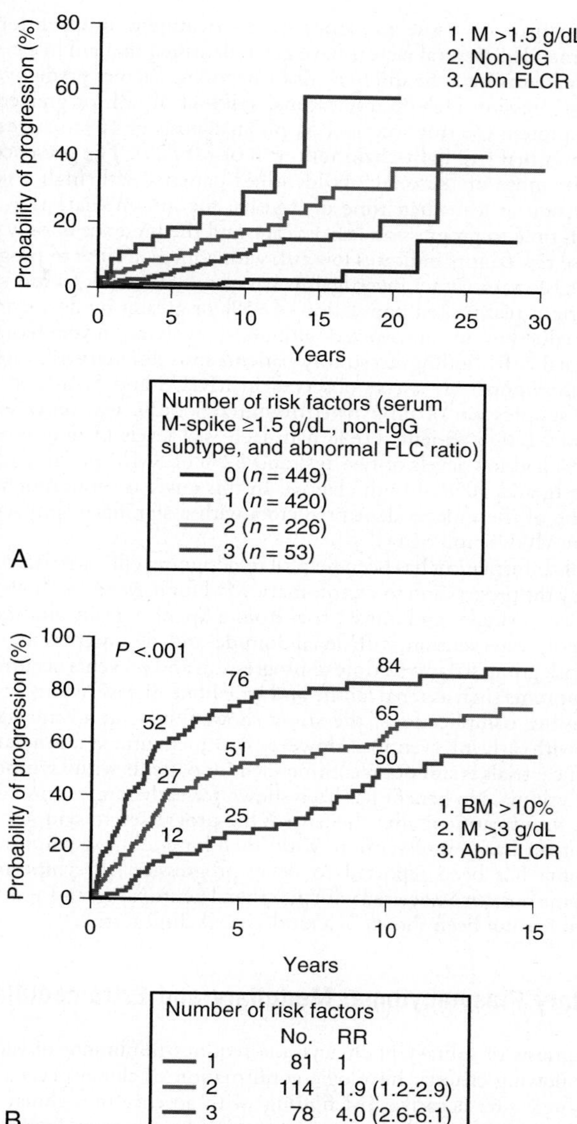

Figure 85-13 KAPLAN-MEIER ESTIMATES OF LIKELIHOOD OF PROGRESSION TO MYELOMA FROM MONOCLONAL GAMMOPATHY OF UNKNOWN SIGNIFICANCE (MGUS) **(A)** OR SMOLDERING MULTIPLE MYELOMA (SMM) **(B).** Estimates are based on risk features identified in MGUS (M spike >1.5 gm/dL, non–immunoglobulin G [IgG] paraprotein, and abnormal [Abn] free light-chain ratio [FLCR]); and in SMM (bone marrow [BM] with >10% plasma cells, M spike >3.0 g/dL, and Abn FLCR). *RR,* Relative risk.

after eliminating competing causes of death. If one of these factors is abnormal, patients will fall into low-intermediate-risk category with 10% absolute risk of progression to myeloma at 20 years. The presence of two abnormal factors will place the patients into high-intermediate-risk group; their absolute risk of progression to MM is 18% at 20 years. Finally, when all three risk factors are abnormal, the patient falls into the high-risk category with an absolute risk of progression of 27% at 20 years.

Asymptomatic myeloma (SMM) is characterized by BM plasmacytosis of 10% or greater or serum paraprotein of 3 g/dL or greater.[26] Asymptomatic myeloma is often diagnosed after a workup for elevated total protein in the serum, proteinuria, or borderline anemia. It may also be discovered incidentally like MGUS. It has been shown that every case of MM is preceded by detection of paraprotein for a minimum of 2 years or more. The rate of progression to MM is 10% per year for the first 5 years, 3% per year for the next 5 years, and 1% per year after 10 years. Because the patient has no symptoms or related organ or tissue impairment, no treatment intervention is recommended. Several factors have been identified that aid in categorizing patients into the different risk categories. Factors predictive of early progression include monoclonal spike of 30 g/L or greater on serum protein electrophoresis, BM plasmacytosis of 10% or greater, and abnormal free light-chain ratio (>8 or <0.125). The presence of three or more of these factors identifies patients with high risk to progression at a median time of 2 years; for intermediate risk, the median time to progression is five years; and the presence of only one of these risk factors indicates low risk with a median time to progression of 10 years. Other investigators have used other risk factors such as aberrant plasma cell population of 95% or greater by flow cytometry, reduction in uninvolved globulins, evolving myeloma, and abnormal MRI findings to stratify patients into different risk categories. Immunoparesis is also observed in MGUS and SMM. In one study, suppression of uninvolved immunoglobulin was observed in 25% of MGUS patients (18% had decreased levels of only one Ig, and 7% had low levels of two Igs) and 52% of SMM patients (22% of one Ig and 30% of both chains). In this analysis, immunoparesis was one of the independent predictors with a significant impact on PFS in MGUS and SMM.

This information has been helpful in designing clinical trials to try to delay the progression to symptomatic MM for patients in a high-risk category. A single randomized trial from a Spanish group has shown that early intervention with lenalidomide and dexamethasone in a high-risk group delays the time to progression and prevents occurrence of symptoms such as renal failure and lytic bone disease. Moreover, by preventing complications, the study showed survival advantage for those with early intervention. However, treatment intervention outside of clinical trials is still not recommended for patients with asymptomatic myeloma. No benefit has been shown for early intervention compared with treatment after the patient has progressed to symptomatic myeloma. Early intervention with thalidomide in asymptomatic myeloma has been reported to delay progression to symptomatic myeloma but was associated with peripheral neuropathy, and a survival benefit has not been shown in a randomized clinical trial.

Solitary Plasmacytoma: Medullary and Extramedullary

A diagnosis of solitary plasmacytoma requires fulfillment of each of the following criteria: histologic confirmation of clonal plasma cells at a single site; negative BM findings with absence of a clonal plasmacytosis; no distant bone involvement; and no anemia, hypercalcemia, or renal impairment. The solitary plasma cytoma could present as a single site of bony lesion (medullary) or in soft tissue outside of the bone (extramedullary). Solitary plasmacytoma of the bone is 40% more common than extramedullary soft tissue plasmacytoma. Solitary plasmacytoma of the bone is most commonly encountered in the axial skeleton (skull, spine, pelvis, ribs, and sternum), accounting for 80% of the cases; the upper and lower extremities account for 15% of the cases. Extramedullary soft tissue plasma cytomas are often associated with mucosal area of the upper aerodigestive passages (80%).

Solitary plasmacytomas are rather uncommon and account for 6% of plasma cell neoplasms. The incidence rate is 0.3 per 100,000 person years in the United States. Similar to MM, the incidence of solitary plasmacytoma increases with age; however, the median age of diagnosis was 62 years for extramedullary plasmacytomas and 65 years for solitary bone plasmacytoma compared with a median age of onset of 69 years for MM in the Surveillance, Epidemiology and End Results (SEER) database. The incidence of solitary plasmacytoma has increased by 10% from 1999 to 2004 relative to 1992 to 2008; the incidence of MM has declined by 3% during the same period.

Patients presenting with solitary plasmacytomas require a complete workup to confirm the diagnosis. They should undergo serum protein electrophoresis, serum immunofixation, serum-free light-chain assay, urine protein electrophoresis, urine immunofixation, a diagnostic BM aspiration and biopsy with flow cytometry to detect clonal plasma cells and detailed skeletal imaging that should include either a PET-CT or a skeletal survey and MRI of the spine and pelvis. One-third of the patients may present with a detectable monoclonal paraprotein in the serum, urine, or both. Persistence of the monoclonal paraprotein after local treatment is predictive of a recurrence of MM. Patients with less than 10% plasma cells in the BM biopsy may be managed for the solitary lesion initially. However, these patients will also progress to MM over the subsequent years of follow-up.

Solitary plasmacytomas are generally treated with local radiation therapy at a dose of 40 to 50 Gy. Depending on the location, small extramedullary soft tissue plasmacytomas may be treated with excision biopsy alone. Solitary plasmacytomas of the bone may require surgical intervention for stabilization followed by local radiation therapy.

The disease-free survival at 10 years is 63% for the entire population of solitary plasmacytomas in the SEER database. The disease-specific survival seemed to plateau at about 80% for extramedullary plasmacytomas compared with 50% for solitary bone plasmacytoma. Less than one-third of solitary extramedullary plasmacytoma patients died of myeloma compared with 58% of the patients with solitary bone plasmacytomas. Progression to myeloma generally occurs within 5 years from initial diagnosis. Patients presenting with medullary plasmacytomas, patients with persistence of a monoclonal paraprotein after treatment for the solitary plasmacytoma, patients with detectable low levels of clonal plasma cells in the BM, patients between 40 and 60 years of age, and patients of African American descent are at higher risk for progression to myeloma. These patients need to be followed closely for the next 5 years.

Symptomatic Myeloma

Patients presenting with symptoms caused by myeloma tumor mass such as anemia, lytic bone disease, hypercalcemia, or renal impairment (CRAB) require systemic therapy. In addition, patients with a low tumor mass but presenting with organ dysfunction caused by a paraprotein or immunodeficiency, such as monoclonal immunoglobulin deposition disease or amyloidosis of an organ, progressive peripheral neuropathy, two are more serious infections (pneumonia, bacteremia) related organ or tissue impairment (ROTI) also warrants initiation of systemic therapy.[21]

Front-line therapy for MM is often predicated on whether patient is eligible, willing, and able to proceed with HDT and SCT. The treatment given before stem cell harvest and transplantation is called induction therapy followed by consolidation with HDT and stem cell rescue. Patients not embarking on HDT are started on initial therapy for 9 to 18 months. Both groups of patients may subsequently receive maintenance therapy.

Induction Regimen and Initial Treatment

Four classes of drugs are frequently used for the treatment of patients with MM: (1) cytotoxic drugs targeting the DNA (melphalan, cyclophosphamide, carmustine [BCNU], doxorubicin, etoposide, cisplatin), and antimitotic agent vincristine), (2) glucocorticoids, (3) immunomodulatory agents (thalidomide and lenalidomide), and (4) proteasome inhibitors (bortezomib). The first two classes of drugs are considered standard chemotherapy because they have been available since the early 1960s. The latter two are called novel agents as they became available in the mid 2000s.

STANDARD CHEMOTHERAPY TREATMENTS

Chemotherapy With Stem Cell–Sparing Agents

Patients considered for stem cell harvest are generally treated with combinations that are stem-cell sparing. Before immunomodulatory agents and proteasome inhibitors became widely available, patients were treated with pulsed dexamethasone alone or in combination with vincristine and Adriamycin (VAD) and cyclophosphamide (CVAD or CVAMP [methylprednisolone substituted for dexamethasone]).

Dexamethasone

Glucocorticoids induce apoptosis in myeloma cells. Glucocorticoids induce IkB production, which then sequesters nuclear factor kappa-B (NFκB), resulting in downregulation of IL-6 and production of other inflammatory cytokines. Dexamethasone 40 mg is administered in a pulsed fashion for 4 days, starting on days 1, 9, and 17 for the first cycle. Some studies have continued this dose and schedule every 35 days, and others have given dexamethasone on days 1 to 4, every other cycle, on a 28-day schedule. Results achieved with pulsed dexamethasone alone compare well against VAD chemotherapy and melphalan and prednisone (MP), with equivalent response rate and OS. Single-agent dexamethasone is no longer advocated as a treatment for newly diagnosed myeloma. However, under selected clinical situations, the use of pulsed dexamethasone is helpful in specific situations, including severe spinal cord compromise, hypercalcemia, and acute renal failure caused by light-chain nephropathy. While patients are on intensive dexamethasone, close monitoring for hyperglycemia and prophylaxis against bacterial, *Pneumocystis carinii* pneumonia, and fungal infection is recommended. Weight gain, mood swings, insomnia, fluid retention, proximal myopathy, and steroids psychosis are known side effects. Cataracts, osteoporosis, and the avascular necrosis of the hips are some of the long-term consequences of steroid exposure.

Vincristine, Adriamycin, and Dexamethasone

Infusional therapy with vincristine and Adriamycin with pulsed dexamethasone is an effective stem cell–sparing induction regimen. Vincristine and doxorubicin were administered by continuous infusion at the doses of 0.4 mg/day and 9 mg/m^2/day along with oral dexamethasone 40 mg/day for 4 days. After 6 to 9 cycles of VAD chemotherapy, the overall response rate (ORR) was 45% to 55%, and the complete response rate was less than 5%. There was no difference in the median PFS (18 months) or OS (3 years) compared with standard alkylating agent treatments (MP, VMCP/VBAP, VBMCP). However, if the induction therapy is followed by consolidation with high-dose melphalan and autologous SCT, substantial improvement in the PFS and OS was observed. Hair loss and the need for catheter placement to administer these vesicant agents have been important limitations on its acceptance by the patients. It is also possible to administer the daily dose of vincristine and Adriamycin as an intravenous push without loss of efficacy or increased toxicity.

Chemotherapy With Alkylating Agents

Alkylating agents melphalan and cyclophosphamide were introduced in the management of MM in the early 1960s. Since the time of introduction, they continue to play a vital role in the treatment of patients with myeloma.

Melphalan and prednisone has been the gold standard of treatment. All new combinations are benchmarked against MP. MP has been given in different doses and schedules for a minimum of 9 to 18 months. Other agents such as cyclophosphamide, carmustine (BCNU), vincristine, and Adriamycin have been successfully combined with MP (VBMCP, VBAP, and so on). Combination therapies improved the response rate but did not change the OS outcomes. MP has a response rate of 50% to 60%, a PFS of 18 months, and OS of 30 to 36 months.

In the 1960s, single agent oral cyclophosphamide and oral melphalan were compared head to head in a randomized, double-blind study and were noted to have equivalent antimyeloma activity. Cyclophosphamide is less stem cell toxic than melphalan. Cyclophosphamide in high doses (2 g/msq up to 6 g/msq) followed by filgrastim has been used for stem cell mobilization, and high doses of melphalan (200 mg/msq) are routinely used as the conditioning regimen in conjunction with autologous SCT. There is a higher incidence of secondary leukemia associated with chronic melphalan therapy (17.4% at 50 months) leading to abandonment of melphalan as maintenance therapy and limiting the exposure to 1 year or less.

Novel Agents

Immunomodulatory Drugs

Thalidomide has both selective cytokine inhibitory activity (SelCID) as well as immunomodulatory (IMiD) activity. A series of compounds were derived from thalidomide: drugs with enhanced immunomodulatory activity (IMiD) or selective cytokine inhibitory activity (SelCID). Immunomodulatory drugs stimulate T-cell proliferation and IL-2 and interferon-γ production, inhibit TNF-α and IL-1β production, and increase IL-10 production by peripheral blood mononuclear cells. Both lenalidomide and pomalidomide are 100- to 1000-fold more potent than thalidomide with respect to their immunomodulatory activity. These molecules modulate the adhesion molecules expressed by the myeloma cells, thereby reducing the interaction between the myeloma cells and stromal cells; they downregulate secretion of inflammatory cytokines, including IL-6, TNF-α, and IL-1β by the stromal cells. IL-6 is a growth factor for myeloma cells. They also downregulate the secretion of VEGF and basic fibroblast growth factor (b-FGF) production by the myeloma cells and stromal cells and thereby reduce the microvessel density in the BM microenvironment. IMiDs stimulate the T lymphocytes to produce IL-2 and γ-interferon and thereby activate NK cells and CD8-positive T cells that are cytotoxic to myeloma cells.

More recently, additional insights into the mechanism of action of thalidomide and IMiDs has been gained with the discovery of thalidomide-binding protein cereblon (CRBN). Human CRBN was originally identified as a candidate gene for an autosomal recessive form of mild mental retardation and is located on chromosome 3 at 3p26.2. It encodes a 442–amino acid protein that is highly conserved from plants to humans. CRBN is widely expressed in the testes, prostate, ovary, placenta, spleen, liver, pancreas, kidneys, small intestine, colon, lungs, skeletal muscle, peripheral blood leukocyte, brain, and retina, where CRBN is located in the cytoplasm, nucleus, and peripheral membranes. Thalidomide interacts directly with CRBN and indirectly with damaged DNA-binding protein 1 (DDB1) through its interaction with CRBN. CRBN forms an E3 ubiquitin ligase complex with DDB1 and Cul4A, affecting downstream targets including interferon regulatory factor 4 (IRF4). CRBN likely plays an important role in binding, ubiquitination, and degradation of factors involved in maintaining functional myeloma cells. Drug resistance to IMiDs is associated with depletion of CRBN.

Thalidomide

Thalidomide–dexamethasone (TD) has been shown to be superior to dexamethasone alone in an international randomized phase 3 clinical trial. TD has an ORR of 63% and PFS of 14.9 months compared with 46% and 6.5 months with pulsed dexamethasone; however, there was no difference in the OS at a median follow-up of 18 months. There was no difference between TD versus VAD as a pretransplant induction regimen. Likewise, TD had a slightly inferior survival outcome compared with MP as first-line therapy in elderly patients. Thalidomide does not overcome poor prognostic genetic features. TD is no longer considered optimum treatment for newly diagnosed patients with MM. Thalidomide is generally prescribed at 200 mg/day. No maximally tolerated dose has been defined for thalidomide; doses as high as 800 mg/day have been used. Major side effects of thalidomide include irreversible peripheral neuropathy that develops after exposure for a period of 6 months or longer. Other

Treatment of Relapsed Multiple Myeloma

Ensure that the patient has a relapse requiring intervention.
- The conversion from a negative immune-fixation analysis to a positive study result is not an indication to initiate salvage therapy. A clear clinical relapse with new or increased evidence of end-organ damage or a substantial or aggressive biochemical relapse as defined by criteria for progressive disease are indications for the initiation of treatment.

Selection of treatment depends on prior therapy received.
- Lenalidomide based
  - Initial treatment with bortezomib–thalidomide
  - Underlying peripheral neuropathy
  - Lenalidomide should be used with caution in patients with renal dysfunction with appropriate dose adjustment
- Bortezomib based
  - Initial treatment with immune-modulatory agents
  - Renal dysfunction
  - Poor hematopoietic reserve
  - Prolonged response (>12 mo) to prior therapy with bortezomib
- Thalidomide based
  - Prior bortezomib–lenalidomide
  - Renal impairment
  - Poor hematopoietic reserve
- Chemotherapy with or without a novel agent combination
  - Progressed on novel agents
  - Rapid, aggressive relapse with high LDH or extramedullary plasmacytomas
- Salvage transplant
  - In transplant-eligible patients, one needs to consider if an SCT was deferred as initial therapy or if the patient had a prolonged remission (>3 years) after the first transplant or has poor hematopoietic reserve and stored stem cells. Transplant may also be considered as a way to reestablish hematopoiesis in select cases

Special considerations
- Rapid relapse, or relapse at multiple sites, or extramedullary sites: chemotherapy with or without combination therapy with a novel agent
- CNS relapse: radiation therapy for localized disease; intrathecal chemotherapy for positive CSF cytology; along with systemic therapy as indicated
- Poor performance status and hematopoietic reserve: oral therapy with low-dose daily cyclophosphamide, thalidomide, and prednisone
- Prior drug exposure and associated toxicity: consider the presence of neuropathy, cytopenias, and advanced and renal dysfunction to decide on agents, their schedules, and their doses

Entry in clinical trials

CNS, Central nervous system; *CSF,* cerebrospinal fluid; *LDH,* lactate dehydrogenase; *SCT,* stem cell transplantation.

serious side effects include DVT and pulmonary embolism when combined with dexamethasone and does require thromboprophylaxis. For patients with no additional risk factors for developing a DVT prophylaxis with a low-dose aspirin (81-100 mg) daily is adequate. Other clinically significant side effects include severe constipation, severe bradycardia, and skin rash. Results with thalidomide combinations in relapsed and newly diagnosed patients are summarized in Tables 85-10 and 11.

Thalidomide has been used in combination with other drugs in newly diagnosed MM patients. Six large randomized clinical trials have been conducted combining melphalan and prednisone with or without thalidomide. Meta-analysis of these six large studies with primary data has shown MPT to be superior to MP alone; the ORR improved by 22% (59% vs. 37%), PFS improved by 5 months (20 months vs. 15 months), and OS improved by 6 months (39 months vs. 33 months) (Table 85-12). MPT is an acceptable front-line treatment for patients older than the age of 65 years. Side effects were higher on the MPT arm. DVT occurred in 6% to 12% versus 1% to 4% of patients, peripheral neuropathy occurred in 6% to 23% of patients versus 0% to 5% of patients, and discontinuation of treatment occurred in 41% to 45% of patients versus 6% to 11% of patients with MP alone.

Thalidomide, Adriamycin, and dexamethasone (TAD) induction therapy followed by SCT and subsequent maintenance with thalidomide was noted to be superior to VAD induction followed by transplant and interferon maintenance in a large randomized trial by the HOVON.

Oral Regimens

Cyclophosphamide, thalidomide, and dexamethasone (CTD) was compared with infusional CVAD chemotherapy for patients eligible for HDT in a large multicenter, randomized phase 3 trial conducted in the United Kingdom (MRC myeloma IX trial). The CTD regimen consisted of cyclophosphamide 500 mg weekly, thalidomide 100 mg/day, and dexamethasone 40 mg for 4 days every other week. The induction chemotherapy was given for a minimum 6 cycles and up to 9 cycles or until maximum response. The postinduction ORR was significantly higher with CTD versus CVAD (82.5% vs. 71.2%; *P* <.0001); likewise complete response rates were also higher with CTD (13% vs. 8.1%; *P* = .0083). The superior response rate of CTD was maintained after autologous SCT; posttransplant CR (50% vs. 37.2%; *P* = .00052). With a median follow-up of 47 months, there was no difference in PFS or OS between the two groups. This establishes CTD as an acceptable induction therapy before transplant.

For elderly patients and patients otherwise ineligible for HDT, CTD was compared with MP. The dose of cyclophosphamide was 500 mg weekly, thalidomide was 50 mg/day, and dexamethasone was 20 mg for 4 days every other week. Both arms were oral regimens. CTD therapy was associated with a superior ORR (63.8 vs. 32.6%; *P* <.0001), and complete response rate (13.1% vs. 2.4%) and very good partial response (VGPR) (16.9% vs. 1.7%). After a median follow-up time of 44 months, PFS and OS were similar between the groups. CTD was associated with higher rates of thromboembolic events, constipation, infection, and neuropathy. This study also illustrated that thalidomide was incapable of improving the outcome of patients with unfavorable genetic markers.

Lenalidomide

Lenalidomide–dexamethasone is an effective combination therapy for the treatment of previously untreated symptomatic myeloma patients. A large open-label, phase 3 randomized trial comparing lenalidomide plus high-dose dexamethasone or lenalidomide plus weekly dexamethasone conducted by the Eastern Cooperative Oncology Group established lenalidomide and dexamethasone as a simple oral regimen that could be used as an induction therapy before transplant or as a first-line therapy without SCT. Administration of lenalidomide 25 mg/day for 3 weeks on and 1 week off along with dexamethasone 40 mg in a pulsed fashion (days 1-4, 9-12, and 17-20) for the first 4 cycles only (high-dose dexamethasone arm) gave a higher response rate of 79% compared with weekly dexamethasone 40 mg (low-dose dexamethasone arm, 60%); however, the high-dose dexamethasone arm was associated with a higher incidence of infection and venous thromboembolism and an inferior 1-year survival rate (87%) compared with the low-dose dexamethasone arm (1-year survival rate, 96%). However, with longer follow-up there was no survival difference between the two arms. Landmark analysis at 4 months has projected a 3-year survival rate of 92% for patients who electively received high-dose melphalan and SCT after 4 cycles of induction

Table 85-10 Thalidomide Regimens in Relapsed or Refractory Multiple Myeloma

Trial	Dose	Patients *(n)*	ORR (%)	Median PFS (mo)	Median OS
Barlogie[55]	100-800 mg	169	30	20% at 2 yr	48% at 2 yr
Yakoub-Agha[56]	100 mg +/– dex 400 mg +/– dex	205 195	14 18		68.8% at 1 yr 72.8% at 1 yr
Neben[57]	100-400 mg	83	20.5	45% at 1 yr	86% at 1 yr
Palumbo[58]	Thal-dex	120	51	11 mo	21 mo
Dimopoulos[59]	Thal-dex	42	55	TTP 4.2 mo	12.6 mo
Kyriakou[60]	CTD	52	79	34% at 2 yr	73% at 2 yr
Garcia-Sanz[61]	CTD	71	57	57% at 2 yr	66% at 2 yr
Offidani[62]	TAD	50	76	17 mo	≈62% at 2 yr

CTD, Cyclophosphamide, thalidomide, and dexamethasone *dex,* dexamethasone; *ORR,* overall response rate; *OS,* overall survival; *PFS,* progression-free survival; *TAD,* thalidomide, adriamycin, and dexamethasone; *Thal,* thalidomide; *TTP,* time to progression.

Table 85-11 Thalidomide Regimens in Newly Diagnosed Multiple Myeloma

Trial	Randomization	Patients *(n)*	ORR (%)	Median PFS (mo)	Median OS (mo)
Rajkumar[63]	TD D	235 235	63 46	14.9 6.5	72% at 2 yr 65% at 2 yr
Ludwig[64]	TD MP	145 143	68 50	16.7 20.7	41.5 49.5
Lokhorst[65]	TAD + SCT VAD + SCT	268 268	71 57	34 25	51% at 5 yr 50% at 5 yr
Palumbo[66]	MPT MP	167 164	76 47.6	21.8 14.5	45 47.6
Facon[67]	MPT MP	125 196	76 35	27.5 17.8	51.6 33.2
Hulin[68]	MPT MP	113 116	62 31	24.1 18.5	44 29
Wijermans[69]	MPT MP	165 168	66 45	33 21	40 31
Waage[70]	MPT MP	182 175	57 40	15 14	29 32

MP, Melphalan and prednisone; *MPT,* MP with thalidomide; *ORR,* overall response rate; *OS,* overall survival; *PFS,* progression-free survival; *SCT,* stem cell transplantation; *VAD,* vincristine, dexamethasone, and Adriamycin.

Table 85-12 MPT Versus MP: Efficacy in Newly Diagnosed Elderly Patients With Myeloma

Three trials (IFM 99,[49] IFM 01,[50] HOVON[51])		>RR, PFS, and OS	
Two trials (GIMEMA,[52] TURKISH[53])		>RR, PFS	
One trial (Nordic[54])		>RR	
RR	64% vs. 37%	(>27%)	
CR	10% vs. 2.5%	(>8%)	
PFS	20.3 vs. 14.9 mo	(6 mo)	HR 0.67
OS	39.3 vs. 32.7 mo	(>6 mo)	HR 0.82

CR, complete response; *HOVON,* Dutch-Belgian Hemato-Oncology Group; *HR,* hazard ratio; *IFM,* International Myeloma Foundation; *MP,* melphalan and prednisone; *MPT,* MP with thalidomide; *OS,* overall survival; *PFS,* progression-free survival; *RR,* relative risk.

therapy; patients who continued on primary therapy had a projected 3-year survival rate of 79%. A retrospective case-control study from a single institution comparing lenalidomide–dexamethasone versus thalidomide–dexamethasone revealed that lenalidomide–dexamethasone was better tolerated, with a higher ORR (80% vs. 61%), VGPR (34% vs. 12%), improved PFS (27 months vs. 17 months), and OS. Addition of clarithromycin to lenalidomide and low-dose dexamethasone resulted in an ORR of 90% and VGPR of 74% and CR of 39% of patients. Thus lenalidomide–dexamethasone is an excellent induction regimen for first-line therapy for newly diagnosed myeloma patients. Results with lenalidomide combinations in relapsed and newly diagnosed patients are summarized in Table 85-13 and 85-14. Lenalidomide has also been combined with MP with its continued use as maintenance (MPRR), and as shown in Table 85-15, it provides superior response and PFS as compared with MP alone.

Bortezomib

Bortezomib, a boron-containing dipeptide, is the first proteasome inhibitor to be introduced for the treatment of MM. Bortezomib is

Table 85-13 Lenalidomide Regimens in Relapsed or Refractory Multiple Myeloma

Trial	Regimen/Dose	Patients (*n*)	ORR (%)	Median TTP (mo)	Median OS
Weber[71]	Lenalidomide + dexamethasone	177	61	11.1	30 mo
	Dexamethasone	176	20	4.7	20 mo
Dimpopoulos[72]	Lenalidomide + dexamethasone	176	60	11.3	NR
	Dexamethasone	175	24	4.7	21 mo
Richardson[73]	Lenalidomide 30 mg once daily	67	18	7.7	28 mo
	Lenalidomide 15 mg twice daily	35	14	3.9	27 mo
Richardson[74]	VRD	36	61	7.7	37 mo
Knop[75]	RAD	69	73	6.2	88% at 1 yr
Morgan[76]	CRD	21	65	5.6	≈80% at 1 yr

CRD, carfilzomib, lenalidomide, dexamethasone; *NR,* not reported; *ORR,* overall response rate; *OS,* overall survival; *RAD,* lenalidomide, adriamycin, dexamethasone; *TTP,* time to progression; *VRD,* bortezomib, lenalidomide, dexamethasone.

Table 85-14 Lenalidomide Regimens in Newly Diagnosed Multiple Myeloma

Trial	Regimen/Dose	Patients (*n*)	ORR (%)	Median PFS (mo)	Median OS
Rajkumar[77]	RD/pulse dexamethasone	21	91	59% at 2 yr	85% at 3 yr
	RD/pulse dexamethasone + SCT	13		83% at 2 yr	92% at 3 yr
Niesvizky[78]	BiRD	72	90	75% at 2 yr	86% at 1 yr
Rajkumar[79]	RD	223	79	38% at 3 yr	87% at 2 yr
	Rd	222	68	43% at 3 yr	75% at 2 yr
Palumbo[80]	MPR	54	81	92% at 1 yr	100% at 1 yr

BiRD, biaxin, lenalidomide, dexamethasone; *ORR,* overall response rate; *PFS,* progression-free survival; *Rd,* lenalidomide, low-dose dexamethasone; *RD,* lenalidomide, high-dose dexamethasone; *SCT,* stem cell transplantation.

Table 85-15 Randomized Studies Comparing Melphalan and Prednisone–Related Regimens

Reference	Regimen	Complete Response	Partial Response	PFS (median mo)	OS (median mo)
Morgan[81]	CTD vs. CVAD	13% vs. 8%	82.5% vs. 71.2%		
San Miguel[43]	MPV vs. MP	30% vs. 4% (*P* <.001)	71% vs. 35% (*P* <.001)	24* vs. 16.6 (*P* <.001)	Not reached vs. 43
Palumbo et al[82]	MPRR vs. MP	18% vs. 5% (*P* <.001)	77% vs. 49% (*P* <.001)	Not reached vs. 13 (*P* = .002)	Not reached

CTD, Cyclophosphamide, thalidomide, and dexamethasone; *CVAD,* cyclophosphamide, vincristine, Adriamycin, and dexamethasone; *MP,* melphalan and prednisone; *MPRR,* MP plus lenalidomide with maintenance lenalidomide; *MPV,* melphalan, prednisone, and vincristine; *NS,* significant difference; *OS,* overall survival; *PFS,* progression-free survival.
*Time to progression.

a specific and reversible inhibitor of the 26S proteasome, binding to the chymotrypsin-like enzymatic site. The incomplete and transient inhibition of the proteasome results in apoptosis of myeloma cells by activation of both caspases 8 and 9 while sparing normal tissue. There is downregulation of NFκB in the myeloma cells, osteoclasts, and surrounding stromal cells. This results in decreased release of inflammatory cytokines in the BM milieu such as IL-6. Bortezomib not only arrests osteclastic activity by reducing sRANKL, decreases c-terminal cross-linking telopeptide of collagen type-I (CTX), and serum levels of tartrate-resistant acid phosphatase (TRAP) type-5b but also induces osteoblasts by decreasing serum dickkopf-1 (Dkk1) as reflected by an increase in bone-alkaline phosphatase and osteocalcin, irrespective of treatment response.

Bortezomib as a single agent induces CR in 10% and results in an ORR of 27% in newly diagnosed myeloma patients; bortezomib is not recommended as a monotherapy. Bortezomib and dexamethasone (B-D) is an excellent induction regimen with an ORR of 88% and CR+ VGPR rate of 19% and 1-year survival rate of 87%. Randomized trial has shown B-D to be superior to VAD as an induction regimen with higher complete response rate (15% vs. 6%) and ORR (79% vs. 63%).[28] After autologous SCT, there is continued advantage for the B-D arm (VGPR or better 54% vs. 37%). Median PFS was 36 months versus 30 months, and 3-year survival rates were 81% versus 77% with a median follow-up of 32 months. Results with bortezomib combination therapy, including relapsed and newly diagnosed patients, are summarized in Tables 85-16 and 85-17. Bortezomib has also been combined with melphalan and prednisone (MPV), and as shown in Table 85-15, after 5 years of follow-up, it provides superior ORR, CR, PFS, and OS compared with MP alone.

Combination of Three or Four Classes of Drugs

It is possible to combine drugs from different classes with nonoverlapping toxicities without compromising the dose to maximize the antitumor effect and eliminate potentially resistant clones to prolong the remission duration. Generally, three-drug combinations have been shown to give the highest ORR and VGPR compared with two-drug regimens (VCD, VRD, VTD).[29,30] Fig. 85-14 summarizes the results with two-, three-, and four-drug regimens and suggests improved responses and a higher incidence of CR using a three-drug regimen (RVD, VCD) with apparently no clear benefit of adding a fourth agent yet. Similar results are also depicted in Fig. 85-14 with MP-based regimens.

Table 85-16 Bortezomib Regimens in Relapsed or Refractory Multiple Myeloma

Trial	Regimen/Dose	Patients (*n*)	ORR (%)	Median TTP (months)	Median OS
Richardson[83]	Bortezomib (SUMMIT)	202	28	7	17 mo
Richardson[84]	Bortezomib (APEX)	333	38	6.2	29.8 mo
	Dexamethasone	336	18	3.5	23.7 mo
Orlowski[85]	Bortezomib	332	41	6.5	65% at 15 mo
	PLD + bortezomib	324	44	9.3	76% at 15 mo
Palumbo[86]	VMPT	30	67	PFS 61% at 1 yr	84% at 1 yr

ORR, overall response rate; *OS*, overall survival; *PFS*, progression-free survival; *PLD*, Liposomal doxorubicin; *TTP*, time to progression; *VMPT*, bortezomib, melphalan, prednisone, thalidomide.

Table 85-17 Bortezomib Regimens in Newly Diagnosed Multiple Myeloma

Trial	Regimen/Dose	Patients (*n*)	ORR (%)	Median TTP (mo)	Median OS
Jagannath[87]	VD	32	88	NA	87% at 1 yr
Harousseau[88]	VD + SCT × 2	240	79	36	81% at 3 yr
	VAD + SCT × 2	242	63	30	77% at 3 yr
Neben[89]	VAD + SCT × 2 + T	172	NA	35.7	84% at 3 yr
	PAD + SCT × 2 + V	182	NA	31.2	73% at 3 yr
Richardson[90]	VRD	66	100	75% at 18 mo	97% at 18 mo
Cavo[91]	VTD + SCT × 2 + VTD	236	93	68% at 3 yr	86% at 3 yr
	TD + SCT × 2 + TD	238	79	56% at 3 yr	84% at 3 yr
San Miguel[92]	VMP	337	71	24	68.5% at 3 yr
	MP	331	35	16.6	54% at 3 yr

MP, Melphalan and prednisone; *NA*, not applicable; *ORR*, overall response rate; *OS*, overall survival; *PFS*, progression-free survival; *SCT*, stem cell transplantation; *TTP*, time to progression; *VAD*, vincristine, dexamethasone, and Adriamycin.

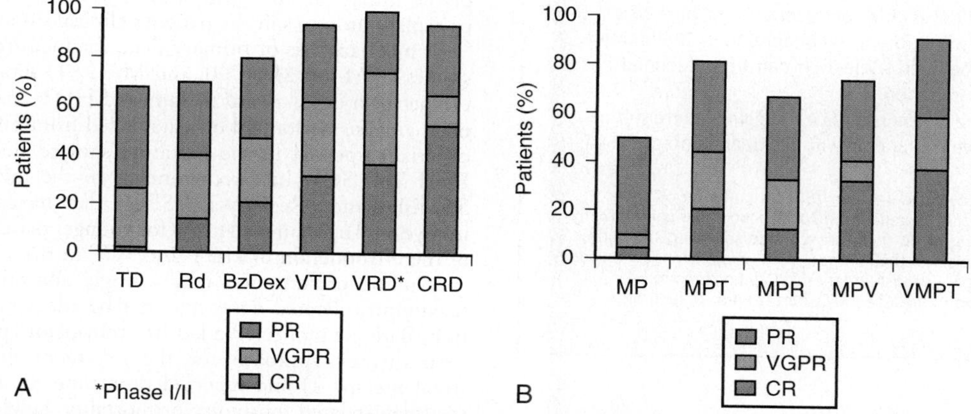

Figure 85-14 PROGRESSIVE IMPROVEMENT IN RESPONSE TO COMBINATION THERAPIES INCORPORATING NEWER AGENTS. The partial response (PR), very good partial response (VGPR), and complete response (CR) rates after induction therapy of newly diagnosed multiple myeloma patients are plotted for common novel agent combinations selected from larger phase III and II studies. **A,** Novel agent backbone. **B,** Melphalan–prednisone backbone. *Bz* or *V,* Bortezomib; *C,* carfilzomib; *Dex,* dexamethasone; *R,* lenalidomide; *T,* thalidomide. *(Data from References 44 to 53.)*

High-Dose Therapy and Consolidation

Tim McElwain introduced high-dose intravenous melphalan for the treatment of MM in 1983. A dose-response effect for melphalan was quite evident in MM. In the 1980s and 90s, HDT with stem cell support was increasingly used to treat younger patients (65 years and younger).

Source of Stem Cells

In the 1980s, BM was harvested from the patient under general anesthesia. This approach has been completely supplanted by the use of peripheral blood stem and progenitor cells. Autologous BM transplant was associated with delayed hematopoietic recovery by 1 week compared with mobilized blood stem cells, resulting in a higher

Treatment of Newly Diagnosed Multiple Myeloma

Confirm that the patient has symptomatic myeloma. Patients with MGUS or SMM should not be treated outside of a clinical trial.

Perform risk stratification using ISS staging, FISH, or cytogenetics, and assessment of renal function and measurement of LDH level to develop long-term plan based on estimate of prognosis. Although initial treatment is not affected by risk category, later consideration of more aggressive consolidation or use of allogeneic SCT in eligible patients can be considered in high-risk younger patients.

Induction: Both transplant-eligible and ineligible patients can be treated with a triple-drug regimen (bortezomib and dexamethasone with lenalidomide, with thalidomide or cyclophosphamide, *or* cyclophosphamide, thalidomide, dexamethasone) for 3 to 6 cycles before transplant or 9 to 12 months for transplant-ineligible patients. For transplant-ineligible patients, additional options include a two-drug regimen (dexamethasone with lenalidomide, with bortezomib, *or* with thalidomide) *or* melphalan containing regimen such as melphalan with prednisone in combination with any of the newer agents, MPT, MPV, or MPR.

Drug Selection should be influenced depending on patient characteristics.

- Renal dysfunction: agents that can be considered for use are bortezomib, cyclophosphamide, thalidomide, and dexamethasone (VCD or VTD)
- Neuropathy: agents that can be considered for use are lenalidomide, cyclophosphamide, and dexamethasone
- Advanced age: consider dose or scheduled attenuation
- Convenience: use of oral vs. intravenous agent regimen

Transplant-eligible patients can undergo a single autologous transplant with melphalan with a second autologous transplant being optional depending on the overall response or on the protocol in which the patient is participating.

Maintenance: After transplant or optimal induction therapy (to best response), patients can receive maintenance with thalidomide, lenalidomide, or bortezomib. For high-risk patients, both bortezomib and lenalidomide or thalidomide combination can be used. Selection can be influenced based on their induction regimen.

Improving complete response rates is a key goal of current trials, but patients can live a long time with residual paraprotein.

FISH, Fluorescent in situ hybridization; *ISS,* International Staging System; *LDH,* lactate dehydrogenase; *MGUS,* monoclonal gammopathy of unknown significance; *MPR,* melphalan, prednisone, lenalidomide; *MPT,* melphalan, prednisone, thalidomide; *MPV,* melphalan, prednisone, bortezomib; *SCT,* stem cell transplantation; *VCD,* bortezomib, cyclophosphamide, dexamethasone; *VTD,* bortezomib, thalidomide, dexamethasone.

transplant-related morbidity and mortality rate of 10% compared with 2% with peripheral blood progenitor cells. Stem cells can be mobilized with chemotherapy alone, chemotherapy and growth factor (G-CSF or GM-CSF), or growth factors alone (G-CSF, G-CSF plus plerixafor). The degree of tumor cell contamination in the peripheral blood stem cell product has had no influence on transplant outcome. Ex vivo manipulations to eliminate tumor cells within the graft have not resulted in any improvement in the depth of response, PFS, or OS. It is preferable to use stem cell–sparing agents as induction therapy before stem cell harvest. Alkylating agent exposure and lenalidomide exposure should be limited to ensure adequate stem cell harvest and complete hematopoietic recovery after transplantation. It is preferable to collect stem cells after the achievement of best antitumor response to induction therapy to minimize tumor cell contamination.

AUTOLOGOUS STEM CELL TRANSPLANTATION

Single High-Dose Therapy With Stem Cell Transplantation Rescue

Several prospective, randomized clinical trials have been performed to define the role of HDT and SCT as a component of front-line therapy for MM patients in the 1990s. Two studies, the IFM 90[31] and MRC VII,[32] reported the superiority of HDT and SCT with respect to response rate, PFS, and OS and led to widespread use of HDT and SCT for patients up to the age of 65 years (Fig. 85-15).[33] However, other studies did not show a survival advantage but did show improvements in the response rate and PFS. One such clinical trial was conducted by the French myeloma autograft group in patients between the ages of 55 and 65 years (MAG 90) and showed a higher response rate (CR + MRD, 36% vs. 20%) and a trend for improved PFS (EFS, 25.3 vs. 18.7 mo; $P = .07$) in favor of the HDT arm but no difference in the OS. The Spanish trial gave induction therapy VBMCP/VBAD for 4 cycles at five weekly intervals; subsequently, responding patients were randomized between HDT and continuation of standard chemotherapy for 8 additional cycles of VBMCP/VBAD. Although the HDT arm had a higher CR rate, there was no difference in PFS or OS. Another trial conducted by the U.S. Intergroup Trial also allowed for induction therapy followed by a randomization of all patients to a single autotransplant versus continued VBMCP therapy for 1 year. This study did not show a difference in the OS between the two arms. In this study, the patients on the standard treatment arm were allowed to receive HDT and SCT after relapse. Results of five large randomized trials comparing standard-dose chemotherapy (SDT) with HDT are summarized in Table 85-18.

Another randomized phase 3 trial in patients younger than the age of 56 years evaluated the role of early versus late transplantation (MAG 91); this study showed that there was no difference in OS. However, the investigator showed that early application of HDT resulted in a prolonged PFS compared with the standard chemotherapy arm; therefore, the time without symptoms, additional treatment, and treatment toxicity was favorable when HDT was applied as part of the initial therapy. This allowed for flexibility in the timing of transplantation to suit the patient's clinical situation and preference.

A meta-analysis of primary data obtained from the three French studies (IFM 90, MAG 90, and MAG 91) showed no difference in OS between the standard therapy and HDT arms. Likewise, another meta-analysis performed on data culled from nine randomized clinical trials reported in the literature showed no survival benefit for HDT and SCT. In direct contrast to the meta-analysis from the Swedish Cancer Registry and SEER, data have shown improvement in 5-year relative survival ratios for younger patients primarily because of the introduction of HDT and SCT in the 1990s.

On the presumption that a single alkylating agent therapy at maximum tolerated doses may not be adequate for disease eradication, Barlogie pioneered a tandem transplant approach as part of his total therapy approach for the treatment of myeloma in 1989 (total therapy 1) and reported promising results without increased treatment-related morbidity or mortality. Single HDT resulted in a CR rate well under 25% in most trials. Addition of TBI, busulfan, cyclophosphamide, or BCNU (BEAM) to melphalan did not result in better outcome. Therefore, investigators tried to improve the results by providing a second consecutive high-dose melphalan and SCT (tandem transplantation).

Four large randomized clinical trials have compared the role of tandem autotransplantation against a single episode of HDT and SCT (Table 85-19). All four studies showed improvement in the depth of response (VGPR) after a tandem transplant; three of the four studies showed improvement in PFS, but only one study showed an improvement in the OS. The French trial, IFM 94,[34] showed the benefit of a second transplant only for patients not in VGPR or better after the first transplantation. In the era of novel agents, a VGPR or better can be obtained before transplantation; therefore, a second transplant is seldom used outside of a setting of a clinical trial (Fig. 85-16).

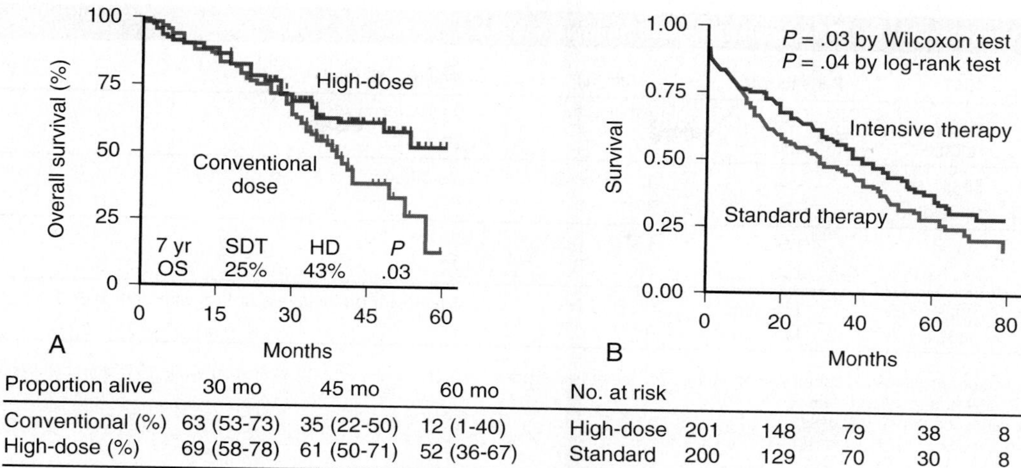

Proportion alive	30 mo	45 mo	60 mo
Conventional (%)	63 (53-73)	35 (22-50)	12 (1-40)
High-dose (%)	69 (58-78)	61 (50-71)	52 (36-67)

No. at risk					
High-dose	201	148	79	38	8
Standard	200	129	70	30	8

Figure 85-15 COMPARATIVE TRIALS OF HIGH-DOSE THERAPY (HDT) VERSUS STANDARD-DOSE CHEMOTHERAPY (SDT). The IFM-90 (Intergroupe Francais de Myelome) **(A)** randomized trials with 200 patients randomized to SDT with VMCP-VBAP versus HDT with melphalan 140 mg/m^2 plus total-body irradiation (800 cGy) and MRC-VII (Medical Research Council) **(B)** trial with 401 patients randomized to SDT with doxorubicin, carmustine, cyclophosphamide, and melphalan or HDT with CVAD (cyclophosphamide, vincristine, Adriamycin, and dexamethasone) followed by melphalan 200 mg/m^2 and stem cell rescue. Significantly longer overall survival was noted with HDT in both studies. *HD,* High dose; *OS,* overall survival. *(Data from Attal M, Harousseau JL, Stoppa AM, et al: A prospective, randomized trial of autologous bone marrow transplantation and chemotherapy in multiple myeloma. Intergroupe Français du Myélome.* N Engl J Med *335:91, 1996 and Child JA, Morgan GJ, Davies FE, et al: Medical Research Council Adult Leukaemia Working Party: High-dose chemotherapy with hematopoietic stem-cell rescue for multiple myeloma.* N Engl J Med *348:1875, 2003.)*

Table 85-18 Results of Large Randomized Study Comparing Standard Dose Therapy Versus High-Dose Therapy

Authors	Therapy	Patients *(n)*	CR (%)	EFS (median mo)	OS (median mo)
Attal et al[93]	Conventional	100	5†	18†	37†
	High-dose	100	22	27	52
Fermand et al[94]	Conventional	96	—	18.7†	50.4*
	High-dose	94	—	24.3	55.3
Blade et al[95]	Conventional	83	11†	34.3†	66.9*
	High-dose	81	30	42.5	67.4
Child et al[96]	Conventional	200	8.5†	19.6†	42.3†
	High-dose	201	44	31.6	54.8
Barlogie et al[97]	Conventional	255	15*	21*	53
	High-dose	261	17	25	58

CR, Complete remission; *EFS,* event-free survival; *OS,* overall survival.
*No significant difference.
†Significant difference.

In the era before introduction of novel agents, the induction regimen had only a minimal role because complete responses were uncommon (<5%) with high-dose dexamethasone or VAD chemotherapy. Thus HDT played a critical role in achieving a favorable CR and VGPR rates and prolonged durability of unmaintained responses. The availability of novel agents has dramatically changed this paradigm. Novel agents have improved VGPR or better before SCT, allowing for posttransplant consolidation and maintenance. Whether novel agents can supplant HDT and SCT is an important question that has yet to be answered.

Induction Therapy With Novel Agents

Randomized clinical trials have shown that thalidomide–dexamethasone is equivalent to VAD chemotherapy. The Dutch HOVON 50 trial compared thalidomide during the induction phase and as maintenance after HDT and SCT. TAD chemotherapy was superior to VAD chemotherapy based on overall response and quality of response before and after HDT and SCT. In addition, maintenance with thalidomide improved the PFS and resulted in a trend toward improved OS. Lenalidomide and dexamethasone have been shown to be useful as an induction regimen before transplantation. But no formal randomized clinical trial has been performed comparing this combination with conventional chemotherapy. Exposure to lenalidomide should be limited to 4 to 6 cycles because it compromises stem cell mobilization.

Bortezomib-Based Induction

Bortezomib–dexamethasone was superior to VAD chemotherapy as an induction regimen. There was improvement in CR and VGPR before and after transplantation, and there was a trend for prolonged PFS but no difference in the OS.[28] The lack of impact on PFS and OS is perhaps attributable to limited bortezomib exposure to a maximum of 4 cycles during the induction phase.

Table 85-19 Single Versus Double ASCT for Newly Diagnosed Multiple Myeloma

Study	ASCT	Patients (*n*)	CR (%)*	Median EFS (mo)	Median OS (mo)
Attal et al[98] (IFM94)	Single	199	42[†] (*P* = NS)	25 (*P* = .03)	48 (*P* = .01)
	Double	200	50[†]	30	58
Fermand et al[99] (MAG95)	Single	94	42* (*P* = NS)	No difference	No difference
	Double	99	37*		
Sonneveld et al[100] (HOVON24)	Single	148	13 (*P* = .002)	20 (*P* = .02)	55 (*P* = NS)
	Double	155	28	22	50
Cavo et al[101] (Bologna 96)	Single	115	35 (*P* = NS)	Significant prolongation of EFS with double SCT	59 (*P* = NS)
	Double	113	48		73

ASCT, Autologous stem cell transplant; *CR,* complete remission; *EFS,* event-free survival; *NS,* not significant; *OS,* overall survival; *SCT,* stem cell transplantation.
*Complete remission + minimum residual disease.
[†]Complete remission + very good partial response.

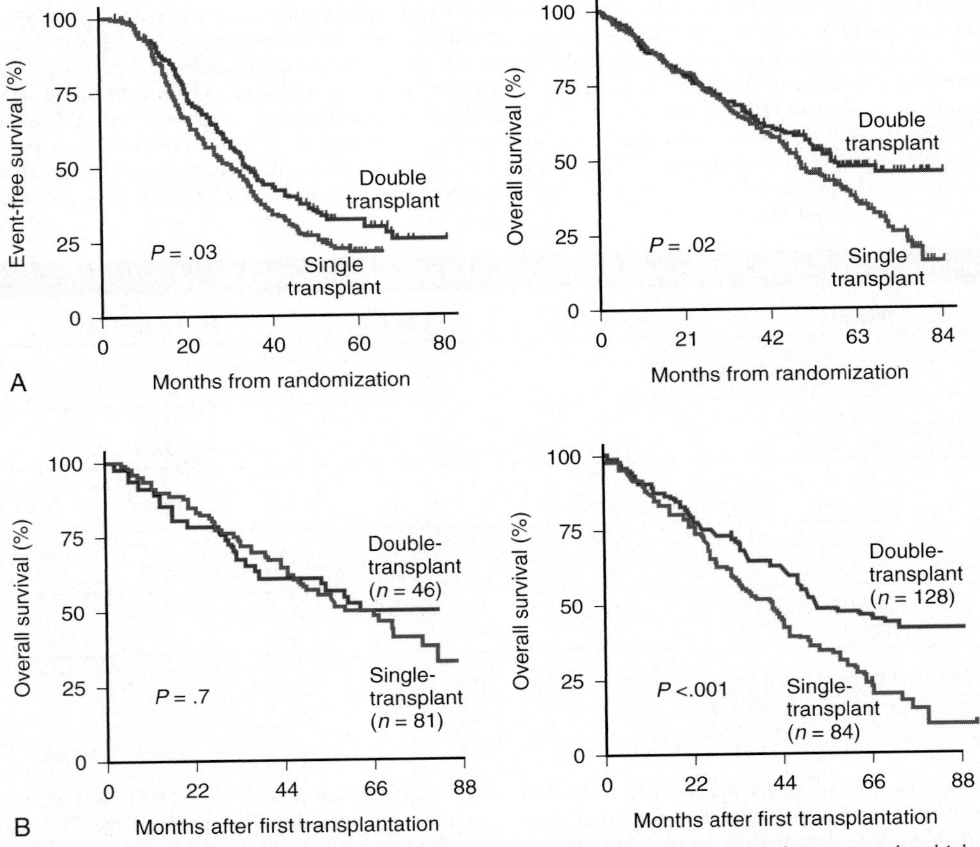

Figure 85-16 **A,** IFM-94 (Intergroupe Francais de Myelome 94) trial comparing a single versus tandem high-dose therapy (HDT). A total of 399 patients were randomized to a single HDT with melphalan 140 mg/m² plus total-body irradiation (800 cGy) versus first HDT with melphalan 140 mg/m² and subsequent second HDT with melphalan 140 mg/m² plus total-body irradiation (800 cGy). Superior event-free and overall survival were noted with tandem HDT. **B,** A subgroup analysis reveals that the survival benefit was observed in those patients not achieving a very good partial response (VGPR) after first transplant *(right)* and not in those with VGPR after first transplant *(left)*. *(From Attal M, Harousseau JL, Facon T, et al: InterGroupe Francophone du Myélome: Single versus double autologous stem-cell transplantation for multiple myeloma.* N Engl J Med *349:2495, 2003.)*

Combining bortezomib with immunomodulatory drugs further improves the outcome before and after SCT. In a large randomized clinical trial of 480 patients conducted by the GIMEMA Italian myeloma network, VTD was shown to be superior to PD for induction therapy and for consolidation after tandem transplantation. VTD induction therapy significantly improved the rate of complete or near-complete response before the transplantation. This higher response rate continued after tandem transplantation and was further augmented by 2 cycles of VTD consolidation as opposed to TD posttransplantation. This increase in the depth of response has translated into a superior PFS. However, increased neuropathy was encountered by the patients on the VTD arm. The French investigators reduce the dose intensity of VTD and confirmed in another randomized trial that 4 cycles of VTD were to be superior to 4 cycles of bortezomib and dexamethasone as an induction regimen before transplantation.[35] There was less neuropathy caused by the adjustment of bortezomib and thalidomide doses. The Spanish group compared TD, VTD, and multiagent chemotherapy as induction therapy and showed that VTD was superior after transplantation. The patients were further randomized to maintenance therapy with VP versus VT, with no difference in the outcome being observed. Results from two large studies using HDT with more than 7 and 12 years of follow-up are shown in Fig. 85-17, suggesting a possibility of a tail in the survival curve with more than 10% to 20% patients remaining disease free or alive beyond 10 years, suggesting a possibility for long-term survival in myeloma.

Allogeneic Stem Cell Transplantation

Allogeneic SCT offers a potential for cure for patients with MM that is mediated by a graft-versus-myeloma effect, tumor-free graft, and potential for donor lymphocyte infusion to combat the residual or recurrent disease. However, the role of allogeneic SCT in MM is limited. Patients are generally older (more than 75% of the patients are older than the age of 55 years), often presenting with comorbidities such as renal impairment, diastolic dysfunction of the heart, and restrictive lung disease. The underlying immunodeficiency associated with this disease is worsened by posttransplant immunosuppression, resulting in a high transplant-related mortality rate with standard myeloablative conditioning regimens. Relapse after allogeneic SCT contributes to the modest efficacy of this approach. Although it could be shown that there are graft-versus-myeloma effects with sustained molecular remissions, it has been difficult to induce graft-versus-myeloma effects while avoiding graft-versus-host disease (GVHD). There have been no convincing survival data to support widespread use of allogeneic SCT outside of a clinical trial.

There has been improvement in 6-month and 2-year survival rates since 1994 compared with the prior era. This improvement in the European Bone Marrow Transplant Registry was attributed to better supportive care measures and patient selection. Reduced-intensity conditioning regimens, with reduction in immediate transplant-related mortality and stable engraftment and use of peripheral blood progenitor cells from the donors with their rapid engraftment kinetics renewed interest in the use of allogeneic SCT for MM. Bensinger et al reported on the long-term results of allogeneic transplantation for MM at the Fred Hutchinson Cancer Research Center spanning 34 years Bensinger et al. Bone Marrow Transpl. 2012:1-6. Among the 144 patients undergoing ablative conditioning regimens, the 2-year, non-relapse transplant mortality rate was 55%; major causes of death included fungal and viral infections, acute respiratory distress syndrome, acute GVHD, and multiorgan failure. The 2-year non–transplant-related mortality rate was 18% among the recipients of nonablative conditioning regimens; the causes of death were mostly chronic GVHD and progressive disease. The 10-year OS rate was 15% for myeloablative regimens compared with 35% for nonmyeloablative regimens. The incidence of acute GVHD was similar (65% + 2%), but the incidence of extensive chronic GVHD was 27% for ablative regimens compared with 67% for nonablative regimens (Table 85-20).

Several studies reported having combined the tandem autologous transplantation approach with mini allogeneic SCT. The Italian group reported superior outcomes for patients receiving an autograft–allograft protocol compared with patients receiving tandem autograft protocols.[36] At a median follow-up time of 46 months, the median OS had not been reached for patients receiving auto–allo transplants compared with 58 months for tandem autotransplants; the EFS was 43 and 33 months, respectively, for the two groups (see Table 85-20). The French group subjected patients with high-risk (β_2-microglobulin >3 mg/L and chromosome deletion 13) to tandem auto transplants or auto–allo transplants based on the availability of human leukocyte antigen–compatible sibling donors. On an intent-to-treat basis, there was no difference in EFS or OS with the trend for better OS in patients treated with tandem autologous SCT. In a recently completed BMT-CTN trial in the United States, there was no difference in outcome between auto–mini allo transplant and tandem autologous transplantation. To increase the effect of community of donor lymphocytes against the tumor cells, vaccination strategies are currently being pursued (Fig. 85-18).

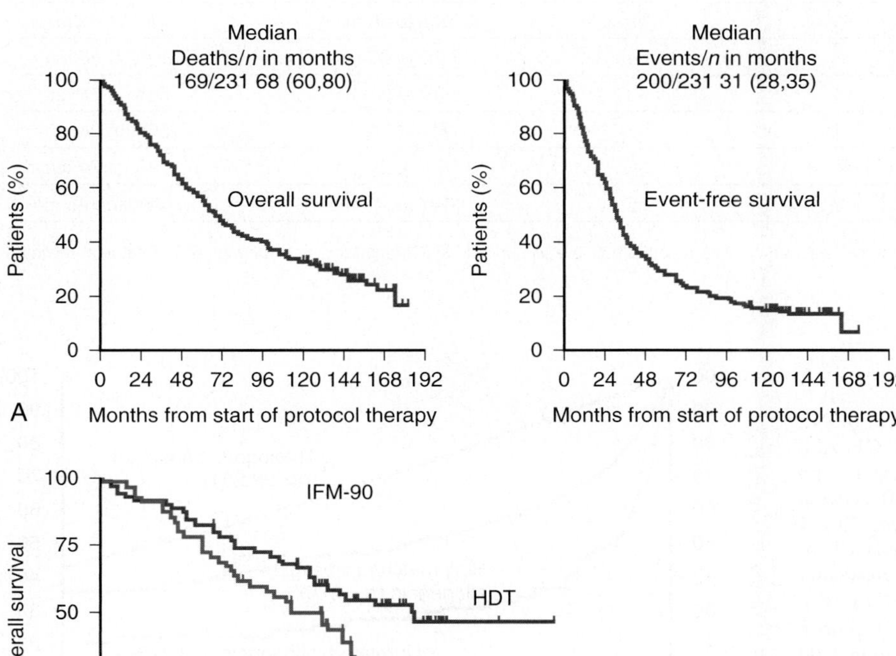

Figure 85-17 **A,** Kaplan-Meier survival estimate in patients receiving total therapy I regimen with tandem transplants after over 12 years of median follow-up (n = 231). There appears to be a plateau in the curve beyond 10 years in event-free survival (EFS). Overall survival (OS) at 10 years is 30%, median progression-free survival (PFS) is 30 months, and median OS is 68 months. **B,** Kaplan-Meier survival estimate in patients treated in the IFM-90 (Intergroupe Francais de Myelome 90) study with patients receiving standard-dose therapy (SDT) versus high-dose therapy (HDT) and single transplant after more than 7 years of median follow-up (n = 200). PFS = 18 vs. 28 mo. Median OS = 44 vs. 57 mo. *(**A** from Barlogie B, Tricot GJ, van Rhee F, et al: Long-term outcome results of the first tandem autotransplant trial for multiple myeloma.* Br J Haematol *135:158, 2006.* ***B** from Harousseau LL: Autologous transplantation for multiple myeloma.* Ann Oncol *19:vii, 128, 2008.)*

Syngeneic Transplantation

Results of syngeneic transplantation are superior to those of autologous and allogeneic SCT. The results are better than autologous transplantation because of lower relapse rates with twin transplantation. This may be related to the lack of tumor cells in the graft or graft-versus-myeloma effect without GVHD. The results of syngeneic transplantation are also superior to those of allogeneic SCT because of a low transplant-related mortality rate and the absence of clinical GVHD. These observations were based on the reports published from two large transplant registries, the Center for International Bone Marrow Transplant Research and European Bone Marrow Transplantation Registry.

Maintenance

Maintenance therapy is the use of ongoing low-intensity chemotherapy to eliminate or suppress the minimal residual tumor clone over a prolonged period of time. Maintenance therapy is administered when the disease is in remission, either undetectable or at a low level. The purpose of maintenance therapy is to prolong remission duration and thereby life expectancy. Maintenance therapy improves the quality of response, supporting the notion that an additional antitumor response during the maintenance phase will be beneficial. Immunomodulatory molecules are well suited for maintenance therapy because they can be administered orally at low doses for a prolonged period of time.[37]

The first two randomized trials published on thalidomide maintenance after autotransplant showed an improvement in PFS and OS. The total therapy II trial randomized patients to thalidomide induction and a maintenance arm versus a no-thalidomide arm; this study showed improvement in PFS and a delayed improvement in OS after 8 years of follow-up. In the HOVON 50 trial, patients were similarly randomized to thalidomide induction followed by thalidomide maintenance after transplant or VAD induction followed by interferon maintenance. This trial also showed improvement in PFS and OS for patients in the thalidomide arm. A meta-analysis of published results to date indicates a significant reduction of the risk for progression with thalidomide maintenance therapy. Outcome did not differ between trials that used thalidomide during the maintenance phase only and those that used thalidomide, both for induction and maintenance treatment. The MRC IX trial had an intensive therapy arm (SCT) and nonintensive arm (no stem cell transplant); after the patients had completed the intensive or nonintensive treatment arm, they were randomized to receive thalidomide maintenance or no maintenance. There was improvement in PFS but no improvement in OS when comparing the two groups. Results of major randomized studies evaluating maintenance therapy are summarized in Table 85-21.

Three large randomized trials have explored the role of lenalidomide as maintenance therapy. There were two studies of maintenance therapy after autologous SCT comparing lenalidomide vs. placebo (CALGB and IFM). A third trial compared 9 cycles of MP alone, MP with lenalidomide and MP with lenalidomide followed my lenalidomide. maintenance. All three studies showed improvement in PFS by 18 months; only the CALGB study showed improvement in OS. There appears to be a slightly increased risk of occurrence of a second malignancy when lenalidomide is administered along with melphalan or immediately after HDT with melphalan. Lenalidomide therapy is also unable to alter the poor prognosis attributed by adverse cytogenetics or FISH results.

Table 85-20 Studies of Myeloablative and Reduced Intensity Allogeneic Stem Cell Transplantation for Newly Diagnosed Myeloma

Authors	Patients (*n*)	TRM (%)	CR (%)	OS (actuarial, mo)	EFS (actuarial, mo)
Gahrton[102]	162	41	44	28% at 84 mo	45% at 60 mo
Bensinger[103]	80	44	36	20% at 54 mo	24% at 54 mo
Alyea[104]	66*	31	NR	39% at 48 mo	23% at 48 mo
Lee[105]	45	38	64	36% at 36 mo	13% at 36 mo
Kroger[106]	17	11	73	74% at 24 mo	56% at 24 mo
Maloney[107]	54	7	57	78% at 24 mo	55% at 24 mo
Giralt[108]	22	40	33	30% at 24 mo	19% at 24 mo
Bruno[109]	58	7	55	Median, 43 mo	Median >46 mo

CR, Complete remission; *DFS,* disease-free survival; *EFS,* event-free survival; *NR,* not reported; *OS,* overall survival; *PFS,* progression-free survival; *TRM,* treatment-related mortality.
*T-cell depleted.

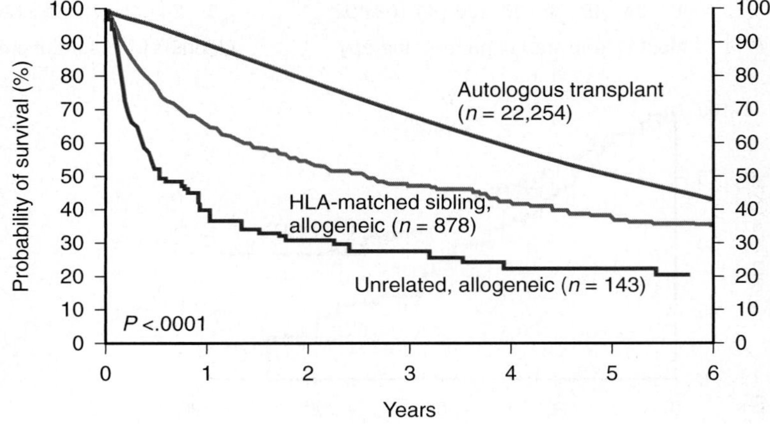

Figure 85-18 CENTER FOR INTERNATIONAL BONE MARROW TRANSPLANT RESEARCH ANALYSIS OF ALL TRANSPLANTS IN MYELOMA. Among 23,197 patients who received an autotransplant for multiple myeloma (MM) between 2000 and 2009, the 3-year probability of survival rate was 70% ± 1%. Allogeneic stem cell transplantation for MM is reserved for patients with high-risk disease, and the majority are performed after an autologous hematopoietic cell transplantation (HCT) with reduced-intensity or nonmyeloablative conditioning regimens. Among the 979 patients who received an allogeneic HCT from 2000 to 2009, the 3-year probabilities of survival were 51% ± 2% for the 827 recipients of human leukocyte antigen (HLA)–matched sibling donor grafts and 26% ± 2% for the 470 recipients of unrelated donor grafts. *(From Pasquini MD, Wang Z: CIBMTR summary slides, 2010. Adapted from* http://www.cibmtr.org.*)*

Bortezomib has also been used in the maintenance setting. Generally, bortezomib maintenance has been restricted to clinical trials in which bortezomib was also used in the induction phase of the treatment. Bortezomib maintenance seemingly improved the outcome in patients with high-risk cytogenetics or FISH results. Bortezomib is given less frequently in the maintenance setting; different studies have used different schedules of administration.

Relapsed Disease

Relapse is defined as reappearance of signs and symptoms of the disease or signs of increasing disease or end-organ dysfunction that are believed to be related to the underlying myeloma.[38a] Patients presenting with symptomatic relapse require treatment intervention. Patients with rapidly rising paraprotein, doubling of the paraprotein within a short interval, also require treatment intervention. Patients with asymptomatic biochemical relapse do not require treatment intervention. Generally, a serum M spike greater than 1 g/dL, Bence-Jones proteinuria greater than 500 mg/day, or serum-free light-chain level greater than 200 mg/L would be a minimum requirement to consider intervention with systemic therapy. Occasionally, myeloma cells may become dedifferentiated or anaplastic and may produce only light-chain components (Bence Jones escape phenomenon) or no paraprotein at all. These patients generally tend to have a more aggressive clinical course. Development of compression fractures and fractures at a site of previous lytic lesion per se need not constitute progression of myeloma. Development of hypercalcemia, progressive anemia, and new or worsening kidney function would merit prompt treatment intervention.

Currently relapsed and refractory disease is defined as having failed three or more lines of prior therapy with previous exposure to all four classes of drugs (cytotoxic agents, immunomodulatory agents, proteasome inhibitors, and glucocorticoids) and progressing on the last line of therapy. These patients have life expectancy of less than 1 year.

There are several considerations in choosing the treatment for patients with relapsed myeloma.[38a] These include disease-related factors such as slow, indolent, or a single site of relapse or rapid and multiple sites of relapse. Patients with a single site of relapse may be amenable to radiation treatment. Special considerations need to be given for patients presenting with extramedullary soft tissue plasmacytomas, CNS relapses, or plasma cell leukemia. Disease presenting with elevated LDH, high β_2-microglobulin, deletions 17p and multiple copies of 1q generally have a poor prognosis. Patients presenting with advanced age, poor performance status, renal impairment, and poor hematologic reserve or concurrent myelodysplastic syndrome from prior therapy present a great challenge for management. The choice of treatment is also predicated on prior drug exposure, whether the relapse is on or off therapy, and ongoing toxicity from prior therapy.

Thalidomide

Thalidomide monotherapy was originally introduced for the treatment of advanced and refractory myeloma. In the initial phase 2 trial, thalidomide was administered at 200 mg/day with increments every 2 weeks up to 800 mg for 169 patients. A partial response or better was noted in 30% of patients with a 2-year EFS of 20% and OS of 48%. A phase 3 trial (OPTIMUM) compared dexamethasone with thalidomide monotherapy at daily doses of 100, 200, and 400 mg. The median times to progression were 6, 7, 8, and 9.1 months, respectively. The response rates and median survival rates were similar in all treatment groups. In a systematic review of 1629 patients with relapsed myeloma treated on 42 uncontrolled phase II trials with thalidomide, a partial response or better was noted in 30% with 1 year survival of 60%, as reported by Glasmacher et al.[38b] Thalidomide has been combined successfully with other conventional chemotherapy agents as well as proteasome inhibitors for improved response rates and better disease control. Thalidomide is especially useful when a patient presents with renal impairment and cytopenias. It is also useful for palliation when combined with oral cyclophosphamide and prednisone in patients with poor performance status.

Lenalidomide

In two large phase 3 randomized trials (MM 009 and MM 010) lenalidomide–dexamethasone was found to be superior to dexamethasone in patients with relapsed myeloma after one to three lines of prior therapy. Updated results with a median follow-up of 48 months showed an ORR of 61%, median time to progression of 13.4 months, duration of response of 16 months, and OS of 38 months. Patients who had more than one line of prior therapy had an ORR of 57%; time to progression was 10.6 months. A median PFS of 9.5 months and OS of 31 months were reported. Patients with moderate or severe renal impairment developed more severe thrombocytopenia, required more frequent dose modifications, and had inferior survival outcomes. Prior exposure to thalidomide did not preclude responses to lenalidomide; however, patients who had relapsed or progressed on thalidomide have a lower response rate (<50%) and a shorter time to progression (7 months). Lenalidomide can be easily combined with conventional chemotherapy as well as bortezomib. Combination therapy results in a higher response rate and better disease control.

Bortezomib

In a large phase 2 trial (SUMMIT) conducted in relapsed and refractory MM, bortezomib monotherapy had an impressive ORR of 28%,

Table 85-21 Randomized Studies Comparing Maintenance Therapy in Myeloma

Reference	Regimen	PFS (median mo)	OS (median mo)
Spencer[110]	Control vs. thalidomide/prednisone	3-yr 23 vs. 42 (*P* <.001)	3-yr 75 vs. 86 (*P* = .004)
Barlogie[111]	Control vs. thalidomide	5 yr 44% vs. 56%† (*P* = 0.01)	5-yr 65%
Attal[112]	Control vs. thalidomide + pamidronate	3-yr 36 vs. 52 (*P* = 0.009)	4-yr 77 vs. 87 (*P* = .04)
Attal[113]	Control vs. lenalidomide	4-yr 22% vs 43%	4-yr 75% vs 73%
Palumbo[114]	MPR vs. MPR-R	4-yr 22% vs 43%	3-yr 65% vs 70%
McCarthy[115]	Control vs. lenalidomide	27 vs. 46	Not reached
Mateos[116]	VP vs. VT	39 vs. 46	5-yr 50% vs 69%

MPR, Melphalan, prednisone, lenalidomide; *MPRR*, MPR with lenalidomide maintenance; *NS*, significant difference; *OS*, overall survival; *PFS*, progression-free survival; *VP*, bortezomib, prednisone; *VT*, bortezomib, thalidomide.
*Survival after 3 years.
†5 year PFS rates.
‡TTP, time to progression.

including 10% complete or near-complete remissions. The median time to progression was 7 months, the duration of response was 12.7 months, and the median survival time was 17 months. Among patients with relapsed myeloma after one to three lines of prior therapy, bortezomib monotherapy had an ORR of 43%, a median time to progression of 6.2 months, a duration of response of 8 months, and a median survival time of 30 months. Bortezomib monotherapy is less effective in patients who have received more than one line of prior therapy. Bortezomib is also synergistic when used in combination with other drugs, including alkylating agents, anthracyclines, immunomodulatory drugs, and dexamethasone. These combinations generally produce higher ORRs in the range of 50% to 80%, with an increasing duration of response and OS. Bortezomib plus pegylated liposomal doxorubicin has been shown to be superior to monotherapy in a large, randomized trial with an improved time to progression (9.3 vs. 6.5 months) and OS. Bortezomib has also been recently used as subcutaneous injection and in a randomized comparison with intravenous administration had identical 42% response in both subcutaneous administration had improved safety profile with reduced incidence of peripheral neuropathy (38% vs. 53%; $P = .044$ of any grade and 6% vs. 16%; $P = .026$ grade 3 or worse).[39]

Carfilzomib

Carfizomib is a tetrapeptide epoxyketone that selectively and irreversibly inhibits the 20S proteasome at the same chymotrypsin-like enzymatic site as bortezomib. In preclinical models it has been shown to overcome bortezomib-resistance. Carfilzomib has been shown to be effective in patients with relapsed multiple myeloma, who had received at least 2 lines of therapy, including bortezomib and an immunomodulatory agent (thalidomide or lenalidomide). In a single arm, multicenter clinical trial enrolling 266 patients with relapsed myeloma, Carfilzomib as a single agent induced an overall response rate of 23%, consisting of 1 complete response, 13 very good partial responses and 47 partial responses. The median response duration was 7.8 months and overall survival was 15.6 months. Most common adverse events included fatigue, anemia, nausea, and thrombocytopenia, dyspnea, diarrhea, and pyrexia. Neuropathy was uncommon (12.4%) and mild (grade 1 or 2). The drug has been combined successfully with other antimyeloma agents such as lenalidomide and dexamethasone (CRD) with greater efficacy, both in relapsed setting as well as in newly diagnosed multiple myeloma. Currently there is an ongoing phase III clinical trial comparing lenalidomide and weekly dexamethasone (Rd) to lenalidomide, weekly dexamethasone plus Carfilzomib. Carfilzomib has been recently approved for the treatment of patients with multiple myeloma who have received at least two prior therapies, including bortezomib and an immunomodulatory agent, and have demonstrated disease progression on or within 60 days of the completion of the last therapy.

Lenalidomide, Bortezomib, and Dexamethasone

As in newly diagnosed patients, a combination of lenalidomide, bortezomib, and dexamethasone[29] is able to achieve responses in relapsed patients as well as patients refractory to either or both agents separately. In a phase I/II study, 38 patients received lenalidomide with or without dexamethasone. Among 36 evaluable patients, 61% achieved a minimal response or better. Among 18 patients who had dexamethasone added, 83% achieved stable disease or better with a median OS time of 37 months. This has established RVD as one of the salvage regimens in relapsed myeloma if this combination has not been used when the patient was newly diagnosed.

Newer Agents

A number of novel agents have been validated using both in vitro and in vivo models.[40] These models have been developed to characterize MM cell–BMSC interactions, as well as signaling pathways controlling growth, survival, drug resistance, or migration within the BM milieu. These studies identified that MM cell growth is mediated via the ERK/MAPK pathway, survival via JAK/STAT signaling, drug resistance via PI3K/Akt signaling, and migration via PKC-dependent signaling cascades. These systems have been used to identify potential novel therapeutic targets and to validate novel targeted therapies (Table 85-22). The immunomodulatory agent pomalidomide and the proteasome inhibitor carfilzomib are two promising drugs. In a phase I/II study, pomalidomide with dexamethasone was shown to have an ORR 34% and minor response or better in 45% of patients. Similar responses were observed in patients who were refractory to both bortezomib and lenalidomide. Other representative novel agents include the histone deacetylase (HDAC) inhibitors vorinostat and panabinostat. A recent phase III study evaluating vorinostat with bortezomib versus placebo and bortezomib has confirmed significant improvement in response with the combination (ORR, 56% vs. 41%; $P < .0001$ and PFS, 7.65 vs. 6.83; $P = .01$).

A similar study evaluating combination of panabinostat with bortezomib versus bortezomib is ongoing. In a phase II study in relapsed or refractory patients, the anti–CS-1 mAb (monoclonal antibody) elotuzumab was evaluated in combination with lenalidomide and dexamethasone and was shown to lead to an 82% ORR; a phase III study evaluating this combination with lenalidomide and dexamethasone is ongoing. CS-1 is a cell surface glycoprotein highly expressed by MM cells irrespective of cytogenetic abnormalities or response to various treatment options. Similarly, a phase I/II study combining perifosine (an Akt inhibitor) with bortezomib with or without dexamethasone has shown a 41% ORR, including a 32% response in bortezomib-refractory patients; a phase III study evaluating this combination with bortezomib alone is ongoing. Other promising targets and agents and the stages of their clinical development are listed in Table 85-22.

The optimal treatment of a relapsed patient requires ensuring that the patient's relapse requires intervention. Approach to therapy is dictated by whether the patient had a transplant or is a transplant candidate, and the selection of possible drug depends on prior therapy received. Additional selection criteria should consider patient characteristics such as age, risk factors, existing comorbidities such as renal failure, and previous toxicities such as neuropathy, and finally patient convenience. Improving complete response rates is a key goal of current trials in relapsed patients as well.

Bisphosphonates

The aminobisphosphonates pamidronate and zoledronate have been investigated in patients with myeloma and bone disease and have been shown to reduce skeletal complications and bone pain. A number of older randomized studies looked at their efficacy in patients with existing bone lesions and evaluated the development of new skeletal-related events. In this regards, pamidronate 90 mg and zoledronic acid 4 mg are equipotent in reducing bone-related problems in MM; the infusion time for zoledronic acid is 15 minutes compared with 1 to 2 hours for pamidronate. A recent large study, MRC IX, evaluated the efficacy of zoledronic acid in a randomized comparison with clodronate. This study in 1960 patients confirmed the efficacy and superiority of zoledronic acid in preventing new SREs in patients both with and without existing bone lesions (Table 85-23) and provided evidence that its continued use beyond 2 years was beneficial[41]; importantly, the study also suggested that zoledronic acid compared with clodronate improves an OS advantage providing for the first time some evidence of its antimyeloma activity (Fig. 85-19).[42] A similar survival advantage has also been reported with pamidronate (21 vs. 14 months; $P = .041$) in patients receiving salvage chemotherapy and pamidronate versus chemotherapy alone. Pamidronate administration alone has also been shown to produce responses or delays in disease progression in occasional patients. The bisphosphonate has multiple actions, including suppression of

Table 85-22 Novel Target in Myeloma, Agents, and Stage of Ongoing Clinical Trials

Target	Agent	Clinical Study Phase	Single Agent (S)/Combination (C)
Cell Surface Targets			
FGF3	Dasatinib	I/II	S
FGF, PDGF	(mAb)TKI258	I	S
CD38	mAb	I	S
CD40	SGN-40 (mAb) HCD122 (mAb)	I/II I	S, C (lenalidomide) S
CD56	huN901-DM1 (C-mAb)	I	S
CS1	HuLuc63 (mAb)	II/III	S, C (lenalidomide, bortezomib)
CD138	BT062 (mAb-DM4)	I	S
RANKL	AMG162 (mAb)	I/II	S
MUC1	AR20.5 (mAb)	I/II	S
BAFFR	LY2127399 (mAb)	I/II	S
CD52	Alemtuzumab (mAb)	II	S
TRAIL	Apo2L/TRAIL (Apo2 ligand) Mapatumumab	I I/II	S S
IGF1/R	IGF1R CP-571 (mAb) EM164 (mAb)	I I	S S
IL-6/R	CNTO328 (mAb)	II/III	S, C (bortezomib)
	Altizumab (mAb)	III	S
VEGF/R	Bevacizumab (mAb) SU5416 Zactima (ZD6474)	II II II	S S S
DKK-1	BHQ-880	I/II	S
ActivinA	ACC001	I/II	S
KIR	IPH101	I/II	S
CXCR3	AMD3100	II	C (bortezomib)
Intracytoplasmic or Nuclear Targets			
CDK	Alvocidib (NSC649890)	I	S
CDK and GSK3 AT7519M	I/II		S, C (bortezomib)
IKK	RTA402	I	S
Akt	Perofosine	III	C (bortezomib)
HDAC	Panabinostat Vorinostat Romidopsin Farnesyltransferase tipifarnib (R115777)	III II/III II/III II	C (bortezomib) C (bortezomib) C (bortezomib) S, C (bortezomib)
HSP90	KOS953 AUY922 IPI504	II II I/II	C (bortezomib) C (bortezomib) C (bortezomib)
Proteasome	Carfilzomib NPI-0052 MLN9708	II/III I I	S, C (lenalidomide) S S
Mitochondria	GCS-100	I/II	C
mTOR	CCI-779 II RAD001 INK128	II II II	C (bortezomib) C (lenalidomide, bortezomib) S
PKC	Enzastaurin	I/II	S, C (bortezomib)
Telomerease	GRN163L	I/II	S, C (bortezomib)

CDK, cyclin-dependent kinases; *CXCR,* C-X-C chemokine receptor; *DKK,* dickkopf-related protein; *HDAC,* histone deacetylase; *IGF,* insulinlike growth factor; *IKK,* I κappa B kinase; *IL-6,* interleukin-6; *KIR,* killer cell immunoglobulin-like receptors; *mAb,* monoclonal antibody; *mTOR,* mammalian target of rapamycin; *PKC,* protein kinase C; *TRAIL,* tumor necrosis factor–related apoptosis-inducing ligand; *VEGF,* vascular endothelial growth factor.
Data collected from National Cancer Institute Clinical Trials website (http://clinicaltrials.gov/), Multiple Myeloma Research Foundation website (http://www.themmrf.org/research-programs/), and the International Myeloma Foundation website (http://myeloma.org/Main.action).

Table 85-23 Cumulative Annual Incidence of First and Subsequent Skeletal-Related Events for the Intention-to-Treat Patients Randomized to Zoledronic Acid Versus Clodronate*

	Skeletal-Related Events		Incidence (95% CI)		Overall Difference (95% CI) Between Clodronic Acid and Zoledronic Acid[†]	*P* for Preceding 12 Months[‡]
	Clodronic acid (*n* = 979)	Zoledronic acid (*n* = 981)	Clodronic acid (*n* = 979)	Zoledronic acid (*n* = 981)		
12 months	451 (46%)	333 (34%)	0.43 (0.38-0.48)	0.33 (0.28-0.37)	0.11 (0.04-0.18)	.0002
24 months	93 (9%)	54 (6%)	0.60 (0.53-0.66)	0.42 (0.36-0.48)	0.18 (0.09-0.26)	.0024
36 months	28 (3%)	16 (2%)	0.69 (0.61-0.78)	0.47 (0.40-0.53)	0.23 (0.12-0.33)	.0089

From Morgan GJ, Child JA, Gregory WM, et al: Effects of zoledronic acid versus clodronic acid on skeletal morbidity in patients with newly diagnosed multiple myeloma (MRC Myeloma IX): Secondary outcomes from a randomised controlled trial. *Lancet Oncol* 12:743, 2011.
CI, Confidence interval.
*Data are number (%) unless otherwise indicated.
[†]*P* <.0001.
[‡]Unadjusted *P* value for the comparison of incidence of skeletal-related events in zoledronic acid group versus clodronic acid group per 12 months (e.g., 24-month *P* value is for incidence between 12 months and 24 months).

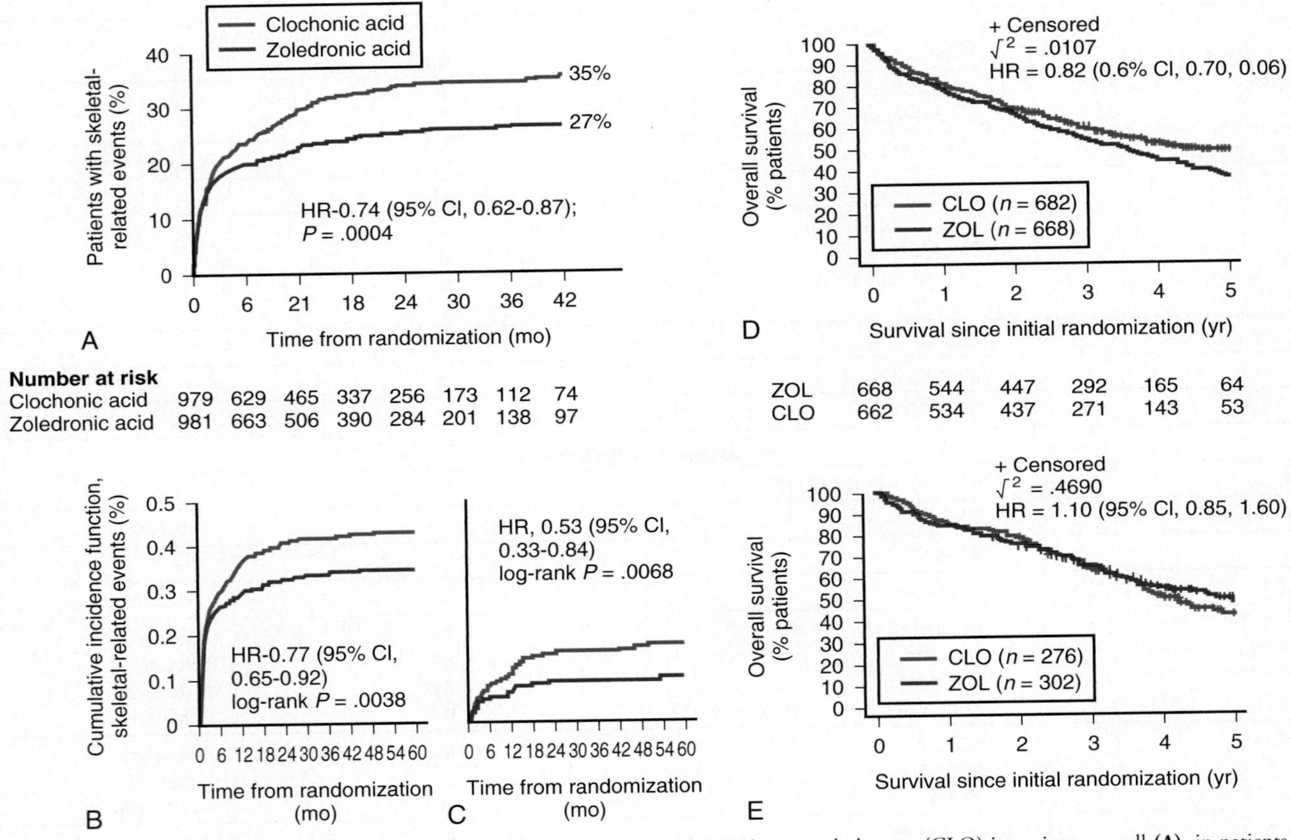

Figure 85-19 **A** to **C,** Time to first skeletal-related event with zoledronic acid (ZOL) versus clodronate (CLO) in patients overall **(A),** in patients with bone lesions at baseline **(B),** and in patients without bone lesions at baseline **(C).** **D** and **E,** Kaplan-Meier analyses of overall survival (OS) with ZOL versus CLO in patients with **(D)** or without **(E)** bone disease or other SRE at baseline. The benefit appears to be predominantly in those with prior SREs. *CI,* Confidence interval; *HR,* hazard ratio. *(Adapted from Morgan GJ, Child JA, Gregory WM, et al: Effects of zoledronic acid versus clodronic acid on skeletal morbidity in patients with newly diagnosed multiple myeloma (MRC Myeloma IX): Secondary outcomes from a randomised controlled trial. 12:743, 2011 and Morgan, GJ, Davies FE, Gregory WM, et al: Effects of induction and maintenance plus long-term bisphosphonates on bone disease in patients with multiple myeloma: The Medical Research Council Myeloma IX Trial.* Blood *119:5374, 2012.)*

osteoclast number and function, inhibition of IL-6 production by stromal cells, inhibition of farnesyl and geranyl–geranyl transferase activity, and immune effects via γ/δ T cells.

Two potential side effects of bisphosphonates—effects on renal function and development of osteonecrosis of the jaw (ONJ)—have limited their very long-term use in the recent past. ONJ is observed in patients with dental infection or procedures after its longer term use. Its frequency has been between 3% and 5%. In one study, 11 of 292 patients (3.8%) with MM developed ONJ. Patients receiving bisphosphonates require a thorough dental checkup before starting therapy and should have frequent dental follow-ups with careful and conservative use of dental procedures. With these precautions, the frequency of ONJ has been reduced. Similarly, measurement of renal function before each bisphosphonate dose and adjustment of dose based on renal function also make use of bisphosphonates safer. A slower administration of bisphosphonates prevents or protects against the development of renal dysfunction. Most recently, recommendations for the duration of bisphosphonate use has been for 2 years with reduction in frequency after that if patients enjoy a good remission. However, in light of the recent MRC-IX study, this recommendation will need revision with suggestion of possible long-term use. Additional bone-directed targets and agents are in development that have the ability to further inhibit osteoclast function (denosumab) and to improve osteoblast activity with bone anabolic effects (DKK-1–BHQ-880 and activin A–ACE-011). These agents are currently under clinical investigation in myeloma.

FUTURE DIRECTIONS

Significant advances have occurred in our understanding of pathobiology of MM that have translated into development of novel therapeutics. Predictive in vitro and in vivo models have been developed to study growth and survival characteristics of MM cells in the context of the BM microenvironment, but more importantly, to preclinically evaluate the efficacy of novel targeted agents. Similarly, there has been an explosion of genomic data covering various genomic correlates, including expression profile, CNA, alternate splicing, miRNA and now whole-genome sequencing and mutational analysis of both expressed genes as well as noncoding regions. Evolving understanding of the epigenomic alterations that affect cell growth, survival, and development of drug resistance is providing clues for novel interventions. For example, MM cell proliferation is now considered to be dependent on the bromodomain and extra-terminal (BET) domain family of bromodomain-containing proteins (BRD2, BRD3, and BRD4), which are novel therapeutic targets. These model systems and our improved understanding have led to new drug developments with seven new agents in advanced phase III studies in myeloma and more than 20 other novel agents in phase I or II studies. The genomic information is being integrated to develop more accurate risk stratification model and to develop personalized medicine to optimize response while avoiding the toxicity of agents that may not be effective in a given patient. Finally, because of these advances, the median survival time of MM patients has increased from 3 years to more than 7 to 8 years, and in a number of individuals, it becomes a chronic disease with curative outcome predicted in a proportion of patients in the near future.

SUGGESTED READINGS

Avet-Loiseau H, Attal M, Campion L, et al: Long-term analysis of the IFM 99 trials for myeloma: Cytogenetic abnormalities [t(4;14), del(17p), 1q gains] play a major role in defining long-term survival. *J Clin Oncol* 30:1949, 2012.

Avet-Loiseau H, Li C, Magrangeas F, et al: Prognostic significance of copy-number alterations in multiple myeloma. *J Clin Oncol* 27:4585, 2009.

Avet-Loiseau H, Minvielle S, Mellerin MP, et al: 14q32 chromosomal translocations: A hallmark of plasma cell dyscrasias? *Hematol J* 1:292, 2000.

Braga WM, Atanackovic D, Colleoni GW: The role of regulatory T cells and TH17 cells in multiple myeloma. *Clin Dev Immunol* 2012:293479, 2012.

Broyl A, Hose D, Lokhorst H, et al: Gene expression profiling for molecular classification of multiple myeloma in newly diagnosed patients. *Blood* 116:2543, 2010.

Carrasco DR, Tonon G, Huang Y, et al: High-resolution genomic profiles define distinct clinico-pathogenetic subgroups of multiple myeloma patients. *Cancer Cell* 9:313, 2006.

Chapman MA, Lawrence MS, Keats JJ, et al: Initial genome sequencing and analysis of multiple myeloma. *Nature* 471:467, 2011.

Decaux O, Lode L, Magrangeas F, et al: Prediction of survival in multiple myeloma based on gene expression profiles reveals cell cycle and chromosomal instability signatures in high-risk patients and hyperdiploid signatures in low-risk patients: A study of the Intergroupe Francophone du Myelome. *J Clin Oncol* 26:4798, 2008.

Dimopoulos M, Kyle R, Fermand JP, et al: Consensus recommendations for standard investigative workup: Report of the International Myeloma Workshop Consensus Panel 3. *Blood* 117:4701, 2011.

Greipp PR, San Miguel J, Durie BG, et al: International staging system for multiple myeloma. *J Clin Oncol* 23:3412, 2005.

Group IMW: Criteria for the classification of monoclonal gammopathies, multiple myeloma and related disorders: A report of the International Myeloma Working Group. *British Journal of Haematology* 121:749, 2003.

Gutierrez NC, Sarasquete ME, Misiewicz-Krzeminska I, et al: Deregulation of microRNA expression in the different genetic subtypes of multiple myeloma and correlation with gene expression profiling. *Leukemia: Official Journal of the Leukemia Society of America, Leukemia Research Fund, UK* 24:629, 2010.

Harousseau JL, Attal M, Avet-Loiseau H, et al: Bortezomib plus dexamethasone is superior to vincristine plus doxorubicin plus dexamethasone as induction treatment prior to autologous stem-cell transplantation in newly diagnosed multiple myeloma: Results of the IFM 2005-01 phase III trial. *J Clin Oncol* 28:4621, 2010.

Hideshima T, Mitsiades C, Tonon G, et al: Understanding multiple myeloma pathogenesis in the bone marrow to identify new therapeutic targets. *Nat Rev Cancer* 7:585, 2007.

Hutchison CA, Batuman V, Behrens J, et al: The pathogenesis and diagnosis of acute kidney injury in multiple myeloma. *Nat Rev Nephrol* 8:43, 2012.

Joshua DE: Biology of multiple myeloma—host-tumour interactions and immune regulation of disease activity. *Hematol Oncol* 6:83, 1988.

Kyle RA, Remstein ED, Therneau TM, et al: Clinical course and prognosis of smoldering (asymptomatic) multiple myeloma. *N Engl J Med* 356:2582, 2007.

Kyle RA, Therneau TM, Rajkumar SV, et al: A long-term study of prognosis in monoclonal gammopathy of undetermined significance. *N Engl J Med* 346:564, 2002.

Kumar S, Flinn I, Richardson PG, et al: Randomized, multicenter, phase 2 study (EVOLUTION) of combinations of bortezomib, dexamethasone, cyclophosphamide, and lenalidomide in previously untreated multiple myeloma. *Blood* 119:4375, 2012.

Landgren O, Kyle RA, Pfeiffer RM, et al: Monoclonal gammopathy of undetermined significance (MGUS) consistently precedes multiple myeloma: A prospective study. *Blood* 113:5412, 2009.

Ludwig H, Pohl G, Osterborg A: Anemia in multiple myeloma. *Clin Adv Hematol Oncol* 2:233, 2004.

Munshi NC, Anderson KC, Bergsagel PL, et al: Consensus recommendations for risk stratification in multiple myeloma: Report of the International Myeloma Workshop Consensus Panel 2. *Blood* 117:4696, 2011.

Nucci M, Anaissie E: Infections in patients with multiple myeloma in the era of high-dose therapy and novel agents. *Clin Infect Dis* 49:1211, 2009.

Prabhala RH, Pelluru D, Fulciniti M, et al: Elevated IL-17 produced by TH17 cells promotes myeloma cell growth and inhibits immune function in multiple myeloma. *Blood* 115:5385, 2010.

Raje N, Roodman GD: Advances in the biology and treatment of bone disease in multiple myeloma. *Clin Cancer Res* 17:1278, 2011.

Richardson PG, Weller E, Lonial S, et al: Lenalidomide, bortezomib, and dexamethasone combination therapy in patients with newly diagnosed multiple myeloma. *Blood* 116:679, 2010.

Salhia B, Baker A, Ahmann G, et al: DNA methylation analysis determines the high frequency of genic hypomethylation and low frequency of hypermethylation events in plasma cell tumors. *Cancer Res* 70:6934, 2010.

Sawyer JR: The prognostic significance of cytogenetics and molecular profiling in multiple myeloma. *Cancer Genet* 204:3, 2011.

Shaughnessy JD, Jr, Zhan F, Burington BE, et al: A validated gene expression model of high-risk multiple myeloma is defined by deregulated expression of genes mapping to chromosome 1. *Blood* 109:2276, 2007.

Tian E, Zhan F, Walker R, et al: The role of the Wnt-signaling antagonist DKK1 in the development of osteolytic lesions in multiple myeloma. *N Engl J Med* 349:2483, 2003.

For complete list of references log on to www.expertconsult.com.

CHAPTER 86

WALDENSTRÖM MACROGLOBULINEMIA AND LYMPHOPLASMACYTIC LYMPHOMA

Steven P. Treon and Giampaolo Merlini

Waldenström macroglobulinemia (WM) is a distinct clinicopathologic entity resulting from the accumulation, predominantly in the bone marrow (BM), of clonally related lymphocytes, lymphoplasmacytic cells, and plasma cells that secrete a monoclonal immunoglobulin M (IgM) protein (Fig. 86-1).[1] This condition is considered to correspond to the lymphoplasmacytic lymphoma (LPL) as defined by the World Health Organization lymphoma classification system.[2] Most cases of LPL are WM, with fewer than 5% of cases made up of IgA, IgG, and nonsecreting LPL.

EPIDEMIOLOGY

Waldenström macroglobulinemia is an uncommon disease, with a reported age-adjusted incidence rate of 3.4 per million among males and 1.7 per million among females in the United States and a geometrical increase with age.[3] The incidence rate for WM is higher among whites, with African descendants representing only 5% of all patients. The incidence of WM may be higher among individuals of Ashkenazi Jewish descent.[4] Genetic factors appear to be important to the pathogenesis of WM. A common predisposition for WM with other malignancies has been raised,[4,5] with numerous reports of familial clustering of individuals with WM alone and with other B-cell lymphoproliferative diseases.[6-10] In a large single-center experience, 26% of 924 consecutive patients with WM had a first- or second-degree relative with either WM or another B-cell disorder.[5] Frequent familial association with other immunologic disorders in healthy relatives, including hypogammaglobulinemia and hypergammaglobulinemia (particularly polyclonal IgM), autoantibody (particularly to thyroid) production, and manifestation of hyperresponsive B cells have also been reported.[10,11] Increased expression of the *bcl-2* gene with enhanced B-cell survival may underlie the increased immunoglobulin synthesis in familial WM.[10] The role of environmental factors in WM remains to be clarified, but chronic antigenic stimulation from infections, certain drugs, and Agent Orange exposures remain suspect. An etiologic role for hepatitis C virus (HCV) infection has been suggested, but in one study, no association could be established using both serologic and molecular diagnostic studies for HCV infection in 100 consecutive WM patients.[12,13]

PATHOBIOLOGY

Cytogenic Abnormalities

Chromosome 6q deletions encompassing 6q21-25 have been observed in up to half of WM patients and at a comparable frequency among patients with and without a familial history.[7,14-16] The presence of 6q deletions has been suggested to distinguish patients with WM from those with IgM monoclonal gammopathy of unknown significance (MGUS) and to have potential prognostic significance, including impacting on progression-free survival (PFS) after treatment, although others have reported no prognostic significance to the presence of 6q deletions in WM.[14,16,17] Other abnormalities observed by cytogenetic or fluorescent in situ hybridization (FISH) analyses include deletions in 13q14, TP53 and ATM, trisomy 4, 12, and 18.[17,18] IgH rearrangements are uncommon in WM and may be helpful in distinguishing cases of WM from IgM myeloma in which IgH switch region rearrangements are a prominent feature.[19]

Mutation in MYD88

A highly recurrent somatic mutation (MYD88 L265P) has recently been identified in WM patients by paired tumor and normal whole-genome sequencing and subsequent confirmation by Sanger sequencing.[20] MYD88 L265P was expressed in tumor cells from 91% of LPL cases, which included patients with IgM- (WM) and IgG-secreting LPL. By comparison, MYD88 L265P was absent in myeloma samples, including IgM myeloma, and was expressed in a small subset (6.5%) of marginal zone lymphoma (MZL) patients, who surprisingly had many WM-related features. The expression of MYD88 L265P occurs in familial and sporadic WM patients at the same frequency. These findings appear to indicate that acquisition of MYD88 L265P is a common transforming event for WM regardless of familial predisposition. Importantly, whereas knock-down of MYD88 decreased survival of MYD88 L265P expressing WM cells, survival was more enhanced by knock-in of MYD88 L265P versus wild-type MYD88. The discovery of a mutation in MYD88 is of significance given its role as an adaptor molecule in Toll-like receptor (TLR) and interleukin-1 receptor (IL-1R) signaling.[21] All TLRs except for TLR3 use MYD88 to facilitate their intracellular signaling. After TLR or IL-1R stimulation, MYD88 is recruited to the activated receptor complex as a homodimer, which then complexes with IRAK4 and activates IRAK1 and IRAK2.[22-24] Tumor necrosis factor receptor associated factor 6 is then activated by IRAK1, leading to nuclear factor kappa-B (NFκB) activation via IκBα phosphorylation.[25] Exposure to inhibitors of MYD88 pathway leads to decreased IRAK1 and IκBα phosphorylation, as well as survival of MYD88 L265P expressing WM cells. These observations are of particular relevance to WM because NFκB signaling is important for WM growth and survival.[26]

Nature of the Clonal Cell

The WM BM B-cell clone shows intraclonal differentiation from small lymphocytes with large focal deposits of surface immunoglobulins to lymphoplasmacytic cells to mature plasma cells that contain intracytoplasmic immunoglobulins.[27] Clonal B cells are detectable among blood B lymphocytes, and their number increases in patients who fail to respond to therapy or who progress.[28] These clonal blood cells possess the peculiar capacity to differentiate spontaneously in vitro culture to plasma cells. This occurs through an IL-6–dependent process in IgM MGUS and mostly an IL-6–independent process in WM patients.[29] All of these cells express the monoclonal IgM present in the blood, and a variable percentage of them also express surface IgD. The characteristic immunophenotypic profile of the lymphoplasmacytic cells in WM includes the expression of the pan B-cell markers CD19, CD20, CD22, CD79, and FMC7.2.[30-32] Expression of CD5, CD10, and CD23 may be found in 10% to 20% of cases and does not exclude the diagnosis of WM.[33]

The phenotype of lymphoplasmacytic cells in WM cells suggests that the clone is a postgerminal center B cell. This phenotype is further strengthened by the results of the analysis of the nature (silent or amino acid replacing) and distribution (in framework or CDR regions) of somatic mutations in Ig heavy- and light-chain variable regions performed in patients with WM cells.[34,35] This analysis showed a high rate of replacement mutations compared with the closest germline genes, clustering in the CDR regions without intraclonal variation. Subsequent studies showed a strong preferential usage of VH3/JH4 gene families, no intraclonal variation, and no evidence for any isotype-switched transcripts.[36,37] These data indicate that WM may originate from an IgM$^+$ or IgM$^+$ IgD$^+$ memory B cell (or both). Normal IgM$^+$ memory B cells localize in BM, where they mature to IgM-secreting cells.[38]

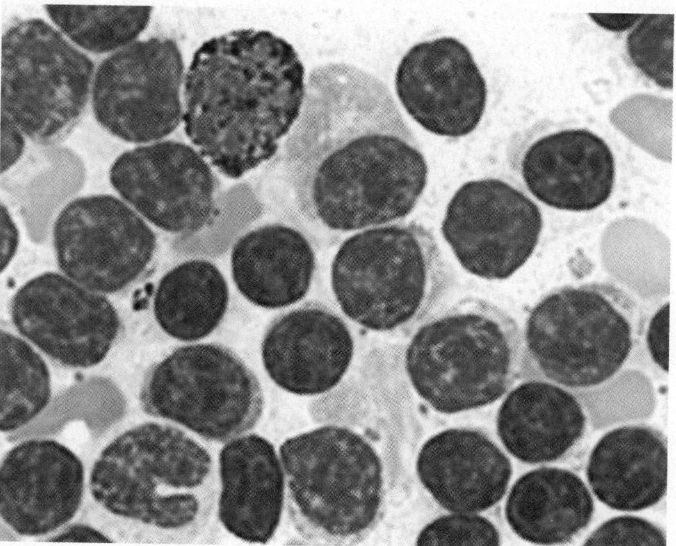

Figure 86-1 ASPIRATE FROM A PATIENT WITH WALDENSTRÖM MACROGLOBULINEMIA DEMONSTRATING EXCESS MATURE LYMPHOCYTES, LYMPHOPLASMACYTIC CELLS, AND PLASMA CELLS.

Bone Marrow Microenvironment

Increased numbers of mast cells are found in the BM of WM patients (Fig. 86-2), wherein they are usually admixed with tumor aggregates.[2,32,39] The role of mast cells in WM has been investigated in one study wherein coculture of primary autologous or mast cell lines with WM LPC resulted in dose-dependent WM cell proliferation or tumor colony formation, primarily through CD40 ligand (CD40L) signaling. Furthermore, WM cells through elaboration of soluble CD27 (sCD27) induced the upregulation of CD40L on mast cells derived from WM patients and mast cell lines, suggesting a microenvironmental support system[39,40] High levels of expression of CXCR4 and VLA-4 in WM cells have been observed.[41] In blocking experiment studies, CXCR4 was shown to support migration of WM cells, and VLA-4 contributed to adhesion of WM cells to BM stromal cells.

CLINICAL MANIFESTATIONS

The clinical and laboratory findings at time of diagnosis of WM in one large institutional study are presented in Table 86-1. Unlike most indolent lymphomas, splenomegaly and lymphadenopathy are prominent in only a minority of patients (≤15%). Purpura is frequently associated with cryoglobulinemia and more rarely with amyloid light-chain (AL) amyloidosis, but hemorrhagic manifestations and neuropathies are multifactorial (see below). The morbidity associated with WM is caused by the concurrence of two main components: tissue infiltration by neoplastic cells and, more importantly, the physicochemical and immunologic properties of the monoclonal IgM. As shown in Table 86-2, the monoclonal IgM can produce clinical manifestations through several different mechanisms related to its physicochemical properties, nonspecific interactions with other proteins, antibody activity, and tendency to deposit in tissues.[42-44]

MORBIDITY CAUSED BY THE EFFECTS OF IMMUNOGLOBULIN M

Hyperviscosity Syndrome

Increased serum IgM levels lead to blood hyperviscosity-related complications.[45] The mechanisms behind the marked increase in the

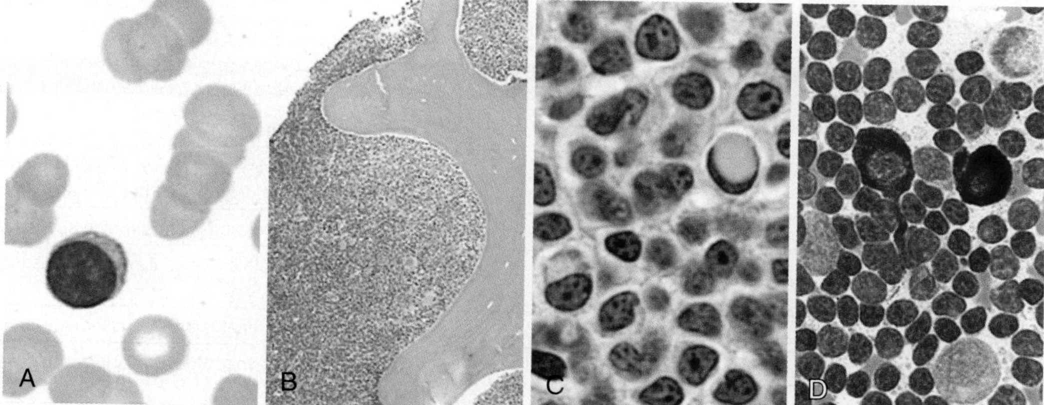

Figure 86-2 LYMPHOPLASMACYTIC LYMPHOMA CONSISTENT WITH WALDENSTRÖM MACROGLOBULINEMIA. The patient was a 78-year-old man who first presented with anemia. Serum electrophoresis demonstrated an immunoglobulin M (IgM) κ monoclonal protein, and quantitative immunoglobulins showed an IgM of 5130 mg/dL. His serum viscosity was elevated at 2.9 centipoise (cP). The peripheral blood smear showed circulating lymphoma cells with slight plasmacytic appearance **(A).** There was also marked rouleaux formation of the red blood cells. The bone core biopsy showed a paratrabecular and interstitial infiltrate of malignant lymphoid cells **(B),** which at higher power included many with intranuclear inclusions or Dutcher bodies (**C,** *center*). The aspirate **(D)** was packed with lymphoplasmacytic cells associated with increased mast cells *(upper left)*. The phenotype was CD19$^+$, CD20$^+$, IgM/κ$^+$ with no CD5, CD10, or CD11c expression.

resistance to blood flow and the resulting impaired transit through the microcirculatory system are rather complex.[45-47] The main determinants are (1) a high concentration of monoclonal IgMs, which may form aggregates and may bind water through their carbohydrate component, and (2) their interaction with blood cells. Monoclonal IgMs increase red blood cell (RBC) aggregation (*rouleaux* formation) and RBC internal viscosity while also reducing deformability. The possible presence of cryoglobulins can contribute to increasing blood viscosity as well as to the tendency to induce erythrocyte aggregation. Serum viscosity is proportional to the IgM concentration up to 30 g/L and then increases sharply at higher levels. Plasma viscosity and hematocrit levels are directly regulated by the body. Increased plasma viscosity may also contribute to inappropriately low erythropoietin production, which is the major cause for anemia in these patients.[48] Clinical manifestations are related to circulatory disturbances that can be best appreciated by ophthalmologic examination, which shows distended and tortuous retinal veins, hemorrhages, and papilledema[49] (Fig. 86-3). Symptoms usually occur when the monoclonal IgM concentration exceeds 50 g/L or when serum viscosity is greater than 4.0 centipoises (cp), but there is a great individual variability, with some patients showing no evidence of hyperviscosity even at 10 cp.[45] The most common symptoms are oronasal bleeding, visual disturbances caused by retinal bleeding, and dizziness that may rarely lead to coma. Heart failure can be aggravated, particularly in elderly adults, owing to increased blood viscosity, expanded plasma volume, and anemia. Inappropriate transfusion can exacerbate hyperviscosity and may precipitate cardiac failure.

Table 86-1 Clinical and Laboratory Findings for 149 Consecutive Newly Diagnosed Patients With the Consensus Panel Diagnosis of Waldenström Macroglobulinemia Presenting to the Dana Farber Cancer Institute

	Median	Range	Institutional Normal Reference Range
Age (yr)	59	34-84	NA
Gender (male/female)	85/64		NA
BM involvement	30%	5%-95%	NA
Adenopathy	16%		NA
Splenomegaly	10%		NA
IgM (mg/dL)	2870	267-12,400	40-230
IgG (mg/dL)	587	47-2770	700-1600
IgA (mg/dL)	47	8-509	70-400
Serum viscosity (cp)	2.0	1.4-6.6	1.4-1.9
Hct (%)	35.0%	17.2%-45.4%	34.8%-43.6%
Plt ($\times 10^9$/L)	253	24-649	155-410
Wbc ($\times 10^9$/L)	6.0	0.3-13	3.8-9.2
B_2M (mg/dL)	3.0	1.3-13.7	0-2.7
LDH	395	122-1131	313-618

BM, Bone marrow; *Ig*, immunoglobulin; *LDH*, lactate dehydrogenase; *NA*, not applicable.

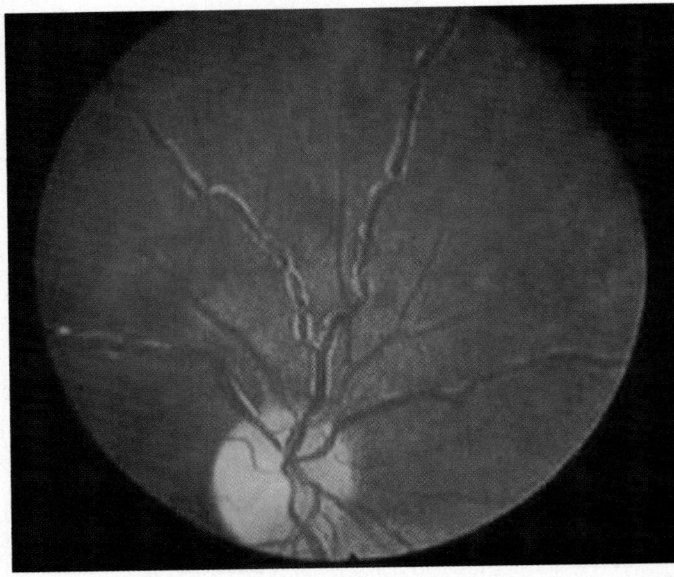

Figure 86-3 FUNDUSCOPIC EXAMINATION OF A PATIENT WITH WALDENSTRÖM MACROGLOBULINEMIA DEMONSTRATING HYPERVISCOSITY-RELATED CHANGES, INCLUDING DILATED RETINAL VESSELS, PERIPHERAL HEMORRHAGES, AND "VENOUS SAUSAGING." *(Courtesy of Marvin Stone, MD.)*

Table 86-2 Physicochemical and Immunologic Properties of the Monoclonal IgM Protein in Waldenström Macroglobulinemia

Properties of IgM Monoclonal Protein	Diagnostic Condition	Clinical Manifestations
Pentameric structure	Hyperviscosity	Headaches, blurred vision, epistaxis, retinal hemorrhages, leg cramps, impaired mentation, intracranial hemorrhage
Precipitation on cooling	Cryoglobulinemia (type I)	Raynaud phenomenon, acrocyanosis, ulcers, purpura, cold urticaria
Autoantibody activity to MAG, GM1, sulfatide moieties on peripheral nerve sheaths	Peripheral neuropathies	Sensorimotor neuropathies, painful neuropathies, ataxic gait, bilateral foot drop
Autoantibody activity to IgG	Cryoglobulinemia (type II)	Purpura, arthralgias, renal failure, sensorimotor neuropathies
Autoantibody activity to RBC antigens	Cold agglutinins	Hemolytic anemia, Raynaud phenomenon, acrocyanosis, livedo reticularis
Tissue deposition as amorphous aggregates	Organ dysfunction	Skin: bullous skin disease, papules, Schnitzler syndrome GI: diarrhea, malabsorption, bleeding Kidney: proteinuria, renal failure (light-chain component)
Tissue deposition as amyloid fibrils (light-chain component most commonly)	Organ dysfunction	Fatigue, weight loss, edema, hepatomegaly, macroglossia, organ dysfunction of involved organs (heart, kidney, liver, peripheral sensory and autonomic nerves)

GI, Gastrointestinal; *GM1*, ganglioside M1; *Ig, immunoglobulin; MAG*, myelin-associated glycoprotein; *RBC*, red blood cell.

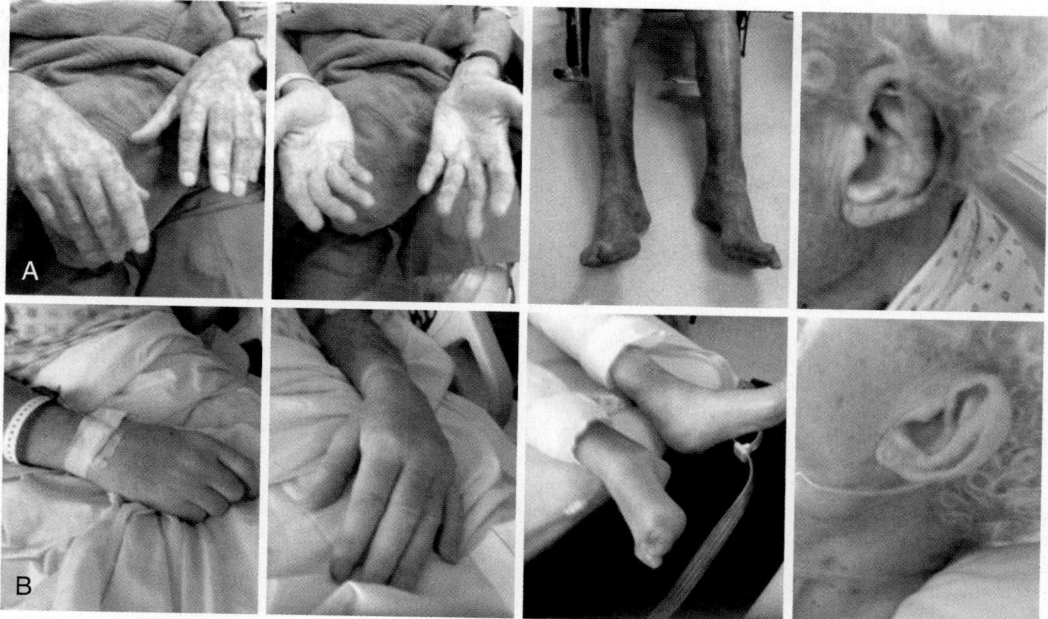

Figure 86-4 CRYOGLOBULINEMIA MANIFESTING WITH SEVERE ACROCYANOSIS IN A PATIENT WITH WALDENSTRÖM MACROGLOBULINEMIA BEFORE **(A)** AND AFTER **(B)** WARMING AND PLASMAPHERESIS.

Cryoglobulinemia

In up to 20% of WM patients, the monoclonal IgM can behave as a cryoglobulin (type I), but it is symptomatic in 5% or fewer of the cases.[50] Cryoprecipitation is mainly dependent on the concentration of monoclonal IgM; for this reason, plasmapheresis and plasma exchange are commonly effective in this condition. Symptoms result from impaired blood flow in small vessels and include Raynaud phenomenon, acrocyanosis, and necrosis of the regions most exposed to cold (e.g., the tip of the nose, ears, fingers, and toes [Fig. 86-4]; malleolar ulcers, purpura, and cold urticaria). Renal manifestations may occur but are infrequent.

Autoantibody Activity

Monoclonal IgM may exert its pathogenic effects through specific recognition of autologous antigens, the most notable being nerve constituents, immunoglobulin determinants, and RBC antigens.

Immunoglobulin M–Related Neuropathy

Peripheral neuropathy has been estimated to occur in 5% to 38% of WM patients.[51-55] The nerve damage is mediated by diverse pathogenetic mechanisms: IgM antibody activity toward nerve constituents causing demyelinating polyneuropathies; endoneurial granulofibrillar deposits of IgM without antibody activity associated with axonal polyneuropathy; occasionally by tubular deposits in the endoneurium associated with IgM cryoglobulin; and rarely by amyloid deposits or by neoplastic cell infiltration of nerve structures.[56] Half of the patients with IgM neuropathy have a distinctive clinical syndrome that is associated with antibodies against a minor 100-kDa glycoprotein component of nerve, myelin-associated glycoprotein (MAG). Anti-MAG antibodies are generally monoclonal IgMκ and usually also exhibit reactivity with other glycoproteins or glycolipids that share antigenic determinants with MAG.[57-59] The anti–MAG-related neuropathy is typically distal and symmetrical, affecting both motor and sensory functions; it is slowly progressive with a long period of stability.[52,60] Most patients present with sensory complaints (paresthesias, aching discomfort, dysesthesias, or lancinating pains), imbalance and gait ataxia owing to lack of proprioception, and leg muscle atrophy in the advanced stage. Patients with predominantly demyelinating sensory neuropathy in association with monoclonal IgM to gangliosides with disialosyl moieties, such as GD1b, GD3, GD2, GT1b, and GQ1b, have also been reported.[61,62] Anti-GD1b and anti-GQ1b antibodies were significantly associated with predominantly sensory ataxic neuropathy. These antiganglioside monoclonal IgMs present core clinical features of chronic ataxic neuropathy with variable presence of ophthalmoplegia or RBC cold agglutinating activity. The disialosyl epitope is also present on RBC glycophorins, thereby accounting for the RBC cold agglutinin activity of anti-Pr2 specificity.[63,64] Monoclonal IgM proteins that bind to gangliosides with a terminal trisaccharide moiety, including GM2 and GalNac-GD1A, are associated with chronic demyelinating neuropathy and severe sensory ataxia that is unresponsive to corticosteroids.[65] Antiganglioside IgM proteins may also cross-react with lipopolysaccharides of *Campylobacter jejuni,* an infection that is known to precipitate the Miller Fisher syndrome, a variant of the Guillain-Barré syndrome.[66] This finding indicates that molecular mimicry may play a role in this condition. Antisulfatide monoclonal IgM proteins associated with sensory or sensorimotor neuropathy have been detected in 5% of patients with IgM monoclonal gammopathy and neuropathy.[67] Motor neuron disease has been reported in patients with WM and monoclonal IgM with anti-GM1 and sulfoglucuronyl paragloboside activity.[68] POEMS (polyneuropathy, organomegaly, endocrinopathy, M protein, and skin changes) syndrome is rarely associated with WM.[69]

Cold Agglutinin Hemolytic Anemia

Monoclonal IgM may present with cold agglutinin activity; that is, it can recognize specific RBC antigens below physiological temperatures, producing a chronic hemolytic anemia. This disorder occurs in fewer than 10% of WM patients[70] and is associated with cold agglutinin titers greater than 1:1000 in most cases. The monoclonal component is usually an IgMκ and reacts most commonly with I/i antigens with complement fixation and activation.[71,72] Mild chronic hemolytic anemia can be exacerbated after cold exposure, but rarely does hemoglobin drop below 70 g/L. The hemolysis is usually extravascular (removal of C3b opsonized cells by the reticuloendothelial system, primarily in the liver) and rarely intravascular resulting from complement destruction of the RBC membrane. The agglutination of RBCs in the cooler peripheral circulation also causes Raynaud syndrome, acrocyanosis, and livedo reticularis. Macroglobulins with the properties of both cryoglobulins and cold agglutinins with anti-Pr specificity have been reported. These properties may have as a common basis the immune binding of the sialic acid–containing carbohydrate present on RBC glycophorins and on Ig molecules. Several other macroglobulins with a variety of antibody activities toward autologous antigens (e.g., phospholipids, tissue and plasma proteins) and foreign ligands have also been reported.

Tissue Deposition

The monoclonal protein can be deposited in several tissues as amorphous aggregates. Linear deposition of monoclonal IgM along the skin basement membrane is associated with bullous skin disease.[73] Amorphous IgM deposits in the dermis determine the so-called IgM storage papules on the extensor surface of the extremities—macroglobulinemia cutis.[74] Deposition of monoclonal IgM in the lamina propria or submucosa of the intestine may be associated with diarrhea, malabsorption, and gastrointestinal bleeding.[75,76] It is well known that kidney involvement is less common and less severe in WM than in multiple myeloma, probably because the amount of light chain excreted in the urine is generally lower in WM than in myeloma and because of the absence of contributing factors, such as hypercalcemia, although cast nephropathy has also been described in WM.[77] On the other hand, the IgM macromolecule is more susceptible to being trapped in the glomerular loops where ultrafiltration presumably contributes to its precipitation, forming subendothelial deposits of aggregated IgM proteins that occlude the glomerular capillaries.[78] Mild and reversible proteinuria may result and most patients are asymptomatic. The deposition of monoclonal light chain as fibrillar amyloid deposits (AL amyloidosis) is uncommon in patients with WM.[79] Clinical expression and prognosis are similar to those of other AL patients with involvement of heart (44%), kidneys (32%), liver (14%), lungs (10%), peripheral or autonomic nerves (38%), and soft tissues (18%). However, the incidence of cardiac and pulmonary involvement is higher in patients with monoclonal IgM than with other immunoglobulin isotypes. The association of WM with reactive amyloidosis (AA) has been documented rarely.[80,81] Simultaneous occurrence of fibrillary glomerulopathy, characterized by glomerular deposits of wide noncongophilic fibrils and amyloid deposits, has been reported in WM.[82]

Manifestations Related to Tissue Infiltration by Neoplastic Cells

Tissue infiltration by neoplastic cells is rare and can involve various organs and tissues, from the BM (described later) to the liver, spleen, lymph nodes, and possibly the lungs, gastrointestinal tract, kidneys, skin, eyes, and central nervous system. Pulmonary involvement in the form of masses, nodules, diffuse infiltrate, or pleural effusions is relatively rare, since the overall incidence of pulmonary and pleural findings reported for WM is only 3% to 5%.[83-85] Cough is the most common presenting symptom followed by dyspnea and chest pain. Chest radiographic findings include parenchymal infiltrates, confluent masses, and effusions. Malabsorption, diarrhea, bleeding, or obstruction may indicate involvement of the gastrointestinal tract at the level of the stomach, duodenum, or small intestine.[86-89] In contrast to multiple myeloma, infiltration of the kidney interstitium with lymphoplasmacytoid cells has been reported in WM,[90] but renal or perirenal masses are common.[91] The skin can be the site of dense lymphoplasmacytic infiltrates, similar to that seen in the liver, spleen, and lymph nodes, forming cutaneous plaques and, rarely, nodules.[92] Chronic urticaria and IgM gammopathy are the two cardinal features of Schnitzler syndrome, which is not usually associated initially with clinical features of WM,[93] although evolution to WM is common. Thus close follow-up of these patients is warranted. Invasion of articular and periarticular structures by WM malignant cells is rarely reported.[94] The neoplastic cells can infiltrate the periorbital structures, lacrimal gland, and retro-orbital lymphoid tissues, resulting in ocular nerve palsies.[95,96] Direct infiltration of the central nervous system by monoclonal lymphoplasmacytic cells as infiltrates or as tumors constitutes the rarely observed Bing-Neel syndrome, which is characterized clinically by confusion, memory loss, disorientation, and motor dysfunction.[97]

LABORATORY MANIFESTATIONS

Hematological Abnormalities

Anemia is the most common finding in patients with symptomatic WM and is caused by a combination of factors, including a mild decrease in RBC survival, impaired erythropoiesis, hemolysis, moderate plasma volume expansion, and blood loss from the gastrointestinal tract. Blood smears are usually normocytic and normochromic, and rouleaux formation is often pronounced. Electronically measured mean corpuscular volume may be elevated spuriously owing to erythrocyte aggregation. In addition, the hemoglobin estimate can be inaccurate (i.e., falsely high) because of interaction between the monoclonal protein and the diluent used in some automated analyzers.[98] Leukocyte and platelet counts are usually within the reference range at presentation, although patients may occasionally present with severe thrombocytopenia. As reported earlier, monoclonal B-lymphocytes expressing surface IgM and late-differentiation B-cell markers are uncommonly detected in blood by flow cytometry. A raised erythrocyte sedimentation rate is almost constantly observed in WM and may be the first clue to the presence of the macroglobulin. The clotting abnormality detected most frequently is prolongation of thrombin time. AL amyloidosis should be suspected in all patients with nephrotic syndrome, cardiomyopathy, hepatomegaly, or peripheral neuropathy. Diagnosis requires the demonstration of green birefringence under polarized light of amyloid deposits stained with Congo red.

Biochemical Investigations

High-resolution electrophoresis combined with immunofixation of serum and urine is recommended for identification and characterization of the IgM monoclonal protein. The light chain of the monoclonal IgM is κ in 75% to 80% of patients. A few WM patients have more than one M component. The concentration of the serum monoclonal protein is very variable but in most cases lies within the range of 15 to 45 g/L. Densitometry should be adopted to determine IgM levels for serial evaluations because nephelometry is unreliable and shows large intralaboratory as well as interlaboratory variation. The presence of cold agglutinins or cryoglobulins may affect determination of IgM levels; therefore, testing for cold agglutinins and cryoglobulins should be performed at diagnosis. If present, subsequent serum samples should be analyzed under warm conditions for determination of serum monoclonal IgM level. Although Bence Jones proteinuria is frequently present, it exceeds 1 g/24 hours in only 3% of cases. Although IgM levels are elevated in WM patients, IgA and IgG levels are most often depressed and do not demonstrate recovery even after successful treatment, suggesting that patients with WM harbor a defect that prevents normal plasma cell development or Ig heavy chain rearrangements.[99,100]

Serum Viscosity

Because of its large size (almost 1,000,000 daltons), most IgM molecules are retained within the intravascular compartment and can exert an undue effect on serum viscosity. Therefore, serum viscosity should be measured if the patient has signs or symptoms of hyperviscosity syndrome. Funduscopy remains an excellent indicator of clinically relevant hyperviscosity. Among the first clinical signs of hyperviscosity, the appearance of peripheral and midperipheral dot and blot–like hemorrhages in the retina is best appreciated with indirect ophthalmoscopy and scleral depression.[49] In more severe cases of hyperviscosity, dot-, blot-, and flame-shaped hemorrhages can appear in the macular area along with markedly dilated and tortuous veins with focal constrictions, resulting in "venous sausaging" as well as papilledema.

Bone Marrow Findings

The BM is always involved in WM. Central to the diagnosis of WM is the demonstration, by trephine biopsy, of *BM infiltration by a lymphoplasmacytic cell population* constituted by small lymphocytes with evidence of plasmacytoid and plasma cell differentiation (see Figs. 86-1 and 86-2). The pattern of BM infiltration may be diffuse, interstitial, or nodular, showing usually an intertrabecular pattern of infiltration. A solely paratrabecular pattern of infiltration is unusual and should raise the possibility of follicular lymphoma.[1] The BM infiltration should routinely be confirmed by *immunophenotypic studies* (flow cytometry or immunohistochemistry) showing the following profile: sIgM$^+$CD19$^+$CD20$^+$CD22$^+$CD79$^+$.[30-32] Up to 20% of cases may express CD5, CD10, or CD23.[33] In these cases, care should be taken to satisfactorily exclude chronic lymphocytic leukemia and mantle cell lymphoma.[1] "Intranuclear" periodic acid–Schiff–positive inclusions (Dutcher-Fahey bodies)[101] consisting of IgM deposits in the perinuclear space and sometimes in intranuclear vacuoles may be seen occasionally in lymphoid cells in WM. An increased number of mast cells, usually in association with the lymphoid aggregates, is commonly found in WM, and their presence may help in differentiating WM from other B-cell lymphomas.[1,2]

Other Investigations

Magnetic resonance imaging (MRI) of the spine in conjunction with computed tomography (CT) of the abdomen and pelvis is useful in evaluating the disease status in WM.[102] BM involvement can be documented by MRI studies of the spine in more than 90% of patients, and CT of the abdomen and pelvis demonstrated enlarged nodes in 43% of WM patients.[102] Lymph node biopsy may show preserved architecture or replacement by infiltration of neoplastic cells with lymphoplasmacytoid, lymphoplasmacytic, or polymorphous cytologic patterns. The residual disease after high-dose chemotherapy with allogeneic or autologous stem cell rescue can be monitored by polymerase chain reaction–based methods using primers specific for the monoclonal Ig variable regions.

DIFFERENTIAL DIAGNOSIS

The differential diagnosis of WM includes other IgM-secreting B-cell disorders, including other B-cell lymphoma subtypes and multiple myeloma. MZL is the most common disease entity with which WM is often confused because of many overlapping clinicopathologic features, including morphologic, immunophenotypic, and cytogenetic features. A recent study found that a mutation in MYD88 (L265P) could be used to differentiate WM wherein it was expressed in over 90% of patients from MZL. The presence of translocations at chromosome 14 involving the immunoglobulin heavy-chain locus is commonly encountered in IgM myeloma, typically t(11;14), although it is absent in WM.[19]

Prognosis

Waldenström macroglobulinemia typically presents as an indolent disease, although considerable variability in prognosis can be seen. The median survival time reported in several large series has ranged from 5 to 10 years,[103-109] but in a recent study of 436 consecutive patients with WM, the median overall survival from time of diagnosis was in excess of 10 years.[110] Age is consistently an important prognostic factor (>60-70 years),[103,104,106,109] but it is often impacted by unrelated morbidities. Anemia, which can be multifactorial, is an adverse prognostic factor in WM, with hemoglobin levels of less than 9 to 12 g/dL associated with decreased survival in several series.[103-105,109] Cytopenias have also been regularly identified as a significant predictor of survival. The number of cytopenias in a given patient may predict survival.[104] Serum albumin levels have correlated with survival in WM patients in certain but not all studies using multivariate analyses.[104,107] High serum β-2 microglobulin (>3-3.5 g/dL) levels,[105,107,109] high serum IgM M protein (>7 g/dL),[109] low serum IgM M protein (<4 g/dL),[107] the presence of cryoglobulins,[103] and the presence of a familial disease background[110] have also been reported to confer adverse outcomes. The presence of 6q deletion as an adverse marker remains controversial.[14,16] A few prognostic scoring systems have been proposed (Table 86-3). Although the use of prognostic markers or scoring systems to make therapeutic decisions remains to be clarified,[106] patients with familial disease predisposition show better outcomes after bortezomib-based therapy.[110]

Therapy

As part of the International Workshops on WM, consensus panels developed guidelines for uniform response criteria in WM.[111,112] The category of minor response was adopted at the Third International Workshop of WM, given that clinically meaningful responses were observed with newer biological agents, and is based on 25% or greater to less than 50% decrease in serum IgM level, which is used as a surrogate marker of disease in WM. At the Sixth International Workshop on WM, the categorical response of very good partial response (VGPR) (i.e., 90% reduction in IgM levels) was adopted given reports of improved clinical outcome associated with VGPR or better response achievement.[113-116] In distinction, the term *major response* is used to denote a response of 50% or greater in serum IgM levels and includes partial or better responses.[112] Response categories and criteria for progressive disease in WM based on consensus recommendations are summarized in Table 86-4.

An important concern with the use of IgM as a surrogate marker of disease is that it can fluctuate independent of the extent of tumor cell killing, particularly with biologically targeted agents such as rituximab, bortezomib, or everolimus.[117-122] Rituximab induces a spike or flare in serum IgM levels that can occur when used as monotherapy and in combination with other agents, including cyclophosphamide, nucleoside analogues, thalidomide, and lenalidomide, and can last for several weeks to months.[117,119,123-126] Bortezomib and everolimus can suppress IgM levels independent of tumor cell killing in certain patients.[120,121,126] Moreover, Varghese et al[127] showed that in patients treated with selective B-cell depleting agents such as rituximab and alemtuzumab, residual IgM producing plasma cells are spared and continue to persist, thus potentially skewing the relative response and assessment to treatment. Therefore, in circumstances in which the serum IgM levels appear out of context with the clinical progress of the patient, a BM biopsy should be considered to clarify the patient's underlying disease burden. Soluble CD27 may serve as an alternative surrogate marker in WM and remains a faithful marker of disease in patients experiencing a rituximab-related IgM flare, as well as plasmapheresis.[40,128]

TREATMENT INDICATIONS

Consensus guidelines on indications for treatment initiation were formulated as part of the Second International Workshop on Waldenström's Macroglobulinemia.[106] Initiation of therapy should not be based on the IgM levels since this may not correlate with either disease burden or symptomatic status.[129,130] Initiation of therapy is appropriate for patients with constitutional symptoms, such as

Table 86-3 Prognostic Scoring Systems in Waldenström Macroglobulinemia

Study	Adverse Prognostic Factors	Number of Groups	Survival
Gobbi et al[103]	Hb <9 g/dL Age >70 yr Weight loss Cryoglobulinemia	0-1 prognostic factors 2-4 prognostic factors	Median: 48 mo Median: 80 mo
Morel et al[104]	Age ≥65 yr Albumin <4 g/dL Number of cytopenias: Hb <12 g/dL Platelets <150 × 10^9/L WBC count <4 × 10^9/L	0-1 prognostic factors 2 prognostic factors 3-4 prognostic factors	5 yr: 87% 5 yr: 62% 5 yr: 25%
Dhodapkar et al[105]	β_2M ≥3 g/dL Hb <12 g/dL IgM <4 g/dL	β_2M <3 mg/dL + Hb ≥12 g/dL β_2M <3 mg/dL + Hb <12 g/dL β_2M ≥3 mg/dL + IgM ≥4 g/dL β_2M ≥3 mg/dL + IgM <4 g/dL	5 yr: 87% 5 yr: 63% 5 yr: 53% 5 yr: 21%
Application of International Staging System Criteria for Myeloma to WM Dimopoulos et al[107]	Albumin ≤3.5 g/dL β_2M ≥3.5 mg/L	Albumin ≥3.5 g/dL + β_2M <3.5 mg/dL Albumin ≤3.5 g/dL + β_2M <3.5 or β_2M 3.5-5.5 mg/dL β_2M >5.5 mg/dL	Median: NR Median: 116 mo Median: 54 mo
International Prognostic Scoring System for WM Morel et al[109]	Age >65 yr Hb <11.5 g/dL Platelets <100 × 10^9/L β_2M >3 mg/L IgM >7 g/dL	0-1 prognostic factors (excluding age) 2 prognostic factors or age >65 yr 3-5 prognostic factors	5 yr: 87% 5 yr: 68% 5 yr: 36%

β_2M, β_2 microglobulin; *Hb,* hemoglobin; *Ig,* immunoglobulin; *NR,* not reached; *WM,* Waldenström macroglobulinemia

Table 86-4 Summary of Updated Response Criteria Adopted at the Sixth International Workshop on Waldenström Macroglobulinemia

Criterion	Abbreviation	Description
Complete response	CR	IgM in normal range and disappearance of monoclonal protein by immunofixation, no histologic evidence of BM involvement, and resolution of any adenopathy or organomegaly (if present at baseline) along with no signs or symptoms attributable to WM; reconfirmation of the CR status is required by repeat immunofixation studies
Very good partial response	VGPR	A ≥90% reduction of serum IgM and resolution in adenopathy or organomegaly (if present at baseline) on physical examination or on CT scan; no new symptoms or signs of active disease
Partial response	PR	A ≥50% reduction of serum IgM and decrease in adenopathy or organomegaly (if present at baseline) on physical examination or on CT scan; no new symptoms or signs of active disease
Minor response	MR	A ≥25% but <50% reduction of serum IgM; no new symptoms or signs of active disease
Stable disease	SD	A <25% reduction and <25% increase of serum IgM without progression of adenopathy or organomegaly, cytopenias, or clinically significant symptoms caused by disease or signs of WM
Progressive disease	PD	A ≥25% increase in serum IgM by protein confirmed by a second measurement or progression of clinically significant findings caused by disease (i.e., anemia, thrombocytopenia, leukopenia, bulky adenopathy or organomegaly) or symptoms (unexplained recurrent fever ≥38.4°C, drenching night sweats, ≥10% body weight loss, hyperviscosity, neuropathy, symptomatic cryoglobulinemia, or amyloidosis) attributable to WM

From Treon SP, Hanzis C, Tripsas C, et al: Bendamustine therapy in patients with relapsed or refractory Waldenström's macroglobulinemia. *Clin Lymph Myeloma Leuk* 11:133, 2011.
BM, Bone marrow; *CT,* computed tomography; *Ig,* immunoglobulin; *WM,* Waldenström macroglobulinemia.

recurrent fever, night sweats, fatigue caused by anemia, or weight loss. The presence of progressive, symptomatic lymphadenopathy or splenomegaly provides additional reasons to begin therapy. The presence of anemia with a hemoglobin value of 10 g/dL or less or a platelet count 100 × 10^9/L or less on this basis of disease is also a reasonable indication for treatment initiation. Certain complications of WM, such as hyperviscosity syndrome, symptomatic sensorimotor peripheral neuropathy, systemic amyloidosis, renal insufficiency, or symptomatic cryoglobulinemia, are also indications for therapy.

TREATMENT OPTIONS

A precise therapeutic algorithm for therapy of WM remains to be defined given the paucity of randomized clinical trials. Active agents include alkylating agents (chlorambucil, cyclophosphamide), nucleoside analogues (cladribine, fludarabine), monoclonal antibodies (rituximab, ofatumumab, alemtuzumab), bortezomib, thalidomide, everolimus, and bendamustine.[129,130] Combination therapy, particularly with rituximab, has been associated with improved clinical outcomes. Individual patient considerations, including the presence of cytopenias, need for more rapid disease control, age, and candidacy for autologous transplant therapy, should be taken into account in making the choice for frontline therapy. For patients who are candidates for autologous transplant therapy, exposure to continuous chlorambucil or nucleoside analogue therapy should be limited given the potential for stem cell damage associated with the use of these drugs. The use of nucleoside analogues may also increase the risk for histologic transformation to diffuse large B-cell lymphoma as well as myelodysplasia and acute myeloid leukemia (AML).[131]

Chlorambucil

Oral alkylating drugs, alone and in combination therapy with steroids, have been extensively evaluated as frontline treatment of WM. The greatest experience with oral alkylating agent therapy has been with chlorambucil, which has been administered on both a continuous (i.e., daily dose schedule) as well as an intermittent schedule. Patients receiving chlorambucil on a continuous schedule typically receive 0.1 mg/kg/day, but with the intermittent schedule, patients will typically receive 0.3 mg/kg for 7 days every 6 weeks. In a prospective randomized study, Kyle et al[132] reported no significant difference in the overall response rates between these schedules, although the median response duration was greater for patients receiving intermittent versus continuous chlorambucil (46 versus 26 months). Despite the favorable median response duration favoring the use of the intermittent treatment schedule, no difference in the median overall survival was observed. Moreover, an increased incidence of developing myelodysplasia and AML with the intermittent (three of 22 patients) versus the continuous (0 of 24 patients) treatment schedule prompted the authors of this study to express preference for use of continuous chlorambucil dosing. The use of steroids in combination with alkylating agent therapy has also been explored. Dimopoulos and Alexanian[133] evaluated chlorambucil (8 mg/m^2) along with prednisone (40 mg/m^2) given orally for 10 days, every 6 weeks, and reported a major response (i.e., reduction of IgM by greater than 50%) in 72% of patients. Non–chlorambucil-based alkylator regimens using melphalan and cyclophosphamide in combination with steroids have also been examined by Petrucci et al[134] and Case et al[135] producing slightly higher overall response rates and response durations, although the benefit of these more complex regimens over chlorambucil remains to be demonstrated. Facon et al[136] have evaluated parameters predicting for response to alkylator therapy. Their studies in patients receiving single-agent chlorambucil demonstrated that age older than 60 years, male sex, symptomatic status, and cytopenias (but, interestingly, not high tumor burden and serum IgM levels) were associated with poor response to alkylator therapy. Additional factors to be taken into account in considering alkylator therapy for patients with WM include necessity for more rapid disease control given the slow nature of response to alkylator therapy, as well as consideration for preserving stem cells in patients who are candidates for autologous transplant therapy.

Nucleoside Analogues

Both cladribine and fludarabine have been extensively evaluated in untreated as well as previously treated WM patients. Cladribine administered as a single agent by continuous intravenous infusion over 2 hours daily infusion or by subcutaneous injections for 5 to 7 days has resulted in major responses in 40% to 90% of patients who received these drugs as primary therapy, but in the salvage setting, response rates have ranged from 38% to 54%.[129-143] Median time for achievement of a response after cladribine ranged from 1.2 to 5 months. The overall response rate with daily infusional fludarabine therapy administered mainly on a 5-day schedule in previously untreated and treated WM patients has ranged from 38% to 100% and 30% to 40%, respectively,[105,144-150] which is similar to the response rates reported with cladribine. The median time to achievement of response for fludarabine was also similar to that reported with cladribine at 3 to 6 months. In general, response rates and durations of responses have been greater for patients receiving nucleoside analogues as front-line agents, although in several of the above studies in which both untreated and previously treated patients were enrolled, no substantial difference in the overall response rate was reported. Myelosuppression commonly occurred after prolonged exposure to either of the nucleoside analogues, as did lymphopenia with sustained depletion of both CD4$^+$ and CD8$^+$ T lymphocytes 1 year after initiation of therapy. Treatment-related mortality from myelosuppression or opportunistic infections attributable to immunosuppression occurred in up to 5% of all treated patients in some series receiving either nucleoside analogue. Factors predicting a response to nucleoside analogues in therapy included age (younger than 70 years), pretreatment hemoglobin greater than 95 g/L, platelets greater than 75,000/mm^3, disease relapsing while off therapy, patients with resistant disease within the first year of diagnosis, and a long interval between first-line therapy and initiation of a nucleoside analogue in relapsing patients. There are limited data on the use of an alternate nucleoside analogue to salvage patients with disease that relapsed while on therapy or relapsed after discontinuation of the particular agent.[143,144] Three of four (75%) patients responded to cladribine to salvage patients who progressed after an unmaintained remission to fludarabine, but only one of 10 (10%) with disease resistant to fludarabine responded to cladribine.[143] However, Lewandowski et al[150] reported a response in two of six patients (33%) and disease stabilization in the remaining patients to fludarabine despite an inadequate response or progressive disease after cladribine therapy. The combination of nucleoside analogues with cyclophosphamide, rituximab, or both has been investigated and is discussed below.

The safety of nucleoside analogues has been the subject of investigation in several recent studies. Thomas et al recently reported their experiences in harvesting stem cells in 21 patients with symptomatic WM in whom autologous peripheral blood stem cell collection was attempted. Autologous stem cell collection succeeded on the first attempt in 14 of 15 patients who received non-nucleoside analogue–based therapy versus two of six patients who received a nucleoside analogue.[151] The long-term safety of nucleoside analogues in WM was recently examined by Leleu et al[131] in a large series of WM patients. A sevenfold increase in transformation to an aggressive lymphoma and a threefold increase in the development of AML or myelodysplasia were observed among patients who received a nucleoside analogue versus other therapies for their WM. A recent meta-analysis by Leleu et al[152] of several trials using nucleoside analogues in WM patients, which included patients who had previously received an alkylator agent, showed a crude incidence of 6.6% to 10% for development of disease transformation and 1.4% to 8.9% for development of myelodysplasia or AML. None of the studied risk factors—gender, age, family history of WM or B-cell malignancies, typical markers of tumor burden and prognosis, type of nucleoside analogue therapy (cladribine versus fludarabine), time from diagnosis to nucleoside analogue use, nucleoside analogue treatment as primary or salvage therapy—as well as treatment with an oral alkylator (i.e., chlorambucil) predicted for the occurrence of transformation or development of myelodysplasia or AML for WM patients treated with a nucleoside analogue.

Monoclonal Antibodies

Rituximab is a chimeric monoclonal antibody that targets CD20, a widely expressed antigen on lymphoplasmacytic cells in WM.[153] The use of rituximab at standard doses (i.e., 4 weekly infusions at 375 mg/m^2) induces major responses in approximately 27% to 35% of previously treated and untreated patients.[154,155] However, patients who achieved even minor responses benefited from rituximab as evidenced by improved hemoglobin and platelet counts and reduction of lymphadenopathy or splenomegaly.[154] The median time to treatment failure in these studies was found to range from 8 to more than 27 months. Studies evaluating an extended rituximab schedule consisting of 4 weekly courses at 375 mg/m^2/wk repeated 3 months later by another 4-week course have demonstrated higher major response rates of 44% to 48% with time to progression estimates of more than 16 to more than 29 months.[156,157]

In many WM patients, a transient increase of serum IgM (IgM flare) may be noted immediately after initiation of rituximab treatment.[117-119] The IgM flare may be related to release of IL-6 by bystander immune in response to binding of rituximab to FcγRIIA receptors and also occurs in response to intravenous immunoglobulin administration in WM patients.[158] The IgM flare in response to rituximab does not herald treatment failure, and although most patients will return to their baseline serum IgM level by 12 weeks, some patients may flare for months despite having tumor responses in their BM. Patients with baseline serum IgM levels of greater than 50 g/dL or serum viscosity of greater than 3.5 cp may be particularly at risk for a hyperviscosity-related event, and in such patients, plasmapheresis should be considered or rituximab omitted for the first few cycles of therapy until IgM levels decline to safer levels.[110] Because of the decreased likelihood of response in patients with higher IgM levels as well as the possibility that serum IgM and viscosity levels may abruptly rise, rituximab monotherapy should not be used as sole therapy for the treatment of patients at risk for hyperviscosity symptoms.

Time to response after rituximab is slow and exceeds 3 months on the average. The time to best response in one study was 18 months.[157] Patients with baseline serum IgM levels of less than 60 g/dL are more likely to respond irrespective of the underlying BM involvement by tumor cells.[156,157] A recent analysis of 52 patients who were treated with single-agent rituximab has indicated that the objective response rate was significantly lower in patients who had either low serum albumin (<35 g/L) or elevated serum monoclonal protein (>40 g/L M-spike). Furthermore, the presence of both adverse prognostic factors was related with a short time to progression (3.6 months). Moreover, patients who had normal serum albumin and relatively low serum monoclonal protein levels derived a substantial benefit from rituximab with a time to progression exceeding 40 months.[159]

The genetic background of patients may also be important for determining response to rituximab. A correlation between polymorphisms at amino acid position 158 in the FcγRIIIa receptor (CD16) and rituximab response has been observed in WM patients. WM patients who carry a valine amino acid (either in a homozygous or heterozygous pattern) at this polymorphic site had a fourfold higher major response rate to rituximab versus patients who expressed phenylalanine in a homozygous pattern.[160] The attainment of better categorical responses (i.e., VGPR or complete response [CR] after rituximab-based therapy) appears also dependent on the presence of at least one valine amino acid at FcγRIIIa-158.[113]

Ofatumumab is a fully humanized CD20-directed monoclonal antibody that targets the small loop of CD20, a target that is different than that of rituximab. A 59% overall response rate was observed in a series of 37 symptomatic WM patients after ofatumumab administration, which included untreated and previously treated patients.[161] Responses were higher among rituximab-naive patients. An IgM flare with symptomatic hyperviscosity was also observed in two patients in this series who required plasmapheresis. Ofatumumab has also been successfully administered to WM patients who demonstrated intolerance to rituximab.[162,163]

The activity of alemtuzumab has also been investigated in WM patients given the broad expression of CD52.[154] A multicenter study was recently completed in symptomatic WM patients who had received a median of two (range, 0-5) prior therapies; 43% had refractory disease.[163] Patients received alemtuzumab intravenously at 30 mg three times weekly for up to 12 weeks after test dosing and received hydrocortisone, acyclovir, and Bactrim or equivalent prophylaxis. The overall response rate in this series was 75% and included major responses in 36% of patients. With a median follow-up of 64 months, the median time to progression was 14.5 months. Hematologic and infectious complications, including cytomegalovirus reactivation, were more common in previously treated patients and indirectly associated with three deaths. Long-term follow-up revealed late-onset thrombocytopenia in four patients at a median of 13.6 months after therapy, which contributed to one death. High rates of response with the use of alemtuzumab were also observed by Owen et al,[164] who reported their preliminary experience in a small series of heavily pretreated WM patients. The median number of prior therapies in this series was four, and similar to this study, patients received up to 12 weeks of therapy (at 30 mg IV three times weekly) after initial dose escalation. Among the seven patients treated with alemtuzumab, five achieved a partial response and one a CR. Disseminated *Aspergillus* and mycobacterial infections contributed to two deaths in this series.

Bortezomib

Bortezomib is a proteasome inhibitor that has been extensively investigated in WM. In a multicenter study, 27 patients received up to 8 cycles of bortezomib at 1.3 mg/m^2 on days 1, 4, 8, and 11.[120] All but one patient had relapsed or refractory disease. After therapy, the median serum IgM levels declined from 4660 mg/dL to 2092 mg/dL (P <.0001). The overall response rate was 85%, with 10 and 13 patients achieving minor (<25% decrease in IgM) and major (<50% decrease in IgM) responses. Responses were prompt and occurred at a median of 1.4 months. The median time to progression for all responding patients was 7.9 (range, 3-21.4+) months, and the most common grade III/IV toxicities occurring in 5% or more of patients were sensory neuropathies (22.2%), leukopenia (18.5%), neutropenia (14.8%), dizziness (11.1%), and thrombocytopenia (7.4%). Importantly, sensory neuropathies resolved or improved in nearly all patients after cessation of therapy. As part of an NCI-Canada study, Chen et al[165] treated 27 patients with 44% being untreated and 56% being previously treated. Patients in this study received bortezomib using the standard schedule until they either demonstrated progressive disease or were 2 cycles beyond a CR or stable disease. The overall response rate in this study was 78%, with major responses being observed in 44% of patients. Sensory neuropathy occurred in 20 patients, five with grade above 3, and occurred after 2 to 4 cycles of therapy. Among the 20 patients developing a neuropathy, 14 patients resolved, and one patient demonstrated a one-grade improvement at 2 to 13 months. In addition to the above experiences with bortezomib monotherapy, Dimopoulos et al[166] observed major responses in six of 10 (60%) previously treated WM patients, and Goy et al[167] observed a major response in one of two WM patients who were included in a series of relapsed or refractory patients with non-Hodgkin lymphoma (NHL). The combination of bortezomib with steroids or rituximab has also been investigated and is discussed later.

Immunomodulatory Agents

Thalidomide as monotherapy and in combination with dexamethasone or clarithromycin has been examined. Dimopoulos et al[168] demonstrated a major response in five of 20 (25%) previously untreated and treated patients who received single-agent thalidomide. Dose escalation from the thalidomide starting dose of 200 mg/day was hindered by development of side effects, including the development of peripheral neuropathy in five patients, obligating discontinuation or dose reduction. Low doses of thalidomide (50 mg orally daily) in combination with dexamethasone (40 mg orally once a week) and clarithromycin (250 mg orally twice a day) have also been examined, with 10 of 12 (83%) previously treated patients demonstrating at least a major response.[169] However, in a follow-up study by Dimopoulos et al[170] using a higher thalidomide dose (200 mg orally daily) along with dexamethasone (40 g orally once a week) and clarithromycin (500 mg orally twice a day), only two of 10 (20%) previously treated patients responded. Thalidomide and lenalidomide have also been investigated in combination with rituximab.

Bendamustine

Bendamustine is a recently approved agent for the treatment of relapsed/refractory indolent NHL. Bendamustine has structural similarities to both alkylating agents and purine analogs.[171] Bendamustine in combination with rituximab has been investigated in both previously untreated, as well as relapsed or refractory WM patients.

Everolimus

Everolimus is an oral inhibitor of the mTOR (mammalian target of rapamycin) pathway, which is approved for the treatment of renal cell carcinoma. The Akt-mTOR-p70 pathway is active in WM, and inhibition of this pathway leads to apoptosis of primary WM cells and WM cell lines.[172,173] Fifty patients with a median of three prior therapies were treated with everolimus in a joint Dana Farber and Mayo Clinic study.[174] The overall response rate was 70%, with 42% of patients attaining a major response. The PFS at 12 months was estimated to be 62%. Grade 3 or higher drug-related toxicities were observed in 56% of patients, with cytopenias constituting the most common. Pulmonary toxicity occurred in 10% of patients. Dose reductions because of toxicity occurred in 52% of patients.

A clinical trial examining the activity of everolimus in previously untreated patients with WM was completed.[175] Although 67% of patients achieved at least a minor response by consensus criteria that rely on paraprotein reduction, IgM discordance to underlying disease burden was seen in up to half of patients in this study. Cytopenias, particularly anemia and thrombocytopenia, were common, and pneumonitis occurred in 15% of patients.

Combination Strategies

Because rituximab is an active and a non-myelosuppressive agent, combination therapy with various chemotherapeutic agents has been extensively explored in WM. The combination of CHOP (cyclophosphamide, doxorubicin, vincristine, prednisone) with rituximab (CHOP-R) was investigated in a randomized frontline study by the German Low Grade Lymphoma Study Group (GLSG) involving 69 patients, most of whom had WM.[175] The addition of rituximab to CHOP resulted in a higher overall response rate (94% versus 67%) and median time to progression (63 versus 22 months) compared with patients treated with CHOP alone. Dimopoulos et al[176] investigated the combination of rituximab, dexamethasone, and oral cyclophosphamide (RCD) as primary therapy in 72 patients with WM. At least a major response was observed in 74% of patients in this study, and the 2-year PFS was 67%. Therapy was well tolerated, but one patient died of interstitial pneumonia. The use of CHOP-R has also been investigated in relapsed or refractory WM patients.[177] Among 13 evaluable patients, 10 patients achieved a major response (77%), including three CR and seven partial response (PR), and two patients achieved a minor response. In a retrospective study, Ioakimidis et al[112] examined the outcomes of symptomatic WM patients who received CHOP-R, CVP-R, or CP-R. Baseline characteristics for all three cohorts were similar for age, prior therapies, BM involvement, hematocrit, platelet count, and serum β-2 microglobulin, although serum IgM levels were higher in patients treated with CHOP-R. The overall response rates to therapy were comparable for all three treatment options: CHOP-R (96%), CVP-R (88%), and CP-R (95%), although more CRs were observed among patients treated with either CVP-R or CHOP-R. Comparison of adverse events for these regimens showed a higher incidence of neutropenic fever as well as treatment related neuropathy in patients receiving CHOP-R and CVP-R versus CPR. These results suggest that in WM, the use of doxorubicin and vincristine may be omitted to minimize treatment-related complications.

Combination therapy with nucleoside analogues has also been investigated as both frontline and salvage therapy. Weber et al[178] administered rituximab along with cladribine and cyclophosphamide to 17 previously untreated patients with WM. At least a partial response was documented in 94% of WM patients, including a CR in 18%. With a median follow-up time of 21 months, no patient has relapsed. Laszlo et al[179] recently evaluated the combination of subcutaneous cladribine with rituximab in 29 WM patients who had either untreated or previously treated disease. Therapy consisted of rituximab on day 1 followed by subcutaneous cladribine 0.1 mg/kg for 5 consecutive days, administered monthly for 4 cycles. With a median follow-up of 43 months, the overall response rate observed was 89.6%, with seven CRs, 16 partial responses, and three minor responses. The therapeutic activity was similar between untreated and previously treated patients. No major infections were observed despite the lack of antimicrobial prophylaxis. In a study by the Waldenström Macroglobulinemia Clinical Trials Group (WMCTG), the combination of rituximab and fludarabine was administered to 43 WM patients, 32 (75%) of whom were previously untreated.[114] The overall response rate was 95.3%, and 83% of patients achieved a major response. The median time to progression was 51.2 months in this series and was longer for patients who were previously untreated and for those achieving at least a VGPR. Hematologic toxicity was common, particularly neutropenia and thrombocytopenia. Two deaths occurred in this study because of pneumonia not attributed to *Pneumocystis carinii* infection. Secondary malignancies, including transformation to aggressive lymphoma and development of myelodysplasia or AML, were observed in six patients in this series. The addition of rituximab to fludarabine and cyclophosphamide has also been explored in the salvage setting by Tam et al[180] wherein four of five patients demonstrated a response. Hensel et al[181] administered rituximab along with pentostatin and cyclophosphamide to 13 patients with untreated and previously treated WM or LPL. A major response was observed in 77% of patients. The addition of alkylating agents to nucleoside analogues has also been explored in WM. Weber et al[178] administered 2 cycles of oral cyclophosphamide along with subcutaneous cladribine to 37 patients with previously untreated WM. At least a partial response was observed in 84% of patients, and the median duration of response was 36 months. Dimopoulos et al[182] examined fludarabine in combination with intravenous cyclophosphamide and observed partial responses in six of 11 (55%) patients with either primary refractory disease or patients who relapsed on treatment. The combination of fludarabine plus cyclophosphamide was also evaluated in a study by Tamburini et al[183] involving 49 patients, 35 of whom were previously treated. Seventy-eight percent of the patients in this study achieved a response, and the median time to treatment failure was 27 months. Hematologic toxicity was commonly observed, and three patients died of treatment-related toxicities. In this study, leukemia developed in two patients, histologic transformation to diffuse large cell lymphoma occurred in one patient, and two cases of solid tumors (prostate and melanoma) were observed. In addition, four of six patients failed to mobilize their stem cells in sufficient numbers to serve as a stem cell graft. Tedeschi et al[184] recently completed a multicenter study of fludarabine, cyclophosphamide, and rituximab in symptomatic WM patients with untreated or relapsed or refractory disease to one course of prior chemotherapy. Treatment consisted of rituximab at 375 mg/m^2 on day 1 and fludarabine at 25 mg/m^2 and cyclophosphamide at 250 mg/m^2 by intravenous administration on days 2 to 4 every 4 weeks. The overall response rate in patients was 89%, with 83% of patients attaining a major remission and 14% a CR. Prolonged neutropenia was observed in up to one-third of patients. With a median follow-up time of 15 months, the median PFS for this study has not been reached.

The combination of bortezomib, dexamethasone, and rituximab (BDR) has been investigated as frontline therapy in patients with WM by the WMCTG. An overall response rate of 96%, major response rate of 83%, and complete remission in 22% was observed with BDR.[115] The updated median PFS in this study was more than 56.1 months. The incidence of grade 3 neuropathy was 30% in this study, which used a twice-a-week schedule for bortezomib administration at a dose of 1.3 mg/m^2. Peripheral neuropathy from bortezomib was reversible in most patients in this study after discontinuation of therapy. An increased incidence of herpes zoster infections was also observed with BDR, prompting the use of prophylactic antiviral therapy. An alternative schedule for bortezomib administration (i.e., weekly at 1.6 mg/m^2) in combination with rituximab or dexamethasone (or both) has been investigated in several studies with overall response rates of 80% to 90% being achieved.[185-187] A lower incidence of peripheral neuropathy was observed in two studies using once-a-week bortzomib.[182,187] The impact of once- versus twice-a-week bortezomib administration on PFS remains to be documented.

The combination of immunomodulatory agents (thalidomide, lenalidomide) with rituximab was investigated by the WMCTG. Thalidomide was administered at 200 mg/day for 2 weeks followed by 400 mg/day, and thereafter thalidomide was continued for 1 year. Patients received four weekly infusions of rituximab at 375 mg/m^2 beginning 1 week after initiation of thalidomide followed by four additional weekly infusions of rituximab at 375 mg/m^2 beginning at week 13. The overall and major response rate was 72% and 64%, respectively, and the median time to progression was 38 months in this series.[124] Dose reduction or discontinuation of thalidomide was common, mainly because of treatment-related neuropathy. The investigators concluded that lower doses of thalidomide (i.e., 50-100 mg/day) should be considered in this patient population. The combination of lenalidomide with rituximab was investigated by the WMCTG with patients receiving lenalidomide 25 mg/day for 3 weeks followed by a 1-week pause for 48 weeks.[125] Patients received 1 week of therapy with lenalidomide, after which rituximab (375 mg/m^2) was administered weekly on weeks 2 to 5 and then 13 to 16. The overall and major response rates in this study were 50% and 25%, respectively, and a median time to progression for responders was 18.9 months. In two patients with bulky disease, a significant reduction in extramedullary disease was observed. However, an acute decrease in hematocrit levels was observed during first 2 weeks of lenalidomide therapy in 13 of 16 (81%) patients with a median absolute decrease in hematocrit of 4.8%, resulting in anemia-related complications and hospitalization in four patients. Despite dose reductions, most patients in this study continued to demonstrate progressive anemia with lenalidomide. There was no evidence of hemolysis or more general myelosuppression with lenalidomide in this study. Therefore, the mechanism for lenalidomide-related anemia in WM patients remains to be determined, and the use of this agent among WM patients should be avoided.

The use of bendamustine in combination with rituximab was explored by Rummel et al[188] as the frontline therapy of WM. As part of a randomized study, patients received 6 cycles of bendamustine plus rituximab (Benda-R) or CHOP-R. A total of 546 patients were enrolled in this study of indolent NHL patients and included 40 patients with WM. Patients on the Benda-R arm received bendamustine at 90 mg/m^2 on days 1 and 2 and rituximab at 375 mg/m^2 on day 1 every 4 weeks. The overall response rate was 96% for Benda-R, and 94% for CHOP-R–treated patients. With a median observation period of 26 months, 20 of 23 (87%) receiving Benda-R versus nine of 17 (53%) receiving CHOP-R remain free of disease progression. Importantly, Benda-R was associated with a lower incidence of grade 3 or 4 neutropenia, infectious complications, and alopecia. In the salvage setting, the outcome of 30 WM patients with relapsed or refractory disease who received bendamustine alone or with a CD20-directed antibody was reported by Treon et al.[189] An overall response rate of 83.3% and a median PFS of 13.2 months were reported in this study. Overall, therapy was well tolerated, although prolonged myelosuppression occurred in patients who received prior nucleoside analogue therapy.

MAINTENANCE THERAPY

A role for maintenance rituximab in WM patients after response to a rituximab-containing regimen was raised in a study examining the outcome of 248 WM rituximab-naive patients who were either observed or received maintenance rituximab.[190] In this retrospective study, categorical responses improved in 16 of 162 (10%) patients not receiving rituximab maintenance and in 36 of 86 (41.8%) patients who received maintenance rituximab after induction therapy. Both PFS (56.3 versus 28.6 months) and overall survival (>120 versus 116 months) were longer in patients who received maintenance rituximab. Improved PFS was evident despite previous treatment status, induction with rituximab alone, or combination therapy. A greater reduction in serum IgM was observed, and hematocrits were higher in patients receiving maintenance rituximab. Among patients receiving maintenance rituximab, an increased number of infectious events, predominantly sinusitis and bronchitis, was observed, but these events were mainly grade 1 or 2.

HIGH-DOSE THERAPY AND STEM CELL TRANSPLANTATION

The use of stem cell transplantation (SCT) therapy has also been explored in patients with WM. Desikan et al[191] reported their initial experience of high-dose chemotherapy and autologous SCT, which has more recently been updated by Munshi et al.[192] Their studies involved eight previously treated WM patients between the ages of 45 and 69 years who received either melphalan at 200 mg/m^2 or at 140 mg/m^2 with total-body irradiation (TBI). Peripheral blood stem cells were successfully collected in all eight patients, but a second collection procedure was required for two patients who had extensive prior nucleoside analogue therapy. There were no transplant-related mortalities, and toxicities were manageable. All eight patients responded, with seven of eight patients achieving a major response and one patient achieving a CR with the duration of response ranging from 5+ to 77+ months. Dreger et al[193] investigated the use of the DEXA-BEAM (dexamethasone, BCNU, etoposide, cytarabine, melphalan) regimen followed by myeloablative therapy with cyclophosphamide and TBI and autologous SCT in seven WM patients, which included four untreated patients. Serum IgM levels declined by more than 50% after DEXA-BEAM and myeloablative therapy for six of seven patients, with PFS ranging from more than 4 to more than 30 months. All three evaluable patients who were previously treated also attained a major response in a study by Anagnostopoulos et al[194] wherein WM patients received various preparative regimens and demonstrated event-free survivals of more than 26, 31, and more than 108 months. Tournilhac et al[195] recently reported the outcome of 18 WM patients in France who received high-dose chemotherapy followed by autologous SCT. All patients were previously treated with a median of three (range, 1-5) prior regimens. Therapy was well tolerated with an improvement in response status observed for seven patients (six PR to CR; one stable disease [SD] to PR), but only one patient demonstrated progressive disease. The median event-free survival for all nonprogressing patients was 12 months. Tournilhac et al[195] have also reported the outcome of allogeneic SCT in 10 previously treated WM patients (ages 35-46 years) who received a median of three prior therapies, including three patients with progressive disease despite therapy. Two of three patients with progressive disease responded, and an improvement in response status was observed in five patients. The median event-free survival for nonprogressing, evaluable patients was 31 months. Of concern in this series was the death of three patients owing to SCT-related toxicity. Anagnostopoulos et al[196] have also reported a retrospective review of WM patients who underwent either autologous or allogeneic SCT, whose outcomes were reported to the International Blood and Marrow Transplant Registry. Seventy-eight percent of patients in this cohort had two or more prior therapies, and 58% of them were resistant to their prior therapy. The relapse rate at 3 years was 29% in the allogeneic SCT group and 24% in the autologous SCT group. Non–relapse-related mortality, however, was 40% in the allogeneic SCT group and 11% in the autologous SCT group in this series.

Kyriakou et al[116] reported on the outcome of WM patients in the European Bone Marrow Transplant (EBMT) registry who received either an autologous or allogeneic SCT. Among 158 patients receiving an autologous SCT, which included primarily relapsed or refractory patients, the 5-year PFS and overall survival rates were 39.7% and 68.5%, respectively. Non–relapse-related mortality at 1 year was 3.8%. Chemorefractory disease, and the number of prior lines of therapy at time of the autologous SCT were the most important prognostic factors for PFS and overall survival. The achievement of a negative immunofixation after autologous SCT had a positive impact on PFS. When used as consolidation at first response, autologous transplantation provided a PFS of 44% at 5 years. In the allogeneic SCT experience from the EBMT, the long-term outcome of 86 WM patients was reported by Kyriakou.[197] A total of 86 patients received allogenic SCT with either a myeloablative (n = 37) or reduced-intensity (n = 49) conditioning regimen. The median age of patients in this series was 49 years, and 47 patients had three or more previous lines of therapy. Eight patients failed prior autologous SCT. Fifty-nine patients (68.6%) had chemotherapy-sensitive disease at the time of allogeneic SCT. Non–relapse-related mortality at 3 years was 33% for patients receiving a myeloablative transplant and 23% for those who received reduced-intensity conditioning. The overall response rate was 75.6%. The relapse rates at 3 years were 11% for myeloablative and 25% for reduced-intensity conditioning recipients. Five-year PFS and overall survival for WM patients who received a myeloablative allogenic SCT were 56% and 62% and for patients who received reduced intensity conditioning were 49% and 64%, respectively. The occurrence of chronic graft-versus-host disease was associated with improved PFS and suggested the existence of a clinically relevant graft-versus-WM effect in this study.

FUTURE DIRECTIONS

Since the initial description of macroglobulinemia by Jan Gosta Waldenström in 1944, the genetic basis for this disease has remained unknown. The recent finding of a highly recurrent somatic mutation (MYD88 L265P) in WM LPL patients provides not only a potentially useful diagnostic tool but also has important implications for therapy of WM. The use of inhibitors that target MYD88 and IRAK signaling induces apoptosis of MYD88 L265P expressing cells and blocks NFκB signaling.[20] These observations are of particular relevance to WM because NFκB signaling is important for WM growth and survival. Blockade of IκBα by proteasome inhibitors is associated with high rates of responses in WM patients, and direct targeting of tonic MYD88/IRAK signaling imposed by MYD88 L265P may therefore provide a novel approach for WM treatment. Such targeting may also circumvent other growth-promoting pathways upstream of NFkB mediated by p38 MAP kinase (MAPK), signal transducers and activators of transcription 3 (STAT3) and Bruton tyrosine kinase (BTK) that may also be dependent on MYD88.

SUGGESTED READINGS

Ghobrial IM, Fonseca R, Greipp PR, et al: The initial "flare" of IgM level after rituximab therapy in patients diagnosed with Waldenström Macroglobulinemia: An Eastern Cooperative Oncology Group Study. *Cancer* 101:2593, 2004.

Ghobrial IM, Xie W, Padmanabhan S, et al: Phase II trial of weekly bortezomib in combination with rituximab in untreated patients with Waldenström Macroglobulinemia. *Am J Hematol* 85:670, 2010.

Hanzis C, Ojha RP, Hunter Z, et al: Associated malignancies in patients with Waldenström's macroglobulinemia and their kin. *Clin Lymphoma Myeloma Leuk* 11:88, 2011.

Ho A, Leleu X, Hatjiharissi E, et al: CD27-CD70 interactions in the pathogenesis of Waldenstrom's macroglobulinemia. *Blood* 112:4683, 2008.

Hunter ZR, Manning RJ, Hanzis C, et al: IgA and IgG hypogammaglobulinemia in Waldenstrom's macroglobulinemia. *Haematologica* 95:470, 2010.

Kimby E, Treon SP, Anagnostopoulos A, et al: Update on recommendations for assessing response from the Third International Workshop on Waldenstrom's macroglobulinemia. *Clin Lymphoma Myeloma* 6:380, 2006.

Kyle RA, Treon SP, Alexanian R, et al: Prognostic markers and criteria to initiate therapy in Waldenström's macroglobulinemia: Consensus panel recommendations from the Second International Workshop on Waldenström's Macroglobulinemia. *Semin Oncol* 30:116, 2003.

Kyriakou C, Canals C, Cornelissen JJ, et al: Allogeneic stem-cell transplantation in patients with Waldenström macroglobulinemia: Report from the Lymphoma Working Party of the European Group for Blood and Marrow Transplantation. *J Clin Oncol* 28:4926, 2010.

Kyriakou C, Canals C, Sibon D, et al: High-dose therapy and autologous stem-cell transplantation in Waldenstrom macroglobulinemia: The Lymphoma Working Party of the European Group for Blood and Marrow Transplantation. *J Clin Oncol* 28:2227, 2010.

Laszlo D, Andreola G, Rigacci L, et al: Rituximab and subcutaneous 2-chloro-2′-deoxyadenosine combination treatment for patients with Waldenstrom macroglobulinemia: Clinical and biologic results of a phase II multicenter study. *J Clin Oncol* 28:2233, 2010.

Leleu XP, Manning R, Soumerai JD, et al: Increased incidence of transformation and myelodysplasia/acute leukemia in patients with Waldenström macroglobulinemia treated with nucleoside analogs. *J Clin Oncol* 27:250, 2009.

McMaster ML, Csako G, Giambarresi TR, et al: Long-term evaluation of three multiple-case Waldenstrom's macroglobulinemia families. *Clin Cancer Res* 13:5063, 2007.

Menke MN, Feke GT, McMeel JW, et al: Hyperviscosity-related retinopathy in Waldenstrom's macroglobulinemia. *Arch Opthalmol* 124:1601, 2006.

Morel P, Duhamel A, Gobbi P, et al: International prognostic scoring system for Waldenstrom macroglobulinemia. *Blood* 113:4163, 2009.

Nobile-Orazio E, Manfredini E, Carpo M, et al: Frequency and clinical correlates of antineural IgM antibodies in neuropathy associated with IgM monoclonal gammopathy. *Ann Neurol* 36:416, 1994.

Owen RG, Treon SP, Al-Katib A, et al: Clinicopathological definition of Waldenström's macroglobulinemia: Consensus Panel Recommendations from the Second International Workshop on Waldenström's Macroglobulinemia. *Semin Oncol* 30:110, 2003.

Rummel MJ, von Gruenhagen U, Niederle N, et al: Bendamustine plus rituximab versus CHOP plus rituximab in the firstline treatment of patients with follicular, indolent and mantle cell lymphomas: Results of a randomized phase III study of the Study Group Indolent Lymphomas (StiL). *Blood* 112, 2008: Abstract 2596.

Schop RF, Kuehl WM, Van Wier SA, et al: Waldenström macroglobulinemia neoplastic cells lack immunoglobulin heavy chain locus translocations but have frequent 6q deletions. *Blood* 100:2996, 2002.

Tam CS, Wolf MM, Westerman D, et al: Fludarabine combination therapy is highly effective in first-line and salvage treatment of patients with Waldenstrom's macroglobulinemia. *Clin Lymphoma Myeloma* 6:136, 2005.

Tournilhac O, Santos DD, Xu L, et al: Mast cells in Waldenstrom's macroglobulinemia support lymphoplasmacytic cell growth through CD154/CD40 signaling. *Ann Oncol* 17:1275, 2006.

Treon SP, Branagan AR, Anderson KC: Paradoxical increases in serum IgM levels and serum viscosity following rituximab therapy in patients with Waldenstrom's macroglobulinemia. *Ann Oncol* 15:1481, 2004.

Treon SP, Branagan AR, Ioakimidis L, et al: Long term outcomes to fludarabine and rituximab in Waldenstrom's macroglobulinemia. *Blood* 113:3673, 2009.

Treon SP, Hanzis C, Tripsas C, et al: Bendamustine therapy in patients with relapsed or refractory Waldenström's macroglobulinemia. *Clin Lymphoma Myeloma Leuk* 11:133, 2011.

Treon SP: How I treat Waldenstrom's macroglobulinemia. *Blood* 114:419, 2009.

Dimopoulos MA, Gertz MA, Kastritis E, et al: Update on treatment recommendations from the Fourth International Workshop on Waldenstrom's Macroglobulinemia. *J Clin Oncol* 27:120, 2009.

Treon SP, Hunter ZR, Aggarwal A, et al: Characterization of familial Waldenstrom's macroglobulinemia. *Ann Oncol* 17:488, 2006.

Treon SP, Ioakimidis L, Soumerai JD, et al: Primary therapy of Waldenstrom's macroglobulinemia with bortezomib, dexamethasone and rituximab: Results of WMCTG Clinical Trial 05-180. *J Clin Oncol* 27:3830, 2009.

Treon SP, Xu L, Zhou Y, et al: Whole genome sequencing reveals a widely expressed mutation (MYD88 L265P) with oncogenic activity in Waldenstrom's macroglobulinemia. *Blood* 118:Abstract 300, 2011.

Treon SP, Yang G, Hanzis C, et al: Attainment of complete/very good partial response following rituximab-based therapy is an important determinant to progression-free survival, and is impacted by polymorphisms in FCGR3A in Waldenstrom macroglobulinaemia. *Br J Haematol* 154:223, 2011.

Swerdlow SH, Campo E, Harris NL, et al, editors: *World Health Organization classification of tumours of haematopoietic and lymphoid tissues.* Lyon, 2008, IARC Press.

For complete list of references log on to www.expertconsult.com.

CHAPTER 87

IMMUNOGLOBULIN LIGHT-CHAIN AMYLOIDOSIS (PRIMARY AMYLOIDOSIS)

Morie A. Gertz, Francis K. Buadi, Steven R. Zeldenrust, and Suzanne R. Hayman

In 1858, Rudolf Virchow described the reaction of amyloid deposits with iodine and sulfuric acid.[1] This reaction was considered a marker for starch; hence Virchow used the term *amyloid,* meaning "starch-like," to describe the deposits. At approximately the same time, Professor Carl Rokitansky in Vienna had recognized lardaceous deposits in the viscera of patients with tuberculosis or syphilis.[2] The white, shiny appearance of these deposits led him to conclude that they were of fat origin. Later, Carl Friedreich recognized that the waxy spleen described by Virchow contained no material structurally similar to cellulose and determined that the deposits were probably albuminoid.[3] Sir Samuel Wilks, the first physician to use bromide in the treatment of epilepsy, reported on a patient who had lardaceous changes of the liver with no obvious cause.[4] This may have been the first reported patient with primary amyloidosis (AL).

Congo red staining of amyloid was introduced by Bennhold in 1922,[5] and in 1927, Divry and Florkin described the green birefringence of amyloid under polarized light.[6] In 1959, Cohen and Calkins[7] recognized that all forms of amyloid had a fibrillar structure when viewed with an electron microscope. In 1968, Eanes and Glenner[8] reported that unlike normal proteins, which have an α-helical configuration, amyloid deposits form a β-pleated sheet, rendering them resistant to the action of solvents. The first purification of amyloid was described by Pras et al[9] in 1968. The first amyloid protein was sequenced in 1970 by Glenner et al,[10] who recognized it as the N-terminus of an immunoglobulin light chain. In 1974, Isobe and Osserman[11] first recognized that the Bence Jones proteins had a role in the pathogenesis of AL.

CLASSIFICATION

All forms of amyloid stain positively with Congo red, and this is the sine qua non for the diagnosis of this disorder. Amyloid deposits appear amorphous and extracellular when stained with hematoxylin and eosin. False-positive results have been reported with Congo red staining, however, and some experience with the technique is desirable.[12] All forms of amyloid are fibrillar in nature; the fibrils are rigid and nonbranching. In the early and mid-20th century, amyloidosis was classified by the anatomic distribution of the amyloid deposits and was assigned to one of three categories.

Familial amyloidosis was recognized by its presentation, which was usually a painful peripheral neuropathy with an autosomal dominant inheritance pattern.[13,14a] Mutations in a number of plasma proteins, including transthyretin (TTR), apolipoprotein AI and AII, fibrinogen A α-chain, and lysozyme, are associated with hereditary systemic amyloidosis. TTR amyloidosis is the most common and is usually associated with peripheral neuropathy. Mutations in the other proteins usually have no neuropathic consequences and instead principally cause renal and cardiac amyloidosis. A completely new form of amyloidosis caused by LECT2 (leukocyte chemotactic factor 2) has recently been described[14b] in a patient presenting with nephrotic syndrome and subsequent azotemia requiring hemodialysis. Over 8 years, 285 renal amyloid samples, of which 31 were unclassifiable by tandem mass spectrometry were found to be LECT2 related in 7.[14c] Isolation of genomic DNA and polymerase chain reaction amplification of LECT2-encoding exons showed no mutations. However, all were homozygous for the G allele encoding valine at position 40 in the mature protein. LECT2-associated renal amyloidosis represents a unique form of renal amyloidosis, especially in Mexican Americans.[14d]

The secondary form of amyloidosis was characterized by an associated long-standing inflammatory disorder. One hundred years ago, this usually represented tuberculosis, leprosy, syphilis, and chronic infection such as bronchiectasis and osteomyelitis. Today in Western countries, amyloidosis is commonly associated with chronic inflammatory polyarthritis syndromes such as ankylosing spondylitis and juvenile rheumatoid arthritis. It is also associated with Castleman disease and Crohn disease. Secondary amyloidosis (AA) is becoming increasingly rare as more effective therapy of inflammatory arthropathies prevents the sustained inflammation necessary for AA to develop.[14e]

Fifty years ago, all forms of amyloidosis that were not secondary or familial were considered "primary." In the original terminology, "primary" meant "idiopathic" and most likely contained a heterogeneous combination of multiple forms of amyloidosis. Today, the term *primary amyloidosis,* or AL, refers to a systemic disorder with amyloid deposits consisting of immunoglobulin light chains or their fragments or heavy chains.

All forms of systemic AL are associated with a clonal disorder of plasma cells, which may range from a small clonal population of 5% plasma cells or less in the bone marrow (BM) to overt multiple myeloma (MM). Table 87-1 contains a modified classification of the more frequently described forms of amyloidosis.

PATHOPHYSIOLOGY

Amyloid fibrils can be produced in vitro by peptic digestion of purified monoclonal human immunoglobulin light chains. The light chains of patients with AL have an abnormal sequence and an abnormal tertiary structure that favors the misfolding into β-pleated sheet configuration. Investigation of the thermodynamic properties of light chains that form fibrils and those that remain stable have shown an inverse relationship between thermodynamic stability and fibrillogenic potential. Structural parameters and overall thermodynamic stability contribute to the fibril-forming propensity of immunoglobulin light chains.[15] When injected into mice, immunoglobulin light chains purified from the urine of patients with AL produce human AL deposits,[16] but light chains from patients with MM (and not AL) do not.

Two-thirds of patients with monoclonal gammopathy of undetermined significance (MGUS) or MM have κ immunoglobulin light chains. Three-fourths of patients with amyloidosis who have a light chain have λ, which reflects the intrinsic "amyloidogenicity" of λ immunoglobulin light chains. The λ_{VI} is always associated with amyloid, suggesting that unique amino acid structures render these proteins amyloidogenic.[17]

A comparison of monoclonal proteins in AL and MM is shown in Fig. 87-1. Amyloid-associated germline gene segments have been identified[18]; the λ_{III} family is found most frequently in amyloidosis. Two germline genes, 3r and 6a, belonging to the λ_{III} and λ_{VI} families contributed equally to encode 42% of amyloid variable λ regions.

Table 87-1 Nomenclature of Amyloidosis

Protein	Precursor	Clinical Characteristics
AL or AH	Immunoglobulin light or heavy chain	Primary or localized; myeloma or macroglobulinemia associated
AA	SAA	Secondary or familial Mediterranean fever, familial periodic fever syndromes
ATTR	Transthyretin	Familial and senile
A fibrinogen	Fibrinogen	Familial renal amyloidosis (Ostertag)
Aβ_2M	β_2-Microglobulin	Dialysis associated; carpal tunnel syndrome
Aβ	ABPP	Alzheimer disease
A Apo A-I/A-II	Apolipoprotein A-I Apolipoprotein A-II	Proteinuria Cardiac Neuropathy
A lysozyme	Lysozyme	GI tract Liver Renal
ALECT2	Renal	

ABPP, Amyloid β protein precursor; *GI*, gastrointestinal; *SAA*, serum amyloid A. From Gertz MA, Lacy MQ, Dispenzieri A: Immunoglobulin light chain amyloidosis (primary amyloidosis, AL). In Gertz MA, Greipp PR, editors: *Hematologic malignancies: Multiple myeloma and related plasma cell disorders.* New York, 2004, Springer-Verlag, p 157. Used with permission of Mayo Foundation for Medical Education and Research.

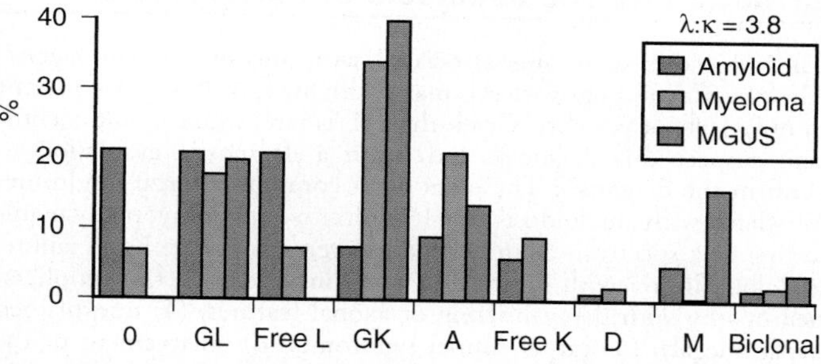

Figure 87-1 DISTRIBUTION OF SERUM MONOCLONAL PROTEIN IN PATIENTS WITH AMYLOIDOSIS (n = 270) OR MULTIPLE MYELOMA (n = 1000). The κ-to-λ ratio in amyloidosis is 1 to 3.6. *0,* No monoclonal protein serum; *A,* monclonal IgA protein in serum; *biclonal,* two different monclonal proteins in serum; *D,* monclonal IgD protein in serum; *GL,* monclonal IgGlambda protein in serum; *GK,* monclonal IgG kappa protein in serum; *free L,* monoclonal lambda light chain in serum; *free K,* monoclonal kappa light chain in serum; *M,* monclonal IgM protein in serum; *GUS,* monoclonal gammopathy of undetermined significance. *(From Gertz MA, Lacy MQ, Dispenzieri A, et al: Transplantation for amyloidosis.* Curr Opin Oncol *19:136, 2007.)*

These same two gene segments have a strong association with amyloidosis and are most likely responsible for the λ light-chain overrepresentation typical of amyloidosis.[18]

The reason that patients with AL present with amyloid disease displaying organ tropism is unknown. The renal tropism of some chains was investigated.[19] Patients with clones derived from the 6a variable λ_{VI} germline gene were more likely to present with renal involvement. Those with clones derived from the 1c, 2a2, and 3r variable λ genes were more likely to present with dominant cardiac and multisystem disease. Patients with variable κ clones were more likely to have dominant liver involvement.[19]

The classification of AL among patients with and without myeloma is usually made on the basis of clinical criteria, but considerable clinical overlap exists. The presence of MM bone disease, such as lytic lesions, multiple compression fractures, or pathologic fractures of long bones, is rare in AL. Patients with AL and renal insufficiency rarely have myeloma cast nephropathy. Renal failure in these patients is usually tubular atrophy from glomerular amyloid and long-standing albuminuria. The percentage of BM plasma cells is useful in making the distinction between AL and myeloma. At Mayo Clinic, we have arbitrarily defined patients as having MM–associated amyloidosis if the BM plasma cells exceed 30%.[20a] Routine Congo red staining of myeloma BM samples is not indicated.[20b] Amyloidosis rarely evolves into overt MM; it occurs in fewer than 0.5% of patients.[20a]

The incidence of amyloidosis is eight per million persons per year and is not increasing with time.[21] Amyloidosis is one-fifth as common as MM but has an incidence similar to those of nodular sclerosing Hodgkin disease, chronic myeloid leukemia, and polycythemia vera.

Chromosomal anomalies are seen often in the BM plasma cells of patients with AL.[22] Studies of BM samples found trisomies involving chromosomes 7, 9, 11, 15, and 18 in 42%, 52%, 47%, 39%, and 33% of patients, respectively. Trisomy X was seen in 13% of women and 54% of men. Monosomy of chromosome 18 was seen in 72%. This aneuploidy supports the neoplastic nature of the disorder even though it is not proliferative over time. Fluorescence in situ hybridization (FISH) analysis of the plasma cells of AL patients showed that 16 of 29 (55%) had a definite immunoglobulin heavy-chain translocation, and five additional patients (17%) had a pattern compatible with heavy-chain translocation.[23] Sixteen of 21 patients were confirmed to have t(11;14)(q13;q32), accounting for 76% of all immunoglobulin heavy-chain translocations.[24a] Seventy percent of AL patients had abnormal cIg-FISH, with the most common abnormalities being IgH translocations (48%)—including t(11;14) [39%], and t(14;16) [2%]—and del13/del13q [30%]. The risk of death for patients harboring the t(11;14) translocation was 2.1.[24b] Fifteen of 16 patients with an 11;14 translocation had cyclin D1 overexpression. In a second study translocation t(11;14) was the most frequent aberration in AL, with 47% versus 26% in MGUS (P = .03), and was strongly associated with the lack of an intact immunoglobulin (P < .001), thus contributing to the frequent light-chain subtype in AL.[24b]

CLINICAL FEATURES

The most common presenting symptoms of amyloidosis are fatigue, dyspnea, edema, paresthesias, and weight loss.[25] The symptoms are generally not specific and not particularly helpful in formulating the differential diagnosis. Weight loss usually results in an investigation for occult malignancy. The fatigue can be misdiagnosed as functional or stress related. Patients with dyspnea on exertion regularly undergo coronary angiography; in most, no coronary artery disease is seen, and the evaluation is halted. Lightheadedness is common but nonspecific. Hypotension is seen in patients with nephrotic syndrome because the hypoalbuminemia results in reduced oncotic pressure and contraction of the plasma volume. In cardiac AL, the stiffened heart has poor diastolic filling.[26a] This results in a reduced cardiac output with a normal ejection fraction on echocardiography. The septal thickening is attributed inappropriately to silent hypertension, and the patient lacks cardiomegaly, all of which conspire to obscure the correct diagnosis.[26b] The stroke volume decreases, resulting in a decrease in systolic blood pressure. Amyloid autonomic neuropathy also leads to orthostatic lightheadedness and occasionally syncope.[27]

The physical findings of amyloidosis can be highly specific but are only present in a minority of patients. Amyloid purpura is typical but is seen in only one-sixth of patients. The purpura occurs above the nipple line and is seen in the webbing of the neck, the face, and the eyelids (Fig. 87-2). The purpura may be subtle and limited to eyelid petechial lesions. Hepatosplenomegaly is seen in 25% of patients but more than 5 cm below the right costal margin in 10% of patients.[28] The presence of macroglossia is highly specific for AL[29]; it is not seen in familial, secondary, or senile systemic amyloidosis. Only one patient in 11 has an enlarged tongue; it can be overlooked because

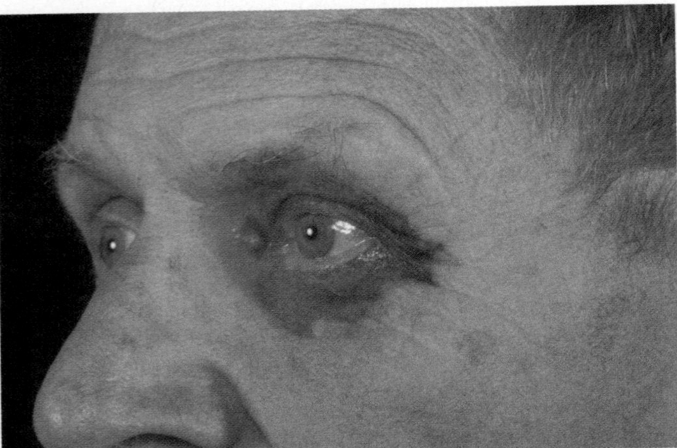

Figure 87-2 CLASSIC PERIORBITAL PURPURA ASSOCIATED WITH AMYLOIDOSIS.

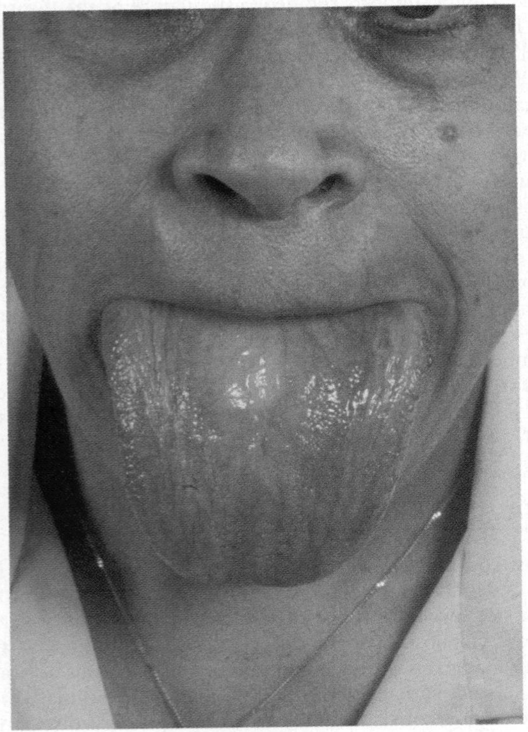

Figure 87-3 MASSIVE ENLARGEMENT OF THE TONGUE CAUSED BY AMYLOID INFILTRATION. This patient had severe obstructive sleep apnea; was unable to swallow solid food; and had obstructed eustachian tubes, leading to bilateral serous otitis media.

the most common finding is dental indentations on the underside of the tongue, which may not be inspected during a routine physical examination. If the tongue is enlarged, the submandibular salivary glands are also palpable (Fig. 87-3), which can be misinterpreted as submandibular lymph nodes. Salivary gland infiltration with amyloid can produce a sicca syndrome, and patients can be misdiagnosed as having Sjögren syndrome.[30]

Patients can be seen with diffuse vascular involvement without obvious visceral disease. Involvement of the small vessels supplying blood to major muscle groups can produce vascular occlusion and ischemic symptoms that include jaw,[31] calf, and limb claudication. Involvement of the coronary arteriolar system can produce true exertional angina without evidence of large vessel coronary disease. In one study, obstructive intramural coronary amyloidosis was found in 63 of 96 patients.[31] Myocardial ischemia was more common in patients with obstructive intramural coronary amyloidosis than those without (86% vs. 52%). Syndromes of myocardial ischemia affected 25% of patients with obstructive intramural coronary amyloidosis.[32] For 11% of these patients, a syndrome of ischemia consisting of acute myocardial infarction or angina was the first manifestation of AL.

Table 87-2 Syndromes in Primary Amyloidosis

Syndrome	Patients (%)
Nephrotic or nephrotic and renal failure	30
Hepatomegaly	24
Congestive heart failure	22
Carpal tunnel	21
Neuropathy	17
Orthostatic hypotension	12

From Gertz MA, Lacy MQ, Dispenzieri A: Amyloidosis. In Mehta J, Singhal S, editors: *Myeloma*. London, 2002, Martin Dunitz Ltd., p 445. Used with permission.

Most patients with AL and cardiac involvement have obstructive intramural coronary amyloidosis and associated changes of myocardial ischemia.[31] The presence of jaw claudication has led to an incorrect diagnosis of polymyalgia rheumatica.[33] Other manifestations of nonvisceral soft tissue infiltration include skeletal muscle pseudohypertrophy, which can produce the shoulder-pad sign.[34] Despite the enlargement of the muscles, patients frequently have diffuse muscular weakness and atrophy.[35] The creatine kinase concentration may be increased, which results in a misdiagnosis of polymyositis or inflammatory myopathy syndrome.

ESTABLISHING THE DIAGNOSIS OF AMYLOIDOSIS

The subjective symptoms associated with amyloidosis are vague.[36] The physical findings with AL may be highly specific but are present in only 15% of patients. Given that AL is rare, when should a clinician suspect this diagnosis and begin a diagnostic evaluation to confirm the diagnosis? The eight most common clinical syndromes associated with amyloidosis are (1) infiltrative cardiomyopathy manifesting as a spectrum from fatigue to overt congestive heart failure, (2) albuminuria with or without renal insufficiency, (3) peripheral neuropathy with demyelinating or axonal features, (4) unexplained hepatomegaly, (5) carpal tunnel syndrome, (6) enlargement of the tongue, (7) weight loss associated with intestinal symptoms of pseudo-obstruction or malabsorption, and (8) "atypical myeloma" (Table 87-2). If any of these syndromes are seen in an adult, AL enters the differential diagnosis.

Because of the presence of a monoclonal protein, patients are often extensively evaluated for MM but are found to have less than 10% plasma cells and no lytic bone lesions, and a diagnosis of AL frequently is not considered by the clinician. These patients are often mislabeled as having MGUS or myeloma with atypical features. By definition, patients with systemic AL have a clonal population of plasma cells that produces the immunoglobulin light chain comprising the amyloid deposits. The finding of a monoclonal protein in a patient with a compatible syndrome would be compelling evidence for pursuing a diagnosis of AL (Fig. 87-4).

If a patient has one of the clinical syndromes outlined above, a sensitive and noninvasive screening test for AL should be used. Simple serum protein electrophoresis is not an adequate screen. The monoclonal proteins in patients with AL are frequently either small or limited to free light chains that do not produce a peak after the electrophoresis. In addition, a high proportion of patients has significant albuminuria, which can obscure the presence of small monoclonal proteins in the urine (Fig. 87-5).

A serious consideration of AL requires immunofixation of serum and urine; urine immunofixation is mandatory because 25% of patients do not have detectable light chains in the serum by immunofixation. By this method, a monoclonal light chain will be detected

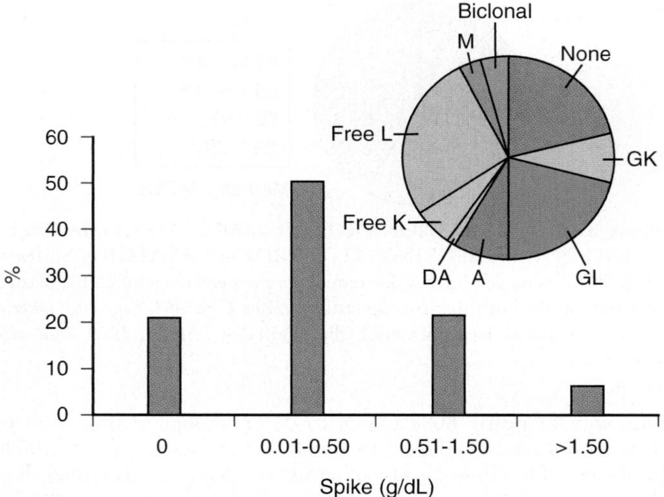

Figure 87-4 SERUM MONOCLONAL PROTEIN CONCENTRATION IN PATIENTS WITH PRIMARY AMYLOIDOSIS. Pie chart shows distribution of serum immunofixation results ($n = 434$). *A,* Monclonal IgA protein in serum; *Biclonal,* two different monclonal proteins in serum; *DA,* monclonal IgD protein in serum; *GK,* monclonal IgG kappa protein in serum; *GK,* monclonal IgG kappa protein in serum; *Free L,* monoclonal lambda light chain in serum; *Free K,* monoclonal kappa light chain in serum; *M,* monclonal IgM protein in serum; *None,* no monoclonal protein serum. *(From Gertz MA, Lacy MQ, Dispenzieri A: Amyloidosis. In Mehta J, Singhal S, editors:* Myeloma. *London, 2002, Martin Dunitz Ltd, p 445. Used with permission.)*

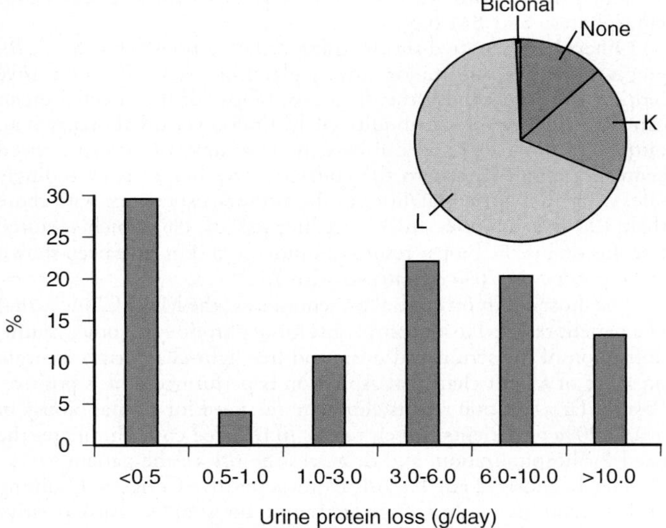

Figure 87-5 DISTRIBUTION OF URINARY PROTEIN EXCRETION IN PATIENTS WITH PRIMARY AMYLOIDOSIS. Pie chart shows results of urine immunofixation ($n = 434$). *Biclonal,* Two different monoclonal proteins in urine; *K,* monoclonal kappa light chain in urine; *L,* monoclonal lambda light chain in urine; *None,* no monoclonal protein urine. *(From Gertz MA, Lacy MQ, Dispenzieri A: Amyloidosis. In Mehta J, Singhal S, editors:* Myeloma. *London, 2002, Martin Dunitz Ltd, p 445. Used with permission.)*

in 90% of patients with AL. Adding the free light-chain nephelometric assay increases the detection rate to 99%. The nephelometric assay for free light chains is more sensitive than immunofixation by at least a factor of 10. Quantification of monoclonal free light chains by nephelometry is more sensitive than immunofixation in serum samples from patients with AL and light-chain deposition disease. This method allows quantification of free light chains in patients who have no detectable serum or urine monoclonal protein.[37]

Immunofixation of serum and urine combined with a free light-chain assay is the best noninvasive screening panel when a patient is seen with a suggestive clinical syndrome. In patients who do not have a detectable light chain in the serum or urine, a BM specimen will almost always demonstrate a clonal population of plasma cells by immunohistochemistry or immunofluorescence. If these study results are negative, the patient does not have amyloidosis (false-positive Congo red stain) or the detected amyloid deposit is localized, or if the amyloid is systemic, then it is secondary or familial.

Virtually all patients with systemic AL have a monoclonal protein in the serum or urine or clonal BM plasma cells. If no immunoglobulin light chain is found in a patient with proven amyloidosis, other types of amyloidosis should be suspected, including familial, secondary, and localized. The presence of a monoclonal protein does not unequivocally prove that the amyloidosis type is AL. Three percent of patients older than 60 years have an incidental MGUS.[38a] It is therefore reasonable to believe that 3% of patients older than 60 years with localized, secondary, and familial amyloidosis have an incidental monoclonal protein in the serum. Case reports exist of patients with low-level monoclonal gammopathies associated with a nonimmunoglobulin form of amyloidosis. The possibility, albeit uncommon, of an incidental monoclonal gammopathy unrelated to the patient's amyloidosis must be kept in mind. The authors have recently reported some of the more common diagnostic errors encountered when a patient is undergoing evaluation for amyloidosis.[38b]

A nephelometric technique for analyzing circulating immunoglobulin light chains in the serum recognizes only free immunoglobulin light chains and not those that are part of the intact immunoglobulin molecule.[39,40] A study of approximately 100 patients using antibodies specific for free immunoglobulin light chains showed a sensitivity of nearly 90% for the nephelometric technique.[41] The sensitivity was the same for patients with κ and λ amyloid. In patients who had a known monoclonal light chain in the urine but negative serum immunofixation results, free light chains were detected in 85% of patients with κ and 80% of patients with λ. In a carefully evaluated group of patients with definite AL who had no detectable monoclonal protein in the serum or urine by immunofixation, a free light chain was found in 86% and a free λ light chain in 30%.[41]

The nephelometric method assists in classification of patients with amyloidosis as having AL.[42] Patients with familial, secondary, or localized amyloidosis are not expected to have an abnormal ratio of free light chains in the serum. If the serum free light-chain assay and serum and urine immunofixation results are all negative or normal, the likelihood of a diagnosis of AL is small.

The free light-chain assay also is useful in assessing the outcome of treatment of amyloidosis. Free light-chain criteria have now been incorporated into the response criteria. The proposed new criteria require a partial response to reflect a greater than 50% decrease in the difference between involved and uninvolved immunoglobulin light chain before and after therapy. A very good partial response would be defined as a difference in the involved and uninvolved immunoglobulin free light chain of less than 4 mg/dL after therapy, and a complete response would be negative immunofixation serum and urine and a normal free light-chain ratio.[43a] Eighty-six patients whose abnormal free light-chain concentration decreased by more than 50% after chemotherapy had a 5-year survival rate of 88% compared with only 39% among patients for whom the free light-chain concentration did not decrease similarly.[43b] The conclusion was that decrease in the free light chain by more than 50% after chemotherapy is associated with a substantial survival benefit.

The amyloid P component is a glycoprotein that comprises as much as 10% of the amyloid fibril by weight.[44] All forms of amyloid contain the P component. The amyloid P component is related structurally to C-reactive protein, an acute-phase reactant used in the screening of patients at risk for coronary artery disease. The amyloid P component is not irreversibly bound to the amyloid fibril but is in dynamic equilibrium with the normal plasma amyloid P component compartment.[45] It is found in all humans and maintains a stable plasma level throughout life.

Radiolabeled amyloid P component—with iodine 123[46] or iodine 131[47]—is a useful imaging agent for identifying amyloid deposits. Serialized serum amyloid P scintigraphic scans have

Table 87-3 Noninvasive Biopsy Results in 325 Patients With Primary Amyloidosis

Finding	No. of Patients (%)
Fat + BM +	202 (62)
Fat + BM −	30 (9)
Fat − BM +	49 (15)
Fat − BM −	44 (14)

BM, Bone marrow.

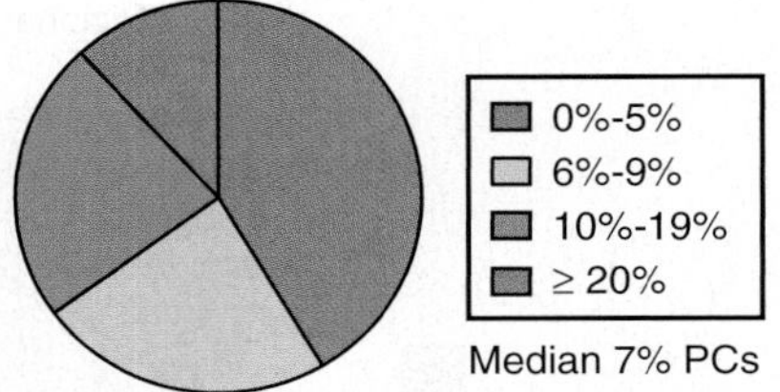

Figure 87-6 DISTRIBUTION OF BONE MARROW PLASMA CELLS IN PATIENTS PRESENTING WITH PRIMARY AMYLOIDOSIS (*n* = 434). *PC,* Plasma cell (each color represents the percentage of clonal plasma cells seen on the bone marrow aspiration). *(From Gertz MA, Lacy MQ, Dispenzieri A: Amyloidosis.* Hematol Oncol Clin North Am *13:1211, 1999. Used with permission.)*

been used to assess the response to therapy and have shown regression of established amyloid deposits after successful interruption of immunoglobulin light-chain production.[48] This scan does not distinguish AL from the other forms of amyloidosis. Imaging indicates deposits in the spleen, liver, and kidneys in 87%, 60%, and 25% of patients, respectively.[49] Because of the cardiac blood pool, this technique is not useful in detecting myocardial amyloid deposits and is usually used in conjunction with echocardiography. The diagnostic sensitivity of serum amyloid P scintigraphy for AL is 90%, and specificity is 93%.[50] Myocardial uptake is not visualized in any patient. Splenic amyloid is present in 80% of patients even though it is rarely detected clinically (15%). Tracer uptake in the liver and kidneys correlates with abnormal liver function and proteinuria. BM uptake is specific for AL but is only seen in 21%.[50]

Plasma clearance of the amyloid P component has been shown to correlate with survival. Rapid plasma clearance is associated with high body burdens of amyloid and shortened survival. Scintigraphic scans have shown that the distribution of amyloid within organs is nonhomogeneous, and imaging studies do not correlate well with the clinical degree of organ dysfunction.[51] Most patients have hepatic involvement by serum amyloid P scan, but palpable hepatomegaly with increased concentration of alkaline phosphatase is seen in no more than 15% of patients. Therapeutic clinical trials of agents that prevent the binding of amyloid P component to the amyloid fibril have been started.[52a] The rationale is that inhibition of P component binding may destabilize the fibrillar structure of amyloid and result in more rapid catabolism by the body. Administration of anti–human-SAP antibodies to mice with amyloid deposits containing human SAP triggers a potent, complement-dependent, macrophage-derived giant cell reaction that swiftly removes massive visceral amyloid deposits without adverse effects. Anti-SAP antibody treatment is clinically feasible because circulating human SAP can be depleted in patients by the bis-d-proline compound CPHPC, thereby enabling injected anti-SAP antibodies to reach residual SAP in the amyloid deposits.[52b]

Although the presence of immunoglobulin free light chains, positive immunofixation results, or positive amyloid P component scans is highly suggestive of the diagnosis of AL, these findings are not substitutes for histologic confirmation of the disease. Amyloidosis is a serious life-threatening disorder, and some of the currently available therapies carry a considerable morbidity and mortality risk. Given the serious prognosis and potential for administering toxic therapies, a biopsy-proven diagnosis is vital. Although the presence of renal, cardiac, hepatic, or peripheral nerve amyloid is easily established by direct biopsy of these tissues, invasive diagnostic biopsies of these tissues are generally not required. Amyloidosis is a widespread disorder at diagnosis, with involvement of blood vessels even in the absence of clinical symptoms. Any biopsy that samples blood vessels can less invasively establish the diagnosis effectively and at a lower risk to the patient.

At the Mayo Clinic, if a patient has a compatible clinical syndrome and screening suggests the presence of a free or monoclonal immunoglobulin light chain, the first diagnostic technique is generally subcutaneous fat aspiration[53] combined with BM biopsy. The fat aspiration procedure performed by the authors' nursing staff is risk free, and no infection at the site of puncture has occurred. Results are generally available in 24 to 48 hours, and the technique has a sensitivity of nearly 80% (Table 87-3). Thorough examination of three fat smears showed a sensitivity of 93% and a specificity of 100% for the test. The clinical utility of fat tissue aspiration was greater than that of a rectal biopsy.[54a] Fat aspiration is the preferred method for detecting amyloidosis, with a sensitivity of 80% using a routine approach and 90% with a thorough assessment by experienced interpreters.[54a] The amount of amyloid in subcutaneous fat tissue in systemic amyloidosis reflects disease severity, as measured by the number of organs involved, and predicts decreased survival independent of other well-known factors.[54b]

A BM biopsy shows amyloid deposits in half of patients if the biopsy specimen contains blood vessels.[55] A BM biopsy is generally required because after a monoclonal protein has been found, determining the percentage of BM plasma cells is vital to exclude the diagnosis of MM (Figs. 87-6 and 87-7, *A*). In the authors' experience, 90% of patients with AL have positive results with a subcutaneous fat aspiration and BM biopsy.

Others have reported success using rectal biopsies[56] (Fig. 87-7, *B*), gingival biopsies, and minor salivary gland biopsies.[57] If noninvasive biopsies do not establish the diagnosis, biopsy of the affected organ can generally be performed quite safely. Endomyocardial biopsy is an outpatient procedure and can be done with low risk in experienced centers. Despite reports to the contrary, liver biopsy is exceedingly safe, with no reported fatalities in the authors' experience with more than 100 liver biopsies and a bleeding risk of 4%, which required transfusion in 2%. Biopsy results of uninvolved skin have been shown to be positive in 70% of patients with AL.[58]

The most common clinical presentation at the Mayo Clinic is that of a patient referred to a nephrologist for nephrotic syndrome. Immunofixation of the serum and urine and free light-chain assay indicate presence of a light chain; fat aspiration is performed and is positive. Positive fat aspiration results eliminate the need for a renal biopsy in nearly 90% of patients, which results in reduced cost, eliminates the need for hospitalization, and decreases the risk to the patient.

The diagnosis of amyloidosis requires positive Congo red staining of tissues, but use of the Congo red stain is not simple.[59] False-positive results have been reported[60] because of overstaining of tissue or misinterpreting Congo red–positive fibrils of collagen and elastin as being amyloid. Conversely, we have seen patients with rectal biopsy specimens that were interpreted as collagenous colitis,[61] only later to be identified as AL. By routine hematoxylin and eosin staining, amyloid deposits in the glomerulus can be misinterpreted as hyalin. In the authors' routine clinical practice, cardiac pathologists prefer the sulfated alcian blue stain[62] for recognition of amyloid deposits in the myocardium. In the authors' peripheral nerve laboratories, pathologists screen biopsy specimens with crystal violet and, if results are positive, subsequently confirm the diagnosis by using Congo red.

DISTINGUISHING PRIMARY AMYLOIDOSIS FROM OTHER FORMS OF AMYLOIDOSIS

After a diagnosis of amyloidosis has been established, it is imperative to be certain that the amyloidosis is of the immunoglobulin

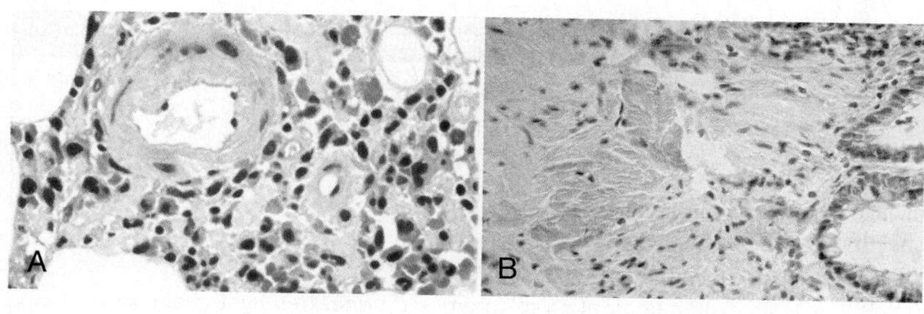

Figure 87-7 A, Bone marrow biopsy specimen showing thickened large and small vessels caused by amyloid deposition. **B,** Rectal biopsy specimen demonstrates amyloid deposits *(left)* with Brunner glands *(right)*. (Congo red; original magnification, ×100.)

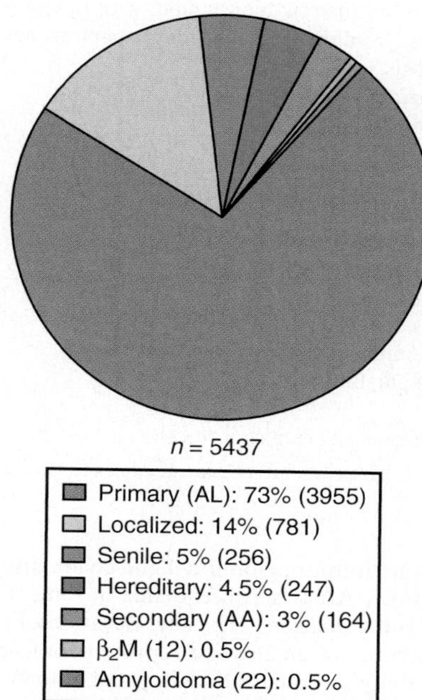

Figure 87-8 DISTRIBUTION OF THE VARIOUS FORMS OF AMYLOIDOSIS SEEN IN PATIENTS AT THE MAYO CLINIC, 1960 TO 2009. *β_2M,* β_2-Microglobulin.

light-chain type. Localized, familial, secondary, and senile systemic forms of amyloid are structurally dissimilar to that in AL, and the therapeutic approach is substantially different for each (Fig. 87-8). Only systemic AL has an underlying BM plasma cell dyscrasia responsible for fibril deposition.

It is possible to misdiagnose hereditary amyloidosis as AL. Among 350 patients with amyloidosis in whom AL was suspected, 34 (9.7%) were found to have mutations consistent with familial amyloidosis, most often fibrinogen-A α-chain mutations and TTR mutations.[63] A low-grade monoclonal gammopathy was detected in eight of the 34 (24%), which easily could have led to a misdiagnosis of AL. A genetic cause should be sought in all patients with amyloidosis in whom AL cannot be unequivocally confirmed.

The possibility of familial amyloidosis with an incidental monoclonal gammopathy must be kept in mind.[63] In 178 consecutive patients referred for amyloidosis, 54 were screened with primers to detect TTR, apolipoprotein, fibrinogen, and lysozyme variants.[64] Three patients had both a monoclonal gammopathy and an amyloid-associated mutation, were thought to have apparent AL and were later found to have hereditary amyloidosis.[64] Techniques to unequivocally identify TTR amyloidosis include immunoaffinity chromatography and immunoprecipitation combined with mass spectrometry.[65] Matrix-assisted laser desorption ionization/time-of-flight mass spectrometry can also quickly detect TTR variants with small changes in molecular weight.[66a] The gold standard for protein identification is mass spectroscopic analysis of the tissue and direct sequencing to identify the amyloid protein, and this is now standard for all pathologic specimens that are Congo red positive at the Mayo Clinic (Fig. 87-9).[66b,66c] The distinction between immunoglobulin and nonimmunoglobulin amyloidosis is important because nonimmunoglobulin amyloidosis does not benefit from chemotherapy and may be amenable to drugs in development including eprodisate,[66d] for slowing the decline of renal function in AA, and tafamidis[66e] has potential utility in the management of senile and familial amyloidosis.

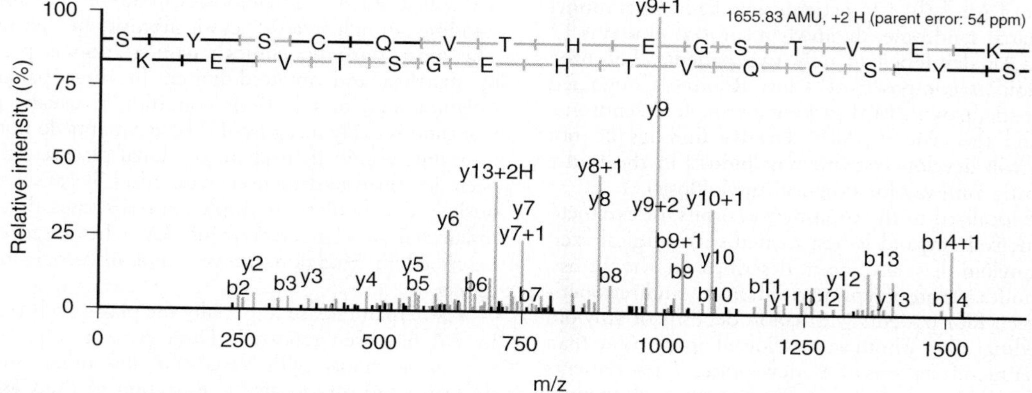

Figure 87-9 MASS SPECTROSCOPIC IDENTIFICATION OF AMYLOID PROTEIN. Mass spectrometry of laser microdissected tissue can be used to type amyloidosis accurately in clinical biopsy specimens. The technology is now the gold standard for protein identification in amyloidosis. *(The image was kindly provided by Dr. Ahmet Dogan of Mayo Clinic. See also Vrana JA, Gamez JD, Madden BJ, et al: Classification of amyloidosis by laser microdissection and mass spectrometry-based proteomic analysis in clinical biopsy specimens.* Blood *114:4957, 2009.)*

Patients with localized amyloidosis can often have serious clinical problems such as hematuria, respiratory compromise, and visual disturbances. Patients with localized amyloidosis do not develop widespread systemic vascular amyloid deposition. Localized forms of amyloidosis most commonly are derived from immunoglobulin light chains, but a BM plasma cell dyscrasia is not present, and it is presumed that there was a localized synthesis of fibrillar material. Most patients with localized amyloidosis have involvement of the respiratory tract, genitourinary tract, conjunctivae, or skin.

Amyloidosis involving the respiratory tract can be divided into tracheobronchial, pulmonary nodular, and pulmonary diffuse interstitial. The first two of these are forms of localized amyloidosis, and the third is a manifestation of systemic AL disease. In tracheobronchial amyloidosis, submucosal deposits (composed of immunoglobulin light chains) can produce obstruction, cough, dyspnea, wheezing, and hemoptysis. The most common site of involvement is the larynx and false vocal cords. The diagnosis is usually established bronchoscopically in a patient who presents with hoarseness. The treatment entails surgical excision[67] or the use of yttrium–aluminum–garnet laser resection of the tissue.[68] If extensive airway obstruction prevents passage of a bronchoscope, external-beam radiotherapy (2000 cGy) can lead to dramatic improvement in symptoms, effort tolerance, bronchoscopic appearance, and forced expiratory volume in 1 second. If amyloidosis involves the pulmonary tissues, it can manifest as solitary nodules.[69] The diagnosis is usually made at thoracotomy or transthoracic needle biopsy because these nodules are noncalcified, and pulmonary malignancy must be excluded.[70]

Amyloid in the urinary bladder, urethra, or ureter is usually localized. Clinically, patients present with hematuria, and the cystoscopic findings of these bladder deposits are usually suspicious for transitional cell cancer.[71] Treatment consists of transurethral resection, fulguration, or partial cystectomy. The authors have experience with the use of intravesicular dimethylsulfoxide (DMSO) and have seen substantial regression of deposits in patients who were not candidates for surgical resection because of extent of disease. Amyloid in the ureter,[72] renal pelvis,[73] and urethra[74] usually presents with obstruction and colicky pain or hematuria; the preoperative diagnosis is usually malignancy. Recognition of ureteral amyloidosis is important because it prevents an unnecessary nephrectomy.

Amyloidosis of the skin can be classified into lichen, macular, or nodular.[75] The first two of these are localized forms of amyloid that never become systemic. Nodular amyloidosis may be a cutaneous manifestation of systemic AL. The deposits in macular and papular amyloidosis appear to be degenerated keratin protein.[76] Local therapy, including dermabrasion, is beneficial. An underlying inflammatory skin condition is usually present. Macular and lichen amyloidosis are benign conditions. Nodular amyloidosis is often an important clinical clue to a more serious life-threatening AL.

Amyloid found in the carpal tunnel may represent either a localized form or be part of AL.[77a] Of 124 patients who had carpal tunnel syndrome as an isolated syndrome, the median survival time was 12 years, and systemic AL developed in only two patients. Localized carpal tunnel amyloid is composed of TTR. Routine Congo red staining of BM in patients with MM lacking an amyloid syndrome is not indicated, and the yield is 1%.[77b] Positive findings do not suggest the patient will develop systemic amyloidosis in the future (see box on Diagnostic Pathway for Primary Amyloidosis).

Amyloid may be localized to the conjunctiva, orbits, or extraocular muscles. Conjunctival amyloid is best treated with surgical excision.[78] Localized amyloid has also been described in the breast, mesenteric lymph nodes, colon polyps, thyroid, ovary, and retroperitoneum. We have seen four patients with colon deposits of amyloid that resulted in bleeding, all of whom were followed up for more than 5 years without other manifestations of AL developing. These patients had no evidence of a plasma cell dyscrasia. Finding traces of amyloid in surgical specimens from total hip arthroplasty is common.[79] Similar deposits can be seen at the time of knee arthroplasty[80] and are never associated with systemic disease.

Secondary amyloidosis also must be distinguished from AL.[81] AA can involve organs in a manner indistinguishable from AL but is not associated with an immunoglobulin light-chain disorder or clonal plasma cell disorder. AA is a consequence of long-standing uncontrolled systemic inflammation. Typically, elevation of the acute-phase proteins in the serum, serum amyloid A protein, or C-reactive protein parallels the activity of the underlying inflammatory process. In underdeveloped countries, AA is common because it can occur after long-standing tuberculosis, lepromatous leprosy, malaria, and untreated syphilis. The most common clinical manifestation of AA is nephrotic-range proteinuria. Therefore, it is not easily distinguished clinically from AL.

Diagnostic Pathway for Primary Amyloidosis

Consider primary amyloidosis in patients with
- Nephrotic-range proteinuria (nondiabetic)
- Cardiomyopathy (no ischemic history)
- Hepatomegaly (no filling defects on imaging)
- Peripheral neuropathy (nondiabetic)

Atypical myeloma

Heighten suspicion
- Immunofixation of serum and urine, free light-chain assay

Confirm diagnosis histologically
- Fat aspirate and marrow biopsy stain with Congo red (90% sensitive); confirm type with mass spectroscopy

Assess prognosis
- Echocardiography required (Doppler important)

NT-pro-BNP and troponin

Treat
- Melphalan and prednisone or dexamethasone
- High-dose steroids
- Stem cell transplantation

Bortezomib + dexamethasone

Melphalan–dexamethasone–lenalidomide

Cyclophosphamide–thalidomide–dexamethasone

Cyclophosphamide–bortezomib–dexamethasone
- Organ transplantation

NT-pro-BNP, N-terminal pro-brain natriuretic peptide.

In the West, AA is rare and found in only 2% of patients with amyloidosis at Mayo Clinic.[82] The most common causes are poorly controlled inflammatory polyarthropathies, including ankylosing spondylitis,[83] juvenile rheumatoid arthritis,[84] psoriatic arthritis,[85] and rheumatoid arthritis.[86] The median duration of the arthritis is 15 years before the diagnosis of amyloidosis, and the underlying cause is usually obvious.[87]

In a 10-year study of 1000 patients with rheumatoid arthritis, 3.1% died of AA.[88] Amyloidosis can be seen in Crohn disease,[89] long-standing bronchiectasis,[90] cystic fibrosis, or chronic osteomyelitis.[91] The most common clinical manifestation is proteinuria followed by diarrhea and amyloid goiter. In these patients, the chronic, inflammatory, or infectious condition is usually present for many years and is easily recognized. These patients do not have a detectable immunoglobulin light chain or clonal plasma cell disorder. AA has been described in drug users who inject illegal substances subcutaneously.[92] The result is multiple skin abscesses that can produce the inflammation characteristic of AA.[93] Instances of AA have been described in Hodgkin disease[94] and in association with renal cell cancer.

Castleman disease (especially the plasma cell variant) complicated by AA has been reported. These patients typically present with a mesenteric mass; with successful abdominal surgery, proteinuria decreases and disappears.[95-97] Resection of the Castleman tumor has been documented to produce regression of the amyloid syndrome, even in advanced cases. AA has been seen in patients with paraparesis as a consequence of chronically infected decubitus ulcers[98] or chronic infection of the urinary tract, a consequence of urinary retention or a long-standing indwelling urinary catheter.[99] At autopsy, AA has been found in more than half of those with sustained spinal cord injuries in excess of 10 years. The presence of an amyloid goiter is characteristic of AA and is rarely seen in the other forms of amyloidosis.

Secondary amyloidosis can also be a consequence of hereditary periodic fevers characterized by recurrence of fever and inflammation separated by symptom-free intervals. Familial Mediterranean fever is the most frequent entity in this group, but hyperimmunoglobulinemia D with periodic fever, tumor necrosis factor receptor–associated periodic syndrome, and cryopyrin-associated periodic syndrome are also seen.[100-102] Effective therapy for inflammatory rheumatic syndromes has led to a decline in the incidence of AA worldwide.[82]

Familial amyloidosis is more common than AA in the United States. A clinical distinction for this variant can be difficult. These patients can present with cardiomyopathy,[103] peripheral or autonomic neuropathy,[104] and nephrotic syndrome.[105] The patients do not have a monoclonal gammopathy or plasma cell dyscrasia unless they have an incidental MGUS. It is important to use immunostains or mass spectroscopic direct sequencing on amyloid-containing tissues in an attempt to determine the protein subunit within the fibril. Typical immunostains include κ and λ immunoglobulin light chain, amyloid A antisera, TTR, fibrinogen, lysozyme, and apolipoprotein.

The most commonly reported forms of familial amyloidosis are a result of mutations of the TTR gene. More than 100 mutations in the TTR gene have been described and are associated with the development of either amyloid peripheral neuropathy or amyloid cardiomyopathy.[106] Half of the patients identified at the Mayo Clinic with familial amyloid polyneuropathy do not have a positive family history, and lack of a family history is not useful in making the distinction.[107] Frequently, the history includes a family member dying of an obscure illness that is suspicious but has not been verified to be amyloidosis. Any patient with amyloidosis who does not have a detectable monoclonal protein or plasma cell dyscrasia should be carefully evaluated for the presence of familial amyloidosis.

Cardiac amyloidosis can be caused by mutations in the TTR gene and can also be seen with deposition of wild-type TTR in the heart.[108] So-called senile systemic amyloidosis usually manifests as amyloid cardiomyopathy in elderly adults. Analysis of the cardiac deposits shows normal TTR that can be found in 8% to 25% of persons older than 80 years.[109] Familial amyloid cardiomyopathy was first recognized 50 years ago in a Danish kindred but has since been detected in pedigrees throughout the world. Onset of symptoms typically begins after age 60 years, which decreases the suspicion of a familial disorder. The clinical manifestations of both senile systemic amyloidosis and familial amyloid cardiomyopathy are quite similar and include congestive heart failure or intractable rhythm disturbances. In one autopsy series, 21% of those older than 90 years had amyloid deposits.[109] Patients with senile systemic amyloidosis are older than those with AL. Proteinuria is generally not present in senile systemic amyloidosis, and the left ventricular wall thickness is substantially greater in senile systemic amyloidosis despite these patients' having less severe heart failure. The median survival has been reported to be 75 months.[110]

An important mutation of the TTR protein at position 122 was described in a 68-year-old African American man.[111] The allele responsible for this mutation is carried by 3.9% of African Americans—1.3 million people in the United States. This mutation is a major cause of cardiac amyloidosis among black Americans.[112] The finding of cardiac amyloidosis in an older adult in the absence of a monoclonal gammopathy should raise the possibility of familial amyloid cardiomyopathy or senile systemic amyloidosis.

Other mutant proteins have been shown to produce amyloidosis. Familial renal amyloidosis has been reported with deposition of a mutant fibrinogen α chain[113] or caused by mutant lysozyme.[114] The clinical course in these patients is more indolent than in patients with nephrotic syndrome caused by AL. The authors have seen such patients with slowly progressive proteinuria for more than a decade without development of extrarenal manifestations of amyloidosis and renal failure. There are no other clinical distinguishing features. Renal amyloidosis has been described in patients with mutations of apolipoprotein A-I[115] and A-II.[116] The clinical presentation is indistinguishable from that of AL; the main difference is the lack of a monoclonal immunoglobulin disorder. LECT2-associated renal amyloidosis represents a unique form of renal amyloidosis, especially in Mexican Americans presenting with proteinuria and renal insufficiency.

Distinguishing familial amyloidosis from AL is critical because liver transplantation has been used successfully in more than 500 patients with familial amyloidosis.[117,118] In the forms of familial amyloidosis caused by mutations of the TTR gene, TTR is produced in only the liver and choroid plexus, and subsequent liver transplantation induced regression of amyloid deposits.[119] The outcome of transplantation appears to be best for patients with a TTR Val30Met mutation. Liver transplantation is not curative in all. Morbidity is high in patients with significant nutritional disability before transplantation or neuronal dropout on a pretransplantation peripheral nerve biopsy. Progressive cardiac amyloidosis after liver transplantation has been reported.[120] The theory is that preexistent amyloid deposits in the myocardium, even when asymptomatic, can serve as the nidus for further deposition of wild-type TTR and progressive cardiac dysfunction and failure.[121]

Early liver transplantation can improve survival in familial amyloid polyneuropathy. For transplant recipients with a modified body mass index (which is multiplied by serum albumin level) greater than 600 $kg/m^2 \cdot L^{-1}$, improved survival has been noted compared with historical control participants without transplantation. It is important for these patients to undergo transplantation when their nutritional status is good.[122] Domino liver transplantation, in which the recipient's liver is in turn given to another recipient, has been used for patients with familial amyloidosis, in one reported case resulting in the transmission of amyloidosis.[123] The authors have seen a patient with hepatic failure from hepatitis C develop amyloid neuropathy 7 years after receiving the liver of a patient with TTR amyloidosis. She was retransplanted within 3 months of histologic proof of amyloidosis.

In summary, any patient with amyloidosis who lacks a monoclonal protein in the serum and urine and does not have a plasma cell dyscrasia should be evaluated for the presence of localized, secondary, senile, or familial amyloidosis. Rarely, a patient with amyloidosis and a monoclonal gammopathy can also have a nonimmunoglobulin form of amyloidosis, and immunohistochemical staining or preferably mass spectroscopic analysis of the amyloid deposits is warranted to exclude this possibility.

CLINICAL PRESENTATION OF PRIMARY AMYLOIDOSIS

A distinct male predominance in amyloidosis has been noted for more than 40 years. In Mayo Clinic patients with AL, 67% are male; males comprise 52% of all MM patients. The median age of patients with amyloidosis seen at Mayo Clinic is 67 years. The median age of patients with AL from Olmsted County, however, is 73 years, which may reflect referral bias of younger patients.

When patients are classified by a dominant organ manifestation, cardiac amyloidosis is the most common and is seen in 37.4% of patients (Fig. 87-10). Overt congestive heart failure is found in half of patients with demonstrable cardiac amyloidosis. The others have manifestations that include fatigue, arrhythmia, or syncope. The widespread use of echocardiography has increased the recognition of cardiac amyloidosis.[124] Dominant renal amyloidosis is seen in 27.8% of patients. The most common manifestation is nephrotic-range proteinuria (albuminuria). Amyloid peripheral neuropathy is seen in 15.3%. Hepatomegaly is found in 17.7% of amyloidosis patients, but liver amyloidosis presenting as the dominant manifestation is seen in only 4.6%. Gastrointestinal (GI) tract amyloidosis manifested by intestinal bleeding, pseudo-obstruction, or diarrhea is seen in 7.1% of patients, and the other patients (7.8%) have a heterogeneous mix of soft tissue, vascular, tongue, periarticular, and pulmonary interstitial amyloidosis.

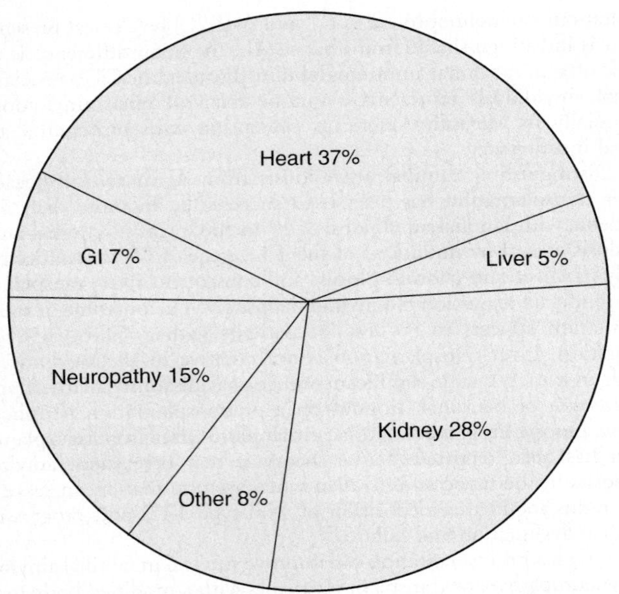

Figure 87-10 DISTRIBUTION OF DOMINANT SYNDROMES IN PATIENTS WITH AMYLOIDOSIS. *GI*, Gastrointestinal.

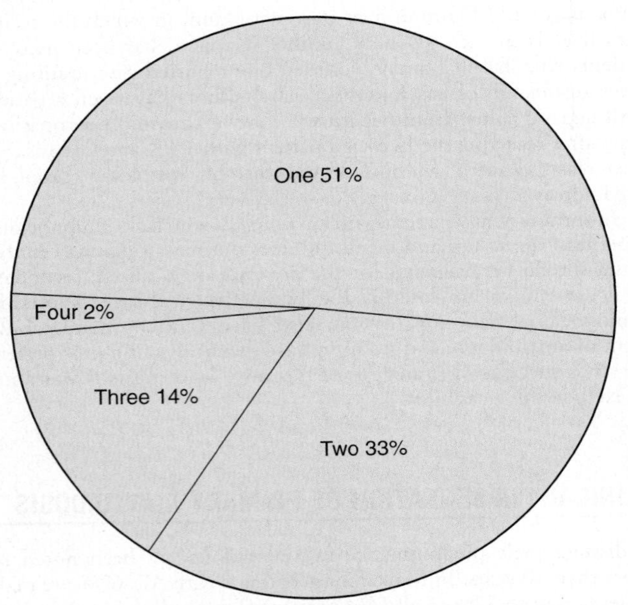

Figure 87-11 NUMBER OF ORGANS INVOLVED AT PRESENTATION IN MAYO CLINIC PATIENTS WITH AMYLOIDOSIS.

In the authors' patient population,[125] 49% presented with two or more organs involved (Fig. 87-11). In assigning a dominant organ of involvement, the designation is occasionally arbitrary because it is often difficult to distinguish which of the organs is responsible for the presenting symptoms.

If presentation with purpura alone is excluded, only 2.3% of patients presented with significant bleeding, 16.4% had carpal tunnel syndrome, and 19.6% had clinically overt congestive heart failure.[126] Symptoms included edema in 44.8% and fatigue in 46.4%. Nephrotic-range proteinuria was seen in 21%, orthostatic hypotension in 12%, lower extremity paresthesias in 34.9%, and weight loss in 51.7%. Anemia is uncommon in AL; 90% of patients have a hemoglobin value greater than 10 g/dL.[126] Only 1.5% of patients had a hemoglobin value less than 8 g/dL, and this was usually a sign of active intestinal tract hemorrhage or the anemia of renal failure. The median platelet count was 257 × 10^9/L; only 5.5% had a platelet count greater than 500 × 10^9/L. Thrombocytosis usually is seen with hepatic amyloidosis and hyposplenism.

A serum creatinine concentration greater than 2 mg/dL is present in 13.6% of patients at presentation.[126] An alkaline phosphatase concentration of two times the institutional normal value, which reflects hepatic involvement, is present in 6.7%. The median number of BM plasma cells is 7% (range, 1%-30%) (see Fig. 87-6); 12% of patients with AL have more than 20% plasma cells in the BM without any other signs of MM. The median 24-hour urine protein loss for all patients was 790 mg/24 hr (see Fig. 87-5). The monoclonal light chain is λ in 70%, κ in 19%, and no monoclonal protein is found in 11%. However, when the immunoglobulin light chain levels and ratios are measured, then fewer than 1% of systemic AL patients fail to have an identifiable light-chain disorder. When an immunoglobulin (Ig) heavy chain was detectable in the serum, it was IgG in 58%, IgA in 10%, and IgM in 8% (see Fig. 87-4). It is important to remember that amyloidosis is associated with IgM monoclonal gammopathies.[127] Waldenström macroglobulinemia has also been reported to be associated with amyloid arthropathy presenting as bilateral symmetric polyarthritis.[128a] Rarely, Waldenström macroglobulinemia is associated with AA amyloidosis, although most patients with macroglobulinemia developing amyloidosis have AL.[128b,128c]

Echocardiographic findings in the entire patient population demonstrate a median septal thickness of 14 mm.[126] The septal thickness is less than 15 mm in 53% and 15 mm or greater in 47%, reflecting a high proportion of patients with cardiac amyloidosis at diagnosis. The median survival of all patients is approximately 12 months. The 2- and 5-year survival rates are 33.6% and 15%, respectively. Variables important in survival prediction include the patient's performance status on the Eastern Cooperative Oncology Group scale, the presence of heart involvement as the dominant syndrome, and the involvement of two or more organs at presentation. Survival in amyloidosis has been steadily improving over the decades.[128d]

Kidney

When free monoclonal light chains are found in the urine, the differential diagnosis of the proteinuria is cryoglobulinemia,[129] amyloidosis, light-chain deposition disease,[130,131] and myeloma cast nephropathy. Immunofixation of the urine is important in the diagnostic evaluation whenever protein is present. Renal involvement is seen in 28% of Mayo Clinic patients,[126] but in the Italian Intergroup, the frequency of renal involvement was nearly 50%.[132] In nondiabetic adults with nephrotic syndrome, amyloid is seen in 12% of biopsies. Survival is associated with the serum creatinine value at diagnosis.[133] The median survival of patients with a creatinine value less than and greater than 1.3 mg/dL was 25.6 and 15 months, respectively. Patients with increased protein excretion do not have shorter survival but do have a shorter time to the development of end-stage renal disease.[134] Fewer than 5% of patients with AL have urinary protein loss less than 150 mg/day. Two-thirds of patients have a light chain detectable in the urine, and two-thirds a detectable light chain in the serum. In AL patients with greater than 1 g of proteinuria, a light chain can be found in as many as 86%. The ratio of κ to λ light chains in patients with nephrotic syndrome is one to five. The median urinary protein loss in κ light-chain amyloidosis is 1.1 g/day; in λ light-chain amyloidosis, it is 4.6 g/day. There is no difference in the frequency of renal insufficiency in κ and λ light-chain amyloidosis.

Long-standing proteinuria results in hypoalbuminemia, which leads to decreased intravascular oncotic pressure. The clinical end result is transudation of fluid into the extracellular space with refractory edema. The use of diuretics can aggravate intravascular volume contraction and hypotension and reduces renal blood flow. In patients with advanced anasarca, bilateral catheter embolization of the renal arteries has been used.[135] Recently, the authors have also placed clips on the ureters laparoscopically to manage a patient with intractable nephrotic syndrome. The continuous loss of protein into the urine produces tubular atrophy and damage. The median time from the

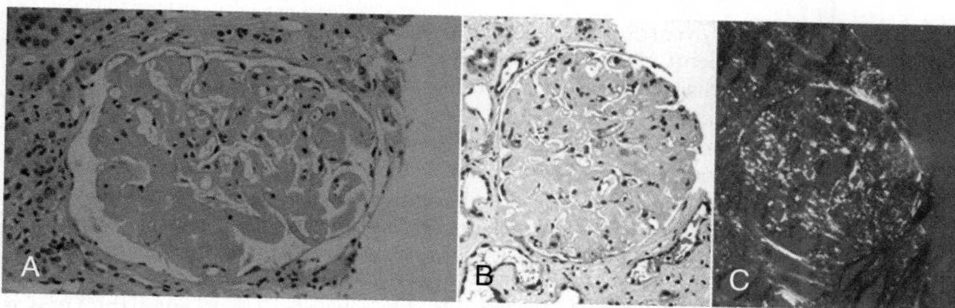

Figure 87-12 A, Amyloid deposits in the glomerulus. Note the amorphous nature that could easily be confused with hyalin degeneration (hematoxylin and eosin; original magnification, ×100). **B,** A second case showing amyloid deposits (×100); **C,** Congo red stain with "apple-green" birefringence (×100).

diagnosis of AL nephrotic syndrome to dialysis is 14 months; the median survival from the start of dialysis in AL patients is 8 months. The cause of death in most patients is the development of cardiac amyloidosis. The authors have not recognized a difference in outcome between patients undergoing hemodialysis and peritoneal dialysis; the 1-year survival rate is 68% after initiation of dialysis. The most important extrarenal complications of AL are heart failure, heart arrhythmias, and hypotension. Dialysis is regularly complicated by hypotension.

The amount of proteinuria is poorly correlated with the extent of amyloid deposits on biopsy (Fig. 87-12). Most patients with AL have normal-sized kidneys by ultrasonography. The urinary sediment shows fat but no casts or red blood cells. In a study of 118 patients with monoclonal gammopathies, 30% of those having a renal biopsy had AL.[136] The median survival time in the group was 24 months, with death largely caused by cardiac amyloidosis. Predictors of survival included age younger than 70 years and high serum calcium and creatinine concentrations at presentation. It is rare for renal amyloidosis to develop if it is not present at diagnosis. The authors have seen four patients in whom nephrotic-range proteinuria developed after cardiac transplantation for amyloidosis. Presumably, in the past, these patients would not have survived long enough for renal amyloidosis to develop.

The cause of the proteinuria in AL is amyloid deposits disrupting the glomerular basement membrane. Immunotactoid (fibrillary) glomerulopathy is a fibrillar deposition in the kidney that can be confused with AL.[137] On electron microscopy, the fibrils of fibrillary glomerulopathy are twice the width of amyloid fibrils, and the deposits do not stain with Congo red. Light-chain deposition disease (Randall type) represents the deposition of nonamyloid immunoglobulin light chains in a granular fashion on the tubular or glomerular basement membrane.[138a] It can produce nephrotic syndrome and renal failure. Amyloidosis and light-chain deposition disease have been reported in the same patient. Light-, light and heavy–, and heavy-chain deposition diseases display essentially similar characteristics, such as involvement of multiple organs, prominent renal involvement with severe renal failure, diabetes-like nodular glomerulosclerosis, marked thickening of tubular basement membranes, and monotypic deposits of Ig light chains (mostly κ) or heavy chains (mostly γ) that feature a non-organized granular, electron-dense appearance by electron microscopy.[138b]

Few reports exist of renal transplantation for AL. In a report on 12 patients, two of whom had AL, four were alive at 2 years, and in two of these four, the renal biopsy showed recurrent amyloid.[139] In another report, 11 patients received transplants, and three showed recurrent amyloid deposits in the allograft at 11, 28, and 37 months.[140] In 45 patients with amyloidosis who received a renal transplant, the 3-year survival rate was 51%, which is inferior to the outcome of renal transplantation for primary renal disease.[141] The estimate for recurrent amyloidosis in a recipient of a renal transplant is approximately 20% at 1 year. On scintigraphy, uptake of radiolabeled serum amyloid was seen in four of 10 renal transplant recipients. Of 22 patients with renal amyloidosis, seven had adrenal insufficiency, and four died of hypoadrenalism.

The authors performed living donor kidney transplantation followed by autologous stem cell transplantation (SCT) for AL patients with end-stage renal disease.[142] Two patients had complications and died 3 and 10 months later. Two patients had development of subclinical acute cellular rejection, and one patient had acute rejection, all reversible. Six patients had successful stem cell harvest, and five underwent SCT with good engraftment. Renal function stabilized after SCT in four and was decreased in one. The feasibility of donor kidney transplant with an autologous SCT for carefully selected patients has been established.[142] It is unclear whether SCT should precede or follow kidney transplantation.[143a] In the United Kingdom, renal transplants were performed in 22 patients with AL. One- and 5-year patient survival rates were 95% and 67% among kidney recipients, respectively. No renal graft failed because of recurrent amyloid during median (range) follow-up of 4.8 (0.2-13.3) years.[143b]

Heart

The extent of cardiac amyloid is the most important factor determining outcome in AL. Patients present with infiltrative cardiomyopathy that leads to restricted ventricular filling and may present with disabling fatigue and unexplained weight loss. These patients have early diastolic dysfunction and no systolic dysfunction.[144] Chest radiography does not show cardiomegaly or pulmonary vascular redistribution. The ejection fraction is preserved on echocardiography. As a result of poor diastolic filling and normal contractility, the ejection fraction is normal, but end-diastolic volume is decreased as a result of poor filling, and this results in low cardiac output.[145] Electrocardiography (ECG) typically shows low voltage, which is frequently overlooked.[146] Patients can be misdiagnosed as having ischemic heart disease because of the pseudoinfarction pattern seen in amyloidosis, with loss of the R wave in leads V1 through V3. Coronary arteriography is commonly performed during evaluation and is invariably normal.[147] Echocardiography shows thickening as a result of infiltration, but this can easily be misinterpreted as concentric left ventricular hypertrophy[148] or asymmetric septal hypertrophy (Fig. 87-13).

A patient with diastolic heart failure or restrictive hemodynamics should be evaluated for the presence of a monoclonal protein in the serum or urine.[149] The noncompliant left ventricle caused by infiltration is referred to as the "stiff heart."[150] There is minimal effect on systolic function, and the ejection fraction is preserved until late in the course of the disease. Echocardiography can be misleading owing to the normal ejection fraction and a lack of focal or segmental wall motion abnormalities.[151] The infiltration of the myocardial wall does result in thickening, but ECG does not show the voltage changes of ventricular hypertrophy. Instead, it shows low voltage or the pseudoinfarction pattern.

Doppler studies are required to assess myocardial function in AL because Doppler echocardiography best demonstrates restriction to inflow during diastole.[152] The Doppler filling patterns closely relate to the extent of amyloid infiltration. Patients with early cardiac amyloidosis show abnormal relaxation. Patients with advanced cardiac AL show a short deceleration time consistent with restrictive physiology. The combination of decreased fractional shortening of less than 20% and a mean left ventricular wall thickness of 15 mm is associated with a median survival time of only 4 months. A short deceleration time on Doppler echocardiography indicates restrictive physiology, and these patients have shortened survival times compared with patients with deceleration times exceeding 150 msec.

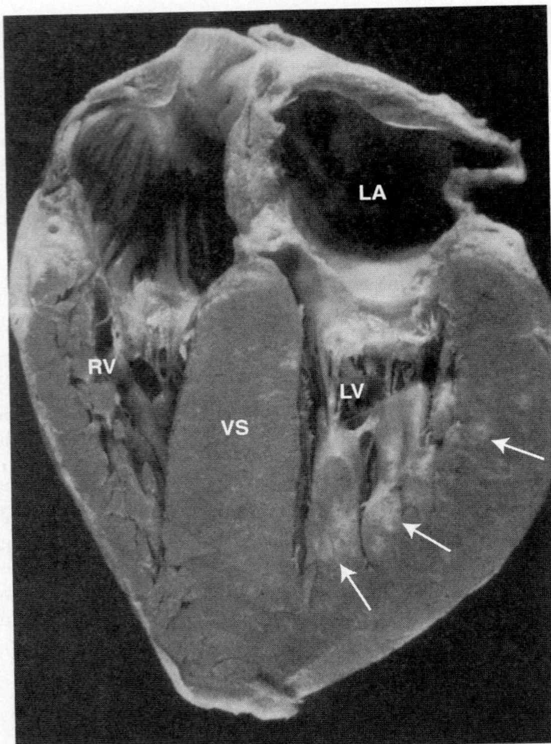

Figure 87-13 AUTOPSY SPECIMEN OF CARDIAC AMYLOIDOSIS. *Arrows* indicate the white deposits of amyloid that Rokitansky thought were "lardaceous." *LA,* Left atrium; *LV,* left ventricle; *RV,* right ventricle; *VS,* ventricular septum.

The recent introduction of echocardiographic strain imaging demonstrated its ability to show functional abnormalities before any morphologic echocardiographic abnormalities were present.[153] When combined with tissue Doppler imaging, cardiac involvement can be detected in early stages.[153a] However, myocardial strain could not differentiate hypertrophic from an infiltrative etiology of a thickened septum.[153b] Magnetic resonance imaging has also been used for early detection of cardiac amyloidosis. The combination of widespread myocardial enhancement on delayed postcontrast inversion recovery T1-weighted images with features of restrictive cardiac disease is highly suggestive.[154a] Late gadolinium enhancement is common in cardiac amyloid and detects interstitial expansion from amyloid deposition. Global transmural or subendocardial late gadolinium enhancement is most common, but suboptimal myocardial nulling and focal patchy late gadolinium enhancement are also observed. LGE-CMR may detect early cardiac abnormalities in patients with amyloidosis with normal left ventricular thickness.[154b]

Sudden death is a well-recognized complication of cardiac amyloidosis.[155] Digoxin has been associated with a risk of sudden death in AL. Digoxin provides rate control in the presence of atrial fibrillation but is unlikely to improve myocardial performance because systolic function is so well preserved in AL.[156] The mainstay of supportive care in cardiac AL is the use of diuretics.[157,158] The presence of orthostatic hypotension and intravascular volume contraction can make diuretic therapy difficult and may cause syncope or an increase in the creatinine value. Pacemaker implantation is commonly required in patients with cardiac amyloidosis and syncope. The use of angiotensin-converting enzyme inhibitors, a standard for the management of heart failure, has an uncertain role in AL. The high frequency of hypotension associated with angiotensin-converting enzyme inhibitors limits their value in AL. The use of implantable cardioverter-defibrillator therapy has been reported. A defibrillator cannot consistently prevent cardiac death from amyloidosis.[159,160a] Sustained ventricular arrhythmias (both monomorphic ventricular tachycardia and ventricular fibrillation) is a mechanism of sudden death in patients with cardiac amyloidosis and suggests that implantable cardiac defibrillator (ICD) therapy may be appropriate in selected patients.[160b]

Of 204 patients with AL seen at the Mayo Clinic, the median septal thickness was 14 mm.[161] The most common echocardiographic features are a thickened right ventricular wall, interventricular septum, and left ventricular free wall. Typically, the left ventricular cavity size is decreased. Cardiac involvement is present on echocardiography in 41% of patients at presentation; overt congestive heart failure is present in 20%. If the interventricular septal thickness is 15 mm or greater, the median survival time is less than 1 year. If the septal thickness is less than 15 mm, the median survival time can approach 4 years. Exercise-induced syncope has been associated with a median survival time of 2 months and is presumed due to complex ventricular arrhythmias.[162] Any patient presenting with symptoms of a cardiomyopathy that does not have a clear-cut ischemic etiology should have immunofixation analysis of the serum and urine and measurement of the free light-chain level performed.

The pseudoinfarction pattern seen on ECG may misdirect the evaluation toward coronary disease. Low voltage is seen on ECG in nearly two-thirds of patients with cardiac AL.[163] Cardiac amyloidosis is characterized by atrial systolic failure and dilatation of the right ventricle. Thickening of the mitral and tricuspid valves is common and is an important clue to the diagnosis. Doppler examination regularly demonstrates clinically insignificant valvular regurgitation.[164] Atrioventricular pacing does not improve cardiac hemodynamics.

Restrictive cardiomyopathy can be confused with pericardial disease causing restriction.[165] Little clinical benefit has been reported from pericardiectomy in patients with AL. An endomyocardial biopsy establishes the diagnosis of AL 100% of the time if at least three biopsy specimens are obtained.[166] Owing to poor contractility, the development of thrombi in the ventricular chambers is common. These can be sources of cardiac emboli resulting in stroke or arterial insufficiency of a lower extremity.[167a] Intracardiac thrombosis occurs frequently in cardiac amyloid patients, especially in those with atrial fibrillation. The risk for thrombosis was increased if the left ventricular diastolic dysfunction and atrial mechanical dysfunction were present. Anticoagulation therapy appears protective. Timely screening in high-risk patients may allow early detection of an intracardiac thrombus. Anticoagulation should be carefully considered.[167b] Atrial standstill in amyloidosis is an indication for long-standing anticoagulation therapy. Rarely, patients can have occlusive deposition of amyloid in small-caliber coronary arterioles. These patients can have ischemic symptoms, including exertional angina and true myocardial infarction.[32] Large-caliber coronary arteries show no abnormalities on angiography. Exercise testing regularly confirms ischemia, but the diagnosis is difficult to establish premortem.

The authors have seen 11 patients who presented with angina or unstable coronary syndromes.[31] Low voltage on ECG was seen in only two, and the median time from symptomatic angina to death was 18 months. Most diagnoses of cardiac AL with coronary artery occlusion were made at autopsy. Obstructive coronary amyloidosis is present in 66% of patients with cardiac involvement. None of these patients have obstruction of epicardial coronary arteries. Myocardial ischemia affects 25% of patients with obstructive intramural coronary amyloidosis. These patients present with ischemia and have normal angiographic studies but have small arteriolar amyloid disease.[31]

All patients with cardiac amyloidosis do not have AL. Familial forms of amyloid cardiomyopathy caused by mutations at position 122 of TTR are commonly seen in older African American men. These patients do not have a monoclonal protein in serum or urine. Senile cardiac amyloidosis is associated with cardiac deposition of wild-type TTR.[168] The echocardiographic features of these forms of cardiac amyloidosis are indistinguishable, and all three show Congo red–positive deposits. One-fourth of patients older than 90 years have amyloid deposits in the heart. Failure to find an immunoglobulin light chain in the serum or urine should redirect the evaluation toward non–light-chain forms of amyloid. Clues to senile systemic amyloidosis include male sex, advanced age, pronounced thickening of the interventricular septum (frequently >20 mm), and TTR immunostaining or protein identification by mass spectroscopy of the endomyocardial biopsy.

Liver

Hepatomegaly is found by physical examination in one-fourth of patients and may be caused by cardiac failure and hepatic congestion. Symptomatic hepatic involvement is present in 16% of patients. The most common clinical presentations are unexplained hepatomegaly accompanied by an increase in serum alkaline phosphatase. There is high concordance between hepatic and renal involvement, and if the liver is involved, the kidney is the next most commonly involved organ. Half of patients with hepatic amyloidosis spill greater than 1 g of protein in the urine over 24 hours. Proteinuria in a patient with hepatomegaly and an increased alkaline phosphatase value is an important clinical clue to the diagnosis of AL.[169]

Four clinical clues permit the prebiopsy recognition of hepatic amyloidosis: (1) presence of proteinuria; (2) monoclonal protein in the serum or urine; (3) Howell-Jolly bodies in the peripheral blood, which reflect splenic replacement with amyloid; and (4) hepatomegaly out of proportion to the degree of abnormality of liver function tests. Most patients have only an increased alkaline phosphatase value. The concentrations of aspartate aminotransferase and alanine aminotransferase are typically less than twice normal at diagnosis. The bilirubin value is normal. The finding of an increased bilirubin value in a patient with hepatic amyloidosis is usually a preterminal finding.[170] Rarely, hepatic amyloidosis occurs with splenic rupture with intraabdominal hemorrhage and, rarely, hepatic rupture.[171] Hepatic rupture has been diagnosed in AL, with computed tomography of the abdomen demonstrating a subcapsular hematoma.[172] At the time of diagnosis of hepatic amyloidosis, the median liver span is 7 cm below the right costal margin; 50% of patients have a span between 5 and 9 cm.[173]

Ten percent of patients with hepatic amyloidosis on liver biopsy do not have palpable hepatomegaly and are diagnosed because of an unexplained increase in alkaline phosphatase.[173] Splenomegaly is seen in 11% of these patients and nephrotic-range proteinuria in 36%. At diagnosis, the median elevation of the alkaline phosphatase value is 2.3 times the upper limit of normal. There is no difference in the ratio of κ to λ light chains in hepatic amyloidosis compared with other forms of amyloidosis.

Liver biopsy is not a high-risk procedure in these patients, and although reports of hepatic rupture have appeared in the literature, the bleeding incidence is 4%, with a transfusion being needed in 2%. The authors recently reported their updated experience with hepatic amyloidosis.[174] Seventy-two percent of patients had involuntary weight loss leading to an evaluation for occult malignancy. Clinicians considered amyloidosis in the differential diagnosis in only 26% before liver biopsy. Predictors of a poor prognosis included heart failure, an elevated bilirubin level, and thrombocythemia.[174]

Cholestatic jaundice is a preterminal finding.[175] Portal hypertension with varices and GI tract bleeding is rarely seen.[176] Presumably, patients succumb to the effects of extrahepatic amyloid deposits before portal hypertension can develop. Ascites is commonly seen but is usually a consequence of concomitant nephrotic syndrome with hypoalbuminemia or of severe congestive heart failure rather than portal hypertension.[177] Liver biopsy shows perisinusoidal and portal deposition in most patients. Vascular involvement of the portal triads is common but not clinically important. The median survival time after diagnosis was 8.5 months.

Radionuclide scintigraphy in amyloidosis is nonspecific, showing irregular distribution of the radionuclide[178] and absence of splenic uptake.[179] This form of imaging is not clinically useful. Angiography is also nonspecific, demonstrating luminal irregularity and abrupt changes in the caliber of the branches of the hepatic artery.[180] The hepatic artery is presumed to be compressed by sinusoidal amyloid deposition. Although liver biopsy is a safe technique, biopsy of the subcutaneous fat or the BM yields a correct diagnosis in 85% of patients, so only a few patients should be subjected to percutaneous liver biopsy.

Patients with hepatic AL have been treated with transjugular intrahepatic portal systemic shunting.[181] This can decrease portal pressures, ascites, and hydrothorax. In one patient, bilateral nephrectomy for uncontrolled nephrotic syndrome resulted in an improvement in liver function and normalization of hyperbilirubinemia.[182] The presence of hepatic involvement in amyloidosis does not adversely affect survival on multivariate statistical analysis. As noted, hepatomegaly may be from causes other than direct infiltration of the organ. In one report, hepatomegaly was caused by passive congestion of the liver without hepatic amyloid deposits in three of nine patients.[183] A second study found that 20% of patients with amyloidosis and palpable hepatomegaly did not have parenchymal amyloid deposits at autopsy.[184]

The presence of hyposplenism on the peripheral blood film is highly specific for a diagnosis of amyloidosis. Conversely, hyposplenism is not a sensitive indicator of splenic involvement.[185] In one report, 12 patients with diffuse splenic involvement at autopsy did not have peripheral blood film evidence of hyposplenism.[185] Technetium scanning can indicate a decrease in splenic blood flow, but this correlates poorly with the findings on the peripheral blood film.

In summary, the cardinal features of hepatic AL are (1) hepatomegaly with increased concentration of alkaline phosphatase and minimal change in aspartate and alanine aminotransferases, (2) proteinuria, (3) a monoclonal light chain in the serum or urine, and (4) hyposplenism on peripheral blood film or technetium scanning.

Gastrointestinal Tract

Anatomic deposits of amyloid are seen in the GI tracts of most patients by screening rectal biopsy or upper endoscopy. These deposits tend to be vascular, are in the submucosa (see Fig. 87-14, *A* and *B*), and are not associated with symptoms or clinical signs. Fewer than 5% of patients with AL present with symptoms referable to the GI tract. The presence of anorexia and weight loss generally is not associated with substantial GI tract deposits, and the cause of the weight loss is unrelated. Malabsorption defined by steatorrhea or a low serum carotene value is seen in fewer than 5% of amyloidosis patients. The symptoms of advanced intestinal amyloidosis include intestinal pseudo-obstruction,[186] and patients have been reported for whom exploratory laparotomy resulted in unnecessary morbidity. Some patients have severe intestinal dysmotility with vomiting and alternating diarrhea and constipation that can be managed only with long-term parenteral nutrition.[187] Abdominal distension and pain are common. Nausea is seen even with fasting. The mechanism underlying GI tract dysmotility can be a consequence of either direct mucosal infiltration or autonomic nerve damage.

The authors reviewed the cases of 19 patients seen at Mayo Clinic with small bowel biopsy-proven AL; these patients represented only

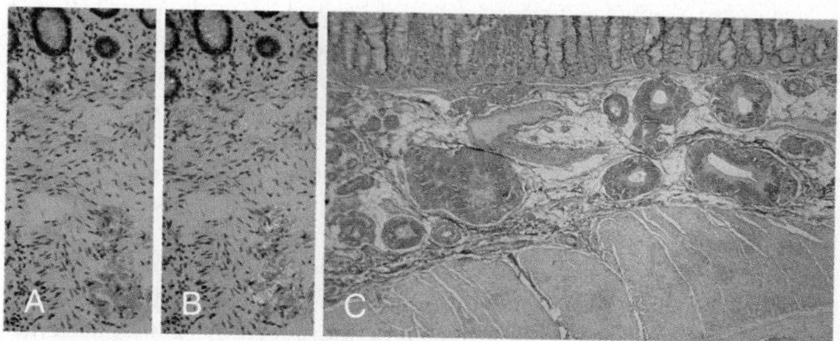

Figure 87-14 A and **B,** Gastrointestinal mucosal biopsies showing vascular amyloid deposits in the submucosa, hematoxylin and eosin and Congo Red stain. **C,** Rectal mucosal biopsy specimen demonstrates marked thickening of submucosal vessels with amyloid deposits. (Congo red; original magnification, ×100.) *(Courtesy Dr. Shu-Yuan Xiao of the University of Chicago.)*

1% of the authors' total patient population with AL.[188] The most common presenting symptoms were diarrhea, anorexia, dizziness, and abdominal pain. The median weight loss was 30 lb. Half had orthostatic hypotension. A prolonged prothrombin time caused by vitamin K malabsorption was seen in 25% of the patients. Depressed levels of factor X were also seen in 25% of patients, but only one patient had less than 30% activity. Less than one-third of the patients had increased serum alkaline phosphatase levels. Only 15% had hepatomegaly.

Barium studies of the upper GI tract showed esophageal dysmotility or gastroesophageal reflux.[189] Dilatation of the small bowel has been seen only rarely. Small bowel barium studies show thickening or nodularity, dilatation with delayed transit, and fluid accumulation. Computed tomography is not helpful, showing mild splenomegaly or lymphadenopathy. Endoscopy demonstrates esophagitis, duodenitis, and gastritis but is frequently normal.[190] The median time from the onset of intestinal symptoms to a histologic diagnosis of AL is 7 months, but in one instance, the diagnosis was delayed by 4 years. Laparotomy was performed in four of 19 patients, and even when the surgical tissue was obtained in three of the four, Congo red stains were not performed initially. The most important features predicting survival were the hemoglobin level at diagnosis and the extent of weight loss. Patients who had weight loss greater than 20 lb had a median survival time of 10 months, and the most common cause of death was nutritional failure (55%). A fourth died of cardiac amyloidosis.

The diarrhea of amyloidosis can be managed with loperamide and diphenoxylate; injections of long-acting octreotide also have been used. Ingested polyethylene glycol appears in the stool of amyloidosis patients 10 times faster than in normal subjects. These patients typically have autonomic neuropathy, which is most likely the cause of rapid transit. The severe chronic diarrhea is mediated by extremely rapid transit of chyme and digestive secretions.[191] The nausea is difficult to manage even with ondansetron. The most common preintestinal biopsy diagnosis is inflammatory bowel disease.

Primary amyloidosis can present as ischemic colitis.[192] In this circumstance, deposits obstruct the vessels of the lamina propria and muscularis mucosa, and this leads to mucosal ischemia with sloughing of the lining and bleeding[193] (Fig. 87-14, *C*). Radiographic studies demonstrate luminal narrowing, thickening of mucosal folds, and ulcerations. The most common site of ischemia is the descending and rectosigmoid colon. Duodenal perforation caused by vascular obstruction has been reported. After intestinal pseudo-obstruction develops, therapy for the underlying amyloidosis does not result in recovery of intestinal motility. Extensive replacement of the muscularis propria by amyloid deposits is particularly prominent in the small intestine.

Nervous System

Amyloid involvement of the peripheral nervous system was first described in 1938.[194] The frequency of neuropathy in AL is 15% to 20%. Most patients are minimally symptomatic, and the clinical picture is dominated by cardiac or renal involvement. If patients present with a predominant neuropathic syndrome, the possibility of a familial amyloidosis syndrome must be kept in the differential diagnosis.[195] A monoclonal protein in the serum or urine would not be expected in patients with nonimmunoglobulin forms of amyloidosis. A diagnosis of amyloid neuropathy can be confirmed by sural nerve biopsy (Fig. 87-15), but most patients with clinical and electromyographic evidence of neuropathy can be diagnosed by a fat aspirate, rectal biopsy, or BM specimen.

The most common symptoms of amyloid neuropathy are paresthesias, muscle weakness, numbness, pain, orthostatic hypotension, urinary retention, and impotence. Syncope is seen in 12% of patients. The peripheral neuropathy has a characteristic dysesthetic feature with distal burning. The lower extremities are involved before the upper extremities in 90% of patients, and symptoms of autonomic failure are seen in two-thirds. Cranial nerve involvement is rare but has been reported.[196] Carpal tunnel syndrome is present in half of patients with neuropathy. One-third have significant weight loss.

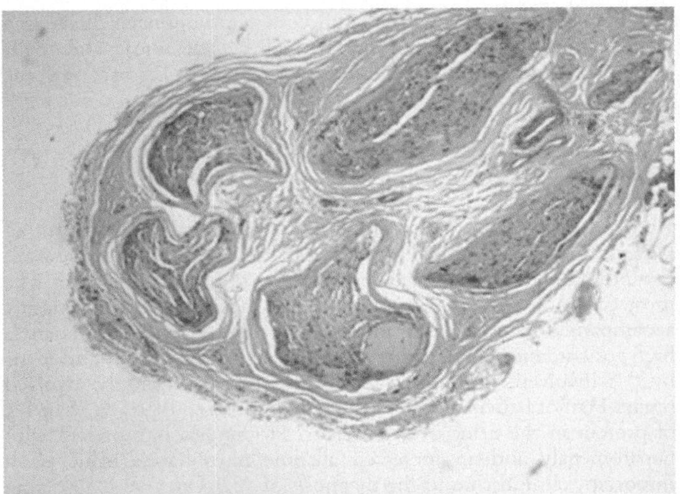

Figure 87-15 SURAL NERVE BIOPSY FOR AMYLOID INVOLVEMENT OF PERIPHERAL NERVOUS SYSTEM. The nodular deposit of pink amorphous material in the bottom center is the amyloid. *(Courtesy Dr. Peter Pytel of the University of Chicago.)*

Atypical presentations of amyloid neuropathy can include mononeuropathy multiplex, painful sensory neuropathy, and primary demyelinating polyneuropathy.[197]

Echocardiography is abnormal in 44% of patients with neuropathy. Renal involvement is uncommon, occurring in only 5%. The neuropathy of AL may be demyelinating and results in an increased concentration of cerebrospinal fluid protein in one-third. Electromyography (EMG) shows decreased amplitude of muscle action potentials, decreased or absent sensory responses, slowing of nerve conduction velocity, and fibrillation potentials.[198] Axonal degeneration is detected by EMG in 96% of patients.

On sural nerve biopsy, deposits of amyloid surround endoneurial capillaries or are found in the epineurium. Examination of teased fibers shows a decrease in myelin fiber density and axonal degeneration.[199] The median survival time of patients presenting with AL neuropathy is 25 months.[200] Standard-dose chemotherapy rarely results in clinical improvement in the neuropathic symptoms. The neuropathy is progressive over time, and three-fourths of patients ultimately have restricted mobility, with one-third becoming bedridden. Survival is predicted by the serum albumin value of these patients at presentation. Patients whose serum albumin concentration is less than 3 g/dL have a median survival time of 18 months compared with 31 months if the albumin value is greater than 3 g/dL.

Associated autonomic neuropathy is an important diagnostic clue to AL as the cause of peripheral neuropathy.[201] Urinary dysfunction is a common manifestation of autonomic failure. Voiding difficulties are caused by detrusor weakness and impaired bladder sensation. There is also evidence of detrusor denervation supersensitivity. This urinary dysfunction implicates postganglionic cholinergic and afferent somatic nerves.[202] Only diabetes mellitus generally produces a substantial autonomic component in patients with peripheral neuropathy.

The diagnosis of AL neuropathy is commonly delayed. The median duration of symptoms before diagnosis is 29 months. It is important that all patients with a peripheral neuropathy of unknown cause have immunofixation of serum and urine and an immunoglobulin free light-chain assay to search for a light chain.

The differential diagnosis of neuropathy associated with a monoclonal protein includes MGUS-associated neuropathy, POEMS syndrome (osteosclerotic myeloma), and cryoglobulinemia. Amyloidosis preferentially causes the loss of small myelinated fibers and unmyelinated fibers. EMG detects changes in large myelinated fibers. Therefore, patients can have symptoms with paresthesias and normal EMG results. The sural nerve biopsy is not 100% sensitive for the diagnosis. Of nine patients who had a sural nerve biopsy, the specimen did not show amyloid in six.[203] Amyloid can deposit proximally in the nerve root and lead to distal demyelination, and amyloid deposits will not be seen in a sural nerve biopsy specimen.

Respiratory Tract

Most patients with histologic deposits of amyloid in the respiratory tract are asymptomatic.[204] Most patients with pulmonary involvement also have cardiac involvement that dominates the clinical picture. If alveolar or interstitial amyloid is present, gas exchange is usually preserved until quite late in the disease.[205] Of 55 patients seen at the Mayo Clinic with lung biopsy proof of amyloidosis, 20 had localized forms of pulmonary amyloidosis, predominantly nodular pulmonary amyloidosis.[206] These patients had a benign prognosis. Patients with tracheobronchial amyloidosis have been treated with neodymium: yttrium–aluminum–garnet laser therapy and external-beam radiotherapy. Thirty-five of the 55 patients had systemic pulmonary AL. These patients presented with radiographic findings of an interstitial or reticulonodular pattern with or without effusion. The median survival time after diagnosis was 16 months. Bronchoscopic lung biopsy was safe and effective and was not associated with bleeding.

Chest radiography in pulmonary AL is nonspecific, showing an interstitial process that can be interpreted as lower lobe fibrosis.[207] Involvement of minor salivary glands is common and results in xerostomia.[208] These patients can be misdiagnosed as having Sjögren syndrome. Patients with amyloidosis associated with an IgM monoclonal protein have a higher prevalence of pulmonary involvement than patients with non-IgM amyloidosis. A monoclonal gammopathy is not associated with tracheal, bronchial, or nodular pulmonary amyloidosis and is seen exclusively in diffuse interstitial amyloidosis. Long-term observation for nodular pulmonary amyloidosis is justifiable. These patients can remain stable for long periods of time without requiring resection of the lung.[209] Patients with dyspnea from interstitial amyloidosis benefit from low doses of prednisone even though this does not produce radiographic change.[210]

At autopsy, pulmonary involvement was reported in 11 of 12 deceased patients.[211] Amyloid deposition was in blood vessel walls and alveolar septa. Of the 12, dyspnea was present in four, and pulmonary amyloidosis was directly responsible for death in only one. Hemoptysis has been reported.[211] Ventilatory failure has been reported caused by muscular infiltration of the diaphragm.[212]

Amyloid infiltration of skeletal muscles and the diaphragm has been reported.[213] Pleural infiltration can produce effusions.[214] Pulmonary hypertension with right-sided cardiac failure can be seen as a rare complication.[215] These patients have occlusive amyloid deposits in the pulmonary arteriolar circulation. None of these patients had echocardiographic evidence of amyloid deposition. In the presence of pulmonary hypertension, the median survival time was 2.8 years. Treatment included calcium channel blockers; however, patients tolerated these medicines poorly owing to concomitant orthostatic hypotension.

Coagulation System

Bleeding is a serious complication of amyloidosis. Factors contributing to the abnormal bleeding include coagulation factor deficiencies, hyperfibrinolysis, platelet dysfunction, and increased fragility of blood vessels.[216] Deficiency of factor X is well recognized.[217] The most common manifestation of bleeding is purpura caused by fragile blood vessels infiltrated with amyloid.[218] Factor X deficiency is seen in fewer than 5% of patients. In a recent review, 8.7% of patients had factor X levels less than 50% of normal; serious bleeding is seen only in those with factor X levels less than 25% of normal.[219] Factor X deficiency is associated with extensive hepatic and splenic amyloidosis. Improvement in factor X levels has been reported with splenectomy,[220] use of oral melphalan and prednisone, and SCT.[221] The use of recombinant human factor VIIa in the management of amyloid-associated factor X deficiency was reported in a 63-year-old woman with levels from 4% to 10% of normal.[222] Recombinant human factor VIIa was administered preoperatively and every 3 hours postoperatively for 48 hours to permit safe splenectomy. This was an effective means of controlling bleeding to allow for definitive surgical intervention.[222] Recombinant factor VIIa has now been widely used to treat intractable life-threatening hematuria and severe bleeding and to support a hemicolectomy.[222-224]

The most common hemostatic abnormality in vitro is prolongation of the thrombin time.[225] This may be related to the low serum albumin values seen in patients with amyloidosis. Others have suggested the presence of an inhibitor to fibrin polymerization. Abnormal platelet aggregation has been reported, as have decreased levels of α_2-plasmin inhibitor and increased levels of plasminogen. Life-threatening bleeding is rare in AL, except for those few patients with severe factor X deficiency or ischemic colitis caused by vascular obstruction. Bleeding in amyloidosis has also been reported as a result of a deficiency of factor V.[226] This deficiency was not caused by acquisition of a factor V inhibitor. The bleeding in this case was fatal and unresponsive to fresh-frozen plasma. At autopsy, massive hepatic deposits of amyloid were seen.[226]

Thirty-six patients underwent extensive coagulation profiling[225]; hemorrhagic manifestations were mild to moderate in nine and severe in only one. The most frequent in vitro abnormalities were prolongation of the thrombin time and reptilase time. Severe depression of factor X was seen in only one. The prothrombin times were prolonged in eight, and the activated partial thromboplastin time was prolonged in 25. None had a lupus anticoagulant.

The authors reviewed the medical records of 2132 patients with AL to identify patients with thromboembolism.[227] They identified 21 men and 19 women with a median age of 65 years. In 11 of 40, thromboembolism preceded the diagnosis of AL. In nine of the 11, the event occurred 1 month or longer before the diagnosis of AL. In 20 of 40 patients, thromboembolism occurred 1 month or more after diagnosis. Twenty-nine had a venous thrombosis, and 11 had arterial clots. Thirty-seven of the 40 patients had an additional risk factor for thrombosis: nephrotic syndrome in 20, immobilization in 13, tobacco in six, heart failure in eight, estrogens in one, obesity in four, aortic aneurysm in one, and prosthetic material in four. Two of the patients had an associated disseminated intravascular coagulation, and five had detectable activated protein C resistance. Eight of the 40 patients died within 1 month after the thrombotic event. Eighteen of the 40 died within 1 year. There were no associations with the type of heavy or light chain.[227]

PROGNOSIS

When a patient has a syndrome compatible with amyloidosis and is found subsequently to have a monoclonal protein or clonal plasma cell population and the diagnosis is confirmed histologically, the next step is to assess prognosis. In a group of 153 patients with AL, the median survival time was 20 months, with a 5-year survival rate of 20%.[228] Patients with congestive heart failure had a median survival time of 8 months and a 5-year survival rate of 2.4%. The best outcome occurred in patients with amyloid neuropathy as the sole manifestation of the disease; they had a median survival time of 40 months and a 5-year survival rate of 32%. Patients may be classified clinically into five groups: heart failure or cardiomyopathy, nephrotic syndrome, peripheral neuropathy, liver, and other. Women have slightly better survival time than men.

In a review of 229 patients with AL, heart failure and orthostatic hypotension were associated consistently with a median survival time of less than 1 year.[25] With heart failure and nephrotic syndrome patients excluded, patients with peripheral neuropathy had a median survival time of 56 months. Jaw claudication can be seen in as many as 9%. These patients have a survival time of 42 months.[229] Patients with jaw claudication have predominantly vascular deposits and sparing of the viscera. They frequently have associated amyloid arthropathy and tongue enlargement.

The presence of hyposplenism on peripheral blood film was associated with a median survival time of 4.4 months, reflecting advanced splenic and hepatic involvement.[230] The median survival time of 80 patients diagnosed by a liver biopsy was 9 months, and the 5-year survival rate was 13%.[169] The cause of death in most patients with amyloidosis was cardiac related—either heart failure or fatal arrhythmia. Echocardiography is important in the assessment of the patient's prognosis.[231] Although only 17% to 20% of patients have heart failure at presentation, nearly 40% have evidence of cardiomyopathy on echocardiography.[232] Early cardiac amyloidosis is characterized by abnormalities of relaxation. Advanced cardiac amyloidosis shows restrictive filling and a shortened deceleration time.[233] With Doppler echocardiography, patients can be divided into two groups on the basis of deceleration time greater or less than 150 msec. The 1-year survival of patients with a deceleration time of 150 msec or less was 49% compared with 92% for a deceleration time greater than 150 msec. Doppler studies of right ventricular function correlate well with the degree of amyloid infiltration.[234]

Findings on renal biopsy have been reported to have prognostic value.[235] A lower percentage of glomerular capillary wall thickening, a higher incidence of amyloid deposits in vessels but not glomerular capillaries, and deposits of IgG and C3 in mesangial and glomerular capillary walls are all associated with a better prognosis. Urinary light-chain excretion and serum creatinine values are also important prognostic indicators. Increased serum creatinine values are associated with a median survival time of 15 months.

Exertional syncope is an ominous finding and is associated with a high incidence of sudden death. This is usually an indication for consideration of an implantable defibrillator. Most patients with exertional syncope die within 3 months.[236]

The plasma cell labeling index measures the proliferative potential of the BM plasma cells in AL. More than 95% of patients with AL have a demonstrable clonal excess of plasma cells in the BM. The median survival time of patients whose plasma cell labeling index was 0 (no proliferative plasma cells) was 30 months. Patients with a plasma cell labeling index greater than 0 had a median survival time of 15 months.[237] Analysis of peripheral blood mononuclear cells in 147 patients with AL showed 16% of the patients to have detectable circulating plasma cells.[238] The median survival time of patients with circulating plasma cells was 10 months compared with 29 months for patients without circulating plasma cells. In a multivariate analysis, the presence of circulating plasma cells and the serum β_2-microglobulin level were independent prognostic indicators of survival.[239]

The median survival time of patients with an increased serum β_2-microglobulin value at presentation was 11 months compared with 33 months in patients with normal β_2-microglobulin values.[240] β_2-Microglobulin value is an independent predictor of survival even in the presence of heart failure and renal failure. When the serum β_2-microglobulin value is combined with the presence or absence of circulating plasma cells, patients can be classified into three separate groups with median survival times of 4 months (circulating cells and increased β_2-microglobulin), 42 months (no circulating cells and normal β_2-microglobulin), and 21 months (one of the two variables abnormal).[239]

The time between diagnosis and referral for evaluation remains an important prognostic variable. When all patients seen at the Mayo Clinic are assessed, the median survival time is 2 years. However, when only patients seen within 1 month of diagnosis are considered, the median survival time decreases to 13 months. This suggests significant referral bias, favoring patients physically able to come to a large amyloidosis treatment center. This information is important when interpreting the results of clinical trials from single centers.[126]

In a multivariate analysis of prognostic factors, the median survival time of the entire group was 12 months, ranging from 4 months for those with overt heart failure to 15 months for those with peripheral neuropathy.[241] Heart failure, urinary monoclonal light chain, hepatomegaly, and MM were all adverse factors influencing survival within 1 year after diagnosis. After the first year, increased serum creatinine concentration, MM, orthostatic hypotension, and a monoclonal serum protein predicted poor survival.[241] Stratification for the impact of variables with an adverse effect on survival is important when comparing studies of therapy among various centers.

Recently, measurement of cardiac biomarkers has been shown to be critically important in assessing the prognosis of patients with amyloidosis. Brain natriuretic peptide (BNP) is a marker of ventricular dysfunction and has been used to assess prognosis in heart failure. When N-terminal pro-BNP (NT-pro-BNP) was quantified at diagnosis in 152 patients with AL and compared with echocardiography results, two groups were distinguished on the basis of NT-pro-BNP levels.[242] Survival was vastly different in patients with elevated and normal NT-pro-BNP levels. This model for assessing prognosis was superior to echocardiography. Serum cardiac troponin value measurements combined with the NT-pro-BNP values were used in the development of a staging system for patients with amyloidosis.[243] Patients who had abnormal values for both parameters (stage III) had a median survival time of 3.5 months; those with normal values for both parameters (stage I) had a survival time of 26.4 months; and those with 1 of 2 abnormal values (stage II), 10.5 months.[243,244a] The staging system using troponins and NT-pro-BNP was subsequently verified in a cohort of patients undergoing SCT.[244] The three stages had median survival times of 66.1, 66.1, and 26.1 months, respectively.[245] Forty-nine percent of transplant patients were in stage I, 38% in stage II, and 13% in stage III. Levels of circulating cardiac biomarkers are the most powerful tool for staging patients with AL undergoing SCT.[245]

Not only has the immunoglobulin free light chain been found to be important in classifying the type of amyloidosis and providing a method for assessing response, it has also been found to be of prognostic value.[244a] Patients with higher baseline free light-chain levels had a significantly higher risk of death. Baseline free light chain correlated with serum cardiac troponin levels, and higher free light-chain levels were associated with more organs with amyloid involvement. The absolute level of free light chain achieved after therapy predicted survival. Normalization of free light-chain level after transplantation predicted both organ response and complete hematologic response. Free light-chain measurements before and after treatment are important predictors of patient outcome.[244a] The overall survival (OS) was shorter among those with a higher dFLC (involved FLC–uninvolved FLC; κ >29.4 mg/dL or λ >18.2 mg/dL using median for cutoff); 10.9 vs. 37.1 months; P <.001. In multivariate analysis, dFLC was independent of other prognostic factors. The type of light chain impacts the spectrum of organ involvement, and the FLC burden correlates with survival in AL.[244b]

In summary, all patients being assessed for amyloidosis require echocardiography, including measures of diastolic performance, ejection fraction, and mitral deceleration time. The serum β_2-microglobulin concentration, the presence of overt congestive heart failure, and circulating plasma cells remain important measures affecting outcome. BNP and troponin levels are an essential part of the diagnostic evaluation of patients with AL.

Patients with uric acid levels greater than 8 mg/dL had a median OS of 9 months from diagnosis compared with 20.3 months for the remaining patients (P <.001). The prognostic value of uric acid was independent of the known cardiac prognostic markers cardiac troponin T (cTnT) and N-terminal propeptide of BNP (NT-ProBNP). Addition of uric acid to these factors allows classification of patients into four groups with significantly different outcomes. Patients with none, one, two, or three of these risk factors (uric acid >8 mg/dL; cTnT >0.035 ng/mL; and NT-pro-BNP >332 pg/mL) had median OS times of 36.6, 29.2, 11.1, and 3.6 months, respectively (P <.001).[244c]

THERAPY

Supportive Therapy for Primary Amyloidosis

Cardiac Amyloidosis

The primary modality of therapy for cardiac AL remains diuretic agents.[246] Diuretics decrease extravascular volume, which reduces the peripheral edema that limits these patients. Diuretic therapy helps decrease preload; filling pressures tend to be extremely high in patients with amyloidosis because of the restriction to cardiac inflow. Diuretic therapy is limited by hypotension, which, if associated with hypoalbuminemia from renal amyloidosis, can be difficult to manage.[247] Furosemide doses of 120 mg three times per day may be necessary for edema control. Metolazone can be beneficial in mobilizing fluid. Spironolactone has been shown to decrease mortality in patients with chronic heart failure, although it has not been specifically tested in amyloid cardiomyopathy. Digoxin has little beneficial effect on the diastolic heart failure seen in amyloidosis[248] but can be useful in controlling heart rate in patients with atrial fibrillation, which is generally difficult to convert to sinus rhythm. Nifedipine and diltiazem can precipitate congestive heart failure in patients with AL.[249,250] The use of angiotensin-converting enzyme inhibitors can reduce the afterload in patients with cardiac amyloidosis and has been shown to decrease mortality in patients with ischemic cardiomyopathy. In addition, lisinopril has been reported to reduce proteinuria in renal amyloidosis.[251a] Forty-five consecutive patients with EMB-documented CA were studied from January 1998 to December 2003. On univariate Kaplan-Meier analysis, New York Heart Association class greater than II, deceleration time less than 150 msec, and β-blocker use were associated with increased mortality (log-rank statistic $P<.001$, $<.05$, and .01, respectively). β-Blocker use cannot be routinely recommended for cardiac AL patients.[251b]

Orthostatic hypotension in amyloidosis can be a major problem.[252] The use of a fitted thigh-high elastic leotard can actually decrease dependence on medications. If medications are necessary, fludrocortisone acetate 0.1 mg two to three times daily can be effective, but it produces some fluid retention and can aggravate supine hypertension.[253] Midodrine can be used in doses ranging from 2.5 to 10 mg two times daily.[254] Dosing should take place during the day to avoid nocturnal supine hypertension. This agent is rapidly absorbed from the intestinal tract, and peak serum values occur in 30 minutes. The maximum recommended dose is 30 mg/day, and the medication comes in 2.5- and 5-mg tablets. If renal insufficiency is present, the dose should be decreased because active metabolites are excreted renally. Adverse effects of midodrine include tachycardia, hypertension, and restlessness. In a patient who did not respond to midodrine and fludrocortisone, subcutaneous erythropoietin resulted in resolution of symptoms related to orthostatic hypotension unassociated with improvement of anemia.[255]

Cardiac transplantation has been used for patients with advanced cardiac AL. A survey of seven patients with a mean age of 46 years reported recurrent amyloidosis in two patients at 3.5 and 4 months, one of whom died 13 months after transplantation.[256] Five patients were alive at 32 months. A follow-up study of 10 patients showed recurrent amyloidosis in the graft in four of nine survivors.[257] One patient with AL survived 9 years after cardiac transplantation.[258] Ten patients (mean age, 54 years) received heart transplants; two died postoperatively, and the mean follow-up time in the remaining eight patients was 50 months. Recurrent amyloid deposits in the cardiac allografts were demonstrable in five patients at 5 to 30 months (median, 12 months) after transplantation. Seven patients died at a median of 32 months; four of the seven died of extracardiac amyloidosis. The 1-year actuarial survival rate was 60%, and the 5-year actuarial survival rate was 30%.[258]

A 47-year-old woman with AL cardiac amyloidosis received a heart transplant followed 6 months later by SCT in an attempt to prevent recurrent disease.[259] The patient died 2 years after SCT, and the myocardium showed mild deposits of amyloid.[259] In 13 cardiac transplant patients with AL at the Mayo Clinic, the actuarial 5-year survival rate was 50%.[260] The authors have performed SCT in 11 patients who were recipients of cardiac transplants; five died and six were alive at 18, 19, 22, 23, 59, and 82 months after SCT.

One study queried the United Network for Organ Sharing database and found 69 patients with amyloidosis who had cardiac transplants.[261] Five operative deaths occurred, and 29 late deaths occurred at a mean follow-up time of 40 months. Nine patients died of amyloid-related complications, and graft vasculopathy developed in one patient. The 1-year survival rate was 84% for men and 64% for women.[261] In a report from the United Kingdom, 24 patients had amyloid heart disease, 17 of whom had AL.[262] The survival rate of 10 patients was 50% at 1 year and 20% at 5 years after heart transplant. Amyloid recurrence in the grafts occurred at a median of 11 months. Extracardiac amyloid contributed to mortality in 70%. Seven patients with AL who also had chemotherapy had 1- and 5-year survival rates of 86% and 64%, respectively. The survival rate was less than after transplant for other indications. Progression of the AL contributed to the increased mortality.[262]

In a single-center report of five patients with cardiac AL, three were dead and two were alive at 60 and 41 months after transplant.[263] Two patients died of sudden death after 23 months and one of multiorgan failure because of progression of AL.[263] Because recurrent amyloidosis is such a common cause of morbidity, the use of SCT to prevent disease recurrence after heart transplantation (HT) has been reported. Five patients had SCTs after heart transplant, and three of the five were well without evidence of recurrent amyloid.[264] Two patients died at 33 and 90 months after heart transplant after relapse of the amyloidosis.[264a] Between 1994 and 2005, 11 patients underwent sequential orthotopic HT followed by autologous peripheral blood SCT for treatment of AL amyloidosis at the Mayo Clinic. Two patients died of complications from the SCT (18% transplant-related mortality). Nine patients survived both the HT and the SCT. Three patients subsequently died from progressive amyloidosis at 66, 56.7, and 55 months after SCT. The 1- and 5-year survival for HT was 82% and 65%. The median survival was 76 months from HT and 57 months from SCT. Two patients died of complications from the SCT (18% transplant-related mortality). Nine patients survived both the HT and the SCT. Three patients subsequently died from progressive amyloidosis at 66, 56.7, and 55 months after SCT. The 1- and 5-year survival rates for HT were 82% and 65%, respectively. The median survival rate was 76 months from HT and 57 months from SCT. HT followed by SCT is feasible and offers the possibility of remission for carefully selected patients with cardiac amyloidosis.[264b]

Renal Amyloidosis

Diuretics can manage the edema of nephrotic syndrome. For patients in whom renal failure eventually develops, hemodialysis support is required. The results of dialysis in AL patients are inferior to those in patients with primary kidney disease.[265] In 61 patients with amyloidosis who had dialysis, 18 died within 1 month after starting therapy, and 43 underwent dialysis for more than 1 month. Younger patients had better 5-year survival times. The most important complications after initiation of dialysis were the subsequent development of cardiac and intestinal amyloidosis. Survival was not different between amyloidosis patients who received hemodialysis and those who received peritoneal dialysis.[265] Two-thirds of the deaths in the patient population were caused by extrarenal amyloidosis progression, primarily cardiac.[133]

The use of lisinopril has been reported to decrease proteinuria in patients with nephrotic syndrome and can result in significant hyperkalemia. Enalapril has been reported to be effective in reducing proteinuria in steroid-resistant nephrotic syndrome.[266] The mechanism of action is thought to be hemodynamic and is potentially effective in amyloidosis as well.

Renal transplantation has been used in patients with AL. Recurrent amyloidosis in the graft remains a major problem, however. The authors have performed renal transplantation in eight patients, six of whom had stem cell harvest; five of them underwent SCT.[142] Stable renal function was present in four. Sequential kidney and SCT is feasible.[142] Others have argued that SCT should precede kidney transplantation in an effort to produce a complete response before placement of the new organ.[143]

Survival is linked to the development of amyloidosis in the graft; it has been estimated that 1-year survivors have a 20% chance of amyloidosis developing in the transplanted kidney. Fifteen patients with renal amyloidosis underwent transplantation and had 42 to 216 months of follow-up (median, 73 months).[267a] The grafts remained normal in all patients whose underlying amyloidogenic disorder had remitted. If the underlying precursor protein production had not remitted, abnormal uptake of radiolabeled serum amyloid P was found, reflecting the development of amyloid in the transplanted kidney. Patients with evidence of renal amyloid by serum amyloid P scan also had evidence of graft dysfunction.[267a]

Three patients were reported who received kidney transplants after monoclonal light-chain synthesis was suppressed by chemotherapy.[267a] The response to chemotherapy was documented by eradication or reduction of immunoglobulin light-chain production. Three patients were alive at 4, 11, and 16 years after transplantation. Renal function in the AL patients remained normal. Renal transplantation is therefore appropriate for patients whose light-chain production can be suppressed.[266] The feasibility of sequential living donor kidney transplantation and autologous SCT for carefully selected patients with end-stage renal disease caused by AL has been established.[142] Disease recurrence remains a problem, particularly for inherited forms of amyloidosis.[267b]

Hepatic Amyloidosis

As is the case for all other types of AL, the mainstay of therapy for hepatic amyloidosis is suppression of the underlying plasma cell clone with chemotherapy. However, liver transplantation has been reported for the management of AL. A 61-year-old man was hospitalized for spontaneous splenic rupture.[268] Shortly after splenectomy, liver failure with jaundice, ascites, and hyponatremia developed. A subsequent hepatorenal syndrome with hepatic encephalopathy developed over 3 weeks. Hepatic transplantation was performed, and the patient was dismissed from the hospital with normal hepatic and kidney function. At 1-year postoperative follow-up, liver function was normal, although a liver biopsy showed amyloid deposits in the hepatic allograft.[268] Another patient with progressive hepatic failure from AL received a liver allograft.[269] The patient had development of recurrent amyloidosis that led to SCT in an effort to suppress amyloid precursor protein production. After a second (tandem) transplantation procedure, the patient had no clinical evidence of recurrent amyloidosis at 28 months. Liver transplantation can be considered for patients with amyloidosis, but suppression of light-chain production is essential to prevent recurrent disease.[269] Liver transplantation is primarily used to manage familial forms of amyloidosis and rarely used as a tool for management of light-chain amyloidosis.

Gastrointestinal Tract Amyloidosis

The most frequent symptoms related to amyloidosis of the GI tract are diarrhea and constipation. In most patients, these are caused by autonomic failure, but in some patients, massive deposits develop in the mucosa and submucosa and result in a malabsorption syndrome. Loperamide, diphenoxylate, tincture of opium, and paregoric are used regularly and produce variable results. Octreotide in a long-acting formulation can decrease diarrhea when given in doses ranging from 10 to 30 mg every 4 weeks for 2 months and then every 4 weeks, according to the response of the diarrhea. Rarely, ostomies are required for diarrhea control. Occasionally, widespread vascular obstruction of blood supply to the bowel develops, leading to massive bleeding and infarction for which surgical intervention is the only option. For nausea, abdominal distension, and pain, cisapride has been reported to provide symptomatic relief.[270]

Noncytotoxic Chemotherapy for Primary Amyloidosis

The primary approach to therapy has been to decrease production of the amyloidogenic light chain with therapy directed against the plasma cell population. DMSO has been used because of in vitro data suggesting an ability to solubilize amyloid deposits.[271] The benefit of DMSO is unproven, and it is infrequently used today to treat amyloidosis.[272] Colchicine has been shown to be effective in the treatment of AA associated with familial Mediterranean fever, a disorder characterized by recurrent peritonitis, pleuritis, synovitis, and rash. Before the introduction of colchicine, the 5-year survival rate of patients with familial Mediterranean fever was 20%. Nephrotic-range proteinuria and dialysis-dependent renal failure developed in these patients. Two double-blind, placebo-controlled trials showed that colchicine was effective in preventing attacks of serositis and reduced the frequency of amyloidosis.[273]

Given the success of colchicine for familial Mediterranean fever amyloidosis,[274] it was used in patients with AL. Fifty-three patients with AL received colchicine and were compared with retrospective control participants.[275a] The median survival time of colchicine-treated patients was 7 months compared with 1 year in melphalan-treated patients.[275a] Today, colchicine is rarely used for AL. Colchicine is not effective for any of the hereditary periodic fever syndromes including hyperimmunoglobulinemia-D with periodic fever, tumor necrosis factor receptor–associated periodic syndrome, and cryopyrin-associated periodic syndrome.[102]

Cytotoxic Chemotherapy for Primary Amyloidosis

The same chemotherapy drugs used to treat amyloidosis have been used for the management of MM. These include oral melphalan and prednisone; oral dexamethasone; and combination chemotherapy, including thalidomide-, lenalidomide-, and bortezomib-based therapies. These therapies can decrease the plasma cell burden to some degree. Many patients die of the disease before adequate time has elapsed to determine if they will achieve a response. The best predictors for early attrition during cycle 1 of chemotherapy were TnT 0.07 µg/L or greater and NT-proBNP 11,939 ng/L or greater. NT-proBNP response underperformed TnT response as a predictor for OS, but both predicted for early protocol attrition and inability to tolerate therapy, rendering a proportion inevaluable for response.[275b] Two prospective, randomized studies have demonstrated a survival benefit for oral melphalan and prednisone compared with colchicine.[276,277] Unfortunately, the median survival time is prolonged to only 17 or 18 months.

Responders to melphalan and prednisone have prolonged survival times compared with nonresponders.[228] Patients who have nephrotic syndrome have a better outcome in terms of response rate than those who have peripheral neuropathy or cardiac involvement. It is unclear whether clinical organ improvement is associated with histologic regression because follow-up biopsies are done infrequently. However, the use of serum amyloid P component scanning has indicated decreased uptake of the isotope at sites of previously known disease, which suggests resolution of the amyloid deposits. Melphalan is leukemogenic, and the risk of myelodysplasia developing is substantial.[278a] The authors identified 10 patients with myelodysplasia or acute myeloid leukemia that directly caused death for eight and transfusion dependency for two. Two of the 10 patients did not have development of myelodysplasia until 144 months after first exposure to alkylating agents. The actuarial risk of myelodysplasia development at 10 years was 18%.[278b]

We have reported that even in the presence of significant cardiac amyloidosis, survival of more than 5 years was seen in eight of 153 patients.[279] All long-term survivors received chemotherapy. All but one had a demonstrable response to chemotherapy. Continuous oral melphalan has been administered as a single agent for patients with cardiac amyloidosis who could not tolerate prednisone or SCT. Seven of 13 evaluable patients achieved a partial hematologic response, three achieved a complete hematologic response, and six survived for longer than 1 year. Continuous low-dose oral melphalan can induce hematologic responses.[280]

Responses to melphalan and prednisone are uncommon if the serum creatinine value exceeds 3 mg/dL, if hyperbilirubinemia is present, or if the alkaline phosphatase value increases to more than four times the institutional normal.[228] In patients who have isolated nephrotic syndrome, a normal serum creatinine value, and a normal

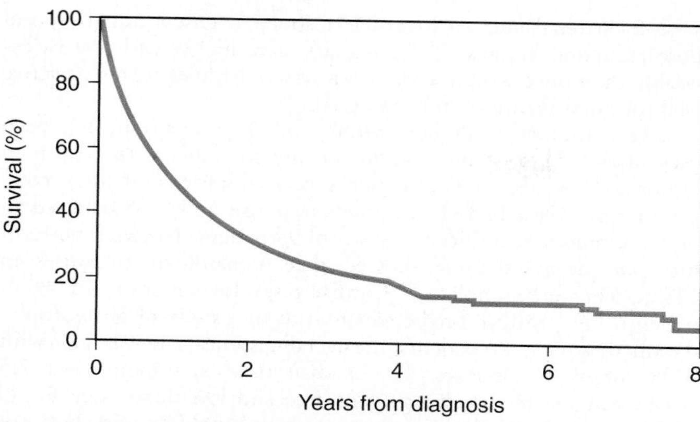

Figure 87-16 OVERALL SURVIVAL OF PATIENTS SEEN AT THE MAYO CLINIC WITH AMYLOIDOSIS.

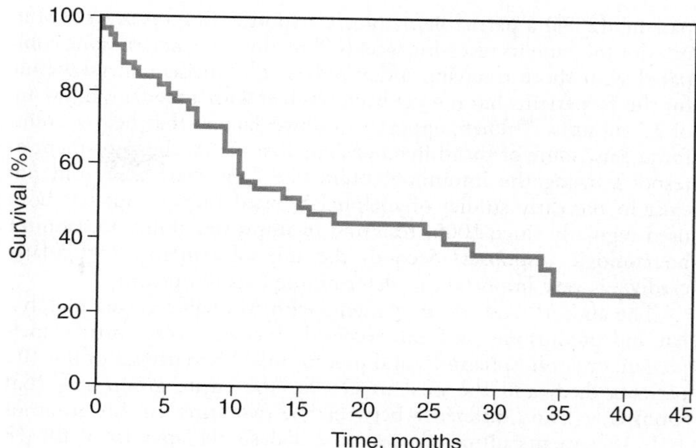

Figure 87-17 SURVIVAL OF 55 PATIENTS WITH AMYLOIDOSIS TREATED WITH HIGH-DOSE DEXAMETHASONE.

echocardiogram, the response rate to melphalan can exceed one-third of patients. It is rare to see symptomatic improvement in peripheral neuropathy after melphalan and prednisone therapy. The median time to response with melphalan is 1 year.[228]

In a 21-year period at the Mayo Clinic, 841 patients with AL were evaluated.[281] The actuarial survival for the 810 patients diagnosed premortem was 51% at 1 year, 16% at 5 years, and 4.7% at 10 years (Fig. 87-16). The authors reported on 30 patients with survival for 10 years after diagnosis, all of whom received melphalan-based therapy.[281] Fourteen had complete eradication of the light chain from serum and urine. Of 10 patients with nephrotic syndrome, four had a greater than 50% reduction in proteinuria. Heart failure, older age, a creatinine value greater than 2 mg/dL, and BM plasma cells greater than 20% were poor prognostic factors for long-term survival.[279,280]

Four patients in whom alkylating agents had failed were treated subsequently with vincristine, doxorubicin (Adriamycin), and dexamethasone (VAD) as a 96-hour infusion.[282] Two of the patients had a 50% decrease in the serum monoclonal protein. The VAD regimen could be considered for patients with AL and has been reported as an induction treatment to decrease the plasma cell burden before SCT.[282] The use of VAD resulted in improvement in patients' conditions, allowing them to receive high-dose chemotherapy and SCT with reduced risk.[282] A series of patients from a single institution had successful use of VAD induction followed by melphalan-based SCT.[283,284]

In a three-arm study that accrued 219 patients over 10 years, patients were randomly assigned to receive colchicine; melphalan and prednisone; or melphalan, prednisone, and colchicine.[276] Patients were stratified by age, sex, and major clinical manifestation of amyloidosis. Half had nephrotic-range proteinuria, and 20% had heart failure. The colchicine group survived a median of 8.5 months, and the melphalan-containing regimens resulted in survival times of 17 months. Similar results were reported in patients treated with melphalan at Boston University.[277] The authors reported on the development of myelodysplasia in 10 of 153 patients who were treated with melphalan for AL.[278] Eight of the 10 died as a result of the myelodysplasia, including acute leukemia and progressive pancytopenia caused by myelodysplasia. This group represents 7% of all patients treated with melphalan; the actuarial risk for survivors at 3.5 years was 21%. The median survival time after the diagnosis of myelodysplasia or acute leukemia was 8 months. As the survival of patients with plasma cell disorders improves, myelodysplasia may be a more common cause of morbidity and mortality for this group.[278b]

In one patient, the diagnosis of amyloidosis was established, and the patient received 28 months of oral melphalan, prednisone, and colchicine.[285] Five years later, he had dialysis-dependent renal failure with no other evidence of amyloidosis and received a renal transplant. He survived for 7 years; pancytopenia developed with BM that showed dysplastic red blood cells but no acute leukemia. Cytogenetics were complex but included a 5q abnormality. Myelodysplasia developed 12 years after his diagnosis of amyloidosis.

High-dose dexamethasone as a single agent given at 40 mg on days 1 to 4, 9 to 12, and 17 to 20 every 5 weeks has been reported.[286] Responding patients received maintenance dexamethasone at 40 mg/day 4 days per month for 1 year. Improvement in amyloid organ involvement was seen in eight of nine patients, and six of seven had a greater than 50% decrease in urinary protein loss with a median time to response of 4 months. Patients with heart failure did not benefit. The median survival time of the cohort was 31 months. In a report on 93 patients treated with this regimen, 2-year OS was 60%, and event-free survival was 52%.[287] Heart failure and β_2-microglobulin levels were the predictors of adverse outcome.[287] The authors treated 19 patients with high-dose dexamethasone therapy,[288] and three showed objective organ response. The median survival time of the entire group was 11.2 months, but three patients were alive at 110, 116, and 119 months. Dexamethasone should be considered as an option for patients who are not suitable candidates for transplantation. Dexamethasone has also been used for patients in whom melphalan therapy had previously failed.[289] The objective response rate was 12% (Fig. 87-17). One patient was alive at 104 months.

Because high-dose dexamethasone therapy can be toxic in patients with AL, a reduced-dose schedule has been reported: 40 mg on days 1 through 4 every 21 days for up to 8 cycles.[290] Overall, eight of 23 patients had a median time to response of 4 months (range, 2-6 months). This regimen has been used as a first-line therapy. This same group reported on the combination of low-dose melphalan and modified high-dose dexamethasone therapy.[290]

Melphalan has been combined with high-dose dexamethasone in patients with AL who were ineligible for SCT, primarily because of cardiomyopathy.[291a] Of 46 patients, a complete response was seen in 15 (33%) and a hematologic response in 31 (67%). Twenty-two patients (48%) showed an improvement in organ dysfunction. There was a strong correlation between hematologic and organ response. If the hematologic response was complete, the organ response rate was 87%. If the hematologic response was greater than 50%, organ function improved in 56%; patients with no hematologic response had no organ functional improvement. The 100-day mortality rate with this regimen was 4%. Cardiac failure resolved in six of 32 patients. The median time to response was 4.5 months, and only 11% had adverse effects.[291a] Using a similar melphalan-and-dexamethasone–based regimen, physicians at Weill-Cornell School of Medicine reported a median survival time of only 10.5 months. Outcomes appear to be strongly linked to the proportion of patients with cardiac amyloidosis.[291b] With melphalan administered parenterally with dexamethasone in patients with immunoglobulin light-chain amyloidosis, the median survival time of 61 patients was 17.5 months. The 3-month mortality rate was 28%.[291c] In Boston, of 48 evaluable patients who survived and returned for follow-up assessment, six patients (13%) achieved a complete hematologic response and 12 patients (25%) a partial hematologic response. Responses were noninferior for patients receiving weekly "low-dose" dexamethasone compared with those receiving 4-day pulses. The median survival time for the 70 patients has not yet been reached with a median follow-up of 17 months.[299d] There appear to be two factors that help account for at least some of this difference. The first is that the assessment of response using the immunoglobulin-free light-chain assay did not exist in the early studies of melphalan-based therapy but has been used regularly since 2005, resulting in improved ability to monitor hematologic responses. Second, the mix of patients, particularly cardiac, is very important in determining overall outcomes.

The authors studied 101 patients with AL; half received melphalan and prednisone, and half received vincristine, carmustine, melphalan, cyclophosphamide, and prednisone.[292] Seventy-six of the 101 patients died, and the median OS for the entire group was 26.4 months, with no difference between the two arms. In this group of 101, 18 patients ultimately required dialysis therapy; 15 of the 18 have since died. The most common cause of death was intractable hypotension related to cardiac involvement while on dialysis. The three surviving dialysis patients have been alive for 87, 94, and 103 months. A myelodysplastic syndrome was documented in eight patients, all of whom have died, including one who received an allogeneic BM transplant. The OS time of these eight patients ranged from 18 to 90 months, with a median of 43 months. The authors also studied 45 patients who received the agent iodo-deoxydoxorubicin and found a response rate of 15%.[293]

Thalidomide has been shown to be active in the treatment of AL. In the initial report, six patients with AL were treated with thalidomide.[294] All patients had renal amyloidosis and were treated previously. The duration of thalidomide therapy was 3 to 9 months (median, 5 months). Four also received oral corticosteroids. An improvement was reported in five patients. Proteinuria decreased by more than 50% in two, and the serum albumin concentration improved in three. Two patients died, and four were alive and remained on therapy.[294]

In another report of 12 patients receiving thalidomide, eight patients had renal, four had cardiac, three had liver, and two had soft tissue amyloidosis.[295] Ten had received prior SCT. The median maximum tolerated thalidomide dose was 50 mg. No patient had a 50% decrease in serum or urine monoclonal proteins. Five of 11 patients had a 25% to 50% improvement. Three patients had stable disease, and three had progressive disease.[295] The authors have found thalidomide difficult to administer, and initial doses should not exceed 50 mg. It is unusual for patients with amyloidosis to tolerate more than 200 mg/day long term, and the toxicity is substantially greater in this population. The authors encountered edema and cognitive difficulties in 75%; dyspnea, dizziness, and rash in 50%; and two deep venous thromboses. The median time on treatment was only 72 days.[296,297]

Thalidomide has been combined with dexamethasone therapy in 31 patients.[298] Forty-eight percent of patients achieved a hematologic response, with 19% complete responses and 26% organ responses. The median time to hematologic response was 3.6 months. Treatment-related toxicity was frequent at 65%.[298]

Lenalidomide has been reported to be useful in the treatment of amyloidosis. A report on 34 patients was recently presented[299a]; eight of the 13 evaluable patients had a measurable response, four to lenalidomide alone. Nine other patients responded when dexamethasone was added. Lenalidomide appeared to be better tolerated than thalidomide.[299a]

Eighty percent of evaluable patients in the first study of bortezomib for amyloidosis had a hematologic response.[299b] Among 18 patients, the hematologic response was 77% with 16% being complete. A phase I dose-escalation study of bortezomib given either twice weekly on days 1, 4, 8, and 11 every 21 days or days 1, 8, 15, and 22 every 35 days reported hematologic responses in 50% of patients. The weekly regimen was associated with lower neurotoxicity. There is a 1-year hematologic progression-free rate of 72.2% and 74.6% and 1-year survival rates of 93.8 and 84%, respectively, for the twice-weekly and once-weekly dose.[299c] Among 70 patients, there were 29% renal and 13% cardiac responses. Discontinuation and dose reduction because of the toxicity were higher with the twice-weekly than once-weekly dose. Both dose schedules represent active well-tolerated regimens in relapsed AL.[299d]

The combination of bortezomib and dexamethasone has been used after SCT as consolidation therapy to improve the depth of response.[299e] Seventeen of 23 patients received bortezomib after transplantation; 74% achieved a complete response, and 58% achieved an organ response. A multicenter study of 94 patients receiving bortezomib and dexamethasone showed that hematologic responses in 71%; 25% were complete.[299f] Cardiac response was seen in 29% of patients. NT-proBNP predicted survival. In a study of bortezomib–dexamethasone in 26 patients, the overall response rate was 54% with 31% complete responses. The median time to response was 7.5 weeks, but the median progression-free and OS times were 5 and 18.7 months, respectively, suggesting short durability with bortezomib combined with dexamethasone. No grade 3 or 4 neuropathy was observed.[299g]

Lenalidomide has been combined with melphalan and dexamethasone.[299h] The maximum tolerated dose of lenalidomide is 15 mg. This three-drug oral combination produced hematologic responses in 58% and complete responses in 42%. The 2-year event-free and OS rates were 54% and 81%, respectively. Lenalidomide has also been combined with cyclophosphamide and dexamethasone in 35 patients.[299i] The hematologic response rate was 60%. In those receiving at least 4 cycles, the response rate was 87%. The OS time was 16.1 months. A randomized study of cyclophosphamide–thalidomide–dexamethasone compared with melphalan–dexamethasone suggested a higher complete response rate with the three-drug regimen, albeit with greater toxicity.[299j] One cautionary note when using lenalidomide or thalidomide in patients with light-chain amyloidosis is that the NT-proBNP appears to rise after the initiation of therapy. Recognition of potential IMID-induced cardiac toxicity is important when these agents are used. High levels of NT-proBNP predict for an inability to tolerate immunomodulatory agents for amyloidosis.[299k,299l]

Pomalidomide, a derivative of thalidomide with structural similarity to thalidomide and lenalidomide, was given to 26 patients in one study. All patients were previously treated. Half received a prior autologous SCT. A prior immunomodulatory agent was given in 12 and prior bortezomib in nine. Nineteen patients evaluable for hematologic response were seen. The overall response rate was seven of 19 (35%). Pomalidomide and dexamethasone is promising for the treatment of amyloidosis. One-year overall and progression-free survival were 77% and 56%, respectively. Pomalidomide was considered effective and safe, including for patients failing prior lenalidomide or thalidomide therapy.[299m]

STEM CELL TRANSPLANTATION FOR PRIMARY AMYLOIDOSIS

The use of high-dose chemotherapy and SCT for patients with amyloidosis remains controversial because this modality of therapy is associated with a high treatment-related mortality (Table 87-4).[300-313] Transplant-related mortality rates can range from 7% to 43%. Moreover, mortality has even been reported during stem cell mobilization using granulocyte colony-stimulating factor (G-CSF); these deaths were attributed to noncardiogenic pulmonary edema,[314] cardiac ischemia, or sudden rhythm disturbances with ventricular fibrillation. The significant visceral organ dysfunction that accompanies amyloidosis places patients at a high risk for complications. The number of organs involved at the time of transplantation is predictive of outcome. Patients who have one organ involved fare better than those who have two, and those who have more than two organs involved have an even poorer outcome.[315] Causes of treatment-related mortality in AL include GI tract bleeding,[316] cardiac rhythm disturbances, and multiorgan failure.

At the Mayo Clinic, high-dose chemotherapy and autologous SCT have been performed in 434 patients with AL. The median age was 57 years. The median serum albumin level was 2.7 g/dL, which

Table 87-4 Results of High-Dose Chemotherapy and Autologous Stem Cell Transplantation for Amyloidosis

Reference	Patients (*n*)	100-Day Treatment-Related Mortality	Overall Survival (Intention to Treat)
Perfetti et al[351]	22	3 (14%)	Median, 68 months
Sanchorawala et al[352]	80	11 (14%)	Median, 57 months
Dimopoulos et al[353]	50	12 (24%)	Median, 22.2 months
Gertz et al[354]	271	27 (10%)	2-year survival, 82%
Frossard et al[355]	16	1 (6%)	Median, 33 months
Mhaskar et al[356]	31	3 (9.8%)	Not given
Girnius et al[357]	16	3 (19%)	Median, 54.5 months
Saba et al[358]	9	7/9 (78%) (3 during mobilization) arrhythmia, CHF, hypotension	2/9 (22%) at >6 months after referral
Sezer et al[359]	1	0	1/1 (100%) at 3 months
Gertz et al[360]	23 (3 never had transplant)	4/20 (20%) pneumonia, multiorgan system failure, sudden death	13/23 (57%) at median of 16 months
Reich et al[361]	4	2/4 (50%) acute MI, diffuse alveolar hemorrhage	2/4 (50%) at 7 and 19 months
Sanchorawala et al[362]	205 (20 never had transplant)	22/185 (12%)	115/152 (76%) at >12 months
Perz et al[363]	13	2/13 (15%)	84% at 2 years
Blum et al[364]	10	0	18.5 months

ARF, Acute renal failure; *CHF,* congestive heart failure; *CMV,* cytomegalovirus; *CR,* complete response; *GI,* gastrointestinal; *MI,* myocardial infarction; *NA,* not available; *PR,* partial response.
Modified from Gertz MA, Lacy MQ, Dispenzieri A: Immunoglobulin light chain amyloidosis (primary amyloidosis, AL). In Gertz MA, Greipp PR, editors: *Hematologic malignancies: Multiple myeloma and related plasma cell disorders.* New York, 2004, Springer-Verlag, p 157. Used with permission of Mayo Foundation for Medical Education and Research.

reflects a high prevalence of nephrotic-range proteinuria. Ten percent of patients had serum creatinine levels greater than 1.8 mg/dL. Alkaline phosphatase levels greater than twice normal, a marker for liver amyloidosis, were observed in 58 (13%) patients. The median serum monoclonal protein concentration was 0.1 g/dL. A serum monoclonal protein component was found in 341 of the 434 patients (79%). The median 24-hour urine protein excretion was 3.7 g/day (interquartile range, 0.28-7.45 g/day). Fifty-six percent had urinary protein loss greater than 3 g/day. Only 8% had monoclonal light-chain excretion of greater than 1 g in 24 hours. One-, two-, and three-organ amyloid involvement was seen in 47%, 39%, and 14% of patients, respectively.

Stem cell mobilization in patients with amyloidosis was achieved with G-CSF alone without prior cytotoxic chemotherapy. The median number of apheresis collections required to collect an adequate stem cell product was 2 (interquartile range, 1-4 apheresis). The median number of $CD34^+$ cells collected was 7.16 × 10(6) CD34 cells (interquartile range, 4.92-9.84 × 106 CD34 cells). Hematopoietic growth factors were not administered after transplantation because of their ability to produce fluid retention in patients with cardiac and renal amyloidosis.

The 100-day mortality rate of these patients was 10.1% (44 of 434 patients), which compares favorably with reports from other institutions where morality rates as high as 40% have been reported.[307a] Mortality rates (before day 100) at the Mayo Clinic have progressively decreased over the years: outcomes of patients treated before January 2006 with those treated from January 2006 to December 31, 2009. Day 100 mortality decreased over this time period from 12% to 7%.[307b] Sixty-six percent of patients received conditioning therapy with melphalan at a dose of 200 mg/m^2, 29% received melphalan at 140 mg/m^2, and the rest received lower doses because of advanced cardiac amyloidosis. The intensity of chemotherapy delivered appears to be predictive of outcome.[317a] Patients receiving full-dose melphalan fare better, although patients selected for full-intensity therapy tend to have less advanced disease and are somewhat younger.[317a] Among 271 patients undergoing SCT, troponin T was a powerful predictor

Guidelines for Exclusion of Patients From Stem Cell Transplantation

Absolute contraindication
- Clinical congestive heart failure
- Total bilirubin >3.0 mg/dL
- Echocardiographic ejection fraction <30%

Troponin T >0.06

Relative contraindication
- Serum creatinine >2.0 mg/dL
- Interventricular septal thickness >15 mm
- Age older than >60 years
- More than two visceral organs involved

From Gertz MA, Lacy MQ, Dispenzieri A: Immunoglobulin light chain amyloidosis (primary amyloidosis, AL). In Gertz MA, Greipp PR, editors: *Handbook of multiple myeloma and related cell disorders.* New York: Springer-Verlag, 2010. By permission of Mayo Foundation for Medical Education and Research.

of treatment-related mortality. Patients with troponin T levels of 0.06 μg/L or higher had a day-100 all-cause mortality rate of 28%. Patients with troponin T levels less than 0.06 μg/L had a day-100 all-cause mortality rate of 7% (P <.001). Troponin T levels should be measured in all patients before transplantation. Those with troponin T levels exceeding 0.06 μg/L should be considered for less toxic therapies until the clinically optimal use of SCT is better defined by randomized clinical trials (see box on Guidelines for Exclusion of Patients From Consideration of Stem Cell Transplantation).[317b]

Bias is inherent in selecting patients for transplantation and the intensity of their conditioning. At the Mayo Clinic, only one-fifth of patients encountered with amyloidosis ultimately go on to receive SCT. Transplant recipients survive longer than patients not selected for transplant. In a case-matched control study, 63 transplant patients were compared with 63 conventionally treated patients matched for age, sex, cardiac function, creatinine, urinary protein loss, and liver involvement. An overall survival advantage for the patients undergoing transplant was observed.[318] In a report from the American Bone Marrow Transplant Registry of 107 patients treated with high-dose chemotherapy and autologous SCT at 48 centers,[319] the 30-day treatment mortality rate was 18%, and the response rate was 34%, with 33% having stable disease.[319] Only 11% of patients had posttransplant disease progression. The projected median survival time was 47 months. Experienced transplant groups appear to be able to achieve similar results as those of centers with a special interest in amyloidosis and transplantation.[320]

The 434 Mayo Clinic patients with amyloidosis received their transplants a median of 4.0 months after histologic diagnosis: one-fourth within 3 months and three-fourths within 6.6 months. The median actuarial survival time for the entire group was 94.9 months. Predictors of survival included weight gain of greater than 2% during stem cell mobilization and an absolute lymphocyte count at day 15 of greater than 500/μL.[321] The number of organs involved appeared to be relevant to successfully predicting outcome (Fig. 87-18). Patients with two-organ involvement have a survival rate of 70% at 60 months; those with three-organ involvement have a median survival time of 58 months. The serum creatinine, troponin-T, and BNP levels (Fig. 87-19) and septal thickness were all significant predictors of outcome.

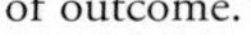

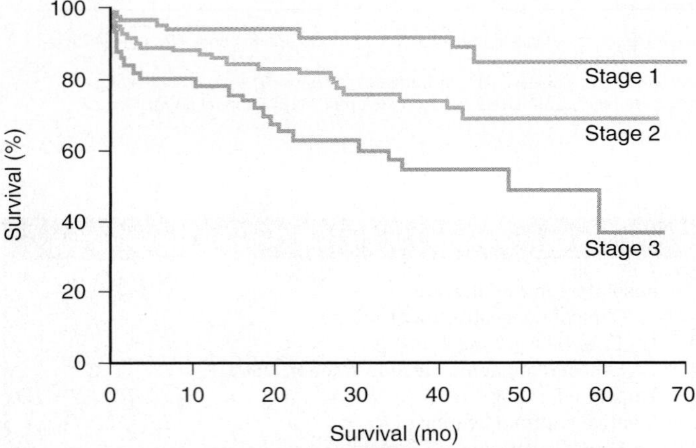

Figure 87-18 KAPLAN-MEIER CURVES ESTIMATING SURVIVAL IN 430 MAYO CLINIC PATIENTS WITH AMYLOIDOSIS ON THE BASIS OF MAYO STAGE AT PRESENTATION.

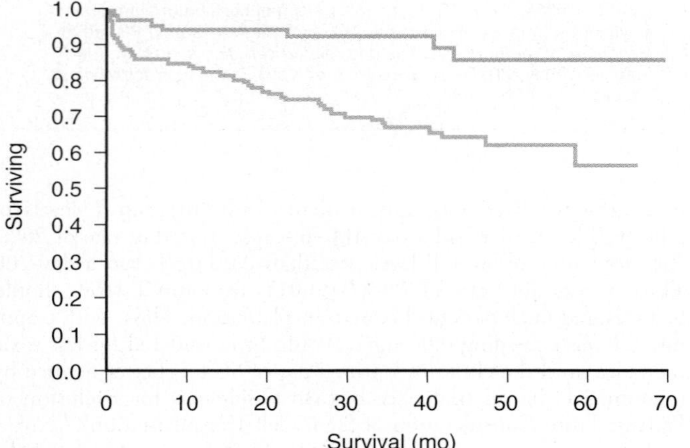

Figure 87-19 KAPLAN-MEIER CURVES ESTIMATING SURVIVAL IN 169 MAYO CLINIC PATIENTS WITH AMYLOIDOSIS ON THE BASIS OF N-TERMINAL PRO-BRAIN NATRIURETIC PEPTIDE (NT-pro-BNP) CONCENTRATION GREATER OR LESS THAN 333 pg/mL (*P* = .002).

Stem cell transplantation has not yet been established as the therapy of choice for patients with amyloidosis. In a French multicenter randomized trial (MAG and IFM Intergroup), patients with amyloidosis received either high-dose chemotherapy and autologous SCT or melphalan–dexamethasone therapy.[322a] The median survival time was 57 months in the melphalan–dexamethasone group and 49 months in the transplant group. Transplant patients received conditioning chemotherapy with either 140 or 200 mg/m^2 of melphalan. The hematologic response rates were similar for both groups (65% vs. 64%). These results suggest that OS may not be superior after SCT compared with melphalan–dexamethasone therapy.[322a] The results of this study must be interpreted with caution because of the short median follow-up (29 months) and high transplant-related mortality (24%). In a published meta-analysis of SCT in AL, transplantation does not appear to be superior to conventional chemotherapy in improving survival in patients with AL. But the quality of evidence is low, indicating a need for well-designed and adequately powered randomized, controlled trials to better address the role of transplantation in AL.[322b]

After transplant, responders to autologous SCT have a superior survival rate compared with nonresponders. OS is linked to pretransplant-free light-chain levels and the number of organs involved.[244,317a] In centers performing SCT, the treatment-related mortality rate has ranged from 6% to 18%, hematologic complete responses from 16% to 50%, and organ responses from 34% to 64%.[323] Organ responses are time dependent and may be delayed for up to 36 months after transplantation. The use of induction therapy with 2 cycles of melphalan and prednisone before SCT did not improve the rate of hematologic or organ response.[324]

Deaths have been reported during stem cell mobilization with cyclophosphamide plus G-CSF or G-CSF alone.[325] Hypoxia and hypotension may develop even in patients without cardiac involvement and may reflect a variant of pulmonary leukostasis syndrome. Excessive fluid accumulation during stem cell mobilization is an important predictor of 1-year survival.[326]

Toxic megacolon is a complication of high-dose chemotherapy.[327] Others have also reported fatal cardiac arrhythmias after infusion of DMSO-cryopreserved stem cell grafts.[328,329] The absolute numbers of CD4$^+$ T cells is significantly reduced after SCT, raising the theoretical risk that serious opportunistic infections will develop after transplantation. In a series of six patients, four had acute renal failure, one had splenic rupture, and one had severe GI bleeding.[330,331] In a multicenter study of 15 transplant patients, there was no treatment-related mortality, and 67% of patients experienced complete hematologic responses, suggesting the feasibility of performing SCT at experienced transplant centers not associated with major amyloidosis referral centers.[332]

Amyloid-related cardiomyopathy is associated with a high rate of early mortality after transplant.[333] The median survival time of patients with cardiac amyloidosis was 2 years. The overall median survival time was 5.5 years, and the relapse rate of complete responders was only 5%.[333]

Most conditioning regimens used to treat patients with AL undergoing transplant include melphalan; currently, melphalan alone is preferred to melphalan plus total-body irradiation. Complete hematologic response rates appear to be related to the dose of melphalan: 55% at 200 mg/m^2 and 35% at 100 or 140 mg/m^2.[2,317a] GI tract bleeding is a frequent complication.[316] It is assumed that amyloid infiltration of the submucosa of the GI tract followed by chemotherapy-induced mucosal erosion leads to exposure of amyloid-laden blood vessels with resultant bleeding.

Despite the high mortality and morbidity associated with transplantation (Table 87-5), the hematologic and organ response rates far exceed the prior experience with conventional-dose melphalan. Improvement in quality of life has also been reported in melphalan-treated patients undergoing SCT.[334] The best responses to transplant are seen in patients who have renal amyloidosis and nephrotic syndrome. The authors believe that the dose of melphalan used for conditioning must be modified according to patient risk factors. Clearly, patients with more than two major organs involved or severe cardiomyopathy are at a high risk when receiving melphalan doses of 200 mg/m^2 (Fig. 87-20). Patients with one or two organs involved, younger patients, and those without advanced cardiac disease are favorable candidates for SCT. A risk-adapted stratification has been useful in selecting patients for therapy and assigning melphalan dose (see box on Risk-Adapted Approach to Chemotherapy Dosing in Stem Cell Transplant Recipients).[317a]

The use of both conventional and high-dose chemotherapy has been shown to normalize factor X deficiency associated with amyloidosis.[335] Dose-intensive melphalan therapy improves nephrotic syndrome in patients with AL, but the benefit is limited to patients achieving eradication of the plasma cell dyscrasia.[336] A randomized study was performed comparing autologous SCT with therapy with 2 cycles of oral melphalan and prednisone followed by SCT.[337] The OS of patients 1 year after randomization was higher for those who went directly to transplantation.

The role of tandem transplants and nonmyeloablative conditioning regimens has yet to be defined in this setting. Tandem transplantation has been reported in four patients, all with nephrotic syndrome.[338,339] Two died, one of sudden death and one, who had sepsis with GI tract bleeding, of complications of renal failure. Two of the patients are alive and in good health.

Patients who receive transplants for AL are highly selected on the basis of age, performance status, number of organs involved, absence of severe cardiomyopathy, and preserved renal function. Dispenzieri et al[340] reviewed an amyloidosis patient database to identify patients who might have been eligible for SCT. The inclusion criteria of biopsy-proven amyloidosis, symptoms of amyloidosis, absence of MM, restrictions on age, and adequate cardiac function led to the selection of 229 of 1288 patients. The median survival time of this group was 45 months, with 5- and 10-year survival rates of 36% and 15%, respectively (Fig. 87-21). Predictors of survival were size of the monoclonal protein component in the urine, number of organs involved (Fig. 87-22), serum alkaline phosphatase value, performance

Risk-Adapted Approach to Chemotherapy Dosing in Stem Cell Transplant Recipients

Good risk
- One or two organs involved
- No cardiac involvement
- Creatinine clearance ≥ 51 mL/min
- Any age

Intermediate risk
- Younger than 61 years old
- One or two organs involved
- Asymptomatic cardiac
- Or compensated cardiac
- Creatinine clearance <51 mL/min

Poor risk
- Three organs involved
- Advanced cardiac involvement

Melphalan dosing: as a function of risk group and age

Good Risk	*Intermediate Risk*	*Poor Risk*
200 mg/m^2 if ≤60	140 mg/m^2 if ≤50	Standard therapy
140 mg/m^2 if 61-70	100 mg/m^2 if 51-60	Clinical trials
100 mg/m^2 if ≥71		

From Gertz MA, Lacy MQ, Dispenzieri A: Immunoglobulin light chain amyloidosis (primary amyloidosis, AL). In Gertz MA, Greipp PR, editors: *Handbook of multiple myeloma and related cell disorders.* New York: Springer-Verlag, 2010. By permission of Mayo Foundation for Medical Education and Research.

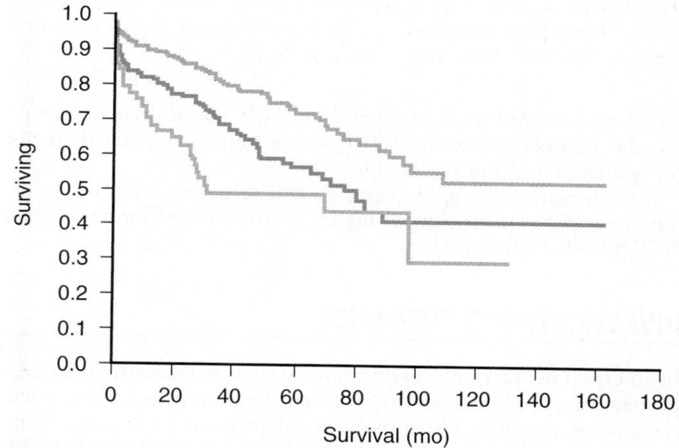

Figure 87-20 SURVIVAL OF PATIENTS WITH AMYLOIDOSIS RECEIVING STEM CELL TRANSPLANTATION ACCORDING TO THE NUMBER OF ORGANS INVOLVED (n = 434).

Table 87-5 Selected Treatment-Related Toxicities (SWOG Grade >2) in Patients With Primary Amyloidosis Who Received Stem Cell Transplantation

	No. of Patients (%)	
Toxicity	**Melphalan, 200 mg/m^2 (n = 23)**	**Melphalan, 100 mg/m^2 (n = 27)**
Nausea or vomiting	19 (83)	14 (52)
Diarrhea	15 (65)	13 (48)
Mucositis	21 (91)	10 (37)
Non-GI bleeding	4 (17)	0 (0)
GI bleeding	5 (22)	2 (7)

GI, Gastrointestinal tract; *SWOG,* Southwest Oncology Group.
Data from Gertz MA, Lacy MQ, Dispenzieri A: Immunoglobulin light chain amyloidosis (primary amyloidosis, AL). In Gertz MA, Greipp PR, editors: *Hematologic malignancies: Multiple myeloma and related plasma cell disorders.* New York, 2004, Springer-Verlag, p 157. Used with permission of Mayo Foundation for Education and Research.

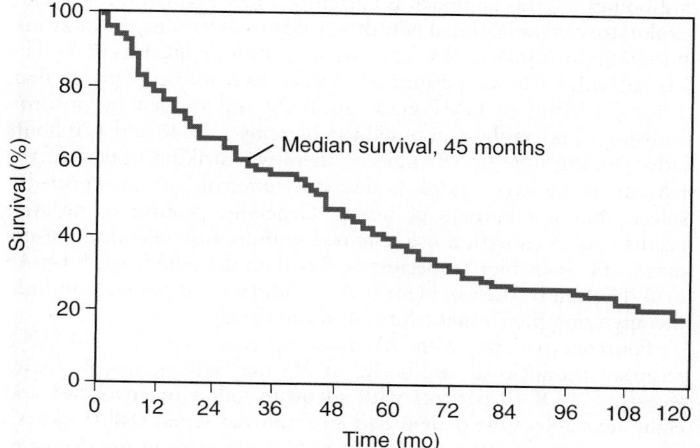

Figure 87-21 KAPLAN-MEIER CURVE ESTIMATING SURVIVAL OF PATIENTS WITH AMYLOIDOSIS WHO WOULD HAVE BEEN ELIGIBLE FOR STEM CELL TRANSPLANTATION BY MAYO CLINIC CRITERIA BUT WERE TREATED CONVENTIONALLY. *(Modified from Dispenzieri A, Lacy MQ, Kyle RA, et al: Eligibility for hematopoietic stem-cell transplantation for primary systemic amyloidosis is a favorable prognostic factor for survival.* J Clin Oncol *19:3350, 2001. Used with permission.)*

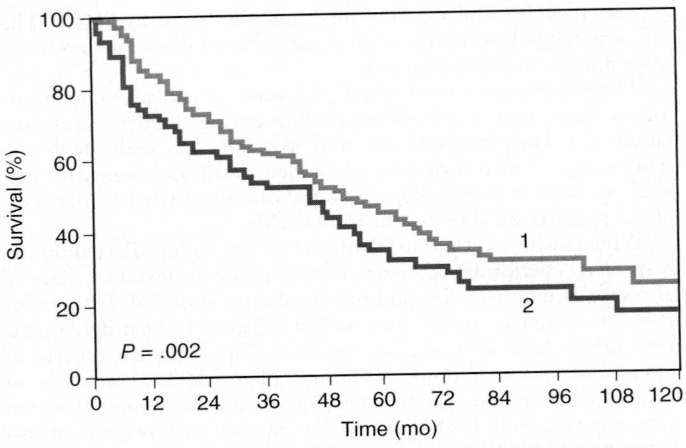

Figure 87-22 KAPLAN-MEIER CURVE ESTIMATING SURVIVAL OF STEM CELL TRANSPLANT–ELIGIBLE PATIENTS WITH AMYLOIDOSIS WHO WERE TREATED CONVENTIONALLY, ACCORDING TO THE NUMBER OF ORGANS INVOLVED AT THE TIME OF DIAGNOSIS. *(Modified from Gertz MA, Lacy MQ, Dispenzieri A: Immunoglobulin light chain amyloidosis [primary amyloidosis, AL]. In Gertz MA, Greipp PR, editors:* Hematologic malignancies: Multiple myeloma and related plasma cell disorders. *New York, 2004, Springer-Verlag, p 157.)*

status, and weight loss. Being eligible for SCT but not actually receiving the transplant was associated with a better outcome than not being eligible for transplantation.

In summary, with appropriate patient selection, SCT is feasible but is associated with risks of higher morbidity and mortality than SCT for other disorders.

INVESTIGATIONAL THERAPIES

In an experimental model in which mice are injected with human AL proteins, amyloidomas result.[341a] When these animals receive injections of an anti–light-chain monoclonal antibody having specificity for an amyloid-related epitope, the amyloidomas rapidly resolve. This monoclonal antibody is directed toward a β-pleated sheet conformational epitope expressed by AL proteins. The amyloidolytic response appears to be associated with the release of proteolytic factors. AL resolution can be induced by passive administration of amyloid-reactive antibodies.[341a] This approach is currently under evaluation. A phase I exploratory investigational new drug study to determine the biodistribution of the fibril-reactive, amyloidolytic murine IgG1 mAb 11-1F4 labeled with I-124 was performed. Patients were infused with less than 1 mg (74 MBq) of GMP-grade antibody and imaged by positron emission tomography-computed tomography scan 48 and 120 hours later. Among nine of 18 subjects, there was striking uptake of the reagent in the liver; lymph nodes; BM; intestine; or, unexpectedly, spleen (but not kidneys or heart). Generally, positive or negative results correlated with those obtained immunohistochemically using diagnostic tissue biopsy specimens. Based on these findings,[124] I-mAb m11-1F4 can be used to identify AL candidates for passive immunotherapy using the chimeric form of the antibody.[341b]

Fourteen patients with AL received etanercept, an anti-TNF receptor monoclonal antibody, at 25 mg subcutaneously twice weekly.[342,343] Of 10 patients with adequate follow-up, two died and eight are stable. One patient had an improved septal wall thickness. Three patients experienced a 25% to 50% decrease in the degree of macroglossia. Two patients with diarrhea had significant improvement. In two of five patients with peripheral neuropathy, disease progression was halted with therapy. Only one patient had adverse effects. Larger studies to further evaluate the role of etanercept in the management of AL are warranted.[342]

Lacy et al[344] reported the use of a dendritic cell–based idiotype vaccination for AL. Ten patients were treated, and five had multiorgan AL. Three had received prior SCTs. One patient had an objective response, with proteinuria decreasing by 95%. One patient had improvement of painful peripheral neuropathy. Specific T-cell proliferative responses to idiotype were detectable in the patient who had a clinical response. Optimizing patients' immune function and response will be the subject of future studies.

Use of antisense oligonucleotides for the inhibition of amyloid immunoglobulin production has been explored.[345a] Antisense oligonucleotides against light-chain complementarity-determining regions prohibited light-chain production. It is possible to design specific complementary oligonucleotides, suggesting that treatment with antisense oligonucleotides could represent a rational approach to improve treatment outcomes in AL.[345a]

Serum amyloid P binds to all forms of amyloid deposits. Drugs have been developed that act as competitive inhibitors of serum amyloid P binding to amyloid fibrils.[52] Such compounds dimerize serum amyloid P molecules, leading to their rapid clearance by the liver and depletion of circulating serum amyloid P. Such agents remove serum amyloid P from human amyloid deposits and may destabilize the existing amyloid fibrils, allowing for their dissolution.[52] Such a therapeutic approach is of great interest. Administration of anti–human-SAP antibodies to mice with amyloid deposits containing human SAP triggers a potent, complement-dependent, macrophage-derived giant cell reaction that swiftly removes massive visceral amyloid deposits without adverse effects. Anti–SAP-antibody treatment is clinically feasible because circulating human SAP can be depleted in patients by the bis-d-proline compound CPHPC, thereby enabling injected anti-SAP antibodies to reach residual SAP in the amyloid deposits. The capacity of this combined therapy to eliminate amyloid deposits should be applicable to all forms of systemic and local amyloidosis.[345b]

DEFINING RESPONSES IN PRIMARY AMYLOIDOSIS

Responses to therapy in patients with AL can be defined by improved organ function or by hematologic responses comparable to those seen in patients with MM.[346a] All patients who have a measurable serum or urine monoclonal protein should be monitored for changes in the size of the monoclonal protein peak after any therapeutic intervention. For patients who have only a free light chain that cannot be quantified, immunofixation is used to determine if the protein is present or absent. The nephelometric free light-chain assay is extremely useful in monitoring patients serially to determine any decrease in circulating free light chain and has made the evaluation of response much easier.[41] FLC response is a more useful measure of hematologic response than M-protein response. It also highlights the importance of achieving at least a 90% reduction in the FLC-diff to improve the outcome of patients with light-chain AL.[346b]

The utility of the free light-chain assay in predicting outcome has been validated as noted earlier in this chapter, with 5-year survival rates of 88% for responders and 39% for nonresponders.[43] In the authors' experience, normalization of the free light-chain level was a better predictor of survival than was achievement of a complete hematologic response or normalization of the free light-chain ratio.[244] These results have been verified in a series of 25 patients with sequential free light-chain analyses.[347] All patients with a normalized κ to λ free light-chain ratio had a good prognosis.[347] The fraction of patients with serum-free light-chain responses has been suggested to be higher in patients receiving high-dose melphalan than in those who receive conventional therapy.[348]

Free light-chain responses also seem to parallel decreases in NT-pro-BNP levels in cardiac responders to therapy. For patients in whom free light chain decreased by more than 50%, the NT-pro-BNP concentration decreased by a median of 48%, but in patients without such a free light-chain decrease, the NT-pro-BNP concentration increased by 47%.[349] The NT-pro-BNP decrease was greater in complete responders than in other responders. The decrease of free light chains translates to a simultaneous decrease of NT-pro-BNP and improved survival. Cardiac function in AL can improve because of a

Table 87-6 Criteria for Amyloid-Related Organ Responses to Treatment*

Response	Progression
Heart	
Decrease of ≥2 mm in mean left ventricular wall thickness from baseline thickness >11 mm	Increase ≥2 mm in wall thickness
Two-class improvement in NYHA class	Two-class worsening in NYHA class
	NT-pro-BNP–based criteria were defined as a decrease or an increase of both >30% and >300 ng/L and a threshold of evaluability based on NT-pro-BNP baseline level >650 ng/L.
Kidneys	
>50% decrease in daily proteinuria without progressive renal insufficiency	>50% increase in daily proteinuria Progressive renal insufficiency
Liver	
A decrease in liver span of >50%	An increase in liver span of >25%
A concomitant decrease of alkaline phosphatase by 50%	An increase of alkaline phosphatase by 50%
Nervous System	
Autonomic: normalization of orthostatic vital signs and symptoms, resolution of gastric atony	Autonomic: progression of orthostatic vital signs and symptoms, increasing gastric atony
Peripheral neuropathy: resolution of symptoms	Peripheral neuropathy: progression of symptoms

NT-pro-BNP, N-terminal pro–brain natriuretic peptide; *NYHA*, New York Heart Association.
*If organ function neither improves nor worsens, it is graded as stable.

decrease in circulating amyloidogenic precursor despite the amount of cardiac amyloid deposits remaining unaltered as measured by echocardiography.[349]

Organ-based response criteria have been defined for patients with amyloid nephrotic syndrome (Table 87-6).[350] Requirements for definition as an "organ response" include a 50% decrease in the 24-hour albumin excretion without an increase in serum creatinine value. For hepatic involvement, a 50% decrease in an increased serum alkaline phosphatase concentration with no increase in liver size is required. Echocardiographic regression of amyloidosis is difficult to assess because of variability in estimates of the interventricular septal wall thickness. Typically, a decrease in septal thickness of at least 2 mm is required. Neurologic responses can be documented by EMG demonstrating improved nerve conduction velocities. A consensus panel has defined what constitutes organ involvement and treatment response in patients with AL.[350]

The consensus panel reconvened in 2010 to update hematologic and organ response criteria. The ability of response criteria to identify patients who died was compared by evaluating the areas under receiver operator characteristic curves based on death at 1 year and by calculating the Harrell C statistic and the Royston explained variation. The category of complete response (negative serum and urine immunofixation, normal FLC κ:λ ratio, and normal BM study results) was unchanged. With respect to cardiac response and progression, NT-pro-BNP–based criteria were defined as a decrease or an increase of both greater than 30% and greater than 300 ng/L, and a threshold of evaluability based on NT-pro-BNP baseline level greater than 650 ng/L was chosen.

The most powerful criteria for PR were those based on dFLC percent decrease, and a 50% cutoff was preferred because of easier clinical use. A definition of VGPR based on dFLC (<40 mg/L) was adopted.

FUTURE DIRECTIONS

Primary amyloidosis is a disease for which therapy remains inadequate. The diagnosis should be suspected whenever a patient is seen with unexplained nephrotic syndrome, heart failure, neuropathy, or hepatomegaly. The first screening test should be immunofixation of serum or urine and the free light-chain assay. If a monoclonal protein is found, BM biopsy and fat aspiration should be performed to obtain tissues for Congo red staining. The prognosis should be assessed by two-dimensional echocardiography and BNP and troponin level measurements. Monitoring therapy includes the use of immunoglobulin free light-chain assays by nephelometry and cardiac biomarkers. Systemic chemotherapy is appropriate for most patients. SCT should be strongly considered if patients fulfill eligibility criteria. The use of solid organ transplantation remains investigational. The ideal treatment of patients with AL remains unknown, but early diagnosis is essential to ensure superior outcome.

ACKNOWLEGEMENT

Portions of this manuscript were originally included in Gertz MA, Lacy MQ, Dispenzieri A, Hayman SR, Kumar S: Transplantation for amyloidosis. *Curr Opin Oncol* 19:136, 2007. Used with permission.

SUGGESTED READINGS

Bellavia D, Abraham RS, Pellikka PA, et al: Utility of Doppler myocardial imaging, cardiac biomarkers, and clonal immunoglobulin genes to assess left ventricular performance and stratify risk following peripheral blood stem cell transplantation in patients with systemic light chain amyloidosis (Al). *J Am Soc Echocardiogr* 24:444, 2011. Epub 2011 Feb 18.

Benson MD, James S, Scott K, et al: Leukocyte chemotactic factor 2: A novel renal amyloid protein. *Kidney Int* 74:218, 2008. Epub 2008 Apr 30.

Benson MD, Teague SD, Kovacs R, et al: Rate of progression of transthyretin amyloidosis. *Am J Cardiol* 2011. [Epub ahead of print].

Blade J, Lonial S, Dimopoulos M, et al; International Myeloma Working Group: International Myeloma Working Group guidelines for serum-free light chain analysis in multiple myeloma and related disorders. *Leukemia* 23:215, 2009. Epub 2008 Nov 20. Review.

Bodin K, Ellmerich S, Kahan MC, et al: Antibodies to human serum amyloid P component eliminate visceral amyloid deposits. *Nature* 468:93, 2010. Epub 2010 Oct 20.

Comenzo RL: How I treat amyloidosis. *Blood* 114:3147, 2009. Epub 2009 Jul 17. Review.

Connors LH, Prokaeva T, Lim A, et al: Cardiac amyloidosis in African Americans: Comparison of clinical and laboratory features of transthyretin V122I amyloidosis and immunoglobulin light chain amyloidosis. *Am Heart J* 158:607, 2009.

Dember LM, Hawkins PN, Hazenberg BP, et al: Eprodisate for AA Amyloidosis Trial Group: Eprodisate for the treatment of renal disease in AA amyloidosis. *N Engl J Med* 356:2349, 2007.

Dispenzieri A, Kyle R, Merlini G, et al: Long-term outcomes of patients with light chain amyloidosis (AL) after renal transplantation with or without stem cell transplantation. *Nephrol Dial Transplant* 2011. [Epub ahead of print].

Kumar SK, Gertz MA, Lacy MQ, et al: Recent improvements in survival in primary systemic amyloidosis and the importance of an early mortality risk score. *Mayo Clin Proc* 86:12, 2011.

Lebovic D, Hoffman J, Levine BM, et al: Predictors of survival in patients with systemic light-chain amyloidosis and cardiac involvement initially ineligible for stem cell transplantation and treated with oral melphalan and dexamethasone. *Br J Haematol* 143:369, 2008. Epub 2008 Aug 4.

Liepnieks JJ, Zhang LQ, Benson MD: Progression of transthyretin amyloid neuropathy after liver transplantation. *Neurology* 75:324, 2010.

Merlini G, Seldin DC, Gertz MA: Amyloidosis: Pathogenesis and new therapeutic options. *J Clin Oncol* 29:1924, 2011. Epub 2011 Apr 11.

Palladini G, Barassi A, Klersy C, et al: The combination of high-sensitivity cardiac troponin T (hs-cTnT) at presentation and changes in N-terminal natriuretic peptide type B (NT-pro-BNP) after chemotherapy best predicts survival in AL amyloidosis. *Blood* 116:3426, 2010. Epub 2010 Jul 19.

Palladini G, Merlini G: Transplantation vs. conventional-dose therapy for amyloidosis. *Curr Opin Oncol* 23:214, 2011.

Palladini G, Russo P, Foli A, et al: Salvage therapy with lenalidomide and dexamethasone in patients with advanced AL amyloidosis refractory to melphalan, bortezomib, and thalidomide. *Ann Hematol* 2011. [Epub ahead of print].

Pinney JH, Lachmann HJ, Bansi L, et al: Outcome in renal Al amyloidosis after chemotherapy. *J Clin Oncol* 29:674, 2011. Epub 2011 Jan 10.

Reece DE, Hegenbart U, Sanchorawala V, et al: Efficacy and safety of once-weekly and twice-weekly bortezomib in patients with relapsed systemic AL amyloidosis: Results of a phase 1/2 study. *Blood* 2011. [Epub ahead of print].

Sanchorawala V, Seldin DC, Berk JL, et al: Oral cyclic melphalan and dexamethasone for patients with Al amyloidosis. *Clin Lymphoma Myeloma Leuk* 10:469, 2010.

Sattianayagam PT, Gibbs SD, Pinney JH, et al: Solid organ transplantation in AL amyloidosis. *Am J Transplant* 10:2124, 2010. doi:10.1111/j.1600-6143.2010.03227.x.

Sipe JD, Benson MD, Buxbaum JN, et al: Amyloid fibril protein nomenclature: 2010 recommendations from the nomenclature committee of the International Society of Amyloidosis. *Amyloid* 17:101, 2010. Epub 2010 Nov 2.

Solomon A, Macy SD, Wooliver C, et al: Splenic plasma cells can serve as a source of amyloidogenic light chains. *Blood* 113:1501, 2009. Epub 2008 Dec 2.

Solomon A, Murphy CL, Westermark P: Unreliability of immunohistochemistry for typing amyloid deposits. *Arch Pathol Lab Med* 132:14, 2008; author reply 14-5.

Tapan U, Seldin DC, Finn KT, Fennessey S, et al: Increases in B-type natriuretic peptide (BNP) during treatment with lenalidomide in AL amyloidosis. *Blood* 116:5071, 2010.

van Gameren II, Hazenberg BP, Bijzet J, et al: Amyloid load in fat tissue reflects disease severity and predicts survival in amyloidosis. *Arthritis Care Res (Hoboken)* 62:296, 2010.

van Gameren II, van Rijswijk MH, Bijzet J, et al: Histological regression of amyloid in AL amyloidosis is exclusively seen after normalization of serum free light chain. *Haematologica* 94:1094, 2009.

Wall JS, Kennel SJ, Stuckey AC, et al: Radioimmunodetection of amyloid deposits in patients with AL amyloidosis. *Blood* 116:2241, 2010. Epub 2010 Jun 3.

For complete list of references log on to www.expertconsult.com.

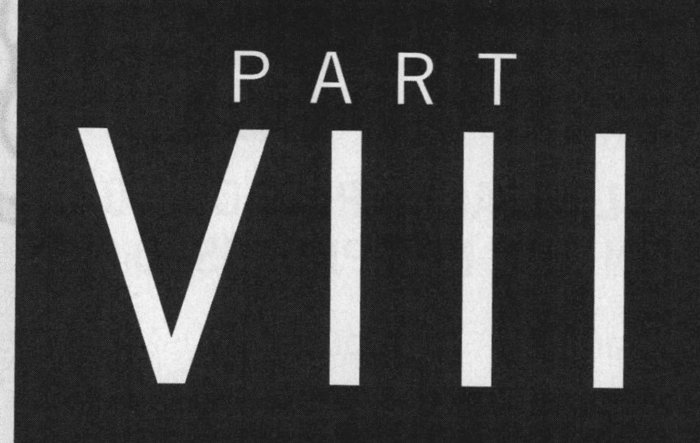

Comprehensive Care of Patients With Hematologic Malignancies

CHAPTER 88

CLINICAL APPROACH TO INFECTIONS IN THE COMPROMISED HOST

Samuel A. Shelburne, Russell E. Lewis, and Dimitrios P. Kontoyiannis

Advances in the supportive care and treatment of hematologic malignancies have markedly improved the life expectancy of afflicted patients, but this progress is increasingly at the expense of developing a wider range of infectious complications often caused by drug-resistant organisms. The clinical approach to infections occurring among hematology patients involves understanding host immune system defects and anatomic barrier disruption that predispose patients to infection (Fig. 88-1). This chapter reviews specific hematologic conditions for their unique host defense defects and associated infections (Table 88-1) and the differential diagnoses of common infectious pathogens (Table 88-2). To demonstrate how periods of predictable anatomic defects combine with severe immune compromise, the prevention, diagnosis, and management strategies for infections occurring in the hematopoietic stem cell transplant (HSCT) recipient are presented as models.[1]

HEMATOLOGIC CONDITIONS PREDISPOSING TO INFECTION

Malignant Hematologic Disorders

Antineoplastic Therapy

During antineoplastic treatment, cytotoxic agents frequently are administered in combination with other immunosuppressive therapies, such as corticosteroids or radiation therapy. Several cytotoxic agents, notably methotrexate, cyclophosphamide, 6-mercaptopurine, and azathioprine, impair cell-mediated immunity. Many of the drugs themselves (e.g., cyclophosphamide) also impair humoral responses and produce quantitative phagocyte defects. Fludarabine, the major first-line therapy for chronic lymphocytic leukemia (CLL), can produce prolonged and profound defects in cell-mediated immunity, thereby increasing susceptibility to *Pneumocystis,* yeast, and herpes group viruses (herpes simplex virus [HSV], varicella-zoster virus [VZV], and cytomegalovirus [CMV]).

The use of monoclonal antibody therapy for hematologic disorders results in dysfunction of particular aspects of the immune system.[2] Rituximab results in a sustained depletion of B lymphocytes for 6 to 9 months and has been specifically associated with reactivation of hepatitis B virus infection.[3] Alemtuzumab administration causes profound lymphopenia and an increased risk for a variety of viral and fungal infections.

Exogenous administration of glucocorticoids leads to increased susceptibility to infection. The degree of immunosuppression and the relative risk for infection depend on the dose and duration of use. The major effect of steroids on granulocyte function is a decrease in chemotactic activity. This accounts, in part, for the clinical observation that the signs and symptoms of severe infections may be masked or greatly reduced in patients receiving steroids. Steroids may enhance susceptibility to infection by means of negative effects on glucose homeostasis, wound healing, skin fragility, monocyte and lymphocyte function, production of cytokines, and humoral immune responses.

Radiation therapy has been associated with granulocyte dysfunction and delayed wound healing. Defects in cell-mediated immunity may persist for more than 1 year after intensive radiation therapy or after HSCT.

Acute Leukemias

In patients with acute leukemias, a major cause of morbidity is infection due to drug-associated mucositis and therapy-induced neutropenia. Most infections occurring during neutropenia are bacterial, but patients with prolonged neutropenia are at additional risk for development of yeast and mold infections. Patients with acute leukemia who progress to advanced therapies, such as hematopoietic cell transplant, have added risk for infections associated with acquired deficiencies in cell-mediated and humoral immunity, such as *Pneumocystis jiroveci* and CMV infections.[1]

Chronic Leukemias

Patients with chronic myeloid leukemia do not have prominent host defense impairments, so infections are limited unless patients proceed to aggressive chemotherapy or HSCT. Host defense defects with tyrosine kinase inhibitors, such as imatinib or dasatinib, have not been well defined. Chemotherapy for blast crisis resembles therapy for acute leukemia. Patients with chronic lymphocytic leukemia (CLL) are predisposed to infection because of immunodeficiency related to the leukemia itself (humoral and cellular immune dysfunction) and to therapy-related immunosuppression.[4] In early B-cell CLL, the infectious risk is mainly related to unbalanced immunoglobulin chain synthesis and resultant hypogammaglobulinemia. In patients with advanced CLL, particularly after the introduction of therapy with purine analogues and monoclonal agents (e.g., rituximab, alemtuzumab), neutropenia and defects in cell-mediated immunity are other factors predisposing to infection. The risk for infectious complications increases with the duration of CLL, reflecting the cumulative immunosuppression related to its treatment. The incidence of infection correlates with the serum levels of immunoglobulins (particularly IgG), which may be further impaired by use of rituximab.

Lymphomas

Hodgkin and non-Hodgkin lymphoma are commonly associated with impaired cell-mediated immunity. The degree of immune impairment may correlate with the extent of disease and often is compounded by administration of immunosuppressive therapy.[3] The intrinsic impairment of cell-mediated immunity in Hodgkin lymphoma can persist even after apparent cure. Splenectomy-related infections occur with sepsis caused by encapsulated bacterial organisms at a median of 22 months but sometimes many years after surgery.

Myelodysplastic Syndrome

Neutrophils and band forms from patients with myelodysplastic syndrome are functionally defective and probably are derived from a

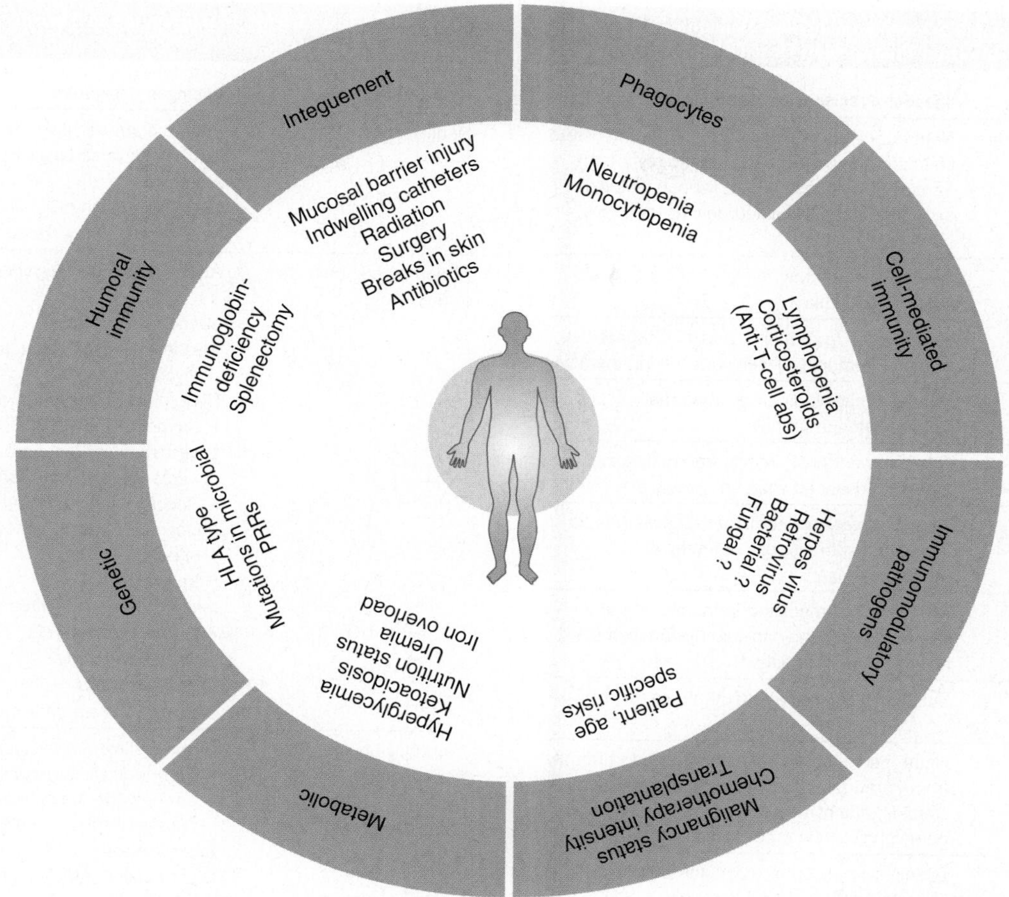

Figure 88-1 CONSTELLATION OF FACTORS CONTRIBUTING TO INCREASED RISK FOR INFECTION IN IMMUNOCOMPROMISED HOSTS.

malignant clone of myeloid precursor cells. Neutrophils from patients with myelodysplastic syndrome have deficiencies in myeloperoxidase, elastase, and integrins. More than half of patients with myelodysplastic syndrome die within 3 years of diagnosis from infections, bleeding complications, or progression to acute leukemia.

Multiple Myeloma

Malignant plasma cells produce a variety of immunomodulatory molecules such as TGF-B which suppress B-cell function, so multiple myeloma is frequently associated with a variety of defects in humoral immunity.[5] Patients having myeloma with IgG paraprotein have an increased rate of catabolism of normal and clonal IgG. They also may have defects in complement and granulocyte function. Cell-mediated immunity is not impaired by the disease but is compromised by corticosteroids or cytotoxic therapy.

Uncommon Malignancies

Patients with hairy cell leukemia develop mycobacterial disease relatively often, especially infection with atypical mycobacteria. Reversal of host cellular immune defects with effective therapy can lead to rapid clinical response with eradication of mycobacterial infection.

Defects in cell-mediated immunity have been postulated to explain the incidence of infection caused by intracellular pathogens in patients with the relatively rare T-cell malignancies mycosis fungoides and T-cell CLL.

Nonmalignant Hematologic Disorders

Aplastic Anemia

This blood dyscrasia is associated with decreased peripheral blood cell counts due to marrow failure. Chronic neutropenia is the main cause of recurrent bacterial and fungal infections among patients. Periodontal infections are particularly common. Treatment of the underlying hematologic disease is required to stop recurrent infections and cure some chronic infections.

Paroxysmal Nocturnal Hemoglobinuria

Patients with paroxysmal nocturnal hemoglobinuria are at some increased risk for bacterial infection due to a deficiency of decay-accelerating factor on the membrane of neutrophils. Modest and progressive granulocytopenia, progression to aplasia or leukemia may compound these risks. Vaccination against meningococcus is required before treatment with the terminal complement inhibitor eculizumab.

Granulocytic Phagocyte Disorders

The clinical approach to infections in patients with granulocytic phagocyte disorders is specific to each of these disorders and is beyond the scope of this chapter. However, chronic granulomatous disease is discussed because patients with this congenital immunodeficiency

Table 88-1 Malignant and Select Nonmalignant Hematologic Diseases and Their Associated Infection-Predisposing Host Defects

Hematologic Condition	Infection-Predisposing Host Defects
Acute myeloid leukemia	Neutropenia; therapies such as dose-intensive chemotherapy and hematopoietic stem cell transplant may result in additional anatomic disruptions, cell-mediated defects, and humoral defects
Acute lymphocytic leukemia	Neutropenia; therapy effects similar to acute myeloid leukemia
Hairy cell leukemia	Neutropenia (also monocytopenia); abnormal humoral immunity; T-cell suppressing therapy
Chronic lymphocytic leukemia	Hypogammaglobulinemia; abnormal cell-mediated immunity
Chronic myeloid leukemia	No prominent host defects unless aggressive therapy, advanced stage, or postsplenectomy
Multiple myeloma	Hypogammaglobulinemia; other host defects may occur with aggressive therapy or advanced stage
Hodgkin/non-Hodgkin lymphomas	Abnormal cell-mediated immunity, therapy-related neutropenia, splenic dysfunction (if splenectomy or radiation)
Myelodysplastic syndromes	Functional or absolute neutropenia
Aplastic anemia	Neutropenia; abnormal cell-mediated immunity from immunosuppressive therapies (e.g., steroids, antithymocyte globulin, cyclosporine, hematopoietic stem cell transplantation)
Paroxysmal nocturnal hemoglobinuria	Deficient Fc receptor may contribute to abnormal cell-mediated immunity
Hemolytic states (thalassemia)	Gallstones may serve as a nidus for infection; splenic dysfunction or splenectomy
Sickle cell disease	Can be neutropenic with aplastic crisis; bone infarcts may serve as a nidus for infection; splenic dysfunction with poor complement activation and opsonization from autosplenectomy

who survive into adulthood are at risk for severe infections. Chronic granulomatous disease is a heterogeneous group of disorders resulting from defective or malfunctioning oxidative metabolism capacity of phagocytes. Recurrent infections with bacteria and fungi are common and occasionally life threatening, despite optimal antimicrobial therapy. Infections with *Staphylococcus* species and *Aspergillus* species can be particularly aggressive.[6] Granulomata may form in response to infection, especially in the gastrointestinal and genitourinary tracts.

Erythrocyte Disorders

Glucose-6-phosphate dehydrogenase deficiency is a sex-linked disorder. Deficiency of this enzyme limits glucose metabolism through the hexose monophosphate shunt, resulting in an abnormal respiratory burst in neutrophils. Bacterial infections can occur if the deficiency is severe.

Hemoglobin Gene Variants

Patients with chronic hemolytic states may develop bilirubin gallstones, which can serve as a nidus for infection. Defects

Table 88-2 Host Defense Impairments and Their Associated Infectious Pathogens

Host Defense Defect	Pathogen Categories
Neutropenia	Enteric gram-negative organisms Gram-positive staphylococci and streptococci Anaerobes Yeast, particularly *Candida* species Molds, particularly *Aspergillus* species
Abnormal cell-mediated immunity	Atypical bacteria: *Legionella, Nocardia* *Salmonella* species *Mycobacteria* (*M. tuberculosis* and atypical mycobacteria) Disseminated infection from live bacilli Calmette-Guérin (BCG) vaccine Environmental fungi, including *Cryptococcus neoformans, Histoplasma capsulatum, Coccidioides immitis* Endogenous yeast, particularly *Candida* species Herpesviruses Infections from live-virus vaccines *Pneumocystis iroveci* *Toxoplasma gondii* *Cryptosporidium* *Strongyloides stercoralis*
Immunoglobulin abnormalities	Gram-positive *Streptococcus pneumoniae, Staphylococcus aureus* Gram-negative *Haemophilus influenzae, Neisseria* species, enteric organisms Enteroviruses Disseminated infections from live-virus vaccines *Giardia lamblia*
Complement abnormalities C3, C5	Gram-positive *S. pneumoniae*, staphylococci Gram-negative *H. influenzae, Neisseria* species, enteric organisms
Complement abnormalities C5–C9	*Neisseria* species
Anatomic Disruption	Pathogen Categories
Oral cavity	α-Hemolytic streptococci, oral anaerobes *Candida* species Herpes simplex virus
Esophagus	*Candida* species, Herpes simplex virus, cytomegalovirus
Lower gastrointestinal tract	Enterococcus, gram-negative enteric organisms, Anaerobes *(Bacteroides fragilis, Clostridium perfringens),* *Candida* species, *Strongyloides stercoralis*
Skin (IV catheter)	Gram-positive staphylococci and streptococci, *Corynebacteria, Bacillus,* Atypical mycobacteria
Urinary tract	Enterococcus, Gram-negative enteric organisms *Candida* species
Splenectomy	Encapsulated organisms: *S. pneumoniae, H. influenzae, Neisseria, Capnocytophaga canimorsus* *Salmonella* (especially sickle cell disease), *Babesia*

in cell-mediated immunity have been described in patients with thalassemia. Patients with sickle cell disease have an increased susceptibility to bacterial infections.[7] Defective alternative complement pathway function, especially in conjunction with asplenia, contributes to the propensity to bacterial infection. Splenic involution results in depressed synthesis of alternate pathway factor(s) of complement and decreased phagocytic clearance of bacteria. Phagocytosis of *Streptococcus pneumoniae* is abnormal, in part because of an inability to use the alternate pathway for C3 fixation as a means of opsonization. An increased risk for *Salmonella* infection appears to be unique to the sickle cell population. Suppurative arthritis can occur after repeated episodes of hemarthrosis among patients with sickle cell disease.

Coagulation Disorders

Hemophilias are sex-linked deficiencies of clotting factor VIII or IX. Septic arthritis should be considered in the differential diagnosis of any hemophiliac with repeated episodes of hemarthrosis whose articular signs and symptoms fail to improve quickly after administration of appropriate coagulation factor replacement. Hemophiliacs who have acquired infection with human immunodeficiency virus (HIV)-1 from plasma-derived factor replacement therapy may develop severe impairment of cell-mediated immunity after this retroviral infection progresses to acquired immunodeficiency syndrome (AIDS).

Blood Groups

The Duffy blood group antigen serves as a receptor for *Plasmodium vivax* to invade erythrocytes. Blood group O is associated with *Helicobacter pylori* infection and an associated increase in peptic ulceration because the Lewis(b) blood group antigen mediates *H. pylori* attachment to human gastric mucosa.

Host Defense Impairment and Associated Infection Issues

Neutropenia

Profound or absolute neutropenia can occur in patients with aplastic anemia or leukemia or from chemotherapy used for treatment of various malignant diseases. Infection rates increase when neutrophil counts fall below 1000/mm^3, but the patient is most at risk for spontaneous infection when the count is below 100/mm (Fig. 88-2). The patient who is neutropenic from cytotoxic therapy can serve as a basic model for predicting infections that could occur in other patients with qualitative or quantitative granulocyte defects.

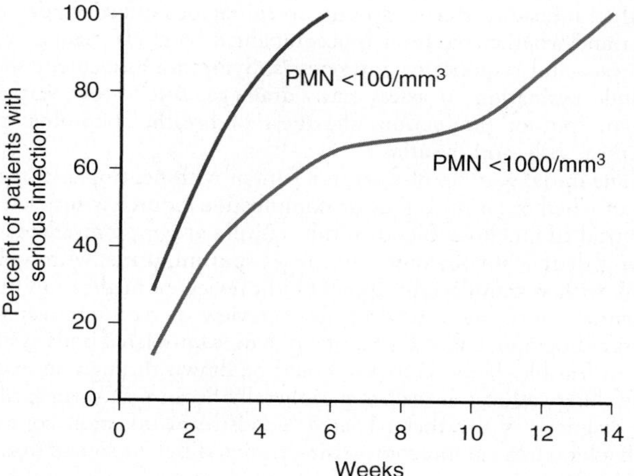

Figure 88-2 RELATIONSHIP OF SEVERITY AND DURATION OF NEUTROPENIA TO THE RISK FOR DEVELOPING A SERIOUS INFECTION. *(Courtesy GE Body.)*

Neutropenia predisposes to the development of bacterial and fungal infections but does not appear to increase the incidence or severity of viral and parasitic infections. Patients with profound and prolonged neutropenia who are at particular high risk for infection (e.g., cytopenic patients with acute myelogenous leukemia and severe mucositis following induction therapy) are likely to benefit from receiving prophylactic antimicrobials.[8,9] However, patients with moderate granulocytopenia (i.e., absolute granulocyte counts in the range from 500 to 2000/mm^3 that are not falling precipitously) should not receive prophylactic antimicrobial agents. Colony-stimulating factors (granulocyte colony-stimulating factor [G-CSF; pegylated filgrastim], granulocyte-macrophage colony-stimulating factor [GM-CSF, sargramostim]) are routinely used in the management of hematologic disorders. A number of functional granulocyte parameters may be enhanced by G-CSF or GM-CSF, including enhanced per-cell phagocytosis, oxidative metabolism, microbicidal activity, and antibody-dependent cytotoxicity.[10] However, G-CSF or GM-CSF administration may decrease the motility of granulocytes, impair in vivo migration, and decrease bacteria-induced chemotaxis. The clinical significance of any of these effects remains to be established but is generally believed to be insignificant in light of the potency of these agents in shortening the depth and duration of therapy-induced neutropenia.

Defects in Cell-Mediated Immunity

Cellular immune dysfunction occurs in patients with lymphoid malignancies, in those with hematologic malignancies undergoing HSCT, and in patients with AIDS. The most frequently encountered pathogens are intracellular organisms because they can survive and even replicate inside macrophages in a nonimmune individual or in the absence of T-cell immunity. Specific pathogens associated with infection in patients with cell-mediated immunity include bacteria (including *Mycobacterium tuberculosis,* atypical mycobacteria, *Salmonella,* streptococci, *Legionella, Nocardia,* and *Listeria*); fungi (including the yeasts *Candida* and *Cryptococcus;* molds such as *Aspergillus;* endemic dimorphic fungi such as *Histoplasma* and *Coccidioides;* and *Pneumocystis*); viruses (including herpes group viruses [HSV, VZV, CMV] and respiratory viruses); and protozoa (*Toxoplasma gondii, Cryptosporidium,* and *Strongyloides stercoralis*).

Patients with defects in cell-mediated immunity or who are about to receive HSCT should undergo risk factor assessment for reactivation of tuberculosis. Patients with a known history of an untreated but positive Mantoux test or interferon-gamma release assay should receive prophylactic isoniazid to prevent reactivation and potential dissemination of tuberculosis. Patients without a prior Mantoux test but with risk factors for tuberculosis should undergo a screening test for latent tuberculosis before starting the conditioning regimen for HSCT.

Patients with defects in cell-mediated immunity are at risk for the development of disseminated infection due to live vaccines, even when the vaccine contains attenuated organisms. Accordingly, these patients should not receive vaccines containing bacillus Calmette-Guérin (BCG), vaccinia/smallpox, measles, mumps, rubella, yellow fever, or oral polio.[11] HSCT recipients are eligible for revaccination with some of the live virus vaccines 2 years after transplantation, provided the patient does not have graft-versus-host disease (GVHD) or is not receiving ongoing pharmacologic immunosuppression (see Chapter 110, Table 110-4).

Defects in the Humoral Immune System

Immunoglobulin and complement are components of the humoral immune system. Immunoglobulin and complement both have associated lytic and neutralizing activities. Patients with primary or secondary defects or deficiencies in humoral immunity are susceptible to recurrent pyogenic infections from polysaccharide-encapsulated bacteria, such as *Streptococcus pneumoniae, Haemophilus influenzae,* and *Neisseria* species. HSCT recipients who continue to receive immunosuppressants more than 100 days after transplantation should be given antimicrobial prophylaxis with coverage for encapsulated bacteria until immunosuppression is discontinued. Patients are also at risk for infections from enteroviruses and *Giardia lamblia*. Patients with low levels of circulating IgG may benefit from intravenous Ig (IVIg) infusions, although the benefit of using of IVIg infusions for routine prophylaxis must be weighed against the expense of this approach.

Abnormalities in Splenic Function

A number of hematologic disorders are complicated by either intrinsic splenic impairment or splenectomy. The spleen removes organisms from the blood that have been ineffectively opsonized by complement, serving an adjunctive role in fighting infection. It is involved in the regulation of the alternate complement pathway, and low levels of immunoglobulin and properdin have been reported in patients after splenectomy. Alternate pathway defects may be particularly important in patients with splenic dysfunction associated with sickle cell disease.

Asplenic or splenectomized patients are at increased risk for serious, frequently fulminant, bacterial infections, primarily for infections caused by *S. pneumoniae, H. influenzae, Neisseria, Babesia,* and *Capnocytophaga canimorsus*. The initial presentation of even overwhelming infection can be subtle, with fever often the only sign. Accordingly, all asplenic patients with underlying hematologic disease who present with fever should be managed initially as potentially septic. Overwhelming infection after splenectomy occurs in approximately 7% of postsplenectomy patients, with 50% of infection-related deaths occurring in the first 3 months. Prophylaxis against pneumococcal infection is used for asplenic patients who are small children or for those with increased immune impairment from malignant disease.

Pneumococcal, *H. influenzae* type b, and meningococcal vaccines should be administered to asplenic patients. Patients with an intact spleen may respond better to pneumococcal polysaccharide vaccine than do splenectomized patients, so immunization is recommended as early as possible before elective surgery. Additionally, immunization before splenectomy can result in protective pneumococcal antibody titers immediately after the operation. For patients with Hodgkin lymphoma, the antibody response to pneumococcal vaccine may not be affected by the timing of immunization relative to splenectomy. Immunizations reduce, but do not eliminate the risk for serious infection with encapsulated bacteria.

Anatomic Alterations in Host Defense

Immunocompromised patients frequently have disruptions in the skin and mucosa, which are important primary physical barriers against endogenous and exogenous sources of infections (Fig. 88-1). Disruption of skin and mucosa may result from invasion by malignant cells, from the effects of chemotherapy or radiation therapy, from use of invasive diagnostic or therapeutic procedures (e.g., intravenous catheters), and from the effects of local infections, such as oral HSV. Such alterations may provide a nidus for microbial colonization, a focus for localized infection, and a portal of entry for systemic invasion. Organisms associated with defects in skin or mucosal surfaces depend on the site of breakdown, local colonizing flora, and other factors. Gram-positive organisms are associated with isolated disruption of the skin from an indwelling intravenous catheter, usually with coagulase-negative staphylococci, but also with *Corynebacterium jeikeium, Bacillus* species, and occasionally atypical mycobacteria.

Gastrointestinal mucosal integrity is frequently disrupted by chemotherapeutic agents. Because the gastrointestinal tract normally is colonized by a multitude of organisms, this state can lead to infection by streptococci, aerobic gram-negative enteric and anaerobic bacteria, and yeast. Mucosal damage can allow normal flora to invade and become pathogens. Lower gastrointestinal ulcerations permit infections by *Bacteroides fragilis* or *Streptococcus bovis*. Oral lesions are associated with HSV reactivation, ulceration, and possible bloodstream infection with other common oral flora such as α-hemolytic streptococci.

The genitourinary tract mucosa may be disrupted by tumors, invasive procedures, or cytotoxic therapy, with subsequent colonization and the potential for local or invasive infection. The most common urinary tract pathogens are enteric gram-negative bacilli, enterococci, and *Candida albicans*. Viral reactivation is common, predominantly from adenovirus and polyomavirus (BK virus), but also from the herpesviruses (HSV and CMV).

The lung, genitourinary tract, biliary tract, and auditory canal are potential sites of mechanical obstruction, increasing the risk for localized infection. Obstruction may lead to stasis of local body fluids, with resultant overgrowth of potentially pathogenic colonizing organisms. Patients with chronic hemolytic states are prone to gallstones that can become a nidus for infection.

Anatomic alteration can predispose to infection simply by providing a nidus for growth of organisms. Many patients with sickle cell anemia and hemophilia have underlying anatomic abnormalities of the bones and joints as a result of vasoocclusive crises causing infarction of marrow, bony cortex, or synovium. In turn, these changes may predispose to infection such as osteomyelitis or arthritis. Decreased local blood flow and increased bacterial adherence may be other contributing factors. Foreign bodies, such as prosthetic devices, can lead to persistent infection after even transient bacteremia.

Infection in Patients With Acute Neutropenia or Lymphopenia Following Chemotherapy or Transplantation

This section outlines predictable infections that can present during acute profound neutropenia/lymphopenia.

Fever

Despite the specific prophylactic measures directed against common pathogens, many fevers occur in neutropenic patients after transplantation or chemotherapy. Fever can be divided into three categories: infectious fever with an obvious source, infectious fever without an obvious source, and noninfectious fever. Risk factor assessment should include knowledge of the temporal relationship to blood product infusions; recent exposure to contagious infection; degree of fever and whether the fever is accompanied by chills, rigors, or diaphoresis; and response to antipyretics. Symptom assessment should include evaluation to assess sinus drainage, sore throat, ear pain, cough, sputum production, shortness of breath, abdominal pain, diarrhea, rash, and dysuria.

The initial workup of fever in a patient with neutropenia, regardless of whether an infectious or noninfectious source is suspected, is identical and includes blood culture, culture of symptom-related sites even if there is no obvious source (e.g., sputum, urine, with/without stool, with/without cerebrospinal fluid), review of medication list for potential contributors to drug fever, review of recent transfusions, chest radiograph, and CT scan of any symptom-related body systems. When feasible, blood cultures should be drawn through an existing indwelling catheter as well as peripherally because this can facilitate the diagnosis of a catheter-related bloodstream infection compared with a bloodstream infection arising from a different source (e.g., the GI tract).[12]

Consensus guidelines on the management of patients with febrile neutropenia have been published.[13] Empiric antibiotics are recommended for all febrile patients with neutropenia, but the type of antibiotics and the site of administration (i.e., hospital vs. outpatient) depends on the severity of immunosuppression, expected duration of neutropenia, and factors related to the local epidemiology and resistance patterns (Fig. 88-3). Patients defined as low-risk using the Multinational Association for Supportive Care in Cancer (MASCC) index can be treated as outpatients, whereas other patients are generally admitted for intravenous therapy.[14] Typical pathogens causing infection in this situation include *Enterobacteriacae, Pseudomonas, Streptococcus,* and *Staphylococcus* spp. Thus antipseudomonal β-lactam antibiotics such as third-generation cephalosporins, piperacillin-tazobactam, and carbapenems are commonly employed as empiric therapy.[15] Vancomycin is administered if staphylococcal disease is suspected or if the patient is clinically unstable while cultures are pending. Severely ill patients are often also treated with an aminoglycoside for the first 48 to 72 hours of illness, although data in support of this approach are lacking.

Therapeutic changes to the antimicrobial regimens are made in response to culture results, but the cultures are negative about 50% of the time (Fig. 88-3). If the patient becomes afebrile, therapy is usually continued for 7 days. Persistent fever after more than 72 hours of empiric therapy suggests an untreated infection. An agent with activity against resistant gram-positive organisms (e.g., vancomycin) should be added at this point if one was not begun initially. If the patient is recovering his or her neutrophil count, no additional changes in antibiotics are typically needed. However, the persistently neutropenic and febrile patient may have an occult fungal infection such as candidiasis or aspergillosis. Thus initiation of empiric antifungal therapy with antimold activity (e.g.,

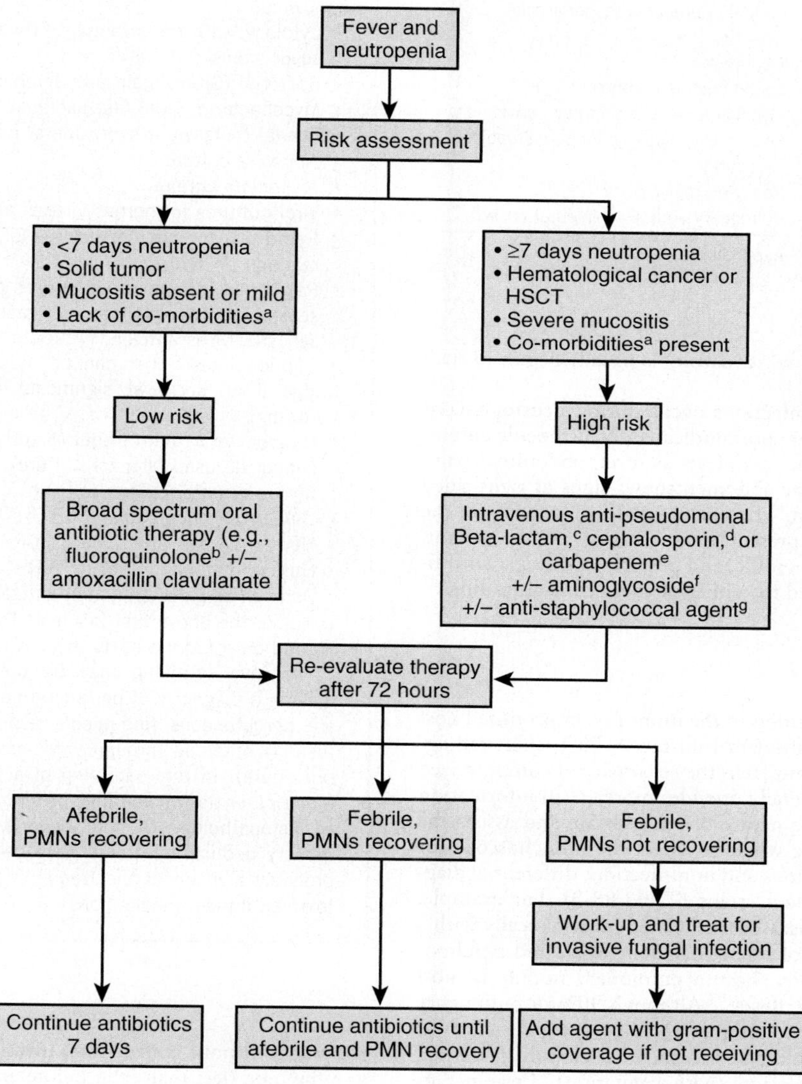

[a] Hypotension, altered mental status, neurologic changes, respiratory failure, abdominal pain, hemorrhage, cardica compromise or new arrythmia, catheter tunnel infection, extensive cellulitis, acute renal or liver failure
[b] Institution sensitivity dependent, ciprofloxacin, levofloxacin, moxifloxacin
[c] Drug selection and dosing institution-specific: piperacillin tazobactam, ticarcillin/clavulanate
[d] Drug selection and dosing institution-specific: ceftazidime, cefepime, [e]imipenem/cilastatin, meropenem, doripenem
[f] Gentamin, tobramycin, or amakacin
[g] Drug selection and instituion institutio-specfic: vancomycin, linezolid, daptomycin, ceftaroline

Figure 88-3 APPROACH TO PATIENT WITH FEVER AND NEUTROPENIA.

Table 88-3 Pulmonary Infiltrates and Their Association With Specific Infectious and Noninfectious Etiologies

Radiologic Sign	Differential Diagnosis
Interstitial infiltrates	Pulmonary edema Diffuse alveolar damage Idiopathic pneumonia syndrome Respiratory viruses: respiratory syncytial virus, parainfluenza, influenza, adenovirus, enterovirus Herpes viruses: cytomegalovirus, herpes simplex virus, varicella zoster virus, human herpes virus type 6 *Pneumocystis* pneumonia
Focal airspace disease	Bacterial pneumonia Fungal pneumonia
Nodules	Fungal pneumonia (aspergillosis) *Nocardia* *Legionella* Septic bacterial emboli Mycobacterial infection (with cavitation) Epstein-Barr virus lymphoproliferative disorder Relapsed malignancy Pulmonary embolism (pleural based)
Halo sign or air crescent sign	Aspergillosis

amphotericin B, caspofungin, voriconazole) is usually begun in such a situation.

Two common anaerobic infections occur during neutropenia at sites where biopsy is difficult or contraindicated. Neutropenic enterocolitis, also known as typhlitis, manifests as fever, abdominal pain, and tenderness. CT scan of the abdomen shows signs of right-sided colonic and ileal inflammation.[16] Excessive soft-tissue swelling of the neck during mucositis can present as a Ludwig angina variant. Broadly active antianaerobic, aerobic, and possibly antifungal antimicrobial agents should be added for either of these clinical findings.

Pulmonary Infiltrates

Pulmonary infections are common in the immunocompromised host (see box on Approach to Pulmonary Infiltrates). Plain chest radiography is a good initial screen but lacks the sensitivity of computerized tomography (CT), which generally provides more useful information in terms of characterizing the nature of an infiltrate and assists the pulmonologist in determining where to direct the bronchoscope for highest yield. A specific infectious and noninfectious differential diagnosis exists for certain radiologic signs (Table 88-3). For example, consolidative focal airspace disease is associated most typically with a bacterial pneumonia. A halo of interstitial changes around a pulmonary nodule or an air crescent above a pulmonary nodule is most likely due to aspergillosis (Fig. 88-4).[17] Although 90% of pulmonary nodules are due to fungal pneumonia (mainly aspergillosis), 10% have various etiologies, including septic bacterial emboli, *Nocardia, Legionella,* mycobacterial infection (with cavitation), Epstein-Barr virus (EBV)–related lymphoproliferative disease, relapsed malignancy, and pulmonary embolism (pleural based). Interstitial infiltrates can be caused by either respiratory viruses during the winter season (except for parainfluenza virus, which is nonseasonal), herpes viruses, *Pneumocystis,* edema, or idiopathic. A complete differential of causes of interstitial pneumonitis (a pulmonary syndrome often associated with HSCT) is given in Chapter 110.

Pulmonary and sinus infections from inhaled molds are more likely to occur as the duration of neutropenia lengthens, particularly beyond an initial 21-day window. For that reason, among HSCT recipients without graft failure, invasive tissue mold infections occur at a low rate (less than 3%) before engraftment because of the environmental preventive measures taken for air filtration. However, if endogenous occult aspergillosis infections are present before HSCT, the infection can rapidly escalate when the immune system is profoundly suppressed by the preparative regimen. This phenomenon manifests as early invasive aspergillosis (before day 40). Therefore patients with hematologic malignancy at risk for occult mold infections in the lungs, sinuses, and at times, the oral cavity should have CT scans of the lungs and sinuses before the onset of any profoundly immunosuppressive regimens, such as HSCT and select nontransplantation regimens. High-risk patients may be given mold-active

Approach to Pulmonary Infiltrates

Pulmonary infiltrates can be divided into three general categories: consolidative, interstitial, and nodular. A consolidative infiltrate may be bacterial, even polymicrobic, so sampling of the infiltrate through sputum or endotracheal tube suctioning for bacterial and fungal cultures is required. If either of these methods does not provide an adequate sample from a consolidative infiltrate, or if these methods do not lead to a diagnosis, "early" (within 72 hours) bronchoscopy is indicated. If interstitial or nodular infiltrates are not peripheral (i.e., within the range of the bronchoscope), they should also be evaluated with timely bronchoscopy. An advantage of bronchoscopy, in addition to the ability to obtain a deep specimen, is that the samples usually are sent for a broad range of diagnostic tests. These tests usually are ordered from preprinted order sheets, which reduce errors. Most preprinted order sheets for bronchoalveolar lavage fluid will test for the following:

- Cytology, with the attendant Fite and Gomori methenamine silver stains
- Bacterial (Gram) stain and aerobic culture
- Mycobacterial (acid-fast bacillus) stain and culture
- Fungal (potassium hydroxide or calcofluor) stain and culture
- *Nocardia* culture
- *Legionella* culture
- Viral cultures for herpes viruses and respiratory viruses
- Rapid test for cytomegalovirus (shell vial or polymerase chain reaction [PCR])
- Rapid test for respiratory viruses during respiratory virus season (pooled respiratory virus shell vial, respiratory syncytial virus antigen, influenza A/B antigen)

Optional tests that can be requested from bronchoalveolar lavage fluid, some at significant extra expense, include the following:

- Mycobacterial stain (requires separate 5-mL volume that cannot be used later for culture)
- *Mycoplasma pneumoniae* PCR
- *Chlamydia pneumoniae* PCR
- Human herpes virus type 6 PCR
- Human metapneumovirus PCR
- *Aspergillus* galactomannan antigen
- Any of the above first-tier tests that your institution does not send on a routine basis (e.g., *Nocardia* or *Legionella*)

Invasive sampling may be the only definitive means for making a diagnosis of peripheral nodules. The two main options are percutaneous fine-needle aspiration or open lung biopsy (usually obtained through video-assisted thoracoscopic surgical procedure). In toto sampling of a lung nodule permits enough material for the whole range of the above diagnostic tests as well as histopathology. Of note, fewer lobectomies of unilateral pulmonary nodular infiltrates have been reported in recent years, probably a result of the frequent use of a broad range of less toxic antifungal medications.

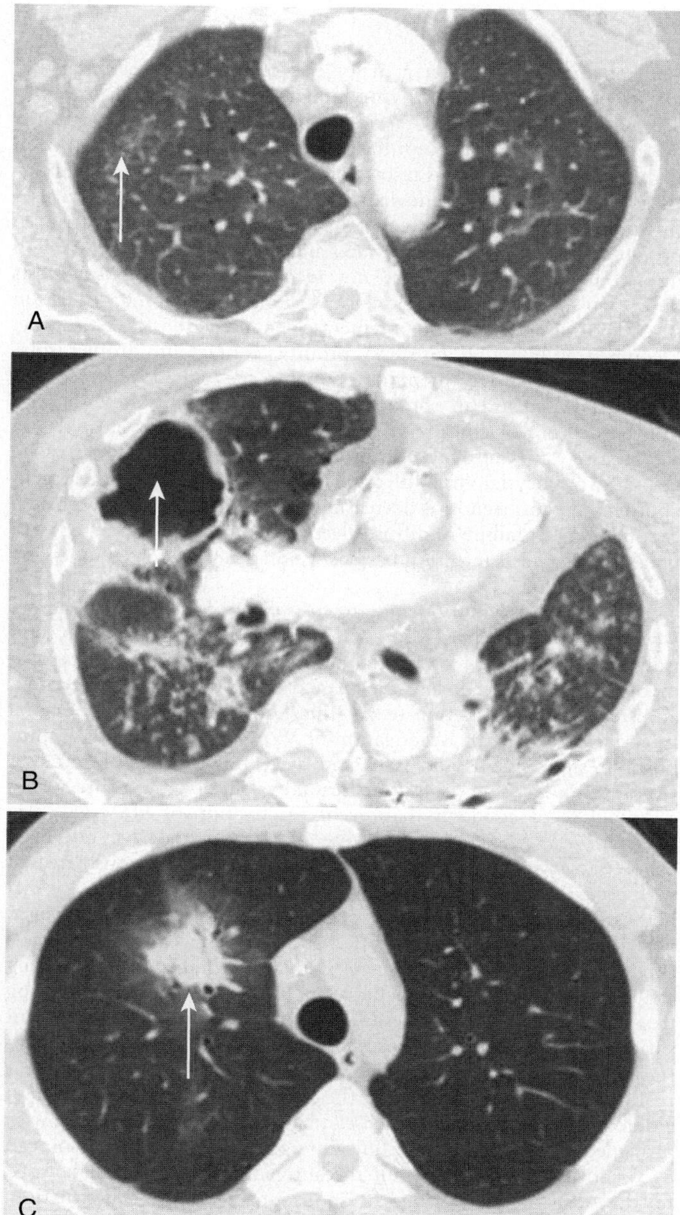

Figure 88-4 CT SCAN EXAMPLES OF DIFFERENT PULMONARY INFILTRATES IN IMMUNOCOMPROMISED PATIENTS. **A,** Diffuse ground-glass opacities in a patient with *Pneumocystis jiroveci* pneumonia. **B,** Cavitary lung lesion in a patient with *Pseudomonas aureginosa* pneumonia. **C,** Lung nodule with halo sign due to *Aspergillus*. For each panel, the *arrow* points to involved pulmonary parenchyma.

antifungal prophylaxis to either prevent or suppress invasive mold infections.

Bacteria

Because bacterial infections cause significant morbidity and mortality in neutropenic patients, broad-spectrum antibacterial prophylaxis is often used during periods of profound neutropenia. The exact agents used vary, but typical agents include a quinolone (e.g., levofloxacin) or a β-lactam (e.g., cefpodoxime). Institutional protocols and resistance patterns drive selection of specific prophylactic agents. Oral prophylaxis regimens are generally discontinued and substituted with intravenous antibacterials with enhanced activity against *Pseudomonas aeruginosa* with the first onset of fever. The use of oral antibiotics among low-risk, neutropenic patients with fever is guided by the use of standardized scoring systems (e.g., MASCC index).[1]

Mucositis, with breakdown of oral and gastrointestinal mucosal barriers, is common during this period. This condition can predispose to sepsis from bacterial and fungal organisms that typically colonize the gastrointestinal tract. The most common serious infections occurring in neutropenic patients with mucositis are bacteremias due to viridans group streptococci and gram-negative bacilli. Such infections are particularly common during the first several weeks following HSCT, so broad-spectrum antimicrobial prophylaxis is generally given during this time period. The propensity of viridans streptococci to develop resistance to quinolones and gram-negative bacilli to be resistant to quinolones and β-lactams means that there is no perfect preventive regimen.

Central venous catheter placement through the skin can lead to blood infection from colonizing gram-positive skin organisms, despite sterile, operative placement of these catheters and antisepsis cleansing procedures.[18] Because the gram-positive bacteremias, including those caused by coagulase-negative *Staphylococcus* species, usually are not immediately life threatening, direct prophylactic coverage often is not immediately provided. During workup of a new fever, some treatment guidelines advocate the administration of vancomycin for several days until blood cultures demonstrate no gram-positive bacteremia. The use of antimicrobial-coated bloodstream catheters can be effective in reducing rates of catheter-related bloodstream infections.

Once a gram-positive bacterial infection is identified, vancomycin therapy is often used empirically until the susceptibility profile is available and targeted therapy can be provided. There are concerns about the efficacy of vancomycin in treating serious *S. aureus* infections because of relative or frank vancomycin resistance. Similarly, if the patient is known to be colonized with vancomycin-resistant enterococcus and the Gram stain indicates gram-positive organisms in chains, therapy for empiric vancomycin-resistant enterococcus is appropriate until the bacterial identification and susceptibility profile is available, usually with daptomycin or linezolid.

Once a gram-negative infection is identified, empiric therapy that includes *Pseudomonas* coverage is continued until the susceptibility profile is available. In the severely neutropenic host, serious gram-negative infections are often treated with combination therapy consisting of a β-lactam plus either an aminoglycoside or a quinolone depending on the antimicrobial sensitivity pattern and patient comorbidities.[15] However, data demonstrating the superiority of combination therapy over β-lactam monotherapy are lacking. The emergence of extended-spectrum β-lactamase producing gram-negative bacilli is a particular concern in patients with significant antimicrobial exposure as are the development of infections with pan-resistant organisms, such as multidrug-resistant *Acinetobacter baumannii* (see box on Treatment of Drug-Resistant Gram-Negative Bacilli). For many infections, the regimen then can be tailored to a single agent and continued for 2 weeks after the last positive culture in clinically responding patients. Therapy with a carbapenem resistant to β-lactamase hydrolysis is required if an organism is isolated that is known to have an inducible β-lactamase enzyme (e.g., *Enterobacter*).

For bloodstream infections, repeat blood cultures should be drawn after 2 to 3 days of effective therapy to ensure that sterilization of the bloodstream has been achieved. Persistently positive blood cultures suggest the development of a deep-seated or endovascular site of infection such as infective endocarditis or suppurative thrombophlebitis. When a bloodstream catheter is proven to be the source of the infection,[12,18] removal of the catheter may be required for most, but not all, infections. At the end of a 14-day treatment course beyond the last positive culture, the patient should be transitioned to an oral gram-negative prophylaxis regimen if still neutropenic.

Antimicrobial agents with anaerobic activity should be added for neutropenic enterocolitis, enlargement of neck soft tissues during mucositis (Ludwig angina variant), or culture-documented anaerobic

Treatment of Drug-Resistant Gram-Negative Bacilli

The widespread use of antibiotic prophylaxis among immunocompromised patients has been associated with the development of antimicrobial drug-resistance, which is especially problematic among gram-negative bacilli. Drug-resistant organisms can colonize the GI tract for prolonged periods of time and emerge to cause serious infections during periods of neutropenia or other medical stress (e.g., following admission to the intensive care unit).

- *Pseudomonas aeruginosa* is the paradigm for drug resistance among gram-negative bacilli and often rapidly develops pan-resistance to antimicrobials. Serious pseudomonal infections are generally treated with two antimicrobial agents, although convincing data supporting this approach are lacking.
- Extended-spectrum β-lactamase (ESBL) production among *Enterobacteriaceae* such as *Escherichia coli* and *Klebsiella pneumoniae* renders these organisms resistant to non-carbapenem β-lactam antibiotics. Treatment is generally with a carbapenem (e.g., meropenem), although a quinolone can sometimes be used.
- The presence of a *Klebsiella pneumoniae* carbapenemase (KPC) can occur among species other than *K. pneumoniae* and creates resistance to all β-lactam antibiotics including carbapenems. Resistance to quinolones is also typical, so therapy is limited to the polymyxins (e.g., colistin), or to tigecycline and the aminoglycosides depending on the organism's antibiotic susceptibility pattern.
- Like *P. aeruginosa, A. baumannii* can develop resistance to all known antimicrobials via a variety of mechanisms. This generally occurs among critically ill patients following prolonged stays in the intensive care unit. Treatment options may include polymyxins and sulbactam, a β-lactamase inhibitor that possesses some activity against drug-resistant *Acinetobacter.*
- *Enterobacter, Serratia,* and *Citrobacter* species can elaborate an AmpC β-lactamase following initiation of β-lactam therapy, which can result in a relapsing infection following an initial response. Thus clinicians treating such infections with penicillins or cephalosporins should closely monitor patients for the emergence of resistance. If resistance does emerge, AmpC-producing organisms can be treated with a carbapenem.
- Patients with multidrug-resistant gram-negative infections should be cared for in such a manner as to minimize spread of these dangerous organisms to other patients. Compliance with infection control protocols is paramount.
- Knowledge of the local epidemiology and antibiogram are important for preemptive and empiric antibiotic choices, especially against gram-negative rods
- A carefully designed and executed antibiotic stewardship program could curtail unnecessary antibiotic use, thereby decreasing antibiotic selection pressure with a resulting decrease in bacterial resistance rates.

infection. Infrequently, tuberculous and nontuberculous mycobacteria are responsible for infections in the bloodstream, catheters, and pulmonary tree. Infections of central catheters or catheter tunnels caused by rapidly growing atypical mycobacterial infections require a high index of suspicion, as well as specific culture media.[19] Organism identification and drug sensitivities may take several weeks. Tuberculous disease can be empirically treated based on risk factors. For patients without risk factors for tuberculosis, recovery of acid-fast bacilli will prompt therapy for suspected nontuberculous mycobacteria, usually with clarithromycin and either a quinolone or ethambutol until specific susceptibility information is available. Tailored therapy is often continued for a minimum of 3 to 6 months.

Viruses

Neutropenia per se is not a major risk factor for developing viral infections but concomitant lymphopenia is common and does predispose to infections with a range of viruses.[20] Respiratory virus infections are seasonal, except for parainfluenza. A frequent pathogen with clinical significance is respiratory syncytial virus, although influenza, parainfluenza, adenovirus, enteroviruses, the herpesviruses (including HHV-6), human metapneumovirus, and rhinovirus also produce diffuse interstitial infiltrates and pneumonitis.[20] HHV-6 and human metapneumovirus are not recovered with the usual tests ordered at the time of bronchoscopy, so a high suspicion for infection is required to order specific polymerase chain reaction (PCR) testing. Documented infection with RSV prompts contact and droplet isolation precautions. Treatment components may include aerosolized ribavirin, IVIg, and in some cases, monoclonal antibody therapy. However, proof of efficacy of these treatments remains elusive, and the disease can cause significant morbidity and mortality.[21] With respiratory syncytial virus infections, aerosolized ribavirin treatment appears safe, and trends of decreasing viral loads have been reported. Secondary graft failure or diffuse alveolar hemorrhage associated with parainfluenza virus infection has been sporadically reported following transplantation.

Patients with lymphopenia are susceptible to a range of herpes virus family infections. Herpes simplex reactivation infections typically manifest as oral or genital ulcers although more widespread involvement can occur and are treated with low doses of acyclovir adjusted for renal function (e.g., 5 mg/kg IV every 8 hours) or oral valacyclovir (1 g bid). Reactivation of VZV can be severe in immunosuppressed persons and is treated with higher doses of acyclovir (e.g., 10 mg/kg IV every 8 hours or oral valacyclovir, 1 g three times a day). Use of acyclovir to prevent reactivation of HSV will also prevent VZV reactivation. Because many patients have not been exposed to acyclovir chronically (except for patients previously treated with recurrent courses of acyclovir for frequent outbreaks of genital herpes), there is little reason to expect resistance to acyclovir. However, HSV infections that appear or persist through acyclovir prophylaxis should be considered acyclovir resistant until viral sensitivity testing can be performed, and consideration should be given to initiating treatment with foscarnet or cidofovir.[22] Reports of acyclovir-resistant varicella are extremely rare. Foscarnet infusions affect calcium homeostasis, so monitoring of ionized calcium and phosphorus levels is required during clinical use of the drug. The major side effect of cidofovir is renal toxicity, which can be reduced to some degree with probenecid and hydration. Clinically significant CMV infection can occur during neutropenia, but the antigenemia test cannot be used for diagnosis or monitoring of response to therapy in this situation, so DNA PCR methods are preferred in that setting.

Human herpesvirus type 6 (HHV-6) is ubiquitous, and reactivation commonly occurs in patients with significant immunosuppression. However, clinically significant disease due to HHV-6 occurs in only a small percentage of patients who have HHV-6 detected in their blood.[23] HHV-6 infection can manifest as fever or pancytopenia. Other recognized clinical syndromes include pneumonitis and encephalitis. Infection is diagnosed by quantitative PCR, although the exact levels of virus that indicate clinically significant disease are not known. Detection of virus in the first 3 weeks following transplantation may be associated with early skin maculopapular rash and acute GVHD, but it can also present without overt clinical symptoms. Prospective large-scale studies are needed to determine the role of HHV-6 infection. HHV-6 has 60% DNA homology with CMV, and treatment of documented infection usually is initiated with induction doses of foscarnet or ganciclovir. Responses to antiviral therapy are not universal, and benefits of foscarnet versus ganciclovir have not been determined.

Cidofovir, when combined with aggressive supportive measures, is considered an adjunct in treatment of BK and adenovirus-associated hemorrhagic cystitis. Similarly, cidofovir can be used to treat disseminated adenovirus infections typically three times a week at 1 mg/kg/day, along with probenicid and hyperhydration.

Fungi

Most yeast infections in immunosuppressed patients are caused by *Candida*.[24] Candidal organisms that colonize the mouth and gut proliferate when antibacterial agents suppress the coexisting bacterial flora population. Guidelines for the treatment of candidiasis have been issued.[25] Patients who are clinically stable generally can be treated with fluconazole unless there has been previous azole exposure or mold infection is also a concern. Unstable patients or those who have been receiving an azole are usually treated with an echinocandin. Prevention of candidemia among allogeneic HSCT recipients is generally achieved with fluconazole. However, fluconazole does not have activity against some nonalbicans *Candida* species (e.g., *C. glabrata, C. krusei*) and all molds (e.g., *Aspergillus, Fusarium,* the Mucorales species). Among patients colonized with yeast species other than *C. albicans* and among heavily pretreated patients who may have incubating mold infection, prophylaxis using a mold-active triazole (e.g., posaconazole) or an echinocandin is preferred.[26]

Although less common than *Candida* infections, mold infections in immunocompromised hosts are a significant source of mortality, with aspergillosis being the most common (Fig. 88-5). Because such infections are difficult to diagnose using standard microbiologic techniques, there has been significant interest in developing more effective screening tests. When used regularly, the serum *Aspergillus* galactomannan ELISA may allow for earlier diagnosis of invasive aspergillosis in some patients.[27] The test is troubled by difficulties with both false-positive and false-negative results and thus needs to be interpreted as part of the overall clinical picture rather than as a standalone diagnostic tool. The development of a fungal infection in a patient receiving voriconazole should raise concern for mucormycosis, which is the second-most common mold infection in many transplant centers. Mucormycosis can rapidly disseminate through the lungs, sinuses, GI tract, and skin, which is uniformly fatal in patients with hematologic malignancies if not diagnosed early and aggressively treated.[28]

Although in vitro antifungal susceptibility testing for yeasts is not as well established as antibacterial testing, susceptibility from bloodstream or invasive isolates can be helpful in the management of infections, especially if the patient will require transition to longer-term oral therapy. Long-term treatment with newer azoles may be valuable in responding patients. Echinocandins cannot be used to treat *Cryptococcus* or Mucorales as monotherapy, but there may be a role for echinocandin in combination treatment for Mucorales. Mucorales species are generally susceptible to amphotericin B and posaconazole, although there are interspecies variations in susceptibility. In the case of mold infections, echinocandin agents may be fungistatic, rather than fungicidal, because interruption of fungal cell wall synthesis is limited to areas of hyphal branch points and growing hyphal tips. Because susceptibility testing for the echinocandin agents is of uncertain reliability, use of an echinocandin after the susceptibility profile has returned should be limited to nonneutropenic patients with uncomplicated candidemia. At present, the efficacy of combination drug therapy is unproven, but such therapy is often used in situations associated with high mortality. Clinical experience, but little clearly documented evidence, supports the value of extended combination antifungal therapy. Molds that often are resistant to amphotericin but may be susceptible to voriconazole or posaconazole include *Fusarium, Scedosporium* or *Pseudallescheria,* and *Trichosporon* (see box on Use of Antifungal Agents in Combination).

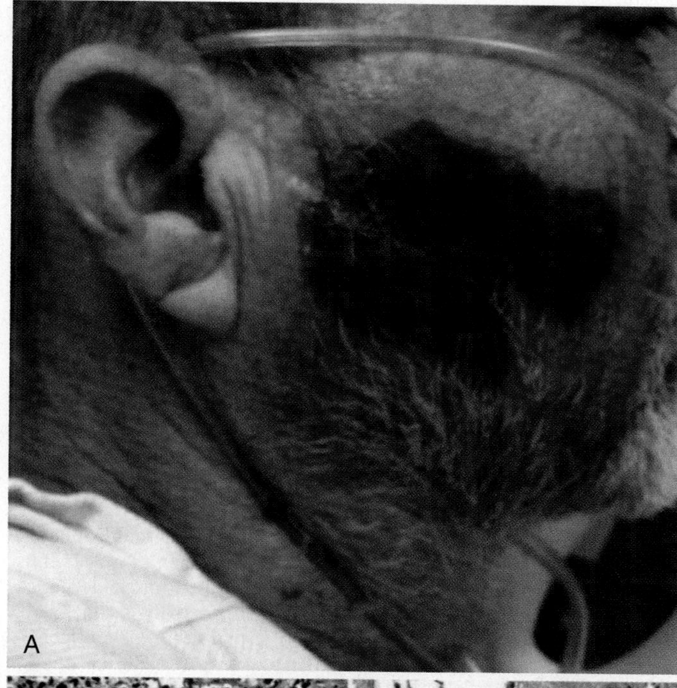

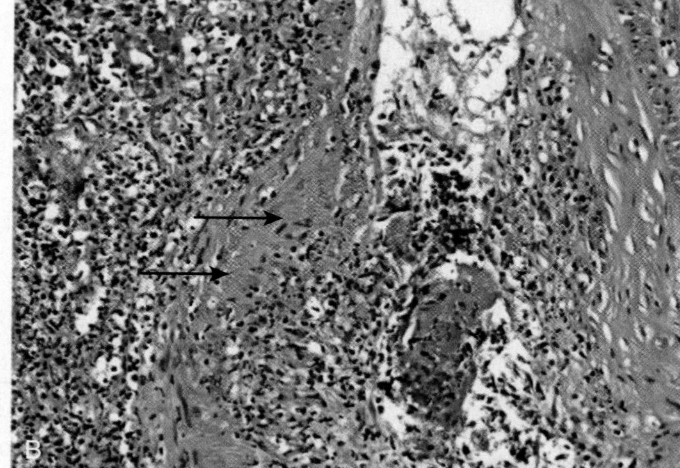

Figure 88-5 EXAMPLES OF ASPERGILLOSIS. **A,** Cutaneous aspergillosis in a patient with lymphoma treated with high-dose steroids. **B,** Invasive aspergillosis with organism invading into blood vessel wall *(black arrows).*

Malignancy-Associated Fever and Drug Fever

Although fever usually indicates the presence of infection, relapsing malignancy, autoimmune-granulomatous, collagen vascular diseases, or immunologic drug reactions can also be sources of fever in the immunocompromised host.[29] Malignancy or drug-associated fevers are the most common causes of persistent noninfectious fevers in cancer patients, but these are "diagnoses of exclusion" that require extensive clinical, radiographic, and microbiologic workup for occult infection until a noninfectious cause is considered most likely. All too often, patients receive escalating empiric broad-spectrum antibiotic therapy during this workup, which should be discouraged in clinically stable patients. Several clinical clues may favor a diagnosis of malignancy-associated fever, including (1) a prior history of fever at the time of initial malignancy diagnosis and (2) response of the fever to a trial of naproxen.[2] Patients with drug-associated fever often appear clinically well with relative bradycardia during periods of fever. Drug fevers typically develop 1 to 3 weeks after the start of a drug (β-lactams, sulfas, vancomycin, and phenytoin are among the most common inciting agents) and resolve, on average, within 48 hours of drug discontinuation unless the patient also has an accompanying rash. Drug-associated fever with rash and liver function test or complete blood count abnormalities (e.g., thrombocytopenia and eosinophilia) are often indicative of more severe reactions that should prompt immediate discontinuation or substitution of the likely offending medications.

Use of Antifungal Agents in Combination

The development of new antifungal drugs gives the clinician more options for prophylaxis and therapy than in previous years. There is an overall level of simplicity to the drug choices once their mechanisms of action are understood. The polyenes, including amphotericin products and the topical agent nystatin, attach onto ergosterol in the fungal cell membrane and are considered fungicidal, because cytoplasm leaks out, and individual cells die. The azoles, including fluconazole, itraconazole, voriconazole, and posaconazole, prevent the formation of new ergosterol. Azoles are considered fungistatic, because removal of the drug permits cell regrowth. Theoretically, use of an azole together with a polyene may have an overall static effect for an established infection as the ergosterol target for the fungicidal polyene is depleted. However, this combination may have advantages in terms of enhanced spectrum of activity. The echinocandins, including caspofungin, micafungin, and anidulafungin, prevent interaction of the catalytic and regulatory subunits of the β-glucan synthesis enzyme, so less β-glucan is formed for the cell wall. The scaffolding for the fungal cell wall is not maintained, and a dividing cell may burst open when trying to extend the new cell wall over daughter cells. The echinocandins are considered fungicidal for yeasts but fungistatic for molds, because drug activity is concentrated at only the tips of the extending hyphae with little effect on less metabolically active subapical compartments of the fungus. Combination therapy may have the most effect when a cell wall agent (an echinocandin) is used together with a cell membrane agent (a polyene or an azole). There is no role for three-drug therapy (an echinocandin, a polyene, and an azole). Aside from cases of cryptococcal meningitis, in which the importance of combination therapy is well established, the benefits of frontline use of combination antifungal for molds remain controversial, although active investigation continues in clinical trials. The value of combination regimens as salvage therapy for refractory mold infections remains uncertain.

INFECTION MANAGEMENT IN THE HEMATOPOIETIC STEM CELL TRANSPLANT RECIPIENT: A MODEL OF SEVERE IMMUNE DEFICIENCY

Infection is a major cause of morbidity and mortality in HSCT recipients. Such patients are susceptible to a wide range of infections, but the risk for a particular infection depends on a multitude of factors, including the type of transplantation, the length of time since transplantation, and the development of GVHD. A summary of common infections occurring in HSCT recipients is shown in Fig. 88-6.

Pretransplantation Prophylactic Techniques in Hematopoietic Stem Cell Transplant Recipients

Over the four decades during which HSCT has evolved, antimicrobial prophylaxis regimens have advanced to prevent common or high-risk infections.[3] This is balanced by problems associated with the preventive regimen, including toxicity, overgrowth of resistant organisms, and sometimes high cost. Algorithms for these preventive regimens evolve with changes in epidemiology, diagnostic methods, and new treatment agents for infections. Despite an overall preventive approach, infections still occur when a severe immune defect persists, when the infecting inoculum of organisms is large, when diagnostic methods are not sensitive enough for early detection, or when infecting agents overcome the effect of the antimicrobial agents. Measures taken to prevent infection in the preengraftment HSCT patient include pretransplantation serostatus blood workup, environmental measures to prevent infection (including frequent handwashing), and common sense.

Assessment of Pretransplantation Serostatus

Current pretransplant serologic testing of donor and recipient includes assaying for latent viruses (herpesvirus antibodies, hepatitis panels, and human T-cell lymphotropic virus antibodies [human

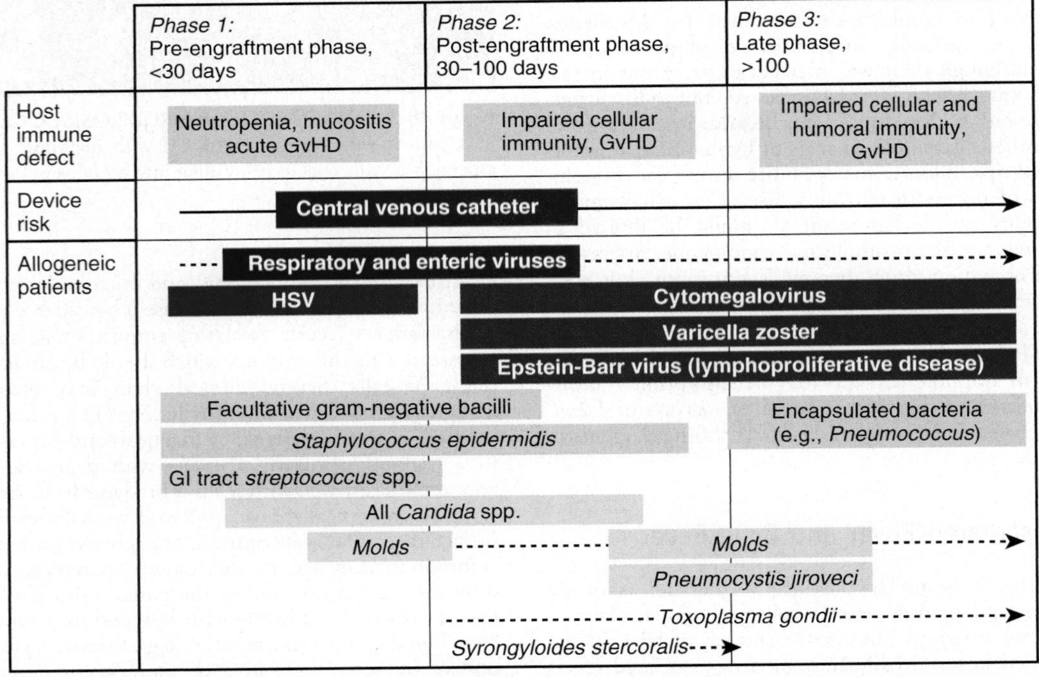

Figure 88-6 TIMING OF INFECTIONS FOLLOWING HEMATOPOIETIC STEM CELL TRANSPLANT. *GVHD,* Graft-versus-host disease.

T-lymphotropic virus I/II and HIV 1/2]) and syphilis. Antibody tests that are checked variably among individual transplantation centers include VZV, EBV, and *Toxoplasma*.

Herpes Simplex Virus

If the antibody test for HSV indicates prior infection or if the patient provides a clinical history of prior HSV infection (i.e., mucosal sores), latent infection exists and has the potential to reactivate during periods of T-cell suppression and neutropenia. This patient requires prophylactic medication (e.g., acyclovir or oral valacyclovir), which targets HSV for the neutropenic phase of transplantation. HSV lesions can appear as black scabs on the outside of the lips, white- to yellow-based ulcers when found on oral mucosa, or as an unusually severe exacerbation of mucositis or esophagitis. HSV prophylaxis administered until recovery from neutropenia may be helpful even in patients receiving nontransplantation chemotherapy such as acute leukemia induction therapy.

Cytomegalovirus

If the candidate is CMV seropositive before transplantation, the recipient should be followed with periodic (usually weekly) diagnostic monitoring tests (e.g., pp65 antigenemia or PCR) for 10 to 20 weeks. No special measures are needed during neutropenia because a detectable circulating white count usually is necessary for reactivation of CMV. If the patient is CMV seronegative before transplantation but the donor is seropositive, the same monitoring algorithm used for the CMV-seropositive patient is needed.

If the donor and recipient are CMV seronegative before transplantation, infection through blood products is possible; therefore exclusive use of CMV-seronegative blood products or other means of preventing CMV seroconversion, such as leukocyte depletion by filtration, are recommended. CMV monitoring should be followed weekly, but the duration of this testing can be shortened by 50%, to 6 to 10 weeks, because late infection in seronegative recipients is uncommon.

Varicella, Human Herpes Virus Type 6, and Epstein-Barr Virus

A history of chickenpox is an adequate surrogate for performing the VZV antibody test. As an alternative to ordering varicella serology on every patient, the test could be ordered in patients with no history of varicella infection or vaccination.

Acyclovir used to prevent reactivation of HSV during neutropenia will also prevent occurrence of clinical VZV infection in most transplantation recipients. Later after transplantation, when acyclovir prophylaxis may have been discontinued, VZV reactivations usually are recognized by their characteristic dermatomal distribution, and treated using acyclovir or valacyclovir.

Serology for HHV-6 is not tested before transplantation because more than 95% of adults are seropositive for the virus. The transplantation recipient receiving minimal herpesvirus antiviral therapy during the transplantation procedure is at risk for reactivation of HHV-6. Whether the CMV-seronegative or HSV-seronegative recipient with a CMV-seronegative donor who ordinarily would receive no antiviral prophylaxis is at highest risk is not known. Additionally, the consequences of asymptomatic and untreated HHV-6 reactivation are not known.

The vast majority of adult patients undergoing transplantation and their donors are EBV seropositive. EBV reactivation is in the differential diagnosis of any new mass, such as enlarged nodes or lung nodules after transplantation (Chapter 52). Now that sensitive quantitative EBV viral load tests and effective treatments, such as rituximab, are available, investigators are monitoring high-risk recipients with quantitative viral load studies.[30]

Hepatitis B and C

Hepatitis B (core antibody, surface antibody, and surface antigen) and hepatitis C serologies are tested in donor and recipient before transplantation. Hepatic dysfunction from either hepatitis B or C after HSCT can lead to life-threatening liver complications, including venoocclusive disease and acute hepatic necrosis. Short-term complications are usually due to hepatitis B, whereas the long-term complication of cirrhosis is due to hepatitis C. The risk for hepatitis in the recipient can be reduced by antiviral therapy for recipients and donors who have detectable viral loads and by transfer of immunity from donor to recipient. A hepatitis-infected individual can be used as a donor if no alternative donor is available or if the intended recipient already is seropositive.

The risk for transmission is small when the hepatitis B–seropositive donor has an undetectable viral load; however, careful follow-up of recipients is recommended. A surface antigen-positive hepatitis B donor with a high viral load should be treated with lamivudine or another agent to reduce the circulating viral load before transplantation. High-circulating hepatitis C viral load in the seropositive donor for a seronegative recipient is an indication for interferon or other antiviral therapy of the donor before HSCT.

If the potential recipient has serologic evidence of infection with hepatitis B or C before transplantation, viral load levels should be checked before and monitored after HSCT. High hepatitis B viral load (>10^5 copies/mL) is the most important risk factor for reactivation in patients positive for surface antigen undergoing HSCT. High-circulating hepatitis B viral load in the intended recipient is an indication for lamivudine. There is no evident correlation between hepatitis C genotype and type or severity of liver disease after transplantation. There is currently no effective therapy for hepatitis C in the HSCT recipient, although new agents are being developed.

Human Immunodeficiency Virus

A positive donor HIV test for a recipient candidate not known to be seropositive is a contraindication for donation. If the screening test for HIV is positive, a Western blot study should be completed to confirm the result because of the potential for false-positive testing.

Syphilis

If the indirect screening test for syphilis returns positive and is confirmed by a direct test, high-dose penicillin treatment should be given for 10 days after transplantation.

Toxoplasma

Historically, 15% of patients who undergo transplantation in the United States are seropositive for *Toxoplasma,* but this percentage may be higher for European centers. The risk for reactivation among seropositive patients is 2%, for an overall incidence of less than 1% of HSCT recipients. It is suspected that low-dose sulfa-based regimens, such as those used to prevent *Pneumocystis* pneumonia, may be effective in preventing *Toxoplasma*.

Review of Commonsense Measures to Prevent Infection

Commonsense measures that should be discussed before transplantation or aggressive nontransplantation chemotherapy include attention to diet, travel, crowds, and pets. Additionally, a history of family or social exposure to tuberculosis should be used to guide whether or not a Mantoux test is applied before therapy.

Diet should be reviewed for herbal supplements or restricted foods. Patients may not recognize that most supplements will have to be discontinued after HSCT. Ground meat products need to be thoroughly cooked so that bacteria, distributed onto meat in the grinding process, are killed. Any fruits or vegetables that cannot be peeled should be washed. Salad bars are associated with occasional transmission of infections. Food products or supplements that inherently contain infectious organisms should be avoided, including undercooked eggs. Blue cheeses have molds spiked into the cheese wheel as they are curing and should be avoided. Soft cheeses carry the potential risk for *Listeria* infection. Yogurt contains *Lactobacillus* that, rather than causing gut problems, has been found to cause infection in other sites, including the lungs after aspiration events.

There are no particular travel restrictions, but strategies to minimize transmission of infectious diseases have been summarized. Some social situations, such as sitting in a crowded movie theater or classroom, increase the risk for acquiring a viral illness. Turning away from individuals who are coughing or sneezing may be helpful in preventing the transmission of infections. Patients need instruction to remember to complete the cycle of infection prevention by washing their hands as soon as possible after being close to such an individual. Given outbreaks of noroviruses (Norwalk-like viruses) on cruise ships and other types of outbreaks (e.g., *Staphylococcus*) commonly associated with the close living quarters during this type of travel, cruise ships should be avoided.

Healthy dogs and cats are considered acceptable pets. However, the immunosuppressed patient should not be responsible for scooping cat litter because of potential *Toxoplasma* cyst exposure. Similarly, the patient should not play in sandboxes because these areas are concentrated sites that feral outdoor cats may use as litter boxes. Because reptiles of many sorts have been reported to be infected with *Salmonella,* patients should not touch these animals or the insides or outsides of their cages or tanks. The heated water of tropical fish tanks carry *Mycobacterium marinum*. *Cryptococcus* and *Chlamydophila* (formerly *Chlamydia) psittaci* can be transmitted from large pet birds.

Environmental Measures to Prevent Infection

Persons entering the patient's room to perform an examination or touch the patient (including visitors as well as health care workers) should wash their hands outside the room. Ideally, the institution will have handwashing sinks in the hallways outside patient rooms for this purpose. During respiratory virus season, the infection control department often adds extra signs to doorways and other places in the wards to remind visitors of the importance of handwashing. Staff and visitors without control of body secretions should not be permitted to have direct patient contact.

Some infectious situations require special isolation procedures. Contact isolation (gloves and gowns) is used for patients with adenovirus, methicillin-resistant *S. aureus,* or *Clostridium difficile* infection. Droplet precautions are added to contact precautions for respiratory virus or varicella infection. Carriers of vancomycin-resistant *Enterococcus* are placed in contact isolation until they meet defined criteria for discontinuation of isolation.

Laminar airflow is a cumbersome and expensive isolation technique that has been largely outmoded with advances in airflow and isolation technology as well as current antimicrobial therapy. Historically, it has been most commonly used for patients with aplastic anemia or those receiving T cell–depleted transplants.

High-efficiency particulate air (HEPA) filtration has replaced laminar airflow as the means for preventing infection through ventilation. With at least 12 air exchanges per hour, HEPA filters are capable of removing particles greater than 0.2 μm in diameter, such as mold spores. Patients often ask whether they should purchase portable HEPA filters for the home or apartment they will occupy after hospitalization. In the broadest sense, this is an extra measure that can be used on an individual basis. If portable HEPA filters are used, they should be obtained for each room that the patient will occupy during the day and night, and each unit should be sized for the individual room. A beneficial effect of HEPA filtration in the outpatient setting has not been demonstrated.

Infection in the Hematopoietic Stem Cell Transplant Recipient Preengraftment

The major risk factors for infection in the preengraftment period include drug-induced mucositis, profound neutropenia, and the presence of indwelling catheters. Thus the major infections observed in this period are due to bacteria that colonize the skin and GI tract (e.g., viridans group streptococci and gram-negative bacilli), *Candida,* and respiratory viruses, especially in the winter months (see Fig. 88-6). Reactivation of latent or partially treated fungal infections can also occur, with *Aspergillus* being well recognized. The propensity of patients to develop such infections has led to widespread use of prophylaxis with an antiviral, antibacterial, and antifungal agent during this time period.

Infection in the Hematopoietic Stem Cell Transplant Recipient After Engraftment

Once engraftment has occurred, the major risk factors for infection include immunosuppression used to treat GVHD and mechanical disruption of mucosal barriers, particular indwelling venous catheters. Viral infections that reactivate after engraftment often are related to defective T cell–mediated immunity and include CMV, adenovirus, and hepatitis viruses. Outpatient HSCT recipients inhale mold spores and *Pneumocystis* cysts from the environment, so common exogenously acquired infections include aspergillosis, mucormycosis, and *P. jiroveci* (previously *carinii*). Bacterial infections associated with defective cell-mediated immunity such as pneumococcosis, nocardiosis, and atypical mycobacterial disease can also occur in association with significant immunosuppression (Fig. 88-6).

Cytomegalovirus

CMV causes significant morbidity and mortality in transplant patients both directly and because of its immunosuppressive effects that predispose patients to concomitant or sequential infection with bacterial and fungal pathogens. Use of prophylactic ganciclovir at engraftment usually is avoided because it leads to myelosuppression and possibly a higher incidence of late CMV disease. Instead, the patient is treated with ganciclovir when weekly PCR or pp65 antigenemia monitoring test meets a positive threshold. Initial viral load levels do not predict disease. CMV infections are treated with an induction ganciclovir regimen followed by approximately 6 weeks of a maintenance regimen (half the induction dose). The duration of induction (1 to 3 weeks) varies by institution, but in general 1 week is used for low-grade infection, 2 weeks for high-grade infection, and 3 weeks for end-organ disease. A rising viral load, when checked weekly during the first month of preemptive therapy, signals the need for continued induction dosing or repeat induction dosing.

When the end-organ manifestation of CMV is pneumonitis (recovery of CMV from a deep lung specimen along with an interstitial infiltrate on chest radiograph), IVIg is added on an every-other-day basis for the duration of induction. When CMV manifests in an end organ other than the lungs, use of IVIg is not as clearly useful. Some centers add IVIg when the patient's total IgG level falls below 400 mg/dL. Dosing schedules vary from IVIg given once weekly for 3 weeks to every other day for the duration of induction, similar to therapy for pneumonitis. Ganciclovir resistance is uncommon, but when it occurs, foscarnet or cidofovir may be used.

Varicella-Zoster Virus

Varicella-zoster virus reactivations from latency (zoster) usually are recognized by their characteristic dermatomal distribution. No temporal pattern is seen, viremia can occur concurrently, and multiple episodes are possible but uncommon. For patients who have been treated for a zoster episode after HSCT, some centers provide acyclovir prophylaxis until 1 year after HSCT. Less common VZV clinical manifestations that can result in severe infection and may require molecular testing or viral culture for diagnosis include hemorrhagic pneumonia, hepatitis, central nervous system disease, thrombocytopenia, and retinal necrosis.

HSCT recipients with a negative or unknown VZV disease history and a significant exposure to active varicella are susceptible to primary VZV infection. For these patients, varicella-zoster immune globulin should be provided within 96 hours of exposure. Patients with positive serology can become clinically reinfected after exposure and should be provided with acyclovir prophylaxis; however, such patients do not require varicella-zoster immune globulin.

Epstein-Barr Virus

EBV causes a spectrum of scenarios after stem cell transplantation, ranging from asymptomatic but detectable viremia, hemophagocytic syndrome, or posttransplant lymphoproliferative disorder (Chapter 52). The incidence of EBV-related complications is higher in mismatched donors, patients with T cell–depleted transplants, and patients receiving intensive immunosuppression (e.g., antithymocyte globulin). Posttransplant lymphoproliferative disorder after allogeneic stem cell transplantation most often is of donor origin. Quantitative EBV viral load diagnostic testing is relatively new and not standardized, so the algorithms for monitoring and initiation of treatment vary. Recognition of greater than 1000 viral copies/mL of blood requires investigation, repeated testing, and possibly treatment, especially in high-risk patients. Direct antiviral agents have limited impact on reducing detectable EBV viral loads. General treatment approaches involve reduction of immunosuppression and rituximab or donor lymphocyte infusion (see Chapter 52).

Invasive Mold Infections

Invasive fungal infections are among the most feared complications of HSCT both because of their high mortality rates and the difficulty in establishing a diagnosis.[4] Among HSCT recipients studied at autopsy, yeast and mold infections were common, seen in more than 25% of deaths. The probability of survival is higher in recent years, likely due to newer and more effective agents, as well as nonmyeloablative conditioning. Posaconazole has been shown to be effective in preventing invasive fungal infections during GVHD, but erratic absorption and the lack of an intravenous formulation limit its efficacy.[5] Mold spores may initiate a localized infection in the lungs or sinuses that, after intensive immunosuppression for GVHD, may disseminate to the skin, abdominal organs, or central nervous system. Treatment of central nervous system infections should include voriconazole, which attains cerebrospinal fluid levels approximately 50% those of plasma or central nervous system tissue levels approximately 200% those of plasma. Infection with Mucorales organisms tends to have later onset than infection with *Aspergillus* (after day 90).[4]

Pneumocystis

The most common presenting symptoms of *Pneumocystis* infection are dyspnea, cough, and fever. Diagnosis requires demonstration of the organism in silver-stained specimens (bronchoalveolar lavage or lung biopsy). Disease occurs by both new infection and activation of latent infection. Most patients present between day 40 and day 80 after HSCT, but cases as early as day 12 and as late as 42 months after HSCT have been reported. Once lymphocyte function is more reconstituted, *Pneumocystis* infections are rare. Prophylaxis options include trimethoprim-sulfamethoxazole, aerosol or intravenous pentamidine, dapsone, and atovaquone. Among patients treated with dapsone after transplantation, increased red blood cell and platelet transfusion requirements are noted. Prophylaxis is generally discontinued 1 to 2 years after HSCT, or later if immunosuppression is ongoing.

Parasitic Infections

Toxoplasma gondii is a ubiquitous pathogen that causes significant morbidity and mortality. Although relatively uncommon, toxoplasmosis is recognized as a cause of cerebral, ocular, and lung disease in immunocompromised patients. Accurate diagnosis of this treatable infection is critical. PCR-based testing has become an adjunct method for diagnosis, occasionally replacing tissue biopsy.

Infection Issues in the Late Posttransplantation Period

Encapsulated Organism Prophylaxis

Penicillin prophylaxis has decreased the incidence of infection-related morbidity and mortality from polysaccharide-encapsulated bacteria (*S. pneumoniae, H. influenzae* type b, *Neisseria meningitidis*). Penicillin-resistant pneumococcal infection has been reported, prompting consideration of alternate prophylaxis, such as a change from penicillins to quinolones. Prophylaxis is generally discontinued 2 years after HSCT, or later if GVHD and immunosuppression are ongoing at the 2-year time point. Once the patient is ready for vaccinations, conjugate pneumococcal, meningococcal, and *H. influenzae* type b vaccines are given.

Vaccination

Recipients of HSCT frequently lose antibody responses to viral and bacterial pathogens previously targeted by childhood vaccination. Although practice varies among transplantation centers, killed-virus vaccines are often given at 1 year after HSCT and live-virus vaccines approximately 2 years after HSCT for patients without GVHD.[6] For adults, Tdap (formulation of reduced-antigen, combined diphtheria-tetanus-acellular pertussis vaccine) has replaced Td (diphtheria-tetanus booster vaccine) as a means for decreasing the adult reservoir of pertussis. For protection against hepatitis, the combined vaccine providing protection against both hepatitis A and B can be used. The efficacy of vaccination is influenced by the time elapsed since transplantation, the nature of the hematopoietic graft, the presence of GVHD, and the use of serial immunization. Guidelines have been published (Chapter 110, Table 110-4).

REFERENCES

1. Parody R, Martino R, Rovira M, et al: Severe infections after unrelated donor allogeneic hematopoietic stem cell transplantation in adults: Comparison of cord blood transplantation with peripheral blood and bone marrow transplantation. *Biol Blood Marrow Transplant* 12:748, 2006.
2. Koo S, Baden LR: Infectious complications associated with immunomodulating monoclonal antibodies used in the treatment of hematologic malignancy. *J Natl Compr Canc Netw* 6:213, 2008.
3. Gea-Banacloche JC: Rituximab-associated infections. *Semin Hematol* 47:198, 2010.
4. Morrison VA: Infectious complications of chronic lymphocytic leukaemia: Pathogenesis, spectrum of infection, preventive approaches. *Best Pract Res Clin Haematol* 23:153, 2010.
5. Pratt G, Goodyear O, Moss P: Immunodeficiency and immunotherapy in multiple myeloma. *Br J Haematol* 138:579, 2007.

6. Song E, Jaishankar GB, Saleh H, et al: Chronic granulomatous disease: A review of the infectious and inflammatory complications. *Clin Mol Allergy* 9, 2011.
7. Ramakrishnan M, Moisi JC, Klugman KP, et al: Increased risk of invasive bacterial infections in African people with sickle-cell disease: A systematic review and meta-analysis. *Lancet Infect Dis* 10:337, 2010.
8. Falagas ME, Vardakas KZ, Samonis G: Decreasing the incidence and impact of infections in neutropenic patients: Evidence from meta-analyses of randomized controlled trials. *Curr Med Res Opin* 24:235, 2008.
9. Engelhard D, Akova M, Boeckh MJ, et al: Bacterial infection prevention after hematopoietic cell transplantation. *Bone Marrow Transplant* 44:470, 2009.
10. Clark OA, Lyman GH, Castro AA, et al: Colony-stimulating factors for chemotherapy-induced febrile neutropenia: A meta-analysis of randomized controlled trials. *J Clin Oncol* 23:4214, 2005.
11. Ljungman P, Cordonnier C, Einsele H, et al: Vaccination of hematopoietic cell transplant recipients. *Bone Marrow Transplant* 44:526, 2009.
12. Mermel LA, Allon M, Bouza E, et al: Clinical practice guidelines for the diagnosis and management of intravascular catheter-related infection: 2009 update by the Infectious Diseases Society of America. *Clin Infect Dis* 49:45, 2009.
13. Freifeld AG, Bow EJ, Sepkowitz KA, et al: Clinical practice guideline for the use of antimicrobial agents in neutropenic patients with cancer: 2010 update by the Infectious Diseases Society of America. *Clin Infect Dis* 52:431, 2011.
14. Baskaran ND, Gan GG, Adeeba K: Applying the Multinational Association for Supportive Care in Cancer risk scoring in predicting outcome of febrile neutropenia patients in a cohort of patients. *Ann Hematol* 87:569, 2008.
15. Paul M, Yahav D, Bivas A, et al: Anti-pseudomonal beta-lactams for the initial, empirical, treatment of febrile neutropenia: Comparison of beta-lactams. *Cochrane Database Syst Rev* CD005197, 2010.
16. Blijlevens NM: Neutropenic enterocolitis: Challenges in diagnosis and treatment. *Clin Adv Hematol Oncol* 7:530, 2009.
17. Georgiadou SP, Sipsas NV, Marom EM, et al: The diagnostic value of halo and reversed halo signs for invasive mold infections in compromised hosts. *Clin Infect Dis* 52:1155, 2011.
18. O'Grady NP, Alexander M, Burns LA, et al: Guidelines for the prevention of intravascular catheter-related infections. *Clin Infect Dis* 52:e193, 2011.
19. Redelman-Sidi G, Sepkowitz KA: Rapidly growing mycobacteria infection in patients with cancer. *Clin Infect Dis* 51:434, 2010.
20. Kumar D: Emerging viruses in transplantation. *Curr Opin Infect Dis* 23:378, 2010.
21. Shah JN, Chemaly RF: Management of RSV infections in adult recipients of hematopoietic stem cell transplantation. *Blood* 117:2763, 2011.
22. Piret J, Boivin G: Resistance of herpes simplex viruses to nucleoside analogues: Mechanisms, prevalence, and management. *Antimicrob Agents Chemother* 55:472, 2011.
23. Agut H: Deciphering the clinical impact of acute human herpesvirus 6 (HHV-6) infections. *J Clin Virol* 52:171, 2011.
24. Kontoyiannis DP, Marr KA, Park BJ, et al: Prospective surveillance for invasive fungal infections in hematopoietic stem cell transplant recipients, 2001-2006: Overview of the Transplant-Associated Infection Surveillance Network (TRANSNET) database. *Clin Infect Dis* 50:1100, 2010.
25. Pappas PG, Kauffman CA, Andes D, et al: Clinical practice guidelines for the management of candidiasis: 2009 update by the Infectious Diseases Society of America. *Clin Infect Dis* 48:535, 2009.
26. Ullmann AJ, Lipton JH, Vesole DH, et al: Posaconazole or fluconazole for prophylaxis in severe graft-versus-host disease. *N Engl J Med* 356:347, 2007.
27. Wheat LJ, Walsh TJ: Diagnosis of invasive aspergillosis by galactomannan antigenemia detection using an enzyme immunoassay. *Eur J Clin Microbiol Infect Dis* 27:251, 2008.
28. Kontoyiannis DP, Lewis RE: How I treat mucormycosis. *Blood* 118:1224, 2011.
29. Zell JA, Chang JC: Neoplastic fever: A neglected paraneoplastic syndrome. *Support Care Cancer* 13:877, 2005.
30. Gulley ML, Tang W: Using Epstein-Barr viral load assays to diagnose, monitor, and prevent posttransplant lymphoproliferative disorder. *Clin Microbiol Rev* 23:366, 2010.

CHAPTER 89

INDWELLING ACCESS DEVICES

Franklin W. Huang and Janet L. Abrahm

Indwelling devices that provide prolonged access to the venous and central nervous systems have permitted novel and more comfortable forms of treatment for children and adults. Indwelling central venous access devices are essential for patients who require frequent withdrawal of blood specimens or administration of blood or blood products, peripheral stem cell apheresis, parenteral nutrition, or infusional therapy with medications such as chemotherapeutic agents, antibiotics, or pain medications. These devices facilitate therapies in the outpatient and home settings. Similarly, through the use of indwelling epidural or intrathecal catheters and Ommaya reservoirs, prolonged access to the cerebrospinal fluid (CSF) may be obtained for the delivery of chemotherapy, antibiotics, antifungal agents, or pain medications. The choice of the appropriate device and application of careful maintenance procedures can minimize the associated complications and maximize the patient's quality of life. As therapies continue to become more intensive, maintenance of adequate, reliable venous access is a critical issue for the management of many patients with hematologic diseases. Since 1973, when the Broviac catheter was first introduced, the sizes and uses of indwelling central venous access devices (CVADs) have expanded dramatically. Although exact numbers are not known, it has been previously estimated that 5 million CVADs are placed in patients in the United States every year.[1] We currently estimate that 5 to 10 million CVADs are placed in patients in the United States every year.

INDWELLING CENTRAL VENOUS ACCESS DEVICES

Chronic venous access devices can minimize the physical and psychologic discomforts of repeated venipuncture; prevent venous thrombosis, phlebitis, and vesicant infiltration; maintain patient mobility; and minimize hospital stays. Certain patients with hematologic diseases are at increased risk for the development of thrombophlebitis from standard (peripheral) intravenous lines and may therefore be best served by an indwelling access device. Factors associated with this increased risk include age of the patient (60 years or older); certain characteristics of the solutions being infused (e.g., hypertonicity of the solution, irritating diluents such as alcohol, highly acidic or alkaline pH, particulate matter in the solution); type of drugs infused (vesicant chemotherapy, certain antibiotics, dexamethasone, furosemide, phenytoin); factors associated with the catheter itself and its insertion (size and composition, traumatic insertion, microbial contamination); and duration of infusion (85% of cases of phlebitis occur 24 to 48 hours after placement of the intravenous line). Because patients with these risk factors or with visibly poor peripheral venous access can usually be identified before therapy begins, early placement of an indwelling device is reasonable. To minimize the occurrence of septic episodes, the devices should be placed before the administration of agents that induce neutropenia. With platelet transfusions, catheters and ports can be safely placed surgically or radiologically in patients whose thrombocytopenia (platelet count less than 50,000/mm^3) is caused by conditions other than disseminated intravascular coagulation.

DEVICE TYPES

Catheters

In all indwelling catheters used for prolonged central venous access, the proximal capped portion of the catheter exits from a subcutaneous tunnel on the chest or abdominal wall while the distal tip is indwelling in a central vein (Fig. 89-1). All catheters are composed of radiopaque elastomeric hydrogel, polyurethane, or silicone elastomer but differ in types of opening and internal diameter. Catheter design varies among manufacturers with some catheters having end openings at the distal tip, others having side openings, and some having end and side openings.

Catheters with a simple opening at the distal tip include those placed at the bedside (i.e., midline catheters and peripherally inserted central catheters [PICC]) and the tunneled Hickman, Broviac, and apheresis catheters, which are surgically inserted. Hickman catheters can have single, double, or triple lumens and have an anchoring cuff in subcutaneous tissue. Broviac catheters have a smaller internal lumen diameter than Hickman catheters and are primarily used in the pediatric setting. Midline catheters, which do not extend into the veins beyond the arm itself, come with single or double lumens. Their use is restricted to nonirritating and nearly isoosmotic therapies and has declined in favor of the more versatile PICCs. PICCs terminate in the superior vena cava (SVC) and are available as single, double, or triple lumen catheters. The tunneled catheters are generally double or triple lumen and extend to the SVC. For apheresis (e.g., for peripheral stem cell harvest), for preoperative exchange transfusions, or for vasoocclusive crisis in patients with sickle cell disease, the catheters used are shorter, with larger lumens, than Hickman catheters to allow for flow of large volumes.

Valved catheters (e.g., Groshong, PASV) are available in a variety of internal diameters and are designed to prevent the reflux of blood into the catheter tip. The valve allows the catheter to be flushed with saline solution rather than with heparin. The PASV has a pressure-sensitive valve at the proximal end, and the Groshong three-position slit valve is adjacent to a closed distal tip. The valve remains closed at rest but opens outward for infusion when positive pressure is applied and opens inward for aspiration when negative pressure is applied. Valved catheters are also available as peripherally inserted devices.

For patients requiring multiple simultaneous therapies (e.g., nutritional support or infusional therapy, along with blood sampling and blood product administration), all the previously mentioned catheters are available with double lumens, and a triple-lumen tunneled catheter is available as well.

Implantable Central Venous Devices (Ports)

In the United States, more than 200,000 ports are implanted annually, and their use is increasing. Ports provide potentially lower infection rates than tunneled central venous catheters (CVCs) and are useful for long-term intermittent access that is needed in outpatient chemotherapy. These totally implantable CVADs consist of single- or dual-lumen ports that may be round, square, oval, or hexagonal and are connected to a radiopaque silicone elastomer or polyurethane catheter (Fig. 89-2). Ports are also available in low profile (less depth) designs. The port includes a self-sealing silicone septum with a body of plastic or metal, both of which can cause an artifact on magnetic resonance imaging (MRI). The artifact effect is greater with stainless steel than with plastic. Many ports now available are MRI compatible. No portion exits onto the chest wall. The port is surgically placed in a subcutaneous pocket, and the catheter is inserted into a central vein. The single or double port is connected to a standard or valved catheter. Ports are available as one- or two-piece systems. The position of the distal tip of the two-piece system is more easily adjusted during insertion because it can be shortened at the port pocket before connection to the reservoir. However, with the two-piece system there is the potential for disconnection of the port from the catheter with resultant infiltration into the port pocket.

The Vortex port is designed with a tangential rather than perpendicular outlet tube to promote more efficient and thorough flushing of the port chamber. This design appears to inhibit buildup of thrombus or drug residuals in the port chamber, resulting in fewer complications than those associated with traditional ports.

Ports that can be placed in the antecubital fossa are also available but less frequently used. The peripherally implanted ports are smaller and flatter than is the standard port. Other implantable devices have self-contained pumps.

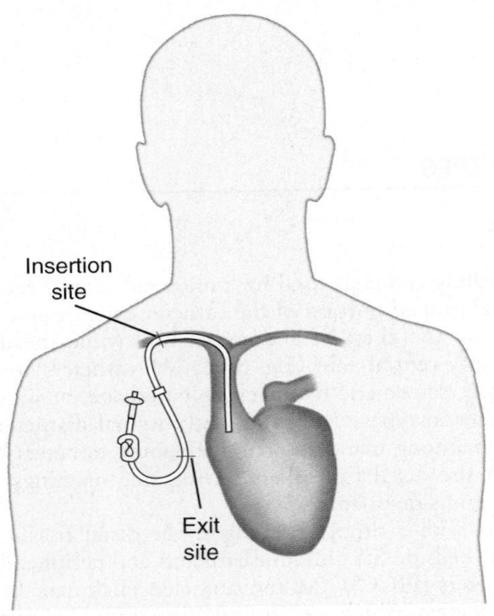

Figure 89-1 Schematic diagram of an indwelling central venous catheter in place. *Insertion site* refers to the insertion of the proximal end of the catheter into the chest wall. Clamp attached to the catheter is shown next to the Luer-Lok cap at the distal end. *(Modified from* Hickman Subcutaneous Port, Use, and Maintenance and How to Care for Your Hickman or Broviac Catheter. *Cranston, RI, Davol Inc.)*

DEVICE CHOICE

Patient characteristics and preference, as well as the duration of use, purposes for which the device is required, and relative complication rates all aid in deciding among the types of catheters and in choosing between catheters and ports (Table 89-1).

Patient Characteristics and Preference

The peripheral devices are helpful in patients with chest wall abnormalities that preclude the use of centrally placed catheters or ports (e.g., subcutaneous carcinoma of the chest wall, open wounds, tracheostomies, or fibrosis induced by radiation therapy).

In patients with a known heparin allergy or who develop heparin-induced thrombocytopenia (HIT), valved catheters that do not require heparin for maintenance are particularly appropriate for patients in whom continuation of a CVAD is necessary. Although

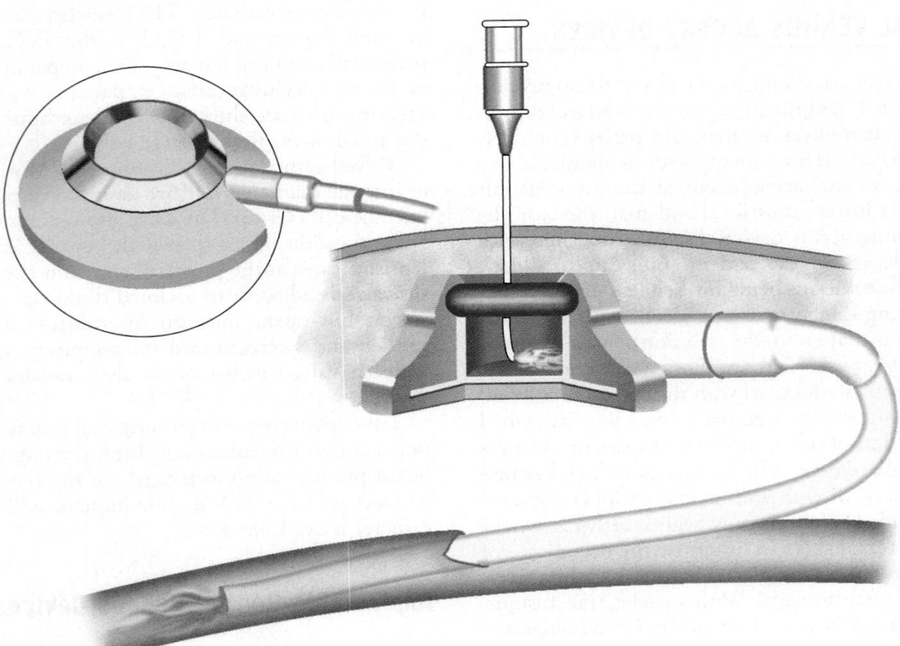

Figure 89-2 Totally implanted Hickman subcutaneous (central venous access) port with a noncoring needle in place. *(Modified from* Hickman Subcutaneous Port, Use, and Maintenance and How to Care for Your Hickman or Broviac Catheter. *Cranston, RI, Davol Inc.)*

Table 89-1 Choices of Indwelling Venous Access Devices

	Duration of Use	Access in Thrombocytopenia?	Uses	Comments
Peripheral port	<3 mo	Yes	Patients with chest wall problems; intermittent access	Not commonly used
Tunneled CVC	>6 mo	Yes	Commonly used in leukemia induction chemotherapy and bone marrow transplant; used for hyperalimentation	Lower risk for infection than with nontunneled CVCs
PICC (peripherally inserted central catheter)	<6 mo	Yes	Can be accessed frequently; rapid infusion, vesicant infusion, hyperalimentation; useful in patients with limited peripheral access	Lower risk for infection than with nontunneled CVCs; can be placed and removed easily at bedside; can be placed in patients with thrombocytopenia (<50,000 plts per microliter) or with elevated INR
Port	>6 mo	No	Prolonged and intermittent access for chemotherapy administration and blood draws	Less infection risk than with catheters; placement and removal by surgery or interventional radiology; can be used for patient with sickle cell disease or hemophilia

rare, HIT from catheter flushes alone has been documented with heparin flush doses as low as 60 units per day. Valved catheters require somewhat less care than standard catheters and may be preferred for patients unable to care for a Hickman or Broviac catheter at home.

Children and adolescents have lower risks for complications with ports than with catheters; indeed, studies have indicated a significantly lower complication rate, especially in the youngest children, when ports are used rather than catheters. Implantable devices have several advantages for children in particular: they are cosmetically acceptable, cause less limitation of activities, are at less risk for accidental dislodgment or damage, and require less care when not in active use. Ports also have a lower rate of infectious complications in adult patients and are especially useful for adults who are unable to care for a catheter or who do not wish to do so, as well as for those who prefer a less visible access device.

Port systems are less successful in patients with hematologic malignancies because these patients are at an increased risk for developing any type of complication such as infection and thrombosis. Ports are also less successful when placed outside the cervical or infraclavicular areas because of factors such as tendencies for groin infections or catheter thrombosis in low-flow vessels. In patients receiving anti-VEGF therapy with bevacizumab, wound healing issues have been reported after port placement and have led investigators to suggest a 2-week period following port placement before initiating bevacizumab therapy.[2,3]

In obese patients and in patients with thrombocytopenia, the subcutaneous location of ports poses a problem. In the obese patient, it may be difficult to access a port placed deep in the antecubital fossa or chest wall. Needle stability may also be an issue for obese patients. If the needle length is not sufficient, it may be displaced or lifted out of the port by shifting flesh (i.e., if the patient lies on the affected side). For the patients with chronic thrombocytopenia (platelet count below 20,000/mm^3), the risk for hematoma associated with recurrent needle punctures required for access makes ports more problematic.

For hemophiliac patients, consensus recommendations for CVADs have been published to help guide clinicians in patient selection. Ports are recommended both for patients with and without inhibitors, in part to minimize infectious risks. CVADs can be advantageous for small children requiring frequent factor infusions, for facilitating home-based treatment and/or prophylaxis, for rapid and reliable response to a spontaneous bleed, or for administration of immune tolerance therapy.[4,5]

For sickle cell patients requiring chronic apheresis red cell exchange, the limited reported experiences have been poor with permanent access devices such as Vortex ports and double/dual ports. Furthermore, ports cannot accommodate the flow rates required by apheresis machines.

Duration of Use

In patients needing only short-term access (usually several weeks to months), PICCs are ideal. The average PICC is in place for 2 to 10 weeks, but some devices have functioned for more than 300 days. In patients needing a longer duration of infusion and more extensive supportive care, surgically placed catheters and ports are generally preferred. Catheters and ports have remained in place safely for months to years. Most ports remain in place until the patient dies. Of 707 ports studied in an oncology population, 72.4% were still in place at the patient's death (2 to 1960 days in use), and only 13.5% of the ports were removed at the end of therapy.

For patients who require continuous daily access such as during stem cell transplantation, tunneled catheters are preferred.

Purpose for Which the Device Is Required

PICCs are used for antifungal/antibacterial therapy, hyperalimentation, or infusion of chemotherapy regimens that may include vesicant agents. Their smaller bore makes them less useful for blood drawing or transfusion. Contraindications to PICCs include ipsilateral local cellulitis, thrombophlebitis, conditions that affect venous return (e.g., lymphedema, previous axillary node dissection, or hypercoagulopathy). Central ports are often considered for outpatient chemotherapy regimens lasting months and reduce the need for venipuncture for routine blood draws and repeated peripheral intravenous catheters.

In general, surgically implanted catheters are more useful than ports or PICCs in patients in whom frequent access to the device or frequent blood drawing or blood product administration is needed. The larger-bore catheters are more useful for blood drawing and blood product administration, because the incidence of clotting after such use is lower with them than with smaller-bore devices. If a port or a PICC is chosen, the catheter with the largest bore is recommended. In the larger-gauge PICCs, which collapse easily, blood drawing is usually more successful if a syringe is used instead of a vacuum tube collection system.

Continuous vesicant infusion may be more safely accomplished with catheters, because they avoid the danger of needle dislodgment and disconnection of the catheter from the septum associated with the implanted ports.

For support during autologous or allogeneic bone marrow transplantation, double- or triple-lumen catheters are the standard of care. In transplantation patients undergoing peripheral stem cell apheresis, silicone apheresis or the largest-bore standard catheters is preferred, because the internal diameter of the smaller catheters may not support the apheresis procedure. The complication rates for the large-bore catheters in transplantation recipients are similar to those of other central venous catheters used for pheresis or transplantation, or both.

RELATIVE COMPLICATION RATES

PICCs cause more phlebitis than tunneled catheters, and earlier reports indicated that the infection rates associated with their use were also higher than those for tunneled catheters. A large analysis of various types of devices shows that PICCs have higher infection rates when used in inpatients as compared with outpatients, and ports appear to have the lowest infection rates overall.[6]

Conflicting data have been reported regarding the relative complication rates seen with tunneled catheters and ports, although the overall complication rate is probably lower for ports than for catheters. Many studies have found significantly higher rates of complications with tunneled catheters than with ports. The only complication that is no more likely with catheters than with ports is catheter occlusion. Patients with ports also reported fewer restrictions in activity and hygiene.

In HIV-infected patients, retrospective studies demonstrate that catheters appear to cause more infectious complications than ports. Hemophiliacs have higher infection rates than the oncology population for external and implanted venous access devices (71% versus 41%). Hemophilia patients with fully implanted CVADs were 31% as likely to develop an infection as those with external devices.[4] The presence of inhibitors seems to increase the infection rate, though the incidence of infection in inhibitor patients with ports was still only 33% of that with external catheters. There has been debate over potential bleeding risks into a port pocket, with associated infectious risk, versus ample risk reduction with newer recombinant hemostatic regimens such as activated prothrombin complex concentrate or rFVIIa. Given these considerations, this metaanalysis supported the use of fully implantable ports for hemophiliacs with inhibitors.

Sickle cell patients may also have higher complication rates of sepsis and thrombosis than the oncology patient. This may be due to the hypercoagulable state and frequent admissions with resultant antibiotic resistant colonization.

In children with cancer, risk factors for CVC-related complications included having a hematologic malignancy and being younger than 6 years of age at time of insertion. Single-lumen Hickman/Broviac catheters had fewer complications and greatest catheter survival, compared with double-lumen catheters or a PASV catheter.

For more details, see box on Choice of Device.

DEVICE INSERTION

Catheters

Catheters can be inserted surgically or nonsurgically. In the hospital, appropriately trained physicians, nurses, or physician assistants generally place midline catheters and PICCs nonsurgically. Insertion failure can occur in 8% to 22% of attempts, although the failure rate decreases with experience. After careful skin preparation using a sterile technique (and for large-gauge introducers, local anesthesia) and under ultrasound guidance, the catheter is inserted 1 to 2 inches above or below the antecubital fossa into the basilic, cephalic, or median cubital vein. PICC catheters are advanced into the superior vena cava (or, less frequently, the axillary, innominate, or subclavian vein) and secured by sutures or sterile tape. Placement above the antecubital fossa is more acceptable to patients and interferes less with patients' activities of daily living. Radiologic confirmation of tip placement should be obtained before initiating therapy.

Tunneled Hickman, Broviac, and valved catheters (and ports) are inserted surgically in an operating suite or minor procedure room, physician's office, radiology suite, or at the bedside. All catheter insertion techniques include creating a subcutaneous tunnel on the anterior chest wall, pulling the catheter up through the tunnel, and positioning the catheter cuff in it, leaving its remaining proximal portion with the Luer-Lok tip exiting from the tunnel on the chest wall (see Fig. 89-1). The distal catheter tip is then usually placed percutaneously or by a cutdown technique into the central circulation through the axillary, subclavian, internal jugular, or cephalic vein and threaded into the superior vena cava under fluoroscopic guidance. Cutdown technique greatly diminishes the possibility of pneumothorax or hemothorax because the vessel is cannulated under direct visualization. Literature from the dialysis population and a retrospective study of oncology patients suggest that there is a lower incidence of symptomatic venous thrombosis when the catheter is inserted through the internal jugular vein.

The catheter position in the superior vena cava at the right atrial junction should be confirmed by chest radiography. In patients expected to need crutches for a prolonged period, catheters should be inserted through the internal or external jugular vein or in the subclavian vein lateral to the midclavicular line to prevent pinching the catheter in the costoclavicular space, which leads to catheter pinch-off and fracture.

No significant differences have been found in time to failure or in infection or obstruction rate of catheters inserted percutaneously ("blind" or landmark technique) rather than under direct visualization. Real-time ultrasound-guided insertion techniques are associated with fewer placement failures and complications compared with landmark techniques. One study of 589 blind placements had a 92% success rate, with 2.9% of catheters requiring repositioning. Especially thin or obese patients are identified as having a higher risk for insertion failure and complications when the landmark technique is used. Other patients at higher risk are those who have had previous major surgery or previous central venous access devices.

Catheters should be inserted by experienced personnel, and complication rates fall with increasing experience in catheter insertion. Increasingly, long-term central venous access devices are placed with interventional radiology techniques. These image-guided techniques have a 99% success rate at a lower cost than surgical placement and with a comparably low infection rate. Placement using interventional radiology is often obtainable in a more timely manner than with surgical placement. If the chest wall or the vessels of the upper body are not usable, an alternative site is the inferior vena cava, which is accessed through the femoral or saphenous vein or by a translumbar approach directly into the inferior vena cava.

Choice of Device

We recommend indwelling venous access devices based on patient characteristics and preference, anticipated duration of use, purpose(s) for which the device is required, and relative complication rates among catheters and ports.

PICCs can be selected when duration of use will be 3 months or less. They are an appropriate choice when patients have chest wall problems, require outpatient-based treatments, and/or have thrombocytopenia. PICCs allow for vesicant infusions, antifungal and antibiotic therapies, and hyperalimentation.

Peripheral ports may be used longer than PICCs, but not longer than 6 months, and they may be chosen for patients with chest wall problems receiving outpatient-based treatments.

Tunneled catheters may be chosen for patients with thrombocytopenia who require frequent access, rapid infusion, or administration of vesicants. Valved catheters that do not require heparin are useful for patients who should not receive heparin. Like peripheral ports, they may be used for up to 6 months.

Of the various devices, central ports allow for the longest duration of use (more than 6 months). They are appropriate for outpatients, particularly children or adolescents, but they may be problematic in patients who are obese, especially if they are thrombocytopenic. They are used for rapid infusions and administration of vesicants and, if they have more than one lumen, for hyperalimentation.

Ports

Ports are inserted with surgical or interventional radiology techniques into the antecubital fossa or the chest or abdominal wall with the patient under local anesthesia. If possible, the port should be placed in the nondominant arm (or in the side of the chest near the nondominant arm) to minimize the probability of needle dislodgment or coring of the port septum during continuous access.

The chest wall ports are placed into a subcutaneous pocket in the infraclavicular space, and the attached catheter is placed under fluoroscopic guidance into the subclavian, jugular, or cephalic vein and threaded through the superior vena cava to the junction with the right atrium (see Fig. 89-2). No portion of the device remains visible.

DEVICE MANAGEMENT

Catheters

Care of nontunneled and tunneled catheters is begun by the nurses and later taught to patients and their families. To minimize infectious complications, it is preferable to assign this responsibility (as well as infusions and blood sampling through the catheter) to nurses who are expert in catheter care and use. Standard procedures are available and should be adopted by each institution, to be followed by all who care for the patient.

Patient and family education in catheter care is required to maintain patency, to prevent damage to the external portion of the catheter, to prevent air embolization, and to reduce the risk for infection. Instructions should cover permissible activities, techniques of dressing changes, heparin instillation, and changing the Luer-Lok plug, as well as emergency care in the event of damage to the external portion of the catheter. This educational program should be started well in advance of patient discharge to ensure patient and family competence; it may be reinforced by an educational booklet, by attendance at a "hands-on" class, or by nurses sent into the home, at least initially, to verify compliance with procedures. Patients with a catheter or port in place should be given written information about the device, as well as a medical alert card, necklace, or bracelet indicating the device's location, the type of access, and a person to contact if problems arise.

Dressing changes for surgically inserted catheters require a sterile technique for 2 weeks after insertion, until fibrous growth into the cuff is complete. The catheter exit site is cleaned with an antiseptic solution. Povidone iodine has been commonly used in the United States, but chlorhexidine-based solutions may be preferable because they have been shown to reduce the risk for catheter colonization and catheter-related bloodstream infection (CRBSI).

A formulation of chlorhexidine with isopropyl alcohol has been approved by the U.S. Food and Drug Administration (FDA) for catheter site use and has been available for over-the-counter purchase since 2005. Sterile dressing changes are done every 3 to 7 days for 2 to 3 weeks after insertion, depending on the dressing materials used (more frequently for povidone iodine and less frequently for chlorhexidine).

The type of dressing, if any, needed to cover the site once the incision is healed is controversial. One prospective, randomized study indicated that when a rigorous cleaning protocol was followed, the incidence of site infection was no different regardless of whether standard gauze and povidone iodine, a transparent polyurethane dressing (e.g., OpSite, Tegaderm) permeable to water vapor, or no dressing was applied. Current guidelines recommend use of either sterile gauze or sterile, transparent, semipermeable dressing. A chlorhexidine-impregnated sponge dressing decreased the risk for catheter colonization and catheter-related infection in a prospective, randomized study. Their use is recommended for temporary short-term catheters in patients older than 2 months of age if the central line–associated bloodstream infection (CLABSI) rate is not decreasing despite adherence to basic prevention measures.

Dressings should be replaced whenever damp, loosened, or soiled. Moisture vapor-occlusive dressings are strongly recommended for patients with tracheostomies or open wounds near the catheter site. After 2 to 3 weeks, a clean technique is used in some institutions for nonneutropenic patients, and an adhesive bandage or small gauze dressing may be used to cover the exit site. More complete guidelines for access and maintenance of surgically inserted catheters are available.

Except with dialysis catheters, the use of antibiotic or iodine ointment to prevent infection at the catheter insertion site is not recommended, because of the potential for promotion of fungal infection and antibiotic resistance.

As a rule, the catheter is not considered to be securely anchored in place until 10 to 21 days after placement, although insertion site stitches are usually removed after 10 days. Even then, catheters should not be allowed to hang freely; instead, they should be taped to the chest wall or inserted into a brassiere cup. A clamp should be immediately available in the event of any breaks in the line. Some manufacturers include a clamp placed on the catheter. Patients should be advised to keep the catheter out of the reach of pets or small children, who could inadvertently dislodge the catheter by pulling on it.

Because a thrombus on the catheter tip can be the nidus for a bacterial or fungal infection, every effort should be made to prevent one from forming. Heparin should be instilled in nonvalved catheters after each episode of blood drawing or blood product administration and when the catheters are not being used for intravenous therapy. A wide variety of flushing regimens are reported in the literature with various concentrations and volumes of heparin and frequencies, although few regimens are based on research. Based on a review of the available research-based practice, a flushing regimen of 5 mL of 10 units/mL heparin one or two times per week is recommended. In one study, twice-weekly flushing, rather than daily, resulted in a 33% decrease in catheter-related bacteremia without an increase in thrombus or intraluminal clots. A further decrease in intraluminal infection rate in immunocompromised, nonneutropenic patients with tunneled catheters may be provided by adding vancomycin to the heparin flush. However, the antibiotic flush has been associated with increased antibiotic resistance and allergic reactions. Recommendations for PICC flushes range from 3 mL of heparin (100 units/mL daily) to 3 mL of 10 units/mL three times per week. The dose of heparin used to flush the catheter should not alter the patient's clotting factors. At a minimum, the flush should be twice the volume of the catheter plus any add-on devices.

The use of the heparin flush alters coagulation tests if blood is drawn through the catheter. The first 10-mL sample shows spurious elevations in levels of fibrin degradation products, prothrombin times, partial thromboplastin times, and spuriously low fibrinogen levels. Elevations in the prothrombin time and partial thromboplastin time will persist in the second 10-mL sample.

Valved catheters require a 5-mL to 10-mL normal saline flush weekly or after use. The Groshong-type valve can be kept in the open position by small clots or solid residues from medications, allowing blood to flow back into the catheter, forming a clot.

Investigators have examined the potential role for using thromboprophylaxis for cancer patients with central venous access devices. The most recent data show no proven role for using mini-dose warfarin or low-molecular-weight heparin despite being shown to be safe and well tolerated in such patients with hematologic malignancies and pronounced thrombocytopenia. Some experts still advocate thrombophylaxis for patients at high risk for developing catheter-related complications. Dalteparin prophylaxis using 5000 international units once daily did not reduce frequency of central venous catheter-related thrombosis in cancer patients.

More detailed guidelines for nursing education and practice regarding maintenance of catheters are available.[7]

Ports

Ports can be used immediately after insertion. However, because postoperative edema and discomfort often delay any attempts at access for several days, patients should be sent from the operating room with the Huber needle in place and ready for use. Incisions should have a dressing until the sutures are removed. If skin closure is accomplished with surgical adhesive, a dressing is not required after the operative day and the site may get wet after the first day, although it may be preferable to delay this longer.

To access a port that has no needle in place, the skin is prepared with antiseptic; povidone-iodine or chlorhexidine is recommended. Anesthetic agents that may be applied include ice or a cold pack for a few minutes, a freezing agent (ethylene dichloride), or topical anesthetic cream (EMLA), which must be applied 1 hour before needle insertion. A 19- to 22-gauge Huber needle (depending on the product to be infused) is inserted (see Fig. 89-2). This steel needle has a deflected point and side opening, designed to prevent coring of the septum. The needle is primed with saline, attached to a saline-containing syringe, and then inserted perpendicular to the septum. Correct placement in the port can be confirmed by aspiration for blood return. However, aspiration for blood may be unsuccessful, usually because the needle is misaligned or because a fibrin sheath has formed, creating a ball-valve effect. If there is no swelling, the port flows well to gravity and there is no other symptom to suggest a potential problem, the needle can be assumed to be correctly placed and the port safely used for nonvesicant infusions. If access is difficult, it may be helpful to palpate the site while comparing it with a recent radiograph. Access may also be accomplished under fluoroscopy if standard technique by palpation is unsuccessful. Detailed accessing procedures for drawing blood and for administering drugs and blood products are available.[7] During use, the port is covered with a sterile dressing. A transparent, occlusive dressing may be preferable to help stabilize the needle and prevent inadvertent dislodgment. Dressing guidelines for external catheters can be followed for ports. The needle is changed weekly. After each use or every 4 weeks, implanted access devices also require heparin instillation or a 20-mL saline flush for valved ports. A variety of heparin concentrations and volumes have been reported. Use and maintenance of the peripheral port are essentially the same as for ports implanted in the chest wall. Ongoing discussion continues regarding optimal maintenance procedures.

DEVICE REMOVAL

Device removal should be considered when it is no longer needed, in part to minimize risks for thrombosis and infection, as well as when complications arise. Nontunneled catheters are removed nonsurgically by applying steady tension. If the catheter appears to be stuck, measures should be taken to reverse vasospasm (e.g., application of warm compresses, flushing with normal saline). If the catheter remains fixed, a cutdown on the venous insertion site to remove thrombotic material is usually effective. Tunneled catheters should be removed by surgical cutdown around the cuff, which should be entirely removed. For cases in which bacterial studies of the internal catheter tip are desired, blunt dissection of the cuff, with transection of the catheter above it and sterile removal of its inner portion, can be performed under local anesthesia. Ports, including the reservoir, catheter, and all suture materials, are removed surgically with the patient under local anesthesia. PICCs can be removed by nursing staff at the bedside.

COMPLICATIONS

Complications of indwelling vascular access devices include those occurring during the initial placement, cutaneous reactions to standard care materials, mechanical problems, phlebitis and infiltration, infection, hemorrhage, catheter occlusion of nonthrombotic or thrombotic origin, and vesicant drug extravasation.

Children

Pediatric-specific studies have cited age (younger than 5 years in one study, younger than 2 years in another), use of multilumen catheters, absence of skin exit site suture, and platelet transfusion at time of insertion as the most common reasons for premature catheter removal. Pediatric cancer patients with external catheters have had more complications requiring device removal compared with port devices from infectious causes and occlusive events.

Initial Placement

Approximately 1% to 4% of patients in whom a central catheter is inserted percutaneously develop a pneumothorax. Other surgical complications include hemothorax, arterial venous or cardiac perforation, brachial plexus injury, air embolism, and pericardial tamponade. After placement of PICCs, the distal tip can be malpositioned and requires replacement or repositioning of the PICC.

Cutaneous Reactions

Approximately 5% of patients develop skin reactions to the products used in caring for the devices. These reactions include erythema, urticaria, exanthematous or purpuric eruptions, and skin peeling or abrasion. These skin abnormalities must be distinguished from exit-site infections by appropriate culturing of the site for bacteria. In uninfected patients, changes in the dressing material, tape, and local skin care regimen are effective in reversing the skin abnormalities. Skin reactions may be compounded when the patient has received radiation therapy to the area covered by the dressing.

Skin erosion over the implanted ports, caused by malnutrition, separated wound edges, local infection, or carcinoma metastatic to the skin, occurs in 3% to 10% of patients, and removal of the port is always required. In very thin patients, the risk for erosion may be lower when a low profile rather than standard depth port is used.

MECHANICAL PROBLEMS

Catheters

Damage to the external segment of the tunneled catheter includes separation between the Luer-Lok connection and the tubing; cracks caused by repeated cross-clamping, if rubber-tipped forceps are not used; and cuts made by scissors mistaken for clamps. Catheter repair kits should therefore be available. Patients should also be instructed to contact their physicians or the oncology nursing staff immediately if the catheter is damaged at home.

Catheter fractures and emboli occur in about 0.2% of subclavian catheter insertions. The internal portion of the catheter usually fractures at the junction of the clavicle and first rib, and angiographic studies reveal the pathognomonic catheter pinch-off sign. Catheter pinch-off occurs when catheters inserted medially to the midclavicular line become compressed by shoulder movements. The resulting fragments migrate to the right heart or pulmonary artery and cause thromboses, cardiac arrhythmias, and fatal emboli; extravasation of fluids, lymph, or vesicant agents may also ensue at the site of breakage. Patients complain of pain or swelling at the port or vein insertion site, chest pain, cough, or palpitations. Catheter fragments are usually retrievable with interventional radiology techniques.

PICC lines can also embolize if they are sheared by needles, sutures, or surgical instruments while they are being inserted. If the fragment cannot be prevented from migrating more proximally by applying local pressure at the break site or by placing a tourniquet proximal to the site, it can be removed by venous cutdown. If it has migrated, percutaneous techniques or a thoracotomy will be required, but some fragments are never retrieved. Apheresis catheters placed in the inferior vena cava can also develop fractures of the external segment, with visible leakage, and they can be repaired using the kits mentioned earlier. Fractures of the internal portion of the catheter, however, require catheter removal. Most of these fractures can be detected by injecting radiologic contrast material through them and observing the flow of the dye fluoroscopically.

Ports

The port may migrate or flip within its pocket because of defective suturing or excessive arm movement or because of manipulation by the patient. This malposition can be surgically corrected.

PHLEBITIS AND INFILTRATION

Phlebitis and infiltration are uncommon complications associated with properly positioned centrally placed access devices but are noted with the peripheral port and in 2.2% to 23% of patients with PICCs. Cancer patients with PICCs have had comparable rates of phlebitis. In a randomized, controlled trial comparing the complications associated with steel needles, short Teflon catheters and PICCs, these findings were noted: PICCs were associated with the highest incidence of phlebitis (27%) and the lowest incidence of infiltration (8.1%); steel needles were associated with the lowest incidence of phlebitis (8%) and the highest incidence of infiltration (45%); Teflon catheters ranked in between PICCs and steel needles, with incidence of phlebitis and infiltration at 19% to 20%. An aseptic phlebitis may occur within the first week after PICC insertion. It can be prevented by administration of nonsteroidal antiinflammatory agents or by treatment with warm compresses applied for 48 to 72 hours. Catheter removal is usually not required.

INFECTION

For a list of important infection-related terms and definitions, see box on Infection.

Incidence

Intravascular devices (IVDs) are the most important cause of hospital-acquired bloodstream infections and are associated with increased hospital costs and length of stay.[6] When expressed as infection rate per 1000 IVD-days, the highest risk exists with peripheral catheters placed by surgical cutdown, followed by peripheral steel needles. The lowest rates of infection are associated with subcutaneous venous ports, either central or peripheral. Cuffed and uncuffed tunneled catheters have lower risks for infection than do untunneled catheters. Cuffed devices share the lower rates of infection with outpatient, PICC and peripheral IV catheters, as well as ports.[9] Increasingly, standardized infection control procedures are being used to help reduce CRBSI, as published by the Centers for Disease Control and Prevention (CDC) in 2011.[9]

Between 1% and 9% of patients experience infection at the exit site, tunnel, or pocket. Exit-site infections appear to be responsible for up to 45.5%; tunnel infections, for up to 22% of all catheter-related infections. Most CRBSIs for catheters in place for less than 10 days are of cutaneous origin from the insertion site, and the organisms gain access extraluminally, whereas for long-term devices in place for more than 10 days, luminal colonization is the major mechanism of CRBSI. Prophylactic antibiotics have not consistently proven beneficial in preventing these infections, and their use is not generally recommended. Catheters and cuffs coated or impregnated with antimicrobial or antiseptic show some promise in decreasing CRBSI and remain an area of investigation. Metaanalyses of randomized controlled trials suggest that these catheters may reduce the risk for CRBSI.[10] The compounds that have been used are minocycline/rifampin and chlorhexidine/silver sulfadiazine, but there are concerns about the emergence of resistant organisms with these catheters. The evidence supporting use of these compounds to reduce risk for CRBSI is equivocal for short-term CVCs and inconclusive for long-term CVCs in place longer than 10 days. Current CDC guidelines recommend use of a chlorhexidine/silver sulfadiazine or minocycline/rifampin–impregnated CVC in patients whose catheter is expected to remain in place for more than 5 days if CLABSI rates are not decreasing at the institution despite a comprehensive strategy.[10]

Infections are generally prevented by meticulous insertion and maintenance techniques. PICCs inserted at the bedside show a higher rate of infection than do those inserted by interventional radiologists, probably because of insertion conditions (aseptic technique at the bedside versus sterile technique in the interventional radiology suite). With maximal barrier precautions, however, catheter insertion at the bedside is associated with no higher infection incidence than is placement in the operating room.

The incidence of device-associated infection varies depending on the type of device inserted and the medical disorder of the patient. Overall, the incidence of midline catheter-associated infections is low and that of tunneled catheters is approximately 1 to 3 per 1000 days of patient use. Cumulative incidence of PICC-related blood stream infections is 1.1 per 1000 PICC-days (range 0.9 to 1.3), but higher in the inpatient setting (2.1 per 1000 PICC-days).[6] The use of multiple-lumen catheters probably increases the infection rate significantly. In one study, the sepsis rate for double- and triple-lumen catheters was comparable at 13% and 16%, respectively, but infections occurred significantly earlier with the triple-lumen catheters (a mean of 54 days versus 141). Fewer catheter-related bacteremias

Infection

Definitions

The Centers for Disease Control and Prevention (CDC) has established the following definitions for catheter- and port-associated infections.[8]

Localized catheter colonization: Significant growth of a microorganism (greater than 15 CFU) from the catheter tip, subcutaneous segment of the catheter, or catheter hub.

Exit-site infection: Erythema, or induration within 2 cm of the catheter exit site, in the absence of concomitant bloodstream infection (BSI) and without concomitant purulence.

Clinical exit-site infection (or tunnel infection): Tenderness, erythema, or site induration of more than 2 cm from the catheter exit site along the subcutaneous tract of a tunneled catheter (i.e., Hickman or Broviac) in the absence of concomitant BSI.

Pocket infection: Purulent fluid in the pocket of a totally implanted intravascular catheter that may or may not be associated with spontaneous rupture and drainage or necrosis of the overlaying skin in the absence of concomitant BSI.

Infusate-related bloodstream infection: Concordant growth of the same organism from the infusate and blood cultures (preferably percutaneously drawn) with no other identifiable source of infection.

Catheter-related bloodstream infection: Bacteremia or fungemia in a patient with an intravascular catheter with at least one positive blood culture obtained from a peripheral vein, clinical manifestations of infections (e.g., fever, chills, or hypotension) and no apparent source for the BSI except the catheter. One of the following should be present: a positive semiquantitative (greater than 15 CFU/catheter segment) or quantitative (greater than 10^2 CFU/catheter segment) culture whereby the same organism (species and antibiogram) is isolated from the catheter segment and peripheral blood; simultaneous quantitative blood cultures with a 3 : 1 ratio for CVC versus peripheral; or differential period of CVC culture versus peripheral blood culture positivity of more than 2 hours.

occur with totally implantable venous access devices (ports) than with tunneled catheters. Several social conditions contribute to greater risk for indwelling venous access device infections, including poor hygiene and lower socioeconomic status. For pediatric cancer patients, increased risk for infection is associated with language barriers that limit parental understanding of how to care for the CVC. The infection rate with implanted ports is lower, 0.0 to 0.1 per 1000 patient-days for ports inserted on the chest wall.

Neutropenic patients, particularly with a hematologic malignancy, have a near 14% greater risk for developing CRBSI. Patients with HIV infection and those receiving a bone marrow transplant have significantly higher rates of catheter- and port-related infections. Patients with hemophilia had a pooled incidence of 0.66 infections per 1000 CVAD days; age greater than 6 years and the use of fully implanted CVADs significantly reduced the risk for infection, whereas the presence of inhibitors significantly increased the risk.[4] For adult patients with sickle cell disease, bacterial infections are a leading cause of mortality, and one study cited a greater incidence of bloodstream infections in younger patients with hemoglobin S (HbS) disease, on transfusion and/or desferrioxamine programs, and in patients with a central venous catheter. Of all episodes of bloodstream infections in these sickle cell patients, 41% were attributed to a venous catheter, and device infection occurred in 77% of patients with tunneled implantable ports.[11]

Patients with acute leukemia have higher rates of infection than do patients with other types of cancer. This is in part because of the higher occurrence of catheter manipulation associated with treatment for acute leukemia; longer periods of neutropenia may also be a factor. Patients with acute leukemia are also at higher risk for developing septicemia as a consequence of prolonged neutropenia. The presence of a CVC increases the risk for infection in the early phases of low-intensity treatment for acute lymphoblastic leukemia (ALL) in pediatric patients.

Organisms

The most common organisms associated with hospital-acquired CRBSI are coagulase-negative staphylococci (37%), *Staphylococcus aureus* (13%), enterococci (13%), and *Candida* (8%).[5] Staphylococcal and candidal organisms adhere to the fibrin or fibronectin sheaths surrounding indwelling catheters, and some staphylococci produce a "slime" that further promotes bacterial proliferation on the catheter surface as the slime protects the organisms from phagocytes, antibodies, and antibiotics. Catheters with siliconized latex and polyvinyl chloride catheters have been shown to have more bacterial adherence than catheters made from other materials. Coagulase-negative staphylococci also adhere to polymer surfaces more readily than other organisms. Other gram-negative organisms, including *Pseudomonas,* also cause infection. *Pseudomonas* is particularly problematic when showering or swimming has been allowed. *Xanthomonas (Stenotrophomonas maltophilia)* infections can be particularly troublesome because of increasing multidrug resistance, formation of biofilm, and their prevalence in immediate post-CVC insertion setting and longer-term indwelling setting. They are more prevalent in cancer patients who have these three independent risk factors: pneumonia, neutropenia at onset of bacteremia, and admission to ICU within 1 month of onset of bacteremia.

A reported 5.4% to 9.9% of infecting organisms are fungal, three-fourths of which are *Candida* species, although nosocomially acquired cutaneous infections with *Aspergillus flavus* have been noted at the sites of insertion and along the subcutaneous tract of Hickman catheters. *Candida* infections in the oncology or bone marrow transplantation population are associated with a high mortality rate. Infection with drug-resistant non–*C. albicans* is increasing in frequency in patients with CVCs. In HIV-positive patients, staphylococci are the most common infecting organisms, but *Pseudomonas* species causing fatal septicemia, other gram-negative organisms, and lactobacilli are increasingly reported. Septicemia due to catheter infection by typical or atypical *Mycobacterium* species has also been noted.

S. aureus is the most common organism infecting ports of patients with hemophilia, especially those with inhibitors. Other implicated organisms in hemophilia patients include *Pseudomonas* species, *Enterobacter cloacae, Escherichia coli, Klebsiella* species, *Serratia liquefaciens,* and *Acinetobacter* species.

In adult sickle cell patients with CVADs, infections were seen with *S. aureus, E. coli, Acinetobacter* species, and *Pseudomonas.*

INDICATIONS FOR REMOVAL

Debate continues over cost-effectiveness and salvage rates for catheters once CRBSI is documented.

Exit-Site and Tunnel Infections

Exit-site infections caused by bacteria rarely require catheter removal for resolution, because most (69% to 100%) respond to antibiotics alone. These infections are most often caused by *S. epidermidis.* Similarly, with implanted ports, infections of the skin pocket have been found to resolve in about 70% of cases without removal of the device.

Tunnel infections or port pocket abscess, by contrast, usually do not respond to antibiotics; they have been reported to resolve without catheter removal in only 25% to 50% of cases. Catheters were removed from all patients with cutaneous *Aspergillus* infection, six of whom recovered after antifungal therapy and local wound care (see box on Infectious Indications for Device Removal). Resolution of leukopenia was required for infection resolution. Similarly, *Mycobacterium* and atypical mycobacterial infection of the tunnel or exit site requires catheter removal as well as excision of infected tissue.

Septicemia

In a patient with septicemia and a catheter or port in place, it is often difficult to determine whether the catheter itself is truly infected or whether the bacteremia is from another source. Quantitative culture is the most sensitive technique, but the semiquantitative roll-plate method is most often used to diagnose catheter-related infections. Both, however, require that the catheter be removed. Quantitative blood culture techniques can be used with a catheter in place. If the

Infectious Indications for Device Removal

Venous Access Devices

Tunnel infection or port pocket abscess
Catheter-related bacteremia caused by *Staphylococcus aureus, Xanthomonas, Pseudomonas* spp, mycobacteria, *Bacillus* and *Corynebacterium* species
Catheter-related fungemia
Septic thrombosis
Endocarditis
Osteomyelitis
Sepsis with signs of shock/persistent end-organ dysfunction
Central venous thrombosis

Central Nervous System Access Devices

Deep catheter track or epidural space infection

From Mermel LA, Farr BM, Sheretz R, et al: Guidelines for the management of intravascular catheter-related infections. *J Intraven Nurs* 24:180, 2001; and
Simon A, Bode U, Beutel K: Diagnosis and treatment of catheter-related infections in paediatric oncology: An update. *Clin Microbiol Infect* 12:606, 2006.

colony count in cultures of blood drawn from the catheter is 5 to 10 times greater than the count in cultures of peripherally drawn blood, the infection is very likely to be catheter-related.[6] For presumed *Candida* infection, it has been suggested that molecular analyses of material from various anatomic sites may help determine the true source of the infection (e.g., sputum versus blood) and prevent needless device removal.

In assessing the cause of infection in a patient with a port, care must be taken not to draw blood for culture through a possibly infected port pocket unless the Huber needle is already in place. Accessing a port through an infected port pocket could introduce organisms into the reservoir and from there into the systemic circulation. To determine whether a port is truly infected, material within the port should also be cultured after it is removed.

When another source is definitely identified, however, the catheters can usually be left in place, because the incidence of hematogenous colonization is low (1%). When there is no thrombophlebitis, even when the catheter is believed to be the source of the infection, or when no source is clearly identified, resolution of bacterial septicemia occurs in 75% of episodes without removal of the catheter.

The possibility of clearing the infection without catheter removal, however, is much lower in patients with septic thrombophlebitis, occluded catheters, exit-site infections, fungal septicemia, or bacteremia due to *S. aureus, Xanthomonas,* or *Pseudomonas*. In other studies, children and adults with catheter-related candidemia had higher rates of treatment failure, secondary complications, and mortality if the catheters were left in place during antifungal treatment. Line removal is recommended when the fungemia is line-related. Successful surgical removal of right atrial thrombi superinfected with *C. tropicalis* or *S. epidermidis* has been reported in several patients, including those with sickle cell anemia. Replacement of catheters on the contralateral side within 1 to 3 days after removal is usually not associated with recurrent catheter infection.

Antibiotic-lock therapy (ALT), with and without concomitant parenteral therapy, has shown success in the prevention and treatment of catheter-related bacteremia when intraluminal infection is likely. In 21 trials of ALT for CRBSI involving long-term catheters, catheter salvage without relapse occurred in 77% of episodes.[8] ALT involves instillation of an antibiotic solution, at a concentration of 1 to 5 mg/mL, into the catheter hub. The solution remains in place for a predetermined amount of time and is withdrawn before the next dose of intravenous antibiotic or medication. ALT itself allows much higher concentration and longer duration of activity of antibiotics at the colonized intraluminal/infected catheter surface without the potential side effects of systemic exposure. It also helps eradicate biofilm-forming bacteria. The goals include prolonging catheter life and reducing patient morbidity and costs associated with catheter-related infections. ALT can also be an option for salvaging venous access when venous access is otherwise limited, and patients have a CRBSI that has not progressed to septicemia and does not involve tissue infection at insertion or tunnel site. ALT has been less effective for treating infections of implantable ports than infections from other types of CVCs.

The most efficacious concentration and duration of ALT remains unclear, although the Infectious Disease Society of America (IDSA) recommends catheter locking for 14 days, with daily changing, in addition to 7- to 14-day systemic administration of antibacterial treatment for uncomplicated catheter-related bacteremias.[8] It should be combined with systemic treatment for at least the first 72 hours. At this time, no evidence-based recommendations are available regarding optimal concentration or intraluminal dwell time. The IDSA does recommend that for vancomycin, concentration should be at least 1000 times higher than the MIC of the microorganism involved and the lock therapy be changed every 48 hours. Combination ALT, including minocycline/vancomycin, minocycline/rifampin, vancomycin/rifampin, is more effective in vitro against biofilm-forming coagulase negative staphylococci. M-EDTA (minocycline plus ethylenediaminetetraacetic acid, or EDTA) has demonstrated activity against gram-positive and gram-negative bacteria, as well as *Candida* species. A randomized control trial is needed to judge its efficacy for long-term CVC infections. In general, ALT has not been as successful for fungal infections. Catheters should be removed in the case of a CRBSI that is due to *S. aureus* or *Candida*.

In existing studies, several factors limit how best to use ALT. These include a lack of data from large, randomized control trials, comparing the efficacy of ALT to systemic antibiotics for treatment of line infections. Additionally, differences in antibiotics used for ALT, heterogeneity in study populations tested, presence or absence of heparin, and inconsistent definitions of catheter-related sepsis further complicate the generalizability of existing data. Overall, it appears ALT alone shortens the length of hospital stay, compared with systemic antibiotic therapy for treatment of line infections.

Hemorrhage

Despite the frequent occurrence of thrombocytopenia in patients with indwelling access devices, few bleeding complications are associated with their placement or with the placement of the larger apheresis catheters. Capillary fragility from prolonged steroid therapy, however, may contribute to perioperative hemorrhage. Pressure dressings and platelet transfusions given pre- and postoperatively usually control local oozing. However, in patients with uncontrolled disseminated intravascular coagulation, excessive bleeding has occurred with catheter insertion; many groups consider disseminated intravascular coagulation an absolute contraindication to catheter placement. In contrast, catheters and ports have been placed without excessive bleeding in patients with hemophilia when factor levels were maintained at 100% preoperatively and for 5 days postoperatively.

CATHETER OCCLUSION

Nonthrombotic Causes

Although a clot is the most common cause of occlusion, inability to aspirate blood from the port or catheter does not necessarily mean that it has clotted. Other causes include a malpositioned Huber needle, catheter abutment against the wall of the vein, catheter kinking, catheter pinch-off, precipitation of drug solutions in the catheter lumen, development of fibrin sheaths, and catheter migration with resultant malposition of the tip. Tip migration secondary to growth, especially during periods of growth spurts, is a problem specific to the pediatric population. Tip placement should be evaluated regularly as the child grows in height. Algorithms for the evaluation and treatment of catheter occlusion are available.

Catheter abutment may resolve by changing the patient's position or by performing a Valsalva maneuver. Pinch-off occurs when the catheter is placed too medially and is compressed between the clavicle and first rib. Repositioning patients with catheter pinch-off often relieves the compression and reestablishes catheter function; however, this is impractical for long-term catheter use, and the catheter usually needs to be repositioned.

Precipitation of incompatible solutions occurs with etoposide, calcium, diazepam, phenytoin, heparin, and total parenteral nutrition (TPN) infusions. Catheter blockage due to precipitation of calcium carbonate was reported at 8 to 24 weeks in 50% of patients with metastatic colon carcinoma receiving once-weekly 24-hour infusions of high-dose 5-fluorouracil (2600 mg/m^2) and leucovorin (500 mg/m^2). Although precipitates may occasionally resolve with warm soaks over the tunnel site, dilute solutions of hydrochloric acid have successfully cleared precipitates from TPN solutions alone or with lipids, etoposide, calcium salts plus sodium bicarbonate, and heparin with incompatible antibiotics. A solution of 0.1 normal HCl to equal the volume of the catheter is instilled and allowed to stand for 20 to 60 minutes. Febrile reactions may occur. Sodium bicarbonate has resolved phenytoin, ticarcillin clavulanate, and oxacillin precipitates. Lipid buildup or occlusions may respond to 70% ethanol instilled for 1 to 2 hours or sodium hydroxide (0.1 N).

Fibrin starts depositing on a catheter within 24 hours of insertion and may be present in as many as 67% of catheters. Withdrawal occlusion secondary to the ball-valve effect of a fibrin sheath accounts for 10% to 57% of catheter occlusions. The fibrin sleeve itself may embolize. Presence of a fibrin sheath increases the risk for infection. Techniques using nonlytic and lytic agents to remove the sheaths have been described. Lytic therapy is discussed later.

Maintaining correct position of the catheter tip can help prevent numerous complications. Catheter migration occurs in 5.5% to 29% of insertions when the subclavian approach is used. Review of the patient's chest radiograph most commonly shows the malpositioned catheter tip to be in the ipsilateral jugular vein, the axillary vein, or the contralateral brachiocephalic vein. When the catheter is in the jugular vein, patients often complain of a whooshing or gurgling sound when the line is flushed. Venous thrombosis can occur as a result of damage to the endothelium, turbulence created by the tip at venous branching points, or insufficient dilution of infusate that causes thrombophlebitis. Catheter erosion through the vessel or cardiac wall can produce extravasation, fistula formation, and pericardial tamponade. Catheters inserted into the left internal jugular or subclavian veins have also eroded into the bronchi; the ensuing venobronchial fistulas were associated with cough, pneumonia, and respiratory failure. Repositioning the catheter can usually be accomplished by interventional radiologists without catheter removal.

PICC malposition is common. PICCs should be well secured at the insertion site to prevent "pistoning" in the vein, which increases the possibility of phlebitis or infection. The catheters can usually be repositioned by trained nurses using simple bedside techniques. Migration of the apheresis catheter in the subcutaneous space also manifests as access failure, because the catheter tip is pulled back to the wall of the inferior vena cava or out of the intravascular space. Intravascular malposition can be corrected by tip deflectors or J-wires.

Thrombosis

Thrombosis can occur in the catheter itself or in the superior vena cava or veins of the upper extremity. While asymptomatic thromboses have been reported in rates up to 60%, most recent studies show an incidence of symptomatic catheter-related deep venous thrombosis (DVT) to be lower than 6%, with similar rates of catheter-related DVT for access achieved through the subclavian and jugular veins. Almost all central indwelling venous access devices become coated with a fibrin sheath within days of insertion, and accordingly, the majority of CVC-related thrombi arise within 30 days of initial placement.[12]

Several potential risk factors for indwelling access catheters in cancer patients have been studied. In a metaanalysis of cancer patients with PICCs or implanted ports, improper catheter tip locations, history of DVT, and subclavian venipuncture insertion technique were associated with increased thrombosis risk.[13] Catheter tip placement has been implicated in the formation of extraluminal thrombosis, with location high in the SVC accounting for a greater incidence of thrombosis than placement in the distal SVC or right atrium (62% to 78% versus 16%). Thrombogenicity was shown to be lesser in silicone and polyurethane CVC compared with polyvinylchloride and polyethylene CVC. Additional risk factors include greater than one attempt at insertion, a previous catheter (with vessel wall trauma and endothelial damage), ovarian cancer, and left-sided insertion site. There were no clear differences in the rate of CVC-related thrombosis with regard to chemotherapy administration methods (push/bolus versus infusion). A threefold increased rate of catheter failure from thrombosis was noted for triple-lumen compared with double-lumen Hickman catheters.

A bidirectional impact of infection and thrombosis has been well documented. One study reported an RR of 17 for developing clinical thrombosis manifestations after an episode of CVC-related infection, with 57% risk after an episode of CVC-associated septicemia versus 27% risk in patients with local CVC-infection only. Even in those patients with subclinical thrombosis, CVC-related infection occurred in 92%, compared with 7% without thrombosis.

Special Populations

For pediatric patients, those who have ALL and are receiving L-asparaginase and external catheters had 3.9-fold higher risk for CVC-thrombosis compared with children who had implanted ports. Children with leukemia, neuroblastoma, and Hodgkin lymphoma with FVL, protein C deficiency, and high lipoprotein (a) levels had a significant association with symptomatic CVC-related thrombosis.

For hemophilia patients, thrombosis has been a relatively rare event. A pooled thrombosis incidence of 0.056 per 1000 CVAD-days has been cited, with no cases documented of superior vena cava syndrome or catheter-associated pulmonary embolism. Furthermore, neither age nor the presence of inhibitors significantly altered the thrombotic incidence. However, because thrombotic complications have been documented less extensively for hemophiliac patients (especially compared with infectious complications), the true extent of subclinical and clinical complications is unknown.

For sickle cell patients, although the condition itself is considered hypercoagulable, it remains unclear how this, coupled with the presence of indwelling access devices, affects the incidence of clinically significant and symptomatic thrombosis.

Patients with multiple myeloma are likely at increased risk for venous thrombosis in the setting of hyperviscosity and treatment with thalidomide or lenalidomide-containing regimens; placing central venous access devices likely increases the risk.[14] Patients with acute promyelocytic leukemia (APML) and high-grade lymphoma also appear to be at higher risk for venous thrombosis.

Spontaneous upper extremity DVT (UEDVT) has been reported to be 2.6-fold to 2.8-fold more likely in patients with active cancer, with the additional presence of an indwelling venous access device increasing the risk further. Clinical UEDVT has been reported to occur in 0% to 9% of patients with chest ports and 2% to 30% with arm ports. Overall, CVADs account for 75% of all cases of UEDVT. Postphlebitic or postthrombotic syndrome following UEDVT among cancer patients range from 4% to 30%.

Most noninvasive methods used for diagnosis of catheter-related thrombosis and/or UEDVT, including duplex ultrasound, Doppler imaging, and plethysmography, have low sensitivity or have not been reliable. Color Doppler duplex sonography, however, has been shown to have sensitivity of 78% to 100% and specificity of 82% to 100% for diagnosis of UEDVT in the setting of peripheral UEDVT (e.g., jugular, distal subclavian, and axillary veins) and in symptomatic patients. Still, the presence of overlying bones may make the visualization and direct assessment via compression techniques difficult. Spiral computed tomography (CT) can be helpful for suspected catheter-related thrombosis involving the brachiocephalic vein or superior vena cava and for those with suspected pulmonary embolus. Magnetic resonance angiography has not proven to be a reliable alternative. Although venography is the gold standard, it is limited by its invasiveness and cost. If venous obstruction is demonstrated, intraluminal versus extraluminal obstruction may be further defined by venography if clinically warranted. In patients with prior central venous catheterization associated with deep venous thrombosis, preprocedural duplex ultrasound may be useful to predict the success of repeat catheter placement.[17]

THERAPY

The clinical significance and course of action are unclear in patients undergoing high-intensity antineoplastic therapy who develop asymptomatic subclavian, or innominate vein thromboses. The majority of catheter-related thromboses are asymptomatic. But patients with symptomatic UEDVT require therapy. They may develop septic thrombophlebitis, superior vena cava syndrome, major long-term upper extremity disability, venous gangrene, and pulmonary emboli. In one retrospective study and review, 12% of patients with catheter-induced UEDVT developed pulmonary emboli, 40% of which occurred in patients receiving anticoagulant therapy. A 16% incidence of pulmonary emboli was found in a prospective study of patients with UEDVT in whom lung scans were performed within 24 hours of venographic diagnosis of the thrombosis.[15]

The National Comprehensive Cancer Network (NCCN) updated guidelines in 2011 for catheter-related UEDVT to help guide clinicians in evaluation and treatment.[16] These guidelines suggest that anticoagulation be used if DVT is present, if the catheter is required, and if there are no contraindications to anticoagulation. Suggested duration of therapy includes all time with the catheter in place or for 3 months, whichever period is longer. If DVT symptoms or presence of clot persist despite this therapy, the catheter should be removed. If anticoagulation is contraindicated, the catheter should be removed, the patient followed for any changes in relative contraindications, and anticoagulation initiated if otherwise permissible. Recommendations for the duration of anticoagulation are a minimum of 3 to 6 months for DVT, 6 to 12 months for pulmonary embolism (PE), and indefinitely if active cancer or persistent risk factors are present.

Management of Catheter Occlusion

Catheter occlusion, whether partial (sluggish flow), complete (inability to infuse or withdraw), or withdrawal type, have all been successfully treated with thrombolytic agents. Streptokinase, urokinase, and recombinant alteplase have all been used. Bolus thrombolytic therapy has reopened occluded catheters in 85% to 90% of episodes, and removal of the catheter is not usually required. No excessive bleeding has been noted, even in patients with hemophilia. Streptokinase is not commonly used because of its antigenic properties and associated allergic and anaphylactic reactions. Urokinase is available in recombinant form and has demonstrated efficacy for lysis of intraluminal thrombosis. Alteplase, a recombinant tissue plasminogen activator (tPA), has demonstrated superiority and is the preferred therapeutic option. A randomized trial comparing bolus urokinase (10,000 units) with tPA (2 mg) suggested marked superiority for tPA. Alteplase is available for catheter clearance in a 2 mg/2 mL vial, a volume sufficient to fill most catheter lumens. The technique is to fill the catheter lumen plus 0.2 mL to ensure that the tPA has close contact with any fibrin/clot at the distal tip of the catheter. It should dwell for 30 minutes to 2 hours and then be withdrawn. An additional dose of 2 mg can be repeated.

For extraluminal thrombi refractory to the bolus administration of thrombolytics, options to dissolve the thrombus include infusions of tPA, urokinase, or streptokinase through a catheter placed at or within the clot. High-dose streptokinase therapy is effective but expensive and is associated with a high incidence of bleeding. It is not recommended for patients with bleeding risks such as thrombocytopenia or mucositis. Infusion of urokinase for 24 to 72 hours restored catheter patency in 74% of patients (81% of those with clots present less than 7 days, and 56% of those with clots present more than 7 days). Infusion into the superficial venous circulation of the involved extremity was not effective. Although a low infusion concentration was used (5000 international units/hour of streptokinase or 500 to 2000 international units/kg/hour of urokinase), a systemic lytic state was documented. Urokinase infusion should not be undertaken in patients with contraindications to systemic fibrinolytic therapy. Another regimen for refractory clots involves an infusion of urokinase (40,000 units/hour) for 6 hours. This regimen led to dissolution of thrombi in 90% of patients; a repeat 6-hour infusion raised the dissolution rate to 95%. Infusions as short as 1 to 3 hours were successful in half of the cases studied. Addition of heparin to the 1- to 12-hour infusion did not improve the results. No bleeding complications were seen. In patients with catheter tips placed below the carina and not adherent to the venous wall, there is a low risk for reocclusion; these catheters need not be removed. Successful clot resolution with urokinase was reported for 50% to 87% of patients.

Once patency is restored, heparin is usually given for 5 to 7 days. Studies have shown an increased risk for recurrent DVT/PE in cancer patients. Currently there is no sound evidence to guide duration of anticoagulant therapy in these patients. The recommended practice is to continue treatment while there is evidence of active cancer and while the patient is receiving antineoplastics.

Vesicant Drug Extravasation

It is very unusual for a spontaneous leak to form in a large-bore catheter, but an attempt to irrigate an occluded catheter with a small syringe can cause a rupture through which the drug can extravasate. Occlusion of the catheter tip by a fibrin sheath may force drugs back up the sheath and through the exit site of the catheter. This so-called backtracking appears to be more common with percutaneously placed access devices.

Leaks may develop if the catheter is disconnected from the reservoir or if the catheter is punctured by mistake by the Huber needle. Outpatients using a port for continuous infusion of chemotherapy can experience drug extravasation if the Huber needle is dislodged from the septum. Even usually nonvesicant drugs can produce skin necrosis severe enough to warrant removal of the port. Use of the Port-A-Cath port, which has a thicker septum than the Mediport and Infus-A-Port devices, has been associated with only a 3% to 4% incidence of extravasation. The thickness of the septum has been postulated to be responsible for the low incidence of needle displacement noted with the Port-A-Cath, but no randomized trials have compared complications associated with the three devices. Selection of an appropriate length Huber needle and securing the needle to the chest wall with tape or a transparent occlusive dressing can provide some protection against dislodgment. If infusion pumps are used, attention must be paid to minimizing tension between the needle and the infusion tubing. See box on Treatment of Vesicant Drug Extravasation.[17]

CENTRAL NERVOUS SYSTEM ACCESS DEVICES

In patients with hematologic disorders, devices that permit chronic access to the CNS are useful for a variety of purposes. The available devices include temporary or permanent epidural catheters, ports with attached silicone elastomer catheters, implanted pumps with attached silicone elastomer catheters, and Ommaya reservoirs. The choice of device is determined by a number of factors, including available routes, duration of therapy, cost, efficacy for the therapy planned (e.g., antineoplastics versus pain medications), and the ability of the patient and family to care for the device.

Treatment of Vesicant Drug Extravasation

Treatment protocols for vesicant drug extravasation, including those recommended by the Oncology Nursing Society, are outlined in Table 89-2. When these protocols were used, 89% of vesicant extravasations were reported to resolve without additional therapy. However, 30% of anthracycline extravasations progressed to ulceration.

At many centers, it is recommended that an extravasation kit be kept in units in which vesicant drugs are given. The kit includes the appropriate medications, as well as order sheets preprinted for immediate use. For most vesicant drugs there is no proved antidote or local care measures. In general, whether an antidote is to be administered through the device or not, as much of the residual drug as possible should be aspirated from the needle, tubing, and tissues. Any antidote may then be administered. If swelling or pain persists for 72 to 96 hours after drug administration, a plastic surgeon should be consulted.

Table 89-2 Management of Vesicant Drug Extravasation

Drug Therapy	Local Care	Antidote Administration
ANTIBIOTICS		
Anthracyclines	Cold/ice pack for 15-20 min qid for 24-48 hr	Administer dexrazoxane (Totect) by IV in a vein away from the extravasation site. Infuse 1000 mg/m² within 6 hr of extravasation on day 1, 1000 mg/m² on day 2, and 500 mg/m² on day 3. Maximum daily dose is 2000 mg. Dimethyl sulfoxide (DMSO) should not be applied, and topical cooling (e.g., ice packs) should be removed 15 min before, and every 15 min during, administration.
Mitomycin-C	Cold/ice pack for 15-20 min qid for 24-48 hr	Topical application of 99% DMSO
VINCA ALKALOIDS		
Vincristine Vinblastine Vindesine Vinorelbine	For all vinca alkaloids, elevate and apply warm pack for 15-20 min at least qid for 24-48 hr	For vinca alkaloids extravasation, inject hyaluronidase subcutaneously, 1 to 6 mL of 150 units/mL solution into area of extravasation in clockwise manner, 1 mL of solution for 1 mL of extravasated drug.
TAXANE		
Paclitaxel	Cold/ice pack 15-20 min qid for 24-48 hr	
ALKYLATING AGENTS		
Mechlorethamine		Mix 1.2 mL of 25% sodium thiosulfate with 8.4 mL of sterile water for injection. Inject 2 mL of antidote for each 1 mg of drug extravasated.
Cisplatin (only if >20 mL of 0.5 mg/mL of concentration infiltrates)		Use sodium thiosulfate as described for mechlorethamine, 2 mL for each 100 mg of cisplatin infiltrated.

From Schulmeister L: Extravasation management: Clinical update, *Semin Oncol Nurs* 27:82, 2011.

Catheters

Local anesthetics alone or combined with fentanyl, other opioids, and medications given through temporary epidural catheters (in place for less than 5 days), have successfully managed the pain and have improved oxygenation in children with sickle cell crisis. Chronic epidural access has become widely available since the development of a permanent epidural catheter that can be placed percutaneously. The catheters are most commonly used for pain control. Some catheters are one piece, and others consist of three pieces: two radiopaque silicone rubber catheters, an epidural segment (1.3-mm outer diameter), and an exteriorized line (3.1-mm outer diameter, 0.68-mm inner diameter) with an external Luer connector and a subcutaneous Dacron cuff and a splice segment that joins the two catheter segments.

Insertion

Catheter insertion is done under local anesthesia or conscious sedation. A paravertebral incision is made at the level of the L2 dorsal spine, and the epidural portion of the catheter is inserted through a 14-gauge Hustead or Tuohy needle to the desired spinal cord level. Epidural placement is verified by fluoroscopy and sensory blockade. The exteriorized line is then tunneled from a subcostal location on the midnipple line around to the lower end of the paravertebral incision, and the splice segment is secured to the two catheters and then to the supraspinous tissue to avoid kinking. A Millex-OR 0.22-μm filter is attached to the Luer connector, and a locking Luer injection cap is connected to the filter.

Access and Management

The catheter can be used immediately. Bolus doses can be given from a syringe, or the catheter can be connected to external pumps that deliver continuous infusion opioid with bolus rescue doses or combinations of opioids and local anesthetics. Only preservative-free solutions should be used. Wound and catheter exit-site cleaning and dressing changes are recommended until the last sutures are removed, usually after 3 weeks. After that, the exit site is cleaned every other day with povidone iodine, and the filter and injection port are changed weekly using sterile technique. More detailed nursing protocols for accessing and managing these catheters and for monitoring patients receiving epidural opioids are available. Patient and family education in catheter care can be effectively supplemented by referral to a home health care or hospice agency.

Complications

Some catheters can remain safely in place for months; however, in rare cases, even temporary catheters can cause serious infections if left in place for days to weeks. Complications include pain during injection, myoclonus, epidural fibrosis, obstruction and dislocation, and infection, as well as complications attributable to the opioids being infused. Patients whose catheters take longer to insert have higher infection rates. Exit-site and superficial catheter track infections occur infrequently (in approximately 10% of patients). The epidural space infection rate has been reported as 1 in 1702 days of catheter use, similar to the infection rate of 1 in 1045 per days of use associated with the Hickman catheter. *S. aureus* and *S. epidermidis* account for two-thirds of all infections. Exit-site and superficial catheter track infections may be cleared without catheter removal, but catheter removal is required for patients with deep catheter track or epidural infections (Table 89-3; also see box on Infectious Indications for Device Removal).

Epidural Ports and Implanted Pumps

Epidural ports (e.g., Port-A-Cath) and implanted pumps (e.g., Infusaid, Medtronic) have also been used to deliver bolus or continuous

Table 89-3 Important Pathogens in Central Venous Access Device–Related Infections

Pathogen	Source	Notable Complications
GRAM-POSITIVE BACTERIA		
S. epidermidis		
Coagulase-negative staphylococci	Hub; skin at exit site of device	Local/systemic and suppurative complications
Methicillin-resistant *Staphylococcus aureus* (MRSA)		
Enterococci, including vancomycin-resistant *Enterococcus* (VRE)	Intestines	Bacteremia, endocarditis
α-hemolytic streptococci	Oropharynx	
GRAM-NEGATIVE BACTERIA		
Pseudomonas aeruginosa	Hospital-acquired	
Klebsiella spp	Urinary Tract	

infusions of opioids into the epidural or intrathecal space to relieve pain of malignant or nonmalignant origin. Intrathecal devices that deliver pain medication have become increasingly sophisticated and offer an alternative for long-term treatment of persistent pain.[18] Consensus guidelines have been published on the selection of patients for intrathecal drug delivery.[19] Subarachnoid infusions using the implanted pumps are recommended as efficacious and cost-effective for patients with a relatively long life expectancy (more than 3 months).

Complications include those previously described for implanted ports, as well as pain on injection of morphine, pump pocket seromas, CSF leaks, CSF hygromas, and postspinal headache. The use of injection ports appears to reduce the rate of complications associated with percutaneously inserted epidural catheters. A retrospective comparison of catheters with or without associated injection ports indicated that those attached to ports became dislodged much less frequently and were associated with half the infection rate per 1000 patient-days. Port removal rates for infection were similar to removal rates of ports used for vascular access (10%). Because the seromas act as growth media for bacterial contamination, they should be monitored carefully. The management of hygromas and postspinal headache is reviewed elsewhere. Ports and pumps can also erode through the skin. Detailed access and management procedures are available for epidural ports and implanted pumps and for monitoring patients receiving opioids through them.

Ommaya Reservoir

The Ommaya reservoir device was first described in 1963 by Ommaya, and with minimal changes, it is still used for access to the spinal fluid within the cerebral ventricle. The reservoir is used to remove CSF for culture, cytology, or measurement of drug levels; to drain cysts in craniopharyngiomas and astrocytomas; to administer antibiotics or antifungal agents; to administer intraventricular chemotherapy to treat leukemic or carcinomatous meningitis; to administer interferon or lymphokine-activated killer cells directly into a tumor; and to administer opioid pain medications.

The device consists of a dome- or mushroom-shaped capsule with a top made of a self-sealing silicone elastomer that can be punctured numerous times without leaking. The flat base of the capsule, by contrast, is composed of firm polypropylene and is not easily punctured. An outlet arm connected to a ventricular catheter is attached at the base, laterally or in the center, extending downward. Capsules range from 12 mm in diameter (for babies) to 30 mm. Those commonly used for adults have an internal volume capacity of 1.45 to 2.4 mL.

Insertion

The Ommaya reservoir is placed subcutaneously by a neurosurgeon. Before insertion, CT is generally required to evaluate ventricular size and placement. Presoaking the device in bacitracin to prevent subsequent infection has been advocated. For placement, the ventricular catheter is passed through a burr hole into the frontal horn of the right lateral ventricle or, if necessary, into that of the left lateral ventricle or the ventricle body. The catheter end is connected to the base or side arm of the capsule, which then is fitted into the burr hole or a subgaleal pocket. The Silastic skirt of the reservoir may be sutured to the periosteum. A postoperative CT scan is suggested to verify the catheter tip position. Stereotactic techniques are used when the ventricle is small or misplaced.

Accessing the Device

The Ommaya reservoir can be used immediately postoperatively for sampling CSF or for injection of drugs. Usually, however, it is not accessed until the third postoperative day. The thoroughly cleaned, gently shaved scalp is prepared with three iodine scrubs, and with the use of a sterile technique, the reservoir is accessed obliquely with a 23- or 25-gauge butterfly needle inserted with the bevel downward. The CSF can be directly aspirated, or antibiotics or chemotherapeutic agents can be administered through a second syringe attached to the butterfly needle. After removal of the needle, the injected medication can be gently pumped into the spinal fluid by emptying the capsule using repeated pressure, but to allow CSF to refill the reservoir, the clinician should avoid steadily compressing the device. After the incision has healed and the stitches have been removed, no special local care or flushing is required. The device can remain in place for months or years. More detailed accessing and management guidelines are available.[2]

Complications

Infection

In general, the Ommaya reservoir has proved very safe, with a complication rate of 9% to 20%, although higher rates were reportedin the past.[20] The most common complication is infection, which occurs in about 1% to 15% of patients, especially those who have undergone radiation therapy or who required a second surgical procedure for revision of the catheter. Most infections have been caused by *S. epidermidis,* but infections from numerous other gram-positive and gram-negative bacteria and fungal organisms have been documented. In general, the device is not removed, and patients are treated as though they had meningitis. For infections with *S. epidermidis,* vancomycin is given intravenously or, in refractory cases, instilled into the reservoir. Removal of the reservoir is sometimes required.

Miscellaneous Complications

Neurologic complications are rare when the catheter is placed into the nondominant ventricle, but a variety of other complications, which occur infrequently, have been reported. These include intraventricular hemorrhage or subdural hematoma shortly after catheter placement; leakage of CSF around the catheter, primarily in patients with increased intracranial pressure, which caused backflow of fluid along the catheter and produced a subgaleal collection; reservoir leaks after repeated use; occlusion by cellular debris or, when a catheter is placed directly into a tumor, by very proteinaceous tumor fluid; obstruction by lodging of the catheter in brain tissue or abutment against a ventricle wall; seizures immediately after injection of medications; white matter disease (leukoencephalopathy or brain necrosis), most often due to methotrexate injection through the Ommaya device, although found with systemic administration of methotrexate as well; and tumor growth around the cannula. In one case, the catheter may have permitted the spread of Burkitt lymphoma cells from the meninges into the cerebral tissue, where the tumor was found.

REFERENCES

1. McGee DC, Gould MK: Preventing complications of central venous catheterization. *N Engl J Med* 348:1123, 2003.
2. Erinjeri JP, Fong AJ, Kemeny NE, et al: Timing of administration of bevacizumab chemotherapy affects wound healing after chest wall port placement. *Cancer* 117:1296, 2011 Mar 15.
3. Zawacki WJ, Walker TG, DeVasher E, et al: Wound dehiscence or failure to heal following venous access port placement in patients receiving bevacizumab therapy. *J Vasc Interv Radiol* 20:624, 2009 May.
4. Valentino LA, Ewenstein B, Navickis RJ, et al: Central venous access devices in haemophilia. *Haemophilia* 10:134, 2004 Mar.
5. Santagostino E, Mancuso ME: Venous access in haemophilic children: Choice and management. *Haemophilia* 16:20, 2010 Jan.
6. Maki R, Kluger DM, Crinich CJ: The risk of bloodstream infection in adults with different intravascular devices: A systematic review of 200 published prospective studies, *Mayo Clinic Proceedings,* Sept 2006, 1159.
7. Camp-Sorrell D, Camp-Sorrell M: *Access device guidelines: Recommendations for nursing practice and education*, Pittsburgh, 2010, Oncology Nursing Society.
8. Mermel LA, Allon M, Bouza E, et al: Clinical practice guidelines for the diagnosis and management of intravascular catheter-related infection: 2009 Update by the Infectious Diseases Society of America. *Clin Infect Dis.* 49:1, 2009.
9. O'Grady NP, Alexander M, Burns LA, et al; and the Healthcare Infection Control Practices Advisory Committee (HICPAC): Guidelines for the prevention of intravascular catheter-related infections. *Clin Infect Dis* 2011. First published online April 1, 2011.
10. Hockenhull JC, Dwan KM, Smith GW, et al: The clinical effectiveness of central venous catheters treated with anti-infective agents in preventing catheter-related bloodstream infections: A systematic review. *Crit Care Med* 37:702, 2009 Feb.
11. Zarrouk V, Habibi A, Zahar J-R, et al: Bloodstream infection in adults with sickle cell disease: Association with venous catheters, *staphylococcus* aureus, and bone-joint infections. *Medicine* 85:43, 2006.
12. Kuter D: Thrombotic complications of central venous catheters in cancer patients. *Oncologist* 9:207, 2004.
13. Saber W, Moua T, Williams EC, et al: Risk factors for catheter-related thrombosis (CRT) in cancer patients: A patient-level data (IPD) meta-analysis of clinical trials and prospective studies. *J Thromb Haemost* 9:312, 2011.
14. Palumbo A, Rajkumar SV, Dimopoulos MA, et al: Prevention of thalidomide- and lenalidomide-associated thrombosis in myeloma. *Leukemia* 22:414, 2008.
15. Monreal M, Raventos A, Lerma R, et al: Pulmonary embolism in patients with upper extremity DVT associated to venous central lines: A prospective study. *Thromb Haemost* 72:548, 1994.
16. Streiff MB, Bockenstedt PL, Cataland SR, et al: NCCN clinical practice guidelines in oncology for venous thromboembolic disease. *J Natl Compr Canc Netw* 9:714, 2011.
17. Schulmeister L: Extravasation management: Clinical update. *Semin Oncol Nurs* 27:82, 2011 Feb.
18. Lawson EF, Wallace MS: Current developments in intraspinal agents for cancer and noncancer pain. *Curr Pain Headache Rep* 14:8, 2010 Feb.
19. Deer TR, Smith HS, Cousins M, et al: Consensus guidelines for the selection and implantation of patients with noncancer pain for intrathecal drug delivery. *Pain Physician* 13:E175, 2010 May-Jun.
20. Sandberg D, Bilsky M, Souweidane M, et al: Ommaya reservoirs for the treatment of leptomeningeal metastases. *Neurosurgery* 47:49, 2000.

CHAPTER 90

NUTRITIONAL ISSUES IN PATIENTS WITH HEMATOLOGIC MALIGNANCIES

Regina S. Cunningham

Nutritional status plays a critical role in predicting risk for the development of human malignancies, affecting responses to therapeutic interventions, and influencing the outcome of disease. Ongoing research has demonstrated that diet can significantly influence the development of hematologic malignancies, and in those who are diagnosed, nutritional status has been correlated with overall survival, chemotherapy response rates, toxicity, quality of life, length of stay, functional status, and cost of care outcomes.[1-8] Nutritional alterations can manifest at any point along the cancer trajectory; they may serve as a harbinger of disease, develop during the treatment process, and often accompany advanced disease. Nutritional alterations in patients with hematologic malignancies can develop as a result of tumor–host interactions, a consequence of cancer treatment, or as a result of psychosocial responses to the disease; most often, the etiology is multifactorial.[9]

SCOPE OF THE PROBLEM

Nutritional problems are common in cancer patients and in those who have survived the disease. Both malnutrition and overnutrition are associated with cancer, but the precise incidence or prevalence of these issues is not well documented. It is estimated that as many as 87% of patients experience weight loss or malnutrition during their trajectory of illness, depending on the site and stage of disease.[8] Approximately 20% of cancer patients die as a result of malnutrition or complications of weight loss rather than from the malignancy itself.[10] The specific incidence of nutritional issues within the hematologic malignancies are not well documented. In general, nutritional alterations are less common among patients diagnosed with hematologic malignancies than in those who have solid tumors. Patients with leukemia are at a relatively low risk for weight loss, but 31% to 48% of patients with non-Hodgkin lymphoma experience significant weight loss.[11] Nutritional deficits have also been reported in myeloma patients undergoing bone marrow transplant. In one study, 61% of patients were found to have altered nutritional status before receiving high-dose chemotherapy.[12] Decreases in lean body mass index (LBMI) have been reported in both adults and children who have been treated with allogeneic stem cell transplantation (aSCT). In a longitudinal study of 82 adult patients with primary hematologic malignancies who underwent aSCT, 38% were found to have LBMIs that were lower than pretreatment levels 4 to 6 years after their transplants had been completed.[13] Decline in body mass index (BMI) over time has also been reported in survivors of pediatric hematologic malignancies after aSCT.[14] Weight loss and diminished nutritional status have been documented in patients with chronic graft-versus-host disease (GVHD), although the frequency and severity has not been well characterized. Patients with advanced GVHD frequently become nutritionally depleted with loss of lean body mass and diminished functional status.[15] One study involving a sample of 93 patients with chronic GVHD found that 43% were malnourished (defined as a BMI of 21.9) and 14% severely malnourished (defined as a BMI of <18.5).[16] Patients with myeloproliferative neoplasms (MPNs) can also experience malnutrition as a result of their disease process. The presence of hypercatabolic symptoms, defined as weight loss, profound fatigue, night sweats, and low-grade fever, at the time of diagnosis is an indicator of adverse prognosis in patients who have primary myelofibrosis.[17] Moreover, in patients with MPNs, long-term complications often include progressive constitutional symptoms, cachexia, and weight loss.[18] A recent study documented that male patients experience greater symptomatology and weight loss and that symptom burden in this population is correlated with decreased quality of life.[19]

Diminished nutritional status in patients with hematologic malignancies can be profound and lead to significant weakness and decline in functional status. Nutritional deterioration and weight loss are associated with poorer responses to treatment and survival outcomes, as well as higher complication rates, longer hospitalizations, greater risk of unplanned hospitalization, higher readmission rates, more disability, and higher overall cost of care.[2,20] In a classic study of the prognostic effects of weight loss among subjects participating in Eastern Cooperative Oncology Group protocols, patients with hematologic malignancies who experienced no weight loss had a median survival approximately twice as long as those who experienced weight loss.[8] From a patient perspective, changes in weight often serve as an ostensible sign of illness and can affect patients' sense of well-being and quality of life. This can be exacerbated when patients develop symptoms as a result of their disease or treatment that have the potential to further impede nutritional intake. Oral pain, hoarseness, nausea, vomiting, mucositis, and unclear speech have all been associated with decreased quality of life scores in patients with cancer.[21,22]

Overnutrition has been identified as a risk factor in the development of hematologic malignancies.[4,23] The relationship between increased BMI and risk for developing both acute and chronic myeloid and lymphoid leukemia has been supported in several large cohort studies as well as meta-analyses. Risk for the development of non-Hodgkin lymphoma, B-cell lymphoma, and multiple myeloma has also been correlated with increased BMI.[24] In addition to the potential etiologic association between overnutrition and hematologic malignancies, obesity may have profound effects on interventions used in the treatment of these diseases. Weight can impact the dose and pharmacokinetics of chemotherapeutic agents, as well as adipocyte metabolism and drug distribution. These factors may be especially important in the setting of hematopoietic stem cell transplantation (HSCT).[25]

Overnutrition has also been reported as an outcome of disease in patients diagnosed with hematologic malignancies.[26,27] Many Childhood Cancer Survivor Study participants are at increased risk for obesity. The etiology of their obesity is likely multifactorial and not well understood.[26] In a retrospective cohort of survivors of childhood acute lymphocytic leukemia (ALL), 1765 adult survivors were compared with 2565 adult siblings on a number of anthropometric outcomes. Findings indicated that subjects who had been treated with cranial radiation therapy at doses of 20 Gy or greater were at greater risk for obesity, particularly female patients who were treated at a younger age. Researchers hypothesized that cranial radiation at a young age may affect the developing hypothalamus and result in leptin-receptor insensitivity.[28] Obesity after a cancer diagnosis is associated with adult-onset diabetes mellitus, hypertension, dyslipidemia, and ultimately cardiovascular disease.[29] Additional research focusing on elucidating the mechanisms for increased weight and preventing obesity in survivors of hematologic malignancies is needed.

ETIOLOGY AND CONTRIBUTING FACTORS

Many factors contribute to nutritional alterations and weight loss in patients with hematologic malignancies. A decrease in oral intake in the setting of increased energy requirements frequently leads to loss of weight. The type and location of tumors may contribute to the development of symptoms that lead to decreased oral intake. Physiologic alterations related to the tumor (e.g., malabsorption or obstruction), tumor–host interactions (anorexia and altered metabolism), and the development of nutrition-impact symptoms associated with cancer treatment (e.g., nausea, vomiting, mucositis, pain, diarrhea) can all contribute to decreased oral intake and the inability to maintain weight. Symptom burden can be profound in patients with hematologic malignancies, especially in those who are receiving complex multimodality therapies.

All types of cancer treatment have the potential to impact nutritional status. The magnitude of this effect depends on the type, dose, intensity, and duration of treatment. Aggressive multimodality therapeutic interventions that include chemotherapy and radiation therapy are frequently used in the setting of hematologic malignancies. Chemotherapy is associated with both direct and indirect effects that have the potential to interfere with nutritional intake. Rapidly dividing cells are most vulnerable to the effects of chemotherapy and radiation. Alterations in the gastrointestinal (GI) tract after these treatments include damage to the mucosal lining of the oral cavity, changes in the length and surface of the intestinal villi, stimulation of neurobiologic pathways controlling nausea and vomiting, and interference with specific metabolic and enzymatic reactions. The extent of radiation-induced nutritional alterations varies according to the anatomic location, dose, and duration of treatment.[30] Surgical interventions may also lead to alterations in nutritional status, although extensive surgical procedures are less common in patients with hematologic malignancies than they are in those with solid tumors.

CANCER- AND TREATMENT-INDUCED ALTERATIONS IN NUTRITIONAL STATUS

Anorexia

Anorexia is defined as loss of desire to eat accompanied by diminished oral intake.[31] Anorexia often accompanies other symptoms that can lead to decreased food intake and are associated with central nervous system regulation of energy intake, such as changes in sense of smell and taste, nausea, vomiting, and early satiety. Approximately 50% of patients newly diagnosed with cancer experience anorexia, and in later stage disease, the prevalence of this symptom approaches 80%.[32] Prolonged anorexia has been reported in recipients of autologous stem cell transplantation (ASCT).[33] Myeloablative conditioning regimens frequently lead to anorexia and poor oral intake. In a prospective study of 147 patients receiving cyclophosphamide, total-body irradiation, and allogeneic stem cell grafts, oral caloric intake was found to be reduced in 92% of subjects. The nadir in oral intake was noted at days 10 to 12 when the median caloric intake was only 3% of basal energy requirements.[34] Anorexia can lead to malnutrition, decreased ability to tolerate treatment, increased toxicity, debilitation, and decreased quality of life.[32]

Anorexia is a complex physiologic phenomenon that is regulated by numerous GI, metabolic, and endocrine mechanisms. Loss of appetite is associated with gastric motor dysfunction[33] as well as the effects of hormones (e.g., leptin, ghrelin), neuropeptides, and cytokines produced by the cancer and the host in response to the disease.[31,35] Cytokines, including tumor necrosis factor-α (TNF-α), interferon-γ (IFN-γ), leukemia inhibitory factor (LIF), interleukin-1 and -6 (IL-1 and -6), and ciliary neurotrophic factor, are thought to play a pivotal role in the stimulation of anorexigenic and orexigenic circuits that regulate intake and body weight.[31]

Loss of appetite may be precipitated by cancer-induced psychologic distress as well. Depression, anxiety, pain or analgesic medication, and situational factors (isolation, dislike of hospital food) may negatively influence food intake. Cancer-related fatigue, the most commonly reported symptom in patients with cancer, has also been associated with diminished food intake. Fatigue often interferes with activities of daily living and may limit the patient's ability to obtain and prepare food. In many patients, anorexia may linger long after cancer treatment has been completed.

Mucositis

Mucositis is a generalized inflammatory response of the mucosal epithelial cells lining the GI tract. The rapidly dividing cells in this area are particularly vulnerable to the effects of treatment with antineoplastic agents. The clinical presentation of mucositis includes painful inflammation, erythema, and ulcerations of the oral mucosa and GI tract.[36,37] The erythematous ulcerative lesions are a consequence of epithelial damage and cell death that is mediated through a complex series of molecular and cellular events associated with chemotherapy or radiation.[38,39] Mucositis usually develops within 5 days of chemotherapy with peak severity in 7 to 10 days.[36,40] Mucositis is commonly reported in patients receiving conventional chemotherapy, and the risk for developing this symptom increases with each subsequent course of therapy.[41] There is substantial variability in the stomatoxicity of chemotherapeutic regimens used to treat hematologic malignancies. In the setting of Hodgkin disease, for example, the incidence of mucositis with the administration of ABVD (doxorubicin, bleomycin, vinblastine, and dacarbazine) is 3%.[42] Patients with acute myeloid leukemia (AML), who receive anthracycline-based regimens, often develop profound myelosuppression and oral mucositis (10%-15%). More aggressive protocols, such as FLAG (fludarabine, cytarabine, and granulocyte colony-stimulating factor [G-CSF]) induce mucosal damage in 50% of patients[43] and in patients receiving myeloablative chemotherapy regimens in preparation for stem cell transplantation, severe mucosal toxicity occurs in 60% to 100%.[44-46] Conditioning regimens that contain melphalan or total-body irradiation are associated with particularly high rates of oral mucositis.[47] Targeted therapies have also been associated with the development of oral complications that may be independent or additive.[37,48] Imatinib mesylate (Gleevac–Gilvec, Novartis), for example, is a TKI that selectively targets platelet-derived growth factor receptor, C-kit, and the abl-bcr fusion gene. Several case reports of patients developing oral lichenoid reactions presenting as erythematous reticular plaques on oral mucosa with or without ulceration have been reported.[49,50]

Recent surveys have indicated that mucositis is a serious toxicity reported by patients undergoing high-dose chemotherapy or chemoradiation.[51,52] Severe pain almost uniformly accompanies mucositis, a factor that can severely limit oral intake and lead to changes in nutritional status. Mucositis is also associated with increased need for total parenteral nutrition and opioid analgesics, longer hospitalizations, and increased risk for infection.[41,53,54]

Preventing or minimizing mucositis is an important goal in patients with hematologic malignancies receiving high-dose chemotherapy. The Multinational Association for Supportive Care in Cancer recommends the use of keratinocyte growth factor-1 (palifermin) at a dosage of 60 μg/kg per day for 3 days before administration of a conditioning regimen of aSCT and for 3 days posttransplant for the prevention of oral mucositis.[47,55] Strong evidence supports the benefits of palifermin in reducing both the severity and duration of oral mucositis as well as decreasing mouth and throat soreness and improving patient function in the setting of aSCT.[56,57] Cryotherapy to prevent oral mucositis in patients receiving high-dose melphalan as a conditioning agent in HSCT is also recommended.[47]

Early Satiety

Early satiety is defined as the desire to eat associated with the subsequent inability to eat (except for small amounts) because of a sense of fullness.[58] In a recent prospective evaluation of more than 1000 patients with advanced cancer, early satiety was ranked among the 10 most common symptoms experienced by patients.[59] Another investigation of patients with MPNs reported that early satiety was experienced by 53% of patients with essential thrombocytosis, 62% of those with polycythemia vera, and 75% of patients who had myelofibrosis.[18] Early satiety often occurs with other symptoms, including anorexia, taste changes, and weight loss.[60] Early satiety contributes to decreased food intake and has been identified as an independent prognostic variable.[59]

Both central and peripheral pathophysiologic mechanisms as well as physical barriers contribute to the development of early satiety. Central influences can alter smell and taste and lead to food aversions as well as diurnal variations in food intake. Satiety is less prominent during the early hours of the day. Peripheral mechanisms underlying early satiety include gastric dysmotility and accommodation as well as the influence of specific gastric and small bowel hormones. Physical barriers that contribute to the development of early satiety include a lack of gastric accommodation and delayed gastric emptying.[60] In patients with MPNs, for example, early satiety may be related to gastric compression that occurs as a result of the striking hepatosplenomegaly that is frequently associated with extramedullary hematopoiesis.

Chemosensory Alterations in Taste and Smell

Alterations in taste and smell are common in patients with cancer and in those receiving chemotherapy. In an investigation of subjects with advanced cancer, 86% of patients reported some type of chemosensory alteration.[61] In another study of 518 patients receiving ambulatory chemotherapy, 66% of patients reported changes in taste and smell. An additional 8% experienced changes in smell without changes in taste.[62] Although this investigation included patients with mixed cancer diagnoses, olfactory changes have been reported among patients receiving high-dose chemotherapy followed by aSCT. In one study of 50 subjects, 26% reported that they experienced increased sensitivity to odors, and 8% reported decreased sensitivity. Other changes affecting smell were reported by 24% of subjects.[63] Altered taste and smell sensors, with diminution of taste and olfactory cues, change the normal references that are important to appetite and intake. Increases in the recognition thresholds for sweet, sour, and salty as well as decreases in the recognition levels for bitter are seen frequently in patients receiving cancer treatment. Such changes can lead to food aversions, which in turn can decrease food intake and lead to malnutrition. Psychosocial factors may also contribute to food aversions. Pleasurable and social aspects of eating can be negatively influenced by alterations in taste or smell, leading to a reduced desire to eat and diminished intake.

Taste alterations are defined as changes in the usual patterns of taste perception that are unique to the individual experiencing the changes.[64] Taste alterations may result in reduced interest in food and decreased oral intake, nutritional compromise, and weight loss. Moreover, because one of the basic qualities of taste is desirable flavor associated with pleasure, changes in taste have also been associated with decrease in quality of life.[63] Although taste alterations are common in patients with cancer, they may be overlooked because of more pressing consequences of disease and treatment. As such, data on incidence, prevalence, and the impact of these symptoms on nutritional status are limited. Changes in taste and smell may be related to effects of tumors, cancer-induced deficiencies of vitamins and minerals, selected chemotherapeutic agents, or the action of cytokines. The perception of taste may be distorted (dysgeusia), which will often be described by patients as rancid, bitter, salty, or metallic. Taste alterations can also include enhanced (hypergeusia), diminished (hypogeusia), or completely absent (ageusia). Dysosmia, or distorted perception of smell, is categorized according to whether it is preceded by something in the environment (parosmia) or happens spontaneously (phantosmia). Dysosmia is often unpleasant and is frequently described by patients as rancid.[61,65]

Cancer Cachexia

Cachexia is a multifactorial syndrome characterized by progressive weight loss, anorexia, asthenia, skeletal muscle and adipose tissue loss, and dysregulated metabolic changes with increased basal energy expenditure that is resistant to conventional nutritional support interventions.[66,67] Cachexia is one of the most profound alterations in nutrition that is observed in patients with cancer, and it is associated with declining performance status, decreased quality of life, and shortened survival. Weight loss in cachexia is caused by depletion of adipose tissue and skeletal muscle mass as well as changes in glucose metabolism.

Body mass is controlled by the balance of energy intake and expenditure. Glucose is the most essential substrate of the human body and is required to support all critical organ functions. In the setting of cachexia, the intake of glucose can be severely compromised by anorexia and other symptoms impacting nutrition. This is exacerbated by cancer-induced changes in glucose metabolism that lead to inefficient production in the setting of increased need.[68] Most cancer cells use glycolysis as the principal method to generate adenosine triphosphate. The increased glucose uptake in tumors is the basis of the [^{18}F] fluorodeoxyglucose positron emission tomography (FDG-PRT) tumor diagnostic method.[69] The reasons for this phenomenon is not clear; it has been hypothesized that it is related to dysfunctional mitochondria, which prevent their use of the tricarboxylic acid cycle, preventing total combustion of pyruvic acid.[70] The result is the conversion of glucose to lactic acid, an extremely inefficient process. Tumor growth requires approximately 40 times more glucose than if it was fully oxidized through the tricarboxylic cycle. In addition, lactate passes from the tumor to the liver, where it is resynthesized into glucose.[71] This may account for an additional loss of energy in cancer patients of about 300 kcal/day.[72]

Changes in protein metabolism and depletion of muscle mass are also features of cancer cachexia. Depletion of skeletal muscle is the result of an imbalance between the rate of protein synthesis and degradation. There is an overall increase in muscle protein catabolism leading to a net loss of muscle mass. Proteolysis-inducing factor (PIF) is a glycoprotein secreted by cachexia-inducing tumors that has been shown to inhibit protein synthesis and stimulate protein degradation directly. PIF is also involved in hepatic gene expression, which can influence the production of cytokines that are implicated in the cachectic process.[73,74] Cachexia is also associated with significant reduction in adipose tissue. This is driven by lipid-mobilizing factor and other tumor–host factors that have direct lipolytic effects.[67] These changes lead to decreased body fat, which is lost more readily than lean tissue.[71]

The pathophysiologic mechanisms underlying cachexia have not been fully elucidated. It is hypothesized that the syndrome is the result of highly complex cell signaling between the tumor and host. Cytokines play an important role in mediating many of the metabolic changes seen in cancer cachexia. Proinflammatory cytokines can modulate gastric motility and emptying either directly through the GI tract or by altering signals that regulate satiety. TNF-α, or cachectin, leads to decreased food intake and wasting. IFN-γ is also produced and has biologic functions that overlap with TNF. Ciliary neurotrophic factor is expressed in skeletal muscle and has been shown to induce cachectic effects and produce acute-phase proteins. LIF and transforming growth factor-β are also produced and are hypothesized to play a role in the development of cachexia.[75-77] Elucidating the molecular mechanisms underlying the development of cachexia is an area of active research. This knowledge is essential to guide the development of rational therapeutics to manage cachexia in the future.

Energy Balance in Cancer

Energy balance is the difference between dietary energy intake and expenditure through physical activity and resting metabolism. It is the result of the complex interaction of diet, physical activity, and genetics. Changes in energy intake are common in patients with hematologic malignancies; they may have increased, normal, or decreased energy expenditure. Increased energy expenditure may result from tumor–host interactions that facilitate changes in metabolism and appetite. Heightened cytokine activity, inefficient metabolic cycles, protein destruction, acute-phase reactions, and inappropriate energy production in response to decreased intake can all lead to increased energy requirements. It is estimated that energy requirements in aSCT recipients may reach 130% to 150% of predicted basal energy expenditure.[78] Patients may also experience infection and fever, which can further increase energy demands. In response to these demands, nutritional needs increase as the body tries to repair damage. Cancer treatments may lead to both increases and decreases in energy expenditure. Many cancer treatments are associated with the development of symptoms that impact oral intake and influence functional status. Most chemotherapeutic agents stimulate the emetic pathways, leading to nausea and vomiting. Specific drugs, such as doxorubicin and cyclophosphamide, are associated with changes in taste and smell perception. Radiation can also damage taste and olfactory receptors. In addition, radiation can damage the salivary glands, causing xerostomia. The lack of saliva creates an extremely dry mouth and makes food consumption very challenging. Patients who develop GVHD can experience profound diarrhea, leading to changes in fluid status and electrolyte balance. All of these changes can lead to decreased energy intake and weight loss. Decreased energy expenditure can also be seen in patients with hematologic malignancies. This may occur as a result of deconditioning from lengthy hospitalizations, decreased physical activity, or changes in metabolic rate resulting from loss of muscle.

Specialized Nutritional Issues in Hematopoietic Cell Transplantation

Hematopoietic stem cell transplantation is a therapeutic intervention used in the management of many hematologic malignancies. HSCT describes a diverse group of interventions, the outcomes of which depend on the type of transplant (autologous, related or unrelated allogeneic), preparative regimen, degree of histocompatibility, stem cell source (bone marrow, peripheral blood, or cord blood), age, type and stage of disease, previous therapy, and nutritional status. One of the major adverse effects of HSCT is malnutrition.[66,79,80] HSCT involves the use of high-dose chemotherapy with or without radiation to eradicate tumor; hematologic rescue is then provided with previously harvested cells. Many of the preparative chemotherapeutic regimens used in HSCT are extremely intense and are associated with severe mucositis, enteritis, painful oral ulcerations, nausea, vomiting, and profound diarrhea. All of these symptoms can lead to diminished oral intake, significant weight loss, and malnutrition. Disruption of the mucosal barrier predisposes patients to the development of infection during the period of neutropenia, which may last for as long as 6 weeks.[66] The development of GVHD can exacerbate these symptoms and complicate the clinical picture with the addition of hepatic and renal insufficiency. Underweight transplant recipients have a greater risk of death in the early posttransplant period as well as greater nonrelapse mortality.[80] Conversely, a shorter time to engraftment and lower probability of developing infection are associated with being well nourished.

Nutritional deficits that develop in transplant patients linger long after completion of the transplant, with as many as 50% of patients not returning to their pretransplant weight at 1 year.[66] According to the American Society for Parenteral and Enteral Nutrition (ASPEN) Clinical Guidelines, all patients undergoing HSCT with myeloablative preparatory regimens are at nutritional risk and should undergo nutritional screening to identify those who require a more extensive nutritional assessment and development of a nutritional care plan. These proactive steps will assist in the early identification of patients who are at risk of developing nutritional alterations and facilitate early intervention for these issues.

NUTRITIONAL SCREENING AND ASSESSMENT

Early intervention is the cornerstone of effective management of nutritional issues in patients with hematologic malignancies. Nutritional screening is an essential preliminary step in the development of a successful nutritional plan. The major goals of nutritional screening are to proactively identify patients who are at risk for malnutrition, prevent or treat malnutrition early, and modify treatment plans as necessary. Both The Joint Commission (TJC) and the ASPEN endorse the identification of patients with actual or potential nutritional issues through a systematic screening process. TJC requires the identification of patients who are at nutritional risk within 24 hours of admission to a hospital, within 14 days of admission to a long-term care facility, and within an organizationally specified time period in the ambulatory and home care settings.[65] ASPEN has developed guidelines that recommend that all patients undergo nutritional screening as a component of their initial assessment.[81]

Nutritional screening tools typically include both objective and subjective data that can be obtained quickly and easily in a busy clinical setting. Objective data should at a minimum include height, weight, weight change, primary diagnosis, and the presence of comorbidities. Subjective components include patient-reported information about symptoms, changes in dietary intake, and activity levels.

The need to efficiently screen for nutritional issues has led to the development of a number of clinical tools. Screening tools should be easy to use, valid, reliable, cost effective, and sensitive. The Patient-Generated Subjective Global Assessment (PG-SGA) has been identified by the Oncology Nutrition Practice Group and the Academy of Nutrition and Dietetics as the standard for nutritional screening in oncology patients. The PG-SGA was adapted from the Subjective Global Assessment specifically for use in the cancer population by Ottery.[82] The form (Fig. 90-1) uses a simple check box format to obtain information from both the patient and the clinician. Each of the patient's subjective responses is scored from 0 (least) to 4 (most) depending on nutritional impact. This score is combined with objective data collected by the clinician, and a total score is calculated. The overall PG-SGA score indicates if a patient is well nourished, suspected of being malnourished, or severely malnourished. An algorithm (Fig. 90-2) outlining nutritional interventions for each of these categories has been developed.

The PG-SGA has demonstrated good construct validity and inter-rater reliability.[83] In a sample of 61 consecutive patients with hematologic malignancies newly admitted to a transplant program, patients completed a battery of standardized supportive care measures, including the PG-SGA. A total of 61% of patients experienced nutritional deficits, indicating the need for attention to nutritional difficulties, before the administration of high-dose therapy and transplantation.[12] In another investigation, the PG-SGA was used to assess nutritional risk among hospitalized cancer patients (49% of whom had a diagnosis of lymphoma). In this setting, the instrument demonstrated 98% sensitivity and 82% specificity of predicting patients who were well nourished, moderately malnourished, or severely malnourished.[84] Nutritional status is often used as a proxy for well being. The PG-SGA has also been used as a predictor of length of stay in patients with hematologic malignancies. In a sample of patients with multiple myeloma, non-Hodgkin lymphoma, B-cell lymphoma, chronic lymphocytic leukemia, and AML who were admitted to the hospital for HSCT, those who were identified as being malnourished at baseline required longer hospitalizations.[85]

Other nutritional screening tools have been effectively used in the oncology setting. The Mini Nutritional Assessment[86] is a screening tool that is completed by clinicians that includes information on weight history, food intake, activity, psychosocial stress, and anthropometric measures. The Malnutrition Screening Tool[87] elicits similar

Text continued on page 1412

Scored Patient-Generated Subjective Global Assessment (PG-SGA)

Patient ID Information

History (Boxes 1-4 are designed to be completed by the patient.)

1. Weight *(See Worksheet 1)*

In summary of my current and recent weight:

I currently weigh about _______ pounds
I am about _________ feet _________ tall

One month ago I weighed about _________ pounds
Six months ago I weighed about _________ pounds

During the past two weeks my weight has:
□ decreased (1) □ not changed (0) □ increased (0)

Box 1 □

2. Food Intake: As compared to my normal intake, I would rate my food intake during the past month as:
- □ unchanged (0)
- □ more than usual (0)
- □ less than usual (1)

I am now taking:
- □ *normal food* but less than normal amount (1)
- □ little solid food (2)
- □ only liquids (3)
- □ only nutritonal supplements (3)
- □ very little of anything (4)
- □ only tube feedings or only nutrition by vein (0)

Box 2 □

3. Symptoms: I have had the following problems that have kept me from eating enough during the past two weeks (check all that apply):
- □ no problems eating (0)
- □ no appetite, just did not feel like eating (3)
- □ nausea (1)
- □ constipation (1)
- □ mouth sores (2)
- □ things taste funny or have no taste (1)
- □ problems swallowing (2)
- □ pain; where? (3) _________
- □ other** (1) ______________________
- □ vomiting (3)
- □ diarrhea (3)
- □ dry mouth (1)
- □ smells bother me (1)
- □ feel full quickly (1)
- □ fatigue (1)

** Examples: depression, money, or dental problems

Box 3 □

4. Activities and Function: Over the past month, I would generally rate my activity as:
- □ normal with no limitations (0)
- □ not my normal self, but able to be up and about with fairly normal activities (1)
- □ not feeling up to most things, but in bed or chair less than half the day (2)
- □ able to do little activity and spend most of the day in bed or chair (3)
- □ pretty much bedridden, rarely out of bed (3)

Box 4 □

Additive Score of the Boxes 1-4 □ **A**

 email: fdottery@savientpharma.com or noatpres1@aol.com

Figure 90-1 PATIENT-GENERATED SUBJECTIVE GLOBAL ASSESSMENT. *(From Ottery FD: Patient-generated subjective global assessment. In McCallum PD, Polisena CG, eds:* The clinical guide to oncology nutrition, *Chicago, 2000, The American Dietetic Association, p 11.)*

Continued

The remainder of this form will be completed by your doctor, nurse, dietitian, or therapist. Thank you.

Scored Patient-Generated Subjective Global Assessment (PG-SGA)

Additive Score of the Boxes 1-4 (See Side 1) ☐ A

Worksheet 1 - Scoring Weight (Wt) Loss

To determine score, use 1 month weight data if available. Use 6 month data only if there is no 1 month weight data. Use points below to score weight change and add one extra point if patient has lost weight during the past 2 months

Wt loss in 1 month	Points	Wt loss in 6 months
10% or greater	4	20% or greater
5-9.9%	3	10-19.9%
3-4.9%	2	6-9.9%
2-2.9%	1	2-5.9%
0-1.9%	0	0-1.9%

Numerical score from Worksheet 1 ☐

5. Worksheet 2 - Disease and its relation to nutritional requirements

All relevant diagnoses (specify) ____________________

One point each:
☐Cancer ☐AIDS ☐ Pulmonary or cardiac cachexia ☐ Presence of decubitus, open wound, or fistula
☐Presence of trauma ☐ Age greater than 65 years ☐Chronic renal insufficiency

Numerical score from Worksheet 2 ☐ B

6. Work Sheet 3 - Metabolic Demand

Score for metabolic stress is determined by a number of variables known to increase protein & calorie needs. The score is additive so that a patient who has a fever of >102 degrees (3 points) and is on 10 mg of prednisone chronically (2 points) would have an additive score for this section of 5 points.

Stress	none (0)	low (1)	moderate (2)	high (3)
Fever	no fever	>99 and <101	≥101 and <102	≥102
Fever duration	no fever	<72 hrs	72 hrs	>72 hrs
Corticosteroids	no corticosteroids	low dose (<10 mg prednisone equivalents/day)	moderate dose (≥10 and <30 mg prednisone equivalents/day)	high dose steroid (≥30 mg prednisone equivalents/day)

Numerical score from Worksheet 3 ☐ C

7. Worksheet 4 - Physical Exam

Physical exam includes a subjective evaluation of 3 aspects of body composition: fat, muscle, & fluid status. Since this is subjective, each aspect of the exam is rated for degree of deficit. Muscle deficit impacts point score more than fat deficit. Definition of categories: 0 = no deficit, 1+ = mild deficit, 2+ = moderate 3+ = severe

Muscle Status:				
temples (temporalis muscle)	0	1+	2+	3+
clavicles (pectoralis & deltoids)	0	1+	2+	3+
shoulders (deltoids)	0	1+	2+	3+
interosseous muscles	0	1+	2+	3+
Scapula (latissimus dorsi, trapezius, deltoids)	0	1+	2+	3+
thigh (quadriceps)	0	1+	2+	3+
calf (gastrocnemius)	0	1+	2+	3+
Global muscle status rating	**0**	**1+**	**2+**	**3+**
Fat Stores:				
orbital fat pads	0	1+	2+	3+
triceps skin fold	0	1+	2+	3+
fat overlying lower ribs	0	1+	2+	3+
Global fat deficit rating	**0**	**1+**	**2+**	**3+**

Fluid Status:				
ankle edema	0	1+	2+	3+
sacral edema	0	1+	2+	3+
ascites	0	1+	2+	3+
Global fluid status rating	**0**	**1+**	**2+**	**3+**

Numerical score from Worksheet 4 ☐ D

Total PG-SGA score ☐

(Total numerical score of A+B+C+D above)

(See triage recommendations below)

Global PG-SGA rating (A, B, or C) = ☐

Clinician Signature ____________________ RD RN PA MD DO Other ___ Date ______

Worksheet 5 - PG-SGA Global Assessment Categories

Category	Stage A	Stage B	Stage C
Weight	Well nourished No wt loss **OR** Recent wt gain	Moderately malnourished ≤5% wt loss in 1 month (or 10% in 6 mos) **OR** Progressive wt loss	Severely malnourished >5% wt loss in 1 month (or >10% in 6 mos) **OR** Progressive wt loss
Nutrient intake	No deficit **OR** Significant recent improvement	Definite decrease in intake	Severe deficit in intake
Nutrition Impact Symptoms	None **OR** Significant recent improvement allowing adequate intake	Present of nutrition impact symptoms (PG-SGA Box 3)	Present of nutrition impact symptoms (PG-SGA Box 3)
Functioning	No deficit **OR** Recent improvement	Moderate functional deficit **OR** Recent deterioration	Severe functional deficit **OR** recent significant deterioration
Physical Exam	No deficit **OR** Chronic deficit but recent improvement	Evidence of mild to moderate loss of muscle mass / SQ fat / muscle tone on palpation	Obvious signs of malnutrition (e.g., severe loss muscle, SQ tissue, possible edema)

Nutritional Triage Recommendations: Additive score is used to define specific nutritional interventions including patient & family education, symptom management including pharmacologic intervention, and appropriate nutrient intervention (food, nutritional supplements, enteral, or parenteral triage).
First line nutrition intervention includes optimal symptom management.

Triage based on PG-SGA point score

0-1	No intervention required at this time. Re-assessment on routine and regular basis during treatment.
2-3	Patient & family education by dietitian, nurse, or other clinician with pharmacologic intervention as indicated by symptom survey (Box 3) and lab values as appropriate.
4-8	Requires intervention by dietitian, in conjunction with nurse or physician as indicated by symptoms (Box 3).
≥9	Indicates a critical need for improved symptom management and/or nutrient intervention options.

Figure 90-1, cont'd PATIENT-GENERATED SUBJECTIVE GLOBAL ASSESSMENT. *(From Ottery FD: Patient-generated subjective global assessment. In McCallum PD, Polisena CG, eds:* The clinical guide to oncology nutrition, *Chicago, 2000, The American Dietetic Association, p 11.)*

Worksheets for PG-SGA Scoring

Boxes 1-4 of the PG-SGA are designed to be completed by the patient. The PG-SGA numerical score is determined using 1) the parenthetical points noted in boxes 1-4 and 2) the worksheets below for items not marked with parenthetical points. Scores for boxes 1 and 3 are additive within each box and scores for boxes 2 and 4 are based on the highest scored item checked off by the patient.

Worksheet 1 - Scoring Weight (Wt) Loss

To determine score, use 1 month weight data if available. Use 6 month data only if there is no 1 month weight data. Use points below to score weight change and add one extra point if patient has lost weight during the past 2 weeks. Enter total point score in Box 1 of the PG-SGA.

Wt loss in 1 month	Points	Wt loss in 6 months
10% or greater	4	20% or greater
5-9.9%	3	10-19.9%
3-4.9%	2	6-9.9%
2-2.9%	1	2-5.9%
0-1.9%	0	0-1.9%

Score for Worksheet 1 = ☐
Record in Box A

Worksheet 2 - Scoring Criteria for Condition

Score is derived by adding 1 point for each of the conditions listed below that pertain to the patient.

Category	Points
Cancer	1
AIDS	1
Pulmonary or cardiac cachexia	1
Presence of decubitus, open wound, or fistula	1
Presence of trauma	1
Age greater than 65 years	1

Score for Worksheet 2 = ☐
Record in Box B

Worksheet 3 - Scoring Metabolic Stress

Score for metabolic stress is determined by a number of variables known to increase protein & calorie needs. The score is additive so that a patient who has a fever of >102 degrees (3 points) and is on 10 mg of prednisone chronically (2 points) would have an additive score for this section of 5 points.

Stress	none (0)	low (1)	moderate (2)	high (3)
Fever	no fever	>99 and <101	≥101 and <102	≥102
Fever duration	no fever	<72 hrs	72 hrs	>72 hrs
Corticosteroids	no corticosteroids	low dose (<10 mg prednisone equivalents/day)	moderate dose (≥10 and <30 mg prednisone equivalents/day)	high dose steroids (≥30 mg prednisone equivalents/day)

Score for Worksheet 3 = ☐
Record in Box C

Worksheet 4 - Physical Examination

Physical exam includes a subjective evaluation of 3 aspects of body composition: fat, muscle, & fluid status. Since this is subjective, each aspect of the exam is rated for degree of deficit. Muscle deficit impacts point score more than fat deficit. Definition of categories: 0 = no deficit, 1+ = mild deficit, 2+ = moderate deficit, 3+ = severe deficit. Rating of deficit in these categories are *not* additive but are used to clinically assess the degree of deficit (or presence of excess fluid).

Fat Stores:				
orbital fat pads	0	1+	2+	3+
triceps skin fold	0	1+	2+	3+
fat overlying lower ribs	0	1+	2+	3+
Global fat deficit rating	**0**	**1+**	**2+**	**3+**
Muscle Status:				
temples (temporalis muscle)	0	1+	2+	3+
clavicles (pectoralis & deltoids)	0	1+	2+	3+
shoulders (deltoids)	0	1+	2+	3+
interosseous muscles	0	1+	2+	3+
scapula (latissimus dorsi, trapezius, deltoids)	0	1+	2+	3+
thigh (quadriceps)	0	1+	2+	3+
calf (gastrocnemius)	0	1+	2+	3+
Global muscle status rating	**0**	**1+**	**2+**	**3+**

Fluid Status:				
ankle edema	0	1+	2+	3+
sacral edema	0	1+	2+	3+
ascites	0	1+	2+	3+
Global fluid status rating	**0**	**1+**	**2+**	**3+**

Point score for the physical exam is determined by the overall subjective rating of total body deficit.

No deficit	score = 0 points
Mild deficit	score = 1 point
Moderate deficit	score = 2 points
Severe deficit	score = 3 points

Score for Worksheet 4 = ☐
Record in Box D

Worksheet 5 - PG-SGA Global Assessment Categories

Category	Stage A Well-nourished	Stage B Moderately malnourished or suspected malnutrition	Stage C Severely malnourished
Weight	No wt loss **OR** Recent non-fluid wt gain	~5% wt loss within 1 month (or 10% in 6 months) **OR** No wt stabilization or wt gain (i.e., continued wt loss)	>5% wt loss in 1 month (or >10% in 6 months) **OR** No wt stabilization or wt gain (i.e., continued wt loss)
Nutrient Intake	No deficit **OR** Significant recent improvement	Definite decrease in intake	Severe deficit in intake
Nutrition Impact Symptoms	None **OR** Significant recent improvement allowing adequate intake	Presence of nutrition impact symptoms (Box 3 of PG-SGA)	Presence of nutrition impact symptoms (Box 3 of PG-SGA)
Functioning	No deficit **OR** Significant recent improvement	Moderate functional deficit **OR** Recent deterioration	Severe functional deficit **OR** Recent significant deterioration
Physical Exam	No deficit **OR** Chronic deficit but with recent clinical improvement	Evidence of mild to moderate loss of SQ fat &/or muscle mass &/or muscle tone on palpation	Obvious signs of malnutrition (e.g., severe loss of SQ tissues, possible edema)

Global PG-SGA rating (A, B, or C) = ☐

Figure 90-1, cont'd PATIENT-GENERATED SUBJECTIVE GLOBAL ASSESSMENT. *(From Ottery FD: Patient-generated subjective global assessment. In McCallum PD, Polisena CG, eds:* The clinical guide to oncology nutrition, *Chicago, 2000, The American Dietetic Association, p 11.)*

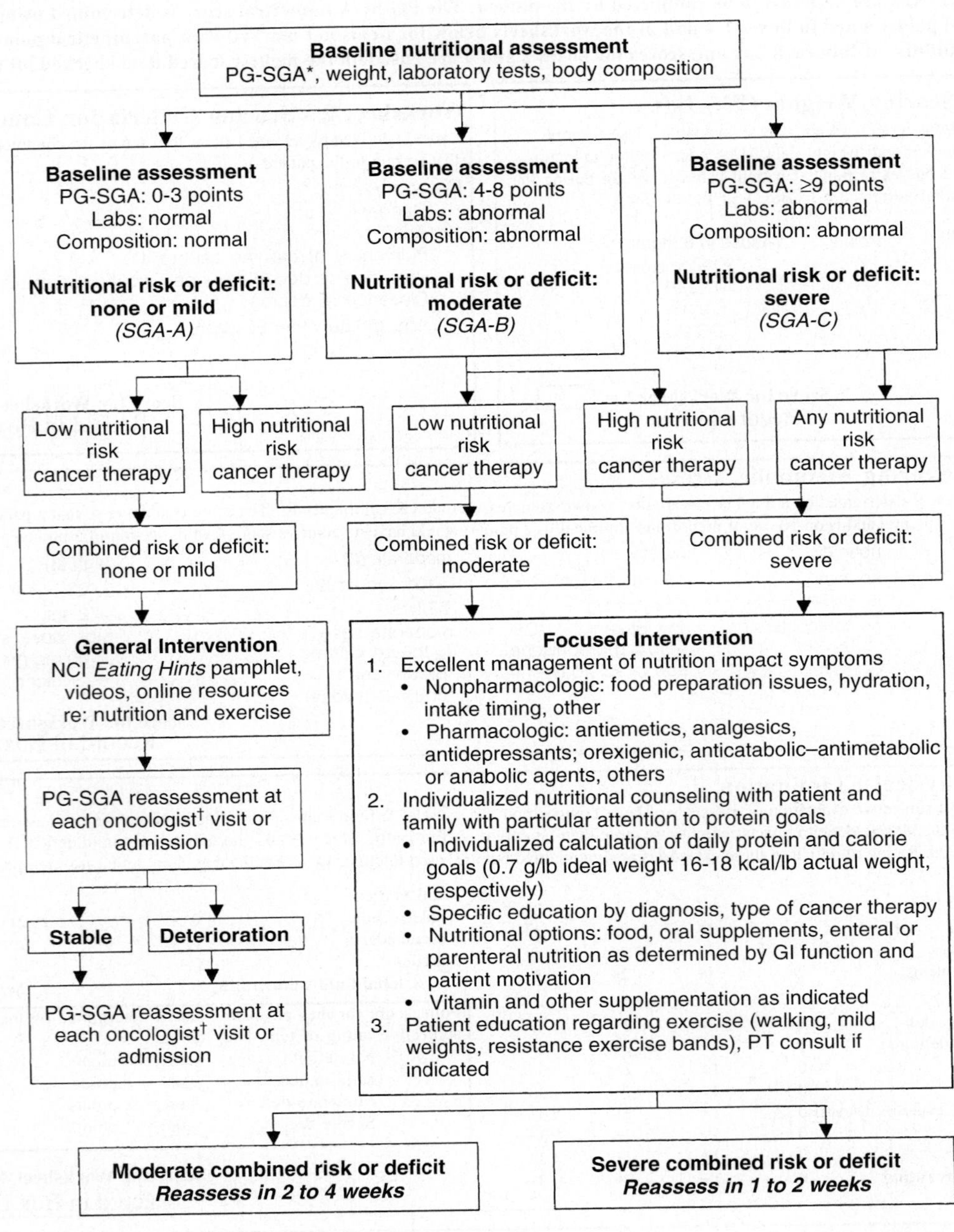

Figure 90-2 ALGORITHM OF OPTIMAL NUTRITIONAL INTERVENTION. *GI,* Gastrointestinal; *NCI,* National Cancer Institute; *PG-SGA,* Patient Generated-Subjective Global Assessment; *PT,* physical therapy; *SGA,* Subjective Global Assessment. *(From Ottery FD: Patient-Generated Subjective Global Assessment. In McCallum PD, Polisena CG, eds:* The clinical guide to oncology nutrition, *Chicago, 2000, The American Dietetic Association, p 11.)*

information and can be completed by medical, nursing, or administrative personnel. Both instruments have established validity and reliability in ambulatory cancer settings.

Nutrition Assessment

Patients meeting screening risk criteria are candidates for nutritional assessment. This is a more comprehensive and detailed evaluation that includes a medical and dietary history, anthropometric measurements, body composition analysis, a review of findings from a nutritionally focused physical examination, specific laboratory data, and assessment for symptoms that have the potential to impact nutritional intake.[88] The purpose of nutrition assessment is to gather data to plan for nutrition interventions. Optimally, trained dietary specialists are responsible for performing comprehensive nutritional assessment, planning nutritional interventions, and systematic reassessment of nutritional status. In practice settings where there is not access to registered dietitians, experienced nurses may perform nutritional assessments.

Anthropometrics

Anthropometrics refers to measurement of the human body in terms of dimensions, proportions, and ratios. Anthropometrics commonly

Table 90-1 Common Terminology Criteria for Adverse Events Version 4.02 Grading for Weight Loss

Adverse Event	1	2	3	4	5
Weight loss definition: A finding characterized by a decrease in overall body weight	5% to <10% from baseline; intervention not indicated	10% to <20% from baseline; nutrition support indicated	≥20% from baseline; tube feeding or TPN indicated	—	—

TPN, Total parenteral nutrition.

Table 90-2 Categories of Body Mass Index

Category	Body Mass Index
Underweight	<18.5
Normal Weight	18.5-24.9
Overweight	25-29.9
Obesity	≥30

Source: National Heart, Blood, and Lung Institute, 2012. http://www.nhlbisupport.com/bmi/.

includes weight, height, and skin-fold thickness; these variables are easy to assess in busy clinical practice settings, are noninvasive, and can be accomplished with minimal cost. Weight and height are the most common forms of serial anthropometric measurement performed in clinical practice settings. The measurement of height and weight in the oncology setting is especially critical because dosing for many therapeutic interventions is based on body surface area. It is essential that height and weight be measured longitudinally from a reliable baseline and that the instruments used for measurement are accurate and precise. Longitudinal measurement provides the temporal context to assess weight change in an individual patient; the time period over which weight change occurs is critical. An involuntary loss of 10% or more of body weight within a 6-month period or 5% or more over 1 month is defined as severe weight loss and is associated with poorer outcomes.[89] Changes in performance status have been associated with a 2.5-kg weight loss over a 6- to 8-week period.[67] The Common Terminology Criteria for Adverse Event (CTCAE) reporting for weight loss is shown in Table 90-1. In clinical practice, lower grades of toxicity are often deemed tolerable. The CTCAE indicates that intervention is not indicated for patients experiencing a weight loss of 5% to 10% or less of body weight (grade 1).[90] Moreover, no time frame is identified in this toxicity assessment. Early intervention is the cornerstone to effective management of nutritional issues in patients with hematologic malignancies. As such, the criteria outlined in Table 90-1 facilitate reactive rather than proactive interventions for patients experiencing weight loss.[89]

Instruments used in anthropometric measurement should be recalibrated and checked for accuracy and precision by the manufacturer or the organization's biomedical engineering group at least every 6 months. Clinical practices should develop clear procedures for the measurement of height and weight so that personnel accountable for these activities are able to obtain this information in an accurate and consistent manner. Patients should be instructed to remove overcoats and shoes as well as heavy objects from their pockets before their weight is assessed. Some patients may not be able to be weighed in a standing position. Chair scales, bed scales, and scales that allow measurement of weight while in wheelchairs should be considered in these situations. Height should be measured using a stadiometer with the patient standing with the feet flat on the floor or platform. Anthropometry often includes calculation of BMI, which is a measure of fat based on height and weight. BMI provides information on whether a patient's weight is within a healthy range (Table 90-2) but does not provide any information on body composition.

Body Composition Analysis

Body composition analysis reflects nutritional intake, loss, and need over time. Unlike assessment of height, weight, and BMI, body composition analysis provides measurement of tissue loss by analyzing two major body compartments, fat-free (or lean body) mass and fat mass. Decreases in fat-free mass are associated with impairments in overall health, function, and quality of life.[91] Methods of assessing body composition include bioelectrical impedance analysis (BIA), dual-energy x-ray absorptiometry (DEXA), and computed tomography (CT). BIA is based on the capacity of hydrated tissues to conduct electrical energy and measures impedance or opposition to the flow of an electrical current through body fluids contained mainly in lean and fat tissue. Impedance is proportional to body water volume. BIA is valid, easy to use, and noninvasive. There may be some inaccuracies in patients who have fluid losses, dehydration, or fluid retention, and for these reasons, it is not an optimal strategy in the cancer population. DEXA is a highly accurate and reproducible method of assessing body composition; it is the reference method for assessment in clinical research settings. DEXA provides noninvasive direct measurement of three components of body composition: fat mass, fat-free mass, and bone mineral mass. Although DEXA is frequently used in cancer to assess bone mineral density, it is not commonly used to assess other aspects of body composition longitudinally. Accessibility, operator skill, cost, and radiation exposure are factors contributing to its limited use in this setting. CT provides assessment of fat-free mass through regional analysis of the third vertebra, which strongly predicts whole body fat and fat-free mass. Because CT scanning is used commonly in cancer patient diagnosis and follow-up, this approach has practical benefits because it can be integrated with routine care. Specific software is required to perform these assessments.[91]

Nutrition Biomarkers

Although there is no gold standard test to assess nutrition status, selected laboratory values are often included as part of a comprehensive nutritional assessment. Many of these values are readily available because they are being collected as part of routine care. Circulating proteins, including albumin, prealbumin, transferrin, and retinol-binding protein, are often used as indicators of nutritional status. C-reactive protein, total lymphocyte count, and serum total cholesterol are also common. Low serum albumin or depressed total lymphocyte counts may be early indicators of protein-energy deficiencies; however, because these laboratory tests are influenced by many other variables, they lack sensitivity and should be used along with other variables in making decisions about patients. The usefulness of serum albumin levels as an indicator of nutritional status, for example, is limited by that fact that it can be influenced by hydration status or the presence of ascites. Serum albumin is also a negative acute-phase reactant, meaning that it is decreased in the presence of inflammation, which occurs in many hematologic malignancies as well as other types of cancer. Some laboratory tests may be normal even when deficits are present. Zinc deficiency, for example, is relatively common, but because zinc is primarily stored in muscle and liver tissues with only a small percentage in the serum, zinc levels may appear normal when stores are actually low.[92] Other levels can be influenced by recent dietary intake or supplements. Serum iron levels, for example, may be elevated by recent food intake, and vitamin C supplementation may lower serum B_{12} levels.

The use of biochemical indices for the assessment of nutritional status in patients with hematologic malignancies undergoing both aSCT and ASCT. aSCT has been investigated. Findings indicated that biochemical indices were not sufficiently reliable in this population of patients because levels were markedly affected by the acute-phase response (measured with acute-phase protein levels) secondary to infections. Prealbumin levels, measured 8 days after completion of the conditioning regimen were, however, helpful about making decisions to start parenteral nutrition (PN) support.[93]

Nutrition Support Strategies

The goals of nutrition support therapy are to ensure adequate intake of calories and protein, minimize symptoms impeding nutritional status, maintain weight, or reverse weight loss, preserve lean body mass, and optimize function and quality of life.[94] Interventions prescribed to support nutrition should be based on the results of nutritional assessment. In addition, the presence of a functional GI tract is an essential consideration in determining a nutritional care plan. Moreover, the patient's ethnicity, culture, preferences, performance status, quality of life, and prognosis, as well as cost effectiveness, should also be taken into account. Interventions may include dietary education and counseling, oral supplementation, nutritional supplements delivered directly into the GI tract, PN, the use of orexigenic or other pharmacologic agents, or some combination of these strategies.

Neutropenic Diets

Neutropenic diets were developed in an effort to decrease infections in neutropenic patients by limiting the introduction of bacteria by food ingestion.[95] The diet evolved from practices used in germ-free protective environments during the 1960s in which patients were isolated and foods sterilized with the goal of preventing colonization by microorganisms.[96] In this environment, patients were able to tolerate higher doses of chemotherapy with less toxicity, including infections.[97] Over the ensuing decades, many of these practices have changed, but the neutropenic diet continues to be part of routine care for patients with low neutrophil counts in many institutions. In a survey of 156 institutions belonging to the Association of Community Cancer Centers, 78% reported the use of restricted diets during periods of neutropenia.[98] Neutropenic diets typically limit consumption of fresh fruits, raw vegetables, aged cheeses, cold meat cuts, fast food, and take-out food. Yogurt and ice cream may also be restricted. These restrictions may limit patient food choices at a time when adequate consumption of calories is critical and contributes to malnutrition. Investigations of the effectiveness of neutropenic diets have not been able to demonstrate appreciable differences between intervention and control groups with respect to the development of febrile neutropenia, neutrophil counts, postchemotherapy filgrastim use, median cycles of chemotherapy,[95] time to major infection, survival,[99] febrile admissions, or gram-negative bacteremia.[100] Without clear evidence, the restrictions concerning diet that are best to recommend are the Food and Drug Administration—approved food safety guidelines available at http://www.foodsafety.gov.[101]

Dietary Education and Counseling

Individualized early dietary education and counseling is correlated with improved nutritional status and body weight. Dietary counseling includes the prescription of a therapeutic diet that is individualized to meet patient needs. Providing education on specific food choices, such as calorie-dense foods, and the management of symptoms that can impact oral intake can be extremely effective. In a review of evidence investigating the effectiveness of nutritional interventions, a summary of seven studies reporting on the effects of dietary counseling and nutritional supplementation on oral intake found that improved caloric intake was reported in all trials.[102] Clinical trials investigating the effects of dietary counseling specific to patients with hematologic malignancies were not identified in the literature.

The use of oral nutrition supplements is an intervention that is frequently suggested for cancer patients. These supplements may be of benefit in increasing caloric intake in patients who are malnourished, particularly those who have BMIs of less than 20. Moreover, in a Cochrane review, the use of supplements with energy and protein was associated with weight gain, shorter hospitalization, and improved survival.[103]

Specialized Nutritional Support Therapy

Specialized nutrition support includes the use of enteral nutrition (EN) and PN. EN refers to the delivery of nutrition through an enteral feeding device inserted into a functioning GI tract. PN refers to the administration of an admixture of nutrients via the intravenous route. The use of these interventions in patients with cancer has been the subject of considerable debate because of the concern that the provision of nutrients may stimulate tumor growth and metastases. EN is associated with improvements in nitrogen balance and consistent weight gain. PN consistently leads to weight gain, increases in body fat, and improved nitrogen balance. Neither EN nor PN has demonstrated improvements in serum protein levels.[66]

Enteral nutrition is recommended in patients with a functioning GI tract in whom oral intake is inadequate to meet energy requirements. Contraindications include a malfunctioning GI tract, severe diarrhea or bleeding, mechanical obstructions or malabsorption, GI fistulas, or intractable vomiting.[81]

ASPEN is a multidisciplinary organization dedicated to improving patient care through the advancement of the science and practice of nutritional support therapy. ASPEN has developed evidence-based guidelines outlining specific recommendations for nutrition support therapy during adult anticancer treatment and HSCT. The ASPEN recommendations for patients receiving anticancer treatment and those for undergoing HSCT are outlined in Tables 90-3 and 90-4, respectively.[66]

The use of nutritional support therapy during routine cancer treatment, including surgery, chemotherapy, or radiation, has not been shown to improve outcome. Nutrition support therapy is appropriate for subsets of these populations who are malnourished or at risk for malnutrition, but this should only be instituted as part of a nutrition care plan that is developed after a formal nutritional assessment is completed. EN and PN can both be used in the setting of HSCT to support nutritional status during the peritransplant period. ASPEN recommends the use of nutrition support therapy for patients undergoing HSCT who are malnourished and who will be unable to consume or absorb adequate nutrients for a prolonged period of time to minimize the complications associated with malnutrition. Seven to 14 days is generally accepted as a prolonged period, although this has not been clearly defined in the literature.[66] It is important to note that PN is also associated with a number of complications, including fluid overload, hepatic dysfunction, subclavian vein thrombosis, delays in platelet engraftment, and catheter-related infections. PN may also diminish appetite. Specific contraindications for using the parenteral approach include a functioning GI tract, the need for nutritional support therapy for a period of less than 5 days, lack of adequate vascular access, hemodynamic instability, anuria, profound metabolic or electrolyte disturbances, and patient or caregiver preference.[81]

Symptom Management

Patients with hematologic malignancies experience a variety of symptoms related to both their underlying disease and treatment process.

Table 90-3 ASPEN Clinical Guidelines: Nutrition Support Therapy During Adult Anticancer Treatment

1. Patients with cancer are nutritionally at risk and should undergo nutritional screening to identify those who require formal nutritional assessment with development of a nutrition care plan.
2. Nutrition support therapy should not be used *routinely* in patients undergoing major cancer operations.
3. Perioperative nutrition support therapy may be beneficial in moderately or severely malnourished patients if administered for 7 to 14 days preoperatively, but the potential benefits of nutrition support must be weighed against the potential risks of the nutrition support itself and of delaying the operation.
4. Nutrition support therapy should not be used *routinely* as an adjunct to chemotherapy.
5. Nutrition support therapy should not be used *routinely* in patients undergoing head and neck, abdominal, or pelvic irradiation.
6. Nutrition support therapy is appropriate in patients receiving active anticancer treatment who are malnourished and who are anticipated to be unable to ingest or absorb adequate nutrients for a prolonged period of time.
7. The palliative use of nutrition support therapy in terminally ill cancer patients is rarely indicated.
8. Omega-3 fatty acid supplementation may help stabilize weight in cancer patients on oral diets experiencing progressive, unintentional weight loss.
9. Patients should not use therapeutic diets to treat cancer.
10. Immune-enhancing enteral formulas containing mixtures of arginine, nucleic acids, and essential fatty acids may be beneficial in malnourished patients undergoing major operations.

ASPEN, American Society for Parenteral and Enteral Nutrition.

Table 90-4 ASPEN Clinical Guidelines: Nutrition Support Therapy During Adult Hematopoietic Cell Transplantation

1. All patients undergoing hematopoietic stem cell transplantation (HSCT) with myeloablative conditioning regimens are at nutritional risk and should undergo nutrition screening to identify those who require formal nutritional assessment with the development of a nutritional care plan.
2. Nutrition support therapy is appropriate in patients undergoing HSCT who are malnourished and who are anticipated to be unable to ingest or absorb adequate nutrients for a prolonged period of time. When parenteral nutrition is used, it should be discontinued as soon as toxicities have been resolved after stem cell engraftment.
3. Enteral nutrition should be used in patients with a functional GI tract in whom oral intake is inadequate to meet nutritional requirements.
4. Pharmacologic doses of parenteral glutamine *may benefit* patients undergoing HSCT.
5. Patients should receive dietary counseling regarding foods that may pose infectious risks and safe food handling during the period of neutropenia.
6. Nutrition support is appropriate for patients undergoing HSCT who develop moderate to severe GVHD accompanied by poor oral intake and/or significant malabsorption.

ASPEN, American Society for Parenteral and Enteral Nutrition; *GI,* gastrointestinal; *GVHD,* graft-versus-host disease; *HSCT,* hematopoietic stem cell transplantation.

Symptoms may occur concurrently or in clusters and cause patients significant distress. The symptom burden is the combined impact of all disease- or therapy-related symptoms on the patient's ability to function. In the hematopoietic population, physical symptoms occur frequently and include pain, mucositis, nausea, vomiting, diarrhea, and delirium.[104] Cancer treatment, particularly aggressive, multimodality interventions, can be extremely stressful for patients and often result in psychosocial distress. Psychologic symptoms occur frequently in patients with hematologic cancers and include anxiety, depression, grief, loss, and feelings of demoralization.[105] Symptom severity and the cumulative effects of symptom clusters can be indicators of nutritional risk.[106] To preserve optimal nutritional intake and function, it is essential that nutrition-impact symptoms be anticipated and proactively managed regardless of the outcome of underlying disease. The management of symptoms that have the potential to interfere with oral intake is a critical component of a nutritional care plan. Selected interventions to manage some of the common nutrition-impact symptoms in patients with hematologic malignancies are shown in Table 90-5.

Pharmacologic Interventions

Current treatments for cachexia include the use of agents that affect either appetite or cachectic mediators or signaling pathways. Empirical evidence supports only a limited number of pharmacologic interventions in the management of anorexia. Corticosteroids are recommended for patients in whom short-term benefit is needed or those with a limited life expectancy. Progestins, such as megestrol acetate, have been extensively studied for their orexigenic effects. More than 15 randomized clinical trials of high-dose progestins have been completed demonstrating statistically significant improvements in appetite and body weight; however, body composition analysis has indicated that the weight gain associated with these agents is related to increased fat and not lean body mass.[71] Cannabinoids and hydrazine sulfate have also been investigated, but in a recent review, the effectiveness of these agents could not be demonstrated.[32] Ghrelin, a neuropeptide released from the stomach in response to fasting, has been shown to stimulate energy intake by approximately 30% in patients with cancer and anorexia without side effects. Further studies are needed to determine if ghrelin increases lean body mass and weight. RC-1291, a ghrelin mimetic, is currently being investigated in the setting of cancer-induced anorexia. This agent has been shown to increase lean body mass and improve hand grip strength; no changes in quality of life or weight have been reported.[71]

Several mediators of cachexia signaling pathways have also been investigated to determine their effect on weight gain and a number of other outcome variables. Eicosapentaenoic acid (EPA) is an essential omega-3 fatty acid that is found in oily fish such as salmon, mackerel, and sardines. EPA has been found to attenuate muscle atrophy and stimulate appetite. Empirical evidence supports stabilization of body weight in patients with cancer, although poor compliance has been an issue for patients participating in these studies. β-Hydroxy-β-methylbutyrate (HBM) is similar to EPA in that it attenuates PIF-induced protein degradation in muscle by downregulating the ubiquitin–proteasome pathway. It also plays a role in the depression of protein synthesis. In placebo-controlled trials, when HBM was administered in combination with L-glutamine and L-arginine, increased body weight and lean body mass were reported, but no change in fat mass was demonstrated.[71]

Thalidomide is a cyclic imide that has been shown to decrease the stability of mRNAs coding for different proinflammatory cytokines, including TNF-α.[107] Thalidomide has now been used in several clinical trials aimed at evaluating its effectiveness in the treatment of cancer-related anorexia and cachexia. In a small preliminary study, thalidomide has been shown to improve symptoms, including nausea, appetite, sensation of well-being, and restedness in the morning.[108] Another early investigation evaluating the use of an isocaloric diet in combination with thalidomide demonstrated increases in body weight and lean body mass in patients with solid tumors. In this study, the agent was well tolerated, with no patients developing neuropathy.[109]

Several other compounds that have the ability to inhibit cytokine production have been investigated for their potential use in the setting of cachexia. Atractylenolide (ATR) is an agent that has been used in Chinese traditional medicine to improve GI symptoms such as nausea, vomiting, and anorexia. Recent evidence has demonstrated its ability to markedly decrease circulating IL-1, and in a randomized,

Table 90-5 Practical Interventions and Patient Education for Nutrition-Impact Symptoms

Symptom	Selected Interventions
Anorexia	Avoid drinking liquids with meals; instead drink liquids in between meals. Avoid large meals; six smaller meals are usually better tolerated. Keep high-calorie, high-protein snacks on hand, such as peanut butter, ice cream, cheese, and granola bars. Avoid consuming empty calories such as sod, fast food, and processed snacks. Stimulate appetite with light exercise, wine or beer (if not contraindicated), orexigenic agents as prescribed. Add extra calories and protein such as butter, skim milk powder, wheat germ, brown sugar, or honey to food.
Mucositis	Avoid tart or citrus foods, tomato-based foods, and pickled or vinegary foods. Avoid spicy foods, hot sauces, and spices such as pepper, cloves, chili powder, and nutmeg; other seasonings such as basil, thyme, and oregano are less irritating and may be better tolerated. Avoid caffeine, alcohol, and tobacco; these substances cause dryness and irritation. Choose soft-textured foods such as creamy puddings, cream soups, custards, soft eggs, cooked cereals, mashed potatoes or other root vegetables, casseroles, ice cream, puddings, and yogurt. Avoid hard, rough foods such as toast, crackers, pretzels, and granola. Moisten dry foods with gravies or sauces.
Nausea	Take antiemetics as prescribed. Eat small, frequent meals rather than three larger meals. Avoid overly sweet, salty, greasy, fried, or rich foods. Consume foods that are not associated with strong odors. Eat dry foods such as saltines, pretzels, or bread sticks every few hours during the day. Rest with the head elevated for at least 1 hour after consuming foods.
Taste changes	Use plastic utensils to minimize a bitter or metallic taste. Substitute high-protein foods for red meats in patients who are experiencing taste aversions to meat. Substitute foods may include fish, poultry, Greek yogurt, milkshakes, high-protein milk, soy products, eggs, cheese, puddings, whole grains, and ice cream. Rinse mouth with water, salt water, tea, or ginger ale before eating to help clear and stimulate taste buds. Use cool rather than warm or hot foods. Freeze foods such as grapes, cherries, watermelon, and oranges for snacks. Use tart flavors such as lemon or citrus; tart hard candies such as lemon drops may reduce bitter or metallic taste. Mints or chewing gum may help get rid of unpleasant tastes in the mouth.
Xerostomia	Drink 8 to 12 beverages per day. Use a straw to drink liquids. Moisten dry food with sauces or gravies. Avoid commercial mouthwashes, alcohol, and acidic beverages. Eat soft or moist foods at cool or room temperature. Take small bites and chew food completely.

From the National Cancer Institute: Eating hints before, during, and after cancer treatment, http://www.cancer.gov/cancertopics/coping/eatinghints/page1/AllPages; and Clegg H, Miletello G: *Eating well through cancer.* Nashville, TN, 2006, Favorite Recipes Press.

nonblinded pilot study involving a small sample of patients with cancer, ATR was shown to significantly increase body weight and arm circumference.[110] Cytokine-neutralizing agents, such as the monoclonal antibody infliximab (Remicade, Janssen Biotech) or soluble receptors such as etanercept (Enbrel, Amgen, Pfizer), which both target TNF-α, are used to treat other chronic inflammatory pathologies and have been shown to increase weight and lean body mass in patients with rheumatoid arthritis. Little information about the use of these agents in the setting of cancer cachexia is available in the literature, although a number of trials are underway. An alternative approach to treating patients with cancer associated cachexia is the use of small molecule inhibitors of Janus kinase 1 (JAK1) and JAK2. Although these drugs are frequently not active against the underlying malignancy, their use in this scenario is directed toward interrupting tumor-associated cytokines that result in cachexia. This approach is currently being explored in patients with far advanced pancreatic cancer. Although these and other molecules that block cytokine production or interfere with the proposed mechanisms of cachexia hold promise, none of them are currently available for routine use in cancer patients. Moreover, the use of these agents in patients with hematologic malignancies will require careful consideration because they have the potential to influence immune response.

FUTURE DIRECTIONS

Hematologic malignancies comprise a heterogeneous group of diseases that entail diverse therapeutic interventions. The malignancies, as well as the interventions used to treat them, are associated with toxicities that can profoundly influence nutritional status. Nutritional issues span the continuum between malnutrition and overnutrition in this population, and both of these alterations have the potential to negatively influence patient outcomes. Additional research on nutritional issues within the hematologic malignancies population is needed. Particular areas of focus should include descriptive work detailing the incidence, prevalence, and etiologies of nutritional issues within patient subgroups as well as investigations of the effectiveness of novel nutrition support interventions and their influence on overall outcomes. Additionally, as emerging therapeutics continue to shift survival rates among these populations, there will be growing need to understand the enduring effects of nutritional alterations on survivors of hematologic malignancies.

SUGGESTED READINGS

Adams LA, Shepard N, Caruso RA, et al: Putting evidence into practice: Evidence-based interventions to prevent and manage anorexia. *Clin J Oncol Nurs* 13:95, 2009.

August DA, Huhmann MB: American Society for Parenteral and Enteral Nutrition (A.S.P.E.N.) Board of Directors. A.S.P.E.N. clinical guidelines: Nutrition support therapy during adult anticancer treatment and in hematopoietic cell transplantation. *JPEN J Parenter Enteral Nutr* 33:472, 2009.

Bernhardson BM, Tishelman C, Rutqvist LE: Olfactory changes among patients receiving chemotherapy. *Eur J Oncol Nurs* 13:9, 2009.

Bozzetti F: Screening the nutritional status in oncology: A preliminary report on 1,000 outpatients. *Support Care Cancer* 17:279, 2009.

Calle EE, Rodrigues C, Walker-Thurmond K, et al: Overweight, obesity, and mortality from cancer in a prospectively studied cohort of U.S. adults. *N Engl J Med* 348:1625, 2003.

Cunningham RS, Huhman MB: Nutritional Disturbances Cancer Nursing Principles and Practice Seventh Edition (2011).

Dewys WD, Begg C, Lavin PT, et al: Prognostic effect of weight loss prior to chemotherapy in cancer patients. Eastern Cooperative Oncology Group. *Am J Med* 69:491, 1980.

Epstein JB, Barasch A: Taste disorders in cancer patients: Pathogenesis, and approach to assessment and management. *Oral Oncology* 46:77, 2010.

Epstein JB, Hong C, Logan RM, et al: A systematic review of orofacial pain in patients receiving cancer therapy. *Support Care Cancer* 18:1023, 2010. Epub 2010 Jun 11.

Gardner A, Mattiuzzi G, Faderl S, et al: Randomized comparison of cooked and noncooked diets in patients undergoing remission induction therapy for acute myeloid leukemia. *J Clin Oncol* 26:5684, 2008. Epub 2008 Oct 27.

Green DM, Cox CL, Zhu L, et al: Risk factors for obesity in adult survivors of childhood cancer: A report from the childhood cancer survivor study. *Clin Oncol* 30:246, 2012. Epub 2011 Dec 19.

Gupta D, Vashi PG, Lammersfeld CA, et al: Role of nutritional status in predicting the length of stay in cancer: A systematic review of the epidemiological literature. *Ann Nutr Metab* 59:96, 2011. Epub 2011 Dec 2.

Inagaki J, Rodriguez V, Bodey GP: Proceedings: Causes of death in cancer patients. *Cancer* 33:568, 1974.

Johansson P, Mesa R, Scherber R, et al: Association between quality of life and clinical parameters in patients with myeloproliferative neoplasms. *Leuk Lymphoma* 53:441, 2012.

Jubelirer SJ: The benefit of the neutropenic diet: Fact or fiction? *Oncologist* 16:704, 2011. Epub 2011 Apr 6.

Keefe DM, Schubert MM, Elting LS, et al: Mucositis Study Section of the Multinational Association of Supportive Care in Cancer and the International Society for Oral Oncology. Updated clinical practice guidelines for the prevention and treatment of mucositis. *Cancer* 109:820, 2007.

Kyle UG, Chalandon Y, Miralbell R, et al: Longitudinal follow-up of body composition in hematopoietic stem cell transplant patients. *Bone Marrow Transplant* 35:1171, 2005.

Lichtman MA: Obesity and the risk for a hematological malignancy: Leukemia, lymphoma, or myeloma. *Oncologist* 15:1083, 2010. Epub 2010 Oct 7.

Luthringer S: Nutritional implications of radiation therapy. In Elliott L, Molseed LL, McCallum P, editors: *The clinical guide to oncology nutrition*, Chicago, IL, 2006, American Dietetic Association, p 88.

Oeffinger KC, Mertens AC, Sklar CA, et al: Childhood Cancer Survivor Study. Obesity in adult survivors of childhood acute lymphoblastic leukemia: A report from the Childhood Cancer Survivor Study. *J Clin Oncol* 21:1359, 2003.

Ottery FD: Definition of standardized nutritional assessment and interventional pathways in oncology. *Nutrition* 12:S15, 1996.

Penna F, Minero VG, Costamagna D, et al: Anti-cytokine strategies for the treatment of cancer-related anorexia and cachexia. *Expert Opin Biol Ther* 10:1241, 2010.

Roeland E, Mitchell W, Elia G, et al: Symptom control in stem cell transplantation: A multidisciplinary palliative care team approach. Part 1: Physical symptoms. *J Support Oncol* 8:100, 2010.

Roeland E, Mitchell W, Elia G, et al: Symptom control in stem cell transplantation: A multidisciplinary palliative care team approach. Part 2: Psychosocial concerns. *J Support Oncol* 8:179, 2010.

Rubenstein EB, Peterson DE, Schubert M, et al: Mucositis Study Section of the Multinational Association for Supportive Care in Cancer; International Society for Oral Oncology. Clinical practice guidelines for the prevention and treatment of cancer therapy-induced oral and gastrointestinal mucositis. *Cancer* 100:2026, 2004.

Scherber R, Dueck AC, Johansson P, et al: The myeloproliferative neoplasm symptom assessment form (MPN-SAF): International prospective validation and reliability trial in 402 patients. *Blood* 118:401, 2011. Epub 2011 May 2.

Strom SS, Yamamura Y, Kantarijian HM, et al: Obesity, weight gain, and risk of chronic myeloid leukemia. *Cancer Epidemiol Biomarkers Prev* 18:1501, 2009.

Tan BH, Fearon KC: Cachexia: Prevalence and impact in medicine. *Curr Opin Clin Nutr Metab Care* 11:400, 2008.

Tisdale MJ: Mechanisms of cancer cachexia. *Physiol Rev* 89:381, 2009.

Vera-Llonch M, Oster G, Ford CM, et al: Oral mucositis and outcomes of allogeneic hematopoietic stem-cell transplantation in patients with hematologic malignancies. *Support Care Cancer* 15:491, 2007. Epub 2006 Dec 1.

Watters AL, Epstein JB, Agulnik M: Oral complications of targeted cancer therapies: A narrative literature review. *Oral Oncol* 47:441, 2011. Epub 2011 Apr 22.

For complete list of references log on to www.expertconsult.com.

CHAPTER 91

PSYCHOSOCIAL ASPECTS OF HEMATOLOGIC DISORDERS

Ruth McCorkle and Elizabeth Cooke

Major changes in the understanding and treatment of cancer have led to increased survival for people diagnosed with hematologic cancers. Regardless of the advances and concomitant survival increase, a diagnosis of a hematologic malignancy can have great impact on the psychosocial aspects of the lives of cancer survivors and their families. Diseases of the blood are perceived as serious and often fatal. Psychologic, existential, cognitive, social, and economic stressors are common experiences for cancer survivors. Despite the increasing attention by providers, policy makers, and the general public on long-term survivorship issues within the past 20 years, ongoing progress must continue to be made in identifying and testing interventions and services to meet the psychosocial aspects of quality cancer care for patients and their families.[1,2] Psychosocial interventions and services are those that enable patients, their families, and health care providers to optimize health care and health care outcomes by managing the psychologic, social, and behavioral aspects of cancer and its consequences.

These psychosocial aspects may be intensified in patients with hematologic malignancies because of their association with an uncertain prognosis, a prolonged treatment course often involving numerous hospitalizations, and the systemic nature of the diseases.[3] Discomfort from painful medical procedures, body image disturbances, central line catheters, sexual dysfunction, and role and relationship disruptions resulting from lengthy hospitalizations and fear of premature death are just a few of the issues that confront patients, highlighting the necessity for monitoring of their psychosocial needs. Involvement with a complex and fragmented health care system, the need for episodic and aggressive treatment, remissions and exacerbation of acute and distressing symptoms, functional limitations, family separation, financial burden, and role disruptions are a few of the issues that characterize the life of patients with hematologic malignancies, not to mention the threat to life imposed by these diagnoses. This chapter provides information on factors that affect psychosocial adjustment among patients with hematologic malignancies, the wide range of psychologic responses that are possible throughout the illness trajectory, and the efficacy of psychosocial interventions and services to minimize distress and promote adaptation. Some practical guidelines regarding patient management and identification of patients who may require formal psychiatric consultation are offered.

ACCOMPANYING TRENDS IN PSYCHOSOCIAL ISSUES

Within the past 25 years there have been significant advances in oncology that have affected the psychosocial care of the cancer patient. The continued advances in quality-of-life research, survivorship, personalized medicine, and quality care initiatives; interest in the reduction of health care disparities, evidence-based medicine, and palliative medicine; and the increasing interest in psychosocial health for patients and caregivers are a few of the changes in cancer care.

Interest in health-related quality of life can be traced back to 1947 with the beginning of the first nonphysiologic outcome measure for cancer: the Karnofsky performance scale. Exponential growth in disease-specific and individual-specific tools for measurement of health-related quality of life continues to this day.[4,5] Since the beginning of the survivorship movement, there has been increasing growth in legislation, education, and advocacy for cancer survivors. The focus on personalized medicine coupled with an interest in decreasing health care disparities has incorporated the idea of tailoring interventions to the needs of individual patients.[6-8] The emergence of palliative medicine, a new specialty that overlaps symptom management and end-of-life care with oncology specialists has made an impact on improving symptoms in oncology patients.[9] The Institute of Medicine report *Cancer Care for the Whole Patient: Meeting Psychosocial Health Needs* lists 10 recommendations related to improving psychosocial health for patients and family members.[10]

CLINICAL COURSE OF HEMATOLOGIC MALIGNANCIES

The incidence, course, treatment, and survival for various hematologic malignancies vary widely. New cases of multiple myeloma are estimated to be 21,700, with dramatic improvements in treatment and 5-year survival rates from 25% in 1975 to 34% in 2003.[11,11a] Myelodysplastic syndromes occur in 5 per 100,000 individuals, and recent prognostic stratification has been able to determine those patients who have increased survival.[12] The median age of onset for chronic myeloid leukemia is 67 years with an estimated 5430 cases diagnosed in the year 2010 with 610 deaths.[13-16] The translocation between chromosomes 9 and 22 results in the Philadelphia chromosome marker for chronic myeloid leukemia. The disease evolves from a chronic phase to an accelerated phase and finally an acute phase, which looks similar to acute leukemia in its presentation and intensity. Recent newer tyrosine kinase inhibitors have transformed the treatment, response, and prognosis for chronic myeloid leukemia.[13-16] Close to 13,780 individuals will be diagnosed with acute myeloid leukemia in 2010 with approximately 10,200 patients dying of the disease.[17] As the population has increased in age, the incidence of acute myeloid leukemia has been also rising.[17] Hodgkin disease is uncommon with an incidence of approximately 9000 cases per year and 1320 deaths per year.[18] The cure rate is 80% with an improved 5-year survival over the past decades.[18] Non-Hodgkin lymphoma is a heterogeneous group of lymphomas with an incidence of 66,000 cases and a death rate of approximately 19,000.[19-21] The incidence has been increasing dramatically in the past decades for two main types of non-Hodgkin lymphoma: B-cell and T-cell lymphomas. A new classification system and better imaging with positron emission tomography–computed tomography (PET-CT) have better tailored the treatment combinations such as chemoimmunotherapy and radioimmunotherapy. In contrast to treatment of many solid cancers, treatment of hematologic malignancies often involves intense regimens, highly technical therapies, lengthy hospitalizations, episodes of high infection risk, periods of unpredictability, and ongoing outpatient monitoring of the patient's condition. A number of patients respond to the curative attempts with long-term remission, remain well, and, after a period, are considered cured. However, some patients have a positive response to a curative attempt but then relapse. Other patients begin treatment with a hope for a cure but do not respond and progressively decline. In some patients, the disease is too far advanced when diagnosed, and they experience a

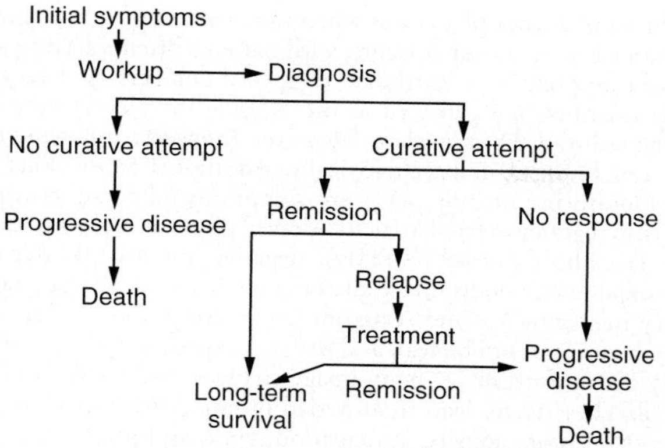

Figure 91-1 CLINICAL COURSE OF A PATIENT WITH A HEMATOLOGIC MALIGNANCY. *(Modified from Lesko LM: Hematopoietic dyscrasias. In Holland JC, editor:* Psychooncology, *New York, 1998, Oxford University Press, p 408.)*

Factors That May Predict Poor Coping in Patients With Cancer

Past psychiatric history
Compliance issues
Demographic factors such as younger age and female sex
Limited social support or difficult social relationships
Recent history of smoking cessation
Substance abuse history
Recent losses
Advanced disease
Uncontrolled symptoms
Pessimistic outlook on life
Multiple obligations
Avoidance coping (escape-avoidance, distancing, and denial)
Lower functional status
Higher regimen-related toxicity
Treatment

rapid progression of their disease. The remainder of this chapter proceeds through the common trajectories associated with hematologic malignancies including diagnosis, treatment, relapse, the end of life, and survivorship (Fig. 91-1).

Time of Diagnosis

Being diagnosed with a hematologic malignancy can be a devastating time of crisis. The time of diagnosis has been described by a cancer survivor as "a lightning bolt through a stop sign."[22] It is a time of intense stress and likened to a personal disaster in the patient's and family's life.[23] Often these patients describe vague symptoms such as fatigue for weeks, even months, or they are treated in urgent care centers for bronchitis or other infections only to be diagnosed with an unexpected catastrophic illness such as leukemia. Weismann and Worden[24] described the first 100 days after diagnosis as an "existential plight." They documented that patient concerns initially focused on existential issues of life and death more than on concerns related to health, work, finances, religion, self, or relationships with family and friends. The period from time of diagnosis through initiation of treatment is characterized by sometimes fast-paced medical evaluation and treatment, the development of new relationships with unfamiliar medical personnel, and the need to integrate a barrage of information that is at best frightening and confusing. Often patients with hematologic malignancies need immediate treatment intervention compared to those patients with solid tumors. But even with the advanced speed of information in this technologic age, patients have difficulty with information integration in a short period of time. Within the context of this anxiety-provoking situation, timely decisions must be made regarding treatment, and patients may feel tremendous responsibility, concern, and isolation during this period.

Initial response to a diagnosis may be profoundly influenced by a person's prior experience with cancer.[25] Those with memories of close relatives with cancer often demonstrate heightened distress, particularly if the relative died or had negative treatment experiences. During the diagnostic and early treatment periods, patients may search for explanations or causes for their cancer and may struggle to give personal meaning to their experience.[26] Because many clinicians are guarded about disclosing information until a firm diagnosis is established, patients may develop highly personal explanations that can be inaccurate and provoke intensely negative emotions. Ongoing involvement and consistent and repeated information from key health care providers help to minimize patients' uncertainty and the development of maladaptive coping strategies based on incomplete or inaccurate information.

Although extreme and sustained psychologic reactions as the first response to a cancer diagnosis are unusual, careful assessment of the nature of the patient's reaction remains important. Initial reactions often are predictive of later adaptation.[27,28] Early assessment by clinicians can help to identify people who are at risk for later adjustment problems and in greatest need of ongoing psychosocial support[29-34] (see box on Factors That May Predict Poor Coping in Patients With Cancer). Although the literature substantiates the devastating psychologic impact of a cancer diagnosis, it is also well documented that many patients cope effectively. Positive coping strategies, such as taking action and finding favorable characteristics in the situation, have been reported as effective. Maintaining optimism[35] and having an active determination to recover have been associated with positive adjustment. Contrary to the beliefs of many clinicians, denial has also been found to assist patients in coping effectively with a diagnosis of cancer, unless used to an excessive degree. With the firm establishment of the cancer diagnosis, planning for treatment begins. If patients have been given a clear explanation of their condition while encouraged to maintain hope, the initial reaction of shock, fear, and desperation can give way to a sense of optimism. Health care providers have an important role in monitoring and possibly mediating psychosocial adjustment. Keeping patients informed and actively involved in their care and being aware of the unique meaning that people may associate with a diagnosis of cancer are vital. Patients who have a pervasive and unyielding negative affect that persists long after the crisis of diagnosis may require ongoing psychosocial monitoring and referral for services and supportive interventions throughout their treatment and disease course.[36]

In addition, family assessment during this phase is vital. Levels of family distress, depression, and anxiety are mediated by the functioning of the family at the time of diagnosis.[37] Studies have shown that caregivers and families share similar rates of psychosocial angst.[37,38] Families who have open expression of feelings and actions have reported lower depression; however, those families who have dysfunctional problem-solving abilities have higher depression.[37] Also, anxiety within the family increases with unclear communication.[37] Both anxiety and depression are easy to assess in patients and family members, and timely referral for assistance during this period may lay a foundation of adequate coping throughout the patient's course of illness. During this time, many providers are conveying large amounts of information. It is not always easy for patients to differentiate the importance of each communication and prioritize their problem-solving behaviors. Consequently, providers must repeat information at each contact and inquire about the patients' and families' understanding of facts and treatment options. Often patients and families describe that they are in a state of numbness and that information is not really processed, understood, or comprehended.

Psychosocial factors are critical parameters in considering which treatment is best for an individual patient. The development of a treatment plan should include information about all aspects of medical/surgical treatments as well as what is known about the psychosocial sequelae. Often, patients react to a diagnosis of cancer with feelings of fear and helplessness. Patients look to the primary oncologist for a curative treatment that also can preserve their quality of life. Patients may feel vulnerable and believe that complete reliance on the oncologist is essential. Combating feelings of helplessness during this period can help patients alleviate painful anxiety. This is best done by a member of the health care team who has established a treatment alliance with the patient. The health care provider must make the patient feel like a partner in all aspects of care. This is especially true regarding decisions about treatment options. Giving information to patients and families often alleviates anxiety and uncertainty because patients feel more in control.

Active treatment of cancer usually initiates another acute phase of the cancer experience. It can occur while a patient is receiving treatment or as a complication of treatment. An important standard of clinical practice, based on extensive research, is to provide patients with information that will prepare them for what to expect during their treatment. Research by Johnson[39] provides convincing evidence that patients who receive specific information about the nature, pattern, and timing of treatment side effects report less disruption in activity than those who are not given this detailed information. Some providers wait until patients complain about potentially expected side effects. When this happens, patients may become skeptical about the completeness or accuracy of any future information given by the person. This threat to undermine a trusting relationship has important implications for decision making, patient choice of care setting in the future, and recommendations made by patients to others who are seeking a source of cancer care.

Often during the treatment phase increasing burdens are placed on the immediate caregiver and family to support the patient's schedule for treatment, multiple admissions, and increasing dependency.[40] The patient may be unable to work, and financial stressors accumulate. Sensitivity and awareness by providers to social, economic, and relationship stresses are needed to assist with referral for social services and other psychologic assistance. Support groups with other patients can be helpful during this time. Evidence clearly indicates that sharing a common experience in a support group can have psychologic benefit.[41]

DECISION FOR HEMATOPOIETIC STEM CELL TRANSPLANTATION

Hematopoietic stem cell transplantation (HSCT) is standard treatment for many high-risk hematologic malignancies and nonmalignant diseases either as part of overall treatment or after relapse. Both autologous and allogeneic transplant numbers are increasing worldwide.[42] The procedure for transplantation is complex and can cause intense psychologic distress and extreme social strain on the patient's caregiver, friends, and family members. Often the psychologic and social issues can be more challenging for the health care team than the medical issues. Because HSCT is an intense and distinctive experience for patients and families and has the potential to cause prolonged psychologic distress unlike other experiences with oncology patients, the issues unique to this population warrant a separate discussion.[43,44]

HSCT patients face physical and psychologic stresses of hospitalization and social isolation for weeks to months during their initial recovery. Consequently, a thorough pretransplant psychosocial evaluation is recommended to identify those patients at risk for development of psychosocial morbidity and to initiate timely interventions to optimize adaptation. Identified risk factors for psychosocial morbidity following transplant include previous psychiatric morbidity, pretransplant compliance issues, pretransplant physical and mental health problems, younger age, female sex, avoidant coping style, recent smoking cessation, lower functioning status on admission, problems with quality and presence of social support before transplant, perception of limited social support, the presence of difficult relationships, and professional integration concerns.[29,31]

The time of transplantation when the infusion of cells occurs can be a special moment for patients, with patients often referring to the date of transplant as a "birthday" or special anniversary date. Often family members are gathered at the bedside to celebrate the long-awaited event of the transplant. However, the weeks following transplant can be difficult psychologically. Additional factors that need close monitoring include persistent symptoms following transplant, increased regimen-related toxicity, slower physical recovery, chronic graft-versus-host disease (GVHD), negative appraisal of the transplant experience, body image disturbance, fears of relapse and secondary malignancies, and sexual function disruption.[44-47] The threat of death continues to be real, and patients experience social isolation, bodily discomfort, major body image changes, and a sense of loss of control. These issues lead to a myriad of emotions, including hope, anger, depression, anxiety, anticipation, guilt, and joy.[44]

Khan et al[48] identified the following common psychiatric diagnoses with inpatient transplant patients: adjustment disorder (40%), depression (23%), generalized anxiety disorder (10%), acute psychotic disorder (10%), delirium (10%), and depressive psychosis (7%). Kishi et al[49] compared inpatient psychiatric consultations among transplant and nontransplant patients. Transplant patients differed on several characteristics: more frequently white, less likely to have a previous psychiatric history, longer time period between admission to consult, more delirium, and more socioeconomic and health-related distress.

Patients are often not prepared for the long, gradual recovery. Patients are more familiar with recovery after surgery that takes days to weeks, and they are unprepared for and overwhelmed with the long recovery that can take weeks to months or even months to years. Typically patients perceived their quality of life to be worse the first year after transplant than before transplant.[50] Patients continue to feel functional limitations, and both autologous and allogeneic patients report common somatic symptoms, especially fatigue, the most common distressing symptom.[51-53] Patients who experience depression the first year have a higher mortality rate.[54] Periods when patients are particularly psychologically vulnerable during the first year include admission workup, directly before transplant, discharge from the inpatient setting, between 3 and 5 months, and between 6 and 9 months.[27,55] Other factors that have been identified as related to psychologic distress and poor health after transplantation include pre-HSCT psychologic and physiologic status, anxiety, depression, poorer quality of life, disease recurrence, negative mood, type of transplant, locus of control, low social support, presence of GVHD, and caregiver/family distress.[44,51,52,56] The financial burden for patients who undergo bone marrow transplantation (BMT) can be overwhelming, including medical expenses for the patient and marrow donor in the case of an allogeneic BMT, potential travel expenses, and loss of income for other family members.[41] Patients and their immediate families often are geographically far from their usual support systems because of the distance to the BMT center. In some cases, family members who have not been close in the past may be forced to interact with each other, leading to additional stress.

Although the literature is clear that most patients return to a productive life with high quality of life, during the first few years after transplantation, patients and family members may continue to experience physical and psychologic sequelae.[57] One study reported that 43% of patients with an average of 3.4 years after transplant had clinically significant global psychologic distress.[58] Despite this distress, only 50% of the patients received mental health services.[59]

Researchers have described the following factors as predictors of poorer quality of life in patients 1 to 5 years after transplant: younger age, long-term sequelae, chronic GVHD, unemployment, lower income, poor functional status, and short follow-up by the treatment center.[50,60] Patient and families are ready to put the experience behind them, only to discover that the experience of transplant has forever changed the patient's outlook, priorities, and family network. Fear of recurrence and feelings of uncertainty related to future relationships, work, and financial strain continue.[41] There is discordance between the patients' pre-HSCT expectations and the everyday symptoms that limit their physical abilities. Besides fatigue, which continues to be the dominant symptom, another distressing issue is cognitive dysfunction as patients return to the workplace or reenter school.[41] Educating patients about some expected common short-term side effects can reduce anxiety. Neurocognitive side effects of treatment can be long term in high-risk patients but are mostly temporary, including diminished concentration, short-term memory loss, decreased speed of information processing and loss of effective problem-solving abilities. Sexuality issues are another area of great concern for patients in the posttransplant period. Barriers for discussion and lack of referrals for supportive services in this area may be related to the patient's embarrassment, the clinician's lack of knowledge, or the focus on other issues that may be interpreted as more critical. Common sexual issues after transplant include vaginal dryness and distressing menopausal symptoms in women and erectile dysfunction in men.[61]

Patients who experience physical symptoms after transplantation may be at risk for long-term psychologic distress.[40] Despite the fact that patients are followed by transplant physicians longer than patients with nonhematologic malignancies, this population often is referred back to primary care physicians 1 to 2 years after transplant. Primary care clinicians do not have the knowledge or experience to recognize physical complications related to the effects of chemotherapy, radiation, and GVHD, so ongoing communication between the providers and the transplant team and center is imperative. Long-term effects may include persistent viral, bacterial, and fungal susceptibility, GVHD, dental caries, muscle atrophy, pneumonitis, gonadal dysfunction, sexual dysfunction, endocrine abnormalities, cataracts, ocular sicca syndrome, reduced bone mass, secondary malignancies, and cognitive dysfunction.[62] In addition to monitoring physical complications, the American Society for Blood and Marrow Transplantation consensus statement recommends annual evaluation of patients' psychologic status. Health care providers must have a high level of vigilance to assess depression in both the patient and family caregiver years after transplant, with clinical assessments recommended annually after transplant. Studies of transplant survivors beyond 10 years indicate possible issues with returning to work, physical fitness, impairment in social functioning and family life, insurance denial, and continued symptoms such as pain, depression, muscle stiffness/cramps, memory/attention problems, sleep disorders, sexual issues, and incontinence.[63,64] In spite of the range of problems, only 9.8% of patients reported accessing psychologic support.[63]

The concept of posttraumatic growth (PTG) after transplantation has been evolving. By definition, the potential for PTG requires that patients experience a stressful event and subsequently experience positive psychologic outcomes or benefits. As early as 1996, Fromm identified that positive sequelae are possible after transplantation, including the development of a new philosophy of life, greater appreciation of life, making changes in personal characteristics, and improving relationships with family and friends.[64a] Potential predictors of PTG among posttransplant patients include good social support, little avoidance coping, younger age, less education, greater use of positive reinterpretation, problem solving, seeking alternative rewards, more stressful appraisal of the experience, and more negatively biased recall of pretransplant levels of psychologic distress.[32,65] Discussing the PTG potential with patients and making referrals for counseling to experienced clinicians who are aware of the potential for PTG are essential.

Although patients report long-term psychosocial effects after transplantation, they may be reluctant to accept help and fail to access psychologic resources and social support.[63] These patients must be encouraged to use resources and seek psychologic support, because this experience may impair the patients' and families' ability to cope with life after transplant. In an article about HSCT patients' experiences with a support group, Sherman et al[41] identified the themes of meaning and changing of perspectives as patients expressed their struggles with redefining themselves, their priorities, and their values. Some patients wanted to change their former values and behaviors. The support group experience may be therapeutic for patients who often do not have physical signs of transplant to the untrained eye but continue to experience increasing or unresolved psychologic and physical issues.[29,40] Sharing a common experience may encourage patients to believe that their symptoms and feelings are not unique and may decrease their feelings of isolation.

Immediate Period Following Diagnosis and Treatment

As the treatment and acute side effects improve and subside, patients often feel that the whirlwind has passed, only to be confronted with uneasy silence. Weeks and months of clinic and physician appointments, infusions, and admissions stop or trickle to a small stream of appointments. Families who have been functioning on a grinding schedule of crisis mode find the change almost paralyzing. Adding to this halt of activity, health care providers have a tendency to limit their contacts when the patients' physical status has stabilized. This is a critical time when psychosocial interventions and supportive services from other members of the health care team must be instituted for patients and family members to deal with the uncertainty and anxiety of waiting. Fears and anxieties change from fighting the disease to returning to life.[66] Because of less contact with the primary treatment oncologists, patients and families may perceive a withdrawal of support from the medical team. Long-term psychosocial health of the patient and family is affected by the meaning ascribed to the cancer experience, fear of recurrence, support of the family, demographic factors, and financial stressors. This transition time is pivotal for patients' long-term quality of life. Surveillance with specific questions to access the need for referrals can have lasting outcomes.

Time of Relapse

The time of recurrence of cancer has been reported to be more distressing for patients and family members than the initial diagnosis. The recurrence of the disease can plunge the patient and family into despair and crisis as they realize that death may occur despite the ongoing fight to live. The psychosocial issues experienced by the person with cancer depend in part on the clinical course of the disease process. As the disease progresses, the person often reports an upsetting scenario that includes uncertainty, frequent pain, diminished functional ability, increased dependence, and disability.[25]

The development of a relapse after a disease-free interval can be especially devastating for patients and those close to them. The medical workup often is difficult and anxiety provoking, and psychosocial problems experienced at the time of diagnosis frequently resurface, often with greater intensity.[25] Shock and depression often accompany relapse and require patients and family members to revaluate the future. In spite of the overwhelming nature of the psychosocial responses, however, most patients do cope effectively with progressive disease, and it is important to recognize that intense emotions do not necessarily equate with maladaptive coping. Investigators studying quality of life in patients with cancer have demonstrated a clear relationship between a person's perception of their quality of life and the presence of discomfort.[67,68] As uncomfortable symptoms increase, perceived quality of life diminishes. An important goal in the psychosocial treatment of patients with advanced cancer centers on optimal symptom management.

An issue that repeatedly surfaces among patients, family members, and professional care providers is the use of aggressive treatment protocols in the presence of relapse and progressive disease. Currently there are newer agents that can induce remission in the face of relapse. In addition, patients and families often request participation in experimental protocols, even when there is little likelihood of extending survival. Controversy continues about the efficacy of such therapies and the role health care providers can play in facilitating patients' choices about participating. Clear communication about treatment goals and expectations will assist in patient and family preparation.

Certain patients respond to investigational treatment with increased hope. It is vital to clarify the values, thoughts, and psychologic reactions of care providers, patients, and families to the delicate issues that evolve if individualized care with attention to the patient's psychosocial needs is to be provided.

Survivorship

The definition of a long-term survivor has evolved over time. Initially, individuals who had survived cancer-free for longer than 5 years were considered "survivors and cured." More recently the term *survivors* has been used to define individuals who have completed the acute phase of illness. Others use the term for all patients initially diagnosed with cancer. Some people would prefer changing the term to "thrivers," champions, or fighters.[69]

Successful treatment of hematologic malignancies has resulted in cure for many patients and progressively longer lives for others. However, longer survival is not without significant psychologic sequelae.[70-75] Innovative and new treatments may produce long-term physiologic consequences, such as infertility, treatment-related toxicity, persistent side effects, and organ system failure that can magnify and exacerbate the psychologic issues initially associated with diagnosis and treatment.[67,68,76] The overwhelming evidence from the literature involving survivors with hematologic malignancies is that, on the average, most do very well after the initial adjustment in the first 1 to 3 years after treatment.[50,71] Most long-term BMT survivors express satisfaction with their quality of life and describe themselves as productive, stable, and well adjusted without significant physical, functional, psychologic, and social problems related to their disease or BMT treatment. However, there is a group of patients with a high rate of psychosocial morbidity who are vulnerable to ongoing and intermittent psychosocial distress. Empiric evidence showed that as many as 9% to 30% of long-term survivors with hematologic malignancies experience significant psychologic distress, including anxiety, depression, and posttraumatic distress symptoms.[72,74,77]

Psychologic aspects of survivorship may include concern over termination of treatment; fear of relapse; preoccupation with somatic symptoms; reentry into previous roles; lingering affinity with death; and financial, job, and insurance difficulties. These issues may manifest in a variety of ways, including denial of past illness, leading to medical compliance issues; ongoing problems with anxiety, panic, and depression; and inability to reenter or modify previous roles. Fear of recurrence by both patients and family members can severely affect quality of life.[66] In her classic article "The Enduring Seasons in Survival," Dow[23] stated that the season of extended survival is dominated by fear of recurrence. In fact, Baker et al[51] showed in a group of cancer survivors that "being fearful my illness will return," "concern about relapsing," "fears about the future," and "difficulty making long-term plans" were a problem 68%, 60%, 58%, and 41% of the time, respectively. Mellon and Northouse[78] found that the strongest predictors of quality of life 1 to 5 years after treatment were concurrent family stressors, family social support, family member fear of recurrence, family meaning of the illness, and patient's employment status.

There is increasing interest in patients' experiences with posttraumatic stress disorder (PTSD). Studies have consistently described a higher incidence of PTSD in patients with hematologic malignancies than in the average population.[79-81] Predictors of PTSD severity among patients with hematologic diagnosis include higher levels of distress and high avoidance coping coupled with low social support.[32] These researchers describe how providers can assess coping and presence of family support and potentially mitigate the effects of a distressing experience with the cancer diagnosis. Considerable evidence indicates that the wide range of surgical, chemotherapeutic, and radiation therapies leaves permanent damage to organs and physiologic functioning and disfigurement across the different hematologic diagnoses (Table 91-1). Health care providers should be mindful of psychologic sequelae among patients, even within the context of remission and a hopeful prognosis, and refer patients and family members to a mental health specialist for further evaluation, as needed.

Table 91-1 Long-Term Consequences of Therapies for Hematologic Cancers

Anxiety
Depression
Fear of recurrence
Disfigurement
Conditioned nausea and vomiting
Unemployment
Denial of life insurance
Denial of health benefits
Increase in life insurance rates
Difficulty changing health care coverage
Breakdown of marriage or relationship
Decline in participation in leisure activities
Diminution of support from others
Disruption in sexual functioning
Fertility

Terminal Stage and End-of-Life Care

Technologic advances in health care have improved the potential for cure of many previously fatal hematologic malignancies. However, many patients still have disease that is unresponsive to treatment, continues to progress, and is considered incurable. When cure is acknowledged to be impossible and alternative efforts to combat the progress of disease are exhausted, patients are recognized as terminally ill or dying. In this situation, some authors advocate a palliative care approach with no active treatment and a shift in the emphasis of medical care from the pursuit of cure to supportive and hospice care, including the provision of care and comfort, control of distressing symptoms, and maintenance of quality of life at an optimal level.[82-84] However, this paradigm currently is shifting in the field of palliative care to one of initiating palliative care alongside curative treatment with the philosophy that it should be implemented across the illness trajectory, with the promotion of quality of life to facilitate relief of suffering.[85] The new World Health Organization definition states: "Palliative care is an approach to care which improves quality of life of patients and their families facing life-threatening illness, through prevention, assessment and treatment of pain and other physical, psychologic, and spiritual problems."[86]

Palliative care began with the hospice movement. Since the concept of hospice was first introduced in England in the 1960s, hospice care has been recognized as the state-of-the-science end-of-life care, and hospice services now are available around the world. However, hospice care has not been integrated into the care of patients dying with hematologic malignancies.[87,88] Despite the strong emphasis on providing end-of-life care in accordance with patients' wishes and empiric studies showing that most terminal patients prefer spending their final days of life and dying at home, hematologic malignancy is the only diagnosis that has been repeatedly and consistently shown to predict hospital death.[89,90]

The reasons for such insufficiency have been attributed to many factors. Manitta et al[91] in their article "Palliative Care and the Hemato-Oncologic Patient: Can We Live Together?" identified barriers between the expectations of two specialities: (1) the dying trajectory can be rapid with more unpredictability and more technology, (2) the various hematologic diagnoses are not uniform in response and treatment, (3) the goals of care can be unclear, (4) the focus on cure can preclude the focus on palliation, (5) lack of knowledge exists among hematologists about palliative care principles, and (6) the health care system does not encourage collaborative care. Health care providers, first and foremost, must examine their own attitudes toward death and dying and avoid imposing their own values on patients and their families. Respecting patient and family wishes, appropriately managing and alleviating distressing symptoms, and providing care tailored to meeting patients' needs can help patients dying of hematologic malignancies reach the end of life with peace and dignity.

FACTORS THAT INFLUENCE PSYCHOSOCIAL ADJUSTMENT

Psychosocial responses to cancer vary widely and are influenced by several factors that clinicians should bear in mind when considering the responses of individual patients. A review of the literature points to key factors that may have an impact on psychosocial adjustment and include individual patient factors, environmental factors, and disease-related factors.

Individual Patient Factors

These factors include demographics, comorbid conditions, previous psychiatric morbidity, previous coping strategies, and stage of the illness. Female sex and younger age have been consistently documented as important predictors for psychosocial adjustment and quality of life for patients with hematologic malignancies.[29,92-94] Also, as the population ages, there are more individuals diagnosed with cancer who already have comorbid diseases.[95,96] These issues complicate treatment decisions and recovery. Patients who have preexisting psychologic issues are acutely at risk for poor psychologic adjustment to the cancer diagnosis.[31,97] Many individual factors are interrelated; for example, a significantly higher anxiety score and more impaired quality of life were observed more in women than in men. The presence of current sleep problems and fatigue were associated with older age at BMT. Poor quality of life after treatment was associated with higher age of the recipient at the time of the transplant, poorer self-image and overall cognitive functioning, and inability to return to work.[73,98-103]

One of the key predictors of psychosocial adjustment to cancer is the psychologic stability of the person before diagnosis. People with a history of poor psychosocial adjustment before development of cancer are at highest risk for psychologic decomposition and should be monitored closely throughout all phases of treatment. This is particularly true of people with a history of a major psychiatric syndrome, psychiatric hospitalization, or both.[31] Also, because a person's coping style is determined relatively early in life and remains stable over time and across situations, it serves as a useful predictor of adjustment to cancer. Several investigators have identified specific personality characteristics, coping strategies, and life experiences that enhance or inhibit positive adjustment to cancer.[104,105] Empiric evidence also demonstrated the beneficial impact of positive coping strategies and personality attributes on long-term survival.[44,106,107] Coping strategies found to be most effective include a "fighting spirit," hopefulness and acceptance of the situation, a belief that life has purpose and coherence, and having a feeling of control over events, resulting in active participation in treatment and engagement in daily life. By contrast, poor adjustment and even PTSD have been associated with avoidant coping strategies, anxious preoccupation and high distraction, prior negative sexual experiences, body image problems, and inhibition in discussing personal and sexual problems.[18] One study showed that patients who smoke are at higher risk for psychiatric morbidity, perhaps due to the potential development of depression and/or anxiety with withdrawal symptoms.[19] It is important to include smoking history in the patient's assessment of substance control use when preparing patients for treatment options.

Environmental Factors

Environmental factors include spouse and family support, other social support, and professional reintegration. The quality of spousal and family relationships has a significant impact on the psychologic health and even mortality of the patient.[108] Social support, network size, satisfaction with social support, and reliance on formal and informal social ties have consistently been found to influence a person's psychosocial adjustment to cancer.[89,90] The ability and availability of significant others in dealing with a diagnosis and discussion of treatment options can significantly affect the patient's view of himself or herself. Patients diagnosed with all types of life-threatening chronic disorders experience a heightened need for interpersonal support. Those who are able to maintain close connections with family and friends during the course of illness are more likely to cope effectively with the disease than are those who are not able to maintain such relationships.[107,109,110]

Traditionally patients are not referred routinely to formal home nursing care at discharge. An initial home visit can be invaluable in assisting patients and families with the transition, in addition to identifying areas in which ongoing assistance is needed. Home care referral can assist families that are increasingly relied on within the current health care system to be the major providers of care outside the hospital.

Disease-Related Factors

Disease-related factors include treatment and toxicity, residual symptoms, appraisal of the disease, treatment and recovery, and fear of relapse. Time interval after treatment has been documented as an important predictor for psychosocial adjustment. Different treatment modalities introduce varying degrees of side effects, symptoms, and impact on quality of life. Significant differences were found between transplant groups with regard to loss of appetite, physical and role functioning, symptom distress, sexual impairment, infertility, mood, and overall quality of life.[27,50,76,103,111-113] Without exception, the greatest difficulties in psychosocial adjustment were observed among patients who underwent allogeneic BMT, followed by autologous BMT recipients, and patients who received conventional or maintenance chemotherapy. The latter groups experienced the least impairment in quality of life and psychologic distress. Patients who underwent transplant also had more psychiatric morbidity if they experienced lower functional status and higher regimen-related toxicity.[31]

Time since BMT or completion of treatment was an important factor for facilitating psychosocial adjustment and improving quality of life. In general, during the first year after BMT, patients perceived their physical and overall well-being as being worst, experienced more anxiety and total mood disturbance, and reported the highest degree of illness intrusiveness in every aspect of life.[27,50,76,103,111-113] With the passage of time, improvements in functional status, quality of life, levels of anxiety, depression, and satisfaction with life were frequently observed after transplant.

Living with a chronic illness often requires continuing care and management by a team of specialists. Use of supportive care services has been related to improved quality of life; therefore it is in the patient's best interest to access services needed for psychologic distress early in the continuum of care.[110] Care usually is provided through follow-up visits to ambulatory or outpatient clinics and consulting rooms, rather than through hospitalization. However, several barriers that may impair the outpatient cancer survivor from accessing health care services include economic and financial constraints.[114] Differentiating a psychiatric complication from expected psychologic responses is imperative.

Although any individual experiencing the crisis of a cancer diagnosis may become clinically depressed or experience a panic attack, most patients do not experience a diagnosable psychiatric condition. Currently the rates of adjustment disorder, depression, anxiety, and PTSD are 40%, 25%, 10%, and 5%, respectively. The ability of health care providers to distinguish expected reactions from more severe psychiatric complications is crucial.

Unfortunately, nonpsychiatric care providers often miss clinically relevant and severe psychiatric syndromes. Being knowledgeable about common symptoms of adjustment disorder, depression, anxiety, and PTSD are helpful. Table 91-2 provides a quick reference; also refer to the *Diagnostic and Statistical Manual of Mental Disorders*.

Table 91-2 Common Symptoms of Psychiatric Disorders

Adjustment Disorder	Depression	Anxiety	Posttraumatic Stress Disorder
The development of emotional or behavioral symptoms in response to an identifiable stressor	Symptoms that are present for a 2-week period and a change from previous functioning	Excessive worry and anxiety for at least 6 months; the person finds it difficult not to worry	The person has been exposed to a traumatic event
1. Marked distress that is in excess of what would be expected for exposure to the stressor 2. Significant impairment in social or occupational functioning	1. Depressed mood most of the day 2. Marked diminished interest or pleasure 3. Significant weight loss or decrease or increase in appetite 4. Insomnia or hypersomnia 5. Psychomotor agitation or retardation 6. Fatigue 7. Feelings of worthlessness or guilt 8. Diminished ability to think or concentrate 9. Recurrent thoughts of death, suicidal ideation, or a plan for suicide	Anxiety and worry have to have three of the six following symptoms: 1. Restlessness 2. Fatigue 3. Difficulty concentrating 4. Irritability 5. Muscle tension 6. Sleep disturbance	1. Reexperiencing symptoms such as images, thoughts, and perceptions 2. Persistent avoidance of stimuli and numbing of general responsiveness 3. Persistent symptoms of increased arousal: sleep issues, anger or irritability, difficulty concentrating, hypervigilance, and exaggerated startle response

Data from American Psychiatric Association: *Diagnostic and statistical manual of mental disorders,* ed 4, Arlington, Va, 2000, American Psychiatric Association.

Another group of patients who are at high risk for developing adjustment problems include those with coexisting severe mental disorders that may include schizophrenia, bipolar disorder, schizoaffective disorder, and obsessive-compulsive disorder. Integrated care of psychiatry and oncology is the best option in treating these patients, first to stabilize the psychiatric illness and then to treat the cancer.[115,116] Good communication, empathy, listening skills, and providing emotional support are all skills that benefit these patients and specifically those who have severe mental illness, who often have a history of disregard and neglect from providers[117] (see box on Screening for Psychologic Distress).

Most patients manifest transient psychologic symptoms that are responsive to support, reassurance, and information about what to expect regarding the cancer course and its treatment. Some require more aggressive psychotherapeutic interventions, such as pharmacotherapy and ongoing psychotherapy. The following guidelines can assist the clinician in identifying those patients who exhibit behavior suggesting the presence of a psychiatric syndrome.

General guidelines designed to assist in distinguishing patients who should be referred for evaluation by a trained psychiatric clinician include the following:

Screening for Psychologic Distress

A number of tools have been developed to screen for psychologic distress, but they have not been consistently incorporated into clinical care.[118,119] One tool that is easy to administer and that patients report as capturing their problems is the *distress thermometer.*[120] The tool is similar to pain measurement scales that ask patients to rate their pain on a scale from 0 to 10 and consists of two parts. The first part is a picture of a thermometer, and patients are asked to mark their level of distress. A rating of 4 or above indicates that a patient has symptoms indicating a need for evaluation by a mental health professional and potentially has a need for referral for services. On the second part, the patient marks items that relate to his or her distress from a six-item problem list (illness-related, family, psychologic, practical, financial, spiritual effects, or other) (Fig. 91-2).[120,121] Lee et al[122] found that the distress thermometer was a useful tool for screening transplant patients before admission. Pretransplant distress appeared to be highly predictive of distress following transplant and was a feasible marker to use to screen patients for distress.

1. History of psychiatric hospitalization or significant psychiatric/personality disorder
2. Persistent refusal, indecisiveness, or noncompliance with regard to needed treatment
3. Persistent symptoms of anxiety and depression that are unresponsive to usual support from health care providers or family members; symptoms may present in the form of constant fear associated with treatment and procedures or excessive crying and feelings of hopelessness that worsen rather than improve with time
4. Abrupt, unexplained change in mood or behavior
5. Insomnia, anorexia, diminished energy out of proportion to expected treatment effects
6. Persistent suicidal ideation
7. Unusual or eccentric behavior or confusion (may be indicative of an organic mental disorder)
8. Excessive guilt and self-blame for illness
9. Evidence of dysfunctional family coping or complex family issues

After referral to a psychiatric specialist, one or a combination of therapeutic modalities may be used. Cancer and its treatment may precipitate an exacerbation of an underlying mental illness to which a patient was predisposed and that may require extensive treatment (e.g., hospitalization for a psychosis, ongoing pharmacotherapy, or psychotherapy). A discussion of these specialized forms of treatment is beyond the scope of this chapter. The reader is encouraged to consult an appropriate standard textbook.[30]

MANAGEMENT OF PSYCHOSOCIAL PROBLEMS

Interventions for these patients center on the uniqueness of the experience. In the initial phase of the experience, 50% of patients have psychologic distress, including both anxiety and depression.[121] A growing body of literature provides evidence that patients may experience PTSD.[123] Increased length of survival from time of diagnosis has highlighted the need for psychopharmacologic, psychotherapeutic, and cognitive and behaviorally oriented interventions to reduce distress, promote adjustment, and improve quality of life for patients with hematologic malignancies. Cognitive behavioral therapy is a promising intervention that has been used with transplant patients and shown to decrease PTSD symptoms and overall distress.[124] Because of the increasing complexity of patient care, a multidisciplinary approach that includes regular avenues and options for communication about patient management and status updates is imperative. Numerous studies have documented the efficacy of a

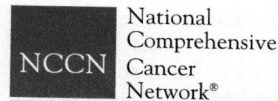

NCCN Guidelines Index
Distress Management TOC
Discussion

SCREENING TOOLS FOR MEASURING DISTRESS

Instructions: First please circle the number (0-10) that best describes how much distress you have been experiencing in

Extreme distress 10

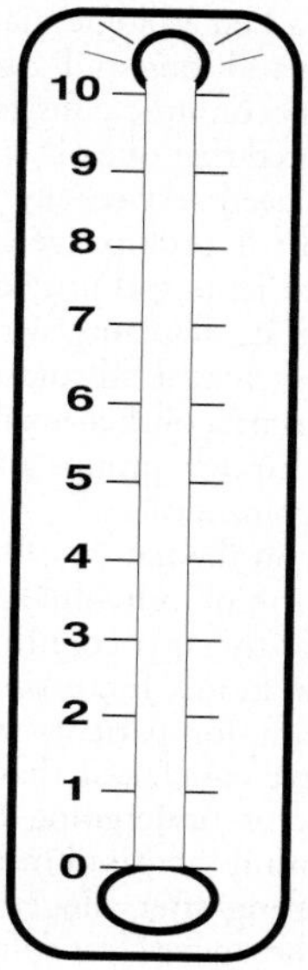

9

8

7

6

5

4

3

2

1

No distress 0

Second, please indicate if any of the following has been a problem for you in the past week including today. Be sure to check YES or NO for each.

YES	NO	Practical Problems
❑	❑	Child care
❑	❑	Housing
❑	❑	Insurance/financial
❑	❑	Transportation
❑	❑	Work/school
❑	❑	Treatment decisions
		Family Problems
❑	❑	Dealing with children
❑	❑	Dealing with partner
❑	❑	Ability to have children
❑	❑	Family health issues
		Emotional Problems
❑	❑	Depression
❑	❑	Fears
❑	❑	Nervousness
❑	❑	Sadness
❑	❑	Worry
❑	❑	Loss of interest in usual activities
❑	❑	**Spiritual/religious concerns**

YES	NO	Physical Problems
❑	❑	Appearance
❑	❑	Bathing/dressing
❑	❑	Breathing
❑	❑	Changes in urination
❑	❑	Constipation
❑	❑	Diarrhea
❑	❑	Eating
❑	❑	Fatigue
❑	❑	Feeling Swollen
❑	❑	Fevers
❑	❑	Getting around
❑	❑	Indigestion
❑	❑	Memory/concentration
❑	❑	Mouth sores
❑	❑	Nausea
❑	❑	Nose dry/congested
❑	❑	Pain
❑	❑	Sexual
❑	❑	Skin dry/itchy
❑	❑	Sleep
❑	❑	Tingling in hands/feet

Other Problems: ______________________

 DIS-A

Figure 91-2 NATIONAL COMPREHENSIVE CANCER NETWORK (NCCN) DISTRESS MANAGEMENT GUIDELINE DIS-A-DISTRESS THERMOMETER. *(From National Comprehensive Cancer Network:* The National Comprehensive Cancer Network 1.2005 Distress Management, *the complete library of NCCN clinical practice guidelines in oncology (CD-ROM), Jenkintown, Pennsylvania, 2005, National Comprehensive Cancer Network.)*

variety of modalities in managing psychosocial problems for such patients. Problems that can be managed effectively include psychologic distress such as anxiety and depression; sexual dysfunction; body image disturbances; noncompliance, pain, and neurologic complications such as delirium and dementia induced by brain metastasis or treatment; anticipatory and posttreatment nausea and vomiting; anorexia and feeding problems; and marital and family difficulties.

Pharmacologic Interventions

Pharmacotherapy, as an adjunct to one or more of the psychotherapies, can be an important aid in bringing psychologic symptoms under control. For patients with excessive anxiety, factors other than a psychologic state must first be evaluated. Metabolic abnormalities, pain, hypoxia, and drug withdrawal states all can present as anxiety. Many common medications and substances are associated with anxiety and depression. Medications such as steroids and antipsychotics, often used to control nausea, can cause anxiety characterized by agitation and motor restlessness. After medical or drug-induced causes for anxiety are ruled out, an anxiolytic agent is the treatment of choice, except for patients who present with panic episodes, in whom tricyclic antidepressants are most efficacious. Medications are most effective when used at adequate dosages and as standing orders. Use of these medications may assist the patient with participating in psychotherapy, which can provide more lasting control over psychologic symptoms. Anxiety that develops in the context of the terminal stages of cancer often results from hypoxia or an untreated pain syndrome. Intravenous morphine sulfate and oxygen usually are effective palliative treatments. All pharmacologic treatments must be monitored for effectiveness and side effects.

Patients commonly demonstrate transient depressive symptoms at various points in the disease trajectory, particularly during the palliative care period when a hope for cure is not possible. In patients who exhibit prolonged or severe depressive symptoms, a major depressive illness must be considered. Depression can be related to a recurrence of a past depressive disorder or the stress associated with treatment, or it can be a result of the illness process or treatment agents. Antidepressant medications are easily administered and are an effective treatment strategy. Disadvantages include the need for repeated visits to health care clinicians to monitor patient response and adjust the dosage, possible adverse side effects and medical reactions, potential use in suicide attempts, and the need for strict adherence to the medication schedule. Patients should be informed that most antidepressant medications must be taken for 3 to 4 weeks before a significant response is achieved. The clinician must be aware that patients at risk for suicide become more energized with medications and appear to look better long before their depressive feelings and suicidal thoughts are relieved. Careful monitoring of suicidal ideation should continue for weeks after the patient appears improved.

A diagnosis of major depression in medically ill patients relies heavily on the presence of affective symptoms such as hopelessness, crying spells, and guilt; preoccupation with death or suicide; feelings of diminished self-worth; and loss of pleasure in most activities, such as being with friends and loved ones. The neurovegetative symptoms that usually characterize depression in physically healthy individuals are not good predictors of depression in the medically ill because disease and treatment can also produce these symptoms. A combination of psychotherapy and antidepressant medication often proves useful in treating major depression.[125] Antidepressant medications may take 2 to 6 weeks to produce their desired effects. Patients may need ongoing support, reassurance, and monitoring in the period before the antidepressant effects of medication are achieved. Patients must be monitored closely by a consistent provider during the initiation and modification of psychopharmacologic regimens.

Psychotropic drugs are highly effective for treatment of anxiety, depression, agitation, and confusion in patients with hematologic malignancies.[126] It is beyond the scope of this chapter to include the current medications recommended for common psychiatric disorders. A comprehensive discussion of psychotropic drugs is summarized in the quick pocketbook reference for oncology clinicians.[126] Medications specific for the management of anxiety, depression, and delirium also are presented.[127]

Psychotherapeutic Modalities

"Returning to normal" is a prominent theme and desired goal in the clinical management of patients but is not always possible for patients with hematologic malignancies.[103,128] Survivors of cancer continue to face challenges with long-term physical and psychologic symptoms long after treatment has ended, and data indicate that they report more contact with mental health providers than do people without cancer.[114] The American Society for Blood and Marrow Transplantation released a joint statement recommending screening and preventive practices for long-term survivors of hematopoietic cell transplantation. The recommendation states that "a high level of vigilance for psychologic symptoms should be maintained. Clinical assessment is recommended throughout the recovery period, at 6 months, 1 year and annually thereafter, with mental health professional counseling recommended for those with recognized deficits."[62] The number of intervention studies designed with the hematologic population is limited; however, growing interest in survivorship is changing the research climate in this area.

Support groups can provide a therapeutic experience for patients and family members. Initial evidence suggests that support groups may help reduce health care costs along with depression, mood disturbance, and psychiatric symptoms in patients.[129] Patients often feel alone in their distress and report that sharing a common experience normalizes their feelings, provides an avenue for emotional support, facilitates dialogue to problem solve, and offers opportunities to learn from other patients. Support groups facilitated by professionals such as social workers, nurses, or psychologists can provide a forum for health and psychologic education and provide patients with printed literature and online community-based resources. Sherman et al[41] found that psychoeducational support groups facilitated by professionals were a helpful strategy for patients' post-HSCT psychologic recovery.

Other modalities have been shown to be effective with patients.[103,104] Studies have consistently shown that relaxation training with or without guided imagery or hypnosis may have some benefit with improving quality of life, symptom management, and anxiety and depression management.[128,130,131] It is a skill taught to patients that takes minimal time. It does, however, require that patients be motivated to learn and practice new techniques and a way of coping. Cognitive therapy/reappraisal, problem solving, and stress management training also have been shown to be helpful in the general cancer population.[123,128,132] Fritzsche et al[131] identified that a considerable need for psychotherapeutic treatment of inpatient hematology patients is best handled by mental health professionals. They described a psychosomatic liaison service that provides psychosocial support for patients with hematologic malignancies, including patients going through transplant. The service screened patients for anxiety, depression, poor coping, quality of life, and psychosocial openness for support and provided psychotherapy, relaxation training, or group therapy as interventions. Although all transplant patients received support from the team, 23% of the hematology patients on the general ward received additional psychosocial interventions.

Other evidence-based interventions that have been found to be helpful in the general oncology population include individual and group counseling, family therapy, and music and art therapy. In comparison to patients with solid cancers, there should be a low threshold for referral for psychosocial support for patients and families faced with a hematologic malignancy because the primary treatment is intense and long and associated with sensitivity to potential barriers such as economic constraints, including loss of insurance. It has been estimated that one of six cancer survivors with mental health problems who need services are unable to access those services due to cost.[114] If cost is prohibitive and referral to a psychologist is not feasible, both patients and providers must investigate other potential providers, such as chaplains, art therapists, music therapists, social workers, and psychiatric advanced practice nurses who might be able to see patients as part of their work responsibilities. Other possibilities include online support groups and advocacy organizations, including local wellness communities.

Depending on the nature of the problem, the treatment modality may take the form of individual psychotherapy, group therapy, family therapy, marital therapy, cognitive or behaviorally oriented therapy, or some combination.[10] Increasing evidence supports use of an aerobic exercise program for patients with hematologic malignancies.[133-135] Researchers have concluded that fatigue and loss of physical performance in patients undergoing BMT may improve with exercise.[134] Others have found increased muscle strength with supervised weight bearing and lifting after allogeneic BMT.[135] Table 91-3 outlines the major psychotherapeutic modalities and their advantages, goals, and indications.

FUTURE DIRECTIONS

The psychosocial issues faced by people diagnosed with and treated for hematologic malignancies are influenced by individual, environmental, and disease-related factors. Because involvement in decision making clearly is a positive aspect of current cancer therapies, great care should be taken to ensure that communication is timely, repeated, relevant, and consistent with the patient's needs, tolerance for information, and comprehension. A multidisciplinary approach is necessary to guarantee the communication of timely and essential information to patients and family members. Patients should be given the opportunity to speak with multiple members of the multidisciplinary treatment team and other patients who have experienced similar management and treatment protocols. Care should be taken to provide needed information from a variety of expert perspectives while respecting the unique characteristics, psychosocial profiles, needs, and desires of each individual. In treatment settings with limited resources, every effort should be made to enlist the help and support of providers and services that can assist patients with treatment decisions and their complex management. Referral to community resources and support services after discharge from the hospital often is helpful, even for patients who cope well with initial treatment.[20]

Most patients undergoing cancer treatment, as well as their families, experience expected periods of psychologic turmoil that occur at transition points along the clinical course of cancer. In a small proportion of patients, more severe psychiatric complications may occur, warranting referral to a psychiatric specialist, including psychiatrists, social workers, psychologists, and psychiatric nurses. Screening for ongoing psychiatric problems must become standard care. A variety of psychotherapeutic modalities are useful for helping patients

Table 91-3 Therapeutic Modalities Useful for Patients and Family Members

Modality	Selected Indications	Goals and Advantages	Comments
Individual psychotherapy	Prolonged adverse reactions to diagnosis, treatment, and other aspects of chronic illness (e.g., anxiety, depression)	Supports patients and enhances ability to cope with distressing feelings Short-term therapy; focused and goal directed	Pharmacology and family involvement are useful adjuncts in some cases.
Support groups	Patients desire contact with others who are experiencing chronic illness	Supports patient and enhances coping ability Patients benefit by observing coping strategies of others Usually does not involve a fee	Expands social network of patients with limited support systems
Family and marital therapy	Relationship problems secondary to illness (e.g., family tension, role changes, conflict, sexual problems)	Assists couples with clarifying problems and facilitates solving them together Addresses role changes in the family system	Problems, issues, and concerns about relationships including children can be addressed.
Mind-body therapies, including progressive muscle relaxation, yoga, guided imagery, Reiki, meditation, hypnosis, and biofeedback	Patients desire assistance with control of pain, anxiety, anticipatory and posttreatment nausea and vomiting, fears associated with medical procedures	Increases sense of control and participation in treatment Individualized to meet patient's preferences and circumstances Time limited and goal directed Evaluated in terms of observable changes in symptoms and self-efficacy	Realistic goals should be stated explicitly. (Some patients may view these therapies as a cancer cure.)

work through the expected psychologic responses to cancer as well as more severe responses.[24] Supportive psychotherapeutic measures should be used routinely because they minimize distress and enhance feelings of control and mastery over self and environment. For these reasons alone, their value in the care of patients with cancer is paramount.

Throughout the clinical course of cancer, the patient's relationship with health care providers and the presence of a supportive social network are important factors that can ensure successful management of the many physical and psychosocial demands imposed by a cancer diagnosis and treatment. As scientific inquiry continues to produce vast but sometimes conflicting information regarding etiology and treatment of cancers, concurrent research regarding the psychosocial aspects of hematologic malignancies is crucial. This line of inquiry will, at the very least, assist in promoting psychosocial well-being in patients and family members faced with an extreme and unexpected life crisis. At best, expanding the knowledge base relative to the psychosocial aspects of cancer may provide some "missing links" regarding psychosocial adaptation and quality of life and the impact of cancer on patients' survival. The Institute of Medicine report that recommends that all cancer care should ensure the provision of appropriate psychosocial health services states that at a minimum, patients must be screened for emotional distress and evaluated for additional services.

SUGGESTED READINGS

Baker F, Denniston M, Smith T, et al: Adult cancer survivors: How are they faring? *Cancer* 104:2565, 2005.

Cooke L, Gemmill R, Kravits K, et al: Psychological issues of stem cell transplant. *Semin Oncol Nurs* 25:139, 2009.

Cooke L, Grant M, Eldredge D: Hematopoietic cell transplantation: The trajectory of quality of life. In Ezzone S, Schmit-Pokorny K, editors: *Blood and marrow stem cell transplantation,* ed 3, Sudbury, Mass, 2007, Jones & Bartlett Publishers, p 391.

Edwards B, Clarke V: The psychological impact of a cancer diagnosis on families: The influence of family functioning and patients' illness characteristics on depression and anxiety. *Psychooncology* 13:562, 2004.

Evan EE, Zeltzer LK: Psychosocial dimensions of cancer in adolescents and young adults. *Cancer* 107:1663, 2006.Haylock PJ: The shifting paradigm of cancer care: The many needs of cancer survivors are starting to attract attention. *Am J Nurs* 106:16, 2006.

Fleishman S, Greenberg D: Pharmacological interventions. In Holland J, Greenberg D, Hughes M, editors: *Quick reference for oncology clinicians: The psychiatric and psychological dimensions of cancer symptom management,* Charlottesville, Va, 2006, IPOS Press, p 26.

Fritzsche K, Struss Y, Stein B, et al: Psychosomatic liaison service in hematological oncology: Need for psychotherapeutic interventions and their realization. *Hematol Oncol* 21:83, 2003.

Hewitt M, Sheldon G, Stovall E: *From cancer patient to cancer survivor: Lost in transition,* Washington, DC, 2006, National Academy Press.

Institute of Medicine (US) Committee on Psychosocial Services to Cancer Patients/Families in a Community Setting; Adler NE, Page AEK, editors: *Cancer care for the whole patient: Meeting psychosocial health needs,* Washington DC, 2008, National Academies Press.

Jacobsen PB, Donovan KA, Trask PC, et al: Screening for psychologic distress in ambulatory cancer patients. *Cancer* 103:1494, 2005.

Jacobsen PB, Sadler IJ, Booth-Jones M, et al: Predictors of posttraumatic stress disorder symptomatology following bone marrow transplantation for cancer. *J Consult Clin Psychol* 70:235, 2002.

Jenks Kettmann JD, Altmaier EM: Social support and depression among bone marrow transplant patients. *J Health Psychol* January 1, 2008 13:39, 2008.

Khan A, Irfan M, Shamsi T, et al: Psychiatric disorders in bone marrow transplant patients. *J Coll Physicians Surg Pak* 17:98, 2007.

Kishi Y, Meller WH, Swigart SE, et al: Are the patients with post-transplant psychiatric consultation different from other medical–surgical consultation inpatients? *Psychiatry Clin Neurosci* 59:19, 2005.

Lim JW, Zebrack B: Social networks and quality of life for long-term survivors of leukemia and lymphoma. *Support Care Cancer* 14:185, 2006.

Lorenz KA, Lynn J, Dy SM, et al: Evidence for improving palliative care at the end of life: A systematic review. *Ann Intern Med* January 15, 2008 148:147, 2008.

Manitta VJ, Philip JAM, Cole-Sinclair MF: Palliative care and the hemato-oncological patient: Can we live together? A review of the literature. *J Palliat Med* 2010/08/01 13:1021, 2010.

McGrath P: End-of-life care for hematological malignancies: The 'technological imperative' and palliative care. *J Palliat Care* 18:39, 2002.

McQuellan R, Danhauer S: Psychosocial rehabilitation in cancer care. In Chang A, Ganz P, Hayes D, editors: *Oncology: An evidence-based approach,* New York, 2006, Springer Verlag, p 1942.

Mellon S, Northouse LL: Family survivorship and quality of life following a cancer diagnosis. *Res Nurs Health* 24:446, 2001.

Miovic M, Block S: Psychiatric disorders in advanced cancer. *Cancer* 110:1665, 2007.

Misono S, Weiss NS, Fann JR, et al: Incidence of suicide in persons with cancer. *J Clin Oncol* October 10, 2008 26:4731, 2008.

Mosher CE, DuHamel KN, Rini CM, et al: Barriers to mental health service use among hematopoietic SCT survivors. *Bone Marrow Transplant* 45:570, 2010.

National Comprehensive Cancer Network: *The National Comprehensive Cancer Network 1.2005 Distress Management,* The Complete Library of NCCN Clinical Practice Guidelines in Oncology (CD-ROM), Jenkintown, Pa, 2005, National Comprehensive Cancer Network.

Patrick DL, Engelberg RA, Curtis JR: Evaluating the quality of dying and death. *J Pain Symptom Manage* 22:717, 2001.

Sherman RS, Cooke E, Grant M: Dialogue among survivors of hematopoietic cell transplantation–Support-group themes. *J Psychosoc Oncol* 23:1, 2005.

Tang ST, McCorkle R: Determinants of place of death for terminal cancer patients. *Cancer Invest* 19:165, 2001.

Zabora J, BrintzenhofeSzoc K, Curbow B, et al: The prevalence of psychological distress by cancer site. *Psychooncology* 10:19, 2001.Hewitt M, Rowland JH: Mental health service use among adult cancer survivors: Analyses of the National Health Interview Survey. *J Clin Oncol* December 1, 2002 20:4581, 2002.

For complete list of references log on to www.expertconsult.com.

CHAPTER 92

PAIN MANAGEMENT AND ANTIEMETIC THERAPY IN HEMATOLOGIC DISORDERS

Kathy J. Selvaggi, Bridget Fowler Scullion, Craig D. Blinderman, and Janet L. Abrahm

Relieving the pain of patients who have hematologic disorders requires a multifaceted approach.[1,2] An understanding of the taxonomy of pain, basic pain pathophysiology, and a systematic evaluation of the pain complaint will provide a rational basis for treatment decisions. After the source of the pain has been identified, appropriate nonpharmacologic and pharmacologic therapies can be initiated. The neurosurgical and anesthetic procedures for the management of cancer pain are not discussed in this chapter; those interested in these techniques are referred to several excellent reviews.[1-4]

TAXONOMY OF PAIN

Although there is no one standardized classification system for cancer pain, several systems have been proposed. Cancer pain syndromes, and thus by analogy, pain syndromes in hematologic disorders, may be classified temporally, pathophysiologically, etiologically, according to distinct clinical-anatomical entities, or any combination thereof. It is important to determine both the etiology and inferred pathophysiology in the assessment of the pain complaint because this may suggest the use of specific therapies. Pain can be categorized as *nociceptive* (somatic or visceral), *neuropathic,* or *idiopathic*. Nociceptive pain is pain that is sustained predominantly by tissue injury or inflammation. Nociceptive somatic pain is described as sharp, aching, stabbing, throbbing, or pressure-like. Nociceptive visceral pain is poorly localized and is usually described as crampy pain (e.g., obstruction of hollow viscus) or as aching and stabbing (e.g., pain secondary to splenomegaly). Neuropathic pain is sustained by abnormal somatosensory processing in the peripheral or central nervous system (CNS). Sensations described as "burning," "shocklike," and "electrical" typically suggest neuropathic pain. On physical examination, patients may have allodynia (pain induced by nonpainful stimuli) and hyperalgesia (increased perception of painful stimuli). In the absence of evidence sufficient to label pain as either nociceptive or neuropathic, we may use the term "idiopathic." However, in patients with hematologic disorders, this term should lead to additional workup and a search for an underlying etiology and pathophysiology.

BASIC PAIN PATHOPHYSIOLOGY

Pain is defined as an unpleasant sensory and emotional experience associated with actual or potential tissue damage or described in terms of such damage. For a patient to feel pain,[1] a signal arising from a noxious stimulus in the periphery must be transmitted to the centers in the brain that create the experience of pain. After activation of peripheral receptors by chemical, thermal, or mechanical stimuli, the signal passes along unmyelinated A-delta or C fibers and enters the spinal cord via the dorsal root ganglion. Chemicals released at the site of tissue injury mediate or modulate the transmission of the pain signal. Arachidonic acid metabolites, bradykinin, adenosine, serotonin, nitric oxide, prostaglandins, and lipoxygenase products have all been identified as playing a role in initiating or increasing the transmission of the pain signal in peripheral nociceptors.

The dorsal horn of the spinal cord is where the peripheral signals are received and modulated. The excitatory amino acids (e.g., glutamate and aspartate) and neuropeptides (e.g., substance P and calcitonin gene-related peptide [CGRP]) enhance transmission of the peripheral signal.[1] But a complex interaction of other neurotransmitters (i.e., γ-aminobutyric acid [GABA], glycine, adenosine, bombesin, cholecystokinin, dynorphin, enkephalin, neuropeptide-Y, neurotensin, substance P, somatostatin, and vasoactive intestinal peptide) determines whether the signal will proceed up the spinothalamic tract.[1] The signals that are transmitted ascend in one of the two contralateral spinothalamic tracts: the paleospinothalamic tract, which mediates the "suffering" and autonomic reactions to pain, or the neospinothalamic tract, which localizes the pain and records its intensity.[1]

Descending pathways originating in the CNS can inhibit transmission of the pain signal. A modulatory network with major relays in the midbrain periaqueductal grey (PAG) and rostral ventromedial medulla (RVM) exerts control over dorsal horn nociceptive transmission and is the central substrate of opioids—both endogenous and exogenous.[5] This major pain-modulating pathway involves regions of the frontal lobe, amygdala, and hypothalamus, all of which have projections to the PAG. The PAG inhibits spinal nociceptive neurons via connections in the RVM and the dorsolateral pontine tegmentum. The neurotransmitters involved in this and other central inhibitory pathways include serotonin, norepinephrine, cholecystokinin, neurotensin, acetylcholine, cannabinoids, and the endogenous opiates β-endorphin, enkephalin, and dynorphin.[5]

Opiate receptors for endogenous and exogenous opioids are present in the dorsal horn of the spinal cord, in those ventromedial thalamic nuclei that transmit signals from the paleospinothalamic tract, the periaqueductal gray, the periventricular diencephalon, and the amygdala.[5] The analgesic affects of opioids is thought to be attributable to the reduction of neurotransmitter release (e.g., glutamate, substance P, and others) from presynaptic nociceptive fibers, as well as postsynaptic inhibition of neurons transmitting the painful signal to the brain.

The *N*-methyl-D-aspartate (NMDA) receptor at the level of the spinal cord plays an important role in chronic painful states. Chronic pain or long-term opioid therapy may result in activation of the NMDA receptors. Activation of the NMDA receptor initiates intracellular processes that lead to several neuronal plastic changes, which in turn result in enduring increases in neuronal excitability.[6] Antagonists of these receptors (e.g., ketamine and dextromethorphan) may enhance analgesia and reduce the amount of opioid analgesics required. Further studies are necessary to determine the clinical role of NMDA antagonists.

Several reviews have described the diverse pathophysiological processes involved in neuropathic pain.[7] Most neuropathic pain syndromes are the result of peripheral nerve injury. After injury, changes occur at the molecular level, within the nerve itself, and within the spinal cord and brain. At the molecular level, there is upregulation in the expression of both tetrodotoxin-sensitive (TTX-S) and tetrodotoxin-resistant (TTX-R) Na channels. These Na channels are the targets for many of the adjuvant medications used to treat neuropathic pain (e.g., local anesthetics, antiarrhythmics, anticonvulsants, and tricyclic antidepressants [TCAs]).[8] Other cellular components that are thought to play a role in neuropathic pain include TRPV-1 channels, N and P/Q type voltage-gated calcium channels, purine receptors (P2X), TrkA, proton receptors, and cannabinoid receptors (CB1, CB2).[7] Additional changes take place within the nerve itself. After injury to peripheral nerves, there is a subsequent change in the phenotype of the nerves by de novo gene expression. Both injured and unaffected nerves develop a sensitivity to a number of factors to which they were previously insensitive and respond to subthreshold stimuli. Such sensitization may lead to ectopic and spontaneous activity in tissue nociceptors, perhaps explaining paroxysmal episodes of pain. A host of chemical and inflammatory mediators further alters the gene expression of nerves, leading to increased sensitivity. At the level of the spinal cord, several processes occur that alter the way sensory nerves function, thus maintaining a pathological pain state. These processes can be described as reorganization, sensitization, and disinhibition.[8] Reorganization refers to the phenomenon of new connections being established in the laminae of the spinal cord (e.g., A-beta fibers, which normally transmit light touch) sprout into lamina II of the dorsal horn, replacing C-fibers which transmit nociceptive information to second order neurons. Dorsal horn neurons also become sensitized as a result of repeated firing from peripheral nerve fibers. The release of substance P, CGRP, and other neuropeptides leads to the activation of the NMDA receptor and release of nitric oxide postsynaptically with subsequent excitation of pain transmission neurons (PTNs). Microglia activation also plays a role in sensitization and maintaining pathological pain states. Finally, disinhibition at the level of the spinal cord is thought to be a result of interneuron death in lamina II, downregulation of GABA and opioid receptors, and increased production of cholecystokinin.[8]

Table 92-1 Common Pain Syndromes in Hematologic Malignancies

Procedure-Related Pain	
Bone marrow biopsy	
Central catheter placement	
Lumbar puncture headache	
Therapy-Related Pain	
Myalgias (e.g., from corticosteroid withdrawal)	
Myopathy	
Oropharyngeal mucositis	
Osteoporosis	
Peripheral neuropathies (e.g., secondary to chemotherapy agents)	
Postherpetic neuralgia	
Visceral pain syndromes (e.g., typhlitis, hemorrhagic cystitis, enteritis)	
Pain from Hematologic Malignancy	
Pain syndrome	Cause(s)
Bone pain	Bone marrow expansion or infiltration
	Bone infarct or necrosis
	Osteomyelitis
	Compression fracture
	Hemarthrosis
Visceral pain	Tumor involvement
	Splenomegaly
	Lymphadenopathy or lymphadenitis
Headache	Meningeal infiltration, infection
	Brain metastasis or primary tumor
Neuropathic pain	Paraproteins with antimyelin properties
	Amyloid infiltration
	Peripheral nerve compression
	Spinal cord compression

EVALUATION OF THE PAIN COMPLAINT

Initial Evaluation

Effective pain management requires a comprehensive assessment of the patient's pain. Pain reports by patients should be believed. The clinical presentation of a patient with chronic pain is very different from that of a patient in acute pain. If a patient does not manifest the common autonomic manifestations of acute pain (e.g., tachycardia, sweating, elevated blood pressure) or facial grimacing, the clinician might doubt that the patient has severe pain. A patient with severe but chronic pain does not manifest these autonomic findings but often is withdrawn, quiet, depressed, or irritable; moves very little spontaneously; and complains of discomfort when moved. When the pain is relieved, these patients often exhibit completely different behaviors, becoming mobile, engaged, and involved with other people. The first component in the assessment is to believe the patient's complaint.

Patient reports of pain are valid, reliable, and reproducible.[1] A variety of assessment tools that can be completed within 5 to 10 minutes are available.[1,9] The pain complaint should be characterized by a number of descriptors, including the pain location, intensity, quality, onset, and duration; location and patterns of radiation; and what relieves or exacerbates the pain and its functional consequences, including how the pain affects the patient's ability to sleep or eat and how it affects physical activity, relationships with others, emotions, and concentration. Most patients with chronic cancer pain also experience periodic flares of pain, or "breakthrough pain."[9] An important subtype of breakthrough pain is "incident pain," which is caused by voluntary activity. The initial evaluation should determine the extent to which the patient has breakthrough pain and if it is provoked by movement (nociceptive) or tends to be paroxysmal in nature (neuropathic). This subjective information, combined with the physical examination and diagnostic studies, may identify a specific pain syndrome and its implied pathophysiology.

In a patient with a hematologic disorder, the cause of pain may be the disease itself, the specific therapy for the disease, diagnostic procedures related to the disease, or unrelated disorders (Table 92-1). Splenomegaly, bone injury (e.g., infarction, infection, hemarthroses, and infiltration), leptomeningeal infiltration, and spinal cord compression frequently accompany hematologic diseases. Chemotherapy and radiation therapy can cause mucositis, typhlitis, hemorrhagic cystitis, and peripheral neuropathy; corticosteroid withdrawal may cause myalgias. Immunosuppression, caused by the diseases themselves or by the therapies used to treat them, may lead to painful infections such as perirectal abscesses, herpetic or candidal esophagitis, and herpes zoster. Patients with sickle cell disease have a number of causes for both acute and chronic pain (Table 92-2).

Distress, however, may arise from non-anatomic sources. The pain complaint may represent the patient's only means of expressing nonspecific feelings of distress to the physician. Chapman recognized three categories of this distress: anxiety, arising from fear of disfigurement or of uncontrollable pain, fear of loss of social position or of self-control, or fear of death; anger at the failure of the physicians to provide a cure; and depression from the loss of physical ability, a sense of helplessness, and the impact of financial problems. In addition to these psychological, social, and financial contributions, spiritual concerns may exacerbate any concomitant painful sensations.[10] Alleviating them may significantly reduce distress and decrease the need for pain medications or other interventions.

For a patient whose complaint of pain does not seem to have a straightforward explanation or who has not responded well to the therapeutic maneuvers outlined in this chapter, additional questions may help evaluate the patient's distress. Some patients may deny the extent of their disease and use the complaint of pain to justify their incapacity. For example, when asked: "How would life be different without the pain?" Such patients may give unrealistic assessments of the extent of their abilities, such as, "If only the pain were gone. ..." Another question that we have found valuable in this situation is: "What do you think is causing your pain?" The patient may not acknowledge the effects of cancer or its treatment on his or her pain. In addition, the answer may reveal hidden fears, resentments, and even distrust of the physician. Finally, when answering the question: "To what extent do you expect your pain to be relieved?" the

Table 92-2 Classification of Pain Syndromes in Sickle Cell Disease

Pain secondary to the disease itself
Acute pain syndromes
Acute chest syndrome
Calculus cholecystitis (pigment stones)
Hand–foot syndrome (in children)
Hepatic crisis
Priapism
Pulmonary infarction
Recurrent acute painful episode
Splenic sequestration (in children)
Chronic pain syndromes
Arthropathies or arthritis
Avascular necrosis
Chronic osteomyelitis
Intractable chronic pain
Leg ulcers
Neuropathic pain
Pain secondary to therapy
Loose prosthesis (in patients after arthroplasty for avascular necrosis)
Opioid withdrawal
Postoperative pain
Pain caused by comorbid conditions

Adapted from Ballas SK. Pain management of sickle cell disease. *Hematol Oncol Clin North Am* 19:785, 2005.

patient may expect that taking one pill each day will provide total relief, but the physician expects that even a multiple-modality pain treatment will relieve only 75% of the pain, thus highlighting the patient's unrealistic expectations of pain treatment.

Sometimes there may be a disparity between the patient's expression of pain and the patient's family or friends' appreciation of the impact of the pain. The following observation may help to begin a conversation around this issue: "You seem to show different feelings about the pain from those your family and friends show. Help me to understand what the pain is like for you and why you think your family and friends feel differently." Patients may come from a cultural background different from the person reporting the pain, and people with cultural differences often report pain very differently.[10] For example, patients from a "stoic" cultural upbringing may not communicate their distress to their spouse; the spouse may then question why the patient needs opioid pain medications (i.e., if the spouse were ill and were in that much pain, he would be sure to talk about it.)

Continued Assessment

A standardized measurement tool, such as a verbal rating scale (VRS) or a visual analog scale (VAS), should be consistently used during follow-up visits.[1,9] These measurements are thought to be more accurate than mere qualitative descriptors, such as: "The pain is better." Using, for example, a scale of 0 (no pain) to 10 (the worst pain one can imagine), a decrease in pain intensity from 10 to 8 indicates that the patient needs a stronger pain medication, but a decrease from 10 to 3 suggests that the current medication regimen is effective. This inference can be confirmed by asking the patient, "Is this level of pain relief acceptable to you?"[1] The ongoing assessment should also pay attention to changes in the phenomenology of the pain, new occurrences of pain, or a change in the location of pain—all of which may suggest progression of disease in the patient with a hematologic disorder.

The successful outcome of pain therapy should be more than simply the lowering of pain intensity scores. Passik and Weinreb developed a useful mnemonic device for the assessment of pain therapy in chronic nonmalignant pain known as the "4 As": analgesia, activities of daily living, adverse events, and aberrant drug-taking behaviors (e.g., repeated dose escalation or noncompliance, hoarding drugs or acquiring drugs from other medical sources). By focusing on these relevant domains in the continued assessment of the pain therapy, the clinician is able to determine if the therapy makes a true difference in the patient's life, stabilizes or improves psychosocial functioning, manages side effects, and provides a means of assessing for aberrant drug behaviors. Ultimately, the goal should be to lower the pain *to a level acceptable to the patient* and to improve the patient's level of functioning.

THERAPY

A major component of pain therapy is an attempt to ameliorate the underlying cause of the pain. Surgery, chemotherapy, radiation therapy, immunosuppression, and antibiotics may all be used. However, the pain can still be treated effectively during diagnostic testing to define the cause, during specific therapy, or after all disease-related therapies are exhausted.

NONPHARMACOLOGIC METHODS OF PAIN MANAGEMENT

Cognitive-Behavioral Interventions

Education and Reassurance

Patients with serious hematologic disorders are often required to undergo extensive diagnostic testing, which can include painful procedures. A rehearsal of the planned test or procedure, including a discussion (or view) of the appearance of the room and the length of time to be spent in the test apparatus, can minimize the patient's anxiety. Such explanations, offered preoperatively, lessen the need for postoperative medication and shorten the patient's hospital stay. If conscious sedation is not planned, a pleasant distraction may be helpful to divert attention from certain procedures (e.g., bone marrow aspiration or biopsy) that take place in the physician's office or in the patient's room. For example, the physician might encourage the patient to bring in a CD or MP3 player with earphones so the patient can listen to a favorite piece of music or a book on tape while the procedure is taking place. Patients can also dissociate themselves[10] from the procedure by concentrating on pleasant memories and thereby diminishing the painfulness of the procedure.

Hypnosis

Hypnosis can be a useful adjunct in the management of pain, including for patients undergoing painful procedures.[10] The hypnotic trance, a state of heightened and focused concentration, allows one to manipulate the perception of pain and diminish sleeplessness, anxiety, and anticipation of discomfort. Hypnotic training of patients with sickle cell anemia or hemophilia decreases the frequency and pain intensity of painful crises or bleeding episodes, respectively. In a controlled trial comparing hypnosis with cognitive-behavioral therapy in relieving mucositis after a bone marrow transplant, patients using hypnosis reported a significant reduction in pain control compared with patients who used cognitive-behavioral techniques.[11]

In the absence of a formal hypnotic induction, words used by a practitioner to describe procedures are very important. For example, the suggestion that skin coolness and numbness will persist after application of an alcohol swab may markedly diminish the discomfort of starting an intravenous line. Using the phrase: "You will feel something; I'm not sure what you will feel because everyone feels this a little differently" in place of "This is going to hurt a lot!" gives the patient permission to alter the sensation and may also diminish the experience of pain.

Cognitive-Behavioral Techniques and Counseling

The cognitive-behavioral approach addresses a number of psychosocial and behavioral factors that contribute to patients' experience of pain.[9,10] These techniques have demonstrated clinical utility for patients with a wide range of chronic pain syndromes. Psychological counseling as part of a multidisciplinary approach to pain treatment provides education, support, and skill development for patients with pain. It can improve patients' abilities to communicate their pain to health care personnel and may be effective in overcoming anxiety and depression. Spiritual counseling may help patients who have lost hope, can find no meaning in their lives, or believe they are being punished or have been forsaken by God.[10] They may interpret their pain in light of these feelings. Through counseling, they can regain a sense of worth and belonging. As they recast the pain in its true light, its intensity is often diminished.

Cutaneous Techniques

Acupuncture, massage, vibration, and applying cold or heat to the skin over injured areas are often very effective. Cold wraps, ice packs, or cold massage using a cup filled with water that has frozen into a solid piece of ice relieve the pain of muscles that are in spasm from nerve injury. Heat from heating pads, hot wraps, or paraffin treatments can soothe injured joints but should not be used over areas of vascular insufficiency. Transcutaneous electrical nerve stimulation (TENS) devices are indicated for patients with dermatomal pain, such as postherpetic neuralgia or radiculopathy from spinal cord compression.[10] For optimal effect, a physiatrist or physical therapist familiar with the device should train the patient in its use. The efficacy of TENS therapy for patients with cancer pain remains controversial.

EMLA, a cream containing two topical anesthetics (2.5% lidocaine and 2.5% prilocaine) is used, especially in children, to decrease the pain of superficial cutaneous procedures (e.g., venous cannulation or skin anesthesia before lumbar puncture, bone marrow aspiration, or biopsy).[10] In adults, it is used before access of implanted vascular access devices or CNS ports. To achieve anesthesia, the EMLA cream must be applied 1 to 1.5 hours before the planned procedure in a mound under a semipermeable dressing such as Opsite or Tegaderm. When EMLA is used as directed, methemoglobinemia has not been a problem even in infants as young as 3 months old. Skin blanching occurs, sometimes exceeding or equaling the frequency of that found with placebo moisturizing cream placed under the occlusive dressing. ELA-Max, a cream containing 4% lidocaine, is available over the counter and is an alternative to EMLA cream. Because it does not contain prilocaine, there is no risk of methemoglobinemia.

Lidocaine patches can be used over areas of hyperesthesia, as can occur in patients with postherpetic neuralgia or nerve entrapment by vertebral body collapse.[10] The patch is applied to the affected area for no more than 12 consecutive hours a day and can be cut to size. Use should be avoided over areas of broken skin and in patients undergoing radiation therapy. Extended application of lidocaine patches has been safely applied for up to 24 hours/day for up to 4 days with minimal systemic absorption in healthy volunteers and in postherpetic neuralgia patients.

Radiation Therapy

Radiation therapy is commonly used in the management of painful bone lesions, spinal cord compression, bulky lymphadenopathy, and symptomatic splenomegaly in patients with hematologic malignancies.[10,12] Radiotherapy is the treatment of choice for local metastatic bone pain in most situations, although patients with underlying pathologic fractures may require surgical fixation before radiotherapy. Randomized trials have shown that single-fraction radiotherapy is as effective as multifraction radiotherapy in relieving pain caused by metastases. However, there are higher rates of retreatment, and single-fraction radiotherapy may not prevent pathological fractures or spinal cord compression.[12] In patients with poor performance status or a short life expectancy, a single dose (8 Gy) of radiation or a hypofractionated course (20 Gy/5 fractions) may be preferable and less burdensome.

Vertebroplasty and Kyphoplasty

Vertebroplasty and kyphoplasty are both minimally invasive techniques used to stabilize vertebral compression fractures and reduce pain. Vertebroplasty is a procedure in which bone cement, usually polymethylmethacrylate, is injected into the vertebral body. With kyphoplasty, a balloon is first inserted into the vertebral body followed by inflation and then deflation before cement is added. Balloon kyphoplasty has been shown to stabilize pathological vertebral fractures caused by multiple myeloma and significantly reduce pain.[13]

Anesthetic Techniques

Trigger-point injections, nerve blocks, and neurolytic procedures are useful for acute and chronic localized pain. After excisional biopsy of an axillary lymph node, for example, a burning, constricting pain in the posterior arm and chest wall may develop; this pain is often promptly relieved by trigger-point injection.

Lymphoma or myeloma may involve the spine and lead to vertebral collapse or pain from progressive disease that is refractory to antineoplastic therapy. Such pain is often particularly difficult to manage. Insertion of temporary or permanent indwelling epidural or intrathecal catheters to deliver opioids, local anesthetic agents, clonidine, or combinations of these and other agents can be very effective, especially in relieving lower thoracic or lumbar spine pain, as well as pelvic and lower extremity pain.[14] Reviews of the indications for and techniques of the anesthetic and neurolytic procedures are available.[4]

PHARMACOTHERAPY

Drugs useful for pain relief include nonopioid analgesics, opioids, and adjuvant analgesics. Most patients require a combination of medications for optimal pain relief (Fig. 92-1).

Nonopioid Analgesics

Nonopioid analgesics should be given to patients with mild to moderate pain.[1,9] Aspirin and nonsteroidal antiinflammatory drugs (NSAIDs), including cyclooxygenase-2 (COX-2) inhibitors, are especially useful as antiinflammatory agents because they decrease local prostaglandin release through the inhibition of COX (though the mechanisms for their analgesic properties are not as clear).[15] Acetaminophen is an effective analgesic but only a weak antiinflammatory agent. Daily intake of acetaminophen should not exceed 4 g because of the potential hepatic toxicity (see box on Management of Severe Pain). It is important to prescribe an adequate dose of acetaminophen or NSAID at regular intervals, switching to another nonopioid analgesic only when maximal doses of the first have become ineffective.[15]

Ketorolac tromethamine (Toradol) is an NSAID of particular value in relieving moderate to severe acute pain.[16] A parenteral dose of 30 mg of ketorolac equals the pain-relieving potency of a parenteral dose of 15 mg of morphine, and acute toxicity is minimal if the total daily dose is under 100 mg. Oral ketorolac is considered less potent. Ketorolac has all of the side effects of the NSAIDs and is not recommended for use beyond 5 days because of an increased risk of renal toxicity. If that degree of pain relief is needed chronically, an opioid agent should be substituted.

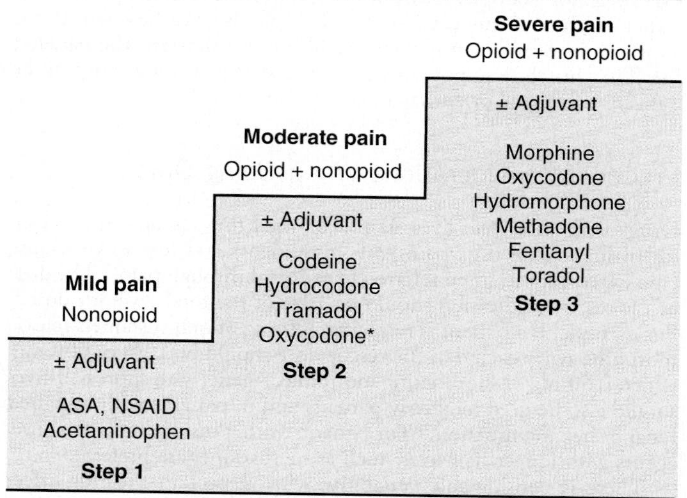

Figure 92-1 STRATEGY FOR PHARMACOLOGIC MANAGEMENT OF PAIN USING THE WORLD HEALTH ORGANIZATION (WHO) ANALGESIC LADDER. Multiagent therapy is usually required for optimal pain management. Patients with mild pain should be started on a nonopioid analgesic, and those with moderate pain should be started on a step 2 opioid. Many patients can benefit from the addition of a nonopioid to the opioid (e.g., for bone pain) or an adjuvant agent to the opioid (e.g., for neuropathic pain). If this combination does not produce adequate relief or the patient presents with severe pain, step 3 opioids should be begun initially. Toradol (Ketorolac) is a nonsteroidal antiinflammatory drug (NSAID) with the pain-relieving potency of a step 3 opioid. Many patients can benefit from the addition of nonopioid analgesics or adjuvants, if indicated. *ASA,* Aspirin; *, oxycodone in combination with products.

Because the NSAIDs can cause renal insufficiency in a significant number of patients, renal function should be assessed 1 or 2 weeks after initiation of any of these agents. NSAIDs should be used with caution in patients with a history of aspirin allergy or asthma because they can precipitate bronchospasm in as many as 20%.[15] Significant edema can occur in patients with cirrhosis or congestive heart failure.[15] The relatively selective COX-2 inhibitors, such as meloxicam, celecoxib, and nabumetone, should not, and apparently do not, cause gastrointestinal side effects with the same frequency as nonselective NSAIDs. If NSAIDs are required in patients with a history of significant gastritis or ulcer disease or who are older than 70 years, COX-2 inhibitors or a concomitant proton pump inhibitor should be considered. Cardiotoxicity is well described in the literature for COX-2 selective inhibitors.[17] Recently, the cardiac risk associated with traditional NSAIDs has been questioned. In a meta-analysis that included naproxen, ibuprofen, diclofenac, and several COX-2 specific inhibitors, ibuprofen and diclofenac demonstrated an increased risk of stroke. Diclofenac was also associated with an increased risk of cardiovascular death. Naproxen was not noted to have risk elevations.[17] The nonopioid analgesics should be continued in appropriate cases when opioid analgesics are added because they can potentiate the pain-relieving effect of the opioid (see Fig. 92-1).[1,9] However, when aspirin or acetaminophen is included in a fixed drug combination (e.g., Percodan, Percocet), toxicities may develop if the patient takes the pills more often than the prescription indicates. The metabolism of salicylates is limited by the capacity of the hepatic microsomal system.[10] After that is saturated, salicylate levels are dependent on renal clearance. Small increases in maintenance doses can lead to serious salicylism. Patients with low albumin levels or acid urine are particularly susceptible to the development of salicylate toxicity.

Management of Severe Pain

Opioid therapy is the cornerstone of management of patients presenting with severe pain. Our practice is to begin with reassurance of patients and their families. We tell them that to relieve the pain as quickly as possible, we will initiate the use of intravenous opioid medications immediately but that we will begin oral pain medication as soon as the pain is well controlled. Without this explanation, patients have misinterpreted a "morphine drip" as an indication that they were considered terminal.

The starting dose is calculated from the patient's current opioid dose (10% of their 24-hour opioid requirement) or weight (e.g., 0.05 mg/kg/hr of morphine). After the opioid bolus dose is administered, the patient should be monitored continuously during dose titration. If the patient was on standing opioid medication, the medication is continued when possible or converted to a continuous infusion if necessary. Pain is reassessed 20 minutes after the patient receives a bolus dose. If the pain remains severe (7, 8, or 9 of 10), a subsequent bolus dose is administered at double the dose. If the pain has decreased to moderate (4, 5, or 6), another bolus at the same dose as the immediately previous dose is used. If the pain score is below 4, the patient is carefully monitored. At 4 to 8 hours, either a continuous infusion is begun or the ongoing infusion rate is adjusted upward based on the amount of opioid taken as boluses during that period. There is no maximal opioid dose; we give whatever is required to relieve the pain. If the patient falls asleep, this is usually an indication that pain relief has been achieved, not that the dose should be lowered. We lower the dose if the respiratory rate falls to below 10 to 12 breaths/min or if there are signs or symptoms of neurotoxicity (e.g., myoclonus).

Agents to prevent side effects are begun along with the opioid. All patients are given a stool softener and an irritant agent such as senna (one or two tablets orally daily to twice daily, up to a maximum of 8 pills per day). If a more laxative effect is needed, lactulose (15-30 mL) or polyethylene glycol (17 g) is added. In opioid-naive patients, prochlorperazine (Compazine 10 mg taken orally two or three times daily) is ordered as needed to treat nausea. In patients with bone or nerve pain, appropriate adjuvants are added.

When pain relief is adequate, the patient is converted to an equivalent dose of oral or transdermal opioid. If morphine is used, for example, the patient will need three times the parenteral dose that was effective (see box on Relative Potencies of Commonly Used Opioids). For example, a patient who requires 10 mg of morphine per hour (i.e., 240 mg/24 hours given intravenously) will need 720 mg/day of the oral sustained-release agent (240 mg every 8 hours). This can also be given orally as 360 mg every 12 hours. Two hours after the long-acting oral opioid is begun, the drip is discontinued. Short-acting immediate-release morphine should be available for rescue dosing at 10% of the total daily dose. For this patient, 60 to 90 mg every 3 to 4 hours is recommended. If the amount of opioid taken as a rescue dose is significant (>25% of the daily dose) for 1 or 2 days, the total dose of long-acting agent is adjusted upward accordingly.

Tramadol, which both weakly inhibits norepinephrine and serotonin reuptake and weakly binds to μ-opioid receptors and has opioid-like side effects but is not an opioid, also relieves mild to moderate pain. A dose of 100 mg is more effective than 60 mg of codeine. Tapentadol also had both μ-receptor agonism and norepinephrine reuptake inhibition. Studied in moderate to severe acute postoperative pain, osteoarthritis and low back pain, doses of 50 to 100 mg every 4 to 6 hours are comparable to oxycodone 10 to 15 mg every 4 to 6 hours with less nausea, vomiting, and constipation.

Opioid Analgesics

Patient Education

Opioid analgesics are the mainstay of therapy for moderate to severe pain of malignant or nonmalignant origin. To ensure patient compliance with an opioid prescription, education of members of the health care team, the patient, and the family is often required to dispel the many misconceptions associated with opioid therapy.[10] Even physicians who are cancer specialists may hesitate to prescribe opioids as needed for patients with severe pain.

Fear of addiction is a common cause of inadequate prescribing of opioids and a barrier to their acceptance by patients.[10] Patient adherence can be improved by providing a full explanation of the differences between addiction and physical dependence along with reassurance that research has repeatedly indicated that patients with malignancies who take opioids do not become addicts.[10] Patients may also fear that if they take opioid medications for moderate pain, the medications will no longer be effective if more severe pain occurs. Because this fear, if unexpressed, can lead to undertreatment, the topic should be addressed even if the patient does not raise the question. A functional goal of therapy, such as returning to a favorite hobby or reinstituting normal activities of everyday life, may enable the patient and the family to accept the opioid. Misconceptions about religious teachings may prevent health care personnel, patients, and their families from giving or accepting adequate pain medication. Catholics, for example, may not be aware of the church's position, as stated in the current catechism, that opioids may be used at the approach of death even if their use ultimately shortens the patient's life. The church does not consider this use of pain medication to be a means of suicide or euthanasia.[10]

Choice of Medication

Because a wide variety of medications are available, pharmacokinetic considerations and side effect profiles should be considered when choosing opioid agents. Intermittent moderate to severe pain lasting hours to several days is amenable to oral analgesics with short half-lives (3-4 hours) with appropriate potency (e.g., immediate-release oxycodone, morphine, hydromorphone [Dilaudid], or oxymorphone [Opana] when available). Severe pain of relatively constant intensity should be treated with oral sustained-release morphine or oxycodone taken every 8 or 12 hours,[1,9] hydromorphone (Exalgo) taken every 24 hours or oxymorphone (Opana ER) taken every 12 hours, methadone taken every 8 hours, or transdermal fentanyl renewed every 48 to 72 hours. Twelve- to 24-hour formulations of oral morphine (e.g., Kadian, Avinza) are available; for patients unable to take pills, the capsule can be opened and the pellets sprinkled on food or suspended in water and given through a feeding tube[10] (see boxes on Relative Potencies of Commonly Used Opioids and Choice of Medication).

Relative Potencies of Commonly Used Opioids

Drug	*Epidural*	*SC or IV (mg)*	*PO (mg)*
Morphine	1	10	30
Codeine		130	200
Oxycodone		N/A	20
Hydromorphone	0.15	1.5	7.5
Methadone*		*	
Oxymorphone		1	10
Levorphanol		2	4
Fentanyl		0.1	N/A
Meperidine (Demerol)†		75	300

IV, Intravenous; *N/A*, not applicable; *PO*, oral; *SC*, subcutaneous.
*Methadone is approximately half as potent orally as it is intravenously. It is usually not given SC because of local irritation. Standard equianalgesic tables do not reflect methadone's potency when used in repeated doses.
†Not recommended for patients with chronic pain.

Practical Considerations When Using Opioids

Drugs with short half-lives should be used for "rescue doses" given for incident pain (i.e., pain with movement) and for between-dose pain exacerbations often referred to as "breakthrough pain." The dose of the rescue medication should be 10% of the total 24-hour dose.[18] For example, if a patient is receiving 300 mg of oral sustained-release morphine twice each day, the rescue dose should be 10% of 600 mg, which is 60 mg of short-acting morphine. Agents with short half-lives should also be used in elderly patients and in patients with impaired renal or hepatic function.[10] For patients with a history of drug abuse, agents with longer half-lives, such as methadone, are preferred.

There is considerable variability with respect to the side effect profile of the various opioids in each patient. Therefore, it is often useful to switch to another agent if a patient is experiencing dose-limiting side effects with the initial opioid chosen. If the patient receiving morphine experiences disabling nausea, the substitution of oxycodone at an equianalgesic dose, for example, should be considered (see box on Relative Potencies of Commonly Used Opioids). Because of incomplete cross-tolerance, the initial dose for patients taking higher doses of opioids should be only half to two-thirds of the calculated equianalgesic dose.[18] In the same patient taking morphine (600 mg/day taken orally), oxycodone should begin at 200 to 300 mg/day (i.e., half or two-thirds of the 400-mg dose that would be equianalgesic). The short-acting rescue medication (20 or 30 mg of oxycodone) can provide relief if this initial dose does not prove adequate.

Although methadone is not a new drug, it is increasingly used for patients with moderate to severe pain. It is by far the least expensive of the opioids; can be given by the oral, rectal, intravenous, or epidural routes; and has particular usefulness in patients with neuropathic pain.[10] Methadone is structurally unrelated to morphine and fentanyl and can be used in the rare case of true allergy to these. It is also helpful when patients have neurotoxic side effects of the high doses of other opioids that are often needed to control severe neuropathic pain. Methadone is an opioid receptor agonist and a presynaptic inhibitor of NMDA.[19] Patients with neuropathic pain and patients taking opioids chronically have increased levels of NMDA receptors in the dorsal horn of the spinal cord. NMDA antagonizes the activity of the opiate receptors. Blocking the NMDA receptors therefore enhances the analgesic effect of externally administered opioids. Ketamine, a pure NMDA antagonist, similarly enhances opioid efficacy but is associated with more cognitive side effects than methadone.

Conversions Between the Transdermal Fentanyl Patch and Morphine

	Morphine (mg/24 hr)	
Fentanyl (mcg/hr)	*Oral*	*IM or IV*
25	50	17
50	100	33
75	150	50
100	200	67
125	250	83
150	300	100

Data from: Miaskowski C, Cleary J, Burney R, et al: *Guideline for the management of cancer pain in adults and children, APS clinical practice guidelines series, No.3.* Glenview, Ill, 2005, American Pain Society.
IM, Intramuscular; *IV*, intravenous.

Methadone interacts with inducers and inhibitors of the cytochrome P450 system. It is extensively metabolized by CYP1A2, CYP3A4, and CYP2D6; the first two are induced by a number of drugs and other substances (e.g., cigarette smoke), and the last enzyme has a genetic polymorphism. Drug levels of desipramine and zidovudine increase when patients are receiving methadone. Drugs that lower the levels of methadone include phenytoin (by 50%), phenobarbital, carbamazepine, rifampicin, and risperidone, each of which has precipitated withdrawal symptoms.[19] Drugs that raise the serum methadone levels include ketoconazole, fluconazole, fluoxetine and fluvoxamine. The selective serotonin reuptake inhibitors (SSRIs) (except venlafaxine) may raise methadone levels in CYP2D6 rapid metabolizers.

Methadone can cause prolongation of the QT interval. A mean methadone dose of 400 mg/day (standard deviation, 283 mg) was found in 17 patients with torsades de pointes. In an evaluation of reports of methadone-related adverse events to the U.S. Food and Drug Administration (FDA), approximately 1% of the greater than 5000 reports were of QT prolongation or torsades de pointes. The median dose was 345 mg with a range of 29 mg to 1680 mg. Drugs that also prolong the QT interval, such as metoclopramide and olanzapine, should be used with caution in patients receiving significant doses of methadone. Gabapentin, the drug used most often as a neuropathic pain adjuvant, does not interact with methadone metabolism.

Other difficulties with using methadone lie in its variable and long biologic half-life and the controversy about its equianalgesic dosing range. Some studies have reported that the equianalgesic dose of morphine to methadone varies as the dose of morphine increases.[10] Dose ratios vary from 4:1 at morphine doses of 30 to 90 mg, to 6:1 at 90 to 300, and to 8:1 at doses of more than 300 mg of morphine. Other studies report a ratio of 20:1 for doses of oral morphine equivalents greater than 1000 mg. Some physicians advise a 3-day conversion to methadone. The first day, the dose of the old opioid is reduced by one-third, and one-third of the calculated dose of methadone is given; the second day, the dose of the remaining opioid is reduced by half, and the dose of methadone is only increased if the patient is experiencing moderate to severe pain; the third day, the old opioid is discontinued, and the standing dose of methadone is adjusted to reflect the rescue doses.[19] When converting patients directly from intravenous fentanyl to intravenous methadone, a conversion ratio of 25 μg/hr of fentanyl to 0.1 mg/hr of methadone has been found in a pilot study to be a safe and effective initial infusion rate.

A new opioid to the U.S. market that is now available in both extended release and immediate release is oxymorphone. Oxymorphone extended release has been found to provide safe and effective pain relief for cancer pain.[20] Oxymorphone extended release is dosed twice daily and is about twice as potent as oxycodone.[21]

Levorphanol, which is chemically similar to dextromethorphan (an NMDA antagonist and cough suppressant), is a potent opioid that may be considered for patients with severe cancer pain. It was originally synthesized as an alternative to morphine more than 40 years ago. It has a greater potency than morphine, approximately five times as potent in its oral formulation. Analgesia is achieved through its agonistic activity at μ, δ, and κ opioid receptors, as well as by its antagonism of NMDA receptors. Levorphanol can be given orally, intravenously, and subcutaneously.

Buprenorphine has long been used to treat patients with addiction as an alternative to methadone. The new buprenorphine patch has been found to be effective in patients with cancer and noncancer pain. Postmarketing surveillance has indicated that 81% of patients achieve good or very good pain relief and about 50% of patients did not require additional medications for breakthrough pain.

Meperidine is eight to 10 times less potent than morphine and has a short duration of action, approximately 2 to 3 hours. Normeperidine, an active metabolite, which induces dysphoria, is excitatory to the CNS and can cause agitation, tremors, myoclonus, and seizures, especially in high doses, with prolonged use, or in renal failure.[10] Normeperidine has a half-life of 13 to 24 hours, which can lengthen with renal failure. The seizure incidence is further increased if the opioid antagonist naloxone (Narcan) must be given. Therefore, meperidine is not recommended for use in patients with long-lasting moderate to severe pain.[1,9]

Routes of Delivery

Opioids can be delivered noninvasively (orally, rectally, transmucosally, or transdermally) or invasively (subcutaneously, intravenously, or by spinal infusion). For patients switched from one route to another such as oral or rectal to parenteral or spinal medication or vice versa the dose must be converted accordingly to avoid overdose or undertreatment (see box on Relative Potencies of Commonly Used Opioids).

Oral Route

Most patients can achieve excellent pain relief with short-acting and/or sustained-release oral opioid preparations. The typical onset of short-acting opioids via the oral route is 45 minutes to 1 hour with a typical duration of action around 3 to 4 hours. When tablets and capsules are not feasible, many liquid forms are available in various concentrations. Some solutions do contain alcohol, which can be irritating to patients with oral lesions.

Rectal Route

Rectal opioids (i.e., morphine, oxymorphone, and hydromorphone) replace subcutaneous injections in patients who are suddenly unable to take oral medications. They have about the same potency and half-life as orally administered agents[10] and must therefore be administered frequently. Oxycodone has been shown to have a similar mean bioavailability but with a large interpatient variability but longer duration of activity (8 hours). Although not approved by the FDA, in single-dose bioavailability studies of sustained-release morphine preparations, despite delayed absorption from the rectal route, total morphine absorption over 24 hours was equivalent, whether the drug was given orally or rectally.[10]

Transdermal Route

The transdermal fentanyl patch delivers the lipophilic fentanyl into the fat-containing areas of the skin. The drug diffuses continuously from the patch's reservoir through a rate-controlling membrane and is absorbed from the skin depot into the bloodstream, where it is rapidly metabolized[10]. The onset of pain relief is delayed about 12 hours, and a relatively constant plasma concentration of fentanyl is not reached until about 14 to 20 hours after the initial patch is placed.[10] Liberal rescue medication must therefore be provided during the first 24 hours of use of the patch. Similarly, if a patient develops signs of fentanyl overdose, naloxone (Narcan) must be given until the skin reservoir has become depleted. About 50% of the drug is still present 24 hours after patch removal. Converting patients from oral or parenteral medication to the patch is easily accomplished[10] (see box on Relative Potencies of Commonly Used Opioids). A new patch is applied every 72 hours, although up to 25% of patients require a new patch every 48 hours.

The transdermal system is an effective method of delivering pain relief for patients with a stable level of chronic moderate to severe pain, no oral route available, or no desire to take pills. Side effects include those caused by the contact adhesive along with those commonly associated with other opioids, but they may be better tolerated than those caused by morphine.

The transdermal system should not be used in patients with sepsis, those experiencing acute pain, those with markedly fluctuating opioid requirements, cachectic patients, or individuals with significant dermatologic insults (i.e., skin graft-versus-host-disease [GVHD] or diffuse varicella). When the patient's temperature rises to 40°C, drug absorption from the skin can increase by as much as 35%. If hepatic function is impaired or sepsis or shock develops and blood flow to the liver decreases, plasma concentrations may rise sharply. Patients with cachexia lack the subcutaneous tissue necessary for formation of a drug reservoir. Lower doses may also be required in elderly patients and in those with respiratory insufficiency.

Transmucosal Route

Transmucosally administered fentanyl induces rapid analgesia with a short duration of effect (≈1 hour) and is an effective treatment in the management of breakthrough pain.[22] Oral transmucosal fentanyl citrate (Actiq), fentanyl buccal tablet (Fentora), fentanyl buccal soluble film (Onsolis), and fentanyl sublingual tablets (Abstral) as well as a fentanyl nasal spray (Ladanza) are the available transmucosal fentanyl products. They have been found to be both efficacious and safe in the treatment of cancer-related breakthrough pain.

Subcutaneous and Intravenous Routes

Subcutaneous or intravenous administration of opioids can provide pain relief in the shortest amount of time with a minimum of oversedation. The drugs can be delivered by portable infusion pump that is initiated or continued in the home.[10] Guidelines for their use are available. Patient-controlled analgesia (PCA) systems for subcutaneous or intravenous drug delivery have the advantage of responding to the individual patient's threshold for pain while eliminating delays when nurses must administer supplemental medication. The pumps can administer a continuous fixed infusion of the opioid chosen and allow the patient to self-administer boluses of additional medication at frequencies chosen by the physician. By recording the additional amounts of self-administered medication, the devices also facilitate the adjustment of the continuous dose required for pain relief.

Spinal Route

Epidural or intrathecal opioid infusions, which may include the option of PCA, can be helpful for select patients. The infused opioids block pain transmission by binding to receptors in the dorsal horn of the spinal cord. Because the drug is being infused in close proximity to the receptors, only a small amount of opioid is needed, and the systemic side effects are reduced. Problems with this delivery system in patients who are not opioid naive include pruritus, respiratory depression, and sedation. If tolerance to the opioid develops and higher doses are required for relief, the incidence of side effects may approach that of systemically administered opioids. Addition of local anesthetic or α-adrenergic agent (e.g., clonidine) or other agents[14] to the epidural opioid infusion allows for fairly rapid lowering of the opioid concentration and reestablishing opioid sensitivity but can cause hypotension.[23]

Adjuvant Analgesics

Adjuvant analgesics are a diverse class of medications, which typically have indications for conditions other than pain. They have analgesic properties and are often used when an opioid regimen alone is unable to provide sufficient analgesia or is associated with dose-limiting side effects.

Neuropathic Pain

Adjuvant agents for patients with neuropathic pain include anticonvulsants, antidepressants, α_2-adrenergic agonists, corticosteroids, topical agents, GABA agonists, and NMDA receptor antagonists.[1,9,10,24] However, the analgesic antidepressants and anticonvulsants are typically preferred for treating neuropathic pain secondary to cancer.[25]

The anticonvulsants gabapentin (Neurontin) and pregabalin (Lyrica) have the fewest side effects and are very effective for patients with neuropathic pain from tumor, peripheral neuropathy from tumor or treatment, and postherpetic neuralgia.[24] Despite their names, they have no effect on GABA but rather bind to the α-2-delta subunit of the N-type calcium channels in neurons within the dorsal horn, thus inhibiting calcium influx and diminishing neuronal hyperactivity. To minimize sedation, doses should be low at first (e.g., gabapentin 100 mg three times daily or 300 mg at bedtime; pregabalin 50 mg twice a day) and should be increased as tolerated every 3 to 5 days until analgesia is achieved. The effective dose of gabapentin varies between 900 and 3600 mg/day in divided doses and that of pregabalin is 150 to 300 mg twice a day. The pharmacokinetics of gabapentin are unique in that it has a ceiling effect related to a saturable transport mechanism in the gut, such that the effects of this drug may plateau during dose escalation.[25] The most common dose-limiting side effect is sedation. Gabapentin and pregabalin need to be renally dosed in patients with decreased creatinine clearance. Peripheral edema related to gabapentin or pregabalin may require diuretics. Pregabalin's gastrointestinal absorption is proportional to the dose throughout the effective dose range, making titration simpler. Other, generally less effective anticonvulsants used for neuropathic adjuvants include phenytoin, carbamazepine, lamotrigine, topiramate, and tiagabine.

The TCAs (e.g., amitriptyline, nortriptyline) are effective agents for neuropathic pain.[10] The TCAs, when used as adjuvant analgesics, are effective faster and at lower doses than when they are used as antidepressants (e.g., amitriptyline is effective within 2-3 days at 50-100 mg/day). However, because of their anticholinergic side effects, they should be started at doses of 10 to 25 mg at bedtime and used with caution in elderly patients and in patients who have cardiac conduction abnormalities or bladder outlet obstruction. Combination therapy with gabapentin and nortriptyline has been shown to be more effective than either drug alone in patients with diabetic neuropathy and postherpetic neuralgia.[26]

Selective serotonin and norepinephrine reuptake inhibitors (SSNRIs; e.g., venlafaxine and duloxetine) have been shown to be analgesic for a number of neuropathic pain syndromes. There is less evidence supporting the use of SSRIs for neuropathic pain.

Corticosteroids given epidurally, intravenously, or orally are useful as antineoplastics (e.g., in leukemia, lymphoma, and myeloma) and can also provide nonspecific relief for patients with spinal cord compression and plexus infiltrations. Doses of 16 to 100 mg of dexamethasone are needed to reduce vasogenic edema in spinal cord compression,[10] but lesser doses (6-20 mg/day) can be helpful in patients with plexus injuries. Patients must be monitored for the development of oral or esophageal candidiasis and steroid-induced delirium.

Bone Pain

Adjuvants for bone pain include NSAIDs, corticosteroids, bisphosphonates, RANK-L inhibitors (e.g., denosumab), and the radiopharmaceuticals strontium chloride (89Sr) and samarium153-lexidronan.[10] Multiple studies have demonstrated the efficacy of bisphosphonates in reducing skeletal complications and pain from bone metastases.[10] Pamidronate and zoledronate are recommended for patients with multiple myeloma and other hematologic malignancies with painful bone lesions. Calcium and sometimes vitamin D supplementation (especially for denosumab) are often needed.[27] Also, the long-term use of bisphosphonates is associated with a small but meaningful risk of osteonecrosis of the jaw.[27] The limitations of radiopharmaceuticals include cost and cytopenias.[10] Given the limited evidence available, a recent Cochrane review did not support the use of calcitonin for control of pain from bone metastases.

Management of Opioid-Related Side Effects

Sedation

The addition of 2.5 to 7.5 mg of dextroamphetamine or methylphenidate[10] (taken orally twice daily) has been shown to reduce opioid-induced sedation and at times allow for escalation of opioid doses without sedation. These medications also improve cognitive function and symptoms of depression. Methylphenidate may also enhance the analgesic effects of opioids.[10] They should be avoided in patients with anxiety, moderate to severe hypertension, agitation, thyrotoxicosis, tachyarrhythmias, severe angina pectoris, and closed-angle glaucoma. Modafinil (Provigil), a novel psychostimulant with a mechanism of action different than the amphetamine derivatives, which is approved for narcolepsy and fatigue related to multiple sclerosis, has also been found to be effective for opioid-related sedation.[10]

Constipation

Constipation is the most common opioid-induced side effect.[9] Laxatives should therefore be given routinely, not on an as-needed (PRN) basis,[1,9,10] to patients treated with any of the drugs listed in the box on Relative Potencies of Commonly Used Opioids. Detailed bowel preparation recommendations can be found, but no regimen has been studied in a controlled fashion. Commonly used stool softeners and stimulants include docusate sodium, senna, lactulose, and polyethylene glycol. A combination of a stool softener and laxative seems to be a rational choice for patients taking chronic opioids (e.g., docusate sodium with senna). Promotility agents most directly counter the mechanism of opioid-induced constipation. Bulk-forming laxatives such as psyllium and methylcellulose should be avoided because they increase stool volume without promoting peristaltic action. For refractory opioid-induced constipation, a trial of oral naloxone, methylnaltrexone, or alvimopan may be initiated.[10] These μ-opioid receptor antagonists act locally to reverse the effects of opioids on the gut. There is minimal systemic absorption with oral naloxone and subsequently a low risk of precipitating opioid withdrawal or worsening pain at low to moderate doses (1.6-12 mg/day). Methylnaltrexone (administered subcutaneously)[10] and alvimopan (oral) do not cross the blood–brain barrier and therefore do not cause opioid withdrawal or worsening pain.

Nausea

Prochlorperazine (10 mg taken two or three times daily) or metoclopramide (10 mg taken three to four times daily) can prevent the nausea that occurs in most patients during the first days of opioid therapy. Relieving constipation or changing the opioid (e.g., from morphine to oxycodone) often eliminates the later development of nausea. Rarely, patients need oral or intravenous ondansetron (8 mg taken two or three times daily).

Respiratory Depression

Naloxone (Narcan), given intravenously, reverses opioid-induced respiratory depression, although repeated doses are often required.[10] Respiratory depression can occur in patients with mild to moderate pain during the initial use of opioids, although it is rare in patients with severe pain and in those chronically receiving opioids. Caution should be exercised before administering naloxone to patients who are chronically receiving opioids to avoid precipitation of severe pain and withdrawal. In such cases, it is inadvisable to administer the usual 0.4 mg/mL dose. Rather, 0.4 mg of naloxone should be diluted with 9 mL of saline and 1 to 2 mL (0.04-0.08 mg) of this dilute mixture given every 2 to 3 minutes until the patient is rousable and breathing at least 10 times/min. Do not give enough to fully waken the patient or withdrawal is likely to ensue.[1] In a comatose patient, endotracheal tube placement is recommended to prevent aspiration from the salivation and bronchial spasm that will be induced.[1] Naloxone should not be administered to an alert patient.

SPECIFIC CLINICAL PROBLEMS

Oral Complications

Oral complications of chemotherapeutic and bone marrow transplant regimens can be frequent causes of pain. A thorough dental evaluation and prompt treatment of infections can minimize the discomfort arising from underlying periodontal disease and caries; secondary bacterial, viral, and fungal infections; and mucositis. Preventive regimens include saline, sodium bicarbonate, chlorhexidine gluconate rinses, acyclovir, antifungals, and ice. Palifermin (keratinocyte growth factor [KGF-1]) is used for the prevention and treatment of mucositis induced by conditioning regimens for hematopoietic stem cell transplants.[10] Amifostine is a thiol compound that is a selective cytoprotective agent approved for salivary gland protection in patients receiving radiation therapy. The use of colony-stimulating factors in the treatment of oral mucositis remains investigational.

Viscous lidocaine (Xylocaine) or a slurry of sucralfate, dyclonine, or Kaopectate in diphenhydramine provides symptomatic treatment of mucositis pain. For individual lesions, benzocaine in Orabase can be helpful. Milk of magnesia, which dries out the mucosa, is not recommended. Recently, GelClair, a bioadherent gel that adheres to the oral surface, creating a protective barrier for irritated tissue, has had mixed results in small clinical trials. The more severe cases, occurring in bone marrow transplant recipients, usually require infusional opioid therapy delivered by standard drip or PCA. Pilocarpine (5-7.5 mg three or four times daily 1 hour before meals) may improve xerostomia from neck irradiation. However, caution is warranted because of reported side effects of glaucoma and cardiac problems. Sugar-free hard candy is also useful for opioid-induced xerostomia and dysgeusia.

Coagulation Disorders

Patients with inherited or acquired disorders of coagulation may have excessive risks of bleeding if aspirin or unselective COX-inhibiting NSAID-containing pain relievers are used.[10] If acetaminophen and celecoxib, which has no measurable effect on platelet function or bleeding, are not effective, these patients may obtain significant relief from the nonacetylated salicylates, salsalate (Disalcid), or choline magnesium trisalicylate (Trilisate), which do not prolong the bleeding time.[10] Because these agents share aspirin's ability to compete with warfarin for albumin binding,[10] the careful monitoring of patients' coagulation parameters is recommended when these drugs are started or stopped.

Postherpetic Neuralgia

Postherpetic neuralgia, defined as pain persisting beyond 4 months from the initial onset of the rash, can be a difficult problem for patients with hematologic disorders and has been the subject of several reviews. The anticonvulsant medications gabapentin and pregabalin are especially useful in reducing the lancinating component of the various pain syndromes generated by this infection.[10] The efficacy of gabapentin was demonstrated in a randomized, double-blind, placebo-controlled study to cause a statistically significant reduction in the average daily pain score compared with placebo. If the patient cannot tolerate gabapentin or pregabalin, amitriptyline is effective in 60% to 70% of patients. Elderly patients, however, often do not tolerate the anticholinergic side effects well. Nortriptyline (Pamelor), a less anticholinergic TCA, may be useful in these patients. Opioid analgesics provide modest pain control. The lidocaine patch (5%) is indicated for the relief of pain associated with post herpetic neuralgia, however, the role of lidocaine gel, or ointment (5% to 10%) has not been established. Topical capsaicin (0.075%), which depletes substance P, has shown efficacy in a multicenter, double-blinded, randomized, placebo-controlled trial.[10] Capsaicin (0.075%) is also used for musculoskeletal discomfort. TENS devices provided relief for 1 year in 50% of postherpetic neuralgia patients, and 30% were pain free at 2 years. Patients with severe pain refractory to these therapies may benefit from a combination of intrathecal methylprednisolone and lidocaine. Acute herpes zoster pain may be diminished by a combination of acyclovir and prednisone.[10]

Sickle Cell Anemia

Patients with sickle cell anemia have chronic and episodic pain despite optimal medical therapy, and 60% of patients with sickle cell anemia will have an episode of severe pain each year. Chronic arthritic pain can be treated with physical therapy and full doses of antiarthritic medication, but some patients require low doses of chronic opioid therapy to maintain independent functioning. Several studies have confirmed the safety and efficacy of long-term opioids in the treatment of pain of nonmalignant origin. In some cases, joint replacement may be required.

When a patient with sickle cell anemia experiences pain, it is important to attempt to define the precise cause of the pain before attributing it to a vaso-occlusive crisis. Acute vaso-occlusive pain may occur along with the chronic pain caused by the long-term complications of compression fractures, avascular necrosis, arthropathies, fractures, avascular necroses, and leg ulcers.[28]

Treating patients with sickle cell pain is complex and requires understanding that much of the pain in adults with this illness is chronic with intermittent, recurring painful episodes. For mild pain, nonopioid therapy such as NSAIDS or acetaminophen with oxycodone or hydrocodone should be considered. However, because of possible compromise of renal blood flow in these patients and the risk of acute renal failure, NSAIDs should probably not be used beyond 5 days.[9] Uncontrolled severe pain accounts for more than 90% of hospital admissions in adults with sickle cell disease. Using short-acting analgesics on an "as-needed basis" exposes the patient to periods of insufficient analgesia, anticipation, and anxiety. Their repeated requests for medication to relieve their ongoing pain may be mistakenly interpreted as "drug-seeking behavior," and they may be unfairly stigmatized. Thus, intravenous analgesics should be started as a continuous infusion or with PCA. When adequate analgesia is obtained, a long-acting opioid, or a sustained-release opioid may be initiated with intermittent use of rescue medication. In adult patients with frequent episodes of painful crisis, the use of long-acting opioid medications reduced visits to the emergency department and hospitalizations and shortened the lengths of stay in hospital. Meperidine should be avoided in this population and has been associated with seizures in 1% to 12% of these patients.

Graft-Versus-Host Disease

For patients who have undergone bone marrow transplantation, GVHD can be a significant problem. The usual triad of GVHD includes hepatitis, dermatitis, and gastroenteritis. Patients are usually unable to take oral, rectal, subcutaneous, or transdermal opioids because of the effects on the skin (GVHD), lining of the gastrointestinal tract (mucositis, infection, and GVHD), and thrombocytopenia. Therefore, pain management with intravenous opioids is a necessity. The intestinal involvement that usually causes the most physical pain includes abdominal cramping and voluminous diarrhea. Treatment often begins with intravenous opioids given through a PCA pump. Addition of octreotide continuous infusion at 50 to100 μg/hr intravenously or intermittent dosing at 500 μg subcutaneously every 8 hours may be effective in decreasing the volume of diarrhea and level of abdominal pain.[10]

Peripheral Neuropathy Caused by Chemotherapy Agents

Several chemotherapy agents used in the treatment of hematologic malignancies can cause painful sensory peripheral neuropathy. The vinca alkaloids, most notably vincristine, are neurotoxic, but they are not always associated with painful neuropathy. Thalidomide, lenalidomide, bortezomib, cisplatin, oxaliplatin, and paclitaxel are all commonly used agents that carry a significant risk of causing painful peripheral neuropathy. The most common mechanism of neuropathy is damage to the axons starting with the most distal branches and is a result of chemotherapy's ability to damage DNA replication, leading to apoptosis. The major manifestations are burning paresthesias of the hands and feet and loss of reflexes. Paclitaxel also causes a motor neuropathy, which predominately affects proximal muscles.

Studies have evaluated numerous agents for prevention of painful peripheral neuropathy, although there have not been any magic bullets. Most of the research has focused on taxane and platinum-based chemotherapy agents. Amifostine and leukemia-inhibitory factor do not prevent neurotoxicity induced by these agents. Magnesium and calcium infusions have been shown to prevent neurotoxic symptoms associated with oxaliplatin without affecting its antitumor activity. Glutathione at doses of 1500 mg/m^2 administered before each dose of oxaliplatin for 12 cycles prevented grade 2 to 4 toxicities compared with placebo with no effect on response rate. Vitamin E has been shown to prevent neurotoxicity associated with cisplatin in small open-label evaluations. Glutamine 10 g three times daily for 4 days has had positive results as a neuroprotective agent in paclitaxel-treated patients. Acetyl-L-carnitine 1 g three times daily has been reviewed in the treatment of cisplatin- and paclitaxel-induced peripheral neuropathy, although no randomized studies have been done.

Treatment of chemotherapy-induced painful peripheral neuropathy includes the usual agents used for patients with neuropathic pain from any etiology (i.e., anticonvulsants, TCAs, and occasionally tramadol or opioids). In addition to treating these painful symptoms of neuropathy, the doses of the chemotherapy often require reduction or even discontinuation of therapy.

Problems of Elderly Patients

Pain management in elderly patients is a highly prevalent problem. It is complicated by difficulties in pain assessment and by the altered pharmacokinetics of opioids and of psychotropic adjuvant medications. Elderly patients may underreport pain.[10] Physicians may ascribe observed limitations in social contacts and physical activities to age-related changes when they are pain-induced limitations.

Elderly patients are particularly susceptible to the side effects of NSAIDs and opioids, and patients taking them should be monitored closely.[10] In elderly patients (70-89 years old), the volume of distribution for opioids is generally smaller, the drugs have longer plasma half-lives, and renal and hepatic clearances are decreased, all of which can prolong the duration of effect. The effective doses for these patients are half to one-fourth of those needed in younger patients. Drugs with short half-lives (e.g., morphine, oxycodone, hydromorphone) should be used, and initial doses should be low. Patients should be monitored carefully for the development of sedation or confusion, especially if they are receiving antihistaminic agents (e.g., famotidine, diphenhydramine), drugs with anticholinergic activity, or hypnotics.

Neuropathic pain syndromes are common in older adults, and the adjuvant analgesics gabapentin and pregabalin are often used. Common side effects include somnolence and ataxia that can be problematic in the geriatric population. Treatment should be initiated at 100 mg of gabapentin or 50 mg of pregabalin at bedtime, and close monitoring for side effects should occur before dose escalation. Acute urinary retention caused by opioids (especially in patients with prostatic hypertrophy) and the hypotension and tachycardia caused by tricyclic compounds can occur more frequently and be more clinically severe in this population. The starting dose of nortriptyline should be low (usually 10 mg at bedtime), and the dose should be slowly increased as tolerated. Treatment of opioid-related urinary retention may include generic Proscar (5 mg/day) in patients with benign prostatic hypertrophy and bethanechol (10 to 50 mg three times daily) to help increase bladder smooth muscle tone.

ANTIEMETIC THERAPY

A number of effective antiemetic therapies are used to prevent the nausea and vomiting induced in patients by treatment of their hematologic disorders with chemotherapy or radiation therapy. These antiemetic therapies markedly improve patients' quality of life. The vast majority of patients can expect complete control of vomiting[29] (see box on Combination Antiemetic Regimens), and most patients also are free of nausea.

PATHOPHYSIOLOGY OF NAUSEA AND VOMITING

Nausea is the subjective sensation that precedes vomiting. It is caused by stimulation of one or more of four sites—the gastrointestinal tract, the vestibular system, the chemoreceptor trigger zone in the area postrema of the floor of the fourth ventricle, or higher centers in the CNS (Fig. 92-2). The gastrointestinal tract can activate the vomiting center by stimulation of mechanoreceptors or chemoreceptors on glossopharyngeal or vagal afferents (cranial nerves IX and X) or by release of serotonin from gut enterochromaffin cells, which in turn stimulates serotonin (5-HT3) receptors on vagal afferents. The vestibular system activates the vomiting center when stimulated by motion or disease (e.g., labyrinthitis) or when sensitized by medication (e.g., opioids). Histamine (H1) and acetylcholine M1 receptors are present on vestibular afferents. Endogenous or exogenous bloodborne toxins may activate chemoreceptors in the area postrema of the floor of the fourth ventricle via dopamine type 2 receptors. Finally, higher CNS centers may activate or inhibit the vomiting center. In addition, there may be direct activation of H1 receptors in the meninges secondary to increased intracranial pressure.

The means by which chemotherapy agents induce vomiting are still incompletely understood, but the most likely mechanism is believed to include stimulation of the chemoreceptor trigger zone.[10] Other causes of nausea and vomiting in hematologic patients include stimulation of the cerebral cortex, gastritis and gastroesophageal reflux disease, delayed gastric emptying, radiation enteritis, constipation, esophageal candidiasis, inner ear processes, hypoadrenalism, hypercalcemia, changes in taste and smell, and anticipatory nausea.[10]

Although the sites of emetic action of the chemotherapeutic agents have not been identified, blocking agents directed against type 3 serotonin receptors (5-HT3 receptors), dopamine (D2) receptors, and neurokinin (NK1) receptors have been effective in inhibiting chemotherapy-induced nausea and vomiting (CINV).[10] Higher centers in the brain, such as the cortex, are also believed to be involved in producing anticipatory nausea and vomiting (ANV). Cognitive therapy, as well as antianxiety and amnesic agents, may provide effective antiemesis.

EVALUATION

Risk factors for developing CINV include age younger than 60 years, female gender, history of motion sickness, and hyperemesis gravidarum.[10] Patients who have a history of alcohol intake of more than five alcoholic drinks per day (>100 g of alcohol) tend to have less nausea and vomiting. This has been studied carefully in patients receiving high-dose cisplatin therapy but has been anecdotally observed in patients receiving other agents.

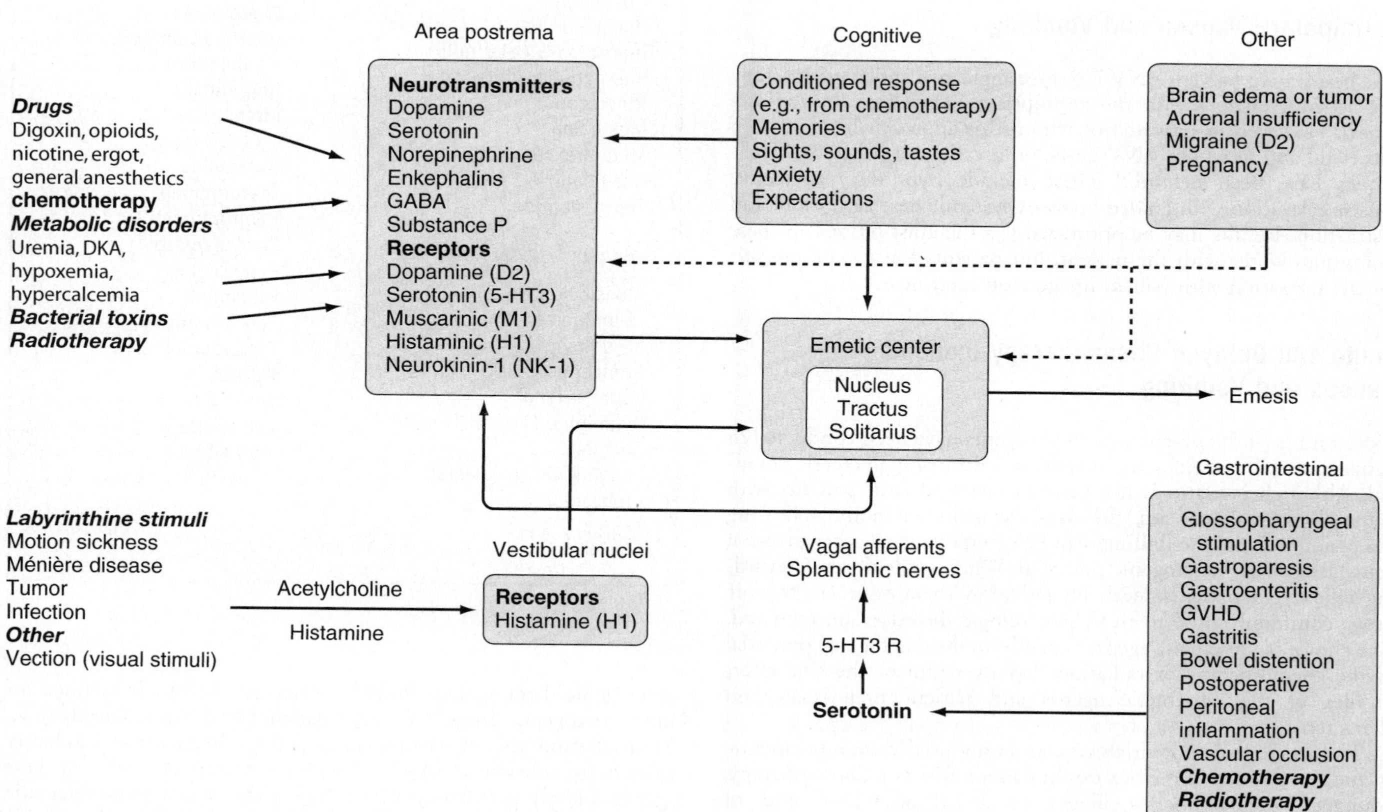

Figure 92-2 PATHOPHYSIOLOGY OF NAUSEA AND VOMITING. *DKA,* Diabetic ketoacidosis; *GABA,* γ-aminobutyric acid; *GVHD,* graft-versus-host-disease; *5-HT3,* serotonin.

Anticipatory Nausea and Vomiting

Anticipatory nausea and vomiting is believed to be a classic conditioned response.[10] Chemotherapy administration (the unconditioned stimulus) results in nausea and vomiting (the unconditioned response). Clinic sights, smells, and sounds are the conditioned stimuli. After frequent pairings of chemotherapy administration and the clinic's sights, smells, and sounds, the responses (nausea and vomiting) can be triggered in the absence of any chemotherapy by the clinic's sights, smells, or sounds or simply by seeing clinic personnel even at a location distant from the site of treatment.

Patients who are at risk for developing ANV are those who have already experienced posttreatment nausea and vomiting. The risk of developing ANV increases with the increasing frequency, severity, and duration of the symptoms. Other possible predisposing factors include susceptibility to motion sickness, awareness of tastes or odors during infusions, younger age, lengthier infusions, greater autonomic sensitivity, and general anxiety or emotional distress.[10]

Acute and Delayed Chemotherapy-Induced Nausea and Vomiting

Acute CINV is defined as nausea, vomiting, or both occurring within 24 hours of administration of the agent. The emetogenic potential of the drugs[29,30] is shown in the box on the Emetic Risks of Chemotherapy. Although most drugs produce emesis 1 to 2 hours after they are given (in patients who have never before received chemotherapy), the onset of emesis from high-dose intravenous cyclophosphamide is delayed until 9 to 18 hours after treatment, and nausea and vomiting from high total doses of cisplatin can occur 24 to 72 hours later.

Emetic Risks of Chemotherapy

High (>90%)

Carmustine (>250 mg/m^2)
Cisplatin (≥ 50 mg/m^2)
Cyclophosphamide (>1500 mg/m^2)
Dacarbazine
Doxorubicin (>60 mg/m^2)
Epirubicine (>90 mg/m^2)
Ifosfamide (≥10,000 mg/m^2)
Mechlorethamine
Streptozocin

Moderate (30%–90%)

Aldesleukin (IL-2) (>12-15 million international units/m^2)
Amifostine (>300 mg/m^2)
Arsenic trioxide
Azacitidine
Bendamustine
Busulfan
Carboplatin
Carmustine (≤250 mg/m^2)
Cisplatin (≤50 mg/m^2)
Clofarabine
Cyclophosphamide (<1500 mg/m^2)
Cytarabine (>200 mg/m^2)
Dactinomycin
Daunorubicin
Doxorubicin (≤60 mg/m^2)
Epirubicin (≤90 mg/m^2)
Idarubicin
Ifosfamide (≤10,000 mg/m^2)
Interferon-α (≥10 million international units/m^2)
Irinotecan
Melphalan
Methotrexate (≥250 mg/m^2)
Oxaliplatin
Temozolomide

Low (10%–30%)

Aldesleukin (IL-2) (≤12 million international units/m^2)
Amifostine (≤300 mg/m^2)
Cabazitaxel
Cytarabine (100-200 mg/m^2)
Docetaxel
Doxorubicin (liposomal)
Etoposide
5-Fluorouracil
Floxuridine
Gemcitabine
Interferon alfa (>5–<10 million international units/m^2)
Ixabepilone
Methotrexate (>50–<250 mg/m^2)
Mitomycin
Mitoxantrone
Paclitaxel
Paclitaxel albumin bound
Pemetrexed
Pentostatin
Pralatrexate
Romidepsin
Thiotepa
Topotecan

Minimal (<10%)

Alemtuzumab
Asparaginase
Bevacizumab
Bleomycin
Bortezomib
Cetuximab
Cladribine
Cytarabine (<100 mg/m^2)
Decitabine
Denileukin diftitox
Dexrazoxane
Fludarabine
Interferon alfa(≤5 million units/m^2)
Ipilimumab
Methotrexate (≤50 mg/m^2)
Nelarabine
Ofatumumab
Panitumumab
Pegaspargase
Peginterferon
Rituximab
Temsirolimus
Trastuzumab
Valrubicin
Vincristine
Vinblastine
Vinorelbine

IL-2, Interleukin.

Adapted from NCCN Guidelines Antiemesis Version 1.2012.

THERAPY

Anticipatory Nausea and Vomiting

The best way to prevent ANV is to give aggressive antiemetic therapy and to treat anxiety with the appropriate agents (see Benzodiazepines). However, in patients for whom this approach has not been successful and in whom ANV develops, a variety of behavioral techniques have been helpful.[10] These include hypnosis, progressive muscle relaxation with guided imagery, systemic desensitization, and distraction. Results may be optimized if a therapist trained in these techniques works with the patient, but patients can use progressive muscle relaxation with guided imagery on their own.

Acute and Delayed Chemotherapy-Induced Nausea and Vomiting

Most studies of the potent antiemetic agents have been conducted in patients receiving therapy with cisplatin, a drug of high emetic potential. Although cisplatin is not generally used to treat patients with hematologic malignancies, the data are included in the following discussion because the findings can be extrapolated to other drugs of equivalent or less emetogenic potential. When available, data regarding efficacy in patients receiving radiation therapy or emetogenic drugs commonly used to treat hematologic disorders are reviewed. The choice of antiemetic agents depends on the emetogenic potential of the chemotherapy or radiation therapy regimen, the side effect profiles of the antiemetic agents and patient preferences and characteristics.

The emetogenic potentials of commonly used chemotherapeutic agents are outlined in the box on the Emetic Risks of Chemotherapy. Younger patients have a higher incidence of CINV and of metoclopramide-related acute dystonic reactions; trismus or torticollis was seen in only 2% of patients older than 30 years of age but in 27% of younger patients. Even if they are receiving only moderately emetogenic therapy, they should be given an antiemetic regimen for high-emetogenic drugs.[29] Younger patients find cannabinoids (e.g., Marinol) more effective than do older patients because they can better tolerate the side effects associated with the therapeutic doses of these agents. Elderly patients also have high risks of extrapyramidal side effects and are more susceptible to anticholinergic and sedating side effects. 5-HT3 receptor antagonists are therefore preferred to regimens containing metoclopramide and diphenhydramine. Patient

Combination Antiemetic Regimens

Highly Emetogenic
Prophylactic

5-HT3 RA PO or IV 30 minutes before chemotherapy each day for the duration of chemotherapy plus
Dexamethasone, 12 to 20 mg PO or IV 30 minutes before chemotherapy each day for the duration of chemotherapy plus
Aprepitant, 125 mg PO 1 hour before chemotherapy (use 12-mg dose of dexamethasone)

To prevent or manage delayed nausea and vomiting after chemotherapy

For 2 to 5 days after chemotherapy:
Dexamethasone, 8 mg PO each day
Aprepitant, 80 mg PO each morning on days 2 and 3 (see above)

Moderately Emetogenic
Prophylactic

5-HT3 RA PO or IV 30 minutes before chemotherapy ±
Dexamethasone 8-12 mg PO or IV 30 minutes before chemotherapy

To prevent or manage delayed nausea and vomiting

Dexamethasone 8 mg PO once daily for days 2 and 3

Low Emetogenic Potential
Dexamethasone 8 mg PO or IV 30 minutes before chemotherapy as needed *or*
Metoclopramide 10-20 mg PO or IV 30 minutes before chemotherapy as needed *or*
Compazine 10 mg PO or IV 30 minutes before chemotherapy as needed

From Kris MG, Hesketh PJ Sommerfield MR, et al: American Society of Clinical Oncology Guideline for Antiemetics in Oncology: Update 2006. *J Clin Oncol* 24:2932.
IV, Intravenous; *PO,* oral; *5-HT3 RA,* serotonin receptor antagonist.

preferences regarding degree of alertness can help the health care provider choose an antiemetic regimen, as can the level of anxiety the provider observes in the patient.

Serotonin Receptor Antagonists: Ondansetron, Granisetron, and Palonosetron

Ondansetron, granisetron, and palonosetron are the best studied of the 5-HT3 receptor antagonists (5-HT RAs). This class also includes the drugs dolasetron and tropisetron. Several studies of patients receiving regimens that included cyclophosphamide, methotrexate, or doxorubicin showed significant efficacy and the superiority of ondansetron over placebo.

Ondansetron also demonstrates efficacy in patients with emesis (induced by non–cisplatin-containing chemotherapy) that has been refractory to standard antiemetics, with complete control achieved in 50% of these patients. When dexamethasone is added, the rate of control is as high as 91%.

Ondansetron effectively prevents nausea and vomiting in patients treated with highly emetogenic agents for acute leukemia or multiple myeloma (i.e., high-dose melphalan) or who are being prepared for bone marrow transplantation with cyclophosphamide and total-body irradiation.[29,30] In the transplantation recipients, 83% of patient-days were without any vomiting or retching, and in another 10%, there were no more than two emetic episodes. Ondansetron is also effective in preventing emesis induced by single- or multiple-fraction radiation therapy.[10] Ondansetron is as effective as high-dose metoclopramide in preventing nausea induced by cisplatin, cyclophosphamide alone, or doxorubicin chemotherapy.

Oral granisetron has shown equivalence to ondansetron in studies of patients receiving cisplatin- or carboplatin-based regimens. In patients receiving moderately emetogenic therapy, oral granisetron with dexamethasone was as effective as intravenous ondansetron and dexamethasone. Oral or intravenous granisetron and dexamethasone were effective in a bone marrow transplantation program in which patients were treated with Cytoxan and total-body irradiation, and these agents, along with oral prochlorperazine, were also effective in patients undergoing peripheral blood stem cell transplantation for which patients received Cytoxan, VP-16 or thiotepa, and cisplatin.

Palonosetron is a second-generation 5-HT3 RA with higher potency, stronger receptor binding activity, and longer half-life than the other drugs in this class.[10] Palonosetron 0.25 mg intravenously has been studied in moderately and highly emetogenic chemotherapy. Several subgroup analyses of the registrational noninferiority trials have been reported in which palonosetron was superior. Current studies seek to find palonesetron's place in therapy. Ondansetron and the other 5-HT3 RAs have far fewer side effects than high-dose metoclopramide. Reports of extrapyramidal reactions are rare,[10] and sedation, dystonic reactions, akathisia (e.g., severe restlessness, "ants-in-the-pants" feeling), and tardive dyskinesias do not occur. Patients can develop constipation, mild headache, and elevated levels of transaminases.

Corticosteroids

The mechanism of the antiemetic action of corticosteroids remains undefined. Corticosteroids are effective when used alone to prevent emesis induced by agents of moderate or low emetogenic potential.[29,30] They are also a useful component of antiemetic therapy regimens that include ondansetron, granisetron, aprepitant, or metoclopramide and add efficacy in randomized controlled trials.[29,30] Dexamethasone and methylprednisolone are the best-studied agents, but no trials have demonstrated the superiority of one corticosteroid over another.

Metoclopramide

Metoclopramide is a substituted benzamide that promotes gastric motility and reduces the emetic activity of chemotherapy agents by blocking dopamine receptors (at low to moderate doses) and 5-HT3 receptors (at high doses) in the chemoreceptor trigger zone. Because of a more favorable side effect profile, 5-HT3 antagonists have replaced high dose metoclopramide. At lower doses (5-10 mg orally or intravenously every 6 hours), metoclopramide is useful in treating mild to moderate and delayed nausea and vomiting. Delivery of the drug on a schedule that maintains adequate levels during expected emesis appears to be important.

The side effects, which may be caused by the interaction of metoclopramide with dopamine receptors, can be quite troublesome. They include akathisia, dystonic reactions (age related), sedation, and diarrhea. Benzodiazepines such as lorazepam and β-blockers such as propranolol can prevent or reverse the akathisia, and diphenhydramine or benztropine can prevent or reverse the dystonias. However, these agents induce additional side effects, including dry mouth and sedation. Short-term, high-dose metoclopramide or long-term use at usual doses has been associated with persistent and disabling movement disorders, especially tardive dyskinesias.

Neurokinin-1 Inhibitors

Substance P can cause emesis, and it appears to play a role in chemotherapy-related nausea and vomiting. Its effects are mediated through NK-1 receptors.[10] Agents that cross the blood–brain barrier and inhibit NK-1 activity (e.g., aprepitant) are more effective than a 5-HT3 RA and dexamethasone alone in moderating acute chemotherapy-related nausea and vomiting, and they are particularly effective in decreasing delayed nausea and vomiting occurring after cisplatin chemotherapy.[10,29] The need for continued dexamethasone with the NK-1 inhibitor has not yet been determined, and comparisons with the metoclopramide and dexamethasone regimen for delayed nausea and vomiting have not yet been performed. Aprepitant is an inhibitor of CYP3A4 and therefore may cause elevation of chemotherapy agents primarily metabolized by this route; however, these elevations are not considered clinically significant, and there are no recommend dose adjustments. Aprepitant can cause significant decreases in the prolongation of the international normalized ratio induced by warfarin. Fosaprepitant, the intravenous prodrug of aprepitant, has demonstrated equivalent efficacy to the 3-day oral regimen as a single dose at 150 mg on day 1.

Combination Antiemetic Therapy

For drugs with low or minimal emetogenic potential, no antiemetic drug may be needed, or a single agent such as dexamethasone or metoclopramide may be sufficient. For drugs with higher emetogenic potential, standard antiemetic treatment usually includes combinations of several antiemetic agents along with agents designed to treat anxiety, cause amnesia, or prevent known side effects. These combinations include a 5-HT3 receptor antagonist such as ondansetron and a corticosteroid such as dexamethasone for moderately emetogenic regimens.[29] For highly emetogenic combination chemotherapy or regimens that include two moderately emetogenic agents, such as cyclophosphamide and Adriamycin, aprepitant (NK-1 inhibitor) should be added to the antiemetic combination.[29] Optional lorazepam may be added for anxiety-related symptoms. It is important to give antiemetic therapy before administering chemotherapy agents and to continue for about 24 to 72 hours after the drugs have been given to prevent emesis.

Benzodiazepines

The benzodiazepine lorazepam has only mild antiemetic activity when used as a single agent. It is used frequently in the treatment and prevention of nausea and vomiting, particularly when anxiety is associated with the nausea and vomiting. It markedly decreases anxiety and the akathisia associated with metoclopramide therapy and induces a dose-related memory loss and marked sedation.

Other Drugs

Other agents that are more active than placebo include the butyrophenones haloperidol and droperidol, the phenothiazine prochlorperazine, and the cannabinoids dronabinol (THC) and nabilone. These agents are less effective drugs than the agents previously mentioned, and all cause sedation. The butyrophenones produce dystonic reactions, akathisia, and occasionally hypotension. The cannabinoids cause ataxia, dry mouth, orthostatic hypotension and dizziness, euphoria or dysphoria, and a feeling of being "high." Scopolamine, a centrally-acting anticholinergic, can be effective for patients with a vertiginous component to their nausea (see box on Combination Antiemetic Therapy). Olanzapine has been shown to improve control of both acute and delayed nausea and vomiting in highly and moderately emetogenic chemotherapy when used in combination with dexamethasone and a 5-HT3 receptor antagonist.

REFERENCES

1. Foley KM: Management of cancer pain. In DeVita VT, Lawrence TS, Rosenberg SA, et al, editors: *DeVita, Hellman, and Rosenberg's Cancer: Principles and practice of oncology*, ed 9, Philadelphia, 2011, Lippincott Williams & Wilkins.
2. McMahon SB, Koltzenberg M, editors: *Wall and Melzack's textbook of pain*, ed 5, Philadelphia, 2006, Elsevier/Churchill Livingstone.
3. Strada EA, Portenoy RK: Nonpharmacologic therapy of cancer pain. *UpToDate online* 19:1, 2011.
4. Kaplan R, Portenoy RK: Interventional approaches to the management of cancer pain. *UpToDate online* 19:1, 2011.
5. Fields, HL, Basbaum AI, Heinricher MM: Central nervous system mechanisms of pain modulation. In McMahon SB, Koltzenberg M, editors: *Wall and Melzack's textbook of pain*, ed 5, Churchill Livingstone, 2006, Elsevier, p 125.
6. Mercadante S, Ferrera P, Villari P, et al: Hyperalgesia: An emerging iatrogenic syndrome. *J Pain Symptom Manage* 26:769, 2003.
7. Pappagallo M, Shaiovo L, Perlov E, Knotkoa H.: Difficult pain syndromes: Bone pain, visceral pain, neuropathic pain. In Berger A, Shuster JL, Von Roenn JH, editors: *Principles and practice of palliative care and supportive oncology*, ed 3, Philadelphia, 2007, Lippincott Williams and Wilkins.
8. Chang VT, Janjan N, Jain S: Update in cancer pain syndromes. *J Palliative Med* 9:1414, 2006.
9. Miaskowski C, Cleary J, Burney R, et al: *Guideline for the management of cancer pain in adults and children, APS clinical practice guidelines series, No.3*, Glenview, Ill, 2005, American Pain Society.
10. Abrahm JL: *A physician's guide to pain and symptom management in cancer patients*, ed 2, Baltimore, 2005, Johns Hopkins University Press.
11 Syrajala K, Cummings C, Donaldson G: Hypnosis or cognitive behavioral training for the reduction of pain and nausea during cancer treatment: A controlled trial. *Pain* 48:137, 1992.
12. Sze WM, Shelley MD, Held I, et al: Palliation of metastatic bone pain: Single fraction versus multifraction radiotherapy—A systematic review of randomized trials. *Clin Oncol* 15:345, 2003.
13. Berenson J, Pfugmacher R, Jarzem P, et al: Balloon kyphoplasty versus non-surgical fracture management for treatment of painful vertebral body compression fractures in patients with cancer: A multicentre, randomized controlled trial. *Lancet Oncol* 12:225, 2011.
14. Stearns L, Boortz-Marx R, Du Pen S, et al: Intrathecal drug delivery for the management of cancer pain: A multidisciplinary consensus of best clinical practices. *J Support Oncol* 3:399, 2005.
15. Rawlins MD: Non-opioid analgesics. In Hanks G, Cherny NI, Christakis NA, et al, editors: *Oxford textbook of palliative medicine*, ed 3, Oxford, UK, 2010, Oxford University Press, p 355.
16. Joishy SK, Walsh D: The opioid-sparing effects of intravenous ketorolac as an adjuvant analgesic in cancer pain: Application in bone metastases and the opioid bowel syndrome. *J Pain Symptom Manage* 16:334, 1998.
17. Trelle S, Reichenbach S, Wandel S, et al: Cardiovascular safety of nonsteroidal anti-inflammatory drugs: Network meta-analysis. *BMJ* 342:c7086, 2011.
18. Portenoy RK: Cancer pain management. *Clin Adv Hematol Oncol* 3:30, 2005.
19. Bruera E, Sweeney C: Methadone use in cancer patients with pain: A review. *J Pall Med* 5:127, 2002.
20. Prommer, E: Oxymorphone: A review. *Support Care Cancer* 14:109, 2006.
21. Gabrail NY, Dvergsten C, Ahdieh H: Establishing the dosage equivalency of oxymorphone extended release and oxycodone controlled release in patients with cancer pain: A randomized controlled study. *Curr Med Res Opin* 20:911, 2004.
22. Zeppetella G, Ribeiro MD: Opioids for the management of breakthrough pain in cancer patients. *Cochrane Database Syst Rev* 25(1):CD004311, 2006.
23. Swarm RA, Cousins MJ: Anaesthetic techniques for pain control. In Hanks G, Cherny NI, Christakis NA, et al, editors: *Oxford textbook of*

palliative medicine, ed 3, Oxford, UK, 2010, Oxford University Press, p 390.
24. Portenoy RK: Adjuvant analgesics in pain management. In Hanks G, Cherny NI, Christakis NA, et al, editors: *Oxford textbook of palliative medicine*, ed 3, Oxford, UK, 2010, Oxford University Press, p 361.
25. McDonald A, Portenoy RK: How to use antidepressants and anticonvulsants as adjuvant analgesics in the treatment of neuropathic cancer pain. *J Support Oncol* 4:43, 2006.
26. Filron I, Bailey JM, Tu D, et al: Nortriptyline and gabapentin, alone and in combination for neuropathic pain: A double-blind, randomized controlled crossover trial. *Lancet* 374(9697):1252, 2009.
27. Kyle RA, Yee GC, Somerfield MR, et al: American Society of Clinical Oncology clinical practice guideline update on the role of bisphosphonates in multiple myeloma. *J Clin Oncol* 25:2464, 2007.
28. Ballas SK: Pain management of sickle cell disease. *Hematol Oncol Clin North Am* 19:785, 2005.
29. Kris MG, Hesketh PJ, Sommerfield MR, et al: American Society of Clinical Oncology guideline for antiemetics in oncology: Update 2006. *J Clin Oncol* 24:2932, 2006.
30. National Comprehensive Cancer Network: Clinical practice guidelines in oncology: Antiemesis, v.1.2012. Available at www.ncc.org/professionals/physician_gls/pdf/antiemesis.pdf. Accessed August 11, 2011.

CHAPTER 93

PALLIATIVE CARE

Kristen G. Schaefer, Janet L. Abrahm, and Joanne Wolfe

Palliative care is specialized care for children and adults with a focus on individual patient and family goals, values, preferences, and expressed needs in the face of serious illness. Palliative care practitioners need to have expertise in communication, in treatment of physical symptoms, and in relieving sources of social, psychologic, and spiritual distress. Each section of this chapter will first review core elements of palliative care for children and then for adults.

PEDIATRIC PALLIATIVE CARE

I just wish that I had armfuls of time.

— *(4-year-old child)*[1]

Pediatric palliative care is an emerging frontier in the comprehensive care of children. The 2003 Institute of Medicine report *When Children Die: Improving Palliative and End-of-Life Care for Children and Their Families*[2] (Table 93-1) highlights its critical importance. In the last few years, a powerful statement by the American Academy of Pediatrics, the findings of a comprehensive British report on children with life-threatening and terminal conditions, and two earlier Institute of Medicine studies set the stage for this seminal report. A comprehensive definition is as follows:

Palliative care for children and young people with life-threatening illness is an active and total approach to care, embracing physical, emotional, social, and spiritual elements. Pediatric palliative care focuses on optimizing quality of life and well-being for patients and families by using expert symptom management, caregiver support and respite, and specialized care at the end of life and in bereavement.

As this field develops, there is much debate about the terms *life-limiting* and *life-threatening.* Life-threatening is a broader concept, in that it includes illnesses for which cure is possible, although the threat of a fatal outcome exists (e.g., childhood malignancies). Of course, an illness may begin as life-threatening and convert into a life-limiting condition, as when a child relapses and curative options no longer exist. Life-limiting conditions are those for which there is no reasonable chance of cure from the outset; even if children survive for years and decades, they will not live out a normal life expectancy.

In addition to end-of-life care for the child (and bereavement follow-up for the family), pediatric palliative care includes care throughout the trajectory of the child's illness, including respite as an important component. Specific issues related to palliative care for pediatric patients and their families include the following[3]:

- Smaller numbers of dying children than adults mean that there is less professional expertise and underrepresentation of children in palliative care protocols.
- The heterogeneity of illnesses, many rare, requires the involvement of many disciplines and specialists.
- Many children have genetic diseases, so there may be more than one affected child in a family.
- The time course of some illnesses is extremely variable. Pediatric palliative care may extend over years, even decades.
- A broad developmental spectrum is represented, including changes in the individual child through time.
- The underlying principles and ethics of palliative care are universal across the life span. However, as in all specialties, children bring with them unique issues and dilemmas.
- A child or adolescent diagnosed with a life-threatening or life-limiting illness throws an assumed sequence out of order. A time of role reversal is expected, when children will care for dying parents. When parents instead find themselves watching their child face death, a sense of tragic absurdity prevails. Not only is time shortened, but its order is shattered. A child or adolescent with a life-threatening illness represents a premature separation to the family. Even before the child has become a differentiated individual through a natural developmental sequence, that child is wrenched away. There is little preparation for separation by death when a psychologic separation has not yet been effected. The adolescent who is beginning to negotiate an independent existence is often the hardest to face when that "moving forward" is irreversibly halted, or at least disrupted. A child has not even had the time to begin to form life goals.[4]
- The necessity for palliative care—the concept and the clinical approach—may emerge at different points in the illness trajectory, depending on the prognosis for the child, the decisions that must be made in choosing treatment options, and always, the management of pain and suffering in the provision of optimal quality of life. One of the foremost goals is to initiate palliative care for children earlier in the illness trajectory—in a proactive manner—so that effective care planning can be implemented. Care of the family, with a particular focus on the young siblings, is a priority.

ADULT PALLIATIVE CARE

Palliative care for adult patients involves the same specialized, interdisciplinary, patient- and family-centered attention to physical comfort, psychologic needs, social and spiritual sources of distress, and the alignment of treatment plans with patients' and families' goals of care. Although often conflated with end-of-life care or hospice care, the specialty aims to improve quality of life for patients throughout the course of serious illness, from diagnosis through the final stages, including simultaneously with life-prolonging or curative therapies.[5] In 2006, hospice and palliative medicine was accepted as a specialty by the American Board of Medical Specialties. In 2007, the Accreditation Council for Graduate Medical Education began accrediting fellowship programs, and the first qualifying examination in hospice and palliative medicine was given in 2008. Emerging evidence suggests that concurrent palliative care in advanced illness can decrease costs and improve outcomes,[6] and patient access to high-quality specialty-level palliative care is becoming standard of care at most academic cancer centers.

Table 93-1 Summary of the Institute of Medicine Report: *When Children Die: Improving Palliative and End-of-Life Care for Children and Their Families*

IMPROVE ORGANIZATION AND DELIVERY OF CARE
Emphasis is placed on the development of care guidelines and protocols in all pediatric settings, the development of regional information programs and resources in rural areas, and policies and procedures for involving children in decision making.
REFORM FINANCING OF PALLIATIVE SERVICES AND HOSPICE CARE
Vast changes in public and private health coverage: add hospice, change eligibility rules, provide outlier payments, extend coverage for counseling family members and for bereavement follow-up.
BETTER PREPARE HEALTH PROFESSIONALS
Create educational experiences and curricula that will provide basic and advanced competence in palliative, end-of-life, and bereavement care.
STRENGTHEN RESEARCH BASE FOR EFFECTIVE CARE
Emphases include appropriate quality-of-life measures, effective symptom management, impact of perinatal death on parents and siblings, impact of sudden death on family and professional caregivers, efficacy of bereavement interventions, models for provision of care, financing alternatives, effective strategies for educating professionals.

From Institute of Medicine: *When children die: Improving palliative and end-of-life care for children and their families,* Washington, DC, 2003, National Academy Press.

Table 93-2 Breaking Bad News

1. Make yourself, the patient, and the family comfortable.
2. Find out what they know.
3. Indicate that you are planning to tell them something that is unpleasant and may be disturbing.
4. Find out whether they want to be told, or whether they want someone else to be told.
5. Find out how much they want to know (i.e., the big picture versus all the details).
6. Tell them in words they can understand, allowing time for questions along the way.
7. Respond to their feelings.
8. Let them know that this is only the first of many discussions with you.
9. Ask them to summarize what they heard you say; ask if they have further questions.
10. Arrange your next meeting with them.

From Abrahm JL: Update in palliative medicine and end-of-life care, *Annu Rev Med* 54:53, 2003.

COMMUNICATION

Good communication can dispel fears of abandonment. Breaking bad news and discussing prognosis with patients with advanced disease are occasions when physicians can demonstrate their commitment to an ongoing partnership with patients and families. Conversations must demonstrate respect for cultural differences[7] and the conviction that growth can occur even at the end of life.[8] If done well, the groundwork will be laid for further discussions of patient hopes and fears, goals, values, and spiritual concerns that form the basis of decisions about resuscitation and artificial life support.

Communication with a child …

> *When I first heard my diagnosis, one question kept going around and around in my head: "How long do I have, Doc?"*
>
> — *(12-year-old child)*[1]

Children with serious hematologic disorders have usually lived with the illness over a prolonged period of months or years. Their knowledge, understanding, and awareness of their precarious life situation is often profound, at physical, cognitive, and emotional levels.

> *The doctors think my bone marrow is fine for now—and for now is for now.*
>
> — *(8-year-old child)*[4]

The protective stance of the past stated that disclosure to the child of his or her prognosis (and even, in some instances, the diagnosis) would cause increased anxiety and fear. Since the 1980s, however, a shift toward open communication has been evident.[9] To shield the child from the truth may only heighten anxiety and cause the child to feel isolated, lonely, and unsure of whom to trust.

In communication with the life-threatened child at any juncture in the illness, the precedent for a climate that enables such honest interchange is created from the time of diagnosis. The individual child's competence and vulnerability serve as the context for decisions regarding disclosure at any point in the illness trajectory. Considerations about what or how much to tell include the child's age, cognitive and emotional maturity, family structure and functioning, cultural background, and history of loss.[1] These same factors apply at the end of life, with extreme sensitivity to how the parents have chosen to inform the child throughout the illness experience, how the child has understood and processed information up to this time, and what the child is now asking—implicitly and explicitly—about his or her situation.

For adult patients with advanced cancer, having had a discussion about end-of-life wishes with one's physician has been shown to correlate with less aggressive medical care near death, earlier hospice referrals, cost savings at the end of life, and improved bereavement adjustment for caregivers.[10] Furthermore, having had conversations about end-of-life wishes is not associated with higher rates of major depressive disorder or more worry. Proactive, direct communication with patients and their families about approaching and managing the end of life can be a satisfying and rewarding part of patient care. However, more training in palliative care clinical and communication skills is needed during hematology/oncology fellowship and in continuing medical education settings to ensure competency in these areas.

Breaking Bad News

Table 93-2 contains an outline of the suggested steps to take when breaking bad news.[11] For patients with advanced disease, the goal is to establish or strengthen trust and reassure them that the physician is committed to caring for them. To do this well, physicians need to believe that they have not failed the dying patient, medicine has.

Prognosis and Decision Making

Surveys of bereaved parents indicate that physician communication about prognosis is not optimal. At the same time, emerging data suggest that bereaved parents consider high-quality communication as the most important value when reflecting on physician quality of care.[12] Parents value clear information that is communicated sensitively and includes the child, when developmentally appropriate. When it comes to discussing prognosis, a majority of parents want as much information as possible.[13] Furthermore, although many parents find prognostic information about their child upsetting, they still want prognosis to be discussed. The data suggest, however, that parents are overly optimistic about the child's chances of cure in comparison to physicians, and this is especially true when the prognosis is uncertain. Being aware of these trends may help physicians to discuss prognosis with greater clarity.

One side of my head says: "Think optimistic." The other side says: "What if this treatment doesn't work?"

— (11-year-old-child)[1]

The child is often aware of the diminishing curative or life-prolonging options that he or she faces. It is at this time that the child may ask anxiously: "What if this medicine doesn't work? What will you give me next?" The child experiences a profound sense of loss of control. It is at this time that families are confronted with a series of decisions regarding the nature and intensity of medical interventions they wish to pursue. This process can be excruciating: they do not want their child to suffer more, yet they often cannot tolerate the thought of "leaving any stone unturned" in the quest for a cure or prolonged time, however minuscule the chance.[14] The physician and team's role shifts from leadership in recommending a curative treatment plan to the clarification of experimental and palliative options and consequences. In most instances, the parents make the decision; however, to varying degrees, the child may be involved in such discussions.[15] Hinds et al[15] have demonstrated that when asked in a sensitive manner, children as young as 10 years of age are able and willing to talk about their experiences and end-of-life decisions.

During the last decade there has been increased recognition of the child's participation in making treatment decisions. Crucial to this process is an assessment of the child's or adolescent's ability to appreciate the nature and consequences of a specific medical decision. This becomes particularly complex when the wishes of the child differ from those of the parents. Because actual assessment tools are only in the early stages of development, professionals must rely exclusively on their clinical judgment to assess children's understanding of the contingencies they are facing. This is often a juncture when input from members of the interdisciplinary team can be crucial: children often express their understanding, awareness, and thoughts about treatment options and living or dying to individuals other than their parents or primary physician.

The following example illustrates the remarkable capacity of a young child to address the transition to palliative care.

A 7-year-old girl told her parents that she was too tired to fight anymore, and that she wanted to give up. She added: "If I have to continue suffering, I would rather be in heaven." These statements were major determinants in the parents' choosing a palliative care plan without any further attempts at life-prolonging treatment. She went home on hospice care and died peacefully several weeks later.[1]

Adult patients and families want to be prepared for the end of life. The vast majority (80% to 98%) want to be able to name someone to make decisions, know what to expect about their physical condition, have financial affairs in order, know that the physician is comfortable talking about death and dying, feel that the family is prepared for their death, have funeral arrangements in place, and have treatment preferences in writing. For this to happen, patients must know how long they are likely to have left to live.[16] Although most patients report wanting prognostic information from their oncologist, patients with advanced refractory disease may not ask about their prognosis, and oncologists often do not initiate the discussion. In one recent observational study, only half of patients were told unambiguous prognostic estimates for mortality or cure during their first oncologic visit for a hematologic malignancy.[17]

There are significant benefits from having a discussion of prognosis with a relatively asymptomatic patient with a limited time left to live and his or her caregivers. Patient preferences for resuscitation are affected by the likely outcome of treatment and by their understanding of their prognosis. It is equally important that patients with very poor prognoses understand how limited they really are. Patients who thought they had a greater than 10% chance of surviving 6 months, for example, usually wanted to be resuscitated. Patients who thought they had a less than 10% chance of surviving 6 months overwhelmingly chose comfort care and did not want to be resuscitated.[18]

Discussions of prognosis can be very painful for clinicians, because they may cause feelings of guilt, failure, or sadness. Clinicians interested in improving their skills may refer to practical educational handbooks[19] and articles that outline how to discuss these issues both with patients who want to know their prognosis and with those who do not or are ambivalent.

Cultural Considerations

Ethnicity, culture, socioeconomic status, religion, and religious background all affect the ways patients experience illness and face death.[20] Autonomy may be expressed in a number of ways. For example, non-Hispanic whites prefer to have immediate family only present, whereas African Americans want their extended family, friends, and pastor. African Americans are also more interested in spiritual concerns, lack of trust, concerns about do not resuscitate (DNR) orders and hospice, allowing adequate time for decisions, and not feeling pressure to make them.[7] The best way to show respect for patient and family views is to individualize the approach with attention to language, religious beliefs/concerns, cultural context, health beliefs, decision-making patterns, and social support/resources. Qualified interpreters should be provided whenever the clinician is not fluent in the patient's language.

Impact on Hope

The rigors of treatment regimens and the physical and emotional demands of the complex care required for advanced disease tend to isolate patients and their families and focus all their hopes on disease remission. They may have forgotten how to hope for anything else. Physicians and the teams they work with can help patients with advanced hematologic diseases develop new kinds of hope by encouraging them to reintegrate into activities that were meaningful before their disease began and they rearranged their lives around treatment schedules. Paradoxically, discussion about limited prognosis is likely to lessen fears of abandonment and strengthen the trust patients have in the oncology team. Most patients hope for time to say their goodbyes, to bring closure to their lives, and to leave their legacies: videos, scrapbooks, letters, and presents for children or grandchildren for events far into the future.

As disease progresses, despite ongoing treatment, patients who have begun to reengage in non–treatment-related activities and who have developed a broader relationship with their physicians are more likely to understand that the physician is not abandoning them when he or she says that the goals of treatment should be comfort. Such patients do not complain that stopping treatment is "waiting around to die" because they have other activities to fill their days.

CAREGIVERS

Families and other nonprofessional caregivers provide the vast majority of care for patients with advanced cancer, which is thought to be worth the equivalent of more than $250 billion dollars a year. Caregivers of patients with advanced illness are stressed by the patient's disability and degree of suffering, the lack of coordination of care, and underlying family, work, or financial pressures.[21,22] Caregiving can take a physical and psychologic toll on the caregivers, with increased prevalence of depression, decrease in self-care and preventive care, and perhaps increased mortality. Providing information and increasing coping skills can improve caregiver knowledge and skill, but even providing respite care has not lessened the sense of burden or depression. As many as 32% of caregivers either have a major psychiatric condition (panic disorder, major depression, posttraumatic stress disorder, or generalized anxiety disorder), or access mental health services after the patients' diagnosis. Caregivers are likely to need the support of many members of the team therefore to continue in their difficult role.

RELIEF OF SUFFERING

Suffering includes physical, psychologic, social, and spiritual dimensions.

Symptom Management in Children

Therapist: If you could choose one word to describe the time since your diagnosis, what would it be?

— *Child: PAIN.*[1]

Maintaining patient comfort is a critical issue throughout treatment, as well as during the end stages of life. Although effective pain control is a hallmark of palliative care, pain is only one of many distressing symptoms.[3] The spectrum of physical symptoms includes (although it is not limited to) dyspnea, fatigue, seizures, loss of appetite, nausea and vomiting, constipation, and diarrhea. Several comprehensive studies,[23] in which bereaved parents were interviewed regarding their children's end-of-life care, indicated that optimal symptom management is still far from being achieved, even in major pediatric teaching centers. More than 10% of parents considered hastening their child's death; this was more likely if the child was in pain.[24] Relief of a child's end-of-life distress may have long-lasting implications for bereaved parents, who are negatively affected by the child's experience of pain years beyond the death.

Psychologic symptoms such as depression and anxiety are also prevalent in children at the end of life.[23] Children also experience existential concerns. Creating opportunity for communication around these sources of distress involves using creative strategies that incorporate the developmental stage of the child. Strategies may involve verbal communication using open-ended questions such as "What are you hoping for?" and "What are you worried about?"

However, many children communicate best through nonverbal means such as artwork and music. Children may be more willing to "talk things over" with puppets or stuffed animals rather than real people. Importantly, euphemistic expressions about death can be confusing or even frightening (for instance, equating death with sleep may result in the child's being afraid of going to bed) and should be avoided.

Needless to say, parents of children with life-limiting conditions also experience distressing symptoms such as anxiety, depression, and spiritual concerns.[25] Recognition by the pediatric clinician may serve families well while the child is alive and during bereavement.

Symptom Management in Adults

Pain and antiemetic therapy for adults is reviewed elsewhere in this volume. Anxiety, depression, delirium, and control of symptoms occurring in the last days of life are reviewed subsequently. Interested readers are referred to other references for reviews of assessment and management of other common troubling symptoms and syndromes in adults (e.g., posttraumatic stress disorder, substance abuse, major psychiatric illnesses, personality disorders, or demoralization).[26,27]

Among social sources of distress are financial concerns and with increasing debility, loss of independence and sense of contribution and efficacy. Worries about burdening the family or that the family will fail them when they really need them may lead patients to request physician-assisted suicide. Social workers are the key team members who can help alleviate or at least ameliorate these sources of distress and can help the caregivers cope.

Physicians should also explore religious and spiritual concerns and understand what rituals will be important at the end of life.[28] Spiritual and existential distress occur when individuals are unable to find sources of meaning, hope, love, peace, comfort, strength, and connection in life or when there is dissonance between their beliefs and what is happening to them. Patients who use "positive" religious coping (e.g., prayer, feeling a sense of connectedness to a religious community, having a positive relationship with God) have been found to have better mental health status, growth with stress and in the spiritual dimension, as well as a better overall quality of life. Patients who use "negative" religious coping (e.g., ascribe their illness to a punishing God or one who has abandoned them) have a poorer quality of life.[28] Clinicians should therefore include either a formal or informal spiritual assessment for all patients diagnosed with life-limiting diseases. Psychologic, spiritual, or religious counseling may be needed to help these patients reconnect and find what they have lost.

PSYCHOLOGIC CONCERNS

As Block[27] states in her 2006 review of psychologic issues in end-of-life care, "grief, sadness, despair, fear, anxiety, loss and loneliness are present, at times, for nearly all patients facing the end of their lives." For patients to cope with the diagnosis and its implications, they need "good communication and trust among patient, family, and clinical team, the ability to share fears and concerns, as well as meticulous attention to physical comfort and psychological and spiritual concerns."[28] For a thorough discussion of the patient assessment (which includes "developmental issues; meaning and impact of illness; coping style; impact on sense of self; relationships; stressors; spiritual resources; economic circumstances; physician-patient relationship"), please refer to Dr. Block's review.

Anxiety and Depression

It is noteworthy that the psychologic states of depression and anxiety are often not recognized as symptoms in children, and in many instances are inadequately addressed. Significant anxiety is found in approximately 25% of adult patients with cancer, and anxiety symptoms can interfere with ability to receive care.[29] Patients with panic disorders, agitated depression, phobias, obsessive-compulsive disorder, delirium, posttraumatic stress disorder, or adjustment disorders can all present with anxiety.[28] Anxiety in dying patients may arise from worries about the future (uncontrolled symptoms, family concerns, or concerns about death), isolation from loved ones, sepsis, hypoxia, metabolic abnormalities, withdrawal from alcohol, opioids or benzodiazepines, drug reactions (e.g., akathisia from metoclopramide, phenothiazines, and butyrophenones; paradoxical agitation from benzodiazepines and olanzapine), and uncontrolled pain. Nonpharmacologic treatments, such as relaxation training, hypnosis, supportive psychotherapy, and counseling, are very effective. Pharmacologic treatments usually include benzodiazepines (e.g., the short-acting lorazepam, starting dose 0.5 to 2 mg every 8 hours as needed; or long-acting clonazepam, starting dose 0.25 to 0.5 mg PO [orally] two times daily), selective serotonin reuptake inhibitors (SSRIs; see later), and, when there is evidence of delirium, neuroleptics (see later).

At least 7% of patients with advanced cancer meet criteria for a major depressive disorder, 41% of whom had a previous history of major depressive disorder.[30] It can be difficult to discern which patients with advanced disease are depressed or grieving. The usual somatic signs of depression or grief (e.g., anorexia, sleep disturbances, fatigue, or weight loss) are common in this population. Depressed patients, however, will be anhedonic and feel worthless, guilty, hopeless, or helpless. Grieving patients, in contrast, are very sad, but they are able to find happiness in some circumstances and can plan for the future.[28] Pain, a past or family history of substance abuse, depression, or bipolar illness are major risk factors for depression. Terminally ill patients responding "Yes" to the screening question "Are you depressed?" are very likely to be confirmed as depressed in a more comprehensive evaluation. Useful follow-up questions include "How do you see your future?" "What do you imagine is ahead for yourself with this illness?" "What aspects of your life do you feel most proud of? Most troubled by?"

As part of the treatment of depression, pain must be brought under control. Counseling can explore patient fears, provide emotional support, and help patients review their lives and find the

Table 93-3 Delirium

Drug	Dose	Comment
ANTIPSYCHOTICS		
Haloperidol	0.5-5 mg PO, IM, subcutaneously, IV	Do not exceed 20 mg in 24 hr Repeat q 2-12 hr prn Maintain the patient on the effective dose (divided into a bid dose), then taper over 2 wk, as tolerated Oral dose is 60%-70% as potent as parenteral dose
Quetiapine	25-200 mg PO qhs	Particularly useful in elderly patients with evening delirium Start 25 mg hs for 3-4 days
Olanzapine	2.5-15 mg PO bid	Start 2.5-5 mg PO bid (2.5 mg for elderly patients); can use q 4-6 hr prn agitation Maintain the patient on the effective dose (divided into a bid dose), then taper over 2 wk, as tolerated; also antiemetic
Chlorpromazine	12.5-50 mg PO/IV/PR	Sedating; in very agitated patients, may repeat q 1-4 hr until sedated
SEDATIVES		
Lorazepam	0.5-2 mg q 1-4 hr	Add to haloperidol/olanzapine for patients with an agitated delirium Tablets can be used PR for terminal delirium
Diazepam	10-30 mg daily	Useful PR for patients unable to take oral medication
Clonazepam	0.5-2 mg bid to tid	Tablets have been used PR for terminal delirium; do not exceed 20 mg/24 hr
Midazolam	30 to 100 mg over 24 hr	IV drip or subcutaneous infusion for terminal delirium

Modified from Abrahm JL: *A physician's guide to pain and symptom management in cancer patients,* ed 2, Baltimore, 2005, Johns Hopkins University Press; and Miovic M, Block S: Psychiatric disorders in advanced cancer, *Cancer* 110:1665, 2007.
bid, Twice a day; *hr,* hour; *hs,* at bedtime; *IM,* intramuscularly; *IV,* intravenously; *PO,* orally; *PR,* rectally; *prn,* as needed; *q,* every; *qhs,* at every bedtime; *tid,* three times a day.

meaning and areas of accomplishment in them. A variety of models of therapy are used, and none has been shown to be superior over the others. The psychostimulants dextroamphetamine and methylphenidate (2.5 to 5 mg, 8 AM and noon; maximum dose 60 mg daily) often act within a few days. The SSRIs are the first choice when immediate onset is not needed because they usually take several weeks to show effect. Useful agents include citalopram (Celexa) and paroxetine (Paxil) (10 mg PO daily initially; maximum 40 mg PO daily); escitalopram (Lexapro) (10 mg PO daily initially; maximum 20 mg PO daily); sertraline (Zoloft) (50 mg PO daily initially, maximum 200 mg PO daily); fluoxetine (5 to 10 mg PO daily initially; maximum 60 mg PO daily); and venlafaxine (Effexor) (37.5 mg PO twice daily initially; maximum 225 mg PO daily). Venlafaxine inhibits norepinephrine, serotonin, and dopamine reuptake. Major side effects of the SSRIs include hyponatremia, sexual dysfunction or loss of libido, and gastrointestinal complaints (e.g., nausea, diarrhea, and foul-smelling flatus). Modafinil may also be an effective adjuvant agent to reduce SSRI-related sedation. The exact mechanism of action of mirtazapine (Remeron) (15 mg PO at bedtime initially; maximum 45 mg PO at bedtime) is unknown.

If the patient is expected to live longer than weeks to a few months, a stimulant and an SSRI should be started simultaneously, and the stimulant can be titrated off several weeks later. Tricyclic antidepressants are less useful in these patients because of their side-effect profile.

If the patient does not respond to first-line agents, a psychiatrist should be consulted. Referral to a psychiatrist is also necessary when the physician is unsure of the diagnosis; the patient is psychotic, confused, or delirious; the patient previously had a major psychiatric disorder; the patient is suicidal or requesting assisted suicide; or there are dysfunctional family dynamics.

Delirium

Delirium occurs in up to 80% of dying patients and can cause distress and anxiety in caregivers.[26] Delirious patients can be agitated, hypoactive, or vacillate between the two. Symptoms of delirium include insomnia and daytime somnolence, nightmares, restlessness or agitation, irritability, distractibility, hypersensitivity to light and sound, anxiety, difficulty in concentrating or marshaling thoughts, fleeting illusions, hallucinations and delusions, emotional lability, attention deficits, and memory disturbances.

Validated delirium screening and severity tools are available, but a comprehensive psychiatric evaluation is recommended to exclude other disorders, such as anxiety, minor depression, anger, dementia, or psychosis. The cause of delirium is often never determined and often multifactorial. Medications, especially opioids, nonsteroidal antiinflammatory drugs, and high-dose corticosteroids, often contribute. Opioid-induced central nervous system toxicities are more common in patients with renal dysfunction, on high doses of opioids for long periods of time, with impaired cognition before starting the opioids, with dehydration, or taking other psychoactive drugs. Other causes include metabolic abnormalities (hypercalcemia, hyperglycemia, or uremia), malnutrition, hypoxia, fever, infection, uncontrolled pain, hepatic failure, primary brain tumor, and brain metastases.

Treatment for delirium should begin while the underlying cause(s) are being treated. In addition to the medications listed in Table 93-3, it is helpful to make the patient's surroundings as familiar as possible, restore aids to hearing and sight if they are needed, reorient the patient frequently, and have family members, friends, or well-known caregivers present.

MANAGEMENT CONCERNS DURING THE LAST DAYS OF LIFE

For some families, there is the possibility of planning ahead and choosing a setting for their child's death—home, hospice, or hospital. The child may express a preference about where he or she feels safe or prefers to be. Clear information about how the child is likely to die and professional support to validate the family's choice are crucial. Even more important is the explicitly stated "permission" from all

Table 93-4 Treatment of Problems at the End of Life

Problem	Agent(s)	Routes, Doses
Baseline pain	Morphine, hydromorphone, oxycodone SL oral concentrates, subcutaneous infusions Fentanyl transdermal	Scheduled; individualized Scheduled; individualized
Breakthrough pain	Concentrated oxycodone or morphine solutions	Intermittent; individualized
"Death rattle"	Scopolamine Hyoscyamine Glycopyrrolate	Transderm Scop patch 1-3 q 3 days; gel 0.125-0.25 SL tid to qid 0.1-0.2 mg IV tid to qid
Dyspnea (anxiety)	Lorazepam	1 mg PO, SL, q 2-4 hr
Dyspnea (other)	Morphine/oxycodone Morphine Chlorpromazine	5-10 mg SL oral concentrate q 2 hr 2-4 mg IV q 1 hr 25-50 mg PO, PR q 4-12 hr
Nausea	Combinations of lorazepam, metoclopramide, dexamethasone, and/or haloperidol	PR q 6 hr; compounded suppositories with desired agents (depending on presumed cause of nausea)
Anxiety	Lorazepam	1 mg PO, SL, q 2-4 hr

Modified from Abrahm JL: *A physician's guide to pain and symptom management in cancer patients*, ed 2, Baltimore, 2005, Johns Hopkins University Press, p 408.
hr, Hour; *IV*, intravenously; *PO*, orally; *PR*, rectally; *q*, every; *qid*, four times a day; *SL*, sublingually; *tid*, three times a day.

members of the professional team that the family may change their choice freely at any time—that all options remain open and that no decision is irrevocable. Although in the current zeitgeist there is strong advocacy for children to die at home, professionals must bear in mind that for some children and families, the hospital is a better option, and that choice must be respected. In the past, siblings were rarely included in these discussions and were often inadequately prepared for the eventuality of a child dying at home. It is only recently that their voices are beginning to be heard.

The Dying Child

Therapist: Are you in any pain? Does anything hurt?
Child: My heart.
Therapist: Your heart?
Child: My heart is broken. I miss everybody.[31]

The distillation of anticipatory grief to its essence marks the imminence of death. At times imperceptibly, at other times dramatically, the child who has been living with the illness is transformed into a dying child.

The end point of the terminal phase is often marked by a turning inward on the part of the child, a pulling back from the external world. Cognitive and emotional horizons narrow, because all energy is needed simply for physical survival. A generalized irritability is not uncommon. The child may talk very little and may even retreat from physical contact. Although such withdrawal is not universal, a certain degree of quietness is almost always evident. The child is pulling into himself or herself, not away from others. This behavior is a normal and expectable precursor to death—a form of preparation for the ultimate separation that lies ahead.[1]

Adults

Physical symptoms that occur in the last week to days before an adult's death include pain, 70%; noisy or moist breathing, restlessness/agitation/delirium, 60%; urinary incontinence or retention, 50%; dyspnea, 20%; and nausea and vomiting, 10%.[26] Patients may also experience fatigue. Hunger and thirst are unusual. Treatments for problems at the end of life are reviewed in Table 93-4. Patient and family wishes and options about the setting for end-of-life care should be explored. Some evidence suggests that patients with cancer who die at home have better quality of life, and their caregivers have better bereavement outcomes than cancer patients who die in the hospital.

Table 93-5 Hospice Services

PERSONNEL
Medical director, nurses, social workers, home health aides, chaplains, volunteers, administrative personnel, medical consultants, occupational therapists, physical therapists, speech therapists, and bereavement counselors.
ITEMS NEEDED FOR PALLIATION OF TERMINAL ILLNESS
Prescription medications Durable medical equipment and supplies Oxygen Laboratory and diagnostic procedures Radiation and chemotherapy Transportation when medically necessary for changes in level of care (i.e., inpatient or "respite" in nursing home)

HOSPICE PROGRAMS

In the United States, most hospice care takes place in the home, although patients can be admitted to nursing homes for brief periods (usually 5 days) to provide a respite for the family caregivers, or to the hospital (usually for up to 14 days) if symptoms cannot be controlled at home. Early referral to hospice improves outcomes, and in many cases hospice is the only effective way to support these patients and families at home at the end of life. The Medicare Hospice Benefit does not require a DNR status, but it does require that the attending physician and the hospice medical director certify that the patient has a prognosis of 6 months or less to live if the disease follows its usual course. Medicare reimburses hospice programs about $150 per day per patient (as of fiscal year 2012) to provide the routine care described in Table 93-5. Therefore the cost of transfusions typically required for many patients with hematologic malignancies, even at the end of life, may make it difficult for hospice programs to enroll patients insured by Medicare alone. Other insurance programs, thankfully, often will allow their patients to receive transfusions and hospice care. Notably, many children are not referred to hospice because their illness experience is inconsistent with hospice specifications—prognosis is uncertain; there is a blending of goals, which can result in more costly health care; and providers lack pediatric expertise. Importantly, the Patient Protection and Affordable Care Act now requires state Medicaid programs to allow children with a life-limiting illness to receive both hospice care and curative treatments concurrently; the full effect of this change remains to be uncovered.

BEREAVEMENT

Bereavement follow-up by the professional team is an intrinsic component of comprehensive pediatric palliative care. Bereaved families often express the sentiment of a double loss: loss of their child and loss of their professional "family"—the treatment team whom they have known and trusted, often over months and years.[2] Parental grief has been recognized as more intense and longer lasting than other types of grief. Contact from a team member after the child's death not only assuages the family's sense of abandonment; the palliative care team can serve a crucial preventive role by identifying families at particular risk and identifying resources for them.[30]

Each bereaved person's loss is unique, but many people manifest similar symptoms of grief, some of which become less persistent as they rebuild their lives. Recurrent intense symptoms typically occur at the anniversary of the death of the patient but can occur at unpredictable times, induced by reminders of the deceased. Just as in the patients described under Anxiety and Grieving, survivors' grief must be differentiated from depression. Survivors appreciate calls or letters from the patient's physician and nurses. For patients enrolled in hospice, a formal bereavement program is offered for the family throughout the first year after the patient's death. After the formal program ends, the bereaved are welcome to continue to participate in any bereavement activities that have been meaningful to them.

At the time of death, survivors may seem numb, confused, or dazed and experience disbelief. By the second month after the death, yearning has replaced disbelief. During the next months, disbelief, depressed mood, and yearning decline gradually, and by 6 months after the death, most people will have accepted the reality of the death and are beginning to think about reengaging in relationships and work, discovering new meaning and purpose. By a year or two, most survivors have accommodated to their loss. They become aware of the changes that must be made if they are to resume old relationships and responsibilities or to establish new ones and risk recurrent loss.

About 10% to 20% of survivors, however, suffer either from depression and/or from a symptom complex previously called *complicated grief*, now identified as *prolonged grief disorder*. Patients with depression manifest symptoms of sadness, anhedonia, and psychomotor retardation, but they are not yearning for the deceased or unable to accept the death. Depressed survivors benefit from counseling and consideration of pharmacologic treatment. Patients with prolonged grief disorder, in contrast, have grief symptoms that last beyond 6 months and cause functional impairments. Such patients are at increased risk for medical and psychiatric illness and should be referred for psychiatric or spiritual counseling. Persons at higher risk for this disorder include those with a history of attachment disorders (childhood abuse, childhood separation anxiety), aversion to lifestyle changes, and being unprepared for the death and unsupported after it. Additional risks include a "dependent, close, confiding" relationship with the deceased. Unfortunately, although there is no randomized controlled trial of a pharmacotherapy that is effective for the extreme grief symptoms, there is a novel effective psychotherapy developed specifically for this disorder that is superior to standard interpersonal psychotherapy.[26]

INTERDISCIPLINARY TREATMENT TEAM

Thank you for giving me aliveness.

— *(6-year-old child)*[1]

Palliative care demands the combined expertise of an interdisciplinary treatment team to address medical, psychologic, social, and spiritual concerns of the child, siblings, parents, and close family. This knowledge-based expertise must be provided within a context of ongoing accessibility and availability to the family, granting them a sense of the team's abiding presence.

Yet, even while providing this steady care for the patient and family, professional caregivers are often experiencing their own distress in a sort of parallel process. The professional often feels anguish and helplessness in witnessing a child endure pain and suffering—physical or psychic. He or she often identifies with the parents of the child. This reaction intensifies when the caregiver is also a parent, especially if his or her healthy child is the same age as the patient. For the caregiver who does not yet have children, the specter of a fatally ill child may loom threateningly. In surveys, medical and nursing staff often cite the personal pain of losing a child as the most difficult experience in their work with dying children. Special attention should be paid to the grief experienced by trainees with little previous experience with death and dying. Interns are in special need of emotional support following a patient's death. Reviewing each death on the next morning's rounds provides the needed debriefing and shows respect for the patient who has died. When possible and it feels appropriate, clinicians can write a card or attend the funeral or memorial service, which may facilitate closure.

For all these reasons, the professionals who engage in this extraordinarily rich and demanding work articulate significant needs for support themselves. Otherwise, the toll of cumulative unresolved grief exacts a heavy toll in their personal and professional lives. A cohesive team and/or the opportunity for individual and group consultation are crucial for those who are intimately engaged in repeated cycles of attachment.

REFERENCES

1. Sourkes B: *Armfuls of time: The psychological experience of the child with a life-threatening illness*. Pittsburgh, 1995, University of Pittsburgh Press, pp 11, 31, 114, 156, 167.
2. Institute of Medicine: *When children die: Improving palliative and end-of-life care for children and their families*. Washington, DC, 2003, National Academy Press.
3. Ullrich C, Duncan J, Joselow M, et al: Pediatric palliative care. In Kliegman RM, Behrman RE, Stanton BF, et al, editors: *Nelson textbook of pediatrics*, ed 19, Philadelphia, 2011, Elsevier.
4. Sourkes B: *The deepening shade: Psychological aspects of life-threatening illness*. Pittsburgh, 1982, University of Pittsburgh Press.
5. Hanks G, Cherny NI, Christakis NA, et al, editors: *Oxford textbook of palliative medicine*, ed 4, Oxford, UK, 2010, Oxford University Press.
6. Temel JS, Greer JA, Muzikansky A, et al: Early palliative care for patients with metastatic non-small-cell lung cancer. *N Engl J Med* 363:733, 2010.
7. Crawley LM, Marshall PA, Lo B, et al: Strategies for culturally effective end-of-life care. *Ann Intern Med* 136:673, 2002.
8. Byock I: *Dying well: The prospect of growth at the end of life*. New York, 1997, Riverhead Books.
9. Jelalian E, Boergers J, Spirito A, et al: Psychologic aspects of leukemia and hematologic disorders. In Nathan D, Orkin S, Ginsburg D, et al, editors: *Nathan and Oski's Hematology of infancy and childhood*, ed 6, Philadelphia, 2003, WB Saunders, p 1671.
10. Wright AA, Zhang B, Ray A, et al: Associations between end-of-life discussions, patient mental health, medical care near death, and caregiver bereavement adjustment. *JAMA* 300:1665, 2008 Oct 8.
11. Mack J, Grier HE: The day one talk. *J Clin Oncol* 22:563, 2004.
12. Mack JW, Hilden JM, Watterson J: Parent and physician perspectives on quality of care at the end of life in children with cancer. *J Clin Oncol* 23:9155, 2005.
13. Mack JW, Wolfe J, Grier HE, et al: Communication about prognosis between parents and physicians of children with cancer: Parent preferences and the impact of prognostic information. *J Clin Oncol* 24:5265, 2006.

14. Bluebond-Langner M, Belasco JB, Goldman A, et al: Understanding parents' approaches to care and treatment of children with cancer when standard therapy has failed. *J Clin Oncol* 25:2414, 2000.
15. Hinds PS, Drew D, Oakes L, et al: End-of-life care preferences of pediatric patients with cancer. *J Clin. Oncol* 284:2476, 2005.
16. Steinhauser KE, Christakis NA, Clipp EC, et al: Factors considered important at the end of life by patients, family, physicians, and other care providers. *JAMA* 284:2476, 2000.
17. Alexande SC, Sullivan AM, Back AL, et al: Information giving and receiving in hematological malignancy consultations. *Psychooncology* 21:297, 2012.
18. Weeks JC, Cook EF, O'Day SSJ, et al: Relationship between cancer patients' predictions of prognosis and their treatment preferences. *JAMA* 279:1709, 1998.
19. Back A, Arnold R, Tulsky J: *Mastering communication with seriously ill patients: Balancing honesty with empathy and hope*, New York, 2009, Cambridge University Press.
20. Smith AK, McCarthy EP, Paulk E, et al: Racial and ethnic differences in advance care planning among patients with cancer: Impact of terminal illness acknowledgment, religiousness, and treatment preferences. *J Clin Oncol* 26:4131, 2008.
21. Hebert R, Schulz R: Caregiving at the end of life. *J Palliat Med* 9:1174, 2006.
22. Dussel V, Bona K, Heath JA, et al: Unmeasured costs of a child's death: Perceived financial burden, work disruptions, and economic coping strategies used by American and Australian families who lost a child to cancer. *J Clin Oncol* 29:1007, 2011.
23. Wolfe J, Grier H, Klar N, et al: Symptoms and suffering at the end of life in children with cancer. *N Engl J Med* 342:326, 2000.
24. Dussel V, Joffe SJ, Hilden JM, et al: Considerations about hastening death among parents of children who die of cancer. *Arch Pediatr Adolesc Med* 164:1, 2010 Mar.
25. Kreicbergs U, Valdimarsdottir U, Onelov E, et al: Care-related distress: A nationwide study of parents who lost a child to cancer. *J Clin Oncol* 23, 2005.
26. Abrahm JL: *A physician's guide to pain and symptom management in cancer patients*, ed 2, Baltimore, 2005, Johns Hopkins University Press.
27. Block SD: Psychological issues in end-of-life care. *J Palliat Med* 9:751, 2006.
28. Balboni TA, Paulk ME, Balboni MJ, et al: Provision of spiritual care to patients with advanced cancer: Associations with medical care and quality of life near death. *J Clin Oncol* 28:445, 2010.
29. Miovic M, Block S: Psychiatric disorders in advanced cancer. *Cancer* 110:1665, 2007.
30. Kreicbergs U, Lannen P, Onelov E, et al: Parental grief after losing a child to cancer: Impact of professional and social support on long-term outcomes. *J Clin Oncol* 25:3307, 2007
31. Contro N, Larson J, Scofield S, et al: Hospital staff and family perspectives regarding quality of pediatric palliative care. *Pediatrics* 114:1248, 2005.

CHAPTER 94

LATE COMPLICATIONS OF HEMATOLOGIC DISEASES AND THEIR THERAPIES

Wendy Landier and Smita Bhatia

There has been a marked improvement in survival for patients with hematologic malignancies over the past three decades. Currently the population of long-term cancer survivors continues to grow; for patients with hematologic malignancies, the 5-year survival is as follows: adult leukemia, 55%; childhood acute lymphoblastic leukemia (ALL), 89%; childhood acute myeloid leukemia (AML), 61%; adult Hodgkin lymphoma (HL), 87%; childhood HL, 96%; adult non-Hodgkin lymphoma (NHL), 69%; and childhood NHL, 87%.[1] It is estimated that there are 11.9 million cancer survivors in the United States, and approximately 952,000 (8%) of these are survivors of hematologic malignancies.[2]

With this success comes the need to consider the long-term morbidity and mortality associated with the treatments responsible for that improvement in survival. The subject of long-term morbidity suffered by cancer survivors has been the topic of numerous reviews.[3-10] To varying degrees, it has been shown that disease- or treatment-specific subgroups of long-term survivors are at risk for developing adverse outcomes, including premature death, second neoplasms, organ dysfunction (e.g., cardiac, pulmonary, gonadal), reduced growth, decreased fertility, impaired intellectual function, difficulties obtaining employment and insurance, and overall reduced quality of life.

Hematopoietic cell transplantation (HCT) is the treatment of choice for patients with hematologic malignancies experiencing disease recurrence after conventional regimens and for those with disease characteristics associated with poor prognosis if treated with conventional chemotherapy and radiation regimens. Complications observed after HCT often have a multifactorial origin encompassing issues related to prior cancer therapy, intensity of the preparative regimen, graft-versus-host disease (GVHD), and other posttransplantation complications.[11-18]

This chapter summarizes select adverse outcomes among individuals treated for hematologic malignancies with conventional therapy alone or with HCT. Recommendations for providing ongoing follow-up care to this population of survivors are also reviewed.

CARDIAC EFFECTS

Anthracyclines are well-known causes of late-onset cardiomyopathy, characterized by increased afterload followed by development of a dilated, thin-walled left ventricle, which eventually becomes poorly compliant. A review of 30 published studies determined that the prevalence of clinically detected anthracycline-related congestive heart failure among survivors treated for cancer during childhood ranged from 0% to 16%.[19] The incidence of anthracycline-induced cardiomyopathy, which is dose dependent, may exceed 30% among survivors who received cumulative doses in excess of 600 mg/m^2.[20] Among children, this report indicated that a cumulative anthracycline dose exceeding 300 mg/m^2 is associated with an 11-fold increased risk for clinical heart failure, compared with a cumulative dose of less than 300 mg/m^2, with the estimated risk for clinical heart failure increasing with time from exposure.[20] Mulrooney et al[21] used the resources offered by the Childhood Cancer Survivor Study and demonstrated that survivors were 5.9 times more likely to report congestive heart failure. Exposure to 250 mg/m^2 or more of anthracyclines and cardiac radiation exposure of 1500 cGy or more increased the relative hazard of congestive heart failure. More recently, a large case-control study from the Children's Oncology Group demonstrates that cumulative anthracycline exposure as low as 101 to 150 mg/m^2 may be associated with a 3.9-fold increased risk for cardiomyopathy.[22]

The incidence of subclinical anthracycline-related myocardial damage has been the subject of considerable interest. A review of the literature on subclinical cardiotoxicity among children treated with an anthracycline found that the reported frequency of subclinical cardiotoxicity varied considerably across the 25 studies reviewed (frequency ranging from 0% to 57%).[19] Steinherz et al[23] reported that 23% of 201 patients who had received a median doxorubicin cumulative dose of 450 mg/m^2 had echocardiographic abnormalities a median of 7 years after therapy. In a group of childhood leukemia survivors who received a median doxorubicin cumulative dose of 334 mg/m^2, progressive elevation of afterload or depression of left ventricular contractility was present in approximately 57% of patients.[24] Because of marked differences in the definition of outcomes for subclinical cardiotoxicity and because of the heterogeneity of the patient populations investigated, it is difficult to accurately evaluate the potential long-term outcomes within anthracycline-exposed patient populations with subclinical findings.

Among anthracycline-exposed patients, the risk for cardiotoxicity can be increased by mediastinal irradiation,[25] uncontrolled hypertension,[26,27] underlying cardiac abnormalities,[28] exposure to chemotherapeutic agents other than anthracyclines (such as cyclophosphamide, dactinomycin, mitomycin C, dacarbazine, vincristine, bleomycin, and methotrexate),[27,29,30] and electrolyte imbalances such as hypokalemia and hypomagnesemia.[31] Risk is also increased for survivors who are female,[32] African American,[33] and those who were very young (<5 years old) at the time of therapy.[34]

Chronic cardiac toxicity associated with radiation alone most often manifests as valvular abnormalities, coronary artery disease, pericardial effusions, or constrictive pericarditis, sometimes in association with pancarditis. This risk is associated with radiation dose and volume and is lifelong; absolute risk increases with length of time since exposure.[35] Although a dose of 40 Gy of total heart irradiation appears to be the usual threshold, pericarditis has been reported after as little as 15 Gy, even in the absence of radiomimetic chemotherapy.[36] Symptomatic pericarditis, which usually develops 10 to 30 years after irradiation, is found in 2% to 10% of patients.[37] Subclinical pericardial and myocardial damage, as well as valvular thickening, may be common in this population.[38] Coronary artery disease has also been reported after radiation to the mediastinum.[39]

HCT recipients are at an increased risk for cardiovascular complications. In allogeneic HCT recipients, risk for premature death resulting from cardiac complications was 2.3-fold that of the U.S. general population.[40] A recent study reported the incidence of coronary artery disease after allogeneic HCT to be 2.2%. Coronary artery disease was the cause of death for 5% of the 60 patients who died in the study population.[41] Tichelli et al[42] described the cumulative incidence and risk factors for cardiovascular events among allogeneic and autologous HCT recipients. The 15-year cumulative incidence of cardiovascular events (coronary artery disease, stroke, and peripheral vascular disease) after allogeneic HCT was 7.5% compared with 2.3% after autologous HCT. Adjusting for age, the risk for cardiovascular event was sevenfold higher among allogeneic HCT recipients, when compared with autologous HCT recipients. Increasing age at HCT was also associated with an increased risk; thus the 20-year cumulative incidence of cardiovascular event was 8.7% for those transplanted at less than 20 years of age; it was 20.2% for those transplanted between 20 and 40 years; and finally it was 50% among those transplanted at ages 40 to 60 years.

Late cardiac dysfunction after HCT is multifactorial in origin. Factors that may increase the risk for its development include pre-HCT therapy with anthracyclines, chest radiation, total body irradiation (TBI), and post-HCT therapeutic exposures to cardiotoxic agents. In addition, there is now increasing evidence that presence of the conventional cardiovascular risk factors (hypertension, diabetes, dyslipidemia, increased body mass index [BMI], physical inactivity, and smoking) could increase the risk for cardiac toxicity in patients already exposed to cardiotoxic agents. Armenian et al[43] used a nested case-control design to examine the independent role of pre-HCT therapeutic exposures, transplantation-related conditioning, and comorbidities (pre- and post-HCT) in the development of late congestive heart failure after HCT. The authors found that anthracycline dose greater than 250 mg/m^2 and two or more cardiovascular risk factors post-HCT were independently associated with an increased risk for late congestive heart failure.[43] Tichelli et al[44] reported the cumulative incidence of first arterial events to be 6% at 15 years after HCT. When patients were stratified by number of cardiovascular risk factors, cumulative incidence of cardiovascular events increased to 17% for those with three or more risk factors, versus 4% for those with two or fewer risk factors. In another report, Armenian et al[45] used a nested case-control study design to identify clinical and treatment-related risk factors for development of late (1+ years after HCT) cardiovascular disease. The authors found the presence of multiple cardiovascular risk factors (two or more of the following: obesity, dyslipidemia, hypertension, and diabetes) after HCT to be associated with a 5.2-fold increased risk for late cardiovascular disease. Furthermore, pre-HCT chest radiation was associated with a ninefold increased risk for coronary artery disease.

Thus HCT recipients are at increased risk for cardiovascular complications, and traditional cardiovascular risk factors are important in modifying that risk. Estimates of dyslipidemia in different cohorts who survived at least 1 year after allogeneic HCT range from 8.9%[41] to 56% (71% of these patients were on immunosuppressive therapy).[46] The presence or absence of ongoing immunosuppressive therapy in allogeneic HCT patients may account for some of the differences in reported risk factor incidence. The Bone Marrow Transplant Survivor Study ascertained the prevalence of self-reported late occurrence of cardiovascular risk factors, in particular, diabetes and hypertension in 1089 HCT survivors, who were not taking immunosuppressants at the time of study participation. Allogeneic HCT recipients were 3.65 times more likely to report diabetes than siblings and 2.06 times more likely to report hypertension compared with siblings. Allogeneic HCT recipients were also 2.3 times more likely than autologous HCT recipients to develop hypertension. TBI was associated with an increased risk for diabetes. This study demonstrated that allogeneic HCT survivors have a higher age- and BMI-adjusted risk for diabetes and hypertension, potentially leading to a higher-than-expected risk for cardiovascular events with age.[47]

Given the known acute and long-term cardiac complications of cancer therapy, prevention of cardiotoxicity is a focus of active investigation. Previous reports have suggested that doxorubicin-induced cardiotoxicity can be prevented by continuous infusion of the drug.[48-50] Lipshultz et al[51] compared cardiac outcomes in children with leukemia receiving bolus or continuous infusion doxorubicin and reported that continuous doxorubicin infusion over 48 hours did not offer a cardioprotective advantage over bolus infusion. Both regimens were associated with progressive subclinical cardiotoxicity. Several other studies have reported no statistically significant difference in echocardiographic characteristics of children with cancer 5 to 7 years after treatment with either continuous infusion (over 6 to 24 hours) or bolus infusion of anthracyclines.[52,53]

Liposome-encapsulated anthracyclines have been explored for their propensity to result in a lower incidence of cardiotoxicity. The premise behind this theory is as follows: liposome-encapsulated anthracyclines escape the capillaries with wide endothelial gaps in the tumor, thus reaching high concentrations in the interstitial fluid of the tumor bed. On the other hand, they are less likely to escape the tight capillary junctions of the heart. Biopsy results have confirmed a low early cardiotoxicity[54] and the relative safety in clinical use.[55]

Agents such as dexrazoxane, which remove iron from anthracyclines, have been investigated as cardioprotectants. Clinical trials of dexrazoxane have been conducted, with encouraging evidence of short-term cardioprotection among children.[56] In a study of 206 children with ALL who were randomly assigned to receive doxorubicin with or without dexrazoxane, Lipshultz et al[57] demonstrated that patients treated with doxorubicin alone were significantly more likely to have elevated troponin T levels, indicative of myocardial injury, than those who received doxorubicin with dexrazoxane. There was no difference in event-free survival at 2.5 years between the two arms. A recent follow-up report of this group at a median of 8.7 years found that event-free survival did not differ significantly between the two groups, and that the risk for second malignancies was not increased.[58,59] Serial echocardiographic measurements during the 4 years after this trial revealed that children treated with doxorubicin and dexrazoxane have less left ventricular fractional shortening and greater left ventricular mass and left ventricular wall thickness over time. Also, the cardioprotective effects appear to be sex specific, with females showing the greatest protective effect. However, comprehensive longer-term follow-up is required to document that dexrazoxane does indeed have a cardioprotective effect, while maintaining comparable event-free survival.[60,61]

Specific recommendations for monitoring, based on age and therapeutic exposure, are delineated within the Children's Oncology Group *Long-Term Follow-Up Guidelines*[62] (COG LTFU guidelines) available at http://www.survivorshipguidelines.org. According to these guidelines, patients exposed to anthracyclines need ongoing monitoring for late-onset cardiomyopathy using serial noninvasive testing (echocardiogram) and physical examination. The frequency of echocardiograms can range from yearly to every 5 years, depending on cumulative anthracycline dose, age at exposure, and treatment with mediastinal radiation. Pregnant women previously treated with anthracyclines should be closely monitored, because changes in volume during the third trimester could add significant stress to a potentially compromised myocardium. In addition to monitoring for cardiomyopathy, survivors who received radiation involving the heart field also need monitoring for potential early-onset atherosclerosis. Heart-healthy lifestyles should be encouraged for all survivors, including implementation of a regular exercise program, dietary recommendations, and screening for dyslipidemia. Joint recommendations for monitoring long-term survivors of HCT by the European Group for Blood and Marrow Transplantation/Center for International Blood and Marrow Transplant Research/American Society for Blood and Marrow Transplantation (EBMT/CIBMTR/ASBMT) suggest that at a minimum, cholesterol and high-density-lipoprotein cholesterol (HDL-C) should be checked at least every 5 years for men starting by age 35 years and women starting at age 45. It is suggested that screening for dyslipidemia should start at age 20 for smokers, patients with diabetes, or patients with a family history of heart disease. Abnormalities (total cholesterol >200 mg/dL or HDL-C <40 mg/dL) should be followed up with a full fasting lipoprotein profile.[63]

PULMONARY EFFECTS

Compromise of pulmonary function among survivors of hematologic malignancies has been reported after conventional therapy for HL[64-66] and leukemia[67,68] and after HCT.[12,13,69] Impairments evident by pulmonary function testing include reductions in total lung capacity (TLC), forced vital capacity (FVC), forced expiratory volume in the first second of expiration (FEV_1), and gas transfer (diffusing capacity of lung for carbon monoxide [DLCO]), suggesting obstructive and restrictive defects. Risk factors include exposure to certain chemotherapeutic agents (particularly bleomycin), radiation to the chest, underlying lung disease, and a younger age at exposure to the pulmonary-toxic therapeutic agents.

Significant late toxicities involving the airway and lung parenchyma, including restrictive and chronic obstructive lung disease and bronchiolitis obliterans, are observed after HCT.[70] Inaba et al[71] measured serial pulmonary function tests before and after HCT at a single institution. The following tests were noted to decline after HCT: FEV_1/FVC, forced midexpiratory flow, TLC, DLCO, residual volume (RV), functional residual capacity, and RV/TLC. Older age at the time of allogeneic HCT was associated with lower FEV_1/FVC, DLCO, and higher RV/TLC. The prognosis is quite dismal, with overall survival of only 13% at 5 years. Bronchiolitis obliterans syndrome is a progressive, insidious lung disease occurring after allogeneic HCT and results in progressive circumferential fibrosis and ultimate cicatrization of the small terminal airways, manifesting as new fixed airflow obstruction (reviewed in Williams et al[72]). Bronchiolitis obliterans has been shown to have a strong correlation with chronic GVHD and has been reported in up to 6% of HCT recipients. Most patients present when the degree of airflow is severe, causing significant dyspnea on exertion and a persistent nonproductive cough. Lung biopsy findings demonstrating damage to the bronchiolar epithelium, obliteration of bronchiolar lumens, inflammation between the epithelium and the smooth muscle, and pulmonary fibrosis are characteristic. The National Institutes of Health definition of bronchiolitis obliterans requires the following: (1) absence of active infection, (2) decreased FEV_1 (<75% of predicted value), (3) evidence of airway obstruction with a ratio of FEV_1 to FVC of less than 0.7, (4) elevated RV of air (>120% of predicted normal), or (5) an expiratory chest computed tomographic (CT) scan or lung biopsy results that reveal air trapping or bronchiectasis. Recommended therapy includes high-dose systemic steroids for a protracted course, with or without the addition of other immunosuppressants. Leukotriene inhibitors have emerged as a potential therapy, because of the elevated levels of leukotrienes implicated in bronchiolitis obliterans.

The COG LTFU guidelines recommend monitoring for pulmonary dysfunction in childhood cancer survivors that includes assessment of symptoms such as chronic cough or dyspnea on annual follow-up. Risks of smoking and exposure to secondhand smoke should be discussed with all patients.[62] The best approach to chronic pulmonary toxicity of anticancer therapy is preventive and includes respecting cumulative dosage restrictions of bleomycin and alkylators, limiting radiation dosage and port sizes, and avoidance of primary or secondhand smoke. Pulmonary function tests and chest x-ray examination are recommended as a baseline upon entry into long-term follow-up for patients at risk, repeated as clinically indicated in symptomatic patients and in those with subclinical abnormalities identified on screening evaluation. Repeat evaluation should also be considered for at-risk patients before general anesthesia. Influenza and pneumococcal vaccines are encouraged in survivors at risk for pulmonary compromise. Joint recommendations for monitoring long-term survivors of HCT by the EBMT/CIBMTR/ASBMT suggest routine clinical assessment at 6 months, 1 year, and annually thereafter; institution of active smoking cessation programs; and pulmonary function tests and focused radiologic assessment at 1 year after allogeneic HCT for patients with signs or symptoms of lung compromise or earlier as clinically indicated. Annual testing is recommended thereafter for patients with recognized defects or appropriate clinical circumstances. For autologous HCT recipients, pulmonary function testing should be performed for those with known deficits before HCT or with those exposed to radiation or other pulmonary toxic agents during or after transplantation. Chest radiographic studies are indicated based on symptoms or abnormal pulmonary function test results.[63]

ENDOCRINOLOGIC EFFECTS

Thyroid

Patients with hematologic malignancies treated with cranial, craniospinal, or mantle irradiation are at increased risk for thyroid complications. Among survivors of HL, and to a lesser extent leukemia, abnormalities of the thyroid gland, including hypothyroidism, hyperthyroidism, and thyroid neoplasms, have been reported to occur at rates significantly higher than those found in the general population.[73-75] Hypothyroidism is the most common nonmalignant late effect involving the thyroid gland. After exposure to radiation at doses above 15 Gy, laboratory evidence of primary hypothyroidism is evident in 40% to 90% of patients with HL and NHL.[74,76,77]

In an analysis of 1791 5-year survivors of pediatric HL (median age at follow-up, 30 years), Sklar et al[73] reported the occurrence of at least one thyroid abnormality in 34% of subjects. The risk for hypothyroidism was increased 17-fold compared with sibling controls; increasing dose of radiation, older age at diagnosis of HL, and female sex were identified to be significant independent predictors of increased risk. The actuarial risk for hypothyroidism for subjects treated with 45 Gy or more was 50% at 20 years after diagnosis of HL. Hyperthyroidism was reported to occur in only 5%.

In another large cohort of 1677 patients with HL treated at Stanford University Hospital between 1961 and 1989 with irradiation involving the thyroid (mean age at diagnosis, 28 years; mean duration of follow-up, 9.9 years), the actuarial risk for developing thyroid disease was 52% at 20 years and 67% at 26 years after treatment. In this population, the actuarial risk for developing overt or subclinical hypothyroidism was 44% by 25 years after therapy; the risk for developing thyroid cancer was 1.7% (15.6 times the expected risk).[74]

Most cases of overt hypothyroidism after HCT result from primary hypothyroidism caused by radiation injury. The incidence of hypothyroidism after HCT depends on the type of myeloablative conditioning regimen, ranging from as high as 90% after exposure to single-dose TBI to 10% to over 50% after fractionated TBI.[15,16]

Thyroid nodules are common in patients treated with neck radiation for HL, but the majority of these do not undergo malignant transformation.[78,79] In a study of 647 children treated for HL, 67 developed thyroid nodules during or after therapy (median time between diagnosis of HL and thyroid nodule was 10.5 years with a range of 0.2 to 24.8 years). All but one of these patients had received neck radiation as part of their therapy, with a median dose to the thyroid of 35 Gy. Seven (10%) of the 67 nodules were malignant.[78]

Growth

Poor linear growth and short adult stature are common complications after successful treatment of hematologic malignancies in childhood. The adverse impact of central nervous system (CNS) irradiation on adult final height among childhood leukemia patients has been well documented, with final heights below the fifth percentile in 10% to 15% of survivors.[80-83] The effects of cranial irradiation appear to be related to age and sex, with females and children younger than 8 years at the time of therapy being more susceptible.[84,85] The precise mechanisms by which cranial irradiation induces short stature are not clear. Disturbances in growth hormone production have not been found to correlate well with observed growth patterns in these patients.[86,87] The phenomenon of early onset of puberty in girls receiving cranial irradiation may play some role in the reduction of final height.[88,89] In childhood, leukemia survivors not treated with cranial irradiation, there are conflicting results regarding the impact of chemotherapy on final height.[81,90]

Impaired linear growth after HCT is likely due to an interaction of multiple factors, including host characteristics (young age), treatment exposures (prior cranial irradiation, TBI), and post-HCT complications, such as chronic GVHD.[16] Findings suggest that final height is unaffected in children who receive busulfan or cyclophosphamide as pretransplant conditioning.[91]

Survivors should be monitored using standardized growth curves until final height is achieved. An endocrine consultation should be obtained for children whose height is less than the third percentile, for those whose height has dipped across two or more percentiles, or whose growth velocity is less than 4 to 5 cm/yr.[85]

Obesity

An increased prevalence of obesity has been reported among survivors of childhood ALL.[92-94] In an analysis from the Childhood Cancer Survivor Study, Oeffinger et al[95] compared the distribution of BMI of 1765 adult survivors of childhood ALL with that of 2565 adult siblings of childhood cancer survivors. Survivors were significantly more likely to be overweight (BMI of 25 to <30) or obese (BMI ≥30). Risk factors for obesity were cranial irradiation, female sex, and age 0 to 4 years at diagnosis of leukemia. Females diagnosed under the age of 4 years who received a cranial radiation dose of more than 20 Gy were found to have a 3.8-fold increased risk for obesity. Obesity has the potential to adversely impact the overall health status in survivors and is associated with insulin resistance, diabetes mellitus, hypertension, and dyslipidemia. Growth hormone deficiency related to cranial radiation may predispose adult survivors of childhood ALL, particularly females, to abdominal obesity[96] and metabolic syndrome.[97]

Gonadal Dysfunction

Treatment-related gonadal dysfunction has been well documented in male and female patients after therapy for hematologic malignancies, and there is a reasonable body of research that provides a basis for counseling patients regarding the long-term gonadal effects of radiation and chemotherapy.

Radiation effects on the ovary are age and dose dependent. It has been estimated that there is a 50% depletion in oocytes after exposure of the ovaries to 2 Gy.[98] Amenorrhea develops in approximately 68% of prepubescent females treated for HL with ovarian doses of 12 to 15 Gy, whereas 100% of adult females older than 40 years of age will sustain irreversible ovarian failure after doses of 4 to 7 Gy.[99] Spinal irradiation for the treatment of childhood leukemia appears to result in clinically significant ovarian damage in some survivors,[100] and cranial irradiation in young girls is associated with an increased risk for premature puberty.[101]

The effects of radiation on testicular function, including germ cell number and Leydig cell function, have been investigated. Reduced sperm production has been observed after testicular doses of 1 to 6 Gy and follows a dose-dependent pattern.[102] Azoospermia has been reported among HL patients with calculated testicular irradiation exposures ranging from 1 to 3 Gy.[103] Testicular doses between 4 and 6 Gy have been associated with prolonged azoospermia and decreased testicular volume.[104] The limited data on the long-term outcomes of very young males treated for HL suggest germ cell effects similar to those seen in older HL patients.[105] Leydig cells, although also affected by radiation in a dose-dependent fashion, require higher exposure levels to sustain damage than those seen for the germ cells.[106] Testicular dose of 24 Gy among prepubertal males have been reported to be associated with delayed pubertal development and abnormal testosterone and gonadotropin levels.[107-109]

Ovarian and testicular damage can also result from chemotherapeutic agents, with alkylating agents showing the strongest association. Effects of chemotherapy on gonadal function are typically sex-, age-, and dose-dependent. The ovaries tend to be less sensitive to the effects of alkylating agent exposure, compared with the testes. Ovarian dysfunction has been well documented in HL patients treated with alkylating agents, singly or in combination (e.g., MOPP regimen consisting of mechlorethamine, vincristine [Oncovin], procarbazine, and prednisolone or a COPP regimen consisting of cyclophosphamide, vincristine [Oncovin], procarbazine, and prednisolone).[105,110-112] MOPP and COPP regimens have been reported to result in azoospermia in more than 90% of exposed males.[113] Even with a reduction in the dose of cyclophosphamide in the hybrid COPP/Adriamycin, bleomycin, and vinblastine (ABV) regimen for HL, the majority of young males are infertile, likely due to the procarbazine component in this regimen.[114] In a study of 6224 male survivors of childhood cancer between ages 15 and 44, those with a diagnosis of hematologic malignancy were significantly less likely to sire a pregnancy compared to sibling controls; those with a diagnosis of HL were least likely to sire a pregnancy (relative risk [RR] of fertility, 0.34; 95% confidence interval [CI], 0.28 to 0.41), followed by NHL (RR, 0.60; 95% CI, 0.48 to 0.74), and leukemia (RR, 0.70; 95% CI, 0.59 to 0.84); P <.001 for all comparisons.[115]

Young boys and adolescent males with aplastic anemia who receive standard-dose cyclophosphamide alone (200 mg/kg) as the pretransplant conditioning regimen appear to retain normal Leydig cell function, as do males who receive busulfan and cyclophosphamide, with normal plasma concentrations of luteinizing hormone and testosterone and normal progression through puberty.[16] Evidence of germ cell damage can occur and is more likely among patients treated after puberty.[116] Semen analyses have been normal in approximately two-thirds of men after high-dose cyclophosphamide, and several men have fathered normal children. Men treated with TBI-based regimens who have not received prior testicular irradiation generally retain normal Leydig cell function, regardless of their age at treatment.[116] Germ cell dysfunction occurs in all men treated with TBI-based regimens, and azoospermia is the rule.

Female patients treated with high-dose cyclophosphamide alone retain normal ovarian function, regardless of age at exposure, although these subjects may be at an increased risk for early menopause as they reach the third decade of life.[117] These individuals can sustain a normal pregnancy resulting in normal offspring. Females treated with busulfan and cyclophosphamide are at very high risks for ovarian failure and premature menopause.[118] The outcome of ovarian function after TBI appears to be determined by the age at exposure. Approximately 50% of prepubertal girls receiving fractionated TBI enter puberty spontaneously, and premature ovarian failure is seen in all patients who are older than 10 years of age when treated with TBI.[16] Pregnancies among survivors of TBI are at an increased risk for spontaneous abortion.[119]

Pregnancy Outcomes

Offspring of survivors of childhood hematologic malignancies do not appear to be at increased risks for cancer or congenital malformations.[120] In a study of 593 adult survivors of childhood ALL, 15.7% (93 of 593) of survivors (mean age, 22.6 years) had given birth to or fathered a total of 140 live-born offspring, compared with 29.8% (122 of 409) of sibling controls (mean age, 25.2 years). There was no significant difference in the rate of birth defects between offspring of survivors (3.6% [5 of 140]) versus sibling controls (3.5% [8 of 228]) (RR, 1.02; 95% CI, 0.34 to 3.05).[121] In a recent review of pregnancy outcomes of participants in the Childhood Cancer Survivor Study,[112] the offspring of survivors were more likely to be premature (born before 37 weeks' gestation) compared with the survivors' female siblings (odds ratio [OR], 1.9; 95% CI, 1.4 to 2.4; P <.001); and the offspring of women who received uterine radiation at a dose of more than 5 Gy were more likely to be small for gestational age (OR, 4.0; 95% CI, 1.6 to 9.8; P = .003). The frequency of premature birth was not related to prior maternal exposure to alkylating agents, but prior exposure to doxorubicin or daunorubicin increased the risk for low birth weight independent of pelvic irradiation history.[112] There were no significantly increased rates of congenital or chromosomal anomalies in the offspring of survivors compared with siblings.[112]

MUSCULOSKELETAL EFFECTS

Osteonecrosis is a painful and debilitating condition that develops when the blood supply to the bone is disrupted, usually in areas of terminal circulation. The condition is believed to be the result of vascular compromise with resultant death of bone and cell tissues or disruption of bone repair mechanisms.[122,123] Osteonecrosis has been reported after conventional therapy for hematologic malignancies, particularly after exposure to dexamethasone between the ages of 10 and 20 years. This complication usually develops during or shortly after completion of therapy but may progress over time.[124-126] Mattano et al[124] described the magnitude of risk and associated risk factors for development of osteonecrosis in children with ALL treated on Children's Oncology Group therapeutic protocols. The cumulative incidence was 9.3% at 3 years; the incidence was higher in older patients (14.2% for patients ≥10 years of age versus 0.9% for patients <10 years of age), and higher among whites than African Americans. Furthermore, the incidence was higher among patients randomized to receive two 21-day dexamethasone courses versus one course.

Osteonecrosis is increasingly being reported among HCT recipients.[127-129] Campbell et al[130] conducted a retrospective cohort study and described the cumulative incidence of osteonecrosis to be 2.9% among autologous HCT recipients, 5.4% among allogeneic HCT recipients, and 15% among unrelated-donor HCT recipients. Among allogeneic HCT recipients, male sex, presence of chronic GVHD, and exposure to cyclosporine, tacrolimus (FK506), prednisone, and mycophenolate mofetil (MMF) rendered patients at increased risk, in particular among patients with a history of exposure to three or more drugs. The mean latency period was 18 months. The hip joint was the most commonly involved joint (80%); however, the knee, wrist, and ankle joints were also affected. The cumulative incidence of surgery (mainly arthroplasty) approached 31% at 1 year from osteonecrosis diagnosis.

Osteopenia (bone density 1 to 2.5 standard deviations [SDs] below mean) or osteoporosis (bone density >2.5 SDs below mean) is commonly seen in survivors of hematologic malignancies.[131-133] Risk factors include therapy with corticosteroids, methotrexate (at higher doses), and cranial irradiation with resultant pituitary insufficiency or gonadal dysfunction. Survivors of HCT are also at increased risk for reduced bone mineral density; identified risk factors in these patients include treatment with corticosteroids for chronic GVHD, prior cranial irradiation (resulting in growth hormone deficiency), and gonadal failure.[16] Lifestyle factors that increase the risk for osteopenia include lack of regular weight-bearing exercise, inadequate calcium and vitamin D intake, smoking, and excessive alcohol consumption.[134,135]

Detection and diagnosis of musculoskeletal sequelae depend largely on anticipating these issues in vulnerable hosts, on taking a careful history, and on performing a thorough physical examination. Pain or a history of fractures may be the only indication of osteonecrosis or osteoporosis. Because of progress with various interventions (including the use of calcium supplementation, calcitonin, bisphosphonates, and hormone replacement in patients with gonadal failure), the COG LTFU guidelines recommend a baseline dual-energy x-ray absorptiometry (DEXA) or quantitative CT scan for survivors 2 or more years following completion of treatment, with repeat studies as clinically indicated.[62] Joint recommendations for monitoring long-term survivors of HCT by the EBMT/CIBMTR/ASBMT suggest a screening dual photon densitometry performed at 1 year after transplantation in adult women or for any patient who has received prolonged treatment with corticosteroids or calcineurin inhibitors.[63] Screening for osteonecrosis is not recommended; however, clinicians should maintain a high level of suspicion for patients with exposure to irradiation or prolonged corticosteroids.

NEUROCOGNITIVE EFFECTS

Among survivors of childhood leukemia, neurocognitive late effects represent one of the more intensively studied topics.[136-139] Early curative regimens for childhood ALL relied heavily on cranial irradiation, usually in doses of 24 Gy.[136] Results from studies of neurocognitive outcomes in early populations of ALL survivors (particularly in younger children) are directly responsible for the marked reduction in the use of cranial irradiation, which is currently reserved for the treatment of very high-risk subgroups or patients with CNS involvement. For the majority of children with ALL, CNS prophylaxis consists of either intrathecal methotrexate or triple intrathecals (i.e., methotrexate, cytosine arabinoside, and hydrocortisone). Kadan-Lottick et al[140] evaluated the neurocognitive function in children with ALL randomized to receive intrathecal methotrexate or intrathecal triples. The two groups performed similarly on tests of full-scale intelligence quotient (IQ), academic achievement, attention/concentration, memory, and visual/motor integration. The study did not show any clinically meaningful differences in neurocognitive functioning between patients previously randomly assigned to intrathecal methotrexate or triple intrathecals. Dexamethasone has been shown to result in better event-free survival than prednisone, presumably due to higher CNS penetration. Kadan-Lottick et al[141] compared the neurocognitive function in children previously randomized to dexamethasone or prednisone in the treatment of childhood ALL. There were no group differences in the distribution of test scores or the parents' report of neurologic complications, psychotropic drug use, and special education.

Neurocognitive deficits, as a general rule, usually become evident within several years after CNS-directed therapy and tend to be progressive in nature. Leukemia survivors treated at a younger age (i.e., less than 6 years of age) may experience significant declines in IQ scores.[142] However, reductions in IQ scores are typically not global but rather reflect specific areas of impairment, such as attention and other nonverbal cognitive processing skills.[143,144] Affected patients may experience information-processing deficits resulting in academic difficulties. These patients are particularly prone to problems with receptive and expressive language, attention, and visual and perceptual motor skills, most often manifested as academic difficulties in the areas of reading, language, and mathematics. Assessment of educational needs and subsequent educational attainment have demonstrated that survivors of childhood leukemia are significantly more likely to require special educational assistance but have a high likelihood of successfully completing high school if they receive appropriate educational services.[145,146] Chemotherapy- or radiation-induced destruction of normal white matter partially explains intellectual and academic achievement deficits.[147] The pathogenesis of CNS damage is only partially understood; evidence suggests that therapy-related direct effects on intracranial endothelial cells and brain white matter, as well as immunologic mechanisms, play roles.

A spectrum of neuropathologic syndromes related to leukoencephalopathy[148] may occur in survivors of childhood hematologic malignancies, including radionecrosis, necrotizing leukoencephalopathy, mineralizing microangiopathy and dystrophic calcification, cerebellar sclerosis, and spinal cord dysfunction, manifesting clinically as ataxia, spasticity, dysarthria, hemiparesis, or seizures. Imaging abnormalities may or may not be evident in these patients. Leukoencephalopathy has been primarily associated with methotrexate-induced injury of white matter. However, cranial irradiation may play an additive role through disruption of the blood-brain barrier, allowing greater exposure of the brain to systemic therapy. Although some abnormalities have been detected by diagnostic imaging studies, the abnormalities observed have not been well demonstrated to correlate with clinical findings and neurocognitive status.

Many survivors of adult-onset hematologic malignancies also experience impairments of neurocognitive function, including memory loss, distractibility, and difficulty performing multiple tasks. These patients may also concurrently suffer from mood disturbances and symptoms that compromise their ability to function adequately, including fatigue and pain.[149]

HCT survivors are also at risk for neurocognitive late effects. Prospective, longitudinal evaluations of intellectual and adaptive functioning of children receiving a transplant have revealed declines in intellectual function, particularly among those less than 6 years of age at transplantation.[150] Among the adult populations, studies in general have reported good levels of function and well-being in long-term survivors of transplantation, although there are increasing reports of fatigue, lack of energy, and sleep problems, which could potentially affect cognitive functioning.[151] Syrjala et al[152] used a prospective longitudinal study design to describe neurocognitive function over 5 years after allogeneic HCT for cancer survivors and compared with matched controls. Ninety-two survivors were tested before HCT, after 80 days, and 1 and 5 years after HCT. Sixty-six case-matched controls received testing at the 5-year time point.[152] A global deficit score summarized overall impairment. Survivors recovered significant cognitive function from posttransplantation (80 days) to 5 years in all tests except verbal recall. Between 1 and 5 years, verbal fluency improved, as did executive function, but motor dexterity did not, remaining significantly below population norms. Using the global deficit score, 41.5% of the survivors had mild or greater deficits, a proportion that was significantly higher than that among the controls (17.5%, $P = 0.007$). For additional information see box on Neuropsychologic Sequelae After Hematopoietic Cell Transplantation in Adults.

The COG LTFU guidelines recommend a baseline neuropsychologic evaluation for patients who received therapy that may affect neurocognitive function. This should be repeated as clinically indicated and at key transition points (e.g., transitioning from grade school to middle/high school); an annual assessment of their vocational or educational progress should also be monitored.[62] Joint recommendations for monitoring long-term survivors of HCT by the EBMT/CIBMTR/ASBMT suggest that all recipients of HCT should undergo clinical evaluation for symptoms or signs of neurologic dysfunction at 1 year after HCT. Additional tests such as neuropsychologic testing may be warranted for those with symptoms or signs.[63]

OTHER TOXICITIES

Ocular Effects

Survivors of hematologic malignancies are at risk for the development of cataracts as a consequence of therapy with corticosteroids, cranial irradiation,[153,154] TBI,[155] or busulfan.[156] Hoover et al[154] evaluated 82 ALL survivors, all of whom received treatment with prednisone (3.4 to 10.2 g/m^2/yr) and cranial irradiation (1800 to 2800 cGy). At a mean of 32 months after completion of therapy, 52% of patients had evidence of posterior subcapsular cataracts; however, there was minimal ocular morbidity in this cohort, with median visual acuity of 20/20 in the affected eyes (range, 20/15 to 20/50). Holmstrom et al[156] studied a cohort of 45 children who were followed for 2 to 10 years after HCT, 95% (20 of 21) of children conditioned with TBI and 21% (5 of 24) of children conditioned with busulfan developed cataracts. Belkacemi et al[157] studied 1063 patients who underwent HCT for acute leukemia; the overall 10-year incidence of cataracts in this group of patients was 50%. Single-dose TBI was associated with a 60% incidence of cataracts, and fractionated TBI was associated with a 43% incidence for those receiving six or fewer fractions, and a 7% incidence for those receiving more than six fractions. Factors independently associated with an increased risk for cataract formation in this cohort were older age (>23 years), allogeneic bone marrow transplantation, higher dose rate (>0.04 Gy/min), and steroid administration for longer than 100 days. Xerophthalmia may also occur as a late complication because of decreased lacrimation resulting from damage to the lacrimal gland during radiation or, in HCT patients, from chronic GVHD.[158] Westeneng et al[159] followed 101 adults up to 24 months after allogeneic HCT and reported ocular GVHD in 54% of patients, manifesting mainly as xerophthalmia and conjunctivitis; blepharitis and uveitis were encountered less often. Tabbara et al[160] reported major ocular complications in 13% of 620 patients (age range 9 to 65 years) after allogeneic HCT; complications included chronic ocular GVHD, corneal ulcers, cataracts, glaucoma, cytomegalovirus retinitis, fungal endophthalmitis, and the acquisition of allergic conjunctivitis from atopic donors.

Audiologic Effects

Survivors of hematologic malignancies who received platinum chemotherapy, those who had cranial irradiation at a young age (especially during infancy),[161] and those who required supportive therapy with aminoglycoside antibiotics[162] are at risk for therapy-related hearing loss. Hearing loss associated with ototoxic agents is generally sensorineural in origin and is usually irreversible. Although a low incidence of hearing loss has been reported in survivors of HCT performed in childhood, the risk is elevated threefold to fourfold over that in the general population.[155] Data are beginning to emerge regarding genetic polymorphisms associated with increased susceptibility to platinum-related hearing loss; these data may prove useful in identifying future patients who are at increased risk for hearing loss as a consequence of platinum-based chemotherapy.[163,164]

Dental Effects

Children whose teeth have not completely developed at the time of cancer treatment are most vulnerable to dental complications, and treatment with chemotherapy during early childhood may result in qualitative problems with enamel and root development.[165,166] However, patients of all ages who received radiation therapy involving the head or neck (including cranial irradiation and TBI) are susceptible to dental complications, most often manifesting as increased susceptibility to dental caries and gingivitis as a result of diminished salivary gland function. Patients who have undergone HCT are at increased risks for dental caries, gum disease, and xerostomia[124]; abnormalities of tooth development are seen in survivors who underwent HCT during childhood.[167] Younger age at transplantation (especially under 6 years) and TBI doses above 10 Gy are associated with the greatest risk.[168]

Hepatic Effects

Although acute hepatic dysfunction may be seen with certain chemotherapeutic agents, including antimetabolites and anthracyclines, there has generally been a low reported incidence of delayed hepatotoxicity in patients receiving these agents.[169] However, recent reports of chronic hepatotoxicity and portal hypertension have emerged in survivors of childhood ALL who received 6-thioguanine–based maintenance therapy,[170-173] and these survivors require long-term surveillance for this complication.[174] Chronic viral hepatitis, resulting from transfusion of contaminated blood or serum products, should be considered in the differential diagnosis of all survivors with

Neuropsychologic Sequelae After Hematopoietic Cell Transplantation in Adults

The few studies describing neurocognitive sequelae in adults undergoing hematopoietic cell transplant (HCT) suggest that these patients are at risk for developing adverse sequelae related to neuropsychologic functioning, such as slowed reaction time, reduced attention and concentration, and difficulties in reasoning and problem solving[247]; memory impairment[240,248-250]; problems with executive functioning and processing speed[248]; and cognitive impairment.[240,247,248] Reduced memory function is associated with older age, longer interval since HCT, chronic graft-versus-host disease, and long-term cyclosporine use.[251] Other predictors include fatigue and poor physical functioning. Lower education level and poorer social functioning appear to impact cognitive performance.[248] It is therefore prudent to query post-HCT patients regarding perceived deficits in neuropsychologic functioning and to refer patients with these problems to a neuropsychologist who is experienced in the follow-up care of HCT patients.

persistently elevated alanine aminotransferase (ALT) levels. Hepatitis C is the most prevalent type of hepatitis seen in survivors transfused before universal screening of the blood supply for this infection (implemented in the United States in July 1992). Cirrhosis and hepatocellular carcinoma are potential sequelae of untreated chronic viral hepatitis and potential causes of morbidity and mortality in this population. In a cohort of 431 pediatric patients in Italy who were diagnosed with leukemia or lymphoma before 1990 and completed treatment before August 1994, 17.2% (74 of 431) were anti–hepatitis C virus (HCV) positive.[175] Hepatocellular carcinoma or progression to liver failure was not seen in this group of patients after a 14-year median follow-up; however, due to the natural history of this disease, a longer follow-up is required to clearly define the risk for chronic HCV infection in this population. In a study of 3721 survivors of HCT,[176] the cumulative incidence of cirrhosis was estimated at 0.6% after 10 years and 3.8% after 20 years. The major risk factor for development of cirrhosis in this cohort was chronic hepatitis C infection, evident in 81% (25 of 31) of patients with cirrhosis. These Seattle investigators estimate that approximately 30% to 35% of their patients transplanted before 1991 were infected with hepatitis C and are at risk for the development of cirrhosis and related complications. In addition, iron overload associated with HCT for hematopoietic malignancies may also be a contributing factor to hepatotoxicity in survivors.[177,178]

Second and Subsequent Malignancies

Second or subsequent malignancies are defined as histologically distinct cancers developing after the occurrence of a first cancer. Second malignant neoplasms are one of the most devastating consequences of cancer therapy. Subsequent malignancies are conventionally categorized into two major types: therapy-related myelodysplastic syndrome and acute myeloid leukemia (t-MDS/AML) or solid tumors. The latency between diagnosis and treatment of the primary cancer and the development of t-MDS/AML is generally short, whereas nonhematopoietic malignancies or solid tumors seem to have a longer latency, and the risk continues to rise for 3 or more decades. The second malignancy experience differs across the age spectrum, in terms of the types of second malignancies observed, magnitude of risk, latency, and the mediating and moderating factors. This is due to the difference in susceptibility of individual tissues at different ages to the genotoxic insult and the presence of lifestyle factors that can modify the risk. A wide variety of factors influence the risk for second malignancies.

Several large epidemiologic studies have attempted to determine the magnitude of the burden of second cancers after adult-onset primary cancer. For example, 470,000 cancer patients registered between 1953 and 1991 in Finland were followed for the development of a second cancer.[179] Overall, the cohort was not at an increased risk for developing a second cancer when compared with the risk for cancer in an age- and sex-matched healthy population. However, patients less than 50 years of age at the diagnosis of their primary cancer were at a 1.7-fold increased risk for developing a second cancer. Another cohort of 633,964 cancer patients diagnosed between 1958 and 1996 in Sweden and followed for the development of subsequent cancers revealed a modestly increased risk (less than twofold), when compared with the general population.[180] A third cohort of 250,000 patients followed for the development of a second cancer in the United States revealed that cancer patients had a 1.3-fold increased risk for developing a second cancer, when compared with the general population.[181] However, when we look at second cancers after cancers in childhood or adolescence, a clearer and somewhat different picture emerges.

Studies following large cohorts of childhood cancer survivors have reported a threefold to sixfold increased risk for a second cancer compared with the background incidence of cancer in the general population, and this risk continues to increase as the cohort ages. Follow-up of a Nordic cohort of 30,880 patients diagnosed with their first cancer at 21 years of age or younger between 1943 and 1987 resulted in the identification of 247 second cancers.[182] The estimated cumulative incidence of second cancers in this cohort was 3.5% at 25 years, and the cohort was at a 3.6-fold increased risk for developing a second cancer when compared with an age- and sex-matched healthy population. A retrospective cohort of 14,359 children diagnosed with common cancers in the United States before the age of 21 years between 1970 and 1986, and surviving at least 5 years, was followed for the development of second cancers by the Childhood Cancer Survivor Study.[183] The estimated 30-year cumulative incidence was 7.9% for second cancer excluding nonmelanoma skin cancers. Overall, the cohort was at a sixfold increased risk for developing a second cancer. The relative risk for developing a second malignancy was significantly increased for survivors of HL (standardized incidence ratio [SIR] = 8.7). However, only 2.6 excess malignancies occurred per 1000 years of patient follow-up; therefore, even though the incidence of a second cancer is greater in those whose first cancer occurred in early life, the annual excess risk for second cancers in this group is still very small. Female sex, older age at diagnosis, earlier treatment era, HL, and treatment with radiation were identified to increase the risk for subsequent malignancies. Finally, childhood cancer survivors are at risk for the development of multiple primary malignancies. Armstrong et al[184] examined the occurrence of multiple subsequent neoplasms in long-term survivors of childhood cancer and reported the cumulative incidence of a third primary malignancy to be 46.9% at 20 years after the second primary malignancy.

The magnitude of risk for subsequent malignant neoplasms after HCT performed in childhood or in adults ranges from fourfold to 11-fold that of the general population. Several host and clinical factors are associated with an increased risk for subsequent malignant neoplasms after HCT. These include age at HCT, pre-HCT exposure to chemotherapy and radiation, exposure to TBI as part of conditioning, infection with oncogenic viruses (Epstein-Barr virus [EBV] and hepatitis B and C viruses [HBV and HCV]), prolonged immunosuppression after HCT, autologous versus allogeneic HCT, and original cancer.[185,186] t-MDS/AML is now the major cause of nonrelapse mortality in patients undergoing autologous HCT for patients with a primary diagnosis of HL or NHL.[187,188] The cumulative probability of t-MDS/AML ranges from 1.1% at 20 months to 24.3% at 43 months after autologous HCT, with a median latency of 12 to 24 months after HCT (range, 4 months to 6 years). Using the World Health Organization classification, two types of t-MDS/AML are recognized, related closely to the therapeutic exposure: alkylating agent/radiation and topoisomerase II inhibitor.[189] The alkylating agent–related t-MDS/AML typically develops 4 to 7 years after exposure. Cytopenias are common. Roughly 65% of the patients present with myelodysplasia; the remaining present with AML but carry myelodysplastic features. Abnormalities involving chromosomes 5 (-5/del[5q]) and 7 (-7/del[7q]) are frequently seen. AML secondary to topoisomerase II inhibitors presents as overt leukemia, without a preceding myelodysplastic phase. The latency is brief, ranging from 6 months to 5 years, and is associated with balanced translocations involving chromosome bands 11q23 or 21q22. The magnitude of risk for solid tumors exceeds twofold that of an age- and sex-matched general population.[190-192] Rizzo et al[191] report the risk for solid tumors in a multiinstitutional cohort of 28,874 allogeneic HCT recipients. Although the overall risk for solid malignancies is twofold that of the general population, the risk reaches threefold among patients followed for 15 or more years after HSCT.[191] Solid timors are unequivocally related to radiation therapy used to treat the primary cancer, they typically have a long latency, and the risk is high among those exposed to irradiation at a young age. Rizzo et al demonstrate that the risk for developing a non–squamous cell carcinoma (SCC) following conditioning radiation is dependent on age at exposure to radiation. Thus, among patients exposed to radiation at age less than 30 years, the risk is ninefold that of the general population, whereas for those older than 30 years, it approaches that of the general population.

Evaluations of large cohorts of patients with childhood ALL entered on Children's Oncology Group therapeutic trials have shown that the cumulative incidence of second and subsequent malignancies approaches 2% at 15 years from diagnosis of ALL.[193,194] CNS tumors, the most common second malignancy observed among survivors of childhood ALL, are predominantly associated with exposure to cranial irradiation.[195] Histologically, radiation-related late-occurring neoplasms include high-grade gliomas, (glioblastomas and malignant astrocytomas), peripheral neuroectodermal tumors, ependymomas and meningiomas, and basal cell carcinomas (BCCs).[193,194,196,197] Other commonly reported second cancers within the population of ALL survivors include thyroid cancer, lymphoma, and t-MDS/AML. Secondary thyroid malignancies, typically papillary carcinoma, are generally associated with radiation exposure to the thyroid gland as part of CNS irradiation, either prophylactic or for treatment of CNS leukemia. Thyroid malignancy has been reported to represent between 6% and 17% of secondary cancers among large cohorts of ALL survivors[193-195] and typically develops 10 or more years from treatment. As is true of de novo thyroid malignancy, the long-term outcome for survivors diagnosed with a secondary thyroid malignancy is excellent. The risk for t-MDS/AML after therapy for ALL is generally low, except among those patients treated with epipodophyllotoxin therapy, where a cumulative risk of 3.8% at 6 years has been reported.[198] t-AML associated with topoisomerase II inhibitors is characterized typically by a shorter latency period (3 to 5 years from therapeutic exposure) than that seen for t-MDS/AML after alkylating agents, lack of a myelodysplastic phase, and the presence of 11q23 rearrangements with mutations in the MLL gene. Epipodophyllotoxin-associated secondary AML depends more on the schedule of drug administration than total cumulative dose.[199]

Survivors of HL clearly represent one of the subgroups of cancer survivors who are at a very high risk for secondary cancer. This is particularly true for patients who received earlier regimens with predominantly radiation-based therapies, for which an approximate 10-fold increased risk has been reported.[195] A number of studies, with cohorts ranging from 499 to 5925 HL patients, have reported cumulative incidence of second malignancies to range from 7.6% at 20 years to 18.0% at 30 years.[195,200-203] Early studies of HL identified the increased risk for t-MDS/AML among patients treated with MOPP-based therapy, which included mechlorethamine and cyclophosphamide.[204,205] These alkylating agent–associated t-MDS/AMLs are characterized by a relatively short latency period, presence of chromosomal abnormalities involving chromosomes 5 and/or 7, and are often preceded by a phase of myelodysplasia.[206] The risk for t-MDS/AML usually does not extend beyond the first 10 to 15 years after therapeutic exposure. Extended follow-up studies of early cohorts have already reported excess risks for lung and gastrointestinal cancers.[207-211] More recent studies, with longer follow-up of cohorts, demonstrate that the most frequently observed solid second malignancies include breast cancer, thyroid cancer, and bone/soft tissue sarcomas.[207,212,213] With extended follow-up of cohorts of young HL survivors, increased risks for common adult carcinomas, including colorectal, lung, and stomach have emerged, and these cancers are being diagnosed at younger ages than observed in the general population.[207] In a large population-based study of solid tumor risk among 18,862 5-year survivors reported to 13 registries, breast, lung, and gastrointestinal cancers accounted for almost two-thirds of the estimated excess number of cases.[214]

Breast Cancer

Breast cancer is the most commonly reported second malignancy among female survivors of childhood Hodgkin lymphoma treated with mantle field irradiation, and the risk remains markedly elevated for many decades after exposure.[195,200-203] An update of the Late Effects Study Group cohort found female survivors to have a 55-fold increased risk for breast cancer compared with the general population, and the cumulative incidence of developing a secondary breast cancer approached 20% at 45 years of age.[207] Moreover, 40% of identified cases were found to have developed contralateral disease. Secondary thyroid cancer, the second most common solid tumor reported among survivors of childhood HL, is strongly associated with radiation therapy, occurs more frequently in females, and is associated with an approximate 36-fold increased risk over the general population. As the cohort of pediatric HL survivors continues to age, it is likely that an increasing number of other forms of malignancy associated with an excess risk will emerge. Using the resources offered by the Childhood Cancer Survivor Study, Inskip et al[215] sought the relation between radiation dose and breast cancer in childhood cancer survivors. The risk for breast cancer increased in a linear fashion with radiation dose, and it reached 11-fold for local breast doses of approximately 40 Gy relative to no radiation. Risk associated with breast irradiation was sharply reduced among women who received 5 Gy or more to the ovaries. Although the risk for breast cancer is elevated among women who received therapy at a young age, the risk declines with age at radiation, such that the relative risks compared with the general population are comparable to those of the general population after age 35. Travis et al[216] developed estimates of cumulative absolute risk for use in counseling patients. For example, the cumulative absolute risks for an HL survivor who was treated at age 25 years with a chest radiation dose of 40 Gy or more without alkylating agents were estimated to be 1.4% after 10 years, 11% after 20 years, and 29% after 30 years.[216] There appears to be a protective effect of early menopause either because of alkylating agents or radiation dose above 5 Gy to the ovaries, suggesting that ovarian hormones play an important role in promoting tumorigenesis once an initiating event has been produced by radiation.[217,218] The 25-year cumulative incidence of breast cancer is reported to be 11% after allogeneic HCT.[219] Allogeneic HCT survivors are at a 2.2-fold increased risk for developing breast cancer, when compared with age- and sex-matched general population. The median latency from HCT to diagnosis of breast cancer is 12.5 years. The incidence is higher among those exposed to TBI (17%) than among those who did not receive TBI (3%). The risk is increased among those exposed to TBI at a younger age.

Thyroid Cancer

Bhatti et al[220] quantified the long-term risk for thyroid cancer associated with radiation treatment among 12,547 5-year survivors of childhood cancer from the Childhood Cancer Survivor Study Cohort. Thyroid cancer risk increased linearly with radiation dose up to 20 Gy, where the relative risk peaked at 14.6-fold. At thyroid radiation doses above 20 Gy, a downturn in the dose-response relationship was observed. Sex, age at exposure, and time since exposure were identified to be significant modifiers of the radiation-related risk for thyroid cancer. HCT recipients are at a 3.3-fold increased risk for thyroid cancer, when compared with age- and sex-matched general population.[221] Age younger than 10 years at HCT, neck radiation, female sex, and chronic GVHD are associated with an increased risk for thyroid cancer. Thyroid cancer develops after a latency of 8.5 years and is associated with an excellent outcome.

Central Nervous System Tumors

Radiation is the most important risk factor for the development of a new CNS tumor. Neglia et al[222] described the dose-response relationship between radiation exposure and development of new primary neoplasms of the CNS. They also described the excess risk over time and the modifying effect of other host and treatment factors. A total of 116 subsequent CNS tumors were included in the analysis.[222] Gliomas occurred a median of 9 years from the original diagnosis; for meningiomas, the latency was 17 years. Radiation exposure was associated with increased risk for subsequent glioma (OR, 6.78) and meningiomas (OR, 9.94). The dose-response relationship for the excess relative risk was linear. For gliomas, the excess relative risk per gray was highest among children exposed at less than 5 years of age. The overall SIR was 8.7 for the gliomas, and the excess absolute risk (EAR) was 1.9 per 1000 person-years.

t-MDS/AML

Several studies have described an increased risk for t-MDS/AML with older age at HCT[185]; pretransplantation therapy with alkylating agents, topoisomerase II inhibitors, and radiation therapy[187]; use of peripheral blood hematopoietic cells; stem cell mobilization with etoposide; difficult stem cell harvests; conditioning with TBI; number of CD34+ cells infused; and a history of multiple transplants.[185,187] Thus t-MDS/AML after autologous HCT is the result of cumulative toxicity that includes pre-HCT chemotherapy (alkylators and topoisomerase II inhibitors), topoisomerase II inhibitors used for stem cell mobilization, and transplantation-related conditioning. The diagnosis of t-MDS/AML after autologous HCT confers a uniformly poor prognosis, with a median survival of 6 months in patients treated with conventional chemotherapy.

Skin Cancer

Among allogeneic HCT recipients, the incidence of BCC is 6.5% at 20 years, whereas that for SCC is 3.4%.[223] TBI increases the risk for BCC especially in younger patients. SCC risk is increased among patients with acute GVHD, whereas chronic GVHD is associated with both BCC and SCC.[224] Immunologic alterations predispose patients to SCC of the buccal cavity particularly, hence the association with chronic GVHD.[223] In patients with prolonged immunosuppression, oncogenic viruses such as human papillomavirus contribute to SCC of the skin and buccal mucosa.[223] Solid tumors commonly seen after HCT include melanoma, cancers of the oral cavity and salivary glands, brain, liver, cervix, thyroid, breast, bone, and connective tissues.[190,191]

The COG LTFU guidelines recommend monitoring for t-MDS/AML with annual complete blood cell count for 10 years after exposure to alkylating agents or topoisomerase II inhibitors.[62] Most other subsequent malignancies are associated with radiation exposure. Screening recommendations include careful annual physical examination of the skin and underlying tissues in the radiation field. Mammography, the most widely accepted screening tool for breast cancer in the general population, may not be the ideal screening tool by itself for radiation-related breast cancers occurring in relatively young women with dense breasts, hence the American Cancer Society recommends including adjunct screening with magnetic resonance imaging (MRI). Thus the following are recommendations for females who received radiation with potential impact to the breast (i.e., radiation doses of 20 Gy or higher to the mantle, mediastinal, whole lung, and axillary fields): monthly breast self-examination beginning at puberty; annual clinical breast examinations beginning at puberty until age 25 years; and a clinical breast examination every 6 months, with annual mammograms and MRI scans beginning 8 years after radiation or at age 25 (whichever occurs later). Screening of those at risk for early-onset colorectal cancer (i.e., radiation doses of 30 Gy or higher to the abdomen, pelvis, or spine) should include colonoscopy every 5 years beginning at age 35 years or 10 years following radiation (whichever occurs last).[62] Joint recommendations for monitoring long-term survivors of HCT by the EBMT/CIBMTR/ASBMT suggest that all recipients of HCT should be advised of risks for subsequent malignancies and encouraged to perform screening self-examinations, such as breast and skin examinations. All patients should be advised to avoid high-risk behaviors, including avoidance of tobacco or excessive unprotected exposure of skin to ultraviolet light.[63]

Late Mortality

Late recurring disease, as well as sequelae of the treatment for hematologic malignancies, can have a direct or indirect impact on overall mortality. Several large studies of late mortality among 5-year survivors of childhood cancer have been conducted.[225-227] In a study of the 5-year survivors in the United States,[227] the probability of survival 30 years from diagnosis was 82%. When compared with the U.S. population, the absolute excess risk for death from any cause was 7.36 deaths per 1000 person-years, and the cohort was at an 8.4-fold increased risk for premature death. Increase in cause-specific mortality was seen for deaths due to subsequent malignancies (standardized mortality ratio [SMR], 15.2), cardiac (SMR, 7.0), pulmonary (SMR, 8.8), and other medical conditions (SMR, 2.6). At 25 years from diagnosis, the death rate due to a subsequent malignancy exceeded that due to all other causes.

Late mortality due to recurrent disease and complications of therapy has also been described among patients who underwent HCT for hematologic malignancies.[188,228] Socie et al[228] reported that among 6691 individuals who underwent allogeneic transplant for hematologic malignancies and were free of disease 2 years after transplantation, the probability of living for 5 more years was 89%. The authors concluded that the disease is probably cured in patients who receive an allogeneic HCT as treatment for AML, ALL, chronic myeloid leukemia (CML), or aplastic anemia and who remain free of their original disease 2 years later. However, for many years after transplantation, the mortality rate among these patients is higher than that in a normal population. Wingard et al[229] described the long-term survival and late deaths after allogeneic HCT, updating the previous study from CIBMTR. The conditional survival at 10 years after HCT was 85%. The chief risk factors for late death were older age and chronic GVHD.[229] Bhatia et al[188] assessed late mortality in 854 survivors who underwent autologous HCT for hematologic malignancies and survived 2 or more years following transplant. After a median follow-up of 7.6 years, the overall survival was 68.8% ± 1.8% at 10 years, and the cohort was found to be at a 13-fold increased risk for late death when compared with the general population. Relapse of primary disease (56%) and subsequent malignancies (25%) were leading causes of late death. On the other hand, among 1479 allogeneic HCT recipients who had survived 2 or more years, the conditional survival probability approached 80%, and the cohort was at a 9.9-fold increased risk for late death, when compared with the general population. Relative mortality decreased with time but remained significantly elevated at 15 years after HCT. Relapse of primary disease and chronic GVHD were the leading causes of premature death.[40] In a recent study, Martin et al[230] described the life expectancy in patients surviving more than 5 years after HCT. Estimated survival of the cohort at 20 years after HCT was 80.4%. Mortality rates remained fourfold to ninefold higher than the expected population rate for at least 30 years after transplantation, yielding an estimated 30% lower life expectancy compared with that in the general population. The leading causes of excess deaths were subsequent malignancies and recurrent disease.

Psychosocial Effects

Survivors of hematopoietic malignancies are at risk for adverse psychosocial outcomes that may affect the overall quality of life, including anxiety, depression, posttraumatic stress disorder, and barriers to accessing the health care system due to problems obtaining health insurance coverage. The impact of cancer therapy on psychosocial functioning is dependent on many variables, including intensity and duration of therapy, treatment-related complications, family functioning, developmental processes, and treatment-specific sequelae such as altered cognitive or physical functioning.[231] An increased risk for adverse socioeconomic outcomes has been associated with younger age and cranial radiation therapy in survivors of childhood acute ALL.[232]

Results from an analysis of 5736 long-term survivors of childhood leukemia and lymphoma demonstrated that although a relatively low proportion reported symptoms indicative of depression (4.6%) and somatic distress (10.8%), they were significantly more likely to report these symptoms when compared with sibling controls.[233] In a study of 6542 childhood cancer survivors (55% of whom were survivors of leukemia/lymphoma), the risk for posttraumatic stress disorder was increased by 4.6-fold, 4.1-fold, and 3.8-fold for survivors of HL, NHL, and leukemia, respectively, compared with sibling controls;

Evaluating Survivors for Potential Late Effects

To diminish the incidence and severity of untoward late effects and to improve the quality of survival for patients with hematopoietic malignancies, systematic evaluation of outcomes with subsequent modification of current and future therapies is required. To decrease late morbidity and mortality rates and to meet the specialized health care needs of this group of patients, ongoing comprehensive follow-up care with attention to early detection and intervention for late effects are essential.

Patients are generally eligible to enter formal long-term follow-up care when the risk for relapse of their primary disease is minimal. For most hematologic malignancies, this occurs when a patient is at least 2 years off therapy. When a patient enters long-term follow-up, the focus of care shifts from vigilant surveillance for disease recurrence to a survivorship model of health maintenance or promotion and management of treatment-related late effects. Effective management of these late effects requires ongoing surveillance, early intervention, and when possible, prevention.

The long-term complications of treatment for which an individual survivor is at risk are determined by several factors, including the patient's diagnosis, age at treatment, specific chemotherapeutic agents received (including cumulative doses), specific radiation fields and doses, therapy-related complications, degree of psychosocial support received, genetic predisposition, and current health-related behaviors (e.g., diet, physical activity, tobacco, and alcohol use).

increased risk was associated with lower educational level (high school or less), lower income (<$20,000 annually), being unmarried, being unemployed, and having had more intensive treatment.[234] Long-term survivors of adult-onset HL report poorer health-related quality of life, primarily in physical health, when compared with a healthy general population.[235] Survivors of HL also appear to be at increased risk for psychosocial distress when compared with acute leukemia survivors; areas of greatest impact for these patients include impaired family and sexual functioning.[236] There is growing interest in the reported occurrences of fatigue and sleep disturbances among cancer survivors, particularly those with HL,[6,237,238] which may contribute to depression.

Fatigue, psychologic distress, psychiatric symptoms, mood disturbances, and sexual difficulties are commonly reported by HCT survivors.[239] Risk factors for impaired health-related quality of life include older age, advanced disease at transplantation, presence of chronic GVHD, and lower level of education. Fatigue and sleep disturbances have been reported in up to 65% of the patient cohorts studied,[240] and sexual disturbances are prevalent in 25% of HCT survivors[241] (see box on Evaluating Survivors for Potential Late Effects).

POTENTIAL LATE EFFECTS BY DIAGNOSIS

Therapeutic approaches to hematologic malignancies vary widely depending on the patient's age at diagnosis, biologic subtype and staging of disease, year (era) of diagnosis, initial response to therapy, and physician/institutional preference. Even though two patients may share an identical diagnosis, their risks for late effects may differ significantly because of differences in therapy, age at exposure to therapy, or pharmacogenetics. General associations of late effects with conventional treatment for common hematologic malignancies are reviewed in Tables 94-1 to 94-3. The risk for specific late effects in survivors who have undergone HCT depends on the conditioning regimen, donor source, complications experienced during the transplantation process, presence or absence of GVHD, and prior cancer therapy. Transplantation-related sequelae have been reviewed throughout the text of this chapter.

Table 94-1 Late Effects Associated With Conventional Therapy for Acute Lymphoblastic Leukemia and Non-Hodgkin Lymphoma

Common Therapeutic Exposures	Potential Late Effects
Vincristine	Peripheral neuropathy, Raynaud phenomenon
Corticosteroids	Cataracts, osteopenia, osteoporosis, avascular necrosis
Asparaginase	No known late effects
Mercaptopurine	Hepatic dysfunction (rare)
Thioguanine	Portal hypertension, hepatotoxicity (when used continuously in maintenance therapy)
Methotrexate (systemic)	Osteopenia, osteoporosis, osteonecrosis, renal dysfunction (rare), hepatic dysfunction (rare)
Methotrexate (intrathecal, high-dose), or cytarabine (high-dose)	Neurocognitive deficits, clinical leukoencephalopathy
Cranial or craniospinal irradiation	Neurocognitive deficits, clinical leukoencephalopathy, cataracts, hypothyroidism, second malignant neoplasm in radiation field (e.g., skin, thyroid, brain), short stature, scoliosis or kyphosis, obesity
Anthracyclines	Cardiomyopathy, arrhythmias, subclinical left ventricular dysfunction, secondary AML
Cyclophosphamide	Hypogonadism, hemorrhagic cystitis, dysfunctional voiding, bladder malignancy, secondary AML or MDS
Blood products	Chronic viral hepatitis, HIV

AML, Acute myeloid leukemia; *HIV*, human immunodeficiency virus; *MDS*, myelodysplastic syndrome.

Table 94-2 Late Effects Associated With Conventional Therapy for Acute Myeloid Leukemia

Common Therapeutic Exposures	Potential Late Effects
Anthracyclines	Cardiomyopathy, arrhythmias, subclinical left ventricular dysfunction, secondary acute myeloid leukemia
Corticosteroids	Cataracts, osteopenia, osteoporosis, avascular necrosis
Asparaginase	No known late effects
Cytarabine (high dose)	Neurocognitive deficits, clinical leukoencephalopathy
Blood products	Chronic viral hepatitis, human immunodeficiency virus infection

Acute Lymphoblastic Leukemia

ALL is a heterogeneous disease. Therapy for ALL ranges from a relatively innocuous, antimetabolite-based approach for low-risk childhood ALL[242] to marrow-ablative therapy followed by HCT for very high-risk disease in all age-groups.[243,244] The risk for long-term complications for individual survivors varies widely and is dependent on

Table 94-3 Late Effects Associated With Conventional Therapy for Hodgkin Lymphoma

Common Therapeutic Exposures	Potential Late Effects
Anthracyclines	Cardiomyopathy, arrhythmias, subclinical left ventricular dysfunction, secondary AML or MDS
Corticosteroids	Cataracts, osteopenia, osteoporosis, avascular necrosis
Bleomycin	Pulmonary dysfunction
Vincristine, vinblastine	Peripheral neuropathy, Raynaud phenomenon
Procarbazine, mechlorethamine, dacarbazine	Hypogonadism, infertility, secondary AML or MDS
Cyclophosphamide	Hypogonadism, infertility, hemorrhagic cystitis, dysfunctional voiding, bladder malignancy, secondary AML or MDS
Mantle irradiation	Hypothyroidism, premature cardiovascular disease, cardiac valvular disease, cardiomyopathy, arrhythmias, carotid artery disease, scoliosis or kyphosis, second malignant neoplasm in radiation field (e.g., thyroid, breast), pulmonary dysfunction
Inverted Y irradiation	Hypogonadism, infertility, adverse pregnancy outcome, second malignant neoplasm in radiation field (e.g., gastrointestinal)
Splenectomy	Acute life-threatening infections
Blood products	Chronic viral hepatitis, HIV

AML, Acute myeloid leukemia; *HIV,* human immunodeficiency virus; *MDS,* myelodysplastic syndrome.

the specific therapy received as well as the patient's age at time of treatment. Potential late effects that may occur as a consequence of conventional therapy for ALL are listed in Table 94-1.

Acute Myeloid Leukemia

Therapy for AML is generally more intense and of shorter duration than that used for treatment of ALL. Higher doses of anthracycline chemotherapy are often employed, as is consolidation therapy with HCT. Typically patients with AML receive less CNS-directed therapy than those with ALL. Examples of potential late effects associated with conventional therapy for AML are listed in Table 94-2.

Hodgkin Lymphoma

Therapy for HL relies on the use of alkylating agents, antitumor antibiotics (including anthracyclines and bleomycin), corticosteroids, and radiation therapy. Some patients may be apslenic as a consequence of the staging procedures performed in the earlier era. Examples of potential late effects associated with conventional therapy for HL are listed in Table 94-3.

Non-Hodgkin Lymphoma

The potential late effects after therapy for NHL are therapy specific and similar to those experienced by survivors of ALL (see Table 94-1). Those patients whose treatment included HCT are, of course, also at risk for transplantation-related sequelae.

Late Effects Research: What Is Needed

Medical Issues Faced by This Population

Premature death
Second malignancies
Organ dysfunction (e.g., cardiac, pulmonary, gonadal)
Impaired growth and development
Decreased fertility
Neurocognitive impairment
Difficulties obtaining employment and insurance
Overall reduced quality of life

Issues to Be Considered by Physicians Providing Care to This Population

Providing long-term follow-up care for cancer survivors
Models of care delivery
- Pediatric oncology-based
- Adult oncology-based
- Community medicine–based

Guidelines for ongoing screening and management
- Screening for potential complications
- Health protective counseling or interventions
- Management of identified complications

Major Clinical and Research Challenges

Cancer survivorship research continually changing because of new:
- Therapeutic agents or combinations of agents
- Radiation oncology techniques
- Surgical procedures
- Supportive care techniques

Future Directions

Much of the available information relates to outcomes within the first decade after treatment, and only minimal data address the longer-term outcomes that may occur later.

Research is needed to more clearly define the survivors at greatest risk for specific outcomes.

Research is needed to identify genetic predispositions to certain key outcomes and the roles of gene-environment interactions.

Research is needed to identify the role of lifestyle choices (e.g., alcohol, tobacco, diet, exercise) in terms of modification of the risks for these late outcomes.

Research is needed to understand the potential long-term impact of cancer therapy to effectively counsel survivors and offer effective intervention strategies to prevent or minimize the impact of adverse late effects.

Interventions are needed to include scientifically valid, evidence-based recommendations for clinical follow-up of survivors, which should include screening for potential late effects and application of proven approaches for health promotion.

Chronic Myeloid Leukemia

Long-term survivors of CML have usually either undergone HCT or are receiving tyrosine kinase inhibitors long-term. Among HCT recipients, there is a significant risk for late effects as a result of the transplantation conditioning regimen, as well as treatment for and sequelae of GVHD.[17] With the transition over the past decade to tyrosine kinase inhibitor therapy for CML as the predominant treatment modality, the long-term effects of these agents will need to be studied in detail in the growing cohort of CML survivors[245] (see box on Late Effects Research: What Is Needed and the section Providing Clinical Care to Survivors).

PROVIDING CLINICAL CARE TO SURVIVORS

A comprehensive treatment summary should be prepared for each patient entering long-term follow-up (Table 94-4) and a copy given to each survivor with instructions to share this information with all health care providers. Survivors should undergo annual comprehensive, multidisciplinary health evaluations (Fig. 94-1) with special attention to the detection of potential late effects specific to the patient's diagnosis and treatment history (Table 94-5). Guidelines for long-term follow-up of survivors of hematologic malignancies and those who underwent hematopoietic cell transplantation in childhood, adolescence, or young adulthood have been developed by the Children's Oncology Group[62] and are available at http://www.survivorshipguidelines.org. Because certain late effects have prolonged asymptomatic intervals before becoming clinically evident (e.g., late-onset congestive heart failure as a result of anthracycline-induced cardiomyopathy), ongoing evaluation is important to identify and provide early intervention for these potential complications. Health education regarding potential health risks and risk-reduction measures should be provided to each survivor. Targeted health education materials related to potential late complications of therapy during childhood, adolescence, or young adulthood have been developed by the Children's Oncology Group[246] and are available at http://www.survivorshipguidelines.org. After completion of each annual evaluation, identified late effects should be systematically recorded, and recommendations for any additional testing and for health maintenance and promotion should be shared with the patient and his or her primary health care provider. To optimize future follow-up care for all survivors, patients should be invited to participate in any relevant research studies for which they are eligible (see box on Late Effects Research: What Is Needed).

FUTURE DIRECTIONS

As treatment for hematopoietic malignancies continues to improve, follow-up care for survivors of these diseases must be provided in a comprehensive manner. To minimize treatment-related sequelae and provide early intervention for identified late effects, the risks of long-term complications for each individual survivor must be evaluated;

Text continued on page 1467

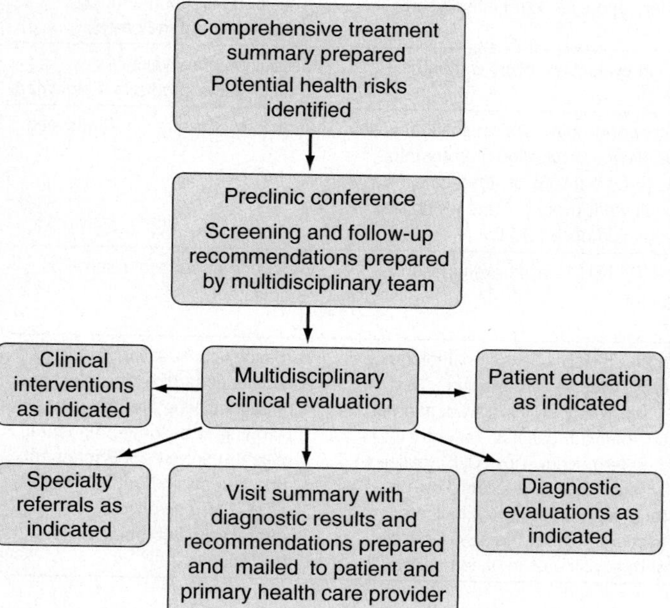

Figure 94-1 ANNUAL COMPREHENSIVE MULTIDISCIPLINARY HEALTH EVALUATION FOR THE CANCER SURVIVOR.

Table 94-4 Comprehensive Treatment Summary

Topic	Specific Information to Include
Demographics	Name Record number or patient identification number Date of birth Sex Race or ethnicity
Diagnosis	Date or age at diagnosis Referring physician or institution Treating physician or institution Presenting symptoms Past medical history Family history (including cancer in first- or second-degree relatives) Physical examination findings at presentation Initial diagnostics (complete blood cell count, chemistry panel, radiographic studies) Diagnostic procedures (biopsies, cytologic studies) Pathology (morphology, histology, cytochemistry, flow cytometry) Cytogenetics Central nervous system status (if applicable) Stage (if applicable) Metastatic sites (if applicable) Initial response to therapy (e.g., rapid early response [RER], slow early response [SER], date first complete remission achieved) Relapse(s) dates, age at relapse(s), relapse site(s)
Treatment	Date of initial treatment (initiated and completed) Date(s) for treatment of relapse (initiated and completed) Final off-therapy date Chemotherapy agents received, including route of administration (list all) Cumulative doses (in mg/m^2) and age at treatment for all alkylators, anthracyclines, and heavy metals Dose ranges for cytarabine and methotrexate (e.g., standard dose versus high dose >1000 mg/m^2) Radiation fields, doses, shielding, age at treatment Surgical procedure(s) Transfusion(s), including all blood or serum products Stem cell transplantation(s), including donor source, preparative regimen, GVHD prophylaxis or treatment
Acute complications	Significant therapy-related complications (e.g., tumor lysis, septic shock, typhlitis, acute GVHD) Significant treatment required for complications (e.g., hemodialysis, amphotericin, aminoglycosides)
Complications after therapy	Significant complications after completion of therapy (e.g., herpes zoster, acute life-threatening infection after splenectomy)

Modified from Children's Oncology Group Summary of Cancer Treatment, 2008. http://www.survivorshipguidelines.org.
GVHD, Graft-versus-host disease.

Table 94-5 Monitoring for Potential Late Effects

Potential Late Effects	Therapeutic Exposure	Recommended Monitoring	Suggested Interventions
Adverse psychosocial effects (e.g., depression, anxiety, posttraumatic stress disorder, limitations in health care access, risky behaviors, psychosocial disability due to pain, fatigue)	Diagnosis and treatment for hematologic malignancy	Clinical interview: yearly	Psychologic or social work consultation if indicated
Dental abnormalities (abnormal tooth development, increased susceptibility to caries and gum disease)	Chemotherapy Cranial irradiation TBI	Dental examination: every 6 months	Professional dental cleaning every 6 months; use of fluoridated toothpaste; topical fluoride applications as indicated; Panorex radiograph before orthodontic or dental procedures for patients treated before completion of tooth development
Peripheral neuropathy Raynaud phenomenon	Vincristine Vinblastine	Neurologic examination if symptomatic	Physical therapy if indicated; advise patient to protect against precipitating factors (e.g., cold environment)
Neurocognitive deficits	Methotrexate (intrathecal, high-dose systemic) Cytarabine (high-dose systemic) Cranial irradiation TBI	Formal neuropsychologic testing: baseline on entry to long-term follow-up; repeat as clinically indicated if evidence of impaired performance Clinical interview yearly, including assessment of educational and vocational progress	Referral for specialized educational services, curricular modifications, or vocational training programs if indicated
Clinical leukoencephalopathy	Methotrexate (intrathecal, high-dose systemic) Cytarabine (high-dose systemic) Cranial irradiation	Clinical evaluation: yearly brain MRI or CT if clinically indicated	Neurology consultation if clinically indicated
Cataracts	Corticosteroids Busulfan Cranial irradiation TBI	Funduscopic examination and visual acuity evaluation: yearly Ophthalmologic examination: yearly for patients who received TBI or cranial radiation ≥30 Gy; every 3 years for cranial radiation <30 Gy	Ophthalmology consultation if abnormalities detected
Xerophthalmia	Chronic GVHD related to HCT	History and eye examination yearly	Artificial tears, ophthalmology consultation if indicated
Xerostomia	Cranial irradiation Chronic GVHD related to HCT	Dental evaluation: every 6 months	Meticulous oral hygiene Artificial saliva products if indicated
Hearing loss	Platinum chemotherapy Aminoglycoside antibiotics Cranial irradiation	History and physical examination: yearly Audiogram: baseline at entry into long-term follow-up, then as clinically indicated; every 5 years for cranial radiation dose ≥30 Gy	Audiology consultation if indicated
Hypothyroidism Thyroid nodules Thyroid malignancy	Cranial, cervical, spinal, mantle, thoracic, or mediastinal irradiation; TBI	Free T_4, TSH, thyroid examination: yearly	Endocrine or surgical referral as indicated
Cardiomyopathy Arrhythmias Subclinical left ventricular dysfunction	Anthracyclines Chest or thoracic irradiation (e.g., mantle, mediastinal)	Detailed history of exertional tolerance (e.g., dyspnea on exertion, chest pain): yearly ECG (for evaluation of QT interval): baseline on entry into long-term follow-up; ECHO: baseline on entry into long-term follow-up, then every 1 to 5 yr as indicated based on age at therapy and total anthracycline or radiation dose	Cardiology consultation if indicated; additional cardiology evaluation of patients who are pregnant or planning to become pregnant if patient received ≥300 mg/m² of an anthracycline, radiation dose ≥30 Gy, or any dose of anthracycline combined with irradiation

Table 94-5 Monitoring for Potential Late Effects—cont'd

Potential Late Effects	Therapeutic Exposure	Recommended Monitoring	Suggested Interventions
Pericarditis Pericardial fibrosis Valvular disease Premature atherosclerotic heart disease	Chest or thoracic irradiation (e.g., mantle, mediastinal)	Consider cardiology consultation 5-10 yr after irradiation to evaluate risk for coronary artery disease in patients who received doses ≥40 Gy Fasting glucose and lipid profiles: every 2 yr	Cardiology consultation if indicated; additional cardiology evaluation in patients who are pregnant or planning to become pregnant if patient received anthracycline combined with radiation, ≥300 mg/m^2 anthracycline, or radiation dose ≥30 Gy
Pulmonary dysfunction (fibrosis, interstitial pneumonitis)	Bleomycin Busulfan Chest/thoracic irradiation TBI Chronic GVHD related to HCT	Pulmonary function testing and chest radiograph: baseline at entry into long-term follow up and as clinically indicated for patients with progressive dysfunction	Pulmonary consultation for symptomatic patients; influenza and pneumococcal vaccine; counsel patients to avoid smoking and avoid scuba diving
Thrombosis Vascular insufficiency Infection of retained cuff or line tract	Central venous catheter	History and physical examination: yearly as clinically indicated	Surgical referral as indicated
Hepatic dysfunction	Mercaptopurine, thioguanine, methotrexate (systemic) HCT	ALT, AST, bilirubin: baseline on entry into long-term follow-up; repeat if clinically indicated	If abnormal results for baseline studies, obtain prothrombin time (to assess hepatic synthetic function) and viral hepatitis screening
Chronic viral hepatitis	Blood products	Hepatitis C antibody and HCV-RNA by PCR: once if transfused before universal screening of blood supply (1992 in the United States) Hepatitis B surface antigen and core antibody: once if transfused before universal screening of blood supply (1972 in the United States)	Gastroenterology or hepatology consultation and annual AFP for patients with chronic hepatitis; hepatitis A and B immunizations in patients lacking immunity
HIV infection	Blood products	HIV-1 and HIV-2 antibodies: once if transfused before universal screening of blood supply (1985 in the United States)	Infectious disease consultation for patients with confirmed infection
Life-threatening infection	Splenectomy Splenic radiation ≥40 Gy Chronic active GVHD	Physical examination at time of febrile illness to evaluate degree of illness and for potential source of infection	Administer parenteral antibiotics and continue close medical observation in patients with temperature >38.3° C (101° F) or other signs of serious infection; immunize with pneumococcal, meningococcal, and HIB vaccines
Iron overload	HCT (and patients requiring multiple red blood cell transfusions)	Serum ferritin: at entry into long-term follow-up	If abnormal, consider chelation, or repeat as clinically indicated until within normal limits
Bowel obstruction Chronic enterocolitis Fistulas and strictures	Abdominal surgery Abdominal or pelvic irradiation Chronic GVHD related to HCT (esophageal strictures, vaginal stenosis)	History and physical examination: yearly and as clinically indicated Serum protein and albumin levels: yearly in patients with chronic diarrhea or fistula	Surgical and gastroenterology consultations as clinically indicated
Renal insufficiency	TBI Abdominal or splenic irradiation Ifosfamide Platinum chemotherapy Methotrexate	Blood pressure: yearly Urinalysis: yearly BUN, creatinine, electrolytes, calcium, magnesium, phosphorus baseline and repeat as clinically indicated	Nephrology consultation for proteinuria, hypertension, progressive renal insufficiency
Hemorrhagic cystitis Bladder fibrosis Dysfunctional voiding Bladder malignancy	Cyclophosphamide Ifosfamide Irradiation of abdomen, pelvis, iliac, inguinal sites	Urinalysis: yearly Voiding history: yearly	Urology consultation for incontinence, dysfunctional voiding, macroscopic hematuria (culture negative)

Continued

Table 94-5 Monitoring for Potential Late Effects—cont'd

Potential Late Effects	Therapeutic Exposure	Recommended Monitoring	Suggested Interventions
Growth hormone deficiency	Cranial irradiation TBI	Height, weight: every 6 months during puberty until growth is complete Obtain bone age in poorly growing children	Endocrine referral for patients failing to follow normal growth curve
Overweight/obesity	Cranial irradiation	BP, growth percentile, BMI: yearly	Endocrine referral as indicated
Metabolic syndrome	TBI	Fasting glucose, lipid profile and insulin level every 2 yr	
Hypogonadism Infertility	Alkylating agents Cranial irradiation Abdominal or pelvic irradiation Testicular irradiation Spinal irradiation >25 Gy TBI	Menstrual history, sexual function, height, weight: yearly Pubertal history, Tanner stage: yearly until maturity FSH, LH, estradiol, or testosterone: baseline at age 13 (females) or 14 (males) or at entry into long-term follow-up and for clinical symptoms of estrogen or testosterone deficiency Semen analysis: as indicated or requested by patient	Endocrine referral for hypogonadal patients (for hormone replacement therapy); reproductive endocrinology referral for patients desiring evaluation of fertility options
Precocious puberty	Cranial irradiation	Physical examination, height, weight, Tanner stage: yearly until maturity LH, FSH, estradiol, or testosterone: as clinically indicated in patients with accelerated pubertal progression Obtain bone age in rapidly growing prepubertal children	Endocrine referral as indicated
Adverse pregnancy outcomes (e.g., spontaneous abortion, premature delivery, low-birth-weight infant)	Irradiation of abdomen, pelvis, iliac, inguinal, para-aortic sites TBI	History: yearly and as clinically indicated	High-risk obstetric care
Osteopenia, osteoporosis	Corticosteroids Methotrexate (high-dose systemic) HCT	Bone-density study (DEXA scan or quantitative CT scan): baseline at entry into long-term follow-up, repeat as clinically indicated	Calcium and vitamin D supplementation; weight-bearing exercise; treatment of exacerbating conditions (e.g., hypogonadism); consider pharmacologic intervention (e.g., bisphosphonates)
Avascular necrosis	Corticosteroids Methotrexate (systemic) HCT	History: yearly; MRI if clinically indicated	Orthopedic consultation if indicated
Scoliosis/kyphosis	Irradiation of trunk (e.g., mantle, spine, abdomen, pelvis)	Physical examination of spine: yearly (every 6 months during pubertal growth spurt) Radiologic imaging of the spine if clinical evidence of scoliosis or kyphosis	Orthopedic referral
Joint contractures	Chronic GVHD related to HCT	Physical examination yearly	Orthopedic referral if indicated
Chronic infection	Chronic GVHD related to HCT	History: yearly	Prophylactic antiinfective agents; infectious disease consultation if indicated
Vitiligo Scleroderma Joint contractures Nail dysplasia Dysplastic nevi Skin cancer Secondary benign or malignant neoplasms in radiation field	Chronic GVHD related to HCT Irradiation (any field)	Physical examination: yearly Careful physical examination, inspection and palpation of irradiated skin and soft tissues: yearly	Dermatology or rehabilitation consultation if clinically indicated Dermatology or surgical referral and radiographs if indicated for any suspicious lesions

Table 94-5 Monitoring for Potential Late Effects—cont'd

Potential Late Effects	Therapeutic Exposure	Recommended Monitoring	Suggested Interventions
Bone malignancies Brain tumor	Cranial irradiation	History and physical examination: yearly Brain MRI: baseline at maturity for all patients and as clinically indicated	Neurosurgical consultation as indicated
Breast cancer	Chest or thorax irradiation ≥20 Gy (mantle radiation field)	Clinical breast examination: yearly until age 25, then every 6 months Mammogram and breast MRI: yearly beginning at age 25 or 8 yr after irradiation (whichever comes last)	Teach breast self-examination; instruct patient to perform monthly self-examination and report changes immediately; surgical consultation if clinically indicated
Gastrointestinal malignancy	Abdominal, pelvic, spinal irradiation ≥30 Gy	Colonoscopy every 5 years beginning 10 years after radiation or at age 35, whichever comes last; or more frequently as clinically indicated	Surgical consultation if indicated
AML (preceding myelodysplastic phase associated with alkylating agents)	Anthracyclines Epipodophyllotoxins Alkylating agents Stem cell priming with etoposide Autologous transplantation for NHL or Hodgkin lymphoma	Physical examination, CBC and differential: yearly for 10 yr after therapy Bone marrow evaluation if clinically indicated	Counsel patient to report fatigue, bruising, bleeding, bone pain

Modified from Children's Oncology Group: *Long-term follow-up guidelines for survivors of childhood, adolescent, and young adult cancers,* version 3.0, 2008, Children's Oncology Group. http://www.survivorshipguidelines.org.

AFP, α-Fetoprotein; *ALT,* alanine aminotransferase; *AML,* acute myeloid leukemia; *AST,* aspartate aminotransferase; *BMI,* body mass index; *BP,* blood pressure; *BUN,* blood urea nitrogen; *CBC,* complete blood cell count; *CT,* computed tomography; *DEXA,* dual-energy x-ray absorptiometry; *ECG,* electrocardiogram; *ECHO,* echocardiogram; *FSH,* follicle-stimulating hormone; *GFR,* glomerular filtration rate; *GVHD,* graft-versus-host disease; *HCT,* hematopoietic cell transplantation; *HCV,* hepatitis C virus; *HIB, Haemophilus influenzae* type B; *HIV,* human immunodeficiency virus; *LH,* luteinizing hormone; *MRI,* magnetic resonance imaging; *NHL,* non-Hodgkin lymphoma; *PCR,* polymerase chain reaction; T_4, thyroxine; *TBI,* total body irradiation; *TSH,* thyroid-stimulating protein; *yr,* year.

however, it is important that these risks are kept in perspective. In reality, most survivors of hematologic malignancies have the potential to lead full lives with excellent performance status and minimal to no physical limitations. The overall goal of follow-up care is to assist each patient in maximizing his or her full potential for a healthy life while balancing the small, but real, risk for potential complications that may arise. Providing this type of ongoing comprehensive follow-up care is an essential service for survivors of hematologic malignancies.

SUGGESTED READINGS

Armenian SH, Meadows AT, Bhatia S: Late effects of childhood cancer and its treatment. In Pizzo PA, Poplack DG, editors: *Principles and practice of pediatric oncology,* ed 6, Philadelphia, 2010, Lippincott Raven, p 1431.

Armenian SH, Sun CL, Francisco L, et al: Late congestive heart failure after hematopoietic cell transplantation. *J Clin Oncol* 26:5537, 2008.

Armenian SH, Sun CL, Mills G, et al: Predictors of late cardiovascular complications in survivors of hematopoietic cell transplantation. *Biol Blood Marrow Transplant* 16:1138, 2010.

Baker KS, Ness KK, Weisdorf D, et al: Late effects in survivors of acute leukemia treated with hematopoietic cell transplantation: A report from the Bone Marrow Transplant Survivor Study. *Leukemia* 24:2039, 2010.

Bhatia S, Constine LS: Late morbidity after successful treatment of children with cancer. *Cancer J* 15:174, 2009.

Bhatia S, Francisco L, Carter A, et al: Late mortality after allogeneic hematopoietic cell transplantation and functional status of long-term survivors: Report from the Bone Marrow Transplant Survivor Study. *Blood* 110:3784, 2007.

Bhatia S, Sather HN, Pabustan OB, et al: Low incidence of second neoplasms among children diagnosed with acute lymphoblastic leukemia after 1983. *Blood* 99:4257, 2002.

Bhatia S, Yasui Y, Robison LL, et al: High risk of subsequent neoplasms continues with extended follow-up of childhood Hodgkin's disease: Report from the Late Effects Study Group. *J Clin Oncol* 21:4386, 2003.

Green DM, Kawashima T, Stovall M, et al: Fertility of male survivors of childhood cancer: A report from the Childhood Cancer Survivor Study. *J Clin Oncol* 28:332, 2010.

Green DM, Sklar CA, Boice JD, Jr, et al: Ovarian failure and reproductive outcomes after childhood cancer treatment: Results from the Childhood Cancer Survivor Study. *J Clin Oncol* 27:2374, 2009.

Hewitt ME, Greenfield S, Stovall E, editors: *From cancer patient to cancer survivor: Lost in transition,* Washington, DC, 2006, The National Academies Press.

Hewitt ME, Weiner SL, Simone JV, editors: *Childhood cancer survivorship: Improving care and quality of life,* Washington, DC, 2003, The National Academies Press.

Hudson MM: Late complications after leukemia therapy. In Pui CH, editor: *Childhood leukemias,* ed 2, Cambridge, 2006, Cambridge University Press.

Landier W, Bhatia S, Eshelman DA, et al: Development of risk-based guidelines for pediatric cancer survivors: The Children's Oncology Group Long-Term Follow-Up Guidelines from the Children's Oncology Group Late Effects Committee and Nursing Discipline. *J Clin Oncol* 22:4979, 2004.

Mulrooney DA, Dover DC, Li S, et al: Twenty years of follow-up among survivors of childhood and young adult acute myeloid leukemia: A report from the Childhood Cancer Survivor Study. *Cancer* 112:2071, 2008.

Oeffinger KC, Mertens AC, Sklar CA, et al: Chronic health conditions in adult survivors of childhood cancer. *N Engl J Med* 355:1572, 2006.

Rizzo JD, Wingard JR, Tichelli A, et al: Recommended screening and preventive practices for long-term survivors after hematopoietic cell transplantation: Joint recommendations of the European Group for Blood and Marrow Transplantation, Center for International Blood and Marrow Transplant Research, and the American Society for Blood and Marrow

Transplantation (EBMT/CIBMTR/ASBMT). *Bone Marrow Transplant* 37:249, 2006.

Rowland JH, Hewitt M, Ganz PA: Cancer survivorship: A new challenge in delivering quality cancer care. *J Clin Oncol* 24:5101, 2006.

Sanders JE: Growth and development after hematopoietic cell transplant in children. *Bone Marrow Transplant* 41:223, 2008.

Sun CL, Francisco L, Kawashima T, et al: Prevalence and predictors of chronic health conditions after hematopoietic cell transplantation: A report from the Bone Marrow Transplant Survivor Study. *Blood* 116:3129, 2010.

For complete list of references log on to www.expertconsult.com.

PART

IX

CELL-BASED THERAPIES

CHAPTER 95

OVERVIEW AND HISTORICAL PERSPECTIVE OF CURRENT CELL-BASED THERAPIES

Leslie E. Silberstein and Helen E. Heslop

The discovery in 1900 by Karl Landsteiner of the ABO blood group system paved the way for transfusion therapy, that is, the ability to safely infuse living blood cells as a therapeutic modality (see Chapters 111 to 123). Thus the discipline began with the collection by venipuncture of whole blood, which required anticoagulation and storage at refrigerated temperatures. These procedures were optimized when it became possible to isolate different cell populations, such as red blood cells, platelets, and granulocytes. The term *blood banking* refers to collection and storage of blood products, both of which are highly regulated by the U.S. Food and Drug Administration (FDA).

The pioneering work by E. Donnall Thomas and others between 1950 and 1970, demonstrating the feasibility of transfusing bone marrow cells (i.e., bone marrow transplantation) as a treatment modality,[1,2] marked the next significant development of cellular therapies (see Chapters 104 to 110). The success of bone marrow engraftment is related to the presence of hematopoietic stem and progenitor cells in the bone marrow; immune cells in the graft, including T cells and NK cells, mediate graft-versus-tumor effects in patients transplanted for hematologic malignancy. Hematopoietic stem cell populations, currently used for therapy of malignant and nonmalignant disease, can be isolated from bone marrow, from (mobilized) peripheral blood, and from umbilical cord blood (see Chapter 96). An exciting new development in hematopoietic stem cell transplantation is the genetic manipulation/transduction of the hematopoietic stem cell to correct hereditary disorders such as the congenital immunodeficiencies and hemoglobinopathies[3] (see Chapter 99).

More recently, the ability to isolate and expand cell populations in culture has led to the evaluation of a number of cell therapy strategies. Only one approach, a dendritic cell vaccine, is currently approved by the FDA in the United States.[4] Infusions of other cells expanded ex vivo or significantly manipulated are conducted as experimental procedures through the FDA's Investigation of New Drug (IND) application process. Many such studies use autologous cells, which do not have a risk for transferring communicable disease but (because they are patient-specific products) make late-stage clinical trials more challenging. The use of allogeneic cells requires careful assessment of donor eligibility because of the risk for infectious disease transmission or transfer of immune reactivity[5] (Table 95-1). Allogeneic cells may also be used to produce a patient-specific product in some clinical settings, such as treatment of relapse postallogeneic transplant in which full HLA matching is required. In other applications, however, third-party cells may have benefits, including the advantage of broad applicability since a larger number of patients can receive a product generated from a single donor.

A broad range of cell types are currently being evaluated in clinical trials (see Chapters 97 to 103) Immune cell populations with distinct biologic properties are being infused to treat cancer and infectious diseases, and some approaches have progressed to late-phase testing (see Chapters 101 to 103). Nonhematopoietic stromal cells from bone marrow have attracted considerable interest recently for use in tissue repair and immunomodulation, largely because of their multilineage differentiation potential and their secretion of cytokines and chemokines (see Chapter 100). Their use, while experimental, is promising. Thus significant experience in cell-based therapies involving hematopoietic/bone marrow–derived cells has evolved, similar to blood banking and transfusion medicine, into a highly regulated discipline with oversight by several regulatory agencies, including the FDA and the NIH Recombinant DNA Advisory Board (see Chapters 97 and 98).

The next frontier of cellular therapies is being driven by the discovery and ability to culture stem cell populations from various other adult tissues (retina, cornea, heart, lung, etc.), embryonic stem cells, and inducible pluripotent stem cells. The therapeutic application of these cell populations, although intensely investigated worldwide, is regarded as preliminary at present.

Table 95-1 Evaluation of Allogeneic Donor for Eligibility to Provide Cell Therapy Product

Evaluation/Test*	Rationale/Purpose
Complete history and physical	To review the donor's medical and social history for risk factors for communicable disease agents and diseases. To review for clinical evidence of risk factors or diseases.
Donor questionnaire	To evaluate risk factors for communicable disease (using uniform donor questionnaire[†] drafted by international task force).
CBC, platelets, differential	To evaluate for evidence of hematologic abnormalities.
Electrolytes, BUN, creatinine, glucose, total protein, albumin, total bilirubin, alkaline phosphatase, ALT, AST, LDH	To evaluate for evidence of liver or electrolyte abnormalities.
ABO typing	To confirm identity.
HLA typing	To conduct HLA matching for some indications. To confirm identity.
HIV-1 antibody, HIV-2 antibody, HIV NAT, HTLV-1/2 antibodies, HBs antigen, HBc antibody, HCV NAT, CMV antibody, serologic test for syphilis (STS), West Nile virus NAT, Chagas disease (if indicated by region)	To exclude communicable disease agents. Must be collected at the time of recovery of the cells or tissue from the donor; or up to 7 days before or after recovery. For donors of peripheral blood stem/progenitor cells, oocytes and bone marrow may be collected for testing up to 30 days.

*The donor eligibility rule requires human cell and tissue products (HCT/Ps) establishments to screen and test cell and tissue donors for risk factors for, and clinical evidence of, relevant communicable disease agents or diseases. Additional IND-specific tests may also be mandated. All facilities need to use FDA-approved testing.

†Foundation for the Accreditation of Cellular Therapy (FACT) Standards: HPC Donor History Questionnaire (http://www.factwebsite.org/Inner.aspx?id=163&terms=donor+questionnaire).

REFERENCES

1. Thomas ED, Lochte HL, Jr, Lu WC, et al: Intravenous infusion of bone marrow in patients receiving radiation and chemotherapy. *N Engl J Med* 257:491, 1957.
2. Thomas ED, Buckner CD, Banaji M, et al: One hundred patients with acute leukemia treated by chemotherapy, total body irradiation, and allogeneic marrow transplantation. *Blood* 49:511, 1977.
3. Hacein-Bey-Abina S, Hauer J, Lim A, et al: Efficacy of gene therapy for X-linked severe combined immunodeficiency. *N Engl J Med* 363:355, 2010. PMC2957288.
4. Cheever MA, Higano CS: PROVENGE (Sipuleucel-T) in prostate cancer: The first FDA-approved therapeutic cancer vaccine. *Clin Cancer Res* 17:3520, 2011.
5. Horowitz MM, Confer DL. Evaluation of hematopoietic stem cell donors. *Hematology Am Soc Hematol Educ Program* 469, 2005.

CHAPTER 96

PRACTICAL ASPECTS OF HEMATOLOGIC STEM CELL HARVESTING AND MOBILIZATION

Scott D. Rowley and Michele L. Donato

Hematopoietic stem cell (HSC) products for autologous or allogeneic transplantation are available from bone marrow, peripheral blood, or umbilical cord blood (UCB) sources. Bone marrow was the original source of cells for transplantation because of the ease and reliability of collecting adequate numbers of cells for transplantation, and it remains the standard with which other sources of HSC are compared.

Peripheral blood stem cell (PBSC) products have virtually replaced bone marrow as the HSC component for autologous transplantation and are widely used for allogeneic transplantation. The rapid engraftment kinetics of PBSC compared with bone marrow is widely recognized. Median times to achieve an absolute neutrophil count greater than 500/μL and platelet transfusion independence after PBSC transplantation typically are approximately 11 to 14 days.[1-3] The improvement in engraftment kinetics reduces the cost of autologous transplantation (Table 96-1).[3-6] Although graft-versus-host disease (GVHD) prophylaxis with posttransplant methotrexate will slow engraftment, the kinetics of engraftment for the allogeneic PBSC recipient is similar to that experienced by the autologous PBSC recipient. A number of phase III studies involving either autologous or allogeneic HSC transplantation have confirmed the more rapid engraftment kinetics for recipients of PBSC (Table 96-2),[7-10] and this effect is not limited to HSC collected from the peripheral blood, because cytokine administration to the patient or donor before marrow harvesting will also increase the number of HSC collected and result in quicker hematologic recovery (Table 96-2).[11-13] The disadvantages to use of PBSC components compared with bone marrow or UCB for autologous or allogeneic transplantation include the usual need for multiple days of collection (especially for autologous transplantation), the inability to collect adequate components from all patients and donors, and a possibly higher risk for chronic GVHD or the occurrence of chronic GVHD that is more difficult to control[14] (see box on Choice of Hematologic Stem Cell Product for Transplantation).

UCB has found an important niche in the treatment of patients undergoing unrelated donor transplantation but who lack an appropriate related or unrelated volunteer donor. The relative immunologic naivete of the donor allows multiple-antigen mismatched transplantation without undue risks for acute or chronic GVHD.[15] The primary limitations of UCB transplantation derive from the small cell dose collected, which can result in a longer time to hematologic recovery and a higher risk for primary engraftment failure.

SELECTION AND EVALUATION OF THE STEM CELL DONOR

Selection of the Stem Cell Donor

The primary selection criterion for the patient undergoing autologous HSC collection and transplantation is the diagnosis of an illness amenable to treatment with a dose-intense regimen requiring HSC support. Extensive prior treatments, especially with marrow-toxic chemotherapy regimens, may preclude successful collection of autologous HSC, which would exclude a patient from this treatment option. In general, however, any comorbid illnesses that would preclude either marrow or PBSC collection would also disqualify the patient from treatment with dose-intensive regimens used in preparation for autologous HSC transplantation.

The selection of the allogeneic HSC donor is more complex. The HLA major histocompatibility complex (MHC) is the primary consideration in selection of a donor for allogeneic HSCT, since its loci contribute significantly to host-versus-graft (HVG, leading to immunologic rejection of donor HSC) responses and to graft-versus-host (GVH, leading to GVHD and GVL) reactions.[16,17] Donor age, gender, and parity are secondary considerations in the selection of an allogeneic HSC donor.[17,18] Mismatching for killer-cell immunoglobulin-like receptor (KIR) ligands may reduce the risk for posttransplant relapse of disease.[19] More than 30% of allogeneic HSC transplants from related or unrelated donors will involve ABO-disparate donor and recipients, and donor and recipient pairs may also differ for other red blood cell antigens, with no clear evidence of deleterious effect on engraftment, survival, or GVHD.[20] Cancer, autoimmune disorders, and genetic diseases such as the hemoglobinopathies can be transmitted to the allograft recipient; thus donor health is an important consideration in donor selection.

Evaluation of HSC Donors

The immediate precollection evaluation of a patient or donor is intended to address the risks of the collection procedure to the donor and the risks for transmission of disease from the donor. The same general donor health criteria apply to both bone marrow and PBSC donors. Patients undergoing autologous HSC collection and transplantation are not at risk for transmitting disease to themselves, but the laboratory must be notified of the infectious disease status of the patient because some viruses, particularly viruses with high infectious potency such as hepatitis B, can cross-contaminate other products stored in the liquid phase of nitrogen. All allogeneic HSC donors must be evaluated using the same criteria currently applied to blood donors, including a targeted history regarding behaviors exposing the donor to virus infection, recent or concurrent illnesses, and medication use.[21-24] This evaluation must be documented in the donor medical record with appropriate documentation of donor suitability in the recipient's medical record before initiation of the transplant conditioning regimen. Older donors will have more comorbid medical conditions, which will increase the risks of the collection procedures, and the risks to the donor with underlying health problems must be fully considered before subjecting the donor to HSC collection. Published standards describe evaluation of the donor for the risk of the donation process, as well as the risk for transmission of disease to the recipient.[21-23] Numerous infectious diseases that would not exclude the donor from blood donation, such as cytomegalovirus, may be transmitted with the allograft. However, donors who otherwise would be excluded for health reasons from donating blood for transfusion (e.g., individuals with a history of viral hepatitis) still may be selected to donate HSC if the needs of the recipient outweigh the risks and consequences of disease transmission. Evaluation by appropriate consultants may be required before donor approval is finalized. Procedures involving donors with acute infectious illnesses

Table 96-1 Costs of Autologous Transplantation by Source of Hematopoietic Stem Cell

Study	No. of Patients	Days to Engraftment: ANC >500/μL	Days to Engraftment: Platelet >20,000/μL	Hospital Stay	Costs
Hartmann et al[3]					
BM	65	12	36.5	31	$28,429
PBSC	64	8	17.5	24	$23,591
Smith et al[4]					
BM	31	14	23	23	$59,314
PBSC	27	11	16	17	$45,792
Vellenga et al[5]					
BM	42	26	18	34	$17,668
PBSC	76	15	13	27	$13,954
van Agthoven et al[6]					
BM	29	15	18	34	e19,000
PBSC	62	10	13	27	e15,008

Choice of Hematologic Stem Cell Product for Transplantation

Virtually all patients undergoing autologous HSC transplantation will have PBSC as the source of HSC, based on the following advantages: ease of collection, greater quantities of HSC (resulting in faster hematologic recovery and shorter and less costly hospital stays), and potentially lower risks for tumor cell contamination of the graft.

The allogeneic donor has a wider range of options, including marrow, PBSC, or UCB products from HLA-compatible or partially compatible related or unrelated donors. The transplant recipient may request a source of cells, but the donor has the right to decide about the method of donation. PBSC products have the greatest quantity of HSC and will result in faster hematologic recovery compared with marrow or UCB transplants. In some reports, PBSC transplantation also results in a survival advantage. However, PBSC transplantation is also associated with a higher risk for difficult-to-control chronic GVHD and may not be appropriate for use in patients who would not benefit from a robust GVL effect, such as those treated for nonmalignant diseases. Umbilical cord blood has the advantage of being immediately available, reducing the time to transplantation. Targeted collection of UCB products from ethnic populations not well represented in donor registries will facilitate treatment of ethnic minority patients. The relative immature immunity of the cord blood donor allows use of HLA mismatched products without an undue increase in GVHD risk. Infusion of two cord blood units may achieve a greater graft-versus-tumor effect, even though one unit will be rejected. The much smaller quantity of HSC in the cord blood product results in slower hematologic recovery, and the adult patient, in particular, may be at greater risk for post-transplant infections because of the relative immature immune system of the donor.

Table 96-2 Randomized Studies Comparing Marrow and PBSC as HSC Sources*

Study	No. of Patients: BM	No. of Patients: PBSC	CD34+ Cell Dose: BM	CD34+ Cell Dose: PBSC	ANC >500/μL: BM	ANC >500/μL: PBSC	ANC >500/μL: p	Platelet >20,000/μL: BM	Platelet >20,000/μL: PBSC	Platelet >20,000/μL: p	Acute GVHD: BM	Acute GVHD: PBSC	Acute GVHD: P
ALLOGENEIC BM VERSUS PBSC													
Blaise et al[7]	52	48	2.4	6.6	21	15	<0.001	21*	13*	<0.001	42%	44%	NS
Bensinger et al[8]	91	81	2.4	7.3	21	16	<0.001	19	13	<0.001	57%	64%	0.35
Couban et al[9]	118	109	2.4	6.7	23	19	<0.001	22	16	<0.001	44%	44%	>0.9
Schmitz et al[10]	116	163	2.7	5.8	15	12	<0.001	20	15	<0.001	39%	53%	0.013
G-BM VERSUS PBSC													
Morton et al[11]	28	29	2.6	7.2	16	14	<0.1	14	12	<0.1	52%	54%	<0.6
AUTOLOGOUS BM VERSUS PBSC													
Beyer et al[1]	23	24	2.5*	13.1*	11	10	<0.01	17	10	<0.01			
Schmitz et al[2]	31	27	Not stated	2.8	14	11	0.005	23	16	0.02			
Hartmann et al[3]	65	64	Not stated	92.7*	12	8	<0.001	27*	12*	<0.001			
G-BM VERSUS PBSC													
Damiani et al[13]	36	19	0.6	3.3	12	11	0.22	13	11	0.24			

ANC, Absolute neutrophil count; *BM*, bone marrow, *G-BM*, granulocyte colony-stimulated bone marrow; *NS*, not significant; *PBSC*, peripheral blood stem cell.
*Shown are number of patients enrolled in each arm of the study, quantity of $CD34^+$ cells × 10^6/kg (CFU-GM × 10^4/kg for reports by Beyer and Hartmann), days after transplantation to achieve a peripheral blood absolute neutrophil count >500/μL and platelet count >20,000/μL (25,000/μL for report by Blaise and 30,000/μL for report by Hartmann), and percentage of patients developing acute graft-versus-host disease.

Evaluation of the Marrow or Peripheral Blood Stem Cell Donor

HSC transplantation involves the infusion of a "blood product," and all donors must be evaluated for risks for disease transmission as per the current criteria for blood donation. Exemptions from criteria that specifically address the risk for disease transmission are permissible, if the risks of excluding an otherwise appropriate donor outweigh the risks for disease transmission to the transplant recipient, who may not have an alternate donor. Informed consent must be obtained for the evaluation and collection procedures. Informed consent also must be specifically obtained for the release of protected donor health information to the transplant recipient, allowing proper informed consent for the transplant to be obtained. Minors and donors not competent to provide consent must be represented by a third party not involved in the care of the recipient. Ideally, similar courtesy will be provided to the adult donor. Donors must also be evaluated for health issues that would increase the risks resulting from the collection procedures. For marrow donors, this includes the risks of anesthesia; for PBSC donors, evaluation should include the risks of mobilization medications and apheresis.

The donor collection facility's standard operating procedures for evaluation of HSC donors must meet FACT/JACIE or AABB guidelines and FDA (or other regulatory agency) standards, and include policies and procedures for the following:

- Education of donor, including education regarding procedures, risks, alternatives, and possible future collections
- Medical history, including special attention to history of autoimmune disorders, arthritis, cardiac and vascular diseases, and history of cancer
- History of high-risk behaviors, such as recent tattoos, body piercing, sexual practices, and travel
- Physical examination, including vein assessment (PBSC donors) and oral examination (marrow donors undergoing inhalational anesthesia)
- Laboratory studies, including verification HLA typing, ABO typing, CBC, chemistry panel, infectious disease panel, urinalysis, ECG, CXR
- Consent for collection procedures and the release of protected health information to the stem cell recipient

should be delayed, if at all possible, because of the risk for disease transmission. Genetic disorders, such as hemoglobinopathies, will be transmitted to the recipient as a direct consequence of stem cell engraftment. Cancer can be transmitted, as illustrated by the transmission of donor leukemia not detected during initial evaluation of the donor,[25] and donors previously treated for cancer should be evaluated for the probability of recurrent disease that could be transferred to the immunocompromised recipient.[26] Collection of PBSC is generally an outpatient procedure conducted in the clinic setting. In contrast, marrow harvesting has the luxury of the intensive support capability of the operating room. PBSC collection should never be viewed as a safer alternative to marrow harvesting for the donor with underlying health problems. Pediatric donors present different challenges, based on the smaller size and varying ages (and ability to cooperate) of the donors (see box on Evaluation of the Marrow or Peripheral Blood Stem Cell Donor).

Use of a donor who does not meet eligibility criteria and who poses a risk for transmission of disease requires appropriate informed consent both from the donor (for disclosure of this confidential health information to the recipient and for counseling of the recipient) and from the recipient (for use of the stem cell product). The potential conflict of interest between protecting donor health and patient needs must be recognized, and preferably, the donor and patient should be represented by different physicians.[27]

Specific Evaluation of Bone Marrow Donors

Anesthesia and blood loss present the greatest risks for serious complications to the bone marrow donor. Most marrow harvesting is performed under general anesthesia, which requires intubation for control of the airway for a surgical procedure performed on a prone patient. Regional (spinal or epidural) anesthesia may not be effectively established, so patients and donors who express a preference for this anesthesia must be counseled about the potential need for general anesthesia. The health assessment must include questioning about a history of joint disease of the cervical spine and mandible and examination of the mouth if general anesthesia requiring intubation is chosen. Patients and donors with comorbid conditions, such as aortic stenosis sensitive to changes in blood volume and blood pressure, may require anesthesia consultation and plans for invasive monitoring during the surgical procedure. A history of marrow fibrosis, pelvic irradiation, or pelvic tumor involvement may exclude a patient from marrow harvesting, although unilateral harvesting from the posterior and iliac crests and aspiration of the sternum may achieve adequate quantities of cells for transplantation.

Specific Evaluation of Peripheral Blood Stem Cell Donors

The PBSC donor is exposed to the risks of cytokine (and chemokine) administration and the risks related to the apheresis procedure, including the risks of central venous catheter insertion and use. No long-term health consequences have been associated with cytokine administration, and the specific toxicities with these agents are described later. Filgrastim may lead to a flare of autoimmune disorders and may increase the risk for blood clots, particularly for donors who are sedentary or who may be traveling shortly after the donation procedures.[28] The PBSC donor must be assessed for venous access before the patient receives conditioning, and consent for use of a central venous catheter must be obtained if the venous access is deemed inadequate for the apheresis procedure.

Specific Evaluation of Umbilical Cord Blood Donors

Evaluation of the donor for UCB donation begins with a history of maternal (and paternal) illness and exposures to infectious diseases. A comprehensive genetic and family history should be obtained. Although linkage between the infant and the product is currently maintained, an update of infant health is not obtained at the time of transplantation, which may be several years after collection. Parental medical history includes specific questions addressing the risks for transmission of hereditary or acquired blood-borne diseases. Testing for infectious diseases is obtained from the mother at the time of collection to minimize loss of product.

Public UCB banks set criteria for the storage of units in order to avoid the collection and storage of UCB units that would not be acceptable for transplantation.[29] Exclusion criteria for potential donors in one multicenter study, for example, included the following: multiple gestation; premature delivery; active chorioamnionitis or sepsis; mother being the recipient of an organ transplant; mother with history of cancer; mother with high-risk behaviors or previously diagnosed with HIV, hepatitis, or syphilis; and mother having active venereal disease such as vaginal herpes simplex and delivering vaginally.

COLLECTION OF BONE MARROW FOR TRANSPLANTATION

Bone Marrow Collection Techniques

Bone marrow typically is harvested from the posterior iliac crests using virtually the same techniques used to obtain diagnostic samples in the clinic. The primary differences between obtaining diagnostic specimens and cell quantities adequate for transplantation are the volume of blood and marrow removed, which requires attention to fluid replacement during the procedure, and the need for appropriate anesthesia. Bone marrow harvesting from healthy donors presents little risk for serious morbidity, permitting the ethical recruitment of allogeneic donors, including unrelated and pediatric bone marrow donors.[21] Multiple aspirations are performed with collection of approximately 5 mL of marrow from each puncture site. If properly spaced, no more than two to three skin puncture sites per side usually are required. Other harvest sites, such as the anterior iliac crests or sternum, can be used, but at increased risk for complications from accidental laceration or perforation of contiguous anatomic structures. For patients with a history of radiation or tumor involvement of one pelvic crest, adequate cells can be harvested from the anterior and posterior crests of the other side.

Marrow is collected in the day surgery suite using either general or regional anesthesia. With proper fluid and blood replacement, overnight hospitalization should not be required. For the healthy donor, the risks for serious complications from either general or regional anesthesia are minimal, although a multivariate analysis of adverse events performed by the National Marrow Donor Program (NMDP) for unrelated donors reported a higher risk for serious adverse events for donors receiving regional anesthesia.[30] Use of spinal or epidural anesthesia avoids the nausea that may occur with general anesthesia, especially for younger women, but hypotension from loss of vascular tone in the lower extremities often occurs as the volume of marrow is collected. General anesthesia is preferable for the donor with comorbid disorders such as cardiovascular or cerebral vascular disease because of the better control of donor airway and lower risk for hypotension during the harvest procedures. Local anesthesia is acceptable only if a very limited harvest is being performed, because local anesthesia does not achieve anesthesia of the marrow space and because large quantities of lidocaine, for example, are cardiotoxic.

Both heparin and acid-citrate-dextran–A (ACD-A) can be used for anticoagulation of bone marrow products. ACD-A decreases the accumulation of lactic acid and may be preferable, especially for products that will be transported or stored for longer periods before infusion or cryopreservation.[31]

Toxicity of Bone Marrow Collection

Anesthesia complications present the major health risk to the donor; marrow aspiration is generally well tolerated, although postharvest discomfort is experienced to some extent by all donors.[32] Complications include hemorrhage and infections at skin puncture sites. Severe hematomas and neuralgias rarely occur, and attention to pelvic anatomy is required to decrease the risk for damage to vessels and nerves lying under or adjacent to the iliac crest harvest sites. Irritation of the sacral nerves may result from needle penetration through the pelvic bone or from blood tracking into the nerve roots and requires several months of convalescence. Localized pain is common, may last for several days, and may require a brief period of medication with opioid/acetaminophen combinations. In a survey of over 9000 donors for unrelated bone marrow transplantation, 82% reported collection site pain, with a median time to recovery of 3 weeks.[30] Pain associated with the anesthesia procedures (throat pain, 33%; postanesthesia headache, 17%) was reported by a large proportion of the donors. Fatigue was reported by 59% of donors. Serious adverse effects were reported for 125 donors (1.35%), with 116 donors reporting serious complications considered to be associated with the collection procedures. Most serious complications ($n = 69$) were due to mechanical injury to tissue, bone, or nerve, and a smaller but similar number ($n = 45$) were related to anesthesia. Infection and grand mal seizure were reported for one donor each. A retrospective survey of donor events reported by the European Group for Blood and Marrow Transplantation described almost 28,000 bone marrow donors, with one death from pulmonary embolism.[33] An additional 12 donors experienced severe adverse events, including four cardiac arrests (three during anesthesia), two episodes of severe hypertension, one pulmonary embolism from heparin-induced thrombocytopenia, one episode of pulmonary edema, one donor with a subdural hematoma, and three events not otherwise specified. This retrospective survey did not include all donors and may have underreported adverse events. This report, furthermore, did not report the experiences of related and unrelated donors separately. The risks reported for healthy donors reported by unrelated donor registries may underestimate the risks faced by donors for related recipients, who may undergo collection despite comorbid illnesses that would preclude participation in an unrelated donor registry. Most donors are able to return to routine activities 1 to 2 days after harvesting, although the recovery time for the 67 donors reporting serious mechanical injury was a median of 10 months (range, 1 to 96 months).[30]

The usual volume harvested from healthy donors is approximately 10 to 15 mL of marrow per kilogram of recipient body weight to achieve the desired nucleated cell and CD34$^+$ cell doses. This results in a blood loss of 800 to 1000 mL for donors providing marrow for an average-sized adult recipient. The quantity of marrow harvested from autologous patients may be greater, reflecting previous chemotherapy given to these patients. Donors for pediatric recipients will lose proportionately less blood. Most patients and donors receive blood transfusions to alleviate symptoms of volume depletion. With proper preharvest autologous blood storage, use of homologous blood for healthy first-time allogeneic donors should be extremely rare. For a blood loss of less than 10 mL/kg of donor weight, salt solutions are acceptable for volume replacement. Colloid solutions, such as hydroxyethyl starch, also can be used to avoid homologous blood transfusion for blood losses between 10 and 20 mL/kg donor weight. Blood transfusion will be required for larger blood losses (>20 mL/kg) or for patients with comorbid illnesses. Homologous blood transfusions must be irradiated to prevent transfusion-associated GVHD in the transplant recipient. Donors undergoing second harvest shortly after the first harvest are more likely to require homologous blood.[23] Oral iron supplements should be considered for healthy donors, particularly for female donors or donors from whom a large blood volume is to be harvested.

COLLECTION OF UMBILICAL CORD BLOOD STEM CELLS FOR TRANSPLANTATION

Cord Blood Collection Techniques

Advantages of this source of HSC include the ability of public cord blood banks to target collections from ethnic minority populations not well represented in the various unrelated donor registries and the relative immaturity of the donor immune system allowing transplantation of HLA mismatched units without overwhelming GVHD. The primary obstacle to the widespread use of cord blood cells is the limited quantity of HSC collected, and one public UCB bank predicted that from less than 5% to less than 38% (depending on the cell dose criterion for transplantation) of the units stored in that bank would be acceptable for transplantation of an 80-kg adult patient.[34] The speed and success of engraftment are predicted by the total nucleated cell dose and, more important, by the quantity of CD34$^+$ cells or infused colony-forming units (CFUs).[35]

UCB is collected from the placental vein after delivery of the infant and transection of the cord, either before delivery of the placenta by the obstetrician or by laboratory personnel after delivery of the placenta.[34] Published reports conflict regarding the volume of UCB collected and the likelihood of obtaining a product inadequate for storage with either in utero or ex utero collection. The timing of cord clamping after delivery of the infant is associated with the volume of cord blood collected, and greater volumes are collected with earlier clamping. Greater cell quantities were found for infants with greater birth weight, but no difference was found based on gender or gestational age. Ethnic background appears to predict the cell quantities, with smaller quantities of cells collected from ethnic minorities compared with whites.[36] UCB usually is collected by cannulation of the umbilical cord veins with aspiration of the blood into a collection bag. Collection of cord blood into open containers results in an unacceptable rate of bacterial contamination. Perfusion of the placenta with salt solutions may increase the cell number collected, but this has not been widely adopted. Many cord blood banks reduce the volume of the product by red cell and plasma depletion to minimize storage space and to reduce possible infusion-related toxicities from mature blood cells contained in unfractionated cord blood units.[37] Bacterial contamination of UCB products is of concern, especially in the collection of products for related donor transplantation by obstetricians with limited or no experience in HSC collection and processing.[38] The identification and evaluation of the donor and the collection techniques used should be viewed as the first step in a manufacturing process with adequately validated procedures, personnel training, quality control, and performance improvement oversight.

COLLECTION OF PERIPHERAL BLOOD STEM CELLS FOR TRANSPLANTATION

Background

The presence of HSC in the peripheral circulation was suggested by animal studies as early as 1951.[39] Although the nature of the survival agent was not recognized at that time, parabiosis experiments demonstrated that some factor in the blood of a healthy animal was able to rescue another animal from the effects of lethal irradiation. Subsequently, a number of animal models demonstrated the presence of HSC in the peripheral blood and the successful use of these cells to rescue animals from the marrow-lethal effects of radiation. The concentration of HSC in the peripheral blood normally is very low, requiring the processing of large quantities of blood to collect the quantity of HSC equivalent to what could be collected in a bone marrow harvest. For this reason, PBSC transplantation initially was limited to a few transplant programs that explored this source of HSC for patients who otherwise were ineligible for marrow harvesting, collecting cells during steady-state hematopoiesis or during the transient increase in circulating HSC that occurred during recovery from marrow hypoplasia-producing chemotherapy.[40-44] These early reports noted that engraftment could be achieved sooner after infusion of PBSC components compared with marrow cell transplantation. However, because of the occasionally limited quantity of HSC that was collected from the peripheral blood, the kinetics of engraftment for some patients was considerably slower (Table 96-3). The effective mobilization of HSC achieved by cytokine or chemokine administration[45-47] and the reliability of same-day flow cytometric analysis in assessing the quality of the collection are the direct bases for the rapid and widespread adoption of PBSC as a source of HSC for transplantation (see box on Mobilization and Collection of Peripheral Blood Stem Cell for Autologous Transplantation).

Cytokine-mobilized PBSC components contain much greater numbers of cells expressing the CD34 antigen ($CD34^+$ cells), which, along with myeloid progenitor cells grown in culture (CFU-GM), serve as surrogate markers for the engraftment capacity of the stem cell component. The dose of $CD34^+$ cells infused predicts the kinetics of engraftment (Figs. 96-1 and 96-2). Patient groups that receive higher quantities show a higher probability of quicker recovery of

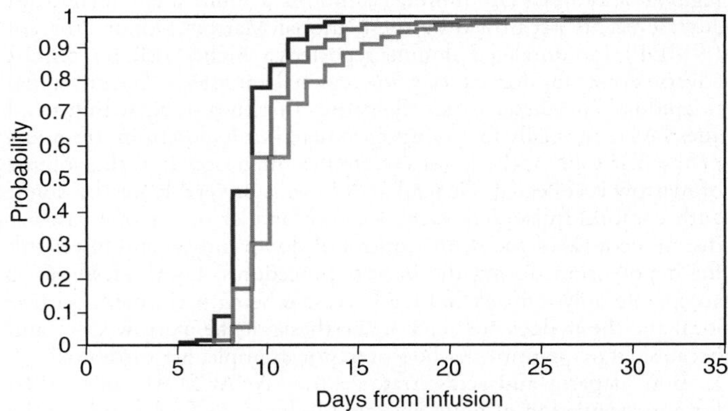

Figure 96-1 Kaplan-Meier probability of achieving $\geq 0.5 \times 10^9$ neutrophils/L for $<5.0 \times 10^6$ (–), >5.0 to 10.0×10^6 (..), and $>10 \times 10^6$ (—) $CD34^+$ cells per kilogram ($P = 0.0001$). *(From Weaver CH, Hazelton B, Birch R, et al: An analysis of engraftment kinetics as a function of the CD34 content of peripheral blood progenitor cell collections in 692 patients after the administration of myeloablative chemotherapy.* Blood *86:3961, 1995.)*

Table 96-3 Relationship Among Mobilization Therapy, Dose of Progenitor Cells, and Engraftment Kinetics for Autologous Peripheral Blood Stem Cell Transplantation

			Progenitor Cell Dose		Engraftment Kinetics	
Author	**No. of Patients**	**Mobilization Therapy**	***CFU-GM (× 10^4/kg)***	***$CD34^+$ Cells (× 10^6/kg)***	***ANC >500/μL***	***Platelet >20,000/μL***
To et al[40]	43	Chemotherapy	86.6	ND	11 (9-17)	13.5* (9-NR)
Fermand et al[41]	8	Chemotherapy	5.5	ND	16 (10-25)	12* (10-28)
Juttner et al[42]	8	Chemotherapy	127.2	ND	11 (9-14)	34 (10-90)
Kessinger et al[43]	10	Steady-state	8.0†	ND	22 (11-58)	23 (14-36)
Nademanee et al[44]	30	Steady-state	ND	1.2	20 (9-458)	31 (8-441)
Nademanee et al[44]	39	G-CSF	ND	6.2	10 (7-40)	15.5 (7-63)
Sheridan et al[45]	29	G-CSF	21.0	ND	6 (4-10)	11 (9-136)
Weaver et al[46]	692	Chemotherapy + G-CSF	30.8‡	9.9‡	9 (5-38)	9 (4-53)*
Bensinger et al[47]	124	Chemotherapy + G-CSF	ND	9.4	11 (4-20)	10 (6-65)

Shown are mean values for progenitor cell quantities infused and median times to achieve the particular endpoint of engraftment. *ANC*, Absolute neutrophil count; *G-CSF*, granulocyte colony-stimulating factor; *ND*, not measured; *NR*, not reached.
*Time to achieve >50,000 platelets/μL
†Colony-forming unit granulocyte-macrophage (CFU-GM) cultures performed on thawed cells.
‡Median value.

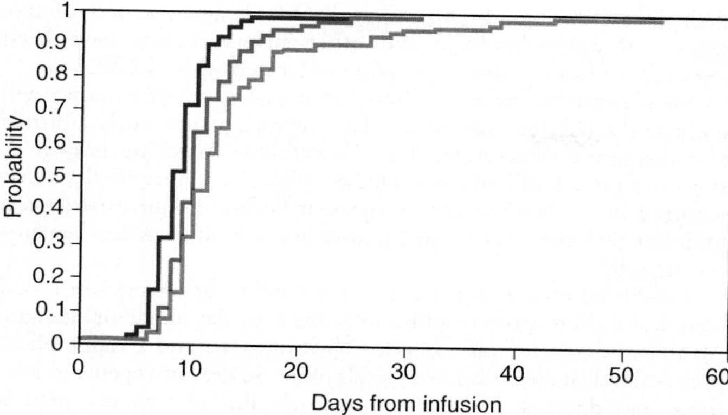

Figure 96-2 Kaplan-Meier probability of achieving ≥20.0 × 10^9 platelets/L for <5.0 × 10^6 (–), >5.0 to 10.0 × 10^6 (..), and >10 × 10^6 (—) CD34$^+$ cells per kilogram (P = 0.0001). *(From Weaver CH, Hazelton B, Birch R, et al: An analysis of engraftment kinetics as a function of the CD34 content of peripheral blood progenitor cell collections in 692 patients after the administration of myeloablative chemotherapy.* Blood *86:3961, 1995.)*

Mobilization and Collection of Peripheral Blood Stem Cell for Autologous Transplantation

Four important considerations when prescribing a mobilization regimen for collection of PBSC for autologous transplantation are as follows: (1) A regimen of chemotherapy followed by G-CSF results in higher numbers of circulating CD34$^+$ cells than will be found with G-CSF alone. (2) The choice of chemotherapy (or cytokine alone mobilization) should be appropriate to the disease and stage of disease for the patient. (3) Each cycle of prior chemotherapy and any previous treatment with radiotherapy will decrease the response to mobilization therapy. (4) Tumor infiltration of the marrow will increase the probability of circulating tumor cells and will decrease the response to mobilization therapy. With these considerations in mind, elective collection of PBSC either before extensive treatment or after a limited number of cycles of debulking chemotherapy should be considered. If tumor contamination is found, additional components can be collected after additional rounds of chemotherapy. The timing of apheresis after chemotherapy and G-CSF mobilization is best guided by measurement of the level of peripheral blood CD34$^+$ cells. Daily or every-other-day quantification of these cells can be initiated after the WBC count reaches 1000/μL. Patients with poor mobilization of CD34$^+$ cells should be considered for large-volume apheresis or addition of plerixafor to reduce the costs associated with daily doses of G-CSF, laboratory testing, apheresis procedures, and cryopreservation. Patients who fail to mobilize may have successful collections if given a short drug holiday before undergoing mobilization with high-dose G-CSF with plerixafor.

neutrophil and platelet counts.[46,47] Although PBSC products containing at least 1 × 10^6 to 2 × 10^6 CD34$^+$ cells per kilogram of recipient weight will achieve hematopoietic stem cell reconstitution, for most patients, cell doses of 2.5 × 10^6 to 5 × 10^6 CD34$^+$ cells per kilogram are desirable, and quicker and more uniform neutrophil and platelet recoveries will be observed with even higher doses.[46,47]

Mobilization of Hematopoietic Stem Cells into Peripheral Blood

The self-renewal and differentiation of HSC is controlled by the surrounding microenvironment of the stem cell niche(s) in which the HSC reside.[48] These niches are composed of a complex three-dimensional architecture of a variety of cell types including sinusoidal endothelial cells, sympathetic nerve fibers, cells of the osteoblastic lineage, macrophages, and mesenchymal stem cells that are responsible for controlling the balance between HSC quiescence, self-renewal, and differentiation. A number of pathways with mutually recognized cellular adhesion molecules and their respective ligands responsible for the spontaneous migration of HSC from the stem cell niche, as well as the multistep process of homing back into the niche, have been identified.[49] The mechanisms by which G-CSF and other cytokines promote mobilization of HSC are being elucidated and appear to be an indirect effect (HSC do not express receptors for G-CSF) on the CXCR4/SDF-1 axis mediated by monocytes and the sympathetic nervous system.[48] The mechanisms of mobilization by chemotherapy and CXCR4 antagonists such as plerixafor are also being determined, and the elucidation of the mechanisms of mobilization and homing may result in more effective harvesting and transplantation techniques.[50]

Cytokine Mobilization

The ability of recombinant hematopoietic cytokines to increase the level of myeloid progenitor cells in the blood, as well as mature blood cells, was reported in 1988 by different groups for both G-CSF and GM-CSF.[51,52] Subsequently, a number of different investigators reported the collection of PBSC from patients using a variety of mobilization regimens, including cytokines alone, cytokine combinations, and combinations of chemotherapy with cytokines (Table 96-2). Various other recombinant human hematopoietic cytokines, including fusion molecules, increase the quantity of CD34$^+$ cells in the peripheral blood, but have not been developed for clinical transplantation.

Granulocyte Colony-Stimulating Factor

G-CSF is the cytokine most commonly used because of its efficacy compared with other cytokines and its relatively benign toxicity profile. Recombinant methionyl human G-CSF (filgrastim) and recombinant human G-CSF (lenograstim) are the two forms of this cytokine available for clinical use.[53] There is slight, if any, difference between these two cytokines in their ability to mobilize PBSC. Watts and colleagues studied 20 healthy volunteers and found that peak levels of CFU-GM in the peripheral blood were 28% higher after treatment with the glycosylated molecule (lenograstim), likely resulting from the higher specific activity of this form.[54] De Arriba and colleagues treated 30 women with breast cancer in a randomized study of these two drugs, using dosages containing bioequivalent units of activity and found no difference in mobilization of CD34$^+$ cells.[55] The two forms have otherwise similar biologic activity and are not further distinguished in this discussion.

Mobilization of Hematopoietic Stem Cells Using Granulocyte Colony-Stimulating Factor

G-CSF is the most potent cytokine currently available for mobilization of HSC. In a randomized study of healthy volunteers comparing G-CSF, GM-CSF, and the combination of both, Lane and colleagues reported an average 0.99% CD34$^+$ cells in the peripheral blood of healthy donors treated with 10 μg/kg/day of G-CSF compared with 0.25% for donors treated with the same dose of GM-CSF.[56] The quantity of CD34$^+$ cells in the peripheral blood before treatment averaged 1.6/μL. After GM-CSF treatment, the level increased to 3/μL, but with G-CSF, the level increased to 61/μL. Each group underwent one leukapheresis on the fifth day of treatment, and the collections from donors treated with G-CSF averaged 119 × 10^6 CD34$^+$ cells compared with 12.6 × 10^6 for the donors treated with GM-CSF.

The appearance of CD34+ cells during administration of G-CSF follows a distinct time course, with the maximal level of CD34+ cells occurring on day 5 after daily G-CSF administration.[57] Smaller numbers of CD34+ are present on days 4 and 6, and the level falls rapidly on subsequent days despite a continual rise in white blood cell (WBC) count.

The number of CD34+ cells collected after G-CSF treatment is proportional to the number of these cells in the peripheral blood before initiation of the cytokine.[17] Although doses as low as 5 mcg/kg/day have been used, there is a dose response to G-CSF, with higher average levels of CD34+ cells achieved with 10 mcg/kg/day compared with 5 mcg/kg/day.[58] With appropriate dosing of allogeneic donors, adequate numbers of CD34+ cells can be collected in one procedure for transplantation of most patients. A similar dose response is observed in autologous patients and may extend to doses as high as 40 mcg/kg/day.[58] An advantage to twice daily dosing of G-CSF has been suggested but not confirmed. Anderlini and colleagues compared administration of 6 mcg/kg given twice daily with 12 mcg/kg given once daily and found no differences in CD34+ cells per liter of blood processed or the yield of CD34+ cells per kilogram collected.[59] In contrast, a second trial enrolling primarily pediatric subjects noted better results with the twice-daily schedule.[60] Patients, especially those previously treated with chemotherapy or radiotherapy, will generally have lower quantities of CD34+ cells mobilized.[50]

Toxicity and Complications of Granulocyte Colony-Stimulating Factor

The toxicity of G-CSF has been most clearly defined in studies of allogeneic donors.[28,61,62] The autologous patient will experience a similar toxicity profile, but with the added complications of the underlying malignancy and its treatment.

Almost all recipients of G-CSF will develop somatic complaints, of which skeletal pain is most prominent (Table 96-4). The somatic complaints are generally tolerable, and few donors will require reduction in dose or discontinuation of the medicine. At present, there appear to be minimal, if any, long-term health risks for the donor. Few serious complications of the mobilization regimen and donation process have been reported.[63] Filgrastim increases spleen size, with a rare patient or donor experiencing splenic rupture. Filgrastim induces a hypercoagulable state, which is of concern for donors (and patients) requiring central venous catheter placement or for those who may have other risk factors for the development of deep venous thrombosis (such as air travel immediately after the collection procedures). Patients with autoimmune disorders may experience a flare-up of their disease during administration of G-CSF, and a variety of case reports of ophthalmologic and other adverse events have been reported for healthy donors or patients treated with G-CSF.

Of concern is the possibility that cytokine administration will increase the risk for marrow dysplasia or malignancy. Although this is a theoretical concern in that the cytokines used are known to stimulate growth of leukemia cells, no clinical evidence (such as that reported in the large registry reviews of healthy donor experiences) indicates that these agents will induce abnormalities in the hematopoietic cell.[63]

G-CSF administration results in a number of changes in blood counts and chemistries in addition to the coagulation factor changes. Alanine aminotransferase, lactate dehydrogenase, and alkaline phosphatase levels increase, and the levels of blood urea nitrogen and bilirubin may decrease.[62] The elevation in alkaline phosphatase level is primarily of bone origin; γ-glutamyl transferase levels remain normal. These abnormalities of serum chemistries resolve within 2 weeks after discontinuation of the medication. G-CSF administration also will result in a decrease in platelet count, especially if the cytokine is administered over 5 to 10 days.[62] WBC counts fall rapidly after discontinuation of G-CSF. In approximately 10% of donors, the WBC count may fall to abnormal levels (but generally still remaining above 1000/μL), reaching a nadir 10 to 14 days after discontinuation of the cytokine before stabilizing at normal levels.

Table 96-4 Incidence of Somatic Complaints for Normal Donors Treated With Granulocyte Colony-Stimulating Factor

	Anderlini et al[28]	Bishop et al[61]	Stroncek[62]
No. of donors	43	41	85
G-CSF dose (mcg/kg/day)	6	5	2-10
Symptoms (%)*			
Malaise	82	83	86
Headache	70	44	28
Fatigue	20	NR	14
Fever	0	27	NR
Chills	NR	22	NR
Nausea	10	22	11

G-CSF, Granulocyte colony-stimulating factor; *NR*, particular complaint not reported in this series.
*Shown are reported proportions of donors experiencing the listed somatic complaint.

Granulocyte-Macrophage Colony-Stimulating Factor

Much of the early experience with the use of hematopoietic cytokines for mobilization of HSC involved GM-CSF and chemotherapy.[52,64] GM-CSF is not as potent as G-CSF,[56,64] although as with G-CSF, there is a dose response in mobilization of PBSC with GM-CSF over a range from 0.3 to 20 mcg/kg/day, without a plateau.[65] In this dose-ranging study, however, the average increase in CFU-GM in the blood at this highest dose level again was only 8.4-fold. In a randomized study comparing GM-CSF with G-CSF, or both drugs used in sequence after chemotherapy administration, patients had faster recovery of counts, required less supportive care including transfusions, and achieved greater collections of CD34+ cells if given one of the G-CSF–containing regimens.[64]

Administration of GM-CSF results in somatic complaints and hepatic function abnormalities similar to those reported after G-CSF administration. In addition, 44% to 80% of patients experience fever, sometimes after each dose, as well as generalized or local skin reactions. Doses greater than 20 mcg/kg/day are poorly tolerated because of fluid retention, pleural and pericardial inflammation, and venous thrombosis. A "first-dose reaction," characterized by hypoxia and hypotension occurring within 3 hours of administration, has been described for some recipients, especially after IV administration.

Other Hematopoietic Cytokines

Recognition of the mobilization potential of G-CSF led many investigators to study other hematopoietic cytokines, including erythropoietin, monocyte–colony-stimulating factor (M-CSF), interleukin-3, PIXY 321 (a fusion molecule), and stem cell factor (SCF) for their capacity to mobilize HSC into the peripheral blood. Used as single agents, these cytokines resulted in only an approximately 5- to 10-fold increase in circulating CFU-GM or CD34+ cells. Only SCF is approved for human use (in Europe), and none of these cytokines are widely used in clinical HSC transplantation.

Chemotherapy Plus Cytokine Mobilization

The number of HSC in the peripheral blood is greatly increased during the early hematologic recovery phase after marrow hypoplasia-producing chemotherapy (Table 96-3). Moreover, chemotherapy plus cytokine generally mobilizes greater numbers of PBSC than either agent alone. This finding was confirmed in a randomized study comparing cyclophosphamide followed by G-CSF versus G-CSF alone, in which higher numbers of CD34 cells were found for the patients treated with the chemotherapy-based regimen.[66] However, no differences in the degree of tumor cell contamination of PBSC components, engraftment kinetics, or survival were found. A wide variety of different chemotherapy regimens has been used successfully for mobilization of HSC into the blood, with cyclophosphamide- or ifosfamide-based regimens being most commonly used. The primary consideration is that the choice of chemotherapy used must meet the treatment needs of the patient. However, the choice of chemotherapy regimen can affect the mobilization of HSC. Demirer and colleagues studied the effect of different chemotherapy regimens for mobilization of HSC for patients with breast cancer.[67] Four regimens were used, all involving CY, but including etoposide with or without cisplatin, or paclitaxel. All patients also received G-CSF. The median quantity of $CD34^+$ cells collected on the first day of apheresis after cyclophosphamide mobilization was 0.9×10^6 per kilogram of patient weight. The addition of etoposide and then of etoposide and cisplatin increased the first-day yield to 8.1×10^6 and 3.5×10^6 $CD34^+$ cells per kilogram, respectively, in separate cohorts of patients. The median number of $CD34^+$ cells harvested on the first day of apheresis after cyclophosphamide plus paclitaxel was 11.1×10^6/kg, and more than 50% of the women mobilized with this last regimen achieved the target dose of $CD34^+$ cells in one apheresis procedure. Of the 100 women studied, 94 achieved the target dose of greater than 5×10^6 $CD34^+$ cells per kilogram. Only four patients failed to reach a lower but acceptable dose of 2.5×10^6 $CD34^+$ cells per kilogram.

Chemokines

Chemokines (chemoattractant cytokines) are a family of approximately 40 related small proteins that influence leukocyte (and malignant cell) migration and function.[68] Chemokines with varying effects on different WBC populations have been identified, as have a number of chemokine receptors. The roles of chemokines and chemokine receptors in the trafficking of HSC into and from the bone marrow compartment are under active investigation.[69]

In a preclinical study, administration to both mice and rhesus monkeys of a modified CXC chemokine GRO-β after 4 days of G-CSF resulted in a fivefold increase in the number of circulating stem and progenitor cells compared with G-CSF alone, with also a much shorter time course of release, measured in hours.[70] Furthermore, more rapid recovery of hematopoietic function was observed for animals given similar quantities of cells collected after administration of the chemokine and cytokine combination. IL-8, a related ligand for the CXCR2 receptor, mobilizes stem cells within 15 to 30 minutes of injection into mice,[71] which appears to involve increased matrix metalloproteinase-9 activity detectable immediately before the appearance of HSC in the peripheral circulation. Murine studies demonstrate a mobilizing effect of the chemokine SDF-1 and its receptor CXCR4 that can be blocked by neutralizing antibodies to either.[71] The bicyclam molecule plerixafor disrupts SDF-1/CXCR4 binding and has been shown to result in mobilization of HSC in murine, canine, and nonhuman transplant models.

Similar signaling pathways are used for mobilization and homing of normal and malignant hematopoietic cells.[72] Although PBSC products collected after G-CSF mobilization generally contain fewer detectable tumor cells than does bone marrow harvested from the same patient, the effects of chemokine treatment on the degree of PBSC contamination and on disease relapse after autologous transplantation remain to be elucidated. For example, acute myelogenous leukemia cells express CXCR4 in varying levels and homing of primary human AML cells into NOD/SCID mice is CXCR4 dependent, similar to normal human stem cells. Similar studies of chemokine control on tumor cell growth, migration, and metastasis are being reported from a number of laboratories.

Plerixafor

Plerixafor is a small molecule inhibitor of CXCR4. Clinical studies of HSC mobilization using plerixafor (AMD3100) with or without G-CSF priming are being reported in both healthy donors and patients undergoing autologous or allogeneic HSC transplantation. In a study involving normal volunteers, a single dose of plerixafor was equal in mobilization of $CD34^+$ cells to administration of a standard 5-day course of G-CSF.[73] However, a single dose of plerixafor given on day 5 of a daily course of G-CSF administration resulted in a further 3.8-fold increase in circulating $CD34^+$ cells (as well as B and T cells, which may be important in allogeneic transplantation). Randomized phase III studies conducted in patients undergoing autologous PBSC transplantation in the treatment of multiple myeloma or non-Hodgkin lymphoma demonstrated a clear increase in $CD34^+$ cells collected by the addition of plerixafor to filgrastim.[74,75] Plerixafor was also effective in remobilization attempts for patients who failed initial collection goals.[76] Plerixafor clearance is proportional to degree of renal function in patients with renal failure.[77] Minor gastrointestinal symptoms appear to be the most common toxicities of this medication.

Strategies for the Patient Who Is Difficult to Mobilize

Most patients achieve the targeted dose of $CD34^+$ cells after processing 20 to 30 L of blood in one to three apheresis procedures. However, approximately 5% to as many as 30% of patients in various series have inadequate collections because only small numbers of HSC are present in the peripheral blood despite the administration of hematopoietic cytokines. Of note, the number of days of apheresis separately predicts the kinetics of neutrophil engraftment beyond the $CD34^+$ cell dose, indicating an undefined measurement of graft quality, probably a reflection of the various quantities of $CD34^+$ cell subsets and $CD34^-$ stem cells.[78] Patient-specific factors predictive of poor mobilization include older age, marrow disease, prior radiotherapy, and prior chemotherapy.[50] Approximately 50% of patients who fail to achieve the targeted dose of $CD34^+$ cells will achieve this goal on a second attempt. High-dose (15 mg/kg bid) G-CSF after a 2- to 4-week drug holiday to allow marrow recovery is one strategy. Combination cytokine therapy is also of potential value in this situation, and the combination of SCF with G-CSF may be effective for patients who reside in countries where SCF is available. The addition of GM-CSF to G-CSF is not of proven value. Initial experience with plerixafor suggests that the agent will often be effective when used in combination with G-CSF for collection of PBSC from patients who failed a prior mobilization attempt.[76] Treatment with a use of cyclophosphamide- or ifosfamide-based mobilizing chemotherapy plus cytokine regimen also will be effective but may be associated with increased toxicity.[79] Bone marrow can be harvested, but the poor mobilization of PBSC predicts for a poor marrow harvest. Patients who fail initial collection attempts frequently will fail subsequent attempts, and transplantation of these patients with a lower dose of $CD34^+$ cells (as low as 1×10^6 $CD34^+$ cells per kilogram) may be an option.

It is preferable to avoid collection failure. Consideration should be given to the prophylactic collection of PBSC early in the course of treatment for patients who later may be candidates for autologous HSC transplantation but who are advised to receive multiple courses of therapy or therapy involving alkylating agents or radiation therapy. HSC can be collected and cryopreserved before extensive therapy while the patient has good marrow function and stored for years without obvious progressive loss of engraftment potential.

Timing of Apheresis

A major problem with chemotherapy-based mobilization regimens is the difficulty in determining the optimal time to commence HSC collection. Apheresis devices can collect only those $CD34^+$ cells actually being released into and circulating in the peripheral blood. It is

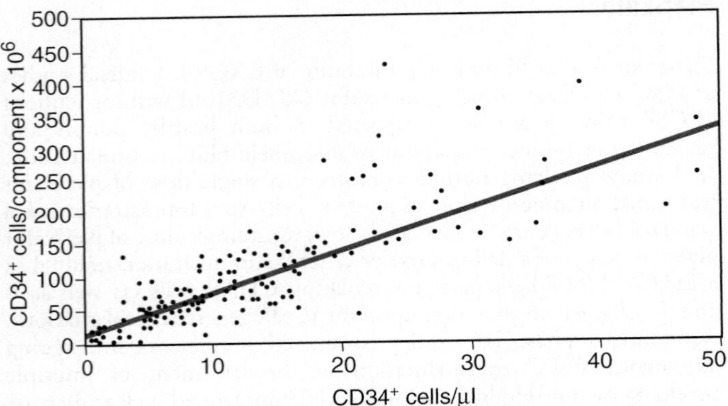

Figure 96-3 Relationship between quantity of CD34$^+$ cells in the peripheral blood and number collected by apheresis using apheresis and flow cytometric techniques. Data shown are limited to peripheral blood CD34$^+$ cell numbers <50.0/µL (n = 157, r = 0.82, P <0.001).

possible to estimate the quantity of CD34$^+$ cells that will be collected during apheresis by multiplying the quantity of CD34$^+$ cells in the blood by the total volume of blood processed during the apheresis procedure and by the efficiency of the apheresis device in collecting these cells. If the device has an efficiency of 50% and the patient undergoes a 10-L exchange, approximately 5×10^7 CD34$^+$ cells will be collected for a peripheral blood level of 10 CD34$^+$ cells per microliter and 5×10^8 CD34$^+$ cells for a blood level of CD34$^+$ cells that is 10-fold higher. Although many protocols call for initiation of apheresis after chemotherapy mobilization when the WBC count has recovered to greater than 1000/µL, there is a poor, if any, correlation between the peripheral blood white cell or mononuclear cell counts and the CD34$^+$ cells in the peripheral blood. Characteristics that suggest a higher CD34$^+$ cell level are a rapidly rising WBC count, shift in differential to immature myeloid cells, circulating nucleated red cells, and platelet transfusion independence. However, it is much more cost effective to obtain an actual measurement of CD34$^+$ cells in the blood and to time the apheresis collection when these cells are present in adequate numbers. Fig. 96-3 shows such a relationship for patients with lower concentrations of CD34$^+$ cells in the peripheral blood and illustrates the very poor collections obtained when the peripheral blood CD34$^+$ count is less than 10/µL. Although there is considerable error in the enumeration of CD34$^+$ cells at levels less than 5/µL, this error is not clinically relevant because even a doubling of the CD34$^+$ cells in this low range still results in a very poor apheresis yield.

The level of CD34$^+$ cells in the peripheral blood at which to start apheresis is a clinical decision. Although levels in the range from 50 to 100/µL or greater will reduce the number of apheresis procedures necessary to achieve a target goal of CD34$^+$ cells, each day's delay in initiating apheresis incurs the costs of additional cytokine administration and blood testing. In some patients who previously have undergone extensive treatment and who may show a slowly rising WBC count, multiple apheresis procedures may be necessary to achieve the target goal. No patient should undergo apheresis if the peripheral blood CD34$^+$ cell count is less than 5/µL (see Fig. 96-3). For patients with CD34$^+$ cell counts in the range from 10/µL to 20/µL, it is possible to process more blood per day using large-volume leukapheresis (LVL) techniques, thereby reducing the numbers of days the patients are required to return to the apheresis unit. Most patients mobilized with chemotherapy have a rising CD34$^+$ cell count in the peripheral blood, so starting apheresis the day after the patient has achieved a desirable CD34$^+$ level generally is feasible.[80]

The timing of apheresis after G-CSF mobilization differs from the timing after chemotherapy and cytokine mobilization. For both patients and healthy donors, the peak concentration of CD34$^+$ cells occurs on day 5 of G-CSF administration (after four daily doses).[57] Lower levels are present on day 4, and the concentration continues to fall after day 6, even if cytokine administration is continued and despite a possible continued rise in WBC count. Thus PBSC collection should be initiated on day 4 or 5 of G-CSF administration. The kinetics of CD34$^+$ cells in the peripheral blood for patients and donors mobilized with G-CSF alone are so reliable that monitoring of peripheral blood levels is not necessary unless there is concern that the patient has failed to mobilize cells and it is practical to obtain the cell count rapidly enough to initiate apheresis on the same day.

Physician Prescription for Apheresis and Peripheral Blood Stem Cell Processing

The attending physician should be aware of apheresis and laboratory procedures in order to maximize the value of PBSC components. The choices of venous access, anticoagulant(s), blood volume processed, target dose of CD34$^+$ cells, and cryopreservation volumes can be individualized. Apheresis unit staff may ask for guidance regarding pain medications, concurrent medications, and blood transfusions (although it is advisable to avoid transfusion during the apheresis procedure because of citrate or other reactions and because changes in the hematocrit may affect the efficiency of the collection). Adequate numbers of CD34$^+$ cells can be collected for more than one cycle of chemotherapy. It is important to communicate with the cryopreservation facility if PBSC components will be used to support more than one cycle of chemotherapy or if DMSO toxicity is of concern, in order to facilitate appropriate packaging of each product. Current cytometric techniques for quantification of CD34$^+$ cells require at least 1 hour of processing, so it may not be practical to prescribe the number of CD34$^+$ cells to be frozen in each bag. However, it is possible to divide the component into the number of bags equaling the number of anticipated infusions so that equal numbers of CD34$^+$ cells will be available for each.

Timing of Apheresis Using Plerixafor

Plerixafor administration results in a rapid mobilization of HSC into the peripheral blood with peak CD34$^+$ cell and CFU-GM concentrations occurring about 6 to 10 hours but with a wide range of activity extending to over 24 hours after administration of a dose of 240 mcg/kg.[81-83] The initial phase III studies demonstrating efficacy of this agent in patients failing to mobilize adequate cells with G-CSF alone required administration of plerixafor about 10 hours before apheresis, followed by daily administration of plerixafor until completion of collections. The broad duration of activity may allow alternate timing schedules and, conceivably, two apheresis procedures after one dose of plerixafor (particularly for patients with renal impairment[77]), although rigorous clinical studies addressing alternate timing schedules have not been performed.

Collection of PBSC by Apheresis

A number of apheresis devices are available for separating HSC from the peripheral blood. The devices may be classified as continuous flow (e.g., Fenwal CS3000, COBE Spectra, Fresenius AS104) or discontinuous flow (e.g., Haemonetics family of equipment). Discontinuous-flow devices have the advantage of requiring only a single venous access. Continuous-flow devices require two access lines for aspiration and return of blood, but they process much larger volumes of blood in a shorter period of time. All apheresis devices collect HSC. The choice of apheresis device used by the collection center depends primarily on the needs and experience of the center. Continuous-flow devices are more efficient in the collection of PBSC and are, accordingly, preferred over discontinuous-flow devices (see box on Physician Prescription for Apheresis and Peripheral Blood Stem Cell Processing).

Apheresis Technology

Apheresis technology is widely used for collection of platelets and other blood products from healthy donors and is considered to be without major risk to the donor. The important safety considerations for PBSC collection are the same as for platelet collection and include the venous access to be used for the procedure, the extracorporeal volume of blood during the procedure, and the solutions administered to the donor. Of note, however, PBSC collection for autologous transplantation involves patients with underlying medical conditions who may require considerable nursing care during the procedure. In a prospective evaluation of 2408 healthy unrelated volunteer donors, apheresis-associated adverse events were reported by 20% of female donors ($n = 964$) and 7% of male donors ($n = 1444$) on the first day of apheresis, falling to 10% and 4%, respectively, on the second day of collection (if performed).[63] Most (51%) of reported adverse events were related to citrate infusion. A smaller proportion of donors (22%) reported problems with venous access. Rare (1%-6% of events) adverse events included hypertension or hypotension, allergic reactions, fatigue, and syncope. The placement of a central venous catheter was required by 17% of female donors and 4% of male donors. Also, larger-volume and repetitive exchanges will result in platelet depletion.[62] The platelet count may reach its nadir several days after completion of the apheresis collections and discontinuation of G-CSF, and donors should be counseled in this regard.

Important caveats are that the donors in this analysis from the unrelated donor registry met strictly defined health criteria and were between 18 and 69 years of age. A higher probability of adverse events may be expected in patients and in donors of older (or younger) age. For example, in an older retrospective publication, Goldberg and colleagues studied the complications occurring during 554 PBSC collections from 75 consecutive patients.[84] Patient diagnoses and the mobilization treatment regimens were varied. All but one patient had subclavian or jugular venous system catheters placed for apheresis. A median of nine collections per patient were performed using a discontinuous-flow apheresis device. The most common problems were related to the venous catheters: 50% of patients developed at least one occlusion. Hypocalcemia occurred in 14.6% of patients and hypotension in 13.3%. Sixteen percent of patients experienced infectious complications during the PBSC collection period.

Staffing of the apheresis unit should be appropriate for the medical condition of the patients undergoing apheresis. Staffing must include nurses familiar with the care of the oncologic patient who may be recovering from marrow hypoplasia complicated by neutropenic fever requiring multiple medications and the care of a central venous catheter. Collection of PBSC by apheresis in the outpatient setting should be performed only after careful review of the medical support requirements for the individual patient or donor, and it should never be assumed to be a safer alternative for the donor or patient with a serious comorbid illness than marrow harvesting conducted in the intensive care setting of the operating room.

Venous Access

Adequate venous access is required for optimal apheresis technique. Continuous-flow apheresis devices require two-lumen access with a stable blood flow capacity generally greater than 20 mL/min. Single-lumen access may be used with discontinuous-flow apheresis devices, although at a much slower rate of blood processing. The great majority (≈95%) of adult male allogeneic PBSC donors have adequate arm veins for the procedure to be conducted "vein to vein," with female donors more likely to require alternate venous access.[63] Some donors, especially those with small veins and undergoing several daily procedures, may require placement of a temporary venous catheter. Venous access for the patient undergoing collection for autologous PBSC transplantation is much more heterogeneous. Vein-to-vein procedures can be performed, even on several consecutive days, with proper phlebotomy technique and postcollection care of the phlebotomy site. Most patients received previous chemotherapy or are proceeding directly to transplantation, conditions for which tunneled access is commonly placed. Ideally, this venous access should be appropriate both for the apheresis procedures and the subsequent transplant. Length, lumen size, and wall stiffness all affect the blood flow that can be achieved through a catheter. For this reason, the commonly used dual-lumen Hickman or Broviac catheters usually are unsuitable for apheresis, as are all subcutaneously placed ports. Most triple-lumen catheters are inadequate because of the small lumen size. If such access is already in place, consideration can be given to replacement with a shorter, stiffer tunneled catheter or to placement of a temporary percutaneous dialysis/apheresis catheter. The catheters designed for dialysis and apheresis have adequate wall thickness to prevent collapse during aspiration of blood as well as a tip design that decreases local recirculation of blood and the resulting decrease in apheresis efficiency. Catheters of 10 F or larger size are appropriate for adult patients. Pediatric patients, whose blood flow rates are considerably slower, may use catheter sizes of 5 to 7 F.[85]

Anticoagulation for PBSC Collection

Anticoagulants are added to the blood during apheresis to prevent clotting of the extracorporeal circuit and clumping of cells in the component. Citrate anticoagulants have a proven record of safety in the apheresis of healthy platelet donors. The major drawback is the risk for a symptomatic decrease in the level of ionized calcium ("citrate toxicity"), especially during processing of large volumes of blood. Citrate ions chelate calcium ions (and other divalent cations such as magnesium), making them unavailable for Ca^{2+}-dependent metabolic reactions. ACD-A contains 10.67 g of citrate per 500-mL volume in the form of trisodium citrate and citric acid. Citrate is diffused throughout the extravascular space, and this diffusion is the first defense against citrate toxicity. The body size and difference in muscle mass between men and women results in an increased risk for citrate toxicity for women in particular and smaller donors in general. Metabolism by liver, kidney, and muscle also reduces the concentration of citrate. Metabolism of citrate becomes more important during prolonged apheresis procedures such as LVL. The initial signs of citrate toxicity include circumoral or acral paresthesias and may progress to nausea, vomiting, loss of consciousness, tetany, and seizures. Because pediatric patients may not be able to relate the initial symptoms of the condition, citrate toxicity should be considered as the cause of any change of behavior, such as crying, during the apheresis procedure. Citrate toxicity is prevented by limiting the quantity of citrate infused either by decreasing the blood flow rate through the apheresis device or changing the blood-to-citrate ratio. The processing of blood of patients experiencing the initial symptoms of citrate toxicity should be temporarily halted until the symptoms abate and then resumed at a slower rate. The benefit of oral calcium supplements for these patients is not certain. Heparin can be used as a replacement for some or all of the citrate, although additional citrate is added to the component bag to prevent clumping of platelets. Some centers that use citrate anticoagulants also administer intermittent or continuous infusions of calcium gluconate during the procedure, especially if large volumes of blood are being processed. However, excessive calcium replacement can induce cardiac dysfunction.

Large-Volume Leukapheresis

The apheresis device has a uniform and fairly reproducible efficiency of collection. Thus for a consistent quantity of blood processed through the machine, the quantity of $CD34^+$ cells collected is directly related to the number present in the peripheral blood. Greater quantities of $CD34^+$ cells can be collected by increasing the number of these cells in the peripheral circulation or by increasing the volume of blood processed by the device. For patients with lower $CD34^+$ cell levels, multiple apheresis procedures will be required to achieve the target dose of $CD34^+$ cells needed for transplantation. An alternate approach is to process the same total quantity of blood but in fewer, longer procedures. LVL is not standardly defined, but in general usage it refers to processing of more than two or three times the patient's blood volume. Typically, the quantity of blood processed is six or more times the patient's blood volume, often 25 to 36 L of blood. The advantage of LVL is that it reduces the number of days of cytokine administration and apheresis, with associated reduced costs of laboratory processing and testing. The apheresis techniques are the same as those used for processing of smaller volumes of blood, although blood flow rates may be increased to reduce the time required. The risks of LVL are the increased time required and the higher risk for citrate (or other anticoagulant) toxicity. Patients will also incur a proportional drop in platelet counts and may become profoundly thrombocytopenic.

Most reports of LVL describe the collection of more $CD34^+$ cells than are calculated to be present in the peripheral blood at the initiation of the apheresis procedure. Most likely, the ongoing release of cells from the marrow replaces those cells removed by apheresis (or returning to the marrow space).[86] Apheresis of $CD34^+$ cells is a three-compartment system consisting of the extracorporeal circuit of the apheresis device (including the collection bag), the peripheral blood, and the marrow. It is not obvious that the apheresis technique itself "mobilizes" $CD34^+$ cells, as suggested by some authors. This phenomenon, if it occurs, may be related to a decrease in divalent cations resulting from the citrate anticoagulant, possibly affecting cell adhesion forces.

Studies at the Fred Hutchinson Cancer Research Center demonstrated a continuous release of $CD34^+$ cells from the marrow (and, presumably, return to the marrow space).[86] Patients having higher levels of $CD34^+$ cells in the peripheral blood appeared to have a greater number of these cells circulating between the marrow and peripheral blood compartments (Table 96-5). In this model the apheresis device merely serves as a siphon, removing these cells from the blood as they are released from the marrow. If this description of $CD34^+$ cell kinetics is accurate, it may be possible to deplete these cells from the blood and marrow by prolonged processing, but probably only if limited numbers of them are present in the marrow compartment. Also, the model suggests that higher blood flow rates used to shorten the apheresis procedure may be counterproductive for patients with low $CD34^+$ cell levels in the blood because of the slower rate of release of $CD34^+$ cells in these patients.

Table 96-5 Replenishment of $CD34^+$ Cells During Large-Volume Leukapheresis*

	CD34+ Cells				
UPN	*Blood (per μL)*	*Blood (Total)*	*Harvested (Total)*	*Released (Total)*	*Released (per min)*
10605	6.5	34.9	123.5	88.6	0.3
10698	15.6	603.3	1438.1	540.8	2.1
10849	30.7	109.7	211.1	62.6	0.3
10920	37.9	214.2	952.8	57.0	1.6
11128	66.1	280.6	1010.8	532.7	1.9

*Shown are numbers of $CD34^+$ cells in the peripheral blood or apheresis component for five patients with acute myelogenous leukemia or multiple myeloma undergoing large-volume leukapheresis after granulocyte colony-stimulating factor (G-CSF) or chemotherapy plus G-CSF mobilization treatment. Blood volumes processed were six times the calculated blood volume of the patient. Peripheral blood stem cell collection was performed on the COBE Spectra. The total number of $CD34^+$ cells in the blood (third column) was calculated from the level of $CD34^+$ cells in the blood and the estimated blood volume of the patient. The total number of $CD34^+$ cells released (fifth column) was calculated from the total number in the apheresis component and the number in the peripheral blood after collection minus the total number in the peripheral blood at the start of the collection procedure. All $CD34^+$ cell quantities (except blood levels reported per μL) are $\times 10^6$. Full data are given in Rowley SD, Yu J, Heimfeld S, et al: Trafficking of CD34+ cells into the peripheral circulation during collection of peripheral blood stem cells by apheresis. *Bone Marrow Transplant* 28:649, 2001.

Pediatric Donors and Patients

PBSC can be collected from pediatric patients, including infants. The special challenges of the pediatric patient arise from the fixed extracorporeal blood volume of the apheresis device, the need for venous catheters for blood access, and the management of a patient who may be unwilling or unable to rest quietly for the period of apheresis. It is especially important in management of the pediatric patient that timing of apheresis be optimal to minimize the number of procedures required to achieve the desired quantity of PBSC. Given these considerations, a number of centers have reported successful collection of PBSC from pediatric patients and donors.

Almost all pediatric patients undergo insertion of a venous catheter adequate for the flow rates expected, although older patients (>12 years) may tolerate vein-to-vein procedures. The whole blood flow rate for the pediatric patient is much reduced compared with that of adult patients, and catheters as small as 5 F may be adequate.

Appropriate management of fluid balance during the apheresis procedure is critical for the smaller patient. The volume of red blood cells contained in the extracorporeal circuit of continuous flow apheresis device could represent 30% to 50% of the red cell mass of a pediatric donor. Although discontinuous-flow devices are appealing because of the feasibility of performing apheresis with a single-lumen venous access, they may result in even higher extracorporeal volumes and should be avoided in the smallest patients. The obvious solution to this problem is to prime the apheresis device with ABO-compatible, irradiated red blood cells (leukocyte-depleted and cytomegalovirus-negative blood may also be desirable) when the blood in the extracorporeal circuit is expected to exceed 15% of the patient's blood volume. Packed red blood cell units can be diluted with saline or albumin (to reduce the loss of plasma protein that may occur). The red cells remaining in the extracorporeal circuit at the completion of the run need not be returned ("rinse-back"), although if performed slowly with monitoring of vital signs, rinse-back may actually increase the hematocrit after the procedure and otherwise reduce the need for red cell transfusions for these patients. For the intermediate-size pediatric patient (weight 25-50 kg), the apheresis device can be primed with a 5% albumin solution. This step will reduce the albumin loss that otherwise would occur. However, clotting proteins and other proteins not contained in this solution may decrease with repetitive apheresis.

The pediatric patient may not exhibit or relate the prodromal symptoms associated with citrate toxicity. Continuous calcium gluconate infusion can be incorporated into the procedure, or heparin can be added to the citrate anticoagulant solution or used as the sole anticoagulant. Sedation of the pediatric patient is usually not necessary, however, and hinders the ability to recognize the symptoms of citrate toxicity. (Some patients may require antihistamine premedication if the apheresis device is primed with red blood cells.) Centers routinely performing pediatric PBSC collection should design an environment conducive to the management of pediatric patients and develop support procedures that recognize the unique physical and cognitive features of pediatric patients.

The range in blood volumes for pediatric donors of differing ages is greater than the range for adult donors. Therefore most centers set a goal for volume processed based on the individual's blood volume instead of a set volume (e.g., two blood volumes versus 6 L of blood) for all patients. The pediatric patient may undergo LVL to achieve the target goal of HSC with fewer procedures. Blood flow rates for pediatric patients are slower than for adults to minimize the risk for citrate reaction. As with adults, the timing of apheresis can be optimized by monitoring the quantity of $CD34^+$ cells in the peripheral blood.

QUALITY CONTROL OF HSC PRODUCTS

Quantity of Bone Marrow Cells for Transplantation

Cell dose normally is used as a surrogate for the stem cell content of the marrow product because the definition of adequate HSC products predated the availability of flow cytometric analysis of HSC content, and nucleated cell counting is the only quality control measure easily performed during the collection procedure. For autologous transplantation, cell doses of 1×10^8 nucleated cells per kilogram are adequate. Based on early reports that smaller quantities increased the risk for engraftment failure, most centers target 3×10^8 nucleated cells per kilogram of recipient weight for allogeneic transplantation. However, those early reports were of patients being treated for aplastic anemia, in which engraftment failure is a more common event. A review of unrelated donor transplantation found that recipients of higher cell doses experienced faster neutrophil and platelet engraftment, as well as better leukemia-free survival.[87] Pretreatment of the marrow donor with either GM-CSF or G-CSF may increase the number of myeloid progenitor cells harvested and decrease the period of posttransplant aplasia to that achievable by PBSC transplantation (see Table 96-2). $CD34^+$ cell dose now is being correlated with transplant outcomes—with more rapid engraftment kinetics, possibly lower transplant-related mortality, and better overall survival, for example, in recipients of allogeneic bone marrow products containing higher quantities of $CD34^+$ cells.[88] This assay should be a routine component of bone marrow product quality control.[88]

Definition of Adequate PBSC Component(s)

The quantity of $CD34^+$ cells in a PBSC component varies greatly and is dependent on the number in the peripheral blood at the time of apheresis, the volume of blood processed, and the efficiency of the apheresis device. Therefore any definition of an adequate component cannot include a set number of $CD34^+$ cells to be contained in any single apheresis component. Instead, one or more components will be collected to meet the appropriate dose of these cells for transplantation. The dose of $CD34^+$ cells required for infusion depends on the intended treatment regimen. For marrow-ablative regimens, increasingly higher $CD34^+$ doses results in greater likelihood of rapid engraftment (Figs. 96-1 and 96-2).[89] Lower doses of $CD34^+$ cells appear satisfactory for nonablative regimens.

Patients who receive a dose of $CD34^+$ cells above a certain threshold will engraft. At lower doses of $CD34^+$ cells, considerable heterogeneity occurs in engraftment speed, especially for platelet engraftment. Why this heterogeneity exists is not known, but it may reflect a weakness in the correlation between $CD34^+$ cells and the cells responsible for engraftment, a greater heterogeneity of $CD34^+$ subsets collected, or perhaps, simply a greater degree of error in the measurement of $CD34^+$ cells at the lower cell concentrations. As the dose of $CD34^+$ cells increases, the engraftment kinetics becomes both more rapid and more consistent for the population studied.[89]

Subset analysis of $CD34^+$ cells may improve the accuracy of predicting neutrophil and platelet engraftment kinetics but does not appear to predict engraftment failure enough to be of clinical utility. Pecora and colleagues reported that the quantity of $CD34^+CD33^-$ cells infused was identified as an independent factor predictive of engraftment kinetics.[90] Dercksen and colleagues reported better correlation between the number of $CD34^+CD33^-$ cells and time to granulocyte engraftment and between the number of $CD34^+CD41^+$ cells and time to platelet engraftment than found with the overall number of $CD34^+$ cells.[91] Coexpression of adhesion molecules is also predictive of hematopoietic recovery, with the same pathways important for both mobilization and homing of HSC.[92] Given the limited range in recovery times when adequate numbers of $CD34^+$ cells are collected and infused, however, this additional information is currently of limited clinical value.

$CD34^+$ cell dose is also predictive of outcome of allogeneic PBSC (and marrow) transplantation.[88] Higher $CD34^+$ cell doses result in better neutrophil and platelet engraftments after either related or unrelated donor transplantation and may correlate with better survival after bone marrow transplantation, but may also be associated with the development of more chronic GVHD.

Management of Donor-Recipient Red Blood Cell Incompatibility

Transplantation of hematopoietic progenitor cells from ABO (or other red cell antigen) incompatible donors occurs in ≈30% of patients undergoing related or unrelated donor allogeneic HSC transplantation.[20] The immunohematologic consequences of red cell incompatible transplantation include delayed red blood cell recovery, pure red cell aplasia, and delayed hemolysis from viable lymphocytes carried in the graft ("passenger lymphocytes"). The risks for these reactions, which may be abrupt in onset and fatal, can be minimized with appropriate graft modifications to remove incompatible red cells and plasma, attention to the pretransplant conditioning and posttransplant immunosuppressive regimens, and prescription of proper blood product support.[20]

Red cell incompatibility is classified into two categories: one in which the recipient has antibodies directed against donor red cells with the potential for acute hemolysis upon infusion of the component (major incompatibility) and one in which the donor has antibodies against the recipient. Although the latter rarely causes difficulty during infusion of incompatible plasma, B lymphocytes carried in the component can form isoagglutinins, resulting in a delayed transfusion reaction 7 to 12 days after transplantation. Although PBSC components have much greater numbers of B cells compared with other HSC products, it is not clear that delayed-type transfusion reactions will be more likely or of greater severity in PBSC recipients. The risk for immediate hemolysis resulting from infusion of incompatible donor red cells is minimized by minimizing the quantity of red cells infused. There is no "safe" quantity of red cells below which the recipient will not experience an immediate transfusion reaction, but fatal reactions appear more likely for recipients of ABO incompatible blood products containing more than 50 mL of red cells.[20] PBSC products collected by apheresis contain only a few milliliters of red blood cells. Bone marrow products can be similarly depleted by processing using an apheresis device. UCB products can be depleted of red cells before cryopreservation to reduce the risk from infusion of ABO incompatible products and to reduce the space requirements for storage.

Tumor Cell Contamination

The probability that tumor cell contamination of HSC product could contribute to relapse was demonstrated by Brenner and colleagues in studies involving the autologous transplantation of genetically marked marrow cells,[93] as well as in individual case reports describing the transmission of malignancy to allogeneic recipients from donors with occult disease at time of harvesting.[25,26] Sensitive immunocytostaining techniques, clonal assays, flow cytometric analysis, and polymerase chain reaction amplification of malignant genetic material detect tumor cells in the autologous PBSC components of many patients with a variety of malignancies.[94] In general, the incidence of contamination (number of patients with positive components) and the level of contamination (number of tumor cells per number of normal cells) is much less for PBSC than for marrow products.

The presence of tumor cells at the time of collection or persisting after ex vivo processing may correlate with the extent of systemic disease or the chemotherapy-sensitivity of disease at the time of cell collection. Whether patients transplanted with autologous PBSC have a lower relapse rate compared with patients receiving bone marrow is not well defined, and appropriate phase III studies of this question will be difficult to design and enroll with patients in light of the other well-defined advantages of PBSC transplantation. In a retrospective study, Sharp and colleagues demonstrated similar probabilities of relapse-free survival in recipients of PBSC or marrow components if the components were free of lymphoma cells.[95] In that study, patients with marrow involvement by lymphoma were assigned to transplantation with PBSC. The authors concluded that PBSC transplantation is a sensible approach to the patient with overt marrow involvement. However, Brugger and colleagues demonstrated that patients with breast cancer involvement of the marrow at the time of chemotherapy mobilization were likely to mobilize tumor cells into the blood. The most disturbing finding of this study is that the tumor cells were detected in the peripheral blood at the same time as CD34$^+$ cells.[96] Similarly, Pecora and colleagues found a relationship between the ability to detect tumors in PBSC components and in bone marrow samples, but they also found a higher incidence of positive PBSC components for patients who required greater numbers of apheresis procedures to achieve the target dose of CD34$^+$ cells.[97] Investigators at The Johns Hopkins Oncology Center found no difference in the incidence of tumor contamination of PBSC components between patients treated with chemotherapy and cytokines and those treated with cytokines alone.[98] Ex vivo purging of tumor cells from PBPC products has not been shown to reduce the risk for relapse after autologous transplantation, either because the techniques are not adequate in depleting minimal residual disease or because patients relapse primarily from endogenous disease surviving the pretransplant conditioning regimen. Patients with marrow involvement may benefit from several cycles of debulking (in vivo purging) chemotherapy before collection of HSC, with the caveat that extensive chemotherapy will also decrease the subsequent yield of PBSC. Tumor cells in the HSC inoculum likely will not benefit the patient, but until further data demonstrating a deleterious effect on transplant outcomes are available, it is advisable that reports of tumor contamination in the collections for individual patients be interpreted with caution.

Microbial Contamination of Hematopoietic Stem Cell Components

Bacterial culture is an essential quality control component in HSC collection and transplantation used to identify errors and breakdowns in manufacturing technique. Skin flora are the bacteria usually isolated, and infusion of culture-positive HSC products is generally without clinical sequelae, although serious infections have occurred after infusion of HSC products contaminated during processing.[38] Culture-positive products need not be automatically destroyed. Any decision regarding the disposition of a culture-positive HSC product must be made by the patient's transplant physician after considering the type of contamination, the anticipated risks from use of the component, and the ability to replace the culture-positive product(s) in a timely manner.

The incidence of culture-positive PBSC components is considerably less than that for marrow. The actual incidence of contamination for all HSC products is likely several times higher than reported, however, because most laboratories will culture only a very small volume of product (≈1 mL). In a retrospective review of 2935 HSC products processed and transplanted at one center, positive microbial products were reported for 1.3% of bone marrow products, 0.7% of PBSC products, and 2.0% of UCB products.[38] Coagulase-negative *Staphylococcus* and *Bacillus* species accounted for 23 of the 38 positive cultures, but *Escherichia coli, Klebsiella pneumonia,* and *Pseudomonas cepacia* were cultured from one product each. The recipient of the *Pseudomonas*-contaminated product subsequently died of complications of *Pseudomonas* sepsis, but no adverse sequelae could be documented for any of the other 34 recipients of culture-positive products. The highest rate of contamination occurred in the UCB products collected for related donor transplantation (5 of 18, 27.8%), likely a reflection of the collection techniques in place at the time, and illustrating the need for strict quality control in the collection and processing of HSC products.

Quantitation of CD34$^+$ Cells

Quantification of CD34 antigen-positive cells by flow cytometry has become the standard of care for management of the PBSC donor because it provides a rapid and clinically relevant assessment of HSC content in the peripheral blood or in the PBSC product. This antigen is found on HSCs (including a variety of subpopulations) and limited populations of other blood cells[99] and can be identified using a variety of commercially available antibodies. If antibodies directly conjugated with dyes are used, the technique requires only about 1 hour of preparation time. Cell viability using propidium iodide (PI) or 7-aminoactinomycin D (7-AAD) exclusion can simultaneously be determined if the cells are analyzed while still fresh, or the cells can be fixed after staining for analysis at a later date. Other antibodies can be added for analysis of CD34 subsets if desired (and if the flow cytometer has proper detectors to detect the different emission wavelengths of the fluorochromes used). A strong correlation exists between the numbers of CD34$^+$ cells and CFU-GM in the sample but with ratios of about 5 : 1 to 20 : 1.[100] Thus CD34 analysis will provide data similar to that obtainable with cell cultures, except that the latter demonstrates the functional viability of the progenitor cells. Mobilized PBPC products contain a heterogeneous mixture of cells including CD34$^+$ cells belonging to different cell subsets. Subset analysis of CD34$^+$ cells will provide additional information regarding early and sustained engraftment after autologous PBPC transplantation but does not appear to be clinically useful for the patient who easily meets the PBSC collection goal.

The major difficulty with analysis of CD34$^+$ cells is the low frequency of these cells. Clinical decisions to initiate apheresis are being made for CD34$^+$ cell levels as low as 10/μL. This may represent a cell frequency that is 0.01% or less of the nucleated cells in the specimen. This enumeration is possible because of multidimensional measurements obtained by flow cytometry. Most cytometers can measure at least five characteristics of each cell, including size, granularity, and the presence of up to three different fluorochromes. Thus the cells of interest can be separated in five-dimensional space, achieving discrimination of cells as rare as 1 : 10,000. The difficulties arise from developing an adequate technique that makes optimal use of the cytometer to measure these rare cells. Sources of errors include (a) sampling of the HSC product, (b) cell counting, (c) cytometer calibration and operation, (d) choice of antibody and fluorochrome, (e) lysis technique, and (f) gating strategy. Moreover, cytometry provides a proportion of cells, which must be multiplied by the cell count to obtain an absolute number. The steps involved in preparing a specimen for cytometry may alter the proportion of cells in the sample, and this error will be translated into an error in the absolute number. Clinically, this imprecision may explain some of the range in engraftment kinetics observed for patients receiving low doses of CD34$^+$ cells.

Progenitor Cell Cultures

Hematopoietic progenitor cells committed to granulocytic (CFU-GM), erythroid (burst-forming unit-erythroid [BFU-E]), or mixed granulocytic and erythroid (CFU-granulocyte, erythrocyte, megakaryocyte, macrophage; CFU-Mix) lineages can be identified using a variety of culture techniques. These techniques require expertise and equipment not available in many clinical laboratories. Other than availability of equipment and expertise, the major limitation is that progenitor cell assays require 10 to 14 days of culture before the results are available. Thus progenitor cell cultures cannot be used in the day-to-day management of the PBSC donor or the immediate quality control of bone marrow products. As with quantitation of CD34$^+$ cells, the lack of a standard culture technique adopted by all laboratories complicates comparisons between laboratories of progenitor cell quantities harvested and infused. The clinical relevance of the culture technique to the transplant population must be determined if the data obtained are to be used in the management of individual patients.

Unlike other measures of component quality, progenitor cell cultures demonstrate the functional potential of the cells. Progenitor cell cultures are the only currently available relevant assay of HSC viability other than actual engraftment of the recipient and should be available at the HSC processing facility for use in quality control or if questions about the viability of a particular component are raised.

SUGGESTED READINGS

Balkwill F: Cancer and the chemokine network. *Nat Rev Cancer* 4:540, 2004.

Barker JN, Byam C, Scaradavou A: How I treat: The selection and acquisition of unrelated cord blood grafts. *Blood* 117:2332, 2011.

Bosi A, Bartolozzi B: Safety of bone marrow stem cell donation: A review. *Transplant Proc* 42:2192, 2010.

Broxmeyer HE: Chemokines in hematopoiesis. *Curr Opin Hematol* 15:49, 2008.

Buell JF, Beebe TM, Trofe J, et al: Donor transmitted malignancies. *Ann Transplant* 9:53, 2004.

Confer DL, Shaw BE, Pamphilon DH: WMDA guidelines for subsequent donations following initial BM or PBSCs. *Bone Marrow Transplant* 46:1409, 2011.

Dettke M, Buchta C, Wiesinger H, et al: Anticoagulation in large-volume leukapheresis: Comparison between citrate versus heparin-based anticoagulation on safety and CD34+ cell collection efficiency. *Cytotherapy* 2012, in press.

DiPersio JF, Micallef IN, Stiff PJ, et al: Phase III prospective randomized double-blind placebo-controlled trial of plerixafor plus granulocyte colony-stimulating factor compared with placebo plus granulocyte colony-stimulating factor for autologous stem-cell mobilization and transplantation for patients with non-Hodgkin's lymphoma. *J Clin Oncol* 27:4767, 2009.

Ehninger A, Trumpp A: The bone marrow stem cell niche grows up: Mesenchymal stem cells and macrophages move in. *J Exp Med* 208:421, 2011.

Heimfeld S: HLA-identical stem cell transplantation: Is there an optimal CD34 cell dose? *Bone Marrow Transplant* 31:839, 2003.

Horowitz MM, Confer DL: Evaluation of hematopoietic stem cell donors. *Hematology Am Soc Hematol Educ Program* 469, 2005.

Kao GS, Kim HT, Daley H, et al: Validation of short-term handling and storage conditions for marrow and peripheral blood stem cell products. *Transfusion* 51:137, 2011.

Kurtzberg J, Cairo MS, Fraser JK, et al: Results of the Cord Blood Transplantation (COBLT) Study unrelated donor banking program. *Transfusion* 45:842, 2005.

Malik S, Bolwell B, Rybicki L, et al: Apheresis days required for harvesting CD34+ cells predicts hematopoietic recovery and survival following autologous transplantation. *Bone Marrow Transplant* 46:1519, 2011.

Miller JP, Perry EH, Price TH, et al: Recovery and safety profiles of marrow and PBSC donors: Experience of the National Marrow Donor Program. *Biol Blood Marrow Transplant* 14:29, 2008.

Pulsipher MA, Chitphakdithai P, Miller JP, et al: Adverse events among 2408 unrelated donors of peripheral blood stem cells: Results of a prospective trial from the National Marrow Donor Program. *Blood* 113:3604, 2009.

Rowley SD, Yu J, Heimfeld S, et al: Trafficking of CD34+ cells into the peripheral circulation during collection of peripheral blood stem cells by apheresis. *Bone Marrow Transplant* 28:649, 2001.

Sacchi N, Costeas P, Hartwell L, et al: Haematopoietic stem cell donor registries: World Marrow Donor Association recommendations for evaluation of donor health. *Bone Marrow Transplant* 42:9, 2008.

Sharma M, Afrin F, Satija N, et al: Stromal-derived factor-1/CXCR4 signaling: Indispensable role in homing and engraftment of hematopoietic stem cells in bone marrow. *Stem Cell Dev* 20:933, 2011.

Solves P, Mirabet V, Perales A, et al: Banking strategies for improving the hematopoietic stem cell content of umbilical cord blood units for transplantation. *Current Stem Cell Research & Therapy* 3:79, 2008.

Thomas ED, Storb R: Technique for human marrow grafting. *Blood* 35:507, 1970.

To LB, Levesque J-P, Herbert KE: How I treat patients who mobilize hematopoietic stem cells poorly. *Blood* 118:4530, 2011.

Weaver CH, Hazelton B, Birch R, et al: An analysis of engraftment kinetics as a function of the CD34 content of peripheral blood progenitor cell collections in 692 patients after the administration of myeloablative chemotherapy. *Blood* 86:3961, 1995.

For complete list of references log on to www.expertconsult.com.

CHAPTER 97

PRECLINICAL PROCESS OF CELL-BASED THERAPIES

Robert Lindblad, Deborah Wood, Traci Heath Mondoro, and Leslie E. Silberstein

The use of cells as more than replacement therapy has become a reality over the course of the past several years. While basic and clinical scientists are developing many new and promising strategies to improve immune reconstitution and transplant outcome, they are dependent on many others to implement these new therapies. Ultimately, implementation of procedures that were successful in the laboratory can be expensive and difficult to scale up to a process that will produce the required dosage with consistent quality for clinical trials. To cope with these issues, many institutions have established specialized cell processing centers; however, a specialized cell processing laboratory and specially trained laboratory staff do not resolve all of the problems associated with scaling a new procedure for a clinical trial. In some cases, equivalent reagents and processes suitable for clinical work are not available.

In addition to the technical challenges of producing clinical grade cells, all of this work must be performed under the Investigational New Drug (IND) process through the U.S. Food and Drug Administration (FDA). The use of any investigational therapy in humans requires an IND, and even if the cellular therapy has been approved, a new IND must be filed if the agent is being tested in new populations or a situation in which the risks are unknown. Novel cell therapies are more than minimally manipulated from their original source, so the FDA must review the procurement, storage, processing, and other manufacturing details as well as the clinical trial design. A study that is not likely to yield interpretable results is considered an unethical study because it places participants at risk without the prospect of either direct or generalizable benefit.

As the field of cellular therapy moved beyond transfusion of blood components and bone marrow transplantation, it became apparent that the preparation of the cellular product was becoming a science unto itself. The isolation and identification of the desired cell population could take months, and the optimization of this process could take years. This did not include the development and validation of potency assays. All of this work is expensive and labor intensive and requires staff qualified to perform at the highest technical level. Even though these tasks are vital to the production process, they are not hypothesis driven, so this type of work does not meet the requirements for National Institutes of Health (NIH) research project grants. One of the review criteria for NIH grant applications and contract proposals is innovation. Work required to validate a scale-up procedure and potency assays is not considered innovative and is not eligible for discovery research that is typically funded through NIH grants. Many investigators perform this translational work by piecing together funding from institutional or philanthropic sources. The National Heart, Lung, and Blood Institute (NHLBI) sponsors the Production Assistance for Cellular Therapies (PACT) program, which provides translational services for cellular therapies or the manufacture of clinical grade cells. The National Institute of Biomedical Imaging and Bioengineering (NIBIB) funds hypothesis-driven research related to technologies, and some investigators have been able to utilize services provided by NIH Clinical and Translational Sciences Awards (CTSA) programs. Regardless of the source of funding, this chapter provides general information about requirements during the preclinical phase of the development of a cellular therapy before it is tested for safety in a clinical trial. Critical elements involved in the stages of cell therapy product development are outlined in Fig. 97-1.

OVERVIEW OF THE CELL THERAPY PRODUCT

Novel cell-based therapy offers great potential for treating a number of currently untreatable disorders and diseases, including immune reconstitution, tissue repair and regeneration, and metabolic support. Cell-based therapies can be derived from a variety of human autologous, allogeneic or xenogeneic tissue sources such as blood, bone marrow, adipose, umbilical cord blood, fetal, embryonic stem cell lines, and induced pluripotent cells. Cellular engineering techniques such as selection, depletion, expansion, and genetic modification can be applied to alter or modify a cell to achieve a desired therapeutic effect. With these novel cell therapies; however, come development, manufacturing, characterization, and testing challenges in generating a safe and effective cell therapy product.

Challenges for Cell Therapy Product and Manufacturing Development

Current good manufacturing practices (cGMP) govern manufacturing processes to ensure consistent manufacture of safe, pure, and potent products.[1] Current good tissue practices (cGTP) govern the methods used in and the facilities used for the manufacture of human cells, tissues, and cellular and tissue-based products (HCT/Ps). cGTPs focus on the prevention of the introduction, transmission, and spread of communicable diseases and other adverse events while preserving product function and integrity.[2]

Biologic Variability

Living biologic products present unique challenges. Cells need to be alive in order to function. With cell-based therapy, inherent patient-to-patient biologic variability and cellular heterogeneity are issues. Cell therapy products are derived from tissue sources that contain multiple cell types. In addition to known "active components," there are known and unknown cell subpopulations that may be considered "contaminants" or "inactive components" or be critical to the biologic function of the product. Evolving characterization and rigorous process control are critical to counter the intrinsic heterogeneity and variability.[3]

Characterization

Cell therapy products are difficult to fully characterize. Critical decisions need to be in the product development stage, and the establishment of a characterization profile should occur early in the process. Successful product development demonstrates that the cell therapy

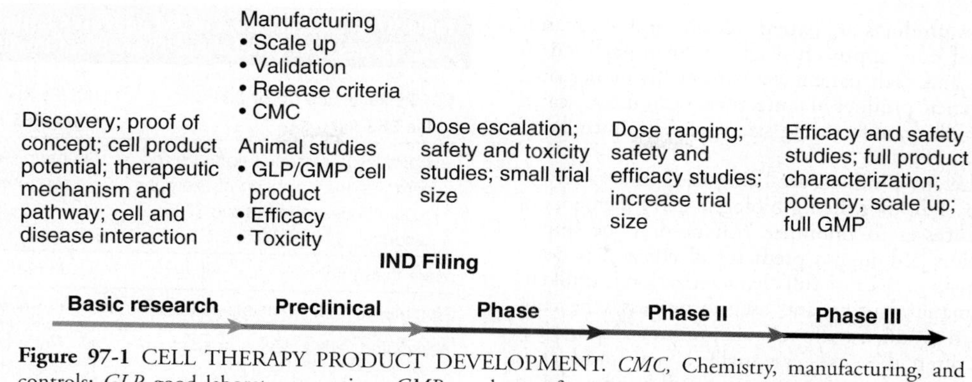

Figure 97-1 CELL THERAPY PRODUCT DEVELOPMENT. *CMC,* Chemistry, manufacturing, and controls; *GLP,* good laboratory practices; *GMP,* good manufacturing practices; *IND,* Investigational New Drug.

product is safe, pure, potent, effective, and stable. Of these five elements, developing a potency assay for cell therapy products is most challenging. Potency measures the product's relevant biologic function. Biologic products are inherently complex, variable, and often heterogeneous, with complex or poorly defined mechanisms of action(s). Despite complex cell engineering processes, the final product may contain both therapeutic and nontherapeutic cells. It is difficult to ascertain if the combination of "active" and "inactive" components contributes to biologic function. Because cells and cell lines are genetically diverse, they may behave differently during manufacturing than they did under experimental conditions. Cell characterization testing, particularly with respect to potency, will evolve and change significantly during preclinical and clinical product development.[4]

Raw Materials

Many types of raw materials are used in cell therapy manufacturing. Such materials include culture media, sera, growth factors, cytokines and "feeder cells" that are used to support cell growth. They may be simple or complex and may remain in the final therapeutic product as active substances or as excipients. They may also be used in the manufacturing process as ancillary products. Raw materials can affect the cell product characteristics. They may be viable, functional, or biologic materials, and all must be qualified. A qualification program for raw materials needs to be implemented to ensure the consistency and quality of raw materials and be designed to address identification and selection of the material, suitability of materials for use in manufacturing, characterization of materials, justification for use of animal-derived materials (e.g., fetal bovine serum), and quality assurance for all materials.[5]

Adventitious Agents

Adventitious agents or contamination may originate from the source (e.g., infected animals or tissues), during cell culture manipulation (e.g., repeated passages and manipulation in the laboratory), or by using contaminated biologic reagents. Unidentified diseases may exist in the use of xenogeneic cells. The range of infectious agents that produce little or no effect in animals may have severe consequences in humans. With xenogeneic materials, rigorous qualification of source animals and primary cell substrates is critical. Also, complex cell engineering procedures may extend over months and can result in an increased risk of contamination and other adverse effects. Quality control of the manufacturing process as well as the final product is necessary. Poor control of production processes can lead to the introduction of adventitious agents or other contaminants or to inadvertent changes in the properties or stability of the biologic product that may not be detectable in final product testing.[6]

Aseptic Processing

Living functional cells are the product, so terminal sterilization is not an option. Therefore, aseptic processing is required. The risk of delivering a contaminated product is increased because of the inability to sterilize the product and that product administration may occur before final sterility testing has been completed. This is why testing for contamination and cross-contamination are implemented as safety measures during the multistep cell processing procedure. The nature of the starting material and processes that involve open or closed manipulations determine the level of a controlled environment to be implemented.

Target Cell Population

Cells of therapeutic interest are often found in small numbers. An important step involves initial isolation or enrichment of a cell population of interest from the tissue source. Several commercial systems are already in use and include the CliniMACs (Miltenyi Biotec), the Sepax (BioSafe SA), and Elutra (CaridianBCT, Inc.) systems. Cell culturing processes are cell type specific. Cells such as T cells can be grown in nonadherent suspension culture where large-scale bioreactors such as bag-based and traditional stirred-tank vessels are used. This culturing system requires a small surface area and can produce a high cell yield. There is a growing interest in ex vivo expansion of adherent cells for a variety of clinical applications. Mesenchymal stromal cells are grown adherently on tissue culture–treated surfaces but require a large surface area to produce on a large scale. Miltenyi culture bags offer a closed system process along with the CLINIcell (MABio). Multilayered flasks have been developed (CellCube and CellSTACK, Corning, Inc.) to address surface area and bioreactors, and microcarrier-based culturing systems are currently in development (SoloHill Engineering, Inc., Ann Arbor, MI).[7]

Autologous Versus Allogeneic Products

Given their unique donor specificity, autologous products are attractive because of their decreased risk of immunologic reactions, bioincompatibility, and communicable disease transmission. However, they are inherently more limited and more variable because of individual patient characteristics and disease state. Use of allogeneic donors is associated with a greater risk than autologous donation because of the risk of infectious disease transmission from the donor to the recipient, the overall risk of an immune response, and donor-to-donor variability. Allogeneic cells have the potential to treat hundreds of patients from a single manufactured lot of cells and can be an "off-the-shelf" product.

Methods used in the production of cell products for clinical therapies depend on the nature of the final product and their targeted population. Autologous products are patient specific and are manufactured using a "scaled out" approach. Cells are manufactured in small volume batches, and each patient constitutes his or her own "lot" of product. Allogeneic product manufacturing can use a "scaled up" approach with a bulk manufacturing strategy to produce larger volume batches.

In summary, cell therapy products are being used in a variety of therapeutic indications. However, living biologics carry elements of risk. Rigid control processes to minimize risk need to be implemented. Characterization, although a predictor of efficacy, is not a predictor of safety or quality. Because full characterization is unlikely, it is imperative that manufacturing and aseptic processes be controlled and consistent to produce a safe reliable product. If manufacturing changes, as is often the case, essentially a new product is created and recharacterization, and repeat testing will be required to assess comparability of those changes.

THE REGULATION OF CELL THERAPY PRODUCTS: THE CENTER FOR BIOLOGICS EVALUATION AND RESEARCH

The Center for Biologics Evaluation and Research (CBER) currently regulates cell therapy products considered as HCT/Ps under two sections of the Public Health Service (PHS) Act.[8,9] Section 361 includes products that require no premarket approval and are consistent with products defined in 21 CFR 1271.10,[10] that is, minimally manipulated, homologous use, not a combination product, and either has no cellular or systemic effect or, if it is active on a cellular or systemic basis, is used in an autologous setting, in an allogeneic setting in first- or second-degree blood relatives, or is for reproductive use. Section 351 of the PHS Act[10,11] includes products that require premarket approval, that is, require data with clinical investigations to be collected for FDA review under an IND application and do not meet the definition of exempt products described above for Section 361 products. Cell therapies that also have a device or scaffold associated with them can be regulated by the Center for Devices and Radiological Health (CDRH) as a consultant to CBER or as the lead center if the scaffold is the primary mode of action. Table 97-1 summarizes regulation of HCT/Ps as 351 and 361 products.

Table 97-1 Determination of 351 and 361 Classification of Human Cells, Tissues, and Cellular and Tissue-Based Products

HCT/Ps Regulated Under 351 of the PHS Act	HCT/Ps Regulated Under 361 of the PHS Act
Require IND premarket approval; do not meet the definition of exempt products described above 361 products; 21CFR 1271	No premarket approval requirement
More than minimally manipulated	• Minimally manipulated, and
Not intended for homologous use	• For homologous use, and
Associated with a device or scaffold*	• Not a combination product, *and* either
Cellular or systemic effect or dependent of metabolic activity of the cells for its primary function	• has no cellular or systemic effect *or* • if it is active on a cellular or systemic basis is used in an autologous setting or in an allogeneic setting in first or second-degree blood relatives or is for reproductive use

HCT/Ps, Human cells, tissues, and cellular and tissue-based products; *IND*, Investigational New Drug; *PHS*, Public Health Service.
*Cell therapies that also have a device or scaffold associated with them can be regulated by the Center for Devices and Radiological Health as a consultant to Center for Biologic Evaluation and Research or as the lead center if the scaffold is the primary mode of action.

THE INVESTIGATIONAL NEW DRUG PROCESS

Presented here is a summary of the basic procedures to file an IND with the FDA. The regulatory pathway to conduct a clinical trial using a cell therapy product involves an IND the majority of the time.

Investigational New Drug Sponsor and Investigator

The *sponsor* of an IND trial is the individual or organization that takes legal responsibility for and initiates the clinical investigation. This may be an individual, an academic institution, the government (the NIH), or a pharmaceutical company. In contrast, the *investigator* is the individual who actually conducts the clinical trial and under whose direction the investigational product is administered. In many small cell therapy clinical trials, the sponsor may in fact also be the investigator so that the trial is conducted under a single individual who is designated as a *sponsor/investigator*.[12]

Requesting a Meeting

Product regulatory development almost always begins with meetings between the sponsor and FDA. Even with the availability of various Guidance Documents, sponsors are rarely in a position to submit a successful IND application with a cellular therapeutic product without direct FDA interactions in order to agree on submission details. The agency has designated meeting types to create a consistent level of support for products under development.

Type A meetings are used to discuss products stalled in the development pathway and products that have been placed on clinical hold after a clinical trial is already underway. Type C meetings are any other meetings not covered under type A or B.[13,14]

Type B meetings (the most common) include several specified time points in the development of a product. These include a pre-IND, end of phase I, end of phase II/pre–phase III, pre–Biological License Application (BLA), Product License Application (PLA), Establishment License Application (ELA), and New Drug Application (NDA) meetings. Under the performance goals set for the FDA, type A meetings should occur within 30 calendar days from receiving the request, type B meetings within 60 days, and type C meetings within 75 days. Information should be submitted to the agency 14 days before the meeting for type A meetings and 30 days before the meeting for type B and C meetings.[14]

Pre–Investigational New Drug Meeting

For cell therapy products, the most critical meeting is the pre-IND meeting. The general format of a pre-IND package that the sponsor sends to FDA 30 days before the meeting will include the proposed clinical protocol and consent, preclinical information, any existing clinical information, a manufacturing section, and hard copies of pertinent references. The closer the pre-IND package parallels the content of the anticipated IND, the more likely a complete review can take place and key questions can be addressed before submitting the IND itself. A list of questions that the sponsor would like the FDA to address and focus the discussion is critical to the success of the meeting. The FDA will specifically address these questions and provide a formal response as part of the meeting minutes. These questions should include issues related to the preclinical testing data; chemistry, manufacturing, and controls (CMC) information; and the clinical protocol.

The sponsor, principal investigator, individual responsible for the preclinical work, and cell manufacturer should attend the pre-IND meeting. The FDA will be represented by reviewers to match these areas. After the pre-IND meeting, the FDA reviewers in general make themselves available for further discussion and clarification or can review a new manufacturing technique or a preclinical study to ensure that the sponsor and the FDA are in agreement regarding the next steps. This process is a collaborative process with the goal of moving the development into the clinical arena as quickly and as safely as possible. Engaging the FDA early on in the IND submission process is recommended to facilitate the IND's overall success. Within CBER, pre-Pre IND meetings are available that are nonbinding, informal scientific discussions between CBER nonclinical (pharmacology/toxicology and manufacturing) reviewers and the sponsor to initiate dialogue at an early stage in the process. This structure reflects CBER's willingness to engage the cell therapy community early in the development process and helps avoid delays caused by a lack of communication.

Investigational New Drug Submission

The submission of the IND will follow the pre-IND meeting must fully address the issues raised at the pre-IND meeting in order to move forward. When the IND is submitted, the FDA has 30 days to respond. The IND may proceed unless the FDA reviewers provide comments or place the IND on hold within that 30-day time limit. Typically, the FDA will have comments and will contact the IND sponsor before the 30-day deadline. The IND submission is organized in a similar fashion to the pre-IND package noted above. Several key sections in the IND are the clinical protocol with appropriate eligibility, end points, stopping rules and dosing justification, the CMC section, and the preclinical section.[12]

Chemistry, Manufacturing, and Control Section

Unlike chemical manufacturers that may produce a massive lot to treat multiple individuals, cell therapies are usually a single lot to treat a single individual. The CMC section of a cellular therapy IND is crucial to the success of an IND submission.[15] From the regulations in 21 CFR 312.23,[16] sufficient information is required to assure the proper identification, safety, quality, and purity of the cell product. The *drug substance* is the starting material(s), including the procurement, process description, and test methods used to determine identity, strength, quality, and purity. The *drug product* is the end product, and its composition, manufacturing methods and packaging, and stability data should be included. Components used in the manufacturing of the IND; active, inactive compendial, and noncompendial excipients should be listed. If available, Certificates of Analysis for reagents not FDA approved should be submitted. The IND/GMP Sliding Scale was developed with the recognition that manufacturing under cGMP is a challenge for early stage cell therapy research. Perceived deviations from standard cGMP can be acceptable with scientific justification and an alternative approach proposed. FDA will not direct the development of the product but will respond to the data-driven suggestions put forward by the sponsor in an IND application.

The format of the information that is included in the CMC section of an IND is described in (CFR 312. 23).[16] Typical problems encountered with submission of CMC sections include:

- Poor organization and key elements missing from the submission.
- Incomplete descriptions of materials and reagents used in the manufacturing process
- Insufficient facility information
- Insufficient details regarding release criteria and tests employed.
- Insufficient standard operating procedures (SOPs)

Pharmacology/Toxicology Section

The pharmacology/toxicology section must support the planned clinical trial. Pharmacology information should describe the pharmacologic effects and mechanism of action in the animal model and provide information on the absorption, distribution, metabolism, and excretion of the product. In cellular therapies, much of this information is not readily measurable. An attempt to organize the preclinical data to address these areas should be made. If this information is not known, it should be stated. Toxicology studies, on the other hand, are critical to the initiation of clinical trials in humans.

Preclinical animal studies in general will be conducted in two species under good laboratory practices (GLP) conditions, including a developed protocol and complete data record keeping. An adequate number of animals, typically of both sexes, and adequate sampling time points are required. The appropriate species include a proof of concept relevant animal model of the appropriate disease or injury and a healthy animal toxicology model. One study must include the same route of administration, the same cell manufacturing technique, and the same product as will be proposed in the clinical study. Deviations from this ideal should be clearly explained and justified scientifically. The pre-pre–IND meeting is the time to decide the acceptable animal models to conduct these studies before embarking on time-consuming, expensive pathways that do not adequately answer the questions to advance the development process.

Cross-Referencing

The FDA permits one IND to cross-reference information that is already on file at the agency. Written authorization must be obtained from the sponsor of the submission that is being cross-referenced. Specific details, including the submission and volume number and the heading and page numbers, should be provided to identify what material is being cross-referenced. This allows FDA reviewers to quickly locate the referenced materials, facilitating the review process.

An Investigational New Drug Hold

After the IND is filed, FDA has 30 days to respond with comments before the IND automatically becomes active. The FDA applies a clinical hold to stop the clinical investigation from proceeding until identified issues are adequately addressed.[17] For new INDs, this represents a failure of the pre-IND process. If the sponsor in the pre-IND meeting presents sufficient detail and asks appropriate questions, then potential hold issues will be addressed before the IND submission. The FDA will put a clinical trial on hold for predefined reasons that include:

- Exposure to unreasonable risk for significant illness or injury
- Clinical investigators are not qualified
- Investigator brochure is misleading, erroneous, or incomplete
- IND does not contain sufficient information to assess risk
- Gender exclusion for a condition that occurs in both men and women

In practice, a clinical hold on cell therapy INDs is applied for several reasons, which include:

- The clinical trial does not provide adequate safety protection, which includes appropriate dosing based on the preliminary clinical or preclinical data, appropriate dose escalation, and appropriate stopping rules for the trial.
- The pre-clinical data do not support the clinical trial based on product manufacturing or route of delivery.
- The manufacturing section has inadequate characterization of the product, inadequate controls over manufacturing, and insufficient details.

These issues should all be addressed in the pre-IND process.

Investigational New Drug Maintenance

When an IND becomes active, future communication with the FDA outside of specific meeting requests occur through the submission of IND amendments. Each submission is sequentially numbered and adds to the overall content of the IND. Amendments are submitted to the IND on a rolling basis and include protocol revisions, expedited safety reports, changes to the manufacturing technique or to the facility, key personnel changes, and any other significant changes to the clinical or manufacturing portions of the IND. Additionally, each IND sponsor is required to submit an annual report. In some cases, the FDA may require more frequent progress reports. Each annual progress report is an opportunity to submit other details regarding the IND that were not submitted during the year. The annual report is due within 60 days of the anniversary date of the IND's becoming active.

When Is a Cell Therapy Product Ready to be Tested in a Clinical Trial?

The ultimate test of the cellular therapy is its performance in human trials. This is the last step of an incredibly complex journey. The cell population has been identified along with a manufacturing method and assays to characterize the consistency and key properties of the product. The manufactured product has been tested in animal models for both proof of concept data, including the route of administration, dosing schemes, and toxicology. The best way to make the transition from animals to humans smoothly is, if possible, to continue working with the same cell processing facility and staff that have been preparing the product throughout the preclinical studies. Good communication among the investigator, the cell processing staff, and the FDA is key for the success of the clinical trial. When this occurs, then it is easier to solve inevitable operational difficulties, attribute adverse events, and solve recruitment problems that may occur during the course of the trial.

Trial Design Considerations

The initial studies are safety based, typically at a single center, exposing few humans to the new therapy and carefully monitoring for adverse effects. As development continues, the clinical trial design can be broken down into two broad areas, scientific and operational. The scientific area includes the clinical questions to be answered and the statistical methods used to answer them. The investigator and the cell processing staff should meet early with statistical staff to determine how to phrase the clinical questions so that they can be answered with the proper end points. If a surrogate end point is proposed, this should be discussed with FDA staff. The method of end point measurement must be determined. Is there an existing validated assay to measure the end point? Is the assay commercially available, and is it FDA approved for clinical use or is it a "research-based" assay? The statisticians will calculate the appropriate sample size that is required to answer the questions with sufficient statistical power. After the sample size has been derived, the investigators must determine if the trial can be conducted at one center or if a multicenter study is needed.

Operational Issues

These are addressed using experience gained from prior clinical trials or may need to be solved through pilot studies or "dry runs" by the manufacturing and clinical staff, including the use of any device needed to deliver the cell therapy product. The first operational details to be worked out are those involving the timing of manufacture and the delivery to the patient. If the trial must be conducted at multiple sites, will there be a central manufacturing site or will processing staff need to be trained at each recruitment site?

Shipping and Administration of Cellular Products

Shipping is considered an extension of storage conditions. Selecting the right vendor is essential to shipping a stable product. The shipping containers purchased must be validated by the laboratory before their use. Transport documentation is a cGTP requirement for traceability of donor to final product purposes [1271.290(e)].[18] The U.S. Department of Transportation has guidance on classifying biologic materials in accordance with 49 CFR 171.[19]

Depending on the type of product, certain postshipment release testing may be indicated before its use. This requires cell therapy expertise at the receiving site or significant training. Shipping validation procedures can be conducted to determine what tests are required for certain products. Establishing postshipment acceptance criteria is critical for the use of many cell therapy products. Practice runs are recommended for shipment of the product, especially if the timing of the administration is crucial. For example, if a product is to be administered during a surgical procedure, it will be important to know the product viability if there are delays in shipment or postshipment testing or the surgical procedure.

In addition to a product meeting, the appropriate release criteria, the product administration process needs to be monitored. Patient baseline and postadministration evaluations are conducted, adverse events are documented, and any deviations from the product administration procedures or processes are recorded. Such documentation can allow the cell processing laboratory to evaluate common elements across different products as well as observe any product-specific trending.

Quality Control and Quality Assurance

A parallel process to the manufacturing process and preclinical studies is quality control (QC) and quality assurance (QA). QA begins before the manufacture of the cellular therapeutic begins. It is based on the manufacturing process and confirms that each step from raw material procurement to product release can be performed in a consistent and regulation-compliant manner. QC is product based and confirms whether or not the final cell therapy product satisfies the preestablished specifications for final release. Managers and third-party auditors are responsible for QA through the development of process documentation, establishing SOPs, conducting audits, and training. Inspectors and area supervisors perform QC by performing and receiving inspection reports at all points throughout the manufacturing process.

Data and Adverse Event Monitoring

In addition to the QC and QA of the cellular therapeutic, there is also the QC of data collection. Case report forms must be tailored to the study and need to be linked to the source data collected during the manufacture and delivery of the cells and throughout the clinical trial. The forms should be tested for ease of completion so that data coming in from the clinical sites will be easy to interpret. Data coordinators and research nurses should be given rigorous training on the completion of these forms and should know how long each form takes to fill out so they will be able to give a reasonable estimate of how many subjects they can follow within a given time period.

Whereas single-center trials are often monitored by an institutional data safety monitoring board (DSMB), multicenter trials typically have a centralized independent DSMB that is often convened by the sponsor (NIH or a pharmaceutical company). A monitoring plan must be developed for the collection and reporting of adverse events to the DSMB and the FDA. This is another step during which good communication is essential. The trial investigator and the cell processing facility must meet regularly to discuss any adverse events, especially events that occur during product administration, to determine if they are attributable to the cellular product or the subject's underlying disease. The FDA and the DSMB must be informed of these events to determine if a prespecified stopping boundary has been crossed.

FUTURE DIRECTIONS

The development of novel cellular therapeutics is a long and complex process. There are many translational steps to be completed before exposure to humans is feasible. These steps range from practical issues such as the shipment of cells to the complicated issues of preclinical studies to be performed in multiple animal models. Investigators need to develop good working relationships with the cell processing facility staff and statistical staff in order to complete an effective clinical trial. All novel cell therapies and established cell therapies for novel indications require an IND application to be filed with the FDA. The key to a successful IND is early and frequent communication with the FDA.

SUGGESTED READINGS

Cell Therapy cGMP Facilities and Manufacturing. Adrian Gee, chief editor, United States, 2009, Springer-Verlag.

Food and Drug Administration, HHS. Guidance for Industry: Eligibility Determination for Donors of Human Cells, Tissues, and Cellular and Tissue-Based Products (HCT/Ps) Final Guidance, 2007.

Guidance for Industry: Guidance for Human Somatic Cell Therapy and Gene Therapy, 1998.

Preti RA: Bringing safe and effective cell therapies to the bedside. *Nat Biotechnol* 23:801, 2005.

REFERENCES

1. U.S. Food and Drug Administration, HHS. 21 Code of Federal Regulations Part 211: Current good manufacturing practice for finished pharmaceuticals.
2. 21 Code of Federal Regulations Part 1271: Human Cells, Tissues, and Cellular and Tissue-Based Products. May 25, 2005.
3. Burger S: GTP/GMP cell engineering for cell and gene therapies. *BioProcess J* 2:1, 2003.
4. Draft Guidance for Industry: Potency tests for cellular and gene therapy products. October 2008.
5. Seaver S: U.S. pharmacopeia. General Information Chapter, Cell and Gene Therapy Products United States, Rockville, Md., 2002.
6. Guidance for Industry: Source animal, product, preclinical, and clinical issues concerning the use of xenotransplantation products in humans. Final Guidance. April 2003.
7. Brandenberger R, et al: Integrating process and product development for the next generation of biotherapeutics. *BioProcess Int*, March 2011.
8. U.S. Food and Drug Administration, Center for Biologics Evaluation and Research: References for the regulatory process for the Office of Cellular, Tissue and Gene Therapies. August 18, 2011.
9. U.S. Food and Drug Administration: FDA History. http://www.fda.gov/oc/history/.
10. 21 Code of Federal Regulations Part 1271 Human Cells, Tissues, and Cellular and Tissue-Based Products, May 2005.
11. U.S. Food and Drug Administration, Center for Biologics Evaluation and Research: About CBER. September 2011.
12. U.S. Food and Drug Administration, Center for Biologics Evaluation and Research: Information on submitting an investigational new drug application. August 2011.
13. U.S. Food and Drug Administration, Center for Biologics Evaluation and Research: Formal meetings with sponsors and applicants for PDUFA products. February 2000.
14. U.S. Food and Drug Administration, Center for Biologics Evaluation and Research: Scheduling and conduct of regulatory review meetings with sponsors and applicants. Version 4. May 2007.
15. U.S. Food and Drug Administration, Center for Biologics Evaluation and Research Guidance for FDA Review Staff and Sponsors: Content and review of chemistry, manufacturing, and control information for human gene therapy investigational new drug applications. April 2008.
16. 21 Code of Federal Regulations Part 312.23: IND content and format. 2005.
17. U.S. Food and Drug Administration, Center for Biologics Evaluation and Research: Issuance of and response to clinical hold letters for investigational new drug applications. Version 3. April 1999.
18. 21 Code of Federal Regulations, Part 1271.290: Tracking from donor to consignee or final disposition. May 2005.
19. 49 Code of Federal Regulations, Part 171: Hazardous materials regulations. 2007.

CHAPTER 98

GRAFT ENGINEERING AND CELL PROCESSING

Adrian P. Gee

The abbreviation *BMT* has changed over the past few years from standing for bone marrow (BM) transplantation to denoting blood and marrow transplantation. This reflects the increased use of hematopoietic progenitor cells (HPCs) derived from cytokine-mobilized peripheral blood. It is fortunate that the abbreviation can also be used to cover stem cells derived from placental and umbilical cord blood, which represent the next new source of cells for transplantation. Other sources, such as adipose tissue, are being discovered, and each may provide cells with specific properties that can be exploited for different applications. The mobilization and collection of hematopoietic stem cells (HSCs) are discussed in Chapter 96. In this chapter, the ex vivo processing of these cells is reviewed. Processing may range from simple depletion of plasma or red blood cells (RBCs) to overcome ABO incompatibilities, to more complex procedures designed to engineer the graft components to enhance engraftment, prevent graft-versus-host disease (GVHD) or to introduce genetic modifications into the cells. Facilities performing these procedures are increasingly involved in other types of cellular therapies. These include provision of cells for adjuvant therapies in the posttransplant setting and to support clinical trials in regenerative medicine. The dramatic growth in these new applications has attracted the interest of regulatory agencies, which have worked hard to develop an appropriate strategy to address a complex new area of medicine. An understanding of the regulations is therefore essential because they are based on the type of cellular therapy product.

REGULATORY ISSUES WITH CELL PROCESSING

Regulation of a fast-moving field, such as cellular therapies, has posed a challenge to the U.S. Food and Drug Administration (FDA) and other national regulatory authorities. However, in the past few years, a risk-based structure has emerged in the USA that has clarified the strategy. In brief, manufacturers of cellular therapy products need to determine whether they fall under Investigational New Drug (IND) regulations, which require manufacturing of the product under good manufacturing practices (GMP); whether they fall under Part 1271 of Title 21 of the Code of Federal Regulations (21CFR) human cells, tissues, and cellular and tissue-based products (HCT/Ps), which require manufacturing of the product under good tissue practices (GTP); or whether they are exempt from both of these regulations.

The newer GTP regulations, which came into effect in May 2005, were established nominally to prevent the introduction, transmission, and spread of communicable diseases by HCT/Ps. This was based on the presumption that the majority of posttransplant infections and admissions to intensive care units were attributable to receipt of contaminated products. The basis of this statement is open to question, but the regulations provide a framework for screening, performing ex vivo processing, storing and distributing HCT/Ps, and providing the FDA with an overview of current activities by an annual registration of collection and processing facilities. The Part 1271 regulations effectively filled a gap in the law that left unregulated HCT/Ps that were minimally manipulated (e.g., were not cultured ex vivo, genetically modified, activated ex vivo), were intended for homologous use, or were not combined with another article (e.g., a matrix or scaffold) for administration. Minimally manipulated HCT/Ps should not exert a systemic effect and should not be dependent on the metabolic activity of living cells for their function. If this was not the case, then the cells should be for autologous use, for use in a first- or second-degree blood relative, or for reproductive use. Cellular products that fall into this classification are referred to as Type 361 products. The Part 1271 regulations do not apply to vascularized organs for transplantation; whole blood or blood components; and, important for this discussion, minimally manipulated BM for homologous use and not combined with another article.

With the exceptions noted, most other cellular therapy and HPC transplant products fall under IND regulations and are referred to as Type 351 products. These products have been cultured ex vivo and transduced or activated ex vivo and therefore are more-than-minimally manipulated. The facility processing these cells is required to operate under GMP. These regulations were originally developed for the pharmaceutical industry to ensure that drugs are manufactured under a controlled and auditable process that ensures their safety, purity, and potency. The FDA has indicated that the application of GMP to cellular therapy products follows a continuum, such that products that are manufactured for a phase I/II clinical trial under IND are not expected to be prepared under full GMP. As the trial proceeds the expectation is that the application of GMP will become more rigorous, such that a phase III product would be extensively characterized and manufactured using a fully validated process.

Implementation of Part 1271 regulations has had an impact on the "routine" laboratory that prepares cells primarily for hematopoietic transplantation. Laboratories that use cells other than BM now must register annually with the FDA; ensure that donors meet eligibility requirements (or document why noneligible donors are used); and manufacture, store, and distribute the cells under GTP. If a laboratory has previous experience manufacturing products for IND studies under GMP conditions, it already will be familiar with most of the features of GTP. In general, these cover personnel, procedures, facilities, environmental control and monitoring, equipment, supplies and reagents, recovery, processing and process controls, process changes, process validation, labeling controls, storage, receipt, predistribution shipment and distribution, records, tracking, and complaints. Implementation of the components of either GMP or GTP operations is a time-consuming process that requires the development, implementation, and maintenance of numerous components and generates a considerable volume of paperwork. Professional societies, such as the Foundation for the Accreditation of Cellular Therapy (FACT) and AABB (formerly the American Association of Blood Banks), have developed an accreditation process that takes into account GTP regulations and provides a framework around which compliance can be built (see Professional Standards).

An exception from the products described above is cord blood. In the United States, cord blood is a licensed product and facilities that prepare and bank cord blood will be required to request a Biologics License Application (BLA). This is permission to introduce or deliver for introduction a biologic product into interstate commerce (21 CFR 601.2). At the time of writing, the first American banks are undergoing this process.

Central to both GMP and GTP regulations is the establishment and maintenance of a quality program. This should ensure that the appropriate regulations are being followed on an ongoing basis; that mechanisms are in place for detecting, reviewing, and remediating errors and deviations from regulations, policies, and procedures; and that an audit program will be developed and implemented. Evidence of the work of the quality program must be documented, and the program should ideally be staffed by individuals who are not involved in hands-on manufacturing of the products.

Holders of INDs must provide the agency with an annual report on the protocol and include a listing of the products administered and those that have been prepared but not used. In addition, cell processing facilities should be prepared to assist in reporting to the FDA information on products that have been associated with severe adverse reactions in the recipients. For Type 361 products, the facility must report, as Biological Product Deviations, any contaminated products that have been administered to a patient.

PROFESSIONAL STANDARDS

The two major accrediting organizations in the United States for cellular therapies are FACT and AABB. Whereas FACT offers accreditation of collection, processing, and clinical use of cellular therapy products, the AABB focuses on collection and laboratory processing. Both organizations inspect based on standards that are published every 18 months to 3 years. In the case of FACT, the standards are published in collaboration with the Joint Committee on Accreditation in Europe (JACIE). FACT also publishes separate standards in collaboration with NetCord that cover cord blood banking. Both organizations have worked to harmonize their standards with American, Canadian, Australasian, and European regulatory agencies; therefore, accreditation by either organization is of great assistance on the pathway to regulatory compliance. A number of other professional organizations accredit particular aspects of operations within the cell processing facility. These include the College of American Pathologists (CAP), which inspects general laboratories, hematology, and flow cytometry; the American Society for Histocompatibility and Immunogenetics (ASHI); and the European Federation for Immunogenetics (EFI), which accredits histocompatibility testing laboratories. Some organizations, such as CAP and StemCell Technologies, also provide proficiency testing services for laboratory staff.

MANIPULATION OF HEMATOPOIETIC STEM CELL TRANSPLANTATION PRODUCTS

Manipulation of a product for HSC rescue is intended to remove a component that is unwanted or may cause adverse effects or to enrich a desired population, such as CD34 cells. As discussed previously, the degree of manipulation may determine the regulations under which the product is manufactured and handled. The FDA defines minimal manipulation as processing that does not alter the relevant biologic characteristics of the cells or tissues. This includes procedures such as RBC and plasma depletion, and cell selection using an approved device. By contrast, more-than-minimal manipulation would include activities such as culture ex vivo, genetic modification, and ex vivo activation.

Routine Minimal Manipulation for Volume Reduction or ABO Incompatibility

The most widely used form of manipulation in the HPC processing facility probably is removal of erythrocytes or plasma (or both) to overcome ABO incompatibility between donor and recipient (Table 98-1). This process is performed using techniques that were developed by the blood banking industry.

Plasma depletion to remove donor antibodies that may react with recipient cells is achieved by centrifugation of the graft, usually in a transfer pack, at approximately 2000 g for 10 minutes at ambient temperature. The pack then is placed in a plasma expresser, which compresses the product bag so that plasma can be forced out and into

Table 98-1 Processing Performed to Address ABO Incompatibilities Between Hematopoietic Stem Cell Donors and Recipients

Recipient ABO Type	Donor ABO Type	Type of Processing
ABO identical	ABO identical	No special processing required
A or B	AB	RBC depletion
O	A/B/AB	RBC depletion
A	B	RBC + plasma depletion
B	A	RBC + plasma depletion
Antibody to RBCs	N/A	RBC depletion
A/B/AB	O	Plasma depletion
AB	A or B	Plasma depletion

N/A, Not applicable; *RBC*, red blood cell.

a separate collection bag. Plasma depletion can also be used to reduce the volume of ABO-compatible grafts when the donor is large and the recipient small.

Red blood cell depletion removes incompatible donor erythrocytes that would stimulate a reaction by the donor upon administration. Most facilities establish a maximum volume of incompatible RBCs that can be infused with HPC; exceeding this limit can result in hemolysis and a transfusion reaction. Depletion of erythrocytes can be achieved most simply by centrifugation. The product is centrifuged at approximately 3000 g for approximately 10 minutes at ambient temperature, and the leukocyte-rich buffy coat is collected at the interface between the plasma layer and the RBCs.

Red blood cell depletion can also be achieved by sedimenting erythrocytes using hydroxyethyl starch (hetastarch). This promotes RBC sedimentation by formation of erythrocyte rouleaux. The hematocrit of the product is first adjusted to 25% by addition of normal saline, and 6% hetastarch (Hespan) is added at a volume:volume ratio of 1:6 to 7. Sedimentation can be performed under gravity or may be accelerated by centrifugation.

The most rigorous erythrocyte depletion is achieved by centrifugation of the collection on a Ficoll-Hypaque density gradient. This process enriches mononuclear cells at the interface between the gradient and the layered cells after centrifugation and depletes erythrocytes, platelets, and granulocytes. As a result of enrichment for mononuclear cells, the overall nucleated cell recovery is lower than with other techniques.

Automated devices are available for preparing buffy coats and density gradient-enriched cells. For larger volumes, the COBE 2991 Cell Processor from Terumo can be used. This requires a minimum volume of 150 mL RBCs for operation and may therefore not be suitable for pediatric processing. It is capable of preparing buffy coats and density separated cell preparations using a functionally closed disposable set.

The COBE Spectra from Terumo is in common use to collect peripheral blood progenitor cells by apheresis. The device is also less widely used in the processing facility to enrich mononuclear cells from BM. A similar procedure and density gradient separation can be performed on the CS3000 separator from Fenwal Blood Technologies.

For smaller starting volumes, the Sepax device from Biosafe can be used (Fig. 98-1). It has found widespread application in cord blood banks for buffy coat preparation (with or without hydroxyethyl starch) and has also been used for volume reduction of peripheral blood progenitor cell collections, density gradient separation of BM and for cell washing. The device has a small footprint, uses functionally closed disposables, and provides a print-out of operations.

Xpress devices for cord blood and marrow processing are available from Thermogenesis. The AXP AutoXpress is designed for enriching

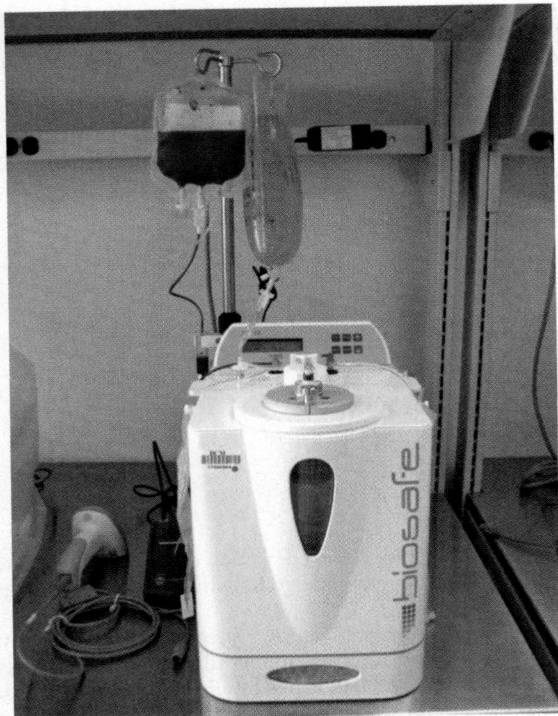

Figure 98-1 THE BIOSAFE SEPAX DEVICE. Used for automated processing of hematopoietic cells.

mononuclear cells from cord blood that is transferred to the processing set, which is then placed into the AXP device. This fits into a centrifuge bucket, and during spinning, the red and mononuclear cells are collected into separate bags and the plasma is retained in the processing set. The MarrowXpress performs a similar procedure on marrow harvests. Both devices provide closed sterile systems, and the XpressTRAK software enables data tracking to assist with regulatory compliance.

Purging of Autologous Grafts

Autologous HPC can be used for recipients lacking a human leukocyte antigen (HLA)-matched related or unrelated donor. It has been proposed that occult viable tumor cells collected with the graft and returned to the patient could act as a source for disease relapse. Gene marking studies have supported this hypothesis. As a result, much effort has been exerted to develop methods for the ex vivo detection and removal of tumor cells from autologous grafts. Techniques have included incubation with chemotherapeutic drugs, such as 4-hydroperoxycyclophosphamide (4-HC), photosensitizing agents, and antisense oligonucleotides. Alternatively, tumor-directed monoclonal antibodies (MAb) can be used to identify the cells and effect their removal. The MAb-coated tumor cells can be eliminated by addition of serum complement or by capturing them on a solid phase, such as a column matrix, a plastic sheet, or magnetic particles. These particles may be large (5 μm diameter) so they can be collected, with the attached tumor cells, in a standard magnetic field. The matrix material may be much smaller, such as nanoparticles or ferrofluids, which coat the cells. These are then collected on a metal matrix placed in a field generated by permanent magnets. Such systems are capable of depleting 4 to 6 logs of tumor cells from a graft. However, even at such high efficiencies, given the limits of our ability to detect residual tumor cells, the clinical value of purging autologous grafts is debatable. There has been a decline in interest in purging techniques because of the potential benefits of a graft-versus-tumor (GVT) effect detected in recipients of allogeneic grafts.

T-Cell Depletion of Allogeneic Products

T cells in HPC grafts have the potential to cause severe or lethal GVHD or potentially to exert a beneficial GVT effect (discussed in Chapter 109). Considerable work has been done to determine whether these opposing effects are produced by distinct subpopulations of T lymphocytes. This would allow ex vivo manipulation of allogeneic grafts to remove differentially the GVHD-producing T cells while sparing those that mediate GVT responses. Various subpopulations of T cells have been identified as candidate effector subpopulations; however, there is no widespread consensus as to which subsets should be targeted.

Methods are available for eliminating T cells from grafts using approaches similar to those used for purging tumor cells. Early approaches included use of soybean agglutinin to aggregate the majority of nonprogenitor cells and rosetting of sheep erythrocytes with T cells to facilitate their removal. Although successful, these techniques are not "FDA friendly" and do not offer the specificity that likely is required to engineer T-cell subpopulations in allogeneic grafts. This is possible by use of MAb directed toward the antigens that currently are used to identify T-lymphocyte subpopulations. The target population then can be removed with high efficiency using immunomagnetic separation, as described previously for purging autologous grafts. The challenge remains to identify the appropriate target T cell populations and to source clinical grade MAb for these procedures. A number of potential target antigens have been identified and separation techniques implemented. They range from pan–T-cell depletions using antibodies to CD3 and CD2, to depletions of helper and cytotoxic T cells using monoclonals against CD4 and CD8, to stimulation and removal of alloreactive populations by targeting activation antigens.

Methods that eliminate or physically remove either T cells or tumor cells from grafts are referred to as *negative selection techniques*. They are affected by variables such as target antigen expression, sensitivity of detection technologies for quantitating separation efficiency, and other technical hurdles. They may be difficult to manipulate to achieve the ideal composition of the graft and the target level of T cells remains to be established, although the figure of 10^5 T cells/kg is generally regarded as the goal to minimize the risk of GVHD while facilitating engraftment. There are also no approved devices for negative selection, so these types of procedures must be performed under an IND.

For many years, the goal was to replace negative selection with a procedure in which HPC populations could be specifically enriched by positive selection. This would effectively deplete T cells and tumor cells from allogeneic and autologous graft, respectively. The problem was the lack of a method for identifying the target HPC until the CD34 antigen was identified on a small population of progenitor cells, including the pluripotent cells required for hematopoietic transplantation. The subsequent availability of monoclonal antibodies directed against this antigen made possible the development of techniques for enrichment of cells. Immobilization of the antibodies on a matrix (e.g., plastic sheets) and cellulose and magnetic particles was used as the primary approach, and a number of devices were commercially developed. The first to achieve FDA approval for use with apheresis products was the Baxter Isolex 300i, which uses Dynal 5-μm magnetic beads as the separation modality and releases $CD34^+$ cells from the beads using a competitive binding peptide. This device was recently withdrawn from the market for this application and is currently under evaluation for use in regenerative medicine protocols.

An alternative is the CliniMACS system (Fig. 98-2), which currently has regulatory approval in Europe but still requires an IND for use in the United States. This uses anti-CD34 nanoparticles to effect separation. The labeling and removal of unbound CD34 reagent is performed manually. The CD34 reagent-treated cells are then processed on the device, where they are retained on a column located in a high-gradient magnetic field. Nonlabeled cells flow through the column and are collected in the negative fraction. The labeled cells are recovered from the column after several automated separation and

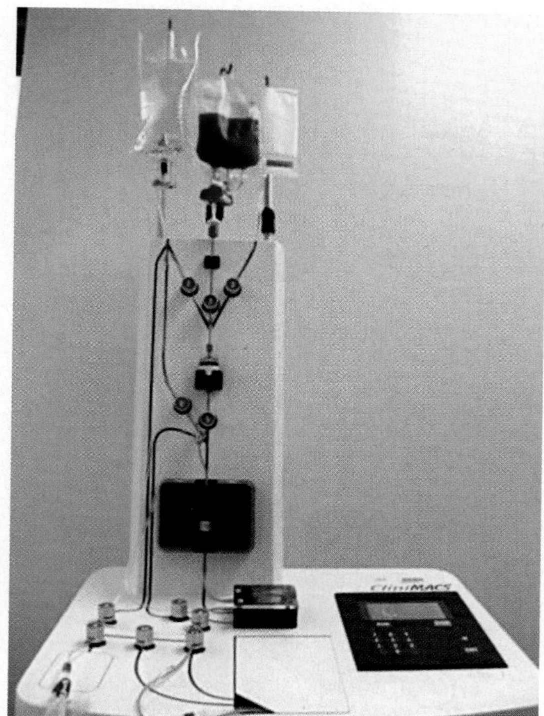

Figure 98-2 MILTENYI CLINIMACS IMMUNOMAGNETIC SEPARATOR. Used for enrichment of hematopoietic progenitor cells and for the selective enrichment or depletion of other cell types.

Table 98-2 Methods Used for T-Cell Depletion of Hematopoietic Grafts

Destruction in Situ	Physical Separation
Monoclonal antibody-based Antibody + complement Immunotoxins (e.g., ricin) Panning and immunoaffinity columns	Monoclonal antibody-based Immunomagnetic separation Negative selection (T-cell removal) Positive selection (CD34 selection) CliniMACs device
Cytotoxic drugs (e.g., 4-HC)	Rosetting with sheep erythrocytes
Photopheresis	Lectins (e.g., soybean agglutinin) Centrifugal elutriation

4-HC, 4-Hydroperoxycyclophosphamide.

washing cycles by removing the magnetic field. The nanoparticles remain on the CD34-positive cells; however, they are biocompatible and may be infused into the recipient. The device normally achieves purities in excess of 90% with yields of approximately 60%. This results in passive depletion of 4 to 6 logs of T cells. The device may be used with a variety of MAb directed against antigens expressed by various types (T, B, and natural killer [NK] cells), potentially allowing it to be used as a platform for multiple types of graft engineering.

Positive selection techniques may also passively deplete from the graft certain cells that could be of potential benefit to the recipient. These include some stromal elements, GVT-mediating T cells, and other subpopulations that may facilitate engraftment. As our understanding of the identity of these populations improves, it may be possible to recover them from the normally discarded negative fraction and add them back to the CD34+ cells or to use them in the posttransplant period as donor leukocyte infusions (see later discussion).

Table 98-2 lists various methods of direct T-lymphocyte depletion and indirect depletion by HPC enrichment.

EVALUATION OF MANIPULATED GRAFTS

Most allograft engineering has focused on T-lymphocyte depletion and has emphasized quantitative versus qualitative removal. The majority of allografts are infused immediately after preparation rather than after cryopreservation and storage. This restricts the types of assays that can be used to evaluate graft composition to those that have a rapid turnaround, and the implications of infusing large numbers of T lymphocytes can be severe or lethal. Therefore, it is important to have available methods that can rapidly enumerate the numbers of T lymphocytes within the graft. Although early methods used detection of E-rosette–forming cells or manual immunofluorescence after staining with pan–T-lymphocyte–directed monoclonal antibody, most laboratories currently rely on flow cytometry. This technology is widely used in routine clinical laboratories; however, some precautions must be taken when it is used for T-depleted allografts.

Flow Cytometry

Accurate enumeration of very small numbers of target cells by cytometry requires rare event analysis. In this technique, large numbers of events must be accumulated and carefully analyzed if reliable data are to be obtained. This approach has been widely adopted for counting $CD34^+$ cells in unfractionated grafts but still is often neglected when enumerating T lymphocytes in depleted grafts. The choice of MAb for detection of the T-lymphocyte population also is critical when a MAb-mediated depletion technology is used. The same MAb should not be used for both depletion and analysis because cells that became coated with the antibody during the depletion phase but were not effectively removed will be blocked from detection. However, they can be detected by adding an anti-immunoglobulin antibody conjugated to a fluorochrome different from the one conjugated to the T-lymphocyte–directed MAb. The most sensitive detection is achieved by using panels of non–cross-blocking anti–T-lymphocyte antibodies directed against a variety of epitopes.

It is important to include a viability stain in the analysis panel. Although this is less crucial when T-lymphocyte depletion is achieved by physical removal of target cells, it is extremely important when in situ elimination methods are used. In these cases, the depleted allograft may contain dead or dying T lymphocytes that will be detected by flow but may not contribute to postinfusion events. Suitable viability stains include propidium iodide and 7-aminoactinomycin (7-AAD). Analysis of cell viability after ex vivo depletion is not straightforward. Cell death may not be expressed immediately but develops in the hours or days after processing and infusion. Under such circumstances, the analysis of apoptotic cells by a combination of Annexin-V staining with 7-AAD may provide a more accurate estimate of cell damage. This approach can be used in combination with simultaneous staining for T-cell surface markers to provide additional information. In some cases, incubating the cells for a period before analysis is advisable (e.g., in the case of depletion by immunotoxins, cells require time to divide to manifest the toxic effects). Stimulation of cells with interleukin-2 (IL-2) and ex vivo culture also has been used to detect functional residual T lymphocytes. In some cases, this method has shown a correlation between the numbers of T lymphocytes in the cultured sample and the development of clinical GVHD in the graft recipient.

Tetramer Analysis

Enumeration of T cells bearing receptors for specific antigens can be achieved using tetramer analysis (Fig. 98-3). In this procedure, soluble versions of heavy chain of major histocompatibility complex (MHC) molecules are synthesized and adopt the appropriate conformation when a synthetic peptide representing the epitope is recognized by the T-cell receptor (TCR) and β2-microglobulin is added. The carboxyl-terminus of the MHC molecule is biotinylated, and four of these peptide/MHC–biotin complexes assemble into a

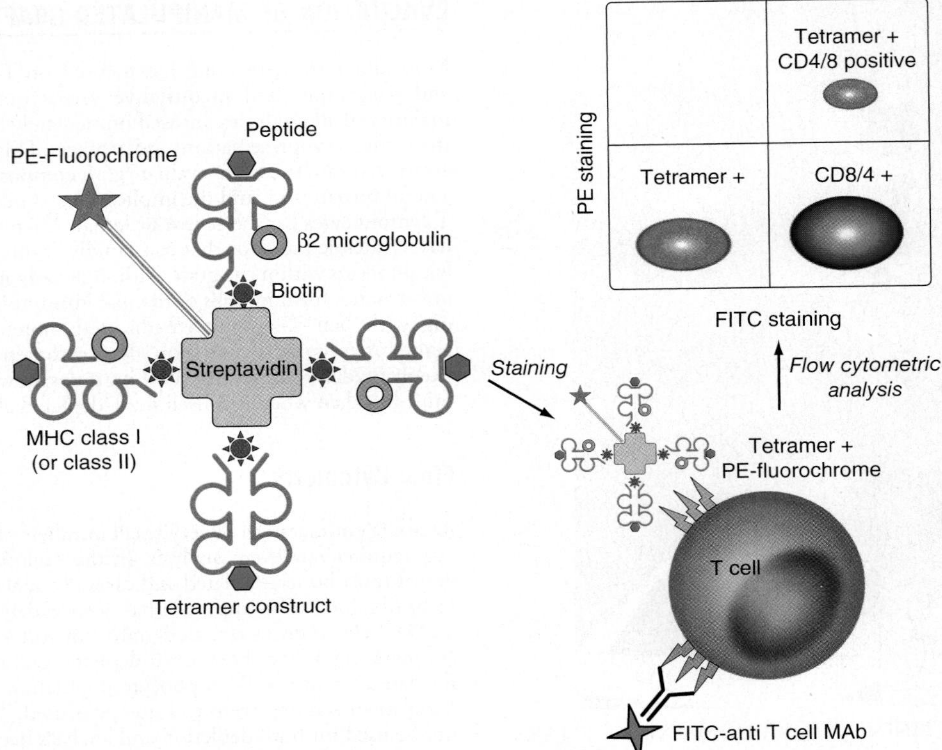

Figure 98-3 TETRAMER STAINING TO DETECT ANTIGEN-SPECIFIC T CELLS (SEE TEXT FOR DETAILS). *FITC,* Fluorescein Isothiocyanate; *MHC,* major histocompatibility complex; *PE,* Phycoerythrin.

tetramer when streptavidin is added. The streptavidin is tagged with a fluorochrome; therefore, T cells reactive with the chosen peptide–MHC complex become fluorescently stained and can be detected by flow cytometry.

Functional Assays

Flow cytometry detects residual cells by their ability to bind monoclonal antibodies. Routine flow does not provide information on the functional capacity of these cells, which may be important when assessing the graft for its potential to mediate GVHD or GVT. For this purpose, a number of assays have been developed. These are not suitable for use as release tests because of their turnaround time, but they can provide retrospective information that may correlate with clinical outcome. They include limiting dilution analysis, in which a range of dilutions of the graft are plated out and assessed for the ability of T cells to form colonies in response to the addition of stimulants, such as phytohemagglutinin (PHA) and IL-2. Based on the proportion of colony-forming wells at the various dilutions, it is possible to determine by the Poisson distribution the number of T cells present in the original graft.

Another approach is use of an enzyme-linked immunosorbent spot (ELISpot) assay in which cells are stimulated to produce an analyte that is characteristic of their normal function. The cells are plated onto a surface that has been coated with an antibody directed against that analyte and incubated for a fixed period. The secreted analyte binds to this antibody, and the cells and any other unbound material are washed away. The surface is incubated with a biotinylated antibody directed against the analyte and washed and incubated with alkaline phosphatase linked to streptavidin. After washing, the plate is incubated with a substrate solution. A blue-black precipitate will appear at sites were the analyte was produced, with each spot representing an analyte-secreting cell. The spots can be enumerated manually or by using an ELISpot reader.

CELLULAR THERAPY PRODUCTS

A number of cellular therapy products, including some that have been genetically modified, are being evaluated in clinical trials (see Chapter 95). These have examined the safety and efficacy of different cell populations, including, but not limited to, unmanipulated leukocyte infusions from HPC donors, cytokine-induced T cells, lymphokine-activated killer (LAK) cells, tumor-infiltrating lymphocytes (TILs), T-regulatory cells, antigen-specific T cells (see Chapter 101), mesenchymal cells (see Chapter 100), dendritic cells (DCs) (see Chapter 103), and NK cells (see Chapter 102). Detailed accounts of the scientific basis for such studies as well as results of clinical trials are given in Chapters 95 and 97. This section focuses on processing and product evaluation issues.

Cells that have been more-than-minimally manipulated must be prepared under GMP conditions. This requires that manufacturing be performed by trained staff following formal standard operating procedures. These procedures will have been submitted to the FDA in the chemistry, manufacturing, and control (CMC) section of the IND application and will specify how the product is prepared, the reagents and materials that will be used, and the criteria for the release of the product for clinical use. Release criteria are test specifications that are designed to ensure that the product is sterile and pure, and they may include assays for functionality. The specific tests for sterility and purity that have been approved by the FDA are described in 21CFR 610.12, and a number of guidances have been issued by the FDA on the use and validation of alternative techniques. The CFR assays are generally considered to be outdated; however, the Agency indicated in June 2011 its intent to amend the sterility test requirements for biologic products. They would eliminate the prescribed methods in CFR 610.12 and allow the use of alternative validated methods. If the proposed test method is an established U.S. Pharmacopeia compendial sterility test, then formal validation is considered to have been already completed. This should considerably simplify and reduce the costs of sterility testing.

In the normal release mechanism for a cellular therapy product, the quality unit reviews the production records and issues a certificate of analysis (CofA) (Fig. 98-4). This document details the testing that was performed together with test method, the testing laboratory, the specification required by the FDA, and the actual results obtained. Routine testing required for most cellular therapy products consists of aerobic, anaerobic, and fungal sterility; endotoxin levels (by Limulus amebocyte method); mycoplasma for ex vivo expanded cells (assayed by the culture method); identity and purity (by flow cytometry and, in some cases, HLA typing); and, for products in later stages of evaluation, functionality (e.g., cytotoxic activity toward target cells or secretion of specific bioactive products). Products that have been transduced with a retroviral vector will also require testing for replication-competent virus. Use of non-FDA approved test methods should be cleared with the FDA at the IND application stage. In most cases, regulatory agencies also like to see some form of stability testing program that evaluates the stability of the cellular product over time in storage in the frozen state and when thawed for administration.

Phase I studies are designed to assess the safety of the product and should include assessment of reactions to infusion, risks for contamination during preparation, and delayed effects after administration. Clinical efficacy is evaluated during phase II/III. At this time, progress should be made toward the development of an in vitro assay for functionality that correlates with clinical efficacy. This can be problematic because most in vitro assays currently used are unreliable as predictors of the clinical value of the product, and some form of surrogate marker has been substituted.

Donor Leukocyte Infusions

The ability of infusions of donor leukocytes (DLI) to mediate antitumor responses was originally described in patients with chronic myeloid leukemia (CML) in hematologic relapse after allogeneic stem cell transplantation (SCT), but lymphomas and Hodgkin disease also are sensitive to the effects of DLI. Remission rates of up to 80% have been reported in CML patients who relapse after transplant. Up to 90% responses have been described in patients with Epstein-Barr virus (EBV)–associated lymphoproliferative disease. Moderate success has been achieved with use of DLI after relapse in other malignancies such as acute myeloid leukemia (15%-40%), low-grade lymphomas (≤60%), and metastatic multiple myeloma (40%-60%). Fewer than 5% of patients with relapsed acute lymphoblastic leukemia respond

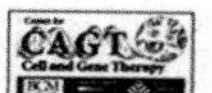

CERTIFICATE OF ANALYSIS

Center for Cell & Gene Therapy, GMP Cell Processing Facility

Baylor College of Medicine, Houston, Texas 77030

Retrovirally Transduced Donor Leukocytes

Depleted of Alloreactive T cells by Anti CD25-Immunotoxin (RFT5-DGA)

Caution: New Drug-Limited by Federal Law to Investigational Use

Properly identify intended Recipient and Component

Recipient Name: DOE, Jane
Recipient MR #: TCH 123456
Recipient CAGT Number: P2669
Donor Name: DOE, John (TCH789101)
Component CAGT Number: C1234.A.61
Date Frozen: 08/21/2011

Store at temperatures below -150°C

TEST	LABORATORY	SPECIFICATION	RESULT
Viability – Cell product (Trypan Blue dye exclusion)	CAGT GMP Facility	> 70% viable	99% viable 08/21/11
Endotoxin – Cell supernatant (LAL assay by Endosafe)	CAGT QC Laboratory	≤ 5.0 EU/ml	<2.0EU/ml 08/25/11
Bacterial Sterility – Cell product Bactec – aerobic Bactec - anaerobic	Clinical Laboratory Services, The Methodist Hospital, Houston	Negative (at 14 days)	Negative 09/05/11 Negative 09/05/11
Fungal sterility – 1st wash Bactec	Clinical Laboratory Services, The Methodist Hospital, Houston	Negative (at 28 days)	Negative 10/21/11
Mycoplasma – Cell product (PCR assay)	CAGT QC Laboratory	Negative	Negative 08/31/11
Phenotyping (Flow cytometry)	CAGT GMP Flow Facility	< 1% CD25+ cells	0.03% CD25+ 08/21/11
Proliferation in Primary Mixed Lymphocyte Culture – Cell Product	CAGT 7th Floor Labs.	<10% proliferation	3% proliferation 08/13/11
Replication-Competent Retrovirus (Extended S+L- assay for GAL-V pseudotyped virus)	Vector Production Facility, University of Indiana	Sample sent for testing	Sent for testing 09/23/11
HLA Typing - Donor blood and Cell product	Donor & Product Histocompatibility & Transplantation Labs. The Methodist Hospital, Houston Houston, TX, USA	Donor A*3101,2407 B*1521,3505 DRB1*1501,1202 DQB1*0602,0301 DRB3*0301 DRB4* DRB5*0101 04/21/09	Product A*24,31 B*15(75)(w6),35(w6) DRB1*12,15 DQB1*03(7),06 DRB3*Pos(52) DRB4*Neg DRB5*Pos(51) 08/25/11

Released for Allogeneic Use by Intended Recipient Only by:

_______________________ Date 11/05/11
James Smith
Quality Assurance

_______________________ Date 11/05/11
Sara Jones
Laboratory Medical Director

Certificate consists of one page – not valid without signatures

Figure 98-4 SAMPLE CERTIFICATE OF ANALYSIS USED FOR THE RELEASE OF CELLULAR PRODUCTS MANUFACTURED UNDER AN INVESTIGATIONAL NEW DRUG.

to DLI alone. Although the etiology is unclear, the reason could be lack of antigenic expression, downregulation of T-cell recognition molecules, or tumor burden at the time of treatment.

The regulatory situation for DLI is complicated and probably is in transition. At present, nonmanipulated DLI are classified as Type 361 products and fall under Part 1271 of 21CFR. It is possible that they will be reclassified as Type 351 products requiring an IND application. Currently, formal release criteria are not required; however, the normal practice is to evaluate T-cell content by flow cytometry and to test for sterility. This may be done by a Gram stain (used for immediate release) accompanied by culture-based methods. These provide results after the product has been infused. Formal procedures should be in place to inform the recipient's physician if a positive test result is subsequently received. The contaminant should be speciated and antibiotic sensitivities obtained and communicated to the physician. DLI that have been manipulated ex vivo in any way (e.g., by targeting them to specific antigens or by transduction with a suicide gene, as described later) will be classified as Type 351 products requiring an IND. These products will require formal release testing as described previously for other cellular therapy products.

Nonspecifically Activated Autologous T Cells

T cells can be expanded ex vivo through polyclonal activation using PHA, anti-CD3 antibody, or a combination of anti-CD3 and anti-CD28 antibodies. Several groups have evaluated whether such expanded T cells have antitumor activity. Faster recovery of lymphocyte counts with improved outcome after autologous transplant observed in non-Hodgkin and Hodgkin lymphoma led to a phase I study evaluating infusion of autologous CD3/CD28 activated cells after a CD34-selected SCT.

Cells prepared for these types of studies are Type 351 products because they are cultured ex vivo and may have undergone some form of activation. Manufacturing must be carried out under GMP, and the clinical studies must be performed under an IND. The IND application must describe in the CMC the procedure for manufacturing the cells and the criteria that will be used to determine whether they can be released for clinical use. Many manufacturing procedures use reagents and materials that are not approved for human use, and the application should include information about these materials and what testing will be performed before they can be used for manufacturing the clinical product. Justification should be provided for the use of nonapproved media and supplements and any potentially undesirable ancillary products, such as antibiotics. Evidence should be provided on the efficacy of their removal before administration of the product.

The release criteria for autologous T-cell products are similar to those described for generic Type 351 products. They include tests for sterility, endotoxin, mycoplasma, and identity and purity (i.e., by flow cytometry); some test of functionality is recommended but is not usually required for phase I studies. A draft of the CoA, which will be used for release, should be included in the IND submission.

Tumor-Infiltrating Lymphocytes

Tumor-infiltrating lymphocytes are cells harvested from tumor sites and are expanded ex vivo with IL-2. As the cells are being expanded, increased tumor specificity is achieved by pulsing the cells with tumor-specific peptides or transducing them with a retrovirus encoding a tumor-specific TCR. A major limitation is that patients must have preexisting lymphocytes that can both respond to tumor and be expanded ex vivo; however, in studies, transfer of these cells led to tumor regression in 50% of lympho-depleted patients with metastatic melanoma.

A number of methods have been developed for isolation of TIL from tumors. They include mechanical disruption, enzymatic treatment, differential centrifugation approaches, and positive immunomagnetic selection. The method of choice depends on the type of tissue from which the cells are to be extracted and the availability of reagents, such as MAb, targeting the T-cell population of interest. As with T-cell depletion of allogeneic grafts, the predominant effector TIL cell population is not fully characterized, and the availability of this information should facilitate the design of more effective separation techniques. A number of approved enzymes and centrifugation media are available, and several companies have suitable MAb that have been prepared under GMP conditions but have not been submitted for FDA approval.

The extracted cells are expanded ex vivo, usually starting in semi-open systems such as cluster plates. The initial populations may be tested in a cytotoxicity assay in an attempt to identify the effector population, which can then be selected for expansion. The expansion phase usually progresses through a number of types of cultures as cell numbers increase. These may progress from plates to T flasks and gas-permeable bags to hollow fiber and culture bag bioreactors. The culture medium contains IL-2 as the primary cytokine, although other agents alone and in combination may be used to promote outgrowth of specific cell subpopulations.

Some investigators have used irradiated tumor cells to restimulate TIL during culture; others have performed selective separations to enrich the effector cells during expansion. Highly characterized tissue culture media, such as the serum-free lymphocyte medium AIM V, have been used for expansion. The goal is to use the simplest medium with the fewest additives that will support growth of functional cells. When possible, the media should be free of animal serum and proteins to simplify the regulatory issues. However, the FDA is aware that complex media and serum combinations may be required to support growth of some cell types and is willing to consider them, particularly if the cells can be washed into an approved carrier for administration.

Initiation of a phase I study using TIL or TIL subpopulations will not require complete characterization of the effector cell population, but some preliminary information should be available that allows quantification of the putative effectors for dosing. In most cases, flow cytometric analysis will be used, and the target antigens may be pan–T-cell markers or specific combinations of T subset markers. When other constituents of the product may adversely affect the activity of effector cells, it may be necessary to set an upper limit for contamination by these cells in the clinical product. Most facilities perform some type of functional assay as a part of the release process, which in the case of TIL may be cytokine release or cytotoxic activity toward tumor cells of the appropriate histologic type.

Allodepleted Cells

The major drawback of DLI is the significant risk of GVHD, which is the most important source of treatment-related mortality. Given that the frequency of tumor or viral antigen-specific T cells in most cases is considerably lower than that of alloreactive T cells, it is necessary to expand antigen-specific T cells ex vivo not only to enhance antitumor activity but also to try to separate GVHD from GVT effect. An alternative method for separating GVHD from GVT effect is to selectively deplete alloreactive donor T cells ex vivo. Selective allodepletion is performed by removing donor T cells that express activation markers after coculture with nonleukemic recipient cells. Activation markers investigated include CD25 and CD69 and the increased sensitivity of activated T cells to photosensitizing dyes. A number of phase I/II studies using immunotoxin directed against CD25 have demonstrated the feasibility of this approach, with accelerated reconstitution of virus-specific and total T-cell numbers and low rates of severe GVHD. Relapse rates remained high in this study, which probably reflects the high-risk nature of the patient population.

Potential recipients of allodepleted cells often receive a CD34-selected HPC graft. As a part of the CD34 selection process, a negatively selected population of cells that includes T cells becomes available. However, this fraction usually is not used as the source of cells for allodepletion. These cells usually have been obtained from donors who received granulocyte-macrophage colony-stimulating factor (GM-CSF) for mobilization of peripheral blood progenitor cells, and during processing for CD34 selection, they were exposed to anti-CD34 monoclonal antibody. Therefore, it is preferable to obtain cells for allodepletion from a peripheral blood draw of the donor before administration of growth factor for mobilization. The T cell–enriched fraction usually is obtained by centrifugation on a Ficoll-Hypaque density cushion. The cells are washed and co-incubated with irradiated recipient mononuclear cells, which act as stimulators. A convenient source for stimulator cells is obtained by generation of a cell line from the donor by infection of his or her peripheral blood mononuclear cells with a laboratory strain of EBV. The co-incubation step produces stimulation of alloreactive donor T cells with resulting expression of activation markers, which then can be targeted to remove the alloreactive population. Methods for elimination include cytotoxic drugs (e.g., methotrexate), anti-CD25 monoclonal antibody conjugated to the toxin ricin, and immunomagnetic selection. All of the regulatory issues associated with the manufacturing and release of Type 351 products apply to allodepleted T-cell products. Release criteria include routine assays for sterility and purity. HLA typing may be included as a confirmation that the cells in the product are of donor origin. Functional assays may include demonstration that the allodepleted cells fail to proliferate when cultured in a primary mixed lymphocyte reaction (MLR). If a suicide gene has been introduced (see below), testing will include demonstration that it can be efficiently activated.

Suicide Gene Transduced Lymphocytes

Although treatment with DLI has led to remission in patients with disease after HSC transplantation, unmanipulated cells also contain alloreactive T cells and can induce GVHD. The incidence of GVHD ranges from 55% to 90% and is associated with a treatment-related mortality rate of about 20%. Approaches that maintain the GVT effect while decreasing the incidence of GVHD have been evaluated and include transduction of donor T cells with a "suicide gene." Genes can be introduced into DLI or alloreactive-depleted cells to express the herpes simplex virus-1 thymidine kinase (HSV-tk). If GVHD develops, ganciclovir is administered to the recipient, resulting in suicide of the transduced donor leukocytes.

Alternative suicide genes based on the dimerization of Fas or Caspase-9 in the apoptotic pathway have been developed to circumvent the problem of immunogenicity of HSV-tk. The inducible Caspase construct also encodes a selection marker, such as CD19, that can be used to enrich the transduced population. In the event that GVHD develops after administration of the Caspase-transduced cells, the suicide activation drug can be administered to the recipient to eradicate the transduced T cells by dimerization of Caspase 9 and activation of the apoptosis pathway.

Antigen-Specific Cytotoxic T Lymphocytes

Two major prerequisites for generating antigen-specific cytotoxic T lymphocytes (CTL) are the identification of appropriate viral or tumor target antigens and the availability of suitable antigen-presenting cells (APCs). After being identified, CTL lines can be generated by coculturing T cells with APC that express the target antigen. The lines are then expanded by restimulation with the antigen of choice and the addition of cytokines such as IL-2.

To generate antigen-specific CTLs, it is necessary to have a good source of APCs and a source of antigen to present to T cells. A variety of APCs have been evaluated, including fibroblasts, monocytes, and DCs, using different sources of antigen, including virus lysate or lysate of antigen-positive cells, peptides, or transduction of the APC, such as lymphoblastoid cells (LCLs) and DC with an immunodominant antigen. Use of lysates as the antigen source can be problematic because they are likely to be variable and difficult to standardize. Alternatively, many processing laboratories may not be experienced in handling virus and virus-infected cells.

Lymphoblastoid cells prepared using laboratory strains of EBV make excellent APCs for use in manufacturing EBV-specific T cells. They present EBV antigens efficiently, and they express high levels of costimulatory molecules. The normal procedure for generating the LCL is co-incubation with EBV derived from the tamarin B95-8 cell line. This line has undergone extensive testing and has been approved for use as a source of "clinical" EBV. The resulting LCLs are cultured in media containing acyclovir to eliminate any residual EBV. The LCLs are used to repeatedly stimulate T cells (as a mononuclear cell fraction of peripheral blood leukocytes), resulting in a population that is directed toward the immunodominant EBV antigens. These CTLs can be frozen while release testing is performed. They are delivered frozen to the bedside, where they are thawed and administered intravenously. Release testing consists of the routine tests described earlier for Type 351 products. For allogeneic CTL, functionality usually is assessed by cytotoxicity assays, which must demonstrate less than 10% killing of autologous PHA blasts.

One limitation of this approach is that expansion of virus-specific T cells to achieve adequate dose levels is extremely time consuming. All of these procedures require several weeks to generate APCs. One means of overcoming this problem is to manufacture banked allogeneic EBV-specific CTLs so that an "off-the-shelf" product is available. Clinical responses have been described for patients who received partially matched allogeneic CTL. The generation of banks of CTL requires careful donor screening and HLA typing and the manufacture of products with a sufficiently wide range of HLA types to allow at least partial matching with the intended recipient.

Natural Killer Cells

Natural killer cells are effectors from the innate immune system that also mediate antiviral and antitumor immunity. Studies have shown that haploidentical NK cells infused after lymphodepleting chemotherapy can have antitumor effects. Most facilities use a simple positive selection with clinical scale immunomagnetic methods involving CD56 selection or CD3 depletion for such products. These procedures must be done under an IND because of lack of commercially available devices and reagents for this indication.

When preparing an IND application for NK cell enrichment, care should be taken to ensure that the MAb used for the selection or depletion are of the highest quality available. CofA for these reagents should be submitted with the IND application, and the agency probably will require detailed information on their manufacturing (i.e., to ensure that the process includes robust procedures for virus inactivation or removal). The same type of information may be required for any ancillary reagents (e.g., buffers and protein sources used to supplement buffers). Preclinical data demonstrating that the enrichment technique is effective should be provided and accompanied by data from clinical scale validation enrichments, providing evidence that the NK cells can be separated with acceptable viability, purity, and yield for the proposed study. The CMC section of the IND application should include information on the methods used to store, label, and administer the cells. Engineered APCs, such as the K562-mb15-41BBL cell line, if used to stimulate NK cells, should initially have been grown and tested as a Master Cell Bank, from which a Working Cell Bank is generated and tested for routine use.

Dendritic Cells

Dendritic cells are powerful APCs that can be used in vitro or in vivo to elicit immune response to the antigen they are presenting. A number of studies have evaluated tumor antigen-primed DCs for treatment of hematologic malignancies and solid tumors. Antigen-primed DCs are used to target T cells in vitro toward specific antigens. These cells then can be used therapeutically to eliminate viruses or tumor cells bearing that antigen. DC can be derived from BM or cord blood and mobilized and resting peripheral blood obtained from normal donors and patients. The normal procedure consists of enriching monocytes from the source material, which has been accomplished by plastic adherence or CD14-based immunomagnetic selection (or by depletion of $CD19^+$ B cells and $CD2^+$ T cells). An alternative approach is use of elutriation to collect an enriched monocyte fraction from the donor. A purpose-built elutriation system for collection of monocytes is available (the Elutra). This method also has been used successfully to enrich monocytes from cryopreserved mobilized apheresis collections.

The monocyte fraction can be cultured in polystyrene tissue culture flasks or gas-permeable bags in culture medium containing IL-4 and GM-CSF) to induce DC differentiation. This is followed by culture in medium containing proinflammatory mediators to accelerate maturation. A number of supplements have been used during this phase, including CD40 ligand or poly(I:C), interferon-α, tumor necrosis factor-α, IL-6, IL-1α, and prostaglandin E_2. Some protocols add proinflammatory mediators at the initiation of the cultures rather than after induction of differentiation. One issue for facilities is finding clinical or GMP-grade cytokines and growth factors. Some sources now are available, and many manufacturers assist investigators by providing information on test procedures and stability information. Attempts have been made to expand DC in serum-free medium with varying degrees of success; improved growth and maturation have generally been obtained in the presence of human AB or autologous serum. Of note, minor changes in composition of the culture medium and even in the type of vessel used for culture have been reported to affect the yield, phenotype, and functional activity of the resulting DCs. Cultured DCs have been effectively transfected using native tumor DNA or lentiviral or adenoviral vectors. The cells can be cryopreserved for later administration or use.

Assessment of DC product usually involves immunophenotyping ($CD1a^+$, $CD80^+$, $CD83^+$) and some type of functional assay (ability to generate an allogeneic T-cell response or response to a recall antigen as measured by proliferation assay) in addition to the standard release assays.

Mesenchymal Stromal Cells

Mesenchymal stromal cells (MSCs) are cells with multilineage potential that have shown efficacy in promoting engraftment and suppressing GVHD. They are also being widely used in regenerative medicine applications. In vitro MSCs are capable of differentiating into bone, cartilage, cardiac and skeletal muscle, neuronal cells, adipose and connective tissue, and tendons. The cells are not inherently immunogenic and do not appear to be recognized by allogeneic T cells or NK cells. They express very low levels of MHC class II and intermediate levels of class I antigens. They appear to be able to suppress in vitro T-cell proliferation and function of both memory T and naive T cells and to inhibit the development of monocyte-derived DCs in vitro.

A number of technical variables affect MSC culture and expansion ex vivo. They include culture medium, passaging density, serum type and concentration, population selection, culture vessel, and use of growth factors. To reduce some of this variability and reduce the costs of preclinical testing, the FDA often encourages investigators to adopt a manufacturing process that is in current clinical trials. The following is a basic procedure. MSCs usually are isolated from BM collected from the iliac crest. The cells are diluted, and the mononuclear fraction is isolated using a Ficoll-Hypaque density cushion. This fraction is plated into culture flasks to enrich for adherent cells. The nonadherent population is removed after approximately 7 days of incubation. The adherent cells are washed and detached by incubation with trypsin/ethylenediaminetetraacetic acid (EDTA) (alternatively, Trypzean, a recombinant form of trypsin, can be substituted) and then cultured and passaged at weekly intervals. In a study designed to optimize culture conditions, the best results were obtained when cells were cultured in low-glucose Dulbecco modified Eagle medium (DMEM)–based media containing 10% fetal bovine serum (human platelet lysate is now frequently substituted) and GlutaMAX instead of l-glutamine. The cells also proliferated better when plated at low cell densities (5000-10,000 cells/cm^2) in Falcon flasks. Use of basic fibroblast growth factor as a growth supplement was found to be effective; however, it caused HLA-DR induction and upregulated HLA class I expression. This did not affect the immunosuppressive capabilities of the cells. An increase in osteogenic and adipogenic potential was noted, but neurogenesis and engraftment support for CD34-positive cells were slightly suppressed. A number of media specifically designed for culture of MSC are commercially available (e.g., STEMPRO MSC-SFM a serum-free formulation from Invitrogen, and Mesencult, a basal culture medium from StemCell Technologies). Various investigators have reported success growing MSCs in serum-free media or using platelet lysate, autologous serum, or human AB serum as alternatives to fetal bovine serum.

Mesenchymal stromal cells can be characterized by their expression of CD105, CD73, and CD90 and their lack of expression of CD45, CD34, CD14 or CD11b, CD79a or CD19, and HLA-DR. They must be plastic adherent under standard culture conditions and must be capable of differentiating into osteoblasts, adipocytes, and chondroblasts in vitro. Differentiation assays involve growing MSCs under conditions that promote differentiation along the specific pathway. For neurogenic differentiation, the medium contains linoleic acid, platelet-derived growth factor, and epidermal growth factor. Neural cells are identified by immunostaining with antibodies against tubulin BIII, synaptophysin, galactocerebroside, neurofilament M, and neuronal nuclei (NeuN). To assess adipogenic potential, the medium contains dexamethasone, isobutylmethylxanthine, and indomethacin. The lipid droplets in the generated adipocytes are visualized by staining with Sudan black IV. Osteogenic differentiation is measured by culturing the cells in medium containing dexamethasone, β-glycerophosphate, and l-ascorbic acid 2-phosphate. Calcium accumulation and alkaline phosphatase activity in the resulting cells is visualized by alkaline phosphatase/Von Kossa staining, and the osteogenic differentiation is measured as the percentage of mineralized area in the total cultured area.

The ability of MSC to suppress an MLR is used as an indication of their immunosuppressive activity. A traditional MLR assay is used; however, in the test wells, the MLR is performed on a layer of MSC seeded the day before. The response traditionally is measured by uptake of tritiated thymidine. Numerous animal assays for MSC are available but are predominantly used in preclinical studies and are not useful as release assays. Release criteria consist of the usual assays for sterility, endotoxin, and mycoplasma, with immunophenotyping for the MSC population. Depending on the intended use of the MSC, the release process may require an assay showing potential for differentiation into a specific lineage or ability to suppress an immune response such as an MLR assay.

Genetically Modified Cell Therapy Products

Many cell therapy approaches involve genetic modification of either APCs or effector cells (see earlier discussion). This therapy requires a source of vector that has been manufactured to meet regulatory requirements. Vector specifications changed markedly after the death of a gene therapy patient in Philadelphia, and they continue to evolve. Manufacturers must maintain close contact with the FDA to ensure that their products meet current specifications. Manufacturing and testing of viral vectors is extremely expensive, and use of genetically modified products requires additional monitoring of recipients. Use of vectors to transduce or transfect cellular therapy products ex vivo usually requires additional testing of the product, which may include detection of replication competent virus and checking the functionality of the introduced vector (by detecting expression of the gene product).

Gene-Modified Tumor Vaccines

Tumor vaccines as an approach to inducing or stimulating immunity have been evaluated. Various techniques have been tested, including use of DCs pulsed with a tumor-associated antigen preparation and use of the entire tumor cells as an immunogen, either unmodified or transduced with immunostimulatory genes, aimed at eliciting a broad-based, robust immune response.

From the manufacturing perspective, the autologous product is much more of a challenge because a stable tumor cell line must be isolated from each patient. This can be an extremely difficult process. Many isolated lines do not expand well in culture, or they change phenotype over time. In some patients, the line cannot be generated; other patients progress clinically before the vaccine is available and are excluded from the study. As a result, the autologous approach has a relatively high "failure rate." The allogeneic cell line approach is technically easier because a line is selected before the study and can be used as the generic immunogen. This line must be tested extensively for infectious agents and should pass the FDA testing criteria for Master and Working Cell Banks. Currently testing of this type costs $100,000 to $200,000 for each line. Scientifically, the drawback is that the selected line may not adequately express the antigen or range of antigens present on each patient's tumor. In addition, the choice of immunostimulatory molecules that are expressed or enhanced by transduction of the cell line may not be those that would most effectively evoke an immune response. These products are relatively expensive to produce, involving not only the costs of testing the tumor cell line but also the expense of manufacturing and testing the vectors used for transduction. However, these are one-time costs because the same vaccine is used for all patients in the study.

Release testing involves testing for sterility, endotoxin, and mycoplasma, with immunophenotyping of the cells and some form of test demonstrating that the line has been effectively transduced (e.g., flow cytometry for CD40 ligand and IL-2 production in the examples described earlier). Because the product will be stored cryopreserved over the course of the study and thawed for administration to each patient, the requirement for an ongoing stability study should be anticipated.

FUTURE DIRECTIONS

The science of hematopoietic transplantation has expanded dramatically over the past 10 years and has stimulated entirely new areas of medicine. New sources of stem cells have been discovered that have expanded the availability of grafts and provided new insights into stem cell biology. This in turn has stimulated the development of regenerative medicine to treat a wide variety of diseases for which there were limited therapeutic options. Time will provide insight as to the efficacy and mechanism of action of these approaches.

An improved understanding of immune responses and the effector cells involved has reinvigorated the field of immunotherapy and made it possible to design treatments that have a more realistic chance of success. Coupled with new laboratory techniques for the manipulation and selection of cells, these therapies are showing promise for the treatment of cancers and viral infections. Gene therapy is recovering from some early setbacks and disappointments to find a place in redirecting immune responses and retargeting cells.

These advances in knowledge coupled to development in technology promise a bright future for engineering specific cell populations to provide targeted therapies.

SUGGESTED READINGS

Professional Standards for Cellular Therapy

AABB Standards for Cellular Therapy Product Services, ed 5, Bethesda, MD, 2011, AABB.

FACT-JACIE International Standards for Cellular Therapy Product Collection: *Processing and Administration*, ed 5, Omaha, NE, 2011, FACT.

NetCord-FACT International Standards for Cord Blood Collection, Processing, and Release for Administration, ed 4, Omaha, NE, 2010, NetCord-FACT.

FDA Regulations: cGMP and cGTP

cGMP in Manufacturing, Processing, Packing, or Holding of Drugs and Finished Pharmaceuticals. Code of Federal Regulations Title 21, Parts 210 and 211.

Human Cells, Tissues, and Cellular and Tissue Based Products. Code of Federal Regulations Title 21, Part 1271.

FDA Guidances on Cellular and Gene Therapy

Guidance for FDA Reviewers and Sponsors: Content and Review of Chemistry, Manufacturing, and Control (CMC) Information for Human Somatic Cell Therapy Investigational New Drug Applications (INDs). U.S. Department of Health and Human Services, Food and Drug Administration, Center for Biologics Evaluation and Research, April 2008.

Guidance for Human Somatic Cell Therapy and Gene Therapy. U.S. Department of Health and Human Services, Food and Drug Administration, Center for Biologics Evaluation and Research, March 1998.

GMP Facilities and Product Manufacturing

Cell Therapy – cGMP Facilities and Manufacturing. Gee AP, editor: New York, NY, 2009, Springer.

Cellular Therapy: Principles, Methods, and Regulations. Areman E, editor: Bethesda, MD, 2009, AABB.

Specific Cell Types: Current Reviews

Overview

Copier J, Bodman-Smith M, Dalgliesh A: Current status and future application of cellular therapies for cancer. *Immunotherapy* 3:507, 2011.

Mesenchymal Stromal Cells

Vemuri MC, Chase LG, Rao MS: Mesenchymal stem cell assays and applications. *Methods Mol Biol* 698:3, 2011.

Dendritic Cells

Delamarre L, Mellman I: Harnessing dendritic cells for immunotherapy. *Semin Immunol* 23:2, 2011.

Natural Killer Cells

Romagne F, Vivier E: Natural killer cell-based therapies. F1000. *Med Rep* 3:9, 2011.

Tumor-Infiltrating Lymphocyte Cells

Park TS, Rosenberg SA, Morgan RA: Targeting cancer with genetically engineered T cells. *Trends Biotechnol* 29(11):550, 2011.

T Cells

Brenner MK, Heslop HE: Adoptive T cell therapy of cancer. *Curr Opin Immunol* 22:251. 2010.

Hanley PJ, Shaffer DR, Cruz CR, et al: Expansion of T cells targeting multiple antigens of cytomegalovirus, Epstein Barr virus and adenovirus to provide broad antiviral specificity after stem cell transplantation. *Cytotherapy* 13:976, 2011.

Kohn DB, Dotti G, Brentjens R, et al: CARs on track in the clinic. *Mol Ther* 19:432, 2011.

T-cell depletion in GVHD: Less is more? *Antin J. Blood* 117:6061, 2011.

Donor Leukocyte Infusions and Suicide Genes

Di Stasi A, Tey S-K, Dotti G, et al: Inducible apoptosis as a safety switch for adoptive cell therapy. *N Eng J Med* 2011 365:1673.

Roddie C, Peggs KS: Donor lymphocyte infusion following allogeneic hematopoietic stem cell transplantation. *Expert Opin Bio Ther* 11:473, 2011.

Tumor Vaccines

Dougan M, Dranoff G: Immune therapy for cancer. *Annu Rev Immunol* 27:83, 2009.

CHAPTER 99

PRINCIPLES OF CELL-BASED GENETIC THERAPIES

David A. Williams

The use of gene transfer to treat human diseases has now efficacious in a limited number of instances. Proof-of-principle successes proven in several monogenic diseases—both hematologic and nonhematologic—have been published and widely publicized in the past decade. Despite these successes, the occurrence of serious adverse events in some trials related to insertional mutagenesis has tempered the enthusiasm accompanying these reports but has also stimulated rapid development of safer vector systems. This chapter discusses the basic biology of vector systems applicable to blood diseases, discusses details of the application of gene therapy to blood diseases using specific trials as examples of this technology, and discusses modifications in vector systems driven by clinical experience that predict future trials. The chapter also discusses the prospects that the evolving field of somatic cell reprogramming may generate alternative cellular targets for genetic engineering.

HEMATOLOGIC DISEASES, CELLULAR TARGETS, AND THE BASIS FOR GENETIC THERAPIES

Gene therapy is defined as the introduction of new genetic material into the cells of an organism for therapeutic purposes. Broadly speaking, two types of gene therapy can be envisioned. The introduction of genetic material into germ cells such that the new DNA can be expected to be passed into the gene pool. This is termed *germline gene therapy* and is currently banned in the United States and around the world. In contrast, introduction of new genetic material into specialized cells of the body with no risk of the new genetic material being passed onto subsequent generations is termed *somatic gene therapy*. The ultimate goal of gene therapy would be to correct a genetic disease by *replacement* of the defective gene in situ. Such gene replacement could be envisioned via a process termed *homologous recombination*. Homologous recombination in mammalian cells is widely practiced in laboratories but up to now has been relatively inefficient. Advantages of this approach would include a reduction in the risk of inadvertent disruption or dysregulation of expression of a critical gene sequence and regulated (appropriate level and distribution) expression of the normal (replaced) gene. However, the frequency of this event (in contrast to random chromosomal integration) in mammalian cells makes therapeutic use of homologous recombination impractical at this point. Methods to effect homologous recombination have improved in the past 5 years and may make this goal attainable in the future.

The requirements for successful application of our current gene transfer technology for treatment of human diseases include knowledge of the abnormal gene sequence responsible for the disease phenotype and the availability of the corresponding normal gene sequence. In addition, the cells responsible for the disease phenotype must be identified and accessible for genetic manipulation. Finally, a means of introducing and expressing the correct gene sequence in cells such that the disease phenotype can be reversed is needed. This latter requirement has been, although effectively accomplished more than 2 decades ago in murine studies, the most difficult to consistently meet in human applications using current gene transfer technology. Since the early development of virus vectors, blood-forming cells have been used as one optimal target for gene transfer studies, and most studies to date use ex vivo approaches to genetic modification. For this purpose, hematopoietic stem and progenitor cells (HPSCs) are isolated, manipulated in the laboratory and administered back to the patient. The advantages of these cells as targets of gene transfer are multiple. First, all blood cells are derived from a common progenitor cell, the hematopoietic stem cell (HSC), which is both long lived in vivo and capable of significant self-renewal. The latter capacity and the pluripotency of HSC is exploited to amplify the genetically manipulated cells into large cell numbers of multiple blood lineages in vivo. There is a long and successful experience in obtaining these stem cells from the bone marrow (BM) and peripheral and umbilical cord blood. There is extensive experience in the use of HSCs in the clinical setting for transplantation, and there is experience in purification of these cells and limited knowledge of the requirements for ex vivo manipulation of the cells. In addition, the experience of HSC transplantation has defined a variety of genetic diseases in which the phenotype can be altered by the successful engraftment of normal allogeneic donor cells. Finally, the blood system is involved as a major dose-limiting organ in cancer therapies and both a target and an effector organ in immune reactions providing a large group of diseases that could theoretically be approached using gene transfer technology. As noted earlier, there are already a large number of monogenic diseases of the blood extensively characterized with more being defined at the molecular level on a regular basis because whole-exome and whole-genome sequencing is being applied to rare disease phenotypes. In addition to HSC targets, another application of gene transfer technology exploits the experience in adoptive T-cell immunotherapy. In this application, T cells (and less well developed to this point, other immune effector cells) are modified ex vivo in an attempt to enhance potency and specificity. This application of gene transfer technology will not be reviewed here.

The field of gene therapy is rapidly evolving. Successes of proof-of-principle small trials have demonstrated the utility of gene transfer approach in a sizable number of patients but in a limited number of diseases. The technology itself is quickly evolving in response to new understanding of viruses, the regulation of gene expression, and gene editing. The application of gene transfer technology to HSC gene therapy has been made possible by exploitation of viruses that have evolved the capacity to efficiently and precisely insert viral genome into cellular chromosomes of infected cells. The field has taken about 25 years to evolve to its current state of clinical application. Although this might be viewed as a slow pace, in reality, this time frame parallels the development of many other novel therapies. This developmental phase also reflects the complexities of the biologic systems involved and the caution required in moving forward in the face of serious adverse events seen in early safety trials. It is indeed an exciting time with respect to the clinical application of gene transfer technology in human diseases.

VECTOR SYSTEMS

The initial impetus to develop gene transfer for human studies derived from the exploitation of oncoretroviruses, mainly murine γ-retroviruses, as vectors for gene delivery in the early 1980s.[1a]

However, over approximately the past 25 years, a multitude of virus vectors have been developed. All vector systems use parts of the virus life cycle in an attempt to increase the frequency and fidelity of gene transfer. Although many vector systems have been developed, retrovirus vectors remain the most used system for human gene therapy trials involving HSC, and this review will focus primarily on this vector system and the closely related lentivirus, foamy virus, and avian virus vectors (reviewed by Touw and Erkeland[1b]). As noted, the majority of trials registered with the Recombinant DNA Advisory Committee (RAC) of the National Institutes of Health use retroviruses with non-integrating adenovirus vectors, adeno-associated virus and nonvirus (liposomes and plasmids) systems making up the second and third largest groups.[2] The latter are primarily focused on immune stimulation trials in cancer and have limited relevance to the use of HPSCs for the treatment of genetic blood diseases.

Retrovirus Vectors

The use of γ-retroviruses as gene transfer vectors takes advantage of the normal virus life cycle. The virus, a membrane-bound particle enclosing a dimer of genomic RNA, gag, and reverse transcriptase proteins, interacts with specific cell surface receptors on the target cell. After entry into the cytoplasm, the virus is uncoated, and the genomic messenger (m) RNA is reverse transcribed into DNA. Subsequent polymerase activity yields a double-stranded (DS) DNA provirus molecule. For γ-retroviruses, transport into the nucleus depends on the loss of the nuclear membrane, which accompanies cell division (see later discussion). Integration of the DS provirus is semirandom in the chromosome, which allows tracking of subsequent progeny cells using molecular analysis of unique integration junctional fragments. The occurrence of insertional activation of oncogenes in several human trials and the subsequent scrutiny of insertion sites in HSC-derived progeny in both murine and human cells using deep sequencing methods have provided a more detailed understanding of subtle but biologically relevant preferences for insertions of these vectors (see later discussion). After being integrated, the provirus can give rise to mRNA leading to encoded protein products. Full-length (genomic) mRNA can also be used as the genomic nucleic acid in newly formed virus particles, which are budded nonlytically from the cell surface after assembly in the cytoplasm of the infected cell. Use of retroviruses for gene delivery depends on the capacity to replace viral genes with other heterologous gene sequences and to provide necessary viral proteins in trans in specialized cell lines, called *packaging cells*. The advanced generation of packaging cells appears to be capable of generating pure stocks of recombinant virus without contaminating wild-type helper virus, an important safety consideration. Indeed, to date in human trials, there have been no reports of inadvertent generation of infectious virus. Thus, this infection with replication-incompetent (ie helper-free) retrovirus vectors would be predicted to yield integration into the targeted cell population but no further spread of virus in the body of the treated patient. The proteins provided in trans for γ-retroviruses are generally gag, reverse transcriptase, and envelope proteins, the latter defining the host range of infection. In summary, the advantages of retrovirus vectors include the high efficiency of stable transfer of intact DNA sequences, the broad range of host cells susceptible to infection by retroviruses, and the ability to generate helper-free recombinant virus.

Despite these advantages, the application of retrovirus vectors to treatment of human blood diseases in early trials was disappointing. In multiple studies, transduction of long-lived and transplantable HSCs has been extremely low. In most studies, the frequency of circulating marked blood cells was too low to effect phenotypic correction of any disease, usually less than 0.1%. The biologic parameters contributing to the poor results in human trials are varied. The major impediments appear to include the low levels of viral receptors on the surface of human HSCs, reducing the efficiency of interaction of virus particles with these target cells,[3-5] and the quiescent nature of the majority of HSC, which hinders the transport of the provirus into the nucleus and thus reduces integration frequency. Practical issues, including the difficulty in obtaining high-titer virus in large-scale preparations required for human trials, have also been noted.

These difficulties have led to various strategies and development of entirely new vector systems, which seek to improve gene transfer methods in human HSCs. These strategies include attempts to increase virus–cell interactions or methods to enhance the chances of successful DNA integration. Different viral envelopes were used to pseudotype recombinant particles to more efficiently target CD34 cells.[6-10] The use of various cell surface markers, such as CD34, to purify the target cell population can also increase the multiplicity of infection at a given virus titer and has been used in clinical transplantation protocols. Thus, the development of antibody-based enrichment of the CD34$^+$ HPSC compartment from human hematopoietic tissues using magnetic column purification provided a rapid, clinically applicable method to further enhance retroviral transduction by increasing the vector to target cell ratio.[11-14] Methods to increase physical interactions between vector particles and target cells include co-localization on fibronectin and centrifugation methods. Where polycations such as polybrene had previously been used to enhance transduction frequencies by negating electrostatic charge repulsion between target cells and viral particles, the characterization of the recombinant CH296 fibronectin fragment (Retronectin has a matrix upon which one could co-localize HSCs and viral particles was a significant advance in the quest to improve CD34$^+$ transduction frequencies.[15-18] Efforts to increase the chances of DNA integration have focused on attempts to increase the number of HSC that are undergoing cell division (primarily the use of cytokines that effect stem cell proliferation). The development of improved in vitro growth media formulations incorporating novel cytokine cocktails achieved the dual aim of promoting HSC division, which is required for transduction with gammaretroviral vectors while minimizing stem cell loss in vitro via apoptosis or differentiation.[19-25] Finally, the use of new virus systems that do not require nuclear membrane disruption (and therefore cell division) for entry of the provirus DNA into the nucleus, including primarily lentivirus vectors but potentially also vectors based on foamy viruses, appears to be the most significant development in the field in the past decade. These newer vector systems will be discussed later.

In addition to the energy in the field that was devoted to advancing stem cell transduction methodology, additional work focused on developing retroviral vectors that would express transgene cassettes at levels that would be high enough to elicit a therapeutic benefit and be resistant to gene silencing. Advances in vector design such as the optimization of long-terminal repeat (LTR) enhancer and promoter elements and viral leader sequences resulted in recombinant vectors that were able to mediate high level transgene expression in both primitive and mature hematopoietic cells.[26-32] As discussed in detail later, although these power promoter and enhancer elements provided robust expression of transgenes, they appear also to be capable of long-range activation of endogenous regulatory sequences as a form of insertional mutagenesis that can have significant deleterious effects. Taken together, these technologic advances served as the platform for the first successful gene therapy trial in humans.

The use of pharmacologic in vivo selection in combination with gene transfer, both in the setting of cancer trials and in genetic diseases, remains a potentially important method to enhance the reconstitution of human recipients with gene-modified blood cells but has not yet gained widespread usage. This approach is reviewed in more detail in a recent publication.[33] General considerations include the need for a particular drug to effect damage to BM stem or progenitor cells. A gene or genes encoding resistance to this agent would need to be identified and resistance in vivo to the agent would need to be demonstrated after overexpression of this gene in BM cells. For applications in cancer therapies, dose intensification of drugs used within chemotherapeutic regimens should improve antitumor efficacy. For noncancer applications (most likely uses attempting co-selection of a nonselectable therapeutic gene in a genetic disease application), the mutagenic potential of the chemotherapy agent must be considered as a risk in relation to the overall benefit of the gene therapy procedure. Several chemoresistance genes and chemotherapy drug combinations are currently under investigation for this application, and encouraging preclinical studies have led to a limited number of early phase human studies in cancer patients.

Lentivirus Vectors

One of the key advances in the gene therapy field in the past decade has been the development of recombinant vectors based on lentiviruses, including human immunodeficiency virus (HIV). These vectors were originally developed after the observation that targets of HIV included more differentiated cells, such as macrophages, that are often also postmitotic, suggesting this group of retroviruses has evolved a method of circumventing the block in infection of gammaretroviruses seen in nondividing cells. Investigators demonstrated lentivirus vectors derived from HIV were capable of infecting nondividing neurons after direct injection into the brain.[34] Subsequently, Naldini et al[35] showed efficient infection of growth arrested cells. As with gammaretroviruses, lentivirus vectors use key viral gene products in trans to generate replication-defective infectious particles carrying the transgene of interest. To date, most lentivirus vectors use vesicular stomatitis virus as envelope sequence, which provides a very broad range of target cells susceptible to lentivirus vector transduction. In the case of lentivirus vectors, viral gag and pol as well as tat and rev proteins expression are required in trans for efficient virus production along with the envelope proteins. These proteins are usually supplied from separate plasmids, and recombinant lentivirus production is today generally created using "four plasmid" systems encompassing all the necessary viral proteins on three plasmids and the transfer vector sequences on the fourth plasmid.[36] In addition to *gag* and *pol,* the transfer vector contains all the virus regulatory sequences required *in cis* for packaging an infectious particle, including the *psi* packaging sequence, integrase, and reverse transcriptase. Thus, generation of high-titer recombinant virus is more complicated than gammaretroviruses.

To reduce the chances of generation of replication competent retroviruses (RCRs), a major safety concern with HIV, most of the nonessential viral sequences were removed from vectors. This included *viv, vpu, vpr,* and *nef* genes and subsequently *tat,* an important regulator of viral transcription. Recombinant vectors generated without these sequences were demonstrated to efficiently infect a variety of cells.[36,37] RCR testing is based on sensitive assays to detect gag protein by p24 immunoassays or polymerase chain reaction. In addition, lentivirus vectors have traditionally been produced using the "self-inactivating design" (SIN) for added safety because of reduced risk of recombination with and subsequent mobilization of endogenous HIV viruses. The transfer vector thus contains a deletion of the 5′ LTR U3 region and are devoid of viral enhancer and promoter sequences. During reverse transcription, the 5′ LTR is replicated, and the integrated provirus is thus devoid of both 5′ and 3′ U3 regions.[38,39] In SIN constructs, the transgene of interest is thus expressed from an internal promoter that can be chosen with varying strengths. This added safety feature ultimately has proven important also to reduce the risk of insertional mutagenesis (see later) by which integration near cellular genes are inadvertently activated by the LTR enhancer sequences of vectors.

Lentivirus vectors were originally developed for use in a wide range of tissues in which cells are largely nondividing. Early work focused on brain,[35,40] retinal cells,[39] liver,[41] pancreatic islets,[42] airway epithelium,[43] and muscle.[41,44] However, it was subsequently appreciated that the requirement of stimulating HSCs into division with various cytokines to effect efficient transduction with gammaretrovirus vectors may have negative effects on engraftment or that a large fraction of HSCs remain quiescent and therefore resistant to transduction during clinical transduction protocols. After several groups reported successful transduction of primitive HSC populations in protocols in which these cells remained resistant to transduction by gammaretroviruses,[45-49] the adaption of lentivirus vectors has now included several recent human trials, and initial results are encouraging. In a trial for adrenoleukodystrophy, long-term "marking" in the myeloid compartment appears to be 10% to 20%, a level that is about 100-fold higher than the marking in the myeloid compartment seen in previous trials in immunodeficiency conditions that used gammaretrovirus vectors.[50] In addition to the safety advantage of SIN vector design used in all lentivirus vectors, there is an additional theoretical advantage of the preference of lentiviruses for integration away from transcription start sites (TSS) of genes in contrast to gammaretroviruses. However, the recent experience with a lentivirus vector used in a single patient with thalassemia,[51] in which abnormal splicing resulted in clonal expansion in the erythroid compartment, suggests that insertion within genes may also have potential adverse effects on endogenous sequences. These trials are described in more detail later. Thus, long-term safety of lentiviruses in human trials remains to be determined, and important aspects of insertional mutagenesis are described in more detail later.

Foamy Virus Vectors

Foamy viruses possess several features that have been exploited to yield vectors for the purpose of transducing HSCs.[52] Foamy viruses are members of the spumaretroviruses family. They have been shown to be endemic retroviruses in a wide range of animals but are not found in humans. These vectors are the largest of the retroviruses (≈14 kb) and thus yield vectors with a capacity to efficiently package large amounts of genetic sequences.[53] The virus has a DNA genome that is reversed transcribed within the virion particle forming a stable preintegration complex within the transduced cell. As with gammaretrovirus vectors, the virus packaging signals have been successfully exploited to allow production of high-titer, replication-free vector stocks.[54] Based on accidental exposure of a limited number of animal care workers, it has been reported that infection of humans with wild-type foamy virus has no pathologic effects.[55] Foamy virus vectors have been used to successfully transduce mouse and human hematopoietic cells. Proof-of-principle work by Hickstein's group has demonstrated correction of canine leukocyte adhesion deficiency using a foamy virus vector expressing CD18 after transduction and infusion of $CD34^+$ cells after submyeloablative conditioning.[56] No human trials have been opened to date using this vector system, but several are planned for the future.

Alpharetroviruses

Retrovirus vectors derived from Rous sarcoma virus, which is a member of the alpharetrovirus family, have been described. Although these vectors maintain genomic integration as part of the viral life cycle, they have attracted recent attention because of their propensity to integrate in a relatively neutral fashion with respect to promoter regions and TSS of genes.[57] In large animal studies, alpharetovirus-transduced HSC-derived progeny demonstrated integrations that were not clustered in gene-rich CpG or TSS regions of the genome.[58,59] The development of a self-inactivating alpharetrovirus with a split-packaging design by Schambach and colleagues has provided proof-of-principle with respect to the capacity to generate high-titer, replication-free vector stocks that use internal promoters to express transgenes in a potentially safer fashion than gammaretrovirus vectors.[60] Such vectors have been demonstrated to efficiently infect murine and human hematopoietic cells at low multiplicity of infection.[60]

EXPERIENCE IN HEMATOLOGIC CLINICAL TRIALS TO DATE

X-Linked Severe Combined Immunodeficiency

Severe combined immunodeficiency (SCID) comprises a number of rare monogenic diseases with the common feature of a block in T-cell differentiation and impaired B-cell and natural killer (NK) cell immunity.[61] Studies of pattern of inheritance, immune function, and genotypes have led to the identification of at least 11 distinct SCID conditions. The most common variant of SCID results from the deficiency in expression or function of the common cytokine receptor γ chain, which is shared by the receptors for interleukin (IL)-2, IL-4, IL-7, IL-9, IL-15, and IL-21. This condition is inherited in a sex-linked fashion (X-linked SCID or SCID-X1) and accounts for 40% to 50% of all SCID cases.[62,63] SCID-X1 is characterized by abnormal development or function of T, B, and NK cells, although B cells are usually present in humans (so called T-minus, B-plus SCID). Survival depends on the reconstitution of T-cell development and function by allogeneic BM transplantation.[64,65] If a genotypically matched family donor is available, HSC transplantation (HSCT) confers greater than 80% chance of long-term survival.[65] The absence of T and NK cells in the patient allows for the engraftment of donor cells without preparative chemotherapy conditioning; thus, this is the treatment of choice with minimal toxicity. When a genotypically matched family member is not available, haploidentical donors (e.g., a parent) or closely matched unrelated donors are used, with varying preference center to center, and a survival rate of 64% to 78% has been reported.[64-68] These inferior outcomes may be attributed to the increased risk of graft rejection or graft-versus-host disease (GVHD), as well as the effects of T-cell depletion, immune suppression causing slower immune reconstitution, or conditioning with increased risk of infection.[69,70] Haploidentical transplants rigorously depleted of T cells, similar to genotypically related transplant, are performed in some institutions without preparative chemotherapy conditioning; however, B-cell reconstitution is poor, and the majority of patients require intravenous immunoglobulin (IVIG) replacement for life.[69,70] Interestingly, spontaneous partial correction of severe T-cell immunodeficiencies, including SCID, has previously been reported, suggesting a selective advantage of wild-type T cells over defective T cells.[71-73]

Two independent gene therapy trials aimed at correcting the immunologic defect of SCID-X1 patients who lack a genotypically matched BM donor have been reported,[74,75] and another has recently been opened for accrual. Thus far, a total of 20 patients have been treated in the reported studies. Despite minor technical differences in the two protocols, the basic design of both gene therapy trials is quite similar: The complete coding region of the human γ chain was cloned into a "first-generation" gammaretroviral vector regulated by the murine leukemia virus (MLV) LTR sequences, which was used to infect BM-derived CD34$^+$ cells in vitro. The transduction occurred in the presence of early acting cytokines (stem cell factor, thrombopoietin, IL-3, and FMS-like tyrosine kinase 3 [FLT 3] ligand) and the CH296 human fragment of fibronectin described earlier. Cells were subsequently infused without prior conditioning or cytoreductive treatment. Minor differences between the two protocols included the uses of a threefold higher concentration of IL-3 and 4% fetal cell serum in the French trial. Additionally, the French investigators used the amphotropic envelope pseudotype compared with the use of gibbon ape leukemia virus (GALV) envelope in the British trial.[74,75] Results in both trials have been extremely encouraging.

In the French trial, 10 children younger than the age of 1 year were enrolled between 1999 and 2002.[74,76] Nine of 10 infants developed normal numbers of T and NK cells, with good immune function.[77] In seven of the nine patients who developed T cells, T-cell counts reached normal levels within 3 months and have remained normal at the time of the last published follow-up.[78] Protective levels of antibodies, including antibody production after immunization, were achieved, and the prophylactic administration of IVIG was discontinued.[77] At almost 8 years after gene therapy, these patients continued to retain a functional immune system, enabling them to live normally.[78]

However, serious adverse events related to gene therapy have been reported in four patients in the French trial, occurring 31 to 68 months after gene therapy,[78-80] and in one patient in the British trial.[75,81] In these patients, untoward effects of viral integration into the genome resulted in T-cell leukemia, leading to the death of one of the four affected patients. Much research has subsequently been directed at elucidating the mechanism responsible for these adverse events. Retroviral integration in the proximity of proto-oncogenes, particularly the LIM domain only 2 (LMO2) promoter, was involved in leukemogenesis in three French patients and one British patient.[78,81] An integration of the unaltered γ chain–encoding viral vector on chromosome 11q13, near the first exon of the *LMO2* gene, led to the unregulated transcription of LMO2, giving rise to a T-cell acute lymphoblastic leukemia (T-ALL)–like lymphoproliferation in the initial two patients.[79] In the patient in the British trial, the integration of the vector 35 kb upstream of the *LMO2* locus cooperated with secondary genetic aberrations, including a gain of function mutation of NOTCH1, a deletion at the CDKN2A tumor suppressor gene locus, and a translocation of the T-cell receptor β region, to give rise to T-ALL.[81] LMO2 is a master regulator of human hematopoiesis that is involved in stem cell growth and is not normally expressed in T cells. However, LMO2 activation has been has been implicated in some cases of human T-cell leukemia.[82] In addition, LMO2 transgenic mice have been shown to develop T-ALL within 10 months.[83] It is increasingly clear that retroviral vectors may "turn on" cellular proto-oncogenes adjacent to their integration site in the genome. The strong promoter or enhancer activity of the retroviral LTR element shows particular propensity to the upregulation of genes neighboring the integration site.[84-86] Multiple studies now indicate that gammaretroviral vectors, such as the vectors used in the two SCID-X1 trials, preferentially integrate into the 5′ end of genes near the TSS.[87] In addition, gammaretroviral vectors have been shown to integrate in or near a number of proto-oncogenes that are actively expressed in human CD34$^+$ cells. When human CD34$^+$ cells were transduced with retroviral vectors ex vivo, 21% of retroviral integrations occurred at recurrent insertion sites ("hot spots"), which were highly enriched for proto-oncogenes and growth-controlling genes.[88] A recent series of papers investigating the vector integration sites in both SCID-X1 trials and the Italian Adenosine Deaminase Deficiency SCID trial observed a greater than random frequency of vector integrations near the TSS of genes that are active in HSCs.[89-91] Interestingly, in the SCID-X1 trial, a skewing of vector integration site distribution in vivo was noted. Compared with retroviral integration sites (RIS) recovered from transduced CD34$^+$ cells, RIS recovered from T cells in vivo 9 to 30 months after transplantation showed an overrepresentation of RIS within or near genes encoding proteins with kinase activity, transferase activity, or proteins involved in phosphorous metabolism. This skewing of RIS in vivo suggests a selection of T cells as a result of viral integration in certain growth- and survival-promoting genes.[89]

Strikingly, in contrast to five cases of insertional mutagenesis in the two SCID-X1 trials, no adverse events have been reported in the 10 patients treated in the Italian ADA-SCID trial despite a similar RIS pattern observed in this patient group.[90] This observation has led to the proposal of a "disease effect" contributing to oncogenesis of γ-chain gene therapy. Woods et al[92] demonstrated lentiviral transduction of $\gamma c^{-/-}$ mice with vectors containing the human common γ chain (cγ) or an inert control gene at very high viral doses. They observed the induction of T-cell malignancies in one-third of the animals receiving cγ transduced cells but not in the control groups. The merit of this very limited study was subsequently challenged, primarily on the basis of a viral dose much higher than that used in clinical scenarios and incomplete data on the pathogenesis of the malignancies, particularly as they relate to the downstream activation level of a key signaling target of the common γ chain, Janus kinase 3 (JAK3), in the tumors.[93,94] In addition, the lentiviral vector used in this study incorporated a hybrid promoter or enhancer element that is extremely powerful and likely to possess a greater transactivating potential than promoter or enhancer elements that would be considered for clinical gene therapy use.[92] More recent occurrence of leukemia in another trial for Wiskcott-Aldrich Syndrome (WAS; see later) using the same vector backbone further challenges the presence of SCID-X1 disease or transgene effects in these leukemias.

In summary, thus far, 5 of 20 patients treated with gene therapy for SCID-X1 have encountered a life-threatening severe adverse event, thought to be triggered by retroviral activation of LMO2 in 4 patients. Four patients were salvaged with chemotherapy, and one patient succumbed to the disease after an unsuccessful allogeneic BM transplantation (BMT). At this point, the use of MLV-based retroviral vectors with LTR promoter enhancer elements intact is viewed as contraindicated in this disease by most investigators in the field. The continued development of safety-enhanced vectors and the validation of these vectors in clinically relevant systems have emerged as a major priority in the field, and an international trial has recently been opened using a gammaretrovirus that is deleted of LTR enhancer elements. Transgene expression is mediated by a weak cellular promoter in this vector. Data suggest that early efficacy is maintained despite lower expression of the IL-2 γ chain.[95]

Adenosine Deaminase Deficiency

Adenosine deaminase (ADA) is a housekeeping enzyme of the purine metabolic pathway that is expressed in all tissues of the body.[96] Deficiency of this enzyme leads to a buildup of toxic metabolites with detrimental systemic effects, including neurodevelopmental deficiencies, sensorineuronal deafness, and skeletal abnormalities. Importantly, ADA deficiency causes abnormal T-, B-, and NK-cell development, resulting in the SCID phenotype. As is the case with the more common SCID-X1, untreated patients generally succumb to severe opportunistic infections in the first year of life. Treatment strategies used to manage affected patients include allogeneic HSCT; enzyme replacement therapy; and more recently, gene therapy.[97] Allogeneic HSCT from a human leukocyte antigen (HLA)–matched family donor offers good immunologic and biochemical correction with 73% survival. However, outcomes after mismatched and haploidentical transplants are less impressive.[65] Likewise, the exogenous replacement of ADA, administered in a polyethylene glycol (PEG) conjugate by intramuscular injection on a weekly or twice-weekly schedule, results in systemic detoxification and immune reconstitution. In the long term, however, about half of the patients receiving PEG-ADA replacement continue to require IVIG infusions, and some patients show a decline in T-cell numbers over time.

A number of gene therapy trials for ADA deficiency were initiated in the early 1990s, targeting retroviral gene transfer into various cell types, including peripheral blood lymphocytes, umbilical cord blood, BM, and CD34[+] selected stem cells.[98-101] These early studies failed to produce clear efficacy. By contrast, more recent studies introduced key modifications to the gene therapy protocol, including the use of a reduced-intensity myelosuppressive conditioning regimen and the withdrawal of concurrent PEG-ADA replacement.[102,103] The Milan-based group of Aiuti and colleagues have reported on their initial experience with 10 children.[90] Patients were conditioned with 4 mg/kg of busulfan before the infusion of transduced cells. The mean age at the time of gene therapy was 2.2 years. All children on this trial are healthy and thriving, with the longest published follow-up time now more than 64 months.[90,97,104] Gene therapy has resulted in a substantial increase of lymphocyte counts and normalization of T-cell function.

Similarly, four patients have been treated in London.[105] One patient that has been reported in detail had been treated with PEG-ADA for 3 years but showed a gradual decline in T-cell numbers despite effective metabolic correction. Because a matched BM donor was not available, the patient was enrolled on the ADA-SCID gene therapy trial. PEG-ADA replacement was stopped 1 month before gene therapy, and the patient was conditioned with a single dose of 140 mg/m^2 of melphalan before the infusion of the transduced BM CD34[+] cells.[103] At the time of the last published follow-up, the patient was 2 years from gene therapy, clinically well, and off prophylactic antibiotic therapy. An increase in T-cell numbers and normalization of the proliferative response have been noted.[97,103] Importantly, no adverse events have occurred thus far in the patients treated for ADA-SCID at these two centers.

Aiuti et al[90] recently published a comprehensive genome-wide analysis of RIS of five patients treated in Milan. This paper analyzed the RIS patterns in CD34[+] cells before infusion as well as RIS in vivo, up to 47 months after gene therapy. As anticipated, a nonrandom proviral integration pattern, favoring TSS and gene dense regions, was observed in the pretransplant cells. RIS observed in vivo in T cells were additionally enriched for TSS, suggesting the occurrence of in vivo selection. More recently, Aiuti and colleagues[104] have demonstrated that cellular genes in the proximity of the proviral integration site are subject to moderate dysregulation in gene modified T-cell clones isolated from patients. However, in contrast to the SCID-X1 trial, no in vivo skewing toward RIS in genes affecting survival, cell cycling, signal transduction, or proliferation were observed, making a clonal dominance effect appear less likely. Interestingly, only one *RIS* was detected at the MDS-EVI1 locus and became undetectable at later time points. This is in contrast to the clonal dominance of *MDS-EVI1* integration sites observed in the X-linked Chronic Granulomatous Disease trial[107] (see later). Additionally, an overrepresentation of RIS was noted in the proximity of the *CCND2* and *LMO2* gene with a total of 5 of 523 RIS recovered in vivo. Notably, the *CCND2* insertions were detected only in the first 2 years of follow-up and not subsequently. *LMO2* insertions were also overrepresented in the pretransplant CD34[+] samples, highlighting the fact that the *LMO2* gene is a hot spot for retroviral integration in human CD34[+] cells.[90] The lack of in vivo expansion of clones carrying LMO2 RIS indicates that this integration site may not be sufficient to mediate clonal dominance and leukemic transformation. Rather, additional cooperating mutations or insertions are required for malignant transformation. The lack of malignant transformation in two ADA-SCID trials may point to the role of the genetic background or the role of the therapeutic transgene introduced into human CD34[+] cells. However, the patient cohort remains relatively small, and follow-up is still short term. Overall, the genotoxicity profile in these two ADA-SCID trials has been sufficiently favorable to continue to recommend this experimental therapy to patients and families lacking a perfectly matched sibling donor. Indeed, this vector and treatment portfolio has been licensed in 2011 to a major pharmaceutical company for clinical development.

Chronic Granulomatous Disease

Chronic granulomatous disease (CGD) is an inherited disorder of phagocyte dysfunction characterized by often life-threatening invasive fungal and bacterial infections and by granuloma formation in vital organs. CGD results from a mutation in one of four subunits of the reduced form of nicotinamide adenine dinucleotide phosphate (NADPH) oxidase of phagocytes. The inability to form microbiocidal oxygen species renders the phagocytes unable to fight invasive infections.[108] Almost 70% of CGD cases result from defects in the X-linked gene encoding gp91^{phox} (X-CGD). With conventional therapy, including lifelong antimicrobial prophylaxis and interferon-γ therapy, the yearly mortality rate of X-CGD remains at 5%.[109] BMT is curative for patients with a perfectly matched sibling donor but remains risky in patients with active infections. Unrelated donor transplantations are not routinely recommended.[110] Thus, the development of a gene therapy approach that uses autologous HSC provides an important therapeutic advance for this patient group. In previous clinical gene therapy trials conducted without myeloreductive conditioning, the engraftment level of gene modified cells remained low.[111]

In 2002, the German group of Grez and colleagues in Frankfurt, Germany, initiated a gene therapy trial of X-CGD. The initial patients received a mild immunosuppressive preparative regimen and failed to engraft significant numbers of gene modified cells. However, 2 years later, low-dose busulfan—modeled on the successful gene therapy trial for ADA-SCID[102]—was incorporated into the preparative regimen, and additional patients were treated.[107] This group of patients has been followed with unprecedented sophistication by the prospective monitoring of integration sites that marks each hematopoietic cell before transplantation and then allows the tracking of these cells in vivo.[107] The initial two patients treated were 26 and 25 years old. Both subjects carried the diagnosis of X-CGD and had failed to clear invasive infections, including a *Staphylococcus aureus* liver abscess and pulmonary aspergillosis with medical treatment. Thus, autologous peripheral blood CD34+ cells were mobilized with granulocyte colony-stimulating factor (G-CSF) and collected. Gene transfer was performed using a gammaretroviral vector SF71gp91^{phox}. This vector, containing the spleen focus-forming virus LTR elements (in contrast to the Moloney MLV LTR in the two SCID trials) was chosen for its ability to achieve high expression levels in transduced HSCs.[112] The in vitro transduction rates in the two patients were 45% and 39.5%, respectively, with a proviral copy number of 2.6 and 1.5 per transduced cell. Proviral integration occurred preferentially in gene-coding regions (47%-52%) and was highly skewed toward the 5-kb sequence surrounding TSS. Moreover, the clonal distribution pattern was not stable over time. Rather, starting 5 months after therapy, a less diverse integration pattern emerged, indicating the appearance of dominant clones.

Clinically, following a period of cytopenia after the conditioning and cell infusion, the initial engraftment rates detected in the peripheral blood were 12% to 13%. Significant improvement in the previously refractory infections was noted 50 to 60 days after therapy. Surprisingly, a gradual increase in the number of gene-corrected cells up to 50% to 60% of all peripheral blood cells was observed, starting around day 150 after transplant. This coincided with increased oxidase activity and occurred in the absence of altered blood counts. These events were accompanied by a selective outgrowth of progenitors carrying vector insertions that activated one of three oncogenes, *PRDM16, SETBP1,* and most notably *MDS-EVI1.* Although all three genes are well-known cancer-associated genes, most clonal outgrowths were exhausted after a few months with the exception of *MDS-EVI1,* which increased to 67% to 90% in both patients approximately 1 year after cell infusion. Of note, the dominant *MDS-EVI1* clones initially did not transgress the boundaries of the normal myeloid pool because these cells remained cytokine dependent in vitro and failed to engraft in immunocompromised mice, suggesting their benign nature.[107] Thus, the expansion of gp91^{phox+} cells, although clearly providing therapeutic benefit during the initial phase, was viewed with mixed feelings by the investigators and the general gene therapy community.

More recent follow-up on these two study patients has been provided.[113,114] Indeed, although gene marking remained high in both patients, downregulation of gene expression was noted as a result of CpG methylation in the viral LTR promoter. As a consequence, gp91^{phox} expression was suppressed, but the capacity of the LTR encoded enhancer to transactivate nearby genes remained intact.[115] One patient died 2.5 years after therapy of severe sepsis.[116] The second patient developed monosomy 7 and myelodysplastic syndrome (MDS) and died after an unsuccessful unrelated donor BMT.[113] Of note, the *EVI1* locus has previously been identified as a common target of retroviral oncogenesis.[84,117] EVI1, which is not detected in normal hematopoietic cells, has been associated with myeloid leukemia and MDS.[118,119] The constitutive overexpression of Evi1 in mouse BM cells has been shown to induce MDS in mice,[120] and data from the CGD trial suggest that dysregulated expression is associated with genomic instability, presumably contributing to the acquisition of additional somatic mutations. Despite these molecular events, the infusion of gene-corrected CD34+ cells was highly effective with regard to clearing refractory pyogenic infections,[107] raising the possibility of using gene therapy to bridge patients with refractory pyogenic infections into eligibility for allogeneic HSCT.

Wiskott-Aldrich Syndrome

Wiskott-Aldrich syndrome (WAS) is an X-linked immunodeficiency caused by inactivating mutations in the WAS protein (WASP). WASP plays a regulatory role in cell signaling and cytoskeletal reorganization in hematopoietic cells.[121] The disease is fatal and is characterized by severe combined immunodeficiency, thrombocytopenia, elevated frequency of tumor formation, eczema, and other autoimmune manifestations.[122] The only currently available curative therapy for WAS is BM transplant, but as with the other primary immunodeficiencies, the availability of suitably matched donors is limiting.[123] A clinical trial for the genetic correction of WAS via retroviral delivery of the WASP cDNA into autologous CD34+ cells was recently reported.[124a] A combination of a relatively high cell dose (8-7 × 10^6 CD34+/kg body weight) and good transduction efficiency led to gene marking across both myeloid and lymphoid lineages. A marked clinical benefit from gene therapy has been reported in one of the patients.[124a] Of particular note is the fact that the architecture of the vector backbone used in this trial is similar to that used in both the CGD and the SCID trials described earlier. That is, the gammaretroviral vector has an intact LTR that contains the enhancer and promoter from the spleen focus forming virus.[124b] Recent reports describe T-cell leukemia from insertional mutagenesis in four patients in this trial (C. Klein, personal communication). Thus, a common molecular etiology in this trial strongly suggests that the initial vector design (intact strong viral LTRs containing enhancer elements that can transactivate promoters over long distances) are unsafe. In addition, the occurrence of T-cell leukemia in a disease other than SCID weakens the argument that the leukemias in X-SCID was related either to the transgene or some unknown disease-specific characteristic. In any regard, use of the "first–generation" MLV backbone in human trials may now be ended.

Childhood Cerebral X-Linked Adrenoleukodystrophy

Childhood cerebral X-linked adrenoleukodystrophy (CCALD) is a fatal neurodegenerative disease that results from progressive neural demyelination within the brain.[125,126] The defective gene that is responsible for the phenotype, adenosine triphosphate–binding cassette D1 (ABCD1), encodes a transmembrane transport protein that is responsible for the shuttling of fatty acids into peroxisomes, where they are subsequently degraded.[127] ALD is characterized by an accumulation of very long chain fatty acids, although the exact pathophysiology of the disease is unknown. Cerebral demyelination is associated with inflammation evident on gadolinium magnetic resonance imaging studies. Most patients progress from no symptoms to a vegetative state and death within 5 years of diagnosis. Allogeneic BM transplant has been found to be therapeutic for cerebral demyelination, presumably because of the infiltration of donor-derived microglia cells into the brain.[128] However, because of the very rapidly progressive nature of the demyelination and the time required to generate mature microglia from transplanted HSCs, BM transplant is most effective when administered as soon after development of demyelination evident by imaging methods as possible.[128] In cases in which CCALD is successfully treated with HSCT, continued progression of the disease occurs for 18 months to 2 years before disease arrest. Myelin inflammation resolves, but lost neurologic function is not regained in successfully treated patients. Because of the time constraints imposed upon finding a suitable HLA-matched donor and the occurrence of GVHD, the genetic correction of autologous BM CD34+ cells is an attractive experimental therapeutic option.

A phase 1 gene therapy trial using a recombinant HIV-1 based lentiviral vector to deliver the ABCD1 cDNA into CD34+ cells has been reported from Paris.[50] In the three patients who have been enrolled to date, a transduction efficiency of 30% to 50% in CD34+ cells was achieved with mean vector copy numbers of 0.6 to 0.7 per cell. Patients were preconditioned with cyclophosphamide and busulfan, and between 9% and 23% multilineage gene marked chimerism has been reported in a follow-up period that extends up to 16 months. In the two patients who have been followed for 16 months after transplant, HSC gene therapy resulted in arrests of neurologic functional loss and resolution of central nervous system inflammation that are similar to those achieved with allogeneic transplant. This trial is particularly noteworthy in that it is the first trial to report reconstitution of BM cells that have been transduced with a recombinant lentiviral vector. Molecular characterization of lentiviral integration sites in engrafting cells indicated that reconstitution was polyclonal, but detailed analysis of genomic loci targeted by this vector has yet to be reported. A multisite, biotechnology-sponsored registration trial is currently being reviewed by regulators in several countries using a similar lentivirus vector in this disease.

β-Thalassemia

A second patient treated in a clinical trial that used a lentiviral vector has recently been reported for the correction of β-thalassemia.[51] Thalassemias result from mutations that attenuate the expression of either the α or β globin chains that compromises hemoglobin synthesis and thus causes ineffective erythropoiesis.[129,130] Because adult hemoglobin consists of a tetramer of two α and two β chains, inherited mutations at the β globin locus cause a mismatch in the ratio of these two chains, thus preventing the correct assembly of the hemoglobin molecule. Clinically, this may result in transfusion-dependent anemia, which in turn can promote the serious side effect of iron overload. In general, disease severity correlates with the degree to which inactivation mutations inhibit β-globin expression. However, other genetic loci can modulate the disease phenotype, for example, by inducing adult expression of the fetal γ-globin gene, which can be efficiently incorporated into functional hemoglobin in place of the β-globin chain.[129,131] In particular, Orkin's group has recently demonstrated that the transcription factor BCL11A plays a major role in switching γ globin off and β-globin expression on during the transition from fetal to adult life.[132] Gene therapy of β-thalassemia is complicated by the requirement for an exact stoichiometry of α- and β-globin chains to facilitate efficient assembly of hemoglobin. Thus, an effective gene therapy vector must be able to facilitate high level expression of β-globin in the range of that mediated by the normal endogenous gene in an erythroid-specific context. Lineage-specific expression of the β-globin chain is particularly important in the context of genetic modification of HSC to prevent high level expression of β globin in nonerythroid hematopoietic lineages.

The lentiviral vector used in the trial mentioned above comprises a SIN configuration with elements from the β-globin LCR driving expression of the β-globin cDNA that has been mutated to enhance β-globin chain stability. Additionally, the vector's expression cassette is flanked by chromatin insulator elements that function to both prevent silencing of the transgene expression cassette by inhibitory chromatin structure surrounding the integration site and to prevent the vector-encoded enhancer from modulating expression of endogenous genes near to the insertion site. An interim report on the findings of the clinical trial describes that in 2007, a single patient with severe transfusion-dependent β-thalassemia major received $CD34^+$ cells transduced with the lentiviral vector described earlier.[51] There was a clear demonstration of clinical efficacy because the patient has been transfusion independent for 15 months. Of note, posttransplant molecular analysis revealed a mild clonal skewing comprising less than 5% of peripheral blood cells. The clone, which harbors a proviral integration within the high-mobility group A2 proteins *(HMGA2)* gene locus, is reported to be stable. Insertion of the provirus into this locus resulted in the production of a 3′ truncated mRNA resulting from the introduction of a cryptic splice acceptor, present in the vector insulator element, into intron 3 of the gene. This truncated mRNA, comprising exons 1 through 3, was expressed at elevated levels because of a loss of negative posttranscriptional regulation by Let-7 miRNAs because the miRNA target sequence in exon 5 was lost. *HMGA2* has been found to be mutated in chromosomal translocations primarily in benign tumors and less often in malignant tumors.[133] Although the clinical implications of this clonal outgrowth are unclear, this event clearly demonstrates that lentiviral vectors can contribute to insertional mutagenesis albeit in this case via modulation of posttranscriptional regulation of gene expression. Indeed, the propensity to insert in coding sequences may lead to an abundance of abnormal mRNA splicing variants.

Several additional trials are planned using a similar approach to express either a sickle-resistant mutated β-globin protein (as earlier), γ-globin, or based on recent data showing "cure" of humanized sickle mice by genetic deletion of BCL11A expressing shRNA against this transcription factor.[134] These trials represent important extensions of the technology from very rare diseases to a disease with a much larger patient population.

INSERTIONAL MUTAGENESIS

From an early stage in the development of retroviral vectors for gene therapy applications, there has been a concern that recombinant vectors could elicit cellular transformation by altering expression of either cellular proto-oncogenes or tumor suppressor genes that are proximal to the genomic integration site. This phenomenon, referred to as insertional mutagenesis, was characterized as a property of wild-type γ-retroviruses. Having greatly reduced the likelihood that retroviral gene therapy vectors could generate replication competent virus, the risk of a recombinant vector being able to transform a cell via insertional mutagenesis was initially perceived by many investigators to be very low.[135] The lack of efficacy in preclinical models using human hematopoietic stem and progenitor ($CD34^+$) cells also shifted emphasis away from the risks of insertional mutagenesis. However, soon after the publication detailing the efficacy of the Paris-based SCID-X1 trial, work emerged from the group of Baum and colleagues[4] that would reestablish the importance of insertional mutagenesis as a significant risk factor in the retroviral-mediated genetic correction of hematopoietic cells and that ultimately predicted the appearance of leukemia in the SCID and WAS gene therapy trials (X-Linked Combined Immunodeficiency, earlier). Baum demonstrated for the first time that a replication incompetent retroviral vector backbone designed for gene therapy applications could cause cellular transformation via insertional mutagenesis in the context of a transplant model of transduced murine HSCs.[84] In this and a subsequent study, it was found that a single retroviral insertion in the vicinity of the ecotropic viral integration site 1 *(EVI1)* gene or the related PR domain containing 16 *(PRDM16)* gene resulted in their overexpression likely because of the influence of the LTR viral enhancer element and was sufficient to initiate a cascade of events resulting in leukemic transformation in vivo.[84,136] Furthermore, a high copy number infection of murine BM with recombinant retroviral vectors was able to facilitate combinatorial hits which caused leukemogenesis.[85] The pattern of cellular genes that combine to promote cellular transformation demonstrated a significant overlap with those that are deregulated in experiments that used replication competent retrovirus vectors to provoke the development of leukemia.[85] Although murine HSCs likely represent a more readily transformed target than their human counterparts, these studies formally established the mutagenic potential of recombinant retroviral vectors intended for gene therapy applications.

Baum's group then made the seminal observation that at low copy number, retroviral-transduced murine HSCs are selectively expanded during transplant dependent upon proviral insertion sites.[86] These nonmalignant dominant clones are enriched for proviral integration sites in the locale of genes encoding signal transduction molecules and growth promoting genes.[86,137] Analysis of mRNA expression levels in these clones revealed that the proviral insertion did indeed alter transcriptional regulation of genes proximal to the integration site and led to the hypothesis that this was a powerful method to identify pro-engraftment genes through positive selection. These observations were found to have direct translational relevance in the gene therapy trial for CGD where the nonmalignant expansion of dominant retroviral transduced clones in two patients was found to correlate with insertional upregulation of growth promoting genes.[107] Subsequent experience with γ-retroviruses used in the clinical trial for WAS confirmed that insertional leukemogenesis in the SCID-X1 trial was not a disease-specific side effect. At least three children in the WAS trial have developed T-cell leukemia.[124a] Thus far, leukemias associated with replication-incompetent retrovirus vectors are associated with insertional activation of known proto-oncogenes by viral promoter and enhancer sequences (reviewed by Kohn et al[138]).

Wild-type and recombinant retroviral vectors (including α, γ, spuma, and lenti) integrate into the host genome in a semirandom manner and demonstrate insertion site biases that are dependent on the accessibility of the insertion site in the target cell and variations in the viral integrase enzyme that depend on retroviral genus.[57,139,140] Gammaretroviruses such as MLV have been shown to exert a clear preference for integration in the region immediately surrounding the TSS of actively transcribed genes.[57,87,141,142] Although lentiviral vectors also demonstrate a preference to integrate within the loci of actively transcribed genes, their integration profile favors sites that are downstream of the TSS within the body of the primary transcript.[57,87,88,143-146]

Using viral chimeras, it has been shown that incorporation of MLV integrase into an HIV-1–based vector alters the integration pattern of the lentivirus to more closely resemble that associated with a gammaretroviral vector.[147] It is possible that this phenomenon results from the binding of the MLV integrase with cell type–specific transcription factors resulting in the recruitment of the preintegration complex to the promoter and enhancer region of actively transcribed genes.[148] This work clearly demonstrates that gammaretroviral and lentiviral vectors have developed distinct mechanisms of integrase-dependent integration that may have an impact on the mutagenic potential of recombinant retroviral vectors. If one considers the possibility of integrating vectors upregulating oncogene expression via either readthrough transcription or enhancer effects on the endogenous promoter, then gammaretroviral vectors could be considered as potentially more mutagenic than lentiviral vectors in this context because of their preference for integration near the TSS. Conversely, preferential integration within the body of the primary transcript may result in lentiviral vectors having a higher probability of interrupting, for example, tumor suppressor gene expression or as noted earlier in the treatment of one patient with thalassemia in altering normal gene splicing. Progress has been made in the development of model systems to functionally evaluate the relative mutagenic potential of different vector systems. However, the model systems developed to date have a clear preference to detect mutagenesis mediated via upregulation of oncogene transcription. It is not clear whether this is a reflection of tumor suppressor gene inactivation being inconsequential as a mechanism of insertional mutagenesis or is a result of bias within the model system. Clearly, the preliminary results from the β-thalassemia trial described earlier demonstrate that lentiviral vectors may mediate insertional mutagenesis via alternate mechanisms.

As noted earlier, other related retroviral vector systems have also been shown to have an integration pattern that is distinct from gammaretroviral vectors and as such may represent a safer vector configuration. Recombinant foamy virus vectors do not preferentially integrate within genes, and their integration pattern does not significantly correlate with actively transcribed genes.[149] Likewise, avian sarcoma leukosis virus vectors do not favor gene-rich regions or TSS as preferred integration sites.[59] However, these novel vectors systems have not been as well characterized as gammaretroviral or lentiviral vectors with regards to safety and efficacy and have not yet been translated to clinical use in the near future.

RECENT MODIFICATIONS OF VECTOR SYSTEMS BASED ON CLINICAL EXPERIENCE

New Cell Targets in Genetic Engineering

Despite recent advances in improving ex vivo manipulation of HSC for the purpose of gene transfer, an ongoing limitation of this technology is the loss of engraftment potential of manipulated cells. This is dramatically emphasized in genetic diseases such as Fanconi anemia, in which the disease process itself leads to a marked reduction in HSC targets and in addition HSCs, which appear to have increased susceptibility to in vitro stress.[150,151] An exciting area of recent research advances that may in the future address this issue and also allow prescreening at the molecular level of insertions to determine safety is the use of embryonic stem (ES) cells. These cells offer exciting possibilities for studying mechanisms of pluripotency; establishing models for disease-specific investigations; and enabling future applications in genetic and cellular therapies, including tissue engineering for regenerative medicine. ES cells can be propagated and expanded in vitro, making them amenable to manipulations, including the genetic correction of molecular defects. ES cells can be differentiated into a number of cells resembling mature cell types in vitro.[152] In theory, cell therapy using donor cells of the same genetic constitution as the recipient may avoid the issues related to the immune barrier of allogeneic transplantation. One of the key ethical and practical barriers to applying ES cell research to human diseases is the need for obtaining human oocytes or embryos for the in vitro generation of ES cell lines.

A key recent finding with potential applications to cell and gene therapy has been the observation that many somatic tissues can be "reprogrammed" into pluripotent stem cells with characteristics of ES cells. These cells have been termed *induced pluripotent stem* (iPS) cells, and direct reprogramming of differentiated somatic cells by gene transfer of a small number of defined transcription factors has been shown to yield cells that are indistinguishable from inner cell mass-derived ES cells. Takahashi et al reasoned that forcing the expression of ES cell–specific genes, particularly transcription factors in somatic cells might induce (reprogram) somatic cells to take on the properties of ES cells, much like factors present in oocytes can reprogram somatic nuclei in mammals.[154] By systematic screening experiments, four factors, including some known to be involved in the process of self-renewal (Oct3/4, Sox2), and others associated with transformation and maintenance of ES cell pluripotency (c-Myc, Klf 4), were identified as sufficient to achieve reprogramming. The resultant cells, termed iPS cells, exhibited key features of ES cells, including the fulfillment of stringent pluripotency requirements.[154-156] This work was subsequently confirmed and expanded upon by other groups describing the application of this technology to human cells.[157-160] Proof-of-concept for the utility of iPS cells in regenerative medicine of inherited blood disorders was recently provided when iPS cells were generated from tail tip fibroblast in a humanized sickle cell anemia mouse model. The genetic sickle hemoglobin defect of the iPS cells was corrected in vitro via homologous recombination. Using established protocols for the differentiation of hematopoietic progenitors from ES cells,[161,162] hematopoietic cells capable of reconstituting lethally irradiated recipient mice were generated.

Transplantation of these cells into irradiated recipients resulted in robust engraftment and amelioration of the sickle cell phenotype in transplant recipients.[163] Reprogramming of a panel of disease-specific human iPS cells, including patients with blood diseases, has been demonstrated.[164] Human iPS cell lines shared defining features with human ES cells, including morphology, proliferation, feeder dependence, surface markers, gene expression, promoter and telomerase activities, in vivo differentiation, and teratoma formation. In analogy to the murine system, the reprogramming viruses are strongly silenced in human iPS cells, indicating that the maintenance of pluripotency does not depend on continuous transgene expression.[157-159] Enforced transgene expression appears to initiate a sequence of stochastic events over several days that eventually induces a small fraction of cells (0.001%-0.5% of cells) to acquire a stable pluripotent state. During direct reprogramming, gradual changes lead to a stable epigenetic state that is indistinguishable from inner cell mass-derived ES cells. For example, the Dnmt3a and Dnmt3b methyltransferases become activated and silence the viral transgenes as endogenous pluripotency factors are transcriptionally reactivated.[165,166] Human iPS cell lines thus represent a novel stem cell population that can be studied with regard to normal and pathologic tissue formation in vitro, enabling disease investigation, drug development, and a platform for producing autologous cell therapies that avoid immune rejection. Moreover, the creation of iPS cells allows the correction of genetic defects and exhaustive molecular characterization at the clonal level before tissue reconstruction. Unfortunately, the genetic transduction with exogenous genes, particularly oncogenes such as *c-MYC* and *KLF4,* and the use of integrating retroviral delivery systems are clear handicaps of this technology with regard to future clinical translation. In addition, to date robust reconstitution of murine hematopoiesis has not been consistently demonstrated and there no successful reports of *in vivo* reconstitution of human hematopoiesis in model systems. These all represent significant barriers to the translation of this powerful technology into human therapies.

One utility of targeting iPS cells for genetic therapies is that these cells can be cloned and expanded, allowing analysis of vector insertion sites before clinical use. In addition, reprogramming has now been accomplished, albeit at lower efficiencies using both nonintegrating vectors and protein transduction.[167-170] Reprogramming has also now been accomplished with the expression of fewer transcription factors,[170,171] most notably without c-Myc. Several laboratories have demonstrated that targeting specific loci is associated with limited or no adverse effects on expression of neighboring genes (reviewed by Sadelain et al[172]). Most notably, targeting of the *AAVS1* locus located on chromosome 19 has been well characterized.[173,174] This locus encodes the *PPP1R1C* gene that is ubiquitously expressed. Insertion at this site appears to provide a "safe harbor" with respect to genotoxicity and allows stable and long-term expression of transgenes in human embryonic stem cells (hHSCs).[173] Finally, Naldini and colleagues[175] have recently demonstrated that targeted insertion into two genomic sites (*IL2RG* and *CCR5*) using zinc-finger technology leads to no detectable alteration in the expression of nearby genes and sustained expression of the transgene cargo. The frequency of directed site-specific integration in primary fibroblasts was as high as 10%.[175] In addition, elegant work by Sadelain and colleagues[176] has demonstrated the feasibility of screening large numbers of iPS-derived clones for both integration in operationally defined safe harbors and for clinically relevant transgene expression using vectors that express globin genes.[176] Thus, this approach offers exciting future applications in treating a variety of human diseases.

Site-Directed Homologous Recombination to Correct Gene Mutations

A long-standing but unrealized goal of genetic therapy has been homologous recombination to affect *replacement* of abnormal disease-causing gene mutations. Although human ES cells theoretically provide an ideal target for such correction,[177-183] gene targeting in these cells has proven difficult. Zinc-finger nuclease (ZFN = mediated DS breaks allow high-efficiency site-specific homologous recombination and has been used to target a number of genes in human cells.[184,185] ZFNs are generated by fusing the FokI nuclease domain to a DNA recognition domain composed of engineered C2H2 zinc finger motifs that specify genomic DNA binding site for the chimeric protein. Compared with standard homologous recombination vectors, one advantage of ZFN is the relatively short stretch of homology needed (500 bp vs. 10-12 kb) to mediate genomic targeting. Binding of two fusion proteins to cognate DNA allows dimerization of the nuclease, leading to generation of a DS DNA break. When donor DNA with homology to sequence flanking the DS break is present, repair occurs with incorporation of the incoming DNA sequence. This system has been successfully used to target genes in multiple species and has recently been demonstrated in both human ES cells and iPS cells to effectively target both expressed and nonexpressed genes with a frequency of 1% to 20%[173,175,186,187] and has been termed *genome editing*. Because the development of a DNA DS break is a prerequisite to ZFN-mediated gene editing and such breaks induce both p53 and HDR, this approach, although attractive, could also have significant "off-target" effects. In addition, if efficiency improves, direct targeting in HSC could also be envisioned.

Other systems that seek to target specific genetic loci have also been described and are at different levels of development. As with ZFN nucleases, these approaches use cellular DNA repair mechanisms to introduce exogenous DNA sequences into the chromosome. Thus, methods to increase the efficiency of targeting by introducing DNA DS breaks, and several methods have exploited endonucleases that target rare DNA sequences to establish these DS breaks. Alternative methods in development include meganucleases[188] and transcription activator–like effector nucleases.[189] Challenges of all of these approaches include efficiency of targeting in primary cells and potential off-target effects on the genome and will likely also depend on technologic advances that allow ex vivo HSC cloning and large-scale expansion. At present, the use of ES or iPS cells is clearly amendable to this approach, but as noted earlier, use of these cells to derive transplantable HSC is a major impediment to clinical utilization.

FUTURE DIRECTIONS

The use of gene transfer to treat human diseases has now been successful in several diseases. Compared with allogeneic BMT, ex vivo gene therapy using autologous cells eliminates the risk of GVHD and in some cases reduces the intensity of preparative regimen required before transplant, which also reduces toxicity. Thus, in some diseases, this therapeutic approach can now be considered an alternative to standard therapy. Insertional mutagenesis, which has resulted in serious adverse events in several trials, has stimulated rapid development of putative safer vector systems that are being tested in human trials but remains a challenge. Rapid progress in molecular technology, such as high-throughput sequencing and the development of new sources of expandable stem cell sources, offers significant potential for ongoing development of gene transfer in regenerative biology for a wide range of human conditions.

ACKNOWLEDGEMENTS

Funding from NIH DK062757, CA113969, AI097628, DK090913, and the NHLBI Gene Therapy Resource Program. I would like to thank members of my laboratory and particularly Michael Milsom and Lars Mueller for helpful discussions and members of the Transatlantic Gene Therapy Consortium for productive collaborations.

SUGGESTED READINGS

Aiuti A, Cassani B, Andolfi G, et al: Multilineage hematopoietic reconstitution without clonal selection in ADA-SCID patients treated with stem cell gene therapy. *J Clin Invest* 117:2233, 2007.

Aiuti A, Slavin S, Aker M, et al: Correction of ADA-SCID by stem cell gene therapy combined with nonmyeloablative conditioning. *Science* 296:2410, 2002.

Bauer TR Jr, Allen JM, Hai M, et al: Successful treatment of canine leukocyte adhesion deficiency by foamy virus vectors. *Nat Med* 14:93, 2008.

Cartier N, Hacein-Bey-Abina S, Bartholomae CC, et al: Hematopoietic stem cell gene therapy with a lentiviral vector in X-linked adrenoleukodystrophy. *Science* 326:818, 2009.

Cavazzana-Calvo M, Hacein-Bey S, de Saint Basile G, et al: Gene therapy of human severe combined immunodeficiency (SCID)-X1 disease [see comments]. *Science* 288:669, 2000.

Cavazzana-Calvo M, Payen E, Negre O, et al: Transfusion independence and HMGA2 activation after gene therapy of human beta-thalassaemia. *Nature* 467:318, 2010.

Gaspar HB, Parsley KL, Howe S, et al: Gene therapy of X-linked severe combined immunodeficiency by use of a pseudotyped gammaretroviral vector. *Lancet* 364:2181, 2004.

Hacein-Bey-Abina S, Le Deist F, Carlier F, et al: Sustained correction of X-linked severe combined immunodeficiency by ex vivo gene therapy. *N Engl J Med* 346:1185, 2002.

Hacein-Bey-Abina S, Von Kalle C, Schmidt M, et al: LMO2-associated clonal T cell proliferation in two patients after gene therapy for SCID-X1. *Science* 302:415, 2003.

Hanna J, Wernig M, Markoulaki S, et al: Treatment of sickle cell anemia mouse model with iPS cells generated from autologous skin. *Science* 318:1920, 2007.

Hirschhorn R, Yang DR, Puck JM, et al: Spontaneous *in vivo* reversion to normal of an inherited mutation in a patient with adenosine deaminase deficiency. *Nat Genet* 13:290, 1996.

Howe SJ, Mansour MR, Schwarzwaelder K, et al: Insertional mutagenesis combined with acquired somatic mutations causes leukemogenesis following gene therapy of SCID-X1 patients. *J Clin Invest* 118:3143, 2008.

Laufs S, Nagy KZ, Giordano FA, et al: Insertion of retroviral vectors in NOD/SCID repopulating human peripheral blood progenitor cells occurs preferentially in the vicinity of transcription start regions and in introns. *Mol Ther* 10:874, 2004.

Li Z, Dullmann J, Schiedlmeier B, et al: Murine leukemia induced by retroviral gene marking. *Science* 296:497, 2002.

Milsom M, Schambach A, Williams DA, et al: Chemoprotective gene delivery. *Viral Therapy of Cancer* 376, 2008.

Miyoshi H, Smith KA, Mosier DE, et al: Transduction of human CD34(+) cells that mediate long-term engraftment of NOD/SCID mice by HIV vectors [In Process Citation]. *Science* 283:682, 1999.

Moritz T, Patel VP, Williams DA: Bone marrow extracellular matrix molecules improve gene transfer into human hematopoietic cells via retroviral vectors. *J Clin Invest* 93:1451, 1994.

Naldini L, Blomer U, Gallay P, et al: In vivo gene delivery and stable transduction of nondividing cells by a lentiviral vector [see comments]. *Science* 272:263, 1996.

Ott MG, Stein S, Schultze-Strasser S, et al: Phase I/II gene therapy study for chronic granulomatous disease: results, lessons and perspectives. *Nat Med* 503, 2007.

Pai SNL, Harris C, Cattaneo F, et al: Somatic gene therapy for x-linked severe combined immunodeficiency using a self-inactivating modified gammaretroviral vector results in an improved preclinical safety profile and early clinical efficacy in a human patient. *Blood (ASH Annual Meeting Abstracts)* 118:164, 2011.

Park IH, Zhao R, West JA, et al: Reprogramming of human somatic cells to pluripotency with defined factors. *Nature* 451:141, 2008.

Porteus MH, Carroll D: Gene targeting using zinc finger nucleases. *Nat Biotechnol* 23:967, 2005.

Sadelain M, Papapetrou EP, Bushman FD: Safe harbours for the integration of new DNA in the human genome. *Nat Rev Cancer* 12:51, 2012.

Sankaran VG, Menne TF, Xu J, et al: Human fetal hemoglobin expression is regulated by the developmental stage-specific repressor BCL11A. *Science* 322:1839, 2008.

Stein S, Ott MG, Schultze-Strasser S, et al: Genomic instability and myelodysplasia with monosomy 7 consequent to EVI1 activation after gene therapy for chronic granulomatous disease. *Nat Med* 16:198, 2010.

Takahashi K, Tanabe K, Ohnuki M, et al: Induction of pluripotent stem cells from adult human fibroblasts by defined factors. *Cell* 131:861, 2007.

Thrasher AJ, Gaspar HB, Baum C, et al: Gene therapy: X-SCID transgene leukaemogenicity. *Nature* 443:E5, discussion E6-7, 2006.

Urnov FD, Miller JC, Lee YL, et al: Highly efficient endogenous human gene correction using designed zinc-finger nucleases. *Nature* 435:646, 2005.

Xu J, Peng C, Sankaran VG, et al: Correction of sickle cell disease in adult mice by interference with fetal hemoglobin silencing. *Science* 334:993, 2011.

Yu J, Vodyanik MA, Smuga-Otto K, et al: Induced pluripotent stem cell lines derived from human somatic cells. *Science* 318:1917, 2007.

For complete list of references log on to www.expertconsult.com.

CHAPTER 100

MESENCHYMAL STROMAL CELLS

Edwin M. Horwitz

Mesenchymal stromal cells (MSCs) are spindle-shaped plastic adherent cells isolated from bone marrow and from many other tissue sources. Although MSCs were first described in the study of bone marrow, little interest in these cells occurred over the subsequent two decades. The remarkable resurgence of interest among hematologists and, in particular, specialists who perform hematopoietic cell transplantation (HCT) represents a full circle in the study of MSC biology and therapy.

It was Alexander Friedenstein, during his pioneering work studying the bone marrow as the organ of hematopoiesis, who first identified the cells that now bear the designation *MSC*.[1] He showed that these cells contributed to the hematopoietic microenvironment and could support hematopoiesis in vitro[2] as well as serving as precursors for osteoblasts.[1] Noting that a small subset of cells demonstrated a high proliferative potential by forming clonal colonies when plated at low density (termed *CFU-F* by Friedenstein in analogy to hematopoietic colony-forming units), Owen proposed the concept of a stromal stem cell that could repopulate the marrow microenvironment as the hematopoietic stem cell can repopulate hematopoiesis.[3-5]

The term *mesenchymal stem cell* was proposed by Arnold Caplan, who hypothesized that this cell could differentiate to a wide variety of mesenchymal tissues and proposed a broad lineage "tree," suggesting that the mesenchymal stem cell could give rise to bone, cartilage, muscle, hematopoietic-supportive stroma, tendon, ligament, adipose, and other connective tissues.[6] This notion attracted the attention of investigators in the emerging arena of regenerative medicine. Despite efforts to exploit MSC-based therapy in hematology, definitive indications of potential clinical benefits have not been obtained; hence the focus of MSC research has shifted to regenerative medicine.[7,8]

Most recently, investigators have recognized the ever-increasing spectrum of cytokines secreted by ex vivo–expanded MSCs, the striking immunomodulatory properties of the cells, and the fact that the mechanism of therapeutic activity in virtually all cases has been through paracrine effects—the release of soluble mediators. Collectively, these observations have spurred a renaissance of MSCs in hematology.

NOMENCLATURE AND THE DEFINING PHENOTYPE

The nomenclature of these cells merits clarification. MSCs have been designed by a wide variety of terms including *marrow stromal cells, marrow stromal fibroblasts,* and most frequently, *mesenchymal stem cells,* which was the basis for the abbreviation *MSC*. The various monikers have created some confusion in the literature, as some would suggest that they refer to different cell types. Although the specific properties of MSCs isolated in the laboratory may vary depending on the methods employed, the assortment of terms, in general, refers to the same heterogeneous population of cells.

The notion that all MSCs that have been isolated and expanded in the laboratory are stem cells remains unproven. *Stem cells* are defined as having the capacity for extensive self-renewal and differentiation to two or more distinct lineages in a physiologically relevant manner. Thus studies are needed to demonstrate that a given cell can undergo self-renewal and give rise to terminally differentiated lineages in situ. Although important studies are emerging, comprehensive unifying data to define a clinically relevant mesenchymal stem cell are yet to be reported.

This idea is not intended to dispel the notion that a mesenchymal stem cell may exist, or at least a stem cell for the bone marrow microenvironment as proposed by Owen. Indeed, emerging data suggest that a rare cell within the population of adherent cells that we designate MSCs or some other, adherent or nonadherent, cell population may be a mesenchymal stem cell. Nonetheless, the unfractionated population of MSCs isolated by plastic adherence does not seem to meet the criteria of a homogeneous population of stem cells. Therefore in 2005, the Mesenchymal and Tissue Stem Cell Committee of the International Society for Cellular Therapy (ISCT) recommended that the term *mesenchymal stromal cell* is a more appropriate designation for this heterogeneous population of cells, maintaining the abbreviation *MSC* for that term and reserving the term *mesenchymal stem cell* for a subset of these (or other) cells that demonstrate stem cell activity in vivo by clearly stated criteria.[9]

Although MSCs have not been proven to be stem cells, they do seem to possess significant clinical potential. Accordingly, a system to easily identify the cells is imperative. Unfortunately, no single clinically validated cell surface marker (analogous to CD34 expression on human hematopoietic stem cells) has been universally accepted, nor is there a single functional assay (analogous to hematopoietic repopulating assays) to define MSCs.

To begin to address this issue, the Mesenchymal and Tissue Stem Cell Committee of the ISCT sought in 2006 to standardize a working definition of MSCs by proposing a set of minimal criteria to denote these cells.[10] First, MSCs must be plastic-adherent when maintained in standard culture conditions. Second, MSCs must express CD105, CD73, and CD90, and they must lack expression of CD45, CD34, CD14 or CD11b, CD79 or CD19, and HLA-DR surface molecules. Third, MSCs must differentiate to osteoblasts, adipocytes, and chondrocytes in vitro (Fig. 100-1). Although novel surface markers expressed by MSCs have been described,[11,12] these criteria remain the most applicable. As new knowledge unfolds, however, these guidelines will likely require modifications; as modifications continue, it is hoped that a simpler system will emerge.

IDENTIFICATION AND PHYSIOLOGIC ROLE OF MESENCHYMAL STEM CELLS

The physiologic cell that corresponds to the isolated and expanded cells is of great interest to investigators of bone marrow biology and may reveal novel therapeutic applications. However, only recently has evidence as to the origins of MSCs begun to emerge.

Sacchetti and colleagues identified a CD146-expressing stromal cell from human bone marrow.[13] In situ, these CD146 cells reside in the subendothelial layer in sinusoidal walls as adventitial reticular cells. CD146 expression is found on all CFU-Fs and their clonal progeny, but on only about 30% of the heterogeneous populations of stromal cells. After isolation and ex vivo expansion, the CD146-expressing cells were capable of forming the hematopoietic microenvironment, including bone and marrow space, in heterotopic locations

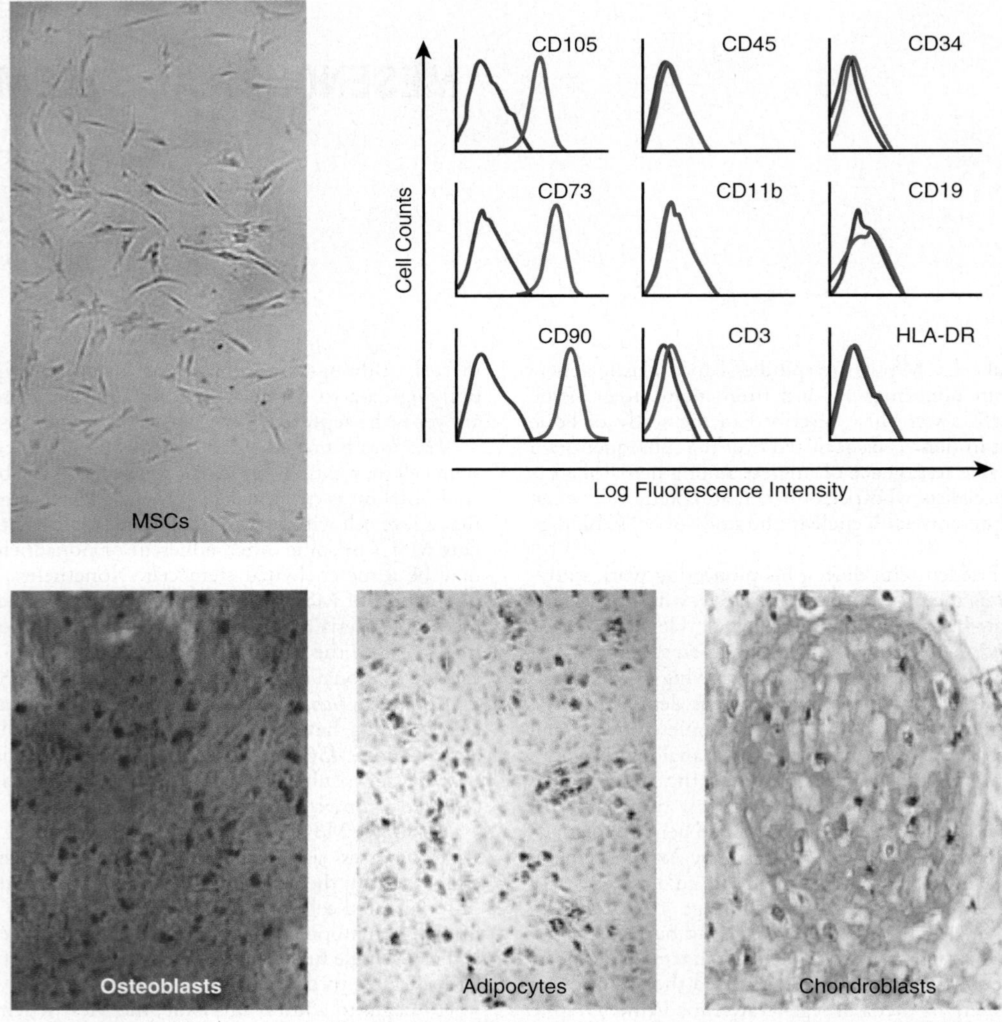

Figure 100-1 A PANEL OF DATA DEMONSTRATING THE DEFINING CHARACTERISTICS OF MSCS: ADHERENCE, IMMUNOPHENOTYPE, AND IN VITRO DIFFERENTIATION. *Top left,* Photomicrograph of undifferentiated MSCs showing the characteristic spindle shape and adherent properties of the cells. Original magnification, × 40. *Top right,* Flow cytometry histograms demonstrating the typical expression pattern of surface antigens (—) and isotype control (——), as indicated. *Bottom,* Immunocytochemical staining demonstrating the differentiation of MSCs into osteoblasts (Alizarin Red stain), adipocytes (Oil Red O stain), and chondroblasts (Alcian Blue stain). *(With permission from Martinez C, Hofmann TJ, Marino R, et al: Human bone marrow mesenchymal stromal cells express the neural ganglioside GD2: A novel surface marker for the identification of MSCs.* Blood *109:4245, 2007.)*

after subcutaneous transplantation into immune deficient mice. Bone was evident at 4 weeks after transplantation. Then capillaries formed and developed into a system of sinusoids similar to human bone marrow. The endothelium of the sinusoids was murine, but the adventitial cells were human, indicating that the transplanted human adventitial cells were capable of self-renewal. Adipocytes were also observed in the developing marrow space. By 8 weeks, murine hematopoietic cells had migrated into and colonized the marrow space of the regenerated bone. Thus the CD146-expressing cells isolated from human bone marrow and accounting for all CFU-Fs seemed to be able to give rise to bone, and the entire bone marrow microenvironment was sufficient to attract primitive hematopoietic cells and support the ensuing hematopoiesis.

Crisan and colleagues reported that CD146-expressing cells exist as pericytes in multiple human organs.[14] These cells expressed typical MSC markers, lacked hematopoietic markers, and differentiated to osteoblasts, adipocytes, and chondrocytes, thereby meeting the criteria for MSCs. Of interest, the cells exhibited myogenic potential in vitro and in vivo. These studies bear resemblance to prior reports suggesting that MSCs isolated from different tissue sources show different gene expression profiles and the expression patterns, in some cases, seem to reflect the tissue from which they were derived.[15] Moreover, these two studies are consistent with the evolving paradigm of MSCs that ostensibly similar cells isolated from different tissues may have markedly different biologic—and therapeutic—potential. Furthermore, it underscores the need to consider the source of MSCs in the development of MSC-based cell therapies.

Although murine MSCs share some characteristics with their human counterparts, they also seem to differ in many ways[16]; hence murine studies of MSC biology must be interpreted with the understanding of potential interspecies differences. Such caution notwithstanding, murine studies have also shed light on the physiologic role of MSCs. Morikawa and colleagues identified a subset of cells from the heterogeneous population of MSCs of murine bone marrow characterized by platelet-derived growth factor receptor α (PDGFRα) and stem cell antigen 1 (Sca 1), termed *PαS cells.*[17] The population was highly enriched for CFU-Fs, expressed common MSC markers, was capable of self-renewal in vitro, and underwent differentiation to osteoblasts, adipocytes, and chondrocytes. Unexpectedly, these cells also seemed to differentiate to endothelial cells. In healthy mice, the cells were found in the perivascular space, similar to the human CD146-expressing cells, which we presume are human MSCs.[13,14] After intravenous transplantation of freshly isolated cells (without ex vivo expansion), the PαS cells gave rise to osteoblasts and adipocytes, as well as perivascular cells, consistent with stem cell–like behavior.

Finally, Mendez-Ferrer and colleagues[18] have identified a nestin-expressing MSC within murine bone marrow. Although the cells were found exclusively in the perivascular region adjacent to bone or within the bone marrow, they were distinct from typical vascular endothelial cells. The nestin-expressing MSCs contained all CFU-Fs and exhibited the differentiation characteristics attributed to MSCs. Of note, the cells were able to undergo self-renewal in serial transplantation, although they were propagated in vitro as nonadherent aggregates termed *mesenspheres*. In vivo, these cells were intimately associated with hematopoietic stem cells and seemed to be critically important for hematopoietic stem cell homeostasis and marrow homing of transplanted hematopoietic stem cells.

These studies illustrate the important, evolving paradigm of mesenchymal stem cells; however, MSCs as agents of cell therapy, after isolation and ex vivo expansion, may bear little biologic resemblance to their physiologic counterparts in situ. Thus the engineered biology of ex vivo–expanded MSCs is critically important to the development of effective cell therapy.

Cell biology of Ex Vivo–Expanded Mesenchymal Stromal Cells for Clinical Cell Therapy

Source

MSCs for clinical applications are most commonly isolated from bone marrow[19] but have also been obtained from adipose tissue,[20,21] umbilical cord blood,[22,23] and placenta.[24] Other reported sources include amniotic fluid[25] and fetal tissues such as lung, liver, and blood.[26] Mobilized peripheral blood cells have been reported as a source of MSCs[27]; however, current consensus is that MSCs do not appreciably circulate in cytokine mobilized or steady-state peripheral blood. Reports of MSCs in umbilical cord blood have also been conflicting; however, recognizing that cord blood unit storage time, volume, and cell count are critical parameters affecting the efficiency of MSC isolation,[23] general agreement now exists that MSCs do reside within cord blood.

Isolation

MSCs are most often isolated by "adherence selection." For bone marrow, mononuclear cells are placed in tissue culture, and the MSCs will adhere to the plastic surface of the tissue culture vessel. The identification of new surface markers has led to the prospective isolation of MSCs using immunomagnetic beads or FACS sorting of freshly prepared mononuclear cell preparations. GD2, CD271, and frizzled-9 have been shown to serve as effective markers for the isolation of MSCs[11,12,28,29]; however, in all cases, culture expansion of the selected cells was required to obtain a sufficient sample for further study. If prospective isolation of MSCs is to become a common practice, a substantial advantage must be demonstrated.

Expansion

MSCs have a remarkable capacity for ex vivo expansion. In standard culture conditions, MSCs isolated by adherence selection demonstrate a population doubling time of about 2 to 5 days[30]; however, plating cell density can impact the expansion potential.[31] Most MSC preparations can be maintained in continuous culture for 4 to 6 months before senescence. MSCs isolated from different species exhibit differing growth potentials. Although human MSCs rapidly expand in culture, murine MSCs expand more slowly. Moreover, different mouse strains show a marked difference in growth and differentiation.[16]

All MSC cultures, at present, require some serum supplementation. Fetal bovine serum is the most commonly used supplement, but the translation of MSCs to the clinics and the report of a clinically significant immune response against fetal bovine serum proteins in one patient who received MSCs[32] has led to the development of human serum supplementation strategies. Human serum containing a platelet lysate[33] is rapidly becoming the principal supplement; however, supplementation with recombinant growth factors with or without human serum is also developing.

Phenotype

The expanded MSC product is a heterogeneous population of cells most easily demonstrated by in vitro adipocyte differentiation, in which only a subset of cells develops cytoplasmic fat globules, and a CFU-F assay, in which a small fraction of cells exhibit a high proliferative, colony-forming potential. However, this assorted population does have some common characteristics. The uniform surface phenotype of MSCs includes expression of CD105, CD73, and CD90, which can be used to define the cells, as well as CD49b, CD49e, and CD166. STRO-1, an IgM monoclonal antibody generated by inoculating mice with human $CD34^+$ cells, binds to human MSCs (or perhaps MSC precursors) in freshly isolated bone marrow but does not bind to murine MSCs or human MSCs in tissue culture.[34] The antigen recognized by STRO-1 has not been identified. The low-affinity nerve growth factor receptor, LNGFR or CD271, is also expressed on human MSCs in freshly harvested bone marrow but not in culture-expanded cells.[28] Ex vivo–expanded MSCs lack expression of hematopoietic and endothelial antigens, CD34, CD45, CD3, CD19, CD14, CD11b, and CD31.

MSCs demonstrate a surface antigen profile predicted to be hypoimmunogenic. At baseline, MSCs express moderate levels of HLA class I molecules but lack expression of HLA class II molecules on the cell surface. Upon stimulation with interferon γ in vitro, class II antigens are found on the cell surface.[35] MSCs do not express the costimulatory molecules CD80, CD86, CD40, and CD40L.[35,36]

One of the most distinguishing characteristics of MSCs, in contrast to other spindle-shaped, plastic-adherent cells, is the capacity for trilineage differentiation in vitro. MSCs differentiate to osteoblasts, chondrocytes, or adipoctyes when cultured under lineage-specific inductive conditions, and the cells can be identified by either tissue-specific immunohistochemical staining (e.g., Oil Red O to identify the cytoplasmic fat globules of adipocytes) or by gene expression.

Secretome

MSCs have an enormous capacity for secretion of soluble mediators, and indeed, it is these mediators that constitute the principal mechanism of biologic/therapeutic activity. MSCs secrete stromal cell–derived factor-1 (SDF-1),[37] which plays a critical role in the homing of hematopoietic stem cells to the marrow niche.[38] In vitro, MSCs constitutively secrete interleukin 6 (IL-6), IL-7, IL-8, IL-11, IL-12, IL-14, IL-15, macrophage colony-stimulating factor (M-CSF), Flt-3 ligand, and stem cell factor (SCF). Upon IL-1α stimulation, MSCs are induced to further express IL-1α, leukemia inhibitory factor (LIF), granulocyte colony-stimulating factor (G-CSF), and granulocyte-macrophage colony-stimulating factor (GM-CSF).[35,39] Finally, MSCs can secrete several chemokine ligands, including CCL2, CCL4, CCL5, CCL20, CX_3CL1, and CXCL8.[40]

It is important to note that the list of cytokines secreted by MSCs is rapidly growing. The secretome of an MSC product is, in part, dependent on the tissue source and the conditions of ex vivo expansion.[15,41] In theory, then, specific tissue sources can be identified, and specific expansion protocols can be developed to generate a secretome that is especially well suited for specific clinical indications. Indeed, exceptionally active investigation continues in the search for as-yet-undescribed cytokines generated by MSCs and processing conditions to induce expression of specific cytokines or other mediators.

Homing and Migration

Ex vivo–expanded, intravenously infused MSCs have been reported to preferentially migrate to sites of tissue damage, and this property can potentially be exploited in regenerative medicine to enhance tissue repair.[42,43] Additionally, these cells seem to migrate to solid tumors and incorporate into the tumor stroma.[44] Whether MSCs inhibit or promote tumor growth is a matter of ongoing debate. Homing does not seem to be important for potential therapeutic activity of MSCs for hematologic applications.

Life Span of Mesenchymal Stromal Cells

The turnover rate of bone marrow MSCs in situ is unknown. More relevant to clinical applications of MSCs is the life span of ex vivo–expanded MSCs after intravenous infusion. Although a definitive answer may be difficult to conclusively prove, three lines of evidence suggest MSCs persist about 6 to 9 months in the recipient. First, Nolta and colleagues infused human IL-3–secreting MSCs into NOD-SCID mice to support human hematopoiesis and were able to detect human IL-3 in the murine serum for up to 9 months.[45] Second, Horwitz and colleagues infused human MSCs into children with osteogenesis imperfecta and observed a striking acceleration of growth velocity over the first 6 months with a far slower rate of growth over the subsequent 6 months.[32] After 1 year, the growth rate approximated the rate before the MSC infusion. Finally, Keating infused autologous MSCs gene-marked with the factor IX cDNA into three adult patients after autologous HSCT for a hematologic malignancy. Gene-marked cells were identified in recipient culture–expanded MSCs obtained from bone marrow aspirations up to 8 months after the MSC infusion. Studies at 12 months were consistently negative.[46]

Immunobiology of Ex Vivo–Expanded Mesenchymal Stromal Cells

Although the specific interactions of MSCs with the immune system and the mechanisms of those interactions remain to be fully elucidated, MSCs clearly have a profound impact on immunity.[47] The field of MSC-mediated immune modulation continues to evolve, but several overriding themes have emerged. First, MSCs interact with all arms of the immune system (Fig. 100-2). Second, there seems to be a dynamic cross-talk between the immune effector cells and MSCs, suggesting that MSCs may play a physiologic role in regulating the immune response. Third, unfortunately, the data are often conflicting, with many reports diametrically opposed to the research of others, indicating the need for additional studies to fully understand the MSC-immune system interaction. The immunomodulatory properties of MSCs may be exploited therapeutically in hematopoietic cell transplantation to suppress graft rejection, treat severe graft-versus-host disease (GVHD), and possibly prevent clinical GVHD. Indeed, the recognition that MSCs can suppress the immune response is what attracted the collective attention of the HCT community.

T Lymphocytes

The first studies to suggest that MSCs may possess inherent immunomodulatory properties were based on the recognition that ex vivo–expanded third-party human MSCs inhibit the proliferation of allogeneic lymphocytes in a mixed lymphocyte reaction.[48] The effect is nonspecific, because MSCs inhibit the proliferation of T cells in response to alloantigens[36,49-51] and mitogens,[48] and it is MHC-unrestricted, based on the fact that both allogeneic and autologous MSCs generate a similar suppression.[36,49,50,52,53] The antiproliferative effect of MSCs has been reported to resemble divisional arrest anergy of activated T cells based on evidence that MSCs induce a cell cycle arrest in the G_1 phase, which persisted after removal of the MSCs from the in vitro culture.[54] In addition to this antiproliferative effect,

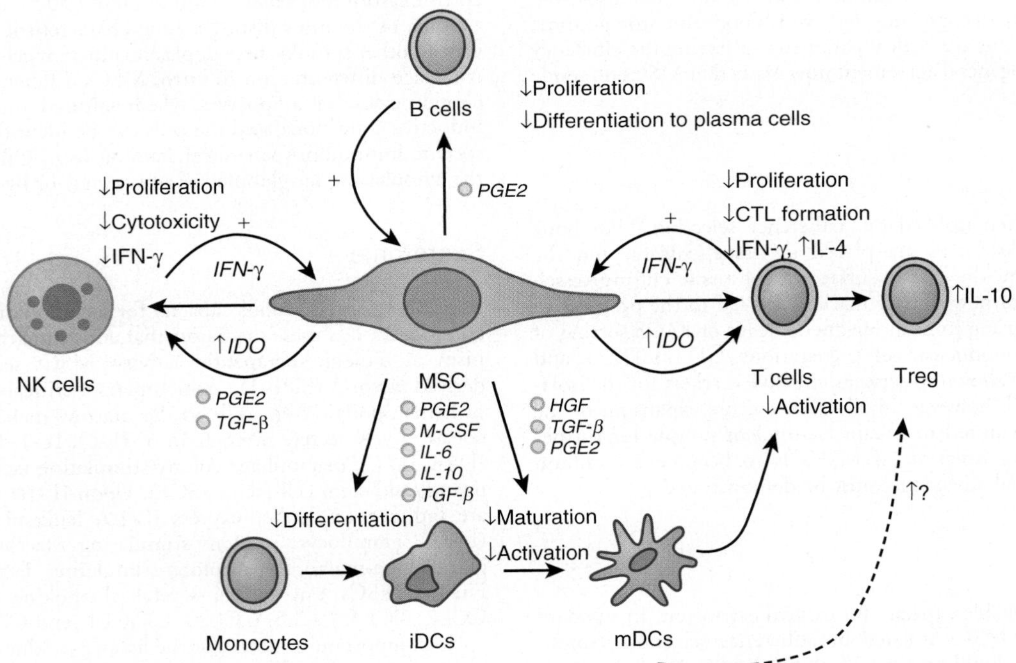

Figure 100-2 A SCHEMATIC REPRESENTATION OF THE PROPOSED IMMUNOMODULATORY EFFECTS OF MESENCHYMAL STROMAL CELLS. *CTL,* Cytotoxic T cell; *HGF,* hepatocyte growth factor; *IDO,* indoleamine 2,3-dioxygenase; *PGE2,* prostaglandin E2; and *TGF-β,* transforming growth factor β. *(With permission from Nauta AJ, Fibbe WE: Immunomodulatory properties of mesenchymal stromal cells,* Blood *110:3499, 2007)*

MSCs may also inhibit the cytotoxicity of T lymphocytes[50] and increase the proportion of $CD4^+CD25^+Foxp3^+$ regulatory T cells, which possess potent immune suppressor activity.[55] Finally, MSCs seem to decrease interferon γ production by Th-1 cells and increase interleukin-4 by Th-2 cells, suggesting a shift from a proinflammatory to an antiinflammatory state.[56]

B Lymphocytes

MSCs also interact with B lymphocytes, although the precise mechanisms are unclear. MSCs seem to inhibit B lymphocyte proliferation in vitro via divisional arrest anergy, impair B lymphocyte maturation and antibody secretion, and decrease the chemotactic properties.[57,58] By contrast, some studies have suggested that MSCs support the survival, proliferation, and differentiation of B lymphocytes to mature, antibody-secreting cells.[59]

NK Cells

MSCs have been reported to inhibit IL-2- and IL-15-induced proliferation of freshly isolated, resting NK cells and prevent the induction of cytotoxic activity and cytokine production; however, proliferation of NK cells preactivated with IL-2 was only partially inhibited.[60,61] Other studies have shown that the cytolytic activity of freshly isolated NK cells is unaffected by MSCs, whereas NK cells cultured with IL-2 and MSCs seem to have reduced, but not absent, cytotoxicity against K562 target cells.[62-64] Of interest, MSCs seem to be highly susceptible to NK cell-mediated lysis due to expression of surface ligands involved in NK cell activation, such as NKG2D and DNAX accessory molecule-1 ligands[60] as well as low-level MHC class I expression.

Dendritic Cells

MSCs can inhibit the differentiation of $CD14^+$ monocytes and $CD34^+$ cells into dendritic cells (DCs), as well as the maturation and function of DCs in vitro.[65-67] MSC coculture inhibited the GM-CSF-, IL-4-induced differentiation of monocytes to DCs, but the inhibition was reversible. MSC-DC coculture also induced mature DCs to downregulate surface expression of CD83, CD1a, CD80, CD86, and HLA-DR, as well as IL-12 secretion. Moreover, MSC-treated DCs showed an impaired capacity to prime allogeneic T cells, consistent with the observation that MSCs direct DCs to acquire a tolerogenic phenotype.

Immune Privilege

MSCs are considered to be immune privileged by many investigators.[68] Indeed, MSCs exhibit a hypoimmunogenic phenotype and do not elicit a T cell–proliferative response in vitro. Moreover, HLA-disparate MSCs can be safely infused into patients and often demonstrate a therapeutic effect, such as in the treatment of GVHD.[69,70] However, it is not strictly correct to infer immune privilege from such data. Immune suppressive activity and immune privilege are distinct biologic properties, and immune suppression does not indicate immune privilege a priori. Murine studies and in vitro studies of human MSCs do not necessarily reflect clinical (in vivo) immune activity, and infusion of allogeneic MSCs into immunosuppressed hosts does not provide data to support (or refute) the immunogenicity of the cells.

Rigorous evaluation of the immune response to allogeneic, HLA-disparate MSCs in immune competent hosts has not yet been reported. However, an early observation suggested that MSCs are recognized by the immune system. Horwitz and colleagues infused gene-marked MSCs into immune-competent children with osteogenesis imperfecta.[32] In this double gene-marking study, MSCs transduced with a nonexpressing retroviral vector were identified in all evaluable patients, whereas MSCs transduced with a vector that expressed neomycin phosphotransferase (neo^R), a bacterial protein, were never found. These data suggest the possibility that the MSCs expressing neo^R were immunologically recognized by the immunocompetent hosts.

The preponderance of current data suggests that MSCs are not intrinsically immune privileged and, in fact, may stimulate an immune response in some conditions. However, MSCs seem to be hypoimmunogenic as a result of their low-level expression of MHC molecules and complete lack of costimulatory molecule expression, and this property may be exploited in a variety of clinical settings. Indeed, the use of allogeneic HLA-unmatched MSCs seems to be safe and does elicit a therapeutic response in some patients.

Risks of Mesenchymal Stromal Cells as Cell Therapy

Malignant Transformation

MSCs invariably undergo ex vivo expansion for all clinical applications. This extensive cell replication raises the possibility of spontaneous transformation to a malignant phenotype, the most serious potential adverse event in a clinical trial. Murine MSCs seem to more readily undergo malignant transformation than do human MSCs,[71] possibly because of their significantly greater susceptibility to chromosomal aberrations and spontaneous mutations with prolonged culture,[72] suggesting such models are not good predictors of transformation of human MSCs in clinical trials.

Although there are several reports of malignant transformation of MSCs in vitro, the two most often cited studies[73,74] have been retracted[75,76] since the authors found their results were due to contamination of the MSC cultures by malignant cell lines. Further studies have confirmed the lack of spontaneous transformation.[77] During ex vivo expansion, MSCs may acquire chromosomal aberrations that have been suggested to predict the likelihood of malignant transformation.[78] However, such theoretical predictions have not been validated, and substantial data to the contrary have been presented.[79,80]

Malignant transformation of MSCs after infusion into human subjects in a clinical trial has never been reported. This may be because it is an exceedingly rare event and there have not yet been sufficient numbers of patients for such an event to occur. Alternatively, the latency for such an event could be quite long. Since MSCs do not seem to survive in the patients for more than 1 year, the likelihood of malignant transformation of ex vivo processed, transplanted MSCs in patients may be significantly less than predicted based on clinical experience with hematopoietic stem cell transplantation,[81] genetically modified hematopoietic stem cells,[82] or karyotype analysis.[80]

It must be emphasized that the field of MSC therapy is relatively young and definitive conclusions are not yet available; however, current opinion favors the notion that malignant transformation is an unlikely outcome and should not impede clinical investigation.

Ectopic Tissue Formation After Systemic Infusion

The potential of MSCs to differentiate to osteoblasts, chondrocytes, and adipocytes in vitro raises the possibility that MSCs may inappropriately differentiate to a mesenchymal tissue, such as bone, after intravenous infusion. Such ectopic tissue formation is thought to be unlikely, because the local environmental cues seem to regulate the differentiation of MSCs. A recent single report of murine MSCs injected into experimentally infracted myocardium demonstrated calcifications at the site of the cell injection.[83] In countless other experimental systems and clinical investigations, however, measurable ectopic tissue formation after systemic infusion of MSCs had never been reported.

Opportunistic Infections

Given the remarkable immune-modulatory capacity of MSCs, there is concern that MSCs may sufficiently suppress patients' immunity, rendering them susceptible to opportunistic infections. Such an outcome has never been reported, and MSCs seem to exert differential effects on alloantigen and virus-specific T-cell responses,[84] suggesting that MSC therapy is unlikely to induce clinically significant increased risk for opportunistic infections.

Mesenchymal Stromal Cells in Hematopoiesis

The principal application of MSC therapy in hematology is directed toward fostering hematopoietic reconstitution, most commonly (at this time) after hematopoietic cell transplantation. However, early promising results are being reported in regard to MSCs as cell-processing reagents for umbilical cord blood hematopoietic stem/progenitor cell expansion before transplantation.

Hematopoietic Cell Transplantation

MSCs were originally considered to be stem cells composing the hematopoietic supportive element of the marrow space and were studied in an effort to rebuild the microenvironment to foster hematopoietic stem cell (HSC) engraftment after allogeneic transplantation. The marrow microenvironment is, in fact, damaged by the chemoradiotherapy preparatory regimen, which likely disrupts the HSC niche,[18,85] thereby contributing to the delay of hematopoietic reconstitution after both autologous and allogeneic HSCT.[86-88] Although we now recognize that MSCs do not appreciably engraft in the host marrow microenvironment after intravenous infusion, the cells may foster engraftment by immune suppressive mechanisms, which could reduce the risk for graft rejection, or facilitate hematopoietic reconstitution by secreting cytokines into the circulation that would promote hematopoiesis reducing the risk for primary graft failure and hasten the time to neutrophil, erythrocyte, and platelet recovery.

Clinical Studies

The first effort to determine whether MSCs can promote engraftment and hematopoietic reconstitution in patients was reported by Koc and colleagues in 2000.[89] Twenty-eight women undergoing autologous HSCT with mobilized peripheral blood cells for advanced breast cancer were infused with 1 to 2.2 × 10^6 ex vivo–expanded MSCs/kg 4 hours before the hematopoietic graft. The MSCs were harvested about a month preinfusion, before the patients underwent mobilization for stem cell collection, and expanded for two to six passages. The median time to attain a neutrophil count greater than 500/μL was 8 days (range, 6 to 11 days), and a platelet count greater than 20,000/μL was 8.5 days (range, 4 to 19 days). Definitive clinical conclusions cannot be drawn from this single arm uncontrolled trial, but the rapid hematopoietic recovery demonstrated the potential of MSCs to enhance reconstitution in patients after autologous HSCT.

Lazarus and colleagues assessed the capacity of ex vivo–expanded MSCs obtained from HLA-identical sibling donors to facilitate hematopoietic recovery after cotransplantation with either bone marrow or peripheral blood stem cells in patients with hematologic malignancies.[90] MSCs were isolated, expanded, and cryopreserved before the initiation of the conditioning regimen. The MSC units were thawed at the bedside and intravenously infused into the patients 4 hours before the hematopoietic stem cell graft. The median hematopoietic cell doses were 3.6 × 10^8 mononuclear cells/kg for bone marrow and 5.0 × 10^6 $CD34^+$ cells/kg for peripheral blood grafts, whereas the MSC dose ranged from 1 to 5 × 10^6 cell/kg for both patient groups. Overall, the median time to attain a neutrophil count of 500/μL was 14 days (range, 11 to 26 days) and to attain a platelet count of 20,000/μL, 20 days (range, 15 to 36 days). Patients receiving peripheral blood grafts demonstrated a more rapid neutrophil recovery (median, 13.5 days) compared with those receiving bone marrow (15.5 days). Although this study also lacked a control cohort of patients, the time to neutrophil recovery of bone marrow appears to be slightly faster than usual. On the other hand, it is less clear whether the time to engraftment of PBSC represents a hastening of hematopoietic recovery.

Haploidentical HSCT in children typically results in rapid hematopoietic reconstitution, often in as little as 10 days[91]. However, primary graft failure/rejection occurs frequently with these highly T cell–depleted grafts, and a second hematopoietic stem cell infusion is often required. Ball and colleagues sought to determine whether MSCs could positively impact engraftment in haploidentical children.[92] Fourteen children underwent transplantation with HLA-disparate $CD34^+$ cells obtained from mobilized peripheral blood. A median of 21.5 × 10^6 $CD34^+$ cells/kg were infused. MSCs were isolated from bone marrow about 5 weeks before HSCT and expanded up to three passages. The ex vivo–expanded cells were infused, either cryopreserved or fresh, at a dose of 1 to 5 × 10^6 cells/kg 4 hours before the hematopoietic stem cell graft. Compared with 47 age-, sex-, and diagnosis-matched historical controls, no difference was found in the time to neutrophil recovery (12 versus 13 days) or the time to platelet (20,000/μL) recovery (10 versus 13 days). However, the time to attain a total leukocyte count of 1 × 10^6/μL was shorter in the MSC group (11.5 days) compared with controls (14.9 days, $P = 0.009$). More important, none of the children receiving MSCs ($n = 14$) experienced graft failure. In contrast, the graft failure rate among the controls was 15%, consistent with published experience.

One of the consistent themes of the preclinical studies is that MSCs are most beneficial at limiting doses of HSCs. This observation suggests that umbilical cord blood transplantation may be the most useful setting for MSC cotransplantation. Umbilical cord units have a threshold cell count for clinical use, since low cell doses increase the risk for graft failure (see Chapter 108). Moreover, the time to neutrophil and platelet reconstitution tends to be longer when umbilical cord grafts are used as compared with other HSC sources.

Based on this rationale, MacMillan and colleagues[93] have cotransplanted parental (haploidentical) MSCs with unrelated umbilical cord blood grafts. Eight patients underwent transplantation with an HLA-matched unrelated umbilical cord graft for a hematologic malignancy. Haploidentical MSCs were isolated from parental bone marrow obtained at the time the patient was referred for transplant and the ex vivo–expanded cells were cryopreserved for storage. MSCs, thawed immediately prior to intravenous infusion, were transplanted at a median dose of 2.1 × 10^6 cells/kg 4 hours before the umbilical cord blood graft. The median umbilical cord blood total nucleated cell dose was 3.1 × 10^7 cell/kg. All patients attained a neutrophil count of 500/μL at a median of 19 days (range, 8 to 28 days) as compared with 86% of historical control patients at a median of 30 days (range, 10 to 59 days). Six of the eight patients attached a platelet count of 20,000/μL at a median of 1.7 months (range, 1.1 to 3.2 months) compared with 79% of historical controls at a median of 2.7 months (range, 1.5 to 6.6).

Two additional studies of cotransplantation of MSCs with umbilical cord blood cells have been reported.[94,95] However, neither was able to show a statistically significant benefit of engraftment or hematopoietic reconstitution, although this may be due to the small sample size in each study.

Of note, MacMillan and colleagues showed a striking, but not significant, reduction of regimen-related toxicity and a corresponding improvement of overall survival. Thus MSCs may find their greatest application in HCT as an ancillary cell therapy to reduce regimen-related toxicity and improve overall survival without directly impacting hematopoietic recovery, consistent with the recent reports that MSCs may confer tissue protection against radiation injury.[96,97]

Three studies have used MSCs to rescue HCT patients after graft failure. Le Blanc and colleagues used MSC therapy to induce hematopoietic recovery in three patients with either primary or secondary graft failure.[98] Meuleman and colleagues rescued two of six patients,[99] and Fouillard and colleagues reported a single patient in which haploidentical MSCs stimulated autologous hematopoietic recovery after primary failure of a mafosfamide-purged autograft.[100] Collectively, these case reports suggest that MSCs may most significantly foster hematopoietic engraftment/reconstitution under "failure" conditions. Thus MSCs may find greater value as an agent to rescue graft failure in contrast to up-front use to promote primary engraftment.

Future Applications

Before MSCs became cell therapy agents, stromal cells were used to generate long-term bone marrow cell cultures. This hematopoietic marrow cell culture methodology is being applied to clinical setting by using MSCs as a "feeder" layer to culture-expand primitive hematopoietic progenitors for transplantation to foster engraftment and promote hematopoietic reconstitution. Early results of an ongoing clinical trial at the MD Anderson Cancer Center[101] show that after double cord blood transplantation, in which 1 unit was expanded ex vivo on a monolayer of MSCs, the median time to neutrophil recovery (>500/μL) was 15 days (range, 9 to 42 days) and the time to platelet recovery (>20,000/μL) was 40 days (range 13 to 62 days). Moreover, 97% of patients attained neutrophil engraftment. Although preliminary, these data represent a marked improvement compared with standard cord blood transplantation.

Mesenchymal Stromal Cells for the Treatment of Graft-Versus-Host Disease

GVHD occurs in HCT when donor T cells recognize the patients' organs (host) as foreign and cell-mediated immune attack ensues. It is one of the most severe complications of allogeneic HCT. The immunomodulatory capacity of MSCs suggests that these cells may be effective agents for the treatment of GVHD.

Based on limited preclinical in vitro data, and without animal models, a 9-year-old boy with severe refractory gut and liver GVHD (after a peripheral blood stem cell transplant from a matched, unrelated donor) was treated with ex vivo–expanded MSCs derived from his haploidentical mother.[69] While continuing to receive prednisolone and cyclosporine, an infusion of 2×10^6 MSCs/kg led to a prompt reduction of his serum bilirubin concentration and stool output (Fig. 100-3). His cyclosporine was then discontinued to enhance a graft-versus-leukemia effect, but this led to an acute exacerbation of his gut and liver GVHD. A second infusion of MSCs (1×10^6 cells/kg) again resulted in rapid reduction of his serum bilirubin and stool output. About 18 months after the MSC infusions, the patient had recurrent GVHD, developed interstitial pneumonia, and died. Despite the unfortunate regimen-related death, this landmark report indicated the potential of MSCs to effectively treat GVHD.

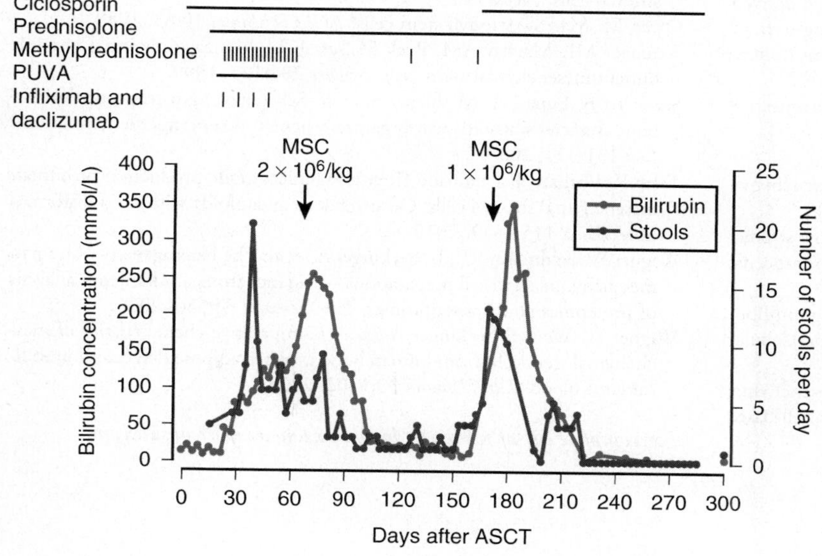

Figure 100-3 CLINICAL COURSE AND IMMUNE SUPPRESSION OF THE FIRST GRAFT VERSUS-HOST DISEASE (GVHD) PATIENT TO BE TREATED WITH MESENCHYMAL STROMAL CELLS. Pharmacologic immune suppression is indicated *(top)*; *arrows* indicate the time of MSC infusions. *ASCT,* Allogeneic stem cell transplantation. *(With permission from Le Blanc K, Rasmusson I, Sundberg B, et al: Treatment of severe acute graft-versus-host disease with third party haploidentical mesenchymal stem cells,* Lancet *363:1439, 2004.)*

Subsequently, many small studies (case series) have been published that mostly support the notion that MSCs may be effective therapy for GVHD; however, the outcomes are highly varied, possibly due to the different MSC expansion protocols and the diversity of patients and treatment schedules. Notably, growth media supplementation with fetal bovine serum or human serum platelet lysate or growth factors with or without serum may alter the immune modulatory capacity of the processed MSC product.

The largest published trial in this area is a phase II multicenter study by the European Group for Blood and Marrow Transplantation to treat steroid-resistant acute GVHD.[70] The study included 55 patients (30 adults, 25 children) with grade II ($n = 5$), III ($n = 25$), or IV ($n = 25$) disease who had failed one to five prior therapies. Patients received a median total dose of ex vivo–expanded bone marrow MSCs of 1.4×10^6 cells/kg patient body weight (range, 0.4 to 9.0×10^6) derived from HLA-identical sibling donor ($n = 5$), haploidentical donors ($n = 18$), or third-party HLA-disparate donor ($n = 69$). Of these 55 patients, 27 received 1 infusion of MSCs, 22 received two infusions, and 6 received three to five infusions, all without MSC-related toxicity. Thirty patients (55%) had a complete response, and nine (16%) had a partial response, yielding an overall response rate of 71%. HLA-matching had no effect on the response. Of note, complete responders had a lower 1-year transplant-related mortality compared with partial responders and nonresponders (37% versus 72%, $P = 0.002$) and a higher overall survival (53% versus 16%, $P = 0.018$). These data portend great use of MSCs for the treatment of GVHD; however, such remarkable results have not yet been reproduced.

The only large, randomized, double-blind, placebo-controlled phase III trial of MSC therapy of steroid-refractory acute GVHD to date was conducted by Osiris Therapeutics, Inc. The study outcome has been released to the public but not published in the peer-reviewed literature. Briefly, patients (n = 260, 28 children) received 2×10^6 MSCs/kg or placebo twice a week for 4 weeks. The durable complete response (primary endpoint) was not statistically different between the treatment and placebo groups (35% versus 30%), and overall survival was not improved; however, the responses specifically in the liver (76% versus 47%, $P = 0.26$) and in the gut (88% versus 64%, $P = 0.018$) were significantly improved.

MSC therapy is also being studied as a component of first-line treatment of acute GVHD. In a trial sponsored by Osiris Therapeutics, Inc., 32 patients with newly diagnosed GVHD were treated with standard corticosteroid therapy and randomized to receive either 2 or 8×10^6. Complete response was observed in 73% of all patients without a difference between the two dose groups.[102] Although these results are encouraging, randomized controlled trials are essential before any assertions can be made regarding the role of MSCs as a component of first-line therapy of acute GVHD.

Of note, the enormous interest in MSCs as treatment for GVHD originated from the report of a single-patient treatment, which took place without a supportive animal model. This sequence of events is quite fortunate for the field because the subsequently published animal data suggest that MSCs may not effectively treat established GVHD, in contradiction to the clinical findings.[103,104] This discrepancy may reflect the substantial difference between mouse and human MSCs,[16] as well as their respective immune systems.[105] Although the role of MSC therapy for GVHD remains to be completely defined, the recognition of clinical benefits warranting further randomized trials underscores the importance of initial pilot clinical trials, as opposed to relying solely on preclinical animal models, to investigate the therapeutic potential of a novel cell therapy product.

FUTURE DIRECTIONS

We are beginning to unravel the highly complex biology of MSCs that will undoubtedly foster effective clinical applications. MSCs hold great promise to facilitate hematopoiesis, as well as hematopoietic reconstitution after HCT. Additionally, MSCs clearly can modulate the immune response, despite our present inadequate understanding of the MSC immune system interaction. Moreover, novel approaches using MSCs as cell therapy in regenerative medicine are emerging.

Two overriding challenges lie ahead. First, we must better understand the mechanism of action for each therapeutic activity and design clinical trials to ensure that the best possible outcomes are being observed. Second, we must conduct numerous early-phase clinical trials to define the potential of MSCs followed by double-blind, placebo-controlled trials published in the peer-reviewed literature to first prove and then validate the clinical utility of MSCs.

SUGGESTED READINGS

Ball LM, Bernardo ME, Roelofs H, et al: Cotransplantation of ex vivo expanded mesenchymal stem cells accelerates lymphocyte recovery and may reduce the risk of graft failure in haploidentical hematopoietic stem-cell transplantation. *Blood* 110:2764, 2007.

Ben-David U, Mayshar Y, Benvenisty N: Large-scale analysis reveals acquisition of lineage-specific chromosomal aberrations in human adult stem cells. *Cell Stem Cell* 9:97, 2011.

Bernardo ME, Zaffaroni N, Novara F, et al: Human bone marrow derived mesenchymal stem cells do not undergo transformation after long-term in vitro culture and do not exhibit telomere maintenance mechanisms. *Cancer Res* 67:9142, 2007.

Buhring HJ, Battula VL, Treml S, et al: Novel markers for the prospective isolation of human MSC. *Ann N Y Acad Sci* 1106:262, 2007.

Caplan AI: Mesenchymal stem cells. *J Orthop Res* 9:641, 1991.

Crisan M, Yap S, Casteilla L, et al: A perivascular origin for mesenchymal stem cells in multiple human organs. *Cell Stem Cell* 3:301, 2008.

Di Nicola M, Carlo-Stella C, Magni M, et al: Human bone marrow stromal cells suppress T-lymphocyte proliferation induced by cellular or nonspecific mitogenic stimuli. *Blood* 99:3838, 2002.

Dominici M, Le BK, Mueller I, et al: Minimal criteria for defining multipotent mesenchymal stromal cells: The International Society for Cellular Therapy position statement. *Cytotherapy* 8:315, 2006.

Doucet C, Ernou I, Zhang Y, et al: Platelet lysates promote mesenchymal stem cell expansion: A safety substitute for animal serum in cell-based therapy applications. *J Cell Physiol* 205:228, 2005.

Fouillard L, Chapel A, Bories D, et al: Infusion of allogeneic-related HLA mismatched mesenchymal stem cells for the treatment of incomplete engraftment following autologous haematopoietic stem cell transplantation. *Leukemia* 21:568, 2007.

Friedenstein AJ, Petrakova KV, Kurolesova AI, et al: Heterotopic of bone marrow: Analysis of precursor cells for osteogenic and hematopoietic tissues. *Transplantation* 6:230, 1968.

Glennie S, Soeiro I, Dyson PJ, et al: Bone marrow mesenchymal stem cells induce division arrest anergy of activated T cells. *Blood* 105:2821, 2005.

Horwitz E, Le BK, Dominici M, et al: Clarification of the nomenclature for MSC: The International Society for Cellular Therapy position statement. *Cytotherapy* 7:393, 2005.

Horwitz EM, Gordon PL, Koo WKK, et al: Isolated allogeneic bone marrow-derived mesenchymal cells engraft and stimulate growth in children with osteogenesis imperfecta: Implications for cell therapy of bone. *Proc Natl Acad Sci USA* 99:8932, 2002.

Karp JM, Leng Teo GS: Mesenchymal stem cell homing: The devil is in the details. *Cell Stem Cell* 4:206, 2009.

Koc ON, Gerson SL, Cooper BW, et al: Rapid hematopoietic recovery after coinfusion of autologous-blood stem cells and culture-expanded marrow mesenchymal stem cells in advanced breast cancer patients receiving high-dose chemotherapy. *J Clin Oncol* 18:307, 2000.

Lazarus HM, Koc ON, Devine SM: Cotransplantation of HLA-identical sibling culture-expanded mesenchymal stem cells and hematopoietic stem cells in hematologic malignancy patients. *Biol Blood Marrow Transplant* 11:389, 2005.

Le Blanc K, Rasmusson I, Sundberg B, et al: Treatment of severe acute graft-versus-host disease with third party haploidentical mesenchymal stem cells. *Lancet* 363:1439, 2004.

Le Blanc K, Samuelsson H, Gustafsson B, et al: Transplantation of mesenchymal stem cells to enhance engraftment of hematopoietic stem cells. *Leukemia* 21:1733, 2007.

Macmillan ML, Blazar BR, DeFor TE, et al: Transplantation of ex-vivo culture-expanded parental haploidentical mesenchymal stem cells to promote engraftment in pediatric recipients of unrelated donor umbilical cord blood: Results of a phase I-II clinical trial. *Bone Marrow Transplant* 43:447, 2009.

Mendez-Ferrer S, Michurina TV, Ferraro F, et al: Mesenchymal and haematopoietic stem cells form a unique bone marrow niche. *Nature* 466:829, 2010.

Meuleman N, Tondreau T, Ahmad I, et al: Infusion of mesenchymal stromal cells can aid hematopoietic recovery following allogeneic hematopoietic stem cell myeloablative transplant: A pilot study. *Stem Cells Dev* 18:1247, 2009.

Morikawa S, Mabuchi Y, Kubota Y, et al: Prospective identification, isolation, and systemic transplantation of multipotent mesenchymal stem cells in murine bone marrow. *J Exp Med* 206:2483, 2009.

Nauta AJ, Fibbe WE: Immunomodulatory properties of mesenchymal stromal cells. *Blood* 110:3499, 2007.

Owen M: Marrow stromal stem cells. *J Cell Sci Suppl* 10:63, 1988.

Pittenger MF, Mackay AM, Beck SC, et al: Multilineage potential of adult human mesenchymal stem cells. *Science* 284:143, 1999.

Sacchetti B, Funari A, Michienzi S, et al: Self-renewing osteoprogenitors in bone marrow sinusoids can organize a hematopoietic microenvironment. *Cell* 131:324, 2007.

Tarte K, Gaillard J, Lataillade JJ, et al: Clinical-grade production of human mesenchymal stromal cells: Occurrence of aneuploidy without transformation. *Blood* 115:1549, 2010.

Wagner W, Feldmann RE, Jr, Seckinger A, et al: The heterogeneity of human mesenchymal stem cell preparations—evidence from simultaneous analysis of proteomes and transcriptomes. *Exp Hematol* 34:536, 2006.

Wagner W, Wein F, Seckinger A, et al: Comparative characteristics of mesenchymal stem cells from human bone marrow, adipose tissue, and umbilical cord blood. *Exp Hematol* 33:1402, 2005.

For complete list of references log on to www.expertconsult.com.

CHAPTER 101

T-CELL THERAPY OF HEMATOLOGIC DISEASES

Gianpietro Dotti and Malcolm K. Brenner

Conventional modalities for treating cancer remain unsatisfactory. Despite the introduction of small molecules that target specific molecular lesions or pathways within the cancer cells, cure rates for many common tumors remain low, while adverse events are still distressingly high. Cancer immunotherapy represents a promising extension of highly targeted cancer therapy with a favorable toxicity profile and excellent pharmacoeconomics. Although most attention has been on the development of monoclonal antibodies, beneficial results with cellular immunotherapy are now being reported.[1-4] Although to date these have primarily been obtained in subjects with lymphoma, melanoma, or neuroblastoma, methodologies are being developed to allow us to extend the tumor range.

Many human tumors express tumor-specific antigens (TSAs) or tumor-associated antigens (TAAs) that can be recognized by the host immune system and induce antitumor cell-mediated and humoral immune responses.[5] Although these responses may be transient and are not always associated with clinical responses, they provide evidence for the existence of tumor-directed immunity in humans that may also have antitumor activity.[1] Several barriers block the development of more effective antitumor immunity in subjects with cancer.[6,7] First, many human tumors express few major histocompatibility complex (MHC) molecules or have poor processing of their potential tumor antigens. Even when TAAs/TSAs are processed and presented, most tumors lack the costimulatory molecules necessary to implement a long-lived and effective immune response. In addition to these passive defenses against immunity, many tumors can "edit" the immune system to their advantage, secreting cytokines such as TGFβ that directly inhibit cytotoxic effector T-cell growth, function, and survival or that favor expansion of IL-4-producing T cells (Th2 cells) or regulatory T cells (Treg) rather than effector T cells.[6] Finally, intensive chemotherapies and radiotherapies can themselves severely reduce immune function by destroying antigen-presenting cells and dividing T lymphocytes.

As our understanding of the molecular basis of tumor immune escape has increased, it has been possible to derive countermeasures that may allow us to induce more potent antitumor immune responses, and that will soon allow us to extend effective therapies to a broad range of common tumors.

TYPES OF CELLULAR IMMUNOTHERAPY

Cellular immunotherapy may be active, using cell-based vaccines derived from tumor cells themselves or antigen-presenting cells expressing TAA/TSA from proteins or peptides, or passive, by direct adoptive transfer of viable immune cells. The former approach relies on the intact afferent and efferent immune system of the host responding to the stimulus with an effective antitumor response, whereas the latter is the cellular equivalent of antibody serotherapy, in which the transferred immune cells are expected to attack the tumor cells directly, albeit with a phase of in vivo expansion, and to subsequently establish a pool of memory cells to provide long-term protection against resurgent disease. Several cell subsets are currently being studied in adoptive transfer protocols, including activated T lymphocytes, tumor-infiltrating T lymphocytes, antigen-specific cytotoxic T lymphocytes (CTLs), natural killer cells, γδ T cells, and natural killer T cells. In this chapter we discuss adoptive transfer of activated T lymphocytes and CTLs.

Adoptive Cell Therapy With T Lymphocytes

In principle, lymphocytes have the ability to traffic through multiple tissue planes and to be self-renewing. These assets, coupled with their ability to destroy tumor or viral infected target cells through a range of mechanisms, make them an appealing resource for adoptive transfer, and a multiplicity of clinical studies using this approach have now been described. Adoptive lymphocyte therapies may use allogeneic or autologous cells, which may be of tightly defined specificity (e.g., T-cell clones) or broad phenotype and activity (e.g., tumor-infiltrating lymphocytes). As we have learned more about the molecular basis of immune recognition and immune regulation, it has become possible to genetically modify the infused lymphocytes to alter their specificity or behavior. In this section we describe examples of each type of adoptive transfer and discuss the relative merits and limitations of each.

Donor Lymphocyte Infusion

It has long been apparent that the curative effects of allogeneic stem cell transplants for many hematologic malignancies can be attributed to a graft-versus-leukemia (GVL) effect largely mediated by the incoming T cells within the donor graft. Thus patients with chronic graft-versus-host disease (GVHD) were well recognized as having a lower probability of relapse than individuals without this unpleasant complication. Similarly, recipients of syngeneic grafts have the lowest rate of GVHD and the highest risk for relapse. In 1990, Kolb et al[8] took advantage of this observation and deliberately infused donor lymphocytes in an attempt to eliminate recurrent disease in patients with chronic myeloid leukemia (CML). Their positive results have been confirmed in multiple studies worldwide, and remission can be induced in over 80% of patients with Epstein-Barr virus (EBV) lymphoma and in more than 50% of CML patients who relapse after transplantation by stopping immunosuppressive treatment or infusing donor lymphocytes.[9] Unfortunately, donor lymphocyte infusion (DLI) is much less effective at treating other types of relapsed leukemias after transplantation, with a 29% remission rate for acute myeloid leukemia and only 5% for acute lymphoblastic leukemia.[10] It is not clear why these differences occur, because all these leukemias present the minor histocompatibility antigens that are likely the targets of this GVL effect, although many minor histocompatibility antigens have yet to be defined. DLI therapy may also produce severe adverse effects, because the frequency of broadly alloreactive effector cells is usually much higher than the frequency of lymphocytes targeted exclusively to the relapsed malignancy. As a consequence, patients receiving DLI often develop GVHD. This complication may be manifested by skin, gut, or liver damage or by pancytopenia if there is significant residual host hemopoietic chimerism. Strategies aimed at retaining the benefits of GVL while preventing GVHD have included the depletion of alloreactive T cells in the donor lymphocyte product and the incorporation of suicide genes into the infused donor T cells so that they may be killed if the GVHD activity exceeds the benefits from GVL.[11] Ultimately, investigators may wish to identify tumor-restricted target antigens on the malignant cells and infuse antigen-specific T cells directed to them.

Infusion of Activated T Lymphocytes

When T cells are polyclonally stimulated, for example by simultaneously cross-linking their CD3 and CD28 receptors by CD3/CD28 monoclonal antibodies on beads, then the cells proliferate. They also secrete tumoricidal cytokines such as tumor necrosis factor-α and can mediate MHC-unrestricted cytotoxicity toward a range of tumor target cells. Efforts have been made to harness these effects by producing large numbers of CD3/CD28-activated T cells for cancer patients and infusing them. Although infusion of CD3/CD28-activated T lymphocytes after autologous stem cell transplant may improve patients' T-cell reconstitution, as yet there is no evidence to suggest improved antitumor activity.[12] In current studies, adoptive therapy is being combined with vaccination with tumor antigens such as the human telomerase reverse transcriptase and the antiapoptotic protein survivin to enhance antitumor activity.[12] Activated T lymphocytes that are additionally primed with interferon-γ and IL-2 (so-called cytokine-induced killer cells) may have superior clinical potential for hematologic malignancies.

Adoptive Immunotherapy With Virus-Specific Cytotoxic T Lymphocytes

Viral infections are one of the commonest causes of morbidity and mortality after stem cell transplant and are more prevalent as the degree of antigen mismatching between donor and recipient is increased. The most common problematic viral infections after stem cell transplant are reactivated herpesviruses, including cytomegalovirus (CMV), which typically causes pneumonitis and hepatitis, and the γ-herpesvirus EBV, which may cause a rapidly fatal lymphoproliferative disease (LPD). In children and recipients of cord blood transplants, adenoviral disease is also common. Adoptive transfer of virus-specific T cells appears to effectively prevent and treat these infections after transplant. Infusion of even small numbers of specific cells (10^6 or less) may be sufficient for benefit, because the lymphodepletion of the immediate posttransplant period is associated with the release of homeostatic cytokines such as IL-7 and IL-15, which augment the expansion of virus-specific T cells when they encounter their antigen.

Donor-Derived Virus-Specific Cytotoxic T Lymphocytes

Walter et al[13] pioneered the use of CMV-specific $CD8^+$ T-cell clones to prevent CMV reactivation in allogeneic hematopoietic stem cell transplant (HSCT) recipients. They activated and expanded donor-derived CTL by coculture with CMV-infected autologous fibroblasts. Neither viremia nor disease activation were detected in any of the treated patients. However, CMV-specific CTL clones did not persist unless there was also recovery of endogenous $CD4^+$ T cells.

We reported the use of donor-derived polyclonal but EBV-specific CTLs to treat and prevent EBV-associated LPD after allogeneic HSCT.[14] Since 1993, over 110 stem cell recipients have received donor-derived EBV-specific CTLs. None of the patients in our prophylaxis group developed posttransplant lipoproliferative disorder, in contrast to an incidence of 11.5% in 44 patients in the control group. Elevated EBV-DNA levels declined within 1 to 3 weeks of first T-cell infusion, and EBV-specific CTLs have also been found effective in 10 of 12 patients with bulky EBV-associated lymphoma. Other groups have confirmed that adoptive immunotherapy with EBV-specific CTLs effectively prevents and treats EBV-LPD after hematopoietic stem cell or solid organ transplant. Improvements in methodology to simplify and accelerate manufacture of these viral-specific CTLs have followed. We have developed a culture method to generate, in a single culture, CTL lines that have antiviral activity for EBV, CMV, and adenovirus and minibioreactors in which to prepare these cells in a closed system.[15] In combination, these techniques allow us to make sufficient CTLs for patient treatment in less than 10 days instead of more than 10 weeks. Other groups have developed even faster techniques, in which T cells activated by viral antigens are selected by columns specific for activation markers such interferon-γ.[16]

Third-Party Allogeneic Virus-Specific Cytotoxic T Lymphocytes

Ideally, virus-specific CTLs should be immediately available from a cryopreserved line. The cost of doing this for each patient at risk is prohibitive, but Haque et al[17] generated a bank of polyclonal EBV-specific CTLs expressing common human leukocyte antigens (HLAs) and gave the best-matched cells to subjects who developed EBV lymphoproliferation after solid organ transplant. More recently they reported results of a phase II multicenter trial in which they treated 33 patients with EBV-LPD with an overall response rate of 64% at 5 weeks and 52% at 6 months. These impressive results have led us to develop a similar multicenter study to evaluate whether these trivirus-specific CTL lines may have similar activity against EBV, CMV, and adenovirus in partially HLA-matched allogeneic patients. The interim analysis of this study confirmed a greater than 80% rate of infection control in 45 recipients of allogeneic stem cell transplant with intractable EBV, CMV, or adenovirus infections.

Adoptive Immunotherapy of Viral-Related Malignancies

The encouraging results of adoptive immunotherapy with EBV-specific CTLs in the immunocompromised host led us to extend this strategy to other EBV-associated tumors (lymphoma and nasopharyngeal cancer) that develop in the immunocompetent subject. Unlike EBV-LPD, which expresses the highly immunogenic viral latency antigens EBV nuclear antigen 1 (EBNA1), EBNA2, and EBNA3, these other EBV tumors express a limited number of poorly processed (EBNA1) or weakly stimulatory (latent membrane protein 1 [LMP1] and LMP2) EBV-derived antigens. We have therefore used CTLs specific for these EBV antigens, beginning with the cells directed to LMP2. The CTLs were generated from patients with Hodgkin disease by using dendritic cells that are engineered to overexpress LMP2. The infusion of polyclonal LMP2-specific T cells containing both $CD4^+$ and $CD8^+$ T cells increases LMP2-specific T-cell responses and lead to complete tumor regression in 8 of 12 patients with EBV-positive lymphoma.[2]

Similar results have been obtained in EBV-associated nasopharyngeal carcinoma (NPC), a tumor that originates from the epithelial cells of the nasopharynx.[18] Like EBV-associated lymphomas, NPCs express the same restricted set of weakly immunogenic viral antigens, including EBNA1, LMP1, and LMP2. Treatment of EBV-positive NPC with polyclonal EBV-specific CTLs has produced complete clinical responses in patients with limited tumor burden.[18] One of the main limitations of treatment of NPC with EBV-specific CTLs is the failure of in vivo expansion of adoptively transferred cells. Thus infusions of these cells may best be given immediately after lymphoreductive chemotherapy, enabling their expansion to be supported by the increased availability of homeostatic cytokines. Alternatively, these cells could be engineered to enhance their "survival" in vivo as discussed in Genetic Modifications of T Cells.

Adoptive Immunotherapy of Non–Viral-Mediated Malignancies

Many different types of tumor-associated or tumor-specific antigens have been described and are reviewed in a National Cancer Institute initiative to prioritize cancer antigens.[5] Among the most widely studied are the tumor testis antigens, which are expressed by a range of tumors, including melanoma. For example, CTL clones specific for melanoma Ag recognized by T cells (MART) have been successfully used to treat patients with metastatic melanoma.[1] Although infused CTLs localized to tumor sites and induced clinical responses, tumor antigen–loss variants were observed in three patients who subsequently relapsed, highlighting the risk for escape mutants when a single clone of CTLs targets a single epitope. In the allogeneic transplant setting ex vivo–expanded donor-derived CTLs have also shown antileukemia activity when directed at minor antigens, although off-target toxicity was observed due to the unexpected presence of the target antigens on lung tissue.[19]

GENETIC MODIFICATIONS OF T CELLS

There is considerable interest in genetically modifying T cells so that they may be used for cancer therapy. Early clinical studies used genetic modification to "mark" the T cell infused so that these cells can be detected by polymerase chain reaction amplification in the peripheral blood or other tissues.[14] More recently, efforts have been devoted to "redirecting" the antigen specificity of T lymphocytes. Most TAAs are self-proteins to which the immune system has limited responsiveness, because of the development of tolerance by clonal deletion or anergy. Hence tumor antigen–specific T cells isolated from patients with cancer may have low-affinity T-cell receptors (TCRs), limiting their cytotoxic activity against tumor cells. Investigators have overcome this limitation by expressing transgenic TCR α- and β-chains of high affinity[20] or by expressing a synthetic chimeric antigen receptor (CAR)[21] that has the binding domains of, for example, a monoclonal antibody, and the endodomains of the T-cell receptor to ensure signaling and T-cell activation once the CAR has been engaged (Fig. 101-1). Finally, interest in genetic modification of T cells has also arisen as a means of incorporating countermeasures to the multiplicity of immune evasion strategies used by potentially immunogenic tumor cells or to enhance the "survival" of T cells in vivo[22] (see Fig. 101-1). Because T lymphocytes can be long-lived cells and may proliferate extensively in vivo, most gene transfer studies have used integrating vectors such as γ-retroviral vectors, lentiviral vectors, or transposon/transposase integrating plasmids.

T Lymphocytes and Gene-Marking Studies

Incorporation of a marker gene in T cells was the first authorized human gene transfer study.[23] In subsequent studies, tumor-infiltrating T lymphocytes and antigen-specific CTLs were transduced with retroviral vectors coding for the neomycin resistance gene (neo) or for a nonfunctional human receptor such as the truncated form of the p75 low-affinity nerve growth factor receptor (LNGFR). These studies indicated that adoptively transferred T cells and antigen-specific CTLs could persist and recirculate for more than 10 years in the peripheral blood.[14] Gene-marked tumor antigen–specific CTLs were also able to reach the tumor microenvironment. There were no adverse events attributable to gene transfer. There are now extensive efforts to develop technologies that will allow more sophisticated in vivo analyses in real time of functional transgenes (such as the thymidine kinase gene) expressed by adoptively transferred T lymphocytes, allowing evaluation of their temporospatial distribution.

Artificial αβ-T-Cell Receptors

The large-scale culture of T lymphocytes to enrich the scanty precursors specific for weak TAAs is often unsuccessful and always tedious. This process can be bypassed by introducing additional TCR genes with predetermined specificity for the weak tumor antigen into a polyclonal population of T cells. Technical improvements in retroviral transduction mean that 30% of polyclonal T lymphocytes can now be induced to express a transgenic TCR for TAAs, including MART1, melanoma antigen (MAGE)3, MDM2, and WT1, for minor histocompatibility antigens such as HA1, and for infectious agents such as human immunodeficiency virus type 1 (HIV-1) and EBV.

Polyclonal T cells expressing transgenic MART1-specific αβ-TCRs have been safely infused in patients with metastatic melanoma after lymphodepleting chemoradiotherapy.[20] Up to 30% of these patients had objective regression of metastatic disease. Similar results have been obtained in patients with metastatic synovial cell sarcomas and melanoma who were given T cells expressing an NY-ESO-1–specific αβ-TCR. Although most of these patients had no severe adverse events, toxicity was observed in patients with metastatic colon carcinoma who received T cells expressing a TCR directed to the carcinoembryonic antigen,[24] due to T cell–mediated damage to

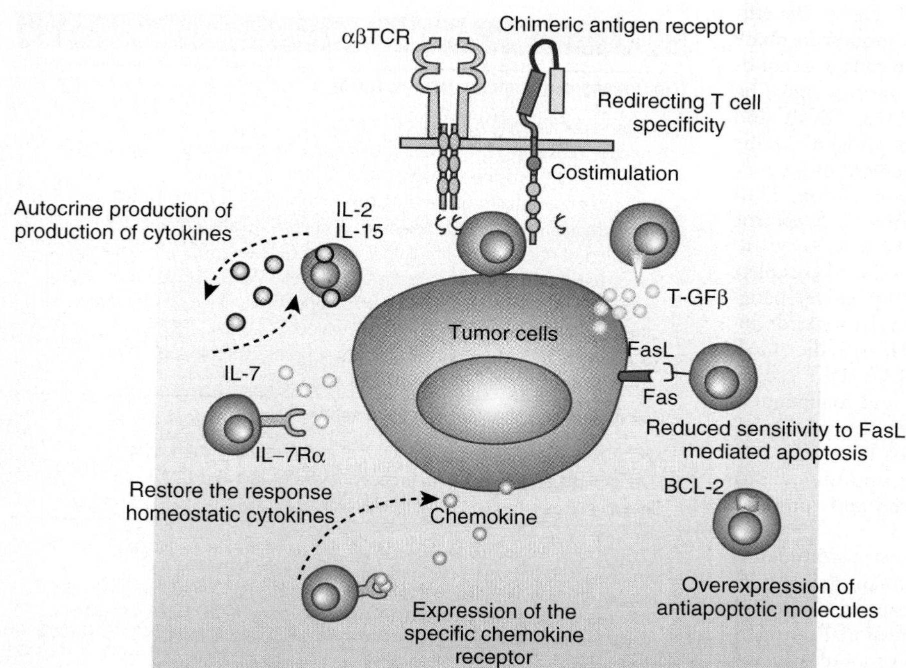

Figure 101-1 GENETIC MODIFICATIONS OF T LYMPHOCYTES FOR ADOPTIVE T-CELL THERAPY. *TCR*, T-cell receptor.

normal gastrointestinal epithelial cells expressing low levels of the target antigen. Thus T cells with high-affinity transgenic TCR may produce "on-target" but "off-organ" toxicities to normal tissues that physiologically express the target antigen at low level. The first TCR gene therapy trial for patients with acute leukemia targeting WT1 is currently recruiting patients.

A major problem of TCR gene transfer is the resulting "cross pairing" between transgenic α- or β-receptor chains and the reciprocal endogenous TCR α- and β-chains, to create loss of function or—and potentially worse—gain of function receptors that may produce autoimmune disease. Although such adverse effects have been elegantly demonstrated in mouse models, human clinical trials have not yet revealed such issues. Investigators have developed several molecular strategies intended to modify the transgenic TCRs to make them less likely to cross pair or to silence the endogenous TCRs.

Chimeric Antigen Receptors

The cytotoxic activity of T cells through their native or transgenic TCR is MHC restricted so that multiple distinct transgenic αβ-TCRs would be required to recognize tumor antigens associated with the multiple MHC polymorphisms in a human population, precluding a "universal" receptor. In addition, tumor cells can downregulate MHC molecules and avoid immune recognition by conventional TCRs. In an attempt to overcome this limitation, MHC-unrestricted artificial CARs have been generated.[25] CARs are usually generated by joining the light and heavy chain variable regions of a monoclonal antibody expressed as a single-chain Fv (scFv) molecule to the transmembrane and cytoplasmic signaling domains derived from CD3ζ-chain or Fc receptor γ chain through a flexible spacer. Thus they combine the antigen specificity of an antibody and the cytotoxic properties of a T cell in a single fusion molecule. Because CARs bind to target antigens in an HLA-unrestricted manner, they are resistant to many of the tumor immune evasion mechanisms, such as downregulation of HLA class I molecules or failure to process or present proteins, used by tumor cells to escape immune attack. First-generation CARs, incorporated the cytoplasmic region (endodomains) from the CD3ζ or the Fc receptor γ chains as their signaling domain.[21] Although these receptors successfully redirected T-cell cytotoxicity, they failed to stimulate T-cell proliferation and survival in vivo, likely because of the lack of appropriate costimulatory signals to T cells following engagement of the CAR. Hence the efficacy of these first-generation CAR T cells has been modest in phase I clinical trials in patients with lymphoma or ovarian cancer. Second-generation CARs were constructed by incorporating signaling domains from costimulatory molecules such as CD28, OX40, and 4-1BB within the endodomain.[26] This improved antigen-specific T-cell activation and expansion as tumor cell engagement of second-generation CARs alone is sufficient to provide costimulation. Thus the incorporation of the CD28 endodomain within a CAR specific for the B cell–associated antigen CD19 enhances the in vivo expansion of T lymphocytes that express this CAR and produced complete responses in lymphodepleted patients with CD19-positive malignancy.[27] A similar study in which a different costimulatory endodomain (4-1BB) was incorporated into the CD19-specific CAR produced even more striking expansion of the CAR-CD19 T cells in vivo and the apparent eradication of both normal and malignant B cells in two of three patients with B-cell chronic lymphocytic leukemia, implying greater potency.[4] As yet we do not know the best costimulatory endodomain(s) to use or whether the optimum choice will be affected by the nature of the target antigen and tumor to which the CAR is directed.

An alternative approach to the incorporation of costimulatory endodomains within the CAR is to express CARs in antigen-specific T cells, which will then also be activated and expanded through engagement of their native αβ-TCR by professional antigen-presenting cells, with attendant costimulation. As a proof of principle we engineered EBV–specific CTLs with a CAR specific for the disialoganglioside antigen GD2a expressed by neuroblastoma cells and infused these cells in EBV-positive patients with neuroblastoma. We found that engineered EBV-specific CTL had better in vivo persistence compared with polyclonally activated T cells engineered with the identical CAR and could be associated with tumor responses, including complete remissions in 3 of 11 patients.[3] Progression-free survival correlated with persistence of CAR T cells.

Engineering T Cells to Overcome Immune Evasion Strategies

One of the main challenges to effective adoptive T-cell therapy is the lack of in vivo expansion and maintenance of ex vivo–manipulated, adoptively transferred T cells because of various tumor-induced immune evasion mechanisms. Gene transfer technologies allow us to modify T cells and restore their functionality in a hostile environment. Table 101-1 and Fig. 101-1 summarize some of the evasion strategies and genetic T-cell modification to counter them that have been described to date. For example, many tumor cells or their associated stroma produce TGFβ, which favors the development of immune tolerance and T-cell anergy, inducing effector T cell growth arrest with induction of Treg cells. Zhang et al[28] demonstrated that transfection of a dominant negative form of TGFβRII (dnTGFβRII) improved the persistence of T cells and that infusion of modified cells eliminated tumor in a mouse prostate cancer model. Subsequently investigators showed that antigen-specific T cells expressing dnTGFβRII were resistant to the antiproliferative effects of TGFβ and retained their effector function in vivo, and such TGFβ-resistant T cells are currently being studied in patients with EBV-associated lymphomas.[29] T cells may also be modified to express cytokine or cytokine receptor genes that mimic the milieu found during lymphoid regeneration and restoration of homeostasis, such as IL-2, IL-7, or IL-15.[22] Although these approaches are effective in preclinical models, we do not know yet how safe or effective these transgenic cytokines and their receptors will be in clinical trials. Other genetic modifications can modulate T-cell survival and apoptosis or render antigen-specific T cells resistant to immunosuppressive drugs and may also enhance the persistence and effectiveness of T-cell therapies.

Table 101-1 Causes of Immunocompromise in Cancer Patients

IMMUNOSUPPRESSION INDUCED BY TUMOR
Antigen-specific $CD4^+/CD8^+$ T-cell tolerance
Defective proximal TCR signaling (decreased expressions of CD3δ chain, $p56^{lck}$, $p59^{fyn}$ tyrosine kinases)
Impairment of antigen-processing machinery (TAP, LMP2, LMP7) or downregulation of MHC molecules and costimulatory molecules
Activation of negative costimulatory signals (CTLA-4, PD-1, B7-H4, BTLA)
Tumor-derived immunosuppressive cytokines (TGFβ, IL-10, VEGF, PGE_2)
Expression of immunomodulatory or proapoptotic molecules by tumor (tryptophan-depleting enzyme IDO, galectin-1, FasL, TRAIL)
Recruitment and expansion of immunosuppressive cell populations (regulatory T cells, myeloid/plasmacytoid dendritic cells)
IMMUNOSUPPRESSION INDUCED BY THERAPY
Neutropenia, depletion and functional impairment of monocytes
Hypogammaglobulinemia (decreased levels of IgA and IgM)
Defective T cell–mediated immune response

BTLA, B- and T-lymphocyte attenuator; *IgA*, immunoglobulin A; *IgM*, immunoglobulin M; *LMP*, latent membrane protein; *MHC*, major histocompatibility complex; *PD-1*, programmed death-1; *PGE_2*, prostaglandin E_2; *TAP*, transporter associated with antigen processing; *TCR*, T-cell receptor; *TRAIL*, tumor necrosis factor–related apoptosis-inducing ligand; *VEGF*, vascular endothelial growth factor.

T Lymphocytes and Transfer of Safety Genes

A major problem of any successful cell therapy is that adverse events produced by the infused cells may persist and worsen if the cells survive and proliferate. A classic example is the GVHD that occurs when allogeneic donor T cells are transferred with the hemopoietic graft. It is also clear, however, that even nonalloreactive T cells may cause serious and even lethal toxicities, particularly if they are genetically modified to target highly expressed self-antigens present on both tumors and normal tissues. Similarly, efforts to enhance the survival and expansion of T cells may lead to uncontrolled expansion of the manipulated T cells, an event that may even occur as a result of retroviral genotoxicity alone. Although malignant transformation has so far been observed only in clinical studies of hemopoietic stem cells transduced by murine oncoretroviral vectors,[30] there is understandable concern that it can potentially occur after the transfer of gene-modified T cells. For all these reasons there has been increasing interest in the incorporation of safety switches or suicide genes in any T cell that is adoptively transferred to humans.

Safety or suicide genes have been best studied in the recipients of DLI in patients with hematologic malignancies relapsed after allogeneic HSC transplantation in order to prevent the occurrence of GVHD. Adequate doses of donor T cells can be safely given only if there is some means by which unwanted alloreactivity can be abrogated in vivo. Over the past 10 years efforts have been made to achieve this aim by genetically modifying T cells through the introduction of suicide genes, of which the herpes simplex thymidine kinase (HSVtk) is the most popular and advanced in term of clinical development, because it is currently in a Phase III clinical trial.[11] HSVtk phosphorylates specific nucleoside analogues, including ganciclovir, to nucleoside monophosphates. These compounds block effective DNA synthesis and kill dividing cells. In several clinical trials this gene has been transferred to donor T lymphocytes, which have then been given to the allogeneic stem cell transplant recipient to prevent or treat relapse.

The approach has had some success. HSVtk gene–modified T cells persist in the circulation in most of the patients and are removed after the administration of ganciclovir, often with an improvement in GVHD.[11] However, several problems remain. HSVtk is a viral protein, and in some patients a cell-mediated immune response against HSVtk is detected, causing undesired premature elimination of transgenic cells. Other drawbacks of HSVtk include the unintended elimination of gene-modified cells when ganciclovir is used for treatment of CMV reactivation, ganciclovir resistance that may occur from truncated HSVtk generated from cryptic-splice donor and acceptor sites, and slow elimination of transgenic cells because HSVtk requires DNA synthesis to be active; such delayed activity may be undesirable if T cells are acutely toxic.

Investigators attempted to overcome some of these limitations by developing new suicide genes based on human molecules that are potentially less immunogenic. T cells expressing human CD20 can be theoretically rapidly eliminated by the infusion of anti-CD20 monoclonal antibodies. Other suicide genes are based on chimeric molecules derived from human proteins that are involved in the apoptotic pathway and modified to be activated by a small molecule (inducible Fas and inducible caspase 9). These inducible molecules activate apoptosis, which produces rapid cell death.

A clinical study has used iCasp9, which consists of the sequence of the human FK506-binding protein (FKBP) with an F36V mutation, connected to human caspase 9 deleted for its endogenous activation and recruitment domain.[31] FKBP12-F36V binds with high affinity an otherwise bioinert small-molecule dimerizing agent (AP1903). In the presence of the drug, the iCasp9 promolecule dimerizes and activates the intrinsic apoptotic pathway leading to cell death. To ensure the suicide gene is expressed in all the infused cells, the construct incorporates a selectable marker gene (CD19). The study infused donor-derived iCasp9 T cells after haploidentical stem cell transplant and if patients developed GVHD, administered a single dose of the dimerizing drug. The investigators observed rapid destruction of more than 95% of the cells with prompt resolution of GVHD.[31]

FUTURE DIRECTIONS

With the approval of the first cell therapeutic for cancer (Dendreon), and the publication of increasing numbers of reports of complete tumor responses after cellular immunotherapy, there is increasing hope that this methodology will finally take its place among other more conventional cancer therapeutics. In addition, the combination of T-cell therapies with agents such as antibodies to T-cell check-point molecules (including CTLA-4[32] and anti-PD-1[33]) that block the immunosuppressive mechanisms of the tumor environment may further increase the clinical potency of T-cell therapies. Much remains to be done to ensure the effectiveness and safety of these cell therapies and to develop economic models to support their development to licensure, but we are confident that well within the next decade this approach will cease being almost entirely experimental and will be considered a significant component of standard cancer therapy.

REFERENCES

1. Rosenberg SA, Restifo NP, Yang JC, et al: Adoptive cell transfer: A clinical path to effective cancer immunotherapy. *Nat Rev Cancer* 8:308, 2008.
2. Bollard CM, Gottschalk S, Leen AM, et al: Complete responses of relapsed lymphoma following genetic modification of tumor-antigen presenting cells and T-lymphocyte transfer. *Blood* 110:2845, 2007.
3. Pule MA, Savoldo B, Myers GD, et al: Virus-specific T cells engineered to coexpress tumor-specific receptors: Persistence and antitumor activity in individuals with neuroblastoma. *Nat Med* 14:1270, 2008.
4. Kalos M, Levine BL, Porter DL, et al: T cells with chimeric antigen receptors have potent antitumor effects and can establish memory in patients with advanced leukemia. *Sci Transl Med* 3, 2011.
5. Cheever MA, Allison JP, Ferris AS, et al: The prioritization of cancer antigens: A national cancer institute pilot project for the acceleration of translational research. *Clin Cancer Res* 15:5337, 2009.
6. Zou W: Immunosuppressive networks in the tumour environment and their therapeutic relevance. *Nat Rev Cancer* 5:274, 2005.
7. June CH, Blazar BR, Riley JL: Engineering lymphocyte subsets: Tools, trials and tribulations. *Nat Rev Immunol* 9:716, 2009.
8. Kolb HJ, Mittermuller J, Clemm C, et al: Donor leukocyte transfusions for treatment of recurrent chronic myelogenous leukemia in marrow transplant patients. *Blood* 76:2465, 1990.
9. O'Reilly RJ, Doubrovina E, Trivedi D, et al: Adoptive transfer of antigen-specific T-cells of donor type for immunotherapy of viral infections following allogeneic hematopoietic cell transplants. *Immunol Res* 38:250, 2007.
10. Kolb HJ: Graft-versus-leukemia effects of transplantation and donor lymphocytes. *Blood* 112:4383, 2008.
11. Ciceri F, Bonini C, Stanghellini MT, et al: Infusion of suicide-gene-engineered donor lymphocytes after family haploidentical haemopoietic stem-cell transplantation for leukaemia (the TK007 trial): A non-randomised phase I-II study. *Lancet Oncol* 10:500, 2009.
12. Rapoport AP, Aqui NA, Stadtmauer EA, et al: Combination immunotherapy using adoptive T-cell transfer and tumor antigen vaccination on the basis of hTERT and survivin after ASCT for myeloma. *Blood* 117:797, 2011.
13. Walter EA, Greenberg PD, Gilbert MJ, et al: Reconstitution of cellular immunity against cytomegalovirus in recipients of allogeneic bone marrow by transfer of T-cell clones from the donor. *N Engl J Med* 333:1044, 1995.
14. Heslop HE, Slobod KS, Pule MA, et al: Long-term outcome of EBV-specific T-cell infusions to prevent or treat EBV-related lymphoproliferative disease in transplant recipients. *Blood* 115:935, 2010.
15. Leen AM, Myers GD, Sili U, et al: Monoculture-derived T lymphocytes specific for multiple viruses expand and produce clinically relevant effects in immunocompromised individuals. *Nat Med* 12:1166, 2006.
16. Rauser G, Einsele H, Sinzger C, et al: Rapid generation of combined CMV-specific $CD4^+$ and $CD8^+$ T-cell lines for adoptive transfer into recipients of allogeneic stem cell transplants. *Blood* 103:3572, 2004.

17. Haque T, Wilkie GM, Jones MM, et al: Allogeneic cytotoxic T-cell therapy for EBV-positive posttransplantation lymphoproliferative disease: Results of a phase 2 multicenter clinical trial. *Blood* 110:1131, 2007.
18. Straathof KC, Bollard CM, Popat U, et al: Treatment of nasopharyngeal carcinoma with Epstein-Barr virus–specific T lymphocytes. *Blood* 105:1904, 2005.
19. Warren EH, Fujii N, Akatsuka Y, et al: Therapy of relapsed leukemia after allogeneic hematopoietic cell transplantation with T cells specific for minor histocompatibility antigens. *Blood* 115:3878, 2010.
20. Morgan RA, Dudley ME, Wunderlich JR, et al: Cancer regression in patients after transfer of genetically engineered lymphocytes. *Science* 314:129, 2006.
21. Eshhar Z, Waks T, Gross G, et al: Specific activation and targeting of cytotoxic lymphocytes through chimeric single chains consisting of antibody-binding domains and the gamma or zeta subunits of the immunoglobulin and T-cell receptors. *Proc Natl Acad Sci USA* 90:724, 1993.
22. Vera JF, Brenner MK, Dotti G: Immunotherapy of human cancers using gene modified T lymphocytes. *Curr Gene Ther* 9:408, 2009.
23. Rosenberg SA, Aebersold P, Cornetta K, et al: Gene transfer into humans—immunotherapy of patients with advanced melanoma, using tumor-infiltrating lymphocytes modified by retroviral gene transduction. *N Engl J Med* 323:578, 1990.
24. Parkhurst MR, Yang JC, Langan RC, et al: T cells targeting carcinoembryonic antigen can mediate regression of metastatic colorectal cancer but induce severe transient colitis. *Mol Ther* 19:626, 2011.
25. Jena B, Dotti G, Cooper LJ: Redirecting T-cell specificity by introducing a tumor-specific chimeric antigen receptor. *Blood* 116:1044, 2010.
26. Sadelain M, Brentjens R, Riviere I: The promise and potential pitfalls of chimeric antigen receptors. *Curr Opin Immunol* 21:223, 2009.
27. Savoldo B, Ramos CA, Liu E, et al: CD28 costimulation improves expansion and persistence of chimeric antigen receptor-modified T cells in lymphoma patients. *J Clin Invest* 121:1826, 2011.
28. Zhang Q, Yang X, Pins M, et al: Adoptive transfer of tumor-reactive transforming growth factor-beta-insensitive CD8+ T cells: eradication of autologous mouse prostate cancer. *Cancer Res* 65:1761, 2005.
29. Bollard CM, Rossig C, Calonge MJ, et al: Adapting a transforming growth factor beta-related tumor protection strategy to enhance antitumor immunity. *Blood* 99:3187, 2002.
30. Hacein-Bey-Abina S, Von Kalle C, Schmidt M, et al: LMO2-associated clonal T cell proliferation in two patients after gene therapy for SCID-X1. *Science* 302:419, 2003.
31. Di Stasi A, Tey SK, Dotti G, et al: Inducible apoptosis as a safety switch for adoptive cell therapy. *N Engl J Med* 365, 2011.
32. Hodi FS, O'Day SJ, McDermott DF, et al: Improved survival with ipilimumab in patients with metastatic melanoma. *N Engl J Med* 363:711, 2010.
33. Topalian SL, Hodi FS, Brahmer JR, et al: Safety, Activity, and Immune Correlates of Anti-PD-1 Antibody in Cancer. *N Engl J Med* 366:2443, 2012.

CHAPTER 102

NATURAL KILLER CELL-BASED THERAPIES

Sarah Cooley, Michael R. Verneris, and Jeffrey S. Miller

The antileukemia effect of allogeneic hematopoietic cell transplantation (allo-HCT) is mediated through both high-dose chemotherapy and immune reactions. Reduced intensity regimens still provide significant protection from relapse, supporting the notion that allogeneic immune effectors can control or eradicate leukemia (or both). Exactly which cell populations account for this graft-versus-leukemia (GVL) effect is not entirely established and may vary among individuals and diseases. Immune cell populations can be mechanistically divided into two broad categories, the innate (natural killer [NK] cells and antigen-presenting cells [APCs]) and adaptive (T cell and B cells) arms of the immune system. Whereas developmentally mature innate immune cells are able to perform their biologic functions, adaptive immune cells generally require antigen presentation, activation, and expansion before they can act. These paradigms are changing. It is becoming increasingly clear that NK cells are capable of memory responses, a function previously ascribed only to the adaptive immune system. Likewise, it appears that adaptive cells can mediate major histocompatibility complex (MHC) unrestricted killing, typically considered a quality of the innate system. Importantly, for optimal function, cells from both arms of the immune system work in concert with other immune cells. Because the antitumor efficacy of conventional cytotoxic agents is limited by off target toxicity and resistance, cell-based therapies provide an attractive alternative. Progress in cytokine biology and improved techniques to separate, expand, and purify cells have transformed the concept of cell-based therapy into a reality. This chapter examines characteristics of innate NK cells and discusses how they may be manipulated to combat infection and treat malignancy, both in transplant and nontransplant settings.

NATURAL KILLER CELL BIOLOGY

Natural killer cells were first functionally recognized in 1975 for their ability to lyse virally infected and tumor targets without prior sensitization. NK cells comprise 10% to 15% of the peripheral blood (PB) lymphocyte pool in normal humans, but they are also found in the bone marrow (BM), spleen, liver, lymph nodes, lungs, and pregnant uterus (Fig. 102-1). Defined phenotypically by the expression of CD56 or NKp46 and a lack of a CD3/T-cell receptor complex, they develop from BM-derived progenitors via distinct developmental stages in secondary lymphoid tissue (SLT)[1] (see Chapter 20). Mature NK cells can be functionally distinguished by CD56 density. The CD56^{dim} subset exhibits potent natural cytotoxicity (killing of class I negative targets) and displays Fc receptors (CD16) that trigger potent activating signals after recognition of immunoglobulin-coated targets, a process called *antibody-dependent cellular cytotoxicity* (ADCC). CD56^{dim} cells also produce cytokines in response to targets or activating receptor ligation. In contrast, CD56^{bright} NK cells are more proliferative and are less cytotoxic. CD56^{bright} cells respond to inflammatory cytokines (interleukin-2 [IL-12], IL-15, and IL-18) to rapidly produce large amounts of interferon-γ (IFN-γ). NK cells also proliferate and become activated in response to IL-2, IL-15, and IL-21. IL-15 is of particular importance for NK cell homeostasis. Transpresentation of IL-15 by IL-15Rα on dendritic cells (DCs) appears to be the physiologic source of cytokine leading to NK activation.[2] Although these cytokines enhance CD56 receptor density on activated cells, they should not be confused with the unique functional properties of steady-state CD56^{bright} cells.

Natural Killer Cell Functions

Natural killer cells provide a link between the innate and adaptive immune systems[3] and play an important role in immune surveillance, pregnancy outcomes, and response to infections (see Fig. 102-1). NK cell function can be divided into seven separate activities that include interaction with autologous DCs, activation, expansion, homing to malignant or virally infected targets, direct cell–cell killing, cytokine production, and eradication of allogeneic DCs. These responses may differ based on the stimulus and the NK cell subset studied. Activated NK cells produce (and often respond to) cytokine and chemokines, including IFN-γ, tumor necrosis factor (TNF), and transforming growth factor β (TGF-β). NK cells express β2 integrins such as LFA-1 and CD2, which bind to molecules such as intercellular adhesion molecule 1 (ICAM-1) and LFA-3. Engagement of other NK activating receptors induces target cell apoptosis via Fas ligand (FasL) and TNF-related apoptosis inducing ligand (TRAIL) pathways or by releasing perforin and granzyme into a small area between the NK cell and the target cells (called the *immune synapse*). These activated NK cells then produce cytokines. It is not completely known whether cytokine production or direct cell killing is physiologically most important for a therapeutic antitumor and antiinfection response. It may be that both functions are required for efficacy.

Natural Killer Cell Receptors

The ability of NK cells to respond to a wide array of targets is regulated by a complex network of surface proteins that comprise the NK receptors (NKRs). These receptors can mediate either activating or inhibitory signals. A recurring theme is that many of these receptors are MHC class I specific. Engagement of MHC class I results in a *reduction* in NK cell function. Thus, recognition of MHC class I, which is ubiquitously expressed by healthy tissues, leads to NK cell tolerance. In contrast, the loss of MHC class I, which occurs during the process of viral infection and malignant transformation, leads to the *lack* of engagement of these inhibitory receptors and in turn permits activation of the NK cell via other receptor–ligand interactions.

Killer Immunoglobulin-like Receptors

The killer immunoglobulin-like receptor (KIR) gene cluster, located on chromosome 19q13.4, encodes for 16 different type I transmembrane molecules in the immunoglobulin (Ig) superfamily. KIR genes contain either two or three extracellular domains (2D or 3D), a transmembrane region and an intracellular domain that is either long (containing inhibitory motifs) or short (containing docking sites for activating molecules). Individuals vary in the number of KIR genes that they have in their genome, and their "KIR content" can be

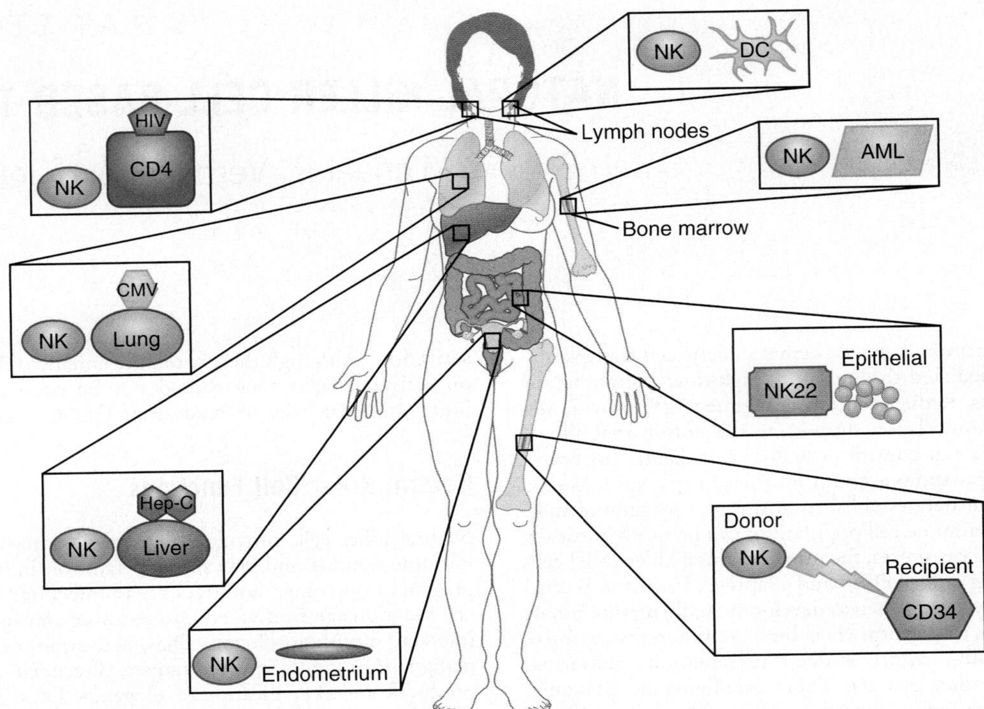

Figure 102-1 ROLES OF NATURAL KILLER (NK) CELLS IN CANCER AND HEALTH. The roles of NK cells in both health and cancer are depicted. NK cells play a critical role in initiation of immune responses by interacting with dendritic cells (DCs), resulting in reciprocal activation of both cell types (i.e., NK cells activate DCs and vice versa). NK-induced DC activation likely also results in the initiation of adaptive immune responses by inducing DCs to present antigens to T cells. Activated NK cells can go on to destroy malignant tissues, including leukemia. In the setting of allogeneic transplantation, NK cells can eradicate recipient stem cells, thereby facilitating allogeneic stem cell engraftment. Emerging data show that a subpopulation of NK cells or similar cells (known as NK22 cells, innate immune effector cells, or lymphoid tissue inducer cells) produce interleukin-22 (IL-22) and interact with lymph node stroma to mediate mucosal immunity and may accelerate immune responses after transplantation. A unique population of uterine NK cells is responsible for the maintenance of pregnancy. Still other roles for NK cells include the surveillance for and response to infectious organisms, including hepatitis virus C, cytomegalovirus (CMV) and human immunodeficiency virus (HIV). *AML,* Acute myeloid leukemia.

simplified into two haplotypes. Each haplotype contains three framework genes (*KIR3DL3, KIR2DL4,* and *KIR3DL2*) and a variable number of activating and inhibitory genes from the centromeric (Cen) or telomeric (Tel) ends of the gene locus. KIR A haplotypes contain five inhibitory receptors (2DL1, 2DL3, 3DL1, 3DL2, and 3DL3) and just one activating receptor (2DS4). KIR B haplotypes contain a variable number of genes but have more activating KIR than A haplotypes.

Inhibitory KIRs bind to self-class I HLA molecules on potential target cells. This interaction suppresses the NK cell effector responses. Inhibitory KIRs recognize polymorphisms of HLA-C and B in a biallelic manner (i.e., C1 vs. C2 and Bw4 vs. Bw6). KIR2DL1, KIR2DL2/KIR2DL3, and KIR3DL1 bind HLA class I C2, C1, and Bw4 alleles, respectively. New data demonstrate the complexity of these inhibitory receptor–ligand interactions because the mere expression of the receptors does not predict the cellular response. The affinity of a given KIR seems to depend on allelic polymorphisms of the individual KIR itself, as well as polymorphisms of the MHC class I protein to which it binds. In some cases, these binding rules are not absolute because KIR2DL2 can bind both HLA-C1 and C2 alleles. Although KIR binding to HLA-A is controversial, some HLA-A alleles (A3 and A11) contain the Bw4 epitope, and some HLA-A alleles in the context of peptide can bind KIR3DL2. Complicating our understanding of the KIR system is the fact that the natural ligands for activating KIR remain unknown. Although some bind MHC molecules at low affinity, it is not known whether MHC functions as the natural ligands in vivo.[4]

Additional Natural Killer Cell Receptors

Several other families of activating and inhibitory receptors influence NK cell function. Some of these bind HLA molecules. The NKG2 family of C-type lectin receptors that heterodimerize with CD94 may be either inhibitory (NKG2A) or activating (NKG2C) and can recognize nonclassical HLA-E. NKG2D does not heterodimerize with CD94 and recognizes stress-induced molecules such as MHC class I polypeptide-related sequence A/B (MICA and MICB) or viral-derived proteins such as the cytomegalovirus (CMV)-related UL binding proteins (ULBP1-6).[5] Additional receptors include the natural cytotoxicity receptors (NCR) NKp30, NKp46 and NKp44, DNAM-1, and Nectin-2 (CD122), 2B4, Ig-like (ILT) receptors, and leukocyte-associated immunoglobulin-like receptor-1 (LAIR-1).[6] These activating receptors are believed to play a role in communication between NK cells and DCs as well as determining whether an NK cell can recognize a target.

Natural Killer Cell Education—The Acquisition of Function, Self-Tolerance and Alloreactivity

A mechanistic explanation for the phenomenon of "hybrid resistance" and "missing self" is derived from the characterization of NK cell inhibitory receptors that recognize self MHC class I.[9,10] In both instances, because they fail to engage inhibitory receptors, target cells lacking self MHC class I expression are sensitive to NK-mediated killing. Thus, NK cells detect either allogeneic cells or disease-associated loss of MHC class I on virally infected or tumor cells.[11] The process by which signals mediated through inhibitory receptors allow NK cells to acquire cytotoxic and cytokine producing functions has been referred to as *NK cell education* or *NK licensing*.[12,13] It has been demonstrated that NK cells lacking both KIR and NKG2A are hyporesponsive and that they cannot become educated until inhibitory receptors are expressed. Importantly, NK cell education may not be fixed. For instance, adoptive transfer of NK cells from β2-microglobulin knock-out mice (that lack MHC class I) into wild-type mice leads to education and an associated gain of function. Conversely, adoptive transfer of fully functional NK cells from wild-type mice into β2-microglobulin knock-out hosts leads to NK hyporesponsiveness.[14,15] Collectively, these data support the model of NK cell education as a dynamic, inherently plastic process in which low-level, tonic interactions may be needed to maintain cytotoxic capacity. It has also been demonstrated that the cumulative strength of inhibitory receptor signaling correlates with functional thresholds. This model, aptly compared with a "rheostat," permits self-tolerance in the normal state and allows for enhanced sensitivity to damage to healthy cells through class I downregulation.[16] Importantly, it must be emphasized that not all acquisition of NK cell function is through NK cell education. NK cells can overcome rules of NK cell education when stimulated by exogenous cytokines or cytokines induced by inflammation. In mice, the importance of inflammation-induced cytokine production leading to enhanced NK function is clearly demonstrated by the ability of NK cells from β2-microglobulin knock-out mice, which are hyporesponsive in vitro to clear murine CMV. In summary, NK education determines the function of NK cells at steady state, but other factors may overcome or even dominate, especially in the setting of disease or when cytokine-stimulated NK cells are adoptively transferred.

Natural Killer Cell Recognition of Tumors

Although the antitumor efficacy of NK cells has been most evident for myeloid malignancies, a wide variety of solid tumors, including breast, ovarian, hepatocellular, colon, neuroblastoma, Ewing sarcoma, rhabdomyosarcoma, and melanoma, are also sensitive to NK cell lysis. The relative resistance of some tumors may be attributable to a higher expression of class I HLA, which inversely correlates with the susceptibility of primary pre-B cell acute lymphoblastic leukemia (ALL) blasts to NK cell lysis.[17] Successful destruction of a target requires co-engagement of NK cell receptors by both inhibitory and activating signals. Accordingly, activating receptors such as NKG2D play an important role in immune surveillance and killing of acute myeloid leukemia (AML) stem cells. Other tumor ligands that correlate with responsiveness to NK cell–mediated killing include DNAM-1 on MDS blasts; CD137 ligand on AML targets; and B7-H3, which protects neuroblastoma from NK lysis. When considering therapeutic uses of NK cells and interventions such as the use of anti-KIR antibodies to promote tumor lysis, it is important to remember that approximately half of NK cells circulating in the PB lack KIR. Therefore, maximum killing of targets such as leukemia blasts may require blockade of other inhibitory receptor interactions, such as NKG2A and LIR-1.

Interleukin-22–Producing Tissue Resident Natural Killer Cells

Mature NK cells arise from progenitors that progress through an orderly series of developmental intermediates, defined as stages I through V on the basis of phenotype and function. Very early human NK cell differentiation occurs in the BM, but shortly thereafter, progenitors migrate to SLTs, where they become stage IV NK cells ($CD56^{bright}$ cells). Through a process not yet defined, stage IV NK cells are then exported from SLTs into the PB, where they terminally differentiate into stage V ($CD56^{dim}$) NK cells. Stage III NK cells represent a small progenitor population that makes up about 0.1% to 0.5% of the mononuclear cells in SLTs. Recent studies show that some stage III cells have the unique ability to produce IL-22 and interact with lymph node stroma.[18] These cells have been given many names, including NK22 cells, lymphoid tissue inducer-like cells, and innate lymphoid cells. IL-22 production by these cells occurs in response to inflammatory cytokines, such as IL-1 and IL-23 and bacterial products. IL-22 acts on epithelial cells, causing them to proliferate and elaborate antibacterial proteins, thereby supporting their role in mucosal immunity. These IL-22–producing NK cells also may play a critical role in lymph node repair after viral infection or chemotherapy-induced injury. They also express high amounts of OX40 ligand important in T-cell memory responses. At present, it is not clear whether they are truly NK progenitors or a separate lineage of terminally differentiated innate lymphoid cells. Either way, discovery of these cells has advanced our understanding of SLT biology, and these cells hold promise for improving SLT repair and immune function after allogeneic HCT.

CLINICAL APPLICATIONS OF NATURAL KILLER CELLS

Determination of Donor Natural Killer Cell Alloreactivity

It is widely accepted that the ability of NK cells to contribute to protection from relapse and infection requires that they be functionally competent and present in sufficient numbers. As already described, NK cells are alloreactive against targets that lack self-HLA ligands for the inhibitory receptors that contributed to their education or licensing. Fortunately, the NK cell repertoire is diverse, allowing NK cell education to occur through multiple receptors. Several models have been developed to predict NK cell alloreactivity. KIR–ligand mismatch or incompatibility, as defined by the Perugia group, predicts that donor-derived NK cells will be alloreactive in the GvH direction when recipients lack C2, C1, or Bw4 alleles that are present in the donor. To predict alloreactivity, the receptor–ligand model also requires knowledge of the expression of a particular inhibitory KIR in the donor. Alternatively, in the KIR–ligand absence model, alloreactive potential is based entirely on the number of KIR ligands a recipient lacks. Because KIR genes have multiple alleles with variable levels of expression and functional activity, alloreactivity may be best determined by evaluating the donor KIR genotype with functional assessments of their KIR phenotype.

The Role of Natural Killer Cells in Hematopoietic Cell Transplantation

After HCT, NK cells are the first lymphocyte population to reconstitute. Engrafted alloreactive NK cells may mediate (1) decreased rates of GVHD by targeting of host APC, (2) improved engraftment by secretion of cytokines and elimination of host immune barriers, (3) decreased rates of relapse, and (4) decreased infectious complications. A seminal report published by the Perugia group demonstrated a beneficial effect of alloreactive NK cells and showed that KIR-ligand mismatched NK cells play a key role in achieving durable remission after T-cell deplete haploidentical transplantation for AML but not ALL. KIR–ligand mismatched donors were associated with improved engraftment and decreased relapse and decreased GVHD.[19] However, in a long-term follow-up of 112 patients, only decreased relapse in patients transplanted while in complete remission and improved disease-free survival were maintained. Subsequent analyses of the role of KIR–ligand mismatching and KIR–ligand absence in different settings have produced mixed results. In umbilical cord blood (UCB) transplantation, the effect of KIR–ligand mismatching on outcomes appears to depend on either the intensity of the preparative regimen or the drugs used (i.e., ATG or not).[20,21] In a 2009 study of 169 children treated with autologous HCT for neuroblastoma, KIR ligand absence was strongly associated with improved survival and decreased risk of disease progression.[22] Inconsistent effects of KIR–ligand mismatch and KIR–ligand absence strategies are likely attributable to differences in the stem cell source, conditioning, degree of T-cell depletion, and post-HCT immunosuppression used, all of which can affect NK cell development, education, and function. Despite this confusion, NK cell effects continue to emerge, implicating them as key effectors reconstituting after transplant capable of protecting against relapse in myeloid malignancies. Similar promise has been demonstrated in pediatric, but not adult, ALL, suggesting that unique interactions between NK cells and targets might account for these differences.

Natural Killer Cell Function After Hematopoietic Cell Transplantation

Despite their high numbers early after transplantation, it is unknown whether these NK cells were fully functional. This question has been explored by several investigators.[23,24] Recently, Foley et al[25] studied simultaneous NK cell functions. They demonstrated that degranulation stimulated by class I negative targets recovered early after transplant, suggesting that NK cells could be educated through either NKG2A or KIR. NK cells from double umbilical cord grafts exhibited CD107a hyperfunction compared with adult unrelated donors (URDs), which may explain the enhanced relapse protection seen in this setting. In marked contrast, IFN-γ production was severely diminished for at least 6 months after HCT, especially in settings of T cell–depleted grafts (even without posttransplant immune suppression) or grafts containing naïve T cells (UCB), suggesting that NK cells require T cells for optimal education. This defect could be rapidly reversed by short-term exposure to IL-15. In addition, and in contrast to CD107a degranulation, IFN-γ production could only be educated through self-KIR (NK cells expressing KIR that encounter their cognate ligand [MHC class I] in the recipient), suggesting a hierarchy of thresholds for different NK effector functions. Last, different conditioning regimens may have varied effects on the tempo of NK and T-cell reconstitution after transplantation and may therefore affect function and impact on clinical outcomes.

Donor Selection Based on Killer Immunoglobulin-like Receptor Genotype

Another approach to capitalize on the beneficial effects of NK cells after HCT is to consider the full KIR genotype of the donors. In a study of 448 patients undergoing myeloablative HLA matched or mismatched URD HCT for AML, the 3-year overall survival was significantly higher after transplantation from a KIR B/x genotype donor (containing at least one B haplotype), irrespective of recipient KIR genotype, with a 30% improvement in relative risk of relapse-free survival.[26] A subsequent analysis of 1409 URD transplant recipients confirmed these findings and refined the beneficial effect of KIR B genes to AML patients. Similar effects were not seen in ALL. Additionally, this later study showed that the most benefit from donor KIR B genotype was localized to genes present in the centromeric part of the KIR locus. The greatest protection from relapse and best disease-free survival, in both HLA-matched and -mismatched transplants, was associated with donors homozygous for this region. Donors could be stratified by KIR into those with best (Cen-B homozygous present in 11% of the population), better (≥2 B defining domains as seen in 20% of the population), or neutral donor KIR genotypes. A publically available calculator to determine this stratification is available online (http://www.ebi.ac.uk/ipd/kir/donor_b_content.html). KIR genotyping as few as three of the best HLA-matched donor candidates should substantially increase the frequency of URD transplants from donors with favorable KIR gene content (from 31% to 79%) in AML.[27] A prospective trial designed to select donors for relapse protection is underway. The benefit of donor KIR B/x has been verified in other studies. The B-haplotype KIR genes 2DL5A, 2DS1, and 3DS1 were associated with an AML-specific fourfold reduction in relapse in a study of 246 T-cell depleted HLA-matched sibling transplants, and KIR B haplotypes were associated with improved survival and reduced TRM in association with less CMV reactivation in otherwise similar patients. A 2010 study of 86 nonmyeloablative, T-cell replete HLA haploidentical HSCTs found a protective effect on relapse, TRM, DFS, and OS when there were mismatches of inhibitory KIR genes between the donor and recipient or when KIR A/A recipients received grafts from donors with at least one KIR B haplotype.[9] In addition to HLA matching, donor selection for KIR genes is a promising strategy to improve outcome after HCT. As recently shown, the benefits of NK cells can be realized in the HLA-matched setting and even in the autologous setting.[10]

Manipulation of Natural Killer Cell Alloreactivity

Another attractive strategy to enhance NK cell alloreactivity is to manipulate the KIR repertoire itself. Therefore, it is of great interest to understand how individual NK cells acquire KIR as they differentiate from stem cells. In general, the stochastic expression of KIR follows the product rule, meaning that the probability of the coexpression of two or more different KIRs equals the product of the individual expression frequencies for those KIRs. The expression frequencies of individual KIRs are independent of MHC class I and are instead established and maintained by a dynamic, yet ill-defined, transcriptional program. Although KIR promoter methylation clearly controls gene expression, other mechanisms are also involved. The Anderson laboratory has identified a number of noncoding RNAs subsequently found to be important in KIR transcriptional regulation.[28] Understanding the molecular mechanisms that underlie KIR expression may help guide the design of novel NK cell strategies with specific KIR repertoires tailored to enhance NK cell efficacy.

Control of Viral Infection

Current studies also support the concept that NK cells play an important role in controlling infections, including those which result in significant morbidity after allogeneic HCT. Interestingly, many observations concerning the development of self-tolerance by NK cells in the context of tumor recognition do not seem to apply in the setting of viral infection. This is likely attributable to a decrease in MHC and an increase in stress-induced ligands on the infected cells, which are recognized by NK cell–activating receptors.[29,30] Some NK cell–activating receptors (NKp44 and NKp46) bind directly to viral epitopes (hemagglutinin), suggesting that they are involved in the control of infections. Likewise, the KIR genotype of donor NK cells appears to also play an important role in control of infections. For example, in a study of donor and recipient CMV seropositive sibling transplants, a 65% reduction in CMV reactivation was observed with donors who had more than one activating KIR gene.[31] Other receptors are also involved in recognition of infectious organisms, including NKG2C. In the solid organ transplant setting, CMV reactivation resulted in an increase in a population of NKG2C$^+$ NK cells.[32] This was not observed in CMV seronegative recipients. The NKG2C$^+$ population was also found to expand in victims of a recent hantavirus outbreak in Sweden, suggesting that specific NK cell subsets are involved in the response to viral infection. Another study of the effect of donor KIR genotype on infections after URD HCT suggests a protective benefit against bacterial infections with donors with the more activating B/x genotype. Interest is growing rapidly in the investigation of the role of NK cells on infection complications.

Adoptive Transfer of Natural Killer Cells

Although methods to exploit the beneficial effects of NK cells engrafting after allo-HCT are increasing, it should be recognized that NK cells are also well suited for adoptive cellular therapies. Many groups tested methods to induce autologous NK cell activity, such as treatment with prolonged, low-dose subcutaneously IL-2, higher dose IV IL-2, and infusions of ex vivo IL-2 activated NK cells. Although these approaches induced in vivo NK cell expansion and function, they were shown by several investigational teams to have only limited clinical efficacy. Therefore, the Minnesota Group pioneered the use of haploidentical NK cell infusions. This approach was based on the likelihood that haploidentical NK cells, educated in the donor, would be mediate stronger GVL reactions because they are not exposed to immunosuppressive mechanisms seen in cancer patients. It was further hypothesized that this would result in a higher frequency of alloreactive NK cells (NK cells with inhibitory receptors functionally educated through a different inhibitory receptor that will not be inhibited by class I expressed by the tumor). The safety and success of NK cell infusions was established in a trial using haplotype mismatched, related-donor NK cell products followed by subcutaneous IL-2 to induce in vivo NK survival and expansion.[33] Successful expansion was achieved only after a lymphodepleting regimen of high-dose cyclophosphamide and fludarabine. Interestingly, complete remissions in AML correlated with in vivo NK expansion and higher proportions of circulating (and functional) NK cells. The importance of the high-dose chemotherapy regimen delivered before NK cell transfer cannot be overstated. Chemotherapy not only creates space for the NK cells to expand but also results in a surge of endogenous IL-15 and IL-7 and transiently prevents recipient T cells from rejecting the allogeneic NK cells. Importantly, the NK cells that expand in vivo in this platform exhibit hyperfunction, either because of the cytokine milieu induced by the lymphodepleting therapy or by the exogenously administered IL-2. This platform allows in vivo expanded NK cells to partially overcome the rules of NK cell education and tolerance, potentially obviating the need to select specific alloreactive NK cell donors. This assumption requires formal clinical testing. Other modifications are currently being explored to improve in vivo expansion or persistence, including the elimination of regulatory T cells that may impair NK function. Adoptive transfer of haploidentical NK cells has been tested in other settings. In a pediatric cohort, recovery of functional donor-derived $CD56^{+}/CD16^{+}$ NK cells that lysed K562 targets mediated strong ADCC activity against neuroblastoma and leukemic blasts by ay +14 after the infusion. The use of NK cell–based therapies to target minimal residual disease is being tested. This preemptive approach is being tested by use of NK cell donor lymphocyte infusions after haploidentical HCT to in adults with AML.[34] A recently published study in pediatric patients used NK cells as consolidation therapy to maintain remissions in a nontransplant setting. This platform is being adapted for testing in elderly AML patients. Additional studies to explore applications in multiple myeloma, lymphoma, and solid tumors are being developed.

FUTURE DIRECTIONS

Several promising strategies to exploit NK cell alloreactivity to treat cancer are in development. These include various approaches to develop in vivo or ex vivo expanded products, manipulations of the host immune system, and strategies to modify the tumor targets to enhance their sensitivity to NK cell–mediated killing (Fig. 102-2). Unlike T cells, haplotype mismatched NK cells can be given without risk of graft-versus-host disease (GVHD). However, adoptive transfer is limited by the cell dose attained from leukopheresis and the current requirement for high-dose lymphodepleting chemotherapy. In vivo expansion, although detectable, is minimal, transient, and appears to require the use of exogenous cytokines such as IL-2, which is associated with significant side effects. The use of IL-15, which is the true homeostatic factor for NK cells, is now being tested in patients receiving adoptively transferred NK cells to treat their acute myeloid leukemia. A major advantage to IL-15 is that unlike IL-2, it does not stimulate regulatory T cells. If it proves safe, the use of IL-15 to stimulate NK cells may overcome the need for high-dose lymphodepleting chemotherapy. Platforms that use IL-2 will likely need to be combined with strategies to deplete host regulatory T cells. Various methods to enrich the NK cell fraction in haploidentical apheresis products are being tested, including depletion of T (CD3) and B (CD19) cells or positive selection for $CD56^{+}$ NK cells. Several investigators are also exploring ex vivo NK expansion using Epstein-Barr virus transformed or modified K562 feeder cells to increase the infused NK cell dose, potentially circumventing the need for in vivo expansion. The use of "off-the-shelf" NK cell lines, such as NK92 and KHYG-1, may provide a large supply of highly cytotoxic NK cells that could be used for repeated infusions. Other approaches using NK cell products derived from UCB stem cells, embryonic stem cells, or induced pluripotent stem cell sources are also being developed. UCB stem cell derived NK cells that produce IL-22 may enhance tissue integrity and improve immune reconstitution after HCT. Alternative forms of activation, such as combining NK cells with either Toll-like receptor agonists or DC vaccines, are also being explored. Other strategies include sensitizing the target cells using chemotherapy (bortezomib or histone deacetylase inhibitors) or, in the case of solid tumors, irradiation. Last, if cytokines such as IL-15 can safely and efficiently expand autologous NK cells in vivo, it may be possible to mimic an allogeneic approach by using antibodies that block inhibitory receptors. Anti-KIR and anti-NKG2A reagents are currently under development and may functionally convert tolerant autologous NK cells into alloreactive antitumor effectors.[35,36]

FUTURE DIRECTIONS

The therapeutic use of NK cells is a promising strategy in both transplant and nontransplant settings. NK cells have the potential to induce graft-versus-tumor effects without the devastating side effects of GVHD. To date, the majority of evidence supporting NK cells as antileukemia effectors has emerged from the allo-HCT literature. However, the complexities of allo-HCT, including variations in preparative regimens, stem cell sources, graft products, and posttransplant immune suppression, as well as disease specific differences, all contribute to the challenge of understanding mechanistic actions of these cells and to designing effective therapies that exploit NK cell alloreactivity. Investigators developing adoptive NK cell strategies are working to establish proof of concept and to develop exportable techniques. Platforms that support robust in vivo or ex vivo NK cell expansion and education, selecting NK donors based on their NK cell receptor genes, manipulation of tumor NK receptor ligand expression, and coordinating interactions with other immune cells are underway at many institutions. Ultimately, combination therapy using several strategies will likely prove most successful. In particular, agents including IL-15 and antibodies to block inhibitory receptors hold great promise.

NK PRODUCT

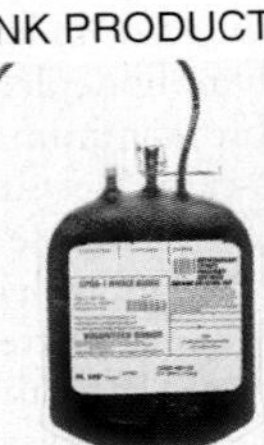

HOST

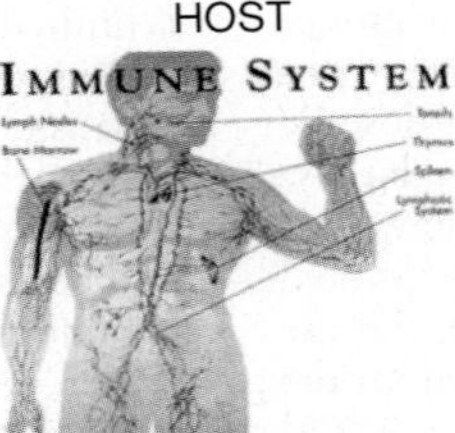

TARGET

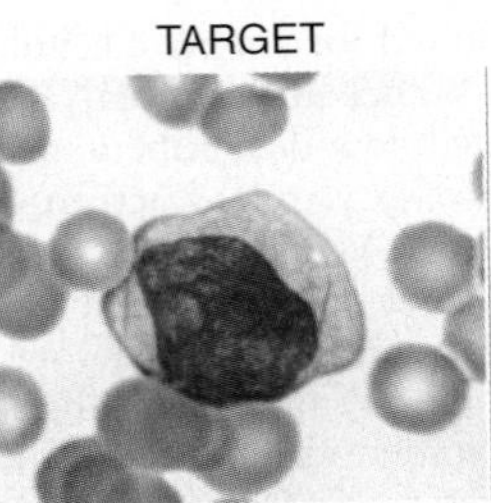

Adult NK cells
Autologous
Allogeneic/haploidentical
UCB/ES/iPS stem cells
Cell lines (NK92 and KHYG-1)

Processing
$CD3^-$ alone
$CD3^-/CD56^+$
$CD3^-/CD19^-$

Ex vivo activation
None
IL-2 or IL-15
Tumor lysates
Lymphoid or K562 feeders

Lympho/myelo depletion
Cytokine sinks
Expansion space

T regulatory cell depletion
Fludarabine/cytoxan
TBI
Cyclosporine
Steroids
Denileukin Diftitox
(anti-CD25)

DC activation
TLR agonists
DC vaccines

Tumor/transformed cells
Infected cells
↑ Activating ligands
↓ Inhibitory ligands

TBI/radiation
Chemotherapy
Bortezomib, HDAC-1
inhibitors
Antibody targeting
(ADCC)

In vivo manipulation
IL-12/IL-15 cytokines
anti-KIR, anti-NKG2A
antibodies

Figure 102-2 MANIPULATIONS TO INCREASE THE EFFECTIVENESS OF ADOPTIVE NATURAL KILLER (NK) CELL THERAPIES. Current approaches to improve the effectiveness of adoptive transfer of NK cells involve a balance between factors from the NK cell product, the host, and the tumor target. The NK cell product can be derived from adult blood and can be autologous (although there is greater concern for "self" major histocompatibility complex inhibition through inhibitory receptors), allogeneic, derived from primitive progenitors, or from NK cell lines; all of which may be more amenable to gene therapy. The optimal product may be the one that gives rise to longer in vivo persistence and survival, which needs formal testing. Use of donor NK cells infused across allogeneic barriers is complicated and clinical trials have been published using each of these manipulations. At a minimum, a T cell–depleted product is needed to prevent graft-versus-host disease. Contaminating B cells have also been shown to contribute to complications such as Epstein-Barr virus–induced lymphoproliferative disease and autoimmune hemolytic anemia as part of a passenger lymphocyte syndrome. It is still unclear whether NK cell products should be administered without activation (fresh or frozen), with interleukin-2 (IL-2) or IL-15 (early in clinical development), or using activation through other mechanisms (tumor cell lysates). Several investigators are exploring ex vivo expansion, a process that requires lymphoblastoid cell line or membrane-bound IL-15 and 41BB-ligand transduced K562 feeders. The success of adoptive transfer is also dependent on host factors that determine whether the recipient is permissive to adoptive transfer. NK cell proliferation depends on lymphodepletion allowing for transient removal of cytokines sinks to free up cytokines such as endogenous IL-15 as well as added myelodepletion that provides space for adoptively transferred cells. Immune barriers to adoptive transfer include an increase in regulatory T cells, especially when IL-2 is administered to the patient, and methods to blunt this inhibitory response may be effective if they do not dampen NK cell function. As NK cells and dendritic cells (DCs) coactivate each other, use of DC vaccines or Toll-like receptor 7 (TLR-7) or TLR-9 agonists that work through DC may be synergistic. Last, a number of manipulations involve the target itself to enhance sensitivity to NK cell adoptive transfer. These manipulations are intended to promote interactions between NK cells and their targets based on known biology to enhance activation interactions, decrease inhibition, or prolong NK cell survival. It is anticipated that a combination of these variables will ultimately be needed for clinical efficacy, and these strategies may need to be tailored to different tumor types. *ADCC,* Antibody-dependent cell-mediated cytotoxicity; *ES,* embryonic stem cells; *HDAC-1,* histone deacetylase 1, *iPS,* induced pluripotent stem cells; *TBI,* total-body irradiation; *UCB,* umbilical cord blood.

REFERENCES

1. Freud AG, Yokohama A, Becknell B, et al: Evidence for discrete stages of human natural killer cell differentiation in vivo. *J Exp Med* 203:1033, 2006.
2. Huntington ND, Legrand N, Alves NL, et al: IL-15 trans-presentation promotes human NK cell development and differentiation in vivo. *J Exp Med* 206:25, 2009.
3. Walzer T, Dalod M, Robbins SH, et al: Natural-killer cells and dendritic cells: "l'union fait la force". *Blood* 106:2252, 2005.
4. Moesta AK, Norman PJ, Yawata M, et al: Synergistic polymorphism at two positions distal to the ligand-binding site makes KIR2DL2 a stronger receptor for HLA-C than KIR2DL3. *J Immunol* 180:3969, 2008.
5. Lopez-Botet M, Angulo A, Guma M: Natural killer cell receptors for major histocompatibility complex class I and related molecules in cytomegalovirus infection. *Tissue Antigens* 63:195, 2004.
6. Moretta L, Bottino C, Pende D, et al: Surface NK receptors and their ligands on tumor cells. *Semin Immunol* 18:151, 2006.
7. Murphy WJ, Kumar V, Bennett M: Acute rejection of murine bone marrow allografts by natural killer cells and T cells. Differences in kinetics and target antigens recognized. *J Exp Med* 166:1499, 1987.
8. Ljunggren HG, Karre K: In search of the 'missing self': MHC molecules and NK cell recognition. *Immunol Today* 11:237, 1990.
9. Symons HJ, Leffell MS, Rossiter ND, et al: Improved survival with inhibitory killer immunoglobulin receptor (KIR) gene mismatches and KIR haplotype B donors after nonmyeloablative, HLA-haploidentical bone marrow transplantation. *Biol Blood Marrow Transplant* 16:533, 2010.
10. Delgado DC, Hank JA, Kolesar J, et al: Genotypes of NK cell KIR receptors, their ligands, and Fcgamma receptors in the response of neuroblastoma patients to Hu14.18-IL2 immunotherapy. *Cancer Res* 70:9554, 2010.

11. Kim S, Poursine-Laurent J, Truscott SM, et al: Licensing of natural killer cells by host major histocompatibility complex class I molecules. *Nature* 436:709, 2005.
12. Raulet DH: Missing self recognition and self tolerance of natural killer (NK) cells. *Semin Immunol* 18:145, 2006.
13. Parham P: Taking license with natural killer cell maturation and repertoire development. *Immunol Rev* 214:155, 2006.
14. Joncker NT, Shifrin N, Delebecque F, et al: Mature natural killer cells reset their responsiveness when exposed to an altered MHC environment. *J Exp Med* 207:2065, 2010.
15. Elliott JM, Wahle JA, Yokoyama WM: MHC class I-deficient natural killer cells acquire a licensed phenotype after transfer into an MHC class I-sufficient environment. *J Exp Med* 207:2073, 2010.
16. Brodin P, Karre K, Hoglund P: NK cell education: Not an on-off switch but a tunable rheostat. *Trends Immunol* 30:143, 2009.
17. Feuchtinger T, Pfeiffer M, Pfaffle A, et al: Cytolytic activity of NK cell clones against acute childhood precursor-B-cell leukaemia is influenced by HLA class I expression on blasts and the differential KIR phenotype of NK clones. *Bone Marrow Transplant* 43:875, 2009.
18. Tang Q, Ahn YO, Southern P, et al: Development of IL-22-producing NK lineage cells from umbilical cord blood hematopoietic stem cells in the absence of secondary lymphoid tissue. *Blood* 117:4052, 2011.
19. Ruggeri L, Capanni M, Urbani E, et al: Effectiveness of donor natural killer cell alloreactivity in mismatched hematopoietic transplants. *Science* 295:2097, 2002.
20. Brunstein CG, Wagner JE, Weisdorf DJ, et al: Negative effect of KIR alloreactivity in recipients of umbilical cord blood transplant depends on transplantation conditioning intensity. *Blood* 113:5628, 2009.
21. Willemze R, Rodrigues CA, Labopin M, et al: KIR-ligand incompatibility in the graft-versus-host direction improves outcomes after umbilical cord blood transplantation for acute leukemia. *Leukemia* 23:492, 2009.
22. Venstrom JM, Zheng J, Noor N, et al: KIR and HLA genotypes are associated with disease progression and survival following autologous hematopoietic stem cell transplantation for high-risk neuroblastoma. *Clin Cancer Res* 15:7330, 2009.
23. Yu J, Venstrom JM, Liu XR, et al: Breaking tolerance to self, circulating natural killer cells expressing inhibitory KIR for non-self HLA exhibit effector function after T cell-depleted allogeneic hematopoietic cell transplantation. *Blood* 113:3875, 2009.
24. Fauriat C, Ivarsson MA, Ljunggren HG, et al: Education of human natural killer cells by activating killer cell immunoglobulin-like receptors. *Blood* 115:1166, 2010.
25. Foley B, Cooley S, Verneris MR, et al: NK cell education after allogeneic transplantation: Dissociation between recovery of cytokine-producing and cytotoxic functions. *Blood* 118:2784, 2011.
26. Cooley S, Trachtenberg E, Bergemann TL, et al: Donors with group B KIR haplotypes improve relapse-free survival after unrelated hematopoietic cell transplantation for acute myelogenous leukemia. *Blood* 113:726, 2009.
27. Cooley S, Weisdorf DJ, Guethlein LA, et al: Donor selection for natural killer cell receptor genes leads to superior survival after unrelated transplantation for acute myelogenous leukemia. *Blood* 116:2411, 2010.
28. Cichocki F, Hanson RJ, Lenvik T, et al: The transcription factor c-Myc enhances KIR gene transcription through direct binding to an upstream distal promoter element. *Blood* 113:3245, 2009.
29. Sun JC, Lanier LL: Cutting edge: Viral infection breaks NK cell tolerance to "missing self". *J Immunol* 181:7453, 2008.
30. Orr MT, Murphy WJ, Lanier LL. 'Unlicensed' natural killer cells dominate the response to cytomegalovirus infection. *Nat Immunol* 11:321, 2010.
31. Cook M, Briggs D, Craddock C, et al: Donor KIR genotype has a major influence on the rate of cytomegalovirus reactivation following T-cell replete stem cell transplantation. *Blood* 107:1230, 2006.
32. Lopez-Verges S, Milush JM, Schwartz BS, et al: Expansion of a unique CD57NKG2Chi natural killer cell subset during acute human cytomegalovirus infection. *Proc Natl Acad Sci USA* 108:14725, 2011.
33. Miller JS, Soignier Y, Panoskaltsis-Mortari A, et al: Successful adoptive transfer and in vivo expansion of human haploidentical NK cells in patients with cancer. *Blood* 105:3051, 2005.
34. Passweg JR, Tichelli A, Meyer-Monard S, et al: Purified donor NK-lymphocyte infusion to consolidate engraftment after haploidentical stem cell transplantation. *Leukemia* 18:1835, 2004.
35. Benson DM Jr, Bakan CE, Mishra A, et al: The PD-1/PD-L1 axis modulates the natural killer cell versus multiple myeloma effect: A therapeutic target for CT-011, a novel monoclonal anti-PD-1 antibody. *Blood* 116:2286, 2010.
36. Lu L, Ikizawa K, Hu D, et al: Regulation of activated CD4+ T cells by NK cells via the Qa-1-NKG2A inhibitory pathway. *Immunity* 26:593, 2007.

CHAPTER 103

DENDRITIC CELL THERAPIES

Karolina Palucka and Jacques Banchereau

The immune system has the potential to eliminate neoplastic cells. Perhaps the most compelling evidence of tumor immunosurveillance in humans is provided by paraneoplastic diseases that associate neurologic disorders to an antitumor response. Onconeural antigens, which are normally expressed on neurons, can also be expressed in breast cancer cells. Some patients develop a strong antigen-specific $CD8^+$ T-cell response that controls tumor expansion but concomitantly results in autoimmune cerebellar degeneration, causing a severe neurologic disease.

The adoptive transfer of cancer antigen-specific effector T cells in patients can result in rejection of established tumors, thereby illustrating the potential of tumor immunotherapy. Ideally, one would like to directly induce efficient tumor-specific T cells through vaccination, including effector T cells able to reject tumors and memory T cells able to prevent tumor relapse. Therapeutic vaccines have two objectives: priming antigen-specific T cells and reprogramming memory T cells, that is, a transformation from one type of immunity to another (e.g., regulatory to cytotoxic). Recent successful phase III clinical trials showing improved survival in patients receiving cancer vaccines have revived this field. Dendritic cells (DCs) are essential in generation of immune responses and as such represent both targets and vectors for vaccination. DCs are a rare cell type that has been discovered by Ralph Steinman in 1973. After 4 decades of research, it is now clear that DCs are at the center of the immune system through their ability to control both tolerance and immunity.

Indeed, murine models demonstrate that the generation of protective anti-tumor immunity depends on the presentation of tumor antigens by DCs.[1,2] There, DCs can capture tumor antigens released from tumor cells, either alive or dying and cross-present these antigens to T cells in tumor draining lymph nodes. This antigen presentation results in the generation of tumor-specific effector T cells that contribute to tumor rejection.[1,2] Thus, DCs represent important targets for therapeutic interventions in cancer.

BASICS OF DENDRITIC CELL BIOLOGY

Dendritic cells are bone marrow–derived cells that seed all tissues (reviewed by Steinman[3]). They are poised to sample the environment and transmit the gathered information to cells of the adaptive immune system (i.e., T cells and B cells).[3,4] In peripheral tissues, DCs capture Ags in the tissues through several complementary mechanisms. DCs launch the immune response by presenting the captured Ag in the form of peptide–major histocompatibility complex (MHC) complexes to naive (i.e., antigen–inexperienced) T cells in lymphoid tissues. Upon interaction with DCs, naive $CD4^+$ and $CD8^+$T cells differentiate into antigen-specific memory T cells with different functions. $CD4^+$ T cells can become Th1, Th2, Th17, or T follicular helper cells (Tfh) that help B cells differentiate into antibody-secreting cells (Tfh) as well as regulatory T cells (Tregs) that downregulate the functions of other lymphocytes. Naive $CD8^+$ T cells can give rise to cytotoxic effector lymphocytes (CTLs).

In the steady state, nonactivated (immature) DCs present self-antigens to T cells, thereby leading to tolerance through either T-cell deletion or differentiation of regulatory/suppressor T cells. These immature DCs have special characteristics, including (1) the ability to efficiently capture antigens, (2) accumulation of MHC class II molecules in the late endosome–lysosomal compartment, (3) low levels of costimulatory molecules expression, (4) a unique set of chemokine receptors that allow their migration to lymphoid tissues (e.g., CCR7), and (5) a limited capacity to secrete cytokines.[5] In contrast, mature antigen-loaded DCs can launch the differentiation of antigen-specific T cells into effector cells with unique functions and cytokine profiles (Fig. 103-1). Indeed, immature DCs promptly respond to environmental signals and differentiate into mature DCs. DC maturation is associated with (1) downregulation of antigen-capture activity; (2) increased expression of surface MHC class II molecules and costimulatory molecules; (3) the ability to secrete cytokines[5]; and (4) the acquisition of CCR7, which allows migration of the DC into the draining lymph node.[5] However, DC maturation does not result in a unique phenotype. Rather, in response to different signals that are provided by different microbes either directly or through the surrounding cells, DCs acquire distinct phenotypes that eventually contribute to diverse immune responses. In addition to cytokines or direct microbial signals, the ligation of CD40 represents an essential signal for the differentiation into fully mature DCs able to launch adaptive T-cell immunity.[6]

DENDRITIC CELL SUBSETS

The type of T-cell response (e.g., helper $CD4^+$ T cell or cytotoxic $CD8^+$ T cell) is at least in part linked with the subset of DCs that presents the antigen to T cells. Humans display two major DC subsets: myeloid DCs (mDCs, also called conventional or classical DCs), and plasmacytoid DCs (pDCs). Blood DC subsets can be distinguished by the differential expression of three surface molecules: CD303 (BDCA-2), CD1c (BDCA-1), and CD141 (BDCA3). $CD303^+$ pDCs represent a front line of antiviral immunity through their ability to secrete large amounts of type I interferon (IFN) in response to virus encounter.[7] Their presynthesized stores of MHC class I may permit a rapid initial $CD8^+$ T-cell response to viral infections. pDCs derived type I IFN may promote the immunogenic maturation of other DC populations, therefore helping in the activation of novel T-cell clones. In their resting state, pDCs are considered as playing an important role in tolerance, including oral tolerance.

Two subsets of blood mDCs can be distinguished by reciprocal expression of CD1c and CD141. Human $CD141^+$ DCs share with mouse $CD8^+$ DCs the high capacity to capture exogenous antigens for presentation on human leukocyte antigen (HLA) class I molecules ("cross-presentation"). $CD141^+$ DCs express XCR1, the receptor for the chemokine XCL1 that is produced by natural killer (NK) cells and activated $CD8^+$ T cells. Thus, mouse $CD8^+$ DCs and human $CD141^+$ DCs are geared up for generation of $CD8^+$ T-cell immunity. In mice, gene ablation studies have shown that the $CD8^+$ subset plays an important role in cross-presentation.[8] However, other human DCs such as epidermal Langerhans cells (LCs)[9] also cross-present antigens. Whether $CD141^+$ blood mDCs are related to DCs subsets in peripheral tissues remains to be determined.

The human skin hosts two main mDC subsets: epidermal LCs and dermal interstitial DCs (dermal DCs) (Fig. 103-2). The dermal

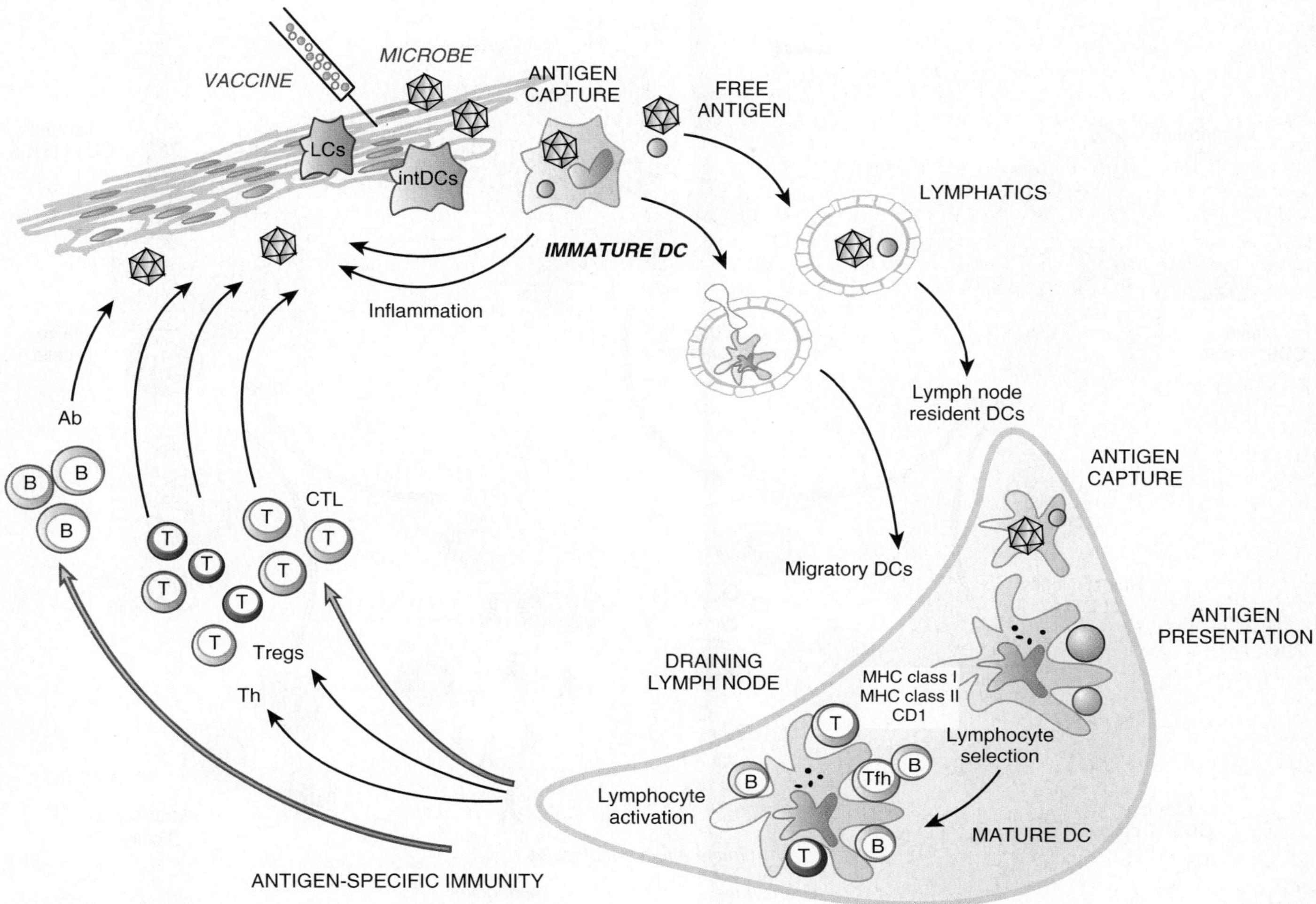

Figure 103-1 LAUNCHING OF THE IMMUNE RESPONSE. Antigen(s) can reach lymph nodes via two pathways. One pathway is via lymphatics, where the antigen is captured by lymph node resident dendritic cells (DCs). The other pathway is mediated by tissue resident DCs. There, immature DCs capture antigens, and DC activation triggers their migration toward secondary lymphoid organs and simultaneous maturation. DCs display antigens in the context of classical major histocompatibility complex (MHC) class I and class II or nonclassical CD1 molecules, which allow selection of rare antigen-specific T lymphocytes. Activated T cells drive DCs toward their terminal maturation, which induces further expansion and differentiation of lymphocytes into effector cells. If DCs do not receive maturation signals, they will remain immature, and antigen presentation will lead to immune regulation, suppression, or both. *CTL,* Cytotoxic effector lymphocyte; *intDC,* interstitial; *Treg,* T regulatory cell.

DCs can be further subdivided into CD1a$^+$ DCs and CD14$^+$ DCs. The authors' studies concluded that human CD14$^+$ DCs can directly help activated B cells as well as induce naive T cells to differentiate into cells with properties of T follicular helper cells (Tfh).[9] They may thus be specialized for the development of humoral responses.[9] On the contrary, LCs are more efficient in cross-presenting peptides from protein antigens to CD8$^+$ T cells and priming CD8$^+$ T cells into potent CTLs.

The DC subsets that sit in tissues under the steady state depend on FLT3 and MCSF-R. However, inflammatory processes such as those initiated by microbial invasion substantially alter the DC compartments. The origin of DCs that are recruited to inflammation sites is still under investigation, but it is clear that monocytes give rise to inflammatory DCs in vivo. Human studies depend on the in vitro exposure of monocytes to different cytokine combinations based on granulocyte macrophage colony-stimulating factor (GM-CSF). GM-CSF can be used together with interleukin-4 (IL-4), IFN-αβ, tumor necrosis factor (TNF), or IL-15 to yield DCs that can activate T cells. The cytokine combination is critical because it results in DCs with different phenotypes and functions. Several of these variants have been administered as vaccines to cancer patients. Another repertoire of tolerogenic DCs can be generated by culturing monocytes with IL-10 or with vitamin A or vitamin D3. Thus, we still need to establish how these distinct DC subsets are related, how they contribute to disease pathogenesis, and how they can be used to design efficient vaccines.

CANCER IMMUNOTHERAPY VIA DENDRITIC CELLS

Immunotherapy is moving to the forefront of cancer therapy owing to recent progresses in the field. For example, an antibody that blocks the function of CTLA-4, a molecule providing negative regulatory feedback in T-cell activation, was approved in 2011 by the U.S. Food and Drug Administration for the treatment of melanoma.[10]

The molecular identification of human cancer antigens has allowed the development of Ag-specific immunotherapy based on different approaches. In one approach, adoptive T-cell therapy (reviewed in[11,12]), autologous antigen-specific T cells are expanded ex vivo and reinfused to patients. The genetic engineering of cancer Ag-specific effector T cells has permitted the generation of promising early clinical data that confirm the therapeutic potential of T cells in cancer. Another approach to Ag-specific immunotherapy is active immunotherapy through immunization (vaccination, i.e., provision

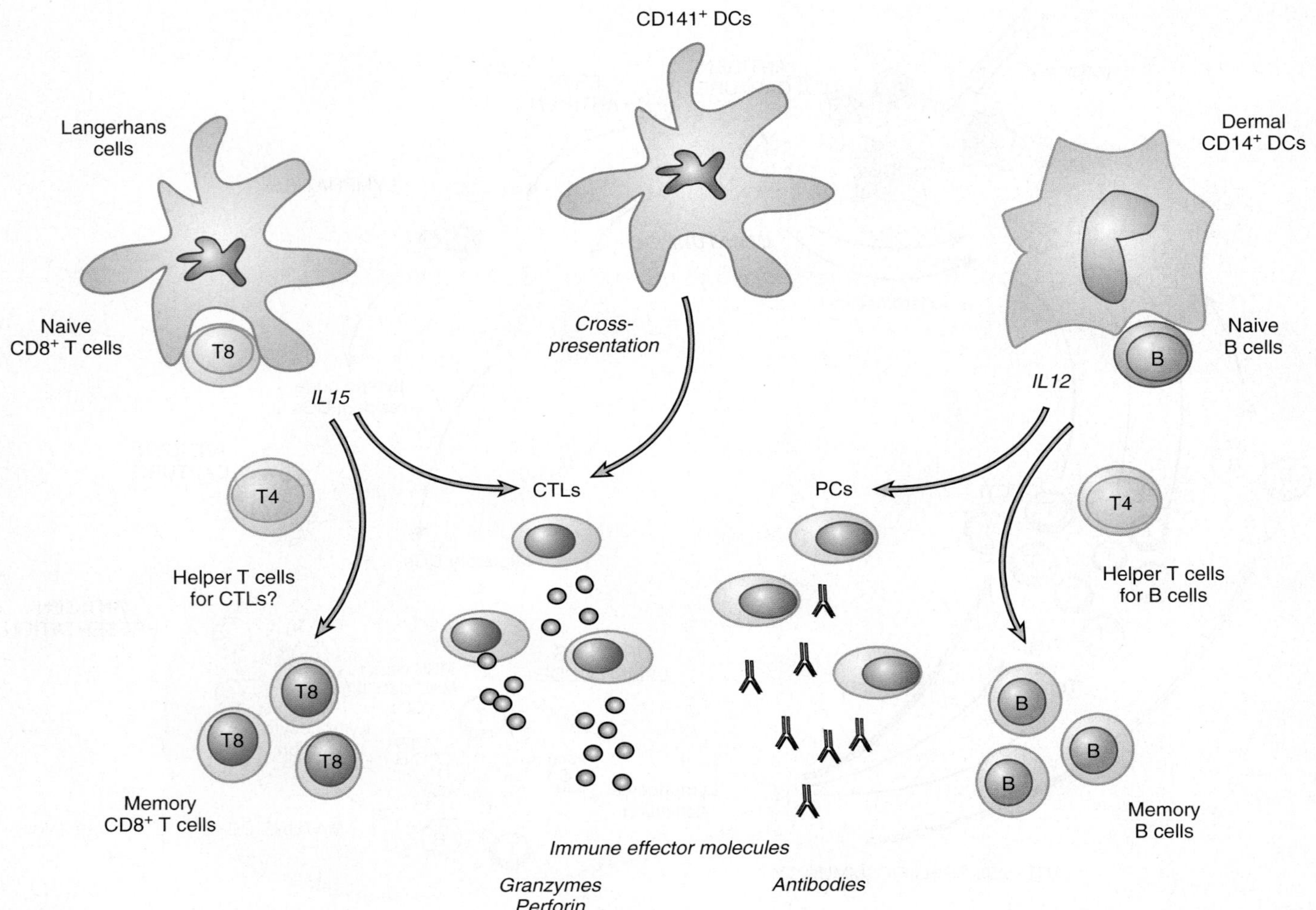

Figure 103-2 DENDRITIC CELL (DC) SUBSETS. The humoral and cellular arms of adaptive immunity are regulated by different human myeloid DC (mDC) subsets. Humoral immunity is preferentially regulated by CD14$^+$ dermal cells (DCs) by means of interleukin-12 (IL-12), which acts directly on B cells and promotes the development of T follicular helper cells (Tfhs). Cellular immunity is preferentially regulated by Langerhans cells (LCs), possibly through IL-15 and a dedicated subset of CD4$^+$ T cells specialized to help CD8$^+$ T cells (cytotoxic effector lymphocyte [CTL] Th cells). Given their capacity to cross-present antigens to CD8$^+$ T cells, CD141$^+$ DCs are likely to be involved in the development of cytotoxic T-lymphocyte responses. CD141$^+$ DCs might also be involved in the development of humoral responses through IL-12 secretion. This hypothesis is supported by mouse in vivo antigen-targeting studies showing that CD8$^+$ DCs, the mouse counterpart of human CD141$^+$ DCs, can induce both cytotoxic T-lymphocyte and humoral responses, although the mechanisms may be different. It will be important to determine whether and how CD141$^+$ DCs are related to LCs and to dermal DCs, and how these DC subsets shape adaptive immunity. *PC,* Plasma cells.

of an antigen together with an adjuvant to elicit an immune response of therapeutic value). Because of their molecular and functional characteristics, DCs are considered "nature's adjuvants." Furthermore, it is now well accepted that vaccine adjuvants (e.g., alum) act via activation of DCs. The progress in our understanding of DC biology will lead to development of next-generation potent cancer vaccines. Current studies aim at generating therapeutic cancer vaccines that are designed to elicit potent CD8$^+$ T-cell immunity able to eradicate tumor cells.

Vaccination via Dendritic Cells

Ex Vivo–Generated Dendritic Cell Vaccines

Dendritic cells generated ex vivo by culturing hematopoietic progenitor cells or monocytes with cytokine combinations have been tested as therapeutic vaccines in cancer patients for more than a decade.[13] These studies concluded that DC-based vaccines are safe and can induce the expansion of circulating CD4$^+$ and CD8$^+$ T cells that are specific for tumor antigens (Table 103-1). Objective clinical responses have been observed in some patients. The clinical response take time to build up, but remissions can be very long lasting.

The selection of tumor antigens for loading the DCs represents an important parameter. Candidate tumor antigens include unique (mutated) antigens and shared nonmutated self-antigens. To generate broadly applicable vaccines, nonmutated self-antigens have often been selected. These, however, present potential shortcomings: (1) the repertoire of high avidity clones might be depleted through negative selection and (2) the existing memory T cells often include regulatory T cells.

Mutated antigens might not display these drawbacks. Cancer vaccines designed to elicit strong immune responses against these mutated antigens will require a fully personalized approach. This represented a considerable challenge a few years ago. Fortunately, the fast development of modern sequencing technologies will allow us to determine the complete repertoire of mutated antigens in the patient's primary tumor and metastasis. This transforming technology might therefore allow us to craft therapeutic vaccines perfectly tailored to the patient's tumor.

Table 103-1 Examples of Clinical Trials Testing Vaccination with Ex Vivo Dendritic Cells

Vaccine/Antigen	Indication	Key Contribution	Reference
GM-CSF/IL-4 DCs with or without HLA-A201 restricted peptides or peptides alone	Metastatic prostate cancer	One of the first studies testing DCs immunogenicity	34
GM-CSF/IL-4 DCs Peptides Tumor lysates Autologous tumor eluted peptides	Stage IV melanoma Renal cancer Malignant glioma	Loading DCs with complex antigen preparations Objective clinical responses	35-37
Blood DCs Idiotype	Multiple myeloma	Immunogenicity Tumor regression	38,39
Mature GM-CSF/IL-4 DCs Peptides	Stage IV melanoma	Well-controlled and validated vaccine manufacture process Testing mature DCs Immunogenicity Objective clinical responses	40
CD34+ HPC-derived DCs Peptides	Stage IV melanoma	First studies to test CD34+HPC-dervied DCs Loading vaccines with a mixture of well-defined peptides Durable immune responses in long-term survivors Objective clinical responses	41,42
FLT3 ligand expanded blood DCs Altered peptides	Advanced CEA+ cancer	Immunogenicity Objective clinical responses	43
Immature GM-CSF/IL-4 DCs	Healthy volunteers	Antigen-specific inhibition of effector T-cell function after injection of immature DCs	44
GM-CSF/IL-4 DCs Tumor lysates	Refractory pediatric solid tumors	Immunogenicity Objective clinical responses	45
Mature cryopreserved GM-CSF/IL-4 DCs	Stage IV melanoma	Immunogenicity	46
DCs loaded with killed allogeneic tumor cells	Stage IV melanoma	Immunogenicity Durable objective clinical responses Long-term survival	47,48
Monocyte-derived DCs Loaded with NK T-cell ligand GalCer	Advanced cancer	Adjuvant effect of NK T-cell activation on CD8+ T-cell immunity	49
Monocyte-derived DCs	Melanoma	In vivo identification of antigen-specific immune response by PET imaging in patients	50
Monocyte-derived DCs	Melanoma	Route of DC administration impacts T-cell activation with intradermal administration showing better responses than intranodal	51
Comparative study CD34+ HPCs derived LCs vs. monocyte DCs	Melanoma	LC-based vaccines stimulated significantly greater tyrosinase-HLA-A*0201 tetramer reactivity than the monocyte DC-based vaccines	52
α-Type 1 polarized monocyte-derived DCs	Glioma	Combination of DC vaccination with poly ICLC to trigger systemic type I INF-driven inflammation	53

CEA, Carcinoembryonic antigen; *DC,* dendritic cell; *FLT,* fetal liver tyrosine; *GalCer,* galactopsylceramide; *GM-CSF,* granulocyte macrophage colony-stimulating factor; *HLA,* human leukocyte antigen; *HPC,* hematopoietic progenitor cell; *polyICLC,* a synthetic complex of carboxymethylcellulose, polyinosinic-polycytidylic acid, and oly-L-lysine double-stranded RNA *IL,* interleukin; *INF,* interferon; *LC,* Langerhans cell; *mDC,* myeloid dendritic cell; *NK,* natural killer; *PET,* positron emission tomography.

Targeting Antigen to Dendritic Cells in Vivo

Dendritic cells can be engaged by delivering antigens directly in vivo using chimeric proteins made of anti-DC receptor antibody fused to a selected antigen (DC targeting). Ralph Steinman and his colleagues demonstrated that the specific targeting of antigens to DCs in vivo results in the elicitation of potent antigen-specific CD4+ and CD8+ T-cell immunity.[14] The induction of immunity necessitates that maturation signals are provided.[14] Otherwise this strategy can result in antigen-specific tolerance, a finding of significant value in the context of autoimmunity. The use of vaccines targeting surface molecules expressed on different DC subsets allowed Steinman and Nussenzweig to formally demonstrate that distinct DC subsets elicit distinct immune responses.[15] There, CD8+ DCs that express the whereas cell surface protein CD205 present delivered antigens in the context of both MHC class I and class II, CD8− DCs, which are positive for the 33D1 antigen, are specialized for presentation on MHC class II.[15] Furthermore, targeting antigen to these distinct receptors on DCs leads to generation of T-cell responses via independent pathways. Thus, DEC-205 expressing DCs generate Th1 response in an IL-12–independent CD70-dependent mechanism, but 33D1+ DCs generate Th1 responses through the classic IL-12[16] pathway. DC targeting is not purely confined to the delivery of an antigenic cargo inasmuch as the engagement of some surface molecules such as Dectin-1, DC-SIGN, and CD40 by targeting antibodies provides activation signals as well. It remains important to determine whether the activation signals might actually polarize the DCs in the desired fashion. Thus, the challenge will be to match the DC surface target and the selected adjuvant with the desired immune outcome, all this in the context of an altered immune system.

IMMUNE AND CLINICAL EFFICACY

Most phase I/II studies have stumbled on two critical issues: (1) how to assess the clinical efficacy of cancer immunotherapy and (2) how to define the correlates (biomarkers) of clinical efficacy. In the early days, the RECIST (response evaluation criteria in solid tumors) criteria that had been designed to assess chemotherapy-based trials were considered critical to assess of clinical efficacy in vaccine and immunomodulation trials.[17] This has recently been challenged because in the early phase of treatment, tumors might increase in size, which might actually reflect the inflammatory process associated with active immune responses and lymphocyte infiltration.

Thus, overall survival might actually be the only objective parameter of clinical efficacy. However, surrogate markers are needed because trials based on overall survival might be exceedingly long. A number of cancer vaccine studies have suggested that the therapeutic vaccination outcome, success or failure, correlates with the vaccine-induced expansion of antigen-specific effector T cells.[18] However the quality, more than the quantity, of the antigen-specific immune response remains one of the key parameters of efficacy.

Indeed, the immunologic goal of vaccination against cancer is to elicit tumor-specific CD8⁺T cell responses that will be sufficiently robust and long lasting to generate durable tumor regression or eradication (or both) as we have already discussed above. Ideally, vaccine-elicited CD8⁺ T cells should (1) be of high avidity and able to recognize peptide–MHC class I complexes on tumor cells; (2) express high levels of granzyme and perforin, molecules essential for cytotoxic activity against cancer cells; (3) be able to traffic into the tumor; and (4) overcome regulatory mechanisms present in the tumor.[19] At least four components of the immune response are necessary for that ideal response to happen: (1) the presence of appropriate DCs, (2) the quality of induced CD4⁺ helper T cells, (3) the elimination or non-activation (or both) of Tregs, and (4) the breakdown of the immunosuppressive tumor microenvironment. Here we will briefly elaborate on the fate of CD8⁺ T cells in the context of DC vaccination. Naive CD8⁺ T cells initiate a CTL differentiation program upon encounter with DCs presenting tumor-derived peptides.[20] A complex system of signals drives the subsequent CD8⁺ T-cell expansion and differentiation, which include costimulatory pathways mediated by co-stimulatory molecules CD80, CD70, and 4-1BB as well as DC-derived cytokines such as IL-12 and IL-15. The quality of CD8⁺ T cell differentiation is further regulated by CD4⁺ T cells[21] through (i) help for the differentiation and expansion of tumor antigen-specific CTLs; (ii) induction of long-term memory CD8⁺ T cells. Unfortunately, CD4⁺ T cells can also suppress CTL differentiation. Thus, Tregs can inhibit CTLs via the secretion of various cytokines including transforming growth factor-β (TGFβ). They can also compete with CD8⁺ T cells for IL-2 via constitutive expression of CD25.[22]

Antigen-specific CTLs must also traffic into the tumor bed, an area that is not clearly understood.[19] A dysregulation of chemokine homeostasis might prevent the CD8⁺T cells from entering the tumor bed. Tumors might also actively repulse CD8⁺ T cell.[23] Finally, the tumor-infiltrating myeloid-derived suppressor cells and Tregs[24,25] might inhibit effector CD8⁺ T-cell functions. The negative cues of the tumor environment can be counteracted by a series of therapeutic modalities. Both antibodies that neutralize cytokines, such as IL-10, IL-13, and TGFβ and antibodies such as anti-CTLA-4 and anti-PD-L1, which block the immune-inhibitory signals in lymphocytes, will represent important contributors to cancer vaccines. Likewise, antibodies such as anti-CD137 that further promote costimulation of effector T cells should be tested in conjunction with vaccination. Just as oncologists currently use different combinations of cytostatic drugs and targeted therapies to treat cancer patients, we foresee the development of clinical protocols combining DC vaccines with individualized adjunct therapies.

"ENDOGENOUS" VACCINATION

The classical cancer therapies that are based on chemotherapy might in fact be effective partly through the engagement of the immune system. For example, chemotherapeutic agents such as anthracyclines and oxaliplatin induce cancer cells to undergo apoptosis, which is associated with cell surface exposure of calreticulin. Surface calreticulin might contribute to the capture of apoptotic bodies by DCs and the elicitation of tumor-specific CD8⁺ T-cell immunity. These T cells might contribute to the elimination of the tumor cells[26] that have not responded to the chemotherapy.

There is now strong evidence that antibody therapy with agents such as anti-CD20 and anti-HER2 involve the adaptive immune system beyond the elicitation of antibody-dependent cytotoxicity (ADCC). Indeed, antibodies against HER2 can enhance cross-presentation of tumor antigens, leading to the break of tolerance against this antigen.[27] Accordingly, patients responding to trastuzumab (Herceptin) show enhanced CD8⁺ T-cell immunity to HER2.[27]

MODULATING DENDRITIC CELLS IN THE TUMOR ENVIRONMENT

Another approach to immunotherapy via DCs is focused on exploiting DCs in the tumor microenvironment (Fig. 103-3). Indeed, DCs are found in most tumors in humans and mice. DCs can sample tumor antigens through the capture of dying tumor cells and through the nibbling of live tumor cells (reviewed in[28]). Tumors can prevent antigen presentation and the establishment of tumor-specific immunity through a variety of mechanisms. By converting immature DCs into macrophages (i.e., through IL-6, and M-CSF [macrophage colony-stimulating factor]), tumors can prevent the priming of tumor-specific T cells. Alternatively, the tumor glycoproteins carcinoembryonic antigen (CEA) and MUC-1 that are endocytosed by DCs stay confined in the early endosomes, therefore preventing efficient processing and presentation to T cells.

Tumors also interfere with DC maturation. First, they can inhibit DC maturation (i.e., through the secretion of IL-10, leading to Ag-specific anergy). Second, tumor-derived factors can alter mDCs maturation so as to yield cells that indirectly help tumor growth ("protumor" DCs). As an example, we have shown that thymic stromal lymphopoietin (TSLP) that is produced by tumor cells induces DCs to express OX40-L that directs the generation of Th2 cells. These skewed CD4⁺ T cells accelerate breast tumor development through the secretion of IL-4 or IL-13. These cytokines prevent tumor cell apoptosis and promote the proliferation of cancer cells indirectly by stimulating tumor-associated macrophages to secrete epidermal growth factor (EGF). A similar pathway operates in pancreatic cancer.[29]

Plasmacytoid DCs that are infiltrating breast carcinomas produce little type I IFN upon TLR ligation.[30] These pDCs induce naive CD4⁺T cells to differentiate into IL-10–producing T cells with suppressive functions. Such inhibition of type I IFN secretion might also impact the generation of effector T cells because DCs require type I IFN signals to cross-present tumor antigens.[1,2] Whether this mechanism explains why pDCs are associated with a poor prognosis[31] remains to be determined.

Finally, DCs can have direct protumor effects. In multiple myeloma, mDCs directly promote the survival and clonogenicity of tumor cells.[32] In ovarian cancer, pDCs contribute to tumor angiogenesis by secreting proangiogenic cytokines.[33] Thus, understanding the functions of DCs in the tumor bed might represent a rich field of investigation. Ultimately, rewiring the "protumor" DCs into "antitumor" DCs might represent a novel approach for cancer immunotherapy.

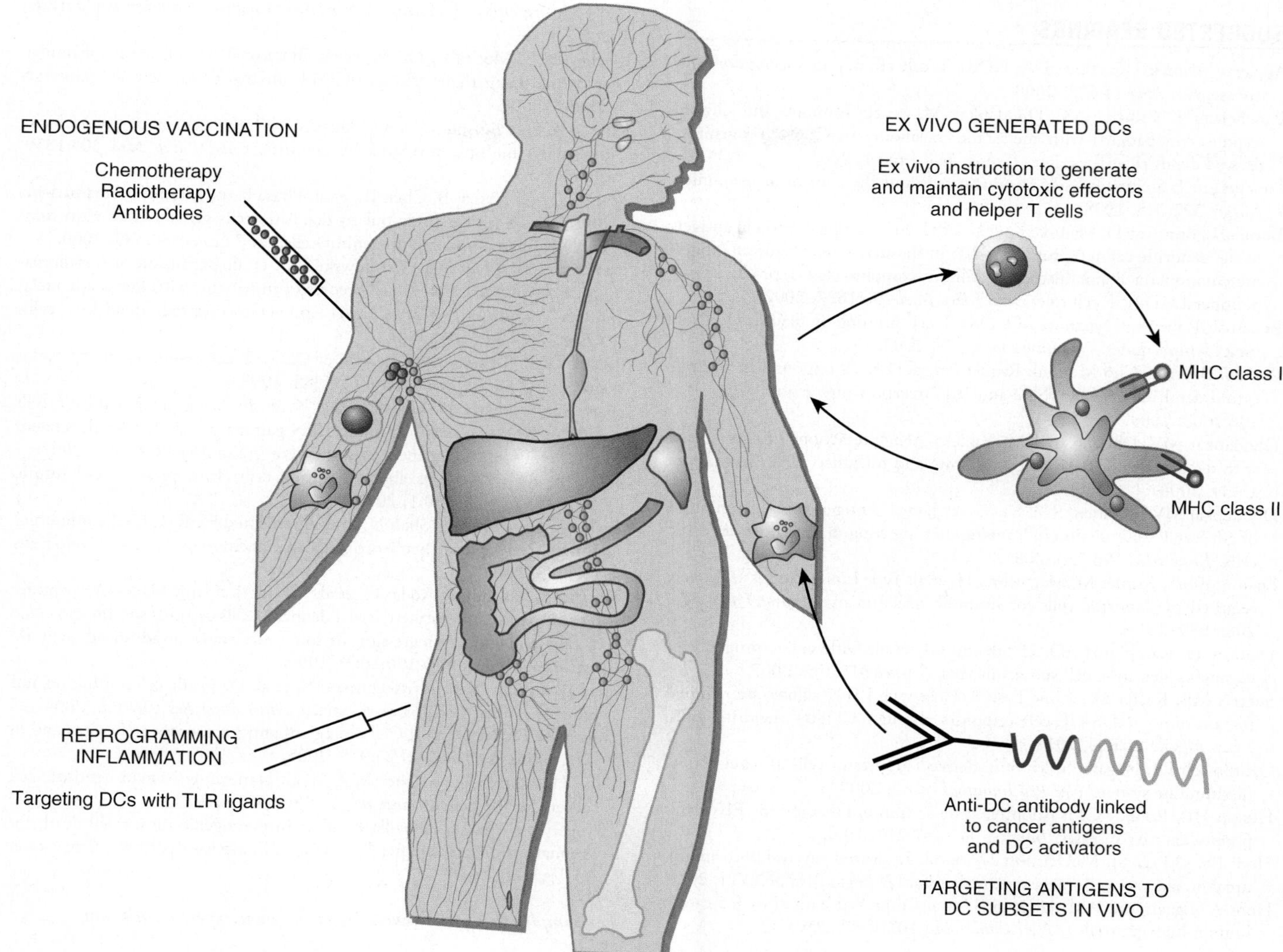

Figure 103-3 DENDRITIC CELLS (DCs) AND CANCER IMMUNOTHERAPY. (1) Random targeting of DCs in "endogenous" vaccination resulting from in vivo antigen release in a process of immunogenic cell death in response to chemotherapy, radiotherapy, or immune modulation approaches targeted at T cells; (2) vaccines based on ex vivo–generated tumor antigen-loaded DCs that are injected back into patients; (3) specific in vivo DC targeting with anti-DC antibodies fused with antigens and with DC activators; and (4) targeting DCs in the tumor environment to reprogram protumor inflammation toward tumor rejection. *MHC,* Major histocompatibility complex; *TLR,* toll-like receptor.

FUTURE DIRECTIONS

Nearly 40 years after their discovery, the importance that DCs has taken in physiology and medicine has been recognized by the award to Ralph Steinman of the Nobel Prize for Medicine and Physiology. Studies performed in the past decade have highlighted the commonalities and uniqueness of the various DC subsets. This new knowledge represents a fertile ground to work on to design better strategies for intervening in numerous clinical situations. The capacity of LCs and CD14$^+$ DCs to preferentially prime cellular immunity and humoral immunity, respectively, has significant implications, most particularly in the context of novel human vaccines. Thus, targeting LCs will be important for the design of vaccines that aim at eliciting strong cellular immunity. Such vaccines might be particularly useful at preventing, and perhaps even treating, chronic diseases, including viral (HIV, hepatitis C virus), bacterial (*Mycobacteria* spp.), and parasitic (malaria) diseases, as well as cancer. The most efficient vaccines might actually be those that will target both CD14$^+$ DCs and LCs, thereby allowing the maximal stimulation of both humoral and cellular immune responses. We foresee that the improved vaccines that target DCs will permit us to treat and prevent many chronic diseases, and likewise, manipulation of DCs will also permit to dampen overly enhanced immune responses as occurs in allergy and autoimmunity, possibly by turning on regulatory mechanisms.

ACKNOWLEDGMENT

We thank all the patients and volunteers who participated in our studies and clinical trials. We thank former and current members of the Institute for their contributions to our progresses. Our studies have been supported by the NIH (P01 CA084514, U19 AIO57234, R01 CA089440, CA078846, and CA140602), the Dana Foundation, the Susan Komen Foundation, the Baylor Health Care System, the Baylor Health Care System Foundation, the ANRS, and the INSERM. KP holds the Michael A. Ramsay Chair for Cancer Immunology Research. Because of space limits, we could cite only a fraction of the vast number of publications.

SUGGESTED READINGS

Appay V, Douek DC, Price DA: CD8+ T cell efficacy in vaccination and disease. *Nat Med* 14:623, 2008.

Banchereau J, Palucka AK, Dhodapkar M, et al: Immune and clinical responses in patients with metastatic melanoma to CD34+ progenitor-derived dendritic cell vaccine. *Cancer Res* 61:6451, 2001.

Banchereau J, Steinman RM: Dendritic cells and the control of immunity. *Nature* 392:245, 1998.

Bonifaz L, Bonnyay D, Mahnke K, et al: Efficient targeting of protein antigen to the dendritic cell receptor DEC-205 in the steady state leads to antigen presentation on major histocompatibility complex class I products and peripheral CD8+ T cell tolerance. *J Exp Med* 196:1627, 2002.

Bousso P, Robey E: Dynamics of CD8+ T cell priming by dendritic cells in intact lymph nodes. *Nat Immunol* 4:579, 2003.

Cao W, Bover L, Cho M, et al: Regulation of TLR7/9 responses in plasmacytoid dendritic cells by BST2 and ILT7 receptor interaction. *J Exp Med* 206:1603, 2009.

Dhodapkar MV, Dhodapkar KM, Palucka AK: Interactions of tumor cells with dendritic cells: Balancing immunity and tolerance. *Cell Death Differ* 15:39, 2008.

Dhodapkar MV, Steinman RM, Krasovsky J, et al: Antigen-specific inhibition of effector T cell function in humans after injection of immature dendritic cells. *J Exp Med* 193:233, 2001.

Diamond MS, Kinder M, Matsushita H, et al: Type I interferon is selectively required by dendritic cells for immune rejection of tumors. *J Exp Med* 208:1989, 2011.

Dudziak D, Kamphorst AO, Heidkamp GF, et al: Differential antigen processing by dendritic cell subsets in vivo. *Science* 315:107, 2007.

Fuertes MB, Kacha AK, Kline J, et al: Host type I IFN signals are required for antitumor CD8+ T cell responses through CD8α+ dendritic cells. *J Exp Med* 208:2005, 2011.

Gabrilovich DI, Nagaraj S: Myeloid-derived suppressor cells as regulators of the immune system. *Nat Rev Immunol* 9:162, 2009.

Heslop HE, Rooney CM: Adoptive cellular immunotherapy for EBV lymphoproliferative diseases. *Immuno Rev* 157:217, 1997.

Hodi FS, O'Day SJ, McDermott DF, et al: Improved survival with ipilimumab in patients with metastatic melanoma. *N Engl J Med* 363:711, 2010.

Hoos A, Eggermont AM, Janetzki S, et al: Improved endpoints for cancer immunotherapy trials. *J Natl Cancer Inst* 102:1388, 2010.

June CH: Principles of adoptive T cell cancer therapy. *J Clin Invest* 117:1204, 2007.

Klechevsky E, Morita R, Liu M, et al: Functional specializations of human epidermal Langerhans cells and CD14+ dermal dendritic cells. *Immunity* 29:497, 2008.

Kukreja A, Hutchinson A, Dhodapkar K, et al: Enhancement of clonogenicity of human multiple myeloma by dendritic cells. *J Exp Med* 203:1859, 2006.

Mackensen A, Herbst B, Chen JL, et al: Phase I study in melanoma patients of a vaccine with peptide-pulsed dendritic cells generated in vitro from CD34(+) hematopoietic progenitor cells. *Int J Cancer* 86:385, 2000.

Paczesny S, Banchereau J, Wittkowski KM, et al: Expansion of melanoma-specific cytolytic CD8+ T cell precursors in patients with metastatic melanoma vaccinated with CD34+ progenitor-derived dendritic cells. *J Exp Med* 199:1503, 2004.

Pardoll DM, Topalian SL: The role of CD4+ T cell responses in antitumor immunity. *Curr Opin Immunol* 10:588, 1998.

Soares H, Waechter H, Glaichenhaus N, et al: A subset of dendritic cells induces CD4+ T cells to produce IFN-gamma by an IL-12-independent but CD70-dependent mechanism in vivo. *J Exp Med* 204:1095, 2007.

Steinman RM: Decisions about dendritic cells: Past, present, and future. *Annu Rev Immunol* 30:1, 2011.

Taylor C, Hershman D, Shah N, et al: Augmented HER-2 specific immunity during treatment with trastuzumab and chemotherapy. *Clin Cancer Res* 13:5133, 2007.

Thurner B, Haendle I, Röder C, et al: Vaccination with Mage-3A1 peptide-pulsed mature, monocyte-derived dendritic cells expands specific cytotoxic T cells and induces regression of some metastases in advanced stage IV melanoma. *J Exp Med* 190:1669, 1999.

Treilleux I, Blay JY, Bendriss-Vermare N, et al: Dendritic cell infiltration and prognosis of early stage breast cancer. *Clin Cancer Res* 10:7466, 2004.

Trombetta ES, Mellman I: Cell biology of antigen processing in vitro and in vivo. *Annu Rev Immunol* 23:975, 2005.

Ueno H, Schmitt N, Klechevsky E, et al: Harnessing human dendritic cell subsets for medicine. *Immunol Rev* 234:199, 2010.

Zitvogel L, Kepp O, Senovilla L, et al: Immunogenic tumor cell death for optimal anticancer therapy: The calreticulin exposure pathway. *Clin Cancer Res* 16:3100, 2010.

For complete list of references log on to www.expertconsult.com.

PART X

TRANSPLANTATION

CHAPTER 104

OVERVIEW OF HEMATOPOIETIC STEM CELL TRANSPLANTATION

Helen E. Heslop

Since the first hematopoietic stem cell transplants (HSCTs) were performed more than 50 years ago, this modality has become a well-established therapeutic option for many hematologic malignancies as well as for bone marrow (BM) failure states, immune deficiencies, and inborn errors of metabolism[1-3] (Table 104-1). The wider application of allogeneic transplantation has been possible because of increased knowledge of the genetic basis of histocompatibility and advances in molecular methodology to more accurately type donors and recipients. In addition, the development of large donor registries and cord blood banks has expanded access to transplant as well as increasing the likelihood that a recipient will find a well-matched donor.[4]

Over the last 20 years, there has also been identification of additional sources of stem cells so that BM, peripheral blood (PB), and umbilical cord blood (UCB) are all widely used in clinical practice to provide long-term hematopoietic reconstitution. The increasing use of reduced-intensity conditioning regimens has made transplant an option for older patients and patients with comorbidities. Finally, there have been improvements in graft-versus-host disease (GVHD) prophylaxis and supportive care during the period of hematopoietic and immune suppression after transplant. Allogeneic HSCT should therefore be considered for patients in whom this procedure is likely to result in superior long-term disease-free survival (DFS) compared with other therapeutic modalities. Potential candidates must also have a suitable source of hematopoietic stem cells (HSCs) available at an appropriate time in the course of the disease.

This chapter provides an overview of HSCT procedures, including conditioning regimens and selection of donor and HSC source and common early and late posttransplant complications. These topics are discussed in depth in Chapters 105 to 110, and the disease specific indications are discussed in the relevant disease chapters (see Table 104-1 for details). Technical aspects of transplant, including HSC harvesting and cell processing, are discussed in Chapters 96 and 98.

ALLOGENEIC TRANSPLANTATION

Allogeneic transplant is a potential treatment for patients with relapsed or high-risk hematologic malignancy as well as for patients with inherited and acquired disorders of the hemopoietic and immune systems. The goal is to replace the recipient's hemopoietic and immune systems with normal HSCs from a closely matched donor whose hematopoietic stem and progenitor cells obtained from donor BM or other sources can home to the recipient's hematopoietic microenvironment and engraft. The major criteria for choosing an allogeneic donor is the degree of histocompatibility between the donor and recipient because the risks of both graft rejection and of GVHD increase with the degree of genetic disparity. The most important determinant of alloreactivity is matching at loci in the major histocompatibility complex (MHC) which includes human leukocyte antigens (HLA), encoded by class I (HLA-A, HLA-B, and HLA-C) and class II (HLA-DR, HLA-DQ, and HLA-DP) genes. HLA molecules were originally defined by serology, but molecular testing is now routine because gene sequencing has revealed multiple alleles for most serologically defined specificities[5] (see Chapter 106). Other determinants include minor histocompatibility antigens, which are naturally processed peptides derived from normal cellular proteins that can stimulate an MHC-restricted response when different polymorphisms are present in donor and recipient. Natural killer (NK) cells may also contribute to alloreactivity, particularly in the setting of haploidentical transplantation. There is also increasing evidence that genetic loci outside of the MHC may influence the risk of transplant complications such as infection or regimen-related mortality and several groups are undertaking genome-wide association assays to define genetic variants that might predict these complications.

The choice of donor for an allogeneic HSCT depends on several factors, including donor choices, the urgency of the transplant, and the patient's disease status. The optimal donor is a matched sibling sharing HLA class I and HLA class II alleles, but because each child inherits one set of paternal and one set of maternal HLA antigens, the likelihood of any sibling matching is only 25%. For patients who lack such donors, other options include a closely matched unrelated or cord donor or a haploidentical family member. Development of high-resolution molecular tissue typing methods and establishment of large donor registries have facilitated transplants from closely HLA-matched unrelated donors. These volunteer donors are healthy individuals between 18 and 60 years of age who fulfill eligibility requirements similar to those applied to blood donors. With increasing registry size, the chance of finding a donor has increased, so that more than 70% of patients can identify an HLA-A, B, C, and DRB1 allele-matched unrelated donor.[6] The likelihood of finding a donor matching at these eight loci (or 10 loci if matching at DQB1 is also included) varies for different ethnic groups and is less for groups with more polymorphism of HLA antigens. The initial results of transplantation from unrelated donors were inferior to those seen after matched sibling transplantation because of increased incidences of graft rejection and of GVHD caused by the greater genetic disparity. Over the past decade, though, results have gradually improved in both single-center and multicenter registry studies, reflecting better donor–recipient matching and advances in GVHD prophylaxis and supportive care.[6] One remaining limitation, though, is the time required to identify and screen an unrelated donor, which can be up to 3 to 6 months. Cord units by contrast can be obtained within 1 week of identifying a suitable matched unit. Haploidentical family donors have the greatest genetic disparity but are usually also rapidly available. Several studies have compared outcomes of cord and haploidentical donor transplants, but they do not show a definitive advantage for either source of HSCs.[7]

AUTOLOGOUS TRANSPLANTATION

Autologous transplant in which the recipient's own HSCs are collected then reinfused after high-dose chemotherapy is used to produce hemopoietic reconstitution after high-dose chemotherapy. This approach allows dose intensification in settings where there is a correlation between dose and tumor response rate and hematopoietic toxicity is a limiting factor for dose intensification. HSCs are harvested and cryopreserved and then reinfused after doses of chemotherapy and radiotherapy that would otherwise be lethal or require a

Table 104-1 Hematologic Disorders Treated by Hematopoietic Stem Cell Transplantation

Hematologic Malignancies	Chapters
Acute lymphoblastic leukemia	64 (pediatric), 65, 105 (adult)
Acute myeloid leukemia	60, 105 (adult), 61 (pediatric)
Myelodysplasia	60, 105 (adult), 62 (pediatric)
Myeloproliferative disorders	62 (pediatric), 69 (myelofibrosis)
Chronic lymphocytic leukemia	76, 105
Chronic myeloid leukemia	62 (pediatric), 66 (adult)
Multiple myeloma	85, 105
Hodgkin lymphoma	74, 105 (adult), 83 (pediatric)
Non-Hodgkin lymphoma	79 (follicular), 80 (mantle cell), 81 (diffuse large B cell), 83 (pediatric), 105 (all types)
Nonmalignant Disorders	
Hemoglobinopathies	
Sickle cell disease	40
Thalassemia	38
Immune deficiencies	
SCID	49
Wiskott Aldrich syndrome	49
Bone marrow failure syndromes	
Aplastic anemia	28
Paroxysmal nocturnal hemoglobulinuria	29
Fanconi anemia and other inherited bone marrow failure syndromes	27
Neutrophil disorders	
Chronic granulomatous disease	48
Histiocytic disorders	
Hemophagocytic lymphohistiocytosis	50
Lysosomal storage diseases	51

SCID, Severe combined immunodeficiency.

prolonged period of recovery. In general, autologous transplant is well tolerated, and data from the Center for International Bone Marrow Transplant Research (CIBMTR) show that the 100-day mortality rate is less than 5%.[8] The major cause of failure after autologous transplant is relapse of the primary disease. One longer-term concern is that recipients of autologous transplant have an increased risk of secondary therapy-related myeloid leukemia or myelodysplastic syndromes (t-MDS/AML) although this may also reflect effects of previous treatment. Indeed, a study which identified a pattern of altered gene expression in patients who developed t-MDS/AML after transplant for lymphoma found that the genetic programs associated with t-MDS/AML are perturbed pre close up transplant.[9]

The most common indications for autologous transplant are currently, myeloma, non-Hodgkin lymphoma (NHL), and Hodgkin lymphoma, in which it has been shown in randomized trials or concluded in evidence-based reviews that dose intensification and hemopoietic rescue result in improved DFS.[10-12] Patients with newly diagnosed myeloma who are considered potential candidates for autologous transplant ASCT are usually treated with 2 to 4 cycles of therapy that usually includes an immunomodulatory agent and a proteasome inhibitor before proceeding to autograft.[13] High- or intermediate-dose melphalan is the most widely used conditioning regimen with patients who are younger than the age of 65 years and do not have significant comorbidities receiving high-dose regimens (200 mg/m^2); older patients or those with comorbidities receive a reduced dose regimen (usually 140 mg/m^2).[14] The optimal post-autograft therapy is under investigation. A multicenter randomized trial showed no advantage for performing tandem autologous non-myeloablative allogeneic HSCT compared with tandem autologous HSCT for patients with standard-risk multiple myeloma,[15] and current studies are comparing tandem autologous transplants with single transplant followed by maintenance with an immunomodulatory agent or proteasome inhibitor.

Both ASBMT and NCCN guidelines recommend autologous transplantation in patients with relapsed or refractory diffuse large B-cell lymphoma,[10,16] as well as selected patients with follicular lymphoma.[11] Several large studies have also showed benefit from consolidating with an autograft after initial therapy in patients with mantle cell lymphoma.[17,18] A number of different myeloablative conditioning regimens are used in patients with NHL with the most common being BEAM (BCNU, etoposide, cytosine arabinoside, and melphalan), often in combination with rituximab.

SOURCE OF HEMATOPOIETIC STEM CELLS

The major sources of stem cells for transplant are BM, mobilized PB, and cord blood.

Autologous Donors

In autologous transplantation, the source of HSCs is mobilized PB in almost all adults and more than 90% of pediatric patients.[8] Cytokine-mobilized PB stem cells (PBSCs) can be harvested either after treatment with recombinant human granulocyte colony-stimulating factor (GCSF) alone or with GCSF given after chemotherapy. In patients who are heavily pretreated and difficult to mobilize, plerixifor, an antagonist of CXCR4 that interferes with adhesion of hematopoietic progenitors in the microenvironment thereby promoting their circulation in the PB, can be used to increase the mobilization of CD34$^+$ stem cells when given in combination with standard GCSF therapy.

The success of HSC mobilization is related to the amount of previous chemotherapy with some drugs such as alkylating agents having a particularly adverse effect on the success of HSC mobilization. The International Myeloma Working Group has therefore recommended early mobilization of stem cells, preferably within the first 4 cycles of initial therapy.[19]

Allogeneic Donors

Bone marrow was the historic source of HSCs for transplant and remains the most widely used source in children. BM can be harvested from the posterior iliac crests of allogeneic donors in amounts up to 10 to 20 mL per kilogram of recipient weight to obtain sufficient HSCs for engraftment. Cytokine-mobilized allogeneic PBSC harvest has become an alternative to BM as a source of HSCs and is now the most widely used source in adults receiving allogeneic transplants. In both single-center randomized studies and CIBMTR registry studies, use of this source of stem cells from matched sibling donors resulted in more rapid engraftment with no increase in acute GVHD. However, there was a higher incidence of chronic GVHD associated with a lower risk of relapse, which translated to improved DFS in patients transplanted for advanced hematologic malignancies. However, this survival benefit was not seen in patients with early stage disease. A recent large, prospective, randomized trial in recipients of unrelated HSCs who were randomized to receive BM versus PB grafts for hematologic malignancies shows no difference in overall survival at 2 years but a higher incidence of chronic GVHD in the recipients who received PB.[20] Longer follow-up is needed to determine if this more frequent development of chronic GVHD will be associated with higher late mortality.

Umbilical Cord Blood

Another alternative source of stem cells is cord blood. There are several large cord banks where cord blood is collected, cryopreserved, and tested for infectious agents in accordance with standards developed by governmental and specialty oversight organizations.[21]This worldwide network for UCB cell procurement, typing, and storage has collected a large inventory of cords and has facilitated more than 20,000 unrelated donor UCB transplants. A major advantage of cord transplant is the immediate availability of cryopreserved units. Cord transplants have slower engraftment, but they also may also induce less GVHD because of the relative naivety of cord T cells. One limitation is the cell count, which can be limiting for individuals weighing more than 50 kg. However, several studies show that double cord blood transplant, with each unit sharing at least 4/6 HLA antigens with the recipient, can overcome this problem and extend the use of cord transplant to larger adult recipients (see Chapter 108).

CONDITIONING REGIMENS

The conditioning regimen has different roles in autologous and allogeneic transplant. In autologous transplant, the aim of the conditioning regimen is to intensify doses of chemotherapy agents that would be limited by hematopoietic toxicity. In allogeneic transplant, the goal of conditioning is to achieve immunosuppression of the recipient sufficient to prevent rejection of the donor BM cells and to destroy residual malignant cells (see Chapter 105). Historically, patients transplanted for malignancy have received intensive fully ablative regimens in which hematopoietic reconstitution would not occur without HSC support. Conditioning regimens are discussed in more detail in Chapter 105, but the most commonly used allogeneic regimens use total-body irradiation (TBI) and cyclophosphamide or chemotherapy alone with combinations such as busulfan and cyclophosphamide. Biologic agents, such as antithymocyte globulin and monoclonal antibodies, may also be included in some regimens to increase immunosuppression. Reduced-intensity conditioning regimens were developed in the late 1990s and are primarily immunosuppressive, relying on graft-versus-leukemia mechanisms to eradicate malignancy. Reduced-intensity conditioning is often used in older patients or patients with comorbidities in whom the toxicity associated with ablative conditioning would be unacceptable. A variety of regimens based on low-dose TBI or fludarabine have been used.

COMPLICATIONS AFTER STEM CELL TRANSPLANTATION

Patients who receive transplants are at risk of a number of short- and long-term complications and require long-term-follow up. Guidelines for screening and monitoring long-term survivors have been published,[22] and there is increasing interest in research to define the quality of life in long-term transplant survivors. Recipients of both allogeneic and autologous transplant have risks of infection during the period of hematopoietic and immune reconstitution and short- and long-term complications from toxicities from the conditioning regimen. Allograft recipients are also at risk of graft failure and GVHD because of the genetic disparity between donor and recipient.

Acute Graft-Versus-Host Disease

GVHD is the most important cause of mortality, morbidity, and diminished quality of life after allogeneic HCT and results from alloreactivity between donor and recipient. The process is initiated by donor T lymphocytes that recognize antigenic disparities between donor and recipient. In the initial phase, chemotherapy or radiation given as part of the conditioning regimen results in production of inflammatory cytokines secreted by damaged host cells.[23] The release of microbial products that are produced by intestinal flora, as well as the release of cytokines by damaged host tissues, lead to the activation of innate immune cells by pathogen recognition receptors such as Toll-like receptors. After infusion of the HSC product, donor T cells become activated by exposure to host antigens and further activate other immune effectors, resulting in secretion of cytokines and clinical manifestations of GVHD. Chronic GVHD is defined as GVHD occurring after day 100 after transplant, although this definition is somewhat arbitrary. Chronic GVHD often occurs in a patient who has had preceding acute GVHD, although it may arise de novo. It targets the skin, liver, and gastrointestinal tract but may also target other organs and shares features with autoimmune diseases such as scleroderma.

Graft Failure

Graft failure results when recipient immune system cells that survive the conditioning regimen are able to eliminate the incoming donor BM. It is uncommon after fully ablative allogeneic HSCT for hematologic malignancies, but higher incidences are seen after reduced-intensity conditioning and when cord blood is the source of HSCs. Other risk factors include the degree of mismatch between donor and recipient, a low nucleated cell dose, and T-cell depletion of the donor product. Patients who experience graft failure may be retransplanted after additional immunosuppressive conditioning, but mortality from infection caused by prolonged neutropenia is significant.

Infections

After engraftment of the donor HSCs, donor-derived cells reconstitute the recipient's immune system. This is usually a rapid process after autologous transplant but is more prolonged after allogeneic transplant and may be further delayed in a recipient who develops GVHD and requires additional immunosuppression. During the early period after HSC infusion, neutropenic patients are at risk for bacterial infection, fungal infection, and infection with respiratory viruses. After engraftment, allogeneic recipients are at risk for viral infection, particularly reactivation of herpes viruses such as cytomegalovirus. Late infectious complications are mainly seen in allogeneic recipients, in whom a major risk factor is chronic GVHD. International consensus guidelines on the management of infections posttransplant have recently been published.[24]

Regimen-Related Toxicity

A number of early and late posttransplant complications are related to the conditioning regimen as well as previous therapies and pretransplant comorbidities. These include pneumonitis, sinusoidal obstruction syndrome, hemorrhagic cystitis, growth impairment, and endocrine abnormalities and are described in Chapter 110.

Secondary Malignancies

After HSCT, recipients have a two- to sevenfold increased risk of developing a secondary neoplasm, with the most frequently seen malignancies being EBV-related posttransplant lymphoproliferative disease (EBV-PTLD), therapy-related AML and myelodysplasia, and a variety of solid tumors.[25,26] As discussed earlier, autologous transplant recipients are at risk of developing therapy-related MDS and AML because of previous therapy as well as transplant conditioning. Recipients of allogeneic transplant have an increased incidence of both PTLD and solid cancers.[25,26]

Treatment of Relapse

Relapse remains a major cause of treatment failure after HSCT for hematologic malignancies, and present treatment options are inadequate.[27] Maneuvers that are commonly used are withdrawal of immune suppression, donor lymphocyte infusions, chemotherapy, and second transplants. Chemotherapy may induce some responses but rarely results in long-term disease control. Increasing knowledge of the molecular basis of graft-versus-tumor responses has stimulated interest in the use of immunotherapy to treat relapse. Infusion of unmanipulated donor lymphocytes can result in significant clinical responses in patients with relapsed CML, but responses are less frequent in other hematologic malignancies.[28] Current research is focusing on targeting minor antigens differentially expressed on hemopoietic cells or lineage-specific antigens, such as Wilm's Tumor 1 (WTI), preferentially expressed antigen of melanoma (PRAME), or proteinase 3.[29] Other immunotherapy approaches under investigation include the administration of antitumor vaccines, NK cells, or immune effectors genetically modified with artificial receptors targeting surface antigens such as CD19 or CD30.[30]

FUTURE DIRECTIONS

An ongoing challenge is to delineate the indications for transplant as new drugs are incorporated in primary therapies for many hematologic malignancies and as risk factors continue to be redefined by new information from genetic sequencing and proteomics studies. The wider use of reduced-intensity transplant offers the prospect of using such transplants as a platform for immunotherapy, and transplant will likely be integrated more closely with other cell therapies such as infusions of NK cells, cytotoxic T cells, and regulatory T cells. The question of optimal stem cell source for patients who lack a matched sibling or 10/10 matched unrelated donor is an open issue as novel regimens to improve outcomes are being evaluated for cord and haploidentical transplants. Finally, there is a need for comparative effectiveness studies that include quality of life measures to compare transplant with other therapeutic options.

REFERENCES

1. Appelbaum FR: Hematopoietic-cell transplantation at 50. *N Engl J Med* 357:1472, 2007.
2. Jenq RR, van den Brink MR: Allogeneic haematopoietic stem cell transplantation: Individualized stem cell and immune therapy of cancer. *Nat Rev Cancer* 10:213, 2010.
3. Copelan EA: Hematopoietic stem-cell transplantation. *N Engl J Med* 354:1813, 2006.
4. Petersdorf EW, Hansen JA: New advances in hematopoietic cell transplantation. *Curr Opin Hematol* 15:549, 2008.
5. Nunes E, Heslop H, Fernandez-Vina M, et al: Definitions of histocompatibility typing terms. *Blood* 118:e180, 2011.
6. Karanes C, Nelson GO, Chitphakdithai P, et al: Twenty years of unrelated donor hematopoietic cell transplantation for adult recipients facilitated by the National Marrow Donor Program. *Biol Blood Marrow Transplant* 14:8, 2008.
7. Brunstein CG, Fuchs EJ, Carter SL, et al: Alternative donor transplantation after reduced intensity conditioning: Results of parallel phase 2 trials using partially HLA-mismatched related bone marrow or unrelated double umbilical cord blood grafts. *Blood* 118:282, 2011.
8. Pasquini MC, Wang Z: Current use and outcome of hematopoietic stem cell transplantation: CIBMTR summary slides. 2012.
9. Li L, Li M, Sun C, et al: Altered hematopoietic cell gene expression precedes development of therapy-related myelodysplasia/acute myeloid leukemia and identifies patients at risk. *Cancer Cell* 20:591, 2011.
10. Oliansky DM, Czuczman M, Fisher RI, et al: The role of cytotoxic therapy with hematopoietic stem cell transplantation in the treatment of diffuse large B cell lymphoma: Update of the 2001 evidence-based review. *Biol Blood Marrow Transplant* 17:20, 2011.
11. Oliansky DM, Gordon LI, King J, et al: The role of cytotoxic therapy with hematopoietic stem cell transplantation in the treatment of follicular lymphoma: An evidence-based review. *Biol Blood Marrow Transplant* 16:443, 2010.
12. Hahn T, Wingard JR, Anderson KC, et al: The role of cytotoxic therapy with hematopoietic stem cell transplantation in the therapy of multiple myeloma: An evidence-based review. *Biol Blood Marrow Transplant* 9:4, 2003.
13. Laubach J, Richardson PG, Anderson K: Hematology: Setting the standard for newly diagnosed multiple myeloma. *Nat Rev Clin Oncol* 8:255, 2011.
14. Palumbo A, Anderson K: Multiple myeloma. *N Engl J Med* 364:1046, 2011.
15. Krishnan A, Pasquini MC, Logan B, et al: Autologous haemopoietic stem-cell transplantation followed by allogeneic or autologous haemopoietic stem-cell transplantation in patients with multiple myeloma (BMT CTN 0102): A phase 3 biological assignment trial. *Lancet Oncol* 12:1195, 2011.
16. Zelenetz AD, Abramson JS, Advani RH, et al: NCCN clinical practice guidelines in oncology: Non-Hodgkin's lymphomas. *J Natl Compr Cancer Netw* 8:288, 2010.
17. Geisler CH, Kolstad A, Laurell A, et al: Long-term progression-free survival of mantle cell lymphoma after intensive front-line immunochemotherapy with in vivo-purged stem cell rescue: A nonrandomized phase 2 multicenter study by the Nordic Lymphoma Group. *Blood* 112:2687, 2008.
18. Damon LE, Johnson JL, Niedzwiecki D, et al: Immunochemotherapy and autologous stem-cell transplantation for untreated patients with mantle-cell lymphoma: CALGB 59909. *J Clin Oncol* 27:6101, 2009.
19. Kumar S, Giralt S, Stadtmauer EA, et al: Mobilization in myeloma revisited: IMWG consensus perspectives on stem cell collection following initial therapy with thalidomide-, lenalidomide-, or bortezomib-containing regimens. *Blood* 114:1729, 2009.
20. Anasetti C, Logan BR, Lee SJ, et al: Increased incidence of chronic graft-versus-host disease (GVHD) and no survival advantage with filgrastim-mobilized peripheral blood stem cells (PBSC) compared to bone marrow (BM) transplants [abstract]. *Blood (Suppl 1)* 118:1, 2011.
21. Warkentin PI: Voluntary accreditation of cellular therapies: Foundation for the Accreditation of Cellular Therapy (FACT). *Cytotherapy* 5:299, 2003.
22. Majhail NS, Rizzo JD, Lee SJ, et al: Recommended screening and preventive practices for long-term survivors after hematopoietic cell transplantation. *Biol Blood Marrow Transplant* 18:348, 2012.
23. Ferrara JL, Levine JE, Reddy P, Holler E: Graft-versus-host disease. *Lancet* 373:1550, 2009.
24. Tomblyn M, Chiller T, Einsele H, et al: Guidelines for preventing infectious complications among hematopoietic cell transplantation recipients: A global perspective. *Biol Blood Marrow Transplant* 15:1143, 2009.
25. Landgren O, Gilbert ES, Rizzo JD, et al: Risk factors for lymphoproliferative disorders after allogeneic hematopoietic cell transplantation. *Blood* 113:4992, 2009.
26. Rizzo JD, Curtis RE, Socie G, et al: Solid cancers after allogeneic hematopoietic cell transplantation. *Blood* 113:1175, 2009.
27. Porter DL, Alyea EP, Antin JH, et al: NCI First International Workshop on the biology, prevention, and treatment of relapse after allogeneic hematopoietic stem cell transplantation: Report from the Committee on Treatment of Relapse after Allogeneic Hematopoietic Stem Cell Transplantation. *Biol Blood Marrow Transplant* 16:1467, 2010.
28. Kolb HJ: Graft-versus-leukemia effects of transplantation and donor lymphocytes. *Blood* 112:4371, 2008.
29. Bleakley M, Riddell SR: Molecules and mechanisms of the graft-versus-leukaemia effect. *Nat Rev Cancer* 4:371, 2004.
30. Kalos M, Levine BL, Porter DL, et al: T cells with chimeric antigen receptors have potent antitumor effects and can establish memory in patients with advanced leukemia. *Sci Transl Med* 3:95ra73, 2011.

CHAPTER 105

INDICATIONS AND OUTCOME OF ALLOGENEIC HEMATOPOIETIC CELL TRANSPLANTATION FOR HEMATOLOGIC MALIGNANCIES IN ADULTS

Parameswaran Hari and Mary Horowitz

Thomas et al[1] first reported long-term leukemia-free survival (LFS) after human leukocyte antigen (HLA) identical sibling hematopoietic stem cell transplantation (HSCT) in some patients with refractory acute leukemia in the 1970s. Since then, allogeneic HSCT has evolved to become a frequently used and effective therapy for many hematologic malignancies. Changes in both HSCT and non-HSCT therapy have modified the indications and applicability of HSCT over time. In chronic myeloid leukemia (CML), HSCT (once the mainstay for cure) is now largely supplanted by molecularly targeted therapy. In recent years, especially after the advent of reduced intensity conditioning in the late 1990s, allogeneic HSCT is increasingly used in older patients and as an effective salvage strategy for patients with lymphoma or myeloma not responding to chemotherapy or autologous HSCT. Transplant-related mortality (TRM), although steadily declining, still remains a challenge. General principles, indications, and optimal timing of allogeneic HSCT for hematologic malignancies and long-term outcomes after HSCT are discussed in this chapter.

Allogeneic HSCT involves administration of a preparative regimen of chemotherapy, immune suppressive drugs, and/or radiation followed by infusion of donor hematopoietic cells. Most patients then receive prolonged (several months) therapy with immune suppressive drugs to prevent or treat graft-versus-host disease (GVHD). The purpose of the preparative or conditioning regimen is twofold: to eradicate malignant cells and to eliminate host immune cells capable of rejecting donor cells. The ability to restore hematopoiesis with donor HSCs permits the administration of substantially higher (myeloablative) doses of cytotoxic therapy than is otherwise possible. Although originally regarded primarily as a way of rescuing patients from therapy-induced bone marrow (BM) aplasia, it is now accepted that graft-versus-tumor (GVT) effects conferred by alloreactive donor cells contribute substantially to cancer eradication and relapse prevention.

PATIENT POPULATION

Accompanying the growth of HSCT, a coordinated, international effort evolved to collect and analyze data on transplant outcomes through the International Bone Marrow Transplant Registry (IBMTR), established in 1972. The IBMTR affiliated with the U.S. National Marrow Donor Program (NMDP) in 2004 to become the Center for International Blood and Marrow Transplant Research (CIBMTR). CIBMTR currently collects data on HSCT outcomes from more than 400 transplant centers worldwide. Approximately 5500 allogeneic transplants performed in patients 18 years of age and older were reported to the CIBMTR in 2009. These data show hematologic malignancies (and premalignant conditions) to be the most common indications for allogeneic HSCT. Acute myeloid leukemia (AML) accounted for 36% of allogeneic HSCTs, acute lymphoblastic leukemia (ALL) for 11%, CML for 3.5%, chronic lymphocytic leukemia (CLL) for 5%, and Hodgkin and non-Hodgkin lymphomas for 18% (Fig. 105-1).

Improved immunosuppression and supportive care and reduced intensity conditioning allowed increased use of allogeneic HSCT for older adults in recent years. Only 4% of allogeneic HSCT recipients from 1987 to 1992 were older than 50 years of age. In 2009, 38% were older than 55 years and 9% were 65 years or older. Allogeneic transplantation in patients without HLA-identical siblings was facilitated by establishment of large unrelated donor registries. In 1987 to 1992, fewer than 10% of HSCTs for hematologic malignancies used unrelated donors; in 2009, this figure was greater than 55%. More transplantation in older adults and increasing use of unrelated donors were the main reasons for the steady growth in allogeneic HSCT over the past 5 years.

CONDITIONING REGIMENS

Historically, conditioning regimens included myeloablative doses of cytotoxic drugs with or without radiation with the dual purpose of tumor cell kill and host immunosuppression. Myeloablative regimens for hematologic malignancies often involve a combination of cyclophosphamide (commonly 60 mg/kg/day for 2 days) and total-body irradiation (TBI) (8-15 Gy, single or fractionated doses). Many regimens substitute busulfan (typically, 4 mg/kg/day for 4 days orally or 3.2 mg/kg/day intravenously) in place of TBI. Posttransplant survival rates with cyclophosphamide and TBI and with cyclophosphamide and busulfan are similar, but there may be advantages for TBI-containing regimens in ALL. Other drugs such as etoposide, melphalan, and cytarabine are sometimes added to or substituted for cyclophosphamide or busulfan in a variety of regimens in efforts to provide better, generally disease-specific, antineoplastic activity. Large prospective trials comparing the efficacy of these regimens are lacking. A CIBMTR study suggested better outcomes in ALL in second complete remission (CR2) with either higher doses of TBI or substitution of cyclophosphamide by etoposide in a standard dose TBI regimen.

High-dose or myeloablative conditioning regimens are associated with significant risk of regimen-related toxicity. Toxicity can be minimized and efficacy improved with careful pharmacokinetic monitoring of certain drugs (e.g., busulfan).[2] Another strategy for lowering TRM is by reducing the dose intensity of the conditioning regimen. This approach uses lower doses of drugs and radiation to facilitate donor cell engraftment and relies more on GVT effects to eradicate malignant cells. The lower doses of cytotoxic agents produce less host tissue damage and less inflammatory cytokine secretion, resulting in less regimen-related morbidity and mortality and, with some regimens, less GVHD. Use of reduced-intensity conditioning regimens greatly increased the applicability of allogeneic HSCT in patients ineligible for HSCT with conventional myeloablative regimens because of age or comorbidities. The development of these novel conditioning regimens produced a major change in practice in the past decade (Fig. 105-2).

The latest consensus criteria published by the CIBMTR distinguish between myeloablative, reduced-intensity, and nonmyeloablative regimens based on the likelihood of the regimen to produce toxicity to the recipient BM (Table 105-1).[3] Myeloablative regimens produce profound and usually irreversible pancytopenia within 1 to 3 weeks and are usually fatal in the absence of stem cell rescue. Nonmyeloablative regimens cause minimal cytopenia and do not necessarily require stem cell rescue for hematopoietic recovery. Reduced

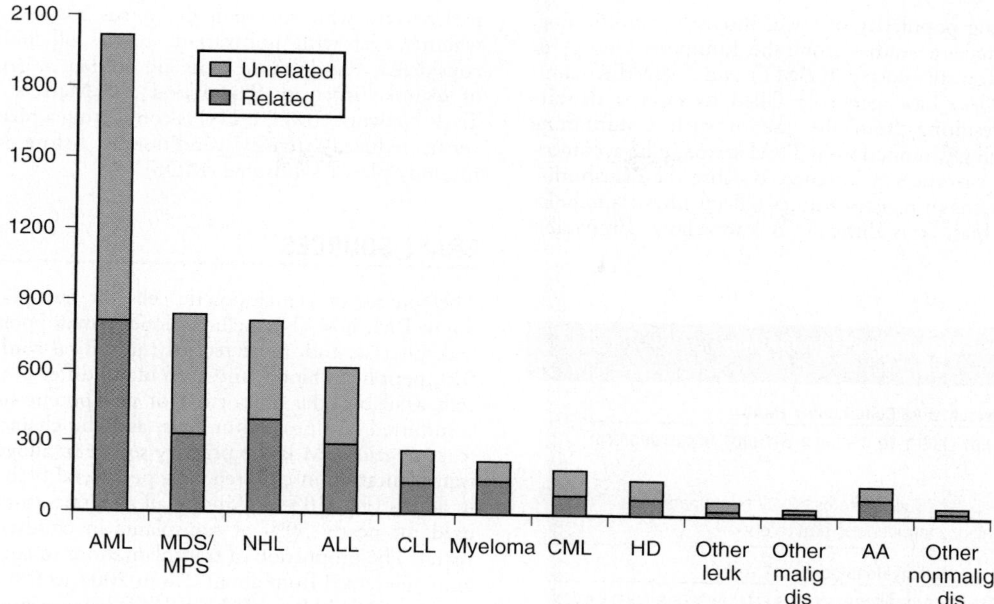

Figure 105-1 INDICATIONS FOR ALLOGENEIC HEMATOPOIETIC STEM CELL TRANSPLANTATION IN ADULTS (U.S. DATA), 2009. *AA,* Aplastic anemia; *ALL,* acute lymphoblastic leukemia; *AML,* acute myeloid leukemia; *CLL,* chronic lymphocytic leukemia; *CML,* chronic myeloid leukemia; *HD,* Hodgkin lymphoma; *MDS,* myelodysplastic syndrome; *MPS,* myeloproliferative disorders; *NHL,* non-Hodgkin lymphoma.

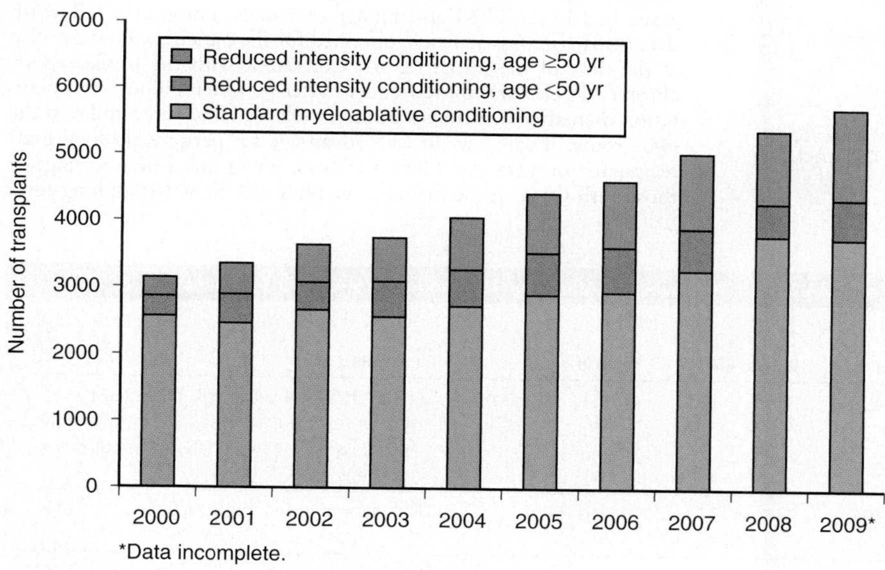

Figure 105-2 CONDITIONING REGIMEN INTENSITY AND PATIENT AGE—CHANGING TREND OVER TIME.

intensity regimens are an intermediate category not fitting well in either of the above because they produce pancytopenia that may recover without stem cell rescue but that is prolonged and, in clinical practice, requires stem cell support. It is important to recognize that these definitions are not based on the biologic effect of the transplant.

Reduced-intensity regimens induce less immune compromise in the immediate post-HSCT setting because the duration and depth of neutropenia are reduced and host-derived immunocompetent cells are not immediately eliminated. Additionally, the faster recovery of a more robust and complex T-cell repertoire and less organ toxicity make reduced-intensity regimens attractive for patients ineligible for conventional high-dose regimens because of advanced age or comorbidities.[4] Whether these benefits outweigh the risks of potentially reduced antitumor effects in patients eligible for high-dose conditioning regimens remains an important research question.

It is generally accepted that reduced intensity regimens allow HSCT to be done in some patients who will not be offered HSCT with myeloablative conditioning. For example, in the United States, the proportion of transplantations done in patients older than 60 years increased from fewer than 5% before 2000 to 12% in 2004 to 2008. Two-thirds of the latter patients received reduced-intensity conditioning regimens. The Seattle consortium described the outcomes of 372 “older” patients (ages 60-75 years) receiving very low-intensity nonmyeloablative regimens.[5] Increasing age was not associated with an increase in organ toxicity or GVHD, and the 5-year survival rate of the entire cohort was 35%. However, reduced-intensity regimens are increasingly used in patients of all ages receiving both related and unrelated donor transplants, as shown in Fig. 105-2. In 2009, about 30% of allogeneic transplantations for hematologic malignancies in patients between 18 and 55 years used reduced-intensity regimens.

Despite the growing popularity of lower intensity conditioning, large retrospective database studies from the European Group for Blood and Marrow Transplantation (EBMT) and CIBMTR (summarized in Table 105-2) have generally failed to show a definite survival advantage resulting from the use of such conditioning regimens. Disappointingly, reduction in TRM seems to be accompanied by a higher risk of cancer recurrence. Because the distribution of conditioning regimens in registry studies reflects physician choice or patient selection bias, it is difficult to know how comparable patients are who receive high- versus reduced-dose regimens and whether, even with multivariate analysis, all confounding factors are considered. Randomized trials are needed to gauge the true impact of regimen intensity. The Blood and Marrow Transplant Clinical Trials Network (BMT CTN) is conducting a phase III study of high- versus reduced-intensity conditioning before HSCT in AML or myelodysplastic syndrome (MDS).

Table 105-1 Consensus Definition of Conditioning Regimen Intensity

Myeloablative Conditioning (MAC)
PROFOUND CYTOPENIA; NOT LIKELY TO RECOVER WITHOUT HEMATOPOIETIC CELL RESCUE
Total-body irradiation ≥5 Gy single dose or ≥8 Gy fractionated
Busulfan >8 mg/kg orally or intravenous equivalent
Nonmyeloablative
MINIMAL CYTOPENIA; AUTOLOGOUS RECOVERY OF HEMATOPOIESIS LIKELY EVEN WITHOUT TRANSPLANT
Total-body irradiation ≤2 Gy ± purine analogue
Fludarabine + cyclophosphamide ± antithymocyte Globulin
Fludarabine + cytarabine ± idarubicin
Cladribine + cytarabine
Total lymphoid irradiation + antithymocyte globulin
REDUCED-INTENSITY CONDITIONING
Regimens that are intermediate between the above categories

Adapted from Bacigalupo A, Ballen K, Rizzo D, et al: Defining the intensity of conditioning regimens: working definitions. *Biol Blood Marrow Transplant* 15:1628, 2009.

GRAFT SOURCES

The sources of hematopoietic cells for transplantation, historically donor BM, now also include blood hematopoietic cells collected by leukapheresis and, more recently, umbilical cord blood. Grafts from BM, peripheral blood, and cord blood differ in the total numbers of cells available, the proportion of pluripotent stem cells to lineage-committed late progenitor cells, and the characteristics of immune reactive cells. BM is the primary source of allogeneic donor cells for transplantation in children, and peripheral blood is the main source in adults (Fig. 105-3). Among all allografts, umbilical cord blood is used for nearly 30% of transplants in children (younger than 20 years). The proportion of transplantations in adults using cord blood grafts increased from about 2% in 2004 to 6% in 2009.

The CIBMTR and the EBMT have examined long-term outcomes after peripheral blood versus BM grafts from HLA-identical siblings in adults with acute and chronic leukemia. The first report, with a median follow-up of 1 year, showed higher chronic GVHD rates in patients receiving peripheral blood grafts. Among patients transplanted for advanced leukemia, those receiving peripheral blood grafts had lower TRM and higher LFS rates. Long-term follow-up data (median, >6 years) were obtained for the patients who were alive at the time of the initial report. Consistent with the initial report, chronic GVHD was more frequent after peripheral blood transplantation than after BM transplantation; relapse rates were similar in the two groups. There was an LFS advantage for peripheral blood graft recipients for advanced CML (33% vs. 25%) but a disadvantage in those with CML in the first chronic phase (41% vs. 61%); long-term

Table 105-2 Retrospective Registry-Based Comparisons of NMA/RIC vs. Myeloablative Allogeneic Hematopoietic Stem Cell Transplantation

Group	Disease	Donor	*n* RIC vs. MAC	TRM RIC vs. MAC	Relapse	Comments
EBMT[33]	MDS or sAML >50	MUD 39%	315 vs. 407	32% vs. 44% at 4 years	41% vs. 33% at 4 years	Survival 31% at 4 years. RIC predicted for greater relapse but lower TRM in multivariate model. Wide variety of different conditioning regimens used.
EBMT[34]	MM	MUD 12%	320 vs. 196	24% vs. 37% at 2 years	27% vs. 54%	TRM lower after RIC but relapse risk is double.
EBMT[35]	AML	Sibling	215 vs. 621	22% vs. 32% at 3 years	45% vs. 27% at 3 years	Relapse rate higher and TRM lower in RIC but OS similar (41% vs. 45%) in both groups.
EBMT[36]	CLL	MUD 22%	73 vs. 82	19% vs. 26%	28% vs. 11%	Similar TRM but higher relapse risk after RIC.
EBMT[37]	HL	MUD 13%	89 vs. 79	23% vs. 46% at 1 year	57% vs. 30%	Relapse rate higher and TRM lower in RIC but OS similar.
CIBMTR[38]	Follicular NHL	Sibling	88 vs. 120	23% in both at 1 year	17% vs. 8%	RIC associated with higher risk of relapse but similar TRM but lower KPS impacted on TRM. OS was similar.
EBMT[39]	ALL	Sibling	127 vs. 449	21% vs. 29%	32% vs. 38%	TRM lower after RIC but higher relapse rate. LFS similar to MAC
CIBMTR[40]	AML or MDS	MUD or sibling	1448 vs. 3731	3-year TRM similar	Lower risk of relapse in myeloablative	Overall and disease-free survival was highest for myeloablative group.

ALL, Acute lymphoblastic leukemia; *AML*, acute myeloid leukemia; *CIBMTR*, Center for International Blood and Marrow Transplant Research; *CLL*, chronic lymphocytic leukemia; *EBMT*, European Group for Blood and Marrow Transplantation; *HL*, Hodgkin lymphoma; *KPS*, Karnofsky performance score; *LFS*, leukemia free survival; *MAC*, myeloablative conditioning; *MDS*, myelodysplastic syndrome; *MM*, multiple myeloma; *MUD*, matched unrelated donor; *NHL*, non-Hodgkin lymphoma; *NMA*, nonmyeloablative; *OS*, overall survival; *RIC*, reduced-intensity conditioning; *sAML*, secondary acute myeloid leukemia; *TRM*, transplant-related mortality.

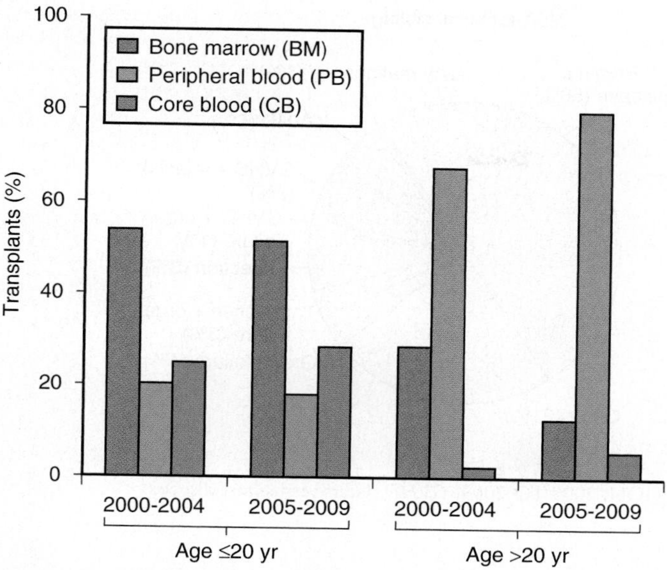

Figure 105-3 ALLOGENEIC STEM CELL SOURCES, BY DONOR TYPE VERSUS DONOR AGE, 2000 TO 2009.

LFS was similar with peripheral blood and BM in patients with acute leukemia. A meta-analysis using data from nine randomized trials of related donor peripheral blood versus BM transplants[6] suggested that patients receiving peripheral blood grafts had faster engraftment, a lower relapse rate if transplanted for hematologic malignancy and higher overall and disease-free survival if transplanted for late-stage disease. However, peripheral blood was also associated with a significantly increased risk of extensive chronic GVHD and conferred no survival advantage for patients with early stage disease. In the unrelated donor setting, a recent CIBMTR analysis of 917 transplants facilitated by the NMDP suggested that survival is similar with BM and peripheral blood grafts but that chronic GVHD is more frequent with peripheral blood. A large prospective randomized trial of 550 unrelated BM versus peripheral blood grafts for hematologic malignancies conducted in the United States by the BMT CTN was recently completed and shows similar findings—no difference in 2-year survival but a higher incidence risk of chronic GVHD in patients receiving peripheral blood.[7]

ALTERNATIVE DONOR TRANSPLANTS

A major obstacle to allogeneic HSCT is donor availability for the majority (70%) of adult patients without an HLA-identical sibling. At this time, identification of a 7/8 or 8/8 HLA-A, B, C, DRB1 allele matched adult donor is possible for about 90% of U.S. patients of white European ancestry, about 70% of those of Asian or Hispanic ancestry, and about 60% of those of African ancestry[8] (see Chapter 106). The unrelated donor search process can be time consuming, raising the risk of disease progression before transplantation can be performed. As a source of HSCs for unrelated donor transplantation, umbilical cord blood offers several advantages (see Chapter 108). It is readily available and entails no risk to the donor. Current data also indicate that HLA-matching criteria for cord blood transplantation need not be as stringent as for adult donor transplantation, greatly increasing the likelihood of finding a suitably matched graft for most patients. The major drawback of cord blood transplants is the limited number of cells in each cord blood unit, leading to slower rates of hematopoietic recovery compared with BM or peripheral blood grafts.

Numbers of cord blood transplants have increased steadily, especially in children but also in adults. Comparative data on cord blood versus adult donor transplantation come from registry studies. A CIBMTR analysis compared HLA-matched (at the allele level for A, B, C, and DRB1) BM transplants with matched and mismatched (intermediate resolution for A and B, allele level for DRB1) cord blood transplants in children with leukemia. The highest survival was in children receiving HLA-matched cord blood, although this group was small. There was no difference in outcome between HLA-matched BM and 5/6 HLA-locus matched cord blood transplants, providing the cord blood nucleated cell dose was greater than 3×10^7/kg body weight of recipient. A retrospective two-center comparative study demonstrated similar 5-year LFS after double cord blood unit, HLA-matched related donor, and HLA-allele matched or 1-antigen mismatched unrelated donor transplantation. At many experienced centers, unrelated donor and cord blood searches are simultaneously performed to ensure timely availability of a graft.

Comparisons of cord blood transplants in adults[9] consistently suggest slower hematopoietic recovery but less GVHD with cord blood grafts. Comparison of adult leukemia patients receiving cord blood versus matched unrelated BM or peripheral blood cell grafts indicated that LFS after cord grafts was comparable with that of 8/8 and 7/8 allele-matched BM or peripheral blood grafts. Results from these studies generally suggest that a one or two HLA-antigen mismatched cord blood graft of appropriate cell dose is an acceptable alternative for patients with hematologic malignancies who need HSCT but do not have an HLA-identical adult donor. Based on current evidence, cord blood grafts in adults are indicated in those without 8/8 matched unrelated donor availability or when transplantation is needed urgently. Patients without a single unit of adequate size may receive 2 units to units to facilitate engraftment.[10] Other approaches to facilitate engraftment with limited cord blood cell doses, including ex vivo cell expansion techniques, are in trials.

Human leukocyte antigen haploidentical donor HSCT (mismatched at 3 loci HLA A, B, and DR; usually parents, siblings, or children of patients) is another option for patients without matched sibling or unrelated donors (see Chapter 107). Despite the potential benefit of a strong GVT effect, the risk of severe GVHD has limited the applicability of haploidentical HSCT. Newer intense immunosuppressive strategies, graft T-cell depletion, and the use of post-transplantation cyclophosphamide have improved the safety of haploidentical transplants. Immediate donor availability and the potential to select donors with a favorable killer immunoglobulin receptor (KIR) phenotype that enhances antileukemia activity are advantages. The BMT CTN conducted two parallel multicenter phase 2 trials in patient with leukemia or lymphoma and no suitable related donors using either double cord blood units or HLA-haploidentical donor BM grafts (BMT CTN 0603) after reduced-intensity conditioning.[10] Survival at 1 year was similar: 54% after cord blood HSCT and 62% after haploidentical BM. Incidences of TRM and relapse after cord blood grafts were 24% and 31%, respectively; corresponding incidences after haploidentical BM grafts were 7% and 45%. Another approach combines a cord blood unit with a haploidentical T cell–depleted peripheral blood graft. Early hematopoietic recovery derives from the haploidentical graft but is later replaced by cord blood cell engraftment.

GRAFT VERSUS MALIGNANCY EFFECTS

Substantial laboratory and clinical evidence indicates that alloreactive cells exhibit potent anticancer activity (see Chapter 109). Barnes and Loutit studied leukemic mice treated with high-dose TBI and compared those receiving syngeneic and allogeneic BM infusions. Mice receiving syngeneic BM died quickly of leukemia; those receiving allogeneic cells survived longer but eventually developed fatal GVHD. Importantly, the allografted mice had no evidence of leukemia at death. Several canine and murine experiments reproduced these results.[11] Mathé and colleagues proposed the term *adoptive immunotherapy* for the antitumor effect of allogeneic cells. Antitumor effects could be specific (i.e., after sensitization of the donor or the donor's cells to antigens present on malignant cells) or nonspecific (i.e., associated with GVHD, an immune reaction of donor lymphocytes against normal and malignant host cells presumably triggered by differences in histocompatibility antigens).[12] The term

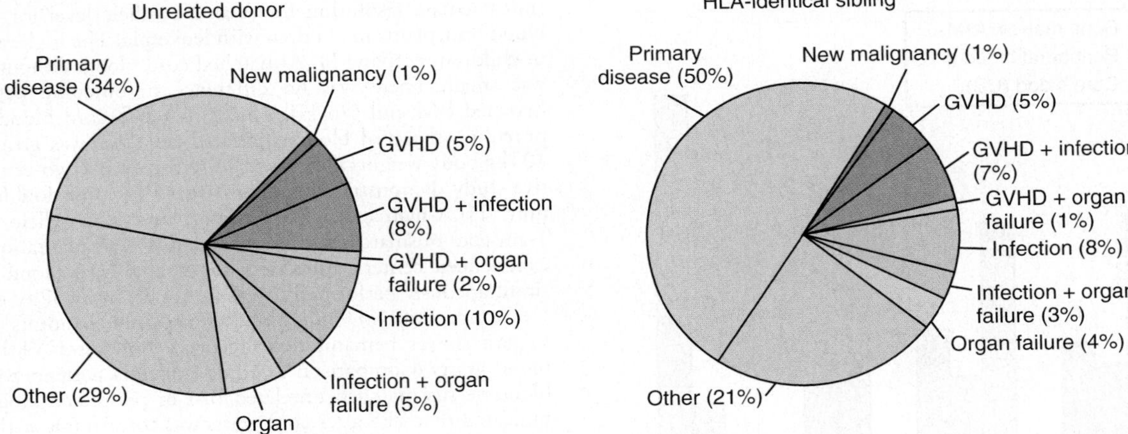

Figure 105-4 CAUSES OF DEATH AFTER TRANSPLANTATION, 2008 TO 2009. *GVHD,* Graft-versus-host diseases.

graft-versus-leukemia (GVL) was coined by Bortin and coworkers[11] to indicate the adoptive immunotherapeutic effect of transplanted allogeneic hematopoietic cells against leukemia cells. In some animal models, the GVL effect could not be distinguished from GVHD, but in others, the two were separable. Clinical evidence for the importance of GVL in eradicating tumor includes (1) a lower incidence of leukemia relapse in allograft recipients with acute or chronic GVHD than in those without GVHD,[12] (2) higher relapse rates after identical twin versus allogeneic HSCT,[12] (3) higher relapse rates after T cell–depleted transplants,[12] (4) durable cytogenetic and molecular remissions induced after posttransplant relapse by infusion of donor leukocytes without other antileukemia therapy,[13,14] and (5) durable remissions achieved after very low doses of conditioning agents (e.g., 200 cGy TBI) and allogeneic HSCT.[15] GVT effects are associated with GVHD, and measures that prevent or suppress GVHD may allow more relapse, but significant anticancer effects are demonstrable even in the absence of clinically significant GVHD, especially in AML and CML. The efficacy of immune-mediated antitumor effects varies by disease; they are most evident in myeloid leukemias and some subtypes of lymphoma.

The role of natural killer (NK) cells in the posttransplant setting is of increasing interest (see Chapter 102). After HSCT, donor-derived NK cells promote engraftment; reduce the risk of GVHD; enhance immune reconstitution; and decrease the risk of relapse, especially in AML.[16] In the physiologic state, NK cells can engage and kill target cells lacking major histocompatibility (HLA) class I molecules. This function is regulated by signaling through the killer-cell immunoglobulin-like receptor (KIR) family. In the allogeneic setting, lack of expression of the inhibitory KIRs' ligand on the recipient's leukemic cells can trigger donor NK cell alloreactivity against leukemia. The KIR family represents a second immunogenetic system inherited independent of HLA that can affect transplant outcomes, especially relapse-free survival in AML. It has been proposed that in the setting of HSCT for AML, KIR genotyping be used in addition to HLA typing by selecting donors with favorable KIR haplotypes.[17] In the setting of haploidentical and T cell–depleted HSCT for myeloid malignancies, donor–recipient KIR ligand mismatching is associated with favorable outcomes in some studies.

PROGNOSTIC FACTORS

Although allogeneic HSCT has efficacy in hematologic malignancies, the procedure carries a substantial risk of morbidity and mortality. TRM may result from toxicity of the pretransplant conditioning regimen to the lung, liver, and other organs or complications of cytopenia, GVHD, and infection related to delayed immune reconstitution, especially in the setting of GVHD or its treatment. The risk of TRM may be 30% or higher in adults receiving unrelated donor transplantation. Additionally, many patients have recurrence of their malignancy despite intensive conditioning and GVL. Primary causes of death after allogeneic transplantation for hematologic malignancy are shown in (Fig. 105-4). The prognosis of transplant recipients is influenced by several factors associated with risk of TRM or cancer recurrence or progression.

Donor Factors

Historically, TRM rates were lower after HLA-identical sibling than after other related or unrelated donor transplants because of less graft failure, faster immune reconstitution, and less GVHD. Considerable progress has been made in reducing the risk of TRM after both HLA-identical sibling and alternative donor HSCT. For matched sibling donor HSCT in AML in CR1, the incidence of TRM decreased from 29% in 1985 to 1989 to about 15% in 2000 to 2004. For unrelated donor HSCT, the incidence of TRM in 1990 to 1994 was 39%, which decreased to 31% by 2000 to 2004.[18] Among alternative donor transplants, those from more closely HLA-matched donors tend to have lower risks of GVHD and TRM. Donor–recipient HLA mismatching is associated with an increased risk of posttransplant complications, including graft rejection, acute and chronic GVHD, and mortality; risks increase progressively with multiple HLA mismatches. With modern molecular HLA typing techniques (allowing selection of more closely HLA-matched donors) and current GVHD prevention strategies, the difference in TRM between HLA-matched sibling and unrelated donor transplantation has narrowed (Fig. 105-5). Using data reported to the CIBMTR in 2009, TRM at day 100 for adults with acute leukemia receiving allografts was 10% overall, 8% for those transplanted in remission, and 14% for those transplanted with active disease. At 1 year, the TRM was 20% overall and 17% and 24% for those in remission and with active disease at HSCT, respectively. The causes of death in the first 100 days posttransplant mainly relate to the primary disease, GVHD, infection, and end-organ damage.

Adoption of molecularly defined HLA matching techniques, calcineurin inhibitor–based GVHD prophylaxis, fungal prophylaxis with azoles, leukocyte reduction of blood products, newer assays for viral reactivation, and pharmacokinetic testing of conditioning drugs are some of the major innovations that have impacted TRM. Stratification and scoring of patient comorbidity and genome-wide analysis for polymorphisms that predict for susceptibility to TRM are currently being explored to develop tailored approaches to HSCT that may make it safer.

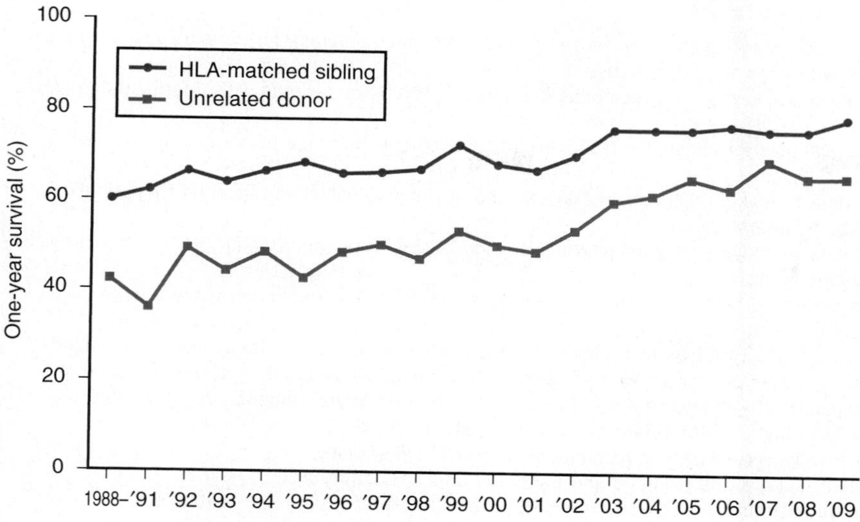

Figure 105-5 ONE-YEAR SURVIVAL AFTER MYELOABLATIVE HEMATOPOIETIC STEM CELL TRANSPLANTATION IN YOUNGER PATIENTS (RELATED VS. UNRELATED DONOR). *HLA,* Human leukocyte antigen.

Timing of Transplantation

In general, HSCT outcomes are better when transplantation is done earlier in the course of a malignancy (see box on Timing of Hematopoietic Cell Transplantation and Transplant Referral). Transplantation for advanced disease is associated with higher risks of both relapse and TRM. High TRM in the setting of advanced disease likely reflects patients' poorer clinical status and the cumulative effects of more extensive prior treatment. Because some hematologic malignancies have an excellent prognosis with nontransplant therapy (e.g., children with standard risk ALL or adults with acute promyelocytic leukemia), appropriate timing of transplantation requires consideration of likely outcomes with transplant and nontransplant therapies. However, even when not used as first-line therapy, transplantation should not be inordinately delayed because patients with refractory disease or severe complications from extensive prior therapy are unlikely to benefit. For patients with diseases potentially curable by allografting, appropriate timing of transplantation should be considered early in planning management strategies. This includes determining the availability of suitable related or unrelated donors. The American Society for Blood and Marrow Transplantation (ASBMT) has developed evidence-based guidelines based on current clinical practice and available literature (available online at http://www.asbmt.org; see boxes on American Society of Blood and Marrow Transplantation Consensus Policy for Allogeneic Hematopoietic Cell Transplantation and Transplant Referral: Guidelines for Transplant Consultation for Hematologic Malignancies).

Timing of Hematopoietic Cell Transplantation and Transplant Referral

- HSCT outcomes are better when performed earlier in the course of hematologic malignancies.
- HSCT for advanced disease is associated with higher TRM and relapse.
- Appropriate timing of HSCT requires consideration of likely outcomes with nontransplant and transplant therapies and the suitability of patient to undergo HSCT.
- Even when not considered as front-line therapy, inordinate delay in HSCT is to be avoided.
- For patients who are potentially curable by allogeneic HSCT, consideration of HSCT should be addressed early in the treatment plan. This includes HLA typing and identification of suitable donors.

Patient- and Disease-Related Factors

Transplant-related mortality is lower and, consequently, survival is higher, in patients who are young, cytomegalovirus (CMV) antibody screen negative, and have good performance scores and no active infection.[19] Age still poses a significant barrier to application of allogeneic HSCT because older patients are at significantly higher risk of regimen-related toxicity and GVHD. Consequently, the median age of transplant recipients is substantially lower than the median age at diagnosis of the diseases for which transplantation is done. Factors associated with increased likelihood of relapse or progression after conventional therapy also predict increased risk of posttransplant relapse or progression. Importantly, patients whose disease does not respond to conventional therapy are significantly less likely to have durable remissions after transplantation than those with responsive disease. However, HSCT may cure a significant proportion of patients with diseases considered incurable with non-transplant therapy.

CLINICAL RESEARCH IN ALLOGENEIC TRANSPLANTATION

The number of HSCTs performed in the United States is increasing at a rate of approximately 5% per year. Only a minority of patients have their transplantations performed in clinical trials. Challenges unique to the field of HSCT, such as small numbers treated at individual centers, the wide variety of indications, and multiple competing risks in the peritransplant period, make it difficult to perform single-center studies. To overcome these challenges, in the United States, a national multicenter transplant study network has been established. The BMT CTN has thus far launched 27 multicenter trials and accrued more than 4000 patients.

Although clinical trials focus on short- and intermediate-term outcomes, there is also a need for long-term follow-up of transplant recipients. Outcomes registries, such as those maintained by the CIBMTR and the EBMT, are important in facilitating additional clinical research. The CIBMTR maintains a large database of clinical information on the outcome of HSCTs performed in 500 transplant centers in nearly 50 countries. The database includes information on more than 350,000 transplant recipients. Data quality and consecutive registration are ensured through extensive computer checks and on-site audits. Data collection is through a web-based data entry program. Some important questions, such as results of HSCT in specific patient groups and rare diseases, analysis of prognostic factors, evaluation of new transplant regimens, comparison of HSCT with nontransplant therapy, and defining intercenter variability in practice and outcome, are difficult to address in randomized trials and can be studied using registry data. Analysis of outcomes after transplantation

American Society of Blood and Marrow Transplantation Consensus Policy for Allogeneic Hematopoietic Cell Transplantation*

Disease State	*Policy Regarding Allogeneic Transplantation*
AML in adults[30]	1. Survival advantage is established for allogeneic HSCT vs. chemotherapy for patients younger than age 55 years with high-risk cytogenetics. 2. Insufficient evidence to routinely recommend allogeneic HSCT for patients with intermediate-risk cytogenetics. 3. No survival advantage for allogeneic HSCT in patients younger than age 55 years with low-risk cytogenetics. 4. Insufficient data to make a recommendation for the use of myeloablative regimens for patients older than age 55 years. 5. Insufficient data to make a recommendation for reduced-intensity conditioning (RIC) followed by HSCT vs. chemotherapy. 6. For patients in second complete remission, allogeneic HSCT is recommended if there is an available donor.
ALL in adults[26]	1. In first CR, allogeneic HSCT as first-choice therapy is appropriate for all risk groups. In younger patients (younger than 35 years), with standard risk, Ph-negative ALL, HSCT results in superior survival compared with chemotherapy. In older (older than 35 years) patients, with standard risk Ph-negative ALL, higher TRM diminishes survival benefits of HSCT. 2. In second CR, allogeneic HSCT is recommended over chemotherapy. 3. There is similar survival after related and unrelated donor HSCT for ALL. 4. RIC may produce similar outcomes to myeloablative, but available data are limited. RIC is appropriate only for patients with ALL in remission and unsuited for myeloablative conditioning.
Diffuse large B-cell lymphoma[31]	1. Survival outcomes are equivalent for autologous and allogeneic HSCT; neither option is recommended over the other. Comparison between the two techniques is biased by different patient selection criteria. 2. Based on limited data, RIC is an acceptable alternative for selected patients who cannot tolerate a myeloablative regimen.
Follicular non-Hodgkin lymphoma[32]	3. Autologous vs. allogeneic HSCT: There are insufficient data to recommend one option over the other because comparison between the two techniques is biased by different patient selection criteria. 4. Based on limited data and expert opinion, RIC is an acceptable alternative approach to myeloablation. 5. Based on expert opinion, matched unrelated donor transplants are considered as effective as matched related donor transplants.
Myeloma	6. Autologous transplant is preferred over allogeneic HSCT based on current evidence. Studies are ongoing to further evaluate the role of allogeneic HSCT.

*Available at http://www.asbmt.org/displaycommon.cfm?an=4.

Transplant Referral: Guidelines for Transplant Consultation for Hematologic Malignancies*

Adult Acute Myeloid Leukemia

High-risk AML, including:

- Antecedent hematologic disease (e.g., myelodysplasia)
- Treatment-related leukemia
- Induction failure

First complete remission with poor-risk cytogenetics or high-risk molecular markers

Second complete remission and beyond

Adult Acute Lymphoblastic Leukemia

First complete remission up to age 35 years

High-risk ALL in those older than age 35 years, including:

- Poor-risk cytogenetics (e.g., Philadelphia chromosome or 11q23 rearrangements)
- High WBC (>30,000-50,000/cu mm) at diagnosis
- CNS or testicular leukemia
- No CR within 4 weeks of initial treatment
- Induction failure

Second complete remission and beyond

Chronic Myeloid Leukemia

- No hematologic or minor cytogenetic response 3 months after imatinib initiation
- No complete cytogenetic response 6 to 12 months after imatinib initiation
- Disease progression, accelerated phase, or blast crisis

Non-Hodgkin Lymphoma

Follicular Lymphoma

- Poor response to initial therapy
- Initial remission duration <12 months
- Second relapse
- Transformation to diffuse large B-cell lymphoma

Diffuse Large B-Cell Lymphoma

- First or subsequent relapse
- First CR for patients with high or high intermediate IPI
- No CR with initial treatment

Mantle Cell Lymphoma

- After initial therapy

Hodgkin Lymphoma

No initial CR

First or subsequent relapse

Multiple Myeloma

After initiation of therapy

At first progression

*Available online at http://www.marrow.org/PHYSICIAN/Medical_Education/Quick_Reference/index.html?src=mdguidelines.

needs an understanding of statistical methodologies such as multistate modeling. Such models involve competing risk problems such as the study of relapse versus death in remission or the complex interrelationships among engraftment, transplant complications (e.g., infection or GVHD), and primary events such as death or relapse.[20] Outcomes registries also provide a platform to analyze the availability, access, and economics of HSCT. A biospecimen repository maintained by the NMDP and associated with the CIBMTR database allows the linkage of clinical and immunologic data for analysis and has led to important insights into transplant immunobiology.

LONG-TERM SURVIVAL AFTER ALLOGENEIC TRANSPLANTATION

Most deaths related to HSCT occur within the first 2 years. However, an analysis of 2-year survivors found that compared with age- and nationality-matched death rates, subsequent survival was still inferior for HSCT recipients.[21] Overall, 85% of 2-year survivors were still alive at 10 years post-HSCT. Late relapse was the major cause of late deaths and was associated with advanced disease at HSCT. Older age and GVHD were the other major predictors of late mortality.

There are now about 250,000 persons surviving 5 years or more after transplantation, and that number is growing. Most 5-year survivors are well, off all immune suppression, and leading normal lives. However, transplant recipients remain at risk for late complications, including late infections, cataracts, abnormalities of growth and development, thyroid disorders, chronic lung disease, and avascular necrosis. There is also an increased incidence of leukemias, myelodysplasia, and solid tumors in transplant recipients compared with the general population. Lifelong surveillance is necessary, as is increased awareness of late complications among the many nontransplant physicians who will care for these patients. Recommended long-term follow-up of HSCT recipients is summarized in the box Recommended Practices for Allogeneic Transplant Recipients in Long-Term Follow-up.

DISEASE-SPECIFIC INDICATIONS FOR ALLOGENEIC TRANSPLANTATION

Acute Myeloid Leukemia

There is general agreement that most patients younger than the age of about 60 years who fail conventional therapy and who have good performance status are best treated with allogeneic transplantation if an appropriate related or unrelated donor is available (see Chapter 60). HSCT is not recommended for those with favorable risk cytogenetics with the possible exception of those with additional mutations in the KIT gene in the setting of core binding factor AML.

The National Comprehensive Cancer Network (NCCN) guidelines,[22] widely used to guide cancer therapy in the United States, distinguishes between patients younger than 60 versus those older than 60 years. Among younger patients, the panel recommended a postremission strategy based on factors such as the expected relapse rates with high-dose cytarabine therapy alone, salvage treatment options at relapse, and patient-specific comorbidities that predict for TRM. The guidelines uniformly endorsed allogeneic HSCT from related or unrelated donors including cord blood HSCT, in first remission for patients with unfavorable cytogenetic or molecular abnormalities, therapy-related AML, or prior myelodysplasia. Also, there was consensus that patients with high-risk features such as an elevated leukocyte count at presentation and those needing more than 1 cycle to achieve a remission be considered for allogeneic HSCT in first remission. Among those older than 60 years, the recommendation was to consider HSCT as an early option in those achieving a complete response and as treatment for induction failure only in patients with low-volume residual disease. For relapsed AML, HSCT was recommended irrespective of age but only after a complete remission was achieved or in the context of a clinical trial. For patients with acute promyelocytic leukemia, the recommendation was to reserve allogeneic HSCT for patients with persistent relapsed disease despite salvage therapy.

The ASBMT's evidence-based policy for allogeneic HSCT in AML recommends HSCT in the relapse setting (after achievement of a second complete remission) and in patients with poor-risk cytogenetics in first remission. The ASBMT guidelines did not routinely recommend allogeneic HSCT for patients with intermediate-risk cytogenetics, myeloablative conditioning for patients older than age 55 years, or use of reduced-intensity conditioning. The NMDP guidelines for transplant evaluation recommend an HSCT consultation for all patients with high-risk AML (defined as AML preceded by another hematologic disorder, treatment-related leukemia, and primary induction failure), those with poor prognostic markers by cytogenetics or molecular studies, and patients in second or subsequent remission.

A systematic review of various national guidelines found the following[23]:

1. Consistent recommendations that patients with relapsed or refractory disease or high-risk cytogenetics be considered for HSCT.
2. Consistent recommendations that patients with good prognosis cytogenetics receive HSCT only after failure of nontransplant therapy.
3. Inconsistent recommendations for patients with intermediate-risk disease or without a family donor regarding transplantation in the first remission.
4. Lack of consensus regarding the efficacy of reduced-intensity conditioning.
5. Most national guidelines recommend a risk-based approach to guide selection of chemotherapy versus transplant approaches using factors such as patient age, comorbid conditions, disease phenotype at diagnosis, and the number of cycles of therapy before remission.

Acute Lymphoblastic Leukemia

Allogeneic HSCT in first remission from related or unrelated donors is generally accepted as the most effective available therapy for patients with Philadelphia chromosome (Ph)-positive ALL. For adults with Ph-negative ALL, the appropriate timing of HSCT is more controversial despite the largest prospective study (MRC/ECOG) and a meta-analysis suggesting a survival advantage for those assigned to transplant in first remission.[24,25] Allogeneic transplantation is currently considered by NCCN expert consensus as the best curative therapy for adult patients with high risk features such Ph+ ALL or those with a poor response to initial induction therapy and among adults with t(4;11) ALL. A recent evidence-based policy statement from the ASBMT recommended allogeneic HSCT for young (younger than 35 years) adults in first remission irrespective of risk group and for ALL in second or higher remission. Related and unrelated donor HSCT were recommended as being similar in outcomes.[26] For those without suitable matched adult donors, cord blood grafts should be considered.

Chronic Myeloid Leukemia

In general, HSCT is indicated for patients whose initial presentation is in blast phase and should be considered for those with a suboptimal response or relapse while taking tyrosine kinase inhibitors (TKIs) (see Chapter 66). HSCT is also a consideration for patients who have bcr-abl mutations that predict for TKI nonresponse. It is important to establish a monitoring plan for early signs of progression and for mutation screening because outcomes are significantly better if HSCT is performed before transformation to advanced disease. Definitions of suboptimal response and failure with TKIs and guidelines

Recommended Practices for Allogeneic Transplant Recipients in Long-Term Follow-up

	6 mo	12 mo	Annual	Comments (*)
Liver				
Liver function tests	√	√	*	Annual check only if previously abnormal or new signs or symptoms
Serum ferritin		√	*	
Respiratory				
Clinical assessment	√	√	√	
Smoking and tobacco avoidance	√	√	√	
Formal pulmonary function tests		√	*	Annual study or imaging as needed in follow-up of prior or new abnormalities
Chest radiograph	*	*	*	
Bone density screening		√	*	High risk: women and those on prolonged steroid or calcineurin inhibitor use
Kidney				
Blood pressure screen	√	√	√	
Proteinuria screen	√	√	*	Annually as needed
BUN and creatinine level	√	√	√	
Nervous System				
Clinical assessment		√	*	Annually as needed
Endocrine				
Thyroid function		√	*	Annually as needed
Gonadal function in postpubertal women		√	√	
Cardiac and Vascular				
Cardiovascular risk factor screen		√	√	
Immune System and Infection Risk				
Encapsulated organism prophylaxis	*	*	*	If on immune suppression or with ongoing GVHD
Pneumocystis prophylaxis	√	*	*	
CMV test	√	√		
Immunizations		√	√	
Endocarditis prophylaxis		*	*	Follow AHA guidelines
Antifungal and antiherpes viral prophylaxis	*	*	*	If on immune suppression or with GVHD; if not, no consensus
Second Cancer Risk				
Cancer risk assessment and education		√	√	
Pap smear		√	√	
Mammography (women older than 40 years)		√	√	
Breast, skin, testes self-examination		√	√	
Clinical screen for second cancers		√	√	
Psychosocial				
Clinical psychosocial and QOL screen	√	√	√	
Sexual function screen	√	√	√	
Dental Assessment	√	√	√	
Ocular				
Clinical evaluation	√	√	√	
Fundus examination		√	*	Annualy as needed
Schirmer test		*	*	If with ongoing GVHD or on immune suppression

AHA, American Heart Association; *BUN*, blood urea nitrogen; *CMV*, cytomegalovirus; *GVHD*, graft-versus-host disease; *QOL*, quality of life.

for monitoring have been developed.[27] In 2011, the NCCN taskforce recommended consideration of HSCT in chronic phase CML for those receiving second-line TKI therapy after failing primary TKI therapy. In this setting, failure to achieve complete hematologic response at 3 months or any cytogenetic response at 6 to 12 months or at least a partial cytogenetic response at 18 months after initiation of therapy or a cytogenetic relapse at any time on therapy were considered indications to proceed to HSCT. For those with CML progression to advanced phase or blast crisis, TKI-based therapy for induction followed by HSCT was recommended. European experts have evolved very similar recommendations and consider HSCT the only curative option for patients in accelerated or blast phase, patients with T315I mutation, and those in chronic phase failing or intolerant of second-generation TKIs.

Chronic Lymphocytic Leukemia

Current NCCN guidelines recommend allogeneic HSCT in chronic lymphocytic leukemia for those of younger age with high-risk disease (TP53 deletion, 11q deletion) in the front-line setting, and for those with CLL relapsing shortly after initial response (<2 years) irrespective of cytogenetics. The EBMT consensus group[28] has recommended allogeneic HSCT as a reasonable treatment option for younger patients with nonresponse, partial responses, or relapse (within 12 months) after purine analogue therapy. Patients who relapse within 24 months after having a response to purine analogue–based combinations and patients with TP53 abnormalities and those with Richter transformation requiring treatment are also considered candidates for transplant evaluation.

Diffuse Large B-Cell Lymphoma

The NCCN guidelines recommend autologous transplantation (after second-line chemotherapy) as the treatment of choice for relapsed or refractory diffuse large B-cell lymphoma. Allogeneic HSCT is a consideration in the context of clinical trials, and in selected situations, such as mobilization failure and persistent BM disease.

Follicular Lymphoma

A systematic review by the ASBMT noted the lack of high-quality evidence regarding indications for allogeneic HSCT in follicular lymphoma. The consensus panel recommended autologous HSCT for relapsed disease or transformed follicular lymphoma. In the allogeneic setting, reduced-intensity conditioning was considered an acceptable alternative to myeloablative regimens. The panel found no differences in outcomes between the use of HLA-identical sibling donors and matched unrelated donors. Given the efficacy of rituximab-based salvage treatments and autologous HSCT for follicular lymphoma, allogeneic HSCT is generally used for patients who have failed, are likely to fail, or are unable to proceed to salvage autologous HSCT. However, late application of allogeneic HSCT may be less effective, especially for chemotherapy-refractory disease. The NCCN guideline panel recommended autologous transplantation in second or third remission as a standard consolidative strategy for relapsed follicular lymphoma. Allogeneic HSCT was a consideration for highly selected patients and those with histologic transformation to a higher grade (especially in the context of a clinical trial).

Mantle Cell Lymphoma

In recent years, reduced-intensity conditioning is the standard approach for allogeneic HSCT for mantle cell lymphoma. Current NCCN guidelines recommend autologous transplantation as an adjunct to initial therapy in eligible patients because it has the potential of establishing durable remission.[29] Expert opinion is that allogeneic HSCT has a limited role as consolidation in chemotherapy-sensitive disease. Given the poor prognosis of recurrent mantle cell lymphoma and the curative potential of allogeneic HSCT, it is a reasonable option for patients relapsing after upfront autologous transplantation and those with chemotherapy-refractory disease.

T-Cell Lymphoma

The NCCN guidelines recommend consideration of allogeneic HSCT in the relapsed or refractory setting in T-cell lymphoma. In cutaneous T-cell lymphoma, allogeneic HSCT is considered in the setting of progressive or refractory stage IIB to IV disease after failure of biologic agents and at least one line of chemotherapy.

Hodgkin Lymphoma

The NCCN guidelines currently consider allogeneic HSCT in progressive or relapsed Hodgkin lymphoma as a category 3 recommendation (major disagreement) and recommend that this treatment should therefore ideally be performed as part of a clinical trial.

Multiple Myeloma

The NCCN guidelines consider allogeneic HSCT with myeloablative conditioning as an accepted option in the setting of a clinical trial, in those responding to primary therapy, and those with primary progressive disease. The guidelines did not recommend allogeneic HSCT with nonmyeloablative conditioning alone as an option. Reduced-intensity conditioning with allogeneic HSCT after autologous HSCT was considered a category 2A recommendation (reflecting uniform NCCN consensus based on lower level evidence, including clinical experience, that the recommendation is appropriate). Allogeneic HSCT in the relapsed setting after a prior autograft was considered a grade 3 recommendation, reflecting major disagreement.

REFERENCES

1. Thomas E, Storb R, Clift RA, et al: Bone-marrow transplantation (first of two parts). *N Engl J Med* 292:832, 1975.
2. Slattery JT, Clift RA, Buckner CD, et al: Marrow transplantation for chronic myeloid leukemia: The influence of plasma busulfan levels on the outcome of transplantation. *Blood* 89:3055, 1997.
3. Bacigalupo A, Ballen K, Rizzo D, et al: Defining the intensity of conditioning regimens: Working definitions. *Biol Blood Marrow Transplant* 15:1628, 2009.
4. Sorror ML, Maris MB, Storer B, et al: Comparing morbidity and mortality of HLA-matched unrelated donor hematopoietic cell transplantation after nonmyeloablative and myeloablative conditioning: Influence of pretransplantation comorbidities. *Blood* 104:961, 2004.
5. Sorror ML, Sandmaier BM, Storer BE, et al: Long-term outcomes among older patients following nonmyeloablative conditioning and allogeneic hematopoietic cell transplantation for advanced hematologic malignancies. *JAMA* 306:1874, 2011.
6. Stem Cell Trialists' Collaborative G: Allogeneic peripheral blood stem-cell compared with bone marrow transplantation in the management of hematologic malignancies: An individual patient data meta-analysis of nine randomized trials. *J Clin Oncol* 23:5074, 2005.
7. Anasetti C, Logan B, Lee SJ, et al: Increased Incidence of Chronic Graft-Versus-Host Disease (GVHD) and No Survival Advantage with Filgrastim-Mobilized Peripheral Blood Stem Cells (PBSC) Compared to Bone Marrow (BM) Transplants From Unrelated Donors: Results of Blood and Marrow Transplant Clinical Trials Network (BMT CTN) Protocol 0201, a Phase III, Prospective, Randomized Trial. *Blood* 118; Ash Annual Meeting Abstracts: Abstract 1, 2011.
8. Gragert L, Maiers M, Williams E, et al: Modeling effective patient-donor matching for hematopoietic transplantation in United States populations. *Human Immunol* 71:S114, 2010.
9. Laughlin MJ, Eapen M, Rubinstein P, et al: Outcomes after transplantation of cord blood or bone marrow from unrelated donors in adults with leukemia. *N Engl J Med* 351:2265, 2004.
10. Brunstein CG, Fuchs EJ, Carter SL, et al: Alternative donor transplantation after reduced intensity conditioning: Results of parallel phase 2 trials using partially HLA-mismatched related bone marrow or unrelated double umbilical cord blood grafts. *Blood* 118:282, 2011.
11. Bortin MM, Truitt RL, Rimm AA, Bach FH: Graft-versus-leukaemia reactivity induced by alloimmunisation without augmentation of graft-versus-host reactivity. *Nature* 281:490, 1979.
12. Horowitz MM, Gale RP, Sondel PM, et al: Graft-versus-leukemia reactions after bone marrow transplantation. *Blood* 75:555, 1990.
13. Porter DL, Roth MS, Lee SJ, et al: Adoptive immunotherapy with donor mononuclear cell infusions to treat relapse of acute leukemia or myelodysplasia after allogeneic bone marrow transplantation. *Bone Marrow Transplant* 18:975, 1996.
14. Collins R Jr, Shpilberg O, Drobyski W, et al: Donor leukocyte infusions in 140 patients with relapsed malignancy after allogeneic bone marrow transplantation. *J Clin Oncol* 15:433, 1997.
15. Maris MB, Niederwieser D, Sandmaier BM, et al: HLA-matched unrelated donor hematopoietic cell transplantation after nonmyeloablative conditioning for patients with hematologic malignancies. *Blood* 102:2021, 2003.

16. Leung W, Iyengar R, Turner V, et al: Determinants of antileukemia effects of allogeneic NK cells. *J Immunol* 172:644, 2004.
17. Cooley S, Weisdorf DJ, Guethlein LA, et al: Donor selection for natural killer cell receptor genes leads to superior survival after unrelated transplantation for acute myelogenous leukemia. *Blood* 116:2411, 2010.
18. Horan JT, Logan BR, Agovi-Johnson MA, et al: Reducing the risk for transplantation-related mortality after allogeneic hematopoietic cell transplantation: How much progress has been made? *J Clin Oncol* 29:805, 2011.
19. Boeckh M, Nichols WG: The impact of cytomegalovirus serostatus of donor and recipient before hematopoietic stem cell transplantation in the era of antiviral prophylaxis and preemptive therapy. *Blood* 103:2003, 2004.
20. Eapen M, Rocha V: Principles and analysis of hematopoietic stem cell transplantation outcomes: The physician's perspective. *Lifetime Data Analysis* 14:379, 2008.
21. Socie G, Stone JV, Wingard JR, et al: Long-term survival and late deaths after allogeneic bone marrow transplantation. Late Effects Working Committee of the International Bone Marrow Transplant Registry. *N Engl J Med* 341:14, 1999.
22. The NCCN GUIDELINE Practice Guidelines in Oncology—v.2.2011. Copyright 2011 National Comprehensive Cancer Network, Inc. Available at: http://www.nccn.org. Accessed [August 01, 2011]. To view the most recent and complete version of the guideline, go online to www.nccn.org. 2011.
23. Hubel K, Weingart O, Naumann F, et al: Allogeneic stem cell transplant in adult patients with acute myelogenous leukemia: A systematic analysis of international guidelines and recommendations. *Leuk Lymphoma* 52:444, 2011.
24. Goldstone AH, Richards SM, Lazarus HM, et al: In adults with standard-risk acute lymphoblastic leukemia, the greatest benefit is achieved from a matched sibling allogeneic transplantation in first complete remission, and an autologous transplantation is less effective than conventional consolidation/maintenance chemotherapy in all patients: Final results of the International ALL Trial (MRC UKALL XII/ECOG E2993). *Blood* 111:1827, 2008.
25. Ram R, Gafter-Gvili A, Vidal L, et al: Management of adult patients with acute lymphoblastic leukemia in first complete remission: Systematic review and meta-analysis. *Cancer* 116:3447, 2010.
26. Oliansky DM, Larson RA, Weisdorf D, et al: The role of cytotoxic therapy with hematopoietic stem cell transplantation in the treatment of adult acute lymphoblastic leukemia: Update of the 2006 evidence-based review. *Biol Blood Marrow Transplant* 18:16, 2011.
27. Baccarani M, Saglio G, Goldman J, et al: Evolving concepts in the management of chronic myeloid leukemia: Recommendations from an expert panel on behalf of the European LeukemiaNet. *Blood* 108:1809, 2006.
28. Dreger P, Corradini P, Kimby E, et al: Indications for allogeneic stem cell transplantation in chronic lymphocytic leukemia: The EBMT transplant consensus. *Leukemia* 21:12, 2007.
29. Rockova V, Abbas S, Wouters BJ, et al: Risk stratification of intermediate-risk acute myeloid leukemia: Integrative analysis of a multitude of gene mutation and gene expression markers. *Blood* 118:1069, 2011.
30. Oliansky DM, Appelbaum F, Cassileth PA, et al: The role of cytotoxic therapy with hematopoietic stem cell transplantation in the therapy of acute myelogenous leukemia in adults: An evidence-based review. *Biol Blood Marrow Transplant* 14:137, 2008.
31. Oliansky DM, Czuczman M, Fisher RI, et al: The role of cytotoxic therapy with hematopoietic stem cell transplantation in the treatment of diffuse large B cell lymphoma: Update of the 2001 evidence-based review. *Biol Blood Marrow Transplant* 17:20, 2011.
32. Oliansky DM, Gordon LI, King J, et al: The role of cytotoxic therapy with hematopoietic stem cell transplantation in the treatment of follicular lymphoma: An evidence-based review. *Biol Blood Marrow Transplant* 16:443, 2010.
33. Lim Z, Brand R, Martino R, et al: Allogeneic hematopoietic stem-cell transplantation for patients 50 years or older with myelodysplastic syndromes or secondary acute myeloid leukemia. *J Clin Oncol* 28(3):405, 2010.
34. Crawley C, Iacobelli S, Björkstrand B, et al: Reduced-intensity conditioning for myeloma: Lower nonrelapse mortality but higher relapse rates compared with myeloablative conditioning. *Blood* 109:3588, 2007.
35. Martino R, Iacobelli S, Brand R, et al: Retrospective comparison of reduced-intensity conditioning and conventional high-dose conditioning for allogeneic hematopoietic stem cell transplantation using HLA-identical sibling donors in myelodysplastic syndromes. *Blood* 108:836, 2006.
36. Dreger P, Brand R, Milligan D, et al: Reduced-intensity conditioning lowers treatment-related mortality of allogeneic stem cell transplantation for chronic lymphocytic leukemia: A population-matched analysis. *Leukemia* 19:1029, 2005.
37. Sureda A, Robinson S, Canals C, et al: Reduced-intensity conditioning compared with conventional allogeneic stem-cell transplantation in relapsed or refractory Hodgkin's lymphoma: An analysis from the Lymphoma Working Party of the European Group for Blood and Marrow Transplantation. *J Clin Oncol* 26:455, 2008.
38. Hari P, Carreras J, Zhang MJ, et al: Allogeneic transplants in follicular lymphoma: Higher risk of disease progression after reduced-intensity compared to myeloablative conditioning. *Biol Blood Marrow Transplant* 14:236, 2008.
39. Mohty M, Labopin M, Volin L, et al: Reduced-intensity versus conventional myeloablative conditioning allogeneic stem cell transplantation for patients with acute lymphoblastic leukemia: A retrospective study from the European Group for Blood and Marrow Transplantation. *Blood* 116:4439, 2010.
40. Luger SM, Ringdén O, Zhang MJ, et al: Similar outcomes using myeloablative vs. reduced-intensity allogeneic transplant preparative regimens for AML or MDS. *Bone Marrow Transplant* 47:203, 2012.

CHAPTER 106

UNRELATED DONOR HEMATOPOIETIC CELL TRANSPLANTATION

Effie W. Petersdorf and Claudio Anasetti

The outcomes of unrelated donor hematopoietic cell transplantation (HCT) have greatly improved as a result of better understanding of the diversity of genes that give rise to host-versus-graft (HVG) and graft-versus-host (GVH) allorecognition. Development of robust typing methods that define functional variation of human leukocyte antigen (HLA) and killer immunoglobulin-like receptor (KIR) genes have greatly accelerated understanding of gene–gene interactions that lead to graft failure, graft-versus-host disease (GVHD), and graft-versus-leukemia (GVL). Elucidation of which HLA molecules are the ligands for KIR receptors of natural killer (NK) cells and discovery of the pivotal role played by NK alloreactivity are opening up new avenues for potential antitumor therapy. Continued growth of registries of volunteer donors worldwide now provides the potential for identifying suitable donors for up to 65% of white patients in need of a transplant. The major challenges are to increase the safety and efficacy of unrelated donor HCT therapy through improved prevention and treatment of GVHD while leveraging control of leukemia through GVL effects. For unrelated HCT to be more widely applied to patients of diverse ethnic and racial backgrounds, more information on permissible HLA mismatches is needed so that mismatched donors can be safely used when matched donors are not available. This chapter chronicles genotyping methods used for donor selection and the clinical results of unrelated donor HCT in the era of DNA typing for HLA and KIR genes. Double cord blood transplantation (CBT) permits almost every patient a transplant when matched cell sources are not available. The relative merit of CBT compared with mismatched unrelated donor transplantation has not been elucidated. Readers are invited to read Chapter 108 for more detailed information on CBT.

VOLUNTEER REGISTRIES

The field of allogeneic transplantation has witnessed a rapid growth in the use of unrelated donors over the past 15 years. In a Center for International Bone Marrow Transplant Research (CIBMTR) survey, unrelated donor transplants accounted for the largest increase among all transplants and for 51% of the allogeneic transplants in the United States. A total of 16,974 transplants were performed yearly, of which 39% were allogeneic and 20% from unrelated donors (http://www.CIBMTR.org). The primary indications for unrelated donor HCT were leukemia (acute myeloid leukemia [AML], acute lymphoblastic leukemia [ALL], myelodysplastic syndrome [MDS], lymphoma, chronic myeloid leukemia [CML], multiple myeloma [MM], and chronic lymphocytic leukemia [CLL]) and nonmalignant disorders. In Europe, unrelated donor transplants also constitute 51% of all allogenic transplants, and they are performed for treatment of leukemia (63%), MDS and myeloproliferative disorders (8%), lymphoma (16%), and nonmalignant disorders (8%).[1] Approximately one-third of allogenic transplants are performed for patients ages 50 years and older.

Unrelated HCT has been made feasible by the establishment of registries of volunteer donors worldwide. The Anthony Nolan Appeal was the first effort to demonstrate the feasibility of donor recruitment. Now known as the Anthony Nolan Research Institute, this registry was the first to promote access to HLA-matched bone marrow (BM) donors for patients around the world. In the United States, early efforts for donor recruitment were spearheaded by individual centers. Growing interest in unrelated donor HCT led the U.S. Congress to authorize the creation of a national registry comprising a network of donor centers, transplant centers, and a national coordinating center through the Transplant Act of 1984. Two years later, a federal contract to establish a national registry was awarded to the National Marrow Donor Program (NMDP) (http://www.nmdp.org). In the Netherlands, Professor Jon J. van Rood led the Europdonor Foundation in the collection of HLA data from donor registries around the world and in the formation of a database of HLA phenotypes known as Bone Marrow Donors Worldwide (BMDW) (http://www.bmdw.org). Continued growth in registry size worldwide has increased the chances that well-matched donors can be identified. The NMDP registers 25,500 new donors each month and more than 300,000 each year (http://www.marrow.org). Today, more than 8 million donors are available through the NMDP, and more than 18 million donors are available through international cooperative agreements with registries around the world (http://www.worldmarrow.org).[2] With this database of 18 million donors, North American white patients have a 62% chance of identifying an 8/8 matched unrelated donor. This number increases to 89% if the donor selection criteria are relaxed to 7/8. The situation is not as favorable for patients of non-European white background. For African Americans, the likelihood of finding an 8/8 matched donor is only 15% and improves to 63% with 7/8 donors. These statistics emphasize that although the total number of donors is climbing, the challenges for the future remain achieving the ideal optimal registry size and composition to improve the odds that every patient in need of a transplant has at least one suitable donor.

The median time from initiation of a formal unrelated donor search to a request for a donation is 51 days (http://www.marrow.org). Although more than half of all U.S. patients who initiate a search will have 10 or more suitably matched NMDP donors, the efficiency of the search process is highly dependent on the racial and ethnic background of the recipient and the composition of the registry. A Dutch study of 549 unrelated donor searches conducted between 1987 and 2000 showcased the differences between median search times for patients of Northwestern and non-Northwestern European descent.[3] Whereas almost 60% of Northwestern European patients received a transplant within a median time of 4.4 months from the start of the search, only 32% of non-Northwestern European patients were able to identify suitable donors, and half did not have a compatible donor. For all patients, the efficiency with which the unrelated donor search is conducted is critical, and guidelines for planning transplantation as well as approaches for surmounting the unique challenges of finding donors are available (http://www.asbmt.org/policystat/policy.html).

DONOR EVALUATION AND SELECTION

Selection of unrelated donors includes consideration for the level of the HLA tissue type match with the recipient and the presence of recipient antidonor antibodies, which place the patient at high risk for nonengraftment. Criteria other than HLA are considered for donor selection when more than one HLA-identical match is available for a given patient. An NMDP analysis designed to study donor variables associated with transplant outcome examined 6978 transplants performed between 1987 and 1999.[4] Improved recipient survival and disease-free survival (DFS) were observed with use of young BM donors; these transplant recipients experienced lower risks of both acute and chronic GVHD. With each increasing decade of donor age, the risk of acute and chronic GVHD increased by 10%. This study did not find any effects of donor gender on engraftment, acute GVHD, or survival. However, transplantation from parous female BM donors was associated with increased risk of chronic GVHD. Among female parous donors, the relative risk was 1.19 with a history of a single pregnancy and increased to 1.40 with two or more pregnancies. In general, larger (male) donors provide larger BM and peripheral blood stem cell (PBSC) doses compared with smaller (female) donors. Donor ABO blood type does not affect the risk of GVHD or mortality. In an NMDP analysis of 7043 transplants performed between 2000 and 2004, the donor–recipient HLA match status and younger donor age were the two variables significantly associated with clinical outcome. In an NMDP analysis of transplants performed through 2007, donor HLA mismatching was confirmed to be significantly associated with transplant outcome, trumping the cytomegalovirus (CMV) serostatus of the donor.[5]

Evaluation of unrelated donors includes a screening medical history, physical examination, and laboratory testing for risks associated with transmissible elements akin to blood transfusion donors. Special focus is placed on risks of transmission of hepatitis, human immunodeficiency virus (HIV), malaria, West Nile virus, transmissible spongiform encephalitis (Creutzfeldt-Jacob disease), and Chagas disease. Donor screening includes blood tests for HIV 1 and 2, hepatitis B virus, hepatitis C virus, *Treponema pallidum,* human T-cell lymphotrophic virus I and II, and CMV.

The importance of a "backup" donor has been increasingly recognized. In a Dutch study of 502 unrelated donor evaluations, 46 were cancelled with 78% deferred because of medical reasons and 22% deferred because of nonmedical reasons.[6] In half of the cases for which a backup donor was already identified, the delay in scheduling the transplant was less than 2 weeks. However, when no backup donor was available, the median delay to transplant was 18 weeks. Identification of backup donors is particularly important for patients with high-risk hematologic malignancies, whose disease tempo does not allow delays in transplantation.

Table 106-1 Common Definitions in Human Leukocyte Antigen Genetics

Term	Definition	Example
Allele	Unique sequence of an HLA gene defined by molecular methods	DRB1*04:01 allele is a unique sequence defined as DR4 by serologic methods
Antigen	Antibody-defined protein	DR4 antigen is a serologically defined protein product of an HLA gene
Haplotype	HLA genes inherited as a chromosomal unit	HLA-A1, HLA-B8, HLA-DR3 is a common haplotype among white populations
Genotype	Molecularly defined HLA allele or sequence	Genotypically matched donor and recipient are identical for the HLA alleles at a given HLA gene (e.g., HLA-DRB1*04:01)
Phenotype	Serologically defined HLA protein or antigen	Phenotypically matched donor and recipient share the same HLA antigen (e.g., HLA-DR4)

HLA, Human leukocyte antigen.

Table 106-2 Polymorphism of Human Leukocyte Antigen Genes

	Antigens	Alleles
HLA-A	24	1698
HLA-B	50	2271
HLA-C	9	1213
HLA-DRB1	15	975
HLA-DQB1	9	158
HLA-DPB1	6	149

Available at http://www.ebi.ac.uk/imgt/hla.
HLA, Human leukocyte antigen.

PROCESS OF IDENTIFYING A SUITABLE UNRELATED DONOR

Human Leukocyte Antigen Typing and Donor Matching in the DNA Era: Genetics of the Human Leukocyte Antigen Complex

The advent of molecular techniques has made possible the definition of unique sequence variants (alleles) that encode each HLA molecule that is recognized by an antibody (antigen; Table 106-1). Polymorphism ensures that a large array of foreign peptides can be presented to the immune system by HLA molecules. As of July 2011, more than 1698 HLA-A, 2271 HLA-B, 1213 HLA-C, 975 HLA-DRB1, 158 HLA-DQB1, and 149 HLA-DPB1 alleles have been defined in diverse human populations (http://www.ebi.ac.uk/imgt/hla; Table 106-2). HLA nomenclature was recently modified to accommodate the steady discovery of new human variants (http://www.ebi.ac.uk/imgt/hla). The HLA prefix is followed by a hyphen to separate the HLA prefix from the gene name (e.g., HLA-A). The gene is listed followed by an asterisk to separate the gene from the unique sequence (HLA-A*). The unique sequence name embodies up to four kinds of information, each delimited by a colon. The first set of numbers after the asterisk and before the first colon correspond to the serologic antigen equivalent (e.g., HLA-A*02 refers to sequences of the HLA-A2 antigen family). The second set of numbers provides the unique protein that correspond to the subtype (HLA-A*02:101). The third set of numbers indicate synonymous substitutions (HLA-A*02:101:01). The last series of numbers give information on noncoding variation often denoting expression (HLA-A*02:101:01:02 N). Letter suffixes are used to denote null alleles (N), low cell surface expression (L), a soluble secreted molecule not present on the surface of the cell (S), a cytoplasmic product not expressed on the cell surface (C), a protein with aberrant expression (A), and a sequence of questionable expression (Q). This new nomenclature has no limits on the number of digits for each of the four categories and in this way obviates the need for constant renumbering.

DNA genotyping was adopted as the standard technique for selection of HLA-matched unrelated donors because unrelated individuals who are matched for HLA antigens may not necessarily share the same HLA sequences. If HLA alleles can be expressed in any combination and if inheritance of alleles were random, then the total estimated number of possible five-locus HLA-A, HLA-B, HLA-C, HLA-DRB1, and HLA-DQB1 genotypes would be more than 1 × 1023. Clinical experience demonstrates that some patients have been able to find a matched donor even in a relatively small file of unrelated donors. Donor identification is successful because HLA alleles are found in association with each other at an observed frequency that exceeds their expected frequency, a phenomenon known as linkage disequilibrium (LD). The probability of identifying a matched donor for a given patient is higher when the patient and donor share

Table 106-3 Definition of Matching for Alleles and Antigens

Designation	Match Status	Examples*	Donor	Recipient
Allele	Antigen matched	HLA-B*44	HLA-B*44	
Allele	Matched	HLA-B*44:02	HLA-B*44:02	
Allele†	Mismatched	Antigen matched	HLA-B*44	
Allele	Mismatched	HLA-B*44:02	HLA-B*44:03	
Antigen‡	Mismatched	Antigen mismatched	HLA-B*44	HLA-B*27
Allele	Mismatched	HLA-B*44:02	HLA-B*27:05	

*Human leukocyte antigen (HLA) alleles and antigens are designated according to the World Health Organization Nomenclature for Factors of the HLA System.
†Defined by DNA sequencing.
‡Defined by serology.

a similar ethnic background. Linked HLA genes are inherited from each parent as a haplotype in classical Mendelian fashion (see Assessment of Human Leukocyte Antigen Haplotypes later). HLA gene and haplotype frequencies provide important data for estimating optimal registry size and composition (http://www.allelefrequencies.net).

Given the polymorphism of allele sequences that encompass variants of a single serologically defined antigen, it is not surprising that antigen-matched donor and patient pairs may differ for their alleles (Table 106-3). A study by the NMDP defined the extent of allele mismatching among serologically typed recipients and their transplant donors.[7] Among HLA-A, HLA-B, HLA-DRB1 serologically matched pairs, as many as 29% encoded allele mismatches at HLA-A, HLA-B, or HLA-DRB1; 89% of HLA-A, HLA-B, HLA-DRB1 allele-identical pairs encoded additional mismatches at HLA-C and HLA-DP. Early donor selection criteria did not include consideration for HLA-C, so many donors who were serologically or even sequence matched for HLA-A and HLA-B antigens were later found to be mismatched at the HLA-C locus. The overall frequency of allele mismatching is lower if the recipient has a common haplotype. Because the frequencies of HLA alleles and haplotypes reflect the ethnicity and race of the patient and donor population, donor–recipient HLA mismatches can be ethnogeographically distinct (http://www.allelefrequencies.net). In white transplant populations, for example, donor–recipient allele disparity is frequent for the A*02, B*27, B*35, B*39, and DRB1*04 allele families.

HUMAN LEUKOCYTE ANTIGEN TYPING METHODS

Serology and Cellular Assays

Serologic reagents have served as the gold standard for HLA antigen typing since the early 1960s. Development of standardized tissue typing reagents and methods of nomenclature for HLA genes have been facilitated by a series of 15 international histocompatibility workshops (Table 106-4). Serologic typing methods use a complement-dependent microcytotoxicity assay with alloantisera containing antibodies against polymorphic HLA specificities. Whereas a public specificity is shared by distinct HLA molecules, a private specificity is unique to a single HLA molecule. HLA molecules can share one or more public epitopes and differ for private epitopes. The combination of HLA antigens of an individual defines their phenotype, and the alleles define their genotype. All serologically defined alloantigens have been characterized at the allele level; however, not all sequenced-defined alleles have an equivalent phenotype studied by serology. Hence, a nomenclature has been developed to translate serologically defined antigens and DNA-defined alleles.

The most commonly used cellular assay for the class II region is the mixed lymphocyte culture (MLC), in which disparity between the donor and the recipient for the antigens encoded by HLA class II region genes (also known as the HLA-D region) leads to lymphocyte activation and proliferation. Although the strength of the proliferation measured in an MLC correlates roughly with the degree of HLA-D region incompatibility, MLC is poorly predictive of GVHD and therefore has limited clinical utility for donor selection.

The limiting dilution assay is a technique for determining the frequency of donor antihost cytotoxic T-lymphocyte precursors and helper T-lymphocyte precursors. These assays have proved useful in predicting the risk of GVHD and mortality before transplantation in some reports and may provide a means for selecting a suitable unrelated donor when more than one equally matched donor is available. High frequencies of cytotoxic T-lymphocyte precursors have been observed with class I donor–recipient mismatching; helper T-lymphocyte precursor has been shown to detect class II disparity. The frequency of donor cytotoxic T-lymphocyte precursor reactivity against recipient targets is correlated with the risk of acute GVHD after unrelated donor HCT when ex vivo or in vivo T-cell depletion is used for GVHD prophylaxis. In T-cell–replete transplantation, significant associations between frequency of cytotoxic T-lymphocyte precursors and acute GVHD have not been identified.

DNA Methods

The advent of polymerase chain reaction (PCR) in the 1980s revolutionized donor typing and matching and has greatly accelerated understanding of the HLA barrier in transplantation. Guidelines for typing volunteer donors using DNA-based methods are available. To transition from serologic to DNA-based methods, development of dictionaries of HLA alleles and antigen equivalents has become a necessity because many donors in the registries have been typed only by serologic assays. Interpretation and use of molecular typing data for donor search and selection has required the development of informatics programs.

Low-resolution DNA-based typing methods can define groups of alleles that are serologic equivalent (e.g., HLA-A*02 is DNA defined and is equivalent to HLA-A2 that is serologically defined). Intermediate-resolution DNA typing methods provide additional information but not to the level of the complete DNA sequence that distinguishes one allele from another (e.g., the information is sufficient to delineate one group of alleles that include HLA-A*0201 and another that include HLA*0205 but cannot definitely assign the allele). High-resolution typing defines the unique DNA sequence of an allele (e.g., HLA-A*0201). The term "6/6" matched refers to recipients and donors who share the same low-resolution-defined HLA-A, HLA-B, and HLA-DR genes. The term "8/8" refers to high-resolution matching at the four loci HLA-A, HLA-B, HLA-C, and HLA-DRB1. When HLA-DQB1 is added, "10/10" refers to high-resolution matching at the five loci. When HLA-DPB1 is added, "12/12" refers to donor–recipient pairs that are allele matched at all six genetic loci.

Several PCR-based HLA typing approaches are widely used by clinical tissue typing laboratories in support of unrelated HCT

Table 106-4 International Histocompatibility Workshops and Conferences

Workshop	Year	Chairman	Venue	Advances
First	1964	D.B. Amos	Durham, NC	Definition of "Hu-L," "LA," and "Four" antigen specificities
Second	1965	J.J. Van Rood	Leiden, The Netherlands	MLC testing
Third	1967	R. Ceppellini	Turin, Italy	Family studies HLA in renal transplantation
Fourth	1970	P. Terasaki	Los Angeles, CA	Definition of 27 HLA-A, HLA-B, and HLA-C specificities
Fifth	1972	J. Dausset	Evian, France	Worldwide typing of 49 populations
Sixth	1975	F. Kissmeyer	Aarhus, Denmark	Description of Dw specificities, Nielsen
Seventh	1977	W. Bodmer	Oxford, England	Definition of DR1-7 specificities HTC testing
Eighth	1980	P. Terasaki	Los Angeles, CA	Definition of HLA-MB (DQ) MT (DR52/53) HLA in renal transplantation and disease association
Ninth	1984	E. Albert W. Mayr	Munich, Germany Vienna, Austria	New class I and II specificities HLA class II in renal transplantation
10th	1987	B. Dupont	Scanticon, NJ New York, NY	Establishment of RFLP/T cell clones and HTC methods Creation of panel of homozygous cell lines
11th	1991	T. Sasazuki K. Tsuji	Yokohama, Japan	HLA class I PCR typing anthropology
12th	1996	D. Charron	Saint-Malo, France Paris, France	Sequencing Class I DNA typing/HLA in medicine
13th	2002	J. Hansen	Seattle, WA Victoria, British Columbia, Canada	Virtual DNA analysis http://www.ihwg.org Identification of SNP markers HLA in anthropology, disease association, HCT
14th	2005	J. McCluskey	Melbourne, Australia	MHC and anthropology, disease, infection, HCT, cancer Nonclassical genes, NK-KIR, cytokine genes http://www.ihwg.org
15th	2008	M. Gerbase and M-E Moraes	Brazil Population Studies, Bioinformatics Tools	

HCT, Hematopoietic cell transplantation; *HLA,* human leukocyte antigen; *HTC,* homozygous typing cells; *KIR,* killer immunoglobulin-like receptor; *MHC,* major histocompatibility complex; *MLC,* mixed lymphocyte culture; *NK,* natural killer; *PCR,* polymerase chain reaction; *RFLP,* restriction fragment length polymorphism; *SNP,* single nucleotide polymorphism.

programs. The sequence-specific primer method uses a panel of primers to amplify the HLA locus or alleles. The PCR products are electrophoresed on a gel, and assignment of an HLA type is made by examining the composite pattern of positive and negative PCR reaction methods.

The sequence-specific oligonucleotide probe hybridization (SSOPH) method uses a solid phase support to immobilize PCR-amplified products. Nonradioactive-labeled oligonucleotide probes are allowed to hybridize to the support. Whereas probes with sequences complementary to the target DNA will hybridize, probes with as few as one nucleotide difference will fail to hybridize. Alternatively, SSOPH methods can use probes that are immobilized to the solid phase support and allow PCR-amplified target DNA to hybridize to the support.

A variation of the SSOPH method is oligonucleotide array technology. Arrays can simultaneously query multiple regions of polymorphisms in many HLA genes. Oligonucleotide probes can be designed to all four potential nucleotides, thereby enabling detection of new sequence polymorphisms with the same sensitivity and specificity as sequencing-based typing. Redundancy of probe sequences allows combinations of alleles to be distinguished in heterozygous individuals. Commercial platforms are now available and provide quality-controlled reagents for high through-put genotyping.[8-10] Finally, sequencing methods provide high resolution of HLA alleles and are the definitive method for characterizing novel HLA sequences.

ASSESSMENT OF THE VECTOR OF MISMATCHING

The "vector" or "direction" of HLA compatibility between a donor and a recipient has biologic relevance in defining the risks of graft failure and GVHD. The concept of the vector was first demonstrated in cases of haploidentical related mismatched transplantation and defines HVG and GVH alloreactivity. Whereas the presence of donor alleles not shared by the recipient determines HVG allorecognition, the presence of recipient alleles not shared by the donor provides the immunologic basis for GVH allorecognition (Table 106-5). "Bidirectional" mismatching refers to the situation in which both HVG and GVH vectors are present at a given HLA locus. "Unidirectional" mismatching describes the situation in which either the donor or the recipient is homozygous for the same allele at the mismatched locus. A unidirectional GVH vector mismatch occurs when the donor is homozygous and the recipient is heterozygous and shares one allele with the donor (e.g., patient DRB1*01:01, *04:10 vs. donor DRB1*01:01, *01:01). A unidirectional HVG vector mismatch

Table 106-5 Vector of Mismatch

Vector	Definition	Examples	
		Donor	Recipient
HVG	Presence of donor alleles not present in the recipient	DRB1*01:01,04:01* DRB1*01:01,04:01†	DRB1*01:01,04:10 DRB1*01:01,01:01
GVH	Presence of recipient alleles not present in the donor	DRB1*01:01,04:01* DRB1*01:01,01:01†	DRB1*01:01,04:10 DRB1*01:01,04:10

GVH, Graft versus host; *HVG*, host versus graft.
*These combinations contain bidirectional (both HVG and GVHD) mismatch vectors.
†Unidirectional mismatches.

Criteria for an Interpretable Study on the Role of Human Leukocyte Antigen Matching in Cases of Unrelated Donor Transplantation

DNA-based methods have become established as the gold standard for HLA testing. Research studies aimed at defining the importance of HLA mismatching in transplant outcome ideally examine donor–recipient transplant pairs that are fully typed for HLA-A, HLA-B, HLA-C, HLA-DRB1, HLA-DQB1, and HLA-DPB1 at the sequence level. In this way, the relative risks of HLA disparity on a given clinical endpoint can be more accurately measured. Many non-HLA variables have an impact on the same clinical endpoints that are also affected by HLA disparity including whether the underlying disease is malignant or nonmalignant, whether the conditioning regimen is ablative or reduced intensity, and the specific regimen used to prevent GVHD. These nongenetic variables may contribute risks that diminish the ability to discern HLA-specific effects and require multivariate models to adjust or stratify for these variables to assess independence of HLA effects on the clinical endpoint of interest. Finally, the study should have sufficient statistical power to detect a significant difference in outcome when one truly exists. Very large numbers of transplants are required to adjust for HLA and non-HLA variables.

occurs when the patient is homozygous and the donor is heterozygous and shares one allele with the patient (e.g., patient DRB1*01:01, *01:01 vs. donor DRB1*01:01, *04:01). Clinical outcomes analyses that evaluate the association between HLA disparity and risk of graft failure or GVHD should specify the vector of incompatibility that is used to define the comparison groups.

ASSESSMENT OF HUMAN LEUKOCYTE ANTIGEN HAPLOTYPES

Patients who are candidates for allogeneic transplantation undergo a pedigree analysis to determine the availability of potential HLA genotypically identical siblings who could serve as a donor. The family study, which includes typing of the propositus' mother, father, and all full siblings, provides an internal verification of the patient's HLA haplotypes. Because HLA genes segregate in classical Mendelian fashion, the probability that a sibling inherits the same parental haplotypes is 25% (genotypically identical). The probability that a sibling inherits one identical paternal or maternal haplotype plus one nonshared haplotype is 50% (haploidentical). The probability of inheriting neither of the same haplotypes is 25% (complete mismatch).

When no related donor is available or suitable, a search for an unrelated donor is initiated. A search of all available international registries today includes consideration of more than 11 million donors worldwide (http://www.nmdp.org; http://www.worldmarrow.org). In the assessment of every unrelated donor, matching for each HLA genetic locus allele is considered. However, gene-by-gene identity for HLA-A, HLA-B, HLA-C, HLA-DR, and HLA-DQ between two unrelated individuals does not necessarily signify that the HLA alleles are linked on the same chromosomal haplotype. Hence, it is possible for two unrelated individuals who share the same HLA genotype to have different HLA haplotypes. The clinical significance of haplotype matching is described next.

CLINICAL IMPORTANCE OF DONOR HLA MATCHING IN CASES OF UNRELATED DONOR HCT

The first successful human allogeneic BM transplantations were performed in 1968. Early clinical experience in allogeneic transplantation identified both HLA and non-HLA factors as important in defining posttransplantation complications. Donor HLA mismatching was identified as a risk factor for graft failure after HCT from relatives. Non-HLA factors associated with an increased risk of graft failure included transplantation of a lower BM cell dose, use of T cell–depleted BM, and transplantation of BM from a cross-match–positive donor (presence of antidonor lymphocyte antibodies in the patient's serum pretransplant). HLA mismatching was also shown to increase the incidence and severity of acute GVHD.

Use of HLA-matched unrelated donors as the source of BM was first applied in the case of a patient with severe aplastic anemia. Durable engraftment and immunologic reconstitution were early barriers to successful unrelated donor HCT. As clinical experience matured and tissue typing methods became more robust, unrelated donor HCT was established as a therapeutic approach for treatment of hematologic disorders when an HLA-identical sibling is not available. DNA-based methods have become established as the gold standard for HLA testing because serologically identical recipients and potential unrelated donors can be mismatched for one or more alleles that are identified by DNA testing methods. Retrospective analysis of transplant donors and recipients that test the hypothesis that allele disparity confers biologic significance on transplant outcome should include examination of pairs that are fully typed for HLA-A, HLA-B, HLA-C, HLA-DRB, HLA-DQB1, and HLA-DPB1 at the sequence level. Many non-HLA variables have an impact on the same clinical endpoints that are also affected by HLA disparity. Hence, multivariable models should adjust for all clinical variables that are known to affect outcome. Finally, the study should have sufficient statistical power to detect a significant difference in outcome when one truly exists. Very large numbers of transplants are required to adjust for HLA and non-HLA variables (see box on Criteria for an Interpretable Study on the Role of Human Leukocyte Antigen Matching in Cases of Unrelated Donor Transplantation). Studies meeting these criteria have demonstrated that patients had superior DFS after HLA-matched unrelated HCT. When allele-matched donors are not available, the criteria for prioritization of mismatched donors come into focus. The current criteria for donor selection are as follows. (1) When feasible, "8/8" HLA-A, HLA-B, HLA-C, and HLA-DRB1 matching predicts for best patient survival. (2) When a matched donor cannot be identified, use of a donor mismatched for a single allele can be considered. Under these circumstances, matching for HLA-DQB1 should also be considered because mismatch for DQB1 alone seems forgiving, but mismatch for DQB1 plus another locus appears to increase mortality. (3) Multiple mismatches are less well tolerated and should be limited. (4) Permissible HLA mismatches have been proposed as defined by polymorphism for selected HLA class I residues that participate in peptide repertoire or direct contact with the T-cell receptor. (5) HLA haplotype matching between donors and recipients may lower the risk of severe acute GVHD. (6) Polymorphisms outside of the classical HLA loci may be clinically significant (Table 106-6).

Table 106-6 Principles of Donor Human Leukocyte Antigen Matching Using High-Resolution DNA Typing Methods

1. When feasible, four-locus HLA-A, HLA-B, HLA-C, and HLA-DRB1 matching is optimal.
2. Although there are no "good" mismatches, HLA-C antigen mismatches are particularly detrimental.
3. Multiple mismatches are less well tolerated and should be limited.
4. Permissible HLA mismatches can be defined by specific class I and class II residues that participate in peptide repertoire or direct contact with the T-cell receptor.
5. Haplotype matching of HLA-A, HLA-B, HLA-C, HLA-DRB1 allele-identical donors and recipients may lower posttransplant risks of clinically severe acute GVHD.

GVHD, Graft-versus-host disease; *HLA,* human leukocyte antigen.

Human Leukocyte Antigen Selection Criteria for Unrelated Donors

DNA typing can uncover additional allele disparity between HLA-A, HLA-B, HLA-DR phenotypically matched unrelated donors and recipients. Both GVHD and mortality are increased with use of phenotypically matched unrelated donors compared with related donor–recipient pairs. The difference in outcome can be attributed in part to the effects of mismatching for HLA-A, HLA-B, HLA-C, and HLA-DRB1 alleles and to the degree of HLA-A, HLA-B, HLA-DRB1 haplotype identity between the donor and recipient. Routine testing of potential donors should include DNA typing for HLA-A, HLA-B, HLA-C, and HLA-DRB1 at the intermediate resolution (antigen-equivalent) level. After the best-matched unrelated donors are identified, routine testing should include allele (sequence)-level typing for these genes. When a matched donor is not available, then the number of mismatches should be limited to one or two, with a single HLA-DQB1 mismatch being the best tolerated.

HUMAN LEUKOCYTE ANTIGEN–MATCHED UNRELATED DONOR HEMATOPOIETIC CELL TRANSPLANTATION

The impact of more complete and precise donor HLA matching is dramatic. Overall survival after transplantation for treatment of AML, MDS, ALL, and CML from an 8/8 matched unrelated donor can approach the results observed after HLA-identical sibling transplantation (http://www.marrow.org). For all modalities, the underlying disease diagnosis and stage of disease at transplantation remain the most important prognostic features that affect DFS. The impact of HLA mismatching with respect to these clinical variables is coming into better focus. The development of reduced-intensity conditioning regimens has expanded the clinical indications of HCT to patients of older age and patients who have underlying medical conditions that preclude the use of myeloablative regimens. The role of HLA mismatching in growth factor-mobilized PBSC unrelated HCT has recently been clarified.[11]

In an analysis of patients transplanted for treatment of acute or chronic leukemia or NHL from HLA-identical siblings, patients positive for HLA-DR15 had lower recurrence of disease posttransplant and improved survival compared with patients who were DR15 negative.[12] Additional reports of HLA associations with GVHD risk after sibling transplantation suggest that the immunogenicity of the specific alleles may directly influence GVHD risk.[13] Because the siblings were HLA identical, these observations cannot be explained by HLA disparity. These data have significance not only in the setting of HLA-identical related HCT but also for unrelated and mismatched related donor HCT. In addition to HLA allele mismatch-specific risk after unrelated HCT, new evidence suggests that risk can arise from mismatching for HLA haplotypes (see Importance of Major Histocompatibility Complex Haplotypes later). The risk associated with haplotype mismatching after unrelated donor HCT can be assessed with haplotyping tools.

SINGLE-LOCUS MISMATCHED UNRELATED HEMATOPOIETIC CELL TRANSPLANTATION

Early studies of patients receiving HLA antigen-matched, MLC-compatible unrelated donor HCT uniformly reported a relatively high incidence of acute GVHD and transplant-related mortality (TRM) compared with transplantations from HLA-identical siblings. The possibility that undetected donor–recipient mismatching for HLA allele variants could be responsible for increased complications in cases of unrelated donor HCT suggested that the safety and success of unrelated donor transplantations could be improved by further advances in HLA typing and donor matching and prompted close examination of serologically identical unrelated transplant pairs using DNA typing methods. The HLA variation that is identifiable using DNA methods is functional. DNA-based methods can detect differences in allele sequences among serologically identical unrelated donor–recipient pairs, and the risk of mortality is increased with mismatching for a single HLA allele. Most posttransplant complications associated with donor HLA mismatching occur within the first 6 months after transplantation, but some occur quite late.

The risks of graft failure, GVHD, and mortality associated with mismatching are not contributed equivalently by all HLA loci. Because DNA-based laboratory methods were first developed for class II genes, clinical information on donor mismatching for HLA-DRB1, HLA-DQB1, and HLA-DPB1 preceded that for HLA-A, HLA-B, and HLA-C. As a result, donor selection criteria included consideration for donor class II matching in the early 1990s followed by refined criteria inclusive of class I (see box on Human Leukocyte Antigen Selection Criteria for Unrelated Donors). Early studies of class II allele matching were performed in study populations typed by serology for class I antigens. As a result, the risks attributed to DRB1 or DQB1 mismatching may have included the risk related to additional undetected class I disparities. In one of the earliest studies of patients with hematologic malignancy transplanted from HLA-A, HLA-B, HLA-DR serologically matched unrelated donors, DRB1 and DQB1 allele mismatching was associated with increased risk of severe acute GVHD. Several large studies extended the findings of class II disparity and risk of clinically significant acute GVHD. An NMDP analysis of 831 CML transplants found that the HLA-DRB1 effects were significant when class II allele matching was evaluated in a good-risk subset of patients transplanted during the first chronic phase from class I serologically matched unrelated donors.

Human Leukocyte Antigen C: Discovery of a Classical Transplantation Antigen

Among the earliest clinical observations implicating class I was the demonstration that HLA-C is capable of eliciting an alloantibody immune response.[14] HLA-C antigens could be recognized by cytotoxic T lymphocytes and present peptides to T cells. Demonstration of HLA-C as a classical transplantation antigen did not occur until the 1990s. HLA-C mismatching was identified as an independent risk factor for graft failure, particularly in patients receiving myeloablative conditioning regimens followed by T cell–replete transplantations for treatment of CML.[15] Increased risk of graft failure was also associated with HLA-A or HLA-B mismatching and low BM cell dose.

The importance of unrelated donor matching for HLA-C was confirmed by several large analyses (Table 106-7). In the NMDP study,[5] DNA from donors and recipients were typed for HLA-A, HLA-B, HLA-C, HLA-DRB, HLA-DQA1, HLA-DQB1, HLA-DPA1, and HLA-DPB1 alleles using high-resolution methods. After accounting for clinical variables and mismatching at HLA-A, HLA-B,

Table 106-7 Impact of HLA-A, B, C, DR Matching on Mortality: 8/8 Model

	Patients (*n*)	Relative Risk	95% Confidence Interval	*P* Value
Matched	1840	1.00	—	—
HLA-A, mismatch	274	1.36	1.17-1.59	<0.0001
HLA-B, mismatch	116	1.16	0.92-1.47	0.20
HLA-C, mismatch	478	1.19	1.05-1.35	0.006
HLA-DR, mismatch	117	1.48	1.19-1.85	0.0005

From Lee SJ, Klein J, Haagenson M, et al: High-resolution donor-recipient HLA matching contributes to the success of unrelated donor marrow transplantation. *Blood* 110:45763, 2007.
HLA, Human leukocyte antigen.

Table 106-8 Importance of HLA Mismatching on Survival After Unrelated Donor Transplantation

	n	Relative Risk (95% Confidence Interval)	*P*
Fully matched (8/8)*	1840	1.00	—
Single mismatch (7/8)	985	1.26 (1.15-1.39)	<.001
A	274	1.36 (1.17-1.58)	<.001
B	116	1.16 (0.92-1.47)	.20
C	478	1.19 (1.05-1.35)	.006
DRB1	117	1.48 (1.19-1.85)	.001
Double mismatch (6/8)	633	1.66 (1.48-1.85)	<.001
A+B	41	1.13 (0.77-1.65)	.53
A+C	130	1.68 (1.37-2.07)	<.001
A+DRB1	20	1.96 (1.19-3.23)	.008
B+DRB1	29	1.51 (1.00-2.27)	.05
B+C	284	1.87 (1.62-2.16)	<.001
C+C	36	1.73 (1.18-2.54)	.005
C+DRB1	72	1.27 (0.96-1.67)	.09
Others	241	—	—
Triple mismatch (5/8)	275	1.64 (1.42-1.91)	<.001
A+B+C	97	1.77 (1.40-2.24)	<.001
A+C+DRB1	20	1.82 (1.11-2.99)	.02
B+C+C	41	1.96 (1.40-2.75)	<.001
B+C+DRB1	48	1.64 (1.19-2.25)	.002
B+B+C	25	0.93 (0.56-1.56)	.79
Others	44	—	—
Quadruple mismatch (4/8)	91	2.05 (1.61-2.60)	<.001
A+B+C+DRB1	23	2.39 (1.51-3.77)	<.001
Others	68	—	—

Data from Lee SJ, Klein J, Haagenson M, et al: High-resolution donor-recipient HLA matching contributes to the success of unrelated donor marrow transplantation. *Blood* 110:4576, 2007.
*HLA-A, C, B, DRB_1.

and HLA-DR, multivariate analysis revealed that HLA-C allele disparity conferred a statistically significantly increased relative risk on mortality (Table 106-8).

Most of the historical data concerning HLA disparity and transplant outcomes were derived from BM as the stem cell source. The use of growth factor–mobilized PBSC has been widely used as the preferred stem cell source for ease of donor collection. A recent analysis of the impact of HLA mismatching in unrelated PBSC transplantation was conducted by the NMDP and CIBMTR.[7] In this series of 1933 transplants, risks associated with donor disparity at HLA-A, -C, and -B and DRB1 were defined ("8/8"). Complete matching was associated with improved 1-year survival compared with any single mismatch ("7/8"). Overall, donor HLA-C antigen mismatching was associated with the worse outcomes compared with HLA-A, HLA-B, or DRB1 mismatching. HLA-C antigen mismatching increased mortality (relative risk [RR], 1.41; $P = .0005$), lowered DFS (RR, 1.36; $P = .001$) and grades III or IV acute GVHD (RR, 1.98; $P < .0001$). HLA-C allele mismatches did not increase risks. HLA-B allele or antigen mismatches were associated with GVHD; there were no statistically significant associations of HLA-A, DRB1, or DQB1 mismatches with transplant outcomes. These data demonstrate that prospective evaluation of unrelated donors should include consideration for compatibility at HLA-C.

Models for Understanding Alloreactivity

HLA-B and HLA-DP have served as models for understanding the structural basis for allorecognition, where specific amino acid residues of class I and II molecules contribute to eliciting the immune response. Donor-derived cytotoxic T lymphocytes isolated from a patient with graft rejection selectively recognized the patient-mismatched HLA-B44 allele (B*4402 vs. B*4403), indicating that class I allele differences may evoke donor–antihost responses and supporting the hypothesis that allelic variants of the same HLA antigen can be functionally relevant.[16] A parallel story emerged for HLA-DP. Population studies have shown that HLA-DP is unique among other HLA genes because of very weak LD between HLA-DP and HLA-A, HLA-B, HLA-C, HLA-DR, and HLA-DQ. As a result, fewer than 20% of HLA-A, HLA-B, HLA-C, HLA-DRB1, and HLA-DQB1–matched unrelated donor pairs are also matched for HLA-DP. Retrospective examination of HLA-DP has required very large transplant populations so that sufficient numbers of HLA-DP matched pairs could be compared with mismatched pairs. Furthermore, the measured effects attributed to single loci in early studies likely measured additive effects of HLA-DP with HLA-A, HLA-B, and HLA-DR. HLA-DP does function as a classical transplantation antigen with respect to GVHD. Mismatching for two DPB1 allele increases the risk of acute GVHD compared with one or no HLA-DP mismatch. Analysis of the structural basis of HLA alloreactivity sheds light on specific epitopes encoded by HLA-DP exon 2 that are responsible for increased GVHD risk.[17] This study showcases the importance of functional studies side-by-side genetic analysis to better understand the residues that define alloreactivity.

The hypothesis that donor–recipient mismatching at certain amino acid substitutions in the class I HLA molecule may be associated with higher posttransplant risks compared with mismatching at other residues was first tested by Ferrara et al.[18] Amino acid mismatching at residue 116 was found to be associated with significantly increased risks of acute GVHD and TRM compared with matching at this residue. Recently, the JMDP has evaluated 5210 Japanese recipients of unrelated donor transplants to identify mismatched residues of HLA-A, -B, -C, -DRB1, -DQB1, or -DPB1 molecules that correlate with clinical outcome.[19] Analysis of each allele-defined mismatch yielded four HLA-A, one HLA-B, seven HLA-C, two HLA-DR/DQ, and two HLA-DP mismatch combinations to be significantly associated with increased posttransplant complications. Each allele was subsequently defined by its putative amino acid sequence, and all polymorphic donor–recipient mismatched positions at each locus were individually analyzed for associations. Donor–recipient mismatching for Tyr9–Phe9 of HLA-A and for Tyr9–Ser9, Asn77–Ser77, Lys80–Asn80, Tyr99–Phe99, Leu116–

Ser116, and Arg156–Leu156 of HLA-C were identified to be clinically significant. When the study group was restricted to pairs matched at HLA-C for positions 77 and 80 that define KIR ligands, donor–recipient mismatching at positions 9, 99, 156, and 163 were found to correlate strongly with GVHD risk. This study demonstrates that mismatching for positions of HLA-A or HLA-C that participate in peptide binding is functional and provides a basis for defining nonpermissive HLA allele mismatches. Of the 10 mismatch combinations associated with GVHD risk, the JMDP explored whether the same mismatch combinations were involved in both GVHD and relapse (GVL effects) or only one.[20] In a population of 4643 transplants, 10 mismatch combinations (four for HLA-C and six for HLA-DPB1) were statistically significantly associated with lowered relapse; however, only a subset were also involved in GVHD. These results suggest that HLA mismatches do not confer equivalent risks to GVHD and relapse and that approaches for separating GVH from GVL may be possible through selected HLA combinations. Statistical models have been developed to predict peptide binding of HLA molecules as an approach to predict HLA alleles that lead to diverse binding of peptide and that may consequently affect T-cell recognition of HLA and its minors.

DOES MISMATCH FOR ALLELES OR ANTIGENS POSE THE SAME RISKS?

With the availability of molecular methods for defining the HLA alleles of transplant recipients and donors, it now is possible to evaluate the impact of the location and number of mismatched amino acid residues as potential factors defining the permissibility of a mismatch. In a single-center study of graft failure after myeloablative unrelated HCT, donor–recipient mismatching for HLA-A, HLA-B, or HLA-C antigens conferred greater risk for graft failure than did single allele mismatches at these loci.[21] Recipient homozygosity for alleles or antigens was also significantly associated with graft failure among patients with a single class I antigen mismatch. Graft failure occurred in one of two homozygous recipients and in none of 47 heterozygous recipients mismatched for a single allele ($P = 0.04$), but graft failure occurred in four of five homozygous recipients and in seven of 51 heterozygous recipients mismatched for a single antigen ($P = 0.004$). The allele and antigen mismatches represented in this study population differed in the number of nonsynonymous substitutions and in the location of the mismatch in the α_1 and α_2 domains of the molecule. Single class I allele disparity encoded from 0 to 14 (median, 2) substitutions in the α_1 and α_2 domains. In contrast, single antigen mismatched pairs had involvement of one to 27 (median, 13) substitutions. These data series, highly enriched for mismatches at HLA-C, suggest that multiple mismatches for residues that affect peptide binding and T-cell receptor contact might have been instrumental in evoking T-cell responses that led to graft failure in these patients.

Two studies have examined allele and antigen mismatches in large populations and the risks conferred by each kind of mismatch on TRM and survival.[5,22] A single-center analysis from Seattle indicated that an isolated allele or antigen mismatch was similarly detrimental to survival. Among low-risk patients, no single-locus mismatch with the exception of HLA-DQ appeared tolerable. HLA-C mismatches were particularly detrimental, whether patients had low- or high-risk malignancy. An analysis by the NMDP measured risks associated with single-locus mismatches in a large population of HLA allele-typed pairs (see Table 106-8).[5] Each HLA-A, HLA-B, HLA-C, or HLA-DRB1 mismatch was found to confer a 9% to 10% lower overall survival compared with a baseline of 8/8 allele matches. Among all single-locus mismatches, disparity for HLA-A or HLA-DRB1 was associated with higher mortality rate than disparity at HLA-B or HLA-C. Mismatching at HLA-A, HLA-B, and HLA-C each was associated with an increased risk of GVHD. As in the previous NMDP analysis, allele and antigen mismatches were similarly detrimental except for the case of HLA-C, in which allele disparities did not contribute to the risk. These data are consistent with the graft failure study discussed earlier in which a predominance of HLA-C mismatches and allele disparities did not contribute to increased risk. In the recent update from the NMDP and CIBMTR,[11] only HLA-C locus mismatches showed a difference between allele and antigen mismatches; HLA-C antigen mismatches conferred a RR of 1.41 for mortality, but C allele mismatches did not increase risk. These studies demonstrate that when measuring the effects of HLA mismatching, large, well-characterized populations are needed, and variables known to affect clinical outcome should be accounted for. Avoidance of HLA-A, HLA-B, HLA-C, and HLA-DRB1 allele mismatches may lower the risks of posttransplant complications.

MULTILOCUS MISMATCHED UNRELATED DONOR HEMATOPOIETIC CELL TRANSPLANTATION

The effects of HLA disparity on risk of graft failure, GVHD, and mortality can be measured by the total number of detectable mismatches. As the number of HLA disparities increases, so does risk for these complications. In the JMDP study of 1298 patients, the overall incidence of graft failure increased with increasing numbers of mismatched HLA loci: 1.7% matched; 4.8%, 4.1%, and 4.8% of single HLA-A/B, HLA-C, and HLA-DR/DQ, respectively; 10.4%, 8.9%, and 6% in two-locus HLA-A/B plus HLA-C, HLA-A/B plus HLA-DR/DQ, and HLA-C plus HLA-DR/DQ, respectively; and 10.6% in three-locus incompatible transplants.[23] In patients who received unrelated donor HCT for treatment of CML,[21] single allele mismatch at HLA-A, HLA-B, or HLA-C did not increase the risk of graft failure compared with matched recipients (2%); however, multiple HLA-A, HLA-B, or HLA-C allele mismatches were associated with a 29% incidence of graft failure.

Quantitative effects of multiple class I, multiple class II, or simultaneous class I and II mismatching can be associated with acute GVHD risk. Pronounced effects of two-locus HLA-DRB1, HLA-DQB1 mismatching on risk of grade III and IV acute GVHD can be discerned (22% matched; 43% single-locus mismatches; 64% two-locus mismatches). In HLA-A, HLA-B, HLA-DR serologically matched unrelated pairs who received unmodified grafts, matching for both HLA-DRB1 and HLA-DQB1 reduced the rate of GVHD from 73% (any mismatch) to 38% (matched for both genes; $P = 0.02$).

JMDP data provide information on the quantitative effects of HLA mismatching on GVHD risk.[23] Not only were multiple class I disparities a risk factor for GVHD, but HLA-C disparity in the presence of mismatching at any other HLA locus (class I, class II, or both) was associated with significantly increased incidence of grades II through IV GVHD: 60.9%, 55.7%, and 64.3% for HLA-C plus HLA-A/B, HLA-C plus HLA-DR/DQ, and HLA-C plus HLA-A/B and HLA-DR/DQ, respectively, compared with 34.5%, 54.9%, 42.7%, and 34.4% for matched, HLA-A/B mismatched, HLA-C mismatched, and HLA-DR/DQ mismatched, respectively. The JMDP experience demonstrates that multilocus mismatching is associated with a decreased rate of survival. In some pediatric series, children tolerate higher degrees of disparity with use of certain immunosuppressive regimens.

IMPORTANCE OF MAJOR HISTOCOMPATIBILITY COMPLEX HAPLOTYPES AND MAJOR HISTOCOMPATIBILITY COMPLEX RESIDENT VARIATION

Currently, gene-by-gene matching between recipients and unrelated donors is performed to approximate the haplotype matching that is feasible between genotypically identical sibling pairs. However, HLA-matched unrelated donors and recipients are not related to one another; therefore, they are described as identical by state. This opens the possibility that genes other than classical HLA may be clinically relevant. The major histocompatibility complex (MHC) is the most diverse region in the human genome known to date. More than 300 loci have been verified within the extended 7.6-megabase (Mb) MHC region have immune function.[24] Hence, current donor matching is performed for less than 5% of the total gene content of the MHC.

In addition to the classical HLA loci, the MHC is residence to the nonclassical *HLA-E, HLA-F, HLA-G, MICA,* and *MICB* genes. Data suggest a role for HLA-E in transplant outcome.[25] Increased risk for bacterial infections and corresponding TRM at day 180 posttransplant were found in recipients transplanted from HLA-E*0101,0101 homozygous unrelated donors. HLA-E*0103,0103 homozygosity among HLA-identical siblings conferred protection against acute GVHD and TRM, leading to increased overall survival. These data point to the potential involvement of the innate immune system in GVHD. New information on *MICA* in transplantation has become available.[26] In a retrospective study of 236 patients transplanted from HLA-matched and -mismatched unrelated donors, 8.4% were mismatched for *MICA*. The presence of *MICA* disparity was associated with higher risk of overall grades II to IV acute GVHD and higher gastrointestinal GVHD independent of HLA mismatching. Because the gastrointestinal epithelium is the sole organ where *MICA* is expressed, the data suggest that *MICA* serves as a classical transplantation antigen.

Mapping with microsatellite (Msat) markers was among the earliest approaches for discovering disease-causing variation in many model systems, including autoimmunity and cancer. Msats provide indirect information because Msats themselves are not functional. Their LD with putative functional genes, however, provides the basis for its application in estimating optimal donor registry size and composition and for donor selection. Studies have used Msats to query the MHC region for novel determinants. Tumor necrosis factor (TNF) variation within the class III region of the HLA complex was associated with lower survival among patients who developed GVHD.[27] These early studies provided key evidence that variation outside of the classical HLA genetic loci both exist and are potentially functional in transplantation.

More recently with the availability of a complete sequence of the MHC, mapping with the use of single nucleotide polymorphisms (SNPs) has provided investigators with a robust tool for disease mapping.[28-31] The MHC is characterized by LD of discrete segments or blocks of sequences that reside between HLA genes. Although the specific content of these blocks is under investigation, donor–recipient matching for these regions is associated with superior clinical outcome. The map of the MHC continues to be refined for both simple variation such as that represented by SNPs to more complex variation, including insertions and deletions (http://www.sanger.ac.uk/HGP/Chr6?MHC). The content of several common HLA haplotypes, including HLA-A1, B8, DR3 and HLA-A2, B DR15, showcases the extreme levels of sequence conservation over long stretches of the MHC, upward of 4 Mb in some haplotypes.[24] This work importantly shows the need for similarly dense sequence information on common as well as rare haplotypes in all ethnicities and racial populations to understand how such variation may be clinically relevant.

How can knowledge of haplotype content facilitate the discovery of new transplantation determinants? The available sequence alignments demonstrate that the classical HLA loci serve as robust markers for the undetected linked variation on the haplotype. To test the hypothesis that the HLA haplotype serves as a tool for querying such areas outside of classical loci, a novel long-range phasing technique has been developed.[32] By physically linking HLA-A with HLA-B with HLA-DR on the same strand of DNA, this technique has been applied to test the hypothesis that HLA-identical unrelated donors and recipients encode different HLA haplotypes, and furthermore, haplotype mismatching is associated with increased posttransplant risks conferred by variation that is linked to the different haplotypes.[33] In this study, a homogeneous population of HLA-A, HLA-B, HLA-C, HLA-DRB1, HLA-DQB1 allele-matched unrelated transplants were characterized using the phasing method. Of these pairs, 20% were found to have different physical linkage of HLA-A, HLA-B, and HLA-DR. Haplotype mismatching was associated with a significantly increased risk of grade III to IV acute GVHD. The increased risk of GVHD was offset by lower relapse, leading to similar overall survival. This study demonstrates that variation linked to the haplotype is functional and that the HLA haplotype can be used as a surrogate marker for GVHD risk.

Fine mapping will entail comprehensive analysis of both simple and complex MHC variation. In this way, comparative sequences analysis of common and rare haplotypes continues to be an important research area.[34] Most recently the JMDP carried out an extensive analysis of three commonly observed HLA haplotypes in their transplant population.[35] This work has provided invaluable information on the degree of conservation within and across haplotypes of the Japanese population and provides insight into the possible genetic basis for differences in GVHD risk among Japanese patients compared with white patients.

KIR RECEPTORS

Elucidation of the genetic diversity of the KIR family of genes and their functional role as receptors for HLA class I offers a novel approach for use of HLA class I mismatched donors to decrease risks of GVHD and relapse. KIRs are inhibitory or activating. Both types are expressed on NK cells and other cell types, including T cells; however, inhibitory KIRs are dominant. *HLA* and *KIR* genes are encoded on chromosomes 6 and 19, respectively, and segregate independently. However, HLA serves a dominant role in selection of the peripheral repertoire of NK cell inhibitory KIRs. Thus, HLA-mismatched siblings, haploidentical relatives, and mismatched unrelated donors have different repertoires of NK cell inhibitory KIRs. In only HLA mismatching pairs can there be the potential for "mismatched ligand." In some HLA-matched and -mismatched pairs, the recipient is missing the appropriate ligands for donor NK cell inhibitory KIR ("missing ligand"). A recipient who lacks the appropriate HLA ligand for the donor KIR will trigger NK-mediated killing of host target cells. In HCT for malignancy, such a combination is desirable because killing of target host leukemia cells would lead to a lower risk of relapse after transplantation. Some pairs of HLA-identical individuals encode distinct KIR sequences and can express distinct KIR on their peripheral NK cells. Recipients lacking the specific HLA ligand for donor KIR could benefit from enhanced antitumor activity after HCT.

The specificity of the dominant inhibitory KIR receptors for its ligand is governed by residues 77 and 80 of HLA-C and by the HLA-Bw4 epitope present on some HLA-B and HLA-A molecules. For HLA-C, ligands are classified into two groups, named C1 and C2. Inhibitory KIR2DL2 and 2DL3 receptors recognize Ser77 and Asn80 present in the following C1 ligands: HLA-Cw1, Cw3 (except Cw*0307, 0310, 0315), Cw7 (except Cw*0707, 0709), Cw8, Cw12 (except Cw*1205,12041/2), Cw13, Cw14 (except Cw*1404), Cw*1507, and Cw16 (except Cw*1602). The KIR2DL1 receptor recognizes Asn at position 77 and Lys at position 80 of the following C2 ligands: HLA-Cw2, Cw*0307, Cw*0315, Cw4, Cw5, Cw6, Cw*0707, Cw*0709, Cw*1205 Cw*12041/2, Cw15 (except Cw*1507), Cw*1602, Cw17, and Cw18. The HLA-Bw4 epitope serves as a ligand for the inhibitory KIR3DL1 receptor. The following HLA-B antigens and alleles are Bw4 positive: B5, B13, B17, B27, B37, B38, B44, B47, B49, B51, B52, B53, B58, B59, B63, B77, B*1513, B*1516, B*1517, B*1523, and B*1524. Based on high-resolution typing of HLA class I alleles of the recipient, the presence or absence of ligands and whether the recipient is C1/C2 heterozygous, C1/C1 homozygous, or C2/C2 homozygous is determined.

The concept of donor NK-mediated killing of recipient antigen-presenting cells was demonstrated in mice and suggested by a study in patients who underwent HLA haplotype-incompatible T-cell–depleted mismatched transplantation for high-risk AML or ALL.[36] These patients received a high $CD34^+$ cell dose and no postgrafting immunosuppression, a regimen that promotes rapid NK recovery. AML patients who received transplants from KIR ligand–mismatched donors had significantly improved 5-year survival rates compared with patients who received KIR ligand–matched transplants (60% vs. 5%; $P = 0.0005$). Donor KIR ligand mismatching was associated with no graft failure, no acute GVHD, and a 0% 5-year probability of relapse in cases of transplantation for AML. Relapse of ALL was not associated with KIR mismatching, presumably because NK cells do not express adhesion receptors to LFA-1–deficient ALL cells. In contrast, KIR ligand mismatching was an independent risk factor for poor transplantation outcome (15.5% incidence of graft failure, 13.7% incidence of acute GVHD, and 75% 5-year probability of relapse). Patients carrying the diagnosis of ALL were not protected against relapse with use of KIR ligand–mismatched donors (90% in KIR ligand matched vs. 85% in KIR ligand mismatched at 5 years).

Three aspects of KIR biology in transplantation have been explored: ligand, allele, and haplotype.

Ligands

Beginning with the earliest studies, the concept of KIR ligand mismatching and KIR ligand absence have received the most attention and have been reproduced in some (but not all) studies. Extension of the original concepts of KIR ligand mismatch in the haploidentical transplant model to HLA-matched sibling donor and unrelated donor populations has yielded heterogeneous results and may reflect the vastly different conditioning and immunosuppressive regimens that promote T-cell and NK-cell reconstitution early after transplantation. In one study, HLA genotypes were analyzed in a large population of T cell–replete unrelated donor transplants.[37] Lower posttransplant relapse was observed among HLA-mismatched recipients who were homozygous for HLA-Bw6 and HLA-C KIR ligand groups. This association was not observed among HLA-matched recipients. A population of T cell–replete allografts for ALL, AML, MDS, and CML was examined, and three groups were established based on HLA genotypes ligand and 14 KIR genes: (1) HLA class I antigen matched (KIR ligand matched), (2) class I antigen mismatched but KIR ligand matched, and (3) mismatch at both HLA class I and inhibitory KIR-ligand mismatched.[38] The overall survival at 1 year posttransplant for these three groups differed significantly (59%, 49%, and 30%, respectively). The mismatched groups had lower overall survival and event-free survival compared with the matched group. Furthermore, the group with both HLA and KIR mismatching had higher relapse and TRM than the other groups. A detrimental effect was observed for patients who lacked inhibitory KIR receptors. Among HLA-matched cases, those who lacked C1 or C2 HLA ligand had lower overall survival rates compared with patients with either present. Patients who lacked C1 or C2 had higher TRM compared with patients who had all ligands present. Therefore, for T cell–replete unrelated donor HCT, inhibitory KIR ligand mismatching and missing inhibitory KIR ligands confer higher risk to patients.

In a side-by-side comparison of missing ligand and mismatched ligand in patients undergoing haploidentical transplantation for the treatment of myeloid diseases, Ruggeri et al[39] confirmed the protective effect of mismatched ligand and not missing ligand on disease recurrence. In a large analysis of patients transplanted from unrelated donors for the treatment of myeloid malignancies, patients with low-risk diseases (first complete remission of AML, first chronic phase of CML, early stage myelodysplastic syndrome), a beneficial effect of missing ligand on lowered disease recurrence was readily apparent in both HLA-matched and -mismatched transplants.[40] The protective effect was diminished in patients with more advanced disease.

A large analysis by the JMDP sheds further light on the importance of KIR ligand matching.[41] This study included 1790 T cell–replete unrelated donor transplants. Donor–recipient HLA-C disparity was associated with reduced relapse among patients with ALL. HLA-DPB1 mismatches were associated with lower relapse among CML transplants. Mismatching for the KIR2DL ligand in the GVH vector was associated with an increased risk of relapse for ALL. An increased risk of rejection was observed for KIR2DL ligand mismatches in the HVG vector. The risk of acute GVHD was increased with disparity for HLA-A, HLA-B, HLA-C, HLA-DPB1, and KIR ligand mismatching in the GVHD vector. Mismatching for HLA-A, HLA-B, HLA-DQB1, and KIR ligand in the GVH vector increased mortality. In summary, this analysis demonstrated an important role for HLA-C, HLA-DPB1, and KIR ligand mismatching in GVHD vector on posttransplant relapse. As a whole, KIR ligand mismatching had adverse effects on acute GVHD and rejection and had no survival benefit for patients undergoing T cell–replete unrelated HCT.

The concepts of KIR ligand absence and mismatching have each been explored retrospectively in patients receiving reduced intensity conditioning and in cord blood transplantation. In a series of patients conditioned with low-dose total-body irradiation with or without fludarabine before HLA matched transplantation, the most robust indicator of lower posttransplant relapse was high donor NK chimerism, a finding observed chiefly among patients with no missing ligands (C1, C2, Bw4 positive).[42] The transplantation of cord blood units provides a model for investigating the mismatch ligand model caused by the very high frequency of HLA-C disparity between the recipient and cord blood unit(s). Two such studies have been conducted and have drawn different conclusions. Ligand mismatched patients who received myeloablative conditioning had higher TRM chiefly because of higher rates of acute GVHD.[43] In contrast, lower relapse rates and better survival associated with ligand mismatching, particularly for patients with AML, have also been described.[44] These studies highlight the need for continued analysis of large, well-characterized populations.

Alleles and Haplotypes

The KIR family of genes displays allelic and haplotypic polymorphism. KIR genes are organized into two broad groups of haplotypes known as "group A" and "group B" haplotypes. Group A haplotypes encode primarily inhibitory receptors and the activating *KIR2DS4* gene. Group B haplotypes tend to exhibit more diversity, encoding more activating genes, including *KIR2DS1, KIR2DS2, KIR2DS3, KIR2DS5,* and *KIR3DS1*. The clinical relevance of KIR haplotypes has been explored and reveals that the number of activating KIR genes is a determinant of relapse and DFS.[45] In this analysis, patients received myeloablative in vivo antithymocyte globulin T cell–depleted unrelated transplants. The study population was evaluated according to the presence of donor group A haplotypes (inhibitory receptors with one activating KIR2DS4) and donor group B haplotypes (more activating *KIRD KIR2DS1, KIR2DS2, KIR2DS3, KIR2DS5,* and *KIR3DS1*). KIR ligand mismatching was associated with significantly higher TRM, lower overall survival, and lower DFS compared with ligand matching. Transplantation from donors with group A *KIR* haplotypes or donors with lower numbers of activating *KIR* genes was associated with reduced relapse and improved DFS among AML/MDS recipients and to lesser extent among CML patients. No haplotype effects were observed in patients with ALL. This study indicates not only that the HLA ligand is an important factor but also that the composition of donor KIR haplotypes (i.e., group A KIR haplotypes) influences the risk of relapse and improved DFS.

The clinical importance of KIR haplotypes and haplotype gene content is beginning to come into focus.[45-49] Clinical outcome after allogeneic transplantation correlates with number (0, 1, 2) donor B haplotypes and not with A haplotypes nor with recipient haplotypes.[46,48,50,51] However, the mechanisms of the B haplotype–associated protective effect is not known. In a study of 1409 patients transplanted for AML or ALL, donors were genotyped for 15 *KIR* genes to define B/x or AA haplotypes. B haplotypes were further distinguished by their specific gene content. Homozygosity for motifs of the B haplotype was strongly associated with lowered relapse and improved DFS after both HLA-matched and -mismatched transplantation for the treatment of AML. As the number of B motifs increased, the risk of relapse decreased, demonstrating a biologic effect of gene/haplotype dose.

If the presence of B haplotypes is associated with lowered relapse, is the protective effect conferred by specific genes *(KIRsDS2, 2DL2),* by absence of genes *(2DL3),* or a combination thereof? New information on activating KIRs may shed some light on potential mechanisms. In a retrospective study of 1087 patients transplanted from HLA-matched or -mismatched unrelated donors for AML, CML, MDS, or ALL using primarily T cell–replete BM as grafting source, KIR3DS1 was genotyped in the donor population and the effect of zero, one, or two copies of the gene was analyzed. As the number of donor copies of KIR3DS1 increased from zero to one to two, the risk of grades II to IV acute GVHD, TRM, and mortality decreased, suggesting a biologic dose effect of 3DS1. The results gave impetus to the study of the B3DS1-positive haplotypes in the study population. To test the hypothesis that the observed putative effects of 3DS1 were associated with 3DS1 or from other haplotype-associated genes, the patient population was further defined according to whether donors possessed no B haplotype or any B haplotype. Although GVHD risk was again lower in B haplotype–positive transplants, the haplotype effect was weaker than the 3DS1 effect; furthermore, possible contribution from 2DS2 among B haplotypes was ruled out by virtue of similar GVHD rates associated with haplotype A-positive transplants. Finally, the presence of the HLA-Bw4 epitope was an independent protective factor for GVHD. Taken together, these observations suggest that clinical outcome is defined by a complex interaction of specific donor activating genes, their gene number, and the target ligand. These observations point to the potential usefulness of prospective integration of recipient and donor KIR genotype information into donor selection to fully maximize NK-driven antileukemic effects.

FUTURE DIRECTIONS

The HLA and KIR genetic systems regulate the transplantation barrier. Clinical outcome after unrelated donor transplantation can be achieved with donor matching for the highly polymorphic HLA loci. When HLA disparity cannot be avoided, judicious selection of a donor with the fewest HLA mismatches and avoidance of certain loci may provide patients with the opportunity for lifesaving transplantation. Disease stage remains a strong predictor of overall transplant outcome, and expediency in timing of transplantation for patients with high-risk disease is paramount. New research avenues include identification of novel MHC resident genetic variation that may contribute to risks of GVHD and TRM and the precise role of the KIR systems in preventing transplant complications and disease relapse.

SUGGESTED READINGS

Allcock RJ, Atrazhev AM, Beck S, et al: The MHC haplotype project: A resource for HLA-linked association studies. *Tissue Antigens* 59:520, 2002.

de Bakker PI, McVean G, Sabeti PC, et al: A high-resolution HLA and SNP haplotype map for disease association studies in the extended human MHC. *Nat Genet* 38:1166, 2006.

Baldomero H, Gratwohl M, Gratwohl A, et al: The EBMT activity survey 2009: Trends over the past 5 years. *Bone Marrow Transplant* 46:485, 2011.

Baron F, Petersdorf EW, Gooley T, et al: What is the role for donor natural killer cells after nonmyeloablative conditioning? *Biol Blood Marrow Transplant* 15:580, 2009.

Baschal EE, Aly TA, Jasinski JM, et al: Defining multiple common "completely" conserved major histocompatibility complex SNP haplotypes. *Clin Immunol* 132:203, 2009.

Brunstein CG, Wagner JE, Weisdorf DJ, et al: Negative effect of KIR alloreactivity in recipients of umbilical cord blood transplant depends on transplantation condition intensity. *Blood* 113:5628, 2009.

Chen C, Busson M, Rocha V, et al: Activating KIR genes are associated with CMV reactivation and survival after non-T-cell depleted HLA-identical sibling bone marrow transplantation for malignant disorders. *Bone Marrow Transplant* 38:437, 2006.

Cooley S, Trachtenberg E, Bergemann TL, et al: Donors with group B KIR haplotypes improve relapse-free survival after unrelated hematopoietic cell transplantation for acute myelogenous leukaemia. *Blood* 113:726, 2009.

Cooley S, Weisdorf DJ, Guethlein LA, et al: Donor selection for natural killer cell receptor genes leads to superior survival after unrelated transplantation for acute myelogenous leukaemia. *Blood* 116:2411, 2010.

Foeken LM, Green A, Hurley CK, et al: Monitoring the international use of unrelated donors for transplantation: The WMDA annual reports. *Bone Marrow Transplant* 45:811, 2010.

Horton R, Gibson R, Coggill P, et al: Variation analysis and gene annotation of eight MHC haplotypes: The MHC Haplotype Project. *Immunogenetics* 60:1, 2008.

Kawase T, Matsuo K, Kashiwase K, et al: HLA mismatch combinations associated with decreased risk of relapse: Implications for the molecular mechanism. *Blood* 113:2851, 2009.

Lee SJ, Klein J, Haagenson M, et al: High-resolution donor-recipient HLA matching contributes to the success of unrelated donor marrow transplantation. *Blood* 110:4576, 2007.

Loacker K, Hortnagl P, Grabmer C, et al: A novel HLA-A allele detected by sequence-based typing: A*68:66. *Tissue Antigens* 78:397, 2011.

McQueen KL, Dorighi KM, Guethlein LA, et al: Donor-recipient combinations of group A and B KIR haplotypes and HLA class I ligand affect the outcome of HLA-matched, sibling donor hematopoietic cell transplantation. *Hum Immunol* 68:309, 2007.

Miller JS, Cooley S, Parham P, et al: Missing KIR ligands are associated with less relapse and increased graft-versus-host disease (GVHD) following unrelated donor allogeneic HCT. *Blood* 109:5058, 2007.

Miretti MM, Walsh EC, Ke X, et al: A high-resolution linkage-disequilibrium map of the human major histocompatibility complex and first generation of tag single-nucleotide polymorphisms. *Am J Hum Genet* 76:634, 2005.

Morishima S, Ogawa S, Matsubura A, et al: Impact of highly conserved HLA haplotype on acute graft-versus-host disease. *Blood* 115:4664, 2010.

Morishima Y, Yabe T, Matsuo K, et al: Effects of HLA allele and killer immunoglobulin-like receptor ligand matching on clinical outcome in leukemia patients undergoing transplantation with T-cell-replete marrow from an unrelated donor. *Biol Blood Marrow Transplant* 13:315, 2007.

Parmar S, Del Lima M, Zou Y, et al: Donor-recipient mismatches in MHC class I chain-related gene A in unrelated donor transplantation lead to increased incidence of acute graft-versus-host disease. *Blood* 114:2884, 2009.

Petersdorf EW, Malkki M, Gooley TA, et al: MHC haploytpe matching for unrelated hematopoietic cell transplantation. *PLoS Med* 4:e8, 2007.

Ruggeri L, Mansusi A, Capanni M, et al: Donor natural killer cell allorecognition of missing self in haploidentical hematopoietic transplantation for acute myeloid leukemia: Challenging its predictive value. *Blood* 110:443, 2007.

Stringaris K, Adams S, Uribe M, et al: Donor KIR Genes 2DL5A, 2DS1 and 3DS1 are associated with a reduced rate of leukaemia relapse rate of leukaemia relapse after HLA-identical sibling stem cell transplantation for acute myeloid leukaemia but not other hematologic malignancies. *Biol Blood Marrow Transplant* 16:1257, 2010.

Symons HJ, Leffell MS, Rossiter ND, et al: Improved survival with inhibitory killer immunoglobulin receptor (KIR) gene mismatches and KIR haplotype B donors after nonmyeloablative, HLA-haploidentical bone marrow transplantation. *Biol Blood Marrow Transplant* 16:533, 2010.

Testi M, Troiano M, Di Luzio A, et al: The novel HLA-C*06:58 allele, identified by sequence-based typing in a Italian family. *Tissue Antigens* 79:80, 2012.

Traherne JA, Horton R, Roberts AN, et al: Genetic analysis of completely sequenced disease-associated MHC haplotypes identifies shuffling of segments in recent human history. *PLoS Genet* 2:e9, 2006.

Venstrom JM, Gooley TA, Spellman S, et al: Donor activating KIR3DS1 is associated with decreased acute GVHD in unrelated allogeneic hematopoietic stem cell transplantation. *Blood* 115:3162, 2010.

Waterhouse M, Pfeifer D, Pantic M, et al: Genome-wide profiling in AML patients relapsing after allogeneic hematopoietic cell transplantation. *Biol Blood Marrow Transplant* 17:1450.e1, 2011.

Willemze R, Rodrigues CA, Labopin M, et al: KIR-ligand incompatibility in the graft-versus-host direction improves outcomes after umbilical cord blood transplantation for acute leukaemia. *Leukemia* 23:492, 2009. Erratum in: Leukemia 23(3):630, 2009.

Woolfrey A, Klein JP, Haagenson M, et al: HLA-C antigen mismatch is associated with worse outcome in unrelated donor peripheral blood stem cell transplantation. *Biol Blood Marrow Transplant* 17:885, 2011.

For complete list of references log on to www.expertconsult.com.

CHAPTER 107

HAPLOIDENTICAL HEMATOPOIETIC CELL TRANSPLANTATION

Bimalangshu R. Dey and Thomas R. Spitzer

PRINCIPLES AND RATIONALE

The complex innate and adaptive human immune systems are well equipped to withstand major antigenic challenges. Transgressing major histocompatibility barriers has been a particularly severe challenge, and the experience of haploidentical hematopoietic cell transplantation (HCT) has underscored the problems of this approach. Our understanding of the basic immunobiology of HCT across major histocompatibility complex (MHC) barriers has increased dramatically over the past 2 to 3 decades; however, the translation of those discoveries into clinical practice has evolved more slowly. The most formidable complications of HCT across human leukocyte antigen (HLA) barriers, namely, graft rejection and graft-versus-host disease (GVHD), have been more effectively prevented and treated with modern pharmacologic interventions and manipulations of the hematopoietic graft[1] (see box on Haploidentical Hematopoietic Cell Transplantation: Why Bother?).

Realization of the potential of allogeneic HCT has one major limitation: the lack of an HLA-matched related donor in the majority of families. The HLA genes are tightly linked and inherited in a genetic unit called a *haplotype*. Haplotypes can be determined by testing for alleles at three loci: HLA-A, HLA-B, and HLA-DR. Every child inherits one haplotype from each parent. Two siblings have a 25% chance of inheriting the same two parental haplotypes and thus of becoming HLA-genotypically identical. There is always an excellent chance of finding a family member who shares with the patient at least one HLA haplotype but differs in the second haplotype. If the donor's different haplotype is by chance phenotypically identical for HLA-A, HLA-B, and HLA-DR to the recipient's, the results of transplantation following HLA-phenotypically matched related donors are comparable to those after HLA-genotypically identical related donors. However, only approximately 30% of patients have an HLA-genotypically or HLA-phenotypically matched related donor. In approximately 60% of cases without a family donor, an HLA-matched unrelated donor can be identified. In reality, in a substantial proportion of situations an unrelated HLA-compatible adult donor cannot be identified in the needed time frame. Related donors matched for one haplotype but mismatched for the alleles of the other haplotype (haploidentical donors) are virtually always readily available.

The successful performance of haploidentical HCT would mean that most patients would have an immediately available donor both for the transplant and potentially for future modulation of the cellular environment by administration of selected donor cell populations. At least in preclinical animal models, a stronger graft-versus-tumor (GVT) effect has been demonstrated when MHC barriers are crossed.[2] A primary reason for treatment failure after HCT for advanced hematologic malignancies, particularly with use of reduced-intensity conditioning, is recurrent malignancy.[3-5] One way to address the risk for relapse would be to capture the potentially more potent GVT effect of a haploidentical transplant. Finally, the lessons of haploidentical HCT will be important for strategies to induce donor-specific tolerance through mixed lymphohemapoietic chimerism.[6,7]

COMPLICATIONS OF HAPLOIDENTICAL HEMATOPOIETIC CELL TRANSPLANTATION

Although the theoretic rationale for haploidentical HCT is clear, the application of this strategy has been limited by three major complications: GVHD, graft rejection, and prolonged immunodeficiency. These problems are discussed as a prelude to the historical clinical experience of haploidentical HCT and the attempts that have been made to overcome these complications.

Graft-Versus-Host Disease

Not surprisingly, the risk for acute (and perhaps chronic) GVHD is substantially higher after T cell–replete haploidentical HCT than HLA-matched related donor transplantation.[8-10] The frequency and severity of a "hyperacute GVHD" syndrome with pharmacologic prophylaxis was well demonstrated by Powles et al[8] in an early experience with T cell–replete haploidentical bone marrow transplantation (BMT) for advanced acute leukemia. Powles et al reported 35 patients with advanced acute myeloid leukemia (AML) or acute lymphoblastic leukemia (ALL) who received one to three HLA antigen–mismatched related BMT following cyclophosphamide/total body irradiation (TBI) or cyclophosphamide/melphalan conditioning and cyclosporine with or without methotrexate GVHD prophylaxis. Twelve of these patients died of a syndrome consisting of pulmonary edema, seizures, intravascular hemolysis, and/or acute renal failure. Ten patients had primary graft failure requiring a second transplant from the same donor. This life-threatening syndrome probably reflects an inflammatory cytokine cascade associated with a potent graft-versus-host alloresponse (or, in some cases, possibly graft rejection) and illustrates the potentially catastrophic consequences of crossing HLA barriers with pharmacologic GVHD prophylaxis alone.

Beatty et al[9] at the Fred Hutchinson Cancer Research Center also showed in an early retrospective analysis of transplant outcomes that the incidence of acute GVHD was significantly higher after one to three HLA antigen–mismatched BMT compared to HLA-genotypically identical sibling donor transplants. Despite a higher incidence of GVHD, however, overall survival was not significantly different following HLA-matched and single antigen–mismatched donor BMT, likely due to a stronger GVT effect of single antigen–mismatched BMT balancing the harmful effects of acute GVHD. Although the number of patients who received a two or three HLA antigen–mismatched transplant was too small to reach meaningful conclusions, the survival of those patients was poor and indicated that the mortality risk of transplants was unacceptably high in donor-recipient pairs with more than a single-antigen mismatch.

Use of ex vivo T-cell depletion of the haploidentical hematopoietic graft can result in a substantially lower incidence of GVHD, albeit in some experiences with a greater risk for engraftment failure.[11] With "megadose" peripheral blood stem cells (PBSCs) obtained by stimulation of the donor with high-dose granulocyte colony-stimulating factor (G-CSF) and vigorous ex vivo T-cell depletion, the probability

Haploidentical Hematopoietic Cell Transplantation: Why Bother?

Haploidentical hematopoietic cell transplantation (HCT) involves related donor-recipient combinations sharing one haplotype who are mismatched for one to three human leukocyte antigens (HLA) on the other haplotype
- Only 30% of patients have an HLA genotypically or phenotypically matched related donor
- Successful haploidentical HCT would mean that most patients would have an immediately available donor
- A more potent graft-versus-tumor (GVT) effect may occur following histoincompatible HCT

Myeloablative Haploidentical HCT: Survival Outcomes—Conclusions in 1985
- Equivalent following HLA-matched and single HLA antigen–mismatched related HCT
- Inferior following two to three HLA antigen–mismatched HCT

Myeloablative Haploidentical HCT: Conclusions in 1997
- For favorable-risk hematologic malignancies
  Haploidentical HCT is associated with inferior survival outcomes
- For intermediate- to high-risk hematologic malignancies
  Single HLA antigen–mismatched related transplant equals matched unrelated-donor transplant
- For intermediate- to high-risk hematologic malignancies
  Two HLA antigen–mismatched related transplant equals single HLA antigen–mismatched unrelated donor transplant

Haploidentical HCT: Conclusions in 2011
Haploidentical HCT is feasible in selected circumstances in which matched donors are unavailable. However, the following problems remain:
- It is unclear whether a stronger graft-versus-leukemia effect occurs
- Graft-versus-host disease (GVHD) and graft rejection are problematic, although becoming more manageable with vigorous T-cell depletion (TCD) and high stem cell dose
- Immune reconstitution, particularly following TCD, is poor

Nonmyeloablative Haploidentical HCT: Rationale
- Reduced early transplant-related mortality
- More candidates for HCT by virtue of age or comorbidity
- Mixed chimeric platform to prevent GVHD and optimize a GVT effect via donor lymphocyte infusion

Nonmyeloablative Haploidentical HCT: Conclusions
- Engraftment occurs in the majority of cases
- GVHD, prolonged immunodeficiency, and disease relapse remain challenging
- Mixed chimerism is achievable and may serve as a platform for adoptive cellular therapy
- Sustained remissions following donor graft rejection are seen and suggest an alternative antitumor mechanism
- Mixed chimerism can be used as a platform for achieving donor-specific solid organ tolerance

of sustained engraftment after haploidentical transplant was high (100/101 patients in one series),[1] and the probability of acute GVHD was very low (8%) in that same series. However, the complications of severe opportunistic infection and disease relapse, reflecting inadequate immune reconstitution, persist with this approach.[12,13]

Graft Rejection

A strong association between the degree of HLA incompatibility and graft failure was well demonstrated by Anasetti et al[14] in an analysis of 269 myeloablative BMTs for leukemia or lymphoma. The overall rate of graft failure for transplants from haploidentical donors was 12.3% compared to 2.0% for transplants from genotypically identical sibling donors. The graft failure rate also correlated with the degree of histocompatibility with 9% and 21% graft failure rates for transplants from single-locus mismatched and two-loci mismatched donors, respectively. Incompatibility at both the B and D loci and a positive crossmatch for antidonor lymphocytotoxic antibody independently predicted graft failure.

With T-cell depletion of bone marrow grafts, graft failure rates after haploidentical HCT have been very high.[15] The problem of graft failure has been overcome in large part by the use of very-high-dose G-CSF–mobilized PBSCs, as discussed in Principles and Rationale.[1] A "veto" function of $CD34^+$ cells and selected $CD8^+$ cells likely has contributed to the high rate of sustained engraftment with this strategy.[16,17]

Nonmyeloablative haploidentical HCT approaches have been explored more recently. Higher rates of graft failure have been observed with T cell–replete bone marrow versus T cell–depleted G-CSF–mobilized PBSCs.[18,19] Posttransplant high-dose cyclophosphamide also has been used to deplete alloreactive (in both the GVH and host-versus-graft directions) T cells with a high rate of sustained engraftment following nonmyeloablative haploidentical BMT.[20]

Prolonged Immunodeficiency

The well-known serious consequences of haploidentical HCT, including relapse and delayed immune recovery with resultant risk for fatal infectious complications, are complicated by the rigorous T-cell depletion that is necessary to prevent fatal GVHD. Delayed immune recovery after T cell–depleted haploidentical HCT has been associated with a very high risk for bacterial, fungal, viral, and other opportunistic infections.[13,21,22] With refinements in transplant strategy, including the use of "megadose" $CD34^+$ cells, the rate of donor engraftment has improved with a very low incidence of GVHD, but infectious complications have remained a substantial problem.[23] In this important study, the mortality from causes other than leukemic relapse was 40%. The high incidence of infectious complications, which occurred despite the use of antibacterial, antifungal, and antiviral prophylaxis, resulted in 59% of all nonleukemic deaths. Of note, $CD4^+$ T-cell counts were below 200/μL for as long as 16 months. Immune recovery was faster in patients who received 10 times as many T cells, but that resulted in an increased incidence of GVHD.[24]

Delayed immune recovery results from the degree of HLA disparity, the low numbers of T cells infused, the use of T cell–depleting serotherapy (e.g., antithymocyte globulin [ATG]), the intensity of the conditioning regimen, and impaired thymic function.[25,26] Development of a fully functional immune system requires recovery of both innate and adaptive immune responses. Whereas the innate system, represented by natural killer (NK) cells, neutrophils, dendritic cells, monocytes, and macrophages, is restored relatively rapidly, the recovery of the adaptive system, represented by a broad functional T- and B-cell repertoire, is markedly delayed following T cell–depleted haploidentical HCT. T-cell reconstitution occurs through two main pathways: early reconstitution via a thymic-independent pathway known as *homeostatic peripheral expansion,* which involves expansion of mature T cells that survive the conditioning and/or are retained within the allograft, and late reconstitution via a thymic-dependent pathway. Although a broad T-cell repertoire presumably resulting from donor precursor cells emigrating from the thymus (i.e., via thymopoiesis) provides optimal T-cell reconstitution, effective immune reconstitution can occur relatively early through homeostatic peripheral expansion alone conferring protection against disease progression and infectious pathogens. However, this recovery is effectively eliminated by T-cell depletion in the haploidentical HCT setting. Impaired thymic function as a result of toxicity of the conditioning regimen or GVHD further contributes to delayed immune recovery.[26-28] Lamb et al[22] demonstrated NK cell recovery as early as 1 month posttransplant, with B- and T-cell recovery at 6 months and more than 2 years, respectively, in patients who received T cell–depleted haploidentical HCT.

HISTORICAL CLINICAL EXPERIENCE OF HAPLOIDENTICAL HEMATOPOIETIC CELL TRANSPLANTATION

The first reported successful allogeneic transplants were performed in children with primary immunodeficiency syndromes who received HLA-matched sibling donor bone marrow.[29,30] Based on this initial encouraging experience, T cell–depleted parental donor haploidentical BMT was attempted. This strategy subsequently was shown to be successful in a number of primary immunodeficiency disorders, including severe combined immunodeficiency disease and Wiskott-Aldrich syndrome.[31,32] Despite the early successes of HLA-matched BMT and the realization that only sustained lymphoid chimerism was necessary for functional cure of these diseases, it was quickly learned that more aggressive conditioning was required to overcome HLA barriers in the haploidentical BMT setting.[33,34]

The early clinical experience with myeloablative T cell–replete BMT with pharmacologic GVHD prophylaxis for treatment of hematologic malignancies was remarkable for a significantly higher incidence of GVHD compared to HLA-matched related donor transplants[9] and a high incidence of early and severe ("hyperacute") GVHD.[8] The comparable survival of patients in the Beatty report who received an HLA-matched versus a single antigen–mismatched donor BMT despite a higher incidence of acute GVHD in the latter patient population was believed to result from a stronger GVT effect of HLA single antigen–mismatched BMT balancing the harmful effects of acute GVHD. Too few patients received a two or three HLA antigen–mismatched transplant to reach meaningful conclusions, but the poor outcomes of those patients suggested that the mortality risk of transplants involving donors who were more than a single-antigen mismatch with their recipient was unacceptably high.

An International Bone Marrow Transplant Registry analysis of transplant outcomes following HLA-matched and HLA-mismatched related and unrelated donor BMT for AML, ALL, and chronic myeloid leukemia (CML) added to our understanding of transplant outcomes according to degree of histocompatibility. In this analysis, transplant-related mortality was significantly higher after a one or two HLA antigen–mismatched related or matched or single antigen–mismatched unrelated donor BMT than after HLA-matched sibling BMT.[10] The large number of patients also permitted an analysis of outcomes according to leukemia status at the time of transplant. Among patients with early leukemia (AML or ALL in first complete remission or CML in chronic phase), transplants from non–HLA-matched related donors were associated with a higher risk for transplant-related mortality than were matched donor transplants. The risk for treatment failure also was higher following alternative donor BMT. For patients with more advanced leukemia, treatment failure risk was similar for HLA-matched donor transplants and single antigen–mismatched related donor transplants and lower than the treatment failure risk following matched unrelated donor and two HLA antigen–mismatched related donor BMT. Although this study demonstrated the importance of leukemia status and the impact of HLA matching on treatment failure risk and survival outcomes, the analysis was limited by the heterogeneous groups of patients (including, for example, both T cell–depleted and T cell–replete transplants) and the exclusive use of serologic methods of HLA typing (thus underestimating the HLA disparity that now can be identified by molecular methods).

Drobyski et al[35] compared the transplant outcomes of 139 patients with hematologic malignancies who underwent T cell–depleted BMT from HLA-matched unrelated, single antigen–mismatched unrelated, and related haploidentical donors. No significant differences in rates of engraftment or cumulative incidences of acute or chronic GVHD were observed among the three groups. Surprisingly, a higher 2-year cumulative relapse probability was observed after haploidentical BMT, and transplant-related mortality risk was higher in both the haploidentical and single antigen–mismatched unrelated donor groups. Overall survival was significantly higher in the HLA-matched unrelated donor group.[35]

RECENT HAPLOIDENTICAL HEMATOPOIETIC CELL TRANSPLANTATION APPROACHES

In an effort to overcome the complications of haploidentical HCT and to improve disease-free and overall survival, a number of strategies have been developed (Tables 107-1 and 107-2). Both myeloablative and nonmyeloablative (reduced-intensity) conditioning regimens have been evaluated. The most successful approaches have been those that address and modulate the T-cell content (or function) of the graft and provide sufficient immunosuppression to allow for sustained engraftment.

Myeloablative Haploidentical Hematopoietic Cell Transplantation: Ex Vivo T-Cell Depletion

An abundant preclinical experience[36] and an early randomized clinical trial in patients undergoing HLA-matched BMT[37] showed that GVHD could be effectively prevented following ex vivo T-cell depletion of the graft. However, increased rates of graft failure and disease recurrence showed important limitations of this strategy.

Mehta et al[38] in a series of haploidentical BMT clinical trials evaluated TBI-based myeloablative conditioning with partial (1 to 1.5 log reduction) T-cell depletion of the allograft and posttransplant cyclosporine-based pharmacoprophylaxis. Ex vivo T-cell depletion was accomplished with either a T10B9 (anti-$\alpha\beta$ T-cell receptor) monoclonal antibody or OKT3 (anti-CD3) monoclonal antibody. Sustained engraftment occurred in more than 90% of their transplants, which was attributable to an intensified conditioning regimen and the incomplete T-cell depletion. The incidence of acute GVHD was low in one report, and an encouraging long-term survival probability of 20% in patients with advanced hematologic malignancy was observed.

Using high numbers of PBSCs to address the problem of graft loss and more vigorous T-cell depletion to prevent GVHD, Aversa et al[23] demonstrated a very low incidence of GVHD and impressive event-free and overall survival probabilities following myeloablative haploidentical HCT in patients with acute leukemia. Conditioning therapy consisted of TBI, thiotepa, fludarabine, and ATG. Ex vivo T-cell depletion was performed using $CD34^+$ cell selection (most recently with a Miltenyi CD34 cell selection device). With "megadose" PBSC containing a median of 13.6×10^6 (range, 5.1 to 29.7×10^6) $CD34^+$ cells/kg, sustained engraftment was reliably achieved with minimal acute or chronic GVHD. In a published experience, 104 patients with AML (n = 67) or ALL (n = 37) received a haploidentical T cell–depleted HCT using this regimen. Engraftment ultimately was achieved in 100 of 101 evaluable patients. Eight patients had grade II or higher acute GVHD, whereas 5 of 70 patients developed chronic GVHD. A 38% nonrelapse mortality risk, predominantly due to opportunistic infection, occurred. Killer immunoglobulin-like receptor (KIR) ligand mismatching in the GVH direction was shown to be associated with strikingly less relapse following transplantation for AML.[39] No difference in relapse probability was observed for ALL, according to KIR ligand compatibility.

Several pediatric experiences have demonstrated high rates of sustained engraftment and a low incidence of GVHD following vigorously T cell–depleted HCT for nonmalignant hematologic disorders and hematologic malignancy.[40-42] Using positive selection of stem cells with $CD34^+$- or $CD133^-$-coated magnetic microbeads or, more recently, depletion of T and B cells using $CD3^-$- and $CD19^-$-coated microbeads, Lang et al[40,41] reported high probabilities of primary engraftment in their patients (highest in the CD3/CD19 group at 91%). Of 63 patients with long-term follow-up transplanted with $CD34^+$- or $CD133^-$-selected cells, 83% achieved stable primary engraftment (which increased to 98% after re-transplant). Grade II to IV acute GVHD occurred in less than 10% of

Table 107-1 Ex Vivo T Cell–Depleted Haploidentical Stem Cell Transplantation

Center	Disease	Conditioning / *GVHD Prophylaxis*	GVHD (%) *Acute*	GVHD (%) *Chronic*	NRM	EFS or DFS/OS
University of South Carolina[38] (N = 201)	AML/ALL	TBI/VP-16/CY/ara-C, ATG, CYA Partial TCD, steroids, ATG/MP	13%	15%	51%	18%/19% at 5 yr
Basel University Hospital[11] (N = 10)	AML/CML/MDS	TBI/VP-16/CY or BU/CY ± ATG CYA ± OKT3	30%	NS	40%	30%/30% at 3-24 mo
University of Perugia (N = 104)[1]	AML/ALL	TBI/TT/FLU/ATG TCD PBSC	8%	7%	40%	48% (AML)* 46% (ALL)*
Multicenter (Canada) (N = 11)[12]	AML	MEL/TT/FLU/ATG TCD PBSC	0%	0%	55%	9%/9% at 9+ mo
Emory University (N = 28)[13]	HM	ATG based TCD PBSC	NS	NS	64%	NS/7%
Children's University Hospital, Teubingen[40] (N = 63)	HM, NMD	TBI or BU + CY/TT ± FLU TCD PBSC	8%	13%	29%	48% at 3 yr (ALL, NHL in CR)/NS
Catholic University of Korea (Seoul)[168] (N = 11)	AML	TBI or MEL + BU/ATG/FLU TCD PBSC	0%	0%	36%	36%/36% at 6 mo
Bristol Children's Hospital[43] (N = 34)	AML/ALL/CML/MDS	TBI/CY ± ATG TCD PBSC ± CYA ± alemtuzumab MMF ± CYA	13%	12%	35%	36%/36% at 6 mo
MD Anderson[56] (N = 28)	HM	TT/MEL/FLU/ATG TCD PBSC	7%	19%	32% (AML/MDS)	42%/42% (low-burden AML/MDS) 0%/0% (high-burden AML/MDS)
Massachusetts General Hospital, Boston[18] (N = 12)	AML, lymphoma	CY, anti-CD2 MAb, thymic XRT CYA (≥35 days) ± ex vivo TCD PBSC	25%	NS	25%	17%/25% at 5-34 mo

ALL, Acute lymphoblastic leukemia; *AML*, acute myeloid leukemia; *ara-C*, cytarabine; *ATG*, antithymocyte globulin; *BU*, busulfan; *CML*, chronic myeloid leukemia; *CR*, complete remission; *CY*, cyclophosphamide; *CYA*, cyclosporine; *DFS*, disease-free survival; *EFS*, event-free survival; *FLU*, fludarabine; *GVHD*, graft-versus-host disease; *HM*, hematologic malignancy; *MAb*, monoclonal antibody; *MDS*, myelodysplastic syndrome; *MEL*, melphalan; *MMF*, mycophenolate mofetil; *mo*, month; *MP*, methylprednisone; *NHL*, non-Hodgkin lymphoma; *NMD*, nonmalignant disease; *NRM*, nonrelapse mortality; *NS*, not stated; *OS*, overall survival; *PBSC*, peripheral blood stem cell; *TBI*, total body irradiation; *TCD*, T-cell depletion; *TT*, thiotepa; *VP-16*, etoposide; *XRT*, irradiation; *yr*, year.
*AML/ALL in remission, EFS only.

patients. Disease-free and overall survival probabilities for patients with nonmalignant disease and hematologic malignancy (non-Hodgkin lymphoma or ALL in complete remission) were 60% and 48%, respectively. A less than 10% incidence of fatal viral infections in recently transplanted patients was observed, suggesting favorable immune reconstitution in this population of pediatric patients.

Marks et al[43] treated 34 children having acute leukemia and other hematologic malignancies with TBI/cyclophosphamide and alemtuzumab or ATG followed by T cell–depleted (either by CD34+ cell selection or ex vivo treatment with alemtuzumab) megadose PBSC transplantation. Cyclosporine as sole GVHD prophylaxis was used only for children who did not receive CD34+ cell–selected grafts. Twenty-four patients (71%) died of relapse or infection. Actuarial overall survival at 2 years was 26%. Of the nine patients with refractory AML, there were no long-term survivors.

The experience with myeloablative ex vivo T cell–depleted (by CD34+ cell selection) "megadose" PBSC transplantation for hematologic malignancy has not been universally favorable. High early nonrelapse mortality rates due to impaired immune reconstitution (resulting in a high incidence of opportunistic infections or recurrent malignancy) have been reported with this approach. Cavazzana-Calvo et al[13] reported a mortality rate of 93% (26 of 28 patients), mostly due to infection or relapse, following ATG-based myeloablative conditioning and high-dose CD34+ cell–selected PBSC transplantation. In a Canadian multicenter trial using myeloablative conditioning and CD34+ cell–selected PBSC grafts, 10 (91%) of 11 patients died of infection or recurrent leukemia.[12] The reasons for the inferior survival outcomes in these trials are unclear but may reflect patient selection (i.e., transplantation of patients with more advanced disease) or modifications of the treatment regimen.

Ex Vivo T-Cell Anergization

Given the impaired reconstitution following nonselective T cell–depleted HCT and based on experiments showing ex vivo induction of alloantigen-specific anergy by coculturing of host and donor bone marrow mononuclear cells in the presence of cytotoxic T-lymphocyte antigen 4 immunoglobulin (CTLA4Ig), Guinan et al[44] conducted a trial of ex vivo anergized haploidentical BMT in an attempt to induce alloantigen-specific tolerance. Anergy was demonstrated by measuring precursor T-cell frequencies before and after ex vivo treatment of the marrow graft. A multiple log decrease in antirecipient precursor helper T-cell frequency was demonstrated after ex vivo anergization. Anti–third party precursor helper T-cell frequency was not significantly changed by ex vivo treatment of the graft. Twelve patients with advanced hematologic malignancy received TBI-based myeloablative conditioning and ex vivo anergized BMT. Three patients developed acute gastrointestinal GVHD. Five of 12 patients were alive and disease free from 4.5 to 29 months following transplant.

Table 107-2 Non–Ex Vivo T Cell–Depleted Haploidentical Stem Cell Transplantation

Center	Disease	Conditioning / GVHD prophylaxis	GVHD (%) Acute	GVHD (%) Chronic	NRM	EFS or DFS/OS
Royal Marsden[8] (N = 35)	AML/ALL	TBI/CY or TBI/MEL CYA ± MTX	80%	18%	34%	NS/31% at 6 mo-3 yr
Boston Children's[44] (N = 24)	Leukemia, NHL, NMD	TBI/CY Ex vivo T-cell anergization	24%	8%	50%	33%/33% at 7 yr
Peking University[170] (N = 250)	AML/ALL	BU/CY/ara-C/MeCCNU/ATG CYA/MTX/MMF	46%	42%	19%-51%	56%-71% (AML) and 25%-60% (ALL) at 3 yr
University of Tokyo[169] (N = 12)	Leukemia, MDS, NHL	TBI/CY/VP-16 or BU/FLU + alemtuzumab CYA/MTX	18%	25%	17%	42%/58%
Asnan Medical Center (Seoul)[171] (N = 83)	Leukemia, MDS	BU/FLU/ATG CYA/MTX	20%	34%	18%	60%/60% (acute leukemia in CR1) 53%/53% (MDS)
Multicenter (Japan)[103] (N = 35)	Leukemia, NHL	Myeloablative (n = 24) Nonmyeloablative (n = 11) Microchimeric NIMA-mismatched donor HCT/tacrolimus ± other drugs	56%	57%	31%	40%/43% at 20 mo
Duke University Medical Center[56] (N = 49)	HM, solid tumors	Alemtuzumab/CY/FLU CYA,MMF	16%	14%	31%	43%/31% at 1 yr
Johns Hopkins[20] (N = 68)	HM, PNH	TBI/CY/FLU post-BMT CY CYA, MMF	34%	13%	15%	26%/36% at 2 yr

ALL, Acute lymphoblastic leukemia; *AML,* acute myeloid leukemia; *ara-C,* cytarabine; *ATG,* antithymocyte globulin; *BMT,* bone marrow transplantation; *BU,* busulfan; *CR,* complete remission; *CY,* cyclophosphamide; *CYA,* cyclosporine; *DFS,* disease-free survival; *EFS,* event-free survival; *FLU,* fludarabine; *GVHD,* graft-versus-host disease; *HCT,* hematopoietic cell transplantation; *HM,* hematologic malignancy; *MDS,* myelodysplastic syndrome; *MeCCNU,* methyl CCNU; *MEL,* melphalan; *MMF,* mycophenolate mofetil; *mo,* month; *MTX,* methotrexate; *NHL,* non-Hodgkin lymphoma; *NIMA,* noninherited maternal antigen; *NMD,* nonmalignant disease; *NRM,* nonrelapse mortality; *NS,* not stated; *OS,* overall survival; *PNH,* paroxysmal nocturnal hemoglobinuria; *TBI,* total body irradiation; *TT,* thiotepa; *VP-16,* etoposide; *yr,* year.

Myeloablative Haploidentical Hematopoietic Cell Transplantation With In Vivo T-Cell Depletion

Because of the very high incidence of GVHD and transplant-related mortality following non–T cell–depleted haploidentical HCT, most of the recent efforts in this field have focused on ex vivo T-cell or T-cell subset depletion. Recently, however, several groups have reported impressive, acceptably low transplant-related mortality and favorable survival probabilities following non–T cell–depleted PBSC transplantation. Common to these strategies, however, has been the use of polyclonal ATG for in vivo T-cell depletion.

Lu et al[45] treated 135 patients having a variety of hematologic malignancies with busulfan, cytarabine, cyclophosphamide, rabbit ATG (on days −5 through −2), and non–ex vivo T cell–depleted bone marrow and/or PBSC transplantation. GVHD prophylaxis consisted of mycophenolate mofetil, cyclosporine, and methotrexate. All patients had full donor chimerism at day 30 posttransplant. The cumulative incidence of grades II to IV acute GVHD was 40%, and the 2-year incidence of transplant-related mortality was 22%. The probability of relapse at 2 years was 18%. Infectious complications included cytomegalovirus virus (CMV) interstitial pneumonitis and hemorrhagic cystitis in 17% and 35% of patients, respectively. Two-year leukemia-free and overall survival probabilities were 64% and 71%, respectively.

Ogawa et al[46] used reduced-intensity conditioning (busulfan, fludarabine, and rabbit ATG) as preparation for two to three HLA antigen–mismatched non–ex vivo T cell–depleted PBSC transplantation in 26 patients with high-risk hematologic malignancies. GVHD prophylaxis consisted of tacrolimus and corticosteroids. Serum-soluble interleukin-2 receptor (sIL-2R) levels were followed, and tapering of corticosteroids was based partly on the results of these assays. Twenty-five of the 26 patients achieved full donor chimerism. Five patients developed grade II acute GVHD, and 5 of 20 evaluable patients developed chronic GVHD. Transplant-related mortality was 15% (4 of 26 patients). $CD4^+$ cell recovery was slow, with a median count greater than 100/μL at 9 months. Fifteen (58%) of the 26 patients were alive and in complete remission at a median of 664 days posttransplant.

The surprisingly low incidence of GVHD in these series compared to historical experiences of non–ex vivo T cell–depleted HCT likely reflects the use of ATG for in vivo T-cell depletion, improved GVHD prophylaxis strategies, and better prevention and treatment of opportunistic infections. The importance of genetic factors (i.e., heterogeneity of the population) and other factors, such as use of donors mismatched for noninherited maternal antigens, remains to be determined in future clinical trials of non–ex vivo T cell–depleted haploidentical transplant.

Nonmyeloablative Conditioning for Haploidentical Hematopoietic Cell Transplantation

Nonmyeloablative (reduced-intensity) conditioning for HCT is associated with significantly less transplant-related morbidity and mortality than is myeloablative conditioning, thus permitting the transplantation of older patients and patients with significant pretransplant comorbidity.[3-5,47] A variety of postulated mechanisms, including less proinflammatory cytokine production and preservation of host "regulatory" cellular elements observed after nonmyeloablative transplants, may account for less clinical evidence of GVHD.[48] A potent GVT effect may be achieved, following either spontaneous or donor lymphocyte infusion (DLI)-induced conversion of mixed to full donor lymphohematopoietic chimerism.[4,49]

NONMYELOABLATIVE HAPLOIDENTICAL HEMATOPOIETIC CELL TRANSPLANTATION STRATEGIES USING IN VIVO T-CELL DEPLETION

Pelot et al[49] showed in murine MHC-mismatched transplant models that mixed lymphohematopoietic chimerism can be reliably induced following nonmyeloablative conditioning, in vivo T-cell depletion with anti-CD4 and anti-CD8 monoclonal antibodies, and thymic irradiation. Remarkably, these mixed chimeric mice are resistant to induction of GVHD following delayed DLI, despite a potent lymphohematopoietic GVH response, which converts their mixed chimerism to full donor hematopoiesis. A more potent GVT effect has been demonstrated in mixed chimeric mice that convert to full donor chimerism after DLI, compared to full donor chimeras given DLI (with the enhanced antitumor effect shown to result from the preservation of host professional antigen-presenting cells).[50,51]

Based on these murine models, a series of haploidentical nonmyeloablative HCT clinical trials have been conducted at the Massachusetts General Hospital. The initial trials involved cyclophosphamide, equine ATG for in vivo T-cell depletion, and pretransplant thymic irradiation.[52] Cyclosporine was given as GVHD prophylaxis and was tapered and discontinued by 5 weeks posttransplant in the absence of GVHD. DLIs were given to patients with mixed chimerism and without GVHD in an attempt to maximize the GVT effect. Because of a high incidence of severe acute GVHD in the initial group of patients, the monoclonal anti-CD2 antibody MEDI-507 was substituted for ATG in an effort to effect a more complete T-cell depletion.[18] A series of protocol changes have since been made, including the use of ex vivo T cell–depleted G-CSF–mobilized PBSCs (rather than bone marrow), changes in the dose and schedule of MEDI-507, and the addition of fludarabine to address the problems of GVHD and graft failure. Mixed "split-lineage" lymphohematopoietic chimerism has been achieved in all of the patients treated with ex vivo T cell–depleted PBSCs, with an early predominance of donor granulocyte chimerism and a much lower percentage of donor T-cell chimerism. In the majority of these patients, mixed chimerism in all lineages has converted to full or nearly full donor chimerism, either with tapering of immunosuppression or following DLI. Although GVHD has occurred in the majority of patients following conversion to full donor chimerism, it has been manageable in most cases. Striking antitumor responses in selected patients with chemorefractory aggressive lymphomas also have been achieved.

An unexpected observation in these clinical trials and HLA-matched nonmyeloablative HCT trials at the Massachusetts General Hospital was that durable antitumor responses in some patients with chemorefractory hematologic malignancies occurred despite loss of the hematopoietic graft.[53] Nine (41%) of 22 patients who received an HLA-matched or haploidentical nonmyeloablative HCT achieved a response after loss of their graft. Six patients were alive from 2.5 to 5.5 years posttransplant; four of these patients were in a sustained complete remission. The observation of ongoing tumor regression following serial DLI in a patient who lost his graft, accompanied by "spikes" in circulating host $CD8^+$ T cells, raised the intriguing possibility that a host-specific antitumor response was induced. In an effort to elucidate the mechanism of these antitumor responses, Rubio et al[54,55] established a murine nonmyeloablative transplant model in which recipient lymphocyte infusions were administered in order to cause rejection of the graft, followed by tumor challenge with host strain-specific malignant cells. A survival benefit was observed in the mice that developed mixed chimerism followed by recipient lymphocyte infusion–induced graft rejection compared to mice that received conditioning only, conditioning and transplant, or conditioning and recipient lymphocyte infusions alone. The antitumor response has been shown to be mediated by recipient lymphocyte infusion–derived interferon-γ–producing $CD8^+$ cells and recipient $CD4^+$ cells.

Rizzieri et al[56] at Duke University Medical Center have used anti-CD52 monoclonal antibody therapy (alemtuzumab) for both ex vivo and in vivo T-cell depletion in a clinical trial of haploidentical nonmyeloablative HCT for hematologic malignancies and selected solid tumors. Conditioning consisted of fludarabine, cyclophosphamide, and alemtuzumab, followed by infusion of alemtuzumab-treated PBSCs. GVHD prophylaxis consisted of mycophenolate mofetil with or without cyclosporine. DLIs were given to patients with persistent disease. Of 49 patients, 8 (16%) developed grade II to IV acute GVHD, and 7 (14%) developed chronic GVHD. Three patients (6%) experienced primary graft failure, and 4 (8%) had secondary graft failure. The complete remission rate was 75%; relapse-free and overall survival probabilities at 1 year were 43% and 31%, respectively.

Nonmyeloablative Haploidentical Hematopoietic Cell Transplantation With Posttransplant High-Dose Cyclophosphamide

Based on canine experiments in which high-dose posttransplant cyclophosphamide was effective in depleting alloreactive T cells in both the GVH and host-versus-graft directions, investigators at Johns Hopkins have performed a series of studies to determine the minimal conditioning needed to achieve stable engraftment after one to three HLA antigen–mismatched BMT. Sixty-eight patients with advanced hematologic malignancies received cyclophosphamide 50 mg/kg intravenously on day 3 (n = 28) or on days 3 and 4 (n = 40) after transplantation.[20] Graft failure occurred in 9 of 66 (14%) evaluable patients and was fatal in 1. The cumulative incidences of grades II to IV and grades III to IV acute GVHD by day 200 were 34% and 6%, respectively. Actuarial overall survival and event-free survival at 2 years after transplantation were 36% and 26%, respectively. More recently this approach has been evaluated in a multicenter study using a conditioning regimen of cyclophosphamide, fludarabine, and 200 cGy of total body irradiation. The 1-year probabilities of overall and progression-free survival in 50 patients after haploidentical marrow transplantation were 62% and 48%, respectively, confirming the exportability of this approach.[57]

Selective Allodepletion

Nonselective depletion of T cells from the allograft before transplantation effectively prevents severe acute GVHD but invariably predisposes the recipient to loss of the graft, disease relapse, and an increased incidence of infectious complications. Unmanipulated T-cell add-backs likely will not be effective in preventing these problems without causing GVHD because the frequency of alloreactive T cells in the peripheral blood is far greater than that of either specific antiviral or antileukemic T cells. One approach to overcoming these adverse outcomes is to selectively deplete the graft of the GVHD-causing alloreactive T cells identified by upregulation of activation markers while conserving cells mediating GVT and antimicrobial immune responses. Several methods of selective removal of alloreactive T cells have been reported that rely on ex vivo stimulation of donor T cells by recipient peripheral blood mononuclear cells in a unidirectional mixed lymphocyte reaction culture. Host-reactive donor T cells can be identified by their expression of activation markers (CD25, CD69, CD71), proliferative potential, or preferential retention of photoactive dyes. They subsequently can be targeted for depletion using a variety of methods, including an immunotoxin,[58,59] immunomagnetic bead separation,[60-63] fluorescence-activated cell sorting,[64,65] photodynamic purging,[66,67] or Fas–Fas ligand–mediated apoptosis.[68] These selective allodepletion methods have yielded 70% to 95% reductions in alloreactivity in vitro, with retention of immune responses against third-party and infectious organisms. Several methods even allow retained alloreactivity against leukemia cells.[66,69-71] Although this promising approach has been shown to be feasible in clinical trials,[72,73] several concerns have been raised, including contamination of recipient peripheral blood mononuclear cells by leukemic cells, loss of antileukemic activity, and induction of clinically significant GVHD. In a clinical trial, Amrolia et al[74] used different cell doses for allodepleted (via immunotoxin) T-cell add-back. At a dose level of 10^5 $CD3^+$ cells/kg, patients exhibited significantly more rapid recovery of T cells at 3 to 5 months after haploidentical HCT than did patients who received 10^4 $CD3^+$ cells/kg. The incidence of GVHD was very low, and the median time to reach a $CD4^+$ cell count greater than 300/μL was 4 months in patients at a dose of 10^5 $CD3^+$ cells/kg compared with more than 6 months in patients at a dose of 10^4 $CD3^+$ cells/kg and 8 months in the series by Eyrich et al[75] without allodepleted T-cell add-back. A similar improvement in immune reconstitution without GVHD has been demonstrated by another group that used photodynamic therapy for selective depletion of alloreactive T cells.[76] Bear in mind that however small the alloreactive T-cell subset of the total T-cell population (<0.1% in the HLA-matched sibling setting; 1% to 5% in the HLA-mismatched setting), their complete elimination may be difficult, and doses of unmanipulated T cells as low as 3 to 10^3 cells/kg can be associated with severe GVHD following haploidentical HCT. Mielke et al[77] at the National Institutes of Health demonstrated that selective depletion of alloreactive T cells preserves a $CD25^-CD4^+Foxp3^+$ fraction of T cells that is capable of undergoing marked expansion posttransplant to regulatory T cells (Tregs), which can provide protection against GVHD.

CHOICE OF DONORS FOR HAPLOIDENTICAL HEMATOPOIETIC CELL TRANSPLANTATION: SPECIAL CONSIDERATIONS

Exploiting KIR Ligand Mismatching in the Graft-Versus-Host Direction

NK-cell alloreactivity in the GVH or host-versus-graft direction can be a powerful means of optimizing the efficacy and safety of haploidentical HCT. NK cells are a unique $CD56^+CD3^-$ cell population composing approximately 10% of peripheral blood lymphocytes[78,79] and are involved in innate antiviral and antitumor immune responses[80-83] (see Chapter 20). They constitute a heterogeneous population of different cell subsets with distinct phenotypic and functional characteristics. The majority (90%) are highly cytotoxic $CD56^{dim}$ cells likely functioning as efficient effector cells, whereas a minority (10%) are immunoregulatory $CD56^{bright}$ cells producing cytokines.[84,85] Following HCT, including haploidentical transplant with selected $CD34^+$ cells, NK cells recover as early as 2 to 3 weeks posttransplant by rapid differentiation from engrafted $CD34^+$ cells.[14,22,86]

The "missing self" recognition concept was hypothesized 2 decades ago by Klas Karre. He suggested that, unlike T and B cells, NK cells are activated by the absence of self-MHC class I molecules on the surface of target cells.[87-90] Expression of self-MHC molecules on target cells delivers an inhibitory signal to NK cells via inhibitory KIRs. In the absence of this inhibitory signal, NK-cell alloreactivity, manifested by NK cell–mediated target cell lysis, proceeds by default. When NK cell–inhibitory receptors are engaged by KIR-specific epitopes, killing is inhibited, whereas killing of target cells occurs when NK cell–inhibitory receptors are not engaged, because of either absence of MHC class I or MHC mismatch. Because virally infected cells and tumor cells downregulate MHC expression to escape adaptive immune surveillance, the ability of NK cells to identify "missing self" is critical in (innate) immune response against viruses and tumor cells.[91,92] Essentially all NK cells express at least one inhibitory receptor that is specific for a self-MHC class I epitope, thereby preventing autoreactivity.[93] NK cells also have activating receptors, most notably NKG2D and NKp46, which can trigger NK-cell alloreactivity when they are engaged by appropriate antigens on virally infected cells and tumor cells.[94-97] Although inhibitory signals are believed to dominate over activating signals, NK-cell activity is regulated by quantitative differences in cumulative inhibitory and activating signals transmitted via KIRs. Therefore the presence or absence of the respective ligands on recipient cells determines if NK cells will be primed to be alloreactive and kill the targets.[79,98]

By selecting haploidentical stem cell donors whose NK cells are not fully inhibited by recipient MHC class I ligands, that is, there is a KIR ligand mismatch in the GVH direction, the graft NK-cell alloreactivity may be used to optimize a GVT effect. As discussed in Myeloablative Haploidentical HCT: Ex Vivo T-Cell Depletion, Ruggeri et al[39,99] found that HLA (KIR ligand) mismatching in the GVH direction following T cell–depleted haploidentical HCT is associated with strong NK-cell alloreactivity leading to (1) a dramatically reduced relapse in patients with AML, (2) a lower rate of graft rejection, and (3) a reduction in GVHD. As supported by their animal studies, the reduction in GVHD is due to donor NK-mediated depletion of host antigen-presenting cells that are crucial in priming alloreactive donor T cells and hence in the pathogenesis of GVHD, and donor NK cells that attack host hematopoietic cells and spare epithelial GVHD target tissues.[39,99,100] The lower rates of graft rejection were shown to be due to donor NK–mediated lysis of host residual T cells, thereby preventing them from rejecting the graft. Furthermore, in their murine transplant model they showed that pretransplant transfer of NK cells into mice improved engraftment after transplantation, allowing durable full donor chimerism following reduced-intensity conditioning. This NK-cell conditioning prevented GVHD well enough to allow for safe infusion of otherwise lethal doses of allogeneic T cells, which were given to facilitate immune reconstitution.

Fetomaternal Microchimerism

Several transplant centers have developed haploidentical HCT strategies based on the principle of tolerance induction as a result of in utero exposure to maternal antigens and the development of long-lasting fetomaternal microchimerism.[101] A large International Bone Marrow Transplant Registry analysis by van Rood et al[102] showed that the incidence of grade II or higher acute GVHD following non–T cell–depleted haploidentical HCT was related to haplotype inheritance. Transplants from a noninherited maternal antigen–mismatched sibling were associated with significantly less acute GVHD. Moreover, transplant-related mortality was significantly higher in transplants from a maternal or a paternal donor. Several Japanese transplant centers have performed non–T cell–depleted transplants following either myeloablative or nonmyeloablative conditioning from microchimeric noninherited maternal antigen–mismatched donors.[103-106] Although the overall incidence of grade II or higher acute GVHD incidence was high (56% of 34 evaluable patients) in one series, a significantly lower risk for acute GVHD was observed in patients who received a transplant from a donor who was noninherited maternal antigen mismatched in the GVH direction.

IMMUNE RECONSTITUTION FOLLOWING HAPLOIDENTICAL HEMATOPOIETIC CELL TRANSPLANTATION

Transfer of a functional lymphohematopoietic system from donor to recipient in a timely fashion determines in large part the eventual success of HCT. Given the problem of delayed immune reconstitution with resultant risk for infectious complications and disease relapse following haploidentical transplantation, particularly after ex vivo T cell–depleted HCT, new strategies are required to limit the severity and duration of this immunodeficiency. Both adoptive cellular therapy approaches and strategies using soluble factors are being investigated (see box on Haploidentical Hematopoietic Cell Transplantation: Ongoing Novel Efforts to Improve Transplant Outcomes).

Immunotherapy involving both cellular and soluble factors can be guided by two distinct concepts: (1) enhancement of general immune reconstitution relative to enhancement of antigen-specific responses and (2) expansion of beneficial cell subsets and depletion of harmful effector cells. New approaches aimed at facilitating engraftment and reducing GVHD while preserving GVT effects have been developed using Tregs and mesenchymal stem cells (MSCs). In mice, two types of regulatory T cells, $CD4^+CD25^+$ T cells (Tregs) and NK T cells (NK Tregs), have been shown to prevent acute GVHD.[107-111]

Haploidentical Hematopoietic Cell Transplantation: Ongoing Novel Efforts to Improve Transplant Outcomes

Selective Allodepletion

- Unmanipulated donor lymphocyte infusions (T-cell add-backs) cause significant graft-versus-host disease (GVHD).
- Selective depletion of specific host-reactive donor T cells (instead of global T-cell depletion) may mediate graft-versus-tumor (GVT) and antimicrobial immune responses without causing significant GVHD.

Cells and Cytokines of Special Appeal (Importance)

Natural Killer Cells

- Natural killer (NK)-cell alloreactivity in GVH direction following T cell–depleted transplant can dramatically reduce leukemic relapse.
- NK-cell alloreactivity in GVH direction can lead to lower rates of graft rejection due to donor NK–mediated lysis of host residual T cells.
- NK-cell alloreactivity in GVH direction can reduce GVHD via donor NK–mediated depletion of host antigen-presenting cells (and sparing of epithelial target tissues).

Immunoregulatory T Cells

- Ex vivo expanded regulatory T cells may inhibit GVHD while enhancing immune reconstitution and facilitating GVT effects.

Mesenchymal Stem Cells

- Ex vivo expanded mesenchymal stem cells have the potential to diminish GVHD while facilitating immune reconstitution.

Cytokines and Chemokines

- A number of cytokines and chemokines and their associated monoclonal antibodies can influence effector cell development, activation, trafficking, and thereby transplant outcomes, including engraftment, GVHD, immune reconstitution, and antitumor effects.

Tregs represent approximately 5% to 10% of peripheral $CD4^+$ T cells in mice and humans and are identified by their capacity to suppress both $CD4^+$ and $CD8^+$ T-cell activation. Tregs have been shown to promote engraftment and reduce acute GVHD without loss of GVT effects.[107,108,112] In murine models, Tregs can be successfully expanded ex vivo by in vitro stimulation with allogeneic splenocytes plus IL-2. When added to the donor inoculum containing alloreactive T cells, the Treg population can prevent GVHD, enhance immune reconstitution, and reduce the risk for infection while the GVT effect is well preserved.[113] There has been considerable interest in developing approaches for expansion of human Tregs to prevent and treat GVHD.[114] Preliminary experience with expanded Tregs in humans is promising with a recent study showing that adoptive transfer of Tregs prevented GVHD in the absence of any posttransplantation immunosuppression and enhanced immunity to opportunistic pathogens.[115]

MSCs, which are multipotential nonhematopoietic progenitors and constitute only 0.001% of nucleated cells in human bone marrow,[116] have been extensively evaluated for their regenerative and immunomodulatory properties. Human MSCs have a high in vitro proliferative potential and have the capacity to differentiate into a number of mesenchymal tissues, such as bone, cartilage, and fat. MSCs have been demonstrated to inhibit T-cell alloreactivity[117-121] and prolong skin allograft survival.[122] In addition, ex vivo expanded MSCs have the potential to prevent and treat acute GVHD when used after HLA-matched or HLA-mismatched HCT.[123,124] Although the exact mechanism of immune modulation by MSC is not clearly defined, they appear to mediate their immunomodulatory effects by inhibiting interferon-γ secretion from Th1 and NK cells, increasing IL-10 secretion from Tregs and increasing IL-4 secretion from Th2 cells, thereby promoting a Th1 to Th2 shift.[120]

Cytokines and Chemokines

A number of cytokines and chemokines and their associated monoclonal antibodies can be applied to influence effector cell development, activation, trafficking, and thereby transplant outcomes, including engraftment, GVHD, immune reconstitution, and antitumor effects.[124-126] Posttransplant use of G-CSF accelerates neutrophil recovery, but studies have shown deleterious effects on immune restoration, namely, by inhibition of NK-cell and T-cell function.[127-129] Given their excellent capacity to enhance in vivo expansion of NK and T cells after T cell–depleted HCT, IL-2[130-133] and IL-18[134] potentially could improve immune reconstitution after haploidentical transplant. However, caution must be taken because, depending on the timing of administration of these cytokines, unfavorable outcomes such as exacerbation of GVHD may occur.[135,136] In one murine model, IL-7 improved immune reconstitution by enhancing thymopoiesis in addition to expanding peripheral T cells, NK cells, NK Tregs, B cells, monocytes, and macrophages.[137] However, in another model this cytokine enhanced the development of acute GVHD.[138] Keratinocyte growth factor has been shown in a murine model to improve thymic and peripheral T-cell recovery after transplant.[139] Monoclonal antibodies specific for selective cytokines and chemokines to prevent GVHD[44,140,141] and optimize GVT effects are being evaluated.[125]

Enhancement of Antigen-Specific Immune Responses

Prevention and treatment of opportunistic viral, fungal, bacterial, and parasitic infections remain formidable challenges after haploidentical HCT. For example, the failure to successfully treat viral infections, which is partly due to the limited number of nontoxic antiviral drugs, constitutes a major cause of treatment failure following haploidentical transplant. Both $CD4^+$ and $CD8^+$ cells are critical in maintaining CMV, Epstein-Barr virus, adenovirus, polyomavirus, and herpesvirus in their latent phase. Therefore adoptive immunotherapy with ex vivo expanded virus-specific cytotoxic T lymphocytes (CTLs) is being explored. Infusion of donor-derived allogeneic CMV-specific T-cell clones into recipients for prevention or treatment of CMV-related disease, without causing GVHD, has shown promising potential.[142-145] These studies also demonstrated that CMV-specific $CD4^+$ cells are important for reconstitution and maintenance of $CD8^+$ CTL responses. Encouraging early results have been achieved when ex vivo expanded allogeneic CTL clones specific for Epstein-Barr virus were used for prophylaxis and management of Epstein-Barr virus–associated diseases, including posttransplant lymphoproliferative disorder.[146-149] The identification of antigens that are specifically expressed by leukemia cells, such as PR1 by CML and AML cells, and can be recognized by T cells has led to successful ex vivo generation of leukemia-specific donor T cells (PR1-CTL) that may promote a GVT effect.[150-152] Notwithstanding the promise of these novel approaches, the large-scale therapeutic potential of adoptive transfer of ex vivo expanded antigen-specific effector cells has not yet been fully realized for a number of reasons. One reason is the short survival of the effector cells, which likely is due to factors intrinsic to the cells themselves or to the host environment into which the cells are infused.

OPTIMIZATION OF GRAFT-VERSUS-TUMOR EFFECT: ADOPTIVE CELLULAR THERAPY VIA DLI

Adoptive cellular immunotherapy using DLI has been shown experimentally and clinically to be a potent means of inducing a GVT effect by converting mixed to full donor chimerism after allogeneic transplant.[153-155] In patients with recurrent CML after HLA-matched HCT, complete clinical and molecular remissions are achieved in the majority of patients following unmodified DLI.[156,157] A high incidence of GVHD (and marrow aplasia) has tempered the use of this approach and has led to a revision of DLI strategies, such as lowering the dose of infused T cells or giving T-cell subsets such as $CD8^+$-depleted DLI.[158] The GVHD risk likely is higher after alternative donor transplantation, and considerably smaller doses of T cells have been used in the haploidentical HCT setting.[159,160] Lewalle et al[159] reported the outcomes of escalating DLI doses after haploidentical transplantation. $CD3^+$ T-cell doses greater than 1×10^4 kg every 3 months (given to convert mixed to full chimerism) caused significant GVHD in recipients of T cell– and B cell–depleted myeloablative haploidentical HCT. Or et al[160] treated 28 patients (6 prophylactic and 22 therapeutic) with HLA-mismatched DLI. The dose range of T cells in the DLI was 1×10^2 to 1.5×10^9 kg. GVHD (median peak grade II) occurred in 13 of the 28 patients. A higher incidence of GVHD unexpectedly occurred in recipients of a 5/6 HLA-matched DLI compared to recipients of a 3/6 HLA-matched DLI. In our nonmyeloablative HCT trial, in which vigorous ex vivo and in vivo T-cell depletion are used, $CD3^+$ T-cell doses greater than 1.0×10^6 cells/kg were given in some circumstances. Because GVHD occurred in the majority of cases (most often skin-limited GVHD), future strategies will use a smaller initial DLI dose.[18] Additional dose-finding studies are required to establish the safest and most effective DLI T-cell dose and schedule following haploidentical HCT. Critical to the success of HCT will be the identification of specific cellular populations that can be administered as adoptive cellular immunotherapy (e.g., pathogen- or tumor-specific CTL) and that are capable of optimizing the separation of GVHD and GVT. An alternative approach that has been evaluated in Europe is to add back donor lymphocytes genetically engineered with a suicide gene to facilitate immune reconstitution and prevent late mortality.[161] In 50 patients who received these cells in a multicenter study, immune recovery appeared to be more rapid, and GVHD occurring in 10 was controlled by induction of the suicide gene.[161]

HAPLOIDENTICAL HEMATOPOIETIC CELL TRANSPLANTATION: NEW APPLICATIONS

Combining Haploidentical Peripheral Blood Stem Cells With Umbilical Cord Blood for Facilitation of Engraftment

Umbilical cord blood transplantation has been complicated by slow hematologic recovery and delayed immune reconstitution due in part to the relatively low number of hematopoietic progenitor cells collected and transplanted. In an attempt to facilitate hematologic recovery and reduce the complications associated with impaired immune recovery, Fernandez et al[162] cotransplanted 11 patients with umbilical cord blood cells and $CD34^+$ cell–selected haploidentical PBSCs. Rapid neutrophil recovery occurred at a median of 10 days (range, 9 to 17 days). Chimerism studies showed a predominance of the haploidentical genotype in the granulocyte and mononuclear lineages early posttransplant, followed by progressive replacement by cells of umbilical cord donor origin. Grade II or higher GVHD occurred in 4 (36%) of the 11 patients. Five of the 11 patients were alive and in complete remission 6 to 43 months posttransplant. Evaluation of immune reconstitution in this patient population demonstrated early recovery of NK cells and B cells and delayed but eventually complete recovery of $CD4^+$ and $CD8^+$ cells.[163]

Specific Tolerance Induction

Induction of donor-specific tolerance has important implications for the field of organ transplantation, which currently is limited by the complications of lifelong immunosuppressive therapy. Multiple preclinical small and large animal models have shown that sustained specific tolerance can be induced after induction of even transient mixed lymphohematopoietic chimerism.[164,165] Based on these preclinical discoveries, we have conducted clinical trials of combined related-donor bone marrow and kidney transplantation for patients with end-stage renal disease. In the first of these trials, combined HLA-matched bone marrow and kidney transplantation was performed in patients with multiple myeloma and end-stage renal disease. This experience was notable for the achievement of complete remissions in four of six patients and the occurrence of renal graft rejection (transient and reversible) in only one patient. All six patients were alive from approximately 3 to 8 years posttransplant.[7,166]

To broaden the application of this strategy, we initiated a trial of combined haploidentical bone marrow and kidney transplantation for patients with end-stage renal disease but no associated malignancy. The preparative therapy is one that we used in earlier trials of haploidentical HCT for hematologic malignancies and was notable for the uniform development of transient mixed chimerism followed by graft rejection.[18] Of the first five patients who received a combined haploidentical bone marrow and kidney transplant, four are no longer receiving immunosuppressive therapy. In vitro evidence of specific tolerance also has been demonstrated.[167]

The proof of the principle of sustained donor-specific tolerance induction through mixed lymphohematopoietic chimerism has been demonstrated clinically. Future trials will include the transplantation of other organs, including cadaveric organs, and the inclusion of fully HLA-mismatched related donors.

FUTURE DIRECTIONS

The promise of haploidentical HCT, specifically the opportunity to offer allogeneic transplantation to virtually everyone who requires it and to take advantage of the powerful GVT effect that it affords, has yet to be fully realized (see box on Haploidentical Hematopoietic Cell Transplantation: Future Direction). Although the complications of severe GVHD and graft rejection have been overcome in large part by the use of "megadose" T cell–depleted hematopoietic progenitor cells, prolonged immunodeficiency remains a formidable problem. Reduced-intensity conditioning has ameliorated early transplant-related morbidity and perhaps mortality but has been associated with a higher relapse probability and no clear advantage in terms of restoration of effective immunity. Vigorous pan–T cell depletion of the graft dramatically reduces the incidence of acute GVHD but delays immune reconstitution, resulting in a high incidence of opportunistic infections and disease relapse.

The future of haploidentical HCT relies on the ability to modulate the cellular content of the graft and the posttransplant cellular environment, to separate GVHD and GVT, and to rapidly restore effective immunity (shown schematically in Fig. 107-1). Strategies such as selective allodepletion of the graft or enrichment for (or

Haploidentical Hematopoietic Cell Transplantation: Future Directions

Approaches involving T-cell depletion or modulation are likely required to prevent severe graft-versus-host disease. Therefore we will need the following:

- Improved immune reconstitution, such as pathogen-specific cytotoxic T lymphocytes (CTLs) and better infectious disease monitoring
- Strategies to prevent disease relapse, such as adoptive natural killer cells, regulatory T cells, and tumor-specific CTLs
- Prospective, multicenter trials to define optimal regimens and post–hematopoietic cell transplantation care

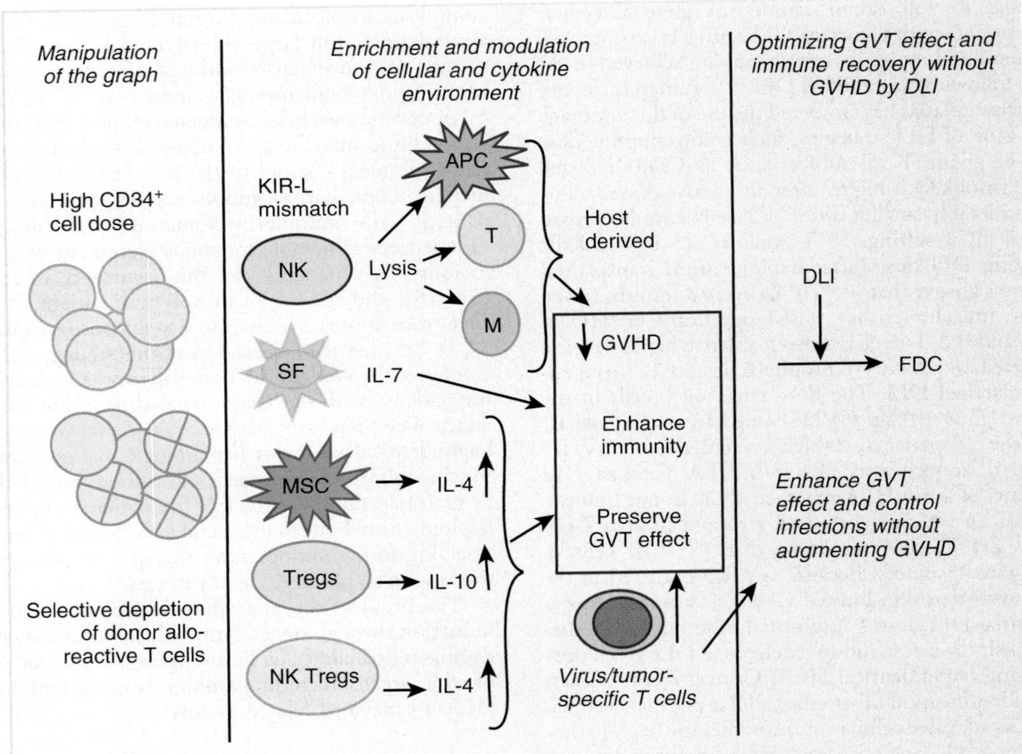

Figure 107-1 SCHEMA OF A STRATEGY TO OPTIMIZE THE OUTCOMES OF HAPLOIDENTICAL HEMATOPOIETIC CELL TRANSPLANTATION. *Manipulation of the graft:* A high CD34$^+$ cell dose will likely improve donor engraftment by overcoming host-mediated resistance; selective ex vivo depletion of donor alloreactive T cells may reduce the incidence of severe acute graft-versus-host disease (GVHD) while preserving a graft-versus-tumor (GVT) effect and improving immune recovery. *Enrichment and modulation of cellular and cytokine environment:* Killer immunoglobulin-like receptor ligand (KIR-L) mismatching in the GVH direction will prompt donor natural killer (NK) cells to promote engraftment by attacking host T cells (T), diminish acute GVHD by depleting host antigen-presenting cells (APC) while eliminating host-derived malignant cells (M). Ex vivo expanded NK cells, mesenchymal stem cells (MSC), regulatory T cells (Tregs), NK Tregs, and soluble factor (SF; IL-7) will further augment donor engraftment, innate and adaptive immune responses, and reduce GVHD while not impairing GVT effects. MSC and NK Tregs, via IL-4 production, will skew donor T cells toward an antiinflammatory Th2 phenotype that is associated with reduced GVHD. *Optimizing GVT effect and immune recovery without GVHD by unmodified donor leukocyte infusion (DLI):* Ex vivo engineered tumor antigen and pathogen (virus)-specific donor-derived T cells (both cytotoxic T lymphocytes and CD4 cells) can be used to prevent and/or treat relapse of an underlying malignancy and opportunistic infections, respectively. In some circumstances, unmodified DLI may be used to convert mixed chimerism to full donor chimerism (FDC), probably enhancing a GVT effect without augmenting GVHD.

addition of) cell populations such as Tregs or MSCs to the graft may achieve effective protection from GVHD while imparting effective antitumor and antiinfective immunity.

Following the transplant, administration of specific cellular populations or soluble factors may affect the separation of GVHD and GVT effect. Unmanipulated DLI may still be considered at certain times to convert the mixed chimerism to full donor hematopoiesis in an effort to achieve an early GVT effect and facilitate early reconstitution. The adoptive transfer of allogeneic cytotoxic T cells that are specific for viral or tumor antigens may be other strategies for addressing the problems of infection and disease relapse. Other cellular populations, such as NK or NK T regs cells or MSC, may favorably influence the balance of GVHD and immune reconstitution. The future of haploidentical transplant depends on our expanding knowledge of the cellular populations and soluble factors that determine the separation of GVHD and GVT effect and our ability to modulate the cellular content of the graft and the post-transplant environment to improve disease-free and overall survival probabilities.

SUGGESTED READINGS

Aggarwal S, Pittenger MF: Human mesenchymal stem cells modulate allogeneic immune cell responses. *Blood* 105:1815, 2005.

Alpdogan O, Schmaltz C, Muriglan SJ, et al: Administration of interleukin-7 after allogeneic bone marrow transplantation improves immune reconstitution without aggravating graft-versus-host disease. *Blood* 98:2256, 2001.

Amrolia PJ, Muccioli-Casadei G, Huls H, et al: Adoptive immunotherapy with allodepleted donor T-cells improves immune reconstitution after haploidentical stem cell transplantation. *Blood* 108:1797, 2006.

Aversa F, Terenzi A, Tabilio A, et al: Full haplotype-mismatched hematopoietic stem-cell transplantation: A phase II study in patients with acute leukemia at high risk of relapse. *J Clin Oncol* 23:3447, 2005.

Barrett J, Gluckman E, Handgretinger R, et al: Point-counterpoint: Haploidentical family donors versus cord blood transplantation. *Biol Blood Marrow Transplant* 17:S89, 2011.

Beatty PG, Clift RA, Mickelson EM, et al: Marrow transplantation from related donors other than HLA-identical siblings. *N Engl J Med* 313:765, 1985.

Brunstein CG, Fuchs EJ, Carter SL, et al: Alternative donor transplantation after reduced intensity conditioning: Results of parallel phase 2 trials using partially HLA-mismatched related bone marrow or unrelated double umbilical cord blood grafts. *Blood* 118:282, 2011.

Cavazzana-Calvo M, Andre-Schmutz I, Dal CL, et al: Immune reconstitution after haematopoietic stem cell transplantation: Obstacles and anticipated progress. *Curr Opin Immunol* 21:544, 2009.

Chen BJ, Cui X, Liu C, et al: Prevention of graft-versus-host disease while preserving graft-versus-leukemia effect after selective depletion of host-reactive T cells by photodynamic cell purging process. *Blood* 99:3083, 2002.

Ciceri F, Bonini C, Stanghellini MT, et al: Infusion of suicide-gene-engineered donor lymphocytes after family haploidentical haemopoietic stem-cell transplantation for leukaemia (the TK007 trial): A non-randomised phase I-II study. *Lancet Oncol* 10:489, 2009.

Di Ianni M, Falzetti F, Carotti A, et al: Tregs prevent GVHD and promote immune reconstitution in HLA-haploidentical transplantation. *Blood* 117:3921, 2011.

Edinger M, Hoffmann P, Ermann J, et al: $CD4^+CD25^+$ regulatory T cells preserve graft-versus-tumor activity while inhibiting graft-versus-host disease after bone marrow transplantation. *Nat Med* 9:1144, 2003.

Fehse B, Frerk O, Goldmann M, et al: Efficient depletion of alloreactive donor T lymphocytes based on expression of two activation-induced antigens (CD25 and CD69). *Br J Haematol* 109:644, 2000.

Guinan EC, Boussiotis VA, Neuberg D, et al: Transplantation of anergic histoincompatible bone marrow allografts. *N Engl J Med* 340:1704, 1999.

Huang XJ, Chang YJ: Unmanipulated HLA-mismatched/haploidentical blood and marrow hematopoietic stem cell transplantation. *Biol Blood Marrow Transplant* 17:197, 2011.

Ichinohe T, Uchiyama T, Shimazaki C, et al: Feasibility of HLA-haploidentical hematopoietic stem cell transplantation between noninherited maternal antigen (NIMA)-mismatched family members linked with long-term feto-maternal microchimerism. *Blood* 104:3821, 2004.

Kanda J, Chao NJ, Rizzieri DA: Haploidentical transplantation for leukemia. *Curr Oncol Rep* 12:292, 2010.

Karre K, Ljunggren HG, Piontek G, et al: Selective rejection of H-2-deficient lymphoma variants suggests alternative immune defence strategy. *Nature* 319:675, 1986.

Le Blanc K, Rasmusson I, Sundberg B, et al: Treatment of severe acute graft-versus-host disease with third party haploidentical mesenchymal stem cells. *Lancet* 363:1439, 2004.

Luznik L, O'Donnell PV, Symons HJ, et al: HLA-haploidentical bone marrow transplantation for hematologic malignancies using nonmyeloablative conditioning and high-dose, posttransplantation cyclophosphamide. *Biol Blood Marrow Transplant* 14:641, 2008.

Mapara MY, Kim YM, Wang SP, et al: Donor lymphocyte infusions mediate superior graft-versus-leukemia effects in mixed compared to fully allogeneic chimeras: A critical role for host antigen-presenting cells. *Blood* 100:1903, 2002.

O'Donnell PV, Luznik L, Jones RJ, et al: Nonmyeloablative bone marrow transplantation from partially HLA-mismatched related donors using post-transplantation cyclophosphamide. *Biol Blood Marrow Transplant* 8:377, 2002.

Peggs KS, Verfuerth S, Pizzey A, et al: Adoptive cellular therapy for early cytomegalovirus infection after allogeneic stem-cell transplantation with virus-specific T-cell lines. *Lancet* 362:1375, 2003.

Powles RL, Morgenstern GR, Kay HE, et al: Mismatched family donors for bone-marrow transplantation as treatment for acute leukaemia. *Lancet* 1:612, 1983.

Ruggeri L, Capanni M, Urbani E, et al: Effectiveness of donor natural killer cell alloreactivity in mismatched hematopoietic transplants. *Science* 295:2097, 2002.

Shlomchik WD, Couzens MS, Tang CB, et al: Prevention of graft versus host disease by inactivation of host antigen-presenting cells. *Science* 285:412, 1999.

Spitzer TR, McAfee S, Sackstein R, et al: Intentional induction of mixed chimerism and achievement of antitumor responses after nonmyeloablative conditioning therapy and HLA-matched donor bone marrow transplantation for refractory hematologic malignancies. *Biol Blood Marrow Transplant* 6:309, 2000.

Sykes M, Preffer F, McAfee S, et al: Mixed lymphohaemopoietic chimerism and graft-versus-lymphoma effects after non-myeloablative therapy and HLA-mismatched bone-marrow transplantation. *Lancet* 353:1755, 1999.

Velardi A, Ruggeri L, Mancusi A, et al: Natural killer cell allorecognition of missing self in allogeneic hematopoietic transplantation: A tool for immunotherapy of leukemia. *Curr Opin Immunol* 21:525, 2009.

For complete list of references log on to www.expertconsult.com.

CHAPTER 108

UNRELATED DONOR CORD BLOOD TRANSPLANTATION FOR HEMATOLOGIC MALIGNANCIES

Doris M. Ponce and Juliet N. Barker

Cord blood (CB) is now routinely used as an alternative stem cell source for unrelated donor allogeneic stem cell transplantation. In the late 1980s, Broxmeyer and colleagues[1] reported that CB is a rich source of hematopoietic stem cells (HSCs) and progenitors, setting the stage for the first related donor CB transplantation (CBT) in 1988.[2] Subsequently, placental blood banking programs were initiated in 1992 to 1993 in New York, Milan, Dusseldorf, and Paris.[3,4] The first unrelated donor CBT was performed in 1993, and the first unrelated donor CBT series were published in 1996.[5,6] Public CB banks have since grown in number with an estimated 600,000 public CB units banked globally.[7] Furthermore, the number of CBT continues to increase with an estimated 20,000 now performed.[7]

The use of CB stem cells has several benefits. Given it is a cryopreserved product, it has rapid accessibility, does not carry the risk of donor unavailability, and has the advantages that the admission of the patient revolves around the patient's readiness for transplantation and not the availability of the donor. Barker et al[8] reported that recipients of CB grafts were transplanted a median of 25 days earlier than unrelated donor transplant recipients. This is particularly advantageous for patients in need of an urgent transplant. Another benefit is the reduced stringency of the required human leukocyte antigen (HLA) match afforded by the naïve neonatal immune system. This has facilitated the extension of transplant access, especially to racial and ethnic minorities. A recent prospective analysis conducted at Memorial Sloan-Kettering Cancer Center (MSKCC) of 525 patients undergoing combined unrelated donor and CB unit searches demonstrated that 53% of patients from European ancestry but only 21% of non-Europeans had a 10/10 HLA-matched unrelated donor identified (P <.001).[9] By contrast, 5-6/6 HLA-matched CB units were identified for a high proportion of all patients (79% of Europeans and 71% of non-Europeans). Of the 269 unrelated volunteer donor transplant recipients, only 23% had non-European origins, but 56% of CBT recipients had non-European ancestry (P<.001) (Fig. 108-1). Thus, CB is frequently able to provide a suitable graft regardless of patient racial or ethnic background.

SINGLE UNIT CORD BLOOD TRANSPLANTATION

Engraftment

Unrelated donor CBT was initiated using single-unit grafts. Studies have demonstrated that higher cell dose and better donor–recipient HLA match are independent factors associated with improved neutrophil engraftment.[10-17] The 1997 Eurocord analysis was the first large series reporting on 143 related and unrelated donor CBT recipients. In unrelated donor CBT recipients, improved neutrophil and platelet engraftment were both associated with a higher total nucleated cell (TNC) dose above the median of 3.7×10^7/kg and donor–recipient HLA match.[10] In 1998, Rubinstein et al[11] confirmed these findings in an analysis of 562 CBT facilitated by the New York Blood Center (NYBC) as did an updated analysis by Gluckman and Rocha in 2004.[15] In 2002, Wagner et al[13] reported that infused CD34$^+$ cell dose was superior to infused TNC dose in determining the success of neutrophil and platelet engraftment in an analysis of 102 CBT (median age, 7.4 years) with recipients of units with less than 1.7×10^5 CD34$^+$ cells/kg having a significantly lower neutrophil engraftment incidence of 72% at a median of 34 days compared with higher cell doses ($P < 0.01$).

These analyses have the limitation that cell dose and HLA match are analyzed separately and yet these graft characteristics must be considered together in the selection of individual units. In 2009, Rocha and Gluckman[18] reported on 925 recipients of single-unit CBT transplanted for malignant disease and found that neutrophil engraftment was related to the number of cells infused (P <.0001) and HLA match with a significant difference between zero and one (81%), two (75%), and three and four (63%) HLA disparities (P = .037). The role of HLA match was partially abrogated by an increase in cell dose except for recipients of highly mismatched grafts. In 2010, Barker et al[17] analyzed the combined effect of TNC dose and donor–recipient HLA match in 1061 single-unit CBT recipients transplanted for hematologic malignancies after myeloablative conditioning. The best neutrophil engraftment was associated with a fully HLA-A, -B antigen, and -DRB1 matched unit or a cryopreserved TNC greater than 10.0×10^7/kg with one or two mismatches. The worst was with a unit with three mismatches or a cryopreserved TNC below 2.5×10^7/kg with one or two mismatches (Fig. 108-2). There was no difference in neutrophil engraftment in recipients of one versus two mismatched units, and in this setting, the TNC dose determined neutrophil engraftment.

Graft-Versus-Host Disease

Single-unit CBT is associated with a lower than expected incidence of graft-versus-host disease (GVHD) for the degree of donor–recipient HLA mismatch, which allows use of units with a less stringent HLA match (i.e., only a 4-6/6 HLA-A, -B antigen, -DRB1 allele match). Incidences of grades II to IV acute GVHD have been reported between 10% and 50% and likely vary according to the GVHD prophylaxis used and the inclusion of antithymocyte globulin in the conditioning.[10,17,19-23] As with the transplantation of adult donors, the major graft determinant of acute GVHD is the HLA match, although with CB, the permissible mismatch is considerably greater than can be tolerated with HSC transplantation from adult donors.

Although an effect of HLA mismatch could not be demonstrated in early series of unrelated donor CBT,[10,11,13,24] the recent large NYBC retrospective analysis of 1061 single-unit CBT recipients demonstrated that recipients of matched CB units had significantly less grade III to IV acute GVHD and that increasing mismatch was associated with a progressively increased risk of severe acute GVHD.[17] There was also an association between the degree of mismatch and chronic GVHD, although this only reached significance in recipients of units with three mismatches.[17] Kurtzberg et al[22] have reported that high-resolution matching at HLA-A, -B, and -DRB1 alleles was protective with significantly higher incidence of grades II-IV (P = .02) and III to IV (P = .02) acute GVHD in recipients of units with less than 5/6 allele match. A recent report by Eapen et al[25] in 803 recipients of single CB units that analyzed the effect of match at HLA-A, -B, -C at intermediate resolution and DRB1 at allele resolution did not show a significant effect of HLA-match for grades II to IV acute GVHD, but high-resolution matching was not examined at HLA class I.

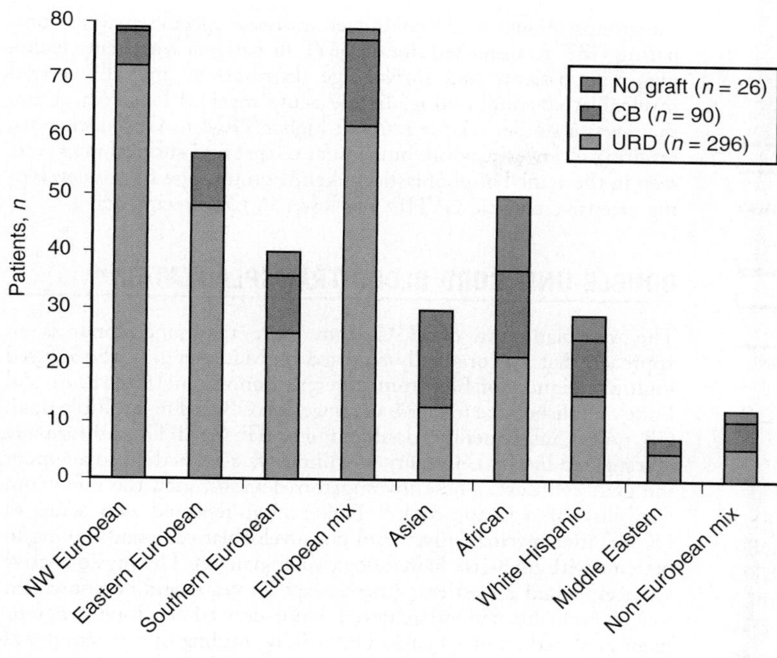

Figure 108-1 COMPARISON OF PATIENT ANCESTRY IN RECIPIENTS OF UNRELATED VOLUNTEER DONOR (URD) OR CORD BLOOD (CB) TRANSPLANTATION, OR THOSE WHO LACKED A SUITABLE GRAFT. *(From Barker JN, Byam CE, Kernan NA, et al: Availability of cord blood extends allogeneic hematopoietic stem cell transplant access to racial and ethnic minorities.* Biol Blood Marrow Transplant *16:1541, 2010.)*

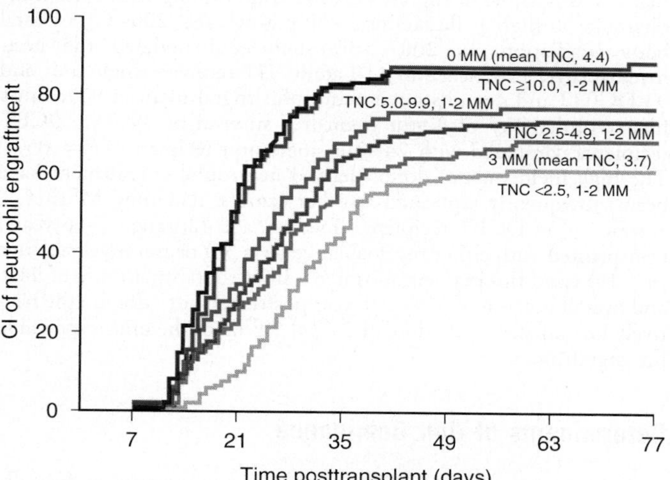

Figure 108-2 NEUTROPHIL ENGRAFTMENT AFTER MYELOABLATIVE SINGLE-UNIT CORD BLOOD TRANSPLANTATION FACILITATED BY THE NEW YORK BLOOD CENTER ACCORDING TO CRYOPRESERVED TOTAL NUCLEATED CELL (TNC) DOSE AND HUMAN LEUKOCYTE ANTIGEN MATCH. *CI,* Cumulative incidence; *MM,* mismatched. *(From Barker JN, Scaradavou A, Stevens CE: Combined effect of total nucleated cell dose and HLA match on transplantation outcome in 1061 cord blood recipients with hematologic malignancies.* Blood *115:1843, 2010.)*

Relapse

During the early years of CBT, there was concern that the neonatal immune system would not adequately protect against relapse. However, multiple series have demonstrated a strong protection against relapse after CBT with the major determinant of relapse being the recipients' disease status.[13,22,23,26] The NYBC series of 1061 single-unit CBT recipients showed no association between HLA match grade and the incidence of relapse, and subgroup analysis in only relapsed patients, only remission patients, and only those who engrafted also failed to demonstrate any association.[17] However, the 2011 analysis of Eapen et al[25] (n = 803) showed a lower relapse incidence after CBT mismatched at more than one loci compared with recipients of units matched at HLA-A, -B, -C and -DRB1, although the number of mismatched loci had no effect. The reason for the disparity in the findings of these two studies is not known, and this area requires further investigation before definitive conclusions can be drawn.

Transplant-Related Mortality and Survival

Early series of single-unit CBT demonstrated high transplant-related mortality (TRM) and consequently poor survival after single-unit CBT. This likely related to the high-risk nature of the patient population and standards of supportive care as well as the characteristics of the transplanted units. Factors such as disease status and recipient cytomegalovirus (CMV) positivity are strong determinants of survival after single-unit CBT.[22] From the standpoint of the graft, both TNC dose and HLA-match influence TRM and survival. In addition to low TNC dose being associated with increased TRM and decreased survival,[10,11,13,17] the 68 adult patient analysis of Laughlin et al[27] and the Wagner et al[13] 102 patient analysis demonstrated a higher $CD34^+$ cell dose (>1.2 and 1.7, respectively) were associated with significantly improved disease-free survival (DFS). Similarly, studies have identified increasing HLA-mismatch is significantly associated with increased TRM and lower survival.[13,17,21] The 2010 NYBC analysis of combined TNC dose and HLA match showed that recipients of 6/6 HLA-matched units had the lowest TRM and best survival regardless of the dose at least within the dose range tested (Fig. 108-3).[17] Recipients of units with 1 HLA-mismatch and a TNC dose 2.5 to 4.9 × 10^7/kg had a similar TRM as those receiving units with two mismatches and a TNC greater than 5.0 ×10^7/kg despite the higher cell dose in the latter group (see Fig. 108-3). Recipients of single units with one or two mismatches and a TNC below 2.5 × 10^7/kg had very high TRM and poor survival.

In the recent 2011 Eapen series evaluating the contribution of HLA-C matching after single unit CBT, patients matched at HLA-A, -B, and -DRB1 had a higher TRM if mismatched at HLA-C (n = 23; hazard ratio [HR], 3.97; P = .18) as compared with those matched at all 4 loci (n = 69).[25] TRM was also higher in 5/6 but 6/8 matched CBT recipients mismatched at one of HLA-A, -B or -DRB1 plus HLA-C (n = 234; HR, 1.70; P = .029) compared with those

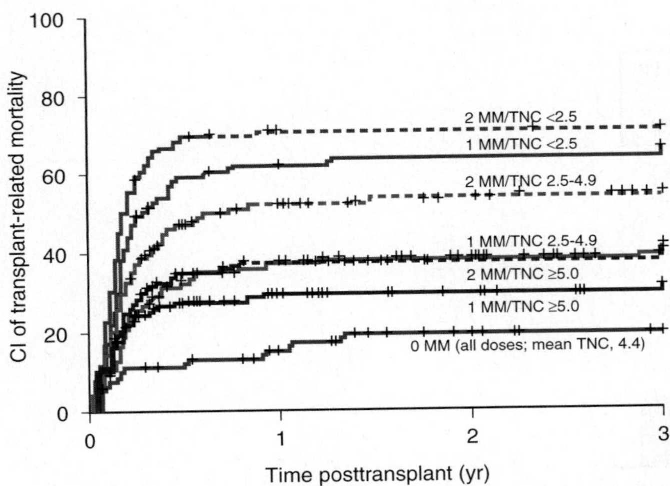

Figure 108-3 CUMULATIVE INCIDENCE (CI) OF TRANSPLANT-RELATED MORTALITY (TRM) ACCORDING TO THE COMBINED TOTAL NUCLEATED CELL (TNC) DOSE AND HUMAN LEUKOCYTE ANTIGEN MISMATCH AFTER SINGLE-UNIT MYELOABLATIVE CORD BLOOD TRANSPLANTATION. *MM,* Mismatched. *(From Barker JN, Scaradavou A, Stevens CE: Combined effect of total nucleated cell dose and HLA match on transplantation outcome in 1061 cord blood recipients with hematologic malignancies.* Blood *115:1843, 2010.)*

who were 5/6 and 7/8 matched (i.e., when there was a single HLA mismatch at -A, -B, or -DRB1 but a match at -C; n = 127). This study suggests that HLA-C matching is an important determinant of survival and should be considered in unit selection algorithms.

Comparison of Single-Unit Cord Blood Transplantation and Adult Donor Allografts

Although the use of CBT as an alternative HSC source has increased substantially, no randomized studies evaluating survival after CBT versus adult donor allografts have yet been reported. Retrospective comparisons have demonstrated varying results depending on whether the series evaluated children or adults and if matched versus mismatched unrelated volunteer donors were included. Selected series are summarized in Table 108-1. In 2007, Eapen and colleagues[21] compared the outcomes of pediatric single-unit CBT with those of unrelated volunteer bone marrow (BM) recipients who were transplanted for the treatment of acute leukemia. Compared with the recipients of 8/8 allele matched unrelated donor BM transplantation (BMT), the 5-year leukemia-free survival in recipients of one or two HLA-mismatched CBT was similar. Notably, however, a significantly higher leukemia-free survival was observed in recipients of 6/6 HLA-matched units. Interestingly, TRM was similar in 6/6 HLA-matched and 5/6 HLA-matched high cell dose compared with that of allele-matched unrelated donor recipients' transplant (P= .0659 and .1332, respectively). By contrast, TRM was higher in recipients of one antigen HLA-mismatched low cell dose and two antigen HLA-mismatched of any cell dose compared with allele-matched unrelated donor recipients (P = .0455 and .0003, respectively).

A similar analysis done in adult patients with acute leukemia demonstrated that single-unit CBT recipients had a higher TRM compared with recipients of 8/8 HLA-matched unrelated donor transplants but a similar TRM to that of 7/8 HLA-mismatched unrelated donor transplant recipients.[23] The Japanese group of Takahashi et al[20] compared CBT recipients with unrelated donor BM or peripheral blood HSC transplantation for the treatment of hematologic malignancies. They demonstrated a slower neutrophil recovery in CBT recipients but a similar rate of neutrophil engraftment. The incidences of grades III to IV acute GVHD and extensive chronic GVHD were higher after unrelated donor transplantation. No differences were demonstrated in TRM, relapse, or DFS between the groups. Atsuta et al[28] conducted a disease-specific analysis comparing CBT to unrelated donor BMT in patients with acute leukemia. The patients had similar age distribution, and all received myeloablative conditioning. In the acute myeloid leukemia group, there was a similar relapse rate but higher TRM in CBT recipients, resulting in lower survival, but similar relapse and survival rates were seen in the acute lymphoblastic leukemia group. The risk of developing extensive chronic GVHD was lower in CBT recipients.

DOUBLE-UNIT CORD BLOOD TRANSPLANTATION

The transplantation of HSC from more than one donor is an approach that was originally reported by Mathé et al,[29] who infused multiple aliquots of BM from different donors. In 1972, Ende and Ende[30] published the first case of allogeneic CBT using multiple small CB units. Subsequently, double-unit CBT (DCBT) was formally investigated by the University of Minnesota as a method to augment the graft cell dose. These investigators demonstrated the safety and feasibility of this approach.[31] Barker et al reported two series of DCBT after myeloablative[32] and nonmyeloablative[33] conditioning in patients with high-risk hematologic malignancies. The myeloablative series evaluated 23 patients (median age 24 years) and demonstrated that all evaluable patients achieved donor-derived neutrophil engraftment at a median of 23 days. The striking finding of this report was the high level of engraftment despite sustained hematopoiesis being mediated by a single donor in nearly all patients and the high 1-year overall survival of 72%. The non-myeloablative series demonstrated that it was possible to engraft CB after conditioning with cyclophosphamide 50 mg/kg, fludarabine 200 mg/m^2, and 200 cGy of total body irradiation. In 2007, Brunstein et al updated the non-myeloablative experience in 110 adults (17 received single-unit and 93 DCBT) and demonstrated neutrophil engraftment in 92% but a higher probability of 3-year event-free survival of 39% in DCBT recipients compared with 24% in single-unit recipients (P = .05).[34] The high incidences of donor-derived neutrophil engraftment have been subsequently replicated at other centers, including MSKCC.[35] A series of 54 DCBT recipients (median, age 42; range, 7-66 years) transplanted with either myeloablative (n = 35) or nonmyeloablative (n = 19) conditioning demonstrated a high engraftment rate of 94% and overall survival of 65% at 1-year posttransplant[35] despite the relatively low infused TNC dose of 2.52×10^7/kg of the unit responsible for engraftment.

Determinants of Unit Dominance

The determinants of DCBT unit dominance remain to be fully elucidated. Better HLA match, ABO group, and higher infused TNC or CD34$^+$ cell doses have not predicted which unit will win. Current evidence suggests that unit dominance is predominantly immune mediated, although unit hematopoietic potential can also play a role (Table 108-2).

Host Factors as Determinants of Unit Dominance

Eldjerou et al[36] were the first to report both in vitro and in vivo studies of DCBT using aliquots of cells from each unit of a clinical double-unit CB allograft and correlation of the laboratory findings with patient engraftment. The experimental design used nonobese diabetic severe combined immunodeficient interleukin-2 receptor gamma null (NOD/SCID/IL2R-γ^{null}) mice and demonstrated that the engrafting unit in the mice correlated with clinical engraftment in 18 of 21 cases (P <.001). Thus, given the concordance of the human and murine engraftment, these findings suggest that unit dominance is not related to host-versus-graft factors. Brunstein et al[37] evaluated the effect of donor-specific anti-HLA antibodies in 126 DCBT recipients and found no correlation with the speed of engraftment or unit dominance. Similar findings have been documented in MSKCC

Table 108-1 Comparison of Single-Unit Cord Blood Transplantation With Adult Donor Hematopoietic Stem Cell Transplantation

Reference	Graft (*n* Patients)	Median Age (yr)	Conditioning (*n* Patients)	Neutrophil Engraftment	II to IV Acute	Chronic GVHD	TRM	Survival
Eapen et al[21]	**503 CBT**							
	35 matched	Unknown	24 TBI, 11 chemotherapy	85% at +42	8/34	10/33	2/35	LFS 60% at 5 years
	1-Ag MM							
	44 high dose		142 TBI, 54 chemotherapy, 5 unknown	80%	62/142	27/147	45/157	LFS 45%
	157 low dose			59%			19/44	LFS 36%
	2-Ag MM 267		208 TBI, 54 chemotherapy, 5 unknown	76%	107/259	38/247	124/267	LFS 33%
	208 BM							
	116 matched	Unknown	98 TBI, 18 chemotherapy	97%	53/116 and 37/116	100/166 and 66/166	24/116	LFS 38%
	MM/166		153 TBI, 13 chemotherapy	97%			51/166	LFS 37%
Takahashi et al[20]	**100 CBT**	38	TBI	91% at +60	52% and 74% at 3 years		9% at 1 year	DFS 70% at 3 years
	71 RD 55 BM 16 PBSC	40	TBI	96%	52% and 69%		13%	DFS 60%
Atsuta et al[28]	**287 CBT**							
	173 AML	38	154 TBI, 19 chemotherapy	77% at +100	32%	28%	33% at 2 years	DFS 36% at 2 years
	114 ALL	34	110 TBI, 4 chemotherapy	80%	28%	37%	24%	DFS 45%
	533 URD							
	311 AML	38	252 TBI, 59 chemotherapy	94%	35%	32%	22%	DFS 54%
	222 ALL	32	204 TBI, 18 chemotherapy	97%	42%	30%	25%	DFS 51%
Eapen et al[23]	**165 CB**	Unknown	90 TBI, 75 chemotherapy	80% at +42	49/162	39/161	55/165 at 2 years	DFS 98/165 at 2 years
	888 PBSC							
	632 matched	Unknown	583 TBI, 305 chemotherapy	96%	303/630	327/632	149/632	DFS 358/632
	265 1-Ag MM				134/256	113/256	93/256	DFS 170/256
	472 BM							
	332 matched	Unknown	321 TBI, 151 chemotherapy	93%	129/ 332	132/332	188/332	DFS 188/332
	140 1-Ag MM				64/139	51/140	80/140	DFS 80/140

Ag, Antigen; *ALL,* acute lymphoid leukemia; *AML,* acute myeloid leukemia; *BM,* bone marrow; *CBT,* cord blood transplantation; *DCBT,* double-unit cord blood transplantation; *DFS,* disease-free survival; *GVHD,* graft-versus-host disease; *LFS,* leukemia-free survival; *MM,* mismatched; *PBSC,* peripheral blood stem cell; *RD,* related donor; *TBI,* total-body irradiation; *TRM,* transplant-related mortality; *URD,* unrelated donor.

DCBT recipients transplanted for hematologic malignancies (J. Barker, unpublished data, 2011). This is further evidence that host factors do not play a major role in unit dominance.

Hematopoietic Potency as a Determinant of Unit Dominance

Although the infused $CD34^+$ cell or colony-forming unit (CFU) dose has not been associated with unit dominance, Scaradavou et al[38] have shown that hematopoietic potential can sometimes determine unit dominance. These investigators evaluated the effect of the percentage of viable $CD34^+$ cells postthaw in 46 DCBT recipients and found that engrafting units almost always had a high $CD34^+$ cell viability greater than 75%, but units with lower $CD34^+$ cell viability were very unlikely to engraft ($P = .0006$). Low $CD34^+$ cell viability also correlated with CFU potential. Thus, one mechanism by which DCBT can favorably influence engraftment is that the infusion of two units increases the chance that at least one unit with engraftment potential will be administered. Interestingly, in the only patient that had graft failure in this series, both units had poor $CD34^+$ cell viability.

Georges et al[39] have confirmed that higher $CD34^+$ cell viability was the only graft variable to predict unit dominance in a canine model of DCBT. By contrast, Eldjerou et al[36] evaluated the hematopoietic potential of each unit in vitro as measured by colony-forming cell and cobblestone area–forming cell content using either mononuclear cells or $CD34^+$ cells, and this did not correlate with clinical unit dominance with the contribution of each unit in co-cultures being concordant with the clonogenic efficiency of that unit when cultured alone. Thus, although $CD34^+$ and CFU dose may not predict unit dominance, damage to the unit as reflected by a low percentage of viable $CD34^+$ cells is associated with impaired engraftment potential in large animal models and humans.

Immune Factors as Determinants of Unit Dominance

Analysis of early DCBT series showed that higher infused $CD3^+$ cell dose correlated with the engrafting unit.[9] This has been subsequently confirmed in recent studies[40] supporting the role of T cells in unit dominance. Murine models have also suggested that an immune mechanism accounts for unit dominance. Kim et al[41] demonstrated that despite each unit engrafting alone, co-infusion of mononuclear

Table 108-2 Potential Determinants of Unit Dominance After Double-Unit Cord Blood Transplantation

Potential Mechanism	Reference	Finding	Implications
Host factors	Eldjerou et al[36]	Unit dominance in mice correlated with clinical engraftment.	Host factors do not influence unit dominance.
	Brunstein et al[37]	Donor specific anti-HLA antibodies had no influence on unit dominance.	
Unit factors Hematopoietic potential	Scaradavou et al[38]	Infused TNC/kg, CD34+/kg, and CFU doses were not associated with unit engraftment. However, units with low CD34+ viability were very unlikely to engraft.	Infused CD34+ cell dose and CFU, CFC, or CAFC content do not directly influence unit dominance, but poor-quality units are very unlikely to engraft in humans.
	Eldjerou et al[36]	In vitro CFC and CAFC content did not correlate with unit dominance.	
Immune factors	Barker et al,[32] Scaradavou et al,[38] Avery et al[40]	Higher infused CD3+ cell dose is associated with unit dominance.	Graft-versus-graft interactions dictate unit dominance.
	Kim et al[41]	DCBT with MNC associated with unit dominance whereas co-engraftment achieved with lineage depletion or MSC infusion.	
	Yahata et al[42]	Mixed chimerism achieved by CD34+ selection.	
	Eldjerou et al[36]	Loss of unit dominance with CD34+ DCBT restored with addition of CD34- cells.	
	Delaney et al[44]	Unmanipulated unit is dominant when co-infused with T-cell depleted expanded CB.	
	Gutman et al[43]	Dominant unit CD8+ T cells directed against the nondominant unit detected in patients with single unit dominance.	
	Avery et al[40]	High level of unit-unit match associated with increased likelihood of co-engraftment.	
	Brunstein et al[45]	Higher prevalence of dual chimerism after Treg infusion.	

CAFC, 5 Cobblestone area-forming cell; *CB,* cord blood; *CFC,* colony forming cell; *CFU,* colony forming unit; *DCBT,* double-unit cord blood transplantation; *MNC,* mononuclear cell; *MSC,* mesenchymal stromal cell; *TNC,* total nucleated cell dose; *Treg,* regulatory T cell.

cells as a double-unit graft was associated with predominance of one CB unit in NOD/SCID mice. Unit dominance could be mitigated (and engraftment of both units achieved) with either lineage depletion of the units or cotransplantation of third-party BM-derived mesenchymal stromal cells. Yahata et al[42] replicated this observation in NOD/SCID/IL2R-γ^{null} mice and found that the co-infusion of mononuclear cells from two CB units resulted in single unit dominance but mixed chimerism could be generated by CD34+ cell selection. Additional experiments by this group extended this observation by demonstrating that unit dominance was T cell–mediated and specifically involved both CD4+ and CD8+ cells. The study of Eldjerou et al[36] found that NOD/SCID/IL2R-γ^{null} murine DCBT resulted in single unit dominance that correlated with clinical engraftment in 18/21 patients. Furthermore, murine DCBT using CD34+ cells was associated with loss of both unit dominance and clinical correlation, and addition of CD34- cells from only one of the two units restored unit dominance but with engraftment being mediated by the origin of the CD34- cells regardless of which unit engrafted in the patient. These findings suggest that unit dominance is an in vivo event that is mediated by graft-versus-graft interactions.

Additional evidence in favor of an immune basis for unit dominance comes from the study by Gutman et al,[43] who identified CD8+ T cells derived from the dominant unit that recognized the nondominant unit were present in the peripheral blood 28 days after transplantation in nine of 10 DCBT recipients engrafting with single units regardless of the conditioning regimen. Interestingly, the three patients who had persistent mixed chimerism also did not develop an alloreactive CD8+ T-cell response. Furthermore, it can be hypothesized that the failure of sustained engraftment of ex vivo expanded CB units in clinical trials of DCBT in which one of two units is expanded is not attributable to failure to expand or maintain sufficient progenitors in the manipulated unit but because the expanded unit is T cell depleted and therefore cannot compete with a T cell replete unmanipulated unit.[44] Moreover, Brunstein et al[45] evaluated the safety of ex vivo expanded regulatory T cells (Tregs) in DBCT recipients and found an increased prevalence of co-engraftment of both units (dual donor chimerism), suggesting that graft-versus-graft interactions could be ameliorated by suppressing T-cell responses.

Clinical data from Avery et al[40] have demonstrated a role of HLA-match in unit dominance. Interestingly, in this analysis of 84 DCBT recipients, the dominant units were not necessarily better HLA matched to the recipient compared with the nondominant unit of a double-unit pair (Fig. 108-4). However, the unit–unit HLA match influenced the length of time the ultimately nonengrafting unit was able to be detected. Specifically, recipients of double-unit grafts in whom the unit–unit HLA match was 7/10 or greater HLA-allele matched were significantly more likely to have initial co-engraftment and transient persistence of the ultimately nonengrafting unit with one patient having sustained engraftment of both units long term. By contrast, recipients of units highly mismatched (<6/10) to each other were more likely to have engraftment with only a single unit. This is likely because of an enhanced unit-versus-unit immune response, whereas closely HLA-matched units are more likely to be relatively tolerant of each other, and in this setting, at least transient co-engraftment is possible.

Taken together, these findings suggest that unit dominance likely involves a complex interplay of hematopoietic potential as suggested by the role of CD34+ cell viability as well as immune factors that are likely T cell mediated because no role for natural killer (NK) cells has been identified to date.[46] Future studies need to elucidate the specific cell population mediating the graft-versus-graft effect in the setting of the transplantation of two units with adequate engraftment potential.

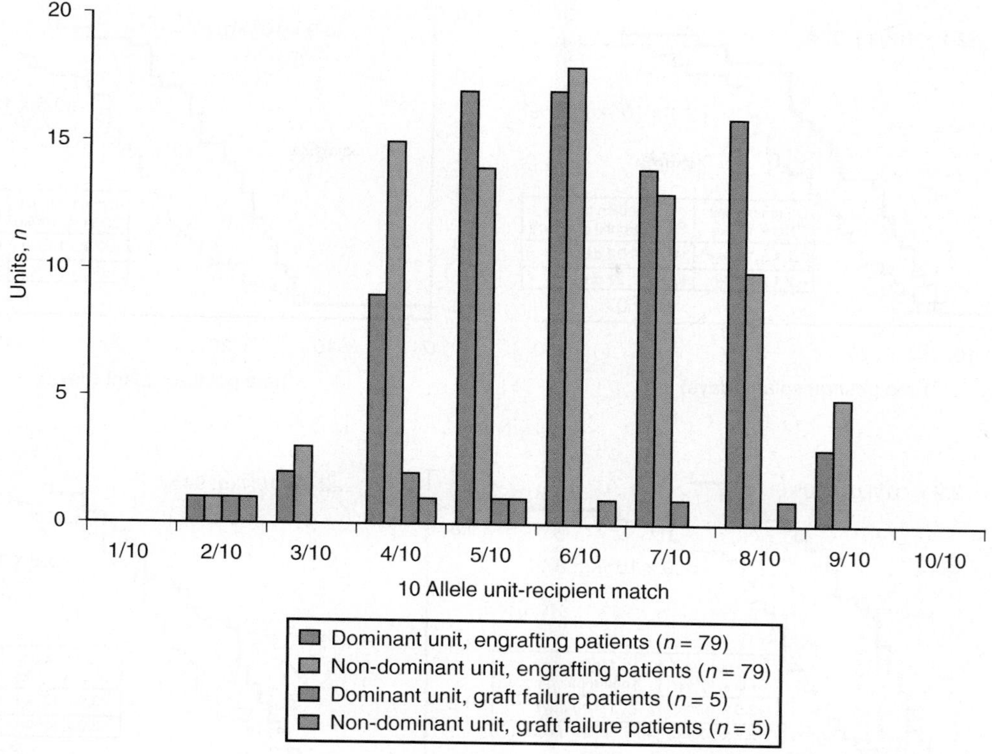

Figure 108-4 INFLUENCE OF HIGH RESOLUTION UNIT-RECIPIENT HUMAN LEUKOCYTE ANTIGEN MATCH ON SUSTAINED DONOR ENGRAFTMENT AFTER DOUBLE-UNIT D BLOOD TRANSPLANTATION ($n = 84$). The engrafting units were not better matched to the recipient. *(From Avery S, Shi W, Lubin M, et al: Influence of infused cell dose and HLAmatch on engraftment after double-unit cord blood allografts.* Blood *117:3277, 2011.)*

Determinants of Speed and Success of Engraftment After Double-Unit Cord Blood Transplantation

The use of double-unit CB grafts is now a standard approach to augment cell dose, although whether DCBT improves engraftment compared with single-unit CBT is yet to be definitively proven. Barker et al[35] reported the analysis of 54 DCBT recipients with hematologic malignancies who received either myeloablative ($n = 35$) or nonmyeloablative ($n = 19$) conditioning and found a high incidence of sustained donor engraftment of 94% (95% confidence interval [CI], 87-100) by day 50 (Fig. 108-5). This is in contrast to the reported engraftment after myeloablative conditioning in single-unit CBT series of 65% to 88%.[13,19,22,23,26,34] The Avery MSKCC series updated their experience in 2011 with the analysis of the influence of infused cell dose on engraftment after DCBT in 84 patients.[40] A high incidence of sustained donor engraftment was achieved among myeloablative ($n = 61$) and nonmyeloablative ($n = 23$) conditioning recipients of 93% and 96%, respectively. Interestingly, sustained donor neutrophil engraftment was mediated by 1 unit in the majority of patients regardless of conditioning intensity. Notably, initial engraftment of both units did not increase the likelihood or speed of neutrophil recovery ($P = .71$), suggesting that this is not the mechanism of enhanced engraftment after DCBT.

This analysis also demonstrated that in recipients of myeloablative conditioning, a higher infused cell dose (TNC, $CD34^+$) and CFU dose of the dominant unit was associated with a higher incidence of sustained donor engraftment and improved speed of neutrophil recovery (Fig. 108-6) whereas the doses of the non-dominant unit had no impact. Neutrophil recovery was faster with all patients engrafting if the dominant unit had a $CD34^+$ cell dose of 0.9×10^5/kg or greater compared with lower cell doses ($P = .0008$). A higher infused total (unit 1 + unit 2) graft TNC and $CD3^+$ cell dose was also associated

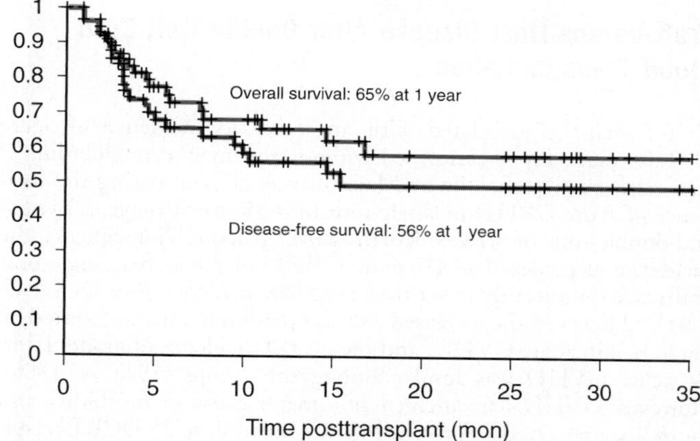

Figure 108-5 KAPLAN-MEIER 1-YEAR OVERALL SURVIVAL AND DISEASE-FREE SURVIVAL AFTER DOUBLE-UNIT CORD BLOOD TRANSPLANTATION ($n = 54$). *(From Barker JN, Abboud M, Rice RD, et al: A "no-wash" albumin-dextran dilution strategy for cord blood unit thaw: high rate of engraftment and a low incidence of serious infusion reactions.* Biol Blood Marrow Transplant *15:1596, 2009.)*

with improved engraftment, suggesting that the nonengrafting unit may help facilitate the engraftment of the dominant unit in a dose-dependent fashion. By contrast, unit–recipient HLA match and unit–unit HLA match evaluated at 6 HLA loci or 10 HLA alleles had no association with engraftment speed or success. As seen in single-unit CBT, however, analysis of large numbers of patients are required to determine the role of HLA match in DCBT engraftment rates.

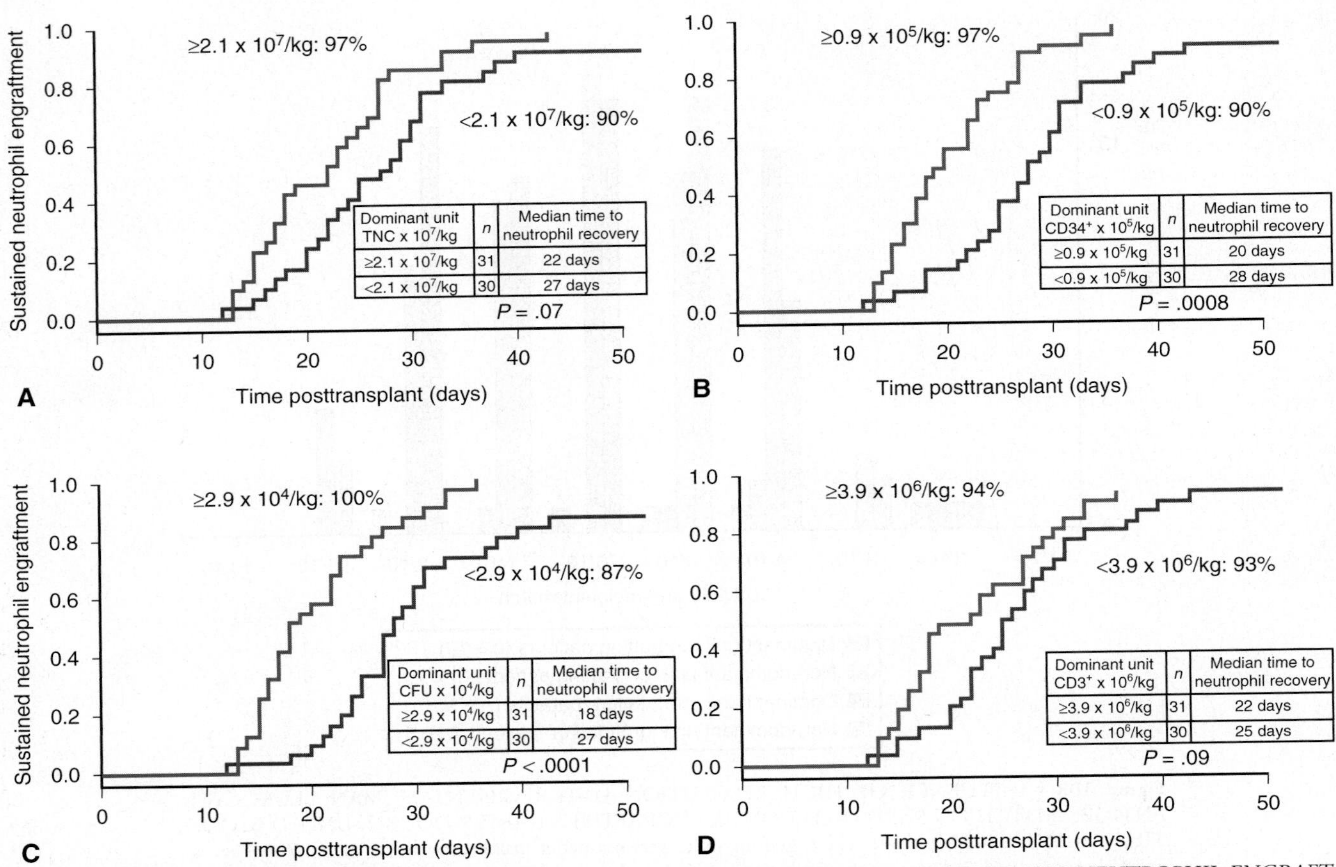

Figure 108-6 RELATIONSHIP BETWEEN THE INFUSED CELL DOSES OF THE DOMINANT UNIT AND NEUTROPHIL ENGRAFTMENT AFTER DOUBLE-UNIT D BLOOD TRANSPLANTATION. **A,** Dominant unit total nucleated cell dose. **B,** Dominant unit CD34⁺ dose. **C,** Dominant unit colony-forming unit dose. **D,** Dominant unit CD3⁺ dose. *(From Avery S, Shi W, Lubin M, et al: Influence of infused cell dose and HLAmatch on engraftment after double-unit cord blood allografts.* Blood *117:3277, 2011.)*

Graft-Versus-Host Disease After Double-Unit Cord Blood Transplantation

DCBT may be associated with an increased incidence of acute GVHD, especially if performed without antithymocyte globulin.[47,48] In a retrospective analysis by MacMillan et al[47] comparing the incidence of acute GVHD in single-unit (n = 80; median age, 23 years) and double-unit (n = 185; median age, 45 years) CBT recipients, the incidence of grades II to IV acute GVHD of 39% after single-unit grafts was significantly lower than the 58% incidence after DCBT (P <.01).[47] However, the increased risk was predominantly accounted by grade II skin acute GVHD, and the overall incidence of grades III to IV acute GVHD was similar among the groups (19% vs. 18%). However, GVHD has emerged as a major cause of morbidity and mortality after DCBT. A recent MSKCC analysis of 75 DCBT recipients demonstrated that GVHD was the second most common cause of TRM after organ failure.[48]

Ponce et al[49] evaluated the incidence and characteristics of GVHD in 101 DCBT recipients with hematologic malignancies. Patients received either myeloablative (n = 76; 75%) or nonmyeloablative (n = 25; 25%) conditioning. GVHD prophylaxis consisted of a calcineurin inhibitor and mycophenolate mofetil, and no patient received antithymocyte globulin. The cumulative incidence of grade II to IV acute GVHD by day 100 was 50% (95% CI, 40-60) with 26% (95% CI, 16-35) having grade III to IV disease. The median onset was 39 days (range, 14-99), and the organ most commonly affected was the gastrointestinal tract followed by the skin. With a median follow-up of 24 months (range, 4.5-60.5), the 1-year cumulative incidence of ongoing late acute or chronic GVHD was 35% (95% CI, 26-45), and the 1-year progression-free survival (PFS) was 65% (95% CI, 56-75). Series of DCBT incorporating antithymocyte globulin have demonstrated lower rates of GVHD. For example, Cutler et al[50] reported an overall incidence of grade II to IV acute GVHD of 9.4% and chronic GVHD of 12.5%. Although the incidence of acute GVHD after DCBT is increased with the omission of antithymocyte globulin in the pretransplant conditioning, its use is associated with a higher risk of serious infections, including serious Epstein-Barr virus (EBV)–related complications,[51] delayed immune reconstitution,[52] and an increased risk of TRM,[34,53] and may also increase the risk of relapse.[54] Thus, better understanding of the pathophysiology of GVHD after DCBT is needed to facilitate improved prevention and treatment of this disease.

Relapse

Multiple retrospective series of DCBT have been associated with a reduced incidence of relapse in patients with leukemia and lymphoma, suggesting an enhanced graft-versus-malignancy effect.[34,53,55] Verneris et al[55] analyzed the risk of acute leukemia relapse in 177 recipients of myeloablative CBT (47% single-unit and 53% double-unit CBT) and found that the 19% relapse risk in DCBT recipients in first or second remission was lower than that 34% relapse risk in single-unit recipients (P = .03). Notably, the lower risk of relapse was not influenced by conditioning regimen, GVHD prophylaxis, engrafting unit–recipient HLA match, infused cell dose, or development of acute or chronic GVHD in multivariate analysis. The University of Minnesota group also analyzed 110 nonmyeloablative CBT recipients (17 single-unit and 93 double-unit grafts) and found a trend toward a reduced relapse risk among those receiving DCBT (30% vs. 41%; P = .07).[13] Eurocord-Netcord investigators have published similar findings in patients with lymphoid malignancies.[53] The

Barker et al 2011 series of 75 DCBT recipients (31% children and 69% adults) transplanted for high-risk acute leukemia or myelodysplasia demonstrated a strikingly low 2-year incidence of relapse of 9% in children and 6% in adults.[56] It is possible that the increased $CD3^+$ cell dose or unit–unit interactions may mediate an enhanced graft-versus-malignancy effect after DCBT. Further investigation of the potential mechanisms accounting for these observations should be a priority.

Transplant-Related Mortality and Survival

The MSKCC series of 75 DCBT recipients of either myeloablative (n = 53; 71%) or nonmyeloablative (n = 22; 29%) conditioning demonstrated that the 2-year TRM of 25% was almost entirely accounted for by patients dying in the first 6 months after transplant.[48] Thus, DCBT recipients who survive the first 180 days were very unlikely to die of transplant-related causes. Interestingly, Sauter et al[57] demonstrated steady immune recovery from day 120, which likely contributes to this protection against late mortality.

The Minnesota series of 177 myeloablative CBT recipients (84 single-unit and 93 double-unit grafts) transplanted for the treatment of acute leukemia demonstrated a 5-year overall rate and DFS of 47% and 46%, respectively.[55] The MSKCC series of 75 DCBT recipients with lymphoid and myeloid malignancies demonstrated a 2-year overall and PFS of 65% and 55%, respectively.[48] Barker et al[56] have evaluated 75 DCBT recipients (23 children and 52 adults) with high-risk acute leukemia, myelodysplasia, and myeloproliferative disorder and found a 2-year DFS of 78% in children and 64% in adults. Multivariate analysis revealed that CMV serostatus was the only significant determinant of DFS. Brunstein et al[58] reported the outcomes of 50 DCBT recipients in a multicenter study of nonmyeloablative CBT for the treatment of hematologic malignancies. The 1-year overall survival and PFS were 54% and 46%, respectively.

Comparison of Double-Unit Cord Blood Transplantation With Adult Donor Allografts

A number of recent retrospective series have shown similar survival after DCBT and adult donor transplantation, supporting the use of double-unit grafts as an alternative stem cell source (Table 108-3). The 2010 combined series of the Fred Hutchinson Cancer Research Center and the University of Minnesota compared DCBT (n = 128), matched related (n = 204), matched unrelated (n = 152), and mismatched unrelated (n = 52) donor recipients for the treatment of acute or chronic myeloid leukemia.[59] They found that neutrophil recovery was delayed at least 1 week but grade II to IV acute GVHD was lower after DCBT. The 2-year TRM was higher in DCBT recipients, but when the analysis was restricted to DBCT recipients with earlier neutrophil engraftment (median <26 days), the TRM incidence was similar among the groups. When compared with adult unrelated donor transplantation, TRM risk was similar. Interestingly, the 5-year DFS was not different by donor type.

Similarly, Ponce et al[48] have compared 75 DCBT recipients with 108 related donor and 184 unrelated donor transplant recipients with hematologic malignancies. They demonstrated that the median time to neutrophil recovery was delayed in myeloablative CBT recipients compared with other stem cell sources. However, the 2-year PFS was similar among the groups (P = 0.573) (Fig. 108-7). These results are striking given the median match of the CB units to the patient was 6/10 (range, 2-9/10) at high resolution and the median infused $CD34^+$ dose was 0.09×10^6/kg/unit. A Eurocord-Netcord analysis compared patients with lymphoid malignancies who received either CBT (44 single-unit and 31 double-unit grafts) or matched unrelated donors (n = 284) after reduced-intensity conditioning.[60] They found a lower incidence of neutrophil engraftment in CBT recipients but similar rates of acute GVHD, TRM, and DFS. Relapse rates were also similar despite more aggressive lymphoid histologies and refractory disease in the CBT group. Overall, these findings are encouraging and suggest the feasibility of conducting a prospective comparison and possibly randomized trials between double-unit CB and adult unrelated donor transplantation.

CORD BLOOD UNIT SELECTION

Efficient search and selection of CB units requires decision making as to what banks to consider and what factors to prioritize in unit selection. The unit selection algorithm currently used at MSKCC is shown in Fig. 108-8.[61] Primary unit selection criteria are based on the prethaw cryopreserved TNC/kg, the unit-recipient HLA match

Table 108-3 Comparison of Double-Unit Cord Blood Transplantation With Adult Donor HSC Transplantation

Reference	Graft/Patients (*n*)	Median Age, Years (range)	Conditioning (Patients, *n*)	Neutrophil Engraftment or Median Days to ANC (range)	II to IV Acute	Chronic GVHD	TRM	Survival (PFS or DFS)
Rodrigues et al[60]	31 DCBT 44 single CBT	44	RIC	85%	33%	37%	28%	34% (2 years)
	284 MUD	48	RIC	98%	31%	48%	30%	34%
Brunstein et al[59]	128 DCBT	25 (10-46)	MA	26 (13-45)	60%	26%	34% (5 years)	51% (5 years)
	204 MRD	40 (12-67)	MA	16 (11-39)	65%	47%	24%	33%
	152 MUD	31 (10-57)		19 (11-39)	80%	43%	14%	48%
	52 MMUD	31 (10-51)		18.5 (8-33)	85%	48%	27%	38%
Ponce et al[48]	75 DCBT	37 (<1-66)	53 MA 22 NMA	93%	43%	28%	25% (2 years)	55% (2 years)
	108 RD	47 (<1-71)	89 MA 19 NMA	100%	Unmodified 27%, TCD 8%	unmodified 31%, TCD 12%	15%	66%
	184 URD	48 (1-71)	156 MA 28 NMA	97%	Unmodified 31%, TCD 12%	unmodified 44%, TCD 19%	27%	55%

ANC, Absolute neutrophil count; *CBT*, cord blood transplantation; *DCBT*, double-unit CBT; *DFS*, disease-free survival; *GVHD*, graft-versus-host disease; *MA*, myeloablative; *MMUD*, mismatched unrelated donor; *MRD*, matched related donor; *MUD*, matched unrelated donor; *NMA*, nonmyeloablative; *PFS*, progression-free survival; *RD*, related donor; *RIC*, reduced intensity conditioning; *TCD*, T cell depleted; *TRM*, transplant-related mortality; *URD*, unrelated donor.

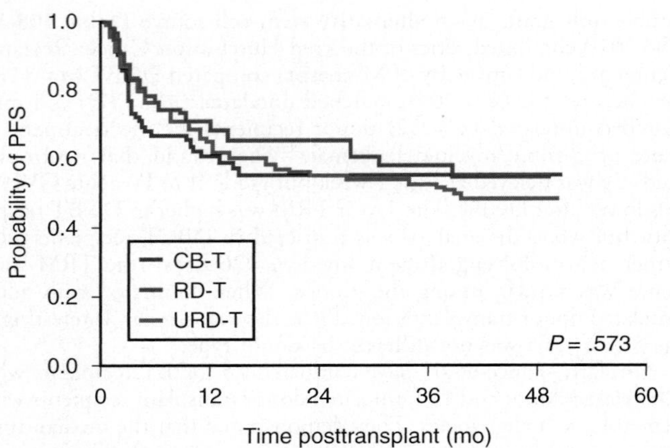

Figure 108-7 TWO-YEAR PROGRESSION-FREE SURVIVAL (PFS) ACCORDING TO HEMATOPOIETIC STEM CELL SOURCE. *CB-T,* Cord blood; *RD-T,* related donor transplantation; *URD-T,* unrelated donor transplantation. *(From Ponce DM, Zheng J, Gonzales AM, et al: Reduced late mortality risk contributes to similar survival after double-unit cord blood transplantation compared with related and unrelated donor hematopoietic stem cell transplantation.* Biol Blood Marrow Transplant *17:1316, 2011.)*

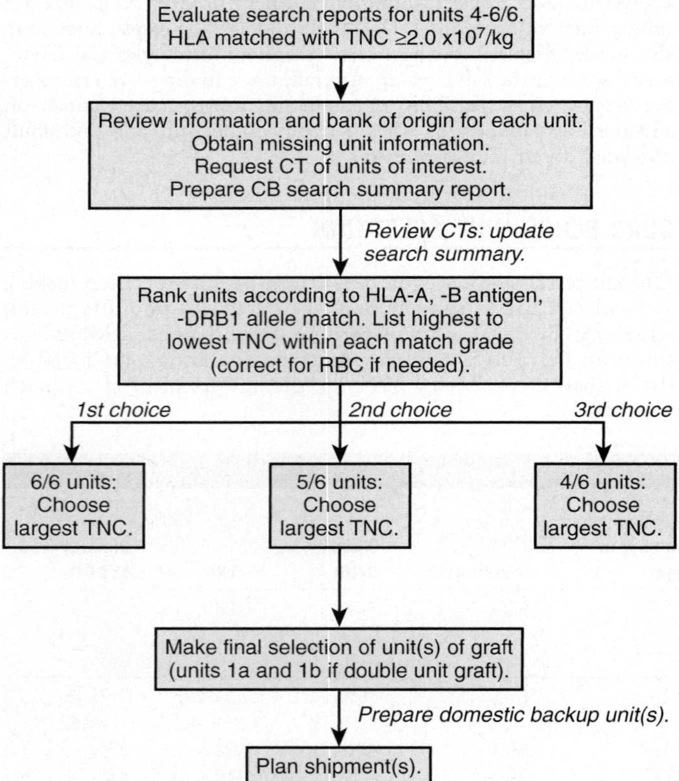

Figure 108-8 CURRENT MEMORIAL SLOAN-KETTERING CANCER CENTER SCHEMA OF HOW TO SELECT CORD BLOOD (CB) UNITS. *CT,* Confirmatory typing; *HLA,* human leukocyte antigen; *RBC,* red blood cell; *TNC,* total nucleated cell. *(From Barker JN, Byam C, Scaradavou A: How I treat: the selection and acquisition of unrelated cord blood grafts.* Blood *117:2332, 2011.)*

(4-6/6 of HLA-A, -B antigen and -DRB1 allele), and the bank of origin based on the authors' experience with the bank and their accreditation. Other factors such as the availability of confirmatory HLA typing on an attached segment and the completeness of maternal infectious disease marker and hemoglobinopathy testing are also taken into account.

The exact threshold for acceptable TNC/kg has yet to be established and varies with HLA match. For example, the 2010 NYBC analysis of single-unit CBT demonstrated that recipients of units with a 6/6 HLA match had the best transplantation outcomes regardless of the cryopreserved TNC dose. By contrast, recipients of 4/6 units required a TNC dose of 5.0×10^7/kg or greater to achieve similar TRM and DFS to that of recipients of 5/6 units with TNC of $2.5\text{-}4.9 \times 10^7$/kg.[17] Although the numbers of DCBT recipients available do not yet permit such analysis, it is likely that similar principles will be found associated with the engrafting unit in DBCT recipients. Indeed, Avery et al[40] have reported that a higher infused TNC and CD34$^+$ cell dose in the engrafting unit of a double-unit pair was strongly associated with the speed and success of neutrophil engraftment. However, because it is not currently possible to predict which unit will predominate at the time of double-unit graft selection, a minimum threshold for each unit of a double-unit graft is needed. Based on the Avery et al analysis, a minimum TNC dose threshold of at least 2.0×10^7/kg is currently recommended in DCBT.

Recent analyses have highlighted new factors to be considered in unit selection. The 2009 NYBC analysis evaluated the impact of fetal exposure to noninherited maternal antigens (NIMAs) on the outcome of CBT.[62] The 79 single-unit CBT recipients that had an HLA-mismatched antigen that was identical to a donor NIMA engrafted earlier and had lower TRM and overall mortality. There was also a lower tendency toward relapse among patients with myeloid malignancies. Subsequently, in 2011, the NYBC analyzed the effect of HLA-mismatch vector in 1202 single-unit CBT recipients.[63] They identified 98 donor–recipient pairs with only unidirectional mismatches (58 in the graft-versus-host direction and 40 in the rejection direction). The graft-versus-host vector group had faster engraftment and decreased TRM and overall mortality compared with the one-bidirectional mismatch reference group, but recipients of rejection only mismatched units had slower engraftment, a higher incidence of graft failure, and higher relapse rates. Also in 2011, Eapen et al[25] reported that HLA-C matching is important in addition to HLA-A, -B, and -DRB1, although how to balance this against TNC dose needs to be further investigated. Finally, the potential importance of antigens in the patients that are shared with inherited paternal antigens (IPAs) in the CB donor that could be a target for maternal T cells has recently been reported as a potential mechanism of reduced relapse after CBT.[64]

The findings concerning the importance of HLA-mismatch vector and HLA-C can be immediately incorporated into CB unit selection algorithms, but incorporation of NIMA and IPA will require banks to provide maternal typing. In addition, although the best available CB unit or units are selected as the graft, it is important to identify and reserve at least one backup unit in the event of problems with unit shipment, mislabeling, problems with thaw, or graft failure.[65,66a,66b] At MSKCC, the authors select at least one domestic unit as backup to ensure the timely infusion of an optimal CB product.

NOVEL STRATEGIES TO ENHANCE ENGRAFTMENT

One of the main limitations of myeloablative CBT is the delayed time to neutrophil recovery compared with the transplantation of related and unrelated donor peripheral blood HSCs. This leads to prolonged hospitalization, higher rates of early infectious complications, and increased early TRM. Thus, strategies to enhance engraftment are of great interest. Studies investigating the infusion of multiple small CB units have not enhanced engraftment.[67,68] Results of direct intra-BM injection of CB have been mixed[69,70] with a study at the University of Minnesota study being abandoned for futility. New approaches focusing on enhancing engraftment are summarized in Table 108-4.

The Spanish group of Fernandez et al[71] evaluated the co-infusion of CD34$^+$ cells from a related haploidentical donor with a single-unit CBT as a "bridge" strategy to shorten the period of posttransplant neutropenia. Subsequently, these investigators updated their

Table 108-4 Potential Strategies to Enhance Cord Blood Engraftment

Strategy	Reference	Protocol	Patients (n)	Median Age (yr)	Neutrophil Engraftment	Platelet Engraftment (≥20,000/mm³)	Outcomes
Co-infusion of HSC	Bautista et al[72]	Single CB units + co-infusion of TCD HSC from haploidentical or third-party donors	55	34	96%; median ANC, 10 days (9-36)	78%; median time, 32 days (13-98)	DFS 47% and OS 56% at 5 years
	Liu et al[73]	Single CB units + co-infusion of TCD HSC from haploidentical related donors	45	50	95%; median ANC 11 days (9-15)	83%; median time, 19 days (15-33)	PFS 42% and OS 55% at 1 year
Stem cell expansion	de Lima et al[76]	CB ex vivo expansion with copper chelator TEPA	10	21	Median ANC, 30 days (16-46); 9/10 patients engrafted	Median, 48 days (35-105) in 6/10 patients	30% survival at 25 months
	Delaney et al[44]	Notch-mediated expansion of CD34⁺ cells	10	27	Median ANC, 16 days (7-34); one patient had primary graft rejection	Unknown	7/10 alive
	de Lima et al[77]	CB ex vivo expansion with MSC	32	35	97%; median ANC, 15 days (9-42)	Median, 40 days (13-62)	OS 40% at 5 years
Stem cell homing	Campbell et al,[81] Christopherson et al[83]	CD26 inhibition	N/A (mice)	N/A	Significant increase in engraftment	Unknown	N/A
	Robinson et al[85]	Fucosylation of CB CD34⁺ cells	N/A (mice)	N/A	Human engraftment detected 1 week earlier and fivefold higher	Unknown	N/A
	Cutler et al[86]	CB treated with PGE_2	11	44	10/11 patients engrafted	Unknown	9/11 alive

ANC, Absolute neutrophil count; *CB,* cord blood; *DFS,* disease-free survival; *HSC,* hematopoietic stem cell; *MSC,* mesenchymal stem cell; *N/A,* not applicable; *OS,* overall survival; *PGE_2,* prostaglandin E_2; *PFS,* progression-free survival; *TCD,* T cell depleted; *TEPA,* tetraethylenepantamine.

experience using mobilized peripheral blood HSCs from either a haploidentical or an unmatched third-party donor to support single-unit CBT.[72] This series included 55 patients with high-risk hematologic malignancies. The median time to neutrophil recovery was 10 days, and there was a high incidence of neutrophil engraftment of 96%; the median time to platelets greater than 20,000/mm³ was 32 days with an incidence of 78%. The cumulative incidence of full CB chimerism was 91% and took a median of 44 days. Grade II to IV acute GVHD developed in 10 patients and grade III to IV acute GVHD in 6 patients. Twenty-two patients died (three relapse, six organ failure, four GVHD, eight infection, one graft failure). The 5-year overall survival and DFS were 56% and 47%, respectively. The van Besien group recently reported similar findings that included 45 patients with hematologic malignancies (47% had refractory or untreated relapse) who received reduced-intensity conditioning followed by transplantation of a single CB unit and CD34⁺ cells from a haploidentical donor.[73] Rapid engraftment was obtained with cumulative incidences for neutrophils and platelets (>20,000/mm³) of 95% at day 50 and 83% at day 100, respectively, with a median time to recovery of 11 days for neutrophils and 19 days for platelets. However, the percentage of host-derived hematopoiesis was 5% by day 180, and four patients had graft failure (two primary and two secondary). The cumulative incidence of grade II to IV acute GVHD was 25%, and the 1-year overall survival and PFS rates were 55% and 42%, respectively.

Cord blood expansion is another approach to enhance neutrophil recovery. Peled et al[74,75] have cultured of CD34⁺38⁻ CB HSCs with a copper chelator tetraethylenepentamide (TEPA) given that cellular copper has been found implicated in the regulation and differentiation of HSC. The group of Shpall conducted a phase I/II clinical trial in which a portion of a single CB unit was cultured with TEPA and cytokines for 21 days and was co-infused to the patient with the unmanipulated portion.[76] The fold expansion for TNC and CD34⁺ were 219 and six, respectively. This methodology was proven to be safe, but time to neutrophil engraftment was not improved (median absolute neutrophil count was 30 days and median to platelets >20,000/mm³ was 48 days).

Delaney et al[44] studied a double-unit CB strategy in which CD34⁺ CB progenitors were expanded using a notch-ligand based culture that resulted in an average expansion of 562- and 164-fold for TNC and CD34⁺ cells, respectively. Thus, the average infused CD34⁺ cell dose from the expanded unit was 6×10^6/kg. The expansion was initiated 16 days before transplantation, and cultures were harvested and co-infused after the infusion of an unmanipulated CB unit. Ten patients with high-risk hematologic malignancies were transplanted. The median CD34⁺ cell dose from the manipulated unit was significantly higher than the unmanipulated CB units (6×10^6/kg vs. 0.24 $\times 10^6$/kg) with a fold expansion for TNC and CD34⁺ of 660 and 160, respectively. An accelerated myeloid engraftment was observed with a median neutrophil recovery in nine of 10 evaluable patients of 16 days (range, 7-34), although one patient had primary graft rejection. The seven surviving patients, however, had sustained donor engraftment mediated exclusively by the unmanipulated unit likely caused by the depletion of T cells in the manipulated unit.

de Lima et al[77] have reported an ex vivo expansion approach of CD34⁺ cells using a mesenchymal stromal cell–based culture derived from either third-party haploidentical family member BM or universal donors. The median expansion for TNC was 14-fold and for CD34⁺ was 40-fold. This method resulted in successful engraftment in 31 of 32 patients with significant shortening of neutropenia (median, 15 days) and platelets engrafted at a median of 40 days. Eleven patients survived for an overall survival of 40% at 1 year. The incidences of grade II to IV and III to IV acute GVHD were 50% and 16%, respectively. Preclinical data with aryl hydrocarbon receptor antagonists[78] and novel cytokines[79,80] with enhanced HSC expansion capacity are promising approaches that are currently under investigation.

Another method to improve engraftment is to enhance stem cell homing to the BM niche. The Broxmeyer group have reported that endogenous CD26 expression negatively regulates the homing and engraftment of stem cells.[81,82] Campbell et al[81] evaluated pre-treated purified CD34+ human CB cells with a CD26 peptidase inhibitor (Ditropin A) and found a significant enhanced engraftment in NOD/SCID mice. Christopherson et al[83] demonstrated that transplantation of either CD34+ or lineage depleted human CB cells in NOD/SCID/B2m-null mice after treatment with a CD26 inhibitor was associated with a significant improvement in the engraftment of long-term repopulating. Moreover, Hidalgo et al[84] found a defect in CB homing that was likely associated to reduced α-1,3-fucosyltransferase expression and activity in CB CD34+ cells, decreasing their ability to bind to P- and E-selectins expressed by the BM vasculature. Subsequently, Robinson et al[85] demonstrated that human CD34+ CB cells fucosylated using a recombinant fucosyl transferase in a murine model exhibited improved engraftment. Cutler et al[86] are investigating the ex vivo treatment of human CB cells with 16,16-dimethyl prostaglandin E2 (FT 1050) as a method to enhance engraftment by improved homing. One advantage of this method is that it only requires 1 to 2 hours of incubation before infusion. An early phase clinical trial is being conducted in adults with hematologic malignancies with 1 of 2 units of a double-unit graft being incubated with the agent.

ADOPTIVE IMMUNOTHERAPY

Cord blood transplantation offers a platform for the investigation of novel immunotherapy strategies to treat viral infections, enhance antitumor responses, and prevent GVHD (Table 108-5). Sun et al[87] have reported the generation of CD4+ EBV-specific cytotoxic lymphocytes from CB, and Park et al[88] have generated CMV pp65-specific T cells from CB. The Bollard group has generated multivirus-specific T cells from CB lymphocytes to prevent and treat CMV, EBV, and adenovirus.[89,90] The efficacy of these cells is currently being evaluated in a phase I trial. The O'Reilly group at MSKCC has investigated the alternative approach of using third-party EBV-specific cytotoxic T lymphocytes to successfully treat EBV associated posttransplant lymphoma in two CBT recipients who failed tapering of immunosuppression and rituximab therapy.[91]

Cord blood transplantation is also being used as a platform to enhance antitumor responses. CB NK cells have demonstrated in vitro and in vivo antileukemic effects. The enhancement of NK cells cytolytic activity by IL-2 exposure in a murine model has been reported by the Xing group.[92] Micklethwaite et al[93] have generated T cells from CB cells with both antiviral activity against CMV, EBV, and adenovirus (multivirus specific cytotoxic lymphocytes) and antileukemic activity by retroviral transduction of chimeric antigen receptors (CAR) for the CD19 molecule expressed in B-cell acute lymphoblastic leukemia. The efficacy of this approach has been demonstrated in vitro, and results of clinical application are awaited with great interest. Brunstein et al[45] have reported the results of a phase I clinical trial of CB derived ex vivo expanded Tregs. Twenty-three nonmyeloablative CBT recipients received Treg infusion(s) manufactured from a third-party CB donor in addition to a double-unit CB graft. This was well tolerated without toxicities. The incidence of grade II to IV aGVHD of 43% was lower than the 61% in the historical control participants ($P = .05$).

Table 108-5 Cellular Therapeutic Strategies to Mitigate Viral Infections, Relapse, and Graft-Versus-Host Disease After Cord Blood Transplantation

Target	Strategy	Results
Antiviral	Multivirus specific CTLs (CMV, EBV, adenovirus)[90]	Lysed antigen-pulsed and virus infected targets
	Third-party EBV-specific CTLs[91]	2 EBV PTLD patients achieved durable CR
Antitumor	IL-2 expansion of CB NK cells[92]	Cytolytic effect in vitro and in vivo against leukemia cells
Antitumor and antiviral	CB derived CTLs against CD19 and viruses (CMV, EBV, adenovirus)[93]	In vitro antileukemic and antiviral effect
GVHD prevention	Infusion of ex vivo expanded CB Treg[45]	23 patients accrued; aGVHD incidence decreased without increase in relapse

aGVHD, Acute graft-versus-host disease; *CB,* cord blood; *CBT,* cord blood transplantation; *CMV,* cytomegalovirus; *CR,* complete remission; *CTL,* cytotoxic T cell lymphocyte; *EBV,* Epstein-Barr virus; *GVHD,* graft-versus-host disease; *IL-2,* interleukin-2; *NK,* natural killer; *PTLD,* posttransplant lymphoproliferative disease; *Treg,* regulatory T cell.

FUTURE DIRECTIONS

Cord blood is a promising alternative HSC source for use in the transplantation of patients with high-risk hematologic malignancies. CBT extends transplant access to patients from ethnic and racial minorities and those in need of urgent transplantation. Furthermore, survival after CBT has greatly improved because of larger CB inventory; possibly better unit quality; and improved conditioning regimens, grafts, and supportive care. Single-unit CBT has been shown to be comparable to unrelated donor transplantation in children,[21] and DCBT has had comparable DFS to the transplantation of adult donor HSC.[48,59,60] CBT should be considered as an immediate alternative in patients with high-risk hematologic malignancies who are candidates for allogeneic HSC transplantation but lack a suitable related donor.

DISCLAIMER

No relevant conflicts of interest to disclose.

ACKNOWLEDGMENT

This work was supported in part by Gabrielle's Angel Foundation for Cancer Research (J.N.B.), the Memorial Sloan-Kettering Cancer Center Society (J.N.B.), the Translational and Integrative Medicine Research Grant (J.N.B.), P01 CA23766 from the National Cancer Institute, and National Institutes of Health.

SUGGESTED READINGS

Avery S, Shi W, Lubin M, et al: Influence of infused cell dose and HLA-match on engraftment after double-unit cord blood allografts. *Blood* 117:3277, 2011.

Barker JN, Byam C, Scaradavou A: How I treat: The selection and acquisition of unrelated cord blood grafts. *Blood* 117:2332, 2011.

Barker JN, Byam CE, Kernan NA, et al: Availability of cord blood extends allogeneic hematopoietic stem cell transplant access to racial and ethnic minorities. *Biol Blood Marrow Transplant* 16:1541, 2010.

Barker JN, Doubrovina E, Sauter C, et al: Successful treatment of EBV-associated posttransplantation lymphoma after cord blood transplantation using third-party EBV-specific cytotoxic T lymphocytes. *Blood* 116:5045, 2010.

Barker JN, Scaradavou A, Stevens CE: Combined effect of total nucleated cell dose and HLA match on transplantation outcome in 1061 cord blood recipients with hematologic malignancies. *Blood* 115:1843, 2010.

Barker JN, Weisdorf DJ, DeFor TE, et al: Transplantation of two partially HLA-matched umbilical cord blood units to enhance engraftment in adults with hematologic malignancy. *Blood* 105:1343, 2005.

Bautista G, Cabrera JR, Regidor C, et al: Cord blood transplants supported by co-infusion of mobilized hematopoietic stem cells from a third-party donor. *Bone Marrow Transplant* 43:365, 2009.

Brunstein C, Barker JN, Weisdorf DJ, et al: Umbilical cord blood transplantation after non-myeloablative conditioning: Impact on transplant outcomes in 110 adults with hematological disease. *Blood* 110:3064, 2007.

Brunstein CG, Fuchs EJ, Carter SL, et al: Alternative donor transplantation: Results of parallel phase II trials using HLA-mismatched related bone marrow or unrelated umbilical cord blood grafts. *Blood* 118:282, 2011.

Brunstein CG, Gutman JA, Weisdorf DJ, et al: Allogeneic hematopoietic cell transplantation for hematological malignancy: Relative risks and benefits of double umbilical cord blood. *Blood* 116:4693, 2010.

Christopherson KW, 2nd, Hangoc G, Mantel CR, et al: Modulation of hematopoietic stem cell homing and engraftment by CD26. *Science* 305:1000, 2004.

Delaney C, Heimfeld S, Brashem-Stein C, et al: Notch-mediated expansion of human cord blood progenitor cells capable of rapid myeloid reconstitution. *Nat Med* 16:232, 2010.

Eapen M, Klein JP, Sanz GF, et al: Effect of donor-recipient HLA matching at HLA A, B, C, and DRB1 on outcomes after umbilical-cord blood transplantation for leukaemia and myelodysplastic syndrome: A retrospective analysis. *Lancet Oncol* 11:653, 2010.

Eapen M, Rocha V, Sanz G, et al: Effect of graft source on unrelated donor haemopoietic stem-cell transplantation in adults with acute leukaemia: A retrospective analysis. *Lancet Oncol* 11:653, 2010.

Eapen M, Rubinstein P, Zhang MJ, et al: Comparison of outcomes after transplantation of unrelated donor umbilical cord blood and bone marrow in children with acute leukemia. *Lancet* 369:1947, 2007.

Eldjerou LK, Chaudhury S, Baisre-de Leon A, et al: An *in vivo* model of double unit cord blood transplantation that correlates with clinical engraftment. *Blood* 116:3999, 2010.

Gutman JA, Turtle CJ, Manley TJ, et al: Single-unit dominance after double-unit umbilical cord blood transplantation coincides with a specific CD8+ T-cell response against the nonengrafted unit. *Blood* 115:757, 2010.

Hanley PJ, Cruz CR, Savoldo B, et al: Functionally active virus-specific T cells that target CMV, adenovirus, and EBV can be expanded from naive T-cell populations in cord blood and will target a range of viral epitopes. *Blood* 114:1958, 2009.

Kurtzberg J, Prasad VK, Carter SL, et al: Results of the Cord Blood Transplantation Study (COBLT): Clinical outcomes of unrelated donor umbilical cord blood transplantation in pediatric patients with hematologic malignancies. *Blood* 112:4318, 2008.

Liu H, Rich ES, Godley L, et al: Reduced-intensity conditioning with combined haploidentical and cord blood transplantation results in rapid engraftment, low GVHD, and durable remissions. *Blood* 118:6438, 2011.

MacMillan ML, Weisdorf DJ, Brunstein CG, et al: Acute graft-versus-host disease after unrelated donor umbilical cord blood transplantation: Analysis of risk factors. *Blood* 113:2410, 2009.

Micklethwaite KP, Savoldo B, Hanley PJ, et al: Derivation of human T lymphocytes from cord blood and peripheral blood with antiviral and antileukemic specificity from a single culture as protection against infection and relapse after stem cell transplantation. *Blood* 115:2695, 2010.

Ponce DM, Zheng J, Gonzales AM, et al: Reduced late mortality risk contributes to similar survival after double-unit cord blood transplantation compared with related and unrelated donor hematopoietic stem cell transplantation. *Biol Blood Marrow Transplant* 17:1316, 2011.

Rocha V, Gluckman E: Improving outcomes of cord blood transplantation: HLA matching, cell dose and other graft- and transplantation-related factors. *Br J Haematol* 147:262, 2009.

Scaradavou A, Smith KM, Hawke R, et al: Cord blood units with low CD34+ cell viability have a low probability of engraftment after double unit transplantation. *Biol Blood Marrow Transplant* 16:500, 2010.

Stevens CE, Carrier C, Carpenter C, et al: HLA mismatch direction in cord blood transplantation: Impact on outcome and implications for cord blood unit selection. *Blood* 118:3969, 2011.

van Rood JJ, Stevens CE, Smits J, et al: Reexposure of cord blood to noninherited maternal HLA antigens improves transplant outcome in hematological malignancies. *Proc Natl Acad Sci U S A* 106:19952, 2009.

Verneris MR, Brunstein CG, Barker J, et al: Relapse risk after umbilical cord blood transplantation: Enhanced graft-versus-leukemia effect in recipients of 2 units. *Blood* 114:4293, 2009.

Wagner JE, Barker JN, DeFor TE, et al: Transplantation of unrelated donor umbilical cord blood in 102 patients with malignant and nonmalignant diseases: Influence of CD34 cell dose and HLA disparity on treatment-related mortality and survival. *Blood* 100:1611, 2002.

Wagner JE, Gluckman E: Umbilical cord blood transplantation: The first 20 years. *Semin Hematol* 47:3, 2010.

For complete list of references log on to www.expertconsult.com.

CHAPTER 109

GRAFT-VERSUS-HOST DISEASE AND GRAFT-VERSUS-LEUKEMIA RESPONSES

Pavan Reddy and James L.M. Ferrara

The ability of allogeneic hematopoietic cell transplantation (HCT) to cure certain hematologic malignancies is widely recognized. An important therapeutic aspect of HCT in eradicating malignant cells is the graft-versus-leukemia (GVL) effect. The importance of the GVL effect in allogeneic HCT has been recognized since the earliest experiments in stem cell transplantation. Forty years ago Barnes and colleagues noted that leukemic mice treated with a subtherapeutic dose of radiation and a syngeneic (identical twin) graft transplant were more likely to relapse than mice given an allogeneic stem cell transplant.[1,2] They hypothesized that the allogeneic graft contained cells with immune reactivity necessary for eradicating residual leukemia cells. They also noted that recipients of allogeneic grafts, though less likely to relapse, died of a "wasting syndrome" now recognized as graft-versus-host disease (GVHD). Thus in addition to describing GVL, these experiments highlighted for the first time the intricate relationship between GVL and GVHD. Since these early experiments, both GVHD and the GVL effect have been studied extensively.[3] This chapter reviews the pathophysiology, clinical features, and treatment of GVHD and summarizes current understanding of the relationships between GVHD and the GVL effect.

GRAFT-VERSUS-HOST DISEASE: CLINICAL AND PATHOLOGIC ASPECTS

Ten years after the work of Barnes and Loutit, Billingham formulated the requirements for the development of GVHD: the graft must contain immunologically competent cells, the recipient must express tissue antigens that are not present in the transplant donor, and the recipient must be incapable of mounting an effective response to destroy the transplanted cells.[4] According to these criteria, GVHD can develop in various clinical settings when tissues containing immunocompetent cells (blood products, bone marrow, and some solid organs) are transferred between persons. The most common setting for the development of GVHD is following allogeneic HCT; without prophylactic immunosuppression, most allogeneic HCTs will be complicated by GVHD. GVHD occurs secondary to mismatches between histocompatibility antigens between the donor and recipient. Matching of the major histocompatibility complex (MHC) antigens hastens engraftment and reduces the severity of GVHD.[5] The MHC contains the genes that encode tissue antigens and were first identified functionally in murine models as transplantation antigens responsible for rejection of tissue grafts. In humans, the MHC region lies on the short arm of chromosome 6 and is called the HLA (human leukocyte antigen) region.[6] The HLA region includes many genes, not all of which are involved in immune activation. It is divided into two classes, class I and class II, each containing numerous gene loci that encode a large number of polymorphic alleles. MHC class I molecules are involved in the presentation of peptides to $CD8^+$ T cells, and class II molecules present peptides to $CD4^+$ T cells.[6]

Each MHC antigen is composed of two polypeptide chains. Class I antigens are made up of a heavy chain that contains the polymorphic regions and the nonpolymorphic light chain, $beta_2$ microglobulin. The class IHLA antigens include HLA A, B, and C antigens. These are expressed on almost all cells of the body at varying densities.[6,7] Both chains of class II antigens contain polymorphic regions and are encoded in the MHC. The class II antigens are further divided into DR, DQ, and DP antigens. Class II antigens are expressed on B cells, dendritic cells, and monocytes, and their expression can be induced on many other cell types following inflammation or injury.[6,8] The determination of HLA types has become much more accurate with molecular techniques that replace earlier serologic or cellular methods. In patients whose ancestry involves extensive interracial mixing, the chances of identifying an HLA identical donor are diminished.[9]

Despite HLA identity between a patient and donor, substantial numbers of patients still develop GVHD because of differences in minor histocompatibility antigens that lie outside the HLA loci. Most minor antigens are expressed on the cell surface as degraded peptides bound to specific HLA molecules, but the precise elucidation of many human minor antigens is yet to be accomplished.[10] In the United States, the average patient has a 25% chance of having an HLA match within his or her immediate family.[9] Patients who lack an HLA-identical family member donor must seek unrelated donor volunteers or cord blood donations.

Acute Graft-Versus-Host Disease

Acute GVHD can occur within days (in recipients who are not HLA-matched with the donor or in patients not given any prophylaxis) or as late as 2 months after transplantation. The incidence ranges from less than 10% to more than 80%, depending on the degree of histoincompatibility between donor and recipient, the number of T cells in the graft, the patient's age, and the GVHD prophylactic regimen.[11] The principal target organs include the immune system, skin, liver, and intestine. GVHD occurs first and most commonly in the skin as a pruritic maculopapular rash, often involving the palms, soles, and ears; it can progress to total-body erythroderma, with bullae formation, rupture along the epidermal-dermal border, and desquamation in severe cases.[11] Gastrointestinal (GI) and liver manifestations often appear later and rarely represent the first and only findings. Intestinal symptoms include anorexia, nausea, diarrhea (sometimes bloody), abdominal pain, and paralytic ileus.[11] Liver dysfunction includes hyperbilirubinemia and increased serum alkaline phosphatase and aminotransferase values. Coagulation studies may become abnormal, and hepatic failure with ascites and encephalopathy may develop in severe cases.[11-13] Hepatic GVHD can be distinguished from hepatic venoocclusive disease by weight gain or pain in the right upper quadrant in the latter.[13] Acute GVHD also results in the delayed recovery of immunocompetence.[11] The clinical result is profound immunodeficiency and susceptibility to infections, often further accentuated by the immunosuppressive agents used to treat GVHD.[11]

Pathologically, the sine qua non of acute GVHD is selective epithelial damage of target organs.[14,15] The epidermis and hair follicles are damaged and sometimes destroyed. Small bile ducts are profoundly affected, with segmental disruption. The destruction of intestinal crypts results in mucosal ulcerations that may be either patchy or diffuse. Other epithelial surfaces, such as the conjunctivae, vagina, and esophagus, are less commonly involved. A peculiarity of GVHD histology is the frequent paucity of mononuclear cell infiltrates;

however, as the disease progresses, the inflammatory component may be substantial. Recent studies have identified inflammatory cytokines as soluble mediators of GVHD and have suggested that direct contact between target cells and lymphocytes may not be required for target cell destruction (see following sections). GVHD lesions are not evenly distributed in the target tissues. In the skin, damage is prominent at the tip of rete ridges; in the intestine, at the base of the crypts; and in the liver, in the periductular epithelium. These areas contain a high proportion of stem cells, giving rise to the idea that GVHD targets may be undifferentiated epithelial cells with primitive surface antigens.[16]

The histologic severity of a given lesion is at best semiquantitative, and consequently the severity of pathologic findings is not used in the grading of GVHD. Because it is often difficult to obtain an adequate tissue biopsy, the physician is left to use clinical judgment. Even on histology, it can be very difficult to distinguish GVHD from other post–bone marrow transplantation (BMT) complications such as drug eruptions or infectious complications.

A recent multicenter phase III trial used an independent committee to assess the presence and severity of GVHD. The incidence of GVHD as determined by investigators was substantially higher than the review committee could confirm.[17] Nevertheless, for an experienced clinician a combination of physical and laboratory findings in the appropriate context provides a working diagnosis of GVHD that is satisfactory to produce a meaningful prognostic scale based on clinical grading system.[18] Standard grading systems generally include clinical changes in the skin, GI tract, liver, and performance status (Table 109-1).[19] Although the severity of GVHD is sometimes difficult to quantify, the overall grade correlates with disease outcome. Whereas mild GVHD (grade I or II) is associated with little morbidity and almost no mortality, higher grades are associated with significantly decreased survival.[19,20] With grade IV GVHD, the mortality rate is almost 100%.[20]

Clinical Features of Acute GVHD

The clinical features, staging, and grading of acute GVHD are summarized in Tables 109-1 and 109-2. In a comprehensive review of patients receiving therapy for acute GVHD, Martin and colleagues[21] found that 81% had skin involvement, 54% had GI involvement, and 50% had liver involvement at the initiation of therapy. After high-intensity (conventional) conditioning, acute GVHD generally occurs within 14-35 days of stem cell infusion. The time of onset may depend on the degree of histocompatibility, the number of donor T cells infused and the prophylactic regimen for GVHD. A "hyperacute" form of GVHD may occur in patients with severe HLA mismatches and in patients who receive T-cell replete transplants without or with inadequate in vivo GVHD prophylaxis.[22] It is, however, important to note that this hyperacute form is pathophysiologically distinct from the hyperacute rejection after solid organ allografting. This form of GVHD is manifested by fever, generalized erythroderma and desquamation, and often edema. It typically occurs about 1 week after stem cell infusion and may be rapidly fatal. In patients receiving more conventional (in vivo) GVHD prophylaxis, such as a combination of cyclosporine (CSP) and methotrexate, the median onset of GVHD is typically 21 to 25 days after transplantation; however, after in vitro T-cell depletion of the graft the onset may be much later.[22] Thus the findings of rash and diarrhea by 1 week after transplantation would very likely be hyperacute manifestations of GVHD if minimal or ineffective prophylaxis were administered; the same kinetics would be very unlikely with the use of calcineurin inhibitors or in vitro T-cell depletion of the stem cell inoculum. A less ominous syndrome of fever, rash, and fluid retention occurring in the first 1 to 2 weeks after stem cell infusion is the "engraftment syndrome." These manifestations may be seen with either allogeneic or autologous transplantation. Although the pathophysiology is poorly understood, it is thought to be due to a wave of cytokine production as the graft starts to recover. This is related to, but distinct from, the "cytokine storm"[23] that is thought to contribute to acute GVHD in that there is no concomitant T cell–mediated attack. This syndrome responds immediately to steroids in most patients, and it typically presents earlier than acute GVHD.[16] In autologous transplantation the differential diagnosis is of little relevance, but in allogeneic transplant recipients it must be distinguished from the hyperacute manifestations of GVHD. A prompt response to steroids would argue in favor of an engraftment syndrome, although some patients with GVHD will also respond.

Skin is the most commonly affected organ (Fig. 109-1). In patients receiving transplants after myeloablative conditioning, the skin is usually the first organ involved, and GVHD often coincides with engraftment. However, the presentation of GVHD is more varied following nonmyeloablative transplants or donor lymphocyte infusions.[24] The characteristic maculopapular rash can spread throughout the rest of the body but usually spares the scalp; it is often described as feeling like a sunburn, tight or pruritic. In severe cases the skin may blister and ulcerate.[25] Histologic confirmation is critical to rule out drug reactions, viral infections, etc. Apoptosis at the base of dermal crypts is characteristic. Other features include dyskeratosis, exocytosis of lymphocytes, satellite lymphocytes adjacent to dyskeratotic epidermal keratinocytes, and dermal perivascular lymphocytic infiltration.[26]

Gastrointestinal tract involvement of GVHD may present as nausea, vomiting, anorexia, diarrhea, and/or abdominal pain.[27] It is a panintestinal process, often with differences in severity between the upper and lower GI tracts. Gastric involvement gives rise to

Table 109-1 Clinical Manifestations and Staging of Acute Graft-Versus-Host Disease

Organ	Clinical Manifestations	Staging
Skin	Erythematous, maculopapular rash involving palms and soles; may become confluent Severe disease: bullae	Stage 1: <25% rash Stage 2: 25% to 50% rash Stage 3: generalized erythroderma Stage 4: bullae
Liver	Painless jaundice with conjugated hyperbilirubinemia and increased alkaline phosphatase	Stage 1: bili 2 to 3 mg/dL Stage 2: bili 3.1 to 6 mg/dL Stage 3: bili 6.1 to 15 mg/dL Stage 4: bili >15 mg/dL
Gastrointestinal tract	Upper: nausea, vomiting, anorexia Lower: diarrhea, abdominal cramps, distension, ileus, bleeding	Stage 1: diarrhea >500 mL/day Stage 2: diarrhea >1000 mL/day Stage 3: diarrhea >1500 mL/day Stage 4: ileus, bleeding

Table 109-2 Glucksberg Criteria for Staging of Acute Graft-Versus-Host Disease*

Overall Grade	Skin	Liver		Gut
I	1-2	0		0
II	1-3	1	and/or	1
III	2-3	2-4	and/or	2-3
IV	2-4	2-4	and/or	2-4

*See Table 109-1 for individual organ staging. Traditionally, individual organs are staged without regard to attribution. The overall grade of GVHD, however, reflects the actual extent of GVHD. To achieve each overall grade, skin disease plus liver and/or gut involvement are required.

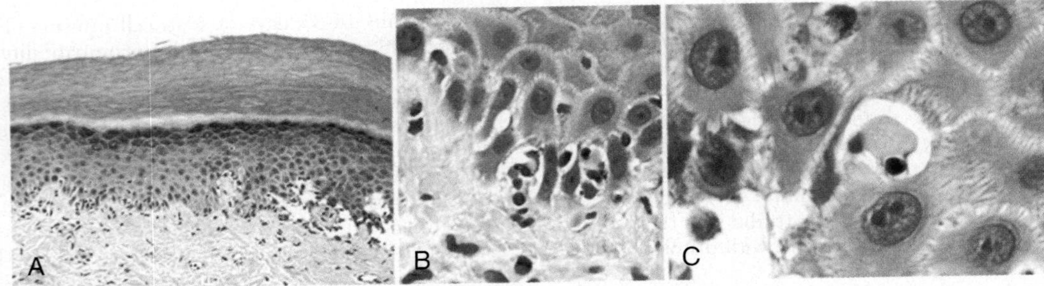

Figure 109-1 GRAFT-VERSUS-HOST DISEASE, SKIN BIOPSY. This 40-year-old man with a history of relapsed Hodgkin lymphoma was status-postallogeneic stem cell transplant with donor lymphocyte infusion. He developed painful oral ulcers and a macular-papular rash on the arms, hand, and chest. The skin biopsy is from the palmar surface of the hand **(A).** It shows a scant lymphoid infiltrate in the dermis with a developing subepithelial blister *(right).* There is basal vacuolar change **(B)** with single lymphocytes in the epithelium, as well as apoptotic keratinocyte accompanied by lymphocytes **(B,** and detail, **C).** *(Courtesy Vesna Petronic-Rosic and Mark Racz, University of Chicago.)*

postprandial vomiting that is not always preceded by nausea. Although gastroparesis is seen after bone marrow transplant, it is usually not associated with GVHD. The diarrhea of GVHD is secretory; significant GI blood loss may occur as a result of mucosal ulceration and is associated with a poor prognosis.[28] In advanced disease, diffuse, severe abdominal pain and distension is accompanied by voluminous diarrhea (>2 liters/day).[20,29]

Radiologic findings of the GI tract include luminal dilatation with thickening of the wall of the small bowel and air/fluid levels suggestive of an ileus on abdominal flat plates or small bowel series. Abdominal computed tomography may show the "ribbon" sign of diffuse thickening of the small bowel wall.[25] Little correlation exists between the extent of disease and the appearance of mucosa on endoscopy, but mucosal sloughing is pathognomonic for severe disease.[30] Nevertheless, some studies have shown that antral biopsies correlate well with the severity of GVHD in the duodenum and in the colon even when the presenting symptom is diarrhea.[30] Histologic analysis of tissue is imperative to establish the diagnosis. The histologic features of GI GVHD are the presence of apoptotic bodies in the base of crypts, crypt abscesses, crypt loss, and flattening of the surface epithelium.[29,31]

Liver function test abnormalities are common after bone marrow transplant and occur secondary to venoocclusive disease, drug toxicity, viral infection, sepsis, iron overload, and other causes of extrahepatic biliary obstruction.[13] The exact incidence of hepatic GVHD is probably underreported because many patients do not undergo liver biopsies. The development of jaundice or an increase in the alkaline phosphatase and bilirubin may be the initial features of acute GVHD of the liver. The histologic features of hepatic GVHD are endothelialitis, lymphocytic infiltration of the portal areas, pericholangitis, and bile duct destruction and loss.[20,32]

Other Organs

Whether GVHD affects organs other than the classic triad of skin, liver, and gut has remained a matter of debate. However, numerous reports suggest additional organ manifestations. The most likely candidate is the lung. Lung toxicity, including interstitial pneumonitis and diffuse alveolar hemorrhage, may occur in 20% to 60% of allogeneic transplant recipients but in fewer autologous transplant recipients. Causes of pulmonary damage other than GVHD include engraftment syndrome (see later), infection, radiation pneumonitis, and chemotherapy-related toxicity (e.g., methotrexate, busulfan).[22,33] At least one retrospective analysis failed to link severe pulmonary complications to clinical acute GVHD per se.[34] The mortality due to pneumonia increases with the severity of GVHD, but this association does not necessarily imply that GVHD, as opposed to immunosuppression given for therapy, is causative.[22] A particular histopathologic syndrome of lymphocytic bronchitis has been attributed directly to GVHD,[33] although this association has not been confirmed by others.

Despite the fact that kidneys and heart can be targets for allogeneic damage as evidenced by their rejection after renal and cardiac transplants respectively, there is no convincing evidence for direct renal or cardiac damage from acute GVHD that is not secondary to drugs or infection. Similarly, neurologic complications are also common after transplantation but most can be attributed to drug toxicity, infection, or vascular insults.

Differential Diagnosis

Acute GVHD ought to be distinguished from any process that causes a constellation of fever, erythematous skin rash with or without low-pressure, and pulmonary edema that may occur during neutrophil recovery. This picture may reflect the dysregulated production of inflammatory cytokines and cellular responses to these molecules, and has been termed engraftment or capillary leak syndrome.[35,36] The picture is most clearly recognized after autologous transplantation where, theoretically, GVHD should not occur. In allogeneic transplant recipients, distinction from acute GVHD is difficult. This engraftment syndrome is thought to reflect cellular and cytokine activities during early recovery of (donor-derived) blood cell counts and/or homeostatic proliferation of lymphocytes, but a precise delineation of the offending cells and mechanisms has not been accomplished. Engraftment syndromes may be associated with increased mortality, primarily from pulmonary failure but also (other) multiorgan dysfunction. Corticosteroid therapy may be effective particularly for the treatment of pulmonary manifestations.[37] The differential diagnosis of skin rashes, diarrhea, and liver function abnormalities can be difficult to resolve. Skin rashes may reflect delayed reactions to the conditioning regimen, antibiotics, or infections; furthermore, histopathologic skin changes consistent with acute GVHD can be mimicked by chemoradiotherapy and drug reactions.[22,38] Diarrhea can be a consequence of TBI, viral infection (especially with CMV and other herpes viruses), parasitic infection, *C. difficile* infection, nonspecific gastritis, narcotic withdrawal, and drug reactions—all of which mimic GVHD of the gut. Liver dysfunction can be due to parenteral nutrition, venoocclusive disease, and viral- or drug-induced hepatitis.

Genetic Basis of Graft-Versus-Host Disease

The graft-versus-host (GVH) reaction was first noted when irradiated mice were infused with allogeneic marrow and spleen cells.[39] Although mice recovered from radiation-induced injury and marrow aplasia, they subsequently died with "secondary disease,"[39] a phenomenon subsequently recognized as acute GVHD. Three requirements for the development of GVHD were formulated by Billingham.[4] First, the graft must contain immunologically competent cells, now recognized as mature T cells. In both experimental and clinical allogeneic HCT, the severity of GVHD correlates with the number of donor T cells transfused.[40,41] The precise nature of these cells and the mechanisms they use are now understood in greater detail (discussed later). Second, the recipient must be incapable of rejecting the transplanted cells (i.e., immunocompromised). A patient with a normal immune system will usually reject cells from a foreign donor. In an allogeneic transplant setting, the recipient is typically immunosuppressed by chemo- and/or radiotherapy before the hematopoietic cell infusion.[42] Third, the recipient must express tissue antigens that are not present in the transplant donor. Thus Billingham's third postulate stipulates that the GVH reaction occurs when donor immune cells recognize disparate host antigens.[4] These differences are governed by the genetic polymorphisms of the HLA system and the non-HLA systems.[42]

HLA Matching

Alloreactive T-cell antigen recognition is characterized by whether the presenting major histocompatibility molecule is matched or mismatched.[43-45] In humans, the MHC is governed by the HLA antigens that are encoded by the MHC gene complex on the short arm of chromosome 6 and can be categorized as class I, II, and III. Class I antigens (HLA-A, B, and C) are expressed on almost all cells of the body.[46] Class II antigens (DR, DQ, and DP) are primarily expressed on hematopoietic cells, although their expression can also be induced on other cell types following inflammation.[46] The incidence of acute GVHD is directly related to the degree of MHC mismatch.[42] The role of HLA mismatching in CBT is more difficult to analyze compared with unrelated donor HCT, because allele typing of CB units for HLA-A, B, C, DRB1, and DQB1 is not routinely performed.[47] Nonetheless, the total number of HLA disparities between the recipient and the CB unit has been shown to correlate with risk for acute GVHD as the frequency of severe acute GVHD is lower in patients transplanted with HLA-matched (6/6) CB units.[47-49]

Minor Histocompatibility Antigens

In the MHC-matched context, as is the case with most clinical allogeneic transplants, donor T cells recognize MHC-bound peptides derived from the protein products of polymorphic genes (minor histocompatibility antigens [MiHAs]) that are present in the host but not in the donor.[10,50-55] Substantial numbers (40%) of patients will develop acute GVHD despite receiving HLA-identical grafts as well as optimal postgrafting immune suppression.[10,42,56] Minor histocompatibility antigens are widely expressed but can differ in their tissue expression.[51,56] This might be one of the reasons for the unique target organ involvement in GVHD. A preponderance of MiHAs, such as HA-1 and HA-2, are expressed on hematopoietic cells, which might account for making the host immune system a primary target for the GVH response and explain the critical role of direct presentation by professional recipient antigen-presenting cells (APCs) in causing antitumor and GVHD responses.[57] By contrast, other MiHAs, such as H-Y and HA-3, are expressed ubiquitously.[56] Minor histocompatibility antigens are not equal in their ability to induce lethal GVHD and instead show hierarchic immunodominance.[58,59] Furthermore, the difference in single immunodominant MiHAs alone is not insufficient for causing GVHD in murine models, although T cells targeting single MiHAs can induce tissue damage in a skin explant model.[60,61] However, the role of specific and immunodominant MiHAs that are relevant in clinical GVHD has not been systematically evaluated in large groups of patients.[62]

Other Non-HLA Genes

Genetic polymorphisms in several non-HLA genes such as in killer-cell immunoglobulin-like receptors (KIRs), cytokines and nucleotide-binding oligomerization domain containing 2 (NOD2) genes have recently been shown to modulate the severity and incidence of GVHD.

KIRs on natural killer (NK) cells that bind to the HLA class I gene products are encoded on chromosome 19. Polymorphisms in the transmembrane and cytoplasmic domains of KIRs govern whether the receptor has inhibitory (such as KIR2DL1, -2DL2, -2DL3, and -3DL1) or activating potential. Two competing models have been proposed for HLA-KIR allorecognition by donor NK cells following allogeneic HCT: the "mismatched ligand" and the "missing ligand" models.[5,63-66] Both models are supported by several clinical observations, albeit in patients receiving very different transplant and immunosuppressive regimens (see Chapters 20 and 102).[64,67-69]

Proinflammatory cytokines, involved in the classic cytokine storm of GVHD (discussed later), cause pathologic damage to target organs, such as the skin, liver, and gastrointestinal tract.[23] Several cytokine gene polymorphisms, in recipients as well as donors, have been implicated. Specifically, tumor necrosis factor (TNF) polymorphisms (TNFd3/d3 in the recipient, TNF863 and TNF857 in donors and/or recipients and TNFd4, TNF-α-1031C, and TNFRII-196R in the donors) have been associated with an increased risk for acute GVHD and TRM.[70,71] The three common haplotypes of the interleukin (IL)-10 gene promoter region in recipients, representing high, intermediate, and low production of IL-10, have been associated with severity of acute GVHD following HLA-matched sibling donor allogeneic HCT.[72] By contrast, smaller studies have found neither IL-10 nor TNF-α polymorphisms to be associated with GVHD following HLA-mismatched CBT.[71,73] Interferon-gamma (IFN-γ) polymorphisms of the 2/2 genotype (high IFN-γ production) and 3/3 genotype (low IFN-γ) have been associated with decreased or increased acute GVHD, respectively.[71,74]

NOD2/caspase-activating recruitment domain 15 (CARD15) gene polymorphisms in both the donors and recipients were recently shown to have a striking association between GI GVHD and overall mortality following related and unrelated donor allogeneic HCT.[75] It is likely that non-HLA gene polymorphisms play differing roles depending on the donor source (related versus unrelated), HLA disparity (matched versus mismatched), graft source (CB versus BM versus peripheral blood stem cells), and the intensity of the conditioning.

PATHOPHYSIOLOGY OF ACUTE GRAFT-VERSUS-HOST DISEASE

It is helpful to remember two important principles when considering the pathophysiology of acute GVHD. First, acute GVHD represents exaggerated but normal inflammatory responses against foreign antigens (alloantigens) that are ubiquitously expressed in a setting where they are undesirable. The donor lymphocytes that have been infused into the recipient function appropriately, given the foreign environment they encounter. Second, donor lymphocytes encounter tissues in the recipient that have been often profoundly damaged. The effects of the underlying disease, prior infections, and the intensity of conditioning regimen all result in substantial changes not only in the immune cells but also in the endothelial and epithelial cells. Thus the allogeneic donor cells rapidly encounter not simply a foreign environment, but one that has been altered to promote the activation and proliferation of inflammatory cells. Therefore the pathophysiology of acute GVHD may be considered a distortion of the normal inflammatory cellular responses that, in addition to the absolute requirement of donor T cells, involves multiple other innate and adaptive cells and mediators.[76] The development and evolution of acute GVHD can be conceptualized in three sequential phases (Fig. 109-2) to provide a unified perspective on the complex cellular interactions and inflammatory cascades that lead to acute GVHD: (1) activation of the antigen-presenting cells; (2) donor T-cell activation, differentiation, and migration; and (3) effector phase.[76] It is important to note that the following three-phase description allows for a unified perspective in understanding the biology. It is not meant to suggest, however, that all three phases are of equal importance or that GVHD occurs in a stepwise and sequential manner. The spatiotemporal relationships between the biologic processes described,

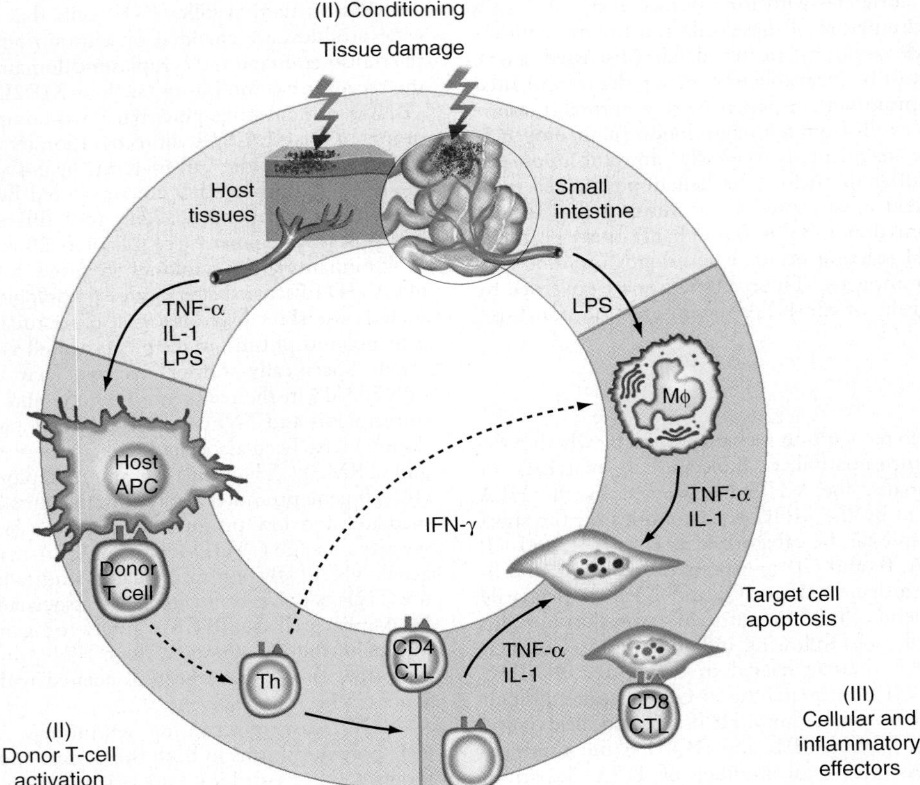

Figure 109-2 PATHOPHYSIOLOGY OF GRAFT-VERSUS-HOST DISEASE. During step 1, irradiation and chemotherapy both damage and activate host tissues, including intestinal mucosa, liver, and the skin. Activated cell hosts then secrete inflammatory cytokines (e.g., TNF-α and IL-1), which can be measured in the systemic circulation. The cytokine release has important effects on APCs of the host, including increased expression of adhesion molecules (e.g., ICAM-1, VCAM-1) and of MHC class II antigens. These changes in the APCs enhance the recognition of host MHC and/or minor H antigens by mature donor T cells. During step 2, donor T-cell activation is characterized by proliferation of GVHD T cells and secretion of the Th1 cytokines IL-2 and IFN-γ. Both of these cytokines play central roles in clonal T-cell expansion, induction of CTL and NK cell responses, and the priming of mononuclear phagocytes. In step 3, mononuclear phagocytes primed by IFN-γ are triggered by a second signal such as endotoxin (LPS) to secrete cytopathic amounts of IL-I and TNF-α. LPS can leak through the intestinal mucosa damaged by the conditioning regimen to stimulate gut-associated lymphoid tissue or Kupffer cells in the liver; LPS that penetrates the epidermis may stimulate keratinocytes, dermal fibroblasts, and macrophages to produce similar cytokines in the skin. This mechanism results in the amplification of local tissue injury and further production of inflammatory effectors such as nitric oxide, which, together with CTL and NK effectors, leads to the observed target tissue destruction in the stem cell transplant host. CTL effectors use Fas/FasL, perforin/granzyme B, and membrane-bound cytokines to lyse target cells.

depending on the context, are more likely to be chaotic and of varying intensity and relevance in the induction, severity, and maintenance of GVHD.

Phase 1: Activation of Antigen-Presenting Cells

The earliest phase of acute GVHD is initiated by the profound damage caused by the underlying disease and infections and further exacerbated by BMT conditioning regimens (which include TBI and chemotherapy) that are administered even before the infusion of donor cells.[77-81] This first step results in activation of the APCs.[8] Specifically, damaged host tissues respond with multiple changes, including the secretion of proinflammatory cytokines, such as TNF-α and IL-1, described as the "cytokine storm."[79,80,82] Such changes increase expression of adhesion molecules, costimulatory molecules, MHC antigens, and chemokines gradients that alert the residual host and the infused donor immune cells.[80] These "danger signals" activate host APCs.[83,84] Damage to the gastrointestinal tract from the conditioning is particularly important in this process because it allows for systemic translocation of immunostimulatory microbial products such as lipopolysaccharide (LPS) that further enhance the activation of host APCs, and the secondary lymphoid tissue in the GI tract is likely the initial site of interaction between activated APCs and donor T cells.[80,85,86] This scenario accords with the observation that an increased risk for GVHD is associated with intensive conditioning regimens that cause extensive injury to epithelial and endothelial surfaces with a subsequent release of inflammatory cytokines and increases in expression of cell surface adhesion molecules.[80,81] The relationship among conditioning intensity, inflammatory cytokine, and GVHD severity has been supported by elegant murine studies.[82] Furthermore, the observations from these experimental studies have led to two recent clinical innovations to reduce clinical acute GVHD: (a) reduced intensity conditioning to decrease the damage to host tissues and thus limit activation of host APC and (b) KIR mismatches between donor and recipients to eliminate the host APCs by the alloreactive NK cells.[65,87]

Host-type APCs that are present and have been primed by conditioning are critical for the induction of this phase; recent evidence suggests that donor-type APCs exacerbate GVHD, but in certain experimental models, donor-type APC chimeras also induce GVHD.[84,88-90] In clinical situations, if donor-type APCs are present in sufficient quantity and have been appropriately primed, they too might play a role in the initiation and exacerbation of GVHD.[91-93] Among the cells with antigen-presenting capability, dendritic cells (DCs) are the most potent and play an important role in the induction of GVHD.[94] Experimental data suggest that GVHD can be regulated by qualitatively or quantitatively modulating distinct DC subsets.[95-100] Langerhans cells were also shown to be sufficient for the induction of GVHD when all other APCs were unable to prime donor T cells, although the role for Langerhans cells when all APCs are intact is dispensable.[101,102] Studies have yet to define roles for other DC subsets. In one clinical study persistence of host DC after day 100 correlated with the severity of acute GVHD, whereas elimination of host DCs was associated with reduced severity of acute GVHD.[92] The allostimulatory capacity of mature monocyte-derived DCs (mDCs) after reduced intensity transplants was lower for up to 6 months compared with the mDCs from myeloablative transplant recipients, thus suggesting a role for host DCs and the reduction in danger signals secondary to less intense conditioning in acute GVHD.[103] Nonetheless this concept of enhanced host APC activation explains a number of clinical observations such as increased risks for acute GVHD associated with advanced-stage malignancy, conditioning intensity, and histories of viral infections.

Other professional APCs such as monocytes/macrophages or semiprofessional APCs might also play a role in this phase.[8] For example, recent data suggest that host-type B cells might play a regulatory role under certain contexts,[104] whereas in other contexts, they were dispensable for GVHD induction. Similarly, host basophils have been shown not to affect the induction or severity of acute GVHD.[105,106] Recent data suggest that radiosensitive hematopoietic-derived APCs may not be obligatory for induction of APCs. Also, host- or donor-type nonhematopoietic stem cells (such as mesenchymal stem cells, endothelial cells, epithelial cells, or stromal cells) can function as APCs in the context of inflammation. The role of these cells in the presence and absence of professional hematopoietic-derived APCs remains to be elucidated.

Phase 2: Donor-T-Cell Activation, Differentiation, and Migration

The infused donor T cells interact with the primed APCs leading to the initiation of the second phase of acute GVHD. This phase includes antigen presentation by primed APCs and the subsequent activation, proliferation, differentiation, and migration of alloreactive donor T cells. After allogeneic HSC transplants, both host- and donor-derived APCs are present in secondary lymphoid organs.[107,108] The T-cell receptor (TCR) of the donor T cells can recognize alloantigens either on host APCs (direct presentation) or donor APCs (indirect presentation).[109,110] In direct presentation, donor T cells recognize either the peptide bound to allogeneic MHC molecules or allogeneic MHC molecules without peptide.[110,111] During indirect presentation, T cells respond to the peptide generated by degradation of the allogeneic MHC molecules presented on self-MHC.[111] Experimental studies demonstrated that APCs derived from the host, rather than from the donor, are critical in inducing GVHD across MiHA mismatch.[8,109] Recent data suggest that presentation of distinct target antigens by the host- and donor-type APCs might play a differential role in mediating target organ damage.[8,112,113] In humans, most cases of acute GVHD developed when both host DCs and donor DCs were present in peripheral blood after BMT.[92]

Costimulation

The interaction of donor lymphocyte TCR with the host allopeptide presented on the MHC of APCs alone is insufficient to induce T-cell activation.[8,114] Both TCR ligation and costimulation via a "second" signal through interaction between the T cell costimulatory molecules and their ligands on APCs are required to achieve T proliferation, differentiation, and survival.[115] The danger signals generated in phase 1 augment these interactions, and significant progress has been made on the nature and impact of these second signals.[116,117] Costimulatory pathways are now known to deliver both positive and negative signals and molecules from two major families: the B7 family and the TNF receptor (TNFR) family play pivotal roles in GVHD.[118] Interruption of the second signal by blockade of various positive costimulatory molecules (CD28, ICOS, CD40, CD30, 4-1BB, and OX40) reduces acute GVHD in several murine models, whereas antagonism of the inhibitory signals (PD-1 and CTLA-4) exacerbates the severity of acute GVHD.[119-125] The various T cell and APC costimulatory molecules and the impact on acute GVHD are summarized in Table 109-3. The specific context and the hierarchy in which each of these signals plays a dominant role in the modulation of GVHD remain to be determined.

T-Cell Subsets

T cells consist of several subsets whose responses differ based on antigenic stimuli, activation thresholds, and effector functions. The alloantigen composition of the host determines which donor T-cell subsets proliferate and differentiate.

CD4⁺ and CD8⁺ Cells

CD4 and CD8 proteins are coreceptors for constant portions of MHC class II and class I molecules, respectively.[126] Therefore MHC class I (HLA-A, -B, -C) differences stimulate $CD8^+$ T cells and MHC class II (HLA-DR -DP, -DQ) differences stimulate $CD4^+$ T cells.[126-129] But clinical trials of $CD4^+$ or $CD8^+$ depletion have been inconclusive.[130] Perhaps this is not surprising, because in the majority of HLA-identical BMT, GVHD is induced by MiHAs, which

Table 109-3 T Cell-APC Interactions

T Cell	APC
ADHESION	
ICAMs	LFA-1
LFA-1	ICAMs
CD2 (LFA-2)	LFA-3
RECOGNITION	
TCR/CD4	MHC II
TCR/CD8	MHC I
COSTIMULATION	
CD28	CD80/86
CD152 (CTLA-4)	CD80/86
ICOS	B7H/B7RP-1
PD-1	PD-L1, PD-L2
UNKNOWN	B7-H3
CD154 (CD40L)	CD40
CD134 (OX 40)	CD134L (OX40L)
CD137 (4-1BB)	CD137L (4-1BBL)
HVEM	LIGHT

HVEM, HSV glycoprotein D for herpesvirus entry mediator; *LIGHT,* homologous to lymphotoxins, shows inducible expression, and competes with HVEM, a receptor expressed by T lymphocytes.

are peptides derived from polymorphic cellular proteins that are presented by MHC molecules.[53] Because the manner of protein processing depends on genes of the MHC, two siblings will have many different peptides in the MHC groove.[53] Thus in the majority of HLA-identical BMT, acute GVHD can be induced by either or both $CD4^+$ and $CD8^+$ subsets in response to minor histocompatibility antigens.[130] The peptide repertoire for class I or class II MHC remains unknown and might even be unique in different individuals.[131] However, it is plausible that only a few of the many of these peptides might behave as immunodominant "major minor" antigens that can potentially induce GVHD. In any event, such antigens remain to be identified and validated in large patient population.

Naive and Memory Subsets

Intriguingly, several independent groups have found that although the naive ($CD62L^+$) T cells were alloreactive and caused acute GVHD, this was not the case for the memory ($CD62L^-$) T cells across different donor/recipient strain combinations.[132-135] Furthermore, expression of naive T-cell marker CD62L was also found to be critical for regulation of GVHD by donor natural regulatory T cells.[136] By contrast, another recent study demonstrated that alloreactive memory T cells and their precursor cells (memory stem cells) caused robust GVHD.[137,138] It remains as yet unknown whether the reduced GVHD potential of memory-type T cells from a naive murine donor, in contrast to their ability to cause greater solid organ allorejection,[139] is a consequence of the intense conditioning regimen and/or altered trafficking or from a restricted repertoire and/or T-cell intrinsic defect.

Regulatory T Cells

Recent advances indicate that distinct subsets of regulatory $CD4^+CD25^+$, $CD4^+CD25^-IL10^+$ Tr cells, γδT cells, DN^- T cells, NK T cells, and regulatory DCs control immune responses by induction of anergy or active suppression of alloreactive T cells.[96,97,140-148] Several studies have demonstrated a critical role for the natural donor $CD4^+CD25^+$ $Foxp3^+$ regulatory T (Treg) cells, obtained from naive animals or generated ex vivo, in the outcome of acute GVHD. Donor $CD4^+CD25^+$T cells suppressed the early expansion of alloreactive donor T cells and their capacity to induce acute GVHD without abrogating GVL effector function against these tumors.[149,150] $CD4^+CD25^+$ T cells induced and/or generated by of immature or regulatory host-type DCs and by regulatory donor-type myeloid APCs were also able to suppress acute GVHD.[96] One of the clinical studies that evaluated the relationship between donor $CD4^+CD25^+$ cells and acute GVHD in humans after matched sibling donor grafts found that in contrast to the murine studies, donor grafts containing larger numbers of $CD4^+$ $CD25^+$T cells developed more severe acute GVHD.[151] These data suggest that coexpression of $CD4^+$ and $CD25^+$ is insufficient because an increase in $CD25^+$ T cells in donor grafts is associated with greater risks for acute GVHD after clinical HCT. Another recent study found that Foxp3 mRNA expression (considered a specific marker for naturally occurring $CD4^+CD25^+$Tregs) was significantly decreased in peripheral blood mononuclear cells from patients with acute GVHD.[152,153] But Foxp3 expression in humans, unlike mice, may not be specific for T cells with a regulatory phenotype.[154] It is likely that the precise role of regulatory T cells in clinical acute GVHD will therefore depend not only on identification of specific molecular markers in addition to Foxp3 but also on the ability for ex vivo expansion of these cells in sufficient numbers. The presence of STAT1 signaling has been shown to enhance Treg-mediated suppression of GVHD.[155] Recent observations have demonstrated key roles for host APCs in the induction and for donor APCs in the sustenance of infused mature Tregs.[156] Several clinical trials are underway in the United States and Europe with attempts to substantially expand these cells ex vivo and use for prevention of GVHD. Emerging data from these trials suggest that donor Tregs can reduce incidence of clinical GVHD and do not prevent engraftment.[157]

Host $NK1.1^+$ T cells are another T-cell subset that has been shown to suppress acute GVHD in an IL-4 dependent manner.[147,148,158] By contrast, donor NKT cells were found to reduce GVHD and enhance perforin-mediated GVL in an IFN-γ dependent manner.[159,160] Recent clinical data suggest that enhancing recipient NKT cells by repeated TLI conditioning promoted Th2 polarization and dramatically reduced GVHD.[148] Experimental data also show that activated donor NK cells can reduce GVHD through the elimination of host APCs or by secretion of transforming growth factor-β (TGFβ) secretion.[160] A murine BMT study using mice lacking SH2-containing inositol phosphatase (SHIP), in which the NK compartment is dominated by cells that express two inhibitory receptors capable of binding either self or allogeneic MHC ligands, suggests that host NK cells may play a role in the initiation of GVHD.[161]

T-Cell Apoptosis

Deletional mechanisms of tolerance fall into two categories: (1) central (thymic) deletion and (2) peripheral deletion.[162] Central deletion is an effective way to eliminate continued thymic production of alloreactive T cells. To this end, lymphoablative treatments have been used as a condition to create a mixed hematopoietic chimeric state in murine BMT models.[163] In this strategy, donor cells seed the thymus and maturing donor-reactive T-cell clones are deleted through intrathymic apoptosis.[164,165] The proportion of the peripheral T-cell repertoire that can respond to allogeneic MHC antigens may play a critical role in the development of tolerance.[166] In the case of MHC-mismatched transplantation, the frequency of alloreactive T cells is at least five orders of magnitude greater than the frequency of peptide-specific T cells responding to a nominal antigen.[166,167] The pathways of T cell apoptosis by which peripheral deletion occurs can be broadly categorized into activation-induced cell death (AICD) and passive cell death (PCD).[166] An important mediator of AICD in T cells is the Fas receptor.[168] Activated T cells expressing the Fas molecule undergo apoptotic cell death when brought into contact with cells expressing Fas ligand. A critical role for Fas-mediated AICD has been clearly demonstrated in attenuation of acute GVHD by several Th1 cytokines.[42]

PCD, or "death by neglect," illustrates the exquisite dependence of activated T cells on growth factors (e.g., IL-2, IL-4, IL-7, and/or IL-15) for survival; apoptotic cell death in this instance is largely due to rapid downregulation of BCL2.[169-171] Transplantation of BCL-XL T cells into nonirradiated recipients significantly exacerbates GVHD; however, no difference in GVHD mortality is observed in animals that have been lethally irradiated.[172] Selective elimination of donor T cells in vivo after BMT using transgenic T cells in which a thymidine kinase (TK) suicide gene is targeted to T cells has also been shown to attenuate the severity of acute GVHD.[172-175] Another recent approach to prevent GVHD is the selective depletion of alloantigen-specific donor T cells by photodynamic cell purging process, wherein donor T cells are treated with photoactive 4,5-dibromorhodamine 123 and subsequently exposed to visible light.[176] Thus several deletional mechanisms have been shown to reduce acute GVHD but the conditions under which one or another of these deletional mechanisms predominate role remain to be determined.

Cytokines and T-Cell Differentiation

APC and T-cell activation result in rapid intracellular biochemical cascades that induce transcription of many genes, including cytokines and their receptors. The Th1 cytokines (IFN-γ, IL-2, and TNF-α) have been implicated in the pathophysiology of acute GVHD.[177-179] IL-2 production by donor T cells remains the main target of many current clinical therapeutic and prophylactic approaches, such as cyclosporine, tacrolimus, and monoclonal antibodies (mAbs) against the IL-2 and its receptor to control acute GVHD.[177,180] However, emerging data indicate an important role for IL-2 in the generation and maintenance of $CD4^+CD25^+$ $Foxp3^+$

Tregs, suggesting that prolonged interference with IL-2 may have an unintended consequence in the prevention of the development of long-term tolerance after allogeneic HCT.[181-184] Similarly, the role of other Th1 cytokines IFN-γ or their inducers as regulators or inducers of GVHD severity depends on the degree of allomismatch, the intensity of conditioning and the T-cell subsets that are involved after BMT.[185-187] Thus although the cytokine storm initiated in phase 1 and amplified by the Th1 cytokines correlates with the development of acute GVHD, early Th1 polarization of donor T cells to HCT recipients can attenuate acute GVHD suggesting that physiologic and adequate amounts of Th1 cytokines are critical for GVHD induction, whereas inadequate production (extremely low or high) could modulate acute GVHD through a breakdown of negative feedback mechanisms for activated donor T cells.[179,187-190] Several different cytokines that polarize donor T cells to Th2 such as IL-4, G-CSF, IL-18, IL-11, rapamycin, and the secretion of IL-4 by NK1.1$^+$ T cells can reduce acute GVHD.[191-198] However, Th1 and Th2 subsets cause injury of distinct acute GVHD target tissues, and some studies failed to show a beneficial effect of Th2 polarization on acute GVHD.[199] Thus the Th1/Th2 paradigm of donor T cells in the immunopathogenesis of acute GVHD has evolved over the last few years, and its causal role in acute GVHD is complex and incompletely understood.

IL-10 plays a key role in suppression of immune responses, and its role in regulating experimental acute GVHD is unclear.[122] Recent clinical data demonstrate an unequivocal association of IL-10 polymorphisms with the severity of acute GVHD.[72] TGF-β, another suppressive cytokine, was shown to suppress acute GVHD but to exacerbate chronic GVHD.[200] The roles of some other cytokines, such as IL-7 (which promotes immune reconstitution) and IL-13 remain unclear.[201-204] The role of IL-17–producing CD4$^+$ T cells (Th17)[205] in GVHD is also unclear at present. Initial studies showed that donor T cells deficient in IL-17A augmented Th1 differentiation and exacerbated acute GVHD.[206] In contrast, another study using a similar model showed that IL-17 contributed to CD4$^+$-mediated GVHD without affecting overall survival rates.[207] In addition, the differentiation of Th17 cells in vitro appeared to cause lethal acute GVHD with severe cutaneous and pulmonary damage.[208] More recently, IL-21, which is known to enhance Th17 cell differentiation while inhibiting the conversion of inducible Tregs from naive T cells,[209] has been shown to increase GVHD-induced injury.[210,211] Consistent with this finding, the abrogation of IL-21 signaling in donor T cells has led to reduced GVHD mortality, which is associated with donor Treg expansion and decreased TNF-α.[212] These conflicting results may be due to variations among the model systems, and further analyses are required to define the role of Th17 cells in GVHD.

CD4$^+$ and CD8$^+$ T Cells

As mentioned previously, in the majority of HLA-matched allogeneic HCTs, acute GVHD may be induced by either or both CD4$^+$ and CD8$^+$ subsets responses to MiHAs.[130] The repertoire and immunodominance of the GVHD-associated peptides presented by MHC class I and class II molecules have not been clearly defined.[131] One approach to retaining the beneficial GVL effects while eliminating the negative effects of GVHD is to selectively deplete subsets of donor alloreactive T cells in the hematopoietic cell inoculums using a TCR Vβ repertoire analysis with CDR3-size spectratyping.[213] More recently, it has been shown that GVL in allogeneic recipients could be restored without GVHD induction when the adoptive transfer of TCR-transduced allogeneic CD8$^+$ T cells was given in combination with PD-L1 blockade.[214]

Naive and Memory T Cells

T cells in murine models can be categorized into naive (CD62L$^+$ CD44$^-$), central memory (CD62L$^+$ CD44$^+$), and terminally differentiated effector/effector memory (CD62L$^-$ CD44$^-$) subsets. Donor naive CD62L$^+$ T cells are the primary alloreactive T cells that drive the GVHD reaction, whereas the donor effector memory CD62L$^-$ T cells do not.[132,133] Of interest, donor Treg cells expressing CD62L are critical to the regulation of GVHD.[136,215] Specifically, it has been shown that CD62L^{hi} Tregs attenuate GVHD and promote allogeneic BM engraftment.[109] The expression of CD62L is important for the migration of Tregs to secondary lymphoid organs, thereby inhibiting the initial expansion of donor T cells.[216] We now know that it is possible to modulate the alloreactivity of naive T cells by inducing anergy with costimulation blockade, deletion via cytokine modulation, or mixed chimerism. Donor effector memory T cells that are nonalloreactive do not induce GVHD, yet are able to transfer functional memory[132] and mediate GVL.[217] In addition, lymphopenia-induced proliferation gives rise to cells that are like memory T cells and enhance the GVL effect after DLI.[218] In contrast, memory T cells that are alloreactive can cause severe GVHD.[137,219,220] However, more recently, Anderson and colleagues demonstrated that enhancing the alloreactivity of effector memory T cells can cause GVHD, although a less severe and possibly more transient GVHD in nature. These findings may be better understood with further analyses that would enable tracking of alloantigen-specific T cells (naive, central memory, and effector memory subsets) in experimental GVHD and GVL models with defined TCR repertoires.

Leukocyte Migration

Donor T cells migrate to lymphoid tissues, recognize alloantigens on either host or donor APCs, and become activated. They then exit the lymphoid tissues and traffic to the target organs and cause tissue damage.[221] The molecular interactions necessary for T-cell migration and the role of lymphoid organs during acute GVHD have recently become the focus of a growing body of research. Chemokines play a critical role in the migration of immune cells to secondary lymphoid organs and target tissues.[222] T-lymphocyte production of macrophage inflammatory protein-1-alpha (MIP-1α) is critical to the recruitment of CD8$^+$ but not CD4$^+$ T cells to the liver, lung, and spleen during acute GVHD.[223] Several chemokines such as CCL2-5, CXCL2, CXCL9-11, CCL17, and CCL27 are overexpressed and might play a critical role in the migration of leukocyte subsets to target organs liver, spleen, skin, and lungs during acute GVHD.[221,224] CXCR3$^+$ T and CCR5$^+$ T cells cause acute GVHD in the liver and intestine.[221,225-227] CCR5 expression has also been found to be critical for Treg migration in GVHD.[228] In addition to chemokines and their receptors, expression of selectins and integrins and their ligands also regulate the migration of inflammatory cells to target organs.[222] For example, interaction between α4β7 integrin and its ligand MadCAM-1 are important for homing of donor T cells to Peyer patches and in the initiation of intestinal GVHD.[85,229] αLβ2/ICAM1, 2, 3 and α4β1/VCAM-2 interactions are important for homing to the lung and liver after experimental HCT.[221] The expression of CD62L on donor Tregs is critical for their regulation of acute GVHD, suggesting that their migration in secondary tissues is critical for their regulatory effects.[108] The migratory requirement of donor T cells to specific lymph nodes (e.g., Peyer patches) for the induction of GVHD might depend on other factors such as the conditioning regimen, inflammatory milieu, etc.[85,230] Furthermore, FTY720, a pharmacologic sphingosine-1-phosphate receptor agonist, inhibited GVHD in murine but not in canine models of HCT.[231,232] Thus significant species differences may also factor in the ability of these molecules to regulate GVHD.

Phase 3: Effector Phase

The effector phase that leads to the GVHD target organ damage is a complex cascade of multiple cellular and inflammatory effectors that further modulate each other's responses either simultaneously or successively. Effector mechanisms of acute GVHD can be grouped into cellular and inflammatory effectors. Inflammatory chemokines expressed in inflamed tissues upon stimulation by proinflammatory effectors, such as cytokines, are specialized for the recruitment of effector cells, such as cytotoxic T lymphocytes (CTLs).[233]

Furthermore the spatiotemporal expression of the cytochemokine gradients might determine not only the severity but also the unusual cluster of GVHD target organs (skin, gut, and liver).[221,234]

Cellular Effectors

CTLs are the major cellular effectors of GVHD.[235,236] The principle CTL effector pathways that have been evaluated after allogeneic BMT are the Fas-Fas ligand (FasL), the perforin-granzyme (or granule exocytosis), and the TNFR-like death receptors (DR), such as TNF-related apoptosis-inducing ligand (TRAIL: DR4, 5 ligand) and TNF-like weak inducers of apoptosis (TWEAK: DR3 ligand).[236-241] The involvement of each of these molecules in GVHD has been tested by utilizing donor cells that are unable to mediate each pathway. Perforin is stored in cytotoxic granules of CTLs and NK cells, together with granzymes and other proteins. Although the exact mechanisms remain unclear, following the recognition of a target cell through the TCR-MHC interaction, perforin is secreted and inserted into the cell-membrane, forming "perforin pores" that allow granzymes to enter the target cells and induce apoptosis through various downstream effector pathways such as caspases.[242] Ligation of Fas results in the formation of the death-inducing signaling complex (DISC) and also activates caspases.[243,244]

Transplantation of perforin-deficient T cells results in a marked delay in the onset of GVHD in transplants across MiHA disparities only, both MHC and MiHA disparities, and across isolated MHC I or II disparities.[236,245-249] However, mortality and clinical and histologic signs of GVHD were still induced even in the absence of perforin-dependent killing in these studies, demonstrating that the perforin-granzyme pathway plays little role in target organ damage. A role for the perforin-granzyme pathway for GVHD induction is also evident in studies employing donor T-cell subsets. Perforin- or granzyme B-deficient $CD8^+$ T cells caused less mortality than wild-type T cells in experimental transplants across a single MHC class I mismatch. This pathway, however, seems to be less important compared with Fas/FasL pathway in CD4-mediated GVHD.[248-250] Thus it seems that $CD4^+$ CTLs preferentially use the Fas-FasL pathway, whereas $CD8^+$ CTLs primarily use the perforin-granzyme pathway.

Fas, a TNF-receptor family member, is expressed by many tissues, including GVHD target organs.[251] Its expression can be upregulated by inflammatory cytokines such as IFN-γ and TNF-α during GVHD, and the expression of FasL is also increased on donor T cells, indicating that FasL-mediated cytotoxicity may be a particularly important effector pathway in GVHD.[236,252] FasL-defective T cells cause less GVHD in the liver, skin, and lymphoid organs.[247,250,252] The Fas-FasL pathway is particularly important in hepatic GVHD, consistent with the keen sensitivity of hepatocytes to Fas-mediated cytotoxicity in experimental models of murine hepatitis.[236] Fas-deficient recipients are protected from hepatic GVHD, but not from other organ GVHD, and administration of anti-FasL (but not anti-TNF) MAbs significantly blocked hepatic GVHD damage occurring in murine models.[236,253,254] Although the use of FasL-deficient donor T cells or the administration of neutralizing FasL MAbs had no effect on the development of intestinal GVHD in several studies, the Fas-FasL pathway may play a role in this target organ, because intestinal epithelial lymphocytes exhibit increased FasL-mediated killing potential.[255] Elevated serum levels of soluble FasL and Fas have also been observed in at least some patients with acute GVHD.[256,257]

The use of a perforin-granzyme and FasL cytotoxic double-deficient (cdd) mouse provides an opportunity to address whether other effector pathways are capable of inducing GVHD target organ pathology. An initial study demonstrated that cdd T cells were unable to induce lethal GVHD across MHC class I and class II disparities after sublethal irradiation.[246] However, subsequent studies demonstrated that cytotoxic effector mechanisms of donor T cells are critical in preventing host resistance to GVHD.[240,258] Thus when recipients were conditioned with lethal dose of irradiation, cdd $CD4^+$ T cells produced similar mortality to wild-type $CD4^+$ T cells.[240] These results were confirmed by a recent study demonstrating that GVHD target damage can occur in mice that lack alloantigen expression on the epithelium, preventing direct interaction between CTLs and target cells.[241]

The participation of another death ligand receptor signaling pathway, TNF/TNFRs, has also been evaluated. Experimental data suggest that this pathway is crucial for GI GVHD (discussed in more detail later). Recently, several additional TNF family apoptosis-inducing receptors/ligands have been identified, including TWEAK, TRAIL, and LTβ/LIGHT, all of which have been proposed to play a role in GVHD and GVL responses.[119,259-265] However, whether these distinct pathways play a more specific role for GVHD mediated by distinct T cell subsets in certain situations remains unknown. Intriguingly, recent data suggest that none of these pathways might be critical for mediating the rejection of donor grafts.[259,266] Thus it is likely that their role in GVHD might be modulated by the intensity of conditioning and by the recipient T-cell subsets. Existing experimental data suggest that perforin and TRAIL cytotoxic pathways are associated with $CD8^+$ T cell–mediated GVL.[236] The available experimental data are strongly skewed toward $CD8^+$ T cell–mediated GVL based on the dominant role of this effector population in most murine GVT models; however, $CD4^+$ T cells can mediate GVL and might be crucial in clinical BMT depending on the type of malignancy and the expression of immunodominant antigens.

Taken together, experimental data suggest some distinction between the use of different lytic pathways for the specific GVHD target organs and GVL, but the clinical applicability of these observations is as yet largely unknown.

Inflammatory Effectors

Inflammatory cytokines synergize with CTLs resulting in the amplification of local tissue injury and further promotion of an inflammation, which ultimately leads to the observed target tissue destruction in the transplant recipient.[267] Macrophages, which had been primed with IFN-γ during step 2, produce inflammatory cytokines TNF-α and IL-1 when stimulated by a secondary triggering signal.[268] This stimulus may be provided through toll-like receptors (TLRs) by microbial products such as LPS and other microbial particles, which can leak through the intestinal mucosa damaged by the conditioning regimen and gut GVHD.[269,270] It is now apparent that immune recognition through both TLR and non-TLRs (such as NOD) by the innate immune system also controls activation of adaptive immune responses.[269,271] Recent clinical studies of GVHD suggested the possible association with TLR/NOD polymorphisms and severity of GVHD.[75,272,273] LPS and other innate stimuli may stimulate gut-associated lymphocytes, keratinocytes, dermal fibroblasts, and macrophages to produce proinflammatory effectors that play a direct role in causing target organ damage. Indeed experimental data with MHC mismatched BMT suggest that under certain circumstances these inflammatory mediators are sufficient in causing GVHD damage even in the absence of direct CTL-induced damage.[88] The severity of GVHD appears to be directly related to the level of innate and adaptive immune cell priming and release of proinflammatory cytokines such as TNF-α, IL-1, and nitric oxide (NO).[42]

The cytokines TNF-α and IL-1 are produced by an abundance of cell types during processes of both innate and adaptive immunity; they often have synergistic, pleiotropic, and redundant effects on both activation and effector phases of GVHD.[179] A critical role for TNF-α in the pathophysiology of acute GVHD was first suggested over 20 years ago because mice transplanted with mixtures of allogeneic BM and T cells developed severe skin, gut, and lung lesions that were associated with high levels of TNF-α mRNA in these tissues.[274] Target organ damage could be inhibited by infusion of anti–TNF-α MAbs, and mortality could be reduced from 100% to 50% by the administration of the soluble form of the TNF-α receptor (sTNFR), an antagonist of TNF-α.[79,82,275] Accumulating experimental data further suggest that TNF-α is involved in a multistep process of GVHD pathophysiology. TNF-α can (1) cause cachexia, a characteristic feature of GVHD; (2) induce maturation of DCs, thus enhancing alloantigen presentation; (3) recruit effector T cells, neutrophils, and monocytes into target organs through the induction of inflammatory chemokines; and (4) cause direct tissue damage by inducing apoptosis and necrosis. TNF-α also involves in donor-T-cell activation directly through its signaling via TNFR1 and TNFR2 on T cells. TNF-TNF1 interactions on donor T cells promote alloreactive T-cell responses and TNF-TNFR2 interactions are critical for intestinal GVHD.[262,276] TNF-α also seems to be an important effector molecule in GVHD in skin and lymphoid tissue.[274,277] Additionally, TNF-α might also be involved in hepatic GVHD, probably by enhancing effector cell migration to the liver via the induction of inflammatory chemokines.[278] An important role for TNF-α in clinical acute GVHD has been suggested by studies demonstrating elevated serum levels or TNF-α or elevated TNF-α mRNA expression in peripheral blood mononuclear cells in patients with acute GVHD and other endothelial complications, such as hepatic venoocclusive disease (VOD).[278-280] Phase I and II trials using TNF-α antagonists reduced the severity of GVHD, suggesting that it is a relevant effector in causing target organ damage.[281,282]

The second major proinflammatory cytokine that appears to play an important role in the effector phase of acute GVHD is IL-1.[42,267] Secretion of IL-1 appears to occur predominantly during the effector phase of GVHD of the spleen and skin, two major GVHD target organs.[283] A similar increase in mononuclear cell IL-1 mRNA has been shown during clinical acute GVHD. Indirect evidence of a role for IL-1 in GVHD was obtained with administration of this cytokine to recipients in an allogeneic murine BMT model. Mice receiving IL-1 displayed a wasting syndrome and increased mortality that appeared to be an accelerated form of disease. By contrast, intraperitoneal administration of IL-1 receptor antagonist (IL-1RA) starting on d 10 posttransplant was able to reverse the development of GVHD in the majority of animals, providing a significant survival advantage to treated animals.[284] However, the attempt to use IL-1RA to prevent acute GBHD in a randomized trial was not successful.[285]

As a result of activation during GVHD, macrophages also produce NO, which contributes to the deleterious effects on GVHD target tissues, particularly immunosuppression.[286] NO also inhibits the repair mechanisms of target tissue destruction by inhibiting proliferation of epithelial stem cells in the gut and skin.[287] In humans and rats, the development of GVHD is preceded by an increase in serum levels of NO oxidation products.[288-290]

Interleukin-6 has also been identified as a critical cytokine that promotes a proinflammatory response during GVHD and inhibits the reconstitution of Tregs.[291] While Tawara and colleagues confirmed an important role for IL-6 in GVHD, their findings were independent of T effector cell expansion or donor Treg responses. It is possible that reduction in GVHD is a consequence of direct reduction in IL-6–induced inflammation and cytopathic damage of the target tissues.[292]

Existing data demonstrate important roles for various inflammatory effectors in GVHD. However, the relevance of currently studied or as yet unknown specific effectors might be determined by other factors, including the intensity of preparatory regimens, the type of allograft, the T-cell subsets and the duration of BMT. In any event, both experimental and clinical data suggest an important role for both the cellular and inflammatory mediators in GVHD-induced target organ damage.

BIOMARKERS OF GRAFT-VERSUS-HOST DISEASE

Emerging data from large datasets have identified and validated biomarkers for acute GVHD. Screening of plasma with antibody microarrays for 120 proteins in a discovery set of 42 BMT patients that revealed eight potential biomarkers for diagnosis of GVHD. The authors then measured by enzyme-linked immunosorbent assay (ELISA) the levels of these biomarkers in samples from 424 BMT patients who were randomly divided into training (n = 282) and validation (n = 142) sets. Logistic regression analysis of these eight proteins determined a composite biomarker panel of four proteins (IL-2Rα, TNFR1, IL-8, and hepatocyte growth factor [HGF]) that optimally discriminated patients with and without GVHD. The receiver operating characteristic area under the curve (ROC AUC) that distinguished these two groups in the training set was 0.91 and 0.86 in the validation set. Cox regression analysis revealed that the biomarker panel predicted survival independently of GVHD severity. These biomarkers did not distinguish organ-specific disease.

An in-depth, unbiased, tandem MS (MS/MS)–based analysis of plasma was able to quantify proteins at low concentrations. The authors chose candidate biomarker proteins with concentrations at least twice as high in pooled samples from 10 BMT patients with histologically confirmed skin GVHD compared with pooled samples from 10 BMT patients without the disease. Among 66 candidate biomarkers, 14 were expressed primarily in the skin. Elafin (also known as peptidase inhibitor-3, skin-derived antileukoproteinase, or trappin-2) emerged as the lead biomarker candidate because suitable antibodies were available for high-throughput screening of plasma samples by ELISA. They validated the biomarker in a large group (492) of allogeneic BMT recipients. Blinded analysis of skin biopsies from 20 patients showed that positive elafin expression, defined as significant staining extending to a depth of more than 50% of the epidermis, was present in 7 of 10 cases of GVHD and in 0 of 10 cases of non-GVHD (P = 0.003). In the large data set, plasma elafin concentrations of patients with GVHD were 3.9 times higher than patients with a non-GVHD rash (P <0.001). When elafin was compared with four previously reported diagnostic biomarkers of systemic acute GVHD (IL-2Rα, TNFR1, IL-8, and HGF), it was the best single biomarker, and the combination of all five biomarkers provided little further information. The prognostic value of the biomarker was also significant because patients with high elafin concentrations at GVHD onset died three times as often as those with low concentrations, and the 5-year overall survival was significantly higher in the low-elafin group: 48% versus 26% (P = 0.01). When survival was modeled simultaneously on elafin concentration, GVHD skin stage at onset, and the other prognostic factors, the association between elafin concentration and risk for mortality remained statistically significant (P = 0.02).

In a follow-up study the authors also identified and validated regenerating islet-derived 3-alpha (REG3α) as a biomarker of gastrointestinal GVHD. Using an identical proteomics approach, they first identified and quantified 562 proteins of which 74 were increased at least two-fold in patients with GVHD. Five proteins (carboxypeptidase N catalytic chain precursor; pancreatic secretory trypsin inhibitor precursor; palladin; lithostathine 1α precursor; and REG3α) were preferentially expressed in the GI tract. They validated the biomarker in samples from 871 allogeneic BMT recipients. Plasma REG3α concentrations were three times higher in patients at the onset of GI GVHD than in all other patients, including those with non-GVHD enteritis. Serum REG3α concentrations were also higher in GI GVHD in an independent validation set of 143 BMT patients from Regensburg, Germany and Kyushu, Japan. In patients with diarrhea caused by GVHD, REG3α concentrations at the onset of GVHD were five times higher than in patients with diarrhea from other causes. REG3α was the best single diagnostic biomarker at the onset of symptoms of lower GI GVHD, and additional biomarkers provided no further increased sensitivity or specificity. Using REG3α at the median concentration provided a positive predictive value (PPV) of 95% and a negative predictive value (NPV) of 32% for GVHD as the etiology of diarrhea. REG3α concentrations were threefold higher at the time of GVHD diagnosis in patients who had no response to therapy at 4 weeks than in patients who experienced a complete or partial response (p <0.001). When patients were divided into two equal groups based on REG3α concentrations, transplant related mortality (TRM) was twice as high in patients with high REG3α group, and this difference remained significant after adjusting for known risk factors of donor type, degree of HLA match, conditioning intensity, age and baseline disease severity (p <0.001). In further analyses, the plasma concentration of REG3α, the clinical severity of GVHD, the histologic severity at GVHD diagnosis independently predicted lack of response to GVHD therapy 4 weeks following treatment and TRM. Patients who had all three risk factors experienced significantly greater NRM than those with any two of the risk factors (86% versus 66%, p <0.001). The integration of clinical stage, histologic grade, and REG3α plasma concentrations into a single grading system will permit better risk stratification and rapid identification of those patients with severe GI damage in whom standard treatment is likely to be insufficient. This study provides potential new insights into the biology of GI GVHD. REG proteins act downstream of IL-22 to protect the epithelial barrier function of the intestinal mucosa through the binding of bacterial peptidoglycans. Intestinal stem cells (ISCs) are principal cellular targets of GVHD in the GI tract, where intestinal flora are critical for amplification of GVHD damage. A leading hypothesis is that ISCs are protected by antibacterial proteins such as REG3α secreted by neighboring Paneth cells into the crypt microenvironment. If death of an intestinal stem cell eventually manifests itself as denudation of the mucosa, the patchy nature of GVHD histologic damage may be explained as the lack of mucosal regeneration following the dropout of individual ISCs. The tight proximity of Paneth cells with ISCs concentrates their secretory contents in that vicinity, so that mucosal barrier disruption caused by stem cell dropout may preferentially allow Paneth cell proteins, including REG3α, to traverse into the bloodstream. Thus the plasma levels of REG3α may serve as a surrogate marker for the cumulative area of these breaches to GI mucosal barrier integrity, a parameter impossible to measure by individual tissue biopsies. Such an estimate of total damage to the mucosal barrier may also help explain the prognostic value of REG3α with respect to therapy responsiveness and NRM.

Less progress has been made with biomarkers for chronic GVHD. One important study, published by the Children's Oncology Group, analyzed candidate biomarkers in 52 patients with extensive chronic GVHD who had participated in a phase III therapeutic trial. Patients were compared for time of onset after BMT (early, 3 to 8 months; late, 9 months or more) with 28 time-matched controls without chronic GVHD. Soluble B-cell activation factor (sBAFF), anti-dsDNA antibody, soluble IL-2 receptor alpha (sIL-2Rα), and soluble CD13 (sCD13) were elevated in patients with early-onset chronic GVHD. sBAFF and anti-dsDNA were also elevated in patients with late-onset chronic GVHD. For the early chronic GVHD group, ROC AUCs were 0.70 for anti-dsDNA (0.66), IL2Rα (0.83), sCD13 (0.77), and sBAFF (0.70). At 90% specificity, the sensitivity was relatively low, ranging between 42% and 53%. A panel of biomarkers slightly improved the diagnostic power. In terms of prognosis, only IL-2Rα demonstrated a significant difference between responders and nonresponders (P = 0.03). These biomarkers need to be validated in much larger cohorts before definitive conclusions can be drawn.

Prevention of Acute Graft-Versus-Host Disease

Elimination of T cells with monoclonal antibodies, immunotoxins, lectins, CD34 columns, or physical techniques are effective at reducing GVHD. A typical unmanipulated marrow transplant entails the infusion of $\approx 10^7$ T cells per kg of recipient weight. A T-cell dose $\leq 10^5$ per kg has been associated with complete control of GVHD.[41] More recently, the combination of very high stem cell numbers and <3 × 10^4CD3 cells/kg allowed haploidentical transplantation without GVHD.[293] Presumably, host immune cells that survive the initial conditioning are responsible for graft rejection. When the stem cell source contains a large numbers of T cells, the GVH reaction further reduces the residual population capable of alloreactivity, thus decreasing graft rejection. To some degree, the higher graft failure rates may be controlled by increasing the intensity of the immunosuppression of the conditioning regimen,[294,295] or adding back T cells.[296] Overall there has been no improvement in survival that can be definitively attributed to T-cell depletion.

Treatment of established GVHD with specific T-cell antibodies has produced mixed results. Although antithymocyte globulin has definite activity in established GVHD, the nonspecific clearance of T cells may result in increased opportunistic infections and no improvement in survival. More specific therapy with humanized anti-IL-2 receptor antibody, daclizumab[297,298] or the humanized anti-CD3 antibody, visilizumab[299,300] are promising, since they offer the potential of selectively removing the activated T cells. However, an increased risk for infection may still be observed.[301]

The first generally prescribed GVHD preventive regimen was the administration of intermittent low-dose methotrexate as developed in a dog model by Thomas and Storb.[302] The principle of this approach was to administer a cell cycle–specific chemotherapeutic agent immediately after the transplant, when the T cells have started to divide after exposure to allogeneic antigens. Subsequently, the addition of antithymocyte globulin, prednisone, or both resulted in incremental improvement in the GVHD rate but no improvement in survival.[303,304] Ultimately, the course of methotrexate was abbreviated and combined with a T-cell activation inhibitor, such as cyclosporine or tacrolimus. The introduction of cyclosporine in the late 1970s was a significant advance in GVHD prevention. A similar agent, tacrolimus, has been shown to provide similar control of GVHD.[305] As a single agent, cyclosporine was about as effective as methotrexate.[306] However, in combination with methotrexate, there was a significant reduction in the incidence of GVHD and an improvement in survival.[307] Subsequent trials of tacrolimus and methotrexate compared with cyclosporine and methotrexate showed no advantage for either combination.[305] The addition of prednisone to the conventional two-drug regimen resulted in similar rates of GVHD and no improvement in survival.[308]

Sirolimus (rapamycin) is a macrocyclic lactone immunosuppressant that is similar in structure to tacrolimus and cyclosporine. All three drugs bind to immunophilins; however, sirolimus complexed with FKBP12 inhibits T-cell proliferation by interfering with signal transduction and cell-cycle progression and can prevent GVHD.[309] Because Sirolimus acts through a separate mechanism from the tacrolimus-FKBP complex (and cyclosporine-cyclophilin complex), it is synergistic with both tacrolimus and cyclosporine. More recently, mycophenolate mofetil (MMF) has been studied. It is the prodrug of mycophenolic acid (MPA), a selective inhibitor of inosine monophosphate dehydrogenase, an enzyme critical to the de novo synthesis of guanosine nucleotide. Since T lymphocytes are more dependent on such synthesis than myeloid or mucosal cells, MPA preferentially inhibits proliferative responses of T cells.[310]

One hypothesis that flows from the three-step model of GVHD posits that reduction of intestinal colonization with bacteria could prevent GVHD. Animal studies in germ-free environments support this notion; GVHD was not observed until mice were colonized with gram-negative organisms.[311] Later, gut decontamination and use of a laminar air flow environment was associated with less GVHD and better survival in patients with severe aplastic anemia.[312] Similarly, studies of intestinal decontamination in patients with malignancies have shown less GVHD in some,[313,314] but not all, studies.[315] Finally, another recent approach to GVHD prevention has been the use of nonmyeloablative conditioning transplants. A less intensive preparative regimen decreases the tissue toxicity and subsequent release of cytokines in animal models.[79,82] Patients generally experience mild toxicity in the initial peritransplant period and develop little or no GVHD, although many develop GVHD later, especially after donor lymphocyte infusions. In fact, the rates of GVHD are often higher than with conventional transplants, and GVHD is associated with a significant portion of the GVL effect.[316-318]

An important role for TNFα in clinical acute GVHD has been suggested by studies demonstrating elevated levels of TNFα in the serum of patients with acute GVHD and other endothelial complications such as venoocclusive disease.[280,319-321] Therapy of GVHD with humanized anti-TNFα (infliximab)[322,323] or a dimeric fusion protein consisting of the extracellular ligand-binding portion of the human TNFα receptor (TNFR) linked to the Fc portion of human IgG1 (etanercept)[324] have shown some promise.[325,326] The second major proinflammatory cytokine that appears to play an important role in the effector phase of acute GVHD is IL-1. Secretion of IL-1 appears to occur predominantly during the effector phase of GVHD in the spleen and skin, two major GVHD target organs.[283] IL-1RA is a naturally occurring pure competitive inhibitor of IL-1 that is produced by monocytes/macrophages and keratinocytes. Of note, the IL-1RA gene is polymorphic, and the presence in the donor of the allele that is linked to higher secretion of IL-1RA was associated with less acute GVHD.[327] Two-phase I/II trials showed promising data that specific inhibition of IL-1 with either the soluble receptor or IL-1RA could result in remissions in 50% to 60% of patients with steroid-resistant GVHD.[328,329] However, a subsequent randomized trial of the addition of IL-1RA or placebo to cyclosporine and methotrexate beginning at the time of conditioning and continuing through day 14 after stem cell infusion did not show any protective effect of the drug, despite the attainment of very high plasma levels.[285,330] Therefore, at least as administered in this study, IL-1 inhibition was insufficient to prevent GVHD in humans. IL-11 was also able to protect the GI tract in animal models and prevent GVHD, but it did not prevent clinical GVHD.[330] Thus not all preclinical strategies successfully translate to new therapies.

Therapy for Acute Graft-Versus-Host Disease

Glucocorticoid steroids are the initial therapy for acute GVHD. The mechanisms by which steroids work are multifactorial; they act as lympholytic agents and inhibit the release of inflammatory cytokines such as IL-1, IL-2, IL-6, gamma interferon, and TNFα. Because of its intravenous availability, methylprednisolone is the steroid most commonly given for acute GVHD. Various dosing regimens have been used, none of which is clearly superior. High-bolus doses (10 to 20 mg/kg or 500 mg/m^2) have higher initial response rates, but flares on tapering and opportunistic infections are common. Both the Seattle and Minnesota transplant groups have found that treatment with steroids was as effective as, or more effective than, other therapies or combination of therapies, with 20% to 40% of patients having durable long-term responses.[331,332] Long-term salvage rates for patients who did not respond to steroids were 20% or less; most patients eventually died from infection, acute GVHD, and/or chronic GVHD. More recently, a randomized trial demonstrated that topical therapy with oral budosenide can have prednisone sparing effects and is efficacious in treatment of GI GVHD.[333] Clinically, two types of failure of corticosteroid treatment of acute GVHD can be distinguished: true steroid resistance (i.e., progression of GVHD symptoms and manifestations while patients are receiving full-dose corticosteroid treatment) and steroid dependence (i.e., reoccurrence [or flare] of GVHD during or after tapering of steroid treatment).[334] In general, the prognosis with true steroid-resistant GVHD is worse than the prognosis of steroid-dependent patients.[334] A comparison of trials dealing with steroid-resistant GVHD is hampered by variable inclusion of both patient groups in many of these trials. A number of agents have been tested, including chemical immunosuppressants such as MMF, ATG, anti-CD3 anti-T cell antibodies, and more specific agents directed against activation or adhesion molecules anti-CD25, anti-CD147, or cytokines or extracorporeal photopheresis.[334,335] To date, there are no randomized trails testing one agent versus the other in this clinical situation. Recent data suggested a role for TNF inhibition when added to steroids in treating GVHD, although a randomized trail failed to demonstrate any difference when compared with the addition of pentostatin or anti-IL2 to steroids and was inferior to the addition of MMF.[325,336]

Targeted elimination of alloreactive T cells has recently been demonstrated to be a safe and efficacious method to mitigate GVHD. Fusion of human caspase 9 to a modified human FK-binding protein that allowed for dimerization when exposed to a synthetic dimerizing drug led to the rapid death of 90% of alloreactive T cells expressing this construct and mitigated acute GVHD in a pilot trial of five patients following haploidentical BMT.[337]

Other Supportive Approaches

Infections are the main cause of death in patients with steroid-refractory acute GVHD, and careful surveillance and control of infections is mandatory in patients with acute GVHD. Fungal infections, especially aspergillosis, are the leading complication. Prophylaxis and early aggressive treatment should be facilitated by the introduction of new azoles (voriconazole, posiconozole) or echinocandins (caspofungin, micafungin), which broaden therapeutic efficacy with acceptable toxicity. Other supplementary approaches have been suggested, such as the use of octreotide[338] and oral beclomethasone (or budesonide) to control large volumes of diarrhea.[333]

CHRONIC GRAFT-VERSUS-HOST DISEASE

Chronic GVHD was initially defined as a GVHD syndrome presenting more than 100 days after transplant; its onset occurred either as an extension of acute GVHD (progressive), after a disease-free interval (quiescent), or with no precedent (de novo).[339,340] Chronic GVHD may be limited or extensive (see Table 109-3). Any grade of acute GVHD increases the probability of chronic GVHD, although no singular pathologic feature of the former predicts the development of the latter. Its incidence ranges from 30% to 60% after transplantation with the bone marrow, although it may be higher after peripheral blood progenitor transplants.[341]

As with acute GVHD, the immune system appears to be affected in all patients, who are highly susceptible to bacterial, viral, fungal, and opportunistic infections. Specific abnormalities of cellular immunity include decreases in the production of antibodies against specific antigens, defects in the number and function of CD4$^+$ T cells, and increases in the number of nonspecific suppressor cells, which further diminish lymphocyte responses. Skin changes resembling widespread lichen planus with papulosquamous dermatitis, plaques, desquamation, dyspigmentation, and vitiligo occur in 80% of patients.[318,342] Destruction of dermal appendages leads to alopecia and onychodysplasia. Severe chronic GVHD of the skin can resemble scleroderma, with induration, joint contractures, atrophy, and chronic skin ulcers. Chronic cholestatic liver disease occurs in 80% of patients and often resembles acute GVHD; it rarely progresses to cirrhosis. Severe mucositis of the mouth and esophagus can result in weight loss and malnutrition. Intestinal involvement, however, is infrequent.[318,342] Chronic GVHD also produces a sicca syndrome, with atrophy and dryness of mucosal surfaces caused by lymphocytic destruction of exocrine glands, usually affecting the eyes, mouth, airways, skin, and esophagus.[25,342,343] The hematopoietic system may also be affected, and thrombocytopenia is an unfavorable prognostic factor in patients with chronic GVHD.[318] Important predictors of unfavorable outcome are progressive onset, lichenoid skin changes, elevated serum bilirubin level, continued thrombocytopenia, and failure to respond to 9 months of therapy.[318,344-346] Among patients with none of these risk factors, 70% are expected to survive, compared with less than 20% with two or more of these risk factors.[346]

Histologic examination of the immune system reveals involution of thymic epithelium, disappearance of Hassall corpuscles, depletion of lymphocytes, and absence of secondary germinal centers in lymph nodes.[343] Pathologic skin findings include epidermal atrophy with changes characteristic of lichen planus and striking inflammation around eccrine units. Sclerosis of the dermis and fibrosis of the hypodermis subsequently develop. GI lesions include localized inflammation of the mucosa and stricture formation in the esophagus and small intestine.[342] Histologic findings in the liver are often similar to those that occur in acute GVHD but are more intense, with chronic changes such as fibrosis and hyalinization of portal triads, obliteration of bile ducts, and hepatocellular cholestasis.[318] The endocrine glands of the eyes, mouth, esophagus, and bronchi show destruction focused on centrally draining ducts, with secondary involvement of alveolar components.[343] Findings of bronchiolitis obliterans, similar to those that occur in rejection of lung transplants, are now generally considered a pulmonary manifestation of chronic GVHD, although the pathogenesis of this process remains unclear.[343]

Clinical Manifestations of Chronic Graft-Versus-Host Disease

Chronic GVHD can present with a plethora of clinical manifestations. Because of its unpredictable pattern and the late onset, when patients are no longer receiving care at their transplant center, the diagnosis is often delayed or not recognized. The staging of chronic GVHD is summarized in Table 109-4. However, consensus criteria recently developed by the National Institutes of Health (NIH) might soon become the standard for diagnosing and evaluating responses for chronic GVHD.[347,348]

Dermatologic

Skin involvement in chronic GVHD presents with varied features. Lichenoid chronic GVHD presents as an erythematous, papular rash that resembles lichen planus with no typical distribution pattern.[25] Scleradermatous GVHD may involve the dermis and/or the muscular fascia and clinically resembles systemic sclerosis. The skin is thickened, tight, and fragile, with very poor wound healing. Either hypo- or hyperpigmentation may occur. In severe cases the skin may become blistered and ulcerate. Hair changes can include increased brittleness, premature graying, and alopecia. Fingernails and toenails may also be affected by chronic GVHD. Destruction of sweat glands can cause hyperthermia.[349]

Ocular

Ocular GVHD usually presents with xerophthalmia or dry eyes. Irreversible destruction of the lacrimal glands results in dryness, photophobia, and burning. Local therapy with preservative-free tears and ointment or the placement of punctal plugs by an ophthalmologist might be required. Conjunctival GVHD, a rare manifestation of severe chronic GVHD, has a poor prognosis.[25,349]

Oral

Oral GVHD causes xerostomia and/or food sensitivity.[349] More advanced disease may cause odynophagia due to esophageal damage and strictures, although esophageal involvement occurs rarely without oral disease. Physical examination may reveal only erythema with a few white plaques, prompting a misdiagnosis of thrush or herpetic infections. Lichenoid changes in advanced disease can cause extensive plaque formation.[25]

Gastrointestinal

Patients with chronic GVHD have GI complaints that mimic other disease states, including acute GVHD, infection, dysmotility, lactose intolerance, pancreatic insufficiency, and drug-related side effects. In one retrospective review of the intestinal biopsies of patients with chronic GVHD and persistent GI symptoms, a majority of patients had evidence of both acute and chronic GVHD, and only 7% of the patients had isolated chronic GVHD.[25,342] Thus although chronic GVHD may involve the GI tract alone, it may be difficult to diagnose in those circumstances without concurrent acute GVHD.

Hepatic

Hepatic disease typically presents as cholestasis with elevated serum levels of alkaline phosphatase and bilirubin. Isolated hepatic chronic GVHD has become more common with the increasing use of donor lymphocyte infusions.[12] Liver biopsy is required to confirm the diagnosis of chronic hepatic GVHD in patients with no other target organ involvement.

Pulmonary

Bronchiolitis obliterans is a late and serious manifestation of chronic GVHD. Patients typically present with a cough or dyspnea.[349] Severe sclerotic disease of the chest wall may also give rise to similar symptoms with no intrinsic pulmonary disease. Pulmonary function tests demonstrate obstructive physiology and a reduction in DLCO. Chest computed tomography results may be normal or may show hyperinflation with a ground-glass appearance. Overall, patients with bronchiolitis obliterans have minimal response to therapy and a very poor prognosis. Patients with chronic GVHD are also at risk for chronic sinopulmonary infections, but symptoms may be minimal.[25]

Hematopoietic

Cytopenias in chronic GVHD are common. This may be a result of stromal damage, but autoimmune neutropenia, anemia, and/or thrombocytopenia are also seen. Thrombocytopenia at the time of chronic GVHD diagnosis is associated with poor prognosis. However, thrombocytopenia posttransplant is a poor prognostic factor regardless of GVHD, and eosinophilia is occasionally seen with chronic GVHD.

Table 109-4 Commonly Administered Drugs for Graft-Versus-Host Disease Prophylaxis and Treatment

Drug	Mechanism	Adverse Effects
Corticosteroids	Direct lymphocyte toxicity; suppress proinflammatory cytokines such as TNF-α	Hyperglycemia; acute psychosis; severe myopathy; neuropathy; osteoporosis; cataract development
Methotrexate (MTX)	Antimetabolite: inhibit T cell proliferation	Significant renal, hepatic, and gastrointestinal toxicities
Cyclosporine A (CSA)	IL-2 suppressor; blocks $Ca2^+$-dependent signal transduction distal to TCR engagement	Renal and hepatic insufficiency; hypertension; hyperglycemia; headache; nausea and vomiting; hirsutism; gum hypertrophy; seizure with severe toxicity
Tacrolimus (FK506)	IL-2 receptor; blocks $Ca2^+$-dependent signal transduction distal to TCR engagement	Similar to CSA
Mycophenolate mofetil (MMF)	Inhibits de novo purine synthesis	Body aches; abdominal pain; nausea and vomiting; diarrhea; neutropenia
Sirolimus	mTOR inhibitor	Thrombocytopenia; hyperlipidemia, TTP
Antithymocyte globulin (ATG)	Polyclonal immunoglobulin	Anaphylaxis; serum sickness

Immunologic

Chronic GVHD is inherently immunosuppressive. Functional asplenia with an increased susceptibility to encapsulated bacteria is common, and circulating Howell-Jolly bodies can be seen on peripheral blood smear. Patients are also at risk for invasive fungal infections and *Pneumocystis carinii* pneumonia (PCP). Hypoglobulinemia is common, and patients with levels below 500 mg/dL should be supplemented with intravenous immunoglobulin.

Musculoskeletal

Fascial involvement in sclerodermatous GVHD is usually associated with skin changes. Fasciitis in joint areas can cause severe restriction of range of motion. Muscle cramps are a common complaint in patients with chronic GVHD, but myositis with elevated muscle enzymes is rare. Many patients with chronic GVHD are on steroid therapy and have low levels of sex hormone posttransplant. Thus avascular necrosis, osteopenia, and osteoporosis are frequent complications.

Although several cases have been described, it is yet to be determined in large studies whether kidneys, which are primary targets in some animal models of chronic GVHD, are also involved.[350] Among the myriad clinical features of chronic GVHD, three definitive signs appear to be risk factors for increased mortality: (1) extensive skin GVHD involving >50% of the body surface area, (2) platelet count of <100,000/μL, and (3)progressive onset and acute GVHD that continues uninterrupted beyond day 100.[351] However, chronic GVHD remains, except in cases with obvious features, a difficult diagnosis; response to therapy is even more difficult to assess. Recent criteria established by NIH consensus conference might prove to be beneficial in establishing uniform guidelines for diagnosis, treatment, and response.[348] The NIH consensus criteria are currently being evaluated.

Differential Diagnosis

The distinction between chronic and acute GVHD has been traditionally based on the time of onset. However, with the advent of low-intensity HCT, that distinction has become less relevant. The NIH Working Group has, in addition to the two main categories of GVHD, added two subcategories. The broad category of acute GVHD includes (1) classic acute GVHD (maculopapular rash, nausea, vomiting, anorexia, profuse diarrhea, ileus, or cholestatic hepatitis), occurring within 100 days after transplantation or DLI (without diagnostic or distinctive signs of chronic GVHD), and (2) persistent, recurrent, or late acute GVHD: features of classic acute GVHD without diagnostic or distinctive manifestations of chronic GVHD occurring beyond 100 days of transplantation or DLI (often seen after withdrawal of immune suppression). The broad category of chronic GVHD includes (1) classic chronic GVHD without features characteristic of acute GVHD and (2) an overlap syndrome in which features of chronic and acute GVHD appear together. In the absence of histologic or clinical signs or symptoms of chronic GVHD, the persistence, recurrence, or new onset of characteristic skin, GI tract, or liver abnormalities should be classified as acute GVHD regardless of the time after transplantation. With appropriate stratification, patients with persistent, recurrent, or late acute GVHD or overlap syndrome can be included in clinical trials with patients who have chronic GVHD.

CHRONIC GRAFT-VERSUS-HOST DISEASE: PATHOPHYSIOLOGY

The pathophysiology of chronic GVHD is generally much less well understood than that of acute GVHD and has undergone less intensive experimental modeling.[25] It is important to recognize that chronic GVHD was originally defined as a temporal rather than a clinical or pathophysiologic entity. The initial clinical reports of chronic GVHD described abnormalities that occurred at least 150 days after stem cell infusion.[352,353] By convention, day 100 after stem cell infusion is used as an arbitrary divider between acute and chronic GVHD. But some manifestations of acute GVHD occur after day 100, and some manifestations of chronic GVHD may occur before day 100. Thus it is preferable to consider the clinical symptoms and signs per se rather than their timing of onset.

Relatively little is known about the pathophysiology of chronic GVHD. This is due in part to the absence of appropriate animal models that can capture the kinetics and the protean manifestation of chronic GVHD.[354] Based on certain clinical features chronic GVHD has been considered to be an autoimmune disease, with some experimental data suggesting that chronic GVHD results from defective central negative selection, which leads to the generation of autoreactive clones that escape tolerogenic mechanisms operating in the periphery.[355,356] This would indicate that the nonpolymorphic antigens expressed in both the donor and recipient rather than MiHA antigens are the likely targets. In contrast to T cells from animals with acute GVHD that are specific for host alloantigens, T cells from animals with chronic GVHD are specific for a public (common) determinant of MHC class II molecules.[357,358] These T cells are considered autoreactive because they recognize public MHC class II determinants that are common to both donor and recipient rather than polymorphic histocompatibility antigens that are specific for the host. The autoreactive cells of chronic GVHD are associated with a damaged thymus, which can be injured by several mechanisms, including acute GVHD, the conditioning regimen, or age-related involution and atrophy. In chronic GVHD the ability of the thymus to delete autoreactive T cells (negative selection) and to induce tolerance is impaired.[25,359,360] However, no clear data exist on the isolation of "autoreactive" donor-derived T-cell clones that equally recognize nonpolymorphic antigens from the donor and recipient cells. This, however, does not directly preclude the existence of a causative role for autoreactive T cells. Chronic GVHD could also be a product of T cells that have undergone relatively chronic antigen stimulation as a result of the presence of inexhaustible and ubiquitous MiHA antigens. Allo-T cells under circumstances of chronic MiHA antigen stimulation can induce syndromes resembling those induced by the chronic antigen stimulation in autoimmune diseases. This concept is also consistent with the proposal of acute GVHD as a risk factor for chronic GVHD. The antigens targeted in chronic GVHD could be the same dominant ones targeted in acute GVHD, but the reactive T cells could be different; for example, they may secrete transforming growth factor-β. However, antigens other than those that were initially immunodominant (even those not initially targeted but introduced through epitope spread of either the nonpolymorphic "autoantigens" or the now-distinct MiHAs) could be important. It is also conceivable that regulatory mechanisms could frequently fail in allo-HCT, resulting in activation and expansion of T cells that recognize both nonpolymorphic and MiHA epitopes. One recent murine study suggested that development of chronic GVHD-like syndrome is target antigen-dependent.[112] Furthermore, chronic GVHD pathogenesis could, in part, be a consequence of T cell priming by donor-derived antigen-presenting cells.[113] In some patient subsets, responses to rituximab, presence of MiHA-specific antibodies, and the presence of chronic GVHD after TCD allo-BMT would indicate that in addition to donor T cells, donor B cells might be a direct effector or might have a role in priming T cells as APCs.[361,362] Given the myriad clinical presentations of chronic GVHD that tend to occur at variable times after HCT, it is possible that separate pathogenic mechanisms are involved in causing distinct manifestations and that no single putative mechanism is sufficient to cause chronic GVHD. Nonetheless, a recent murine model demonstrated a pathogenic role for donor B cells and alloantibody production in causing experimental chronic GVHD.

THERAPY FOR CHRONIC GRAFT-VERSUS-HOST DISEASE

Chronic GVHD has a major impact on both quality of life and survival, frequently involves multiple organs, and necessitates prolonged immunosuppressive therapy.[363] One report noted that 15% of cancer-free patients were still receiving immunosuppressive therapy after 7 years.[364] The more severe forms of chronic GVHD are clearly associated with a lower disease-free survival. Thus the potential benefit of a graft-versus-leukemia effect is shadowed by significant treatment-related mortality.[364]

Current therapies for chronic GVHD are of limited efficacy, and there is no long-term satisfactory regimen for patients who do not respond to front-line steroid-based therapy. Indeed, no medication has been approved by the Food and Drug Administration (FDA) for use in chronic GVHD. The lack of standardized response criteria to measure therapeutic efficacy poses a major obstacle to pursuing therapeutic trials in chronic GVHD. Overall survival and/or discontinuation of systemic immunosuppression are accepted long-term endpoints in chronic GVHD trials. The recent NIH-sponsored consensus project provided, for the first time, a set of standardized measures and definitions to use as response criteria in chronic GVHD.[347,348] Nonetheless, these recommendations are yet to be tested and validated in prospective studies. The NIH consensus conference has defined response measures classified in two main groups: clinician-assessed and patient-reported (Table 109-5).[354]

The prevention of acute GVHD has not consistently resulted in a lower incidence of chronic GVHD. A clear example is the use of reduced-intensity transplants, consistently associated with a lower incidence of acute GVHD but with no major impact on chronic GVHD.[258,365] The extended use of GVHD prophylaxis with cyclosporine, or variations in the cyclosporine dosage used, showed no beneficial effects on the incidence of chronic GVHD.[363,366] The addition of thalidomide to cyclosporine and methotrexate prophylaxis, the administration of IV Ig, and early treatment based on biopsy findings of subclinical GVHD in an attempt to preemptively treat chronic GVHD were unsuccessful.[363] The most commonly used therapies to treat chronic GVHD are cyclosporine A (CSA) and prednisone. Sullivan and colleagues[367] reported that prednisone alone is superior to prednisone plus azathioprine for primary treatment of patients with chronic GVHD. However, in patients classified as high-risk on the basis of platelet counts below 100,000/μL, treatment with prednisone alone resulted in only 26% 5-year survival. When a similar group of patients was treated with alternating-day CSA and prednisone, 5-year survival exceeded 50%.[368] A recent randomized study of 287 patients with extensive GVHD found no statistically significant difference in nonrelapse death at 5 years or in cumulative incidence of secondary therapy at 5 years when prednisone alone was compared with prednisone plus CSA.[25] For chronic GVHD that recurs or fails to respond to initial therapy, there is no standard treatment. Experimental therapies currently under evaluation include psoralen plus ultraviolet light A, MMF, thalidomide, total lymphoid irradiation, Plaquenil, extracorporeal photopheresis, pentostatin, and acetretin.[344] (Table 109-4 lists the commonly used GVHD drugs and their side effects.)

Table 109-5 National Institutes of Health Chronic Graft-Versus-Host Disease Measures

Measure	Clinician-Assessed	Patient-Reported
CHRONIC GVHD-SPECIFIC CORE MEASURES		
Signs	Organ-specific measures	Not applicable
Symptoms	Clinician-assessed symptoms	Patient-reported symptoms
Global rating	Mild, moderate, or severe 0 to 10 severity scale 7-point change scale	Mild, moderate, or severe 0 to 10 severity scale 7-point change scale
CHRONIC GVHD NONSPECIFIC ANCILLARY MEASURES		
Function	Grip strength 2-minute walk time	Patient-reported function
Quality of life	—	Patient-reported health-related quality of life

SYNGENEIC GRAFT-VERSUS-HOST DISEASE

A GVHD-like syndrome that is usually self-limited and predominantly affects the skin can occur in recipients of syngeneic or autologous transplants.[369] It is also possible that some of the reported cases of syngeneic GVHD have reflected a mistaken assumption that the donor was syngeneic without extensive molecular confirmation. The condition manifests primarily as a rash that usually responds promptly to corticosteroid therapy. Although the level of severity may be grade II or III, the disease generally resolves promptly with the administration of glucocorticoids and is not life-threatening. Virtually all patients in whom a GVHD-like syndrome develops after syngeneic transplantation have been prepared with intensive conditioning regimens, usually involving irradiation. Experimental studies suggest that such conditioning is essential for the induction of thymic dysfunction, which is necessary for the development of the disease. Generation of autoreactive cells (a defect in thymic negative selection) and elimination of regulatory cells appear to be the requirements for the development of this disease. An additional hypothesis is that in some individuals maternal cells transmitted to them during their fetal development remain present throughout adult life.[370] These observations suggest the possibility that in some instances small numbers of HLA-incompatible cells (derived from the donor's mother) may be transmitted with HLA-identical transplants. Transplacentally transferred maternal cells may also play a role in the development of neonatal GVHD.[370]

Transfusion-Associated Graft-Versus-Host Disease

Most blood products administered to immunocompromised patients are now irradiated or at least leukocyte-depleted to avoid the transfusion of viable alloreactive T cells. With most homologous blood products, the MHC incompatibility between donor and recipient results in rapid clearance of transfused T cells by the recipient's immune system. However, occasionally, transfusions from donors who are homozygous for one of the recipient's MHC haplotypes are not recognized as foreign by the recipient.[371-373] These cells can survive, "engraft," and mount an immunologic attack against the unshared haplotype in the patient, resulting in transfusion-induced GVHD.[373] Transfusion-associated GVHD differs from GVHD occurring after transplantation in terms of kinetics and manifestations (i.e., with transfusion-associated GVHD, the recipient marrow is a major target).[372] Since the number of stem cells in the offending blood product is inadequate, there is no hemopoietic recovery from donor cells. This syndrome is generally fatal as a result of refractory pancytopenia and/or other organ involvement.

GRAFT-VERSUS-LEUKEMIA RESPONSES

The GVL response after allogeneic HCT results from the immunologic attack of the host tissue and, by extension, the leukemia (i.e., the tumor). This response represents a potent form of immunotherapy that circumvents some of the "immunoediting" mechanisms used by tumor cells to develop in the hosts. The power of the alloimmune response to eliminate malignancy was first reported more than 50 years ago in experimental models by Barnes et al.[1] However, GVL as its own entity and its close association with GVHD were not established until another 15 years later.[374]

Clinical Features

Clinical evidence that the donor graft mediates important antileukemic effect comes from higher relapse rates for recipients of syngeneic stem cells than for recipients of HLA-matched sibling grafts.[375] These findings have also been confirmed in a multicenter analysis of HCT recipients with acute myelogenous leukemia (AML) in first remission and subsequent retrospective analyses by the International Bone Marrow Transplant Registry (IBMTR).[376-378] The second IBMTR analysis also showed that the magnitude of this GVL effect is greater for patients with CML and AML and not statistically significant for patients with acute lymphoblastic leukemia (ALL) in first remission.[379,380]

Several case reports of patients with relapse of leukemia after allogeneic HCT noted remissions of the malignancy either after abrupt withdrawal of immunosuppression or during a flare of acute GVHD.[381-384] Patients who develop GVHD after allogeneic HCT experience relapse less frequently than similar patients who do not develop clinical disease. GVHD is protective against relapse both for HCT recipients with advanced leukemia[385-387] and for patients who receive transplants in earlier stages of malignancy.[388] Additional analyses also suggest that the magnitude of the GVL effect appears to be disease- and stage-specific.[387-389] Initial reports suggested that chronic GVHD was most protective against relapse,[387] but other analyses demonstrate that acute GVHD is also protective.[388] Based on these reports, newer trials of immunotherapy are designed to include cessation of immunosuppressive therapy (without taper) to induce a GVL reaction for patients whose malignancy has relapsed after HCT. Furthermore, Childs and colleagues demonstrated that the graft-versus-tumor effect also plays an important role in inducing remissions from a nonhematologic malignancy, renal cell carcinoma.[390]

Another line of clinical evidence regarding the GVL effect of allogeneic HCT and its tight linkage to GVHD comes from the studies employing T-cell depletion of the donor graft. Donor T cells included in the stem cell graft are critical for acute GVHD, and T-cell depletion by various strategies is one of the most successful means of reducing the incidence and severity of GVHD after allogeneic HCT.[27,391-396] Unfortunately, although T-cell depletion results in less treatment-related morbidity and mortality, improved overall survival rates have not been reliably demonstrated. This failure is due in large part to a reciprocal increase in the subsequent relapse rate after T-cell depletion, as well as to graft failure and other complications.[389,397,398] T-cell depletion increases relapse rates particularly in CML.[388,389,399] This observation provides further strong, albeit indirect, evidence that allogeneic donor T cells are important mediators not only of GVHD, but also of the GVL properties of the allogeneic stem cell graft. Finally, the most compelling evidence of donor T cells in mediating GVL comes from the observations made from donor lymphocyte infusions (discussed later). The induction of GVL is a complex process.

Genetic Basis

The immunotherapeutic effect that occurs in allo-BMT setting is primarily mediated by allogeneic donor T or NK cells directed against the alloantigens shared by the recipient tumor and target tissues and/or tumor-specific antigens that have the advantage of not being subjected to tolerance mechanisms by the host tumor.[56,400,401] Understanding of the exquisite specificity of T cell responses led to attempts to identify specific antigens that are responsible for the GVL effect. Much of the focus has been on the identification of (1) certain oncogenic viral proteins (because these are absent in normal cells but expressed by transformed tumor cells [certain EBV peptides such as EBNA-1, LMP-1, LMP, LCL]), (2) antigens that are expressed in a tissue-specific fashion (melanoma specific proteins), and (3) proteins that are overexpressed in tumors (WT1, proteinase 3, survivin, telomerase reverse transcriptase, CYPB1, and HER2/neu).[53,56] Although these antigens are specific, most T-cell responses to these antigens are limited because of the poor immunogenicity of these proteins, expression on normal cells, defects in the processing or presentation of tumor antigens, or production of factors that disable T-cell responses. Thus clinical attempts to obtain high specificity of T-cell responses have been offset with difficulties in obtaining enough sensitivity and vice versa. Furthermore, given the current concepts of stem cell origins of leukemia and cancers, identification of the immunogenic proteins that are specifically expressed in the malignant stem cells and harnessing T cell responses to those antigens will be needed for the optimal GVL effect to cure malignancy.[402,403]

In contrast to the tumor-specific or tumor-associated antigens discussed earlier, alloantigens are not subjected to tolerance mechanisms. Vaccination strategies with autologous T cells using tumor-associated or tumor-specific antigens have yielded disappointing clinical antitumor responses.[404] By contrast, allogeneic HCT has met with remarkable GVL responses perhaps owing to recognition of minor alloantigens in addition to the tumor-associated antigens.[405] This concept has been demonstrated by recent murine studies, which showed that alloantigen on the tumor cells is required for GVL responses and that the principal targets of GVL are the immunodominant allogeneic MiHAs rather than the tumor-associated antigens.[60,90] Thus T cells specific for MiHA antigens could provide for a potent GVL effect. Significant progress has been made in the identification of MiHAs that are specifically expressed in the host hematopoietic tissues and therefore might allow for a GVL response without causing GVHD.[53] Together, these results suggest that in addition to tumor-specific proteins, expression of alloantigens and cognate interactions between donor T cells and the tumor tissues are required for the effective induction of the majority of GVL responses. However, T cells specific for some MiHAs are also responsible for GVHD, and a means of consistently separating the beneficial GVL effect from GVHD has not yet been clinically achieved.

KIR Polymorphisms

The two competing models described earlier, the "mismatched ligand" and the "missing ligand" models for HLA-KIR allorecognition, have been supported by clinical observations of GVL responses in different patient and transplant populations.[65,66] The former model has been shown to separate GVL and GVHD responses in the context of TCD haploidentical HCT for AML.[46,67] Even though this model is supported by elegant laboratory studies, it was found to be invalid for ALL and also for AML after unrelated donor HCT with immunosuppression.[67] Recent retrospective clinical data suggest that GVHD and GVL can be separated by the "missing ligand" model in CML/AML and MDS patients after TCD HLA identical sibling HCT.[46,66,69] Further validation of either models by clinical prospective studies and a better understanding of the balance between the inhibitory and activating receptor-ligand interaction of the NK cells are needed to adequately exploit the interface between HLA-KIR genetics to separate GVHD from GVL (see Chapter 102).[64,406]

Immunobiology of Graft-Versus-Leukemia Responses

Given the tight association of clinical GVHD and GVL, as well as the common biologic principles governing these responses after allogeneic HCT, it is important to discuss the similarities and distinctions between them in the context of the three cellular phases of GVHD.[407]

Phase 1: Activation of APCs

The concept that tumor eradication after allogeneic HCT might not require toxic chemoradiotherapy and could be achieved primarily by the immunotherapeutic effect from the GVL responses has led to the clinical development of nonmyeloablative HCT for hematologic and nonhematologic malignancies.[408] Phase 1 is characterized by the development of cytokine storm–generated danger signals from the conditioning regimen and the subsequent activation of APCs.[407] Experimental data suggested that the reduction in conditioning would attenuate the cytokine storm, lead to the development of mixed donor-host chimerism, and confine the GVH response primarily to secondary lymphoid organs, thus cause less severe GVHD without impairing GVL responses.[409-411] However, nonmyeloablative HCT has delayed the kinetics but did not reduce the overall incidence of GVHD and a significant number of patients either failed to respond or relapsed.[22] Furthermore, recent murine and human studies have suggested that homeostatic expansion of T cells in a lymphopenic environment induced by conditioning (as opposed to mere immunosuppression) improves the antitumor efficacy of adoptively transferred syngeneic or autologous T cells by increasing the availability of space, enhancing the memory responses, and reducing the competition for homeostatic cytokines (such as IL-7 and IL-15) for transferred T cells while eliminating regulatory T cells.[412-414] Thus low-intensity HCT clearly demonstrates the principle of GVL effect, but the roles of cytokine storm and homeostatic expansion of allogeneic T cells in shaping the intensity of GVL responses are not known.

Host and donor APCs are critical for the induction and severity of GVHD.[8] Activation of APCs is the key step in phase 1 of GVHD.[407] Significant progress has been made in understanding the role of APCs in GVL. Recent experimental evidence has demonstrated a crucial role for professional host APCs in the induction of GVL responses mediated by donor T cells, even when the tumor cells showed some features of APCs.[90,415] Tumors that merely express costimulatory molecules may still be unable to stimulate an effective immune response because of their various "immunoediting" processes that cause ineffective antigen presentation.[416] However, when the tumor cell itself functions as a professional APC, as with CML, it can generate an effective GVL response.[417,418] By contrast, cancers such as acute leukemias that seldom differentiate into APCs generate poor GVL responses. Data also demonstrated that given sufficient time and a low tumor burden, cross-presentation of tumor-associated antigens and/or alloantigens by professional donor APCs can occur and may promote or sustain GVL responses by maintaining or expanding alloreactive T cells after initial priming on host APCs.[90,418] This concept is consistent with clinical GVL responses in CML in which the final stage of a GVL response to CML may be the result of donor T cells responding not directly to the small number of CML stem cells or progenitors (which would be undifferentiated and therefore poor APCs) but to tumor antigens cross-presented on professional donor APCs. Emerging data suggest that enhancing such cross-presentation is sufficient to elicit effective GVL responses against acute or advanced leukemia. These data, however, suggest that GVL responses generated after low intensity conditioning may not be as robust as those after full intensity HCT and highlight the need for a clearer understanding of the effects of cytokine storm and lymphopenia generated danger signals on the activation of APCs in mediating GVL.

Phase 2: Donor T Cell Activation

The core of GVL responses, as with GVHD, is also dependent on the activation of appropriate numbers of T cells. The "second" signals from professional APCs (or certain tumor cells that function as effective APCs) are critical for generating an effective GVL response.[230] Several of the costimulatory pathways that modulate GVHD have also been evaluated in mediating GVL responses. Blockade of CD28 costimulation preserved GVL responses but reduced GVHD in murine studies.[419] However, when the tumor cells also expressed B7 molecules, such blockade reduced the GVL responses.[417] Ex vivo blockade of CD40-CD40L interaction has been shown to reduce GVHD by generating Tregs but still preserve GVL. By contrast, blockade of the 4-1BB pathway reduced both GVHD and GVL.[123] The other costimulatory molecules (OX40 and ICOS) and the inhibitory molecules (CTLA-4 and PD-1) also modulate antitumor responses.[124,125] A better understanding of the context (i.e., low intensity or DLI) and the hierarchy of timing, duration, and extent of costimulatory requirements of donor T cell subsets might allow for balancing the intensity of GVL and GVHD responses. Clinical and experimental evidence suggest that donor T cell numbers correlate with the severity of GVHD and GVL responses. T cell–depleted (TCD) grafts had reduced GVHD but increased disease relapse, suggesting a role for T-cell numbers in GVL responses as well.[420] Clinical attempts to separate GVHD and GVL by regulating allogeneic T-cell dose have met with limited success. For example, administration of 1×10^5 T cells/kg after HLA-matched sibling transplantation did not mediate GVL effects and yet was associated with a measurable incidence of GVHD. Thus infusion of right numbers of donor T cell effectors is crucial for GVL responses.[420] This has been demonstrated by durable responses that are observed in CML and other malignancies after donor leukocyte infusion (DLI, see later), despite the experimental evidence that host APCs stimulate a stronger GVL response than do donor APCs.[90,418] This could be because, clinically, DLI is almost always given without immunosuppression to an individual who has not developed GVHD either from the chemical immunosuppression or physical removal of donor T cells from the allograft. This lack of immunosuppression after DLI increases the likelihood of a GVH response, and DLI is almost always associated with clinical GVHD. The delivery of additional allogeneic effector cells in DLI also increases the effector: target ratio compared with the time of initial HCT. The latter is also clinically demonstrated by a more effective GVL response to DLI against minimal residual disease (BCR-ABL positivity by PCR) compared with the response against high leukemic burden (e.g., blast crisis) in CML patients.[418] Thus DLI provides the proof in principle for the concepts that sufficient T-cell numbers and appropriate antigen presentation are required for both GVHD and an effective GVL response.

T-Cell Subsets

Most experimental studies have implicated donor $CD8^+$ T cells as the primary mediators of GVL, but there are no clinical data for $CD8^+$-mediated GVL responses in the absence of CD4 T cells.[56,236,418] Moreover, some clinical data suggest a role for greater CD4-mediated GVL responses without an increase in GVHD after allogeneic HCT and DLI.[415,421-424] But it is unclear whether $CD4^+$ T cell–initiated GVL responses occur in the absence of generation of MiHA specific $CD8^+$ T cells. Given the critical requirement of alloantigens for most GVL responses, the specific requirement of CD4 and/or CD8 T cells for GVL and GVHD is likely to be determined by the expression of the relevant immunodominant MiHAs and/or tumor-associated proteins. Therefore it is unlikely that GVHD and GVL responses can be separated under all circumstances merely by depletion of either subset of alloreactive T cells. However, experimental data suggest it might be possible to separate GVHD and GVL when certain donor T-cell subsets are either depleted or infused (DLI) at appropriate interval after transplant.[415] But the optimal time interval, if any, after clinical HCT is yet to be determined.

Because of recent identification and understanding of the role of various T-cell subsets in mediating immune responses, depletion of specific T-cell subsets to separate GVHD and GVL remains an area of active investigation. For example, recent experimental data suggest that CD62L expressing naive T cells home to secondary lymph nodes and are critical for initiating GVHD.[133] By contrast, CD62L negative effector memory T cells with enhanced reactivity to recall antigens mediated GVL responses with minimal GVHD.[133] An important caveat to these data is the fact that the lack of a priori knowledge of the repertoire of human memory T cells would make it difficult to predict whether these cells might cross-react only with tumor-associated antigens or with the recipient's alloantigens. Using CD62L status alone as determinant of GVHD potential can also have other unintended consequences; recent studies have demonstrated that its expression is critical for the regulation of GVHD by Tregs (see later). Moreover, it is not known whether the behavior of human memory T cells parallels that of murine memory T cells in their migratory, functional, and cytolytic capabilities. Although Tregs reduce antitumor immunity in murine models and in human subjects experimental data suggest that administration of donor-type Tregs either at the time of HCT or when delayed reduced GVHD but preserved $CD8^+$-mediated perforin-dependent GVL responses.[425,426] Similar preservation of experimental GVL was also observed by harnessing donor NKT function with GCSF analogues.[159,160] However, it remains unclear whether these observations are valid after clinical HCT when the GVL responses might not be entirely dependent on CD8 T cells.

T-Cell Migration

It is conceivable that manipulation of these interactions to focus the alloimmune response to lymphohematopoietic tissues would enhance GVL responses but not GVHD. For example, blockade of CCR9 ligand TECK or CCR5 and CCL17 may prevent the migration of donor T cells to GI tract and skin respectively, but preserve GVL.[221] Pharmacologic manipulation with the immunosuppressive agent FTY720 has recently provided the proof in principle for this approach.[231] Given the redundancy, strategies to modulate the chemokine biology for separation of GVHD and GVL will require greater understanding of these networks in modulating the migration not only of specific T-cell subsets but also of the other immune cells in the context of different conditioning regimens.

Phase 3: Effector Phase of GVL

The effector arm of GVL is also characterized primarily by the antigen-specific cellular components and less by the inflammatory components of alloresponse. Experimental data demonstrate that neutralization of IL-1α reduced GVHD but preserved GVL.[283] By contrast, donor TNF-α secretion contributes to both GVHD and GVL effects, and in some cases, antagonism of TNF-α reduced GVHD and GVL responses.[427-429] Nonetheless, antagonism of nonspecific inflammatory effectors (such as either IL-1 or TNF-α) appears to regulate GVHD to a greater extent than GVL responses after experimental allogeneic HCT.[429]

Several lines of experimental and clinical data demonstrate that antigen-specific donor T-cell subsets and NK cells are the key effectors of GVL.[56] The cytotoxic pathways that are operative in the NK and T cell–mediated antitumor responses have been well characterized.[56] Fas ligand–mediated CTL of tumor targets is used by both NK and T (mostly Th1) cells, but most murine experiments with FasL-deficient donor T cells suggested that FasL is a key effector molecule for causing GVHD but not GVL.[236] However, one study found that FasL is required for $CD4^+$–mediated GVL against myeloid leukemia.[430,431] By contrast, even though perforin-mediated CTL pathways are also used by T (mostly Th2) and NK cells, experimental data with perforin-deficient donor T cells demonstrated a loss of GVL with a diminution in the severity of GVHD.[236] In some other experimental models, perforin was required only for GVL but not for GVHD.[236] Recent data showed that TRAIL-mediated CTL had no effect on GVHD severity but was required for optimal GVL.[260] Therefore strategies that increase donor T cell TRAIL expression or enhance the susceptibility of tumors to TRAIL-mediated CTL (such as HDAC inhibitors) may promote a robust GVL effect without exacerbating GVHD.[432-434] Thus a significant progress has been made in recent understanding of the CTL pathways employed by donor T cells for GVL responses, but the role and context of use of these pathways by donor NK and NKT cells after allogeneic HCT are not known.

DONOR LEUKOCYTE INFUSIONS

Until recently, the evidence for an important GVL effect in clinical transplantation was strong but largely circumstantial. The use of DLI to treat relapses after allogeneic HCT has now provided direct evidence of the GVL effect.[435-437] Kolb and colleagues first reported three patients with relapsed CML who achieved complete cytogenetic remission after treatment with IFN-α and DLI from the original donors.[438] Subsequently, these findings have been confirmed in several reports.[439-441] Two large retrospective studies of DLI have been reported from Europe and North America.[437,442] Although the treatment protocols varied slightly among institutions, the results have been remarkably consistent. When results from these trials are combined, the complete remission rate for patients treated for relapsed CML is consistently 60% to 80%.[435] In many patients with CML, the response to DLI is not immediate. The average time to obtain a molecular remission is between 4 to 6 months, but disease free survival after DLI depends on the stage of CML.[443,444] Complete cytogenetic and molecular responses are achieved in almost 80% of patients treated with either early relapse (cytogenetic or molecular) or hematologic relapse of chronic phase.[380] Patients with more advanced CML (accelerated phase or blast crisis) are less likely to respond. Two recent analyses suggest that the outcome after unrelated DLI is similar to matched sibling DLI in CML patients.[437,442]

DLI has also produced remissions in acute leukemias. Several retrospective studies have reported response rates in AML ranging from 20% to 65%.[380,442,445-447] A prospective study of 65 patients with advanced myeloid leukemia who received cytarabine and GCSF-primed DLI showed that 47% of the patients achieved complete remission, with an overall survival of 19% at 2 years.[448] A recent EBMT analysis of DLI in patients with relapsed AML showed a response rate of 41%, which did not change if chemotherapy was used before DLI.[449] Generally, DLI produces lower response rates and higher relapse rates in patients with AML than in those with CML.[380,418,442,445-447] Extramedullary relapses at multiple regions that are usually not considered sanctuary sites for leukemia have been observed after DLI.[447]

Although GVL responses to ALL after allogeneic HCT have been noted, DLI for ALL has generally been ineffective.[399] Reports both from Europe and the United States found little benefit for DLI in ALL patients.[418,442,445,446] Furthermore, Ruggeri and others found that following TCD haploidentical HCT where the donors had antirecipient NK cells, the probability of relapse was 85% for ALL in contrast with 0% for AML.[67,450]

The experience with DLI for other hematologic malignancies such as NHL and multiple myeloma (MM) is much more limited. Case reports and small series demonstrate responses to DLI in patients with posttransplant relapses of low-grade lymphoma and CLL and also after low-intensity HCT.[451,452] In MM, complete responses to DLI were observed in 25% of the patients in two small series.[418,453,454] DLI has also been shown to induce complete remission in a majority of patients with posttransplant lymphoproliferative disorders (PTLD) after allogeneic HCT.[439,455] Viral infections may be treatable with DLI, and adoptive immune therapy with T cells specific for EBV and CMV have been shown to both treat and prevent these complications.[456-460]

Complications of Donor Leukocyte Infusions

Adoptive immunotherapy with DLI causes significant morbidity. The major complications are myelosuppression and GVHD. Myelosuppression with anemia and/or thrombocytopenia and/or leucopenia and/or pancytopenia occurs in 34% of the patients.[444] Marrow aplasia presumably results from the destruction of host leukemia cells before recovery of normal donor hematopoiesis. This idea is supported by the observation that patients treated with donor MNC infusions for cytogenetic or molecular relapse rarely experience pancytopenia.[437] Occasionally, marrow aplasia has been persistent,[439,440,461] although this toxicity has been successfully reversed with the infusion of additional donor stem cells in some patients.[439,440] If pancytopenia is associated with chronic GVHD, then immunosuppression might be the most appropriate therapy.[462] Acute GVHD and chronic GVHD have been the major direct complications from DLI. In retrospective and prospective studies, acute or chronic GVHD has been reported in 40% to 60% of evaluable patients. In most studies, GVHD correlates with GVL activity and response.[437,442] In the North American analysis, over 90% of complete responders developed acute GVHD, and 88% of responders developed chronic GVHD. Of 23 patients who did not experience GVHD, only 3 achieved a complete remission. In 92 patients who had no response, only 35% had acute GHVD and only 13% had chronic GVHD. In the EBMT analysis, 41% of DLI recipients developed grade II to IV acute GVHD.[437] It should be noted, however, that many patients who fail to respond to GVL induction will die shortly of progressive disease and may not survive long enough for GVHD to develop. This is particularly important for patients with acute leukemia. It is also important to emphasize that a number of complete responses were seen in patients without any sign of GVHD. The GVL effect in the absence of clinical GVHD provides important evidence for GVL activity separate from GVHD.

In general, GVHD that occurs after DLI has been mild to moderate and has been responsive to immunosuppressive therapy. This observation is important since the dose of T cells often administered with DLI may be 10- to 100-fold higher than the T-cell dose administered at the time of transplant, and DLI is given without additional immunosuppression. At the time of transplant, toxicity is unacceptable if immunosuppression is withheld or if a dose of donor T cells similar to that used for DLI is given (to augment GVL).[463,464] This may be because the effects of GVHD are more tolerable when separated from the acute transplant toxicity. GVHD can be stimulated and exacerbated by the cytokine storm that may accompany transplantation. Tissue damage from the intensive conditioning regimen, infections, and other physiologic insults results in a cascade of events that ultimately augments the GVHD reaction.[23] When GVHD is induced independently of other transplant related toxicity, it may be more manageable with appropriate immunosuppression. Nevertheless, in some cases DLI-induced GVHD may be quite severe; as shown in Table 109-2, 20% to 35% of DLI recipients can be anticipated to develop grade III or IV acute GVHD. Furthermore, acute GVHD has contributed to death in almost 10% of patients.[465] Chronic GVHD occurs in 30% to 60% of recipients of unmanipulated DLI.

It is notable that the clinical presentation of GVHD after DLI is somewhat different from that after myeloablative allogeneic HCT. For instance, the onset of GVHD may be later after DLI. The median time to onset of acute GVHD is approximately 32 to 42 days[442,466] compared with a median time to onset of 16 to 20 days following myeloablative T cell–replete transplantation.[305,467] Therefore not only can the severity of GVHD be influenced by the use of intensive conditioning, but the tissue damage and inflammatory cytokine release may influence the pace of GVHD development as well. This possibility is supported by the finding that time to onset of acute GVHD is also delayed following reduced intensity transplantation.[468] The target organs of acute GVHD following DLI are the same as those seen following HCT, but the clinical manifestations may differ. A hepatic variant of liver GVHD characterized by marked elevations of serum aminotransferase levels more than 10 times the upper limit of normal was observed in 11 of 73 (15%) patients who received DLI at Johns Hopkins University.[318] Characteristic skin, liver, and intestinal acute GVHD manifestations can be seen following DLI, but their frequency and severity has not been well described. In a study of 81 patients who received DLI for relapse, mixed chimerism, or prophylaxis following reduced-intensity HCT, skin, liver, and intestinal GVHD developed in 26%, 8%, and 14%, respectively.[469] Likewise, characteristic findings of chronic GVHD can be seen following DLI,[469] and on occasion both acute and chronic GVHD can develop simultaneously following DLI.[470]

In recent years, DLI has been used in the context of reduced-intensity allogeneic HCT. When conditioning is minimal and GVHD has not already occurred, DLI is often required to either reverse mixed chimerism or treat persistent disease.[469,471,472] GVHD after DLI following nonmyeloablative setting develops 19% to 45% of the time, whereas chronic GVHD develops 28% to 34% of the time. In two studies of a combined 134 subjects who received DLI after reduced-intensity transplantation, 37 (28%) patients developed acute GVHD, 15 (11%) developed grade III or IV GVHD, and 8 (6%) died from GVHD.[469,471] There was no statistically significant relationship between DLI dose and GVHD in either study. The clinical features of GVHD after DLI following reduced-intensity HCT are similar to the GVHD that occurs after DLI is used to treat relapse following myeloablative HCT. The similarity between GVHD after DLI in either setting suggests that the reduction of tissue damage associated with either no chemotherapy (as in DLI for relapse following prior myeloablative HCT) or reduced-dose chemotherapy (as in DLI after reduced-intensity HCT) may be an important common theme.

It is likely that effector cells responsible for the GVL and GVHD effects of HCT will similarly be responsible for the GVL effect associated with DLI, although this assumption has not been formally proven. The administration of select subsets of donor mononuclear cell fractions is the ideal setting in which to dissect the cellular mechanisms responsible for GVL induction, and strategies that delay the infusion of these various cellular subsets will help define the mechanisms and enhance the efficacy of DLI.

FUTURE DIRECTIONS

Complications of HCT, particularly GVHD, remain major barriers to the wider application of allogeneic HCT for a variety of diseases. Recent advances in the biology of genetic polymorphisms, the chemocytokine networks, several novel cellular subsets including regulatory T cells, and the direct mediators of cellular cytotoxicity have led to improved understanding of this complex disease process. Animal studies show that modulation of several mediators of the complex GVHD cascade may be able to reduce the undesirable inflammatory aspects of GVHD while preserving the benefits of GVL. However, most of the laboratory observations remain to be studied in well-controlled clinical trials. Multiple cellular effectors may be involved in GVL, although donor T-cell recognition of host antigens is an important element of this process. Cellular immunotherapy such as DLI offers a strategy for separating GVHD and the GVL effect. Both experimental and clinical data suggest that posttransplantation cellular immunotherapy can be performed relatively safely and effectively, and optimization of patient selection, cell dose, and timing of administration may all serve to limit toxicity and enhance the potential GVL effects.

SUGGESTED READINGS

Alousi AM, Weisdorf DJ, Logan BR, et al: Etanercept, mycophenolate, denileukin or pentostatin plus corticosteroids for acute graft vs. host disease: A randomized phase II trial from the BMT CTN. *Blood* 114:511, 2009.

Anasetti C, Beatty PG, Storb R, et al: Effect of HLA incompatibility on graft-versus-host disease, relapse, and survival after marrow transplantation for patients with leukemia or lymphoma. *Hum Immunol* 29:79, 1990.

Baker MB, Altman NH, Podack ER, et al: The role of cell-mediated cytotoxicity in acute GVHD after MHC-matched allogeneic bone marrow transplantation in mice. *J Exp Med* 183:2645, 1996.

Billingham RE: The biology of graft-versus-host reactions. *Harvey Lect* 62:21, 1966-67.

Bortin MM, Rimm AA, Saltzstein E: Graft-versus-leukemia: Quantification of adoptive immunotherapy in murine leukemia. *Science* 173:811, 1973.

Den Haan JM, Sherman NE, Blokland E, et al: Identification of a graft versus host disease-associated human minor histocompatibility antigen. *Science* 268:1476, 1995.

Dickinson AM, Middleton PG, Rocha V, et al: Genetic polymorphisms predicting the outcome of bone marrow transplants. *Br J Haematol* 127:479, 2004.

Edinger M, Hoffmann P, Ermann J, et al: $CD4^+CD25^+$ regulatory T cells preserve graft-versus-tumor activity while inhibiting graft-versus-host disease after bone marrow transplantation. *Nat Med* 9:1144, 2003.

Glucksberg H, Storb R, Fefer A, et al: Clinical manifestations of graft-versus-host disease in human recipients of marrow from HL-A-matched sibling donors. *Transplantation* 18:295, 1974.

Goulmy E, Schipper R, Pool J, et al: Mismatches of minor histocompatibility antigens between HLA-identical donors and recipients and the development of graft-versus-host disease after bone marrow transplantation. *N Engl J Med* 334:281, 1996.

Herve P, Wijdenes J, Flesch M, et al: Anti-TNF alpha monoclonal antibody (B-C7) in the treatment of severe forms of acute GvHD. *Blood* 76:544a (abstr.), 1990.

Hill GR, Ferrara JL: The primacy of the gastrointestinal tract as a target organ of acute graft-versus-host disease: Rationale for the use of cytokine shields in allogeneic bone marrow transplantation. *Blood* 95:2754, 2000.

Kolb H, Mittermuller J, Clemm C, et al: Donor leukocyte transfusions for treatment of recurrent chronic myelogenousleukemia in marrow transplant patients. *Blood* 76:2462, 1990.

Korngold R, Sprent J: Negative selection of T cells causing lethal graft-versus-host disease across minor histocompatibility barriers. Role of the H-2 complex. *J Exp Med* 151:1114, 1980.

Laughlin MJ, Eapen M, Rubinstein P, et al: Outcomes after transplantation of cord blood or bone marrow from unrelated donors in adults with leukemia. *N Engl J Med* 351:2265, 2004.

Lowsky R, Takahashi T, Liu YP, et al: Protective conditioning for acute graft-versus-host disease. *N Engl J Med* 353:1321, 2005.

Martin PJ, Weisdorf D, Przepiorka D, et al: National Institutes of Health Consensus Development Project on Criteria for Clinical Trials in Chronic Graft-versus-Host Disease: VI. Design of Clinical Trials Working Group report. *Biol Blood Marrow Transpl* 12:491, 2006.

Nikolic B, Lee S, Bronson R, et al: Th1 and Th2 mediate acute graft-versus-host disease, each with distinct end-organ targets. *J Clin Invest* 105:1289, 2000.

Petersdorf EW, Hansen JA, Martin PJ, et al: Major-histocompatibility-complex class I alleles and antigens in hematopoietic-cell transplantation. *N Engl J Med* 345:1794, 2001.

Ratanatharathorn V, Nash RA, Przepiorka D, et al: Phase III study comparing methotrexate and tacrolimus (prograf, FK506) with methotrexate and cyclosporine for graft-versus-host disease prophylaxis after HLA-identical sibling bone marrow transplantation. *Blood* 92:2303, 1998.

Reddy P, Maeda Y, Liu C, et al: A crucial role for antigen-presenting cells and alloantigen expression in graft-versus-leukemia responses. *Nat Med* 11:1244, 2005.

Riddell SR, Watanabe KS, Goodrich JM, et al: Restoration of viral immunity in immunodeficient humans by the adoptive transfer of T cell clones. *Science* 257:238, 1992.

Shlomchik WD, Couzens MS, Tang CB, et al: Prevention of graft versus host disease by inactivation of host antigen-presenting cells. *Science* 285:412, 1999.

Shulman HM, Sharma P, Amos D, Fenster LF, McDonald GB: A coded histologic study of hepatic graft-versus-host disease after human bone marrow transplantation. *Hepatology* 8:463, 1988.

Storb R, Deeg HJ, Whitehead J, et al: Methotrexate and cyclosporine compared with cyclosporine alone for prophylaxis of acute graft versus host disease after marrow transplantation for leukemia. *N Engl J Med* 314:729, 1986.

van Bekkum DW, Roodenburg J, Heidt PJ, et al: Mitigation of secondary disease of allogeneic mouse radiation chimeras by modification of the intestinal microflora. *J Natl Cancer Inst* 52:401, 1974.

Weiden PL, Flournoy N, Thomas ED, et al: Antileukemic effect of graft-versus-host disease in human recipients of allogeneic-marrow grafts. *N Engl J Med* 300:1068, 1979.

Wekerle T, Kurtz J, Ito H, et al: Allogeneic bone marrow transplantation with co-stimulatory blockade induces macrochimerism and tolerance without cytoreductive host treatment. *Nat Med* 6:464, 2000.

Wysocki CA, Panoskaltsis-Mortari A, Blazar BR, et al: Leukocyte migration and graft-versus-host disease. *Blood* 105:4191, 2005.

For complete list of references log on to www.expertconsult.com.

CHAPTER 110

COMPLICATIONS AFTER HEMATOPOIETIC STEM CELL TRANSPLANTATION

Navneet S. Majhail and Daniel J. Weisdorf

The high-dose therapy used in hematopoietic cell transplantation (HCT) results in toxicities induced directly by the treatment and secondarily by the prolonged immunodeficiency and extended recovery process. Identification of risk factors for particular complications allows the design of risk-specific supportive care regimens that may reduce the rates of morbidity and mortality accompanying transplantation. HCT-related complications can be broadly classified into infections, early noninfectious complications (within 3 months of HCT), late noninfectious complications (after 3 months of HCT), and graft-versus-host disease (GVHD) (Table 110-1).

INFECTIONS

Infections are among the foremost causes of nonrelapse mortality in HCT recipients and can cause significant morbidity, both in the early and late transplant period (Table 110-2). Immune defects occurring in the posttransplant period can be divided into predictable phases based on time from engraftment (sustained absolute neutrophil count >500/μL), with characteristic infections in each phase (Fig. 110-1). Antimicrobial prophylaxis regimens tailored to address the risk for specific infections during these time periods are effective in decreasing the incidence of posttransplant opportunistic infections (Table 110-3). Evidence-based guidelines for preventing infectious complications among HCT recipients have been published and can be used as a reference for determining infection risk and assigning antimicrobial prophylaxis for an individual patient.[1]

Engraftment generally occurs within 7 to 14 days in autologous and 14 to 28 days in allogeneic HCT recipients. Recipients of grafts from unrelated donors (URDs) or umbilical cord blood (UCB) tend to engraft later compared to sibling donors; more importantly 5% to 10% of unrelated-donor and 5% to 20% of UCB grafts may fail to engraft, leading to prolonged neutropenia and extended transfusion dependence. The main risk factors for infection during this preengraftment phase are disruption of mucocutaneous barriers and indwelling venous catheters. Bacterial infections can occur in up to 30% of transplant recipients during this initial period and usually arise from normal flora of the skin (coagulase-negative *Staphylococcus*), oropharynx, and gastrointestinal tract (viridans streptococci, *Enterococcus* spp., and enteric gram-negative bacilli).[2] Colonizing yeasts or molds also invade because of neutropenia and disruption of normal host flora and can lead to systemic mycotic infections (most often *Candida* spp. or *Aspergillus* spp.) in 10% to 15% of patients.[3] Reactivation of herpesviruses can occur in the absence of prophylaxis.

The predominant defects seen in the early to late postengraftment period are impairments of cellular and humoral immune systems.[4] This state of underlying severe immune dysfunction is enhanced and prolonged by acute and chronic GVHD and by corticosteroids and by the immunosuppressive agents used for GVHD prevention and treatment.[5,6] The incidence of late opportunistic infections is much lower in autologous HCT recipients because of quicker immune reconstitution and the lack of immunosuppressive drugs. Immune reconstitution can take up to 2 years to fully recover in allogeneic HCT recipients. Patients with chronic GVHD can be functionally asplenic and be at risk for infections by encapsulated bacteria. In addition, chronic GVHD patients on long-term immunosuppression are susceptible to fungi (*Aspergillus* spp., *Candida* spp., and *Pneumocystis jiroveci*) and viruses (cytomegalovirus [CMV] and varicella-zoster virus [VZV]).[7] Additional factors that can delay immune reconstitution include donor-recipient human leukocyte antigen (HLA) disparity, graft manipulation with depletion of T cells in vitro or using antithymocyte globulin (ATG) or alemtuzumab in vivo, and use of URDs and possibly UCB as a graft source.[5,8,9] Antimicrobial prophylaxis should continue beyond the initial posttransplant period, typically for at least 3 to 6 months after cessation of all immunosuppression, especially in patients being treated for chronic GVHD. Some centers use total T-cell ($CD3^+$) and particularly $CD4^+$ cell levels as surrogate markers of T-cell immunity and to guide decisions regarding antimicrobial prophylaxis. Supplemental intravenous immunoglobulin (Ig) has been considered for patients with persistent hypogammaglobulinemia (IgG levels <400 mg/dL), but its prophylactic use is costly, does not prolong survival or prevent late infections, and may impair humoral immune reconstitution.[10,11] Patients with GVHD and those with indwelling venous access who undergo dental procedures should receive antibiotics similar to use for endocarditis prophylaxis.[12] Published guidelines are available for immunization of HCT survivors (Table 110-4).[1]

Based on the type and dose of conditioning chemotherapy and radiation, recipients of nonmyeloablative or reduced-intensity conditioning (NMA/RIC) regimens can exhibit varying degrees of myelosuppression.[13] The incidence of bacterial infections is lower in NMA/RIC recipients due to the shorter duration of posttransplant neutropenia.[14] However, the degree of lymphodepletion tends to be comparable to that seen with myeloablative regimens, and the risks of invasive aspergillosis and CMV reactivation remain unchanged.[15-18]

Among UCB HCT recipients, neutrophil engraftment and immune reconstitution can be delayed and a higher incidence of bacterial and viral infections in the early, but not later, posttransplant period has been reported.[19] The incidence of CMV reactivation ranges from 20% to 50%, but organ involvement by CMV is infrequent.[20,21] Recipient CMV serostatus is the most important predictor of CMV disease in this setting. UCB transplantation is associated with lower risks of chronic GHVD. Although detailed studies are lacking, the incidence of late infections using UCB grafts may be lower than what is seen after URD HCT. Overall, the risk for serious infections among children receiving UCB grafts is comparable to that of URD marrow and is lower than that of a T cell–depleted graft source.[22] Among adult UCB HCT recipients, the incidence of infections is higher in the early posttransplant period; however, infections do not clearly compromise the risks for overall and nonrelapse mortality compared to URD HCT.[22]

The approach to managing posttransplant infections is generally similar to that for infections in patients with cancer, especially leukemia (see Chapter 88). However, certain infections, particularly those due to viruses and fungi, are unique to the HCT population and are discussed in further detail here.

Febrile Neutropenia

A large proportion of patients develop fever in the early posttransplantation period, though an infectious pathogen is identified in only

Table 110-1 Major Complications of Hematopoietic Cell Transplantation

	Complication	Incidence
Infections	Bacterial infections	
	Gram-positive bacteremia	20%-30%
	Gram-negative bacteremia	5%-10%
	Viral infections	
	Cytomegalovirus	5%-40% in high-risk patients*
	Herpes simplex virus	5%-10% in seropositive patients
	Varicella-zoster virus	10%-50% in seropositive patients
	Respiratory viruses	10%-20%
	Fungal infections	
	Candida	5%-10%
	Aspergillus and other molds	5%-15%
	Pneumocystis jiroveci	<1%
	Other infections	
	Toxoplasma gondii	2%-7% in seropositive patients
Early noninfectious complications (0-3 mo)	Regimen-related toxicity	
	Mucositis	60%-75%
	Hemorrhagic cystitis	5%-10%
	Venoocclusive disease	5%-40%
	Pneumonitis	10%-20%
	Alveolar hemorrhage	5%-10%
	Graft failure	2%-10%
	Adverse drug reactions	Common
Late noninfectious complications (>3 mo)	Organ-specific late effects	
	Cataracts	25%-40%
	Hypothyroidism	30%-50%
	Sterility/hypogonadism	50%-90%
	Growth disturbances	30%-50% in prepubertal children
	Osteoporosis/avascular necrosis	5%-20%
	Malignant relapse	Variable
	Second cancers	2%-12%
Graft-versus-host disease	Acute	20%-50% with related donors, 40%-90% with unrelated donors, 20%-50% with UCB
	Chronic	20%-40% with related donors, 40%-70% with unrelated donors, 20%-40% with UCB

Mo, Month; *UCB,* umbilical cord blood.
*Cytomegalovirus (CMV)-seropositive hematopoietic cell transplantation recipients or CMV-seronegative recipients with a CMV-seropositive donor.

50% of patients. Fever may also be due to tissue inflammation (oropharyngeal or enteric mucositis), transfusions, amphotericin (though now used less frequently), or other drug fever. Bacterial infections due to aerobic bacteria such as viridans streptococci and enteric gram-negative bacilli are the primary concern during this neutropenic phase, although there is also an ongoing risk for infections with yeasts. Prophylactic strategies can include suppressive antimicrobials, against both bacteria and fungi.

Empiric therapy with broad-spectrum antibiotics is usually started at fever onset along with appropriate clinical and microbiologic evaluation. Choice of antibiotics depends on prior and current antibiotic usage modified by local resistance patterns and can be based on recommendations available for the treatment of febrile neutropenia in general cancer patients.[23] Among patients with persistent febrile neutropenia, that is, fever without an identified focus that continues despite 3 to 5 days of appropriate broad-spectrum antibiotics, invasive fungal infections should be considered.[24] Initiating empiric antifungal therapy with mold-active agents such as voriconazole, caspofungin, or amphotericin is generally recommended at this stage.[25] The choice of agent is dependent on prior exposure to antimold agents for prophylaxis where resistant species (e.g., *Zygomycetes*) may emerge. Empiric mold-specific therapy can be started earlier in patients who have experienced prolonged periods of neutropenia before HCT (e.g., patients with myelodysplastic syndromes). Repeated vigorous investigation to identify sources of infection (e.g., with computed tomographic [CT] scan of the chest and sinuses), even for fever recurring after initial defervescence, is essential. Although administration of myeloid growth factors (granulocyte colony-stimulating factor [G-CSF] or granulocyte-macrophage colony-stimulating factor [GM-CSF]) reduces the duration of neutropenia and accelerates engraftment, it has not been demonstrated to reduce mortality from early posttransplant infections.[26]

Cytomegalovirus Infection

Epidemiology and Risk Factors

Despite the introduction of effective antiviral therapies, CMV infection continues to be a major cause of infection-related morbidity and mortality in HCT recipients.[27] The risk for CMV reactivation spans both the early and late transplant period, especially in patients with GVHD on prolonged immunosuppression. Although the incidence of early CMV disease with organ involvement has declined to 3% to 6% with the use of empiric antiviral drug therapy directed by routine surveillance with CMV deoxyribonucleic acid (DNA) polymerase chain reaction (PCR) or antigenemia testing, late-onset CMV infection is still seen in up to 20% to 40% of patients.[28-30]

Seropositivity of the recipient is the most important risk factor for CMV infection in HCT recipients, and reactivation of latent virus is

Table 110-2 Common Infections in Hematopoietic Cell Transplant Recipients

Pathogen	Risk Period After HCT (wk)	Risk Factors	Common Clinical Syndromes	Treatment
Gram-positive cocci	1-4	Neutropenia Mucositis Central venous catheters Skin breakdown	Bacteremia	Antibiotics based on susceptibility testing
Enterobacteriaceae spp.	1-4	Neutropenia Skin breakdown GI mucosal breakdown	Bacteremia	Antibiotics based on susceptibility testing
Clostridium difficile	1-8	Antibiotics	Colitis	Metronidazole Oral vancomycin
Encapsulated bacteria*	>12	Chronic GVHD Chronic immunosuppression	Sinusitis Pneumonia	Antibiotics based on susceptibility testing
Candida spp.	1-4	Neutropenia Skin breakdown GI mucosal breakdown	Candidemia Mucocutaneous Hepatosplenic	Azoles Echinocandins Amphotericin
Aspergillus spp.	1-4 >8	HLA disparity CMV infection Acute or chronic GVHD Chronic immunosuppression High-dose corticosteroids	Sinusitis Pulmonary nodules or infiltrates	Mold specific azoles Echinocandins Amphotericin
Pneumocystis jiroveci	>4	Chronic GVHD Chronic immunosuppression	Pneumonia	TMP-SMX Dapsone Pentamidine
Cytomegalovirus	>4	Recipient or donor seropositivity HLA disparity Acute or chronic GVHD Chronic immunosuppression	Viremia Enteritis Interstitial pneumonitis	Ganciclovir Foscarnet Valganciclovir
Herpes simplex virus	1-4	Recipient seropositivity	Oropharyngeal Esophagitis	Acyclovir Valacyclovir Foscarnet
Varicella-zoster virus	>4	Recipient seropositivity History of chickenpox HLA disparity Acute or chronic GVHD Chronic immunosuppression	Cutaneous Interstitial pneumonitis Hepatitis	Acyclovir Valacyclovir Foscarnet
Epstein-Barr virus	>4	HLA disparity T-cell depletion	Viremia PTLD	Rituximab Reduce immunosuppression Virus-specific T cells Cytotoxic chemotherapy

CMV, Cytomegalovirus; *GVHD,* graft-versus-host disease; *GI,* gastrointestinal; *HCT,* hematopoietic cell transplantation; *HLA,* human leukocyte antigen; *PTLD,* posttransplant lymphoproliferative disorder; *TMP-SMX,* trimethoprim-sulfamethoxazole; *wk,* week.
*Includes *Streptococcus pneumoniae, Haemophilus influenzae,* and *Neisseria meningitidis.*

Table 110-3 Recommended Antimicrobial Prophylaxis Against Common Infections

Pathogen	Preventing Early Disease (0-100 Days After HCT)	Preventing Late Disease (>100 Days After HCT)
Bacterial infections	No specific recommendations*	Antibiotics (based on local resistance patterns) to prevent infections due to encapsulated bacteria (*Streptococcus pneumoniae, Haemophilus influenzae,* and *Neisseria meningitidis*) in patients on chronic immunosuppression
Cytomegalovirus	Prophylaxis or preemptive treatment with ganciclovir or valganciclovir in high-risk patients†	Preemptive treatment with ganciclovir or valganciclovir in high-risk patients†
Herpes simplex virus	Acyclovir in seropositive patients	Acyclovir in patients with recurrent HSV infections
Yeast infections	Fluconazole	Fluconazole in patients on chronic immunosuppression
Mold infections	No specific recommendations‡	No specific recommendations*
Pneumocystis jiroveci	Trimethoprim-sulfamethoxazole (preferred) or dapsone or pentamidine	Trimethoprim-sulfamethoxazole (preferred) or dapsone or pentamidine in patients on chronic immunosuppression

HCT, Hematopoietic cell transplantation; *HSV,* herpes simplex virus.
*Limited data exist favoring fluoroquinolones such as levofloxacin. No impact on infection-related mortality.
†Cytomegalovirus (CMV)-seropositive HCT recipients or CMV-seronegative recipients with a CMV-seropositive donor.
‡Limited data available. Prospective testing of voriconazole and posaconazole suggests possible benefit as prophylaxis. No impact on mold-related mortality.

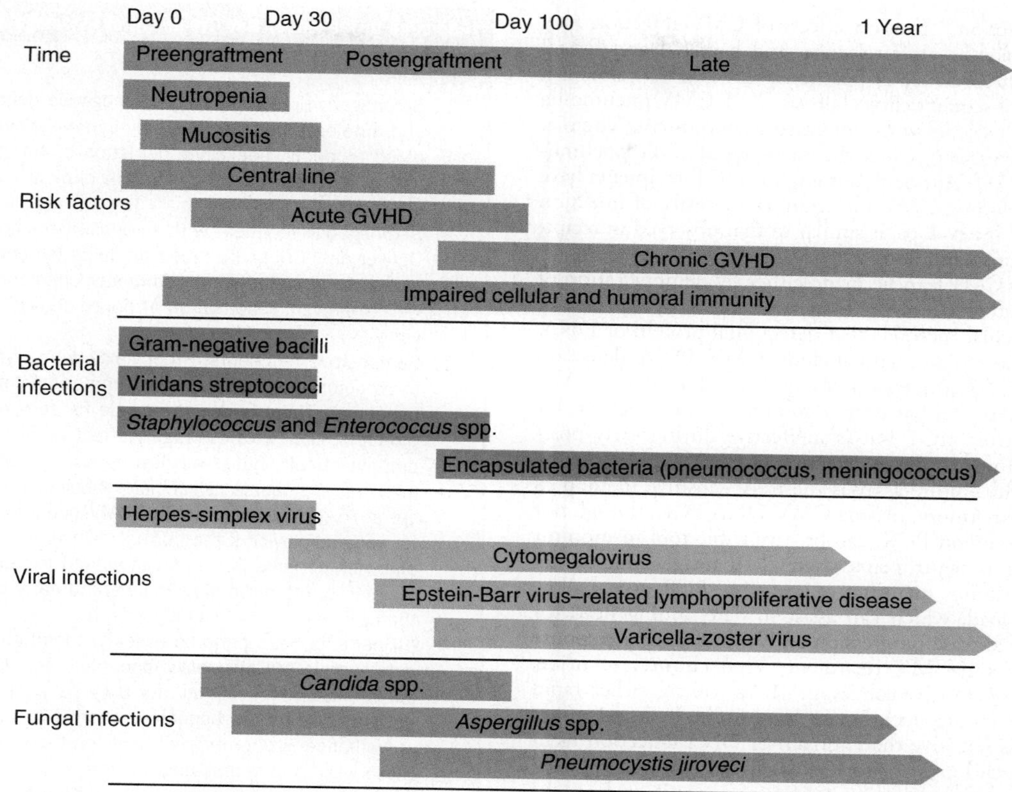

Figure 110-1 COMMON INFECTIONS IN HEMATOPOIETIC CELL TRANSPLANTATION RECIPIENTS. *GVHD,* Graft-versus-host disease.

Table 110-4 Recommended Vaccinations for Hematopoietic Cell Transplantation Recipients

Vaccine*	Time After HCT to Initiate Vaccine	No. of Doses†
Pneumococcal conjugate	3-6 mo	2-3‡
DTaP§	6-12 mo	3
Haemophilus influenzae type b conjugate	6-12 mo	3
Inactivated poliovirus	6-12 mo	3
Recombinant hepatitis B	6-12 mo	3
Inactivated influenza	4-6 mo	1-2 yearly‖
Measles, mumps, and rubella virus (live)	24 mo	1-2¶
Varicella-zoster	24 mo	1¶

DTaP, Diphtheria and tetanus toxoids and acellular pertussis vaccine; *HCT,* hematopoietic cell transplantation.
*Vaccinations are deferred in patients with chronic graft-versus-host disease (GVHD) until discontinuation of immunosuppression.
†A minimum of 1-month interval between doses is suggested.
‡Following the primary series of three pneumococcal conjugate vaccine (PCV) doses, a dose of the 23-valent pneumococcal polysaccharide vaccine (PPSV23) to broaden the immune response might be given. For patients with chronic GVHD who are likely to respond poorly to PPSV23, a fourth dose of the PCV should be considered instead of PPSV23.
§DTaP is preferred; however, tetanus toxoid, reduced diphtheria toxoid, and acellular pertussis vaccine (Tdap) can be used if DTaP is not available.
‖For children younger than 9 years of age, two doses are recommended yearly between transplant and 9 years of age.
¶Not recommended less than 24 months post-HCT, in patients with active GVHD, and in patients on immune suppression. In children, two doses of measles, mumps, and rubella virus vaccine live are favored. Lower viral-dose vaccines (varicella vaccine live [Varivax], not zoster vaccine live [Zostavax]) may be preferred as potentially safer.

the most important mechanism resulting in CMV disease.[30-32] Nearly all CMV infections (<5%) in seronegative recipients are the result of exogenous exposure (primary CMV infection), either from a seropositive stem cell donor or from cellular blood products from CMV-seropositive donors. The possibility of false-negative serology before HCT should also be considered in patients with early CMV reactivation. CMV infection and especially end-organ disease is also more frequent following allogeneic HCT, with CMV infections occurring in less than 5% of autograft recipients.[33,34] However, autologous HCT recipients who have previously received T-cell suppressive therapies (e.g., fludarabine, alemtuzumab) can be at high risk for CMV infection. Among patients undergoing allogeneic transplantation, the risk may be greater with URD compared to related donors.[35] Although the prevalence of donor seropositivity is nearly zero in UCB grafts, the risk for posttransplant CMV infection may be similar because recipient CMV status is still the predominant risk factor for infection, although the CMV-naïve UCB graft confers no latent protective immunity against CMV.[21,22] Other factors that delay immune reconstitution may also increase the risk for CMV infection, including older recipient age, increasing donor-recipient HLA mismatch, acute and chronic GVHD, and need for prolonged immunosuppression, especially with high-dose corticosteroids.[28,33,36-38] CMV reactivation posttransplantation may also be modulated by natural killer (NK) cell activity through donor activating killer immunoglobulin-like receptors.[39]

Clinical Presentation and Diagnosis

The most common manifestation of CMV infection is asymptomatic reactivation noted by screening antigenemia or DNA PCR testing. CMV organ infection and disease are most often pneumonia and enteritis. CMV is the most common specific cause of interstitial pneumonitis and is responsible for up to 50% of all cases.[40] Infection at other sites such as retinitis, hepatitis, and central nervous system disease are less common and are usually seen in late-onset or persisting CMV infection.[28] Indirect effects of CMV infection may include increased risks for graft rejection and bacterial and fungal superinfection.[28,30] The presence of posttransplant CMV viremia is a strong predictor of subsequent clinical disease.[38,41,42] CMV pneumonia develops in 60% of patients with untreated asymptomatic viremia, and treatment of viremia can reduce the incidence of CMV pneumonia to less than 5%.[41,43-45] Although autologous HCT recipients have a lower risk for developing CMV infection, the severity of infection (e.g., pneumonia), if it develops, is similar to that observed in recipients of allogeneic transplantation.

The diagnosis of CMV can be made either by demonstration of characteristic cytopathic effects in tissue culture or by the use of more-sensitive molecular methods that detect viral protein or DNA. Commonly used molecular assays include CMV DNA detection methods, and the pp65 antigenemia assay. Detection of the CMV pp65 antigen in leukocytes has been a commonly used method for CMV surveillance after HCT but is ineffective during early post-HCT leukopenia. However, direct detection of CMV DNA either by PCR or DNA hybrid capture assay is the most sensitive method to detect CMV.[46-49] Furthermore, plasma CMV DNA PCR, though not as sensitive as whole blood PCR, can be a valuable tool to monitor CMV during periods of neutropenia when CMV antigenemia testing is unreliable. In addition, quantitative real-time PCR assays allow estimation of viral load, which can assist in determining need for therapy and risk for disease progression and in monitoring response among patients on anti-CMV treatment. Viral cultures of urine, saliva, blood, or bronchioalveolar lavage (BAL), using either rapid shell-vial or routine culture techniques, have limited clinical utility because they are less sensitive than antigen or DNA detection techniques and take much longer to report. Shell-vial cultures of CMV from BAL fluid are less specific for CMV pneumonia and can be positive in asymptomatic seropositive patients without pneumonia who are shedding CMV in oral or respiratory secretions.[50] Despite this lack of specificity, even in asymptomatic people, finding CMV in BAL fluid is a strong predictor for the development of subsequent CMV pneumonia, and such patients should be treated.

Prevention and Treatment

For seronegative recipients, the use of seronegative donors and CMV-safe blood products is the mainstay of prevention of CMV disease (see box on Approach to Prevention and Treatment of Cytomegalovirus Infection). For high-risk patients (seropositive recipients or seropositive donors of seronegative recipients), two general strategies can be used, both of which have been effective in reducing early CMV infection rates to less than 10%.[28,44,45,51-53] The first is the "preemptive" approach, which involves prompt treatment of early CMV viremia with ganciclovir, valganciclovir, or foscarnet before it can lead to clinical disease. The second is the "general prophylaxis" approach, in which all at-risk patients are treated with antiviral prophylaxis. The former approach requires availability and frequent scheduled use of reliable and rapid early diagnostic tests. The latter approach can reduce the rate of early CMV infection but does not affect mortality or the risk for late CMV infection and is associated with a higher incidence of ganciclovir-induced myelosuppression.[45,51,54] Both approaches require aggressive surveillance to allow prompt detection of infection. High-dose acyclovir or valacyclovir, although not as effective as ganciclovir, also reduces the incidence of CMV viremia, but continued surveillance for CMV is still required with prompt initiation of preemptive therapy with ganciclovir or foscarnet when viremia develops.[55-58] Unlike ganciclovir, which has to be administered intravenously, its prodrug valganciclovir, has excellent oral bioavailability and is often used for prophylaxis and preemptive therapy of CMV infection among HCT recipients.[59-62] Because autologous HCT recipients have a lower risk for CMV disease, the preemptive approach to preventing CMV infection is usually sufficient. Surveillance for CMV is continued weekly until at least day 100 posttransplant for high-risk patients and is continued longer in patients with chronic GVHD on high-dose immunosuppression.

Approach to Prevention and Treatment of Cytomegalovirus Infection

Prevention

1. Seronegative recipient with seronegative donor (allogeneic and autologous): Transfuse only cytomegalovirus (CMV)-safe blood products. Leukocyte depletion by filtration and blood from CMV-seronegative donors are clinically equivalent alternatives.
2. Seronegative recipient with seropositive donor (allogeneic): Deliver only CMV-safe blood products (seronegative or leukocyte depleted), but administer chemoprophylaxis as well to prevent reactivation of donor-derived endogenous virus.
3. Seropositive recipients: Prophylaxis with acyclovir appears to be somewhat useful. Use of immunoglobulin may be beneficial. There is no proven role for seronegative blood products. Ganciclovir is highly effective when given prophylactically but is myelosuppressive. Patients who must interrupt the course of ganciclovir because of leukopenia are at risk for development of CMV pneumonia. Ganciclovir (or valganciclovir) is the current best prophylaxis in high-risk patients but is not indicated for autologous recipients. Intensive surveillance and early preemptive therapy may be equivalently effective.
4. All patients need periodic (weekly) monitoring for CMV antigenemia or CMV deoxyribonucleic acid (DNA) polymerase chain reaction for 8 to 12 weeks posttransplantation. Longer-duration (beyond 12 weeks) surveillance is appropriate for allograft recipients, especially those with graft-versus-host disease.

Treatment

1. Asymptomatic infections (allogeneic and autologous): Ganciclovir or valganciclovir treatment of asymptomatic infection detected in blood or bronchioalveolar lavage (BAL), by either molecular detection or antigenic methods, is recommended to prevent the development of CMV pneumonia. Intensive induction treatment (2 weeks) followed by a maintenance phase of 5 days/wk therapy for an additional 4 to 8 weeks is necessary.
2. CMV pneumonia: Ganciclovir in combination with immunoglobulin is recommended. This should be instituted promptly. Once the disease has progressed to cause respiratory failure and ventilator dependence, survival is limited.

No Treatment

1. Empiric CMV therapy for interstitial pneumonitis is not indicated in seronegative recipients with seronegative graft and blood donors. Diagnostic evidence of CMV infection should be obtained.
2. Empiric CMV therapy for interstitial pneumonitis is also not indicated in patients whose BAL is negative for CMV by direct staining and molecular testing. However, BAL CMV studies have a small (<5%) false-negative rate, and close follow-up and monitoring is still required.
3. Asymptomatic CMV viruria does not require therapy but does need close follow-up and serial blood viral testing for surveillance of systemic disease.

CMV disease, especially pneumonia, must be diagnosed and treated promptly because it remains associated with very high rates of mortality.[33] The combined use of ganciclovir and immunoglobulin has been the most successful treatment for CMV pneumonia, with resolution in 50% to 75% of non–ventilator dependent patients.[33,63,64] Prolonged therapy (>2 months) with the combination is indicated because shorter treatment regimens have been associated with recurrence of CMV pneumonia. Foscarnet can be effective in clinical settings in which ganciclovir fails or is associated with excess toxicity, usually myelosuppression.[65] Although treatment is generally similar, with ganciclovir or foscarnet plus immunoglobulin, CMV enteritis, hepatitis, and retinitis are variably responsive.[28,66] The efficacy of valganciclovir for treatment of CMV organ disease is being investigated. Adoptive cellular therapies (using approaches to enhance NK or infuse CMV-targeted T cells) are also being explored.[67-69] Although rare, CMV antiviral resistance can occur, and ganciclovir or foscarnet can be used as alternative drugs for second-line therapy. Cidofovir can be considered when disease progresses despite treatment with ganciclovir and foscarnet, and a liposomal formulation with good oral bioavailability is being studied.

Other Viral Infections

Primary and reactivation infections of other herpesviruses can occur after transplantation. Herpes simplex virus (HSV) infection is uncommon with the use of acyclovir or valacyclovir prophylaxis in serologically positive patients. Acyclovir-resistant HSV infection can occur in patients given low-dose prophylaxis or intermittent treatment and recipients of T cell–depleted grafts[70]; Foscarnet is the drug of choice for resistant disease with cidofovir reserved as an alternative agent. VZV reactivation can occur in 30% to 50% of HCT recipients with previous exposure to VZV and can be effectively prevented or delayed by acyclovir prophylaxis. Acyclovir prophylaxis has been suggested for the first year after transplantation for VZV-seropositive autologous and allogeneic HCT recipients; patients with chronic GVHD need to continue prophylaxis for the duration of their immunosuppression.[1,71]

HCT recipients can be prone to community-acquired respiratory viral (CRV) infections with influenza, parainfluenza, and respiratory syncytial virus (RSV). Because upper respiratory infections can progress to more-serious lower respiratory infections and certain CRVs can be treated, appropriate diagnostic testing (e.g., nasopharyngeal swabs) should be considered to identify the virus if possible. Zanamivir or oseltamivir can be used for chemoprophylaxis and treatment of influenza. Aerosolized ribavirin can be considered in patients with RSV infection, especially if they are early posttransplantation or have lower respiratory tract involvement.

Adenovirus infections can occasionally occur after allogeneic HCT, especially among recipients of T cell–depleted grafts and in patients with GVHD.[72] Human polyomavirus type I, also known as BK virus, can cause hemorrhagic cystitis in the early posttransplant period.[73] Urine PCR can identify BK virus and distinguish it from hemorrhagic cystitis caused by other infections (e.g., adenovirus) and urotoxic agents (e.g., cyclophosphamide). Quinolone antibiotics suppress BK virus replication in vivo and in vitro and may have a role as prophylaxis in patients at high risk for hemorrhagic cystits.[74] Intravesical or intravenous cidofovir has been used for the treatment of BK virus hemorrhagic cystitis.[11]

Fungal Infections

Invasive fungal infections are among the leading causes of mortality in HCT recipients. The vast majority of fungal infections in this setting are caused by yeasts (*Candida* spp.) or molds (*Aspergillus* spp.).

Candida Infections

Candida albicans has been the leading cause of yeast infections in HCT recipients, but the current widespread use of azole prophylaxis in the early transplant period has led to the emergence of a variety of non-*albicans* species, such as *Candida tropicalis, Candida krusei,* and *Candida glabrata,* as important pathogens.[75] These yeasts are normal inhabitants of the skin and the oral and gastrointestinal mucosa. Breakdown of these mucosal surfaces due to radiation and chemotherapy, compounded by neutropenia in the preengraftment period, can greatly increase the risk for invasion and systemic infections. Presence of indwelling central venous catheters and alteration of normal surface flora due to antibiotics are additional risk factors for *Candida* infections.[3,76]

Clinical manifestations can range from localized mucocutaneous to disseminated deep-tissue infection. A high index of suspicion is needed for the diagnosis of *Candida* infections, especially in patients with persistent febrile neutropenia, because blood cultures are usually not very sensitive for isolation and identification of *Candida* spp. Oral and esophageal candidiasis frequently occurs in the early posttransplant period and should be treated aggressively because they can serve as portals for subsequent systemic infection. Venous catheter infections can be difficult to eradicate with antifungal agents alone and necessitate removal of the central line. Patients with candidemia are also at risk for endovascular infections such as endocarditis and thrombophlebitis. Hepatosplenic candidiasis is the most common manifestation of disseminated candidiasis but is increasingly rare with widespread use of effective anti-*Candida* azoles and echinocandins. Specific signs or symptoms related to organ involvement may be absent, and the diagnosis frequently has to be made by abdominal CT scan imaging.

Prophylaxis with fluconazole is recommended in the preengraftment and early postengraftment period, especially among allogeneic HCT recipients.[1,77,78] In patients who are at high risk for mold infections, caspofungin, micafungin, voriconazole, or posaconazole can be considered because they have antimold activity.[79-83] *C. krusei* and *C. glabrata* are intrinsically resistant to fluconazole and other agents (e.g., posaconazole, voriconazole, or micafungin) should be preferred for prophylaxis in patients colonized with fluconazole-resistant *Candida* species. Itraconazole is another active agent, but its use is limited by its tolerability, absorption, and toxicities. Cross-resistance to azoles can occur among *Candida* species. Antifungal agents for treatment of suspected or known invasive candidiasis include voriconazole or posaconazole, echinocandins, or an amphotericin formulation, especially when infection occurs in the setting of ongoing fluconazole prophylaxis.[78]

Aspergillus Infections

Most mold infections in HCT recipients are due to *Aspergillus fumigatus, Aspergillus flavus,* and *Aspergillus niger,* which gain entry through breakdown of mucosal surfaces or through the nasal passages and respiratory tract. *Aspergillus* infections can occur early after HCT (during the neutropenic phase) or later, especially complicating the immunosuppression associated with acute or chronic GVHD.[84,85] Risk factors for *Aspergillus* infections include allogeneic (more than autologous) HCT, prolonged neutropenia, and GVHD.[18,84-86] Transplantation for diseases that cause extended neutropenia pretransplantation (e.g., chronic granulomatous disease, aplastic anemia, and myelodysplastic syndrome [MDS]) also increases the risk. Prior history of *Aspergillus* infection has also been observed to be a risk factor for reactivation after HCT.[87]

Aspergillus occurring in the posttransplant setting can be difficult to diagnose premortem. Hence a high index of suspicion and an aggressive approach are required to establish its diagnosis and initiate therapy. Because the nasal passages and tracheobronchial tree are the most common portals of entry for *Aspergillus* spp., these two sites are also the most common sites of infection. Sinusitis is frequently symptomatic, and more advanced disease can be associated with erosion and necrosis of surrounding structures. Pulmonary manifestations typically include nodular infiltrates, usually distributed along the lung periphery, with pleuritic pain or cough as an initial symptom. Frank consolidation (with a halo sign on CT scan) or cavitary lesions can be seen in more advanced stages of pulmonary involvement. *Aspergillus* has angioinvasive properties and can present with hemoptysis or with intravascular dissemination to the skin or brain.

Blood cultures have a very low sensitivity in detecting *Aspergillus,* and diagnosis has to rely on demonstration of typical fungal morphology on culture or histopathology or on tests to detect fungal components or nucleic acids. Nasal and bronchial washings for *Aspergillus* also may not be sensitive, and lung biopsy may be required to obtain a definitive diagnosis.[88] The galactomannan assay is an enzyme-linked immunosorbent assay to detect the *Aspergillus* cell wall glycoprotein; it has a high specificity but low sensitivity for diagnosing invasive aspergillosis and has not been reproducible in well-designed trials.[89-91] Molecular methods for diagnosis, including PCR for *Aspergillus* DNA, are also undergoing development.[92] More-invasive evaluations (e.g., fine-needle aspiration or biopsy) are often needed to confirm the presence of *Aspergillus* in suspicious lesions identified on clinical examination or imaging studies.[93]

The use of high-efficiency air filters has reduced the nosocomial acquisition of *Aspergillus,* at least during the early neutropenic phase when isolation measures are used.[75] The optimal pharmacologic strategy for primary prophylaxis against aspergillosis in HCT recipients is not well defined.[94] Posaconazole has been shown to be effective for prophylaxis in HCT recipients with GVHD.[95] Itraconazole is also effective, but side effects limit its use.[80] A large randomized trial showed no difference in fungal-free survival between voriconazole and fluconazole in HCT recipients at low risk for disease progression or early HCT mortality, although there was a trend toward fewer *Aspergillus* infections and less empiric antifungal use in voriconazole recipients.[83] Inhaled or low-dose intravenous amphotericin has not been shown to be effective for primary prophylaxis.[94,96,97] In patients with a previous history of invasive aspergillosis, secondary prophylaxis with a mold-specific azole (e.g., oral voriconazole or posaconazole) or parenteral echinocandins or amphotericin preparation is recommended, possibly for the duration of intensive immunosuppression.[94] Therapy with a mold-specific azole, an echinocandin, or an amphotericin preparation should be initiated in patients with invasive aspergillosis or in high-risk patients with persistent febrile neutropenia. Azoles and echinocandins have a more favorable side-effect profile compared to amphotericin formulations. Patients with disease progressing on a single antimold drug might need combination therapy with two antimold agents. The role of adjunctive measures such as cytokine growth factors, immunoglobulin infusion, or granulocyte transfusion remains undefined.

EARLY NONINFECTIOUS COMPLICATIONS

High-dose chemotherapy and radiation regimens are used before transplantation for their antineoplastic and immunosuppressive effects. However, these treatments can damage host tissue, resulting in significant morbidity.[98] Early HCT-associated complications can frequently simulate infections or be compounded by concurrent infections. In addition, because epithelial tissue repair may be delayed by ongoing neutropenia and local microinvasive infection, delay in hematopoietic engraftment can exaggerate and prolong these toxicities.

Graft Failure

Failure to establish hematologic engraftment (primary graft failure) and loss of an established graft (late graft failure) are serious complications of both autologous and allogeneic HCT. Delayed or poor graft function can exaggerate and prolong the risks of infection and can increase the risk for peritransplant mortality. Failure to engraft can occur if insufficient hematopoietic progenitors are infused. A minimum of approximately 2×10^4 colony-forming cells from marrow per kilogram recipient weight are needed to establish autologous engraftment. This is accomplished by infusing approximately 1×10^8 autologous marrow mononuclear cells per kilogram. Most investigators recommend infusion of a minimum of at least 2×10^8 mononuclear cells per kilogram to ensure establishment of an allogeneic graft. UCB-derived hematopoietic grafts can engraft with a lower number of cells.[99] Stem cells and progenitors can be damaged by cryopreservation or by ex vivo purging, and additional cells are required if intensive purging, especially with alkylators, is performed, though currently this approach to autograft preparation is uncommon. Selection of $CD34^+$ cells as a technique for tumor cell depletion does not compromise engraftment, unless the quantitative cell losses through selection are excessive.

The use of hematopoietic stem cells and progenitors harvested from the blood by apheresis instead of the bone marrow has become widely prevalent, both for autologous and allogeneic HCT. Autologous blood hematopoietic cell grafts are collected after mobilization of marrow-derived progenitors into the blood by cytokine (G-CSF or GM-CSF) therapy or during recovery from myelosuppressive chemotherapy, often in combination with growth factors.[100-103] Progenitor content of blood or marrow grafts is assayed by quantitation of mononuclear cells expressing the hematopoietic progenitor–associated surface marker CD34. Peripheral graft mobilization can be further enriched by the use of plerixafor, an inhibitor of CXCR4 that releases cells from the marrow.[104,105] Allogeneic grafts are mobilized from healthy donors using growth factors alone, nearly exclusively using G-CSF, though early experience with plerixafor has been reported.[106,107]

Graft failure is uncommon if 2×10^6 $CD34^+$ cells/kg or more are collected, cryopreserved, and later infused as an autologous graft.[101,102] The minimum CD34 content for an allogeneic graft is less well defined, but more than 5×10^6 $CD34^+$ cells/kg is frequently cited as a target collection for a sibling donor allograft.[108-110] Mobilized peripheral blood–derived stem cells yield satisfactory and more rapid trilineage hematopoietic recovery than grafts from marrow-derived cells.[110-113] Similar to marrow grafting, late graft failure is possible, but unlikely (<5%) after transplantation using peripheral blood–derived stem cells. Infusion of a sufficient graft cell dose (nucleated or $CD34^+$ cells) may be the most important controllable factor to limit the risk for graft failure.

Recipient myelofibrosis or splenomegaly can interfere with engraftment. Splenomegaly can delay hematologic recovery, presumably because both progenitors and mature blood cells are sequestered in the spleen.[114] The presence of moderate to severe myelofibrosis also delays engraftment, perhaps because of faulty homing of stem cells in the marrow microenvironment.[115,116]

Posttransplantation therapy can jeopardize engraftment. Graft failure or poor graft function has been associated with use of methotrexate, ATG, acyclovir, ganciclovir, trimethoprim-sulfamethoxazole (TMP-SMX), and mycophenolate mofetil (MMF). Posttransplant complications such as CMV, human herpesvirus-6 or fungal infections, and acute and chronic GVHD can also compromise successful engraftment.

Allogeneic HCT, especially using unrelated or mismatched donors, poses unique engraftment problems. Transplants between siblings completely matched at HLA-A, HLA-B, and HLA-DR loci are rarely (1% to 3%) associated with graft failure; however, the probability of graft failure in the related-donor transplantation setting increases to near 10% with greater degrees of donor-recipient HLA incompatibility.[117-120] The problem is frequent (5% to 15%) in the URD setting, where primary or secondary graft failure may occur even after transplantation from donors well matched at the HLA-A, HLA-B, HLA-C, and HLA-DR loci.[119-122] In some cases, failure of URD stem cells to engraft may result from reactivity against other important histocompatibility determinants, including HLA-C.[123] Early failure of an allogeneic graft can be accompanied by emergence of cytotoxic T lymphocytes of host origin, presumably representing immune-mediated graft rejection.[124,125] T-lymphocyte depletion of donor marrow performed as GVHD prophylaxis can also adversely affect engraftment, even from matched sibling donors.[118,126] Ex vivo marrow manipulation can deplete stem cells. T-cell depletion can also render the graft immunoincompetent and functionally less capable of preventing graft rejection.

Compared to related or URD allografts, time to neutrophil recovery is significantly delayed in patients receiving UCB grafts. In addition, the overall incidence of graft failure is somewhat greater.[127-130] The most critical determinants of engraftment following UCB transplantation are both HLA matching and cell dose, and units with a total nucleated cell dose of at least 2.5×10^7 cells/kg or more have a greater probability of successful engraftment.[129-131] Because each UCB unit has a limited number of hematopoietic progenitor cells, methods to overcome this limitation of cell dose are being investigated. These include transplantation using multiple UCB units, ex vivo expansion to increase the number of progenitor cells, and intra–bone marrow injection of the graft. Increasing overall cell dose with transplantation of two UCB units can lead to successful engraftment, especially in adults.[99,132-134]

The use of recombinant G-CSF or GM-CSF, which stimulates myelopoiesis, has improved the treatment of graft failure.[135] Improvement in myelopoiesis can be seen in 50% to 60% of patients with poor graft function within 14 to 21 days after initiation of growth factor therapy. Myeloid growth factor therapy can increase peripheral blood leukocyte recovery but has little effect on platelet reconstitution. Recombinant human thrombopoietin receptor agonists are now available, although their efficacy and safety profile in HCT recipients is uncertain and parallel experience in treating chemotherapy-induced thrombocytopenia suggests that they will be ineffective. Limited experience suggests the value of recombinant erythropoietin in reducing red blood cell transfusion needs.[136]

A second stem cell infusion can be useful if graft failure occurs. In the case of a failed autograft, infusion of previously harvested and frozen marrow or blood cells frequently reestablishes functional hematopoiesis and hematologic improvement. In the case of graft failure after related-donor transplantation, a second infusion of donor marrow or cytokine-stimulated peripheral blood stem cells may allow successful engraftment.[137] Sometimes, due to the presumption of immune-mediated rejection, reconditioning with reduced doses of cytotoxic agents or further immunosuppression with ATG, corticosteroids, or cyclosporine is used to prepare the recipient for a second infusion.

The treatment of graft failure after URD transplantation poses special problems. Unrelated donors may not be available for a second marrow harvest or blood stem cell apheresis. In experimental settings in which graft failure risks are high, it may be prudent to store autologous stem cells from patients undergoing URD transplantation, though this is rarely done. The original donor is unavailable in recipients of unrelated UCB grafts and the only treatment option for graft failure in this setting is a second transplant using cells from a different UCB or volunteer adult donor (related or unrelated) second allograft, or reinfusion of autologous back-up cells if available. Because of variability in the circumstances and donor options available, there are few clear data on the outcomes of second allografts in these situations.[138-140]

Sinusoidal Obstruction Syndrome

Sinusoidal obstruction syndrome (SOS), also known as hepatic veno-occlusive disease (VOD), is a serious liver disorder characterized by jaundice, ascites, fluid retention, and hepatomegaly that complicates up to 5% to 50% of HCTs. The differing incidence is based upon stringency of the definition of the clinical diagnosis (see box on Sinusoidal Obstruction Syndrome).[141-144] The primary initiating event is thought to be portal hypertension due to obstruction of hepatic sinusoids and venules, which secondarily leads to damage to surrounding centrilobular hepatocytes.[145-147] Chemotherapy and total body irradiation (TBI) used in pretransplant conditioning regimens produce sinusoidal endothelial injury. Subsequent deposition of fibronectin and factor VIII/von Willebrand factor at the site of damaged endothelium can lead to activation of the coagulation system and subsequent sinusoidal obstruction.[148] Such changes are often associated with depressed plasma protein C levels and other signs of procoagulant activity, including lower antithrombin III levels and elevated factor VIII and fibrinogen levels.[149-153] Cytokines such as tumor necrosis factor (TNF)-α and alterations in the levels of nitric oxide and matrix metalloproteinases may also have a role in its pathogenesis.[154-157]

Sinusoidal Obstruction Syndrome

Diagnostic Criteria for Sinusoidal Obstruction Syndrome

Bilirubin level of 2 mg/dL or above before day 21 after hematopoietic cell transplantation (HCT) and at least two of the following: (1) hepatomegaly or right upper quadrant pain, (2) ascites, or (3) weight gain of more than 5% over baseline.

Sinusoidal obstruction syndrome (SOS) is a clinical diagnosis; liver ultrasound with Doppler studies or liver biopsy can support or confirm the diagnosis.

Risk Factors

Pretransplant Factors

- Prior hepatic inflammatory disease (e.g., chronic hepatitis B or C, nonalcoholic steatohepatitis, alcoholic hepatitis)
- Prior hepatic fibrotic disease (e.g., cirrhosis)
- Extensive pre-HCT chemotherapy
- Prior exposure to gemtuzumab ozogamicin
- Prior liver irradiation

Transplant-Related Factors

- Conditioning regimen (e.g., myeloablative total body irradiation or busulfan-based regimens)
- Exposure to other agents (e.g., sirolimus, itraconazole)

Prognostic Factors

Adverse prognostic factors include development of multiorgan failure, rapid increase in weight, and rapid increase in bilirubin level.

Treatment

More than 70% of patients will recover spontaneously from SOS with supportive care. However, mortality rates are over 80% for patients with severe SOS. Treatment options, especially for patients with more severe SOS, include the following:

Pharmacologic

- Ursodeoxycholic acid (prophylaxis)
- Defibrotide (investigational—prophylaxis and treatment)
- Low-dose heparin and low-molecular-weight heparin (prophylaxis)
- Tissue plasminogen activator (investigational—prophylaxis and treatment)
- Antithrombin III (investigational—prophylaxis and treatment)

Nonpharmacologic

- Supportive care with management of multiorgan failure
- Transjugular intrahepatic portosystemic shunt (TIPS)
- Liver transplantation

Risk factors associated with the development of SOS include history of pretransplant hepatitis or liver injury, intensive preparative regimens, increased TBI dose and dose rate, and increased busulfan dose.[141-144,147,158-161] SOS may also be more frequent after mismatched related or URD transplantation.[142-144] Prior therapy with gemtuzumab ozogamicin also increases the risk for posttransplant SOS.[162] Sirolimus has also been shown to increase the risk for SOS after myeloablative allogeneic HCT, particularly using busulfan-based regimens.[163]

Signs of SOS usually occur within 1 month after hematopoietic graft infusion but may be recognized much sooner, even during administration of the preparative regimen. Clinical evidence of VOD includes hyperbilirubinemia, tender hepatomegaly, ascites, and weight gain.[141,143,147] More advanced stages can be associated with encephalopathy along with renal, pulmonary, and multiorgan failure. The diagnosis of SOS is primarily based on clinical criteria that include presence of jaundice with either hepatomegaly, weight gain, and/or ascites within 2 to 3 weeks of stem cell infusion.[141,164] However, other causes of hyperbilirubinemia and weight gain early after transplantation (e.g., drugs, hepatitis, capillary leak, cardiac failure, and salt and colloid overloading) can complicate the differential diagnosis, particularly for milder or less abrupt presentations of these symptoms. Percutaneous or transabdominal needle biopsy of the liver is hazardous in severely thrombocytopenic transplant recipients and should be avoided. Transvenous biopsies may provide sufficient histologic material for diagnosis and may allow determination of hepatic wedge pressure product (greater than 10 mm is associated with SOS) but may be associated with hemorrhagic complications as well.[165] Ultrasonographic Doppler flow studies demonstrating reversal of portal flow or a higher portal vein resistive index have been suggested as a noninvasive means of confirming the diagnosis, but their validity has recently been questioned.[166-168] SOS can be graded from mild to severe depending on the degree of hyperbilirubinemia and weight gain, and severe SOS is almost universally fatal within several weeks of onset.[143,169]

Effective methods for prevention and treatment of SOS have not been defined. Limited understanding of the cellular and microvascular pathophysiology of SOS has confounded development of more rational approaches to its prevention and treatment. Possible approaches include preventive therapy with low-dose heparin,[170-172] prostaglandin E,[173] pentoxifylline (a TNF-α blocking agent),[174,175] or ursodiol,[176,177] although none has proved effective in carefully performed prospective trials. Recombinant tissue plasminogen factor has been used successfully to treat established SOS; however, thrombolytics are associated with substantially increased risk for hemorrhage.[178-181] Transjugular intrahepatic portosystemic shunts have also been used with some success.[182,183] Early experience with defibrotide, a single-stranded polyribonucleotide with fibrinolytic, antithrombotic, and antiischemic properties, has been favorable with 30% to 40% of patients with severe SOS achieving complete resolution and improvement in survival.[184-187] Its efficacy in the prophylaxis and management of severe SOS is currently being investigated in larger clinical trials.

Interstitial Pneumonitis

Interstitial pneumonitis is a common and frequently fatal complication, affecting up to 35% of allogeneic transplant recipients, although advances in supportive care have led to substantial reductions in this risk.[188,189] Interstitial pneumonitis is notably less common after autografting.[190] It is characterized by diffuse, nonbacterial interstitial inflammation accompanied by hypoxemia, dyspnea, and nonproductive cough, sometimes with fever. Risk factors associated with the development of interstitial pneumonitis include use of methotrexate for GVHD prophylaxis, older age at transplant, severe GVHD, interval from diagnosis of hematologic disease to HCT of 6 months or greater, poor pretransplant performance status, and use of higher TBI dose rate (>4 cGy/min).[188,189] Remarkably, in one study, the reported risk for interstitial pneumonitis was 8% when none of these risk factors was present, compared to 94% when all six factors were present.[188] It has been hypothesized that URD transplantation is more immunosuppressive and thus associated with more severe opportunistic infections and greater risk for interstitial pneumonitis, but this has not been rigorously investigated.

The course of interstitial pneumonitis is often catastrophic, manifesting with rapidly progressive tachypnea, hypoxemia, and hemodynamic compromise. Therefore therapeutic intervention most frequently occurs before the return of definitive results of diagnostic tests and must be initiated based on the assessment of clinical risk factors and the underlying clinical setting (see box on Approach to Interstitial Pneumonitis).

Infectious Causes of Interstitial Pneumonitis

Infections are the most common cause of interstitial pneumonitis in HCT recipients. CMV and *Aspergillus* are the most common infections associated with interstitial pneumonitis and have been discussed earlier in this chapter. Other important though relatively uncommon infections to consider are *Pneumocystis jiroveci* and RSV and similar respiratory viruses.

Pneumonitis caused by *Pneumocystis* has a typical bilateral distribution with a "butterfly" pattern on chest radiograph and prominent hypoxemia and rarely causes pleural effusions.[191] The previously reported 5% to 15% risk for *Pneumocystis* pneumonia has been largely eliminated by routine use of prophylaxis with TMP-SMX (first choice), dapsone, or inhaled pentamidine.[192,193] Prophylaxis with TMP-SMX virtually eliminates *Pneumocystis* pneumonia from the differential diagnosis, but only if patient compliance with therapy is certain. Diagnosis requires cytologic evaluation of silver-stained preparations of BAL cells or sputum, although transbronchial lung biopsy may slightly increase the diagnostic yield of a bronchoscopic examination. *Pneumocystis* pneumonia is effectively treated with high-dose TMP-SMX or parenteral pentamidine. Prophylaxis against *Pneumocystis* pneumonia should be continued through the period of immunosuppression (6 months to 1 year posttransplantation) and for the duration of any therapy for chronic GVHD.

RSV is a potentially fatal cause of interstitial pneumonitis and typically occurs in the fall and winter months.[194] RSV should be suspected if the patient presents a history of rhinorrhea and if RSV has been frequently recognized in the community or in the hospital. Diagnosis can be made by rapid antigen testing on nasal washings or BAL specimens. Because of the possibility of horizontal transmission, patients with RSV should be isolated. Inhaled ribavirin is used for treatment of RSV-associated pneumonia.[195] Other community-acquired viruses, such as parainfluenza or influenza, can also cause interstitial pneumonitis in the transplant recipient. Their presentation is clinically indistinguishable from RSV, though parainfluenza pneumonitis is not seasonal and may be seen year-round. Yearly influenza vaccination for HCT recipients and especially their household contacts may be effective in reducing risks for this infection.

Noninfectious Causes of Interstitial Pneumonitis

Idiopathic Interstitial Pneumonitis

Idiopathic interstitial pneumonitis is a diagnosis of exclusion based on typical findings and ruling out infectious causes. Its timing is somewhat earlier than other causes of interstitial pneumonitis, typically occurring within the first 2 to 7 weeks after HCT.[40,196,197] The recognized risk factors for idiopathic interstitial pneumonitis include older age at transplant, extensive pretransplant chemotherapy, high-dose cyclophosphamide, TBI (higher total dose and dose rate), blood transfusions, administration of methotrexate, and GVHD.[198-201]

The observation that idiopathic interstitial pneumonitis is as frequent among syngeneic as among allogeneic recipients and has an equally high incidence in T cell–depleted grafts suggests that immunosuppression is less of a risk factor for idiopathic interstitial pneumonitis than it is for infectious interstitial pneumonitis.[202,203] Clinical observations support a toxic cause for idiopathic interstitial pneumonitis and radiation-induced lung damage appears to be the major contributor, especially the use of high-dose TBI.[204,205] Effective therapy has not been established, although high-dose corticosteroids are often administered. Inflammatory cytokines, including interleukin(IL)-1 and TNF-α, have been implicated in lung injury.[206,207] Etanercept, a TNF-α–binding protein has been reported to improve lung function in patients with idiopathic interstitial pneumonitis, particularly if administered before the need for mechanical ventilation. Its use is currently undergoing evaluation in clinical trials.[208,209]

Approach to Interstitial Pneumonitis

The presentation of interstitial pneumonitis after hematopoietic cell transplantation (HCT) should be considered an urgent medical situation, and empiric broad-spectrum therapy must be initiated early. The choice of therapy is influenced by the following:

1. Timing: Within the first 3 weeks after HCT, interstitial pneumonitis is more likely to be idiopathic (including diffuse alveolar hemorrhage) or fungal than due to cytomegalovirus (CMV) infection. Beyond 6 weeks, idiopathic pneumonitis is unusual, and the cause is more likely infectious. *Pneumocystis jiroveci* pneumonia is rare beyond 1 year after transplantation except in patients with ongoing chronic graft-versus-host disease (GVHD). Respiratory syncytial virus (RSV) infections are seasonal (fall and winter), and community outbreaks can be prevalent. Influenza is also seasonal, whereas parainfluenza can occur year-round.
2. CMV serology and prophylaxis: If a seronegative recipient has received a seronegative graft and noninfective (seronegative or leukocyte-depleted) blood, CMV pneumonia is unusual. Seropositive recipients are at higher risk, although with ganciclovir or other antiviral prophylaxis, the risk is markedly reduced. Other prophylactic regimens for CMV, such as acyclovir or intravenous immunoglobulin, have still been associated with significant risk for serious CMV infection in the seropositive recipient. Serial negative testing for CMV antigenemia or deoxyribonucleic acid (DNA) polymerase chain reaction (PCR) makes CMV pneumonitis less likely.
3. Prolonged neutropenia: This factor is associated with infectious causes, particularly with fungal pneumonias.
4. Type of transplant: Diffuse alveolar hemorrhage is less frequently seen in patients undergoing autologous HCT. CMV pneumonia is unusual (2% to 3%) in autologous recipients, but it still has a high case fatality rate. All infectious causes are more common after allogeneic HCT. More-intensive conditioning regimens (e.g., higher total body irradiation, carmustine) are associated with more frequent pneumonitis.
5. Compliance and prophylaxis: A thorough assessment of what prophylaxis the patient has actually been receiving (e.g., trimethoprim-sulfamethoxazole, penicillin, CMV prophylaxis, transfusions outside the transplant center) is critical to assess risk.
6. Chest radiograph: The pattern and distribution of the infiltrate may narrow the differential diagnosis. Cardiac enlargement or pleural effusions may suggest pulmonary edema. A chest computed tomographic scan is useful, especially if nodularity, pleural involvement, or cavitary lesions (possibly fungal) are suspected.
7. Epidemiology: Identification of the causes of other recent cases can be most helpful with infections that are horizontally transmitted (e.g., RSV) or have common environmental risk factors (e.g., *Aspergillus* infection associated with construction).
8. Bronchoalveolar lavage (BAL): This can be extremely useful to establish a specific diagnosis or to exclude others. CMV rarely causes pneumonia without positive BAL findings (either direct staining of CMV-associated antigens in BAL cells or DNA PCR). BAL also usually detects RSV, *Pneumocystis jiroveci,* and other respiratory viruses, though not as rapidly, but is required to identify alveolar hemorrhage. It is less sensitive for diagnosis of fungal pneumonias.
9. Lung biopsy: Although this is the gold standard for definitive diagnosis of most of the possible causes of interstitial pneumonitis, it can often be avoided through the use of the clinical diagnostic measures listed. It may be necessary for the definitive diagnosis of fungal pneumonias, pulmonary changes associated with chronic GVHD (bronchiolitis obliterans), or idiopathic interstitial pneumonitis. Either bronchoscopic (transbronchial) biopsy, open surgical biopsy, or video-assisted thoracoscopic surgery can be performed. Transbronchial biopsies are insufficient for other than very diffuse processes and carry risks for bleeding and/or pneumothorax. The surgical approaches are more invasive, but more often definitive.
10. Ventilator therapy: Progressive respiratory failure after HCT is rarely reversible, especially in adults. Although aggressive diagnostic and therapeutic measures are essential, some centers offer patients and their families the option of foregoing mechanical ventilatory support if survival is not expected. Preliminary discussion of this possible complication in pretransplant patient counseling can facilitate decision making if respiratory failure does occur.

Diffuse Alveolar Hemorrhage

Alveolar hemorrhage is a clinical syndrome of acute onset of pulmonary infiltrates and hypoxemia with a progressively bloodier BAL on bronchoscopy.[210] Alveolar hemorrhage due to noninfectious causes has been called diffuse alveolar hemorrhage, but it is often difficult to distinguish it from infection-associated pulmonary hemorrhage, especially in the early posttransplant period.[211] The reported incidence of diffuse alveolar hemorrhage ranges from 2% to 5% in autologous and 5% to 10% in allogeneic HCT recipients.[210-214] Its pathogenesis is not known, but it most likely develops as result of a complex interaction of a variety of factors, including alveolar injury from radiation and chemotherapy, inflammatory damage due to neutrophils and cytokines, and underlying infections. Older age at transplant, use of allogeneic donor source, and GVHD are risk factors for this syndrome.[211,213] The risk is reportedly similar with nonmyeloablative and myeloablative conditioning regimens, but this has not been confirmed.[212] Onset typically occurs within the first 3 months of transplantation with dyspnea, and cough, although late-onset alveolar hemorrhage is not uncommon. Hemoptysis is usually absent, and bronchoscopy with BAL is required to confirm the diagnosis and to exclude infectious causes. This syndrome is very serious, and the majority of patients develop severe respiratory failure with mortality rates of more than 70%.[211,214] Hemorrhage occurring in the periengraftment period is associated with a better outcome compared to later-onset hemorrhage. Treatment includes correction of any coagulopathy and aggressive ventilatory support. High-dose corticosteroids have been used for its management, but their efficacy has not been clearly proven.[210,211,214] Small case series have reported the successful use of recombinant factor VIIa and aminocaproic acid, but their efficacy needs to be confirmed in clinical trials.[215-217] Cytokine antagonists (e.g., etanercept) might have a therapeutic role that is being investigated in clinical trials.

LATE NONINFECTIOUS COMPLICATIONS

Improvements in transplantation techniques and supportive care have led to an increasing number of long-term HCT survivors. Among HCT recipients who remain disease-free through 2 to 5 years posttransplantation, probability of survival over the next 10 to 20 years is more than 80%.[218-220] These survivors remain at risk for late transplant-associated complications, which can include organ-specific dysfunction, second cancers, infections due to ongoing immunodeficiency, and functional impairments and changes in quality of life (Table 110-5).[221-228] Guidelines for screening and prevention of late effects in HCT survivors have been published.[12] In addition, following general population guidelines for screening and prevention of cancers and chronic diseases and promoting a generally healthy lifestyle is recommended for all HCT survivors.

Table 110-5 Selected Late Complications of Hematopoietic Cell Transplantation

Complication	Risk Factors	Monitoring and Prevention
Endocrine		
Hypothyroidism	TBI/radiation	Periodic assessment of thyroid and gonadal function
Hypogonadism	Chronic GVHD	
Growth retardation	Chemotherapy	
Ocular		
Cataracts	TBI/radiation	Periodic eye examination
Keratoconjunctivitis sicca	Corticosteroids Chronic GVHD	
Oral		
Dental caries	TBI/radiation	Periodic dental assessment
Dry mouth	Chronic GVHD	
Cardiovascular		
Coronary artery disease	TBI/radiation	Periodic clinical evaluation
Cerebrovascular disease	Chemotherapy	Modification of risk factors
Respiratory		
Bronchiolitis obliterans	TBI/radiation	Periodic clinical evaluation
Interstitial pneumonitis	Chronic GVHD Infections	Smoking cessation
Hepatic		
Cirrhosis	Hepatitis B or C	Periodic liver function tests
Iron overload	Transfusions	Serum ferritin level
Renal		
Nephropathy	TBI/radiation	Periodic serum creatinine and urinalysis
	Chemotherapy Cyclosporine	Control hypertension
Skeletal		
Osteoporosis	TBI/radiation	Periodic bone densitometry
Avascular necrosis	Corticosteroids	
Second cancers	TBI/radiation	Periodic cancer screening
	Chemotherapy Chronic GVHD	

GVHD, Graft-versus-host disease; *TBI*, total body irradiation.

Organ-Specific Late Effects

A multitude of pre-, peri- and post-HCT factors determine a patient's overall risk for developing specific late complications. Risk factors include age at the time of HCT, sex, and lifestyle factors such as tobacco use. In addition, patients may have preexisting comorbidities such as chronic renal failure that can be exacerbated by chemotherapy, radiation, and other medications they receive to treat their malignancy and during HCT. Exposure to chemotherapy and radiation as part of the initial treatment of the underlying hematologic disorder or as part of the conditioning regimen given before HCT also can contribute to organ-specific complications. Allogeneic HCT recipients who develop GVHD require long-term, and at times lifelong, treatment with glucocorticoids, calcineurin inhibitors (e.g., cyclosporine or tacrolimus), or other immunosuppressive agents and can be prone to developing medication-related side effects, infections, and second malignancies, especially those associated with chronic immunodeficiency.

Although any organ system can be involved, certain organs have a greater predilection for late-onset problems post-HCT. Cataracts develop in more than one-third of patients by 5-years posttransplantation and often require surgical therapy.[229] Hypothyroidism can be seen in up to 50% and hypogonadism in up to 90% of HCT survivors.[230-232] The majority of HCT survivors become permanently sterile, although HCT without TBI can be fertility sparing in nearly one-third of men and women.[231,233] Prepubertal children may retain fertility, although secondary sexual development may be delayed. Up to 50% of children undergoing HCT also develop growth retardation.[234] Musculoskeletal complications, including osteoporosis and avascular necrosis, can be particularly debilitating. An increased incidence of cardiovascular events and diabetes has also been reported.[225,235] The risk for most organ-specific late complications continues to increase with time, and continued surveillance for these problems is indicated in all HCT survivors.

Second Cancers

Secondary cancers are a rare but devastating complication of HCT. They account for 5% to 10% of deaths among greater-than-2-year survivors. These malignancies can be broadly categorized as posttransplant lymphoproliferative disorders (PTLDs), hematologic malignancies, and solid cancers.[236-238]

PTLDs comprise a heterogeneous group of lymphoid proliferations, primarily involving B lymphocytes that develop as a result of uncontrolled Epstein-Barr virus (EBV) infection. They occur almost exclusively in allogeneic HCT recipients, with an overall incidence rate of 1% to 2%; they typically manifest soon after transplantation with more than 80% of cases diagnosed within the first year.[236,237,239] Because T cells play an important role in preventing proliferation of EBV-infected lymphocytes, removal of T cells from the hematopoietic graft source is a strong risk factor for PTLD.[240] A greater degree of immunosuppression, such as that resulting from GVHD and use of grafts from unrelated or HLA-mismatched donors, also increases the risk for PTLD. Treatment of PTLD is often challenging, and available treatments are not very effective. Withdrawal of immunosuppression is usually attempted first but can be difficult in patients with active GVHD. Treatment options include antiviral therapy with acyclovir or ganciclovir, multiagent chemotherapy, anti-CD20 monoclonal antibody rituximab, or infusion of EBV-specific cytotoxic lymphocytes. Because PTLD is associated with high mortality rates, active surveillance for EBV reactivation in high-risk settings and initiation of preemptive therapy, often with rituximab, is currently under investigation.

Secondary myelodysplastic syndrome (MDS) and acute myeloid leukemia (AML) can be seen in 5% to 15% of autologous HCT recipients but are extremely rare among allogeneic HCT recipients. They usually occur following a latency period of 2 to 5 years.[236,237,241] Bone-marrow evaluation can show cytogenetic abnormalities characteristic of other treatment-induced AML/MDS (e.g., balanced translocations to 11q23, monosomy of 5q and 7q or multiple, complex chromosomal aberrations). Risk factors for secondary MDS/AML include older age at transplant; the type, intensity, and duration of pre-HCT chemotherapy (especially alkylating agents); and use of TBI. Outcomes are very poor and long-term survival rates are less than 20%, sometimes following a second allograft for this new malignancy.

Secondary solid cancers have a latency period of 3 to 5 years following HCT. Subsequently, their incidence continues to rise with time and is higher than what may be expected in age- and sex-matched general populations. Their cumulative incidence ranges from 1% to 2% at 5 years, 2% to 6% at 10 years, and 4% to 15% at 15 years posttransplantation.[13,236,237] Younger age at

Table 110-6 Screening Guidelines for Common Cancers After Hematopoietic Cell Transplantation

Site	Screening Recommendations
Breast	Mammogram annually starting at age 40; in women who have received ≥20 Gy to the chest region begin at age 25 or 8 years after radiation, whichever is later
Cervix	Papanicolaou test every year (for regular Papanicolaou test) or every 2 years (for liquid-based Papanicolaou test); may screen every 2 to 3 years after age 30 if patient has three consecutive normal tests
Colorectal	Beginning at age 50, fecal occult blood annually and/or flexible sigmoidoscopy every 5 years, or double-contrast barium enema every 5 years, or colonoscopy every 10 years; certain high-risk groups (e.g., patients with inflammatory bowel disease) may need earlier initiation and more frequent screening
Lung	Yearly pulmonary examination with imaging as appropriate
Oral	Yearly oral cavity examination
Thyroid	Yearly thyroid examination
Skin	Yearly skin examination

transplantation, use of TBI, and chronic GVHD are important risk factors for solid cancers. Solid cancers at a variety of sites have been reported, including cancers of the head and neck, liver, brain and nervous system, thyroid, and bone and connective tissue. Because there is no plateau in the incidence of secondary solid cancers after HCT, their overall risk has not been completely realized, and longer follow-up than what is currently available is needed before the true magnitude of risk will become apparent. Lifelong cancer screening is recommended for all HCT survivors according to established guidelines (Table 110-6).[12]

Quality of Life After Transplantation

Despite the early morbidity associated with HCT, the majority of transplant survivors attain high levels of physical and psychologic quality of life (QOL) and return to full-time employment by 3 to 5 years posttransplant.[224,242-249] However, up to 20% to 40% of long-term survivors continue to have functional, psychologic, and cognitive impairments years after HCT.[227,250,251] The major risk factors for poor QOL are older age and advanced disease at transplantation, chronic GVHD, and presence of medical late effects.[243,244,246,252] Although chronic GVHD is a strong predictor of poor QOL, the overall health and functional status improves with resolution of GVHD and eventually reaches a level comparable to that seen in patients with no history of chronic GVHD.[252,253] Sex-specific differences in QOL have also been observed, with females more likely to report impairments in psychologic and sexual domains.[243,254] Cognitive deficits, particularly involving executive function, memory, and motor skills, have been reported in 30% to 60% of HCT survivors.[250,255-259] The risk for developing these neuropsychologic sequelae is increased in patients receiving transplantation at an older age, use of TBI-based conditioning regimens, and cyclosporine.

GRAFT-VERSUS-HOST DISEASE

GVHD is a clinicopathologic syndrome of T cell–mediated alloreactivity that commonly occurs as a complication of allogeneic HCT and leads to significant morbidity and mortality (also see Chapter 109). It is usually classified as acute GVHD or chronic GVHD.[260] Acute GVHD is further classified as classic acute GVHD (onset ≤100 days) and persistent, recurrent, or late-onset acute GVHD (onset >100 days). In the absence of clinical features characteristic of acute GVHD, chronic GVHD is called classic chronic GVHD. When features of both acute and chronic GVHD appear together, it is classified as overlap syndrome, based upon a consensus conference–proposed definition.

Current understanding of the pathogenesis of GVHD suggests that alloreactive donor T lymphocytes recognize histocompatibility antigens on host cells and initiate secondary inflammatory injury, leading to the clinical symptoms of GVHD.[261,262] This alloreactive response can be initiated or accelerated by conditioning regimen–induced tissue injury with release of proinflammatory cytokines, primarily IL-1 and TNF-α.[263-266] GVHD is more frequent and more severe in recipients of partially matched or histoincompatible transplants, suggesting that major histocompatibility complex–encoded molecules may be the prime antigenic targets initiating the alloreactive T-cell response.[120,122,267] Minor histocompatibility antigens also play an important role in its pathogenesis, especially in HLA-identical sibling donor grafts.[268] Activated donor-derived T cells produce IL-2 and interferon-γ, expand and differentiate into effector cells, and recruit mononuclear phagocytes and neutrophils, which ultimately yield host tissue destruction, primarily through apoptosis.[261,262,265,269-271] T cell–depletion of the graft reduces the risk for acute and chronic GVHD, albeit at the cost of increasing risks for disease relapse due to blunting of the graft-versus-tumor response.[272,273] Alternative mechanisms may also be involved in the pathogenesis of chronic GVHD, including autoreactivity, loss of self-tolerance, and B-cell dysregulation.[261,274,275]

Acute Graft-Versus-Host Disease

Risk Factors and Clinical Features

Up to 50% of patients receiving HLA-identical sibling-donor and up to 90% of patients receiving URD HCT develop acute GVHD.[120,122,267,276] Donor-recipient HLA disparity is the most important risk factor for acute GVHD.[120,277] Additional risk factors include increasing recipient and donor age,[267,276,278,279] use of alloimmunized donors such as parous women,[278,279] and HCT from unrelated instead of sibling donors.[120,278] Use of peripheral blood stem cells instead of bone marrow as graft source may be a particular risk for chronic GHVD.[280,281] Among recipients of UCB, acute GVHD occurs in 20% to 60% of patients; incidence of acute GVHD, though of only moderate severity, may be higher among recipients of double UCB transplantation.[282-285]

The skin, liver, and gastrointestinal tract are the most common sites of GVHD. Acute GVHD of the skin is characterized by a maculopapular rash that, when severe, can lead to bullae or even resemble toxic epidermal necrolysis. Hepatic involvement manifests as cholestatic hepatitis with marked elevation of serum bilirubin and alkaline phosphatase levels but usually only mild transaminase alterations. In the intestine, upper gastrointestinal tract GVHD can produce nausea, vomiting, and anorexia, whereas small bowel and colon GVHD produces large-volume secretory diarrhea. The diagnosis is clinical but frequently requires histologic confirmation to distinguish it from other frequent toxicities in the early posttransplantation period (e.g., hypersensitivity drug rash, drug-induced cholestasis, SOS, or infectious enteritis). The histologic hallmark of acute GVHD is apoptosis of the proliferative and regenerative cell layer of the epidermis, intestinal or biliary epithelium.

Acute GVHD is graded according to the organs involved (skin, liver, or gastrointestinal tract) and the extent (stage) of each organ involvement.[286,287] Mild to moderate (grade I or II) GVHD is characterized by limited organ involvement and carries an excellent prognosis. Severe (grade III or IV) GVHD has extensive multiorgan involvement with significant morbidity and poor survival, commonly progresses to chronic GVHD, and is associated with an increased risk for secondary opportunistic infections.[288,289]

Prophylaxis of Graft-Versus-Host Disease

The most effective techniques for GVHD prevention have involved ex vivo depletion of donor T lymphocytes, most often coupling immunologic recognition (monoclonal anti–T cell antibodies) with depletion techniques (immunomagnetic beads, complement cytotoxicity, or toxin immunoconjugates). Although vigorous T cell–depletion prevents acute GVHD, it also increases the risk for graft failure and neoplastic relapse after transplantation.[272]

Pharmacologic immunosuppression administered in the first several months after transplantation can prevent or blunt the initiating T-cell recognition and proliferative response that triggers GVHD and can allow development of immune system tolerance and complete lymphohematopoietic chimerism. Methotrexate, corticosteroids, ATG, cyclosporine, tacrolimus, MMF, and sirolimus have been used for prophylaxis of GVHD and have successfully reduced both the frequency and the severity of clinical GVHD.[276,288,290-298] Despite the potential role of inflammatory cytokines in initiation and amplification of GVHD, clinical blockade of IL-1, IL-2, or TNF-α has not been effective in GVHD prophylaxis.[299-301]

Treatment of Acute Graft-Versus-Host Disease

Therapy for acute GVHD requires both immunosuppression to blunt the T cell–induced tissue injury and appropriate supportive care. Corticosteroids are the mainstay of initial therapy for acute GVHD.[288,298,302,303] GVHD involving limited areas of the skin can be treated with topical corticosteroids alone. Oral beclomethasone can be used to treat early-stage GVHD of the upper gastrointestinal tract.[304] Corticosteroids (1 to 2 mg/kg/day prednisone) are initial therapy for more advanced GVHD and have response rates of 30% to 50%.[305-307] Alternative treatment regimens include cyclosporine or ATG alone or in combination with corticosteroids; however, no regimen has shown a consistent increase in response rates or improvement in survival compared to corticosteroids alone.[305,308,309] In a recent large randomized phase II trial comparing corticosteroids with MMF, pentostatin, etanercept, or denileukin diftitox, efficacy and toxicity data suggested the combination of MMF and corticosteroids to be most promising.[310] This combination is presently being tested in a phase III trial compared to corticosteroids alone for treatment of acute GVHD. Other investigational therapies include sirolimus, alemtuzumab, and infusion of mesenchymal stem cells. Prognosis is serious for patients with steroid-resistant disease, which is GVHD that does not respond to initial therapy with corticosteroids. Up to 10% to 40% of patients will respond to salvage therapy with ATG or other drugs such as sirolimus, tacrolimus, MMF, pentostatin, or cyclosporine, either as single agents or in combination.[311-314] Monoclonal antibodies and immunotoxins directed against T cells or inflammatory cytokines have been investigated, although their effectiveness has not been demonstrated outside of small case series. Specific agents with reported activity in steroid-refractory acute GVHD include pentostatin,[315] etanercept and infliximab (TNF-α receptor blockers),[316-318] daclizumab and denileukin diftitox (IL-2 receptor inhibitors),[319-321] and visilizumab (anti-CD3 antibody).[322] Extracorporeal photochemotherapy has also been reported to have some efficacy in cutaneous and hepatic steroid-refractory acute GVHD.[323] In addition to effective immunosuppression, successful management of acute GVHD involves attention to supportive care, particularly skin care, nutrition, and limitation of polypharmacy-associated drug interactions. Infections are a leading cause of death in patients with GVHD, and attention should be paid to infection surveillance and prophylaxis.

Chronic Graft-Versus-Host Disease

Risk Factors and Clinical Features

Chronic GVHD is a complex syndrome in recipients of allogeneic HCT that occurs later, typically between 3 to 7 months posttransplant, although it can also begin before 3 months and even beyond 2 years. Its incidence ranges from 30% to 50% in HLA-matched sibling donor transplants to 50% to 70% in HLA-matched URD transplants, and it is the leading cause of nonrelapse late mortality in allogeneic HCT survivors.[223,324-328] Recipients of UCB grafts have risks that are lower compared to matched adult URD HCT and comparable or even lower compared to matched related-donor HCT recipients.[99,282,283] Chronic GVHD occurs most frequently in patients with preceding acute GVHD but can also manifest de novo without any preceding acute GVHD. The distinction between classic chronic GVHD and overlap syndrome requires attention to clinical symptoms and signs.

Acute GVHD is the most important risk factor for development of subsequent chronic GVHD.[327,329] Use of mismatched or unrelated donors and transplantation using peripheral blood–derived hematopoietic stem cells instead of bone marrow also increases its risk.[280,328,330,331] Other reported risk factors for chronic GVHD include older recipient age, use of a female donor, CMV seropositivity, high graft $CD34^+$ cell count, treatment with donor lymphocyte infusion, and underlying diagnosis of chronic myeloid leukemia or aplastic anemia.[325-329] Similar to acute GVHD, in vitro or in vivo T cell–depletion of the graft can reduce the incidence of chronic GVHD.[292,332-334]

Chronic GVHD can affect any organ system; however, certain pathognomonic clinical signs and symptoms have to be present for establishing its diagnosis (Table 110-7).[260] Other clinical manifestations, though not diagnostic of chronic GVHD, can be characteristic, but they may resemble acute GVHD as well. Additional investigations, including biopsies, might be needed to verify the diagnosis and to rule out other causes, such as infections, drug effects, and malignancies.[335] The skin, mouth, eyes, and liver are the most commonly involved sites of chronic GHVD. The cutaneous manifestations resemble autoimmune disease and can include poikiloderma, lichen planus–like eruptions, or scleroderma (sclerosis). An inflammatory dermatitis can progress to severe dermal and periarticular fibrosis with loss of skin appendages (hair and sweat glands) as well as significant skin tightness, fasciitis, and loss of joint flexibility. Additional manifestations include dry eyes and dry mouth, which can resemble Sjögren syndrome clinically and histologically; enteritis with anorexia,

Table 110-7 Common Clinical Manifestations of Chronic Graft-Versus-Host Disease

Organ System	Clinical Manifestations
Cutaneous	Poikiloderma, lichen planus, dermal sclerosis, morphea-like features, hypopigmentation or hyperpigmentation, ichthyosis, nail dystrophy, onycholysis
Ocular	Keratoconjunctivitis sicca, conjunctivitis, corneal ulcerations
Oral	Lichen planus, hyperkeratotic plaques, xerostomia, mucosal atrophy, ulcers, restriction of mouth opening from sclerosis
Pulmonary	Bronchiolitis obliterans, bronchiolitis obliterans–organizing pneumonia
Gastrointestinal	Esophageal web and strictures, malabsorption syndrome, exocrine pancreatic insufficiency
Hepatic	Cholestasis
Genitourinary	Vaginal stenosis or scarring, lichen planus
Musculoskeletal	Fasciitis, joint contractures from sclerosis, myositis or polymyositis, arthritis
Hematopoietic	Thrombocytopenia, eosinophilia, lymphopenia, hemolytic anemia, hypogammaglobulinemia

early satiety, malabsorption, weight loss and failure to thrive, or esophageal dysmotility or stricture; and cholestatic (or sometimes hepatitic) jaundice. Pulmonary involvement in the form of bronchiolitis obliterans is an uncommon manifestation but can be particularly debilitating and dangerous. In addition, the profound immune dysfunction associated with chronic GVHD due to hypogammaglobulinemia, impaired cellular immunity, and functional asplenia, greatly increases the risk for secondary infections from bacteria, viruses, and fungi. After the onset of chronic GVHD, 25% to 40% of patients die within 2 years, often of secondary infections.[324,325,327]

Chronic GVHD can be classified as mild, moderate, or severe depending on the number of organs involved and the degree of individual organ involvement.[260] In general, factors associated with an adverse prognosis include thrombocytopenia, progressive onset from acute GVHD, poor performance status, lack of response to initial therapy, and extensive skin or lung involvement.[324,325,336]

Treatment of Chronic Graft-Versus-Host Disease

Although acute GVHD is one of the strongest predictors for chronic GVHD, strategies to limit acute GVHD, such as prolonging or intensifying initial immunosuppression, have not been consistently effective in preventing subsequent chronic GVHD.[337,338] As with acute GVHD, the specific immunosuppressive therapy for chronic GVHD is most often corticosteroids, usually in combination with cyclosporine.[339,340] The ongoing and long-lasting nature of the syndrome demands that reduced doses and, if possible, alternate-day steroid therapy be used to minimize chronic complications of prolonged corticosteroid therapy. Typical corticosteroid regimens start with daily prednisone 1 mg/kg/day, and responding patients are tapered down to 0.5 to 1 mg/kg every other day and continued on this dose for 6 to 9 months beyond any active GVHD symptoms, followed by a slow withdrawal of immunosuppression. Longer therapy may be required for some patients, and early withdrawal of therapy has been frequently accompanied by flares of chronic GVHD. Salvage therapies, including high-dose corticosteroids, sirolimus, tacrolimus, MMF, thalidomide, azathioprine, and hydroxychloroquine, have been tried with limited response rates.[326] Newer approaches currently being investigated as potential therapies for chronic GVHD include modulation of T-cell function, B-cell depletion, induction of immune tolerance, and cytokine blockade.[337] Small uncontrolled studies have reported the use of pentostatin, alemtuzumab, and ATG to inhibit T-cell function and rituximab to eliminate B cells with response rates of 30% to 50%.[298,332,334,341,342] T-cell immunomodulation using extracorporeal photopheresis has been shown to have some activity, especially in sclerotic cutaneous chronic GVHD.[343,344] Preliminary studies using daclizumab, etanercept, and infliximab for blockade of the cytokine-mediated inflammatory response have also shown short-term responses.[316,345] The treatment of chronic GVHD demands particular attention to prophylaxis and aggressive therapy of secondary opportunistic infections. Most successful strategies for treating chronic GVHD incorporate long-term reduced-dose immunosuppressive therapy, aggressive antimicrobial prophylaxis, and supportive care. Strategies are being studied that favor development of donor-derived regulatory T cells (Tregs), which may facilitate the development of immunologic tolerance, including avoidance of calcineurin inhibitors (cyclosporine or tacrolimus) or photopheresis.

FUTURE DIRECTIONS

Complications of HCT are one of the major barriers to the wider application of transplantation for a variety of diseases. The impact of newer transplantation modalities, including the use of nonmyeloablative or reduced-intensity conditioning regimens, alternative donor transplantation with UCB, and incorporation of immune-based therapies within transplantation regimens, on early and late complications are areas of vigorous current investigation. Better tools to predict the risk for post-HCT complications and nonrelapse mortality are needed as well.[346,347] Genomic and proteomic approaches to HCT complications are being investigated to monitor and predict complications.[348,349] Although they are some years from use in clinical practice, these approaches could have many potential applications in transplantation, including prediction of risk for complications and GVHD, refining donor selection, and use of pharmacogenomic data to individualize conditioning regimens and immunosuppression, all to improve the safety and effectiveness of HCT.

SUGGESTED READINGS

Arfons LM, Tomblyn M, Rocha V, et al: Second hematopoietic stem cell transplantation in myeloid malignancies. *Curr Opin Hematol* 16:112, 2009.

Armenian SH, Sun CL, Kawashima T, et al: Long-term health-related outcomes in survivors of childhood cancer treated with HSCT versus conventional therapy: A report from the Bone Marrow Transplant Survivor Study (BMTSS) and Childhood Cancer Survivor Study (CCSS). *Blood* 118:1413, 2011.

Boeckh M, Ljungman P: How we treat cytomegalovirus in hematopoietic cell transplant recipients. *Blood* 113:5711, 2009.

Corey L, Boeckh M: Persistent fever in patients with neutropenia. *N Engl J Med* 346:222, 2002.

Ferrara JL, Levine JE, Reddy P, et al: Graft-versus-host disease. *Lancet* 373:1550, 2009.

Filipovich AH, Weisdorf D, Pavletic S, et al: National Institutes of Health consensus development project on criteria for clinical trials in chronic graft-versus-host disease: I. Diagnosis and staging working group report. *Biol Blood Marrow Transplant* 11:945, 2005.

Freifeld AG, Bow EJ, Sepkowitz KA, et al: Clinical practice guideline for the use of antimicrobial agents in neutropenic patients with cancer: 2010 Update by the Infectious Diseases Society of America. *Clin Infect Dis* 52:427, 2011.

Gooley TA, Chien JW, Pergam SA, et al: Reduced mortality after allogeneic hematopoietic-cell transplantation. *N Engl J Med* 363:2091, 2010.

Ho VT, Revta C, Richardson PG: Hepatic veno-occlusive disease after hematopoietic stem cell transplantation: Update on defibrotide and other current investigational therapies. *Bone Marrow Transplant* 41:229, 2008.

MacMillan ML, Weisdorf DJ, Brunstein CG, et al: Acute graft-versus-host disease after unrelated donor umbilical cord blood transplantation: Analysis of risk factors. *Blood* 113:2410, 2009.

Majhail NS: Secondary cancers following allogeneic haematopoietic cell transplantation in adults. *Br J Haematol* 154:301, 2011.

Majhail NS, Parks K, Defor TE, et al: Diffuse alveolar hemorrhage and infection-associated alveolar hemorrhage following hematopoietic stem cell transplantation: Related and high-risk clinical syndromes. *Biol Blood Marrow Transplant* 12:1038, 2006.

McDonald GB: Hepatobiliary complications of hematopoietic cell transplantation, 40 years on. *Hepatology* 51:1450, 2010.

Panoskaltsis-Mortari A, Griese M, Madtes DK, et al: An official American Thoracic Society research statement: Noninfectious lung injury after hematopoietic stem cell transplantation: Idiopathic pneumonia syndrome. *Am J Respir Crit Care Med* 183:1262, 2011.

Pappas PG, Kauffman CA, Andes D, et al: Clinical practice guidelines for the management of candidiasis: 2009 update by the Infectious Diseases Society of America. *Clin Infect Dis* 48:503, 2009.

Rizzo JD, Curtis RE, Socie G, et al: Solid cancers after allogeneic hematopoietic cell transplantation. *Blood* 113:1175, 2009.

Rizzo JD, Wingard JR, Tichelli A, et al: Recommended screening and preventive practices for long-term survivors after hematopoietic cell transplantation: Joint recommendations of the European Group for Blood and Marrow Transplantation, the Center for International Blood and Marrow Transplant Research, and the American Society of Blood and Marrow Transplantation. *Biol Blood Marrow Transplant* 12:138, 2006.

Sun CL, Francisco L, Baker KS, et al: Adverse psychological outcomes in long-term survivors of hematopoietic cell transplantation: A report from the Bone Marrow Transplant Survivor Study. *Blood* 118:4723, 2011.

Sun CL, Francisco L, Kawashima T, et al: Prevalence and predictors of chronic health conditions after hematopoietic cell transplantation: A report from the Bone Marrow Transplant Survivor Study. *Blood* 116:3129, 2010.

Tomblyn M, Chiller T, Einsele H, et al: Guidelines for preventing infectious complications among hematopoietic cell transplantation recipients: A global perspective. *Biol Blood Marrow Transplant* 15:1143, 2009.

Upton A, Kirby KA, Carpenter P, et al: Invasive aspergillosis following hematopoietic cell transplantation: Outcomes and prognostic factors associated with mortality. *Clin Infect Dis* 44:531, 2007.

van Burik JA, Brunstein CG: Infectious complications following unrelated cord blood transplantation. *Vox Sang* 92:289, 2007.

van Burik JA, Weisdorf DJ: Infections in recipients of blood and marrow transplantation. *Hematol Oncol Clin North Am* 13:1065, 1999. viii.

Walsh TJ, Anaissie EJ, Denning DW, et al: Treatment of aspergillosis: Clinical practice guidelines of the Infectious Diseases Society of America. *Clin Infect Dis* 46:327, 2008.

Weisdorf D: GVHD—the nuts and bolts. *Hematology Am Soc Hematol Educ Program* 62, 2007.

Wingard JR: The changing face of invasive fungal infections in hematopoietic cell transplant recipients. *Curr Opin Oncol* 17:89, 2005.

Wingard JR, Carter SL, Walsh TJ, et al: Randomized, double-blind trial of fluconazole versus voriconazole for prevention of invasive fungal infection after allogeneic hematopoietic cell transplantation. *Blood* 116:5111, 2010.

Wingard JR, Majhail NS, Brazauskas R, et al: Long-term survival and late deaths after allogeneic hematopoietic cell transplantation. *J Clin Oncol* 29:2230, 2011.

Yanik GA, Ho VT, Levine JE, et al: The impact of soluble tumor necrosis factor receptor etanercept on the treatment of idiopathic pneumonia syndrome after allogeneic hematopoietic stem cell transplantation. *Blood* 112:3073, 2008.

For complete list of references log on to www.expertconsult.com.

PART XI

TRANSFUSION MEDICINE

CHAPTER 111

HUMAN BLOOD GROUP ANTIGENS AND ANTIBODIES

Connie M. Westhoff, Jill R. Storry, and Beth H. Shaz

Pretransfusion testing includes ABO and Rh type and antibody screening to determine whether a patient has an unexpected red blood cell (RBC) antibody. If the antibody screen is positive, an identification panel is performed to identify the specificity of the antibody. Unexpected antibodies can be clinically significant causing hemolysis (e.g., acute or delayed hemolytic reaction) after transfusion of RBCs carrying the reciprocal antigen, or can be insignificant. The clinical significance of an antibody is assessed by correlating the serologic information with clinical experiences reported in the literature and with the patient's medical history. Notably, the majority of clinically significant antibodies (outside the ABO system) are in response to RBC antigen exposure either through transfusion or pregnancy. Other antibody characteristics that are used to predict clinical significance include immunoglobulin class and in vitro characteristics such as strength of reactivity and titer; however, no foolproof method exists to predict the clinical significance. For antibodies with well-known clinical significance, antigen-negative blood is selected for transfusion. Predicting clinical significance is more difficult when a patient has an antibody to a novel or rare high-prevalence antigen and requires a transfusion but antigen-negative blood is not available.

ERYTHROCYTE BLOOD GROUP ANTIGENS

Erythrocyte blood group antigens are polymorphic, inherited, carbohydrate or protein structures located on the surface of the RBC membrane. There are more than 300 blood group antigens, most of which are included in 30 different blood group systems (Table 111-1). The protein antigens are primarily located on integral transmembrane proteins, but a few are on glycosylphosphatidylinositol (GPI)–linked proteins (Fig. 111-1). Some antigens are carbohydrates attached to proteins or lipids, some require a combination of a specific portion of protein and carbohydrate, and a few antigens are carried on proteins that are adsorbed from the plasma. Many of the proteins carrying blood group antigens reside in the erythrocyte membrane as complexes with other proteins.

Recognition of a new blood group antigen begins with discovery of an antibody. When an individual whose RBCs lack an antigen is exposed to RBCs that possess the antigen, he or she may mount an immune response and produce antibodies that react with the antigen. Depending on the characteristics of the antibody and the number and topology of antigens in the RBC membrane, the interaction in vivo between antibody and antigen may result in removal of antibody-coated red cells by the reticuloendothelial system or in hemolysis if complement is activated.

In blood group testing, most assays are designed to detect antibody-antigen binding with clumping of the RBCs as the detectable endpoint. The ability to detect and identify blood group antigens and antibodies has contributed significantly to current safe supportive blood transfusion practice, to the appropriate management of pregnancies at-risk for hemolytic disease of the fetus and newborn (HDFN), and to management of hematopoietic progenitor cell and solid organ transplantation.

Terminology

Some blood group systems bear the family surname in which the antibody was first discovered (Kell, Kidd, Duffy, etc.), with abbreviations to indicate antigens (K/k, Jk^a/Jk^b, and Fy^a/Fy^b etc.). Others have been given letter designations (A, B, D, M, N, etc.). A committee for terminology of RBC surface antigens and alleles, organized by the International Society of Blood Transfusion (ISBT), works to standardize terminology of new blood group antigens and the coding alleles.

DNA-Based Typing for Blood Group Antigens

The majority of genes encoding blood group antigens have been identified and cloned,[1] and the molecular basis of most blood group antigens has been determined.[2,3] Details concerning the alleles associated with blood group antigens are found on the ISBT nomenclature and the Blood Group Antigen Gene Mutation Database (BGMUT) websites (www.ncbi.nlm.nih.gov/gv/mhc/xslcgi.cgi?cmd=bgmut/home; www.isbtweb.org/working-parties/red-cell-immunogenetics-and-blood-group-terminology/). Knowledge of the genes has advanced understanding of the structure and function of the components carrying antigens and resulted in an appreciation of diseases associated with loss of expression of some blood groups—for example, null phenotypes (Table 111-1). Of importance, knowledge of the gene has made it possible to perform DNA analyses to predict the serologic phenotype, to determine gene dosage (zygosity), to perform noninvasive fetal typing, and to type for numerous blood group antigens in a single assay.

Although the simple hemagglutination test remains the principal assay for RBC antigen typing for ABO and Rh, antibody screen, and compatibility testing; genotyping for minor blood group antigens has become commonplace in several clinical situations (Table 111-2). These include determination of the extended blood group phenotype in patients who are multiply transfused, which avoids false typing due to contaminating donor RBCs and aids determination of antibody specificity. This approach is also preferred in patients with strongly DAT-positive RBCs, as well as for typing for antigens when no serologic reagents are available and for fetal typing from amniocytes or from free DNA present in the maternal plasma. In these instances and others (Table 111-2), hemagglutination is not helpful and genomic analysis is a useful adjunct to routine testing. High-throughput genotyping systems have enabled blood centers to screen donors for a large number of antigens in a single assay.

Blood Group Antibodies

The common causes of immunization against blood group antigens are transfusion, pregnancy, transplantation, or occasionally, practices such as sharing needles. "Naturally occurring" antibodies are not a result of RBC exposure; rather, microbes encountered by way of the

Table 111-1 Blood Group Systems, Antigens, Expression, and Disease Associations

ISBT System Name (Number)	Gene Name (ISBT)	Predicted Topology (Number of Amino Acids AA)	Component Name	Principal Associated Blood Group Antigens (null phenotype)	Present in Other Tissue	Disease Association	Function
ABO (001)	*ABO*	Glycosyl-transferases Type II (354 AA)	Carbohydrate	A, B, AB, A1 (group O)	Secretions, platelets, broad tissue distribution	Altered in some hematologic disorders, leukemia	Glycosylation
MNS (002)	*GYPA (MN)* *GYPB (Ss)*	Type I (131 AA) Type I (72 AA)	GPA GPB	M, N, S, s, U, Vw; $M^k M^k$ lack GPA and GPB; En(a–) lack GPA; S–s–U– lack GPB	Renal endothelium and epithelium	Decreased *P. falciparum* invasion May be receptor for *E. coli*	Negative charge on sialic acid; receptor for microbes
P (003)	*A4GALT*	Galactosyl-transferase Type II (353 AA)	Carbohydrate	P1, Pk (P1–, PP1Pk–)	Lymphocytes, granulocytes, monocytes, platelets	Receptor *E. coli* and *Parvovirus-B19* Miscarriage	Glycosylation
Rh (004)	*RHD* *RHCE*	Multipass—12 spans (417 AA)	RhD RhCE	D, C, E, c, e, G, V/VS (Rh_{null} syndrome)	RBC-specific	Hemolytic anemia; stomatocytosis Reduced expression and mosaicism in hematologic malignancies	Structural link to underlying cytoskeleton
Lutheran (005)	*LU*	Type I IgSF (597 AA) (557 AA)	Lutheran glycoprotein B-CAM	Lu^a, Lu^b, Lu3, Au^a, Au^b (recessive Lu(a–b–))	Broad tissue distribution Not on lymphocytes, granulocytes, monocytes or platelets	Increased expression possibly involved in vasoocclusion in sickle cell disease	Possibly adhesion; may mediate intracellular signaling Binds to laminin
Kell (006)	*KEL*	Type II (732 AA)	Kell glycoprotein	K, k, Kp^a, Kp^b, Ku, Js^a, Js^b (K_0 or K_{null})	Broad tissue distribution Bone marrow, fetal liver, testes, brain, heart, skeletal muscle	Depressed in McLeod syndrome (see XK)	Cleaves big endothelin 3 to ET-3 (a potent vasoconstrictor)
Lewis (007)	*FUT3 (LE)*	Not endogenous to RBCs Type II (361 AA)	Carbohydrate Adsorbed from plasma	Le^a, Le^b, Le^{ab}, Le^{bh}, ALe^b, BLe^b (Le(a–b–))	Saliva and body fluids Blood cells, GI, skeletal muscle, kidney, adrenal	Increased expression in fucosisdosis	Fucosyl transferase
Duffy (008)	*DARC (FY)*	Multipass—7 spans (338 AA)	Fy glycoprotein	Fy^a, Fy^b, Fy3, Fy6 (Fy(a–b–))	Broad tissue distribution Endothelial and epithelial cells, Purkinje cells, colon, lung, spleen, thyroid, thymus, kidney	*Plasmodium vivax* receptor RBC null-resistant to *P. vivax*	Chemokine receptor
Kidd (009)	*SLC14A1 (JK)*	Multipass—10 spans (389 AA)	Kidd glycoprotein	Jk^a, Jk^b, Jk3 (Jk(a–b–) or Jk_{null})	Kidney: vasa recta endothelium Renal medulla	Urine concentrating defect	Urea transport
Diego (010)	*SLC4A1 (DI)*	Multipass—14 spans (911 AA)	Band 3, AE1 (anion exchanger 1)	Di^a, Di^b, Wr^a, Wr^b, (1 reported—transfusion dependent; predicted to be incompatible with life)	Kidney: intercalated cells of distal and collecting tubules	Southeast Asian ovalocytosis, hereditary spherocytosis, renal tubular acidosis	Anion transport CO_2/HCO_3^- exchange
Yt (011)	*ACHE (YT)*	GPI-linked (557 AA)	Acetyl-cholinesterase	Yt^a, Yt^b	Brain, muscle, nerves	Absent from PNH III RBCs	Enzymatic

Continued

Table 111-1 Blood Group Systems, Antigens, Expression, and Disease Associations—cont'd

ISBT System Name (Number)	Gene Name (ISBT)	Predicted Topology (Number of Amino Acids AA)	Component Name	Principal Associated Blood Group Antigens (null phenotype)	Present in Other Tissue	Disease Association	Function
Xg (012)	*MIC2 (XG1)*	Type I (180 AA) (163 AA)	Xg[a] glycoprotein	Xg[a]	The antigen may be restricted to RBC, but CD99 has broad tissue distribution		Adhesion molecule
Scianna (013)	*ERMAP (SC)*	Type I (475 AA)	ERMAP	Sc1, Sc2, Sc3, Rd (Sc –1, –2, –3)			Possible adhesion
Dombrock (014)	*ART4 (DO)*	GPI-linked (314 AA)	Do glycoprotein; ART 4	Do[a], Do[b], Gy[a], Hy, Jo[a] (Gy(a–))	Lymphocytes, spleen, lymph notes, GI, ovary, testes, heart, liver	Absent from PNH III RBCs	Enzymatic
Colton (015)	*AQP1 (CO)*	Multipass—6 spans (269 AA)	Aquaporin	Co[a], Co[b], Co3 (Co(a–b–))	Broad tissue distribution Kidney, liver, gallbladder, eye, capillary endothelium	Monosomy 7, congenital dyserythropoietic anemia	Water transport
Landsteiner-Wiener (016)	*ICAM4 (LW)*	Type I IgSF (241 AA)	LW glycoprotein ICAM-4	LW[a], LW[b], LW[ab] (LW(a–b–))		Depressed in some malignant diseases; decreased in Rh_{null} syndrome	Ligand for integrins
Chido/Rodgers (017)	*C4A, C4B (CH/RG)*	Not endogenous to RBC (1191 AA)	C4A; C4B	Ch1, Ch2, Rg1	Adsorbed from plasma	Certain phenotypes increased susceptibility to autoimmune conditions and infections C4-deficient predisposes for SLE	Part of the complement cascade
H (018)	*FUT1(H)*	Fucosyl-transferase Type II (365 AA)	Carbohydrate	H (Bombay O_h)	Broad distribution Soluble—all fluids except CSF in secretors	Decreased in some tumor cells Increased in hematopoietic stress	Glycosylation
Kx (019)	*XK (XK)*	Multipass—10 spans (444 AA)	XK glycoprotein	Kx (McLeod)	Fetal liver, adult skeletal muscle, brain, pancreas, heart	X-linked midlife onset neuropathy, elevated CPK, muscular dystrophy, acanthocytosis; sometimes associated with CGD	Transport; possible neuro-transmitter
Gerbich (020)	*GYPC (GE)*	Type I (128 AA) (107 AA)	GPC GPD	Ge2, Ge3, Ge4 (Leach phenotype)	Fetal liver, renal endothelium	Hereditary elliptocytosis, hemolytic anemia, receptor *P. falciparum*	Structural Interacts with protein 4.1 and p55
Cromer (021)	*CD55 (CROM)*	GPI-linked (347 AA)	DAF	Cr[a], Tc[a], Tc[b], Tc[c], Dr[a], Es[a], IFC (Inab)	Vascular endothelium Epithelial GI, GU, CNS Soluble form in plasma and urine	Absent from PNH III RBCs Dr[a] is receptor for uropathogenic *E. coli*	Complement regulation; binds C3b; disassembles C3/C5 convertase

Table 111-1 Blood Group Systems, Antigens, Expression, and Disease Associations—cont'd

ISBT System Name (Number)	Gene Name (ISBT)	Predicted Topology (Number of Amino Acids AA)	Component Name	Principal Associated Blood Group Antigens (null phenotype)	Present in Other Tissue	Disease Association	Function
Knops (022)	*CR1 (KN)*	Type I (1998 AA)	CR1	Kn[a], Kn[b], McC[a], Sl[a], Yk[a], KCAM (no nulls reported)	Blood cells, glomerular podocytes, follicular dendritic cells	Antigens depressed in certain autoimmune and malignant conditions	Complement regulation; binds C3b and C4b; mediates phagocytosis
Indian (023)	*CD44 (IN)*	Type I (341 AA)	Hermes antigen	In[a], In[b]	Wide tissue distribution	1 case—congenital dyserythropoietic anemia	Binds hyaluronic acid; mediates adhesion of leukocytes
Ok (024)	*BSG (OK)*	Type I IgSF (248 AA)	Basigin	Ok[a]	All cells tested	Receptor *Plasmodium falciparum*	Possible adhesion
RAPH (025)	*MER2*	Multipass—4 spans (253 AA)	CD151	MER2 (Raph–)	Fibroblasts	Absence associated with renal disease and kidney failure	
JMH (026)	*SEMA-L (JMH)*	GPI-linked (656 AA)	Semaphorin 7A	JMH		Absent from PNHIII RBCs	Adhesion molecule
I (027)	*GCNT2*	*N*-acetyl-glucosaminyl-transferase type II (400 AA)	Carbohydrate	I (I– or i adult)	Broad tissue distribution	Cataracts in Asians	Glycosylation
Globoside (028)	*B3GALT3 or βGalNAcT1*	*N*-acetyl-galactosaminyl-transferase type II (331 AA)	Carbohydrate (Gb_4, globoside)	P (P–) P[k] and p	Broad tissue distribution Placenta (trophoblasts and interstitial cells)	Receptor *E. coli* and *Parvovirus-B19* Spontaneous abortion	Glycosylation
GIL (029)	*AQP3 (GIL)*	Multipass—6 spans (292 AA)	AQP3	GIL (GIL–)	Board tissue distribution Kidney, prostate, GI tract, spleen, skin, eye		Glycerol/ water/ urea transport
RHAG (030)	*RHAG*	Multipass—12 spans (409 AA)	Rh-associated glycoprotein	RHAG1 or Duclos, RHAG2 or Ol[a], RHAG3 or DL, RHAG4 (Rh_{null} regulator)	RBC-specific but homologs RhBG, RhCG in kidney, liver, skin, GI tract	Hereditary overhydrated stomatocytosis	Ammonia transport

IgSF, Immunoglobulin super family; *ISGN*, International Society for Gene Nomenclature; *type I*, protein with a single pass through the RBC lipid bilayer with its amino terminus to the outside of the cell; *type II*, protein with a single pass through the RBC lipid bilayer with its amino terminus to the inside of the cell.

Table 111-2 Uses of DNA-Based Genotyping Assays for Transfusion Medicine

- Type patients who have been recently transfused
- Type RBCs coated with immunoglobulin
- Type patients with AIHA (to select antigen-negative RBCs for transfusion and absorption of autoantibodies when searching for under-lying alloantibodies)
- Type RBCs when commercial antisera are not available
- Type for numerous blood group antigens in a single assay
- Identify weak D and partial D (to determine candidate for Rh immune globulin or avoid use of limited Rh-negative donor supply)
- Resolve blood group typing discrepancies
- Determine paternal zygosity for *RHD* and HPA
- Type fetus to determine risk for HDFN or NAIT

digestive tract and other mucosal surfaces regularly (e.g., anti-A, -B,) or sometimes (e.g., anti-M, -P, -P[k], -P1, -Le[a], -Le[b], -I, -IH) result in production of antibodies with these specificities. These are the most common antibodies present in children and nontransfused male patients and are primarily IgM. These multivalent IgM antibodies directed to carbohydrate antigens optimally bind and directly agglutinate to RBCs at temperatures below 37° C. Most are not clinically significant (outside of ABO). Exceptions occur if the antibody is reactive at 37° C and/or has an IgG component. Antibodies that are considered not to be clinically significant unless the antibody reacts in tests performed at 37° C include those to A1, P1, M, N, Lu[a], Le[a], Le[b], I, IH, and Sd[a] antigens.

In contrast, antibodies occurring following immunization to protein antigens such as those in the Rh, Kell, Kidd, and Duffy blood group systems are primarily of the IgG isotype that react at 37° C and are detected by the indirect antiglobulin test (IAT). These bivalent antibodies optimally bind to, but do not directly agglutinate, RBCs at 37° C. The addition of an antiglobulin reagent (i.e.,

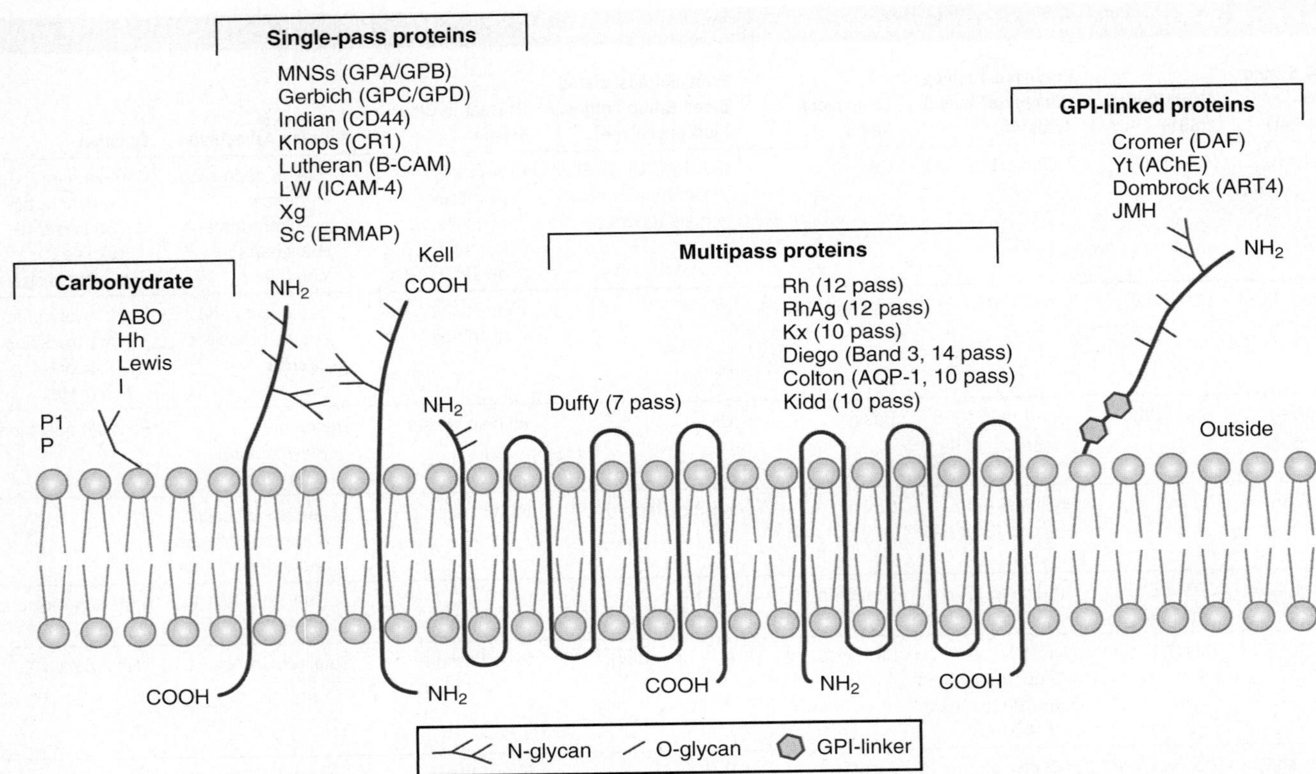

Figure 111-1 MODEL OF BLOOD GROUP PROTEINS IN THE RED BLOOD CELL (RBC) MEMBRANE. Schematic representation of the RBC molecules that carry blood group antigens and the predicted structure. These include carbohydrates, single and multipass proteins, and GPI-linked proteins in the RBC membrane.

antihuman IgG, also known as Coombs serum) is required to induce RBC agglutination. Most of these are clinically significant antibodies, with the exception of antibodies to Knops (KN), Chido/Rodgers (CH/RG) and JMH systems (Table 111-3 summarizes the immunoglobulin class and clinical significance associated with alloantibodies; see also box on Indirect Antiglobulin Test and Direct Antiglobulin Test).

Antibodies recognizing antigens in the ABO system are by far the most clinically significant and are present in nearly all individuals who lack the antigen (they typically appear by 4 months of age). Other clinically significant antibodies occur in the following approximate order, from the most to the least commonly encountered in transfusion practice: anti-D, anti-K, anti-E, anti-c, anti-Fy^a, anti-C, anti-Jk^a, anti-S, and anti-Jk^b. Clinically significant antibodies occur in 2% to 3% of immunized patients[4] but have a higher incidence of 35% to 55% in patients undergoing chronic transfusion.[5-8] The frequency of antibody production depends on the antigen immunogenicity and prevalence of the antigen in a population.

Compatibility Procedures and Location of Antigen-Negative Blood

Manual tube or gel-column methods based on agglutination of RBCs are the most common serologic assays performed in transfusion medicine laboratories.

ABO

Commercially available mouse monoclonal anti-A and anti-B are used to determine ABO type, and these reagents directly agglutinate RBCs at room temperature. To confirm the RBC ABO reactivity, the

Indirect Antiglobulin Test and Direct Antiglobulin Test

The indirect antiglobulin test (IAT) is used to detect alloantibodies in patient sera, or RBCs coated with antibody in vitro following incubation at 37° C, for example, antibody screening and identification, antigen typing, and crossmatching with donor RBCs. After incubation, unbound antibodies are removed from the RBCs by washing with saline, and an antiglobulin reagent containing either antihuman IgG or a mixture of antihuman IgG and monoclonal antihuman complement is added. Agglutination of all cells suggests the presence of an antibody to a high-prevalence antigen or the presence of an autoantibody; differential reactivity suggests the presence of antibodies to one or more specific RBC antigens.

The direct antiglobulin test (DAT) is used to detect the presence of antibody or complement (or both) on the surface of RBCs in vivo such as autoantibodies coating the patient's cells in warm autoimmune hemolytic anemia, cold hemagglutinin disease, or alloantibodies coating the patient's cells in immediate or delayed transfusion reactions or hemolytic disease of the fetus and newborn. Patient RBCs obtained in ethylenediaminetetraacetic acid (EDTA) are washed with saline and then incubated with a commercial antiglobulin reagent containing antihuman IgG or antihuman complement or a mixture of the two. Antiglobulin reagents containing anti-IgM or anti-IgA are available in specialized centers to detect coating of RBCs in vivo by antibodies of these isotypes.

Table 111-3 Characteristics of Some Blood Group Alloantibodies (Listed in Approximate Order of Clinical Significance)

Antibody Specificity	IgM	IgG	Clinical	
			Transfusion Reaction	HDFN
ABO	Most	Some	Immediate; mild to severe	Common; mild to moderate
H in Bombay	Most	Some	Immediate; mild to severe	Rare; Mild
Rh	Some	Most	Immediate/delayed; mild to severe	Common; mild to severe
RhAG	Rare	Most	Immediate/delayed; mild to severe	Mild to severe
Kell	Some	Most	Immediate/delayed; mild to severe	Mild to severe
Kidd	Few	Most	Immediate/delayed; mild to severe	Rare; mild
Duffy	Rare	Most	Immediate/delayed; mild to severe	Rare; mild
S	Some	Most	Delayed/mild	Rare; mild to severe
s	Rare	Most	Delayed/mild	Rare; mild to severe
U	Rare	Most	Immediate/delayed; mild to severe	Rare; severe
PP1P^k	Most*	Most*	Immediate; Mild to severe	Mild to severe†
Vel	Most*	Most*	Immediate/delayed; Mild to severe	Mild to severe
Diego	Some	Most	Delayed; none to severe	Mild to severe
Colton	Rare	Most	Delayed; mild	Rare; mild to severe
Lutheran	Some	Most	Delayed	Rare; mild
Dombrock	Rare	Most	Immediate/delayed; mild to severe	Rare; mild
M	Some	Most	Delayed (rare)	Rare; mild to severe
N	Most	Rare	None	None
LW^a	Rare	Most	Delayed; none to mild	Rare; mild
Yt^a	Rare	Most	Delayed (rare); none to mild	None
Ch/Rg	Rare	Most	Anaphylactic (rare)	None
JMH	Rare	Most	Delayed (rare in genetic variants); none to mild	None
P1	Most	Rare	None (Rare)	None
Le^a	Most	Few	Immediate (Rare)	None
Le^b	Most	Few	None	None
I	Most	Rare	None None to mild in I adults	None
Knops	Rare	Most	None	None
Xg^a	Rare	Most	None	None

HDFN, Hemolytic disease of the fetus and newborn.
*Most examples of these antibodies are both IgM and IgG.
†Seldom hemolysis of fetal cells but high incidence of recurrent spontaneous abortions.

plasma is tested for the presence of the corresponding agglutinins by testing with commercially available group A1 and group B RBCs. In both tests, agglutination is macroscopically visible.

Rh

Patient and donor RBCs are routinely tested for the presence of the D antigen in the Rh system. Reagents containing monoclonal anti-D that directly agglutinate D-positive RBCs (Rh-positive) suspended in saline at room temperature are commonly used for testing. Testing for expression of a weak D antigen on RBCs is required for donor centers, but is usually not performed on patient samples. Exceptions include typing the RBCs of a newborn when the mother is D-negative to determine whether she is a candidate for Rh immune globulin (RhIG) (see box on Rh Immune Globulin).

Antibody Screening

Patient plasma is incubated at 37° C with commercially available reagent RBCs of known antigen type. After incubation, unbound antibodies are removed by washing with saline, and an antiglobulin reagent containing either antihum an IgG (AHG), or a mixture of antihuman IgG and antihuman complement, is added. If the test is positive, the specificity of the antibody is determined by testing the plasma against a panel of different reagent RBCs (usually 10) varying in antigen phenotype (e.g. antibody identification).

Compatibility Testing

Once a patient is actively immunized to an RBC antigen and produces a clinically significant alloantibody, the patient is considered

Rh Immune Globulin

RhIG is a human plasma–derived hyperimmunoglobulin product consisting of IgG antibodies to D antigen that is administered to D-negative pregnant women who are at risk for D sensitization. RhIG is administered (a) at 28 weeks gestational age, (b) when there is a risk for fetal maternal hemorrhage through amniocentesis, trauma, or other procedures, and (c) postpartum in the case of a known or potential D-positive newborn or fetus. RhIG is sometimes administered outside of pregnancy to D-negative patients who receive D-positive blood products, most commonly platelet products. This is primarily considered for females of childbearing potential when the formation of anti-D has serious consequences. (Because the risk for D alloimmunization from platelet transfusion is less than 4%, the majority of D-incompatible platelets are given without RhIG administration.) RhIG in significantly higher doses is used to treat immune thrombocytopenic purpura (ITP) in patients who are D-positive and have not been spleenectomized.

For prevention of D-sensitization in the United States, 300 mcg are routinely administered, but dosing is increased if there is evidence of large fetal-maternal hemorrhage (300 mcg for every 15 mL of RBC exposure). The dose is calculated based on the estimated volume of D-positive RBCs from Kleihauer-Betke or flow cytometry testing. RhIG should be given within 72 hours, which was the time period for the original studies, but should not be withheld if not administered within this time period. Adverse events to low doses used to prevent D immunization include fever, chills, and pain at the injection site. Rarely, hypersensitivity reactions are noted. RhIG doses used to treat ITP are substantial: 50 mcg/kg for hemoglobin values ≥10 g/dL and 25 to 40 mcg/kg when hemoglobin is 8 to 10 g/dL. Adverse events include possible anemia, hemolysis, disseminated intravascular coagulopathy, and rarely, death.

immunized for life and should be transfused with antigen-negative RBCs, even if the antibody is no longer detectable. Patients with passively acquired antibody (e.g., neonates with maternal antibody; recipients of plasma and platelet products or Rh immune globulin) need to be transfused with antigen-negative RBCs only while the passive antibody is present. Selection of blood for transfusion to patients with alloantibodies requires typing of donor units for the corresponding antigen to identify antigen-negative units and crossmatch of the selected units with the patient's plasma. Antigen-negative units are provided by, or can be located by, most donor centers. Provision of antigen-negative blood will to some extent depend on the prevalence of the target antigen(s) in the donor population. Transfusion service staff is vital for communication between the patient's physician and/or consultant transfusion medicine specialist in order to determine the immediate and ongoing transfusion needs of the patient and to ensure that antigen-negative blood is available as appropriate. Understanding the risks and benefits of transfusion is important, as well as understanding the potential clinical significance of the antibody and the urgency of transfusion. When a patient's antibody is directed at a high-prevalence antigen, it is important to test siblings in the quest for compatible blood and to urge the patient to donate blood for long-term storage when clinical status permits. In hemolytic anemia due to warm-reactive autoantibodies, compatibility may be difficult to demonstrate. In this scenario, the important issue is to be sure that there are no clinically significant alloantibodies underlying the warm reactive autoantibodies.

Prevention of Alloimmunization

Transfusion management of patients who require chronic transfusion therapy, in particular patients with sickle cell disease, has been the subject of debate.[9-12] Many programs attempt to reduce or prevent alloimmunization by prophylactic transfusion of blood that is antigen-matched for C, E, and K. Some do antigen matching for these antigens and more, once the patient makes an antibody (Table 111-4). No consensus exists at present as to the best approach, although the goal is to prevent hemolytic or delayed transfusion reactions, which are known to be underreported because they can manifest as a sickle cell crisis.

Table 111-4 Approaches to Supplying Red Blood Cell Products to Prevent Alloimmunization in Patients with Sickle Cell Disease or Other Transfusion-Dependent Anemia

Phenotype or genotype for clinically significant antigens before transfusion
Provide phenotype-matched blood for C, E, and K prophylactically
Provide blood negative for the major antigens that the patient lacks after the patient makes an antibody

Blood Group Disease Association

The absence of some blood group antigens and their carrier molecules can result in disease. For example, an absence of the Rh and RhAG proteins causes stomatocytosis[13] and anemia, termed *Rh_{null} syndrome*. The absence of Xk protein is associated with the *McLeod syndrome.* RBCs and white blood cells from patients with leukocyte adhesion deficiency II (also known as *congenital disorder of glycosylation type II*) lack antigens that are dependent on fucose. The RBCs have the Le(a–b–) Bombay phenotype and the white blood cells lack siayl-Le^x, which explains the high white blood cell count and infections in these patients. Hemagglutination is a simple test that can be used to diagnose these syndromes. In patients with paroxysmal nocturnal hemoglobinuria, a proportion of the RBCs will lack antigens carried on GPI-linked proteins. Other associations between blood group antigens and diseases are summarized in Table 111-1.

Diseases associated with antibodies to blood group antigens include hemolytic disease of the newborn, warm autoimmune hemolytic anemia, cold hemagglutinin disease and paroxysmal cold hemoglobinuria. Hemagglutination is a valuable aid in diagnosis of these conditions.

Blood Group Systems

Presented here is a brief description of the most clinically relevant blood group systems in approximate order of clinical significance. For further information and prevalence of blood group antigens in different populations, refer to specialized texts such as *Human Blood Groups, The Blood Group Antigen Facts Book,* and the AABB *Technical Manual.*[2,3,14]

Carbohydrate Blood Groups

ABO and H

The ABO blood group system is by far the most clinically significant, because of the presence of naturally occurring IgM antibodies (and sometimes IgG). The original observation by Landsteiner that certain human erythrocyte suspensions were agglutinated by other human sera led to the recognition of ABO polymorphism. This initial observation is still the cornerstone of modern transfusion practice more than a century later.

Antigens and Their Synthesis. ABH antigens occur on glycoproteins and glycolipids and are synthesized in a stepwise fashion by glycosyltransferases that sequentially add specific monosaccharides in specific linkages to a growing oligosaccharide precursor chain (reviewed in Clausen and Hakomori[15]). The terminal sugar

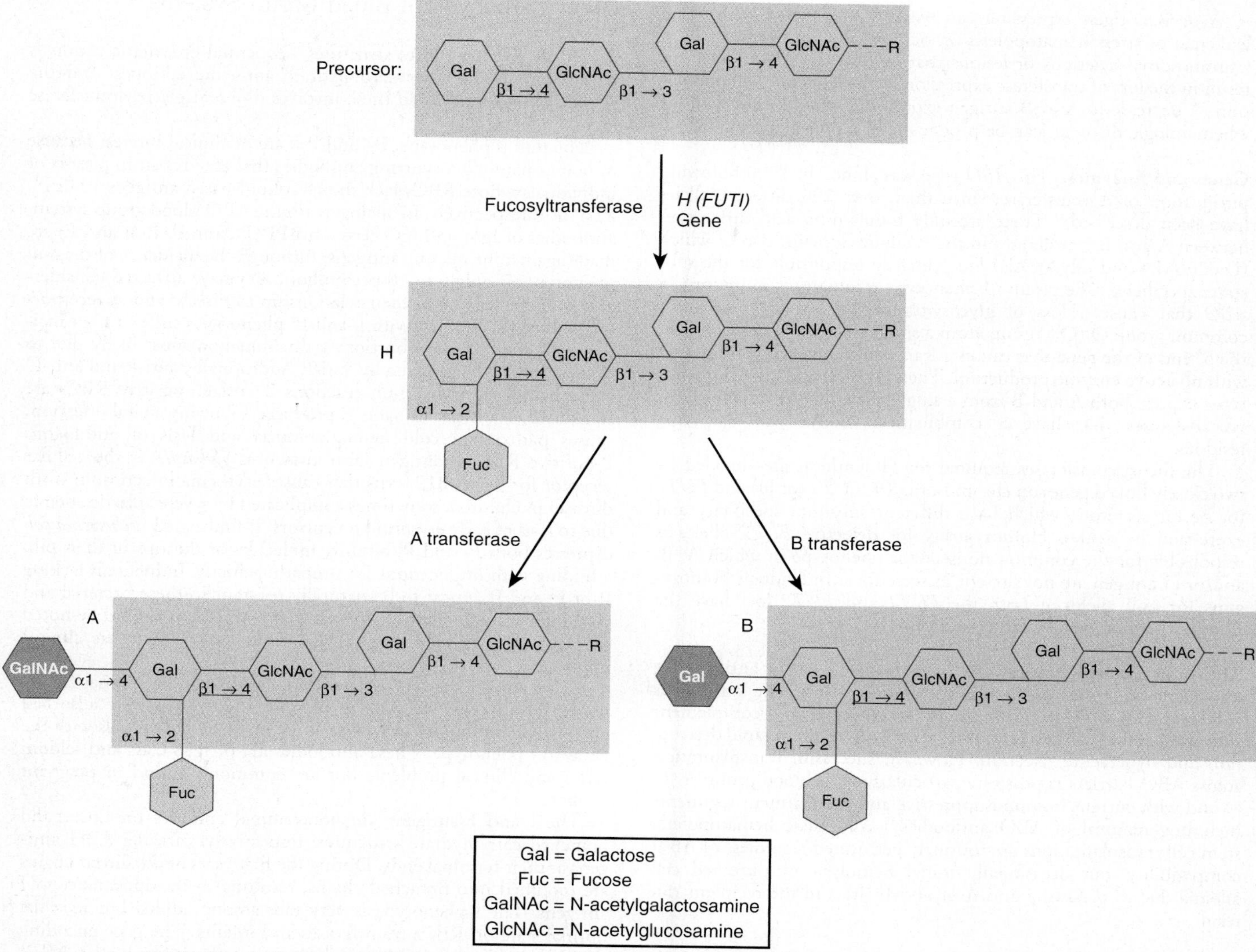

Figure 111-2 BIOCHEMICAL STRUCTURES OF ABH ANTIGENS. Schematic representation of the terminal portions of the carbohydrate structures carrying the H, A, and B antigens on RBCs.

determines antigen specificity (Fig. 111-2). Group O individuals have H antigen only, the terminal sugar of which is fucose, and this is the precursor substrate for A and B antigens. Group O individuals have defective A or B transferases. The A and B transferase enzymes differ only by the nature of the monosaccharide added to the chain. *N*-acetyl-D-galactosamine is added by A-transferase, and D-galactose is added by B-transferase. In clinical practice, four ABO phenotypes (A, B, O, and AB) are discriminated. In addition, two common variations of group A—A_1 and A_2—can be distinguished. The differences between A_1 and A_2 phenotypes are quantitative and qualitative. Not only is the A_1 transferase more efficient in converting H to A antigen (approximately 5 times more A sites per RBC on A_1 RBCs than on A_2 RBCs), it also has the capacity to make A_1 antigen on the repetitive A epitope. Quantitatively normal ABH expression also requires the branching of carbohydrate chains, which is performed by the blood group I enzyme. Some H antigen precursor remains on A and B RBCs in this order: $A_2 > B > A_2B > A_1 > A_1B$.

Inherited and Acquired ABH variants. In addition to the main ABO types, there are many other inherited phenotypes with a weaker expression of the specified antigen, for example, A_3, A_x, A_{el}, B_3, B(A), and cis-AB. This can cause problems in determining the ABO blood group, but for patients needing immediate transfusion, the selection of group O red cells and AB plasma products is an option. In blood donors, if very weak expression of A or B antigens is not detected, the major risk is that the red cells may be transfused to a patient whose antibodies may cause accelerated destruction of the transfused cells.

Rare Bombay (O_h) phenotype RBCs (first reported in Bombay, India) lack H antigen and, consequently, A and B antigens. Other variants with weak H expression on RBCs, with or without H in secretions, also occur (para-Bombay) and have been reviewed.[16] Of clinical relevance, potent anti-H with the same hemolytic potential as anti-A and anti-B can be produced by Bombay individuals. Anti-H is often found in para-Bombay individuals but is generally not a potent antibody. HDFN due to anti-H has not been reported.

Acquired B antigen is a rare phenomenon that results from the action of bacterial deacetylase, an enzyme that can remove an acetyl group from the A-terminal sugar, *N*-acetylgalactosamine. Galactosamine is similar to galactose, the B-specific terminal residue, and anti-B reagents can cross-react with the deacetylated structure. Acquired B can occur in individuals suffering from gram-negative infections of gastrointestinal origin or carcinoma and can be clinically significant if a patient's blood group is misinterpreted and group AB blood is transfused. Other polyagglutinable states (e.g., T, Tn, Tk) are detected by naturally occurring antibodies found in the serum of most people; these can be identified by a panel of lectins.

A or B antigen expression can weaken in patients with acute leukemia or stress hematopoiesis or, occasionally, during pregnancy. Chromosomal deletions or lesions that involve the ABO locus can result in the loss of transferase expression in the leukemic cell population. A decrease in A or B antigen expression, when found without a hematologic disorder, can be prognostic of a preleukemic state.

Genes and Enzymes. The *ABO* gene was cloned in 1990 following purification of A transferase; since then, over 200 different alleles have been described.[17] There are only four amino acid differences between A and B transferases in the catalytic domain, two of which (Leu266Met and Gly268Ala) are primarily responsible for the substrate specificity. The group O phenotype results from mutations in *ABO* that cause a loss of glycosyltransferase activity. The most common group O (O_1) results from a single nucleotide deletion near the 5′ end of the gene that causes a frameshift and early termination with no active enzyme production. The rare B(A) and cis-AB phenotypes express both A and B from a single allele due to variant glycosyltransferases that have a combination of A- and B-specific residues.

The fucosyltransferases required for H synthesis are encoded by two closely linked genes on chromosome 19, *FUT1* (or H) and *FUT2* (or *Se* for secretor), which have different substrate specificity and expression in tissues. Homozygosity for defective *FUT2* alleles is responsible for the common nonsecretor phenotype in which A, B, and/or H antigen are not present in secretions. Individuals homozygous for null alleles at both the *FUT1* and *FUT2* loci have the Bombay phenotype (see earlier section).

ABO and Transplantation. As tissue antigens, ABO antigens are important in solid organ transplantation. Recipient antibodies will react with antigens on the transplanted organ, and complement activation at the surface of endothelial cells can result in rapid destruction and hyperacute rejection. However, successful transplantation across ABO barriers is possible, particularly with blood group A_2 to O and with current immunosuppressive and pretreatment regiments including removal of ABO antibodies.[18] Allogeneic hematopoietic stem cell transplantations are routinely performed regardless of ABO compatibility, but occasionally initial hemolysis or pure red cell anemia due to persisting anti-A or anti-B titers in the recipient can result.

Antibodies. Anti-A and anti-B are found in the sera of individuals who lack the corresponding antigens. They are produced in response to environmental stimulants, such as bacteria. These antibodies are produced after birth, reaching a peak at 5 to 10 years of age, and declining with increasing age. The antibodies are mostly IgM and can activate complement, which in conjunction with the high density of ABO antigen sites on RBCs, are responsible for the severe, life-threatening transfusion reactions that may result following ABO-incompatible transfusions. In contrast, HDFN caused by ABO antibodies is usually mild because (1) placental transfer is limited to the fraction of IgG anti-A and anti-B found in maternal serum, (2) ABH antigens are not fully developed on fetal RBCs because of a lack of fully branched carbohydrate chains, and (3) tissue ABH antigens provide additional targets for the antibodies.

Platelets have intrinsic A, B, and H antigens; thus ABO incompatibility can decrease the post-transfusion platelet increment, but this is usually not of clinical significance.[19] However, platelets from donors with an A_2 phenotype lack both A and H antigens. Approximately 20% of group A platelets would be from A_2 donors and would be appropriate for "universal" use. Platelets from A_2 donors may also be a superior product for patients undergoing A/O major mismatch allogeneic progenitor cell transplantation.[17]

Potent anti-H (along with anti-A and anti-B) found in O_h (Bombay) individuals will destroy transfused RBCs of any ABO group, so these individuals must be transfused only with H– RBCs. In contrast, anti-H identified in individuals with low expression of H antigen, notably A_1B and A_1, is usually IgM, reacts only at lower temperatures, and is thus clinically insignificant.

Other Carbohydrate Blood Group Systems

As for all glycoconjugate structures, sequential enzymatic action is required to build other carbohydrate antigenic epitopes, and the genetic background of all these involves different glycosyltransferase loci.

The null p phenotype, P_2^k and P_1^k, are of clinical interest because of potent naturally occurring antibodies that are present in plasma of individuals whose RBCs lack the glycolipid-based antigens P1/P/P^k, P1/P or P, respectively. In analogy with the ABO blood group system, antibodies of IgM and IgG class (anti-PP1P^k, anti-P1P, or anti-P) are made against the missing antigens. Although the incidence of the null phenotypes is only 5 to 10 per million, they have attracted considerable interest because of their relationship to disease and as receptors for pathogens. Women with p and P^k phenotypes suffer a high incidence of spontaneous abortion, a phenomenon most likely due to destruction of the placenta by anti-P. Additionally, anti-P and anti-P^k cause hemolytic transfusion reactions if antigen-positive RBCs are transfused. Transient autoanti-P, produced following a viral infection, causes paroxysmal cold hemoglobinuria and lysis of autologous P-positive RBC. P antigen (also known as *globoside*) is the cellular receptor for parvo-B19 virus that causes erythema infectiosum (fifth disease) in children, sometimes complicated by severe aplastic anemia due to lysis of early erythroid precursors. P-fimbriated *Escherichia coli* expresses both P- and P^k-binding molecules at the tips of their pili, a finding with implications for uropathogenicity. Individuals lacking P, or P^k and P, appear to be naturally resistant to these bacterial and viral infections. In contrast to anti-P and anti-P^k, it should be noted that anti-P1 is a cold-reactive agglutinin that seldom has clinical importance.

Lewis antigens are fucosylated glycolipids that are synthesized by nonerythroid cells, circulate in plasma, and are passively adsorbed onto RBC. Antibodies to Lewis can be made by individuals with the Le(a–b–) phenotype. These antibodies are of IgM class and seldom cause any clinical problems but are commonly found in pregnant women.

The i and I antigens are nonterminal epitopes on linear and branched carbohydrate structures, respectively, carrying ABH antigens at their terminal ends. During the first years of life, linear chains are modified into branched chains, resulting in the appearance of I antigens. The i phenotype is very rare among adults, but it is the normal state on RBCs from fetuses and infants. The gene encoding the I-branching β-1,6-*N*-acetylglucosaminyltransferase (GCNT2) has three alternative forms of exon 1 with common exons 2 and 3. Mutations in exon 2 or exon 3 silence *GCNT2* and give rise to the form of the i phenotype that is associated with cataracts in Asians. Mutations in exon 1C silence the gene in erythrocytes (but not in other tissues) and lead to the i phenotype without cataracts.

Alloanti-I made by a person with the rare i adult phenotype can be clinically significant and cause destruction of transfused I-positive RBCs. However, the sera of all I-positive individuals contain autoanti-I that is clinically benign and reactive only at or below room temperature. In contrast, cold hemagglutinin disease is characterized by a high titer of complement-fixing monoclonal anti-I, which causes in vivo hemolysis and hemolytic anemia. The titer and thermal range of autoanti-I is often increased following infection with *Mycoplasma pneumoniae*. If transfusion cannot be avoided, donor RBCs should be transfused through a blood warmer.

Protein Blood Groups

Rh, RhAG, and LW Blood Group Systems

The Rh system is second only to the ABO system in importance in transfusion medicine. Rh antigens, especially D, are highly immunogenic; thus in most countries, blood for transfusion is tested and labeled with the D antigen type (Rh-positive or Rh-negative) and D– recipients are transfused with D– RBC products.

Three systems for naming Rh antigens have been used. Two are shown in Table 111-5, which indicates the incidence of the common

Rh haplotypes present in different ethnic groups. The Fisher-Race nomenclature was based on the premise that there were three closely linked genes (D, C/c, and E/e), whereas the Wiener nomenclature (Rh-Hr) was based on the belief that a single gene encoded multiple factors (antigens). Although it is now well-established that two genes, *RHD* and *RHCE,* encode the Rh proteins, the Fisher-Race (D, C/c, and E/e) terminology is often preferred for written communication; for spoken communication, a modified version of the Wiener nomenclature is preferred. Uppercase *R* indicates that D antigen is present and use of a lowercase *r* (or "little r") indicates that it is absent. The C or c and E or e antigens carried with D are represented by subscripts: 1 for Ce (R_1), 2 for cE (R_2), 0 for ce (R_0), and Z for CE (R_z). The presence of these antigens without D is represented by a superscript: prime for Ce (r′), double-prime for cE (r″), and y for CE (r^y). This terminology allows one to convey the common Rh antigens (the phenotype) with a single term. The third system of numeric designations is not widely used in the laboratory, with a few exceptions (Rh17, Rh32, Rh33).

Genes, Proteins, Antigens, and Phenotypes. The Rh proteins are designated RhD (encoded by *RHD*), which carries the D antigen, and RhCE (encoded by *RHCE*), which carries the CE antigens (either ce, cE, Ce, or CE). RhD differs from the various forms of RhCE by 32 to 35 amino acids. RhD and RhCE are not glycosylated but form a complex in the RBC membrane with RhAG (Rh-associated glycoprotein). Other proteins present in the Rh-complex are CD47 (an integrin-associated protein), LW, and glycophorin B. The Rh-complex also associates with band 3 (the anion exchanger) as a macro-complex in the membrane.

The D-negative (Rh-negative) phenotype is prevalent in whites (15%-17%), less likely in African Blacks (3%-5%), and rare in Asians (<0.1%). The absence of D in Europeans is due primarily to a deletion of the *RHD* gene. African Blacks and rare D-negative whites and Asians carry a *RHD* gene that is silenced by a variety of molecular events.[3]

RBCs with weak D have D antigen but at lower levels than normal because of one or more amino acid changes that are often predicted to be in the intracellular or transmembrane regions of RhD. The majority of individuals with a weak D phenotype can safely receive D-positive blood and do not make anti-D.[18]

Partial D antigens (previously called *D categories* or *D mosaics*) are caused either by point mutations in *RHD*, resulting in amino acid changes that alter D epitopes, or by replacement of *RHD* nucleotides or exons by the equivalent part of *RHCE.* RBCs with a partial D antigen may have strong or weak expression of the D antigen but have altered or missing D epitopes. Because patients with partial D antigens can make anti-D to the D epitopes they lack, they ideally should receive D-negative blood and women of childbearing potential are candidates for Rh immune globulin. In practice, most type as D-positive and are recognized only after they make anti-D. Some monoclonal D typing reagents can classify some partial D phenotypes as D negative (partial DVI) in direct testing. *RHD* genotyping is very useful to distinguish partial D in order to prevent D alloimmunization and to avoid unnecessary Rh immune globulin injection (see box on Weak or Variable D Typing).

Several phenotypes, including D– –, Dc– and DC^w–, have an enhanced expression of D antigen and no, or variant, CE antigens. They are caused by replacement of portions of *RHCE* by *RHD.* The RhD sequences in RhCE, along with a normal RhD, explain the enhanced D and account for the lack, or reduced expression, of CE antigens. Immunized individuals with these CE-depleted phenotypes can make antibodies to high-prevalence Rh antigens.

C and c antigens differ by four amino acids, but only residue Ser103Pro is predicted to be extracellular. E and e differ by one amino acid, Pro226Ala. The RhD and various combinations of RhCE proteins (ce, Ce, cE, and CE) are typical for the majority of white transfusion recipients. However, Rh proteins in other ethnic groups often carry additional polymorphisms, particularly in individuals of African descent, and this fact often complicates transfusion in patients with sickle cell disease. For example, the RBCs of more than 30% of blacks are VS+ because of a Leu245Val substitution in Rhce, and expression of this antigen is associated with variant expression of e antigen. Many other amino acid changes in Rhce, as well as in RhD, are associated with production of Rh antibodies in patients with sickle cell disease. RH genotyping by DNA methods allows enhanced Rh antigen matching of patients and donors and is particularly important in patients who present with Rh antibodies reacting with all, or the majority, of cells tested.

The Rh_{null} phenotype is very rare and occurs on two genetic backgrounds: the "regulator" type, caused by mutations in RHAG, which encodes Rh-associated glycoprotein, and the "amorph" type, caused by mutations in *RHCE* on a D- (deleted *RHD*) background. Rh_{null} RBCs are stomatocytic, fragile, and associated with anemia.

Antibodies. Most Rh antibodies are IgG and do not activate complement. As a result, primarily extravascular hemolysis, rather than intravascular hemolysis, occurs in transfusion reactions involving Rh antibodies. The antibodies are almost always due to RBC immunization from pregnancy or transfusion and usually persist for years. Anti-D can cause severe transfusion reactions and HDFN, but the incidence of anti-D has decreased with the prophylactic use of Rh immune globulin. Most Rh antibodies should be considered as having the potential to be clinical significant for HDFN and transfusion reactions. If serum antibody levels fall below detectable levels, subsequent exposure to the antigen characteristically produces a rapid secondary immune response. Autoantibodies in the sera of patients

Table 111-5 Prevalence of the principal Rh Haplotypes

Fisher-Race Haplotype	Modified Weiner Haplotype	Incidence (%) White	African Black	Asian
Rh-POSITIVE				
DCe	R_1	42	17	70
DcE	R_2	14	11	21
Dce	R_0	4	44	3
DCE	R_Z	<0.01	<0.01	1
Rh-NEGATIVE				
ce	r	37	26	3
Ce	r′	2	2	2
cE	r″	1	<0.01	<0.01
CE	r^y	<0.01	<0.01	<0.01

Weak or Variable D Typing

Clinically significant D sensitization potentially results in a pregnancy with a fetus at risk for hemolytic disease of the fetus and newborn and hemolytic transfusion reactions if transfused with D-positive RBCs. Individuals with RBCs that express a partial D antigen are at risk for D-sensitization, whereas those with weak D antigen are usually not at risk. These cannot be distinguished by serologic reactivity, because either may present as weak or moderately positive or give variable results with anti-D reagents. Particularly in the prenatal setting, RHD genotyping should be done to distinguish weak D from partial D. Women with weak D expression are not at risk for clinically significant D sensitization and therefore are not candidates for RhIG prophylaxis. In contrast, individuals with partial D lack D epitopes and have produced clinically significant anti-D and should receive RhIG prophylaxis. RHD genotyping avoids unnecessary treatment with RhIG in women with weak D antigen.

with warm autoimmune hemolytic anemia (AIHA), as well as in some cases of drug-induced autoimmune hemolytic anemia, appear to demonstrate relative specificity to high-prevalence Rh antigens, although other members of the Rh complex have not been ruled out (see box on Transfusion Management of Patients With Warm Autoimmune Hemolytic Anemia).

RHAG Blood Group System

RhAG glycoprotein, encoded by *RHAG,* is highly similar to the RhD and RhCE proteins. It carries four blood group antigens: two of high prevalence (RHAG1 and 3) and two of low prevalence (RHAG 2 and 4). Antibodies to RHAG4 cause HDFN. RhAG is important for erythrocyte ion balance in RBCs and is required for the expression of RhD and RhCE proteins forming the core of the Rh-complex.

Transfusion Management of Patients With Warm Autoimmune Hemolytic Anemia

Patients with warm autoimmune hemolytic anemia may present with jaundice, fatigue, and anemia, or they may show no overt clinical manifestations. The antibody screen and antibody identification panel will show all RBCs positive (panagglutinin) with anti-IgG in the indirect antiglobulin test. The autocontrol (patient's own plasma and RBCs) will also be positive.

History: A transfusion history should be obtained to differentiate these results from a hemolytic transfusion reaction or hemolysis due to an alloantibody.

DAT: A direct antiglobulin test should be performed with anti-IgG and -C3. In clinically significant hemolysis, the DAT is usually strongly positive.

Eluate: If patient has been recently transfused (3-4 months), an eluate should be prepared from the patient cells to remove the antibody(ies); the eluate should be tested to determine specificity. The eluate is usually reactive with all cells when tested by the IAT with anti-IgG.

Phenotype: Type the patient's RBCs for minor blood group antigens (Cc, Ee, K, Jka/b, Fya/b, Ss) if the patient has not been recently transfused. When possible, IgM typing reagents are used because the patient's own antibody-coated RBCs may result in false-positive typing. Some laboratories are able to remove the IgG from the RBCs and perform a phenotype. Alternatively, genotyping for minor blood group antigens including $Do^{a/b}$ antigens (there is no serologic reagent) can be performed.

Adsorption: Adsorb the serum autoantibody onto the patient's own RBCs to test for underlying alloantibody if the patient has not been recently transfused (3-4 months). If the patient has been recently transfused or if the low hematocrit results in insufficient autologous RBCs, perform alloadsorption with well-characterized RBCs (usually three with known antigen profiles). Test the adsorbed serum for underlying alloantibodies.

Crossmatch: Perform with neat and with adsorbed plasma. Crossmatch performed with neat plasma will usually be incompatible.

Communication: Inform ordering physician of reactivity and of delay in receiving crossmatched RBCs. Provide emergency-release RBCs if patient's clinical situation warrants. Inform the physician that the patient may hemolyze transfused RBCs similar to hemolysis of his or her own RBCs.

Transfusion: Consider providing RBC units negative for minor antigens that the patient also lacks (consider matching for Cc, Ee, K, Jka/b, Fya/b, Ss). This potentially enables RBC units to be available before completion of the antibody identification testing. Transfusion with antigen matched units potentially allows continued transfusion without need for auto- or alloadsorption unless signs and symptoms of RBC destruction occur or there is a change in reactivity in antibody screening or the DAT.

LW Blood Group System

Rh and LW are independent blood group systems but have a phenotypic relationship. In adults, D-positive RBCs have a stronger expression of LW antigen than D-negative RBCs, and anti-LW can be confused with anti-D. Transient loss of LW antigens from RBCs has been described in pregnancy and in patients with diseases, particularly Hodgkin's disease, lymphoma, leukemia, sarcoma, and other forms of malignancy. Loss of LW antigens is usually associated with the production of antibodies that appear to be alloanti-LW.

Kell and Kx Systems

The Kell glycoprotein is highly folded through multiple intrachain disulfide bonds and is covalently linked to XK protein in the RBC membrane. Kell is highly polymorphic due to single amino acid substitutions in the glycoprotein that account for 33 of 34 antigens described to date. The K antigen is remarkably immunogenic for differing from wild-type (small k) by only one amino acid, and it appears that loss of an N-glycan exposes the peptide, thereby rendering it immunogenic.

Inherited weak expression of Kell antigens occurs with amino acid changes in the protein, termed K_{mod} phenotype, and occurs with Kp^a in cis, and in the McLeod phenotype.[19] Transient depression of Kell system antigens occurs in autoimmune hemolytic anemia, in microbial infections, and in two cases of idiopathic thrombocytopenia purpura. The lack of Kell antigens (the K_0 or K_{null} phenotype) is caused by several different gene defects.

HDFN due to anti-K can result in severe neonatal anemia, and unlike anti-D, maternal antibody titers and amniotic bilirubin levels are not good predictors of the severity of the disease. Kell antigens are expressed very early during erythropoiesis, and anti-K has been shown to suppress erythropoiesis in vitro. This may explain the low level of bilirubin observed in cases of neonatal anemia; thus Doppler screening of the fetal middle cerebral artery peak systolic velocity is used to monitor anemia. Other unusual consequences of Kell antibodies include risk for fetal thrombocytopenia and neutropenia.

McLeod Syndrome. This uncommon syndrome is associated with the loss of expression of Kx protein due to mutations and deletions in the *XK* gene.[20,21] The syndrome, which is X-linked and manifests only in males, may be underdiagnosed. The physical characteristics, which often develop only after the fourth decade of life, include muscular and neurologic problems. A minority of patients with chronic granulomatous disease (CGD) also have the McLeod phenotype as a result of X-chromosome deletions encompassing both genes. Carrier females have two populations of RBCs (one of the McLeod phenotype and one of normal phenotype).

Duffy Blood Group System

The Duffy (FY) glycoprotein is a promiscuous chemokine receptor found on RBCs and on endothelial cells in the kidney and brain that binds a family of chemotactic and proinflammatory peptides from the CXC (IL-8, MGSA) and the CC (RANTES, MCP-1, MIP-1) classes. The physiologic role of FY is clear, but on RBCs the receptor may allow RBCs to act as scavengers for excess chemokines. FY is also a receptor to which *Plasmodium vivax* merozoites can bind to invade RBC and cause malaria.

Antigens. The Fy^a and Fy^b antigens differ by a single amino acid (Gly42Asp) located on the N-terminal extracellular domain of the FY glycoprotein and is responsible for the common Fy(a+b−), Fy(a−b+) and Fy(a+b+) phenotypes. The null Fy(a−b−) phenotype is rare in most ethnic groups, but it is common in people of African and Arabian origins. The null phenotype most often results from a mutation in the promoter region of *FY* that disrupts a binding site for the erythroid transcription factor GATA-1 and results in loss of FY on RBCs.[22] Because the erythroid promoter controls expression only in erythroid cells, FY expression in other tissues is unaffected. All individuals of African origin with a mutated GATA box to date have been shown to carry *FYB* and therefore Fy^b is expressed on nonerythroid tissues. This explains why Fy(a–b–) individuals make anti-Fy^a but not anti-Fy^b. Fy(a–b–) due to a mutated GATA box on an *FYA* allele has been found in Papua New Guinea, another malaria-endemic region.

Antibodies. FY antigens are much less immunogenic than Rh and K. Anti-Fy^b is less common than anti-Fy^a, and both antibodies can cause DHTR and rarely HDFN. Anti-Fy3 is made by Fy(a–b–) individuals who may lack FY protein on all cells.

Kidd Blood Group System

The Kidd (JK) blood group protein was implicated in urea transport when RBCs lacking the antigens were shown to resist lysis in 2 M urea. The protein is present in RBCs and kidney medulla and is a constitutive urea transporter, but failure to express Kidd does not result in an overt clinical syndrome; the only observed manifestation is a reduced capacity to concentrate urine.[23]

Antigens. The Jk^a and Jk^b antigens differ by a single amino acid (Asp280Asn) and are responsible for the common Jk(a+b–), Jk(a–b+) and Jk(a+b+) phenotypes. The Jk(a–b–) or Jk_{null} phenotype is uncommon and occurs with greater incidence in Polynesians, Asians, and Finns. The silent alleles in Polynesians/Asians have splice-site or missense mutations in *JKB* alleles that abolish expression of Jk^b, and large deletions and premature stop codons in *JKA* alleles have been found in Caucasian Jk_{null} pedigrees. Weakly expressed variants of Jk^a and Jk^b antigen are found.

Antibodies. JK antibodies are responsible for at least one-third of cases of delayed hemolytic transfusion reactions. The antibodies often drop to undetectable levels or react only with cells that are homozygous for the antigen and escape detection in the sensitized patient's serum before transfusion. JK antibodies only rarely cause HDFN, and if they do, it is typically not severe. Anti-Jk3, sometimes referred to as anti-Jk^{ab}, is produced by Jk(a–b–) individuals, and rare donors must be located for transfusion.

MNS System

M and N antigens are carried on alternative forms of glycophorin A (GPA), whereas S and s antigens are carried on alternative forms of glycophorin B (GPB). M/N and S/s are homologous proteins encoded by adjacent genes and consequently show linkage disequilibrium in inheritance of the antigens. The MNS system is highly polymorphic and most of the 46 antigens are the result of amino acid substitutions or rearrangements between *GYPA* and *GYPB*. Persons who are S–s– are usually of African origin who also lack the high-prevalence U antigen due to a deletion of *GYPB* or express variant weak U antigen as a result of an altered form of *GYPB*.

Antibodies. Anti-S, -s, and -U are usually IgG and can be clinically significant antibodies. Anti-M and anti-N can be naturally occurring, may be reactive at room temperature or below, and are often clinically insignificant.

Other Protein Antigens

Antibodies to antigens in the following systems are less common than those described earlier in this chapter, and information regarding their general clinical significance is summarized in Table 111-3.

Lutheran System

Lutheran (Lu), along with Secretor, provided the first example of autosomal linkage in humans, the first example of autosomal crossing over, and the first indication that crossing over in humans is more common in females than in males. The Lutheran system consists of four antithetical pairs of antigens and 12 independent high-prevalence antigens. The Lu(a–b–) phenotype is rare, but in the majority of individuals, it is due to heterozygosity for silencing mutations in the *EKLF/KLF1* gene.[24] KLF1 is a transcription factor that regulates many erythroid-specific genes, and the expression of antigens in other blood group systems (e.g., Knops, Indian) is also affected.

Antibodies. Antibodies in this system are rarely encountered because the antigens are not highly immunogenic. They are usually IgG and give characteristic agglutinates surrounded by unagglutinated RBCs. They can cause mild transfusion reactions, but do not typically cause HDFN. Anti-Lu3 is found in the serum of immunized people of the rare recessive Lu(a–b–) phenotype, and the antibody is usually IgG and may cause a delayed transfusion reaction or HDFN. Blood with the Lu(a–b–) phenotype should be used for transfusion of patients with these antibodies.

Diego System

The Diego (Di) blood group antigens are on band 3, the red cell anion exchanger (AE1), one of the most abundant erythrocyte glycoproteins. Band 3 forms complexes with many other proteins in the cell membrane and is important for RBC stability. The Diego blood group system contains 2 antithetical pairs of antigens and 18 low-prevalence antigens. Di^b antigen has a prevalence of greater than 99.9%, but Di^a is rare in most populations. Exceptions include South American Indians (Di^a occurs in 54% of this population) and North American Indians, approximately 12% of whom are Di(a+).

Antibodies. Diego antibodies are usually IgG and do not bind complement. These antibodies have caused transfusion reactions (usually delayed) and HDFN. Autoantibodies to band 3 are common in patients with warm autoimmune hemolytic anemia.

Yt Blood Group System

The Yt system was named in 1956 when an antibody was found in the serum of patient whose last name was Cartwright. Yt^a occurs with a prevalence of more than 99% in random blood samples, and Yt^b is found with a prevalence of approximately 8%, except in Israelis, in whom it has a prevalence of 20% or higher.

Antibodies. Yt antibodies usually are IgG and do not bind complement. These antibodies have caused delayed transfusion reactions but not HDFN.

Scianna Blood Group System

The Scianna (Sc) antigens are expressed by the RBC adhesion protein, erythrocyte membrane-associated protein (ERMAP). Sc1 is a high-prevalence antigen (prevalence ≈99.9%), and Sc2 is a low-prevalence antigen (1%); there are five other Scianna antigens.

Antibodies. Scianna antibodies are usually IgG, and some bind complement. These antibodies have not caused transfusion reactions, and although they have caused a positive DAT in cord RBCs, they have not caused HDFN. Several examples of autoanti-Sc1 have been reported, some reactive in tests using patient serum but not plasma. Autoanti-Sc3–like antibodies have been described in one patient with lymphoma and in one patient with Hodgkins disease whose RBCs had suppressed Sc antigens.[2]

Dombrock Blood Group System

Dombrock (Do) antigens are carried on a GPI-linked glycoprotein that is a member of the mono-ADP-ribosyltransferase family (ART4), although Do has no demonstrable enzyme activity on the RBC. The Dombrock blood group system consists of two antithetical antigens, Do^a and Do^b, and six other antigens of high prevalence. The null phenotype is Gy(a−).

Antibodies. Do^a and Do^b antigens are poor immunogens, and anti-Do^a and anti-Do^b are rarely found as single specificities. Antibodies in the Do system are usually IgG and do not bind complement. These antibodies have caused delayed transfusion reactions and a positive DAT but no clinical HDFN.

Colton Blood Group System

The Colton antigens are carried on aquaporin-1 (AQP-1), the first water channel protein characterized in mammals, and are also found in the kidney. The function of AQP-1 in RBCs may be to rehydrate rapidly after shrinking in the hypertonic environment of the renal medulla. Co^a has a prevalence of 99.9%, its antithetical antigen Co^b has a prevalence of 10%, and Co3 and Co4 are present on all RBCs except those of the very rare Co(a−b−) null phenotype. Apparently healthy propositi with the Co(a−b−) phenotype and AQP-1 deficiency have RBCs with an 80% reduction in the ability to transport water. The residual water transport in these RBCs may be through another member of the water channel protein family, AQP-3, which transports water, glycerol, and urea, and carries the blood group antigen GIL.

Antibodies. Antibodies in the Colton system are usually IgG and some bind complement. The antibodies have caused delayed transfusion reactions and HDFN.

Gerbich Blood Group System

The Gerbich system antigens are carried on glycophorin C (GPC) and glycophorin D (GPD). There are six high-prevalence antigens and five low-prevalence antigens. The two glycoproteins are products of the *GYPC* gene. The gene consists of four exons, and the smaller GPD is generated by the use of an alternative translation initiation site.

Antibodies. The antibodies may be immune or naturally occurring. Most are IgG, and some of these bind complement. Some antibodies may be IgM. Although some antibodies have caused delayed transfusion reactions, others have been benign. Clinical HDFN has not been reported, but the antibodies have been eluted from DAT-positive cord RBCs.

Cromer Blood Group System

The Cromer antigens are carried on decay-accelerating factor (DAF, CD55), a complement control protein attached to the RBC membrane through GPI-linkage. Cromer is a system of two sets of antithetical antigens ($Tc^a/Tc^b/Tc^c$ and WES^a/WES^b), 13 high-prevalence antigens, and three low-prevalence antigens. The Cr(a−) phenotype is the least rare of the negative phenotypes, and with the exception of one Spanish-American woman, all people with Cr(a−) RBCs are black. Most of the other phenotypes are exceedingly rare.

Antibodies. Antibodies in the Cromer system are usually IgG and do not bind complement. The antibodies have caused mild delayed transfusion reactions but not HDFN.

Knops Blood Group System

The Knops blood group antigens are carried on complement receptor 1 (CR1). Kn^a, Sl^a, and McC^a antigens are fairly common and have a similar prevalence (>90%) in different populations; however, Sl^a is present on RBCs of 98% of whites, but on only 60% of African Americans. Typing for Knops system antigens can be challenging because of the low level of expression on the RBCs in some disease processes gives false-negative results. RBC CR1 is important in the processing of immune complexes, binding them for transport to the liver and spleen for removal from the circulation. The CR1 copy number per RBC (and thus antigen strength) is reduced in SLE, cold agglutinin disease (CAD), PNH, hemolytic anemia, insulin-dependent diabetes mellitus, acquired immunodeficiency syndrome, some malignant tumors, and any condition associated with increased clearance of immune complexes. CR1 (the Sl^a antigen in particular) may act as a receptor for the malarial parasite *Plasmodium falciparum*; thus the Sl(a−) phenotype may provide selective advantage.[25]

Antibodies. Antibodies in the Knops system are usually IgG, and they do not bind complement. The antibodies do not cause transfusion reactions or HDFN, and once identified, they can usually be ignored for clinical purposes. Identification may be complicated by the fluctuation of antigen expression on RBCs. In the Knops system, anti-Kn^a is the most common antibody in whites, and anti-Sl^a is the most common in African Americans.

Indian Blood Group System

The antigens of the Indian system are carried on CD44. CD44 has a diverse range of biologic functions involving cell-cell and cell-matrix interactions in cells other than RBCs. It is an adhesion molecule in lymphocytes, monocytes, and some tumor cells. CD44 binds to hyaluronate and other components of the extracellular matrix and is also involved in immune stimulation, as well as signaling between cells.[26] In^b is a common antigen, and In^a is rare in white persons but has a prevalence of 4% in Indians, 10% in Iranians, and nearly 12% in Arabs.

Antibodies. Antibodies in the Indian system are usually IgG and do not bind complement. Some antibodies may directly agglutinate RBCs, but the reactivity is greatly enhanced by the IAT. These antibodies have caused decreased RBC survival and a positive DAT in the neonate but not HDFN. A severe, delayed, hemolytic transfusion reaction due to anti-In^b has been reported.

Chido/Rodgers Blood Group System

Although the Ch and Rg antigens are readily detected on RBCs, they are located on the fourth component of complement (C4), which becomes bound to RBCs from the plasma. In complement activation through the classical pathway, C4 becomes bound to the RBC membrane and undergoes further cleavage; ultimately, a tryptic fragment, C4d, remains on the RBC. This C4d glycoprotein carries the Ch/Rg blood group antigens. The antigens are stable in stored serum or plasma, and the phenotypes of this system are most accurately defined in plasma by agglutination inhibition tests.

Antibodies. Antibodies in the Ch/Rg system are usually IgG, do not activate complement, and are considered benign. Considerable variation may be common in the reaction strength obtained with different RBC samples. Although these antibodies do not generally cause transfusion reactions, they have caused anaphylactic reactions.[27] The antibodies have not caused HDFN.

REFERENCES

1. Lögdberg L, Reid ME, Zelinski T: Human blood group genes 2010: Chromosomal locations and cloning strategies revisited. *Transfus Med Rev* 25:36, 2011.
2. Reid ME, Lomas-Francis C: *Blood Group Antigen FactsBook*, ed 2, San Diego, 2004, Academic Press.
3. Daniels G: *Human Blood Groups*, ed 2, Oxford, 2002, Blackwell Science Ltd..

4. Heddle NM, Soutar RL, O'Hoski PL, et al: A prospective study to determine the frequency and clinical significance of alloimmunization post-transfusion. *Br J Haematol* 91:1000, 1995.
5. Rosse WF, Gallagher D, Kinney TR, et al: Transfusion and alloimmunization in sickle cell disease. *Blood* 76:1431, 1990.
6. Aygun B, Padmanabhan S, Paley C, et al: Clinical significance of RBC alloantibodies and autoantibodies in sickle cell patients who received transfusions. *Transfusion* 42:37, 2002.
7. Vichinsky EP, Earles A, Johnson RA, et al: Alloimmunization in sickle cell anemia and transfusion of racially unmatched blood. *N Engl J Med* 322:1617, 1990.
8. Cox JV, Steane E, Cunningham G, et al: Risk of alloimmunization and delayed hemolytic transfusion reactions in patients with sickle cell disease. *Archives of Internal Medicine* 148:2485, 1988.
9. Afenyi-Annan A, Willis MS, Konrad TR, et al: Blood bank management of sickle cell patients at comprehensive sickle cell centers. *Transfusion* 47:2089, 2007.
10. Wayne AS, Kevy SV, Nathan DG: Transfusion management of sickle cell disease. *Blood* 81:1109, 1993.
11. Ness PM: To match or not to match: The question for chronically transfused patients with sickle cell anemia. *Transfusion* 34:558, 1994.
12. Osby M, Shulman IA: Phenotype matching of donor red blood cell units for nonalloimmunized sickle cell disease patients: A survey of 1182 North American laboratories. *Arch Path Lab Med* 129:190, 2005.
13. Bruce LJ, Guizouarn H, Burton NM, et al: The monovalent cation leak in overhydrated stomatocytic red blood cells results from amino acid substitutions in the Rh-associated glycoprotein. *Blood* 113:1350, 2009.
14. Roback JD, Grossman BJ, Harris T, et al, editors: *Technical Manual*, ed 17, Bethesda, Md, 2011, American Association of Blood Banks.
15. Clausen H, Hakomori S: ABH and related histo-blood group antigens; immunochemical differences in carrier isotypes and their distribution. *Vox Sang* 56:1, 1989.
16. Oriol R, Candelier JJ, Mollicone R: Molecular genetics of H. *Vox Sanguinis* 78:105, 2000.
17. Storry JR, Olsson ML: The ABO blood group system revisited: A review and update. *Immunohematology/American Red Cross* 25:48, 2009.
18. Rydberg L: ABO-incompatibility in solid organ transplantation. *Transfus Med* 11:325, 2001.
19. Curtis BR, Edwards JT, Hessner MJ, et al: Blood group A and B antigens are strongly expressed on platelets of some individuals. *Blood* 96:1574 2000.
20. Cooling LL, Kelly K, Barton J, et al: Determinants of ABH expression on human blood platelets. *Blood* 105:3356, 2005.
21. Flegel WA: Homing in on D antigen immunogenicity. *Transfusion* 45:466, 2005.
22. Chou ST, Westhoff CM: The role of molecular immunohematology in sickle cell disease. *Transfus Apher Sci* 44:73, 2011.
23. Danek A, Rubio JP, Rampoldi L, et al: McLeod neuroacanthocytosis: Genotype and phenotype. *Ann Neurol* 50:755, 2001.
24. Russo DCW, Lee S, Reid ME, et al: Point mutations causing the McLeod phenotype. *Transfusion* 42:287, 2002.
25. Tournamille C, Colin Y, Cartron JP, et al: Disruption of a GATA motif in the *Duffy* gene promoter abolishes erythroid gene expression in Duffy-negative individuals. *Nature Genet* 10:224, 1995.
26. Sands JM, Gargus JJ, Frohlich O, et al: Urinary concentrating ability in patients with Jk(a-b-) blood type who lack carrier-mediated urea transport. *J Am Soc Nephrol* 2:1689, 1992.
27. Singleton BK, Burton NM, Green C, et al: Mutations in EKLF/KLF1 form the molecular basis of the rare blood group In(Lu) phenotype. *Blood* 112:2081, 2008.

CHAPTER 112

PRINCIPLES OF RED BLOOD CELL TRANSFUSION

Melissa M. Cushing and Paul M. Ness

The clinical practice of transfusion medicine has evolved substantially since the discovery of the ABO system around 1900. Two technologic advances set the stage for clinical practice through blood component therapy. First, the introduction of a safe and effective anticoagulant-preservative solution (suggested by Loutit and Mollison) allowed for the preservation of blood products. Second, in the mid-1960s, the introduction of plastic blood bags by Walter and Murphy, combined with the ability to store blood for extended periods, created opportunities to use transfusions in varied clinical settings. With these discoveries, the era of modern component therapy began. Today, approximately 15 million units of blood are transfused each year in the United States; whole blood transfusions account for only 0.03% of total transfusions. This chapter reviews component therapy, appropriate red blood cell (RBC) transfusion practice in a variety of clinical settings, the clinical implications of red blood cell storage, and existing and emerging alternatives to allogeneic red blood cell transfusions.

RED BLOOD CELL COMPONENTS

Modern transfusion medicine practice aims at providing the specific component of the blood required, rather than whole blood: red cells for oxygen-carrying capacity, plasma for coagulation proteins, and platelets for microvascular bleeding. The component therapy approach allows for optimal use of a limited community resource. Today, the clinician wishing to increase the patient's oxygen-carrying capacity is more likely to use a red blood cell concentrate than whole blood, although there may still be situations in which whole blood, if available, is appropriate. For particular clinical applications, several modifications can be made to red blood cell products to render them depleted of leukocytes or plasma. Red blood cells can also be frozen for long-term storage (Table 112-1).

Whole Blood

A unit of whole blood is collected in CPDA-1 anticoagulant, giving it a shelf life of 35 days and a volume of approximately 510 mL (450 mL of blood plus 63 mL of CPDA-1). Within 24 hours of collection, the platelets and granulocytes are dysfunctional, and several plasma coagulation factors have fallen.

Whole blood has the advantage of correcting simultaneous deficits in oxygen-carrying capacity and blood volume. Therefore whole blood is useful in the management of trauma or in surgical cases involving extensive blood loss. In this setting, whole blood has two distinct advantages: (a) it provides colloid osmotic pressure and coagulation factors not supplied by crystalloid solutions and (b) it does not expose the recipient to red blood cells and plasma from different donors.

The goal of using whole blood for all cases of concomitant red blood cell and volume deficit is difficult to achieve in practice. Most indications for whole blood transfusion are now well managed exclusively with blood component therapy, but the use of fresh whole blood has persisted in military settings. In the civilian setting, the simultaneous need for volume and oxygen-carrying capacity can usually be met by combining red cells with crystalloid or colloid solutions. In some cases of trauma and cardiovascular surgery, platelet transfusion may be indicated to combat microvascular bleeding from dilutional thrombocytopenia or bypass-associated platelet dysfunction. The transfusion of platelets usually supplies the equivalent of several units of relatively fresh plasma so that there is often no reason for further donor exposure by the administration of thawed plasma.

There has been recent renewed interest in fresh whole blood for patients with severe coagulopathy and shock. Few prospective trials have compared fresh whole blood to component therapy. The potential advantages of fresh whole blood when compared with component therapy are a relative increase in hemoglobin (Hb) concentration, coagulation factors, and platelets. In addition, fresh products avoid all of the negative effects of storage and processing. However, fresh whole blood is often not leukoreduced or irradiated. Furthermore, the completion of standard infectious disease testing before transfusion may not be possible within the time frame. Published randomized controlled studies of fresh whole blood in adults are lacking, but research is underway to determine potential indications and optimal storage temperature and duration.

Red Blood Cells

Red blood cells (also referred to as *packed red blood cells* or *red blood cell concentrates*) are obtained from whole blood after removal of most of the plasma for the production of frozen plasma or platelets, or both. At most blood centers, the red blood cells are then mixed with 100 mL of an additive nutrient solution that extends the storage period to 42 days and results in flow properties similar to those of whole blood.

Red blood cells are the product of choice for the correction of an isolated defect in oxygen-carrying capacity, as in cases of chronic anemia. In addition, red blood cells rather than whole blood are used for the emergent transfusion of patients of unknown ABO type. Concentrated group O red blood cells are transfused after the plasma containing isohemagglutinins is removed to prevent potential hemolysis of the recipient's red blood cells.

Leukocyte-Reduced Red Blood Cells

Leukocyte-reduced red blood cells (LRRCs) can be prepared by a variety of methods, resulting in differing degrees of white blood cell removal. Early techniques of preparation involved centrifugation or washing with saline, whereby the buffy coat was repeatedly removed. Currently, the most widely used method of leukoreduction is filtration, which can be performed either in the laboratory or at the bedside. The various filters on the market result in greater than 99% leukocyte reduction while depleting less than 10% of the red blood cells. Blood bags with in-line filters allow prestorage leukoreduction.

The major indication for the use of LRRCs is the prevention of the febrile nonhemolytic transfusion reaction, the most common adverse effect of transfusion, particularly in multiply transfused

Table 112-1 Red Blood Cell Components: Characteristics and Indications

Component	Characteristics	Indications
Whole blood	High volume; good flow	Combined red cell/volume deficit (massive hemorrhage; exchange transfusion)
Red blood cells	Lower volume Higher hematocrit	Red cell deficit
Leukocyte-reduced red blood cells	Good flow in AS	Prevention of febrile reactions Reduction of alloimmunization Reduction of immunomodulatory effects
Washed red blood cells	Plasma depletion Must use within 24 hours	Prevention of severe allergic reactions Prevention of anaphylaxis in IgA deficiency
Frozen red blood cells	Long-term storage Plasma and leukocyte depletion Must use within 24 hours of thawing	Rare donor unit storage Autologous storage for postponed surgery

patients or multiparous females. These reactions are believed to be mediated by antibodies directed against leukocyte antigens (HLA or granulocyte-specific antigens). Depletion of leukocytes to less than 5×10^6 has been shown to prevent, or at least ameliorate, such reactions in most patients. Increasing evidence suggests that cytokines play a role in causing these reactions. Because cytokines may be released from leukocytes during storage, prestorage leukoreduction procedures are the preferred mode of leukoreduction.

A second important indication for LRRCs is the prevention of alloimmunization to HLA antigens that can adversely affect post-transfusion platelet increments, such as in oncology patients undergoing chemotherapy. This approach will be effective only if leukoreduced platelets are also used. According to current AABB standards, the total leukocyte number must be less than 5×10^6 when intended for this purpose. With the introduction of third-generation leukoreduction filters for both red blood cells and platelets, this goal is achievable. A multicenter study known as TRAP showed that the use of leukoreduction filters for platelet products significantly decreased the rate of alloimmunization, but did not completely eliminate the problem.

A third indication for the use of LRRCs is to prevent transfusion-related immunomodulation (TRIM), which is of particular concern in the postoperative period. A large metaanalysis previously demonstrated that patients who receive a blood transfusion are more likely to experience a postoperative infection than patients not transfused. This effect has been found to be dose-dependent and is thought to be mediated by suppression of the patient's immune function. The mechanism of TRIM has yet to be defined, but multiple theories have been proposed. It has been suggested that immunologically active white blood cells or soluble biologic response modifiers released from white blood cells during storage downregulate the recipient's immune function. Alternative theories suggest that soluble mediators that circulate in allogeneic plasma may have an immune modulatory effect. Universal leukoreduction has been found by some studies, but not by others, to mitigate the immunomodulatory effect of allogeneic transfusions.

Washed Red Blood Cells

Red blood cells are washed using isotonic saline solutions by either automated or manual techniques. Automated techniques are more efficient, but there is always some degree of red blood cell loss with each wash cycle. When the washing is performed in an open system, the resulting product must be transfused within 24 hours because of concerns over potential bacterial contamination.

The primary aim of washing is to remove plasma proteins, although some leukocytes and platelets are removed simultaneously. The major indication for washed red blood cells is the prevention of severe allergic transfusion reactions, thought to be mediated by recipient antibodies (most likely IgE) to donor plasma proteins. Washing is recommended when reactions are recurrent and severe, even in the face of steroid and antihistamine administration. In IgA-deficient patients who have preformed antibody to IgA, IgA-containing plasma can cause anaphylaxis. Multiple cell washes may be required to remove the contaminating plasma protein.

Irradiated Red Blood Cells

Red blood cells are irradiated with a minimum dose of 25 Gy. Red cells expire 28 days after irradiation or the original expiration date, whichever is sooner. A method is used to ensure that irradiation has occurred with each batch. The primary aim of irradiation is to prevent the rare, but often fatal risk for transfusion-associated graft-versus-host disease (TA-GVHD) by the abrogation of the proliferative potential of donor T lymphocytes. Graft-versus-host disease can occur after the transfusion of immunologically competent donor lymphocytes, usually to an immunoincompetent recipient. Some patient populations with indications for irradiated products include neonates, patients with hematologic malignancies, stem cell transplant recipients, and patients with congenital immune deficiencies. There is still much debate among experts regarding which additional patient populations may be at risk for TA-GVHD. It has been suggested that a policy of universal blood component irradiation could prevent TA-GVHD in patients with currently unsuspected risks, including advanced age, unrecognized immune deficiencies in the recipient, or unsuspected donor-recipient immune similarities.

Frozen Red Blood Cells

Red blood cells can be frozen (with glycerol, used as a cryoprotective agent) and stored in liquid nitrogen or mechanical freezers. The required concentration of glycerol depends on the rate and the temperature of freezing. The freezing process destroys other blood constituents, except for a small percentage of immunocompetent lymphocytes. Red blood cells are prepared for transfusion by thawing and washing away the glycerol using a series of progressively less hypertonic saline solutions, allowing glycerol to diffuse gradually from the cells to prevent hemolysis. The cells are resuspended in an isotonic saline solution containing glucose. The extensive washing removes approximately 99.9% of the plasma as well as cellular debris.

Red blood cells can be stored in the frozen state for at least 10 years with good viability. After thawing and washing, storage is typically limited to 24 hours because of the open system. Frozen cells have been shown to maintain prefreezing ATP and 2,3-DPG levels. To maintain these factors at high levels, the standard is to freeze within 6 days of collection. When it is necessary to freeze older units, rejuvenation with a solution containing pyruvate, glucose, phosphate, and adenine has provided excellent results. The major indication for frozen red blood cells is the stockpiling of rare donor units for patients who have developed alloantibodies. Some patients with rare phenotypes can make autologous donations that can be frozen for later use. Cells from autologous donors can be frozen if more units are required than can be collected in the 42-day liquid storage period or if surgery is postponed. Because of the high cost and cumbersome nature of freeze-thaw procedures, other uses of frozen red blood cells are somewhat difficult to justify.

APPROPRIATE TRANSFUSION PRACTICE IN VARIOUS CLINICAL SETTINGS

The response to red blood cell transfusion varies from patient to patient. In the absence of increased red blood cell destruction or sequestration, 1 unit of red blood cells can be expected to increase the hemoglobin level by 1 g/dL or the hematocrit level by approximately 3%. This rise is usually not fully realized until approximately 24 hours after transfusion, when the plasma volume has had time to return to normal. On the basis of a half-life of approximately 57.7 days for donor red blood cells, Mollison and associates calculated that an average-sized adult requires 24 mL of red blood cells per day to maintain a given hematocrit level, assuming no red blood cell production. Patients with red cell aplasia require approximately 2 units of red blood cells every 2 weeks.

Several factors can adversely affect the survival of transfused red blood cells. Hemolysis, caused by either immune red blood cell damage or mechanical trauma, shortens the survival of transfused cells, much as it shortens the survival of the patient's own cells. Hypersplenism can lead to initial sequestration as well as increased destruction of red blood cells. Continued blood loss is another obvious cause of suboptimal response to transfusion. It should also be emphasized that transfusion suppresses erythropoiesis, so that the net result of transfusion may be less than expected if transfusions are administered on a chronic basis.

Chronic Anemia

As a rule, signs and symptoms attributable to anemia are unlikely to develop at a hemoglobin level of greater than 7 or 8 g/dL. When the anemia is of gradual onset, the body's compensatory mechanisms for maintaining oxygen delivery to the tissues come into play. Both cardiac output and intracellular 2,3-DPG increase, and thus oxygen unloads at a lower oxygen saturation of hemoglobin. When chronic anemia is due to red blood cell destruction, the healthy bone marrow responds by increasing production up to sixfold.

Red blood cell transfusion is always symptomatic and supportive rather than definitive therapy for anemia. Transfusion should be used only when there is no definitive treatment for the underlying cause or when the severity of the anemia and the clinical manifestations in the patient make it impossible to wait for the effects of the treatment to be realized.

Generalizations about whether or when to transfuse red blood cells, and how many, are difficult to make and are usually inappropriate. The clinical impact of anemia varies, depending on its pathogenesis, rate of onset, the presence or absence of accompanying hypovolemia, and most important, the individual patient. The hemoglobin level at which a given individual manifests the signs and symptoms of anemia relates, in part, to underlying health status, cardiorespiratory reserve, and activity level.

Perioperative Period

Many generalizations have been made about the appropriate transfusion management of acute blood loss, often with little hard data to support the arguments. One rule of thumb is that blood loss of 10% or less of total blood volume requires no replacement therapy at all; loss of up to 20% can be replaced exclusively with crystalloid solutions; and loss of greater than 25% generally requires red blood cell transfusion to restore oxygen-carrying capacity, along with crystalloid and sometimes colloid solutions to restore intravascular volume to maintain perfusion. For years, the figure of 10 g/dL of hemoglobin had been used as the gold standard for the red blood cell transfusion trigger during the perioperative period, but 7 g/dL is now more commonly used. Each case must be evaluated individually on the basis of clinical signs and symptoms, rather than on the basis of laboratory values. If the cardiovascular system is healthy and the degree of hypoperfusion is not significant, good tissue oxygenation can be maintained at much lower hemoglobin levels. A National Institutes of Health consensus conference suggested that many surgical patients do not need transfusion unless the hemoglobin level falls to less than 7 g/dL. Given that red blood cell transfusion should be tailored to individual needs, the question arises as to whether there is any readily available, objective measurement that can be used to determine how low the hemoglobin level can safely be allowed to fall before red blood cell transfusion is initiated.

Global hemodynamic parameters do not always correlate with microvascular perfusion. Assessment of tissue oxygenation at the microvascular level would help evaluate the effectiveness of a red cell transfusion, evaluate the effect of red cell storage on end-organ perfusion, and provide data about when to transfuse. Several general methods are available to evaluate the microcirculation and include direct assessment using image techniques and indirect methods of assessment, such as measures of microvascular oxygen availability and function. Direct assessment can be performed using laser Doppler flowmetry, imaging of the microcirculation, intravital microscopy, orthogonal polarization spectral imaging, and sidestream dark-field imaging. Assessments of oxygen availability include oxygen electrodes, reflectance spectrophotometry, and near-infrared spectroscopy. The techniques described are currently considered research tools and are not available in routine clinical practice. Many have yet to prove reliable and reproducible in the clinical setting. Further, some are useful only in specific organ systems and do not reflect the global oxygenation of the patient. To be useful at the bedside, a technique must be technically simple, rapid, and noninvasive without large interoperator variation. Such a device has yet to become available.

The Society of Thoracic Surgeons and the Society of Cardiovascular Anesthesiologists published clinical practice guidelines that identified six variables that increased a patient's risk for postoperative blood transfusion: advanced age, low preoperative red blood cell volume, preoperative antiplatelet or antithrombotic drugs, reoperative or complex procedures, emergency operations, and noncardiac patient comorbidities. The report recommended developing institution-specific protocols to screen for high-risk patients and apply blood conservation interventions, such as erythropoietin or antifibrinolytic administration, intraoperative blood salvage or normovolemic hemodilution, and institution-specific blood transfusion algorithms supplemented with point-of-care testing.

Randomized clinical trials have evaluated the effects of different transfusion thresholds in the surgery setting; however, the thresholds used in the studies differ widely. Many of the studies found no difference in outcome. Most studies were not powered to adequately evaluate clinically important outcomes. Few included more than 100 patients. The Transfusion Requirements in Critical Care (TRICC) trial included 838 ICU patients who were randomized to a restrictive transfusion strategy (transfused at Hb 7 g/dL) or liberal strategy (transfused at 10 g/dL). The 30-day mortality was slightly lower in the restrictive group (18.7% versus 23.3%), but not significantly lower. The FOCUS trial (Functional Outcomes in Cardiovascular Patients Undergoing Surgical Hip Fracture Repair), a 2600-patient, multicenter randomized trial designed to determine whether patients with cardiovascular disease or cardiovascular risk factors undergoing surgical repair of the hip benefit from a lower or higher transfusion trigger, has recently completed. The results suggest that patients do not benefit from liberal transfusion therapy.

The possibility of immunomodulation by allogeneic transfusions in humans was first suggested more than 30 years ago when improved renal allograft survival was reported in pretransplant transfusion recipients. A potential link between allogeneic transfusion and an increased rate of cancer recurrence and postoperative infection was first raised in the 1980s, and numerous retrospective and prospective observational studies supporting these contentions have been reported in the literature since that time. These studies, as well as reports from investigations with opposing data, have been analyzed in numerous reviews on the topic. Studies in experimental animals have also yielded contradictory results. Research using animal models and human subjects on the specific immunomodulatory effects of transfusion has consistently pointed to depression of cell-mediated immunity, although the specific defects seen have varied. The mediators of these immunomodulatory effects appear to be leukocytes present in cellular blood components, including whole blood and red blood cells. Several well-designed, prospective, randomized controlled trials comparing transfusion of leukoreduced blood components or autologous blood with transfusion of unmodified allogeneic blood components have reported inconclusive results. Although controversy exists about whether red cell transfusions produce immunomodulatory effects, such as cancer recurrence or perioperative surgical infections, the use of leukoreduced red cell components has been advocated as a means to mitigate the effects of transfused white cells.

Red Blood Cell Transfusion in Neonates

In neonates it is convenient to consider periodic, small-volume transfusion separately from massive transfusion situations. The trigger for transfusion and the optimal type of component are very different in the two settings. The potential adverse effects may be quite distinct.

Low-volume red blood cell transfusion is rarely indicated in full-term infants unless acute blood loss has occurred at birth or an intrauterine situation has led to prenatal anemia. In contrast, premature infants are frequent recipients of transfusions. In the intensive care setting, the premature infant is subjected to frequent blood sampling, and iatrogenic anemia may necessitate transfusion. Anemia of prematurity is also a well-recognized entity; premature infants have a slightly lower Hb value at birth. In addition, the postnatal decline in Hb occurs earlier and is more pronounced in premature infants. The mechanism for anemia of prematurity appears to involve a relatively lower output of erythropoietin in response to a given degree of anemia. This phenomenon is attributed in part to the fact that the liver, rather than the kidney, is the major site of erythropoietin production in these infants. Although some practitioners have considered this degree of anemia to be physiologic, the benign nature of this condition remains controversial.

Another debate among neonatologists concerns the triggers for red blood cell transfusion, as in what clinical signs and symptoms are valid reflections of poor tissue oxygenation. Congestive heart failure and severe pulmonary disease are generally accepted indications for transfusion, but recurrent apnea, tachypnea, tachycardia, and failure to thrive are also used as transfusion triggers. In recent times, the rate of transfusion and the donor exposure rate of premature infants have consistently declined. These changes, however, reflect improvements in patient care (e.g., microtesting methods resulting in less iatrogenic blood loss; the use of surfactant resulting in decreases in respiratory distress) and the use of a single unit to supply one infant over a longer period rather than being attributable to changes in the transfusion trigger. The prolonged use of single units has become possible with the advent of the sterile docking technology, which preserves the full shelf life of the unit of red blood cells, as well as with the accumulating solid evidence that fresh blood is not necessary for low-volume transfusions in neonates, because supernatant potassium and decreased pH are not of concern in this setting. Two recent studies have provided additional information about the relative risks and benefits of using restrictive rather than more liberal criteria for very-low-birth-weight infants. One study showed that a liberal transfusion practice resulted in more infants receiving transfusion but conferred little evidence of benefit. The other study showed a lower risk for apnea and major brain injury for the liberal transfusion arm of the study. Therefore the safest transfusion trigger in the preterm infant still remains unclear and further studies are indicated. Most institutions assess the clinical situation and consider the postnatal age and whether a neonate has oxygen requirements when determining the need for a red blood cell transfusion.

The dose of an RBC transfusion in a neonate can vary by institution between 5 to 20 mL/kg. Few studies have assessed the optimal dose in this patient population, and further studies are needed. Paul and colleagues compared 10 and 20 mL/kg and found that the larger volume did not cause impaired pulmonary function. Wong and colleagues demonstrated that extra transfusion episodes could be avoided with 20 mL/kg versus 15 mL/kg, without any additional risk to the patient. Many transfusion services now routinely use red blood cells stored in additive solutions for low volume red blood cell transfusion and thus prefer a dose of 20 mL/kg to account for the lower hematocrit of an additive unit.

Finally, several trials of erythropoietin therapy in premature infants have been undertaken. The administration of relatively high-dose erythropoietin has been shown to raise hemoglobin levels and reticulocyte counts in healthy premature infants, but the effect in sicker neonates is unclear. Although transfusion exposure was decreased, the significance of this observation is diminished, given the promise of new strategies for limiting transfusions and donor exposure. The high cost and the increased risk for retinopathy associated with erythropoietin treatment does not justify its use in this patient population.

In the case of massive transfusion, the situation differs. There have been marked increases in massive transfusion in recent years in full-term as well as premature infants. Hemolytic disease of the newborn remains a prominent indication for exchange transfusion; however, the recent use of intravenous immune globulin to decrease red cell antibody levels in newborns has decreased the necessity of this procedure. The two triggers for exchange are (a) rapidly rising levels of unconjugated bilirubin that may lead to kernicterus and permanent central nervous system damage and (b) congestive heart failure secondary to severe anemia. Exchange transfusion is especially beneficial in cases of hemolytic disease of the newborn because it clears the bilirubin and the offending antibody from the circulation and removes antibody-coated red blood cells before lysis, while providing a source of red blood cells lacking the offending antigen. A two-blood-volume exchange is commonly performed by using a fresh unit of blood concentrated to a final hematocrit level of approximately 50%. In cases of hyperbilirubinemia resulting from other causes (e.g., that associated with liver immaturity in premature infants), phototherapy is the treatment of choice because its effects are usually more sustained, and exchange transfusion is used only for cases of marked elevations. Extracorporeal membrane oxygenation and open-heart surgery are two other situations in which the neonate may be exposed to large volumes of allogeneic red blood cells. The extracorporeal membrane oxygenation circuit requires a prime with red blood cells, as do many of the types of extracorporeal circuits used for cardiopulmonary bypass.

Although accumulating evidence supports the safety of using red blood cell units of any age and with any preservative solution for low-volume transfusions in neonates, the same transfusion policies may not apply to massive transfusion. Newborn physiology is unique in several ways that may have implications for massive transfusion therapy. The newborn does not handle metabolites in a mature fashion. Renal immaturity may lead to problems in clearing potassium or acid from stored red blood cells, and the immature liver may not catabolize citrate efficiently. These problems are accentuated and protracted in the premature infant. To address the concern about potassium load, fresh (<5 days old) or washed red blood cells are often used, although the necessity of this practice is actively debated. Fresh blood may also be preferred because of its higher 2,3-DPG levels and better red blood cell integrity. The citrate problem is probably best handled by using slow infusion rates, because the use of bicarbonate or calcium replacement to counteract the acid load or calcium-chelating effects of citrate is controversial. Finally, the use of red blood cells stored in the newer preservative solutions (CPDA-1, Adsol, Nutricel, Optisol) is avoided by some authorities because of the risk for renal damage and renal stones due to adenine metabolites. If CPD red blood cells are not available, the additive solution can be removed and the cells washed. Red blood cells preserved in additive solutions also have a lower hematocrit, which must be taken into account in making calculations for exchange transfusion.

The humoral and cellular immune systems of the neonate are immature, especially in the premature infant. There is a small but real risk for transfusion-induced graft-versus-host disease in premature infants receiving red blood cell transfusions and in the fetus undergoing intrauterine transfusion. Irradiation of red blood cells should be performed in both settings. Another risk of transfusion in low-birth-weight (<1500 g) premature infants is the development of clinical cytomegalovirus (CMV) infection in infants of cytomegalovirus-seronegative mothers. CMV-safe blood, either CMV seronegative or leukoreduced, should be provided to these infants.

Novel ideas to decrease donor exposure in neonates include delayed cord clamping in premature infants and autologous cord blood transfusion. One review of 10 delayed cord clamping studies demonstrated lower transfusion requirements in the delayed versus early clamped group. However, a randomized controlled trial by Strauss found no difference in transfusion needs between delayed versus early clamped groups. A few studies have looked at autologous cord blood transfusions in neonates. One study found that the amount of blood harvested was insufficient to cover all transfusions in low-birth-weight infants. In addition, studies have demonstrated that blood processing problems, bacterial contamination and costs are all barriers to the routine collection and autotransfusion of cord blood.

RED BLOOD CELL PRESERVATION AND STORAGE

The first key to the storage of blood is a stable, minimally toxic anticoagulant with preservative properties. During the early 1900s, it was recognized that citrate met these criteria. Citrate is slightly more toxic than heparin, especially when given rapidly and in large amounts, but citrate has preservative action that heparin lacks. Citrate has the added advantage of not causing systemic anticoagulation in the recipient.

The other factor essential for long-term storage is a mechanism to maintain cell viability and function. Fresh transfused red blood cells have a good survival rate in the recipient's circulation, with a destruction rate approximately equal to that of the recipient's own cells: 1% per day.

Discoveries during the past 2 decades have raised clinical concern regarding the efficacy and risks of RBC transfusion. Changes within the RBC and its supernatant during RBC storage have been associated with reduced tissue oxygenation and other adverse effects in patients receiving red blood cell components stored for extended periods. The biochemical, structural, and functional changes are collectively termed the *red cell storage lesion*. The alterations found with the storage lesion, along with the clinical implications, will be discussed in this section.

Biochemical Changes Associated With Red Blood Cell Storage

Adenosine Triphosphate Levels

Adenosine triphosphate (ATP) levels appear to be a major determinant of red blood cell viability. The drop in cellular ATP levels during storage has been correlated with increased cell rigidity and with loss of membrane lipid, leading to decreased red blood cell life span. For this reason, most efforts to extend red blood cell storage have focused on ways to maintain intracellular ATP levels. First, dextrose was introduced into the citrate solution (citrate-phosphate-dextrose [CPD]: 21 days), and then adenine was added (CPDA-1: 35 days). Three additive solutions containing additional dextrose and adenine (Nutricel, or AS-3) or dextrose and adenine plus mannitol (Adsol, or AS-1) and (Optisol, or AS-5) allow extension of the maximum storage time to 42 days (Table 112-2). The majority of today's red blood cell supply is stored in an additive solution.

Table 112-2 Biochemical Changes in Stored Red Blood Cells

Variable	CPDA-1 Fresh	CPDA-1 35 Days	Adsol 35 Days
In vivo survival (at 24 hours) (%)	100	<71.0	<88.0
pH	<7.5	<6.7	<6.7
ATP (% initial)	100	<45.0	<76.0
2,3-DPG (% initial)	100	<10.0	<10.0
Plasma K^+ (mEq/L)	5.1	<78.5	<49.0

Data from Zuck TF, Bensinger TA, Peck CC, et al: The in vivo survival of red cells stored in modified CPD with adenine: report of a multi-institutional cooperative effort. *Transfusion* 17:34, 1977; and Moore GL, Peck CC, Sohmer RR, et al: Some properties of blood stored in anticoagulant CPDA-1 solution: a brief summary. *Transfusion* 21:135, 1981.

2,3-Diphosphoglycerate Levels

Stored red blood cells must also maintain their capacity to deliver oxygen. It was not until 1967 that the central role of 2,3-diphosphoglycerate (2,3-DPG) in releasing oxygen from oxyhemoglobin was recognized. Attention was then focused on ways to maintain high levels of 2,3-DPG in stored blood cells. The first anticoagulant introduced on a large scale, acid citrate-dextrose, was ineffective because of its low initial pH; however, the subsequently developed CPD, with its higher initial pH and slower fall in pH, was superior. CPDA-1 and additive solutions have not further improved 2,3-DPG maintenance. Although 2,3-DPG depletion of stored red blood cells is known to decrease oxygen delivery, the clinical significance of this finding is unclear. 2,3-DPG levels in stored blood cells are rapidly regenerated in vivo, rising to greater than 50% of normal within several hours and to normal within 24 hours. Although a patient with normal cardiac status should be able to compensate by increasing cardiac output to maintain normal oxygen delivery until 2,3-DPG levels are regenerated, an improvement in 2,3-DPG preservation in stored red blood cells is still desirable.

Citrate

Infusion of large volumes of blood with citrate anticoagulant over a short period may cause plasma citrate levels to reach the toxic range. The primary concern is the cardiovascular effects of hypocalcemia caused by chelation of calcium by citrate. The risk for citrate toxicity is exacerbated by liver dysfunction or liver immaturity. Despite these theoretical considerations, there is little documented evidence of clinical citrate toxicity, and the problem can usually be prevented by slower infusion. If large amounts of blood have to be infused over a very short period, administration of calcium gluconate can be considered, but whether the benefits justify the risk is controversial.

Potassium

Another issue with prolonged storage is the excess potassium in the red blood cell supernatant that could potentially cause cardiac arrhythmias. At a storage temperature of 4° C, the red blood cell sodium-potassium pump is essentially nonfunctional, and intra- and extracellular levels gradually equilibrate. In addition, hemolysis results in increased potassium in the supernatant. However, because the total volume of plasma in red blood cell concentrates is low (approximately 70 mL), the total potassium burden is only approximately 5.5 mEq at product expiration. Practically speaking, the potassium load is rarely a clinical problem except in the setting of preexisting hyperkalemia and renal failure. In this situation, fresher units of red blood cells or washed red blood cells can be used.

DEHP

Since their introduction in the 1960s, plastic blood bags used for storing red blood cells have been made from polyvinylchloride containing the lipophilic plasticizer di(2-ethylhexyl)phthalate (DEHP), which confers pliability. The safety of DEHP has been questioned for years owing to its tendency to leach from the bag and to be present at levels of 50 to 70 mg/L in stored red blood cells. The storage of RBCs in bags made of polyvinyl chloride plasticized with DEHP has caused more concern recently because of the reported association between DEHP exposure and impaired development of the male genital tract. One of the benefits of the use of DEHP for red blood cell storage is the prevention of hemolysis. DEHP leaches out from the plastic bag and intercalates and stabilizes the red cell membrane. Shorter storage lessens the load of DEHP delivered to the recipient. Although there are potential replacement plasticizers, DEHP is most commonly used since the exposure to DEHP through transfusion is generally felt to be less than through other environmental exposures.

Storage Length of Red Blood Cells

Current Status

The current expiration time of a red blood cell unit stored in an additive solution is 42 days. The allowable storage time is regulated by the FDA and requires (1) the recovery of at least 75% of red cells transfused 24 hours after infusion and (2) less than 1% hemolysis, both at the end of the storage limit. There is no criterion based on the clinical ability of transfused red cells to oxygenate tissue. The 2009 National Blood Collection and Utilization Survey reported that the mean age of red blood cell units at transfusion was 18.2 days.

Many variables affect the age of a specific red blood cell unit at transfusion. The blood group of the unit will impact the length of storage. Group O units tend to be issued quickly because of their universal compatibility; as a result, Group O units are often issued with a shorter age. Group B and AB tend to be stored the longest. Transfusion service type will also affect the overall age of red blood cell units at the time of transfusion. Busy tertiary care hospitals tend to transfuse some of the oldest units since they may receive units returned from smaller community centers that did not expect to use them before their outdate. Hospitals that have blood refrigerators outside the blood bank tend to age units in the refrigerators because it is cumbersome to rotate the units out frequently. Hospitals with high crossmatched-to-transfused ratios also tend to have older units on their shelves.

Red Cell Storage Lesion

The red blood cell storage lesion includes all the changes that occur to blood components during blood bank storage. The lesion includes biochemical and structural changes to the red cell, as well as changes that occur in the storage supernatant. The structural changes include red cell membrane loss that leads to the reversible evolution of the shape of the red cell from a biconcave disc to a spheroechinocyte. After this stage, further red cell membrane loss becomes irreversible and microvesicles are produced. Red cell vesicles are quickly cleared by macrophages as a result of exposed negatively charged lipids. The infusion of a large amount of red cell vesicles during a red blood cell transfusion may overwhelm the reticuloendothelial system and cause a proinflammatory and prothrombotic response. The shape changes are also associated with a rheologic effect, including increased viscosity and reduced flow within the capillaries, leading to decreased tissue perfusion. Many of the biochemical and structural changes, aside from vesiculation, are reversible when the red blood cells enter human circulation where pH, ATP levels, and 2,3 DPG levels are normal.

Older red cells become more susceptible to oxidative damage, although this change generally occurs at a lower rate during in vitro conditions than in vivo because of the lower storage temperature. However, during a transfusion the human circulation is confronted by a bolus of equally damaged red blood cells that may overwhelm the reticuloendothelial system. Irradiated cells are exposed to additional oxidative stress that can damage red cell protein and lipid. White blood cells in the component also break down during storage and release proteases and lipases. Lysophospholipids and glycosidases are produced. Glycosidases may remove sialic acid and other sugars from the red cell membrane and can cause increased binding of stored red cells to endothelial cells and potentially contribute to endothelial inflammation. Increased lysophospholipids, such as platelet activating factor, have been found in units that have caused transfusion-related acute lung injury (TRALI).

Clinical Relevance of the Red Cell Storage Lesion

Retrospective or prospective observational studies in many diverse patient populations have suggested numerous adverse events that may be associated with prolonged red blood cell storage, including increased risk for mortality, postoperative infection, multiorgan failure, deep venous thrombosis, or increased length of stay in the ICU or hospital. The observational studies on this topic have a number of significant limitations. First, larger volumes of RBC transfusion predict worse outcomes. Patients who are transfused larger volumes are statistically more likely to receive older RBCs. Second, confounding factors may not be recognized and discounted in nonrandomized studies. Third, individual methodologies in the presently available studies have varied markedly. Some studies have looked at the effect of mean storage age of all units transfused on outcome, and some have broken storage time into categorical groups (i.e., is storage less than 14 days safer than storage beyond 14 days). In addition, studies have not used a single definition for "older" units; some have defined older units as greater than 14 days, greater than 21 days, or greater than 28 days. The definitions of age have not been based on either clinical or microcirculatory relevance or related to the feasibility and practicality of blood collection. Most studies have been designed for convenience and feasibility; a study of red cell storage age with a definition of an older red blood cell unit as greater than 14 days of storage is achievable given current hospital inventories. Although 14 days is close to the average age of RBCs stored in a blood bank, from a blood collection and inventory management perspective, an expiration time of 14 days would be disastrous for both hospitals and blood collection facilities. Authorities have argued that studies should be designed to measure storage age differences between lengths of storage that would be achievable given current inventory levels and those that would be feasible during times of difficulties in donor recruiting.

Published studies have focused on three patient groups that consume large numbers of RBC components: cardiac surgery, trauma, and critical care patients. A publication on the effect of red blood cell storage age on hematopoietic transplant recipients has also been recently published. The cardiac surgery studies have confirmed the previous finding that large numbers of red blood cell transfusions are associated with adverse outcomes, largely reflecting the patient's underlying condition. If the number of units transfused is controlled for, the effect of the RBC storage lesion is difficult to discern in cardiac studies. The majority of studies in cardiac and trauma patients addressing red blood cell storage duration have reported negative outcomes with longer storage, but none has been both large and randomized, and even multivariate analysis cannot separate all potential confounding effects. Unlike in cardiac surgery and trauma, there have been three prospective, randomized trials addressing the storage lesions in ICU patients. Adverse effects with longer storage were not demonstrated in these studies.

Although the randomized prospective trial seems to be the only option to determine the clinical consequences of the red blood cell storage lesion, conducting a well-designed trial is not an easy task. Limited blood bank inventories to supply the longer and shorter storage duration arms, difficulty in consenting patients, and the difficulty in selecting outcome measures to study have plagued the previously attempted studies.

Three large, multicenter, randomized, double-blinded trials are underway in North America investigating three different patient groups. The Age of Blood Evaluation (ABLE) study will investigate the effect of leukoreduced red blood cells stored 7 days or less versus leukoreduced standard-issue red blood cells on 90-day all-cause mortality. Investigators will attempt to enroll 2510 adult subjects receiving their first red blood cell unit in an intensive care unit. The study is powered to detect a 5% absolute risk reduction. A second study, the Age of Red Blood Cells in Premature Infants (ARIPI), is a double-blinded study that will evaluate the effectiveness of RBCs stored no longer than 7 days versus standard-issue red blood cells in 450 neonates requiring transfusions. The primary outcome for this study will be a composite measure of major neonatal morbidities. The study is powered to detect a 15% absolute risk reduction. Finally, the Red Cell Storage Duration Study (RECESS) will evaluate 1434 pediatric and adult subjects undergoing complex cardiac surgical procedures who are likely to require red blood cell transfusion. Subjects will be randomized to receive red blood cell units stored either for 10 or fewer days or for 21 or more days. Randomization will occur only if the blood bank has enough units of red blood cells of both storage times to meet the crossmatch request. The primary outcome is the change in the multiple organ dysfunction score (MODS) since a mortality outcome would have required too many patients.

The published studies evaluating whether adverse clinical consequences are associated with prolonged red blood cell storage have yet to satisfactorily answer this important question in any patient population. The anticipated publication of the three randomized, controlled studies in the coming years may provide an answer to this question in a specific patient population; until these results are available, clinicians should continue to use red cells for their permissible storage period. It is important to remember that if one of these studies does find worse outcomes with longer storage age duration, many questions and obstacles will remain before this issue can be resolved. If proven, the adverse clinical effects will most likely apply not only to the patient population studied, but to all patients. Further, the current red blood cell inventory almost always meets hospital needs with a 42-day RBC expiration period but is not currently equipped to meet the needs of a less than 7-day inventory, or even a less than 21-day inventory. Finally, although it is logical to expect that there is a limit to red blood cell storage, beyond which the risks of transfusion outweigh the benefits of transfusion, none of the randomized studies just described is designed to determine this limit.

ALTERNATIVES TO ALLOGENEIC RED CELL TRANSFUSIONS

There are many alternatives to standard allogeneic red cell transfusions for a patient requiring elective surgery (Table 112-3). Potential alternatives include banking autologous units before the surgery, acute normovolemic hemodilution, pharmacologic therapies (i.e., erythropoietin or fibrinolysis inhibitors), perioperative salvage, virally inactivated donor red cells, or blood substitutes. All current options have their own unique benefits and drawbacks, and some of these alternatives are not yet available. In cases where an emergency transfusion is needed, the first three options would not be possible, because they all require significant planning. Only virally inactivated components and red cell substitutes (both of which are still works in progress) would be available for unanticipated transfusion needs.

Table 112-3 Alternatives to Standard Allogeneic Transfusions

Hemodilution
Intraoperative autologous transfusion
Perioperative blood salvage
Lower transfusion trigger
Pharmacologic therapies
Pathogen inactivation
Red cell substitutes
Stem cell–derived red blood cells

Autologous Blood Transfusion

Advantages of Autologous Blood Transfusion

The substitution of autologous blood components for those collected from other (allogeneic) donors eliminates transfusion-transmitted diseases such as hepatitis and acquired immunodeficiency syndrome. Immunologic complications related to the transfusion of foreign cells, including hemolysis and febrile reactions to white blood cells, are also prevented. Other advantages, though possible, are less clearly established. For example, erythropoiesis may be sufficiently stimulated in the repeatedly bled autologous donor to hasten recovery from postoperative anemia. Intraoperatively salvaged red blood cells are spared the acquired membrane defects (storage lesion) and 2,3-diphosphoglycerate deficiencies of refrigerated red blood cells.

An important drawback to these techniques is their increased expense, in contrast to the simpler allogeneic transfusions they replace. In addition, the availability of autologous components may result in their use in situations where transfusion might not have otherwise been considered. Patients with suboptimal compensatory erythropoiesis and donation-induced anemia at the time of surgery are also more likely to be given transfusions. Based on the current level of viral safety in blood components in the developed world, the use of autologous blood has dropped significantly from times when viral testing was not available or reliable.

Some patients and their families ask for directed blood donations, hoping to select blood donors that are known to them and presumably have less risk. This practice has not been shown to have any medical benefit, may cause reduced or delayed blood availability, and should not be considered a worthwhile transfusion alternative.

Preoperative Autologous Blood Collection

The typical volunteer allogeneic blood donor is allowed to give 1 unit of blood no more than once every 8 weeks, to prevent iron deficiency. However, provided that bone marrow erythropoiesis can be stimulated and satisfactory iron supplies maintained, blood can be collected as frequently as once a week from an autologous donor. Although the shelf life of refrigerated red blood cells is limited to 42 days, frozen storage for up to 10 years is possible at less than −65° C, using glycerol as a cryopreservative.

From a cardiovascular standpoint, phlebotomy is well tolerated by a variety of seemingly high-risk donors, including older adults, children, pregnant women, and patients with coronary artery disease. By contrast, anemia frequently develops during the donation interval and limits the number of autologous units that can be collected. In addition to marginal iron stores, erythropoietin levels often do not increase during the donation interval, probably because the hematocrit level of most donors is not allowed to fall to less than 30%. This situation may be improved by the administration of the recombinant growth hormone erythropoietin to autologous donors. The use of preoperatively donated autologous blood has also been reported for a variety of surgical procedures, including radical prostatectomy; hysterectomies and other gynecologic procedures; colorectal, biliary, and gastric surgery; orthopedic surgery; and neurosurgery.

Autologous blood has been safely collected from women during pregnancy for use during childbirth. Nevertheless, the transfusion rate at delivery is quite low (<2.5% in many institutions), and most autologous donations are unused. Long-term (frozen) storage of autologous red blood cells in the absence of a planned transfusion episode is largely ineffective and expensive.

Intraoperative Blood Salvage

Cell salvage occurs in three phases: collection, washing, and reinfusion. RBCs are collected from the operative field using a dedicated double-lumen suction device. One lumen suctions blood from the operative field, and the other lumen adds heparinized saline to the salvaged blood. The anticoagulated blood then passes through a filter and is collected in a reservoir. If less than 1 L of blood is collected, further processing is foregone and the collected blood is discarded.

In most circumstances the contents in the bag can be washed to remove free hemoglobin, surgical irrigant solutions, and other debris. Instruments are available that include both a reservoir for collecting salvaged blood and a centrifugal washer. Large aliquots (>500 mL) can be fully washed in as little as 3 minutes. As a result of this speed, autologous blood salvage has become practical in situations in which blood loss may be extremely rapid, such as trauma or liver transplantation.

The hematocrit level of unwashed blood is typically low because of dilution from irrigating surgical fluids and some degree of mechanical hemolysis. Free hemoglobin levels are sometimes greater than 1000 mg% in unwashed blood, and hemoglobinemia and hemoglobinuria may occur after the transfusion, although renal sequelae are surprisingly low. Despite this evidence of red blood cell injury, the survival rate of ^{51}Cr-labeled salvaged cells is normal in most patients studied.

Many potential complications are associated with cell salvage, such as nonimmune hemolysis, air embolus, febrile nonhemolytic transfusion reactions, mistransfusion, coagulopathy, and contamination with drugs. Transfusion of salvaged blood has resulted in coagulation abnormalities, including hypofibrinogenemia, prolonged prothrombin time and partial thromboplastin time, elevated fibrin degradation products, and thrombocytopenia. These coagulation abnormalities most likely reflect the characteristics of the salvaged blood itself, which, after exposure to serosal surfaces, becomes deficient in coagulation factors and platelets and, in the case of unwashed blood, has high levels of fibrin degradation products (Table 112-4).

Fat, fibrin, bone fragments, and microaggregates often contaminate salvaged autologous blood. However, infusion of unwashed blood has not been proved harmful in either animals or humans, possibly because routine blood filters remove most particulate material. Other contaminants, such as heparin, topical antibiotics, hemostatic agents, and biologic substances such as tissue enzymes, can be at least partially removed by washing. Complete removal of bacteria is also not possible, even when the salvaged blood is washed with antibiotics. Thus collection of blood from a contaminated site (e.g., with intestinal contents) is usually considered to be contraindicated; in fact, manufacturers contraindicate the use of cell salvage in cases in which there is potential contamination of salvaged blood with enteric contents. However, in recent years this viewpoint has been reconsidered, because studies have found that autotransfusion of microbiologically contaminated salvaged blood have demonstrated no adverse outcomes or increase in postoperative infectious complications. Tumor cells have been found in blood salvaged during cancer operations and many practitioners consider cancer another contraindication; others believe that filtration would remove salvaged tumor cells.

Approximately one-half the blood lost during surgery can be salvaged. The rest is usually irretrievably absorbed in drapes and sponges or damaged during collection. The use of salvaged autologous blood has been associated with a 50% reduction in allogeneic blood use in orthopedic procedures such as spinal surgery and hip replacement and is also effective in vascular surgical procedures such as aortic reconstruction. Autologous salvage has been a useful adjunct in the treatment of some Jehovah's Witnesses, whose literal acceptance of the Bible includes abstention from routine allogeneic blood transfusions.

Both the canister systems and red blood cell processors used to collect intraoperative autologous blood can also be employed to collect postoperative blood drainage, such as that from the mediastinum after open heart surgery, from the knee or hip after orthopedic procedures, or from the peritoneal cavity after hepatic injury. Because blood salvaged from a serosal cavity has little residual fibrinogen and platelets, clotting is not a problem, and the addition of anticoagulants is usually unnecessary. Shed mediastinal blood after open-heart surgery contains high levels of cardiac muscle enzymes, especially creatine kinase, as well as lactate dehydrogenase from hemolyzed red blood cells. Therefore reinfusion of shed blood results in elevated levels of both enzymes, which can confound the diagnosis of myocardial infarction in the postoperative period. Reinfusion of shed mediastinal blood has been shown to reduce the need for allogeneic transfusions.

Hemodilution

The collection of autologous blood during surgery for later reinfusion at the end of the procedure was first suggested in open-heart operations, in which it was hoped that a supply of platelets undamaged by exposure to the membrane oxygenator might reduce the incidence of coagulopathies. Hemodilution itself reduces red blood cell loss: a patient with a hematocrit level of 45% and 2 L blood loss during surgery loses roughly 900 mL of red blood cells, but one with a hematocrit level of 20% from hemodilution loses only 400 mL of red blood cells. Hemodilution is less expensive to accomplish than preoperative autologous blood donation and may be the only option available when surgery is performed in nonelective settings. Proponents claim that the induced anemia may even be beneficial to the patient, in that oxygen delivery at a hematocrit level of 30% is enhanced by an increased cardiac output resulting from the decreased blood viscosity.

Reductions in allogeneic blood needs have been reported after marked intraoperative hemodilution (after the hematocrit is lowered by 50%). More modest hemodilution (e.g., removal of 2 U of blood at the beginning of surgery) is also beneficial, according to some

Table 112-4 Autologous Blood Salvage Systems* Characteristics of Collected Blood

System	Hardware	Software	Hematocrit	Free Hemoglobin	Platelet Count	Coagulation Factors	Fibrin Degradation Products
Collection without washing	Rigid plastic container	Plastic bag	Low (25%)	Very high (200 mg%)	Low (100,000/mm^3)	Low (35%-75%)	High (300 mg%)
Collection followed by washing	Integral or separate blood cell processor	Disposable plastic bowl and tubing	High (60%)	Low (<50 mg%)	Very low (10,000/mm^3)	Absent (0%)	Absent (0%)

Data from Noon GP: Intraoperative autotransfusion. *Surgery* 84:719, 1978; and Silva R, Moore EE, Bar-Or D, et al: The risk: benefit ratio of autotransfusion-comparison to banked blood in a canine model. *J Trauma* 24:557, 1984.

*Typical results of laboratory tests are shown. Transfusion of large volumes of salvaged blood results in similar alterations in these tests in the recipient.

investigators but the amount of red cells saved is small. Furthermore, one group has provided evidence that hemodilution may jeopardize patients at risk for ischemic myocardial injury. More research is needed to establish the safety, efficacy, and ideal protocols for this form of blood conservation. Future availability of blood substitutes could facilitate augmented hemodilution for some patients who are expected to have large volumes of blood loss or who refuse blood transfusions.

BLOOD SUBSTITUTES

The search for blood substitutes began when our early scientific ancestors tested alternatives to human blood, including animal blood, milk, and wine. Modern research into the use of animal blood includes the work by Amberson and colleagues, who reported the successful use of a bovine hemosylate for exchange transfusions in cats and dogs. Further work revealed that human and bovine hemosylates caused renal dysfunction in human recipients. The suspected cause of this nephrotoxicity was the stromal lipid component of the RBC membrane. The logical next step in the search for the ideal substitute was the development of stroma-free hemoglobin (hemoglobin tetramer). Unfortunately, in 1978, Savitsky and colleagues demonstrated renal dysfunction, hypertension, and abdominal pain using stroma-free hemoglobin in healthy volunteers. It was hypothesized that these adverse events were due to the instability of the hemoglobin tetramer. Since then, efforts have been made to produce stabilized products with desirable oxygen off-loading characteristics and extended intravascular retention times.

Today, the U.S. blood supply is safe and has sufficient capacity to meet most patient needs. There is room for considerable improvement, however, in supply levels and risk reduction. The gap continues to narrow between a shrinking donor pool (owing to willingness and/or ability) and increasing transfusion requirements of an aging population. The threat of new and emerging infections results in the vulnerability of human-derived oxygen carriers. The continuous battle against emerging infectious disease underscores the risk for a tainted blood supply and depletion of transfusion resources. Theoretically, the ideal red cell substitute would solve both of these issues (Table 112-5). Many attempts have been made to develop red cell substitutes in the past, but no product has been able to fulfill all of the aforementioned criteria or meet the Food and Drug Administration's requirements of purity, potency, and safety. No licensed red cell substitute is available.

TYPES OF RED CELL SUBSTITUTES

It is important to differentiate between "blood substitutes" and red cell substitutes. Red cell substitutes are oxygen carriers and do not replace all components and functions of blood, for example, coagulation factors and white blood cells. Two main categories of oxygen carriers show promise as red blood cell substitutes: perfluorocarbons (PFCs) and hemoglobin-based oxygen carriers (HBOCs).

Table 112-5 The Ideal Red Cell Substitute

Delivers oxygen (and maybe enhances delivery)
Does not transmit disease
Does not have immunosuppressive effects
Available in abundant supply
Universally compatible (no need to type and crossmatch)
Prolonged shelf life and stable at a range of temperatures
Similar in vivo half-life to the red blood cell
Available at a reasonable cost
Easy to administer
Able to access all areas of the human body (including ischemic tissue)
Effective on room air or ambient conditions

Perfluorocarbons

Perfluorocarbons are chemically and biologically inert artificial fluorinated organic fluids that are immiscible in water and have a high solubility for oxygen. The amount of dissolved oxygen in PFC is directly related to the ambient oxygen tension—unlike Hb, gas molecules are not chemically bound to PFC but are absorbed and released by simple diffusion. Products require oxygen inhalation by the patient, because the oxygen delivery capacity is less than 30% of normal blood. PFCs have been shown to reduce the need for RBC transfusion, but have been associated with an increase in stroke rates. Although some PFCs are still being investigated, no major trials are currently ongoing and no licensed products are available in the United States.

Hemoglobin-Based Oxygen Carriers

The stroma of the red cell causes many of the problems in allogeneic human red cell transfusions. The red cell membrane ultimately fails and limits the shelf life. The red cell membrane also contains the antigens that limit compatibility. Unfortunately, initial efforts to develop HBOCs that focused on unmodified Hb failed—unmodified tetramers naturally dissociate into dimers outside of the RBC. This unmodified tetrameric Hb is associated with renal toxicities, gastrointestinal effects, and vasoconstriction.

The HBOCs currently in clinical development are stroma-free and engineered to produce desirable oxygen dissociation characteristics as well as an adequate in vivo half-life with minimal toxicities. Stroma-free Hb has a very high oxygen affinity compared with native Hb in an RBC because of a lack of 2,3-DPG. Furthermore, the Hb tetramer is such a small molecule that the kidney rapidly removes it.

Four different methods have been suggested to avoid toxicities: stabilization, polymerization, conjugation, and Hb vesicles. HBOC can be prepared from different Hb sources. Human Hb would not alleviate supply concerns, because the amount of outdated human blood is likely to be inadequate to make large supplies of HBOC. Bovine Hb has been used as a source of hemoglobin because of its naturally low oxygen affinity and its ability to be directly polymerized (to avoid renal excretion) without prior manipulation. Bovine Hb has a molecular structure similar to human Hb but has enhanced oxygen unloading in ischemic tissue. Unlike human Hb, which is regulated by 2,3-DPG, the affinity of bovine Hb is partially regulated by serum chloride ions. Although this product removes the constraint of using human donated red blood cells, there are uncertainties about using bovine Hb because of its potential to transmit disease (e.g., bovine spongiform encephalopathy) and its potential immunogenicity.

Researchers have explored options for recombinant sources of Hb. These products are either developed in microorganisms (*Escherichia coli*, yeast) or in transgenic plants or animals. A first-generation product developed in *E. coli* was discontinued because of vasoconstrictive effects in animals. At the current time, recombinant Hb is still within preclinical development.

Two HBOC products remain in advanced clinical development: Hemopure (Biopure Corp, Cambridge, Mass) and Hemospan (Sangart, San Diego, Calif). HBOCs have recently faced significant challenges in proving their safety and efficacy in late-phase clinical trials. Hemopure has been used to treat surgical anemia in South Africa since 2001; however, since April 2011 this product has not been available.

Limitations

Several shortcomings in HBOC have emerged across the class. Although molecular size has increased enough to prevent immediate removal by the kidney, the molecules are still seen as foreign in the recipient and quickly cleared by the reticuloendothelial system. The plasma half-life is generally 24 hours or less, thus unlikely to have a role in patients with chronic anemia.

The safety of red cell substitutes remains a serious concern. Although cross-linking and polymerizing Hb subunits have reduced the incidence of nephrotoxicity, problems with vasoconstriction and pressor effects have not been completely eliminated. Vasoconstrictive responses, including increased systemic and pulmonary arterial pressures, are thought to result from the binding of nitric oxide to Hb. Free Hb is a scavenger of nitric oxide (NO); NO plays a key role in vasomotor control, specifically vasodilation, and its removal by Hb results in a vasoconstrictive effect leading to hypertension (systemic and pulmonary). In addition, Hb interaction and scavenging of NO also leads to decreased blood flow, increased release of proinflammatory mediators, a loss of platelet activation, and gastrointestinal effects, such as dysphagia.

A large metaanalysis by Natanson and colleagues identified 16 randomized controlled trials in which adult patients received HBOC therapeutically. The analysis reviewed the association between HBOC and the risk for myocardial infarction and mortality in clinical trials. The study included five different HBOCs in the analysis and reported a 30% increase in risk for death and threefold increase in risk for myocardial infarction when all HBOC trials were pooled. The metaanalysis has been criticized for including trials of varying methodologies performed on heterogeneous patient populations in different settings with different controls. The authors of the metaanalysis in turn criticized U.S. government oversight, as well as the transparency and timeliness in reporting the results of the HBOC clinical trials. The editorial that accompanied the publication of the metaanalysis in the *Journal of the American Medical Association* recommended that further Phase III trials of HBOC not be conducted until the mechanisms and potential toxicities are better understood. The effects may be due to the interaction of hemoglobin and nitric oxide, a concern not fully appreciated in the early days of blood substitute research but potentially addressed by the expansion of knowledge about NO and mitigating its effects.

In January 2009, after the metaanalysis was published, Northfield Laboratories reported the results of their multicenter controlled trial assessing survival of injured patients resuscitated with an HBOC versus intravenous fluids starting at the scene of injury. The study included 714 patients at 29 urban Level I trauma centers. No significant difference was seen in day 30 mortality between the two arms of the study. Allogeneic blood use was lower in the HBOC arm. The incidence of multiple organ failure and serious adverse events was higher in the HBOC arm, but this was not clinically significant. Although some of the data from the randomized trial suggested that the product was not inferior to transfused blood, the FDA did not approve a license application and the product is no longer being developed.

The immunogenicity of HBOC is still being studied. Because human hemoglobin has been chemically modified, it may trigger an immune response in humans. Bovine Hb has an even greater chance of causing immunogenicity in humans because of its substantial differences from the protein structure of human Hb. To date, no serious immune or allergic responses have been reported, but most patients have only had single-incident exposures to these products, usually over short periods of time. Animal studies by manufacturers have not demonstrated a problem.

Potential Clinical Applications

Red blood cell substitutes have many potential applications. One of the most compelling would be use for resuscitation during military and civilian traumas. In developing a specific plan to avoid the consequences of blood unavailability after national disasters involving large-scale injuries, blood substitutes could play a key role as an immediate treatment option. In addition to these acute emergency situations, numerous less urgent applications exist in which oxygen carriers might provide a viable solution to difficult situations, including augmenting perioperative hemodilution, transfusion of patients who refuse human blood components because of religious beliefs, transfusion of patients with rare blood types or antibodies to high incidence antigens, organ preservation for transplant surgery, and transfusion in patients with autoimmune hemolytic anemia in whom it is difficult to detect underlying antibodies.

Patients with hemoglobinopathies constitute a unique population that might receive added benefits from red cell substitutes versus donor red cells. These patients tend to be chronically transfused and also seem to be at a higher risk for becoming alloimmunized per unit transfused compared with the general population. The universal compatibility of red cell substitutes would be ideal to protect these patients from further alloimmunization and the risks of delayed hemolytic transfusion reactions.

A number of successful cases of red cell substitutes used in Jehovah's Witnesses have been reported. For religious reasons, many Jehovah's Witnesses have refused blood transfusions, even in cases of life-threatening blood loss. Fractions derived from blood are not prohibited by the religion; the decision is left to the individual as a "matter of conscience." Many Witnesses accept and even seek out blood substitutes. Severe anemia in a Jehovah's Witness makes a blood substitute a very attractive therapeutic option as a bridge to provide oxygen transport until the patient's own endogenous production can compensate for the anemia.

Patients with autoimmune hemolytic anemia are another population that may benefit from a safe and effective red blood cell substitute. It is often difficult to find compatible blood for patients with this disease because the autoantibody can make it difficult to detect coexisting alloantibodies. The universal compatibility would allow red cell substitutes to become an important bridge for patients until compatible blood could be found.

The Future of Red Cell Substitutes

Proving the benefit of red cell substitutes in clinical trials has not been easy for a number of reasons. First, in order to reduce use of donor red blood cells, we must prove that the risks presented by HBOC or PFC are not greater than those of blood transfusions. This fact has not been established. Second, without specific transfusion triggers or guidelines, it is difficult to establish whether a transfusion has actually been avoided. Finally, the goal of reducing transfusion-related expenses may not be achievable because initially, HBOCs are likely to be very expensive.

Red cell substitutes have a promising potential value for transfusion services—the increased availability of blood components and the removal of donor and contamination safety risks. However, much remains to be accomplished before these goals can be achieved; in fact, little progress has been made in recent years, and red cell substitute development may have even taken a step backwards. On the other hand, our increasing knowledge about the interactions of Hb and NO may lead to pharmacologic means to avoid some of the apparent toxicity of HBOCs.

Red Blood Cells Derived From Stem Cells

In the context of potential future blood shortages due to an increase in aging patients requiring transfusion support and a decreasing percentage of the aging population available to donate, as well as the possibility that prolonged red blood cell storage may prove to be more detrimental to a patient than beneficial, the need for a new source of red blood cells to replace the voluntary blood donor supply is urgent. Blood substitutes will not answer this need in the near future. The generation of cultured red blood cells from amplified stem cells could meet this need, and this method is currently under development by researchers worldwide.

Umbilical cord blood is an accessible source of stem cells with proliferative capacity; however, the proliferation is not infinite, requiring a system of production in batches. Giarratana and colleagues recently reported the first transfusion of cultured RBCs derived from umbilical cord stem cells into a human; the survival of the cells was similar to that of native red blood cells. Stem cells cultured from umbilical cords would necessitate the use of cord blood banks and would still be dependent on human donation. Alternatively, embryonic stem cells and induced pluripotent stem (iPS) cells can be maintained indefinitely in culture, thus providing an unlimited source of cells. Like embryonic stem cells, iPS cells are capable of in vitro self-renewal and differentiation into cell types from all germ layers. Additionally, iPS cells possess an advantage over embryonic cells in that they pose no ethical dilemma and can be selected based on known phenotypes. Researchers have been able to demonstrate that iPS cells can differentiate into terminally mature and fully functional red blood cells. A number of challenges must be overcome before we have an unlimited supply of clinical-grade red blood cells. The ideal choice for the initial cell type (hematopoietic stem cell, erythroblast, etc.) remains to be determined. The method of reprogramming the cells must be established to avoid the risk for potential mutation and tumor development (although this is less problematic with red blood cells because they are enucleated and can be safely irradiated) while still ensuring the functionality of the end product. Finally, the use of good manufacturing process (GMP) conditions for mass amplification and production seems to be the greatest hurdle to date. Under current culture conditions, Mazurier and colleagues reported that they were able to produce only the equivalent of 1 mL of a red blood cell unit. The problem is related to the percentage of iPS cells susceptible to erythroid commitment and their amplification. A number of strategies are under development to solve this crucial problem. Until mass amplification is possible, the iPS cells could be developed, not as an unlimited supply, but as a source of cells expressing a rare blood group used to treat alloimmunized patients with rare blood types.

SUGGESTED READINGS

Ashworth A, Klein AA: Cell salvage as part of a blood conservation strategy in anesthesia. *British Journal of Anaethesia* 105:401, 2010.

A succinct review of the principles, risks, benefits, and complications of cell salvage in various patient populations.

Bell EF, Strauss RG, Widness JA, et al: Randomized trial of liberal versus restrictive guidelines for red blood cell transfusion in preterm infants. *Pediatrics* 115:1685, 2005.

Blajchman MA: Transfusion immunomodulation or TRIM: What does it mean clinically? *Hematology* 10:208, 2005.

A concise overview of transfusion immunomodulation.

Dzik WH, Anderson JC, O'Neill EM, et al: A prospective, randomized clinical trial of universal WBC reduction. *Transfusion* 42:1114, 2002.

Goodnough LT, Rudnick S, Price TH, et al: Increased preoperative collection of autologous blood with recombinant human erythropoietin: A controlled trial. *N Engl J Med* 321:1163, 1989.

Hebert PC, Wells G, Blajchman MA, et al: A multicenter, randomized controlled clinical trial of transfusion requirements in critical care. *N Engl J Med* 340:409, 1999.

The TRICC trial is a large study of 838 ICU patients transfused at liberal or restrictive transfusion thresholds.

King KE, Ness PM: Treatment of autoimmune hemolytic anemia. *Semin Hematol* 42:131, 2005.

Kirpalasni H, Whyte RK, Andersen C, et al: The premature infants in need of transfusion (PINT) study: A randomized, controlled trial of a restrictive (low) versus liberal (high) transfusion threshold for extremely low birth weight infants. *J Pediatr* 149:301, 2006.

Klein HG: Transfusion-associated graft-versus-host disease: Less fresh blood and more gray (Gy) for an aging population. *Transfusion* 46:878, 2006.

Mazurier C, Douay L, Lapillonne H: Red blood cells from induced pluripotent stem cells: Hurdles and developments. *Current Opinion in Hematology* 18:249, 2011.

A well-written update on the current status of research on developing an unlimited supply of red blood cells from a stem cell source.

Meryman HT, Hornblower M: A method for freezing and washing red blood cells using high glycerol concentration. *Transfusion* 12:145, 1972.

Natanson C, Kern SJ, Lurie P, et al.: Cell-free hemoglobin-based blood substitutes and risk of myocardial infarction and death, a meta-analysis. *JAMA* 299:2304, 2008.

Ness PM, Bourke DL, Walsh PC: A randomized trial of perioperative hemodilution versus transfusion of preoperatively deposited autologous blood in elective surgery. *Transfusion* 32:226, 1992.

Ness PM, Cushing MM: Oxygen therapeutics: Pursuit of an alternative to the donor red blood cell. *Arch Pathol Lab Med* 131:734, 2007.

An overview of the red blood cell substitutes in development with a focus on risks and clinical trials.

NIH Consensus Conference: Perioperative red blood cell transfusion. *JAMA* 260:2700, 1988.

Paglino JC, Pomper GJ, Fisch GS, et al: Reduction of febrile but not allergic reactions to RBCs and platelets after conversion to universal prestorage leukoreduction. *Transfusion* 44:16, 2004.

Sehgal LR, Sebala LP, Takagi I, et al: Evaluation of oxygen extraction ratio as a physiologic transfusion trigger in coronary artery bypass graft surgery patients. *Transfusion* 41:591, 2001.

Tinmouth A, Fergusson D, Yee IC, et al: Clinical consequences of red cell storage in the critically ill. *Transfusion* 46:2014, 2006.

TRAP Study Group: Leukocytic reduction and ultraviolet B irradiation of platelets to prevent alloimmunization and refractoriness to platelet transfusions. *N Engl J Med* 337:1861, 1997.

A landmark study describing the benefit of leukoreduction in preventing alloimmunization.

U.S. Department of Health and Human Services: *The 2009 national blood collection and utilization survey report*, Washington, DC, 2011, USDHHS, Office of the Assistant Secretary for Health. Available at http://www.hhs.gov/ash/bloodsafety/2009nbcus.pdf. This report provides national estimates of the blood collection and utilization activities in the United States in 2008.

Vamvakas EC: Pneumonia as a complication of blood product transfusion in the critically ill: Transfusion-related immunomodulation (TRIM). *Crit Care Med* 343:S151, 2006.

Von Lindern JS, Brand A: The use of blood products in perinatal medicine. *Seminars in Fetal and Neonatal Medicine* 13:272, 2008.

An overview discussing transfusion guidelines and recommendations for further research for the most common transfusion indications (red blood cells, platelets, and granulocytes).

CHAPTER 113

PRINCIPLES OF PLATELET TRANSFUSION THERAPY

Richard M. Kaufman

PLATELET COLLECTION AND MANUFACTURING

Platelet products are either prepared from whole blood donations (platelet concentrates) or are collected by apheresis (single donor platelets [SDPs]). In the United States, whole blood–derived platelet concentrates are made using the platelet-rich plasma (PRP) method. First, a whole blood unit is separated by gentle centrifugation (slow spin) into red blood cells (RBCs) and PRP. The PRP is then centrifuged a second time (hard spin) to isolate one platelet concentrate plus one unit of plasma. Each platelet concentrate contains approximately 5.5 × 1010 platelets suspended in a plasma volume of approximately 50 mL. In Europe and Canada, the alternate buffy coat method is used to produce platelet concentrates. Platelets are stored at room temperature under continuous gentle agitation for up to 5 days. To prepare an adult dose of platelets for transfusion, four to six platelet concentrates are pooled together.

Apheresis platelet units are collected from a single platelet donor by continuous flow centrifugation using an automated device. A high volume of whole blood is processed through the machine, and the platelets are retained in a sterile collection bag. By American Association of Blood Banks (AABB) standards, an apheresis platelet unit should contain a minimum of 3 × 1011 platelets,[1] a dose that is approximately equivalent to six pooled platelet concentrates. Current devices allow many different combinations of blood products to be collected during a single apheresis donation, such as 1 unit of platelets plus 1 unit of RBCs. Apheresis platelet units generally contain less than 1 × 106 white blood cells (WBCs) per unit; thus, they meet the current AABB definition for leukoreduced blood products (<5 × 106 WBCs/unit).[1] Although apheresis platelets cost more to produce than whole blood–derived platelet concentrates, they have become increasingly popular. In the United States in 2006, approximately 1.5 million therapeutic doses of platelets were provided as apheresis platelets, and only 216,000 doses were administered as whole blood–derived platelet concentrates.[2]

Apheresis platelets provide some (limited) advantages over whole blood–derived platelet concentrates. Radiolabeling studies indicate that apheresis platelets circulate longer in vivo than pooled concentrates,[3] most likely reflecting gentler handling and less platelet activation during collection. Recipients of apheresis platelets are exposed to fewer donors per transfusion (one donor vs. six as with a pool of platelet concentrates), so in principle, apheresis platelets should pose a lower risk of viral transmission than whole blood–derived platelets. However, given that the per unit transfusion-transmission risks for HIV and hepatitis C virus have been cut to approximately one in 2,000,000,[4] the viral safety advantage of apheresis platelets over whole blood–derived platelets is marginal. Data from surveillance culture studies suggest that apheresis platelets may be less likely than platelet concentrates to become contaminated with bacteria.[3] At one time, it was predicted that apheresis platelets would be less likely than pooled concentrates to provoke platelet alloimmunization by virtue of exposing recipients to fewer unique donor human leukocyte antigens (HLAs). This hypothesis was not confirmed empirically, however.[5] Although they express surface HLA class I antigens, platelets appear to be rather poor immunogens. HLA alloimmunization to platelets primarily appears to be triggered by contaminating WBCs within a platelet unit. Thus, alloimmunization is not platelet dose dependent, and simply providing leukoreduced platelet units prevents most cases of immune-mediated platelet refractoriness.[5]

PROPHYLACTIC PLATELET TRANSFUSION

The vast majority of platelet units are transfused prophylactically to prevent bleeding in nonbleeding patients rather than to treat active bleeding. Before 1960, platelet transfusions were not widely available, and death from hemorrhage was common among patients with leukemia who received chemotherapy. In 1962, Gaydos and colleagues[6] published a seminal study demonstrating a relationship between platelet count and likelihood of bleeding. After this study was published, prophylactic platelet transfusion rapidly became standard practice. Of note, no specific platelet transfusion trigger was suggested by the authors based on their data. Regardless, a platelet count of 20,000/μL was widely adopted as the standard prophylactic platelet transfusion trigger.

Later studies suggested that a lower transfusion trigger would be as effective as a trigger of 20,000/μL. Slichter and Harker,[7] for instance, performed RBC radiolabeling studies in thrombocytopenic patients who were not receiving platelet transfusions. They demonstrated that only patients with platelet counts below 5000/μL had significantly elevated fecal RBC loss.[7] Years later, several clinical studies directly challenged the 20,000/μL trigger. Platelet transfusion triggers of 10,000/μL versus 20,000/μL were compared directly in three randomized prospective studies of patients with acute leukemia.[8-10] All of these studies, as well as large nonrandomized prospective trials,[11,12] demonstrated no increased risk of bleeding when a trigger of 10,000/μL is used.

Prophylactic Platelet Dosing

There are currently thought to be two distinct clearance mechanisms for platelets. Most platelets undergo senescence after circulating in the peripheral blood for 8 to 10 days. But there is also evidence for a second clearance route in which there is a fixed daily loss of platelets that occurs independent of platelet age. Platelets exiting the circulation via this second route are postulated to function in maintaining vascular integrity.[13] This small fixed daily platelet requirement has been estimated to be 7.1 × 109 platelets/L/day. In principle, a low dose of platelets could be used to meet this daily requirement. This hypothesis was tested directly by the Platelet Dosing (PLADO) study published in 2010. A total of 1272 patients undergoing hematopoietic stem cell (HSC) transplantation or chemotherapy were randomly assigned to receive low-, medium-, or high-dose platelets for a morning count of 10,000/μL or lower. The risk of spontaneous bleeding was not increased until patient platelet counts fell to 5,000/μL or lower. No differences were observed in bleeding rates among the three treatment groups, supporting the concept that few platelets are required to maintain hemeostasis. Although significantly fewer total platelets were transfused to patients in the low-dose group, platelet transfusions were required more frequently.[14]

Prophylactic Platelets for Invasive Bedside Procedures

At present, there have been no large randomized trials evaluating the need for platelet prophylaxis before invasive bedside procedures such as lumbar puncture. However, retrospective data provide reassurance that moderate thrombocytopenia does not pose a serious risk for performing such procedures. Howard et al[15] reviewed the records of 956 consecutive pediatric patients with newly diagnosed acute lymphoblastic leukemia who underwent lumbar puncture. No serious hemorrhagic complications were observed after 5223 lumbar punctures, including 170 procedures that were done when the platelet count was 11,000 to 20,000/μL. The authors concluded that prophylactic platelet transfusion was unnecessary in patients with platelet counts above 10,000/μL. Lumbar punctures were performed in only 29 patients with platelet counts of 10,000/μL or less, making it difficult to assess the risk of bleeding in patients with very low platelet counts. A similar, albeit much smaller, retrospective study examined the same issue in adult patients with acute leukemia.[16] No hemorrhagic complications were observed after 195 lumbar punctures, including 35 that were done with platelet counts of 20,000 to 30,000/μL. For other common bedside procedures such as central venous catheter placement, platelet counts of 20,000 to 30,000/μL are generally considered to be adequate, although, again, data from prospective studies are unavailable.

Prophylactic Platelets for Major Surgical Procedures

There are currently no data from randomized trials addressing the question of what constitutes an adequate platelet count before surgery. Retrospective studies, though, suggest that patients with platelet counts of 50,000/μL or higher are not at excess bleeding risk during surgery. Bishop and colleagues[17] reported a series of 95 patients with acute leukemia who underwent 130 surgical procedures with platelet counts of less than 50,000/μL. Intraoperative blood loss exceeded 500 mL in only 7% of cases. No relationship was seen between the preoperative platelet count and surgical blood loss. These data suggest that prophylactic platelet transfusions need not be administered before surgery when the preoperative platelet count is at least 50,000/μL. This rule of thumb is thought to apply to most types of surgery (cardiac, orthopedic, and so on). For a few types of surgeries, though, requiring a higher platelet count (70,000-100,000/μL) is traditional, although no published data currently exist either to support or refute this approach. These settings include neurosurgery, retinal surgeries, and other procedures in which the risk is not that the patient may exsanguinate but rather that even a minor bleed might cause clinically significant damage in a vulnerable vital structure such as the brain.

THERAPEUTIC PLATELET TRANSFUSION

A small number of studies published in the 1970s and early 1980s suggested the idea of using a purely therapeutic platelet transfusion strategy—transfusing platelets only to treat active bleeding rather than administering prophylactic platelets in thrombocytopenic patients. This concept was revived recently by Wandt and colleagues,[18] who reported a series of 140 HSC transplants in which no prophylactic platelets were given to clinically stable patients regardless of platelet count unless the patient had World Health Organization (WHO) grade II or higher bleeding. Patients deemed to be clinically unstable (defined as fever >38.5°C, infection, or known coagulation factor disorder) were given prophylactic platelet transfusions for platelets less than 10,000/μL. No WHO grade III or IV bleeding was observed. Grade II bleeding was seen in 26 transplants (19%). No clinically relevant bleeding was seen in the remaining 114 of 140 patients (81%). The first 60 patients in this study were compared with 60 historical control participants who were transfused with prophylactic platelets for a platelet count of less than 10,000/μL. The total number of platelets transfused was only 111 in the therapeutic group compared with 237 in the historical control group. Thus the therapeutic strategy was quite effective in this study. Randomized trials directly comparing therapeutic versus prophylactic platelet transfusion strategies are currently ongoing.

ADVERSE EFFECTS OF PLATELET TRANSFUSION

Infectious Risks

Platelets are associated with the same range of infectious pathogens as any other blood component, but septic transfusion reactions caused by bacterially contaminated units comprise a unique risk of platelet transfusion. Over time, improvements in donor screening virtually eliminated the risk of transfusion transmission of hepatitis B virus, hepatitis C virus, and HIV. The risk of septic transfusion reactions remained fairly constant over this same time period, so eventually, platelet bacterial contamination became, by default, the most frequent infectious risk of transfusion. Unlike other blood components, which are stored either refrigerated or frozen, platelets are stored at room temperature. The reason is that if platelets are refrigerated before transfusion, they are cleared rapidly from the recipient's circulation.[19] Although room temperature storage allows transfused platelets to circulate in vivo, it has the downside of promoting bacterial growth. Because of this risk, platelet storage is ordinarily limited to only 5 days, making platelet inventory management extremely challenging.

In the 1990s, numerous studies demonstrated that contaminating bacteria, usually representing skin flora from the donor, could be cultured out of approximately one of 3000 platelet units. Clinically apparent septic transfusion reactions were thought to occur after approximately 1 of 25,000 platelet transfusions, although there is considerable uncertainty around this point estimate.[20] In response to the issue, the AABB developed the following standard:

5.1.5.1 The blood bank or transfusion service shall have methods to limit and detect or inactivate bacteria in all platelet components. Standard 5.6.2 applies [skin disinfection].[1]

How this standard is being met varies by facility. Many blood collection centers have begun routinely culturing platelet units using an automated culture system. The BacT/ALERT system (BioMerieux), used by many centers, works by continuously monitoring for bacterial production of CO_2 within culture bottles. Platelet units are sampled on the day after collection. The samples are cultured for a period of time, typically 24 hours, and if the cultures fail to produce abnormal levels of CO_2, the product is released into inventory. Overall, culture-based bacterial screening appears to have decreased, but not eliminated, the risk of septic reactions.[21] Rapid, point-of-issue tests that can be used to test the sterility of a platelet unit just before issue have also been developed. Reducing the bacterial risk further may ultimately require alternative approaches, such as pathogen reduction. Pathogen inactivation systems, using photosensitive dyes or ultraviolet (UV) light, can provide up to 6 logs of killing of spiked virus or bacteria within 1 unit of platelets or RBCs. Although such systems have been used in Europe and elsewhere, at this time, no pathogen inactivation system is licensed for use in the United States.

Allergic and Febrile Nonhemolytic Transfusion Reactions

The typical RBC unit contains approximately 20 mL of plasma. Platelet units contain far more plasma, approximately 200 mL on average. There are multiple potential adverse effects associated with this large plasma content. First, allergic transfusion reactions are frequently associated with platelet transfusion. Allergic reactions to platelet transfusions occur when the recipient has a preexisting allergy to a plasma protein component. Allergic reactions can range from mild, uncomplicated urticarial reactions to full-blown anaphylaxis.

Febrile nonhemolytic reactions, defined as an increase in temperature of more than 1°C, may also be seen after platelet transfusion. In an elegant study, Heddle and colleagues[22] demonstrated that the plasma component of platelet units, rather than the cellular component, causes most reactions. Cytokines that accumulate during product storage have been implicated.

ABO and Hemolytic Reactions to Platelets

Whenever possible, platelet units are assigned so as to match the donor plasma with recipient RBC type. For example, a type A patient would ordinarily receive type A or AB platelets, which do not contain anti-A antibody. When platelet inventories are constrained, however, it is a frequent practice to provide ABO-incompatible platelets. For example, a type A patient can receive type O platelets, containing anti-A. The passive transfusion of donor anti-A or anti-B to a patient rarely results in a clinically apparent reaction. Occasionally, however, hemolysis may be observed. Most often, this occurs with units from type O donors, who occasionally have high titer anti-A, anti-B, or anti-A,B antibody. In a typical type O adult, the titer of circulating anti-A is on the order of one in 128 to one in 256. Some donors, for unclear reasons, have anti-A titers of one in 10,000 or higher. Recipients of products from donors with high-titer anti-A (and less frequently, anti-B) rarely do have clinically apparent hemolysis, and a small number of fatalities have been reported. This is considered to be a low-risk event, but it may be on the rise in the United States because of the increased number of single-donor apheresis platelet units used. One strategy to deal with this issue is to measure the anti-A/B titer on all platelet donors; components exceeding a threshold titer are assigned to type-specific recipients. An alternate strategy is to gently reduce the load of plasma in a platelet unit before transfusing the unit to a non–ABO-identical recipient.

Transfusion-Related Acute Lung Injury

Transfusion-related acute lung injury (TRALI) is an acute respiratory distress syndrome associated with the transfusion of any plasma-containing blood component, including platelets. Most cases of TRALI appear to be precipitated by the passive transfusion of donor anti-HLA or (less commonly) antineutrophil antibody. It is believed that products containing higher volumes of plasma such as fresh-frozen plasma (FFP) and apheresis platelets carry a higher risk of TRALI. Approximately one-third of female blood donors have circulating anti-HLA antibody because of prior sensitization during pregnancy. To help mitigate against the risk of TRALI, many countries, including the United States, now produce FFP from the blood of male donors only. Although this strategy has been relatively easy to apply to FFP production, female platelet donors are still needed to ensure an adequate platelet supply. A variety of strategies are being implemented to screen female platelet donors for anti-HLA antibody and to defer women who are antibody positive.

Rh(D) Sensitization

The Rh(D) antigen is the most immunogenic RBC protein antigen. More than 80% of individuals who are Rh(D) negative will form an anti-D antibody after a single Rh(D)-positive RBC transfusion.[23] Anti-D antibodies are associated with both hemolytic transfusion reactions and hemolytic disease of the fetus and newborn. For this reason, it is standard practice to provide Rh(D)-negative individuals exclusively with Rh(D)-negative RBC units. Platelet units contain a small number of contaminating RBCs. In the case of platelet concentrates, approximately 0.3 to 0.5 mL RBCs may be present. Current apheresis platelets contain far fewer RBCs (≈0.0002 to 0.0007 mL per unit). Ordinarily, Rh(D)-negative platelet units are given to Rh(D)-negative recipients. However, inventory constraints frequently force blood banks to provide Rh(D)-positive platelet products to Rh(D)-negative recipients. Transfusion of such units is associated with a low but nonzero risk of sensitization and formation of anti-D. Anti-D antibody formation can be prevented by administering Rh immune globulin, as is done to prevent fetomaternal Rh sensitization in Rh(D)-negative mothers of Rh(D)-positive children. The risk of sensitization is especially low among Rh(D)-negative immunocompromised patients transfused with Rh(D)-positive platelets (e.g., hematopoietic stem cell transplantation patients). In this setting, the value of Rh immune globulin (RhIG) prophylaxis appears to be marginal.

PLATELET REFRACTORINESS

Causes of Refractoriness to Platelet Transfusion

Platelet refractoriness is defined as an inappropriately low platelet increment after repeated platelet transfusions. It can be caused by nonimmune or immune factors (Table 113-1). The most commonly reported nonimmune causes of platelet refractoriness include fever, sepsis, bleeding, splenomegaly, and disseminated intravascular coagulation. In a subset of cases, platelet refractoriness is immune mediated. Platelets express HLA class I antigens, ABO antigens, and several platelet-specific antigens. Any of these molecules may potentially serve as an immune stimulus in a transfusion recipient. Whereas antibodies directed against HLA molecules are responsible for most cases of immune-mediated platelet refractoriness, antibodies to the human platelet antigens (anti-HPA antibodies) are less frequently implicated.

Diagnosis of Platelet Refractoriness

Because fewer than half of all platelet-refractory patients have demonstrable anti-HLA or antiplatelet antibodies,[24] evaluation of both an immediate response to platelet transfusion and an 18- to 24-hour posttransfusion platelet survival is needed to help establish the cause of platelet refractoriness. Platelet counts obtained from 10 minutes to 1 hour after transfusion that repeatedly fail to demonstrate a corrected count increment of more than 5000/μL usually indicate immune-mediated platelet refractoriness.[25] If the 10-minute to 1-hour posttransfusion platelet count shows a reasonable increment but the platelet count falls back to baseline by 18 to 24 hours, a nonimmune mechanism of refractoriness may be presumed (see Table 113-1). In cases of suspected immune-mediated refractoriness, HLA antibody screening (panel reactive antibody [PRA]) provides valuable supporting evidence that allosensitization has occurred.[26] A patient with a PRA greater than 70% may be considered to be "severely immunized" and a good candidate for HLA-matched platelets (below).

Table 113-1 Causes of Refractoriness to Platelet Transfusion

Nonimmune
Fever
Sepsis
Drug associated
Active bleeding
Splenomegaly
Disseminated intravascular coagulation
Veno-occlusive disease
Immune
Anti-HLA antibodies
Anti-HPA antibodies
ABO mismatch
Drug-dependent antibodies

HLA, Human leukocyte antigen; *HPA,* human platelet antigen.

Detection of Anti–Human Leukocyte Antigen Antibodies

Several assays are available to detect the presence of anti-HLA class I antibodies in the serum of alloimmunized patients. Years ago, the most commonly used test was the lymphocytotoxicity assay (LCA). The results of the LCA correlate well with the response to platelet transfusion. However, this assay does not detect anti-HLA antibodies that do not activate complement. The anti-HLA antibodies can also be detected using an HLA-specific solid-phase enzyme-linked immunosorbent assay, glycoprotein-specific monoclonal antibody-specific immobilization of platelet antigens, or flow cytometric detection of antibody binding to beads coated with purified HLA antigens. The flow cytometry–based methodology has significantly improved sensitivity over LCA and, similar to solid-phase assays, it can detect both complement-fixing and non–complement-fixing antibodies.[27]

Detection of Antiplatelet Antibodies

The most commonly used methods for detection of anti-HPA antibodies are solid-phase assays using purified platelet antigens for detection of antibody specificity. However, testing for anti-HPA antibodies is not typically performed in the workup of platelet refractory patients, mainly because the importance of these antibodies in causing clinical refractoriness is not well established.

Prevention of Alloimmunization

Although they express HLA class I antigens, platelets themselves are fairly weak immunogens. It has been shown that contaminating leukocytes in platelet products are primarily responsible for stimulating HLA antibody formation in platelet transfusion recipients.[28] Thus removing WBCs from blood products (leukoreduction) is an essential means of preventing alloimmunization and subsequent platelet refractoriness. The definitive study showing this was the Trial to Reduce Alloimmunization to Platelets (TRAP study),[5] which compared alloimmunization rates in 530 newly diagnosed patients with acute myeloid leukemia randomized to receive unmodified, pooled platelet concentrates (control); filtered, pooled platelet concentrates (F-PC); filtered single-donor apheresis platelets (F-AP); or UV-B-irradiated pooled platelet concentrates (UVB-PC). Anti-HLA antibodies were detected in 45% of control participants compared with 17% to 21% of patients receiving modified platelets. A total of 13% of control group patients became platelet refractory versus only 3% in the F-PC group, 4% in the F-AP group, and 5% in the UVB-PC group.

Management of Platelet-Refractory Patients

When platelet refractoriness has been demonstrated, several strategies may facilitate achieving therapeutic platelet increments in vivo (Table 113-2). A trial of ABO-matched, fresh (1-2 days old) platelets may be helpful. In cases of immune-mediated refractoriness, a trial of HLA-matched platelets,[29] antigen-negative platelets, or crossmatched platelets should be considered. The basic principles for selection of HLA-matched platelets are outlined in Table 113-3. In most cases, alloimmune refractory patients will show some degree of response to HLA-matched platelets.[30] Because of the high degree of polymorphism of the HLA loci, it is often not possible to find perfect HLA-A and -B locus matches, leading to the use of platelets mismatched at one or more loci (Table 113-4). In general, transfusion of grade A- or BU-matched platelets can result in an increase in platelet count that is superior to platelet increment obtained using either crossmatched platelets or platelets with different degrees of HLA mismatching (BX, C, or D). Examples of different categories of matches are provided in Figure 113-1. An additional step that may help in finding compatible platelets is flow cytometric detection of anti-HLA antibody specificity using single HLA antigen–coated beads. This information can be used to find donors that may be HLA mismatched with the recipient but whose platelets lack the antigens to which the patient has specific antibodies. Furthermore, family members may be considered as platelet donors in addition to the available pool of HLA-matched volunteer donors. As an alternative to HLA antigen matching, patients may benefit from receiving donor platelets that are crossmatch compatible with the patient's serum. The major benefit of crossmatching is a potentially larger pool of donors that would have been excluded by strict HLA antigen matching. Also, platelet crossmatching may be helpful in cases of refractoriness caused by antibodies directed against platelet-specific antigens.

The most challenging cases are the rare instances involving immune-refractory patients who are actively bleeding and HLA-matched platelets or crossmatched platelets are either ineffective or

Table 113-2 Management of the Platelet-Refractory Patient

Obtain 10-minute to 1-hour posttransfusion platelet count on two occasions.

If there is an appropriate increment in platelet count after a single platelet transfusion, continue to transfuse random platelets and treat nonimmune factors associated with decreased platelet survival such as sepsis and DIC, discontinue offending drugs, and so on.

If the 10-minute to 1-hour posttransfusion platelet counts demonstrate no platelet increment (or only a marginal increment), obtain the patient's HLA type and screen the patient for the presence of anti-HLA antibodies (panel reactive antibody test).

While awaiting HLA antigen typing and antibody screening results, consider transfusion of "fresh" (<3 days old) ABO-matched platelets.

If PRA shows less than 20% reactivity, continue with "fresh" ABO-matched random platelets.

If PRA shows more than 20% reactivity, obtain anti-HLA antibody specificity. Use the recipient's HLA typing information to locate grade A or B matched platelet units for transfusion. Avoid transfusion of platelets containing antigens against which the recipient has antibodies. Consider recruiting recipient's family for platelet donation.

Transfusion of crossmatch-compatible platelets is an option if there is a poor response to grade A- or B-matched platelets or if the recipient has antibodies to platelet-specific antigens.

All HLA-matched or crossmatched platelet units must be irradiated before transfusion to prevent transfusion-associated GVHD.

DIC, Disseminated intravascular coagulation; *GVHD,* graft-versus-host disease; *HLA,* human leukocyte antigen; *PRA,* panel reactive antibody.

Table 113-3 Traditional Platelet Selection Guidelines for Refractoriness Caused by Alloimmunization

ABO antigens are expressed on platelets. Consider transfusion of ABO-matched platelets while awaiting the recipient's HLA type and antibody specificity

Platelet matching for the recipient's HLA A and HLA B antigens is important.

Platelet matching for the recipient's HLA C antigens is not essential.

Determine the antigen specificity of recipient's antiplatelet antibodies and try to transfuse antigen negative platelets.

Some HLA antigens may be weakly expressed on platelets. Consider giving platelets mismatched for those antigens (e.g., HLA B12 and its splits B44, B45)

If HLA-matched platelets are unavailable, consider transfusion of platelets mismatched for HLA antigens that are serologically cross-reactive with the recipient's HLA antigens.

If platelets mismatched for serologically cross-reactive antigens are not effective, matching for HLA-associated antigen systems such as Bw4/Bw6 may be helpful.

HLA, Human leukocyte antigen.

Table 113-4 Grades of Human Leukocyte Antigen–Matched Platelets

Match Grade	Description
A	4-antigen match (donor and recipient match at both HLA-A and -B loci)
B1U	1 antigen unknown or blank (e.g., donor is: A2, –; B5, 27)
B1X	1 cross-reactive group*
B2UX	1 antigen blank and 1 cross-reactive*
C	1 mismatched antigen present
D	≥2 mismatched antigens present
R	Random

Adapted from Brecher ME, editor: *Technical manual,* ed 15, Bethesda, Md, 2005, American Association of Blood Banks.
*The clusters of human leukocyte antigen (HLA) that share antigenic epitopes can be classified into cross-reactive antigen groups. Antibodies recognizing one HLA molecule within the group cross-react with other members of the same group.

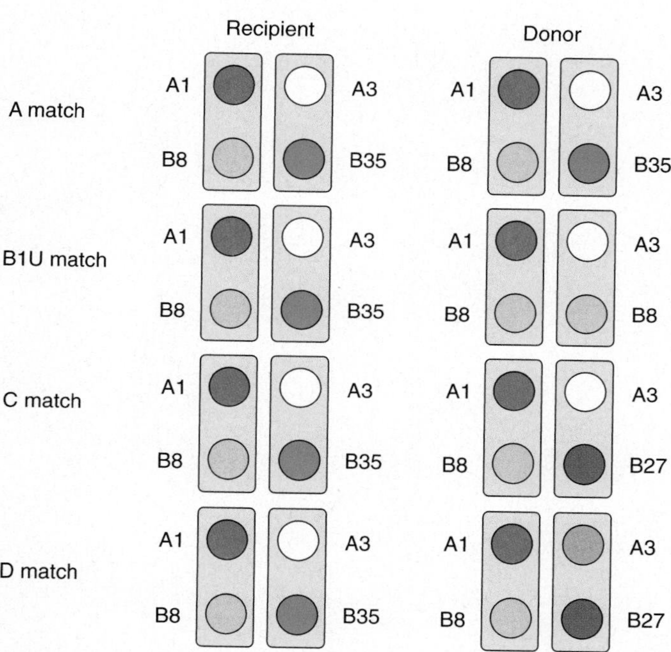

Figure 113-1 EXAMPLES OF DONOR–RECIPIENT PAIRS ON THE BASIS OF HUMAN LEUKOCYTE ANTIGEN MATCH.

unavailable. In such cases, patients are typically transfused with repeated doses of random HLA-incompatible platelets during hemorrhagic episodes. The efficacy of this practice is unclear.

REFERENCES

1. Carson TH, editor: *Standards for Blood Banks and Transfusion Services,* ed 27, Bethesda, MD, 2011, AABB.
2. Whitaker BI: *The 2007 Nationwide Blood Collection and Utilization Survey Report,* Bethesda, MD, 2007, AABB.
3. Ness P, Braine H, King K, et al: Single-donor platelets reduce the risk of septic platelet transfusion reactions. *Transfusion* 41:857, 2001.
4. Stramer SL: Current risks of transfusion-transmitted agents: A review. *Arch Pathol Lab Med* 131:702, 2007.
5. The Trial to Reduce Alloimmunization to Platelets Study Group: Leukocyte reduction and ultraviolet B irradiation of platelets to prevent alloimmunization and refractoriness to platelet transfusions. *N Engl J Med* 337:1861, 1997.
6. Gaydos LA, Freireich EJ, Mantel N: The quantitative relation between platelet count and hemorrhage in patients with acute leukemia. *N Engl J Med* 266:905, 1962.
7. Slichter SJ, Harker LA: Thrombocytopenia: Mechanisms and management of defects in platelet production. *Clin Haematol* 7:523, 1978.
8. Heckman KD, Weiner GJ, Davis CS, et al: Randomized study of prophylactic platelet transfusion threshold during induction therapy for adult acute leukemia: 10,000/microL versus 20,000/microL. *J Clin Oncol* 15:1143, 1997.
9. Rebulla P, Finazzi G, Marangoni F, et al: For the Gruppo Italiano Malattie Ematologiche Maligne dell'Adulto: The threshold for prophylactic platelet transfusions in adults with acute myeloid leukemia. *N Engl J Med* 337:1870, 1997.
10. Zumberg MS, del Rosario ML, Nejame CF, et al: A prospective randomized trial of prophylactic platelet transfusion and bleeding incidence in hematopoietic stem cell transplant recipients: 10,000/L versus 20,000/microL trigger. *Biol Blood Marrow Transplant* 8:569, 2002.
11. Gmur J, Burger J, Schanz U, et al: Safety of stringent prophylactic platelet transfusion policy for patients with acute leukaemia. *Lancet* 338:1223, 1991.
12. Rebulla P, Finazzi G, Marangoni F, et al: For the Gruppo Italiano Malattie Ematologiche Maligne dell'Adulto: The threshold for prophylactic platelet transfusions in adults with acute myeloid leukemia. *N Engl J Med* 337:1870, 1997.
13. Hanson SR, Slichter SJ: Platelet kinetics in patients with bone marrow hypoplasia: Evidence for a fixed platelet requirement. *Blood* 66:1105, 1985.
14. Slichter SJ, Kaufman RM, Assmann SF, et al: Dose of prophylactic platelet transfusions and prevention of hemorrhage. *N Engl J Med* 362:600, 2010.
15. Howard SC, Gajjar A, Ribeiro RC, et al: Safety of lumbar puncture for children with acute lymphoblastic leukemia and thrombocytopenia. *JAMA* 284:2222, 2000.
16. Vavricka SR, Walter RB, Irani S, et al: Safety of lumbar puncture for adults with acute leukemia and restrictive prophylactic platelet transfusion. *Ann Hematol* 82:570, 2003.
17. Bishop JF, Schiffer CA, Aisner J, et al: Surgery in acute leukemia: A review of 167 operations in thrombocytopenic patients. *Am J Hematol* 26:147, 1987.
18. Wandt H, Schaefer-Eckart K, Frank M, et al: A therapeutic platelet transfusion strategy is safe and feasible in patients after autologous peripheral blood stem cell transplantation. *Bone Marrow Transplant* 37:387, 2006.
19. Murphy S, Gardner FH: Effect of storage temperature on maintenance of platelet viability: Deleterious effect of refrigerated storage. *N Engl J Med* 280:1094, 1969.
20. Hillyer CD, Josephson CD, Blajchman MA, et al: Bacterial contamination of blood components: Risks, strategies, and regulation: Joint ASH and AABB educational session in transfusion medicine. *Hematol Am Soc Hematol Educ Program* 575, 2003.
21. Eder AF, Kennedy JM, Dy BA, et al: Bacterial screening of apheresis platelets and the residual risk of septic transfusion reactions: The American Red Cross experience (2004-2006). *Transfusion* 47:1134, 2007.
22. Heddle NM, Klama L, Singer J, et al: The role of the plasma from platelet concentrates in transfusion reactions. *N Engl J Med* 331:625, 1994.
23. Klein HG, Anstee DJ: *Mollison's blood transfusion in clinical medicine,* ed 11, Malden, MA, 2005, Blackwell Publishing Ltd.
24. Yankee RA, Graff KS, Dowling R, et al: Selection of unrelated compatible platelet donors by lymphocyte HL-A matching. *N Engl J Med* 288:760, 1973.
25. Daly PA, Schiffer CA, Aisner J, et al: Platelet transfusion therapy: One-hour posttransfusion increments are valuable in predicting the need for HLA-matched preparations. *JAMA* 243:435, 1980.
26. Lee EJ, Schiffer CA: Serial measurement of lymphocytotoxic antibody and response to nonmatched platelet transfusions in alloimmunized patients. *Blood* 70:1727, 1987.

27. Pei R, Wang G, Tarsitani C, et al: Simultaneous HLA Class I and Class II antibodies screening with flow cytometry. *Hum Immunol* 59:313, 1998.
28. Saarinen UM, Kekomaki R, Siimes MA, et al: Effective prophylaxis against platelet refractoriness in multitransfused patients by use of leukocyte-free blood components. *Blood* 75:512, 1990.
29. Moroff G, Garratty G, Heal JM, et al: Selection of platelets for refractory patients by HLA matching and prospective crossmatching. *Transfusion* 32:633, 1992.
30. Heal JM, Blumberg N, Masel D: An evaluation of crossmatching, HLA, and ABO matching for platelet transfusions to refractory patients. *Blood* 70:23, 1987.

CHAPTER 114

HUMAN LEUKOCYTE ANTIGEN AND HUMAN NEUTROPHIL ANTIGEN SYSTEMS

Ena Wang, Sharon Adams, David F. Stroncek, and Francesco M. Marincola

This chapter reviews human leukocyte antigen (HLA) and human neutrophil antigen (HNA) systems. A general background of the structure, function, and nomenclature of both systems and their relevance in clinical hematology is presented. Analysis of HLA gene products is applied in clinical settings (1) to select compatible donor-recipient pairs for transplantation, (2) to select HLA-compatible single-donor platelet products for thrombocytopenic patients refractory to standard transfusion of random pooled platelets, (3) to screen for genetic factors that may contribute to the prevalence of diseases, and (4) for forensic purposes in which the identity of individuals may contribute to solving legal disputes or criminal investigations. In addition, we discuss new applications that have broadened the relevance of HLA in the area of immune pathology. HLA phenotypes determine the suitability of patients for epitope-specific immunization. Tetrameric HLA/epitope complexes (tHLA) allow enumeration of antigen-specific T-cell responses. Furthermore, molecular identification of T-cell epitopes associated with distinct diseases and characterization of the communication between immune effector cells through HLA–HLA ligand interactions extend the relevance of HLA to biologic fields. These biologic fields encompass natural killer (NK) and cytotoxic T-cell function, antigen recognition in the context of infection, autoimmunity, graft-versus-neoplasia (GVN) effect, and autologous cancer rejection. Finally, the recognition that polymorphism extends to other protein families relevant to immune pathology including cytokines, their receptors, and killer cell–inhibitory receptors has broadened the significance of immunogenetics beyond HLA. Thus this chapter emphasizes the importance of viewing human pathologic conditions through the kaleidoscopic complexity of human polymorphism.

GENETICS, STRUCTURE, AND FUNCTION OF HLA MOLECULES

HLAs embrace a family of genes clustered in the short arm of chromosome 6 as the human version of the major histocompatibility complex (MHC), initially identified in mice as responsible for graft rejection between genetically unrelated strains (transplantation antigens).[1] Credit for the description of the human MHC goes to three individuals. In 1952, Jean Dausset observed that serum of individuals who had received several transfusions contained hemagglutinins specific for donors' leukocytes. In 1958, Rose Payne noted that the only requirement for the development of hemagglutinins against leukocytes was a history of previous transfusion or pregnancy and concluded that these antibodies were directed against antigens on the surface of circulating leukocytes. This conclusion was concomitantly and independently confirmed by Jon van Rood, who observed that multiple pregnancies immunize mothers against leukocytes leaked from the fetus into the mother's circulation. Based on these discoveries, the term *human leukocyte antigen* was subsequently adopted.[2] It should be clarified, however, that this historical name is misleading. Neither is HLA molecule expression limited to leukocytes nor do they display, in natural conditions, antigenic behavior. In fact, several are expressed by most somatic cells, and, rather than being antigens, they chaperone protein bioproducts to the cell surface for recognition by T cells. There is, however, some substance to the name, because HLAs, by virtue of being densely packed on the cell surface, are exposed to recognition in a foreign environment such as allotransplantation or xenoinfusion performed to induce anti-HLA antibodies as diagnostic reagents.

ORGANIZATION OF THE HLA GENES

HLA genes constitute a string of coding sequences that regulate the expression of molecules with similar but not identical function. Residing in a region that spans approximately 4000 kilobases of the short arm of chromosome 6 (Fig. 114-1),[3] HLA contains several genes and pseudogenes characterized by sequence homology and functional similarity. Of them, 47 are officially recognized by the World Health Organization nomenclature committee[4] and include classic HLA class I and class II genes associated with antigen processing such as PSMB8 and PSMB9 (proteasomal units) or TAP1 and TAP2 associated with peptide transport. Both HLA and HLA-associated genes can be physically grouped into three subregions according to chromosomal location. In centromeric to telomeric direction, the first is HLA class II region comprising the α-and β-chains of HLA-DR, -DQ, -DP, -DM, and -DO as well as TAP and PSMB. Sandwiched between the class II and class I region, class III region encodes for functionally unrelated genes such as complement components, heat shock proteins, and tumor necrosis factor. The reason for their genetic link to the HLA complex is unknown, but their immunologic function seems more than coincidental. The class I region is most telomeric and includes HLA-A, -B, and -Cw loci; the nonclassic HLA-E, -F, and -G loci; and several pseudogenes.

General terminology separates HLA genes into classic and nonclassic. Classic HLA genes have been well characterized and are clearly associated with presentation of antigen to immune cells. They are further subdivided into class I (HLA-A, -B, -C) and class II (HLA-DR, -DQ, and -DP). In general, HLA class I and II genes have very similar structure and function.[5,6] They contain six to eight exons coding for functionally distinct domains (Fig. 114-2). The first exon encodes a leader sequence; the following exons (exons 2 to 4) are highly polymorphic and encode extracellular domains responsible for peptide binding and T cell–antigen receptor (TCR) engagement. Because they are exposed on the cell surface, these domains are also responsible for alloreactivity. The last exons encode a conserved transmembrane and small intracellular domains whose function is unclear.

Only the heavy chain of HLA class I is encoded in the MHC region. Genes encoding HLA-A, -B, and-C contain three exons coding for α_1, α_2, and α_3 extracytoplasmic domains, one transmembrane, and three cytoplasmic domains (Fig. 114-3). The associated class I light chain, β_2-microglobulin, is encoded on chromosome 15.[7] By contrast, the HLA class II molecule is composed of a heterodimer of an α-chain and a β-chain encoded in the MHC region. Although the genetics are different, the protein product is structurally similar to HLA class I, with two helices resulting in the antigen-presenting part of the molecule (Fig. 114-4).

All DR molecules use DRA for α-chains but can use alleles coded by DRB1, DRB3, DRB4, or DRB5 for β-chains. DP, DQ, DM, and DO molecules are the product of DPA1 and DPB1, DQA1 and DQB1, DMA and DMB, and DOA and DOB genes, respectively.

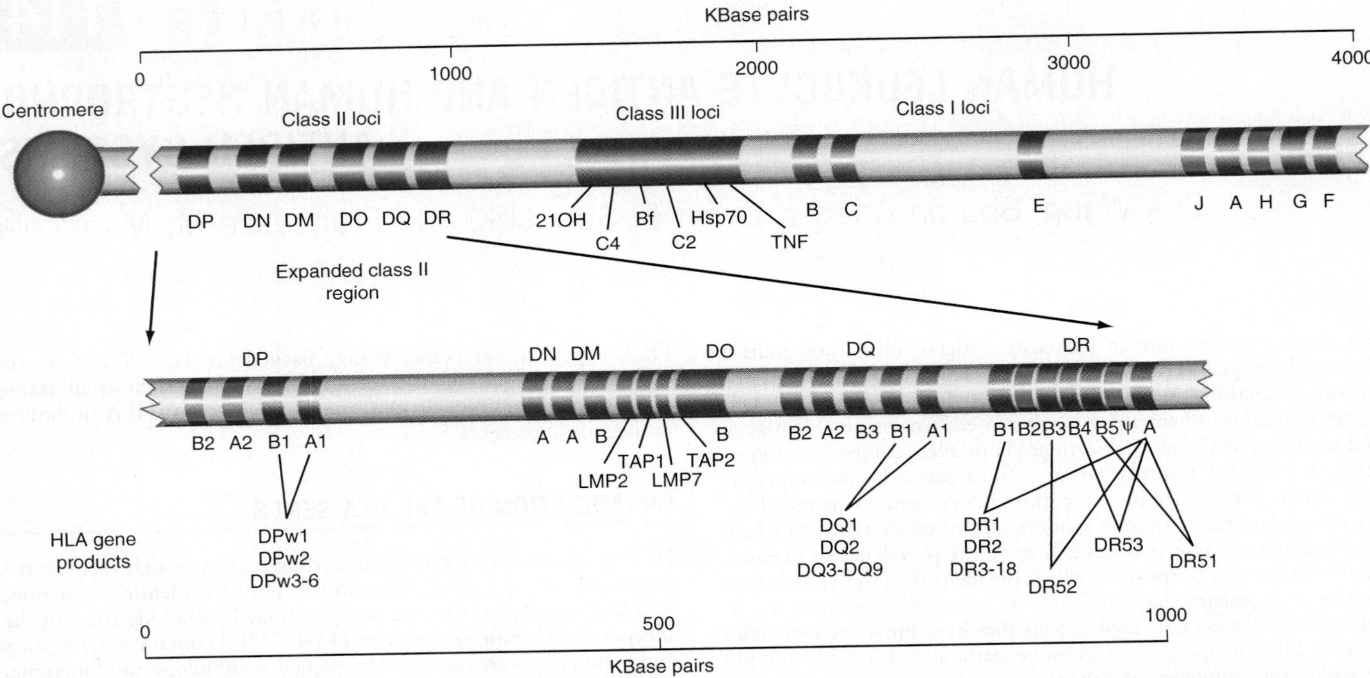

Figure 114-1 PHYSICAL MAP OF THE HUMAN LEUKOCYTE ANTIGEN (HLA) GENETIC COMPLEX, ILLUSTRATING THE CLUSTERS OF GENES ACCORDING TO THE CLASS OF ENCODED GENE PRODUCTS. The symbol ψ represents four DRB pseudogenes, designated 7, 8, and 9. Other pseudogenes are shown in *gray*.

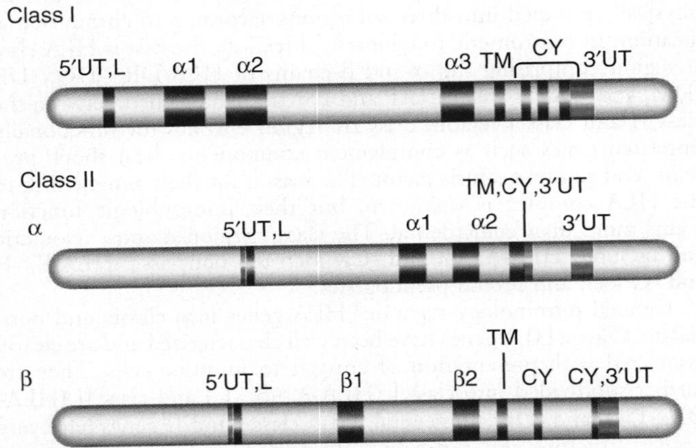

Figure 114-2 ORGANIZATION OF CLASS I AND II MAJOR HISTOCOMPATIBILITY COMPLEX (MHC) GENES. *5′UT* and *3′UT,* Untranslated regions in the 5′ and 3′ ends of the gene; *α, β,* exons encoding extracellular domains; *CY,* exon encoding cytoplasmic tail; *L,* leader sequence; *TM,* transmembrane exon. *(From Germain RN, Malissen B: Analysis of the expression and function of class-II major histocompatibility complex-encoded molecules by DNA-mediated gene transfer,* Annu Rev Immunol *4:281, 1986.)*

HLA DRB1 locus is expressed in all HLA haplotypes (the set of HLA alleles derived from the same parental chromosome and therefore genetically linked). However, only one other HLA DR locus is present in each individual chromosome. Thus each haplotype can have either DRB5 (DR1 haplotype); DRB3, -B4, or -B5 loci (DR2 haplotype); DRB4 locus (DR4 and DR7 haplotype); or none (DR8 and DR10 haplotype).[3]

INHERITANCE AND LINKAGE DISEQUILIBRIUM

Because of their proximity within a short chromosomal distance, HLA genes are inherited en bloc from each parent unless a

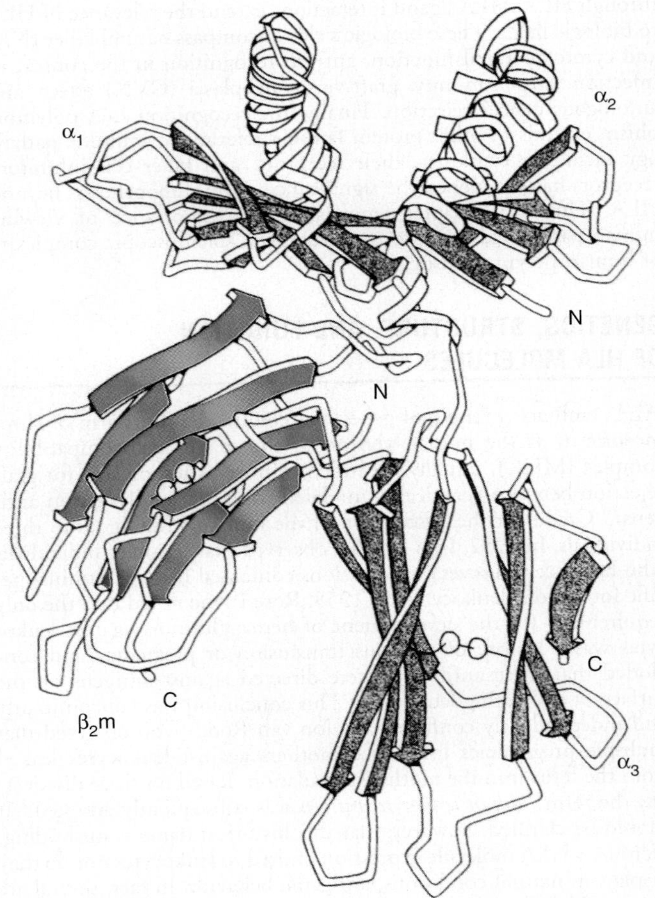

Figure 114-3 THREE-DIMENSIONAL CONFIGURATION OF HLA-A2, MODELED FROM X-RAY CRYSTALLOGRAPHIC STUDIES. *HLA,* Human leukocyte antigen. *(From Bjorkman PJ, Saper MA, Samraoui B, et al: Structure of the human class I histocompatibility antigen, HLA-A2,* Nature *329:506, 1987.)*

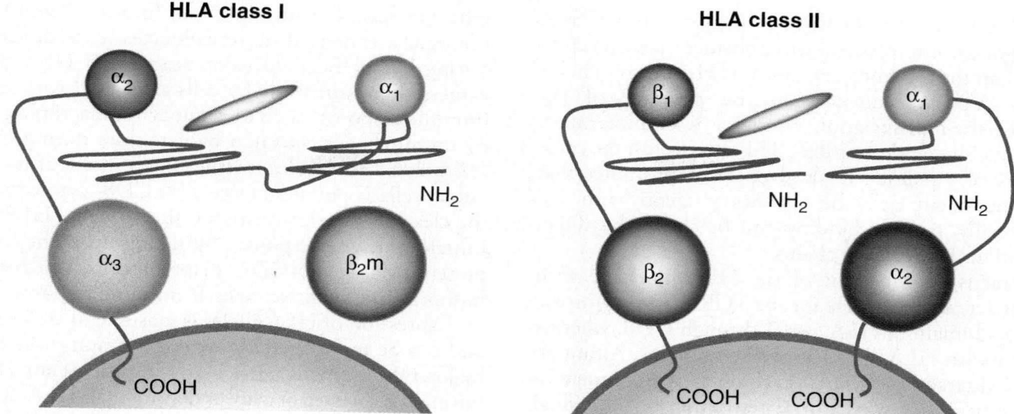

Figure 114-4 SCHEMATIC DIAGRAM OF HUMAN LEUKOCYTE ANTIGEN (HLA) CLASS I AND CLASS II MOLECULES POINTING TO THEIR STRUCTURAL SIMILARITY. In both HLA classes, two immunoglobulin-type domains reside close to the cell membrane (α_3 and β_2m for class I and α_2 and β_2 for class II). The other two domains project toward the extracellular milieu with α-helices (α_1 and α_2 for class I and α_1 and β_1 for class II) and a platform of parallel β-sheets that form a peptide-binding groove.

recombinant event occurs. Thus each HLA haplotype behaves as a unit and is transmitted through generations according to mendelian principles. Because there are four possible genotypes (two from each parent), the probability of genotypic identity between two siblings is 25%. Most HLA phenotypically identical siblings are also HLA genotypically identical, because the genetic pool of derivation is restricted to the parents. In 2% of cases, recombinant HLA haplotypes (a set of genes derived partially from two chromosomes through recombination) deviate from this rule.

The occurrence of HLA haplotypes within a population with a frequency higher than expected from the prevalence of individual alleles is called *linkage disequilibrium.* In large populations, gene frequencies achieve equilibrium within a few generations unless selective pressure influences individuals' survival and mating capacity (Hardy-Weinberg principle). In equilibrium, gene prevalence is maintained based solely on its frequency. Thus, assuming that there were 18, 36, and 8 alleles for the HLA-A, -B, and -C loci, respectively (number of alleles known when this example was described[2]), theoretically $18 \times 36 \times 8 = 5184$ HLA class I allelic combinations or haplotypes would be possible. Adding HLA class II genes to the calculation yields an astronomical number, making unlikely the identification of two HLA-matched individuals. However, individual alleles occur with different frequency, and an allele that occurs with high frequency is predominant in a given population, such as HLA-A2 in whites and A24 or A11 in Asians.[8] Because predominant alleles come with the related haplotype, most theoretical permutations never occur, and the chances of identifying matched individuals are much higher than theoretically possible.

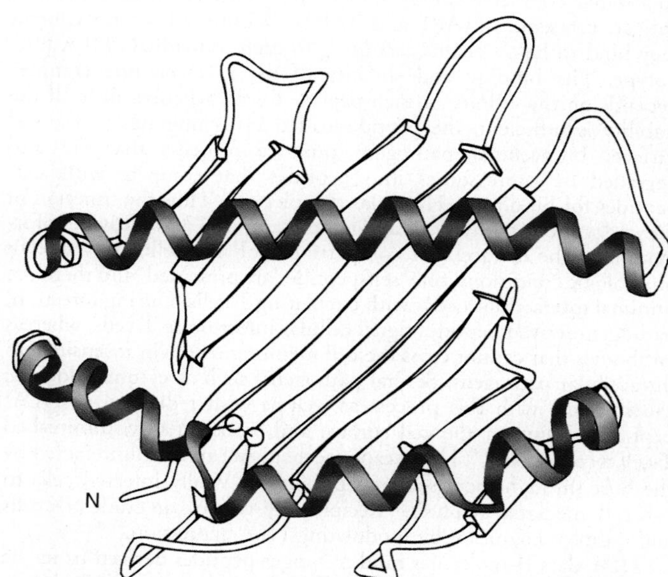

Figure 114-5 SCHEME OF THE PEPTIDE GROOVE OF A HUMAN LEUKOCYTE ANTIGEN (HLA) CLASS I MOLECULE, FORMED BY THE α_1 AND α_2 DOMAINS AT THE SIDE AND THE β-SHEETS AT THE BOTTOM. The view is looking down on the vertically oriented molecule: the T-cell receptor point of view. *(From Bjorkman PJ, Saper MA, Samraoui B, et al: Structure of the human class I histocompatibility antigen, HLA-A2,* Nature *329:506, 1987.)*

STRUCTURE OF THE HLA CLASS I AND II

The structure of HLA molecules and their relationship with their natural ligand, the TCR, has been well characterized by crystallography.[9-11] HLA molecules are heterodimer glycoproteins belonging to the immunoglobulin superfamily with common features (see Fig.114-4). This includes two α-helical domains protruding toward the extracellular milieu. Between them lies a flat surface formed by β-sheet structures that contributes to the formation of a groove accommodating peptides generated from intracellular (HLA class I) or extracellular proteins (HLA class II) (Fig. 114-5). The helices/peptide complex is exposed for TCR recognition. Because HLA polymorphism is clustered within the α-helixes and β-sheets domains, peptides display variable affinity for distinct HLA alleles.[12,13] It has been proposed that a given peptide can bind to closely related alleles, and HLA superfamilies with similar binding characteristics have been described.[14-16] However, peptide binding to related but distinct HLA alleles is associated with conformational dissimilarity caused by differential interaction with variant residues in the binding groove.[17] The TCR interaction with HLA required for productive engagement spans a surface including the peptide and portions of the α- and β-helix.[11,18-20] This double requirement of interaction between TCR and HLA/peptide complex represents the structural basis for HLA restriction. Degenerate and promiscuous TCR recognition of peptides presented by distinct HLA alleles within the same superfamily has also been described.[21] Although this concept holds in general, several exceptions can be expected because single amino acid variants in the HLA molecule may disallow binding of a peptide[22] or may not be permissive to TCR engagement.[23,24]

The binding affinity of a given peptide for an HLA allele can be predicted through algorithms that compile available information to identify amino acid residues that fit distinct pockets of the HLA groove.[12,25] Several algorithms implement this information with experimental testing based on the refolding capability of HLA heavy chains exposed to known peptide sequences in the presence of β_2-microglobulin and/or their dissociation rates (see www.bimas.dcrt.nih.gov or www.uni-tuebingen.de/uni/kxi). This is based on the principle that the affinity of a peptide for a given HLA promotes that stability of the noncovalent assembly of heavy chain with β_2-microglobulin.[12,26] Finally, peptide binding can be shown by direct elutriation from purified HLA heavy chains.[13,27]

Beyond the interactive component of the HLA molecule with TCR, other domains act as coreceptors for the TCR. CD8$^+$ cytotoxic T cells bind to the α_3-domain of HLA class I through CD8, whereas CD4$^+$ T cells interact with HLA class II–specific domains. Although the coreceptor-TCR interaction is not an absolute requirement in most cases, it determines HLA class I or II restriction of individual T cells.[28]

Specific to HLA class I is the assembly with β_2-microglobulin on stabilization in the presence of high-affinity peptides derived from the cleavage of intracellular proteins (endogenous pathway of antigen presentation).[29] Most peptides derive from degradation of self-protein in the cytosol by proteasomes (PSMB) and other proteases.[30] Soluble peptides (9 to 10 amino acids long) are then chaperoned into the endosomal compartment by transporter molecules associated with antigen processing (TAP1 and TAP2). Within this compartment, they bind to heavy chains according to each individual's HLA phenotype. The binding and stability of the HLA-peptide complex depends on the affinity of each peptide for a particular allele. If the stability is sufficient, the peptide-loaded HLA migrates to the cell surface. Intracellular pathogens produce proteins that are also degraded by proteasomes into peptides that compete with self-peptides for binding to HLA class I molecules. Thus the function of the endogenous pathway of antigen presentation is to provide information to the extracellular compartment of intracellular events. In physiologic conditions, only self-peptides are presented, and therefore minimal interactions occur with circulating T cells. During infection, pathogen-derived peptides signal cellular infection to T cells, whereas antibodies that cannot cross the cell membrane remain insensitive to intracellular pathogens. Several pathogens, such as cytomegalovirus, can interfere with this process as well as with reduction of HLA/peptide density on the cell surface and, consequently, diminished T-cell recognition.[31,32] This escape mechanism can be counteracted by the host through increased susceptibility of virally infected cells to NK cell–mediated cytolysis.[33] Reciprocally, viruses can evade NK cells and escape recognition by modulating HLA expression.[34-36]

HLA class II molecules bind to longer peptides derived from the metabolism of molecules endocytosed from the extracellular compartment (exogenous pathway of antigen presentation).[29] This is a specialized process used by professional antigen-presenting cells such as macrophages and dendritic cells. HLA class II molecules are assembled within the endosomal compartment where they are composed of a heterotrimer. This includes the α- and β-chains plus a short invariant chain that stabilizes the molecule by occupying its groove while chaperoning its migration to the endosomal compartment where exogenous antigen is processed. Upon uptake, the exogenous antigen undergoes limited proteolysis in the membrane-bound acidic endosomal compartment (MHC class II peptide-loading compartment, MIIC). Upon entering the MIIC, the pre-HLA class II complex is degraded, and antigenic peptides are loaded with the help of the nonclassic HLA-DM molecule.[37]

EXPRESSION OF HLA MOLECULES

There are genetic and structural differences between the two classes of HLA alleles. The most striking difference is functional, because HLA class I molecules are expressed by most nucleated cells with the exception of germinal cells, whereas HLA class II molecules are expressed mainly by specialized antigen-presenting cells.[38,39] HLA class I molecules are also expressed by platelets.[40] They are responsible for refractoriness after multiple transfusions[41-44] and sufficiently, though minimally, expressed by reticulocytes to be targets of alloantibodies during hemolytic transfusion reactions.[45] HLA class II proteins are expressed constitutively by cells associated with the initiation of the immune response, such as monocytes, macrophages, and B cells,[46] or by immune cells activated by cytokines during inflammation. Thus HLA class I molecules instruct the host about the condition of individual cells as potential targets for CD8$^+$ cytotoxic T cells responsible for clearing the organisms of altered cells. HLA class II molecules initiate immune responses by taking up pathogen components and presenting them to CD4$^+$ helper T cells, which can in turn initiate humoral and facilitate cellular immune responses.

Expression of HLA alleles is sensitive to environmental conditions and can be modulated by cytokines among which interferons play a major role.[47] This is particularly important for HLA-B and HLA-C normally expressed at a lower density than HLA-A but which are more sensitive to cytokine induction.[48,49] In addition, HLA class II molecules can be expressed by most cells following cytokine stimulation.[50,51] Thus the ability of cells to present antigen in association with HLA is strongly influenced by the surrounding environment. This might explain why chronic inflammation induced by alloreactions during graft-versus-host disease (GVHD) may facilitate the presentation of tumor-specific antigens by tumor cells with consequent development of GVN effect. In addition, it might explain how systemic administration of proinflammatory cytokines such as interleukin-2 may stimulate immune responses by increasing the antigen-presenting ability of cells within the tumor microenvironment.[52]

HLA POLYMORPHISM AND ITS CLINICAL SIGNIFICANCE

A striking characteristic of the HLA system is its extreme polymorphism.[53] By chance, most individuals are heterozygote and therefore carry two different alleles for each HLA gene that, being codominant, are equally expressed on the cell surface. Because everybody carries three HLA class I (-A,-B, and -C) and three HLA class II (-DR, -DQ, and -DP) genes, most individuals (with the exception of homozygotes) express six different HLA class I and six different HLA class II molecules on the surface of their cells. This has important functional implications, because HLA polymorphism is clustered in domains of the HLA molecule associated the peptide binding and interaction with the TCR. Thus most individuals have a broad repertoire of molecules capable of presenting different pathogen components to immune cells. Therefore it is believed that HLA polymorphism improves the chances of a given species of surviving infection.[54] This paradigm is difficult to demonstrate in human pathologic conditions in which the natural history of infectious diseases rarely correlates with HLA phenotype. An exception is the strong association between HLA-B*5701 and lack of progression to acquired immunodeficiency syndrome of individuals infected with human immunodeficiency virus (HIV).[55] Associations have been observed between HLA phenotype and predisposition for nasopharyngeal carcinoma.[56,57] This is of particular interest because nasopharyngeal carcinoma is a virally induced cancer against which T cells can mediate immune surveillance. HLA associations have also been described with less consistency for other virally driven tumors, such as cervical carcinoma,[58] or immunogenic tumors, such as melanoma.[59,60]

The difficulty in demonstrating conclusive associations between infectious disease and HLA in humans could be caused by the successful implementation of antigen presentation through a broad repertoire of HLA genes, which could compensate for each other in limitations in antigen presentation. Chickens carry a single MHC locus, and their susceptibility to infection appears to be clearly related to MHC. For instance, Kaufman et al[54] have shown that chickens carrying a particular Bf (the only MHC class I gene in chickens) allele are fully protected from Rous virus–induced sarcomas, because this allele (B-f12) can bind several antigenic peptides from its proteins. On the contrary, chickens homozygous for B-f4 are killed by the same infection, because this allele cannot bind peptides from sarcoma virus proteins.[54]

HLA polymorphism is the basis of alloimmunization, because most individuals are likely to have different HLA molecules on the surface of their cells. Hundreds of HLA alleles have been identified through high-resolution typing, making the chances of two individuals having identical HLA phenotypes extremely low. Thus partial mismatches are commonly accepted in transplantation cases, which are at the root of hyperacute, acute, and chronic rejections. Hyperacute rejection is caused by preformed antibodies against donor HLA alleles in patients presensitized by multiple transfusions.[61] Acute and chronic rejection result from a combination of humoral and cellular immune reactivity toward HLA alleles of the donor.[62,63] In addition to allosensitization, HLA alleles can mediate GVHD, whereby hematopoietic cells derived from the grafted tissue recognize and reject the host tissues. They do this by identifying polymorphisms of intracellular proteins of the host (minor histocompatibility antigens) presented in association with donor-recipient matched HLA alleles.

NONCLASSIC MHC AND MHC CLASS I CHAIN-RELATED MOLECULES

Besides the three ubiquitously expressed highly polymorphic classic HLA class I molecules, humans encode three relatively conserved nonclassic, selectively expressed (HLA-E, -F, and -G) MHC class I genes (also known as MHC-Ib). These evolved at different rates in primates reflecting differential involvement in the modulation of immune responses.[4,64,65] In addition, these molecules are characterized by unique patterns of transcription, protein structure, and immunologic function.[66]

The MHC class I–related chain genes (MICA and MICB) are located within the MHC region and are characterized by high polymorphism (more than 50 alleles so far identified).[67] The molecules encoded by these genes do not appear to bind peptides or associate with β_2-microglobulin. Their polymorphic variants are not concentrated around the peptide-binding groove, yet they seem to have functional significance, because most mutations are nonsynonymous, suggesting selective pressure as a driving force. Their tissue distribution is restricted to epithelial and endothelial cells and fibroblasts. It appears that MIC genes modulate the function of NK and CD8$^+$ T cells by binding the NKG2D stimulating receptor.[68] Also, MIC genes have been implicated in transplant rejection because alloantibodies against them are often found in transplant recipients that may exert complement-mediated cytotoxicity against endothelial cells from the graft.

Other unusual MHC-like molecules are present in the genome and have disparate functions, including presentation of lipid antigens (CD1), transport of immunoglobulins (Fc receptor), and regulation of iron metabolism (hemochromatosis gene product).[69] Contrary to classic MHC class I genes that are constitutively expressed, nonclassic MHC and MIC gene expression is dependent on stimulation by proinflammatory cytokines.[70] In addition, two nonclassic MHC class II proteins (HLA-DM and HLA-DO) have been described that function as mediators of peptide exchange by stabilizing empty MHC class II molecules.[37] Finally, it is possible that several nonclassic MHC molecules whose function is to present peptides to lymphocytes may be present throughout the genome. Because of their limited polymorphism, however, these genes may have evolved to serve specialized presentation functions.[71]

Characterized by low polymorphism, the regulation of HLA-G expression follows a nonclassic behavior. Aberrant cytokine-responsive regulatory sequences[72-74] may be responsible for its predominant expression by trophoblasts that do not express other HLA proteins.[75] It may also account for its low levels in a variety of human tissues.[76] Lack of responsiveness to common immunostimulatory pathways (NF-κB, interferon-γ, or CIITA) is most pronounced in HLA-G cells and is shared by other nonclassic MHC such as HLA-E.[77] Also, HLA-G is expressed in a variety of cancers.[72] It is hard to know what the relevance of HLA-G expression is, because it can occur in various membrane-bound or soluble isoforms with distinct functional characteristics.[72] Functional isoforms that include the α-1 and α-2 domains bind and present peptides from cytoplasmic proteins.[78] Because of the minimal polymorphism, however, the repertoire of peptides presented is likely to be limited, suggesting that peptide binding is necessary to stabilize the molecule rather than being involved in antigen presentation.

Functionally, HLA-G is thought to modulate the function of NK cells through interactions with their inhibitory receptors.[79] In addition, the HLA-G leader sequence contains a peptide that can bind and stabilize the expression of HLA-E, which, in turn, inhibits NK cells.[80] Because the HLA-G–derived leader peptide has the strongest affinity for HLA-E (among all HLA class I molecules), it is likely that HLA-G is a powerful direct and indirect inhibitor of NK cells, reducing the risk for cardiac rejection[81] or inducing immune escape of cancer cells.[72] Although much has been published about the immunoregulatory role of HLA-G, its true function remains mysterious, principally because of discordant findings reported by various groups.[73] With the goal of achieving consensus, a workshop was recently organized to standardize methods of analysis of HLA-G.[66]

HLA-E is minimally polymorphic,[4] binds hydrophobic peptides from other HLA class I leader sequences, and interacts with CD94/NKG2 lectin-like receptors present predominately on NK and partially on CD8$^+$ T cells.[82-85] The peptide binding is highly specific and stabilizes the HLA-E protein, allowing its migration to the cell surface. Thus surface density of HLA-E is an indirect reflection of the number of HLA class I alleles expressed by a cell.[86] The interaction of HLA-E with CD94/NKG2 protects HLA-E–expressing cells from killing. Cells damaged by viral infection or neoplastic degeneration may lose HLA class I expression. As a backup mechanism of protection, reduced HLA class I expression results in decreased expression of HLA-E, leading to vulnerability to NK cells.[87] Some viruses express mimic peptides that bind and stabilize HLA-E so that, although classic MHC molecules are downregulated, HLA-E expression is maintained, allowing the pathogen to simultaneously escape CD8$^+$ T- and NK-cell killing.[88]

The function of HLA-F remains enigmatic. Its transcriptional regulation is closest to classic HLA molecules in that it can be induced by NF-κB, interferon regulatory factor-1, and class II trans-activator.[89] However, contrary to classic HLA molecules, HLA-F is predominantly empty, mostly intracellular, with a restricted pattern of expression.[90] Its tissue distribution appears to be limited to B cells, and therefore it is mostly found in lymphatic organs.[90] Structural studies suggest that HLA-F is a peptide-binding molecule and may reach the cell surface under favorable conditions when a suitable peptide is present.[91] Once on the cell surface, HLA-F may interact with the effector-cell receptors IL-T2 and IL-T4, as suggested by HLA-F tetrameric complexes–binding studies.[91] Thus it is possible that in specific yet unknown conditions, HLA-F may modulate the function of immune effector cells similarly to HLA-E and HLA-G.

NON-HLA POLYMORPHISM AND ITS CLINICAL SIGNIFICANCE

Although this chapter is dedicated to HLA, it would be incomplete without mentioning the increasingly recognized polymorphisms of other immune modulators. The significance of non-HLA polymorphism is evidenced by the development of GVHD in the presence of HLA identical matching among relatives. As recently summarized,[92] three general areas of polymorphism are being investigated: NK cell–receptor genes, minor histocompatibility antigens, and cytokines. Over the last decade, much progress has been made in identifying the mechanisms of action of NK cells. A major breakthrough was made in the discovery of HLA class I–specific inhibitory receptors and in the role that they play in the regulation of NK function with consequent effects on the eradication of hematologic malignancies, prevention of graft rejection, or induction of GVHD.[93] NK cells recognize HLA molecules via killer immunoglobulin-like receptors (KIRs). The regulation of NK cell function by KIRs is further

Table 114-1 HLA Class I Alleles Recognized by Different Killer Immunoglobulin-Like Receptors

KIR	HLA Class I Allele	Amino Acid Sequence Motif
P58.1 (KIR2DL1)	HLA-C2, -C4, -C5, -C6	Asn 77, Lys 80
P58.2 (KIR2DL2/3)	HLA-C1, -C3, -C7, -C8	Ser 77, Asn 80
P70 (KIR3DL1)	HLA-Bw4 public specificity	Aa 77-83
P140 (KIR3DL2)	HLA-A3, -A11	
(KIR2DL4)	HLA-G	

Aa, Amino acid; *Asn*, asparagine; *HLA*, human leukocyte antigen; *KIR*, killer immunoglobulin-like receptor; *Lys*, lysine; *Ser*, serine.

discussed in Chapter 12. KIRs are glycoproteins encoded by at least 17 different genes located on chromosome 19q13.4.[94] All human KIR genes derive from a gene encoding three immunoglobulin (Ig)-like domains (D0, D1, and D2) and a long cytoplasmic tail. However, the KIRs genes are diverse and may encode either two or three Ig-like domains and either a long or short cytoplasmic tail (Table 114-1). The long cytoplasmic tails contain one or two immunoreceptor tyrosine-based inhibition motifs.[95] Although KIR molecules with long cytoplasmic tails inhibit NK cytotoxicity, those with short tails do not. The names given to KIR genes are based on the molecule that they encode. The first digit corresponds to the number of Ig-like domains in the molecule and a *D* denotes domain. The D is followed by either an *L* for long cytoplasmic tail or *S* for short cytoplasmic tail or *p* for a pseudogene. The last digit indicates the number of the KIR gene.[96]

Expression of KIR in individual NK cells is complex because NK cells may express several members of the KIR family. The number of KIR genes in each haplotype varies among individuals. The most common haplotype is known as group A, which is made up of six genes (2DL1, 2DL2 or 2DL3, 3DL1, 3DL2, 2DS4, and 2DL4). Various KIR genes can recognize different HLA-A, HLA-B, and HLA-C molecules. HLA-C antigens can be divided into two groups based on polymorphisms at amino acid positions 77 and 80 of their class I heavy chains. One group has asparagine (Asn) at position 77 and lysine (Lys) at 80 and the other has serine (Ser) at 77 and Asn at 80. Some KIRs recognize HLA-C antigens with Asn 77 and Lys 80, whereas other KIRs recognize HLA-C antigens with Ser 77 and Lys 80. The polymorphism at position 80 is most important. Another group of KIR reacts with HLA-B antigens that carry specific combinations of amino acids at positions 77 and 83 of the heavy chain that forms HLA-Bw4. Because a single KIR can interact with multiple HLA class I alleles, KIR recognition of HLA class I molecules is degenerate. Another NK inhibitory receptor (CD94-NKG2A) recognizes the nonclassical HLA-E molecule. In addition, each of the KIR genes is extensively polymorphic.

Because the genes for KIR, HLA, and CD94-NKG2A are located in separate chromosomes, they segregate independently and consequently individuals can carry genes for KIR for which there is no correspondent HLA ligand.[97] Because HLA-E is expressed in all individuals, NK cells that bear the CD94-NKG2A receptor are not alloreactive. Because the specificity of KIR for their ligands is broad and each individual carries several KIRs, it is likely that in most cases all NK cells of a given person express at least one KIR that is specific for a self-HLA class I allele. Thus in autologous settings, NK cells kill only aberrant cells that have lost HLA class I expression. By contrast, NK cells can kill allogeneic cells that do not express HLA class I alleles recognized by their KIR. Thus, by knowing the KIR repertoire of a given transplant recipient and the HLA type of the donor, it would theoretically be possible to predict the likelihood of an NK-mediated alloreaction. Importantly, it appears that alloreactive NK cells undergo proliferation on exposure to the stimulatory cells and therefore can preferentially expand in the presence of allogeneic tissue. NK cells also express activating receptors that are responsible for their lytic activity. Although the identity of the ligands for these receptors has not been identified, it is possible that they are expressed primarily by activated or proliferating cells. It is therefore possible that during the inflammatory process induced in allogeneic conditions, normal cells can become activated by cytokines and express ligands, which are responsible for NK activation in the absence of HLA class I molecules reactive with the inhibitory receptors.[93] The relevance of KIR in transplantation has been well studied in the context of haploidentical hematopoietic transplantation. In this case, several combinations are possible: NK cells from the graft express KIRs that do not interact with the donor's HLA (graft-versus-host alloreactivity). It seems that the presence of graft-versus-host reactive NK cells associated with incompatibilities between donor and recipient (especially HLA-Cw families) has favorable effects on the outcome of acute myeloid leukemia.[98] Alternatively, a good match may be present between graft NK and host HLA as well as between host NK and graft HLA. In such a case, no alloreactivity occurs. Finally, the graft's HLA type may be unsuitable for the host's NK repertoire, and the host's reactivity may lead to graft rejection. Alloreactive grafted NK cells seem to prevent GVHD while inducing GVN.[93]

Like HLA, KIR genes are polymorphic, and their variability is clustered in positions likely to affect the overall structure of the molecule. The relevance of KIR gene polymorphism in the outcome of bone marrow transplantation (BMT) is unclear. It appears that the risk for GVHD is highest in the context of unrelated BMT when the recipient KIR genotype is included in the donor KIR genotype.[99] These results show that compatibility between KIR genotypes themselves may influence the outcome of BMT.

The minor histocompatibility antigens (mHags) are represented by polymorphic molecules whose peptides containing variant sequences are presented by HLA alleles. They have been shown to be targets of cytotoxic T cells, which can lyse leukemia cells.[98,100] In addition, some mHags are selectively expressed by neoplastic cells.[101] At present, little is known about the identity of mHag epitopes in the context of various HLA types and their significance in the development of GVHD and GVN.

Cytokines are another large family of molecules associated with antigen recognition, graft rejection, and GVHD. Their polymorphism is becoming an important area of investigation in the context of transplantation, autoimmunity, and cancer.[102] Polymorphic sites reside in regulatory regions so that genetic variants are associated with high or low production of a given cytokine rather than differences in its function. A Web site compiles information about cytokine polymorphism (www.bris.ac.uk/Depts/PathAndMicro/services/GAI/cytokine4.htm). Although no consensus has been achieved yet, several studies have shown associations between various cytokine genotypes and propensity toward disease and transplant outcome. These studies have been summarized elsewhere.[92,103] A strong association was recently noted between a low interleukin-10 producer genotype and a tendency to develop melanoma and prostate cancer.[104,105]

HLA NOMENCLATURE

The history of the HLA system nomenclature was summarized by Sir Walter Bodmer who, together with Ruggero Ceppellini, was primarily involved in its development.[106] It began as HL-A, for *human leukocyte locus A.* With the recognition that HLA molecules are encoded by more than one locus, the A came to stand for *antigen* and a locus designation was added after HLA (i.e., HLA-A, -B, -C, -D, etc.).[2] From then on, the World Health Organization has updated on a quarterly basis. The most recent update was assigned in January 2012, as seen in Table 114-2.[4] At present two systems are used. An immunologically defined nomenclature is based on the identification of HLA antigens on the surface of leukocytes. Therefore HLA phenotypes described by immunologic methods are conventionally called *HLA antigens.*[107] The second system is based on the molecular identification of nucleotide sequences in genomic deoxyribonucleic acid (DNA), and results are conventionally referred to as *HLA alleles.*

Table 114-2 Name of Genes in the HLA Region Considered by the WHO Nomenclature Committee

Name	Previous Equivalents	Molecular Characteristics	No. of Alleles January (2012)
HLA-A	–	Class I α-chain	1757
HLA-B	–	Class I α-chain	2338
HLA-C	–	Class I α-chain	1304
HLA-E	E, "6.2"	Associated with class I 6.2-kBa Hind III fragment	10
HLA-F	F, "5.4"	Associated with class I 5.4-kBa Hind III fragment	22
HLA-G	G, "6.0"	Associated with class I 6.0-kBa Hind III fragment	47
HLA-H	H, AR, "12.4", HLA-54	Pseudogene association with class I 5.4-kBa Hind III fragment	12
HLA-J	cda 12, HLA-59	Pseudogene association with class I 5.9-kBa Hind III fragment	9
HLA-K	HLA-70	Pseudogene association with class I 7.0-kBa Hind III fragment	6
HLA-L	HLA-92	Pseudogene association with class I 9.2-kBa Hind III fragment	5
HLA-X	–	Class I gene fragment	0
HLA-DRA	DRα	DR α-chain	7
HLA-DRB1	DRβI, DR1B	DR β_1 determining specificity for DR1, DR2, DR3, etc.	1052
HLA-DRB2	DRβII2	Pseudogene with DRβ-like sequence	1
HLA-DRB3	DRβIII, DR3B	DR β3 determining DR52, Dw24, w25, -26 specificity	57
HLA-DRB4	DRβIV, DR4B	DR β4 determining DR53 specificity	15
HLA-DRB5	DRβV, DR5B	DR β5 determining DR52, Dw24, w25, -26 specificity	19
HLA-DRB6	DRBX, DRBσ	Pseudogene found in DR1, DR2, and DR10 haplotypes	3
HLA-DRB7	DRBψ1	Pseudogene found in DR4, DR7, and DR9 haplotypes	2
HLA-DRB8	DRBψ2	Pseudogene found in DR4, DR7, and DR9 haplotypes	1
HLA-DRB9	M 4.2 β exon	Pseudogene isolated fragment	1
HLA-DQA1	DQα1, DQ1A	DQ α-chain as expressed	47
HLA-DQB1	DQβ1, DQ1B	DQ β-chain as expressed	162
HLA-DOA	DNA, DZα, DOα	DO α-chain	8
HLA-DOB	DOβ	DO β-chain	9
HLA-DMA	RING 6	DM α-chain	4
HLA-DMB	RING 7	DM β-chain	13
HLA-DPA1	DPα1, DP1A	DP α-chain as expressed	33
HLA-DPB1	DPβ1, DP1B	DQ β-chain as expressed	152
TAP1	ABCB2, RING4	ABC (ATP-binding cassette) transporter	12
TAP2	ABCB3, RING 11	ABC (ATP-binding cassette) transporter	12
MICA	PERB 11.1	Class I chain–related gene	80
MICB	PERB 11.2	Class I chain–related gene 18	33

Data from Marsh SGE, Albert AD, Bodmer WF, et al: Nomeclature for factors of the HLA system, 2010. *Tissue Antigens* 75:291, 2010.
ATP, Adenosine triphosphate; *HLA*, human leukocyte antigen; *WHO*, World Health Organization.

Because molecular typing has higher resolution, it has gained increasing popularity.

IMMUNOLOGICALLY DEFINED HLA NOMENCLATURE

Immunologically defined nomenclature follows this rule: HLA separated by a hyphen from a capital letter identifying the locus encoding distinct HLA class I (-A, -B, -C) or class II (-DR, -DQ, -DP) antigens. The letter is followed by a number that identifies a serologic family of alleles sharing epitopes recognized by alloantibodies or alloreactive cytotoxic T cells. With improved understanding of the molecular genetics of the HLA region, various appendages have been removed from the HLA nomenclature. For instance, the letter *w* was used to indicate a provisional assignment, and this has been discontinued, but it is occasionally added to HLA-C antigen nomenclature to distinguish it from complement genes; DP and DW also maintained this letter to reinforce the dependency of their immune identification predominantly through cellular techniques. Finally, HLA-Bw4 and -Bw6 retain the *w* to emphasize that the public epitopes are shared by several HLA-B and some HLA-Antigens. More recently, a bridge between immunologic and molecular nomenclature has been proposed whereby HLA antigens that encompass a single gene product can be assigned a two-digit numeric extension corresponding to the molecular nomenclature for that allele.[108]

SEQUENCE-DEFINED ALLELIC NOMENCLATURE

The 10th International Histocompatibility Workshop recommended in 1987 a sequence-based nomenclature[108a] to describe alleles not distinguishable by immunologic methods. Since then, the number of HLA alleles has rapidly increased. As of January 2012, a total of 7130 alleles for HLA exist. This is a drastic increase from the original numbers established in 2003. Other designations are summarized in Table 114-2. HLA designates molecules belonging to the human MHC followed by the locus (-A, -B, etc). Alleles are then identified after an asterisk (*). Each HLA allele name has a unique number corresponding to up to four sets of digits separated by colons. The length of the allele designation is dependant on the sequence of the allele and that of its nearest relative. All alleles receive at least a four digit name, which corresponds to the first two sets of digits, longer names are only assigned when necessary. The digits before the first colon describe the type, which often corresponds to the serological antigen carried by an allotype. The next set of digits are used to list the subtypes, numbers being assigned in the order in which DNA sequences have been determined. Alleles whose numbers differ in the two sets of digits must differ in one or more nucleotide substitutions that change the amino acid sequence of the encoded protein. Alleles that differ only by synonymous nucleotide substitutions (also called silent or non-coding substitutions) within the coding sequence are distinguished by the use of the third set of digits. Alleles that only differ by sequence polymorphisms in the introns or in the 5′ or 3′ untranslated regions that flank the exons and introns are distinguished by the use of the fourth set of digits.[108b] A four-digit number is used in which the first two digits refer to the original serologic family (e.g., HLA-A2 serologically would be HLA-A*02). Often numbers are missing because an original assignment was revoked (e.g., this is why there is no HLA-A*24:01). When silent mutations are identified (variation in nucleotide sequence that does not translate into changes in amino acid sequence), the name of the allele remains identical, but another two digits are added to designate a variant that has no functional significance. New sequences are submitted to European Molecular Biology Laboratory (EMBL; www.ebi.ac.uk/Submissions/index.html), GenBank (www.ncbi.nlm.nih.gov/Genbank/index.html), or DNA Data Bank of Japan (DDBJ; http://www.ddbj.nig.ac.jp/submission-e.html).

Requirements for new allele naming were described by Marsh et al.[4] The World Health Organization committee also made recommendations about naming alleles with aberrant expression such as HLA-G isoforms and KIR. Some alleles are identifiable at the genomic level but are not translated into protein (pseudogenes). These are indicated by the addition of an *N* (for null) following the numerical designation of the allele. Mutations inducing a reduction of expression are marked by *L* (low expression). An *S* denotes alleles expressed as soluble secreted molecules, such as HLA-B*44:02:01:02S characterized by an intronic variant that disallows the expression of the transmembrane domain of the HLA molecule and is therefore only in soluble form. Differential splicing of HLA-G leads to production of membrane-bound and soluble forms, which are respectively denoted by a lowercase *m* or *s* before HLA. Limited cytoplasmic expression is denoted by *C* and aberrant expression by *A*. Finally, KIR polymorphism will be classified by a new system that is in preparation.[4,97,109] A nomenclature system for cytokine polymorphism has not yet been developed.[110]

HLA TYPING IN CLINICAL HEMATOLOGY AND DETERMINATION OF COMPATIBILITY HLA TYPING

Originally HLA typing was done primarily in support of transplantation or transfusion needs with the purpose of identifying histocompatibility through the best match between donor and recipient. Allosensitization of recipients previously exposed to heterologous cell products is tested by identifying alloreactive antibodies in serum, and crossmatch procedures are performed to grade compatibility of candidate donor-recipient pairs. In addition, HLA testing has been applied to identify links between a given disease and the genetic makeup of its carriers.[111] Strong associations are exemplified by birdshot uveitis (a disease occurring exclusively in HLA-A29 individuals),[112] type 1 diabetes and other autoimmune diseases,[113-115] or long-term survival of HIV-infected individuals.[55] These studies evaluated the role that genetic background may have contributed over environmental factors.[111,116] HLA associations are thought to be caused by the differential ability of distinct alleles to present immunogenic epitopes[112,113] or by the close linkage to the HLA class III region where potent immunomodulators such as tumor necrosis factor-α are located.[117] It has also been suggested that HLA associations may be predictors of immune responsiveness of cancer to immune therapy.[60] However, such associations have remained quite difficult to reproduce.[118] HLA typing is requested for enrollment of patients into and interpretation of immunization protocols,[24] because specific HLA-epitope combinations require high-resolution typing.[22,119]

Serologic testing takes advantage of fetomaternal sensitization. In mammals, the progeny carries a full haplotype of paternal origin, and pregnant women may develop antibodies against the paternal haplotype. Maternal serum samples are collected at term and characterized by testing their ability to kill HLA-bearing repository cell lines of known phenotype in the presence of complement (complement-dependent cytotoxicity [CDC]).[120] Then CDC is used for HLA typing by exposing circulating cells expressing HLA class I (most cells) and class II (predominantly B cells) antigens from the individual (to be typed to previously characterized sera or monoclonal antibodies).[121] Conversely, already typed repository cell lines are used in CDC to identify alloantibodies in sera of sensitized individuals. The fraction of cell lines killed by the sera roughly grades the intensity of allosensitization or panel reactive antibody (PRA) reactivity. Some antibodies activate complement and kill with poor efficiency, known as the *cytotoxicity-negative absorption-positive (CYNAP) phenomenon.*[122] As judged by cytotoxicity testing, CYNAP may underestimate allosensitization. By modifying CDC with the addition of antihuman antibodies suitable for complement activation, CYNAP can be circumvented (augmented CDC). In this case, however, relatively innocuous antibodies can cause overestimation of clinically relevant allosensitization.[123] Other methods identify alloantibodies, including immobilization of HLA molecules on solid surface to capture soluble antibodies[124-126] and flow cytometry using a spectrum of microbeads loaded with known HLA alleles.[127,128] An interlaboratory comparison of serum screening for HLA-antibody determination suggested that enzyme-linked immunosorbent assay and flow cytometry yield higher PRA activity values compared with CDC or augmented CDC.[125] However, the study suggested a lack of consistency among participant laboratories, leaving unsolved the question of which method most accurately defines clinically relevant allosensitization, and a panel of various methods may be most informative.[72]

Complement-dependent cytotoxicity is declining in interest in the United States because most laboratories are switching to easier-to-handle and higher-resolution molecular methods. However, immunologic methods remain valuable to characterize functional aspects of HLA because molecular methods cannot define whether an HLA allele is expressed nor, at least until recently,[129] grade allosensitization. Thus it is likely that immunologic methods will continue to complement molecular methods in the future.[129]

The usefulness of conventional serologic typing has been limited by the availability of allele-specific sera. Most importantly, because antibodies identify structural differences on the surface of HLA molecules, variants caused by nucleotide polymorphism in nonexposed areas such as the peptide-binding groove of the HLA heavy chain are not detectable. However, these differences are of functional significance because they determine the specificity and affinity of peptide binding[130,131] and T-cell recognition of self and allogeneic target cells.[23,132] DNA-based typing directly determines the sequence,[133] and its resolution is limited only by the number of allele-specific probes used to identify an ever-growing number of alleles (see www.anthonynolan.com/HIG/index.htm). Various polymerase chain reaction (PCR)-based methods have been described, among which sequence-specific primer[133,134] and sequence-specific oligonucleotide probe[135,136]–based methods are the most universally used. The rich nature of HLA has led to proportionally increasing complexity of the assays used to cover all possible alleles. As a consequence, accurate HLA typing for donor and recipient matching in transplantation has become increasingly complex and burdensome. In addition, because of the important role that HLA molecules play in antigen presentation and the stringency of the relationship between epitope and associated HLA allele, high-resolution typing is increasingly requested for appropriate enrollment of patients into immunization protocols aimed at the enhancement of T-cell responses.[137] Therefore high-resolution HLA typing is increasingly in demand in clinical and experimental settings.

Although oligonucleotide-based methods could theoretically discriminate any known polymorphic site, they have two major limitations. First, they require a specific PCR reaction for each allele investigated. Because each individual has only two alleles for each locus, a disproportionately large number of PCR reactions must be performed to cover all possible polymorphisms to identify the two borne by the individual tested. Because both methods are based on specific interactions with known oligonucleotide sequences unique to a particular allele, they cannot identify unknown polymorphisms unless the variation occurs within the region spanned by one of the oligonucleotides used in the assay. Because of these limitations, interest is growing for definitive typing methods that yield conclusive information about the identity of the alleles typed. The most comprehensive method is sequence-based typing. Unfortunately, its use has been limited by the cost of equipment and reagents and by the high level of expertise and time required for the interpretation of each typing. More recently, high-throughput, robotic, sequence-based typing has been developed that allows sequencing of hundreds of genomic fragments each day.[138-140] However, even sequence-based typing has some technical limitations. Some combinations of HLA class I and class II alleles result in ambiguous allele combinations that require additional testing for resolution.[141] Finally, new methods based on high-density array technology are being developed that may allow extensive typing of known and unknown polymorphisms on microchips.[142,143]

High-resolution methods yield high-resolution information of an individual's HLA type. However, the wealth of information is counterbalanced by increased difficulty in identifying suitable HLA alleles during donor-recipient pairing or accrual into immunization protocols restricted to specific HLA-epitope combinations. Thus at present clinicians are faced with the daunting task of applying high-resolution typing results of unclear relevance to clinical settings.[144]

TESTING FOR ALLOSENSITIZATION AND DETERMINATION OF COMPATIBLE RECIPIENT-DONOR PAIRS

Any cell-containing product transfused or transplanted between different individuals should be compatible in an ideal situation. Yet, in most cases, histocompatibility is not prospectively sought. Thus patients with multiple exposures to blood products often become reactive to various antigens, including HLA. Transplant candidates often develop prior alloreactivity following transfusion of platelet concentrates contaminated with leukocytes, even though the incidence of allosensitization is much less because of leukodepletion of blood products. Alloreactivity must be documented before transplantation, because alloreactive patients can still undergo transplantation, provided that the donor has no mismatched HLA antigens reacting with the patient's antibodies. Patients who have received repeated platelet transfusions may become allosensitized and consequently refractory to further transfusions unless HLA-compatible platelets are used. Obviously the best compatibility consists of identical matching. It is often impossible to identify a perfectly matched unrelated donor, particularly in the case of rare HLA types. Thus other strategies are adopted to identify the best possible match or compatible mismatch. Selection of unrelated donor-recipient pairs is carried out through typing with serologic, cellular, and molecular methods.[145] The chances of identifying compatible donors based on full or partial HLA matching have become increasingly low with the increasing resolution of the typing methods.[144] To broaden compatibility, matching criteria of donor-recipient pairs are based on shared public epitopes assigned to cross-reactive groups (CREGs)[146] or shared amino acid polymorphisms defined through sequence information (Table 114-3).[147] The preexistence of alloantibodies restricts the identification of compatible donors even further. Highly sensitized recipients with PRA activity exceeding 85% of tested specificities (generally between 30 and 60) represent a particularly challenging group.[148] An alternative approach to the exclusion of alloreactive determinants is the inclusion of acceptable antigen mismatches expressed in a panel of cells that give negative reactions with the recipient sera,[149] which extends the repertoire of possible donors. All these are fundamental tools for the identification of nonrelated, not fully matched donor-recipient pairs. Unfortunately, even these compromises often fail to identify a suitable match.

Duquesnoy[148] recently described a molecularly based algorithm to identify histocompatible pairs called HLAMatchmaker. This method focuses on the structural basis of HLA class I polymorphism so that compatible HLA mismatches can be identified without extensive serum screening. This algorithm is based on the principle that short amino acid sequences (triplets) characterizing polymorphic sites of the HLA molecules are critical components of allosensitizing epitopes. Such amino acids reside in the α-helices and β-loops of the heavy chain. Because each HLA molecule expresses a characteristic string of these determinants, it is possible to characterize each molecule according to the linear sequence of amino acid triplets present on its surface. Based on the reasonable assumption that none of the triplets present in the HLA repertoire of the recipient is self-immunogenic, it is possible through a process of electronic recombination to identify donors with HLA alleles different from the recipient's but containing exclusively shared triplets. These HLA alleles will be compatible, because they do not contain any epitope absent in the recipient.

In theory, a large number of triplets could occur if polymorphisms were randomly distributed. However, most HLA molecules span conserved domains, and only a total of 142 different polymorphic triplets designate serologically defined HLA-A, -B, and -C antigens.[148] Triplet polymorphism can occur in 30 locations on HLA-A, 27 in HLA-B, and 19 in HLA-C chains. Because the HLAMatchmaker algorithm includes interlocus comparison, it is possible to accumulate the information into a single database. Among the 142 polymorphic triplets, 29 are polymorphic for one class I locus but monomorphic for another class I locus. Such polymorphic triplets cannot be immunogenic because they are always present on the patient's own HLA antigens, whereas the remaining 113 triplets have immunogenic potential. With this algorithm, it is possible to significantly broaden the number of molecularly matched HLA alleles and significantly increase the chances of identifying a compatible donor, particularly in those cases in which the recipient has a rare HLA phenotype. In addition, HLAMatchmaker considers triplets that are present in the panel cells that give negative reactions with the recipient's serum. These negative panel cells can be expected to share antigens with the patient's, but other HLA antigens may be present and contain mismatched triplets apparently not immunogenic for that patient. Such triplets are therefore acceptable and can be added to the algorithm for the identification of possible donors. Thus HLAMatchmaker assesses HLA compatibility at a molecular level by determining whether or not a triplet in a given position of a mismatched HLA antigen is also found in the same position in any of the recipient's own HLA-A, HLA-B, and HLA-C molecules. A shared triplet in the same position on a mismatched HLA antigen cannot elicit a specific antibody response in that patient. This hypothesis needs future testing, because this strategy might represent a revolutionary tool for the identification of potential donors. Preliminary verification of the algorithm in a series of high-PRA renal patients suggested that this is a proper strategy at least in highly sensitized renal transplantation candidates waiting for unrelated donors.[150] HLAMatchmaker is also effective at selecting an optimal HLA-typed platelet component for alloimmunized thrombocytopenic patients.[151]

A new version of HLAMatchmaker considers so-called eplets and is based on the structural definitions of functional epitopes on well-characterized protein antigens that have been complexed with anti-

Table 114-3 Population Frequencies of Major Cross Reactive or Determinants Present on HLA-A and -B Gene Products

Major Cross-Reactive Group	Public Epitope	Associated Private Epitopes	Approximate Epitope Frequency (%)*
1C	1p	A1, 3, 9 (23, 24), 11, 29, 30, 31, 36, 80	79
	10p	A10 (25, 26, 34, 43, 66), 11, 28 (68, 69), 32, 33, 74	
2C	28p	A2, 28 (68, 69), 9, 17	70
	9p	A2, 28 (68, 69), 9 (23, 24)	
	17p	A2, B17 (57, 58)	
5C	5p	B5 (51, 52), 18, 35, 53, 78	50
	21p	B5 (51, 52), 15 (62, 63, 75, 76, 77), 17 (57, 58), 21 (49, 50), 35, 53, 70 (71, 72), 73, 74, 78	
7C	7p	B7, 8, 41, 42, 48, 81	54
	22p	B7, 22 (54, 55, 56), 27, 42, 46	
	27p	B7, 13, 27, 40 (60, 61), 47	
8C	8p	B8, 14 (64, 65), 16 (38, 39), 18	38
12C	12p	B12 (44, 45), 13, 21 (49, 50), 40 (60, 61), 41	44
Bw4	Bw4	B13, 27, 37, 38, 47, 49, 51, 52, 53, 57, 58, 59, 63, 77, A24, 25, 32	79
Bw6	Bw6	B7, 8, 18, 35, 39, 41, 42, 45, 46, 48, 50, 54, 55, 56, 60, 61, 62, 64, 65, 67, 71, 72, 73, 75, 76, 78, 81	87

*North American white populations of European origin.

body.[152] Eplets represent amino acid residue configurations within a 3- to 3.5-Å radius of each polymorphic residue on the HLA molecular surface. Many eplets correspond to triplets, but eplets represents a more complete repertoire of structurally defined epitopes.

THE HLA MOLECULES AS ANTIGENS AND HLA ALLOIMMUNIZATION

By no means are HLA molecules antigenic in physiologic condition (with the exception of maternofetal alloimmunization). However, because of their high density on the surface of cells, they can become highly immunogenic in the nonphysiologic event in which cells from different individuals are exposed to another person's immune system. The mechanism or mechanisms leading to allosensitization are believed to follow two pathways. The first pathway mimics the one followed during most immune reactions in which antigen is up taken by antigen-presenting cells and presented to autologous lymphocytes (indirect pathway). In this case the donor's HLA molecules are processed into peptides through the exogenous pathway of antigen presentation and presented to autologous T cells as linear peptides.[153,154] This pathway is believed to be responsible for the development of alloantibodies as well as T-helper cell responses, but its role in the development of cytotoxic T-cell responses remains unclear. Because this pathway depends on the presentation of donor HLA molecules by recipient HLA alleles, it may explain why the humoral response to HLA class I allodeterminants correlates with the HLA phenotype of the responder.[155] The indirect pathway of HLA allorecognition has been associated with allograft rejection.[156] Because the function of HLA molecules is to present antigenic determinants to T cells, it could be easily envisioned how minor changes in their structure could be misinterpreted as antigenic epitopes. Intact HLA molecules residing on the surface of donor cells are a perfect target for T cell–mediated allorecognition (direct pathway) either through the direct cytotoxic effect of T cells against target cells or by the activation of helper T cells, through HLA class II engagement, which leads to stimulation of antibody-mediated immune responses.[157]

Humoral responses mediated most frequently by IgM are predominant in the sensitization to infrequent allogeneic exposure, because they require smaller amounts of antigenic material. T-cell responses become more manifest in the context of transplantation in which the persistence of the allogeneic stimulus allows the expansion and sustenance of alloreactive cytotoxic T cells. Antibodies and TCR have different requirements for their engagement, which means epitopes recognized by T cells and antibodies are different. Antibodies require interaction with a small structure, including a limited number of amino acids; thus any sequence combination on the surface of an HLA allele not present in the individual exposed to the alloreaction may represent an epitope. T cells have much lower binding affinity for their ligand and require a complete interaction with the peptide as well as the α– and β–helices of the HLA class I heavy chain.[11] Although several B-cell epitopes recognized by antibodies can be identified in a given HLA molecule, generally the whole HLA molecule is necessary for T cell–dependent allorecognition. Definition and topographic mapping of epitopes defined by serologic or cellular methods has revealed distinct regions of hypervariability in the α-1 and α-2 domains of the class I heavy chains and in the α-1 and β-1 domains of class II molecules.[158] Two types of antibody-defined epitopes can be identified according to their frequency among HLA alleles. Private epitopes are almost but not totally unique for a single serologically defined HLA antigen and are used for typing. These epitopes are generally shared by all molecular alleles present in that given family, and fine differences among alleles within a general family cannot be distinguished by antibodies. Public epitopes are more widely distributed and cluster distinct serologic families into groups. These epitopes bear an immunodominant character. Immune sera that identify public epitopes have been considered predictive of major CREGs with the idea that alloreactivity among patients belonging to the same CREG may be less likely (see Table 114-3). The predictive value of CREGs in transplant outcome or platelet transfusion results, however, remains to be demonstrated.

Not all subjects who have been exposed to alloantigens develop alloantibodies, and in fact exposure to low doses of donor-specific HLA antigens through donor transfusion may have a beneficial effect on graft survival.[159] Obviously, the degree of compatibility in the context of allosensitization may vary according to the degree of mismatch between donor and recipient. In addition, alloantibodies are one aspect of alloreaction that does not take into account cellular responses. These have been more difficult to document, although they are likely to play an important role in the context of acute transplant rejection. Several hypotheses have been discussed about the reason or reasons for the capriciousness of allosensitization, including the presence of regulatory immune responses or cytokine-mediated immunosuppression. Currently the mechanism modulating the quality and quantity of alloimmunity remains elusive, and different aspects of this algorithm are discussed ad hoc in this chapter, with particular attention to molecularly defined algorithms for the prediction of histocompatibility.[129,148,160,161]

Clearly, HLA matching is beneficial in patients undergoing renal transplantation. An analysis of more than 150,000 recipients receiving transplants in different centers participating in the Collaborative Transplant Study showed that a complete mismatch (6 HLA-A+B+DR) had a 17% lower survival expectation than no mismatch ($P<0.0001$).[162] Matching was particularly beneficial in patients with highly reactive preformed alloantibodies. The same study suggested that high-resolution matching based on molecular typing improved graft survival. Similar results were observed in cases of cardiac transplantation in which HLA matching yielded significantly better results ($P<0.0001$). This is particularly important because donor hearts are currently not allocated according to HLA match in most centers. In cases of liver transplantation, HLA matching was not beneficial.[163]

Donor-specific hyporesponsiveness has been particularly well documented in the context of renal allotransplantation and may limit the need for immunosuppression. A recent randomized study suggested that pretransplant donor transfusions improved the survival of cadaver kidney grafts in patients receiving modern immunosuppressive regimens, but the mechanism remains unclear.[164,165] Although most centers currently do not implement deliberate blood transfusions, the usefulness of this approach needs to be investigated further.

Approximately 5% to 10% of platelet transfusions are given to patients who have been previously exposed to HLA class I–expressing heterologous cells and are reactive to HLA antigens. Such patients are refractory to random-donor platelets and must be given HLA-matched or semimatched plateletpheresis components.[41-44] However, a provision of HLA-matched platelets does not always improve platelet recovery and survival. Possibly, the ineffective platelet transfusion is in part caused by unrecognized HLA mismatches between the donor and recipient resulting from the low-resolution methods used for typing, and higher resolution methods have been advocated. It is currently controversial whether or not molecularly based HLA typing confers an advantage over serologic typing, and this principle was recently questioned in the context of hematopoietic cell transplantation.[166,167]

HLA AS A FUNCTIONAL MEDIATOR OF GRAFT-VERSUS-HOST DISEASE AND/OR GRAFT-VERSUS-NEOPLASIA EFFECT

Allogeneic or syngeneic bone marrow transplantation is used predominately for the treatment of hematologic malignancies[168-170] and other hematologic disorders such as aplastic anemia,[171] thalassemia,[172] or myelodysplastic syndrome.[173] This strategy can induce long-term disease-free survival in chronic myelogenous leukemia patients.[168,169] The objective of bone marrow transplantation in cases of malignancy is to cure the patient by eradication of the neoplastic cells with myeloablative chemotherapy followed by restoration of hematopoiesis through the transplantation of normal hematopoietic stem cells derived from HLA-compatible normal donors. This strategy is characterized by the insurgence of an immune reaction toward the host's normal cells (GVHD),[174-176] which is often associated and preferentially targets neoplastic cells (GVN effect).[177-184] Both the GVHD and the GVN effect occur in the presence of a full HLA match; thus the HLA molecules are not targets of allosensitization themselves but present polymorphic molecules expressed by the recipient's cells recognized by the grafted immune cells.

GRAFT-VERSUS-HOST DISEASE

GVHD represents the alloimmune reaction of donor lymphocytes against normal cells of the recipient. GVHD occurs predominantly in association with hematopoietic progenitor cell transplantation (HPCT) compared to other types of transplants because the hematopoietic transplant is enriched of immune cells. Myeloablative therapy is generally administered before transplantation and, as a consequence, in most cases prevents graft rejection. GVHD is a major complication of HPCT, and a fine balance between GVHD and graft rejection is maintained by modulating the level of posttransplantation immunosuppression.[184] In addition, other major disturbances associated with HPCT, such as overwhelming infection, leukemia, or tumor relapse, and other regimen-related morbidities are strongly influenced by the treatment of GVHD. With the advent of nonmyeloablative HPCT for the treatment of nonhematologic diseases such as solid tumors, GVHD has reached a predominant role because of its close association with GVN effect.

T-cell depletion has been advocated for the prevention of GVHD by decreasing the probability of cellular and humoral alloresponses.[185,186] This strategy decreases the occurrence of GVHD but is associated with an increased risk for graft rejection and tumor or leukemia relapse.[184] In fact, Weiden et al[187] observed that survivors of severe acute GVHD had a significantly lower incidence of tumor relapse compared with patients who did not experience GVHD. This association appeared mandatory, and it was believed that the beneficial GVN reaction was inseparable from GVHD.

The risk for GVHD increases with genetic distancing between donor and recipient. Thus recipients of transplants from HLA-identical twins have a lesser chance of developing GVHD than recipients of transplants from HLA-unrelated donors and from donors with only a partial HLA match.[188,189] Interestingly, however, although the genetic closeness between donor and recipient appears to decrease the risk for GVHD, it also decreases the therapeutic benefit, with increased chances of tumor relapse.

GRAFT-VERSUS-NEOPLASIA EFFECT

It was originally observed that a beneficial collateral effect of GVHD was the rejection of neoplastic cells by the donor immune system in the context of hematologic malignancies (graft-versus-leukemia effect).[177] It was rapidly recognized that the graft-versus-leukemia effect could play a powerful therapeutic role in the treatment of refractory malignant disorders, including some solid tumors (graft-versus-tumor effect).[181] Because the biology and clinical principles underlining the two effects are likely similar, for simplicity, in this chapter we coin a unifying term: *graft-versus-neoplasia effect.* Indeed, there is a perception that the GVN reaction is the most potent form of tumor immunotherapy currently in clinical use. Its mechanism of action is still poorly understood. T cells definitely play a fundamental role in the initiation and maintenance of the alloreaction toward neoplastic cells.[190] A sevenfold increase in the chance of relapse was noted in patients with chronic myelogenous leukemia who received a T cell–depleted BMT as compared with a subset of patients who had received a T cell–repleted BMT but did not develop GVHD.[185,186] This result suggested that GVHD is a biologic entity different from GVN effect. In addition, on leukemia relapse, administration of donor lymphocyte infusion could reinduce clinical remission.[191] Finally, leukemia-specific $CD8^+$ T cells have been identified in circulating lymphocytes at the time of leukemia regression.[192] NK cells play an additional role in mediating this phenomenon, and clinical data suggest that mismatch of NK receptor and ligands during allogeneic BMT can be used to enhance the GVN effect.[93,193] Appreciation of the GVN effect has led to the development of nonmyeloablative stem cell transplants designed to immunosuppress the host to a level sufficient to permit engraftment of the donor immune cells to generate GVN without inducing the serious complications associated with myeloablation.[184] The GVN effect has gained popularity in the last decade to the point that allogeneic-based immunotherapeutic approaches have been advocated for several nonhematologic malignancies.[184] The rationale is largely based on the assumption that the immune cell repertoire capable of recognizing cancer cells in the allogeneic context is broader than in the autologous system. Donor

T cells can target not only tumor-specific antigens but also allelic variants of these antigens; mHag; and, in the case of HLA-mismatched transplants, HLA antigens disparate from the donor expressed by the tumor cells.[194-196] Although there are several theories about how the GVN effect occurs, it remains unclear why allo-T cells have a better chance of targeting tumor cells in an allogeneic context as compared with the natural insurgence of antitumor immunity described for several solid tumors.

HLA AND T CELL–DIRECTED IMMUNIZATION

The last decade has witnessed remarkable progress in the identification and mapping of T-cell epitopes for various infectious diseases and cancer. In particular, progress was made in mapping HLA-associated epitopes for HIV, cytomegalovirus, and Epstein-Barr virus.[197-200] In addition, the molecular identification of tumor-associated antigens has yielded a large number of epitopes that could be used to immunize against neoplasia.[201] A comprehensive discussion of these topics is beyond the scope of this chapter, but we address a few points framing the relevance of HLA in the context of T cell–directed immunization.

The identification of T-cell epitopes led to two major areas of clinical investigation. The first is active-specific immunization to prevent or treat ongoing infections or cancer. The second is the harvest and in vitro expansion of immunization-induced T cells for adoptive transfer. In general, active immunization has proved successful in inducing epitope-specific T cells easily detectable among circulating lymphocytes.[119,202-204] However, often the immunization-induced enhancement of T-cell function is not associated with clinical improvement. Although the reason for the clinical ineffectiveness of immunization-induced T cells is unclear, it has been postulated that they may be quantitatively[203] or qualitatively[205] inadequate for eradicating disease. Therefore a second strategy is being pursued whereby the number of antigen-specific T cells is amplified in vitro for autologous or donor-derived adoptive transfer. This second strategy has met some promising success in the context of ganciclovir-resistant cytomegalovirus infection,[206] Epstein-Barr virus–induced posttransplantation lymphoproliferative disorders,[207] and metastatic melanoma.[208]

Whether delivered as a primary form of therapy or to prime in vivo T cells for further ex vivo expansion, epitope-specific vaccination encounters the major limitation of a stringent requirement for HLA allelic association. Although superfamilies of HLA alleles may share epitopes,[14,15] in practical terms, clinically relevant HLA-epitope associations are restricted to few peptide-allele combinations for a given protein.[22] Patients considered for enrollment in immunization protocols are best served by high-resolution HLA typing to exclude subtypes with unproven immunogenic potential for a given epitope. To bypass the stringent HLA requirements demanded by epitope-specific vaccination, whole-antigen delivery is suggested. This is based on the assumption that the epitope repertoire of a protein can be adjusted to distinct HLA phenotypes by a cellular process of self-selection naturally coupling peptides to HLA according to binding affinity. Although theoretically indisputable, in practice the truth of this assumption depends on the efficiency with which individual molecules are processed and presented in association with distinct HLA alleles. Even in these settings, high-resolution typing is desirable because it allows accurate interpretation of immunization results by allowing a comparison between the detailed genetic makeup of the individual receiving the vaccine and his or her antigen-specific immune response. It is likely that in the future HLA laboratories will receive increasing demands for high-resolution, definitive typing for appropriate patient enrollment and for subsequent interpretation of immune responses.

MONITORING IMMUNE RESPONSES WITH TETRAMERIC HLA-PEPTIDE COMPLEXES

A growing understanding of the molecular immunology of T-cell interactions with HLA/epitope complexes in the context of infectious disease, virally induced malignancies, and spontaneous tumors as well as interest in their treatment with T cell–directed vaccines has generated more attention to the issue of using accurate methods to quantify ex vivo the extent of antigen-specific immune responses.[209] The most commonly used assays available for the enumeration of antigen-specific T cells include tHLA; intracellular fluorescence-activated cell sorter staining for cytokine expression on cognate stimulation; detection of cytokine release by enzyme-linked immunospot assay; and quantitative real-time PCR, recently reviewed by Keilholz et al.[210] tHLAs are complexes of four HLA molecules combined with a specific peptide and bound to a fluorochrome (Fig. 114-6). These complexes bind to complementary TCR and identify antigen-specific T

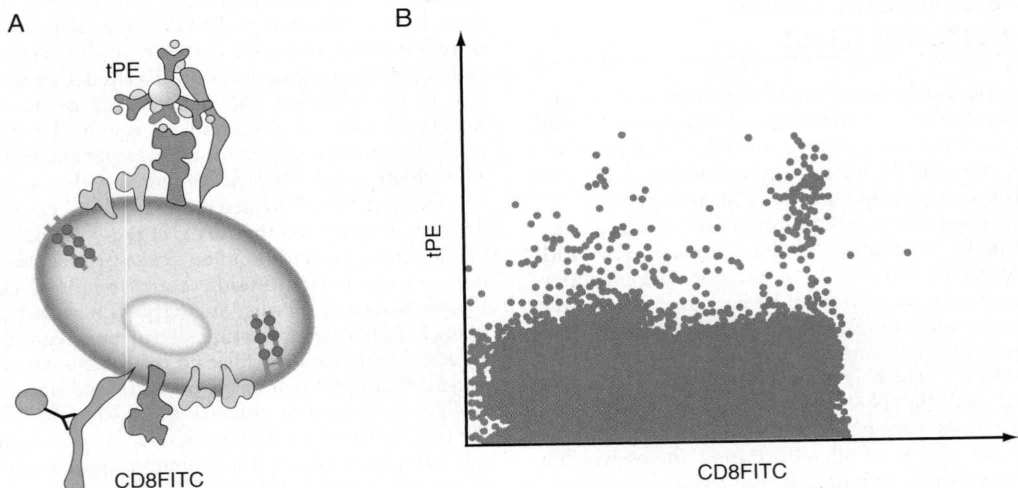

Figure 114-6 SCHEMATIC REPRESENTATION OF THE MECHANISM OF BINDING OF TETRAMERIC PEPTIDE/HUMAN LEUKOCYTE ANTIGEN COMPLEXES (THLA) TO ANTIGEN-SPECIFIC T CELLS. **A,** Binding of tHLA to T-cell receptor. The tHLA consists of four HLA/peptide complexes identical to the ones recognized by the T cell on the surface of live cells. Each HLA molecule is modified to contain one biotin molecule that serves as a bridge for binding to tetravalent streptavidin molecules fluorescently labeled. **B,** Actual fluorescence-activated cell sorter (FACS) analysis result of CD8$^+$, tHLA-positive T cells. *(Modified from Monsurro V, Nargosen D: Immunotracking of specific cancer vaccine CD8 lymphocytes,* ASHI Q *26:100, 2003.)*

cells,[211] measuring cellular responses against specific epitopes with sensitivity as low as 1 in 5000 CD8+ T cells. To synthesize tHLA molecules, soluble HLA heavy chains containing a biotinylation site and recombinant β_2-microglobulin are synthesized and purified. They are then refolded in the presence of the specific epitope, and the monomer is isolated by gel filtration and is biotinylated. Fluorescent streptavidin is added to induce tetramerization. An aliquot of tetramers is added to the peripheral blood mononuclear cells together with other antibodies for a more detailed characterization of antigen-specific T cells.[205] Analysis is performed using a flow cytometer. Because of the specificity of vaccines, the patient's HLA type and specific peptide must be identified and synthesized to provide the adequate tetramer. Pentameric HLA/peptide complexes have recently become available and in some laboratories have replaced the use of tHLA.

Analysis of tHLA offers many potential advantages over other T-cell assays. This method is quantitative and enables an estimation of the avidity between TCR and peptide-loaded HLA class I molecules. tHLA staining does not kill the labeled cells, allowing sorting of subpopulations by flow cytometry for additional analysis or expansion for adoptive transfer. With tHLA specific T cells can be analyzed from blood samples without the prerequisite of in vitro culture, and all specific cytotoxic T lymphocytes are detected, regardless of their functional status.[203,205,212]

HLA SUMMARY

The relevance of HLA in clinical pathology has broadened from its role as a predictor of allosensitization to a mediator of GVHD and GVN. The understanding of action mechanisms in various nonclassic HLA genes as well as KIR has opened a new field. The study examining the function of the innate immune response in the context of transplantation and other immunopathologies is a result of this. Together with HLA, immunogenetics is rapidly growing, driven by the realization that polymorphism is the hallmark of human immunopathology as its spans mHag, KIR, cytokines, and their receptors. Each of these is interwoven in an intricate array of interdependent functions that cannot be discounted. Modern methods should be able to adopt high-throughput systems for the parallel assessment of all these variables when addressing the genetic makeup of an individual in correlation with the natural or therapeutic history of his or her disease. The comparison of donor and recipient protein profiling and cytokine polymorphism may offer insights into the rejection mechanism when matched-donor grafts are used. Finally, the increased use of T cell–directed immunization is driving renewed interest in high-resolution typing of HLA molecules to allow a more accurate interpretation of clinical and immunologic results.

HUMAN NEUTROPHIL ANTIGENS AND THEIR CLINICAL SIGNIFICANCE

Lalezari et al described the first granulocyte antigens. These antigens were designated *N* for neutrophil. Each antigen system was described alphabetically, and each allele was described numerically in order of discovery. They identified NA1 in 1966 and its allele, NA2, in 1972.[213,214] In 1971, Lalezari et al[215] described another granulocyte antigen, NB1. Reports of several other granulocyte antigens followed.

A new nomenclature was established in 1998 by the International Society of Blood Transfusion Working Party (Table 114-4).[216] In this nomenclature, antigen systems are referred to as *human neutrophil antigens,* or HNA. The antigen systems—that is, the polymorphic forms of the immunogenic proteins—are indicated by integers, and specific antigens within each system are designated alphabetically by date of publication. Alleles of the coding genes are named according to the Guidelines for Human Gene Nomenclature. Neutrophil antigens NA1 and NA2 became HNA-1a and HNA-1b in the new nomenclature, and NB1 became HNA-2a.

Table 114-4 International Society of Blood Transfusion Nomenclature

Antigen System	Antigens	Location	Former Name	Alleles
HNA-1	HNA-1a	FcγRIIIb	NA1	FCGR3B*1
	HNA-1b	FcγRIIIb	NA2	FCGR3B*2
	HNA-1c	FcγRIIIb	SH	FCGR3B*3
HNA-2	HNA-2a	CD177 (NB1 gp)	NB1	CD177*1
HNA-3	HNA-3a	70-95 kDa gp	5b	Not defined
HNA-4	HNA-4a	CD11b (CR3)	Mart(a)	CD11B*1
HNA-5	HNA-5a	CD11a (LFA-1)	Ond(a)	CD11A*1

CR3, C3bi receptor; *gp,* glycoprotein; *HNA,* human neutrophil antigen; *LFA-1,* leukocyte function–associated antigen-1.

Neutrophil antigens were first characterized using clinically important alloantibodies and autoantibodies. Most often, neutrophil-specific alloantibodies are directed toward antigens in the HNA-1 or HNA-2 systems. The availability of many different alloantibodies and monoclonal antibodies to HNA-1 and HNA-2 antigens has allowed the characterization of these antigen systems. In addition, three other antigen systems have been partially characterized, HNA-3, HNA-4, and HNA-5. The serology, biochemistry, molecular biology, and clinical significance of these antigens are reviewed here.

THE HNA-1 ANTIGEN SYSTEM

Expression of HNA-1 Antigens

HNA-1 antigens are expressed only on neutrophils. HNA-1 antigens are located on the low-affinity Fc-γ receptor IIIb (FcγRIIIb), CD16.[217-220] FcγRIIIb, HNA-1a, HNA-1b, and HNA-1c antigens are expressed on all segmented neutrophils, approximately one-half of neutrophilic metamyelocytes, and approximately 10% of neutrophilic myelocytes.[221] Neutrophil expression of FcγRIIIb and HNA-1 antigens are diminished by the treatment of neutrophils with stimulants such as complement component C5a and chemotaxin F-met-leu-phe or granulocyte colony-stimulating factor (G-CSF). Soluble Fc γ RIIIb is present in plasma, and it has the same HNA-1 polymorphisms found on neutrophils. Fc γ RIIIb released from granulocytes is the source of the soluble Fc γ RIIIb and HNA-1 antigens.[222]

Biochemistry

Fc γ RIIIb is a glycoprotein with 233 amino acids and is glycosylphosphatidylinositol (GPI) anchored.[217-220] Its molecular weight is 50 to 80 kDa, and the glycoprotein has *N*-linked carbohydrate side chains. HNA-1a form of Fc γ RIIIb is 50 to 65 kDa, the HNA-1b form of Fc γ RIIIb is 65 to 80 kDa, and the heterozygous form is 50 to 80 kDa. Differences in *N*-glycosylation account for the differences in molecular mass.

Molecular Biology

Fc γ RIIIb and the HNA-1 antigens are encoded by the FCGR3B gene located on chromosome 1q23-24 within a cluster of two families of Fc γ R genes, FCGR2 and FCGR3. The FCGR3 family is made up of FCGR3A and FCGR3B. FCGR3B is highly homologous to FCGR3A, which encodes Fc γ RIIIa. Only four nucleotides differ between FCGR3B and FCGR3A (Table 114-5). The most important difference between the two genes is a C to T change at 733 in

Table 114-5 Nucleotide Differences Among the Genes Encoding the HNA-1a, HNA-1b, and HNA-1c Antigens of Fcγ RIIIb Base Pair Position

Gene	141	147	227	266	277	349	473	505	559	641	733
FCGR3B*1	AGG	CTC	A**A**C	GCT	GAC	**G**TC	GAC	CAC	GTT	TCT	TGA†
FCGR3B*2	AG**C**	CT**T**	AGC	GCT	**A**AC	ATC	GAC	CAC	GTT	TCT	TGA†
FCGR3B*3	AG**C**	CT**T**	AGC	G**A**T	**A**AC	ATC	GAC	CAC	GTT	TCT	TGA†
FCGR3A	AGG	CTC	AGC	GCT	GAC	ATC	G**G**C	**T**AC	**T**TT	T**T**T	**C**GA

HNA, Human neutrophil antigen.
*N-Glycosylation site.
†Stop codon.
Note: Differences among genes are in bold.

FCGR3B that creates a stop codon. As a result, FCGR3A has 21 more amino acids than FCGR3B, and FCGR3A is a transmembrane rather than GPI-anchored glycoprotein. Fc γ RIIIa is not recognized by antibodies specific to HNA-1 antigens, but the similarities between FCGR3A and FCGR3B complicate genotyping of HNA-1 alleles.

HNA-1a, -1b, and -1c Polymorphisms

The neutrophil-specific HNA-1 antigen system is made up of the three alleles, HNA-1a, -1b, and -1c.[223] The antigens are also known as NA1, NA2, and SH (see Table 114-4). The gene frequencies of the three alleles vary widely among different racial groups. Among whites, the frequency of the gene encoding HNA-1a, FCGR3B*1, is between 0.30 and 0.37, and the frequency of the gene encoding HNA-1b, FCGR3B*2, is from 0.63 to 0.70.[224-228] In Japanese and Chinese populations, the FCGR3B*1 gene frequency is from 0.60 to 0.66, and the FCGR3B*2 gene frequency is from 0.30 to 0.33.[217,219-221,224,226-228] The gene frequency of the gene encoding HNA-1c, FCGR3B*3, also varies among racial groups. FCGR3B*3 is expressed by neutrophils in 4% to 5% of whites and 25% to 38% of African Americans.[229]

The FCGR3B*1 gene differs from the FCGR3B*2 gene by only five nucleotides in the coding region, at positions 141, 147, 227, 277, and 349 (see Table 114-5).[217-220] Four of the nucleotide changes result in changes in amino acid sequence between the HNA-1a and HNA-1b forms of the glycoprotein. The fifth polymorphism at 147 is silent. The glycosylation pattern of the protein differs between the two antigens because of two nucleotide changes at bases 227 and 277. HNA-1b form has six *N*-linked glycosylation sites, and HNA-1a form has four glycosylation sites.

The gene encoding the HNA-1c form of Fc γ RIIIb, FCGR3B*3, is identical to FCGR3B*2 except for a C to A substitution at nucleotide 266 resulting in an alanine to aspartate change at amino acid 78 of Fc γ RIIIb (see Table 114-5).[223] In many cases, FCGR3B*3 exists on the same chromosome with a second or duplicate FCGR3B gene.[223,230] One group has found that in Danish people, FCGR3B*3 always exists as a duplicate gene in association with FCGR3B*1.[231] However, in other populations duplicate FCGR3B*3 genes were associated with both FCGR3B*1 and FCGR3B*2.

Several other sequence variations in FCGR3B have been described.[226] These chimeric alleles have single-base substitutions involving one of the five single-nucleotide polymorphisms that distinguish FCGR3B*1 and FCGR3B*2. FCGR3B alleles that more closely resembled FCGR3B*2 were found more often in African Americans than in whites or Japanese.[226]

FC γ RIIIB Deficiency

Blood cells from patients with paroxysmal nocturnal hemoglobinuria lack the GPI-linked glycoproteins, and their granulocytes express reduced amounts of Fc γ RIIIb and the HNA-1 antigens.[220] Genetic deficiencies of granulocyte Fc γ RIIIb and HNA-1 antigens have also been reported. With inherited deficiency of Fc γ RIIIb, the FCGR3B gene is deleted along with an adjacent gene, FCGR2C.[225,232] Among white subjects the incidence of individuals homozygous for FCGR3B deletion is about 0.1%.[233,234] However, among Africans and African Americans the incidence is much higher; in one study, 3 of 126 Africans were found to be FCGR3B deficient,[229] and, in another, 1 of 53 was found to be FCGR3B deficient.[226]

Function of HNA-1 Antigens

The low-affinity Fc-γ receptors link humoral immunity to cellular immune function; specifically, Fc γ Rs on effector cells recognize cytotoxic IgG molecules and immune complexes containing IgG molecules. Polymorphisms in Fc γ RIIIb affect neutrophil function. Neutrophils that are homozygous for HNA-1b have a lower affinity for IgG3 than granulocytes homozygous for HNA-1a.[235] Neutrophils from people who are homozygous for HNA-1b phagocytize erythrocytes sensitized with IgG1 and IgG3 anti-Rh monoclonal antibodies and bacteria opsonized with IgG1 at a lower level than granulocytes homozygous for HNA-1a.[236,237]

Clinical Relevance of FC γ RIIIB Deficiency

Despite the important role of Fc γ RIIIb in neutrophil function, deletion of the entire Fc γ RIIIB gene does not cause major clinical problems, and most people with Fc γ RIIIb deficiency are healthy. However, too few patients have been studied to identify a slight increase in susceptibility to infection or autoimmune disease due to Fc γ RIIIb deficiency. In a study of 21 people with Fc γ RIIIb deficiency, 2 were found to have autoimmune thyroiditis and 4 had multiple episodes of bacterial infections.[232] Other smaller studies and case reports have found that despite their Fc γ RIIIb deficiency, all individuals, except for the one person with systemic lupus erythematosus, were healthy, had no circulating immune complexes, and showed no increased susceptibility to infections.

FCGR3B Polymorphisms and Disease Associations

Several studies suggest that FCGR3B polymorphisms affect the incidence and outcomes of some autoimmune and inflammatory diseases, but the results seem contradictory. Children with chronic immune thrombocytopenia purpura are more likely to be FCGR3B*1 homozygous than control subjects,[238] but Spanish patients with systemic lupus erythematosus are more likely to be FCGR3B*2 homozygous.[239] Myasthenia gravis is more severe in FCGR3B*1 homozygous patients,[240] but multiple sclerosis is more benign in FCGR3B*1 homozygous patients.[241] Patients with chronic granulomatous disease who are FCGR3B*1 homozygous are less likely to develop major gastrointestinal or genitourinary tract infectious complications than heterozygous and FCGR3B*2 homozygous chronic granulomatous patients.[242] Because FCGR3B is clustered with FCGR3A and

FCGR3B on chromosome 1q22, it is possible that some of these findings may be caused in part by linkage disequilibrium among Fc receptors.

THE HNA-2 ANTIGEN SYSTEM

HNA-2 system has one well-described allele, HNA-2a. It was previously known as NB1.[215] Monoclonal antibodies specific to HNA-2a have been clustered as CD177.

Expression of HNA-2a

HNA-2a is neutrophil-specific antigen. It is expressed only on neutrophils, neutrophilic metamyelocytes, and myelocytes.[221,243] HNA-2a is unique in that it is expressed on subpopulations of neutrophils. The mean size of the HNA-2a–positive subpopulation of neutrophils is 45% to 65%.[244-246] The expression of HNA-2a is greater on neutrophils from women than men.[246,247] The size of the HNA-2a–positive subpopulation of neutrophils from women is approximately 60%, compared with approximately 50% for men. The expression of HNA-2a falls with age in women but remains constant in men.[246] Neutrophil expression of HNA-2a is greater in pregnant women than in healthy female blood donors.[247] The surface expression of HNA-2a is slightly upregulated by treatment with the chemotactic peptide F-met-leu-phe.[244] The administration of G-CSF to healthy subjects for several days increases the proportion of neutrophils expressing HNA-2a to near 90%.[248]

NB1 Glycoprotein Biochemistry

The glycoprotein carrying HNA-2a, NB1 glycoprotein, is located on neutrophil plasma membranes and secondary granules[244,249] and is linked to the plasma membrane via a GPI anchor.[244] Although some GPI-anchored proteins are shed by F-met-leu-phe–treated neutrophils, NB1 glycoprotein is not, nor is soluble NB1 glycoprotein present in plasma.[244] The molecular weight of NB1 glycoprotein is 58 to 64 kDa, and it contains *N*-linked carbohydrate side chains.[244,249]

Molecular Biology

The gene encoding NB1 glycoprotein, CD177, is located on chromosome 19q13.31, and its coding region consists of 1311 bp that code for a protein of 416 and a signal peptide of 21 amino acids.[250,251] The predicted protein has two cysteine-rich domains, three potential *N*-linked glycosylation sites, and a potential ω-site for attachment of the GPI anchor.[250] This gene belongs to the Ly-6 snake toxin superfamily. Other genes in this family include urokinase-type plasminogen activator receptor (uPAR) (CD87) and decay-accelerating factor (CD59).

Two different groups sequenced CD177 independently. One group sequenced it as the gene encoding HNA-2a and called the gene NB1,[250] and the other group sequenced it as a gene overexpressed in granulocytes from people with polycythemia rubra vera and called the gene PRV-1.[252] The NB1 and PRV-1 alleles differ at only 4 bp.[250] Bettinotti et al[253] used Human Genomic Project databases to characterize the structure of the PRV-1 and NB1 genes. They described the intron and exon structure of NB1, but they found only one gene homologous to both PRV-1 and NB1, suggesting that they are alleles of the same gene that they called CD177. In addition, they found a pseudogene homologous to exons 4 through 9 of CD177.[253]

Polymorphisms

HNA-2a is expressed on neutrophils by approximately 97% of whites, 95% of African Americans, and 89% to 99% of Japanese.[246,254,255] HNA-2a has been reported to have an allele, NB2; but the product of this gene cannot be reliably identified with alloantisera, and no monoclonal antibody specific for NB2 has been identified.[256]

HNA-2a negative neutrophil phenotype is caused by a CD177 transcription defect.[257] HNA-2a genes from two women with HNA-2a–negative neutrophils who produced HNA-2a–specific alloantibodies have been studied, and CD177 complementary DNA (cDNA) sequences were present in both women.[257] However, all neutrophil CD177 messenger ribonucleic acid (mRNA) contained accessory sequences that were considered to be introns. HNA-2a–negative phenotype was the result of different off-frame insertions at the RNA level, resulting in NB1 gp deficiency in neutrophils.[257]

Role of NB1 Glycoprotein in Neutrophil Function

The role of CD177 in neutrophil function is unknown. In some studies HNA-2a may have a role in the adhesion of neutrophils to endothelial cells.[258] Upregulation of HNA-2a after F-met-leu-phe stimulation, HNA-2a internalization on antibody cross-linking, and activation of the respiratory burst after binding of HNA-2a antibodies to HNA-2a–bearing neutrophils suggest a possible role as receptor molecule.[259]

Clinical Relevance of HNA-2 Antigens

The rare women who produce HNA-2a–specific alloantibodies and who lack NB1 glycoprotein are healthy. The expression of HNA-2a is reduced on neutrophils from people with paroxysmal nocturnal hemoglobinuria and chronic myelogenous leukemia.[243] It is unknown whether the lack of expression of HNA-2a on neutrophils from patients with paroxysmal nocturnal hemoglobinuria or chronic myelogenous leukemia has any clinical significance. CD177 mRNA is overexpressed by neutrophils from patients with polycythemia rubra vera and essential thrombocytosis.[252,260] Some groups are using quantitative real-time PCR to measure neutrophil CD177 mRNA levels to assist with the diagnosis of polycythemia rubra vera and essential thrombocytosis. Patients with essential thrombocytosis and increased CD177 mRNA levels have been reported to have increased risk for thrombocytosis and bleeding.[261] Patients with polycythemia rubra vera and essential thrombocytosis have been found to have gain of function mutations in the gene encoding Janus kinase-2 (JAK2)[262-266] and the increased expression of CD177 mRNA in neutrophils from these patients may be secondary to the JAK2 mutation.

HNA-3 ANTIGEN SYSTEM

HNA-3 antigen system has one antigen, HNA-3a, that was previously known as 5b. HNA-3a is expressed by neutrophils, lymphocytes, platelets, endothelial cells, kidney, spleen, and placental cells. HNA-3a has a gene frequency of 0.66 and is located on a 70- to 95-kDa neutrophil glycoprotein.[267] The gene encoding HNA-3a has not yet been cloned, and the nature and function of the 70- to 95-kDa glycoprotein is unknown. Although the biologic role for this system has not been established, several cases of transfusion-related acute lung injury (TRALI) have been associated with transfusion of plasma containing anti-5b.[268,269]

HNA-4 AND HNA-5 ANTIGEN SYSTEMS

HNA-4 and HNA-5 antigens are located in the β_2-integrins. Each antigen system contains only a single antigen, HNA-4a and HNA-5a, respectively. HNA-4a antigen was previously known as Mart(a). HNA-4a was defined by an antibody in the sera of three nontransfused multiparous blood donors. The antigen was shown to have autosomal dominant inheritance and has a phenotype frequency of 99.1% in white subjects. HNA-4a has been located on the αM chain (CD11b) of the C3bi receptor (CR3) and is caused by a single nucleotide substitution of G to A at position 302.[270] The substitution would be predicted to result in an arginine to histidine polymorphism at amino acid 61. The significance of the antibody is unknown, and none of the infants of the three multiparous women with anti–HNA-4a showed evidence of neonatal alloimmune neutropenia.

A second polymorphism of the β_2-integrins, HNA-5a, was first described as Ond(a). A chronically transfused man with aplastic anemia became alloimmunized to HNA-5a. HNA-5a was found to be expressed on the αL integrin unit, leukocyte function–associated antigen-1 (LFA-1) (CD11a), and is caused by a G to C single nucleotide substitution at position 2446. This change predicts an amino acid change of arginine to threonine at amino acid 766.[270]

CLINICAL SIGNIFICANCE OF ANTIBODIES TO NEUTROPHIL ANTIGENS

Alloimmune Neonatal Neutropenia

During pregnancy, mothers can become alloimmunized to neutrophil antigens. Maternal IgG directed to neutrophils can cross the placenta and destroy the neonate's neutrophils. Maternal alloimmunization to neutrophil antigens can occur in utero and affect the first child. Most neonates experience isolated neutropenia, but the cytopenias are self-limiting and resolve as the antibody is cleared. The alloimmunized mothers produce and carry the antibodies; but the antibodies do not react with the mother's blood cells or tissues, and they have normal neutrophil counts. Antibodies to neutrophil-specific antigens HNA-1a, HNA-1b, and HNA-2a most commonly cause neonatal alloimmune neutropenia (Table 114-6).[267,271] Antibodies to HNA-1c and HNA-3a rarely cause alloimmune neonatal neutropenia. Mothers with FcγRIIIb deficiency have produced FcγRIIIb-specific antibodies that caused neonatal neutropenia.[234,267,271]

Newborns with alloimmune neutropenia are usually asymptomatic. Most often, the neutropenia is detected in the first week of life when the neonate becomes febrile or develops an infection and a neutrophil count is done. Typically the counts are 0.100 to 0.200 × 10^9/L. Some neonates have normal neutrophil counts the first day of life, but they become neutropenic on their second day.[271] White blood cell count, platelet count, and hemoglobin level are usually normal; but eosinophilia or monocytosis may be present. If a bone marrow biopsy is performed, it often shows normal numbers of erythroid progenitors and megakaryocytes with hyperplasia of myeloid progenitors.

The clinical course is quite variable. An occasional infant is asymptomatic, but almost all affected children have an infection. The most common infections are umbilicus infections, skin infections, abscesses, and respiratory tract infections. Less commonly, infants experience otitis media, urinary tract infections, and gastroenteritis. Serious infections such as sepsis, pneumonia, and meningitis can occur. The duration of the neutropenia may be as short as a few days or as long as 28 weeks.[271] The mean duration of neutropenia is about 11 weeks.[271]

For an asymptomatic child, no immediate treatment may be required. Prompt and aggressive antibiotic treatment of children with fevers or other signs of infections is indicated. Intravenous immunoglobulin has a limited role in the treatment of neonatal alloimmune neutropenia. Approximately half the patients treated have a transient increase in count lasting only a few days. The use of G-CSF to treat alloimmune neutropenia has also had mixed results. The administration of G-CSF elevates the neutrophil count in some but not all neonates.[271]

Table 114-6 Specificities of Antibodies in Alloimmune Neonatal Neutropenia

Antigen	$N = 18$[211,271]	$N = 48$[253,267]
HNA-1a	28%	10%
HNA-1b	22%	8%
FcγRIIIb	0%	8%
HNA-2a	11%	2%
HNA-3a	0%	2%
Unknown	0%	15%
HLA class I[251,271]	11%	54%
Negative	28%	38%

HLA, Human leukocyte antigen; *HNA,* human neutrophil antigen.

AUTOIMMUNE NEUTROPENIA OF CHILDHOOD

Autoimmune neutropenia has been well described in children.[272-275] Typically the onset of the autoimmune neutropenia of children begins at 8 months of age, but children between 1 and 36 months of age can be affected. Most studies found that neutrophil counts recover spontaneously by the age of 5 years, with a median of 13 to 20 months of neutropenia.[272-275]

In most cases, children presented with severe neutropenia, having neutrophil counts less than 0.5 × 10^9/L. Monocytosis has been reported to occur in up to 38% of patients. Results of bone marrow biopsies in affected patients usually show normal to hypercellular marrow with a decreased number of mature granulocytes. Febrile episodes and infections, including bacterial skin infections, otitis media, respiratory tract infections, and urinary tract infections, are common. Life-threatening complications are rare.

Antibodies to neutrophils can be detected in up to 98% of affected patients. If an antibody specificity is identified, the antibodies are almost always specific to epitopes located on FcγRIIIb. The antibodies are directed to HNA-1a in 10% to 46% of patients, to HNA-1b in 2% to 3% of patients, and rarely to FcγRIIIb epitopes expressed by granulocytes from all donors.[273,274]

Autoimmune neutropenia has been treated with corticosteroids, intravenous immunoglobulin, and G-CSF. Approximately half the patients responded to intravenous immunoglobulin, but neutrophil counts remained elevated for only 1 week.[273] Almost all the patients responded to G-CSF and 75% to corticosteroids, and neutrophil counts remained elevated as long as the drugs were given.

TRANSFUSION REACTIONS

Antibodies to neutrophil and HLA antigens can cause febrile nonhemolytic transfusion reactions and TRALI. Before the widespread transfusion of leukocyte-reduced blood components, approximately 0.5% of transfusions were associated with febrile nonhemolytic transfusion reactions, and leukocyte antibodies are a common cause of these reactions. These febrile reactions are caused by the interaction of leukocyte antibodies in the transfusion recipient with leukocytes contained in the transfused blood components. These reactions can be prevented by the use of components that have been filtered to remove leukocytes.

A more serious type of transfusion reaction associated with leukocyte antibodies is the acute noncardiac pulmonary edema, or TRALI. This entity is characterized by acute respiratory distress that usually occurs within 4 hours after a transfusion. These reactions are characterized by dyspnea, hypoxia, and bilateral pulmonary infiltrates on chest radiograph without cardiomegaly or pulmonary vascular congestion. The mortality rate associated with TRALI is approximately 5%.[276] Of patients with TRALI, 80% have rapid resolution of pulmonary infiltrates and return of arterial blood gas values to normal within 96 hours after the initial respiratory insult. However, pulmonary infiltrates have persisted for at least 7 days after the transfusion reaction in 17% of TRALI patients.

TRALI has been associated with both neutrophil and HLA antibodies. Antibodies reported in these reactions include HNA-1a, HNA-1b, HNA-2a, HNA-3a, and HLA class I and II antibodies. Most of these cases involve the passive transfusion of the offending antibody in donor plasma, as contrasted with the reactivity of the recipient's antibody with donor leukocytes to cause febrile nonhemolytic reactions. Retrospective studies involving antibodies to HNA-3a have implicated blood components from single donors with anti-HNA-3a in several TRALI cases.[269]

GRANULOCYTE TRANSFUSIONS

Granulocyte transfusion recipients sometimes produce antibodies specific to HNA-1a, HNA-1b, and HNA-2a. The transfusion of granulocytes to patients with these antibodies can result in febrile transfusion reactions and pulmonary transfusion reactions.[277] HPCT recipients who produce HNA-2a antibodies as a result of granulocyte transfusions have experienced marrow graft failure.[278]

NEUTROPHIL ANTIGENS SUMMARY

Two neutrophil antigen systems, HNA-1 and HNA-2, have been well described, and three others, HNA-3, HNA-4, and HNA-5, have been described in part. HNA-1 antigens are located on FcγRIIIb, and antibodies to these antigens are frequently implicated in autoimmune and alloimmune neutropenia. HNA-2a is located on NB1 glycoprotein, and antibodies to HNA-2a are found in patients with alloimmune and autoimmune neutropenia. The gene expressing this protein is overexpressed by neutrophils in patients with polycythemia rubra vera. Antibodies to HNA-3a are rare; but relative to other neutrophil antibodies, may be more frequently associated with cases of TRALI. The significance, if any, of HNA-4a and HNA-5a antibodies is uncertain.

SUGGESTED READINGS

Braun WE: Update in kidney transplantation: Increasing clinical success, expanding waiting lists. *Cleve Clin J Med* 69:501, 2002.

Bux J, Behrens G, Jaeger G, et al: Diagnosis and clinical course of autoimmune neutropenia in infancy: Analysis of 240 cases. *Blood* 91:181, 1998.

Bux J, Jung KD, Kauth T, et al: Serological and clinical aspects of granulocyte antibodies leading to alloimmune neonatal neutropenia. *Transfus Med* 2:143, 1992.

Childs R, Srinivasan R: Advances in allogeneic stem cell transplantation: Directing graft-versus-leukemia at solid tumors. *Cancer J Sci Am* 8:2, 2002.

Daser A, Michinson H, Michinson A, et al: Non-classical-MHC genetics of immunological disease in man and mouse: The key role of proinflammatory cytokine genes. *Cytokine* 8:593, 1996.

Dawkins RL, Degli-Esposti MP, Abraham LJ, et al: Conservation versus polymorphism of the MHC in relation to transplantation, immune responses and autoimmune disease. In Klein J, Klein D, editors: *Molecular evolution of the major histocompatibility complex*, Berlin, 1991, Springer-Verlag, p 391.

De Haas M, Kleijer M, van Zwieten R, et al: Neutrophil FcγRIIIb deficiency, nature, and clinical consequences: A study of 21 individuals from 14 families. *Blood* 86:2403, 1995.

Duquesnoy RJ, Marrari M: HLAMatchmaker: A molecularly based algorithm for histocompatibility determination. II. Verification of the algorithm and determination of the relative immunogenicity of amino acid triplet-defined epitopes. *Hum Immunol* 63:353, 2002.

Hennecke J, Wiley DC: T cell-receptor-MHC interactions up close. *Cell* 104:1, 2001.

Kim CJ, Parkinson DR, Marincola FM: Immunodominance across the HLA polymorphism: Implications for cancer immunotherapy. *J Immunother* 21:1, 1997.

Kissel K, Santoso S, Hofmann C, et al: Molecular basis of the neutrophil glycoprotein NB1 (CD177) involved in the pathogenesis of immune neutropenias and transfusion reactions. *Eur J Immunol* 31:1301, 2001.

Matzinger P: An innate sense of danger. *Semin Immunol* 10:399, 1998.

Opelz G, Vanrenterghem Y, Kirste G, et al: Prospective evaluation of pretransplant blood transfusion in cadaver kidney recipients. *Transplantation* 63:964, 1997.

Opelz G, Wujciak T, Dohler B, et al: HLA compatibility and organ transplant survival: Collaborative transplant study. *Rev Immunogenet* 1:334, 1999.

Parker KC, Bednarek MA, Coligan JE: Scheme for ranking potential HLA-A2 binding peptides based on independent binding of individual peptide side-chains. *J Immunol* 152:163, 1994.

Petersdorf EW, Hansen JA, Martin PJ, et al: Major-histocompatibility-complex class I alleles and antigens in hematopoietic-cell transplantation. *N Engl J Med* 345:1794, 2001.

Petz LD, Garratty G, Calhoun L, et al: Selecting donors of platelets for refractory patients on the basis of HLA antibody specificity. *Transfusion* 40:1446, 2000.

Stroncek DF, Skubitz KM, McCullough J: Biochemical nature of the neutrophil-specific antigen NB1. *Blood* 75:744, 1990.

Velardi A, Ruggeri L, Moretta A, et al: NK cells: A lesson from mismatched hematopoietic transplantation. *Trends Immunol* 23:438, 2002.

For complete list of references log on to www.expertconsult.com.

CHAPTER 115

PRINCIPLES OF NEUTROPHIL (GRANULOCYTE) TRANSFUSIONS

Ronald G. Strauss

Current cytapheresis technology permits collection of large numbers of several types of blood leukocytes (e.g., neutrophils, hematopoietic progenitors/stem cells, and lymphocytes) from either healthy donors (allogeneic use) or patients (autologous use)—who often are stimulated with recombinant cytokines such as granulocyte colony-stimulating factor (G-CSF)—to be used for transfusion and transplantation or for further processing (e.g., ex vivo expansion and genetic manipulation). Polymorphonuclear neutrophils (PMNs) are granulocytic leukocytes that are collected from healthy donors and issued as a standard blood component (granulocytes, pheresis). This chapter analyzes the use of neutrophil (i.e., granulocyte) transfusions (GTX) as an adjunct to antimicrobial drugs in the treatment and prevention of progressive infections in patients with severe neutropenia or PMN dysfunction.

Life-threatening infections with bacteria, yeast, and fungus continue to be a consequence of severe neutropenia ($<0.5 \times 10^9$/L blood PMNs), most commonly occurring after intense chemotherapy of hematopoietic progenitor cell (HPC) transplantation, and disorders of PMN dysfunction such as chronic granulomatous disease. The most frequent clinical situation today is neutropenic fever and infection following intense chemotherapy or HPC transplantation given to treat hematologic malignancies. Neutropenic infections cause considerable morbidity, occasionally are fatal, and add considerable cost to the management of these patients. However, because of improved antifungal prophylaxis and therapy following HPC transplantation, severe fungal infections often occur after neutrophil engraftment (i.e., due more to longer-standing immunodeficiency), and neutrophil transfusions (GTX) of course are not warranted during this later time in the posttransplant period. Thus the number of patients with severe fungal infections, for whom GTX previously were considered, has decreased—further questioning the need in some physicians' opinions for GTX therapy.

Previous attempts to prevent infections in severely neutropenic patients by transfusing PMN concentrates (i.e., prophylactic GTX) achieved only questionable success. Although rates of certain infections were significantly reduced by prophylactic GTX, many adverse effects, such as pulmonary infiltrates and cytomegalovirus infections, were reported, and GTX were expensive. Thus prophylactic GTX have gained little support over the years. Similarly, use of therapeutic GTX to resolve existing infections has not gained lasting acceptance, despite many reports documenting significant benefit. This lack of enthusiasm for GTX can be explained by the continuing development of new and very effective antimicrobial drugs to prevent and treat infections and by the availability of recombinant hematopoietic growth factors and peripheral blood hematopoietic progenitor cell (PBHPC) transfusions—both of which hasten patient recovery from myelotoxic therapy and thereby shorten the period of risk for neutropenic infections. The lack of familiarity of some oncology and transplant physicians with the markedly improved modern PMN concentrates available for transfusion today plus the lack of definitive clinical trials with modern GTX undoubtedly limit use of GTX.

Historically, PMN concentrates were collected for transfusion from unstimulated donors or those stimulated only with corticosteroids and contained woefully inadequate numbers of PMNs. Currently, very large numbers of PMNs can be collected from normal donors using G-CSF plus corticosteroid marrow stimulation followed by large-volume leukapheresis, during which several liters of donor blood are processed. In this chapter the historical and modern experiences with GTX are reviewed, and the current technology of PMN collection is discussed.

THERAPEUTIC GRANULOCYTE TRANSFUSIONS IN NEUTROPENIC PATIENTS' HISTORICAL EXPERIENCE

In the third edition of this book, 34 papers were reviewed that reported the therapeutic use of GTX—collected before the advent of G-CSF donor stimulation—in severely neutropenic patients ($<5 \times 10^9$/L blood PMNs). Data were tabulated (Table 115-1) according to the index infection that prompted GTX therapy. Patients were counted only once (e.g., patients with septicemia were listed only in the septicemia group, even if they had another infection, such as pneumonia). As an exception, all patients with invasive fungal infections were counted together because it was impossible to accurately separate sepsis, pneumonia, sinusitis, and so forth into distinct categories. All patients given GTX for a designated type of infection were enumerated in the "Treated" column. The treated patients, those for whom the actual course and mortality of the index infection could be clearly documented, were enumerated again in the "Evaluable" column. GTX therapy was considered successful if so stated by the authors. Combining data from multiple reports of varying experimental design admittedly is of limited value for drawing firm conclusions, and it was done simply to document the breadth of historical reported experience.

To obtain more definitive information regarding efficacy of historical GTX (i.e., collected without G-CSF), the seven controlled studies were analyzed in more detail.[1-7] In these seven studies, the response of infected neutropenic patients to treatment with GTX plus antibiotics (study group) was compared with that of comparable patients given antibiotics alone and evaluated concurrently (control group). The design, size, and results of these seven studies are presented in Tables 115-2 and 115-3. Three of the seven studies reported a significant overall benefit for GTX.[4-6] In two additional studies,[1,3] overall success was not demonstrated for GTX, but certain subgroups of patients were found to benefit significantly. Some measure of success for GTX was evident in five of the seven controlled studies. However, this success was counterbalanced by four studies that were negative in some respect—two totally[2,7] and two partially negative.[1,3]

An explanation of these inconsistent results is evident on critical analysis of the adequacy of GTX support (see Table 115-3). Patients in the three successful trials received relatively high doses of PMNs (generally $\geq 1.7 \times 10^{10}$/day).[4-6] Donors were selected to be erythrocyte AND leukocyte compatible. By contrast, the four controlled studies yielding negative results can legitimately be criticized. Two of the four studies with negative conclusions used PMNs collected by filtration leukapheresis for some patients.[1,3] It is now known that such PMNs are defective, and they are no longer transfused. In the negative studies using PMNs collected by centrifugation leukapheresis,[2,3,7] the dose was extremely low (0.41 to 0.56×10^{10} per concentrate). As another factor, investigators in two of the four negative studies[1,7] made no provision for the possibility of leukocyte alloimmunization, because donors were selected solely on the basis of erythrocyte compatibility. Finally, control subjects responded reasonably well to antibiotics alone in three of the four negative studies,[1,3,7] suggesting that some patients fared so well with conventional treatment that they had no apparent need for additional therapeutic modalities.

These impressions from the seven controlled GTX trials have been analyzed by formal meta-analysis,[8] with conclusions that the dose of PMNs transfused and the survival rate of the nontransfused control subjects were primarily responsible for the differing success rates of the historical studies. In clinical settings in which the survival rate of nontransfused control subjects was low, study subjects benefited from receiving adequate doses of GTX—prompting the authors to suggest that severely neutropenic patients with life-threatening infections should be considered to receive GTX given in adequate doses.[8]

Table 115-1 Infectious Problems in Neutropenic Patients Treated With Historical Granulocyte Transfusions in 34 Studies

Type of Infection	Treated	Evaluable	Success Rate (%)
Bacterial septicemia	298	206	127/206 (62)
Sepsis organism unspecified	132	39	18/39 (46)
Invasive fungus and yeast	83	77	28/77 (36)
Pneumonia	120	11	7/11 (64)
Localized infections	143	47	39/47 (83)
Fever etiology unknown	184	85	64/85 (75)

Table 115-2 Results of Seven Controlled Studies Evaluating Historical Therapeutic Granulocyte Transfusions in Neutropenic Patients

		Study Group		Control Group	
Investigators	*Success*	*N*	*Survival (%)*	*N*	*Survival (%)*
Higby et al[5]	Yes	17	76	19	26
Vogler and Winton[6]	Yes	17	59	13	15
Herzig et al[4]	Yes	13	75	14	36
Alavi et al[1]	Partial	12	82	19	62
Graw et al[3]	Partial	39	46	37	30
Winston et al[7]	No	48	63	47	72
Fortuny et al[2]	No	17	78	22	80

MODERN EXPERIENCE

Bacterial, fungal, and yeast infections occur frequently in patients with severe neutropenia or PMN dysfunction, and when these infections fail to promptly respond to antimicrobial drugs, they pose a major challenge for which modern therapeutic GTX offer a possible answer. Recipients of HPC transplants—particularly marrow transplant patients—often become severely neutropenic and exhibit PMN dysfunction shortly after transplant. Importantly, they manifest defective cellular and humoral immunity for months after transplantation. Altered immunity is particularly profound when the HPC graft is T-lymphocyte depleted to diminish graft-versus-host disease. Hence all types of infection pose a threat, with fungal and yeast infections being major problems. In a series of 1186 marrow transplant patients, 10% developed a noncandidal fungal infection, with only 17% of infected patients surviving. When the marrow graft is depleted of T lymphocytes, the rate of infection is increased twofold to sevenfold above that occurring with standard bone marrow transplantation.

Data are insufficient to determine the proper role of GTX in treating fungal/yeast infections (which are of the greatest importance). Historical case reports, experimental studies in animals, and experience in treating patients with chronic granulomatous disease have supported the efficacy of GTX in fungal infections. In contrast, a large clinical study reported that GTX collected in the pre–G-CSF era were of no benefit in treating fungal and yeast infections in 87 bone marrow transplant patients, 50 of whom received GTX. Although this study was a retrospective review with several shortcomings that must be interpreted cautiously, as pointed out later, the poor response of invasive fungal infections in neutropenic patients to even modern GTX is supported by recent reports.

At this time, no randomized clinical trials of therapeutic GTX collected after G-CSF donor stimulation have been completed and reported to establish the efficacy or potential toxicity of modern GTX. One randomized controlled clinical trial of therapeutic GTX collected following G-CSF donor stimulation has been reported, but it was closed before completion with less than 50% of patients entered because of futility (i.e., poor enrollment).[9] Moreover, the design of the trial was less than ideal, because donors were stimulated only with G-CSF without combination with corticosteroids, resulting in relatively low PMN doses, and GTX were given only every other day, rather than daily. However, five case reports (Table 115-4) and six uncontrolled studies of multiple patients (Table 115-5) will be reviewed.[10-20]

Clarke et al[10] and Catalano et al[12] each reported single patients (see Table 115-4) with aplastic anemia undergoing HPC transplantation with fungus infections that responded favorably to strikingly different doses of PMNs. Similarly, Ozsahin et al[13] and Bielorai et al[14] each reported single patients (see Table 115-4) with chronic

Table 115-3 Design of Seven Controlled Studies Evaluating Historical Therapeutic Granulocyte Transfusions in Neutropenic Patients

Investigators	Randomized?	Collection Method	Dose (× 10[10])	Schedule	HLA*	WBC*
Higby et al[5]	Yes	Filtration	2.2	Daily	No	Yes
Vogler and Winton[6]	Yes	Centrifugation	2.7	Daily	Yes	Yes
Herzig et al[4]	Yes	Filtration	1.7	Daily	No	Yes
		Centrifugation	0.4	Daily	No	Yes
Alavi et al[1]	Yes	Filtration	5.9	Daily	No	No
Graw et al[3]	No	Filtration	2.0	Daily	No	Yes
		Centrifugation	0.6	Daily	No	Yes
Winston et al[7]	Yes	Centrifugation	0.5	Daily	No	No
Fortuny et al[2]	No	Centrifugation	0.4	Daily	No	Yes

HLA, Human leukocyte antigen; *WBC,* white blood cell.
*Donors selected to be compatible with recipient either by HLA typing (A and B loci matched, at least in part) or by leukocyte crossmatching.

Table 115-4 Case Reports of Modern Therapeutic Granulocyte Transfusions Using Neutrophils Collected From Granulocyte Colony-Stimulating Factor–Stimulated Donors in Neutropenic Patients

Investigators	PMNs × 10^{10} per Each GTX	Stimulation	Leukapheresis	Outcomes
Clarke et al[10]	5.3*	G-CSF 5-10 mcg/kg	Dextran 10 L processed	One patient with fungus recovered
Catalano et al[12]	1.9	G-CSF 300 mcg/dose	Not described	One patient with fungus recovered
Ozsahin et al[13]	3.1	G-CSF 5 mcg/kg	Hetastarch 5-7 L processed	One patient with fungus recovered
Bielorai et al[14]	7.0*	G-CSF 5 mcg/kg	Not described	One patient with fungus recovered
Bielorai et al[15]	4.8-6.8	Not described	Not described	One patient with vancomycin-resistant *Enterococcus* recovered

G-CSF, Granulocyte colony-stimulating factor; *GTX,* granulocyte transfusions; *PMN,* neutrophil.
*Assumptions made because PMN dose expressed × 10^{10} unclear in these reports. Dose calculated that would be given to a 70-kg recipient for Clarke et al and Bielorai et al.

Table 115-5 Groups of Neutropenic Patients Treated With Modern Therapeutic Granulocyte Transfusions Using Neutrophils Collected From Granulocyte Colony-Stimulating Factor–Stimulated Donors

Investigators	PMNs × 10^{10} per Each GTX	Stimulation	Leukapheresis	Outcomes
Hester et al[11]	4.1	G-CSF 5 mcg/kg	Pentastarch 7 L processed	60% (9 of 15) Success with fungus (11 patients) and yeast (4 patients)
Grigg et al[16]	5.9*	G-CSF 10 mcg/kg	Dextran 10 L processed	100% (3 of 3) Success with bacterial infection 0% (0 of 5) Success with progressive fungus 67% (2 of 3) Success with stable fungus
Peters et al[17]	3.5*	G-CSF 5 mcg/kg -or- Prednisolone	Hetastarch 6.4 L processed	82% (14 of 17) Success with bacterial infection 54% (7 of 13) Success with fungal infection
Price et al[18]	8.2	G-CSF 600 mcg/kg -plus- Dexamethasone 8 mg	Hetastarch 10 L processed	100% (4 of 4) Success with bacterial infection 0% (0 of 8) Success with invasive fungus 57% (4 of 7) Success with yeast infection
Lee et al[19]	5.1-10.6	G-CSF 5 mcg/kg -and/or- Dexamethasone 3 mg/m^2	Pentastarch 6-10 L processed	40% (10 of 25) Success with multiple-organism infections
Hubel et al[20]	4.6-8.1	G-CSF 600 mg/kg -with or without- Dexamethasone 8 mg	Hetastarch or pentastarch 10 L processed	55% (unrelated donor) Success with bacterial infection 75% (family donor) Success with bacterial infection 0% (unrelated donor) Success with yeast infection 40% (family donor) Success with yeast infection 15% (unrelated donor) Success with fungal infection 25% (family donor) Success with fungal infection

G-CSF, Granulocyte colony-stimulating factor; *GTX,* granulocyte transfusions; *PMN,* neutrophil.
*Assumptions made because PMN dose expressed × 10^{10} unclear in these reports. PMN dose calculated using values for range of leukocytes collected, percentage of collected cells being myeloid, and volume of units collected (Grigg et al). Dose calculated that would be given to a 70-kg recipient for Peters et al.

granulomatous disease and fungal infections that responded favorably to GTX during the transplantation period. Bielorai et al[15] reported a single patient with acute leukemia and sepsis with progressive, antibiotic-resistant bacteria whose infection cleared slowly with GTX. It is impossible, in these single reports of very complicated patients, to firmly ascribe the good outcome to the GTX.

Hester et al[11] transfused 15 patients with hematologic malignancies and infections (see Table 115-5). PMNs were collected from donors stimulated only with G-CSF and selected without regard for leukocyte compatibility. Although GTX were successful in most patients, it was not possible to distinguish responses of fungus versus yeast infections. Lee et al[19] transfused 25 patients with hematologic malignancies, many of whom were infected with multiple organisms. PMNs were collected from donors stimulated with G-CSF alone (66% of donors), G-CSF plus dexamethasone (25% of donors), or dexamethasone alone (8% of donors). Of patients with sepsis, 50% (2 of 4) responded favorably, and 38% (8 of 21) of patients with progressive localized infections responded favorably. Grigg et al[16] transfused 11 patients (see Table 115-5). Eight patients had hematologic malignancies and progressive infections—five of the eight undergoing progenitor cell transplantation and three receiving chemotherapy. Three additional patients who were undergoing progenitor cell transplantation had stable fungus infections. PMNs were collected from donors stimulated only with G-CSF and selected without regard for leukocyte compatibility. Success was excellent for bacterial and stable fungus infections but was quite poor for progressive fungus infections with organ dysfunction—a troubling pattern reported by others.[18]

Peters et al[17] transfused 30 patients (see Table 115-5) with hematologic disorders—18 undergoing HPC transplantation. PMNs were collected from donors stimulated with G-CSF or prednisolone and selected without regard for leukocyte compatibility. The exact PMN dose transfused is uncertain because values from 0.9 × 10^{10} to 14.4 × 10^{10} can be calculated from data reported, and it was impossible to distinguish the success of GTX from G-CSF–stimulated versus prednisolone-stimulated donors. However, the outcome of bacterial infections appeared to be superior to that of fungus infections.

Price et al[18] transfused 19 patients (see Table 115-5) with hematologic malignancies, 16 who had received HPC transplants and 3 who were pretransplantation recipients. PMNs were collected from donors stimulated with G-CSF and dexamethasone. Although donors were selected without regard for leukocyte compatibility, recipients were documented not to exhibit evidence of leukocyte alloimmunization at study entry. Bacterial infections responded well, and yeast infections responded modestly. Despite very high PMN doses, success for invasive fungus infections was dismal.

Lee et al[19] transfused 25 patients with hematologic malignancies. Many were infected with multiple organisms. Donors were stimulated with G-CSF plus dexamethasone (25%), G-CSF alone (66%), or dexamethasone alone (8%). Of septic patients, 50% (2 of 4) responded favorably, and 38% (8 of 21) of patients with localized infections responded.

Hubel et al[20] expanded the study of Price et al[18] to a total of 74 patients (see Table 115-5) with HPC transplants. Controls were 74 historical patients not given GTX. Donors were either family members or unrelated individuals stimulated with G-CSF with or without dexamethasone. Comparative favorable responses varied with family versus unrelated donors but were approximately 70% for bacterial, 50% for yeast, and 20% for fungal/mold infections—values similar to the historical control patients not given GTX.

The report of Safdar et al[21] is not presented in Table 115-5 because many aspects of the patients and their infections are quite heterogeneous. The study was a case-control retrospective analysis of 491 cancer patients with candidemia—29 given GTX and 462 not. Donors were stimulated with G-CSF plus dexamethasone, and GTX were given either daily or on alternate days. Not all patients were evaluable, but unexpectedly only 35% of patients given GTX resolved their infections versus 67% of those not given GTX ($p < .001$). However, death ascribed to candidemia was almost identical: 48% in the GTX group and 45% in the control patients.

No firm conclusions can be drawn from these somewhat anecdotal and very heterogenous reports of modern therapeutic GTX for several reasons: (1) the only randomized control trial was not completed and was of very questionable scientific design, and in most other reports no concurrent control subjects were included (i.e., randomly assigned to receive no GTX or GTX from donors stimulated only with corticosteroids); (2) the number of patients reported was quite small; and (3) PMN collection methods and GTX transfusion schedules were variable, with a broad range of PMN doses transfused. On the basis of these preliminary findings—acknowledging the many shortcomings—bacterial infections appeared to respond well to modern GTX, and relatively mild fungus and yeast infections responded modestly well, whereas serious/invasive fungus infections with tissue damage resisted even the large doses of PMNs transfused with modern GTX.[16-18] The precise role of modern therapeutic GTX, collected from donors stimulated with G-CSF plus corticosteroids, in the management of infected, neutropenic, oncology/transplant patients awaits definition by well-designed randomized clinical trials.

EXPERIENCE IN INFANTS AND CHILDREN

Most patients with congenital disorders of PMN dysfunction have adequate numbers of blood PMNs, but they are susceptible to serious infections because their PMNs fail to kill pathogenic microorganisms. Patients with severe forms of PMN dysfunction are relatively rare, and no randomized clinical trials have been reported to establish the efficacy of therapeutic GTX in their management. Firm recommendations about the use of GTX to treat patients cannot be made. However, several patients with chronic granulomatous disease, complicated by progressive life-threatening fungal infections, have been reported to benefit. Because of the possibility of alloimmunization to leukocyte and red blood cell antigens plus the other risks of allogeneic transfusions, such as pulmonary reactions and transfusion-transmitted infections, therapeutic GTX are recommended only for progressive infections that cannot be controlled with antimicrobial drugs. Because of lifetime problems with infections, prophylactic GTX are impractical.

Neonates (infants within the first month of life) are another group of patients who may suffer life-threatening bacterial infections caused, at least in part, by PMN dysfunction and neutropenia. Neutropenia must be viewed differently in neonates than in older patients. In older infants and children, GTX are considered usually when the blood PMN count falls to less than 0.5×10^9/L. By contrast, because normal neonates exhibit a physiologic neutrophilia compared to normal PMN counts in older children and adults, absolute blood PMN counts as high as 3.0×10^9/L (i.e., relative neutropenia) might prompt consideration of GTX in neonates.[22] The mechanism of neutropenia cannot always be identified, but in some infants a marked decrease in the marrow PMN storage pool can be demonstrated. For example, storage pool neutrophils (metamyelocytes and segmented PMNs) account for 26% to 65% of all nucleated cells in normal marrow, but in some neonates with sepsis, this value will be less than 10% of nucleated marrow cells.

Six controlled trials have assessed the role of GTX in treating neonatal infections. Although four of the six found a significant benefit for GTX, the controlled studies, when assessed by meta-analysis, were insufficiently homogeneous to permit clear recommendations regarding the efficacy of GTX.[8] The varying dose of PMNs transfused was identified as the primary reason for disagreements in results among studies. When leukapheresis PMN concentrates with higher doses of PMNs were transfused, GTX were beneficial. When buffy coats with lower doses of PMNs were transfused, GTX were not beneficial.[8] The role of therapeutic GTX for neonatal infections is unclear at present and, because they are transfused only rarely at this time, they will not be discussed further. However, the possible roles of immunoglobulin and cytokine therapies for neonatal sepsis will be discussed later.

PROPHYLACTIC GRANULOCYTE TRANSFUSIONS IN NEUTROPENIC PATIENTS

Based on historical reports, prophylactic GTX were of marginal value. In 12 reports, benefits were few, whereas risks and expenses were substantial. However, some measure of success was found in 7 of 12 studies; the remaining 5 studies failed to show a benefit for prophylactic GTX. In none of these five negative studies were large numbers of PMNs obtained from matched donors and transfused daily. In a situation analogous to that for the negative therapeutic GTX trials, the failure of prophylactic GTX might be explained, at least in part, by inadequate transfusions (see box on Collection and Transfusion of Neutrophil Concentrates).

The role of modern prophylactic GTX (i.e., from G-CSF–stimulated donors) has not been established by definitive clinical trials. However, two factors suggest possible success: (1) because of the rapid recovery from myeloablation, hastened by peripheral blood HPC transplantation plus treatment of patients with recombinant growth factors such as G-CSF, the period of severe neutropenia may be as short as 1 week; and (2) this relatively brief period of severe neutropenia might literally be eliminated by transfusing large doses of PMNs collected from donors stimulated with G-CSF plus corticosteroids. A few studies have begun to explore this possibility (Table 115-6).

Bensinger et al[23] transfused seven allogeneic marrow recipients with PMNs collected from their HLA-identical or syngeneic marrow donors after G-CSF stimulation. Because donors experienced leukapheresis on consecutive days, collection techniques were quite variable in terms of quantities of hydroxyethyl starch infused and liters of donor blood processed—thus the number of PMNs collected varied from 0.3 to 14.4×10^{10}. Recipients received an average of 7.6 GTX while awaiting marrow recovery, and recipients were given 5 mcg/kg G-CSF daily to maintain a mean blood PMN count of

Table 115-6 Modern Prophylactic Granulocyte Transfusion Studies Using Neutrophils Collected From Granulocyte Colony-Stimulating Factor–Stimulated Donors in Hematopoietic Progenitor Cell Transplant Recipients

Investigator	PMNs × 10^{10} Per Each GTX	Stimulation	Leukapheresis	Outcomes
Bensinger et al[23]	4.2	G-CSF 3.5-6 mcg/kg	Variable	Not reported
Adkins et al[24]	4.1 (day 1) 5.1 (day 3) 6.1 (day 5)	G-CSF 5 mcg/kg × 5 Days posttransplant	Hetastarch 7 L processed Days 1, 3, and 5	60% (6 of 10) afebrile 40% (4 of 10) febrile 3 culture positive
Adkins et al[25]	5.6 (day 2) 7.0 (day 4) 8.5 (day 6) 9.9 (day 8)	G-CSF 10 mcg/kg	Hetastarch 7 L processed Days 2, 4, 6, and 8	Reduction of fever and antibiotics if no leukocyte antibodies

G-CSF, Granulocyte colony-stimulating factor; *GTX,* granulocyte transfusions; *PMN,* neutrophil.

Collection and Transfusion of Neutrophil Concentrates

To ensure adequate numbers and quality of polymorphonuclear neutrophils (PMNs) for transfusion, PMNs must be collected from stimulated donors by automated leukapheresis using an erythrocyte sedimenting agent, such as hydroxyethyl starch. A major limitation of granulocyte transfusion (GTX) efficacy has been the inability to transfuse adequate numbers of perfectly functioning PMNs. Under the stress of a severe bacterial infection, the marrow of an otherwise healthy adult will produce between 10^{11} and 10^{12} PMNs in 24 hours. Granulocyte concentrates collected from healthy donors who are not stimulated with corticosteroids or granulocyte colony-stimulating factor (G-CSF) will contain between 0.2 and 0.8 × 10^{10} PMNs—a woeful number equal to approximately 1% of a healthy marrow's output. Hence donor stimulation is mandatory to achieve even a hope of a reasonable PMN dose per GTX.

Donor stimulation using only properly timed corticosteroids (≥24 hours before leukapheresis, NOT immediately before) will increase the yield to approximately 2 × 10^{10} PMNs. Stimulation with G-CSF, alone or in combination with corticosteroids, will produce higher but variable PMN yields. Yields of 4 to 8 × 10^{10} PMNs are achieved regularly, and posttransfusion blood PMN counts frequently increase to 1 to 3 × 10^9/L, with PMNs detected in the recipient's bloodstream for several hours after GTX. Currently PMN donors are optimally stimulated using 300 to 480 mcg G-CSF given subcutaneously plus 8 mg dexamethasone taken orally approximately 12 hours before beginning leukapheresis.[26] Recent reports suggest that adrenal corticosteroids might cause posterior subcapsular cataracts in PMN donors. Although these reports are not in total agreement, it seems logical to include this cautionary information in donor consent forms or to stimulate PMN donors using only G-CSF—accepting lower PMN doses with the last option.[27]

Each institution must assess local needs. If, despite optimal antimicrobial and other supportive therapy, neutropenic patients suffer significant morbidity or mortality from infections, GTX should be considered. Once therapeutic transfusions have been prescribed, they must be given effectively (≥2 × 10^{10} PMNs per dose with corticosteroid stimulation, ≥4 × 10^{10} PMNs per dose with G-CSF, and never <1 × 10^{10} PMNs per dose). Transfusions are continued until the infection has resolved or until blood PMNs have risen above 1.0 × 10^9/L in the absence of further GTX. It seems logical that patients with evidence of alloimmunization (platelet refractoriness, leukocyte antibodies, repeated febrile transfusion reactions, or posttransfusion pulmonary infiltrates) should receive GTX collected from donors selected to be leukocyte compatible by human leukocyte antigen matching and/or leukocyte crossmatching. However, it has not been clearly shown that attempts to improve leukocyte antigen compatibility do in fact increase the success of GTX in alloimmunized patients—particularly when modern GTX from G-CSF–stimulated donors are transfused. Granulocyte concentrates should be transfused as soon as possible after collection because PMN functions begin to deteriorate rapidly. Some delay between collection and transfusion is inevitable, and granulocyte concentrates are usually stored briefly at 22° C, with little or no agitation. It is highly desirable to transfuse granulocyte concentrates within 6 hours of collection; they should not be given if more than 24 hours old.

0.95 × 10^9/L measured 24 hours posttransfusion. The goals of this study were to evaluate the feasibility and safety of collecting and transfusing PMNs from G-CSF–stimulated donors; patient outcomes were not reported.

Adkins et al[24] transfused 10 allogeneic marrow recipients with PMNs collected from their HLA-matched sibling marrow donors (see Table 115-6). Leukapheresis was performed on days 1, 3, and 5 posttransplant, and GTX were infused. Recipients were given 7.5 mcg/kg G-CSF every 12 hours until blood PMNs were greater than or equal to 1.5 × 10^9/L. Recipient blood PMNs were maintained at greater than 1.5 × 10^9/L throughout the 5 days of posttransplant GTX. By comparison, a historical group of control recipients treated with G-CSF, but no GTX, exhibited lower mean blood PMN counts of less than 0.5 × 10^9/L posttransplant. Prophylactic GTX seemed promising in this setting and perhaps would have been even more effective (i.e., higher recipient blood PMN counts and fewer infections) if given daily.

In another study, Adkins et al[25] transfused 23 autologous peripheral HPC recipients with PMNs collected from first-degree relative donors (see Table 115-6). Leukapheresis was performed on posttransplant days 2, 4, 6, and 8, and GTX were infused. Recipients were given 5 mcg/kg G-CSF daily until the blood PMN count was greater than or equal to 1.5 × 10^9/L. Recipients were studied for the effects of lymphocytotoxic antibodies (i.e., leukocyte alloimmunization) on GTX effectiveness. The 15 recipients who did not exhibit lymphocytotoxic antibodies during the 10-day study period experienced a mean of 4.1 febrile days and required 7.3 days of antibiotics. Values for the eight recipients with lymphocytotoxic antibodies were less desirable—6.3 febrile days and 10.5 days of antibiotics. Rates of documented infections were not reported.

No firm conclusions can be drawn from these reports of modern prophylactic GTX because (1) no nontransfused control subjects were included, (2) few patients were studied, and (3) most patients were given GTX every other day, rather than daily—possibly providing a lower-than-optimal dose of PMNs. Modern prophylactic GTX appear promising, but their efficacy, potential adverse effects, and economic analysis await definition by randomized clinical trials.

ALTERNATIVE OR ADDITIVE MEASURES TO GRANULOCYTE TRANSFUSIONS

Patients with severe neutropenia, particularly those undergoing intense chemotherapy or HPC transplantation, exhibit a variety of abnormalities in multiple body defense mechanisms, most of which cannot be corrected by GTX. Consequently infections that occur in these patients often occur after the period of severe neutropenia and accordingly do not respond to GTX. To bolster body defenses, a number of additional therapies have been evaluated—two of which are the use of recombinant myeloid growth factors (i.e., cytokines) and intravenous immunoglobulin (IVIg).

Recombinant myeloid growth factors such as G-CSF and granulocyte-macrophage colony-stimulating factor (GM-CSF) are glycoprotein cytokines that enhance the production, differentiation, and function of myeloid cells. As previously reviewed, studies of cytokine production in neonates have yielded conflicting results, with investigators reporting values that are higher than, equal to, or lower than adult values. Generally the dysregulation of expression and production of hematopoietic cytokines in neonates contributes to quantitative and qualitative myeloid abnormalities that lead to decreased availability and function of blood PMNs. Several trials of G-CSF and GM-CSF, used to prevent and to treat neonatal sepsis, have been reported. Although most studies have shown some benefit, such as improved production and function of PMNs, reduction in the incidence of infections and/or mortality has not been convincingly shown.

In older children and adult patients, G-CSF and GM-CSF have been used to accelerate marrow recovery after chemotherapy and to successfully diminish the rate of acquired infections and the need for prolonged hospitalization. In contrast to success in preventing neutropenic infections, the role of G-CSF and GM-CSF in treating already established infections is not as firmly documented. Regardless of solid evidence, these growth factors frequently are given to patients with neutropenia and severe infections, and it seems reasonable to consider adding therapeutic GTX when severe bacterial, yeast, or fungal infections are progressing in neutropenic patients, despite the use of appropriate antibiotics plus recombinant cytokines (see box on Author's Approach to Therapeutic Granulocyte Transfusions).

The use of IVIg to prevent or to treat neonatal sepsis has appeal because this therapy may correct developmental abnormalities/delays of humoral immunity and neutrophil function. In studies of experimental infections, IVIg proved beneficial by increasing opsonic activity and by improving PMN kinetics. Although the precise role of IVIg in the management of human infants is controversial, this therapy has been given (with mixed results) to prevent and to treat infections. Most prophylactic studies evaluating IVIg to prevent infections have documented few positive effects, but a few have reported true benefit. In contrast, several therapeutic studies reported benefit from adding IVIg to antibiotics during the treatment of neonatal infections. However, the data remain insufficient to justify the routine use of IVIg as standard therapy to prevent and/or treat infections in all extremely low-birth-weight preterm infants.

Author's Approach to Therapeutic Granulocyte Transfusions

Indicated for severe bacterial, yeast, or fungal infection in a neutropenic patient (<0.5 × 10^9 polymorphonuclear neutrophils [PMNs]/µL blood) when the infection progresses despite optimal antimicrobial therapy.

Collect PMNs (4 to 8 × 10^{10}) from allogeneic blood donors, as follows:

1. Stimulate neutrophilia by giving the donor 300 to 480 mcg of granulocyte colony-stimulating factor (G-CSF) subcutaneously 12 hours before beginning leukapheresis, with or without 8 mg dexamethasone orally 12 hours before beginning leukapheresis.
2. Process 10 L of donor blood using a continuous-flow blood separator with citrated hydroxyethyl starch solution infused throughout the collection.

Transfuse one granulocyte concentrate (4 to 8 × 10^{10} PMNs) daily until bone marrow recovery (blood PMNs >1.0 × 10^9/L without granulocyte transfusion) or clinical resolution of infection.

REFERENCES

1. Alavi JB, Root RK, Djerassi I, et al: A randomized clinical trial of granulocyte transfusions for infection in acute leukemia. *N Engl J Med* 296:706, 1977.
2. Fortuny IE, Bloomfield CD, Hadlock DC, et al: Granulocyte transfusion: A controlled study in patients with acute non-lymphocytic leukemia. *Transfusion* 15:548, 1975.
3. Graw RG, Jr, Herzig G, Perry S, et al: Normal granulocyte transfusion therapy. *N Engl J Med* 287:367, 1972.
4. Herzig RH, Herzig GP, Graw RG, Jr, et al: Successful granulocyte transfusion therapy for gram-negative septicemia. *N Engl J Med* 396:702, 1977.
5. Higby DJ, Yates JW, Henderson ES, et al: Filtration leukapheresis for granulocytic transfusion therapy. *N Engl J Med* 292:761, 1975.
6. Vogler WR, Winton EF: A controlled study of the efficacy of granulocyte transfusions in patients with neutropenia. *Am J Med* 63:548, 1977.
7. Winston DJ, Ho WG, Gale RP: Therapeutic granulocyte transfusions for documented infections: A controlled trial in 95 infectious granulocytopenic episodes. *Ann Intern Med* 97:509, 1982.
8. Vamvakas EC, Pineda AA: Meta-analysis of clinical studies of the efficacy of granulocyte transfusions in the treatment of bacterial sepsis. *J Clin Apheresis* 11:1, 1996.
9. Seidel MG, Peters C, Wacker A, et al: Randomized phase III study of granulocyte transfusions in neutropenic patients. *Bone Marrow Transplant* 42:679, 2008.
10. Clarke K, Szer J, Shelton M, et al: Multiple granulocyte transfusions facilitating unrelated bone marrow transplantation in a patient with very severe aplastic anemia complicated by suspected fungal infection. *Bone Marrow Transplant* 16:723, 1995.
11. Hester JP, Dignani MC, Anaissie EJ, et al: Collection and transfusion of granulocyte concentrates from donors primed with granulocyte stimulating factor and response of myelosuppressed patients with established infection. *J Clin Apheresis* 10:188, 1995.
12. Catalano L, Fontant R, Scarpato N, et al: Combined treatment with amphotericin-B and granulocyte transfusion from G-CSF-stimulated donors in an aplastic patient with invasive aspergillosis undergoing bone marrow transplantation. *Haematologica* 82:71, 1997.
13. Ozsahin H, von Planta M, Muller I, et al: Successful treatment of invasive aspergillosis in chronic granulomatous disease by bone marrow transplantation, granulocyte colony-stimulating factor-mobilized granulocytes, and liposomal amphotericin-B. *Blood* 92:2719, 1998.
14. Bielorai B, Toren A, Wolach B, et al: Successful treatment of invasive aspergillosis in chronic granulomatous disease by granulocyte transfusions followed by peripheral blood stem cell transplantation. *Bone Marrow Transplant* 26:1025, 2000.
15. Bielorai B, Neumann Y, Avigad I, et al: Successful treatment of vancomycin-resistant *Enterococcus* sepsis in a neutropenic patient with G-CSF-mobilized granulocyte transfusions. *Med Pediatr Oncol* 34:221, 2000.
16. Grigg A, Vecchi L, Bardy P, et al: G-CSF stimulated donor granulocyte collections for prophylaxis and therapy of neutropenic sepsis. *Aust N Z J Med* 26:813, 1996.
17. Peters C, Minkov M, Matthes-Martin S, et al: Leucocyte transfusions from rhG-CSF or prednisolone stimulated donors for treatment of severe infections in immunocompromised neutropenic patients. *Br J Haematol* 106:689, 1999.
18. Price TH, Bowden RA, Boeckh M, et al: Phase I/II trial of neutrophil transfusions from donors stimulated with G-CSF and dexamethasone for treatment of patients with infections in hematopoietic stem cell transplantation. *Blood* 95:3302, 2000.

19. Lee J-J, Chung I-J, Park M-R, et al: Clinical efficacy of granulocyte transfusion therapy in patients with neutropenia-related infections. *Leukemia* 15:203, 2001.
20. Hubel K, Carter RA, Liles WC, et al: Granulocyte transfusion therapy for infections in candidates and recipients of HPC transplantation: A comparative analysis of feasibility and outcome for community versus related donors. *Transfusion* 42:1414, 2002.
21. Safdar A, Hanna HA, Boktour M, et al: Impact of high-dose granulocyte transfusions in patients with cancer with candidemia. *Cancer* 101:2859, 2004.
22. Strauss RG: Current status of granulocyte transfusions to treat neonatal sepsis. *J Clin Apheresis* 5:25, 1989.
23. Bensinger WI, Price TH, Dale DC, et al: The effects of daily recombinant human granulocyte colony stimulating factor administration on normal granulocyte donors undergoing leukapheresis. *Blood* 81:1883, 1993.
24. Adkins D, Spitzer G, Johnston M, et al: Transfusions of granulocyte-colony-stimulating factor-mobilized granulocyte components to allogeneic transplant recipients: Analysis of kinetics and factors determining posttransfusion neutrophil and platelet counts. *Transplantation* 37:737, 1997.
25. Adkins DR, Goodnough LT, Shenoy S, et al: Effect of leukocyte compatibility on neutrophil increment after transfusion of granulocyte colony-stimulating factor-mobilized prophylactic granulocyte transfusions and on clinical outcomes after stem cell transplantation. *Blood* 95:3605, 2000.
26. Liles WC, Rodger E, Dale DC: Combined administration of G-CSF and dexamethasone for the mobilization of granulocytes in normal donors: Optimization of dosing. *Transfusion* 40:642, 2000.
27. Strauss RG, Johnson AT: Cataracts and corticosteroids in granulocyte donors. *Transfusion* 51:904, 2011.

CHAPTER 116

PRINCIPLES OF PLASMA TRANSFUSION: PLASMA, CRYOPRECIPITATE, ALBUMIN, AND IMMUNOGLOBULINS

Matthew S. Karafin, Christopher D. Hillyer, and Beth H. Shaz

Plasma and its derivatives are valuable resources, but cost, risk of infectious disease transmission (although rare), and other adverse effects mandate their appropriate use. Plasma can be separated from red blood cells (RBCs) through centrifugation of whole blood at the time of collection or can be collected by apheresis as a single product or as a byproduct of platelet or RBC apheresis. Plasma can be processed into derivatives through cold ethanol fractionation (method of Cohn). In this chapter, the features and uses of plasma products, which include fresh-frozen plasma (FFP); plasma frozen within 24 hours of phlebotomy (PF24); thawed plasma; and plasma derivates, including cryoprecipitate-reduced plasma, cryoprecipitate, albumin, intravenous immunoglobulin (IVIG), and intramuscular immunoglobulin, are discussed. The use of plasma-derived clotting factor concentrates as well as coagulation factor concentrates that are genetically engineered as therapy for specific clotting factor deficiencies are discussed in Chapter 118.

PLASMA PRODUCTS

Plasma is the acellular, fluid compartment of blood, and it consists of 90% water; 7% protein and colloids; and 2% to 3% nutrients, crystalloids, hormones, and vitamins. The protein fraction contains the soluble clotting factors: fibrinogen; factor XIII; von Willebrand factor (vWF); factor VIII primarily bound to its carrier protein vWF; and the vitamin K–dependent coagulation factors II, VII, IX, and X. Clotting proteins are the constituents for which transfusion of plasma is required. Plasma products include FFP, PF24, and thawed plasma, which can be used interchangeably. Notably, FFP and PF24 are both termed FFP in some countries outside of the United States.

Fresh-Frozen Plasma and PF24

Plasma frozen at −18° C or colder within 8 hours of donation (6 hours with the use of some storage bags after apheresis collection) can be labelled as FFP. This product may be stored up to 1 year before use, at which time it is thawed at 30 to 37°C over 20 to 30 minutes. A second type of frozen plasma, the most commonly used in the United States, is PF24 plasma, which is also thawed at 30 to 37C before use. PF24 is frozen at −18° C or colder within 24 hours of collection. If either product is not immediately used it can be stored for 24 hours at 1 to 6°C. The difference between FFP and PF24, using historic data, is a reduction in the following factors: fibrinogen, 12%; factor V, 15%; factor VIII, 23%; and factor XI, 7%. More recently, a direct comparison between FFP and PF24 mean factor activity immediately after thaw revealed the following changes in activity levels: factor II, 0%; factor V, +1%; factor VII, −16%; factor VIII, −15%; factor IX, +6%; factor X, 0%; vWF antigen activity, +34%; vWF : Ristocetin cofactor activity, +22%; fibrinogen, +29 mg/dL; Antithrombin, 0%; protein C, −19%; and protein S, −5%. A disintegrin and metalloproteinase with a thrombospondin type 1 motif, Member 13 (ADAMTS13) activity level is also equivalent in FFP, PF24, and cryoprecipitate-reduced plasma (discussed below). All of the factors evaluated in this study reveal that PF24 immediately after thaw had activities above the minimum activity required for safe surgical hemostasis (factor II, 97%; factor V, 86%; factor VII, 89%; factor VIII, 66%; factor IX, 88%; factor X, 94%; vWF : Ristocetin cofactor activity, 123%; fibrinogen, 309 mg/dL). Therefore, studies support that FFP and FP24 can be used interchangeably.

Thawed Plasma

Even after 1 day, coagulation factors are well maintained in thawed FFP and PF24 stored at 1 to 6° C for up to 5 days, termed *thawed plasma*. Studies show that during 5 days of storage, most clotting factors, including ADAMTS13, remain stable. However, evidence shows that activity levels fall for factors V, VII, and VIII. A review by Eder and Sebock revealed that at day 5, factor V, VII, and VIII activity levels fell from day 1 on average by 16%, 20%, and 41%, respectively, if the FFP was derived from whole blood, and 9%, 4%, and 14%, respectively, if the FFP was derived via apheresis. Although some recent evidence suggests that thrombin generation may be slower in 5-day-old thawed plasma, the decrease in clotting factor activity for both FFP and PF24 is generally not considered to be of clinical significance because the mean factor activity levels for 5-day-old thawed plasma remain above the minimum activity required for safe surgical hemostasis (on average, FFP: factor V, 67%; factor VII, 70%; factor VIII, 43%; PF24: factor V, 59%; factor VII, 77%; and factor VIII, 48%). Stored thawed plasma improves patient care and is more cost effective, due to decreased wastage, than frozen plasma because no preparation time is required. This difference consequently results in a decreased turnaround time and a substantially reduced wastage rate.

Cryoprecipitate-Reduced Plasma

Cryoprecipitate-reduced plasma, also known as cryosupernatant or cryoreduced plasma, is the remaining supernatant after the removal of cryoprecipitate from FFP, which is subsequently refrozen. This product is deficient in factor VIII, factor XIII, vWF, fibrinogen, and fibronectin. Cryoprecipitate-reduced plasma is only indicated in the treatment of patients with thrombotic thrombocytopenic purpura (TTP) and thus cannot be used interchangeably with thawed plasma, FFP, or FP24.

Solvent-Detergent Plasma

Solvent-detergent plasma is a product manufactured from 2500 or fewer pooled plasma products that has been treated with solvent (tri-η-butyl phosphate)/detergent (triton X-100) to inactivate lipid-enveloped viruses (HIV, hepatitis B, hepatitis C). The product is distributed in 200-mL containers and frozen at −18° C with a shelf life of 1 year. This product has approximately 50% loss of protein S and approximately 10% loss of other factors. SD plasma is approved for use by the U.S. Food and Drug Administration (FDA) but is no longer sold in the United States; however, SD plasma is available in other countries. Other pathogen-reduction methods have also been developed, including amotosalen photochemical treatment, riboflavin-treated plasma, and methylene blue-treated plasma. Studies in Europe show that these methods are also quite effective at reducing the risk of viral contamination, but none is currently FDA approved.

Recovered and Source Plasma (Plasma for Manufacture)

Some plasma products are not used clinically but are used for further manufacturing into plasma derivatives. These products include recovered plasma (liquid plasma and "plasma") that are derived from whole blood and are sent to a manufacturer from a collection facility through a "short supply agreement." Liquid plasma (which can be used clinically) is defined as plasma that is separated from whole blood at any time during storage at 1 to 6° C up to 5 days after the whole blood expiration date. *Plasma* is defined as liquid plasma that is frozen at −18° C or colder with a frozen shelf-life of 5 years. Source plasma, an FDA licensed product, is collected by apheresis, which is intended for further manufacturing. The Plasma Protein Therapeutics Association promotes safe collection and manufacturing practices of plasma derivatives.

Indications

Most guidelines consistently support plasma transfusions for correcting multiple acquired coagulation factor deficiencies, as seen in liver failure, disseminated intravascular coagulation (DIC), massive transfusion, reversal of warfarin effect, and certain indications as a replacement fluid in therapeutic plasma exchange (Table 116-1). There is no current evidence-based laboratory value "trigger" for plasma administration, and any recommendation needs to be weighed against the patient's presence, or risk, of bleeding.

Plasma is typically indicated when the prothrombin time (PT) or partial thromboplastin time (PTT) is greater than 1.5 to 1.7 times normal paired with the presence of bleeding or anticipated bleeding. A variable response to plasma can be largely explained by the nonlinear, exponential relationship between clotting factors activity levels and coagulation test results (Fig. 116-1).

Audits of recent transfusion practices have consistently demonstrated that plasma product use is inappropriately high. Recent estimates suggest up to 83% (reported range, 10%–83%) of plasma transfusions are not administered according to published guidelines. The most commonly cited reason for plasma administration is a preprocedural elevation in coagulation studies. This indication is not evidence based, especially when the coagulation abnormality is mild to moderate. Moreover, plasma should not be used as a volume expander or as a source of nutrients. Clinical situations in which plasma transfusions are used are further defined in the following sections.

Table 116-1 Indications for Plasma Product Transfusion

Indicated
Multiple acquired coagulation factor deficiency
Replacement of an inherited single plasma factor deficiency for which no coagulation factor concentrate exists
Liver failure
Massive transfusion
Disseminated intravascular coagulation
Rapid reversal of warfarin effect
Plasma infusion or exchange for thrombotic thrombocytic purpura and other thrombotic microangiopathies, diffuse alveolar hemorrhage, and catastrophic antiphospholipid syndrome
Not Indicated
Immunodeficiency
Burns
Wound healing
Volume expansion
Source of nutrients

Liver Failure

Patients with severe liver disease may have low levels of the vitamin K–dependent clotting factors (II, VII, IX, and X). These patients develop a prolonged PT and PTT. In addition, the thrombin time (TT) may be prolonged and fibrin split products may be elevated, and in later stages, the fibrinogen level may decrease. Hemorrhage, most often secondary to an anatomic lesion, may be complicated by the coagulopathy resulting from these abnormalities.

Plasma transfusions are indicated during bleeding if the coagulation test results are abnormal. In the absence of anatomic lesions, bleeding does not usually occur until the PT is greater than 16 to 18 seconds or the PTT is greater than 55 to 60 seconds. Plasma products are not recommended prophylactically before a surgical challenge or liver biopsy unless these values are exceeded. In fact, the PT and PTT are poor predictors of surgical bleeding, and mild abnormalities in these coagulation tests may be impossible to correct even with infusion of large quantities of plasma. A recent randomized controlled trial revealed that intranasal desmopressin was both less expensive and as effective as plasma transfusion for patients with liver disease with international normalized ratios (INRs) between 2 and 3 undergoing minor surgery. Orthotopic liver transplantation complicated by preexisting severe liver disease, lack of clotting factor synthesis during the anhepatic stage, massive packed RBC transfusion, and DIC may require large volumes of plasma. Transfusion should be guided by clinical assessment of bleeding, coagulation test results, and thromboelastographic changes.

Massive Transfusion

Massive transfusion is generally defined as receiving 10 or more units of RBCs within 24 hours (or one blood volume). Trauma patients

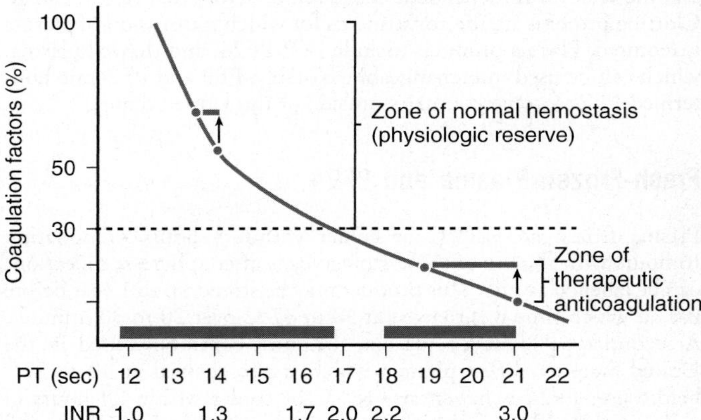

Figure 116-1 RELATIONSHIP BETWEEN FACTOR ACTIVITY LEVELS AND COAGULATION STUDIES. The general relationship between the concentration of coagulation factors and the result of prothrombin time (PT) and international normalized ratio (INR) studies. The normalization of modest elevations in the INR required much larger volumes of plasma than would be expected, and modest doses of plasma can result in marked changes in the INR when markedly elevated. The cause of this phenomenon can be explained by the nonlinear, exponential relationship between coagulation factor concentration and standard coagulation test results. As shown, small increases of coagulation factors correlate with marked changes in coagulation studies when coagulation factors are depleted. The opposite is true when the coagulation factors are at higher concentrations. *(Adapted from Kor DJ, Stubbs JR, Gajic O: Perioperative coagulation management; Fresh frozen plasma.* Best Pract Res Clin Anaesthesiol *24: 51, 2010.)*

may arrive at the hospital with a prolonged PT (termed acute trauma-induced coagulopathy, early trauma-induced coagulopathy, or acute coagulopathy of trauma). Early trauma-induced coagulopathy is associated with increased mortality and increased use of blood products. Trauma patients can also develop a secondary coagulopathy, termed the *lethal triad,* secondary to dilutional coagulopathy, acidosis, and hypothermia. The dilutional coagulopathy is secondary to the administration of crystalloid and RBCs without coagulation factor support. Studies have shown that the early use of plasma and platelets in trauma patients undergoing massive transfusion appears to decrease the incidence of secondary coagulopathy (lethal triad) and improve survival in these patients.

Some experts have previously argued that plasma should be used only in the context of abnormal coagulation study results in massively bleeding patients. However, recent studies have shown that this may not be the most effective approach. Because of the rapidity required to treat severely bleeding patients, standardized hospital-based massive transfusion protocols providing predetermined ratios of RBCs, plasma, cryoprecipitate, and platelets until the hemorrhage is controlled are in use and have been associated with improved survival. Furthermore, massive transfusion protocols identify who is responsible for different aspects of the patient's care, what laboratory tests should be ordered and when, and what blood products should be prepared and at what intervals. Currently, there is no optimal protocol. Some protocols are laboratory based, others have preset blood product volumes and ratios, and some others integrate both. Importantly, hospitals develop these protocols using a multidisciplinary team, defining quality measures with periodic review to adjust the protocols based on new evidence and data.

The optimal ratio of RBC to plasma products in the context of massive transfusion is under active investigation. Multiple studies in both the military and civilian literature have shown a reduction in morbidity and mortality with a transfusion ratio of 1 unit of plasma for every 1 to 3 RBC units transfused in the context of severe posttraumatic bleeding. To date, the sum of available evidence supports the use of this more aggressive plasma transfusion strategy, but survivorship bias remains a concern because of the retrospective nature of most of the studies to date, and some recent studies do not show benefit. Moreover, one European group has recently suggested that the use of prothrombin complex concentrate (PCC) and fibrinogen concentrates, instead of plasma, provides a safer alternative for massive transfusion patients. When published, data from the recently completed Prospective Observational Study of Massive Transfusion Trial (PROMTT), an observational trial including massively transfused trauma patients in 10 civilian trauma centers, will greatly advance knowledge regarding optimization of transfusion ratios.

In the recent past, trauma patients would be provided primarily crystalloid and albumin followed by component transfusion therapy based on specific transfusion "triggers." A hemoglobin below 8 g/dL for RBCs, PT above 1.5 times normal for plasma, platelet count below 50,000/μL for platelet transfusions, and fibrinogen below 100 g/dL for cryoprecipitate were often used. These "triggers" have now been incorporated as part of some massive transfusion protocols as algorithms to guide therapy. In these protocols, component therapy is guided by rapid and regular laboratory value correlation. To improve the speed by which one can address coagulation abnormalities, some protocols now use thromboelastography (TEG) or other point-of-care tests. TEG technology provides a dynamic and global assessment of the coagulation process and can provide rapid assessments of the patient's platelet function, coagulation cascade, and fibrinolysis. The mechanism underlying TEG technology and the interpretation of TEG data are beyond the scope of this chapter. Currently, sufficient data are lacking to universally recommend the use of TEG in massive transfusion protocols.

Massive transfusion in other conditions, such as liver, cardiac, or orthopedic surgery and obstetric hemorrhage, likely has a different pathophysiology; thus transfusion management of these patients may be different than for trauma patients. Studies exploring the use of massive transfusion protocols in these situations are lacking, but institutions should have policies in place for rapid availability of blood products and laboratory testing.

Disseminated Intravascular Coagulation

Disseminated intravascular coagulation may be secondary to sepsis, liver disease, hypotension, surgery-associated hypoperfusion, trauma, obstetric complications, leukemia (usually promyelocytic), or underlying malignancy. Successful treatment of the underlying cause is paramount. Recent guidelines suggest that plasma should not be initiated based on abnormal laboratory results alone. Rather, patients with DIC and bleeding, those requiring invasive procedures, and those at risk for bleeding complications should be given plasma in amounts sufficient to correct or ameliorate the coagulopathy or hemorrhagic diathesis. Large volumes of plasma are often necessary to correct the coagulation defect in these patients, and a dose of 30 mL/kg has been suggested. However, in patients with severe liver disease, bleeding, and DIC, plasma infusions often fail to normalize the PT and PTT.

Rapid Reversal of Warfarin Effect

Warfarin inhibits the hepatic synthesis of vitamin K–dependent clotting factors (factors II, VII, IX, and X) by blocking the recovery of the form of vitamin K that is active in the carboxylation of these proteins. Warfarin therapy induces functional deficiencies of these factors, which correct within 48 hours after the discontinuation of warfarin if diet and vitamin K absorption are normal.

The use of plasma in the context of warfarin anticoagulation is well established. Plasma is generally not indicated for warfarin reversal when the patient is not bleeding and when the patient has an INR below 9 because vitamin K administration corrects the coagulopathy in 12 to 18 hours. In patients anticoagulated with warfarin who have active bleeding, require emergency surgery, or have serious trauma, however, the deficient clotting factors can be immediately provided by PCC or plasma transfusions. Plasma use may not be optimal in all situations of warfarin-induced bleeding, though, because large volumes of plasma might be required for adequate warfarin reversal, and lengthy infusion times, especially in those who are volume sensitive, might delay needed surgical intervention.

Consequently, in Europe, PCC should be chosen as first-line therapy for rapid reversal of warfarin anticoagulation, especially if volume overload is a concern. In the United States, though, PCCs do not contain adequate factor VII levels and thus likely need to be paired with plasma transfusions for optimal efficacy. The volume of plasma needed when combined with PCC is still less than that needed when plasma is used alone. Studies have shown that PCC can reverse warfarin-induced coagulopathy faster than plasma or vitamin K alone. However, it is not yet known whether more rapid improvements in coagulation variables afforded by PCC or plasma translate into clinical benefits for the patient (i.e., reduced bleeding) without an increased risk of thromboembolic events. In addition to PCC and plasma, some recent reports support the use of recombinant FVIIa for warfarin reversal in the context of head trauma. Also, INR levels need to be closely followed to ensure that warfarin reversal is sustained.

Thrombotic Thrombocytopenic Purpura and Other Indications During Plasma Exchange

In patients with TTP, plasma exchange with plasma as the replacement fluid is lifesaving. Plasma infusion or exchange is also critical in the treatment of individuals who have congenital TTP. Plasma exchange has decreased the mortality of TTP from more than 90% to less than 10%. Six randomized control trials have demonstrated that plasma exchange is most effective in patients who have an autoantibody to ADAMTS13. This is attributable to both the removal of a patient's plasma containing the inhibitor coupled with the addition of donor plasma containing the functional vWF-cleaving protease. The FDA has approved the use of cryoprecipitate-reduced plasma for TTP. Some authorities advocate the use of cryoprecipitate-reduced plasma as a first-line therapy for TTP. However, in 2001, the North American TTP Group published a multicenter prospective randomized trial comparing exchange transfusion with plasma and cryoprecipitate-reduced plasma for the initial treatment of TTP, which demonstrated equal efficacy between plasma- and cryoprecipitate-reduced plasma for the initial therapy in TTP.

Plasma exchange is not an established indication for individuals with diarrhea associated hemolytic uremic syndrome (HUS). Plasma exchange with plasma replacement fluid, however, is currently indicated in HUS secondary to a genetic deficiency of complement factor (or plasma infusion) or autoantibody to factor H. Although no randomized control trials have been done to date evaluating the effect of plasma exchange for these cases of HUS, plasma exchange has been theoretically proposed to effectively remove the potentially causative autoantibody or mutated circulating complement regulator while replacing absent or defective complement regulators.

Plasma exchange with plasma replacement may be indicated in other thrombotic microangiopathies. Some medications cause thrombotic microangiopathies, which require plasma exchange. Current examples include ticlopidine and clopidogrel and potentially cyclosporine or tacrolimus. Lastly, plasma exchange with plasma replacement may also be used in the treatment of thrombotic microangiopathy associated with stem cell transplantation and in catastrophic antiphospholipid syndrome.

Plasma as replacement fluid, either partially or completely, for plasma exchange is used in other diseases with risk of hemorrhage caused by the resulting coagulopathy, such as diffuse alveolar hemorrhage, liver failure, and periperatively.

Prophylactic Use of Plasma

Studies have shown that prophylactic administration of plasma to recipients with an INR of 1.5 or less is unlikely to produce a clinical benefit and unnecessarily exposes patients to the risks of plasma transfusion. A number of randomized control trials and meta-analyses have evaluated the efficacy of the prophylactic use of plasma products to reduce the risk of bleeding. One trial, the Northern Neonatal Nursing Initiative Group Trial, randomized 776 neonates and evaluated whether plasma transfusion prophylaxis could prevent intraventricular hemorrhage compared with volume expanders (gelofusin or dextrose saline). In a second large randomized clinical trial, 275 patients were randomized to see whether plasma transfusions could prophylactically prevent bleeding in acute pancreatitis patients. Neither large study showed clinical benefit of prophylactic plasma use. In one systematic review, 55 other randomized clinical trials were reviewed and evaluated. Only 17 of these 55 involved a control group that did not receive plasma. Overall, similar to the two largest studies, the results of these randomized control trials failed to show evidence for the efficacy of prophylactic plasma use across multiple clinical and laboratory outcomes. Similarly, a second meta-analysis evaluated 25 independent studies of minor surgical procedures and found that there was no significant difference in bleeding risk between those who did and did not have a coagulopathy. Despite this evidence, current recommendations still indicate that a pretransfusion INR of 1.6 or above be used as a transfusion trigger because the prophylactic use of plasma is theoretically justified when the clinical risk of bleeding is greater than potential harms of using plasma.

Dosage

One unit of plasma derived from a unit of whole blood contains 200 to 280 mL. When plasma is collected by apheresis, as much as 800 mL can be obtained from one individual ("jumbo" plasma units), but the majority of units clinically used have a volume around 250 mL. If larger units are substituted, then the number of units prepared will decrease proportionally. On average, there is 0.7 to 1 unit/mL of activity of each coagulation factor per milliliter of plasma and 1 to 2 mg/mL of fibrinogen. The appropriate dose of plasma may be estimated from the plasma volume, the desired increment of factor activity, and the expected half-life of the factor being replaced (i.e., factor VII has a half-life of only 4-6 hours, and thus plasma doses should be repeated every few hours if replacing factor VII in a patient with factor VII deficiency). Alternatively, the plasma dosage may be estimated as 10 to 15 mL/kg and ideally should be ordered as the number of milliliters to be infused. The frequency of administration depends on the clinical response to the infusion and correction of laboratory parameters. Moreover, plasma infusions should be given as close to the time as it is needed to allow for its maximum hemostatic effect if given preprocedure.

Compatibility

Plasma is screened for unexpected RBC antibodies during product testing and should be ABO-type compatible for transfusion. Notably, group AB plasma is universally compatible with all patients, and group O plasma is only compatible with patients with group O RBCs.

Adverse Events

Plasma transfusion is associated with a number of infectious and noninfectious adverse events. Transfusion-transmitted diseases traditionally include HIV, hepatitis B, and hepatitis C (see Chapter 121), which are currently rare. Noninfectious risks include allergic reactions, transfusion-related acute lung injury (TRALI), transfusion-associated circulatory overload (TACO), and hemolytic reactions (see Chapter 120).

Transfusion-Related Acute Lung Injury

Transfusion-related acute lung injury is noncardiogenic pulmonary edema associated with the transfusion of blood products. TRALI is caused by neutrophil and pulmonary endothelial activation, usually caused by transfused donor white blood cell (WBC) antibodies, including human leukocyte antigen (HLA) antibodies and human neutrophil antigen (HNA) antibodies. These donor antibodies react with the recipient's WBCs in the pulmonary vasculature, causing leukoagglutination, activation of the complement cascade, cytokine release, and pulmonary edema. Approximately 5% of TRALI is caused by the opposite mechanisms, which are recipient WBC antibodies against transfused donor WBCs. Nonimmune mechanisms are also postulated to mediate TRALI, including bioactive lipids and CD40 ligand (see also Chapter 120). Lastly, certain patients are at increased risk for TRALI including those with high interleukin-8 levels, liver surgery, chronic alcohol abuse, shock, higher peak airway pressure while being mechanically ventilated, current smoking practice, and positive intravascular fluid balance.

Multiple strategies have been implemented to reduce the risk of TRALI. First, donors implicated in prior TRALI reactions are deferred from further blood donation. Second, multiparous female donors can be tested for HLA and HNA antibodies, and blood products with high-volume plasma (i.e., plasma and apheresis platelets) are not made from those with high-titer antibodies. Third, plasma supplied to hospitals for transfusion can be from male or never pregnant female donors; the parous female plasma is diverted for fractionation. Currently, these strategies have significantly reduced the risk of TRALI without significantly reducing blood product availability.

Allergic Reactions

Allergic transfusion reactions occur when preformed recipient antibodies bind to transfused allergens. Allergic transfusion reactions occur in approximately 1% to 3% of plasma transfusions. Anaphylactic reactions occur in approximately one in 20,000 to 50,000 transfusions. The majority of allergic transfusion reactions are mild. Mild reactions consist of urticaria with or without generalized pruritus or flushing. More severe symptoms include hoarseness, stridor, wheezing, dyspnea, hypotension, gastrointestinal symptoms and shock. Mild reactions can be treated with antihistamines, and more severe reactions can be treated with epinephrine, H1-receptor antagonists, and steroids (see also Chapter 120).

Transfusion-Associated Circulatory Overload

Transfusion-associated circulatory overload results from vascular fluid volume overload after the transfusion of blood products and is most common in very young or elderly patients with cardiac dysfunction or positive fluid balance. Studies show that the mean age of patients who develop TACO range from about 70 to 85 years. Additional known risk factors for TACO include larger volumes of transfusion, a greater plasma transfusion volume, and a faster transfusion rate. The incidence of TACO is unknown, but it is increasingly recognized clinically. Studies have reported the incidence to range from 1 in 356 to one in 10,000 blood products transfused or 1% to 8% of transfusion recipients, depending on the study population and data collection methodology, and is currently associated with a mortality rate of 5% to 15% in the United States.

Symptoms include dyspnea, orthopnea, cough, chest tightness, cyanosis, hypertension, and headache. Symptoms usually present at the end of transfusion but may occur up to 6 hours after transfusion. Diagnosis is based on the presence of cardiogenic pulmonary edema. Management includes discontinuing transfusion, diuretic therapy, oxygen supplementation, and sitting the patient upright. Avoiding rapid transfusion can prevent TACO unless clinically indicated. Transfusions should be administered slowly, usually 1 mL/kg/hr, particularly in patients at risk for TACO.

CRYOPRECIPITATE

Cryoprecipitate is prepared from 1 unit of FFP thawed at 1 to 6°C. The precipitate is then refrozen and stored at −18° C or colder for 1 year. Cryoprecipitate, volume of 10 to 15 mL, contains 80 to 100 units of factor VIII, 100 to 250 mg of fibrinogen, and 50 to 60 mg of fibronectin as well as vWF and factor XIII.

Cryoprecipitate takes 10 to 15 minutes to thaw at 30 to 37°C and then requires pooling before infusion. Prepooled (pooled before storage) cryoprecipitate products are now available, easing the burden of preparation on the transfusion services. After being pooled and thawed, cryoprecipitate is maintained at 20 to 24°C and outdates in 4 hours (6 hours if unpooled or pooled in a closed system).

Indications

Cryoprecipitate is used predominately to treat bleeding associated with fibrinogen or factor XIII deficiency (Table 116-2). Cryoprecipitate should not be used to treat vWF, factor VIII, and factor XIII deficiencies because virally inactivated factor concentrates are available. Similar to plasma, recent studies also indicate that cryoprecipitate is not used appropriately in clinical practice. One large audit, for instance, demonstrated that across 25 Canadian hospitals and 4370 units of cryoprecipitate transfusions, only 24% of transfusions were considered appropriate, and 34% of cryoprecipitate transfusions were deemed inappropriate according to published guidelines.

Table 116-2 Administration of Cryoprecipitate

Indicated
Fibrinogen deficiency
Massive transfusion
Reversal of thrombolytic therapy
Congenital afibrinogenemia
Dysfibrinogenemia
Factor XIII deficiency
Possibly Indicated
Uremic bleeding
Amniotic fluid embolism (used as last resort to replace depleted fibronectin)
Snake bites

Fibrinogen Deficiency

Fibrinogen deficiency is the primary indication for cryoprecipitate transfusion. The deficiency may be attributable to congenital afibrinogenemia or dysfibrinogenemia, severe liver disease, DIC, or massive transfusion. Patients with the latter indications often have concomitant decreases in clotting factor levels and require the coadministration of plasma products. It is important to obtain fibrinogen measurements because levels below 100 mg/dL cause prolongation of the PT and PTT despite adequate clotting factor replacement. Very low levels of fibrinogen occur during liver transplantation, during which transfusion support with cryoprecipitate is vital.

A specific purified human fibrinogen concentrate is now available and may represent a safer alternative for direct fibrinogen replacement in isolated fibrinogen deficiencies, such as inherited hypofibrinogenemia. Fibrinogen concentrates undergo viral inactivation and have a standardized fibrinogen content; these are used preferentially over cryoprecipitate in some countries, but studies have not demonstrated a clinical benefit over cryoprecipitate. In the United States, fibrinogen concentrate is FDA approved for treatment of bleeding in patients with congenital fibrinogen deficiency.

Fibrin Glue or Sealant

Fibrin glue or sealant results from the mixture of a fibrinogen source (from plasma, platelet-rich plasma, or allogeneic or autologous cryoprecipitate) with a thrombin source (bovine, human, or recombinant). The enhanced local hemostasis achieved by the sealant product is through the action of thrombin on fibrinogen. "Fibrin glue" is a non–FDA-approved thrombin and fibrinogen preparation, and it has been widely used in Europe many years. Fibrin and thrombin sealants are FDA-approved alternatives to fibrin glue and are advantageous over locally made fibrin glues because of standard dosing. Fibrin- and thrombin-containing glues or sealants can be used for multiple surgical purposes, including as a topical hemostat (creating a blood clot to halt bleeding), as a sealant (agents to prevent leakage of potentially nonclotting fluids, such as cerebrospinal fluid), or as an adhesive (bonds different tissues together). Multiple fibrin- or thrombin-containing products are now FDA approved for use.

The safety profile of each product differs depending on the product components and source. Bovine thrombin has been reported to cause anaphylaxis (because of bovine allergies), coagulopathy through formation of antibodies to factor V or II, and rarely death because of severe systemic hypotensive reactions. Consequently, bovine products have an FDA-mandated black box warning on their package inserts. Pooled human plasma sources have the potential risk of viral or prion disease transmission. Reports indicate that hepatitis A and parvovirus B19 are particularly difficult to remove from these products despite current cleansing and filtration methods, and it is recommended that patients be counseled about this risk. Some human plasma products also contain synthetic aprotinin, which is a potential source of allergic reactions. Recombinant products, although eliminating the risk of infectious transmission or antibody formation, may also cause allergic reactions because of the hamster or snake proteins used to manufacture the products. Lastly, autologous fibrin glue preparations have been used, and the infectious risks (e.g., HIV and hepatitis) associated with the use of heterologous fibrin glue are eliminated by replacement with the autologous source but are resource intensive.

Alternatively, albumin mixed with glutaraldehyde has been used to form both an effective sealant and adhesive. The FDA has currently approved one albumin-based product to seal large blood vessel anastomoses and to reattach layers of the aorta in the context of an aortic dissection. Other successful reported uses include as a sealant in breast cancer surgery and to reduce air leaks in lung volume reduction procedures. Side effects of this compound can be significant, however, and include nerve and muscle necrosis, sinoatrial node damage, calcium metabolism abnormalities, mucosal and skin irritation, adhesive emboli, limitation of aortic growth, and pseudoaneurysms.

Uremic Bleeding

Abnormal bleeding is a common complication of uremia and is primarily attributable to platelet dysfunction and defective interaction with endothelium. Use of cryoprecipitate as a source of vWF has been speculated to correct the platelet dysfunction. However, cryoprecipitate has been shown not to affect platelet aggregation in vitro but does shorten the bleeding time. In 1980, a single study published in the *New England Journal of Medicine* led to the widespread, but temporary, use of cryoprecipitate for the treatment of uremic bleeding. Since that time, variable response reports have been published. Numerous alternative strategies are currently available for the prevention and treatment of uremic-type bleeding including dialysis, erythropoietin, RBC transfusion, desmopressin, and conjugated estrogens, and as such, cryoprecipitate is now rarely used in the prevention or treatment or uremic bleeding.

Massive Transfusion

Although most studies regarding massive transfusion evaluate the use of platelets and plasma, some recent studies suggest that regular doses of cryoprecipitate also help improve survival. One recent study found that a high transfusion ratio involving cryoprecipitate in 214 massive transfusion patients resulted in improved 30-day survival (66% vs. 41%). Another key study found that maintaining a 0.2 g or greater fibrinogen-to-RBC unit ratio resulted in a significantly higher survival rate (76% vs. 48%). They also recommended that 10 units of cryoprecipitate be used for every 10 units of RBCs. Because of survivor bias in these studies, further prospective clinical studies need to be performed to verify these findings. Consequently, although still under investigation, current data tentatively support the use of cryoprecipitate in the context of massive transfusion protocols; however, cryoprecipitate is indicated in the treatment of hypofibrinogenemia.

Dosage

The dosage of cryoprecipitate is calculated on the basis of the amount of fibrinogen present in 1 unit of cryoprecipitate, the plasma volume, and the desired increment. The difficulty in determining the correct amount to administer is primarily attributable to variability in the fibrinogen content of cryoprecipitate secondary to variability in donors and component processing and preparation. The goal of therapy should be to maintain the measured fibrinogen at greater than 100 mL/dL. Consequently, it is estimated that a dose of 8 to 10 units of cryoprecipitate will increase the fibrinogen in a 70-kg adult by 50 to 70 mg/dL. The dosing frequency should be determined based on clinical and laboratory responses because factor XIII and fibrinogen are very stable proteins. Specifically, the half-life of fibrinogen is 4 days, and factor XIII has a half-life of 9 days.

Compatibility

Cryoprecipitate can contain minimal anti-A or anti-B antibodies and, as such, ABO and D compatibility is not necessary for most adult and pediatric patients.

Adverse Events

Cryoprecipitate has similar adverse event risk as other blood products, including transfusion-transmitted diseases, hemolytic reactions, and allergic reactions. Because it contains less plasma and no leukocytes, febrile and allergic reactions are less likely to occur.

ALBUMIN

Albumin, an important plasma protein, contributes primarily to the maintenance of plasma colloid oncotic pressure; it is also involved in the transport of numerous substances, such as unconjugated bilirubin, various hormones, and drugs. The human body content of albumin is 4 to 5 g/kg and is responsible for 80% of the osmotic pressure of human plasma. It is clinically available in four forms: 5% solution in saline; 25% solution in distilled water; albumin conjugated with polyethylene glycol (PEG); and purified protein fraction (PPF), which is 5% total protein (88% albumin and 12% globulins). These products are heat treated, and albumin has not been documented to transmit infectious diseases. (A single outbreak of transfusion-associated hepatitis B occurred with PPF formulation of albumin in 1973.)

Indications

A decrease in measured plasma albumin is found in many situations and is often not a clinically significant concern. Mild edema caused by hypoalbuminemia does not require albumin therapy. However, inadequate synthesis, as seen in severe liver disease and severe malnutrition, or excessive loss, as seen in nephrotic syndrome and protein-losing enteropathy, can lead to significant hypoalbuminemia with intravascular volume depletion, anasarca, ascites, and pleural effusions. Historically, albumin had a broader use (i.e., nutritional support, correction of hypoalbuminemia, volume replacement), but recent studies support its benefit in fewer situations, including nephrotic syndrome resistant to potent diuretic therapy, after large-volume paracentesis, and in ovarian hyperstimulation syndrome (OHSS) (Table 116-3).

Intravascular Volume Expansion

As noted, albumin provides the majority of plasma colloid oncotic pressure. Infused albumin provides colloid oncotic pressure; however, 50% of the infused protein is lost to the extravascular fluid compartment within 4 hours. Crystalloid may also provide volume expansion and is more quickly redistributed into total body fluids. Studies investigating the use of albumin in various situations, including volume expansion during and after surgery, as priming solution in cardiopulmonary bypass, or in maintaining colloid oncotic pressure, found no clinical benefit compared with controls. In 1998, the Cochrane Injuries Group performed a systematic review of randomized control trials in albumin treatment of critically ill patients and concluded that there was no evidence that albumin reduces mortality in patients with hypovolemia, burns, or hypoalbuminemia. They suggested that albumin increases mortality. On the basis of their findings, the group recommended that hypoalbuminemia be eliminated from the list of indications and called for a large randomized trial to assess the effect of albumin on mortality, which has yet to be performed. However, several small prospective studies have argued that albumin is at least clinically equivalent to saline or plasma for intravascular volume resuscitation in some clinical settings.

Thus, the conclusion that albumin has no use in the context of volume expansion and hypoalbuminemia is not definitive.

Table 116-3 Administration of Albumin

Indicated
After large-volume paracentesis
Nephrotic syndrome resistant to potent diuretics
Ovarian hyperstimulation syndrome
Volume or fluid replacement in plasmapheresis
Possibly Indicated
Adult respiratory distress syndrome
Cardiopulmonary bypass pump priming
Fluid resuscitation in shock, sepsis, or burns
Neonatal kernicterus or hyperbilirubinemia
To reduce enteral feeding intolerance
Not Indicated
Correction of measured hypoalbuminemia or hypoproteinemia
Nutritional deficiency, total parenteral nutrition
Preeclampsia
RBC suspension
Simple volume expansion (surgery, burns)
Wound healing
Investigational
Cadaveric renal transplantation
Cerebral ischemia
Stroke
Common Usages
Serum albumin <20 g/dL
Nephrotic syndrome, proteinuria, and hypoalbuminemia
Labile pulmonary, cardiovascular status
Cardiopulmonary bypass, pump priming
Extensive burns
Plasma exchange
Hypotension
Liver disease, hypoalbuminemia, diuresis
Protein-losing enteropathy, hypoalbuminemia
Resuscitation
Intraoperative fluid requirement >5–6 L in adults
Premature infant undergoing major surgery

RBC, Red blood cell.

Cirrhosis

The use of albumin in patients with cirrhosis dates to before 1950. In this setting, albumin is recommended for temporary improvement in hyponatremia; spontaneous bacterial peritonitis; or prevention of the complications associated with paracentesis, including volume shifts and hyponatremia. Several studies demonstrated that after large-volume paracentesis (>5 L), hyponatremia and renal insufficiency were improved with albumin infusion compared with other volume-expanding agents. Moreover, a single randomized control trial of albumin use in cirrhotic patients with spontaneous bacterial peritonitis revealed that albumin administration with antibiotics resulted in reduced mortality and a reduced risk of renal failure compared with antibiotic use alone. Recent studies with albumin infusions have also been done in end-stage liver disease patients for hypoalbuminemia. However, results are less encouraging, with studies indicating no additional benefits or reduction in morbidity.

Nephrotic Syndrome

Albumin has been used to increase colloid oncotic pressure with the intention of increasing diuresis via increasing vascular pressure at the level of the glomerulus. Several studies have shown that albumin use in this context have resulted in no clinical benefit. However, other studies have suggested that albumin use is associated with increased hypertension, respiratory distress, and electrolyte abnormalities. Consequently, the current recommended use of albumin for nephrotic syndrome patients is limited to patients in whom diuretic therapy is poorly tolerated or ineffective or in those with massive ascites or anasarca.

Ovarian Hyperstimulation Syndrome

This syndrome is usually a result of iatrogenic administration of human chorionic gonadotrophin (hCG) to induce ovulation. OHSS is typified by enlarged ovaries, which release vascular endothelial growth factor that can result in increased capillary permeability. This in turn leads to a fluid shift out of the intravascular compartment to the abdominal or pleural spaces, resulting in ascites and hypovolemia. In the most severe form, the patient can develop tense ascites, oliguria, dyspnea, hemodynamic instability, and thromboembolism. Treatment includes fluid restriction, analgesics, and close monitoring; occasionally, hospitalization may be necessary.

Mild OHSS occurs in approximately one-third and moderate to severe in approximately 5% of women receiving exogenous hCG. Increased risk of OHSS includes young age, low body weight, polycystic ovarian syndrome, high dose hCG, high or rapid rise in estradiol level, and previous history of OHSS. In addition, the risk is proportional to the number of developing follicles and number of oocytes retrieved. Moderate to severe OHSS can be mitigated by closely monitoring women during treatment and subsequently withholding or reducing hCG administration when a large number of intermediate-size developing follicles is present or when estradiol levels are elevated.

In 2011, the Cochrane Collaboration systematically reviewed eight randomized clinical trials of albumin administration in OHSS, and concluded that there is only a borderline statistically significant decrease in the incidence and severity of OHSS when albumin was administered during oocyte retrieval in high-risk women. In contrast, the meta-analysis further revealed that the use of hydroxyethyl starch (HES) resulted in a markedly decreased incidence of severe OHSS. Additionally, Bellver et al published a large randomized trial that demonstrated no difference in moderate to severe OHSS when 40 g of albumin was administered after the retrieval of 20 or more oocytes. Only one (nonrandomized) study to date has compared human albumin and 6% HES. This study concluded in 16 patients with severe OHSS that patients who received HES had a higher urine output, needed less abdominal paracentesis, and drainage of pleural effusions and had a shorter hospital stay than patients who received albumin. Therefore, although still clinically used, albumin may be inferior to other therapies in the prevention of OHSS.

Therapeutic Apheresis

Albumin is the replacement fluid of choice for many therapeutic apheresis indications, particularly therapeutic plasma exchange. Albumin compared with plasma replacement for plasma exchange, reduces the risk of adverse events during apheresis procedures by reducing the risk of viral transmission, allergic reactions, and TRALI compared with plasma use (see Plasma section.) Albumin can also be used in combination with saline during apheresis procedures, but excessive use of saline results in hypotensive reactions. Albumin is also indicated if large (>15% of the total blood volume) blood volumes are removed to prevent hypotensive reactions in other therapeutic apheresis procedures (leukapheresis, plateletpheresis).

Although albumin is generally well tolerated in therapeutic apheresis patients, albumin use can result in significant hypotension, bradycardia, and flushing in patients receiving angiotensin-converting enzyme inhibitor (ACE) therapy. ACE inhibitors prevent patients' ability to metabolize bradykinins that are present in the albumin and activated during the apheresis procedure. In patients taking ACE inhibitors, symptoms can be prevented by using plasma as the replacement fluid or halting ACE inhibitor use and delaying the start of apheresis therapy.

Dose

The volume and speed of administration should be determined by the patient's volume status, condition, and response to the product. A typical adult dose is 25 g, which may be repeated in 15 to 30 minutes. In a 48-hour period, the maximum dose is 250 g. In the pediatric population, albumin dose again depends on the patient's condition, but 0.5 to 1.0 g/kg/dose with a maximum dose of 6 g/kg/day could be used as a general guideline. Albumin 5% is oncotically equivalent to normal human plasma. Albumin 25% provides less infusion volume per amount of albumin and is usually administered to patients with fluid or sodium intake restriction. Albumin 25% expands the blood volume by 3.5 times by drawing fluid into the intravascular space. Five percent Albumin is used for therapeutic apheresis replacement fluid; volume administered depends on volume being replaced during the procedure.

Adverse Effects

Albumin is a plasma derivative used widely and associated with rare adverse reactions. Allergic reactions, including urticaria, may be encountered. Changes in vital signs (heart rate, blood pressure, respiration rate), nausea, emesis, and fever or chills have also been rarely reported. Volume overload and dilutional anemia as well as hypocalcemia may occur. Albumin has not been associated with transfusion-transmitted diseases.

INTRAVENOUS IMMUNOGLOBULIN

Intravenous immunoglobulin (IVIG) is prepared by fractionation of large pools of human plasma. Numerous preparations are available in the United States and throughout the world. Each preparation is slightly different and has theoretical advantages and disadvantages and specific licensed indications. Ideally, IVIG should contain each immunoglobulin G (IgG) subclass; retain Fc receptor activity; have a normal half-life; demonstrate virus neutralization, opsonization, and intracellular killing; and have antibacterial capsular polysaccharide antibody. Furthermore, vasoactive impurities should be absent, and no transmissible infectious agents should be present. The uses of IVIG have been extensively reviewed, and the number of theoretical and accepted uses for IVIG are rapidly expanding.

Indications

Intravenous immunoglobulin is indicated for replacement of immunoglobulins or for its immunomodulatory effects. Currently, there are six FDA-approved indications for IVIG treatment: primary immunodeficiency, pediatric HIV infections, secondary immunodeficiency in chronic lymphocytic leukemia (CLL), idiopathic thrombocytopenic purpura (ITP), Kawasaki disease, and allogeneic stem cell transplantation in patients older than 20 years of age. Some of the FDA indications are no longer applicable, such as in patients with CLL and HIV, given better medications. IVIG is also considered first-line therapy for multiple other conditions, such as Guillain-Barré syndrome, chronic inflammatory demyelinating polyradiculoneuropathy (CIDP), neonatal alloimmune thrombocytopenia (NAIT), posttransfusion purpura, myasthenia gravis, and stiff-person syndrome (Table 116-4). An exhaustive review of all of the known established and investigational uses for IVIG cannot be reasonably summarized in this chapter. For further information, some excellent

Table 116-4 Administration of Intravenous Immunoglobulins

Indicated
Primary immunodeficiency syndromes
Common variable immunodeficiency
X-linked agammaglobulinemia
SCID
Ataxia-telangiectasia
Wiskott-Aldrich syndrome
IgG subclass deficiency
CMV-interstitial pneumonia after BMT
GVHD after bone marrow transplantation
Persistent deficit in antibody production after BMT
Secondary hypogammaglobulinemia
Chronic inflammatory demyelinating polyneuropathy
Chronic lymphocytic leukemia (hypogammaglobinema, high risk for infections)
Guillain-Barré syndrome
ITP
Inflammatory myopathies
Mucocutaneous lymph node syndrome (Kawasaki disease)
Pediatric HIV infection
Parvovirus infection
Stiff-person syndrome
Possibly Indicated
Antiphospholipid syndrome in pregnancy
Autoimmune hemolytic anemia (warm type unresponsive to prednisone)
Factor VIII inhibitors (refractory)
Graves ophthalmopathy
Immune neutropenia
Multiple myeloma (stable disease, high risk for infections)
Myasthenia gravis
Pemphigus
Systemic lupus erythematosus (refractory, severe, active)
Thrombocytopenia refractory to platelet transfusion
Vasculitis (refractory to standard therapy)
Solid organ transplantation (kidney)
Hemolytic disease of the fetus and newborn
Investigational
Acquired von Willebrand disease
Amyotrophic lateral sclerosis
Burn patients
Chronic fatigue syndrome
Fetomaternal alloimmune thrombocytopenia
GVHD
HIV infection
Immune-mediated aplastic anemia
Inflammatory bowel disease
Intractable childhood epilepsy
Multiple sclerosis
Neonatal sepsis
Prevention of nosocomial postoperative infections
Prophylaxis in transplant recipients against CMV infection
Recurrent unexplained spontaneous abortions
Rheumatoid arthritis
Dilated cardiomyopathy
Postpartum cardiomyopathy
Myocarditis
Chronic idiopathic pericarditis
Neonatal hemochromatosis
Parvovirus B19 infection

BMT, Bone marrow transplantation; *CMV,* cytomegalovirus; *GVHD,* graft-versus-host disease; *IgG,* immunoglobulin G; *ITP,* idiopathic thrombocytopenic purpura; *SCID,* severe combined immunodeficiency.

reviews are cited in the Suggested Readings. A brief summary of some of the more well-established uses of IVIG are presented in the following section.

Primary Immunodeficiency Syndromes

Patients with primary congenital immunodeficiency syndromes have been treated with intramuscular immunoglobulin for the past 30 years. The use of intramuscular immunoglobulin has certain disadvantages, including delayed absorption, delivery of inadequate amounts because of small muscle mass, and pain at the injection site. IVIG overcomes these disadvantages and when used prophylactically in patients with primary immunodeficiency has been demonstrated to reduce the number of febrile and infectious episodes as well as improve survival rate. IVIG use in IgG subclass deficiencies is also beneficial.

Chronic Lymphocytic Leukemia

Chronic lymphocytic leukemia may be associated with hypogammaglobulinemia and complications of repeated bacterial infections. IVIG decreases the incidence and severity of bacterial infections in CLL patients with hypogammaglobulinemia and has become accepted prophylactic therapy.

Bone Marrow Transplantation

The use of prophylactic IVIG or cytomegalovirus (CMV)–IVIG in CMV-negative bone marrow (BM) transplant recipients during the first 100 days after transplant has been demonstrated to reduce the incidence of symptomatic CMV-associated disease, including CMV interstitial pneumonia, in some trials. Because of the high cost of this treatment and the increasing use of prophylactic ganciclovir, IVIG is currently not indicated for the prophylaxis of CMV infections in BM transplant recipients. In established CMV interstitial pneumonia, IVIG in combination with ganciclovir has been shown to reduce the mortality rate and has become the recommended treatment modality. Its role in preventing severe graft-versus-host disease (GVHD) is unclear. Prolonged IVIG therapy during GVHD prevention may suppress humoral immunity recovery.

Pediatric Human Immunodeficiency Virus Infection

The defects in humoral and cellular immunity observed in children with HIV infection predispose them to life-threatening bacterial infections. Studies previously demonstrated that the administration of IVIG to HIV-infected children can reduce the incidence and severity of bacterial infections as well as the frequency of hospitalization. More recently, studies have shown that IVIG does not improve outcome likely because of improved medications for HIV and HIV-associated infections.

Idiopathic Thrombocytopenic Purpura

Intravenous immunoglobulin and Rh immune globulin are routinely and effectively used in the treatment of acute and chronic ITP. IVIG significantly raises the platelet count within 5 days in adults with chronic ITP and in children with acute ITP. The mechanism of action of IVIG in ITP is unknown; one postulation is that Fc receptor blockade decreases the removal of antibody-coated platelets. Other proposed mechanisms include suppressed antiplatelet antibody synthesis, increased antiviral immunity, and blockage by antiidiotypic antibodies. In general, IVIG induces responses in most patients within 1 to 2 days. Responses are of variable duration and are rarely sustained, although maintenance therapy may be of some value. IVIG may be effective in chronic ITP refractory to corticosteroids or splenectomy and may show greater efficacy in conjunction with corticosteroids.

Although IVIG has shown equal efficacy with corticosteroids in pediatric acute ITP and in 75% of adults with chronic ITP, because of the transient responses and high cost, its use is justified only in clinical situations requiring rapid elevation of platelet count or if standard therapy has failed. IVIG is therefore indicated in acute bleeding episodes or before urgent surgery, including splenectomy; in patients at high risk of intracranial hemorrhage; and in those in whom corticosteroids are contraindicated or ineffective. IVIG has also been used to treat ITP during pregnancy, postinfectious thrombocytopenia, ITP associated with HIV infection, and neonatal thrombocytopenia. Intravenous anti-D immune globulin (also known as Rh immune globulin) has demonstrated efficacy in Rh-positive, nonsplenectomized individuals with ITP. It has been suggested that the mechanism of action may involve a shift in the immune-mediated destruction from platelets to the antibody-coated RBCs.

Kawasaki Disease

Patients with mucocutaneous lymph node syndrome (Kawasaki disease) have been treated with aspirin with or without concomitant IVIG administration. Coronary artery aneurysm, a serious complication of this disease, was significantly reduced in the IVIG-treated group. However, in a multicenter retrospective survey of all children treated with Kawasaki disease, persistent or recrudescent fever after their first course of IVIG was associated with a statistically significant risk of treatment failure. Furthermore, IVIG retreatment in those patients with persistent fever after IVIG treatment failure was approximately 60%. Current randomized trials are now being done to compare the efficacy of newer, and perhaps better, therapies, such as infliximab (anti–tumor necrosis factor-α). To date, these randomized control studies show that infliximab is at least as safe and as efficacious as IVIG in these refractory patients. One retrospective review has even suggested that infliximab might result in faster resolution of fever and fewer days of hospitalization compared with IVIG. Although studies are still ongoing, IVIG may soon be replaced by alternative therapies in this refractory patient population.

With regard to the pathogenesis of Kawasaki disease, decreased peripheral blood lymphocyte apoptosis has been demonstrated. Therefore, the effect of IVIG in Kawasaki disease has been postulated to partially reverse inhibited lymphocyte apoptosis.

Solid Organ Transplantation

The presence of high-titer reactive antibodies against incompatible graft HLA or ABO antigens increases the risk of early solid organ, antibody-mediated graft rejection and mortality, especially in kidney and cardiac transplants. For some patients who have HLA antibodies to undergo transplantation, these antibodies must be removed or decreased. Although morbidity and mortality can be reduced by selecting an adequately cross-matched donor, IVIG with or without plasma exchange has also been shown to decrease sensitization of incompatible antigens in patients awaiting renal and cardiac transplantations. In addition, IVIG with or without plasma exchange is used in the treatment of biopsy-proven antibody-mediated rejection. One review discussed three randomized control trials that investigated the use of IVIG for renal transplantation and revealed a trend in improvement in desensitization rates and a statistically significant decrease in time to transplant for patients treated with IVIG, superior graft survival rate in kidney transplant patients desensitized with IVIG, and a lower rate of recurrent acute rejection with IVIG compared with OKT3. Consequently, current consensus renal transplant guidelines indicate that IVIG is a useful treatment modality for desensitization of patients with HLA antibodies and in patients with acute rejection.

Randomized trials have not yet been performed for ABO incompatible kidney transplants, or heart, liver, or lung transplants. Moreover, there is a paucity of data for transplant outcomes, and current studies have small numbers without data on donor-specific antibody levels. Current guidelines assert that there is insufficient evidence to make a recommendation for or against the routine use of IVIG for desensitization in these transplants.

Aplastic Anemia Secondary to Parvovirus

Parvovirus B19 infection can result in severe anemia and reticulocytopenia, especially in immunocompromised individuals and individuals with sickle cell disease or thalassemia, and the use of IVIG is considered first-line therapy in the treatment of these patients (typical dose, 0.5 g/kg weekly for 4 weeks).

Chronic Inflammatory Demyelinating Polyradiculoneuropathy

Chronic inflammatory demyelinating polyradiculoneuropathy is a chronic disorder resulting in demyelination of peripheral nerves that result in weakness and sensory changes. Equivalent outcomes have been observed in the treatment of CIDP with IVIG (reported dose, 2.0 g/kg given over 2 to 5 days once each month), plasma exchange, or glucocorticosteroids. The decision as to which treatment to use is made on an individual basis, balancing the risks and benefits of each treatment modality.

Dermatomyositis

Dermatomyositis is a chronic inflammatory disorder that results in progressive weakness and rash. IVIG (typical dose, 2.0 g/kg per month administered over 2-5 days) results in improved muscle strength and neuromuscular symptoms.

Guillain-Barré Syndrome (Acute Inflammatory Demyelinating Polyneuropathy)

Guillain-Barré syndrome is an acute demyelinating peripheral neuropathy affecting both motor and sensory nerves. IVIG (typical dose, 2.0 g/kg given over 1 to 5 days) is likely equivalent to TPE in improving disability and shortening the time to improvement.

Hypogammaglobulinemia Associated With Multiple Myeloma

Multiple myeloma is a monoclonal B-cell (plasma cell) disorder with clinical symptoms arising as a result of plasma cell infiltration of the BM, monoclonal Ig in the blood and urine, and immunosuppression. IVIG has shown to be beneficial in preventing serious infections in plateau-phase multiple myeloma or other hematologic malignancy, when the patients have hypogammaglobinemia, at doses of 0.4 g/kg every 3 weeks.

Immunoglobulin M Paraproteinemic Demyelinating Neuropathy

Paraproteinemic demyelinating neuropathy is a chronic disorder resulting in decreased sensory and motor function, similar to CIDP, in association with monoclonal immunoglobulins. One placebo-controlled trial demonstrated that IVIG may improve short-term morbidity, but the remainder of the available evidence is mixed. The use of IVIG for this condition has recently fallen out of favor with current consensus groups.

Inclusion Body Myositis

Inclusion body myositis is an inflammatory myopathy resulting in chronic muscular weakness. Randomized trials using IVIG appear to result in short-term improvement in strength scores and improved swallowing in patients with inclusion body myositis and is equivalent to treatment with glucocorticosteroids in one small clinical study. The use of IVIG for this condition has also recently fallen out of favor with current consensus groups because of the lack of known sustained benefit for patients with this condition.

Lambert-Eaton Myasthenic Syndrome

Lambert-Eaton myasthenic syndrome results from antibodies to the neuromuscular junction, leading to autonomic dysfunction. One randomized control trial reveals that IVIG significantly improves generalized central and peripheral muscle strength and decreases serum calcium channel antibody titers. A total dose of 2.0 g/kg given over 2 to 5 days is a recommended initial treatment.

Multifocal Motor Neuropathy

Multifocal motor neuropathy is a chronic progressive disorder resulting in primarily hand weakness. IVIG is now considered a first-line treatment for this condition, and improved strength can be seen at a dose of 2.0 g/kg over 2 to 5 days.

Multiple Sclerosis

Multiple sclerosis is a chronic progressive or relapsing and remitting disorder characterized by brain white matter demyelination. There are two published meta-analyses, and several randomized controlled clinical trials in patients with relapsing-remitting multiple sclerosis using a wide range of IVIG doses that demonstrate the success of IVIG in reducing the number of exacerbations and disability in patients with relapsing-remitting multiple sclerosis compared with placebo. However, no studies to date have compared IVIG with standard therapies, and one clinical trial (PRIVIG trial) has raised doubt that IVIG is effective as a routine treatment. Consequently, IVIG is considered a viable second-line option for patients who fail, decline, or are unable to tolerate standard immunomodulatory therapies such as B-interferon and glatiramer acetate.

Myasthenia Gravis

Myasthenia gravis is a chronic neurologic autoimmune disorder characterized by weakness and fatigue upon repetitive skeletal muscle use that improves with rest. IVIG has been used successfully as a short-term measure for acute severe exacerbations of myasthenia gravis at a dose of 2.0 g/kg given over 2 to 5 days and appears comparable to plasma exchange. A definitive randomized control trial comparing the two treatment modalities has not been done, however.

Neonatal Alloimmune Thrombocytopenia

Neonatal alloimmune thrombocytopenia is a rare condition that results from maternal platelet alloantibodies against the fetal or neonatal platelets resulting in neonatal or fetal thrombocytopenia. Studies evaluating the use of IVIG for NAIT are limited but unlikely to improve because of the rarity of the condition. The treatment of NAIT during pregnancy is maternal administration of 1.0 g/kg IVIG weekly as a first-line therapy beginning at 20 to 24 weeks of gestational age with or without the use of glucocorticosteroids. Moreover, the neonate may need to receive IVIG and platelet transfusions after delivery at a dose of 1.0 g/kg to increase fetal platelet counts to prevent intracerebral hemorrhage.

Hemolytic Disease of the Fetus and Newborn

Hemolytic disease of the fetus and newborn (HDFN) results from maternal RBC alloantibodies binding to fetal or neonatal RBCs and may result in hemolysis, leading to anemia or hydrops fetalis and death depending on the severity. Two meta-analyses reveal that IVIG significantly reduces the need for exchange transfusions in patients with HDFN. IVIG is now consequently recommended at a dose of 0.5 to 1.0 g/kg to treat newborns with HDFN if there is established jaundice and a rising total serum bilirubin despite phototherapy. In addition, maternal IVIG infusion (with or without therapeutic plasma exchange) has been used in severe cases of HDFN in which treatment must occur before the ability to perform intrauterine transfusions.

Posttransfusion Purpura

Posttransfusion purpura (PTP) is a rare complication of transfusion that results in acute, profound thrombocytopenia secondary to platelet antibodies that destroy both transfused and autologous platelets. Although the evidence evaluating the effect of IVIG in these patients is limited to multiple case reports, the available evidence suggests that IVIG should be a first-line therapy for this condition. PTP treatment with IVIG at a dose of 1.0 g/kg over 2 days may result in a rapid increase in platelet count.

Sepsis and Septic Shock in Adults

The use of IVIG in adult patients with bacterial sepsis or septic shock is potentially beneficial. One randomized control trial revealed that in intensive care unit patients with intraabdominal sepsis and shock, IVIG with antibiotics was superior to antibiotics with albumin in improving patient survival. Encouraging results have also been identified in patients receiving IVIG for streptococcal toxic shock syndrome, but further studies are currently needed.

Stiff-Person Syndrome

Stiff-person syndrome is a neurologic disorder associated with truncal and limb rigidity and heightened sensitivity. One small randomized control trial suggests that IVIG could play a positive role in improving stiffness and sensitivity symptoms. Currently, IVIG is considered a second-line therapy for those who fail or cannot tolerate GABAergic medications. A dose of 2.0 g/kg given over 2 to 5 days is the current recommended starting dose.

Dosage

The dosage and frequency for IVIG varies significantly depending on the age of the patient and the clinical indication. Many typical dosages are described in the preceding section. In general, patients require 200 to 800 mg/kg IV every 3 to 4 weeks to achieve adequate IgG levels if immunodeficient (usually 500 mg/dL) and needing protection against infection. Initially, serial IgG level determination may allow the physician to individualize the dose and schedule. These are affected by the recovery, half-life, redistribution, and catabolism of IVIG, which vary from product to product and patient to patient. Patients with ITP are usually initially treated with 400 to 1000 mg/kg/day for 2 to 5 consecutive days with a maximum dose of 2.0 g/kg. Maintenance doses of 400 to 1000 mg/kg/dose every 3 to 6 weeks is recommended in some patients (particularly children) based on clinical response and platelet count. Kawasaki disease is treated with 2.0 g/kg as a single dose in combination with aspirin.

Adverse Effects

Infusions of IVIG should be started slowly, and patients should be closely monitored. If the initial rate (0.5 mL/kg/hr) is well tolerated, the rate can be increased gradually, but not more than eightfold. Fever, headache, nausea, vomiting, fatigue, backache, leg cramps, urticaria, flushing, elevation of blood pressure, and thrombophlebitis may be seen. Adverse events have been reported in 2% to 10% of infusions. IgA-deficient patients may have IgG anti-IgA antibodies, which can cause anaphylactic reactions. This complication is rare and may be avoided by using products with a lower concentration of IgA. Aggregated IgG may produce chills, nausea, flushing, chest tightness, and wheezing. Rarely, IVIG preparations contain RBC antibodies that can produce hemolysis or interfere with serologic evaluations, including RBC compatibility testing. IVIG treatment may produce a positive direct antiglobulin test (DAT), and positive hepatitis and CMV serologies. Serum sickness can also occur. Lastly, high-dose IVIG therapy has been associated with thrombosis, reversible acute renal failure, TRALI, and aseptic meningitis. Improved manufacturing processes currently in place render IVIG free of enveloped and nonenveloped viruses.

HYPERIMMUNE IMMUNOGLOBULIN PRODUCTS

Hyperimmune globulins are concentrated immune globulins with specificity for a specific antigen or group of antigens. These products are manufactured in a similar manner to that used for IVIG product production. However, donors for these specific products are unique in that they have high titers for the Ig specificity of interest. The donor high titers can be achieved via natural immunity, prophylactic immunization, or target immunization, depending on the antibody of interest. These products are generally used to provide passive immunity for a variety of conditions that are described in more detail in the following sections (Table 116-5).

Antithymocyte Globulin

Antithymocyte globulin is a purified concentrated globulin made from hyperimmune serum of horses immunized with human T lymphocytes. ATG is used in renal transplant patients as an adjunct therapy in the treatment of graft rejection. It is also used in patients with aplastic anemia who are not candidates for BM transplantation.

Table 116-5 Hyperimmune and Intramuscular Immunoglobulins

ATG
Botulism immunoglobulin
CMV immunoglobulin
Hepatitis A immunoglobulin
Hepatitis B immunoglobulin
Rabies immunoglobulin
RSV immunoglobulin
Rh(D) immunoglobulin
Tetanus immunoglobulin
Vaccinia immunoglobulin
Varicella-zoster immunoglobulin
Western equine encephalitis immunoglobulin

ATG, Antithymocyte globulin; *CMV*, cytomegalovirus; *RSV*, respiratory syncytial virus.

Hyperimmune Immunoglobulin

Hyperimmune globulin is used to prevent the development of specific clinical disease or alter its symptomatology. Hepatitis B immunoglobulin is used to provide passive immunity to hepatitis B virus associated with needle stick exposure or sexual contact with hepatitis B surface antigen–positive individuals, after liver transplantation for prevention of recurrence, and prevention of hepatitis B vertical transmission. Other hyperimmunoglobulins include botulism, CMV, hepatitis A, rabies, respiratory syncytial virus, tetanus, vaccinia, and varicella-zoster virus immunoglobulins.

Rh Immunoglobulin

Rh immunoglobulin has two primary indications, prevention of D antigen alloimmunization and treatment of ITP. Rh immunoglobulin is given to D-negative mothers after potential exposure to fetal D positive RBCs, such as after abortion or amniocentesis, as well as at 28 weeks gestational age and postpartum if the child proves to be D positive. The therapeutic effect is thought to be caused by antibody feedback with T-cell suppression of the B-cell clone responsible for the formation of anti-D antibody. Rh immunoglobulin can also be given to prevent immunization in D-negative individuals given D-positive blood products, such as platelets.

Rh immunoglobulin is dosed to adequately prevent D immunization. In the United States, 300 μg are administered after an event resulting in maternal–fetal hemorrhage, at 28 weeks and postpartum. Doses are increased for evidence of large maternal–fetal hemorrhage (300 μg for every 15 mL of RBC exposure). This dosing is also used in the prevention of D alloimmunization after receipt of RBC-containing blood products. Rh immunoglobulin should be given within 72 hours after RBC exposure. Adverse events to low doses, such as those used to prevent D immunization, include fever, chills, and pain at the injection site. Rarely, hypersensitivity reactions are noted.

Rh immunoglobulin doses are substantially higher for the treatment of ITP. They are 50 μg/kg for hemoglobin 10 g/dL or greater and 25 to 40 μg/kg when hemoglobin is 8 to 10 g/dL. Rh immunoglobulin use in ITP is indicated in D-positive patients with intact spleens. Adverse events at high doses of Rh immunoglobulin include hemolysis, DIC, and rarely death.

SUGGESTED READINGS

Toy P, Gajic O, Bacchetti P, et al: Transfusion related acute lung injury: Incidence and risk factors. *Blood* 119:1757, 2012.

AABB: *Standards for blood banks and transfusion services*, ed 27, Bethesda (MD), 2011, AABB.

Allford SL, Hunt BJ, Rose P, et al: British Society of Haematology: Guidelines on the diagnosis and management of thrombotic microangiopathic haemolytic anaemias. *Br J Haematol* 120:556, 2003.

Bechtel BF, Nunez TC, Lyon JA, et al: Treatments for reversing warfarin anticoagulation in patients with acute intracranial haemorrhage: A structured literature review. *Int J Emerg Med* 4:40, 2011.

Buchanan GR, Journeycake JM, Adix L: Severe chronic idiopathic thrombocytopenic purpura during childhood: Definition, management, and prognosis. *Semin Thromb Haemost* 29:595, 2003.

Callum JL, Karkouti K, Lin Y: Cryoprecipitate: The current state of knowledge. *Transfus Med Rev* 23:177, 2009.

Cardigan R, Lawrie AS, Mackie IJ, et al: The quality of fresh-frozen plasma produced from whole blood stored at 4° C overnight. *Transfusion* 45:1342, 2005.

Eder AF, Sebok MA: Plasma components: FFP, FP24, and thawed plasma. *Immunohematology* 23:150, 2007.

Hillyer CD, Shaz BH, Zimring JC, et al: *Transfusion medicine and hemostasis: Clinical and laboratory aspects,* St Louis, 2009, Elsevier.

Holland LL, Brooks JP: Toward rational fresh frozen plasma transfusion: The effect of plasma transfusion on coagulation test results. *Am J Clin Pathol* 126:133, 2006.

Ketchem L, Hess JR, Hiippala S: Indications for early fresh frozen plasma, cryoprecipitate, and platelet transfusion in trauma. *J Trauma* 60:S51, 2006.

Kor DJ, Stubbs JR, Gajic O: Perioperative coagulation management: Frozen plasma. *Best Pract Res Clin Anaesthesiol* 24:51, 2010.

Levi M, Toh CH, Thachil J, et al: Guidelines for the diagnosis and management of disseminated intravascular coagulation. *Br J Haematol* 145:24, 2009.

Liumbruno G, Bennardello F, Lattanzio A, et al: Recommendations for the use of albumin and immunoglobulins. *Blood Transfus* 7:216, 2009.

Nakazawa H, Ohnishi H, Okazaki H, et al: Impact of fresh-frozen plasma from male-only donors versus mixed-sex donors on postoperative respiratory function in surgical patients: A prospective case-controlled study. *Transfusion* 49:2434, 2009.

Newburger JW, Takahashi M, Gerber MA, et al: Diagnosis, treatment, and long-term management of Kawasaki disease: A statement for health professionals from the Committee on Rheumatic Fever, Endocarditis, and Kawasaki Disease, Council on Cardiovascular Disease in the Young, American Heart Association. *Pediatrics* 114:1708, 2004.

Pantanowitz L, Kruskall M, Uhl L: Cryoprecipitate patterns of use. *Am J Clin Pathol* 119:874, 2003.

Roback JD, Caldwell S, Carson J, et al; American Association for the Study of Liver; American Academy of Pediatrics; United States Army; American Society of Anesthesiology; American Society of Hematology. *Transfusion* 50:1227, 2010.

Robinson P, Anderson D, Brouwers M, et al: IVIG Hematology and Neurology Expert Panels: Evidence-based guidelines on the use of IVIG for hematologic and neurologic conditions. *Transfus Med Rev* 21:S3, 2007.

Finfer S, Bellomo R, Boyce N, et al: SAFE study investigators: A comparison of albumin and saline for fluid resuscitation in the ICU. *N Engl J Med* 350:2247, 2004.

SAFE study investigators: Saline or albumin for fluid resuscitation in patients with traumatic brain injury. *N Engl J Med* 357:874, 2007.

Sandler SG: The status of pathogen-reduced plasma. *Transfus Apher Sci* 43:393, 2010.

Scott E, Puca K, Heraly J, et al: Evaluation and comparison of coagulation factor activity is fresh-frozen plasma and 24-hour plasma at thaw and after 120 hours of 1-6C storage. *Transfusion* 49:1584, 2009.

Shaz BH, Stowell SR, Hillyer CD: Transfusion-related acute lung injury: From bedside to bench and back. *Blood* 117:1463, 2011.

Shehata N, Palda VA, Meyer RM, et al: The use of immunoglobulin therapy for patients undergoing solid organ transplantation: An evidence based practice guideline. *Transfus Med Rev* 24:S7, 2010.

Spotnitz WD, Burks S: Hemostats, sealants, and adhesives II: Update as well as how and when to use the components of the surgical toolbox. *Clin Appl Thromb Hemost* 16:497, 2010.

Stanworth SJ: The evidence-based use of FFP and cryoprecipitate for abnormalities of coagulation tests and clinical coagulopathy. *Hematology* 179, 2007.

Stanworth SJ, Brunskill S, Hyde CJ, et al: What is the evidence base for the clinical use of FFP? A systematic review of randomized controlled trials. *Br J Haematol* 126:139, 2004.

Szczepiorkowski ZM, Winters JL, Bandarenko N, et al: Guidelines on the use of therapeutic apheresis in clinical practice: Evidence-based approach from the apheresis applications committee of the American Society for Apheresis. *J Clin Apher* 25:83, 2010.

Udi N, Yehuda S: IVIG-indications and mechanisms in cardiovascular disease. *Autimmun Rev* 7:445, 2008.

CHAPTER 117

PREPARATION OF PLASMA-DERIVED AND RECOMBINANT HUMAN PLASMA PROTEINS

David B. Clark

The development of large-scale methods for the preparation of human plasma proteins began more than 70 years ago soon after the outbreak of World War II. The U.S. Armed Forces issued an urgent request to the medical community for 300,000 units of human whole blood or plasma, which appeared to be an impossibly large amount at the time. Thinking that albumin could be used instead of plasma, Dr. Edwin J. Cohn of Harvard Medical School drew together a task force of investigators who developed methods for the fractionation of plasma based on differential precipitation of various proteins with ethanol. After an unsuccessful attempt to use bovine plasma, Cohn was able to obtain a supply of human plasma from the American Red Cross. Although albumin was the only product distributed during the war, the remaining plasma fractions were carefully preserved, and other preparations, including fibrinogen and immunoglobulins, were soon developed. This was the beginning of the plasma fractionation industry.

PLASMA FRACTIONATION

Beginning in the post–World War II era and continuing to the present, major improvements have occurred in the preparation of human plasma protein products. Most large-scale manufacture of plasma-derived products is still based on modifications of the original method developed by Cohn's group supplemented by more selective purification techniques to produce a wide variety of products. In addition, genetic engineering technology has allowed recombinant human plasma proteins to be produced in cell culture systems and transgenic animals. This chapter describes current methods and future directions for the preparation of plasma-derived and recombinant human plasma proteins for clinical use, primarily for products available in the United States.

Plasma is estimated to contain approximately 10,000 different proteins, most of which have yet to be identified. One of the unique features of plasma fractionation is the ability to produce multiple products from a single raw material. Plasma for fractionation is derived from two sources, either directly by plasmapheresis, termed source plasma, or as a byproduct of whole blood donation, termed recovered plasma. The plasma is usually shipped frozen as individual units from local blood or plasma collection centers to a central processing plant.

At the plant, sufficient units to produce typically 2000- to 3000-L pools are thawed slowly at 1° to 5° C to produce cryoprecipitate, a cold-insoluble fraction that contains significant amounts of factor VIII, von Willebrand factor (vWF), fibrinogen, fibronectin, and factor XIII, along with a number of other proteins present in smaller quantities. The cryoprecipitate is usually recovered by centrifugation. The cryo-supernatant or cryo-poor plasma may be treated with a chromatographic media to capture the factor IX complex or antithrombin (AT) before it enters the Cohn process. There it goes through a series of precipitations as the ethanol concentration is increased in steps from 8% to 40% at specific combinations of pH, ionic strength, protein concentration, and cold temperature. The precipitates and supernatants are separated either by the traditional continuous-flow centrifugation or in large-scale filter presses. The method provides both relatively pure fractions containing albumin and immunoglobulins, which need minimal additional processing, as well as fractions enriched in other proteins, which are used as the starting materials for further purification. Fig. 117-1 shows a schematic of the ethanol process.

The first precipitate, fraction I at 8% alcohol, contains factor VIII, fibrinogen, and other poorly soluble proteins. Fractions II and III are precipitated together and contain the immunoglobulins, which are separated in a subsequent series of precipitations to produce fraction II, essentially pure immunoglobulins. Because many of the fraction I proteins are removed in the cryoprecipitate, some manufacturers do not produce a separate fraction I. Instead they collect a combined fraction I + II + III. Fraction IV, produced from the supernatant of fraction (I+)II + III, is sometimes produced in two subfractions. Fraction IV-1 contains the vitamin K–dependent (VKD) clotting factors, AT and α_1-proteinase inhibitor (API), whereas fraction IV-4 contains transferrin, haptoglobin, and some of the albumin. Fraction V is almost pure albumin.

PRODUCT SAFETY

Ensuring the safety of plasma products depends on a complex system that starts with donor selection and carries all the way through to the patient receiving the product. The system is highly redundant so that a failure in one area may be compensated for by another.

Donor Selection, Screening, and Testing

Product safety starts with donor selection. Gone are the days when anyone could be a donor, with prisons and mental hospitals providing much of the country's plasma. Plasma collection centers screen their potential donors rigorously, both for medical history and any social behaviors that might put them at risk of infection. Plasma products licensed in the United States are only produced from plasma collected from U.S. donors in U.S. Food and Drug Administration (FDA)–licensed establishments.

Every donation is tested for a number of different viral diseases by a battery of tests, again with redundancy. Sensitive antigen and antibody tests are followed by NAT testing (nuclear amplification or nucleic acid testing, a form of polymerase chain reaction), which can detect extremely small numbers of virus particles. Because of the "window period" between the time a donor is infected and the time antibodies or viruses can be detected in his or her plasma, most manufacturers also hold donations for at least 60 days until a donor has returned for a repeat donation. If the repeat donation still tests negative several weeks later, there is a high likelihood that the first donation is safe. In addition to FDA oversight, many manufacturers and collection agencies belong to the Plasma Protein Therapeutic Association (PPTA), which has strict quality regulations to help ensure the safety of donated plasma.

Viral Inactivation and Removal Processes

Maximizing the safety of the incoming plasma is only the first step. Viral inactivation and removal methods are now incorporated into

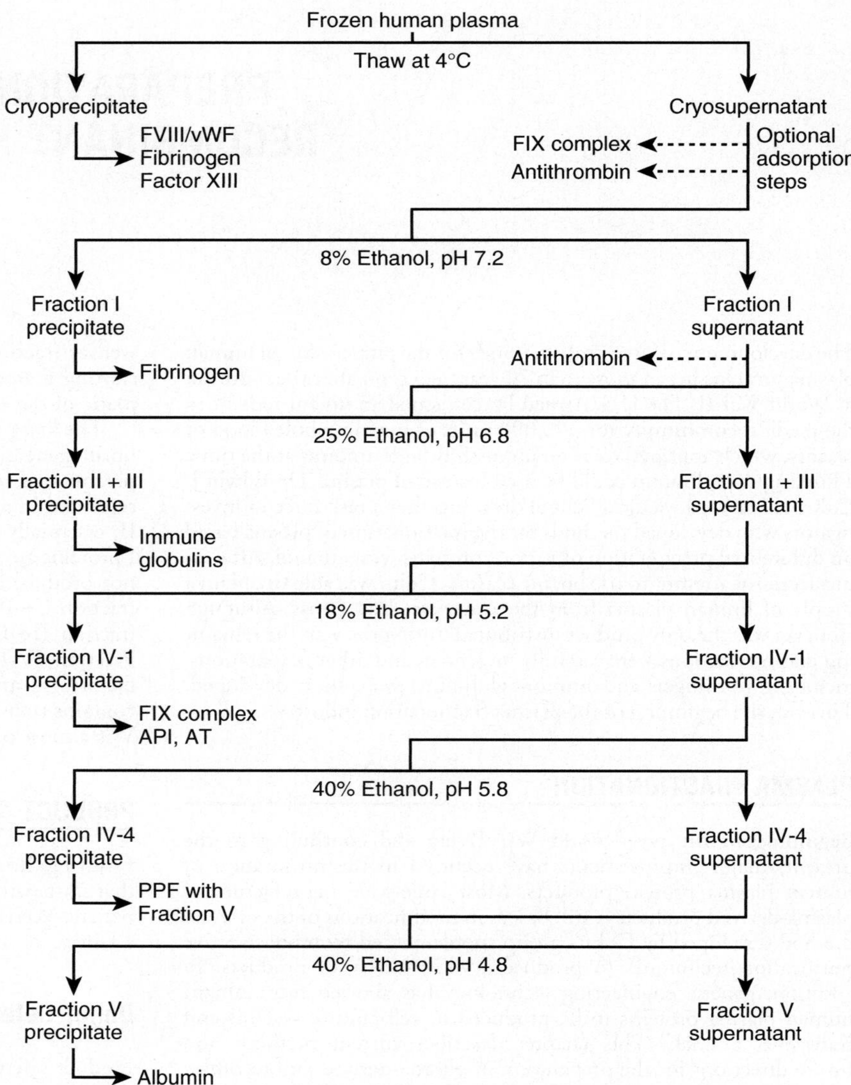

Figure 117-1 SCHEMATIC OF A TYPICAL PLASMA FRACTIONATION PROCESS. The *dashed lines* show optional steps. *API,* α_1-Proteinase inhibitor; *AT,* antithrombin; *FIX,* factor IX; *FVIII,* factor VIII; *PPF,* plasma protein fraction.

all purification processes. One of the early methods, still used today, was pasteurization of albumin; otherwise, except for donor screening and testing, most other early products had no antiviral treatment. That all changed with the AIDS crisis in the early 1980s, when many in the hemophilia community became infected with HIV from clotting factor concentrates.

Since then, many viral inactivation and removal methods have been developed, including various types of heat treatment, solvent and detergent treatment, and nanofiltration. Manufacturers have also realized that many of their purification methods remove viruses, which works well as long as they take steps to protect the treated products from recontamination. Many of those steps also remove prions, the agents of the transmissible spongiform encephalopathies.

The bottom line in all of this is that modern plasma-derived products are extremely safe, as shown both theoretically and by actual experience over the past 25 years. Still, many patients and physicians prefer recombinant products because of their perceived greater safety in terms of the future unknown, emergent virus.

PLASMA PRODUCTS

The following sections provide information about the plasma-derived and recombinant plasma protein products available in the United States in 2011. Additional details, including manufacturing and viral reduction methods, are listed in the tables for most products. The manufacturing methods were taken from prescribing information sheets provided with each product and from the published literature. However, most manufacturers consider their processes proprietary, so some descriptions are not very detailed.

FRESH-FROZEN PLASMA

Whole plasma is still used to treat various conditions, including as a source of coagulation proteins that are not available in purified form and for replacement of significant blood loss. Plasma from a single donor that has been separated from the red blood cells, placed in a freezer within 8 hours after phlebotomy, and stored at 18°C or less is labeled as fresh-frozen plasma (FFP). FFP undergoes essentially the same donor screening and donation testing as plasma for fractionation, but it is not treated for viral inactivation or removal. However, it still has a low risk of infectious disease transmission.

ALBUMIN AND PLASMA PROTEIN FRACTION

Albumin remains one of the major products of human plasma fractionation. Literally tons of albumin have been isolated and millions of units have been infused. Albumin recovered in very pure form in fraction V is pasteurized in the final vial for 10 hours at 60°C with sodium acetyltryptophanate and sodium caprylate added as stabilizers.

Albumin is a commodity product, with little to distinguish one manufacturer's product from another's. There are small differences in purity, but those are only clinically relevant in rare cases. Three albumin products are manufactured in the United States: albumin (human) 25% solution, albumin (human) 5% solution, and plasma protein fraction (PPF) (human). In albumin (human), more than 96% of the protein content must be albumin, but PPF, obtained by co-precipitating fraction IV-4 with fraction V, has a lower purity of greater than 83% albumin. PPF is more economical to produce than albumin, but the rapid infusion of PPF has been associated with hypotensive episodes.

IMMUNE GLOBULINS AND HYPERIMMUNE GLOBULINS

Since the early 1950s, immune globulin products have been prepared from Cohn fraction II + III by the method developed by Oncley, a collaborator of Cohn. The Oncley process uses additional ethanol precipitations to remove lipoproteins, immunoglobulin A (IgA), IgM, and other plasma proteins, leaving fraction II, which contains purified IgG. Whereas immune globulin is prepared from the plasma of unselected normal donors, hyperimmune globulins are prepared from the plasma of donors with high antibody titers against specific antigens (e.g., rho(D), hepatitis B, rabies, and tetanus). These donors may be identified during convalescent periods after infection or transfusion, or they may be specifically immunized to produce the desired antibodies. The immune globulin products are listed in Tables 117-1 and 117-2.

Intravenous Immune Globulin Concentrates

The original immune globulin concentrates, initially termed immune serum globulin and currently immune globulin (human), were administered by the intramuscular route, with the associated problems of limited injectable volume, poor bioavailability, and discomfort at the injection site. Intravenous (IV) injection of immune serum globulin causes serious clinical reactions, which are attributed to complement-activating aggregates in these products.

To overcome these limitations, immune globulin intravenous (human) (IGIV) products were developed using a variety of methods to remove or inactivate anticomplementary aggregates. Today most

Table 117-1 Immune Globulin Products*

Generic Name	Manufacturer or Distributor	Product Name (Product Form)	Purity IgA Content	Production Methods (Formulation)[†]	Virus Inactivation or Removal
Immune globulin (human)	Talecris	GamaSTAN S/D (15%-18% solution)	≥96% GG IgA: N/A	CP/CEF (glycine)	Purification steps, S/D, TSE
Immune globulin intravenous (human)	Baxter Healthcare	Gammagard S/D, S/D treatment IgA <2.2 µ/mL in a 5% solution (lyophilized)	≥90% GG IgA <2.2 µg/mL	CP/CEF, IEC (albumin, glycine, glucose, and PEG)	Purification steps, S/D
		Gammagard S/D, S/D treated, IgA <1 µ/mL in a 5% solution (lyophilized)	≥90% GG IgA <1 µg/mL	CP/CEF, IEC (albumin, glycine, glucose, and PEG)	Purification steps, S/D
		Gammagard liquid (10% solution)	≥98% GG IgA ≈37 µg/mL	CP/CEF, IEC (glycine)	S/D, NF, low pH
	Bio Products Laboratory/FFF Enterprises	Gammaplex, 5% liquid (5% solution)	>95% GG IgA <10 µg/mL	CP/CEF, IEC (glycine, sodium acetate, and P80)	S/D, NF, low pH
	CSL Behring	Carimune NF, nanofiltered, lyophilized preparation (lyophilized)	≥96% GG IgA: N/A	CP/CEF, pH 4/pepsin treatment (sucrose)	Purification steps, NF, low pH, DF, TSE
		Privigen, 10% liquid (10% solution)	≥98% GG IgA ≤25 µg/mL	CP/CEF, FAF, IEC (L-proline)	low pH, DF, NF, TSE
	Instituto Grifols/ Grifols Biologicals	Flebogamma 5% DIF (5% solution)	≥97% GG IgA ≤50 µg/mL	CP/CEF, PEG PPTN, IEC (D-sorbitol and PEG)	Purification steps, PEG PPTN, low pH, PST, S/D, NF
		Flebogamma 10% DIF (10% solution)	≥97% GG IgA ≤100 µg/mL	CP/CEF, PEG PPTN, IEC (D-sorbitol and PEG)	Purification steps, PEG PPTN, low pH, PST, S/D, NF, TSE
	Octapharma USA	Octagam, 5% liquid preparation (5% solution)	≥96% GG IgA ≤200 µg/mL	CP/CEF, CHR (maltose)	Purification steps, low pH, S/D
	Talecris	Gamunex-C, 10% caprylate/chromatography purified (10% solution)	≥98% GG IgA ≈46 µg/mL	CP/CEF, FAF, IEC (glycine)	Purification steps, FAF, DF, low pH, TSE
Immune globulin subcutaneous (human)	CSL Behring	Hizentra, 20% liquid (20% solution)	≥98% GG IgA ≤50 µg/mL	CP/CEF, FAF, IEC (L-proline and P80)	Low pH, DF, NF, TSE
		Vivaglobin, 16% liquid (16% solution)	≥96% GG IgA ≤1.7 µg/mL	CP/CEF, FAF (glycine)	Purification steps, PST

CHR, Chromatography (specific method not available); *CP/CEF*, cryoprecipitation/cold ethanol fractionation; *DF*, depth filtration; *FAF*, fatty acid fractionation; *GG*, gamma globulin; *IEC*, ion-exchange chromatography; *IgA*, immunoglobulin A; *N/A*, not available; *NF*, nanofiltration; *P80*, polysorbate 80; *PEG*, polyethylene glycol; *PPTN*, precipitation; *PST*, pasteurization (heat treatment in solution); *S/D*, solvent/detergent; *TSE*, validated for removal of transmissible spongiform encephalopathies. Various forms of filtration and ultrafiltration are common in plasma fractionation, so those steps are not listed.

*These products were marketed in the United States in 2011. Data were obtained from manufacturers, distributors, and available literature.

[†]Not including NaCl.

Table 117-2 Hyperimmune Globulin Products*

Generic Name	Manufacturer or Distributor	Product Name (Product Form)	Purity IgA Content	Production Methods (Formulation)†	Virus Inactivation or Removal
Botulism immune globulin intravenous (human)	MassBioLogics and Cangene/ FFF Enterprises Sponsored by California Department of Public Health	BabyBIG (lyophilized)	Antibotulism type A toxin ≥15 IU/mL antibotulism type B toxin ≥2.0 IU/mL % GG: N/A IgA: N/A	CEF (sucrose)	Purification steps, S/D, NF
Cytomegalovirus immune globulin intravenous (human)	CSL Behring	Cytogam, liquid formulation, S/D treated (5% solution)	Anti-CMV: N/A % GG: N/A IgA: N/A	CP/CEF (sucrose and albumin)	S/D
Hepatitis B immune globulin (human)	Biotest Pharmaceuticals	Nabi-HB, S/D treated and filtered (5% solution)	Anti-HBs >312 IU/mL % GG: N/A IgA ≤40 μg/mL	CEF (glycine and P80)	Purification steps, S/D, NF
	Talecris	HyperHEP B S/D, S/D treated (15%-18% solution)	Anti-HBs ≥220 IU/mL % GG: N/A IgA: N/A	CP/CEF (glycine)	Purification steps, S/D, TSE
Hepatitis B immune globulin intravenous (human)	Cangene/Cangene BioPharma	HepaGam B (5% solution)	Anti-HBs >312 IU/mL % GG: N/A IgA <40 μg/mL	IEC (maltose and P80)	Purification steps, S/D, NF
Rabies immune globulin (human)	Sanofi Pasteur	Imogam Rabies-HT, (10%-18% solution)	Anti-rabies ≥150 IU/mL % GG: N/A IgA: N/A	CEF (glycine)	Purification steps, PST
	Talecris	HyperRAB S/D, S/D treated (15%-18% solution)	Anti-rabies ≈150 IU/mL % GG: N/A IgA: N/A	CP/CEF (glycine)	Purification steps, S/D, TSE
Rh_o(D) immune globulin (human)	Ortho-Clinical Diagnostics	RhoGAM Ultra-Filtered PLUS (300 μg) (1500 IU) (5% solution)	Anti-D: 1500 IU/dose ≥98% GG IgA <15 μg/dose	CEF (glycine and P80)	Purification steps, S/D, NF
		MICRhoGAM ultra-filtered PLUS (50 μg) (250 IU) (5% solution)	Anti-D: 250 IU/dose ≥98% GG IgA <15 μg/dose	CEF (glycine and P80)	Purification steps, S/D, NF
	Talecris	HyperRHO S/D full dose, S/D treated (15%-18% solution)	Anti-D ≥1500 IU/dose % GG: N/A IgA: N/A	CEF (glycine)	Purification steps, S/D, TSE
Rh_o(D) immune globulin intravenous (human)	Cangene/Cangene BioPharma	WinRho SDF (liquid)	Anti-D ≈1150 IU/mL % GG: N/A IgA ≈5 μg/mL	IEC (maltose and P80)	Purification steps, S/D, NF
	CSL Behring	Rhophylac (3% solution)	Anti-D = 750 IU/mL ≥95% GG IgA <5 μg/mL	CP, IEC, AH (albumin and glycine)	Purification steps, S/D, NF
Tetanus immune globulin (human)	Talecris	HyperTET S/D, S/D treated (15%-18% Solution)	Tetanus antitoxin ≥250 μ/vial % GG: N/A IgA <5 μg/mL	CEF (glycine)	Purification steps, S/D, TSE
Vaccinia immune globulin intravenous (human)	Cangene	CNJ-016 (4%-7% frozen solution)	Anti-vaccinia ≥3300 U/mL % GG: N/A IgA <40 μg/mL	IEC (maltose and P80	Purification steps, S/D, NF

AH, Aluminum hydroxide adsorption; *CMV,* cytomegalovirus; *CP/CEF,* cryoprecipitation/cold ethanol fractionation; *GG,* gamma globulin; *HBs,* hepatitis B surface antigen; *HT,* heat treated; *IEC,* ion-exchange chromatography; *IgA,* immunoglobulin A; *NF,* nanofiltration; *P80,* polysorbate 80; *PST,* pasteurization (heat treatment in solution); *S/D,* solvent/detergent; *TSE,* validated for removal of transmissible spongiform encephalopathies. Various forms of filtration and ultrafiltration are common in plasma fractionation, so those steps are not listed.

*These products were marketed in the United States in 2011. Data were obtained from manufacturers, distributors, and available literature.

†Not including NaCl.

intramuscular immune globulin usage is limited to hyperimmune products. Although immune globulin products tend to be self-protecting from viral transmission because of the large pools of antibodies they contain, infections have occurred, and as a result, all manufacturers have incorporated viral inactivation or removal steps in the production of IGIV.

The development of IGIV has permitted the administration of much higher doses, with a subsequent expansion in immunoglobulin therapy. Although immune globulin products were originally also considered commodity products, the increased usage has led manufacturers to distinguish their products in various ways. As shown in the tables, products are available in both lyophilized and liquid forms, with various strengths and purities. IgA content and product formulation are also distinguishing factors.

Subcutaneous Immune Globulin Concentrates

The first patient treated for primary immune deficiency was actually given subcutaneous injections of immunoglobulins. However, as already described, intramuscular and later IV injection became the preferred methods. Recently, however, two immune globulin concentrates for subcutaneous injection, termed immune globulin subcutaneous (human), have been marketed. These products are intended for patients who have problems with IV infusion.

COAGULATION FACTOR CONCENTRATES

Transfusion of whole blood was shown in the mid-1800s to curtail bleeding in patients with hemophilia, and by 1940, bleeding episodes were being routinely treated with plasma. However, large amounts of plasma were needed, and this method of therapy could not provide normal levels of coagulation factors without producing hypervolemia. The development of more highly purified plasma-derived coagulation factor concentrates and more recently of recombinant concentrates has resulted in dramatic increases in quality of life and life expectancy for patients with hemophilia. Hemophilia treatment is a large market, and the development of improved coagulation factor concentrates continues to be a major focus of research.

FACTOR VIII CONCENTRATES

Factor VIII is the protein that is missing or defective in patients with hemophilia A. Factor VIII concentrates, generically termed antihemophilic factor (AHF) (human), for the treatment of hemophilia A have evolved from cryoprecipitates to very-high-purity plasma-derived products to recombinant products. The various AHF concentrates available in the United States are listed in Table 117-3.

Table 117-3 Antihemophilic Factor and von Willebrand Factor Concentrates*

Generic Name	Manufacturer or Distributor	Product Name	Specific Activity[†]	Production Methods	Virus Inactivation or Removal
Antihemophilic factor (human)	Baxter	Hemofil M, monoclonal purified	2-22 ≈2000[‡]	CP, CAP, IAC, IEC	Purification steps, S/D
	Talecris	Koate-DVI, S/D treated and heated in final container at 80°C	9-22 ≈50[‡]	CP, AH, PEG PPTN, glycine PPTN, SEC	Purification steps, S/D, HT
	CSL Behring	Monoclate-P, factor VIII:C pasteurized, monoclonal antibody purified	4-10 >3000[‡]	CP, CAP, AH, IAC, AC	Purification steps, PST
Antihemophilic factor/vWF complex (human)	CSL Behring	Humate-P	1-2 ≈40[‡] vWF/FVIII =2.4	CP, AH, glycine PPTN, NaCl PPTN	Purification steps, PST
	Grifols Biologicals	Alphanate	≥5 ≈150[‡] vWF/FVIII ≥0.4	CP, PEG PPTN, AC, NaCl PPTN;	Purification steps, S/D, HT, Lyo, TSE
vWF/coagulation factor VIII complex (human)	Octapharma/ Octapharma USA	Wilate	≥60 vWF/FVIII =1.0	CP, AH, IEC, SEC	Purification steps, S/D, HT
Antihemophilic factor (recombinant)	Baxter	Recombinate	2-20 >4000[‡]	CHO, IAC, IEC	Purification steps
	Bayer (also distributed as Helixate FS by CSL Behring)	Kogenate FS	2600-6800	BHK, IEC, IAC, IMAC	Purification steps, S/D, TSE
Antihemophilic factor (recombinant), plasma/ albumin-free method	Baxter	Advate	4000-10,000	CHO, IAC, IEC	S/D
Antihemophilic factor (recombinant), plasma/ albumin free	Wyeth	XYNTHA (B domain deleted)	5900-9900	CHO, IEC, AC, SEC	Purification steps, S/D, NF

AC, Affinity chromatography; *AH,* aluminum hydroxide adsorption; *BHK,* baby hamster kidney cell culture; *CAP,* cold acid precipitation; *CHO,* Chinese hamster ovary cell culture; *CP,* cryoprecipitation; *HT,* dry heat treatment; *IAC,* immunoaffinity chromatography; *IEC,* ion-exchange chromatography; *IMAC,* immobilized metal affinity chromatography; *Lyo,* lyophilization; *NF,* nanofiltration; *PEG,* polyethylene glycol; *PPTN,* precipitation; *PST,* pasteurization (heat treatment in solution); *S/D,* solvent/detergent; *SEC,* size exclusion chromatography; *TSE,* validated for removal of transmissible spongiform encephalopathies; *vWF,* von Willebrand factor. Various forms of filtration and ultrafiltration are common in plasma fractionation, so those steps are not listed.

*These concentrates were marketed in the United States in 2011. Data were obtained from manufacturers, distributors and available literature. All products are lyophilized.

[†]IU-factor VIII/μg of total protein.

[‡]Before addition of human albumin.

Cryoprecipitate

In a landmark discovery for hemophilia A treatment, cryoprecipitate was found in the mid-1950s to contain much of the factor VIII activity of the original plasma. By 1965, single-donor cryoprecipitate with factor VIII concentrations five to 30 times that of plasma became widely available for use in the treatment of patients with hemophilia A. Single-donor cryoprecipitate is still available from many blood banks but does carry a risk of viral transmission.

Intermediate- and High-Purity Antihemophilic Factor Concentrates

The development of AHF concentrates purified approximately 3000-fold over plasma was the next significant advance in the treatment of hemophilia A. Cryoprecipitate was used as the starting material, and a variety of methods were developed to remove fibrinogen, immunoglobulins, and other contaminating proteins. These were the mainstay of hemophilia A treatment for many years and are still available, their chief advantage being lower cost. Some of these products are also indicated as a source of vWF, which circulates in a complex with factor VIII. Products purified 5000- to 20,000-fold over plasma were subsequently developed using various chromatographic methods, but they have primarily been supplanted by immunoaffinity-purified products in the United States.

Immunoaffinity-Purified Concentrates

The next major advance in the preparation of AHF concentrates was the use of murine monoclonal antibodies (mAbs) immobilized on a chromatographic column for the purification of factor VIII. Factor VIII concentrates partially purified by conventional means are applied to an immunoaffinity column that binds either factor VIII directly or the factor VIII–vWF complex. The columns are washed extensively to remove unwanted proteins and then eluted with a solution that disrupts the antibody binding. A final chromatography step removes the harsh elution solutions as well as any mAb that might have leached off the column to produce a factor VIII concentrate that is essentially pure before the addition of albumin as a stabilizer.

Recombinant Antihemophilic Factor Concentrates

One of the remarkable early accomplishments of molecular biology was the elucidation of the structure of factor VIII, its molecular cloning, and the successful production of two recombinant human factor VIII products, Recombinate and Kogenate. Because proper posttranslational processing is essential for factor VIII functionality, the products are produced in mammalian cells, either baby hamster kidney (BHK) cells or Chinese hamster ovary (CHO) cells. The CHO cells used to produce Recombinate also coexpress recombinant vWF, which helps to stabilize the factor VIII and substantially increase its recovery from the culture medium, but is completely removed by subsequent processing. Recombinant factor VIII is purified by various combinations of immunoaffinity chromatography, ion-exchange chromatography, and gel filtration.

One of the major driving forces for development of recombinant products is viral safety; they are seen as inherently safer because they are not produced from plasma. However, the first generation of recombinant products used animal-derived proteins and sera in their cell culture media and in the production of the monoclonal antibodies used for purification, plus human albumin to stabilize the products in the final vial, all potential sources of viral contamination. With this in mind, manufacturers went still further to develop recombinant products completely free of human and animal proteins, both in their production processes and in their formulations. Most current production methods for recombinant products also incorporate viral inactivation or removal procedures for an added measure of safety.

One of the potential benefits of recombinant technology is the ability to design completely new proteins that do not occur in nature, ones that potentially perform better or are easier to produce than their natural counterparts. The factor VIII molecule is a multidomain complex consisting of a heavy chain with A1, A2, and B domains and a light chain consisting of A3, C1, and C2 domains. Previous research had shown that the B domain is not necessary for coagulant activity, so a B domain–deleted product, ReFacto, was developed. Eliminating the B domain, which is highly glycosylated, increased the expression of the molecule as much as 20-fold over full-length factor VIII. ReFacto was subsequently replaced by Xyntha after several improvements, including replacing immunoaffinity purification with a synthetic peptide ligand affinity column.

FACTOR IX CONCENTRATES

Factor IX is the protein that is missing or defective in patients with hemophilia B. Two types of plasma-derived factor IX concentrates are available today: factor IX complex, which contains significant amounts of the other vitamin K-dependent (VKD) clotting factors, and coagulation factor IX (human), a preparation substantially free of these other proteins. A recombinant product, coagulation factor IX (recombinant) is also available. The factor IX concentrates available in the United States are listed in Table 117-4.

Factor IX Complex Concentrates

The VKD proteins are serine proteases that include clotting factors II, VII, IX, and X and the anticoagulants protein C and protein S. Because of their similar structures, they tend to co-purify by most of the methods used to isolate them from plasma. Thus the original factor IX products for treatment of hemophilia B were mixtures of the VKD proteins. Because the protein in highest concentration in these products is prothrombin (factor II), they have also been identified as prothrombin complex concentrates (PCCs); however, factor IX complex is the generic name in the United States.

The VKD proteins were originally adsorbed from either cryo-poor plasma or fraction IV-4 using tricalcium phosphate. Later, ion exchange chromatography resins were used with cryo-poor plasma with the advantage that the supernatant plasma can then be further fractionated by the Cohn method for the production of immune globulins, albumin, and other products with little loss in yield.

Coagulation Factor IX Concentrates

With the widespread use of factor IX complex, it became apparent that serious thromboembolic episodes and acute myocardial infarction were major complications of its infusion, especially when used in large quantities for extended periods, such as for surgical procedures and in patients with liver disease. The cause of the thrombogenicity has not been conclusively determined, but the problem led to the development of more highly purified concentrates that are essentially free of the other VKD clotting factors. These products are designated coagulation factor IX (human). Of the two products available in the United States, one is prepared by immunoaffinity chromatography using a monoclonal antibody to factor IX, and the other is purified by heparin affinity chromatography. These preparations have proven to be largely nonthrombogenic in clinical use.

Recombinant Factor IX Concentrates

A recombinant coagulation factor IX, BeneFIX, has also been developed. It is produced in cell culture by CHO cells that also coexpress furin, a protease that enhances the ability of the cells to remove the amino-terminal propeptide. The factor IX protein secreted into the cell culture medium is purified using several chromatography steps. As

Table 117-4 Factor IX and Other Coagulation Factor and Anticoagulant Concentrates*

Generic Name	Manufacture or Distributor	Product Name	Specific Activity[†]	Purification Methods	Virus Inactivation or Removal Methods
Factor IX complex	Baxter	Bebulin VH, vapor heated	2	CP/CEF, IEC	VHT
	Grifols Biologicals	Profilnine SD, S/D treated	4	CP/CEF, IEC	Purification steps, S/D
Coagulation factor IX (human)	CSL Behring	Mononine, monoclonal antibody purified	≥190	CP/CEF, IEC, IAC, HIC	Purification steps, CT, UF
	Grifols Biologicals	AlphaNine SD, S/D treated/virus filtered	≥150	CP/CEF, IEC, BCA, AC	purification steps, S/D, NF
Coagulation factor IX (recombinant)	Wyeth	BeneFIX	≥200	CHO, IEC, AC, IMAC	NF
Anti-inhibitor coagulant complex	Baxter	FEIBA NF, nanofiltered and vapor heated	N/A	CP/CEF, IEC, surface activation	Purification steps, VHT, NF
Coagulation factor VIIa (recombinant)	Novo Nordisk	NovoSeven RT, room temperature stable	N/A	BHK, autocatalytic activation, IEC, IAC	Purification steps
Fibrinogen concentrate (human)	CSL Behring	RiaSTAP	N/A	CP, AH, glycine PPTN	Purification steps, PST
Factor XIII concentrate (human)	CSL Behring	Corifact	N/A	CP/CEF, AH, VC, IEC	Purification steps, PST
Antithrombin III (human)	Talecris	Thrombate III	N/A	CP/CEF, AC	PST, TSE
Antithrombin III (recombinant)	GTC Biotherapeutics/ Lundbeck	ATryn	>99% AT	TGM, AC, IEC, HIC	Purification steps, HT, NF
Protein C concentrate (human)	Baxter	CEPROTIN	N/A	CP/CEF, IAC, IEC	Purification steps, P80, VHT
Drotrecogin alfa (activated [activated protein C])	Eli Lilly	Xigris	N/A	HCC, TA, IAC	None

AC, Affinity chromatography; *AH,* aluminum hydroxide adsorption; *AT,* antithrombin; *BCA,* barium citrate adsorption; *BHK,* baby hamster kidney cell culture; *CHO,* Chinese hamster ovary cell culture; *CP/CEF,* cryoprecipitation/cold ethanol fractionation; *CT,* chemical treatment; *HCC,* human cell culture; *HIC,* hydrophobic interaction chromatography; *HT,* heat treatment; *IAC,* immunoaffinity chromatography; *IEC,* ion-exchange chromatography; *IMAC,* immobilized metal affinity chromatography; *N/A,* not available or not applicable; *NF,* nanofiltration; *P80,* polysorbate 80; *PPTN,* precipitation; *PST,* pasteurization; *S/D,* solvent/detergent; *TA,* thrombin activation; *TGM,* transgenic goat milk; *UF,* ultrafiltration; *TSE,* validated for removal of transmissible spongiform encephalopathies; *VHT,* vapor heat treatment. Various forms of filtration and ultrafiltration are common in plasma fractionation, so those steps are not listed.
*These concentrates were marketed in the United States in 2011. Data were obtained from manufacturers, distributors, and available literature.
[†]IU-factor IX/μg of total protein.

with the latest generation AHF products, BeneFIX is produced without human or animal proteins and includes a nanofiltration step to remove any viruses that might be present. The final product has been shown to be structurally and functionally similar to plasma-derived factor IX. However, it has a lower recovery when infused into patients, apparently because of differences in posttranslational glycosylation.

OTHER COAGULATION AND ANTICOAGULANT CONCENTRATES

Now that the risk of infection has essentially been eliminated, the major complication in hemophilia treatment is the development of inhibitors, antibodies directed against factor VIII or factor IX. Low-titer inhibitors can usually be saturated by administering large amounts of factor VIII or factor IX, but this is not an effective therapy for higher-titer inhibitors. There are two primary means of treating bleeding in inhibitor patients, both based on administration of activated clotting factors. Many of the clotting factors circulate as inactive zymogens that are only activated as needed in the coagulation cascade.

Factor IX complex was known to be somewhat effective in preventing bleeding in inhibitor patients, possibly because it contains small amounts of activated clotting factors. That may be the same reason that it can be thrombogenic, but that idea has not been proven conclusively. Based on that information, two activated factor IX complex products were developed, one of which, FEIBA, is still available. FEIBA, which is named for factor eight inhibitor bypassing activity, is generically named anti-inhibitor coagulant complex and is indicated for inhibitor treatment in both hemophilia A and B.

The hypothesis that administration of activated clotting factors can bypass inhibitors also led to the development of NovoSeven, a recombinant activated factor VII concentrate. NovoSeven is produced in tissue culture in BHK cells and purified by ion-exchange and immunoaffinity chromatography. It spontaneously activates during the final ion-exchange chromatography steps. NovoSeven has been extensively studied and is currently the most widely used option for inhibitor treatment, especially for patients who have never been exposed to plasma-derived products. However, both FEIBA and NovoSeven do carry a risk of thromboembolic complications. FEIBA and NovoSeven are listed in Table 117-4.

von Willebrand disease (vWD), caused by missing or abnormal vWF, is actually the most commonly inherited coagulation disorder. vWF is a large protein that circulates in a complex with factor VIII. It stabilizes factor VIII in the bloodstream but also has coagulation functions of its own. There are several types of vWD, some of which behave similarly to hemophilia A because of the missing protection for factor VIII. Several intermediate-purity viral-inactivated AHF concentrates that contain significant amounts of vWF are also indicated for replacement therapy for vWD. These vWF/AHF concentrates are listed in Table 117-3.

Fibrinogen is the final protein in the coagulation cascade. It is cleaved by thrombin to form fibrin, a protein that naturally self-associates to form a clot. RiaSTAP is a plasma-derived concentrate for replacement therapy in fibrinogen-deficient patients that is made from the concentrated fibrinogen in cryoprecipitate. Interestingly, fibrinogen was also one of the first plasma products used, but it was soon taken off the market because it almost universally transmitted viral infections. RiaSTAP is pasteurized (heat treated) in solution for 20 hours at 60°C, twice as long as the typical treatment for pasteurized plasma products. Significant viral removal has also been demonstrated for its purification process, and the resulting product is considered safe.

Factor XIII does not participate directly in the coagulation cascade but instead stabilizes the final clot by cross-linking the fibrin molecules. Factor XIII deficiency is rare and is characterized by weak clots prone to rebleeding. Patients deficient in factor XIII have hemarthroses and deep tissue bleeds. Before the availability of factor XIII concentrates, patients were usually treated with plasma or cryoprecipitate, both of which carry a risk of viral infection. Corifact, the only factor XIII product available in the United States, is purified from cryoprecipitate and employs a unique process step using Vitacel, a wheat-based vegetable fiber, to remove fibrinogen, after which the factor XIII is further purified by ion exchange chromatography. The final product is pasteurized. RiaSTAP and Corifact are listed in Table 117-4.

Anticoagulant Concentrates

Antithrombin III, now generally just called antithrombin (AT), is an anticoagulant. As its name suggests, it inhibits thrombin (activated factor II), but it also inhibits the activated forms of factors IX, X, XI, and XII. It belongs to the serpin family named for their activity as serine protease inhibitors. Heparin is a cofactor that increases the native activity of AT significantly, from 500- to 1000-fold for factor Xa inhibition up to one million–fold for factor IXa inhibition. The clinical utility of heparin as an anticoagulant is because of its cofactor activity; in the absence of AT, heparin has little effect.

The affinity of AT for heparin is also used to purify the protein by affinity chromatography on an immobilized heparin column. Thrombate III, the only plasma-derived product currently on the U.S. market, is purified by heparin affinity chromatography from Cohn fraction IV-1, but as shown in Figure 117-1, AT is also found in cryo-poor plasma or Cohn fraction I supernatant. ATryn, a recombinant AT, was the first recombinant human plasma protein produced in transgenic animals to be approved anywhere. It is made in the milk of goats and also purified by heparin affinity chromatography. The two available AT concentrates are listed in Table 117-4.

Protein C is a serine protease with a structure similar to clotting factors II, VII, IX, and X, but it is an anticoagulant that cleaves activated factors V and VIII. Patients deficient in protein C are susceptible to thrombosis. One plasma-derived protein C concentrate, CEPROTIN, is available. A recombinant human activated protein C, Xigris, is also available, but it is not indicated for treatment of protein C–deficient patients. It is intended for treatment of severe sepsis, but its efficacy is controversial. The two protein C products are listed in Table 117-4.

Fibrin Sealant and Thrombin

Fibrinogen and thrombin are also used as topical hemostatic agents, together as fibrin sealant and as stand-alone thrombin concentrates. The fibrin sealant and thrombin products available in the United States are listed in Table 117-5.

Fibrin sealant uses the clot-forming reaction of thrombin and fibrinogen to form a physiological glue or sealant that has become widely used in surgical procedures. All three fibrin sealant products on the U.S. market are made from human plasma–derived fibrinogen and thrombin. Fibrinogen is purified directly from cryoprecipitate followed by further purification steps. ARTISS and TISSEEL contain a plasmin inhibitor, synthetic aprotinin, which is a non–animal-sourced product, to delay clot lysis. EVICEL contains a more highly purified fibrinogen component that has minimal plasmin activity and therefore does not contain a clot lysis inhibitor. Both fibrinogen preparations contain residual factor XIII for clot stabilization, and additional factor XIII is recruited from the patient's bloodstream during use.

Table 117-5 Fibrin Sealants and Thrombin Concentrates*

Generic Name	Manufacturer or Distributor	Product Name (Product Format)	Purification Methods	Virus Inactivation or Removal Methods
Fibrin sealant (human)	Baxter	ARTISS (frozen solution and lyophilized powder)	Fibrinogen: CP, OS Thrombin: IEC, CA	Both components: purification steps, VHT, S/D
		TISSEEL (frozen solution and lyophilized powder)	Fibrinogen: CP, OS Thrombin: IEC, CA	Both components: purification steps, VHT, S/D
	OMRIX/Ethicon	EVICEL (frozen solution)	Fibrinogen: CP, AH, HIC, AC Thrombin component: CP, IEC, CA	Fibrinogen component: S/D, PST Thrombin component: S/D, NF
Absorbable fibrin sealant patch	Nycomed/Baxter	TachoSil (lyophilized [equine collagen sponge coated with fibrinogen, thrombin, and albumin])	Fibrinogen: CP, glycine PPTN, AH, HIC, AC Thrombin: CP, CHR, AS, CTA Albumin: CEF	Fibrinogen and thrombin: purification steps Albumin: PST Collagen: low pH, GI Final product: GI
Thrombin, topical U.S.P. (bovine origin)	GenTrac/King Pharmaceuticals (Pfizer)	Thrombin-JMI (lyophilized)	Thrombin: BP, IEC, thromboplastin activation, NF Bovine thromboplastin: GBL, MHA, AS	Purification steps, NF, TSE
Thrombin topical (human)	OMRIX Biopharmaceuticals/ Ethicon	EVITHROM (frozen solution)	CP, IEC, CA	S/D, NF
Thrombin, topical (recombinant)	ZymoGenics	RECOTHROM (lyophilized)	CHO, enzymatic activation, AC, IEC	S/D, NF

AC, Affinity chromatography; *AH,* aluminum hydroxide adsorption; *AS,* ammonium sulfate precipitation; *BP,* bovine plasma; *CA,* calcium activation; *CEF,* cold ethanol fractionation; *CHO,* Chinese hamster ovary cell culture; *CHR,* chromatography (specific method not available); *CP,* cryoprecipitation; *CTA,* citrate activation; *GBL,* ground bovine lung tissue; *GI,* gamma irradiation; *HIC,* hydrophobic interaction chromatography; *IEC,* ion-exchange chromatography; *MHA,* magnesium hydroxide gel adsorption; *NF,* nanofiltration; *OS,* other steps, not specified; *PPTN,* precipitation; *PST,* pasteurization; *S/D,* solvent/detergent; *TSE,* validated for removal of transmissible spongiform encephalopathies; *VHT,* vapor heat treatment. Various forms of filtration and ultrafiltration are common in plasma fractionation, so those steps are not listed.
*These concentrates were marketed in the United States in 2011. Data were obtained from manufacturers, distributors, and available literature.

Thrombin is purified from prothrombin (factor II) in the factor IX complex captured by ion exchange from cryosupernatant plasma. Prothrombin is autocatalytically activated to thrombin in the presence of calcium. Both the fibrinogen and thrombin components are also treated for viral inactivation and removal.

Three stand-alone thrombin products are also available for use in promoting topical hemostasis. For years, bovine thrombin was the standard of care for such use; however, research has suggested that it may have been responsible for postsurgical hemostatic problems in some patients. The cause was apparently contamination with bovine factor V, against which some patients developed antibodies that cross-reacted with their own human factor V. Most bovine thrombin products were taken off the market, but Thrombin-JMI, the sole remaining bovine product, was instead further purified to reduce bovine factor V to undetectable levels. A plasma-derived human thrombin product, EVITHROM, was also developed, which is the same thrombin used in EVICEL fibrin sealant.

A recombinant human thrombin product, RECOTHROM, is another example of a bioengineered protein. The VKD clotting factors contain a domain called the Gla region that is rich in a unique amino acid, γ-carboxyglutamic acid (Gla). The posttranslational modifications required to produce the Gla residues are a rate-limiting step in the production of all of the VKD proteins in cell culture. Presence of the Gla region is absolutely necessary for the function of most of the clotting factors but not for thrombin. Therefore, the Gla-less molecule prethrombin-1 is actually produced in the CHO cells, with a significant increase in production rate. Prethrombin-1 is activated to thrombin using a proprietary enzyme system. RECOTHROM behaves similarly to human and bovine thrombin in clinical use.

PLASMA PROTEINASE INHIBITORS

The proteinase inhibitors that are present in human plasma play critical roles in the regulation of the coagulation, fibrinolytic, complement, and kinin cascade systems. Most of these inhibitors have similar amino acid and structural properties and are members of a superfamily of proteins called serpins (serine proteinase inhibitors). AT, an anticoagulant, was discussed earlier. Two other proteinase inhibitors, API and C1 esterase inhibitor, are also available for treatment of deficient patients. These concentrates are listed in Table 117-6.

α_1-Proteinase Inhibitor

α_1-Proteinase inhibitor (human), also known as α_1-antitrypsin, was the first of the serpins to be isolated and characterized. Although the protein was originally named for its antitrypsin activity, its primary physiologic function appears to be the inhibition of neutrophil elastase in the lung. Patients with hereditary deficiencies of this inhibitor develop pulmonary emphysema and liver disease. API replacement therapy is indicated for chronic treatment of individuals with hereditary deficiency. However, even with four products available, the supply is tight because of the limited amount ultimately available from plasma. One issue is the poor efficiency of IV administration. It is estimated that only approximately 2% of the infused API ends up in the lung. Studies have suggested that aerosol delivery of API directly into the lungs by inhalation would be efficacious and could replace IV administration because of its lower cost and greater convenience. API is also a good candidate for recombinant production.

C1 Esterase Inhibitor

C1 esterase inhibitor acts as a regulator in the complement and fibrinolytic systems and as an inhibitor of factor XIIa and kallikrein. Its name comes from its inhibition of the complement proteins C1r and C1s. Patients deficient in C1 esterase inhibitor are at risk for attacks of hereditary angioedema. Two plasma-derived C1 esterase inhibitor concentrates were licensed in the United States in 2008 and 2009 after being available in Europe for a number of years. CINRYZE is indicated for prophylactic replacement therapy for prevention of hereditary angioedema, while Berinert is only indicated for acute treatment of hereditary angioedema. The products are listed in Table 117-6, but detailed descriptions of their manufacturing processes are not available.

FUTURE DIRECTIONS

New Plasma-Derived Concentrates

With licensure of a number of new products in the past few years, including protein C, vWF, factor XIII and C1 esterase inhibitor, the United States is catching up with Europe and other parts of the world. Concentrates of factor VII and factor XI are also available elsewhere.

Table 117-6 Alpha$_1$-Proteinase Inhibitor and C1 Esterase Inhibitor Concentrates

Generic Name	Manufacturer or Distributor	Product Name (Product Format)	Potency* Specific Activity (SA)	Purification Methods	Virus Inactivation or Removal Methods
Alpha$_1$-proteinase inhibitor (human)	Baxter	Aralast NP, S/D treated, nanofiltered (lyophilized)	≥16 mg API/mL ≥0.55 mg/mg-protein	CP/CEF, PEG PPTN, $ZnCl_2$ PPTN, IEC	Purification steps, S/D, NF
	CSL Behring	Zemaira (lyophilized)	≈50 mg API/mL ≥0.7 mg/mg-protein	CP/CEF, EXTN, DST, IEC, HC	PST, NF
	Kamada/Baxter	GLASSIA (liquid)	20 mg/mL SA: N/A	CP/CEF, CHR	S/D, NF
	Talecris	Prolastin-C (lyophilized)	≈50 mg API/mL ≥0.7 mg/mg-protein	CP/CEF, PEG PPTN, IEC	Purification steps, S/D, NF, TSE
C1 esterase inhibitor (human)	CSL Behring	Berinert (lyophilized)	N/A	HIC, IEC, AS	Purification steps, PST
	Sanquin Blood Supply Foundation/ViroPharma Biologics	CINRYZE (lyophilized)	N/A	CHR, PEG pptn	Purification steps, PST, NF

AC, Affinity chromatography; *ADS,* adsorption (no further details available); *AH,* aluminum hydroxide adsorption; *API,* α_1-proteinase inhibitor; *AS,* ammonium sulfate precipitation; *BP,* bovine plasma; *CA,* calcium activation; *CEF,* cold ethanol fractionation; *CHO,* Chinese hamster ovary cell culture; *CHR,* chromatography (specific method not available); *CP/CEF,* cryoprecipitation/cold ethanol fractionation; *CTA,* citrate activation; *DST,* dithiothreitol and silicon dioxide treatment; *EXTN,* extraction (specific details not available); *GBL,* ground bovine lung; *GI,* gamma irradiation; *HC,* hydrophobic chromatography; *IEC,* ion-exchange chromatography; *MHA,* magnesium hydroxide gel adsorption; *N/A,* not available; *NF,* nanofiltration; *PEG,* polyethylene glycol; *PPTN,* precipitation; *S/D,* solvent/detergent; *VHT,* vapor heat treatment. Various forms of filtration and ultrafiltration are common in plasma fractionation, so those steps are not listed.

*These concentrates were marketed in the United States in 2011. Data were obtained from manufacturers, distributors, and available literature.

Several other proteins in plasma would be potentially useful as therapeutic products, including butyrylcholinesterase for reversal of succinylcholine-induced apnea and treatment of cocaine overdose and other coagulation factors and inhibitors, such as factors X and XII and protein S. However, the prevalence of these disorders is small, so they would be true orphan drugs with limited markets. There are also potential improvements that can be made to current plasma-derived and recombinant concentrates. In addition to enhanced purification and viral clearance methods, products can be made more user friendly. For instance, prophylactic treatment of hemophilia A and B currently requires infusions every 2 or 3 days because of the short natural half-lives of the proteins in the circulation. Several companies are developing factor VIII and IX products with longer half-lives by coupling the molecules to polyethylene glycol, the immunoglobulin Fc domain, or albumin.

Alternate delivery systems could also potentially improve the utility of many products. Delivery of clotting factors by inhalation, ingestion, and subcutaneous injection has been explored. As mentioned earlier, several studies have looked at aerosol delivery of API. Production of fibrin sealant in a powder form that could be sprinkled on a wound has also been studied.

Recombinant Plasma Protein Concentrates

Almost all plasma proteins licensed for human use have been cloned and expressed in biologically active form in animal cells in the laboratory, and several have been developed into licensed products, as described earlier. The main advantages of recombinantly produced proteins include freedom from human viruses and a potentially unlimited supply. AT has already been produced in the milk of transgenic animals, and others such as API, which are required in relatively large amounts, are also candidates. Transgenic cows, goats, pigs, and sheep can produce large quantities of human proteins, typically 1 to 10 g/L in milk. In contrast, animal tissue culture systems routinely produce substantially less protein, typically 0.01 to 0.1 g/L.

Recombinant proteins can also be produced in modified forms that may give them advantageous new properties such as increased potency, longer half-lives, or varied specificity. One product already available is B domain–deleted factor VIII described earlier.

SUGGESTED READINGS

General Overviews of Plasma Products and Production Methods

Burnouf T: Modern plasma fractionation. *Transfus Med Rev* 21:101, 2007.

Farrugia A, Robert P: Plasma protein therapies: Current and future perspectives. *Best Pract Res Clin Haematol* 19:243, 2006.

Hooper JA: Intravenous immunoglobulins: Evolution of commercial IVIG preparations. *Immunol Allergy Clin North Am* 28:765, 2008.

Key NS, Negrier C: Coagulation factor concentrates: Past, present, and future. *Lancet* 370:439, 2007.

Ofosu FA, Freedman J, Semple JW: Plasma-derived biological medicines used to promote haemostasis. *Thromb Haemost* 99:851, 2008.

Thiele T, Steil L, et al: Proteomics of blood-based therapeutics, a promising tool for quality assurance in transfusion medicine. *Biodrugs* 21:179, 2007.

Recombinant Plasma Products

Burnouf T: Recombinant plasma proteins. *Vox Sang* 100:68, 2011.

Grillberger L, Kreil TR, et al: Emerging trends in plasma-free manufacturing of recombinant protein therapeutics expressed in mammalian cells. *Biotechnol J* 4:186, 2009.

Houdebine LM: Production of pharmaceutical proteins by transgenic animals. *Comp Immunol Microbiol Infect Dis* 32:107, 2009.

Pipe SW: Hemophilia: New protein therapeutics. *Hematology Am Soc Hematol Educ Program* 2010: 203, 2010.

Pipe SW: Recombinant clotting factors. *Thromb Haemost* 99:840, 2008.

Safety of Plasma Products

Cai K, Gierman TM, et al: Ensuring the biologic safety of plasma-derived therapeutic proteins: Detection, inactivation, and removal of pathogens. *BioDrugs* 19:79, 2005.

Dolan G: Clinical implications of emerging pathogens in haemophilia: The variant Creutzfeldt-Jakob disease experience. *Haemophilia* 12:16, 2006.

Jorquera JI: Safety procedures of coagulation factors. *Haemophilia* 13:41, 2007.

MacLennan S, Barbara JA: Risks and side effects of therapy with plasma and plasma fractions. *Best Pract Res Clin Haematol* 19:169, 2006.

Turner ML, Ludlam CA: An update on the assessment and management of the risk of transmission of variant Creutzfeldt-Jakob disease by blood and plasma products. *Br J Haematol* 144:14, 2009.

History of Plasma Product Production

Cohn EJ, Strong LE, et al: Preparation and properties of serum and plasma proteins. IV. a system for the separation into fractions of the protein and lipoprotein components of biological tissues and fluids. *J Am Chem Soc* 68:459, 1946.

Palmer JW: The evolution of large-scale human plasma fractionation in the United States. In Sgouris JR, Rene A, editors: *Proceedings of the Workshop on Albumin,* Washington, DC, 1976, DHEW Publication No. (NIH) 76-925, US Government Printing Office.

CHAPTER 118

TRANSFUSION THERAPY FOR COAGULATION FACTOR DEFICIENCIES

Elizabeth Roman, Peter J. Larson, and Catherine S. Manno

This chapter reviews products available to treat deficiencies of plasma coagulation proteins. The development of blood component therapy and subsequently protein concentrates that are enriched in particular coagulation factors and other proteins made possible the effective treatment of bleeding episodes in patients with hemophilia and other diatheses. In the 1940s, a collaborative effort funded by the U.S. government was undertaken among protein scientists with the goal of rapidly developing a method to isolate albumin from human plasma to provide a lyophilized intravascular volume expander for use in the military. As part of this effort, Dr. Edwin Cohn developed an ethanol fractionation procedure that was amenable to large-scale manufacture.[1] Building on the foundation of the Cohn fractionation procedure (see Chapter 117), the first coagulation factor concentrates were developed in the mid-1960s and provided a safer and more effective treatment for patients with the X-linked coagulation deficiencies, hemophilia A and B. Given the limited human plasma resource as a raw material for production of all but a few coagulation protein concentrates, manufacturers of human plasma–based products attempt to derive the maximum yield from each pool of plasma. Manufacturers of plasma-derived products strive to maximize the therapeutic potential of pooled human plasma by deriving more products from these processes.

Development of recombinant products has been fueled by concerns of infectious disease transmission through the human plasma resource. Currently licensed products are produced in mammalian cell culture to optimize necessary posttranslational modifications required for biologic activity. These recombinant expression processes are complicated and expensive. Transgenic recombinant technology is currently being explored as a way to decrease or eliminate reliance on the human plasma resource and the technically rigorous production of recombinant proteins using mammalian cell culture methods.

HEMOPHILIA A AND B

The hemophilias are X-linked disorders caused by deficiencies of either factor VIII (hemophilia A, or classic hemophilia) or factor IX (hemophilia B, or Christmas disease). The genes for these coagulation factors are located in close proximity on the long arm of the X chromosome. Whereas hemophilia A affects one in 10,000 males, hemophilia B affects one in 30,000. This difference in incidence is roughly correlated with the size of the genes, and more than 30% of cases arise from spontaneous mutations.

The major morbidity of the severe hemophilias A and B is arthropathy, developing over the course of years in untreated or undertreated adults as a result of recurrent spontaneous joint bleeding. The major cause of hemorrhagic mortality is bleeding into critical closed spaces (e.g., intracranial or retroperitoneal).[2] Central nervous system (CNS) bleeding occurs in 3% to 14% of patients, and mortality from CNS hemorrhage ranges from 20% to 50%[3-5] with neurologic sequelae (including seizures, motor impairment, or mental retardation) observed in 40% to 50% of survivors.[3] CNS bleeding episodes occur predominantly in patients with severe disease (<1% factor level).[3] A more detailed discussion of the hemophilias and the molecular biology of factors VIII and IX can be found in Chapters 137.

TRANSFUSION THERAPY OF HEMOPHILIA A AND B

History of Transfusion for Hemophilia

Transfusion was first proposed by Schönlein and his student Hopf in 1832 as a treatment for "bleeders" who were suffering from exsanguinating hemorrhage, and these two were likely the first to have used the term *Haemophilie* to describe the disease.[6,7] The first effective transfusion-based intervention for hemophilia is credited to Samuel Lane who, in 1840, infused 10 to 12 oz of fresh human blood into a 12-year-old boy with postoperative hemorrhage after eye surgery for correction of a squint.[8] Subsequently, a variety of interventions using the infusion of human and animal blood and blood derivatives were used in the therapy of hemorrhage in patients with congenital bleeding diatheses (Table 118-1). Citrated plasma was first used in 1923 for the treatment of hemophilia by Feissly to overcome a major ABO incompatibility in a father-to-son transfusion.[9] Development of modern blood banking in the 1930s and expansion of transfusion during and after World War II allowed for more widespread use of whole blood and subsequently frozen plasma in the treatment of hemophilia. Because of limited availability, the use of whole blood and components of whole blood for the treatment of hemophilia and other diseases was initially confined to larger metropolitan areas. In addition, volume constraints with the infusion of whole blood and plasma made the achievement of high plasma levels of coagulation factors (>5%) difficult.[10]

The advent of modern transfusion therapy for hemophilia came with the observation that the cold-insoluble precipitate remaining after thawing of frozen plasma at 4 °C contains high concentrations of factor VIII.[11] Application of this procedure to the separation of components of whole blood[12] allowed for the production of a low-volume blood product known as *cryoprecipitate.* Cryoprecipitate derived from a single whole blood collection contains approximately 125 U of factor VIII and quickly replaced frozen plasma as the therapy of choice for the treatment of bleeding episodes in hemophilia A in the 1960s. The availability of cryoprecipitate made the treatment of bleeding episodes by patients in their homes, rather than at a hospital, a reality. In addition, the development of quantitative assays for factor VIII[13] and for factor IX[14] meant that the two diseases could now be distinguished and effects of transfusion therapy on circulating levels of factors could be more accurately assessed.

Before the discovery of plasma cryoprecipitate, significant advances had been made in the fractionation of plasma using ethanol,[1] glycine,[15] polyethylene glycol,[16] a combination of glycine and polyethylene glycol,[17] and calcium or barium[18-20] to precipitate plasma proteins. These techniques, in conjunction with cold precipitation of frozen plasma, laid the groundwork that resulted in the production of the first factor VIII and factor IX concentrates for clinical use.[17,19] These concentrates could be lyophilized and stored at temperatures up to 4 °C with extended stability. Infusion of factor concentrates resulted in high circulating levels of factor VIII and factor IX without the complication of volume overload and paved the way for intensive infusion therapy for serious and life-threatening bleeding complications such as intracranial, retroperitoneal, and retropharyngeal hemorrhages and major surgery. Because they were produced from large pools of single plasma donations (>1000), initial concentrates were

Table 118-1 Development of Transfusion Therapy for Hemophilia

1832	Schönlein proposes transfusion for exsanguination[7]
1840	Lane transfuses whole blood to stop postoperative bleeding in hemophilia[8]
1905	Weil reports use of human serum to treat hemophilia[109]
1911	Addis fractionates plasma by acid method[110]
1923	Feissly uses citrated plasma in ABO-mismatched father-to-son transfusion for hemophilia[9]
1930s-1940s	Development of modern blood banking. Availability of whole blood and frozen plasma for therapy (allows levels of approximately 5%)
1946	Cohn develops ethanol fractionation of plasma[1]
1949	Graham uses FFP in canine hemophilia model[111]
1945-1960	Fractionation of plasmas with AHF activity
1952	Biggs distinguishes hemophilia B from hemophilia A[14]
1953	Graham, Langdell, and Brinkhous develop quantitative assays to measure AHF[13,112]
1958	Barium precipitation of plasma to enrich for factor IX[18,113]
1963	Wagner uses glycine precipitation to partially purify factor VIII
1964	Pool develops clinically useful cryoprecipitate for factor VIII deficiency (allows levels of >20%)[12]
1966	Johnson uses PEG to partially purify factor VIII[16]
1967	Brinkhous develops glycine and PEG method to produce large-scale high potency factor VIII product (allows levels of 100%)[17]
1965-1970	Home infusion therapy
1969	Hoag produces large-scale prothrombin complex concentrate for factor IX deficiency[19]
1970s	HBsAg assay is developed
1978-1985	HIV contaminates blood supply and factor concentrates
1979-1986	Heat treatment of factor concentrates reduces transmission of hepatitis B and HIV[23,24]
1985	Assay for HIV is licensed
1982	Immunoaffinity method of purification for factor VIII[114,115]
1986	S/D method of treating infusible protein solutions to inactivate enveloped viruses[116,117]
1992-1993	First recombinant factor VIII concentrates are licensed[30,118]
1998	Recombinant factor IX concentrate is licensed[119]
1999	Nucleic acid amplification testing of blood donors
1999	Recombinant factor VIIa approved for hemophilia A and B with inhibitor
2007	Recombinant factor VIIa approved for acquired hemophilia
2011	First plasma-derived factor XIII product approved by the FDA

AHF, Human antihemophilic factor; *FDA*, Food and Drug Administration; *FFP*, fresh-frozen plasma; *HBsAg*, hepatitis B surface antigen; *PEG*, polyethylene glycol; *S/D*, solvent/detergent.

nearly universally contaminated with viral pathogens such as hepatitis B and non-A, non-B hepatitis (hepatitis C).[21] Initial attempts to attenuate viral transmission using pasteurization and dry heat, instituted by manufacturers in the late 1970s and early 1980s,[22,23] were found to limit the transmission of hepatitis B. Eventually, these techniques were found to inactivate the human immunodeficiency virus (HIV).[24-26] Before the widespread application of these techniques, however, the majority of patients with severe hemophilia treated with concentrates between 1978 and 1985 were infected with HIV and hepatitis C virus. This tragic consequence of infusion therapy helped fuel the development of modern strategies to reduce the risk of viral transmission by products derived from human plasma. These strategies include (1) careful screening of potential donors for risk factors leading to infection with transfusion-transmissible infections, (2) more vigilant surveillance of the blood donor base for the appearance of new pathogens, (3) development and implementation of testing specific for markers of infectious agents, (4) purification strategies that reduce viral load in final products, and (5) physical and chemical viral inactivation methods to treat infusible products. Finally, development and refinement in techniques of molecular biology in the 1970s and 1980s resulted in the cloning of the genes for many plasma proteins, including factor VIII and factor IX.[27-29] Within the next decade, the production and licensure of biologically active recombinant factor VIII and factor IX products had become a reality.[30-33] Concentrates of these recombinant products have been shown to be effective and have not been associated with the transmission of pathogens. Further development of recombinant products centers on the removal of all human and animal proteins in the production and formulation of products to further reduce the risk of their inadvertent contamination with emerging pathogens, such as variant prions,[34,35] and newly discovered agents, such as hepatitis G virus and other transfusion transmitted viruses.[36,37] In addition, episodic supply constraints incurred in the manufacture of recombinant proteins in mammalian cell culture systems resulting in supply shortages of recombinant factor VIII[38] have led to greater interest in transgenic production of human plasma proteins compared with mammalian cell culture. With transgenic systems, raw material from which the protein of interest is purified (milk, plant tissue) can be produced in abundance.

Attenuation of Pathogens in Blood-Derived and Other Biologic Products

The development of factor VIII and factor IX concentrates in the 1960s improved the life expectancy of patients with hemophilia from approximately 11 years (before effective transfusion therapy) to nearly normal.[39] Experience with these first-generation concentrates, however, showed that they invariably transmitted the viral agents responsible for hepatitis B and hepatitis C,[21] which are associated with chronic hepatitis with attendant morbidity and mortality, including cirrhosis and hepatocellular carcinoma. Although efforts were being directed at methods to attenuate these known hepatitis viruses during the late 1970s and early 1980s,[22,23] HIV contaminated the human blood supply. More than 70% of patients in many countries and 30% to 40% of hemophilia patients worldwide were infected with HIV.[40-43] The devastating effects of both HIV and chronic hepatitis in the hemophilia patient population provided a major impetus for the improvement in viral safety of all infusible products derived from human and, in the case of porcine factor VIII, animal blood. More recently, concern about the prion agents responsible for transmissible spongiform encephalopathies such as Creutzfeldt-Jakob disease (CJD), variant CJD, and bovine spongiform encephalopathy, as well as newly identified viral agents in the blood supply,[36,37] have reinforced the need for continued surveillance and further refinements in the production of products for the treatment of hemophilia. This attention has also been focused on recombinant products because nearly all currently licensed products use added human or animal protein in fermentation or as stabilizers during purification or formulation. Table 118-2 lists agents that are potential contaminants of human

Table 118-2 Viruses Implicated in Transfusion of Plasma-Derived Products

Virus	Nucleic Acid Human Disease	Human Disease	Known Transmission by Blood	Lipid Enveloped	Size (nm)	Reduction/Inactivation
HIV	RNA	Yes (AIDS)	Yes	Yes	100-120	S/D
HBV	DNA	Yes (acute and chronic hepatitis)	Yes	Yes	40-45	S/D
HCV	RNA	Yes (acute and chronic hepatitis)	Yes	Yes	40-60	S/D
Parvovirus B19	DNA	Yes (fifth disease, transient erythroblastopenia of childhood, chronic anemia in immunocompromised patients)	Yes	No	18-20	Incompletely by heat; nanofiltration
HAV	RNA	Yes	Yes	No	25-30	Incompletely by heat
Hepatitis G	RNA	No	Yes	Yes		?S/D
TTV	DNA	No	Yes	No		?S/D
HHV-8	DNA	Kaposi sarcoma	Unknown			
SEN V	DNA			No		
TSE (prion)	Peptide	Yes (CJD)	Unknown	N/A	250 kd	Unknown

Data from Teitel J: Transmissible agents and the safety of coagulation factor concentrates. World Federation of Hemophilia: Facts and Figures 7:1,118 1999; and Allain JP: Emerging viruses in blood transfusion and Allain JP: Emerging viruses in blood transfusion. *Vox Sang* 78:243, 2000.
CJD, Creutzfeldt-Jakob disease; *HAV*, hepatitis A virus; *HHV-8*, human herpesvirus 8; *N/A*, not applicable; *S/D*, solvent/detergent; *SEN V*, SEN virus; *TSE*, transmissible spongiform encephalopathy; *TTV*, torque teneo virus.

plasma. Other viruses such as cytomegalovirus and human T-lymphotropic virus type I (HTLV-1) are transmissible primarily by cellular blood products.

Although ideal, the absolute removal of infectious agents in transfusable products may be unattainable and in fact may be unnecessary because the primary goal is to make them noninfectious. Practically, this can be accomplished by reducing the levels of the contaminating agent below the level of infectivity. The most relevant agents, viruses and prions, are small and therefore difficult to separate from protein components of plasma. Some pathogens are resistant to currently used methods of inactivation. In addition, as exemplified by HIV and prions, new agents may periodically emerge in the human population by crossing species barriers. Unless detected rapidly, newly emerging agents have the potential for global dissemination, especially if they are transmitted by transfusion of contaminated blood products. Despite these limitations, the safety of infusible products derived from human or animal sources (which includes cultured mammalian cells expressing recombinant protein) can be optimized by reducing the initial viral load in the source material (human plasma, culture medium, or transgenic material). With human plasma, this is accomplished by screening to limit potentially infected donors, by removal and inactivation of infectious agents, and by prospective surveillance of all products and recipients of products that potentially may become contaminated. Progress continues in technology to reduce virus transmission; nanofiltration, an example of this, allows for more than 4 to 6 log reduction of viruses through size exclusion by filtering the solution through membranes with extremely small poor size (15-40 nm) and without denaturing plasma proteins.[44] Nonenveloped viruses such as hepatitis A and parvovirus B19, both smaller than 30 nm, can be effectively removed by nanofiltration. Benefix (Pfizer) undergoes nanofiltration.

Current discussions in the medical, health economic, and patient communities center around achieving an appropriate balance between safety and costs given that plasma-derived products on the market today are extremely safe with regard to pathogen transmission.[45]

Infusion Regimens and Dosing for Hemophilia

The mainstay of therapy for hemophilia involves the treatment of bleeding episodes with the infusion of products capable of replacing the missing factor VIII or IX. This so-called on-demand therapy is effective in staunching hemorrhage but not before tissue damage has occurred. Bleeding is especially destructive in the synovium, where a vicious cycle develops in which the initial bleed results in a proliferative inflammatory response and hypertrophy of synovial tissues that then become more susceptible to further trauma and bleeding. The result in the short term is repeated bleeds into the same joint, referred to as a "target joint," and eventually chronic joint destruction or hemophilic arthropathy. Patients with chronic arthropathy often require surgical intervention, including synovectomy, debridement, joint replacement, or even joint fusion.

With the availability of factor concentrates that allowed for the attainment of high plasma levels of factor VIII or IX, prophylactic therapy became possible. This approach was pioneered by Swedish treaters who have demonstrated that the use of prophylactic regimens,[46] wherein trough factor levels are maintained at greater than 1% of normal, reduces the incidence of arthropathy and CNS hemorrhage.[45] Greater availability of virally safe factor concentrates has allowed for the initiation of prophylactic regimens in early childhood. This "primary" form of prophylaxis has become the standard of care in developed countries. For prophylaxis, the National Hemophilia Foundation Medical and Scientific Advisory Council recommends infusion of factor VIII 25 to 50 units/kg three times a week or every other day for hemophilia A and factor IX 40 to 100 units/kg two or three times a week for hemophilia B.[47] Prophylaxis is not universally practiced, however, owing to the high cost of factor concentrates, the requirement for frequent intravenous (IV) infusion, and the need for placement of central venous catheters in some patients, especially small children, to obtain IV access. Use of central catheters is attended by the risks of catheter-induced septic and thrombotic complications.

To understand how prophylaxis is currently being instituted in the United States, a survey of hemophilia treatment centers was conducted: 62 centers responded, and 32% (or 20 centers) initiated prophylaxis on a once-weekly schedule, 21% (13 centers) on a twice-weekly schedule, and 47% on a thrice-weekly schedule.[48] This survey demonstrated the diversity in practice and deviation from the recommendation from the National Hemophilia Foundation. Alternative schedules for prophylaxis have been investigated. For example, the Canadian Hemophilia Primary Prophylaxis Study, a small, prospective, multicenter study, evaluated a tailored prophylaxis regimen in 25 patients with severe hemophilia A; patients were started at 50 units/kg once a week and were escalated to 30 units/kg twice weekly and then 25 units/kg on alternate days if one of the three situations occurred: development of a target joint, four bleeds in 3 months, or

Table 118-3 Dosing Regimens for Bleeding and Prophylaxis in Hemophilia

Site	Factor Level (%)	Dose Hemophilia A (U/kg)	Dose Hemophilia B (U/kg)	Duration of Treatment	Comments
Joint	30-70	15-35	30-70	1-3 d	Splinting, temporary splinting, no weight bearing
Life threatening (e.g., intracranial, retropharyngeal, retroperitoneal)	80-100	40-50	80-100	10-14 d	Antifibrinolytic therapy with retropharyngeal bleeds
Soft tissue	30-50	15-25	30-50	2-5 d	Higher levels can be used for compartment syndrome
Surgery	80-100	40-50	80-100	10-14 d (or shorter for minor procedures)	Significant blood loss can occur into large muscles of the lower extremity and the iliopsoas
Oral	20-50	10-25	20-50	1-2 d	Antifibrinolytic therapy
Gastrointestinal*	30-100	15-50	30-100	2-3 d	Should be evaluated for source
Genitourinary†	30-50	15-25	30-50	1-2 d	Avoid antifibrinolytic therapy
Prophylaxis‡	50	25	50	qod or 3×/wk	Steroids may be useful

Data from DiMichele D: Hemophilia 1996. New approach to an old disease. *Pediatr Clin North Am* 43:709, 1996; Mannucci PM: Haemophilia treatment protocols around the world: Towards a consensus. *Haemophilia* 4:421, 1998; and Lusher J: *Treatment of congenital coagulopathies,* 1999, AABB Press.
qod, Every other day.
*Depending on severity.
†Painless spontaneous hematuria often requires no treatment other than fluid intake. Persistence requires treatment and evaluation.
‡Use of a schedule of 25 U/kg qod and a dose of 40 U/kg with an interval of 2 days between the next dose may increase compliance by decreasing infusions to three per week.

five or more bleeds occurred into any one joint. This seemed to be well tolerated, resulting in 1.2 bleeds per year while maintaining good joint function; long-term follow-up of tailored prophylaxis is needed, but it may be a cost-effective and central line–sparing option.[49]

Dosing regimens for the treatment of bleeding episodes in hemophilia and for prophylactic regimens have evolved paralleling the availability of high-concentration pathogen-safe replacement products. Although no universal regimen for treatment has been established, certain trends prevail. In general, for non–life-threatening bleeding episodes, the goal of therapy is to achieve a plasma factor VIII or IX level of between 30% and 100%. For life-threatening bleeds or prophylaxis for surgical procedures, the goal is a level of 100% to be maintained by repeated bolus infusions or continuous infusion for a duration of 10 to 14 days or longer, depending on the severity of the bleed or surgical intervention.

The majority of prophylaxis regimens aim at achieving a trough factor level of approximately 1%. Prophylactic regimens can be "primary," instituted in young children to prevent bleeding episodes, especially hemarthroses that result in chronic arthropathy, or "secondary," in which limited or prolonged periods of prophylactic therapy are instituted after a serious bleed or the development of repeated bleeding into a single joint (target joint). A prospective randomized trial evaluating the safety and efficacy of a preemptive approach using once-weekly dosing before the first bleed to reduce inhibitor formation is currently in the planning stages.[50]

To prevent the development of a target joint and chronic arthropathy, many hemophilia treatment centers have recently adopted a regimen of two, three, or more infusions after a hemarthrosis. Specific dosing regimens for bleeding episodes have been developed by treaters and treatment centers. Although slight variations in indications and target plasma levels of factor VIII and factor IX among treatment centers exist, representative dosing regimens are similar and are presented in Table 118-3.[51-53]

Venous Access in Hemophilia Patients

Parents of young hemophilia patients are taught how to administer factor preparations through a butterfly needle until the patient is old enough and can be taught to self-infuse. Alternatively, visiting nurse services obtain peripheral access for some patients. Factor administration via peripheral veins can be very challenging in infants and in patients who require frequent IV therapies, such as those with inhibitors; therefore, more permanent venous access is required in some patients. Options for venous access include externally tunneled or fully implantable catheters or arteriovenous fistulas (AVFs). Hemophilia practitioners differ in their approach to venous access; one survey indicated that central venous access devices are widely used in 89% of centers and avoided in 11%.[48] Complications such as infections and thrombosis limit the life of a device and add to the morbidity of the patient. From a meta-analysis of 48 studies, the incidence of infection was 0.66 per 1000 catheter-days. A multivariate analysis of these data showed that the presence of an inhibitor was associated with an increased risk of infection; additionally, they demonstrated that the risk of infection with a fully implantable device was one-third that of an external device.[54] In one prospective study of catheter-related deep venous thrombosis (DVT) in boys with hemophilia, 69% of children had a DVT when screened and 81% at the 2-year rescreening.[55] One study of 38 hemophilia patients confirmed that AVF is feasible, with complications in 34% of the patients; this group suggests that in patients with inhibitors, AVF should be considered the first line for venous access because they frequently require long-term, daily administration of factor.[56] In deciding on access for a patient, practitioners should address the risks and benefits of each type of device on an individual basis.

TREATMENT OF HEMOPHILIA

Products Available for Treatment of Factor VIII Deficiency

Products available for the treatment of bleeding episodes or prophylaxis against bleeding in patients with hemophilia A include DDAVP (1-deamino 8-d arginine vasopressin), a vasoactive peptide that stimulates release of stored factor VIII, and infusible products containing exogenous factor VIII protein. These may be blood components, concentrates purified from blood plasma, or concentrates containing recombinant factor VIII protein.

DDAVP

The preferred product for treatment of patients with mild or moderate hemophilia A is the synthetic octapeptide DDAVP, a vasopressin analog. DDAVP causes a release of factor VIII (and von Willebrand factor [vWF]) from endothelial cells, raising plasma factor VIII by approximately threefold (range, two- to 12-fold) in patients with hemophilia in whom the disease is caused by decreased production or secretion of a functional protein or a protein that has decreased activity. To be effective, DDAVP relies on a partial quantitative deficiency of factor VIII; thus, patients with severe hemophilia will not benefit from its use if the causative mutation results in no synthesis, secretion, or a protein with no activity. In a retrospective study assessing response to a DDAVP challenge in mild or moderate hemophilia, 57% of patients with mild hemophilia had a positive response, and several who failed the initial challenge had a response after a mean of 6 years, increasing the response rate to 71% in the mild group.[57] The response to DDAVP in an individual patient is typically reproducible, and an effective response must be documented before its routine use or as prophylaxis for bleeding in surgical procedures (see box on 1-Deamino 8-D Arginine Vasopressin Trial). IV and intranasal preparations are available. The IV product has been used in a subcutaneous route of administration. The intranasal preparation more easily allows a patient to administer the compound on an as-needed basis in a home therapy regimen. The phenomenon of tachyphylaxis, the decreased effectiveness of repeated doses of the compound, occurs after several, typically three, consecutive doses.

Injectable DDAVP (Sanofi Aventis) is available in 4 μg/mL. The recommended dose is 0.3 μg/kg, mixed in 30 mL normal saline (for children <10 kg, 10 mL normal saline), infused intravenously slowly over 30 minutes. This dose can be repeated after 12 to 24 hours. DDAVP nasal spray Stimate (CSL Behring) is available in a metered-dose pump that delivers 0.1 mL (150 μg) per activation (spray). The dose is one activation for patients weighing less than 50 kg and two activations in separate nostrils for those weighing more than 50 kg. Generally, only three consecutive doses of DDAVP should be used unless otherwise advised by an experienced hemophilia treater. Because DDAVP is a vasopressin analog, there is a risk of fluid retention with its use. Changes in fluid balance can result in hyponatremia and seizures, especially when DDAVP is used in individuals on nonfluid-restricted or salt-restricted diets (e.g., elderly or very young patients or surgical patients undergoing fluid replacement with solutions with concentrations <0.9% sodium). For this reason, DDAVP is not recommended for children younger than 2 years of age. Caution is advised with the use of DDAVP in patients at risk for arterial thrombosis because there have been reports of myocardial infarction and cerebral thrombosis with its use.[58]

1-Deamino 8-D Arginine Vasopressin Trial

1. Collect citrated plasma from the patient immediately before DDAVP infusion for testing with the postinfusion blood specimen.
2. Administer DDAVP intravenously (0.3 μg/1 kg) in 25 to 50 mL normal saline.
3. Wait approximately 30 minutes after the infusion, carefully observing the patient for possible adverse side effects (increased blood pressure, facial flushing, signs or symptoms of hyponatremia).
4. Collect post-DDAVP infusion specimen in sodium citrate at 60, 120, and 240 minutes.
5. Compare the pre- and post-DDAVP FVIII:C and vWF:Ag levels to confirm a therapeutic response, threefold increase from baseline (for mild or moderate hemophilia, response is defined as twofold increase in FVIII:C levels or an absolute level above 0.31 U/mL at 1 hour).[57]

Factor VIII Concentrates

In developed countries, the current standard of care for the treatment and prevention of bleeding episodes in patients with severe hemophilia A and in patients with mild or moderate disease who do not respond to DDAVP is the infusion of recombinant human factor VIII. Recovery of recombinant factor VIII ranges from 1.5% to 2.5%/IU/kg so that dosing assumes a rise in plasma factor VIII activity of 2% for every 1 IU/kg infused. Available concentrates are optimized to enhance viral clearance during purification and undergo one or more viral inactivation steps during manufacture. Plasma-derived FVIII concentrates, treated with multiple purification and viral inactivation steps, are also available and have an excellent recent record of safety.

Intermediate- and High-Purity Plasma-Derived Concentrates

Intermediate-purity plasma-derived concentrates are prepared from cryoprecipitated plasma or fresh-frozen plasma (FFP), from which factor VIII is further purified using precipitation, gel permeation, ion exchange, or affinity chromatography, often in combination. Specific factor VIII coagulant activity in these products ranges from 2 to more than 100 IU/mg of protein, and many of the methods used also copurify significant amounts of vWF, making them useful for the treatment of some patients with von Willebrand disease (vWD; see later discussion on treatment of vWD). More highly purified plasma-derived concentrates are produced using heparin ligand or immunoaffinity purification methods and have specific activities ranging from 140 to greater than 3000 IU/mg. To stabilize the factor VIII molecule, the majority of these products are formulated by adding human albumin before lyophilization.

Highly purified recombinant factor VIII concentrates have been licensed in North America, Europe, and Japan since the early 1990s. These are either full-length or B domain–deleted molecules (the B domain is not required for activity in coagulation) that are expressed in mammalian cell culture (Chinese hamster ovary or baby hamster kidney cell lines) and are purified using immunoaffinity techniques. The development of these recombinant products was fueled primarily by concerns regarding safety of the human blood donor pool and the viral epidemics that occurred within the hemophilia population with the use of early plasma-derived products. As with highly purified plasma-derived factor VIII concentrates, the first-generation recombinant products are formulated with added albumin as a stabilizer. More recently introduced "second generation" products (Kogenate FS, Bayer, Refacto, Pfizer) have been developed that stabilize the factor VIII molecule with nonprotein excipients.[59-61] Third-generation products (Advate, Baxter, Xyntha, Pfizer) do not have human proteins or other additives in the cell culture or as a stabilizer. Recombinant production methods that do not rely on the human plasma resource theoretically should provide for unlimited supply.

Plasma/Cryoprecipitate

In communities where virally inactivated factor VIII concentrates are not available, cryoprecipitate provides an effective alternative to therapy with concentrates for hemophilia A and vWD patients. Cryoprecipitate is a small-volume product (10-15 mL) enriched in factor VIII, vWF, fibrinogen, fibronectin, and factor XIII. Dosing can be calculated assuming approximately 80 to 150 IU of factor VIII per bag of cryoprecipitate (derived from a 450-mL single whole blood donor collection unit). Thus, a typical 1750-IU dose (50% correction for a 70-kg patient) would require between 10 and 21 bags or units. The limitations of cryoprecipitate therapy are (1) lack of a viral inactivation step in manufacture of the component and (2) lack of convenience, because multiple units must be pooled into a large volume (≈70-100 mL) for infusion. FFP and whole blood provide less desirable alternatives because adequate therapy with both of these products suffers from the limitations described for cryoprecipitate, and their use often results in intravascular volume overload. Solvent/detergent (S/D)–treated FFP product is available in some countries. ABO group–specific S/D plasma is prepared by S/D treatment (TNBP and Triton ×100) of a pool of up to 2500 donors. After removal of the solvent and detergent components, 200-mL aliquots are refrozen for infusion.

Products Available for Treatment of Factor IX Deficiency

Factor IX Concentrates

As with replacement therapy for factor VIII deficiency, intermediate- and high-purity products derived from plasma for the treatment of factor IX deficiency are available, as well as a single recombinant factor IX product. All of these concentrates also undergo at least one viral inactivation or exclusion step in manufacture. The volume of distribution of factor IX is approximately twice the plasma volume. This can be explained in part by the affinity of factor IX for type IV collagen present in the extracellular matrix.[62] Recovery of factor IX after infusion is therefore approximately 1%/IU/kg. The recovery observed with recombinant factor IX is approximately 20% lower than that observed with plasma-derived factor IX.[63] This is likely due to differences in posttranslational modifications between recombinant factor IX and plasma-derived factor IX.

Intermediate-purity factor IX products are generally purified from plasma using anion-exchange chromatography or calcium or barium precipitate adsorption. These methods select for proteins that contain highly negatively charged epitopes. The vitamin K–dependent (VKD) coagulation factors, by virtue of their gamma-carboxyglutamic acid (gla) rich domains, are such proteins; thus, these techniques copurify varying amounts of the other VKD coagulation factors, factor VII, factor X, and prothrombin with factor IX. Hence, the products are referred to as *prothrombin complex concentrates* (PCCs). The levels of vitamin K proteins in these products vary and can be obtained from the manufacturer. In addition, the PCCs are contaminated with trace amounts of activated forms of VKD factors. The presence of these activated factors is the likely explanation for thromboses that have occurred with the use of these intermediate-purity products, typically in the setting of postoperative immobility or hepatic dysfunction.[64] To minimize the risk of thrombosis with the use of PCCs, it is advisable to achieve a peak factor IX level no higher than 50%.[65] Some clinicians add small amounts of heparin to infusions of these products to prevent thrombosis, and some manufacturers have formulated PCCs with heparin or antithrombin III.

High-purity factor IX products are produced from plasma using techniques of ligand affinity or immunoaffinity chromatography and typically have specific activities greater than 150 IU/mg. Three single high-purity recombinant factor IX products have been licensed in the United States (Alphanine, Grifols; Mononine, CSL Behring; and BeneFIX, Wyeth). Because specific products have different recovery results, consulting the package insert and performing recovery studies are recommended; for example, one IU BeneFIX/kg will increase the circulating activity of factor IX by 0.8 ± 0.2 and 0.7 ± 0.3 IU/dL in adults and pediatric (younger than 15 years old) patients, respectively.[66] Also, the initial dose of BenFIX should be given under direct medical supervision because the potential for an allergic reaction is significant.[66] Thrombotic complications have not been reported with these high-purity products; some thrombotic events have been associated with continuous administration, which is not an approved method.[66] In patients with a history of allergy and inhibitors, an irreversible nephrotic syndrome has been reported during immune tolerance induction.[67]

In communities where factor IX concentrates are not available, plasma may provide a means of replacing factor IX in hemophilia B patients during bleeding episodes. Each unit of FFP derived from a 450-mL whole blood collection contains approximately 200 IU of factor IX. Replacement to therapeutic levels of factor IX with FFP is difficult because of the complication of volume overload. In some areas, S/D plasma provides a virally inactivated alternative to FFP.

Other Useful Adjuncts for Treatment of Bleeding in Hemophilia A and B

The antifibrinolytic agents tranexamic acid and ε-aminocaproic acid (EACA) (Amicar, Xanodyne Pharmaceuticals, Inc) are sometimes used in conjunction with clotting factor replacement therapy or DDAVP in the treatment of bleeding that occurs with hemophilia and other bleeding disorders. These agents interact with the lysine-binding site of plasminogen and enhance its activation. The more important effect of lysine analogs is that their occupancy of this site inhibits binding of the zymogen, plasminogen, to fibrin, which is necessary for full fibrinolytic activity. Antifibrinolytics are useful in the setting of mucosal bleeding and may substantially reduce the need for clotting factor concentrates in the setting of oral mucosal bleeding with tooth extractions. These agents are administered preoperatively and continued postoperatively until wound healing occurs. Although tranexamic acid is more potent, it is less readily absorbed when given orally. Tranexamic acid is administered at 25 mg/kg orally or 10 mg/kg intravenously preoperatively, and therapy can be continued postoperatively using oral rinses with a 5% solution. EACA is used at a dose of 100 mg/kg preoperatively followed by 100 mg/kg every 6 hours either orally or intravenously (maximum dose, 24 g/day). Dosing of EACA should be reduced in patients with renal insufficiency.

INHIBITORS OF FACTOR VIII AND FACTOR IX

A major complication in the treatment of patients with hemophilia is the development of inhibitory antibodies against the infused factors that interfere with factor activity. Rarely, antibodies may develop that do not affect activity but increase clearance of factor VIII or factor IX. The incidence of factor VIII inhibitors is approximately 30%, and inhibitors typically develop within the first 20 exposures to replacement therapy.[68,69] Well-designed prospective studies of the use of recombinant factor VIII in previously untreated patients revealed that many of these inhibitors are low titer and transient in nature.[31,32] Patients with low-titer, transient inhibitors can be managed with increased doses of factor VIII. Inhibitors to factor IX occur less frequently, with an estimated incidence of approximately 1% to 3%.[70] Patients with factor IX antibodies may have anaphylactic reactions when treated with high-purity products.[71,72]

Patients with high-titer inhibitors to either factor VIII or factor IX do not usually achieve hemostasis after factor replacement and thus present a treatment challenge. Treatment of patients who develop inhibitors involves two approaches: (1) acute treatment of bleeding episodes and (2) immune tolerance induction therapy, whereby the patient is treated frequently (often daily) with factor VIII or factor IX in an effort to suppress the production of inhibitors by the immune system (similar to allergic desensitization therapy).

Treatment of acute bleeding episodes can be accomplished by two methods. For patients with low-titer inhibitors (<5 Bethesda units [BU], a laboratory measurement of inhibitor activity), hemostasis can be accomplished with large doses of factor VIII or factor IX (e.g., as high as 200 IU/kg given at frequent intervals) in an effort to neutralize or "override" the circulating inhibitor. A neutralization approach is usually ineffective for patients with high-titer inhibitors (>5-10 BU) and is expensive because of the large amounts of factor required. These patients and patients with low-titer inhibitors who fail to respond to override therapy can be treated using products that act to "bypass" the inhibitor. The only current bypass agents include activated prothrombin complex concentrates (FEIBA, Baxter Bioscience) (aPCC), which contain factors VII, X, and prothrombin in addition to factor IX that enhance production of thrombin generation by activating the coagulation pathway at points further down than the factor VIIIa/factor IXa step. FEIBA is used as first-line treatment of bleeding episodes in patients with inhibitors by some treaters even though the concentrate is derived from human plasma.

Recombinant activated factor VII (rFVIIa) (NovoSeven, Novo Nordisk) product was licensed in Europe and the United States with an indication for use as a bypass agent in the treatment of inhibitors in patients with hemophilia A and hemophilia B. This product has the advantage of being the only recombinant product available for the treatment of bleeding episodes in patients with inhibitors. The dose of rFVIIa is 90 µg/kg. Recombinant factor VIIa is administered every 2 hours compared with every 8 to 12 hours for PCCs or activated PCCs. Thrombosis has also been reported with the use of rFVIIa[73,74] and PCCs.

Despite the success achieved with immune tolerance induction regimens (80%-90%),[75] "bypass" agents will still be needed in patients undergoing tolerization because an interval potentially as long as 2 to 3 years exists between the time that induction is initiated and the inhibitor is suppressed. Bleeding episodes that occur before achievement of tolerance usually require treatment with one or other of the bypassing agents.

Recently, Leissinger et al[76] demonstrated in hemophilia A patients with high titer inhibitors the superiority of prophylactic thrice-weekly FEIBA (Baxter) at 85 units/kg over on-demand therapy in a prospective, randomized, crossover study with a 3-month washout between the two arms, which were each 6 months, and prevented progression of joint disease in high-titer inhibitor patients; this regimen is recommended for prophylaxis in high-titer inhibitor patients (see box Treatment of Life-Threatening Bleeding Episodes in Patients With Inhibitors Against Factor VIII or Factor IX).

Treatment of life-threatening bleeds in the context of a high-titer inhibitor represents a significant challenge. The infusion of non–factor VIII concentrates, when the inhibitor titer precludes the use of factor VIII, is less effective than treatment with factor VIII concentrates and is difficult to monitor because plasma factor VIII levels are of no value. Adjunctive therapies are frequently used in this setting to lower the titer of the antibody to allow for treatment of the patient with factor VIII concentrates. Aggressive regimens are used in which circulating antibodies are depleted using plasmapheresis or staphylococcal protein A immunoadsorption, and reduction of antibody production is attempted using immunomodulatory agents such as steroids, cyclophosphamide, and IV infusion of gamma globulin (IgG).[77-80] These strategies for acutely reducing antibody titers are also used by some hemophilia treaters at the outset of immune tolerance induction. A study sponsored by the National Heart, Lung, and Blood Institute evaluated the safety and efficacy of rituximab in reducing inhibitor levels in hemophilia A patients[81]; the study was completed, and the results are pending.

Treatment of Life-Threatening Bleeding Episodes in Patients With Inhibitors Against Factor VIII or Factor IX

Concentrates

1. Factor VIII containing concentrates in high doses (as high as 150-200 IU/kg) if inhibitor titer is low (<5-10 BU) or if neutralization can be demonstrated with high doses. High-dose continuous infusion of factor VIII (≈10 IU/kg/hour) after a high-dose bolus may be useful.
2. Recombinant factor VIIa. Dose is 90 µg/kg (or a dose up to 320 µg/kg) administered every 2 hours. Risk of thrombosis exists with this product.
3. Activated PCCs at a dose of 50 to 75 IU/kg every 8 to 12 hours. Risk of thrombosis exists with this product.

Immunomodulation

1. Antibody depletion
   a. Plasmapheresis
   b. Extracorporeal immunoadsorption of plasma (staph protein A column therapy and other methods)
2. Suppression of antibody production
   a. High-dose steroids (equivalent of prednisone 80 mg/day)
   b. Cyclophosphamide (10-15 mg/kg load and 2-3 mg/kg/day)
   c. IV immunoglobulin (1 g/kg daily for 2 days)
   d. More aggressive regimens that may include vincristine, azathioprine, cyclosporine, or interferon-γ

Conservative Measures

1. Immobilization
2. Compression
3. Local application of hemostatic agents
4. Antifibrinolytics
5. Avoid venipunctures, intramuscular injections, arterial puncture, and lumbar punctures
6. Avoid use of medications that inhibit platelet function
7. DDAVP may be effective in some patients with low titer inhibitors

VON WILLEBRAND DISEASE

von Willebrand disease is an autosomal dominant bleeding disorder first described by Erik von Willebrand in 1926, who named this bleeding diathesis *pseudohemophilia*. vWD is relatively common, with a prevalence of up to 2% of the general population.[82] The penetrance and severity of the disease vary depending on the type of vWD (type 1, 2, or 3); the specific mutation; the number of affected genes; the patient's blood type; and numerous drug, hormonal, and stress-related parameters. These factors, particularly the subtype of vWD and the patient's response to DDAVP, influence the recommended treatment for acute bleeding episodes or for prophylaxis against bleeding.

Although the disease had been described in the 1920s, the primary defect had earlier been attributed to either platelets or the vessel wall. An understanding of the missing protein in vWD and its relationship to factor VIII was not appreciated until the 1950s. Correction of the defect with transfusion of plasma, but not with platelet concentrates alone, defined the disease as one involving a missing plasma protein factor (vWF), not a platelet or vessel wall defect.[83] A correlation between vWD and factor VIII activity had previously been observed—the observation that a plasma fraction from patients lacking factor VIII (hemophilia A) could correct the defect in vWD in addition to the autosomal inheritance pattern, which helped further differentiate hemophilia A from vWD.[83] A more detailed discussion of clinical features and pathophysiology of vWD and the molecular biology of vWF can be found in Chapters 140.

Transfusion Therapy for von Willebrand Disease

The specific treatment for vWD varies with the bleeding symptoms and signs and with the subtype of vWD. Treatment is guided further by laboratory results indicating the potential success of increasing vWF with DDAVP and the clinical experience with a particular patient and his or her natural biologic family members who have vWD. When possible, attempts should be made to treat the patient without exposing him or her to plasma-derived products.

Non–Protein-Based Treatment

DDAVP is a synthetic octapeptide homolog of vasopressin that results in the release of stored vWF from Weibel Palade bodies of the endothelium (see section on treatment of hemophilia A). DDAVP is often effective for type 1 disease and may be useful in certain patients with type 2 disease. It is not appropriate for use in patients with type 3 disease in whom no stores of vWF exist. Before the use of DDAVP, a DDAVP trial should be conducted to document its efficacy in an

Table 118-4 Other Coagulation Deficiencies

Factor	Incidence	Inheritance	Chromosome	Half-Life	Target Plasma Level	Treatment Product*
I (fibrinogen)	1-2/10⁶		4	2-4 days	50-100 mg/dL	Concentrates
Afibrinogen		AR				Cryoprecipitate
Hypofibrinogen		AR or AD				
Dysfibrinogen		AR or AD				
II (prothrombin)	<1/10⁶	AD	11	3 days	30%	PCCs Plasma
V	1/10⁶	AR	1	36 hours	25%	Plasma
VII	2/10⁶	AR	13	3-6 hours	25%	rFVIIa Concentrates PCCs Plasma
X	2/10⁶	AR	13	40 hours	10%-25%	PCCs Plasma
XI		AR or AD	4	80 hours	20%-40%	Concentrates Plasma
XIII	<1/10⁶	AR	1.6	9 days	5%	Concentrates Cryoprecipitate Plasma

Data from Cohen AJ and Kessler: Treatment of inherited coagulation disorders. *Am J Med* 99:675, 1995.
AD, Autosomal dominant; *AR,* autosomal recessive; *PCC,* prothrombin complex concentrates.
*Products are listed in order of viral safety.

individual patient. The trial is performed as described for hemophilia A. The phenomenon of tachyphylaxis is also observed when DDAVP is used to treat vWD. For bleeding that does not respond to DDAVP or in patients in whom a poor response is observed with DDAVP, other modalities (typically protein based) must be used.

As described for hemophilia A, the antifibrinolytic agent EACA or tranexamic acid are often administered in the setting of dental surgery to inhibit fibrinolysis. Care should be taken when these agents are administered in patients with a predisposition to thrombosis.

Estrogens upregulate vWF synthesis and may be useful especially in women. Therapy with estrogens should also help ameliorate menorrhagia in affected symptomatic patients.

Plasma-Protein–Based Therapy

Factor VIII Concentrates

Some intermediate-purity factor VIII concentrates are manufactured from plasma using methods that copurify significant amounts of vWF. Many of the products listed in Table 118-4 contain vWF. Humate-P (ZLB Behring), Alphanate (Grifols USA), and Wilate (Octapharma), which is 1:1 vWF:RCo/factor VIII, are currently licensed for the treatment of vWD. Others, including Koate-DVI (Talecris Biotherapeutics), have been tested in vitro and in vivo for their potential use in therapy for vWD.[84-86] The multimeric pattern of vWF in these concentrates varies, and no product has the pattern of multimers that is present in normal plasma.[85] Because many of these products are effective clinically, the importance of these differences in multimer pattern remains to be determined. In addition, when using multiple doses of these products, factor VIII and vWF:RCo should be monitored because there is an increased risk of thrombotic events with the accumulation of factor VIII.

von Willebrand Factor Concentrates (Plasma Derived and Recombinant)

Several chromatography-purified plasma-derived concentrates enriched in vWF have been studied by manufacturers in Europe.[87,88] Preliminary reports suggest that these are amenable to viral inactivation steps and may be effective both in vitro and in vivo.[85] To date, none of these have been developed as widely licensed products. Recombinant vWF has been successfully isolated from a number of expression systems and partially characterized, but a recombinant product for the treatment of patients has not yet been developed clinically.

Cryoprecipitate

Cryoprecipitate had been the mainstay of plasma-based therapy for bleeding in patients with vWD until the availability of virally inactivated intermediate-purity factor VIII concentrates with preserved functional vWF protein. These factor VIII concentrates are the products of choice for the treatment of bleeding in patients with types 1 and 2 vWD who are unresponsive to DDAVP and for bleeding in patients with type 3 vWD. Owing to the small potential for viral contamination of cryoprecipitate, manufacture of which does not include steps to inactivate viral pathogens, cryoprecipitate is currently indicated only when virally safe concentrates containing vWF are unavailable.

ACQUIRED FACTOR VIII AND VON WILLEBRAND FACTOR DEFICIENCY

Antibodies that inhibit the activity of factor VIII can develop in previously normal patients. Most of these patients have no underlying disease; however, factor VIII antibodies can arise in the setting of autoimmune disorders or in the postpartum period. Although approximately one-third of inhibitors disappear spontaneously, the mortality rate among affected patients is significant.

In adults, acquired vWD is a rare autoimmune disorder that can occur in association with other autoimmune disorders or lymphoproliferative disease. Antibody may interact with the epitopes on vWF required for its normal activity or result in increased clearance of antibody–vWF complexes.

In children, acquired vWD is extremely rare but has been reported in the context of Wilms tumor, hypothyroidism, and congenital heart disease and some medications; with treatment of the underlying disorder, vWF normalizes.

Treatment

Therapy for those patients with relatively high inhibitor titers (>5 BU) includes bypassing agents (FEIBA or rFVIIa) to stop bleeding and immunosuppression to reduce inhibitor levels. Plasmapheresis or immunoadsorption can be used to reduce the circulating levels of inhibitors. Immunosuppressive agents and IV immunoglobulin (IgG) are useful adjuncts to abrogate production of the autoantibody. DDAVP can also be effective in some patients with low-titer inhibitors. Unlike inhibitors that develop with hemophilia A, exposure to factor VIII usually does not result in increased antibody titers.[89] Conservative measures to control hemorrhage should also be used in conjunction with the above, including immobilization and compression, topical or local hemostatic agents, and antifibrinolytic therapy. The use of venipunctures, intramuscular injections, and drugs with platelet inhibitory activity should be minimized or avoided.

OTHER COAGULATION PROTEIN DEFICIENCIES

Approximately 15% of inherited bleeding disorders are caused by deficiencies of coagulation factors other than factor VIII, factor IX, or vWF. Inherited deficiencies of fibrinogen and factors II, V, VII, X, XI, and XIII may result in bleeding, requiring treatment. The genes for these factors are not located on the X chromosome; thus, two gene defects are typically required for symptomatic disease. Consanguinity is frequent in affected kindreds. The characteristics of these deficiencies are presented in Table 118-4. Hereditary deficiencies of factor XII, prekallikrein, and high-molecular-weight kininogen have not been described to result in bleeding diatheses.

The mainstays of therapy for these disorders are cryoprecipitate (for fibrinogen deficiency) and plasma. In some countries, concentrates enriched in the missing protein have been available. An S/D-treated pooled plasma product is also available in some regions. Pooled S/D-treated plasma has the advantage over FFP in that it is virally inactivated but has the drawback of exposing the patient to a large number of donors (2500) with each dose.

Fibrinogen Deficiency

Bleeding disorders can result from low to absent levels of fibrinogen (hypofibrinogenemia or afibrinogenemia) or a protein with abnormal function (dysfibrinogenemia). The inheritance pattern for the former is autosomal recessive and for the latter is autosomal dominant. Dysfibrinogenemias can result in bleeding or hypercoagulability. The gene for fibrinogen is located on chromosome 4. Because fibrinogen is required for the formation of a fibrin clot, it is surprising that afibrinogenemic patients survive gestation and birth. Diagnosis is made when patients present with bleeding from the umbilical stump, intracranial hemorrhage, or mucosal bleeding. Hemarthroses can occur but are less common than observed with the hemophilias. Wound healing may be delayed. Increased incidence of fetal wastage in patients with afibrinogenemia and hypofibrinogenemia is observed, and term gestation is rarely achieved without replacement of fibrinogen.[90-92] Because the substrate for clot formation, fibrinogen, is missing or deficient, the prothrombin time (PT), activated partial thromboplastin time (aPTT), thrombin clotting time (TCT), and coagulation assays that have fibrin formation as their end points are all prolonged. Replacement of fibrinogen is accomplished with cryoprecipitate with a goal of achieving a plasma level between 50 and 100 mg/dL and at least 60 mg/dL for maintenance of pregnancy.[92] Each bag of cryoprecipitate contains approximately 200 to 300 mg of fibrinogen. The biologic half-life of fibrinogen is between 2 and 4 days. Virally inactivated fibrinogen concentrates are available in Europe, China, and Japan (Japan Green Cross, Aventis, LFB). Adverse reactions to treatment include the development of fibrinogen antibodies; allergic reactions; and, paradoxically, thrombosis.

Prothrombin Deficiency

Congenital prothrombin deficiency is a rare autosomal recessive disorder estimated to be present at a rate of 0.5 cases per million. Disease has been described with both homozygous and heterozygous defects (including compound heterozygotes). Hemorrhagic symptoms include bruising; intracranial, mucosal, and deep tissue bleeding; and menorrhagia. Hemarthroses are rare. Correlation between bleeding and prothrombin levels is poor. No reports of a prothrombinemia appear in the literature, suggesting that complete lack of the protein is incompatible with normal development. Both the PT and the aPTT time are prolonged, and the thrombin time is normal. Treatment of prothrombin deficiency includes plasma at a dose of 15 to 20 mL/kg followed by 3 mL/kg every 12 to 24 hours to achieve levels of approximately 30%. The half-life of prothrombin is approximately 3 days. Prothrombin complex concentrates contain prothrombin and other VKD factors and can be used to treat prothrombin-deficient patients who are undergoing major surgery or life-threatening bleeds. Caution should be exercised because these have been associated with thrombosis.

Factor V Deficiency

Inherited deficiency of factor V occurs in fewer than one per 1,000,000 people with an autosomal recessive inheritance pattern (homozygous or compound heterozygous), resulting in factor V levels less than 20%. Symptoms include bleeding from the umbilical stump and mucous membranes, ecchymoses, menorrhagia, postpartum bleeding, and intracranial hemorrhage. Hemarthroses can occur but are less common than with severe hemophilia. No factor V–enriched plasma concentrates are available. Because factor V is in the common pathway of coagulation, in deficiency states, both the PT and the aPTT are prolonged. Treatment of bleeding involves the infusion of plasma at 15 to 20 mL/kg with a goal of achieving levels of 20%. The half-life of factor V is approximately 36 hours. Because platelets contain stored factor V,[93] they have been used to treat bleeding. Platelet infusion may result in the production of platelet-specific antibodies.

Factor VII Deficiency

Factor VII deficiency occurs in approximately one in 500,000 people. Severe bleeding occurs with levels below 5%, and symptoms in severely affected patients are similar to those observed with severe hemophilia. Intracranial hemorrhage may occur in up to 16% of cases and in neonates after vaginal delivery. The PT is prolonged, but the aPTT and thrombin time are normal. Prothrombin complex concentrates contain factor VII and may provide a benefit over plasma because they are virally inactivated. As with the use of these products for factor VIII and factor IX inhibitors, thrombosis has been reported. Several plasma-derived factor VII concentrates have been developed and have been used to treat congenital deficiency. Recombinant activated factor VII concentrate is effective in the treatment of bleeding with a congenital factor VII deficiency.[94-97] Inhibitors to factor VIIa have developed in patients with congenital factor VII deficiency.[94]

Factor X Deficiency

Congenital deficiency of factor X is a rare condition resulting from homozygous or compound heterozygous defects in the autosomal genes for factor X located on chromosome 13. Bleeding is correlated with factor X levels, and symptoms include epistaxis, menorrhagia, hemarthrosis, intracranial hemorrhage, hematuria, and umbilical cord bleeding. Because factor X is a component of prothrombinase (the first step in the common pathway), diagnosis is suggested by both a prolonged PT and a prolonged aPTT but a normal TCT. Treatment is with plasma products (FFP or S/D-treated plasma) at approximately 10 to 15 mL/kg followed by 5 mL/kg every 24 hours with a goal of plasma factor X activity levels of 20%. No factor X–specific concentrates are available, but PCCs contain variable amounts of factor X. As with the use of PCCs for other indications, the risk of thrombosis is increased. Currently, a Phase III, multicenter study to investigate the pharmacokinetics, safety, and efficacy of a high purity factor X (Bio Products Laboratory) is accruing patients with moderate to severe factor X deficiency.[98]

Factor XI Deficiency

Congenital factor XI deficiency (sometimes called hemophilia C) is an autosomal disorder with a recessive pattern of inheritance and is particularly common in Ashkenazi Jews in whom two specific mutations account for the approximately 8% prevalence of an abnormal factor XI gene.[95,96] The factor XI gene is located on chromosome 4. Bleeding symptoms are variable and include postsurgical or traumatic bleeding or heavy menses in women. Spontaneous hemorrhage is not typical of the disorder, and this characteristic distinguishes the disorder from hemophilia A and B. Plasma levels of factor XI do not correlate with bleeding symptoms unlike the factor levels in hemophilia A and B. The aPTT is prolonged with factor XI deficiency; PT and thrombin time are normal. Patients with factor XI deficiency are usually treated before surgical procedures with a goal of factor XI levels between 30 and 45 U/dL.[95] Plasma (FFP and S/D-treated plasma) provides the mainstay of therapy, and dosing takes into consideration the long half-life of 60 to 80 hours; however, some patients may have difficulty tolerating the large fluid volume of FFP. Although the half-life of factor XI in S/D plasma is comparable to that of FFP, decreased levels of factor XI in the product (≈30%-50%) have been reported.[97] Two virally reduced or inactivated factor XI concentrates have been developed using affinity chromatography or cation-exchange chromatography.[99] These two concentrates, licensed in France (Hemoleven, LFB Biomedicaments France) and England (FXI concentrate Bio Products Laboratory), are not available in the United States, although the factor XI concentrate from France can be obtained through compassionate use in the United States.[100] Both have been demonstrated to be effective, but there have been reports of thromboembolic complications with their use, presumably because of contaminant activated factor IX. Both products are now formulated with antithrombin and heparin, but caution is advised with their use in elderly patients and in patients with preexisting cardiovascular disease. Doses should not exceed 30 U/kg and peak factor XI should not exceed 100 U/dL.[101]

Because bleeding occurs in patients with factor XI deficiency more often in settings in which fibrinolysis is more active (oral mucosa, urinary tract), antifibrinolytic agents can be useful adjuncts in the treatment of such bleeding episodes or used as sole agents to prevent bleeding with dental procedures. Fibrin glue can provide a useful adjunct or be used solely in topical bleeding (dental extractions, circumcisions). DDAVP has been reported as useful for the prevention of surgical bleeding in factor XI deficiency.[102] The mode of effect of DDAVP is unclear but is likely due to the coexistence of mild vWF deficiency.

Factor XIII Deficiency

Factor XIII is a transglutaminase that catalyzes the cross-linking of γ-glutamyl and ε-lysyl groups of fibrin monomers, stabilizing the forming clot by decreasing its susceptibility to fibrinolysis. Inherited deficiency of factor XIII is autosomal recessive and results from defects in the genes for the two subunits of factor XIII located on chromosome 1 (B subunit) and chromosome 6 (A subunit). The majority of reported defects involve the A subunit. Umbilical bleeding in homozygotes may be observed at birth. Soft tissue bleeds, hemarthroses, excessive intracranial bleeding (relative to other coagulation deficiencies), pseudotumors, and bleeding during surgery are observed in affected patients. Surgery is also complicated by poor wound healing. Affected male patients may have oligospermia, and female patients may have recurrent miscarriages. Coagulation screening test results (PT, aPTT, and TCT) are normal. Solubility of clots is increased with factor XIII deficiency; thus, the diagnosis can be made by incubating clots in the presence of solubilizing agents such as 5 M urea or 1% to 2% chloroacetic acid. Factor XIII has a long half-life (9-15 days). Previously, FFP (2-3 mL/kg) or cryoprecipitate (1 bag/10-20 kg) were the only options for treating patients with factor XIII deficiency. However, in February 2011, the first plasma-derived factor XIII concentrate (Corifact, CSL Behring) was approved by the U.S. Food and Drug Administration for prophylaxis; this concentrate is given intravenously to maintain a trough level of 5% to 20% with the initial recommended dose being 40 IU/kg every 28 days.[103] Because of the long half-life of factor XIII, replacement can be used on a prophylactic basis (dosing every 3-4 weeks) to prevent intracranial hemorrhage and other bleeding episodes. The United Kingdom Haemophilia Centre Doctors' Organisation's current guidelines recommend that because the incidence of cerebral hemorrhage is so high, all patients with severe factor XIII deficiency should receive prophylaxis at diagnosis, and it should be considered in some moderate and mild as well.[104] Dosing with factor XIII concentrate is 10 to 75 IU/kg every 4 to 6 weeks, with lower doses for prophylaxis and higher doses for the treatment of bleeding episodes. Recombinant FXIII-A2 was found in phase I testing to be safe and potentially effective for replacement in patients with FXIII deficiency and is currently in clinical trials.[105]

OTHER PLASMA-DERIVED PROTEIN CONCENTRATES

As discussed in Chapter 117, plasma fractionation processes also allow for the isolation of plasma components other than the coagulation proteins. Immunoglobulins are isolated by a variety of techniques from the Cohn fraction II-III. α_1-Antitrypsin and antithrombin are produced from fraction IV. As with other VKD proteins, protein C may be isolated from Cohn fraction II.

Anticoagulant Proteins (Protein C and Antithrombin)

Brief mention should be made of plasma-derived concentrates enriched in protein C and antithrombin III. These products have been used for a variety of indications, but both are licensed for the treatment of congenital deficiencies that result in thrombosis. Protein C concentrate has also been used in the treatment of purpura fulminans with meningococcemia. Antithrombin in combination with defibrotide has been used for the successful treatment of venoocclusive disease in patients who develop this complication after undergoing bone marrow transplantation,[106] heparin resistance in patients undergoing cardiopulmonary bypass, and sepsis. Additionally, antithrombin has been used in patients with acute lymphoblastic leukemia who are receiving asparaginase. Early studies showed some efficacy in using activated protein C to treat sepsis.[107] However, a recent update of a Cochrane review reported that in five randomized controlled trials, including 5101 patients, activated protein C did not decrease the risk of death and was associated with an increased risk of bleeding.[108] Its utility for other indications is not yet known.

Immunoglobulins

The use of immunoglobulins (both IV and hyperimmune products) for a variety of diseases is discussed elsewhere in this book.

α_1-Protease Inhibitor (Antitrypsin)

α1-Protease inhibitor (or antitrypsin) concentrates (Prolastin, Bayer Healthcare LLC; Aralast, Baxter Biosciences; Zemaira, ZLB-Behring) are available for the prophylactic treatment of people with congenital deficiency of α_1-antitrypsin. α_1-Antitrypsin inhibits neutrophil elastase, which is thought to be responsible for the alveolar damage resulting in emphysema. These replacement products, administered intravenously, are presumed to act to delay the progression of congenital emphysema associated with this protease inhibitor deficiency.

FUTURE DIRECTIONS

Virally safe plasma-derived concentrates have been developed that are enriched in a variety of coagulation and other proteins. Initially, refinements in techniques of plasma fractionation formed the basis for the development of these concentrates as an improvement over the use of blood component therapy (whole blood, plasma, and cryoprecipitate). Plasma-derived protein concentrates were first developed for the treatment of the more common hemophilias A and B. Subsequent refinements were made to reduce and then eliminate the transmission of viral and other pathogens present in the human plasma pool while increasing product purity. Techniques in molecular biology and heterologous expression of mammalian proteins have allowed for the production of some proteins, most notably factor VIII and factor IX, without reliance on the limited plasma resource. These plasma-derived and recombinant concentrates have supplanted the use of plasma or cryoprecipitate for the treatment of some congenital and acquired deficiencies of soluble plasma factors and have decreased or eliminated the attendant risks of allergic reactions, volume overload, and pathogen transmission. For patients on home infusion regimens, protein concentrates also have the benefit of increasing patient convenience because infusion volumes are small relative to blood component therapy. Although the development of high-purity, virally safe concentrates to treat other plasma protein deficiencies that are currently treated with blood components is technically feasible, such development is limited by the very small numbers of patients with these disorders. In the future, the development of products produced in transgenic animals holds the promise of producing large quantities of recombinant proteins, thus making available more of these lifesaving products for use clinically.

SUGGESTED READINGS

Bolton-Maggs PH, Perry DJ, Chalmers EA, et al: The rare coagulation disorders–review with guidelines for management from the United Kingdom Haemophilia Centre Doctors' Organisation. *Haemophilia* 10:593, 2004.

Bray GL, Gomperts ED, Courter S, et al: A multicenter study of recombinant factor VIII (recombinate): Safety, efficacy, and inhibitor risk in previously untreated patients with hemophilia A. The Recombinate Study Group. *Blood* 83:2428, 1994.

Ehrenforth S, Kreutz W, Scharrer I, et al: Incidence of development of factor VIII and factor IX inhibitors in haemophiliacs. *Lancet* 339:594, 1992.

Horowitz B, Wiebe ME, Lippin A, Stryker MH: Inactivation of viruses in labile blood derivatives. I. Disruption of lipid-enveloped viruses by tri(*n*-butyl)phosphate detergent combinations. *Transfusion* 25:516, 1985.

Leissinger C, Gringeri A, Antmen B, et al: Anti-inhibitor coagulant complex prophylaxis in hemophilia with inhibitors. *N Engl J Med* 365:18, 2011.

Lusher JM, Arkin S, Abildgaard CF, et al: Recombinant factor VIII for the treatment of previously untreated patients with hemophilia A: Safety, efficacy, and development of inhibitors. Kogenate Previously Untreated Patient Study Group. *N Engl J Med* 328:453, 1993.

Nilsson IM, Berntorp E, Zettervall O: Induction of immune tolerance in patients with hemophilia and antibodies to factor VIII by combined treatment with intravenous IgG, cyclophosphamide, and factor VIII. *N Engl J Med* 318:947, 1988.

Roberts H: The treatment of hemophilia: Past tragedy and future promise. *N Engl J Med* 321:1188, 1989.

Schwartz RS, Abildgaard C, Aledort L, et al, Group TRFVS: Human recombinant DNA derived antihemophilic (factor VIII) in the treatment of hemophilia A. *N Engl J Med* 323:1800, 1990.

United Kingdom Haemophilia Centre Doctor's Organization: Guidelines on the selection and use of therapeutic products to treat haemophilia and other hereditary bleeding disorders. *Haemophilia* 9:1, 2003.

White GC, Beebe A, Nielsen B: Recombinant factor IX. *Thromb Haemost* 78:261, 1997.

For complete list of references log on to www.expertconsult.com.

CHAPTER 119

HEMAPHERESIS

Diarmaid Ó Donghaile and Harvey G. Klein

Bloodletting is an ancient therapy, fashionable, albeit unproved, and practiced well into the 19th century. About the time that scientific skepticism began to temper the widespread use of therapeutic phlebotomy, a new technique for blood removal, apheresis, appeared in the research laboratory. The term *apheresis*, derived from a Greek verb meaning "to take away or withdraw," was coined to describe removal of one component of blood with return of the remaining components to the donor. Like phlebotomy, apheresis was used first to treat patients but later became more important for collecting blood components for transfusion. Increasingly, apheresis techniques are used to collect cell populations from the peripheral blood of healthy donors and patients for purposes of hematopoietic stem/progenitor cell (HPC) transplantation and immune cell therapies. Annually in the United States, more than 50,000 units of peripheral blood stem cells (PBSCs) and therapeutic cellular therapy products are collected at hospital and blood center apheresis facilities.[1]

PRINCIPLES OF APHERESIS

The principal objective of apheresis is efficient removal of some circulating blood component, either cells (cytapheresis) or some plasma solute (plasmapheresis). For most disorders, the treatment goal is to deplete the circulating cell or substance directly responsible for the disease process. Apheresis can also mobilize cells and plasma components from tissue depots. For example, lymphocytes may be mobilized from the spleen and lymph nodes of some patients with chronic lymphocytic leukemia (CLL), and low-density lipoproteins (LDLs) can be removed from tissue stores in patients with familial hypercholesterolemia. Apheresis also appears to mobilize $CD34^+$ cells from extravascular depots in peripheral blood stem/progenitor cell (PBSC) donors, resulting in collection of more than twice as many $CD34^+$ cells than estimated based on pre-apheresis peripheral blood cell counts (Fig. 119-1). Apheresis may have other, less obvious effects. Lymphocyte depletion may modify immune responsiveness in some disease states, possibly by disturbing the control mechanisms of cellular immune regulation. Plasmapheresis enhances splenic clearance of immune complexes in certain autoimmune disorders. When therapeutic effect is judged by clinical improvement rather than by efficiency of solute removal, apheresis is more often a helpful adjunct than a form of first-line therapy.

Several mathematic models formulated for different clinical conditions describe the kinetics of apheresis. Removal of most blood constituents follows a logarithmic curve (Fig. 119-2). This model assumes that the substance removed is neither synthesized nor degraded substantially during the procedure, remains within the intravascular compartment, and mixes instantaneously and completely with any plasma replacement solution. When the goal of plasmapheresis is to supply a deficient substance, for example, the cleavase ADAMTS13 in the treatment of thrombotic thrombocytopenic purpura (TTP), replacement follows logarithmic kinetics similar to those developed for solute removal. From Fig. 119-2, it is evident that removal of 1.5 to 2.0 volumes will reduce an intravascular substance by approximately 80% and that processing larger volumes results in little additional gain. Specific cell removal with centrifugal automated cell separators depends on the number of cells available, the volume of blood processed, the efficiency of the particular instrument, and the separation characteristics of the different cells. Most commercially available instruments remove platelets and lymphocytes extremely efficiently. Granulocytes and other mononuclear cells, including HPCs from peripheral blood, cannot be cleanly separated from other cells by standard centrifugal apheresis equipment (Fig. 119-3). Optimal harvesting of these cells requires special techniques such as stimulating the donor with corticosteroids or cytokines and adding sedimenting agents to enhance cell separation.

Whereas the model above accurately estimates removal of cells and large proteins such as fibrinogen and immunoglobulin M (IgM), removal of smaller solutes such as IgG and albumin-bound drugs is less efficient. Transfer of these moieties from the extravascular to the intravascular compartment depends both on diffusion along a concentration gradient and on active transport. The rate of clearance can be calculated using diffusion coefficients, sieving coefficients, and lymphatic flow rate, although in practice this degree of accuracy is rarely necessary.

TECHNOLOGY AND TECHNIQUES

The plasmapheresis technique that originated in the animal laboratory required manual resuspension of red blood cells (RBCs) and posed a substantial risk of microbial contamination of the components being reinfused. With the introduction of sterile, disposable, interconnected plastic blood bags, plasmapheresis became relatively safe and easy. However, manual apheresis proved too inefficient and labor intensive for collecting large component volumes and raised concerns that the separated units of RBCs might be reinfused accidentally into the wrong donor or patient. The introduction of automated online blood cell separators solved these problems. Automated apheresis instruments use microprocessor technology to draw and anticoagulate blood, separate components either by centrifugation or by filtration, collect the desired component, and recombine the remaining components for return to the patient or donor. The equipment contains disposable plastic software in the blood path and uses anticoagulants containing citrate or combinations of citrate and heparin that do not result in clinical anticoagulation of the patient or donor. Most instruments function well at blood flow rates of 30 to 80 mL/min and can operate from peripheral venous access or from a variety of multilumen central venous catheters. Newer therapeutic apheresis devices are smaller and more automated, allowing for implementation of more safety functions and improved portability.

Because the ideal method for treating disorders mediated by abnormal plasma components is to remove the offending substance selectively, a variety of online filtration and column adsorption techniques have been introduced or proposed. Ligands bound to a column matrix may be relatively nonspecific chemical sorbents, such as charcoal or heparin, or specific ligands, such as monoclonal antibodies and recombinant protein antigens. Two such columns are commercially available: one using staphylococcal protein A and the other using negatively charged dextran sulfate cellulose beads. Staphylococcal protein A has high affinity for the Fc portion of IgG1, IgG2, and IgG4 and for immune complexes containing these IgG subtypes. This column is approved for use in therapeutic apheresis procedures for patients with chronic immune thrombocytopenia and selected adult

Cell type	Blood concentration			Cell content			Apparent volume of distribution	
	Initial	End	% change*	Blood†	Product‡	Fraction§	Liters	No. of blood volumes
CD34 Cells								
25 L	0.077	0.045	–45	3.8	7.9	2.3	25.9	5.3
15 L ×2	0.078	0.039	–50	3.9	8.1	2.3	22.2	5.1

* Percentage change, end vs. iniial
† Estimated initial content in peripheral blood
‡ Total product content
§ Total product content divided by estimated initial content in peripheral blood. l, liters. CD34 cell concentration in 10^9/L, CD34 cell content x 10^8 cells.

Figure 119-1 TWENTY HEALTHY MOBILIZED DONORS UNDERWENT EITHER A SINGLE LARGE VOLUME LEUKAPHERESIS PROCEDURE OF 25 L OR TWO CONSECUTIVE-DAY SMALLER VOLUME PROCEDURES OF 15 L EACH. In both study groups, more than twice as many CD34 cells were collected than the estimated total content of these cells in the peripheral blood before apheresis, providing evidence for the existence of a large extravascular pool of peripheral blood stem cells (PBSCs), which becomes accessible to collection by leukapheresis. *(Modified from Bolan CD, Carter CS, Wesley RA, et al: Prospective evaluation of cell kinetics, yields and donor experiences during a single large-volume apheresis versus two smaller volume consecutive day collections of allogeneic peripheral blood stem cells,* Br J Hematol *120:801, 2003, by permission of the authors.)*

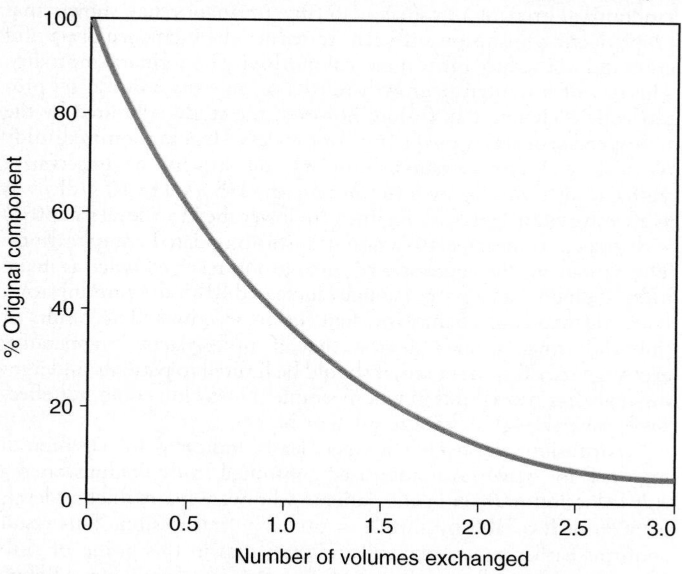

Figure 119-2 RELATIONSHIP BETWEEN VOLUMES REMOVED BY APHERESIS AND PERCENTAGE OF THE TARGET COMPONENT REMAINING. The relation is valid for blood volumes during red blood cell exchange or for plasma volumes during plasmapheresis if the target solute remains primarily within the intravascular compartment.

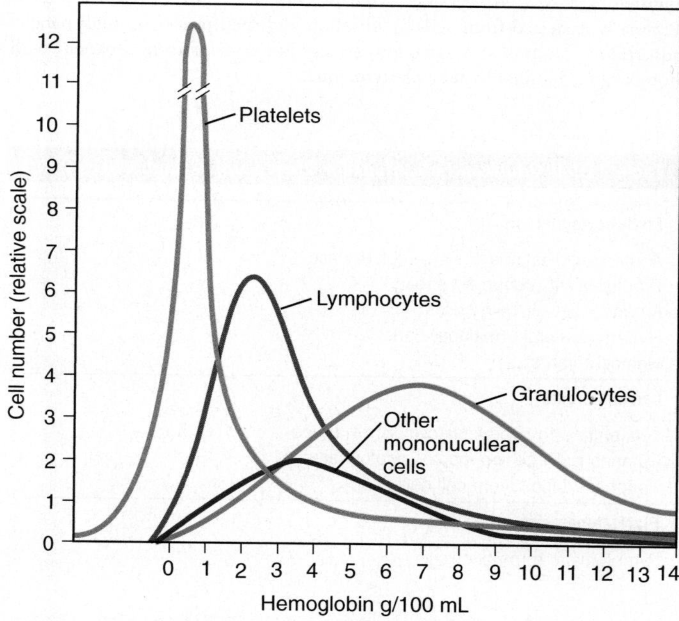

Figure 119-3 SCHEMATIC DISTRIBUTION OF CELLS AT THE COLLECTION PORT OF A CENTRIFUGAL CELL SEPARATOR. The number and percentage of each cell type collected can be varied by adjusting the site of collection along the interface or by changing centrifugal force, blood flow rate, or rate of cell removal.

patients with rheumatoid arthritis. The dextran sulfate cellulose columns selectively remove LDL, very-low-density lipoprotein, and lipoprotein (LP^a), and have proved effective in managing patients with homozygous hypercholesterolemia who have not responded to diet and cholesterol-lowering drug therapy (Fig. 119-4). A similar technique, heparin-induced extracorporeal lipoprotein precipitation, uses low pH and negatively charged heparin to precipitate lipoproteins and remove the precipitate by filtration online (H.E.L.P. Plasmat Futura, Braun Medical). Apheresis technology has also been adapted for extracorporeal phototherapy of patient leukocytes (photopheresis) to treat cutaneous T-cell lymphoma and to modulate the pathologic immune response in graft-versus-host disease (GVHD), solid organ transplant, and autoimmune diseases (see later discussion).

THERAPEUTIC CYTAPHERESIS

Common indications for therapeutic cell removal are listed in Table 119-1. Most of these procedures entail simple apheresis of the patient's peripheral blood with diversion for discarding the affected RBC, white blood cell (WBC), or platelet fraction. Special apheresis technologies have been approved, such as photopheresis devices, that divert a cell fraction that is photochemically treated in the extracorporeal circuit and returned to the patient's circulation, and apheresis immunoabsorption columns, which selectively remove immunoglobulins in the plasma by binding to a solid matrix.

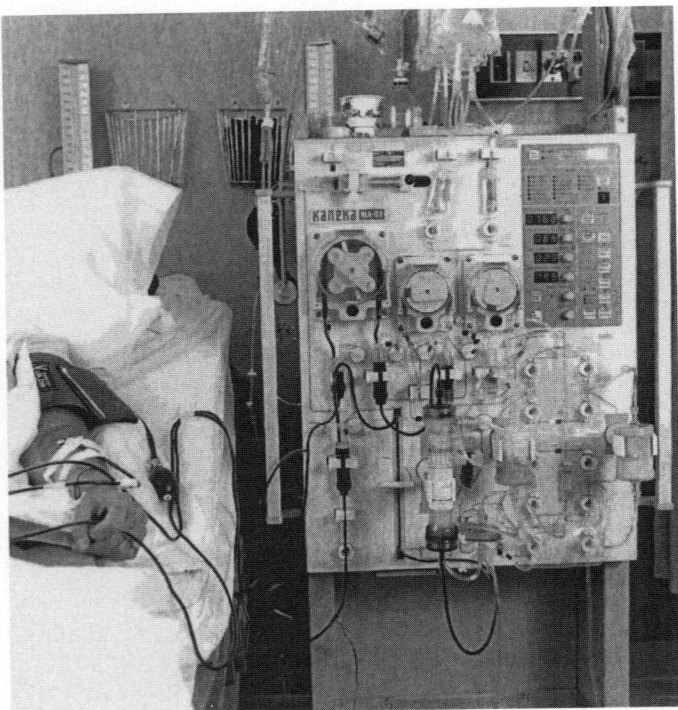

Figure 119-4 TWO-STAGE THERAPEUTIC PLASMAPHERESIS. Plasma is separated from cells by filtration and then passed through parallel adsorption columns to remove low-density lipoproteins from a patient with homozygous familial hypercholesterolemia.

Table 119-1 Common Indications for Therapeutic Cytapheresis

Erythrocytapheresis
Acute complications of sickle cell disease
Prophylaxis for recurrent stroke
Frequent severe pain crises
Hyperparasitemia (malaria, babesiosis)
Hemochromatosis
Leukapheresis
Leukemia with hyperleukocytosis syndrome
Cutaneous T-cell lymphoma (photopheresis)
Peripheral blood stem cell collection
Plateletpheresis
Symptomatic thrombocytosis

Erythrocytapheresis

Red blood cell exchange (erythrocytapheresis) is used most often to manage or prevent the acute vasoocclusive complications of sickle cell disease. Compared with manual exchange transfusion, mechanical cell separators offer the advantages of speed and ease and reduce the risks of rapid blood volume alteration and increased blood viscosity that may occur with simple transfusion. Automated procedures can be performed with all centrifugal instruments and programmed procedures allow accurate prediction of target hemoglobin concentration and percent hemoglobin A (HbA) at the conclusion of the procedure. A single volume exchange will remove about two-thirds of the circulating cells. Sickle cell anemia occurs in individuals who are homozygous for a single mutation in codon 6 of the β-globin gene, resulting in substitution of a single amino acid. Although the defect appears simple, the pathophysiology of the vasoocclusive crises is complex, involving hemoglobin polymerization, change in cell shape, adhesion to endothelial cells, dysregulated nitric oxide homeostasis, and release of free hemoglobin and inflammatory cytokines.[2] Clinical manifestations vary from patient to patient. The rationale behind exchange transfusion involves improving tissue oxygenation, reducing hemolysis, and preventing microvascular sickling by diluting the patient's abnormal RBCs, simultaneously correcting anemia and favorably altering whole blood viscosity and rheology. No clinical data support a single optimal level of HbA; however, as few as 30% of transfused cells markedly decrease blood viscosity. At mixtures of 50% or greater, resistance to membrane filterability approaches normal. In nonemergency situations, such levels can often be achieved with a simple transfusion regimen. For simple and exchange transfusions, raising the level of Hb A to between 60% and 70% while lowering the level of Hb S to 30% is generally efficacious, although even higher levels of HbA may be required to treat an ongoing crisis. Clinical indications for exchange transfusion in patients with sickle cell anemia remain controversial, with limited controlled study data available. Simple transfusion has been shown to improve renal concentrating ability and splenic function in young sickle cell patients; exchange transfusion improves exercise tolerance and reverses the periodic oscillations in cutaneous blood flow associated with this disease. Such observations have encouraged the use of exchange transfusion for acute complications of sickle cell disease such as acute chest syndrome, priapism, cerebrovascular accident, and hepatic and retinal infarction. Exchange transfusion for sickle cell patients has also been used for prophylaxis during pregnancy and before surgery, although prophylactic transfusion in these settings is controversial. The only randomized trial of transfusion during pregnancy has shown that prophylactic transfusion sufficient to reduce the incidence of painful crises did not reduce other maternal morbidity or perinatal mortality. The risk of intrauterine growth restriction may be reduced by prophylactic exchange transfusion; however, the study is limited by the retrospective observational nature of the data.[3] In a randomized study of sickle cell disease patients undergoing surgery, a conservative simple transfusion regimen (to increase the Hb level to 10 g/dL) was as effective as an aggressive regimen (to lower the Hb S level to <30%) with respect to perioperative non–transfusion-related complications. The patients in the aggressive regimen group received twice as many units of blood, had a proportionally increased RBC alloimmunization rate, and had more hemolytic transfusion reactions. The results of this and other studies suggest that if prophylactic preoperative exchange transfusion is used, it should be limited to patients undergoing high-risk procedures in whom simple transfusion could not effectively raise the Hb A level to 70% or higher.

Transfusion prophylaxis is now clearly indicated for children at high risk for stroke. A randomized controlled study demonstrated a risk reduction of 90% in the patients who were maintained at levels of 30% or less HbS by simple or exchange transfusion. This result confirms earlier experience and indicates that in this group of children with sickle cell anemia, transfusion therapy should begin before the first event and continue indefinitely. A second trial then addressed whether transfusion could be safely discontinued because of the cumulative long-term risks of iron overload from simple transfusion and RBC alloimmunization. After 10 months of randomization, half of the patients who discontinued transfusion had developed abnormalities, including reversion to abnormal transcranial Doppler findings and a small number of strokes, necessitating and early conclusion to the trial. Furthermore, long-term erythrocytapheresis may be preferable for patients at high risk for stroke who have developed iron overload to levels associated with organ damage. Exchange transfusion, although relatively safe and convenient, carries all the complications of RBC transfusion. Patients are exposed to a large number of donors and are at a small but significant risk of contracting hepatitis and other bloodborne infections. As many as 33% of all patients develop alloantibodies, and life-threatening delayed hemolytic transfusion reactions have been reported. In addition, an immunohematologic study of multiply transfused sickle cell patients shows that 85% of heavily transfused patients are alloimmunized to human leukocyte antigens (HLAs), platelet-specific antigens, or both. Most centers avoid inducing nonhemolytic transfusion reactions and HLA alloimmunization by using leukocyte-depleted RBCs. Extended RBC phenotyping at diagnosis and provision of phenotypically matched blood, when practical, can reduce the risk of RBC alloimmunization and associated hemolytic transfusion reactions. Despite the removal of RBCs during exchange, most patients remain in positive iron balance, although iron accumulation is slow and chelation is rarely required to prevent transfusional hemosiderosis.

Other indications for RBC exchange are rare. The procedure has been used for patients with overwhelming RBC parasitic infections, such as severe and complicated malaria and babesiosis. In malaria, exchange transfusion may have at least three beneficial effects. An automated exchange rapidly decreases the concentration of circulating parasites while improving the rheologic properties of the blood by replacing the infected RBCs. The exchange may also reduce levels of proinflammatory cytokines and may help sustain life until conventional therapy and natural immunity take effect. Although the efficacy of this therapy has not been evaluated by controlled trials, prospective studies and review of published cases suggest the use of erythrocytapheresis for parasitemia greater than 10% to 15% or even less in selected patients such as those with cerebral malaria or pulmonary edema. Case reports document RBC exchange in such diverse conditions as carbon monoxide poisoning and G6PD-deficient hemolysis.

Automated RBC removal with volume replacement (isovolemic hemodilution) can be performed rapidly and safely in polycythemic subjects. This maneuver should be reserved for polycythemic patients with an urgent clinical indication to lower the hematocrit (e.g., evolving thrombotic stroke) for which standard single-unit manual phlebotomy might be inadvisably slow. Automated double RBC apheresis technology has more recently been used to treat individuals with hereditary hemochromatosis. This procedure removes excess iron more rapidly than manual phlebotomy and may be more tolerable to patients because of the lower frequency of maintenance procedures required (Fig. 119-5). Emerging data from patients randomized to simple phlebotomy versus therapeutic erythrocytapheresis indicates a potential 74% reduction in the total number of procedures in the latter group.[4]

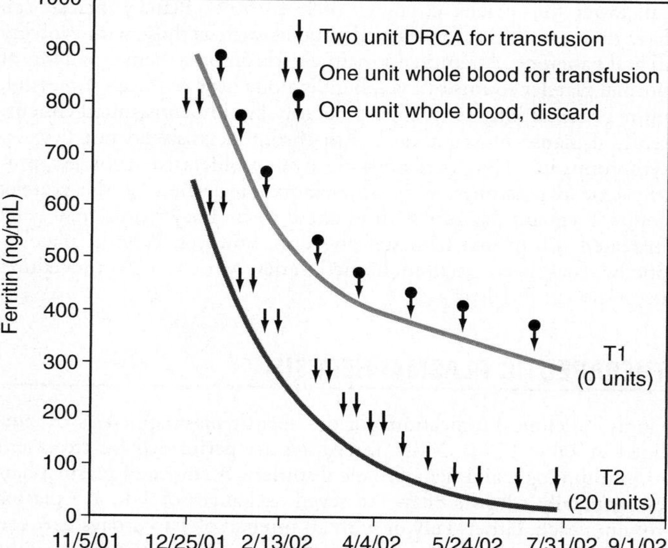

Figure 119-5 ONE TWIN WAS TREATED WITH MANUAL PHLEBOTOMY (T1) AND THE OTHER WITH DOUBLE RED BLOOD CELL APHERESIS (DRCA) (T2). In the same time period, ferritin levels declined more rapidly and to lower levels in the twin treated with double red blood cell apheresis. *(Unpublished data from Bolan CD, Leitman SF, with permission of the authors.)*

Leukapheresis

Therapeutic leukapheresis has been used most successfully to help manage patients with acute leukemia and extremely high WBC numbers, so-called acute hyperleukocytic leukemia (AHL). When the fractional volume of leukocytes (leukocrit) exceeds 20%, blood viscosity increases and leukocytes can interfere with pulmonary and cerebral blood flow and compete with tissue for oxygen in the microcirculation. Investigations of the expression and function of adhesion receptors in leukemic cells and the role of adhesion molecules in leukocyte-induced acute lung injury in sepsis suggest that the pathophysiology of leukostasis in AHL may also be related to interactions between leukemic blasts, platelets, and endothelial cells mediated by locally released adhesion molecules. A single-volume leukapheresis procedure generally reduces the WBC count by 20% to 50%, depending on the differing sedimentation characteristics of the specific blast cell population. Ordinarily, leukapheresis is initiated in a patient with acute myeloid leukemia (AML) or in the accelerated phases of chronic myeloid leukemia (CML) when the blast count exceeds 100,000/mm^3 or when rapidly rising blast counts are higher than 50,000/mm^3, especially when evidence of central nervous system or pulmonary symptoms appears. The threshold for initiation of leukapheresis in patients with acute lymphocytic leukemia (ALL) is generally higher (WBC count >200,000/mm^3). Leukostatic syndromes do not occur when concentrations of well-differentiated lymphocytes exceed even several million/mm^3.

Although leukapheresis may be effective in numerically reducing the number of circulating blasts, the evidence for clinical benefit is less certain. The data are controversial because of a lack of a randomized controlled trial and reliance on retrospective studies. Leukapheresis may reduce early death (ED) rates but does not improve the overall survival of patients with AML.[5] Trials reporting reduction in ED need to be interpreted with caution because one retrospective cohort study associated leukapheresis with a poorer outcome attributed to a delay in commencing chemotherapy.[6] Therefore, leukapheresis should not delay other immediate measures for treatment of patients with AHL include infusion of intravenous (IV) fluids, administration of hydroxyurea, and uricosuric medication with urinary alkalization, and correction of coagulopathy and thrombocytopenia.

Mechanical cytoreduction for managing other leukemic processes has limited value. Although repeated leukapheresis has adequately reduced the WBC count in a series of patients with CML, the median patient survival rate was not significantly different from that of similar patients treated with conventional chemotherapy. Chronic leukapheresis can provide acceptable control of the peripheral WBC count in clinical situations such as pregnancy, when cytotoxic agents may best be avoided, but cytoreduction alone does not appear to alter the course of CML. In a limited series of patients leukapheresis in combination with interferon has successfully controlled the disease until therapy with tyrosine kinase inhibitors could begin after delivery.[7] Some studies of patients with CLL suggested short-term clinical benefit, but long-term support of patients when the disease is refractory to chemotherapy does not appear to prolong life.

Lymphocyte removal by apheresis has also been used to modify immune responsiveness in patients with autoimmune diseases and to enhance solid organ allograft survival and reverse solid organ graft rejection, but evidence of clinical efficacy in these situations is sparse. Removal of large numbers of lymphocytes over a period of a few weeks can suppress peripheral lymphocyte counts in patients with rheumatoid arthritis for up to 1 year and can alter skin test reactivity and lymphocyte mitogen responsiveness to a variety of stimulants. Selected patients experience a modest but significant reduction in disease activity; however, the subset of patients who may derive substantial benefit from this therapy is difficult to identify. Because leukocytes are a major source of inflammatory cytokines implicated in the pathogenesis of inflammatory bowel diseases (IBD), nonpharmacologic methods for selective leukoreduction have been developed to treat these chronic, relapsing, lifelong disorders. Although IBD respond to a variety of drug regimens, leukapheresis may have a role as a "steroid-sparing" agent for patients who develop toxicity from long-term steroid use. Cellsorba removes leukocytes by extracorporeal filtration. Granulocyte-monocyte apheresis (Adacolumn) selectively adsorbs cells through columns filled with cellulose beads.[8] Clinical trials using Adacolumn technology have promising results in the treatment of ulcerative colitis, with remission rates in excess of 70% compared with conventional medical therapy. The studies are limited, however, by high risk of bias and inclusion of predominantly Japanese patients, limiting how results may be applied to western populations with different genetic and environmental factors.[9] Because the optimum course of therapy is yet to be defined, recent trials have investigated the safety and efficacy from weekly to procedures on a daily basis.[10]

Photopheresis, although not strictly a "cell removal" procedure, involves an automated extracorporeal photochemotherapy (ECP) treatment that includes leukapheresis, extracorporeal photoactivation with a light-sensitizing agent, 8-methoxypsoralen (8-MOP) and ex vivo ultraviolet A irradiation, and reinfusion of the leukocyte fraction (Fig. 119-6). The light-sensitizing agent is delivered directly to the extracorporeal leukocyte fraction, which may reduce the adverse effects such as nausea and vomiting associated with oral administration. The mechanism of action of photopheresis is unclear but may involve induction of apoptosis in pathogenic T lymphocytes and induction of a dendritic cell–mediated cytotoxic T-cell response. This therapy has minimal toxicity and is highly effective in the treatment of patients with advanced cutaneous T-cell lymphoma. Patients who present with the erythrodermic form and circulating malignant cells have the best clinical response. Photopheresis is typically performed once or twice a month, with symptomatic patients with higher circulating tumor burden benefiting from a more intense regimen.[11] Other disorders reported to respond to photopheresis therapy include cardiac and other solid organ graft rejection, and GVHD after stem cell transplantation in patients who do not respond to standard immunosuppressive therapy. Patients with chronic extensive GVHD should be considered for treatment, with best responses observed in cutaneous, mucous membrane and liver forms of the disease. Treatment commonly involves a trial of two ECP treatments on consecutive days every 2 weeks followed by an evaluation at 3 months. A response may facilitate a reduction in immunosuppression ("steroid sparing") with continued photopheresis.[11]

Acute rejection in cardiac transplantation occurs in 25% of recipients in the first year. In 30% to 50% of cases, acute rejection is T cell mediated. Prospective studies have shown benefit of photopheresis in prevention of rejection.[12] In the case of lung transplant, utility has only been studied retrospectively. Chronic rejection is manifest as bronchiolitis obliterans syndrome, presenting as progressive dyspnea and airflow limitation. ECP is associated with a reduction in rate of decline in lung function with progressive disease.[13] The acute adverse effects of photopheresis include skin erythema, low-grade fever, and transient hypotension. Anemia caused by incomplete reinfusion of RBCs may occur in patients undergoing long-term photopheresis.

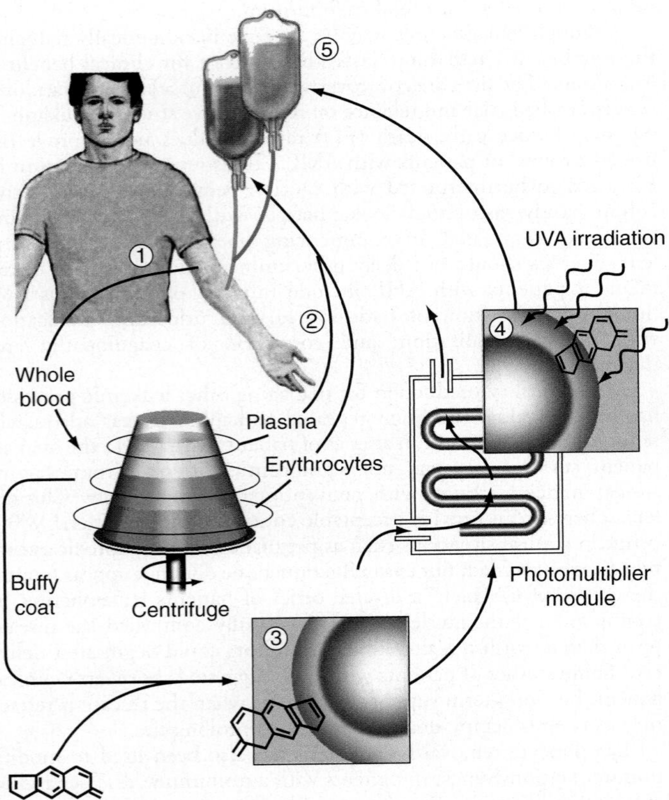

Figure 119-6 OVERVIEW OF A PHOTOPHERESIS PROCEDURE. (1) Vascular access is achieved by placement of a peripheral intravenous line or through a temporary central venous catheter. Whole blood is withdrawn from the patient, mixed with an anticoagulant solution, and pumped to a centrifuge, where it is separated into plasma, red blood cell, and mononuclear cell (buffy coat) fractions by elutriation. (2) After the collection of each mononuclear cell fraction, the uncollected red blood cells and plasma are pumped from the plasma/return bag through a blood filter and returned to the patient. (3) The mononuclear cell fractions are mixed with 8-methoxypsoralen and then (4) pumped through a sterile cassette surrounded by ultraviolet A (UVA) bulbs, resulting in a controlled rate and amount of UVA exposure. (5) The treated cell fraction is filtered and returned to the patient.

Plateletpheresis

Therapeutic plateletpheresis is generally reserved for patients with myeloproliferative disorders and hemorrhage or thrombosis associated with an increase in circulating platelets. Many centers consider using plateletpheresis when the patient's peripheral platelet count is greater than $10^6/mm^3$, although no consistent relationship between the level of platelet elevation and the occurrence of symptoms has been found and no generally accepted assay of platelet dysfunction predicts which patients are at risk. A single cytapheresis procedure can lower the platelet count by 30% to 50%. Plateletpheresis can have dramatic effects for selected patients such as those with evolving digital gangrene. Attempts to maintain thrombocythemic patients at normal platelet counts by cytapheresis alone have not been successful; more practical long-term chemotherapy should be instituted concurrently. Because most patients with thrombocytosis do not develop symptoms, including patients with myeloproliferative disorders, prophylactic plateletpheresis is unwarranted regardless of the platelet count. Pregnant patients with essential thrombocythemia may be at increased risk of first trimester abortion, however. Periodic plateletpheresis has been used in limited series, with weekly procedures necessary until delivery.

THERAPEUTIC PLASMAPHERESIS

Common clinical indications for therapeutic plasmapheresis are outlined in Table 119-2. Most procedures are performed for treatment of immunologic and hematologic disorders. A course of plasmapheresis generally consists of five to seven exchanges of 1 to 1.5 plasma volumes each, either daily or with an interval of 1 to 2 days between procedures, although the course of therapy varies depending on the specific disease indication and rate and duration of response.

Several expert committees have published practice guidelines for using plasmapheresis in a wide variety of disease states.[14,15] Some of the least controversial indications for plasmapheresis are supported by small series of uncontrolled cases that rely on some objective clinical or laboratory measurement of patient improvement.

Table 119-2 Common Indications for Therapeutic Plasmapheresis

Hematologic Diseases (Including Blood Cell–Specific Autoimmune Diseases)
Thrombotic thrombocytopenic purpura
Idiopathic thrombocytopenic purpura (immunoabsorption)
Hyperviscosity
Posttransfusion purpura
Cold agglutinin syndrome
ABO-mismatched marrow transplant (recipient)
Autoimmune Diseases
Cryoglobulinemia
Rheumatoid arthritis (immunoadsorption, lymphoplasmapheresis)
Myasthenia gravis
Goodpasture syndrome
Guillain-Barré syndrome
Chronic inflammatory demyelinating polyneuropathy
Metabolic Diseases
Homozygous familial hypercholesterolemia (selective adsorption)
Refsum disease
Other
Drug overdose and poisoning

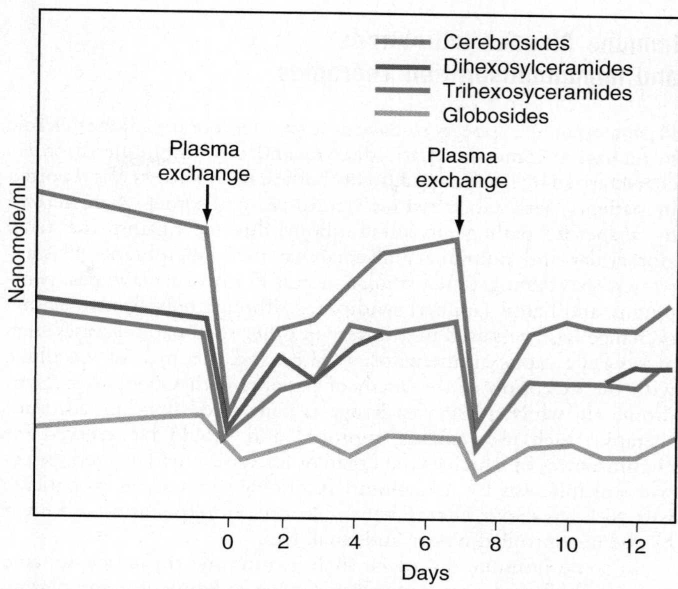

Figure 119-7 PLASMA EXCHANGE TO REMOVE PLASMA NEUTRAL GLYCOLIPIDS IN A PATIENT WITH FABRY DISEASE. The plasma lipid recovery curve appears to be biphasic, reflecting initial reequilibration from tissue stores and subsequent new synthesis of that glycolipid.

Hematologic Indications

Two of the most common indications for plasmapheresis are treatment of TTP and treatment of clinical syndromes associated with paraproteinemias. Plasma exchange with fresh-frozen plasma (FFP) replacement has been estimated to improve survival rates of patients with TTP from 10% to more than 75%. Comprehensive reviews of the clinical and laboratory evaluation and treatment of patients with suspected TTP, including management with plasma exchange therapy, have been published.[16] Treatment usually involves daily single-volume plasma exchange with both frequency and duration of treatment guided by clinical response and continued until the platelet count is above 150,000/μL and lactate dehydrogenase is near normal for 2 to 3 consecutive days. The persistence of schistocytes on the peripheral blood smear does not preclude weaning or discontinuation of treatment. Typically, patients should respond within 2 or 3 days of beginning treatment. In acutely unwell patients, escalating the intensity of plasma exchange to twice daily may be necessary.[17] Despite initial reports of improved response rates in certain patients, recent experience suggests that the use of cryoprecipitate-poor plasma may not be more effective than the use of standard FFP as a specific replacement fluid for plasma exchange in patients with TTP. The effectiveness of plasma exchange in this setting may derive from removal of antibody to or replacement of the von Willebrand factor–cleaving zinc metalloprotease, ADAMTS13. However, patients with clinical features of TTP and only moderate ADAMTS13 deficiency or even normal activity may respond to plasma exchange. Plasma exchange for hematopoietic progenitor cell transplant recipients exhibiting clinical features of TTP, now generally referred to as transplantation-associated thrombotic microangiopathy (TAM), has proved far less efficacious. This syndrome likely differs in pathogenesis from classic TTP in many aspects, including the absence of severe ADAMTS13 deficiency, the spectrum of clinical symptoms, and the lack of evidence of systemic microthrombus formation. Furthermore, plasma exchange has been unsuccessful in reversing most cases of TAM.

Small, uncontrolled studies and extensive clinical experience support the use of plasmapheresis as an adjunctive therapy for patients with paraproteinemia and hyperviscosity syndrome and with some paraproteinemias in the absence of hyperviscosity. Comprehensive reviews describing the rationale and treatment schedules for plasmapheresis in patients with a variety of paraproteinemias, including cryoglobulinemia and Waldenström macroglobulinemia, and other hematologic-oncologic indications, have been published. Waldenström macroglobulinemia manifests as a lymphoplasmacytic lymphoma with a monoclonal IgM protein in the plasma. Because IgM is a large molecule and resides predominantly in the intravascular space, as little as one apheresis procedure will result in improvement in symptoms. Recurrence of symptoms and rising plasma viscosity will determine the need and frequency of repeated exchanges.

Low-Density Lipoprotein Apheresis and Other Metabolic Disease Indications

Evidence that cutaneous lesions and vascular lesions regress in individuals with familial hypercholesterolemia as LDL levels are controlled by plasmapheresis has encouraged the use of apheresis column absorption procedures in patients with homozygous disease and in poorly controlled heterozygous patients. LDL apheresis is a procedure for removing apolipoprotein B–containing lipoproteins from the blood by a variety of techniques, including dextran sulfate cellulose adsorption, immunoadsorption, and heparin-induced extracorporeal precipitation. Short-term safety and efficacy have been demonstrated. Patients have now been treated successfully for several years; however, additional experience with this therapy will be required to prove long-term benefit for refractory hypercholesterolemia and coronary artery disease for heterozygotes in particular.[18] In 36 homozygous children in two studies, 20% to 22% developed new aortocoronary lesions or showed progression of existing lesions while on apheresis despite impressive reductions in mean LDL cholesterol.[19,20] Side effects such as malaise, shivering, and pain at the phlebotomy site are common, but mild and the treatments are generally well tolerated. Patients with severe hypertriglyceridemia are at risk of developing acute pancreatitis. Plasma exchange appears to reduce the episodes of recurrent episodes by an average 67% but requires continuation of medical therapy.

Simple plasma exchange may be used in patients with other inherited metabolic diseases, such as Refsum disease. The frequency of exchange depends primarily on total body burden, rate of synthesis, and plasma concentration of the solute to be removed (Fig. 119-7). Less evidence exists to support a role for repeated treatments in these diseases.

Immune Disease Indications and Immunoadsorption Therapies

Plasma exchange appears to have at least a temporary adjunctive role in managing some rheumatic diseases and other immune disorders characterized by circulating autoantibodies. Early success was reported in patients with Goodpasture syndrome, a disorder characterized by a specific pathogenic autoantibody directed against the renal glomerular and pulmonary alveolar basement membrane. Plasmapheresis has demonstrated similar success in myasthenia gravis, pemphigus, and Eaton-Lambert syndrome. Although nonselective plasma exchange has been used in a variety of other rheumatic diseases such as systemic lupus erythematosus (SLE) and rheumatoid vasculitis, with the exception of treatment of patients with Goodpasture syndrome (in which plasma exchange is considered first-line adjuvant therapy), such use remains unproved and should be reserved for circumstances in which a vital organ or life itself is endangered. Selective leukapheresis by Adacolumn technology in a series of patients with SLE has shown clinical benefit, but trial interpretation is limited by the uncontrolled nature and small size.

In some immune disorders, such as immune thrombocytopenic purpura (ITP) and immune inhibitors to coagulation proteins, plasma exchange may be helpful during a catastrophic event, but in general, benefit of nonselective plasma exchange therapy is not established.

Plasma exchange appears to be a useful therapeutic option in renal transplant patients threatened with refractory humoral rejection and is now widely used to overcome ABO and HLA incompatibilities between renal transplant patients and their only available donors. Several studies have shown successful reversal of acute humoral rejection mediated by HLA-specific donor antibody using a combination of plasmapheresis and IV immune globulin (IVIG), which is superior to high dose IVIG alone.[21] A conditioning regimen consisting of pretransplant plasmapheresis, immunosuppressive medications, and low-dose cytomegalovirus immune globulin effectively reduces donor-specific antibody and isoagglutinin titers with and without posttransplant splenectomy and anti-CD20 treatment. The strength of donor-specific antibodies is also important and can be determined by titration, but greater sensitivity and specificity may be obtained using Luminex flow-bead technology. Patients with strong anti-HLA antibodies have increased mean bead fluorescence and were more likely to have acute rejection; however, the introduction of peritransplantation apheresis reduced this from 66% to 7%.[22]

Plasma exchange has also been used to treat patients with focal segmental glomerulosclerosis, both for primary disease refractory to standard immunosuppressive therapy and for treatment of patients with recurrent disease after renal transplantation.

Two immunoadsorption columns have been approved in the United States for removal of autoantibodies to factor VIII or factor IX (Immunosorba staphylococcal protein A–agarose column) and treatment of ITP and rheumatoid arthritis (Prosorba staphylococcal protein A–silica column). Several case series describe the use of immunoadsorption for patients with immune inhibitors to factor VIII or factor IX. A phase III, multicenter, sham-controlled randomized study of staphylococcal protein A column immunoadsorption shows a significant increase in clinical response in adult patients with longstanding rheumatoid arthritis. Sparse published evidence exists to support the use of immunoadsorption therapy in patients with chronic ITP refractory to standard medical management.

Plasmapheresis is effective first- or second-line therapy in selected patients with certain neurologic disorders. Controlled clinical trials of plasmapheresis have demonstrated efficacy in at least two of the polyradiculoneuropathies. In Guillain-Barré syndrome, plasmapheresis should be considered when patients are unable to walk independently or require mechanical ventilation. However, IVIG alone may be equally effective and is more readily available.[15] Periodic plasmapheresis may be necessary in patients with a chronic inflammatory demyelinating neuropathy. Because the long-term prognosis varies, plasmapheresis may be used in conjunction with steroids and IVIG. Rapid deterioration may occur upon discontinuation.

Multiple sclerosis (MS) is a relapsing and progressive disorder with demyelination of the central nervous system white matter. Patients who present with acute fulminant demyelination may benefit from early plasma exchange, particularly when they fail to respond to high-dose corticosteroids.[23] The majority of patients have a relapsing-remitting form of the disease, and plasmapheresis may be of benefit. Unfortunately, for chronic progressive forms of MS, plasma exchange has been constantly been shown to be ineffective.

REPLACEMENT FLUIDS FOR PLASMA EXCHANGE

The success of therapeutic apheresis procedures seldom depends on the composition of the replacement solution that is used; the single exception is TTP (discussed in the previous section). With therapeutic plasmapheresis for most other disorders, the primary function of the replacement solution is to maintain intravascular volume. Additional requirements include restoration of important plasma proteins, maintenance of colloid osmotic pressure, maintenance of electrolyte balance, and preservation of trace elements lost during a prolonged course of plasmapheresis procedures. In moderately well-nourished patients, homeostatic mechanisms normally obviate the need for precise plasma replacement, and 5% albumin in normal saline or combinations of albumin and crystalloid are usually sufficient. Commonly used is 60% to 80% replacement by colloid, with the crystalloid component consisting of a combination of normal saline and an anticoagulant. Patients with clinical conditions such as hypotension, hypoalbuminemia, or preexisting coagulopathies should receive solutions prepared specifically to meet their individual requirements. Routine supplementation with calcium, potassium, or immunoglobulins is unnecessary. However, for large-volume apheresis procedures to collect PBSCs, IV calcium supplementation is beneficial (discussed in the following section). Because less than 500 mL is removed during most cell collection procedures and therapeutic cell depletions, no volume replacement beyond the anticoagulant and saline priming solution is required. Problems of decreased availability and high cost of albumin have led some centers to develop protocols for alternatives to plasma derived volume expanders, such as hydroxyethyl starch (HES), for full- or partial-volume replacement with plasma exchange. One center has used a combination of 3% HES and 5% albumin mixture successfully, but patients did experience mild adverse events more frequently than historical control participants.[24] Although such solutions are generally well tolerated, extensive replacement with HES in patients undergoing longer courses of plasmapheresis, especially those with impaired renal function, can result in diffuse tissue accumulation of the larger starch molecules (acquired lysosomal storage).

COMPLICATIONS OF THERAPEUTIC APHERESIS

Automated apheresis is a minimal-risk procedure for normal healthy donors. The current generation of blood cell separators is remarkably reliable and equipped with sensitive detection and alarm systems to alert the operator to potential problems. Nevertheless, serious morbidity and rare deaths have been associated with therapeutic procedures. In most reports, deaths are related to either complications associated with the use of central venous access catheters or to cardiac and respiratory problems in patients who were critically ill before apheresis; in the latter, the contributory role of the apheresis procedure is often questionable. The most common adverse effects of therapeutic apheresis are citrate-induced hypocalcemia, allergic reactions (usually to donor plasma or other blood components), vasovagal reactions, and hypovolemia. If transient paresthesia and mild vasovagal events are excluded, approximately 5% of all therapeutic apheresis procedures have medical complications. The frequency of adverse reactions is influenced by the experience of the operator and the nature of the patient population being treated. Expected and predictable effects of therapeutic apheresis include alterations in laboratory parameters caused by removal and dilution by replacement fluids. A

5% to 15% decrease in hemoglobin and hematocrit, a 20% to 30% decrease in platelet count, and mild transient increase in leukocyte count are commonly observed. Significantly but transiently abnormal coagulation test results are often observed (recovery generally occurs within 48 hours after a single-volume exchange procedure), as well as clinically insignificant decreased levels of other plasma proteins after serial plasma exchange procedures. The most common adverse effect of both donor and therapeutic apheresis procedures is symptomatic hypocalcemia caused by infusion of calcium-chelating citrate ions in the anticoagulant, and if used as replacement fluid, anticoagulated donor plasma. Hypocalcemia is usually manifested by mild perioral or acral paresthesia, or both, requiring no intervention other than slowing the reinfusion rate. The benefit of oral calcium supplements in this setting is questionable, although the practice is widespread. Hyperventilation may exacerbate the symptoms of hypocalcemia. More severe citrate toxicity is uncommon; signs may range from involuntary carpopedal spasm, nausea, and vomiting to frank tetany with spasm in other muscle groups, including life-threatening laryngospasm and grand mal seizure. Severe toxicity is most commonly experienced by small patients, particularly women, when the blood flow rate is rapid and the procedure is prolonged beyond a few hours. Symptoms correlate inversely with the level of ionized calcium. Extremely low concentrations of ionized calcium are encountered routinely in therapeutic procedures that process more than 15 L of blood. Acute severe hypocalcemia leading to fatal cardiac arrhythmia has been reported in patients who have undergone apheresis. Controlled infusions of 10% calcium gluconate or calcium chloride are effective in the management of these complications. Because metabolism of citrate occurs predominantly in the liver and kidney, patients with conditions affecting these organs are at increased risk for severe citrate reactions. Studies of therapeutic plasma exchange procedures and of PBSC donations performed with and without calcium gluconate or calcium chloride infusion show the effectiveness of continuous calcium infusion for the prevention of mild to moderate citrate toxicity (Fig. 119-8). A study of plateletpheresis donors documented sustained effects of citrate infusion on bone metabolism demonstrated by changes in alkaline phosphatase, osteocalcin, parathyroid hormone, and 1,25-dihydroxyvitamin D levels, suggesting the potential for long-term effects on bone metabolism in these donors. Magnesium, another divalent cation, is also bound by citrate. Despite decreases in serum ionized magnesium levels to 39% below baseline, clinical effects are not typically observed even during large-volume leukapheresis procedures. The most severe allergic complications occur when plasma is used as the replacement solution, and this risk increases with repeated exposure. Allergic reactions to ethylene oxide, an agent used in the sterilization of plastic disposable equipment, have been reported. IV diphenhydramine is usually effective in managing allergic reactions; premedication with steroids and precautions against anaphylaxis may be necessary for sensitized individuals. Atypical (hypotension and flushing) and anaphylactic reactions have been reported in patients receiving angiotensin-converting enzyme inhibitors undergoing different apheresis procedures, including immunoadsorption with staphylococcal protein A columns. These medications should be discontinued for at least 24 hours before apheresis. Unlike donors undergoing apheresis for donation of RBCs, platelets, or plasma, donors undergoing apheresis for collection of therapeutic granulocytes are stimulated with steroids and granulocyte colony-stimulating factor (G-CSF) before donation. The well-known association of long-term steroid treatment and posterior subcapsular cataracts has not been believed to be relevant in the context of short-term steroid stimulation for donor granulocyte mobilization. However, an increased number posterior subcapsular cataracts was detected in two small studies and in 100 granulocyte donors compared with age-matched plateletpheresis donors, suggesting that granulocyte donors may be at increased risk for certain types of cataract formation. Repeated steroid stimulation for granulocyte collection warrants regular ophthalmologic examination and close follow-up.[25] Serious complications indirectly associated with therapeutic apheresis include adverse consequences of large-needle vascular access; namely, retroperitoneal or pericardial hemorrhage, pneumo- or hemothorax, thrombosis, nerve damage, and infection. A retrospective review of 381 therapeutic plasma exchange procedures at one institution reported an approximately 1% incidence of severe complications, all of them related to central venous catheters.

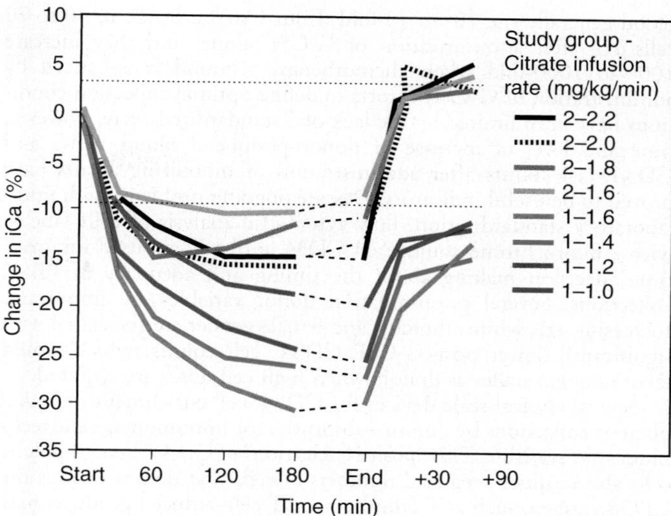

Figure 119-8 LEVELS OF IONIZED CALCIUM (iCa) ARE MARKEDLY LOWER IN PROCEDURES PERFORMED WITHOUT PROPHYLACTIC Ca INFUSION AND REMAIN BELOW THE REFERENCE RANGE 90 MINUTES AFTER COMPLETION OF APHERESIS. *Dotted lines* indicate upper and lower limits of the reference range. *Open symbols* represent procedures without prophylactic Ca; *solid symbols* represent those with Ca infusion. *Dashed lines* between 180 minutes and end-procedural values (End) reflect varying procedure duration. *(From Bolan CD, Cecco SA, Wesley RA, et al: Controlled study of citrate effects and response to i.v. calcium administration during allogeneic peripheral blood progenitor cell donation.* Transfusion *42:935, 2002, used by permission).*

HEMOPOEITIC STEM CELL COLLECTION

Blood cell separators developed for hemapheresis are used to collect peripheral blood cells for cellular therapy. The most common application of apheresis technology for cell therapy indications is the collection of HPCs from peripheral blood after administration of recombinant hematopoietic growth factor or chemotherapy, or both, to "mobilize" large numbers of HPCs into the circulation. The collected mononuclear cell fraction contains a subset of progenitor cells that, on infusion, can home to and reconstitute the bone marrow in patients who receive ablative radiation or chemotherapy or both. Similarly, donor leukocytes are obtained from leukapheresis procedures may be used for donor lymphocyte infusion or subject to further processing for immunotherapy.

Peripheral Blood Stem Cells

Pluripotent HPCs, and quite possibly primordial hematopoietic stem cells capable of reconstituting the bone marrow and the immune system, have long been known to circulate in the peripheral blood. Numerous studies have confirmed the potential for rapid and durable engraftment of PBSCs mobilized into the circulation by hematopoietic growth factors harvested by large-volume leukapheresis procedures and subsequently administered to patients with marrow aplasia after high-dose chemotherapy. The concentration of hematopoietic stem cells in the peripheral blood can be increased by the administration of cytokines such as G-CSF and granulocyte-macrophage colony-stimulating factor (GM-CSF) and by the administration of chemotherapy. $CD34^+$ hematopoietic cell numbers in the peripheral blood generally rise 20- to 40-fold (from 1 to 3 cells/μL to 40 to 70 cells/μL) after administration of G-CSF alone, and they increase 100- to 1000-fold when chemotherapy rebound is enhanced by administration of G-CSF. Efforts to define optimal collection conditions have been limited by the lack of a standardized assay; however, time and level of increase of donor peripheral blood WBC and $CD34^+$ cell counts after administration of mobilizing agents have proved to be useful indicators. Despite ongoing problems with interlaboratory standardization, flow cytometric analysis of cells labeled with a fluorochrome-conjugated CD34 antibody are used for "real-time" decision making about the timing and adequacy of PBSC collections. Several prestimulation donor variables are important. Increasing age, white ethnicity, and female gender are associated with significantly lower post–G-CSF $CD34^+$ cell counts, which would favor younger males as donors when high cell doses are required.[26]

Several clinical scale devices for $CD34^+$ cell enrichment of leukapheresis collections by immunoabsorption or immunomagnetic techniques are available. This "positive selection" of $CD34^+$ hematopoietic cells also results in reduced numbers of cells that do not express the CD34 antigen, such as T lymphocytes. T cell–reduced products may confer a lower risk of GVHD, and the ability to produce apheresis products enriched for $CD34^+$ cells facilitates graft manipulations for experimental cell therapies such as ex vivo expansion of $CD34^+$ cells. However, some studies suggest a higher incidence of engraftment failure and possibly delayed immune reconstitution in certain patient populations when transplants are performed with highly purified CD34-selected, T cell–depleted products.

Several problems have slowed enthusiastic universal adoption of PBSC transplants for all recipients. Concerns remain regarding the hypothetical long-term effects of exposure of healthy donors to growth factors. The possible risks of donor G-CSF administration and leukapheresis must be weighed against less evidence of benefit of PBSCs compared with bone marrow (or against the rapid availability of cord blood) for pediatric recipients. Also, some clinical data suggest the possibility that allogeneic PBSC transplant may result in more frequent chronic GVHD in certain patient populations than occurs with bone marrow transplant without obvious reciprocal benefit with regard to graft-versus-leukemia effect. For allogeneic donors, the discomfort and inconvenience of multiple-day cytokine administration may be a significant deterrent. Most donors experience some degree of malaise and bone pain, and some donors require hospitalization for more serious adverse reactions to G-CSF administration. A large prospective trial of the National Marrow Donor Program found female donors at greater risk of apheresis adverse events and more frequently required central line insertion.[27] Splenic enlargement occurs commonly, and several instances of splenic rupture have been reported. Citrate toxicity is a common complication of PBSC collections; although usually mild and transient, it may be severe and even life threatening in some individuals (see previous section). Venous access requires large-bore multilumen catheters, and these appear particularly susceptible to clotting, especially when patients receive recombinant cytokine stimulation. Hemorrhage, especially in thrombocytopenic patients, is another potentially severe complication of central venous catheter placement.

Some patients who have received multiple prior cycles of chemotherapy and a small proportion of normal healthy donors, referred to as "poor mobilizers," fail to respond adequately to mobilization regimens. In this circumstance, Plerixafor, a reversible CXCR4 antagonist that can block the adhesion of HPCs to the bone marrow stroma can enhance collections by releasing these cells into the circulation. In a randomized controlled trial, the combination of G-CSF and Plerixafor resulted in a significantly higher proportion of patients with non-Hodgkin lymphoma achieving their target cell dose in fewer apheresis days.[28] Similar success is achieved with multiple myeloma patients achieving a 4.8-fold increase peripheral blood CD34 cell count compared with 1.7-fold with G-CSF alone.[29] Emerging evidence indicates that Plerixafor may be administered to rescue collections for patients who mobilize poorly with G-CSF alone; however, the optimum timing for administration has not yet been determined.[30]

Patient Management Issues for Therapeutic Apheresis

Important issues to consider when preparing a patient for therapeutic apheresis, for monitoring the patient during the procedure, and for managing the patient after removal from the apheresis device include:

Preparation

- Volume considerations—Calculate volume to be processed or exchanged; order replacement solutions; assess patient volume status. A blood prime may be necessary for children who weigh less than 25 kg.
- Vascular access—Assess need for apheresis line placement. Note that not all large catheters are suitable for apheresis procedures.
- Medications—Evaluate impact of medications (Coumadin, platelet inhibitory agents, angiotensin-converting enzyme inhibitors) and indications to suspend certain medications. Albumin-bound medications may be depleted by apheresis.
- Cell counts—Patient may require transfusion for preprocedure anemia or thrombocytopenia.
- Electrolytes—Assess risks for citrate toxicity; order calcium replacement solutions if indicated.

Procedure

- Volume considerations—Monitor replacement fluids (saline-to-albumin ratio). Rapid infusion of refrigerated solutions may cause hypothermia.
- Vascular access—Observe for impaired, intermittent, or obstructed flow. Kinked tubing can result in hemolysis.
- Medications—Limitations on blood or citrate flow rate caused by symptomatic citrate-induced hypocalcemia may necessitate addition of anticoagulant to the final apheresis product or inclusion of heparin in the anticoagulant regimen.
- Cell counts—Consider the impact of very high or low cell counts on device settings and procedure efficiency.
- Electrolytes—Continually monitor for adverse citrate effects; bolus or continuous intravenous calcium administration may be required.

Postprocedure Management

- Volume considerations—Review net volume balance and consider additional infusion or administration of diuretic if needed.
- Vascular access—The decision to remove the apheresis catheter should include the possibility of additional apheresis or procedures; monitor for complications associated with maintenance or removal of venous catheter.
- Medications—Determine when to restart medications; consider the impact of transiently reduced coagulation factor levels.
- Cell counts—The patient may require transfusion for postprocedure thrombocytopenia; monitor cumulative red blood cell and platelet loss after repeated procedures.
- Electrolytes—Assess for imbalance postprocedure with attention to ionized calcium and magnesium as indicated by symptoms.

PEDIATRIC HEMAPHERSIS

Therapeutic apheresis in pediatrics poses a particular challenge. The indications for apheresis in children are limited by a lack of clinical trial data in this population. Therefore, the evidence for therapy in many diseases is extrapolated from trials in adults despite differing patient physiology and an age-dependent presentation and natural history of the disease. For example, hemolytic uremic syndrome is more common in children and responds to supportive care; at the other spectrum of this disease, TTP is more common in adults and necessitates plasma exchange.

Similarly, the mechanics of apheresis was developed for adults and therefore designed for their larger circulating blood volume. Therefore, depending on the size of the child, modifications to the apheresis procedure may be necessary. Central venous catheters are required in most circumstances because the caliber of peripheral venous access is too small in most circumstances to permit adequate blood flow.

Technical Aspects

In pediatric apheresis, maintenance of isovolemia is essential to prevent circulatory compromise, particularly in an acutely ill patient who may have some degree of cardiac or renal impairment. The beginning and end of the apheresis procedure involves negative and positive intravascular fluid shifts, respectively. Typically, this has negligible impact on an adult's circulation but can represent a substantial proportion of the total blood volume (TBV) of an infant. The volume of the patient's blood required to fill the apheresis tubing and circuit at the start of the procedure is the extracorporeal volume (ECV). Symptomatic hypovolemia is possible when this exceeds 15% of TBV. For example, when the ECV is 400 mL, this represents 8% of the TBV in a 70-kg patient but may be as much as 35% for a 15-kg infant. Therefore, modification of the apheresis procedure is necessary if this is to be performed safely in infants and children.

In adults, the apheresis circuit is primed with saline, which is then diverted to the collection or waste bag. One option permits return of saline prime to the patient, which may be useful for larger children. For children who weigh less than 25 kg, a prime with RBCs is often necessary to prevent intravascular volume depletion. RBCs are chosen over pure crystalloid solutions alone to prevent a RBC deficit. This is important for patients sensitive to a drop in intravascular RBC volume. Upon completion, fluids remaining in the apheresis circuit, typically returned to the adult patient, are not returned in pediatrics to avoid a positive fluid shift causing fluid overload.

Pediatric Apheresis

The majority of apheresis procedures in children are erythrocytapheresis for patients with sickle cell disease and mononuclear cell collections for HPCs to be used in conjunction with high-dose chemotherapy. Plasma exchange is infrequently indicated apart from uncommon neurologic disorders. For example, pediatric autoimmune neuropsychiatric disorders associated with streptococcal infection (PANDAS) and Sydenham chorea (SC) are autoimmune neuropsychiatric disorders that occur rarely after infection with group A β-hemolytic streptococcal infections. Circulating immune factors may be part of the pathogenesis of these diseases because both respond to IVIG and plasmapheresis. In a small randomized study, 50% of patients with SC also responded to plasmapheresis, and although superior to corticosteroids, treatment with IVIG had the best response, with 72% of patients having a reduction in symptoms of chorea.

REFERENCES

1. Whitaker BL, Henry RA: *The 2007 National Blood Collection and Utilization Survey Report*, Washington DC, 2007, US Department of Health and Human Services.
2. Kato GJ, Gladwin MT, Steinberg MH: Deconstructing sickle cell disease: Reappraisal of the role of hemolysis in the development of clinical subphenotypes. *Blood Rev* 21:37, 2007.
3. Gilli SC, De Paula EV, Biscaro FP, et al: Third-trimester erythrocytapheresis in pregnant patients with sickle cell disease. *Int J Gynecol Obstet* 96:8, 2007.
4. Rombout-Sestrienkova E, Noord PAHv, Reuser E, et al: Therapeutic Erythrocytapheresis (TE) versus Phlebotomy (P) in the treatment of Hereditary Hemochromatosis (HH) patients: Preliminary results from an ongoing randomized clinical trial (NCT 00202436). *Tranfus Apher Sci* 40:135, 2009.
5. De Santis GC, de Oliveira LCO, Romano LGM, et al: Therapeutic leukapheresis in patients with leukostasis secondary to acute myelogenous leukemia. *J Clin Apher* 26:181, 2011.
6. Chang M-C, Chen T-Y, Tang J-L, et al: Leukapheresis and cranial irradiation in patients with hyperleukocytic acute myeloid leukemia: No impact on early mortality and intracranial hemorrhage. *Am J Hematol* 82:976, 2007.
7. Klamová H, Marková M, Moravcová J, et al: Response to treatment in women with chronic myeloid leukemia during pregnancy and after delivery. *Leuk Res* 33:1567, 2009.
8. Vernia P, D'Ovidio V, Meo D: Leukocytapheresis in the treatment of inflammatory bowel disease: Current position and perspectives. *Tranfus Apher Sci* 43:227, 2010.
9. Thanaraj S, Hamlin PJ, Ford AC: Systematic review: Granulocyte/monocyte adsorptive apheresis for ulcerative colitis. *Aliment Pharmacol Ther* 32:1297, 2010.
10. Yamamoto T, Umegae S, Matsumoto K: Daily granulocyte and monocyte adsorptive apheresis in patients with active ulcerative colitis: A prospective safety and feasibility study. *J Gastroenterol* 46:1003, 2011.
11. Scarisbrick JJ, Taylor P, Holtick U, et al: On behalf of the Photopheresis Expert G. U.K. consensus statement on the use of extracorporeal photopheresis for treatment of cutaneous T-cell lymphoma and chronic graft-versus-host disease. *Br J Dermatol* 158:659, 2008.
12. Marques MB, Schwartz J: Update on extracorporeal photopheresis in heart and lung transplantation. *J Clin Apher* 26:146, 2011.
13. Morrell MR, Despotis GJ, Lublin DM, et al: The efficacy of photopheresis for bronchiolitis obliterans syndrome after lung transplantation. *J Heart Lung Transplant* 29:424, 2010.
14. Szczepiorkowski ZM, Winters JL, Bandarenko N, et al: Guidelines on the use of therapeutic apheresis in clinical practice–evidence-based approach from the Apheresis Applications Committee of the American Society for Apheresis. *J Clin Apher* 25:83, 2010.
15. Cortese I, Chaudhry V, So YT, et al: Evidence-based guideline update: Plasmapheresis in neurologic disorders. *Neurology* 76:294, 2011.
16. George JN: How I treat patients with thrombotic thrombocytopenic purpura: 2010. *Blood* 116:4060, 2010.
17. Nguyen L, Li X, Duvall D, et al: Twice-daily plasma exchange for patients with refractory thrombotic thrombocytopenic purpura: The experience of the Oklahoma Registry, 1989 through 2006. *Transfusion* 48:349, 2008.
18. Thompson GR: Recommendations for the use of LDL apheresis. *Atherosclerosis* 198:247, 2008.
19. Hudgins LC, Kleinman B, Scheuer A, et al: Long-term safety and efficacy of low-density lipoprotein apheresis in childhood for homozygous familial hypercholesterolemia. *Am J Cardiol* 102:1199, 2008.
20. Kolansky DM, Cuchel M, Clark BJ, et al: Longitudinal evaluation and assessment of cardiovascular disease in patients with homozygous familial hypercholesterolemia. *Am J Cardiol* 102:1438, 2008.
21. Lefaucheur C, Nochy D, Andrade J, et al: Comparison of combination Plasmapheresis/IVIg/anti-CD20 versus high-dose IVIg in the treatment of antibody-mediated rejection. *Am J Transplant* 9:1099, 2009.
22. Akalin E, Dinavahi R, Friedlander R, et al: Addition of plasmapheresis decreases the incidence of acute antibody-mediated rejection in sensitized patients with strong donor-specific antibodies. *Clin J Am Soc Nephrol* 3:1160, 2008.
23. Llufriu S, Castillo J, Blanco Y, et al: Plasma exchange for acute attacks of CNS demyelination: Predictors of improvement at 6 months. *Neurology* 73:949, 2009.
24. Agreda-Vásquez GP, Espinosa-Poblano I, Sánchez-Guerrero SA, et al: Starch and albumin mixture as replacement fluid in therapeutic plasma exchange is safe and effective. *J Clin Apher* 23:163, 2008.
25. Clayton JA, Vitale S, Kim J, et al: Prevalence of posterior subcapsular cataracts in volunteer cytapheresis donors. *Transfusion* 51:921, 2010.
26. Vasu S, Leitman SF, Tisdale JF, et al: Donor demographic and laboratory predictors of allogeneic peripheral blood stem cell mobilization in an ethnically diverse population. *Blood* 112:2092, 2008.

27. Pulsipher MA, Chitphakdithai P, Miller JP, et al: Adverse events among 2408 unrelated donors of peripheral blood stem cells: Results of a prospective trial from the National Marrow Donor Program. *Blood* 113:3604, 2009.
28. DiPersio JF, Micallef IN, Stiff PJ, et al: Phase III prospective randomized double-blind placebo-controlled trial of plerixafor plus granulocyte colony-stimulating factor compared with placebo plus granulocyte colony-stimulating factor for autologous stem-cell mobilization and transplantation for patients with non-Hodgkin's lymphoma. *J Clin Oncol* 27:4767, 2009.
29. DiPersio JF, Stadtmauer EA, Nademanee A, et al: Plerixafor and G-CSF versus placebo and G-CSF to mobilize hematopoietic stem cells for autologous stem cell transplantation in patients with multiple myeloma. *Blood* 113:5720, 2009.
30. Basak GW, Mikala G, Koristek Z, et al: Plerixafor to rescue failing chemotherapy-based stem cell mobilization: It's not too late. *Leuk Lymphoma* 52:1711, 2011.

CHAPTER 120

TRANSFUSION REACTIONS TO BLOOD AND CELL THERAPY PRODUCTS

Jacquelyn D. Choate, Robert W. Maitta, Christopher A. Tormey, YanYun Wu, and Edward L. Snyder

A *transfusion reaction* can be defined as any untoward reaction that occurs as a consequence of infusion of blood or cell therapy products. Transfusion reactions can be classified as acute or delayed. Acute reactions occur during the transfusion or within several hours after its completion. Delayed transfusion reactions occur at any point after this time frame; for example, delayed hemolytic transfusion reactions typically present days after the transfusion. Other types of delayed reactions may present long after the actual transfusion—months or even years later, as in the case of some transfusion-transmitted diseases. From 2005 to 2010, there were 307 transfusion related fatalities reported to the FDA.[1] This chapter will review various types of transfusion reactions (Table 120-1).

HEMOLYTIC TRANSFUSION REACTIONS

Hemolytic transfusion reactions are caused by the immune-mediated lysis of transfused red blood cells (RBCs). Immune-mediated hemolysis can be classified according to the timing of the reaction (acute or delayed) and by site of hemolysis (intravascular or extravascular). The four types of hemolytic transfusion reactions are acute intravascular, acute extravascular, delayed intravascular, and delayed extravascular (Table 120-2).[1,2]

ACUTE INTRAVASCULAR HEMOLYTIC TRANSFUSION REACTIONS

Acute reactions are those that occur within minutes after incompatible RBCs are transfused into a patient who already possesses the corresponding antibody. Because ABO antibodies are naturally occurring (and primarily IgM class or a mixture of IgG and IgM class), infusion of ABO-incompatible blood is the most likely cause of a clinically significant acute intravascular hemolytic transfusion reaction. However, other complement-fixing antigen-antibody systems, such as alloantibodies with specificity for the Jk[a] (Kidd) blood group system, can also produce these reactions in situations where they are undetectable in the pretransfusion sample. Such a reaction could occur, for example, after transfusion of A RBCs into an O recipient who has significant amounts of circulating anti-A. Although the titer and avidity of the antibody affect the extent of the hemolytic reaction, the clinical severity of an incompatible RBC transfusion is greatly influenced by the degree of complement activation and cytokine stimulation. The transfused incompatible RBCs undergo complement-mediated osmotic lysis, producing hemoglobinemia and hemoglobinuria. The sine qua non of an acute intravascular hemolytic transfusion reaction is the presence of red plasma and red (dark) urine.

It is critical to distinguish, as quickly as possible, hemoglobinuria and hemoglobinemia resulting from an acute hemolytic transfusion reaction from similar signs due to other causes. Hemoglobin in the urine can be confused with myoglobin or with hematuria from a urinary tract source. Hemoglobinemia caused by non-immune-mediated lysis can result from mechanical hemolysis from an improperly collected blood sample. The direct antiglobulin test (DAT) usually becomes positive in an immune hemolytic reaction (if tested before all the incompatible RBCs are destroyed); preparation of an antibody eluate is often necessary to identify the presence of an offending IgG antibody. An elution is a procedure that chemically separates the bound antibody from the RBCs and concentrates it so that it may be identified.

If time is lost in making a clinical diagnosis, a mild treatable reaction can quickly turn into one that is life threatening. An acute intravascular hemolytic transfusion reaction is a true medical emergency. Initial clinical symptoms can include fever and chills, shortness of breath, chest pain, dizziness, and back or flank pain. Some patients report feeling pain or warmth ascending from the site of infusion, or a feeling of anxiety or "impending doom." Acute transfusion reactions can quickly progress to shock and acute renal failure. In an ABO-incompatible transfusion reaction, activation of the complement cascade occurs with release of C3a and C5a (anaphylatoxins 1 and 2, respectively). Fixation of the C5b-9 complement membrane attack complex produces pores in the RBC membrane, resulting in osmotic lysis. Antibody-coated RBC stroma produced during an immune hemolytic transfusion reaction induces renal vasoconstriction, resulting in acute tubular necrosis. Another contributing cause of ischemic renal failure involves the release of free plasma hemoglobin. It has been shown that cell-free hemoglobin binds tightly to nitric oxide. Endothelium-derived relaxing factor, a powerful vasodilator, is composed in part of nitric oxide. By binding to nitric oxide, free plasma hemoglobin blocks relaxing factor and prevents renal vasodilation. This also promotes renal vasoconstriction and renal tubular ischemia, with eventual tubular necrosis. Many patients, curiously even anephric patients, often complain of lower back pain. It is speculated that this symptom is caused by ischemic muscle pain or vasospasm, rather than by kidney pain from developing renal failure. In addition to complement components, cytokines and interleukins (ILs) also play a role in the clinical symptom complex, including fever, associated with acute intravascular hemolytic transfusion reactions. For example, IL-1β, IL-6, and tumor necrosis factor-α (TNF- α) have pyrogenic activity; IL-8 is a neutrophil chemotactic and activating factor. These four cytokines have been generated in various in vitro models of intravascular hemolysis and IgG-mediated RBC incompatibility. The clinical variability of hemolytic transfusion reactions is likely explained by the relative balance of cytokine production in the transfusion recipient. Factors that increase the circulating levels of proinflammatory cytokines and chemokines often result in more severe reactions.

Laboratory Evaluation

Laboratory findings include hemoglobinuria, hemoglobinemia, and a haptoglobin level that is low to undetectable. During the hemolytic episode, the bilirubin (especially indirect bilirubin) usually increases only to 2 to 3 mg/dL if the patient has normal liver function. Elevations of bilirubin to 20 to 30 mg/dL are not seen in otherwise normal patients, even with florid hemolysis. Very elevated bilirubin levels are seen only in patients with concurrent hepatocellular disease, such as viral hepatitis or hepatic carcinoma. Because of the lysis of RBCs, levels of lactate dehydrogenase (LDH) may rise markedly. If the patient shows no signs of vasomotor instability and if hemostatic and

Table 120-1 Types of Acute Transfusion Reactions

Reaction Type	Presenting Signs and Symptoms
Acute intravascular hemolytic	Fever, chills, dyspnea, hypotension, tachycardia, flushing, vomiting, back pain, hemoglobinuria, hemoglobinemia, shock
Acute extravascular hemolytic	Fever, indirect hyperbilirubinemia, posttransfusion hematocrit increment lower than expected
Febrile reaction	Fever, chills
Allergic (mild)	Urticaria, pruritus, rash
Anaphylactic	Dyspnea, bronchospasm, hypotension, tachycardia, shock
Hypervolemic	Dyspnea, tachycardia, hypertension, headache, jugular venous distention
Septic	Fever, chills, hypotension, tachycardia, vomiting, shock
Transfusion-related acute lung injury	Dyspnea, decreased oxygen saturation, fever, hypotension

Table 120-2 Hemolytic Transfusion Reactions: Serologic Presentation

Type	Antibody Detectable Initially	Primary Antibody Type	Degree of Complement Binding	Example
Acute intravascular	Yes	IgM	Full (C1-9)	ABO system
Acute extravascular	Yes	IgG	None/partial	Rh system
Delayed intravascular	No	IgG	Full (C1-9)	Kidd system
Delayed extravascular	No	IgG	None/partial	Duffy system

renal function is unchanged 24 to 36 hours after the incompatible transfusion, the episode can be considered to be over, with serious sequelae unlikely.

Therapy

Initial therapy consists of immediately stopping the transfusion, maintaining a patent intravenous line, cardiorespiratory support, and ensuring a brisk diuresis. Increasing renal blood flow is the best way to prevent acute oliguric renal failure. Usually, 0.9% NaCl or some other suitable crystalloid solution is infused to maintain a urine output of 100 mL/hour for approximately 24 hours. Diuretics, such as furosemide, also can be used and are preferred by some to infusion of mannitol to increase intravascular volume. Mannitol, if chosen, must be used with caution; if acute tubular necrosis (ATN) occurs before mannitol infusion, pulmonary edema may occur as a result of the acute increase in intravascular volume secondary to fluid expansion. Similarly, excessive crystalloid infusion should be avoided in patients with fluid overload, including those patients with congestive heart failure. Renal damage must be minimized, however, and increasing renal blood flow helps to prevent anuric renal failure. The mechanisms responsible for the beneficial effect of increased renal blood flow likely include increased clearance of free hemoglobin, resulting in decreased binding of nitric oxide, and a return of more physiologic control of renal vasodilation. Creatinine and blood urea nitrogen

Workup of an Acute Intravascular Hemolytic Transfusion Reaction

If an acute transfusion reaction occurs:

1. Stop blood component infusion immediately.
2. Maintain intravenous access with a suitable crystalloid or colloid solution.
3. Monitor/maintain blood pressure and heart rate.
4. Maintain an adequate airway.
5. Give a diuretic or institute fluid diuresis, or both.
6. Obtain blood and urine studies for the transfusion reaction workup.
7. Blood bank workup of suspected transfusion reaction:
   - Check paperwork to ensure correct blood component was transfused to the correct patient.
   - Observe plasma for hemoglobinemia.
   - Perform direct antiglobulin test.
   - Repeat compatibility testing (crossmatch).
   - Repeat other serologic testing as needed (ABO, Rh).
   - Analyze urine for hemoglobinuria.

If intravascular hemolytic reaction is confirmed:

8. Monitor renal status (BUN, creatinine).
9. Monitor coagulation status (prothrombin time, partial thromboplastin time, fibrinogen).
10. Monitor for signs of hemolysis (lactate dehydrogenase, bilirubin-total/direct, haptoglobin).
11. If sepsis is suspected, culture as appropriate.

(BUN) should be closely monitored; dialysis may be necessary for treatment of oliguric acute renal failure. Support of blood pressure and respiration may require the use of vasopressors, bronchodilators, and when necessary, intubation. High doses of dopamine cause vasoconstriction and should be avoided unless required to support the patient's blood pressure. Disseminated intravascular coagulation (DIC) can occur in severe cases. The prothrombin time, partial thromboplastin time, and fibrinogen level should be closely monitored (see box on Workup of an Acute Intravascular Hemolytic Transfusion Reaction).

ACUTE EXTRAVASCULAR HEMOLYTIC TRANSFUSION REACTION

In an extravascular hemolytic transfusion reaction, complement is either not fixed at all or is fixed only to C3b. In either situation, because of the nature of the antigen-antibody reaction, complement activation with fixation of the C5b-9 complex does not occur. This presentation is commonly associated with Rh antibodies, but can be seen with any number of non-ABO antigen-antibody complexes. The presence of IgG bound to the RBCs or C3b fixation results in an extravascular reaction because the antibody-coated cells are cleared by the IgG receptors in the spleen or the C3b receptors in the liver. In these circumstances, RBC lysis does not occur in the intravascular space. Because of the lack of generation of C3a or C5a, an extravascular hemolytic transfusion reaction does not usually present as a clinical emergency. It is characterized by development of a positive DAT due to recipient RBC alloantibodies binding to the incompatible circulating donor RBCs. Moreover, an increase in indirect bilirubin, an increase in LDH, a decrease in hematocrit, a decrease in haptoglobin, and an increase in colorless urine urobilinogen can occur, but hemoglobinuria and hemoglobinemia are rarely present. The patient typically remains clinically stable; renal failure, shock, and hemostatic abnormalities, such as DIC, are rarely seen unless the amount of incompatible blood infused is excessive. However, patients often have a low-grade fever, probably from the generation of IL-1 or other proinflammatory cytokines.

When an extravascular hemolytic transfusion reaction is suspected, the diagnostic test of choice is a DAT with an eluate. The eluate is performed to identify the antibody coating the RBCs. The positive DAT result reflects the patient's antibody (or antibodies) coating the incompatible donor RBCs. Because this is not an autoantibody (or antibodies), the patient's own RBCs are not usually involved in the reaction.

Typically, an acute extravascular hemolytic transfusion reaction requires no special therapeutic intervention. Maintaining a good urine output and monitoring renal and hemostatic function are usually sufficient. The patient characteristically recovers in a few days as the offending donor RBCs are cleared from the circulation. The pathogenic alloantibody can often be identified in the patient's serum/plasma. These extravascular acute reactions may occur if the patient's pre-existing alloantibody was missed by the blood bank during the antibody screening process, if a wrongly labeled sample was used, if the unit of blood was labeled for the wrong patient, or if the unit was hung, in error, on the wrong patient.

DELAYED HEMOLYTIC REACTIONS

The pathogenesis of a delayed intravascular transfusion reaction is similar to that described for an acute intravascular hemolytic reaction.[2,3] However, in the delayed type, the patient develops the antigen-antibody reaction some time (usually at least 3-10 days) after the transfusion. The process occurs more slowly and is less likely to present as a clinical emergency. Hemoglobinuria and hemoglobinemia can occur but often are less pronounced than with an acute intravascular reaction. This probably is due to the continual and gradual removal of antibody-coated RBCs as the antibody titer rises and by the more gradual generation of C3a and C5a. The same serologic diagnostic and treatment concepts used for an acute intravascular hemolytic reaction apply here. However, the need for acute intervention is much less likely. Initiating a diuresis and monitoring renal and hemostatic function may be sufficient.

Delayed extravascular hemolytic transfusion reactions occur as well and are, in fact, the most common presentation resulting from an anamnestic antibody response. Such antigen-antibody reactions often involve the Rh system. The clinical presentation is similar to that of an acute extravascular reaction: the patient often has no acute sequelae such as shock or DIC, but may present with a fever, a falling hematocrit, and the development of a new DAT with a positive eluate. Because these reactions are typically mild in nature, they are usually addressed with supportive care only.

One final note regarding the serologic evaluation of a transfusion reaction: posttransfusion testing may be complicated and difficult to interpret because of the possibility of autoantibodies or the involvement of medications. In such circumstances, referral to the pretransfusion specimen is often helpful (because the DAT or other testing may show positive results in these specimens). In cases of more complex evaluations, consultation with an expert serologist is recommended to better detect and identify new alloantibodies in the patient's serum, which may be responsible for a hemolytic transfusion reaction.

FEBRILE NONHEMOLYTIC TRANSFUSION REACTIONS

A febrile nonhemolytic transfusion reaction (FNHTR) is suspected when a transient temperature rise of 1° C or more occurs during or after transfusion and when no other cause for the fever can be identified.[3] In addition to fever, FNHTRs are often associated with shaking chills. In fact, shaking chills can also manifest without a concomitant fever, an atypical or "afebrile" FNHTR. In these cases, temperature increases may be masked by antipyretic premedication. Febrile reactions are likely mediated in part by cytokines released in response to antibody-leukocyte or antibody-platelet interactions. Cytotoxic or agglutinating antibodies having human leukocyte antigen (HLA) specificity, neutrophil specificity, or platelet specificity may be present in the recipient's plasma and react against antigens present on transfused donor lymphocytes, granulocytes, or platelets.[4] Conversely, donor plasma may contain the offending antibody that can react with the corresponding cellular antigens in the recipient's blood. The febrile reaction is mediated largely by the release of cytokines such as IL-1β, IL-6, and TNF-α from macrophages, monocytes, granulocytes, or lymphocytes. IL-1 (endogenous pyrogen), through prostaglandin PGE_2 synthesis, probably stimulates the thermoregulatory center of the hypothalamus to produce fever. Other mediators such as macrophage inflammatory proteins (e.g., MIP-1) may also participate in the febrile response, but this reaction is not mediated through prostaglandin synthesis. CD154 (CD40 ligand) derived from platelets may also be involved in febrile reactions by inducing cyclooxygenase-2 and PGE_2.[5]

Studies have shown that generation of cytokines does occur in units of blood during storage and that such generation is directly proportional to the leukocyte count of the unit and the duration of storage. Use of third-generation prestorage leukocyte reduction filters can lower the incidence of febrile reactions.[6] However, proinflammatory cytokines are not removed by bedside blood filters, and they enter the circulation. Prevention of cytokine generation by prestorage leukoreduction is more efficient and effective than is scavenging of the biologic response modifiers by using bedside filtration technology.

The frequency of febrile reactions for a non-leukoreduced unit has been estimated to be 6.8 per 100 units RBCs transfused and 2.2 per 100 units platelet transfused.[3] With the advent of prestorage leukoreduction these risks have been decreased to about 0.09 to 1.1 per 100 units RBCs transfused and 0.04 to 1.56 per 100 units platelet transfused. Reactions are most commonly seen in recipients who have been exposed to multiple white cell or platelet antigens. Oncology patients are at risk as a result of frequent transfusions, as are multiparous women who may have received multiple exposures during pregnancy and childbirth. Both of these groups of patients can form multiple HLA-, granulocyte-, or platelet-specific antibodies that will react with white cells or platelets upon subsequent exposure. Antigen-antibody reactions are capable of stimulating cellular activation with resultant complement fixation, cytokine generation, and activation of other biologic response modifiers.

Laboratory Evaluation

The workup of a febrile reaction must be undertaken promptly, because fever may also be the first sign of other, more severe reactions, including acute hemolysis or sepsis. A hemolytic transfusion reaction may be ruled out by reconfirming the ABO and Rh type of the patient and the donor unit, repeating crossmatching to confirm patient-donor compatibility, evaluating the results of the pretransfusion and posttransfusion direct antiglobulin tests, evaluating the serum for hemolysis, and rechecking the accuracy of paperwork. The posttransfusion DAT should yield negative findings, because FNHTRs do not involve RBC alloantibodies.

As laboratory testing is being completed, the workup should extend beyond the blood bank to include bedside patient evaluation. Fever and chills also may be caused by drugs or underlying diseases, or they may be associated with infection or inflammation. Neutropenic fever often complicates the clinical picture in patients undergoing high-dose chemotherapy, a population of patients likely to undergo repeated RBC or platelet transfusions. To rule out a septic transfusion reaction, blood cultures of the patient and the blood product should be considered, especially if the patient has very high fever or shows signs of sepsis (see later text for a more in-depth discussion of septic transfusion reactions). The difficulty lies in knowing when to order blood cultures, because they are expensive and there is a 3% incidence of false-positive cultures as a result of contamination during culturing. Most routine hospital blood banks do not have the expertise or reagents needed to identify specific HLA, platelet, or granulocyte antibodies. Accordingly, the diagnosis of an FNHTR is usually made as a diagnosis of exclusion without isolating an identifiable antibody.

Treatment and Prevention

Fever from an FNHTR usually responds to antipyretics, including aspirin, nonsteroidal antiinflammatory drugs (NSAIDs), and acetaminophen. For thrombocytopenic adult patients, acetaminophen is the antipyretic of choice. Aspirin and NSAIDs should be avoided in thrombocytopenic patients, because they further compromise platelet function because of their inhibitory effects on platelet cyclooxygenase. Diphenhydramine is not indicated for treatment of febrile reactions.

For patients with no history of febrile reactions, routine premedication is unnecessary. Those with a history of febrile reaction may be premedicated with acetaminophen or an NSAID. Those patients with severe reactions despite premedication may require more intensive pharmacotherapy, including hydrocortisone 1 to 2 hours before transfusion. Patients with severe shaking chills can be treated with meperidine, which can stop shaking chills almost immediately. Febrile reactions after granulocyte transfusions and, less frequently, after platelet transfusions can be so severe that hypotension and cardiovascular collapse may occur.

Prevention of febrile reactions when pharmacologic therapy fails relies on the use of leukocyte-depleted blood components. Several leukocyte depletion techniques are available. Centrifugation can remove approximately 70% of the leukocytes in a unit of blood; cell washing or use of frozen deglycerolized RBCs can remove up to 95% of contaminating white cells. Older microaggregate blood filters can reduce leukocyte content by approximately 1 to 2 logs (90%-93%). Third-generation leukocyte-depletion RBC filters are more useful for preventing febrile reactions.[7] They can remove up to 4 logs (99.99%) of white cells, often lowering the level of white cells in a unit of blood from 10^9 to 10^5. They also may be useful for preventing or delaying the onset of HLA alloimmunization. Leukocyte depletion platelet filters are also available. Recommendations for usage of leukocyte-depleted blood components are published. Data show that a patient who has had one febrile transfusion reaction has a 1 in 8 chance of having another one. Individuals with a history of recurrent severe febrile reactions should have notations made in their blood bank record to ensure future use of leukocyte-reduced components. Although clearly indicated for patients with multiple and recurrent febrile reactions, some physicians still question whether leukodepleted blood products should be used for all patients.

ALLERGIC AND ANAPHYLACTIC TRANSFUSION REACTIONS

Allergic Reactions

Allergic transfusion reactions are believed to be most commonly caused by infusion of plasma proteins (e.g., haptoglobin) against which recipients have formed IgE or IgG class antibodies.[3,8] The allergic manifestations produced vary. They can include erythema with associated mild to extensive urticaria and mild to intense pruritus; severe vasomotor instability; bronchospasm; and anaphylaxis. A patient who develops hives and a mild allergic reaction during a blood transfusion usually does not progress to a more severe anaphylactic reaction after infusion of additional blood from the same unit. The severity of allergic transfusion reactions is not necessarily dose related.

The exact nature of the antibodies involved in the various types of allergic reactions is unclear. The mild allergic reactions are usually IgE mediated, but other classes of immunoglobulins may also be involved; anaphylactic reactions are most often IgE mediated.[3,7] Allergic reactions are believed to be mediated by histamine. Histamine can be released through the antigen-antibody interactions involving antibodies present in recipients against donor antigens or via antibodies passively transferred from donor against recipient antigens. Histamine can also be passively transferred from donors to recipients by transfusion of stored blood components. Allergic transfusion reactions are quite common, occurring in approximately 1% of all transfusions. Most of these reactions start with pruritus, followed by the development of hives. At this point, the transfusion should be stopped and the patient given 25 to 50 mg of diphenhydramine, if there are no medical contraindications and if the patient had not already been maximally premedicated. After a short interval, the transfusion can resume, but only if the rash decreases or the hives disappear and the patient feels well without signs of fever, chills, or vasomotor instability; re-initiation of transfusion is possible in most cases because such allergic symptoms are not likely to recur. The risk for transfusion-transmitted disease posed by infusion of another unit of blood is greater than the risk posed by continuing a transfusion that has produced only mild urticaria.

Allergic transfusion reactions do not generally recur, but patients who have had more than one mild allergic reaction should continue to receive routine units and may be premedicated with diphenhydramine or other H_1 blockers (e.g., ranitidine). Washed RBCs or plasma-reduced platelets can be used to prevent severe recurrent reactions. Leukocyte depletion or microaggregate filters are of no value because the plasma protein passes through the filter. Corticosteroids, provided in advance of a transfusion, also may be useful in patients with serious recurrent reactions unless contraindicated.

Although it is convenient to characterize a transfusion reaction as being purely febrile or allergic, in reality there is often a mix of the two symptoms, and the reaction is designated according to the predominant clinical sign.

Anaphylactic Reactions

Although any number of proteins can mediate severe allergic reactions, it has been observed that plasma containing IgA, when transfused to patients with IgG or IgE class anti-IgA antibodies, is the most common cause of anaphylactic transfusion reactions. It is not routine to test a patient's plasma for IgG or IgE class anti-IgA, and such assays are not readily available. This type of reaction may also occur in patients with deficiency of other plasma proteins such as haptoglobin. Anaphylactic reactions are often associated with severe hypotension, respiratory distress, and even cardiovascular collapse. As such, these reactions can be life threatening and may require intubation, pressor agents, and use of potent antiallergic medications (e.g., epinephrine) to overcome the severe symptoms. If a clear cause for an anaphylactic reaction is found (e.g., an anti-IgA antibody in an IgA deficient recipient), then the use of product washing is appropriate. In addition, for patients with evidence of severe or recurrent allergic/anaphylactic reactions, a combination of H_1 and H_2 blockers may be more effective for treatment and premedication, and again, the addition of corticosteroids may be necessary if not otherwise contraindicated.

HYPOTENSIVE TRANSFUSION REACTION

A less recognized, but occasionally severe acute transfusion reaction is isolated hypotension during or immediately following a blood product infusion.[3] The classic presentation of such acute hypotensive reactions includes (a) a drop in blood pressure (often >30 mm Hg) as the main symptom and (b) hypotension occurring within minutes of the start of the transfusion and resolving quickly after the stop of the transfusion. This type of transfusion reaction was initially reported after transfusion of platelets administered through some types of bedside leukoreduction filters. Later, it was also reported in other types of blood products including plasma and RBCs. The pathogenesis of this syndrome appears to be related to the activation of the contact pathway (prekallikrein converting to kallikrein) induced in plasma by the negatively charged surface of some leukoreduction filters. Kallikrein activation stimulates the conversion of high-molecular-weight kininogen to bradykinin. Notably, these reactions have also been reported in cases where leukoreduction filters were used before storage, indicating that bradykinin generation may occur via pathways other than via bedside filtration alone. The syndrome is often much more severe in patients already taking angiotensin-converting enzyme (ACE) inhibitors. ACE is identical to kininase II, which is responsible for degrading bradykinin. Blockage of the kininase II degradation of bradykinin by ACE inhibitors results in a prolonged bradykinin half-life and a reaction that can be very severe.

Hypotensive transfusion reactions are typically self-limited, as discussed above, since the hypotension often resolves upon cessation of transfusion. For patients with prolonged hypotension, the use of fluids to increase blood pressure may be warranted. Finally, although rare, pressors may also be indicated for patients with blood pressures unresponsive to simple fluid infusion alone.

INFECTIOUS COMPLICATIONS OF TRANSFUSION

Septic Transfusion Reactions

Bacterial contamination of stored blood can pose grave risks to the recipient. Bacteria can enter the blood bag during venipuncture (as a result of inadequate skin preparation), during component preparation, or through the collection of blood from a donor with an occult infection or asymptomatic bacteremia.[3] Bacteria that grow optimally at refrigerated blood bank temperatures (1° C to 6° C), including *Pseudomonas, Yersinia, Enterobacter,* and *Flavobacterium,* are organisms commonly associated with a contaminated unit of RBCs. Platelet concentrates, stored at room temperature, are also known to be subject to bacterial contamination; several reports have described fatal septic transfusion reactions due to platelets containing *Salmonella* or *Staphylococcus.* Units of blood that are contaminated need not be obviously discolored, malodorous, or clotted; by simple visual inspection, it is extremely difficult to determine whether a unit is contaminated. However, Kim and coworkers[9] reported that visual inspection, including comparison of the blood bag segmented tubing with that of the blood bag itself, can occasionally identify units of RBCs likely to be bacterially contaminated.

Patients who receive a unit of contaminated blood may develop high fever, rigors, skin flushing, abdominal cramps, myalgias, DIC, renal failure, cardiovascular collapse, and cardiac arrest. Clinically, the patient can present in shock. These reactions may be immediate, or there may be a delay of several hours before the symptom complex becomes apparent. Reaction to infusion of a unit of contaminated blood is most often distinguishable from an FNHTR by the former's more severe clinical presentation and from intravascular hemolytic transfusion reactions by the absence of characteristic hemoglobinuria and hemoglobinemia. Shock in a septic transfusion reaction is attributable to endotoxin produced by gram-negative bacteria. The presence of bacteria alone, however, can also cause many of these symptoms. The symptom complex often is attributable, in part, to cytokines and interleukins that are generated in vitro in the contaminated, stored blood. These biologic response modifiers produce severe reactions in vivo after transfusion.[3,7] For example, nitric oxide, produced locally in smooth muscle by the synergistic action of TNF-α, IL-1, and interferon-γ, probably mediates refractory hypotension and vasoplegia associated with septic shock.

If, during transfusion, a patient who appeared well suddenly develops rigors and shock, infusion of an infected component should be considered. If on further evaluation this diagnosis is still considered likely, the patient should be treated immediately, because delay significantly contributes to the chance of a fatal outcome. Blood pressure, heart rate, respirations, and renal blood flow need to be supported. Blood infusion should be stopped the moment any transfusion reaction is suspected, and appropriate samples should be sent to the blood bank for a DAT and other studies. Cultures of the untransfused blood remaining in the blood bag should be obtained because they may be diagnostic. Broad-spectrum antibiotics should be started immediately if infusion of contaminated blood is suspected and continued until the culture results are reported. Although these reactions are rare, they can be fatal. Because of the decrease in viral transmission by blood transfusion, septic transfusion reactions now account for a significant portion of the transfusion-related infections in the United States.[10] Data from the BaCon (Bacterial Contamination of Blood) study showed that from 1998 to 2000, the rate of transfusion-transmitted bacteremia was 9.98 per million single-donor platelets, 10.64 per million pooled platelets, and 0.21 per million RBC units; the rate of fatal reactions was 1.94 per million single-donor platelets, 2.22 per million pooled platelets, and 0.13 per million RBC units, respectively. To decrease the likelihood of a septic unit of platelets being transfused, the expiration date of units of platelet concentrate has been rolled back by the FDA, from a previously licensed 7-day storage period to the current licensed 5-day outdate. To further reduce the risk for bacterial transmission through platelet transfusion, the American Association of Blood Banks (AABB) mandated in 2004 that platelet concentrates be tested for bacterial contamination.[11] There are two bacterial detection systems approved by the U.S. Food and Drug Administration (FDA)[1] to be used for screening of blood components. Since the implementation of the mandatory bacterial testing for platelets, FDA data indicate that the mortality associated with septic transfusion reactions in the United States has dramatically decreased, although the risks for septic transfusion reaction have not been eradicated.

Transfusion Transmitted Diseases

With improvement of donor testing, especially NAT testing, the risk for transfusion-transmitted diseases has decreased dramatically. The current risks are approximately 1 : 1,900,000 for HIV, 1 : 137,000 for HBV, and 1 : 1,000,000 for HCV.[12] However, the risk is never zero. Moreover, there are emerging pathogens, such as babesiosis,[13] that may pose risks to the blood supply. It would be expensive and impossible to screen all potential pathogens to protect the blood supply. To improve blood safety, new technologies such as pathogen inactivation have been developed.[14,15] There are several platforms of pathogen-inactivation technologies. The principle of most pathogen inactivation is that agents added to blood components modify DNA or RNA templates, making them inaccessible to DNA or RNA polymerase, thereby inactivating pathogens (viruses, bacteria, and parasites) and also inactivating white blood cells. Pathogen-inactivation compounds that have been studied include alkylating compounds, binary ethyleneimine-like compounds, riboflavin, and methylene blue. Preclinical studies and phase III clinical trials have shown promising results in the efficacy and safety of pathogen inactivation agents. There are pathogen-inactivation systems approved for plasma and platelets in Europe. As of this date, the FDA has not licensed any pathogen inactivation technologies in the United States.

TRANSFUSION-RELATED ACUTE LUNG INJURY (NONCARDIOGENIC PULMONARY EDEMA)

Transfusion-related acute lung injury (TRALI), has become the leading cause of transfusion-related death reported to the FDA.[1,16] Even though TRALI represented 47% of reported fatalities to the FDA for the period of 2005 to 2010, the number of cases has continued to decrease in trend. The high percentage of TRALI cases may be alarming, but they are in part due to increased awareness of its clinical presentation. Symptoms of TRALI may range from mild dyspnea to severe noncardiogenic pulmonary edema, with symptoms and signs that include dyspnea, oxygen desaturation, respiratory failure, chills, fever, and hypotension. Most patients require oxygen support, and many may require mechanical ventilation. TRALI may develop within 1 to 6 hours of starting a transfusion and is not associated with an elevation in cardiac pressure.[16,17] The chest radiograph may reveal pulmonary edema pattern (bilateral infiltrates). In addition, there is respiratory insufficiency with decreased O_2 saturation, but without development of elevated left-side cardiac pressure. Copious amounts of fluid are produced in the lungs, as is characteristic of hypervolemia; however, the noncardiogenic reaction usually follows infusion of volumes of blood too small to produce fluid overload. Silliman and associates[18,19] postulated that TRALI consists of a "two-hit" event, the first "hit" being a weakened underlying clinical condition that leads to the sequestration and priming of neutrophils in the lung tissue and the second being the transfusion of blood products containing human leukocyte antibodies (class I and II) that activate the neutrophils already present in the pulmonary parenchyma, leading to edema.[17] Complement and monocyte activation with aggregation of white blood cells also may occur when leukoagglutinins present in the recipient react with leukocytes contained in the infused donor blood. As a result of the HLA antigen-antibody reaction, the activated leukocytes express adhesive molecules on their surface (CD11/CD18), which then permit the leukocytes to attach to the cell membrane of the pulmonary endothelial cells and migrate to the interstitial space between the pulmonary capillaries and the alveolar epithelium. Once in the interstitial space, the neutrophils degranulate and through enzymatic digestion produce capillary dehiscence that results in fluid filling the alveolar sacs. Pulmonary leukostasis with pulmonary edema thus occurs as a result of microvascular occlusion and capillary leakage. Complement-activated granulocytes also produce oxygen radicals that damage pulmonary endothelial cells, resulting in a further increase in pulmonary vascular permeability and additional passage of fluid into alveolar spaces. Recently, it has been reported that aged blood products may accumulate bioactive lipids and soluble mediators, such as CD40L, that hamper the chemokine scavenging ability of erythrocytes as a result of reduction in the expression of the Duffy antigens, and this may represent a second hit in the two-hit model.[20] Rodent model systems for TRALI have also been described, and some of these models suggest a role for platelets in TRALI.[21] Work is ongoing in order to elucidate the different mechanisms leading to this symptomatology, which may be a final common pathway from a variety of initiating insults.

Because a definitive diagnosis of TRALI usually requires that cardiac monitoring (Swan-Ganz) catheters be in place, TRALI is difficult to diagnose outside the operating room or intensive care unit. When a patient shows signs of noncardiogenic pulmonary edema, the infusion should be immediately stopped, as it would be with all other reactions. These HLA/neutrophil antigen-antibody reactions may be idiosyncratic and often do not recur. Because of the inherent difficulty in differentiating TRALI from other competing diagnoses such as circulatory overload and the patient's underlying pulmonary status, efforts have been made to develop consensus guidelines to diagnose TRALI.[22]

The removal of leukocyte antigens from units of RBCs or platelets using leukocyte reduction filters may be helpful; and in other instances, washing RBCs may prove useful. Treatment is symptomatic (Table 120-3). Donors who are implicated in moderate to severe TRALI reactions should not be maintained as blood donors. In November 2006, the AABB made further recommendations to implement TRALI risk reduction.[23] It is, however, controversial regarding the optimal approach for TRALI risk reduction. Because their serum may contain high titers of leukoagglutinating antibodies, deferral of blood donors who are multiparous women and blood donors who have been transfused multiple times or have leukoagglutinating antibodies in serum has been used for TRALI risk reduction. This approach may be justified because TRALI reactions may originate when antibody titers are above certain threshold.[16] The exclusion of these donors may have merit since data continue to indicate that using male-only plasma leads to a significant reduction in TRALI cases.[24]

Table 120-3 Diagnosis of Transfusion-Related Acute Lung Injury

Onset	Within 6 hours of start of transfusion
Frequency	1:1000 to 1:4500 transfusions (probably underreported)
Signs and symptoms	Decreased O_2 saturation, fever, hypotension, tachypnea, dyspnea, diffuse pulmonary infiltrates, normal cardiac pressures (requires Swan-Ganz catheter), copious amounts of pulmonary edema fluid
Pathogenesis	HLA/granulocyte-specific antibodies (usually of donor origin) reacting with recipient leukocytes. Activates recipient neutrophils; stimulates complement activation; generates CD11/18 on the polymorphonuclear neutrophil surface, resulting in pulmonary capillary adherence and diapedesis and eventual pulmonary capillary leak syndrome. The latter is associated with generation of proteolytic enzymes and toxic O_2 metabolites, which cause endothelial cell damage. Neutrophil priming lipids may also play a role.
Diagnosis	Chest radiograph; blood gases; blood for HLA or antineutrophil antibodies
Differential diagnosis	Fluid overload; septic transfusion; anaphylaxis
Treatment	STOP TRANSFUSION! Provide ventilatory support (administer O_2, intubate as needed), support blood pressure, administer steroids; diuretics are of *no* value.

TRANSFUSION-ASSOCIATED CIRCULATORY OVERLOAD

Transfusion-associated circulatory overload (TACO) results from hydrostatic transudate accumulation in the lungs and should be considered in patients who, during a blood infusion, develop sudden onset of dyspnea, jugular venous distention, tachycardia, congestive heart failure, or other signs of fluid overload.[3] Unless a patient is actively hemorrhaging, blood should never be infused rapidly, because the acute expansion of a patient's intravascular volume may exceed the capacity of the cardiovascular system to compensate, resulting in fluid overload. Likewise, rapidly transfusing an anemic patient who is euvolemic and not actively bleeding produces no benefit and may cause harm. This caveat applies to transfusion of any blood component. Patients with compromised cardiopulmonary status may not tolerate acute blood volume expansion and may develop right- or left-sided heart failure. This is especially true for infants and the elderly. If symptoms occur, the transfusion should be stopped and the patient's blood volume reduced, either by diuretics or by phlebotomy. If there is a concern that the patient may not tolerate infusion of a full unit of blood or component within the 4-hour period allotted for infusion of blood components, the blood bank can divide the product into smaller portions, which can be transfused in aliquots. As a general guide, infusions in nonbleeding adults should occur at less than 2 to 3 mL/kg/hour. The rate should be lowered to 1 mL/kg/hour for patients at risk for fluid overload. Diuretics may be given to patients with compromised cardiopulmonary status before transfusion. Diagnostically, if the patient improves with diuretics, it is suggestive of TACO.

The initial stages of transfusion-induced hypervolemia may be difficult to distinguish from hemolytic transfusion reaction, FNHTR, allergic reaction, or TRALI. The absence of hemoglobinuria and hemoglobinemia and the absence of a positive posttransfusion DAT result should serve to distinguish the reaction from one caused by immune hemolysis. Likewise, the absence of fever, chills, or urticaria should help distinguish TACO from the febrile or allergic types of reactions. The clinical use of laboratory testing such as N-terminal pro-brain natriuretic peptide (NT-proBNP) may aid in the diagnosis; when NT-proBNP is elevated, it is highly sensitive and specific for TACO and makes other diagnoses in the differential much less likely.[25]

OTHER ADVERSE EFFECTS OF TRANSFUSION

Transfusion-Associated Graft-Versus-Host Disease

Transfusion-associated graft-versus-host disease (GVHD) occurs when immunologically competent lymphocytes are introduced into an immunoincompetent host who cannot destroy the donor lymphocytes. The immunocompetent donor lymphocytes engraft, recognize the host as foreign, and then attack host tissues. GVHD occurs after allogeneic bone marrow transplantation and, less often, after transfusion of nonirradiated cellular blood components, especially when the blood donor and recipient share some HLA antigens.[3] There is an increased danger from posttransfusion GVHD, in part because of the frequent failure of physicians to recognize the risk. Another major factor, however, is the propensity of the donor's lymphocytes to produce recipient bone marrow aplasia. In GVHD after bone marrow transplantation, the bone marrow is of donor origin, and bone marrow aplasia does not occur. In posttransfusion GVHD, however, the donor's lymphocytes attack the bone marrow of recipient/host origin, producing aplasia.

Posttransfusion GVHD is fatal in more than 90% of cases, primarily because of aplasia of the recipient's bone marrow. It may occur 8 to 10 days after transfusion with a marked pancytopenia, as well as multiorgan involvement of GVHD such as skin and liver. The signs and symptoms include nausea, vomiting, anorexia, fever, watery diarrhea, liver dysfunction, and rash. Patients often die of infection and bleeding within 3 to 4 weeks. There is no effective treatment, with the possible exception of bone marrow transplantation, if posttransfusion GVHD is recognized early and if a suitable donor can be found in a short time. Reports have shown that haploidentical directed donor units of blood may produce fatal posttransfusion GVHD even in immunocompetent recipients. The use of irradiated blood (2500 cGy) is thus recommended in clinical situations in which posttransfusion GVHD is considered likely, such as when patients receive directed blood transfusions from their relatives. Leukocyte-reduction filters should not be used as prophylaxis against GVHD, because the exact number of leukocytes needed to produce the disease is not known with certainty. Case reports of fatal GVHD in patients who received leukoreduced, but not irradiated, blood have been published. Several articles have addressed this subject. Irradiation of RBCs produces a membrane defect, however, which causes slow leakage of potassium and hemoglobin. Accordingly, the FDA ruled that irradiated units of RBCs shall have an outdate not to exceed 28 days from the time of irradiation. GVHD continues to be a rare but extremely serious complication of blood transfusion. Although it is controversial, prophylactic irradiation is usually not indicated for patients with human immunodeficiency virus (HIV) infection (see box on Risk Groups for Transfusion-Associated Graft-Versus-Host Disease).

Risk Groups for Transfusion-Associated Graft-Versus-Host Disease

Risk Well Defined

- Congenital T-cell defects (known or suspected)
- Immunologic immaturity (fetus or premature infant)
- Intrauterine transfusion
- Neonates undergoing intrauterine exchange transfusion or extracorporeal membrane oxygenation
- Acquired T-cell defects
- Bone marrow or peripheral blood stem cell transplant recipients (allogeneic or autologous)
- Hodgkin disease
- Haplotype sharing between donor and recipient
- Transfusions from blood relatives
- HLA-matched platelets

Risks Identified but Not Clearly Defined

- Hematologic malignancies (other than Hodgkin disease)
- Solid tumors
- Immunologic immaturity or prematurity (in the context of small-volume transfusion)
- Certain immunosuppressive agents such as fludarabine

Risks Not Identified

- Acquired immunodeficiency syndrome (AIDS)
- Aplastic anemia (except in setting of bone marrow transplantation or immunosuppressive therapy)

Posttransfusion Purpura

Posttransfusion purpura (PTP) is a rare and self-limiting thrombocytopenia occurring 5 to 10 days posttransfusion in patients lacking a specific platelet antigen, usually PLA1 (HPA-1a).[3] These patients often have a history of sensitization with prior transfusions or pregnancies. After resensitization by the transfusion, patients can develop potent antibodies against the platelet-specific antigen that they are lacking but which is present on donor platelets. These platelet antibodies often have a high titer and can fix complement. As a result, the transfused platelets and the patient's own platelets are also destroyed through the adsorption of the antigen or immune complexes on their own platelets. A concurrent autoimmune process may also involve destruction of the recipient's own platelets, as shown in one case report of a positive antibody against the patient's own platelets. The thrombocytopenia can be marked with a platelet count falling below 10,000/μL. The onset is sudden, although self-limited, and usually resolves in 2 weeks. Intravenous immunoglobulin (IVIg) appears to be an effective treatment, although plasma exchange, steroids, and splenectomy can also be useful. Patients with acute bleeding and needing platelet support should receive platelets without the platelet-specific antigen, if at all possible. If random donor platelets are given, patients can develop severe reactions, including allergic reactions. Recurrence of PTP is rare.

Hypothermia

Hypothermia can occur with rapid infusion of large quantities of refrigerated (1° C-6° C) blood, such as in cases of rapid and massive transfusions.[3] Data have shown that rapid infusion of blood (1 unit every 5 minutes) may lower the temperature of the sinoatrial node to less than 30° C, at which point ventricular fibrillation may occur. Use of warming devices for some trauma patients may reduce the incidence of coagulopathies associated with major trauma and also help to overcome cardiac complications. Most transfusions need not be given this rapidly. For routine transfusion, blood does not have to be warmed. Indeed, overwarming a unit of blood can cause RBC thermal injury and produce hemolysis, DIC, or shock.

If blood is to be warmed, the temperature must be monitored and kept below a level that could cause hemolysis. Usually, this is less than 42° C. Heating blood under running hot tap water or heating in a microwave device is unacceptable; microwave devices produce hot spots that can cause hemolysis.

Electrolyte Toxicity

Citrate, a component of the preservative solution used in blood storage, functions as an anticoagulant by chelating calcium and interfering with the coagulation cascade.[3] Rapid transfusion of citrated blood can be associated with a drop in ionized calcium levels. Citrate-containing blood products, however, are routinely infused without any problem, because the citrate is rapidly metabolized to bicarbonate. In patients with normal liver function, citrate infusion is very unlikely to produce reactions. Mild to severe citrate toxicity can be seen, however, in individuals undergoing therapeutic apheresis when large volumes of citrated RBCs or plasma are reinfused.

The effects of hypocalcemia range from mild circumoral paresthesias to frank tetany. However, severe citrate toxicity, even with massive transfusion, is very rare. More commonly, the reaction is mild and self-limiting and can be treated by merely slowing the rate of reinfusion. If prolonged QT intervals or signs of tetany are seen, calcium can be administered. Infusion of calcium itself, however, may be associated with the development of ventricular arrhythmias and cardiac arrest. Calcium need not be infused routinely, even after large-volume blood transfusions. However, it may be prudent to monitor calcium status in patients undergoing massive transfusion and at risk for hypocalcemia due to citrate toxicity. Under no circumstances should calcium be added to a unit of blood, because it would recalcify the unit and cause clots to form in the bag. In patients with signs of hypocalcemia associated with infusion of citrate, such as in apheresis, correction of the hypocalcemia often requires infusion of magnesium, as well. Signs of hypocalcemia are often better treated with intravenous calcium infusion, because oral calcium carbonate supplements may be ineffective. In addition to the effects on calcium, the metabolism of citrate also can result in a metabolic alkalosis due to the generation of large amounts of bicarbonate.

Hypomagnesemia, presumably due to chelation of magnesium by citrate, has also been reported. Actual clinical complications of transfusion-induced hypomagnesemia, however, have not been well documented, other than in the cases of cytapheresis.

Hyperkalemia due to infusion of stored blood is a rare occurrence. Although hyperkalemia is often thought to be a problem in massive transfusion, in reality development of hypokalemia is of greater concern. With storage, leakage of potassium from RBCs to the extracellular fluid occurs. However, after infusion, the RBCs reverse the biochemical storage lesion by restoring the Na-K ATP membrane pump, and intracellular potassium levels are restored. As the citrate is metabolized to bicarbonate, the blood becomes alkalotic, contributing to hypokalemia. In massive transfusion, it is not uncommon for this to result in the need for administration of potassium. Extracellular potassium increases at the rate of approximately 1 mEq/day during the first few weeks of storage. If this presents a concern for neonates or patients with renal failure, fresher or washed blood can be requested. As there is increased potassium leakage from RBCs after exposure to 25 Gy of radiation to prevent posttransfusion GVHD, a maximum 28-day shelf life from the day of irradiation is imposed on this blood component.[11] Ammonia toxicity, previously a concern with stored blood, rarely presents problems.

Iron Overload

One milliliter of red blood cells contains 1 mg of iron. A unit of blood with 250 mL of RBCs thus contains approximately 250 mg of iron, and 4 units of blood contain 1 g of iron, roughly the amount stored in the bone marrow. Men and nonmenstruating women lose only approximately 1 mg of iron each day. Continued use of transfusion therapy in individuals with an extravascular type of hemolytic anemia, such as those with thalassemia or sickle cell anemia, in which iron is not lost from the body but is recycled, can thus result in the accumulation of excessive tissue stores of iron. Over long periods, the iron that is stored in parenchymal cells results in death of the cell and eventual organ failure.[26] Iron chelation therapy, such as that with deferoxamine, is now widely used and is often able to maintain patients with chronic hemolytic anemia in negative iron balance. The availability of oral iron chelaters such as deferasirox and deferiprone provides an alternative mode of iron chelation therapy.[27]

Air Emboli

Since the replacement of evacuated glass bottles by plastic blood bags, the risk for air embolism from phlebotomy or transfusion has virtually disappeared from transfusion practice. Air, however, still may be pumped into patients by the roller pumps contained in various transfusion devices, especially apheresis machines and intraoperative salvage machines.[28] All such devices currently manufactured, however, contain air-in-line sensors. However, any operators using this equipment must be well trained and remain alert to the potential risk for air embolization at all times while the patient is being treated. Patients who receive air intravenously experience acute cardiopulmonary insufficiency. The air tends to lodge in the right ventricle, preventing blood from entering the pulmonary circulation. Acute cyanosis, pain, cough, shock, and arrhythmia may occur, and death may result unless immediate action is taken. The patient should be placed head-down on the left side; this usually displaces the air bubble from the pulmonary valve. Use and removal of central lines may also pose a risk for air embolism.

Complications Associated With Massive Transfusion

Patients requiring massive transfusion (frequently defined as the transfusion of one whole blood volume within a 12- to 24-hour period of time) are critically ill with multiple medical issues. Common problems associated with massive transfusion include coagulopathy, hypothermia, and metabolic abnormalities; hypothermia and metabolic abnormalities are discussed earlier in this chapter.

Coagulopathy of massive transfusion is a multifactorial hemostatic disorder that can have devastating consequences.[29,30] Classically, the coagulopathy associated with massive transfusion was thought to be attributable solely to consumption of factors due to ongoing hemorrhage and/or dilution due to the large volume of fluids and RBCs typically infused. However, the understanding of hemostasis in massive transfusion has recently expanded to include a form of coagulopathy that occurs *before* coagulation factors and platelets are consumed. This so-called early coagulopathy, described primarily in the setting of trauma, is driven by tissue hypoperfusion and increased fibrinolysis.[29] Early coagulopathy is not likely to respond to traditional transfusion therapy and may only be resolved with restoration of circulatory capacity and inhibition of fibrinolysis.

Despite enhancements in our understanding of early coagulopathy, platelet/coagulation factor dilution and consumption still remain outstanding problems in the setting of massive transfusion. Patients undergoing large-scale transfusion must be regularly monitored for hematocrit, platelet count, prothrombin time/INR, partial thromboplastin time, and fibrinogen. Reasonable goals to promote hemostasis in the setting of massive transfusion are to maintain (1) Hct >25%, (2) platelets >50,000 /µL, (3) INR <1.7, and (4) fibrinogen ≥100-150 mg/dL.[29,30] Therefore it is imperative that clinicians provide more than just RBCs to their massively bleeding patients. To better ensure a more appropriate provision of plasma and platelet products, many facilities have developed rigorous protocols consisting of preset numbers of RBC, FFP, and platelet units that are immediately issued upon requests for massive transfusion. Such protocols, developed in conjunction with surgical and trauma services, can drastically improve blood product provision and outcomes in the setting of massive transfusion. Although massive transfusion protocols are useful tools to combat coagulopathy, there remains much controversy regarding the numbers of plasma and platelet products that should be provided to patients transfused with large volumes of RBCs. Trials and reports from military trauma centers have promoted use of massive protocols based around a 1:1:1 ratio of RBC units:plasma units : platelets. Data from combat theaters suggest that such ratios are successful in avoiding the coagulopathy of massive transfusion and ultimately lead to improved survival.[31] Despite these data, it is unclear whether such approaches are relevant to noncombat, civilian hospitals, which frequently issue massive transfusions for wide-ranging indications such as surgical complications, large gastrointestinal or retroperitoneal hemorrhages, or blunt trauma.[32]

Complications Associated With Hematopoietic Progenitor Cell Infusion

Hematopoietic progenitor cells (HPCs), the most widely used cell therapy products, may be derived from bone marrow, peripheral blood, and cord blood. As with regular blood transfusions, the infusion of HPCs carries the risk of the same typical types of transfusion reactions. However, additional risks are associated with HPC infusion, such as those related to the cryopreservatives used and the complex cellular components collected.[3] For many reactions, it may be difficult to identify the causative agent. Moreover, because of the often-irreplaceable nature of HPC products, higher infectious risks may be unavoidable. Only those reactions that are unique or more problematic for HPC infusions are discussed in this section. See Table 120-4 for summary.

DMSO Toxicity

The most common reactions to HPC have been attributed to dimethyl sulfoxide (DMSO), the most widely used cryopreservative.[3,33] A variety of symptoms may be associated with DMSO infusion. A garlic odor commonly accompanies DMSO infusion, and nausea and vomiting are often reported with DMSO-cryopreserved HPC infusions. Additional DMSO-related symptoms include flushing, coughing, chest tightness, dyspnea, abdominal pain, hypotension, hypertension, cardiac toxicity (such as bradycardia and other arrhythmias), and rarely, neurologic toxicity (such as syncope and transient encephalopathy). Some cases of DMSO toxicity are thought to be due to the release of histamine. Agents such as diphenhydramine have been used for the treatment and prevention of DMSO-related toxicity. Antiemetic agents such as prochlorperazine have been useful for ameliorating nausea and vomiting. Most clinical services have protocols in place to limit the volume of DMSO that can be infused, such as setting an upper infusion limit of 1 g/kg/day, dividing HPC infusion doses, or washing HPC products to remove DMSO (this, however, may result in cellular loss).

RBC Engraftment and Hemolysis

Although ABO and non-ABO blood groups are not obstacles to successful HPC transplantation, these antigens (and their corresponding antibodies) do create some problems during the transplant period. When considering incompatibilities within the ABO system, three scenarios are possible: (1) antibodies present in the recipient that interact with incompatible cells present in the graft (major incompatibility), (2) antibodies present in the plasma-portion of the graft that mediate hemolysis of recipient RBCs (minor incompatibility), or (3) antibodies present in both the recipient and the donor that may interact with incompatible RBCs (bidirectional, or two-way, incompatibility).[3] It has been previously shown that both major and bidirectional ABO incompatibility can result in delayed progenitor cell engraftment. In such cases, it is postulated that anti-ABO antibodies may mediate a suppressive effect on RBC precursors expressing these antigens, leading to reticulocytopenia and prolonged anemia. In the most severe form of this process, HPC recipients can develop pure RBC aplasia, a condition wherein bone marrow shows a virtual absence of immature erythroid elements more than 3 months posttransplantation. In cases of either delayed engraftment or pure RBC aplasia, patients are often dependent on RBC transfusions for prolonged periods of time in order to maintain adequate oxygen-carrying capacity.

Another risk factor associated with HPC infusion is the possibility for RBC hemolysis. Both ABO and non-ABO antibodies are capable of mediating RBC lysis. In such conditions, preformed antibodies in either the recipient or HPC plasma can cause accelerated clearance of incompatible RBCs by either intra- or extravascular mechanisms. Presentation of hemolytic transfusion reactions immediately after HPC infusion is no different from that of typical transfusion reaction. Policies and protocols should be in place to prevent postinfusion HPC-related hemolysis—for example, plasma depletion of HPC products (in cases of minor mismatch and bidirectional ABO incompatibility), limiting the infusion of incompatible RBCs (in cases of major mismatch and bidirectional ABO), hydration of patients, and others.

Although delayed hemolysis is rarely clinically significant in major ABO mismatched HPC transplant, clinically significant delayed hemolysis is commonly reported in minor and bidirectional ABO-incompatible HPC transplants. As a result of donor lymphocyte engraftment, typically occurring 1 to 2 weeks after HPC infusion, donor ABO antibodies can cause hemolysis of residual recipient RBCs. This delayed hemolysis is typically clinically evident with decreased hemoglobin, increased indirect bilirubin, increased LDH, and decreased haptoglobin, and patients often require RBC transfusion. Sometimes, the hemolysis can be massive and result in multi-organ failure and death. Thus it is important to monitor patients for hemolysis after minor and bidirectional ABO incompatible HPC infusion. Timely support and treatments such as RBC exchange can be provided for massive hemolysis if it occurs.

Infectious Complications

As a result of an underlying bacteremia during collection, or contamination through collection, processing, storage, thawing, and sampling, some HPC products may harbor microbial organisms

Table 120-4 Common Hematopoietic Progenitor Cell Infusion Reactions

Types	Presentations	Treatment and Prevention
DMSO toxicity	Halitosis, nausea, vomiting, flushing, coughing, chest tightness, dyspnea, abdominal pain, hypotension, hypertension, cardiac toxicity (such as bradycardia and other arrhythmias), and rarely neurologic toxicity, such as syncope and transient encephalopathy	Antihistamine Antiemetics Limiting DMSO infusion volume
ABO mismatch	Hemolysis at the time of infusion Delayed RBC engraftment (major mismatch and bidirectional) Delayed hemolysis (minor mismatch and bidirectional)	Plasma depletion of HPC products (in cases of minor mismatch and bidirectional ABO incompatibility) Limiting the infusion of incompatible RBC (in cases of major mismatch and bidirectional ABO) Hydration of patients Other supportive care if necessary RBC transfusion support Monitor for RBC engraftment Modify immunosuppression RBC transfusion support Monitor for hemolysis Hydration, RBC exchange, and other supportive care if massive hemolysis

capable of mediating septic reactions during or immediately after HPC infusion.[2] Such reactions may manifest with high fever, tachycardia, hypotension, nausea, or vomiting and, in severe cases, can progress to a shock-like state. Patients experiencing such symptoms should be treated with broad-spectrum antibiotics to cover both gram-positive and gram-negative organisms.[34] Transfer of the patient to an intensive care setting is also prudent because mechanical respiration and additional supportive measures (e.g., pressors) may be necessary to prevent a cardiovascular collapse.

Fortunately, the bacterial contamination of an HPC unit is often known well in advance of an actual HPC infusion. This is because many HPC products are cultured at the time of collection and processing. As such, clinical teams can be well-prepared for such reactions. In such circumstances, preventative measures include provision of preinfusion antibiotics to cover the documented organism(s) and close patient surveillance during and after infusion. The infusion of the product in a monitored setting may be warranted. One additional option would be to avoid infusion of a contaminated unit altogether. This is possible if a patient has multiple, separate HPC products available for infusion. Clinical and transplant teams can preferentially infuse noncontaminated HPC units first, saving the contaminated unit as a "last resort" should the graft fail.

Other Infusion Complications Related to HPC Products

In addition to the problems related to DMSO and ABO mismatches, other adverse reactions sometimes occur with the use of HPC products.[3] Nausea and vomiting are frequently reported with infusion of freshly collected HPC products such as fresh marrow. Fever and chills are commonly seen with cryopreserved HPC; these have been speculated to be caused by the cellular debris and cytokines contained in HPC products. Antipyretics and steroid premedication may be used for prevention. Severe adverse reactions to HPC infusion (such as cardiac arrest and neurologic symptoms, including loss of consciousness and seizure) have been linked to high granulocyte counts in HPC products.

Respiratory problems are increasingly being recognized as an important cause of morbidity and morality in the setting of HPC infusion. Although many of these are late-onset problems (e.g., infectious complications associated with immunosuppression occurring days or weeks after transplantation), some pulmonary issues will arise acutely during HPC infusion. The National Marrow Donor Program (NMDP) issued a report in 2010 regarding seven patients who experienced hypertension, chest pain, and decreased oxygen saturation after infusion of cord blood.[35] Even though no clear cut cause-effect relationship was established, some recommendations were made, including minimizing thaw to infusion time, filtering HPC products with standard 150-250 micron blood filters, avoiding very high infusion rate, and others. In addition, the classic pulmonary complications encountered during HPC infusion may resemble TRALI in that they are typically associated with dyspnea, hypoxemia, a low-grade fever, and bilateral pulmonary infiltrates, all occurring within a short time after initiation or completion of infusion. Some authors have attributed these problems to a noncardiogenic capillary leak syndrome that appears to be independent of cardiac function, similar to the proposed pathophysiology of TRALI.

Patients demonstrating signs or symptoms of respiratory distress during HPC infusion must be treated aggressively. The first response should be to stop the HPC infusion and provide immediate respiratory support in the form of oxygen. If the patient does not recover with these measures, or if the situation worsens, then consideration may be given to intubation to prevent respiratory failure. The provision of corticosteroids or other immunosuppressive agents is not likely to be of benefit for such reactions. It may also be prudent to investigate whether the patient's symptoms are related to circulatory overload rather than arising from noncardiogenic pulmonary edema. This distinction may be accomplished by measuring plasma levels of brain-natriuretic peptide (BNP). If BNP is elevated, then the patient's symptoms may be attributable, in part, to volume overload and a trial of diuresis is likely warranted.

National Healthcare Safety Network

The National Healthcare Safety Network (NHSN) is a national program of combined governmental and private sector agencies designed to evaluate and track transfusion reactions and other adverse effects associated with infusion of blood products and derivatives. Similar programs exist in other countries, including the United Kingdom and France. The Hemovigilance Module, the first protocol release of the Biovigilance Component of NHSN, was developed through a public-private partnership between the Centers for Disease Control and Prevention (CDC) and subject matter experts convened by AABB. The Hemovigilance Module is designed for transfusion services staff in health care facilities to monitor recipient adverse reactions and quality-control incidents related to blood transfusion.

The Hemovigilance Module provides standard criteria and definitions to participating facilities to report adverse events related to blood transfusion that will result in aggregate data suitable for trend analyses and benchmarking. Participating facilities can analyze their data independently within NHSN and will be able to compare their data with national aggregate rates in a confidential manner through NHSN in the future.

The following transfusion reaction categories are used to identify types of adverse events related to blood transfusion:

- Allergic
- Acute hemolytic
- Delayed hemolytic
- Delayed serologic
- Febrile nonhemolytic
- Hypotensive
- Posttransfusion purpura
- Transfusion associated circulatory overload (TACO)
- Transfusion-associated dyspnea
- Transfusion-associated graft versus host disease
- Transfusion-related acute lung injury (TRALI)
- Transfusion-transmitted infection

Transfusion reactions are further classified by their severity and imputability—that is, the likelihood that the reaction is attributable to infusion of the blood product being investigated. Protocols, forms, and enrollment information are available online (http://www.cdc.gov/nhsn/bio.html).

SUGGESTED READINGS

American Association of Blood Banks (AABB): Appendix II, *TRANFUSION*, August 2009 Supplement Fact Sheets, http://www.aabb.org/resources/bct/eid/Pages/appendix2.aspx.

American Association of Blood Banks (AABB): Association Bulletin #06-07: Transfusion-Related Acute Lung Injury, in AABB PulsePoint. 2006.

American Association of Blood Banks (AABB): Transfusion-transmitted diseases. http://www.aabb.org/resources/bct/bloodfacts/Pages/fabloodtrans.aspx.

Benjamin R, McCullough J, Mintz PD, et al: Therapeutic efficacy and safety of red blood cells treated with a chemical process (S-303) for pathogen inactivation: A Phase III clinical trial in cardiac surgery patients. *Transfusion* 45:1739, 2005.

Benumof J: Minimizing venous air embolism from reinfusion bags [comment]. *Anesthesiology* 91:1962, 1999.

Davenport R, Burdick M, Moore SA, et al: Cytokine production in IgG-mediated red cell incompatibility [comment]. *Transfusion* 33:19, 1993.

Davenport RD: Hemolytic Transfusion Reactions. In Popovsky MA, editor: *Transfusion Reactions*, Bethesda, Md, 2007, AABB Press, p 1.

Gilliss B, Looney M: Experimental models of transfusion-related acute lung injury. *Transfus Med Rev* 25:1, 2011.

Hardy J, de Moerloose P, Samama C: The coagulopathy of massive transfusion. *Vox Sang* 89:123, 2005.

Jensen PD, Jensen FT, Christensen T, et al: Relationship between hepatocellular injury and transfusional iron overload prior to and during iron chelation with desferrioxamine: A study in adult patients with acquired anemias. *Blood* 101:91, 2003.

Kim D, Brecher M, Bland L, et al: Visual identification of bacterially contaminated red cells. *Transfusion* 32:221, 1992.

King K, Shirey RS, Thoman SK, et al: Universal leukoreduction decreases the incidence of febrile nonhemolytic transfusion reactions to RBCs. *Transfusion* 44:25, 2004.

Kleinman S, Caulfield T, Chan P, et al: Toward an understanding of transfusion-related acute lung injury: Statement of a consensus panel [comment]. *Transfusion* 44:1774, 2004.

Kuehnert M, Roth VR, Haley NR, et al: Transfusion-transmitted bacterial infection in the United States, 1998 through 2000. *Transfusion* 41:1493, 2001.

Maggio A, Filosa A, Vitrano A, et al: Iron chelation therapy in thalassemia major: A systematic review with meta-analyses of 1520 patients included on randomized clinical trials. *Blood Cells Mol Dis* 47:166, 2011.

Menitove J: *Standards for Blood Banks and Transfusion Services*, Bethesda, MD, 2011, AABB Press.

Phipps R, Kaufman J, Blumberg N: Platelet derived CD154 (CD40 ligand) and febrile responses to transfusion. *Lancet* 357:2023, 2001.

Popovsky M: *Popovsky MA: Transfusion Reactions*, Bethesda, Md, 2007, AABB Press.

Sachs UJ, Wasel W, Bayat B, et al: Mechanism of transfusion-related acute lung injury induced by HLA class II antibodies. *Blood* 117:669, 2011.

Shimada E, Tadokoro K, Watanabe Y, et al: Anaphylactic transfusion reactions in haptoglobin-deficient patients with IgE and IgG haptoglobin antibodies. *Transfusion* 42:766, 2002.

Sihler K, Napolitano L: Complications of massive transfusion. *Chest* 137:209, 2010.

Silliman C, Paterson AJ, Dickey WO, et al: The association of biologically active lipids with the development of transfusion-related acute lung injury: A retrospective study [comment]. *Transfusion* 37:719, 1997.

Simon T, Snyder EL, Solheim BG, et al: *Rossi's Principles of Transfusion Medicine,* Philadelphia, 2009, Lippincott: Williams & Wilkins.

Snyder E, McCullough J, Slichter SJ, et al: Clinical safety of platelets photochemically treated with amotosalen HCl and ultraviolet A light for pathogen inactivation: The SPRINT trial. *Transfusion* 45:1864, 2005.

Tobian A, Sokoll LJ, Tisch DJ, et al: N-terminal pro-brain natriuretic peptide is a useful diagnostic marker for transfusion-associated circulatory overload. *Transfusion* 48:1143, 2008.

U.S. Food and Drug Administration: Vaccines, Blood & Biologics: Fatalities reported to FDA following blood collection and transfusion: Annual summary for fiscal Year 2010. http://www.fda.gov/BiologicsBloodVaccines/SafetyAvailability/ReportaProblem/TransfusionDonationFatalities/ucm254802.htm.

Vlaar A, Hofstra JJ, Determann RM, et al: The incidence, risk factors, and outcome of transfusion-related acute lung injury in a cohort of cardiac surgery patients: A prospective nested case-control study. *Blood* 117:4218, 2011.

Vlaar A, Straat M, Juffermans N: The relation between aged blood products and onset of transfusion-related acute lung injury. A review of pre-clinical data. *Clin Lab* 57:267, 2011.

Wiersum-Osselton J, Middleburg RA, Beckers EA, et al: Male-only fresh-frozen plasma for transfusion-related acute lung injury prevention: Before-and-after comparative cohort study. *Transfusion* 51:1278, 2011.

Wyman TH, Bjornsen AJ, Elzi DJ, et al: A two-insult in vitro model of PMN-mediated pulmonary endothelial damage: Requirements for adherence and chemokine release. *Am J Physiol Cell Physiol* 283:C1592, 2002.

For complete list of references log on to www.expertconsult.com.

CHAPTER 121

TRANSFUSION-TRANSMITTED DISEASES

Louis M. Katz and Jay E. Menitove

Adverse reactions following blood transfusion reflect immunologic, pathophysiologic, and microbiologic events. This chapter presents information about transfusion-associated viral, bacterial, parasitic, and prion infections and emerging agents. Transfusion-transmitted infection risk mitigation through blood donor screening and blood testing strategies are presented.[1] The box discussions provide insights into interventions aimed at reducing risk from known and emerging threats and new technologies for reducing or eliminating microbial contamination. Red cell, platelet, and plasma transfusion represent important therapeutic modalities for appropriately selected patients. Awareness of the hazards of transfusion and the rate at which these events occur should enable physicians to better determine the benefit : risk ratios when prescribing transfusions.

HEPATITIS VIRUSES

The hepatitis viruses can be classified according to their predominant modes of transmission, parenteral and enteric, with the parenterally transmitted agents, hepatitis B virus (HBV) and hepatitis C virus (HCV) dominating concerns about transfusion transmission because many individuals unknowingly infected with these agents become asymptomatic chronic carriers and may make blood donations.

Hepatitis B

HBV is a deoxyribonucleic acid (DNA) virus in the family Hepadnaviridae. The infective virion is known as the Dane particle and has surface and core components, surface antigen (HBsAg) and core antigen (HBcAg), respectively. Epitopes on the viral surface provide a basis for epidemiologic studies and consist of the HBsAg "a," d/y, and w/r determinants. Recombinant vaccines containing the "a" determinant confer protective immunity to a high proportion of vaccinees and are dramatically altering the incidence and prevalence of HBV infection in the general population where they are in wide use and consequently in the donor population.

The average incubation period (the time from infection to liver enzyme elevation and symptomatic hepatitis) is 59 days (range, 5 to 12 weeks) but may be as long as 6 months. Symptoms, which occur in 30% to 50% of infected persons age 5 years and older, include fatigue, anorexia, nausea, vomiting, jaundice, dark urine, light stools, arthralgias, rashes, vasculitis, and glomerulonephritis. The risk for progression to chronic infection is inversely related to age at infection. HBV infection becomes chronic in more than 90% of infants, 25% to 50% of children 1 to 5 years of age, and less than 5% of older children and adults. Approximately 5% of the U.S. population has serologic evidence of prior HBV infection (antibodies against HBcAg [anti-HBc] reactive). From the mid-1980s through 2008, with increasing immunization in early childhood, the incidence of acute HBV infection has fallen nearly an order of magnitude from more than 11 cases per 100,000 to 1.3. There were an estimated 800,000 to 1.4 million U.S. residents with chronic HBV infection in 2006.

Based largely on data from parenteral exposures of health care workers, HBV is 100 times more infective than human immunodeficiency virus (HIV) and 10 times more infective than HCV. The predominant mode of transmission to adults and adolescents is through sexual contact. Forty percent have infected partners, 15% are males having sex with other males, injecting drug users account for 14% of cases, and one-third have no identifiable risk.

HBsAg is detectable in blood approximately 4 weeks (30 to 60 days) after infection. Subsequently, immunoglobulin M (IgM) anti-HBc antibodies appear coincident with symptom onset. High viral titers (10^{10} genomes/mL) present at that time decline subsequently. HBsAg persists transiently in acute infections for up to 4 months (average 63 days). Antibodies against HBsAg (anti-HBs) develop subsequently and protect against reinfection. Some anti-HBc–positive and anti-HBs–negative carriers have circulating HBV DNA, and this pattern defines so-called occult HBV infection. Although anti-HBs confers immunity to reinfection, sufficient virus remains in the liver to transmit HBV following liver transplant from anti-HBs–positive donors and to cause reactivation under intense immunosuppression.

Blood donors in the United States are queried for a history of hepatitis and risks associated with hepatitis and screened for HBsAg and anti-HBc. The use of HBV nucleic acid testing (NAT) in minipools, though not required as of mid-2011, is nearly universal. The risk for HBV transmission per unit in the United States was 1 per 280,000 to 355,000 donations using very sensitive HBsAg testing and is only modestly decreased with minipool NAT (Table 121-1).[2,3] Most contemporary HBV transfusion-transmitted infections are attributable to blood donations from asymptomatic donors during acute infection preceding the development of detectable HBsAg. During this "window period," HBV replicates relatively slowly with a doubling time of HBV viral load of approximately 2.6 days. Rare cases are due to HBV variants not detectable by HBsAg testing. With current routine testing for HBsAg and anti-HBc, the addition of HBV NAT in minipools will have a small impact on residual HBV risk because contemporary HBsAg tests approach the sensitivity of minipool NAT. Among 3.7 million blood donors to the American Red Cross during 2008, 1 per 6028 were infected with HBV. Of these, 604 had positive HBsAg, with or without HBV DNA (1 per 6117), and only 9 were identified solely by NAT in minipools (1 per 410,540). NAT on individual donation aliquots has the potential to reduce the risk for transfusion-transmitted HBV further by detecting newly infected donors slightly earlier than the HBsAg tests licensed for blood donor screening. The costs of performing individual donation NAT for HBV, combined with declining HBV incidence associated with population-based vaccination and the low rate of clinical morbidity in most transfused populations, suggest it is not cost-effective by usual criteria.

Manufacturers of NAT donor screening assays have now included HBV DNA in Food and Drug Administration (FDA)–licensed multiplex platforms (with HIV and HCV), eliminating an important operational barrier to its implementation, leading to widespread use. The Blood Products Advisory Committee at FDA endorses the use of HBV DNA testing, although there has been no formal guidance from that agency at the time of this writing.

There is evidence that some HBsAg assays will not detect all S gene variants of HBV. Donors in the United States are screened universally for both HBsAg and anti-HBc, and increasingly with NAT; this makes it likely that a mutant strain of HBV would be

Table 121-1 Risk for Transfusion-Transmitted Diseases in the United States

Pathogenic Agent or Disease	Average Estimated Risk Per Unit
Hepatitis A	Rare
Hepatitis B	<1/350,000-1/470,000 (assuming MP NAT implemented)
Hepatitis C	1/1,935,000
Human immunodeficiency virus	1/1,467,000
Human T-lymphotropic viruses 1, 2	1/2,400,000
Cytomegalovirus	Infrequent
Parvovirus B19	Rare
West Nile virus	Rare
Malaria	3 cases per year
Babesiosis	>160 transfusion-associated cases reported
Chagas disease	Rare
Creutzfeldt-Jakob disease	4 vCJD transfusion-associated cases reported
Bacterial contamination:	
Red cells	1/30,000
Septic reaction	1/500,000-1/10,000,000
Platelets	1/3000-1/8000
Septic reaction	1/15,000-1/100,000
Emerging infections: Dengue virus Chikungunya virus Pandemic influenza viruses (see Dengue, in text, for added language on pandemic flu) (H5N1, H1N1)	Risk unknown

MP, Minipool; *NAT*, nucleic acid test; *vCJD*, new variant Creutzfeldt-Jakob disease.

detected in the United States. An exception might be an individual with an S gene variant who presents in the early stages of acute hepatitis before the development of anti-HBc, although NAT should detect all these donors.

Hepatitis D

Hepatitis D Virus (HDV) was originally called the delta agent. It is a defective ribonucleic acid (RNA)–containing passenger virus that requires active synthesis of HBsAg to act as a "helper" for assembly of HDV virions. As many as 10% of HBV infections are accompanied by HDV worldwide. Its prevalence is very low in the United States but higher in injection drug users. HDV superinfection of chronic HBV carriers is associated with worsened chronic sequelae and with fulminant hepatitis. Screening for HBV acts synergistically to prevent transfusion-associated HDV cases by identifying donors that are coinfected with HBV and HDV.

Hepatitis C

HCV is an RNA virus in the family Flaviviridae, genus Hepacivirus There are six genotypes that share similar epidemiology, pathogenesis, and natural histories. In the United States, genotypes 1, 2, and 3 cause 75%, 10%, and 10% of infections, respectively. Genotype 1 responds relatively poorly to traditional treatment regimens using interferon and ribavirin compared with 2 and 3, but recent approval of HCV protease inhibitors promises to improve these rates. HCV is distinguished by a low rate of recognized acute infection and by a high rate of chronic infection, with substantial morbidity and mortality over long periods of observation as a result. In the United States there are an estimated 3.2 million chronic infections.

The most common source of HCV acquisition is injection drug use. The prevalence of HCV in U.S. adults (20 to 59 years old) with any history of illicit injection drug use is greater than 45%. Other risks include blood transfusion before donor serologic screening began in 1990, a high lifetime number of sex partners, and exposure in health care settings, including through dialysis. Fifteen percent to 30% of patients report no risk factors in large series. Vertical transmission occurs to 3% to 7% of infants of mothers with active infections. In contrast to HBV, sexual transmission is an inefficient route of infection, but was found to be the most likely mode of transmission of HCV among HIV-infected men who have sex with men in New York City. Among blood donors, 0.072% have confirmed positive HCV test results.

At most 20% to 30% of newly infected persons develop recognizable symptoms during acute HCV infection. Chronic infection develops in 75% to 85% of persons infected after 45 years of age and in 50% to 60% of those infected as children or young adults. Chronic HCV infection progresses to cirrhosis in 15% to 30% over 30 years of observation. Hepatocellular carcinoma occurs in 1% to 4% per year in those with cirrhosis. HCV is among the most prevalent causes of chronic hepatitis, cirrhosis, and primary liver cancer in the developed world and is the most common indication for liver transplantation in the United States, resulting in around 2400 procedures annually.

The risk for posttransfusion HCV infection declined progressively with the introduction of surrogate markers for non-A, non-B hepatitis in the 1980s (alanine aminotransferase and anti-HBc) and of serologic testing for HCV antibodies in May 1990, followed sequentially by improved serologic testing and NAT. The seronegative-window period for the first-generation HCV antibody test extended to 6 months from infection, but was reduced to 82 and 70 days with second- and third-generation assays, respectively. NAT further reduced the window period to 10 to 25 days. The risk per unit declined from an estimated 1 per 276,000 units to 1 per 1,935,000 units, and residual risk estimates from the incidence-window period model using serologic data have been confirmed using NAT.

NAT is labor and resource intensive, so HCV NAT deployment was dependent on the use of so-called minipools, created by combining aliquots from 16 to 24 donations (currently 6 to 16). Loss of test sensitivity due to sample pooling was tolerable given the rapid increase or burst of HCV viremia before antibody seroconversion (estimated doubling time of 10.8 hours in that period) and the high titer of viremia during the 40- to 50-day plateau phase preceding antibody seroconversion. Although minipool NAT has been implemented successfully and with moderate yield in many developed countries, it is expensive and its cost-effectiveness low in comparison to other medical interventions.

As an alternative to NAT assays, enzyme immunoassays (EIAs) have been developed that detect HCV core antigen in serum or plasma, either as an individual analyte in parallel with antibody assays or as HCV antigen-antibody combination assays. These tests reduce the preseroconversion-window period and are being adopted in some developing countries. They are less sensitive than HCV NAT and are not approved for blood donor screening in the United States.

The remarkable advances in safety achieved by the introduction and successive improvements in the clinical sensitivity of HCV assays have greatly reduced transfusion-associated HCV cases. Nonetheless, some newly infected individuals demonstrate fluctuations in HCV RNA, at times below NAT detection thresholds before antibody seroconversion. This likely explains some of the low residual risk for transfusion-transmitted HCV infection despite the ongoing combination of HCV antibody and RNA testing.

The seroprevalence of HCV, the prolonged interval between infection and clinical manifestations, and the relatively high rate of HCV clinical sequelae prompted blood collection facilities and hospitals to conduct "look-back" notification of previous recipients of blood given by donors found on subsequent donations to be HCV infected. Look back was subsequently made mandatory in companion rules from FDA and the Centers for Medicare and Medicaid Services. In general, HCV look-back programs found half or fewer of targeted transfused individuals alive, but were able to find both seropositive and RNA-positive recipients who were unaware of their status. In one study the cost to find a seropositive recipient who was unaware of his or her infection was $3146.

Hepatitis A

The hepatitis A virus (HAV), a nonenveloped picornavirus, is transmitted predominantly by the fecal-oral route, with an average incubation period of 28 days (range, 15 to 50 days) with signs or symptoms persisting for less than 2 months. The incidence of HAV infection in the United States fell by 76% from the period 1990 to 1997 to 2003 after the recommendation for targeted immunization of members in high-risk communities. Populations at risk include those in areas where extended community outbreaks occur and children living in states that have high and intermediate rates of disease, staff and residents of closed communities, close personal contacts of cases, the staff and parents of children in day-care centers and those with common-source exposure to infected food or water. For many sporadic cases there is no recognized source. HAV is self-limited with no chronic carrier state, but approximately 10% to 15% of infected individuals develop a more prolonged or relapsing illness. It is the most frequent cause of hepatitis among children under 11 years of age.

Transfusion-related transmission, although rare, is due to a blood donation from a recently infected, asymptomatic, viremic individual. The peak viremia occurs 2 weeks before onset of jaundice or elevation of hepatocellular enzymes and persists for a median period of 42 days (range, up to 59 days). The virus is quite resistant to many inactivation procedures, including the pathogen-reduction procedures being developed for cellular blood components (e.g., psoralens or riboflavin, both with ultraviolet [UV] irradiation) and fresh-frozen plasma (solvent/detergent and methylene blue). Transmission by clotting-factor concentrates treated with the solvent/detergent pathogen-reduction process occurred in the 1990s, and low risk persists despite the lack of HAV infection among hemophilia patients treated in the early 2000s.

An indefinite deferral for a clinical history of viral hepatitis after age 11 years is required in the United States (regardless of the specific viral agent). Because most viral hepatitis in the United States before 11 years is HAV, with its relatively brief and self-limited viremia, individuals with a history of hepatitis before the age of 11 are allowed to donate on the assumption they had HAV. A 120-day deferral is recommended after exposure to HAV during community outbreaks to prevent transfusion transmission. In vitro screening for HAV is not done.

Hepatitis E

The hepatitis E virus (HEV) is an RNA virus that is endemic in Southeast and Central Asia, Japan, the Middle East, North and West Africa, and Brazil and causes epidemics associated with fecally contaminated water. Sporadic infections occur in other developed countries. It usually causes a self-limited illness but can be lethal in pregnant women, their fetuses, and patients with chronic liver disease. Transfusion-related transmission was postulated on the basis of cohort studies in endemic countries that showed a high prevalence of anti-HEV among transfused patients. Blood transmission is rare but has been reported from endemic areas, and rarely in nonendemic regions, presumably resulting from an extended asymptomatic viremia. Transfusion-transmitted HEV has not been reported in the United States or most other developed countries, and screening is not under active consideration.

Non–A-E Hepatitis

Cases of posttransfusion hepatitis are still seen occasionally despite donor screening and recipient diagnostic testing for known hepatitis viruses, causing speculation that undiscovered hepatitis agents exist. Likewise, a small but consistent percentage of community-acquired hepatitis cases test negative for known hepatitis viruses, some cirrhosis is classified as "cryptogenic," an etiologic agent for hepatitis-associated aplastic anemia eludes description, and the cause of some cases of acute liver failure remains elusive. Several candidate agents have been proposed as non–A-E hepatitis viruses.

GBV-C (initially called hepatitis G virus [HGV]) is a flavivirus with no confirmed disease association that is transmitted parenterally, including frequently from transfusion. Of interest, GBV-C infection may delay progression of disease in those coinfected with HIV, which has led to studies of the interactions of these viruses.[4]

From 1% to 4% of U.S. blood donors are viremic compared with 15% to 20% of injection drug users who have detectable GBV-C RNA. Infection occurs frequently among those infected with HCV and HIV. More people have antibodies against the E2 envelope protein, in the absence of RNA, suggesting viral clearance. GBV-C has not been shown to cause liver disease or other morbidity, and hence there is no consideration of donor screening at this time.

The torque teno virus (TTV) complex is a genetically diverse group of nonenveloped DNA viruses in the family Circoviridae, which was discovered in 1997. They cause viremia, and they are transmitted by transfusion, but they cause no recognized liver disease or other clinical illness. Initial studies indicated a prevalence of viremia of 1% to 2% in North American blood donors, but recent studies targeting more diverse TTV variants have identified viremia in the majority of healthy donors, suggesting these agents are commensal and nonpathogenic. SEN virus (SENV), another member of the Circoviridae, was described using degenerate polymerase chain reaction (PCR) primers while working with TTV. After an initial report associating SENV variants in two patients with transfusion-associated non–A-E hepatitis, subsequent epidemiologic studies have failed to link SENV with clinical hepatitis. Thus GBV-C, TTV, and SENV do not represent clinically relevant hepatitis viruses, but it is anticipated that identification of new putative viral hepatitis agents will continue; the role and possible relationship of such agents to presumed non–A-E posttransfusion hepatitis awaits their discovery and analysis.

RETROVIRAL INFECTION

Human Immunodeficiency Virus

The human immunodeficiency viruses type 1 and type 2 (HIV-1 and HIV-2), pathogenic retroviruses of the family Retroviridae, genus Lentivirus, are the etiologic agents of the acquired immunodeficiency syndrome (AIDS). Molecular characterization divides HIV-1 into three groups: group M (main), group O (outliers), and group N (non-M/O). Group M subtype B infections predominate in the United States; only 3% of HIV-positive blood donors have non-B strains. Very rare group O infections have been detected in the United States among patients who were born, lived, or had sexual contact in endemic regions of West and Central Africa. HIV-2 infected persons in the United States, in contrast to those with HIV-1, are infected after heterosexual transmission from West African emigrants or residents. HIV-2 is less likely to cause AIDS and represents less than 1% of HIV cases diagnosed annually in the United States

Tests used currently for screening blood donors detect infection with all of these viruses.[5] Testing for HIV-1 began in 1985, for

HIV-2 in 1991 to 1992 (although HIV-1 tests before that time detected most HIV-2 infections) and for HIV-1 group O in 2003 to 2009.

Both serologic testing and NAT are performed on every blood donation. Antibody testing, implemented in early 1985, becomes positive, on average, 21 days after infection. NAT detects HIV RNA at a minimum concentration of 5.5 copies per milliliter; donor RNA screening has been performed since 1999. As is done for HCV because of the rapid ramp-up of viremia, the exquisite sensitivity of NAT, operational and cost-containment considerations, donor-testing laboratories pool aliquots from several donations (minipools) rather than test individual donations as is done for serologic tests. RNA is detected 5.6 to 9.0 days following infection, thereby substantially closing the seronegative-window period between HIV exposure and virus detection. Rare genetic variants of HIV may escape NAT detection when nucleotide sequence changes affect NAT primer or probe binding sites, but the vast majority of the these infections will be detected serologically.

To interdict donations in the window period between exposure and test positivity, each blood donor is asked at each donation about exposure risks using questions developed in the early to mid-1980s, subsequent to the first reports of AIDS in hemophiliacs and transfusion recipients. These initial interventions targeted blood donations from homosexually active men and injection drug users, substantially reducing the transmission risk between 1983 and 1985. Four transfusion transmissions have been documented subsequent to NAT testing, three before 2002 and one in 2008.[6] Modeling suggests a residual risk for HIV transmission persists at approximately one transmission per 1.5 million to 2.1 million donations, because NAT cannot detect HIV infection during the immunosilent 9-day eclipse phase between infection and test reactivity and due to very rare processing and quarantine procedure errors. Fourth-generation tests, under development, that combine HIV antibody and HIV antigen testing detect almost 90% of infections detected by NAT. Their role in future testing algorithms is unclear at this time, but their greatest utility may be in resource-constrained settings where NAT is not feasible.

The continued permanent lifetime deferral in the United States (and other countries) of men who have had sex with men even once since 1977 may be inappropriate from a risk-benefit perspective in light of improvements in donor testing. These stringent policies are being relaxed in some countries (e.g., Australia and the United Kingdom).[7] Reluctance to revise this policy in North America in pursuit of a zero-risk blood supply arises from unwillingness to accept any course of action that results in even a de minimis increased risk for transmission (see box on Blood Safety Decision Making).

Human T-Lymphotropic Virus-1 and Virus-2

Human T-lymphotropic virus-1 (HTLV-1) and HTLV-2 are closely related deltaretroviruses with 60% to 70% sequence homology and shared tropism for T lymphocytes. In contrast to HIV, HTLV is rarely present in cell-free plasma and shows little active replication in infected humans. HTLV-1 is distributed worldwide, with endemic foci in southern Japan, the Caribbean, certain parts of South America, Africa, the Middle East, and Melanesia. HTLV-2I is endemic among Amerindians in both North and South America and African Pygmies. An epidemic of HTLV-2I infections has occurred over the past 40 to 50 years among intravenous drug users in the United States, Brazil, and Europe. Transmission of both HTLV-1 and HTLV-2 occurs by parenteral exposures, sexual contact, and by vertical transmission from mother to child during pregnancy and breastfeeding.

Diseases associated with HTLV-1 infection include adult T-cell leukemia/lymphoma (ATL), HTLV-associated myelopathy/tropical spastic paraparesis (HAM/TSP), lymphocytic pneumonitis, uveitis, polymyositis, and arthritis. HTLV-2 does not appear to cause hematologic malignancy but has been associated with HAM/TSP and linked to a higher rate of common infections such as acute bronchitis, pneumonia, and urinary tract infections, suggesting a subtle immunomodulatory effect of the virus.[11]

ATL occurs in only 1% to 5% of infected persons following a latent period of decades. The illness is characterized by malignant lymphocytosis and leukemia, lymphadenopathy, hepatomegaly, abnormal liver function test results, splenomegaly, skin lesions, bone lesions, and hypercalcemia. HAM/TSP occurs in approximately 2% of individuals infected with HTLV-1 and HTLV-2. Patients with transfusion-associated HAM/TSP develop neurologic symptoms rather more rapidly, at a median of 3.3 years after transfusion. This illness is characterized by slowly progressive chronic spastic paraparesis, lower limb weakness, urinary incontinence, impotence, sensory disturbances, low back pain, hyperreflexia, and impaired vibration sense.

Blood donor screening for HTLV-1 antibodies began in 1988, and a more sensitive combination HTLV-1/2 EIA that detects close to 100% of HTLV-2 infections was introduced in 1998. The prevalence of true positive HTLV markers decreased approximately 10-fold during the 1990s to 0.01% in 2001 and has remained at this level. The rate is threefold higher in female compared to male donors. Incident infections are rare in repeat donors, an observation that has led to one-time testing of donors in some European countries, but an incidence of three per million donor years of follow-up is felt by some to be too high for adoption of this strategy in the United States. Cell-free components such as plasma and cryoprecipitate do not transmit HTLV, and less than 30% of infected cellular components transmit. The residual risk for transfusion-associated HTLV infection using contemporary serologic testing is approximately 1 per 2.4 million donations. The contribution of blood-donor serologic testing to this low residual risk is confounded by the effect of effective leukoreduction that reduces HTLV-1 copy numbers in red blood cells (RBCs) by up to 6 logs, to below the infectious dose of 10^7 to 10^8 infected cells per unit (one of a number of arguments used in support of universal leukoreduction of blood components).

The deferral, notification, and counseling of healthy blood donors after a repeatedly reactive screening test for HTLVs is problematic, and tens of thousands have been affected since screening started. The vast majority of such tests are false positive, and there are no licensed confirmatory tests available for the HTLVs, leaving donor-testing laboratories to use unlicensed and largely unregulated supplemental tests to explicate reactive screening results. Recognizing this deficiency, the FDA approved an algorithm that accepts nonreactivity, on further testing of the original donation, using a second licensed donor-screening test from a different manufacturer as evidence that infection is absent. Alternatively, if the second screening with an alternate test is not done, donors may continue to donate as long as subsequent donations are negative on the original screening test. This complex algorithm resolves many false-positive screening results, but there remain a large number of notifications for false-positive reactivity, and it does not address the issue of the most appropriate counseling messages for false-positive donors. This frequently results in a mixed message to donors that they are uninfected based on available test results, but that they are nevertheless deferred from future blood donation.

HUMAN HERPESVIRUS INFECTIONS

Human herpesviruses (HHVs) are enveloped, structurally complex double-stranded DNA viruses that cause common infectious diseases. Primary infection is followed by lifelong carrier states and the possibility of reactivation. They are classified in three subfamilies, Alphaherpesvirinae, Betaherpesvirinae, and Gammaherpesvirinae, of which the latter two contain the herpesviruses that are of greatest concern from a transfusion medicine standpoint. Members of the Alphaherpesvirinae subfamily, herpes simplex viruses (HSVs) and varicella-zoster virus (VZV), rarely if ever cause transfusion-transmitted infections. Transfusion-transmitted cytomegalovirus is well recognized. Transmissions of EBV, HHV-6, HHV-7, and HHV-8 by blood appear to be rare or nonexistent in the United States.

Blood Safety Decision Making

Most consider the blood supply in the developed world to be at its highest historical safety level. This reflects incremental improvements in donor selection and history screening, blood testing, and process control that span four decades. For years, blood collection professionals and government regulators formulated blood safety policy decisions on the premise that a zero-risk blood supply was achievable. In part, this reflects the perceived tardy transfusion medicine community's response in the early 1980s to the emergence of human immunodeficiency virus (HIV) in the blood supply and the recognition (of) the scope and severity of posttransfusion non-A, non-B hepatitis (subsequently hepatitis C [HCV]) following that. It reflects also the "dread fear" associated with transfusion-associated HIV. This visceral reaction occurs when devastating, unpredictable, and stigmatizing events threaten potential victims who have minimal avoidance discretion. This fear was validated by numerous transfusion-related HIV cases. It was amplified by widely publicized lawsuits, indictments, and criminal convictions of health ministers and policy makers in the 1980s and 1990s (*l' affaire du sang contaminé* in France addressing HIV and Canada's Royal Commission of Inquiry on the Blood System into blood collection agencies' response to non-A, non-B hepatitis risk).

Not surprisingly, from the 1980s until now, donor deferrals and blood-testing interventions have been rapidly, successively, and additively implemented for emerging and theoretical risks. Collection facilities introduced anti-HBc and alanine aminotransferase (ALT) testing as surrogates for non-A, non-B hepatitis, HIV p24 antigen testing, then nucleic acid testing (NAT) for hepatitis C, HIV, extensive deferrals for the risks attending transmissible spongiform encephalopathies (TSEs,) NAT for West Nile virus (WNV) and hepatitis B, and antibody testing for *Trypanosoma cruzi*. The cost-benefit estimates for some of these interventions exceeded by orders of magnitude generally accepted thresholds but did not deter their adoption. For example, the costs per quality-adjusted life-year proximate to implementation include HIV NAT, $1,966,000; HCV NAT, $1,830,000; WNV NAT, $520,000 to $897,000; human T-lymphotropic virus (HTLV) antibody testing, $63,000,000; and *T. cruzi* antibody testing, $2,123,000 (Fig. 121-1). It is unlikely that this reactive approach can be sustained in the current health care–reform environment.

Application, after HIV entered the blood supply, of a stringent form of the precautionary principle (originally promulgated for environmental protection, not transfusion safety) pushed decision making toward avoidance of all risks. The precautionary principle promotes implementation of measures to mitigate risk even if evidence of a risk is incomplete. It is supposed to be tempered by proportionality; that is, any measures adopted are to be proportional to the risk and with those used in similar circumstances, but some have argued that this has not been the case with blood safety measures, at least by the metric of cost-benefit. Nevertheless, although in potential conflict with evidence-based decision making, this approach resonated with policy advocates charged with transfusion safety. The impact on transfusion safety is mixed. In retrospect, the implementation of HIV p24 antigen testing in the mid-1990s despite enormous studies demonstrating its lack of utility was extreme. Likewise, the recent decision to defer donors with chronic fatigue syndrome, based on a single study, to prevent xenotropic murine leukemia virus–related virus (XMRV) transmission was not necessary. Continued lifetime deferral of men having sex with men even once since 1977 is seen by many to be discriminatory in light of increasingly sensitive in vitro tests and alternative approaches to other risk behaviors. In contrast, when the risk for transfusion transmission of vCJD was theoretical, modeling was used to balance any such danger against the impact of broad donor deferrals on the adequacy of the blood supply and to arrive at a policy decision. Some argue that the magnitude of risk does not justify the stringency of donor criteria and number of resulting deferrals given the tiny risk in a country that is not bovine spongiform encephalopathy (BSE) endemic, but the process was rational and should perhaps be seen as a precedent that "an acceptable risk" is estimable.

Hemovigilance programs, such as the Serious Hazards of Transfusion (SHOT) in the United Kingdom and others in Canada, France, and a fledgling program in the United States, have emerged, supplying evidence about a much broader range of transfusion hazards than just infections. For example, a data-driven decision to minimize plasma transfusions from potentially alloimmunized female donors resulted in a dramatic reduction in transfusion-related acute lung injury in the United Kingdom, and early studies in the United States are consistent with this effect.

These systems provide an opportunity for monitoring the risks and benefits of new initiatives, (e.g., proactive pathogen reduction). Pathogen-reduction processes (see box on Pathogen Reduction) offer the opportunity to abrogate most of the residual risk for all of the historically important transfusion-transmitted infections, bacterial contamination, babesiosis, malaria, WNV, and Chagas disease. Pathogen reduction could eliminate the often lengthy, reactive, iterative paradigm of emergence of a new pathogen in the population, recognition of a material threat to transfusion recipients, development of donor-deferral strategies followed by development and refinement of test systems that has characterized our historical approach. Critically, broadly active pathogen-reduction processes offer a layer of protection against unsuspected emergence of new agents. If already in use, they would need only to be validated as active against a new agent or appropriate model agents. The challenge to precautionism is balancing the impact of pathogen reduction on product quality and the potential long-term toxicities that may not be apparent in premarketing clinical trials against the unquantified probability that new agents will emerge and threaten enough morbidity to make pathogen reduction clinically and economically feasible.[8]

More recently, as cost pressures for health care increase, transfusion professionals are questioning whether the zero-risk paradigm remains relevant. A consensus conference held in Toronto in October 2010 addressed concerns about "safety at any cost" and inconsistent decision-making practices affecting the blood supply.

The conference's consensus statement potentially portends a paradigm change toward risk-based decision making: risk identification, risk assessment, risk management, and risk communication.[9] Risk will never be zero, and there is now a realization that cost considerations,[10] politics, ideology, and public opinion cannot be ignored. Further policy making considerations will likely take these factors into account, balancing risk, safety, stakeholder interest, and overall impact on public health.

Cytomegalovirus

Cytomegalovirus (CMV), a betaherpesvirus, infects a wide range of cell types, including leukocytes of the monocyte-macrophage lineage and their progenitors. The former represents the preeminent source of transfusion-transmitted infection. Consequently, acellular blood components (plasma, cryoprecipitate) do not transmit CMV, and effectively leukocyte-depleted cellular components do so rarely.

Primary CMV infection in immunocompetent individuals is usually community acquired, often asymptomatic or associated with a mild, self-limited infectious mononucleosis syndrome. After virtually all infections, latent virus persists permanently in cellular reservoirs, allowing lifelong reactivation, and in the setting of transfusion or transplantation, the potential for viral transmission via unmanipulated cellular blood products, and allografts.

In immunosuppressed patients, CMV infection can cause severe morbidity and mortality from pneumonitis, hepatitis, gastroenteritis,

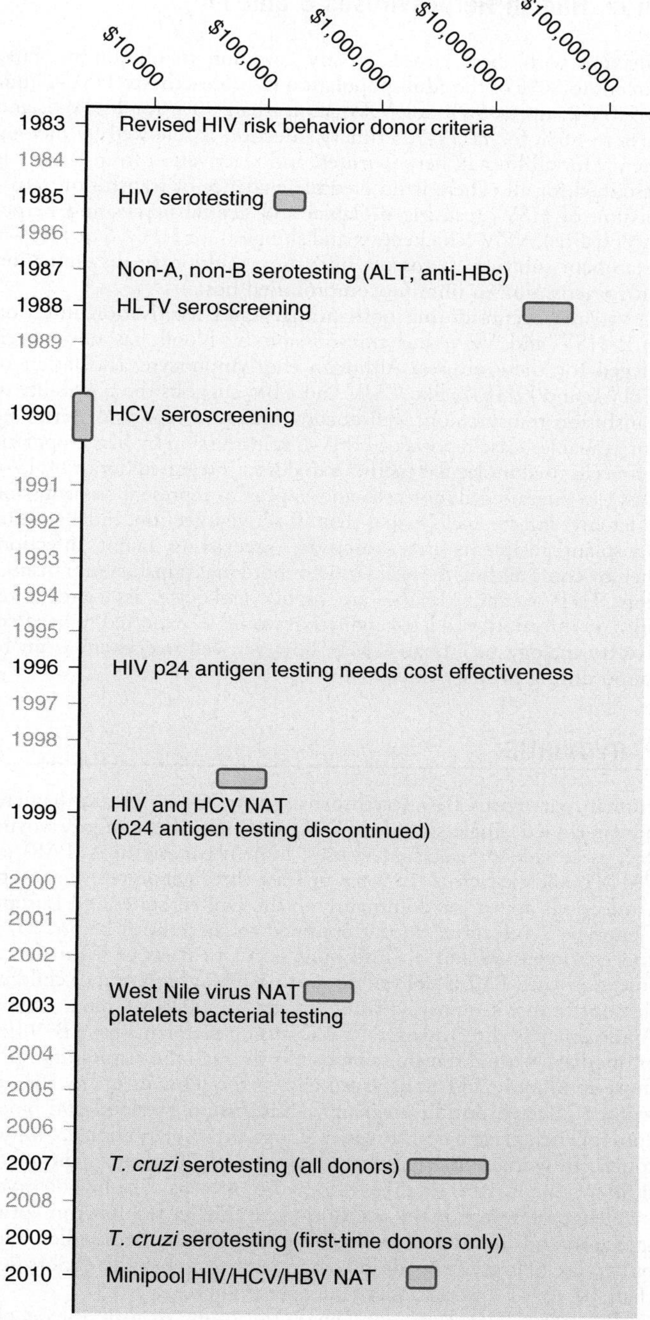

Figure 121-1 VARIOUS SAFETY MEASURES INTRODUCED DURING THE PAST THREE DECADES ENHANCED TRANSFUSION SAFETY. The x-axis displays costs associated with these advances per quality-adjusted life-year (QALY). Hepatitis C virus (HCV) seroscreening saves costs. Estimates for platelet bacterial culturing and human immunodeficiency virus (HIV) p24 antigen testing are not available. *ALT,* Alanine aminotransferase; *anti-HBc,* antibodies against HBcAg; *HBV,* hepatitis B virus; *HLTV,* human T-lymphotropic virus; *NAT,* nucleic acid testing; *T. cruzi, Trypanosoma cruzi.*

retinitis, and other inflammatory conditions. CMV infection in low-birth-weight infants is associated with sepsis-like syndromes, respiratory distress, and liver and bone marrow dysfunction. Their infections can be acquired in utero, from breast milk, or from transfusion. Reported infant morbidity varies considerably but can approach 50%

Table 121-2 Patients Benefiting From Cytomegalovirus Risk–Reduced Blood Components*

Infants <1200 g with CMV-seronegative mothers
Seronegative autologous and allogeneic (CMV-seronegative donors) stem cell transplant recipients
Seronegative stem cell transplant candidates
Seronegative recipients of seronegative solid organ transplants
Seronegative pregnant women
Fetuses receiving intrauterine transfusions
Immunosuppressed patients receiving granulocyte transfusions
HIV-seropositive/CMV-seronegative patients

CMV, Cytomegalovirus; *HIV,* human immunodeficiency virus.
*CMV risk–reduced components include CMV-seronegative and leukocyte-reduced components.

of seronegative low-birth-weight infants receiving unscreened, non-leukoreduced blood. CMV-seronegative marrow transplant patients are also susceptible to CMV infection, with approximately 30% of those infected developing symptomatic CMV disease before the adoption of routine monitoring for CMV antigen or nucleic acid in transplant recipients with provision of preemptive antiviral therapy. Seronegative solid organ transplant recipients are also susceptible to symptomatic transfusion-transmitted CMV infections. CMV-seronegative HIV-infected patients, although fewer in number, are another group at risk for transfusion-transmitted primary CMV infection. The reported risk for (usually asymptomatic) CMV infection in seronegative immunocompetent patients who receive non–leukocyte reduced cellular blood components unscreened for presence of CMV antibodies is approximately 1%. In contrast, the historical risk for CMV infection in immunosuppressed recipients receiving CMV-unscreened, non–leukocyte reduced blood components varies from 13.5% to 53.3%.

In the United States, in the population-based National Health and Nutrition Examination Survey (NHANES) III study, 58.9% of individuals more than 5 years old were seropositive, indicating prior CMV infection. The prevalence is age dependent, rising to over 90% in octogenarians, and is also dependent on race/ethnicity and other demographic indices. Such high seroprevalence rates mean that timely provision of components from seronegative donors from some donor populations can be challenging.

Selection of CMV seronegative and/or leukocyte-reduced blood components for susceptible patient groups has markedly reduced the risk for transfusion-transmitted CMV infection. Neither method is fail-safe in preventing transfusion-associated CMV transmission, however, and the place of one or both methods to supply "CMV-safe" blood components is an open controversy. In a metaanalysis of 11 controlled trials in allogeneic marrow transplantation 12 of 829 recipients of seronegative units versus 24 of 878 receiving leukoreduced but unscreened units developed CMV infections.[12] Pooling of data from three studies of seronegative or leukocyte reduced components, in comparison with CMV unscreened components, demonstrated statistically identical 93.1% and 92.3% reduced risks of CMV infection, respectively. Clinical outcomes would not be expected to be different in the setting of CMV antigen or DNA monitoring and preemptive antiviral therapy, but this has not been demonstrated in a rigorous study.

Current practice in the United States is diverse. Sixty-five percent of respondents to a recent survey considered leukoreduction and serologic screening to be equivalent, but practices for individual patient populations were divergent. In particular, clinicians caring for neonates were more likely to require serologic screening. In the absence of clear-cut scientific data and interpretation, the American Association of Blood Banks (AABB) recommends that each institution review its internal policies for blood use in patients vulnerable to CMV infection. Table 121-2 lists patient populations for whom use of "CMV risk–reduced" components, that is, CMV seronegative, leukocyte reduced, or both, are thought to be beneficial. The failure of clinicians to recognize recipients requiring CMV-safe transfusion and to request such components is an argument that has been advanced in support of universal leukoreduction. If leukocyte reduction is chosen as a means to reduce the risk for CMV transmission, components prepared by prestorage leukocyte reduction should be selected because leukocyte removal by this method is more reliable than bedside filtration, probably related to much more stringent process controls in blood collection facilities.

NAT on blood donors for CMV genomic sequences in plasma is discussed as an approach for additional risk reduction, because rare blood donors present with window-period infections before emergence of CMV antibody and their donations might be detected for diversion from at-risk recipients. Current NAT assays do not seem to be more effective than serologic screening in detecting latently infected healthy blood donors, because CMV DNA was not reproducibly detected in a cohort of 514 unequivocally seronegative samples. Any consideration of additional testing is complicated by the absence of randomized studies using contemporary leukoreduction methods and by our lack of understanding of the clinical impact of transfusion-transmitted CMV in an era of CMV monitoring and treatment.

EPSTEIN-BARR VIRUS (HHV-4)

Epstein-Barr virus (EBV), a gammaherpesvirus, is the causative agent of heterophile antibody-positive infectious mononucleosis and is etiologically associated with Burkitt lymphoma, nasopharyngeal carcinoma, and posttransplant lymphoproliferative disease. Transfusion transmission of the virus is unusual because more than 90% of the adult population is infected, and second infection is prevented by host virus-specific cytotoxic T lymphocytes, capable of lysing EBV-infected B lymphocytes when viral peptides are expressed on the lymphocyte surface. Rare cases of transfusion-transmitted EBV presenting as infectious mononucleosis have been described in immunocompetent recipients and in immunosuppressed patients following solid organ transplantation. Aggressive EBV-associated lymphoproliferative disorders have been observed in patients with immune injury after cord blood stem cell transplantation but have not been documented following transfusion. B lymphocytes are the likely source of transfusion-transmitted EBV infection, so leukoreduction is an attractive strategy to prevent infection in transfusion recipients. Nonclinical studies suggest that leukoreduction is capable of removing detectable EBV DNA from platelet concentrates and RBCs.

Kaposi Sarcoma Herpesvirus (HHV-8)

HHV-8 is a gammaherpesvirus causally linked to Kaposi sarcoma, primary effusion lymphoma, and multicentric Castleman disease. It is highly cell-associated with lymphocytes and monocyte-macrophages. Although generally spread person to person, including sexually, it has been shown to be transmitted by transplantation. There is convincing evidence of HHV-8 transmission by transfusion in sub-Saharan Africa, where the seroprevalence of HHV-8 among blood donors is 40%, and fresh, nonleukoreduced blood transfusions are commonly used. The seroprevalence of HHV-8 among U.S. blood donors has been reported to be as high as 20% to 25%, but a multicenter study using well-characterized antibody tests on donations from five representative U.S. regions estimated a seroprevalence of only 3.5% and showed no evidence of viremia by PCR. The possibility has been raised that transfusions in the United States have transmitted HHV-8, but subsequently reported studies comparing transfused patients with untransfused controls are not suggestive. Similar to what has been established for CMV infection, it is assumed that widespread leukocyte reduction in the United States mitigates the risk for HHV-8 transmission by transfusion, but this has not been proven in a rigorous trial.

Other Herpesviruses (Herpes Simplex, Varicella-Zoster Virus, Human Herpesviruses 6 and 7)

Infection with these viruses is very common to ubiquitous. Fifty percent to 80% of the adult population is seroreactive to HSV-1 and/or HSV-2, up to 95% for VZV, more than 90% for HHV-6, and 70% to 90% for HHV-7. Primary infection is followed by lifelong latency for all human herpesviruses, and reactivation from latency is described for all. There is no credible evidence of transfusion transmission of HSVs (causing orolabial and genital herpes and herpes encephalitis), VZV (chickenpox and shingles), or HHV-6 or HHV-7 (exanthem subitum or roseola infantum, multiorgan dissemination with reactivation in immunocompromised hosts).

Viremia occurs during both primary and reactivation infection with HSV and VZV, but transmission by blood has never been alleged for these viruses. Although the lymphocyte association of HHV-6 and HHV-7, like CMV and EBV, suggests the possibility of transfusion transmission, well-documented case reports or series are not available. Case reports of HHV-6 transmission by hematopoietic stem cells used molecular methods to detect integrated donor HHV-6 DNA in engrafted donor cells and appear to represent transmission of latently infected cells rather than of active infection. Furthermore, transplant recipients may reactivate preexisting latent infection, thereby confounding the evaluation of potential transfusion transmission. HHV-6 and HHV-7 are highly leukocyte associated after primary infection, and leukoreduction would be expected to be effective by analogy to human CMV; however, cell-free viremia can be found during primary infection.

PARVOVIRUS

Human parvovirus B19 (erythrovirus) is a 19- to 23-nm-diameter nonenveloped, single-stranded DNA virus from the family Parvoviridae, as are adeno-associated viruses, human parvovirus 4 (PARV4), PARV5, and bocavirus. B19 has at least three genotypes. Genotype 1 infections appear predominantly in the United States and Europe. Genotype 2 infections appear confined to those born before 1973, and genotypes 3a and 3b infections occur in parts of West Africa. Infection with B19 is ubiquitous, with 50% of high school children demonstrating seropositivity, increasing to 90% in older adults. Approximately three-quarters of transfusion recipients have B19 IgG antibodies. Natural transmission occurs through the respiratory route most commonly and transplacentally to the fetus in up to 30% of women infected during pregnancy. Transfusion of blood and blood components, plasma derivatives, and organ transplantation are minor routes. In women infected during weeks 9 to 20 of pregnancy, fetal death occurs in 10% to 15% from hydrops fetalis. The low observed incidence of infection in transfusion recipients results from prior infection and immunity, coinfusion of neutralizing antibodies, and/or because of low viral loads in components from healthy donors (less than 10^5 to 10^6 International Units per milliliter).

Parvovirus B19 causes erythema infectiosum, or fifth disease, oligoarthritis, and neurologic and myocardial infections. Following acute infection, viral replication leads to extremely high-titer viremia that declines at the time of IgM seroconversion approximately 9 days following infection. B19 may persist in bone marrow, liver, tonsils, and skin of healthy persons with no recognized clinical significance, and low levels of B19 DNA have been amplified from the blood of healthy people for several years after primary infection. The virus is highly tropic for erythroid progenitor cells using the P blood group antigen, or globoside, as its receptor, causing aplastic crises in patients with sickle cell anemia, other inherited hemolytic diseases, and conditions associated with decreased RBC survival, malaria, and HIV/AIDS. Acute infection impairs erythropoiesis for 7 to 10 days, with complete cessation for 3 to 7 days, resulting in hemoglobin decreases. Persistent infection, causing red cell aplasia, occurs in those who fail to develop neutralizing antibodies to the viral capsid protein 1. In these patients, the virus continues to circulate at high titer, greater than 10^{12} genome copies per milliliter. Patients at risk for persistent infection include those receiving intense chemotherapy and immunosuppression, organ transplant recipients, and those with HIV. Infection in these groups tends to respond favorably to intravenous immunoglobulin infusions.

B19 virus–impaired erythropoiesis appears to be multifactorial. B19 virus nonstructural protein 1 (NS1) mediates apoptosis; an 11-kDa protein perturbs signal transduction and induces apoptosis. B19 virus DNA activates Toll-like receptor 9 inhibiting cell growth and is toxic for infected cells.

Blood and plasma-derivative transmission involves donations during the transient 1- to 2-week high-titer viremic period. The prevalence of B19 viremia has been reported as 0.003% to 0.84% in blood and plasma donors. In one study, 43% of blood donations had low-titer viremia (less than 10^3 International Units/mL). In a study involving more than 12,100 B19 DNA–tested blood donations, given to surgical patients with a 78% pretransfusion B19 IgG seroprevalence, no B19 transmissions occurred from transfusions containing less than 10^6 International Units/mL. Hence most blood transfusion recipients are at low risk for an infectious exposure.[13]

By contrast, recipients of plasma-derived products made from manufacturing pools of thousands of donations have a significant risk because the virus survives partitioning, ethanol fractionation, and other antiinfective measures applied to derivatives, and a single high-titer viremic donation can overcome the neutralizing activity of antibody in the pool. Recipients of coagulation concentrates are at highest risk, whereas those of intravenous immunoglobulin and albumin are less so in cohort studies of prevalence. In one report 14% of viremic plasma donors had titers between 10^4 and 10^7 genome equivalents per milliliter, and one in 13,000 had titers greater than 10^7. In observational studies, seroconversion occurred among recipients of plasma derivatives with high titers, $10^{7.5}$ to $10^{8.5}$ International Units/mL, treated with the solvent/detergent pathogen-reduction technique, suggesting that the protective effect of neutralizing anti-B19 antibodies is exceeded in the presence of high viral loads (see box on Pathogen Reduction). Solvent/detergent pathogen-reduction treatment is ineffective in preventing B19 transmission in hemophilia patients receiving factor concentrates. Freeze-drying and dry-heat treatment (80° C [176° F] for 72 hours) inactivate more than 4.7 logs B19, but this is not always sufficient to prevent transmission. Fortunately, clinical morbidity from plasma derivative infections is minimal. Of note, PARV4 and PARV5 have been detected in pooled plasma derivative samples, but the clinical significance is not known.

Currently, plasma derivative manufacturers use "in-process" NAT to identify and remove source (paid donor) and recovered (untransfused plasma from volunteer whole-blood donations) plasma units with parvovirus B19 DNA titers greater than 10^4 International Units/mL. Approximately 1 per 10,000 plasma units is withheld from further processing. For volunteer whole-blood donors, 1 per 6,000 to 1 per 16,000 have titers greater than 10^6 International Units/mL. Because individual whole-blood donations rarely cause recognized parvovirus infection, testing of single red cell units, platelets, or plasma for transfusion for B19 DNA is not currently required, although some advocate use of B19-tested blood components for those potentially at risk, including pregnant women, neonates, those with reduced RBC survival, and immunocompromised patients.

WEST NILE VIRUS

West Nile virus (WNV) is a mosquito-borne lipid-enveloped RNA virus in the Japanese encephalitis complex of the Flaviviridae. Transmitted bird-to-bird primarily by culicine mosquito vectors, human infections occur incidentally. The first cases were identified in the West Nile district of Uganda in 1937. Subsequently outbreaks occurred in the Middle East, South Africa, and Europe. The first North American cases appeared in New York City in 1999. Starting in July 2000, WNV cases spread to the Mid-Atlantic states. This was followed in the next 3 years by transcontinental dissemination. During the summer of 2002, a model suggesting a significant risk for WNV infection in blood donors was published,[16] and then four recipients of organ allografts from a single donor developed neuroinvasive WNV infection. Infection of the organ donor was traced to donor blood transfused before death from trauma. The model and this case provoked a multidisciplinary effort, successfully engaging the blood community, the manufacturers of blood donor–screening NAT platforms, and public health officials and regulators to develop and deploy, under an investigational new drug (IND) exemption, high-throughput screening tests in the 10 months before the 2003 transmission season began. WNV test implementation represents the benchmark for responsiveness to a serious emerging transfusion-transmitted infection in the United States.

In 2003, 9862 clinical WNV cases were reported and more than 1000 healthy blood donors tested positive. In 2004, case reports declined in the Northeast but extended westward into Arizona and Southern California. In 2005, more than 2800 clinical cases were reported, with approximately 25% occurring in California, relatively high activity in South Dakota, Nebraska, Louisiana, and Illinois, and low activity in the Northeast. In 2006, approximately 400 viremic blood donors were identified, and more than 4050 cases occurred. Subsequently WNV activity was reported in Washington state for the first time, and high rates of infection were noted in Idaho, California, Nebraska, Illinois, Louisiana, and the Dakotas; more than 340 blood donors had positive test results. By 2010, fewer than 150 blood donors tested positive with the highest frequencies in New York, Texas, Arizona, and California.

WNV viremia appears 1 to 3 days after a bite of an infected mosquito. In contrast to HIV and HCV, peak WNV levels are low (median 3500 copies/mL compared to 10^5 to 10^7 copies for HIV and HCV). In cohort studies of blood donors with positive WNV RNA tests, only 29% to 61% (retrospectively) describe any symptoms before or after donation consistent with WNV infection, compared to 3% to 20% of those not infected, demonstrating that the donor history is neither sensitive nor specific enough to prevent transfusion transmission.[17] Testing for antibodies also will not prevent transmission because IgM antibodies appear a median of 14 days and IgG antibodies a median of 17 days after infection and infectivity disappears rapidly with the development of antibody. These data explain the selection of WNV NAT for the testing strategy. To maximize efficiency, donors' samples were tested in minipools containing aliquots from 6 to 16 donors, as is done for HCV, HBV, and HIV.

Despite minipool NAT, six transfusion-associated WNV cases occurred during 2003. The implicated donors had low-level antibody-negative viremia that escaped detection in the minipool (i.e., diluted) samples. Subsequently test performance has improved, and, more critically, blood collection organizations have developed strategies to switch to NAT on individual donation aliquots in areas experiencing high WNV activity. One transfusion-associated case occurred in 2004 and one in 2006. Of the 30 cases reported before 2006, all implicated donations tested WNV IgM-antibody negative. The last reported transmission was in 2008 when a blood donor was missed from a collection facility using less-stringent regional WNV activity criteria for triggering a conversion to individual donation testing.

DENGUE VIRUSES

This mosquito-borne infection is of great interest as an emerging pathogen with the potential to spread by transfusion. Forty percent of the world's population live in areas with risk for dengue, including many areas visited by U.S. travelers. It has spread rapidly in Latin America and the Caribbean since the 1980s. Dengue is endemic in Puerto Rico, the U.S. Virgin Islands, and American Samoa, and there have been outbreaks in Hawaii, Texas, and Florida during the last 10 years. Dengue is caused by four related flaviviruses spread person to person by *Aedes aegypti* and *Aedes albopictus,* which are present in 16 and 35 states, respectively, in the United States.

Most infections are asymptomatic, but illness ranges from undifferentiated fever to classic break bone fever and severe dengue (dengue hemorrhagic fever and dengue shock syndrome). An approximately

Pathogen Reduction

Our approach to new transfusion-transmitted infections is intrinsically reactive. We await disease emergence and identification of the new agent, develop an understanding of the infection's risk factors, devise donor deferrals, and then implement screening assays. Before deploying a sensitive and specific test, morbidity and mortality will accumulate. This reactive strategy will continue unless more broad-reaching interventions are brought forward. Pathogen-reduction technology (PRT) offers a proactive strategy to address new threats; these technologies involve physical, chemical, and photochemical treatments of blood components to inactivate or decrease viral, bacterial, and parasite infectivity.[14]

Beginning in the 1980s, heat treatment, nanofiltration, and solvent/detergent treatment eliminated or reduced viral transmission in products derived from large-scale plasma fractionation such as albumin, immunoglobulin, and hemostatic factor concentrates.

In the past decade, attention turned to whole blood–derived components: frozen plasma, platelets, and red cells. For these, PRT utilizes methylene blue and visible light treatment for plasma; amotosalen (psoralen) and ultraviolet A (UVA) light, and riboflavin (vitamin B_2) and UVB and UVA light for plasma and platelets; and riboflavin/UV light and S303 (a labile alkylating compound) for red cells. Many European countries use PRT for platelets and plasma. None is implemented in North America at this time.

Amotosalen/UVA and riboflavin/UV have advanced furthest in investigation in North America. They provide significant antiviral activity against all agents for which tests are performed currently, human immunodeficiency virus (HIV), hepatitis B and C, human T-lymphotropic virus (HTLV), West Nile virus, *Trypanosoma cruzi,* and cytomegalovirus. PRT also inactivates agents causing bacterial contamination of platelets; inactivates white blood cells to prevent transfusion-associated graft-versus-host disease; decreases formation and release of cytokines during storage, reducing febrile, nonhemolytic transfusion reactions; and abrogates white blood cell–induced alloantibody (e.g., human leukocyte antigen (HLA) antibody) formation mitigating alloimmune platelet refractoriness.

Adverse events linked to PRT relate to toxicity and cost. Toxicity affects cell function and recipient safety. Solvent/detergent-treated frozen plasma products prepared commercially in pools of 500 to 2500 donations distributed in the 1990s had reduced α_2-antiplasmin, antitrypsin, and protein S levels. They were associated with deep venous thrombosis in patients with liver disease and, in 2002, withdrawn by the manufacturer. A reformulated product used in Europe has not been associated with these events but has not been submitted for regulatory approval in the United States. Solvent/detergent is not active against hepatitis A or parvovirus. Because solvent/detergent disrupts lipid membranes, it cannot be used with cellular components.

Methylene blue and visible light inactivates pathogens in plasma by targeting nucleic acids. However, it alters fibrinogen structure. Because it damages cell membranes, methylene blue is not used for platelets or red cells. It is not effective against hepatitis A or parvovirus and is not recommend for treatment of thrombotic thrombocytopenic purpura.

Amotosalen/UVA and riboflavin/UVB also target nucleic acids. Treated plasma retains 72% to 77% of fibrinogen and factor VIII levels, greater than 80% of protein S and α_2-antiplasmin, and 96% of ADAMTS13 (a disintegrin and metalloproteinase with thrombospondin motifs 13). Platelets treated with these technologies have approximately 30% lower 1-hour posttransfusion corrected-count-increments than control platelets.[15] In clinical trials, mild and moderate bleeding frequency is increased, but not severe bleeding complications; and the time between transfusions and total platelet transfusions has not generally been different. It is unclear whether a proportion of platelets is impaired (in which case, platelet dose escalation would ameliorate concerns about lower corrected count increment) or all platelets are affected (increasing the dose would be insufficient). Pulmonary toxicity similar to transfusion-related acute lung injury (TRALI) has been reported in clinical trials and in animal model experiments in which UV light has been implicated. Previous clinical trials in red blood cells (RBCs) were halted because of non-symptomatic immunoreactivity against S303–induced red cell neoantigens and are being resumed with a reformulated process. Preliminary reports suggest riboflavin/UV causes functional impairment in red cells stored nearest the 42-day expiration date.

Toxicity relates also to residual chemical contamination. However, amotosalen and its products are removed before infusion, and chemical removal is unnecessary for riboflavin-treated blood components.

Cost-effectiveness studies project $1.3 million per quality-adjusted life-year (QALY) for PRT whole blood and $1.4 million per QALY for PRT platelets and plasma. This is costly, but consistent with NAT for HIV, and these analyses do not integrate the risk- or cost-benefit of mitigating an unanticipated emerging pathogen.

The toxicity issues likely will be resolved through technical adjustments. Cost, presumably, would decrease following large-scale implementation.

Interest in PRT remains high because it reduces sepsis-related platelet transfusion complications; inactivates parasites such as *Babesia microti,* and *Plasmodium falciparum;* mitigates risks associated with recognized emerging pathogens such as dengue and chikungunya viruses; and proactively decreases threats from unknown, emerging pathogens.

7-day viremia is a feature of both asymptomatic and symptomatic infection, and asymptomatic blood donors from Hong Kong, Singapore, and Puerto Rico have transmitted dengue to blood recipients. Although such reports are limited, compared to the high rates of vector-borne infection, there is no systematic surveillance for transfusion-transmitted dengue and its recognition in the face of widespread outbreaks is problematic.[18] Viremic, well donors have been identified in Brazil, Central America, and Puerto Rico using NAT and antigen detection tests. Rates of donor viremia in Puerto Rico are comparable to those found in U.S. donors during the most active WNV seasons.

The current risk for dengue from transfusion in the United States relates mainly to return of infected, asymptomatic or presymptomatic travelers to the United States from endemic areas (blood products imported to the mainland from Puerto Rico during dengue activity are screened). A 3- to 14-day incubation period precedes symptom onset. Deferral for travel to malarious areas (1 year for a U.S. native) offers some protection, but a large proportion of dengue-affected areas frequently visited from the United States are malaria-free and donor-travelers to those areas can introduce the virus into the community and the blood supply. Careful surveillance and a high index of suspicion when sustained febrile illness occurs following transfusion are required to recognize transfusion dengue. Preliminary data on travelers from the United States to dengue-endemic destinations that are malaria-free suggest that 2- to 4-week deferral for travel to dengue-affected areas may have a greater adverse impact on blood donation than current malaria deferrals. The conditions for sustained spread of dengue exist in large areas of the United States: a source of infection from travelers and immigrants; a susceptible population; and competent vectors. Whether the recently identified outbreaks in the United States will continue or increase, and whether sustained transmission will begin is unknown. Transfusion-transmitted dengue has been identified by one group as one of the three highest-priority emerging infections posing a potential threat to transfusion recipients

Emerging Infections

The experiences with human immunodeficiency virus (HIV), new variant Creutzfeldt-Jakob disease (vCJD), and West Nile virus (WNV) have made it clear that planning for the emergence of new pathogens that may threaten the blood supply is critical in order to shorten the interval from emergence to mitigation. To that end, the characteristics of pathogens likely to enter the blood supply must be understood. These include the ability of the agent to establish an asymptomatic blood-borne phase, to survive under contemporary processing and storage conditions, to establish infection by the intravenous route, and to cause significant morbidity in a transfusion recipient.

Using these characteristics and a review of contemporary literature, the Transfusion Transmitted Diseases Committee of the American Association of Blood Banks (AABB), from 2005 to 2009 produced a compendium of infectious agents that might become relevant to transfusion medicine and attempted to prioritize those that were identified.[19] A series of 68 fact sheets was developed. The fact sheets provide transfusion medicine professionals and clinicians with an overview of the agents' phylogeny, epidemiology, clinical characteristics, and interventions that might be useful to protect the safety of the blood supply. Three agents were included in the highest priority stratum: *Babesia* sp., dengue viruses, and the vCJD prion; a section on each is included in this chapter. The fact sheets are freely available online, cover many of the agents discussed in this chapter, and are to be updated when required.

Since the original publication, several new monographs have been added, reflecting an ongoing "horizon-scanning" initiative designed to alert the medical community to potential threats. These include yellow fever and the yellow fever vaccine viruses after the latter was transmitted to blood recipients when recent vaccine recipients failed to divulge that information during blood donation, and xenotropic murine leukemia virus–related virus after alleged associations with prostate cancer or chronic fatigue syndrome/myalgic encephalitis were published (see box on Xenotropic Murine Leukemia Virus–Related Virus). Other fact sheets have been updated and rereleased to capture relevant new information. The availability of these materials to the transfusion medicine and general medical communities is meant to increase awareness that unexpected infections in transfusion recipients should trigger consideration of that source and to provide background allowing the rational consideration of approaches to avert and minimize their spread.

in the United States and Canada and has been the subject of discussions at the FDA's Blood Products Advisory Committee (see box on Emerging Infections).

PANDEMIC INFLUENZA A

There was interest in the transfusion safety implications of influenza A even before the swine origin A-H1N1pandemic of 2009-2010.[22b] Viremia in donors, and the potential for infection of recipients were discussed during meetings of an AABB pandemic influenza planning task force as early as 2008, based on old literature demonstrating the virus in the blood of experimentally infected volunteers and case reports of viral dissemination during human infection with highly pathogenic avian A-H5N1 virus. Subsequent studies have failed to identify influenza viruses in donors drawn in U.S. communities during periods of high seasonal influenza activity or in donors with the onset of influenza-like illness immediately following donations.[22c] The current consensus is that pandemic influenza is not likely a threat to blood recipients, but that disruption of the blood supply in a severe pandemic is a more important possibility requiring careful advance planning.

Xenotropic Murine Leukemia Virus–Related Virus

The alleged association of the gammaretrovirus xenotropic murine leukemia virus–related virus (XMRV) with chronic fatigue syndrome/myalgic encephalomyelitis (CFS/ME) is paradigmatic of the difficulties inherent in the real-time assessment of potential and emerging transfusion-transmissible infections. A group of CFS/ME patients and controls were evaluated using polymerase chain reaction (PCR), virus isolation, serology, and immunohistochemistry.[20] Evidence of the virus's presence was strongly associated with the clinical diagnosis, culturable virus was found in plasma, and the issue of transfusion transmission was appropriately raised.

Multiple subsequent studies from other groups over the ensuing 2 years failed to confirm the presence of XMRV in a variety of populations. Several publications suggested that PCR contamination might underlie some positive results, and data now suggest that XMRV arose as a recombinant of two murine leukemia viruses during passages in nude mice, all suggesting the initial findings to be artifact.[21]

Absent definitive data or scientific consensus, an interdisciplinary task force from the transfusion medicine, research, advocacy, and regulatory communities was formed within 2 months of the original publication to assess potential risks to transfusion recipients and to identify policy alternatives.[22a] The U.S. blood community currently provides educational materials to prospective donors, asking those with a medical diagnosis of CFS/ME to refrain from donation at least while the data are accumulating. A scientific working group convened under the auspices of the National Heart, Lung, and Blood Institute (NHLBI) to establish a scientific agenda with reference to risks from transfusion and to facilitate appropriate research.

Two federal advisory committees, the Health and Human Services Secretary's Advisory Committee on Blood Safety and Availability and the Food and Drug Administration's Blood Products Advisory Committee held briefings and hearings during 2010 to 2011 to review the available data and make policy recommendations. By this writing a consensus has emerged that XMRV is not a human pathogen in either CFS or prostate cancer (where it had originally been described); however, concerns expressed by CFS/ME advocates and the two advisory committees have provided momentum for continued exclusion of these donors. The rationales are that donation may be harmful even to recovered CFS/ME patients and that donors with a history of CFS should be excluded on the general principle that it is a syndrome of unknown etiology that may pose some threat to transfusion recipients.

BACTERIAL CONTAMINATION

Bacterial contamination of red cell and platelet components occurs primarily as a result of incomplete skin disinfection at the donor phlebotomy site, where bacterial populations survive in skin appendages below the accessible surface and contaminate skin plugs made by the phlebotomy needle that enters the blood bag. Transient asymptomatic bacteremia at the time of blood donation, a break in technique during pooling the contents of or sealing blood containers, disruption of blood bag integrity or its contamination during manufacturing are other rare sources. Bacterial proliferation occurs more rapidly in platelet concentrates stored at room temperature than in red cells maintained at 4° C (39.2° F).

The rate of bacterial contamination in allogeneic platelets was estimated at 1 per 1000 to 3000 units with life-threatening septic reactions occurring in 1 per 15,000 to 100,000 recipients before routine implementation of culture-based tests to detect bacteria in apheresis platelets in 2004. These tests reduced contamination rates to approximately 1 per 5000 to 8500 platelet units. Clinical septic reactions occur in approximately 30% of recipients receiving contaminated platelets. Bacterial contamination was responsible for 33 of 267 transfusion-related deaths reported to the FDA from 2005 to 2009.[23] Only acute hemolytic reactions and transfusion-related acute lung injury (TRALI) were responsible for more. Further, there is consensus that these reactions are badly underrecognized and underreported. Culturing fails to detect 50% to 75% of contaminated units. This undetected contamination occurs largely because minimal bacterial levels present when cultures are obtained yield culture aliquots without bacteria. Subsequently the few bacteria remaining in the blood bag can grow out during storage, producing transfusions with significant bacterial levels. To minimize this, collection facilities generally hold apheresis platelets for approximately 24 hours after collection before sampling for culture to allow low bacterial inocula to proliferate, improving the sensitivity of culture. In addition, improved skin antisepsis and diversion for laboratory testing of the first 15 to 30 mL of blood, which contain the skin plug, provide further reduction of contamination rates, transfusion reactions, and fatality rates by lowering the bacterial load that otherwise would enter the final component container.

Septic transfusion reactions should be suspected when one or more of the following occur within 1 to 4 hours of transfusion: temperature elevations greater than 1° to 2° C (1.8° to 3.6° F), chills and rigors, tachycardia more than 120 beats per minute or an increase of 40 beats per minute, or an increase or fall in systolic blood pressure of greater than 30 mm Hg. Additional signs and symptoms can include nausea, vomiting, diarrhea, bleeding, oliguria, or septic shock. Septic transfusion reactions may be confused with hemolytic transfusion reactions, febrile, nonhemolytic transfusion reactions, or TRALI.

Platelet concentrates contaminated with *Escherichia coli, Staphylococcus aureus, Staphylococcus epidermidis, Serratia marcescens,* and *Streptococcus* species account for most fatal reactions. *Propionibacterium acnes* is a frequent culture isolate from platelets during storage but is not believed to be responsible for a significant number of reactions. The bacterial dose in platelet concentrates and species virulence correlate with the clinical outcome. Bacterial concentrations greater than 10^6 colony-forming units (CFU)/mL are more likely to result in severe reactions or fatalities. Alternatively, low concentrations, 10^4 or fewer CFU/mL of skin organisms, frequently elicit no reaction. Endotoxin elaboration by gram-negative organisms is associated with the most severe reactions.

In addition, bacteria grow at variable rates. *S. epidermidis* grows slowly, and *P. acnes* requires on average 69 hours for detection. Because collection agencies continue bacterial culturing until the platelet unit expiration date or detection of growth, there is further opportunity to intercept released platelets that have not been transfused and to alert physicians about the potential risk for bacterial contamination in cases where the units have been administered. However, the vast majority of septic reactions are associated with false-negative culture tests due to sampling insufficiency as noted earlier.

Before the mid-1980s, platelet concentrates were stored for 7 days. Following reports of septic reactions, the shelf life was reduced to 5 days to decrease the interval during which bacteria could proliferate. In the United States, blood suppliers distributed platelets from 2005 to 2008 with a 7-day shelf life following enrollment in an FDA-mandated postmarket surveillance study (Post Approval Surveillance Study of Platelet Outcomes, Release Tested [PASSPORT]) that included testing for bacterial contamination by a sensitive culture method. Initial experience suggested that extended platelet storage coupled with bacterial testing substantially decreased platelet loss from outdating. However, the PASSPORT study found 1 per 4329 tested platelet products with negative bacterial cultures had bacterial growth when tested at the end of storage, 7 days later.[24] Septic reactions occurred in approximately 1 per 25,000 platelet transfusions; some following infusion of 3-day stored platelets, most with those stored 4 days or longer, leading to reinstatement of the 5-day platelet shelf life.

Alternative methods for detecting bacterial contamination include point-of-release testing in the hospital transfusion service. Considered a supplement to culture-based testing, this assay can be used shortly before issuing platelets for transfusion to detect units missed by early culture. This rapid qualitative immunoassay tests for the presence of conserved bacterial antigens (gram-negative lipopolysaccharide and gram-positive lipoteichoic acid). In one report using this test, 1 per 3000 platelet doses contained gram-positive organisms when issued 3 or more days after collection.[25] Other methods, under development, for mitigating septic platelet events include microcolorimetry, bacterial spore biosensors, real-time PCR, flow cytometry, and detection of other bacterial cell wall constituents. Pathogen-reduction technology using psoralens or riboflavin plus UV light provides an opportunity for inactivating multiple pathogens before they can proliferate.

Red blood cell bacterial contamination rates approximate 1 per 30,000 units with adverse clinical outcomes occurring in 1 per 500,000 transfusions and fatalities occurring at a rate of 1 per 10 million. Most septic reactions occur in units stored for 4 weeks or longer, reflecting the delayed growth of bacteria at 4° C (39.2° F).

Bacteria isolated from contaminated red cell units include *S. marcescens, E. coli, Pseudomonas* species (especially *Pseudomonas fluorescens*), and *Yersinia enterocolitica.* The latter two are psychrophilic and well known to proliferate in the cold. Gram-positive skin saprophytes account for most of the organism-contaminating platelet concentrates, with the remaining attributed to gram-negative organisms associated with occult bacteremia.

Immediate recognition of a platelet or red cell septic reaction and immediate discontinuation of the transfusion, supportive care, and antibiotic administration are the mainstays of therapy. Prevention relies on careful donor selection and scrupulous adherence to aseptic techniques and precautions from component collection, processing, transport, and storage to transfusion at the bedside. The Gram stain reveals bacteria in platelet concentrates contaminated with more than 10^5 to 10^6 CFU/mL.

Donors of platelet units contaminated with *Streptococcus bovis* or *Streptococcus infantarius* have been associated with colonic polyps and colon cancer.

SPIROCHETE INFECTIONS

Syphilis

U.S. blood banks first screened donors with a serologic test for syphilis in 1938, and screening has been a regulatory requirement since 1958. It was the first test mandated for U.S. donors and stood alone before the discovery of the Australia antigen almost two decades later. More than 100 transfusion syphilis cases were published before World War II, and many more certainly occurred. The last alleged case of transfusion-transmitted syphilis in the United States, however, was in 1966. Since then, hundreds of millions of components have been transfused in this country without another recognized case. There are multiple explanations for the disappearance of transfusion-transmitted syphilis in addition to testing: (1) the dramatic decline in the incidence of early syphilis in the United States over the decades, more than an order of magnitude, reducing the reservoir of donors able to transmit; (2) the end of direct donor-to-recipient transfusion combined with the loss of viability of *Treponema pallidum* in stored blood—the latter attributed to poor survival in refrigerated red blood cells and to the high oxygen tension in platelets stored at higher temperatures; (3) the ubiquitous administration of antibiotics for trivial to serious viral, bacterial, and noninfectious clinical syndromes, especially to those sick enough to be transfused; (4) donor deferral for behavioral correlates of syphilis risk (e.g., male sex with males, occurrence of recent sexually transmitted infection in donors, exchange of drugs or money for sex, injection drug use); (5) passive surveillance for transfusion-transmitted syphilis compounded by the failure of recognition by physicians (who may have never seen syphilis, venereal or otherwise); and (6) donor illness during spirochetemia severe enough to prevent their presentation to donate blood or causing deferral. The relative contributions of each of these factors are unquantified.

Most blood collection facilities screen donors with an automated test for detecting treponemal antibodies (e.g., *T. pallidum* hemagglutination assay[TPHA]) and confirm reactive assays using reference methods like the *T. pallidum* particle agglutination (TPPA) assay or fluorescent treponemal antibody, absorbed (FTA-abs) test. Approximately 50% of donors with confirmed positive test results have evidence of a treated syphilis infection. Donations with reactive syphilis tests are generally discarded. Blood centers defer donors with positive confirmatory tests for 1 year and then may restore donor eligibility after the donor provides evidence of appropriate treatment for syphilis and has a negative nontreponemal serologic test result. Persistent false-positive reactions on nontreponemal tests (e.g., rapid plasma reagin [RPR]) occur in healthy donors and with a wide variety of infectious diseases other than syphilis, after some immunizations, with autoimmune disease and other chronic inflammatory disease, and have increasing prevalence with increasing age.

The vast majority of contemporary reactive STS results in donors are biologic false positives, unrelated to syphilis, especially where nontreponemal assays are used (<1% confirmed during 2008, data on file Mississippi Valley Regional Blood Center). Many true positives are the "serologic scar" of remote (often treated) infection and pose no risk to blood recipients. A recommendation to discontinue donor screening for syphilis was made in 1985 but not acted upon initially because of the perception that the STS might be functioning as a surrogate for HIV or other transfusion-transmissible viruses.[26] This hypothesis has been rejected, but, because the role of STS in the elimination of transfusion syphilis is unclear, syphilis testing continues. Although small PCR studies of reactive donors have been universally negative, rabbit inoculation studies using samples from confirmed reactive donors will likely be required to eliminate syphilis testing, and it seems unlikely the resources will be found to do a study of the required size.

Lyme Disease

Borrelia burgdorferi is the spirochete that causes Lyme disease, the most frequent vector-borne infection in North America and Europe. The agent was discovered in 1977 during investigations of an arthritis cluster in Connecticut children. Cases reported in the United States doubled between 1992 and 2006 to almost 20,000. Geographic distribution of cases is highly focused with the majority of reported cases occurring in 10 northeast and north central states. *Ixodes scapularis*, the black-legged tick, transmits *B. Burgdorferi* in those areas, and *Ixodes pacificus*, the western black-legged tick, transmits the infection along the Pacific coast. The ticks feed predominantly in late spring and early summer during the nymph stage. Emergence has been associated with environmental changes that increase deer and rodent reservoir populations and changing residential patterns putting humans in more intimate contact with the tick vectors. Rodents are the reservoir. Although deer are not infected, they transport and maintain the ticks. Birds may also play a role in transporting the vector ticks.

The characteristic erythema chronicum migrans ("bull's-eye") rash is present in 70% to 80% of cases within 30 days of infection. The wide variety of clinical findings includes malaise, fatigue, headache, myalgias, large joint arthralgias and arthritis, and neurologic and cardiac signs and symptoms. These may not immediately suggest Lyme disease in the absence of a typical rash or known tick exposure. Serologic testing supports the clinical diagnosis. Unfortunately, poor specificity is recognized with many screening methods, and a two-step approach using a sensitive EIA or immunofluorescence assay (IFA) followed by a confirmatory, more specific, immunoblot is recommended by the Centers for Disease Control and Prevention.

B. burgdorferi spirochetemia occurs in 44% of patients with clinical Lyme disease and peaks 7 to 10 days after tick bite. The spirochete can survive in red cells, platelets, and frozen plasma for at least the duration of their routine storage. Transfusion transmission of *B. burgdorferi* has been demonstrated in a murine model. Despite these observations, no human transfusion-associated cases have been reported. This may reflect the relatively short spirochetemic phase and deferral of donors with nonspecific illness or signs and symptoms of Lyme borreliosis. Although there are no official standards or guidance, it would be prudent for individuals with a history of Lyme disease to be deferred until well and treatment has been completed.

Other Tick-Borne Bacteria

The rickettsia that cause human monocytic ehrlichiosis (HME) and human granulocytic anaplasmosis (HGA; formerly human granulocytic ehrlichiosis) are intracellular bacteria that survive in stored blood. *Ehrlichia chaffeensis* causes HME and is transmitted to humans by Lone Star tick (*Amblyomma americanum*) bites. Most cases occur in the south central and southeastern United States. *Anaplasma phagocytophilum* causes HGA and occurs predominately in the northeastern and upper midwestern areas of the United States. *I. scapularis* and *I. pacificus* (the Lyme borreliosis vector) transmit the organism. Signs and symptoms include fever, chills, and headache, often associated with thrombocytopenia, leukopenia, and increased liver enzyme levels. Intracellular aggregates appear in monocytes in the HME, and inclusions appear in granulocytes in HGA. Seroprevalence studies in blood donors in Wisconsin and Connecticut report 0.5% to 3.5% seropositivity for *A. phagocytophilum* antibodies.

Two cases of transfusion-transmitted HGA from asymptomatic donors have been recognized after nonleukoreduced RBC transfusion. The RBCs had been stored for 30 and 15 days before transfusion. In a study of heavily tick-exposed military recruits in Arkansas, which included a look back to 10 blood recipients of units from soldiers infected with *E. chaffeensis* and *Rickettsia rickettsii* (the agent of Rocky Mountain spotted fever [RMSF]), no clinical illness occurred in recipients. One possible RMSF seroconversion was reported.

There is a single case report of transfusion-associated RMSF that involved a donor developing symptoms 3 days postdonation. The recipient developed symptoms 6 days posttransfusion.

Both *Ehrlichia* and *Anaplasma* spp. are white blood cell–associated, and leukoreduction has been proposed to mitigate their impact. The infectivity of *Orientia tsutsugamushi*, the rickettsial agent of scrub typhus, is reduced by up to 10^5 by filtration leukoreduction, but infectious *E chaffeensis* survived in refrigerated red cells and could be isolated from the packed RBCs after filtration. Tick-borne RBC pathogens like *Babesia* and Colorado tick fever virus are unlikely to be affected by leukoreduction.

PARASITIC INFECTIONS

Malaria

Five *Plasmodium* species (*Plasmodium falciparum, Plasmodium vivax, Plasmodium ovale, Plasmodium malariae and Plasmodium knowlesi*) and occasionally others cause the protozoan disease malaria. In 2008, 243 million cases occurred worldwide, with most in sub-Saharan Africa. Other endemic areas include parts of Asia and South America and more limited areas in Mexico, Central America, and the Caribbean. Of 1478 imported cases in the United States in 2009, 735 were acquired in Africa, 142 in Asia/Western Pacific, and 103 in the Americas.[27] West Africa accounted for most cases associated with Africa, and Honduras, Haiti, and Guyana for most of the cases from the Americas. During 2009, only two cases were acquired in Mexico, both *P. vivax*. In 2003, eight autochthonous infections occurred in Palm Beach, Florida; but none subsequently. Vectorial transmission, overwhelmingly the most common route, is by the bite of an infected female *Anopheles* mosquito. *Anopheles* mosquitoes generally feed between dawn and dusk, thereby limiting the risk to tourists who usually visit malaria areas during daylight hours. Almost three-quarters of those who acquired malaria were visiting friends or relatives in endemic areas. Missionaries and business travelers represent fewer than 20% of infected U.S. citizens. Leisure travelers make up the small remainder. Two other routes are more rare, congenital and induced malaria. The latter includes the intentional parenteral transmission of malaria as was done for treatment of neurosyphilis in the remote past and more recently for Lyme borreliosis, transmissions during injection drug use, and transmission by transfusion.

P. falciparum accounts for 40% to 46% of U.S. cases detected recently, *P. vivax* 11% to 20%, and *P. malariae* and *P. ovale* approximately 2% each. For the remainder most are undetermined with a few mixed-species infections. *P. knowlesi* has not yet been reported.

Seventy percent of imported cases in the United States occurred among returning travelers who were visiting friends or relatives, ethnically and racially distinct from the majority population of the United States (where malaria is not endemic), who return to their homelands (countries where malaria is endemic) to visit friends or relatives. The region of origin is very relevant to measures designed to prevent malaria transmission by transfusion because many of these individuals are semi-immune and therefore can be parasitemic while asymptomatic. In contrast, donors without malarial immunity who travel to endemic areas and become infected are nearly always symptomatic when they are parasitemic and would not be accepted as blood donors. Malaria symptoms occurred within 1 month of arrival in the United States in 84% of those infected with *P. falciparum* and 56% of those with *P. vivax* in 2009. The latter represents almost all cases of relapsing malaria. No acute onsets involving the four most frequent *Plasmodium* species occurred at an interval greater than 1 year.

Ninety-eight transfusion cases have been recognized and reported in the United States since 1963. During the past 10 years there have been 17 (0 to 3 per year) including 1 in 2007, none in 2008, and 2 in 2009. In the majority of these 98 the case would have been prevented had the extant donor deferral criteria been appropriately applied.

The incubation period for transfusion-associated malaria ranges from 8 to 90 days. *P. falciparum* has the shortest time, mean 17 days (range, 8 to 36 days) and *P. malariae* the longest, mean 50 days (range, 8 to 90 days). Most cases involved RBC or whole-blood transfusion, although a few transmissions from platelet transfusions have occurred, presumably related to RBC contamination. Transmission from frozen plasma has not been reported.

Current strategies for reducing the low risk for transfusion transmission in the United States involve deferral of residents of nonendemic areas who have traveled to malaria-endemic regions during the previous 12 months, those with residence in endemic areas for 3 years since their last potential exposure in such regions, and those with a history of malaria for 3 years after resolution. Apart from incomplete elicitation of malaria risk history, residual risk remains because transfusion transmissions of *P. falciparum*, *P. vivax*, and *P. ovale* have been reported 13, 27, and 7 years, respectively, after departure from malarious areas. Because *P. malariae* infection can persist for more than 70 years without symptoms, elimination of transfusion-induced malaria is a practical impossibility. At this time, licensed in vitro screening for at-risk donors using antibody tests, antigen detection, or NAT are unavailable in the United States. It is not clear that the limited commercial potential of assays to be used on a relatively small fraction of donors will justify the investment required to pass the stringent regulatory requirements of a blood donor screening assay. Donor deferral guidelines are undergoing review to reduce the loss of more than 60,000 potential donors with travel to areas of Mexico where the malaria risk is minimal. Removing the restriction for these donors would increase donations and might promote greater attention to more effective screening or travelers at higher risk.[28]

Babesiosis

Babesia species that infect humans include *Babesia microti*, *Babesia duncani* (previously WA1 type), *Babesia divergens* (limited primarily to Europe), *B. divergens*–like (MO1 and EU1), and *Babesia venatorum*. *B. microti*, an intraerythrocytic protozoan, causes most human infections. The white-footed mouse, *Peromyscus leucopus*, serves as the reservoir and the deer or black-legged tick, *I. scapularis* (also the vector of Lyme borreliosis and HGA), as the vector. Transmission follows bites from infected ticks, primarily nymphs, from May through early September. The defined transmission period has less relevance for transfusion transmission because asymptomatic blood donors can be infected chronically.[29] Most cases occur in Massachusetts and its coastal islands, Rhode Island, Connecticut, New York, New Jersey, Wisconsin, and Minnesota. This geographic range has expanded recently, attributed to expansion of white-tailed deer, *Odocoileus virginianus*, populations. Although not a competent host, deer provide a blood meal and transportation for adult ticks to new areas.

The vast majority of both vectorial and transfusion-associated *Babesia* cases involve *B. microti*. *B. duncani* infections include those previously designated WA1. *B. divergens* cases occur predominately in Europe. Most infected patients had splenectomies before infection. Cattle serve as the reservoir and *Ixodes ricinus* ticks the vector. There are no reports of transfusion-associated *B. divergens* infections.

The incubation period varies from 1 to 9 weeks. The severity of illness associated with *Babesia* infections relates more to the infected individual's immune status than the *Babesia* species. The very young, older adults, persons who have had a splenectomy, and those with hereditary hemolytic disorders are at greatest risk for morbidity and mortality. Approximately one-third of infected subjects remain asymptomatic, and parasitemia may persist for more than 2 years. Typical symptoms resemble malaria and include fever, headache, chills, sweats, and arthralgia, myalgia, malaise, nausea, diarrhea, and hemolytic anemia. Parasitemia levels vary from 1% to 2% in otherwise healthy hosts to 85% in immunocompromised and asplenic patients. Case fatality rates approximate 5%.

Case reports of transfusion-associated *Babesia* infections include units stored for 35 days. *Babesia* transmission has been reported following transfusion of cryopreserved red cells, and four cases involve whole blood–derived platelet transfusions presumably contaminated with red cells. At least 159 transfusion-associated *B. microti* cases have occurred, primarily in endemic regions, but cases in nonendemic states reflect the interstate movement of both blood components and blood donors and highlight the high index of suspicion required to recognize cases.[30] More than three-quarters of the reports occurred during the past decade. The all-cause mortality rate approaches 19%. There are three cases involving *B. duncani*, and single cases have been reported from Japan (*B. microti*-like) and Germany.

Risk estimates of transfusion transmission vary over such an extremely wide range as to provide little utility. They are likely to be underestimates due to failure to recognize the infection or its relationship to a recent transfusion. Babesiosis has been made a nationally notifiable infection and included in the nascent biovigilance network of the National Healthcare Safety Network, so more accurate measurements of transfusion risk may become available in the future.

Febrile patients must be queried for a transfusion history and babesiosis considered when transfusion has occurred. Diagnostic laboratory evaluation includes blood smear examination, which requires differentiation of *Babesia* sp. from *Plasmodium* infections. Tetrad or "Maltese cross" forms are diagnostic for *Babesia* but occur infrequently. Serologic testing is under development. Indirect immunofluorescence antibody testing is the current test of choice for identifying persons with low-level parasitemia such as patients with chronic infections but may remain positive after resolution or cure of babesiosis. PCR testing may be more sensitive for detecting acute infections before seroconversion.

In the absence of an FDA-licensed test, mitigation of transfusion transmission involves deferral of potential donors with a history of *Babesia* infection. Questioning donors about tick exposure or tick bite has no predictive value as a donor-screening question. One blood center conducts tests under an IND exemption using IFA and NAT to screen donations intended for immunosuppressed patients considered at highest risk for *Babesia* infection complications such as neonates, pediatric patients with sickle cell disease, and pediatric oncology patients. IFA is being used by another system in highly endemic regions. An attractive alternative is the adoption of pathogen-reduction technologies.

Leishmaniasis

Phlebotomine (Old World) and *Lutzomyia* (New World) sand-fly bites transmit *Leishmania* infections to humans in most of the tropical and subtropical world. Trypanosomatidae of various species cause visceral infection (*Leishmania donovani, Leishmania infantum,* and others, kala-azar) and cutaneous and mucocutaneous infections (*Leishmania tropica, Leishmania major, Leishmania mexicana, Leishmania braziliensis,* and others that go by a variety of local names). In addition, transplacental, sexual, and transfusion transmissions occur.[31] The promastigote form of the parasite resides in the gastrointestinal tract of sand flies and is inoculated into humans through a skin bite. In humans, promastigotes are phagocytosed by monocytes, where they transform into amastigotes that reproduce and reside in macrophages and the reticuloendothelial system. Organisms in monocytes and free amastigotes are released during refrigerated storage, transform back into extracellular promastigotes, and mediate transfusion transmission. *L. tropica* also survives in monocytes contained in frozen red cell preparations and in platelet concentrates stored at room temperature. At least 10 cases of transfusion-associated leishmaniasis attributed to *L donovani* have been reported in endemic areas, mostly in young children or neonates. A probable case of platelet transfusion–transmitted *L. donovani* was reported in India. A presumed case of transfusion-transmitted *L. mexicana* in a renal transplant recipient was mistakenly diagnosed as Chagas disease because of serologic cross-reactivity between *Trypanosoma cruzi* and *Leishmania. L. infantum* DNA was amplified from 6% of peripheral blood mononuclear cells of blood donors with *Leishmania* antibodies in the Balearic Islands. Several animal model studies also demonstrate transmission by blood transfusion.

Asymptomatic infections occur frequently in healthy donors exposed in endemic areas, and the organisms may circulate in peripheral blood more than 1 year following exposure. Foxhounds infected with *Leishmania* species have been found in 18 U.S. states and 2 Canadian provinces, but transmission has not extended to humans.

Following reports of *L. tropica*–related viscerotropic leishmaniasis in veterans of Operation Desert Storm, between August 1990 and December 1992, those serving in that theater of operations were deferred from blood donation for 1 year. The deferral period reflected the development of fever, malaise, abdominal pain, and intermittent diarrhea up to 7 months after return to the United States. *L. tropica* was found in the bone marrow of seven patients and in the lymph nodes in one. When intracellular amastigotes were seen in the peripheral blood of the one patient in whom this was studied following reports of cutaneous and visceral leishmaniasis among troops involved in the Afghanistan and Iraq wars, a similar 1-year deferral following departure from Iraq and Afghanistan was implemented. The military continues to enforce lifetime deferral for any clinical history of *Leishmania* infection.

The possibility of transmission to humans during military deployment and travel and the large number of military personnel returning from Iraq and Afghanistan raise concerns about future transfusion transmission. To date, there are no cases of transfusion-transmitted leishmaniasis in the United States. The widespread use of leukocyte reduction filters may have a beneficial role because these filters reduce both intracellular and extracellular parasite concentrations by 3 to 4 logs.

Toxoplasmosis

Toxoplasmosis is caused by the obligate intracellular protozoan parasite *Toxoplasma gondii*, whose usual host is the domestic cat. The parasite is transmitted by exposure to cat feces, by eating raw or undercooked pork, goat, lamb, beef, or wild game, and congenitally. In NHANES (1999-2004) 24.8% of foreign-born U.S. residents age 12 to 49 years of age, compared with 8.2% of U.S.-born residents, had serologic evidence of infection and perhaps half with antibody harbor parasites in tissue. Transfusion-associated disease has been described in immunocompromised patients receiving granulocyte concentrates from donors with chronic myelocytic leukemia who would not qualify as blood donors currently. One possible transfusion-related case involves a platelet transfusion. Red cells and frozen plasma transmission have not been reported.

Chagas Disease

The protozoan parasite *T. cruzi* causes Chagas disease. The infection is widespread in Latin America; approximately 8 to 10 million people are affected worldwide. Humans become infected when bitten by *T. cruzi*–infected insects of the Reduviidae family (triatomine, assassin, kissing, or chinch bugs). Congenital transmission from mother to fetus, organ transplantation, and blood transfusion are recognized routes as well. Once infection occurs, low-level, intermittently detectable parasitemia usually persists for life. Treatment with benznidazole or nifurtimox can reduce the risk for chronic sequelae. Eighteen mammalian species in the United States can be infected, including armadillos, opossums, and raccoons, and vectors are present in the lower two-thirds of the country, but autochthonous vector transmission is rare. An estimated 300,000 people in the United States and Canada are infected with *T. cruzi*; most are immigrants from Latin America. *T. cruzi* organisms remain viable in whole blood stored at refrigerator temperatures for 18 days, for longer than 8 months in citrated blood samples stored at room temperature, and following freezing and thawing. In South America, approximately 13% to 49% of recipients of parasitemic blood become infected. There has been concern that additional transfusion-associated Chagas disease cases will occur as immigration increases to the United States from Central and South America.

American trypanosomiasis, or Chagas disease, consists of an acute phase that varies from asymptomatic to manifestations that include fever, skin rash, and conjunctivitis with palpebral edema, lymphadenopathy, and hepatosplenomegaly. The acute phase usually resolves in 4 to 8 weeks unless severe myocarditis or meningoencephalitis intervenes. The latter is associated with fatal outcomes. Intracellular *T. cruzi* amastigotes remain in cardiac and skeletal muscle following the acute phase. Following an indeterminate stage of undetermined duration, chronic disease occurs in 20% to 30% of infected patients, manifesting as cardiac disease (initially conduction and left ventricular wall abnormalities), megacolon, or achalasia. Diagnosis is made on clinical and serologic grounds most often. Xenodiagnosis, hemoculture, and nucleic acid amplification tests are also available.

Risk factors for transfusion-transmitted *T. cruzi* infection include birth or residence in endemic regions such as Central America, South America, or Southeastern Mexico; living in dwellings with palm leaf–thatched roofs or mud walls, where vector insects reside; oral intake of contaminated foodstuffs; and receipt of unscreened blood transfusions in Latin America. Among donors who lived in poor housing or received a blood transfusion in endemic areas, 3% to 4% had *T. cruzi* antibodies. One study, conducted in California in the 1990s, found that 1 per 340 blood donors had a risk factor for Chagas disease. A large survey conducted from 1994 to 1998 in Los Angeles and Miami among immigrant blood donors from endemic areas found *T. cruzi* seroprevalence rates of 1 per 7500 and 1 per 9000, respectively. However, none of the 18 recipients in this survey who received blood from a seropositive donor, and who were available for testing, had evidence of infection.

A look-back study involving blood donations in Mexico made before determining the donors were *T. cruzi*–seropositive, found four of nine recipients of subsequently determined seropositive whole blood or platelets to be seropositive.

Since 1987, 30 years before testing started in the United States, seven cases of transfusion-associated Chagas disease were reported in the United States and Canada; symptoms developed 2 to 3 months after transfusion. In six cases, platelets were the implicated component; and the unit in the seventh case was not identified. In each of the six cases, the implicated donor emigrated from a *T. cruzi*–endemic region (Bolivia, Mexico, Paraguay, and Chile) between 16 and 33 years before the implicated donation. *T. cruzi* may separate with platelets, or room-temperature storage may favor parasite survival. In addition, acute Chagas disease has been reported in organ transplant recipients.

The assumed increasing prevalence of *T. cruzi*–infected blood donors with immigration into the United States from Latin America, the reports of transfusion-associated cases, and some autochthonous infections triggered efforts to mitigate the risk for transfusion-transmitted Chagas disease in the United States. Questioning donors about region of birth or extended stay and transfusion in Chagas-endemic areas interdicts 75% of infected donors but would result in deferral of large numbers of noninfected donors. Leukocyte reduction by filtration decreases *T. cruzi* transmission in a mouse model by 50% to 70%. Pathogen-reduction techniques successfully decrease *T. cruzi* viability in plasma (used currently in Europe) and cellular products.

Serologic screening, used for many years in Latin America, was chosen as the preferred strategy for the United States. The first serologic test for screening blood donors, based on a *T. cruzi* whole-parasite lysate, achieved FDA licensure in December 2006, and voluntary screening commenced in early 2007. Approximately 1 per 30,000 donations showed confirmed reactive serologic results, a lower prevalence than estimated. In 2010, the FDA licensed a second assay that uses chimeric recombinant antigens. Seropositive donors are overwhelmingly immigrants from *T. cruzi*–endemic countries with asymptomatic chronic infections, although a small number of seropositive donors may have acquired the infection in the United States via vertical transmission from infected immigrant mothers, or very rarely by autochthonous vectorial transmission.

Look-back studies involving recipients of prior donations from those found positive for *T. cruzi* antibodies on a subsequent donation showed rates of transfusion transmission much lower than predicted. Only two occurred (0.8%), both from the same apheresis platelet donor born in Argentina, among 253 recipients tested. In light of these findings, testing donors is now required only once rather that at each donation.[32] Concern that those tested once might contract *T. cruzi* during travel or within the United States seems unfounded in that no seroconversions have been observed in more than 4 million blood donors during 6 million person-years of follow-up. The unexpectedly low rate of transmission may relate to differences in blood component processing and storage in the United States compared with Latin America, some underrepresentation of platelet donors in the look backs completed to date, or other biases.

TRANSMISSIBLE SPONGIFORM ENCEPHALOPATHIES

The transmissible spongiform encephalopathies (TSEs, prion diseases) are rare, lethal neurodegenerative diseases caused by nucleic acid-free proteins called PrP^{TSE}, as distinguished from the normal cellular protein, PrP^{C}. The existence of additional factors has not been excluded, but current consensus supports the involvement of infectious proteins. PrP^{TSE} is an abnormal conformation of PrP^{C} that induces transformation (recruitment) of additional PrP^{C} to PrP^{TSE}, resulting in deposits of insoluble aggregates in central nervous system tissue followed by progressive dementia and other characteristic neurologic findings. Classic Creutzfeldt-Jakob disease (CJD) is diagnosed at a rate of one case per million population per year worldwide. It occurs as sporadic CJD, vertically transmitted familial diseases caused by germline mutations in the human PRNP gene (e.g., fatal familial insomnia and Gerstmann-Straüssler-Scheinker syndrome), iatrogenically transmitted infection (e.g., from dura mater implantation, contaminated surgical equipment, injection of human pituitary-derived growth hormone, or corneal transplant) and can be spread horizontally (Kuru associated with consumption of human brain during ritual cannibalism is of historical interest).

There are no documented cases of transfusion transmission of sporadic CJD, the familial or iatrogenic forms, and cohort studies of intensively transfused patient groups have failed to establish any epidemiologic association. In an ongoing look-back effort, no cases of CJD have been observed among 461 recipients (of whom 85 were still alive as of December 31, 2008) of blood components from 40 donors subsequently diagnosed with CJD. A case-control study of CJD patients, compared to control patients with CJD ruled out, found a fivefold increased risk for CJD with a history of transfusion more than 10 years before TSE onset, but the authors recognized critical sources of bias in their methods and their findings are unconfirmed. Nevertheless, as a result of the iatrogenic transmissions and long incubation period of the disease (as demonstrated in growth hormone transmissions), concern arose in the mid-1990s that CJD transmission could occur from asymptomatic donors to transfusion or derivative recipients. This theoretical risk resulted in lifetime donor deferral requirements for iatrogenic exposure to or a family history of classical CJD.

Like classical CJD, variant CJD (vCJD) is a fatal, degenerative neurologic disease. It occurs in younger patients than classic CJD and has distinctive clinical, radiographic, histopathologic, and biochemical features. The first reports of vCJD from the United Kingdom were published in 1996. The etiologic agent is the same prion that causes bovine spongiform encephalopathy (BSE or "mad cow disease"). Transmission of the BSE prion to humans occurred by consumption of beef and other bovine products containing infectious neural or reticuloendothelial tissue. In the United Kingdom the vCJD epidemic followed a massive epidemic of BSE in the 1980s and 1990s. The latter was traced to the recycling of material from dead sheep and cattle (offal) into feed for cattle. This practice was banned in 1988, and the vCJD outbreak subsided after a peak of 28 cases in 2000. The number of new vCJD diagnoses in the United Kingdom rose steadily in the first few years after 1995 from 3 in 1995 to 28 in 2000, but decreased since then to 5, 5, 5, 1, 3, 3, and 2 from 2005 to July 2011, by which time 175 (172 deaths, 3 living) definite or probable cases of vCJD had been reported in the United Kingdom. An additional 49 cases have been diagnosed elsewhere, mostly in France and several other European countries. A few cases have been identified outside Europe, including 3 cases in the United States (2 associated with exposure in the United Kingdom and 1 in Saudi Arabia), 2 from Canada, and 1 each from Japan, Taiwan, and Saudi Arabia. Most but not all of the patients with non-European cases had more than 6 months' exposure in the United Kingdom during the BSE epidemic. Although it appears that the vCJD outbreak is waning (and is much smaller than initially feared), concern persists that there could be a second wave of the epidemic due to delayed onset of the disease in infected individuals. This is based in part on observations of abnormal prion protein accumulation in random surgical tissue samples in the United Kingdom, which may represent preclinical vCJD disease. In one retrospective study, 3 of 12,674 appendectomy and tonsillectomy specimens from persons 20 to 29 years of age were positive. Furthermore, a critical polymorphism at codon 129 of the PrP^{C} gene coding for methionine or valine leads to variation in the susceptibility to and incubation period of human TSEs. All of the clinical cases reported to date are methionine homozygotes. Because only 37% of the general British population is homozygous for methionine, and are maximally susceptible to vCJD, a larger population (52%) of heterozygotes and valine homozygotes (11%) may be at risk for asymptomatic infection in a prolonged incubation period.

Four transfusion-transmitted infections with the vCJD prion have been reported in the United Kingdom. Although they may have developed vCJD independent of transfusion, this possibility is regarded highly unlikely based on epidemiologic and statistical considerations. Three of the four cases were diagnosed with clinical vCJD 6.5, 7.8, and 9 years after receiving non–leukocyte reduced red blood cells or a blood component from two different donors who developed clinical symptoms of vCJD 40 and 21 months after donating. These three with symptomatic disease were homozygous for methionine at codon 129. The fourth case was heterozygous (methionine/valine) and had no clinical signs or symptoms of vCJD at death from unrelated causes, but had abnormal prion protein aggregates in lymphoid (but not neural) tissues at autopsy and was considered to have preclinical infection. Five years before death the recipient received non–leukocyte reduced red blood cells from a donor who developed clinical vCJD 18 months after donating. These four cases represent

6% of the 66 U.K. recipients who received blood components from 18 different donors subsequently diagnosed with vCJD (and an estimated 23% of exposed methionine homozygotes). In light of these cases and animal transfusion experiments, TSE transmission and disease from transfusion is no longer regarded as a theoretical event. A single case report epidemiologically links exposure to plasma derivates to transmission to a recipient.

Prion-removal strategies (e.g., affinity filters) remain under evaluation, especially in the United Kingdom, but none is expected to be suitable for consideration for use in the United States in the immediate future. There are no blood donor–screening tests for vCJD, leaving risk mitigation dependent on removal of donors that could have asymptomatic infection. Initially, primarily on the basis of the prominent distribution of vCJD prion in reticuloendothelial tissue compared to classic PrP^C, on subsequent reports of animal and human infection by transfusion, and then on the early observation that nearly all cases of vCJD were associated with potential exposure in the United Kingdom or to U.K. bovine products, the FDA adopted and has modified donor-deferral policies sequentially since 1999.[33] The first called for indefinite deferral of donors who had spent more than 6 months in the United Kingdom from 1980 to 1996, before control of the food chain and of recipients of bovine insulin from the U.K. Models predicted that this would remove approximately 90% of the risk at a "cost" of deferring approximately 5% of otherwise eligible donors. These were subsequently expanded to include U.S. military personnel and their dependents who spent certain durations on bases in the European Union where U.K. beef was imported during the BSE epidemic and recipients of transfusions in the United Kingdom and France during the peak risk periods of their BSE epidemics. Experience at U.S. blood centers has largely confirmed the donor loss predictions of the FDA models. Exclusions for potential exposures in Saudi Arabia are under consideration.

Chronic wasting disease (CWD) of deer and elk is prevalent at rates as high as 15% in cervid populations in multiple areas of the United States and Canada. Concern has been expressed that, given the popularity of hunting, there may be risk for exposure to and infection with the CWD prion during handling or consumption of infected animals. Apparent clusters of classic CJD in hunters have been alleged, but on full evaluation have not been shown to have a relationship to the CWD agent. There is currently no plan to intervene for this theoretical risk in hunters who donate blood beyond hygienic measures when handling cervids or their tissues.

FUTURE DIRECTIONS

The residual risk for transmitting HIV, hepatitis B, and hepatitis C approaches 1 per 2 million units transfused, an extremely low rate. In contrast, platelet septic events occur at a frequency of 1 per 15,000 to 100,000 units. Transmission of known, emerging infectious agents such as dengue, *B. microti,* and those currently unrecognized remain problematic. Continued safety of the blood supply requires constant vigilance, early detection, reporting of untoward events, and excellent communication and cooperation between those providing blood components and those prescribing them.

REFERENCES

1. Busch MP: Cooley Award Lecture. Transfusion-transmitted viral infections: Building bridges to transfusion medicine to reduce risks and understand epidemiology and pathogenesis. *Transfusion* 46:1624, 2006.
2. Stramer SL, Wend U, Candotti D, et al: Nucleic acid testing to detect HBV infection in blood donors. *N Engl J Med* 364:236, 2011.
3. Zou S, Stramer SL, Notari EP, et al: Current incidence and residual risk of hepatitis B infection among blood donors in the United States. *Transfusion* 49:1609, 2009.
4. Xiang J, Wunschmann S, Diekema DJ, et al: Effect of coinfection with GB virus C on survival among patients with HIV infection. *N Engl J Med* 345:704, 2001.
5. Brennan CA, Yamaguchi J, Devare SG, et al: Expanded evaluation of blood donors in the United States for human immunodeficiency virus type 1 non-B subtypes and antiretroviral drug-resistant strains: 2005 through 2007. *Transfusion* 50:2707, 2010.
6. Centers for Disease Control and Prevention: HIV transmission through transfusion—Missouri and Colorado, 2008. *MMWR Morb Mortal Wkly Rep* 59:1335, 2010.
7. Seed CR, Kiely P, Law M, et al: No evidence of a significantly increased risk of transfusion-transmitted human immunodeficiency virus infection in Australia subsequent to implementing a 12-month deferral for men who have had sex with men". *Transfusion* 50:2722, 2010.
8. Kleinman Steven, Cameron C, Custer B, et al: Modeling the risk of an emerging pathogen entering the Canadian blood supply. *Transfusion* 50:2592, 2010.
9. Bennett JL, Blajchman MA, Delage G, et al: Proceedings of a Consensus Conference: Risk-Based Decision Making for Blood Safety. *Transfus Med Rev* 25:267, 2011.
10. Jackson BR, Busch MP, Stramer SL, et al: The cost-effectiveness of NAT for HIV, HCV, and HBV in whole-blood donations. *Transfusion* 43:721, 2003.
11. Murphy EL, Glynn SA, Fridey J, et al: Increased prevalence of infectious diseases and other adverse outcomes in human T lymphotropic virus types I- and II-infected blood donors. Retrovirus Epidemiology Donor Study (REDS) Study Group. *J Infect Dis* 176:1468, 1997.
12. Vamvakas EC: Is white blood cell reduction equivalent to antibody screening in preventing transmission of cytomegalovirus by transfusion? A review of the literature and meta-analysis. *Transfus Med Rev* 19:181, 2005.
13. Kleinman Steven H, Glynn SA, Lee TH, et al: A linked donor-recipient study to evaluate parvovirus B19 transmission by blood component transfusion. *Blood* 114:3677, 2009.
14. Aubuchon JP, Prowse CV, editors: *Pathogen inactivation: The penultimate paradigm shift*, Bethesda Md, 2010, AABB Press.
15. Seghatchian J, Hervig T, Putter JS: Effect of pathogen inactivation on the storage lesion in red cells and platelet concentrates. *Transfus Apher Sci* 45:75, 2011.
16. Biggerstaff BJ, Petersen LR: Estimated risk of West Nile virus transmission through blood transfusion during an epidemic in Queens, New York City. *Transfusion* 42:1019, 2002.
17. Zou S, Foster GA, Dodd RY, et al: West Nile fever characteristics among viremic persons identified through blood donor screening. *J Infect Dis* 202:1354, 2010.
18. Tomashek KM, Margolis HS: Dengue: A potential transfusion-transmitted disease. *Transfusion* 51:1654, 2011.
19. Stramer SL, Hollinger FB, Katz LM, et al: Emerging infectious disease agents and their potential threat to transfusion safety. *Transfusion* 49:1S, 2009.
20. Lombardi VC, Ruscetti FW, Das Gupta J, et al: Detection of an infectious retrovirus, XMRV, in blood cells of patients with chronic fatigue syndrome. *Science* 326:585, 2009.
21. Paprotka T, Delviks-Frankenberry KA, Cingöz O, et al: Recombinant origin of the retrovirus XMRV. *Science* 333:97, 2011.

22a. Klein HG, Dodd RY, Hollinger FB, et al: AABB Interorganizational Task Force on XMRV. Xenotropic murine leukemia virus-related virus (XMRV) and blood transfusion: Report of the AABB interorganizational XMRV task force. *Transfusion* 51:654, 2011.

22b. Likos AM, Kelvin DJ, Cameron CM, et al; National Heart, Lung, Blood Institute Retrovirus Epidemiology Donor Study-II (REDS-II): Influenza viremia and the potential for blood-borne transmission. *Transfusion* 47:1080, 2007.

22c. Stramer SL, Collins C, Nugent T, et al: Sensitive detection assays for influenza RNA do not reveal viremia in US blood donors. *J Inf Dis* 205(6):886, 2012.

23. Food and Drug Administration: Fatalities reported to FDA following blood collection and transfusion. Annual summary for fiscal year 2010. pp. 1–12. Available at http://www.fda.gov/BiologicsBloodVaccines/SafetyAvailability/ReportaProblem/TransfusionDonationFatalities/ucm254802.htm. Accessed 29 Aug. 2011.
24. Dumont Larry, Kleinman S, Murphy JR, et al: Screening of single-donor apheresis platelets for bacterial contamination: The PASSPORT study results. *Transfusion* 50:589, 2010.

25. Jacobs Michael, Smith D, Heaton WA, et al: Detection of bacterial contamination in prestorage culture negative apheresis platelets on day of issue with the PGD test. *Transfusion* 51:2573, 2011.
26. Zou S, Notari EP, Fang CT, et al: Current value of serologic test for syphilis as a surrogate marker for blood borne viral infections among blood donors in the United States. *Transfusion* 49:655, 2009.
27. Mali S, Tan DR, Arquin PM: Malaria surveillance—United States, 2009. *MMWR Surveill Summ* Vol 60:1, Apr 2011. No 3.
28. Spencer Bryan, Kleinman S, Custer B, et al: Deconstructing the Risk for Malaria in United States Donors Deferred for Travel to Mexico. *Transfusion* 51:2398, 2011.
29. Leiby David: Transfusion-Transmitted *Babesia* spp.: Bull's-Eye on *Babesia microti*. *Clin Microbiol Rev* Vol 24:14, Jan 2011. No.1.
30. Herwaldt BL, Linden JV, Bosserman E, et al: Transfusion-associated babesiosis in the United States: A description of cases. *Ann Intern Med* 155:509, 2011.
31. Cardo Lisa J: Leishmania: Risk to the blood supply. *Transfusion* Vol 46:1641, Sep 2006.
32. Food and Drug Administration: Guidance for industry: Use of serological tests to reduce the risk of transmission of *Trypanosoma cruzi* infection in whole blood and blood components intended for transfusion. 12/2010. Available at http://www.fda.gov/BiologicsBloodVaccines/GuidanceComplianceRegulatoryInformation/Guidances/Blood/ucm235855.htm. Accessed 23 August 2011.
33. Food and Drug Administration: Revised preventive measures to reduce the possible risk of transmission of Creutzfeldt-Jakob disease (CJD) and variant Creutzfeldt-Jakob disease (vCJD) by blood and blood products. May 2010. Available at http://www.fda.gov/BiologicsBloodVaccines/GuidanceComplianceRegulatoryInformation/Guidances/Blood/default.htm. Accessed 16 Aug 2011.

CHAPTER 122

TRANSFUSION MEDICINE IN HEMATOPOIETIC STEM CELL AND SOLID ORGAN TRANSPLANTATION

Richard M. Kaufman

HEMATOPOIETIC STEM CELL TRANSPLANTATION

The array of hematopoietic stem cell transplantation (HSCT) approaches used to treat patients with malignant or nonmalignant diseases has continued to grow in complexity. In concert, the scope of transfusion medicine has expanded to support the development of novel hematopoietic stem cell therapies. Hematopoietic stem cells are currently obtained from three sources: bone marrow (BM), mobilized peripheral blood stem cells (PBSCs), and umbilical cord blood (UCB). After harvesting, and before infusion into the patient, stem cell products undergo a variety of manipulations in the laboratory, ranging from simple processing (e.g., red blood cell [RBC] depletion, freezing) to sophisticated graft engineering (e.g., T-cell depletion, retroviral transduction). Like conventional blood components, hematopoietic stem cell products are prepared in rigorously controlled environments using good manufacturing practices.

The focus of this section is on the unique issues involved with providing optimal transfusion support to the HSCT patient. After myeloablative conditioning and stem cell transplantation, there is a 1- to 4-week period of pancytopenia when patients require multiple RBC and platelet transfusions. In general, the criteria for transfusion after HSCT mirror those of other clinical settings, but the magnitude of support required may be great. Frequent platelet transfusions are given to prevent bleeding, and as a result, alloimmunization and platelet refractoriness are important concerns. Switching of ABO blood groups occurs commonly in the allogeneic HSCT patient population, posing unique problems to the blood bank and transfusion service. Because HSCT patients are typically highly immunocompromised, strategies are needed to prevent transfusion-transmitted cytomegalovirus (CMV) disease and transfusion-associated graft-versus-host disease (TA-GVHD).

ENGRAFTMENT AND BLOOD COMPONENT SUPPORT AFTER HEMATOPOIETIC STEM CELL TRANSPLANTATION

The level of transfusion support required by a particular patient after HSCT is dictated largely by the kinetics of engraftment and subsequent hematopoietic reconstitution. A key parameter affecting the engraftment rate is the source of stem cells used (Fig. 122-1). In the 1990s, several randomized trials demonstrated the superiority of PBSC- over BM-derived stem cells in terms of faster platelet and neutrophil recovery for patients undergoing autologous HSCT.[1] More rapid recovery using PBSCs rather than BM was later documented in the allogeneic HSCT setting as well. On average, neutrophil recovery (neutrophil count $>0.5 \times 10^9$/L) occurs 2 to 6 days earlier when PBSCs versus BM are used as the source of stem cells. Similarly, platelet recovery (platelet count $>20 \times 10^9$/L) occurs 5 to 8 days earlier after PBSC transplantation than after bone marrow transplantation (BMT).[2] One reason for the faster engraftment of PBSC products is that the cellular composition of PBSCs and BM is very different. PBSC products contain approximately threefold more $CD34^+$ cells and 10-fold more mature T cells than BM products.

There is a strong relationship between the $CD34^+$ cell dose administered and the speed of hematopoietic recovery. Faster engraftment rates have translated into decreased blood component usage. For example, Haas et al[3] reported that autologous PBSC transplant patients given more than 2.5×10^6 $CD34^+$ cells/kg received significantly fewer platelet transfusions than patients receiving less than 2.5×10^6 $CD34^+$ cells/kg (median of 4 versus 13 platelet units). In addition to the higher numbers of $CD34^+$ cells in PBSC products, there are multiple qualitative factors that differ between PBSC- and BM-derived stem cells, including cell surface molecule expression, metabolic activity, clonogenicity, and cell cycle status.[4] What impact these factors have on engraftment remains incompletely understood.

Several clinical factors may affect the rate of hematopoietic recovery and transfusion requirements after HSCT. Accelerated platelet recovery has been associated with a higher pretransplantation platelet count and receiving a graft from a human leukocyte antigen (HLA)–identical sibling donor. Factors associated with delayed platelet recovery include prior radiation therapy, the presence of fever, hepatic venoocclusive disease, GVHD, and the use of posttransplantation granulocyte colony-stimulating factor or granulocyte-macrophage colony-stimulating factor. The use of recombinant human erythropoietin (rHuEPO) has been shown to accelerate RBC recovery and decrease RBC transfusion requirements among allogeneic HSCT patients. The particular conditioning regimen that is used also affects hematopoietic recovery. In particular, nonmyeloablative transplantation protocols predictably result in decreased transfusion requirements.[5]

Although PBSC products are currently the most commonly transplanted source of stem cells, the use of UCB transplants for both pediatric and adult recipients has continued to grow rapidly. One reason is that only about 30% of patients requiring HSCT have an HLA-matched related donor. Precise HLA matching has been demonstrated to be significantly less important for UCB products than for BM or PBSCs. Also, UCB transplants are associated with a lower rate of GVHD. A primary disadvantage of UCB is the lower $CD34^+$ cell content of these products. The currently accepted minimum cell dose of a UCB unit is 2.0×10^7 nucleated cells/kg at the time of freezing, about one order of magnitude lower than the threshold for PBSC or BM transplant.[6] The lower cell content of UCB has been linked to significantly slower hematopoietic recovery. For this reason, UCB transplants using two (or sometimes more) grafts simultaneously are often performed, particularly in adult patients. Time to recovery aside, outcomes of transplants with UCB have compared favorably with BM. Rocha et al[6] reported that mortality was similar among adults with acute leukemia who received either HLA-mismatched UCB (n = 98) or HLA-matched BM (n = 584). Acute GVHD was lower among the UCB recipients. Laughlin et al[7] likewise found that among adult patients with leukemia, recipients of HLA-mismatched BM and HLA-mismatched UCB grafts had similar rates of treatment-related mortality, treatment failure, and overall mortality.

The growth in UCB banking has created the (potential) advantage of rapidly available grafts to patients requiring transplantation. The University of Minnesota, for example, has reported that the search for a UCB unit typically takes approximately 1 day, compared with 3 to 4 months for a PBSC or BMT donor. It is possible that the ability to provide UCB grafts quickly will translate into better patient outcomes, but this has not been proven to date. In recent years, considerable efforts have been made to standardize UCB-banking

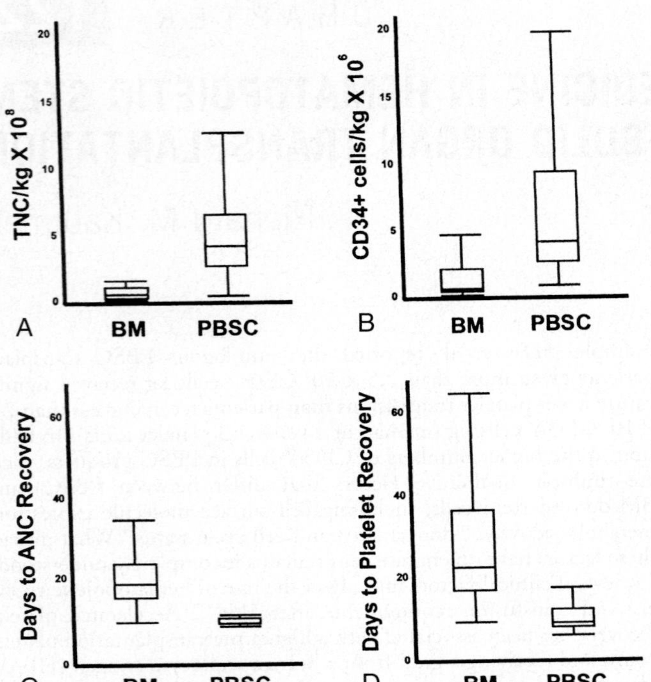

Figure 122-1 COMPARISON OF PERIPHERAL BLOOD STEM CELL (PBSC) PRODUCTS WITH BONE MARROW (BM). BM (n = 187) and PBSCs (n = 104) were collected from autologous donors at the Dana-Farber Cancer Institute and Brigham and Women's Hospital from 2000 through 2002. **A,** The total nucleated cell (TNC) content (TNC/kg recipient weight) was significantly higher in PBSC products (median, 4.2×10^8 nucleated cells/kg) than in BM products (0.5×10^8 nucleated cells/kg). **B,** The $CD34^+$ cell content of PBSC products was also significantly higher compared with BM (median, 4.3×10^6 $CD34^+$ cells/kg versus 0.5×10^6 $CD34^+$ cells/kg). **C,** Reconstitution of neutrophils (absolute neutrophil count [ANC] >0.5×10^9/L) occurred more rapidly in recipients of PBSCs (median, 10 days) compared with BM (median, 18 days). **D,** Similarly, platelet recovery (platelet count >20×10^9/L) was more rapid in PBSC recipients (median, 11 days versus 27 days for BM recipients). *(Courtesy G. Kao, Dana-Farber Cancer Institute, Boston, Mass.)*

practices. The Food and Drug Administration (FDA) has driven the concept that all human cellular or tissue-derived therapies, regardless of source, need to fit into an established regulatory framework and must meet the same essential requirements for donor screening and good tissue practices. Two U.S. accrediting agencies, the American Association of Blood Banks (AABB) and the Foundation for the Accreditation of Cellular Therapy (FACT), have developed standards for collecting, testing, processing, and storing UCB samples, with the intent of ensuring the quality of UCB products provided.

ABO-INCOMPATIBLE HEMATOPOIETIC STEM CELL TRANSPLANTATION

In approximately 20% of allogeneic HSCT, ABO incompatibility exists between the donor and recipient.[8] ABO incompatibility is classified as major (the recipient has ABO antibody directed against donor RBCs), minor (the donor has ABO antibody directed against recipient RBCs), or both (major-minor). In most cases, the clinical impact of donor-recipient ABO incompatibility on HSCT is minimal. ABO incompatibility does not appear to affect overall patient survival, graft rejection, or GVHD. Nevertheless, clinically significant hemolytic complications resulting from ABO incompatibility occasionally do occur.

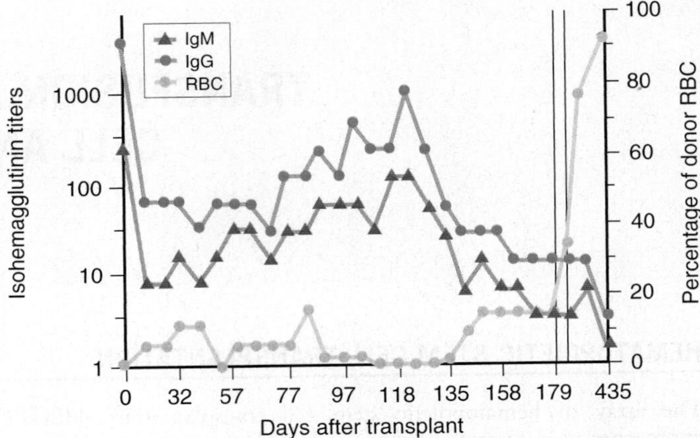

Figure 122-2 DELAYED RED BLOOD CELL (RBC) RECONSTITUTION IN THE RECIPIENT OF A MAJOR ABO-INCOMPATIBLE STEM CELL TRANSPLANT. The appearance of mature RBCs corresponded to declining antidonor isohemagglutinin titers. This patient remained RBC transfusion dependent for 12 months after transplantation. *Ig,* Immunoglobulin. *(From Maciej Zaucha J, Mielcarek M, Takatu A, et al: Engraftment of early erythroid progenitors is not delayed after non-myeloablative major ABO-incompatible hematopoietic stem cell transplantation.* Br J Haematol *119:740, 2002.)*

In major ABO-incompatible HSCT (e.g., group A donor → group O recipient), two types of hemolytic complications may be seen. Immediately on infusion, mature donor RBCs contained within the stem cell product may be destroyed by preformed ABO antibody in the recipient. The usual practice is to reduce the volume of RBCs contaminating major ABO-incompatible stem cell products to less than 10 mL. This manipulation effectively eliminates most immediate hemolytic reactions.

The second potential hemolytic complication of major ABO-incompatible HSCT is that recovery of the recipient's RBC counts may be delayed, in some cases dramatically (Fig. 122-2). This condition is a form of pure red cell aplasia (PRCA).[9] PRCA is characterized by peripheral blood reticulocytopenia and the absence of histologically detectable erythroid precursors in the bone marrow of the recipient. Peripheral-blood ABO antibody titers are characteristically elevated. Red cell transfusion dependence may last for several months after the recovery of platelets and granulocytes. Although red cell *reconstitution* is delayed in these cases, red cell *engraftment* is not. Using in vitro colony assays, the presence of early erythroid progenitors can be demonstrated in the bone marrow at the same time after transplantation as myeloid progenitors.[10] Early erythroid progenitors do not express ABO antigens and appear to survive normally in the bone marrow. On undergoing differentiation, the erythroid precursors begin expressing ABO antigens and are targeted by host ABO antibodies. It has been proposed that PRCA associated with major ABO-mismatched HSCT may be more likely to occur in the setting of nonmyeloablative SCT, because host hematopoiesis may be relatively preserved.[11] A higher PRCA rate in nonmyeloablative SCT has not been observed consistently, however, perhaps because of differences in treatment regimens. The optimal therapy for PRCA after major ABO-incompatible HSCT has not been defined. Various treatment modalities used with variable success have included plasma exchange, corticosteroids, rHuEPO, antithymocyte globulin, donor lymphocyte infusion, rituximab, and discontinuation of cyclosporine.

Minor ABO-incompatible HSCT (e.g., group O donor → group A recipient) has been associated with immediate hemolysis from passively transfused donor ABO antibody and with delayed hemolysis caused by ABO antibodies produced by mature donor lymphocytes contained in the graft. Minor ABO incompatibility does not affect overall rates of graft rejection, GVHD, or patient survival. Depletion of donor plasma in the graft generally eliminates the problem of immediate hemolysis caused by passively transfused ABO antibody. The more serious potential problem is the passenger lymphocyte syndrome, in which mature donor lymphocytes engraft in the host and produce anti-A or anti-B antibodies that bind to and cause the destruction of circulating host RBCs (Fig. 122-3). This complication typically occurs 1 to 3 weeks after transplantation and is heralded by a positive direct antiglobulin test and a fall in hematocrit level. Rarely, hemolysis may be massive. Standard practice is to transfuse group O or donor group RBCs to dilute the recipient red cells and to monitor patients closely for clinical and laboratory evidence of hemolysis. Exchange transfusion has been performed in this setting but is usually unnecessary.

Less is known about ABO incompatibility with respect to UCB transplantation versus PBSC transplantation or BMT. Recent case series, however, suggest that PRCA and other isoagglutinin-mediated potential adverse consequences of ABO-incompatible stem cell transplantation are far less likely to occur with UCB than with the other stem cell sources. Tomonari et al,[12] for example, reported 0 cases of PRCA among 21 major and 18 major-minor ABO-mismatched UCB recipients. Zero of 29 recipients of minor ABO-incompatible UCB transplants developed immune hemolysis in their series. Similarly, Snell et al[13] reported that 0 of 14 minor ABO-incompatible UCB recipients developed immune hemolysis, compared with 14 of 25 contemporaneous patients who developed immune hemolysis after receiving a minor ABO-incompatible PBSC transplant.

The blood bank places specific RBC and plasma restrictions on patients undergoing ABO-incompatible HSCT (Table 122-1). RBCs are selected to be compatible with donor and recipient plasma, and plasma products are selected to be compatible with donor and recipient RBCs. These practices are begun on day 0 of HSCT or earlier if feasible. ABO antigens are widely expressed on endothelial tissues; HSCT recipients therefore may be considered ABO chimeras even after full RBC recovery.

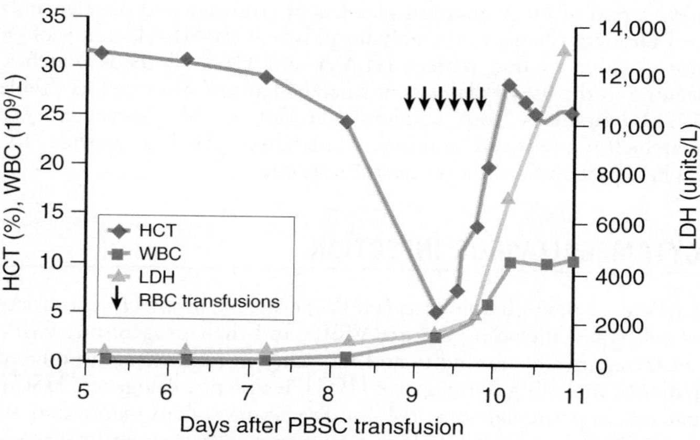

Figure 122-3 SEVERE HEMOLYSIS IN THE RECIPIENT OF A MINOR ABO-INCOMPATIBLE STEM CELL TRANSPLANT. Serologic testing revealed that donor-type anti-A isoagglutinins caused the hemolysis. *HCT,* Hematocrit; *LDH,* lactate dehydrogenase; *RBC,* red blood cell; *WBC,* white blood cell. *(From Bolan CD, Childs RW, Procter JL, et al: Massive immune haemolysis after allogeneic peripheral blood stem cell transplantation with minor ABO incompatibility.* Br J Haematol *112:787, 2001.)*

Table 122-1 Examples of Transfusion Restrictions After ABO-Incompatible Hematopoietic Stem Cell Transplantation

ABO Type			Transfusion Restriction	
Donor	***Recipient***	***Type of Mismatch***	***Red Blood Cell***	***Plasma***
A	A	None	A or O	A or AB
A	O	Major	O	A or AB
O	B	Minor	O	B or AB
A	B	Major-minor	O	AB

PROPHYLACTIC PLATELET TRANSFUSIONS

Most platelet transfusions administered to cancer patients are given prophylactically rather than to control active bleeding. In the past, a platelet count of 20,000/mm^3 was generally used as a transfusion "trigger." Later studies have supported the concept that prophylactic platelet transfusions can safely be provided using even lower platelet thresholds, with associated inventory and cost savings. In an observational study of acute leukemia patients, Gmur et al[14] demonstrated that the platelet transfusion threshold could be set safely at 5000/mm^3 for patients without fever or bleeding, and at 10,000/mm^3 for patients with such signs. Platelet transfusion triggers of 10,000/mm^3 versus 20,000/mm^3 were compared directly in two randomized, prospective studies of patients with acute leukemia.[15,16] Both of these studies and a third nonrandomized, prospective study[17] demonstrated no increased risk for bleeding when a trigger of 10,000/mm^3 was used. All of these trials included provisions for transfusing thrombocytopenic patients at higher platelet counts if associated risk factors for bleeding (e.g., fever) were present. Relatively few studies have directly examined prophylactic platelet transfusion specifically in the setting of HSCT. Nevertheless, the 10,000/mm^3 trigger has been widely applied to the HSCT patient population, and it appears to be safe for patients lacking associated clinical factors (e.g., infection, GVHD). Frequently these clinical factors are more important determinants of bleeding risk than the platelet count alone.

The widespread use of a 10,000/mm^3 transfusion trigger is believed to have helped conserve the overall platelet supply. A potential complementary approach is one of optimizing the dose of prophylactic platelets transfused. A randomized controlled trial designed to empirically determine the optimal prophylactic platelet dose was reported by the Transfusion Medicine/Hemostasis Clinical Trials Network.[18] In this study, termed *PLADO* (PLAtelet DOsing), thrombocytopenic patients were randomized to receive either medium-dose (standard) (2.2×10^{11} platelets/m^2), low-dose (1.1×10^{11} platelets/m^2), or high-dose (4.4×10^{11} platelets/m^2) prophylactic platelets. The primary end point, World Health Organization grade 2 or higher bleeding, was observed in 71%, 69%, and 70% of the patients in the low-, medium-, and high-dose groups, respectively (i.e., there were no significant differences between the groups). Although low-dose platelets provided effective prophylaxis, patients in the low-dose group did require more platelet transfusions (median of five versus three for the medium-dose and high-dose group patients, $P<0.001$). An alternative strategy, using therapeutic rather than prophylactic platelet transfusions, is currently under investigation.

ALLOIMMUNIZATION AND PLATELET REFRACTORINESS

Because HSCT patients typically receive large numbers of transfusions with cellular blood products, they are at risk for becoming alloimmunized to HLA antigens. Although graft failure associated with histocompatibility differences between donor and recipient is usually attributed to rejection by host T lymphocytes, host antibodies may also mediate graft failure by complement-mediated cytotoxicity or by antibody-dependent cell-mediated cytotoxicity. To prevent graft failure and platelet refractoriness, it is important to prevent HLA alloimmunization in patients who are possible candidates for HSCT. In particular, blood transfusions from the potential stem cell donor should be avoided because of the risk for sensitizing the patient to HLA and non-HLA antigens.

Platelet refractoriness may be defined as the failure to achieve an adequate platelet increment after two or more platelet transfusions (Table 122-2). A number of nonimmune factors have been linked to

Table 122-2 Causes of Platelet Refractoriness

Patient Factor	Clinical Effects	Blood Bank
Alloimmunization	Fever	ABO match
Bone marrow transplantation	Sepsis	Platelet storage time
Gender	Splenomegaly	Platelet cross-match
Circulating IVIG	Clinical bleeding	HLA match
Transfusion number	RBC use DIC Neutropenia	

Modified from Friedberg RC, Donnelly SF, Boyd JC, et al: Clinical and blood bank factors in the management of platelet refractoriness and alloimmunization, *Blood* 81:3428, 1993.
DIC, Disseminated intravascular coagulation; *HLA,* human leukocyte antigen; *IVIG,* intravenous immunoglobulin G; *RBC,* red blood cell.

Table 122-3 Degree of HLA Matching for HLA-Matched Platelets

Match Grade	Description	Examples of a Donor Phenotype for Recipient Who Is A1,3;B8,27
A	Four-antigen match	A1,3;B8,27
B1U	No mismatch present	A1,-;B8,27
B1X	One cross-reactive group	A1,3;B8,7
B2UX	One antigen blank and one cross-reactive	A1,-;B8,7
C	One mismatched antigen	A1,3;B8,35
D	Two or more antigens mismatched	A1,32;B8,35

Data from Vengelen-Tyler V: *Technical manual,* ed 12, Bethesda, Md, 1996, American Association of Blood Banks Press.
HLA, Human leukocyte antigen.

platelet refractoriness, including fever, sepsis, disseminated intravascular coagulation, drugs (e.g., amphotericin), bleeding, splenomegaly, hepatic venoocclusive disease, and GVHD. In a subset of cases, platelet refractoriness is caused by alloimmunization. Platelets express HLA class I antigens, relatively low levels of ABO antigens, and several platelet-specific antigens. All of these molecules are potential targets of an immune response. Antibodies directed against HLA molecules are responsible for most cases of immune-mediated platelet refractoriness. Notably, less than half of all platelet-refractory patients have demonstrable antiplatelet or anti-HLA antibodies. Platelet counts obtained at 10 minutes to 1 hour posttransfusion that repeatedly fail to demonstrate an adequate corrected count increment usually indicate an immune mechanism of platelet destruction.[19] If the 10-minute to 1-hour posttransfusion platelet count shows a reasonable increment, but the platelet count falls back to baseline by 18 to 24 hours, a nonimmune mechanism of refractoriness may be presumed. Demonstrating the presence of HLA antibodies in the recipient provides a second important line of evidence for immune refractoriness.

Although platelets express class I HLA antigens, platelets themselves are poor immunogens. Preclinical studies in rodent models suggested that white blood cells (WBCs) contaminating platelet products are the cells primarily responsible for stimulating an anti-HLA immune response in platelet transfusion recipients. It was hypothesized that removing WBCs from platelet products could prevent alloimmunization and platelet refractoriness. This was subsequently shown to be true in human studies. The definitive study was the multicenter prospective Trial to Reduce Alloimmunization to Platelets (TRAP study),[20] which compared alloimmunization rates in 530 newly diagnosed acute myeloid leukemia (AML) patients randomized to receive unmodified, pooled platelet concentrates (control); filtered, pooled platelet concentrates (F-PC); filtered single-donor apheresis platelets (F-AP); or ultraviolet B (UVB)–irradiated pooled platelet concentrates (UVB-PC). Anti-HLA antibodies were detected in 45% of controls, compared with 17% to 21% of patients receiving modified platelets. Thirteen percent of control group patients became platelet refractory, compared with only 3% in the F-PC group, 4% in the F-AP group, and 5% in the UVB-PC group.

Current filtration and apheresis technology can yield blood products with less than 10^6 residual leukocytes. It is standard practice to provide patients requiring long-term blood component support with leukoreduced products. Leukoreduction provides the additional benefit of reducing CMV risk in susceptible patients and of reducing the rates of febrile nonhemolytic transfusion reactions. The benefits in the HSCT patient population are clear; whether prestorage leukoreduced products need to be provided to all patients is controversial. Blood suppliers in many European countries and Canada have moved to providing exclusively prestorage leukoreduced products. Suppliers in the United States have made efforts to do the same, although universal prestorage leukoreduction is currently not mandated by the regulatory agencies (e.g., FDA, AABB) overseeing blood transfusion practices.

Once platelet refractoriness has been demonstrated, several strategies may help in obtaining therapeutic platelet increments in vivo. If refractoriness is nonimmune in nature (e.g., sepsis), the underlying cause must be treated. A trial of ABO-matched, fresh (1 to 2 days old) platelets may be helpful. In cases of immune-mediated refractoriness, a trial of HLA-matched platelets or crossmatched platelets may be indicated. Owing to the polymorphism of the HLA loci, it is often not possible to find perfect HLA-A and HLA -B locus matches, leading to the use of platelets mismatched at one or more loci (Table 122-3). Grade A (four antigens matched) or BU (three antigens matched/one antigen unknown) matched platelets provide the highest probability of a successful response.

CYTOMEGALOVIRUS INFECTION

CMV is a human herpesvirus (HHV-5) capable of infecting a variety of cell types, including mature WBCs and their progenitors. CMV causes significant morbidity and mortality in immunocompromised patients, including seronegative HSCT recipients. Allogeneic HSCT patients in particular are at risk for developing serious manifestations of CMV disease, which include pneumonitis, gastroenteritis, hepatitis, encephalitis, and retinitis. CMV disease is considerably less common in the autologous transplant setting. When a patient who is CMV seropositive at baseline undergoes HSCT, CMV disease occurs primarily as a result of reactivation of latent virus. In those cases in which the HSCT donor is seropositive and the recipient is seronegative, CMV transmission may occur by means of the stem cell product. When both donor and recipient are seronegative, CMV infection results primarily from the transfusion of infectious blood components.[21]

Serologic screening of blood products is currently the most effective means of reducing the risk for transfusion-transmitted CMV. The infrequent CMV infections still seen in part represent limitations of the serologic testing methodologies, such as donations made in the preseroconversion window period. Because the seroprevalence of CMV in various communities ranges from 40% to 80%, it is logistically difficult for blood banks to maintain an inventory of CMV-seronegative components. As an alternative to serologic screening, leukoreduction of blood components using filtration or other means has been used to render blood products "CMV safe." The AABB defines leukoreduced products as containing less than 5×10^6 WBCs. In 1995, Bowden et al[22] reported a large prospective study of 502 seronegative marrow transplant patients randomized to receive seronegative or filtered blood products to test the hypothesis that these methods are equivalent in preventing CMV transmission. In the primary statistical analysis, there were no significant differences in the rates of CMV infection (1.3% versus 2.4%) or CMV disease (0% versus 2.4%) between the seronegative and filtered arms, respectively. The primary analysis excluded patients who seroconverted within the first 21 days of HSCT, based on the premise that they most likely would have been infected with CMV before transplantation. Complicating the interpretation of this study is that a secondary analysis of all patients seroconverting between days 0 and 100 showed a significantly worse outcome for patients in the filtered arm: 2.4% of patients in the filtered arm developed CMV disease, compared with 0% in the seronegative arm. Moreover, five of the six patients in the filtered arm who developed CMV disease progressed to fatal pneumonia. There were no deaths in the seronegative arm. Another confounding factor is that bedside filtration was used, which was subsequently shown to suffer from a relatively high rate of failure. Later methods would be expected to provide better and more consistent leukoreduction. Nevertheless, patients receiving leukoreduced blood showed a low level (2.4%) of CMV infection, which is in keeping with the historical figures of 1% to 4% CMV seroconversion with the use of CMV-seronegative components. The investigators conclude by stating: "We believe that the results of this study justify abandoning the maintenance of dual inventories of seronegative and unscreened blood products. The need to perform serologic screening of blood products of CMV could be eliminated altogether."

Given the previous considerations and the data associating filtered RBC units with an increased risk for CMV infection in HSCT patients, it remains unclear whether leukoreduced products are equivalent to seronegative products for the prevention of CMV transmission. It is certain that leukoreduction is extremely effective in decreasing CMV transmission, and the use of leukoreduced CMV-safe products as a substitute for seronegative products has become an accepted practice standard. Overall, although transfusion-transmitted CMV remains a problem in the HSCT population, the rates seen using seronegative or leukoreduced products are far lower than they have been in the past, in large part because of improvements in surveillance and preemptive therapy.

TRANSFUSION-ASSOCIATED GRAFT-VERSUS-HOST DISEASE

TA-GVHD is a devastating complication of blood transfusion primarily affecting immunocompromised patients, including patients undergoing allogeneic or autologous HSCT. The basic mechanism underlying TA-GVHD is that viable, immunocompetent lymphocytes in a blood product engraft and proliferate in the transfusion recipient. The donor lymphocytes attack host tissues, including skin, liver, intestine, and marrow. Signs and symptoms generally appear 7 to 10 days after transfusion. Patients typically present with fever, rash, elevated liver function test results, and nausea, vomiting, and diarrhea. Severe, refractory pancytopenia often develops as well, in most cases leading to the patient's death. The pancytopenia seen differentiates TA-GVHD from classic GVHD after HSCT. Whereas TA-GVHD involves immune rejection of host marrow cells, the marrow is spared in classic GVHD, because donor and recipient BM are selected to be HLA compatible. In most cases, TA-GVHD is fatal within 3 to 4 weeks of transfusion, with most patients dying from complications of marrow failure (i.e., bleeding or infection).

TA-GVHD occasionally occurs in completely immunocompetent patients. In these cases, the mechanism is a "one-way" HLA match, in which the transfusion recipient shares an HLA haplotype with a donor who is homozygous for that haplotype. The transfused lymphocytes are recognized as self by the host immune system and are not rejected. The recipient's cells, however, are seen as foreign by the infused lymphocytes, leading to a GVH response. Shared HLA haplotypes are more likely to occur among first-degree family members and in population groups with limited HLA heterogeneity. In the United States, the risk for transfusion of blood from HLA-homozygous donors to unrelated HLA-heterozygous patients is estimated to be approximately 1 in 7174. In Japan, a more genetically homogeneous population, the risk is much greater (1 in 874).[23] The incidence of TA-GVHD in the United States is clearly much lower than would be expected based on HLA considerations alone. Although underreporting may play a role, it is likely that other factors, including the use of blood that is stored for up to 6 weeks (with decreased leukocyte viability) and the rejection of HLA-homozygous cells based on minor transplantation antigens, also are factors.

There is no effective therapy for TA-GVHD. Fortunately, TA-GVHD is effectively prevented by γ-irradiation of blood products before transfusion. One case of TA-GVHD has been documented after irradiation with 1500 rad, and previous studies suggest that irradiation to 2000 rad is required to reduce mitogen-responsive lymphocytes by 5 to 6 logs compared with nonirradiated controls. Based on these observations, irradiated blood products are required to receive 2500 rad (25 Gy) to the central part of the container, with 1500 rad (15 Gy) as the minimum dose to any other point. Cellular blood products are required to be irradiated for the following situations: recipients identified to be at risk for TA-GVHD, donations made by blood relatives of the recipient, and donors selected to be HLA-matched with the recipient. At this time, it is recommended that only cellular blood products and fresh plasma be irradiated. TA-GVHD has not been reported to be caused by transfusion of plasma or cryoprecipitate that has been frozen and thawed.

SOLID ORGAN TRANSPLANTATION

Transfusion medicine is integral to the success of any solid organ transplantation program. The role of the transfusion medicine specialist and hematologist focuses on blood group compatibility, histocompatibility, transfusion and coagulation support, and adjunctive treatment of humoral rejection. Improved surgical technique and advances in prevention of allograft rejection have led to tremendous growth in solid organ transplantation during the past decade. During 2002, for example, 25,700 solid organ transplantations were performed, including more than 14,000 kidney, 5000 liver, 2000 heart, and 1000 lung transplantations in the United States. The annual report of the United Network for Organ Sharing (UNOS) is available on the Internet (http://optn.transplant.hrsa.gov/data/annualreport.asp). The availability of multiple drugs to prevent organ rejection, including prednisone, cyclosporine (Sandimmune, Neoral, SangCya), tacrolimus (Prograf, FK506), mycophenolate mofetil (CellCept), daclizumab (Zenapax), antithymocyte globulins (Atgam, Thymoglobulin, murine monoclonal antibodies (Orthoclone OKT3) and rapamycin (Rapamune), has extended graft and patient survival. Designed to suppress T-cell activation and cytokine release, these drugs are not cytotoxic agents and lack direct marrow toxicity.

IMMUNOHEMATOLOGY AND SOLID ORGAN TRANSPLANTATION

Renal Transplantation

Pretransplantation Blood Transfusion

Numerous studies documented that pretransplantation blood transfusions promoted prolonged renal allograft survival. As a result, deliberate use of random donor transfusions before cadaver donor renal transplantation and donor-specific transfusions before living-related donor transplants became widespread. A proportion of deliberately transfused patients became HLA alloimmunized, however, and the resulting HLA incompatibility eliminated them as candidates for transplantation. The introduction of cyclosporine in the 1980s led to improved graft survival, and the benefit of pretransplantation transfusions became more difficult to document. As a result, the practice of pretransplant transfusion was abandoned.

ABO Compatibility

ABO compatibility between donor antigens and recipient antibodies is critical for successful renal transplantation. ABH antigens are richly expressed on vascular endothelial cells and renal cells and are excreted in the urine. As a result, ABO-incompatible grafts are at high risk for humoral rejection, and transplantation against ABO barriers has traditionally been contraindicated. Because group O recipients are restricted to group O donors, several experimental protocols have investigated the use of group A_2 donors (who express group A antigens at approximately one-fourth the strength of group A_1 individuals) for group O or group B recipients with low-titer anti-A antibodies.[24] Protocols aimed at allowing renal transplantation across the ABO barrier typically involve pretransplant plasmapheresis or immunoadsorption to remove anti-ABO antibodies, in combination with immunosuppressive agents and careful monitoring of antibody titers. Short-term results with such protocols have in some cases been encouraging. In some cases, high titers of anti-ABO antibody can continue to circulate in the recipient—but without corresponding damage to the antigen-positive transplanted organ. This phenomenon, termed *accommodation,* is not well understood.

HLA Compatibility

The importance of serologic HLA compatibility between donor antigens and recipient antibodies is well established for renal transplantation. Recipients who express warm-reactive antibodies to HLA class I antigens of the donor are at risk for hyperacute rejection characterized by complement activation, intravascular coagulation in the graft, organ ischemia, and necrosis that may occur within minutes of establishing blood flow to the graft. Several techniques are used for HLA crossmatching, and there is controversy regarding which method has the highest predictive value. Standards of the American Society for Histocompatibility and Immunogenetics require that the final crossmatch employ a technique with greater sensitivity than the basic microlymphocytotoxicity test. Such techniques may use longer incubation times, more wash steps, an antiglobulin reagent, B-cell targets, dithiothreitol, or flow cytometry.

Recognition of the importance of HLA-serologic compatibility led to the practice of monthly HLA antibody screening of serum from HLA-sensitized patients awaiting kidney transplants. Antibody specificities that are identified are recorded, and the corresponding antigens avoided when allocating suitable kidney allografts. Some programs also consider compatibility results using archived sera when allocating allografts to recipients who are known to be HLA sensitized. Analysis of recipient HLA specificities has revealed that identification of antibodies directed against common "public antigens" may be more clinically meaningful than antibodies to private HLA antigens. Understanding the exact value of HLA matching for long-term graft acceptance is complicated by the power of immunosuppressive medications, the polymorphism of the HLA system, variable response to different loci within the major histocompatibility complex, and the confounding effects from minor histocompatibility antigens. Studies of the precise value of matching have yielded conflicting results; nevertheless, consideration of the extent of match remains a high priority in organ allocation. Deoxyribonucleic acid (DNA)–based HLA typing continues to advance understanding of the role for HLA matching in renal transplantation.

Routine practice does not require HLA matching of donor and recipient when allocating cadaver kidneys. However, retrospective studies of graft survival have suggested that certain HLA mismatches are associated with a higher incidence of rejection, and large retrospective analyses have provided evidence that greater degrees of HLA matching between the donor and recipient result in longer graft survival. Although not all have agreed that matching improves outcomes, the potential benefits have prompted organ banks to allocate cadaver organs based on the degree of HLA match rather than simply on the results of HLA-compatibility testing. However, matching cadaver organs to distant recipients may carry the disadvantage of prolonged cold-ischemia time. As a result, allocation based on HLA matching combined with limitation of cold-ischemia time is used. Despite the beneficial effects of HLA matching, matched cadaver transplants do not survive as well as matched living-related transplants. The difference may reflect not only injury to the graft during preservation but also the influence of histocompatibility mismatches not recognized by existing HLA-typing techniques.

Liver Transplantation

ABO Compatibility

Ordinarily the donor liver must be ABO compatible with the recipient. Transplantation of ABO-incompatible livers has occurred by error or under urgent circumstances, with limited success. ABO-incompatible liver transplants may occur more frequently in pediatric cases when a compatible donor organ is unavailable and recipient blood group alloantibodies are poorly developed. Data from the UNOS scientific registry found that ABO mismatch was among the strongest independent predictors of adverse outcome after emergency liver transplantation. The immune response to ABO-incompatible grafts is consistent with a pattern of hyperacute rejection. No standards exist regarding transfusion support for ABO-incompatible grafts, but the use of RBCs and fresh frozen plasma (FFP) compatible with both donor and recipient would seem desirable.

Hemolytic Antibodies of Donor Origin

Passenger lymphocytes that accompany a graft may continue to secrete antibodies directed against blood group antigens during the early postoperative period. If the recipient's native red cells or transfused red cells express the matching antigen, a Coombs-positive hemolytic anemia may appear approximately 1 week after transplant.[25] Although the direct antiglobulin test may only be weakly reactive, rather brisk hemolysis typical of complement fixing ABO antibodies can occur. Acute renal failure from intravascular hemolysis in this setting is rare but has been reported.

Approximately 30% of patients transplanted with ABO-compatible but nonidentical livers have been reported to develop postoperative hemolysis mediated by anti-ABO antibodies produced by passenger lymphocytes. Hemolysis has also been reported to result from non-ABO blood group antigens but is most commonly seen when the donor is group O and the recipient is group A_1. Posttransplant hemolysis has been reported after all types of major solid organ transplants, including liver, kidney, heart-lung, spleen, and pancreas. It is most common after liver transplantation, probably by virtue of the greater number of passenger lymphocytes that accompany this large organ. This phenomenon is uncommon after kidney transplantation because of UNOS policies that reserve group O donors for group O recipients. The diagnosis is confirmed by testing an eluate made from the patient's red cells against non–group O target cells—a test not routinely done by the blood bank in the evaluation of a positive direct antiglobulin test. Treatment consists of transfusion with cells compatible with donor and recipient antibodies. Red cell exchange is usually not required, and the condition is generally self-limited because donor lymphocytes are deleted posttransplant.

Alloantibodies to Red Cell Antigens

Patients with clinically significant alloantibodies directed against red cell antigens outside the ABO system pose a unique problem in the setting of the massive transfusion requirements that unpredictably accompany liver transplantation. Depending on the availability of antigen-negative donor units, one strategy is to begin surgery with antigen negative–compatible red cells and then allow transfusion to "wash out" recipient alloantibody before switching to antigen-positive red cells. Approximately one blood volume of antigen-negative units can be reserved for the end of the case to reconstitute the patient with compatible blood for the postoperative period. Antibody washout can be roughly predicted from the presurgical antibody titer as measured by twofold serial dilution. Each blood volume of transfusion reduces the titer by one dilution. For example, an antibody that reacts at 1 : 16 titer requires roughly four blood volumes of transfusion to wash out.

Heart and Lung Transplantation

Cardiac transplantation has become an established therapy for life-threatening cardiac dysfunction, including coronary disease, cardiomyopathy, and congenital cardiac defects. One-year patient survival rates of approximately 85% and 5-year survival rates of 70% have been achieved through the use of effective immunosuppressive regimens, improved recipient selection criteria, the use of heart-assist devices to bridge the waiting time between diagnosis and transplantation, the development of percutaneous endomyocardial biopsy for improved detection of early rejection episodes, and more effective management of postoperative infectious complications. As a result of these improvements, research has shifted from short-term problems such as acute rejection to those factors influencing long-term morbidity-free survival.

Cadaver lung transplants and living-related partial lung transplants have been used in the treatment of a variety of end-stage pulmonary diseases, including cystic fibrosis, emphysema, and α_1-antitrypsin deficiency. A variety of techniques have been developed to prevent rejection of the bronchial anastomosis between donor and recipient. Combined heart-lung transplants are infrequent and are used in the treatment of congenital heart disease with Eisenmenger syndrome or primary pulmonary hypertension.

ABO Compatibility

Because ABO antigens are present on cardiac endothelial tissue, ABO compatibility of donor and recipient is a prerequisite for heart transplantation. ABO is a major determinant of waiting time for heart and lung transplant recipients, with group O recipients consistently requiring longer waiting times. As with other solid organ transplants, ABO-compatible but ABO-nonidentical allografts are used. However, ABO-identical transplants may have a better overall survival than ABO-compatible but ABO-nonidentical grafts. ABO-incompatible heart transplants are absolutely contraindicated in adults because of the risk for hyperacute rejection. However, many successful ABO-incompatible heart transplants have been performed in infants.[26] The infant immune system does not produce T cell–independent antibodies, and early ABO-incompatible heart transplantation produces tolerance in the recipient to donor blood group A or B antigens. The primary mechanism underlying this tolerance appears to be specific elimination of donor-reactive B lymphocytes. Thus a type O infant who receives a type A heart transplant will typically have normal levels of circulating anti-B antibody, but not the usually expected anti-A antibody later in life.

HLA Compatibility

The clinical significance of HLA-antibody testing in cardiac and lung transplantation remains controversial, and surveyed practices show a lack of consensus. Recipients with HLA antibodies to donor antigens do not experience hyperacute rejection, and some studies have reported no adverse outcomes despite incompatible crossmatches at the time of transplantation. However, most studies have found that patients with HLA antibodies, detected by a pretransplantation HLA crossmatch or by a highly panel reactive antibody (PRA), have a higher frequency of rejection episodes in the first months after transplantation. Whether this reflects a direct effect of HLA antibodies or represents a marker of recipient cellular immune responsiveness is not resolved. For example, in a review of 500 cardiac transplants at the Cleveland Clinic, sensitized patients (PRA >10%) had a 1-year graft survival of 76% compared with 89% for nonsensitized patients (P = 0.02).[27] As with renal transplants, some studies have suggested that antibodies to class I HLA antigens or antigens specific to the donor are more important predictors for early rejection episodes. Other studies have not found HLA antibodies to play a critical role in graft rejection.

Xenoantibodies

Naturally occurring xenoantibodies in humans represent a major immunologic barrier to xenotransplants. Similar to ABO antibodies, xenoantibodies are directed against sugar epitopes, including α-galactose found on the cells of all mammals other than humans and Old World monkeys. Antibodies to α-galactose fix complement avidly and produce a potent hyperacute rejection. As a result, strategies to overcome this immune barrier have been directed against the level of antibody and against prevention of complement activation.

TRANSFUSION MEDICINE SUPPORT FOR SOLID ORGAN TRANSPLANTATION

Specialized Blood Components

Cytomegalovirus–Reduced Risk Blood

The implications of CMV infection are different in solid organ transplant recipients compared with bone marrow transplant recipients. After solid organ transplantation, the recipient's immune system is not chimeric, and immunosuppression is less extensive than that required for allogeneic marrow transplantation. As a result, solid organ recipients appear to have better immunity against infections such as CMV, which cause less postoperative morbidity.

Most serious CMV infections result from primary transmission from the donor allograft rather than from blood transfusion. CMV-seronegative recipients of CMV-seropositive allografts are therefore at greatest risk for posttransplantation infection regardless of blood transfusion therapies. When the recipient is CMV seropositive, reactivation infection is more common than transfusion-transmitted disease. Second-strain infection can occur from the allograft but has not been reported as a result of transfusion. This may result from the fact that the allograft is retained whereas blood donor leukocytes are largely apoptotic and cleared shortly after transfusion. When the organ donor or the recipient is CMV positive, the use of CMV-negative blood components should be considered investigational.

However, when both donor and recipient are CMV negative, CMV–reduced risk blood is indicated for lung transplantation. CMV–reduced risk blood is defined as blood from CMV-seronegative donors or leukoreduced blood—either of which can effectively prevent CMV transmission by transfusion. CMV–reduced risk blood is not generally used for adult liver transplant cases because of the large number of products required. CMV–reduced risk blood products are not a strict requirement among most solid organ recipients. For example, Preiksaitis et al[28] reported the incidence of postoperative CMV among CMV-seronegative recipients who were supported with CMV-untested and nonleukoreduced blood components. Although postoperative CMV was very common (131 [85%] of 154) when the organ allograft was CMV seropositive, CMV syndromes were at near background levels (3 [2.4%] of 127) when organ donor and recipient were CMV seronegative despite the use of blood components that were not CMV–reduced risk. Among the different categories of transplantation, the incidence of postoperative transfusion-associated CMV was 0 of 57 (0%, renal), 0 of 29 (0%, heart), 2 of 20 (10%, liver), and 1 of 6 (16.7%, lung).[28] Current interest has centered on the use of PCR for the early detection of CMV infection as a guide to the preemptive use of ganciclovir.

γ-Irradiated Blood Components

Patients undergoing solid organ transplantation are not known to be at increased risk for TA-GVHD. As a result, γ-irradiated cellular blood components are not currently required for solid organ transplant recipients preoperatively or postoperatively. Because γ-irradiation results in dramatic elevation of plasma potassium levels in stored red cells, irradiated and stored red cells may increase the risk for hyperkalemic cardiac arrest at the time of massive transfusion.

Massive Transfusion During Liver Transplantation

Orthotopic liver transplantation (OLT) has become the treatment of choice for life-threatening end-stage hepatic failure. Successful OLT requires a close working relationship between the surgical team, anesthesia services, and blood services because the operation sometimes requires spectacular quantities of blood support. Improved surgical technique, use of venovenous bypass for those cases in which the vena cava is interrupted, argon laser–directed electrocoagulation, and better preservative solutions for storing the donor liver ex vivo have contributed to decreased transfusion requirements during surgery. One-year and 5-year patient survival rates are approximately 85% and 75%, respectively.

Causes of Bleeding

Intraoperative transfusion requirements for OLT cannot be predicted on the basis of preoperative coagulation screening. Rather, the presence of severe portal hypertension, previous right upper quadrant surgery, vascular abnormalities of the portal vein, poor left ventricular function, pulmonary hypertension, poor nutritional state, or comorbid diseases are the most important predictors of massive transfusion and decreased survival. Prior transjugular intrahepatic portosystemic stent-shunt does not appear to adversely affect surgical outcomes during OLT.

OLT requires a difficult right upper quadrant dissection of the recipient hepatic bed, which can be complicated by severe portal hypertension, friable collateral vessels, adhesions from prior procedures, or inflammation from the patient's underlying disease. Removal of the liver requires isolating the blood supply of the organ and clamping and cutting the portal vein, hepatic artery, common bile duct, and the hepatic vein or the inferior vena cava above and below the liver. The period after the recipient hepatectomy and before reestablishing blood flow to the new graft is referred to as the *anhepatic phase of surgery* and is the period of greatest risk.

Patients who require OLT usually have multiple hemostatic abnormalities associated with acute or chronic liver failure. Decreased coagulation factors, splenomegaly with thrombocytopenia, dysfibrinogenemia, and chronic fibrinolysis with elevated fibrin split products may all be present in varying combinations. Some patients develop a profound intraoperative fibrinolysis. Tissue plasminogen activator (tPA)—presumably released from recipient blood vessels or from the vessels of the graft in response to shock, acidosis, pharmacologic pressors, ischemia, or preservation injury—circulates in high concentration. Normally cleared by the liver, tPA released during and immediately after the anhepatic phase of surgery is not cleared from the bloodstream. As a result, tPA activity can reach 10 to 100 times normal levels, and a pathologic systemic lytic state ensues. A sudden decrease in all coagulation factors occurs with particularly marked declines in fibrinogen and factor VIII. Proteolysis of von Willebrand factor may also occur. Less severe cases may not demonstrate systemic lysis but may lyse clot at sites of previous hemostasis. As the liver allograft begins to function, tPA is rapidly cleared and fibrinolysis decreases.

Transfusion Support During Liver Transplantation Surgery

A rapid transfusion device designed to deliver large volumes of blood components in a rapid fashion is essential for OLT. These devices consist of a sterile holding reservoir, high-capacity blood filter, roller pump, in-line blood warmer, and air detection device. Blood is pumped through large-bore catheters placed in the antecubital or central veins. Intraoperative blood recovery devices are a useful adjunct to blood support during OLT, particularly in cases requiring massive transfusion. Blood suctioned from the operative field is anticoagulated with citrate and collected in a sterile holding reservoir. The shed blood is then centrifuged, the supernatant discarded, and the residual packed red cells washed with saline. The saline-suspended packed red cells may then be pumped to the rapid transfusion device or transferred to a plastic blood collection bag for later reinfusion.

OLT demands careful but aggressive component therapy guided by the clinical course and the results of intraoperative coagulation monitoring. Serial intraoperative hematocrit and coagulation monitoring using a limited number of tests with rapid turnaround time provides valuable information for rational blood component management. Some OLT centers monitor coagulation using thromboelastography—a method that measures whole blood coagulation by impedance to an oscillating cylinder. Other programs use traditional measurements such as the prothrombin time, fibrinogen concentration, and platelet count. Either method of monitoring is valuable, provided that testing is done serially, results are reported rapidly, changes are correlated in the operating room with the clinical picture, and abnormalities are interpreted by someone with experience in the coagulopathy of OLT.

Red cell support must be given in consideration of the competing needs of other patients. Probably as a consequence of postoperative immunosuppression, Rh-negative individuals transfused with Rh-positive blood at the time of transplantation are not likely to make anti-D. Nevertheless, Rh-negative women of childbearing age without anti-D are initially supported in many programs with a reasonable number of D-negative units and then switched to D-positive cells should more blood be needed. In some programs, Rh-negative males and females who are not of childbearing potential are treated from the outset with Rh-positive blood. Because many OLT patients are massively transfused, delayed hemolytic transfusion reactions in the postoperative period if directed against high-frequency antigens can result in dramatic hemolysis.

The use of FFP, platelet concentrates, and cryoprecipitate is guided by the clinical course and by the results of intraoperative monitoring. Although care must be given to prevent dilutional coagulopathy, it is not necessary to mix equal ratios of red cells and FFP or platelet concentrates. Reasonable goals of component therapy in the absence of fibrinolysis or other complications include an international normalized ratio (INR) of less than 2 or 2.5, a platelet count higher than 50,000 to 100,000/μL, and a fibrinogen concentration more than 100 mg/dL. Antifibrinolytic agents are indicated during or shortly after the anhepatic phase of surgery in those patients who demonstrate a systemic lytic state. A loading dose and continuous infusion of ε-aminocaproic acid, tranexamic acid, or aprotinin has been used with success. Hourly bolus doses have also been used. Tranexamic acid or aprotinin each reduced operative blood loss during liver transplantation when studied in randomized, prospective, placebo-controlled trials. Because the routine use of antifibrinolytics may result in thrombotic complications in some patients, our program uses antifibrinolytics for those patients who show evidence of fibrinolysis. Recombinant activated factor VII has been used to promote hemostasis during liver transplantation. Randomized controlled trials, however, have failed to demonstrate a favorable effect on blood loss.[29,30] For all patients, local hemostasis provided by meticulous and advanced surgical skill remains critically important.

Metabolic Complications of Massive Transfusion During Liver Transplantation Surgery

Patients undergoing massive transfusion during OLT are susceptible to all the major complications of massive transfusion, including hypothermia, dilutional coagulopathy, electrolyte imbalance, pulmonary dysfunction, and transfusion-transmitted infections. OLT patients are uniquely at risk for life-threatening hypocalcemia as a result of citrate toxicity. Magnesium is also chelated by citrate, and low magnesium concentrations may accompany massive transfusion during OLT surgery. Because the liver is the main organ for citrate metabolism and because OLT patients can receive very rapid infusions of large volumes of FFP that is rich in Na_3-citrate, the quantity of citrate infused per kilogram body weight per minute can quickly exceed the rate of citrate removal. Citrate toxicity is more pronounced if concomitant renal failure is present because the kidney is the major site of citrate excretion. The principal effects of citrate toxicity are cardiovascular. An initial blunted response of cardiac output to left-ventricular volume loading is followed by hypotension resulting from poor cardiac output and decreased systemic vascular resistance. If misinterpreted as hypotension due to hypovolemia, a more rapid transfusion of citrate-rich blood components will worsen cardiac output. Citrate toxicity is aggravated by hypothermia and hyperkalemia. Because a widened QTc interval on the electrocardiogram has low specificity and poor predictive value, intraoperative monitoring of the ionized calcium level is essential during OLT. Untreated severe depression of the ionized calcium or magnesium results in bizarre electrocardiographic disturbances and fatal arrhythmias.

Plasmapheresis and Photopheresis

The indications for plasmapheresis in transplantation patients remain poorly defined and not established by controlled clinical trials. Preoperative plasmapheresis or blood exchange is able to lower titers of ABO antibodies, especially those of the immunoglobulin M (IgM) class. Plasmapheresis is less effective at reducing titers of HLA antibodies, which are largely IgG in nature. Plasmapheresis has been reported to successfully treat some patients with postoperative HLA-mediated humoral rejection of renal allografts. Photopheresis refers to a treatment in which blood passes along an extracorporeal circuit and is exposed to a photoactive chemical (psoralen) plus ultraviolet light. Used initially in the treatment of Sézary syndrome, photopheresis has been applied to the treatment of solid organ transplant rejection unresponsive to standard therapy. Uncontrolled studies have reported success in cardiac, renal, lung, and liver transplants.

REFERENCES

1. Hartmann O, Le Corroller AG, Blaise D, et al: Peripheral blood stem cell and bone marrow transplantation for solid tumors and lymphomas: Hematologic recovery and costs. A randomized, controlled trial. *Ann Intern Med* 126:600, 1997.
2. Bensinger WI, Martin PJ, Storer B, et al: Transplantation of bone marrow as compared with peripheral-blood cells from HLA-identical relatives in patients with hematologic cancers. *N Engl J Med* 344:175, 2001.
3. Haas R, Mohle R, Fruhauf S, et al: Patient characteristics associated with successful mobilizing and autografting of peripheral blood progenitor cells in malignant lymphoma. *Blood* 83:3787, 1994.
4. McCullough J, McKenna D, Dadidlo D, et al: Issues in the quality of umbilical cord blood stem cells for transplantation. *Transfusion* 45:832, 2005.
5. Weissinger F, Sandmaier BM, Maloney DG, et al: Decreased transfusion requirements for patients receiving nonmyeloablative compared with conventional peripheral blood stem cell transplants from HLA-identical siblings. *Blood* 98:3584, 2001.
6. Rocha V, Labopin M, Sanz G, et al: Transplants of umbilical-cord blood or bone marrow from unrelated donors in adults with acute leukemia. *N Engl J Med* 351:2276, 2004.
7. Laughlin MJ, Eapen M, Rubinstein P, et al: Outcomes after transplantation of cord blood or bone marrow from unrelated donors in adults with leukemia. *N Engl J Med* 351:2265, 2004.
8. Worel N, Greinix HT, Schneider B, et al: Regeneration of erythropoiesis after related- and unrelated-donor BMT or peripheral blood HPC transplantation: A major ABO mismatch means problems. *Transfusion* 40:543, 2000.
9. Dahl D, Hahn A, Koenecke C, et al: Prolonged isolated red blood cell transfusion requirement after allogeneic blood stem cell transplantation: Identification of patients at risk. *Transfusion* 50:649, 2010.
10. Maciej Zaucha J, Mielcarek M, Takatu A, et al: Engraftment of early erythroid progenitors is not delayed after non-myeloablative major ABO-incompatible haematopoietic stem cell transplantation. *Br J Haematol* 119:740, 2002.
11. Bolan CD, Leitman SF, Griffith LM, et al: Delayed donor red cell chimerism and pure red cell aplasia following major ABO-incompatible nonmyeloablative hematopoietic stem cell transplantation. *Blood* 98:1687, 2001.
12. Tomonari A, Takahashi S, Ooi J, et al: Impact of ABO incompatibility on engraftment and transfusion requirement after unrelated cord blood transplantation: A single institute experience in Japan. *Bone Marrow Transplant* 40:523, 2007.
13. Snell M, Chau C, Hendrix D, et al: Lack of isohemagglutinin production following minor ABO incompatible unrelated HLA mismatched umbilical cord blood transplantation. *Bone Marrow Transplant* 38:135, 2006.
14. Gmur J, Burger J, Schanz U, et al: Safety of stringent prophylactic platelet transfusion policy for patients with acute leukaemia. *Lancet* 338:1223, 1991.
15. Heckman KD, Weiner GJ, Davis CS, et al: Randomized study of prophylactic platelet transfusion threshold during induction therapy for adult acute leukemia: 10,000/μL versus 20,000/μL. *J Clin Oncol* 15:1143, 1997.
16. Rebulla P, Finazzi G, Marangoni F, et al, for the Gruppo Italiano Malattie Ematologiche Maligne dell'Adulto: The threshold for prophylactic platelet transfusions in adults with acute myeloid leukemia. *N Engl J Med* 337:1870, 1997.
17. Wandt H, Frank M, Ehninger G, et al: Safety and cost effectiveness of a 10×10^9/L trigger for prophylactic platelet transfusions compared with the traditional 20×10^9/L trigger: A prospective comparative trial in 105 patients with acute myeloid leukemia. *Blood* 91:3601, 1998.
18. Slichter SJ, Kaufman RM, Assmann SF, et al: Dose of prophylactic platelet transfusions and prevention of hemorrhage. *N Engl J Med* 362:600, 2010.
19. Daly PA, Schiffer CA, Aisner J, et al: Platelet transfusion therapy. One-hour posttransfusion increments are valuable in predicting the need for HLA-matched preparations. *JAMA* 243:435, 1980.
20. The Trial to Reduce Alloimmunization to Platelets Study Group: Leukocyte reduction and ultraviolet B irradiation of platelets to prevent alloimmunization and refractoriness to platelet transfusions. *N Engl J Med* 337:1861, 1997.
21. Bowden RA, Sayers M, Fluornoy N, et al: Cytomegalovirus immune globulin and seronegative blood products to prevent primary cytomegalovirus infection after marrow transplantation. *N Engl J Med* 314:1006, 1986.
22. Bowden RA, Slichter SJ, Sayers M, et al: A comparison of filtered leukocyte-reduced and cytomegalovirus (CMV)-seronegative blood products for the prevention of transfusion-associated CMV infection after marrow transplant. *Blood* 86:3598, 1995.
23. Ohto H, Yasuda H, Noguchi M, et al: Risk of transfusion-associated graft-versus-host disease as a result of directed donations from relatives. *Transfusion* 32:691, 1992.
24. Nelson PW, Landreneau MD, Luger AM, et al: Ten-year experience in transplantation of A2 kidneys into B and O recipients. *Transplantation* 65:256, 1998.
25. Ramsey G: Red cell antibodies arising from solid organ transplants. *Transfusion* 31:76, 1991.

26. West LJ, Pollock-Barziv, SM, Dipchand AI, et al: ABO-incompatible heart transplantation in infants. *N Engl J Med* 344:193, 2001.
27. Bishay ES, Cook DJ, El Fettouh H, et al: The impact of HLA sensitization and donor cause of death in heart transplantation. *Transplantation* 70:220, 2000.
28. Preiksaitis JK, Sandhu J, Strautman M: The risk of transfusion-acquired CMV infection in seronegative solid-organ transplant recipients receiving non-WBC-reduced blood components not screened for CMV antibody (1984 to 1996): Experience at a single Canadian center. *Transfusion* 42:396, 2002.
29. Lodge JP, Jonas S, Jones RM, et al: Efficacy and safety of repeated perioperative doses of recombinant factor VIIa in liver transplantation. *Liver Transpl* 11:973, 2005.
30. Planinsic RM, van der Meer J, Testa G, et al: Safety and efficacy of a single bolus administration of recombinant factor VIIa in liver transplantation due to chronic liver disease. *Liver Transpl* 11:895, 2005.

CHAPTER 123

PEDIATRIC TRANSFUSION MEDICINE

Cassandra Josephson and Steven R. Sloan

An essential element of treating various neonatal and pediatric disorders is transfusion of blood components. In order to provide excellent patient care for children it is paramount that clinicians have specific knowledge about blood-bank testing, blood-product components, specific transfusion indications, and potential adverse events.

PEDIATRIC BLOOD BANKING

Blood and Blood Components

Several different blood components, including whole blood, reconstituted whole blood, red blood cells (RBCs), platelets, plasma, and cryoprecipitated antihemophilic factor may be available from a blood bank for transfusion. The availability of specific component types varies between blood suppliers.

- Whole blood is infrequently used and may not be available from a particular blood bank or blood supplier, but it may be available on request and is used by some pediatric cardiac surgery services. Whole blood contains all RBCs, plasma, platelets, and an anticoagulant preservative solution containing citrate, phosphate, dextrose, and possibly adenine.
- RBC units mostly contain RBCs but also contain some plasma and a preservative solution. Most RBC units contain an additive preservative solution that includes some combination of adenine, dextrose, and mannitol. Additive solutions are safe for relatively small (≤20 mL/kg) transfusions. There are concerns over the safety of these additives given in large transfusions to neonates, and their safety in this setting has never been proven in a randomized clinical trial. In view of this concern, some blood banks provide nonadditive RBC units or wash additive units intended for large transfusions to neonates. Because many blood centers provide only additive RBC units and washing an RBC unit takes approximately 1 hour, blood banks have been unable to supply RBC units without additives in many situations. Thus many institutions now have significant experience transfusing large volumes of additive RBC units to neonates and have not noticed any problems.
- Two types of platelet units are available in the United States, although any one blood bank or hospital may stock only one of these types. These two types, whole blood–derived platelets (platelets) and platelets collected by apheresis (pheresis platelets), differ in their size. A platelet unit contains approximately 5.5 to 10 × 10^{10} platelets in about 50 mL, whereas a pheresis platelet unit contains at least 3 × 10^{11} platelets in about 200 mL. It is often easier to use platelet units for small children because pheresis platelets usually need to be prepared as aliquots to provide the correct dose. However, many blood centers exclusively provide only one type of platelet component.
- Plasma is traditionally stored as fresh frozen plasma (FFP) and contains all of the clotting factors and plasma proteins. Although some plasma components are not frozen quickly enough or are thawed for too long before transfusion to be called FFP in the United States, these components still contain all the necessary clotting factors.
- Cryoprecipitate is prepared from plasma and contains high concentrations of fibrinogen.

Because pediatric patients require smaller doses of blood components, they often require only a portion of a component.

- RBCs are stored refrigerated and hence can be prepared in aliquots as needed if the blood bank has the necessary equipment. Alternatively, the blood center can collect RBC units into a collection system in which additional bags are attached for dispensing aliquots. Whole blood is also stored refrigerated, but its use is very limited and it is almost never prepared in aliquots.
- Platelets and pheresis platelets are stored at room temperature under constant agitation and can be prepared in aliquots when needed in the blood bank if the blood bank has the necessary equipment and supplies. However, 1 unit of whole blood–derived platelets does not contain many doses, even for infants, and most blood banks do not find it worthwhile to prepare a unit of platelets in aliquots.
- Plasma is stored frozen, and preparing as aliquots after thawing is not practical or helpful because the plasma remaining after preparing an aliquot is not likely to be used. However, many blood centers will prepare plasma aliquots before freezing.
- Because even small infants rarely require less than 1 unit of cryoprecipitate, this component is rarely prepared in aliquots.

Directed Donations

Families often prefer to donate blood for their children using a process known as directed donations, and some blood banks permit this. If this is done without medical reason, it offers no benefit and there may be increased risks. Although directed donors need to go through the same screening and infectious disease–testing process as all allogeneic blood donors, some studies suggest that directed donors have a slightly higher risk for infectious disease transmission.

In addition, directed donors may be a poor choice for immunologic reasons. For example, if a neonate has alloimmune thrombocytopenia or anemia, the pathologic antibody is a passively acquired maternal antibody directed against inherited paternal antigens. In this case, blood donated by the father would be recognized by the antibody in the baby's circulation and cleared just as the neonate's own platelets are cleared. Another example in which immune concerns make directed donors a poor choice involves transplants. Some patients may require a future tissue or bone marrow transplant, and blood relatives often serve as the best donors for such transplants. However, prior transfusions from relatives may sensitize the patient's immune system to antigens present on the tissues of blood relatives, complicating those potential tissue or bone marrow transplants.

TECHNICAL CONSIDERATIONS/MECHANICAL DEVICES

The small size of pediatric patients necessitates smaller transfusions administered at slower rates. As a result, the transfusion process is subject to the introduction of multiple steps. As mentioned earlier, aliquots of components often need to be prepared. This can be performed with the use of blood collected into collection bags interconnected with sterile tubes. Alternatively, additional containers can be attached to a standard blood component by using a sterile docking device, which produces a sterile weld between the two separate tubing sets. The details of when and where such preparation of aliquots occurs depend on the blood collection sets, the blood component, and the equipment and procedures available at the blood center and hospital blood bank.

Blood components must be filtered to remove microaggregates before transfusion. For an adult patient, this is normally accomplished by transfusing the component through a filter contained within the blood administration set. Although these standard blood administration sets are acceptable for all transfusions, they are not ideal for transfusing small patients because 20 to 40 mL of the component is lost in the dead space of the administration set. Pediatric microaggregate filters with much smaller dead space are available, and these are often used in the blood bank to filter an aliquot before transfusion.

Another issue concerns the standard transfusion rate for nonbleeding patients. The transfusion rate is generally no more than 5 mL/kg/hr. For infants, this corresponds to a lower rate than can be regulated by most standard infusion pumps. Hence such a transfusion is usually performed with the use of a syringe pump, and the blood component aliquot must be transferred to a syringe for the transfusion. Although various procedures can be used for this transfer, one of the simplest and safest is one in which the blood bank transfers an aliquot from the original unit through a pediatric microaggregate filter directly into a syringe. The blood bank dispenses the syringe, and the clinical staff administers the transfusion directly from the syringe and does not need to filter the component.

Table 123-1 Guidelines for Transfusion of Red Blood Cells in Infants Less Than 4 Months of Age

1. Hematocrit <20% with low reticulocyte count and symptomatic anemia (tachycardia, tachypnea, poor feeding)
2. Hematocrit <30% and
   a. On <35% oxygen hood, or
   b. On oxygen by nasal cannula, or
   c. On continuous positive airway pressure and/or intermittent mandatory ventilation on mechanical ventilation with mean airway pressure <6 cm of water, or
   d. With significant tachycardia or tachypnea (heart rate >180 beats per minute for 24 hours or respiratory rate >80 breaths per minute for 24 hours)
   e. With significant apnea or bradycardia (more than six episodes in 12 hours or two episodes in 24 hours requiring bag and mask ventilation while receiving therapeutic doses of methylxanthines), or
   f. With slow weight gain (<10 g/day observed over 4 days while receiving >100 kcal/kg/day)
3. Hematocrit <35% and
   a. On >35% oxygen hood, or
   b. On continuous positive airway pressure/intermittent mandatory ventilation with mean airway pressure >6-8 cm of water
4. Hematocrit <45% and
   a. On extracorporeal membrane oxygenation (ECMO), or
   b. With congenital cyanotic heart disease

RBC, Red blood cell.

TRANSFUSION MEDICINE: GENERAL INDICATIONS AND DOSING

Indications for RBC Transfusion in Neonates, Children, and Adolescents

Neonates Less Than 4 Months Old

RBC transfusions are more commonly administered to hospitalized neonates than any other patient age-group, and RBCs are the component most often transfused in this population. When approximately 10% of the neonate's blood volume has been lost, RBC transfusion should be considered. Symptomatic anemia is the major indication for simple transfusion. When the venous hemoglobin is less than 13 g/dL in the first 24 hours of life, an RBC transfusion should be considered. A transfusion dose of 10-15 mL/kg of RBCs should yield an increase in the neonate of 3 g/dL of hemoglobin after transfusion. Two recent randomized clinical trials in premature infants examining restrictive versus liberal RBC transfusion practices have not resolved the controversy of when RBC transfusion is indicated in the neonatal intensive care unit patient.[1,2] Therefore most guidelines, several published over the past 15 to 20 years, continue to be based on experience rather than evidence-based medicine (Table 123-1).

Older Infants, Children, and Adolescents

RBC transfusion indications for infants older than 4 months and for young children are similar to adults. However, there are several noteworthy differences between children and adults: total blood volume, ability to tolerate blood loss, and age-specific hemoglobin levels (Table 123-2). In infants, RBC transfusions are primarily given for surgical losses, anemia of chronic diseases, and malignancies. Infants inherently have lower hemoglobin levels than adults. Consequently, infants remain asymptomatic at lower hemoglobin concentrations, especially if the anemia occurs gradually. Even with these physiologic differences, general transfusion-trigger guidelines for pediatric intensive care unit patients are similar to those for adults, with a transfusion trigger of 7 g/dL of hemoglobin for hemodynamically stable patients being shown to be safe for these patients.[3] This threshold also has been found to be safe for hematopoietic progenitor cell (HPC) transplant patients.[4] Dosing of RBCs is the same as for infants less than 4 months of age, 10 to 15 mL/kg despite the fact that more concentrated RBC units are often used for infants less than 4 months old.

Table 123-2 Guidelines for Transfusion of Red Blood Cells in Patients More Than 4 Months of Age

1. Emergency surgical procedure in patient with significant postoperative anemia
2. Preoperative anemia when other corrective therapy is not available
3. Intraoperative blood loss ≥15% total blood volume
4. Hematocrit <21%-24%
   a. In perioperative period, with signs and symptoms of anemia
   b. While on chemotherapy/radiotherapy
   c. Chronic congenital or acquired symptomatic anemia
5. Hematocrit <21%, hemodynamically stable patients >3 days old in the pediatric intensive care unit
6. Acute blood loss with hypovolemia not responsive to other therapy
7. Hematocrit <40% and
   a. With severe pulmonary disease
   b. On ECMO
8. Sickle cell disease and
   a. Cerebrovascular accident
   b. Acute chest syndrome
   c. Splenic sequestration
   d. Aplastic crisis
   e. Recurrent priapism
   f. Preoperatively when general anesthesia is planned (target hemoglobin 10 mg/dL)
9. Chronic transfusion programs for disorders of RBC production (e.g., β-thalassemia major and Diamond-Blackfan syndrome unresponsive to therapy)

Modified from Roseff SD, Luban NLC, Manno CS. Guidelines for assessing appropriateness of pediatric transfusion. *Transfusion* 42:1398, 2002 and Wong CC, Luban NLC: Intrauterine, neonatal, and pediatric transfusion. In: Mintz PD, ed: *Transfusion therapy: Clinical principles and practice,* ed 2. Bethesda, Md., 2005, AABB Press, p 159.
ECMO, Extracorporeal membrane oxygenation; *RBC*, red blood cell.

Platelets

Platelet transfusion support in neonates less than 4 months of age, those older than 4 months, children, and adolescents is usually intended as a prophylactic strategy to prevent bleeding (Table 123-3). More often in preterm neonates, platelet transfusions are performed for a therapeutic indication with platelet counts less than 50,000/μL during active bleeding. The prophylactic platelet transfusion thresholds in this group of patients are quite controversial and based primarily on expert consensus rather than evidenced-based medicine. In sharp contrast to adults, who rarely have severe bleeding as a complication until their platelet counts fall below 10,000/μL, preterm infants with other complicating illnesses may bleed at higher platelet counts. The increased risk may be secondary to (1) lower levels of plasma coagulation factors, (2) natural anticoagulants that potentiate thrombin inhibition, (3) intrinsic or extrinsic platelet dysfunction, and (4) increased vascular fragility. Platelet counts and function in older children are similar to those of adults, and the indications for platelet transfusions do not differ from the indications for adults.

Frozen Plasma and Cryoprecipitate

Frozen plasma is used in preterm and term infants most commonly to treat multiple factor deficiencies (vitamin K–dependent factors II, IV, IX, and X as well as proteins C and S), hemorrhagic disease of the newborn, or vitamin K deficiency (Table 123-4). ABO compatibility of the unit is especially important in pediatrics because transfused antibodies can reach high concentrations in infants and children with very small plasma volumes. Dosing is the same for neonates less than 4 months of age and those older: 10 to 15 mL/kg. The expected result is an increase in all factor activity by 15% to 20% unless there is a marked consumptive coagulopathy.

Cryoprecipitate is used primarily to treat disorders resulting from a decrease or dysfunction of fibrinogen or factor XIII deficiency. These indications are similar to those for adults. The important part for children is that it takes only a small volume of cryoprecipitate to increase the fibrinogen. One unit of cryoprecipitate is usually sufficient to achieve hemostatic levels in infants and even less than that in preterm infants. In children 1 to 2 units/10 kg is the dose. The expected rise in fibrinogen should be 60 to 100 mg/dL, assuming 100% recovery. When being administered to infants, cryoprecipitate should also be ABO compatible for the same reasons as mentioned for frozen plasma.

Table 123-3 Guidelines for Transfusion of Platelets in Neonates and Older Children

PLATELET COUNT <150,000/ML

1. Platelet count 5000-10,000/μL with failure of platelet production
2. Platelet count <30,000/μL in neonate with failure of platelet production
3. Platelet count <50,000/μL in stable premature infant
   a. With active bleeding, or
   b. Before an invasive procedure with failure of platelet production
4. Platelet count <100,000/μL in sick premature infant
   a. With active bleeding, or
   b. Before an invasive procedure in patient with DIC

WITHOUT THROMBOCYTOPENIA

1. Active bleeding with qualitative platelet defect
2. Unexplained excessive bleeding during cardiopulmonary bypass
3. Patient receiving ECMO with
   a. Platelet count <100,000/μL
   b. Higher platelet counts and bleeding

DIC, Disseminated intravascular coagulation; *ECMO,* extracorporeal membrane oxygenation.

Granulocytes

Neonatal granulocyte transfusions for sepsis remain unclear. Granulocytes are sometimes transfused for patients older than 4 months, although the benefit has not been clearly demonstrated in trials with modern antimicrobial therapy. The rationale in this population is that granulocytes may help support patients with persistent neutropenia or granulocyte dysfunction in the context of bacterial and/or fungal infection. The minimum dose of granulocytes for larger children and adults is 1×10^{10} cells/kg. The following are guidelines for transfusion of granulocytes to neonates and older children: (1) neonates or children with neutropenia or granulocyte dysfunction (e.g., chronic granulomatous disease) with bacterial sepsis and lack of responsiveness to standard therapy, and (2) neutropenic neonates or children with fungal disease not responsive to standard therapy (see Chapter 115).

TRANSFUSION MEDICINE: INDICATIONS IN UNIQUE PEDIATRIC POPULATIONS

Hemolytic Disease of the Fetus and Newborn

Hemolytic disease of the fetus and newborn (HDFN) occurs when the mother's immune system recognizes a foreign, paternally inherited antigen on fetal erythrocytes. The incidence of HDFN dramatically declined after the introduction of Rh immune globulin to prevent sensitization of the mother to RhD. Although introduction of Rh immune globulin has prevented most cases of HDFN due to RhD sensitization, it has not totally eliminated HDFN due to RhD or reduced HDFN due to other antibodies.

Table 123-4 Guidelines for Transfusion of Frozen Plasma and Cryoprecipitate in Neonates and Older Children

FROZEN PLASMA

1. Support during treatment of DIC
2. Replacement therapy
   a. When specific factor concentrates are not available, including but not limited to, antithrombin, protein C or S deficiency, and factor II, factor V, factor X, and factor XI deficiencies
   b. During therapeutic plasma exchange when FFP is indicated (cryoprecipitate-poor plasma, plasma from which the cryoprecipitate has been removed)
3. Reversal of warfarin in an emergency situation, such as before an invasive procedure with active bleeding

Note: Frozen plasma is not indicated for volume expansion or enhancement of wound healing

CRYOPRECIPITATE

1. Hypofibrinogenemia or dysfibrinogenemia with active bleeding
2. Hypofibrinogenemia or dysfibrinogenemia, undergoing an invasive procedure
3. Factor XIII deficiency with active bleeding or undergoing an invasive procedure in the absence of factor XIII concentrate
4. Limited directed-donor cryoprecipitate for bleeding episodes in small children with hemophilia A (when recombinant and plasma-derived factor VIII products are not available)
5. In the preparation of fibrin sealant
6. von Willebrand disease with active bleeding:
   Cryoprecipitate is used in von Willebrand disease only when both of the following are true:
   a. 1-Deamino-8-D-arginine vasopressin is contraindicated, not available, or does not elicit response
   b. Virus-inactivated plasma-derived factor VIII concentrate (which contains von Willebrand factor) is not available

DIC, Disseminated intravascular coagulation; *FFP,* fresh frozen plasma.

Blood-bank studies are critical in the diagnosis of this syndrome in both fetuses and newborns. Most significant cases of HDFN are due to antibodies outside of the ABO system. These antibodies will be detected in the blood of the pregnant or postpartum woman. Also necessary for the diagnosis, the corresponding antigens would be present on fetal or newborn erythrocytes, or predicted to be present on fetal erythrocytes based on molecular testing of fetal deoxyribonucleic acid (DNA). The direct antiglobulin test (DAT) of the fetal or newborn's erythrocytes should be positive. Additional testing is performed to determine the severity of fetal anemia, if present.

Although antibody titers are used to help predict the severity of the disease during pregnancy, they are generally not useful in the newborn. After birth, the severity of the anemia and the resulting hyperbilirubinemia serve as markers for the severity of the HDFN. Rates of rise in bilirubin level are most helpful in determining whether an exchange transfusion will be necessary, with increases of 8 to 13 µmol/L/hr despite phototherapy indicating that exchange transfusion will likely be necessary.[5]

RBCs transfused in utero to the fetus need to be compatible with the ABO type of the fetus and mother and hence are usually blood group O. They need to lack the antigen(s) to which the mother has made antibodies, and they need to be crossmatch compatible with her serum. The RBCs should be irradiated to prevent transfusion-associated graft-versus-host disease (TA-GVHD) and cytomegalovirus (CMV) safe to minimize the risk for transfusion-transmitted CMV. Relatively fresh RBCs also are usually chosen for these transfusions.

Reconstituted whole blood is usually used for neonatal exchange transfusions. The blood is prepared by removing most of the preservative solution from an RBC unit and adding plasma, usually so that the final hematocrit is 40% to 45%. Intrauterine transfusions are irradiated, and most institutions will select CMV-safe units (leukoreduced and/or CMV seronegative).

Neonatal Alloimmune Thrombocytopenia

The pathophysiology of neonatal alloimmune thrombocytopenia (NAIT) is similar to that of HDFN in that both involve immune-mediated attack and destruction of fetal and neonatal blood cells by the mother's immune system. Unlike HDFN, NAIT often affects a woman's first pregnancy. In addition, the antigens involved are due to polymorphisms on platelet-specific proteins. Although a variety of antigens can be implicated, the human platelet antigen-1 (HPA-1) protein is most frequently implicated in whites, with approximately 80% to 90% of cases being due to women who lack the HPA-1a antigen making antibodies against HPA-1a that is expressed on fetal platelets. When NAIT is suspected, maternal serum can be tested for antibodies to platelet antigens, and the parent's platelet antigens can be determined by testing their platelets or by molecular means in which their platelet antigens are indirectly determined from their DNA. An affected infant or fetus may require platelet transfusions. Although random platelets may be of some transient benefit, antigen-negative units are best. Maternal platelets lack the antigen, but the plasma contains the pathogenic antibody, which means that if maternal platelets are used, they should be washed before transfusion. Alternatively, antigen-negative units may be available. Indeed, major blood centers usually have HPA-1a-negative units available.

Extracorporeal Membrane Oxygenation

Extracorporeal membrane oxygenation (ECMO) is an intervention in which whole blood is removed from the patient's venous circulation and circulated through a machine to remove carbon dioxide and replenish oxygen before it is returned to the patient. This prolonged intervention is reserved for patients with more than 80% mortality risk and those who have been unresponsive to conventional ventilator support and medical treatment but still potentially have a reversible outcome. In neonates and children, ECMO has become a lifesaving therapy in the treatment of multiple disorders; Table 123-5[6] lists indications for ECMO support in neonates and children. Standardized guidelines for transfusion practice have not been established, resulting in individualized centers establishing their own criteria. Bleeding during ECMO is a common complication and may be caused by any of the following factors necessary for operating the ECMO circuit or resulting from the thrombogenic surface of the circuit: (1) systemic heparinization, (2) platelet dysfunction, (3) thrombocytopenia, (4) other coagulation defects, and (5) nonendothelial cell surface lining the circuitry. It is recommended that hospital transfusion services and ECMO staff be in close communication to agree on local protocols to ensure safe, efficient, and consistent care (Table 123-6 provides an example protocol from one institution).[6] Blood products for ECMO are typically ABO and Rh specific and crossmatch compatible for priming. The RBC units are hemoglobin S negative, relatively fresh, between 5 and 7 days old, irradiated, and CMV seronegative and/or leukoreduced.

Table 123-5 Indications for Extracorporeal Membrane Oxygenation for Neonates and Pediatric Patients

NEONATAL
Meconium aspiration
Respiratory distress syndrome
Persistent pulmonary hypertension
Congenital diaphragmatic hernia
Sepsis
PEDIATRIC
Bacterial pneumonia
Viral pneumonia
Acute respiratory distress syndrome
Burns
Inhalation injuries
Near drowning
Sepsis

Trauma

Transfusion management of a trauma patient often must be guided by the patient's estimated blood loss and associated signs and symptoms, such as hypotension or tachycardia. This topic has been the source of significant controversy in recent years, with retrospective studies from the U.S. military suggesting that ratios of 1 : 1 to 1 : 2 of plasma : RBCs and similar ratios of platelets : RBCs transfused during early treatment improves outcomes. Although there is significant criticism concerning inherent limitations in the retrospective nature of these studies, these transfusion strategies have been adopted by many adult trauma centers. Although some have advocated adopting similar protocols for pediatric trauma centers, this has occurred in only a few places, most likely because there are little data on transfusions in pediatric trauma patients.[7]

Hemoglobinopathies

In patients with sickle cell disease (SCD), chronic transfusion therapy has been shown to reduce the risk for both primary and secondary stroke, by decreasing the hemoglobin S content of the patient's blood, as well as achieving a reduction in sickling, suppression of erythropoiesis, and preventing an increase in blood viscosity.[8] The risk for recurrent stroke has been reduced to less than 10% if hemoglobin levels are maintained between 8 and 9 g/dL and hemoglobin S levels below 30%. Simple or partial-exchange transfusion therapy can achieve this goal when performed approximately every 3 to 4 weeks. Chronic erythrocytapheresis has also been used for this therapy with

Table 123-6 Blood Product Protocols for Extracorporeal Membrane Oxygenation

Clinical Scenario	Urgency	Products	Blood Groups	Storage
Cardiac arrest	5-10 min	2 units RBCs	O-negative RBCs	<14 days, AS
ECMO circuit disruption	5-10 min	2 units RBCs	O-negative RBCs	<14 days, AS
Progressive septic shock, nonneonate	30 min	2 units RBCs	O-negative RBCs or type specific	<10 days, any preservative
Neonate transferred for ECMO	1-2 hr	2 units RBCs 1 unit FFP 1 unit platelets	O-negative RBCs AB plasma	<10 days, CPD or CPDA-1
Cardiac ICU	30-60 min	2 units RBCs	Type specific	<7 days, AS
Gradual respiratory or cardiac failure on conventional support	Hours-days	2 units RBCs	Type specific	<10 days, CPD

Modified from protocols developed at The Children's Hospital of Philadelphia. Friedman DF, Montenegro LM: Extracorporeal membrane oxygenation and cardiopulmonary bypass. In: Hillyer CD, Strauss RG, Luban NLC, editors: *Handbook of pediatric transfusion medicine*, London, 2004, Elsevier Academic Press, p 181.
AS, additive solution unit is acceptable; *CPD*, citrate phosphate dextrose; *CPDA-1*, citrate phosphate dextrose adenine; *ICU*, intensive care unit; *RBC*, red blood cell.

an added mission to mitigate iron overload complications. Chronic transfusion treatment for stroke most times is an indefinite therapy, that is, once the patient is placed on it, cessation is not possible because it has been shown to lead to recurrent stroke.[9] Table 123-2 describes other indications for patients with SCD needing either simple or chronic RBC transfusion therapy. Products for patients with SCD should be screened at a minimum for hemoglobin S and should be leukocyte reduced to reduce the risk for febrile nonhemolytic transfusion reactions and to reduce the risk for human leukocyte antigen (HLA) alloimmunization resulting in platelet refractoriness that can complicate possible stem cell transplantation.

In children with SCD, it also is critically important to prevent the alloimmunization to minor RBC antibodies, because, in most children with severe SCD, RBC transfusion is the only therapy available to treat the multiple manifestations of SCD. Overall, the SCD patient has higher rates of alloimmunization than other chronically transfused patient groups. The antibodies are produced against common Rh, Kell, Duffy, and Kidd system antigens. Many sickle cell treatment centers perform thorough phenotype analysis of a patient's red cells before initiating transfusion therapy. This testing helps to reduce the rate of alloimmunization by allowing preferential selection of phenotypically similar units.[10] However, particularly for patients who are not yet alloimmunized, this process remains controversial because phenotypically compatible units may be difficult to obtain and expensive.[11] The most common protocol followed for nonalloimmunized patients is pretransfusion phenotypic matching for C, E, and K antigens to prevent alloimmunization. In addition, some centers extend the protocol so that once patients have developed a red cell antibody, extension of matching to additional red cell antigens (Fy, Jk, S) is often used to prevent further alloimmunization. Furthermore, a recent retrospective study in children with SCD undergoing matched-sibling donor-related bone marrow transplantation demonstrated a decrease in RBC transfusion requirements during transplant when they received phenotypically minor RBC antigen–matched units.[12]

The benefits of RBC transfusion therapy in SCD disease must constantly be weighed against the costs (e.g., iron overload, RBC alloimmunization, and increased donor exposure risks of erythrocytapheresis). As a result of these issues, some clinicians have proposed that a clinically successful course of transfusions that maintains the hemoglobin S below 30% could, after several years, be transitioned to a strategy of more limited transfusions with a hemoglobin S target of 40% to 50% to reduce the risks for iron overload.[8] Patients with SCD may also be at risk for life-threatening delayed hemolytic transfusion reactions, the development of autoantibodies, and "hyperhemolytic" syndrome (a phenomenon that occurs after RBC transfusion when the patient's hemoglobin level unexpectedly decreases after transfusion and the cells that are destroyed are both the allogeneic and autologous cells). The mechanism is not well characterized.

Thalassemia

Thalassemia with severe anemia is usually treated with chronic transfusion therapy to improve tissue oxygenation and suppress extramedullary erythropoiesis in the liver, spleen, and bone marrow. This approach mitigates many of the complications caused by the ineffective erythropoiesis. In contrast to chronic transfusion regimens used to treat SCD, most β-thalassemia major patients requiring chronic transfusion therapy start at a very young age and require lifelong treatment. The treatment goals in this population are characterized by (1) increasing oxygen-carrying capacity by anemia correction, (2) preventing progressive hypersplenism, (3) suppression of endogenous erythropoiesis, and (4) reduction of gastrointestinal absorption of iron.[13] The target hemoglobin levels are usually 8 to 9 g/dL, where normal growth and development can occur in these patients. Supertransfusion protocols aim for higher target hemoglobin levels (11 to 12 g/dL) to reduce organomegaly from extramedullary hematopoiesis. Iron overload is a potential complication of this RBC transfusion protocol that cannot be prevented and must be treated with chelation therapy beginning early in childhood. RBC alloimmunization in this population is estimated at approximately 16%, which is half that of the rate for patients with SCD.[14] Phenotypic-matching protocols are used in some locations to prevent RBC alloimmunization, but data supporting or refuting this practice are scant.

Autoimmune Hemolytic Anemia

Autoimmune hemolytic anemia in children occurs predominantly in young children, with a median age of 3.8 years, and 53% are associated with other immunologic diseases, according to one study.[15] This study also found that 74% of the cases had DAT results that were positive for immunoglobulin G (IgG) and C3d. Like adult cases, most cases of autoimmune hemolytic anemia in children have antibody reactivity with all screening cells and all RBCs on antibody identification panels (i.e., positive indirect Coombs tests).

Children also may develop autoimmune hemolytic anemia associated with a Donath-Landsteiner antibody, an antibody that is rarely seen in adults. Classically the Donath-Landsteiner antibody is associated with paroxysmal cold hemoglobinuria, a disease in which patients developed paroxysms of hemoglobinuria following exposure to cold temperatures.[16] Although this is often true, this classic syndrome is not always seen in children with the Donath-Landsteiner antibody. The syndrome often develops following an infection such as a respiratory infection.

The Donath-Landsteiner antibody is an IgG antibody that binds erythrocytes, usually recognizing the P antigen, at cold temperatures (<20° C [68° F]) and fixes early components of complement. The fixed complement does not cause significant hemolysis at cold temperatures, but when the cells are warmed, the entire complement complex binds and lyses the erythrocytes. Initial testing in the blood bank may be entirely normal or may reveal a positive DAT for C3. The Donath-Landsteiner antibody can be detected only by special testing in which the patient's plasma is incubated with erythrocytes in cold temperatures followed by warm temperatures (see Chapter 44).

Hematopoietic Cellular Transplant Patients

Transfusion support for HPC transplant patients is similar to that for adult patients, although there are few published studies on transfusion of pediatric HPC transplant patients. RBC transfusions are generally not needed in these patients whose hemoglobin level is at least 7 g/dL.[4] No studies in the modern era have been published on platelet transfusions in these patients, but use of a transfusion trigger of 10,000 platelets/μL, like that used for adults, seems reasonable for those patients without a significant bleeding risk other than thrombocytopenia.

Apheresis

Pediatric apheresis is used for many of the same indications as for adults. However, additional aspects need to be considered in treating pediatric patients. Many children require vascular access through a central vein because the peripheral veins of many children are too small. In addition, peripheral access requires patients to remain seated with the limited arm movement for the procedure duration, and younger patients are often unable to comply with this given that procedures usually last at least 2 hours. During the procedures, children are more susceptible to symptomatic hypocalcemia from citrate anticoagulation. For this reason, some pediatric centers use heparin to anticoagulate patients, although prophylactic cation replacement can successfully prevent most symptoms in pediatric apheresis patients.[17] Apheresis procedures subject the patient to volume shifts, which are usually a loss of less than 200 mL of fluid during the procedure and a gain of up to 300 mL at the end of the procedure. The actual fluid shifts depend on the machine, the procedure, and the parameters for that procedure. In some cases, the volume shifts may be too large to be safe for the patient. In these cases, most machines can be primed with 5% albumin, an RBC unit, or reconstituted whole blood. Using a prime solution, it is possible to minimize fluid shifts so that the patient is effectively volume neutral for the entire procedure. Procedures to accomplish this are usually only available at centers that perform apheresis on relatively large numbers of pediatric patients.

Special Processing and Prevention of Adverse Events in Pediatric Patients

In pediatric transfusion medicine, special processing of blood products is performed more often than in adults. This is especially true in the preterm infant population, specifically in very low-birth-weight (VLBW) infants weighing less than 1500 g and extremely low-birth-weight infants weighing less than 1000 g.

Leukocyte-Reduced Blood Components

Leukoreduced cellular blood products are used in greater than 80% of blood components transfused to children in the United States, despite a paucity of clinical studies in children.[18] The rationale behind the use in pediatric patients has primarily been extrapolated from adult studies. Leukoreduction is performed to reduce transmission of CMV, decrease HLA alloimmunization,[19] and decrease febrile nonhemolytic transfusion reactions. From an evidence-based medicine approach, leukoreduction still remains controversial, because transfusion reactions in neonates younger than 4 months of age occur infrequently and infants rarely become HLA alloimmunized due to their immature immune system. Nonetheless, one known benefit of leukoreduced cellular products is reduction in the risk for transfusion-transmitted CMV.[20] In Canada, Fergusson et al[21] evaluated clinical outcomes of premature infants weighing less than 1250 g, before and after nationwide implementation of universal leukoreduction, revealing no changes in mortality or rate of bacteremia. However, the study revealed a decrease in retinopathy of prematurity, bronchopulmonary dysplasia, and length of hospitalization after implementation.[21]

Cytomegalovirus-Seronegative Blood Components

The provision of CMV-seronegative blood products to certain pediatric populations is based on prevention of transfusion transmission of CMV. The residual risk for transfusion-transmitted CMV in adults has been estimated to be between 1% and 3%. In preterm neonates, transfusing CMV-seronegative blood components has been shown to be extremely effective in reducing the risk for CMV infection in multitransfused infants weighing less than 1200 g born to seronegative mothers.[22] Based on this study primarily, it is recommended that infants born to CMV-seronegative mothers receive CMV–reduced risk blood for transfusions. The accepted strategies for CMV–reduced risk transfusions are CMV-seronegative or CMV-leukoreduced products. Many neonatologists in the United States combine the strategies, hoping to improve prevention of transfusion-transmitted CMV. However, in 2001 the Canadian Consensus Conference did not issue a recommendation for a combined use of leukoreduction plus CMV-seronegative allogeneic blood for low-birth-weight (LBW) infants. The combined approach for prevention of transfusion-transmitted CMV was recommended for the following groups: transfusions to CMV-seronegative pregnant women, intrauterine fetal transfusions, and CMV-seronegative allogeneic bone marrow transplantation recipients. Nonetheless, the scientific question of whether the combined strategy reduces the risk for transfusion-transmitted CMV in any vulnerable population is yet to be answered. Currently a large prospective birth cohort study in VLBW infants is under way to estimate the incidence of transfusion-transmitted CMV in LBW infants who receive CMV-seronegative plus leukoreduced blood products to evaluate the effectiveness of this coupled strategy.

Irradiation

Mortality rates associated with TA-GVHD are as high as 80% to 90%, with no effective treatments once it has occurred. As a result, identifying neonates and children who are either immunoincompetent or immunosuppressed is paramount, so irradiation of cellular components can be performed to prevent this noninfectious serious hazard of transfusion. There are differing expert opinions and practices in this area, and local protocols based on patient populations, equipment available, and best practices at each institution should be followed. The following are some guidelines for neonates and older children in this area: (1) premature infants with birth weight less than 1200 g, (2) any child with known or suspected cellular immune deficiency (e.g., severe combined immunodeficiency), (3) any child with significant immunosuppression due to chemotherapy or radiation treatment, (4) any child who receives blood components from blood relatives, and (5) any child who receives HLA-matched or crossmatched platelet components.

Washing

Washing is usually performed to reduce the risk for adverse reactions related to plasma, anticoagulant-preservative solutions, and high levels of potassium. Neonates and children in specific situations may require this intervention, but it should not be a routine practice. Washing, resulting in the removal or reduction of plasma, becomes critical when transfusing maternal blood to treat either hemolytic disease of the newborn or NAIT because the plasma contains the offending antibodies. Indeed, use of maternal blood for these patients is not recommended.

Volume Reduction

Volume reduction of plasma in a closed system is primarily a technique used in premature infants who have renal ischemia or compromised cardiac function. However, it is also employed for infants and children who may receive ABO-mismatched platelet transfusions, because several deaths have been reported in the literature of children who have received out-of-group platelets (e.g., O platelet pheresis to A recipient).[23]

Reconstitution of RBCs for Neonatal Exchange Transfusion

When the RBCs are being prepared for a neonatal exchange transfusion, the component choice and expected potential physiologic effects must be taken into consideration. Usually RBCs are resuspended in ABO-compatible thawed FFP. Typically, RBCs that are less than 5 to 7 days old and stored in citrate phosphate dextrose adenine (CPDA-1) solution are chosen to avoid high levels of potassium. Units provided are hemoglobin sickle negative to avoid potential for intravascular sickling and CMV seronegative to prevent transfusion-transmitted CMV; irradiation is performed to prevent TA-GVHD. The irradiation should be performed just before the exchange to minimize the potentiation of the potassium storage lesion. The glucose load during an exchange transfusion has been noted to be high; therefore it is recommended that in the first few hours of the exchange the infant's glucose levels be monitored.

The expected amount of RBCs needed for an infant double-volume exchange transfusion is approximately 1 unit of RBCs depending on the patient's weight. A final hematocrit of approximately 45% to 60% should be the target for the product. The reconstituted blood must be adequately mixed to maintain the intended hematocrit throughout the exchange transfusion.

When the exchange transfusion is being performed, a standard filter and inline blood warmer are recommended. A rule of thumb for withdrawal and infusion of blood during the exchange is usually no more than 5 mL/kg body weight or 5% of the infant's blood volume is to be removed and replaced during a 3- to 5-minute cycle. The exchange should be performed at a slow pace, so as to not cause sudden hemodynamic changes that can result in cerebral blood flow shifts in intracranial pressure, precipitating an intraventricular hemorrhage.[24] The expected total time for a double-volume exchange transfusion is typically around 1½ to 2 hours.

REFERENCES

1. Bell EF, Strauss RG, Widness JA, et al: Randomized trial of liberal versus restrictive guidelines for red blood cell transfusion in preterm infants. *Pediatrics* 115:1685, Jun 2005.
2. Kirpalani H, Whyte RK, Andersen C, et al: The Premature Infants in Need of Transfusion (PINT) study: A randomized, controlled trial of a restrictive (low) versus liberal (high) transfusion threshold for extremely low birth weight infants. *J Pediatr* 149:301, Sep 2006.
3. Lacroix J, Hebert PC, Hutchison JS, et al: Transfusion strategies for patients in pediatric intensive care units. *N Engl J Med* 356:1609, Apr 19 2007.
4. Lightdale JR, Randolph AG, Tran CM, et al: Impact of a conservative red blood cell transfusion strategy in children undergoing hematopoietic stem cell transplantation. *Biol Blood Marrow Transplant* 18:813, 2012.
5. Wennberg RP, Depp R, Heinrichs WL: Indications for early exchange transfusion in patients with erythroblastosis fetalis. *J Pediatr* 92:789, May 1978.
6. Friedman DF, Montenegro LM: Extracorporeal membrane oxygenation and cardiopulmonary bypass. In Hillyer CD, Strauss RG, Luban NLC, editors: *Handbook of pediatric transfusion medicine,* London, 2004, Elsevier Academic Press, p 181.
7. Dehmer JJ, Adamson WT: Massive transfusion and blood product use in the pediatric trauma patient. *Semin Pediatr Surg* 19:286, Nov 2010.
8. Adams DM, Schultz WH, Ware RE, et al: Erythrocytapheresis can reduce iron overload and prevent the need for chelation therapy in chronically transfused pediatric patients. *J Pediatr Hematol Oncol* 18:46, Feb 1996.
9. Adams RJ, Brambilla D: Discontinuing prophylactic transfusions used to prevent stroke in sickle cell disease. *N Engl J Med* 353:2769, Dec 29 2005.
10. Vichinsky EP, Luban NL, Wright E, et al: Prospective RBC phenotype matching in a stroke-prevention trial in sickle cell anemia: A multicenter transfusion trial. *Transfusion* 41:1086, Sep 2001.
11. Castro O, Sandler SG, Houston-Yu P, et al: Predicting the effect of transfusing only phenotype-matched RBCs to patients with sickle cell disease: Theoretical and practical implications. *Transfusion* 42:684, Jun 2002.
12. McPherson ME, Anderson AR, Haight AE, et al: Transfusion management of sickle cell patients during bone marrow transplantation with matched sibling donor. *Transfusion* 49:1977, Sep 2009.
13. Olivieri NF: The beta-thalassemias. *N Engl J Med* 341:99, Jul 8 1999.
14. Thompson AA, Cunningham MJ, Singer ST, et al: Red cell alloimmunization in a diverse population of transfused patients with thalassaemia. *Br J Haematol* 153:121, Apr 2011.
15. Aladjidi N, Leverger G, Leblanc T, et al: New insights into childhood autoimmune hemolytic anemia: A French national observational study of 265 children. *Haematologica* 96:655, May 2011.
16. Eder AF: Review: Acute Donath-Landsteiner hemolytic anemia. *Immunohematology* 21:56, 2005.
17. Bolan CD, Yau YY, Cullis HC, et al: Pediatric large-volume leukapheresis: A single institution experience with heparin versus citrate-based anticoagulant regimens. *Transfusion* 44:229, Feb 2004.
18. Fergusson D, Hebert PC, Barrington KJ, et al: Effectiveness of WBC reduction in neonates: What is the evidence of benefit? *Transfusion* 42:159, Feb 2002.
19. Leukocyte reduction and ultraviolet B irradiation of platelets to prevent alloimmunization and refractoriness to platelet transfusions. The Trial to Reduce Alloimmunization to Platelets Study Group. *N Engl J Med* 337:1861, Dec 25 1997.
20. Gilbert GL, Hayes K, Hudson IL, et al: Prevention of transfusion-acquired cytomegalovirus infection in infants by blood filtration to remove leucocytes. Neonatal Cytomegalovirus Infection Study Group. *Lancet* 1:1228, Jun 3 1989.
21. Fergusson D, Hebert PC, Lee SK, et al: Clinical outcomes following institution of universal leukoreduction of blood transfusions for premature infants. *JAMA* 289:1950, Apr 16 2003.
22. Yeager AS, Grumet FC, Hafleigh EB, et al: Prevention of transfusion-acquired cytomegalovirus infections in newborn infants. *J Pediatr* 98:281, Feb 1981.
23. Josephson CD, Castillejo MI, Grima K, et al: ABO-mismatched platelet transfusions: Strategies to mitigate patient exposure to naturally occurring hemolytic antibodies. *Transfus Apher Sci* 42:83, Feb 2010.
24. Bada HS, Chua C, Salmon JH, et al: Changes in intracranial pressure during exchange transfusion. *J Pediatr* 94:129, Jan 1979.

PART XII

Hemostasis and Thrombosis

CHAPTER 124

OVERVIEW OF HEMOSTASIS AND THROMBOSIS

Jeffrey I. Weitz

Hemostasis preserves vascular integrity by balancing the physiologic processes that maintain blood in a fluid state under normal circumstances and prevent excessive bleeding after vascular injury. Preservation of blood fluidity depends on an intact vascular endothelium and a complex series of regulatory pathways that maintains platelets in a quiescent state and keeps the coagulation system in check. In contrast, arrest of bleeding requires rapid formation of hemostatic plugs at sites of vascular injury to prevent exsanguination. Perturbation of hemostasis can lead to bleeding or thrombosis. Bleeding will occur if there is failure to seal vascular leaks either because of defective hemostatic plug formation or because of premature breakdown of the plugs. In contrast, thrombosis may occur if prothrombotic stimuli are unregulated.

Thrombosis can occur in arteries or veins and is a major cause of morbidity and mortality. Arterial thrombosis is the most common cause of acute coronary syndromes, ischemic stroke, and limb gangrene, but thrombosis in the deep veins of the leg leads to the postthrombotic syndrome and to pulmonary embolism, which can be fatal.

Most arterial thrombi form on top of disrupted atherosclerotic plaques because plaque rupture exposes thrombogenic material in the plaque core to the blood.[1] This material then triggers platelet aggregation and fibrin formation, which results in the generation of a platelet-rich thrombus that temporarily or permanently occludes blood flow. Whereas temporary occlusion of blood flow in coronary arteries may trigger unstable angina, persistent obstruction causes myocardial infarction. The same processes can occur in the cerebral circulation, where temporary arterial occlusion may manifest as a transient ischemic attack and persistent occlusion can lead to a stroke. Likewise, critical limb ischemia can occur if there is superimposed thrombosis on ruptured atherosclerotic plaques in the major arteries supplying blood to the lower extremities.

In contrast to arterial thrombi, venous thrombi rarely form at sites of obvious vascular disruption. Although they can develop after surgical trauma to veins or secondary to indwelling venous catheters, they usually originate in the valve cusps of the deep veins of the calf or in the muscular sinuses, where there is stasis.[2] Sluggish blood flow in these veins reduces the oxygen supply to the avascular valve cusps. Hypoxemia induces endothelial cells lining the valve cusps to express adhesion molecules, which tether tissue factor-bearing leukocytes and microparticles onto their surface. Tissue factor–bearing leukocytes and microparticles adhere to these activated cells and induce coagulation. Impaired blood flow exacerbates local thrombus formation by reducing clearance of activated clotting factors. Calf vein thrombi that extend into the proximal veins of the leg can dislodge and travel to the lungs to produce pulmonary embolism.[3]

Arterial and venous thrombi contain platelets and fibrin, but the proportions differ. Arterial thrombi are rich in platelets because of the high shear in the injured arteries. In contrast, venous thrombi, which form under low shear conditions, contain relatively few platelets and consist mostly of fibrin and trapped red blood cells. Because of the predominance of platelets, arterial thrombi appear white, but venous thrombi appear red, reflecting the trapped red cells.

The antithrombotic drugs used for prevention and treatment of thrombosis target components of thrombi, and include antiplatelet drugs, which inhibit platelets; anticoagulants, which attenuate coagulation; and fibrinolytic agents that induce fibrin degradation (see Chapter 151). With the predominance of platelets in arterial thrombi, strategies to inhibit or treat arterial thrombosis focus mainly on antiplatelet agents, although in the acute setting, strategies often include anticoagulants and fibrinolytic agents. When arterial thrombi are occlusive and rapid restoration of blood flow is required, mechanical and pharmacologic methods enable thrombus extraction, compression, or degradation (see Chapter 145). Although rarely used for this indication, anticoagulants can also prevent recurrent ischemic events after acute myocardial infarction. Anticoagulants are the mainstay for prevention and treatment of venous thromboembolism because fibrin is the predominant component of venous thrombi (see Chapter 144). Antiplatelet drugs are less effective than anticoagulants because of the limited platelet content of venous thrombi. Selected patients with venous thromboembolism benefit from fibrinolytic therapy—for example, patients with massive or submassive pulmonary embolism achieve more rapid restoration of pulmonary blood flow with systemic or catheter-directed fibrinolytic therapy than with anticoagulant therapy alone. Selected patients with extensive deep vein thrombosis in the iliac or femoral veins also may have a better outcome with catheter-directed fibrinolytic therapy or mechanical thrombus extraction in addition to anticoagulants (see Chapter 145).

This chapter provides an overview of hemostasis and thrombosis and highlights the processes involved in platelet activation and aggregation, blood coagulation, and fibrinolysis.

HEMOSTATIC SYSTEM

The major components of the hemostatic system are the vascular endothelium, platelets, and the coagulation and fibrinolytic systems.

Vascular Endothelium

A monolayer of endothelial cells lines the intimal surface of the circulatory tree and separates the blood from the prothrombotic subendothelial components of the vessel wall (see Chapter 125). As such, the vascular endothelium encompasses about 10^{13} cells and covers a vast surface area. Rather than serving as a static barrier, the healthy vascular endothelium is a dynamic organ (Fig. 124-1) that actively regulates hemostasis by inhibiting platelets, suppressing coagulation, promoting fibrinolysis, and modulating vascular tone and permeability.[4] Defective vascular function can lead to bleeding if the endothelium becomes more permeable to blood cells, if vasoconstriction does not occur, or if premature degradation of hemostatic plugs opens seals in the vasculature.

Platelet Inhibition

Endothelial cells synthesize prostacyclin and nitric oxide and release them into the blood.[4] These agents not only serve as potent vasodilators but also inhibit platelet activation and subsequent aggregation

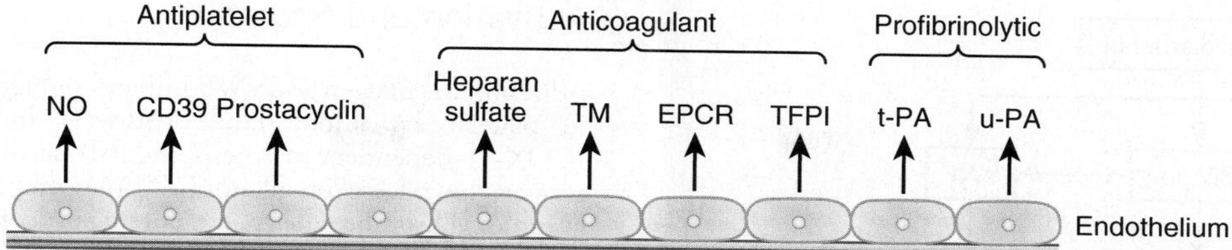

Figure 124-1 THE ANTITHROMBOTIC FUNCTIONS OF THE ENDOTHELIUM. The healthy endothelium has (1) antiplatelet activity because of synthesis and release of prostacyclin and nitric oxide (NO) and expression of CD39, a membrane-associated ectoADPase; (2) anticoagulant activity because of heparan sulphate proteoglycan-mediated activation of antithrombin and expression of thrombomodulin (TM) and endothelial protein C receptor (EPCR), which are involved in protein C activation, and surface-bound tissue factor pathway inhibitor (TFPI); and (c) profibrinolytic activity because of release of tissue and urokinase-type plasminogen activator (t-PA and u-PA, respectively).

by stimulating adenylate cyclase and increasing intracellular levels of cyclic adenosine monophosphate (cAMP). In addition, endothelial cells express CD39 on their surface, a membrane-associated ecto-adenosine diphosphatase (ADPase). By degrading ADP, which is a platelet agonist, CD39 attenuates platelet activation.

Anticoagulant Activity

Intact endothelial cells play an essential part in the regulation of thrombin generation through a variety of mechanisms. Endothelial cells produce heparan sulfate proteoglycans, which bind circulating antithrombin and accelerate the rate at which it inhibits thrombin and other coagulation enzymes. Tissue factor pathway inhibitor (TFPI), a naturally occurring inhibitor of coagulation, binds heparan sulfate on the endothelial cell surface.[5] Administration of heparin or low-molecular-weight heparin (LMWH) displaces glycosaminoglycan-bound TFPI from the vascular endothelium, and released TFPI may contribute to the antithrombotic activity of these drugs.

Endothelial cells regulate thrombin generation by expressing thrombomodulin and endothelial cell protein C receptor (EPCR) on their surfaces. Thrombomodulin binds thrombin and alters this enzyme's substrate specificity such that it no longer acts as a procoagulant but becomes a potent activator of protein C (see Chapter 129). Activated protein C serves as an anticoagulant by degrading and inactivating activated factor V and factor VIII (factors Va and VIIIa, respectively), key cofactors involved in thrombin generation. Protein S acts as a cofactor in this reaction, and EPCR enhances this pathway by binding protein C and presenting it to the thrombin–thrombomodulin complex for activation. In addition to its role as an anticoagulant, activated protein C also regulates inflammation and preserves the barrier function of the endothelium.[6]

Fibrinolytic Activity

The vascular endothelium promotes fibrinolysis by synthesizing and releasing tissue-type and urokinase-type plasminogen activator (t-PA and u-PA, respectively), which initiate fibrinolysis by converting plasminogen to plasmin (see Chapter 129). Endothelial cells in most vascular beds synthesize t-PA constitutively. In contrast, perturbed endothelial cells produce u-PA in the settings of inflammation and wound repair.

Endothelial cells also produce type 1 plasminogen activator inhibitor 1 (PAI-1), the major regulator of both t-PA and u-PA. Therefore, net fibrinolytic activity depends on the dynamic balance between the release of plasminogen activators and PAI-1. Fibrinolysis localizes to the endothelial cell surface because these cells express annexin II, a coreceptor for plasminogen and t-PA that promotes their interaction. Therefore, healthy vessels actively resist thrombosis and help maintain platelets in a quiescent state.

Vascular Tone and Permeability

In addition to synthesizing potent vasodilators, such as prostacyclin and nitric oxide, endothelial cells also produce a group of counter-regulatory peptides known as endothelins that induce vasoconstriction. Endothelial cell permeability is influenced by the connections that join endothelial cells to their neighbors. Macromolecules traverse the endothelium via patent intercellular junctions, by endocytosis, or through transendothelial pores. Vasodilatation, severe thrombocytopenia, and high doses of heparin can increase endothelial permeability, which may contribute to bleeding. Activated protein C may also contribute to the barrier function of the endothelium.

Platelets

Platelets are anucleate particles released into the circulation after fragmentation of bone marrow megakaryocytes (see Chapter 126). Because they are anucleate, platelets have limited capacity to synthesize proteins. Thrombopoietin, a glycoprotein synthesized in the liver and kidneys, regulates megakaryocytic proliferation and maturation as well as platelet production. After they enter the circulation, platelets have a life span of 7 to 10 days.

Damage to the intimal lining of the vessel exposes the underlying subendothelial matrix. Platelets home to sites of vascular disruption and adhere to the exposed matrix proteins (see Chapter 127). Adherent platelets undergo activation and not only release substances that recruit additional platelets to the site of injury but also promote thrombin generation and subsequent fibrin formation (Fig. 124-2). A potent platelet agonist, thrombin amplifies platelet recruitment and activation. Activated platelets then aggregate to form a plug that seals the leak in the vasculature.[7] An understanding of the steps in these highly integrated processes helps pinpoint the sites of action of the antiplatelet drugs and rationalizes the utility of anticoagulants for the treatment of arterial thrombosis and venous thrombosis.

Adhesion

Platelets adhere to exposed collagen and von Willebrand factor (vWF) and form a monolayer that supports and promotes thrombin generation and subsequent fibrin formation. These events depend on constitutively expressed receptors on the platelet surface, $\alpha_2\beta_1$ and glycoprotein (GP) VI, which bind collagen, and GPIbα and GPIIb/IIIa ($\alpha_{IIb}\beta_3$), which bind vWF. The platelet surface is crowded with receptors, but those involved in adhesion are the most abundant: every platelet has about 40,000 to 80,000 copies of GPIIb/IIIa and 25,000 copies of GPIbα. Receptors cluster in cholesterol-enriched subdomains, which render them more mobile, thereby increasing the efficiency of platelet adhesion and subsequent activation (see Chapter 127).

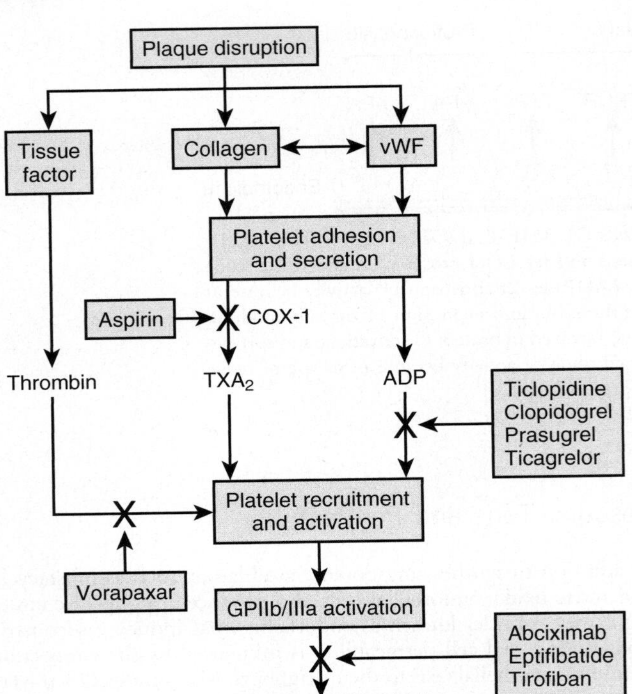

Figure 124-2 SITES OF ACTION OF ANTIPLATELET DRUGS. Aspirin inhibits thromboxane A_2 (TXA_2) synthesis by irreversibly acetylating cyclooxygenase-1 (COX-1). Reduced TXA_2 release attenuates platelet activation and recruitment to the site of vascular injury. Ticlopidine, clopidogrel, and prasugrel irreversibly block $P2Y_{12}$, a key adenosine diphosphate (ADP) receptor on the platelet surface; ticagrelor is a reversible inhibitor of $P2Y_{12}$. Apciximab, eptifibatide, and tirofiban inhibit the final common pathway of platelet aggregation by blocking fibrinogen and von Willebrand factor (vWF) binding to activated glycoprotein (GP) IIb/IIIa. Vorapaxar inhibits thrombin-mediated platelet activation by targeting protease activated receptor-1 (PAR-1), the major thrombin receptor on platelets.

Under low shear conditions, collagen can capture and activate platelets on its own. Captured platelets undergo cytoskeletal reorganization that causes them to flatten and to adhere more closely to the damaged vessel wall. Under high shear conditions, however, collagen and vWF must act in concert to support optimal platelet adhesion and activation. vWF synthesized by endothelial cells and megakaryocytes assembles into multimers that range from 550 to more than 10,000 kDa. When released from storage in the Weibel-Palade bodies of endothelial cells or the α-granules of platelets, most of the vWF enters the circulation, but the vWF released from the abluminal surface of endothelial cells accumulates in the subendothelial matrix, where it binds collagen via its A3 domain. This surface-immobilized vWF can simultaneously bind platelets via its A1 domain. In contrast, circulating vWF does not react with unstimulated platelets. This difference in reactivity likely reflects vWF conformation; whereas circulating vWF is in a coiled conformation that prevents access of its platelet-binding domain to vWF receptors on the platelet surface, immobilized vWF assumes an elongated shape that exposes its A1 domain. In this extended conformation, large vWF multimers serve as the molecular glue that tethers platelets to the damaged vessel wall with sufficient strength to withstand higher shear forces.[8] Large vWF multimers provide additional binding sites for collagen and heighten platelet adhesion because platelets have more vWF receptors than collagen receptors. Adhesion to collagen or vWF results in platelet activation, the next step in platelet plug formation.

Activation and Secretion

Adhesion to collagen and vWF initiates signaling pathways that result in platelet activation. These pathways induce cyclooxygenase-1 (COX-1)–dependent synthesis and release of thromboxane A_2, and trigger the release of adenosine diphosphate (ADP) from storage granules. Thromboxane A_2 is a potent vasoconstrictor, and similar to ADP, locally activates ambient platelets and recruits them to the site of injury. This process results in expansion of the platelet plug. To activate platelets, thromboxane A_2 and ADP must bind to their respective receptors on the platelet membrane. The thromboxane receptor (TP) is a G-protein coupled receptor that is found on platelets and on the endothelium, which explains why thromboxane A_2 induces vasoconstriction as well as platelet activation.[9] ADP interacts with a family of G protein–coupled receptors on the platelet membrane. Most important of these is $P2Y_{12}$, which is the target of the thienopyridines, but $P2Y_1$ also contributes to ADP-induced platelet activation, and maximal ADP-induced platelet activation requires activation of both receptors. A third ADP receptor, $P2X_1$, is an adenosine triphosphate (ATP)–gated calcium channel. Platelet storage granules contain ATP as well as ADP; ATP released during the platelet activation process may contribute to the platelet recruitment process in a $P2X_1$-dependent fashion.

Although TP and the various ADP receptors signal through different pathways, they all trigger an increase in the intracellular calcium concentration in platelets. This in turn induces shape change via cytoskeletal rearrangement, granule mobilization and release, and subsequent platelet aggregation. Activated platelets promote coagulation by expressing phosphatidylserine on their surfaces, an anionic phospholipid that supports assembly of coagulation factor complexes (see Chapter 128). After being assembled, these clotting factor complexes trigger a burst of thrombin generation and subsequent fibrin formation. In addition to converting fibrinogen to fibrin, thrombin amplifies platelet recruitment and activation and promotes expansion of the platelet plug. Thrombin binds to protease-activated receptors types 1 and 4 (PAR1 and PAR4, respectively) on the platelet surface and cleaves their extended amino-termini, thereby generating new amino-termini that serve as tethered ligands that bind and activate the receptors (Fig. 124-3). Whereas low concentrations of thrombin cleave PAR1, PAR4 cleavage requires higher thrombin concentrations.[10] Cleavage of either receptor triggers platelet activation.

In addition to providing a surface on which clotting factors assemble, activated platelets also promote fibrin formation and subsequent stabilization by releasing factor V, factor XI, fibrinogen, and factor XIII (see Chapter 127). Thus, there is coordinated activation of platelets and coagulation, and the fibrin network that results from thrombin action helps anchor the platelet aggregates at the site of injury. Activated platelets also release adhesive proteins, such as vWF, thrombospondin, and fibronectin, which may augment platelet adhesion at sites of injury, as well as growth factors, such as platelet-derived growth factor (PDGF) and transforming growth factor-β (TGFβ), which promote wound healing. Platelet aggregation is the final step in the formation of the platelet plug.

Aggregation

Platelet aggregation links platelets to each other to form clumps. GPIIb/IIIa mediates these platelet-to-platelet linkages. On nonactivated platelets, GPIIb/IIIa exhibits minimal affinity for its ligands. Upon platelet activation, GPIIb/IIIa undergoes a conformational transformation, which reflects transmission of inside-out signals from its cytoplasmic domain to its extracellular domain.[11] This transformation enhances the affinity of GPIIb/IIIa for its ligands; fibrinogen; and, under high shear conditions, vWF (see Chapter 127). Arginine–glycine–aspartic acid (RGD) sequences located on fibrinogen and vWF, as well as a platelet-binding lycine–glycine–aspartic acid (KGD) sequence on fibrinogen, mediate their interaction with GPIIb/IIIa. When subjected to high shear, circulating vWF elongates and exposes its platelet-binding domain, which enables its interaction with the

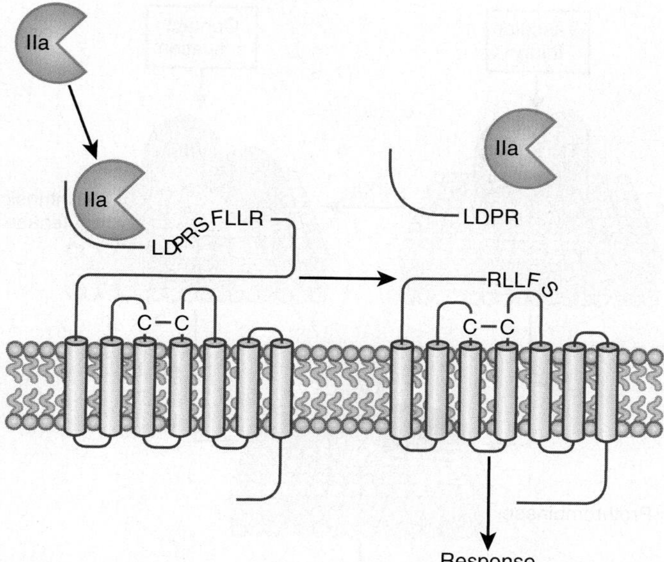

Figure 124-3 ACTIVATION OF PROTEASE-ACTIVATED RECEPTOR (PAR)-1 BY THROMBIN. Thrombin (IIa) binds to the amino terminus of the extracellular domain of PAR-1, where it cleaves a specific peptide bond. Cleavage of this bond generates a new amino-terminus sequence that acts as a tethered ligand and binds to the body of the receptor, thereby activating it. Thrombin then dissociates from the receptor. Analogs of the first five or six amino acids of the tethered ligand sequences, known as thrombin receptor agonist peptides, can independently activate PAR-1.

conformationally activated GPIIb/IIIa. Divalent fibrinogen and multivalent vWF molecules serve as bridges and bind adjacent platelets together. After being bound to GPIIb/IIIa, fibrinogen and vWF induce outside–inside signals that augment platelet activation and result in the activation of additional GPIIb/IIIa receptors, creating a positive feedback loop. Because GPIIb/IIIa acts as the final effector in platelet aggregation, it is a logical target for potent antiplatelet drugs (see Chapters 132 and 151). Fibrin, the ultimate product of the coagulation system, tethers the platelet aggregates together and anchors them to the site of injury.

Coagulation

Coagulation results in the generation of thrombin, which converts soluble fibrinogen to fibrin. Coagulation occurs through the action of discrete enzyme complexes, which are composed of a vitamin K-dependent enzyme and a non-enzyme cofactor, and assemble on anionic phospholipid membranes in a calcium-dependent fashion (see Chapter 128). Each enzyme complex activates a vitamin K–dependent substrate that becomes the enzyme component of the subsequent complex. Together, these complexes generate a small amount of thrombin, which amplifies its own generation by activating the non-enzyme cofactors and platelets, which then provide an anionic surface on which the complexes assemble. The three enzyme complexes involved in thrombin generation are extrinsic tenase, intrinsic tenase, and prothrombinase (Fig. 124-4). Although extrinsic tenase initiates the system under most circumstances, the contact system also plays a role in some situations.

Extrinsic Tenase

This complex forms upon exposure of tissue factor-expressing cells to the blood.[12] Tissue factor exposure occurs after atherosclerotic plaque rupture because the core of the plaque is rich in cells that express tissue factor. Denuding injury to the vessel wall also exposes tissue factor constitutively expressed by subendothelial fibroblasts and smooth muscle cells. In addition to cells in the vessel wall, circulating monocytes and monocyte-derived microparticles (small membrane fragments) also provide a source of tissue factor. When tissue factor–bearing monocytes or microparticles bind to platelets or other leukocytes and their plasma membranes fuse, tissue factor transfer occurs. By binding to adhesion molecules expressed on activated endothelial cells or to P-selectin on activated platelets, these tissue factor-bearing cells or microparticles can initiate or augment coagulation.[13] This phenomenon likely explains how venous thrombi develop in the absence of obvious vessel wall injury.

Tissue factor is an integral membrane protein that serves as a receptor for factor VIIa. The blood contains trace amounts of factor VIIa, which has negligible activity in the absence of tissue factor.[12] With tissue factor exposure on anionic cell surfaces, factor VIIa binds in a calcium-dependent fashion to form the extrinsic tenase complex, which is a potent activator of factors IX and X. After being activated, factor IXa and factor Xa serve as the enzyme components of intrinsic tenase and prothrombinase, respectively.

Intrinsic Tenase

Factor IXa binds to factor VIIIa on anionic cell surfaces to form the intrinsic tenase complex.[14] Factor VIII circulates in blood in complex with vWF. Thrombin cleaves factor VIII and releases it from vWF, converting it to its activated form.[15] Activated platelets express binding sites for factor VIIIa. After being bound, factor VIIIa binds factor IXa in a calcium-dependent fashion to form the intrinsic tenase complex, which then activates factor X. The change in catalytic efficiency of factor IXa–mediated activation of factor X that occurs with deletion of individual components of the intrinsic tenase complex highlights their importance. Absence of the membrane or factor VIIIa almost completely abolishes enzymatic activity, and the catalytic efficiency of the complete complex is 10^9-fold greater than that of factor IXa alone.[14] Because intrinsic tenase activates factor X at a rate 50- to 100-fold faster than extrinsic tenase, it plays a critical role in the amplification of factor Xa and subsequent thrombin generation (see Chapter 128).

Prothrombinase

Factor Xa binds to factor Va, its activated cofactor, on anionic phospholipid membrane surfaces to form the prothrombinase complex. Activated platelets release factor V from their α-granules, and this platelet-derived factor V may play a more important role in hemostasis than its plasma counterpart.[16] Whereas plasma factor V requires thrombin activation to exert its cofactor activity, the partially activated factor V released from platelets already exhibits substantial cofactor activity. Activated platelets express specific factor Va binding sites on their surface, and bound factor Va serves as a receptor for factor Xa. The catalytic efficiency of factor Xa activation of prothrombin increases by 10^9-fold when factor Xa incorporates into the prothrombinase complex.[14] Prothrombin binds to the prothrombinase complex, where it undergoes conversion to thrombin in a reaction that releases prothrombin fragment 1.2 (F1.2). Plasma levels of F1.2, therefore, provide a marker of prothrombin activation.

Fibrin Formation

The final effector in coagulation is thrombin. Thrombin converts soluble fibrinogen into insoluble fibrin. Fibrinogen is a dimeric molecule, each half of which is composed of three polypeptide chains—the Aα, Bβ, and γ chains. Numerous disulfide bonds covalently link the chains together and join the two halves of the fibrinogen molecule (Fig. 124-5). Electron micrographic studies of fibrinogen reveal a trinodular structure with a central E domain flanked by two D

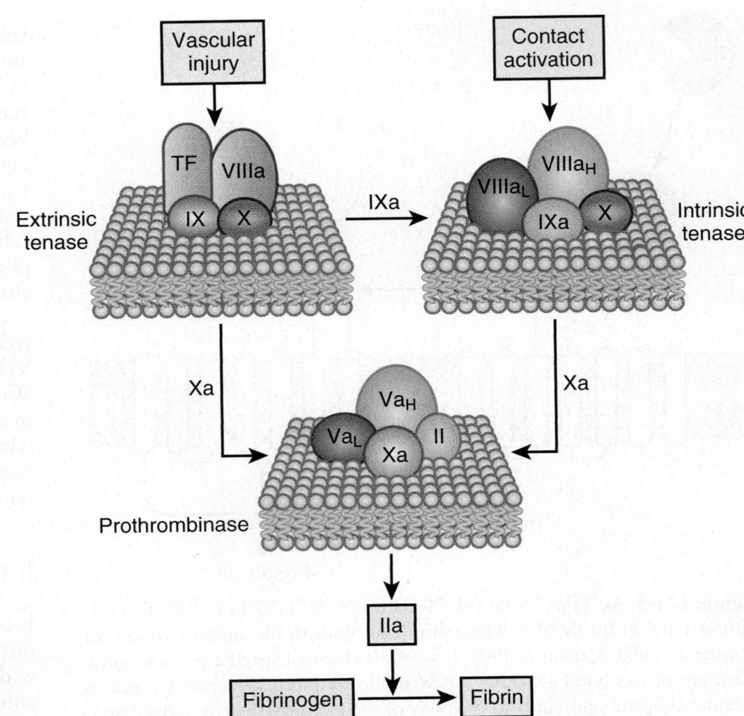

Figure 124-4 COAGULATION SYSTEM. Coagulation occurs through the action of discrete enzyme complexes, which are composed of a vitamin K–dependent enzyme and a non-enzyme cofactor. These complexes assemble on anionic phospholipid membranes in a calcium-dependent fashion. Vascular injury exposes tissue factor (TF), which binds factor VIIa to form extrinsic tenase. Extrinsic tenase activates factors IX and X. Factor IXa binds to factor VIIIa to form intrinsic tenase, which activates factor X. Factor Xa binds to factor Va to form prothrombinase, which converts prothrombin (II) to thrombin (IIa). Thrombin then converts soluble fibrinogen into insoluble fibrin.

domains. Crystal structures show symmetry of design with the central E domain, which contains the amino termini of the fibrinogen chains, joined to the lateral D domains by coiled-coil regions.

Fibrinogen circulates in an inactive form. Thrombin binds to the amino termini of the Aα and Bβ chains of fibrinogen, where it cleaves specific peptide bonds to release fibrinopeptide A and fibrinopeptide B and generates fibrin monomer (see Fig. 124-5). Because they are products of thrombin action on fibrinogen, plasma levels of these fibrinopeptides provide an index of thrombin activity. Fibrinopeptide release creates new amino termini that extend as knobs from the E domain of one fibrin monomer and insert into preformed holes in the D domains of other fibrin monomers. This creates long strands known as protofibrils, consisting of fibrin monomers noncovalently linked together in a half-staggered overlapping fashion.[17]

Noncovalently linked fibrin protofibrils are unstable.[17] The stability of the fibrin network is enhanced by platelets and procoagulant cells.[18] Platelets not only bind fibrin via GPIIb/IIIa and promote the formation of a dense fibrin network, but they also release factor XIII. By covalently cross-linking the α and γ chains of adjacent fibrin monomers, factor XIIIa stabilizes the fibrin in a calcium-dependent fashion and renders it relatively resistant to degradation. Factor XIII circulates in blood as a heterodimer consisting of pairs of A and B subunits. The active and calcium binding sites on factor XIII are localized to the A subunit. Platelets contain large amounts of factor XIII in their cytoplasms, but platelet-derived factor XIII consists only of the A subunits (see Chapter 127). Both plasma and platelet factor XIII are activated by thrombin.

Contact Pathway

Current thinking is that tissue factor exposure represents the sole pathway for activation of coagulation and that the contact system—which includes factor XII, prekallikrein, and high-molecular-weight kininogen—is unimportant for hemostasis because patients deficient in these factors do not have bleeding problems (see Chapter 139). The physiologic role of factor XI is more difficult to assess because the plasma level of factor XI does not predict the propensity for bleeding (see Chapter 139). Although the capacity of thrombin to feed back and activate platelet-bound factor XI may explain this phenomenon, platelet-derived factor XI may be more important for hemostasis than circulating factor XI.

We cannot ignore the contact pathway, however, because coronary catheters and other blood-contacting medical devices, such as stents or mechanical valves, likely trigger clotting through this mechanism. Factor XII bound to the surface of catheters or devices undergoes a conformational change that results in its activation. Factor XIIa converts prekallikrein to kallikrein in a reaction accelerated by high-molecular-weight kininogen, and factor XIIa and kallikrein then feedback to activate additional factor XII. Factor XIIa propagates coagulation by activating factor XI (Fig. 124-6).

In addition to its role in device-related thrombosis, the contact pathway may also contribute to the stability of arterial and venous thrombi.[19,20] DNA and RNA released from damaged cells in atherosclerotic plaques activates factor XII, and mice given DNA- or RNA-degrading enzymes exhibit attenuated thrombosis at sites of arterial injury. Polyphosphates released from activated platelets also activate factor XII and may provide another stimulus for contact pathway activation. Mice deficient in factor XII or factor XI form small unstable thrombi at sites of arterial or venous damage, suggesting that factor XII and factor XI contribute to thrombogenesis (see Chapter 139). It is unknown whether the same is true in humans. Patients with unstable angina have increased plasma levels of factor XIa, but it is unclear whether this reflects activation by factor XIIa or by thrombin. Although the contribution of the contact pathway to thrombin generation remains uncertain, the final product of coagulation is fibrin. Hemostasis depends on the dynamic balance between the formation of fibrin and its degradation. The fibrinolytic system mediates fibrin breakdown.

Fibrinolytic System

Fibrinolysis initiates when plasminogen activators convert plasminogen to plasmin, which then degrades fibrin into soluble fragments. Blood contains two immunologically and functionally distinct plasminogen activators, t-PA and u-PA. Whereas t-PA mediates intravascular fibrin degradation, u-PA binds to a specific u-PA receptor

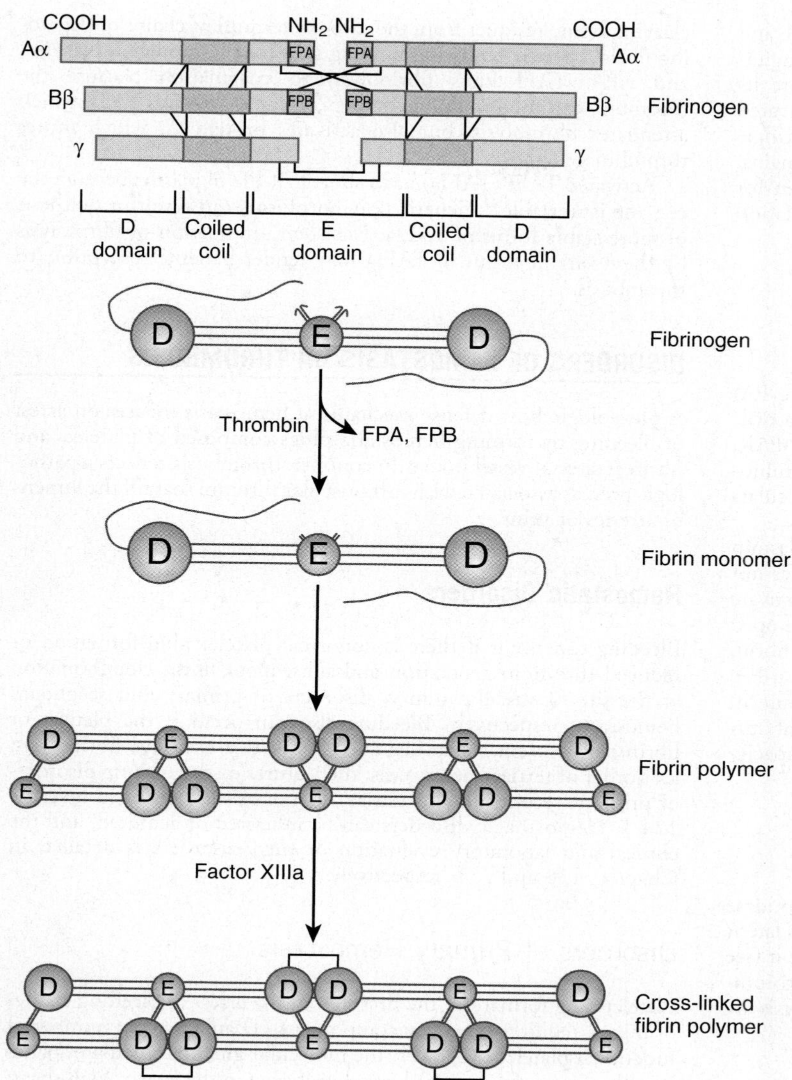

Figure 124-5 FIBRINOGEN STRUCTURE AND CONVERSION OF FIBRINOGEN TO FIBRIN. A dimeric molecule, each half of fibrinogen is composed of three polypeptide chains—the Aα, Bβ, and γ chains. Numerous disulfide bonds *(lines)* covalently link the chains together and join the two halves of the fibrinogen molecule to yield a trinodular structure with a central E domain linked via the coiled coil regions to two lateral D domains. To convert fibrinogen to fibrin, thrombin cleaves specific peptide bonds at the amino (NH_2) termini of the Aα and Bβ chains of fibrinogen to release fibrinopeptide A (FPA) and fibrinopeptide B (FPB), thereby generating fibrin monomer. Fibrin monomers polymerize to generate protofibrils arranged in a half-staggered overlapping fashion. By covalently cross-linking α and γ chains of adjacent fibrin monomers, factor XIIIa stabilizes the fibrin network and renders it resistant to degradation.

(u-PAR) on the surface of cells, where it activates cell-bound plasminogen. Consequently, pericelluar proteolysis during cell migration and tissue remodeling and repair are the major functions of u-PA.[21]

Regulation of fibrinolysis occurs at two levels (see Chapter 129). PAI-1, and to a lesser extent, PAI-2, inhibit the plasminogen activators, and α_2-antiplasmin inhibits plasmin. Endothelial cells synthesize PAI-1, which inhibits both t-PA and u-PA, whereas monocytes and the placenta synthesize PAI-2, which specifically inhibits u-PA. Thrombin-activated fibrinolysis inhibitor (TAFI) also modulates fibrinolysis and provides a link between fibrinolysis and coagulation.[22] Whereas thrombosis can occur if there is impaired activation of the fibrinolytic system, excessive activation leads to bleeding. Therefore, a review of the mechanisms of action of t-PA, u-PA, and TAFI is worthwhile.

Mechanism of Action of Tissue Plasminogen Activator

Tissue plasminogen activator, a serine protease, contains five discrete domains: a fibronectin-like finger domain, an epidermal growth factor (EGF) domain, two kringle domains, and a protease domain. Synthesized as a single-chain polypeptide, plasmin readily converts t-PA into a two-chain form. Single- and two-chain forms of t-PA convert plasminogen to plasmin. Native Glu-plasminogen is a single-chain polypeptide with a Glu residue at its amino-terminus. Plasmin cleavage at the amino-terminus generates lysine–plasminogen, a truncated form with a Lys residue at its new amino terminus.[21] t-PA cleaves a single peptide bond to convert single-chain glutamine- or lysine–plasminogen into two-chain plasmin composed of a heavy chain containing five kringle domains and a light chain containing the catalytic domain. Because its open conformation exposes the t-PA cleavage site, lysine–plasminogen is a better substrate than glutamic acid–plasminogen, which assumes a circular conformation that renders this bond less accessible.

Tissue plasminogen activator has little enzymatic activity in the absence of fibrin, but its activity increases by at least three orders of magnitude when fibrin is present. This increase in activity reflects the capacity of fibrin to serve as a template that binds t-PA and plasminogen and promotes their interaction. Whereas t-PA binds to fibrin via its finger and second kringle domains, plasminogen binds fibrin via its kringle domains. Kringle domains are loop-like structures that bind Lys residues on fibrin. As fibrin undergoes degradation, more Lys residues are exposed, which provide additional binding sites for t-PA and plasminogen. Consequently, degraded fibrin stimulates t-PA activation of plasminogen more than intact fibrin.

α_2-Antiplasmin rapidly inhibits circulating plasmin by docking to its first kringle domain and then inhibiting the active site.[21] Because plasmin binds to fibrin via its kringle domains, plasmin generated on the fibrin surface resists inhibition by α_2-antiplasmin. This phenomenon endows fibrin-bound plasmin with the capacity to degrade fibrin. Factor XIIIa cross-links small amounts of α_2-antiplasmin onto fibrin, which prevents premature fibrinolysis.[18]

Similar to fibrin, annexin II on endothelial cells binds t-PA and plasminogen and promotes their interaction. Cell-surface gangliosides and α-enolase also may bind plasminogen and promote its activation by altering its conformation into the more readily activated open form. Plasminogen binds to endothelial cells via its kringle domains. Lipoprotein a, which also possesses kringle domains, impairs cell-based fibrinolysis by competing with plasminogen for cell-surface binding. This phenomenon may explain the association between elevated lipoprotein a levels and atherosclerosis.

Mechanism of Action of Urokinase-Type Plasminogen Activator

Synthesized as a single-chain polypeptide, single-chain u-PA (scu-PA) has minimal enzymatic activity. Plasmin converts scu-PA into a two-chain form that is enzymatically active and capable of binding u-PAR, the u-PA receptor on cell surfaces. Further cleavage at the amino-terminus of two-chain u-PA yields a truncated, lower-molecular-weight form that lacks the u-PAR binding domain.

Two-chain forms of u-PA readily convert plasminogen to plasmin in the absence or presence of fibrin.[21] In contrast, scu-PA does not activate plasminogen in the absence of fibrin, but it can activate fibrin-bound plasminogen because plasminogen adopts a more open and readily activatable conformation when immobilized on fibrin. Similar to the higher-molecular-weight form of two-chain u-PA, scu-PA binds to cell surface u-PAR, where plasmin can activate it. Many tumor cells elaborate u-PA and express u-PAR on their surfaces. Plasmin generated on these cells endows them with the capacity for metastasis.

Mechanism of Action of TAFI

Thrombin-activated fibrinolysis inhibitor, a procarboxpeptidase B–like molecule synthesized in the liver, circulates in blood in a latent form where thrombin bound to thrombomodulin can activate it (see Chapters 128 and 129). Unless bound to thrombomodulin, thrombin activates TAFI inefficiently.[22] TAFIa attenuates fibrinolysis by cleaving lysine residues from the carboxy termini of chains of degrading fibrin, thereby removing binding sites for plasminogen, plasmin, and t-PA. TAFI links fibrinolysis to coagulation because the thrombin–thrombomodulin complex not only activates TAFI, which attenuates fibrinolysis, but also activates protein C, which mutes thrombin generation.

Activated TAFI (TAFIa) has a short half-life in plasma because the enzyme is unstable.[22] Genetic polymorphisms can result in synthesis of more stable forms of TAFIa. Persistent attenuation of fibrinolysis by these variant forms of TAFIa may render patients susceptible to thrombosis.

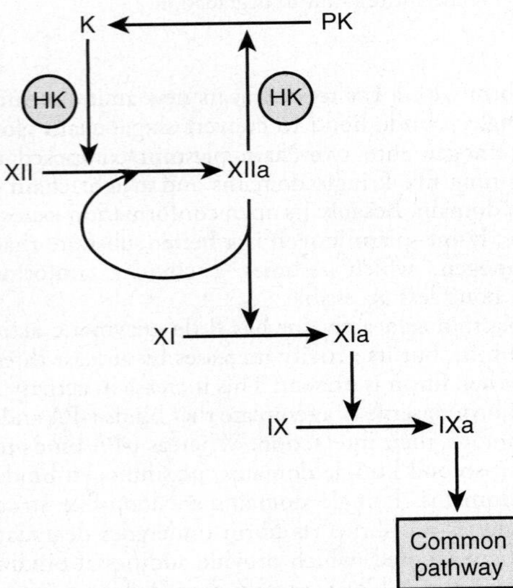

Figure 124-6 CONTACT SYSTEM. Factor XII (XII) is activated by contact with negatively charged surfaces. XIIa converts prekallikrein (PK) to kallikrein (K) and can feed back to activate more XII. Likewise, XIIa also can feed back to amplify its own generation. About 75% of circulating PK is bound to high-molecular-weight kininogen (HK), which localizes it to anionic surfaces and promotes PK activation. XIIa propagates clotting by activating XI, which then activates IX. The resultant IXa assembles into the intrinsic tenase complex, which activates X to initiate the common pathway of coagulation.

DISORDERS OF HEMOSTASIS OR THROMBOSIS

A physiologic host defense mechanism, hemostasis focuses on arrest of bleeding by forming hemostatic plugs composed of platelets and fibrin at sites of vessel injury. In contrast, thrombosis reflects a pathologic process associated with intravascular thrombi that fill the lumens of arteries or veins.

Hemostatic Disorders

Bleeding can occur if there is abnormal platelet plug formation or reduced thrombin generation and subsequent fibrin clot formation at the site of vascular injury; disorders of primary and secondary hemostasis, respectively. Bleeding also can occur if the platelet or fibrin clot is prematurely degraded because of excessive fibrinolysis; a disorder of tertiary hemostasis, the features distinguishing disorders of primary, secondary, and tertiary hemostasis are outlined in Table 124-1. Hemorrhagic disorders can be inherited or acquired, and the clinical and laboratory evaluation of such disorders is detailed in Chapters 130 and 131, respectively.

Disorders of Primary Hemostasis

Platelet plug formation, the first step in the arrest of bleeding at sites of injury, requires three key components (1) an adequate number of functional platelets; (2) vWF, the molecular glue that mediates platelet adhesion to the damaged vessel wall even in the face of high shear; and (3) a normal blood vessel that constricts in response to injury (Table 124-2). Because the platelet plug provides the first line of defense against bleeding, patients with disorders of primary hemostasis often present with immediate bleeding after injury and petechiae, pinpoint hemorrhages, may be noted. In addition to skin bleeding,

Table 124-1 Comparison of the Features of Disorders of Primary, Secondary, or Tertiary Hemostasis

Features	Primary	Secondary	Tertiary
Components involved	Platelets, vWF, and vessel wall	Coagulation	Fibrinolytic factors
Site of bleeding	Skin and mucocutaneous and soft tissues	Muscles, joints, and deep tissues	Wounds and genitourinary tract
Physical findings	Petechiae and ecchymoses	Hematomas and hemarthroses	Hematuria and menorrhagia
Timing of bleeding	Immediate	Delayed	Delayed
Inheritance	Autosomal dominant	Autosomal or X-linked recessive	Autosomal recessive

vWF, von Willebrand Factor

Table 124-2 Disorders of Primary Hemostasis

Components Affected	Causes
Platelets	Quantitative or qualitative platelet disorders
vWF	Inherited or acquired deficiency or dysfunction of vWF
Vessel wall	Vasculitis or abnormalities of connective tissue supporting the vasculature

vWF, von Willebrand factor

Table 124-3 Disorders of Secondary Hemostasis

Component Affected	Causes
Coagulation factors	Congenital deficiency, autoantibodies, increased consumption, or drugs that attenuate thrombin generation or thrombin activity
Fibrinogen	Decreased production; increased consumption or synthesis of an abnormal protein
	Impaired fibrin polymerization because of fibrin(ogen) degradation products or paraproteins
Fibrin cross-linking	Congenital or acquired factor XIII deficiency

mucocutaneous bleeding, which may manifest as epistaxis, bleeding gums, or hematochezia, is common as is excessive menstrual bleeding in women (see Chapter 130).

Disorders of primary hemostasis may be inherited or acquired.[23] Thrombocytopenia or congenital or acquired disorders of platelet function are common causes of bleeding. Thrombocytopenia can be the result of decreased production, which can occur because of failure, infiltration, or fibrosis of the bone marrow (see Chapters 27 and 28); increased platelet destruction; or abnormal distribution because of platelet pooling in the spleen (see Chapter 134). Increased destruction of platelets can occur via immune mechanisms, such as immune thrombocytopenic purpura (ITP), alloimmune thrombocytopenia, posttransfusion purpura and drug-induced thrombocytopenia (see Chapter 133), or nonimmune mechanisms, which include microangiopathic disorders, such as thrombotic thrombocytopenic purpura and hemolytic uremic syndrome (see Chapter 136), as well as consumption because of activation of coagulation, such as occurs with disseminated intravascular coagulation (see Chapter 141).

Platelet function disorders include disorders of (1) platelet adhesion, such as von Willebrand disease (see Chapter 140) and Bernard-Soulier syndrome (see Chapter 127); (2) thromboxane synthesis; (3) secretion, such as alpha or dense granule deficiency or aspirin-like secretion defects; (4) aggregation, such as Glanzmann thrombasthenia (see Chapter 127); or (5) procoagulant activity (Scott syndrome) in which the platelets fail to support clotting factor complex assembly (see Chapter 128). Acquired disorders of platelet function can occur in patients taking drugs that impair platelet function, such as aspirin or nonsteroidal antiinflammatory drugs, or in patients with uremia, paraproteins, or myelodysplastic or myeloproliferative disorders (see Chapter 132).

Bleeding can also occur with inflammation or malformations of the blood vessels or abnormalities of the connective tissue supporting the blood vessels. Inflammatory disorders include Henoch-Schonlein purpura (see Chapter 152) and the vasculitis that occurs with paraproteins or cryoglobulins or in patients with systemic lupus erythematosus or other immune disorders.[24] Hereditary hemorrhagic telangiectasia is an inherited disorder associated with malformations of the capillaries. Telangiectatic vessels can often be seen in the oral and nasal cavities of patients with this disorder and bleeding episodes, primarily from the nose and gastrointestinal tract, are common. Abnormalities of the connective tissue matrix supporting the blood vessels include Marfan syndrome, Ehlers-Danlos syndrome, and pseudoxanthoma elasticum.[25] Patients with these disorders frequently report easy bruising.

Disorders of Secondary Hemostasis

Secondary hemostasis depends on rapid generation of sufficient amounts of thrombin to generate a fibrin mesh that not only consolidates the platelet aggregates that form at sites of vascular injury but is also stable enough to provide a barrier that prevents leakage of blood from the damaged blood vessel.[18] Secondary hemostasis can be compromised by (1) impaired thrombin generation because of congenital or acquired deficiencies of coagulation factors or cofactors or intake of drugs that inhibit one or more steps in the coagulation pathways, (2) congenital or acquired fibrinogen deficiency or dysfunction, or (3) impaired cross-linking of fibrinogen because of congenital or acquired deficiency of factor XIII (Table 124-3).

Examples of inherited deficiencies of coagulation factors include hemophilia A and B, deficiencies of factor VIII and factor IX, respectively (see Chapter 137). Because of redundancy in the coagulation system, only patients with a factor VIII or factor IX level less than 1% have severe disease characterized by spontaneous bleeding or bleeding with minimal trauma. Whereas those with factor levels between 1% and 5% have an intermediate phenotype, patients with factor VIII or IX levels above 5% usually have mild disease and bleed only with trauma or surgery. The frequency of bleeding episodes in patients with severe hemophilia can be reduced by prophylactic administration of the appropriate factor concentrate; such treatment is also administered to those with hemophilia who have overt bleeding or in preparation for surgery or other major interventions. Management of hemophilia becomes more complicated if patients develop inhibitory antibodies that attenuate or abolish the activity of the infused factor (see Chapter 138). Congenital deficiencies of prothrombin (factor II), factors V, VII, X, or XI (hemophilia C) or fibrinogen are less common causes of bleeding (see Chapter 139). In contrast, deficiencies of components of the contact pathway (factor XII, high-molecular-weight kininogen, and prekallikrein) are not associated with bleeding. The clinical and laboratory evaluation of such patients are detailed in Chapters 130 and 131, respectively, and their treatment is outlined in Chapter 116.

Acquired deficiencies of coagulation factors can result from decreased synthesis because of severe liver disease, vitamin K deficiency or intake of drugs that interfere with vitamin K metabolism, consumption because of excessive activation of coagulation (e.g., disseminated intravascular coagulation; see Chapter 141), or accelerated clearance caused by adsorption by paraproteins or amyloid (see Chapters 85 and 86) or caused by autoantibodies that shorten the half-life or attenuate or abolish clotting factor activity.

Congenital disorders of fibrinogen include absence or low levels of fibrinogen (afibrinogenemia and hypofibrinogenemia, respectively) or synthesis of a dysfunctional protein (dysfibrinogenemia). Acquired disorders of fibrinogen include decreased synthesis or production of an abnormal fibrinogen and increased fibrinogen consumption or the presence of inhibitors that interfere with fibrin polymerization, such as paraproteins or autoantibodies, particularly in patients with systemic lupus erythematosus or other immune disorders or elevated levels of fibrin(ogen) degradation products.

Stabilization of fibrin requires cross-linking of the α and γ chains of adjacent fibrin monomers to yield a polymer that is resistant to premature breakdown. Factor XIIIa, a transglutaminase, performs this function by catalyzing the condensation of lysine residues on one chain with glutamic acid residues on another chain.[26] Congenital or acquired deficiency of factor XIII can impair cross-linking, resulting in bleeding. The hallmarks of severe factor XIII deficiency include umbilical stump bleeding in the neonatal period (see Chapter 152); intracranial hemorrhage with little or no trauma; recurrent soft tissue hemorrhages; and, in women, recurrent spontaneous miscarriages.

Table 124-4 Disorders of Tertiary Hemostasis

Component Affected	Causes
Plasminogen activators	Increased t-PA or u-PA release in the GU tract or other tissues
Plasmin	Deficiency of PAI-1 or α_2-antiplasmin, resulting in an increased plasmin concentration
Plasminogen activation	Enhanced plasminogen activation secondary to activation of coagulation by procoagulants, such as cancer cells, artificial surfaces, or snake venoms

GU, Genitourinary; *PAI-1*, plasminogen activator inhibitor 1; *t-PA*, tissue plasminogen activator; *u-PA*, urokinase-type plasminogen activator.

Disorders of Tertiary Hemostasis

Tertiary hemostasis depends on the generation of plasmin, which degrades fibrin and restores blood flow in damaged vessels. Premature lysis of fibrin in hemostatic plugs can lead to bleeding; this can occur systemically or can be localized (Table 124-4). Systemic fibrinolysis that occurs in the absence of activation of coagulation, so-called primary hyperfibrinolysis, is rare but can occur with inherited deficiency of PAI-1 or α_2-antiplasmin, the inhibitors of the plasminogen activators and plasmin, respectively; advanced liver disease; and some snake bites. More commonly, systemic hyperfibrinolysis is secondary to activation of coagulation by procoagulants such as tissue factor (e.g., in patients with metastatic cancer) or artificial surfaces (e.g., in cardiopulmonary bypass surgery or with cardiac assist devices). Examples of localized hyperfibrinolysis include menorrhagia or hematuria after prostatectomy triggered by excessive plasmin generation induced by the high concentrations of t-PA and u-PA in the uterus and genitourinary tract, respectively.

Thrombotic Disorders

Thrombosis may occur in arteries, in the chambers of the heart, or in the veins. Factors contributing to thrombosis in these sites include endothelial injury or activation, reduced blood flow, and hypercoagulability of the blood, the so-called Virchow triad.

Arterial Thrombosis

Most arterial thrombi occur on top of disrupted atherosclerotic plaques. Plaques with a thin fibrous cap and a lipid-rich core are most prone to disruption. Erosion or rupture of the fibrous cap exposes thrombogenic material in the lipid-rich core to the blood and triggers platelet activation and thrombin generation. The extent of plaque disruption and the content of thrombogenic material in the plaque determine the consequences of the event regardless of whether it occurs in the cerebral circulation (see Chapter 147), the coronary circulation (see Chapter 148), or the major arteries of the legs (see Chapter 150), but host factors also contribute. Breakdown of regulatory mechanisms that limit platelet activation and inhibit coagulation can augment thrombosis at sites of plaque disruption.

Decreased production of nitric oxide and prostacyclin by diseased endothelial cells can trigger vasoconstriction and platelet activation. Proinflammatory cytokines lower thrombomodulin expression by endothelial cells, which promotes thrombin generation, and stimulate PAI-1 expression, which inhibits fibrinolysis.

Products of blood coagulation contribute to atherogenesis, as well as to its complications (see Chapter 146). Microscopic erosions in the vessel wall trigger the formation of tiny platelet-rich thrombi.[27] Activated platelets release PDGF and TGFβ, which promote a fibrotic response. Thrombin generated at the site of injury not only activates platelets and converts fibrinogen to fibrin but also activates PAR-1 on smooth muscle cells and induces their proliferation, migration, and elaboration of extracellular matrix. Incorporation of thrombi into plaques promotes plaque growth, and decreased endothelial cell production of heparan sulfate—which normally limits smooth-muscle proliferation—contributes to plaque expansion.[27] The multiple links between atherosclerosis and thrombosis have prompted the term atherothrombosis (see Chapter 146).

Intracardiac Thrombosis

Thrombi can form in the left ventricle after transmural myocardial infarction or with an aneurysm or dyskinetic ventricle or in the left atrial appendage, particularly in patients with atrial fibrillation (see Chapter 149). Damage to the endothelium after myocardial infarction and abnormal blood flow are the major triggers for left ventricular thrombus formation. With rapid atrial fibrillation, there also is stasis and turbulent blood flow in the left atrial appendage, which is a long, blind-ended trabeculated pouch.[28] This may lead to localized activation of endothelial cells and subsequent loss of their anticoagulant phenotype, a process amplified by adhesion of leukocytes and subsequent elaboration of proinflammatory cytokines. The generation of thrombin creates a local hypercoagulable state that likely promotes thrombus formation on the abnormal endothelium. Embolization of these thrombi to the brain is a common cause of ischemic stroke and is the major cause of mortality and morbidity in patients with atrial fibrillation.

Venous Thrombosis

The causes of venous thrombosis include those associated with hypercoagulability, which can be genetic or acquired, and the mainly acquired risk factors, such as advanced age, obesity, or cancer, which are associated with immobility (see Chapters 142 and 144). Inherited hypercoagulable states and these acquired risk factors combine to establish the intrinsic risk of thrombosis for each individual.[2] Superimposed triggering factors, such as surgery, pregnancy, or hormonal therapy, modify this risk, and thrombosis occurs when the combination of genetic, acquired, and triggering forces exceed a critical threshold.[29]

Some acquired or triggering factors entail a higher risk than others. For example, major orthopedic surgery, neurosurgery, multiple trauma, and metastatic cancer (particularly adenocarcinoma) are associated with the highest risk; prolonged bed rest, antiphospholipid antibodies (see Chapter 143), and the puerperium period are associated with an intermediate risk; and pregnancy, obesity, long-distance travel, and the use of oral contraceptives or hormonal replacement therapy are mild risk factors. Up to half of patients who present with venous thromboembolism before the age of 45 years have inherited hypercoagulable disorders—so-called thrombophilia (see Chapter 142)—particularly those whose event occurred in the absence of risk factors or with minimal provocation, such as after minor trauma or a long-haul flight or with estrogen use.[30]

REFERENCES

1. Lippi G, Franchini M, Targher G: Arterial thrombus formation in cardiovascular disease. *Nat Rev Cardiol* 8:502, 2011.
2. Reitsma PH, Versteeg HH, Middledorp S: Mechanistic view of risk factors for venous thromboembolism. *Arterioscler Thromb Vasc Biol* 32:563, 2012.
3. Morris TA: Natural history of venous thromboembolism. *Crit Care Clin* 27:869, 2011.
4. van Hinsbergh VW: Endothelium: Role in regulation and coagulation and inflammation. *Semin Immunopathol* 34:93, 2012.
5. Crawley JT, Lane DA: The haemostatic role of tissue factor pathway inhibitor. *Arterioscler Thromb Vasc Biol* 28:233, 2008.

6. Danese S, Vetrano S, Zhang L, et al: The protein C pathway in tissue inflammation and injury: Pathogenic role and therapeutic implications. *Blood* 115:1121, 2010.
7. Nieswandt B, Pleines I, Bender M: Platelet adhesion and activation mechanisms in arterial thrombosis and ischaemic stroke. *J Thromb Haemost* 9:92, 2011.
8. Di Stasio E, De Cristofaro R: The effect of shear stress on protein conformation: Physical forces operating on biochemical systems: The case of von Willebrand factor. *Biophys Chem* 153:1, 2010.
9. Hechler B, Gachet C: P2 receptors and platelet function. *Purinergic Signal* 7:293, 2011.
10. Adams MN, Ramachandran R, Yau MK, et al: Structure, function and pathophysiology of protease activated receptors. *Pharmacol Ther* 130:248, 2011.
11. Bennett JS, Moore DT: Regulation of platelet beta 3 integrins. *Haematologica* 95:1049, 2010.
12. Owens AP 3rd, Mackman N: Tissue factor and thrombosis: The clot starts here. *Thromb Haemost* 104:432, 2010.
13. Owens AP 3rd, Mackman N: Microparticles in hemostasis and thrombosis. *Circ Res* 108:1284, 2011.
14. Mann KG: Thrombin generation in hemorrhage control and vascular occlusion. *Circulation* 124:225, 2011.
15. Fay PJ: Factor VIII structure and function. *Int J Hematol* 83:103, 2006.
16. Fager AM, Wood JP, Bouchard BA, et al: Properties of procoagulant platelets: Defining and characterizing the subpopulation binding a functional prothrombinase. *Arterioscler Thromb Vasc Biol* 30:2400, 2010.
17. Lord ST: Molecular mechanisms affecting fibrin structure and stability. *Arterioscler Thromb Vasc Biol* 31:494, 2011.
18. Wolberg AS: Plasma and cellular contributions to fibrin network formation, structure and stability. *Haemophilia* 16:7, 2010.
19. Gailani D, Renne T: The intrinsic pathway of coagulation: A target for treating thromboembolic disease? *J Thromb Haemost* 5:1106, 2007.
20. Muller F, Renne T: Novel roles for factor XII-driven plasma contact activation system. *Curr Opin Hematol* 15:516, 2008.
21. Schaller J, Gerber SS: The plasmin-antiplasmin system: Structural and functional aspects. *Cel Mol Life Sci* 68:785, 2011.
22. Heylen E, Willemse J, Hendriks D: An update on the role of carboxypeptidase U (TAFIa) in fibrinolysis. *Front Biosci* 17:2427, 2011.
23. Broos K, Feys HB, DeMeyer SF, et al: Platelets at work in primary hemostasis. *Blood Rev* 25:155, 2011.
24. Eby C: Pathogenesis and management of bleeding and thrombosis in plasma cell dyscrasias. *Br J Haematol* 145:151, 2009.
25. Malfait F, DePaepe A: Bleeding in the heritable connective tissue disorders: Mechanisms, diagnosis and treatment. *Blood Rev* 23:191, 2009.
26. Komaromi I, Bagoly Z, Muszbek L: Factor XIII: Novel structural and functional aspects. *J Thromb Haemost* 9:9, 2011.
27. Borissoff JI, Spronk HM, ten Cate H: The hemostatic system as a modulator of atherosclerosis. *N Engl J Med* 364:1746, 2011.
28. Watson T, Shantsila E, Lip GY: Mechanisms of thrombogenesis in atrial fibrillation: Virchow's triad revisited. *Lancet* 373:155, 2009.
29. Tchaikovski SN, Rosing J: Mechanisms of estrogen-induced venous thromboembolism. *Thromb Res* 126:5, 2010.
30. Anderson JA, Weitz JI: Hypercoagulable states. *Crit Care Clin* 27:933, 2011.

CHAPTER 125

THE BLOOD VESSEL WALL

Aly Karsan and John M. Harlan

The vasculature plays a major role in conveying and distributing hematopoietic cells, nutrients, gases, metabolites, and various chemical mediators.[1] The interior of the vessel wall is lined by the endothelium, comprising more than 1012 endothelial cells, covering a surface of approximately 500 m^2 and weighing approximately 1 kg in total.[2,3] The endothelium forms a continuous monolayer at the interface between blood and tissue. Thus it contributes significantly to sensing and transducing of signals between blood and tissue, trafficking of hematopoietic cells, and maintenance of a nonthrombogenic surface permitting flow of blood. Normally quiescent with cell turnover measured on the order of years, endothelial cells have a remarkable capacity to proliferate and vascularize tissues in physiologic (menstrual cycle) and pathologic (tumorigenesis, diabetic retinopathy) situations.[4] The endothelium is critical for initiating and potentiating the inflammatory response. The pathogenesis of several disorders, such as atherosclerosis, hypertension, diabetic angiopathy, and microangiopathic hemolytic anemias, involves dysfunction of the endothelial lining. The complexity and the vast array of its functional responses have led to the description of the endothelium as a distributed organ.[5] This chapter provides a conceptual framework of the structure and development of the vessel wall and the physiologic functions of the endothelium as it relates to the hematopoietic system.

STRUCTURE OF THE VESSEL WALL

The circulatory system has traditionally been divided into the macrovasculature (vessels >100 μm in diameter) and the microvasculature.[6] The arterial system transports blood to tissues, resists changes in blood pressure proximally, and regulates blood flow distally. Veins return blood to the heart and act as capacitance vessels because they contain approximately 70% of the total blood volume. Venules with luminal diameters less than 50 μm are structurally similar to capillaries.[6] Capillaries and microvessels in general are particularly important in the exchange of gases, macromolecules, and cells between blood and tissue. Although large vessels play an important role in maintaining vascular tone, a significant proportion of peripheral resistance arises from the capillaries.[7] Capillary endothelial cells also have a metabolic role, as in the conversion of angiotensin and hydrolysis of lipoproteins. Finally, sprouting of new vessels is initiated in the microvasculature.

Macrovasculature

Large vessels are composed of three layers: intima, media, and adventitia.[6,8] The intima comprises the endothelium and the subendothelium. The endothelial cells of large vessels contain a distinct rod-shaped organelle, measuring approximately 3 μm × 0.1 μm, called the Weibel-Palade body.[9] Ultrastructural studies indicate the presence of a single membrane around the Weibel-Palade body with tubular structures within. This organelle contains von Willebrand factor (vWF), and P-selectin has been reported to be present on the surrounding membrane.[10-12] The abluminal face of the endothelium rests on a basement membrane, which supports the endothelial cell and can act as a secondary barrier against the extravasation of blood.[2] The subendothelial matrix contains occasional smooth muscle cells and scattered macrophages. Both smooth muscle cells and endothelial cells contribute to the extracellular matrix (ECM) of the intima.[13,14] In large vessels, the media is separated from the intima by a layer of elastin, the internal elastic lamina. The medial layer is composed primarily of concentric layers of smooth muscle cells and their secreted matrix, which is a complex mix of glycoproteins and proteoglycans. This layer is responsible for the structural integrity of the wall and for maintaining vascular tone. Mutations of the fibrillin-1 gene, a microfilament protein in elastic fibers, result in disruption of the media in Marfan syndrome.[12] Defects of type III collagen can cause aortic rupture in patients with Ehlers-Danlos syndrome type IV.[14] An attenuated band of elastic fibers, the external elastic lamina, separates the adventitia from the media. The adventitia is composed of loose connective tissue, and the outer portion of the media contains small nerves and nutritive blood vessels, the vasa vasorum. The external limit of the adventitial layer is loosely defined and becomes continuous with the surrounding connective tissue of the organ.[6,8]

Microvasculature

Capillaries and postcapillary venules are composed of two cell types: endothelial cells and pericytes.[15] Pericytes and endothelial cells are invested with a basement membrane and, depending on the vascular bed, variable amounts of matrix separate the two cell types. Both cell types contribute to secretion of basement membrane proteins. Long pericyte processes extend over the abluminal surface of the endothelial cell, and reciprocal extensions of the endothelial cell make contact with the pericyte. Pericytes and endothelial cells communicate via gap junctions.[16] A variety of functions has been ascribed to the pericyte, including[15,17,18] (1) a contractile function, which regulates blood flow; (2) multipotential capabilities resulting in differentiation to adipocytes, osteoblasts, phagocytes, and smooth muscle cells; and (3) regulation of capillary growth. The best evidence probably exists for the last function. In animal models[19,20] and human disease (diabetic microangiopathy, hemangiomata),[21] a lack of pericytes is associated with microaneurysms and disordered microvasculature. In addition, there is a temporal correlation between pericyte contact and cessation of vessel growth in wound healing,[22] and pericyte contact suppresses endothelial cell migration and proliferation in vitro.[15]

Endothelial Structure and Function

In contrast to circulating blood cells and vascular smooth muscle cells but similar to epithelial cells, the endothelium exhibits polarity manifested by the asymmetric distribution of cell surface glycoproteins and by the unidirectional secretion of some ECM proteins and chemical mediators.[23,24] Although in cultured endothelial cells, an apical–basal polarity is established before confluence, intercellular junctions may have a role in maintaining the asymmetry in vivo.[23,25]

Four types of intercellular junctions between adjacent endothelial cells have been described[25,26]: tight junctions, gap junctions, adherens junctions, and syndesmos. Their distribution varies along the vascular tree, with tight junctions occurring more frequently in the larger arteries and brain vasculature, correlating with a more stringent requirement for permeability control. The molecular structure of endothelial tight junctions is similar to that of epithelial cells, consisting of a network of fibrils, with the integral membrane components composed of occludin, claudin-5, and junctional adhesion molecules (JAMs), which associate with various structural and signaling proteins on the cytoplasmic face.[27] The distribution of gap junctions tends to follow that of tight junctions. Connexin 37, connexin 40, and connexin 43 are gap junction proteins that have been detected in endothelial cells. Gap junctions mediate communication between adjacent endothelial cells and between endothelial cells and pericytes or smooth muscle cells; they also may contribute to the endothelial barrier. Adherens junctions are formed by transmembrane glycoproteins called cadherins, which make the link between cell-to-cell contacts and the cytoskeleton. Several different types of cadherins are expressed in endothelial cells. The endothelial-specific cadherin vascular endothelial cadherin (VE-cadherin [cadherin-5]) is expressed on virtually all types of endothelium.[26] Similar to other cadherins, VE-cadherin forms homotypic contacts with VE-cadherin on adjacent cells. Within the cell, VE-cadherin complexes with catenins, which, through other proteins, contact the actin cytoskeleton. Homotypic engagement of VE-cadherin results in density-dependent inhibition of endothelial proliferation, which appears to be mediated by association of vascular endothelial growth factor receptor 2 (VEGFR-2) with VE-cadherin, thereby sequestering VEGFR-2 at the membrane and preventing its internalization into signaling compartments.[28] The structure of the fourth type of junction, the syndesmos, is not well elucidated.

Other membrane proteins that are located at interendothelial junctions include platelet endothelial cell adhesion molecule 1 (PECAM-1), which may be important in directing the formation of junctions, and the integrins (particularly $\alpha 2\beta 1$ and $\alpha 5\beta 1$).[29] In addition to the functions listed previously, intercellular contacts are important in maintaining cell survival.[30]

On the luminal side, endothelium is exposed to blood elements and, under pathologic conditions, to circulating molecules such as cytokines and bacterial products. Engagement of endothelial receptors by these humoral factors activates a well-described series of responses. including the recruitment and transmigration of leukocytes and changes in endothelial cell coagulant activity (see The Endothelium as a Nonthrombogenic Surface). Biomechanical forces resulting from pulsatile blood flow have been shown to mediate striking changes in endothelial morphology and metabolism. Vessels must withstand three types of physical forces: radial distension (tension), longitudinal stretch, and tangential shear stress. In response to flow (shear stress), endothelial cells reorganize their cytoskeletal architecture, rearrange focal contacts at the basal surface, and align in the direction of flow.[31-33] Some endothelial cell responses following exposure to physical forces occur within seconds, such as activation of potassium channels and increased release of nitric oxide (NO), resulting in vasodilation. Other endothelial cell responses to flow are related to changes in gene expression and occur after a delay of a few hours. Elements in the promoters of various adhesion molecule and growth factor genes have been shown to contain sequences that respond to shear stress (in a positive or negative fashion) and have been referred to as the shear stress response element.[31-33]

Endothelial cells vectorially secrete certain ECM proteins to the abluminal face. The matrix molecules that are secreted by endothelium include several types of collagen, elastin, fibronectin, laminins, and proteoglycans (e.g., heparan sulfate, dermatan sulfate). The exact composition of the subendothelium varies with location in the vascular tree, age, and disease states.[2,14,34] Endothelial cells bind to the ECM via heterodimeric cell surface glycoproteins—the integrins—which link and integrate matrix proteins to the cytoskeleton at sites referred to as focal contacts.[35] The integrins detected in resting endothelium include $\alpha 6\beta 1$, $\alpha 5\beta 1$, $\alpha 2\beta 1$, and $\alpha v\beta 3$.[36] Interestingly, endothelial cells express integrins on luminal as well as abluminal surfaces.[36] The ECM serves several important functions: (1) it serves as a barrier to macromolecules in the event of disruption of the endothelium; (2) it sequesters growth factors and mediates their high-affinity binding to endothelial cells (e.g., heparan sulfate binds to fibroblast growth factor [FGF]); and (3) it acts as a counterstructure for the binding of endothelial cell integrins.[14,34,37] This binding of endothelial cells to the ECM serves at least four purposes: (1) Whereas certain matrix molecules provide a physical scaffold, others act as haptotactic agents, inducing endothelial cells to migrate.[14] (2) Clustering of integrins at focal adhesion contacts by certain matrix molecules can transduce survival or differentiation signals by causing phosphorylation of various proteins and lipids.[37] Whereas fibronectin and vitronectin provide survival signals, laminins appear to signal differentiation.[38-40] (3) By maintaining cell shape, integrin-mediated cell spreading provides an antiapoptotic signal independent of direct integrin-initiated signal transduction.[41] (4) By anchoring the cell, the matrix provides a mechanism whereby blood flow at the luminal surface of the endothelium creates shear stress, which also transmits signals to cells.[31]

Endothelial Heterogeneity

Despite their common features, quiescent endothelial cells in vivo represent a widely heterogeneous population, with their phenotype depending on vessel caliber and location. Exposure to different physical forces (e.g., arteries vs. veins) and the different functions served by vessels of different caliber are reflected in different endothelial phenotypes.[42] However, study of the molecular basis of the heterogeneity of these different populations is just beginning. Experiments using serial analysis of gene expression and in vivo delivery of phage display peptide libraries have revealed organ- and tumor vasculature–specific molecules that will help to elucidate the molecular basis of endothelial heterogeneity.[43-45] Within the microvasculature is a structural heterogeneity of capillaries, depending on the organ supplied. Even within a single organ, endothelial cells exhibit different phenotypes, depending on their functional role. When microvessels from different organs are harvested and cultured in vitro, they lose some of their distinctive characteristics with progressive passaging. Some specialization of the different endothelial cells can be retained if they are cocultured with cells or matrix from the organ from which they are derived. Thus matrix proteins, soluble factors from the organ, or heterotypic contacts with parenchymal cells or pericyte or smooth muscle cells are believed to be important factors in specifying endothelial cell phenotype.[46] Conversely, emerging evidence indicates that endothelial cells in turn provide instructive morphogenic cues during organogenesis and in adults.[47] Specific examples of microvessels found in hematopoietic tissues are discussed in the following sections.

High Endothelial Venules

Lymphocyte migration into secondary lymphoid sites, such as lymph nodes, Peyer patches, and chronically inflamed nonlymphoid tissues, occurs at specialized postcapillary venules.[48] The endothelial cells of these venules exhibit a plump or cuboidal morphology (hence the name high endothelial venule), display intense biosynthetic activity, and are encircled by a continuous basal lamina. They secrete a thick glycocalyx of which a proportion is glycosylation-dependent cell adhesion molecule 1, a ligand for L-selectin.[49] CD34 is another high endothelial venule "addressin" on peripheral lymph node endothelial cells. Endothelium of mesenteric lymph nodes and Peyer patches express mucosal addressin cellular adhesion molecule 1 (MAdCAM-1) as a ligand for L-selectin and $\alpha 4\beta 7$ integrin. Expression of these different addressins may recruit specific subpopulations of lymphocytes to different lymphoid tissues (i.e., they facilitate the "homing" of lymphocytes). Several other proteins, including the chemokine receptor DARC (Duffy antigen receptor for chemokines) and the antiadhesive matrix protein Hevin, have been identified as being preferentially expressed by the high endothelial venule.[50] Tight junctions are present at intermittent spots, and extensive overlap between the membranes of adjacent cells prevents macromolecules from interendothelial transit. However, when lymphoid cells transit to the high endothelial venule, there is a temporary breach in the barrier.[49] Evidence suggests that the high endothelial venule not only plays a critical role in homing and recruitment of immune cells but also can influence the outcome of the immune response.[51]

Bone Marrow Sinuses

Much less is known about the bone marrow (BM) sinuses than about the high endothelial venule. The BM sinus endothelial cell is flat, in contrast to that of the high endothelial venule, and the basal lamina is discontinuous. It has been suggested that hematopoietic cells traverse pores present at attenuated areas of the endothelium rather than moving by an interendothelial route.[52] Clearly, the BM sinus endothelial cell is specialized given the regulated egress of cells from the BM. For example, if a red blood cell (RBC) that still is nucleated begins to enter the circulation, the body of the cell is allowed to cross and is released as a reticulocyte, while the nucleus is retained extravascularly. The adventitial reticular cell (similar to a pericyte) is also thought to play an important role in controlling hematopoietic cell egress.[53] Stromal cell–derived factor 1 (SDF-1, also called CXCL12) and chemokine receptor CXCR4 interactions are essential for stem cell homing, mobilization, and transendothelial migration into the BM.[54,55] SDF-1 activates the integrins lymphocyte function-associated antigen 1 (LFA-1 [$\alpha L\beta 2$]), very late antigen 4 (VLA-4 [$\alpha 4\beta 1$]), and very late antigen 5 (VLA-5 [$\alpha 5\beta 1$]). Whereas vascular cell adhesion molecule 1 (VCAM-1), which is expressed on BM endothelial cells (and spleen endothelial cells in the mouse), appears to be the major BM addressin for hematopoietic progenitor cells expressing VLA-4, intercellular adhesion molecule 1 (ICAM-1) binds LFA-1.[55,56] Endothelial selectins also have been implicated in promoting hematopoietic progenitor homing to the BM.[57] Factors such as CD44, cytoskeletal rearrangement, and matrix metalloproteinases (MMPs) are other key players in the homing process related to the endothelium.[55] The BM endothelium also is involved in regulating hematopoiesis (see Relationship Between Vascular Development and Hematopoiesis).

VASCULAR DEVELOPMENT AND DIFFERENTIATION

The human embryo develops a vascular system by the third week, when its nutritional needs are no longer met by diffusion.[58] Vascular development proceeds in several ways. Vasculogenesis is the process whereby blood vessels form de novo from the differentiation of mesodermal precursors. Angiogenesis is the outgrowth of new capillaries from preexisting vessels and is thought to be the major mode of new vessel development in the adult. Arteriogenesis, or collateral development, is the rapid enlargement of preexisting collateral arterioles after occlusion of a supply artery. Lymphangiogenesis is the development of lymphatic vessels, which are required for transportation of extravasated lymph and lymphoid cells. Finally, in some neoplasms, tumor cells rather than endothelial cells form vascular channels or a portion of some vessels, a process termed *vasculogenic mimicry*.[59] A similar nonendothelial cell lining of vascular channels can be created by placental cytotrophoblasts forming hybrid fetal–maternal vessels in the endometrium.[59]

Vasculogenesis

Vasculogenesis in the yolk sac proceeds initially by the differentiation of mesodermal cells into angioblasts.[60] Angioblasts are vascular cells that express some, but not all, endothelial markers. These cells arise from mesodermal cells resting on the endoderm (splanchnopleuric mesoderm) but not from the mesoderm adjacent to the ectoderm (somatopleuric mesoderm). Thus it is believed that whereas the endoderm positively regulates vascular development, the ectoderm negatively regulates vasculogenesis. Organs that are primarily of ectodermal origin (e.g., brain and kidney) are vascularized by angiogenesis and not by vasculogenesis. The mesodermal cells migrating outward from the endoderm form primitive structures termed *blood islands*. Whereas the cells at the center of the blood island are hematopoietic precursors, those arranged peripherally are angioblastic precursors. Vasculogenesis within the embryo begins shortly after that in the yolk sac, again in close association with endoderm.[61] However, except for a region on the ventral aspect of the embryonic aorta, intraembryonic vascular development occurs in solitary angioblasts rather than blood islands. Angioblasts differentiate in situ and form primary capillary plexuses with lumens, or they migrate and fuse with other angioblasts or capillaries. Fusion of angioblasts or blood islands results in the formation of a capillary plexus that undergoes extensive remodeling over the developmental period.[60]

Vasculogenesis in the Adult

Although initially said to occur primarily in the embryo, vasculogenesis may also play a role in promoting vascular development in adults. The identification of circulating BM-derived vascular precursors and the demonstration that these precursors can integrate into the vasculature at sites of angiogenesis describe an adult form of de novo vessel development.[62] Two distinct BM-derived precursors with the ability to differentiate into vascular cells have been identified: (1) accumulating evidence points to a single precursor, the hemangioblast, which can differentiate into either hematopoietic or endothelial cells,[63] and (2) a multipotent nonhematopoietic adult progenitor cell, which is thought to represent a BM mesenchymal stem cell. When injected intravenously into adult mice, these mesenchymal stem cells differentiated into vascular cells, hematopoietic cells, and several epithelial cell types.[64,65] Both types of multipotential precursor populations express CD133, a cell surface marker that is lost upon further maturation.[66] However, only the hemangioblast expresses CD34. Whether mesenchymal stem cells are able to circulate and thus contribute to neovascularization outside the BM remains to be shown. Various stresses, including neoplasia, sepsis, burns, and trauma, have been suggested to induce mobilization of BM-derived endothelial precursors, which express CD133, CD34, and VEGFR-2.[66] Cytokines that reportedly induce mobilization of BM-derived endothelial precursors include VEGF-A and granulocyte macrophage colony-stimulating factor (GM-CSF).[66] The contribution of BM-derived vascular precursors to angiogenic vessels in tumors is highly variable, depending on the study, the model used, and the tumor cell type used.[67] The degree of endothelial precursor incorporation into the angiogenic vasculature is highly controversial; several groups suggest negligible, if any, involvement by distant precursors.[67] The problem arises in part from the poor definition of a circulating endothelial precursor cell. Many, if not all, of the markers used to define this rare cell population are shared with hematopoietic stem or progenitor cells, and the distinction between the endothelial and hematopoietic precursor has not been rigorously addressed in the majority of studies. More recent work has suggested that BM-derived, perivascular CD11b+ hematopoietic cells secreting angiogenic cytokines have been misidentified as endothelial precursor cells.[68,69]

Angiogenesis

In a normal adult, angiogenesis occurs primarily in the female reproductive system. However, angiogenesis is a process that has a major impact in several pathologic situations. Probably the best-known and studied example of pathologic neovascularization occurs during tumor progression. Angiogenesis also is important in chronic inflammation, ischemia, and wound healing.

Capillary sprouts from the existing microvasculature form secondary to an inciting stimulus that results in increased vascular permeability, accumulation of extravascular fibrin, and local proteolytic degradation of the basement membrane.[70-72] Endothelial cells overlying the disrupted region become "activated," change shape, and extend elongated processes into the surrounding tissue. Filopodia extending from the specialized endothelial cells at the tip of the vascular sprout guide the migration of the nascent vessel.[73] Directed migration toward the angiogenic stimulation results in the formation of a column of endothelial cells. Just proximal to the migrating tip of the column is a region of proliferating endothelial cells. These proliferating cells cause an increase in the length of the sprout. In the region of proliferation, up to 20% of endothelial cells may enter the cell cycle. This is in marked contrast to quiescent endothelium, of which less than 0.01% of cells are cycling. Proximal to the proliferative zone, the endothelial cells undergo another shape change, adhere tightly to each other, and begin to form a lumen. Evidence suggests that endothelial lumina arise through the formation and fusion of intracellular vacuoles.[74] Secondary sprouting from the migrating tip results in a capillary plexus, and fusion of individual sprouts at their tips closes the loop and circulates blood into the vascularized area. Activated macrophages and platelets, by secreting growth factors, cytokines, proteases, and protease inhibitors, can influence all phases of the angiogenic process.[75]

The morphologic features described are characteristic of sprouting angiogenesis. *Intussusceptive microvascular growth* refers to vascular network formation by insertion of interstitial tissue columns, called tissue pillars or posts, into the vascular lumen and subsequent growth of these columns, resulting in partitioning of the vessel lumen. The mechanisms of intussusceptive angiogenesis are less well described, but hemodynamic factors appear to be involved.[76]

Recruitment of Periendothelial Cells

Whether formed by vasculogenesis or angiogenesis, maturation of new vessels requires recruitment of smooth muscle cells or pericytes to reestablish vessel integrity. Periendothelial cells provide structural support, assist in production of the ECM, provide contractile function so as to modulate vessel caliber, and maintain the cells in a quiescent state. Genetically altered mice that fail to invest their vessels with pericytes develop microaneurysms.[19] In embryos, periendothelial cells are thought to be derived from locally available mesenchymal cells as endothelial cells invade organ rudiments. Local derivation of periendothelial cells may be one mechanism that allows for tissue-specific phenotype of the vasculature.[15] Evidence suggests that embryonic endothelial cells may transdifferentiate into vascular smooth muscle cells.[77] Evidence also indicates that some periendothelial cells are derived from the neural crest during embryogenesis and from BM-derived precursors in adults.[78-81] Although some studies have shown pericytes to be potential antivascular targets for tumor therapy,[80,82] other work has suggested that pericytes act to limit tumor metastasis.[83]

Extracellular Matrix

It is thought that whereas interstitial collagens (e.g., collagen I) and provisional plasma-derived fibronectin–fibrin matrices stimulate endothelial tubular morphogenic events, laminin-rich matrices lead to endothelial differentiation and stabilization events.[75] Mice deficient in fibronectin die during embryogenesis and show vascular defects. Type I collagen-deficient mice die of circulatory failure just before birth. Although most tumor vessels are covered by basement membrane, this layer has multiple structural abnormalities consistent with ongoing vascular activation in tumors.[84] ECM proteins or their proteolytic fragments have been shown to inhibit angiogenesis.

Dissolution of the underlying matrix by MMPs and heparanases allows endothelial cells to migrate at the initiation of angiogenesis.[85,86] Matrix-bound growth factors are also released as a consequence of ECM degradation. The balance between positive and negative regulators is the basis of tight control in this process. Tissue plasminogen activator (t-PA) and urokinase plasminogen activator, by generating plasmin, can activate collagenases and other MMPs. Plasminogen activator inhibitors (PAIs) may block angiogenesis at this step. Action of the MMPs is required for angiogenesis, and the tissue inhibitors of MMPs regulate their function.[87]

Cell Adhesion Molecules

Of the various classes of cell adhesion molecules involved in angiogenesis, the integrins have been the most studied.[14,88,89] Although it is universally accepted that integrins and integrin ligands function in angiogenesis, their exact actions remain unclear. In particular, substantial controversy surrounds the role of $\alpha v\beta 3$ integrin.[14,88,90] Immunohistochemical studies localize this integrin to the tips of sprouting vessels. Neutralizing antibodies abrogate angiogenesis and induce vascular cell apoptosis in vivo. However, mice lacking αv show extensive angiogenesis, and mice and humans (Glanzmann thrombasthenia) lacking $\beta 3$ integrin also show normal angiogenesis. Notwithstanding the discrepancies outlined, preclinical studies have validated $\alpha v\beta 3$ and potentially other integrins ($\alpha v\beta 5$, $\alpha 1\beta 1$, $\alpha 2\beta 1$, $\alpha 5\beta 1$, $\alpha 6\beta 4$) as therapeutic antiangiogenic targets, and clinical trials with combination therapy are currently in progress.[91] One of the integrin receptors for fibronectin, $\alpha 5\beta 1$, has been shown to be necessary for vascular development, and $\alpha 2\beta 1$ seems important for the formation of tubes by endothelial cells in vitro. However, there likely is a dynamic regulation of $\beta 1$ integrins during angiogenesis because constitutive activation of this integrin inhibits endothelial sprouting in vitro and angiogenesis in vivo.[92] The junctional proteins VE-cadherin and PECAM-1, and possibly JAM-1, are expressed early in development and have a role in assembling the vasculature.[28,93,94]

Guidance Molecules

Similar to the nervous system, the vascular system forms a highly ordered, branching network. The ordering of this patterned network is dependent on multiple attractive and repulsive cues, many of which are common to both the nervous and vascular systems.[95,96] Whereas VEGF165 acts as an attractive cue to the tip cell of the endothelial sprout, Netrin1 signals to UNC5b on the vasculature act as a repulsive cue. Other guidance pathways implicated in vascular patterning and angiogenesis are ephrinB2–EphB4, plexinD1–semaphorin, and Slit–Robo interactions, as well as the neuropilins. Patterning and specification of small arteries along peripheral nerves in the skin of the embryonic limb involves nerve-derived VEGF; in other situations, neuronal patterning is dependent on the vasculature.[97,98] Thus the congruent patterning of the neural and vascular systems likely is caused by use of common signals and may require cross-talk between the two systems.

Remodeling, Regression, and Apoptosis

Even though the vasculature is laid down before circulation begins, hemodynamic forces are important for maintenance and remodeling. Most of the vessels laid down during vasculogenesis regress or are remodeled. After neovascularization (e.g., during wound healing), the vessels regress when no longer needed. A chronic decrease in blood flow results in narrowing of the vessel lumen. This change in vessel caliber is dependent on an intact and functional endothelium.[99] Remodeling, which involves loss of some vessels as well as changes in lumen diameter and wall thickness, requires both cell death and proliferation (as well as remodeling of the ECM). In addition to survival signals transmitted by integrins, shear stress is important for endothelial survival and vessel healing after injury.[100-102] Oxygen tension is important in vascular maintenance. Hypoxia increases levels of VEGF, which provides signals for vessel maintenance and neovascularization.[103] Hyperoxia, on the other hand, inhibits VEGF expression, which leads to regression and death of retinal vessels.[104] In some models, regression of vessels occurs by apoptosis of vascular cells.[105,106] Endothelial cells express several antiapoptotic molecules to maintain viability when quiescent and when stressed.[107,108] Most likely, an intricate balance between cell death and proliferation is maintained by activators and inhibitors of both processes.

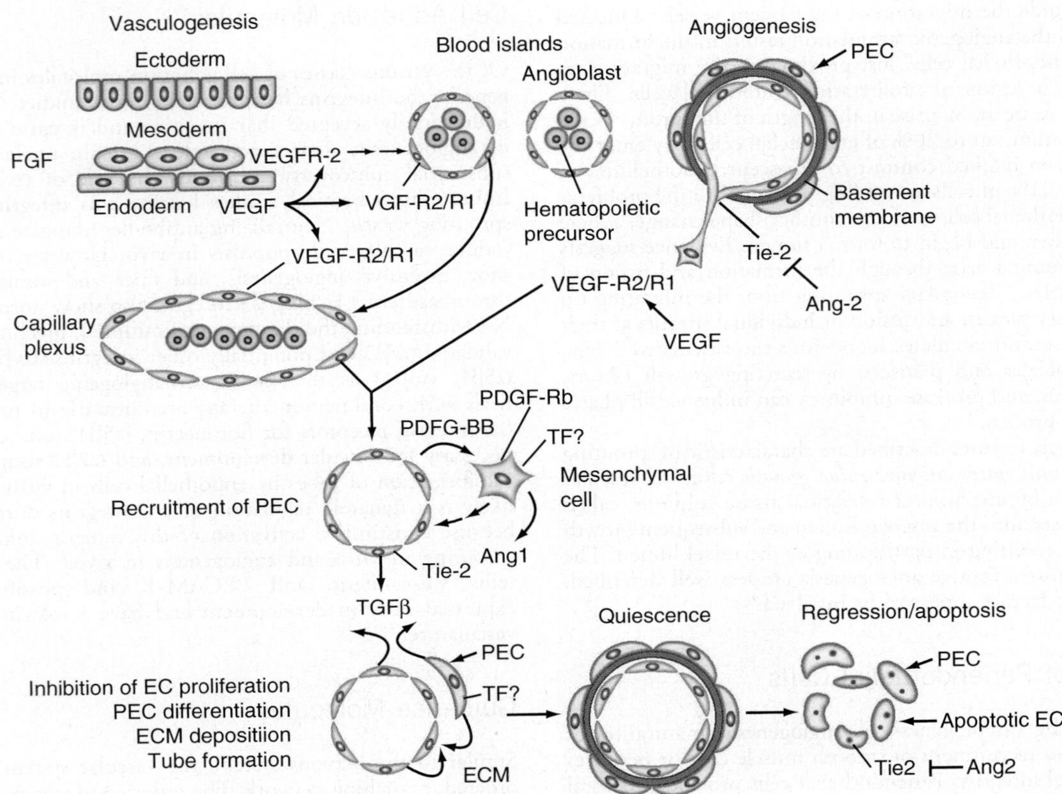

Figure 125-1 MODEL FOR VASCULAR DEVELOPMENT. The role of secreted proteins and membrane receptors in vascular development is highlighted, but other factors such as cell adhesion molecules and extracellular matrix components also contribute significantly. *Ang,* Angiopoietin; *ECM,* extracellular matrix; *FGF,* fibroblast growth factor; *PDGF,* platelet-derived growth factor; *PEC,* periendothelial cell (smooth muscle cell, pericyte); *TF,* tissue factor; *TGFβ,* transforming growth factor-β; *VEGF,* vascular endothelial cell growth factor; *VEGF-R,* vascular endothelial cell growth factor receptor.

Role of Ligand–Receptor Interactions

Numerous factors regulate vascular development and differentiation in a positive or negative fashion. Some of the key molecules and their receptors are discussed here. A model for vascular development is shown in Fig. 125-1.

Inducers of Angiogenesis

Fibroblast Growth Factors

The role of FGFs in vascular development remains murky.[109-111] Because of possible functional redundancy in the numerous family members, assigning specific roles to the various members of the FGF family has been difficult. Evidence suggests that FGF receptors signal an inductive pathway by upregulating VEGFR-2 in differentiating mesoderm before vascular morphogenesis.[111-113] FGF2 may induce neovascularization in adults indirectly through activation of the VEGF–VEGFR pathway.[114]

Vascular Endothelial Growth Factors

Six members of the VEGF family have been identified[70,109,111,115-119]: VEGF-A (also called vascular permeability factor), VEGF-B, VEGF-C, VEGF-D, VEGF-E (a viral ortholog), and placental growth factor. Three members of the receptor tyrosine kinase family[109,118,119]—VEGFR-1 (flt-1), VEGFR-2 (flk-1/KDR), and VEGFR-3 (flt-4)—respond differentially to individual members of the VEGF family. In addition, the coreceptors for VEGF, neuropilin 1 and neuropilin 2, have been identified on arterial and venous endothelial cells, respectively. Neuropilin 1 is a coreceptor for VEGFR-2 that enhances binding of the VEGF-A isoform VEGF165 to VEGFR-2.[118] VEGF-A functions as a homodimer. However, it also heterodimerizes with VEGF-B and placental growth factor, and it has a crucial dose-dependent effect on vasculogenesis.[70,109,111,118,119] Whereas VEGF-A binds VEGFR-1 and VEGFR-2, VEGF-C binds VEGFR-2 and VEGFR-3. Whereas placental growth factor specifically activates VEGFR-1, VEGF-E binds only VEGFR-2.[111,118,119] Lack of VEGFR-2 prevents the development of endothelial cells and a hematopoietic system because cells lacking VEGFR-2 do not reach the correct location to form blood islands.[120] Mice that have been rendered deficient for VEGFR-1 have normal hematopoietic progenitors and abundant endothelial cells, but they do not form capillary tubes or functional vessels.[121] Both VEGFR-2– and VEGFR-1–deficient mice die at an early embryonic stage, as do neuropilin 1– and neuropilin 2–deficient mice. In von Hippel-Lindau disease, development of hemangioblastomas may be caused by stabilization of VEGF mRNA.[122] VEGF is also believed to play a key role in propagating tumor angiogenesis. Whereas tip cell migration has been shown to be dependent on a gradient of VEGF-A, endothelial proliferation in the lengthening vascular stalk is dependent on the absolute concentration of VEGF-A, although both processes require VEGFR-2.[73] Finally, injection of VEGF is capable of relieving limb ischemia by the generation of collateral vessels.[72] Whereas VEGF appears to collaborate with the angiopoietins (Angs) to stimulate vascular development, VE-cadherin acts to temper the VEGF response.[28]

Angiopoietins

The Ang family of secreted glycoproteins comprises four members: Ang1 to Ang4. All four bind to Tie2, a receptor tyrosine kinase.[123-126] Whereas Ang1 and Ang4 act as agonists of Tie2, Ang2 and Ang3 function as antagonists of Tie2.[126] However, the action of Ang2 is context dependent, and in some environments, it may behave as an agonist.[126] Binding of Ang1 to Tie2 results in tyrosine phosphorylation of Tie2 and promotes endothelial cell survival but not proliferation.[123,126] Early in development, Ang1 is found mainly in the myocardium surrounding the endocardium, but it also becomes expressed in the mesenchyme surrounding developing vessels.[123] Disruption of either Ang1 or its receptor Tie2 in the mouse results in embryonic lethality because of similar defects.[124,127] These mice die at a slightly later stage than do VEGFR-deficient mice. Although endothelial cells are present, they have a lack of vascular complexity and a scarcity of periendothelial cells. Reciprocal interactions between the endothelial cells and surrounding matrix and mesenchyme appear to be disrupted. An activating Tie2 mutation in humans causes vascular malformations that show a disproportionate number of endothelial cells compared with smooth muscle cells, resulting in dilated, tortuous vascular channels in certain tissues.[128] Mice engineered to overexpress Ang2 specifically in their vasculature show embryonic lethality and vascular defects that are reminiscent of those seen in Ang1- or Tie2-null embryos.[125] In one proposed model, Ang1–Tie2 coupling mediates vascular maturation by sustaining endothelial cell–periendothelial cell–matrix interactions and may be involved in maintaining endothelial cell quiescence. Because Ang2 is found only at sites of vascular remodeling, Ang2 loosens matrix contacts, thus allowing access and responsiveness to angiogenic factors such as VEGF.[125,126] In the absence of growth factors, disruption of the vessel architecture by Ang2 may result in vascular cell apoptosis and vessel regression. However, Ang2-deficient mice are born alive, and the major defect appears to be lymphatic development.[126] Thus, despite major advances, the data are conflicting. The response of endothelial cells to the Angs likely is context dependent and endothelial cell type specific.[126]

Tie1 is a receptor tyrosine kinase that exhibits structural similarities to Tie2. A ligand for Tie1 has not yet been identified.[109,129] Disruption of the Tie1 gene in mice results in lethality at a much later point in development; Tie1-null mice may survive up to birth.[127,130] Tie1$^{-/-}$ mice die of hemorrhage and edema, implicating Tie1 in signaling the control of fluid exchange across capillaries and in maintenance of vessel integrity under hemodynamic stress. Chimeric mice that express Tie1$^{-/-}$ and Tie1$^{+/-}$ endothelial cells show underrepresentation of Tie1$^{-/-}$ cells in vessels primarily derived by angiogenesis but not in embryonic vessels derived by vasculogenesis, suggesting a differential function for Tie1 in angiogenesis.[131] Evidence also implicates a role for Tie1 in combination with Ang1 in establishing vascular polarity.[132]

Platelet-Derived Growth Factors

The platelet-derived growth factor (PDGF) family is composed of four chains. PDGF-A and PDGF-B can associate in a homodimeric or heterodimeric fashion.[133] Similarly, the receptors α and β are receptor tyrosine kinases that can form homodimers or heterodimers. PDGF-BB can bind the receptors PDGFR-ββ or PDGFR-αβ, but PDGFR-ββ binds only PDGF-BB and not PDGF-AA or PDGF-AB.[109] Mice that are null for PDGF-B die perinatally of renal, hematologic, and cardiovascular abnormalities.[134] The large vessels and heart of these mice are dilated, and microvessels exhibit microaneurysms because of a lack of pericytes.[19,134] PDGFR-β knock-out mice do not show an overtly abnormal cardiovascular phenotype, but generation of chimeric mice demonstrates that PDGFR-β$^{-/-}$ cells are underrepresented in all muscle lineages (smooth, cardiac, and skeletal).[135,136] Thus, it appears that PDGF-BB elaborated by the endothelial cell provides a signal to recruit mesenchymal periendothelial cells as part of the maturation process of vascular morphogenesis. Two novel PDGF chains, PDGF-C and PDGF-D, have been identified.[137] PDGF-CC can bind PDGFR-ββ or PDGFR-αβ, exhibits greater mitogenicity of mesenchymal cells than does PDGF-AA, and promotes wound repair. PDGF-DD activates PDGFR-ββ and possibly PDGFR-αβ. PDGF-DD expression has been found to be elevated in the serum of patients with various types of tumors and has been shown to have transforming and angiogenic activity.[137]

Transforming Growth Factors β

Members of the transforming growth factor-β (TGFβ) family are multifunctional homodimeric peptides with diverse effects on cell proliferation, migration, differentiation, adhesion, and expression of cell adhesion molecules and ECM.[109,138,139] They are secreted as inactive precursors. After being activated, they transmit signals to cells by binding heteromeric complexes of type I and type II serine/threonine kinase receptors. In most cell types, the type I receptor engaged by TGFβ is activin receptor-like kinase 5 (ALK5). However, in endothelial cells, TGFβ can bind and signal through ALK5 and ALK1.[140] Contact between endothelial cells and periendothelial cells is required for production of active TGFβ.[15] Mice lacking TGFβ or TGFβ receptor type II exhibit similar defects in vasculogenesis and hematopoiesis.[138,139] Endothelial proliferation is not affected, but poor contacts between endothelial cell and mesothelial layers in embryos of TGFβ$^{-/-}$ mice result in a disorganized and reduced vascular network lacking capillary tubes. Mutations in two TGFβ receptors, ALK1 and the accessory TGFβ receptor endoglin, have been linked to the vascular disorder hereditary hemorrhagic telangiectasia.[140] Disruption of TGFβ signaling likely plays a role in the telangiectasia seen in this disorder.

Notch

The Notch family is composed of four receptors (Notch1 through Notch4) and five ligands (Jagged1 and Jagged2 and Delta-like 1 [Dll1], Dll3, and Dll4). Ligand engagement results in a series of proteolytic clips that release the Notch intracellular domain, which then translocates to the nucleus where it effects transcriptional activation via the DNA-binding protein CSL (also called RBP-Jκ or CBF1).[141] Gene targeting studies have revealed a critical role for Notch1, Dll1, Dll4, and Jagged1 in vascular development and remodeling.[141] Dll4–Notch1 signaling between endothelial cells within the angiogenic sprout serves to restrict tip cell formation in response to VEGF.[142-144] Consequently, inhibition of Dll4 in adult mice results in increased endothelial proliferation, sprouting, and branching and increased tumor vascularity.[145,146] However, the vasculature is disorganized and poorly perfused; thus Dll4 blockade inhibits tumor growth in several models.[145,146]

Coagulation Factors

Tissue factor (TF) is a member of the cytokine receptor superfamily. In addition to its role in initiating coagulation as a cofactor for factor VII, TF may be involved in intracellular signaling. TF knockout mice have abnormalities of their large vessels and microvasculature secondary to defects in mesenchymal cell and periendothelial cell accumulation and function.[20] Elevated TF expression in various tumors and the associated angiogenic endothelium has been reported.[147] Expression of mutant oncogenes (K-*ras,* EGFR) or tumor suppressor genes (PTEN, p53) leads to increased TF expression and activity, and this may link tumor angiogenesis and the hypercoagulable states manifested in cancer.[147] Abnormal development of the vasculature also affects 50% of mice that are deficient in factor V. The affected mice die in utero, and the 50% embryonic lethality is similar to that observed in thrombin receptor–deficient mice that die without obvious coagulation defects.[148] Factor V–dependent generation of thrombin may be important for early vascular development by signaling through the thrombin receptor.[149] Thrombin can promote angiogenesis through a mechanism that is independent of fibrin formation.[149,150] Studies have suggested that thrombin can stimulate release of angiogenic factors (e.g., VEGF-A) from tumor cells and platelets as well as induce VEGFR-2 on endothelial cells.[150]

Clinical trials have revealed that treatment with low-molecular-weight heparins improves the survival time of cancer patients receiving chemotherapy, an effect that appears to be independent of the anticoagulant properties of the low-molecular-weight heparins.[151,152] Although antiangiogenic effects of specific heparanase-generated fragments of unfractionated heparins have been demonstrated in vitro, the mechanism of the antitumor effect remains to be defined.

The potential involvement of fibrinolytic factors in angiogenesis has been mentioned. Interestingly, fragments 1 and 2 of prothrombin have been reported to inhibit angiogenesis, and various other fragments of coagulation and fibrinolytic proteins also may inhibit angiogenesis.[153]

Other Factors

Various other families of ligand–receptor pairs play a role in angiogenesis. They include ephrin-Eph, Wnt-frizzled, and sonic hedgehog-smoothened. Various chemokines have been shown to modulate angiogenesis in either a positive or negative fashion.

Inhibitors of Angiogenesis

As with the angiogenesis inducers, multiple factors have been reported to negatively regulate vascular morphogenesis.[72,153] Of interest is a class of endogenous angiogenesis inhibitors that are fragments of larger proteins that have little or no angiogenesis-related activity in their intact form. They include fragments of ECM proteins such as fibronectin, collagen type IV α3 chain (tumstatin), and collagen type XIII (endostatin), as well as coagulation protein fragments such as plasminogen (angiostatin) and antithrombin.[153] The mechanism of action of these protein fragments depends on the particular polypeptide, but the functional effect usually is inhibition of endothelial proliferation or induction of apoptosis.[153-155] Other endogenous inhibitors include interferons, chemokines, and interleukin-12 (IL-12).

More than 100 compounds are in clinical trials attempting to cause regression of tumors by inhibiting angiogenesis.[156] These compounds can be broadly divided into those that act directly by targeting the angiogenic endothelial cell and those that act indirectly by targeting activators of angiogenesis. The latter category includes targeting of oncogenes (e.g., mutant EGFR or Her2) because many aberrantly activated oncogenes have been shown to induce expression of angiogenic factors. The first clear-cut evidence of efficacy in clinical trials of an angiogenic inhibitor for tumor therapy came from regimens directed against the VEGF pathway (e.g., bevacizumab).[157,158] Because of the short improvement in overall and progression-free survival with the addition of VEGF inhibitors over standard chemotherapy, it is likely that heterogeneity and inherent instability of tumor cell populations result in the selection of malignant cells that feed their vasculature through factors other than VEGF. In this regard, use of indirect angiogenic inhibitors still suffers from the likelihood of tumors becoming resistant to the therapy.

Whether the mechanism of action of these inhibitors is truly caused by the abrogation of a functional vascular supply is an open question. VEGF inhibitors "normalize" the aberrant, leaky tumor vasculature. Other than in renal cancer, VEGF inhibitors have shown effect only when used in combination chemotherapy regimens, which has led to the proposal that VEGF pathway inhibition improves vessel functionality and perfusion, thus facilitating delivery of chemotherapeutic agents.[157,158] VEGF–VEGFR signaling also acts in autocrine fashion within some tumor cell populations, raising the possibility that positive outcomes may have as much to do with direct tumor kill as with an antiangiogenic effect. Finally, as with organogenesis, the vasculature may provide a juxtacrine or paracrine role in supporting tumor viability and proliferation independent of the provision of a circulatory system for delivery of nutrients and oxygen.[47]

Some of the more common side effects observed with use of VEGF-A inhibitors were not predicted a priori but may be understandable in retrospect. For instance, hypertension and arterial thrombosis are common side effects. Two possible reasons may explain the hypertensive side effect. One is that VEGF directly activates endothelial nitric oxide synthase (eNOS) and thus may be responsible in part for basal production of NO.[159] Another potential explanation is that podocyte-derived VEGF is required for proper glomerular function throughout life.[47] Heterozygous loss of podocyte VEGF results in hypertension and proteinuria in adult mice.[47] Given that proteinuria is also commonly seen in patients treated with VEGF inhibitors, the latter explanation would tie two of the side effects seen. The reasons for arterial thrombosis are less obvious. Because arterial circulation is more dependent on VEGF, it is possible that arterial endothelial apoptosis serves as a nidus for localized activation of coagulation and platelet aggregation. Apoptotic endothelial cells have been shown to increase thrombin-generating capacity and bind to unactivated platelets and leukocytes.[160-162]

More recently the use of PDGF inhibitors to target pericytes has been shown to be a potentially effective antiangiogenic strategy, particularly in combination with antiendothelial (anti-VEGF) molecules.[80,82] "Metronomic" or low-dose, frequent scheduling of traditional cytotoxic agents also is reported to have an antiangiogenic effect and has proven efficacious in animal studies.[163] Antivasculogenic therapy directed against recruitment of BM-derived vascular precursors may have a role in future cancer therapeutic regimens, but thus far the evidence is weak at best.[66]

Arteriogenesis

Arteriogenesis is a term coined to distinguish the development of collateral vessels in adults from the process of angiogenesis.[164,165] Remodeling of a preexisting collateral arteriole is thought to be caused by flow-induced changes secondary to occlusion of a supply artery. The consequent increase in shear stress through the collateral arteriole activates endothelial cells, resulting in monocyte recruitment and infiltration into the media. Elaboration of various cytokines, growth factors, and proteases from monocytes and endothelial cells causes matrix degradation, smooth muscle cell proliferation, and rapid enlargement of the preexisting arteriole. Factors thought to promote arteriogenesis include FGF-2, placental growth factor, PDGF-BB, TGFβ1, monocyte chemoattractant protein 1, and GM-CSF.[165,166]

Lymphangiogenesis

The lymphatics comprise a low-flow, low-pressure system that collects extravasated fluid from the tissues and transfer it back to the venous system via the thoracic duct. Lymphatic vessels also serve an immune function by transporting lymphoid and antigen-presenting cells to lymphoid organs.[167] Lymphatic vessels share features with blood vessels, but they also exhibit differences. Lymphatic vessels develop shortly after blood vessels and may arise de novo from precursor mesenchymal cells (lymphangioblasts) in a process akin to vasculogenesis.[168] Alternatively, other studies suggest that specific venous endothelial cells differentiate to lymphatic endothelium in response to signals that have yet to be determined.[169] VEGF-C and VEGF-D, by activating VEGFR-3 and Ang2 potentially through Tie2 activation, are growth factors necessary for lymphatic vessels.[170] The α9β1 integrin also is necessary for proper lymphatic development, and the homeobox transcription factor Prox1 appears to induce transdifferentiation of venous to lymphatic endothelial cells.[169-171] Lymphedema can be caused by congenital defects, parasitic (filariasis) or neoplastic obstruction, or surgical resection. Congenital lymphedema (Milroy disease) is linked to inactivating mutations of VEGFR-3.[167] Whether lymphatic vessel density in human tumors correlates with disease progression is not clear, but in animal models, induction of lymphangiogenesis by VEGF-C or VEGF-D promotes lymph node metastasis.[167]

Relationship Between Vascular Development and Hematopoiesis

Hematopoietic cells and endothelial cells are intertwined in several ways. First, there is the likely existence of a common precursor (see Vasculogenesis above). Second, the endothelium is intimately involved in hematopoiesis, having a supportive role structurally and nutritionally. Finally, the endothelium organizes the controlled egress and ingress of hematopoietic cells in hematopoietic and other tissues. The last issue is covered in Interaction of Blood Cells With the Vessel Wall section.

Bone marrow stromal cells secrete cytokines, produce ECM, and are in direct cellular contact with hematopoietic cells, thereby providing a microenvironment suitable for hematopoietic proliferation, differentiation, and self-renewal.[172] Many studies demonstrate the supportive role of endothelium in hematopoiesis.[173-175] The physical proximity of endothelium and hematopoietic precursors within the BM and the requirement of blood cells to transit BM endothelium to reach the circulation is presumptive evidence of an important role for endothelium. BM endothelial cells constitutively express high levels of IL-6, stem cell factor, granulocyte colony-stimulating factor, and GM-CSF.[173] Both yolk sac and BM endothelial cells support long-term proliferation and differentiation of hematopoietic cells in vitro.[173] However, endothelial cells also have been reported to inhibit hematopoiesis.[176]

Significant evidence now indicates that hematopoietic stem and progenitor cells are not randomly distributed in the BM but rather are spatially and possibly physically associated with the endosteum and the blood vessels.[175] Functional differences between the osteoblastic and vascular niches have been described. It has been suggested that whereas the osteoblastic niche maintains quiescence of hematopoietic stem cells, stem and progenitor cells that are activated for differentiation and mobilization reside at the vascular niche.[174] Translocation of megakaryocyte progenitors to the vicinity of the BM sinuses is sufficient to induce megakaryocyte maturation and platelet production.[175] However, a study has identified CXCL12 (SDF-1)-abundant reticular cells that are located in close proximity to the sinusoidal endothelium as well as the endosteum.[177] The authors confirmed that the CXCL12–CXCR4 signaling axis is required for maintenance of hematopoietic stem cells in the BM, and these findings raise the possibility that the vascular and osteoblastic niches may not be that different.[177] In all likelihood, endothelial cells and osteoblasts, in concert with other stromal cells, provide a finely tuned system to modulate hematopoiesis in the BM such that differentiation, proliferation, and self-renewal occur in a regulated fashion.

Human endothelial cells have been reported to express receptors for IL-3, stem cell factor, erythropoietin, and thrombopoietin and show functional responses to IL-3 and erythropoietin.[178-180] The shared responses to growth factors, combined with the importance of macrophages in angiogenesis and the production of cytokines by monocytes and macrophages, suggest that hematopoietic cells play a reciprocal role in maintaining the endothelium.

PHYSIOLOGIC FUNCTIONS OF THE ENDOTHELIUM

The Endothelium as a Barrier

The microvessels (capillaries and postcapillary venules) act as the exchange vessels of the circulation. However, as with other endothelial functions, vessel permeability is dependent on the type of vessel and its location. Movement of lipophilic and low-molecular-weight hydrophilic substances between blood and tissue is virtually unimpeded, but the vessels are selectively permeable to macromolecules. This semiselective barrier is necessary to maintain the fluid balance between intravascular and extravascular compartments, yet antibodies, hormones, cytokines, and other molecules must have access to the interstitial space for the initiation and potentiation of various processes, including inflammation, immune response, and wound repair.

Movement of macromolecules across the vessel wall is governed by (1) hydrostatic and oncotic pressure gradients; (2) physicochemical properties of the molecule, such as size, shape, and charge; and (3) properties of the barrier. The barrier of the vessel wall is formed by the cellular components, endothelial cells, and pericytes, as well as by the charge and compactness of the matrix components, glycocalyx, and basement membrane. Macromolecules can pass either directly through the endothelial cell (transcellular path) or between adjacent endothelial cells (paracellular path). Surprisingly, the mechanisms of macromolecular movement remain controversial, and data generated by physiologists, morphologists, and cell biologists have not been consolidated in a model that satisfies the findings of the different groups.[181]

To explain cellular transport in endothelium, physiologists have proposed the existence of two sets of "pores" based on experiments measuring the movement of dextran and other macromolecules—a small pore of radius 3 to 5 nm for transport of water and small hydrophilic molecules and a large pore of radius 25 to 60 nm for macromolecular transport.[181-183] Although water mainly moves across the continuous endothelium via the paracellular route, a significant proportion (≤40%) can traverse the endothelium via the transcellular route by water-transporting membrane channels, the aquaporins.[184] Macromolecular transport into cells can proceed by receptor-mediated systems, such as clathrin-coated pits, in which the molecules usually are targeted to the lysosome, but may be transported through the cell. Alternatively, molecules can be moved across the cell by plasmalemmal vesicles or caveolae, which are abundant in capillary endothelial cells. Caveolae are 50- to 100-nm membrane invaginations that can participate in transcytosis as well as in the translocation of glycosylphosphatidylinositol-linked proteins into the cytoplasm and in transmembrane signaling.[185] Because of the known leakiness of tumor microvasculature, investigators have studied these microvessels and identified a structure designated the vesiculovacuolar organelle.[186] These organelles are grapelike clusters of interconnecting uncoated vesicles and vacuoles that span the entire thickness of vascular endothelium, thereby providing a potential transendothelial connection between the vascular lumen and the extravascular space.[186] Interestingly, their function is enhanced by injection into normal skin of VEGF, which is known to increase the permeability of vessels.[186] Localization of caveolin to vesiculovacuolar organelles suggests that this structure is a fusion of caveolae.[186]

During inflammation, binding of neutrophils to the endothelium results in the generation of oxidants that can mediate endothelial cell injury and increase permeability.[187] Upon adhesion of neutrophils to the endothelium, leukocyte CD18 (β2 integrin)-mediated signals trigger the release of the neutrophil cationic protein called heparin-binding protein/CAP37/azurocidin, which in turn induces formation of gaps between endothelial cells and macromolecular efflux.[188] Thrombin, an inflammatory mediator, can increase endothelial permeability by several mechanisms resulting from activation of its receptor on endothelial cells.[189-191] First is an increase in transcellular vesicular permeability. Second is increased paracellular permeability that results from phosphorylation of endothelial cell nonmyosin light chains and contractile activity generated by movement of actin and myosin filaments past each other. The contraction and retraction of endothelial cells are accompanied by "loosening" of intercellular junctions and focal integrin contacts with the ECM. Finally, thrombin may alter the repulsive effect of the negatively charged glycocalyx. An increase in paracellular permeability may result from alteration of cell–cell contacts present at tight junctions and adherens junctions secondary to posttranslational modification of components of these junctions such as claudins and VE-cadherin.[181] Pericyte contractility also has been hypothesized as a mechanism for increasing permeability in inflammatory states.[191]

The Endothelium as a Nonthrombogenic Surface

The molecular mechanisms of hemostasis and thrombosis are addressed in Chapters 115 and 116 and 118 through 120. This

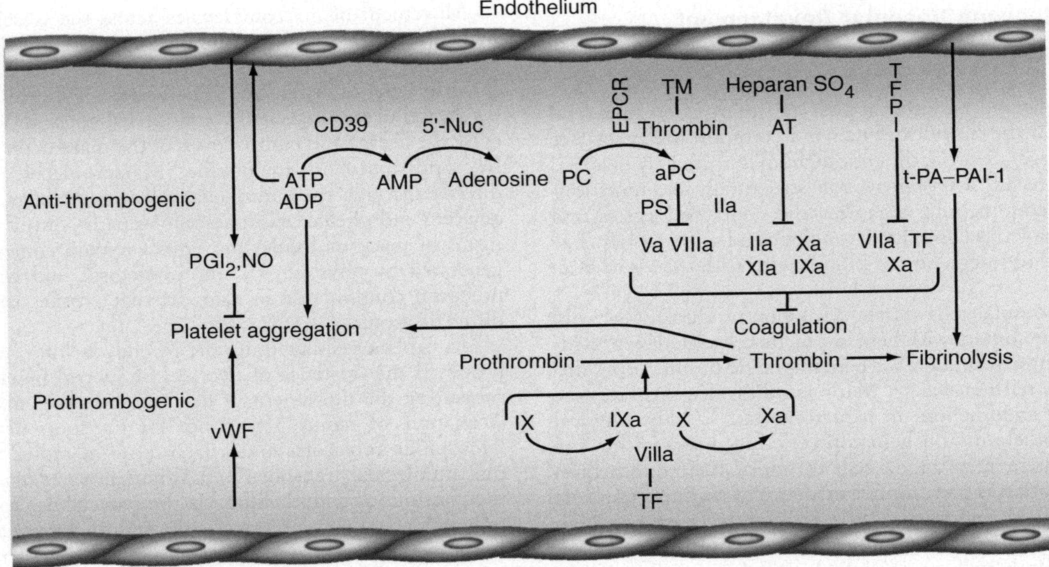

Figure 125-2 OVERVIEW OF ENDOTHELIAL FUNCTION IN COAGULATION. *ADP,* Adenosine diphosphate; *AMP,* adenosine monophosphate; *AT,* antithrombin; *ATP,* adenosine triphosphate; *EPCR,* endothelial protein C receptor; *5′-Nuc,* ecto-5′-nucleotidase; *NO,* nitric oxide; *PAI-1,* plasminogen activator inhibitor 1; *PC,* protein C; *PGI_2,* prostaglandin I_2 (prostacyclin); *PS,* protein S; *TF,* tissue factor; *TFPI,* tissue factor pathway inhibitor; *TM,* thrombomodulin; *t-PA,* tissue plasminogen activator; *vWF,* von Willebrand factor.

section places the endothelium in the appropriate context in these processes. An overview of endothelial cell contributions to the anticoagulant and procoagulant states is shown in Fig. 125-2. Normal unperturbed endothelium presents a nonthrombogenic surface to the circulation by inhibiting platelet aggregation, preventing the activation and propagation of coagulation and enhancing fibrinolysis.[192-196] These activities are accomplished by both passive and active processes. Conversely, when injured or under inflammatory conditions, the endothelium may become procoagulant.

When in close proximity to endothelial cells, platelets become unresponsive to agonists. This inhibition of platelet aggregation is accomplished by secretion of prostacyclin (prostaglandin I2 [PGI_2]) and NO and by surface expression of an ecto-adenosine phosphatase (ADPase)/CD39/nucleoside triphosphate diphosphohydrolase (NTPDase-1).[195,197] Prostacyclin is synthesized mainly by vascular endothelial and smooth muscle cells as a product of arachidonic acid metabolism. It inhibits platelet activation, secretion, and aggregation, as well as monocyte interactions with endothelial cells. It also causes vascular smooth muscle cell relaxation. NO similarly has a wide range of functions, including inhibition of platelet adhesion, activation, and aggregation. Most of the NO released from endothelial cells is elaborated abluminally, where it acts on the smooth muscle cell to cause vasodilation. However, some NO may enter the lumen and thereby diffuse into platelets. Prostacyclin and NO can act synergistically to reverse platelet aggregation.[195] The released platelet agonist, adenosine diphosphate (ADP), can be inactivated by endothelial membrane-associated CD39.[197] Metabolism of adenosine triphosphate (ATP) and ADP to adenosine monophosphate (AMP) by CD39 eliminates platelet recruitment and returns platelets to their resting state. Adenosine, which is generated by hydrolysis of AMP by ecto-5′-nucleotidase, acts to inhibit platelet aggregation and cause vasodilation. ATP/ADP can stimulate purinoreceptors on endothelial cells, resulting in synthesis and release of PGI_2 and NO.[198]

Endothelial cells use three main pathways to inhibit thrombin generation and limit coagulation[192,194,199,200]:

1. Antithrombin system: Heparan sulfate proteoglycans are secreted onto the luminal surface of endothelial cells and into the subendothelium. Heparan sulfates are capable of binding and activating antithrombin III, thereby accelerating inactivation of several procoagulant serine proteases, including thrombin, factor Xa, and factor IXa.
2. Protein C[201]: Thrombomodulin on the surface of endothelial cells binds thrombin. This coupling inhibits the coagulant properties of thrombin and increases its affinity for protein C, which it cleaves and activates. Activation of protein C by the thrombin–thrombomodulin complex is augmented by its binding to the endothelial cell protein C receptor. Protein S, which is thought to be synthesized primarily by the endothelial cell, acts as a cofactor for protein C but itself also has anticoagulant properties. Independent of the presence of activated protein C, free protein S is able to inhibit the prothrombinase and intrinsic tenase complexes and interact directly with factors Va and VIIIa.
3. Tissue factor pathway inhibitor (TFPI)[202]: TFPI is a Kunitz-type serine protease inhibitor that modulates TF-initiated coagulation. TFPI binds to and directly inhibits the TF–factor VIIa–factor Xa complex. It is mainly produced by and bound to endothelial cells, likely to surface glycosaminoglycans. There is also a plasma pool bound to low-density lipoprotein (LDL).

If coagulation occurs despite the many anticoagulant mechanisms, endothelial cells also provide proteins to promote fibrinolysis.[194] Endothelium is a major source of t-PA.[203,204] Approximately 40% of t-PA is bound to its inhibitor, PAI-1, which is also secreted by endothelial cells. Stresses such as exercise, acidosis, hypoxia, shear forces, increased venous pressure, and thrombin cause release of t-PA[203,204] and presumably activate plasminogen. Receptors for plasminogen and t-PA are present on the endothelial cell surface, allowing for effective localized production of fibrinolytic activity.

Although intact endothelium is necessary to maintain blood in a fluid state and inhibit coagulation under normal conditions, injured endothelium can rapidly downregulate its anticoagulant functions and become procoagulant even without overt vascular damage as occurs with trauma or surgery. Further tissue injury or vascular pathology also leads to exposure of the underlying matrix, which is procoagulant by virtue of its binding to and activation of platelets. Endothelial cells that have been induced to undergo apoptosis in vitro become procoagulant. Apoptotic endothelial cells expose phosphatidylserine on their surface and downregulate their anticoagulant properties. Apoptotic endothelial cells and vascular smooth muscle cells also increase thrombin formation in recalcified citrated plasma, and apoptotic endothelial cells show increased adhesion to unactivated platelets.[160,161,205] Thrombosis resulting from procoagulant changes induced by endothelial apoptosis could contribute to the pathogenesis of diverse diseases.[206]

Even without endothelial death, perturbation of the vascular lining by inflammatory mediators could tip the balance such that the endothelium converts from a nonthrombogenic to a procoagulant surface because of downregulation of anticoagulant properties as well as induction of procoagulant properties. For example, the setting of acute inflammation is associated with increased release of vWF, platelet-activating factor, and fibronectin, all of which may potentiate thrombus formation. Tumor necrosis factor (TNF), IL-1, and lipopolysaccharide can increase the expression of PAI-1 in endothelial cells with downregulation or no change in t-PA levels, thereby impairing fibrinolysis. TNF, IL-1, and lipopolysaccharide also have been shown to downregulate thrombomodulin as well as to induce expression of TF on cultured endothelial cells. However, whether endothelial cells express TF on their luminal surfaces in vivo is controversial.[207] More recently, circulating microparticles generated by leukocytes and vascular cells have been shown to be a source of bloodborne TF and to contribute to coagulation.[208] Although most microparticles probably are derived from platelets and monocytes, endothelial-derived microparticles may be an important source of circulating TF under conditions of drastic activation.[208,209]

Control of Vascular Tone

Control of vascular tone is orchestrated primarily by a balance between endothelium-derived vasodilators (NO, PGI_2, and endothelium-derived hyperpolarizing factor [EDHF]) and vasoconstrictors (endothelin-1 [ET-1] and superoxide). In addition to inhibiting platelet aggregation, NO and PGI_2 act as vasodilators.[210,211] NO is produced by conversion of L-arginine to L-citrulline by NO synthase (NOS). Three forms of NOS exist: a constitutive NOS in neuronal tissue; an inducible enzyme found in macrophages and other cells that plays a role in NO-induced cytotoxicity; and a constitutively active endothelial form, NOSIII (eNOS).[212] The inducible form of NOS also is present in endothelial cells and may be responsible for the uncontrolled vasodilation seen in septic shock.[212] Injection into the forearm of L-arginine analogues that inhibit NOS causes substantial vasoconstriction. Conversely, eNOS-deficient mice are hypertensive, suggesting that NO release is crucial for maintaining basal vasodilation.[210,211] The major physiologic stimulus for continuous production of NO in vivo is shear stress. The action of NO on platelets (antiaggregatory), endothelial cells, and smooth muscle cells (relaxation) is caused by activation of guanyl cyclase and formation of cyclic guanosine 3′,5′-cyclic monophosphate. Whereas NO is quite unstable, the formation of *S*-nitrosothiols in the presence of oxygen and thiols provides a stable reservoir of NO.[213] Hemoglobin is an avid scavenger of NO, which may account for the vasoconstriction observed with administration of cell-free, hemoglobin-based RBC substitute.[214] Physiologically, however, *S*-nitrosohemoglobin acts as a regulator of blood flow. Deoxygenation is accompanied by an allosteric change in *S*-nitrosohemoglobin that releases the NO group, relaxing blood vessels to bring blood flow in line with local oxygen requirements.[215]

Prostacyclin (PGI_2), on the other hand, does not appear to have as global a role in vasodilation as does NO. PGI_2 is synthesized mainly by endothelial cells and acts locally at sites of injury. It may counterbalance the vasoconstriction induced by the platelet-produced arachidonic acid metabolite thromboxane A_2 (TXA_2). Most PGI_2 is released luminally, where it has an antiplatelet effect. Whereas prostacyclin transduces a cellular signal by increasing the levels of cyclic AMP (cAMP), TXA_2 signals via the phosphoinositol pathway and lowering of cAMP levels. Synthesis of prostaglandins begins by the action of cyclooxygenases (COX-1 and COX-2) on arachidonic acid. Aspirin inhibits COX irreversibly in both platelets and endothelial cells. However, the clinical effect is seen primarily in platelets for two reasons.[211,212] One reason is that platelets, being nonnucleated, cannot synthesize new COX, but endothelial cells can. Therefore, TXA_2 synthesis recovers only when new platelets enter the circulation, but COX production by endothelial cells restores PGI_2 levels within a few hours. The second reason is that platelets encounter orally administered aspirin before it is deacetylated by the liver and diluted by the venous circulation.

Early experimental evidence suggested that endothelial cells release other relaxing factors (i.e., EDHF), which act by increasing the membrane potential of smooth muscle cells. Hyperpolarization of isolated coronary arteries occurs in the presence of an arginine analogue, a NOS inhibitor, and indomethacin, a COX inhibitor, suggesting that EDHF, NO, and prostanoids contribute differentially to relaxation in human coronary arteries.[216] The nature of EDHF is unclear, but it encompasses different biologic mechanisms. These mechanisms involve an increase in intracellular calcium concentration, the opening of calcium-activated potassium channels, and the hyperpolarization of endothelial cells, resulting in an endothelium-dependent hyperpolarization of smooth muscle cells.[217] Smooth muscle cell hyperpolarization may occur through direct myoendothelial electrical coupling or through accumulation of potassium ions in the intercellular space. Findings suggest that EDHF represents cytochrome P450-linked arachidonate metabolites in some blood vessels but also lipoxygenase derivatives and hydrogen peroxide.[217]

Endothelin-1 is a 21-amino-acid peptide, released preferentially at the abluminal surface of endothelial cells, that exhibits potent vasoconstrictor activity.[218,219] Of the three known ETs, only ET-1 is produced by endothelial cells. At least two receptors (ET-A and ET-B) bind to all three ETs. Whereas ET-A is abundantly expressed on smooth muscle cells, ET-B is predominantly expressed on endothelial cells. The vasoconstrictor activity of ET-1 is preferentially mediated by ET-A receptors on smooth muscle cells. Engagement of ET-B on endothelial cells by ET-3 may paradoxically cause a transient vasodilation. Little evidence indicates that ET-1 plays a role in essential hypertension, but it might contribute to pregnancy-induced hypertension and may play a role in reperfusion injury after ischemia.[219] ET-1 does appear to play a role in pulmonary arterial hypertension, and the dual ET receptor antagonist bosentan has been approved for treatment of this disease.[220]

Another seemingly important regulator of vascular tone is the superoxide anion.[210,221] The source of this free radical may be the endothelium itself or inflammatory cells that have been recruited to sites of injury or inflammation. Interaction of superoxide radicals and NO produces peroxynitrite and reduces the concentration of NO. Peroxynitrite can oxidize LDL and deleteriously modify other proteins, thereby causing endothelial dysfunction. Increased production of superoxide inhibits synthesis of PGI_2 but not that of TXA_2.[221]

The endothelium expresses angiotensin-converting enzyme at its surface; this enzyme converts angiotensin I to angiotensin II, a potent vasoconstrictor. The interaction among ET, angiotensin II, and α-adrenergic agonists in the pathogenesis of hypertension is complex.[222] An altered balance of the vasoactive substances described in this section has been proposed to cause endothelial dysfunction and the attendant vascular pathology observed in atherosclerosis, hypertension, and diabetes mellitus. Alteration of vascular function in these diseases then may perpetuate endothelial dysfunction and, consequently, worsen disease.

Interaction of Blood Cells With the Vessel Wall

Leukocytes

In the absence of any inflammatory stimulus, neutrophils circulate freely and do not interact significantly with the endothelium. This contrasts with continuous, low-level physiologic traffic of monocytes and lymphocytes across the vessel wall. Monocytes emigrate from the bloodstream to develop into tissue macrophages that may exhibit tissue- or organ-specific functions. To maintain immune surveillance of tissue, lymphocytes recirculate between blood and lymphatics, gaining entrance to the latter at the high endothelial venule of postcapillary venules in lymphoid tissue.

Intravital microscopic studies have established a sequence of events involved in leukocyte emigration at extravascular sites of inflammation. Under conditions of flow, leukocytes first tether to and then roll along the endothelium of postcapillary venules adjacent to the site of inflammation. Some of the rolling leukocytes are activated and adhere firmly. The adherent leukocytes migrate along the endothelial surface and diapedese between endothelial junctions to enter the extravascular tissue. These steps in emigration tethering, rolling, activation, firm adhesion, and diapedesis also are involved in lymphocyte emigration at high endothelial venules. They result from the interaction of distinct leukocyte and endothelial receptors in an adhesion cascade (Fig. 125-3; see Chapter 16).[223,224] Rolling is observed only under flow conditions and is the consequence of shear forces acting on the leukocyte and adhesive interactions between selectin receptors and their glycoconjugate counterstructures.[225] It is initiated primarily by activation of the endothelium by extravascular stimuli such as bacterial-derived products or by endogenous mediators produced by the endothelium or cells in tissue. Early on, rolling is mediated by endothelial P-selectin, which is rapidly translocated from Weibel-Palade bodies to the luminal surface, and L-selectin on leukocyte microvilli. E-selectin is involved only at later time points because it is not constitutively expressed by endothelium but rather is induced over hours by de novo synthesis.

For leukocytes to circulate freely, their integrin receptors must be minimally adhesive, but they also must be able to increase binding rapidly at sites of inflammation. After being tethered to endothelium by selectin interactions, leukocyte integrin receptors are activated by endothelial membrane-expressed platelet-activating factor, endothelial membrane-bound chemokines, or locally secreted chemoattractants. Activation of leukocyte integrins involves changes in receptor affinity or affinity-independent receptor clustering,[226] which promotes firm adhesion to endothelial ligands, which are members of the immunoglobulin gene superfamily (IgSF). These IgSF ligands are constitutively expressed (ICAM-1, ICAM-2), further upregulated (ICAM-1), or induced (VCAM-1) by inflammatory mediators (Table 125-1). Although these activation-dependent increases in leukocyte

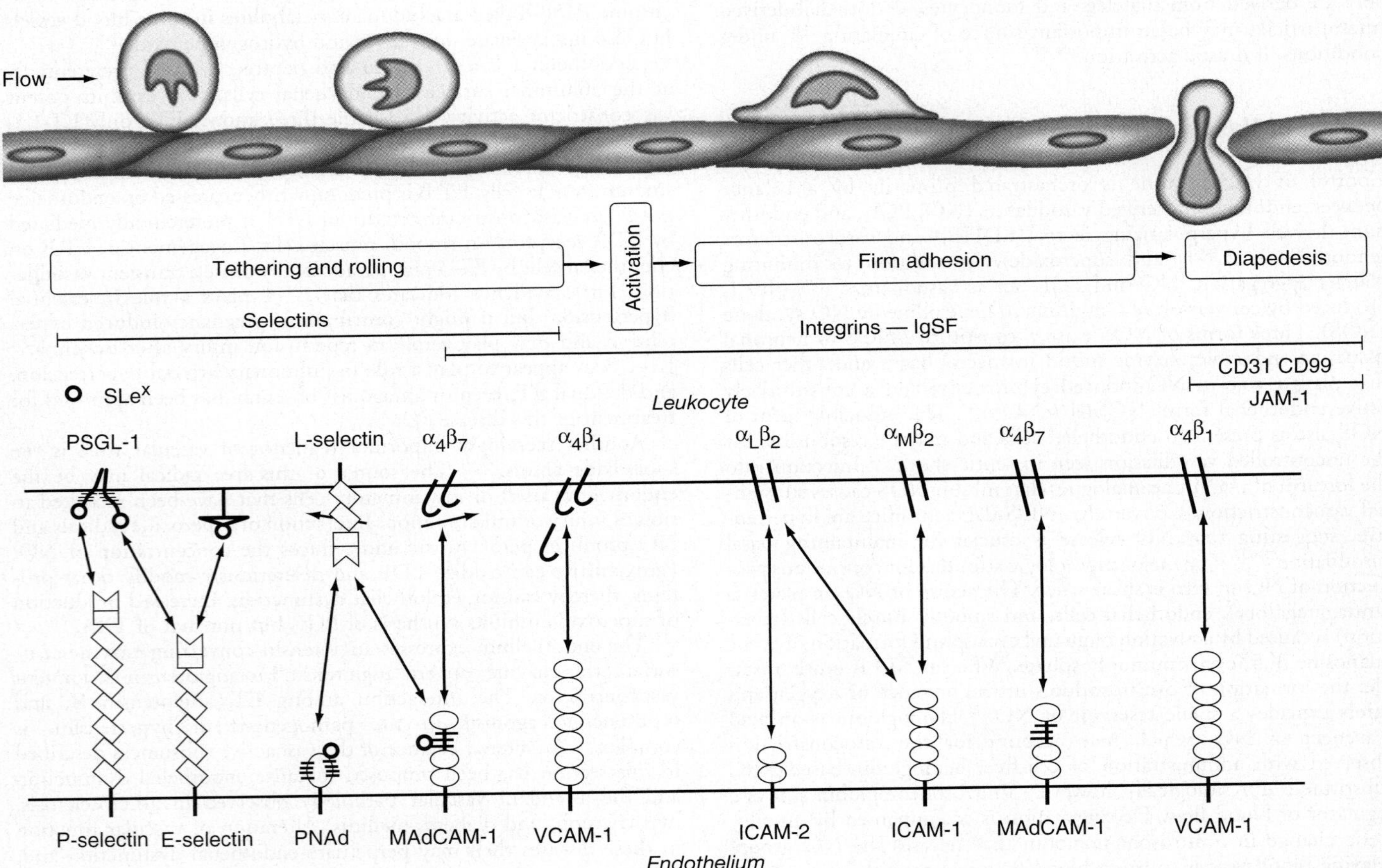

Figure 125-3 ADHESION CASCADE. Under conditions of flow, leukocytes first tether to endothelial ligands and then roll along the vessel wall. Tethering is mediated predominantly by interaction of P-selectin and L-selectin with their cognate glycoconjugate ligands. P-selectin binds to sialyl Lewis X (SLe^x) and sulfate residues expressed on P-selectin glycoprotein ligand 1 (PSGL-1). L-selectin binds to an uncharacterized ligand(s) on inflamed endothelium and to sulfated SLe^x-like moieties on peripheral node addressin (PNAd) and mucosal addressin cell adhesion molecule 1 (MAdCAM-1) on high endothelial venules. E-selectin, $\alpha_4\beta_1$ (very late antigen 4 [VLA-4]), and $\alpha_4\beta_7$ stabilize rolling initiated by P-selectin and L-selectin. E-selectin recognizes SLe^x on PSGL-1 and other glycoproteins or glycolipids. After tethering and rolling, leukocyte integrin receptors are activated, most often by chemoattractants (e.g., chemokines) via G protein–coupled receptors. After activation, integrin receptors engage endothelial immunoglobulin gene superfamily ligands to promote firm adhesion. Leukocyte $\alpha_L\beta_2$ (leukocyte function antigen 1 [LFA-1]) binds to intercellular adhesion molecules 1 and 2 (ICAM-1 and ICAM-2), $\alpha_M\beta_2$ (macrophage 1 [Mac-1]) to ICAM-1, $\alpha_4\beta_1$ (VLA-4) to vascular cell adhesion molecule 1 (VCAM-1), and $\alpha_4\beta_7$ to MAdCAM-1. The adherent leukocyte then migrates across endothelium to interendothelial junctions, where it diapedeses between endothelial cells via leukocyte integrin receptors and their endothelial immunoglobulin gene superfamily ligands as well as endothelial junctional proteins such as CD31, CD99, and junctional adhesion molecule 1 (JAM-1).

Table 125-1 Endothelial Cell Activation*

Agonist	Response
Thrombin	Secretion of vWF, P-selectin, TFPI, and PDGF Synthesis of PAF, IL-8, IL-6, and E-selectin
IL-1β, TNF-α, LPS	Synthesis of adhesion molecules (ICAM-1, VCAM-1, E-selectin), chemokines (IL-8, MCP-1), cytokines (IL-6, CD40), procoagulant proteins (TF, PAI-1, t-PA, u-PA), and cytoprotective molecules (A1, IAP) Downregulation of anticoagulant proteins (TM)
Reduced/disturbed shear stress	Increased expression of proinflammatory genes (e.g., VCAM-1, ICAM-1, MCP-1)
VEGF	Decreased eNOS activity Increased expression of cytoprotective genes (A1, MnSOD), Ang2, COX-2

Ang, Angiopoietin; *A1,* Bcl-2 homologue; *COX-2,* cyclooxygenase 2; *eNOS,* endothelial nitric oxide synthase; *IAP,* inhibitor of apoptosis protein; *ICAM,* intercellular adhesion molecule; *IL,* interleukin; *LPS,* lipopolysaccharide; *MCP,* monocyte chemoattractant protein; *MnSOD,* manganese superoxide dismutase; *PAF,* platelet-activating factor; *PAI,* plasminogen activator inhibitor; *PDGF,* platelet-derived growth factor; *TF,* tissue factor; *TFPI,* tissue factor pathway inhibitor; *TM,* thrombomodulin; *TNF,* tumor necrosis factor; *t-PA,* tissue plasminogen activator; *u-PA,* urokinase-type plasminogen activator; *VCAM,* vascular cell adhesion molecule; *VEGF,* vascular endothelial growth factor; *vWF,* von Willebrand factor.
*Selected agonists and responses. Many other stimuli (e.g., lipoproteins, hypoxia, microbes, and microbial products) have been reported to upregulate or downregulate various endothelial responses.

integrin binding to endothelial IgSF ligands are necessary for shear-resistant firm adhesion, subsequent leukocyte migration over the endothelium requires reversible adhesion caused by cyclic modulation of receptor avidity.[227]

There are several caveats regarding the current multistep model of initial selectin-mediated rolling and subsequent integrin-mediated firm adhesion.[228] First, selectin-mediated rolling is not a prerequisite for emigration under conditions of reduced flow, as might occur at sites of inflammation.[229] Second, the model was developed from observations in the systemic microcirculation, where leukocyte emigration occurs in postcapillary venules under relatively low shear forces. However, selectins do not appear to play a major role in neutrophil emigration in the pulmonary microcirculation, where emigration occurs predominantly in capillaries,[230] or in the liver microvasculature, where leukocytes emigrate primarily in sinusoids.[231] Third, under some conditions leukocytes are able to tether and roll via receptors other than selectins and α4 integrins (e.g., CD44[232] or VAP-1[233]). Finally, several other adhesion pathways have been implicated in leukocyte adhesion to endothelium in vitro, and their roles in the adhesion cascade in vivo remain to be defined.[228]

When adherent, leukocytes migrate upon the endothelial luminal surface. Upon encountering an intercellular junction, some leukocytes diapedese between endothelial cells, enter extravascular tissue, and then migrate to the site of inflammatory or immune reaction.[234,235] This process of transendothelial migration uses leukocyte integrin interactions with endothelial IgSF ligands[236] and several junctional proteins, including PECAM-1 (CD31),[237] JAM-1,[238] and CD99.[239] Diapedesis involves signaling by the leukocyte to the endothelial cell that triggers opening of endothelial cell junctions.[240] Although leukocyte migration is primarily paracellular (i.e., through endothelial cell–cell junctions), under certain circumstances, leukocytes may emigrate by a transcellular pathway.[241]

Leukocyte recruitment is terminated by several mechanisms. Whereas E-selectin and P-selectin are removed from the endothelial cell surface by endocytosis,[242] L-selectin is cleaved from leukocytes by a membrane protease.[243] Decay of cytokine, chemokine, or chemoattractant generation leads to gradual resolution of endothelial adhesion molecule expression and integrin activation. Locally expressed mediators, such as NO,[244] TGFβ,[245] and Fas ligand,[246] also inhibit further leukocyte adhesion to endothelium.

The adhesion molecules involved in leukocyte trafficking from bloodstream to tissue have emerged as important therapeutic targets. Extensive preclinical studies showed that blockade of leukocyte or endothelial adhesion molecules was efficacious in diverse disease models,[247] prompting the development of adhesion antagonists for clinical trials in a variety of diseases. However, results were disappointing overall, with many unsuccessful clinical trials of various adhesion antagonists in multiple disease indications.[248,249] Moreover, the report of progressive multifocal leukoencephalopathy, a rare viral infection of the central nervous system, in several patients treated with the α4-integrin antagonist natalizumab[250] highlights the risks of targeting molecules that are pivotal in host defense and repair as well as in disease. Nevertheless, the potential of antiadhesion therapy is demonstrated by the approval of two integrin antagonists: efalizumab for treatment of psoriasis[251] and natalizumab for treatment of multiple sclerosis.[252]

Platelets

Similar to neutrophils, unactivated platelets do not interact with unperturbed endothelium. After a vascular injury that produces endothelial denudation or retraction, platelets rapidly adhere to the exposed subendothelium. As discussed in greater detail in Chapters 115 and 116, at high shear rates, this initial adhesion does not require platelet activation and involves platelet glycoprotein Ib/V/IX (GPIb-V-IX) binding to vWF in the subendothelial matrix and platelet GPVI binding to collagen in the injured arterial wall. Platelet activation occurs after adhesion, leading to platelet spreading mediated by integrin receptors binding to matrix components and aggregation mediated by fibrinogen binding to GPIIb/IIIa (αIIbβ3).

Evidence indicates that platelets can bind directly to activated endothelium in vivo via endothelial P-selectin[253] and PECAM-1[254] and to roll on venular endothelium via interaction of platelet GPIbα and endothelial P-selectin.[255] Platelets have been shown to bind to high endothelial venules in vivo via platelet P-selectin.[256] In vitro platelets can adhere to intact endothelium via a platelet GPIIb/IIIa-dependent bridging mechanism involving platelet-bound adhesive proteins and the endothelial cell receptors ICAM-1, αVβ3 integrin, and GPIbα.[257] Platelet adhesion to intact endothelium via these various pathways may contribute to thrombus formation in the circulation and may provide a link between thrombosis and inflammation in diseases such as atherosclerosis.[258] Platelet–endothelial interactions also may contribute to the pathogenesis of thrombotic thrombocytopenic purpura. Normally, ultralarge vWF remains attached to endothelium via P-selectin until it is cleaved by the plasma metalloproteinase ADAMTS-13 (a disintegrin and metalloproteinase with thrombospondin). Failure of this mechanism in thrombotic thrombocytopenic purpura because of a deficiency of ADAMTS-13 may lead to spontaneous platelet adhesion to endothelium and microvascular thrombosis.[259]

Red Blood Cells

Plasmodium falciparum-infected and sickled RBCs interact significantly with endothelium, and these adhesive interactions are thought to play an important role in the pathogenesis of human diseases.

Among the human malarial parasites, only *P. falciparum* modifies the surface of the parasitized RBs so that asexual parasites and gametocytes are able to adhere to the vascular endothelium.[260,261] Binding of trophozoite- and schizont-infected RBCs to endothelium not only allows the parasite to escape destruction in the spleen but also may contribute to the pathogenesis of cerebral malaria.[261,262] Multiple endothelial adhesion receptors have been implicated in mediating cytoadherence of infected RBCs, including P-selectin, ICAM-1, VCAM-1, and CD36.[263]

Binding of young sickled RBCs to postcapillary endothelium with secondary trapping of poorly deformable, often irreversibly sickled cells is thought to be an important pathogenic factor in vasoocclusive events.[264] Several interactions between sickle RBC receptors and endothelial ligands have been described, including $\alpha 4\beta 1$/VCAM-1[265]; $\alpha 4\beta 1$/Lutheran blood group (basal cell adhesion molecule)[266]; and ICAM-4/$\alpha V\beta 3$.[267] The adhesive proteins thrombospondin and vWF promote adhesion by serving as bridging factors between various sickle RBC and endothelial adhesion molecules. In addition to direct adhesion to endothelium, sickle RBC binding to adherent leukocytes has been proposed as a mechanism for sickle cell vascular occlusion.[268] As with leukocyte adhesion to endothelium in inflammatory and immune disease, drugs targeting sickle RBC adhesive interactions with endothelial cells or leukocytes may prove useful in preventing or treating vasoocclusive crises.

Endothelial Cell Activation and Dysfunction

Although once viewed as a passive barrier between blood and tissue, the endothelium now is evident to be a dynamic and heterogeneous organ that responds to diverse stimuli, ranging from coagulation proteins and cytokines to hemodynamic forces and growth factors. Activation of endothelial cells induces a complex proinflammatory and prothrombotic phenotype as well as expression of certain cytoprotective genes (see Table 125-1).[269,270] Multiple transcription factors, particularly nuclear factor-κB[271] and early growth response 1,[272] regulate these responses.[269] Endothelial activation undoubtedly is an important event in host defense and repair, but it also may contribute to the pathogenesis of diverse diseases, ranging from sepsis[273] to atherosclerosis.[274]

Endothelial dysfunction is characterized by a reduction in the bioavailability of vasodilators, particularly NO, leading to impairment of endothelium-dependent vasodilation, or by an increase in endothelium-derived contracting factors.[275] Endothelial dysfunction is prominent in atherosclerosis but also has been described in diabetes, preeclampsia, hypertension, uremia, and other diseases. In a broader sense, endothelial dysfunction encompasses proinflammatory and procoagulant changes as well as apoptotic cell death.[206,276,277]

A number of noninvasive approaches for assessing endothelial function in vascular diseases have been developed. Endothelial vasodilatory responses can be evaluated by high-resolution ultrasound measurement of flow-mediated vasodilation or by plethysmography of changes in forearm blood flow during reactive hyperemia.[278] Endothelial activation can be assessed in plasma by circulating markers such as soluble endothelial adhesion molecules (e.g., sVCAM-1, sICAM-1, sE-selectin) and endothelial coagulation proteins (e.g., vWF and thrombomodulin)[279] or endothelial microparticles.[280] Circulating endothelial cells reflect significant vascular damage or cell death.[281]

SUGGESTED READINGS

Aird WC: Spatial and temporal dynamics of the endothelium. *J Thromb Haemost* 3:1392, 2005.

Carmeliet P: Blood vessels and nerves: Common signals, pathways and diseases. *Nat Rev Genet* 4:710, 2003.

Conway EM, Collen D, Carmeliet P: Molecular mechanisms of blood vessel growth. *Cardiovasc Res* 49:507, 2001.

Coultas L, Chawengsaksophak K, Rossant J: Endothelial cells and VEGF in vascular development. *Nature* 438:937, 2005.

De Palma M, Naldini L: Role of haematopoietic cells and endothelial progenitors in tumour angiogenesis. *Biochim Biophys Acta* 1766:159, 2006.

Harrison DG, Widder J, Grumbach I, et al: Endothelial mechanotransduction, nitric oxide and vascular inflammation. *J Intern Med* 259:351, 2006.

Hebbel RP, Yamada O, Moldow CF, et al: Abnormal adherence of sickle erythrocytes to cultured vascular endothelium: Possible mechanism for microvascular occlusion in sickle cell disease. *J Clin Invest* 65:154, 1980.

Kerbel R, Folkman J: Clinical translation of angiogenesis inhibitors. *Nat Rev Cancer* 2:727, 2002.

Lapidot T, Dar A, Kollet O: How do stem cells find their way home? *Blood* 106:1901, 2005.

Luster AD, Alon R, von Andrian UH: Immune cell migration in inflammation: Present and future therapeutic targets. *Nat Immunol* 6:1182, 2005.

Mehta D, Malik AB: Signaling mechanisms regulating endothelial permeability. *Physiol Rev* 86:279, 2006.

Minami T, Aird WC: Endothelial cell gene regulation. *Trends Cardiovasc Med* 15:174, 2005.

Petri B, Bixel MG: Molecular events during leukocyte diapedesis. *FEBS J* 273:4399, 2006.

Pober JS, Min W: Endothelial cell dysfunction, injury and death. *Handb Exp Pharmacol* 135, 2006.

Rafii S, Lyden D, Benezra R, et al: Vascular and haematopoietic stem cells: Novel targets for anti-angiogenesis therapy? *Nat Rev Cancer* 2:826, 2002.

Rak J, Milsom C, May L, et al: Tissue factor in cancer and angiogenesis: The molecular link between genetic tumor progression, tumor neovascularization, and cancer coagulopathy. *Semin Thromb Hemost* 32:54, 2006.

Schofield L, Grau GE: Immunological processes in malaria pathogenesis. *Nat Rev Immunol* 5:722, 2005.

Shih T, Lindley C: Bevacizumab: An angiogenesis inhibitor for the treatment of solid malignancies. *Clin Ther* 28:1779, 2006.

Yin T, Li L: The stem cell niches in bone. *J Clin Invest* 116:1195, 2006.

Yonekawa K, Harlan JM: Targeting leukocyte integrins in human diseases. *J Leukoc Biol* 77:129, 2005.

For complete list of references log on to www.expertconsult.com.

CHAPTER 126

MEGAKARYOCYTE AND PLATELET STRUCTURE

Joseph E. Italiano, Jr., and John H. Hartwig

Platelets are small anucleate fragments that are formed from the cytoplasm of megakaryocytes and have a characteristic discoid shape. To assemble and release platelets, megakaryocytes become polyploid by endomitosis and follow a maturation program that results in the conversion of the bulk of their cytoplasm into multiple long processes called *proplatelets*. To produce its quota of 1000 to 2000 platelets, a megakaryocyte may protrude as many as 10 to 20 proplatelets, each of which begins as a blunt protrusion that over time thins and branches repeatedly. Platelets form selectively at the ends of proplatelets. As platelets develop, their content of granules and organelles is delivered to them in a stream of individual particles moving from the megakaryocyte cell body to the nascent platelet buds at the proplatelet tips. Platelet formation can be arbitrarily divided into two phases. The first phase takes days to complete and requires megakaryocyte-specific growth factors. Massive nuclear proliferation to 16 to 32 × N and enlargement of the megakaryocyte cytoplasm occur as the platelet is filled with cytoskeletal proteins, platelet-specific granules, and sufficient membrane to complete the platelet assembly process. The second phase is relatively rapid and can be completed in hours. During this phase, megakaryocytes generate platelets by remodeling their cytoplasm first into proplatelets, then preplatelets, which undergo fission to generate discoid platelets.

MEGAKARYOCYTE DEVELOPMENT

Endomitosis

Hematopoietic stem cells, which are endowed with the genetic capacity to differentiate into multiple lineages, are induced down the pathway to become megakaryocytes by their exposure to certain growth factors.[1] Megakaryocytes become polyploid (i.e., 4N, 16N, 32N, 64N) through repeated cycles of DNA replication without cell division.[2-5] Normally ploidy ranges from 4 to 64 times the haploid DNA complement, but the majority of cells fall within three ploidy classes (8N, 16N, and 32N), with 16N being dominant (Fig. 126-1).[6,7] Ploidy number appears to be a predetermined event, possibly signifying genetic diversity among megakaryocyte populations. Megakaryocyte polyploidization results in a functional gene amplification whose likely function is an increase in protein synthesis.[8] This process, called *endomitosis,* is a shortened mitosis caused by a block in late anaphase.[9,10]

Whereas cells undergoing diploid mitoses proceed through cytokinesis and complete abscission division, megakaryocytes exhibit regression of the cleavage furrow and reenter G_1 as polyploid cells.[1] During polyploidization of megakaryocytes, the nuclear envelope breaks down, and an abnormal spherical mitotic spindle forms. The spindle has attached chromosomes that align from a position equidistant from the spindle poles. Sister chromatids segregate and move toward their respective poles (anaphase A). However, the spindle poles fail to move apart and do not undergo the microtubule-driven separation typically observed during anaphase B. Individual chromatids are not moved to the poles, and subsequently a single nuclear envelope encapsulates the entire set of sister chromatids.[9,10] In most cell types, checkpoints and feedback controls ensure that DNA replication and cell division are tightly coupled. Megakaryocytes appear to be an exception to this rule, indicating they have managed to deregulate this process. Proposed mechanisms for regulating endomitosis include a reduction in mitosis-promoting factor[11,12] or decreased expression of cyclin B.[12-15] Cyclins appear to play a critical role in directing endomitosis. Cyclin D3 is overexpressed in the G_1 phase of maturing megakaryocytes,[16] but a triple knockout of cyclins D1, D2, and D3 in mice does not appear to affect megakaryocyte development.[17] In contrast, cyclin E-deficient mice exhibit a profound defect in megakaryocyte development.[18] The molecular programming involved in endomitosis is characterized by the mislocalization or absence of at least two critical regulators of mitosis: the chromosomal passenger proteins Aurora-B/AIM-1 and survivin. AIM-1, a serine/threonine kinase in the Aurora family that is implicated in mitosis, is downregulated as megakaryocyte polyploidization occurs, suggesting its loss may lead to the abortive mitosis and polyploidization.[19,20] One explanation for endomitosis could be inhibition of microtubule-based forces in anaphase B. Spindle pole separation during anaphase B is believed to be powered by the sliding of antiparallel interdigitating microtubules past each other[21] by the mitotic kinesin-like protein 1 that localizes at regions of overlapping microtubules during anaphase B and has been shown to slide microtubules past one another in vitro.[22] Therefore lack of spindle pole separation during endomitosis may result from failure of megakaryocytes to undergo normal spindle orientation and/or the absence of signals that localize or activate a kinesin motor molecule that provides force for sliding.

Cytoplasmic Maturation

Megakaryocytes, the largest of the hematopoietic cells, undergo a pronounced cytoplasmic maturation to attain their large volumes (15,000 fL). Cytoplasmic maturation begins during endomitosis and increases considerably after all DNA amplification has ended (Fig. 126-2). Megakaryocytes enlarge dramatically as they mature, reaching sizes of 100 to 150 μm in diameter in culture and in bone marrow. During this process, the megakaryocytic cytoplasm rapidly fills with platelet-specific proteins, organelles, and membrane systems that ultimately are subdivided and packaged into platelets (Fig. 126-3). Their cytoplasmic space expands and, except for the most cortical regions, becomes densely filled with internal membranes that subsequently serve as the repository for the plasma membrane to be regurgitated for coating proplatelets as they extend.[23] This internal membrane system is one of the most striking features of a mature megakaryocyte and has been referred to as the demarcation membrane system (DMS). The DMS, first described by Yamada[24] in 1957, consists of an extensive, tortuous, branching network of membrane channels composed of flattened cisternae and tubules. Initially, the DMS was proposed to play an essential role in platelet formation by defining preformed "platelet territories" or "platelet fields" within the megakaryocyte cytoplasm.[25,26] Release of individual platelets was postulated to occur by massive fragmentation of the megakaryocyte cytoplasm along DMS fracture lines between these fields. However, studies demonstrating that platelets are

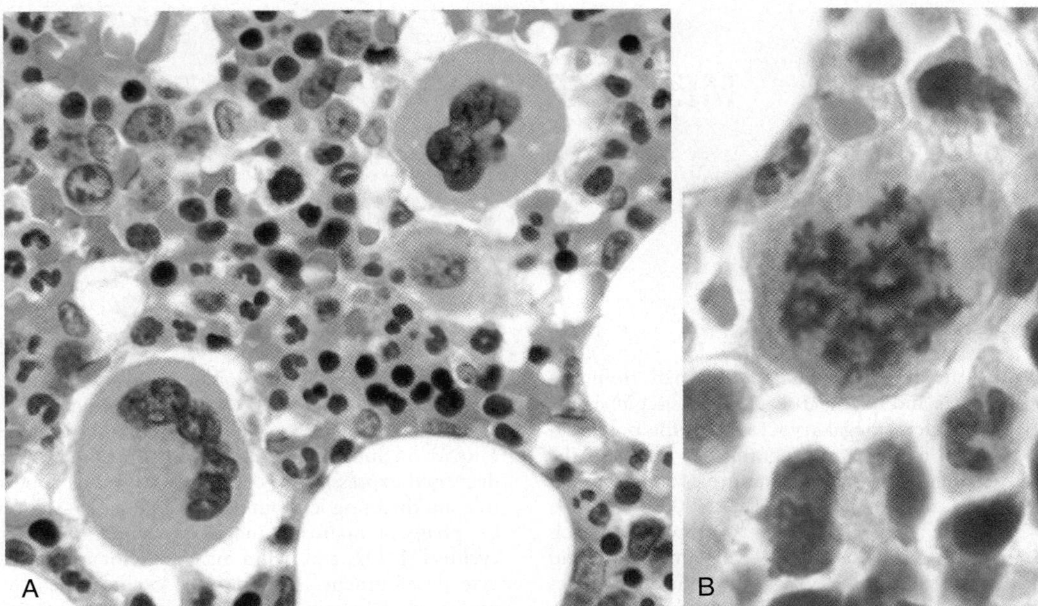

Figure 126-1 POLYPLOID MEGAKARYOCYTES IN THE BONE MARROW. Large polyploid megakaryocytes are seen in the bone marrow on a typical hematoxylin- and eosin-stained slide and are recognized by their abundant pink cytoplasm and large nuclei **(A)**. The degree of polyploidization is difficult to determine. Rarely, megakaryocytes can be seen in mitosis **(B),** and when chromosomes are aligned in metaphase plates, the high ploidy level become quite apparent. In the mitotic figure illustrated, the megakaryocyte is a 16N form with eight 2N metaphase plates.

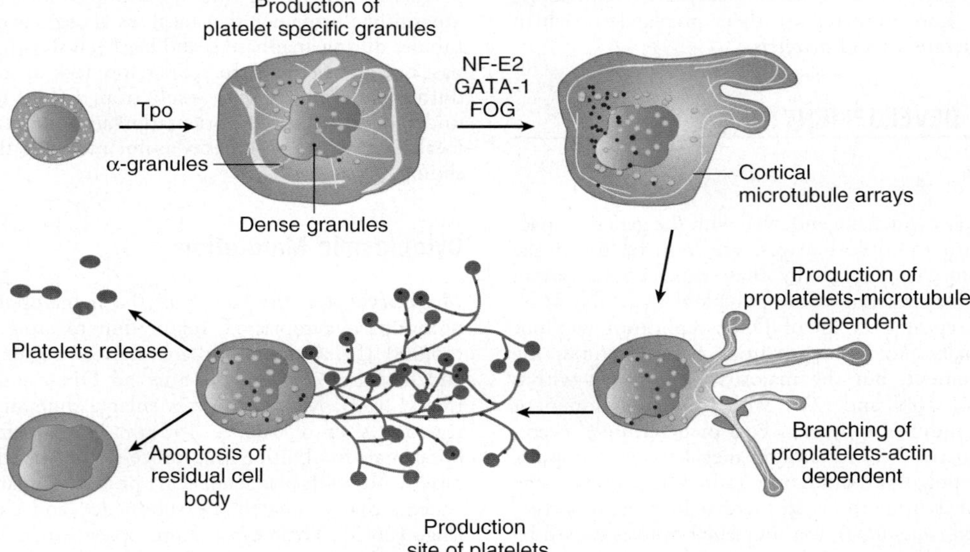

Figure 126-2 SUMMARY OF THE MAJOR EVENTS THAT LEAD TO PLATELET FORMATION AND RELEASE FROM MEGAKARYOCYTES. Hematopoietic stem cells are converted into megakaryocytes by exposure to the specific growth factor thrombopoietin (TPO). TPO initiates a maturation program that amplifies the megakaryocyte DNA and leads to synthesis of platelet-specific proteins. In particular, cytoskeletal elements, membrane systems, and receptor proteins are made in bulk, and the megakaryocyte becomes filled with platelet-specific granules. Platelet production begins when microtubules aggregate in the cell cortex, and one pole of the megakaryocyte spontaneously elaborates pseudopodia. These begin as large blunt pseudopodia, which subsequently thin and branch into proplatelets. The branching reaction is dependent on a localized assembly of actin and is inhibited by drugs that disrupt actin filaments. Platelets are assembled primarily at the ends of the proplatelets. Intracellular organelles are delivered to the platelet buds along microtubule tracks in the shafts. Platelets are released from the ends of proplatelets.

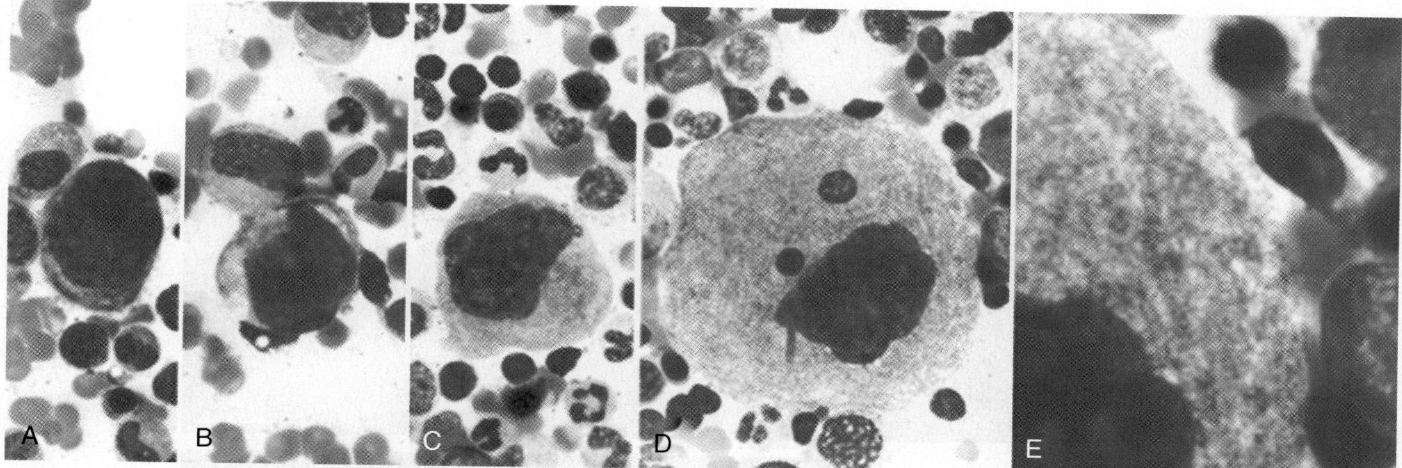

Figure 126-3 PLATELET PRODUCTION IN THE MEGAKARYOCYTE. **A,** Immature polyploid megakaryoblast with little differentiation. **B,** Megakaryocyte with early Golgi zone. **C,** Early platelet production in cytoplasm. **D,** Late-stage megakaryocyte with abundant internal membranes, organelles, and platelet-specific proteins. **E,** Early formation of demarcation membranes.

primarily assembled and released from proplatelet ends (see Platelet Formation, later in this chapter) are inconsistent with this notion and indicate instead that the DMS functions predominantly as a membrane reserve for proplatelet formation.[23] Direct visualization of mature DMS containing phosphatidylinositol 4,5-bisphosphate suggests that it is the source of proplatelet membranes.[2] Maturing megakaryocytes, like other granulated cells, contain an abundance of ribosomes and rough endoplasmic reticulum, where protein synthesis occurs. During this phase of megakaryocyte development, the cytoplasm fills with cytoskeletal proteins, platelet-specific receptors and secretory granules, and normal cellular organelles such as mitochondria and lysosomes.

One of the hallmark features of the mature megakaryocyte is its abundance of platelet-specific secretory granules. The two specific granules destined for platelets are α-granules and dense granules. α-Granules, the more abundant and larger of the two (200 to 500 nm in diameter), contain proteins that enhance platelet adhesion, promote cell-cell interactions, regulate angiogenesis, and stimulate vascular repair. α-Granules store matrix proteins and contain glycoprotein receptors in their membranes (Fig. 126-4, *A*). The bulk of cellular P-selectin and a portion of $\alpha_{IIb}\beta_3$ and the glycoprotein Ib/IX/V complex (GPIb-IX-V, a receptor for von Willebrand factor [vWF]) are expressed in the membranes of α-granules. Adhesion molecules within the granules include vWF, fibrinogen, fibronectin, vitronectin, and thrombospondin. α-Granule proteins can derive from different sources. Some proteins, such as α-thromboglobulin and vWF, are synthesized by megakaryocytes. However, fibrinogen, also a major component of α-granules, is not synthesized by megakaryocytes and is taken up from plasma by an endocytic mechanism requiring fibrinogen binding by $\alpha_{IIb}\beta_3$. Although little is known about the intracellular trafficking of proteins in megakaryocytes, experiments using cryosectioning and immunoelectron microscopy suggest that multivesicular bodies are an essential intermediate stage in the formation of platelet α-granules. During megakaryocyte development, large (≈0.5 μm) multivesicular bodies undergo a gradual transition from granules containing 30- to 70-nm internal vesicles to granules containing secretion concentrates.

The second and smaller type of platelet granule is the dense granule. Platelets contain relatively few dense granules, which are approximately 150 nm in diameter. Dense granules have electron opaque cores and function primarily to recruit additional platelets to sites of vascular injury. Dense granules contain the soluble activating agents serotonin and ADP as well as divalent cations. When the megakaryocyte reaches a certain point of maturation, proplatelet production begins, and granules are sent into the proplatelets destined for platelets.

REGULATION OF MEGAKARYOCYTE DEVELOPMENT

The development of megakaryocytes and the process of platelet biogenesis occur within a complex bone marrow environment where both cytokines and adhesive interactions play an essential role. Megakaryocytes are imprisoned within the subendothelial layer of the bone marrow sinuses where development and platelet biogenesis are regulated at multiple levels by several cytokines. Thrombopoietin (Tpo), which is synthesized in bone marrow and liver, is the principal regulator of thrombopoiesis. Tpo also plays a central role in hematopoietic stem cell survival and proliferation. Circulating levels of Tpo induce proliferation and maturation of megakaryocyte progenitors by binding to the c-Mpl receptor and signaling induction. Tpo regulates all stages of megakaryocyte development, from the hematopoietic stem cell stage through cytoplasmic maturation. Tpo increases platelet production by increasing both the number and size of individual megakaryocytes. c-Mpl activation is regulated by a complex array of signaling molecules that turn on specific transcription factors (see Transcriptional Regulation of Platelet Formation, later in this chapter) to drive megakaryocyte proliferation and maturation. Although Tpo appears to function as the main regulator of megakaryocyte development, it is not exclusive in this action. The cytokine stem cell factor, granulocyte-macrophage colony-stimulating factor, FLT ligand, interleukin (IL)-3, IL-6, IL-11, and erythropoietin also can regulate megakaryocyte development but appear to function mainly in concert with Tpo. Mice that lack Tpo or its receptor c-Mpl have approximately 15% of the normal platelet count. The discovery of Tpo in 1994 and the development of primary megakaryocyte or mouse embryonic stem cell cultures that can be induced to faithfully reconstitute platelet formation have provided systems for studying megakaryocytes in the act of making platelets in vitro. Megakaryocytes isolated from mouse fetal liver and incubated with Tpo for 4 to 5 days mature into huge polyploid cells that are capable of generating and releasing large numbers of platelets. In a similar fashion, mouse embryonic stem cells can be induced to mature into large polyploid megakaryocytes in the presence of stromal cells and Tpo, IL-6, and IL-11. This process requires 10 to 12 days, during which the conversion of embryonic stem cells into hematopoietic stem cells very likely occurs in the first half of the time period and the maturation of hematopoietic stem cells into proplatelet-producing megakaryocytes in the second half. Human embryonic stem cells can be coaxed to differentiate into mature megakaryocytes,[3] although the process takes several more days in culture. Recently, platelets have been generated from human induced pluripotent stem cells in culture using a doxycycline-controlled c-MYC expression vector.[4]

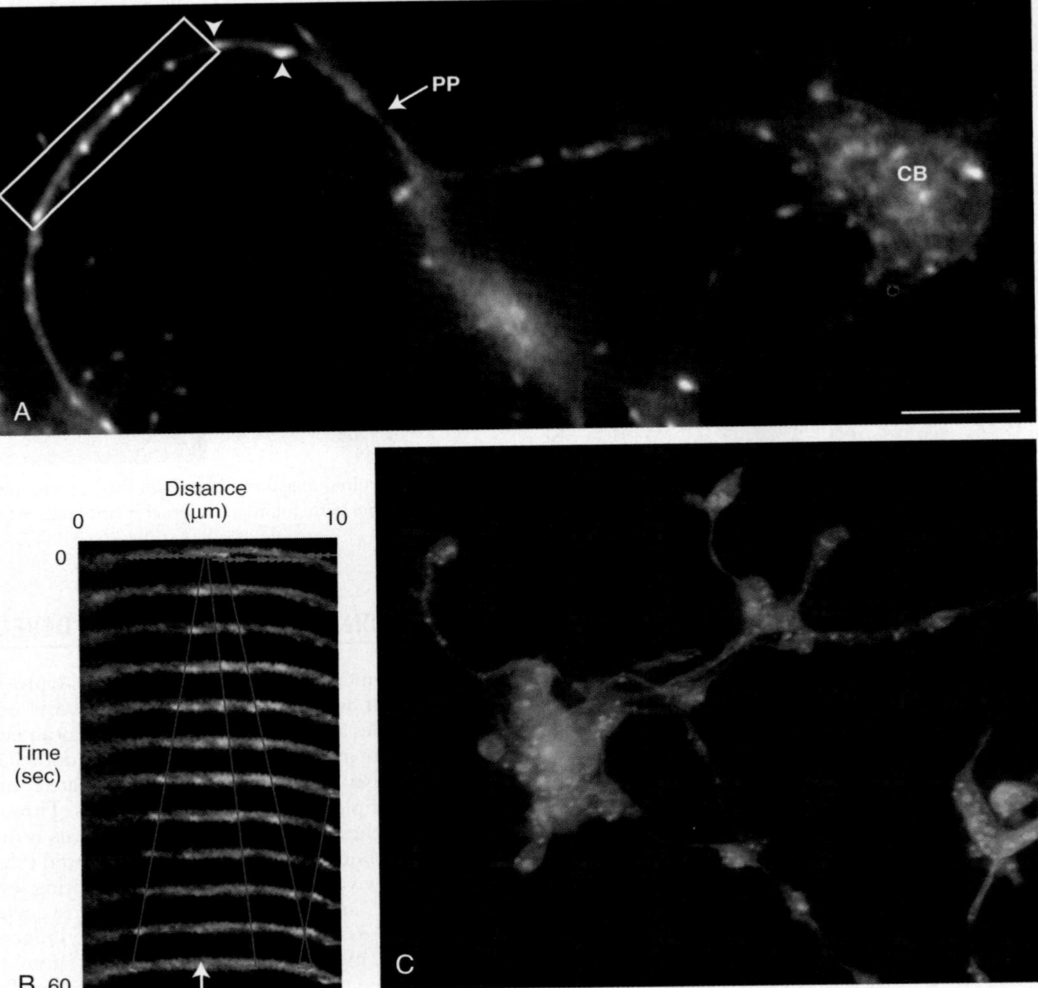

Figure 126-4 MICROTUBULE DYNAMICS DURING PROPLATELET FORMATION. **A,** Visualization of plus-end microtubule assembly in living megakaryocytes expressing end-binding protein 3 (EB3)–green fluorescent protein (GFP). First frame from the time-lapse sequence (shown in **B**) of a living megakaryocyte that was retrovirally directed to express EB3-GFP. The cell body (CB) is at the right of the micrograph, and proplatelets (PP) extend to the left. EB3-GFP labels growing microtubule plus ends in a characteristic "comet" staining pattern that has a bright front and a dim tail. **B,** The kymograph shows movement over time. Images are every 5 seconds. EB3-GFP comets undergo bidirectional movements in proplatelets, demonstrating that microtubules are organized as bipolar arrays. Some EB3-GFP comets move toward the tip and are highlighted in green; others that move toward the cell body are highlighted in *red.* **C,** Distribution of α-granules in megakaryocytes and proplatelet projections visualized by fluorescence microscopy. α-Granules are stained with Alexa 568 *(red)*–labeled anti–von Willebrand factor antibodies. The proplatelets have been co-stained with Alexa 488 *(green)* antitubulin antibodies to highlight the microtubules.

PLATELET FORMATION

Proplatelets and the Cytoskeletal Mechanics of Platelet Formation

The discovery of Tpo and the development of megakaryocyte cultures that reconstitute platelet formation in vitro have allowed visualization of megakaryocytes in the act of forming platelets.[5] The actual mechanical process of platelet production begins when mature megakaryocytes start to elaborate proplatelets (see Fig. 126-2 and Fig. 126-5). This process is distinguished by the erosion of one pole of the megakaryocyte cytoplasm (see Fig. 126-5). Multiple thick pseudopodia are extended and subsequently elongate to yield thin tubules. As these slender tubules grow, they branch repeatedly and develop periodic densities along their length that impart a beaded appearance.[5,6] The first insight into the cytoskeletal mechanics of platelet formation dates from the work of Tablin and colleagues, who showed that proplatelet formation is dependent on microtubules; that is, proplatelet elaboration is inhibited by microtubule poisons. Microtubule poisons are effective because the extension of proplatelets from the megakaryocyte is mediated by the assembly of microtubules and their reorganization into cortical bundles. Cortical bundles align in the shafts of proplatelets, and proplatelet elongation is driven by sliding movements between overlapping microtubules composed of these bundles.[7] The microtubule bundles form loops at the end of each proplatelet, and ultimately a single microtubule is rolled into a coil at the proplatelet end to define the platelet territory. Cytoplasmic tubulin in solution is an αβ dimer that reversibly polymerizes into microtubules, which are long, hollow cylinders with an outer diameter of 25 nm. Several studies reveal an essential role in platelet biogenesis for β_1 tubulin, a divergent and lineage-specific β tubulin, which is a major component of the megakaryocyte proplatelet cytoskeleton and marginal microtubule coil of the platelet. β_1 Tubulin, which is expressed exclusively in platelets and megakaryocytes during the late stages of megakaryocyte development, is essential for the

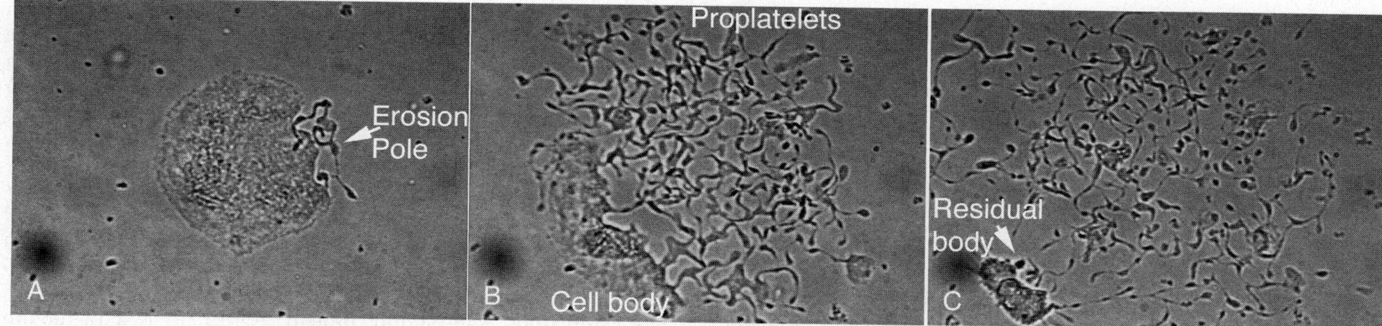

Figure 126-5 FORMATION OF PROPLATELETS BY A MOUSE MEGAKARYOCYTE. Time-lapse sequence of a maturing megakaryocyte showing the events that lead to elaboration of proplatelets in vitro. **A,** Platelet production begins when the megakaryocyte cytoplasm starts to erode at one pole *(arrow)*. **B,** The bulk of the megakaryocyte cytoplasm has been converted into multiple proplatelet processes that continue to lengthen and form swellings along their length. These processes are highly dynamic and undergo bending and branching. **C,** Once the bulk of the megakaryocyte cytoplasm has been converted into proplatelets, the entire process ends in a rapid retraction that separates the released proplatelets from the residual cell body.

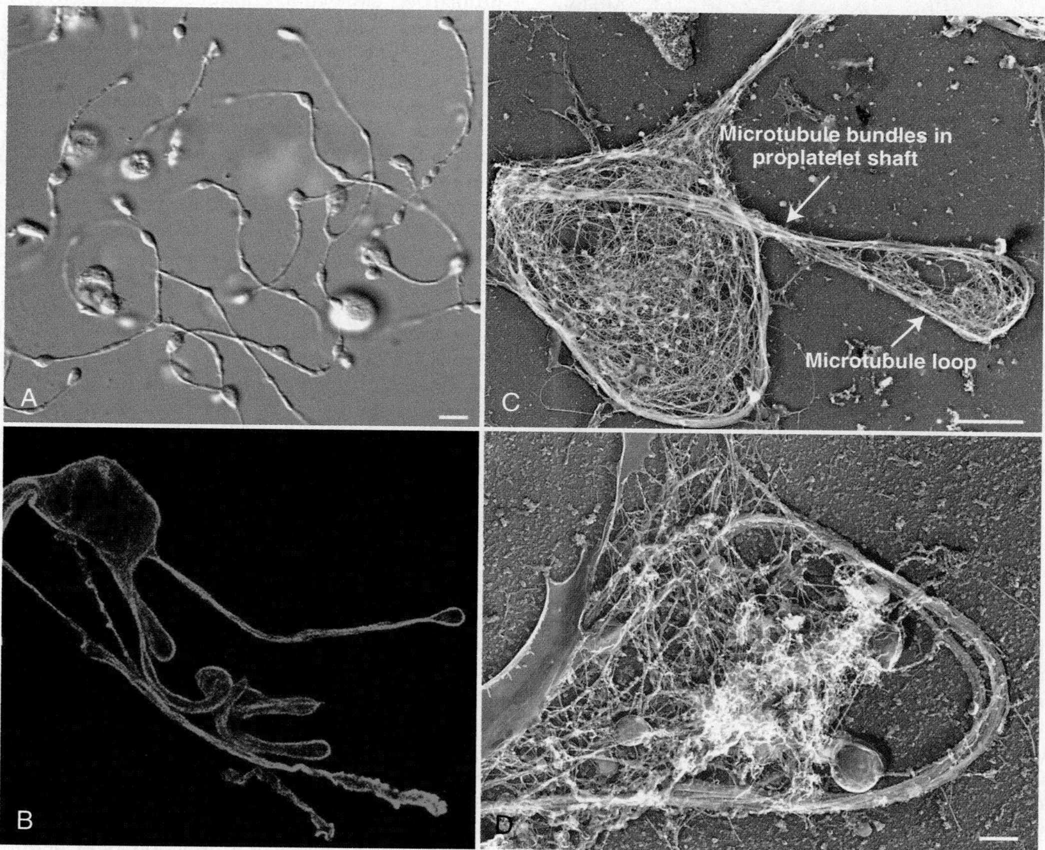

Figure 126-6 STRUCTURE OF PROPLATELETS. **A,** Differential interference contrast image of proplatelets elaborated by mouse megakaryocytes in culture (bar = 5 μm). **B,** Staining of proplatelets with Alexa 488 antitubulin IgG reveals that the microtubules line the shaft of the proplatelet and form loops at the proplatelet tips (bar = 5 μm). **C** and **D,** Organization of microtubules in the tips of proplatelets. **C,** Microtubules form bundles in the proplatelet shafts (bar = 2 μm). **D,** Microtubules loop in the proplatelet ends and reenter the proplatelet shafts (bar = 0.2 μm).

production of normal numbers of platelets, as well as for the discoid shape of platelets. The evidence supporting the role of β_1 tubulin in these processes comes from several sources. First, mRNA subtraction between wild type and NF-E2–deficient megakaryocytes demonstrates that β_1 tubulin is a downstream effector of the megakaryocyte transcription factor NF-E2 and is absent from NF-E2-deficient megakaryocytes. Second, genetic elimination of the β_1-tubulin gene in mice results in thrombocytopenia.[6] Third, megakaryocytes isolated from β_1-tubulin knock-out mice fail to form proplatelets in vitro and instead extend only a small number of blunt protrusions.

The first event that signals proplatelet production is the consolidation of microtubules into large bundles at the megakaryocyte cortex that subsequently are reorganized into parallel bundles in the shafts of the proplatelets (Fig. 126-6).[8] Microtubule bundles are thick near the body of the megakaryocyte as they enter the proplatelet shaft but become progressively thinner throughout the shaft, such that only 5 to 10 microtubules remain at the end of the proplatelet. Of note, the microtubule bundles that run down the proplatelet shaft make characteristic U turns in the tips and reenter the shaft, forming teardrop-shaped structures (Fig. 126-7). This creates a bipolar orientation of

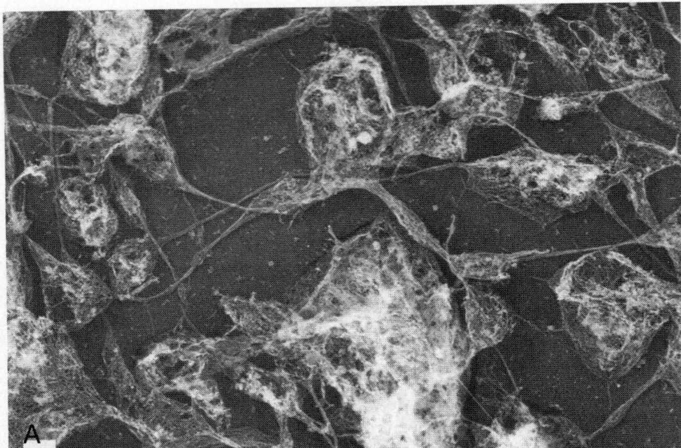

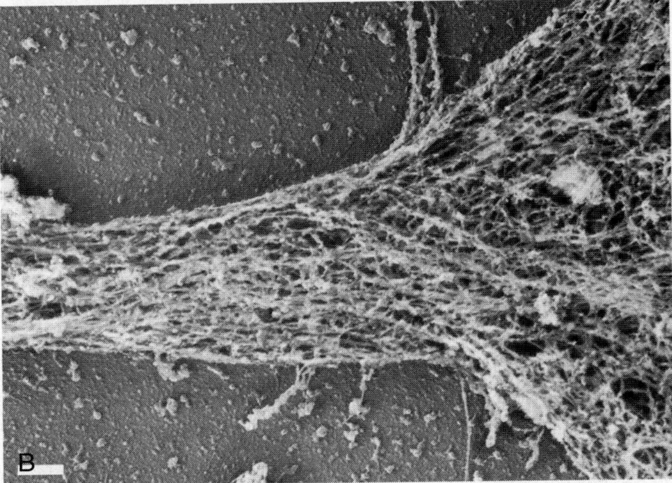

Figure 126-7 MEMBRANE SKELETON OF THE PROPLATELET. Representative electron micrographs of the detergent-insoluble proplatelet cytoskeleton. Proplatelets were permeabilized with 0.75% Triton X-100, 5 μM phallacidin, and 0.1% glutaraldehyde. Examination through electron microscopy reveals that the plasma membrane of the proplatelet tube is supported by a fibrous membrane skeleton that is similar in structure to the membrane skeleton of mature platelets. **A,** This low-magnification field shows that an intact membrane skeleton laminates the underside and extends along the entire length of proplatelets (bar = 1 μm). **B,** High magnification, three-dimensional electron micrograph of the proplatelet membrane skeleton demonstrating it to consist of a lattice-like network of elongated filamentous strands, similar in nature to the spectrin-based network in red blood cells and platelets. The membrane skeleton continuously laminates the underside of the proplatelet. A cytoplasmic bridge is shown *(left)* linking to a swelling *(right)* (bar = 200 nm).

bundles in the vicinity of the proplatelet tip, a geometry required to explain the bidirectional granule and organelle traffic observed in proplatelets. The looped arrangement of microtubules in proplatelet tips also constrains the elongation mechanism used to grow proplatelets because of an insufficient number of free microtubule ends to nucleate this reaction.

Direct visualization of microtubule dynamics in living megakaryocytes using green fluorescent protein (GFP) technology has provided insights into how microtubules orient to power proplatelet elongation (see Fig. 126-4, *A* and *B*). End-binding protein 3 (EB3), a microtubule plus end-binding protein associated only with growing microtubules, fused to GFP was retrovirally expressed in murine megakaryocytes and used as a marker to locate microtubule plus ends and to follow plus end dynamics.[7] Immature megakaryocytes without proplatelets use a centrosomal-coupled microtubule nucleation/assembly reaction, which appears as a prominent starburst pattern when visualized with EB3-GFP. Microtubules assemble only from the centrosome and grow outward into the cell cortex, where they turn and run parallel to the cell edges. Just before proplatelet production begins, however, centrosomal assembly ends and microtubules release and consolidate into the cortex as bundles. Fluorescence time-lapse microscopy of living, proplatelet-producing megakaryocytes expressing EB3-GFP reveals that as proplatelets elongate, microtubules assemble continuously throughout the entire proplatelet. EB3-GFP studies also reveal that microtubules polymerize in both directions in proplatelets—that is, toward both the tips and cell body, demonstrating that microtubules composing the bundles have a mixed polarity. The cytoplasmic Ran-binding protein, RanBP10, is a β_1-tubulin binding protein that appears to regulate the assembly of proplatelet microtubules.[9] Even though microtubules are continuously assembling at their plus ends in proplatelets, polymerization per se does not provide the force for proplatelet elongation. First, the rates of microtubule polymerization (average 10.2 μm/min) are approximately 10-fold faster than the proplatelet elongation rate. Second, proplatelets elongation continues when microtubule polymerization is blocked with drugs that inhibit net assembly, suggesting an alternative mechanism for proplatelet elongation. Third, proplatelets possess an inherent microtubule sliding mechanism. Cytoplasmic dynein, a minus-end microtubule molecular motor protein, localizes along the microtubules of the proplatelet and appears to directly contribute to microtubule sliding because inhibition of dynein through disassembly of the dynactin complex prevents proplatelet formation. Microtubule sliding can be reactivated in detergent-permeabilized proplatelets. Adenosine triphosphate, known to support the enzymatic activity of microtubule-based molecular motors, activates elongation in permeabilized proplatelets that contain dynein and its regulatory complex dynactin. Thus dynein-facilitated microtubule sliding appears to be the key event driving proplatelet elongation.

Nascent platelets assemble at the bulbous ends of proplatelets as defined by the rolling of a single microtubule into a coil having the same diameter as the coil found in the mature platelet. Given that maturation of the platelet is limited to these sites, efficient platelet production requires a large number of proplatelet ends. Megakaryocytes use a unique mechanical process to repeatedly bifurcate the shafts of the proplatelet, thereby amplifying the number of ends. To accomplish this task, the shaft of elongating proplatelets is bent on itself and a new proplatelet grows out of the bend; a process that results in bifurcation of the shaft. Whereas proplatelet elongation is mediated by microtubules, actin mediates the bending and branching of proplatelet shafts. Actin filament assemblies decorate branch points, and agents that disrupt actin assembly, such as the cytochalasins, abolish proplatelet branching. One possibility is that proplatelet bending and branching are regulated by the actin-based molecular motor myosin. Myosin II is an ATPase motor that makes up 2% to 5% of the total platelet protein. Myosin II binds to actin filaments and generates force for contraction. Each myosin has two heads and a long, rod-like tail whose function is to permit the molecules to assemble into bipolar filaments. Of interest, a mutation in the tail domain of the nonmuscle myosin heavy chain A gene in humans results in several disorders, including May-Hegglin anomaly, Sebastian syndrome, and Fechtner syndrome. These rare autosomal platelet disorders are characterized by thrombocytopenia with giant platelets. Recent findings have implicated myosin IIA in restricting proplatelet production until megakaryocytes attain full maturity. The loss of myosin IIA function through targeted gene disruption in mice, through dominant inhibitory mutations in humans, or by manipulation of cultured megakaryocytes appears to accelerate proplatelet production. Consequently, platelet production is inefficient and produces platelets that vary extensively in shape, content, and diameter. These findings also suggest that the Rho-ROCK-myosin light chain pathway regulates myosin IIA.

In addition to playing an essential role in proplatelet elongation, the microtubules lining the shafts of proplatelets serve a secondary function: transport of membrane, organelles, and granules into proplatelets and assembling platelets at proplatelet ends (see Fig. 126-4, *C*). Organelles are sent individually from the cell body into the proplatelets, where they move bidirectionally until they are captured at proplatelet tips.[14] Immunofluorescence and electron microscopic studies indicate that organelles are intimately associated with microtubules, and actin poisons do not diminish organelle motion. Thus movement appears to involve microtubule-based forces. Bidirectional organelle movement is conveyed in part by the bipolar arrangement of microtubules within the proplatelet because kinesin-coated latex beads move in both directions over the microtubule arrays of permeabilized proplatelets. Of the two major microtubule motors, kinesin and cytoplasmic dynein, only the plus end-directed kinesin is localized in a pattern similar to organelles and granules and is likely responsible for transporting these elements along microtubules. It appears that a twofold mechanism of organelle and granule movement occurs in platelet assembly: first, organelles and granules travel along microtubules, and second, the microtubules themselves slide bidirectionally in relation to other motile filaments, indirectly moving organelles along proplatelets in a piggyback manner.

Although the roles of microtubules and actin filaments in proplatelet development have been extensively studied, our understanding of the function of the membrane skeleton has only recently been established. High-resolution electron microscopy reveals that proplatelets have a dense spectrin-based membrane skeleton similar in structure to that of mature blood platelets. Nonerythroid spectrin subunits, alpha-II and beta-II spectrin, are predominately expressed in mouse megakaryocytes, proplatelets, and platelets, but erythroid alpha-I and beta-I spectrin isoforms are also expressed (see Fig. 126-6).[15] Assembly of spectrin tetramers is required for development of the demarcation membrane system and proplatelet elaboration, because expression of a spectrin tetramer–disrupting construct in megakaryocytes inhibits both processes. Furthermore, integration of this spectrin-disrupting construct into a permeabilized proplatelet system quickly destabilizes proplatelets, resulting in massive blebbing and swelling. Spectrin tetramers also stabilize the barbell-like shapes of the penultimate stage in platelet production (see later). Taken together, these studies suggest a role for spectrin in different steps of megakaryocyte development through its participation in the formation of demarcation membranes and in the maintenance of proplatelet structure.

Platelet Maturation at the Proplatelet Tip

Platelet maturation at proplatelet tips finalizes when a single microtubule detaches from the microtubule bundle and is rolled into a coil. To complete construction of mature platelets, once the fundamental cytoskeletal components have been delivered to and assembled in the platelet buds, the buds must fill with their organelle and granule content.

Granules are sent to nascent platelets on the microtubule tracks of the proplatelets. The concentration of this cargo in the platelet occurs by an end-trapping mechanism as granules and organelles, which enter the nascent platelet, continue to move in the tip but do not return to the proplatelet shaft.

Release of Mature Platelets

Details of how mature platelets release from the proplatelet tips are beginning to come into focus. In vitro, maturation of proplatelets ends in a rapid retraction that separates a variable portion of the proplatelets from the residual cell body, leaving behind a naked, denuded nucleus (see Fig. 126-5, *C*). Activation of apoptotic pathways in the cell body has been shown to be coincident with this event. Junt and colleagues have used intravital fluorescence microscopy to visualize proplatelet production in the opened cranial marrow cavity of living mice.[16] Yellow fluorescent protein (YFP)–labeled megakaryocytes were seen to protrude proplatelets and release megakaryocyte fragments into the marrow sinusoids of living mice. Notably, these anucleate fragments typically exceed platelet dimensions, suggesting that platelet morphogenesis continues in the circulation. In line with these observations, we have recently identified a previously unrecognized intermediate stage in platelet formation and release, which we termed the *preplatelet*.[17] Preplatelets are defined as discoid cells (3 to 10 microns) that retain the capacity to convert into barbell-shaped proplatelets and undergo fission into platelets. The conversion of preplatelets to barbell proplatelets is powered by microtubule-based forces. It is likely that the microtubule motors that drive proplatelet extension are involved in aspects of platelet release, as well as in the process of microtubule coiling. Sliding of an uncoiled portion of the microtubule relative to the rigid microtubule bundle in the proplatelet tip would provide a simple mechanism to effect platelet release and would explain the variable morphology of a small but reproducible percentage (<5%) of dumbbell-shaped platelets that are present in blood. Recently, it was demonstrated that individual human platelets have the innate capacity to duplicate and form new cell bodies that undergo fission into platelets.[18] The morphologic similarities between platelets that form new cell bodies and preplatelets are striking. Whether or not newly released platelets exhibit a preplatelet phenotype, which allows them to form barbell-shapes and divide again, is not clear.

Location of Platelet Release

Megakaryocytes are produced in the bone marrow, and some undergo fragmentation into platelets in this location. It has been suggested that, by extending into the bone marrow sinusoids, proplatelets provide a mechanism for extension into the bone, allowing release of platelets directly into the circulation.[19,20] Megakaryocytes have been identified in intravascular sites within the lung, leading to a theory that some platelets are formed from their parent cell in the pulmonary circulation.

Transcriptional Regulation of Platelet Formation

Megakaryocyte development and platelet formation are controlled by the coordinated action of transcription factors that specifically turn on the genes of megakaryocyte precursors or suppress the expression of genes that support other cell types.[21] Gene-targeting studies in mice have identified several genes that are crucial for megakaryocyte development and platelet formation. Leading the list of transcription factors that play an essential role in megakaryocyte maturation and platelet biogenesis is the basic leucine zipper heterodimer NF-E2. NF-E2 is a protein composed of a ubiquitously expressed 18- to 20-kd small-Maf subunit and a p45 subunit that is restricted to erythroid and megakaryocytic lineages. Although NF-E2 was postulated to be a transcription factor that specifically drove the expression of genes essential for erythropoiesis, mice lacking p45 NF-E2 do not exhibit defects in erythropoiesis. Instead, mice deficient in the p45 subunit or two of the small-Maf subunits die of hemorrhage shortly after birth because of a complete lack of circulating platelets. Although megakaryocytes undergo normal endomitosis and proliferate in response to Tpo, mice deficient in p45 NF-E2 produce increased numbers of megakaryocytes that are larger than normal, contain fewer granules, exhibit a highly disorganized DMS, and fail to generate proplatelets in vitro, a phenotype indicative of a late block in megakaryocyte maturation. Therefore NF-E2 appears to control the transcription of a limited number of genes involved in cytoplasmic maturation and platelet formation. Shivdasani and colleagues generated a subtracted cDNA library enriched in transcripts downregulated in NF-E2 knock-out megakaryocytes. Using this approach, these investigators have started to identify the downstream targets of NF-E2 and analyzed their role in the terminal stages of megakaryocyte differentiation. Putative transcriptional targets of NF-E2 include β_1 tubulin, thromboxane synthase, and proteins that regulate inside-out signaling via $\alpha_{IIb}\beta_3$ integrin. The zinc finger protein GATA1 is also a transcription factor that plays a critical role in driving the expression of genes essential for megakaryocyte maturation. However, unlike NF-E2, which appears to drive the later stage of megakaryocyte development, GATA1 functions at multiple stages of development. Initially, GATA proteins were thought to regulate red blood cell maturation because genetic disruption of the GATA1 gene in mice results in embryonic lethality because of a block in erythropoiesis. However, several more recent observations also implicate GATA1 as a regulator of megakaryocyte differentiation. First, forced expression of GATA1 in the early myeloid cell line 416b induces megakaryocyte differentiation. Second, Shivdasani and colleagues used targeted mutagenesis of regulatory elements within the GATA1 locus to generate mice with a selective loss of GATA1 in the megakaryocyte lineage. These knockdown mice expressed sufficient levels of GATA1 in erythroid cells to circumvent the embryonic lethality caused by anemia. GATA1 deficiency in megakaryocytes leads to severe thrombocytopenia. Platelet counts are reduced to approximately 15% of normal, and the small number of circulating platelets are round and significantly larger than usual. These mice have increased numbers of small megakaryocytes that exhibit an accelerated rate of proliferation. The small cytoplasmic volume of GATA1-deficient megakaryocytes typically contains an excess of rough endoplasmic reticulum, very few platelet-specific granules, and an underdeveloped or disorganized DMS, suggesting that maturation of megakaryocytes is arrested in GATA1-deficient megakaryocytes.

A family with X-linked dyserythropoietic anemia and thrombocytopenia due to a mutation in GATA1 has been described. A single nucleotide substitution in the amino-terminal zinc finger of GATA1 inhibits the interaction of GATA1 with its essential cofactor, friend of GATA1 (FOG). Although megakaryocytes in affected family members are abundant, they are unusually small and exhibit several abnormal features, including an abundance of smooth endoplasmic reticulum, an underdeveloped DMS, and a lack of granules. These observations suggest an essential role for the FOG1-GATA1 interaction in thrombopoiesis. Genetic elimination of FOG in mice unexpectedly resulted in specific ablation of the megakaryocyte lineage, suggesting a GATA1-independent role for FOG in the early stages of megakaryocyte development; GATA1 and FOG are required for megakaryocyte generation from a common bipotential progenitor.

Several knock-out mice also indicate a role for additional transcription factors in megakaryocyte development. Mice carrying a null mutation in Fli-1, a member of the ETS family of winged helix-turn-helix transcription factors that bind purine-rich sequences in gene promoters, exhibit defects in megakaryocyte development. Megakaryocytes cultured from mice lacking Fli-1 contain reduced numbers of α-granules, disorganization of the demarcation membranes, and a reduction in size. Mice lacking the hematopoietic zinc finger (Hzf) protein, a transcription factor that is predominantly expressed in megakaryocytes, have reduced numbers of α-granules in megakaryocytes and platelets. Therefore Hzf may regulate the transcription of genes involved in the synthesis of α-granule components and/or their packaging into α-granules. SCL, a basic helix-loop-helix transcription factor initially identified in a subset of human T-cell leukemia with multilineage characteristics, also appears to be critical for megakaryopoiesis. Deletion of SCL in mice indicates this transcription factor is required for proper erythroid and megakaryocyte development.

PLATELETS

Structure of the Resting Platelet

Megakaryocyte development culminates in the release of mature discoid platelets having dimensions of approximately 3.0 × 0.5 μm and a cytoplasmic volume of 7 fL.[22] The evolutionary explanation for the discoid shape of the platelet is unknown. Discoid shape may permit more efficient flow or dispersion of clot-promoting elements or may simply reflect the microtubule-based mechanism by which platelets are produced. In humans, platelets, once released from the ends of proplatelets, normally circulate for 7 to 10 days. Given that nearly 1 trillion platelets circulate in an adult human, each day an adult produces approximately 100 billion platelets.

The precise morphology of newly released platelets is unknown. However, when released into the circulation or maintained in culture, platelets have a very reproducible structure. Although they are heterogeneous in size, presumably because of changes in size as they age, platelets have discoid shapes with flat, featureless surfaces (Fig. 126-8, *A*, and Fig. 126-9, *A*) that are interrupted only by pit-like openings into the open canalicular system (OCS). The OCS is an extensive system of internal membrane conduits that serves as a passageway to the outside world into which granular contents are released. It also is a reservoir of plasma membrane, membrane receptors, and proteins. For example, approximately 30% of the thrombin receptors are localized in the OCS of the resting platelet, awaiting movement to the surface when the cells are activated. Although contiguous with the plasma membrane, not all proteins on the cell surface can enter the OCS. Factors controlling movement into the OCS remain to be defined but likely depend on the actin cytoskeleton. Entry restriction, however, occurs at the necks of OCS infoldings. The third function of the OCS is to serve as a source of redundant plasma membrane for cell spreading. OCS membrane initially is disgorged to the surface following cell activation. When cells are activated in solution, much of this membrane is subsequently reabsorbed into the remnants of the OCS.

A small thin zone of cytoplasm separates the plasma membrane of the resting platelet from a marginal microtubule coil and the general intracellular space, which contains all inclusion bodies and the internal cytoskeleton of the cell. This zone is filled with the spectrin-based membrane skeleton (see Fig. 126-9, *A*). Beneath this zone sits a microtubule coil. Then follows the cytoplasmic space, which is filled with filaments of actin that embed granules, organelles, the OCS, and other specialized membrane systems such as smooth endoplasmic reticulum.

Platelets actively recruit other blood-borne cells to areas of vascular damage by releasing mediators packaged in intracellular granules (described earlier in Cytoplasmic Maturation) that initiate secondary homeostatic interactions and that express a "sticky" apical surface after the platelets adhere. In the resting platelet, granules are juxtaposed together and are in intimate association with the membranes of the OCS. The release reaction of platelet granules differs from that of other cells. Granules rarely fuse with the plasma membrane; instead they exocytose into the OCS. Platelets also contain lysosomes and a few mitochondria, which are easily identified under the electron microscope by their internal system of membrane cristae.

Cytoskeleton of the Resting Platelet

Although both microtubule- and actin-based forces have been considered in the elaboration and branching of proplatelets, respectively, it is the integration of the microtubule and actin cytoskeletal elements that uniquely defines the shape of the mature platelet. One of the most distinguishing features of the resting platelet is its marginal microtubule coil (see Fig. 126-8). αβ-Tubulin dimers assemble into microtubule polymers under physiologic conditions. In resting platelets, tubulin is equally divided between dimer and polymer fractions. In many cell types, αβ-tubulin subunits are in a dynamic equilibrium with microtubules such that reversible cycles of assembly-disassembly of microtubules are observed. Microtubules are long, hollow polymers (24 nm in diameter) that are responsible for many types of cellular movements, such as segregation of chromosomes during mitosis and transport of organelles across the cell. The microtubule ring of the resting platelet, initially characterized in the late 1960s by White and Krivit, was described as a single microtubule approximately 100 μm long and is coiled 8 to 12 times inside the periphery of the platelet. However, recent work suggests that the marginal band is highly dynamic and consists of multiple microtubules with mixed polarity that undergo constant assembly and disassembly.[23] This may accommodate the shrinkage of microtubule coil diameters that occurs

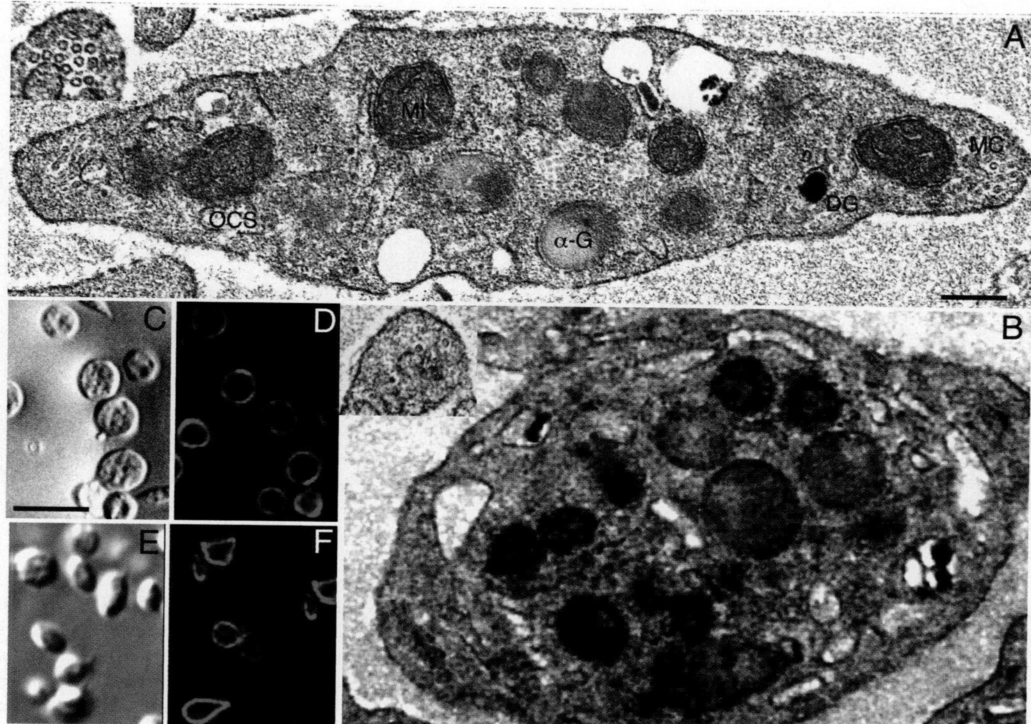

Figure 126-8 STRUCTURE OF NORMAL MOUSE PLATELETS **(A, C, D)** COMPARED WITH PLATELETS LACKING β_1 TUBULIN **(B, E, F). A,** Electron micrograph of a resting mouse platelet. This platelet was sectioned through its thin axis. The cut plane reveals the microtubule coil (MC) at the cell periphery. The inset shows a high-magnification cross-section through the microtubule coil of the resting platelet. The microtubule is wound 11 times in this platelet, forming the coil. The cytoplasmic space embeds mitochondria (MT), α-granules (α-G), and dense granules (DG). The spaces created by the open canalicular system (OCS) are apparent. **B,** Electron micrograph of a thin section through a platelet isolated from a mouse lacking β_1 tubulin (bar = 0.2 μm). Platelets from these animals are spherical **(E)** and have only a rudimentary microtubule coil *(inset)*. In this platelet the microtubule is twisted twice. **C,** Differential interference contrast image of resting platelets shows them to be flat discs. **D,** Microtubule coil of the resting mouse platelet. Staining of fixed mouse platelets with Alexa 488 antitubulin IgG reveals the microtubule coil. This coil resides at the periphery of the platelet. **E,** Differential interference contrast image of platelets lacking β_1 tubulin. **F,** Staining of fixed mouse β_1-tubulin–deficient platelets with Alexa 488 antitubulin IgG reveals the coil is defective and bent in a number of places throughout the platelets. (**C** through **F** are the same magnification; bar = 5 μm.)

with aging of platelets. The primary function of the microtubule coil is to maintain the discoid shape of the resting platelet. Disassembly of platelet microtubules with drugs such as vincristine, colchicine, or nocodazole causes platelets to become round and to lose their discoid shape. Cooling the platelets also causes disassembly of the microtubule coil and loss of the discoid shape. Mice lacking β_1 tubulin, the major hematopoietic β-tubulin isoform, produce platelets that lack their characteristic discoid shapes and have defective marginal bands. Genetic elimination of β_1 tubulin in mice results in thrombocytopenia with circulating platelet counts below 50% of normal. β_1-Tubulin–deficient platelets are spherical in shape, apparently due to shortened marginal bands with fewer coilings. Whereas normal platelets possess a marginal band that consists of 8 to 12 coils, β_1-tubulin knock-out platelets contain only 2 to 3 coils. A human β_1-tubulin functional substitution (AG→CC) inducing both structural and functional platelet alterations has been described. Of note, the Q43P β_1-tubulin variant was found in 10.6% of the general population and in 24.2% of 33 unrelated patients with undefined congenital macrothrombocytopenia. Electron microscopy revealed enlarged spherocytic platelets with a disrupted marginal band and structural alterations. Platelets with the Q43P β_1-tubulin variant showed mild platelet dysfunction, with reduced ATP secretion, thrombin receptor-activating peptide (TRAP)–induced aggregation, and impaired adhesion to collagen under flow conditions.[24] A more-than-doubled prevalence of the β_1-tubulin variant was observed in healthy subjects not undergoing ischemic events, raising the possibility that the variant confers an evolutionary advantage and a protective cardiovascular role.

Actin is the most abundant of all the platelet proteins, with 2 million molecules expressed per platelet. Of these molecules, 800,000 assemble to form the 2000 to 5000 linear actin polymers that exist in the resting cell (see Fig. 126-9, *A*). The remainder of the actin is maintained in storage as a 1 : 1 complex with β_4 thymosin, which can be converted to filaments during platelet activation to drive cell spreading. All evidence indicates that the filaments of the resting platelet are interconnected at various points into a rigid cytoplasmic network because platelets express high concentrations of actin cross-linking proteins, including filamin and α-actinin.[7] Both filamin and α-actinin are homodimers in solution. Three filamin genes are located on chromosomes 3, 7, and X. Filamin A (X) and filamin B (3) are expressed in platelets. Filamin A is expressed at more than 10-fold higher levels than is filamin B. Filamin subunits are elongated strands composed primarily of 24 repeats, each approximately 100 amino acids in length and folded into IgG-like β-barrels. Each strand has an amino-terminus actin-binding site that shares homology with other actin-binding proteins, two rod domains that are end-to-end assemblies of the repeat units, interrupted by two hinge domains between repeats 15 and 16, and 23 and 24, and a C-terminus self-association site (Fig. 126-10, *B*). Subunits assemble to form V-shaped bipolar molecules—that is, the self-association site is the vertex of the

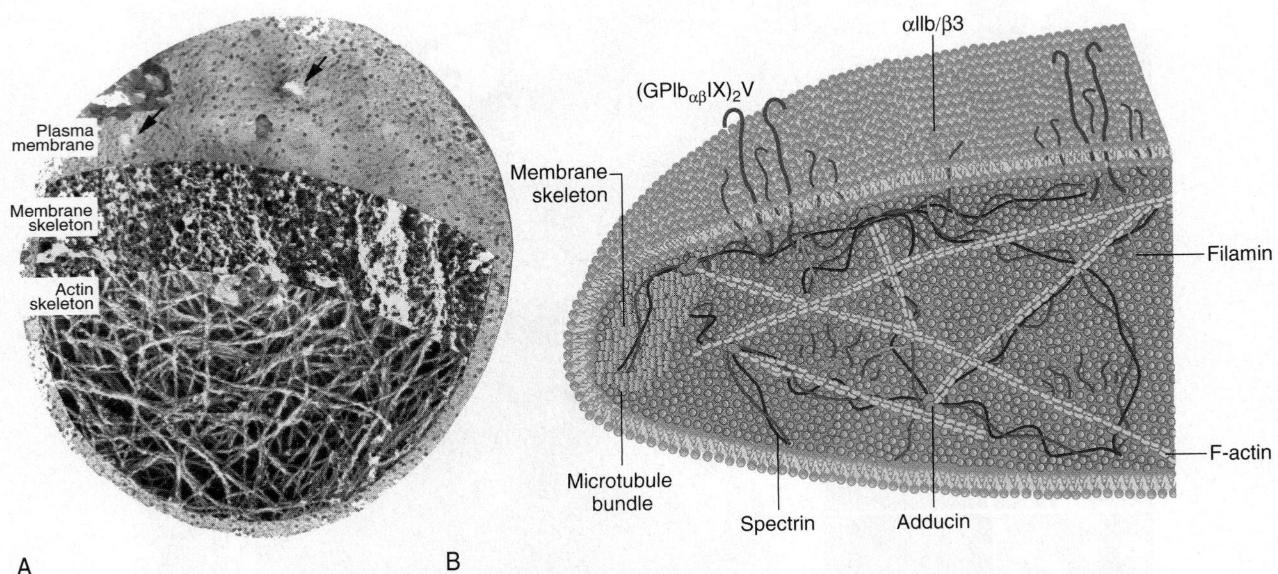

Figure 126-9 STRUCTURE OF THE RESTING HUMAN BLOOD PLATELET AND ITS ACTIN-BASED CYTOSKELETON. **A,** Composite illustrating the major actin cytoskeletal layers of the resting platelet. *Plasma membrane:* The plasma membrane of the resting cell is flat and featureless, except for periodic invaginations that lead into the open canalicular system (OCS) *(arrows). Membrane skeleton:* The plasma membrane of the platelet is supported by a submembranous spectrin-based skeleton. This network is composed primarily of spectrin molecules, which are tetramers with actin binding sites at the ends. Actin filament ends dock on spectrin to complete the network. The association between spectrin and F actin is promoted by adducin. *Actin cytoskeleton:* As discussed earlier, the spectrin network is both directly and indirectly attached to the underlying actin filaments. Filament ends interconnect spectrin molecules, whereas the filamin links run from the filament sides to the plasma membrane receptor (GPIb$_{\alpha\beta}$IX)$_2$V. The cytoplasmic space has a dense filling of actin filaments. Actin filaments from the cell center radiate outward. As the filaments approach the plasma membrane, they turn and run in parallel with it. The actin filaments have been decorated using myosin subfragment 1 (S1), which gives them a twisted cable-like appearance in frozen samples. Myosin S1 labeling reveals the polarity of the actin filament. "Pointed" and "barbed" ends are definable. The ends of actin filaments are bound by the ends of spectrin molecules on the edges of the membrane network *(arrowhead)*. A microtubule coil composed of a single long microtubule resides just beneath the plasma membrane at the periphery of the thin axis of the platelet (not shown) (bar = 0.5 μm). **B,** Schematic showing the structural features of the resting blood platelet cytoskeleton. Resting cells have discoid shapes. Structural elements that support this shape are (1) a marginal microtubule coil, (2) a spectrin-based membrane skeleton, and (3) a rigid network of cross-linked cytoplasmic actin filaments (only a small number of the actin filaments have been added to this illustration so that they will not obscure the rest of the structures in the cell). Platelets have a specialized membrane skeleton composed of spectrin, actin, and many associated proteins. Spectrin tetramers (200 nm long and 5 nm wide) have actin filament-binding sites at each molecular end. The membrane skeleton is held in compression between the plasma membrane and the cytoplasmic actin by filamin connections from the sides of actin filaments to the cytoplasmic tails of GPIbα subunit of the membrane glycoprotein complex that binds to von Willebrand factor (GPIbαβIX)$_2$V complex. Greater than 98% of the barbed ends of actin filaments are capped by adducin and capZ in the resting platelet.

V, and the actin-binding sites are on the free ends. Inclusion of the first hinge in filamin depends on alternative RNA splicing. Filamin now is recognized to be a prototype "scaffolding molecule" that collects binding partners and localizes them adjacent to the plasma membrane. Partners bound by filamin members include the small GTPases RalA, Rac, Rho, and Cdc42, with RalA binding in a GTP-dependent manner; the exchange factors Trio and Toll; kinases such as PAK1; phosphatases; and transmembrane proteins. Most partner proteins are bound within the C-terminus portion of filamin.

Central to the structural organization of the resting platelet is an interaction between filamin and the cytoplasmic tail of the GPIbα subunit of the GPIb-IX-V complex.[26] The second rod domain (repeat 17) of filamin has a binding site for the cytoplasmic tail of GPIbα. The interaction between filamin A and GPIbα occurs at the atomic level. Repeat 17 of filamin A has a groove between certain β-sheet strands that forms a pocket for the GPIbα tail (see Fig. 126-10). Binding between filamin A and GPIbα is driven by entropic forces, and the alignment and specificity are provided by large residues that create a lock-and-key fit between the two molecules. Whereas the interaction between one filamin A subunit and GPIbα has affinity of approximately 10 μM, high-affinity binding (10 nM) occurs when each filamin A subunit in a molecule and both GPIbα chains in a vWF receptor are engaged. Studies have shown that the bulk of platelet filamin (>90%) is in complex with GPIbα. This interaction has three consequences. First, it positions filamin's self-association domain and associated partner proteins at the plasma membrane while dangling filamin's actin binding sites into the cytoplasm. Second, because a large fraction of filamin is bound to actin, it aligns the GPIb-IX-V complexes on the surface of the platelet over the underlying filaments (see Fig. 126-9, *B*). Third, because the filamin linkages between actin filaments and the GPIb-IX-V complex pass through the pores of the spectrin lattice, it restrains the molecular movement of the spectrin strands in this lattice and holds the lattice in compression. The filamin-GPIbα connection is essential for the formation and release of discoid platelets by megakaryocytes; platelets lacking this connection are large and fragile and are produced in low numbers. However, the role of the filamin-vWF receptor connection in platelet construction is unknown. Because a low number of Bernard-Soulier platelets form and release from megakaryocytes, it can be argued that this connection is a late event in the maturation process and is not required for platelet shedding. Both filamin and GPIbα are synthesized early, but linkage between the two may not occur until later, perhaps as late as the final stages of platelet shedding.

Aside from the erythrocyte, the platelet is the only cell whose membrane skeleton has been visualized at high resolution. Like the

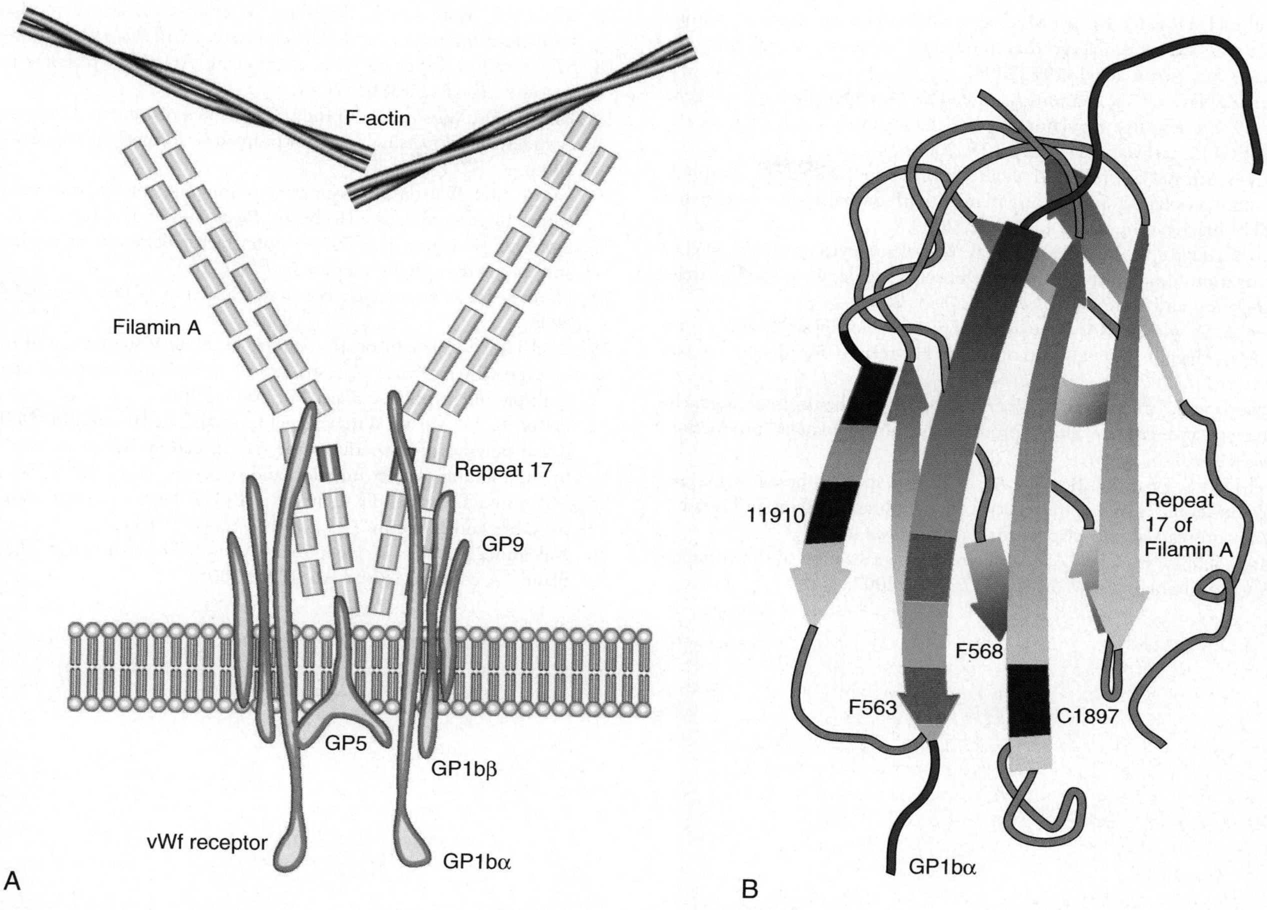

Figure 126-10 INTERACTION OF FILAMIN A WITH THE VON WILLEBRAND FACTOR RECEPTOR (vWFR). **A,** Model showing the orientation of filamin A when interacting with the GPIbα chain of the vWFR and cytoplasmic actin filaments. For tight binding of filamin A to vWFR, both GPIbα chains of the receptor must be engaged by a single filamin A molecule. **B,** Ribbon diagram showing the interface between filamin A repeat 17 and the filamin A binding region of the GPIbα tail (residues 556-577). Critical residues that provide the lock-and-key interaction between the two domains are indicated.

erythrocyte, the platelet membrane skeleton is a self-assembly of elongated spectrin strands (see Fig. 126-9) that interconnect through binding to actin filaments. Platelets express approximately 2000 spectrin molecules. Although considerably less is known about how the spectrin-actin network forms and is connected to the plasma membrane in the platelet relative to the erythrocyte, certain differences between the two membrane skeletons have been identified. First, the spectrin strands composing the platelet membrane skeleton interconnect using the ends of long actin filaments instead of short actin oligomers. These ends arrive at the plasma membrane originating from filaments in the cytoplasm. Hence the spectrin lattice is assembled into a continuous network by its association with actin filaments. Second, tropomodulins are not expressed at sufficiently high levels, if at all, to have a major role in capping the pointed ends of the platelet actin filaments. Instead, biochemical experiments have revealed that a substantial number (≈2000) of these ends are free in the resting platelet. Third, although little tropomodulin protein is expressed, α adducin and γ adducin are abundantly expressed and appear to cap many of the barbed ends of the filaments composing the resting actin cytoskeleton. Adducin is a key component of the membrane skeleton, forming a triad complex with spectrin and actin. Capping of barbed filament ends by adducin also serves the function of targeting them to the spectrin-based membrane skeleton, because the affinity of spectrin for adducin-actin complexes is greater than for either actin or adducin alone. Platelet glycoproteins involved in attaching spectrin to the membrane remain to be defined.

REFERENCES

1. Bluteau D, Lordier L, Di Stefano A, et al: Regulation of megakaryocyte maturation and platelet formation. *J Thromb Haemost* 7:227, 2009.
2. Schulze H, Korpal M, Hurov J, et al: Characterization of the megakaryocyte demarcation membrane system and its role in thrombopoiesis. *Blood* 107:3868, 2006.
3. Lu SJ, Li F, Yin H, et al: Platelets generated from human embryonic stem cells are functional in vitro and in the microcirculation of living mice. *Cell Res* 11.
4. Takayama N, Nishimura S, Nakamura S, et al: Transient activation of c-MYC expression is critical for efficient platelet generation from human induced pluripotent stem cells. *J Exp Med* 207:2817, 2010.
5. Italiano JE, Jr, Lecine P, Shivdasani RA, et al: Blood platelets are assembled principally at the ends of proplatelet processes produced by differentiated megakaryocytes. *J Cell Biol* 147:1299, 1999.
6. Schwer H, Lecine P, Tiwari S, et al: A lineage-restricted and divergent b tubulin isoform is essential for the biogenesis, structure and function of mammalian blood platelets. *Curr. Biol* 11:579, 2001.
7. Patel S, Richardson J, Schulze H, et al: Differential roles of microtubule assembly and sliding in proplatelet formation by megakaryocytes. *Blood* 106:4076, 2005.
8. Patel S, Hartwig J, Italiano J, Jr: The biogenesis of platelets from megakaryocyte proplatelets. *J. Clin. Invest* 115:3348, 2006.

9. Schulze H, Dose M, Korpal M, et al: RanBP10 is a cytoplasmic guanine nucleotide exchange factor that modulates noncentrosomal microtubules. *J Biol Chem* 283:14109, 2008.
10. Chen Z, Naveiras O, Balduini A, et al: The May-Hegglin anomaly gene MYH9 is a negative regulator of platelet biogenesis modulated by the Rho-ROCK pathway. *Blood* 110:171, 2007.
11. Eckly A, Strassel C, Freund M, et al: Abnormal megakaryocyte morphology and proplatelet formation in mice with megakaryocyte-restricted MYH9 inactivation. *Blood* 113:3182, 2009.
12. Leon C, Eckly A, Hechler B, et al: Megakaryocyte-restricted MYH9 inactivation dramatically affects hemostasis while preserving platelet aggregation and secretion. *Blood* 110:3183, 2007.
13. Chen Z, Shivdasani RA: Regulation of platelet biogenesis: Insights from the May-Hegglin anomaly and other MYH9-related disorders. *J Thromb Haemost* 7:272, 2009.
14. Richardson J, Shivdasani R, Boers C, et al: Mechanisms of organelle transport and capture along proplatelets during platelet production. *Blood* 106:4066, 2005.
15. Patel-Hett S, Wang H, Begonja AJ, et al: The spectrin-based membrane skeleton stabilizes mouse megakaryocyte membrane systems and is essential for proplatelet and platelet formation. *Blood* 2011.
16. Junt T, Schulze H, Chen Z, et al: Dynamic visualization of thrombopoiesis within bone marrow. *Science* 317:1767, 2007.
17. Thon JN, Montalvo A, Patel-Hett S, et al: Cytoskeletal mechanics of proplatelet maturation and platelet release. *J Cell Biol* 191:861, 2010.
18. Schwertz H, Koster S, Kahr WH, et al: Anucleate platelets generate progeny. *Blood* 115:3801, 2010.
19. Larson MK, Watson SP: A product of their environment: Do megakaryocytes rely on extracellular cues for proplatelet formation? *Platelets* 17:435, 2006.
20. Larson MK, Watson SP: Regulation of proplatelet formation and platelet release by integrin alpha IIb beta3. *Blood* 108:1509, 2006.
21. Dore LC, Crispino JD: Transcription factor networks in erythroid cell and megakaryocyte development. *Blood* 2011.
22. Hartwig JH. The platelet: Form and function. *Semin Hematol* 43:S94, 2006.
23. Patel-Hett S, Richardson JL, Schulze H, et al: Visualization of microtubule growth in living platelets reveals a dynamic marginal band with multiple microtubules. *Blood* 111:4605, 2008.
24. Freson K, De Vos R, Wittevrognel C, et al: The β1-tubulin Q43P functional polymorphism reduces the risk of cardiovascular disease in men by modulating platelet function and structure. *Blood* 106:2356, 2005.
25. Nakamura F, Stossel TP, Hartwig JH. The filamins: Organizers of cell structure and function. *Cell Adh Migr* 5:160, 2011.
26. Nakamura F, Pudas R, Heikkinen O, et al: The structure of the GP1b-filamin A complex. *Blood* 107:1925, 2005.

CHAPTER 127

MOLECULAR BASIS FOR PLATELET FUNCTION

Charles S. Abrams and Edward F. Plow

Platelets ordinarily circulate in blood vessels as individual cells that do not interact with other platelets or other cell types. A transition from this nonadhesive to an adhesive state can be rapidly initiated if platelets are exposed to a stimulatory agonist. A depiction of the platelet adhesive reactions that may be initiated in response to an injury to a blood vessel wall, as exemplified by rupture of an atherosclerotic plaque, is shown in Fig. 127-1. Disruption of the endothelial cell lining of the vessel exposes constituents within the subendothelial matrix, including a variety of adhesive proteins that can support initial platelet attachment. After attachment, platelets may undergo a spreading reaction that permits formation of multiple tight contacts between the cell surface and the matrix. These additional contacts may be critical for stabilizing the association of the platelets with the matrix in flowing blood. In conjunction with these adhesive reactions, the cells encounter agonists in the microenvironment that can trigger platelet secretion. The platelet secretory response results in the release of the contents of intracellular storage granules. Granule constituents include substances, such as adenosine diphosphate (ADP), that can stimulate circulating platelets and endow them with new adhesive properties. Stimulated platelets interact with one another during platelet aggregation to form an effective plug that seals the injured vessel wall and prevents excessive blood loss. This series of platelet responses—attachment, spreading, secretion, and aggregation—is essential for the hemostatic function of platelets. However, if these same events occur on an injured endothelial cell or on the surface of a disrupted atherosclerotic plaque, they can lead to the formation of an occlusive platelet-rich thrombus. At the other extreme, abnormalities in platelet adhesive reactions of either a genetic (e.g., Glanzmann thrombasthenia or Bernard-Soulier syndrome) (see Chapters 132 and 133) or an acquired origin (e.g., drug induced thrombocytopenia) (see Chapters133 and 135) can result in bleeding. Thus, platelet adhesive reactions and secretion are central events in health and disease processes; bleeding, hemostasis, and thrombosis are in delicate balance and are regulated by these platelet functions.

This chapter addresses the molecular basis of platelet adhesive reactions and secretory responses. Great strides have been made in defining the mechanisms that govern these functional responses. At the heart of these platelet responses are ligand–receptor interactions. Indeed, the platelet has often served as a model cell type for studying ligand–receptor interactions and establishing basic mechanisms of cell adhesion and secretion.

MOLECULAR BASIS OF PLATELET ADHESION

Studies in vitro, particularly under flow conditions (i.e., in closed chambers that permit whole blood or isolated components to flow across a selected matrix at selected shears) and in vivo studies using transgenic mouse models in which specific molecules have been deleted, mutated, or overexpressed illustrate the complexity of the reactions leading to thrombus formation, growth, and stabilization. For simplicity, we have dissected these events, but in reality, they occur rapidly and in an overlapping fashion.

Substrates for Platelet Attachment and Spreading

Some of the major subendothelial matrix proteins that support platelet attachment or spreading reactions are listed in Table 127-1. From the extent of this list, it is clear that the platelet can adhere to a variety of substrates when the endothelium is disrupted. To maintain hemostasis, the endothelium must create an effective barrier that prevents circulating platelets from reaching the matrix and initiating thrombus formation. In addition to serving as a physical barrier, endothelial cells synthesize and elaborate components, such as prostaglandin I_2, nitric oxide, and enzymes (CD39/CD73) that are involved in metabolism of ADP. These components prevent platelet activation and impart a nonthrombogenic character to the normal endothelium (see Chapter 129).

Studies of mice deficient in individual matrix proteins have documented that multiple adhesive proteins are involved in the formation, growth, and stabilization of platelet-rich thrombi.[1-4] Several considerations affect the role of individual matrix constituents in mediating platelet adhesion:

1. Not all of the adhesive proteins listed in Table 127-1 support the same spectrum of platelet adhesive responses. For example, under some conditions, platelets attach to, but do not spread on, laminin,[1] but von Willebrand factor (vWF) and fibronectin support cell attachment and spreading.[5-8] Collagen not only supports the attachment and spreading of platelets but can also induce a secretory response.[9] Of the multiple forms of collagen, types I, III, and VI are particularly important in supporting platelet adhesion.
2. A wealth of evidence indicates that the phenotypic properties of endothelial cells from different blood vessels vary and that the composition of the subendothelial matrix also varies. Even within the same vessel, the characteristics of its endothelial cells may differ. Areas of turbulent flow, which occur at bifurcations of vessels, are prone to development of atherosclerotic lesions, and shear-responsive elements in the promoters of certain genes can lead to changes in the expression of endothelial proteins[10,11] and alterations in their adhesive properties.[12,13] Thus, particular proteins may play a dominant role in supporting platelet adhesion in certain blood vessels.
3. Shear rate in flowing blood, which varies depending on vessel caliber, influences platelet adhesion. Shear is particularly important in defining the contribution of vWF to platelet adhesion. Patients with von Willebrand disease (see Chapter 140) have a bleeding diathesis, attesting to the importance of vWF in supporting platelet function. However, in vitro experiments demonstrate a role for vWF in platelet adhesion at high but not at low shear rates.[6,14,15] By contrast, fibronectin plays a role in platelet adhesion both high and low shear rates.[16,17] Despite these differences, both proteins have been implicated in thrombus formation.[4,14]
4. Many adhesive proteins interact with each other. For example, vWF, fibronectin, and thrombospondin all bind to collagen,[18-20] although they exhibit variable reactivity depending on the collagen

Table 127-1 Some of the Major Subendothelial Matrix Constituents That Support Platelet Adhesion

Matrix Constituent	Comment
Collagens	Large family of proteins with certain members supporting platelet adhesion, aggregation, and secretion
von Willebrand factor	Large multimeric protein critical for the hemostatic function of platelets
Fibronectin	Dimeric or multimeric protein that supports attachment and spreading of platelets
Thrombospondin-1	Trimeric protein exhibiting both adhesive and antiadhesive properties
Laminins	Proteins supporting platelet attachment
Microfibrils	A fibular bundle of protein constituents found in certain matrices

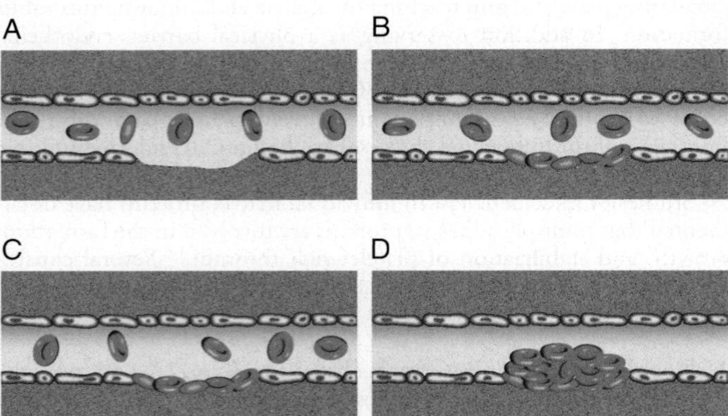

Figure 127-1 HEMOSTATIC RESPONSE OF PLATELETS TO INJURY. **A,** Disruption of the endothelial cell lining of the blood vessel exposes constituents of the subendothelial matrix. **B,** Platelets attach to and spread on matrix constituents. **C,** Platelet secretion may be initiated. **D,** Released platelet constituents can activate additional platelets, which aggregate with one another to form a thrombus.

types. These interactions may bridge platelets to matrix proteins or they may modulate the adhesive properties of a matrix protein.

5. Several of the adhesive proteins are found in platelet secretory granules or in plasma, as well as being matrix constituents. Whereas vWF and fibronectin are present in all three locations, thrombospondin is a major platelet granule constituent.[21,22] Proteins from all three sources—the matrix, the platelet, and the plasma—contribute to platelet adhesion. The adhesive proteins derived from each of these sources may be functionally distinct because they are not structurally identical. For example, the extent of vWF and fibronectin multimerization differs between molecules derived from plasma and those of the matrix. With fibronectin, the splice forms of molecules derived from plasma are different from those in platelets.[23]
6. Matrix proteins are subject to degradation by a variety of proteolytic enzymes. Such proteolysis can modulate the adhesive properties of the matrix proteins. In some cases, degradation exposes cryptic adhesive sequences that can interact with additional platelet adhesion receptors.[24,25]

Overall, the subendothelial matrix should be viewed as a dynamic and mutable interface that provides multiple substrates to support platelet adhesion.

Table 127-2 Platelet Receptors for Adhesive Proteins

Ligand	Receptor(s)	Other Common Designations
Collagen	GPIa-IIa, $\alpha_2\beta_1$ GPIIb-IIIa, $\alpha_{IIb}\beta_3$ GPIV GPVI	VLA-2 GPIIIb, CD36
Fibrinogen	GPIIb-IIIa, $\alpha_{IIb}\beta_3$ Vitronectin receptor, $\alpha_V\beta_3$	
Fibronectin	GPIc-IIa, $\alpha_5\beta_1$ GPIIb-IIIa, $\alpha_{IIb}\beta_3$	VLA-5
Thrombospondin	Vitronectin receptor, $\alpha_V\beta_3$ GPIV Integrin-associated protein	GPIIIb, CD36 IAP
Vitronectin	Vitronectin receptor, $\alpha_V\beta_3$ GPIIb-IIIa, $\alpha_{IIb}\beta_3$	
von Willebrand factor	GPIb-V-IX GPIIb-IIIa, $\alpha_{IIb}\beta_3$	
Laminin	GPIc-IIa region, $\alpha_6\beta_1$	VLA-6

GP, Glycoprotein; *VLA,* very late antigen.

Platelet Adhesion Receptors

The individual adhesive proteins serve as ligands for specific receptors on the platelet surface (Table 127-2). Because several nomenclature systems have been used to identify the membrane proteins of the platelet, the same receptor may have multiple designations. One of the most widely used systems designates the membrane proteins according to their electrophoretic mobility on polyacrylamide gels. Under these conditions, higher-molecular-weight proteins migrate more slowly. Separation by this technique gives rise to glycoprotein (GP) I, II, III, and so on, with GPI having the highest molecular weight. With more discriminating gel systems, additional proteins were identified in the GPI position, hence GPIa, GPIb, and GPIc, and so forth.[26] Even these distinctions require further refinement; for example, there are at least three distinct polypeptides in the GPIc position. Several of the membrane proteins on the platelet surface exist as noncovalent complexes; thus, GPIb-V-IX-V, GPIc-IIa, and GPIIb-IIIa can be regarded as single-membrane proteins. Because several of these membrane proteins are members of the integrin family of adhesion receptors (see later discussion), the integrin nomenclature is often used. For example, GPIc-IIa is referred to as $\alpha_5\beta_1$ and GPIIb-IIIa as $\alpha_{IIb}\beta_3$. Other nomenclature systems have arisen from the fact that several platelet membrane proteins are also found on the surface of other cell types where they have been assigned different names. This forms the basis of the VLA (very late antigens) designations for some platelet membrane proteins. Likewise, certain proteins may also have extracellular matrix (ECM) or leukocyte differentiation antigen (CD) designations. Finally, some receptors have been named based on their function (e.g., the vitronectin, fibrinogen, and fibronectin receptors). Although functional designations are appropriate from a descriptive standpoint, at least two membrane proteins on platelets serve as receptors for vitronectin, fibrinogen, and fibronectin (see Table 127-2), and several platelet constituents have been referred to as collagen receptors (see later discussion). With the exception of the CD identifications, these latter nomenclature systems are rarely used compared with the GP and the integrin nomenclature, but they may be encountered in the older platelet literature. Beyond creating a nomenclature complexity, redundancy of platelet receptors endows the cell with the capacity to form multiple contacts with a single matrix constituent; thus, a single ligand may initiate several distinct functional responses by engaging different receptors.

The Integrin Family of Adhesion Receptors

Many of the adhesive protein receptors on platelets are members of the integrin family. It is estimated that half of the surface area of an activated platelet is occupied by integrins. The integrins are a broadly distributed family of heterodimeric (two subunits) cell surface molecules that share certain structural, immunochemical, and functional properties.[27-35] The ß subunits, of which eight are highly homologous, exhibit at least 35% to 45% identity at the primary amino acid sequence level and store a common structural organization. The α subunits, of which 18 are known, are also similar to one another but exhibit less extensive sequence homology.[36,37]

The α subunits fall into two categories, those with and those without I (A) domains. Integrin I domains are inserted domains of about 200 amino acids and are frequently involved in ligand binding of those integrins containing them.[38] As it turns out, only one of the major integrins on platelets, α2β1, a collagen receptor, contains an I domain in its α subunit. The α subunits are synthesized as single-chain polypeptides; some, such as αIIb, are proteolytically processed to a two-chain form.[39-42] Each β subunit forms a noncovalent complex with an α subunit to form a functional adhesive protein receptor. A single β subunit can combine with several α subunits.

Platelets express two major β subunits, β_1 and β_3 (low levels of β_2 have been reported, but this finding requires confirmation),[43] and five α-subunits (Table 127-3). Of the integrins expressed on blood cells, $\alpha_{IIb}\beta_3$ is the most narrowly distributed and is restricted predominantly to platelets and megakaryocytes. $\alpha_{IIb}\beta_3$ plays a prominent role in platelet aggregation and many other platelet responses, including the association of platelets with tumor cells, an interaction important for metastasis.[44-46]

Role of Glycoprotein Ib-V-IX in Platelet Adhesion

GPIb-V-IX is a notable example of a cell surface molecule involved in platelet adhesion that is not a member of the integrin family.[47] Platelets from patients with Bernard-Soulier syndrome lack GPIb-V-IX; these patients have a marked bleeding diathesis[48-50] (see Chapter 132). A major role of GPIb-V-IX in hemostasis can be traced directly to its function as a receptor for vWF. vWF is composed of multiple functional domains, including the 24kDa A1 domain that binds the amino-terminus of GPIbα and interacts, along with the A3 domain, with matrix constituents, such as collagen and microfibrils[18,51-57] (see Chapter 140). Thus, by associating with matrix proteins, vWF directly mediates rapid and reversible platelet adhesion that promotes the rolling of these cells along the surface of injured vasculature.[58] This rolling may transiently bridge the cells to subendothelial matrix components until a more stable adhesive bond forms. Integrins are the most likely receptors responsible for the stable platelet-adhesive bond that permanently halts the rolling of the platelet. In vitro, vWF does not interact directly with platelet GPIb, although such interactions can be induced by ristocetin, an antibiotic, or botrocetin (a snake venom peptide). Altered forms of vWF, such as asialo-vWF (which lacks sialic acid residues) and bovine vWF, can directly interact with platelets.[59-61] High shear serves as the physiologic counterpart of ristocetin or botrocetin in humans by altering vWF conformation and enabling this high-affinity interaction.[62,63] Such high shear stress can be attained in the microcirculation or in stenotic arteries.

Several laboratories have reported the structures of the vWF A1 domain, as well as A1 domain mutants that interact with the GPIβα complex.[64-66] The globular vWF A1 domain interacts with the amino-terminus of GPIbβα. The vWF-binding region of GPIbα is composed of two ß-loops, which flank a backbone composed of eight leucine-rich repeats. This entire interaction depends on displacement of the termini of the vWF A1 domains, an event that likely occurs under shear conditions that exist at sites of vascular injury. The interaction is complex and is best described as a "flex bond."[67] One state of the bond is seen at low forces, and a second and more stable state of the bond develops only at higher forces, such as those in the arterial system. This specialized type of interaction likely explains why the high shear in arteries promotes platelet plug formation.

The role of GPIb in hemostasis is not restricted to vWF binding. GPIb also serves as a binding site for thrombin,[68,69] and this activity may play an important role in the generation of platelet microparticles and procoagulant activity.[70-73] GPIb also is a target for certain drug-induced platelet antibodies[74] and is a counterreceptor for αMβ2 (CD11b/18, Mac-1), a leukocyte integrin, an interaction that promotes the formation of platelet-leukocyte conjugates.[75] The entire primary structures of GPIb,[76,77] GPIX,[78] and GPV[79] were determined by cDNA cloning approaches in the 1980s. GPIb is composed of a heavy chain (α) and a light chain (β), and both span the platelet membrane. GPIbα, which associates with the cytoskeleton within the platelet,[48,80-82] is susceptible to proteolysis, and a large proteolytic fragment, glycocalicin, can be detected in the plasma of some patients with thrombocytopenic disorders.[83] GPIX is a small, single-chain polypeptide with a molecular weight of 20,000 Da. The contribution of GPIX to the function of GPIb-V-IX is uncertain. GPV, which also is deficient in Bernard-Soulier platelets, forms a loose association with GPIb-V-IX.[50,70,71] Platelets from mice deficient in GPV exhibit enhanced sensitivity to thrombin, which may reflect a role of GPV in controlling the thrombin binding function of GPIb.[84] An important consequence of GPIb-V-IX occupancy by vWF is the induction of intracellular signaling events that ultimately lead to activation of $\alpha_{IIb}\beta_3$ and subsequent platelet aggregation[48,85] (see later discussion). Such communication between adhesion receptors is a repeating theme for platelets as well as for other cells. Key events in the communication among platelet receptors may include changes in the phosphorylation of the cytoplasmic tails of GPIb-V-IX and their association with the signaling molecule 14.3.3.[86,87]

Table 127-3 Platelet Integrins

Integrin	Major Ligands
$\alpha_2\beta_1$ (GPIa-IIa, VLA-2)	Collagen
$\alpha_5\beta_1$ (GPIc-IIa, VLA-5)	Fibronectin
$\alpha_{IIb}\beta_3$ (GPIIb-IIIa)	Fibrinogen, fibronectin, vitronectin, von Willebrand factor, CD40L
$\alpha_V\beta_3$ (Vitronectin receptor)	Fibrinogen, fibronectin, vitronectin, von Willebrand factor, thrombospondin, osteopontin
$\alpha_6\beta1$ (GPIc-IIa region)	Laminin

GP, Glycoprotein; *VLA,* very late antigen.

Collagen Receptors

Subendothelial collagen has long been recognized as an important initiator of platelet responses, serving both as a substrate for platelet adhesion and as a potent platelet agonist. Three different receptors have been implicated in the platelet responses to collagen.[88] First is the GPIb-V-IX complex mentioned above. Second is α2β1 (also known as VLA-2, platelet GPIa-IIa), a member of the integrin family of adhesion receptors that primarily serves as an anchor by which platelets attach to collagen that is exposed after disruptions of the vascular endothelium.[89] A patient with an acquired deficiency of this integrin exhibited a mild bleeding diathesis.[90,91] In addition to binding collagen with high affinity, α2β1 also binds laminins, E-cadherins, matrix metalloproteins, C1q, echovirus, and rotavirus. The identification of a patient with a mild bleeding diathesis who had normal amounts of α2β1 but reduced platelet glycoprotein VI (GPVI) suggested that GPVI also serves as a collagen receptor,[92] at least under low shear conditions. Platelets from mice lacking GPVI on the surface of their platelets exhibit absence of collagen-induced platelet activation and a profound reduction in collagen adhesion.[93] Deficiency of platelet GPVI can be induced by inactivating the GPVI or the FcRγ genes. The latter forms a complex with GPVI and is required for its surface expression.[91] In contrast, α2β1 serves primarily as an auxiliary receptor for platelet adhesion to collagen and only functions as an agonist receptor under unusual circumstances.[89]

Experiments using receptor-blocking antibodies heterologously expressed receptors, and genetically altered mice have elucidated the roles of each of these proteins.[89,93-96] Platelet adhesion to collagen is a multistep process (Fig. 127-2). Initially, platelets adhere to collagen-immobilized vWF via platelet GPIb-V-IX. Although this interaction is rapid, it is transient. Consequently, the interactions repeatedly form and break, thereby causing the platelet to slowly roll along the surface of vWF that is immobilized upon exposed collagen. Ultimately, GPVI interacts directly with collagen, a low-affinity interaction that is a potent stimulus for intracellular signaling pathways. As a result of this signaling cascade, α2β1 is induced to bind collagen with high affinity, thereby forming a stable interaction. Thus, the interaction of platelets with collagen is complex. Whether pharmacologic inhibition of either platelet collagen receptor is of therapeutic benefit is unknown.

CLEC2 Adhesion Receptor

As described earlier, adhesion of platelets to a tear in the vascular system involves the binding of platelet GPIb-V-IX and α2β1 receptors followed by intracellular signaling initiated by GPVI. CLEC2[97] is a recently identified type II transmembrane receptor with C type lectin-like extracellular domains encoded by genes within the genomic natural killer (NK) receptor complex. CLEC2 is highly and selectively expressed on platelets, although it is also found on neutrophils.[98,99] Initially described as the receptor responsible for platelet activation by the snake venom rhodocytin, CLEC2 was later identified as the receptor responsible for platelet activation by the transmembrane glycoprotein podoplanin.[99] Activation of CLEC2 by podoplanin induces a series of platelet signaling events similar to those induced by collagen after it binds to the GPVI receptor. Recent work has demonstrated that infusion of antibodies against CLEC2 into mice affords them with significant protection against occlusive thrombus formation.[100] Rational drug design approaches could exploit this knowledge to develop specific CLEC2 inhibitors.

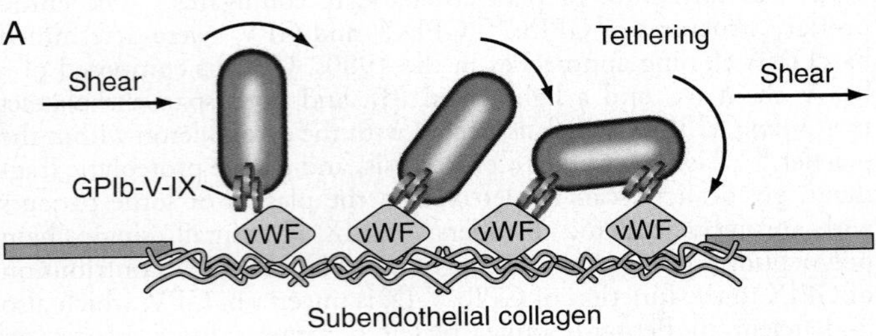

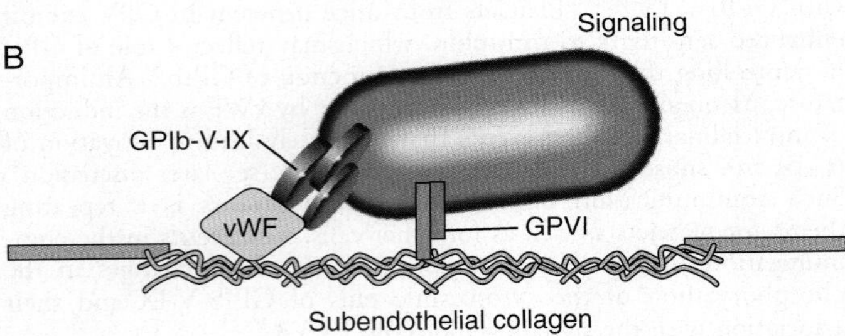

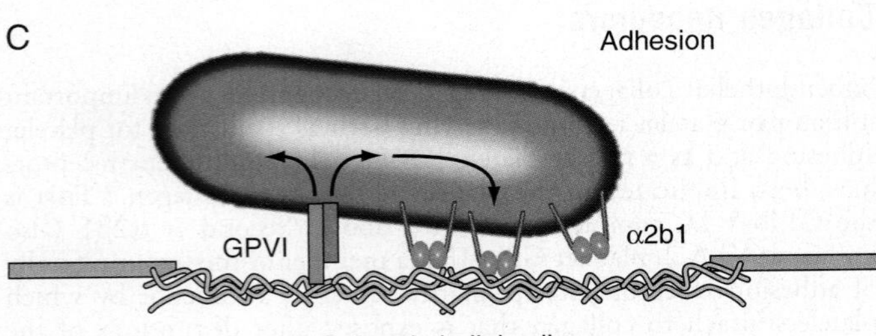

Figure 127-2 ADHESION TO COLLAGEN IS A MULTISTEP PROCESS. **A,** After being exposed to an injured vessel wall, von Willebrand factor (vWF) adheres to subendothelial collagen, where it undergoes a conformational change that allows it to bind to the platelet receptor glycoprotein (GP) Ib-V-IX. This rapidly formed bond is quickly broken and reestablished, causing the platelet to roll along the injured vessel wall. **B,** The rolling process slows platelet transit and allows the platelet signaling receptor, GPVI, to bind collagen. **C,** This induces a cascade of signaling events that ultimately activate the integrin, α2β1. The final association between the platelet and collagen is stable and allows the platelet to firmly adhere to the vessel wall.

Reorganization of the Actin Cytoskeleton

One of the more dramatic events during platelet activation is the metamorphosis that occurs when platelets adhere and spread on exposed collagen fibrils or become activated in the circulation by soluble factors such as thrombin or ADP. In both cases, platelets lose their distinct discoid shape and acquire an irregular morphology with multiple filopodial projections.[101] This transformation is associated with and largely attributable to cytoskeletal rearrangements within the platelet.[102] The proteins are arranged in three major structures: a cytoplasmic actin network, a rim of membrane-associated cytoskeleton, and a marginal band consisting of a microtubule coil.[103] Together these structures lend support to the platelet plasma membrane and give shape to both resting and activated platelets. The capacity to rapidly reorganize these structures allows the platelet to firmly adhere to breaks in the blood vessel wall under conditions of shear found within the arterial vascular system.

The cytoplasmic actin network is composed of actin filaments and associated proteins. Actin is a 42-kDa protein that accounts for as much as 20% of total platelet protein.[103] In resting platelets, 40% to 50% of the actin is filamentous F-actin, and the remainder is globular monomeric G-actin.[104,105] The shift that increases the proportion of F-actin to 70% to 80% during platelet activation involves a coordinated sequence of events in which the actin filaments in resting platelets are severed and the resultant smaller fragments are used as the nidus for new, longer actin filaments. This process is regulated in part by the increase in the levels of a phosphoinositide (phosphatidylinositol 4,5 bisphosphate [PIP2]) that accompanies platelet activation.[106-109] At the same time, myosin is phosphorylated by myosin light chain kinase and becomes associated with F-actin, thereby forming filaments that are anchored to the platelet plasma membrane by attachment (via actin-binding protein) to the GP Ib-V-IX complex.[110,111]

The cytoskeletal rim is composed of actin, filamin, P235 (talin), vinculin, spectrin, α-actinin, and several membrane glycoproteins. Filamin is an elongated 280-kDa protein that is present in platelets and functions as an actin binding protein.[112] In resting platelets, filamin is part of a semirigid array that helps to maintain the platelet's discoid shape and limits the lateral movement of GPIb.[80,113,114] This role is analogous to that performed by spectrin in erythrocytes.[81] When platelets are activated, actin filaments form and attach to actin-binding protein. Later, the rising cytosolic Ca^{2+} concentration activates calpain, which cleaves actin-binding protein, severing the link to GPIb.[113,115,116] Recent evidence in genetically engineered mice has also demonstrated that the synthesis of PIP2 is critical for stable adhesion of the actin cytoskeleton to the cell membrane.[109] Available data suggest that this anchoring of the cell membrane to the underlying cytosketelon is mediated, at least in part, by talin (as discussed in the section Activation of $\alpha_{IIb}\beta_3$.).

The third major structural element in platelets is the marginal microtubule band.[103] This microtubule coil is a single tightly wound polymer of tubulin that encircles the platelet perimeter and helps to maintain its discoid shape.[117] During platelet activation, the microtubule coil contracts. Although it has been proposed that contraction of the marginal band is required for stable adhesion of platelets under arterial shear pressures, this concept remains controversial.[118,119]

PLATELET SECRETION

The foregoing discussion has emphasized the adhesive functions of platelets in mediating the physical closure of breaks in blood vessels. Another important function of platelets is the release of a variety of substances that stimulate or inhibit platelets or other blood and vascular cells, covalently modify the thrombus to affect its mechanical properties, regulate coagulation, contribute to cell adhesive events, and modulate the growth of cells of the vessel wall. Thus, the platelet is not simply the stop plug of the vasculature but also has the capacity to signal its presence in a thrombus and modify the hemostatic response. In addition, although platelets are anucleate, they contain mRNA and can synthesize some proteins.[120,121] Although such synthesis had long been regarded as a vestigial activity of megakaryocytes, recent data indicate that platelets synthesize a restricted repertoire of proteins that are related to apoptosis and inflammation,[122] the so-called platelet "transcriptome."[121] Most of the substances that are actively and selectively secreted from platelets are packaged in preformed storage granules or are synthesized de novo from membrane phospholipids. Platelets contain three types of granules: (1) dense granules that contain platelet agonists that serve to amplify platelet activation, (2) α granules that contain proteins that enhance the adhesive process, and (3) lysosomal granules that contain glycosidases and proteases that have an unclear function in platelet biology.[123] In addition, factors in the platelet cytoplasm can have effects on thrombus structure or on vascular cell growth; they are released as a result of minor degrees of platelet lysis during hemostasis. Some of these factors and their intraplatelet sources are illustrated in Fig. 127-3, *A*.

Dense Granules

The dense bodies and platelet membranes are a source of rapidly secreted mediators. These mediators are either quickly inactivated or promptly diffuse away from the site of the thrombus, so they function for only a brief period of time. Their rapid effects on surrounding cells serve to modulate the behavior of platelets, as well as the behavior of vessel wall cells (particularly with regards vascular tone).

Platelets contain approximately three to eight dense granules, which are the most rapidly secreted platelet organelles.[124] These granules contain and upon activation release ADP (which is a potent agonist that recruits other platelets) as well as adenosine triphosphate (which is an agonist for other cells of the blood).[125,126] Additionally, they release biogenic amines such as serotonin, which can influence vascular tone, and divalent cations. The physiologic role of released dense body calcium is not clear; however, it may serve to ensure that there is sufficient calcium for the calcium-dependent enzymes involved in coagulation or cross-linking of fibrin.

α Granules

A large number of plasma proteins involved in cell adhesion and coagulation are also present in platelet α granules. Some of the

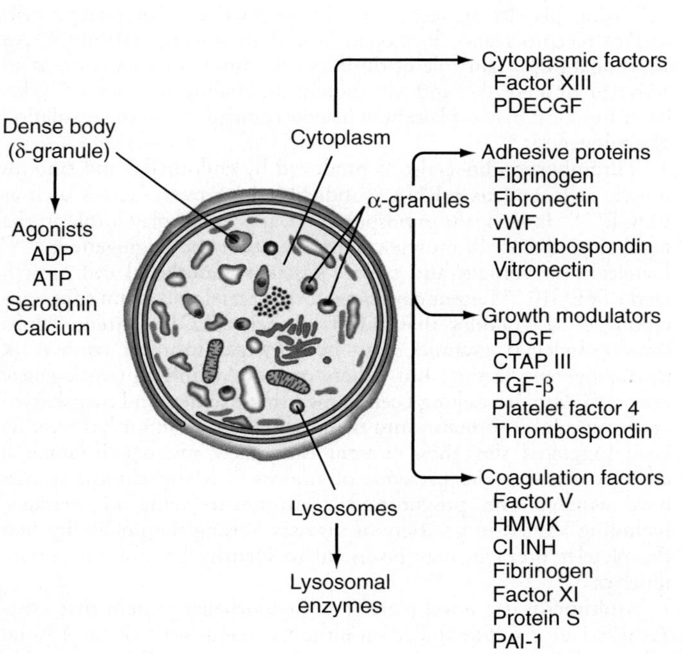

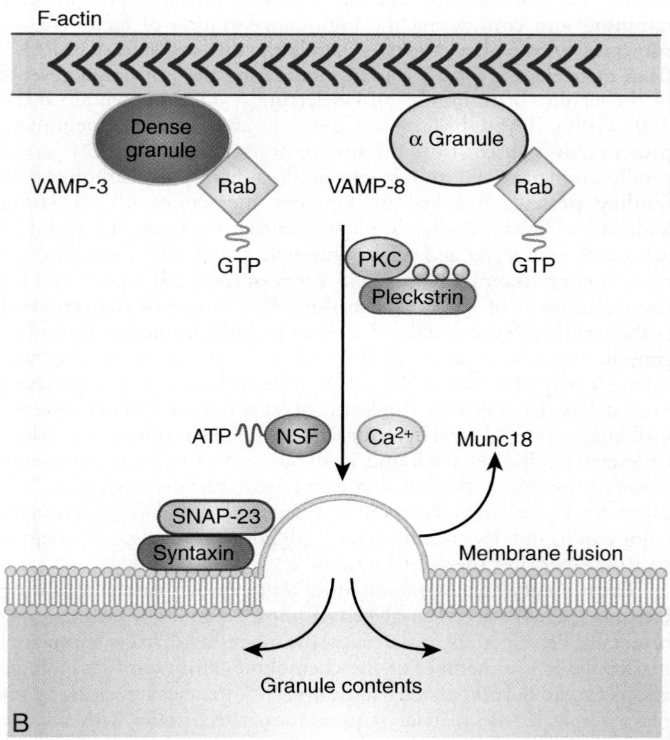

Figure 127-3 **A,** SUBSTANCES RELEASED BY PLATELETS AND THEIR INTRAPLATELET SOURCES. Illustrated are some of the bioactive substances released from dense bodies, α granules, lysosomes, the cytoplasm, and the platelet membrane. *C1 INH,* C1 inhibitor; *CTAP,* connective tissue activating peptide; *HETE,* hydroxyeicosatetraenoic acid; *HMWK,* high-molecular-weight kininogen; *PAF,* platelet-activating factor; *PAI-1,* plasminogen activator inhibitor-1; *PDECGF,* platelet-derived endothelial cell growth factor; *PDGF,* platelet-derived growth factor; *TGF-B,* transforming growth factor-b; *vWF,* von Willebrand factor. **B,** In resting platelets, the actin cytoskeleton needs to be disassembled before platelet secretion. Secretion of α and dense granules occurs through a complex signaling pathway dependent on small GTPases, protein kinases, phosphorylated pleckstrin, and members of the SNARE (soluble *N*-ethylmaleimide-sensitive factor attachment protein receptor)/SNAP (soluble NSF attachment protein) family. These signaling pathways are highly homologous to those used during neuronal cell exocytosis. *ATP,* Adenosine triphosphate; *GTP,* guanosine-5'-triphosphate; *NSF,* N-ethylmaleimide-sensitive fusion; *PKC,* protein kinase C; *VAMP-8,* vesicle-associated membrane protein 8.

proteins found within α granules are only synthesized in megakaryocytes (e.g., β thromboglobulin and platelet factor 4), but others are less specific for platelets and megakaryocytes. Platelets contain approximately 80 α granules that contain adhesive plasma proteins including vWF, fibrinogen, fibronectin, and vitronectin, as well as the platelet and cellular adhesive protein thrombospondin-1.[22,127] Platelet vWF is concentrated in the platelets; megakaryocytes synthesize it[128]; and the platelet form is enriched in the larger, presumably more hemostatically effective multimers.[129] Megakaryocytes clearly take up fibrinogen, but its biosynthesis in megakaryocytes remains controversial.[130] Platelet fibronectin appears to be enriched in alternatively spliced forms that are relatively lacking in plasma,[23] suggesting a possible role for platelet fibronectin in events such as matrix assembly. Vitronectin is present in platelets[131]; however, its concentration suggests that it is passively taken up from plasma. Nevertheless, recent studies have suggested a role for platelet and plasma vitronectin in thrombus formation.[132,133] Plasminogen activator inhibitor type 1 (PAI-1) binds vitronectin,[134] and these two proteins are released in complex.[135] Consistent with this observation, mice lacking vitronectin, PAI-1, or both proteins have a similar deficiency in thrombus formation.[136] A wide variety of procoagulant and anticoagulant enzymes and cofactors have been reported in platelet granules. Although controversial,[137] it appears that megakaryocytes synthesize factor V,[138-140] and more factor V is found in platelet α granules[141] than can be accounted for by nonspecific uptake from plasma. Moreover, platelet factor V is distinct from plasma factor V[142] and plays an important role in platelet prothrombinase assembly.[143] Platelets also contain protein S[144] and PAI-1.[145] Protein S is a cofactor for activated protein C (see Chapter 129), and PAI-1 is an inhibitor of urokinase and tissue plasminogen activators (see Chapter 129). The concentration of these proteins in platelets suggests that platelets may be a favored site for the anticoagulant action of activated protein C, a tempting idea considering the high concentration of factor Va, its substrate, on the platelet surface. Similarly, the local release of PAI-1 from platelets may play a role in modulating the fibrinolytic events in the vicinity of thrombi.[146,147] P-selectin[148-151] (also known as GMP-140, GPIIa, PADGEM, and CD62) is an α-granule membrane protein that is absent from the surface of resting platelets. It is structurally similar to E- and L-selectin,[152] a family of carbohydrate-binding proteins involved in adhesive interactions of circulating leukocytes. Platelet P-selectin plays a central role in mediating interactions of monocytes and neutrophils with platelets.[152] These interactions are important for "cross-talk" between these cell types[153] and for the recruitment of leukocytes to thrombi.[154] Some of the proposed pathogenetic roles of platelet P-selectin include promoting thrombogenesis,[154] platelet–tumor cell interactions,[155] and monocyte recruitment. It may also play a physiologic role in leukocyte phagocytosis of platelets. In addition, P-selectin plays a role in leukocyte–vessel wall interactions[151,156] and hemostasis.[157] Increased numbers of platelet–leukocyte conjugates are found in the plasma of patients with acute coronary events; a finding consistent with platelet activation.[158,159] However, P-selectin and its counterreceptor, PSGL-1 (P-selectin glycoprotein ligand-1), on leukocytes[160] are not the only ligand–receptor pair that mediates these interactions.[161]

The most abundant component of α granules is platelet activating factor[162] (alkyl-2-acetyl-*sn*-glycero-3-phosphocholine), which was originally described as a platelet activator released from stimulated mast cells. It is a member of the chemokine family, and its biologic effects extend beyond platelet activation.[163-165] Platelet activating factor plays a role in the platelet sequestration that occurs with allergic injury, but it is produced by other cells as well as platelets. Is it possible that local generation of this mediator contributes to platelet recruitment or to some of the vascular phenomena associated with hemostasis.

Platelet α granules contain Gas6 (growth-arrest specific gene 6), a vitamin K–dependent protein with homology[166,167] to protein S that serves as a ligand for growth factor receptors, such as Axl.[168] Because platelet express the Axl receptor, it is speculated that secreted Gas6 functions to accelerate platelet recruitment and activation. Consistent with this concept, mice lacking Gas6 have a platelet defect.[142,166]

Platelets are the major peripheral blood source of β-amyloid precursor protein (APP).[169] APP is a membrane protein, thought to be localized to α granules,[170] that serves as the precursor of the approximately 40 residue peptides found in amyloid deposits in the brains of patients with Alzheimer disease. APP is a protease inhibitor and is processed by proteolytic cleavage. Its capacity to inhibit factors Xa, XIa, and IXa[171,172] suggests that it may function as a natural anticoagulant. Platelets contain a wide variety of peptides and proteins, primarily in α granules, that can modulate the growth and patterns of gene expression of cells of the vessel wall. The first of these to be described was platelet-derived growth factor[173] (PDGF), which has three isoforms and two distinct receptors on smooth muscle cells and fibroblasts.[174] PDGF probably plays an important role in the smooth muscle cell proliferation that may occur after platelet interaction with the vessel wall. In fact, platelet-secreted PDGF may play a critical role in angiogenesis.[175] The PDGF receptors are transmembrane tyrosine kinase–type receptors, and signal transduction from these receptors[176] is similar to that from other tyrosine kinase receptors, such as the insulin and epidermal growth factor receptors. Another α-granule growth factor is connective tissue activating peptide (CTAP) III, which stimulates fibroblast proliferation. CTAP III is the likely precursor of β thromboglobulin,[177] and its structure is related to another α-granule protein, platelet factor 4. Both platelet factor 4 and CTAP III are members of a large protein family involved in growth control and inflammation.[178] Although interleukin-1 is expressed on the surface of activated platelets,[179] its origin is unclear.

Transforming growth factor (TGF)-β was first isolated from platelets,[180] and platelets are a rich source of this peptide mediator, which is a potent stimulus for the biosynthesis of matrix molecules and their receptors. TGF-β has complex effects on cell proliferation, stimulating some cells and inhibiting others. In addition, thrombospondin-1 is present in and secreted from platelet α granules. Released thrombospondin-1 is believed to play a role in stabilizing platelet aggregates via its interaction with platelet cell-surface receptors and fibrinogen bound to integrin αIIbβ3.[181] An additional important role of thrombospondin-1 is its function as an activator of TGF-β[182] and as a potent antiangiogenic factor.[183] This latter function may explain how platelets contribute to the regulation of angiogenesis.[184]

Thrombospondin-1 also is produced by endothelial and smooth muscle cells, and its mRNA is inducible by growth factors such as PDGF.[185,186] Indeed, thrombospondin-1 appears to play a role in the regulation of smooth muscle cell proliferation and angiogenesis.[187-189] Platelets also contain and secrete vascular endothelial cell growth factor (VEGF).[190] Recent data suggest that platelets contain subpopulations of α granules that differ in their VEGF content. Thus, some platelet α granules may be enriched in their content of proangiogeneic factors, but others contain mainly antiantiogeneic factors.[191] Also, it has long been known that platelets and megakaryocytes can take up proteins into their α-granules,[192] and it has recently been suggested that their content can reflect microenvironmental changes, such as the presence of tumors.[193] Many clinical studies have assessed the prognostic or diagnostic value of markers, including VEGF, in a variety of diseases, raising the possibility that the platelet protocol may be useful to identify or monitor certain illnesses.

Multimerin is a novel platelet and endothelial protein that exists as massive disulfide-linked multimers composed of a 155-kd subunit.[194,195] Multimerin has a repeating structure, and its sequence contains the adhesive Arg-Gly-Asp-Ser motif, central coiled-coil sequences, several epidermal growth factor-like motifs, and a globular domain that is similar to the protein binding domain found in complement C1q and type VIII and X collagens.[196] Multimerin binds the coagulation protein factor V and its activated form, factor Va. In platelets but not in plasma, all of the biologically active factor V is complexed with multimerin.[197] Multimerin may also have functions as an extracellular matrix or adhesive protein. This large granule protein may play important roles in platelet procoagulant activity and in platelet adhesion.

Lysosomal Granules and The Platelet Cytosol

Platelets contain a few primary and secondary lysosomes[33,123] whose enzymes are released, but platelets are probably a minor source of lysosomal hydrolases in the blood compared with neutrophils. Nevertheless, mention should be made of platelet-associated heparatinase,[198] which can cleave vascular endothelial cell surface glycosaminoglycans to produce an antiproliferative fragment.

Factor XIII, a transglutaminase that catalyzes the formation of isopeptide bonds between the γ-glutaminyl residues and the E amino groups of lysines, forming stable covalent cross-links between proteins, is contained in the platelet cytosol.[199] It is likely that small quantities of platelet factor XIIIα are released into thrombi and serves to cross-link fibrin and to cross-linking fibronectin[200] and α_2-antiplasmin[201] onto fibrin (see Chapter 129). Platelet factor XIII may also play a role in cross-linking and stabilizing cytoskeletal elements.[202,203] Also, transglutaminases have been implicated in the signaling events associated with occupancy of G protein–coupled receptors,[204,205] and many of the agonist receptors, which activate platelets, are members of this family.

Secretion

The secretion of platelet granules occurs through mechanisms analogous to those required for the exocytosis of granules from neurons and mast cells. Platelet secretion is triggered by a variety of strong agonists such as thrombin. Induction of secretion by weak agonists (e.g., ADP) occurs when the cells are brought into close contact, such as occurs during aggregation.[123,206,207] The latter secretory mechanism is clearly dependent on thromboxane A_2 (TXA_2) generated as a consequence of arachidonic acid release.

Granule Exocytosis

As noted previously, the two morphologically prominent platelet storage granules, α granules and dense bodies, contain a variety of substances important in platelet function. Because these granules have a limiting membrane, it is likely that the final secretory event involves exocytosis[208] (i.e., fusion of the secretory granule membrane with the plasma membrane). This has been observed in dense body secretion.[209,210]

Identification of the role of the soluble *N*-ethylmaleimide-sensitive factor attachment protein receptor (SNARE) complex in neuronal cell exocytosis has advanced our understanding of platelet secretion. Platelets have the three basic components of SNARE machinery: t-SNAREs (target receptors), v-SNAREs (vesicle-associated membrane receptors), and soluble components (including NSF and NSF-attachment proteins).[123,207] Through a pathway involving Rab-GTPase, protein kinase C (PKC), and intracellular calcium, the SNARE machinery regulates the association and subsequent fusion of vesicles with membranes (see Fig. 127-3, *B*). Mice deficient in one of these SNAREs, VAMP-8 (vesicle-associated membrane protein 8), exhibits defective platelet secretion,[211,212] and certain single nucleotide polymorphisms in VAMP-8 have been associated with increased susceptibility to acute myocardial infaction.[213] Recent evidence has demonstrated that pleckstrin, a substrate of PKC, is a critical mediator of this process.[214] In mouse platelets lacking pleckstrin, secretion in response to PKC-dependent signaling pathways is lacking because of a failure of the membranes of the granules to fuse with the cellular membrane.

Mention should also be made of platelet microparticles. These vesicles are shed from the membrane of stimulated platelets. In addition to membrane lipids, they are enriched in certain platelet membrane proteins,[215] which enables their detection by flow cytometry.[216] Microparticles are highly procoagulant, and they may contribute to the thrombotic complications associated with heparin-induced thrombocytopenia (see Chapter 135),[217] and their presence in blood has been correlated with coronary artery disease.[218-221]

In addition to the outward movement of granules toward the cell surface, it is clear that there is also substantial inward membrane traffic in platelets.[222-225] This inward traffic serves to clear adhesive and procoagulant proteins from the cell surface and hence limit prothrombotic events.[226]

Eicosanoids and Arachidonate

In addition to exocytosis of platelet granules, the passive release of TXA_2 from platelets is another mechanism by which platelet activation is amplified. Eicosanoids are formed from the arachidonate released from membrane phospholipids by phospholipase A2 during platelet activation.[227-229] Because the availability of arachidonate is the rate-limiting step in this process, phospholipase A2 is tightly controlled. Platelet phospholipase A2 is stimulated by the rise in the cytosolic Ca^{2+} that accompanies platelet activation.

After being released from membrane phospholipids, arachidonate can be metabolized to $TXA_2$by cyclooxygenase-1 (COX-1).[230] Aspirin acetylates COX-1, causing it to be irreversibly inactivated.[231] Because platelets lack the ability to synthesize significant amounts of protein, inactivation of COX-1 by aspirin blocks TXA_2synthesis until new platelets are formed. However, there may be a subset of patients who are "aspirin resistant," although the molecular basis of this disorder and a universally accepted definition are elusive.[232,233] Aspirin resistance can lead to undermedication of patients and therefore an increased risk for recurrent thrombotic events. Nonsteroidal antiinflammatory drugs also inactivate COX-1 but without covalently modifying the enzyme.[234]

After forming, TXA_2 can diffuse across the plasma membrane and activates other platelets through signaling pathways. This leads to platelet shape change, aggregation, secretion, phosphoinositide hydrolysis, protein phosphorylation, and an increase in cytosolic Ca^{2+} while having little effect on cyclic AMP formation (see Chapter 132).[235] Similar to ADP, TXA_2 amplifies the initial stimulus for platelet activation and recruits additional platelets. This process is effective locally but is limited by the short half-life of TXA_2, which confines the spread of platelet activation to the vicinity of the injury.

MOLECULAR BASIS OF PLATELET AGGREGATION

Aggregation Response of Platelets

Platelets in blood, in plasma, or as an isolated cell population do not interact with one another. If an appropriate agonist is added, rapid platelet aggregation ensues. Some of the agonists that initiate this response are listed in Table 127-4. Of particular physiologic relevance

Table 127-4 Common Platelet Aggregating Agonists

Agonist	Comment
Adenosine diphosphate (ADP)	Released from platelet α granule; acts synergistically with many other agonists
Thrombin	Formed by activation of the coagulation system
Collagen	In subendothelial matrix
Epinephrine	May allow for hormonal regulation of hemostasis
Calcium ionophore	Not naturally occurring; mobilizes calcium in platelets
Arachidonate and its metabolites	Active metabolites are formed and released from stimulated platelets
Serotonin	Released from platelets; may primarily sensitize platelets to other agonists
Platelet-activating factor	Lipid mediator produced by other cells that can activate a variety of cells, including platelets

are the platelet-derived agonists—ADP, serotonin, platelet activating factor, and arachidonate metabolites—that provide a means for stimulated platelets to recruit additional cells; collagen, which supports platelet adhesion and secretion as well as aggregation; thrombin, which links platelets and the blood coagulation system in thrombus formation; epinephrine, which permits hormonal regulation of platelet function; and vWF upon its binding to GPIb-V-IX. These agonists activate platelets by interacting with specific receptors, many being members of the G protein–coupled receptor class. Receptor occupancy triggers a complex series of intracellular reactions (detailed in Chapter 132) that ultimately converge to a set of common steps that permit the cells to aggregate. Platelet aggregation is energy dependent and can be distinguished on this basis from platelet agglutination induced by ristocetin or certain platelet antibodies.

At normal blood concentrations of 1 to 3 × 10^8/mL, platelet suspensions are opalescent. On addition of an agonist, a stirred suspension of normal platelets aggregates and a decrease in turbidity is observed. Platelet aggregometers, which monitor the change in light transmission through platelet suspensions, are used extensively in clinical laboratories to evaluate platelet function (see Chapter 131). Certain instruments also provide simultaneous measurements of other platelet functions, such as secretion.[206] Although the information gained from aggregometry can be extremely useful, aggregation in vitro does not necessarily reflect platelet function in vivo. In particular, clinical bleeding and the aggregation response of platelets do not necessarily coincide. This disparity reflects the importance of platelet adhesion in thrombus formation, a reaction that is not detected by aggregometry. For this reason, instruments that measure platelet adhesion under shear or provide more quantitative information are sometimes used to monitor antiplatelet therapy.[236-238] Nonetheless, aggregometry remains the mainstay of the clinical coagulation laboratory.

A typical aggregometer tracing obtained with a suspension of isolated human platelets is shown in Fig. 127-4, *A*. From this pattern, the three essential components required for this functional response can be identified. The first component is the *platelet agonist.* The agonist used in Fig. 127-4 is ADP. This agonist induces platelet shape change from discoid to a more spherical form, a transition that can be detected in the aggregometer as a decrease in light transmission. This transformation is not a prerequisite for platelet aggregation;

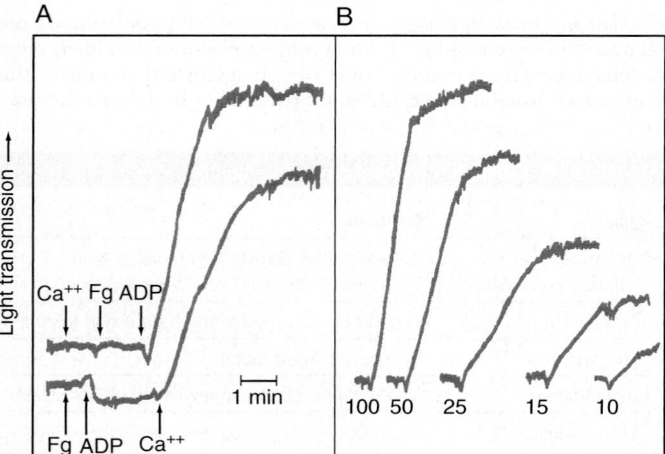

Figure 127-4 AGGREGATION RESPONSE OF HUMAN PLATELETS. **A,** To aggregate, isolated human platelets require divalent ions (Ca^{2+}), an agonist (adenosine diphosphate [ADP]), and an adhesive protein (fibrinogen [Fg]). Shape change is observed as a slight decrease in light transmission induced by ADP and is followed by an increase in transmission as the platelets aggregate. **B,** Both the rate and extent of platelet aggregation depend on the concentration of fibrinogen. The concentration of fibrinogen (in μg/mL) is indicated below each tracing.

epinephrine aggregates platelets but does not induce a shape change that is recordable by conventional aggregometers. At the molecular level, shape change reflects a reorganization of the actin cytoskeleton. The second component is *divalent cations.* Calcium and magnesium, as well as other (but not all) divalent cations, support platelet aggregation.[239-241] The third component is *fibrinogen.* Fibrinogen is not only a major plasma protein but is also present in and secreted from platelets[242,243] (see Chapter 118). By virtue of its capacity to form fibrin and support platelet aggregation, fibrinogen plays a dual role in thrombus formation. These activities, as well as the contribution of fibrinogen to blood viscosity, are believed to account for the increased risk of cardiovascular disease associated with elevated levels of fibrinogen.[244-246] In addition, certain single nucleotide polymorphisms in fibrinogen also have been associated with an increased risk of cardiovascular stroke in some but not all studies.[247-249] The dependence of platelet aggregation on fibrinogen concentration is evident from the tracings illustrated in Fig. 127-4, *B*.

Although not evident by conventional aggregometry, vWF plays a central role in platelet aggregation and in the more complex process of thrombus formation, which entails platelet adhesion as well as aggregation. The role of vWF in platelet aggregation becomes apparent in certain pathologic circumstances such as platelet-type von Willebrand disease and type IIB von Willebrand disease (see Chapter 140).[250-254] In the setting of vascular injury in vivo, it is clear that both molecules, fibrinogen and vWF,[1-3] as well as other identified and as yet unidentified plasma and platelet molecules[4,255] contribute to thrombus formation and stability.

Molecular Mechanisms Involved in Platelet Aggregation

The basis for the requisite roles of the agonist, calcium, and fibrinogen and vWF in platelet aggregation is now well understood at a molecular level. Fibrinogen and vWF are ligands for integrin αIIbβ3. Absence or dysfunction of this integrin on the surface of platelets leads to Glanzmann thrombasthenia, a condition characterized by absent platelet aggregation. Further evidence for the critical role of αIIbβ3 in platelet aggregation and thrombus formation comes from genetically modified mice that are unable to express this receptor. These mice are unable to form a thrombus.[256] In contrast, mice that lack ligands for this receptor can still form a thrombus,[1-4] although increased bleeding may be observed. An agonist is necessary to convert αIIbβ3 from its resting state on circulating platelets in which the integrin is unable to bind its plasma protein ligands to an activated state in which ligands bind rapidly. All of the platelet agonists listed in Table 127-4 can initiate platelet aggregation through this pathway. Calcium is needed for fibrinogen and vWF binding to activated αIIbβ3. Activation of αIIbβ3 by agonists is very rapid; the receptors become fully competent to bind fibrinogen or vWF seconds after platelets encounter an appropriate agonist. More than 40,000 fibrinogen molecules can be bound to the platelet surface via αIIbβ3.[239,257-259] Fibrinogen is a dimer and vWF a multimer. By virtue of their repeating and large structures, these ligands can bind to αIIbβ3 on adjacent platelets and bridge the cells together, leading to formation of platelet aggregates.[241,260-263]

$\alpha_{IIb}\beta_3$: Structure–Function Relationships

The resting platelet has 40,000 to 80,000 copies of $\alpha_{IIb}\beta_3$ on its surface,[264] and platelet activation can produce a further 10% increase in this number as a result of expression of internal receptor pools.[265] Each $\alpha_{IIb}\beta_3$ is capable of binding one fibrinogen molecule. $\alpha_{IIb}\beta_3$ is a typical integrin composed of an α and a β subunit, which combine to form a heterodimer.[34,36] The α subunit, α_{IIb} (GPIIb), is expressed primarily by cells of the platelet/megakaryocyte , although expression by various solid tumors and mast cells has also been reported.[266-268] The β_3 subunit, GPIIIa, forms a complex not only with α_{IIb} but also with the α_V subunit to form $\alpha_v\beta_3$.[269] $\alpha_v\beta_3$ is expressed by a variety of cell types, including platelets, megakaryocytes, and endothelial cells.[270-272] These two sister receptors bind many of the same ligands and antagonists, but their specificities are not identical.[273] Complete amino acid sequences of both α_{IIb} and β_3 subunits were deduced from their cDNAs sequences.[37,40] The carbohydrate side chains and disulfide linkages were also located.[274-277] α_{IIb} is synthesized in megakaryocytes as a single chain but becomes proteolytically processed to the two-chain form during its transit to the cell surface.[278]

Structural biology studies have provided significant insights into the molecular basis for the functions of $\alpha_{IIb}\beta_3$ and $\alpha_V\beta_3$. The crystal structure of the extracellular domain of $\alpha_V\beta_3$ was solved with and without a bound peptide ligand (see later discussion).[279,280] A schematic model illustrating the domain organization derived from these crystal structures is shown in Fig. 127-5. The extracellular domain of each subunit is composed of several domains, and at least one domain from each subunit directly contacts bound ligand. The primary ligand contact domain in the α subunit is termed the β-propeller domain. It is composed of seven "blades" and homologous structures are found in G proteins. In the β subunit, an A domain, also referred to as an I domain, contacts ligand. The β propeller and A domain come into close proximity to form a globular head that is apparent in electron micrographs of isolated $\alpha_{IIb}\beta_3$.[281] Within the A domain of the β_3 subunit are three divalent cation binding sites, and one of these, termed the metal ion-dependent adhesion site (MIDAS), is intimately involved in ligand binding. One of the coordination sites for the cation bound within the MIDAS can be provided by an aspartic acid within the ligand. Thus, occupancy of the MIDAS cation establishes the role for divalent ions in ligand binding and platelet aggregation (see Fig. 127-5). Located within the α_{IIb} and β_3 stalks, which extend out from the globular head, is a "genu," which allows bending so that the head domain can approach the cell membrane. It was this bent structure that was observed in the $\alpha_V\beta_3$ crystal structures. Subsequently, several crystal structures of portions of the extracellular domain of αIIbβ3 also were solved.[282] Structures with antagonists bound to the receptor illustrate how low molecular weight ligands bind to $\alpha_{IIb}\beta_3$.

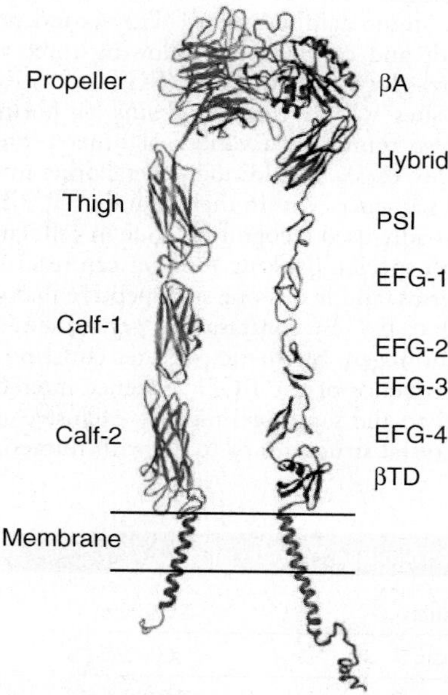

Figure 127-5 MODEL SHOWING THE STRUCTURAL ORGANIZATION OF A β3 INTEGRIN. The model is based on the crystal structure of the extracellular domain of $\alpha_V\beta_3$ and the cytoplasmic tails on the nuclear magnetic resonance (NMR) structure of $\alpha_{IIb}\beta_3$. *(Adapted from Xiong JP, Stehle T, Goodman SL, et al: Integrins, cations and ligands: Making the connection. J Thromb Haemost 1:1642, 2003 and Qin J, Vinogradova O, Plow EF: Integrin bidirectional signaling: A molecular view.* PLoS Biol *2:e169, 2004.)*

Structures for the transmembrane domains and the cytoplasmic tails also are available.[283-287] The transmembrane segment of each subunit is composed of an α helix,[287-289] and these transmembrane helices interact with each other.[290] Two recent structures of the transmembrane helices are similar but differ in the region where α_{IIb} enters the cytosol, one showing an inverse turn[288] and the other indicating a helical region that extends into the cytosol.[289] This distinction is important because this segment is reported to be the binding site for several molecules that regulate integrin-mediated signaling and may or may not be available for such interactions. Regardless, it is clear that the regions proximal to the cytosolic membrane of both α_{IIb} and β_3 are helical, and these helices interact weakly with each other. The dissociation of this "CT membrane complex" is a key regulatory event in integrin activation.[284]

Activation of $\alpha_{IIb}\beta_3$

$\alpha_{IIb}\beta_3$ activation is initiated by a platelet agonist and involves transmission of a signal induced by engagement of the agonist receptor to the cytoplasmic tail of the integrins. The signal is then transmitted from the cytoplasmic tail through the transmembrane helices and ultimately induces a change in the extracellular domain to render the integrin functional. The signaling process responsible for this transformation is referred to as "inside-out" signaling.[291-293] Although a model depicting the structural basis of inside-out signaling has emerged, many specific details have yet to be resolved. An integrin activator binds to the cytoplasmic tail of $\alpha_{IIb}\beta_3$ and disrupts the complex between the subunits.[284,294,295] The dissociation triggers a conformational change that is transmitted into transmembrane segments and disturbs their interaction.[290] These events are then transmitted to the extracellular region, allowing for acquisition of ligand competence. Within the transmembrane region, disassembly of the intramolecular interactions between helices initiates homo-oligomerization between like subunits.[287,290,296] Consequently, the integrin heterodimers become clustered. Such clustering in itself can lead to or enhance activation by enhancing the avidity of the clustered extracellular domains for ligand or by altering the conformation of the extracellular domain.[297-299]

The crystal structures of the extracellular domain of $\alpha_V\beta_3$ revealed bent structures with the head domain in proximity to the cell membrane.[279] This configuration was unanticipated because most electron micrographs suggested that the head domain resided at the end of long, straight stalks.[281] These seemingly disparate results were reconciled by a "switchblade" hypothesis, which suggests that there is sufficient flexibility that the integrin can either assume a bent or an extended conformation. Detailed micrographic studies supported the notion that the integrin can transition between these extreme states and can also assume an intermediate state between the fully bent and fully extended conformation. It was further suggested that the extended conformation coincided with the activated integrin and that in the bent state, the integrin was resting. This model provided an attractive mechanism to account for activation of $\alpha_{IIb}\beta_3$ in particular and integrins in general.[299] However, in a subsequent crystal structure, a fibronectin fragment was observed bound to $\alpha_V\beta_3$ in a bent conformation.[300,301] Thus, even though $\alpha_{IIb}\beta_3$ may transition from bent to extended conformation, this change contributes to but may not be essential for ligand binding. Most likely, the integrin can exist in several conformational states that are in equilibrium; ligand binding is favored with the extended conformation of the integrin with an open headpiece but can occur with intermediate states, including forms that are still in a bent conformation.[298] From crystal structures of $\alpha_{IIb}\beta_3$, with or without bound ligands, differences are noted in the positioning of helices and in divalent ions in the β_3 A domain as well as movements of domains adjacent to the β_3 A domain. Movements of these structural elements may locally regulate ligand binding.[282]

Talin, a large (270 kDa) cytoskeletal protein, has been strongly implicated in integrin activation.[302,303] It is composed of a *N*-terminal FERM-like domain, the talin-head (talin-H) of about 47 kDa, and a long C-terminal rod domain.[304] Talin-H consists of three subdomains, including the F3 subdomain, that resembles a phosphotyrosine binding (PTB) subdomain. This subdomain harbors the sites that interact with the β_3 cytoplasmic tail of integrins to induce integrin activation. In fact, talin-H interacts with two sites in the cytoplasmic tail of the β_3 subunit: the NPLY sequence in the midsegment of the cytoplasmic tail and a sequence in the membrane proximal region.[303,305-311] Talin binding to the membrane proximal site in the β_3 cytoplasmic tail displaces it from its complex with the α_{IIb} cytoplasmic tail, and this "unclasping" triggers integrin activation.[306,307,312,313] Mice containing point mutations in the talin-binding regions of β_3 exhibit a bleeding phenotype.[314,315] Talin-H also contains a membrane binding site, and interaction with the intermembrane region enhances the affinity of talin for the integrin, which is essential for activation. The talin rod harbors sites that mediate its interaction with the actin cytoskeleton. This linkage occurs either by direct binding to actin or indirectly through viculin or α-actinin.[316-318] These contacts allow talin to bridge between the integrin and the cytoskeleton of the cell, a linkage that is also critical for integrin induced outside-in signaling.

Intact talin exists in an autoinhibited state in unstimulated cells where interactions between the rod and talin-H domains prevent binding to the β_3-cytoplasmic tail. Talin becomes activated via several mechanisms, including binding of phosphoinositides[319] or RIAM (rap1 interacting adaptor molecule)[320] and by proteolytic cleavage by calpain.[302] Several other proteins are known to bind to the β_3 cytoplasmic tail. Some of these appear to compete with talin, thereby dampening integrin activation. Notable in this regard are Dok1, which bind to the NPLY sequence, and filamin, which binds to a more C-terminal site, but still inhibits integrin activation.[313,321-323]

Although studies in model systems, cells, and mice have established a pivotal role for talin in integrin activation,[324] it is evident that talin alone is not sufficient for integrin activation in physiologic settings.[325,326] Evidence from mice and humans has shown that the kindlin family members are also essential for integrin activation.[327-329] There are three kindlins in humans. Kindlin-1 deficiency in mice and humans results in a skin disease, Kindler syndromes, frequently associated with gastrointestinal problems.[330,331] Kindlin-2 deficiency has not been described in humans and is embryonically lethal in mice.[332,333] Kindlin-2 is the most broadly distributed of the kindlins. Kindlin-3 is particularly relevant to $\alpha_{IIb}\beta_3$ activation. It is found in hematopoietic cells and endothelial cells.[334,335] Its deficiency in mice leads to death shortly after birth, and the primary manifestations of its deficiency are bleeding, an inability to mount an inflammatory response, and osteopetrosis.[336] These same manifestations have been noted in the few reported cases of kindlin-3 deficiency in humans, although the penetrance of the abnormalities is variable. This deficiency is referred to as LADIII, LADI variant, or IADD (integrin activation deficiency disease).[328,329] In humans as well as in mice, the bleeding associated with kindlin-3 deficiency is a consequence of the inability of platelets to aggregate, which in turn arises from an inability to activate integrin $\alpha_{IIb}\beta_3$. The failure of leukocyte of transmigration reflects the inability to activate β_2 integrins, and the bone defects may be a consequence of an inability to activate one or both of these subfamilies of integrins. β_1 integrin activation can also be dysfunctional. Thus, the activation of at least three major integrin subfamilies is kindlin-3 dependent. In model cell systems, kindlins do not induce integrin activation but appear to cooperate with talin to enhance integrin activation (i.e., talin and kindlins are integrin co-activators).[325,326]

Kindlins exhibit many similarities with talin. Similar to talin, kindlins are FERM domain containing proteins, and like talin, the F_3 subdomain of kindlins interacts with integrin β subunits.[326,332,337] The unique signature of kindlins is the interruption of their FERM domains by an inserted plecksin homology (PH) domain. PH domains are frequently involved in lipid binding, and the PH domains of kindlins possess this function.[338,339] Thus, also similar to talin, kindlins interact with membranes, and the PH domain is not the only membrane binding site in kindlins. Distinct from talin is the sites within integrin β subunits that bind integrins.[326] As noted earlier, one of the talin binding sites in the β_3 cytoplasmic tail is the NPLY[747] sequence. Kindlin binding to the β_3-cytoplasmic tail involves the NITY[759], which is very close to the C-terminus of T[762]. Both tyrosine residues are targets for phosphorylation, which occurs as a consequence of ligand binding and outside-in signaling. Phosphorylation of Y[747] decreases, but does not preclude, talin binding[322]; phosphorylation of Y[759] prevents kindlin-2 binding to the β_3 cytoplasmic tail.[340] Although the role of talin in integrin activation by dissociation of the cytoplasmic tail complex is clear, the mechanism by which kindlins influence integrin activation remains to be resolved.

Several mechanisms can be envisioned to explain how fibrinogen binding to $\alpha_{IIb}\beta_3$ results in platelet aggregation. The simplest explanation is that a single fibrinogen molecule, by virtue of its dimeric structure, bridges two $\alpha_{IIb}\beta_3$ molecules symmetrically on adjacent platelets. Indeed, evidence can be cited to support this possibility.[341-343] Because multiple sites within each fibrinogen molecule can be recognized by $\alpha_{IIb}\beta_3$ (see later), asymmetric variations of direct bridging can be envisioned. Still another possibility is that changes subsequent to fibrinogen binding are required for platelet aggregation. Irreversible fibrinogen binding,[241] conformational changes in bound fibrinogen[216,344] and in occupied $\alpha_{IIb}\beta_3$,[345] clustering of fibrinogen/$\alpha_{IIb}\beta_3$,[346] and additional interactions of the receptor with the cytoskeleton of the cells[347-349] occur after initial binding of fibrinogen to platelets. Moreover, a series of intracellular signaling events is initiated and propagated as a result of receptor occupancy and platelet aggregation, including tyrosine and serine/threonine kinase and phosphatase activation.[291,292] These events are referred to as "outside-in" signaling. Whether such postreceptor occupancy events play a direct role in platelet aggregation is unknown, although circumstances have been described in which fibrinogen binds to $\alpha_{IIb}\beta_3$ without inducing platelet aggregation,[291] and mice with mutations in the tyrosine phosphorylation sites in the β_3 subunit exhibit reduced thrombus stability,[350] which implies a role for outside-in signals in platelet aggregation.

Recognition Specificity and Antagonism of $\alpha_{IIb}\beta_3$

Linear amino acid sequences define the recognition specificity of $\alpha_{IIb}\beta_3$ (Table 127-5). One peptide corresponds to the extreme COOH-terminus of the γ chain,[341,351] one of the three constituent chains of fibrinogen. The recognized amino acid sequence may involve only six amino acid residues.[352] The second peptide includes four amino acids and contains the following three amino acids in sequence: arginyl-glycyl-aspartic acid (RGD).[353-356] RGD sequences occur on two sites within the Aα chains of fibrinogen.[357] RGD sequences are also found on a variety of other proteins, including several that bind to $\alpha_{IIb}\beta_3$. In addition, several other integrin receptors recognize RGD sequences within their ligands.[34,358-361] Thus, the RGD sequence is a broadly used recognition code in cellular adhesive reactions. RGD with specific flanking residues can react selectively with individual integrins, and it was one such peptide that was crystallized in complex with $\alpha_V\beta_3$[280] By contrast, the γ-chain sequence appears to be unique to fibrinogen. Synthetic peptides containing either the γ-chain peptide sequence or the RGD sequence interact directly with $\alpha_{IIb}\beta_3$ and bind to the same or mutually exclusive sites within the receptor.[362,363] Crystal structures of $\alpha_{IIb}\beta_3$ with mimetics of these two

Table 127-5 Recognition Peptides of $\alpha_{IIb}\beta_3$*

Peptide Designation	Structure†
Fibrinogen γ chain	-XXKQAGDV
RGD	RGDX

*The naturally occurring sequences in human fibrinogen; S (serine) or F (phenylalanine) at the COOH-terminus of the two RGD sequences within the α-chain; and H (histidine) –H-L (leucine) –G-G-A at the NH_2-terminus of the γ-chain peptide.
†Amino acids: A, alanine; D, aspartic acid; G, glycine; K, lysine; Q, glutamine; V, valine; X, one of several amino acids.

peptide sequences suggest a similar binding mechanism,[282] but allosteric effects of additional binding sites cannot be excluded,[364] and allosteric inhibitors of ligand binding to integrins have been identified.[365] The preponderance of evidence indicates that the COOH-terminus of the γ chain is critical for fibrinogen binding to $\alpha_{IIb}\beta_3$.[366-368] Nevertheless, in the design of $\alpha_{IIb}\beta_3$ antagonists, the RGD sequence has often served as the starting compound because of its smaller size.[369] Identification of these two sequences does not exclude the possibility that other sequences are involved in fibrinogen binding to $\alpha_{IIb}\beta_3$. Indeed, there is evidence supporting this concept.[370]

Fibrinogen is not the only ligand that binds to $\alpha_{IIb}\beta_3$. Several other adhesive proteins that can serve as ligands are listed in Table 127-2. All of these adhesive proteins contain at least one RGD sequence, and RGD peptides interfere with the binding of fibronectin[353,356] and vitronectin[371] to platelets. Because plasma fibrinogen concentrations are 10-fold higher than its dissociation constant for $\alpha_{IIb}\beta_3$, under physiologic conditions, the receptor is nearly saturated with fibrinogen. Thus, fibrinogen is the dominant ligand for $\alpha_{IIb}\beta_3$ in this environment. However, all of these ligands, except fibrinogen, are found in subendothelial cell matrices, and these other interactions may dominate in this microenvironment. Because vWF is bound to platelets via GPIb-V-IX, it resides in close proximity to $\alpha_{IIb}\beta_3$ on the platelet surface, and this proximity may favor its engagement by $\alpha_{IIb}\beta_3$. In addition to its role in platelet aggregation, $\alpha_{IIb}\beta_3$ may also be involved in platelet adhesion, particularly in stabilizing cell–matrix interactions.[372] It may be in this latter function that other $\alpha_{IIb}\beta_3$ ligands play a key role. Thrombospondin-1 associates with the surface of resting and stimulated platelets.[373-375] On the surface, it plays an auxiliary role in platelet aggregation by stabilizing platelet aggregates.[376] This activity may arise from its capacity to bind to fibrinogen.[181,377] Several candidate receptors for thrombospondin have been proposed,[348,378-381] and the interaction may be mediated by a complex of several of these candidate receptors, including CD36, integrin-associated protein, and $\alpha_{IIb}\beta_3$.[382] Complexation of $\alpha_{IIb}\beta_3$ with other platelet membrane proteins CD9,[383-385] CD40L,[255] and Gas6[166] also may play a role in controlling its activation and ligand-binding functions and platelet responses in general. Increasing evidence indicates that a number of these and other membrane proteins in platelets influence the adhesive responses of platelets in vitro and in vivo.[386]

Throughout the 1980s, a number of compounds were described that bound to $\alpha_{IIb}\beta_3$ and inhibited platelet aggregation. Furthermore, it was noted that bleeding in patients with Glanzmann thrombasthenia tended to be relatively mild. Taken together, these observations prompted the notion that $\alpha_{IIb}\beta_3$ would be and attractive target for antiplatelet drugs. Antagonists included monoclonal antibodies, small peptide ligands, and nonpeptidic ligand mimetics. Representatives of these classes of antagonists were evaluated in various animal models of thrombosis and in large clinical trials.[387-394] Three such agents, all intravenous drugs, ultimately were approved for patient usage by U.S. Food and Drug Administration. Abciximab is a Fab fragment of a humanized monoclonal antibody; eptifibitide is a cyclic peptide based on the sequence of a snake venom peptide; and tirofiban is a nonpeptide that was designed with RGD as a starting structure (see Chapter 148). Although all three $\alpha_{IIb}\beta_3$ antagonists continue to be used, particularly in patients undergoing primary percutaneous coronary interventions for acute myocardial infarction, the need for $\alpha_{IIb}\beta_3$ antagonists has declined with the introduction of more potent oral antiplatelet drugs.[395-398] There was great optimism that orally active $\alpha_{IIb}\beta_3$ antagonists would be of benefit. A number of drugs were developed with excellent pharmacokinetic properties. However, when tested in clinical trials, they proved to be ineffective or even detrimental.[399] The reason for the failure of these oral antagonists is not fully understood. One explanation is that patients were underdosed to avoid safety issues, but this would not in itself explain the detrimental effects. It has also been suggested that these drugs may leave $\alpha_{IIb}\beta_3$ in an activated state when they dissociate from the receptor.[400] Regardless of the explanation, the initial clinical trials dampened the effort to develop orally active $\alpha_{IIb}\beta_3$ antagonists, and all such programs were abandoned.

SUGGESTED READINGS

Cybulsky MI, Gimbrone MA, Jr: Endothelial expression of a mononuclear leukocyte adhesion molecule during atherogenesis. *Science* 251:788, 1991.

Davies PF: Endothelial transcriptome profiles in vivo in complex arterial flow fields. *Ann Biomed Eng* 36:563, 2008.

Davies PF, Civelek M, Fang Y, et al: Endothelial heterogeneity associated with regional athero-susceptibility and adaptation to disturbed blood flow in vivo. *Semin Thromb Hemost* 36:265, 2010.

Denis C, Methia N, Frenette PS, et al: A mouse model of severe von Willebrand disease: Defects in hemostasis and thrombosis. *Proc Natl Acad Sci U S A* 95:9524, 1998.

Engvall E, Ruoslahti E, Miller EJ: Affinity of fibronectin to collagens of different genetic types and to fibrinogen. *J Exp Med* 147:1584, 1978.

Ginsberg MH, Du X, Plow EF: Inside-out integrin signalling. *Curr Opin Cell Biol* 4:766, 1992.

Ginsberg MH, O'Toole TE, Loftus JC, et al: Ligand binding to integrins: Dynamic regulation and common mechanisms. *Cold Spring Harb Symp Quant Biol* 57:221, 1992.

Ginsberg MH, Xiaoping D, O'Toole TE, et al: Platelet integrins. *Thromb Haemost* 70:87, 1993.

Grinnell F, Hays DG: Cell adhesion and spreading factor. Similarity to cold insoluble globulin in human serum. *Exp Cell Res* 115:221, 1978.

Holmbäck K, Danton MJS, Suh TT, et al: Impaired platelet aggregation and sustained bleeding in mice lacking the fibrinogen motif bound by integrin alpha IIb beta 3. *EMBO J* 15:5760, 1996.

Houdijk WP, de Groot PG., Nievelstein PF, et al: Subendothelial proteins and platelet adhesion. von Willebrand factor and fibronectin, not thrombospondin, are involved in platelet adhesion to extracellular matrix of human vascular endothelial cells. *Arteriosclerosis* 6:24, 1986.

Houdijk WP, Sakariassen KS, Nievelstein PF, et al: Role of factor VIII-von Willebrand factor and fibronectin in the interaction of platelets in flowing blood with monomeric and fibrillar human collagen types I and III. *J Clin Invest* 75:531, 1985.

Leytin VL, Gorbunova NA, Misselwitz F, et al: Step-by-step analysis of adhesion of human platelets to a collagen-coated surface defect in initial attachment and spreading of platelets in von Willebrand's disease. *Thromb Res* 34:51, 1984.

McCarty OJ, Calaminus SD, Berndt MC, et al: Von Willebrand factor mediates platelet spreading through glycoprotein Ib and alpha(IIb)beta3 in the presence of botrocetin and ristocetin, respectively. *J Thromb Haemost* 4:1367, 2006.

Mumby SM, Raugi GJ, Bornstein P: Interactions of thrombospondin with extracellular matrix proteins: Selective binding to type V collagen. *J Cell Biol* 98:646, 1984.

Nagel T, Resnick N, Atkinson WJ, et al: Shear stress selectively upregulates intercellular adhesion molecule-1 expression in cultured human vascular endothelial cells. *J Clin Invest* 94:885, 1994.

Ni H, Denis CV, Subbarao S, et al: Persistence of platelet thrombus formation in arterioles of mice lacking both von Willebrand factor and fibrinogen. *J Clin Invest* 106:385, 2000.

Ni H, Yuen PS, Papalia JM, et al: Plasma fibronectin promotes thrombus growth and stability in injured arterioles. *Proc Natl Acad Sci U S A* 100:2415, 2003.

Paul J, Schwazbauer JE, Tamkun JW, et al: Cell-type-specific fibronectin subunits generated by alternative splicing. *J Biol Chem* 261:12258, 1986.

Pfaff M, Aumailley M, Specks U, et al: Integrin and Arg-Gly-Asp dependence of cell adhesion to the native and unfolded triple helix of collagen type VI. *Exp Cell Res* 206:167, 1993.

Pfaff M, Gohring W, Brown JC, et al: Binding of purified collagen receptors (alpha 1 beta 1, alpha 2 beta 1) and RGD-dependent integrins to laminins and laminin fragments. *Eur J Biochem* 225:975, 1994.

Phillips DR, Agin PP: Platelet plasma membrane glycoproteins. Evidence for the presence of nonequivalent disulfide bonds using nonreduced-reduced two-dimensional gel electrophoresis. *J Biol Chem* 252:2121, 1977.

Plow EF, D'Souza SE, Ginsberg MH: Consequences of the interaction of platelet membrane glycoprotein GPIIb-IIIa (alpha IIb beta 3) and its ligands. *J Lab Clin Med* 120:198, 1992.

Sadler JE: Von Willebrand factor assembly and secretion. *J Thromb Haemost* 7:24, 2009.

Sakariassen KS, Bolhuis PA, Sixma JJ: Human blood platelet adhesion to artery subendothelium is mediated by factor VIII-von Willebrand factor bound to the subendothelium. *Nature* 279:636, 1979.

Santoro SA, Cowan JF: Adsorption of von Willebrand factor by fibrillar collagen—implications concerning the adhesion of platelets to collagen. *Coll Relat Res* 2:31, 1982.

Tomlinson MG, Calaminus SD, Berlanga O, et al: Collagen promotes sustained glycoprotein VI signaling in platelets and cell lines. *J Thromb Haemost* 5:2274, 2007.

Weiss HJ, Turitto VT, Baumgartner HR: Effect of shear rate on platelet interaction with subendothelium in citrated and native blood. I. Shear rate—dependent decrease of adhesion in von Willebrand's disease and the Bernard-Soulier syndrome. *J Lab Clin Med* 92:750, 1978.

Wencel-Drake JD, Painter RG, Zimmerman TS, et al: Ultrastructural localization of human platelet thrombospondin, fibrinogen, fibronectin, and von Willebrand factor in frozen thin section. *Blood* 65:929, 1985.

Wencel-Drake JD, Plow EF, Zimmerman TS, et al: Immunofluorescent localization of adhesive glycoproteins in resting and thrombin-stimulated platelets. *Am J Pathol* 115:156, 1984.

For complete list of references log on to www.expertconsult.com.

CHAPTER 128

MOLECULAR BASIS OF BLOOD COAGULATION

Kathleen Brummel-Ziedins and Kenneth G. Mann

Blood is the principal vehicle delivering oxygen and nutrients to the various tissues and organs of the body. Blood flow and the integrity of the vasculature are essential to life itself. The hemostatic process has evolved to provide damage recognition and protection from blood loss after perforation of the vasculature while at the same time preventing the systemic activation of the clotting system. However, pathologic occlusions are associated with dysregulation of the intravascular system, resulting in venous or arterial thrombosis. The fine line between vascular occlusion and hemostasis is defined by the complex interplay between pro- and anticoagulant materials provided by the blood, the vasculature, and subvascular elements. The appropriate functions occur as a consequence of intense focal development and regulation of enzymatic activity at sites of vascular injury.

The development of the inventory of components involved in plasma clotting were initially based on the most abundant procoagulant plasma proteins, notably prothrombin and fibrinogen, and extended during the past century with the identification of genetic abnormalities that led to bleeding and deviations in laboratory tests that evolved as the inventory of congenital defects expanded. In some instances, laboratory test results indicating a defect in the procoagulant system were not mirrored by hemostatic pathology. In a similar fashion, the congenital defects associated with thrombosis led to discovery of anticoagulant proteins in blood and vascular counterparts associated with their presentation and activation.

The functional connections between procoagulant "factors" were developed by mixing and matching plasmas associated with different hemostatic disorders. This inventory and its connectivity were ratified and expanded by experiments performed with transgenically mutated mice.

The dynamics of the plasma coagulation process as expressed are a consequence of the molar concentrations of the pro- and anticoagulant components in blood and the vasculature and the kinetic processes associated with the dynamics of both the activation and functions of the various proteins associated with the process.

The initial result of the activation of the procoagulant hemostatic process is the formation of a fibrin–platelet plug that forms the temporary seal of the vascular perforation in hemostasis. The generation of an occlusive fibrin–platelet plug blocking further flow through an element of the vasculature is thrombosis. In both instances, the fibrin–platelet scaffold is ultimately removed and substituted by vascular repair, new cells, and connective tissue. In thrombosis, the platelet–fibrin plug is removed mechanically or by biochemical intervention to restore flow to the flow-starved vascular bed.

The elements of clotted fibrinogen–platelet plug are dissolved by the fibrinolytic system, a tightly regulated dynamic system involving enzyme activation, feedback regulation, and blockade by a potent series of inhibitors. Just as there is an interplay between the pro- and anticoagulant components that brings about a blood clot in hemostasis, similar mechanisms occur when blood clots are dissolved via the fibrinolytic process, which is essential for tissue repair. This review describes the components of the pro- and anticoagulant system and the pro- and antifibrinolytic system and the interplay between these systems. The common feature of both systems is the focal presentation of activity that is dependent on the presentation of surface bound enzymatic complexes that can cleave their respective substrates.

Blood coagulation can best be understood if viewed as a choreographed system that starts from an inventory of the key players, the relationship or connectivity of these players, and the dynamic catalytic processes. These processes together keep blood in a fluid state but primed to react to vascular injury in an explosive manner. Therefore, following sections describe the process of blood coagulation in terms of the inventory, the connectivity, and then the dynamics.

INVENTORY: PROCOAGULANT, ANTICOAGULANT AND FIBRINOLYTIC PROTEINS, INHIBITORS AND RECEPTORS

Putting together an inventory of the blood coagulation components is still an ongoing process, but what we currently know to date began from initial observations that were made in the fifth century and recorded in the Babylonian Talmud. It was noted that if two male children died of bleeding after circumcision, the third should not be circumcised.[1] Over the centuries, many more hypotheses were made regarding what happens to blood when it escapes from the body.[2,3] The realization that clots stem blood loss only occurred in the 18th century.[2,3] The existence of thrombin, the key enzyme in blood coagulation, was recognized in the 19th century.[2,4]

In 1905, Paul Morawitz proposed the classic theory of coagulation.[5] He hypothesized that in the presence of calcium and thromboplastin, prothrombin was converted to thrombin, which in turn converted fibrinogen to the fibrin clot. These clotting factors were subsequently assigned Roman numerals, factor I (fibrinogen), factor II (prothrombin), factor III (thromboplastin; tissue factor membrane), and factor IV (calcium).[6] As more coagulation factors were introduced, they were assigned consecutive Roman numerals. The activated forms are distinguished by a lower case "a" after their Roman numeral designation. Therefore, the activated form of factor V becomes factor Va.

More complex descriptions of the coagulation system were as a "cascade" or "waterfall". Macfarlane[7] and Davie and Ratnoff[8] proposed that in an intrinsic pathway, involving only plasma, blood coagulated by a sequence of events in which the reactions occurred in a defined series leading to fibrin clot formation. Over the past 6 decades, the Morawitz/Davie and Macfarlane pathways have been significantly expanded (Fig. 128-1). Each reaction shares a similar mechanism in which an inactive zymogen protein is converted to an active enzyme and each "enzyme" is a surface bound multiprotein complex consisting of a surface, divalent calcium ions (Ca^{2+}), a protease, and a cofactor. Although some facets of these initial descriptions are still valid, the emerging concept of coagulation and fibrinolysis centers on a complex network of highly interwoven concurrent processes. Procoagulant and fibrinolytic events occur simultaneously with many positive and negative feedback loops regulating the processes.

To fully understand the multiple simultaneous processes that occur to effect a hemostatic response, we will first inventory the key procoagulant, anticoagulant, and fibrinolytic participants. The inventory sections discuss vitamin k–dependent protein family,

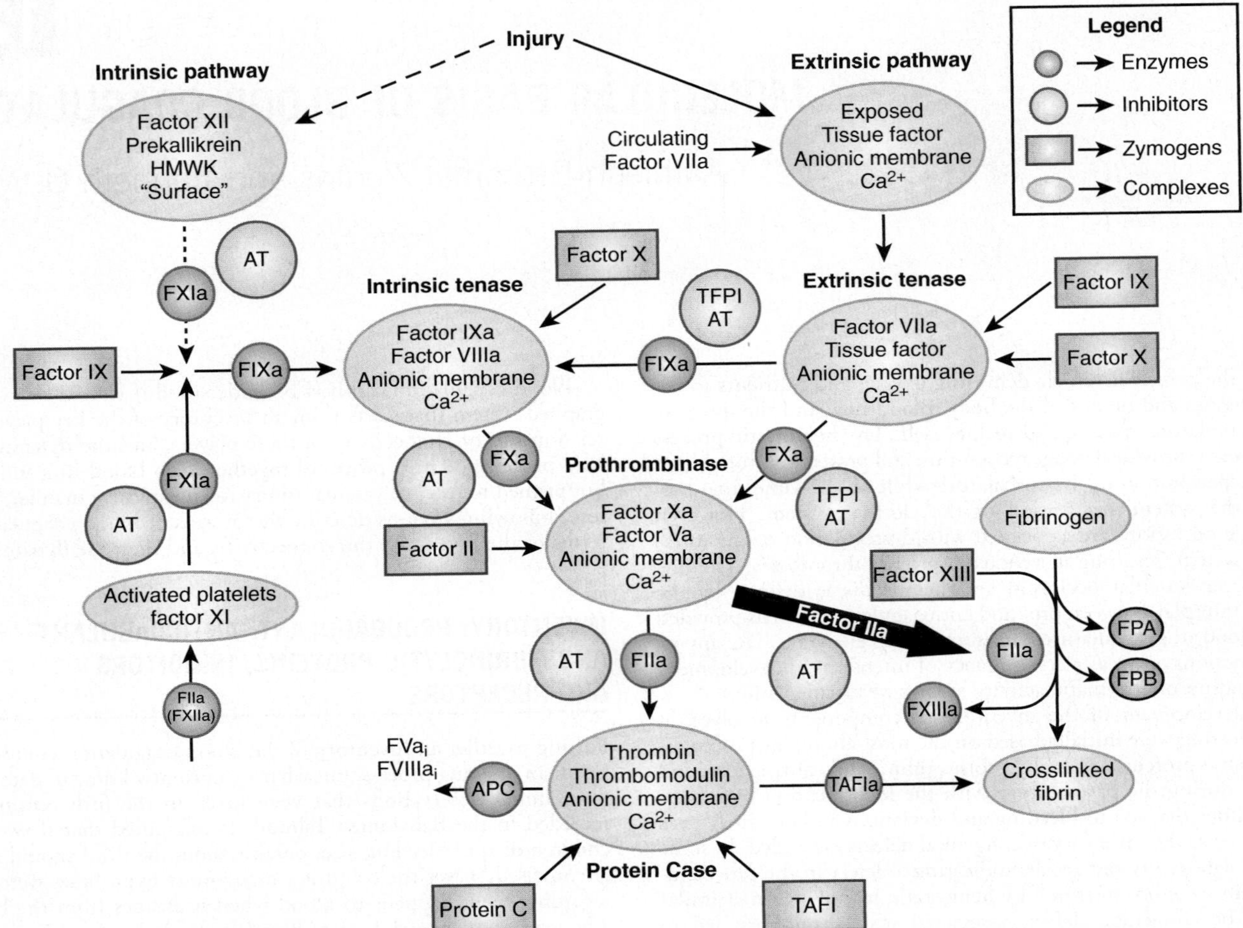

Figure 128-1 OVERVIEW OF HEMOSTASIS. Coagulation is initiated via two pathways, the primary extrinsic pathway *(right)* and the accessory (historically called the *contact* or *intrinsic pathway*) *(left)*. An illustration of the multistep processes are as follows: enzymes *(small circles)*, inhibitors *(large circles)*, zymogens *(boxes)*, or complexes *(ovals)*. The accessory pathway has no known bleeding etiology associated with it; thus, this path is considered accessory to hemostasis. Upon injury to the vessel wall, tissue factor, the cofactor for the extrinsic tenase complex, is exposed to circulating factor VIIa and forms the vitamin K–dependent complex extrinsic tenase. Factor IX and factor X are converted to the serine proteases factor IXa (FIXa) and factor Xa (FXa), which then form the intrinsic tenase and prothrombinase complexes, respectively. The combined actions of intrinsic and extrinsic tenase and the prothrombinase complexes lead to an explosive burst of thrombin (IIa). Thrombin not only functions as a procoagulant but also acts as an anticoagulant when complexed with the cofactor thrombomodulin in the protein Case complex. The product of the protein Case reaction, activated protein C (APC), inactivates the cofactors factors Va and VIIIa. The cleaved species, factors Va_i (FVa_i) and $VIIIa_i$ ($FVIIIa_i$), no longer support the respective procoagulant activities of the prothrombinase and intrinsic tenase complexes. When thrombin is generated through procoagulant mechanisms, thrombin cleaves fibrinogen, releasing fibrinopeptides A and B (FPA and FPB, respectively), and activates factor XIII to form a cross-linked fibrin clot. Thrombin–thrombomodulin also activates thrombin-activatable fibrinolysis inhibitor (TAFI), which delays fibrin degradation by plasmin. The procoagulant response is downregulated by the stoichiometric inhibitors tissue factor pathway inhibitor (TFPI) and antithrombin (AT). TFPI serves to attenuate the activity of extrinsic tenase, the trigger of coagulation. AT directly inhibits thrombin, FIXa, and factor Xa. The accessory pathway provides an alternate route for the generation of factor IXa. Thrombin has also been shown to activate factor XI. *HMWK,* High-molecular-weight kininogen.

cofactor proteins, the intrinsic accessory pathway proteins, endothelium, platelets, proteinase inhibitors, clot proteins, and fibrinolysis proteins.

The Vitamin K–Dependent Protein Family

Vitamin K–dependent proteins, synthesized in the liver, play a central role in blood coagulation through either procoagulant or anticoagulant mechanisms. The vitamin K–dependent protein family includes the zymogen procoagulant factors VII, IX, X, and prothrombin and the anticoagulants protein C, protein S, and protein Z (Fig. 128-2 and Table 128-1). Except for protein S and protein Z, after cleavage to their active forms these proteins are serine proteases related to the trypsin and chymotrypsin superfamily. Peptide bond cleavage at specific sites converts the vitamin K–dependent zymogens to their active serine protease forms. All share noncatalytic domains, each of which is characterized by highly conserved regions that fold, independently from the rest of the molecule, into a characteristic three-dimensional shape. The domains of the vitamin K–dependent proteins are illustrated in Fig. 128-2. Several reviews have been written on vitamin K–dependent proteins.[9-11]

Vitamin K is essential for the biosynthesis of these clotting factors by participating in the cyclic oxidation and reduction of the enzyme that converts 9 to 13 amino-terminal glutamate residues to γ-carboxy glutamate (Gla; see Fig. 128-2) (for reviews, see References 9 and 12-14). This posttranslational modification to form Gla residues adds a net negative charge to the molecules that enables the vitamin

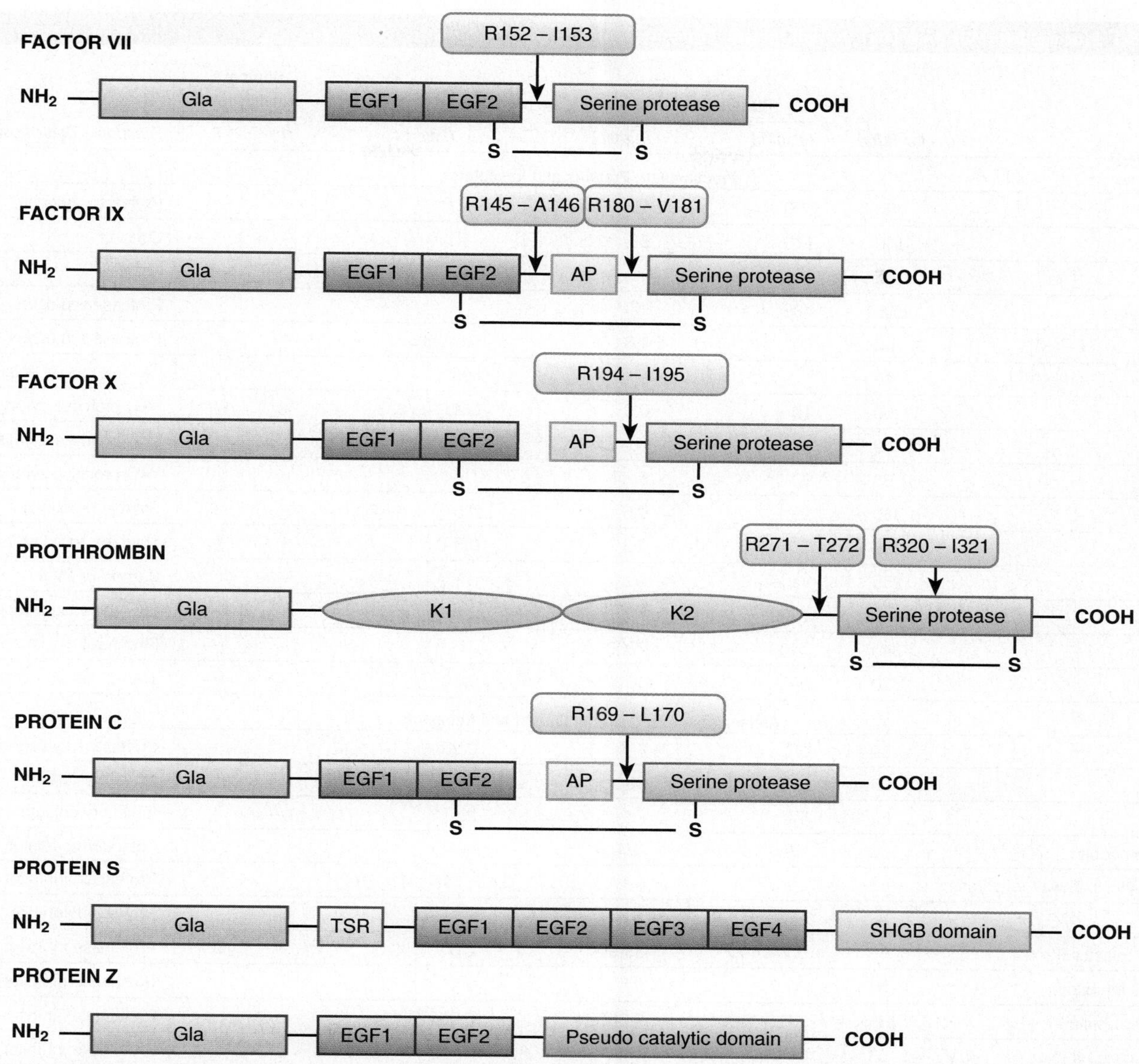

Figure 128-2 SCHEMATIC REPRESENTATION OF THE VITAMIN K–DEPENDENT PROTEINS. The vitamin K–dependent proteins can be divided into two classes, procoagulant (factors II, VII, IX, and X) and anticoagulant (protein C, protein S, and protein Z). The building blocks for these proteins include an NH_2-terminal Gla domain, consisting of nine to 13 Gla residues, followed by either an epidermal growth factor (EGF)–like domain in factor VII, factor IX, factor X, protein C, protein S, and protein Z or a kringle (K) domain in prothrombin. In protein S, a thrombin-sensitive region (TSR) precedes the EGF domain. Active sites are contained within the serine protease domain. Cleavage sites for the conversion of zymogens to their active forms are designated by *arrows;* activating proteases are placed in *boxes* above the *arrows*. Factor IX, factor X, and protein C are activated by proteolytic removal of an activation peptide (AP). Protein S, which is not a serine protease precursor, contains a sex hormone–binding globulin–like domain (SHGB) at the COOH-terminus. Protein Z also contains a "pseudo catalytic domain" in the COOH- terminus and does not function as a serine protease. Disulfide bonds (-S-S-) critical to the integrity of the two-chain zymogens or active forms are presented.

K–dependent proteins to interact with Ca^{2+} and a membrane surface.[15,16] Blocking the formation of the Gla residues is the basis for anticoagulant therapy with coumarin (warfarin) derivatives, such as warfarin, which are chemically similar in structure to vitamin K (Fig. 128-3). The Ca^{2+} binding association with this modification is also the basis for the anticoagulant activity of sodium citrate, a calcium chelator, found in the blue top vacuum tubes used for clinical laboratory testing of clotting activity. The level of inhibition achieved with the same dose of warfarin varies among patients. Increased sensitivity to warfarin has been identified in patients when started after surgery.[17,18] Factors affecting the level of anticoagulation include dietary intake of vitamin K; liver function; concomitant medications that either reduce or enhance the warfarin effect[19]; common polymorphisms in the vitamin K epoxide reductase complex subunit 1 (VKORC1), which is responsible for vitamin K reduction; and polymorphisms in CYP2C0, which affect warfarin metabolism (for reviews, see References 20 and 21). Therefore, genotyping may be helpful to personalize starting doses of warfarin. Ultimately, proper monitoring of warfarin therapy is essential. This is done using the prothrombin time (PT) with the assay sensitivity corrected using the international normalized ratio.[22,23]

The NH_2-terminal Gla domains are followed by either a kringle domain in factor II or an epidermal growth factor–like domain (EGF) in factor VII, factor IX, factor X, protein C, protein S, and protein Z (see Fig. 128-2). Protein S is not a serine protease precursor and instead contains a thrombin-sensitive region before the EGF

Table 128-1 Procoagulant, Anticoagulant, and Fibrinolytic Proteins, Inhibitors, and Receptors

Protein	*Mr (kDa)*	Plasma Concentration *(nmol/L)*	*(μg/mL)*	*Plasma Half-Life (Days)*	Clinical Phenotype* *H*	*T*	*Functional Classification*
Procoagulant Proteins and Receptors							
Factor XII	80	500	40	2-3	–		Protease zymogen
HMWK	120	670	80		–		Cofactor
LMWK	66	1300	90				Cofactor
Prekallikrein	85/88	486	42				Protease zymogen
Factor XI	160	30	4.8	2.5-3.3	+/–		Protease zymogen
TF	44			N/A			Cell-associated cofactor
Factor VII	50	10	0.5	0.25	+	+/–	VKD protease zymogen
Factor X	59	170	10	1. 5	+		VKD protease zymogen
Factor IX	55	90	5	1	+		VKD protease zymogen
Factor V	330	20	6.6	0.5	+	+	Soluble procofactor
Factor VIII	285	0.7	0.2	0.3-0.5	+	–	Soluble procofactor
vWF	255	Varies	10		+		Carrier for FVIII
Factor II	72	1400	100	2.5	+	–	VKD protease zymogen
Fibrinogen	340	7400	2500	3-5	+	+/–	Structural clot protein
Factor XIII	320	94	30	9-10	+	+/–	Transglutaminase zymogen
Anticoagulant Proteins, Inhibitors, and Receptors							
Protein C	62	65	4	0.33		+	Proteinase zymogen
Protein S	69	300	20	1.75		+	Inhibitory cofactor
Protein Z	62	47	2.9	2.5	+/–		Inhibitory cofactor
Thrombomodulin	100	N/A	N/A	N/A			Cofactor/modulator
Tissue factor pathway Inhibitor	40	1-4	0.1	6.4×10^{-4}–1.4×10^{-3}			Proteinase inhibitor
AT	58	2400	140	2.5-3			Proteinase inhibitor
Heparin cofactor II	66	500-1400	33-90	2.5	+	+/–	Proteinase inhibitor
Protein C inhibitor	57	90	5	1			Proteinase inhibitor
α_2-Macroglobulin	735	2700-4000	2-3000	0.002			Proteinase inhibitor
α_1-Proteinase inhibitor	53	28,000-65,000	1500-3500	6			Proteinase inhibitor
EPCR							Receptor
Fibrinolytic Proteins, Inhibitors, and Receptors							
Plasminogen	88	2000	200	2.2			Proteinase zymogen
t-PA	70	0.07	0.005	0.00167			Proteinase zymogen
u-PA	54	0.04	0.002	0.00347			Proteinase zymogen
TAFI	58	75	4.5	0.00694		+	Carboxypeptidase
FSAP	64	190	120				Fibrinolytic zymogen
PAI-1	52	0.2	0.01	<0.00694			Proteinase inhibitor Proteinase inhibitor
PAI-2	47/60	<0.070	<0.005	–			Proteinase inhibitor
α-Antiplasmin	70	500	70	2.6	+		Proteinase inhibitor
u-PAR	55						Cell membrane receptor

AT, Antithrombin; *EPCR,* endothelial protein C receptor; *FSAP,* factor VII–activating protease; *HMWK,* high-molecular-weight kininogen; *LMWK,* low-molecular-weight kininogen; *N/A,* not applicable; *PAI-1,* plasminogen activator inhibitor-3; *TF,* tissue factor; *t-PA,* tissue plasminogen activator; *u-PAR,* urokinase plasminogen activator receptor; *VKD,* vitamin K-dependent; *vWF,* von Willebrand factor.

*Clinical phenotype; the expression of either hemorrhagic or thrombotic phenotype in deficient individuals; ^{1}H, Hemorrhagic disease/ hemophilia; T, thrombotic disease/ thrombophilia; +, presence of phenotype; –, absence of phenotype; ±, some individuals present with the phenotype, and others do not.

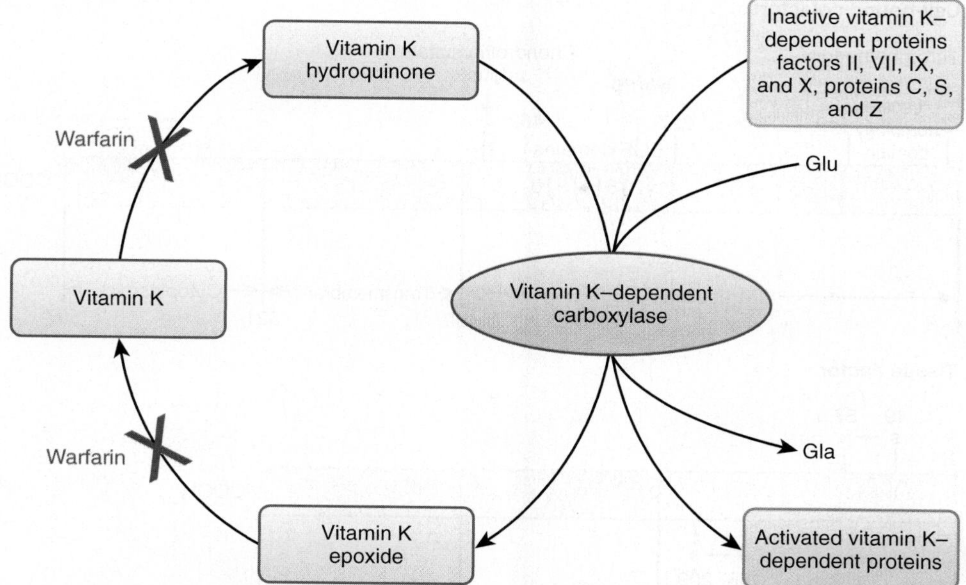

Figure 128-3 VITAMIN K–DEPENDENT PROCESS AND WARFARIN EFFECT. Schematic representation of the mechanism of γ-carboxy glutamate (Gla) generation by a vitamin K–dependent reaction cycle to produce an active protein is illustrated. The regeneration of vitamin K hydroquinone by the vitamin K–dependent reductases is inhibited by warfarin.

domain and a sex hormone–binding globulin–like domain (SHBG) in the COOH- terminus.[24] Protein Z contains a "pseudo catalytic domain" in the COOH- terminus and does not function as a serine protease enzyme.[25]

Vitamin K–dependent protein complexes are essential for establishing hemostatic balance (Fig. 128-4). Each complex is composed of a serine protease enzyme, a cofactor that functions as a surface receptor or enhancer for the enzyme Ca^{2+}, and a negatively charged membrane surface provided by activated or damaged cells (e.g., endothelial cells, monocytes, and platelets). There are four vitamin K–dependent complexes: the extrinsic tenase complex (factor VIIa–tissue factor), the intrinsic tenase complex (factor IXa–factor VIIIa), the prothrombinase complex (factor Xa–factor Va), and the anticoagulant protein Case complex (thrombin–thrombomodulin).

When the serine protease is associated with its respective cofactor on an appropriate membrane surface with Ca^{2+}, the specific reactions occur at a rate that is 10^4 to 10^9 fold faster than that of protease–substrate combination alone.[26] One way to visualize the importance of the assembly of these macromolecular complexes in the formation of the hemostatic plug is to note that if a healthy person takes 4 minutes for his or her blood to clot, then in the absence of membrane and cofactor, blood clot formation would take approximately 3.8 years.

Cofactor Proteins

There are two categories of procoagulant cofactor proteins; the cell-bound cofactors (tissue factor and thrombomodulin) and the soluble plasma-derived procoagulant procofactors (factor V and factor VIII with its circulating carrier von Willebrand factor [vWF]).

Cell-Bound Cofactors

Tissue Factor

Tissue factor is a transmembrane protein that functions as a nonenzymatic cofactor for factor VIIa in the extrinsic tenase complex[27] (for reviews, see References 28 and 29) (Fig. 128-5, *A*). In the absence of injury or inflammatory stimuli, tissue factor is not expressed on cellular surfaces in direct contact with circulating blood (for a review,

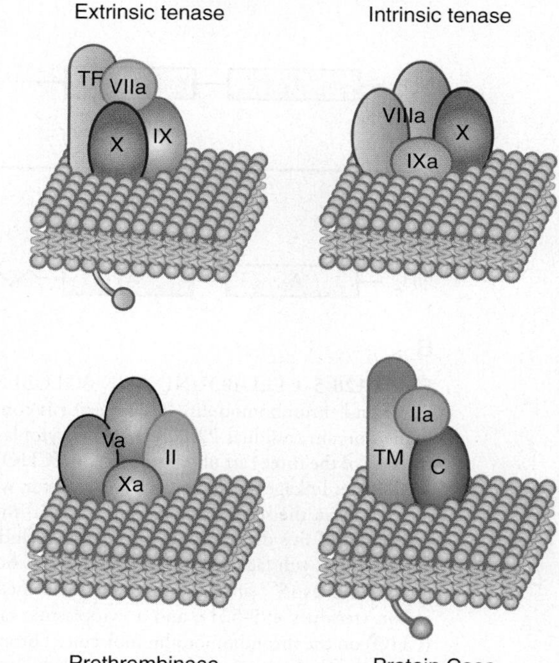

Figure 128-4 VITAMIN K–DEPENDENT COMPLEXES. Three procoagulant complexes (extrinsic tenase, intrinsic tenase, and prothrombinase) and one anticoagulant complex (protein Case) are illustrated. Each membrane complex consists of a vitamin K–dependent serine protease (factor VIIa [VIIa], factor IXa [IXa], factor Xa [Xa], or thrombin [IIa]) and a soluble or cell surface–associated cofactor (factor VIIIa [heavy and light chain VIII_H and VIII_L], factor Va [heavy and light chain V_H and V_L] tissue factor [TF], or thrombomodulin [TM]). Each serine protease is shown in association with the appropriate cofactor protein and zymogen substrate(s) on the membrane surface. The membrane serves as a scaffold for the coagulation reactants, enhancing the reaction rates by 10^4- to 10^9-fold.

Cell-bound cofactors

Thrombomodulin

Chondroitin sulfate adducts

Lectin homology domain

6 149 227 462 S

EGF domains

1 2 3 4 5 6

COOH

Extracellular Transmembrane Cytoplasmic

1 499 521 557

Tissue Factor

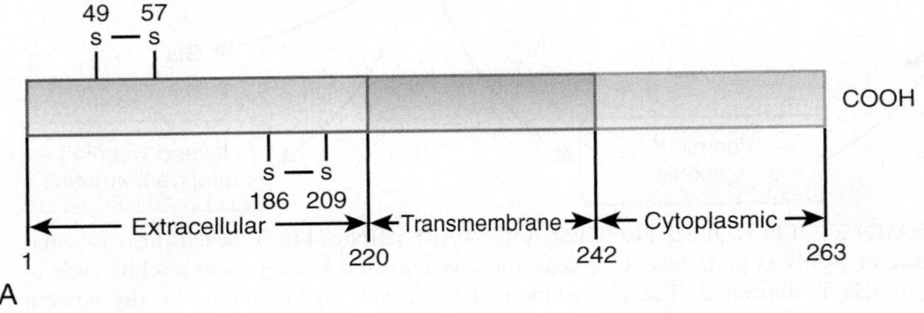

Soluble plasma procofactors

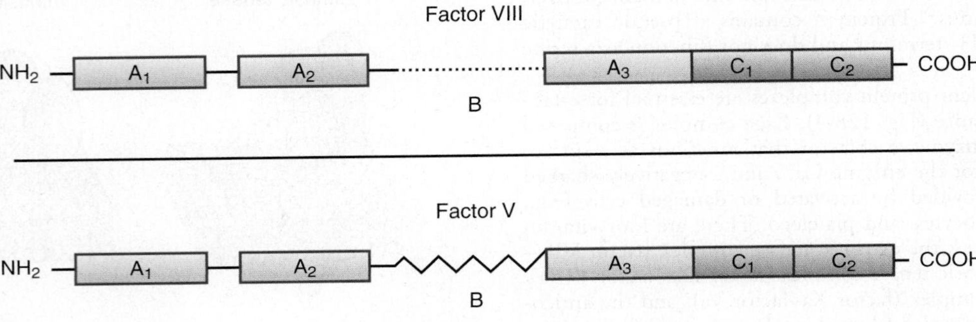

Figure 128-5 CELL-BOUND AND SOLUBLE COFACTOR STRUCTURES. **A,** Cell-bound cofactors: tissue factor and thrombomodulin. Tissue factor is composed of an extracellular domain (residues 1-219), a transmembrane domain (residues 220-242), and a cytoplasmic domain (residues 243-263). Two disulfide bonds (S-S) and the sites of the three carbohydrate moieties (CHO) are identified by amino acid residue. One cysteine (C^{245}) contains a thiol ester linkage to a fatty acid. Tissue factor, which is the cofactor for factor VIIa in the extrinsic tenase complex, is exposed on the subendothelial surface after injury. Thrombomodulin is an endothelial cell-surface glycoprotein composed of five distinct domains. These include a lectinlike domain (residues 6-149), a domain containing six epidermal growth factor (EGF)–like regions (residues 227-462), a small extracellular domain rich in threonine and serine residues (S^{472} and S^{474} have been identified as sites of chondroitin sulfate adducts), a membrane-spanning region (residues 499-521), and a cytoplasmic tail (residues 522-557). There are nine known glycosylation sites (CHO) on the thrombomodulin molecule. Thrombomodulin functions as the cofactor in the protein Case complex and assists in the generation of activated protein C. **B,** Soluble plasma procofactors: factor VIII and factor V. The linear domain structures (A1-A2-A3-C1-C2) are illustrated with *horizontal arrows* bracketed by the beginning and ending amino acid number. Thrombin (IIa) and activated protein C (APC) cleavage sites are shown with *vertical arrows*. The B regions (factor V, residues 709-1545; factor VIII, residues 740-1689) are represented by the *cross-hatched regions.*

see Reference 30). Presentation of tissue factor to the circulation is the event that triggers the primary procoagulant pathway of coagulation[31-33] (see Fig. 128-1). There are no known mutations or deficiencies of human tissue factor, and tissue factor deletion in mice is lethal during embryonic development,[34] leading to the speculation that tissue factor is essential for life.

Tissue factor activity is primarily regulated by controlling its presentation. The commonly accepted sources of functional tissue factor are the subendothelium exposed upon vascular damage or monocytes stimulated by cytokines. However, there is controversy regarding the source and presentation of active tissue factor and whether functional tissue factor circulates in blood in healthy and pathologic states.[35-40] Microparticles (bloodborne tissue factor) are generally defined as submicron-sized cell-derived membrane fragments produced in response to activation or apoptosis. Its role in hemostasis is still debated.[28,35,41,42]

Thrombomodulin

Thrombomodulin is a type 1 transmembrane protein constitutively expressed on the surface of vascular endothelial cells (see Fig. 128-5, *A*). Thrombomodulin is a high-affinity receptor for all thrombin forms and acts as a cofactor for the thrombin-dependent activation of protein C.[43] The endothelial cell protein C receptor (EPCR) provides cell-specific binding sites for both protein C and activated protein C (APC).[44-47] When bound to thrombomodulin, thrombin's procoagulant activities (e.g., its capacity to generate fibrin, and activate factor V, factor VIII, factor XI, and platelets) are neutralized, and the rate of inactivation of thrombin by antithrombin is increased.[48-50] The generation of APC by the thrombin–thrombomodulin complex leads to the inactivation of the procoagulant cofactors, factor Va and factor VIIIa, thus suppressing thrombin formation.[51,52] Thrombin–thrombomodulin, or the protein Case (see Fig. 128-4) complex, also has an antifibrinolytic role via the activation of the fibrinolysis inhibitor, thrombin activatable fibrinolysis inhibitor (TAFI) (for reviews, see References 53-56).

Thrombomodulin activity on the surface of endothelial cells is decreased by inflammatory cytokines,[57,58] and this decrease may contribute to the hypercoagulation characteristic of inflammatory states.

Soluble Plasma Procofactors

Factor V

Factor V is a large single-chain glycoprotein (GP) that circulates in human plasma (see Table 128-1 and Fig. 128-5, *B*) and is also contained in the α-granules of human platelets, with approximately 18% to 25% of the total factor V found in platelets.[59] The procofactor factor V is proteolyzed by α-thrombin to the active cofactor factor Va.[60] Factor Va functions both as a factor Xa receptor and positive modulator of factor Xa catalytic potential in the prothrombinase complex (see Fig. 128-4).[61] Factor Va is proteolytically inactivated by activated protein C (APC).[62,63] The importance of this regulatory mechanism is demonstrated by the "APC resistance" syndrome associated with factor V^{Leiden}.[64,65] Individuals with factor V^{Leiden} have a G to A substitution at nucleotide 1691 in the factor V gene that results in an Arg^{506}→Gln mutation at the protein level.[66] Factor Va^{Leiden} has normal cofactor activity as part of the prothrombinase complex. However, unlike normal factor Va, factor Va^{Leiden} is more slowly inactivated by APC. The Arg^{506}→Gln mutation hinders the first step in the series of inactivating cleavages by APC. Cleaved factor Va^{Leiden} retains limited cofactor activity and continues to promote thrombin generation. The identification, role in coagulation, and overall importance of factor V in hemostasis have been described in numerous reviews.[61,67]

Factor VIII

The soluble procofactor factor VIII, or antihemophilic factor (see Fig. 128-5, *B*), circulates in plasma in complex with the large multimeric protein vWF.[68] vWF acts to regulate the plasma concentration of factor VIII. Factor VIII interaction with vWF requires the NH_2^- and $COOH^-$ termini of the factor VIII light chain (A3, C1, and C2 domains), although a specific vWF-binding site has been identified at residues 1673 to 1684 on the light chain.[68-71] Factor VIII is activated by thrombin cleavage at three sites (Arg^{372}, Arg^{740}, Arg^{1689}) to generate the heterotrimeric cofactor factor VIIIa.[72] The vWF-binding site is removed from the factor VIII protein by thrombin cleavage at Arg^{1689}. After forming, vWF–free factor VIIIa forms a complex with the serine protease factor IXa, Ca^{2+} and a membrane (provided by platelets), resulting in the intrinsic tenase (see Fig. 128-4). Factor VIIIa function is downregulated by the relatively rapid dissociation of the noncovalently associated A2 subunit, which is produced by the cleavages required for activation. Factor VIII is homologous (40% identity) to the procofactor factor V.[73]

Deficiency of factor VIII, or hemophilia A, is a well-characterized bleeding disorder linked to the X chromosome.[74] Hemophilia A, therefore, occurs almost exclusively in males at a frequency of one in 5000 to one in 10,000 males.[75]

Von Willebrand factor

von Willebrand factor has several key roles in coagulation and is also contained in the α-granules of human platelets.[76] vWF is a large adhesive GP that circulates in plasma as a heterogeneous mixture of disulfide-linked multimers that range in size from dimers (M_r = 600,000) to extremely large multimers of more than 20 million KDa. vWF has binding sites for factor VIII, heparin, collagen, platelet GPIb, and platelet GPIIb-IIIa.[77-90] vWF acts as the bridge between platelets to promote platelet aggregation. The primary platelet binding site for vWF is the GPIb-IX-V receptor complex. GPIb-IX-V is an active receptor on unstimulated platelets and serves to promote platelet aggregation and adhesion to vWF in the absence of platelet activation.[91]

von Willebrand factor is a structural protein and is part of the subendothelial matrix. Endothelial cells secrete vWF multimers, which are larger than those found circulating in plasma.[92] The function of these large multimeric forms of vWF is to bind to and agglutinate blood platelets under high shear conditions. These large multimers of vWF are degraded by a specific metalloprotease called a disintegrin and metalloproteinase with a thrombospondin type 1 motif, member 13 (ADAMTS)-13.[93-95] In familial and acquired thrombotic thrombocytopenic purpura, ultra-large vWF multimers are correlated with defective ADAMTS-13 activity.[96]

ABO blood type has a significant influence on vWF levels, with individuals of types A, B, or AB blood having much higher levels of vWF than those with type O blood.[97,98] vWF is also known for its role in ristocetin-induced platelet agglutination,[99,100] which is the basis of clinical assays for von Willebrand disease, a fairly common disorder that is estimated to occur in 1% to 2% of the general population (see Chapter 140).[101-104] vWF is also an acute phase reactant, and vWF levels are elevated as a result of stress, pregnancy, or surgical trauma.[105-108]

The Intrinsic Accessory Pathway Proteins

The designation "intrinsic accessory pathway" emerged as the relationship between genetic deficiencies and bleeding phenotypes was established (see Fig. 128-1). Deficiencies of proteins associated with the intrinsic or accessory pathway (factor XII, prekallikrein, and high-molecular-weight kininogen [HMWK]) are not ordinarily associated with excessive bleeding, even after surgical challenge.[109-111] In contrast, deficiencies of the protein components of the extrinsic or primary pathway (prothrombin and factors V, VII, VIII, IX, and X) can lead to severe bleeding diatheses.[112-116] The physiologic role of the accessory pathway is therefore not clearly understood.[117]

Although the intrinsic pathway proteins have no defined role in normal hemostasis, these accessory pathway factors are thought to play a key role in disseminated intravascular coagulation (DIC) associated with the systemic inflammatory response syndrome[118,119] and in the promotion of thrombus stability[117,120,121] and may be a new target to control pathologic coagulation.[122] Also, the accessory pathway is important in cardiopulmonary bypass because of contact between blood components and synthetic surfaces.[119] Recent evidence suggests that biologic activation of the contact pathway system may be accomplished through assembly of these proteins on endothelial cell membranes and that prekallikrein is activated by an endothelial cell membrane cysteine protease rather than by factor XII.[123,124] Extracellular RNA derived from damaged or necrotic cells has also been found to participate in the activation of proteases of the contact pathway by providing a procoagulant cofactor template for factor XII- or XI-induced contact activation.[125] Polyphosphates, linear inorganic polymers of 60 to 100 phosphate residues, released from platelets have also been shown to activate fXII.[126]

In principle, factor XI represents an intersection point for the two pathways. Individuals with factor XI deficiency (hemophilia C) have a variable bleeding phenotype upon surgical challenge,[127,128] therefore establishing an essential role for factor XI in hemostasis. During the coagulation process, factor XIa formation appears to be catalyzed by thrombin as part of a positive feedback loop stemming from thrombin generation.[129] Factor XIa then functions in the propagation phase of thrombin generation in association with the primary pathway by activation of factor IX.[130]

Three proteins, factor XII, prekallikrein, and HMWK, are required for activity of the intrinsic or accessory pathway. Factor XII and prekallikrein are zymogens that are activated to generate serine proteases, and HMWK is a nonenzymatic procofactor (Fig. 128-6). The activation of this pathway in vitro is accomplished when factor XII autoactivates to factor XIIa upon exposure to foreign surfaces, including kaolin, dextran sulfate, and sulfatides.[131-133] The substrates for factor XIIa, prekallikrein, and factor XI exist in noncovalent complex with HMWK and become activated to kallikrein and factor XIa, respectively.[134] Positive feedback loops exist in which kallikrein cleaves HMWK, thereby releasing bradykinin and allowing more prekallikrein and factor XI to associate and activate.[135] This pathway is also negatively regulated by the cleavage of HMWK by factor XIa.[136]

Proteinase inhibitors

Proteinases, enzymes that hydrolyze peptide bonds, are found in a wide array of biologic systems, including the blood coagulation process (clot formation and fibrinolysis), digestive system, apoptotic cascades, and the immune system. To keep these systems in balance between activation and inhibition, a complex system of proteinase inhibitors has evolved. In blood, proteinase inhibitors constitute a significant percentage of circulating proteins. In general, proteinases that activate the coagulation and fibrinolytic cascades have highly defined substrate specificities. Coagulation is kept in check through the action of several specific and broad-spectrum proteinase inhibitors. Specific clot formation inhibitors are antithrombin, tissue factor pathway inhibitor (TFPI), heparin cofactor II, and protein C inhibitor. Together specific and broad-spectrum inhibitors function to localize, limit, and control hemostasis (see Chapter 129).

Antithrombin

Antithrombin is a member of the serpin proteinase inhibitory family and circulates in blood as a single-chain GP[137] (see Table 128-1; Fig. 128-7). Congenital antithrombin deficiency exhibits an autosomal dominant pattern of inheritance, with an incidence of 1 in 2000 to 1 in 5000.[138] Individuals with this deficiency have partial expression of antithrombin and are prone to venous thromboembolic disease.[139] The complete absence of antithrombin is lethal.

Antithrombin has a broad spectrum of inhibitory activity with most of its target proteases participating in the coagulation cascade (see Fig. 128-1). It is primarily an inhibitor of the serine proteases thrombin, factor Xa, factor IXa, factor VIIa–tissue factor, factor XIa, factor XIIa, kallikrein, and HMWK.[140-142] Heparin and heparan sulfate potentiate these reactions, and heparin is used for the prevention and treatment of thrombosis. When antithrombin is complexed with heparin, its rate of inhibition of several coagulation proteases is accelerated by up to 10,000-fold. The general mechanism of inhibition involves reaction of the active site of the enzyme with a peptide loop structure (the reactive center loop) of antithrombin, forming a tight, equimolar (1 : 1) complex. Inactivation proceeds through covalent bond formation between antithrombin and the protease followed by inactivating structural rearrangements of both antithrombin and the protease.

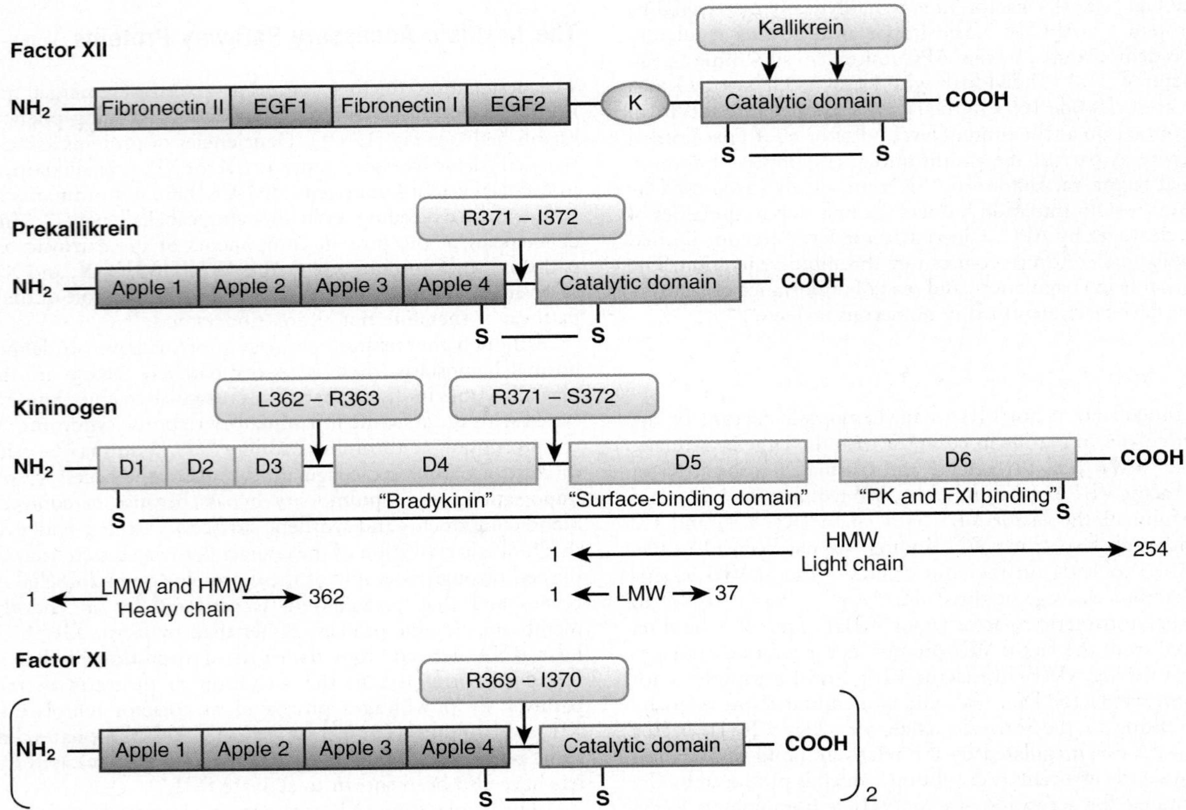

Figure 128-6 SCHEMATIC REPRESENTATION OF THE ACCESSORY PATHWAY (INTRINSIC) PROTEINS. Factor XII, prekallikrein, kininogen, and factor XI are shown with their various domains depicted. Cleavage sites for activation are identified with an *arrow,* and with the specific amino acid residues of the site shown. Key interchain disulfide bonds (S-S) are included. For the kininogens, *horizontal arrows* indicate the amino acid residues defining heavy and light chain regions of the activated forms of the cofactors. Factor XI is illustrated as a monomer. *EGF,* Epidermal growth factor; *HMW,* high molecular weight; *LMW,* low molecular weight.

Tissue factor pathway inhibitor

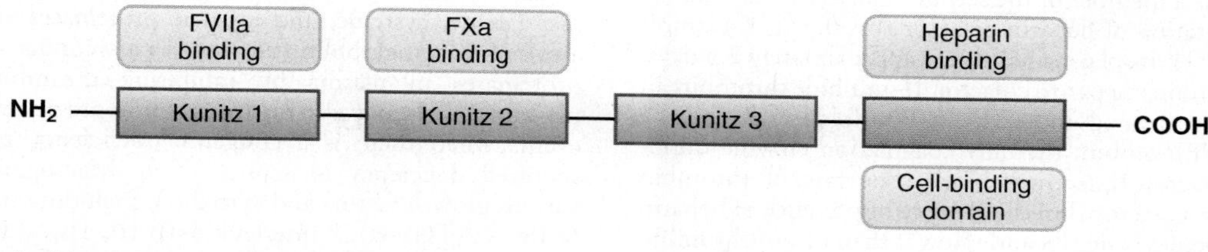

Antithrombin

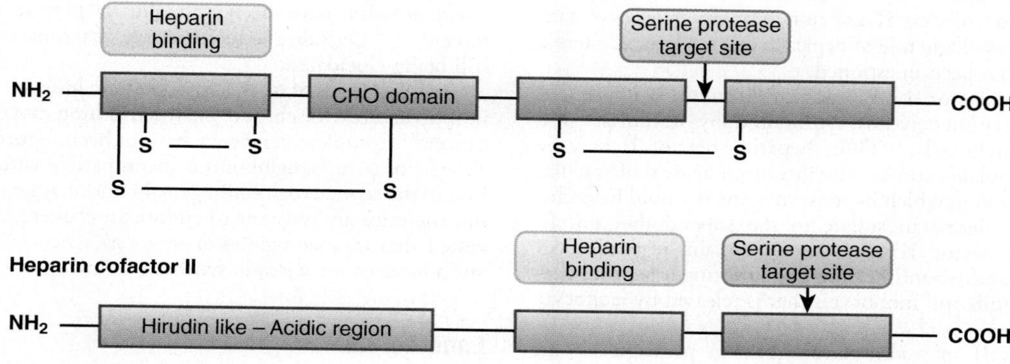

Protein C inhibitor

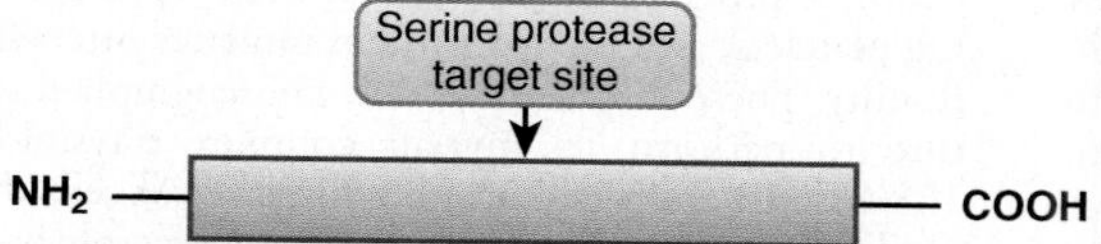

Figure 128-7 SCHEMATIC REPRESENTATION OF SEVERAL PROTEINASE INHIBITORS. Tissue factor pathway inhibitor (TFPI) contains three Kunitz domains. TFPI inhibits the serine proteases factor VIIa (FVIIa) and factor Xa (FXa), shutting down the extrinsic pathway of coagulation. Kunitz 1 domain binds factor VIIa, and Kunitz 2 domain binds factor Xa. The COOH-terminus of TFPI contains a basic region, the cell-binding domain, which binds to heparin. Antithrombin (AT) contains two intrachain disulfide bonds (-S-S-) in its NH_2-terminus and one in its COOH-terminus with a carbohydrate-rich domain (CHO) in between. The region of interaction between the active sites of target proteases and AT is illustrated (reactive center loop). Heparin binding occurs in the NH_2-terminus and enhances the rate of inhibition of serine proteases. Heparin cofactor II (HCII) inhibits thrombin. Structurally, the inhibitor contains an NH_2-terminus hirudin-like region, a heparin or dermatan sulfate binding region, and a reactive center loop. The reactive site is shown at Leu^{444}. Protein C inhibitor (PCI) is a serine protease inhibitor that inhibits several proteases, including activated protein C (APC), thrombin, and factor Xa. It is also a potent inhibitor of the thrombin–thrombomodulin complex. The reactive bond (Arg^{354}) in the reactive center loop is shown.

Antithrombin also displays antiproliferative and antiinflammatory properties that primarily derive from its ability to inhibit thrombin. In addition, latent or cleaved forms of antithrombin have antiangiogenic activities.[143]

Tissue Factor Pathway Inhibitor

Tissue factor pathway inhibitor, formerly called extrinsic pathway inhibitor or lipoprotein-associated coagulation inhibitor, is a multivalent Kunitz-type plasma proteinase inhibitor. It circulates in plasma as a heterogeneous collection of partially proteolyzed forms[144-147] (see Table 128-1 and Fig. 128-7). Up to 90% of circulating TFPI is found associated with lipoproteins, primarily low-density lipoprotein.[144,148,149] Parenteral TFPI is cleared from the circulation mainly by the liver and has an unusually short half-life (minutes) compared with other proteinase inhibitors.

Many reviews of TFPI have been published.[150-160] The importance of TFPI in blood coagulation is best illustrated through transgenic mice with complete TFPI deficiency; the deficiency is embryonic lethal.[154] However, this lethality in mice can be rescued by heterozygous or homozygous factor VII deficiency.[161] This implies that diminishing the level of factor VII lessens the need for TFPI-mediated inhibition of the factor VIIa–tissue factor coagulation pathway during embryogenesis.[161] Similarly, the combination of low normal TFPI with factor V Leiden is lethal.[162,163] Mice with combined heterozygous TFPI deficiency and homozygous apolipoprotein E deficiency develop more extensive atherosclerosis burden,[164] raising the possibility that TFPI contributes to protection from atherosclerosis, as well as serving as a regulator of thrombosis.

Tissue factor pathway inhibitor is the principal stoichiometric inhibitor of the extrinsic factor tenase complex (factor VIIa–tissue factor).[165] Effective TFPI inhibition of the factor VIIa–tissue factor complex depends on the presence of factor Xa. Thus, inhibition of the extrinsic factor tenase by TFPI occurs only after significant factor IXa and factor Xa formation. Inhibition by TFPI is achieved by formation of the stable quaternary, by tissue factor–factor VIIa–TFPI–factor Xa complex, and by formation of the factor Xa–TFPI complex directly.

Heparin Cofactor II

Heparin cofactor II is a member of the serpin family (see Fig. 128-7). The plasma concentration of heparin cofactor II is 0.5 to 1.4 μmol/L[166,167] (see Table 128-1). Its plasma half-life is approximately 2.5 days. Similar to antithrombin, heparin cofactor II inhibits thrombin in a reaction that is accelerated more than 1000-fold by heparin.[168] However, unlike antithrombin, the only coagulation enzyme inhibited by heparin cofactor II is thrombin.[169] The rate of thrombin inhibition by heparin cofactor II in the absence or presence of heparin or heparin-like molecules is significantly slower than by antithrombin under similar conditions. Considering that the plasma concentration of heparin cofactor II is 25% to 50% that of antithrombin and that low levels of heparin cofactor II are not strongly associated with thrombosis,[170] the physiologic role of heparin cofactor II as a systemic thrombin inhibitor has been questioned.

In vitro, heparin cofactor II inhibition of thrombin is accelerated by dermatan sulfate proteoglycans synthesized by fibroblasts and vascular smooth muscle cells.[171] Thus, heparin cofactor II may be uniquely suited to regulate extravascular thrombin in areas of vascular endothelium disruption in which heparin cofactor II would be exclusively stimulated by dermatan sulfate in the subendothelium. In addition, heparin cofactor II may participate in regulation of acute inflammation and wound healing by harboring a peptide chemotactic for neutrophils and monocytes that is released by leukocyte proteolysis.[172]

Heparin cofactor II may also have a role in protection from thrombosis during pregnancy. Increased levels of dermatan sulfate in the maternal and fetal circulation[173] along with increased levels of heparin cofactor II in pregnant women have been reported.[174,175] Low levels of thrombin–heparin cofactor II complexes are detected in normal plasma samples; elevated levels were detected in patients with DIC.[176] Although inherited deficiency of heparin cofactor II has been associated with thrombosis, this is not always the case.[177-179]

Protein C Inhibitor

Protein C inhibitor is a member of the serine proteinase inhibitor family and is also known as plasminogen activator inhibitor-3 (PAI-3). It circulates in blood at a concentration of 5 μg/mL[180,181] (see Table 128-1 and Fig. 128-7) and is cleared from the circulation with a half-life of 1 day. When in complex with a target (e.g., APC), it is cleared from circulation with a $t_{1/2}$ of 20 minutes.[182]

Protein C inhibitor is considered a nonspecific inhibitor in that its targets range from procoagulant (serine proteinases), anticoagulant, and fibrinolytic enzymes to plasma and tissue kallikreins, the sperm protease acrosin, and prostate-specific antigen.[183,184] The major target of protein C inhibitor, as its name suggests, appears to be APC.[182,185,186] Protein C inhibitor has been shown to regulate TAFI activation by inhibiting the thrombin–thrombomodulin complex.[187] Its importance as a dual regulator of coagulation and fibrinolysis remains unresolved.[188,189] Other targets for protein C inhibitor include human plasma kallikrein,[190] factor XIa,[190] factor Xa, and thrombin. Because there are no documented patients with a deficiency to date, the actual function of protein C inhibitor in vivo has yet to be elucidated.

α_2-Macroglobulin

α_2-Macroglobulin is a nonspecific proteinase inhibitor that targets a broad spectrum of protease substrates. It is present in human plasma at concentrations ranging from 2 to 4 μmol/L (2-3 mg/mL). α_2-Macroglobulin can also be found at higher concentrations in extravascular fluids.[191] This protease inhibitor can be produced in a variety of cells, including hepatocytes, fibroblasts, and macrophages.[192,193] Human α_2-macroglobulin circulates in plasma as a tetramer.[191-198] α_2-macroglobulin has a unique mechanism of action, which accounts for its broad specificity. The initial step involves the "bait region" of α_2-macroglobulin.[199] After proteolysis in this bait region, α_2-macroglobulin undergoes conformational changes that trap the proteinase inside the molecule.[199] Consequently, α_2-macroglobulin inhibits a broad range of proteinases. It is distinctive in its capacity to inhibit members from each of four mechanistic classes of proteinases (serine, cysteine, and aspartic proteinases and metalloproteinases). α_2-Macroglobulin functions as a secondary inhibitor of serine proteinases in plasma by inhibiting thrombin, kallikrein, and plasmin.[200,201] It may also be important in preventing thromboembolic events when there is a congenital deficiency of antithrombin or acquired deficiency in sepsis.[202,203] α_2-Macroglobulin also inhibits various growth factors and cytokines, including transforming growth factor-α (TGF-α),[204] interleukin-1β (IL-1β),[205] IL-6,[206] acidic fibroblast growth factor,[207] basic fibroblast growth factor,[207] tumor necrosis factor-α (TNF-α),[208] and IL-2.[209] Polymorphisms identified in α_2-macroglobulin have been thought to play a role in Alzheimer disease.[210-212] Overall, the biologic role of α_2-macroglobulin in vivo is still being elucidated.

Reduced levels of α_2-macroglobulin in humans have been observed in individuals with chronic obstructive lung disease[213] and metastatic cancer.[214] Complete deficiency has not been reported, suggesting that absence of α_2-macroglobulin is incompatible with survival. Inactivation of the α_2-macroglobulin gene in mice has no obvious phenotype, but the mice are resistant to endotoxin challenge.[215] It has been suggested that α_2-macroglobulin serves as a neutralizer of TGF-α and an inducer of nitric oxide synthesis in mice.[216]

Endothelium

Blood cells and the vasculature are crucial to normal hemostasis. Multiple processes involving components of the vessel wall, circulating platelets, and plasma protein moieties interact to maintain blood fluidity. These must be precisely choreographed to allow the vasculature to perform its myriad complex physiologic activities (Fig. 128-8). The endothelium, the thin layer of cells that lines the interior of blood and lymphatic vessels, plays a key role because of its strategic interface among organs, tissues, and circulating blood. The cells that form the endothelium are called *endothelial cells,* those in direct contact with blood are called *vascular endothelial cells,* and those in direct contact with lymph are known as *lymphatic endothelial cells.* Vascular endothelial cells line the entire circulatory system (from the heart to the capillaries).

The endothelium varies in morphology and physiologic function in different parts of the vasculature. This complex cellular network not only provides a structural barrier to contain flowing blood but also regulates blood pressure; vascular tone; permeability; and processes involving other cells such as smooth muscle cells, leukocytes, and platelets, and deposits an intricate basement membrane and extracellular matrix.[217] In addition, the endothelium is involved in inflammatory and immune responses and angiogenesis.[218] Defects in vascular endothelium function, therefore, have profound physiologic implications. Excessive bleeding can result from structural abnormalities of the endothelial cell layer or supporting matrix. Impaired expression or secretion of PAI-1 by the endothelium likewise promote bleeding through increased fibrinolytic activity.[219] Conversely, endothelial cells are also involved in mediating processes that promote atherosclerotic plaque formation and thrombotic pathologies.[220]

The early work of Ware and Seegers[221] identified the phospholipid requirements for coagulation. The biologic elements contributing to the phospholipid include damaged vascular tissue activated platelets and inflammatory cells. The contributions of the membrane to the formation and expression of procoagulant complexes are essential. However, the nature of the membranes that support procoagulant reactions is poorly understood. Mechanically damaged cells can provide the anionic membrane bilayer inner leaflet phospholipids, which can support general procoagulant complex formation; however, more subtle cellular activation events also generate selective complex forming sites on intact cells. Activated platelet membranes express individual binding sites for the factor IXa–factor VIIIa and factor Xa–factor Va complexes. Hemorrhagic pathology is therefore associated with thrombocytopenia and is also displayed in a rare disease, Scott syndrome, which appears to result from the improper

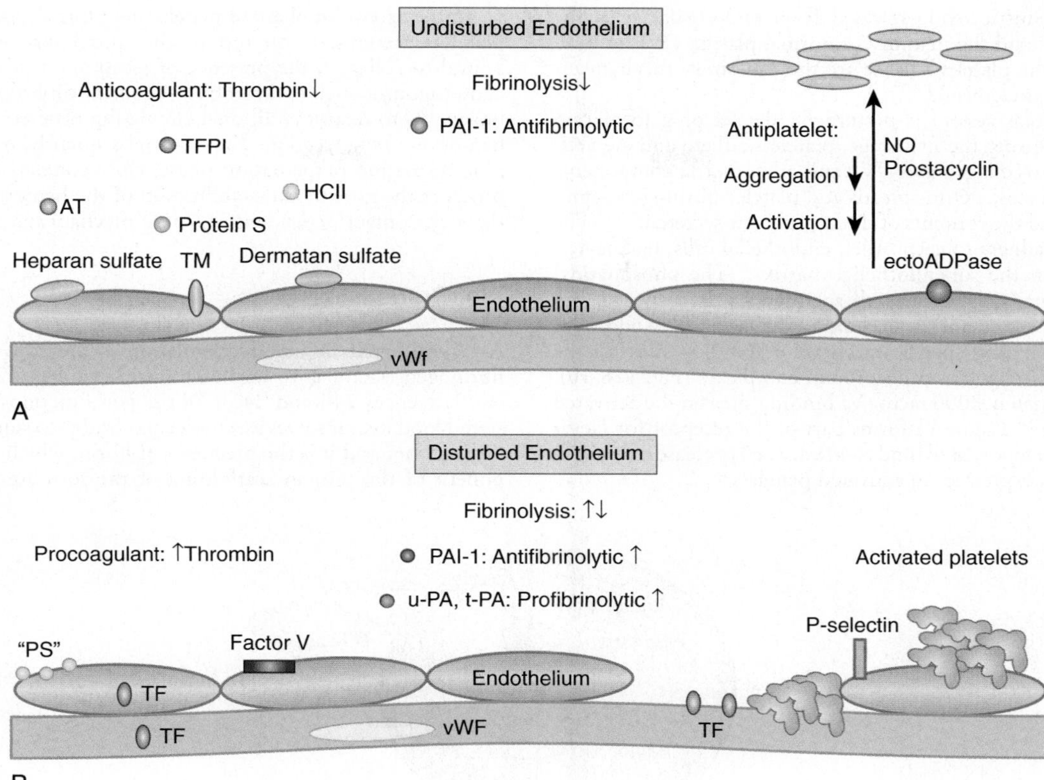

Figure 128-8 SCHEMATIC OF THE CHANGES THAT OCCUR TO THE ENDOTHELIUM UPON INJURY. Under normal conditions in the absence of injury or chemical stimulus **(A),** *the undisturbed endothelium* actively down regulates thrombin generation through production of tissue factor pathway inhibitor (TFPI), antithrombin (AT), protein S, heparan sulfate, thrombomodulin (TM), and dermatan sulfate. The undisturbed endothelium is also antifibrinolytic and secretes plasminogen activator inhibitor-1 (PAI-1). In the absence of a stimulus, the endothelium likewise prevents platelet activation, secretion, and aggregation through production of nitric oxide (NO), prostacyclin, and the membrane-associated protein ectoADPase. When the *endothelium is disturbed* **(B),** the endothelium becomes procoagulant and accelerates thrombin formation by exposing or expressing anionic phospholipid ("PS"), tissue factor (TF), and factor V. The fibrinolytic response is modulated by the release of both antifibrinolytic and profibrinolytic molecules. Urokinase plasminogen activator (u-PA) and tissue plasminogen activator (t-PA) are profibrinolytic and serve to activate plasminogen; PAI-1 inhibits both enzymes and is antifibrinolytic. Platelet activation, secretion, and aggregation are also promoted under conditions in which the endothelium is disrupted. von Willebrand factor (vWF) in the subendothelial matrix is exposed, allowing platelets to attach to the surface of the vessel. P-selectin likewise promotes platelet attachment.

presentation of these platelet binding sites.[222] Binding sites have also been reported on a number of peripheral blood cells, especially activated monocytes. The vascular endothelium itself can provide binding sites after stimulation by cytokine growth factors.[223] The endothelium also provides the anticoagulant thrombomodulin, TFPI and heparan sulfate. The endothelial cell protein C receptor provides cell-specific binding sites for both protein C and APC.[44,224] Endothelial cell protein C receptor is down-regulated by TNF-α.[44] Monocytes appear to express specific binding sites for APC that are distinct from the endothelial cell protein C receptor.[225] The cell-expressed binding sites may be important in the antiinflammatory properties of APC.[46]

A further consequence of damage to the endothelium is the release of pathologic quantities of vWF, which promote platelet aggregation and adhesion to the subendothelium and thus the formation of potentially fatal thrombi. Endothelial dysfunction is also linked with hypertension, diabetes, obesity, and hyperlipidemia.

Platelets

Platelets, or thrombocytes, are vital to procoagulant events and contribute to the fibrinolytic process as well. They are small, irregularly shaped clear cell fragments, which are derived from megakaryocytes. The average lifespan of a platelet is approximately 5 to 9 days. Platelets are at the balance of bleeding or clotting events: when platelet numbers are low (thrombocytopenia), excessive bleeding can occur, and when platelet numbers are high (thrombocytosis), thrombosis can occur. Disorders that reduce the number of platelets but typically cause thrombosis instead of bleeding are heparin-induced thrombocytopenia and thrombotic thrombocytopenic purpura.

Similar to the endothelium, the undisturbed platelet presents a nonthrombogenic surface. Important components of platelet physiology are surface adhesion protein complexes and the platelet secretory granules: α-granules, lysosomes, and dense granules. Contents of the α-granules include procoagulant and adhesive proteins such as fibrinogen, fibronectin, thrombospondin, vWF, P-selectin, HMWK, platelet factor 4, osteonectin, factor V,[59] and factor XI.[226] Other α-granule contents, α_1-antitrypsin, protein S, TFPI, and platelet inhibitor of factor XI are involved in anticoagulant activities.[227-229] The α-granule also contains proteins that meditate both pro- and antifibrinolytic processes. These proteins include plasminogen, α_2-antiplasmin, factor XIII, and PAI-1.[230-234] In the unstimulated platelet, the granule contents remain internalized and anionic phospholipid is sequestered in the inner leaflet of the plasma membrane. Prostaglandin I2 (prostacyclin) and nitric oxide released from endothelial cells, the presence of CD39, and the inability of normal plasma vWF to bind spontaneously to the platelet surface are the inhibitory mechanisms that keep platelets unactivated.[235]

When the vascular system is perturbed, platelet plug formation occurs in stages. During the first stage, platelets adhere and are activated by exposure to collagen and vWF and other matrix components (Fig. 128-9). The cytoskeleton spreads and platelet-fibrinogen aggregates are formed and the contents of the granules are secreted.[236-238] The activated platelets adhere to each other, endothelial cells, leukocytes, and components of the subendothelial matrix.[239] The phosphatidyl serine (PS) rich internal face of cell membranes are exposed and present a highly procoagulant surface to the circulation.[240] In addition, activated platelets express specific receptors or binding sites for the assembly of the procoagulant multiprotein complexes (Fig. 128-10). There are approximately 3000 factor Va binding sites on the activated platelet membrane.[241] Factor Va forms part of the receptor for factor Xa. Factor Xa is also reported to bind to effector cell protease receptor-1 (EPR-1) molecules expressed on activated platelets.[241-244]

In the extension phase of platelet plug formation, where activated platelets accumulate on top of the initial monolayer of platelets bound to collagen, the presence of receptors on the platelet surface allows agonists such as thrombin, adenosine diphosphate, and thromboxane A_2 to recruit additional circulating platelets into the growing hemostatic plug (see Fig. 128-10). Subsequently, during the platelet plug formation perpetuation phase, close contacts between platelets promote the growth and stabilization of the hemostatic plug, in part through contact-dependent signaling mechanisms.[235]

Clot Proteins

A central event in blood coagulation is the conversion of soluble fibrinogen (factor I) to insoluble fibrin (see Fig. 128-1; for reviews, see References 245 and 246). Fibrinogen functions in hemostasis to stem blood loss. It serves as a molecular bridge to support interplatelet aggregation, and it is the precursor of fibrin, which is the main component of the protein scaffolding of the forming hemostatic plug.

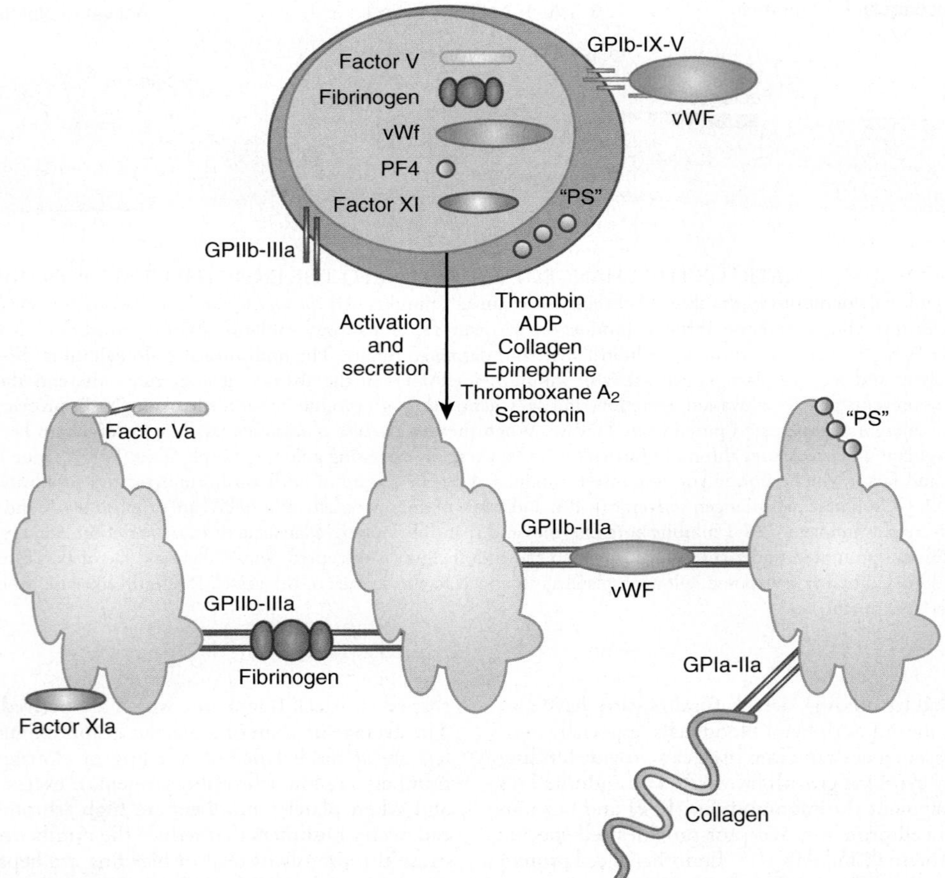

Figure 128-9 SCHEMATIC OF PLATELET ACTIVATION, SECRETION, AND AGGREGATION. Platelets have multiple functions in hemostasis. They serve as reservoirs of factor V, fibrinogen, von Willebrand factor (vWF), platelet factor 4 (PF4), and factor XI. Platelets also contribute a significant portion of the anionic phospholipid ("PS") necessary for membrane-dependent complex formation and function. In the unstimulated state, proteins and other molecules are sequestered in the platelet granules. Anionic phospholipid is found only in the inner leaflet of the platelet membrane and is not exposed to flowing blood. The glycoprotein (GP) Ib-IX-V complex, which recognizes vWF, is an active receptor, but the GPIIb-IIIa receptor, which recognizes a variety of molecules, including fibrinogen and vWF, is not active. The GP Ib-IX-V receptor likely allows unstimulated platelets to attach to exposed subendothelial vWF, thereby promoting procoagulant events before platelet activation. Upon activation by a variety of agonists, platelets secrete granule contents, become activated and bind factor V/Va and factor XI/XIa, and expose anionic phospholipid. The GPIIb-IIIa receptor serves to link platelets to each other and the vessel wall. Collagen receptors, such as GPIa-IIa, promote both platelet activation and aggregation. *ADP,* Adenosine diphosphate.

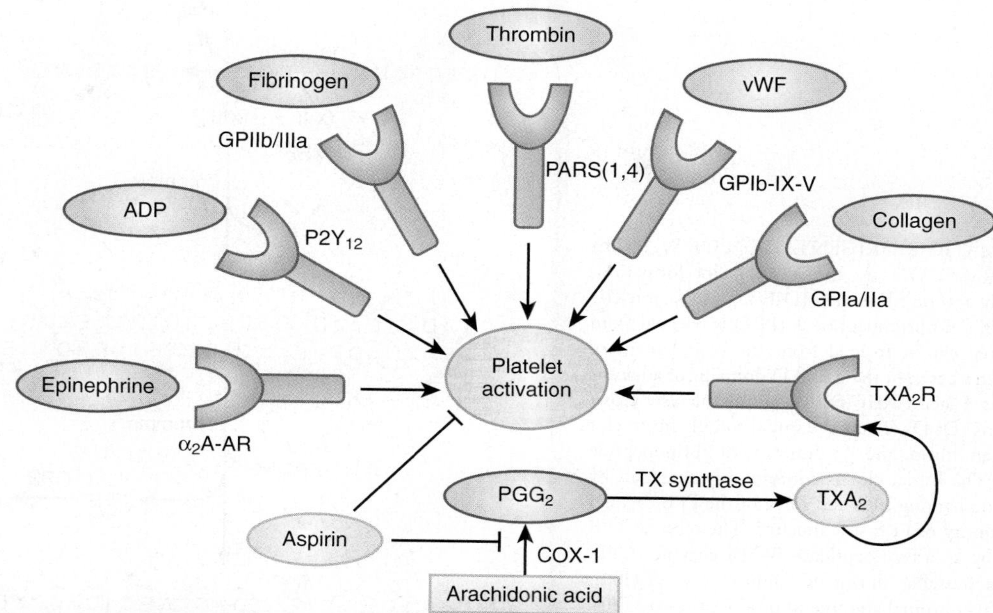

Figure 128-10 SELECTED PLATELET RECEPTOR TARGETS AND THEIR RESPECTIVE INHIBITORY AGENTS. When a platelet encounters a break in the endothelium, it encounters molecules that trigger its activation, such as collagen, thromboxane A_2 (TXA_2), adenosine diphosphate (ADP), and thrombin. The ability of platelets to adhere, aggregate, respond to agonists, aid in coagulation, and bind fibrin are all processes mediated by the plasma membrane glycoproteins of the platelet. The platelet glycoprotein (GP) IbIX-V constitutes the receptor for von Willebrand factor (vWF). GPIa/IIa mediates platelet–collagen interactions. GPIIb/IIIa is a receptor for fibrinogen. $P2Y_{12}$ is a chemoreceptor for ADP. The α_2A-adrenergic receptor (α_2A-AR) is expressed on platelets and binds the naturally occurring ligand epinephrine. Cyclooxygenase-1 (COX-1) is responsible for the formation of prostaglandins and thromboxane. COX-1 converts arachidonic acid to prostaglandin G_2 (PGG_2). Aspirin irreversibly inhibits COX-1.

Platelet aggregation critically depends on fibrinogen binding to activated platelets via the platelet fibrinogen receptor GPIIb/IIIa as well as fibrin adhesion (see Fig. 128-10). Fibrinogen/fibrin also regulates thrombin activity by interactions that include the proteolytic cleavage by thrombin of fibrinopeptides[247,248] to form a fibrin clot and thrombin exosite binding to fibrin, which potentially limits the diffusion of thrombin, thereby regulating clot propagation. The structure, stability, and duration of insoluble fibrin are controlled by an interplay between fibrin formation and fibrinolysis, which includes other molecular and cellular components.

The description of fibrinogen activation and fibrin assembly has been based on studies using citrated plasmas or purified proteins. The three main players in fibrinogen to fibrin conversion are the enzyme thrombin, the substrates fibrinogen and the cross-linking tranglutaminase factor XIII. Fibrinogen is composed of six polypeptide chains (two Aα, two Bß, and two γ chains) that form two symmetrical half molecules (three chains each) with the NH_2 termini crosslinked to each other. The outside two domains of fibrinogen are composed of the Bß and γ chains and designated as the D domain. The central domain that contains the NH_2-termini of all the chains is designated as the E domain. From x-ray crystallographic data, fibrinogen has a trinodular structure aligned as D–E–D domains (Fig. 128-11).

The kinetics of fibrinogen cleavage by thrombin results in the hydrolysis of Arg–Gly bonds removing small, polar amino terminal fragments (fibrinopeptides [FPs]) from the NH_2-terminal of the Aα and Bß chains Fig. 128-11.[249,250] Cleavage at the Arg–Gly bond of the Aα chain releases FPA and forms fibrin I. The release of two FPA peptides exposes a site in the E domain that interacts with a site in the D domain to form overlapping fibrils. Subsequent cleavage of the Arg–Gly bond on the Bß-chain releases FPB to form fibrin II, presumably increasing lateral aggregation of the protofibrils.[251]

An important enzyme for the structure and stability of the fibrin clot is the transglutaminase factor XIIIa.[252-254] Its function is to cross-link fibrin and other adhesive proteins, including integrin receptors providing a stable network. Only the Aα chain and the γ chain, which has donor (Gln) and acceptor (Lys) sites, participate in cross-linking of adjacent glutamyl and lysyl residues by factor XIIIa.[251,255-257]

Fibrinogen also is required for competent inflammatory reactions. Fibrinogen is an acute phase reactant whose levels increase during inflammation.[258,259] In these situations, fibrinogen functions as a bridging molecule in cell–cell interactions.[260,261] Fibrin and fibrinogen constitute a matrix that modulates cellular responses in a variety of cell types, including endothelial cells, epithelial cells, leukocytes, platelets, and fibroblasts. Cellular receptors that bind fibrinogen and fibrin include the integrins $\alpha_{IIb}ß_3$, $\alpha_Vß_3$, and $\alpha_5ß_1$, and the cellular adhesion molecules intercellular adhesion molecule-1 and vascular endothelial cadherin.[262-265]

Fibrin clot based assays have been extensively used in the clinical diagnosis of bleeding disorders. Two in vitro plasma tests, the PT[266,267] and the activated partial thromboplastin time (aPTT),[268] segregate the coagulation process into tissue factor initiated or surface contact processes, respectively. The aPTT, which initiates coagulation by the introduction of a foreign surface, only examines the biologic constituents intrinsic to plasma. This assay is sensitive to isolated or combined deficiencies of factor XII, HMWK, prekallikrein, factor XI, factor VIII, factor IX, factor X, factor V, prothrombin, and fibrinogen. The PT assay is based on initiating coagulation via an extrinsic source of tissue factor (thromboplastin). The PT assay is sensitive to isolated or combined deficiencies of factor VII, factor X, factor V, prothrombin, and fibrinogen. Although these in vitro clotting assays help establish a basis for hemostasis, abnormal test results are not always mirrored by human pathology associated with bleeding or thrombosis.

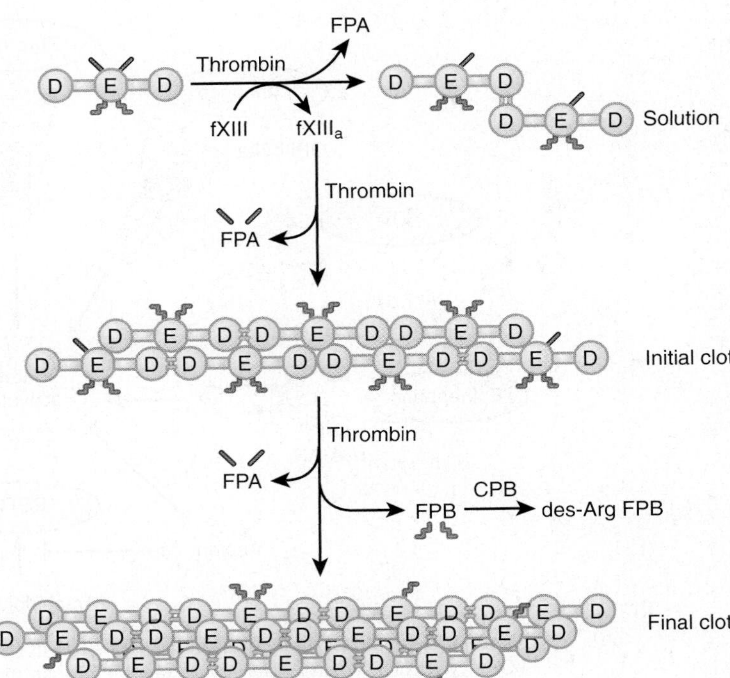

Figure 128-11 SCHEMATIC REPRESENTATION OF WHOLE-BLOOD FIBRIN FORMATION. At the start of clot formation, thrombin simultaneously acts on fibrinogen (D-E-D) and factor XIII (fXIII). A portion (≈40%) of fibrinopeptide A (FPA) is released from fibrinogen, and an initial clot is formed from the complementary overlap of the exposed sites between the E and D domains of adjacent fibrin molecules. Activated factor XIII (fXIIIa) simultaneously cross-links adjacent D domains (D=D). Thus, the initial soluble fibrin clot is composed of fibrinogen, fibrin, and γ-γ dimers with fibrinopeptide B (FPB) still attached. The initial clot is continuously acted on by thrombin, releasing the remaining FPA and some of the FPB to yield a final clot with the majority of FPB still attached. The released FPB is selectively acted on by a carboxypeptidase B–like enzyme (CPB, potentially thrombin activatable fibrinolysis inhibitor a [TAFIa]) which cleaves the carboxyl terminal arginine to produce des-Arg FPB. The significance of this cleavage is still unclear. *(From Brummel KE, Butenas S, Mann KG: An integrated study of fibrinogen during blood coagulation.* J Biol Chem *274(32):22862-72280, 1999, with permission.)*

Fibrinolysis Proteins

Clot formation is integrated with clot dissolution (fibrinolysis). Fibrinolysis, the elimination of blood clots, has two types, primary fibrinolysis and secondary fibrinolysis. Whereas primary fibrinolysis is a normal body process, secondary fibrinolysis is the breakdown of clots due to a medicine, a medical disorder, or some other cause.

The biochemical mechanisms of clot dissolution center on fibrin specific activation of plasminogen to plasmin. The key proteins involved are plasminogen, the plasminogen activators tissue plasminogen activator (t-PA) and urokinase plasminogen activator (u-PA), and the inhibitors (PAI-1, α_2-antiplasmin, and TAFIa). Plasminogen is the inactive precursor of the enzyme plasmin, which is the primary catalyst of fibrin degradation (Fig. 128-12).[269] The process of plasminogen activation can occur through three distinct pathways: (1) the intrinsic activator system (analogous to the contact system of blood coagulation), (2) the extrinsic activators (t-PA and u-PA), and (3) an exogenous activator system involving pharmacologic agents (fibrinolytic drugs). The primary pathway used in vivo appears to be the extrinsic pathway. However, both the intrinsic as well as exogenous activator systems can play important roles in human disease.

t-PA and u-PA, secreted by the endothelium, have unique structures and properties that affect the specificity and rate of plasmin generation (see Fig. 128-12).[270] After being generated, plasmin digests fibrin in a pattern that produces a collection of degradation products, including fragment X; fragment Y; and the core fragments, fragments D and E. The first step in degrading fibrin is the removal of the α chains, thus exposing the coiled coils. As these coils are cleaved, different sized fragments are released.[271] Fibrinogen is represented as a trinodular structure (D-E-D domains) with each E domain and D domain separated by a coiled coil domain. Upon formation of fibrin crosslinks occur between alternating molecules of fibrin at the D domain (D=D). Plasmin degrades fibrin releasing various sized fragments, the smallest of which is the D=D or D-dimer (M_r=180,000). The largest of these fragments is XXD, X=D–E–D, with a mass of 595,000.[272,273] Elevated levels of D-dimer are found in the blood of patients with various thrombotic and thrombolytic disorders.[274] These circulating fragments are cleared by other proteases or by the kidney and liver.

Inhibitors of the Fibrinolytic System

Plasminogen activation in blood is primarily inhibited by PAI-1, which targets u-PA and t-PA. PAI-1 also has a role in tissue remodeling by interfering with vitronectin-dependent processes of cell adhesion and migration.[275] Congenital deficiency of PAI-1 is rare with homozygous individuals displaying abnormal bleeding in response to trauma.[276] Platelets contribute to the fibrinolytic process by binding t-PA and plasminogen and supporting plasmin generation. Increased levels of plasma PAI-1 delay fibrin removal by shortening the functional lifetime of plasminogen activators, thereby shifting hemostasis to a more thrombotic state.[277]

TAFI is a plasma zymogen with homology to procarboxypeptidases A and B (see Fig. 128-12).[55,278-280] Activation of TAFI yields the exopeptidase (TAFIa) with carboxypeptidase B–like substrate specificity. TAFIa catalyzes the removal of basic amino acids (arginine, lysine) from the COOH-termini of polypeptides. The activation of many of the cofactors and zymogens of the coagulation and fibrinolytic cascades results in the generation of functional proteins with COOH-terminus arginine or lysine residues. COOH-terminus lysine residues that appear in fibrin fragments degraded with plasmin have been identified as the major substrates for TAFIa. The physiologic activator of TAFIa is the thrombin–thrombomodulin complex, thus defining TAFIa as a coagulation-dependent activity.[281] Because TAFIa functions as an attenuator of fibrinolysis,[53] an adequate rate of TAFIa generation appears critical for the stabilization of the blood clot. Plasmas with specific deficiencies in the coagulation pathway exhibit reduced rates of thrombin production, decreased levels of TAFIa, and premature clot lysis.[257,282,283]

Fibrinolytic drugs are often given after a myocardial infarct or ischemic stroke to dissolve the fibrin clot blocking the coronary or cerebral artery. Fibrinolytic drugs are also used in massive pulmonary embolism. Antifibrinolytics, such as aminocaproic acid (ε-aminocaproic acid) and tranexamic acid, are used as inhibitors of fibrinolysis.

CONNECTIVITY AND DYNAMICS IN HEMOSTASIS

In the healthy state, the hemostatic system is relatively quiescent with the vascular endothelial cells, the blood, and the extravascular tissue

Plasminogen

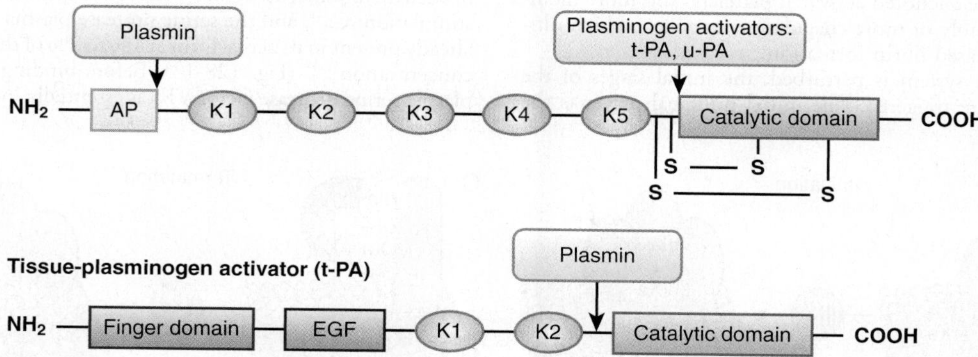

Single chain-urokinase plasminogen activator (sc-uPA)

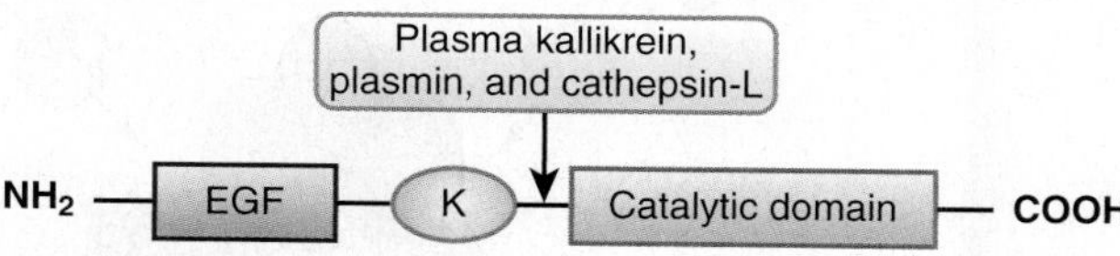

Thrombin activatable fibrinolysis inhibitor (TAFI)

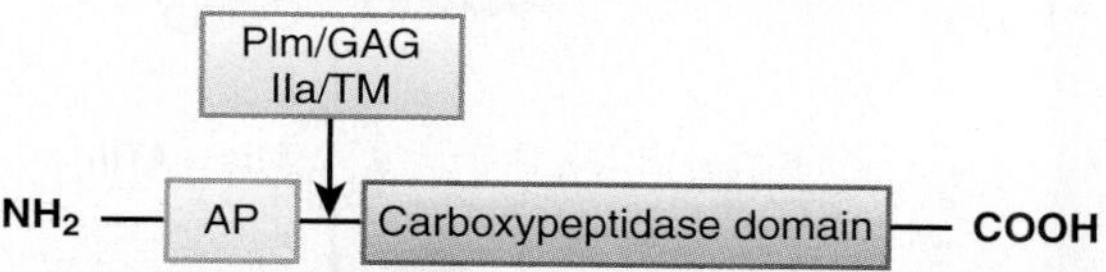

Figure 128-12 SCHEMATIC OF FIBRINOLYTIC PROTEINS. *Plasminogen* is the inactive precursor of the enzyme plasmin, which is the primary catalyst of fibrin degradation. The domain structure of human plasminogen is represented by Kringle domains (K1–K5), a catalytic domain, and the *arrows* indicate the sites of proteolytic cleavage by plasmin, elastase, and plasminogen activators (tissue plasminogen activator [t-PA] and urokinase plasminogen activator [u-PA]). Disulfide bonds are illustrated by S-S. The t-PA molecule is a serine proteinase and consists of an A and B chain. The A chain consists of a fibronectin fingerlike domain, an epidermal growth factor (EGF)–like domain, and two kringle domains. The kringle 2 domain and the finger domain of t-PA are involved in the binding of t-PA to fibrin. The B-chain of t-PA contains the active site catalytic triad. Single-chain t-PA is an efficient plasminogen activator in the presence of fibrin and is converted to the two-chain form by cleavage of the peptide bond between R^{275} and I^{276}. This cleavage is performed primarily by the action of plasmin during fibrinolysis. *Single-chain u-PA* (sc-uPA) is a serine protease and is an ineffective catalyst. Plasmin or plasma kallikrein can hydrolyze the K^{158}-I^{159} peptide bond, converting sc-uPA into the fully active two-chain form (two-chain urokinase-type plasminogen activator). u-PA is composed of an EGF domain (EGF), a single kringle domain, a connecting peptide region, and the serine protease-type catalytic domain. *Thrombin activatable fibrinolysis inhibitor (TAFI):* Activation of TAFI (TAFIa) yields an exopeptidase with carboxypeptidase B–like substrate specificity. TAFIa delays fibrinolysis by cleaving COOH-terminus Arg (R) or Lys (K) residues made available as a consequence of partial plasmin digestion of the fibrin clot. Removing these residues attenuates the self-amplifying mechanism of fibrin-based plasmin formation wherein partial plasmin proteolysis of fibrin increases the number of binding sites (COOH-terminal lysines) available for efficient plasminogen activation. TAFI contains an activation peptide region and a carboxypeptidase domain. It is activated by the thrombin–thrombomodulin complexes (IIa.TM) and plasmin–glycosaminoglycan complexes (Plm/GAG) by hydrolysis of the R^{92}–A^{93} bond.

functioning to maintain fluidity. Blood platelets remain in a quiescent state because of the endothelial cell lining of the blood vessel being an active anticoagulant that secretes small molecules and enzymes. The endothelium also provides constituent anticoagulant proteins, which inhibit the blood coagulation system. These vascular anticoagulant systems are both passive and dynamic in nature and function in cooperation with plasma components. The blood supplies pro- and anticoagulant proteins in the plasma and platelets, which contribute to the coagulation reaction. If the endothelium becomes damaged, the pro- and anticoagulant levels become imbalanced, and cells that should remain in the blood can leak through blood vessels into adjacent body tissue, which triggers a response. The dimensions of the response are relevant to the injury. The extravascular compartment and blood interact to rapidly produce a vigorous local coagulation response, which attenuates blood loss and initiates the vascular repair process in four phases: initiation, propagation, termination, and elimination and fibrinolysis.[284-286]

Initiation

If vascular injury occurs, a measured response is triggered in that the extent of damage regulates platelet and fibrin deposition. Activated platelets provide the membrane surfaces upon which coagulation enzymes can be anchored, assembled, and expressed. Therefore, the activated platelet membrane, provides both an initiating and limiting component to the extent of a coagulation reaction.[287] More vascular damage produces more anchored activated platelets, and more membrane allows the assembly of more coagulation enzymes, which ultimately results in increased fibrin formation.

When the vascular system is perturbed, the initial stages of the hemostatic response are triggered. The initial principal player is the extrinsic tenase complex (tissue factor–factor VIIa), which is composed of a cell membrane; tissue factor exposed by vascular damage or cytokine stimulation; Ca^{2+}; and the serine protease plasma factor VIIa, which is already present in its active form at 1% to 2% of the factor VII zymogen concentration[53,288] (Fig. 128-13). Before binding to tissue factor, the plasma serine protease factor VIIa is essentially inert from the catalytic

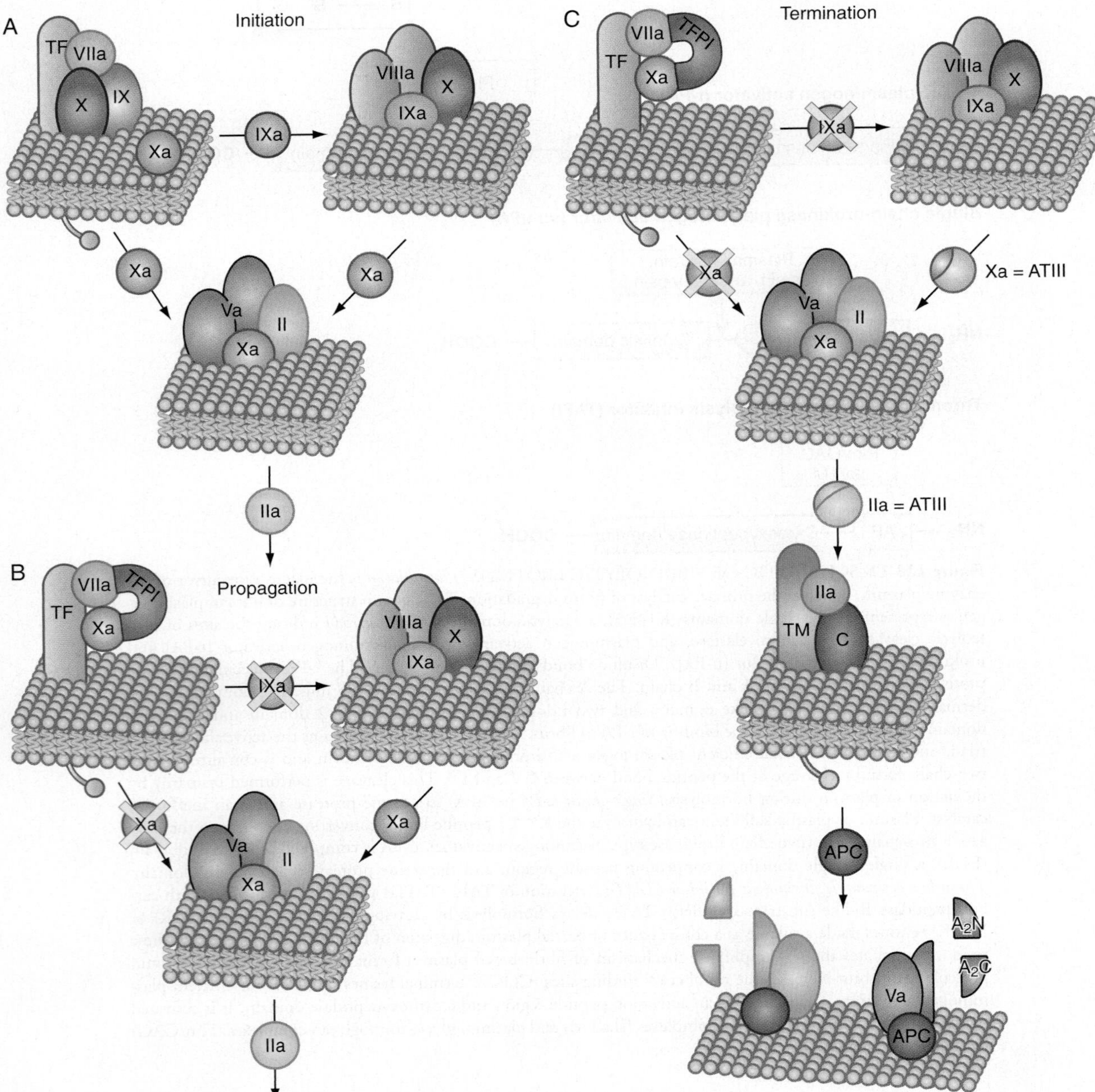

Figure 128-13 REGULATION OF THE DYNAMIC PROCOAGULANT RESPONSE. Initiation **(A)** propagation **(B)** and termination **(C)** of thrombin generation and the procoagulant response are illustrated. Four vitamin K–dependent complexes are shown: extrinsic tenase, intrinsic tenase, prothrombinase, and protein Case. The procoagulant response is regulated by the stoichiometric inhibitors antithrombin (AT) and tissue factor pathway inhibitor (TFPI). AT inhibits thrombin, factor Xa, and factor IXa that are free in solution. TFPI inhibits both factor Xa and the factor VIIa–tissue factor (TF)–factor Xa complex. Activated protein C (APC) generated from the protein Case complex (thrombomodulin [TM]–thrombin [IIa]) inactivates FVa and FVIIIa by proteolysis of their heavy chains. Low levels of thrombin are required to initiate clot formation (initiation phase) and trigger the coagulation cascade response (propagation phase). The enzymes, cofactors, and inhibitors act together to generate a hemostatic response that can be divided into an initiation phase and a propagation and termination phase. During the initiation phase, factors X and IX are converted to their respective serine proteases factor Xa and factor IXa; low levels of thrombin are subsequently generated by factor Xa. This thrombin then can activate platelets and the procofactors factors V and VIII, which stimulate further thrombin generation during the propagation phase. Thrombin generation is attenuated by shutting down the initiation phase by means of the stoichiometric inhibitor of the extrinsic tenase complex, TFPI, followed by AT, which directly inhibits thrombin and factors Xa and IXa. *(From Mann KG:* Coagulation explosion. *Vermont Business Graphics, Burlington, Vermont, 1997, with permission.)*

perspective and thus impervious to the abundant protease inhibitors in plasma.[289] Factor VII also competes with factor VIIa for tissue factor binding, thus serving as a negative regulator that buffers the overall reaction.[290,291] Factor VII activating protease (FSAP) has also been shown to activate factor VII in the absence of tissue factor.[292-294] The physiologic function of FSAP still is unclear but most recently has been suggested to be involved in inflammation (for a review, see Reference 295). The extrinsic tenase complex (tissue factor–factor VIIa) activates low levels of the zymogens factor X and factor IX to their respective serine protease enzymes factor Xa (≈10 pM) and factor IXa (≈1 pM).[296,297] Factor X is the more efficient and abundant substrate.[298,299]

The extrinsic tenase complex is under tight supervision by TFPI, which can bind both the complex and the product factor Xa (see Fig. 128-13).[300,301] TFPI, present in low abundance in blood, is released from the vasculature by heparin.[302] If the initiating procoagulant stimulus is sufficient to overcome the level of this anticoagulant response, a threshold is exceeded and downstream complexes can be formed.

The limited amounts of factor Xa that escapes inhibition by TFPI and antithrombin bind to available membrane sites and can activate tiny amounts of prothrombin to thrombin (see Fig. 128-13).[303] The time period in which factor Xa directly generates picomolar amounts of thrombin[304] is referred to as the *initiation phase* of blood coagulation (Fig. 128-14). During the initiation phase, circulating blood cells and procoagulant proteins are activated,[305] the procoagulant elements necessary for the full procoagulant response are generated, and a

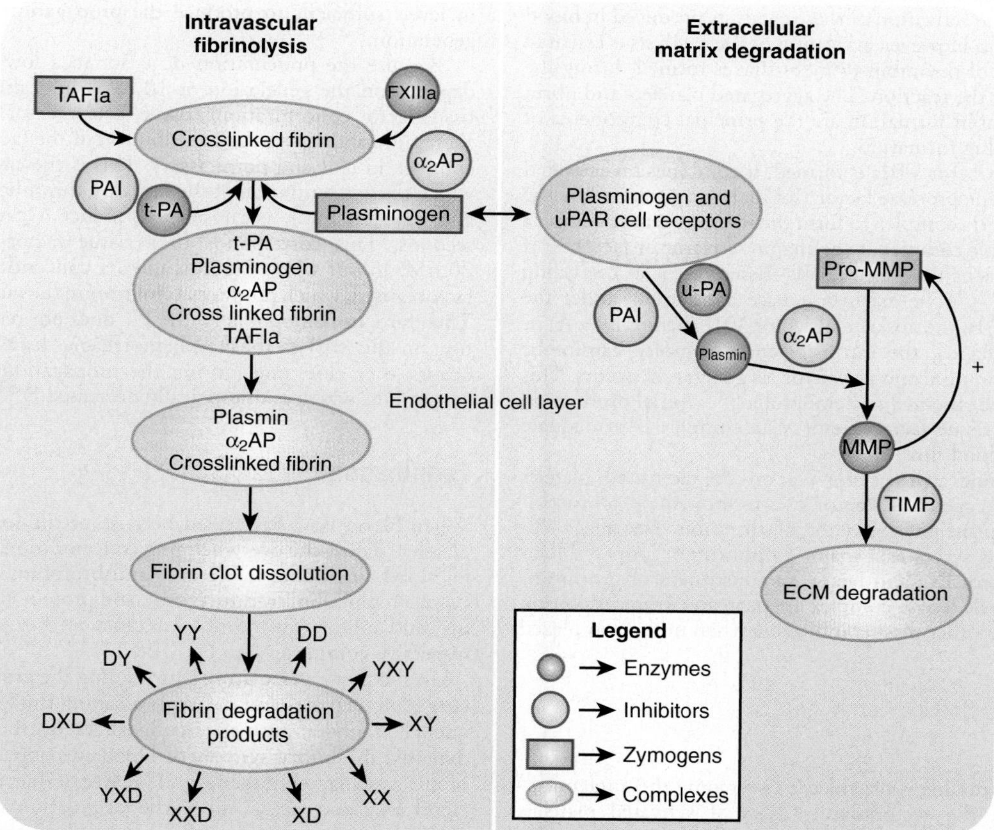

Figure 128-14 SCHEMATIC OF THE DYNAMIC INTERACTION BETWEEN THE PROTEINS AND INHIBITORS OF FIBRINOLYSIS. Cross-linked fibrin formation is integrated with fibrin clot dissolution and degradation of its products. Two pathways are shown, intravascular fibrinolysis and extracellular matrix, separated by an endothelial cell layer. The enzymes *(red circles),* inhibitors *(blue circles),* zymogens *(green boxes),* and complexes *(large yellow ovals)* are illustrated in a simplified form to show this multicomponent process. The key proteins of the fibrinolytic system *(left panel)* are plasminogen, the plasminogen activator tissue type plasminogen activator (t-PA), plasminogen activator inhibitors (PAI), α_2-antiplasmin (α_2-AP) and thrombin activatable fibrinolysis inhibitor (TAFI), and the transglutaminase activated factor XIII (FXIIIa). t-PA and plasminogen both bind to the fibrin surface, crosslinked by FXIIIa, where t-PA is an effective catalyst of plasminogen conversion to plasmin. Initially, plasmin proteolysis of fibrin generates new COOH terminus lysine residues, which function as higher affinity binding sites for plasminogen, setting up an amplifying loop of plasminogen activation. Formation of activated TAFIa results in removal of the plasmin-generated COOH-terminus lysine residues, thus suppressing the rate of fibrin lysis. Opposing these events are antifibrinolytic mechanisms. Soluble and cross-linked α_2-AP complexes with plasmin rendering it inactive. PAI rapidly reacts with t-PA thus reducing the concentration of the plasminogen activator. Fibrin degradation occurs by plasmin cleavage at the D-E-D domains of fibrin polymers to yield a variety of polymers as illustrated (for a definition of the D-E-D domain, see Fig. 128-11). Plasminogen can cross the endothelial cell layer and become converted to plasmin by the urokinase type plasminogen activator (u-PA) *(right panel).* Plasmin can convert latent matrix metalloproteinases (pro-MMP) to their active form (MMP). MMPs themselves can act in a positive feedback mechanism to convert pro-MMP to more MMP, which ultimately degrade the extracellular matrix. Plasmin-mediated effects are inhibited by PAI and α_2-AP. MMP-mediated effects are inhibited by tissue inhibitors of metalloproteinases (TIMP).

preliminary fibrin network is formed.[306] Although this process is inefficient, this initial thrombin is essential for the acceleration of the process by serving as the activator of platelets through cleavage of protease activated receptors (PAR1 and PAR4)[307] and the activation of the procofactors factor V and factor VIII.[129] Thrombin also activates factor XI to factor XIa[130], initiating the accessory pathway that enhances factor IX activation.[308]

In analyses of tissue factor–induced activation of the coagulation process in whole blood, the initial period of thrombin generation (based on levels of thrombin–antithrombin complexes) illustrates that most catalyst formation occurs before fibrin clot formation (see Fig. 128-14).[305] The small amount of thrombin that is generated during the initiation phase is from the extrinsic factor tenase and is able to activate platelets,[309] factor XIII,[310] factor V,[311] and factor VIII[312] and release some fibrinopeptide A and fibrinopeptide B[263] from fibrinogen to form fibrin. Less than 2% of the final thrombin produced is required to achieve the activation of these catalysts produced in blood to form the initial clot. However, activation of the catalysts is essential to generate the bulk of thrombin (≈95%) that is formed during the propagation phase of the reaction. The aggregated platelets and fibrin resulting from thrombin formation are the principal components of the initial vascular plug formation.

After the cofactor factor VIIIa is formed, it combines on activated platelets with the serine protease factor IXa that was generated by the tissue factor–factor VIIa complex to form the intrinsic tenase complex (see Fig. 128-13). This complex is the major activator of factor X; it is 50-fold more efficient than factor VIIa–tissue factor in catalyzing factor X activation.[299,313] The extrinsic tenase complex is under the control of TFPI.[314,315] In the absence of factor VIII (hemophilia A) or factor IX (hemophilia B), the intrinsic tenase complex cannot be assembled; thus, no amplification of factor Xa generation occurs. This is the principal defect observed in hemophilia[316,317]: initial production of factor Xa by the tissue factor–factor VIIa complex is inadequate to efficiently stem blood flow.

Factor Xa combines with factor Va on the activated platelet membrane surfaces at specific receptor sites to form the prothrombinase complex; the principal generator of thrombin (see Fig. 128-13).[318,319] This process serves as a major amplification loop of blood coagulation. The factor IXa and factor Xa constituent of prothrombinase and the intrinsic tenase complex are protected from inhibition by antithrombin and other plasma inhibitors when in the complexed form.

Propagation

When a sufficient stimulus is provided to overcome the antagonist–inhibitor threshold, the accumulating mass of activated platelets will support increasing intrinsic tenase and prothrombinase complex formation on their surfaces through specific platelet receptors, and the local inhibitor concentrations are overwhelmed (see Fig. 128-13). These platelet-bound catalysts execute the propagation phase of the reaction, during which massive amounts of thrombin are produced.[320] This phase of thrombin generation continues, independent of the initially presented tissue factor, as long as there is a continuous supply of blood to deliver new plasma procoagulant reactants, platelets, and fibrinogen to the site of perforation in the vascular endothelium.

Important to the formation of the prothrombinase complex is the generation of factor Xa. Factor Xa is a unique regulatory enzyme in that it is formed through both the intrinsic tenase and the extrinsic tenase complexes. Under normal conditions, the concentration of factor Xa is the rate-limiting component of the prothrombinase complex. The other components of the complex, platelets (membrane surface binding sites), and the cofactor (factor Va) are activated rapidly to produce a surplus that is ready for action.[318] The coagulation mechanism can become sensitive to factor V or platelets when confronted with congenital deficiencies, thrombocytopenia, platelet pathology, or pharmacologic interventions.[321,322]

The initial factor Xa is generated via the tissue factor–factor VIIa complex during the initiation phase. Additional factor Xa is then generated by the intrinsic tenase complex (factor IXa–factor VIIIa–membrane–Ca^{2+}). Initially, the concentration of the factor VIIa–tissue factor complex is higher than the concentration of the factor VIIIa–factor IXa complex, which requires activation and assembly. As time progresses, the contribution of the intrinsic tenase complex to factor Xa generation exceeds that of the extrinsic tenase.[323] The intrinsic tenase complex is kinetically more efficient and activates factor X at a 50- to 100-fold higher rate than the extrinsic tenase complex.[299,324,325] The burst of factor Xa that is generated overcomes the levels of factor Xa inhibitors, such as TFPI, and achieves maximal prothrombinase activity and propagation of the procoagulant response.[162,314] The bulk of thrombin (≈95%) is formed during the propagation phase after fibrin clot formation.[305,326] Without the intrinsic tenase complex being formed, as occurs in hemophilia A or B, factor Xa is not generated in levels sufficient to produce the propagation phase of thrombin generation.[316,327]

Because the presentation of a clot in a low tissue factor model depends on the generation of 10 to 30 nM thrombin,[305,326] at high tissue factor concentrations, tissue factor–factor VIIa generate factor Xa rapidly and masks the contribution of the factor VIIIa–factor IXa complex in clot end point assays. This is the case for the PT[266,267] in which the concentration of the initiator, thromboplastin (tissue factor and phospholipid), is chosen to produce a clot time of 11 to 15 seconds. This corresponds to a tissue factor concentration over 20 nM. In our whole-blood studies, a concentration of 5 pM tissue factor is used, which produces a clot time in the range of 5 minutes.[305,326] Therefore, in hemophilia A, the PT does not reflect a change in clot time in this well-established hemorrhagic disease. The major defect occurs after clot time, during the propagation phase of thrombin generation, which is dramatically decreased.[316,320,328]

Termination

When blood flow has ceased because of the formation of a fibrin–platelet "dam," the overwhelming concentration of inhibitors present in blood, including TFPI and antithrombin, heparin cofactor II, α_2-macroglobulin, α_1-antitrypsin, and protein C inhibitor, can "catch up" and inhibit the various reactants as they dissociate from their respective complexes (see Fig. 128-13).[150,314,329-331]

In the intact vasculature surrounding the growing thrombus, procoagulant enzymes and cofactors escaping the wound site are rapidly quenched under normal circumstances by the stoichiometric and dynamic inhibitory systems of blood in cooperation with elements of the vascular endothelium. The free serine proteases (thrombin, factor IXa, and factor Xa) of the coagulation system in the plasma environment are rapidly inhibited by the surplus of antithrombin molecules. The reaction is accelerated by the interaction of antithrombin with heparan sulfate proteoglycans presented constitutively on the surface of vascular endothelial cells.[332]

Any thrombin escaping from the wound site may bind resident thrombomodulin molecules constitutively expressed by vascular endothelial cells. Thrombomodulin-bound thrombin is converted from a procoagulant enzyme to an anticoagulant enzyme.[333,334] The thrombin–thrombomodulin complex (protein Case) activates protein C, which in turn downregulates the intrinsic factor tenase and prothrombinase procoagulants by cleaving factor VIIIa and factor Va, respectively. The rates of APC inactivation of factors Va and VIIIa are enhanced by protein S. TAFI is also activated by protein Case and serves to delay clot lysis (for reviews, see Reference 53 and 335). Cleavage of factor Va by APC and inhibition of thrombin generation also reduces thrombin–thrombomodulin–mediated TAFI activation.[336]

When operating properly, this system of blood leakage attenuation displays the appropriate level of procoagulant required to obstruct blood loss but is precluded from systemic activation of the coagulation system. The converse to hemostasis occurs when the damaging insult for the vasculature is internal to the vessel lumen.[337]

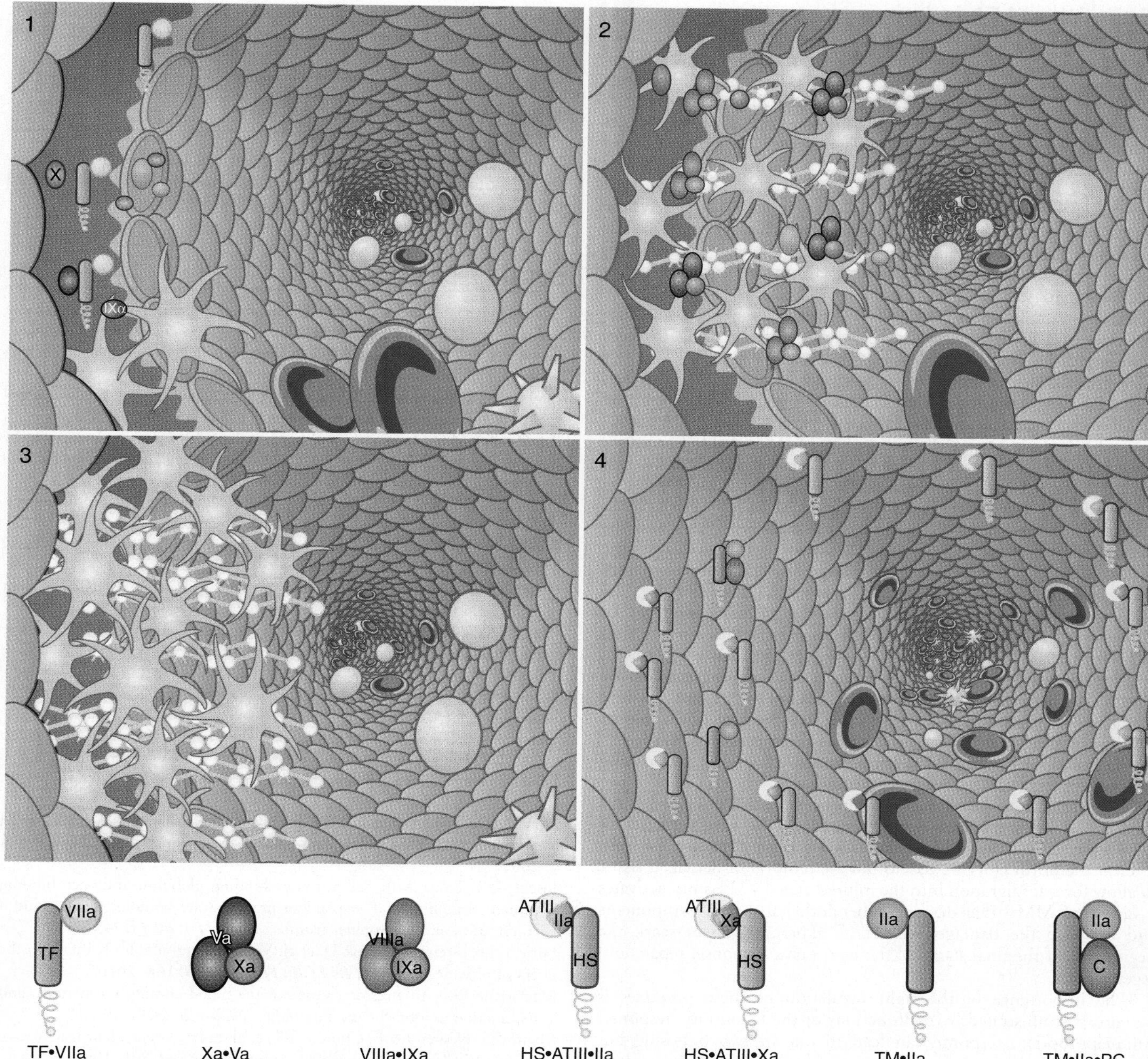

Figure 128-15 SCHEMATIC OF THE DYNAMIC EVENTS DURING TISSUE FACTOR–INITIATED BLOOD COAGULATION. A cross-section of a blood vessel showing the luminal space, endothelial cell layer, and extravascular region is presented at the site of a perforation. The blood coagulation process in response is depicted in four stages. *Extrinsic tenase* complex, TF (tissue factor) •VIIa; *prothrombinase* complex, Xa•Va; *intrinsic tenase*, VIIIa•IXa; AT (antithrombin)–endothelial cell heparan sulfate (HS) proteoglycan complex bound to thrombin or fXa, HS•AT•(IIa or Xa); protein C bound to thrombomodulin–thrombin, TM•IIa•PC.

Stage 1. Perforation results in delivery of blood, and with it circulating factor VIIa and platelets, to an extravascular space rich in membrane-bound TF. Platelets adhere to collagen and von Willebrand factor associated with the extravascular tissue, and TF binds factor VIIa, initiating the process of factor IX and factor X activation. Factor Xa activates small amounts of prothrombin to thrombin, which activates more platelets and converts factor V and factor VIII to factor Va and factor VIIIa.

Stage 2. The reaction is propagated by platelet-bound intrinsic tenase and *prothrombinase* with the former being the principal factor Xa generator. Initial clotting occurs and fibrin begins to fill in the void in cooperation with activated platelets.

Stage 3. A barrier composed of activated platelets ladened with procoagulant complexes and enmeshed in fibrin scaffolding is formed. The reaction in the now filled perforation is terminated by reagent consumption, attenuating further thrombin generation, but functional procoagulant enzyme complexes persist because they are protected from the dynamic inhibitory processes found on the intravascular face.

Stage 4. View downstream of the perforation. Enzymes escaping from the plugged perforation are captured by antithrombin–heparan complexes, and the protein C system is activated by residual thrombin binding to endothelial cell thrombomodulin, initiating the dynamic anticoagulant system. These intravascular processes work against occlusion of the vessel despite the continuous resupply of reactants across the intravascular face of the thrombus. *(From Orfeo T, Butenas S, Brummel-Ziedins KE, Mann KG: The tissue factor requirement in blood coagulation.* J Biol Chem *280(52):42887-42896, 2005, with permission.)*

Elimination and Fibrinolysis

The hemostatic or pathologic thrombus is structurally composed of aggregated platelets and crosslinked fibrin. The steps in thrombin generation of a crosslinked fibrin clot are shown diagrammatically in Fig. 128-11. Other plasma proteins and blood cells are also trapped within the clot. Clot formation is integrated with clot dissolution by plasmin to maintain hemostatic balance. The plasminogen system has two roles: t-PA generates plasmin at the fibrin surface and governs fibrin homeostasis, and u-PA binds to a cellular u-PA receptor (u-PAR) and generates pericellular plasmin, which plays an important role in tissue remodeling and cellular migration.[338,339] The latter function is, to a great extent, mediated by plasmin activation of matrix metalloproteinases (MMPs), which degrade ECM. t-PA and u-PA are secreted by vascular endothelial cells[340,341] and are regulated by cellular cytokines and components produced during the clotting cascade, including thrombin.

In the absence of fibrin, t-PA is a poor enzyme.[342-344] However, both t-PA and plasminogen bind to the fibrin surface with a resulting 100-fold enhancement in plasminogen activation. Thus, t-PA activation of fibrinolysis is primarily initiated by and localized to fibrin.[342,344] The digestion of fibrin by plasmin[345] is seen in Fig. 128-14 and further described under the section Fibrinolysis Proteins.[274,345-348]

Fibrinolysis is regulated primarily by PAI-1,[349,350] PAI-2,[351] α_2-antiplasmin, and TAFI.[352] The antagonism between PAI-1 and the plasminogen activators u-PA and t-PA provides a threshold response of the fibrinolytic process in much the same way as the procoagulant–anticoagulant balance provides an activation threshold for the clotting process.[353-356] α_2-Antiplasmin is the primary inhibitor of plasmin.[357-359] Plasmin, when bound through its lysine binding sites to fibrin, reacts more slowly with α_2-antiplasmin than when free in solution because α_2-antiplasmin interacts with plasma plasmin by binding to the lysine binding sites.[357-361] In contrast, α_2-antiplasmin, bound covalently by factor XIIIa to the Aα chain of fibrin, blocks plasmin binding and appears to decrease plasminogen activation.[362] TAFIa functions in vitro as an antifibrinolytic factor by suppressing the positive feedback pathway of fibrinolysis.[255,256,336]

The elimination phase begins the process of tissue repair by dissolving the fibrin–platelet clot generated in the earlier phases of hemostasis. The damaged vascular tissue not only requires plasmin to clear the fibrin clot but also to initiate removal of damaged tissue to allow for cell migration into the injured area.[363,364] Plasmin activates a variety of MMP that degrade subendothelial matrix components and extricate the damaged tissue.[364,365] These processes mark the beginnings of the final stages of the hemostatic response, repair, and regeneration.

The importance of the tight regulation of these processes is perhaps best illustrated by malfunctions of the hemostatic response. An inappropriate response can lead to one of two opposing but equally undesirable outcomes. Failure to form a sufficient hemostatic plug to arrest blood flow subsequent to vascular injury can result in pathologic hemorrhage. Excessive clot formation or failure to efficiently lyse a clot may result in thrombosis with consequent vascular obstruction. Under normal circumstances, the vascular endothelium together with the aforementioned positive and negative feedback loops within the procoagulant pathways prevent these negative outcomes by actively controlling the coagulation process until a triggering stimulus of sufficient magnitude threatens vascular integrity (Fig. 128-15). Initiation of the procoagulant response also initiates the fibrinolytic response simultaneously with repair and regeneration processes.

FUTURE DIRECTIONS

This chapter describes the process of blood coagulation (extrinsic and intrinsic pathway) by dividing it into sections based on procoagulant, anticoagulant and fibrinolytic enzymes, cofactors, and inhibitors in the overall process of fibrin formation and fibrin dissolution. When all of the players are present, the overall process of blood coagulation and fibrinolysis is best described as a dynamic threshold-limited, complex, intertwined process that together promotes hemostasis.

ACKNOWLEDGEMENTS

We the authors would like to thank Matthew Gissel, George Forguites, and Stacia Rymarchyk for their assistance in the preparation of this chapter. This work was funded by NIH 46703.

SUGGESTED READINGS

Bandyopadhyay PK: Vitamin K-dependent gamma-glutamylcarboxylation: An ancient posttranslational modification. *Vitam Horm* 78:157, 2008.

Berkner KL: Vitamin K-dependent carboxylation. *Vitam Horm* 78:131, 2008.

Brenner B, Kuperman AA, Watzka M, et al: Vitamin K-dependent coagulation factors deficiency. *Semin Thromb Hemost* 35:439, 2009.

Brinkhous KM: A short history of hemophilia, with some comments on the word "hemophilia". In Brinkhous KM, Hemker HC, editors: *Handbook of hemophilia*, New York, 1975, American Elsevier.

Butenas S, Orfeo T, Brummel-Ziedins KE, et al: Tissue factor in thrombosis and hemorrhage. *Surgery* 142:S2, 2007.

Butenas S, Orfeo T, Mann KG: Tissue factor in coagulation: Which? Where? When? *Arterioscler Thromb Vasc Biol* 29:1989, 2009.

Chatrou ML, Reutelingsperger CP, Schurgers LJ: Role of vitamin K-dependent proteins in the arterial vessel wall. *Hamostaseologie* 31:251, 2011.

Cosgriff SW: The effectiveness of an oral vitamin K in controlling excessive hypothrombinemia during anticoagulant therapy. *Ann Intern Med* 45:14, 1956.

Davie EW, Ratnoff OD: Waterfall sequence for intrinsic blood clotting. *Science* 145:1310, 1964.

Garcia AA, Reitsma PH: VKORC1 and the vitamin K cycle. *Vitam Horm* 78:23, 2008.

Hirsh J: Optimal intensity and monitoring warfarin. *Am J Cardiol* 75:39B, 1995.

Hirsh J, Dalen J, Anderson DR, et al: Oral anticoagulants: Mechanism of action, clinical effectiveness, and optimal therapeutic range. *Chest* 119:8S, 2001.

Joseph DR, Baker ME: Sex hormone-binding globulin, androgen-binding protein, and vitamin K-dependent protein S are homologous to laminin A, merosin, and Drosophila crumbs protein. *FASEB J* 6:2477, 1992.

Lurie Y, Loebstein R, Kurnik D, et al: Warfarin and vitamin K intake in the era of pharmacogenetics. *Br J Clin Pharmacol* 70:164, 2010.

Macfarlane RG: An enzyme cascade in the blood clotting mechanism, and its function as a biochemical amplifier. *Nature* 202:498, 1964.

Mann KG, Nesheim ME, Church WR, et al: Surface-dependent reactions of the vitamin K-dependent enzyme complexes. *Blood* 76:1, 1990.

Morawitz P: Die chemie der blutgerrinnung. *Ergebn Physiol* 4:307, 1905.

Nelsestuen GL, Kisiel W, Di Scipio RG: Interaction of vitamin K dependent proteins with membranes. *Biochemistry* 17:2134, 1978.

Nelsestuen GL, Shah AM, Harvey SB: Vitamin K-dependent proteins. *Vitam Horm* 58:355, 2000.

Nemerson Y, Repke D: Tissue factor accelerates the activation of coagulation factor VII: The role of a bifunctional coagulation cofactor. *Thromb Res* 40:351, 1985.

Oldenburg J, Marinova M, Muller-Reible C, et al: The vitamin K cycle. *Vitam Horm* 78:35, 2008.

Owen CA: Older concepts of blood coagulation. In Nichols WL, Bowie EJ, editors: *A history of blood coagulation*, Rochester, MN, 2001, Mayo Foundation for Medical Education and Research, p 7.

Owen CA, Jr: *A history of blood coagulation*, Rochester, MN, 2001, Mayo Foundation for Medical Education and Research.

Prowse CV, Esnouf MP: The isolation of a new warfarin-sensitive protein from bovine plasma. *Biochem Soc Trans* 5:255, 1977.

Ratnoff OD: The evolution of knowledge about hemostasis. In Ratnoff OD, Forbes CD, editors: *Disorders of hemostasis*, Philadelphia, 1996, W.B. Saunders Company, p 1.

Schulman S, El Bouazzaoui B, Eikelboom JW, et al: Clinical factors influencing the sensitivity to warfarin when restarted after surgery. *J Intern Med* 263:412, 2008.

Schwalbe RA, Ryan J, Stern DM, et al: Protein structural requirements and properties of membrane binding by gamma-carboxyglutamic acid-containing plasma proteins and peptides. *J Biol Chem* 264:20288, 1989.

Stafford DW: The vitamin K cycle. *J Thromb Haemost* 3:1873, 2005.

Williams JC, Mackman N: Tissue factor in health and disease. *Front Biosci (Elite Ed)* 4:358, 2012.

Wright IS: The nomenclature of blood clotting factors. *Thromb Diath Haemorrh* 7:381, 1962.

For complete list of references log on to www.expertconsult.com.

CHAPTER 129

REGULATORY MECHANISMS IN HEMOSTASIS

Charles T. Esmon and Naomi L. Esmon

Regulation of hemostasis can be divided into two areas: events that promote coagulation and events that inhibit this process.

KEY EVENTS IN THE PROMOTION OF COAGULATION

Key events that initiate and propagate coagulation are the redistribution of negatively charged phospholipids to the cell surface and the exposure of tissue factor to the blood. The appropriate negatively charged phospholipids, primarily phosphatidylserine, can arise as a result of either cellular activation with strong agonists like thrombin together with collagen in the case of platelets or tissue damage or death.[1,2] The negatively charged phospholipids promote the activation of factors X and IX by the tissue factor–factor VIIa pathway, the activation of prothrombin by factors Va and Xa, and the activation of factor X by factors VIIIa and IXa (see Chapter 128). In addition, it has been suggested that oxidation of a specific disulfide in tissue factor is important for expression of its procoagulant activity, a process that may be regulated by protein disulfide isomerase,[3,4] although this concept remains controversial.[5-8]

Normally tissue factor is not present on cells in contact with blood. Tissue factor is found on extravascular cells surrounding the blood vessel so that a potent procoagulant surface is exposed when the endothelium is breached. This helps to seal the breach.[9] Intravascularly, inflammatory stimuli can induce tissue factor synthesis and expression on leukocytes, particularly monocytes, providing a mechanism for the initiation of coagulation.[10] This response likely contributes to disseminated intravascular coagulation (DIC). Animal studies suggest that this coagulation response plays a role in innate immunity and prevents the dissemination of infectious agents.[11-14]

Other key events that can play a major role in the pathogenesis of thrombosis, at least in animal models, involve the release of intracellular components, including ribonucleic acid (RNA) and polyphosphates. These can trigger activation of factor XII, which initiates coagulation via the contact pathway. Although factor XII does not appear to contribute to hemostasis,[15] it drives several models of thrombosis, including pulmonary embolism[16] and myocardial infarction.[17]

Polyphosphates are stored in the dense granules of platelets and when released, contribute to the procoagulant potential of the platelet.[16] In regions of cellular death or severe inflammation, histones released from the tissue can bind to these polyphosphates, increasing the procoagulant activity more than 20-fold.[18] Heparin analogues can block polyphosphate stimulation of coagulation by histones.[18,19] In addition, neutrophils in hyperinflammatory environments can release their nuclear contents to form neutrophil extracellular traps (NETs). These NETs are effective in killing bacteria and other pathogens[20] and also provide a potent agonist for the activation of platelets and the development of thrombi.[19,21] Interestingly, heparin, an anticoagulant often used in the setting of inflammation, can disrupt the NETs and diminish the activation of platelets by histones and NETs.[19,21]

INHIBITION OF COAGULATION BY NATURAL ANTICOAGULANTS

There are three major natural anticoagulant mechanisms that serve to limit the coagulation process. These are tissue factor pathway inhibitor (TFPI), which blocks the initiation of coagulation by tissue factor-factor VIIa[22]; the antithrombin-heparin mechanism, which inhibits thrombin and factors VIIa, Xa, and IXa[23]; and the protein C pathway, which inactivates factors Va and VIIIa.[24]

Tissue Factor Pathway Inhibitor

TFPI is a complex molecule composed of three similar domains related to a protease inhibitor type known as a Kunitz inhibitor.[25,26] To inhibit the tissue factor–factor VIIa complex, the Kunitz-1 domain of TFPI binds factor VIIa, whereas the Kunitz-2 domain binds factor Xa, either because the factor X is activated on tissue factor[25,27] or (probably less effectively) by first reacting with factor Xa in solution and then inhibiting factor VIIa bound to tissue factor, thus blocking the initiation of coagulation (Fig. 129-1). The carboxy terminal portion of TFPI is very basic,[25] potentially facilitating interaction with the endothelium. Protein S, discussed in greater detail later, can augment the activity of TFPI[28] by increasing the rate of TFPI inactivation of factor Xa.[29]

TFPI exists in two forms, α and β, both found largely associated with the endothelium.[30] TFPIα is the intact form. In contrast, TFPIβ lacks the Kunitz-3 domain and the region that is C-terminal to this domain. TFPI in plasma is associated with lipoproteins and has considerably lower activity. Cellular TFPI is localized to intracellular granules and is found on the endothelial cell surface. Heparin can release TFPI from the endothelium.[31,32] It is unclear whether TFPI released from the endothelium contributes to the antithrombotic activity of heparin. Most likely, TFPIα is the most abundant form, but TFPIβ can bind to the endothelium via a glycosylphosphatidylinositol linkage, which appears to increase its inhibitory activity.[30] Incubation of endothelium with phospholipase D results in the release of both forms of TFPI, suggesting that either both forms are bound via the glycosylphosphatidylinositol linkage or, more likely, that a glycosylphosphatidylinositol–anchored TFPI binding partner is responsible for TFPI retention on the endothelium.[33]

The physiologic importance of TFPI is highlighted by the fact that gene deletion results in embryonic lethality apparently because of thrombosis and subsequent hemorrhage.[34]

Antithrombin

Antithrombin is the major inhibitor of the coagulation proteases thrombin, factor VIIa, factor Xa, and factor IXa. Antithrombin is a member of a large class of protease inhibitors referred to as serine

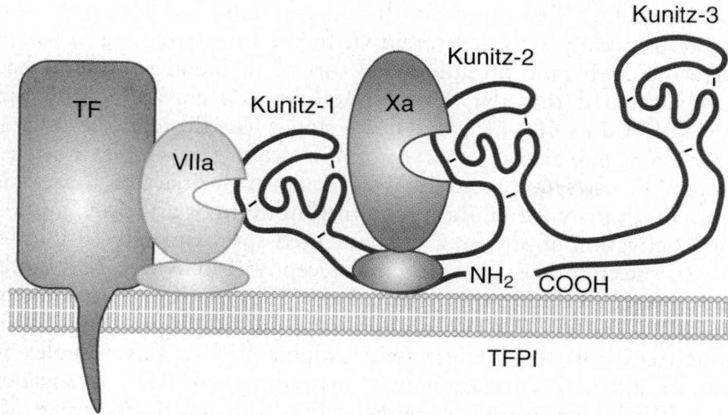

Figure 129-1 TISSUE FACTOR PATHWAY INHIBITOR (TFPI) FUNCTION. TFPI has three Kunitz domains, two of which function as protease inhibitors. The Kunitz-1 domain is responsible for inhibition of factor VIIa (VIIa) that is bound to tissue factor (TF). The Kunitz-2 domain inhibits factor Xa (Xa) either in solution or while the newly formed Xa is still associated with the activation complex. Inhibition of Xa concentrates TFPI in the vicinity of VIIa and facilitates VIIa inactivation. The complex dissociates when calcium ions are removed. *(From Esmon CT: Coagulation. In Fink MP, Abraham E, Vincent J-L, et al, editors:* Textbook of critical care, *ed 5, Philadelphia, 2005, Elsevier, p 165.)*

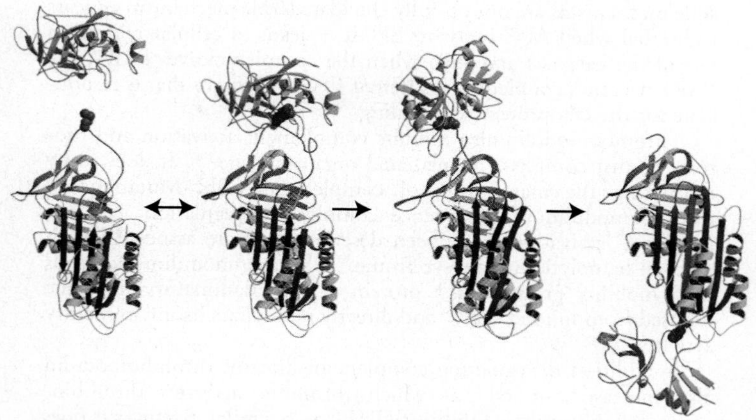

Figure 129-2 COMPLEX FORMATION BETWEEN A SERPIN AND AN ENZYME. Inactivation of trypsin by antitrypsin is shown. The mechanism of inhibition is the same for thrombin inhibition by antithrombin. To the left is the serpin with the major β-sheet A in blue and the reactive center loop with the scissile bond residue in red. The second section shows the formation of a Michaelis complex between the inhibitor and the enzyme, which results in the formation of a covalent inhibitor enzyme complex. The third section shows the complex with the cleaved reactive center loop. The final event is insertion of loop 4 (red) with linked enzyme into the β-sheet A with concomitant denaturation and inactivation of the enzyme (section 4). *(Modified from Huntington JA: Shape-shifting serpins—Advantages of a mobile mechanism.* Trends Biochem Sci *31:427, 2006.)*

protease inhibitors and abbreviated serpins.[35] Antithrombin forms a very tight complex with these proteases. This reaction is rather slow with a half-life in the order of 30 seconds in plasma. Heparin markedly accelerates the reaction, thus accounting for most of its anticoagulant activity. There is a "bait" region in antithrombin that is involved in its interaction with the proteases. In the absence of heparin, this bait region is only partially available to the protease, resulting in the slow inhibition. Heparin binding to antithrombin induces a conformational change in antithrombin that enhances protease access to the bait loop[36,37] (Fig. 129-2).

In addition to the conformational change in antithrombin, heparin has additional roles in the inhibition of coagulation proteases.

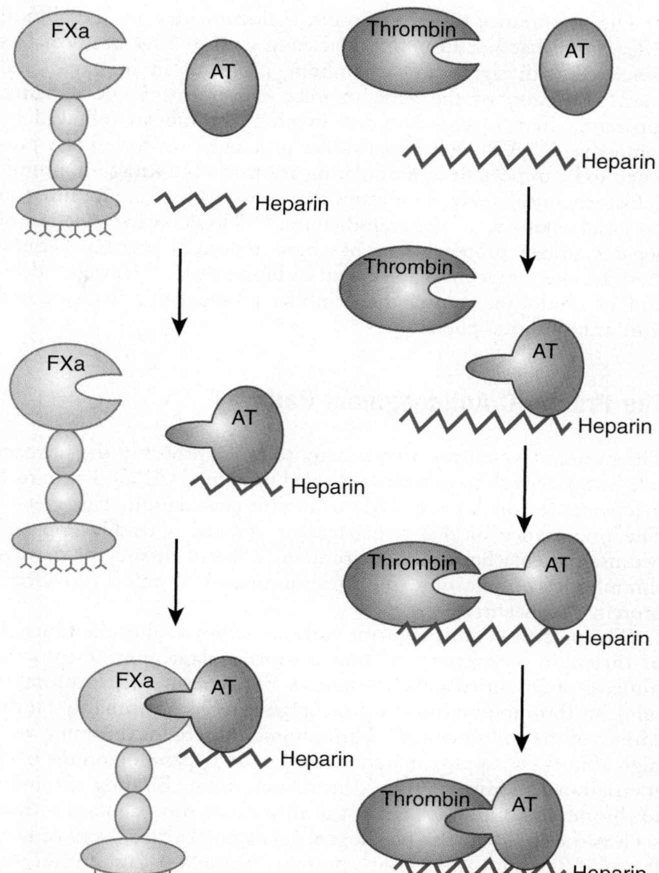

Figure 129-3 THE SIZE DEPENDENCE OF HEPARIN FUNCTION. Unfractionated heparin can simultaneously bind to both antithrombin (AT) and thrombin. This bridges the two together in what is commonly referred to as a template mechanism. This bridging is essential for rapid inactivation as is the binding to antithrombin, which induces a conformational change in antithrombin that is necessary but not sufficient for rapid thrombin inhibition. For factor Xa (FXa) inhibition, the conformational change in antithrombin is sufficient to induce rapid inactivation without an absolute need for bridging between the molecules. The only requirement for heparin here is that it contains the unique pentasaccharide sequence that mediates its binding to antithrombin, as is characterized by fondaparinux. Once the AT enzyme complex forms, heparin rapidly dissociates from the newly formed complex. *(Modified from Esmon CT: Coagulation. In Fink MP, Abraham E, Vincent J-L, et al, editors:* Textbook of critical care, *ed 5, Philadelphia, 2005, Elsevier, p 165.)*

High-molecular-weight (unfractionated) heparin can bind to both antithrombin and the protease, creating a situation where both reactants are brought into close proximity, thus increasing the reaction rate.[38] This function is of variable importance with different proteases of the cascade. It is essential for thrombin inhibition,[36,38] but plays a less important role in the inhibition of factor Xa[39] (Fig. 129-3). High-molecular-weight heparins accelerate factor Xa inhibition somewhat better than low-molecular-weight forms, but in contrast to most of the other heparin-mediated inhibitory functions, the additional acceleration gained by the high-molecular-weight forms is dependent on calcium ions.[39] It is of interest that as heparins become processed to generate lower-molecular-weight fractions, such as enoxaparin, the capacity to promote thrombin inhibition versus factor Xa inhibition decreases. With the smallest functional form of heparin, the synthetic pentasaccharide fondaparinux, the ability to augment thrombin inhibition is almost completely lost, while good inhibition of factor Xa is maintained.[40] Although heparin is a potent antithrombin-dependent anticoagulant, it is not effective against clot-bound thrombin[41] or the factor Va–factor Xa complex assembled on membrane surfaces.[42]

The importance of antithrombin is documented by the clinical observation that antithrombin deficiency, even to 50% of normal, is associated with significant thrombotic problems in humans[43] and mice.[44] Deletion of the gene in mice causes embryonic lethality, apparently in a mechanism that involves thrombosis followed by hemorrhage.[45] Although heparin-like proteoglycans have been proposed to be important in modulating antithrombin function, immunohistochemical analysis indicates that most of these are localized to the basolateral side of the endothelium.[46,47] No definitive deletion of heparin sulfate proteoglycans has been reported, possibly because there are alternative mechanisms for its biosynthesis.[48] However, deletion of ryudocan, another heparin-like proteoglycan, is associated with a thrombotic phenotype.[45]

The Protein C Anticoagulant Pathway

The protein C pathway serves many roles,[49,50] probably the primary role being to work to generate activated protein C (APC) that in turn inactivates factors Va and VIIIa to inhibit coagulation (Fig. 129-4). The importance of this anticoagulant activity is readily apparent because patients born without protein C die in infancy of massive thrombotic complication (purpura fulminans)[51,52] unless provided a protein C concentrate.[53,54]

The protein C anticoagulant pathway serves to alter the function of thrombin, converting it from a procoagulant enzyme into the initiator of an anticoagulant response.[49] This occurs when thrombin binds to thrombomodulin, a proteoglycan receptor primarily on the surface of the endothelium.[49] Thrombomodulin binds thrombin with high affinity (K_d approximately 1 to 10 nM), depending on the post-translational modifications of thrombomodulin. Binding thrombin to thrombomodulin blocks most of thrombin's procoagulant activity such as the ability to clot fibrinogen,[55] activate platelets,[56] and activate factor V[55] but does not prevent thrombin inhibition by antithrombin.[57] The thrombin-thrombomodulin complex gains the ability to rapidly activate protein C. In the microcirculation, where there is a high ratio of endothelial surface to blood volume, it has been estimated that the thrombomodulin concentration is in the range of 100 to 500 nM.[49,58] Thus a single pass through the microcirculation effectively strips thrombin from the blood, initiates protein C activation, and holds a coagulantly inactive thrombin molecule in place for inhibition by antithrombin or protein C inhibitor.[59] Activation of protein C is augmented approximately 20-fold in vivo by the endothelial cell protein C receptor (EPCR).[60] EPCR binds both protein C and APC with similar affinity (K_d approximately 30 nM).[61] The EPCR-APC complex is capable of cytoprotective functions (see later), but at least with soluble EPCR, this complex is not an effective anticoagulant.[62] Instead, when APC dissociates from EPCR, it can interact with protein S to inactivate factors Va and VIIIa and thus inhibit coagulation[63] (see Fig. 129-4). Factor V increases the rate at which the APC–protein S complex inactivates factor VIIIa.[63]

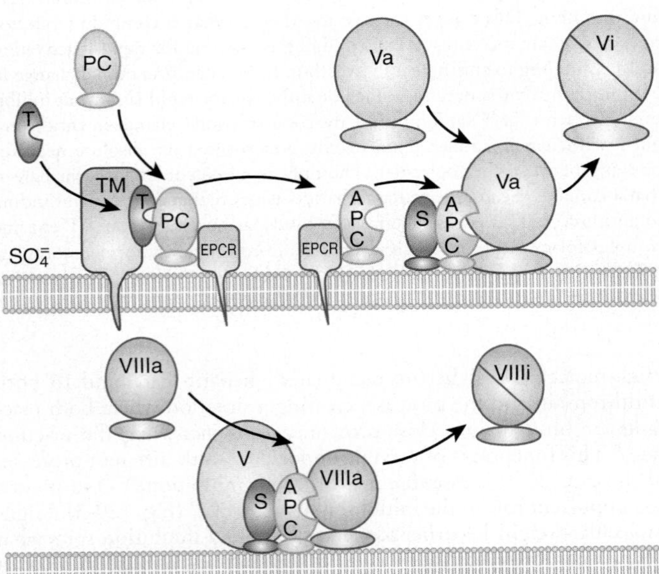

Figure 129-4 THE PROTEIN C ANTICOAGULANT PATHWAY. Thrombin (T) binds to thrombomodulin (TM) and activates protein C (PC). The activation is augmented by protein C binding to the endothelial cell protein C receptor (EPCR). Both protein C and activated protein C (APC) bind reversibly to EPCR. When APC dissociates from EPCR, it binds to protein S (S) and this complex inactivates factors Va (Va and Vi) and VIIIa (VIIIa and VIIIi). In the case of factor VIIIa, factor V (V) also increases the inactivation rate. *(From Esmon CT: Coagulation. In Fink MP, Abraham E, Vincent J-L, et al, editors:* Textbook of critical care, *ed 5, Philadelphia, 2005, Elsevier, p 165.)*

The ability of EPCR to bind both APC and protein C has interesting ramifications. By binding protein C, EPCR augments the conversion to APC and leaves the receptor "filled" with the active protease. APC bound to EPCR can cleave and activate protease activated receptor 1,[64] generating cytoprotective responses that are not only antiapopototic[50] and antiinflammatory[50] but also enhance endothelial cell barrier function.[65] Of interest, thrombin can cleave this same receptor, generating responses that are proinflammatory[66] and lead to loss of endothelial cell barrier function.[50] Although the responsible mechanisms are not yet fully elucidated, one mechanism appears to be that when APC binds to EPCR, it leads to cellular relocation out of the caveolae and then when the complex cleaves PAR1, the PAR1 becomes coupled to a different G (G1) protein that is responsible for the cytoprotective signaling.[67]

Thrombomodulin also inhibits complement activation and protects against complement-mediated organ damage.[68,69] It does so by facilitating the inactivation of complement C3b. Mutations in thrombomodulin that influence complement regulation, but not protein C activation, have been described and are associated with atypical hemolytic uremic syndrome.[69] Thrombomodulin also binds high mobility group box 1 protein, a proinflammatory molecule released from injured cells,[70] and directly neutralizes its inflammatory activity.[71]

In addition to regulating complement directly, thrombomodulin also increases the rate at which thrombin activates thrombin-activatable fibrinolysis inhibitor (TAFI) to a similar extent as it does protein C. TAFI is a procarboxypeptidase B–like enzyme that once activated, releases C-terminal lysine (Lys) and arginine (Arg) residues (with a kinetic preference for Arg).[72,74] C-terminal Lys residues on fibrin enhance fibrin degradation by serving as plasminogen– and tissue plasminogen activator–binding sites. Consequently, their removal by activated TAFI (TAFIa) attenuates clot lysis.[75]

Importantly, many vasoactive peptides, including complement anaphylatoxin C5a and bradykinin, have a C-terminal Arg residue that when removed results in the loss of biologic function.[72,76] Animal studies have suggested that TAFIa is a major mechanism by which these peptides are inactivated.[76]

Regulation of the Protein C Pathway

More than any other regulatory pathway except tissue factor, the protein C pathway is sensitive to regulation by inflammatory mediators (Fig. 129-5). Tumor necrosis factor-α and IL-1β downregulate thrombomodulin both in cell culture[49] and in at least some patients with sepsis.[77,78] Downregulation of thrombomodulin has been observed in animal models of diabetes,[79] inflammatory bowel disease,[80,81] reperfusion injury in the heart,[82] over human atheroma,[83] and in villitis,[84] in addition to sepsis.[77]

In patients with antiphospholipid syndrome, the protein C pathway can also be the target of autoantibodies that can inhibit pathway function and contribute to thrombosis.[85] Antibodies against

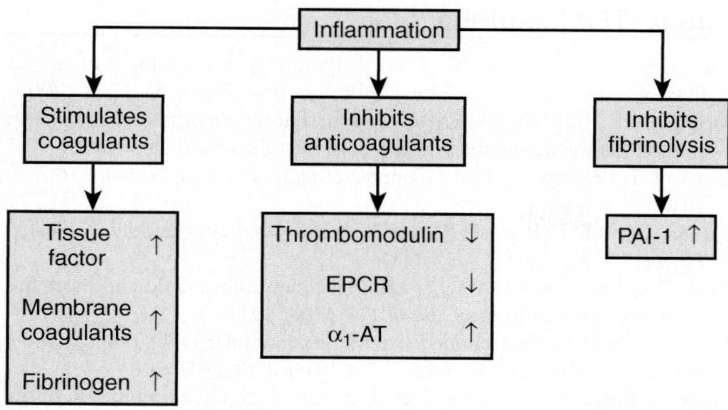

Figure 129-5 THE IMPACT OF INFLAMMATION ON THE REGULATION OF COAGULATION. Inflammatory mediators, such as TNF-α, downregulate thrombomodulin, the endothelial cell protein C receptor (EPCR), and vascular heparin-like molecules, resulting in a decrease in the natural anticoagulant pathways. *α_1-AT,* an inhibitor of APC, is upregulated. These same mediators upregulate tissue factor, triggering coagulation. Complement activation leads to the expression of procoagulantly active lipids on membrane surfaces, which facilitates the amplification of the response. Inflammation also leads to increased plasminogen activator inhibitor 1 (PAI-1) levels, resulting in downregulation of the fibrinolytic pathway. *α_1-AT,* α_1-Antitrypsin. *(Modified from Xu J, Lupu F, Esmon CT: Inflammation, innate immunity and blood coagulation.* Hamostaseologie *30:6, 2010.)*

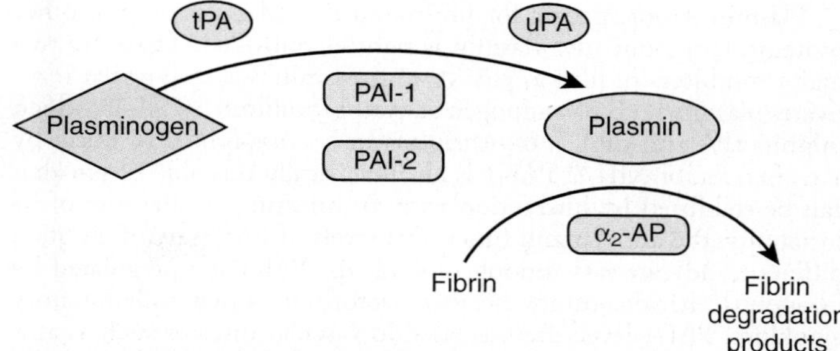

Figure 129-6 SCHEMATIC REPRESENTATION OF THE FIBRINOLYTIC SYSTEM. *α_2-AP,* α_2-Antiplasmin; *PAI,* plasminogen activator inhibitor; *tPA,* tissue plasminogen activator; *uPA,* urokinase plasminogen activator.

every protein involved in the pathway have been detected in selected patients. In addition, antibodies against β2-glycoprotein I, a hallmark of this syndrome, have been shown to inhibit the anticoagulant function of APC.[86] Those antibodies that activate endothelial or other cells and promote a prothrombotic state[87] or impair fibrinolysis[88] may also contribute to thrombosis.

Disease Modulation by Activated Protein C

APC can improve survival or organ function in animal models of inflammatory bowel disease,[79,89] diabetes,[79] myocardial reperfusion injury,[81] stroke,[90-92] and sepsis,[93] the latter being true for humans as well.[94] One of the complications of APC treatment in patients with sepsis is an increased risk for bleeding. In animal models of sepsis, mutant forms of APC that retain their cytoprotective activity, but have reduced anticoagulant activity, have been shown to reduce mortality.[95] These mutants have not been tested in humans.

Trauma results in massive injury, much of this to the microvasculature. To stem the thrombotic risk, protein C is activated. This occurs primarily in the microcirculation where, because of the vast surface to blood volume ratio,[49] the thrombomodulin concentration is extremely high.[49,96] Consequently, high levels of APC are generated in the microcirculation. This may contribute to the coagulopathy that is frequently observed in trauma patients.[97] Protein C levels decline, apparently because of the robust activation, and the APC is postulated to cause a systemic anticoagulant response, which exacerbates the coagulopathy.[97,98] In animal models of trauma, blocking protein C leads to organ dysfunction and death, whereas selectively blocking the anticoagulant activity of APC, but preserving cytoprotective activity, reduces the coagulopathy and improves survival.[99]

Protein S

Protein S circulates in two forms, free protein S and protein S that is tightly but reversibly bound to C4-binding protein, a regulatory protein of the complement system.[100-102] The APC cofactor function of protein S is blocked when it binds to C4-binding protein.[103] When protein S levels decrease in disease, the ratio of free and functional protein S relative to the inactive bound form decreases. Therefore, it is important to measure protein S activity as well as the antigen levels.[104]

Protein S accelerates factor Va inactivation. Importantly, it also alters the cleavage site preference on factor Va. Inactivation of factor Va requires cleavage of two bonds, one at 506 and the other at 306.[105] In a common dimorphism known as factor V Leiden, the cleavage site at 506 is mutated such that the Arg residue at 506 is replaced with a glutamine (Gln).[106] This mutation results in APC resistance and is associated with an increased risk for thrombosis.[24] Cleavage at 506 results in partial loss of factor Va activity, whereas cleavage at 306 results in complete loss of activity. Protein S accelerates the cleavage of the 306 bond, thereby reducing the impact of the factor V Leiden mutation.[107] In addition, factor V enhances APC-mediated inactivation of factor VIIIa,[63] whereas factor V Leiden lacks this ability.[108]

Protein Z and Protein Z–Dependent Protease Inhibitor

Protein Z is a vitamin K–dependent protein that works in concert with protein Z–dependent protease inhibitor and inhibits factor Xa, thereby attenuating coagulation.[109] Deletion of the protein Z gene in mice with factor V Leiden leads to a prothrombotic phenotype.[110] A possible association between genetic defects in protein Z–dependent protease inhibitor and thrombosis has been reported.[111]

REGULATION OF FIBRINOLYSIS

Fibrinolysis is the process by which fibrin clots are dissolved, either through natural mechanisms or with the aid of pharmaceutical interventions. Plasmin is the serine protease that solubilizes fibrin. Plasmin is generated by the activation of its precursor plasminogen either by natural activators, tissue plasminogen activator (tPA),[112] the major activator in the circulation, or urokinase plasminogen activator (uPA)[113] (Fig. 129-6), or by administration of recombinant tPA or streptokinase, a bacterial protein that promotes plasmin generation and aids in dissemination of the bacteria.[13] Staphylokinase, a protein from *Staphylococcus aureus,* is similar to streptokinase and also has been examined as a potential therapeutic.[114]

Fibrin plays an active role in its own degradation because it binds plasminogen and tPA, thereby concentrating them on the fibrin surface and promoting their interaction. The resultant plasmin cleaves fibrin and exposes C-terminal Lys residues that serve as additional plasminogen and tPA binding sites. TAFIa attenuates fibrinolysis by releasing these C-terminal Lys residues.[74] Furthermore, Lys analogues, such as ε-aminocaproic acid or tranexamic acid, bind to tPA and plasminogen. Consequently, these Lys analogues can be used to treat patients with hyperfibrinolysis and can reduce bleeding complications.[115]

Plasmin is not specific for fibrin and degrades a variety of other proteins. Consequently, plasmin is tightly controlled. There are two major inhibitors of fibrinolysis: α_2-antiplasmin,[116] a serpin that inactivates plasmin, and plasminogen activator inhibitor 1 (PAI-1), which inhibits tPA and uPA.[117] α_2-Antiplasmin is cross-linked to fibrin by activated factor XIII.[116] PAI-1 is an intrinsically unstable serpin that can be stabilized by interaction with vitronectin.[118,119] Because of its instability, the antigen and functional levels of PAI-1 are often quite different and can vary among individuals. PAI-1 is upregulated by lipopolysaccharide, tumor necrosis factor, and other inflammatory cytokines. PAI-1 levels are increased in vascular diseases such as atherosclerosis and in metabolic syndrome, sepsis, and obesity.[117] Increased levels of PAI-1 result in decreased fibrinolytic activity, which increases the risk for thrombosis. PAI-1 is also stored in platelets and is released with platelet activation.[117] Platelet-derived PAI-1 may limit the degradation of platelet-rich thrombi, such as those that trigger acute coronary syndromes.

Overall the fibrinolytic system is dynamic and responsive to local phenomena, such as platelet-derived PAI-1, as well as to systemic alterations like obesity and inflammation.[117] In this sense, the fibrinolytic control mechanisms share many similarities with the control of coagulation, in which similar considerations affect their function.

SUGGESTED READINGS

Binder BR, Christ G, Gruber F, et al: Plasminogen activator inhibitor 1: Physiological and pathophysiological roles. *News Physiol Sci* 17:56, 2002.

Delvaeye M, Noris M, De Vriese A, et al: Thrombomodulin mutations in atypical hemolytic-uremic syndrome. *N Engl J Med* 361:345, 2009.

Esmon CT: Far from the heart: Counteracting coagulation. *Nat Med* 16:759, 2010.

Esmon CT, Xu J, Lupu F: Innate immunity and coagulation. *J Thromb Haemost* 9:182, 2011.

Fuchs TA, Bhandari AA, Wagner DD: Histones induce rapid and profound thrombocytopenia in mice. *Blood* 118:3708, 2011.

Fuchs TA, Brill A, Duerschmied D, et al: Extracellular DNA traps promote thrombosis. *Proc Natl Acad Sci U S A* 107:15880, 2010.

Hackeng TM, Sere KM, Tans G, et al: Protein S stimulates inhibition of the tissue factor pathway by tissue factor pathway inhibitor. *Proc Natl Acad Sci U S A* 103:3106, 2006.

Huntington JA: Serpin structure, function and dysfunction. *J Thromb Haemost* 9:26, 2011.

Piro O, Broze GJ Jr: Comparison of cell-surface TFPIalpha and beta. *J Thromb Haemost* 3:2677, 2005.

For complete list of references log on to www.expertconsult.com.

CHAPTER 130

CLINICAL APPROACH TO THE PATIENT WITH BLEEDING OR BRUISING

Catherine P.M. Hayward

Bruising and bleeding problems are common reasons for a hematology referral.[1] The management of an acute bleed (e.g., life-threatening hemorrhage from an acquired factor VIII inhibitor, an anticoagulant drug, or a postpartum hemorrhage) should be the first priority because diagnostic test results are often not immediately available. Most assessments of bruising and bleeding symptoms are not urgent, but they can be challenging because individuals without bleeding problems often experience bleeding symptoms (e.g., bruising with trauma, nosebleeds).[1-3] Furthermore, most individuals referred for assessment of bleeding problems have experienced some bleeding symptoms.[3] In addition, many individuals referred for bleeding symptoms have bleeding disorders; consequently, there is a high pretest probability for a bleeding disorder among such patients.[3]

Some referrals for bleeding disorder assessments are for asymptomatic problems (e.g., abnormal coagulation tests due to vitamin K deficiency, evaluation of a familial bleeding problem after diagnosis of other relatives). Mild bleeding symptoms (e.g., bruising, nosebleeds, possible abnormal bleeding with prior surgery) are more common than severe symptoms (e.g., severe bleed from anticoagulant therapy, life-threatening postpartum hemorrhage) among referred individuals. Sometimes the bleeding symptoms reflect an underlying bone marrow disorder (e.g., bleeding and thrombocytopenia due to leukemia or a platelet function defect induced by a myelodysplastic or myeloproliferative syndrome). Some causes of bleeding, such as vitamin C deficiency (scurvy), are rare in developed countries. For all assessments for bleeding or bruising, it is important to assess symptoms that are concerning to the patient and/or physician and the range of bleeding symptoms/problems that the person has or has not experienced when considering possible causes.[1,3] The next step is to formulate a differential diagnosis and plans for bleeding symptom management (e.g., control of menorrhagia), including strategies to minimize future bleeding risks.[3]

Fig. 130-1 provides a general guide to the steps in a clinical assessment. Bleeding-history assessment tools provide a detailed framework to evaluate the medical history and to determine which symptoms should be considered more suspicious of an underlying bleeding problem.[4-8] Unfortunately, none of the published bleeding-history assessment tools has been prospectively validated for ruling in, or ruling out, a bleeding disorder at the time of an initial assessment for bleeding problems[4] (see box on Influences on Presenting Problems). A very high bleeding score is consistent with a bleeding problem.[4-7,9] However, there is overlap of scores for individuals with and without bleeding problems.[4,5] These tools provide evidence that some bleeding symptoms are uncommon unless there is a bleeding disorder (e.g., joint bleeds, bruises that are as large or larger than an orange or that track downward).[2,4,7,8] Nonetheless, further research is needed to develop tools with acceptable utility for ruling in or ruling out bleeding disorders at the time of an initial assessment (see box on Case 1: Illustration of a Mild, Inherited Bleeding Problem).

Some bleeding symptoms, such as menorrhagia or nosebleeds, are not specific to any particular type of bleeding problem.[1,3,7] Bleeding can be triggered or exacerbated by therapies for atherosclerotic disease (aspirin and/or $P2Y_{12}$ inhibitors, inhibitors of $\alpha_{IIb}\beta_3$), venous thrombotic disease (prophylaxis or treatment with anticoagulants), inflammatory states (e.g., treatment with prednisone or other glucocorticoids) and pain (prescription or nonprescription use of nonsteroidal antiinflammatory drugs [NSAIDs]).[1,3] Bruising can also reflect topical corticosteroid use and/or age-related changes in the skin (i.e., senile purpura).[1,3]

Without treatment, severe bleeding disorders typically cause abnormal bleeding with all major hemostatic challenges. On the other hand, bleeding may not occur with every challenge in persons with mild defects and lower bleeding risks (e.g., those with a 5- to 10-fold increased risk for bleeding). Age influences the bleeding history by increasing the likelihood of exposures to hemostatic challenges and the development of sequelae such as arthropathy in patients with severe hemophilia.[6,7] A severe bleed with surgery that is unexplained may be considered suspicious of a bleeding problem. However, if the person reports that prior challenges did not result in bleeding, this narrows down the possibilities to a mild inherited bleeding disorder, an acquired bleeding disorder, or an iatrogenic condition (e.g., bleeding while on anticoagulant therapy or a technical problem during surgery that caused bleeding). A bleeding-disorder assessment needs to consider both familial and personal bleeding symptoms (see box on Case 2: Illustration of the Importance of Assessing Both Personal and Familial Bleeding Problems).

The timing of bleeding with challenges is evaluated to assess whether the bleeding problem reflects a common bleeding disorder, such as von Willebrand disease, a platelet function disorder, an undefined mucocutaneous bleeding problem, or a rarer cause, such as a defect or deficiency in a coagulation factor or fibrinolytic protein[1,3] (see box on Case 3: Illustration of the Importance of Assessing Bleeding Problems Over Time; see also boxes on Cases 1 and 2). Although patients will often know whether bleeding began on the day of a challenge, their recall of timing details is often better when procedures were done without general anaesthesia (e.g., dental extractions, biopsies).[1,3,7] Bleeding within a few hours or on the same day of a challenge (e.g., surgery or dental extraction) is most suggestive of a defect involving von Willebrand factor or platelets.[1,3,7] Delayed bleeding (beginning 1 or more days after a challenge) is most suggestive of a coagulation or fibrinolytic defect (see boxes on Cases 1 and 2).[1,3,7] However, the onset of some bleeding, such as postpartum hemorrhage, can be delayed in persons with von Willebrand disease or platelet function disorders.[1,3,10-14] Postpartum bleeding may be absent in mild bleeding disorders because pregnancy increases the levels of some hemostatic proteins, including fibrinogen and von Willebrand factor. Bleeding during pregnancy, after implantation, is uncommon with most bleeding disorders, although it can be severe in individuals with bleeding disorders who develop placental abruption (e.g., from an untreated fibrinogen disorder or factor XIII deficiency). Intracranial bleeding in a child may suggest a severe defect or deficiency of factor XIII, a coagulation factor deficiency, or a fibrinolytic inhibitor, but other conditions should be considered if the diagnostic tests for these conditions are negative.

EPIDEMIOLOGY

An understanding of the epidemiology of bleeding problems requires distinction between symptoms that rarely represent a pathologic condition and do not require investigation or therapy (e.g., isolated "easy bruising") and those that are more suspicious, require treatment, and/

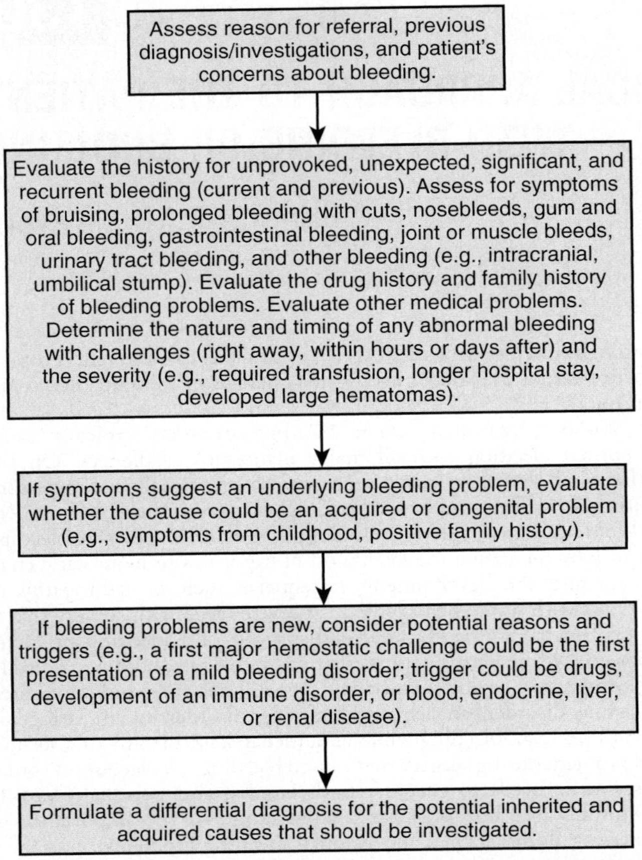

Assess reason for referral, previous diagnosis/investigations, and patient's concerns about bleeding.

↓

Evaluate the history for unprovoked, unexpected, significant, and recurrent bleeding (current and previous). Assess for symptoms of bruising, prolonged bleeding with cuts, nosebleeds, gum and oral bleeding, gastrointestinal bleeding, joint or muscle bleeds, urinary tract bleeding, and other bleeding (e.g., intracranial, umbilical stump). Evaluate the drug history and family history of bleeding problems. Evaluate other medical problems. Determine the nature and timing of any abnormal bleeding with challenges (right away, within hours or days after) and the severity (e.g., required transfusion, longer hospital stay, developed large hematomas).

↓

If symptoms suggest an underlying bleeding problem, evaluate whether the cause could be an acquired or congenital problem (e.g., symptoms from childhood, positive family history).

↓

If bleeding problems are new, consider potential reasons and triggers (e.g., a first major hemostatic challenge could be the first presentation of a mild bleeding disorder; trigger could be drugs, development of an immune disorder, or blood, endocrine, liver, or renal disease).

↓

Formulate a differential diagnosis for the potential inherited and acquired causes that should be investigated.

Figure 130-1 STEPS TO EVALUATE BLEEDING AND BRUISING PROBLEMS.

Influences on Presenting Problems

When evaluating a bleeding history, it is important to recognize that the presenting problems are influenced by the following:

1. The nature and severity of the defect, the presence of a single or multiple risk factors for bleeding
2. Whether the bleeding problem is congenital or acquired
3. Antecedent exposures to hemostatic challenges (such as surgery, dental extraction, menses, and childbirth) and the risk for bleeding with each of these challenges
4. The presence of other medical problems (e.g., renal, liver, or thyroid disease), including anemia
5. Variability in the bleeding symptoms experienced by individuals without bleeding problems (e.g., nosebleeds, bruising) and by individuals with known bleeding disorders, even within families with the same defect
6. Local factors (e.g., vascular lesions, diverticular disease, or cancerous lesions in the gastrointestinal tract)
7. Treatments that increase the risk for bleeding (e.g., nonsteroidal antiinflammatory drug [NSAID] use for pain control, anticoagulant therapy, etc.)
8. Whether treatments were used to prevent or control bleeding, or if they reduced bleeding when prescribed for other reasons (e.g., reduced menstrual bleeding while on oral contraceptives to prevent pregnancy)

Case 1: Illustration of a Mild, Inherited Bleeding Problem

A 77-year-old man who is starting treatment for multiple myeloma was discovered to have a prolonged activated partial thromboplastin time (aPTT). Review of his records indicated that the abnormality was present on a previous admission for spinal cord compression, which was treated with surgery. He required 4 units of packed red blood cells several days after this surgery because of delayed postoperative bleeding. There was no other bleeding history. He was found to have mild factor IX deficiency, unrelated to the myeloma, and his daughter proved to be a carrier of this defect.

Case 2: Illustration of the Importance of Assessing Both Personal and Familial Bleeding Problems

A 22-year-old woman was referred for evaluation of a possible platelet disorder. She had a history of menorrhagia (3 to 4 days out of 7 days of flow were heavy when not on treatment), prolonged nosebleeds in childhood, and hematuria only with urinary tract infections. She did not have thrombocytopenia, and she had no exposure to major hemostatic challenges. Her father, uncle, and grandfather had a striking bleeding history, and two of them had thrombocytopenia. The bleeding in her relatives included joint bleeds with trauma and severe, delayed-onset bleeding after trauma and surgery (usually more than a day later), which continued for weeks despite platelet transfusions. One of these relatives reported no bleeding when he had a tooth extracted while receiving fibrinolytic inhibitor therapy. Although menorrhagia is not specific to any one type of bleeding disorder, the delayed bleeding in affected relatives suggests a possible autosomal dominant disorder and either a fibrinolytic defect or a factor deficiency (the latter had been excluded in previous tests of the affected relatives). Because of the history of thrombocytopenia, joint bleeds, and delayed bleeding, which did not respond well to platelet transfusions, testing was done for the Quebec platelet disorder. The referred patient and her relatives were confirmed to have this disorder by genetic testing for duplication mutation of the urokinase plasminogen activator gene. This case illustrates the importance of evaluating both the personal and family bleeding history and highlights the fact that bleeding-symptom severity can vary among affected family members, in part because of their different exposures to challenges and treatments.

Case 3: Illustration of the Importance of Assessing Bleeding Problems Over Time

A 72-year-old man was referred for evaluation of a severe bleed after receiving a single dose of low-molecular-weight heparin for unconfirmed deep vein thrombosis. He had a history of a similar bleeding episode several years previously while on warfarin treatment for atrial fibrillation. There was no other bleeding history, and the patient subsequently developed a spontaneous iliopsoas bleed. He had undergone numerous surgeries earlier in life without any bleeding problems, and there was no family history of bleeding. The bleeding history suggested the possibility of an acquired bleeding problem, possibly acquired von Willebrand disease or an acquired factor deficiency. Diagnostic testing indicated that he had acquired factor XIII deficiency. This case illustrates the fact that more than one risk factor for bleeding can coexist: in this case, several exposures to anticoagulants triggered bleeding in a patient with an acquired factor deficiency. On initial treatment of his iliopsoas bleed with factor XIII concentrates there was partial neutralization of the infused factor followed by accelerated clearance, consistent with acquired factor XIII deficiency secondary to an autoantibody.

or are highly predictive of a bleeding problem.[1,3] Some individuals have multiple risk factors for bleeding (e.g., low von Willebrand factor levels, exposure to drugs that inhibit platelet function after a surgical procedure associated with a high risk for bleeding).[3] Although some symptoms, such as nosebleeds, easy bruising, and menorrhagia, are quite prevalent in the general population (10% or more report these symptoms), these problems are more frequent and more severe in individuals with bleeding disorders.[1-4,7,10,15,16] Menorrhagia requiring treatment is common among women, and it can be life-threatening in severe bleeding disorders.[11,15,17,18] With moderate or severe disorders, there is less debate about the disease prevalence than there is for milder disorders (e.g., type 1 von Willebrand disease) where there is ongoing debate about the diagnostic criteria that define a pathologic abnormality.[10] There is less information on the prevalence of disorders that require complex tests for diagnosis and have many potential causes (e.g., platelet function disorders). Undefined disorders (definite bleeding problems despite normal or nondiagnostic test findings) have emerged to be a common cause of mucocutaneous bleeding.[19,20]

The process of a referral for bleeding makes it quite likely that the person has had some bleeding symptoms that may or may not reflect an underlying congenital or acquired bleeding problem.[1,3] Because of this referral bias, the prevalence of bleeding disorders in tertiary referral clinics is much higher than in the general population. The prevalence of inherited bleeding disorders in the general population is quite low (from 0.00023% to over 1% for von Willebrand disease, with much lower estimates based on studies of bleeding disorder–clinic cases compared with those derived from population screening using higher cutoffs to define quantitative deficiencies; 0.005% to 0.01% for hemophilia; and much lower for other coagulation factor deficiencies). Consequently, unselected screening is not recommended.[1,3,10,21] Founder effects in populations can alter the prevalence of both common and rare inherited bleeding disorders.

A person with a first-degree relative with an autosomal dominant bleeding problem, or a sibling with a recessively inherited disorder, has a higher pretest probability for an inherited bleeding disorder.[7,10] When assessing the relative of someone with a positive family history of a bleeding problem, it is important to realize that the person may have the same condition or a different bleeding problem.[7] Furthermore, it is common for affected family members to show some variability in the severity of their bleeding symptoms.[7,10] Index cases typically have more bleeding symptoms.[1,4] Accordingly, laboratory investigations are often used to assess family members at high risk, even in the absence of a remarkable personal bleeding history.

Common bleeding disorders that are inherited as autosomal dominant traits include von Willebrand disease, many common platelet function disorders (including secretion defects, MYH9-related disorders, gain-of-function disorders such as platelet-type von Willebrand disease and Quebec platelet disorder), and dysfibrinogenemia.[1,3,10,16] Because the diagnostic criteria for mild von Willebrand disease have changed,[10] a positive family history often requires reevaluation.

X-linked bleeding disorders include hemophilia A, hemophilia B, and X-linked congenital platelet disorders (e.g., Wiskott-Aldrich syndrome or thrombocytopenia due to GATA1 mutations).[1,3,16] X-linked disorders typically affect males but can affect women with skewed X-chromosome inactivation or Turner syndrome. Recessively inherited bleeding disorders are the most rare, and their prevalence is highest in populations in which consanguinity is culturally accepted.[22]

Acquired bleeding problems are common, and the most frequent cause is a drug-induced defect.[1,3] Drugs that alter hemostasis may cause bleeding on their own or unmask symptoms from a mild or moderate underlying bleeding disorder.[1,3,23] Drug-induced problems to consider include the following: (1) use of prescription or nonprescription NSAIDs that transiently inhibit platelet cyclooxygenase-1 (COX-1) (patients may not recall taking these drugs if they received them after a surgical procedure[3,23]); (2) aspirin or $P2Y_{12}$ or $\alpha_{IIb}\beta_3$ inhibitors used for acute or chronic prevention or treatment of cardiovascular disorders; (3) anticoagulants prescribed for the prevention or treatment of venous thromboembolic disease, atrial fibrillation, or acute management of atherosclerotic disease; (4) antidepressant medications (e.g., serotonin reuptake inhibitors), which may cause bruising symptoms; and (5) glucocorticoid therapy.[1,20,24,25] Some dietary practices affect platelet function (e.g., use of fish oil supplements, ingestion of herbal supplements with aspirin-like properties), as can acute alcohol intoxication.[3,16]

Among adults with von Willebrand disease, factor VIII deficiency, and factor XIII deficiency, about 10% of the cases are due to an acquired, autoantibody-induced deficiency state. Autoimmune causes of other bleeding disorders include immune thrombocytopenia, immune-mediated platelet dysfunction (more commonly due to antibodies against glycoprotein IbIXV or $\alpha_{IIb}\alpha_3$), and acquired factor V deficiency.[1,3] Bone marrow disorders are associated with an increased risk for autoimmune or nonimmune bleeding problems, including thrombocytopenia, secondary platelet function defects of diverse etiology (e.g., acquired forms of dense granule deficiency, Glanzmann thrombasthenia, or Bernard-Soulier syndrome), or acquired von Willebrand disease.[16] Acquired bleeding problems can also accompany the development of renal disease, liver disease, hypothyroidism, or Cushing syndrome.[1,3]

PATHOBIOLOGY

There are many different components of the hemostatic, fibrinolytic and vascular response to injury that are important for prevention and control of bleeding (see Chapters 123, 124, 125, 127, and 128). Normal hemostasis requires platelet adhesion to collagen and aggregate formation at sites of tissue injury, which requires von Willebrand factor and other adhesive proteins; the initiation of coagulation by tissue factor; followed by amplification and propagation of coagulation to generate thrombin and convert fibrinogen to fibrin. It also requires stabilization of fibrin through the cross-linking actions of activated factor XIII. The activation of fibrinolysis (which is important for wound healing) is part of the normal response to tissue injury and repair. Fibrinolysis is retarded by platelets (which release large quantities of stored plasminogen activator inhibitor 1 [PAI-1]) and accelerated by deficiencies or defects in PAI-1 or α_2-antiplasmin, gain-of-function defects in plasminogen activators, and pathologic states that increase fibrinolysis. The interdependence of hemostatic mechanisms explains why a failure of platelet adhesive mechanisms (e.g., from defects in platelet number or function or von Willebrand disease) may cause persistent, delayed, and/or recurrent bleeding from a wound site, particularly if initial hemostasis was inadequately managed. That activation of fibrinolysis occurs during hemostasis explains why fibrinolytic inhibitors are often effective for treating diverse bleeding problems (e.g., menorrhagia and bleeding from oral/nasal surgical or dental procedures) in patients with conditions from von Willebrand disease and platelet disorders to factor deficiencies and fibrinolytic defects. Some individuals with severe nosebleeds or gastrointestinal bleeds from platelet function disorders (e.g., Glanzmann thrombasthenia) that are refractory to platelet transfusions (because of development of antibodies) may respond to treatment with recombinant factor VIIa.

Hemostasis is also influenced by other factors, such as anemia. The red cell concentration in blood influences platelet margination, which allows platelets to adhere to the injured vessel wall. Accordingly, anemia can worsen bleeding. Some disorders of hemostasis reflect defects in the vessel wall. For example, hereditary hemorrhagic telangiectasia (which does not always present with obvious skin or oral vascular lesions)[26] can cause troublesome bleeding from sites where the vascular malformations are located. These lesions can cause recurrent epistaxis, gastrointestinal bleeding, and less commonly, intracranial or pulmonary hemorrhage typically without causing bleeding with surgical procedures or menorrhagia.[1,3]

CLINICAL MANIFESTATIONS

Age of Presentation and Extent of Symptoms

Inherited bleeding disorders can present at any age, but if severe, a bleeding disorder typically presents at a younger age.[1,3,6,7,27] Milder disorders can present at any age and may require a significant hemostatic challenge to come to medical attention, often a major surgical procedure or a dental extraction.[1,3,6,7,27] Women with mild, moderate, or severe inherited bleeding disorders may present with troublesome bleeding at the onset of menses or with childbirth-related bleeding.[1,3,7,27] When the bleeding risks are only mildly increased (e.g., low von Willebrand factor levels without other defects, a mild inherited platelet secretion defect), there may be a history of bleeding with some, but not all, hemostatic challenges.[1,3,10]

The severity of a bleeding disorder affects the number, severity, and type of manifestations. Numerical scores, derived from standardized bleeding-history assessment tools, show considerable overlap among subjects with different disease severities.[4] Although use of a standardized tool has been recommended by the International Society on Thrombosis and Haemostasis,[5] the tool has yet to be prospectively validated for use in clinical practice.

Family History and Syndromic Disorders

It is important to consider that the family history for an inherited bleeding disorder is influenced by the disorder severity and the mode of inheritance and whether there is a single or multiple bleeding disorders in the family. The family history is often negative if the cause is an acquired problem, such as iatrogenic bleeding from anticoagulant therapy or a technical problem complicating a surgical or dental procedure.[1] The family history is typically positive when the disorder is autosomal dominant and has high penetrance.[3,7,10] The family history is negative in individuals with novel mutations and in those with recessive disorders unless there are affected siblings or many affected relatives from consanguinity or founder effects. Individuals with mild disorders who have never had a hemostatic challenge may be referred after another family member is identified to have a bleeding problem or if the person has bleeding after a significant hemostatic challenge.[1,3] Early identification of a disorder may alter the natural history, particularly if treatment is given before hemostatic challenges.[7]

Some patients have other clinical problems that suggest the possibility of a syndromic disorder (e.g., albinism or a history of delayed pigmentation, hearing loss, nephritis, absent radii) or an alternative diagnosis (e.g., hyperextensibility due to Ehlers-Danlos syndrome).

Bruising, Petechiae, and Other Skin Changes

Bruising (which reflects bleeding into the skin) is a very commonly reported bleeding symptom.[3,4,7,10,16] Bruising is reported more frequently by women than men.[2]

Some bruising symptoms are more suggestive of a bleeding problem than others. For example, bruises from bleeding disorders often occur after minimal or no recalled trauma.[3,4,7,10,16] Bruises that are unusually large (e.g., as big or bigger than an orange) or lumpy or that migrate (i.e., track downward to the feet over time) are consistent with more extensive bleeding into cutaneous or subcutaneous tissues and are more specific, but not highly sensitive, for bleeding disorders.[4,7,10] When bruises are large or multiple, patients may hide them (by wearing pants and long-sleeve shirts) to avoid being questioned. Severe bruising symptoms may lead to lifestyle changes (e.g., avoidance of sports or other activities that increase the risk for bruising).[7] When there is significant swelling with a bruise, imaging (e.g., by ultrasound) may be necessary to exclude bleeding into deeper tissues.

Bruising symptoms (that are normal or abnormal) can fluctuate, depending on activity levels and exposure to drugs or trauma that increase bruising risks (e.g., increased bruising when moving house, traveling, or engaging in physical sports; bruising in a toddler who just started walking; worsened bruising after initiating antidepressant therapy). Like normal bruising, bruising from bleeding disorders usually occurs at sites that are commonly exposed to trauma (e.g., lower limbs, outer hips, arms). However, bruising with acquired hemophilia A may be extensive and involve other regions (e.g., the trunk). This type of bruising is probably autoantibody related because it does not occur in congenital hemophilia, even if there is an inhibitor.

An examination of the skin sometimes reveals bruising associated with skin pigmentation changes from iron deposition. This is typical of repeated bleeds in persons with severe platelet function disorders or moderate to severe forms of von Willebrand disease. These pigment changes are typically localized to sites of recurrent trauma (e.g., anterior shins), and the distribution (which can be spotty) helps to distinguish the finding from the pigmentation associated with venous stasis.

Petechiae and/or oral blood blisters are typical of severe thrombocytopenia and are less commonly seen in other conditions, including severe platelet function disorders. Scurvy can cause perifollicular hemorrhages (often on the shins), bruising, and gum bleeding, typically with associated swelling and redness. Schamberg disease is a pigmented purpuric dermatitis that does not represent a bleeding problem and can be mistaken for petechiae. Early lesions of purpura fulminans, from congenital deficiency of protein C or protein S, may be mistaken for bruises, but the age of the patient and the distribution of the lesions help to establish the diagnosis. Skin bleeding from minor lesions (e.g., skin cancers) can be unusually troublesome for patients with a severe bleeding disorder.

Epistaxis

Epistaxis is a commonly reported bleeding symptom that does not always reflect a bleeding disorder, even when the bleeding is frequent and/or requires medical interventions.[2-5,7] Although nosebleeds can be due to mucocutaneous bleeding disorders (e.g., platelet or von Willebrand factor problems), they can also be due to severe deficiencies of common pathway coagulation factors (e.g., congenital deficiency of factor V, factor X, or prothrombin), fibrinolytic defects (PAI-1 or α_2-antiplasmin deficiency, increased platelet urokinase plasminogen activator [uPA] from Quebec platelet disorder) or hereditary hemorrhagic telangiectasia.* Nosebleeds, from bleeding disorders or other causes, are often worse in childhood.

When the volume of bleeding from the nose is large, the patient may experience passage of clots, anteriorly and posteriorly, sometimes with melena. Although nosebleeds are not specific to bleeding disorders, it is important to ask about them because severe nosebleeds can be disabling for some individuals with bleeding disorders, such as von Willebrand disease.[3,10]

Gum Bleeding and Bleeding With Loss of Primary Teeth

Gum bleeding can be problematic with inherited or acquired bleeding disorders that affect platelets or von Willebrand factor, although it more frequently reflects gum disease.[1,3,10,22] Severe bleeding with the loss of primary teeth is also suspicious of an underlying bleeding disorder.*

Gastrointestinal Bleeding

Gastrointestinal bleeding can complicate a bleeding disorder, but it is rarely the presenting problem, and it requires investigation to determine the source of the bleeding.[1,3,4,10] Gastrointestinal bleeding can be severe with hereditary hemorrhagic telangiectasia.[26]

Challenge-Related Bleeding

The assessment of challenge-related bleeding is an important part of taking a bleeding history. Bleeding related to accidental trauma may

*References 1, 3, 7, 10, 16, 22.

be more difficult to evaluate than bleeding associated with surgery or dental procedures because accidental trauma often causes bleeding, and it is difficult to determine whether the extent of bleeding was excessive.[7] In addition, large wounds may continue to bleed until sutured.

A history of bleeding with surgical or dental procedures can include being told that there was excessive bleeding by a dentist, physician, or other health care worker and/or experiencing: excessive oozing or drainage from incision or extraction sites; wound hematomas; delayed wound healing; bleeding requiring repeated surgery, suturing of an extraction site, an admission to hospital, a longer hospital stay, and/or transfer to the intensive care unit; and receiving blood transfusions, drugs, and/or factor replacement for hemorrhage control.[1,3,7] Patients may not spontaneously report some symptoms, such as extensive bruising around surgical incisions. Occasionally an operative report or other medical document provides important confirmation that there was abnormal bleeding with surgery (e.g., an operative note that documents generalized oozing during a procedure and greater-than-expected total blood loss).[1,3] Iatrogenic reasons (e.g., oozing vessels that were not cauterized or ligated) should be considered when there is a history of an isolated bleeding episode.

Many individuals undergo dental extractions at some point in their life. Bleeding that persists beyond the first day, or that becomes problematic one or more days after a dental extraction, should be considered suggestive of a bleeding disorder.[1,3] Severe bleeding with dental cleaning should be considered suggestive of a congenital or an acquired bleeding disorder (e.g., von Willebrand disease or a platelet function disorder).

In individuals with a moderate-to-severe bleeding problem, bleeding after surgery, dental procedures, or a severe throat infection can lead to airway compromise, whereas bleeding from a surgical or traumatic limb injury can lead to compartment syndrome.[1,3,28]

Bleeding Symptoms Restricted to Women

Women with bleeding disorders experience more bleeding than men because of the hemostatic challenges associated with menses and childbirth.[17,29] Such women are also at increased risk for developing endometriosis and hemorrhage from ovarian cysts.[17,29] They may also report troublesome bruising or bleeding with sexual activity.

Menorrhagia is a fairly common manifestation of bleeding disorders, and the hemostatic cause can be von Willebrand disease, a platelet disorder, or a defect in coagulation or fibrinolysis.[7,16,17,29] However, menorrhagia can be due to other causes, such as fibroids.[3,18,29] Menorrhagia from inherited bleeding disorders is often long-standing, but it can be influenced by treatments. Accordingly, it is important to ask about menses when on, and not on, treatment. Menorrhagia can develop as a manifestation of an acquired bleeding problem (e.g., from acquired von Willebrand disease or anticoagulant therapy for deep vein thrombosis).

In general, it is more helpful to ask women quantitative or categorical questions about menses, rather than qualitative questions (e.g., are/were your menstrual periods heavy?). Questions to consider include the following: How many days of bleeding do you have with your typical menstrual periods? How many days of this bleeding was heavy flow? On your heavy days of flow, did you soak through sanitary products in an hour or less? What treatments have you taken for heavy periods? When you were not on treatment, how many days of bleeding (and how many days of heavy flow) did you have with a typical menstrual period? Were your periods like this when they first began, or did the heavy-flow problems start later in your life?

Menses up to 7 days in total duration, with 2 to 3 days of heavy flow, can be considered normal.[4,5,7,17,29] Although influenced by the absorbency of the products used, soaking through sanitary products in less than an hour is suspicious of menorrhagia, as is doubling up on products because of heavy flow and gushing and flooding accidents. Dysmenorrhea is common among women with bleeding disorders, and the passage of large blood clots (which reflect increased flow), which is typically painful, suggests the possibility of a bleeding disorder.[5] Pictorial bleeding-assessment tools (which are not applicable to an initial consultation visit) can be helpful to document menorrhagia and responses to treatment.[11,29]

Postpartum hemorrhage is rarely due to an underlying bleeding problem, and it can be complicated by a profound acquired coagulopathy, typically with severe fibrinogen depletion.[12-14] On the other hand, excessive or prolonged bleeding after childbirth or pregnancy loss can be problematic for some women with bleeding problems.[10,12] In addition, severe fibrinogen disorders and factor XIII deficiency compromise carrying a pregnancy to term and need to be excluded if the patient has unexplained pregnancy losses that are associated with hemorrhagic placental abruption[3] (see box on Case 4: Evaluation of an Isolated Symptom—Recurrent Pregnancy Loss With Bleeding).

During the first week after childbirth, the bleeding (lochia) is typically characterized by brighter red flow than a normal period. Afterward, the flow usually lightens and continues for up to 6 weeks postpartum. Flow can be heavier, or persist longer, in women with bleeding disorders.[10,12]

Anemia Related to Bleeding

A history of anemia and/or prior treatment with iron replacement is frequently reported by women with bleeding disorders.[3,17] Pallor of the palms is often observed when the hemoglobin is below 10 g/dL. Anemia is uncommon in individuals with bleeding disorders unless there is acute bleeding or chronic persistent bleeding leading to iron deficiency that compromises red cell production. Many women with bleeding disorders and menorrhagia have low iron stores, but not anemia. Low iron stores may also reflect ongoing gastrointestinal bleeding (overt or occult), which if present, requires investigation even if there is a known congenital or acquired bleeding problem. Some bleeding disorders (e.g., platelet disorders from GATA1 mutations) are associated with anemia and thrombocytopenia.

Joint Bleeds and Muscle Bleeds

Joint bleeds and bleeding into muscles (e.g., iliopsoas bleeds) are uncommon bleeding symptoms that suggest a severe coagulation defect or a fibrinolytic disorder.[1,3,6,7] However, bleeding into a joint after an injury or an orthopedic (e.g., arthroscopic) procedure can be experienced by persons with other types of bleeding disorders.[1,3,6,7] In patients with severe factor deficiencies, the clinical assessment should evaluate for symptoms and signs of arthropathy and muscle wasting and if relevant, neurologic sequelae complicating compartment syndrome bleeds.

Case 4: Evaluation of an Isolated Symptom—Recurrent Pregnancy Loss With Bleeding

A 32-year-old woman was referred for evaluation of a low fibrinogen level in the setting of an acute placental abruption, resulting in a third pregnancy loss (this time in the third trimester). She had no prior bleeding history apart from having suffered three placental abruptions associated with severe bleeding that required transfusion. The family history was negative for bleeding problems. She had previously been investigated for thrombophilia but had not been tested for a bleeding disorder. The low fibrinogen level persisted over many months (levels of approximately 90 mg/dL), suggesting that the defect was inherited. She received fibrinogen concentrate for two subsequent pregnancies, which she carried to term and delivered without bleeding problems. This case illustrates the need to consider inherited disorders when the bleeding symptoms are unusual and severe, even if there is only one bleeding symptom. It also illustrates that prognosis is dependent on diagnosis and treatment.

Subdural and Intracranial Hemorrhage

A newborn or child presenting with spontaneous intracranial hemorrhage or a large cephalohematoma should be investigated for severe underlying bleeding disorders, such as thrombocytopenia, hemophilia, factor XIII deficiency, other coagulation factor deficiencies, or a severe defect in platelets or von Willebrand factor.[1,3-5] Trauma-related subdural or intracranial hemorrhages can also be manifestations of a severe bleeding disorder.[1,3-5] In adults, thrombotic strokes are more frequent than hemorrhagic strokes, although hemorrhagic strokes appear to predominate with some bleeding disorders (e.g., Quebec platelet disorder[7]), and they can be complications of antithrombotic drug treatment.

Hematuria

Urinary tract bleeding with an infection is a commonly reported symptom, whereas spontaneous (or unexplained) hematuria can complicate hemophilia and other bleeding disorders, such as Quebec platelet disorder.[3,7,28]

Bleeding at Birth, Age-Related Changes in Bleeding, and Very Rare Bleeding Symptoms

Many individuals cannot answer questions about bleeding at the time that they were born. Nonetheless, bleeding from the umbilical stump or a cephalohematoma at birth can be symptoms of a bleeding disorder.[6,7] Menarche can cause a marked increase in bleeding in women with inherited or acquired bleeding problems. Some individuals with inherited bleeding disorders report a reduction in their bleeding symptoms as they age, which could reflect lifestyle adaptation and age-related increases in hemostatic protein levels (e.g., von Willebrand factor or fibrinogen) and thrombin generation. Increases in bleeding with aging can suggest an acquired problem (see box on Case 5: Illustration of Changes in Bleeding Problems Over Time).

Some types of bleeds are quite rare among individuals with bleeding disorders, including spontaneous hemorrhage into the spleen, which can lead to rupture (see box on Signs of Active or Recent Bleeding).

LABORATORY MANIFESTATIONS

The general investigations that are appropriate for most assessments of bleeding problems include (1) a complete blood count (to establish if there is thrombocytopenia or anemia), (2) an assessment for a low ferritin level to evaluate for iron deficiency (less commonly associated with microcytosis or anemia; deficit should be corrected if bleeding risks are increased), (3) a blood group and antibody screen, particularly for individuals with prior pregnancies or transfusions and upcoming surgery or major dental procedures, and (4) tests of renal function (creatinine) if antifibrinolytic therapy will be considered because the dosage is dependent on renal function or if an MYH9-related disorder is suspected (see box on The Laboratory Manifestations of Bleeding Disorders). The bleeding time test is no longer recommended, due to its technical limitations and poor sensitivity to common bleeding disorders.[3,16] Electrolyte levels merit monitoring when repeated doses of desmopressin therapy are given and/or if the fluid balance is difficult to assess. Tests of liver function are warranted if the person has risks for transfusion-acquired, chronic liver disease. Tests for liver and thyroid disease (particularly hypothyroidism) can be helpful if the history suggests an acquired bleeding problem of unknown etiology. Screening for Cushing syndrome (24-hour urine test for free cortisol) should be restricted to patients with acquired bleeding problems that suggest this possibility (e.g., bleeding associated with obesity, the development of type 2 diabetes, hypertension, striae, and/or changes in physical appearance).

Case 5: Illustration of Changes in Bleeding Problems Over Time

A 65-year-old woman presented for urgent evaluation of a bleeding problem, requiring treatment for a symptomatic, expanding subdural hematoma. She had been previously diagnosed with type 1 von Willebrand disease but indicated that she had no bleeding problems (despite many challenges) until she reached 30 years of age, when she began to experience increasing problems with bruising, menorrhagia, and challenge-related bleeding, including severe gum bleeds with routine dental cleaning. An activated partial thromboplastin time (aPTT) had been performed and was elevated. The testing confirmed a low level of factor VIII (14%) and a low level of ristocetin cofactor activity (less than 10%). The patient was given emergency treatment with plasma-derived von Willebrand factor concentrate containing factor VIII. Intravenous γ-globulin was given because she had a very poor response to replacement, suggesting rapid clearance of von Willebrand factor and factor VIII. Her von Willebrand factor and factor VIII levels increased above normal within 24 hours of the intravenous γ-globulin treatment, consistent with acquired von Willebrand disease. Additional tests indicated that she had an immunoglobulin G (IgG) paraprotein without evidence of myeloma. Several features of her presentation suggested that her von Willebrand disease was probably acquired and not due to type 1 von Willebrand disease (which is more common): her increasing bleeding symptoms over time and lack of bleeding problems during childhood or early adulthood, her very low level of factor VIII (due to its clearance with von Willebrand factor), the IgG paraprotein, her poor response to von Willebrand factor replacement, and her excellent response to intravenous γ-globulin. She has since been managed with intermittent intravenous γ-globulin treatment.

Signs of Active or Recent Bleeding and Conditions Associated With Bleeding

Although findings from the physical examination in bleeding disorders are often normal, it is important to look for signs of active or recent bleeding, including the following:

1. Petechiae, perifollicular hemorrhages (typical of scurvy)
2. Oral blood blisters, particularly if the patient has thrombocytopenia
3. Ecchymoses, hematomas, and skin pigmentation changes due to recurrent bleeds
4. Signs of active bleeding from a site of trauma or an incision, including excessive blood loss into drains
5. Sequelae of previous bleeds in individuals known or suspected to have a severe bleeding disorder, such as muscle wasting and arthropathy, neurologic abnormalities from prior intracranial or compartment syndrome bleeds
6. Pallor due to anemia: the palms are usually notably pale when the hemoglobin is less than 10 g/dL
7. Signs of an underlying hematologic disorder, such as lymphadenopathy and/or splenomegaly
8. Signs of acute or chronic liver disease, such as jaundice, hepatomegaly, spider nevi, palmar erythema, or Dupuytren contractures
9. Signs of an endocrine disorder, such as hypothyroidism or Cushing syndrome
10. Vascular lesions such as telangiectasia on the face or buccal mucosa, which can suggest hereditary hemorrhagic telangiectasia
11. Hyperextensibility if the bleeding history suggests Ehlers-Danlos syndrome as a potential diagnosis
12. Signs that suggest a syndromic bleeding disorder (albinism, hearing impairment, absent radii)

The Laboratory Manifestations of Bleeding Disorders

The laboratory manifestations of bleeding disorders can include abnormalities from the following:

1. The underlying hemostatic defect
2. Bleeding complications (e.g., anemia, iron deficiency, a coagulopathy of hemodilution after resuscitation for a massive bleed, development of red cell antibodies after transfusion)
3. False-positive abnormalities (e.g., prolonged activated partial thromboplastin time [aPTT] due to an incidental mild factor XII deficiency that occurs in about 1 of 200 patients or a lupus anticoagulant, which can be a transient finding in about 5% of ill, hospitalized patients)
4. Extremes of normal variation (e.g., mildly low von Willebrand factor levels in an individual who is blood group O, absent secondary aggregation with epinephrine in adjusted platelet rich–plasma aggregation studies).

The investigations for a bleeding problem typically also include screening tests (prothrombin time, activated partial thromboplastin time [aPTT], thrombin clotting time, and fibrinogen level), which are inexpensive tests, that detect acquired coagulopathies much more commonly than they detect inherited bleeding disorders because of differences in prevalence. These investigations are useful as a baseline for individuals at risk for developing a dilutional coagulopathy from bleeding and as initial investigations of a possible inherited or acquired coagulation disorder. Abnormalities, if detected, require further evaluation to determine if the cause is a fibrinogen disorder or a deficiency of one or more coagulation factors. Screening tests for von Willebrand disease are warranted for individuals with a personal or familial history of mucocutaneous bleeding.[10] Platelet function disorders should be evaluated by aggregation tests and tests for dense granule release, if available, because these tests are useful for assessing common bleeding disorders.[20,30] Chapters 131 and 132 provides more detail on the specific diagnostic tests that are appropriate for a laboratory workup of bleeding problems.

DIFFERENTIAL DIAGNOSIS OF BRUISING AND BLEEDING

The initial differential diagnosis should focus on three major categories (Table 130-1): deciding whether there is (1) no bleeding disorder, (2) a possible bleeding disorder (equivocal bleeding history and nondiagnostic laboratory findings), or (3) a definite bleeding disorder.

There are many potential inherited and acquired causes of definite bleeding problems (summarized in Tables 130-2 and 130-3). The history should be evaluated to determine if the problems suggest a defect in the initial control of bleeding (e.g., defects in platelet adhesion from von Willebrand disease or a platelet problem) or if there are delayed bleeding problems that suggest a defect in a coagulation factor or a fibrinolytic protein. Laboratory findings are important for distinguishing undefined bleeding problems from von Willebrand disease and platelet function disorders, because their symptoms are quite similar.[1,3,19,20,30]

Acquired bleeding problems due to drugs are often diagnosed solely by the medical history (i.e., acquired bleeding problems that occurred while taking a medication that inhibits coagulation or platelet function), although laboratory testing can be useful to rule out other causes. The subject's medical history and laboratory findings are helpful to determining if there is a possibility of acquired bleeding problems from a bone marrow disorder, liver disease, renal failure, or an endocrine disorder (e.g., hypothyroidism or, less commonly, Cushing syndrome)

Table 130-1 Differential Diagnosis of Bleeding Problems

Major Categories	Comments
No bleeding disorder	Symptoms do not reflect a bleeding disorder and have another explanation (e.g., a surgical bleed, not due to a bleeding disorder).
Possible bleeding disorder	The laboratory findings are nondiagnostic, and the bleeding history is considered equivocal (e.g., unexplained serious bleed with one surgical procedure; unexplained menorrhagia without other bleeding problems).
Definite bleeding disorder, undefined or indeterminate type	The bleeding history is consistent with a bleeding disorder; however, the laboratory findings are nondiagnostic. Commonly the bleeding history resembles mild to moderate defects in platelet function or von Willebrand factor. The diagnosis should only be made once an adequate evaluation for common bleeding disorders (e.g., for von Willebrand disease and platelet aggregation and release defects) is completed. If testing is not complete, the classification should indicate the types of conditions excluded or not excluded, for example: mild mucocutaneous bleeding problem, von Willebrand disease excluded, mild mucocutaneous bleeding problem, platelet release defects not yet excluded.
Definite bleeding disorder with a defined cause	The symptoms and laboratory findings are considered diagnostic of a bleeding disorder. Tables 130-2 and 130-3 summarize many of the potential inherited and acquired causes.

PROGNOSIS

The prognosis for bleeding problems depends on the severity of the nature of the hemostatic defect, exacerbating factors, and whether these problems can be readily corrected (e.g., vitamin K to correct a deficiency, discontinuing aspirin) or if they require hemostatic therapies, such as factor concentrates and/or drugs (e.g., desmopressin, tranexamic acid, or aminocaproic acid). Life expectancy is generally normal unless there is a severe bleeding disorder (e.g., severe hemophilia) or a complication (e.g., transfusion-acquired chronic hepatitis or human immunodeficiency virus [HIV]). The prognosis for some rare disorders significantly improves after puberty (e.g., factor IX Leyden). A few show progressive worsening over time (e.g., development of aplasia from congenital amegakaryocytic thrombocytopenia, transformation of thrombocytopenia from an inherited RUNX1 mutation into myelodysplasia or acute myeloid leukemia). Other disorders (e.g., acquired hemophilia) may go into complete remission after immunosuppressive treatment with risk for later relapses.

Mild platelet function disorders, mild type 1 von Willebrand disease, and many common undefined conditions that cause mucocutaneous bleeding usually respond sufficiently well to prophylactic desmopressin therapy, which is given to prevent bleeding with major surgical and dental procedures or bleeding with childbirth. Nonetheless, it is important to have a specific diagnosis to manage situations in which desmopressin therapy is insufficient to control bleeding.

Women with bleeding disorders have a similar prognosis to men, although they often have a greater burden of symptoms due to menorrhagia and childbirth-related bleeding.[1,3] Their outcomes with pregnancy and childbirth are often similar to individuals without bleeding disorders provided that they receive treatment to control bleeding with delivery.[1,3] However, some disorders have sufficiently good outcomes with childbirth that treatment for uncomplicated childbirth is not required (e.g., for Quebec platelet disorder).[7,28] Childbirth plans for women with bleeding disorders requires consideration of the

Table 130-2 Differential Diagnosis of Congenital Bleeding Disorders

Disorder	Comments
Fibrinogen deficiency or dysfunction	Deficiencies can be mild-moderate hypofibrinogenemia or severe afibrinogenemia. Fibrinogen function is abnormal in dysfibrinogenemias, which can present with bleeding, thrombosis, or both. Fibrinogen levels can be reduced in some dysfibrinogenemias.
X-linked coagulation factor deficiencies—hemophilia	Presentation is influenced by the degree of deficiency. Factor VIII deficiency is more common than factor IX deficiency. If factor VIII is low, von Willebrand disease needs to be excluded as the cause.
Rarer, coagulation factor deficiencies	Deficiencies can affect factors XI, V, II, VII, or X, and the presentation is dependent on the severity of the deficiency. Hereditary deficiencies of multiple coagulation factors are rare (e.g., of factors V and VIII, or multiple vitamin K–dependent coagulation factors for congenital defects impairing γ-carboxylation) and can easily be excluded by measuring multiple factors.
Fibrinolytic defects	Causes include disorders caused by loss of function, such as α_2-antiplasmin or PAI-1 deficiency, and by gain-of-function defects, such as Quebec platelet disorder (overexpression of urokinase plasminogen activator in megakaryocytes).
von Willebrand disease	Causes include quantitative (partial type 1 to severe type 3) and qualitative defects (loss of function in type 2M and 2A, gain of function in type 2B and platelet-type). Type 1 von Willebrand disease can be confused with low von Willebrand factor levels (e.g., due to blood group O).
Platelet disorders	These conditions can affect platelet number, function, or both. The most common type of platelet function disorder is a platelet secretion defect, which may or may not also impair aggregation responses. Disorders of platelet function are commonly subclassified by the nature of the defect, such as the following: 1. Defects of membrane receptors for adhesive proteins (e.g., Glanzmann thrombasthenia and Bernard-Soulier syndrome) or agonists (e.g., $P2Y_{12}$ deficiency) 2. Defects of signaling or secretion (the largest subcategory) 3. Cytoskeletal defects (e.g., MYH9-related disorders) 4. Storage pool disorders (e.g., gray platelet syndrome, dense granule deficiency, αγ-storage pool deficiency, Quebec platelet disorder) 5. Defects of procoagulant function (e.g., Scott syndrome)
Vascular disorders	Congenital vascular malformation, including hereditary hemorrhagic telangiectasia, Ehlers-Danlos syndrome

options for pain management and avoidance of procedures, such as spinal or epidural anesthesia, to limit bleeding risks unless the defect can be readily corrected.

THERAPY

An individual's bleeding history is an important consideration whenever formulating therapeutic plans to control and minimize bleeding risks. Some symptoms do not warrant therapy (e.g., bruising), whereas treatment is important for controlling menorrhagia and for preventing and limiting challenge-related bleeding (e.g., from major or minor surgery and dental procedures, and traumas). For severe disorders, prophylactic treatment is warranted to prevent spontaneous bleeding and to limit challenge-related bleeding, which can be severe. The focus of therapy for some acquired conditions (e.g., acquired hemophilia) is immunosuppressive therapy to achieve a remission while managing any acute bleeding that warrants therapy. For individuals with mild bleeding disorders, who have undergone multiple prior surgical procedures without bleeding, it may be appropriate to have treatment available (e.g., desmopressin on "standby") that is to be administered if and when abnormal bleeding occurs, provided that the procedural-related risks of bleeding are small and readily managed (e.g., biopsy under local anaesthetic) while waiting for the medication to have an effect.

For women with bleeding disorders, there are general treatments that can be considered for symptomatic management regardless of the type of bleeding disorder. For example, options for menorrhagia management include oral contraceptives, antifibrinolytic drugs, and hormone-releasing intrauterine devices. When menorrhagia limits lifestyle and further pregnancies are not desired, surgical options (endometrial ablation, hysterectomy) may be preferred options, particularly when menopause is not imminent.

General management of bleeding often includes supportive care, correction and prevention of anemia (e.g., iron replacement for iron deficiency), and immunization against viruses that may be acquired by blood transfusion (e.g., hepatitis A and B) (see box on Case 6: Illustration of Changes in Bleeding Outcomes With Treatment). If the patient is immobilized or is undergoing a procedure with significant risks for thrombosis, there should be plans for anticoagulant therapy if the defect can be corrected during this treatment (e.g., by factor replacement therapy for hemophilia or von Willebrand disease, fibrinolytic inhibitor therapy for Quebec platelet disorder) or for alternative thromboprophylaxis if this is not possible (e.g., use of venous compression devices without anticoagulant drugs if the treatment will provide only brief hemostatic correction [e.g., desmopressin, platelet transfusions]). Other measures to limit bleeding risks from bleeding disorders, with surgery, include the avoidance of intramuscular injections, spinal and epidural anesthesia, and NSAIDs for pain management. In older individuals with bleeding disorders and symptomatic atherosclerotic disease (e.g., angina), aspirin therapy may be appropriate, with increased vigilance for signs and symptoms of significant bleeding.

For more information on therapies for specific disorders, see the chapters on hemophilia (Chapters 137 and 138), rare coagulation factor deficiencies (Chapter 139), von Willebrand factor (Chapter 140), and platelet disorders (Chapter 132).

FUTURE DIRECTIONS

The development of a bleeding-assessment tool with sufficient utility to distinguish persons with bleeding disorders from those without significant bleeding problems could improve the clinical assessment of bleeding disorders. There is a need for more information on the genetic causes of common disorders (e.g., type 1 von Willebrand disease, common platelet function disorders such as secretion defects) to further understand bleeding disorder pathogenesis and bleeding risks.

Table 130-3 Differential Diagnosis of Acquired Bleeding Problems

Disorder	Comments
Drug induced	Aspirin, NSAIDs, other platelet function inhibitors (e.g., $P2Y_{12}$ and $\alpha_{IIb}\beta_3$ inhibitors), anticoagulants, fibrinolytic drugs, and antidepressants are common causes
Acquired factor deficiencies	The causes can be immune (e.g., acquired factor VIII deficiency, acquired factor V deficiency) or nonimmune. Reductions in multiple factors can result from vitamin K deficiency, treatment with vitamin K antagonists, liver disease, hemodilution, and rarely snakebites. Severe acquired hypofibrinogenemia is commonly due to a postpartum coagulopathy or severe liver disease. Prothrombin deficiency occurs with some lupus anticoagulants. Amyloidosis can cause an acquired factor X deficiency, which may be associated with reductions in other coagulation factors synthesized in the liver if the liver is involved.
Disseminated intravascular coagulation	The manifestations can include thrombocytopenia, consumption of coagulation factors, including fibrinogen, and impairment of hemostatic mechanisms from the fibrin/fibrinogen degradation products. Causes are wide ranging and include postpartum consumptive states, prostate and other cancers, and snakebites.
Acquired von Willebrand disease	The cause can be immune (often in association with an IgG paraprotein) or nonimmune (e.g., increased proteolysis of von Willebrand factor with stenotic aortic valvular disease).
Immune thrombocytopenia	Bleeding is usually influenced by the extent of the thrombocytopenia. Some autoantibodies interfere with platelet membrane receptor function, causing bleeding disproportionate to the thrombocytopenia.
Non–drug induced, acquired platelet function disorders	The cause can be immune (see earlier) or nonimmune, typically from bone marrow disorders, although secretion defects can be secondary to Cushing syndrome or hypothyroidism.
Liver disease	Liver disease can cause thrombocytopenia, deficiencies of coagulation factors, hypofibrinogenemia and dysfibrinogenemia, and increased fibrinolysis. In mild liver disease, factor VII and sometimes factors XI and XII are low. Fibrinogen is often increased in early liver disease, and if low, the finding suggests severe liver disease.
Renal disease	Anemia is an important predictor of uremic bleeding. Uremic bleeding is typically associated with severe renal impairment.
Hypothyroidism	Hypothyroidism can cause an acquired von Willebrand disease and acquired defects in platelet function.
Cushing syndrome	This syndrome should be suspected when there are symptoms and findings suggestive of Cushing syndrome or treatment with systemic or topical glucocorticoids.
Surgical bleeding	This is often a diagnosis of exclusion, although the procedural notes sometimes document that a technical problem was encountered that led to abnormal bleeding.
Vitamin K deficiency	Newborns are at risk, as are individuals with malabsorption and/or receiving broad-spectrum antibiotics that reduce vitamin K production by reducing gut bacteria. Older adults are also at greater risk for developing vitamin K deficiency, due to reduced stores from poorer intake of vitamin K. If the patient does not respond to parenteral vitamin K, other causes should be considered.
Vitamin C deficiency (scurvy)	This diagnosis should be considered when there is lethargy with skin and gum bleeding (perifollicular hemorrhages, gum bleeding with swelling). The condition is rare in developed countries. The cause is usually a very poor diet or malabsorption.

IgG, Immunoglobulin G; *NSAID,* nonsteroidal antiinflammatory drug.

Case 6: Illustration of Changes in Bleeding Outcomes With Treatment

A 38-year-old woman was evaluated for a bleeding disorder. Her family physician had already excluded the possibility of von Willebrand disease. The patient had a long-standing history of massive bruises, often without recollection of trauma, prolonged nosebleeds requiring medical attention since early childhood, prolonged bleeding from minor cuts, and severe bleeding requiring blood transfusions with many surgical procedures. She had a history of recurrent iron deficiency anemia, menorrhagia requiring medical therapies, and immediate postpartum bleeding. Her father had a history of bleeding problems, but the cause of the bleeding problem in the family was unknown. The history suggested an inherited disorder, possibly a platelet function disorder or a form of von Willebrand disease. The testing indicated that she had a platelet secretion defect with multiple aggregation abnormalities, with no evidence of von Willebrand disease. She underwent additional surgical procedures, using desmopressin treatment to reduce her bleeding risks, with no abnormal bleeding. Her menorrhagia was controlled with tranexamic treatment. She self-administered desmopressin treatment to control nosebleeds, with good effect. This case illustrates that treatment affects bleeding outcomes and the importance of evaluating for common defects in hemostasis.

REFERENCES

1. Greaves M, Watson HG: Approach to the diagnosis and management of mild bleeding disorders. *J Thromb Haemost* 5:167, 2007 .
2. Mauer AC, Khazanov NA, Levenkova N, et al: Impact of sex, age, race, ethnicity and aspirin use on bleeding symptoms in healthy adults. *J Thromb Haemost* 9:100, 2011.
3. Hayward CP: Diagnosis and management of mild bleeding disorders. *Hematology Am Soc Hematol Educ Program* 423, 2005.
4. Tosetto A, Castaman G, Rodeghiero F: Bleeding scores in inherited bleeding disorders: Clinical or research tools? *Haemophilia* 14:415, 2008.
5. Rodeghiero F, Tosetto A, Abshire T, et al: ISTH/SSC bleeding assessment tool: A standardized questionnaire and a proposal for a new bleeding score for inherited bleeding disorders. *J Thromb Haemost* 8:2063, 2010.
6. Biss TT, Blanchette VS, Clark DS, et al: Quantitation of bleeding symptoms in children with von Willebrand disease: Use of a standardized pediatric bleeding questionnaire. *J Thromb Haemost* 8:950, 2010.

7. McKay H, Derome F, Haq MA, et al: Bleeding risks associated with inheritance of the Quebec platelet disorder. *Blood* 104:159, 2004.
8. Mauer AC, Barbour EM, Khazanov NA, et al: Creating an ontology-based human phenotyping system: The Rockefeller University bleeding history experience. *Clin Transl Sci* 2:382, 2009.
9. Marcus PD, Nire KG, Grooms L, et al: The power of a standardized bleeding score in diagnosing paediatric type 1 von Willebrand's disease and platelet function defects. *Haemophilia* 17:223, 2011.
10. Nichols WL, Hultin MB, James AH, et al: Von Willebrand disease (VWD): Evidence-based diagnosis and management guidelines, the National Heart, Lung, and Blood Institute (NHLBI) Expert Panel report (USA). *Haemophilia* 14:171, 2008.
11. James AH: Women and bleeding disorders. *Haemophilia* 16:160, 2010.
12. Chi C, Bapir M, Lee CA, et al: Puerperal loss (lochia) in women with or without inherited bleeding disorders. *Am J Obstet Gynecol* 203:56, 2010.
13. Siboni SM, Spreafico M, Calo L, et al: Gynaecological and obstetrical problems in women with different bleeding disorders. *Haemophilia* 15:1291, 2009.
14. Kadir RA, Kingman CE, Chi C, et al: Is primary postpartum haemorrhage a good predictor of inherited bleeding disorders? *Haemophilia* 13:178, 2007.
15. Philipp CS, Faiz A, Heit JA, et al: Evaluation of a screening tool for bleeding disorders in a U.S. multisite cohort of women with menorrhagia. *Am J Obstet Gynecol* 204:209, 2011.
16. Hayward CP: Diagnostic evaluation of platelet function disorders. *Blood Rev* 25:169, 2011.
17. James AH, Kouides PA, Abdul-Kadir R, et al: Evaluation and management of acute menorrhagia in women with and without underlying bleeding disorders: Consensus from an international expert panel. *Eur J Obstet Gynecol Reprod Biol* 158:124, 2011.
18. Kouides PA: Bleeding symptom assessment and hemostasis evaluation of menorrhagia. *Curr Opin Hematol* 15:465, 2008.
19. Mezzano D, Quiroga T, Pereira J: The level of laboratory testing required for diagnosis or exclusion of a platelet function disorder using platelet aggregation and secretion assays. *Semin Thromb Hemost* 35:242, 2009.
20. Hayward CP, Pai M, Liu Y, et al: Diagnostic utility of light transmission platelet aggregometry: Results from a prospective study of individuals referred for bleeding disorder assessments. *J Thromb Haemost* 7:676, 2009.
21. McHugh J, Holt C, O'Keeffe D: An assessment of the utility of unselected coagulation screening in general hospital practice. *Blood Coagul Fibrinolysis* 22:106, 2011.
22. Borhany M, Pahore Z, Ul Qadr Z, et al: Bleeding disorders in the tribe: Result of consanguineous in breeding. *Orphanet J Rare Dis* 5:23, 2010.
23. Masso Gonzalez EL, Patrignani P, Tacconelli S, et al: Variability among nonsteroidal antiinflammatory drugs in risk of upper gastrointestinal bleeding. *Arthritis Rheum* 62:1592, 2010.
24. Loewen P, Dahri K: Risk of bleeding with oral anticoagulants: An updated systematic review and performance analysis of clinical prediction rules. *Ann Hematol* 90:1191, 2011.
25. Chen WT, White CM, Phung OJ, et al: Association between $CHADS_2$ risk factors and anticoagulation-related bleeding: A systematic literature review. *Mayo Clin Proc* 86:509, 2011.
26. McDonald J, Bayrak-Toydemir P, Pyeritz RE: Hereditary hemorrhagic telangiectasia: An overview of diagnosis, management, and pathogenesis. *Genet Med* 13:607, 2011.
27. Mikhail S, Kouides P: Von Willebrand disease in the pediatric and adolescent population. *J Pediatr Adolesc Gynecol* 23:S3, 2010.
28. Hayward CP, Rivard GE: Quebec platelet disorder. *Expert Rev Hematol* 4:137, 2011.
29. Peyvandi F, Garagiola I, Menegatti M: Gynecological and obstetrical manifestations of inherited bleeding disorders in women. *J Thromb Haemost* 9:236, 2011.
30. Pai M, Wang G, Moffat KA, et al: Diagnostic usefulness of a lumi-aggregometer adenosine triphosphate release assay for the assessment of platelet function disorders. *Am J Clin Pathol* 1363:350, 2011.

CHAPTER 131

LABORATORY EVALUATION OF HEMOSTATIC AND THROMBOTIC DISORDERS

Alvin H. Schmaier

The clinical laboratory evaluation is an integral part of the diagnosis and management of patients with hemostatic/thrombotic disorders. A clinical hematologist when challenged by patients with hemostatic/thrombotic disorders is as good as the laboratory that serves him or her for diagnosis and management. This chapter provides a critical practical approach to the diagnosis and management of bleeding and clotting disorders. The latter activity is a new use of laboratory resources for what until the present era has mostly been a diagnostic facility.

Physiologic hemostasis is the sum of protein (coagulation, fibrinolytic, and anticoagulation) and cellular (platelets, endothelial cells, and leukocytes) elements working in concert to staunch the bleeding at sites of vascular injury without occlusive thrombosis. There is no one assay for hemostatic integrity. For example, a patient with Glanzmann thrombasthenia has abnormal platelet function but normal blood coagulation studies. Another patient with factor VIII deficiency has prolonged surface-activated blood coagulation tests, but normal platelet function. Both patients are hemostatically incompetent. The cellular elements, platelets, endothelial cell, and leukocytes localize physiologic hemostasis and provide proteins and peptides that contribute to the process. The proteins of the blood coagulation system lead to thrombin formation. The role of the fibrinolytic system is to lyse clots formed by thrombin. The role of the anticoagulation system is to regulate all the enzymes of the coagulation and fibrinolytic systems so that no excess clotting or bleeding occurs. The sum of these elements leads to the hemostatic plug (Fig. 131-1). Thus the present approach to patients with bleeding disorders is to evaluate the plasma proteins of the hemostatic, fibrinolytic, and anticoagulation systems and platelet number and function that contribute to this process.

For decades the proteins of the hemostatic system have been referred to as the "coagulation cascade" based on the waterfall hypothesis of Ratnoff and Davies[1] and MacFarland,[2] who almost simultaneously reported a sequence of proteolytic reactions starting with factor XII (Hageman factor) activation and ending with formed thrombin proteolyzing fibrinogen to form a clot. However, upon introduction, this hypothesis for physiologic hemostasis was untenable because it was known that factor XII deficiency is not associated with bleeding.[3] By the mid-1970s, the cofactors for factor XII activation (prekallikrein and high-molecular-weight kininogen) were identified, and deficiencies of these proteins also were not associated with a bleeding state.[4-6] In 1977, Osterud and Rappaport[7] recognized that factor VIIa is able to activate factor IX to factor IXa. Later Broze[8] recognized that the kinetics of tissue factor pathway inhibitor (TFPI) were such that, under physiologic circumstances, the factor VIIa/tissue factor complex cannot directly activate factor X, because of the presence of TFPI, but must go through factor IX activation. If this is the case, how does factor XI, whose deficiency is associated with bleeding, become activated independent of factor XIIa? In 1991, Gailani and Broze[9] proposed that formed thrombin cycles back to activate factor XI, resulting in amplification of activation of thrombin formation. Presently, physiologic hemostasis is believed to be an interacting system initiated by factor VIIa and tissue factor activation and amplification of several zymogens that become serine proteases (Fig. 131-2; see Chapter 128). Although the material just presented has become a cohesive hypothesis for physiologic coagulation activation, clinical laboratory testing of the proteins of coagulation is not based on this current understanding—it follows the Ratnoff and Davies hypothesis.

The clinical laboratory assays used to examine the proteins of the coagulation system are based on the original surface-activated coagulation cascade hypothesis.[1,2] Although these tests do not represent physiologic hemostasis, they are useful for diagnosis of defects in coagulation proteins and potential bleeding disorders. Thus the clinician must understand the distinction between physiologic coagulation, fibrinolysis, and anticoagulation contributing to hemostasis and the diagnostic tests that are used to measure these systems. The first part of this chapter describes the assays used to measure blood coagulation–protein bleeding disorders. Understanding these assays is an approach to recognizing a potential bleeding abnormality in a patient. In addition to diagnosis of a bleeding disorder, the coagulation laboratory has the potential to assist the physician in patient management by monitoring changes in the degree of activated blood coagulation.

When faced with a bleeding patient, the hematologist must use an analytic diagnostic approach to determine the cause of the bleeding. Most recognized bleeding states are caused by one of three defects: a defect or deficiency in a plasma protein, a defect in platelet number or function, or a defect in platelet–vessel wall interactions (i.e., an abnormality in the adhesive interactions between platelets and the vessel wall), as in defects associated with the presence or function of von Willebrand factor. Collagen and platelet glycoprotein VI (GPVI) also participate in adhesive interactions, but GPVI deficiency is not a hemostatic disorder.

When approaching the diagnosis of a coagulation protein defect in a patient, understanding the mechanism is paramount. Any coagulation protein defect can be a true protein deficiency, an abnormal protein that cannot participate in its physiologic function(s), or an inhibitor directed against the active site of the protein or one that induces enhanced clearance of the protein. In general, inhibitors to a coagulation protein are immunoglobulins, although abnormal production of endogenous heparin, fibronectin, or cryoglobulins has been reported as the source of acquired inhibitors to coagulation proteins.[10] An abnormal coagulation protein can result from missense, deletion, or translocations of its deoxyribonucleic acid (DNA). Last, enhanced clearance of coagulation proteins usually occurs as a result of an antibody-protein complex that is recognized as foreign and thus removed from the circulation.[11] The resultant increased clearance of the protein results in a deficiency of the protein. Thus clinical laboratory testing, when available, should focus on measuring the presence of the protein by antigen and its functionality by a variety of assays.

In general, hemarthrosis and spontaneous soft-tissue and intramuscular hemorrhage characterize defects of coagulation proteins, such as hemophilia A and B (factors VIII and IX deficiency). Soft-tissue petechiae, purpura, or ecchymoses characterize von Willebrand disease or platelet number or functional disorders. However, distinguishing the potential mechanism for bleeding can be difficult. History and physical examination are important components of the hemostatic workup (see Chapter 130) but are inadequate for specific diagnosis of bleeding or clotting disorders. Thus the clinical laboratory is essential for definitive diagnosis of a blood coagulation protein defect leading to bleeding.

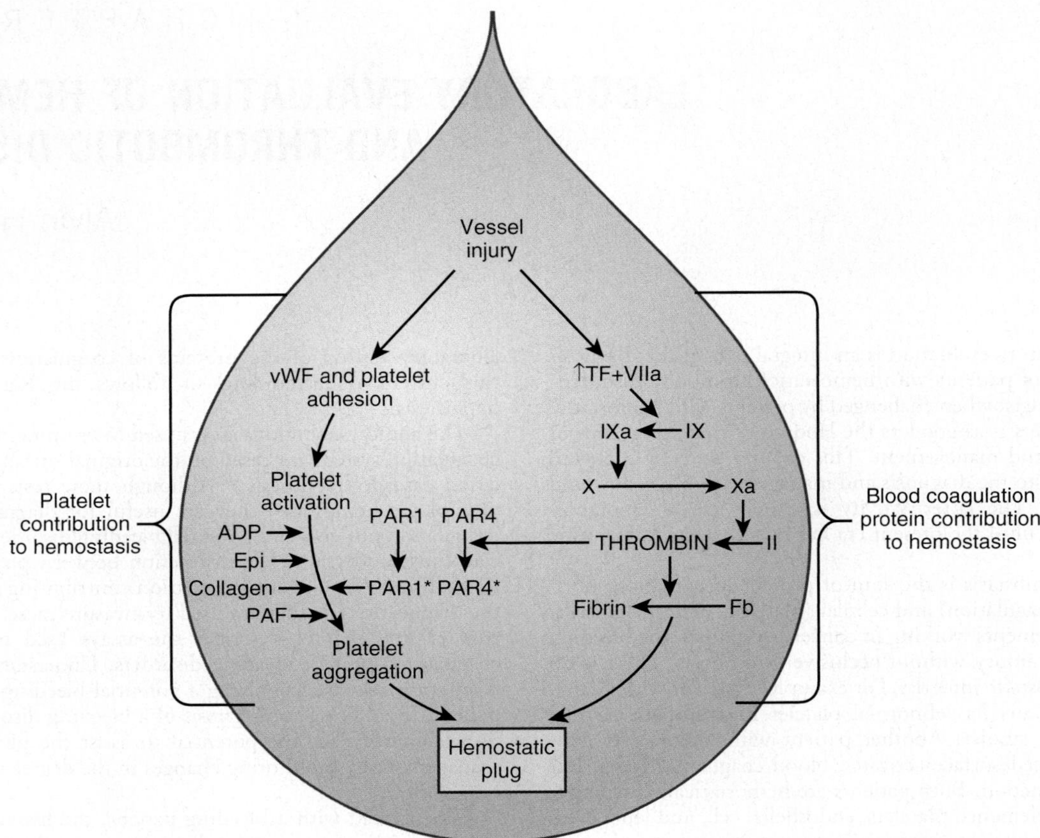

Figure 131-1 SCHEMATIC DIAGRAM OF HEMOSTASIS. Two equally important arms of activity contribute to physiologic hemostasis. The platelet contribution to hemostasis is as follows: When a vessel is injured, exposing collagen, platelets adhere to the injury site via von Willebrand factor (vWF) and, in high-shear areas, glycoprotein VI (not shown in figure). Upon adherence, the platelets are activated and release their granule contents. Released adenosine diphosphate (ADP) and other granule contents recruit more platelets to the injury site. Simultaneously at the site of injury, subendothelial cell tissue factor (TF) is upregulated and with activated factor VII (VIIa) activates factor IX to activated factor IX (IXa) and, sequentially, factor X to activated factor X (Xa) and prothrombin (II) to thrombin. Exposed collagen also allows for factor XII autoactivation and generation of additional thrombin in the milieu of activating platelets (not shown in figure). Thrombin stimulates more platelets, enhancing the platelet plug. Thrombin also proteolyzes fibrinogen to form fibrin monomer, which then polymerizes into a fibrin clot. These events occur on or about the activated platelet surface. *Epi,* Epinephrine; *Fb,* fibrinogen; *PAF,* platelet-activating factor; *PAR,* protease-activated receptor.

CLINICAL SCREENING ASSAYS IN HEMOSTATIC TESTING TO DETECT COAGULATION PROTEIN DEFECTS

In the practice of clinical hemostasis, there are no good global assays for measuring physiologic tissue factor–initiated hemostasis. The three assays most commonly used to examine the proteins of the blood coagulation system are (1) the activated partial thromboplastin time (aPTT) induced by surface (contact) activation of factor XII, (2) the prothrombin time (PT) induced by the addition of excess tissue factor, and (3) the thrombin clotting time (TCT), a test of fibrinogen integrity or inhibitors of the added thrombin. In the aPTT assay, surface or contact activation of the blood coagulation system occurs because factor XII associates with the reagent's negatively charged substances, such that the protein changes shape to allow its autoactivation and subsequent initiation of the cascade of proteolytic reactions seen in the coagulation system.[12-14] These phenomena are the basis of the Ratnoff and Davies hypothesis for activation of the coagulation system. This test measures more proteins (factor XII, prekallikrein, high-molecular-weight kininogen) than those necessary for physiologic hemostasis. In the PT assay, addition of excess tissue factor creates a nonphysiologic change in the normal stoichiometric relationship of coagulation factors, thereby allowing factor VIIa to overcome the inhibitory effect of TFPI and favoring direct activation of factor X to factor Xa without the usual physiologic requirement to proceed through factor IX activation. In the TCT assay, exogenous thrombin is added to examine the integrity of its major substrate, fibrinogen.

When all three assays are performed simultaneously on a sample of plasma, the results indicate almost all of the diagnostic categories for a blood coagulation protein bleeding state. It is most useful to perform a diagnostic evaluation at one time with a complete panel of assays rather than a series of piecemeal studies. The former approach provides a complete snapshot of the patient's blood coagulation parameters, which is best for diagnosis. Patient conditions usually are dynamic, so piecemeal evaluations often miss evolving clinical states. The three screening tests are performed as follows:

1. *Activated partial thromboplastin time.* To perform this assay, equal parts of a negatively charged surface and phospholipid mixture and patient plasma are incubated for more than 5 minutes. Calcium chloride is added to 30 mM to recalcify citrated plasma,

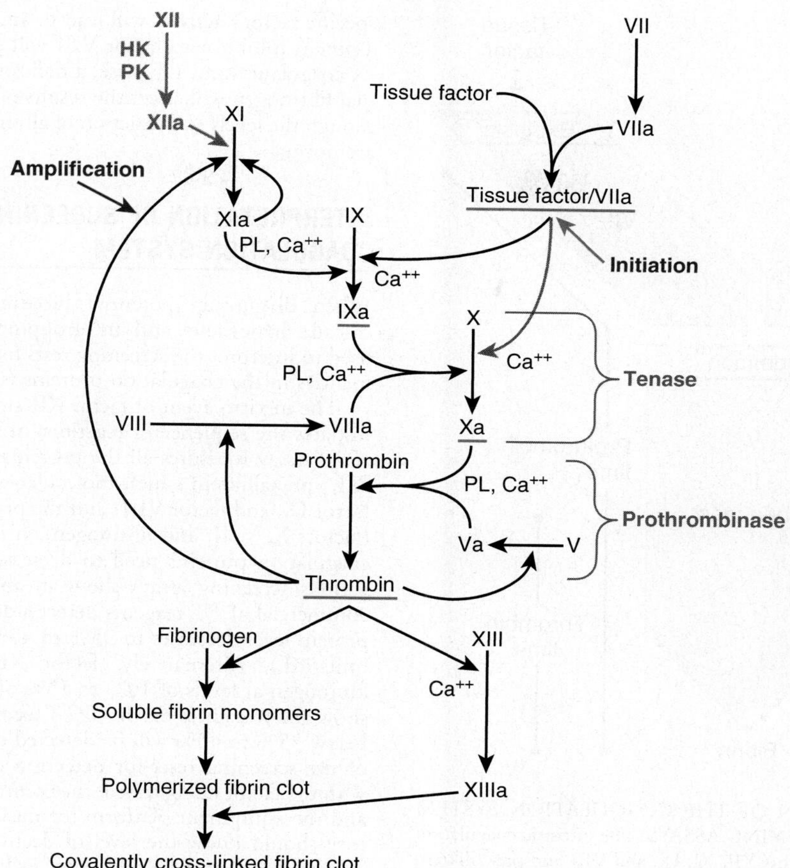

Figure 131-2 SCHEMATIC DIAGRAM OF PHYSIOLOGIC HEMOSTASIS. Formation of the tissue factor–activated factor VII complex (TF/VIIa) results in factor IX activation to activated factor IX (IXa). TF/VIIa does *not* normally activate factor X directly *(brown line)*. Activated factor IX activates factor X to activated factor X (Xa) in the presence of activated factor VIII (VIIIa), which must have been formed from some prior thrombin activation of factor VIII (tenase). Activated factor X in the presence of activated factor V (Va) activates prothrombin to thrombin (IIa) (prothrombinase). Thrombin proteolyzes fibrinogen to form a fibrin clot. If more thrombin is needed, thrombin can activate factor XI to activated factor XI (XIa), which then activates more factor IX to factor IXa, which makes more activated factor X and thrombin. If more thrombin-induced clot formation is needed, thrombin also activates carboxypeptidase U to form a thrombin-activatable fibrinolysis inhibitor (TAFI) that inhibits fibrinolysis (pathway not shown). Factor XI also can be activated by activated factor XII, which is formed secondarily by the constitutive activation of prekallikrein (PK) in the presence of high-molecular-weight kininogen (HK) by contact activation in collagen-exposed injured vessels. These latter mechanisms are *not* constitutive for physiologic hemostasis. However, in nonphysiologic states, such as sepsis, clot formation in the intravascular compartment, or cardiopulmonary bypass, activated factor XII can activate factor XI to initiate hemostasis with thrombin formation. This latter mechanism is the basis of the activated partial thromboplastin time, a major screening test for hemostatic disorders. *PL,* Phospholipid. *(Modified from Schmaier AH, Miller J: Coagulation and fibrinolysis. In McPherson RA, Pincus MR, editors:* Henry's clinical diagnosis and management by laboratory methods, *ed 22, Philadelphia, 2011, Elsevier, p 785.)*

and the time required for clot formation is measured. The aPTT assay assesses the coagulation proteins of the intrinsic and common pathways (Fig. 131-3).[15]

2. *Prothrombin time.* To perform this assay, tissue thromboplastin (tissue-derived or recombinant human tissue factor), phospholipid, and patient plasma are incubated for more than 5 minutes. The plasma then is recalcified by the addition of calcium chloride to 30 mM, and the time required for clot formation is measured. The PT assay assesses the coagulation proteins of the extrinsic and common pathways (see Fig. 131-3).[16] The sensitivity of the assay is based on similarity of the tissue factor used in the assay to human tissue factor (see Interpretation of Screening Tests of the Coagulation System).
3. *Thrombin clotting time.* To perform this assay, purified thrombin is added to plasma, and the time to clot formation is measured. It is a direct measure of the conversion of fibrinogen to fibrin (see Fig. 131-3). When performing this assay, it is essential to use the minimal amount of α-thrombin (3000 units/mg specific activity)

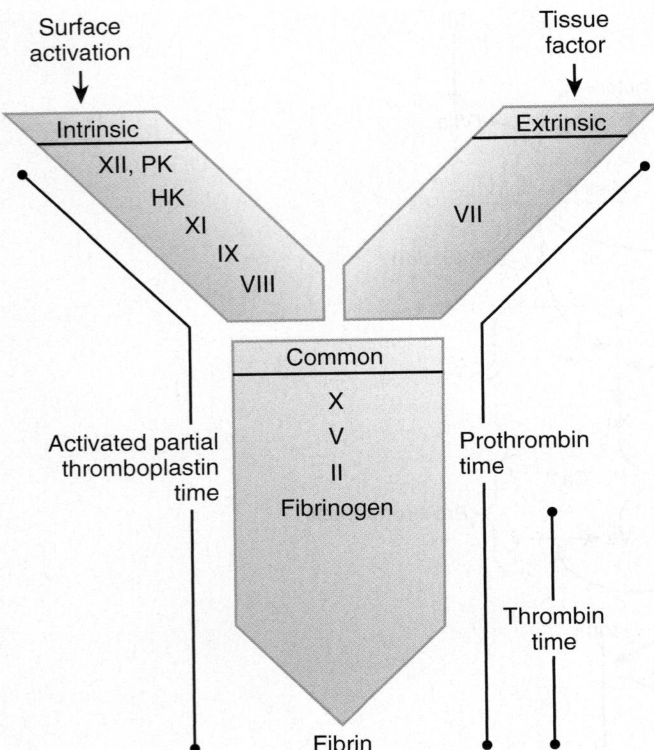

Figure 131-3 ORGANIZATION OF THE COAGULATION SYSTEM BASED ON CURRENT SCREENING ASSAYS. The intrinsic coagulation system consists of the protein factors XII, XI, IX, and VIII and prekallikrein (PK) and high-molecular-weight kininogen (HK). The extrinsic coagulation system consists of tissue factor and factor VII. The common pathway of the coagulation system consists of factors X, V, and II and fibrinogen (I). The activated partial thromboplastin time requires the presence of every protein except tissue factor and factor VII. The prothrombin time requires factors VII, X, V, and II, and fibrinogen. The thrombin clotting time only tests the integrity of fibrinogen. *(Modified from Schmaier AH:* Approach to the bleeding patient. *In Schmaier AH, Petruzzelli LM, editors:* Hematology for the medical student, *Philadelphia, 2003, Lippincott Williams & Wilkins, p 79.)*

that will reproducibly "clot" fibrinogen, usually 2 to 6 units/mL, aiming for approximately 20 seconds with pooled normal plasma to achieve maximal sensitivity for a clinically useful assay.[17,18] This assay is distinguished from the clottable fibrinogen assay (Clauss assay) by the amount of thrombin used (50 units/mL in the Clauss assay).[19]

The results of these assays allow the 40-year-old cascade hypothesis to guide the clinician to a practical differential diagnosis of what protein(s) may be affected. In the coagulation cascade hypothesis, coagulation proteins are classified as members of the intrinsic system, the extrinsic system, or the common pathway (see Fig. 131-3).

All coagulation assays examine the rate of clot formation. In these assays, a sequence of proteolytic reactions takes place, leading to thrombin formation and its proteolysis of fibrinogen. Proteolysis of fibrinogen results in clot formation with precipitation of soluble proteins that are detected by either increased impedance or turbidity or decreased optical clarity, based on the instrumentation used to measure the result. Any defect along the pathway to clot formation will give an abnormal (i.e., a delayed time) result. Furthermore, because a series of reactions must occur to result in the final clot formation, any substance (e.g., inhibitory antibodies, heparinoids, anticoagulants) that interferes with the assay downstream from a specific factor's activity will lead to an abnormal result. For example, a potent inhibitor to factor VIII will give an abnormal factor XI or IX coagulant assay. Likewise, a deficiency of fibrinogen or an abnormal fibrinogen will affect the results of the aPTT and PT assays even though the levels and function of all the upstream coagulation factors are normal.

INTERPRETATION OF SCREENING TESTS OF THE COAGULATION SYSTEM

When diagnosing potential bleeding disorders, the coagulation cascade hypothesis and its grouping of coagulation proteins are used to interpret the screening tests for various deficiencies or abnormalities in the coagulation proteins (see Fig. 131-3).

The in vitro event of factor XII autoactivation in the aPTT assay initiates the sequence of reactions of the coagulation cascade.[1,2] The aPTT assay measures all the proteins of the intrinsic system (factor XII, prekallikrein, high-molecular-weight kininogen, factor XI, factor IX, and factor VIII) and the proteins of the common pathway (factors X, V, II, and fibrinogen). It is important to realize that the coagulation proteins need to decrease to different levels before the various screening assays show an abnormality. For example, most commercial aPTT reagents detect a decrease in factor VIII when the protein level decreases to 35% to 45% of normal (i.e., 0.35 to 0.45 units/mL). Alternatively, factor XII and high-molecular-weight kininogen at levels of 10% to 15% of normal will only just begin to show abnormalities on the aPTT assay.[20,21] Similarly, factor VII levels below 35% to 40% will be detected on the PT assay. The sensitivity of the screening tests for detection of specific abnormalities varies with the factor being tested, the commercial reagent used in the assay, and the equipment platform for measurement. Each clinical laboratory should know the level of decrease for each coagulation factor that produces an abnormal aPTT or PT with their current equipment and reagents.[22]

The PT assay measures the extrinsic pathway of coagulation, which consists of activated factor VII (factor VIIa) and the proteins of the common pathway (factors X, V, II, and fibrinogen).[16] The PT assay also is used to monitor warfarin therapy.[23,24] In this capacity, the test reporting has been modified so that it can be interpreted universally. Because of the plethora of commercially available PT reagents and coagulation instruments, it is impossible for physicians to know normal values for the PT from any given laboratory. A convention called the international normalized ratio (INR) was developed to standardize the reporting of PT for patients taking warfarin.[23] INR = (patient's PT/mean laboratory control PT)^{ISI}, where ISI (international sensitivity index) for a reagent is a measure of the responsiveness of a given thromboplastin to reduction of the vitamin K–dependent coagulation factors. The reliability of the PT decreases as the ISI of the thromboplastin reagent increases and the therapeutic range for the PT diminishes.[24] The ISI is provided by each manufacturer based on the degree of variation of the thromboplastin from the World Health Organization (WHO) reference thromboplastin that has an arbitrarily assigned value of 1. The orthogonal regression slope of the calibration line for any thromboplastin is determined by z, the logarithm of a PT per second determined with the WHO standard, and x, the logarithm of PT in seconds determined with the test preparation, according to the equation $z = a_1 + b_1x$, where $b_1 = m +$ square root of $m^2 + 1$ and $a_1 = z - b_1x$ (see Pollar[24] for meaning of m in these equations). Manufacturer determination of ISI requires a minimum of 20 normal donors and 60 samples of patients stable on warfarin therapy with INRs from 1.5 to 5.0.[24] The higher the ISI, the less sensitive the thromboplastin. Human recombinant thromboplastin gives an ISI value of approximately 1.0. In practice, the term *INR* has become common parlance to describe all PT changes from normal. In reality, it should be used only to characterize the degree of PT prolongation of a plasma sample from a patient on warfarin.

TCT only measures the ability of exogenous thrombin to proteolyze (clot) fibrinogen. It only assesses fibrinopeptide A and B release

Table 131-1 Laboratory Evaluation of Abnormalities of Coagulation Protein aPTT and PT Screening Tests

Long aPTT, Normal PT	Long PT, Normal aPTT	Long aPTT and PT
ASSOCIATED WITH BLEEDING		**THINK MEDICAL STATES (COMMON)**
Factor VIII (male only)	Factor VII (rare)	
Factor IX (male only)	†Slight defects in factors XI, X, II, V and dysfibrinogenemias	Anticoagulants
		DIC
Acquired inhibitors to factor VIII		Liver disease
Amyloid adsorbed factor IX		Vitamin K deficiency
		Massive transfusion
Factor XI		
NOT ASSOCIATED WITH BLEEDING		Antibodies to factor V
Factor XII	**SINGLE FACTOR DEFICIENT**	
Prekallikrein	Perform specific inhibitor assay	**COMMON PATHWAY**
High-molecular-weight kininogen		**DEFICIENCIES (RARE)**
Lupus anticoagulant		Factors X, V, II
		Dysfibrinogenemias
SINGLE FACTOR DEFICIENT		
Perform specific inhibitor assay		**SINGLE FACTOR DEFICIENT**
		Perform specific inhibitor assays
MULTIPLE FACTORS DEFICIENT		
Pan-inhibitor* (e.g., lupus anticoagulant, immunoglobulin)		**MULTIPLE FACTORS DEFICIENT**
		Pan-inhibitors

aPTT, Activated partial thromboplastin time; *DIC,* disseminated intravascular coagulation; *ISI,* international sensitivity index; *PT,* prothrombin time.
*Pan-inhibitor: general description of a nonspecific inhibitor that can be an immunoglobulin (e.g., lupus anticoagulant, myeloma protein) or natural substance (heparin, fibronectin, amyloid) that binds coagulation proteins and interferes with their function.
†This occurs with more sensitive PT reagents, ISI ≈1.0.

from fibrinogen and fibrin polymerization. A prolonged TCT, as indicated by values outside the 95% confidence interval for the time to clot of a population of 20 or more normal donors, suggests reduced fibrinogen levels (usually <100 mg/dL), abnormal fibrinogen function, or the presence of an inhibitor of thrombin.

Knowing what each test measures, the clinician can use the following approach to evaluate bleeding risk in patients who have prolonged values in one or more of these assays (Table 131-1). For example, if a patient has an isolated prolonged aPTT, determination of the patient's risk to bleed begins with the addition of historical information (see Chapter 130). If isolated prolongation of the aPTT is associated with bleeding, then the differential diagnosis in decreasing likelihood of frequency is factor VIII, factor IX, or factor XI deficiency. Factor VIII and IX deficiencies are sex linked and usually are seen only in males; factor XI deficiency is autosomal recessive and is seen in males and females (see Chapters 137 and 139 for a full discussion). If the aPTT alone is prolonged and the patient has no history of bleeding, the most common cause is a lupus anticoagulant (see Chapter 143). The specific proteins of the intrinsic coagulation system associated with a prolonged aPTT but no bleeding history in decreasing frequency are factor XII, prekallikrein, and high-molecular-weight kininogen deficiency (Table 131-2). All of these defects are autosomal recessive and rare. Knowing about these latter three proteins is essential to evaluating a prolonged aPTT, even though the patient is not at bleeding risk. It also is important to recognize these protein defects so that patients do not undergo unnecessary plasma replacement therapy. Information indicates that factor XII and high-molecular-weight kininogen contribute to the extent of thrombosis independent of hemostasis.[25,26] In flowing blood under high shear with collagen exposure, factor XII autoactivation contributes to the extent of fibrin/platelet clot formation.[25,27,28] Thus factor XII influences thrombosis risk but not hemostasis.

Table 131-2 Clinical Peculiarities of Coagulation Protein Screening Tests

Long aPTT, Normal or Long PT, No Bleeding	Normal aPTT, PT, With Bleeding
LONG APTT ONLY	
Factor XII deficiency	Factor XIII deficiency or inhibitor
Prekallikrein deficiency	α_2-Antiplasmin deficiency or defect
High-molecular-weight kininogen	Plasminogen activator inhibitor deficiency or defects
Lupus anticoagulant	α_1-Antitrypsin Pittsburgh defect
LONG APTT AND PT	
Dysfibrinogenemia with fibrinopeptide B–release defect	
Lupus anticoagulant	

aPTT, Activated partial thromboplastin time; *PT,* prothrombin time.

Individuals can have acquired disorders that inhibit specific coagulation factors and increase their risk for bleeding. The clinical laboratory phenotype of these patients depends on the protein to which the coagulation protein inhibitor is directed. The most common severe acquired coagulation protein inhibitor is a spontaneous antibody inhibitor to factor VIII that is seen in both males and females (see Chapters 137 and 138). Patients with the disorder present with bleeding and a long aPTT. Characteristically this inhibitor is seen in older adult patients, patients with B-cell malignancies, patients with connective tissue disorders such as systemic lupus erythematosus, and women postpartum. Patients are managed acutely with replacement therapy (high-dose factor VIII, activated vitamin K–dependent coagulation factor concentrates, or recombinant factor VIIa), but long-term management may require immunosuppression with cyclophosphamide (Cytoxan) and prednisone and/or rituximab.[29,30] Management decisions in these patients are influenced by the severity of bleeding and the height of the titer of the inhibitor to factor VIII as determined by the Bethesda assay.[31-33] The Bethesda assay is a uniform procedure to perform an assay to detect a specific inhibitor to a blood coagulation protein. It requires a 2-hour incubation at 37° C of test plasma with normal plasma. Inhibitor titer is determined by the degree of dilution of test plasma to obtain a factor level of 50% normal. A complete discussion on performance and interpretation of this assay is seen in Schmaier and Miller.[34]

Alternatively, an isolated PT prolongation associated with bleeding usually indicates factor VII deficiency (see Chapter 139). Patients usually have partial factor VII defects since a complete deficiency is incompatible with life.[35] At times, defects in some common pathway proteins (fibrinogen and factors II, V, and X) may first appear as an isolated PT prolongation; if severe, these latter protein defects will yield prolonged PT and aPTT results. The reason for the former is that more sensitive PT reagents, those with an ISI of approximately 1, detect the defect before the aPTT.

In general, defects in the common pathway proteins (fibrinogen and factors II, V, and X) usually result in a prolonged PT and aPTT. When confronted with laboratory results demonstrating a prolonged PT and aPTT, the hematologist should first consider clinical situations that can affect these tests, such as anticoagulation therapy, disseminated intravascular coagulation (DIC), liver disease, vitamin K deficiency, or massive transfusion.[36,37] These general medical conditions are the most common causes of abnormal results in the two screening tests. Anticoagulation, unless the patient is faking medical illness, and massive transfusion are excluded by history.[38] Vitamin K deficiency is rare except in patients who are receiving warfarin therapy, are nutritionally depleted alcoholics, are having intravenous replacement without vitamins, have bacterial overgrowth in the gastrointestinal tract as result of antibiotic therapy, or, very rarely, have defects in transport proteins or enzymes for metabolism (see Chapter 128). There are several mechanisms by which liver disease can contribute to a prolonged aPTT and PT. Prekallikrein, factor XI, factor VII, and factor V are the first proteins to be decreased in liver disease. Abnormal fibrinogens often are produced in liver disease.[39] The TCT detects defects in fibrinopeptide A and B release, as well as polymerization defects. The reptilase time uses a snake venom enzyme to "clot" fibrinogen by liberating only fibrinopeptide A.[40] An abnormal TCT with a normal reptilase time indicates a fibrinopeptide B–release defect, an abnormality that gives very long aPTT and PT values but is not associated with bleeding (see Table 131-2).[18] The reptilase time also will not be altered by the presence of heparin and can be used to determine if a prolonged aPTT and TCT are the result of heparin.[38]

In addition to these general medical conditions, acquired disorders can present with the clinical laboratory phenotype of a prolonged PT and aPTT. Acquired deficiencies or inhibitors are also seen in a number of medical conditions. Systemic amyloidosis is associated with decreases in plasma factor X or IX as a result of adsorption of the coagulation proteins onto the amyloid protein.[41] In the former condition, the PT and aPTT may be affected; in the latter, only the aPTT is affected. Hypergammaglobulinemic states seen with multiple myeloma or Waldenström macroglobulinemia (immunoglobulin M) can be associated with inhibitors to coagulation protein function.[42] Dysfibrinogenemias are common in these patients because fibrinogen binds immunoglobulin.[18] These phenomena are recognized by performing specific factor assays against the one or more proteins affected at multiple dilutions of the patient's plasma. In general, as the factor assay is performed at lower dilutions (e.g., 50%, 25%, and 10% of normal plasma), the degree of inhibition of the coagulation factor reduces, suggesting that as the plasma is diluted, the effect of the inhibitor is lost. This coagulation test pattern is characteristic of a specific inhibitor to a coagulation protein.

Another acquired inhibitor that influences coagulation protein reactions is the lupus anticoagulant (see Chapter 143). This inhibitor represents antibodies directed to epitopes of proteins bound to certain phospholipids.[43] Lupus anticoagulants variably interfere with the aPTT and PT. Detection of the degree of interference depends on the nature of the commercial reagent. Characteristically a lupus anticoagulant will have a greater effect on a coagulation assay as the reagents, not protein, in the assay are diluted out.[44] For example, the degree of prolongation of PT or aPTT in a plasma sample will be greater at 1:50 dilution and 1:500 dilution of the assay reagent in a patient with a lupus anticoagulant than in a patient with a specific inhibitor to a coagulation protein.[44,45] In the latter case, the inhibitor level will change only when the patient's plasma, not the reagent for the assay, is diluted. Specific criteria have been developed to recognize lupus anticoagulants.[43,46,47] In general, assays that have some dilution of the coagulation reagent (dilute PT or tissue thromboplastin inhibition assay, dilute aPTT, dilute Russell viper venom time, or kaolin clotting time) are useful but are not specifically diagnostic for the condition.[43,45,46] Correction of the defect with excess phospholipids or platelet membranes is an additional characteristic of the disorder noted on clot-based assays.[43,48] However, no clot-based assay is diagnostic for lupus anticoagulants. All criteria also emphasize that the diagnosis is one of exclusion.[43,48] Serologic testing examining for antibodies to cardiolipin or β_2-glycoprotein I is additional immunologic testing the laboratory can use to meet criteria for diagnosis of antiphospholipid antibodies.[43] As indicated in Chapter 143, the serologic criteria for diagnosis of antiphospholipid antibody syndrome is assay evidence for a lupus anticoagulant or antibodies to phospholipids by any procedure that is positive when tested twice with a minimum 3-month hiatus between examinations.[43]

FACTOR-SPECIFIC COAGULATION PROTEIN TESTING

All specific coagulation factor assays of the intrinsic system (factor XII, prekallikrein, high-molecular-weight kininogen, factors XI, IX, and VIII) are measured via one-stage assays using aPTT as the assay platform.[15,49-51] These assays became readily available because of accessibility of specific factor–deficient plasma. For example, a factor VIII assay uses a mixture of aPTT reagent, factor VIII–deficient plasma, and patient (test sample) plasma. After incubation for more than 5 minutes, the time to clot is initiated by recalcification with calcium chloride. All coagulation factors of the extrinsic system and common pathway (factors VII, X, V, and II) are measured in assays using PT as the platform.[16,50,51] For example, a factor X assay is a mixture of PT reagent that contains tissue factor (thromboplastin), factor X–deficient plasma, and patient (test sample) plasma. After incubation for more than 5 minutes, the time to clot is initiated by addition of calcium chloride. The amount of factor present in a given patient sample is determined by comparing the patient sample against a standard curve made with 10% to 100% pooled normal plasma using the factor-deficient plasma and aPTT or PT reagent.

Coagulation-based assays are sensitive and specific. They are simpler to perform than antigen assays for each of the coagulation proteins. Additional assays such as the TCT and reptilase time specifically examine the integrity of fibrinogen.[17,39] Coagulation-based assays examine the function of the protein, antigen assays establish its presence, and, combined, these assays may detect protein with reduced function, but normal antigen levels. This pattern is classic for production of an abnormal molecule. Such a situation commonly arises when examining fibrinogen. The most useful means for determining the presence of an abnormal fibrinogen (dysfibrinogenemia) is to measure clottable fibrinogen and fibrinogen antigen on the same sample.[18,52] If fibrinogen clottability is less than 90% of the amount of fibrinogen antigen, the protein produced probably is functionally abnormal.[39,52] If performed for other coagulation proteins, antigen assays would aid in the diagnosis of abnormal proteins as well.[52]

Chromogenic assays also are used to measure certain enzymes (factor VIII, factor Xa, thrombin, plasmin, activated protein C) and various plasma protease inhibitors (antithrombin, α_2-antiplasmin, C1 inhibitor, plasminogen activator inhibitor). In general, chromogenic assays precisely measure the activity of the protein of interest. However, a coagulant-based assay for a protein (e.g., protein C) will provide a more global result of its (e.g., anticoagulant) function. The drawback of coagulant-based assays is that the levels or function of other proteins influence the results. For example, a heterozygous factor V Leiden polymorphism gives an abnormal protein C coagulant assay but will have no influence on protein C activity if performed by chromogenic assay. The ability to neutralize the enzymatic activity of factor Xa or thrombin is the most reliable way to assay for the plasma level of anticoagulants, such as low-molecular-weight heparins (LMWHs) or unfractionated heparin (UFH), respectively.[52] Anti–factor Xa chromogenic assays provide the most reliable means to measure fondaparinux or rivaroxaban, provided each has its own standard curve. The direct thrombin inhibitors (argatroban, bivalirudin, hirudin, or dabigatran) can be assayed in plasma using an antithrombin chromogenic assay. With each agent, a unique standard curve using that drug also needs to be established by the individual laboratory.[53] Alternatively, an ecarin clotting assay can be established to measure direct thrombin inhibitors provided that a standard curve with each agent is constructed.[54] A dilute thrombin clotting time using dabigatran calibrators can also be used to determine plasma concentrations of dabigatran.

PRACTICAL APPROACH TO THE BLEEDING PATIENT WITH A COAGULATION PROTEIN DEFECT

Patients with abnormal results on coagulation assays can be evaluated by the differential diagnosis of an isolated aPTT abnormality, PT abnormality, or both. When presented with a prolonged coagulation assay, the differential diagnosis often is between a true deficiency and an inhibitor to a specific coagulation protein. Two approaches can be used to obtain a specific diagnosis.

A common practice when approaching the problem of determining specific coagulation factor defects begins with a mixing test of patient and normal plasma. Mixing studies based on the PT or aPTT are interpreted based on the fact that a 50% level of any coagulation factor alone gives normal PT and aPTT values. Both of these screening assays have hyperbolic curves, that is, a decrease in any one factor does not lead to a linear prolongation of either of the two assays. At 50% levels of any coagulation factor, global clotting assays will fall in the normal range.[55] Only with values less than 50% of specific factors will the PT and aPTT begin to prolong. The sensitivity of the PT and aPTT to prolongation with lowering of clotting factors varies depending on the factor and the reagent made by the manufacturer.[22] Thus if patient plasma is mixed 1:1 with normal plasma, the PT or aPTT should be normal if no factor is present in the patient plasma. If the mixture does not correct to normal, something in the patient plasma is interfering with the function of the protein in normal plasma.

Because screening assays for inhibitors are not standardized, a mixing study is a weak assay fraught with misinterpretation and, in many ways, is a much less attractive initial approach. Almost no studies provide evidence-based laboratory procedures for inhibitor screening assays. Some approaches to the use of mixing studies were developed for testing for lupus anticoagulants, which have their own peculiar aspects.[45-48] Critical issues in performing mixing studies is the ratio of patient plasma to normal plasma (1:1 to 4:1), the time of incubation from mixing to assay (immediate to 2 hours), and the assays used for measuring results (PT, aPTT). One critical investigation examined the sensitivity and specificity of mixing studies for assessing factor deficiencies and anticoagulants.[56] Patient and normal plasma were incubated at 37° C for 1 hour before assay in a ratio of 1:1 or 4:1 patient to normal plasma. On an aPTT mix of 1:1 with percent correction of 70% to 75% calculated using a specific formula (see reference for formula), the sensitivity and specificity in recognizing a factor deficiency or anticoagulant were 100% and 33% or 33% and 100%, respectively. When the percent correction was 50% calculated from a ratio of 4:1 patient to normal in the plasma mix for the aPTT, the sensitivity and specificity in recognizing a factor deficiency or anticoagulant improved to 88% and 100% or 100% and 88%, respectively.[56] Likewise, on a PT mix of 1:1 with a percent correction of 70% to 75% calculated using a specific formula (see reference for formula), the sensitivity and specificity in recognizing a factor deficiency or anticoagulant were 95% and 50% or 50% and 95%, respectively. When the percent correction was greater than 40% calculated from a ratio of 4:1 patient to normal in the plasma mix for the PT, the sensitivity and specificity in recognizing a factor deficiency or anticoagulant improved to 96% and 100% or 100% and 96%, respectively.[55] Further studies showed that assays performed after an immediate mix had lower sensitivity and specificity than those done after 1-hour incubation at 37° C. These investigations show the variability of mixing studies test performance and the pitfalls in translating their information into meaningful diagnostic data. Usually it takes 1 day to get inhibitor screening results back, hence delaying diagnosis. However, determining that an inhibitor is present only indicates that additional factor assays must be performed to isolate the specific protein against which the inhibitor is directed. With the identification that the level of a specific protein is low, specific inhibitor studies are needed to confirm the diagnostic impression and determine the inhibitor titer so that management can be planned.

As a second approach to diagnosis of a coagulation protein defect, the abnormal factor can be identified by performing all relevant coagulation factor assays indicated by the abnormal PT and aPTT. If any one test value is decreased, then a specific coagulation factor inhibitor assay for that factor can be performed. One can argue that an excess number of specific assays is being performed, but in most developed clinical institutions these assays are automated and can be performed more efficiently in batch fashion than piecemeal with sequential ordering. The value of such an approach is the shortened time to a specific diagnosis. If more than one factor is found to be low using such an approach, then efforts are made to determine the global reason for the result. Finding a decrease in a single factor by any initial approach requires more effort to perform assays for a specific factor inhibitor. One general approach to a specific inhibitor study can be performed by mixing various ratios of patient plasma to normal plasma (e.g., 1:1, 2:1, 4:1, 1:2, 1:4), incubating the samples for 2 hours at 37° C, and then assaying the level of the specific factor in the mixture.[57] Simultaneously, the patient plasma and normal plasma used in the mixing study are incubated under the same conditions. At the time of assay, the percent activities of the specific factor under study in the normal plasma, patient plasma, and each of the mixtures are obtained. If the *observed value* at any given ratio of patient plasma to normal plasma is less than the calculated *expected value* of mixing the two plasmas in the various ratios (e.g., 1:1, 2:1, 1:2), then one can conclude that an inhibitor present in patient plasma was transferred to the normal plasma sample. For example, if there is 100% activity (1 unit/mL) of the factor being studied in an undiluted sample, a 1:1 dilution of normal plasma with factor-deficient plasma should give an activity level of approximately 50%. If the same normal plasma was incubated 1:1 with patient plasma and the activity was 32%, one should conclude that something in the patient plasma transferred and inhibited the factor's activity in normal plasma, which is the definition of an inhibitor. This approach is a general, nonquantitative method for assessing a coagulation factor inhibitor.

An alternative specifically quantitative method for determining inhibitors to any coagulation factor can be developed for all coagulation factors using a modification of specific inhibitor assays used to characterize factor VIII inhibitors (Bethesda assay).[31-33] This approach is preferred because it standardizes assay performance and method for reporting inhibitor assay results. Given the vagaries of general mixing studies for inhibitors, my approach has been to determine if a single coagulation factor is affected when the screening tests are abnormal and then determine if there is a specific inhibitor to the activity of that factor using a standardized approach to a specific factor inhibitor assay.[31-33]

SCREENING TESTS USED TO RECOGNIZE PATIENTS WITH DISORDERS OF PLATELET NUMBER OR FUNCTION

Recognition of platelet function disorders is critical to any hemostatic evaluation (see Chapters 130, 132, and 161). Knowing the platelet count is essential because thrombocytopenia alone may increase bleeding risk. Obtaining a detailed medication history from patients is important to ascertain the mechanism of action of each agent and its possible influence on assays for platelet function. It is clinically not useful to document abnormal platelet function in a patient taking interfering medication. Screening tests for platelet function testing have been developed; each has advantages as well as disadvantages. The screening tests for platelets are as follows:

1. *Platelet count.* This assay measures the number of platelets in 1 μL of blood. It is used to exclude a quantitative platelet defect as the cause of a bleeding disorder. Causes of thrombocytopenia are discussed in Chapters 134 to 136.
2. *Bleeding time.* To perform this assay, the forearm is pierced, and the time until bleeding stops is measured. Specific devices have been manufactured to perform this assay. The bleeding time is a very qualitative assay influenced by technique, skin characteristics, platelet count, and platelet function.[58] It should only be performed by experienced technologists. In general, it should not be performed on any patient with a platelet count less than 100,000/μL because a low platelet count alone can lead to prolongation of the bleeding time. The bleeding time assay is not a good predictor of surgical bleeding.[59,60] It is seldom useful when performed on a hospitalized patient. However, in the outpatient setting for an individual who has a bleeding history and is not taking any medications, an abnormal bleeding time may provide useful information. It may predict whether more costly von Willebrand factor studies and platelet aggregation and secretion studies will be useful for the diagnosis of a bleeding state. If thrombocytopenia is not present, the differential diagnosis of the long bleeding time includes von Willebrand disease and platelet function defects. However, one can equally argue that a normal bleeding time does not exclude von Willebrand disease or platelet function defect. Patients with Ehlers-Danlos syndrome, osteogenesis imperfecta, and scurvy may have variable prolongation of bleeding times that are not necessarily due to platelet dysfunction.[61-63]
3. *High-shear platelet function analyzers.* Several automated platelet function analyzers have come into use as screening tests for platelet function abnormalities. They have been proposed as replacements for the bleeding time as a diagnostic assay. Each method is unique to and should be evaluated against the wide range of congenital and acquired platelet function disorders before it is accepted as a screening assay. One product, the platelet function analyzer PFA-100 (Siemens, Deerfield, Ill), has been best evaluated and is most widely used.[63-65] In citrated whole blood, the PFA-100 measures the "closure time" required for platelets to adhere to agonist-coated membranes and aggregate under high shear stress (5000 to 6000/sec). It is a novel technology and not analogous to the bleeding time or light transmission platelet aggregometry. Two cartridges are available: collagen–adenosine diphosphate (ADP) and collagen-epinephrine coated membranes. Platelet function is measured as a function of the time needed to occlude the aperture, termed "closure time." Abnormal closure times are longer than the mean values of laboratory-specific values for normals. Each laboratory that uses this technology must determine its own normal values because of influences of different collection tubes and anticoagulant concentrations. Test results can only be interpreted as normal or abnormal. The assay does not make a specific diagnosis (e.g., von Willebrand disease). The PFA-100 may be useful to screen for individuals with von Willebrand disease, Glanzmann thrombasthenia, and Bernard-Soulier syndrome but may be less sensitive to primary platelet secretion defects and storage pool disorders.[66-70] Any abnormality detected by the PFA-100 requires specific testing for von Willebrand disease and platelet function disorders for diagnosis.

INTERPRETATION OF SCREENING TESTS OF PLATELET FUNCTION

Abnormalities on one or more of the screening tests in a patient with a normal platelet count usually suggests von Willebrand disease or a defect in platelet function. Of note, von Willebrand disease or platelet function defects leading to bleeding can be present even with normal results for one or both of the screening assays. At present, no screening assay can exclude the diagnosis of von Willebrand disease or a platelet function defect. If the clinical history is compelling but the screening test results are normal, more definitive von Willebrand factor or platelet function testing is needed. Likewise, if screening test results for platelet function abnormalities are abnormal, the consulting physician has the onus to diagnose or exclude von Willebrand disease or a platelet function defect. Thus once medication or nonprescription drug use is excluded, more sophisticated, specifically diagnostic studies for von Willebrand disease and a platelet function defect are needed for most patients requiring invasive procedures. In general, I do not use the bleeding time or PFA-100 to screen patients for von Willebrand disease or platelet function defects on consultation. If clinically appropriate, complete von Willebrand factor and platelet function studies are performed. In general, 1 of 10 patients in this diagnostic category have a platelet function defect. The majority of individuals fall into the category of von Willebrand disease. Von Willebrand disease is discussed in Chapter 140. Its diagnosis is made by abnormal results for studies of von Willebrand antigen, von Willebrand factor activity (ristocetin cofactor assay and collagen-binding assay), and von Willebrand factor multimers. Some patients with von Willebrand disease also have a reduced factor VIII assay, presenting with a long aPTT. Certain subtypes of patients with von Willebrand disease (type IIB or platelet-type) have a lower threshold to agglutinate and aggregate to ristocetin (0.3 to 0.6 mg/mL) in platelet-rich plasma; normal individuals do not respond to this concentration of ristocetin. However, all normal persons respond to 1.0 mg/mL and higher concentrations of ristocetin added to platelet-rich plasma.

In addition to evaluation for von Willebrand disease, individuals with an abnormal bleeding time or PFA-100 result may require evaluation with platelet aggregation studies. Two forms of platelet aggregation studies are available: light transmission aggregometry in platelet-rich plasma and impedance aggregometry in platelet-rich plasma or whole blood. Light transmission aggregometry in platelet-rich plasma is the gold standard of platelet function testing[71]; impedance aggregometry is less well characterized.[72] Whole-blood impedance aggregometry to some extent is a screening study as well. When performed in conjunction with platelet secretion, either of ATP or serotonin, light transmission aggregometry can be diagnostic of several well-characterized platelet function defects and can characterize defects in others (see Chapters 127 and 132). The procedures for light transmission aggregometry have been reviewed.[73-75] Because of the wide variability in how light transmission aggregometry is performed in clinical laboratories, efforts have been made to develop minimal standards for the performance of platelet function testing in clinical laboratories.[76,77] In light transmission aggregometry, the absence of platelet aggregation in response to physiologic platelet agonists is indicative of Glanzmann thrombasthenia (defects in integrin $\alpha_{IIb}\beta_3$), whereas absent agglutination/aggregation in response to ristocetin suggests Bernard-Soulier syndrome (defects in glycoproteins Ib, IX, and V) or von Willebrand disease. Platelet storage pool disorders can be diagnosed if platelet light transmission aggregometry is performed simultaneously with studies that include measurement of proteins within or released from platelet α-granules or dense granules or measurement of granule membrane proteins (e.g., P-selectin) that become surface expressed after cell activation. Platelet activation defects, such as that induced by aspirin, can be diagnosed as well using this combination of techniques (see Chapter 132). Finally, with appropriate monoclonal antibodies, flow cytometry is used to completely examine the surface expression of platelet glycoproteins and the activation state of the cell.[78] It is important to realize that evaluation of all important platelet receptors, granule release, and formation of activated platelet receptors is adequately performed by flow cytometry, supplanting the need for platelet aggregation and secretion studies.

BLEEDING DISORDERS NOT RECOGNIZED BY SCREENING TESTS FOR COAGULATION PROTEINS OR PLATELETS

A few rare bleeding disorders are not recognized by routine blood coagulation and platelet screening tests (see Table 131-2). These entities include, in order of frequency, factor XIII defects, α_2-antiplasmin defects, plasminogen activator inhibitor 1 defects, and α_1-antitrypsin Pittsburgh. Factor XIII deficiency can be congenital or acquired, especially after isoniazid therapy.[79] α_2-Antiplasmin defects and plasminogen activator inhibitor 1 defects produce hyperfibrinolytic states as a result of reduced inhibition of plasmin and tissue plasminogen activator or urokinase, respectively.[80-82] α_2-Antiplasmin deficiency can be acquired in acute leukemia or other activated coagulation states.[81] Deficiency or abnormal forms of plasminogen activator inhibitor 1 also are associated with a bleeding state.[81] α_1-Antitrypsin Pittsburgh is an exceedingly rare bleeding disorder caused by a mutation in antitrypsin that results in potent thrombin inhibition, preventing clot formation.[83]

OTHER ACTIVITIES FOR HEMOSTASIS LABORATORIES

Thrombosis Evaluation

In addition to the diagnosis of bleeding disorders, the hemostasis laboratory is important in the evaluation of prothrombotic states (see Chapter 142). Evaluation of prothrombotic states serves the patient in many ways. In individuals with idiopathic thrombosis, recognition of a specific molecular or protein defect may be important in determining the duration of anticoagulant therapy. Certain prothrombotic states (e.g., antithrombin, protein C, and protein S deficiencies; antiphospholipid antibody syndrome) may confer higher risk for recurrence and thus suggest long-term anticoagulation after the first event. Less severe prothrombotic states (e.g., factor V Leiden and prothrombin 20210 polymorphisms, functional defects in fibrinogen and plasminogen) do not in themselves confer high risk for thrombosis but when conjoined with another risk factor may confer higher risk. Knowing this information helps patients engage in risk modification activity (e.g., stop taking oral contraceptives). Finally, 18% of patients without a family history of thrombosis and 30% to 40% of patients with a family history may have an identifiable molecular or protein risk factor for venous thrombosis.[84] This information helps many patients deal with anticoagulant management issues after they present with idiopathic thrombosis.

Monitoring Acute Hemostatic and Thrombotic Conditions

In addition to the diagnosis of hemostatic and thrombotic disorders, the coagulation laboratory has the function of monitoring patient therapy. Patients receiving UFH and warfarin are monitored using the aPTT and INR, respectively. New monitoring roles are being established for these facilities. This section is divided into two parts: monitoring of anticoagulation therapy and measurement of activated coagulation.

Anticoagulation monitoring is an increasingly larger activity of hemostasis laboratories. In addition to UFH and warfarin monitoring using clot-based assays, LMWH monitoring is an important activity in hospitalized patients. This monitoring is especially important in patients who are obese, in those who have renal function compromise, and in patients before elective surgery.[85] Anti–factor Xa assays for monitoring LMWHs can be developed against each agent using the WHO's LMWH for the standard curve.[53] Each of the new anticoagulants (fondaparinux, dabigatran, rivaroxaban) requires unique standard curves for assay development on the appropriate chromogenic assay.

Monitoring of activated coagulation states and their amelioration with treatment is another activity of the specialized hemostatic laboratory. The classic activated coagulation state is DIC (see Chapter 141). DIC is a clinicopathologic state associated with tissue destruction as a result of infectious, traumatic, obstetric, malignant, and connective tissue disorders. The two forms of clinical presentation are an *acute* form that is a hyperfibrinolytic state and a *subacute* form that is more indolent. In the acute form, aPTT and PT are elevated, and the fibrinogen and platelet count are low. In the subacute form, aPTT, PT, and platelet count may be normal or slightly low, and fibrinogen count can be normal or even elevated. Finding a prolonged PT and aPTT with a reduced fibrinogen and platelet count usually indicates DIC in the hospitalized patient until proven otherwise.[86] This clinical laboratory phenotype of DIC most probably results from a secondary hyperfibrinolytic state and is the form of DIC most commonly recognized. The biochemical diagnosis of DIC then is simplified to finding evidence of simultaneous thrombin and plasmin formation. The D-dimer is a plasmin-proteolyzed fragment of insoluble, cross-linked fibrin.[87,88] It is a confirmatory assay for DIC in the appropriate clinical condition. Insoluble fibrin results from thrombin cleavage of soluble fibrinogen and cross-linking of fibrin by thrombin/activated factor XIII. Presently a scoring system to aid in the diagnosis of DIC is available.[89] D-dimer elevation characterizes DIC but is not specific for it. Assay results are positive in patients in postoperative states, with resolving hematomas, and after large-vessel or pulmonary thrombosis. Positive results of a D-dimer assay also have become an adjunct to the clinical diagnosis of pulmonary embolism.[90]

In addition to DIC (see Chapter 141), other hematologic states such as antiphospholipid antibody syndrome (see Chapter 143), heparin-induced thrombocytopenia and thrombosis syndrome (see Chapter 135), and warfarin–skin necrosis with protein C deficiency (see Chapter 129) also are activated blood coagulation states. Physicians may find that monitoring the degree of the activated blood coagulation state is useful as a guide to therapy. In addition to the D-dimer, other assays that could be used to monitor an activated blood coagulation state include prothrombin fragment 1.2, thrombin-antithrombin complexes, or thrombin generation assays.

Finally, heparin-induced thrombocytopenia presents unique opportunities to coagulation laboratory testing for both diagnosis and monitoring of the activated blood coagulation state. Laboratory diagnosis and monitoring the effectiveness of therapy for heparin-induced thrombocytopenia is discussed in detail in Chapter 135.

SUGGESTED READINGS

Field JJ, Fenske TS, Blinder MA: Rituximab for the treatment of patients with very high-titre acquired factor VIII inhibitors refractory to conventional chemotherapy. *Haemophilia* 13:46, 2007.

H58-A—Platelet Function Testing by Aggregometry: Approved guideline, Wayne, Pa, 2008, Clinical and Laboratory Standards Institute.

Hayward CPM, Harrison P, Cattaneo M, et al: Platelet function analyzer (PFA)-100 closure time in the evaluation of platelet disorders and platelet function. *J Thromb Haemost* 4:312, 2006.

Jennings LK, White MM: Platelet aggregation. In Michelson AD, editor: *Platelets,* ed 2, Amsterdam, 2007, Elsevier, p 495.

Kearon C, Ginsberg JS, Douketis J, et al: Canadian Pulmonary Embolism Diagnosis Study (CANPEDS) Group: An evaluation of D-dimer in the diagnosis of pulmonary embolism: A randomized trial. *Ann Intern Med* 144:812, 2006.

Michelson AD, Linder MD, Barnard MR, et al: Flow cytometry. In Michelson AD, editor: *Platelets,* ed 2, Amsterdam, 2007, Elsevier, p 545.

Moffat KA, Ledford-Kraemer MR, Nichols WL, et al: Variability in clinical laboratory practice in testing for disorders of platelet function: Results of two surveys of the North American Specialized Coagulation Laboratory Association. *Thromb Haemost* 93:549, 2005.

O'Donnell MJ, Kearon C, Johnson J, et al: Preoperative anticoagulation activity after bridging low-molecular-weight heparin for temporary interruption of warfarin. *Ann Intern Med* 146:184, 2007.

Zhou L, Schmaier AH: Platelet aggregation testing in platelet-rich plasma: Description of procedures with the aim to develop standards in the field. *Am J Clin Pathol* 123:172, 2005.

For complete list of references log on to www.expertconsult.com.

CHAPTER 132

ACQUIRED DISORDERS OF PLATELET FUNCTION

Reyhan Diz-Küçükkaya and José A. López

Acquired disorders of platelet function are among the most common hematologic abnormalities, a reflection of the sensitivities of platelets to external and internal perturbations. The clinical challenge in evaluating acquired disorders of platelet function is to determine whether observed derangements in platelet function pose a threat to the patient. Although platelet function can be altered to predispose to either hemostatic or thrombotic disorders, this chapter deals primarily, but not exclusively, with platelet disorders that may compromise hemostasis. We attempt also to guide clinicians in trying to determine the clinical importance of these disorders, but the marked variations in bleeding risks associated with any particular disorder of platelet function make this a difficult task. Bleeding in patients with acquired platelet dysfunction is likely to occur less frequently and predictably than in those affected by severe inherited platelet disorders such as Bernard-Soulier syndrome or Glanzmann thrombasthenia and may manifest only in the setting of trauma or surgery or in the presence of additional hemostatic defects.

The laboratory evaluation of these patients may illuminate these disorders (see Chapter 131) but may offer little concrete guidance in management. Acquired platelet defects (Table 132-1) often exhibit abnormal laboratory test results, such as a prolonged closure time on a platelet function analyzer or abnormal aggregation in response to added agonists. Historically, the bleeding time was used to evaluate bleeding risk in patients with jaundice or uremia; but it measures hemostasis only in one vascular bed (the skin) and bears inherent interoperator variability. These platelet assays are useful as research tools; however, defects as quantified by laboratory tests, including the bleeding time, do not correlate precisely with the risk of bleeding and thus are not predictive of bleeding in these patients. Additionally, some acquired platelet disorders increase the risk of thrombosis rather than bleeding, a risk for which there is currently no effective screening test. Last, tests that depend on assessing the functions of platelets ex vivo do not assess the contributions of labile substances from the endothelium (see Chapter 125) and occasionally (as in platelet aggregometry) lack the component of flow, a key component of in vivo platelet function.

DRUGS, FOODS, AND ADDITIVES THAT AFFECT PLATELET FUNCTION

The most common causes of acquired platelet dysfunction are drugs. In a large prospective study, 5649 unselected adult patients were screened preoperatively for hemostatic defects with activated partial thromboplastin time (aPTT), prothrombin time (PT), platelet counts, platelet function analyzer (PFA-100) testing, and a questionnaire regarding bleeding history.[1] Bleeding history was positive in 628 patients (11.1%), and impaired hemostasis was verified in 256 (40.8%) of these patients. Of these 256 patients, 162 (63.28%) were found to have acquired platelet dysfunction. Antiplatelet drugs or nonsteroidal antiinflammatory drugs (NSAIDs) were responsible for the acquired platelet dysfunction in 147 patients and antibiotics in 10 patients.

Numerous drugs affect platelet function (Table 132-2). For several, inhibition of platelet function is their intended effect (Fig. 132-1); for most, platelet dysfunction is an unintended and undesired side effect. Drug-induced platelet function abnormalities do not usually cause a clinically significant problem in healthy individuals. However, these drugs may increase the bleeding risk with interventions (e.g., surgery, biopsy), trauma, or in the presence of other hemostatic defects, such as those associated with cirrhosis or uremia. Antiplatelet agents are discussed more fully in Chapter 151. For all of these drugs, their effects on platelet function are defined by an abnormality of platelet aggregation, but their contribution to a risk of excessive bleeding is definitively established only for aspirin, clopidogrel, ticlopidine, and inhibitors of $\alpha_{IIb}\beta_3$ function.

ANTIPLATELET DRUGS

Aspirin

Aspirin has been in routine use worldwide for more than 100 years and is still by far the most common agent associated with platelet dysfunction.[2] The antipyretic and analgesic effect of willow bark was first recorded by Galen. In 1826 and 1828, Leroux and Buchner isolated a compound from willow bark that they called *salicin* (which means *willow* in Latin).[3] In 1897, a German chemist, Felix Hoffman from the Bayer Company, inspired by his father's severe arthritis and the untoward side effects of salicylic acid, discovered a method to convert salicylic acid, the active compound in willow bark, to a compound with less gastrointestinal (GI) toxicity, acetyl salicylic acid (aspirin).[4] However, with Hoffmann's subsequent synthesis of heroin from morphine, commercial development of aspirin was relegated to the back burner for a number of decades.[5] Aspirin was widely used for rheumatic fever in the 1940s. In the 1950s, case reports and uncontrolled studies were published suggesting that aspirin could prevent myocardial infarction and stroke.[5,6] The clinical importance of the antithrombotic effect of aspirin was clearly demonstrated in a study of 22,071 physicians who received either 325 mg of aspirin or placebo every other day over the course of 5 years.[7] Those receiving aspirin had a 44% decreased incidence of myocardial infarction. In a large meta-analysis, it was shown that aspirin reduced death from vascular events by 15% and nonfatal vascular events by 30%.[7] The primary mechanism by which aspirin impairs hemostasis is through irreversible acetylation of the enzyme cyclooxygenase-1 (COX-1), an early enzyme in the synthetic pathway that produces the potent platelet agonist, thromboxane A_2 (TXA_2). Because platelets have no nuclei and therefore retain only a limited capacity to synthesize new proteins, a single low dose of aspirin (40-100 mg) or as little as 10 mg taken daily for 1 week can completely inhibit TXA_2 production and therefore impair the function of a cohort of platelets for their circulating life span. Aspirin also acetylates the isoform of COX present in endothelial cells, COX-2; COX-2 acetylation blocks synthesis of prostacyclin, a strong inhibitor of platelet function.[8] However, COX-2 is markedly less sensitive than COX-1 to inhibition by aspirin,[2] and endothelial cells, unlike platelets, are able to synthesize new enzymes quite rapidly.[9]

Platelets exposed to aspirin either in vivo or in vitro predictably demonstrate impaired aggregation in response to epinephrine, adenosine diphosphate (ADP), arachidonic acid, and low concentrations of collagen and thrombin,[10] a result of defective TXA_2 production.

Table 132-1 Acquired Disorders of Platelet Function

Drugs, Foods, and Additives
Drugs: see Table 132-2
Food and additives: omega-3 fatty acids, ethanol, ginger, onion, garlic, black tree fungus, *Gingko biloba*, cumin, turmeric, tonic water, caffeine, others
Clonal Disorders
Clonal hematologic diseases
Myeloproliferative neoplasms
Paroxysmal nocturnal hemoglobinuria
Paraproteinemias
Leukemias and myelodysplastic syndromes
Solid tumors
Systemic Metabolic Disorders
End-stage renal disease
Liver diseases
Diabetes and hyperlipidemias
Platelet Dysfunction Related With Extracorporeal Circuits Miscellaneous
Hypothermia
Disseminated intravascular coagulation

Table 132-2 Drug-Induced Platelet Dysfunction

Anti-Platelet Drugs
COX inhibitor: aspirin
ADP receptor antagonists
Thienopyridines: clopidogrel, ticlopidine, prasugrel
Nonthienopyridines: ticagrelor, cangrelor
$\alpha_{IIb}\beta_3$ inhibitors: abciximab, eptifibatide, tirofiban
PDE inhibitors
Nonselective PDE inhibitors: pentoxifylline, caffeine, theophylline
PDE3 inhibitors: cilostazol, milrinone, anagrelide
PDE5 inhibitors: dipyridamole, sildenafil
Adenyl cyclase stimulators: epoprostenol, iloprost, beraprost
Drugs that adversely affect platelet function
NSAIDs: ibuprofen, naproxen, indomethacin
Cardiovascular agents
Calcium channel blockers: nifedipine, diltiazem, verapamil
β-Blocker: propranolol
Vasodilators: nitrates, nitroprusside
Diuretic: furosemide
Angiotensin II receptor antagonist: losartan
Antibiotics: β-lactams, amphotericin, hydroxychloroquine, nitrofurantoin
Psychiatric drugs: TCAs, fluoxetine, chlorpromazine, promethazine, trifluoperazine
Oncologic drugs: mithramycin, daunorubicin, BCNU, asparaginase, vincristine
Anesthetics: dibucaine, procaine, halothane
Plasma expanders: dextran, hydroxyl ethyl starch
Heparins and thrombolytic agents
Miscellaneous: clofibrate, statins, cocaine, ketanserin, radiographic contrast agents, antihistamines, immunosuppressive drugs

ADP, Adenosine diphosphate; *BCNU*, carmustine; *COX*, cyclooxygenase; *NSAID*, nonsteroidal antiinflammatory drug; *PDE*, phosphodiesterase; *TCA*, tricyclic antidepressant.

These agonists have therefore been defined as *weak* agonists, requiring that TXA_2 diffuse out of the platelet, bind to its receptor on the platelet membrane, and reinforce aggregation by promoting secretion from α and dense granules. Aspirin-treated platelets stimulated with these agonists demonstrate only a primary, reversible wave of aggregation without granule secretion. Stronger agonists (high concentrations of thrombin and collagen) do not require TXA_2 synthesis to cause platelet secretion and irreversible aggregation, which probably accounts for the observation that hemostasis in healthy aspirin-treated subjects is usually normal. Aspirin is a very effective antiplatelet agent when it is used long term even in small doses. In randomized controlled studies, aspirin has been shown to be effective in reducing the risk of ischemic stroke or transient ischemic attack at a dose of 50 mg/day and of unstable angina and severe carotid artery stenosis at 75 mg/day.[11-13] Higher doses of aspirin do not further reduce risk.

Aspirin may also have COX-independent actions that may affect coagulation. At the site of microvascular injury, platelets bind to exposed collagen, and coagulation is initiated by tissue factor concurrently. It was reported that low-dose aspirin (30 mg/day for 7 days) decreased thrombin formation in healthy volunteers.[14] Undas et al[11] used the same microvascular injury model and showed that aspirin at 75 mg/day for 7 days decreased the velocity of prothrombin consumption by 29%, thrombin generation by 29% and delayed both activation and maximum cleavage of factor XIII by thrombin. Interestingly, it was demonstrated that high cholesterol levels (>240 mg/dL) impair the antithrombotic effect of low-dose aspirin in a microvascular injury model.[5]

In contrast to the antiplatelet effect of aspirin, which appears unrelated to the dose above small threshold doses, GI mucosal toxicity is dose related.[15] The mechanism of mucosal injury appears to be distinct from the effect on hemostasis, involving ionic trapping of aspirin within gut mucosal cells[16] and diminished synthesis of protective gut prostaglandins.[17,18] The inhibitory effect of even a single dose of aspirin on gastric prostaglandin synthesis is prolonged, with one study showing that gastric COX activity was still 57% suppressed 72 hours after a single 325-mg dose of aspirin.[19] Bleeding may originate from discrete ulcers or diffuse mucosal damage and is more common to arise from the upper GI tract. The risk of bleeding is increased even with doses of aspirin as low as 10 to 30 mg/day[20]; the protective effect of resistant coatings is unproved.[21] Recently, a nitric oxide–donating form of aspirin (NCX-4016) has been shown to enhance the cardioprotective effect of aspirin while sparing the GI tract.[22] The GI risk of aspirin is increased in elderly adults (older than 65 years of age) and in those with concomitant medical conditions, such as cardiovascular disease, as well as in those taking certain other medications, such as other NSAIDs.[21] Aspirin appears to delay the healing of gastric ulcers, possibly because it interferes with the release of growth factors from platelets, such as endostatin and vascular endothelial growth factor.[23]

Aspirin treatment was also associated with a small but significant increase in mucocutaneous bleeding as evidenced by easy bruising, hematemesis, melena, epistaxis, and an increased frequency of blood transfusion. Because low doses have been shown to be effective in preventing thrombosis, it is likely that the risk of bleeding can be reduced while maintaining an antiplatelet effect.

The response to aspirin therapy varies among individuals. Every day, the human body can produce approximately 10×10^{11} platelets, and this production can increase 10-fold if needed. The life span of platelets is 8 to 10 days, and every day nearly 10% to 12% of the platelets are replaced by new platelets. The capacity of the bone marrow to produce new platelets, the aspirin dosage, the aspirin exposure time (spot doses or regular use), and individual parameters may be different among individuals. The antiplatelet effect of aspirin can be screened by light-transmission aggregometry, flow cytometry, PFA-100, or other automated platelet aggregometers such as VerifyNow.

Assays of Aspirin Effect on Platelets

Light transmission aggregometry (LTA) measures platelet aggregation in response to various agonists. Although LTA is the gold standard for evaluating platelet functions, clinical use of LTA in screening of antiplatelet therapy is limited because of cost, complex assay procedures, and the need for expert interpretation. Flow cytometry assays

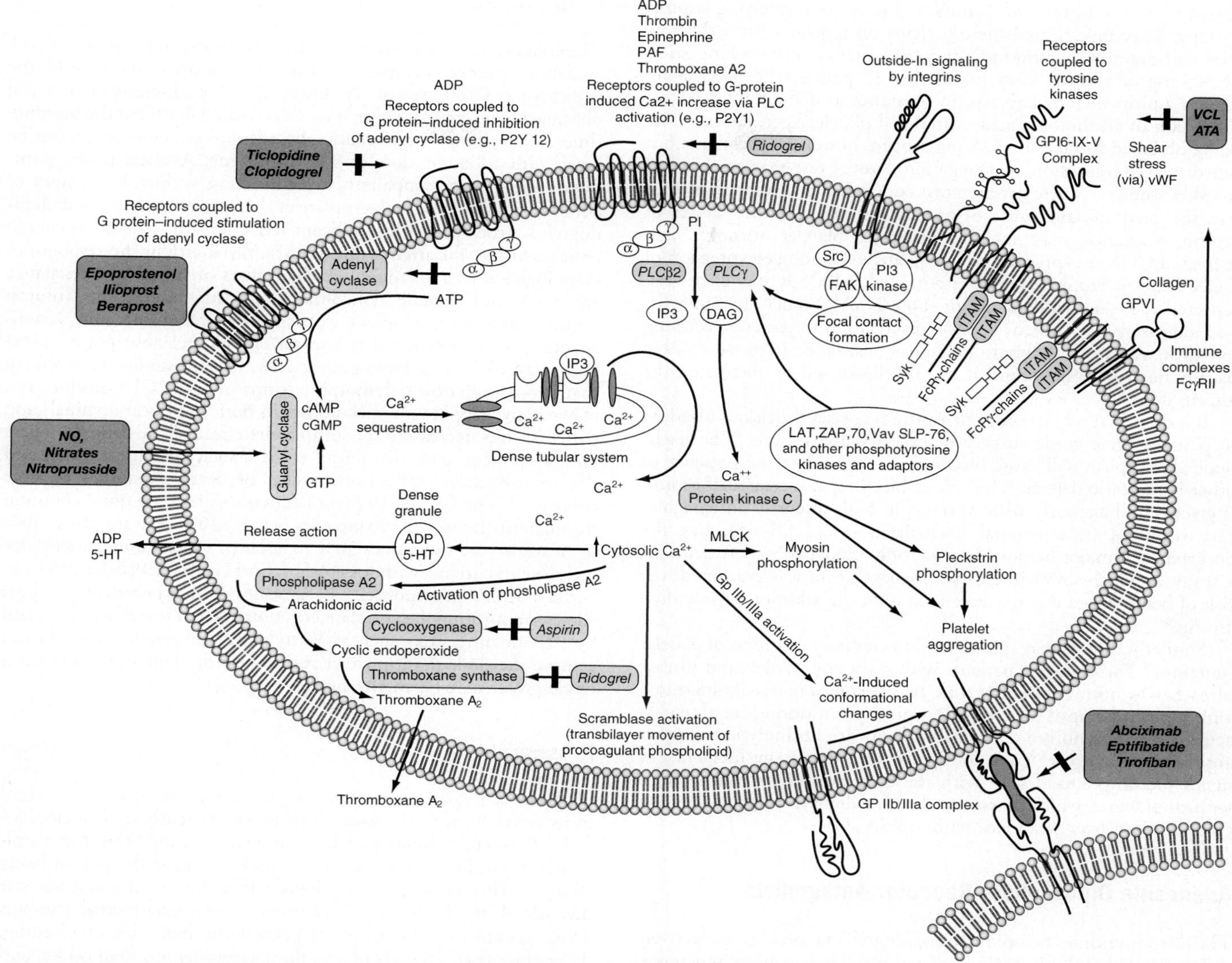

Figure 132-1 MECHANISM OF INHIBITION OF PLATELET FUNCTION BY VARIOUS DRUGS. Some of the drugs shown, such as Ridogrel, VCL (rA1 domain of von Willebrand factor), and ATA (aurin tricarboxylic acid), are not now used clinically. *ADP,* Adenosine diphosphate; *ATP,* adenosine triphosphate; *cAMP,* cyclic adenosine monophosphate; *cGMP,* cyclic guanyl monophosphate; *DAG,* diacylglycerol; *GP,* glycoprotein; *GTP,* guanyl triphosphate; *5-HT,* serotonin (5-hydroxytryptamine); *IP3,* inositol triphosphate; *ITAM,* immunoreceptor tyrosine-based activation motif; *MLCK,* myosin light chain kinase; *NO,* nitric oxide; *PAF,* platelet activating factor; *PI,* phosphatidylinositol; *PLA2,* phospholipase A2; *TXA*$_2$, thromboxane A$_2$; *vWF,* von Willebrand factor.

measure platelet surface glycoproteins, platelet activation markers, and platelet–leukocyte interactions using whole blood or platelet suspensions. The major limitations of flow cytometry analysis are the cost and need for expert interpretation. PFA-100 is an alternative to the bleeding time. This test assays platelet function under flow using two disposable cartridges, one coated with collagen–ADP and one coated with collagen–epinephrine. Citrated blood passes through an aperture within a coated membrane at the end of the cartridge, and the time for occlusion of this aperture is measured. Prolongation of the closure time is indicative of a defect in either platelets or von Willebrand factor (vWF).

VerifyNow is another cartridge-based system designed to assay platelet aggregation in the presence of antiplatelet drugs; the aspirin response is assessed by aggregation in response to arachidonic acid. The percentage of affected platelets (designated as aspirin reaction units [ARU]) determines the sensitivity to aspirin.[24,25]

The issue of aspirin resistance is hotly debated, with reported incidence rates varying from 0% to 57%.[26,27] How aspirin resistance is defined (clinical or laboratory) is important for clinical management. Clinical resistance is a definition applied to patients who experienced a new thrombotic event while receiving regular and effective-dose aspirin therapy. Because arterial thrombosis is a multifactorial process, the inhibition of one pathway of platelet activation may be insufficient to prevent thrombosis. Therefore, clinical resistance is mostly regarded as “drug failure.”

Laboratory aspirin resistance is more complicated. In some patients, aspirin may not produce the expected effects on one or more screening laboratory tests. COX-1 gene polymorphisms (A842G, C50T, nucleotide changes designated) or platelet integrin α2 or β3 polymorphisms have been investigated in these patients, with conflicting results.[27-30] More recently, Voora et al[30] screened 11 single nucleotide polymorphisms (SNPs) reported to be associated with aspirin resistance in 3449 patients with coronary disease. They reported that none of these SNPs were associated with clinical or laboratory aspirin resistance. They suggested that use of these SNPs for guiding more aggressive aspirin therapy was not justified.

The most important issue in determining whether laboratory aspirin resistance is real is compliance: Schwartz et al[31] evaluated 190 patients with a history of coronary disease and receiving aspirin therapy. They investigated these patients on regular aspirin therapy, after withdrawal of aspirin for 7 days, and after an observed ingestion of 325 mg of aspirin. They found that 17 patients (9%) receiving regular aspirin therapy had aspirin resistance as defined by defective inhibition of arachidonic acid–stimulated platelet aggregation. After being observed to take the 325 mg aspirin, however, all patients but one displayed inhibition of aggregation. Similar results were observed in other studies.[32] These investigators concluded that noncompliance was the predominant cause of aspirin resistance. Other causes of aspirin resistance may include increased platelet turnover and increased COX-1 expression in new platelets[33] and overexpression of COX-2 in macrophages and endothelial cells.[34] It has also been reported that concomitant use of some NSAIDs such as ibuprofen and naproxen may prevent COX-1 inactivation in patients receiving low-dose aspirin.[25,35] Laboratory aspirin resistance in these cases is usually dose-dependent, and it can be eliminated by increasing the aspirin dose.[36]

It is clear that regular usage of aspirin increases the risk of bleeding in patients undergoing surgery or experiencing trauma. The likelihood that aspirin will cause bleeding is increased in the presence of other hemostatic defects. The risk of bleeding is increased if aspirin is given simultaneously with warfarin in high-intensity anticoagulation regimens (international normalized ratio, 3.0-4.5), but the occurrence of major hemorrhage was only moderately increased.[37] In a study in which lower intensity anticoagulation was examined, the risk of hemorrhage was not increased with the addition of low-dose aspirin.[38]

Similarly, aspirin may unmask mild hereditary disorders of platelet function.[39] For example, patients with mild von Willebrand disease often have a normal bleeding time that becomes markedly increased with aspirin therapy.[39] Conversely, aspirin given during treatment of acute coronary syndromes in combination with fibrinolytic and other antithrombotic agents does not appear to increase the incidence of major bleeding episodes,[40,41] with the exception of its combination with clopidogrel, which is associated with a slight increase in bleeding complications over treatment with aspirin alone.[42]

Adenosine Diphosphate Receptor Antagonists

The thienopyridines ticlopidine, clopidogrel, and prasugrel selectively and irreversibly inhibit ADP-mediated platelet activation and aggregation.[43] The use of ticlopidine has been greatly curtailed because of serious side effects such as agranulocytosis, thrombocytopenia, and thrombotic thrombocytopenic purpura.[44] ADP activates platelets by raising the concentration of cytoplasmic Ca^{2+} through influx from the extracellular fluid and mobilization from internal stores and by decreasing the concentration of intracellular cyclic adenosine monophosphate (cAMP) coupled to inhibition of adenylyl cyclase. ADP receptors can be divided into two groups: the G protein–coupled receptors, termed *P2Y,* and the ionotropic receptors, *P2X.* Platelets contain two P2Y receptors, $P2Y_1$ and $P2Y_{12}$, complexed to the heterotrimeric G proteins G_q and G_{i2}, respectively. ADP binding to $P2Y_1$ is necessary for platelet aggregation but is not sufficient. Rather, $P2Y_1$ is responsible for ADP-induced platelet shape change, and its engagement by ADP triggers a transient aggregatory response. $P2Y_{12}$, coupled to inhibition of adenylyl cyclase, mediates the amplification of the aggregation response and increases thrombus stability.[45] The thienopyridine derivatives have no effects on arachidonic acid metabolism and hence act synergistically with aspirin to inhibit platelet function.

The thienopyridines are all prodrugs of similar structure that produce active metabolites that bind irreversibly to $P2Y_{12}$, inhibiting ADP-mediated aggregation for up to 10 days after withdrawal of the drug, paralleling the platelet life span.[46] Because most platelet agonists require ADP for their full activity, the thienopyridines inhibit platelet activation by all agonists except strong agonists at high concentrations.[47] They have a further hypothetical advantage over aspirin in that they inhibit shear-induced platelet aggregation.[48]

Clopidogrel

Clopidogrel is administered orally. Approximately 15% of the absorbed prodrug is converted to its active form in the liver by the cytochrome P450 system. At lower doses of clopidogrel, the full pharmacologic effect requires 4 to 7 days, often doubling the bleeding time. When a rapid therapeutic effect is desired, clopidogrel can be given with a loading dose of 300 to 600 mg. At these doses, clopidogrel significantly impairs platelet function within 90 minutes of administration.[44,49-51] Dual antiplatelet therapy with aspirin and clopidogrel is associated with significant reductions of ischemic events in patients at risk for arterial thrombosis. Variability in the response to clopidogrel is well documented. The causes of clopidogrel resistance are many and include noncompliance; drug interactions (proton pump inhibitors may affect clopidogrel metabolism); and various genetic polymorphisms that control clopidogrel absorption, metabolic activation, and biological activity. Several studies have shown that loss-of-function polymorphic forms of CYP2C19 produce less of the active clopidogrel metabolites in both healthy individuals and patients, thus decreasing the antiplatelet effect of the drug.[52,53] These polymorphisms were also found to be associated with an increased risk of myocardial infarction, stroke, or death in studies of large cohorts.[54,55] The CYP2C19 loss-of-function alleles are quite common throughout the world (frequencies being ≈30% in Europeans, 40% in Africans, and more than 50% in Asians).[56] Increasing the clopidogrel dose in patients with loss-of-function CYP2C19 alleles produces better antiplatelet responses.[57] Because of the high prevalence of these alleles, monitoring the antiplatelet action of clopidogrel may be useful by LTA or other tests such as VerifyNow.[24] In patients who do not achieve the desired antiplatelet response with clopidogrel, prasugrel or ticagrelor may be an alternative.

Prasugrel

Prasugrel is a third-generation oral thienopyridine that is converted to its active form in the liver much more efficiently than is clopidogrel.[58] Prasugrel inhibits platelets more consistently than does clopidogrel, regardless of the CYP2C19 allele status of the person being treated.[54] This advantage over clopidogrel comes with a cost because the risk of major bleeding is elevated in prasugrel-treated patients. Three groups of patients are at particularly high risk of bleeding: those older than 75 years of age, those weighing less than 60 kg, and patients with history of stroke or transient ischemic attack.[59]

Ticagrelor

The chemical structure of ticagrelor is distinct from those of the thienopyridines. Ticagrelor is a cyclopentyltriazolo-pyrimidine that inhibits the ADP receptor reversibly and noncompetitively. Ticagrelor is given orally and is metabolized by the liver cytochrome P450 system to the active metabolite, which has a half-life of approximately 12 hours. The recommended dose is 100 mg twice daily. Ticagrelor has some advantages over thienopyridines such as rapid action, reversible and consistent antiplatelet effect with only a small increase in the risk of bleeding, and efficacy in patients with genetic resistance to clopidogrel. The major adverse side effect is dyspnea, which is of unknown mechanism. The drug was recently approved in the United States for the treatment of acute coronary syndromes.[60,61]

Platelet $\alpha IIb\beta 3$ (Glycoprotein IIb/IIIa) Inhibitors

A myriad of pathways lead to platelet aggregation, the final common step being activation of the major platelet integrin $\alpha_{IIb}\beta_3$ to a ligand-competent form, which can bind multivalent ligands such as fibrinogen or vWF to cross-link the platelets into an aggregate. Conventional antiplatelet agents such as aspirin and clopidogrel each inhibit only one pathway leading to platelet aggregation, aspirin preventing thromboxane production and clopidogrel blocking ADP receptors. Dual therapy with aspirin and clopidogrel improves the clinical benefit of antiplatelet therapy, but aggregation is still able to proceed through the action of other agonists such as thrombin. Because $\alpha_{IIb}\beta_3$ engagement is required for aggregation through all pathways, blocking this receptor inhibits platelet aggregation more effectively.

Inhibitors of $\alpha_{IIb}\beta_3$ work selectively and competitively to inhibit platelet aggregation.[62] These agents are intended to produce a transient effect akin to the defect in Glanzmann thrombasthenia, but there are important differences between the drug effect and the disease.

$\alpha_{IIb}\beta_3$ inhibitors have been used in tens of thousands of patients with various forms of cardiovascular disease. Although these agents share many similarities in their pharmacodynamics and therapeutic effects, they also have a number of clinically important pharmacokinetic differences.

Abciximab

The first $\alpha_{IIb}\beta_3$ inhibitor approved for clinical use, abciximab (ReoPro), is a human-murine chimeric Fab fragment of a monoclonal antibody that targets the β_3 subunit of $\alpha_{IIb}\beta_3$ and therefore also reacts with another integrin that shares the β_3 subunit, $\alpha_V\beta_3$. Although $\alpha_{IIb}\beta_3$ expression is restricted to megakaryocytes and platelets, $\alpha_V\beta_3$ is expressed on platelets; at low levels; and in cells of the vascular wall, including endothelial cells and fibroblasts.[63] The clinical relevance of this cross-reactivity is unclear. Abciximab administered intravenously as a standard 0.25 mg/kg bolus blocks approximately 80% of surface $\alpha_{IIb}\beta_3$ and inhibits platelet aggregation to a similar extent, although the extent of inhibition is variable.[62] This level of blockade increases the bleeding time only mildly.[64] The bleeding time only becomes markedly prolonged when receptor blockade exceeds 90%. After the bolus dose, abciximab is infused at 0.125 g/kg/min for 12 hours. Several trials have established this as a clinically effective regimen.[62] Plasma levels of free abciximab drop rapidly after its administration, with an initial half-life of approximately 30 minutes. Most of the drug is bound to platelets. This explains why patients with thrombocytosis may require larger weight-adjusted doses of abciximab to attain a therapeutic antiplatelet effect[65] and why patients with lower platelet counts treated with the usual dose of abciximab display more profound platelet inhibition. Abciximab is not excreted in the urine and is probably metabolized by the reticuloendothelial system at the time platelets (with bound abciximab) are cleared from the circulation. The dose of abciximab does not have to be adjusted in patients with renal impairment. Although a daily platelet turnover rate of 10% would predict that no abciximab would be detected in blood after 10 days of its administration, platelet-bound abciximab has been observed up to 3 weeks after its initial administration, suggesting platelet-to-platelet redistribution of the drug or release of new platelets from megakaryocytes that had previously bound the drug. Several in vitro and in vivo studies confirm abciximab's ability to exchange between platelets.[66] Because of the low plasma levels of unbound abciximab, the drug's inhibitory effect can be rapidly reversed by platelet transfusion; and hemostasis should be normal when the concentration of infused platelets exceeds 50,000/μL, as it is in normal individuals. However, because of abciximab's ability to redistribute to the newly transfused platelets, the platelet-bound abciximab may produce a gradual inhibitory effect on the infused platelets[66]; in severe or refractory bleeding, it may be necessary to infuse a very large dose of platelets, sufficient to leave 50% of $\alpha_{IIb}\beta_3$ receptors free, a number shown to be sufficient for normal hemostasis in studies of Glanzmann thrombasthenia heterozygotes. Without platelet transfusions, platelet aggregation generally returns to baseline levels within 12 to 24 hours after discontinuing abciximab.

Eptifibatide

Eptifibatide (Integrilin) is a cyclic heptapeptide based on the Lys-Gly-Asp (KGD) sequence found in barbourin, a platelet-inhibitory disintegrin from the venom of the Southeastern Pigmy rattlesnake, *Sistrurus miliarius barbouri.*[67] Barbourin differs from other integrin-binding proteins with the Arg-Gly-Asp (RGD) canonical sequence in that the arginine is conservatively substituted by lysine, a change that renders the protein a specific inhibitor of $\alpha_{IIb}\beta_3$.[67] Eptifibatide incorporates the KGD sequence within a cyclic seven-member peptide of high potency. Eptifibatide differs pharmacokinetically from abciximab in several important ways.[62] For example, unlike abciximab, intravenous eptifibatide infusion produces high levels of unbound drug because of its lower affinity for the receptor. Platelet transfusions therefore are not a good method for acutely reversing eptifibatide's antiplatelet effect because the newly transfused platelets are rapidly inhibited. However, its short plasma half-life (≈2.5 hours) allows for rapid clearance of eptifibatide and the reversal of its antiplatelet effect when administration is discontinued. Platelet aggregation returns to normal in approximately 4 hours, with the bleeding time normalizing within 1 hour.[62]

Tirofiban

Tirofiban (Aggrastat) is a peptidomimetic agent based on the RGD sequence, with a pharmacokinetic profile similar to that of eptifibatide.[62] Tirofiban antagonizes $\alpha_{IIb}\beta_3$ and does not cross-react with $\alpha_V\beta_3$.[68] As with eptifibatide, the maximum antiplatelet effect is seen at concentrations that leave a high concentration of unbound drug in the plasma.[62] Therefore, platelet transfusions are not often effective in reversing tirofiban's antiplatelet effect. However, its half-life is even shorter than that of eptifibatide (≈2 hours), and its antiplatelet effect is reversed rapidly after discontinuation of infusion.

The major adverse effects of $\alpha_{IIb}\beta_3$ inhibitors are thrombocytopenia and bleeding complications. Up to 5% of patients receiving abciximab may experience mild thrombocytopenia (<100,000/μL), and 1% may develop profound thrombocytopenia (platelet count <20,000/μL).[69,70] The incidence of severe thrombocytopenia is lower with tirofiban and eptifibatide, being approximately 0.2%.[70-72] A decrease in the platelet count is appreciable within the first hours after administration. It is therefore essential that a platelet count be obtained 2 to 4 hours after initiating treatment. Most patients with severe thrombocytopenia respond well to platelet transfusions and their platelet counts usually recover within 5 days, although they may take more than 1 week to do so. Because patients receiving abciximab frequently also receive heparin, heparin-induced thrombocytopenia (HIT) must be excluded. Ethylenediaminetetraacetic acid (EDTA)–dependent pseudothrombocytopenia should also be considered and ruled out by examination of a blood smear for the presence of platelet aggregates. Many patients require readministration of abciximab, raising the possibility that antibodies against the drug will complicate therapy. The safety of readministration was studied systematically in the ReoPro Readministration Registry.[69] The study found that abciximab readministration has a high clinical success rate and is not associated with hypersensitivity reactions, excessive bleeding, or death, and the incidence of thrombocytopenia is no greater than that seen in patients receiving abciximab for the first time. However, thrombocytopenia tended to be profound, relatively refractory to platelet infusion, and more often delayed. It is therefore recommended that clinicians obtain a second platelet count 24 hours after the readministration of abciximab and that they maintain a high index of suspicion for the delayed development of abciximab-induced thrombocytopenia.

Bleeding complications are quite common, especially in the inguinal area, where the femoral artery has been breached during procedures. Rates of major bleeding vary between 0.7% and 5.2% in different randomized controlled studies.[71,72] Intracranial bleeding is very rare (0.09%).[72] Bleeding risk increases in patients older than 65 years of age; in patients weighing less than 50 kg; in patients taking anticoagulant, antiplatelet, or thrombolytic therapies; and in patients with inherited or acquired bleeding disorders such as hemophilia and uremia, respectively.[72,73] Assessment of the risks and appropriate selection of the patients will decrease major bleeding complications in patients using glycoprotein (GP) IIb/IIIa inhibitors.

Phosphodiesterase Inhibitors

Elevation of cAMP and cyclic guanosine monophosphate (cGMP) inhibits many pathways involving platelet activation, including shape change, $\alpha_{IIb}\beta_3$ activation, and degranulation. Phosphodiesterases (PDEs) catalyze degradation of cAMP and cGMP, thus preventing platelet inhibition. Eleven PDE isoforms have been described, and three are expressed in platelets: PDE2, PDE3, and PDE5.[74] Many PDE inhibitors have antiplatelet effects.

Nonselective Phosphodiesterase Inhibitors

These include the methylxanthines caffeine (1,3,7-trimethylxanthine), theophylline (1,3-dimethylxanthine), and pentoxifylline (3,7-dimethyl-1-(5-oxohexyl)xanthine). Caffeine, at a dosage of 250 mg orally three times a day for 1 week, was demonstrated to reduce platelet aggregation in healthy subjects.[75]

PDE3 inhibitors are anagrelide, cilostazol, and milrinone. Although anagrelide inhibits platelet aggregation in vitro, it surprisingly also inhibits megakaryocyte maturation and proliferation and causes thrombocytopenia in humans by a mechanism that is poorly understood.[76] Anagrelide is used to treat essential thrombocytemia.[77]

Cilostazol is a cyclic nucleotide PDE inhibitor with both platelet inhibitory and vasodilatory effects; its current clinical use for peripheral vascular disease in the United States was preceded by its use in Japan and other Asian countries. In addition to selectively inhibiting PDE, cilostazol also inhibits adenine nucleotide uptake, a property not shared with other PDE inhibitors that further enhances its antiplatelet activity.[78]

Milrinone inhibits platelet aggregation and shape change. The drug is used for congestive heart failure.

PDE5 Inhibitors

Dipyridamole has several biologic effects, including PDE inhibition, targeting the PDE5 isoform that degrades cGMP.[79] It also enhances the release and prevents the breakdown of prostaglandin I_2 (prostacyclin).[80] Primarily used for prevention of stroke, its usefulness was demonstrated by a meta-analysis of recent randomized trials showing that the combination of dipyridamole (particularly the modified release form) and low-dose aspirin was more effective than aspirin alone in secondary prevention of vascular events after transient ischemic attack or stroke.[81] Dipyridamole has been associated with a significantly increased risk of GI bleeding when used either as a single agent or in combination with aspirin.[82]

Recently, inhibitors of PDE5 have become popular in the treatment of erectile dysfunction.[83] PDE5 is expressed in platelets, and its inhibition results in increases in the level of platelet cGMP, an effect similar to the effect of the well-known inhibitor of platelet function, nitric oxide. One study examined the activation response of platelets drawn from patients taking sildenafil (Viagra) when stimulated with either ADP or low-dose thrombin. The results showed significantly reduced activation to ADP in sildenafil-treated platelets, suggesting that the drug impairs selected pathways of platelet function in vivo. Several reports of sildenafil-associated bleeding have appeared, including epistaxis,[84,85] hemorrhoidal bleeding,[86] spontaneous intracranial hemorrhage,[87] and acute variceal bleeding.[88]

Adenyl Cyclase Stimulators or Prostacyclin Analogues

Epoprostenol (the synthetic salt of prostacyclin), prostacyclin (iloprost), and an orally active stable analogue (beraprost) are prostacyclin-like agents in clinical use. Despite the potent inhibition of platelet aggregation by prostacyclin in vitro, the effects on the bleeding time are minimal and inconsistent. These drugs are used for pulmonary arterial hypertension and peripheral artery disease.[89]

PERIOPERATIVE MANAGEMENT OF PATIENTS RECEIVING ANTIPLATELET THERAPY

The widespread use of antiplatelet therapies in patients with arterial disease or at risk for developing arterial diseases increases the risk of both spontaneous bleeding and surgical and traumatic bleeding.[90,91] For example, several studies have demonstrated that aspirin increases blood loss and transfusions in patients undergoing surgery.[64,91-95] Discontinuation of antiplatelet therapy before surgery has to be balanced against the increased risk of arterial thrombosis, as was seen in patients who had recent coronary stent implantation.[96] Optimal management of surgical bleeding risk in patients on platelet inhibitors thus requires consideration of patient features (both thrombosis risk and comorbidities), the reasons for antiplatelet therapy, the dose and the modality of drugs (single, dual, or triple antiplatelet therapy), individual responses to the drugs (noncompliance, the presence of aspirin or clopidogrel resistance), and the type of surgery to be performed.

Patients on antiplatelet therapy can be divided into two groups according to the risk of thrombotic complications. Low-risk patients include those receiving single antiplatelet therapy (usually low-dose aspirin) for primary prophylaxis of arterial disease. The high-risk group includes patients having had a recent (within 3-6 months) myocardial infarction, stroke, or peripheral arterial thrombosis and patients who have had recent implantation of a coronary stent.[95] Patients with coronary stents need special attention and may be considered to be at very high risk for thrombosis and death. Endothelization of bare metal stents requires 4 to 6 weeks but could take up to 1 year for drug-eluting stents. Dual therapy with aspirin plus clopidogrel is recommended for 12 months.[64,97,98] Other high-risk patients are patients receiving combined antiplatelet therapy, such as aspirin plus dipyridamole for stroke prevention and aspirin plus cilostazole for peripheral arterial disease. Approximately 6% to 8% of patients taking combined antiplatelet therapy for coronary artery disease also receive oral anticoagulants due to cardiac rhythm or valve problems.[91,97] For patients taking aspirin and undergoing minor dental, dermatologic, or cataract surgery, current guidelines recommend that aspirin not be stopped during these procedures because bleeding can be readily controlled with local hemostatic agents.[64,92,97] There are only limited data for patients taking clopidogrel in such situations; the decision as to whether to discontinue the drug should be made according to the individual patient's risks. In major surgical procedures such as cranial, spinal, abdominal, urological, major orthopedic or thoracic surgical operations, or posterior chamber eye surgery, antiplatelet therapy should be stopped according the patient's thrombosis risk. Aspirin and clopidogrel irreversibly inhibit platelets; restoration of normal platelet hemostasis thus requires a few days after cessation of the drug. For *patients at low risk for cardiovascular events,* guidelines published by the American College of Chest Physicians (ACCP) suggest stopping antiplatelet treatment 7 to 10 days before surgery[99]; others recommend waiting 5 to 7 days after the last dose.[64,92,97] The ACCP guidelines also suggest resuming aspirin or clopidogrel 12 to 24 hours after surgical bleeding has ceased. In patients at *moderate to high risk* for cardiovascular events (except patients with recent stents) who require noncardiac surgery or coronary artery bypass, the ACCP guidelines recommend continuing aspirin around the procedure but stopping clopidogrel at least 5 days before surgery.[64,92,97] *In patients with recent coronary stent placement,* elective surgeries should be deferred at least 6 weeks in those with bare metal stents and for at least 6 months in those with drug-eluting stents.[99] The risk of major adverse events, which are primarily cardiac, is very high (≤45%) in patients who have recent coronary stent placement.[92] This enhanced risk is not merely a consequence of stopping antiplatelet therapy. Hypoxia, hypercoagulability, and inflammatory responses caused by the operation are also associated with stent thrombosis and adverse cardiac events in these patients. If surgery is required, it is recommended that both aspirin and clopidogrel be continued.[64,91,97] If the operation is associated with a high risk of bleeding and the consequence of bleeding is likely to be dire (as in intracranial operations), the risk of bleeding must be balanced against the risk of thrombosis during the perioperative period. Clopidogrel may be stopped for 1 week in these situations.[91,92]

In patients taking vitamin K antagonists, bridge therapy with short-acting anticoagulants may prevent perioperative thrombosis without excessive bleeding. Replacement of aspirin with unfractionated or low-molecular-weight heparin is not recommended because heparins do not protect against myocardial infarction or stent thrombosis.[64,97] Replacement of aspirin or clopidogrel with short-acting $\alpha_{IIb}\beta_3$ inhibitors beginning 5 days before the planned surgery may decrease bleeding complications while minimizing the thrombotic risks. The short half-lives of tirofiban and eptifibatide may allow use of these drugs until 4 hours before surgery.

For emergency surgeries with a high risk of bleeding, there is no time to stop antiplatelet therapy. In these cases, platelet transfusions, antifibrinolytic agents (tranexamic acid and epsilon aminocaproic acid), and desmopressin (DDAVP) may help to control excessive bleeding.[64,91,97]

Although the ACCP guidelines recommended against the routine use of platelet function assays to monitor the antiplatelet effects of aspirin and clopidogrel,[64] there is no consensus on this topic.

Other Drugs that Adversely Affect Platelet Function

Nonsteroidal Antiinflammatory Drugs

In addition to aspirin, many other drugs used for their antiinflammatory and analgesic properties can cause platelet dysfunction.[100] As with aspirin, their mechanism of action appears to be the inhibition of COX-1; but in contrast to aspirin, these agents only temporarily affect COX-1 function, inhibiting the enzyme only as long as the active drug circulates. Among these agents, therefore, only drugs such as piroxicam, which has a plasma half-life of more than 2 days,[101] affect platelets for more than a few hours. As with aspirin, the most sensitive indication of impaired platelet function is the inhibition of in vitro platelet aggregation and secretion. These agents prolong the bleeding time minimally and transiently or not at all, consistent with the bleeding time being a less sensitive measure of the aspirin-induced defect.[100] The platelet function analyzer–100 more reliably detects the defect, manifested as a prolonged clotting time with the collagen/epinephrine cartridge.[102]

Reports of bleeding correlate with the effects of these agents on platelet function, suggesting that they increase the risk for excessive bleeding less than aspirin. As with aspirin, they may increase the bleeding times in patients with severe hemophilia, but in two studies, therapeutic doses of ibuprofen had no effect on the bleeding time in 19 of 20 patients with hemophilia.[103] Therefore, the clinical approach to patients taking any drug that can inhibit COX-1 should be similar, but the reversibility of the effect of NSAIDs provides an added margin of safety when these agents are used. Because of the increased bleeding risk, these drugs should be stopped before surgery. The timing for cessation of NSAIDs is based on the half-lives of the individual drug. Indomethacin, ibuprofen, ketoprofen, and diclofenac all have short half-lives (2-6 hours), and discontinuing these drugs 1 day before surgery is sufficient. Naproxen, sulindac, diflunisal, and celecoxib have intermediate half-lives (7-15 hours) and should be stopped 2 or 3 days before surgery. Nabumetone, meloxicam, piroxicam have very long half-lives (>20 hours). The ACCP guidelines recommend discontinuing these drugs 10 days before surgery.[64] Analgesics such as acetaminophen and sodium or choline salicylate, do not inhibit platelet function and have no adverse effects on hemostasis.[103]

Cardiovascular Drugs

Administration of nitroglycerin, isosorbide dinitrate, or nitroprusside can decrease platelet aggregation and secretion in vitro, but their effects in vivo are minimal and inconsistently observed.[100] The mechanism of platelet inhibition appears to involve the production of nitric oxide from the drug, with concomitant increases in platelet cAMP and, more markedly, cGMP.[104] α-Adrenergic receptor blockers such as propranolol, metoprolol, nebivolol, and pindolol have also been shown to inhibit platelet aggregation, apparently through mechanisms independent of α-adrenergic receptor blockade.[105,106] Several of these agents have been shown to blunt platelet aggregation to ADP and collagen[107] and to decrease platelet TXA_2 production in response to agonists.[105] Blunting of serotonin uptake by platelets and inhibition of the response to serotonin have also been demonstrated. There are numerous reports of antiplatelet effects of calcium channel blockers, such as nifedipine, verapamil, and diltiazem. Most of these studies demonstrated inhibition of platelet aggregation in vitro when high concentrations (micromolar) of the drug were used with washed platelets. This effect is mainly with epinephrine as the agonist, and it does not appear to be related to inhibition of calcium ion influx. Proposed mechanisms include inhibition of epinephrine binding to α_2-adrenergic receptors, inhibition of the platelet response to TXA_2, and inhibition of serotonin-induced aggregation. In therapeutic doses, the calcium channel blockers do not prolong the bleeding time. At high concentrations, quinidine can act as an antagonist of platelet α_2-adrenergic receptors. In one report, a patient taking 800 mg of quinidine and 650 mg of aspirin daily developed melena and generalized petechiae with a normal platelet count and a bleeding time over 35 minutes.[108] In a subsequent study in two healthy volunteers, quinidine caused a mild prolongation of the bleeding time that was apparently potentiated by aspirin. Quinidine and its stereoisomer, quinine, can also impair hemostasis by inducing drug-dependent antibodies that cause thrombocytopenia.

The commonly used antihypertensive drug losartan, an angiotensin II receptor antagonist, interacts with the TXA_2 receptor and inhibits thromboxane-dependent platelet adhesion and aggregation.[109]

Antibiotics

Antibiotics can also affect platelet function.[100] Those implicated most often are the penicillins and cephalosporins, which share a β-lactam ring structure. Some of these drugs produce predictable dose- and duration-related effects on the bleeding time.[110-112] Because the effect on bleeding time is seen only in patients who are receiving large parenteral doses of antibiotics, this is a potential problem only for hospitalized patients. In a study of 74 hospitalized patients with a consistently prolonged bleeding time, the likely cause was penicillin in 39 patients (30 patients were receiving >15,000,000 U/day of penicillin G, and nine were receiving 6-8 g/day of ampicillin) and aspirin or related drugs in seven patients.[112]

The structural properties that cause some, but not all, penicillins and cephalosporins to affect platelet function are unknown. The side chain structure alters the antibacterial and pharmacologic properties of the penicillins and cephalosporins and may also determine their effects on platelet function. It is postulated that the antibiotic associates with the platelet plasma membrane via a lipophilic mechanism where it perturbs receptor–agonist interactions or signal transduction.[113] The characteristic laboratory findings are a prolonged bleeding time and abnormal platelet aggregation studies that occur after several days of high-dose parenteral therapy.[111,112] These abnormalities do not usually subside until several days after the antibiotic is discontinued.

The frequency of clinically important bleeding in patients taking β-lactam antibiotics is low and is not predicted by a prolonged bleeding time; consequently, the causal relation to antibiotic treatment is unproved.[114] For each report implicating an antibiotic as a cause of hemorrhage, many more patients receive the same antibiotics in large doses without bleeding complications.[114]

In conclusion, antibiotic-induced platelet dysfunction appears to have little clinical importance, and the potential effect on platelet function should not be a consideration when choosing antibiotics. An exception to this rule may be moxalactam. The frequency of clinically important hemorrhagic complications with moxalactam appears to be higher than with other antibiotics.[114] This drug has been demonstrated to inhibit ADP- and collagen-induced platelet aggregation in a dose-dependent fashion and to decrease TXA_2 generation,[115] which suggests that, similar to aspirin, it acts on the thromboxane synthesis pathway. Furthermore, in contrast to most other β-lactam antibiotics, moxalactam contains a methylthiotetrazole-leaving group that has been implicated in the inhibition of synthesis of the vitamin K–dependent coagulation factors.[116] Therefore, moxalactam-induced bleeding may be caused by the combination of deficiencies in vitamin K–dependent coagulation factors and impaired platelet function.

Nitrofurantoin, an antibiotic structurally unrelated to the β-lactam antibiotics, may mildly prolong the bleeding time and impair platelet aggregation at plasma concentrations in excess of 20 μM.[117] Nitrofurantoin is not known to cause clinical bleeding.

Psychiatric Drugs

Platelets from patients taking tricyclic antidepressant drugs (imipramine, amitriptyline, nortriptyline) or phenothiazines (chlorpromazine, promethazine, trifluoperazine) may exhibit impaired in vitro aggregation and secretion responses to ADP, epinephrine, and collagen, but this effect is not associated with an increased risk for bleeding.[100] There are numerous reports of antiplatelet effects of the widely used selective serotonin reuptake inhibitors (paroxetine, sertraline, fluoxetine, citalopram), which may block the only means of platelet serotonin uptake for storage[118-122]; the effect of these drugs in decreasing platelet serotonin levels has been documented.[123,124] Prolonged bleeding times,[125] excessive bruising,[126] and defective platelet aggregation have all been noted in patients taking fluoxetine.[127] Additionally, the risk of GI bleeding is increased in patients taking serotonin reuptake inhibitors, particularly when they are combined with NSAIDs.[128] Further evidence of the antiplatelet effects of serotonin reuptake inhibitors, especially those that bind the serotonin transporter with high affinity, is a reduction in the risk of myocardial infarction with these drugs compared with other antidepressants or no drugs at all.[129]

Oncologic Drugs

Administration of mithramycin has been associated with decreased platelet aggregation, a prolonged bleeding time, and mucocutaneous bleeding.[130] Daunorubicin and bis-chloroethyl-nitrosourea can both inhibit platelet aggregation and secretion when added to platelet-rich plasma, but these effects do not appear to be clinically important.[100] Vincristine inhibits platelet aggregation by interfering with the microtubule network.[131]

Anesthetics

Although some local and general anesthetic agents have been shown to inhibit platelet functions in vitro, this effect is generally produced at high drug concentrations.[132,133] Procaine inhibits calcium and P-selectin release from platelet storage pools.[134] Dibucaine is a calpain activator, induces platelet apoptosis, and inhibits platelet functions.[135] At usual doses, halothane reversibly inhibits platelet aggregation.[136]

Plasma Expanders

Dextrans are partially hydrolyzed branched polysaccharides of glucose. Of the two preparations in clinical use, dextran 70 has an average molecular mass of 70-75 kDa and dextran 40 has an average molecular mass of 40 kDa. Both preparations are effective plasma expanders and can affect platelet function, but the high-molecular-weight molecules have a greater effect on hemostasis.[137] Dextran infusion also impairs platelet aggregation and platelet procoagulant activity and can cause a modest reduction in plasma vWF concentration. However, dextran has no effect on platelet function when added directly to platelet-rich plasma in vitro.[138] Because of its effects on platelet function, dextran was explored as an antithrombotic agent, but it is no longer used for this purpose.

Hydroxyethyl starch, known as *hetastarch,* is a synthetic glucose polymer with an average molecular weight of 450,000 (range, 10,000-1,000,000) that is also used for plasma expansion. Hetastarch use has been associated (albeit inconsistently) with abnormal platelet function, and this appears to be more evident with the higher-molecular-weight forms.[139] Similar to dextran, it can prolong the bleeding time, particularly if administered at doses higher than 20 mL/kg in a 6% solution, and predisposes to bleeding if administered simultaneously with heparin or in the presence of a preexisting hemostatic defect.[140]

Heparins and Thrombolytic Agents

Although heparin is best known for its anticoagulant effect and its association with HIT and thrombosis (see Chapters 135 and 151), it also has the potential to affect platelet function. Heparin can bind to the platelet surface,[141] cause platelet aggregation and secretion,[142] and impair vWF-dependent platelet function.[143] Heparin can also increase the bleeding time.[144] Whether these phenomena contribute to heparin-induced bleeding is unknown. The prolonged bleeding time is probably the result of inhibition of thrombin generation, analogous to the slight but significant increase in bleeding times seen in patients with hemophilia.[136]

Paradoxically, heparin is also capable of inducing the association of vWF with the GPIb complex.[145] Whether this is restricted to certain individuals or occurs only at certain heparin doses is unclear, but it raises the possibility that this mechanism may contribute to heparin-induced thrombosis.

Bleeding during therapy with plasminogen activators is predominantly caused by fibrin degradation, hypofibrinogenemia and increased levels of fibrin(ogen) degradation products, usually in the setting of structural lesions. At pharmacologic concentrations, streptokinase, urokinase, and tissue plasminogen activator (t-PA) may also impair platelet function through several potential mechanisms, all related to excessive production of plasmin.[146] First, high levels of fibrin(ogen) degradation products and low levels of fibrinogen may impair platelet aggregation. Second, the binding of plasminogen to the platelet surface may facilitate its conversion to plasmin.[147] Plasmin can degrade GPIbα (thereby impairing the interaction of the platelet with vWF[148]) and fibrinogen (thereby dispersing platelet aggregates).[149] Third, plasmin can inhibit platelet aggregation by blocking the release of arachidonic acid from platelet membranes, thereby limiting TXA_2 production.[150] The clinical importance of these observations is unknown.

In addition to decreasing platelet function, plasmin has been shown to directly activate platelets,[151-154] an effect that may contribute to vessel reocclusion after t-PA treatment for myocardial infarction.[155] Platelet activation is the result of plasmin-mediated cleavage of protease-activated receptors (PAR), particularly PAR4.[156]

Miscellaneous

The statins, which inhibit 3-hydroxy-3-methylglutaryl coenzyme A reductase, are widely used in patients with dyslipidemia.[157] These agents reduce the risk of cardiovascular events through a variety of mechanisms, including reducing the risk of atherothrombosis. Among its antithrombotic effects are decreases in platelet reactivity, brought about by its beneficial effects on endothelial cells, with increased production of nitric oxide and prostacyclin, and by direct effects on platelets.[158] Membrane cholesterol content, which is lowered by the statins, has been correlated with platelet reactivity,[159,160] with studies demonstrating that the content of cholesterol in platelet membranes correlates with localization of important adhesive and agonist receptors within membrane microdomains known as lipid rafts.[161,162]

Statins, in addition to lowering plasma and membrane cholesterol levels, also reduce the activity of stimulatory signaling pathways involving the small guanyl triphosphate (GTP)–binding proteins Ras, Rho, and Rac, which require posttranslational prenylation to be targeted to cell membranes. Statins inhibit protein prenylation.[163] No bleeding complications have been associated with statin use, but a substudy of the Platelet Receptor in Ischemic Syndrome Management (PRISM) trial showed that their sudden withdrawal in the setting of acute coronary syndrome was associated with an increased cardiac risk compared with that in patients who continued to receive statins (relative risk, 2.93) or never received statins.[164] This increase in cardiac events was partially attributed to increased platelet reactivity mediated through direct and indirect mechanisms. A recent meta-analysis found no correlation between statin therapy and increased intracranial hemorrhage.[165]

Clofibrate, another lipid-lowering drug, diminishes platelet responsiveness to ADP, collagen, and epinephrine when given to patients with type II hyperbetalipoproteinemia and can diminish the responsiveness of normal platelets to ADP and epinephrine in vitro.[100]

Cocaine accounts for more drug-related visits to emergency departments in the United States than any other drug except alcohol. Its use is associated with a large increase in the incidence of myocardial infarction in individuals who are otherwise at low risk, and it has been hypothesized that cocaine-induced platelet aggregation is a major contributor to this risk.[166] In vitro, however, cocaine inhibits platelet aggregation in response to several agonists and dissociates preformed aggregates.[167]

Ketanserin, which has been studied for its potential to prevent atherosclerotic complications, decreases platelet aggregation in response to serotonin. Antihistamines, some radiographic contrast agents, and immunosuppressive drugs can also impair platelet aggregation. The mechanisms responsible for these effects are unknown.

Foods and Food Additives

Certain foods and food additives can have important effects on platelet function, particularly when consumed in large quantities. In a classic study published in 1979, Dyerberg and Bang[168] reported that Greenland Eskimos on traditional diets had markedly prolonged bleeding times compared with gender- and age-matched Danish control subjects (mean, 8.1 min vs. 4.8 min, respectively), and they correlated this finding with an impaired secondary wave of platelet aggregation to ADP and collagen and high plasma levels of ω-3 fatty acids. The proposed mechanisms by which ω-3 fatty acids (eicosapentaenoic acid, C20:5ω-3; and docosahexaenoic acid, C22:6ω-3) interfere with platelet function is through competition with arachidonic acid for the 2-acyl position of membrane phospholipids or access to COX-1.[169,170] ω-3 Fatty acids not only reduce TXA_2 synthesis in response to platelet agonist stimulation by competing with the substrate arachidonic acid but also by producing inhibitory eicosanoids. The latter mechanism was substantiated in the original study of Eskimos by the demonstration that administration of aspirin decreased the bleeding time in all subjects tested but not to normal levels.[168] Additionally, ω-3 fatty acids may increase the production of antiaggregatory prostaglandins by cells in the vessel wall.[168]

Ethanol, one of the most commonly and excessively ingested substances in the world, acts synergistically with aspirin to prolong the bleeding time.[171] In addition, ethanol acts cooperatively with agents that block binding of fibrinogen to $\alpha_{IIb}\beta_3$ to further reduce platelet aggregation in response to several agonists, an effect not solely the result of reduced TXA_2 generation.[172] Ethanol may also impair collagen-induced platelet aggregation, secretion, arachidonate mobilization, and TXA_2 formation, but it did not inhibit platelet adhesion to deendothelialized rabbit aortae.[173]

Other food components or additives may also affect platelet function and increase the risk of minor bleeding. Easy bruising after eating Chinese food has been attributed to a platelet inhibitory effect of black tree fungus.[174] A component of onion extract can inhibit platelet arachidonic acid metabolism.[175] Ajoene, a component of garlic, is an inhibitor of fibrinogen binding to platelets and platelet aggregation.[176] Extracts from frequently consumed spices—cumin, turmeric, and clove—can decrease platelet thromboxane production and inhibit platelet aggregation.[177]

It can be concluded that platelets are sensitive to a variety of therapeutic and dietary compounds.[100] However, an increased risk for clinically important bleeding has been demonstrated only for aspirin and agents specifically designed to inhibit platelet function. Reports of increased bleeding with all other agents must be viewed with caution. Despite this qualification, it is prudent for clinicians to have a thorough understanding of the antiplatelet effects of prescribed drugs and to always consider the potential impacts of drug- or diet-induced platelet dysfunction, particularly in patients with coexisting hemostatic defects.

CLONAL DISORDERS

Hematological Clonal Disorders

Myeloproliferative Neoplasms

According to the 2008 World Health Organization classification, the Philadelphia chromosome–negative myeloproliferative neoplasms (MPNs) include polycythemia vera (PV), essential thrombocythemia (ET), primary myelofibrosis (PMF), chronic neutrophilic leukemia, chronic eosinophilic leukemia, mast cell disease, and unclassified MPN.[178] Of these, PV, ET, and PMF are the most common MPNs and share several features. All three disorders are characterized by bone marrow hypercellularity and megakaryocytic hyperplasia, and megakaryocyte clustering. Chronic MPNs are clonal disorders, with the molecular lesion involving a hematopoietic stem cell. Thus, even when the phenotype is dominated by excessive proliferation of erythrocytes, such as in PV, the platelets are also products of the abnormal clone. In 2005, several laboratories identified an important causative mutation in MPNs, which results in a single, relatively conserved amino acid change (V617F) in the signaling protein Janus kinase 2 (JAK2).[179-183] This gain-of-function mutation is not present in the germline but is acquired in hematopoietic stem cells and increases the sensitivity of hematopoietic precursors to stimulation by erythropoietin and thrombopoietin, accounting for the increased red cell and platelet counts observed in the MPNs. Although the presence of the JAK-2 V617F mutation establishes the diagnosis of MPN and excludes secondary causes of erythrocytosis and thrombocytosis, this mutation does not discriminate among PV, ET, and PMF. It is estimated that the prevalence of the JAK-2 V617F mutation is 95% to 98% in patients with PV and 50% to 60% in those with ET or PMF (see Chapters 67-69).[184,185] After the demonstration of the importance of cell growth and proliferation pathways in MPNs, several other mutations in these pathways were described in MPN patients who are Philadelphia chromosome and JAK2 V617F negative. Mutations in exon 12 of JAK2 are associated with erythrocytosis, and are found in approximately 3% of PV patients. Mutations in MPL, the receptor for thrombopoietin, cause thrombocytosis and are found in 3% of patients with ET and 5% to 10% of those with PMF. Other mutations associated with MPNs affect TET-2, ASXL1, IDHCBL, LNK, EZH2, and IKZF1.[178,185,186]

The MPNs are characterized by varying degrees of leukocytosis or thrombocytosis; patients with PV often have a markedly elevated hematocrit. Particularly in PV and ET, thrombosis or bleeding accounts for a high percentage of the associated morbidity of the disorders, with thrombosis being the most common. Thrombosis in patients with PV and ET can involve arteries, veins, or the microcirculation, but arterial thrombosis is the most common.[187] Microcirculatory disturbances such as erythromelalgia, a syndrome of erythema and burning pain, particularly in the fingers, are more frequently seen with ET and result from platelet-rich arteriolar microthrombi that can lead to ischemia and gangrene. Bleeding in patients with PV and

ET is primarily mucocutaneous. Some bleeding episodes can in part be attributed to thrombosis, such as variceal bleeding resulting from thrombosis-induced portal hypertension.[188] However, bleeding tendencies in these patients can be worsened by aspirin, which is sometimes given to reduce the risk of thrombosis.

In the European Collaboration on Low-dose Aspirin in Polycythemia study, 633 (38.4%) of the 1638 PV patients enrolled had a history of thrombotic events. Of these, approximately three-quarters were arterial, and one-quarter were venous. Of the 164 patients who died during the study, thrombosis accounted for 41% of the deaths and bleeding for only 7%. Excessive bleeding, particularly with surgery, was particularly common in uncontrolled PV patients with an increased whole-blood viscosity and high hematocrit.[189]

The rates of thrombotic and hemorrhagic complications in ET have been studied in 21 retrospective cohort trials, reviewed by Barbui and colleagues.[188] At the time of diagnosis, the rates of thrombosis ranged from 9% to 84%, but rates of hemorrhage ranged from 3.9% to 63%. As in patients with PV, age older than 60 years and a history of prior thrombosis predicted the risk of recurrent thrombosis.[190]

Several intrinsic platelet function defects have been associated with the MPNs, but their clinical importance is uncertain. These may result, at least in part, from an increased sensitivity of the platelets to activation, a potential consequence of the JAK2 gain-of-function mutation. For example, a study demonstrated an increased risk of thrombosis in patients with chronic MPD when the mutant kinase was detected in platelets or in platelets and granulocytes.[191] Likewise, the JAK2 mutation in platelets correlated with increased platelet expression of tissue factor and P-selectin, decreased expression of CD41 and CD42b, and increased quantities of platelet–neutrophil aggregates, all indicators of a hyperreactive platelet phenotype.[192] Panova-Noeva et al[193] evaluated the platelets from 140 patients with MPN (80 ET, 60 PV) for global procoagulant potential by measuring thrombin generation and expression of tissue factor and P-selectin on the platelet surface. They found that patients with the JAK2 V617F mutation had the highest values for thrombin generation and platelet tissue factor and P-selectin expression. These findings correlated with JAK2 V617F allele burden.[193]

The platelets of patients with MPNs can show various morphologic abnormalities, including variations in size and shape, as well as reduced numbers of secretory granules. Platelet survival may be decreased in ET. The most common platelet abnormality is decreased aggregation and secretion in response to agonists, particularly epinephrine, ADP, and collagen.[194] These abnormalities are not simply the result of the high platelet count because patients with reactive thrombocytosis have functionally normal platelets.[195] In what may appear to be a paradox, some patients demonstrate spontaneous in vitro platelet aggregation in platelet-rich plasma. The significance of this phenomenon is unknown because it can also be seen in normal individuals. Decreased platelet aggregation or secretion and decreased procoagulant activity may be caused by decreased (1) agonist-induced release of arachidonic acid from membrane phospholipids, (2) conversion of arachidonic acid to prostaglandin endoperoxides or lipoxygenase products, (3) platelet responsiveness to TXA_2, (4) dense-granule or α-granule contents, or (5) α_2-adrenergic receptors. Some of the described abnormalities may also be a consequence of platelet activation in vivo or ex vivo during platelet preparation.

Specific platelet membrane abnormalities have also been reported, including deficiencies of: glycoproteins Ib and IX, causing an acquired form of the Bernard-Soulier syndrome[196]; receptors for prostaglandin D_2[197]; c-*MPL* receptors[198]; and an increased number of Fc receptors.[199] Because MPDs are clonal in origin, the abnormal platelets may arise from a clone of abnormal megakaryocytes.[200] Alternatively, the findings may be the result of platelet hyperreactivity and previous activation.[192] It is important to emphasize several features about the platelet function defects reported in MPNs. First, no defect has consistently predicted the risk for bleeding or thrombosis. Second, no defect is unique to, and therefore predictive of, a particular MPN. Third, their relative frequency varies widely. Therefore, the clinical importance of the abnormalities of platelet function in MPNs is unknown.

The bleeding time is prolonged in a small percentage of patients with MPNs, but bleeding complications can occur even in patients with normal bleeding times. Bleeding problems are mostly associated with the administration of antiplatelet or cytoreductive drugs. Acquired von Willebrand syndrome may also cause mucocutaneous bleeding in patients with extreme thrombocytosis or may complicate surgical interventions in nonbleeding patients. In acquired von Willebrand syndrome, the largest multimers of vWF are absent, presumably as a consequence of their adsorption to binding sites on the elevated numbers of platelets.[201-205] In a prospective study of MPN patients, the incidence of acquired von Willebrand syndrome was 11%.[206] Although increased adsorption of plasma vWF multimers by platelets is the cause of the syndrome and decreased vWF:RCo/Ag or vWF:collagen binding/Ag ratio was found in patients with extreme thrombocytosis,[205] acquired von Willebrand syndrome has also been described in patients with platelet counts between 120 and 135 × 10^9/μL.[206] The diagnostic criteria for acquired von Willebrand syndrome are the same as those for hereditary von Willebrand disease.

Routine plasma coagulation tests, such as the PT and aPTT, may be falsely prolonged in MPN patients if the red blood cell mass is increased. Because the plasma volume in these patients is reduced, it is important to adjust the citrate concentration in the tubes used to collect the blood for coagulation testing.

Management

In MPN patients, risk stratification systems are used to predict complications and survival. Two large studies have established age and a history of thrombosis as important risk factors for thrombosis in PV and ET patients.[207,208] Patients who are younger than 60 years of age and have no history of thrombosis are classified as "low risk," and those with a history of thrombosis or an age older than 60 years are classified as "high risk" for thrombosis. In low-risk ET or PV patients, the presence of extreme thrombocytosis (>1000 × 10^9 platelets/L) is associated with a higher risk for bleeding.[185,193,209] Besides age and history of thrombosis, other factors associated with shortened survival in patients with PV and ET include leukocytosis, the presence of the JAK2 mutation, and anemia. The International Prognostic Scoring System (IPSS) uses five criteria for risk assessment in PMF: age older than 65 years, the presence of constitutional symptoms, anemia (hemoglobin <10 g/dL), leukocytosis (>25 × 10^9/L), and the percentage of circulating blast cells (>%1). Recently, a "Dynamic IPSS" (DIPSS) score was introduced, which also considers transfusion requirements, thrombocytopenia (<100 × 10^9/L), and karyotype abnormalities as risk factors. According to the DIPSS, PMF patients are classified as low risk (no risk factors), intermediate risk (1-3 risk factors), and high risk (>4 risk factors); the higher the risk, the shorter the survival time in PMF patients.[210]

The main goals of the therapy are to decrease peripheral cell counts, restore hemostasis, and prevent thrombosis or bleeding. Low-risk ET patients are treated with low-dose aspirin; hydroxyurea should be added for high-risk ET-patients. Published guidelines recommend that all patients with PV be phlebotomized to maintain the hematocrit below 45%.[211] In low-risk PV patients, phlebotomy and low-dose aspirin therapy are used. Hydroxyurea is added for high-risk PV patients. For PV and ET, patients who are intolerant of or reluctant to use hydroxyurea, potential alternatives include α-interferon, anagrelide, and busulphan. Although recent studies suggested that pegylated α-interferon produces high rates of both hematologic and molecular responses with low toxicity in patients with ET and PV,[212,213] side effects were more common than with hydroxyurea (affecting 96% of the patients) and resulted in discontinuation of therapy in 22% of the patients.

One study compared hydroxyurea plus aspirin with anagrelide plus aspirin for the prevention of the thrombotic complications in ET patients.[214] Anagrelide was originally developed as a platelet inhibitor but was found to lower platelet counts by inhibiting the proliferation and differentiation of megakaryocytes.[215-217] Anagrelide is more expensive than hydroxyurea. Both regimens achieved good long-term control of platelet counts, but patients in the anagrelide group were much more likely to experience both thrombotic and hemorrhagic complications and to progress to myelofibrosis. Inexplicably, those in the anagrelide group experienced more venous thrombosis. The mortality rate was similar in the two treatment groups. This study reinforces the recommendation that hydroxyurea and aspirin should be the first-line therapy for high-risk patients, on the basis of efficacy, safety, and cost. Low-risk PMF patients are treated according to signs and symptoms; hydroxyurea is useful for treatment of symptomatic splenomegaly, androgens or thalidomide for anemia, and aspirin for thrombocytosis. Because of their poor prognosis, patients with more than two risk factors should be treated aggressively with hematopoietic stem cell transplant. Recently, ruxolitinib, a JAK inhibitor, was approved for the treatment of intermediate- and high-risk PMF patients.

Patients with thrombocytosis should be evaluated for acquired von Willebrand disease. In those with low (<30%) ristocetin cofactor activity, aspirin or other antiplatelet agents should be avoided because of the bleeding risk. In these patients, cytoreductive therapy is recommended to treat bleeding symptoms. Because cytoreductive therapy requires days or weeks to lower the blood counts, additional interventions should be used in patients with active bleeding. DDAVP was only effective in 21% of these patients because of tachyphylaxis or reduced vWF storage in the endothelium.[205] High-dose vWF concentrates and factor VIIa may be useful in MPN patients with severe bleeding. Local therapies should be considered, such as anti-ulcer therapy for active peptic ulcers, antifibrinolytic agents, and laser coagulation for nasal bleeding.

Paroxysmal Nocturnal Hemoglobinuria

Paroxysmal nocturnal hemoglobinuria (PNH) is another clonal disorder that involves all blood cells. The hematopoietic stems cells and their progeny are defective in the synthesis of the glycosylphosphatidylinositol attachments required for some membrane proteins, leading to a defect in all glycosylphosphatidylinositol-linked proteins on blood cells,[218] including platelets.[219] Thrombosis is a leading cause of mortality in PNH, affecting at least half of these patients and preferentially targeting the hepatic veins.[75] Several mechanisms have been proposed to explain this association, but it is unclear whether platelets play an important role.[220] The platelet function abnormalities described in PNH range from hypersensitivity to agonists to dysfunction. One study showed platelets to be hypersensitive to epinephrine, ADP, and collagen, as judged by their abilities to aggregate and to release ^{14}C serotonin.[221] The total release of nucleotides was also markedly increased over normal with all aggregating agents. By contrast, another study examining platelets from PNH patients showed them to be profoundly hyporeactive, as measured by defective clot formation, adhesion, and aggregation.[222] This finding was interpreted as being a consequence of chronic overstimulation of the platelets while they circulate.

Platelet activation and increased platelet microparticle formation have also been demonstrated in PNH patients.[221,223] Nevertheless, a strong correlation exists between thrombosis and the number of circulating abnormal neutrophil clones.[224] It is likely that the number of abnormal granulocyte clones reflects the number of abnormal platelet clones.[225] Warfarin prophylaxis in patients with high numbers of abnormal clones significantly reduces the thrombotic risk and carries minimal bleeding risk in patients who are not thrombocytopenic. In an open-label study of eculizumab, a humanized monoclonal antibody against human complement C5 that prevents assembly of the membrane attack complex on the cell surface, there was more than a 10-fold reduction in thromboembolic events in treated patients compared with untreated patients.[226] Eculizumab reduced arterial and venous thrombotic episodes even in those taking antithrombotic medications. These encouraging results may herald a new era of therapy for PNH patients because eculizumab has also been shown to decrease transfusion requirements, reduce fatigue, and improve general well-being.[227] The major limitation to this therapy is its high cost.

Paraproteinemias

Although thrombotic complications can occur in patients with dysproteinemias because of hyperviscosity, bleeding complications also are seen. Platelet dysfunction is observed in approximately one-third of patients with immunoglobulin A (IgA) myeloma or Waldenström macroglobulinemia, in 15% of patients with IgG myeloma, and occasionally in patients with benign monoclonal gammopathy.[228,229] Additional hemostatic problems in these patients can be caused by the hyperviscosity syndrome,[230] a heparin-like coagulation inhibitor,[231] acquired von Willebrand syndrome,[205] or complications of amyloidosis (e.g., acquired factor X deficiency[232] or enhanced fibrinolysis[233]). Patients may have markedly abnormal results on laboratory tests (e.g., a prolonged thrombin time) with no evidence of clinical bleeding.[228]

Abnormalities of platelet function correlate with the concentration of the plasma paraprotein. Myeloma proteins can inhibit all platelet functions (aggregation, secretion, procoagulant activity, and clot retraction), and normal platelets can acquire these defects when incubated with the purified monoclonal immunoglobulin.[234] In some cases, specific interactions of the monoclonal protein have been described. One IgA myeloma protein inhibited the ability of a suspension of aortic connective tissue to aggregate normal platelets.[235] The bleeding time and bleeding symptoms of the patient from whom this paraprotein was isolated were corrected when the IgA myeloma protein was removed by plasmapheresis. One patient had a fatal hemorrhage from an IgG1κ paraprotein that bound GPIIIa (β_3 integrin) and inhibited platelet aggregation.[236] A number of reports have described acquired von Willebrand disease in patients with myeloma, benign monoclonal gammopathy, or chronic lymphocytic leukemia.[237] In some patients, the plasma concentration of vWF was decreased; in others, the larger multimers were deficient. The myeloma protein may interact with vWF and accelerate its clearance from plasma or interfere with its binding to platelet GPIb.

Easy bruising, epistaxis, periorbital purpura (in patients with amyloidosis), and GI hemorrhage are the most common bleeding symptoms associated with the paraproteinemias. Because bleeding appears to be related to high plasma paraprotein concentrations,[238] chemotherapy for the underlying plasma cell neoplasm should be given to effect a longer lasting reduction of the paraprotein. In emergency situations, plasmapheresis should be performed expeditiously; the effectiveness of this therapy can be evaluated by amelioration of bleeding symptoms. Intravenous immunoglobulin (IVIG) infusions are effective in controlling bleeding symptoms in patients with plasma cell dyscrasias and acquired von Willebrand disease. IVIG may produce a clinical and laboratory response in 12 to 72 hours, and the effect usually persists for 1 to 3 weeks. In patients with severe bleeding, IVIG can be combined with plasmapheresis, DDVAP, and infusions of vWF concentrates or factor VIIa.[205,206,229,237]

LEUKEMIAS AND MYELODYSPLASTIC SYNDROMES

Bleeding in patients with the leukemias and myelodysplastic syndromes (MDS) is almost always caused by thrombocytopenia, but abnormalities of platelet function have also been described. In acute myeloid leukemia and its variants, platelets may be larger than normal, abnormally shaped, and vary in their granule numbers. Abnormal platelet structure and function have been described, especially in association with acute megakaryoblastic leukemia (FAB M7),[239,240] with one study describing three patients with decreased aggregation to collagen, ADP, epinephrine, and the thromboxane analogue U46619, along with a decreased platelet serotonin content.[241] Platelet abnormalities can also be found in the MDS, with defective aggregation and glass bead retention most often associated with hypolobulated megakaryocytes and the 5q$^-$ syndrome.[242] Abnormal platelet function has also been described in association with B-cell malignancies, such as hairy cell leukemia, which can persist after splenectomy,[243] and with chronic lymphocytic leukemia,[244] in which the platelets exhibit reduced responses to glycoprotein VI agonists, such as collagen and convulxin.

SOLID TUMORS

Bleeding complications in patients with cancer are related to decreased platelet production due to bone marrow infiltration, the myelosuppressive effects of chemotherapy and radiotherapy, sepsis, disseminated intravascular coagulopathy, microangiopathic hemolytic anemia; drug-induced thrombocytopenia; immune thrombocytopenia or hypersplenism. Although several defects of platelet functions have been described in cancer patients, none is specific.[245]

SYSTEMIC METABOLIC DISORDERS

End-Stage Renal Disease

The pathogenesis of the hemorrhagic diathesis in patients with end-stage renal disease (ESRD) is complex. Factors such as platelet function abnormalities caused by uremic toxins, anemia, hemodialysis procedures (both the artificial circulation and the use of anticoagulation), and decreased drug clearance may impair hemostasis.

The recognition of severe hemorrhage as a distinct complication of renal failure is generally attributed to Reisman's description in 1907 of two patients with Bright disease who had severe and generalized bleeding.[246] Reisman proposed that the cause was "a toxin analogous to the hemorrhagins of snake venom." However, the bleeding in Reisman's patients may have reflected any number of other associated conditions.[246] Others observed a "tendency to hemorrhage" in patients with chronic glomerulonephritis in the predialysis era, and the descriptions of epistaxis and menometrorrhagia[247] suggested a primary platelet abnormality. Nevertheless, in the era before dialysis, death in patients with chronic renal failure occurred primarily from hyperkalemia and pulmonary edema.[248] After dialysis became an established treatment, the major causes of death were infection and the underlying cause of the renal failure. Hemorrhage caused 6 of 100 deaths in one series, but additional factors could have contributed in each case.[248] The current prognosis for patients with ESRD is excellent, with a significant proportion surviving past 10 years and some reported to survive up to 3 decades on hemodialysis.[249] Bleeding problems were not mentioned in this discussion, and bleeding was not considered in reviews published in the past 25 years on the clinical course and management of patients with chronic renal failure. However, bleeding and thrombosis in patients with chronic uremia continue to be discussed.[250]

A more objective indication of the rarity of a significant bleeding diathesis in patients with renal failure is the extensive experience with percutaneous renal biopsy. In a study of 1000 consecutive percutaneous renal biopsies performed at the Mayo Clinic, 69 patients had hematuria, which cleared within 2 days in 50 patients.[251] Hypertension was a more significant factor than the bleeding time in predicting the occurrence of this complication.[251] Another study of 183 consecutively performed renal biopsies reported three episodes of hemorrhage that required surgical intervention; all were the results of needle lacerations of the kidney or spleen.[252] In an analysis of 5120 renal biopsies performed at 15 institutions, there were no deaths, and severe bleeding complications appeared to be related to anomalous vessels, heparin anticoagulation, or the presence of amyloid in the kidney.[253] Reports of bleeding with other invasive procedures in patients with chronic renal disease are rare, but they suggest that bleeding complications are uncommon after abdominal surgery, liver and bone marrow biopsies, and tooth extractions.[254]

By contrast, GI tract hemorrhage is a common complication and frequent cause of death in patients with acute renal failure, and patients with chronic renal failure account for a significant proportion of patients undergoing endoscopy for upper GI bleeding.[255] Experimental data suggest that chronic uremia renders the gastric mucosa susceptible to acid injury.[256] More than 90% of patients with renal failure and GI bleeding have an anatomic diagnosis at endoscopy: Angiodysplasia is most common, but peptic lesions (gastric or duodenal ulcer, erosive esophagitis, gastritis, or duodenitis) also are frequent findings.[255] Rectal ulcers can also cause sudden, massive lower GI hemorrhage.

These observations suggest that serious, spontaneous hemorrhage is uncommon in patients with chronic renal failure. Nevertheless, platelet dysfunction is believed to constitute the primary hemostatic abnormality in uremia,[257] consistent with the common findings of easy bruising, epistaxis, gingival bleeding, and prolonged bleeding after venipuncture or trauma in patients with uremia. Descriptions of bleeding in uremia have often focused on the laboratory phenomena of abnormal platelet aggregation or a prolonged bleeding time rather than actual hemorrhagic episodes in patients.[250] As with the drug-induced disorders of platelet function discussed earlier, in uremia abnormal platelet function on laboratory tests is far more common than clinically important bleeding. Thus, laboratory evaluation of platelet function may not be a good predictor of the risk of hemorrhage.

Platelet aggregation studies are frequently abnormal in uremic patients, but these abnormalities do not correlate with the severity of the renal failure or with the occurrence of bleeding.[258] The bleeding time may also be prolonged in uremia and does not necessarily correlate with the severity of the renal failure.[258] Furthermore, controversy exists as to whether the bleeding time is a useful predictor of risk for clinically important bleeding.[259,260] One study found no difference in bleeding complications whether or not a bleeding time was performed before renal biopsy.[261]

Anemia, which does correlate with the severity of renal failure, is an independent cause of a prolonged bleeding time.[262-265] The relationship of the hematocrit to the bleeding time was first discerned in 1910 by Duke, who found that the bleeding time in thrombocytopenic patients was corrected by transfusion of fresh whole blood, but when thrombocytopenia recurred, the bleeding time was not as prolonged in the presence of a higher hematocrit.[266] Furthermore, it has been noted that bleeding times can be prolonged with severe anemia caused by deficiency of vitamin B_{12} or iron and can be corrected with red blood cell transfusions.[262] Therefore, severely anemic patients with chronic renal failure would be expected to have prolonged bleeding times. The relationship of the bleeding time to hematocrit in uremic patients has been confirmed by its correction with the transfusion of red blood cells and by treatment with erythropoietin.[264,267] There was a suggestion that bleeding symptoms also improved with correction of the anemia. It is believed that the association between anemia and a prolonged bleeding time reflects the tendency of red blood cells to displace the less dense platelets to the periphery of the cylindrical blood vessel, where the platelets are poised to survey the vascular wall for defects.[268]

In contrast to the studies of platelet function performed to understand the possible increased risk for bleeding in patients with chronic renal failure, the coagulation and fibrinolytic systems have been interrogated to understand the increased risk for thrombotic complications, a major cause of mortality.[250] Although the data are inconsistent, markers of increased activation coagulation are often seen in patients with uremia, suggesting the presence of a prothrombotic state.[250,269]

Even though the anemia of renal failure appears to be the major cause of the prolonged bleeding time, there is also evidence of abnormal platelet function. Platelet aggregation abnormalities persist when the hematocrit is normalized by red blood cell transfusion[263,264] or erythropoietin treatment.[270] The defects appear to result from intrinsic defects of the platelets and from substances in the plasma capable of inhibiting the function of normal platelets. Deficiencies in the number of GPIb complexes in uremic platelets have been reported, the number inversely correlating with the creatinine level.[271] Consistent with this finding, another study demonstrated that defective ristocetin-induced platelet aggregation of uremic platelet-rich plasma was not corrected by resuspending the platelets in normal platelet-poor plasma. Likewise, uremic platelets suspended in normal plasma were defective in their adhesion to deendothelialized rabbit vessels at high shear, a test of the competency of the interaction between GPIb and vWF.[272] Conversely, the same study demonstrated that plasma factors also influence platelet function by showing that normal platelets suspended in uremic plasma acquired an adhesion defect possibly related to an abnormal interaction of vWF with the subendothelium. This led to the suggestion that vWF may be abnormal in uremia. Two studies have demonstrated normal to elevated vWF antigen and activity (measured as ristocetin cofactor activity) in uremic patients but decreased levels of the largest, most hemostatically active multimers,[273,274] reflected in one study as a decreased ratio of activity to antigen level compared with the vWF from normal subjects.[273] Taken together, the various studies consistently indicate that the first step of platelet adhesion at sites of vessel wall injury is abnormal, a defect that could be clinically significant if coupled with other defects of platelet function.

The platelets of uremic patients frequently exhibit reduced fibrinogen binding, aggregation, and secretion in response to a wide variety of agonists. This abnormality may persist when the platelets are removed from uremic plasma, and in some studies, uremic plasma has induced these defects in normal platelets. Uremic platelets may also exhibit a reduction in several of the biochemical responses necessary for aggregation and secretion, including the rise in cytoplasmic calcium ion concentration, release of arachidonic acid from membrane phospholipids, conversion of arachidonic acid to TXA_2, and dense-granule and α-granule secretion. Abnormal cytoskeletal assembly and deficient tyrosine phosphorylation have also been noted in uremic platelets, abnormalities only partially corrected by dialysis.[275]

The accumulation of dialyzable platelet-inhibitory substances in the plasma of uremic patients has long been recognized. The ability of uremic plasma to inhibit platelet function was demonstrated by Horowitz and colleagues,[276] who showed reduced ADP-induced platelet aggregation and a prolonged Stypven clotting time, a measure of platelet procoagulant activity. This activity, previously called *platelet factor 3,* is vital for the support of coagulation factor complex assembly on the platelet surface and requires externalization of the anionic phospholipid phosphatidylserine. One uremic substance with platelet inhibitory properties described by Horowitz and coworkers[277] was guanidinosuccinic acid, which accumulates in uremic plasma as an alternative byproduct of L-arginine metabolism,[260] a consequence of the inhibitory effect of high urea levels on enzymes of the urea cycle. Similar to L-arginine, guanidinosuccinic acid is a precursor of nitric oxide, which is produced in increased quantities in the endothelial cells and platelets of uremic patients and experimental animals.[260] Consistent with an important role for nitric oxide in uremia, infusion of the nitric oxide synthesis inhibitor monomethyl L-arginine reduced the bleeding time in uremic rats.[278] Furthermore, suppression of nitric oxide production appears to correlate with the benefit of conjugated estrogens in improving the bleeding time in uremia.[279] Increased expression of vascular prostacyclin has also been described in uremic rats, a factor that would further depress in vivo platelet function.[280]

Dialysis itself may be associated with alterations in platelet function. For example, hemodialysis may cause transient increases in the bleeding time and reduced responsiveness of platelet to agonists in vitro,[281] and chronic hemodialysis and peritoneal dialysis are associated with an increase in reticulated platelets, suggesting accelerated platelet turnover.[282] Of the two forms of dialysis, hemodialysis appears to have the greatest effect on platelet function, with one study noting abnormal cytoskeletal assembly and defective tyrosine phosphorylation to thrombin stimulation in the platelets of patients on hemodialysis, parameters that returned almost to normal with the institution of ambulatory peritoneal dialysis.[275] The cause of the defect associated with hemodialysis is likely to be the chronic low-level platelet activation associated with the procedure. In particular, polymerization and depolymerization of actin, release of granule proteins and their binding to the platelet surface, and shedding of membrane proteins may render the platelets relatively refractory to activation.

As would be expected, platelets from uremic patients may be unusually sensitive to medicines that decrease platelet function. Aspirin has been reported to produce a greater prolongation of the bleeding time in uremic patients than in controls, an effect that may be attributable to more than the irreversible inhibition of COX-1.[283] Similarly, β-lactam antibiotics that prolong the bleeding time may also have a greater effect in uremic patients and may increase the risk of bleeding, particularly those antibiotics cleared by the kidney.[100,265]

Mild thrombocytopenia in chronic renal failure likely reflects a combination of decreased marrow production and shortened platelet survival.[265] However, a platelet count below 100,000/μL should alert the physician to the possibility of a systemic disease, such as multiple myeloma, systemic vasculitis, hemolytic uremic syndrome, preeclampsia, or renal allograft rejection, or an adverse reaction to a drug, such as heparin. Erythropoietin deficiency can also contribute to the hemostatic defect of uremia. Consistent with this concept, defective tyrosine phosphorylation in uremic endothelial cells is restored when erythropoietin is added.[284]

Management of Uremic Bleeding

Prolonged bleeding times and abnormal platelet aggregation studies are common findings in uremic patients, but they do not always predict an increased risk for hemorrhage or constitute an indication for transfusion or therapeutic intervention. If a patient with abnormal platelet function and a long bleeding time requires an invasive procedure, such as a kidney or lung biopsy or a laparotomy, and has no history to suggest an increased risk for bleeding, it may be less risky to perform the procedure without specific treatment to correct the platelet defect than to delay the intervention and attempt to normalize the laboratory values.

When therapy is indicated, the best strategy to improve hemostasis is to perform dialysis. Dialysis improves platelet function, normalizes the prolonged bleeding time, and reduces the risk of bleeding. For example, intensive dialysis decreases the occurrence of acute GI bleeding, a major cause of morbidity and mortality in patients with acute renal failure. Peritoneal dialysis and hemodialysis are equally effective, but evidence of in vivo platelet activation is only seen in patients treated with hemodialysis.

If bleeding does complicate a procedure, the cause is most likely structural and the bleeding should be managed as it would be in patients without renal failure. However, angiodysplasia and erosive esophagitis are more common causes of upper GI bleeding in uremic patients than in those with normal renal function.[255] Patients with chronic renal failure who present with hemorrhage should be evaluated as are other bleeding patients; uremia should not be assumed to be the cause of bleeding.

Apart from intensive dialysis, several treatment modalities have been reported to shorten the bleeding time and improve hemostasis, but well-controlled studies are lacking. Therefore, therapy for bleeding in patients with chronic renal failure should take into consideration the severity of bleeding, the anticipated severity of the hemostatic risk from surgery or trauma, and the risks of the therapy.

Options include DDAVP, which can be given intravenously or subcutaneously at a dose of 0.3 mg/kg. Such treatment has been reported to shorten the bleeding time in 50% to 75% of uremic patients. This correction occurs within 30 to 60 minutes and lasts for up to 4 hours, correlating with increases in the overall plasma concentration of vWF and in the fraction of vWF consisting of higher-molecular-weight multimers. DDAVP has been reported to be effective in preventing surgical bleeding in uremic patients, but controlled trials of its efficacy are lacking. Side effects of DDAVP are uncommon but may include facial flushing, mild tachycardia, water retention, hyponatremia (sometimes severe enough to cause seizures), arterial thrombosis, and memory loss. DDAVP stimulates the release of vWF from endothelial cells, which may account for its therapeutic effect, but other mechanisms may be involved, including a direct priming effect on the platelets.

Increasing the hematocrit, either by red blood cell transfusion or by treatment with recombinant human erythropoietin, can correct the bleeding time and possibly reduce the tendency to bleed. It has also been proposed that in addition to localizing the platelets along the vessel wall, erythrocytes facilitate activation of platelets by releasing ADP, a contribution diminished by anemia.[285]

Conjugated estrogens have also been reported to shorten prolonged bleeding times in uremic patients and to correct the bleeding diathesis.[286] Even a single 50-mg dose of oral conjugated estrogen (Premarin) may be effective. In support of this, conjugated estrogens have been shown to shorten the prolonged bleeding time in uremic rats.[280] The correction of the bleeding time in this model was abolished by the nitric oxide precursor L-arginine, and administration of estrogens to uremic rats decreased the expression of nitric oxide synthase. These findings suggest that the estrogen effect on hemostasis in uremia might be mediated by changes in nitric oxide synthesis.

Some studies have reported that cryoprecipitate infusions shorten the bleeding time in patients with uremia, but others have not; it is unlikely that the benefit justifies the risk.

Liver Disease

The bleeding diathesis observed with fulminant or end-stage liver disease is multifactorial, with contributing causes including thrombocytopenia, anemia, deficiencies in liver-synthesized coagulation factors, and excessive fibrinolysis.[287,288] Patients with chronic liver disease and hepatic cirrhosis of various causes have been reported to have prolonged bleeding times, and these disorders may be associated with other platelet function abnormalities possibly related to a decrease in GPIb.[289] Although some have shown an association between prolonged bleeding time and GI hemorrhage in some studies of cirrhotic patients,[290] others showed that the bleeding time and platelet aggregation abnormalities correlated best with the degree of thrombocytopenia,[291] suggesting that no specific platelet function defect exists in liver disease. An aspirin-like defect has been reported in patients with severe liver disease, with defective aggregation and TXA_2 production.[292] Interestingly, one study showed that platelets obtained from the portal circulation of patients with hepatocellular cancer on a background of cirrhosis showed decreased and delayed aggregation in response to collagen compared with circulating platelets.[293] In addition to portal hypertension and esophageal varices, this finding raises the possibility that localized vascular bed factors (including increased prostacyclin) may contribute to variceal bleeding.

Because patients with cirrhosis often have a complicated hemostatic picture that includes thrombocytopenia, decreased fibrinogen levels, and prolonged prothrombin and aPTTs, one might expect this to uniformly produce a severe bleeding diathesis. However, recent studies have shown that the hemostatic defects in these patients are at least partially compensated through several mechanisms. The potential to bleed because of thrombocytopenia is reduced because vWF levels are often elevated and a disintegrin and metalloproteinase with a thrombospondin type 1 motif, member 13 (ADAMTS13) activity is decreased,[294,295] perhaps as a consequence of decreased synthesis by hepatic stellate cells. The decreased concentrations of procoagulant factors are balanced by the decreased concentrations of anticoagulant proteins.[296] Dysfibrinogenemia produces a less severe hemostatic defect because of decreased plasminogen levels.[297,298] This balance may easily be tipped in either direction, favoring either bleeding or thrombosis.

Although patients with cirrhosis may have platelet dysfunction, it is usually not associated with serious bleeding. Bleeding in these patients cannot be predicted with routine diagnostic tests, such as the platelet count and PT.[299]

In addition to bleeding, thrombotic episodes are not uncommon in patients with cirrhosis. In advanced cirrhosis, portal or mesenteric thrombosis may occur, possibly because of stasis in the portal system. Underlying thrombotic disorders may increase the thrombosis risk; examples of these include hereditary thrombophilia, MPNs, and nonalcoholic fatty liver disease. Another factor that increases the risk of thrombosis in patients with liver disease is excessive replacement with fresh-frozen plasma or administration of procoagulants. In conclusion, patients with liver disease are at increased risk for both bleeding and thrombosis, and these complications cannot be predicted with routine tests. Controlled studies are required both to better predict these risks and to help guide the management of these complications.

PLATELET DYSFUNCTION RELATED WITH EXTRACORPOREAL CIRCUITS

Although cardiopulmonary bypass (CPB) is accompanied by decreased plasma levels of coagulation factors and increased fibrinolytic activity, abnormal platelet function is also a prominent observation in these patients. A fall in the platelet count and platelet dysfunction are seen in most patients undergoing bypass surgery with either a bubble or a membrane oxygenator.[300] Typical findings after bypass surgery include a prolonged bleeding time (longer than expected for the degree of thrombocytopenia), decreased platelet aggregation, decreased platelet agglutination in response to ristocetin, and depletion of platelet α-granule and dense granule contents.[300] Despite these abnormalities, excessive bleeding is uncommon, occurring only in about 5% of patients. Bleeding, usually manifesting as excessive chest tube drainage (defined as >100 mL/hr), has many causes, including surgical complications, excessive protamine dosing, heparin rebound, and possibly platelet function abnormalities.[301-305]

As with hemodialysis, the platelet defect caused by CPB is most likely a consequence of platelet activation and fragmentation within the extracorporeal circuit. The severity of the platelet abnormalities correlates with the duration of the bypass procedure.[306,307] With uncomplicated surgery, platelet function returns to normal in 1 hour[306]; however, a much longer time may be required in some patients,[308] and the platelet count typically does not return to normal for several days.[305] Thrombocytopenia is caused by hemodilution and deposition of platelets on the bypass circuit and, to a lesser extent, sequestration of damaged platelets in the liver. Platelet dysfunction during bypass may be caused by reversible adhesion and aggregation of platelets on fibrinogen adsorbed from plasma onto the bypass circuit material, mechanical trauma and shear stress, cardiotomy suction, trace concentrations of circulating thrombin and ADP, complement activation, hypothermia, blood conservation devices; bypass priming solutions; and, with bubble oxygenators, exposure of platelets to the blood–air interface.[100] CPB consistently induces the formation of platelet fragments, or membrane *microparticles,* evidence that the platelet surface membrane is subjected to severe mechanical stress and activation during the procedure.[307] Thus considerable platelet activation and aggregation occur during CPB, which leads to deleterious effects from substances released from the platelets and the new adhesive molecules exposed on their surfaces, and renders the platelets relatively refractory to activation by agonists.

Another surgical cause of platelet dysfunction relates to the use of deep hypothermic circulatory arrest in some surgeries. This procedure involves cooling the vital organs to temperatures between 15°C and 22°C (59°F and 71.6°F) for the purpose of neuroprotection during complex surgeries of the aortic arch or intracerebral aneurysms.[309] During the period of deepest hypothermia, the circulation is stopped, making for bloodless surgical fields. Complications of deep hypothermic circulatory arrest include coagulopathy and neurologic sequelae, with evidence that the latter problem may involve hypothermic activation of platelets and formation of microaggregates.[310] Treatment with $\alpha_{IIb}\beta_3$ inhibitors, such as eptifibatide or tirofiban, may improve neurological outcomes by preventing microvascular occlusion.[310]

A study on the use of aspirin in patients undergoing coronary artery bypass grafting indicates that earlier practices of avoiding platelet inhibitors may in fact lead to increased morbidity of all types, ranging from death to ischemic complications involving the heart, gut, and kidneys.[311] Administration of aspirin within 48 hours of surgery reduced the risk of dying by one-third and the risk of nonischemic complications by approximately two-fifths. In the same study, it was noted that the patients who received either platelets or antifibrinolytic therapy to reduce postoperative bleeding were at increased risk for adverse complications and death. Thus, except in the setting of acute hemorrhage with evidence of platelet dysfunction, platelet transfusion should be avoided. Likewise, it is perhaps best to treat patients with aspirin soon after bypass surgery to decrease the incidence of deleterious effects. In addition to the known benefit of aspirin in reducing the risk of graft occlusion in patients undergoing coronary artery bypass grafting, early institution of aspirin also is warranted for patients who have undergone CPB for other reasons and in whom aspirin therapy is not otherwise contraindicated.

When postoperative blood loss is greater than anticipated, it can be treated with DDAVP after cessation of bypass, but most clinical trials have not demonstrated a beneficial effect of this agent.[312,313] Benefits of DDAVP were more apparent in patients undergoing more complex cardiac surgical procedures. Potential risks of DDAVP include hyponatremia, hypotension, and thrombosis.[312]

Attempts have been made to prevent platelet activation during bypass surgery in humans and experimental animals by infusion of prostaglandin E_1 or prostacyclin. By increasing the platelet concentration of cAMP and reducing platelet responsiveness, these agents reduce the risk of thrombocytopenia and platelet dysfunction.[314] However, the hypotensive properties of these agents limit their usefulness. Antifibrinolytics (tranexamic acid, ε-aminocaproic acid, aprotinin) have been shown to reduce blood loss after CPB.[315] Aprotinin has been studied for its potential to protect platelets from activation by thrombin, plasmin, and other proteases generated during CPB. At high doses, aprotinin appears better than either ε-aminocaproic acid or desmopressin at reducing postoperative blood loss and is at least as good as tranexamic acid.[316] However, aprotinin has been reported to increase mortality and renal toxicity after CPB. These findings resulted in its withdrawal from the market. However, the European Medicines Agency recently lifted this suspension in Europe.

MISCELLANEOUS

Hypothermia

Hypothermia is defined as core body temperature below 35°C or 95°F and is classified as mild (32-35°C or 90-95°F), moderate (28-32°C or 82-90°F), severe (20-28°C or 68-82°F), and profound (below 20°C or 68°F). Major causes of hypothermia are exposure to cold weather or immersion in cold water, but hypothermia can also be caused by dehydration, severe trauma, massive transfusion, head injury, burns, sepsis, and drugs (e.g., alcohol, sedatives, hypnotics). Age is an important risk factor because elderly adults and newborns are particularly prone to hypothermia. Hypothermia is also intentionally induced in some cardiac operations (see the section on extracorporeal circulation).

Mild hypothermia is usually well tolerated, but mortality increases when the core body temperature falls below 20°C. In animals, hypothermia causes thrombocytopenia because of platelet sequestration in the spleen and liver. Hypothermia inhibits platelet aggregation in response to thrombin and thromboxane, increases platelet expression of P-selectin, and decreases expression of the GPIb-IX-V complex.[317] Both the thrombocytopenia and the functional defects are reversible, returning to normal when the body temperature normalizes.

DISSEMINATED INTRAVASCULAR COAGULATION

Disseminated intravascular coagulation is sometimes associated with acquired storage pool disease, believed to be the result of chronic platelet stimulation and resulting in the formation of so-called *exhausted platelets.*[318] The elevated levels of fibrin(ogen) degradation products and reduced fibrinogen concentrations, which are hallmarks of this disorder, may lead to reduced platelet function. Although fibrin(ogen) degradation products can impair platelet aggregation in vitro, the concentrations required to do so are unlikely to be generated in vivo.[319] Platelet dysfunction only occurs with severe hypofibrinogenemia because only small amounts of fibrinogen are needed to saturate the fibrinogen receptors on platelets.[320]

ANTIPLATELET ANTIBODIES

Immunoglobulins may bind to platelets in a specific or nonspecific fashion and can disrupt platelet function. In conditions such as immune thrombocytopenic purpura (ITP), systemic lupus erythematosus (SLE), and platelet alloimmunization, the antibodies can trigger accelerated platelet destruction and subsequent thrombocytopenia. Surviving platelets, known as *stress platelets,* display enhanced function.[321] Indeed, bleeding times in ITP may be shorter than expected for the degree of thrombocytopenia. Sometimes, however, the hemorrhagic tendency is out of proportion to the degree of thrombocytopenia or persists after the platelet count returns to normal, suggesting that the bound antibody may perturb platelet function. Immune thrombocytopenia is common; significantly impaired hemostasis caused primarily by antibody-mediated platelet dysfunction is not. In one study, 3 of 49 patients with ITP whose platelet counts had recovered after therapy with either corticosteroids or splenectomy continued to display elevated bleeding times and persistence of mucocutaneous hemorrhage.[322]

In some patients with ITP or SLE, platelet dysfunction may be suspected because mucocutaneous bleeding symptoms occur despite platelet counts that are usually sufficient for normal hemostasis (>50,000/μL), and the bleeding time may be longer than expected for the degree of thrombocytopenia. Patients with antiplatelet antibodies may exhibit defective platelet function in vitro even if they do not have prolonged bleeding times or clinical symptoms of excessive bleeding, a situation similar to that which occurs with aspirin ingestion or with renal disease. For example, in two studies, 13 of 19 patients with ITP demonstrated impaired platelet aggregation to ADP, epinephrine, or collagen.[323,324] In two other studies, 22 of 35 patients with SLE were found to have decreased platelet aggregation in response to these agonists.[325,326] The platelet function abnormalities appear to be antibody mediated because IgG purified from the plasma or eluted from the platelets of these patients inhibit the aggregation of normal platelets.

Platelet antibodies may affect several aspects of platelet function. The most frequently observed abnormality is absence of platelet aggregation in response to low concentrations of collagen and absence of the second wave of irreversible aggregation in response to ADP or epinephrine. This pattern is identical to the abnormalities caused by aspirin, described earlier. In ITP and SLE, the abnormal aggregation may be related to a reduction in the contents of dense- and α-granules or to an activation defect manifested by diminished synthesis of TXA_2.

Autoantibodies or alloantibodies usually impair the function of the antigen against which they are targeted. For example, alloantibodies (e.g., anti-Pl^{A1}) and autoantibodies that bind to $\alpha_{IIb}\beta_3$ produce a syndrome similar to Glanzmann thrombasthenia.[327-331] These antibody-associated thrombopathies can be severe. It is not surprising that many of the antiplatelet antibodies target $\alpha_{IIb}\beta_3$ because this is the most abundant receptor on the platelet surface and required for all aggregation responses.[332] Antibodies that target GPIb have also been described, in one case producing a syndrome of severe refractory thrombocytopenia and a functional defect resembling that observed in Bernard-Soulier syndrome.[333] An interesting aspect of antibodies against GPIb is their association with more severe thrombocytopenia than that observed with antibodies directed against other antigens.[334] This finding is consistent with the observations that anti-GPIb antibodies inhibit megakaryopoiesis[335] and proplatelet formation in vitro.[336] Autoantibodies that target GPIa (integrin α_2),[337,338] GPIV,[338] and GPVI[339,340] have also been described.[339,341]

Platelet-activating antibodies have been described. Of particular interest is the report of a patient who presented with immune thrombocytopenia and an antibody against CD9 (a member of the tetraspanin protein family) that was capable of activating normal platelets.[342] After recovery of the platelet count, the patient relapsed, this time with an antibody described against the platelet Fc receptor, FcγRIIA. The latter antibody blocked the capacity of the first antibody to activate platelets, confirming that activation involved stimulation of the Fc receptor.

Platelets that have been activated and induced to secrete but have not been incorporated into aggregates are likely to be refractory to platelet agonists and deficient in secretory granule contents, essentially leading to an acquired storage pool deficiency, which has also been described in association with autoantibodies.[343]

SUGGESTED READINGS

Cipollone F, Rocca B, Patrono C: Cyclooxygenase-2 expression and inhibition in atherothrombosis. *Arterioscler Thromb Vasc Biol* 24:246, 2004.

Cryer B, Feldman M: Effects of very low dose daily, long-term aspirin therapy on gastric, duodenal, and rectal prostaglandin levels and on mucosal injury in healthy humans. *Gastroenterology* 117:17, 1999.

Diaz-Buxo JA, Donadio JV, Jr: Complications of percutaneous renal biopsy: An analysis of 1,000 consecutive biopsies. *Clin Nephrol* 4:223, 1975.

Diener HC, Cunha L, Forbes C, et al: European Stroke Prevention Study. 2. Dipyridamole and acetylsalicylic acid in the secondary prevention of stroke. *J Neurol Sci* 143:1, 1996.

Feldman M, Shewmake K, Cryer B: Time course inhibition of gastric and platelet COX activity by acetylsalicylic acid in humans. *Am J Physiol Gastrointest Liver Physiol* 279:G1113, 2000.

Fiorucci S, Del SP: NO-aspirin: Mechanism of action and gastrointestinal safety. *Dig Liver Dis* 35:S9, 2003.

Harker LA, Slichter SJ: The bleeding time as a screening test for evaluation of platelet function. *N Engl J Med* 287:155, 1972.

Hedner T, Everts B: The early clinical history of salicylates in rheumatology and pain. *Clin Rheumatol* 17:17, 1998.

Koscielny J, Ziemer S, Radtke H, et al: A practical concept for preoperative identification of patients with impaired primary hemostasis. *Clin Appl Thromb Hemost* 10:195, 2004.

Kyrle PA, Westwick J, Scully MF, et al: Investigation of the interaction of blood platelets with the coagulation system at the site of plug formation in vivo in man—effect of low-dose aspirin. *Thromb Haemost* 57:62, 1987.

Lee M, Cryer B, Feldman M: Dose effects of aspirin on gastric prostaglandins and stomach mucosal injury. *Ann Intern Med* 120:184, 1994.

Ma L, Elliott SN, Cirino G, et al: Platelets modulate gastric ulcer healing: Role of endostatin and vascular endothelial growth factor release. *Proc Natl Acad Sci U S A* 98:6470, 2001.

Mackowiak PA: Brief history of antipyretic therapy. *Clin Infect Dis* 31:S154, 2000.

Mielke CH, Jr: Aspirin prolongation of the template bleeding time: Influence of venostasis and direction of incision. *Blood* 60:1139, 1982.

Mielke CH, Jr: Influence of aspirin on platelets and the bleeding time. *Am J Med* 74:72, 1983.

Mielke CH, Jr, Kaneshiro MM, Maher IA, et al: The standardized normal Ivy bleeding time and its prolongation by aspirin. *Blood* 34:204, 1969.

Miner J, Hoffhines A: The discovery of aspirin's antithrombotic effects. *Tex Heart Inst J* 34:179, 2007.

O'Laughlin JC, Hoftiezer JW, et al: Does aspirin prolong bleeding from gastric biopsies in man? *Gastrointest Endosc* 27:1, 1981.

Patrono C, Coller B, Dalen JE, et al: Platelet-active drugs: The relationships among dose, effectiveness, and side effects. *Chest* 119:39S, 2001.

Risk of myocardial infarction and death during treatment with low dose aspirin and intravenous heparin in men with unstable coronary artery disease. The RISC Group. *Lancet* 336:827, 1990.

Roderick PJ, Wilkes HC, Meade TW: The gastrointestinal toxicity of aspirin: An overview of randomised controlled trials. *Br J Clin Pharmacol* 35:219, 1993.

Rodgers RP, Levin J: A critical reappraisal of the bleeding time. *Semin Thromb Hemost* 16:1, 1990.

Sibilia J, Ravaud P, Marck G: [Risk factors for gastrointestinal bleeding associated with low-dose aspirin]. *Presse Med* 32:S9, 2003.

Steering Committee of the Physician's Health Study Research Group: Final report of the aspirin component of the ongoing physicians' health study. *N Engl J Med* 321:129, 1989.

Undas A, Brummel K, Musial J, et al: Blood coagulation at the site of microvascular injury: Effects of low-dose aspirin. *Blood* 98:2423, 2001.

Undas A, Brummel-Ziedins KE, Mann KG: Antithrombotic properties of aspirin and resistance to aspirin: Beyond strictly antiplatelet actions. *Blood* 109:2285, 2007.

Wallace JL, Ma L: Inflammatory mediators in gastrointestinal defense and injury. *Exp Biol Med (Maywood)* 226:1003, 2001.

Weiss HJ, Aledort LM: Impaired platelet-connective-tissue reaction in man after aspirin ingestion. *Lancet* 2:495, 1967.

Weksler BB: Regulation of prostaglandin synthesis in human vascular cells. *Ann N Y Acad Sci* 509:142, 1987.

Wolfe MM, Lichtenstein DR, Singh G: Gastrointestinal toxicity of nonsteroidal antiinflammatory drugs. *N Engl J Med* 340:1888, 1999.

For complete list of references log on to www.expertconsult.com.

CHAPTER 133

DISEASES OF PLATELET NUMBER: IMMUNE THROMBOCYTOPENIA, NEONATAL ALLOIMMUNE THROMBOCYTOPENIA, AND POSTTRANSFUSION PURPURA

Donald M. Arnold, Christopher Patriquin, Lisa J. Toltl, Ishac Nazi, James Smith, and John Kelton

Platelets are anucleate cells that are required for primary hemostasis. Platelets have a life span of 7 to 10 days in circulation, after which time they are cleared by the cells of the reticuloendothelial system (RES), including the spleen. Platelet production is stimulated by thrombopoietin (TPO), a hormone that is constitutively secreted by the liver, which binds to its receptor c-Mpl on platelets, hematopoietic progenitor cells, and bone marrow (BM) megakaryocytes. When TPO is bound to c-Mpl, it is internalized, degraded, and removed from the circulation; thus, when the platelet count is low, free TPO levels are high, and more platelets are produced; when platelet counts are high, circulating TPO levels are low, and platelet production declines. This primitive feedback system is very effective at maintaining the platelet count at a stable level.

Immune-mediated platelet disorders disrupt normal regulation of platelet number because of cell-mediated or antibody-mediated platelet destruction or megakaryocyte injury. Antibodies that target self (autoimmune) or nonself (alloimmune) antigens on platelets can cause severe thrombocytopenia. Immune thrombocytopenia (ITP) is characterized by autoantibodies directed against platelet glycoproteins. Neonatal alloimmune thrombocytopenia (NAIT) is an example of a thrombocytopenic syndrome caused by platelet alloantibodies. Posttransfusion purpura (PTP) has features of both allo- and autoantibodies. These platelet disorders have related features yet are distinct clinical syndromes (Table 133-1). The pathophysiology, clinical manifestations, and management of each of these disorders are discussed in this chapter.

IMMUNE THROMBOCYTOPENIA

Immune thrombocytopenia is a common autoimmune disease characterized by low platelet count levels that can be associated with an increased risk of bleeding. Increased platelet destruction resulting from platelet autoantibodies is the hallmark of ITP. Recently, however, it has become evident that relative platelet underproduction is also an important feature of this disorder. Conventional treatments, including corticosteroids, intravenous immunoglobulin (IVIG), immunosuppressant drugs, and splenectomy, are aimed at preventing platelet destruction. TPO receptor agonists, a new class of medications that work by increasing platelet production, represent the most significant advance in ITP management since the first description of the efficacy of IVIG in the early 1980s. In addition to changing the paradigm as to the pathogenesis of ITP, this milestone set the stage for clinical trials of TPO receptor antagonists and was the catalyst for key papers including the report of an international working group on the standardization of terminology in 2009[1] and the development of the American Society of Hematology (ASH) Guidelines on diagnosis and management of ITP in 2011.[2]

Epidemiology

The natural history of ITP is different in children and adults. For the majority of children, ITP presents acutely and resolves within several weeks even in the absence of intervention. Seasonal variability suggests that a viral infection may trigger the disease in many children. Conversely, adult-onset ITP tends to be insidious in onset and is characterized by a chronic or remitting and relapsing course.

Incidence and Prevalence of Childhood Immune Thrombocytopenia

The incidence of acute ITP in children is estimated at 1.9 to 6.4 per 100,000 per year. Nearly 70% of childhood ITP occurs between the ages of 1 and 10 years with the peak prevalence between 4 and 6 years. Most studies in children report an overall male predominance in early childhood and equalization or reversal to female predominance in older children. Reported prevalence estimates are 12.6 per 100,000 for girls and 9.3 per 100,000 for boys in the older age groups.

Adult Immune Thrombocytopenia

Incidence estimates for adult-onset ITP are reported to be between 1.6 to 3.9 per 100,000 per year.[3] A retrospective analysis from the United Kingdom described a bimodal distribution for men, with peak incidences before the age of 18 years and between 75 and 84 years of age. Relatively stable incidence rates were found in women up to the age of 60 years with a steady increase thereafter. The incidence of ITP has been reported to double in patients after age 60 years.

The overall prevalence of ITP in adults has been estimated at 9.5 per 100,000, ranging from 4.1 per 100,000 in younger ages (19-24 years) to 16 per 100,000 in older age groups (55-64 years). Other investigations have reported male and female prevalence rates of 16.6 and 27.2 per 100,000 adults, respectively, for those ages 18 to 64 years, with rates increasing significantly after the age of 65 years. The prevalence in women is reported to be nearly double that in men; however, this trend is attenuated in older age groups and may revert to a male predominance after the age of 65 years. Indeed, the prevalence of ITP in older men is reported to be as high as 38.3 per 100,000. Adult incidence and prevalence rates may reflect a true increase in risk of disease with age or measurement bias because of a higher likelihood of discovering incidental thrombocytopenia with more frequent medical visits.

Table 133-1 Antibody-Mediated Thrombocytopenic Disorders Caused by Autoantibodies (Immune Thrombocytopenia), Alloantibodies (Neonatal Alloimmune Thrombocytopenia) or Potentially Both (Posttransfusion Purpura)

	Immune Thrombocytopenia	Neonatal Alloimmune Thrombocytopenia	Posttransfusion Purpura
Immune reaction	Autoimmune	Alloimmune	Features of both allo- and autoimmunity
Incidence	Five per 100,000 population	40 per 100,000 births (or one per 2,500)	One per 100,000 blood transfusions
Principal antigenic target	GPIIb/IIIa	HPA-1a	HPA-1a plus autoantigens
Nature of the antibody	Intermittent	Persistent (past 1 year)	Persistent often at high titers
Mode of sensitization	Autoantibody	Alloantibody	Features of allo- and autoantibodies
Sensitizing event	Mostly unknown; some viral illnesses, chronic infection	Exposure to fetal platelet antigens early in first pregnancy	Blood transfusion (RBCs or platelets) 5-10 days earlier
Bleeding frequency	Uncommon	Common	Very common
Epidemiology	Higher incidence in children and elderly adults; female predominance in early adulthood	Majority affects fetus or newborn carrying the HPA-1a antigen	Almost all are HPA-1bb women sensitized by previous transfusion or pregnancy

GP, Glycoprotein; *HPA*, human platelet antigen; *RBC*, red blood cell.

Pregnancy

Thrombocytopenia commonly occurs during pregnancy. Incidental thrombocytopenia of pregnancy is the most common cause followed by pregnancy-related vascular disorders and pregnancy-associated ITP.[4]

Incidental thrombocytopenia of pregnancy (also called gestational thrombocytopenia) may represent a physiological state. It is characterized by mild thrombocytopenia with platelet counts generally greater than 70 × 10^9/L, occurs late in pregnancy, and is clinically insignificant for the mother or baby. Treatment is not required.

Pregnancy-related vascular disorders are the next most common cause of thrombocytopenia during pregnancy. These disorders include preeclampsia, microangiopathy (including the HELP syndrome, which is characterized by hemolysis, elevated liver enzymes, and a low platelet count), and acute fatty liver. Platelet counts tend to be mildly reduced, and hypertension and other features are invariably present.

Immune thrombocytopenia is an uncommon cause of thrombocytopenia in pregnancy, and when mild, it can be difficult to distinguish from incidental thrombocytopenia of pregnancy. Differences are that pregnancy-associated ITP may present early, thrombocytopenia can be severe, and platelet counts typically increase after ITP-specific therapies such as IVIG or corticosteroids. During pregnancy, platelet count thresholds for instituting ITP treatment are the same as those for women who are not pregnant; in the absence of bleeding, treatment is rarely indicated unless the platelet count is below 20 × 10^9/L. Although vaginal deliveries are thought to be safe for mothers with ITP, even if the platelet count is very low, most clinicians attempt to maintain the count above 20 to 30 × 10^9/L. Epidural anesthesia is not recommended unless the platelet count is above 70 to 80 × 10^9/L, although this practice is operator driven and based on little evidence. IVIG and corticosteroids are generally safe in pregnancy, but corticosteroids can be associated with hypertension and other morbidities. Splenectomy is rarely indicated during pregnancy because most women can successfully be managed with less aggressive therapy. Immunosuppressant medications, such as azathioprine, have been used in pregnancy but should be reserved for refractory pregnancy-associated ITP with bleeding. The risk of severe thrombocytopenia in the newborn caused by passive transfer of maternal antiplatelet autoantibodies is estimated at approximately 10%.

Pathophysiology

Immune thrombocytopenia is caused by increased platelet destruction and impaired platelet production. Until recently, the pathogenesis of immune-mediated thrombocytopenia was mainly attributed to platelet-reactive autoantibodies. However, it is now evident that the pathophysiology of ITP is more complex and involves alterations in cellular immunity and immune-mediated megakaryocyte injury.

The antibody hypothesis began with evidence implicating a plasma factor in the blood of patients with ITP. In one of the first experiments, William Harrington infused blood from ITP patients into normal volunteers and observed a decrease in the platelet counts in most recipients.[5] This circulating "factor" was later identified as an immunoglobulin (IgG) that bound to the surface of platelets. In further studies, investigators were able to quantify platelet-associated IgG (PAIgG) on or inside platelets; however, this test failed to discriminate between immune and nonimmune thrombocytopenia. Assays that detect antibodies directed against specific platelet glycoproteins (GPs), specifically GPIIb/IIIa or GPIb/IX, exhibit improved specificity but have sensitivities that range from 55.4% to 66%. Autoantibodies against platelet GPs target those cells for rapid destruction in the RES, particularly the spleen. Peptides released from phagocytosed platelets may be processed and presented to specific T cells, which in turn stimulate B cells to produce additional platelet autoantibodies. This process, known as epitope spreading, may explain why patients may have autoantibodies targeting a variety of different platelet antigens in their serum.

In ITP, platelet production does not compensate for the increased platelet destruction, suggesting that BM megakaryocytes may also be impaired. Evidence supporting reduced platelet production comes from at least two sources. First, studies using radiolabeled autologous platelets demonstrate normal or reduced platelet turnover in ITP.[6] Second, the capacity of TPO receptor agonists to raise the platelet counts in patients with ITP[7] indicates reduced production. Megakaryocytes also express GP receptors, which may render them targets of ITP autoantibodies. Indeed, in vitro studies have shown suppression of megakaryocyte growth and maturation by the IgG fraction of ITP plasma, which may explain why platelet production is decreased. The mechanisms invoked to explain the development of thrombocytopenia in the face of platelet autoantibodies include opsonization and clearance, direct activation of complement, or cellular destruction via apoptosis.

In addition to the effect of autoantibodies, cytotoxic T cells from ITP patients may exert direct cytolytic effects on platelets. Patients with active ITP but without detectable platelet autoantibodies have $CD8^+$ T cells that induce platelet lysis in vitro. In contrast, $CD8^+$ T cells from patients in remission do not show significant platelet reactivity. Furthermore, $CD3^+$ cells from ITP patients exhibit increased expression of genes involved in cell-mediated cytotoxicity such as tumor necrosis factor-α (TNF-α), perforin, and granzyme A and B relative to control participants, and $CD8^+$ T cells exhibit increased expression of FasL (Fas–Fas ligand) and TNF-α.

In the broadest sense, autoimmunity develops because of a breakdown in regulatory checkpoints that occurs during development or maturation of the immune system.[8] Although the events that trigger a loss of self-tolerance to platelet GPs and the development of ITP are largely unknown, ITP patients exhibit immune alterations, which may explain why they develop autoreactivity to platelet antigens. These include dysfunctional cellular immunity because of Th0/Th1 polarization, decreased regulatory T cells, and autoreactive platelet-specific cytotoxic T cells. In addition, ITP patients can have increased circulating levels of cytokines and soluble factors that promote the survival of self-reactive T and B cells, including BAFF (B-cell activating factor), APRIL (a proliferation-inducing ligand), and BIM (Bcl-2 interacting mediator of cell death). Alterations in proteins involved in proapoptotic pathways designed to delete self-reactive T cells, such as Fas, interferon (IFN)-γ, interleukin (IL)-2 receptor β (IL2RB), Bax, and caspases 8 and A20, have also been demonstrated.

Infection is another stimulus for the formation of platelet reactive autoantibodies. Cross-reactive antibodies (molecular mimicry) have been best described with infections with *Helicobacter pylori,* HIV or hepatitis C virus (HCV). *H. pylori*-associated ITP is discussed later.

Clinical and Laboratory Features

Thrombocytopenia

Thrombocytopenia is the defining feature of ITP. The international working group on standardization of terminology in ITP established a platelet below 100×10^9/L as the cutoff for the diagnosis (Table 133-2).[1] The rationale behind this decision was that patients with mild thrombocytopenia (150-100 $\times 10^9$/L) have a low risk (≈7%) of developing a persistent platelet count of less than 100×10^9/L; platelet counts slightly below 150×10^9/L may be normal for certain ethnic groups, and mild thrombocytopenia may be caused by physiological processes, such as occurs during pregnancy. Nonetheless, primary ITP remains a diagnosis of exclusion, and as such, investigations are aimed at ruling out nonimmune causes, including pseudothrombocytopenia, myelodysplastic syndrome, thrombotic microangiopathies, splenomegaly, or hereditary thrombocytopenia and secondary immune causes such as infection, concomitant autoimmune disease, or lymphoproliferative disorders.

Immune thrombocytopenia may be primary or secondary. Primary ITP, which was previously known as "idiopathic" but is now referred to as "immune thrombocytopenia" (see Table 133-2), occurs for unknown reasons. Secondary ITP is important to recognize because treatment of the underlying cause is often necessary to increase the platelet count. Examples are ITP occurring in the setting of drugs, lymphoproliferative disease, or HIV or *H. pylori* infection.

Molecular mimicry between the highly antigenic *H. pylori* CagA protein and platelet antigens is the suspected mechanism of *H. pylori*–associated ITP.[9] In most patients, *H. pylori* can be successfully eradicated with a 1- to 2-week course of clarithromycin (500 mg twice daily), amoxicillin (1000 mg twice daily), and pantoprazole or omeprazole (20 mg twice daily); however, the effect of *H. pylori* eradication on platelet count levels is variable. In a meta-analysis that included 788 patients, *H. pylori* eradication resulted in platelet counts that were 34×10^9/L higher than those in untreated control participants and 52×10^9/L higher than those in treated patients whose *H. pylori* was not eradicated. Another systematic review evaluating 696 patients reported that 42.7% of treated patients achieved platelet counts above 100×10^9/L; however, the effect was highly dependent on geographical location with the beneficial effect mainly observed in patients from Japan.[10] Evidence-based guidelines for the investigation and management of ITP recommend against routine screening for *H. pylori* in patients presenting with ITP because of the low yield of testing and the low likelihood of a platelet count increase with eradication. However, testing may be warranted in endemic countries where a high response rate to *H. pylori* eradiation has been demonstrated.

Table 133-2 Standardized Terminology and Definitions for Immune Thrombocytopenia Proposed by the International Working Group (Vicenza Consensus Conference) in 2009

Terminology	Definition
ITP	Immune thrombocytopenia (rather than idiopathic or immune thrombocytopenic purpura)
Platelet threshold for ITP diagnosis	<100×10^9/L
Primary ITP	ITP with no associated cause (diagnosis of exclusion)
Secondary ITP	ITP in the setting of an underlying cause such as drugs, HIV, or SLE
Newly diagnosed ITP	Designation for patients at diagnosis (rather than "acute" ITP).
Persistent ITP	Sustained or recurrent thrombocytopenia lasting 3-12 months
Chronic ITP	Thrombocytopenia lasting >12 months
Complete response	Achievement of a platelet count of ≥100×10^9/L in the absence of bleeding
Response	Achievement of a platelet count of ≥30×10^9/L and at least a twofold increase from baseline in the absence of bleeding
Refractory ITP	Failure to achieve a response or relapse after splenectomy* and requirement for treatment(s) to minimize the risk of clinically significant bleeding.

ITP, Immune thrombocytopenia; *SLE,* systemic lupus erythematosus.
*Splenectomy failure may not be applicable in children.

Clinical Outcomes: Mortality, Bleeding, and Quality of Life

Most commonly, patients with ITP present with asymptomatic thrombocytopenia. Although some patients bleed with platelet counts less than 30×10^9/L, many do not. Bleeding symptoms characteristic of ITP ("platelet-type bleeding") include skin bleeding (i.e., bruises, nonpalpable purpura, or petechiae), oral hemorrhagic blood blisters (purpura) or oral petechiae; epistaxis, menorrhagia, or gastrointestinal bleeding. The most feared complication is intracerebral hemorrhage.

In children, large prospective registries indicate a rate of intracerebral hemorrhage that ranges from 0% to 0.2% in the first 6 months after ITP diagnosis.[11] In adults, the risk of life-threatening bleeding is higher but remains low. In a retrospective cohort study spanning 7 years, two of 117 (1.7%) adults with chronic ITP developed intracerebral hemorrhage. In a pooled analysis of ITP patients with platelet counts persistently below 30×10^9/L, the estimated rate of fatal bleeding was 0.02 to 0.04 cases per patient-year, and age older than 60 years was a risk factor.[12]

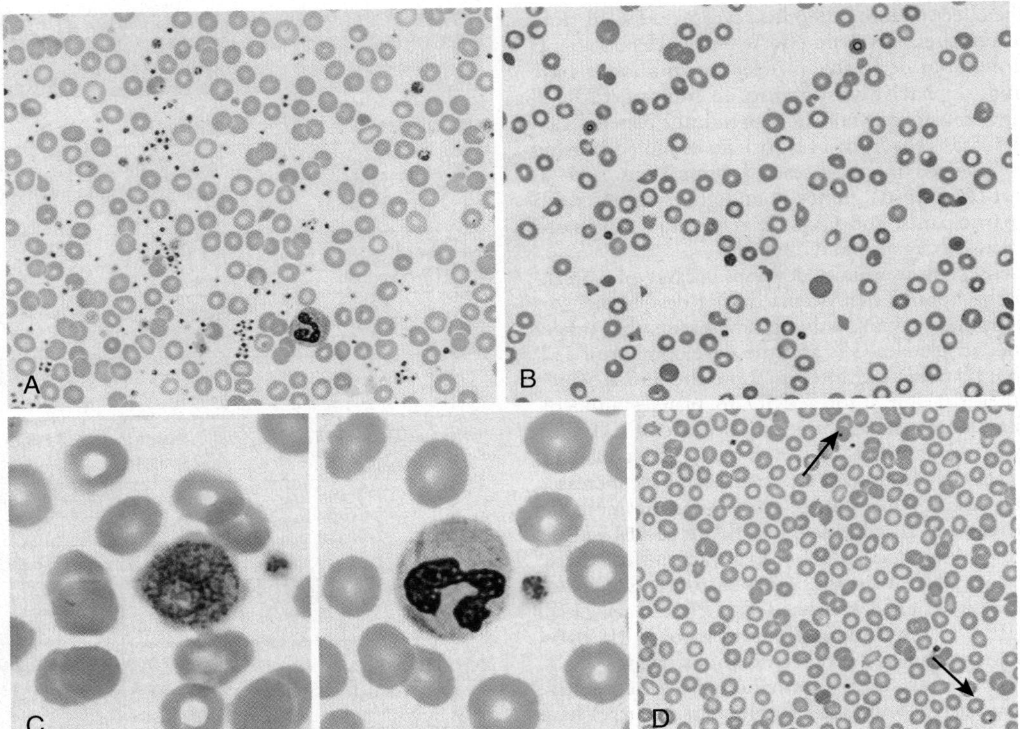

Figure 133-1 BLOOD FILM EXAMINATIONS FROM PATIENTS WITH THROMBOCYTOPENIA. **A,** Pseudothrombocytopenia showing marked platelet clumping. **B,** Schistocytes (fragmented red blood cells) and reticulocytosis in a patient with thrombotic thrombocytopenic purpura. **C,** Macrothrombocyte *(left panel)* and neutrophil-containing cytoplasmic inclusions (Döhle bodies, *right panel*) in a patient with May-Hegglin anomaly. **D,** A patient with immune thrombocytopenia with low platelets and postsplenectomy Howell-Jolly bodies *(arrows).*

Chronic ITP has been associated with a risk of death that is up to four times higher than that in the general population. ITP patients are more likely to die of bleeding, infection, and hematologic malignancies.[13] Some deaths are attributable to adverse effects of treatment rather than the disease. Quality of life in patients with ITP is lower than that of the general population, which is at least partially because of high prevalence of fatigue that appears to be independent of platelet count levels.

Investigations of Patients With Suspected Immune Thrombocytopenia

Patients presenting with newly identified thrombocytopenia require a careful history and physical examination to uncover potential underlying causes of thrombocytopenia and to assess the risk of bleeding. A complete blood count and review of the blood film is required for all patients with thrombocytopenia (Fig. 133-1). In adults (and in children at risk), HIV and HCV testing should be routinely performed; however, there are insufficient data to support screening for antinuclear antibodies or antiphospholipid antibodies unless other signs and symptoms of systemic lupus erythematosus or antiphospholipid antibody syndrome are present. BM aspiration and biopsy should be reserved for patients with abnormalities affecting other cell lines such as anemia, leukopenia, or macrocytosis. For patients with typical ITP, a BM examination is unnecessary to confirm the diagnosis. Quantitative immunoglobulin levels may be helpful in children to exclude common variable immune deficiency.

Treatment

Although data from clinical studies support the use of corticosteroids for newly diagnosed patients, treatment recommendations beyond first line are based mainly on expert opinion and consensus. Recently, the American Society of Hematology published guidelines for the management of ITP using GRADE methodology to assess levels of evidence associated with each recommendation.[2] Aligned with these guidelines, the authors have proposed a staircase model to illustrate a rational approach to ITP treatment, wherein therapies build on each other, often cumulatively in a stepwise fashion starting from the least toxic (Fig. 133-2). Important areas of uncertainty are optimal treatment of patients who fail first-line therapy and development of decision aids to help patients decide among splenectomy, rituximab, or TPO receptor agonists (see box on First-Line Therapy).

First-Line Therapy

An 8-year-old girl is brought to the emergency department because her mother noticed bruising on her legs. She has had a sore throat and fever for the past 7 days but is otherwise well and not taking any medications. On physical examination, there are a few small bruises on her legs but no petechiae on her skin or purpura in her mouth. Neurologic examination findings are normal, and the spleen is not palpable. The platelet count is 23 $\times 10^9$/L. The presumed diagnosis is ITP without significant bleeding; thus the decision is made to observe the child in the hospital with no specific treatment. The next day, the platelet count is 33 $\times 10^9$/L. On day 2, it is 37 $\times 10^9$/L, and the child is discharged home. One week later, the platelet count is 66 $\times 10^9$/L, and 1 month later, it is up to 155 $\times 10^9$/L.

Observation

The vast majority of children with ITP who have either no bleeding or mild bleeding (skin bleeding only) can safely be managed with

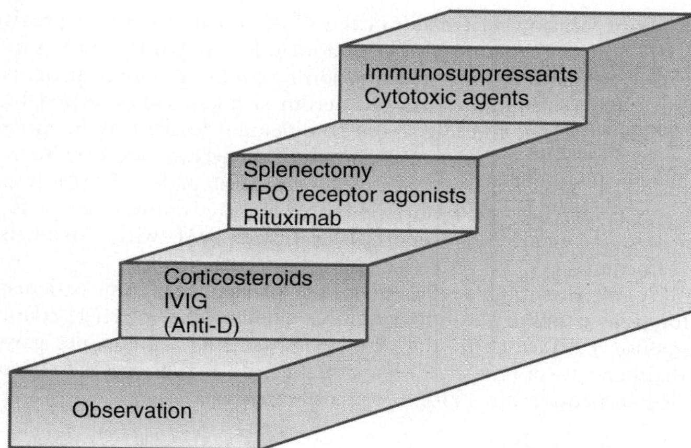

Figure 133-2 STAIRCASE MODEL OF IMMUNE THROMBOCYTOPENIA (ITP) TREATMENT. Therapies build on each other, often cumulatively, in a stepwise fashion starting from the least toxic. After a period of observation, corticosteroid-based treatment is the accepted first-line therapy. Splenectomy, rituximab, and thrombopoietin (TPO) receptor agonists may be reasonable second-line therapy. Rituximab is not currently licensed for ITP. TPO receptor agonists are indicated for patients with ITP who have failed previous therapies, including splenectomy. *(Modified with permission from Arnold DM, Kelton JG: Current options for the treatment of idiopathic thrombocytopenic purpura.* Semin Hematol *44:S12, 2007.)*

observation alone. This recommendation is based on prospective studies demonstrating a low risk of serious bleeding after initial presentation in children and recognition that up to 80% of cases of childhood ITP resolve within 6 months without treatment. A randomized trial that compared prednisone with observation alone in children with ITP who had platelet counts between 10 and 29 × 10^9/L and had no evidence of bleeding demonstrated no significant difference in the number of days with severe thrombocytopenia (2 and 4 days, respectively). However, if patients present with bleeding, such as epistaxis or mucosal hemorrhage, treatment is required. For adults, a period of observation is also reasonable if there is no evidence of bleeding and the platelet count is above 20 × 10^9/L. However, most adults eventually require treatment because spontaneous remissions are rare in this population. To reflect current practice, the ASH 2011 guidelines recommend using a platelet count below 30 × 10^9/L as the threshold for starting treatment.

Corticosteroids

The conventional initial dose of prednisone is 1 to 2 mg per kg for 2 to 4 weeks followed by tapering over a several week period when the platelet count responds. In general, 60% to 70% of adults with acute ITP achieve an initial response; even higher response rates are reported in children. Rates of sustained response (platelet count >100 × 10^9/L at 6 months) with corticosteroids are generally low and vary from 20% to 47%. With longer follow-up, the risk of relapse is high in adults who sustained an initial complete remission with corticosteroids. Low-dose prednisone (0.5 mg/kg per day followed by a taper) may be as effective as the conventional dose for initial treatment of ITP, but long-term remission rates with either dose remain unsatisfactory. The optimal duration of prednisone treatment and the optimal tapering schedule have not yet been adequately determined.

High-dose dexamethasone, typically administered at a dose of 40 mg/day for 4 consecutive days, has also been evaluated in ITP patients. Uncontrolled cohort studies suggest that this treatment may be effective. In one study that included 125 adults with ITP, almost 40% had a sustained response that lasted 2 to 5 years.[14] Repeated cycles of high-dose dexamethasone (once per month for 6 months) may result in even higher rates of durable remissions, although this effect may simply reflect the total corticosteroid exposure. High-dose dexamethasone can be difficult to tolerate; common side effects include weakness, insomnia, and impaired cognition. Controlled trials comparing prednisone with high-dose dexamethasone are needed.

Intravenous Immunoglobulin and Anti-D

The predominant mechanism of action of high-dose IVIG and anti-D is thought to be via RES blockade. Individuals with low plasma IgG levels exhibit more rapid clearance of sensitized red blood cells (RBCs) (indicating enhanced RES capacity) than those with high levels of plasma IgG, such as those achieved with high-dose IVIG. A competitive model of RES clearance would also explain why anti-D administration to Rh-positive individuals is effective in ITP because IgG-sensitized RBCs compete for Fc receptor occupancy. Other potential explanations for the efficacy of IVIG or anti-D include anti-idiotypic antibodies, stimulation of pro- and anti-inflammatory cytokines, up- or downregulation of various Fc receptors, and the induction of soluble immune complexes. In a mouse model of ITP, transfer of IVIG-primed dendritic cells recapitulated the effect of IVIG.[15]

Based on the results of a meta-analysis of randomized controlled trials in children (n = 410), the probability of achieving a platelet count above 20 × 10^9/L at 48 hours is lower with corticosteroids than with IVIG (relative risk, 0.74; 95% confidence interval [CI], 0.65-0.85).[16] Similar results have been observed in adults. Common side effects of IVIG include headache, hypertension, and chills. Hemolysis and neutropenia are rare side effects.

Anti-D has been compared with IVIG in children, and the two agents have similar efficacy provided that anti-D is given in high doses (75 μg/kg). Hemolysis invariably occurs after anti-D administration, and rarely, intravascular hemolysis can have a fatal outcome. Consequently, the Food and Drug Administration has issued a black box warning about the safety of anti-D, and the drug has been removed from certain European markets. In general, the use of anti-D is restricted to nonsplenectomized patients who are Rh positive and have a negative direct antiglobulin test result.

Second-Line Therapy

The choice of treatment for patients who relapse after first-line therapy or who fail to respond is controversial. Although splenectomy has been the treatment of choice for many years, rituximab and TPO receptor agonists are currently being evaluated as viable alternatives. Patient preference and access to medications are important considerations.

Splenectomy

Splenectomy was first proposed in 1913 and was subsequently shown to be an effective means of raising the platelet count in most ITP patients. Results of numerous studies indicate that approximately two-thirds of splenectomized patients achieve a response, generally within days.[17] Despite the high success rate with splenectomy, however, patients and physicians are often divided on the desirability of this approach. Identification of predictors of success of splenectomy has only identified younger age as an indicator. Some investigators have found a correlation between response to IVIG and that to splenectomy, and in some studies, evidence of radiolabeled platelet sequestration in a splenic pattern was associated with a good response to splenectomy.

With currently available minimally invasive surgical techniques, complications after splenectomy are uncommon. The overall mortality rate is approximately 1% after laparotomy and about 0.2% after laparoscopic splenectomy. The most frequent perioperative complications are pneumonia, subphrenic abscess or pleural effusion (4%), major bleeding (1.5%), and thromboembolism (1%). With laparoscopic techniques, patients have less postoperative pain, shorter hospital stays, and fewer wound complications.

Because the spleen is involved in clearance of encapsulated bacteria, asplenic individuals are at risk for infection with *Streptococcus pneumoniae, Neisseria meningitides,* and *Haemophilus influenzae type b* and therefore should receive these vaccinations at least 2 weeks before splenectomy. Poor compliance and vaccine failures contribute to the ongoing risk of serious postsplenectomy infections, which are associated with a 50% to 70% mortality rate.

The lifetime risk of overwhelming postsplenectomy infection is estimated to be 3% with the risk being higher in children younger than 15 years of age and in patients with hematologic malignancies. In a population cohort study of 3812 splenectomized patients in Denmark, the risk of any infection requiring hospitalization was highest in the first 90 days after splenectomy but remained 2.5 times higher than that in the general population thereafter.[18] The risk was lower when the comparison group was nonsplenectomized ITP patients, suggesting that many of the hospitalizations may be attributable to the underlying condition.

Rituximab

Rituximab is an anti-CD20 monoclonal antibody that targets and destroys CD20$^+$ B lymphocytes, some of which are presumably involved in autoantibody production. Rituximab has been widely used in patients with various autoimmune diseases, including ITP, and data correlating cellular profiles with clinical outcomes suggest that its effect may be attributable to improvement in T-cell function and reversion of T-cell abnormalities, downstream effects of B-cell depletion. The effect of rituximab on platelets, autoantibodies requires further study.

In a systematic review of 19 observational studies that enrolled 313 ITP patients of whom 46.2% were not splenectomized, rates of complete response (platelet count >150 × 10^9/L) and overall response (platelet count >50 × 10^9/L) with rituximab were 43.6% (95% CI, 29.5%-57.7%) and 62.5% (95% CI, 52.6%-72.5%), respectively, after a median follow up of 9.5 months.[19] The typical rituximab dose was 375 mg/m^2 administered by intravenous infusion once weekly for 4 consecutive weeks. The median time to response was 5.5 weeks, and responses lasted a median of 10.5 months. Other observational studies have reported lower rates of durable remissions, ranging from 24% at 12 months to 35% at 57 months.

Several completed or ongoing clinical trials have evaluated rituximab as adjuvant therapy for newly diagnosed or relapsed ITP before splenectomy. A pilot randomized trial of 60 nonsplenectomized adults receiving standard of care (which consisted mostly of corticosteroids and/or IVIG) reported no difference between rituximab and placebo for the composite endpoint of platelet count above 50 × 10^9/L, significant bleeding or requirement for rescue treatment after 6 months. Another randomized trial that included 103 treatment-naive adult patients reported that 31 of 49 (63%) patients in the rituximab plus dexamethasone group and 19 of 52 (36%) patients in the dexamethasone alone group achieved a platelet count of 50 × 10^9/L or higher after 6 months without rescue treatment (absolute risk reduction 27%; 95% CI, 8%-46%).[20] In a prospective observational study of 60 nonsplenectomized adult patients with ITP who had a median of 2 prior therapies, 24 (40%) achieved a platelet count above 50 × 10^9/L and at least twice their inclusion value at 1 year, and 20 (33%) maintained their platelet count response at 2 years with rituximab treatment. Low-dose rituximab (100 mg per week for 4 weeks) has been shown to be biologically active in ITP, but the frequency of durable responses is modest.

Rituximab has also been evaluated in a small number of children with chronic ITP. Variable response rates have been reported ranging from 31% to 69%, with sustained responses observed in 43% of patients after a median of 20 months.

Minor infusion-related side effects of rituximab occur in approximately 30% of patients with ITP and include hypotension, rash, sore throat, fever, and rigors. Fatal infusion reactions are rare in patients treated for autoimmune diseases. Serum sickness, characterized by arthropathy, fever, and low serum complement levels, may be more common in children than in adults and often necessitates drug interruption. Progressive multifocal leukoencephalopathy (PML) is a rapidly fatal neurologic syndrome caused by reactivation of latent JC virus in the brain. Rare reports have linked PML with rituximab treatment.[21]

Overall, rituximab has been shown to be effective in some patients. However, rituximab rarely produces a sustained platelet count response. Consequently, the 2011 ASH treatment guidelines gave rituximab a weak (grade 2C) recommendation for patients who have failed corticosteroids, IVIG, or splenectomy.

Thrombopoietin Receptor Agonists

Drugs aimed at increasing platelet production by stimulating the c-Mpl receptor have been investigated for the treatment of thrombocytopenia. Initial studies with recombinant human TPO and pegylated recombinant human megakaryocyte growth and development factor (PEG-rHuMGDF) were halted because of the development of cross-reactive antibodies against endogenous TPO with the pegylated formulation, which led to severe and sustained thrombocytopenia in healthy volunteers. These findings prompted the development of second-generation TPO receptor agonists that have no sequence homology to endogenous TPO. Two such drugs are approved for the treatment of patients with chronic ITP, romiplostim (Nplate, Amgen) and eltrombopag (Promacta/Revolade, GlaxoSmithKline). These agents have demonstrated efficacy even in some patients with refractory disease. Platelet counts generally remain elevated as long as the drugs are continued; when they are stopped, platelet counts tend to rapidly fall back to baseline thrombocytopenic levels.

Romiplostim (administered as a once-weekly subcutaneous injection) is a synthetic peptibody consisting of four peptides linked to an IgG Fc fragment. The molecule binds the c-Mpl receptor at the same location as endogenous TPO and stimulates megakaryocyte proliferation and platelet production through intracellular Janus kinase/signal transducer and activator of transcription (JAK/STAT) and mitogen-activated protein kinase (MAPK) signaling. In a phase III trial, a durable platelet count response (defined as the achievement of a platelet count of 50 × 10^9/L or higher for 6 or more of the last 8 weeks of treatment) was achieved in 41 of 83 patients (49.4%) receiving romiplostim compared with one of 42 (2.4%) patients receiving placebo.[22] In a subsequent randomized trial that compared romisplostim with standard of care treatment, romiplostim was associated with a higher rate of platelet count responses, fewer treatment failures, fewer splenectomies, less bleeding, and better quality of life.[23] Weekly doses of romiplostim range from 1 to 10 µg/kg; most patients achieve a suitable response with a dose of 3 µg/kg. Weekly doses are titrated up or down, depending on the platelet count response, to maintain the platelet count in the appropriate range (30-100 × 10^9/L).

Eltrombopag (administered as a tablet once daily) is a small molecule, nonpeptide TPO receptor agonist that activates c-Mpl by binding to the transmembrane domain. In contrast to romiplastim, eltrombopag does not compete with circulating TPO for binding to c-Mpl. In a phase III trial, the odds of responding to eltrombopag were approximately eight times higher than with placebo throughout the 6-month treatment period.[24] Durable responses were achieved in 57 of 95 patients (60%) receiving maintenance eltrombopag compared with four of 39 patients (10%) receiving placebo. The time to response was 1 to 2 weeks (similar to romisplostim) with a minimal need for dose titration.

A recent systematic review summarizes the data from randomized trials of TPO receptor agonists. The authors concluded that although romiplostim and eltrombopag were each associated with platelet count responses, neither significantly improved the rate of severe, life-threatening or fatal bleeding compared with standard of care.[25] This review highlights the need for patient focused outcomes in ITP trials.

TPO receptor agonists are generally well tolerated but have been associated with headache, fatigue, and insomnia. Both drugs have rarely been linked to the development of bone marrow reticulin in patients with ITP; however, this abnormality resolves with discontinuation of the drug, and stem cell disorders have not been reported. TPO receptor agonists have also been associated with thromboembolic events (independent of platelet count), although follow-up analyses have questioned the strength of this association. One study of eltrombopag in patients with advanced liver disease and secondary thrombocytopenia was stopped early because of an increase in the frequency of portal vein thrombosis. Eltrombopag has been associated with serum liver test abnormalities in approximately 10% of patients. Long-term follow-up data for patients treated with these agents are limited (see box on Long-Term Follow-Up).

Treatment of Refractory Immune Thrombocytopenia

As suggested by the International Working Group on standardization of terminology in ITP, the term *refractory ITP* is used to define patients who have failed splenectomy or relapsed thereafter and either exhibit severe thrombocytopenia or have a risk of bleeding that necessitates therapy (see Table 133-2).[1]

Evidence to help guide management of patients with chronic refractory ITP after splenectomy is limited, and treatment has been mainly unsatisfactory. However, TPO receptor agonists provide a new and effective option for this challenging group of patients. The overarching principals of therapy for this population are (1) the goal of treatment is to prevent bleeding with the achievement of a stable, although not necessarily normal, platelet count, and (2) combination therapy may be more effective than treatment with a single agent.

In randomized trials, the response of splenectomized patients to treatment with TPO receptor agonists is less than that of nonsplenectomized patients; however, the difference is small, and response rates in splenectomized patients approach 50%. Although some patients included in the trials had failed up to 5 prior therapies, the results may not be applicable to all patients with refractory ITP seen in clinical practice.

Before the availability of TPO receptor agonists, a systematic review identified rituximab, azathioprine, and cyclophosphamide as agents most often associated with complete responses in patients with refractory ITP.[26] Good response rates have also been reported with the combination of cyclosporine, azathioprine, and CellCept or with the combination of IVIG, intravenous methylprednisolone, vincristine, or IV anti-D followed by maintenance therapy with danazol and azathioprine. Other treatment options include low-dose or alternate-day corticosteroids, repeated doses of IVIG, high-dose chemotherapy, or dapsone. High-dose chemotherapy and stem cell transplantation have also been used successfully in this population, and with the advent of less toxic regimens, this treatment modality may soon become a more acceptable option for selected patients with severe refractory ITP.

Long-Term Follow-Up

The best treatment of patients with ITP who fail first-line therapy remains controversial and depends on the severity of symptoms, side effect profile, and patient preference. Splenectomy has been used for many years and is the treatment option most likely to be associated with durable remissions. Rituximab may achieve a platelet count response in up to 60% of patients, but responses are rarely sustained past 6 to 12 months. TPO receptor agonists (romiplostim or eltrombopag) are associated with a platelet count response in up to 60% of patients as long as treatment is maintained. These drugs are generally well tolerated; however, long-term safety data beyond 5 years are not yet available.

NEONATAL ALLOIMMUNE THROMBOCYTOPENIA

Neonatal alloimmune thrombocytopenia is an uncommon but serious thrombocytopenic disorder that can cause fetal or neonatal bleeding resulting in death or disability. It is important to recognize this disorder because treatment prevents recurrence in subsequent pregnancies. With NAIT, intracranial bleeding can occur during the neonatal period or in utero, in which case the diagnosis is first suspected after an abnormal fetal ultrasonography. The incidence has been estimated to range from one to two in 1000 births; however, it is often underdiagnosed.

Clinical Presentation

Thrombocytopenia may be severe in infants affected by NAIT; often the platelet count is less than 10 to 20 × 10^9/L shortly after birth. The differential diagnosis is broad and includes septicemia, hypoxia, and birth trauma, among other factors (Table 133-3). Typically, NAIT presents as severe thrombocytopenia, possibly with associated bleeding, in an otherwise healthy neonate with no other explanation for the low platelet count. The thrombocytopenia often worsens hours or days after delivery, likely reflecting increased RES function in the newborn, particularly within the lungs. Without treatment, thrombocytopenia may last for days, but occasionally, it can be severe and can persist for many weeks. Bleeding symptoms range from petechiae and bruising to gastrointestinal or intracranial hemorrhage. Overall, bleeding occurs in up to 20% of neonates with NAIT and has been documented early in pregnancy. For infants with severe thrombocytopenia, mortality estimates of 10% have been reported, and infants with intracranial bleeding may be left with developmental delays and severe, lifelong neurologic deficits.

Table 133-3 Differential Diagnosis of Thrombocytopenia in Newborns

Perinatal hypoxemia
Placental insufficiency
Congenital infection
- Sepsis
- Toxoplasmosis
- Rubella
- Cytomegalovirus

Autoimmune
- Maternal immune thrombocytopenia
- Maternal systemic lupus erythematosus

Disseminated intravascular coagulation
Maternal drug exposure
Congenital heart disease
Hereditary thrombocytopenia
- MYH9 macrothrombocytopenia (including May-Hegglin anomaly)
- Thrombocytopenia absent radii syndrome
- Amegakaryocytic thrombocytopenia
- Wiskott-Aldrich syndrome
- Fanconi anemia

Hemangioma with thrombocytopenia
- Kasabach-Merritt syndrome

Bone marrow infiltration
- Congenital leukemia

Pathophysiology

Fetal and neonatal thrombocytopenia in NAIT is caused by the clearance of IgG-sensitized platelets by maternal alloantibodies directed against platelet-specific antigens. The syndrome can be considered analogous to the destruction of fetal RBCs in hemolytic disease of the newborn (HDN) but with a number of differences. Perhaps most importantly, NAIT often presents in a first pregnancy because of maternal sensitization to paternally derived antigens expressed on fetal platelets. In contrast, it is distinctly uncommon for HDN to occur in a first pregnancy without previous sensitization. This difference suggests that unlike RBCs, transplacental passage of fetal platelets or platelet antigens into the maternal circulation occurs early in pregnancy. Another difference is that pregnant women at risk for HDN (e.g., those who are Rh negative) can be identified early by screening, and treatment with anti-Rh immune globulin reduces the risk of sensitization. To date, screening programs for NAIT have not been widely deployed because women at risk are not readily identifiable before sensitization has occurred, and therapies of proven benefit are not currently available. Screening programs for NAIT continue to be an active area of research (see box on Neonatal Alloimmune Thrombocytopenia Versus Hemolytic Disease of the Newborn).

Laboratory Investigation of Suspected Neonatal Alloimmune Thrombocytopenia

The diagnosis of NAIT is established by documenting the presence of a platelet-specific antigen incompatibility between mother and infant (or mother and father) and the presence of maternal antiplatelet alloantibodies directed against the incompatible antigen (Fig. 133-3).[27]

Neonatal Alloimmune Thrombocytopenia Versus Hemolytic Disease of the Newborn

NAIT can be viewed as the platelet equivalent of HDN with some important differences: (1) maternal sensitization by fetal platelet antigens can occur early in the first trimester, (2) NAIT can affect first pregnancies, (3) women at risk for NAIT are not easily identifiable before sensitization and thus are not amenable to universal screening programs, and (4) a specific therapy that targets prevention of platelet antigen sensitization is lacking (e.g., Rh-immune globulin that target RBC antigen exposure).

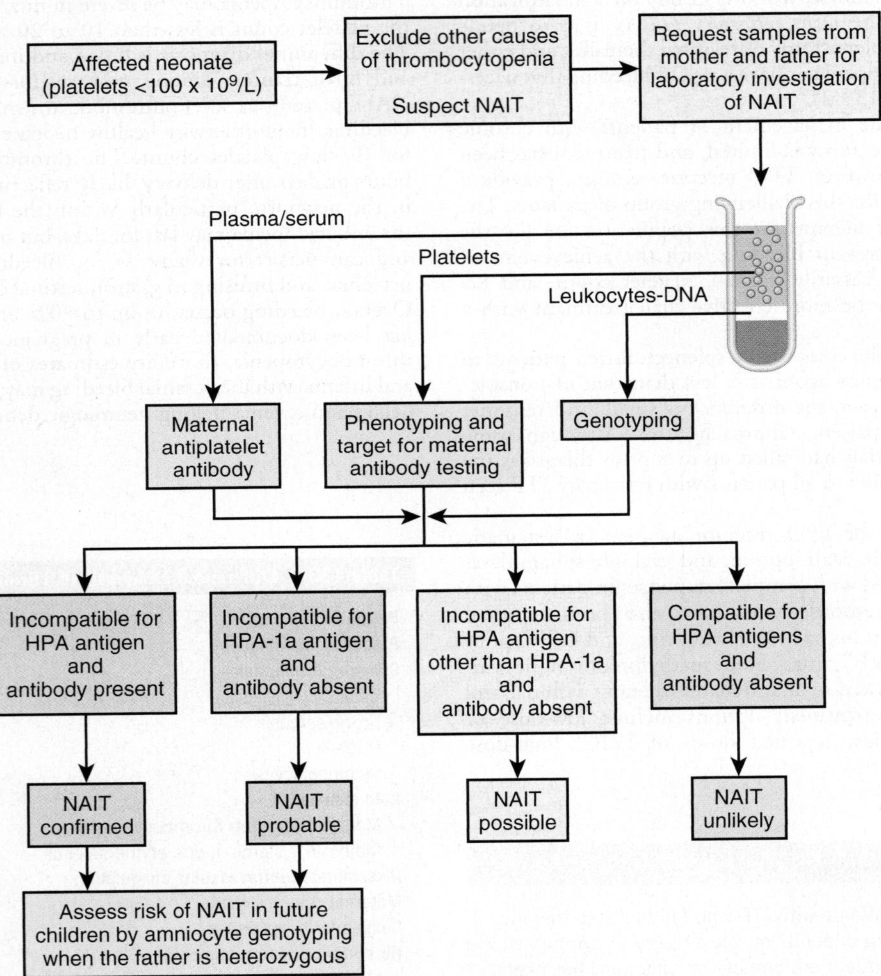

Figure 133-3 DIAGNOSTIC TESTING ALGORITHM FOR INVESTIGATION OF NEONATAL ALLOIMMUNE THROMBOCYTOPENIA (NAIT) AND MANAGEMENT RECOMMENDATIONS BASED ON RESULTS OF TESTING (CURRENTLY USED BY THE ONTARIO PROVINCIAL PLATELET LABORATORY AT MCMASTER UNIVERSITY PLATELET IMMUNOLOGY REFERENCE LABORATORY, 2012). Maternal blood samples are tested for platelet antigens (phenotyping and polymerase chain reaction genotyping) and platelet alloantibodies. Amniocentesis and fetal genotyping are recommended when the father is known to be heterozygous for the incompatible antigen. *HPA,* Human platelet antigen. *(Modified from Arnold DM, Smith JW, Kelton JG: Diagnosis and management of neonatal alloimmune thrombocytopenia.* Transfus Med Rev *22:255, 2008, with permission.)*

Consequently, diagnosis requires allele-specific genotyping to identify maternal–fetal (or maternal–paternal) antigenic mismatch using polymerase chain reaction technology. Serologic confirmation, which requires the documentation of maternal alloantibodies, is more difficult for two reasons. First, *the technology is complex, and relatively few laboratories perform these tests.* In general, most commercial assays detect platelet alloantibodies directed against only a limited number of antigens. This limitation necessitates the use of more specific assays, such as monoclonal antibody immobilization of platelet antigen assays or antigen capture assays.[28] Even these tests are limited by the lack of the monoclonal antibodies required to capture the target protein. An alternative method uses radioimmunoprecipitation, which can detect all of the known alloantibodies described to date. *Second, a proportion of women have no detectable antibodies using currently available laboratory methods.* For example, up to 25% of human platelet antigen-1a (HPA-1a)–negative women with NAIT have no detectable anti–HPA-1a antibody. The explanation for this observation is uncertain.

Alloantibodies recognize epitopes on platelet GPs that are defined by genetic polymorphisms. To date, all of these antigens are the result of single nucleotide polymorphisms or in-frame deletions of the codon. Consequently, platelet typing using genetic analysis is relatively straightforward. The majority of platelet alloantigens occur on GPIIIa, which is the most abundant platelet glycoprotein (50,000-75,000 copies per platelet). GPIIIa, also known as β3, forms a heterodimer with platelet GPIIb to form the integrin $\alpha_2\beta_3$, which serves as the binding site for fibrinogen and enables platelet aggregation.

The most common platelet alloantigen implicated in NAIT is the alloantigen HPA-1a. This important alloantigen is defined by a leucine (HPA-1a) to proline (HPA-1b) substitution at amino acid 33 on GPIIIa. Maternal incompatibility to HPA-1a is implicated in more than 80% of women with NAIT. These women lack the common HPA-1a antigen (i.e., their genotype is HPA-1bb) and during pregnancy, they are immunized with fetal HPA-1a antigen, which is inherited from the father.

The next most commonly implicated antigens in NAIT are HPA-5a5b on glycoprotein Ia/IIa and HPA-15a15b on the glycosylphosphatidylinositol–anchored protein, CD109. Only six of the 17 platelet antigen systems have been defined by maternal alloantibodies to both alleles; these include the HPA 1, 2, 3, 4, 5, and 15 systems. There are a number of other very-low-frequency alleles, the majority of which are expressed on platelet GPIIb/IIIa and are usually found within a single family. Frequently, discrepancies for human leukocyte antigen (HLA) and ABO, which are also expressed on platelets, are found during the course of investigations for NAIT; however, it is unclear whether these are of any clinical consequence.

Management

Management of Infants After Delivery

When NAIT is suspected and depending on the platelet count, treatment should be initiated even before confirmatory test results are available. It is important to appreciate that moderate or severe thrombocytopenia at birth (20-50 × 10^9/L) can worsen over the next few days. Treatment should be initiated immediately if thrombocytopenia is severe (platelets <20 × 10^9/L); if there are petechiae or purpura; or if there is evidence of serious bleeding, such as intracranial bleeding on cranial ultrasonography. The initial treatment is high-dose IVIG (1-2 g/kg), which will increase the platelet count in most infants.[29] Platelet transfusions should also be given if the thrombocytopenia is severe and there is evidence of bleeding. Ideally, platelet products for transfusions should be alloantigen compatible. However, if these are unavailable, random donor platelets can be used because they produce adequate increases in the platelet count.[30]

Antenatal Management of the Mother

Women with a previously affected infant with NAIT are at high risk of having another affected infant. Consequently, careful management in subsequent pregnancies is required. Similar to HDN, the disorder is often more severe in subsequent pregnancies than it is in the first. The exception is if the father is heterozygous for the implicated platelet antigen, in which case antigenic testing can be performed by amniocentesis to determine if the fetus is at risk and whether treatment is required.

Antenatal treatment options for at-risk mothers during subsequent pregnancies range from careful observation to IVIG with or without corticosteroids to fetal blood sampling (FBS) and intrauterine platelet transfusion. Invasive strategies that include FBS are associated with a high rate of complications, including fetal death and premature labor; thus a noninvasive approach is often recommended.

The mainstay of antenatal therapy for women with a previously affected infant is high-dose IVIG (1-2 g/kg) administered weekly throughout pregnancy starting at approximately 20 to 24 weeks of gestation. A systematic review summarizing the results of four randomized trials that included 206 women compared weekly IVIG with a variety of other therapies, including alternate dosing of IVIG or IVIG plus corticosteroids.[31] Although no definitive conclusions could be drawn, most clinicians use IVIG for antenatal treatment. Corticosteroids (prednisone or dexamethasone) given in combination with IVIG should be considered for mothers at high risk, such as those with a previously affected infant with intracranial hemorrhage or severe thrombocytopenia or if the response to IVIG is suboptimal.

Fetal Monitoring During Pregnancy

Serial ultrasonography is indicated for fetal surveillance. This provides a simple, noninvasive method for identifying fetal bleeds at an early stage. FBS by percutaneous cannulation of the umbilical or intrahepatic vein may be a way of capturing high-risk fetuses, identifying those who require treatment, and monitoring response to therapy. However, FBS is technically challenging and is associated with significant morbidity and mortality. In one study, 6% of FBS procedures were associated with complications, including fetal death from exsanguination and premature induction of labor.[32] Furthermore, a platelet transfusion protocol based on the detection of fetal thrombocytopenia would necessitate frequent FBS procedures because of the short (7-day) life span of transfused platelets. Because the risks associated with FBS exceed the benefits, routine FBS is not recommended.

Mode of Delivery

There is no evidence that planned cesarean section is safer than uncomplicated vaginal delivery for infants with NAIT. Nonetheless, planned cesarean section delivery can ensure that personnel and resources, including antigen-compatible platelet transfusions, are available without delay.

Population Screening for Neonatal Alloimmune Thrombocytopenia

Universal NAIT screening programs for all pregnant women are not currently available because of the difficulty in identifying at-risk women early and the lack of specific and proven treatments. One study screened 100,448 pregnant women and offered those with HPA-1a antibodies early cesarean section together with compatible platelet transfusions.[33] This approach identified 161 affected infants, of whom three (6%) died or had an intracranial bleed, compared with 10 of 51 infants (20%) born to mothers who were not screened.

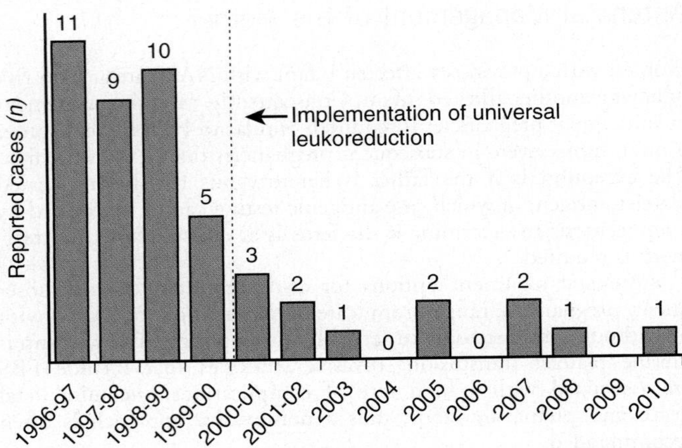

Figure 133-4 CONFIRMED CASES OF POSTTRANSFUSION PURPURA (PTP) REPORTED BY THE UK SERIOUS HAZARDS OF TRANSFUSION (SHOT) SURVEILLANCE PROGRAM. Universal leukoreduction was implemented in late 1999, which coincides with a decrease in new cases of PTP. *(Adapted from Knowles S (ed) and Cohen H on behalf of the Serious Hazards of Transfusion (SHOT) Steering Group.* The 2010 Annual SHOT Report (2011), *with permission.)*

These results are encouraging, and additional studies of NAIT screening programs are ongoing.

POSTTRANSFUSION PURPURA

Posttransfusion purpura is a rare thrombocytopenic syndrome that is provoked by an alloimmune response against human platelet antigens, most frequently HPA-1a. It occurs in patients—usually women—who have been previously sensitized to platelet-specific antigens and who develop a severe immune reaction after exposure to platelets or platelet antigenic material in blood transfusions.

Epidemiology

Posttransfusion purpura is rare with an estimated incidence of one to two per 100,000 transfusions. Data from the Serious Hazards of Transfusion surveillance program in the United Kingdom indicate a decrease in the incidence of PTP in the past decade (Fig. 133-4).[34] This trend may reflect the move to universal leukoreduction of blood products, which was implemented in 1999. The average number of cases of PTP in the years before (1996-1999) and after (2000-2005) universal leukoreduction was 10.3 and 2.3 cases per year, respectively. Since then, there has also been a shift from RBC concentrates to platelet concentrates as the inciting transfusion event, which may be attributable to the reduction in platelet contamination of RBC products with leukoreduction methods (see box on Clinical Presentation of Posttransfusion Purpura).

Approximately 85% of PTP episodes occur in women, almost all of whom have a history of pregnancy. In a report of 61 patients, the sensitizing event among women was pregnancy alone in 58%, pregnancy or transfusion in 34%, and transfusion alone in 7.5%. Men had associated transfusion histories in 55%; some had no known exposure. PTP has not been reported in children.

Clinical Presentation

Posttransfusion purpura presents as severe thrombocytopenia (platelets <10 × 10^9/L) and bleeding, which may include petechiae, purpura, mucosal hemorrhage, hematuria, or intracranial bleeding. The thrombocytopenia is often refractory to platelet transfusion even with antigen-negative platelets, although this treatment is indicated for patients with bleeding, for whom mortality rates range from 5% to 20%. The thrombocytopenia occurs 7 to 10 days after blood transfusion and typically resolves within weeks. Occasionally, thrombocytopenia may persist for months. Other causes of thrombocytopenia that can mimic PTP include primary ITP, drug-induced ITP, sepsis, disseminated intravascular coagulation, and thrombotic thrombocytopenic purpura. However, the temporal association with blood transfusion and the severity of the bleeding suggest the diagnosis. Patients with PTP may present with features that overlap with heparin-induced thrombocytopenia (HIT), and positive HIT test results in the context of anti-HPA antibodies have been reported. However, thrombocytopenia is less severe with HIT, and severe bleeding is rare.

Clinical Presentation of Posttransfusion Purpura

On postoperative day 8 after spinal surgery, a 43-year-old woman has a platelet count of 3 × 10^9/L. During the operation, she received 3 units of non–leuko-reduced packed RBCs because of intraoperative bleeding. She is receiving intravenous ampicillin and prophylactic doses of the low-molecular-weight heparin dalteparin. On physical examination, she has extensive oral mucosal purpura and petechiae on both lower extremities. HIT testing results (anti-PF4/heparin enzyme-linked immunosorbent assay and serotonin release assay) are negative. The ampicillin is stopped, and she is treated with IVIG (2 g/kg) and platelet transfusions. Three days later, the platelet count is 4 × 10^9/L, and the patient develops melena. The presumed diagnosis is posttransfusion purpura; therefore, HPA-1a–negative platelets and high-dose parenteral corticosteroids are administered, and daily plasma exchange is initiated. One week later, the thrombocytopenia and bleeding symptoms resolve. Platelet antibody testing reveals the presence of anti–HPA-1a antibodies.

Diagnosis

The majority of patients with PTP lack the common HPA-1a platelet antigen (i.e., have the HPA-1bb genotype) and have been sensitized by previous pregnancies or transfusions. These sensitizing events result in the development of anti–HPA-1a alloantibodies, the detection of which can be used for serologic diagnosis. Anti–HPA-1a antibodies may persist for many years in these patients.

Pathophysiology

Platelets contain abundant amounts of GPIIb/IIIa. Consequently, even small numbers of platelets or platelet microparticles in RBC concentrates can be immunogenic and lead to the development of PTP. Genotypic analyses indicate that HLA-II alleles DRB3*0101 and DQB1*0201 are associated with PTP, a situation analogous to NAIT. The frequency of immunization depends on platelet alloantigen discrepancy plus the presence of certain immune response genes.

The most intriguing feature of PTP is that the patient's own compatible platelets are destroyed. Furthermore, platelet reactive antibodies can be eluted from both antigen-positive and -negative platelets. Although the mechanism is still poorly understood, potential explanations for this "innocent bystander" phenomenon include immune complex formation, passive antigen adsorption, and autoantibody formation.

Theoretically, immune complexes may form if the anti–HPA-1a antibodies bind soluble antigen. Immune complexes may then bind to platelets through Fc receptors, causing platelet destruction. Alternatively, platelet alloantigens contained within the transfused blood product may be passively adsorbed onto autologous platelets, thereby converting them from antigen-negative to -positive cells and rendering them targets for immune destruction. Anti–HPA-1a antibodies have been shown to induce platelet activation through release of platelet-derived RANTES (regulated on activation, normal, T-cell expressed and secreted), a proinflammatory and immunomodulatory chemokine involved in multiple immunologic processes, including immunoglobulin synthesis and regulation of T-helper 1/T-helper 2 (Th1/Th2) cytokine homeostasis. In some patients with PTP, alloantibodies have been shown to interfere with the platelet–fibrinogen interaction, thereby increasing the risk of bleeding.

The induction of specific anti-HPA alloantibodies could in turn initiate the formation of platelet-reactive *autoantibodies*. Pan-reactive antibodies can be found when the platelet count is at its lowest level, and serologic analyses in PTP cases demonstrate the presence of reactive IgG and IgM antibodies against GPIIb/IIIa, GPIX, and GPIa/IIa. However, only HPA-specific IgG antibodies persist.[35]

Management

Treatment of PTP should be initiated even before serologic test results for anti–HPA-1a are available. The primary goal of treatment is to abbreviate the period of severe thrombocytopenia and minimize the risk of bleeding. Multiple treatments are often administered simultaneously or in rapid succession.

Patients with PTP require supportive treatment and rapid management of bleeding if it occurs. Nonessential transfusions should be avoided. The mainstay of therapy is high-dose IVIG, which usually results in an increase in the platelet count after 3 or 4 days.[36] High-dose corticosteroids have also been used to suppress RES phagocytosis and reduce IgG synthesis. Patients with bleeding should be transfused with HPA-1a–negative platelets. HPA-1a–positive platelet transfusions are generally ineffective and theoretically may stimulate further antibody production. Patients with PTP appear to be at increased risk for transfusion reactions such as fever, dyspnea, and allergic reactions. Plasma exchange should be considered in patients who do not respond to IVIG.

REFERENCES

1. Rodeghiero F, Stasi R, Gernsheimer T, et al: Standardization of terminology, definitions and outcome criteria in immune thrombocytopenic purpura of adults and children: Report from an international working group. *Blood* 113:2386, 2009.
2. Neunert C, Lim W, Crowther M, et al: The American Society of Hematology 2011 evidence-based practice guideline for immune thrombocytopenia. *Blood* 117:4190, 2011.
3. Terrell DR, Beebe LA, Vesely SK, et al: The incidence of immune thrombocytopenic purpura in children and adults: A critical review of published reports. *Am J Hematol* 85:174, 2010.
4. Burrows RF, Kelton JG: Fetal thrombocytopenia and its relation to maternal thrombocytopenia. *N Engl J Med* 329:1463, 1993.
5. Harrington W, Minnuch V, Hollingsworth JW, et al: Demonstration of a thrombocytopenic factor in the blood of patients with thrombocytopenic purpura. *J Lab Clin Med* 38:1, 1951.
6. Ballem PJ, Segal GM, Stratton JR, et al: Mechanisms of thrombocytopenia in chronic autoimmune thrombocytopenic purpura. Evidence of both impaired platelet production and increased platelet clearance. *J Clin Invest* 80:33, 1987.
7. Imbach P, Crowther M: Thrombopoietin-receptor agonists for primary immune thrombocytopenia. *N Engl J Med* 365:734, 2011.
8. Goodnow CC, Sprent J, Fazekas de St GB, et al: Cellular and genetic mechanisms of self tolerance and autoimmunity. *Nature* 435:590, 2005.
9. Takahashi T, Yujiri T, Shinohara K, et al: Molecular mimicry by Helicobacter pylori CagA protein may be involved in the pathogenesis of H. pylori-associated chronic idiopathic thrombocytopenic purpura. *Br J Haematol* 124:91, 2004.
10. Stasi R, Sarpatwari A, Segal JB, et al: Effects of eradication of Helicobacter pylori infection in patients with immune thrombocytopenic purpura: A systematic review. *Blood* 113:1231, 2009.
11. Kuhne T, Buchanan GR, Zimmerman S, et al: A prospective comparative study of 2540 infants and children with newly diagnosed idiopathic thrombocytopenic purpura (ITP) from the Intercontinental Childhood ITP Study Group. *J Pediatr* 143:605, 2003.
12. Cohen YC, Djulbegovic B, Shamai-Lubovitz O, et al: The bleeding risk and natural history of idiopathic thrombocytopenic purpura in patients with persistent low platelet counts. *Arch Intern Med* 160:1630, 2000.
13. Portielje JE, Westendorp RG, Kluin-Nelemans HC, et al: Morbidity and mortality in adults with idiopathic thrombocytopenic purpura. *Blood* 97:2549, 2001.
14. Cheng Y, Wong RS, Soo YO, et al: Initial treatment of immune thrombocytopenic purpura with high-dose dexamethasone. *N Engl J Med* 349:831, 2003.
15. Siragam V, Crow AR, Brinc D, et al: Intravenous immunoglobulin ameliorates ITP via activating Fc gamma receptors on dendritic cells. *Nat Med* 12:688, 2006.
16. Beck CE, Nathan PC, Parkin PC, et al: Corticosteroids versus intravenous immune globulin for the treatment of acute immune thrombocytopenic purpura in children: A systematic review and meta-analysis of randomized controlled trials. *J Pediatr* 147:521, 2005.
17. Kojouri K, Vesely SK, Terrell DR, et al: Splenectomy for adult patients with idiopathic thrombocytopenic purpura: A systematic review to assess long-term platelet count responses, prediction of response, and surgical complications. *Blood* 104:2623, 2004.
18. Thomsen RW, Schoonen WM, Farkas DK, et al: Risk for hospital contact with infection in patients with splenectomy: A population-based cohort study. *Ann Intern Med* 151:546, 2009.
19. Arnold DM, Dentali F, Crowther MA, et al: Systematic review: Efficacy and safety of rituximab for adults with idiopathic thrombocytopenic purpura. *Ann Intern Med* 146:25, 2007.
20. Zaja F, Baccarani M, Mazza P, et al: Dexamethasone plus rituximab yields higher sustained response rates than dexamethasone monotherapy in adults with primary immune thrombocytopenia. *Blood* 115:2755, 2010.
21. Carson KR, Evens AM, Richey EA, et al: Progressive multifocal leukoencephalopathy after rituximab therapy in HIV-negative patients: A report of 57 cases from the Research on Adverse Drug Events and Reports project. *Blood* 113:4834, 2009
22. Kuter DJ, Bussel JB, Lyons RM, et al: Efficacy of romiplostim in patients with chronic immune thrombocytopenic purpura: A double-blind randomised controlled trial. *Lancet* 371:395, 2008.
23. Kuter DJ, Rummel M, Boccia R, et al: Romiplostim or standard of care in patients with immune thrombocytopenia. *N Engl J Med* 363:1889, 2010.
24. Cheng G, Saleh MN, Marcher C, et al: Eltrombopag for management of chronic immune thrombocytopenia (RAISE): A 6-month, randomised, phase 3 study. *Lancet* 377:393, 2011.
25. Zeng Y, Duan X, Xu J, et al: TPO receptor agonist for chronic idiopathic thrombocytopenic purpura. *Cochrane Database Syst Rev* CD008235, 2011.
26. Vesely SK, Perdue JJ, Rizvi MA, et al: Management of adult patients with persistent idiopathic thrombocytopenic purpura following splenectomy: A systematic review. *Ann Intern Med* 140:112, 2004 .
27. Arnold DM, Smith JW, Kelton JG: Diagnosis and management of neonatal alloimmune thrombocytopenia. *Transfus Med Rev* 22:255, 2008.
28. Warner MN, Moore JC, Warkentin TE, et al: A prospective study of protein-specific assays used to investigate idiopathic thrombocytopenic purpura. *Br J Haematol* 104:442, 1999.
29. Mueller-Eckhardt C, Kiefel V, Grubert A, et al: 348 cases of suspected neonatal alloimmune thrombocytopenia. *Lancet* 1:363, 1989.
30. Kiefel V, Bassler D, Kroll H, et al: Antigen-positive platelet transfusion in neonatal alloimmune thrombocytopenia (NAIT). *Blood* 107:3761, 2006.
31. Rayment R, Brunskill SJ, Soothill PW, et al: Antenatal interventions for fetomaternal alloimmune thrombocytopenia. *Cochrane Database Syst Rev* CD004226, 2011.

32. Berkowitz RL, Kolb EA, McFarland JG, et al: Parallel randomized trials of risk-based therapy for fetal alloimmune thrombocytopenia. *Obstet Gynecol* 107:91, 2006.
33. Kjeldsen-Kragh J, Killie MK, Tomter G, et al: A screening and intervention program aimed to reduce mortality and serious morbidity associated with severe neonatal alloimmune thrombocytopenia. *Blood* 110:833, 2007.
34. Williamson LM, Stainsby D, Jones H, et al: The impact of universal leukodepletion of the blood supply on hemovigilance reports of posttransfusion purpura and transfusion-associated graft-versus-host disease. *Transfusion* 47:1455, 2007.
35. Taaning E, Tonnesen F: Pan-reactive platelet antibodies in post-transfusion purpura. *Vox Sang* 76:120, 1999.
36. Mueller-Eckhardt C, Kiefel V: High-dose IgG for post-transfusion purpura-revisited. *Blut* 57:163, 1988.

CHAPTER 134

THROMBOCYTOPENIA CAUSED BY PLATELET DESTRUCTION, HYPERSPLENISM, OR HEMODILUTION

Theodore E. Warkentin

Thrombocytopenia is defined as a platelet count below the lower limit of the normal range (≈150 × 10^9/L). Sometimes an expanded definition of thrombocytopenia is appropriate. For example, an abrupt drop in the platelet count can signify the onset of a platelet-destructive process such as heparin-induced thrombocytopenia (HIT) or bacteremia even if the platelet count remains above 150 × 10^9/L. This is especially relevant in the second or third week after surgery because patients usually have platelet counts that peak at levels two to three times greater than their usual preoperative value (postoperative thrombocytosis).

In the clinical evaluation of a patient with thrombocytopenia, three questions must be asked. First, could the patient have pseudothrombocytopenia? Second, what is the most likely explanation for the thrombocytopenia? And third, what are the risks posed by the causative disorder and the severity of the thrombocytopenia? For example, severe thrombocytopenia caused by drug-dependent antibodies or platelet-reactive autoantibodies is often associated with bleeding. By contrast, thrombocytopenia caused by HIT antibodies or attributable to disseminated intravascular coagulation (DIC) secondary to adenocarcinoma is associated with thrombosis. Often, the underlying cause of the thrombocytopenia (e.g., bacteremia, cancer, cirrhosis), rather than the thrombocytopenia itself, poses the greater risk.

Thrombocytopenia can be caused by any of four general mechanisms: (1) platelet underproduction, (2) increased platelet destruction or consumption, (3) platelet sequestration, and (4) hemodilution. Platelet underproduction usually occurs in association with underproduction of other blood cell lines, which results in bicytopenia or pancytopenia. Thrombocytopenia caused by increased platelet destruction develops when the rate of platelet loss surpasses the ability of the bone marrow (BM) to produce platelets and may be caused by immune or nonimmune mechanisms (Table 134-1). Thrombocytopenia from platelet sequestration is caused by redistribution of platelets from the circulation into an enlarged splenic vascular bed. Hemodilution is characterized by a decrease in the number of platelets, as well as red and white blood cells (WBCs) as a result of the administration of colloids, crystalloids, or platelet-poor blood products.

In the postoperative period, platelet count changes reflect several processes, including initial hemodilution (immediate platelet count decrease) and increased platelet consumption (first 2 to 4 days), at which point the platelet count begins to rise due to increased platelet production; when the platelet count reaches its postoperative peak—usually about 14 days after surgery—platelet production decreases somewhat, and the platelet count returns to baseline (Fig. 134-1).[1] In addition to usual mechanisms, the differential diagnosis of thrombocytopenia in pregnancy includes some unique causes (Table 134-2).

APPROACH TO PATIENTS WITH THROMBOCYTOPENIA

History and Physical Examination

Certain information should be ascertained, including (1) the location and severity of bleeding (if any); (2) the temporal profile of the hemostatic defect (acute, chronic, or relapsing), particularly the temporal relationship with potential proximate triggers (e.g., new drug, recent infection); (3) the presence of symptoms of a secondary illness, such as a neoplasm, infection, or an autoimmune disorder such as systemic lupus erythematosus (SLE); (4) history of recent medication use, alcohol ingestion, or transfusion; (5) presence of risk factors for certain infections, particularly human immunodeficiency virus (HIV) infection or viral hepatitis; and (6) family history of thrombocytopenia (see Chapter 133).

As part of the physical examination, evidence of hemostatic impairment should be sought, as well as secondary causes of thrombocytopenia. The signs of platelet-related bleeding include petechiae and purpura (see Chapter 130). Petechiae typically occur in the dependent regions of the body or on traumatized areas. Spontaneous mucous membrane bleeding (wet purpura), epistaxis, and gastrointestinal bleeding indicate a more serious hemostatic defect. Although petechiae are common in patients whose platelet counts are less than 10 to 20 × 10^9/L, most patients with platelet counts over 50 × 10^9/L have no signs of hemostatic impairment. The physical examination may provide an explanation for the thrombocytopenia. For example, enlarged lymph nodes may indicate a viral infection, such as infectious mononucleosis or HIV infection, or a neoplastic process. An enlarged spleen raises the possibility of hypersplenism.

Timing of Onset and Severity of Thrombocytopenia

Many thrombocytopenic disorders—particularly those involving an immune pathogenesis—exhibit characteristic temporal features that can aid in the diagnosis. For example, if the platelet count begins to fall 5 to 10 days (median, 6-7 days) after starting a new drug or after a blood transfusion and reaches a nadir of less than 20 × 10^9/L a few days later, the diagnosis of drug-induced immune thrombocytopenia (D-ITP) or posttransfusion purpura (PTP), respectively, should be considered (Fig. 134-2).[2] Patients with these disorders typically have mucocutaneous bleeding and are at risk for fatal intracranial hemorrhage.

A similar temporal profile is also characteristic of typical-onset HIT, although there the platelet count only falls below 20 × 10^9/L in 10% of affected patients (see Fig. 134-2); in approximately 80% of patients, the platelet count nadir ranges from 20 to 150 × 10^9/L, and in the remainder, the platelet count nadir never falls below 150 × 10^9/L despite a large reduction in the platelet count. When the platelet count falls abruptly after drug administration, the possibility of rapid-onset thrombocytopenia caused by preexisting drug-dependent antibodies should be considered, as is well described with HIT. Indeed, so-called rapid-onset HIT is the presenting feature of this adverse drug reaction in 25% to 30% of cases. Rapid-onset thrombocytopenia is also a feature of glycoprotein (GP) IIb/IIIa antagonist-induced immune thrombocytopenia.

Occasionally, thrombocytopenia worsens in the first few days after surgery; this can occur in multiorgan system failure (e.g., cardiogenic or septic shock) (see Fig. 134-2). If the platelet count falls to very low levels and is accompanied by microangiopathic hemolysis, the possibility of postoperative thrombotic thrombocytopenic purpura (TTP) should be considered.[3]

Mild to moderate platelet count declines that occur soon after transfusion of blood products are common and can be explained by

Table 134-1 Mechanisms of Platelet Destruction or Consumption

Type of Thrombocytopenia	Specific Example(s)
Immune Mediated	
Autoantibody-mediated platelet destruction by RES	Primary and secondary idiopathic (immune) ITP*
Alloantibody-mediated platelet destruction by RES	NAIT,* PTP,* PAT; alloimmune platelet transfusion refractoriness*
Drug-dependent, antibody-mediated platelet destruction by RES	Drug-induced immune ITP (e.g., quinine) (see Figure 134-5)
Platelet activation by binding of IgG Fc of drug-dependent IgG to platelet FcγIIa receptors	HIT
Non–Immune Mediated	
Platelet activation by thrombin or proinflammatory cytokines	DIC*; septicemia or systemic inflammatory response syndromes
Platelet destruction via ingestion by macrophages (hemophagocytosis)	Infections, certain malignant lymphoproliferative disorders
Platelet destruction through platelet interactions with altered vWF†	TTP,* HUS*
Platelet losses on artificial surfaces	CPB,* use of intravascular catheters
Decreased platelet survival associated with cardiovascular diseases	Congenital and acquired heart disease, cardiomyopathy, PE

CPB, Cardiopulmonary bypass surgery; *DIC,* disseminated intravascular coagulation; *HIT,* heparin-induced thrombocytopenia; *HUS,* hemolytic uremic syndrome; *IgG,* immunoglobulin G; *ITP,* Idiopathic (immune) thrombocytopenic purpura; *NAIT,* Neonatal alloimmune thrombocytopenia; *PAT,* passive alloimmune thrombocytopenia; *PE,* pulmonary embolism; *PTP,* posttransfusion purpura; *RES,* reticuloendothelial system; *TTP,* thrombotic thrombocytopenic purpura; *vWF,* von Willebrand factor.
*See Chapter 133 for a discussion of thrombocytopenia in these disorders.
†Although platelet destruction is not directly caused by antibodies, immune mechanisms can explain altered vWF (e.g., autoimmune clearance of vWF-cleaving metalloprotease).

hemodilution; however, a marked platelet count fall after transfusion may be the result of passive alloimmune thrombocytopenia (PAT) or sepsis because of contaminated blood products (see Fig. 134-2).

Other characteristic temporal features of thrombocytopenia include postenterohemorrhagic *Escherichia coli*–associated hemolytic uremic syndrome (HUS; thrombocytopenia and microangiopathic hemolysis that begin approximately 1 week after a prodromal diarrheal illness) and fungemia-associated thrombocytopenia (onset, 1-3 weeks after complex illness involving indwelling catheters and broad-spectrum antibiotic usage). In contrast, thrombocytopenia of insidious onset that progresses over several years suggests chronic liver disease, with evolution to progressive portal hypertension and associated splenomegaly (e.g., cirrhosis secondary to alcohol or hepatitis C) or a slowly progressive BM disorder (e.g., myelodysplasia).

Laboratory Evaluation

Laboratory evaluation of patients with thrombocytopenia is summarized in Table 134-3 (also see Chapter 131). The blood film is examined to exclude pseudothrombocytopenia, which is characterized by in vitro platelet clumping. This phenomenon, which is evident in approximately one in 1000 blood samples, is most often caused by naturally occurring GPIIb/IIIa ($\alpha_{IIb}\beta_3$)-reactive autoantibodies that induce aggregation of platelets in the presence of the calcium-chelating anticoagulant ethylenediamine tetraacetic acid

Table 134-2 Differential Diagnosis of Thrombocytopenia in Pregnancy

Incidental thrombocytopenia of pregnancy (gestational thrombocytopenia)
Preeclampsia or eclampsia*
DIC secondary to:
- Abruptio placentae
- Endometritis
- Amniotic fluid embolism
- Retained fetus
- Preeclampsia or eclampsia*

Peripartum or postpartum thrombotic microangiopathy
- TTP
- HUS

DIC, Disseminated intravascular coagulation; *HUS,* hemolytic uremic syndrome; *TTP,* thrombotic thrombocytopenic purpura.
*Preeclampsia or eclampsia usually is not associated with overt DIC.

(EDTA). Because the platelet aggregates are not counted by the electronic particle counter, the automated platelet count appears falsely low. The correct platelet count usually can be determined by collecting the blood into sodium citrate or heparin or by performing the count on nonanticoagulated finger prick samples; maintaining the blood sample at 37°C often attenuates platelet clumping. EDTA-dependent pseudothrombocytopenia has no pathologic significance other than potentially placing a patient in jeopardy for inappropriate treatment of thrombocytopenia that does not exist. A much less common (one in 10,000 blood samples) antibody-mediated pseudothrombocytopenic disorder is platelet satellitism, in which rosette-like clusters of platelets surround neutrophils. This entity is produced by immunoglobulin G (IgG) antibodies that recognize EDTA-induced cryptic epitopes on both platelet GPIIb/IIIa and neutrophil FcγIII receptors.

Bone marrow examination can be helpful for assessment of platelet production, particularly if megakaryocytes are reduced in number or abnormal in appearance. Examination of the BM can be diagnostic in some disorders (e.g., leukemia, metastatic tumor, Gaucher disease, megaloblastic anemia).

Elevated platelet-associated IgG (PAIgG) can be detected in patients with either immune or nonimmune thrombocytopenia; therefore, this assay is not useful diagnostically. In contrast, GP-specific platelet antibody assays, such as the monoclonal antibody immobilization of platelet antigens (MAIPA) assay or antigen capture enzyme immunoassay, are relatively specific for detection of autoimmune thrombocytopenic disorders. These assays can also be adapted for detection of drug-dependent GP-reactive antibodies.

When the mechanism of chronic thrombocytopenia is unclear, an autologous platelet survival study using ^{111}In-labeled platelets may be informative. Three patterns can be seen: (1) normal platelet survival and recovery (underproduction), (2) marked reduction in the platelet life span (increased destruction), and (3) reduced recovery but a normal or near-normal life span (sequestration). However, platelet survival studies are rarely performed in practice.

Therapy

The risk of bleeding in patients with thrombocytopenia can be reduced by avoiding drugs that impair hemostasis (e.g., alcohol, antiplatelet agents, anticoagulants) and invasive procedures (e.g., intramuscular injections). If drug-induced thrombocytopenia is suspected, as many medications as possible should be stopped. Life-threatening bleeding episodes should be treated with platelet transfusion regardless of the mechanism of the thrombocytopenia.

The underlying cause and anticipated natural history of the thrombocytopenic disorder influence the decision about prophylactic platelet transfusion. As a general rule, patients with chronic thrombocytopenic disorders characterized by increased platelet destruction (e.g., chronic ITP) or chronic underproduction (e.g., aplastic anemia

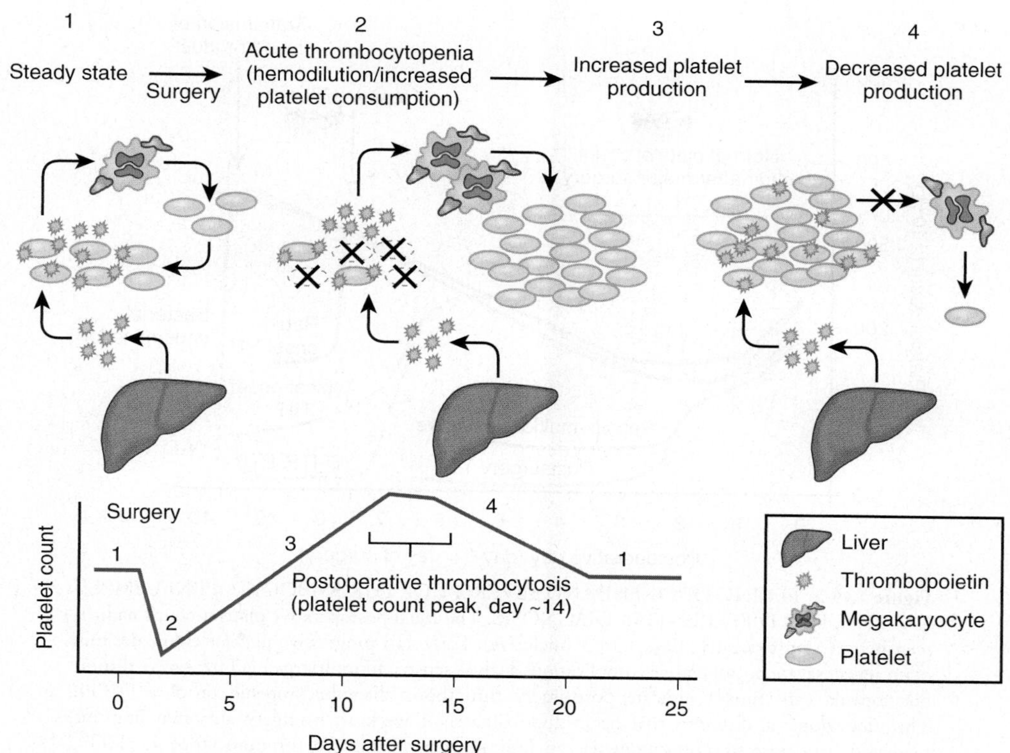

Figure 134-1 POSTSURGERY PLATELET COUNT CHANGES. Initial platelet count declines result from hemodilution and increased platelet consumption, with the platelet count nadir occurring between days 1 to 4 (median, day 2). There is constitutive production of thrombopoietin (TPO) by the liver. TPO binds to platelets and megakaryocytes via a specific receptor (c-Mpl, not shown), and receptor-bound TPO is removed from circulation and degraded. The level of circulating TPO is thus inversely related to the mass of platelets and megakaryocytes. In early postsurgery thrombocytopenia, fewer TPO binding sites are available, resulting in high free TPO levels, which stimulates megakaryocyte proliferation and differentiation and leads to increased platelet production. With subsequent thrombocytosis, the high platelet mass acts as a "sink" for removing TPO, with decreased stimulus for platelet production. Thus, after acute postsurgery thrombocytopenia, TPO levels rise about twofold, leading to increased platelet production that begins on days 2 to 4, with resulting thrombocytosis that generally peaks at approximately day 14 (postoperative thrombocytosis) and returns to baseline by about day 21. *(Reprinted, with modifications, with permission, from Arnold DM, Warkentin TE: Thrombocytopenia and thrombocytosis. In Wilson WC, Grande CM, Hoyt DB, editors:* Trauma: Critical care, *vol 2. New York, 2007, Informa Healthcare, p 983.)*

or myelodysplasia) can tolerate long periods of severe thrombocytopenia without major bleeding. In addition, prophylactic platelet transfusions can trigger alloimmunization against human leukocyte antigen (HLA) or platelet antigens, thereby jeopardizing future therapeutic platelet transfusions. Consequently, prophylactic platelet transfusions are seldom indicated for such patients except when they are at risk of bleeding because of trauma or major surgery. When platelets are given, the platelet count should be maintained above 50 $\times 10^9$/L. Invasive procedures such as thoracentesis, paracentesis, and liver biopsy are not usually associated with excess bleeding if the platelet count is greater than 50 $\times 10^9$/L.

Prophylactic platelet transfusions should not be given to patients with strongly suspected or confirmed HIT, TTP, or HUS because they may exacerbate platelet-mediated thrombotic complications, and, particularly with HIT, mucocutaneous bleeding is uncommon. However, bleeding in the setting of severe thrombocytopenia may justify platelet transfusion even in these disorders.

ANATOMY AND PHYSIOLOGY

The Spleen: Anatomy and Function

The spleen is a small, well-perfused organ that receives about 5% of the total cardiac output. In adults, the spleen weighs between 150 to 200 g and measures approximately 11 cm in length.

The anatomy of the spleen is uniquely suited for its function; progressive branching of the splenic artery into trabecular and central arteries helps separate the plasma from the cellular elements (see Chapter 162). The central arteries arise perpendicularly from the trabecular arteries and skim the plasma layer from the cells. Soluble antigens in the plasma are delivered to the white pulp, where phagocytic cells process them and antibody production is initiated.

A cell-rich, hemoconcentrated fraction of the blood is delivered to the red pulp. Some of this blood flows directly to the splenic veins (the closed system), but most moves into the splenic cords (the open system). Here, the cellular elements percolate through a meshwork of reticulum fibers, reticuloendothelial cells, and supporting cells to reach the splenic sinuses. The cells enter the sinuses by passing through narrow fenestrations in the basement membrane of the endothelial cells lining the sinuses. The blood exits through the splenic vein into the portal system. Because the veins in the portal system lack valves, any increase in portal pressure is transmitted to the splenic microcirculation.

The spleen plays a number of important roles. It is the largest lymphoid organ in the body and contributes to host defense by clearing microorganisms and antibody-coated cells. The spleen also is important for antibody synthesis, especially antibodies directed against soluble antigens. The filtering function of the spleen includes (1) culling (removal of damaged or senescent cells and bacteria), (2) pitting (removal of red blood cell [RBC] inclusion bodies or parasites), and (3) remodeling (reticulocyte sequestration and

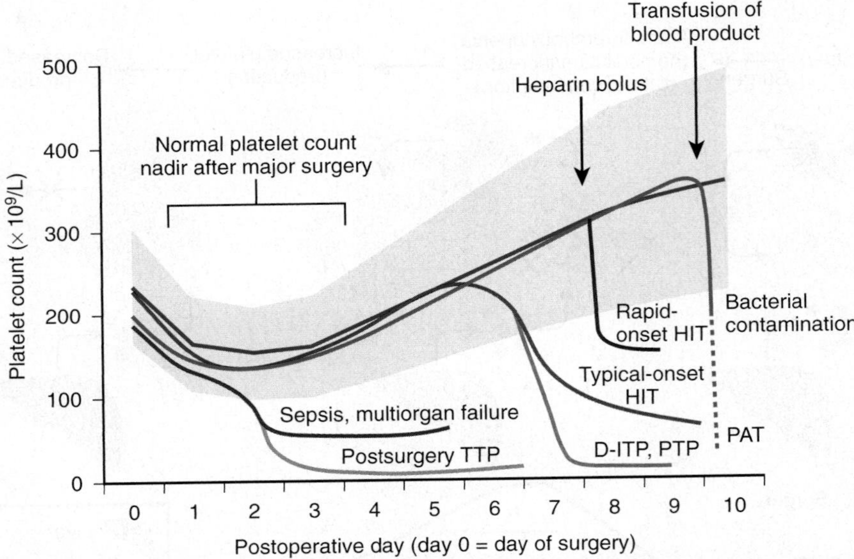

Figure 134-2 TIMING OF ONSET AND SEVERITY OF THROMBOCYTOPENIA: IMPLICATIONS FOR DIFFERENTIAL DIAGNOSIS. The usual postoperative platelet count nadir is seen between postoperative days 1 to 3 (inclusive). Early and progressive platelet count declines often reflect severe postoperative complications such as sepsis and multiorgan failure; severe thrombocytopenia can (rarely) indicate postsurgery thrombotic thrombocytopenic purpura (TTP). Thrombocytopenic disorders that begin approximately 1 week after surgery are often immune mediated: moderate thrombocytopenia can indicate heparin-induced thrombocytopenia (HIT), both "typical onset" or (if heparin is not being given) "delayed onset"; very severe thrombocytopenia can indicate drug-induced immune thrombocytopenic purpura (D-ITP) or (rarely) posttransfusion purpura (PTP). An abrupt decline in platelet count after receiving a heparin bolus in a patient who has received heparin within the past 7 to 100 days can indicate "rapid-onset" HIT; thrombocytopenia that begins abruptly after transfusion of a blood product can indicate sepsis from bacterial contamination or (rarely) passive alloimmune thrombocytopenia (PAT) caused by transfusion of platelet-reactive alloantibodies. *(Reprinted, with permission, from Greinacher A, Warkentin TE: Acquired non-immune thrombocytopenia. In: Marder VJ, Aird WC, Bennett JS, et al, editors:* Hemostasis and thrombosis: Basic principles and clinical practice, *ed 6. Philadelphia, 2012, Lippincott Williams & Wilkins, in press.)*

maturation). The spleen also acts as a reservoir of platelets (accommodating about one-third of the platelet mass in normal individuals). By contrast, the human spleen contains less than 2% of the total red RBC mass, although in some animals (dogs and cats), the spleen is a much more important RBC reservoir.

Physiologic Platelet Sequestration

Radiolabeled platelet studies have shown that approximately 30% of the total platelet mass exists as a freely exchangeable pool in the spleen. Because the normal platelet life span is 9 to 10 days, platelets spend approximately one-third of their lives, or 3 days, within the spleen. In patients with hypersplenism, as many as 90% of the platelets can be found in the spleen.

After labeled platelets are injected, accumulation is apparent in both the liver and the spleen. An initial, irreversible phase of hepatic uptake occurs. This equilibrates during the first 5 minutes and may reflect hepatic clearance of platelets damaged during the labeling procedure. Simultaneously, there is a slow increase in activity over the spleen that peaks in about 20 minutes. Splenic platelet uptake is thus dependent on input (spleen blood flow) and output (clearance).

The splenic platelet pool size can be decreased and the platelet count increased with intravenous infusions of epinephrine in normal persons and in patients with splenomegaly. By contrast, isoprenaline increases the pool size. Splenic blood flow increases with increasing spleen size, although perfusion (flow per unit of tissue volume) falls. Blood flow can be increased in some inflammatory disorders (e.g., SLE) without an increase in spleen size. A marked increase or decrease in splenic perfusion alters the proportion of platelets within the spleen.

Fig. 134-3 shows why approximately 30% of the platelets are normally present in the spleen.[1] Because about 5% of cardiac output goes to the spleen and because the average splenic transit time (i.e., the time for the platelet to pass through the spleen) is approximately 10 minutes—compared with the usual average time of 1 minute for a platelet to make a complete circulatory pass—the proportion of platelets within the spleen is approximately one-third (i.e., 5% × 10 min : 95% × 1 min, or a ratio of 50 : 95, or ≈1 : 2). With hypersplenism, the splenic blood flow can increase up to fivefold (i.e., from 5% to 25% of total blood flow). Thus, even without an increase in splenic transit time, 70% or more of the platelets can be exchangeably sequestered within the spleen.

The most important determinant of the splenic platelet pool is the spleen size. The measurement of spleen size can thus be helpful in predicting the degree of thrombocytopenia expected from excess platelet pooling in the spleen. For example, if the splenic platelet pool is 90% (i.e., 10% outside the spleen), the platelet count will be reduced by a factor of 7 (because normally, 70% of platelets lie outside the spleen). Consequently, and as a general rule, even if the spleen is massively enlarged, severe thrombocytopenia ($<20 \times 10^9$/L) is rarely seen. On the other hand, mild thrombocytopenia may be explained by mild splenomegaly that may not be detectible on physical examination but can be seen with imaging studies.

Table 134-3 Laboratory Tests Used to Investigate a Patient With Thrombocytopenia

Test	Rationale
Common Tests	
CBC	Isolated thrombocytopenia usually is caused by platelet destruction, but involvement of all cell lines suggests underproduction or sequestration
Examination of the blood film	Pseudothrombocytopenia (platelet clumps) Toxic changes and granulocyte "left shift" suggest septicemia Atypical lymphocytes suggest viral infection RBC fragments suggest TTP or HUS Parasites (e.g., in malaria) White cell inclusions suggest hereditary macrothrombocytopenia
Blood cultures	Bacteremia, fungemia
ANA test	Systemic lupus erythematosus
Direct antiglobulin test	Exclude immune hemolysis accompanying ITP (Evans syndrome)
Coagulation assays	
aPTT, PT (INR), thrombin time, fibrinogen, D-dimer assay	DIC
LA assay (nonspecific inhibitor), anticardiolipin and anti-β_2-glycoprotein I assays	aPL antibody syndrome
Serum protein electrophoresis; IgG, IgM, IgA levels	ITP associated with lymphoproliferative disorder (monoclonal); hypersplenism associated with chronic hepatitis (polyclonal)
HIV serologic studies	HIV-associated thrombocytopenia
BM aspiration, biopsy	Assess megakaryocyte numbers and morphology; exclude primary BM disorder
Specialized Tests	
GP-specific platelet antibody assays (e.g., MAIPA)	Relatively specific assay for primary and secondary ITP
Drug-dependent increase in platelet-associated IgG	Specific assay for D-ITP
Drug-dependent platelet activation test (e.g., platelet serotonin release assay) or PF4–heparin (or PF4-polyanion) ELISA	HIT
Radionuclide platelet lifespan study with imaging (e.g., ^{111}In platelet survival study)	Define the mechanism of thrombocytopenia; identify an "accessory" spleen postsplenectomy

ANA, Antinuclear antibody; *aPL,* antiphospholipid; *aPTT,* activated partial thromboplastin time; *CBC,* complete blood count; *DIC,* disseminated intravascular coagulation; *D-ITP,* drug-induced immune thrombocytopenia; *ELISA,* enzyme-linked immunosorbent assay; *GP,* glycoprotein; *HIT,* heparin-induced thrombocytopenia; *HIV,* human immunodeficiency virus; *HUS,* hemolytic uremic syndrome; *IgG,* immunoglobulin G; *INR,* international normalized ratio; *ITP,* idiopathic (immune) thrombocytopenic purpura; *LA,* lupus anticoagulant; *MAIPA,* monoclonal antibody immobilization of platelet antigens; *PF4,* platelet factor 4; *PT,* prothrombin time; *RBC,* red blood cell; *TTP,* thrombotic thrombocytopenic purpura.

PATHOLOGIC PLATELET SEQUESTRATION: HYPERSPLENISM

Definition

Hypersplenism is a syndrome characterized by splenomegaly and any or all of the following cytopenias: anemia, leukopenia, or thrombocytopenia. Implicit in the definition is that the cytopenias will correct after splenectomy. Although splenomegaly is almost always present in hypersplenism, many patients with splenomegaly do not have hypersplenism. The hypersplenism usually is the result of an identifiable pathological process, but rarely, the cause of the splenomegaly remains elusive, and the hypersplenism is termed *primary.*

Pathogenesis

A list of disorders producing splenomegaly and hypersplenism is presented in Table 134-4. An increase in the size of the spleen can be caused by several mechanisms. Increased workload of the spleen can be caused by immunologic stress (infection, inflammation, or an autoimmune disorder) or by increased RBC removal (RBC membrane disorders, hemoglobinopathies). Portal hypertension also increases the size of the spleen, producing congestive splenomegaly. Benign and malignant infiltrative disorders may increase splenic size (infiltrative splenomegaly) and cause hypersplenism. Some of these disorders produce thrombocytopenia by more than just hypersplenism (e.g., BM infiltration with tumor, immune-mediated platelet clearance). Thus the demonstration of an enlarged spleen does not necessarily mean that the cytopenias are caused solely by hypersplenism.

Thrombocytopenia of hypersplenism is caused primarily by increased splenic platelet pooling. A massively enlarged spleen can hold more than 90% of the total platelet mass. In the absence of altered platelet production, the total body platelet mass usually is normal, and the platelet life span is near normal. Usually, the splenic transit time remains normal (≈10 minutes), but the absolute number of platelets retained within the enlarged spleen is increased. All of these platelets remain part of the exchangeable pool. In hypersplenism, the thrombocytopenia is moderately severe (platelet counts of 50×10^9/L to 150×10^9/L). Severe thrombocytopenia ($<20 \times 10^9$/L) suggests another diagnosis. Therefore, it is unusual for patients with hypersplenism to have evidence of hemostatic impairment attributable to thrombocytopenia or to need specific interventions to raise the platelet count. Plasma volume expansion occurs in hypersplenism, but hemodilution plays a relatively minor role in the thrombocytopenia. In some patients with advanced liver disease, impaired hepatic production of thrombopoietin may contribute to thrombocytopenia in addition to hypersplenism.

The neutropenia of hypersplenism is caused by an increase in the marginated granulocyte pool, a portion of which is located in the spleen. The neutropenia of hypersplenism usually is asymptomatic.

Diagnosis

Thrombocytopenia is likely to be caused by hypersplenism when (1) splenomegaly is present, (2) the thrombocytopenia is mild to moderate in severity, (3) moderately reduced neutrophil and low-normal hemoglobin levels are found, and (4) no or minimal evidence for impaired hematopoiesis is observed on BM examination. Ultrasonography, computed tomography, and radionuclide imaging are of comparable sensitivity for documenting splenomegaly, and an imaging study should be performed if splenomegaly is not evident on physical examination. The mean platelet volume often is slightly decreased in hypersplenism, but this finding is not sufficiently specific to be diagnostically useful. An ^{111}In-labeled platelet survival study can be diagnostic of hypersplenism, demonstrating reduced platelet recovery and a normal platelet life span. Determining the cause of the splenomegaly usually is the most important issue.

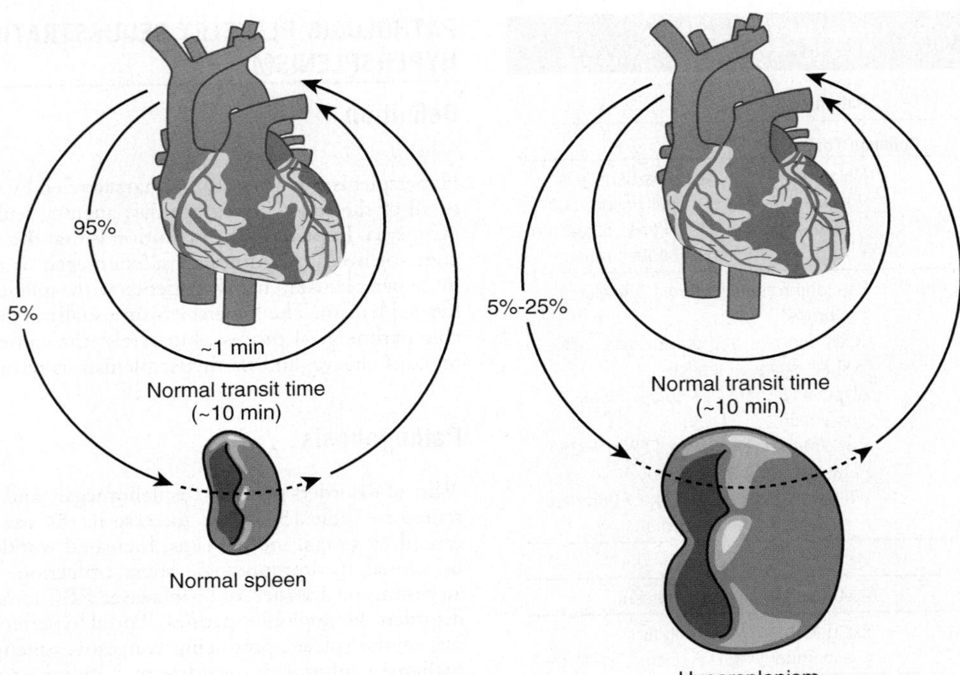

Figure 134-3 PHYSIOLOGIC AND PATHOLOGIC PLATELET SPLENIC SEQUESTRATION. Normally, about 5% of cardiac output is to the spleen; however, a platelet that enters the spleen spends about 10 minutes there (splenic transit time =10 min). In contrast, it usually takes only about 1 minute for a platelet to make a circulatory pass elsewhere. Thus about one-third of the platelets at any one time are located within the spleen: (5% × 10 min):(95% × 1 min), or an approximate 1 : 2 ratio. In hypersplenism, the splenic blood flow can increase by a factor of 5, that is, from 5% to 25% of total blood flow per minute. Thus, even without increase in splenic transit time, up to 70% or more of the platelets can be exchangeably sequestered within the spleen. *(From Arnold DM, Warkentin TE: Thrombocytopenia and thrombocytosis. In: Wilson WC, Grande CM, Hoyt DB, editors:* Trauma: Critical care, *vol. 2. New York, 2007, Informa Healthcare USA, p 983.)*

Therapy

Several maneuvers can improve or correct the cytopenias attributable to hypersplenism, including total or partial splenectomy; partial splenic embolization; and, in patients with congestive splenomegaly, surgical or transjugular intrahepatic portosystemic shunting. However, cytopenias secondary to hypersplenism thrombocytopenia in particular are almost never of sufficient severity to justify treatment. Consequently, the decision to perform one of these interventions usually depends on other considerations. For example, splenectomy should be considered for relief of pain or early satiety associated with massive splenomegaly (e.g., in myelo- or lymphoproliferative disorders) or for splenomegaly of unknown origin (for investigation of possible splenic lymphoma).

Short-term complications from splenectomy include infections, bleeding, and thromboembolism. The major long-term risk associated with splenectomy is overwhelming septicemia; this risk can be reduced by vaccination. All patients should be vaccinated against pneumococci, meningococci, and *Haemophilus* spp. at least 2 weeks before elective splenectomy. Moreover, "booster" doses of pneumococcus and meningococcus vaccines are recommended after 5 years.[4,5] Splenectomy for congestive hypersplenism in the setting of portal hypertension is associated with high morbidity and mortality rates. Splenectomy also is associated with high morbidity (50%) and mortality (10%-15%) rates in myeloid metaplasia and does not alter the natural history of this disorder. Thus splenectomy usually is performed for palliation of intractable symptoms.

Splenectomy in Gaucher disease usually corrects the cytopenias, relieves abdominal discomfort, and improves growth in children. Partial, rather than total, splenectomy has been used in an attempt to avoid shifting the deposition of glucocerebroside from the spleen to the bones. Often, however, splenomegaly and hypersplenism recur after partial splenectomy. Enzyme replacement therapy can reduce the morbidity from hypersplenism (see Chapter 162).

DRUG-INDUCED THROMBOCYTOPENIC SYNDROMES

Many drugs can cause thrombocytopenia. Some drugs (e.g., anticancer chemotherapeutic agents, valproic acid) cause dose-dependent thrombocytopenia, generally through myelosuppressive mechanisms. An important disorder encountered by hematologists is unexpected thrombocytopenia caused by immunologic (idiosyncratic) mechanisms.[6,7] The frequency of these reactions varies considerably among drugs and ranges from very rare (<1 in 10,000) for commonly used drugs such as acetaminophen, indomethacin, naproxen, quinine or quinidine, and trimethoprim–sulfamethoxazole (TMP-SMX) to common (1%-5%) for other drugs such as gold and unfractionated heparin (UFH).

Immunologic drug-induced thrombocytopenia can occur through different mechanisms (Fig. 134-4). For example, thrombocytopenia can occur when the Fab terminus of the pathogenic IgG binds to a complex composed of drug (or drug metabolite) and a platelet membrane component (typically, platelet GPIIb/IIIa or GPIb/IX/V). The Fc portions of the pathogenic IgG molecules do not bind to platelets but interact with Fc receptors on phagocytic cells of the reticuloendothelial system, which ingest the platelets, leading to accelerated platelet clearance. Severe thrombocytopenia (platelet counts <20 × 10^9/L) typically is observed (see Fig. 135-3 in Chapter 135). This mechanism is exemplified by quinine- and quinidine-induced thrombocytopenia. Sometimes the Fab terminus binds to a neoepitope on platelet GPIIb/IIIa induced by the drug, and the drug itself is not

Table 134-4 Differential Diagnosis of Splenomegaly and Hypersplenism

Infections
ACUTE
Viral (viral hepatitis, infectious mononucleosis, CMV infection)
Bacterial (septicemia, salmonellosis, brucellosis, splenic abscess)
Parasite (toxoplasmosis)
SUBACUTE AND CHRONIC
Subacute bacterial endocarditis
Tuberculosis
Malaria
Kala-azar
Fungal disease
Inflammation
Felty syndrome
SLE
Serum sickness
Rheumatic fever
Sarcoidosis
ALPS
Congestive Splenomegaly
INTRAHEPATIC
Cirrhosis
EXTRAHEPATIC
Portal vein obstruction
Splenic vein obstruction
Hepatic vein occlusion (Budd-Chiari syndrome)
CHRONIC PASSIVE CONGESTION
Heart failure
Hematologic Disorders
RBC disorders: hemolytic anemias, thalassemia, sickle cell disorders
Neoplasia
MALIGNANT
MPDs
Myeloid metaplasia
Polycythemia rubra vera
Essential thrombocythemia
Chronic leukemia
Chronic myeloid leukemia
Chronic lymphocytic leukemia
Hairy cell leukemia
Lymphoma
Acute leukemia
Malignant histiocytosis
BENIGN
Hamartoma
Hemangioma
Lymphangioma
Fibroma
Storage Diseases
Gaucher disease
Niemann-Pick disease
Miscellaneous
Amyloidosis
Cysts

ALPS, Autoimmune lymphoproliferative syndrome; *CMV,* cytomegalovirus; *MPD,* myeloproliferative disorder; *RBC,* red blood cell; *SLE,* systemic lupus erythematosus.

part of the neoepitope. This mechanism is exemplified by the GPIIb/IIIa receptor antagonist eptifibatide. Rarely, some drugs may induce the formation of typical platelet GP-reactive autoantibodies (e.g., gold-induced thrombocytopenia or acute ITP after administration of certain vaccines).

Another distinct form of drug-induced thrombocytopenia is exemplified by HIT (see Chapter 135). In this disorder, the Fab portion of the pathogenic IgG binds to platelet factor 4 (PF4), an α-granule protein that is immunogenic when complexed to heparin or certain other polyanions. The Fc portions of the IgG molecules bind to platelet FcγIIa receptors, initiating intense platelet activation (see Fig. 134-4). Perhaps because HIT is a platelet activation syndrome or because of the relatively low number of HIT antibodies that bind to platelet surfaces, the thrombocytopenia is typically mild to moderate rather than severe (see Fig. 135-3 in Chapter 135).

Finally, drug-induced antibodies can explain thrombocytopenia by unusual mechanisms. For example, the antiplatelet agents ticlopidine and clopidogrel are rare causes of TTP, possibly because drug-dependent antibodies form against the von Willebrand factor (vWF)–cleaving metalloprotease ADAMTS13 (a disintegrin and metalloproteinase with a thrombospondin type 1 motif, member 13). Quinine is another cause of microangiopathic hemolysis, although in this situation, the terms *HUS* and *DIC* are often used, reflecting the prominent renal failure or coagulation abnormalities, respectively, observed in some affected patients.

DRUG-INDUCED IMMUNE THROMBOCYTOPENIA

A large number of drugs can cause a syndrome that mimics acute ITP (D-ITP); however, there are relatively few drugs for which causation is well established on both clinical and serologic grounds (Fig. 134-5).[8,9] Typically, severe thrombocytopenia (platelet count usually $<20 \times 109/L$), together with petechiae and purpura, develops within approximately 1 week (although occasionally much longer) after initiation of therapy with the responsible drug. D-ITP is much less common than HIT. For example, a relatively "common" cause of this syndrome is trimethoprim-sulfamethoxazole (co-trimoxazole), even though it occurs in only approximately one in 25,000 patients who receive this drug combination.

Important exceptions to these generalizations occur with immune thrombocytopenia that results from GPIIb/IIIa receptor antagonists; these reactions are relatively common (affecting about 0.5%-1% of patients) and usually occur within hours of first use as a result of preexisting, naturally occurring antibodies. Another exception is carbimazole-induced thrombocytopenia, in which mild thrombocytopenia is explained by the presence of relatively small quantities of the platelet GP target (platelet endothelial cell adhesion molecule-1 [PECAM-1]) on the platelet surface. Besides the atypical immune-mediated syndromes of HIT and GPIIb/IIIa antagonist thrombocytopenia, the most common drugs (in absolute terms) implicated in the causation of classic D-ITP syndrome are quinine (outpatients) and vancomycin (inpatients).[10]

Pathogenesis

Drug-dependent binding of the Fab component of IgG to platelet GP leads to platelet destruction. This occurs because the IgG-sensitized platelets are recognized by Fc receptors of phagocytic cells. For quinine- and quinidine-induced immune thrombocytopenia, both the GPIIb/IIIa and GPIb/IX/V complexes have been implicated as targets for the drug-dependent IgG (see Fig. 134-4). By contrast, for sulfa antibiotic- and naproxen-induced immune thrombocytopenia, the GPIIb/IIIa complex is predominantly involved. Sometimes, drug metabolites form the antigen rather than the parent drug. A trimolecular complex is formed among IgG Fab, the drug (or metabolite), and the platelet GP. In contrast to HIT, platelet Fc receptors are not involved in D-ITP pathogenesis. Drug-dependent IgG binding

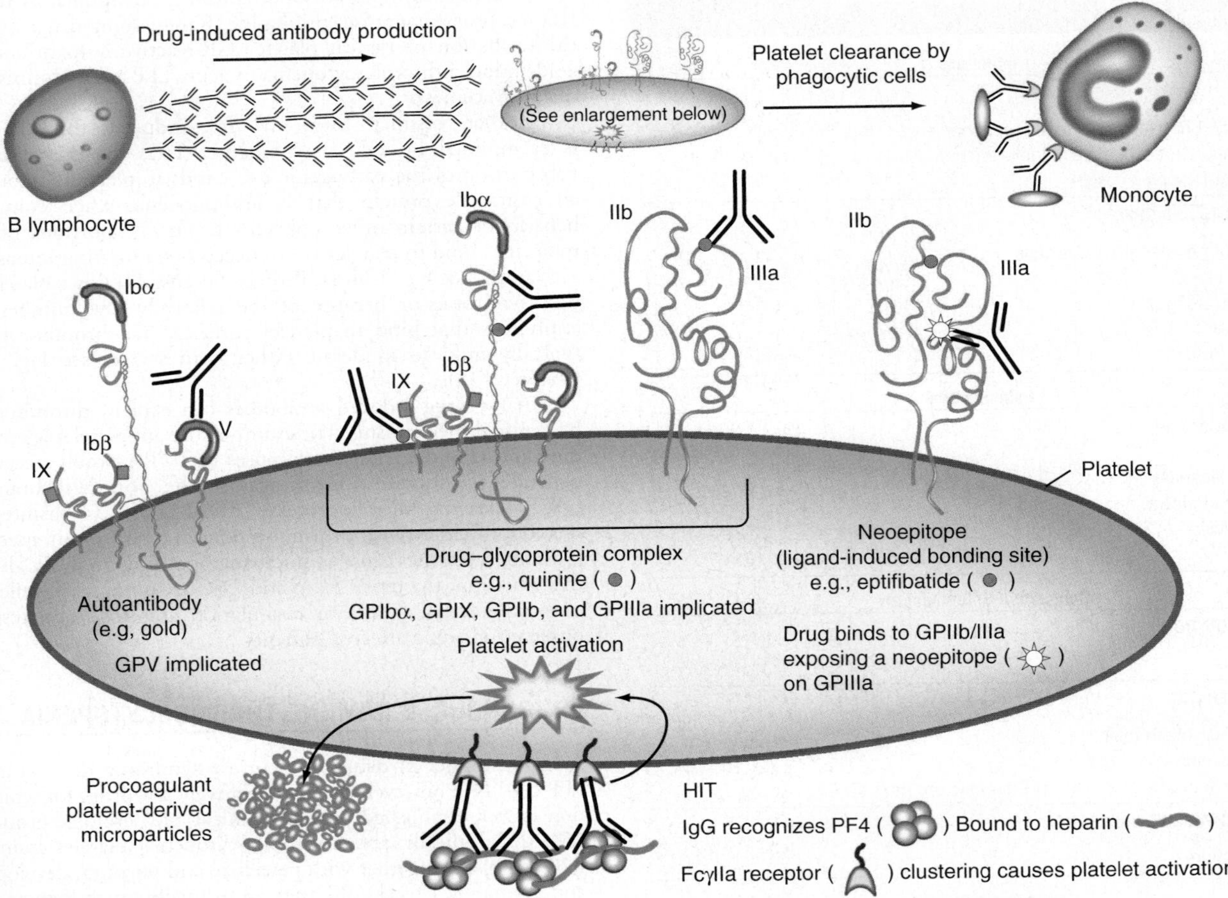

Figure 134-4 MECHANISMS OF DRUG-INDUCED IMMUNE THROMBOCYTOPENIA. Four immune thrombocytopenic syndromes are illustrated. On the *bottom* of the schematic platelet, heparin-induced thrombocytopenia (HIT) is illustrated, indicating that immunoglobulin G (IgG) antibodies bind to complexes of platelet factor 4 (PF4) and heparin, with the Fc regions of the antibodies binding to the platelet FcγIIa receptors, resulting in platelet activation (including generation of procoagulant, platelet-derived microparticles). On the *top* of the schematic platelet, three mechanisms are illustrated that lead to increased platelet clearance by phagocytic cells. From left to right, these are (1) autoantibody-induced immune thrombocytopenia (e.g., gold-induced antiglycoprotein V [GPV] antibodies). (2) drug-dependent antibodies reactive against drug (or drug metabolite)–platelet glycoprotein complex(es) (e.g., quinine-induced thrombocytopenia in which drug-dependent antibodies against GPIbα, GPIX, GPIIb, and GPIIIa have been implicated, resulting in an antibody/drug/glycoprotein ternary complex), and (3) antibodies against neoepitope(s) formed in the presence of a drug (e.g., eptifibatide-induced immune thrombocytopenia caused by formation of ligand-induced binding site elsewhere on the GPIIb/IIIa complex after eptifibatide binding). Note that preexisting (naturally-occurring) antibodies can explain abrupt-onset thrombocytopenia in a patient receiving eptifibatide for the first time.

is remarkably heterogeneous with respect to binding affinity, number of binding sites per platelet, and the range of drug concentrations required. A recent study of quinine-induced immune thrombocytopenia identified two different types of antibodies: quinine-dependent antibodies that bound to platelets in the presence of drug and quinine-specific antibodies that reacted with quinine-conjugated albumin.[11] The pathophysiological implications of this latter group of antibodies remains unclear.

The fundamental mechanism that accounts for antibody formation in a small proportion of patients is unknown. One group has proposed that drug-dependent platelet-reactive antibodies are derived from a pool of naturally occurring autoantibodies with inherently weak (nonpathologic) affinity for certain platelet membrane GPs (Fig. 134-6).[6,11] However, if a certain drug is able to enhance antibody–antigen interaction, and if B cells expressing such antibodies are induced to proliferate and undergo affinity maturation in such a patient, the resulting antibody can destroy the platelets in the presence of the drug.

Clinical Features

Patients with D-ITP typically present with petechiae, purpura, and severe thrombocytopenia (platelet count often <20 × 10^9/L). Systemic symptoms, such as fever and chills, may occur in patients with abrupt-onset thrombocytopenia. Usually, the thrombocytopenia becomes clinically apparent 1 to 2 weeks after initiation of the drug, but the thrombocytopenia can start after a patient has been taking a drug for several years. Typically, the platelet count begins to rise in a few days after discontinuation of the implicated drug, but occasionally several weeks are required for recovery, possibly because of the generation of drug-independent IgG (platelet autoantibodies).

Sometimes drug exposure is relatively obscure. Among outpatients, the physician needs to inquire about potential exposure to quinine. Quinine is widely available—as an ingredient in tonic water, for example, as an additive to street drugs, and in some countries as therapy for leg cramps. Vancomycin is a relatively common cause of D-ITP in hospitalized inpatients; most often this results from the

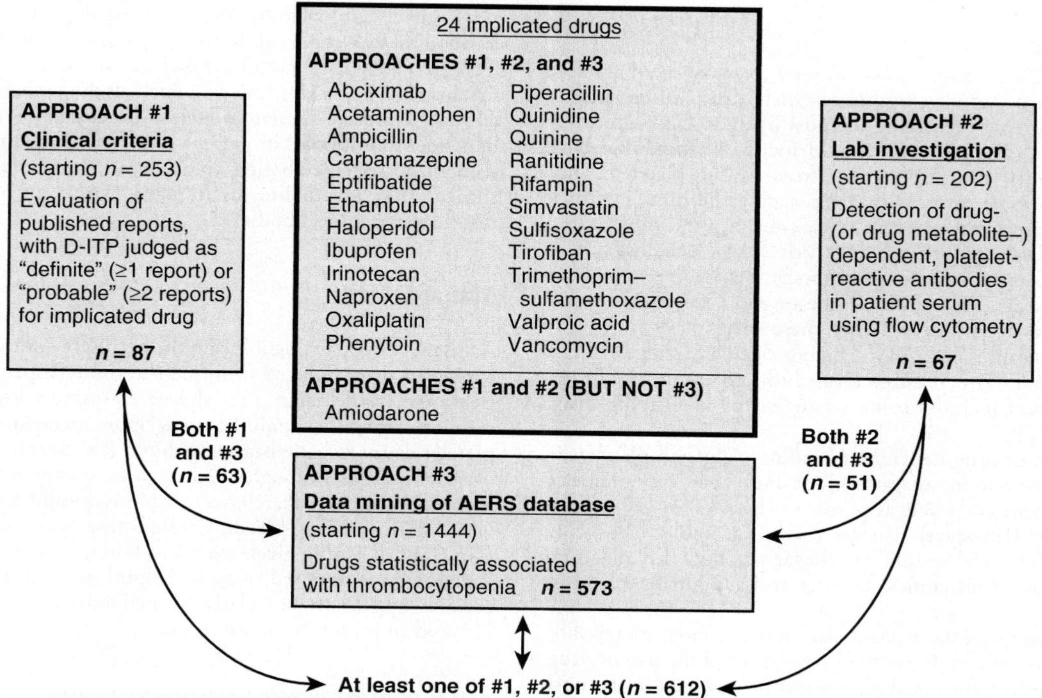

Figure 134-5 TWO DOZEN DRUGS WITH STRONG EVIDENCE FOR CAUSING DRUG-INDUCED IMMUNE THROMBOCYTOPENIA (D-ITP) SYNDROME. Three different approaches were used to adjudicate drugs as possibly causing D-ITP. The *central box* lists the 23 agents identified using all three methods plus one drug (amiodarone) implicated by only the first two methods. The categories "Both #1 & #3" and "Both #2 and #3" include the 23 patients who were identified using all three approaches. The numbers of drugs implicated by only one of the three approaches were 23, 15, and 482 for approaches #1, #2, and #3, respectively. *AERS,* Adverse Event Reporting System. *(Adapted from Warkentin TE, Anderson JAM: DITP causation: 3 methods better than 1?* Blood *116:2002, 2010.)*

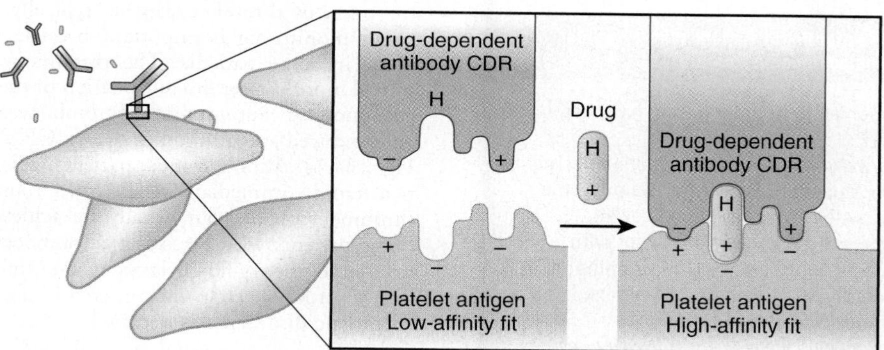

Figure 134-6 MODEL FOR BINDING OF DRUG-DEPENDENT ANTIBODIES TO PLATELET GLYCOPROTEIN (GP) EPITOPES. Antibodies capable of causing drug-dependent thrombocytopenia react weakly with an epitope on a target GP. The binding affinity (K_A) for this interaction is too low to allow a sufficient number of antibody molecules to bind in the absence of the drug ("low-affinity fit"). The drug contains structural elements that are complementary to a negatively charged site on the GP and a hydrophobic site (H) on the complementarity-determining region (CDR) of the antibody. The drug interacts with these sites to improve the fit between the two proteins, increasing the K_A to a value that permits binding to occur at levels of antibody, antigen, and drug achieved in the circulation after ingestion of the drug ("high-affinity fit"). *(From Aster RH, Bougie DW: Drug-induced immune thrombocytopenia.* N Engl J Med *357:580, 2007. Copyright Massachusetts Medical Society. Reprinted with permission.)*

usual intravenous administration, but some reports have implicated exposure via orthopedic cement or with peritoneal administration of vancomycin.

Rarely, distinct drug-dependent IgG molecules destroy RBCs or WBCs in addition to platelets. For example, both platelet- and leukocyte-reactive quinidine-dependent IgG molecules have been detected in a patient with quinidine-induced bicytopenia. Sometimes the immune process is directed against a pluripotent hematopoietic stem cell, resulting in pancytopenia accompanied by BM aplasia or hypoplasia (e.g., gold-, carbamazepine-, or quinidine-induced pancytopenia). A BM aspirate should be performed in patients with suspected drug-induced bicytopenia or pancytopenia because a hypoplastic BM may be indicative of drug-induced aplastic anemia.

Diagnosis

A high index of clinical suspicion is required to make the diagnosis. Moreover, clinicians need to evaluate which drug (often among several that the patient is receiving) is most likely to explain a diagnosis of D-ITP.[8,12-14] The clinician should focus on drugs that have been started 5 to 10 days before the onset of the platelet count decrease (Fig. 134-7, *A*). Also, with drugs such as quinine, in which there may be intermittent exposure (e.g., consumption of "gin and tonic"), a very recent exposure (previous 1 or 2 days) usually explains the abrupt onset of symptomatic thrombocytopenia.

After the physician has identified one or more potential agents, the next step is to determine whether these drugs have previously been implicated as causes of D-ITP. The box Search Strategies When Investigating Patient With Possible Drug-Induced Immune Thrombocytopenic Purpura includes some strategies for identifying drugs implicated in D-ITP.

Demonstration of drug-dependent binding of IgG to platelets in vitro can be important for diagnosis (see Fig. 134-7, *B*). Labeled immunoglobulin-specific probes (e.g., phase II assays) or GP capture techniques (phase III assays) can be used (see Table 134-3). In other cases, D-ITP test results are negative, but the diagnosis still seems likely based on clinical features and supporting literature (Fig. 134-8).

There are certain caveats in diagnostic testing. First, metabolites must sometimes be used to detect the IgG instead of the parent drug. Second, the target drug (or metabolite) must be included in the wash buffer used in these assays. Third, despite these maneuvers, the sensitivity of in vitro assays is relatively low, and the diagnosis of drug-induced immune thrombocytopenia often must be made on clinical grounds. Sometimes the diagnosis is confirmed by inadvertent or deliberate reexposure to the suspected drug. However, deliberate drug challenge is not often performed because of its potential risk.

Search Strategies When Investigating a Patient With Possible Drug-Induced Immune Thrombocytopenic Purpura

Four sources of information as to whether a drug has been implicated as a cause of D-ITP:

- **PubMed search** (http://www.ncbi.nlm.nih.gov/pubmed): [name of drug] and [thrombocytopenia]. By way of example, the author encountered a patient who developed severe thrombocytopenia 5 days after starting treatment with mirtazapine (see Fig. 134-8). Searching [mirtazapine] and [thrombocytopenia] identified one report[12] of mirtazapine-induced D-ITP syndrome.
- **Drug-induced thrombocytopenia website** (http://www.ouhsc.edu/platelets/ditp.html): Investigators at the University of Oklahoma published a comprehensive survey of drugs implicated in D-ITP using clinical criteria[13]; a website maintained by these investigators is updated every 2 years.
- **Database from drug-dependent platelet-reactive antibody testing** at the BloodCenter of Wisconsin, 1995-2010 (http://www.ouhsc.edu/platelets/InternetPostingLab2_18_11Frames.htm): the BloodCenter of Wisconsin maintains a website reporting its experience in detecting drug-dependent platelet-reactive antibodies.[14]
- **Combined approach that uses clinical criteria,[13] laboratory criteria,[14] and Adverse Event Reporting System.[8]** Figure 134-5 lists two dozen drugs for which convincing clinical and laboratory evidence exists.[8,9] To review the comprehensive list of all drugs investigated in this study,[8] interested readers can consult the online supplemental table (http.bloodjournal.hematologylibrary.org/content/suppl/2010/06/08/blood-2010-03-276691.DC1/TableS1.pdf).

A novel approach to identify drug-dependent platelet-reactive antibodies was reported by investigators at the Milwaukee Blood Center.[15] They used nonobese diabetic/severe combined immunodeficient (NOD/SCID) mice (which lack xenoantibodies, thereby allowing infused human platelets to circulate) to identify drug-dependent antibodies in patient sera, including antibodies that only recognize drug metabolites (presumably, mice produce the same or similar drug metabolites as humans, which are recognized by the drug-dependent antibodies).

Management

As many drugs as possible should be discontinued in patients with suspected drug-induced immune thrombocytopenia. If further drug treatment is necessary, an alternate, immunologically non–cross-reactive substitute should be used. Spontaneous improvement in the platelet count usually begins within a few days of discontinuing the offending drug, although in some cases, complete recovery may take 2 weeks or longer. Platelet transfusions should be given to patients with life-threatening bleeding. High-dose intravenous immunoglobulin (IVIG), 1 g/kg given over 6 to 8 hours, with a second dose 1 or 2 days later if required, may be helpful in some situations. Corticosteroids appear to be relatively ineffective for treatment of drug-induced immune thrombocytopenia.

GOLD-INDUCED THROMBOCYTOPENIA

Gold-induced immune thrombocytopenia occurs in as many as 1% to 3% of treated patients. A genetic predisposition is suggested by the association with HLA-DR3, which is found in approximately 85% of affected patients. The thrombocytopenia typically occurs during the first 20 weeks of therapy before a total of 1000 mg of gold has been given. Rarely, the thrombocytopenia begins much later, sometimes several months after discontinuation of the gold. Although the onset of thrombocytopenia typically is abrupt, regular platelet count monitoring is important because an early diagnosis can be made in some patients. The thrombocytopenia often persists for several months after discontinuation of the gold, probably because of gold-induced autoimmune thrombocytopenia (drug-independent gold-induced autoantibodies against GPV have been implicated) (see Fig. 134-4). Although most patients will eventually respond to corticosteroids, immediate, albeit often transient, correction of severe thrombocytopenia can usually be achieved with high-dose IVIG. Some patients with persisting thrombocytopenia benefit from splenectomy or use of gold-chelating agents (dimercaprol, *N*-acetylcysteine). The disorder is rarely encountered because the use of gold to treat rheumatic disorders has declined.

DRUG-INDUCED AUTOIMMUNE THROMBOCYTOPENIA

Certain drugs other than gold have been reported to initiate autoimmune thrombocytopenia (e.g., levodopa, procainamide).[4] Because the pathogenic antibodies are by definition drug independent, however, it is difficult to establish causation. The mumps–measles–rubella (MMR) vaccine can rarely (≈one in 40,000) cause a severe but generally self-limited thrombocytopenia that is clinically and serologically indistinguishable from childhood acute ITP; MMR vaccination of unimmunized children with ITP and revaccination of children with prior ITP does not lead to recurrent thrombocytopenia.[16]

DRUG-INDUCED IMMUNE THROMBOCYTOPENIA OF RAPID ONSET

A rapid onset of thrombocytopenia (within hours) can occur if a patient with preexisting drug-dependent antibodies is (re)exposed to the drug. This situation is relatively common in HIT (≈25% of

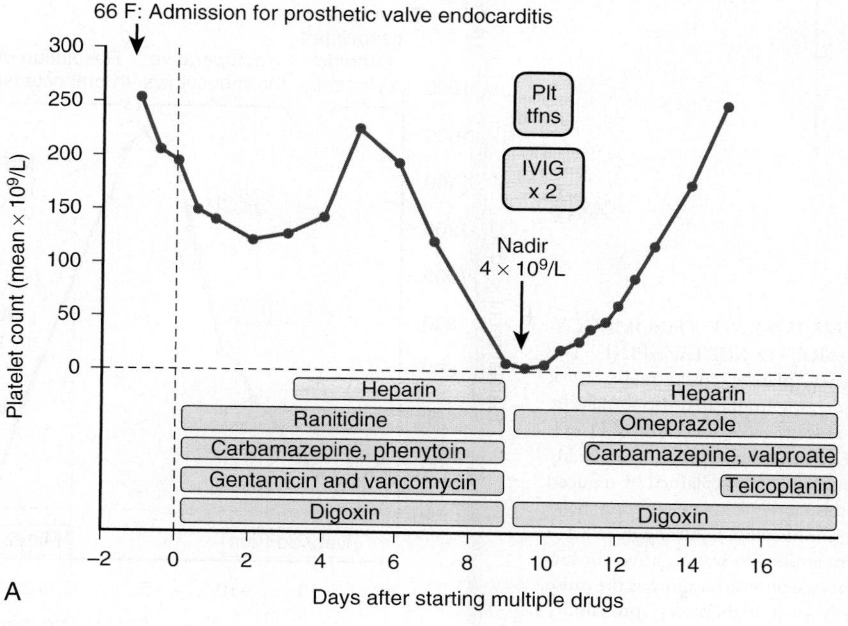

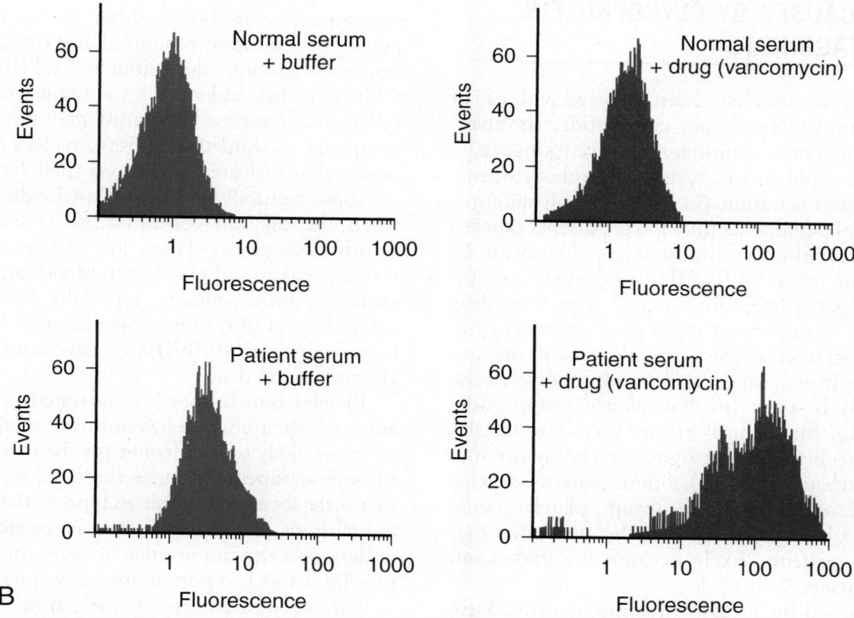

Figure 134-7 DRUG-INDUCED IMMUNE THROMBOCYTOPENIA (D-ITP) SECONDARY TO VANCOMYCIN. **A,** Timeline of D-ITP. A 66-year-old woman was admitted for prosthetic valve endocarditis 5 months after undergoing mitral valve replacement. The initiation of multiple new drugs and the onset 6 days later of progressively severe thrombocytopenia (platelet count nadir, 4×10^9/L on day 9) suggested D-ITP syndrome. However, the timing fit several drugs (ranitidine, carbamazepine, phenytoin, gentamicin, vancomycin, and digoxin). **B,** Drug-dependent binding of antibodies was demonstrated using patient serum and vancomycin. Also, test results for heparin-induced thrombocytopenia antibodies was negative. Thus the diagnosis of vancomycin-induced D-ITP syndrome was made based on clinical and serological grounds. The patient received treatment with high-dose intravenous immunoglobulin (IVIG) and platelet transfusions. *Plt tfns,* Platelet transfusions.

patients identified)[17] because repeated treatment with heparin is common and heparin use itself can result in the complication (HIT-associated thrombosis) that might lead to further use of heparin. Because HIT antibodies are transient, however, rapid-onset HIT occurs in patients with recent heparin exposures, usually within the past 100 days.[17] By contrast, repeated episodes of quinine-induced thrombocytopenia of abrupt onset can occur many months or even years apart because these antibodies persist for much longer. Thrombocytopenia of rapid onset is commonly seen with GPIIb/IIIa receptor antagonists (see next section).

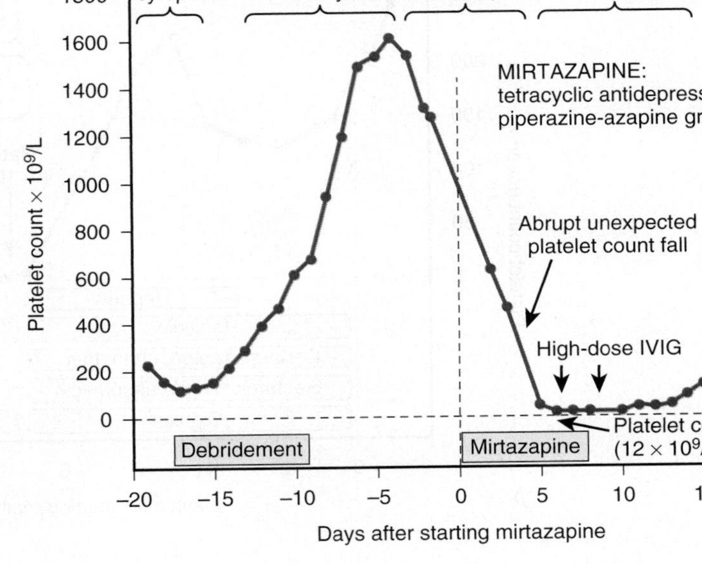

Figure 134-8 DRUG-INDUCED IMMUNE THROMBOCYTOPENIA (D-ITP) SECONDARY TO MIRTAZAPINE. The onset of severe thrombocytopenia (platelet count nadir, 12×10^9/L) on day 6 of mirtazapine therapy implicated this tetracyclic antidepressant of the piperazine-azapine group as a cause of D-ITP syndrome. The very rapid platelet count fall (which was already manifest on day 5 of mirtazapine therapy) is explained by reduced platelet production (because the patient's platelet count was declining from postoperative thrombocytosis). Although in vitro testing for mirtazapine-dependent antibodies was negative, the low sensitivity of these assays does not rule out mirtazapine as the cause of D-ITP syndrome, particularly in a high pretest probability scenario such as this.

THROMBOCYTOPENIA CAUSED BY GLYCOPROTEIN IIB/IIIA RECEPTOR ANTAGONISTS

Several thrombocytopenic syndromes have been reported with use of GPIIb/IIIa receptor antagonists (abciximab, eptifibatide, tirofiban) administered during percutaneous coronary interventions (e.g., angioplasty, stenting): (1) rapid-onset, severe thrombocytopenia within 12 hours of drug administration (in 0.4%-2% of patients), (2) rapid-onset pseudothrombocytopenia (in ~1% of patients exposed to abciximab [ReoPro]), (3) rapid-onset thrombocytopenia within 12 hours of a second exposure to a GPIIb/IIIa antagonist, and (4) delayed-onset thrombocytopenia beginning 5 to 7 days after drug administration (rare).[18] The frequency of rapid-onset thrombocytopenia is higher among patients who receive a second course of therapy, especially if it follows the initial exposure by only a few weeks. Thrombocytopenia typically is severe (median platelet count nadir, ~5×10^9/L to 10×10^9/L), but clinical effects vary dramatically, ranging from absence of petechiae or other signs of bleeding (in 50% of patients) to fatal hemorrhage (in <5%). Some patients develop anaphylactoid reactions accompanying the abrupt platelet count declines. Some investigators have proposed that the antibodies may cause thrombosis in some patients, likely because the pathogenic antibodies also activate platelets.[19]

These syndromes are caused by at least three mechanisms. First, antibodies of IgG (and possibly IgM) class can bind to neoepitopes on the GPIIb/IIIa complex generated by these drugs (or their metabolites)—that is, ligand-induced binding sites (see Fig. 134-4). Up to 5% of humans and nonhuman primates have naturally occurring IgG antibodies that will bind to GPIIb/IIIa receptors in the presence of drug, which could explain why rapid-onset thrombocytopenia occurs so frequently with these agents. A second mechanism is applicable to abciximab, a chimeric Fab fragment comprised of murine GPIIb/IIIa-reactive sequences and human framework sequences. Interestingly, although a high frequency of normal persons (74%) have antibodies that recognize platelets coated with abciximab, these "normal" antibodies were shown to differ from those detected in patients in whom thrombocytopenia developed after a second exposure to abciximab: whereas the pathogenic antibodies recognized murine sequences within abciximab, the "normal" (nonpathogenic) antibodies were specific for the carboxyl terminus (papain cleavage site) of Fab fragments prepared from normal human IgG. Drug-dependent antibodies also can be generated about 1 week after exposure. The antibodies differ among patients with respect to the precise neoepitopes recognized and display variable degrees of cross-reactivity among the different GPIIb/IIIa receptor antagonists ("fibans"); this explains why a repeat treatment course with another GPIIb/IIIa receptor antagonist may not necessarily cause thrombocytopenia. A third mechanism involves eptifibatide-dependent antibodies that activate platelets via their FcγIIa receptors.[19]

Some naturally occurring antibodies only bind to GPIIb/IIIa when the calcium concentration is low, thus explaining pseudothrombocytopenia—falsely low platelet count estimates caused by ex vivo aggregation of platelets in blood samples collected into calcium-chelating anticoagulants, especially EDTA. The rare syndrome of delayed-onset thrombocytopenia after brief exposure might result from high-titer GPIIb/IIIa-reactive antibodies that bind even in the absence of the drug.

Platelet transfusions are indicated in patients who are bleeding, although their efficacy has not been established. Platelet transfusions are most likely to be effective for the treatment of abciximab-induced thrombocytopenia because the drug binds so tightly to GPIIb/IIIa that little abciximab is free to bind to the transfused platelets. Platelet transfusions are not indicated in pseudothrombocytopenia, which underscores the importance of reviewing the blood film when a low platelet count is reported after treatment with one of these agents.

Various in vitro assays using flow cytometry or enzyme-linked immunosorbent assay (ELISA) have been developed to detect these antibodies. Because some pathogenic antibodies are naturally occurring, it is theoretically possible to identify patients at high risk for rapid-onset thrombocytopenia in elective situations (see box on Approach to Patients With Thrombocytopenia Following Percutaneous Coronary Interventions).

MISCELLANEOUS DRUG-INDUCED THROMBOCYTOPENIC SYNDROMES

Drug-Induced Thrombotic Microangiopathy

Several drugs can trigger a syndrome of thrombocytopenia, fragmentation hemolysis, and renal failure known as *drug-induced thrombotic microangiopathy*. This syndrome has been established for quinine, in which multiple quinine-dependent antibodies reactive against platelets, RBCs, leukocytes, and endothelial cells have been reported.

Approach to Patients With Thrombocytopenia Following Percutaneous Coronary Interventions

Four diagnoses should be considered in patients who develop thrombocytopenia within minutes or a few hours after a percutaneous coronary intervention (PCI) and have received one or more of the following agents: (1) platelet GPIIb/IIIa inhibitor (e.g., abciximab, eptifibatide, tirofiban), (2) heparin, or (3) iodinated contrast agent.

- **GPIIb/IIIa inhibitor–induced pseudothrombocytopenia.** The patient has no symptoms or signs of bleeding, and platelet aggregates are seen in the blood film. The platelet count is falsely reported as low by the automated particle counter, which fails to count aggregated platelets. No treatment is required.
- **GPIIb/IIIa inhibitor–induced thrombocytopenia.** The platelet count falls abruptly, often to profoundly reduced levels (typical nadir, <20 × 10^9/L). Hemostatic impairment is variable, ranging from no petechiae to fatal hemorrhages; occasionally, patients develop anaphylactoid reactions or even associated thrombosis. Treatment involves stopping all platelet antagonists and anticoagulants and giving platelets if the patient has signs of bleeding. Prophylactic platelet transfusions also can be considered if the platelet count is very low (e.g., <10 × 10^9/L). Testing for drug-dependent antibodies can be accomplished using flow cytometry or ELISA.
- **Rapid-onset HIT.** In patients who have preexisting HIT antibodies because of recent heparin exposure (generally within the past 100 days), rapid-onset HIT can occur when heparin is given during PCI. This is much less common than GPIIb/IIIa inhibitor–induced thrombocytopenia or pseudothrombocytopenia, so presumptive treatment of HIT with a nonheparin anticoagulant is rarely indicated in this situation. The platelet count nadir is usually much higher than with GPIIb/IIIa inhibitor–induced thrombocytopenia.
- **Radiocontrast-induced ITP.** Very rarely, patients who have previously received iodinated contrast can develop abrupt-onset, severe thrombocytopenia after exposure to contrast during PCI. Platelet transfusions (with or without high-dose IVIG) are appropriate for a bleeding patient.

Immune mechanisms could also be present when TTP-like illnesses are associated with drugs such as ticlopidine, clopidogrel, and simvastatin; for example, autoantibodies against vWF-cleaving metalloproteinase have been identified in ticlopidine-induced TTP. Treatment is with plasmapheresis, as for more typical TTP. Typically, affected patients recover, although some require short-term hemodialysis.

Although a similar syndrome may be caused by mitomycin, gemcitabine, cyclosporine, and tacrolimus, it should be noted that many patients who receive these drugs have an underlying illness (e.g., gastric adenocarcinoma, BM transplantation, collagen vascular disease) that itself can be complicated by thrombotic microangiopathy; moreover, high cumulative doses of the implicated drug have usually been received, suggesting a distinct, perhaps nonimmune pathogenesis. Furthermore, these patients tend to be less responsive to plasma exchange than those with idiopathic TTP.

Drug-Induced Disseminated Intravascular Coagulation

On rare occasions, quinine causes severe thrombocytopenia accompanied by marked coagulation abnormalities indicative of DIC. This syndrome overlaps that of quinine-induced thrombotic microangiopathy, and the explanation for the prominent coagulopathy is unknown. Although all patients with HIT have biochemical evidence of increased thrombin generation, only about 10% to 20% have overt DIC; however, these patients often present with large and small vessel thrombosis.

Nonidiosyncratic Drug-Induced Thrombocytopenia

Most antineoplastic drugs produce dose-dependent pancytopenia because of their effect on hematopoietic cells, including megakaryocytes and their progenitor cells. Typically, the platelet count nadir occurs at a predictable time after treatment, and the count then quickly recovers. Unexpectedly severe or prolonged thrombocytopenia in patients receiving chemotherapy should suggest alternate explanations (e.g., idiosyncratic thrombocytopenia caused by another drug).

Mild to moderate thrombocytopenia develops in approximately 20% of patients who take valproic acid (an antiepileptic agent); bleeding symptoms are uncommon. The mechanism of thrombocytopenia in this setting is unknown, but the condition appears to be nonidiosyncratic because the risk of thrombocytopenia correlates strongly with serum concentrations of valproic acid metabolite.[20] Amrinone is another agent that can cause mild, dose-dependent thrombocytopenia.

Rapid Nonimmune Drug-Induced Thrombocytopenia

Some drugs produce rapid but generally mild and transient drops in the platelet count. These drugs include heparin, protamine, bleomycin, hematin, desmopressin (particularly in patients with type 2B von Willebrand disease), and porcine factor VIII. The mechanisms for thrombocytopenia in these syndromes are obscure.

Drug Hypersensitivity Reactions

Mild to moderate thrombocytopenia is sometimes observed in patients with systemic drug hypersensitivity reactions. Comorbid clinical features can include generalized rash, fever, cholestasis, and leukopenia. Allopurinol, isoniazid, sulfasalazine, and phenothiazine drugs, among others, have been implicated in these reactions.

Thrombocytopenia Secondary to Biologic Response Modifiers

Use of purified or recombinant biologic response modifiers such as interferon, interleukin-2, and certain colony-stimulating factors has resulted in severe, reversible thrombocytopenia in some patients. Antilymphocyte globulins also can produce severe thrombocytopenia.

OTHER CAUSES OF DESTRUCTIVE THROMBOCYTOPENIA

Incidental Thrombocytopenia of Pregnancy

Maternal thrombocytopenia occurs in 4% to 8% of pregnancies.[21] Most affected women are healthy and have no history of thrombocytopenia, and their thrombocytopenia is incidentally detected by routine blood testing. The cause of the mild reduction in platelet count (~75 × 10^9/L to 150 × 10^9/L) is believed to represent a leftward shift in the normal platelet count range during pregnancy related to one or more of hemodilution, reduced platelet production, or increased platelet turnover.[21] This condition is benign and is not associated with an increased risk for maternal bleeding or neonatal thrombocytopenia. Accordingly, no special maneuvers are indicated in these women, and the route of delivery should be determined by obstetric indications. Epidural anesthesia is believed to be safe if the platelet count is at least 75 × 10^9/L.

Preeclampsia and Eclampsia

Preeclampsia is characterized by the onset of hypertension and proteinuria during pregnancy, especially in a primigravida near term. Preeclampsia complicates approximately 5% of pregnancies, and the frequency is higher in black women. Thrombocytopenia occurs in up to 50% of preeclamptic patients, and its severity generally parallels that of the underlying preeclampsia.[21] A subset of patients with preeclampsia has microangiopathic hemolysis, elevated liver enzymes, and low platelets, widely known as the HELLP syndrome. This condition usually indicates severe preeclampsia and is associated with a higher risk of fetal and maternal complications, including maternal hepatic rupture. Repeated clinical and laboratory assessment of these patients is important because this syndrome can mimic other life-threatening complications of pregnancy, such as overt DIC, TTP, septicemia, and acute fatty liver of pregnancy.

Increased platelet destruction is the mechanism for the thrombocytopenia in preeclampsia. However, activation of the coagulation system is relatively modest, suggesting that thrombin generation may not be a major driver of the thrombocytopenia. Endothelial dysfunction (e.g., impaired nitric oxide synthesis) is a potential explanation for increased platelet turnover in preeclampsia.

Pharmacologic control of hypertension and rapid delivery are the treatments for preeclampsia and usually result in resolution of the thrombocytopenia within a few days. If delivery is not an option, treatment with bed rest and aggressive antihypertensive therapy has been reported to result in an improved platelet count. However, the clinical course is markedly variable, and some patients develop life-threatening organ failure. Plasmapheresis has been used in some patients, especially if there is evidence of thrombotic microangiopathy and organ dysfunction. Plasma exchange would seem appropriate for patients whose clinical picture has features that overlap with those of TTP.

Infection

Infection is a common cause of thrombocytopenia, occurring in approximately 50% to 75% of patients with bacteremia or fungemia and in almost all patients with septic shock or DIC. Even when caused by bacteremia, the thrombocytopenia generally is mild to moderate in severity and usually is not accompanied by significant coagulation abnormalities or bleeding. The likelihood of laboratory evidence for DIC increases as the platelet count falls below 50 × 109/L. The mechanisms for thrombocytopenia in septicemia in the absence of DIC are uncertain but could include chemokine-induced macrophage ingestion of platelets (hemophagocytosis[22]) and direct activation of platelets by endogenous mediators of inflammation (e.g., platelet-activating factor) or certain microbial products. In rare situations, platelet-reactive autoantibodies are implicated. Various explanations for thrombocytopenia in different types of infection are listed in Table 134-5.

Unexplained thrombocytopenia in a hospitalized patient warrants studies to exclude infection, such as blood cultures. Prompt recognition and treatment of the infection constitute the most important therapy because platelet count recovery tends to parallel the resolution of the infection. Prophylactic platelet transfusions are generally not required unless the platelet count falls below 10×10^9/L or comorbid clinical features increase the likelihood of serious bleeding (e.g., concomitant coagulopathy, an invasive procedure, uremic platelet dysfunction). The use of heparin for patients with septic shock and DIC is controversial. However, heparin may be of benefit in patients with clinical evidence of DIC and microvascular thrombosis (e.g., acral tissue ischemia or necrosis). The possibility of acquired protein C deficiency complicating acute DIC also should be considered in septic patients with purpura fulminans, such as that secondary to meningococcemia, in whom treatment with vitamin K, plasma, and possibly recombinant activated protein C could be beneficial.

Thrombocytopenia in patients infected with HIV poses a special diagnostic problem because there are many potential explanations for the thrombocytopenia (see Chapter 159). These include immune platelet destruction, impaired platelet production secondary to HIV infection of megakaryocytes, drug-induced myelosuppression (commonly implicated drugs include zidovudine, ganciclovir, and trimethoprim-sulfamethoxazole), HIV-associated thrombotic microangiopathy, hypersplenism, and BM infiltration by tumor or opportunistic infections. Platelet kinetic studies have shown a complex interaction of decreased platelet production, increased platelet destruction, and splenic platelet sequestration. Immune mechanisms for platelet destruction include antibodies that cross-react with GPIIb/IIIa complexes ("molecular mimicry") and immune complexes containing IgM antiidiotype antibodies (which could explain the paradox of high levels of platelet-associated IgG and IgM with low serum levels of platelet-reactive antibodies). Anti-HIV therapy (e.g., zidovudine, HAART) often raises the platelet count in patients with HIV-associated thrombocytopenia. Most patients with HIV-associated thrombocytopenia respond to conventional treatments for ITP, including corticosteroids; splenectomy; IVIG; and, particularly, anti-D.

Table 134-5 Mechanisms for Thrombocytopenia Complicating Infections

Mechanism for Thrombocytopenia	Selected Example(s)*
Increased Platelet Destruction	
DIC	Meningococcemia
Hemophagocytosis	Septicemia, EBV infection
Platelet-reactive autoantibodies (acute)	Varicella, subacute bacterial endocarditis (rare)
Platelet-reactive autoantibodies (chronic)	HIV infection
HUS	Verocytotoxin-producing *Escherichia coli, Shigella* spp., HIV infection
Antibodies against platelet-adsorbed microbial antigens	Malaria
Hypersplenism	
Acute	Disseminated *Mycobacterium avium* infection in HIV infection
Chronic	Viral chronic active hepatitis, malaria
Decreased Platelet Production	
Replacement of BM by granulomas	Ehrlichiosis, tuberculosis
Infection of megakaryocytes	HIV infection
Transient virus-induced aplasia	Parvovirus B19 infection (erythroblastopenia predominates)
Multiple Mechanisms	
Platelet destruction plus hypersplenism	Recurrent malaria
Increased platelet destruction, decreased platelet production, hypersplenism	Chronic HIV infection

*References can be found in Hoffman R, Benz EJ Jr, Shattil SJ, et al, eds: *Hematology: Basic Principles and Practice*, ed 3. New York, 2000, Churchill Livingstone.
BM, Bone marrow; *DIC*, disseminated intravascular coagulation; *EBV*, Epstein-Barr virus; *HUS*, hemolytic uremic syndrome.

Systemic Lupus Erythematosus

Immune-mediated thrombocytopenia, which occurs in as many as 25% of patients with SLE, is associated with a twofold increased risk of organ damage events. Many different types of platelet–IgG interactions are described (e.g., antiglycoprotein, antiglycolipid, β_2-glycoprotein I (β_2GPI)–containing immune complexes). In addition, antithrombopoietin, anti–c-Mpl (thrombopoietin receptor), and anti-CD40 ligand autoantibodies have been reported. Multiple causes for thrombocytopenia—increased platelet destruction, hypersplenism, and even impaired platelet production related to antibody-induced megakaryocytic hypoplasia—have been reported. The predominant explanation for thrombocytopenia in SLE remains unknown.

Several thrombocytopenic syndromes are seen in patients with SLE. For many patients, the thrombocytopenia is chronic, resembling ITP, and is the predominant clinical manifestation of the lupus. Often, these patients have a prolonged bleeding time despite mild thrombocytopenia. Some thrombocytopenic patients with SLE have antiphospholipid (aPL) antibodies and are at increased risk for thrombotic rather than bleeding complications (see Chapter 143). Acute, severe thrombocytopenia can be a prominent feature in patients with a severe multisystem exacerbation of lupus. Rarely, patients with SLE develop an illness that closely resembles TTP or HUS; these patients should be treated with plasma exchange. Thrombocytopenia as a feature of SLE-associated, viral-induced macrophage activation syndrome has been reported.

Treatment of the thrombocytopenia of SLE is similar to that of ITP (see Chapter 143). Corticosteroids constitute the first line of therapy, but many patients do not respond or require high doses. High-dose IVIG may be useful in patients who are bleeding to transiently increase the platelet count. Before resorting to splenectomy, one could try danazol (an attenuated androgen) in doses of 200 to 800 mg/day. Higher doses can cause hepatitis. Typically, several weeks are required before a benefit is seen. Splenectomy probably is as effective in achieving platelet count remission in SLE as in ITP. Patients with refractory thrombocytopenia sometimes benefit from more aggressive therapies, such as azathioprine, intermittent-pulse cyclophosphamide, plasmapheresis synchronized with pulse cyclophosphamide, cyclosporine, thrombopoietin mimetics, or rituximab.

Antiphospholipid Syndrome

Antiphospholipid syndrome (APS; see Chapter 143) is characterized by occurrence of one or more clinical events (e.g., venous, arterial or small vessel thrombosis, pregnancy loss, preterm delivery for patients with severe preeclampsia or placental insufficiency) associated with IgG, IgM, or IgA antibodies that recognize a complex of one or more protein cofactors (e.g., β_2GPI, annexin V, prothrombin, protein C, protein S) bound to negatively charged phospholipid.[23] Many patients (30%-50%) with this syndrome have thrombocytopenia, which is typically mild and intermittent; approximately 15% have autoimmune hemolysis. The APS should be considered in patients who develop idiopathic lower limb or abdominal vein (mesenteric, renal, adrenal) thrombosis, cerebral venous (dural sinus) thrombosis, cardiac valvulitis, nonatheromatous arterial thrombosis (especially thrombotic stroke in a patient younger than 50 years of age), dermal microvascular thrombosis (acrocyanosis, digital ulceration or gangrene, livedo reticularis), or acute multiorgan failure associated with DIC or widespread thrombosis of the microvasculature (catastrophic APS).

The mechanism of the prothrombotic tendency in patients with APS remains elusive, but interference with endothelial cell function, impaired fibrinolysis, antibody-mediated platelet activation, formation of endothelial microparticles, interference with thrombin and factor Xa degradation by antithrombin, disturbance in the protein C anticoagulant pathway or anticoagulant activity of β_2GPI all have been described. Disruption of the antithrombotic annexin V antithrombotic "shield" by aPL antibodies has been proposed to explain pregnancy losses through placental vascular thrombosis. Evidence indicates that thrombocytopenia in patients with APS is associated with platelet GP-reactive autoantibodies.

Antiphospholipid antibodies are detected by either of two methods: (1) solid-phase ELISA with purified phospholipids (usually cardiolipin) as target antigens or (2) a "functional" assay for so-called lupus anticoagulant (LA) activity, shown by demonstrating inhibition of certain phospholipid-dependent coagulation assays, such as the aPTT or the Russell viper venom time. Although aPL antibodies frequently are detected in patients with SLE, they also can be found in patients with other autoimmune disorders, malignancy, or infections or as a complication of certain drugs (e.g., procainamide). Often no associated condition is identified ("primary" APS). aPL antibodies of low titer are sometimes found in normal persons, particularly elderly individuals, or during normal pregnancy. Autoantibody "cluster" studies show that anticardiolipin, LA, and anti–double-stranded DNA antibodies occur together more often than with other SLE-associated autoantibodies (e.g., anti-Sm, anti-Ro, anti-RNP).

There are intriguing parallels between the APS and HIT: in both disorders, the antibodies are directed at a protein target (β_2GPI and PF4, respectively) bound to a negatively charged species (anionic phospholipid and heparin, respectively). For both, high-titer IgG antibodies that result in a positive "functional" test result (LA activity and HIT-IgG–induced platelet activation, respectively) are most likely to be associated with clinical disease. Both disorders are characterized by the paradox of thrombocytopenia associated with increased risk for venous and arterial thrombosis.

To help physicians diagnose the APS, clinical and laboratory criteria have been developed. The laboratory criteria include the presence of anticardiolipin, anti-β_2GPI, or LA antibodies (moderate- to high-titer IgG or IgM) on two or more occasions at least 12 weeks apart. The major clinical criteria are thrombosis and complications of pregnancy. Thrombosis can involve large arteries or veins or small vessels within any organ. The complications of pregnancy include one or more unexplained deaths of normal fetus(es) after week 10 of gestation or premature births (before 34 weeks) or more than three spontaneous abortions before week 10 of gestation. Some experts advocate for thrombocytopenia to be included within the criteria for APS.[24]

Specific treatment for the thrombocytopenia is not usually required. For many patients, long-term anticoagulant or antiplatelet therapy, or both, are needed to prevent recurrent thrombosis. For patients with recurring pregnancy losses and aPL antibodies, randomized trials have documented the benefit of low-dose aspirin combined with either low-dose UFH or low-molecular-weight heparin (LMWH).

Malignancy

Thrombocytopenia complicating malignant disorders most frequently results from antineoplastic treatment or BM replacement by tumor. However, certain thrombocytopenic syndromes have been associated with malignancy, including autoimmune thrombocytopenia, DIC, and thrombotic microangiopathy.

Immune thrombocytopenia attributable to platelet GP-reactive autoantibodies can complicate neoplastic lymphoproliferative diseases such as Hodgkin disease, non-Hodgkin lymphoma, chronic lymphocytic leukemia, and multiple myeloma. Sometimes the thrombocytopenia responds to treatment of the neoplasm, although in some patients (particularly those with Hodgkin disease), the thrombocytopenia is indistinguishable from ITP and is not related to the activity of the lymphoma.

Disseminated intravascular coagulation occurs in certain malignancies, particularly adenocarcinomas of the pancreas, stomach, lung, colon, breast, and prostate. Some patients present with venous or, less commonly, arterial thrombosis as the first clinical manifestation of their malignancy. In these patients, the presence of thrombocytopenia is an important clue that should prompt investigations for DIC, such as measurement of fibrinogen or D-dimer levels. In the author's experience, the platelet count typically rises to normal or even elevated levels with heparin therapy because heparin ameliorates the DIC process; however, recurrent thrombocytopenia and thrombosis can occur within hours of discontinuing the heparin therapy. Cancer patients with DIC and venous thrombosis also are at increased risk for warfarin-associated venous limb gangrene. The role of various tumor-associated procoagulant substances—such as "cancer procoagulant" (a 68-kd cysteine proteinase that activates factor X independently of tissue factor/factor VIIa) and cancer-associated tissue factor (which is expressed on tumor cells, as well as circulating microparticles[25])—suggest pathophysiologic parallels with microthrombosis in HIT because both cancer-associated DIC and acute HIT are risk factors for phlegmasia cerulean dolens and venous limb gangrene during anticoagulation with warfarin. Thus cancer patients with DIC should receive heparin (especially LMWH) rather than warfarin anticoagulation (see box on Diagnostic Considerations in the Patient With Limb Ischemia and Thrombocytopenia in Chapter 135). DIC with hemorrhagic manifestations is characteristically seen in some patients with prostate cancer and in many patients with acute promyelocytic leukemia. It is crucial to recognize promyelocytic leukemia because treatment with all-*trans*-retinoic acid produces differentiation of the malignant cells, thereby rapidly reducing the life-threatening bleeding risks attributable to hyperfibrinolysis.

A destructive thrombocytopenic disorder that resembles HUS or TTP has been described in patients with advanced cancer. In some patients, mitomycin, gemcitabine, or other drugs may have contributed to the microangiopathy. DIC usually is not present. Some patients respond transiently to plasmapheresis, but for many, response to any therapy is poor.

Macrophage Activation (Hemophagocytic) Syndrome

The macrophage activation (or hemophagocytic) syndrome comprises a heterogeneous group of disorders characterized by variable cytopenias and morphologic evidence of macrophage phagocytosis of RBCs, granulocytes, and platelets; hyperferritinemia, hypercytokinemia, and sepsis-like features are characteristic, with potential for evolution to fatal multiple organ failure.[26] Some adult patients have an aggressive disease characterized by high fever, weight loss, prominent hepatosplenomegaly, severe pancytopenia, elevated liver enzymes, and often a terminal infection. Both T- and B-cell lymphomas can explain such a dramatic syndrome. However, similar patients with fulminant illness have been described after otherwise unremarkable bacterial or viral infections (particularly those caused by Epstein-Barr virus). In children, the high mortality rate associated with hemophagocytic lymphohistiocytosis warrants aggressive treatment, including antineoplastic chemotherapy and BM transplantation. Nonneoplastic but nonetheless severe hemophagocytosis can be seen in patients with certain infections (e.g., babesiosis, ehrlichiosis, HIV infection), as well as in patients with rheumatologic disorders (SLE, Still disease, ankylosing spondylitis). Laboratory indicators of macrophage activation syndrome include markedly elevated ferritin,[27] high levels of soluble CD163 and CD25, and morphologic evidence of hemophagocytosis. Treatment should be directed at the underlying illness. Early administration of corticosteroids and high-dose γ-globulin (IVIG) appears to benefit some patients with nonneoplastic macrophage activation syndrome.

Solid Organ and Bone Marrow Transplantation

Thrombocytopenia commonly occurs during episodes of solid organ allograft rejection. It is possible that platelet activation and deposition in the transplanted organ vasculature contribute to the rejection process. Antirejection therapies can also cause thrombocytopenia through increased platelet destruction (antilymphocyte globulin) or BM suppression (azathioprine). Posttransplantation HUS develops in approximately 5% of renal transplant recipients and in even fewer recipients of liver or heart transplants. Although cyclosporine sometimes is implicated in HUS, it usually can be safely resumed after recovery.

Early, severe thrombocytopenia caused by BM-ablative therapy invariably accompanies BM transplantation (BMT). Platelet count recovery to greater than 50×10^9/L is more rapid (16 vs. 35 days) in patients receiving autologous mobilized peripheral blood progenitor cells than in those undergoing autologous BMT. Severe persistent thrombocytopenia despite recovery of RBCs and WBCs is relatively common after BMT or peripheral blood transplantation; autoimmune thrombocytopenia has been implicated in some patients. Late-onset thrombocytopenia after BMT that responds to corticosteroids, IVIG, and splenectomy also has been attributed to autoimmune thrombocytopenia. Rarely, transplantation-associated alloimmune thrombocytopenia can be caused by donor–recipient incompatibility involving platelet-specific alloantigens such as Pl^{A1} (HPA-1a) or Br^{a} (HPA-5b).

A syndrome of thrombocytopenia, RBC fragmentation, and renal impairment can occur in as many as 10% of patients undergoing BMT, usually beginning 3 to 12 months after transplantation (BMT-associated thrombotic microangiopathy). The pathogenesis remains obscure; reduced ADAMTS13 levels have not been implicated. The hematologic abnormalities can be mild and remit spontaneously, although patients often have residual azotemia and hypertension. More severely affected patients usually do not benefit from plasmapheresis. The syndrome has a poor overall prognosis, and many patients die irrespective of any intervention.

Cardiopulmonary Bypass Surgery

Excess bleeding is a common problem in patients who undergo heart surgery using cardiopulmonary bypass. Many of these patients receive blood transfusions, and approximately 5% require reoperation for postoperative bleeding.

Thrombocytopenia and transient platelet dysfunction (see Chapter 161) are observed in virtually every patient. Typically, the platelet count falls by 35% to 65%, primarily as a result of hemodilution but also because of bleeding and losses within the extracorporeal perfusion device. Because patients invariably receive heparin during cardiac surgery and have often received heparin in the remote or recent past, immune HIT is frequently considered in the differential diagnosis of early-onset and persisting postcardiac surgery thrombocytopenia; however, HIT is an unlikely explanation for thrombocytopenia even when anti-PF4/heparin antibodies are positive.[28]

The bleeding time rises markedly during heart surgery (to greater than 30 minutes) but usually improves to less than 15 minutes shortly after surgery and to normal several hours later. By contrast, the thrombocytopenia persists for 3 to 4 days followed by recovery of the platelet count to values exceeding the preoperative baseline.

The pathogenesis and clinical significance of the hemostatic defect in these patients remain uncertain, but the explanation probably is multifactorial. Studies have described transient, *intrinsic* defects in platelet function. These defects include decreased in vitro platelet aggregation, decreased platelet surface membrane proteins, selective depletion of platelet α-granules, and evidence of in vivo platelet activation and platelet vesiculation. The platelet dysfunction in heart surgery also is attributable to an *extrinsic* platelet defect resulting from thrombin inhibition by the high doses of heparin. Furthermore, an important role for hyperfibrinolysis in the pathogenesis of bleeding is shown by elevated D-dimer levels in bleeding patients, as well as the efficacy of antifibrinolytic agents in the prevention and treatment of heart surgery–associated bleeding. Other factors in some patients include residual heparin effect after bypass (including heparin rebound) and preoperative use of aspirin. Treatment of platelet dysfunction after cardiopulmonary bypass is discussed in Chapter 161.

THROMBOCYTOPENIA ASSOCIATED WITH CARDIOVASCULAR DISEASE

Congenital Cyanotic Heart Disease

Thrombocytopenia caused by a decrease in platelet life span occurs in some patients with severe cyanotic congenital heart disease and is approximately related to the severity of the polycythemia. Bleeding occurs in a few patients and can be related to platelet function defects, coagulopathy, or hyperfibrinolysis. Reducing the hematocrit by phlebotomy sometimes helps to correct the hemostatic defects.

Valvular Heart Disease

Increased platelet turnover is common in valvular heart disease, and some patients have mild thrombocytopenia. The pathogenesis of the platelet consumption is not well understood, but the defect could be related to increased platelet–vWF interactions at high shear. Indeed, high-molecular-weight multimers of vWF are reduced in some of these patients, which could explain why bleeding from gastrointestinal angiodysplasia in patients with aortic stenosis (Heyde syndrome) typically resolves after aortic valve replacement.[29] Thrombocytopenia secondary to consumptive coagulopathy can be seen in intracardiac thrombosis associated with valvular heart disease.

Pulmonary Vascular Disorders

Disorders characterized by pulmonary hypertension can be accompanied by thrombocytopenia, the pathogenesis of which is poorly defined. Thrombocytopenia can occur in association with pulmonary embolism,[30] possibly as a result of DIC. When evaluating such patients, the clinician should inquire about current or recent heparin exposure because HIT and pulmonary embolism are strongly associated.

HEMODILUTION AND PLATELET CONSUMPTION AFTER SURGERY

Platelet count declines of 30% to 70% occur universally after major surgery and reflect the combined effects of hemodilution and increased platelet consumption. Such hemodilution-associated thrombocytopenia is especially prominent after cardiac surgery and is proportional to the amount of fluids (crystalloid, colloid, blood products) administered. The platelet count fall is abrupt and is evident a few hours after surgery. Dilutional coagulopathy also occurs, which is responsible for the minor to moderate increases in coagulation test results that occur transiently after surgery.

Perioperative hemodilution is also usually accompanied by increased platelet consumption related to the effects of surgery. This helps to explain why the postsurgery platelet count usually continues to decline over the next 1 to 3 days, with the postoperative nadir (lowest platelet count value) usually occurring at a median of postoperative day 2, with a range between postoperative days 1 to 4 (Fig. 134-9).[2] Subsequently, there is a rise in the platelet count that peaks at approximately day 14 at levels often two to three times the patient's preoperative baseline before it returns to baseline over the next 2 weeks (≈day 28). As described earlier in this chapter (see Fig. 134-1), these platelet count changes reflect thrombopoietin physiology.

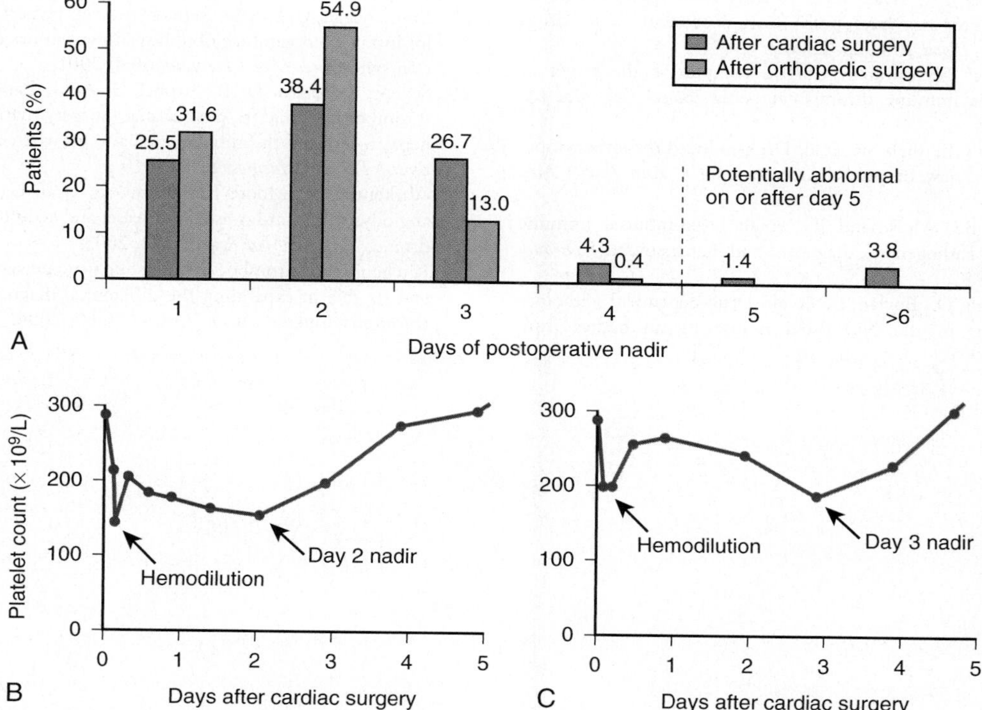

Figure 134-9 EARLY POSTOPERATIVE PLATELET COUNT DECLINES. **A,** Distribution of early postoperative count nadirs. For both orthopedic and cardiac surgery patients, day 2 represents the most common day for the postoperative platelet count nadir to occur (data exclude day 0); beyond postoperative day 4, it is likely that a superimposed thrombocytopenic disorder is occurring. **B** and **C,** Representative post–cardiac surgery platelet count declines. Both patients illustrate early hemodilution effects (day 0) and subsequent additional early platelet count declines with nadirs of day 2 **(B)** and day 3 **(C)**. Neither patient received platelet transfusions. *(From Greinacher A, Warkentin TE: Acquired non-immune thrombocytopenia. In: Marder VJ, Aird WC, Bennett JS, et al, editors:* Hemostasis and thrombosis: Basic principles and clinical practice, *ed 6. Philadelphia, 2013, Lippincott Williams & Wilkins [in press].)*

REFERENCES

1. Arnold DM, Warkentin TE: Thrombocytopenia and thrombocytosis. In Wilson WC, Grande CM, Hoyt DB, editors: *Trauma: Critical care (vol. 2)*, New York, 2007, Informa Healthcare USA, pp 983.
2. Greinacher A, Warkentin TE: Acquired non-immune thrombocytopenia. In Marder VJ, Aird WC, Bennett JS, et al, editors: *Hemostasis and thrombosis: Basic principles and clinical practice*, ed 6. Philadelphia, 2013, Lippincott Williams & Wilkins (in press).
3. Saltzman DJ, Chang JC, Jimenez JC, et al: Postoperative thrombotic thrombocytopenic purpura after open heart operations. *Ann Thorac Surg* 89:119, 2010.
4. Centers for Disease Control and Prevention (CDC): Updated recommendation from the advisory committee on immunization practices (ACIP for revaccination of persons at prolonged increased risk for meningococcal disease. *MMWR Morb Mortal Wkly Rep* 58:1042, 2009.
5. Centers for Disease Control and Prevention (CDC): Advisory Committee on Immunization Practices: Updated recommendations for prevention of invasive pneumococcal disease among adults using the 23-valent pneumococcal polysaccharide vaccine. (PPSV23). *MMWR Morb Mortal Wkly Rep* 59:1102, 2010.
6. Aster RH, Bougie DW: Drug-induced immune thrombocytopenia. *N Engl J Med* 357:580, 2007.
7. Warkentin TE: Drug-induced immune-mediated thrombocytopenia—from purpura to thrombosis. *N Engl J Med* 356:891, 2007.
8. Reese JA, Li X, Hauben M, et al: Identifying drugs that cause immune thrombocytopenia: An analysis using 3 distinct methods. *Blood* 116:2127, 2010.
9. Warkentin TE, Anderson JAM: DITP causation: 3 methods better than 1? *Blood* 116:2002, 2010.
10. Von Drygalski A, Curtis BR, Bougie DW, et al: Vancomycin induced immune thrombocytopenia. *N Engl J Med* 356:904, 2007.
11. Bougie DW, Wilker PR, Aster RH: Patients with quinine-induced immune thrombocytopenia have both "drug-dependent" and "drug-specific" antibodies. *Blood* 108:922, 2006.
12. Liu X, Sahud MA: Glycoprotein IIb/IIIa complex is the target in mirtazapine-induced immune thrombocytopenia. *Blood Cell Mol Dis* 30:241, 2003.
13. George JN, Raskob GE, Shah SR, et al: Drug-induced thrombocytopenia: A systematic review of published case reports. *Ann Intern Med* 129:886, 1998.
14. Aster RH, Curtis BR, McFarland JG, et al: Drug-induced immune thrombocytopenia: Pathogenesis, diagnosis, and management. *J Thromb Haemost* 7:911, 2009.
15. Bougie DW, Nayak D, Boylan B, et al: Drug-dependent clearance of human platelets in the NOD/scid mouse by antibodies from patients with drug-induced immune thrombocytopenia. *Blood* 116:3033, 2010.
16. Mantadakis E, Farmaki E, Buchanan GR: Thrombocytopenic purpura after measles-mumps-rubella vaccination: A systematic review of the literature and guidance for management. *J Pediatr* 156:623, 2010.
17. Warkentin TE, Kelton JG: Temporal aspects of heparin-induced thrombocytopenia. *N Engl J Med* 344:1286, 2001.
18. Aster RH, Curtis BR, Bougie DW, et al: Thrombocytopenia associated with the use of GPIIb/IIIa inhibitors: Position paper of the ISTH working group on thrombocytopenia and GPIIb/IIIa inhibitors. *J Thromb Haemost* 4:678, 2006.
19. Gao C, Boylan B, Bougie D, et al: Eptifibatide-induced thrombocytopenia and thrombosis in humans require FcγRIIa and the integrin β3 cytoplasmic domain. *J Clin Invest* 119:504, 2009.
20. Nasreddine W, Beydoun A: Valproate-induced thrombocytopenia: A prospective monotherapy study. *Epilepsia* 49:438, 2008.
21. McCrae KR: Thrombocytopenia in pregnancy. *Hematology Am Soc Hematol Educ Program* 2010:397, 2010.
22. François B, Trimoreau F, Vignon P, et al: Thrombocytopenia in the sepsis syndrome: Role of hemophagocytosis and macrophage colony-stimulating factor. *Am J Med* 103:114, 1997.
23. Ruiz-Irastorza G, Crowther M, Branch W, et al: Antiphospholipid syndrome. *Lancet* 376:1498, 2010.
24. Cervera R, Tektonidou MG, Espinosa G, et al: Task force on catastrophic antiphospholipid syndrome (APS) and non-criteria APS manifestations (II): Thrombocytopenia and skin manifestations. *Lupus* 20:174, 2011.
25. Manly DA, Wang J, Glover SL, et al: Increased microparticle tissue factor activity in cancer patients with venous thromboembolism. *Thromb Res* 125:511, 2010.
26. Emmenegger U, Reimers A, Frey U, et al: Reactive macrophage activation syndrome: A simple screening strategy and its potential in early treatment initiation. *Swiss Med Wkly* 132:230, 2002.
27. Emmenegger U, Frey U, Reimers A, et al: Hyperferritinemia as indicator for intravenous gammaglobulin treatment in reactive macrophage activation syndromes. *Am J Hematol* 68:4, 2001.
28. Selleng S, Malowsky B, Strobel U, et al: Early-onset and persisting thrombocytopenia in post-cardiac surgery patients is rarely due to heparin-induced thrombocytopenia, even when antibody tests are positive. *J Thromb Haemost* 8:30, 2010.
29. Warkentin TE, Moore JC, Anand SS, et al: Gastrointestinal bleeding, angiodysplasia, cardiovascular disease, and acquired von Willebrand syndrome. *Transfus Med Rev* 17:272, 2003.
30. Kitchens CS: Thrombocytopenia due to acute venous thromboembolism and its role in expanding the differential diagnosis of heparin-induced thrombocytopenia. *Am J Hematol* 76:69, 2004.

CHAPTER 135

HEPARIN-INDUCED THROMBOCYTOPENIA

Theodore E. Warkentin

Heparin-induced thrombocytopenia (HIT) is the most important drug-induced immune-mediated cytopenia for several reasons. First, heparin is a widely used anticoagulant (see Chapter 151). Second, HIT is relatively common, occurring in approximately 1% to 3% of postoperative patients and 0.2% to 0.5% of medical patients who receive unfractionated heparin (UFH) derived from porcine intestine for 7 to 14 days.[1] Third, HIT frequently causes life- and limb-threatening venous or arterial thrombosis. Finally, there are several pitfalls of HIT management, including the potential for thrombocytopenia and/or thrombosis to worsen despite stopping heparin, the high risk for warfarin-associated microthrombosis (most often manifesting as venous limb gangrene), and the potential for failure of approved direct thrombin inhibitor (DTI) therapy because of the confounding of activated partial thromboplastin time (aPTT)-monitored dosing that results from HIT-associated coagulopathies.

HIT is caused by platelet-activating immunoglobulin G (IgG) antibodies that bind to multimolecular complexes of platelet factor 4 (PF4) bound to heparin.[2,3] Although anti-PF4/heparin antibodies are frequently triggered by heparin therapy, relatively few patients develop clinically evident HIT. Indeed, a major current problem with HIT is its "overdiagnosis"[4]: only 5% to 10% of patients who are referred for antibody testing have a serologic profile that supports a diagnosis of HIT.[5] The challenge for the clinician is to discern which of the (many) patients who develop thrombocytopenia in association with heparin therapy really have HIT, a conundrum magnified by the observation that at most 50% of anti-PF4/heparin antibody–positive patients have "true" HIT, as indicated by the presence of platelet-activating IgG antibodies.[1,5]

EPIDEMIOLOGY

Table 135-1 lists risk factors for HIT. The highest risk for HIT is seen in patients with multiple interacting risk factors (e.g., females given postoperative thromboprophylaxis with UFH for 2 weeks [frequency approximately 5%]).[6] Even higher frequencies (approximately 10%) are reported in patients with ventricular assist devices who are receiving therapeutic doses of UFH. Ironically, even though the risk for HIT appears to be somewhat higher in women (odds ratio, 1.5 to 2.0),[6] HIT is rare in pregnancy, particularly with the use of low-molecular-weight heparin (LMWH). The synthetic antithrombin-binding sulfated pentasaccharide, fondaparinux, although similarly immunizing as LMWH, is much less likely than LMWH to cause HIT, likely because fondaparinux does not usually increase the platelet-activating potential of HIT antibodies.[7] Indeed, fondaparinux appears to be an effective treatment for HIT (discussed later).

Only a minority of patients who form anti-PF4/heparin antibodies following heparin treatment develop clinically evident HIT.[2,3] The proportion of antibody-positive patients who develop HIT ranges from as high as one-third (e.g., post–orthopedic surgery thromboprophylaxis with UFH) to as few as 1 in 50 (post–cardiac surgery patients).[1,2] Notably, the risk for HIT in post–cardiac surgery patients who receive UFH thromboprophylaxis is only approximately 1% even though as many as 50% to 80% of patients develop detectable anti-PF4/heparin antibodies within 2 weeks of surgery.[1] In general, those at highest risk for HIT are the subgroup of patients whose anti-PF4/heparin antibodies evince strong platelet-activating properties in vitro.[2,3] However, patient-dependent susceptibility factors are also important, because at most only half of all patients who form platelet-activating antibodies develop HIT.

PATHOBIOLOGY

Fig. 135-1 illustrates several features of HIT pathogenesis. Heparin binds reversibly and saturably to platelets and can weakly activate platelets in vitro through potentiation of $\alpha_{IIb}\beta_3$-mediated outside-in signaling.[8] In general, the direct platelet-activating effects of heparin, as well as its immunogenicity, are proportional to its molecular mass and degree of sulfation; consequently, LMWH is less likely to cause HIT than UFH.[1,2,6]

Platelet activation by HIT antibodies occurs because platelet-activating HIT-IgG cross-link platelet FcγIIa receptors.[1-3] The HIT antigens reside on large multimolecular complexes formed between cationic PF4—a member of the CXC subfamily of chemokines—and anionic heparin. A unique laboratory characteristic of HIT is that high heparin concentrations (10 to 100 units/mL) inhibit platelet activation by the pathogenic IgG[9]; this laboratory feature is exploited in diagnostic testing for HIT (see Diagnosis).

There is a characteristic timeline that underlies the HIT immune response (Fig. 135-2).[3] Formation of pathogenic IgG antibodies is surprisingly fast, even in patients who have never previously been exposed to heparin. Bacterial cell walls—which are negatively charged—bind PF4, and there is evidence that bacterial infection could be responsible for preimmunization against PF4-dependent antigens.[10] This could explain both the high frequency of anti-PF4/heparin immunization and of clinical HIT (i.e., HIT could represent a misdirected antibacterial immune response).[10] Although heparin-treated patients can form heparin-dependent antibodies of the IgM or IgA subclass, these are unlikely to cause HIT.[1-3]

Excess thrombin generation contributes to the pathogenesis of some of the unusual sequelae of HIT, which can include venous thromboembolism,[11] warfarin-associated venous limb gangrene,[12] and overt (decompensated) disseminated intravascular coagulation (DIC). Increased thrombin generation in HIT is triggered by the shedding of procoagulant microparticles from platelets activated by HIT antibodies, as well as by the expression of tissue factor by endothelial cells or monocytes activated by HIT antibodies (see Fig. 135-1).[13]

As noted, thrombocytopenia develops in only a minority of patients who form HIT antibodies.[1] The variable risk for HIT in different patient populations may reflect variations in the susceptibility of platelets to activation by HIT-IgG and/or differences in the levels and immunoglobulin class composition of HIT antibodies.[2,3] Poorly defined clinical factors also influence the risk for HIT, which occurs more often in surgical patients than in medical or obstetric patients.[6] Major trauma was more likely than minor trauma to be associated with HIT antibody formation and clinical HIT in one study.[14] There is indirect evidence that formation of stoichiometrically optimal complexes of PF4/heparin influences the risk for

Table 135-1 Risk Factors for Heparin-Induced Thrombocytopenia

Heparin type:	Unfractionated > low-molecular-weight heparin > fondaparinux
Patient type:	Postoperative (major > minor surgery) > medical > obstetric/pediatric
Dose*:	Prophylactic dose > therapeutic dose > flushes
Duration:	11-14 days† > 5-10 days > 4 days or fewer
Sex:	Female > male

*Importance of heparin dose is uncertain because of confounding effect of patient type (e.g., postoperative patients tend to receive prophylactic-dose heparin whereas medical patients [e.g., with venous thromboembolism] are more likely to receive therapeutic-dose heparin); nevertheless, reported frequencies of heparin-induced thrombocytopenia (HIT) are relatively high in patients given postoperative prophylactic-dose heparin.
†Heparin exposure beyond 14 days does not usually increase the risk of HIT beyond that of an 11- to 14-day exposure.

immunization.[15] The clinical situation influences the type of HIT-associated thrombosis: venous thromboembolism typically develops in orthopedic patients with HIT, whereas thrombosis develops equally often in arteries and in veins in cardiovascular patients with HIT.[1]

CLINICAL AND LABORATORY MANIFESTATIONS

Most patients with HIT have moderate thrombocytopenia; The median platelet count nadir is approximately 60 × 10^9/L; for 90% of patients, the platelet count nadir is greater than 20 × 10^9/L (Fig. 135-3).[16] In the rare patient whose platelet count falls to less than 10 × 10^9/L, there is often evidence of DIC, and red cell fragments and circulating normoblasts may be evident on examination of the blood smear. Thrombosis can occur in HIT patients when there is a 30% or greater decrease in the platelet count, even if the platelet count nadir never falls below 150 × 10^9/L.[1]

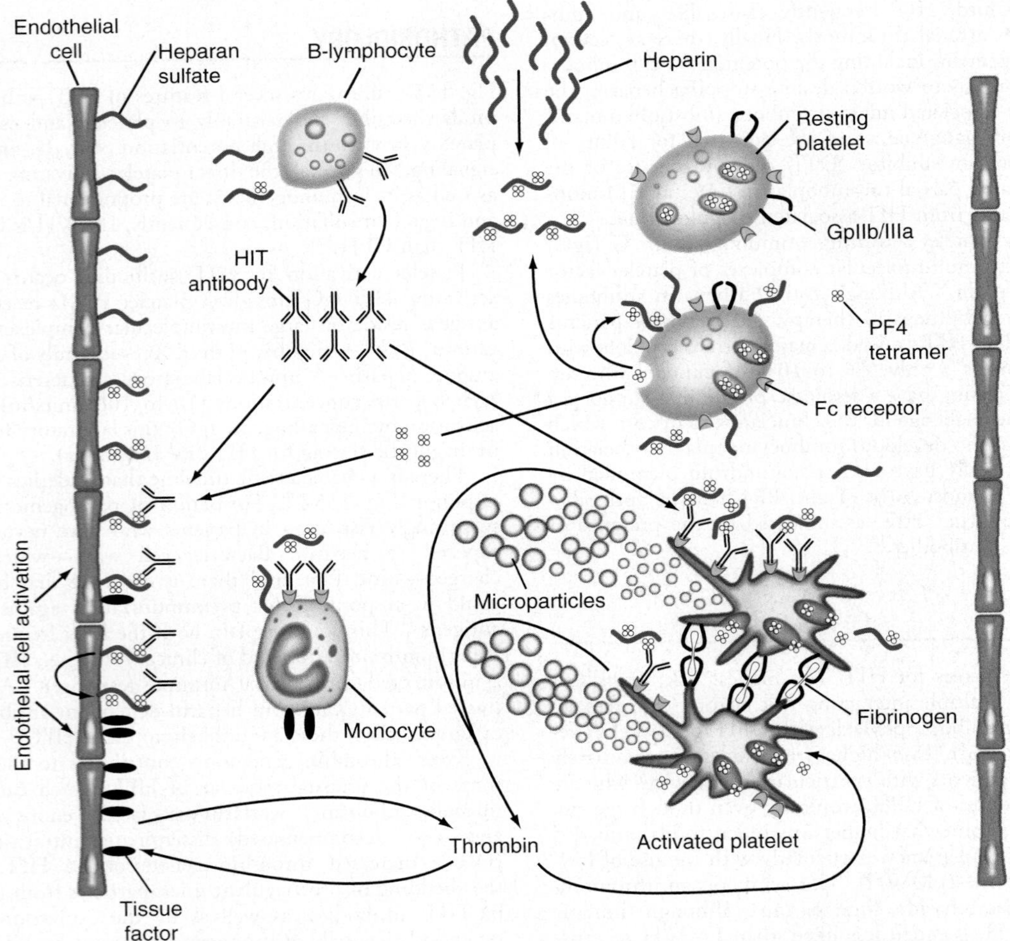

Figure 135-1 PATHOGENESIS OF HEPARIN-INDUCED THROMBOCYTOPENIA (HIT). Heparin produces mild platelet activation, resulting in release of platelet factor 4 (PF4) from platelet α-granules and the formation of immunogenic PF4/heparin complexes. B lymphocytes generate IgG immunoglobulins that recognize the PF4/heparin complexes; the Fc "tails" of the IgG bind to platelet FcγIIa receptors, resulting in Fc receptor clustering and consequent "strong" platelet activation. Platelet-derived microparticles are generated that accelerate thrombin generation. The HIT antibodies also recognize PF4 bound to endothelial heparan sulfate, leading to immunoinjury that causes endothelial activation. Recent evidence suggests that HIT antibodies also activate monocytes. The greatly increased thrombin generation observed in HIT helps to explain its association with venous and arterial thrombosis, as well as some of its unusual clinical features (e.g., warfarin-induced venous limb gangrene, decompensated disseminated intravascular coagulation), and also provides a rationale for treatments that control thrombin generation (e.g., with indirect [antithrombin-dependent] or with direct thrombin inhibitors). *(Reprinted with permission from Greinacher A, Warkentin TE: Treatment of heparin-induced thrombocytopenia: An overview. In Warkentin TE, Greinacher A, editors:* Heparin-induced thrombocytopenia, *ed 4, New York, 2007, Informa Healthcare USA, p 287.)*

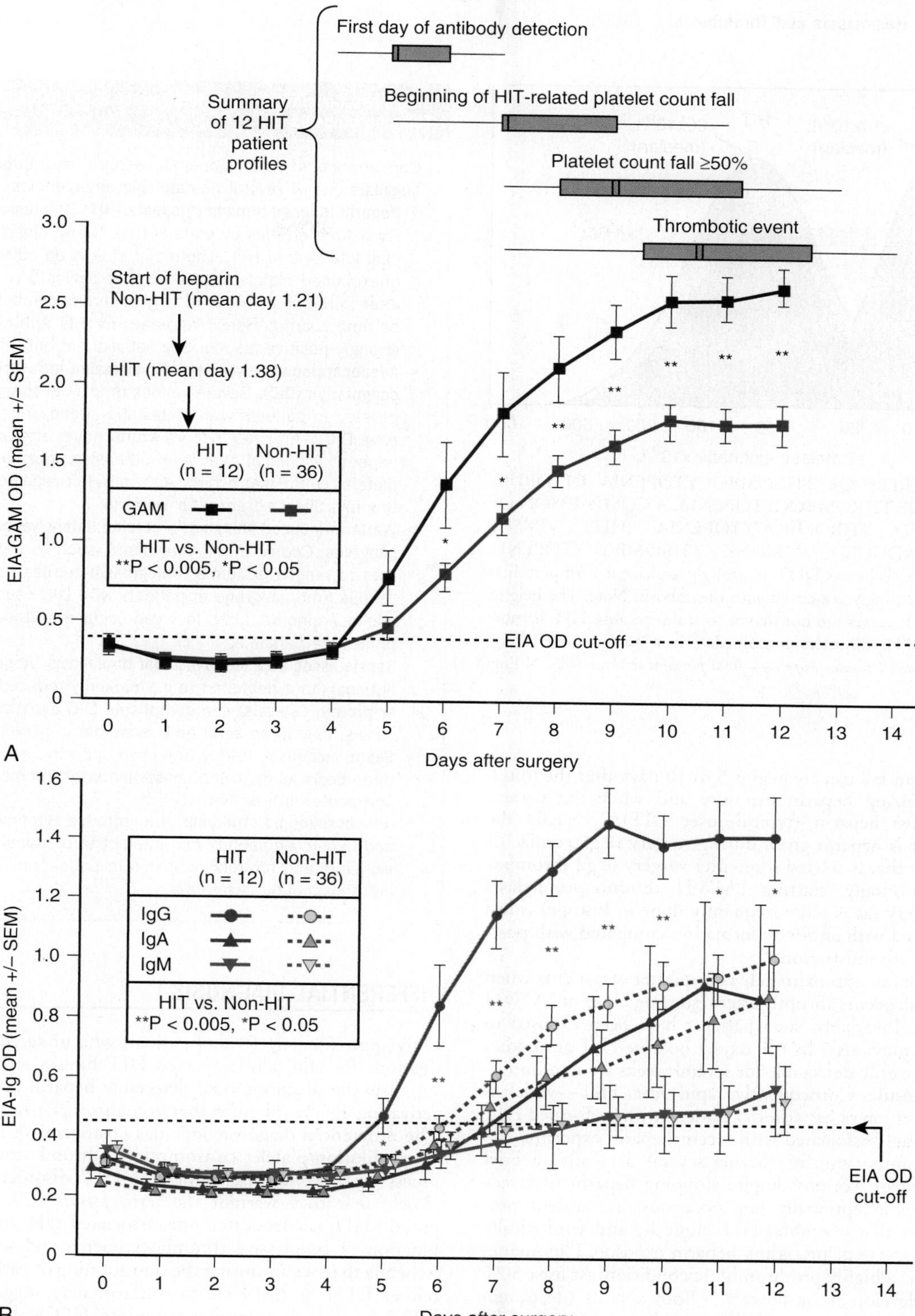

Figure 135-2 CHARACTERISTIC TIMELINE OF HEPARIN-INDUCED THROMBOCYTOPENIA (HIT). Anti-PF4/heparin antibodies (by enzyme immunoassay [EIA]) per postoperative day in 12 patients with HIT and 36 seropositive non-HIT control patients. **A,** Mean (±standard error of the mean [SEM]) optical density (OD) of anti-PF4/heparin antibodies detected using commercial immunoassay (EIA-GAM) that detects antibodies of all three immunoglobulin classes (IgG, IgA, IgM). HIT patients are indicated by ‑■‑, and seropositive non-HIT controls by ‑■‑. On each day beginning on postoperative day 6, there is a significant difference in the mean of the OD levels between the patients with HIT and the seropositive non-HIT controls ($P < .05$ by nonpaired t test). At the top of the figure, summary data for 12 HIT patient profiles are shown for four key events (first day of antibody detection, beginning of HIT-related platelet count fall, platelet count fall ≥50%, and thrombotic event), summarized as median *(small purple squares within rectangles)*, interquartile range *(rectangles)*, and range *(ends of thin black lines)*. **B,** Mean (±SEM) OD values of anti-PF4/heparin antibodies detected using an in-house immunoassay (EIA-Ig) that detects antibodies of the individual immunoglobulin classes, IgG *(red circles)*, IgA *(green triangles)*, and IgM *(blue inverted triangles)* for HIT *(solid symbols)* and non-HIT *(open symbols)*. On each postoperative day beginning on day 5, there is a significant difference in the mean of the OD units for the IgG immunoassay between the patients with HIT and the seropositive non-HIT controls (**$P < .005$ for days 6 to 10; *$P < .05$ for days 5, 11, and 12). *(From Warkentin TE, Sheppard JI, Moore JC, et al: Studies of the immune response in heparin-induced thrombocytopenia.* Blood *113:4693, 2009.)*

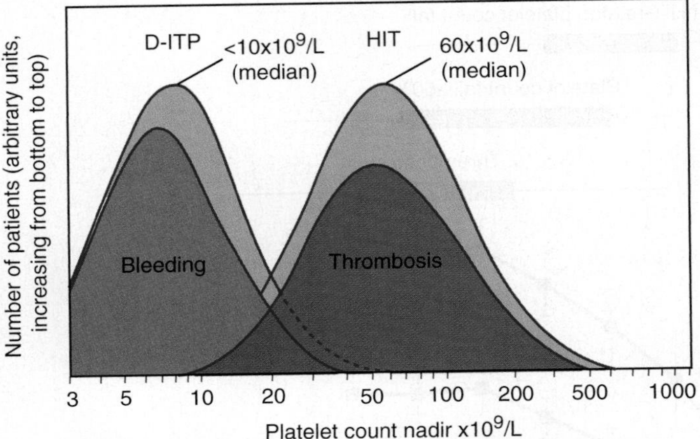

Figure 135-3 SEVERITY OF THROMBOCYTOPENIA IN DRUG-INDUCED IMMUNE THROMBOCYTOPENIA: A COMPARISON OF HEPARIN-INDUCED THROMBOCYTOPENIA (HIT) VERSUS OTHER DRUG-INDUCED IMMUNE THROMBOCYTOPENIA (DITP) DISORDERS. Whereas DITP is strongly associated with petechiae and purpura, HIT is strongly associated with thrombosis. Note: The heights of the DITP and HIT curves are not drawn to scale, because HIT is more common than all DITP disorders combined. *(From Warkentin TE: Drug-induced immune-mediated thrombocytopenia—from purpura to thrombosis.* N Engl J Med *356:891, 2007.)*

The platelet count fall usually begins 5 to 10 days after the initiation of an immunizing heparin exposure and while the patient continues to receive heparin (typical-onset HIT).[17] Usually the immunizing trigger is heparin given during surgery (e.g., cardiac or vascular surgery) or that is started soon after surgery (e.g., thromboprophylaxis). Interestingly, starting LMWH thromboprophylaxis before elective surgery (as is more frequently done in Europe) is less likely to be associated with antibody formation compared with postoperative first-dose administration.[15]

HIT is recognized in approximately one-quarter of patients when the platelet count fall occurs abruptly after restarting UFH or LMWH (rapid-onset HIT). Invariably, such patients have been exposed to heparin within the previous 5 to 100 days,[17] because HIT antibodies are transient and are only detectable for several weeks after an immunizing heparin exposure. Consequently, rapid-onset HIT—which is caused by administration of heparin to a patient with preformed HIT antibodies—is strongly associated with recent heparin exposure.

Sometimes, thrombocytopenia occurs several days after a brief exposure to heparin or worsens despite stopping heparin (delayed-onset HIT).[18,19] On exceptionally rare occasions, a transient prothrombotic disorder that resembles HIT clinically and serologically occurs without an apparent preceding heparin exposure ("spontaneous" HIT).[20] HIT is a highly prothrombotic condition: At least 50% of HIT patients develop thrombosis.[1,11,16] Both venous (deep vein thrombosis and/or pulmonary embolism) and arterial (especially aortic and iliofemoral arterial thrombosis, stroke, or myocardial infarction) thrombosis can occur.[11] Other complications include necrotizing skin lesions at the sites of subcutaneous heparin injection and acute inflammatory/cardiorespiratory (anaphylactoid) or transient memory disturbances after intravenous heparin bolus administration to sensitized persons. Unexplained hypotension or abdominal pain in a patient with HIT suggests bilateral adrenal hemorrhagic infarction, which can lead to acute adrenal failure; the hemorrhagic adrenal necrosis is the result of adrenal vein thrombosis.

Patients with HIT have an unusual predisposition to develop ischemic limb necrosis. Indeed, approximately 5% to 15% of such patients develop some degree of limb necrosis necessitating amputation. Occasionally multiple limbs are involved (see the box on Diagnostic Considerations in the Patient With Limb Ischemia and Thrombocytopenia).

Diagnostic Considerations in the Patient With Limb Ischemia and Thrombocytopenia

Concurrence of limb ischemia/necrosis and thrombocytopenia suggests one of several hematologic emergencies:

- **Heparin-induced thrombocytopenia (HIT).** Occlusion of large lower-limb arteries by platelet-rich "white clots" is characteristic of HIT. The major clue is an otherwise unexplained platelet count fall that begins 5 or more days after initiation of heparin. Urgent thromboembolectomy may be limb sparing. Sensitive assays for HIT antibodies give strongly positive results. See subsequent entry for warfarin.
- **Adenocarcinoma-associated disseminated intravascular coagulation (DIC).** Severe venous or arterial thrombosis can develop in patients with metastatic adenocarcinoma who have DIC. This often occurs within hours after stopping heparin. A clinical clue is an otherwise unexplained rise in platelet count that occurs with initial or repeated heparin therapy. See next entry for warfarin.
- **Warfarin-induced phlegmasia cerulea dolens/venous limb gangrene.** Coumarin anticoagulants, such as warfarin, can lead to venous ischemia (phlegmasia cerulea dolens) or venous limb gangrene in patients with DIC caused by HIT or adenocarcinoma. Limb loss can occur even though the limb pulses are palpable.
- **Sepsis-associated microvascular thrombosis.** Acquired natural anticoagulant depletion (e.g., markedly reduced antithrombin or protein C levels) can complicate DIC associated with sepsis, leading to acral limb ischemia or necrosis.
- **Septic embolism.** Rarely, infective endocarditis or aneurysmal thrombosis leads to the constellation of thrombocytopenia and acute limb ischemia.
- **Antiphospholipid syndrome.** Autoimmune thrombocytopenia and hypercoagulability can interact to produce acute limb ischemia and thrombocytopenia in patients with antiphospholipid syndrome.

DIFFERENTIAL DIAGNOSIS

Only approximately 10% of patients who undergo laboratory investigations for clinically suspected HIT have a serologic profile that supports the diagnosis (i.e., detectable heparin-dependent, platelet-activating IgG antibodies that recognize PF4/heparin complexes).[5] The differential diagnosis includes postoperative thrombocytopenia (hemodilution/platelet consumption), thrombocytopenia of critical illness, and septicemia. Some non-HIT disorders mimic HIT so closely that they warrant the term *pseudo-HIT.* One example of pseudo-HIT is adenocarcinoma-associated DIC, in which the combination of progressive thrombocytopenia and severe venous limb ischemia that occurs during the transitioning of patients from heparin (either UFH or LMWH) to warfarin may suggest a diagnosis of HIT.[21] Another disorder that can mimic HIT is the antiphospholipid syndrome: here, thrombocytopenia, thrombosis, and a false-positive PF4-dependent enzyme immunoassay (EIA) due to anti-PF4 (not anti-PF4/heparin) antibodies can be present.[22]

CLINICAL SCORING SYSTEMS

The pretest probability of HIT can be estimated using validated scoring systems. The 4 Ts system represents a mnemonic that is based on *T*hrombocytopenia, *T*iming (of onset of thrombocytopenia or thrombosis), *T*hrombosis (or other clinical sequelae of HIT), and no o*T*her explanation for thrombocytopenia, with each of the 4 Ts scoring as an integer of 0, 1, or 2 points, based upon the likelihood of HIT (thus the maximum score is 8 points) (Table 135-2).[23] The presence of platelet-activating HIT antibodies is unlikely (< 3%) with

Table 135-2 4Ts Scoring System: Estimating the Pretest Probability of Heparin-Induced Thrombocytopenia

	Points (0, 1, or 2 for Each of Four Categories: Maximum Possible Score = 8)		
	2	*1*	*0*
Thrombocytopenia (acute)	Platelet fall > 50% (nadir ≥20 × 10^9/L) and no surgery within preceding 3 days	Nadir, 10-19 × 10^9/L; or any 30%-50% fall; or, > 50% fall within 3 days of surgery	Nadir, < 10 × 10^9/L; or any < 30% fall
Timing* of platelet count fall, thrombosis, or other sequelae	Clear onset between days 5-10; or ≤1 day (if prior heparin exposure in the past 5-30 days)	Consistent with day 5-10 fall, but not clear (e.g., missing platelet counts); or ≤1 day (heparin exposure within past 31-100 days); or platelet fall after day 10	Platelet count fall begins in ≤4 days without recent heparin exposure
Thrombosis or other clinical sequelae	New proven thrombosis; skin necrosis†; anaphylactoid reaction after IV heparin bolus; adrenal hemorrhage	Progressive or recurrent thrombosis; erythematous skin lesions†; suspected thrombosis (awaiting confirmation with imaging)	None
OTher cause for thrombocytopenia not evident	No other explanation for platelet count fall is evident	Possible other cause is evident	Definite other cause is present
Pretest probability score: 6-8 = HIGH; 4-5 = INTERMEDIATE; 0-3 = LOW			

Reprinted, with permission, from Warkentin TE: Clinical picture of heparin-induced thrombocytopenia. In Warkentin TE, Greinacher A, editors: *Heparin-induced thrombocytopenia*, ed 4, New York, 2007, Informa Healthcare USA, pp 21-66.
IV, Intravenous.
*First day of immunizing heparin exposure considered day 0; immunizing heparin is usually that given during or soon after surgery (e.g., unfractionated heparin [UFH] during cardiac surgery is more immunogenic than UFH given during preceding acute coronary syndrome or with heart catheterization); the day the platelet count *begins* to fall is considered the day of onset of thrombocytopenia.
†Skin lesions occurring at heparin injection sites.
The scoring system shown here has undergone minor modifications from previously published scoring systems.

a low score (≤3 points), but relatively probable (approximately 50%) with a high score (≥6). An intermediate score (4 or 5) indicates a clinical profile compatible with HIT, but also with other disorders, such as sepsis; here the frequency of platelet-activating HIT antibodies is still only approximately 10% to 20%.

A newer scoring system is called the HIT Expert Probability (HEP) score (Table 135-3).[24] In the initial evaluation (not yet independently validated), a HEP score of 4 points or higher indicated an approximately 50% probability of HIT, whereas a score of 3 points or lower was associated with only a 3% probability of HIT.

It is uncertain whether one scoring system offers advantages over the other. In general, low scores in either system indicate a low probability of HIT, whereas high scores indicate at most a 50 : 50 chance of HIT. Thus laboratory testing is crucial to establish a diagnosis of HIT.

LABORATORY DIAGNOSIS

Assays for HIT antibodies can be classified as platelet "activation" (or "functional") and PF4-polyanion "antigen" assays (or immunoassays). Activation assays that measure serotonin release from ^{14}C-labeled, washed platelets (i.e., the serotonin-release assay [SRA]) are quite sensitive and specific for detecting clinically significant HIT antibodies.[25] Important quality control maneuvers include the selection of platelet donors whose platelets respond well to Fc receptor stimulation, as well as the inclusion of negative and positive HIT sera of variable reactivity to ensure that the test platelets identify weaker HIT sera. The characteristic activation profile produced by HIT serum includes increased platelet activation at low heparin concentrations (0.05 to 0.3 units/mL), but background platelet activation at high heparin concentrations (10 to 100 units/mL).[9] Strong platelet activation induced by HIT sera even in the absence of pharmacologic heparin is a feature of delayed-onset HIT and may generally indicate more severe HIT.[18]

Three enzyme(-linked) immuno(sorbent) assays (EIAs or ELISAs) are commercially available for detecting antibodies that recognize PF4 bound to heparin, to the polyanion, polyvinyl sulfonate, or to PF4 (from platelet lysate) bound to protamine. These assays are very sensitive for detecting HIT antibodies but are much more likely than washed platelet activation assays to detect clinically insignificant anti-PF4/heparin antibodies.[2,3,5] Thus results of laboratory tests must be interpreted in the clinical context—that is, HIT is a "clinicopathologic" syndrome.[4] Activation and antigen assays are not 100% concordant, and there are advantages if reference laboratories are able to perform both types of assay. In general, serum or plasma from patients with clinical HIT have strongly positive assay results, whereas clinically insignificant antibodies give weaker results.[2,5] Indeed, if the EIA yields only a weakly positive result (e.g., 0.45 to 1.0 absorbance units), the corresponding probability of "true" HIT is 5% to 10% at most. In contrast, if the EIA yields a strongly positive result (> 2.0 units), the probability of HIT exceeds 90%.[5] Table 135-4[25] provides evidence from three studies supporting the greater diagnostic specificity of the SRA compared with the EIA: importantly, EIA+/SRA− status does *not* support a diagnosis of HIT.

PROGNOSIS

Approximately half of all patients with SRA+ HIT have clinically evident thrombosis at the time of initial diagnosis of HIT.[11] Among patients without thrombosis at diagnosis, there appears to be a high risk (approximately 25% to 50%) for subsequent thrombosis if heparin is simply discontinued.[11] It is increasingly accepted that further anticoagulation is indicated in most patients strongly suspected as having "isolated" HIT[26,27]—that is, HIT recognized because of thrombocytopenia rather than because of HIT-associated thrombosis.

THERAPY

Although it is standard practice to discontinue heparin in patients strongly suspected of having HIT, including stopping heparin "flushes" of intravascular catheters (with substitution of saline flushes), heparin cessation is not necessarily beneficial, for two reasons: (1) heparin likely has an anticoagulant effect even in patients with HIT, and (2) HIT antibodies often cause ongoing platelet activation

Table 135-3 HIT Expert Probability (HEP) Scoring System

Clinical Feature	Score
1. Magnitude of fall in platelet count (measured from peak platelet count to nadir platelet count since heparin exposure)	
a. < 30%	−1
b. 30%-50%	1
c. > 50%	3
2. Timing of fall in platelet count	
For patients in whom typical-onset HIT is suspected	
a. Fall begins < 4 days after heparin exposure	−2
b. Fall begins 4 days after heparin exposure	2
c. Fall begins 5-10 days after heparin exposure	3
d. Fall begins 11-14 days after heparin exposure	2
e. Fall begins > 14 days after heparin exposure	−1
For patients with previous heparin exposure in last 100 days in whom rapid-onset HIT is suspected	
f. Fall begins < 48 hr after heparin reexposure	2
g. Fall begins > 48 hr after heparin reexposure	−1
3. Nadir platelet count	
a. ≤ 20 × 10⁹/L	−2
b. > 20 × 10⁹/L	2
4. Thrombosis (Select no more than one)	
For patients in whom typical-onset HIT is suspected	
a. New VTE or ATE ≥ 4 days after heparin exposure	3
b. Progression of preexisting VTE or ATE while receiving heparin	2
For patients in whom rapid-onset HIT is suspected	
c. New VTE or ATE after heparin exposure	3
d. Progression of preexisting VTE or ATE while receiving heparin	2
5. Skin necrosis	
a. Skin necrosis at subcutaneous heparin injection sites	3
6. Acute systemic reaction	
a. Acute systemic reaction after intravenous heparin bolus	2
7. Bleeding	
a. Presence of bleeding, petechiae, or extensive bruising	−1
8. Other causes of thrombocytopenia (Select all that apply)	
a. Presence of a chronic thrombocytopenic disorder	−1
b. Newly initiated nonheparin medication known to cause thrombocytopenia	−2
c. Severe infection	−2
d. Severe DIC (defined as fibrinogen < 100 mg/dL and D-dimer > 5.0 mcg/mL	−2
e. Indwelling intra-arterial device (e.g., IABP, VAD, ECMO)	−2
f. Cardiopulmonary bypass within previous 96 hr	−1
g. No other apparent cause	3

Reprinted, with permission, from Cuker A, Arepally G, Crowther MA, et al: The HIT Expert Probability (HEP) Score: A novel pre-test probability model for heparin-induced thrombocytopenia based on broad expert opinion, *J Thromb Haemost* 8:2642, 2010.

ATE, Arterial thromboembolism; *DIC*, disseminated intravascular coagulation; *ECMO*, extracorporeal membrane oxygenation; *HIT*, heparin-induced thrombocytopenia; *IABP*, intra-aortic balloon pump; *VAD*, ventricular assist device; *VTE*, venous thromboembolism. In its initial evaluation, a HEP score of ≥4 points indicated an approximately 50% probability of HIT, whereas a score of ≤3 points was associated with only a 3% probability of HIT.

Table 135-4 Frequency of Thrombocytopenia (> 50% Platelet Count Fall) Among EIA+ Patients (Polyspecific or IgG-Specific Assay) Who Received Heparin (UFH or LMWH): A Comparison of SRA+ versus SRA− Status

SRA Status	Positive in Polyspecific EIA (IgG/A/M)	Positive in IgG-Specific EIA
A. Post–orthopedic surgery		
SRA+	12/24	12/24
SRA−	0/58	0/16
P	< 0.0001	0.0009
B. Venous thromboembolism		
SRA+	4/4	4/4
SRA−	0/15	0/6
P	0.0003	0.0048
C. Post–cardiac surgery		
SRA+	4/11	NA
SRA−	0/152	NA
P	< 0.0001	NA

Reprinted, with modifications, with permission, from Warkentin TE: How I diagnose and manage HIT, *Hematology Am Soc Hematol Educ Program* 2011:143, 2011.

EIA, Enzyme immunoassay; *LMWH*, low-molecular-weight heparin; *NA*, not available; *SRA+*, positive in the serotonin-release assay; *SRA−*, negative in the serotonin-release assay; *UFH*, unfractionated heparin.

The data are consistent with the SRA having a high sensitivity for heparin-induced thrombocytopenia (> 95%); the specificity of the SRA depends on the clinical situation but in most circumstances is at least 90%. Patients in studies A and B were tested in both the polyspecific and IgG-specific assays.

and hypercoagulability in the absence of pharmacologic heparin. In addition, HIT antibody levels can decline even with continued heparin. The recognition that patients with HIT have increased thrombin generation[12] provides a rationale for use of nonheparin anticoagulant agents that rapidly inhibit thrombin or its generation.

Currently there are two types of anticoagulant therapeutic approaches that are commonly used to treat HIT: (1) long-acting indirect (i.e., antithrombin-dependent) factor Xa inhibitors (danaparoid, fondaparinux), and (2) direct thrombin inhibitors (recombinant hirudin, argatroban, bivalirudin).[19] In the author's opinion, indirect factor Xa inhibitors—although not approved in the United States for treatment of HIT—are the preferred treatment option for HIT, because they have numerous advantages over DTIs (Table 135-5).[19] In addition, because approximately 90% of patients suspected of HIT do not have HIT,[5] another advantage for indirect factor Xa inhibitors is that these agents—unlike DTIs—are safe and effective for prevention and treatment of thrombosis in numerous non-HIT settings.

Indirect Factor Xa Inhibitors: Danaparoid and Fondaparinux

Danaparoid is an anticoagulant heparinoid (mixture of glycosaminoglycans) with predominant inhibitory activity against factor Xa that is effective for treating HIT; however, danaparoid was never approved for HIT treatment in the United States (although it was approved in many other countries, including Canada and the European Union) and was discontinued in the United States in April 2002. Danaparoid was shown to be safe and effective for treatment of HIT in an open-label randomized controlled trial (versus dextran 70) and in a retrospective comparison against ancrod (defibrinogenating snake venom) and/or vitamin K antagonist therapy.

In recent years, however, physicians have increasingly been using fondaparinux as off-label therapy for HIT. The advantages of fondaparinux include its long half-life, the fact that it does not require coagulation monitoring nor does it influence the aPTT or international normalized ratio (INR), its low potential to cross-react with HIT antibodies, and low cost. In addition, because relatively few patients with suspected HIT actually have this diagnosis, the wide experience with fondaparinux and its approval for the prevention and treatment of thrombosis in non-HIT settings constitute other advantages. To date, the experience with fondaparinux to treat HIT has been favorable, including the treatment of patients with SRA+ HIT (Table 135-6).[28-33] Also, fondaparinux is much less likely than UFH or LMWH to precipitate rapid-onset HIT in patients who have unrecognized HIT antibodies.[34] Although fondaparinux thromboprophylaxis has been associated with rare cases of de novo HIT,[28] this should not deter from its use as a potential treatment of HIT because the potential to trigger immunization is "dissociated" from whether an

Table 135-5 Comparison of the Two Classes of Anticoagulants Used to Treat Heparin-Induced Thrombocytopenia

	Indirect (AT-Dependent) Factor Xa Inhibitors: Danaparoid, Fondaparinux	Direct Thrombin Inhibitors: r-Hirudin (Lepirudin, Desirudin), Argatroban, Bivalirudin
Half-life	√ Long (danaparoid, 25 hr*; fondaparinux, 17 hr): reduces risk of rebound hypercoagulability	Short (< 2 hr): potential for rebound hypercoagulability
Dosing	√ Both prophylactic- and therapeutic-dose regimens†	Prophylactic-dose regimens are not established (exception: subcutaneous desirudin)
Monitoring	√ Direct (anti-Xa levels): accurate drug levels obtained	Indirect (aPTT): risk for DTI underdosing due to aPTT elevation caused by non-DTI factors, including HIT-associated DIC
Effect on INR	√ No significant effect: thus simplifies overlap with warfarin	Increases INR: argatroban > bivalirudin > r-hirudin; complicates warfarin overlap
Protein C pathway	√ Adverse effect unlikely (with reduced thrombin generation, there will be less thrombin to activate protein C)	Thrombin inhibition could impair thrombin-mediated activation of protein C pathway
Reversibility of action	√ Irreversible inhibition: AT forms covalent bond with factor Xa	Irreversible inhibition only with r-hirudin
Efficacy and safety in non-HIT settings	√ Treatment and prophylaxis of VTE (danaparoid, fondaparinux) and ACS (fondaparinux)	Not established for most non-HIT settings (exception: bivalirudin established for PCI)
Platelet activation	√ Danaparoid inhibits platelet activation by HIT antibodies	No effect
Inhibition of clot-bound thrombin	No effect	√ Inhibition of both free and clot-bound thrombin
Drug clearance	Predominantly renal	Variable (predominantly hepatobiliary: argatroban; predominantly renal: r-hirudin)
Cost	√ Relatively low‡	Relatively high‡

Reprinted, with modifications, with permission, from Warkentin TE: Agents for the treatment of heparin-induced thrombocytopenia, *Hematol Oncol Clin North Am* 24:755, 2010.
ACS, Acute coronary syndrome; *aPTT,* activated partial thromboplastin time; *AT,* antithrombin; *DIC,* disseminated intravascular coagulation; *DTI,* direct thrombin inhibitor; *HIT,* heparin-induced thrombocytopenia; *INR,* international normalized ratio; *PCI,* percutaneous coronary intervention; *VTE,* venous thromboembolism.
Check mark (√) indicates favorable feature in comparison of drug classes (author's opinion).
*For danaparoid, half-lives of its anti-thrombin (anti-IIa) and its thrombin generation inhibition activities (2-4 hr and 3-7 hr, respectively) are shorter than for its anti-Xa activity (approximately 25 hr).
†Although therapeutic dosing is recommended for HIT, availability of prophylactic-dose regimens increases flexibility when managing potential non-HIT situations.
‡Another cost consideration is that a patient can be discharged to home on subcutaneous danaparoid or fondaparinux, whereas an additional 5-7 in-hospital days may be required for DTI-warfarin overlap before discharge from hospital.

Table 135-6 Fondaparinux for Treatment of Acute Heparin-Induced Thrombocytopenia

Study	N	N With HITT (%)	Mean Platelet Count Nadir ($\times 10^9$/L)	Thrombosis Rate	Amputation Rate*	Major Bleeding
Kuo and Kovacs[29]	5	5 (100%)	43	0%	0%	0%
Lobo et al[30]	7	6 (86%)	66	0%	1/7 (14%)	0%
Grouzi et al[31]	24	14 (58%)	66†	0%	1/24 (4%)	0%
Warkentin et al[32]	16	9 (56%)	79	0%	1/16 (6%)	1/16 (6%)
Goldfarb and Blostein[33]	8	6 (75%)	56	0%	0%	0%
Pooled data (above five studies)	60	40 (67%)	66	0/60 (0%)	3/60 (5%)	1/60 (2%)

HITT, Heparin-induced thrombocytopenia and thrombosis (in this context, the thrombosis preceded treatment with fondaparinux).
*In all patients with limb amputations, ischemic limb necrosis was judged to have been present before fondaparinux therapy.
†The mean platelet count nadir excludes two patients with myeloproliferative disorder who had baseline thrombocytosis.

anticoagulant potentiates antibody-induced platelet activation,[7] and fondaparinux has low potential to exacerbate HIT.[34] Dosing information for danaparoid and fondaparinux is shown in Table 135-7.

In theory, oral direct factor Xa inhibitors, such as rivaroxaban (approved in the United States for thromboprophylaxis after knee or hip replacement surgery), should be effective for treatment of HIT. However, there is no experience with rivaroxaban for this indication as of yet.

Direct Thrombin Inhibitors: Recombinant Hirudin (Lepirudin, Desirudin), Bivalirudin, Argatroban

The recombinant hirudin–derivative lepirudin (Refludan) is a 65-amino-acid polypeptide that inactivates thrombin by forming a tight, noncovalent 1 : 1 complex with it. Lepirudin is approved for the treatment of HIT-associated thrombosis in the European Union, the United States, and elsewhere.[26] Lepirudin is renally excreted, and the drug must be avoided (or the dosage substantially reduced) in patients with renal failure. With normal renal function, the half-life of intravenously administered lepirudin is about 80 minutes. Coagulation monitoring is performed using the aPTT (target aPTT, 1.5 to 2.5 times the baseline value). In the treatment of HIT-associated thrombosis, lepirudin reduced a composite end point (encompassing new thrombosis, limb amputation, and all-cause mortality) from 40.0% (in historical controls) to 19.2% (pooled data from the HAT-1, -2, and -3 trials; analysis from start of treatment).[26] The end point of new thrombosis was reduced from 25.3% to 7.0%. Major bleeding complications were seen in about 15% of patients

Table 135-7 Treatment Schedules for Danaparoid and Fondaparinux

Anticoagulant	Therapeutic Dosing Protocol for HIT-Associated Thrombosis*	Anticoagulant Monitoring	Clearance	Half-life (hr)	Comment
Danaparoid	Initial bolus, 2250 units[†] IV; accelerated infusion (400 units/hr × 4 hr, 300 units/hr 4 hr; then 200 units/hr IV, subsequently adjusted by anti–factor Xa levels)	Anti–factor Xa levels (target, 0.5-0.8 units/mL)	Renal (minor)	25	Widely approved for HIT treatment (although not in the United States); not available in the United States; low risk for in vivo cross-reactivity; prophylactic-dose therapy[‡] may be appropriate when clinical suspicion for HIT is low
Fondaparinux	7.5 mg[§] subcutaneous once daily	Anti–Xa factor levels (target levels not well established)	Renal (major)	17	Not approved for HIT treatment (although increasingly used as off-label therapy). Prophylactic-dose therapy[‖] may be appropriate when clinical suspicion for HIT is low, or if there is renal insufficiency

HIT, Heparin-induced thrombocytopenia; *IV*, intravenous.
*Therapeutic dosing is usually appropriate for strongly suspected or confirmed HIT (including "isolated" HIT, i.e., HIT without apparent thrombosis), or when thrombosis is documented.
[†]Adjust IV danaparoid bolus for body weight: < 60 kg, 1500 units; 60-75 kg, 2250 units; 75-90 kg, 3000 units; > 90 kg, 3750 units.
[‡]Prophylactic-dose regimen, 750 units subcutaneous every 8 hr (for renal failure, reduce to 750 units every 12 hr).
[§]Five milligrams for body weight < 50 kg and 10 mg for body weight > 100 kg; the author sometimes gives 10 mg as the first and/or second dose (rather than 7.5 mg) for severe HIT. Because HIT treatment is usually started in the afternoon, the author usually gives the second dose (and subsequent doses) at 8 AM (i.e., the interval between first and second doses is often only 14-20 hr rather than 24 hr), which helps to achieve steady-state therapy more quickly. Dose reduction and anti–factor Xa monitoring (if available) is appropriate if being used in a patient with renal insufficiency.
[‖]Prophylactic-dose regimen, 2.5 mg subcutaneous every day (assumes normal renal function).

(compared with 6.7% in historical controls), or approximately 1% per treatment day. The high rate of bleeding prompted recommendations to administer initial doses lower than those recommended in the package insert, even in patients with normal renal function.[26] In patients with isolated HIT (an off-label indication), lepirudin given in "prophylactic" doses (0.1 mg/kg/hr intravenously without an initial bolus, and adjusted to an aPTT of 1.5 to 2.0 times baseline) was associated with new thrombosis in only 4.4% of patients. This lower-dose regimen also seems appropriate for patients with HIT-associated thrombosis.[26] Similarly low rates of thrombosis have been observed in postmarketing studies of treatment of lepirudin for isolated HIT. Fatal anaphylactic reactions have been reported in patients reexposed to lepirudin. These reactions occur in as many as 1 in 400 patients after intravenous bolus administration. This is another reason to avoid bolus dosing in most clinical situations. The manufacturer discontinued lepirudin (April, 2012), but it may remain available in some jurisdictions via another manufacturer.

Another recombinant hirudin, desirudin (Iprivask) is available in the United States, where it is marketed for thromboprophylaxis after hip replacement surgery (dose, 15 mg twice daily by subcutaneous injection in patients with normal renal function). There is minimal experience with desirudin in patients with HIT.

Bivalirudin (Angiomax) is a 20-amino-acid thrombin inhibitor modeled after hirudin that is composed of two peptide fragments that recognize the active site of thrombin and its fibrinogen-binding site, linked by a tetraglycine spacer. The half-life of bivalirudin is about one-third that of lepirudin (25 versus 80 minutes), and only minor dose adjustments are needed in patients with renal insufficiency because bivalirudin is only partially cleared by the kidneys. It is approved as an alternative to heparin in patients undergoing percutaneous coronary intervention (PCI), including those with HIT. Its short half-life and predominantly extrarenal elimination are reasons why it is an option for intraoperative anticoagulation in patients undergoing cardiac surgery, when heparin is contraindicated because of acute or recent HIT. Experience using bivalirudin off-label to treat HIT outside the PCI setting is limited. Anaphylaxis has not been reported.

Argatroban (marketed as argatroban in the United States and as Novastan elsewhere) is a small-molecule (527-Da) Direct thrombin inhibitor (DTI) that undergoes predominantly hepatobiliary excretion and is therefore suitable for use without dose adjustment in patients with renal failure (the dose is reduced by three-quarters in patients with hepatic insufficiency). Argatroban is approved in the United States for both treatment and prevention of thrombosis in HIT. It is given in the same dosage for both indications (usual starting infusion rate of 2 mcg/kg/min without an initial bolus). However, as with lepirudin, lower starting doses are usually given (e.g., 0.5 to 1.2 mcg/kg/min), especially in critically ill patients. Argatroban (in substantially higher doses) is also approved for anticoagulation during PCI in patients with acute HIT or a history of HIT. Its half-life is 40 to 50 minutes. Argatroban prolongs the INR more than lepirudin or bivalirudin, and a higher-than-usual target INR during warfarin cotherapy (which depends on the thromboplastin reagent used to measure the INR) can be expected (see Caveats in Treatment of Heparin-Induced Thrombocytopenia). Argatroban reduced the frequency of a composite end point (new thrombosis, limb amputation, and all-cause mortality) from 56.5% (in historical controls) to 43.8% and 41.5% in two studies of patients with HIT complicated by thrombosis; new thrombosis event rates were reduced from 34.8% to 19.4% and 13.1%, respectively.[26] In patients with isolated HIT, argatroban reduced the rate of new thrombosis from 22.4% to 6.9%, and the combined event rate of new thrombosis, limb amputation, and all-cause mortality from 38.8% to 26.9%.[26] Dosing information for the parenteral DTIs is shown in Table 135-8.

In theory, dabigatran, an oral thrombin inhibitor, should also be effective for treatment of HIT. However, the drug has not yet been tested for this indication.

Caveats in Treatment of Heparin-Induced Thrombocytopenia

Warfarin and other vitamin K antagonists (coumarins) should not be used during the acute thrombocytopenic phase of HIT.[12] A particularly high-risk situation is HIT associated with deep vein thrombosis, especially if there is overt (decompensated) DIC. If such patients are treated with warfarin, there is a risk for progression to venous limb gangrene.[12,26,27] The laboratory marker for this unusual syndrome is a high INR (generally, greater than 4.0), which corresponds to the combination of a marked reduction in the level of protein C together with increased thrombin generation (as evidenced by elevated levels of thrombin-antithrombin complexes) during warfarin therapy.[12] Although warfarin (in theory) should be safe in a patient whose

Table 135-8 Treatment Schedules for Lepirudin, Desirudin, Bivalirudin, and Argatroban

Anticoagulant	Dosing Protocol for HIT-Associated Thrombosis	Anticoagulant Monitoring*	Clearance	Half-Life (min)	Comment
Lepirudin	No bolus; initial infusion rate: 0.05-0.10 mg/kg/hr[†‡]	1.5-2.5 × baseline aPTT	Renal[‡]	80	Approved dosing regimen (not shown) is too high; risk for anaphylaxis, especially on reexposure; minor prolongation of INR (compare to argatroban)
Desirudin	Not established	aPTT	Renal	120	Half-life shown is for subcutaneous administration; minimal experience for treating HIT
Bivalirudin	No bolus; initial infusion rate: 0.15-0.20 mg/kg/hr	1.5-2.5 × baseline aPTT	Enzymic (80%); renal (20%)	25	Off-label treatment for HIT (although approved for PCI in patient with HIT); minor prolongation of INR (compared with argatroban)
Argatroban	No bolus; initial infusion rate: 2 mcg/kg/min	1.5-3.0 × baseline aPTT	Hepatobiliary	40-50	Initial dose 0.5 mcg/kg/min in hepatic insufficiency[§]; moderate or marked prolongation of INR, which complicates overlap with warfarin anticoagulation

aPTT, Activated partial thromboplastin time; *HIT,* heparin-induced thrombocytopenia; *INR,* international normalized ratio; *PCI,* percutaneous coronary intervention.
Dosing protocols shown are appropriate for most patients with strongly suspected or confirmed HIT whether or not complicated by thrombosis. (Dosing for bivalirudin and argatroban is substantially different when given for PCI.)
*Generally the patient's baseline aPTT should be used for calculating target range, when appropriate; otherwise the mean laboratory normal range can be used.
[†]This dosing protocol differs from the package insert (which advises initial bolus of 0.4 mg/kg and initial infusion rate [assuming normal renal function] of 0.15 mg/kg/hr); however, this dosing regimen is now considered too high.[26]
[‡]Major dose reduction in renal insufficiency is required (e.g., lepirudin starting infusion rate, 0.05 mg/kg/hr for serum creatinine 90-140 μmol/L; starting infusion rate, 0.01 mg/kg/hr for serum creatinine 140 to 400 μmol/L; and starting infusion rate 0.005 μmol/L for serum creatinine > 400 μmol/L, with frequent aPTT monitoring [every 4 hr until steady state is achieved, then at least once daily]).[26]
[§]Reduced initial dosing (e.g., 0.5-1.2 mcg/kg/min) is also appropriate in patients in intensive care units, with cardiac failure, or post–cardiac surgery).

thrombin generation is controlled (e.g., using a DTI), it is important to delay the initiation of warfarin until there is substantial resolution of the thrombocytopenia (to more than $150 \times 10^9/L$).[26,27] Warfarin treatment should be delayed because its prolongation of the aPTT may result in *underdosing* of the DTI, and because stopping the DTI before resolution of the HIT during warfarin overlap can lead to limb loss due to fulminant venous limb gangrene.[4,19]

Several case observations suggest that aPTT confounding of DTI therapy can be a factor explaining progression of thrombosis in patients with severe HIT.[4,19] For example, patients can develop progressive thrombocytopenia and HIT-associated consumptive coagulopathy despite stopping heparin (Fig. 135-4). In such patients, aPTT monitoring of DTI therapy can fail because a brief course of DTI can abruptly lead to supratherapeutic aPTT levels—not because of anticoagulant overdosing but because of the combination of DTI and consumptive coagulopathy—and interruption/cessation of DTI therapy can be associated with rapid progression of microvascular thrombosis. In this setting, factor Xa inhibitors (danaparoid, fondaparinux) may be more effective because they do not require aPTT monitoring. Alternatively, DTI levels can be measured directly, but these assays are rarely performed in North American laboratories.

Using sensitive assays for HIT antibodies, LMWH reacts similarly to UFH in vitro. Furthermore, because LMWH can lead to worsening of clinical HIT, these agents should not be used to treat HIT.[26,27]

Although primary treatment for HIT should include an anticoagulant that inhibits thrombin or reduces its generation, certain treatment adjuncts can be used in special situations. These include surgical thromboembolectomy, high-dose intravenous immunoglobulin, antiplatelet drugs such as aspirin, and plasmapheresis.

These caveats, along with recommendations for management of patients with suspected HIT, are summarized in the box on Diagnosis and Treatment of Heparin-Induced Thrombocytopenia.

PREVENTION

The frequency of platelet count monitoring in patients receiving heparin should reflect the overall risk of HIT (i.e., the preparation, the dose, and the clinical situation).[26] At least alternate-day platelet count monitoring should be considered in patients at relatively high risk for developing HIT (e.g., after orthopedic or cardiac surgery). Monitoring at least two or three times a week should be considered for patients at moderate risk for developing HIT (e.g., medical patients receiving UFH, postoperative patients receiving UFH flushes or LMWH). The frequency of HIT is low with LMWH,[1,6] particularly in medical patients or during pregnancy, and routine platelet count monitoring may not be required in such settings.[26] In addition, HIT rarely begins 14 or more days after initiation of a course of heparin,[17] so routine monitoring beyond this period is not required. A recent consensus conference[27] recommended somewhat less intensive platelet count monitoring than advised in this paragraph.

ANTICOAGULATION AND PREVIOUS HEPARIN-INDUCED THROMBOCYTOPENIA

HIT antibodies are transient and usually are undetectable several weeks or a few months after an episode of HIT.[17] If HIT antibodies are no longer detected, it is appropriate to use heparin for a brief indication in situations where other anticoagulants have drawbacks (e.g., cardiac surgery).[17,26,27] Heparin should be avoided preoperatively (e.g., argatroban or bivalirudin can be used for heart catheterization). Patients with acute or recent HIT who require urgent heart surgery and still have detectable antibodies have been successfully treated with alternate anticoagulant approaches (e.g., bivalirudin, lepirudin, or heparin plus an antiplatelet agent such as epoprostenol or tirofiban), but each of these approaches has disadvantages. For example, the high dose of lepirudin regimen needed for cardiac surgery requires monitoring with the ecarin clotting time, a test that is not widely available, and patients can develop severe bleeding if renal failure occurs; epoprostenol causes hypotension, and there is limited experience with its use in cardiac surgery. Bivalirudin is the most promising agent for use in cardiac surgery, but special surgical and anesthesiologic maneuvers are required (because bivalirudin undergoes proteolysis, thus posing a risk for clotting of stagnant blood in the extracorporeal circuit).

A diagnostic and therapeutic approach to HIT[23] is shown in the box on Diagnosis and Treatment of Heparin-Induced Thrombocytopenia.

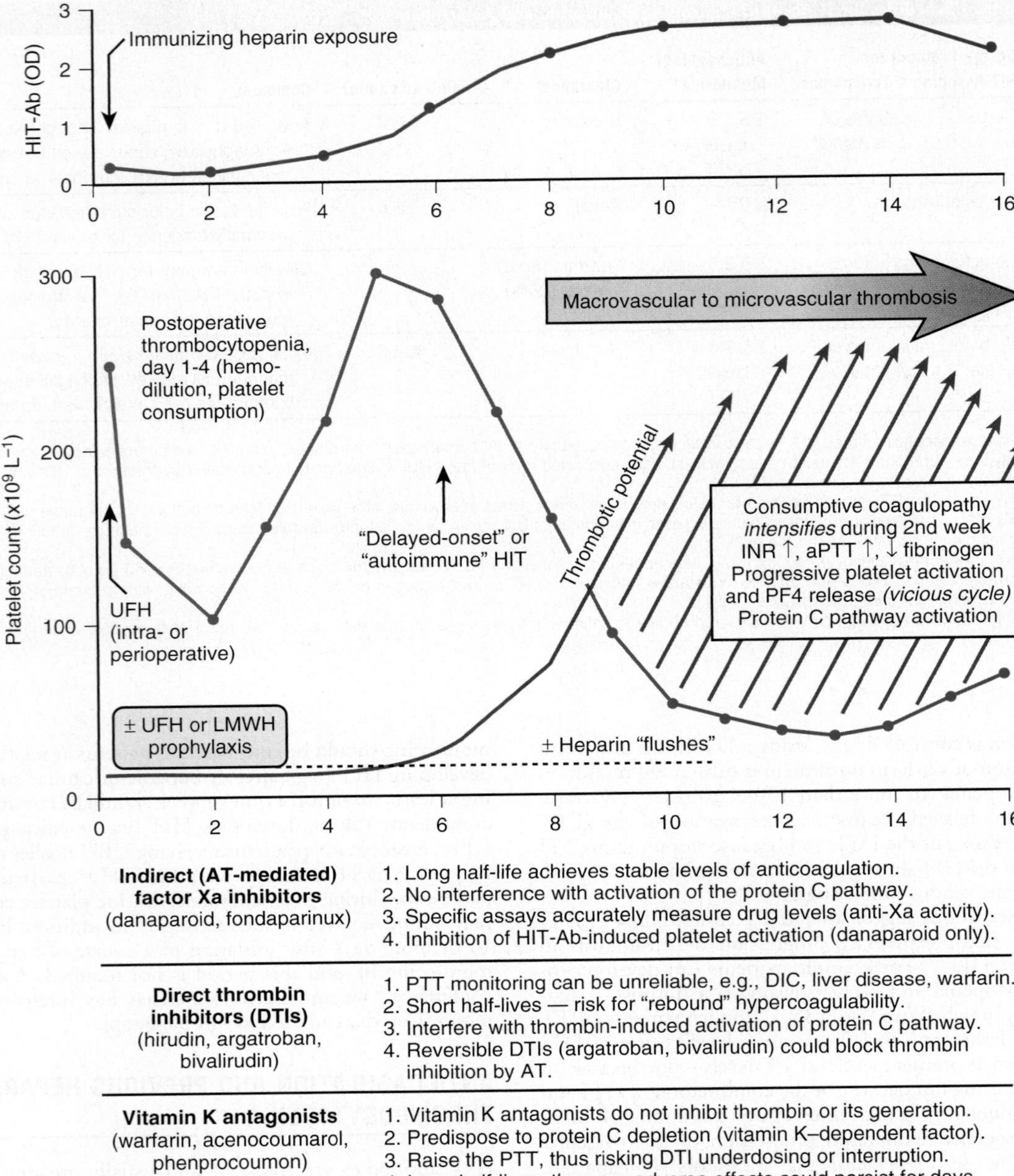

Figure 135-4 CONCEPTUAL FRAMEWORK OF HEPARIN-INDUCED THROMBOCYTOPENIA (HIT): FOCUS ON HEPARIN-*IN*DEPENDENT PLATELET ACTIVATION AND DELAYED-ONSET ("AUTOIMMUNE") HIT. The *upper panel* shows the timeline of HIT antibody (HIT-Ab) formation, as judged by optical density (OD) units in an anti–platelet factor 4 (PF4)/polyanion enzyme immunoassay (EIA). The *middle panel* illustrates a platelet count decline in the absence of heparin (or with small amounts of heparin, e.g., heparin flushes) indicating delayed-onset HIT, with intensification of HIT-associated hypercoagulability from day 7 to 14, especially after stopping heparin. Patients with this clinical profile often have HIT-associated consumptive coagulopathy (overt disseminated intravascular coagulopathy [DIC]), and are at risk for confounding of activated partial thromboplastin time (aPTT)-monitored direct thrombin inhibitor (DTI) treatment. The *lower panel* compares different classes of anticoagulant for expected effects on HIT-associated hypercoagulability, including the risk for aPTT confounding in the setting of HIT-associated DIC. *AT,* Antithrombin; *INR,* international normalized ratio; *LMWH,* low-molecular-weight heparin; *PTT,* partial thromboplastin time; *UHF,* unfractionated heparin. *(From Warkentin TE: Agents for the treatment of heparin-induced thrombocytopenia.* Hematol Oncol Clin North Am *24:755, 2010.)*

Diagnosis and Treatment of Heparin-Induced Thrombocytopenia

Heparin-induced thrombocytopenia (HIT) should be clinically suspected when thrombocytopenia occurs during (or soon after) heparin therapy and the temporal profile of the decrease in platelet count is consistent with immune sensitization to heparin. Four relevant questions—the 4 Ts—should be asked:

Thrombocytopenia: Does the patient have thrombocytopenia? A greater than 50% fall in the platelet count can indicate HIT even if the platelet count has not fallen to below 150 × 10^9/L. (Note: Severe thrombocytopenia, such as a platelet count below 10 × 10^9/L, is rarely caused by HIT.)

Timing: Is the timing of the platelet count fall consistent with immune sensitization? In HIT the platelet count usually begins to fall 5 to 10 days after starting heparin (first day of heparin is day 0); a more rapid fall in the platelet count can occur if the patient is already sensitized from heparin exposure within the past 100 days.

Thrombosis: Does the patient have thrombosis or other sequelae of HIT? (Note: In addition to venous and arterial thrombosis, patients with HIT can develop necrotizing skin lesions at heparin injection sites or systemic inflammatory or cardiorespiratory reactions that begin 5 to 30 minutes after an intravenous [IV] heparin bolus).

OTher: Are there other explanations for the thrombocytopenia? HIT is less likely when there is compelling clinical evidence for another cause of the thrombocytopenia, such as positive blood cultures.

Steps in Management of Clinically Suspected Heparin-Induced Thrombocytopenia

1. Confirm that thrombocytopenia is present (repeat complete blood cell count [CBC]), test for disseminated intravascular coagulation (DIC), and test for HIT antibodies, preferably using a platelet activation test such as the serotonin-release assay (SRA).
2. Assess clinically and radiologically for thrombosis (e.g., compression ultrasound for lower-limb deep venous thrombosis).
3. Stop all heparin, including heparin flushes and possibly use of heparin-coated intravascular catheters (catheters left in situ for several days may not have much residual heparin).
4. Initiate treatment with an alternative anticoagulant, generally in therapeutic doses if HIT is strongly suspected (options: danaparoid,*† fondaparinux,*‡ lepirudin,§ argatroban, bivalirudin*).
5. Although initial treatment decsions are made on clinical grounds, results of testing for HIT antibodies can influence subsequent treatment, including the decision to resume heparin if HIT has been ruled out using one or more sensitive assays for HIT antibodies.

Caveats

- Do not use low-molecular-weight heparin to treat HIT.
- Do not start (or continue) warfarin or other coumarins until the platelet count has returned to normal (greater than 150 × 10^9/L), and give only in low initial doses (warfarin, 5 mg or less) and overlap with a parenteral anticoagulant for at least 5 days.
- Do give vitamin K (e.g., 5 to 10 mg IV over 30 to 60 minutes) if HIT is diagnosed after warfarin has already been given, so as to reduce risk for coumarin necrosis and to avoid underdosing of direct thrombin inhibitor (DTI) because of activated partial thromboplastin time (aPTT) prolongation by warfarin.
- Beware of confounding of aPTT-monitored DTI therapy in patients with severe HIT complicated by HIT-associated consumptive coagulopathy (DIC) or who have other explanations for an elevated aPTT, such as warfarin therapy, liver disease, or antiphospholipid syndrome.
- Do not give prophylactic platelet transfusions (platelet transfusions are appropriate if the patient is bleeding or if there is diagnostic uncertainty).

*Not approved for treatment of HIT in the United States (except, in the case of bivalirudin, for anticoagulation during percutaneous coronary intervention).
†Withdrawn from the U.S. market, but available in many other countries.
‡Fondaparinux is not approved for treatment of HIT, but case series suggest that it is at least as effective as DTI therapy; moreover, the risk for bleeding with fondaparinux is likely to be lower than that with DTI therapy and fondaparinux costs less than the other agents. Also, there is greater experience with fondaparinux than DTIs for prevention and treatment of thrombosis in non-HIT situations, and only approximately 10% of patients with suspected HIT actually have the disorder. Fondaparinux also avoids the risk for confounding of aPTT-monitored DTI therapy. The author is a proponent of the use of fondaparinux to treat HIT.[25,28,32,34]
§Lepirudin discontinued by the manufacturer, April 2012; however, it may continue to be available through another manufacturer (Cellgene, U.K.)/distributor (Pharmore, Germany).

REFERENCES

1. Lee DH, Warkentin TE: Frequency of heparin-induced thrombocytopenia. In Warkentin TE, Greinacher A, editors: *Heparin-induced thrombocytopenia,* ed 4, New York, 2007, Informa Healthcare USA, p 67.
2. Warkentin TE, Sheppard JI, Moore JC, et al: Laboratory testing for the antibodies that cause heparin-induced thrombocytopenia: How much class do we need? *J Lab Clin Med* 146:341, 2005.
3. Warkentin TE, Sheppard JI, Moore JC, et al: Studies of the immune response in heparin-induced thrombocytopenia. *Blood* 113:4963, 2009.
4. Warkentin TE: HIT paradigms and paradoxes. *J Thromb Haemost* 9:105, 2011.
5. Warkentin TE, Sheppard JI, Moore JC, et al: Quantitative interpretation of optical density measurements using PF4-dependent immunoassays. *J Thromb Haemost* 6:1304, 2008.
6. Warkentin TE, Sheppard JI, Sigouin CS, et al: Gender imbalance and risk factor interactions in heparin-induced thrombocytopenia. *Blood* 108:2937, 2006.
7. Warkentin TE, Cook RJ, Marder VJ, et al: Anti-platelet factor 4/heparin antibodies in orthopedic surgery patients receiving antithrombotic prophylaxis with fondaparinux or enoxaparin. *Blood* 106:3791, 2005.
8. Gao C, Boylan B, Fang J, et al: Heparin promotes platelet responsiveness by potentiating αIIbβ3-mediated outside-in signaling. *Blood* 117:4946, 2011.
9. Sheridan D, Carter J, Kelton JG: A diagnostic test for heparin-induced thrombocytopenia. *Blood* 67:27, 1986.
10. Greinacher A, Holtfreter B, Krauel K, et al: Association of natural anti-platelet factor 4/heparin antibodies with periodontal disease. *Blood* 118:1395, 2011.
11. Warkentin TE, Kelton JG: A 14-year study of heparin-induced thrombocytopenia. *Am J Med* 101:502, 1996.
12. Warkentin TE, Elavathil LJ, Hayward CPM, et al: The pathogenesis of venous limb gangrene associated with heparin-induced thrombocytopenia. *Ann Intern Med* 127:804, 1997.
13. Rauova L, Hirsch JD, Greene TK et al: Monocyte-bound PF4 in the pathogenesis of heparin-induced thrombocytopenia. *Blood* 116:5021, 2010.
14. Lubenow N, Hinz P, Thomaschewski S, et al: The severity of trauma determines the immune response to PF4/heparin and the frequency of heparin-induced thrombocytopenia. *Blood* 115:1797, 2010.
15. Warkentin TE, Cook RJ, Marder VJ, et al: Anti-PF4/heparin antibody formation post-orthopedic surgery thromboprophylaxis: The role of non-drug risk factors and evidence for a stoichiometry-based model of immunization. *J Thromb Haemost* 8:504, 2010.
16. Warkentin TE: Drug-induced immune-mediated thrombocytopenia—from purpura to thrombosis. *N Engl J Med* 356:891, 2007.
17. Warkentin TE, Kelton JG: Temporal aspects of heparin-induced thrombocytopenia. *N Engl J Med* 344:1286, 2001.

18. Warkentin TE, Kelton JG: Delayed-onset heparin-induced thrombocytopenia and thrombosis. *Ann Intern Med* 135:502, 2001.
19. Warkentin TE: Agents for the treatment of heparin-induced thrombocytopenia. *Hematol Oncol Clin North Am* 24:755, 2010.
20. Warkentin TE, Makris M, Jay RM, et al: A spontaneous prothrombotic disorder resembling heparin-induced thrombocytopenia. *Am J Med* 121:632, 2008.
21. Warkentin TE: Venous limb gangrene during warfarin treatment of cancer-associated deep venous thrombosis. *Ann Intern Med* 135:589, 2001.
22. Pauzner R, Greinacher A, Selleng K, et al: False-positive tests for heparin induced thrombocytopenia in patients with antiphospholipid syndrome and systemic lupus erythematosus. *J Thromb Haemost* 7:1070, 2009.
23. Lo GK, Juhl D, Warkentin TE, et al: Evaluation of pretest clinical score (4 T's) for the diagnosis of heparin-induced thrombocytopenia in two clinical settings. *J Thromb Haemost* 4:759, 2006.
24. Cuker A, Arepally G, Crowther MA, et al: The HIT Expert Probability (HEP) Score: A novel pre-test probability model for heparin-induced thrombocytopenia based on broad expert opinion. *J Thromb Haemost* 8:2642, 2010.
25. Warkentin TE: How I diagnose and manage HIT. *Hematology Am Soc Hematol Educ Program* 2011:143, 2011.
26. Warkentin TE, Greinacher A, Koster A, et al: Treatment and prevention of heparin-induced thrombocytopenia: American College of Chest Physicians Evidence-Based Clinical Practice Guidelines (8th edition). *Chest* 133:340S, 2008.
27. Linkins LA, Dans AL, Moores LK, et al: Treatment and prevention of heparin-induced thrombocytopenia. Antithrombotic Therapy and Prevention of Thrombosis, 9th ed: American College of Chest Physicians Evidence-Based Clinical Practice Guidelines.. *Chest* 141:e495S, 2012.
28. Warkentin TE: Fondaparinux: Does it cause HIT? Can it treat HIT? *Exp Rev Hematol* 3:567, 2010.
29. Kuo KHM, Kovacs MJ: Successful treatment of heparin-induced thrombocytopenia with fondaparinux. *Thromb Haemost* 93:999, 2005.
30. Lobo B, Finch C, Howard A, et al: Fondaparinux for the treatment of patients with acute heparin-induced thrombocytopenia. *Thromb Haemost* 99:208, 2008.
31. Grouzi E, Kyriakou E, Panagou I, et al: Fondaparinux for the treatment of acute heparin-induced thrombocytopenia: A single-center experience. *Clin Appl Thromb Hemost* 16:663, 2010.
32. Warkentin TE, Pai M, Sheppard JI, et al: Fondaparinux treatment of acute heparin-induced thrombocytopenia confirmed by the serotonin-release assay: A 30-month, 16-patient case series. *J Thromb Haemost* 9:2389, 2011.
33. Goldfarb MJ, Blostein MD: Fondaparinux in acute heparin-induced thrombocytopenia: A case series. *J Thromb Haemost* 9:2501, 2011.
34. Warkentin TE, Davidson BL, Büller HR, et al: Prevalance and risk of preexisting heparin-induced thrombocytopenia antibodies in patients with acute VTE. *Chest* 140:366, 2011.

CHAPTER 136

THROMBOTIC THROMBOCYTOPENIC PURPURA AND THE HEMOLYTIC UREMIC SYNDROME

Keith R. McCrae, J. Evan Sadler, and Douglas B. Cines

In 1925, Moschowitz described a 16-year-old girl who died of a previously undescribed illness characterized by microangiopathic hemolytic anemia, petechiae, hemiparesis, and fever. Postmortem examination revealed numerous hyaline thrombi, most prevalent in the terminal arterioles and capillaries of the heart and kidneys. In 1936, four similar cases were reported by Baehr and colleagues, who proposed that the hyaline thrombi were secondary to agglutinated platelets; in 1947, Singer suggested that the term *thrombotic thrombocytopenic purpura (TTP)* be used to describe this disorder. In 1955, Gasser used the term *hemolytic uremic syndrome (HUS)* to describe a related syndrome that consisted of Coombs-negative hemolytic anemia, thrombocytopenia, and renal failure. These disorders are now referred to as *thrombotic microangiopathies (TMA),* based on their shared features of microangiopathic hemolytic anemia, thrombocytopenia, and microvascular thrombotic lesions.

Although the clinical and pathologic features of TTP and HUS may overlap, recent scientific advances have demonstrated that the pathogenesis of these disorders differs. Several pathogenesis-based classification schemes for thrombotic microangiopathies have been developed; one example incorporated in recent guidelines developed by the British Committee for Standard in Haematology and the British Transplantation Society is illustrated (Table 136-1).

EPIDEMIOLOGY

Thrombotic Thrombocytopenic Purpura

Idiopathic TTP (not precipitated by a defined event or exposure) occurs with an estimated annual incidence of 3.7 to 11 cases per million, but it appears to be increasing, perhaps the result of increased awareness. TTP has a female/male ratio of 3 : 2 and a peak incidence in the fourth decade. Additional risk factors include obesity and African ancestry, which is also associated with an increased risk for relapse. Nonidiopathic TTP (defined as TTP associated with a known precipitant, such as hematopoietic stem cell transplant [HSCT]) appears to be more common. TTP occurs in 1 in 1600 to 1 in 5000 individuals treated wih ticlopidine. In contrast, the estimated incidence of TTP is 12 per million clopidogrel-treated patients. Other drugs associated with nonidiopathic TTP include the calcineurin inhibitors gemcitabine and mitomycin-C, as well as quinine, cyclosporine, and tacrolimus.

HSCT-associated TTP affects between 0.5% and 76% of transplant patients. The wide variation in incidence likely reflects diagnostic uncertainty and a lack of universally accepted criteria, as well as the effects of posttransplant infection, DIC, and other morbidities that mimic TTP. Pregnancy is another common precipitating factor for TTP (12% to 31% of individuals). TTP develops most frequently in the second or third trimester, with the decrease in ADAMTS13 levels and increase in von Willebrand factor (vWF) and factor VIII that occur in normal pregnancy perhaps acting as precipitants. TTP has also been reported in approximately 0.3% of HIV-infected patients, usually in those with advanced disease.

Congenital TTP, also known as *Upshaw-Schülman syndrome,* is considerably less common than idiopathic TTP. A recent study describing the natural history of congenital TTP in Japan identified 43 cases ranging in age from childhood to 79 years. Of these cases, 42% were diagnosed during childhood, 36% between the ages of 15 and 45 (all female, most commonly presenting during pregnancy), and 12% beyond age 45.

Hemolytic Uremic Syndrome

Two primary variants of HUS are described based on epidemiologic patterns. Most common is "typical" HUS, often referred to as *Stx-HUS* because of its association with infection by bacteria that express Shiga or Shiga-like toxins. "Atypical" HUS may occur in sporadic or familial patterns.

Stx-HUS

Stx-HUS ("typical," "epidemic," "childhood," diarrhea-associated, or Shiga toxin–producing *E. coli* [STEC]–associated) accounts for at least 90% of all cases. In one study conducted in the United States, the median age of patients with Stx-HUS was 4 years; 55% of patients were younger than 5 years of age, 33% between 5 and 17 years, 6% between 18 and 44 years, and 6% older than 45 years of age. STEC accounts for 80% to 86% of cases in the United States and Europe. The major reservoir of STEC is domestic cattle; approximately 2% to 3% harbor STEC in their gastrointestinal tract at the time of slaughter, and meat can become contaminated during processing. The organism has also been isolated from deer, sheep, goats, horses, dogs, birds, and flies. Outbreaks are often associated with ingestion of inadequately cooked ground beef, although contamination of poultry, cheese, fruits, and vegetables has also been reported. Other cases have been attributed to ingestion of contaminated water or unpasteurized apple cider or milk. The incidence of Stx-HUS may be increasing as a result of developments in food-production methods. Industrial farming generates large quantities of potentially contaminated manure that periodically enters streams, where it can contaminate feed and uncooked vegetables. A recent outbreak of HUS in Northern Germany that affected more than 3000 individuals was caused by STEC O104:H4; the reservoir of pathogenic *E coli* was bean sprouts with evidence of intrahousehold transmission. Carriage of STEC may be asymptomatic, and fecal-oral transmission may contribute to spread in day care centers, nursing homes, and petting zoos. Aerosolization in barns has been implicated in outbreaks at fairs.

The relationship of Stx to human disease was first recognized in 1983 based on the identification of *E. coli* strain O157:H7 as the cause of two outbreaks of hemorrhagic gastroenteritis. Over 100 additional STEC strains have been identified. STEC strains are also associated with sporadic, nonepidemic cases of HUS. The disease occurs more frequently during summer and autumn in temperate climates. Infection by Shiga toxin–producing *Shigella dysenteriae* serotype 1 is associated with HUS in developing countries and carries a higher mortality.

Table 136-1 Proposed Classification Scheme for Thrombotic Microangiopathies

ADVANCED UNDERSTANDING OF ETIOLOGY
Infection induced
Shiga and verocytotoxin (Shiga-like toxin)–producing bacteria
Streptococcus pneumoniae
Disorders of complement regulation
Genetic disorders of complement regulation
Acquired disorders of complement regulation, for example anti-FH antibody
ADAMTS13 abnormalities
ADAMTS13 deficiency secondary to mutations
Autoantibodies against ADAMTS13
Defective cobalamine metabolism
Quinine induced
ETIOLOGY NOT FULLY UNDERSTOOD
HIV
Malignancy
Drugs
Pregnancy
Systemic lupus erythematosus and antiphospholipid antibody syndrome

Adapted from Taylor CM, Machin S, Wigmore SJ, et al: Clinical Practice Guidelines for the management of atypical haemolytic uraemic syndrome in the United Kingdom. *Br J Haematol* 148:37, 2009.

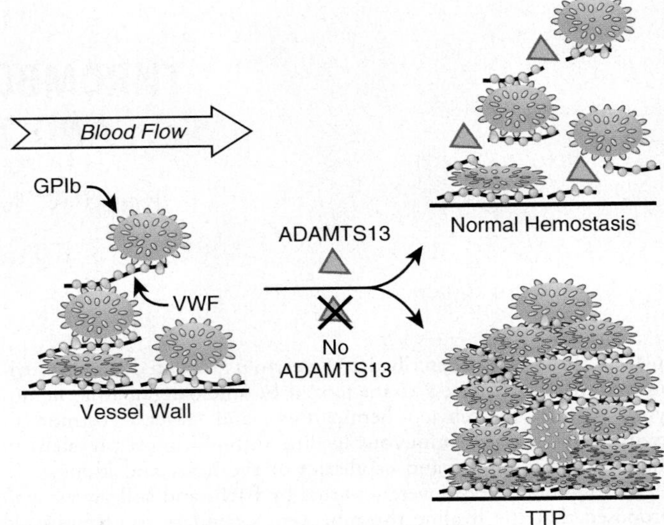

Figure 136-1 PATHOGENESIS OF IDIOPATHIC THROMBOTIC THROMBOCYTOPENIC PURPURA CAUSED BY ADAMTS13 DEFICIENCY. Multimeric vWF adheres to endothelial cells or to connective tissue exposed in the vessel wall. Platelets adhere to vWF through platelet membrane GP1b. In flowing blood, vWF in the platelet-rich thrombus *is stretched* to form extended linear polymers and cleaved by ADAMTS13, limiting thrombus growth. If ADAMTS13 is absent, vWF-dependent platelet accumulation continues, eventually causing microvascular thrombosis and TTP. *(Reproduced from Sadler JE: von Willebrand factor, ADAMTS13, and thrombotic thrombocytopenic purpura.* Blood *112:11, 2008, with permission.)*

Atypical HUS (aHUS)

aHUS is a form of systemic TMA in which renal failure develops in the absence of an obvious precipitating factor. Although sometimes referred to as "adult" HUS, 60% of cases occur in children. However, aHUS only accounts for 5% to 10% of all childhood HUS. Seventy percent of children have their first episode before 2 years of age, 25% of these developing before 6 months, an age at which Stx-HUS is very uncommon. Childhood aHUS is equally prevalent in males and females, with a slight female preponderance in adults. Though aHUS is generally not associated with a prodrome of bloody diarrhea, a history of recent gastroenteritis may be obtained from up to 30% of patients. Abnormalities in complement regulation, most commonly due to mutations in complement regulatory proteins, have been implicated in 70% of cases. Inheritance is autosomal with approximately 50% penetrance. TMA that complicates bone marrow transplantation, immunosuppressive medication, and chemotherapy resembles aHUS, although it is likely that the pathogenesis of these other disorders differs.

Though aHUS is less common than TTP, the fact that up to 16% of patients included in large TTP series required dialysis demonstrates that these disorders can be indistinguishable on clinical grounds. The incidence of aHUS in the United States has been estimated at 2 per million. More than 1000 patients with aHUS investigated for complement abnormalities have been identified through registries in Europe and the United States.

PATHOBIOLOGY

TMA is a syndrome in which different pathogenic pathways lead to vascular endothelial injury. In Stx-HUS, endothelial injury is caused by Shiga toxin and inflammatory cytokines, perhaps inciting disease with increased frequency in individuals with specific genetic predispositions. In most patients with TTP or aHUS, an inciting event may not be obvious but may involve viral infections, surgery, or other perturbations in vascular function and inflammation.

TTP

Most patients with TTP exhibit inherited or acquired deficiency of ADAMTS13, leading to increased levels of "unusually large" vWF multimers that induce platelet aggregation in the microvasculature. Endothelial cells secrete unusually large vWF multimers that may adhere to cell surfaces and promote platelet attachment or enter the circulation and promote intravascular platelet aggregation. Under high shear, vWF multimers elongate along the endothelium and promote platelet adhesion through interactions with platelet glycoprotein (GP) Ib; shear stress–induced conformational changes also enhance the susceptibility of vWF to enzymatic cleavage. ADAMTS13 regulates the activity of vWF by cleaving the most hemostatically active high-molecular-weight multimers; failure of this feedback mechanism may lead to the microvascular thrombosis, tissue ischemia, and infarction characteristic of TTP (Fig. 136-1). However, the factors that trigger sporadic episodes of TTP by causing endothelial damage or activation remain undefined. Moreover, some patients develop TTP despite normal levels of circulating ADAMTS13, while patients with congenital deficiencies of ADAMTS13 may not develop TTP until adulthood, or not at all. The latter observations suggest that ADAMTS13 deficiency should be considered an important predisposing factor, but not the sole cause of this syndrome. This concept is supported by studies of ADAMTS13-deficient mice, in which a TTP-like syndrome develops spontaneously in some genetic backgrounds (high vWF levels) but requires a triggering factor, such as Shiga toxin, in other strains.

Inherited ADAMTS13 Deficiency

Upshaw-Schülman syndrome is an autosomal recessive form of TTP first linked to vWF by Moake, who found unusually large vWF multimers in the plasma of patients with chronic relapsing TTP. He proposed that the patients lacked a plasma enzyme that cleaves these unusually large multimers and that the abnormal multimers then caused uncontrolled intravascular platelet aggregation, thrombosis, and tissue infarction. Subsequently, a plasma metalloprotease was discovered that degrades vWF multimers by cleaving the Tyr[1605]-Met[1606] bond in the vWF subunit that is lacking in patients with Upshaw-Schülman syndrome.

The vWF protease has been purified from plasma, cloned, and found to be a member of the ADAMTS (a disintegrin-like and metalloprotease [reprolysin type] with thrombospondin type 1 motif) family of metalloproteases (Fig. 136-2). Genome-wide linkage analysis showed that Upshaw-Schülman syndrome is caused by mutations in the ADAMTS13 gene on chromosome 9q34.

ADAMTS13 is synthesized mainly by hepatic stellate cells but also in vascular endothelial cells and renal glomerular podocytes. Small amounts of functional ADAMTS13 are present in platelets. Deletion, splice site, frameshift and missense mutations that cause Upshaw-Schülman syndrome have been found in almost all structural domains of ADAMTS13 (see Fig. 136-2). Expression studies have shown that missense mutations usually prevent the secretion of ADAMTS13, although some also impair catalytic activity.

Acquired ADAMTS13 Deficiency

Almost all patients with nonfamilial, idiopathic TTP have an acquired severe reduction or absence of ADAMTS13 activity (<5%), usually associated with autoantibody IgG inhibitors. Some of the reported variation in ADAMTS13 activity levels may reflect inclusion or exclusion of patients with acute renal failure or other preexisting conditions. For example, severe ADAMTS13 deficiency was found in 18 of 48 adults with idiopathic TMA unselected for renal function, but it was seen in 22 of 22 patients without acute anuric renal failure. Acquired severe ADAMTS13 deficiency (<5%) is rare in other settings, with the possible exception of severe hepatic insufficiency or sepsis. For example, ADAMTS13 levels below 5% were found in 17 of 109 patients with sepsis-induced DIC. More modest decreases (typically >40%) occur in newborns and among adults with cirrhosis, chronic renal insufficiency, pregnancy, connective tissue diseases, and various inflammatory conditions; none had levels below 6%. Therefore severe ADAMTS13 deficiency appears to be specific for TTP in the appropriate clinical setting.

Antibodies against ADAMTS13 have been reported in 59% to 100% of patients with acquired severe ADAMTS13 deficiency. This variability probably reflects differences in assay sensitivity. Some antibodies promote ADAMTS13 clearance without inhibiting activity.

Other Mechanisms of Potential Relevance to TTP

ADAMTS13 levels are normal in some cases of idiopathic TTP, and in almost all cases of TMA associated with stem cell or organ transplantation, cancer, infections, severe hypertension, and certain drugs. Therefore mechanisms other than ADAMTS13 deficiency can cause thrombotic microangiopathy, and various studies have implicated direct endothelial injury, platelet activation, and alterations in blood clotting as contributory factors. Evidence in support of these mechanisms include the demonstration of (1) increased levels of circulating endothelial proteins (thrombomodulin, PAI-1, vWF) and endothelial cell microparticles in TTP plasma; (2) circulating antiplatelet and antiendothelial cell antibodies, some of which may bind CD36 and impair ADAMTS13 binding to endothelial cells; (3) increased levels of circulating platelet-derived microparticles; (4) induction of microvascular endothelial cell apoptosis by plasma from patients with idiopathic, HIV-associated, or ticlopidine-associated TTP; (5) increased

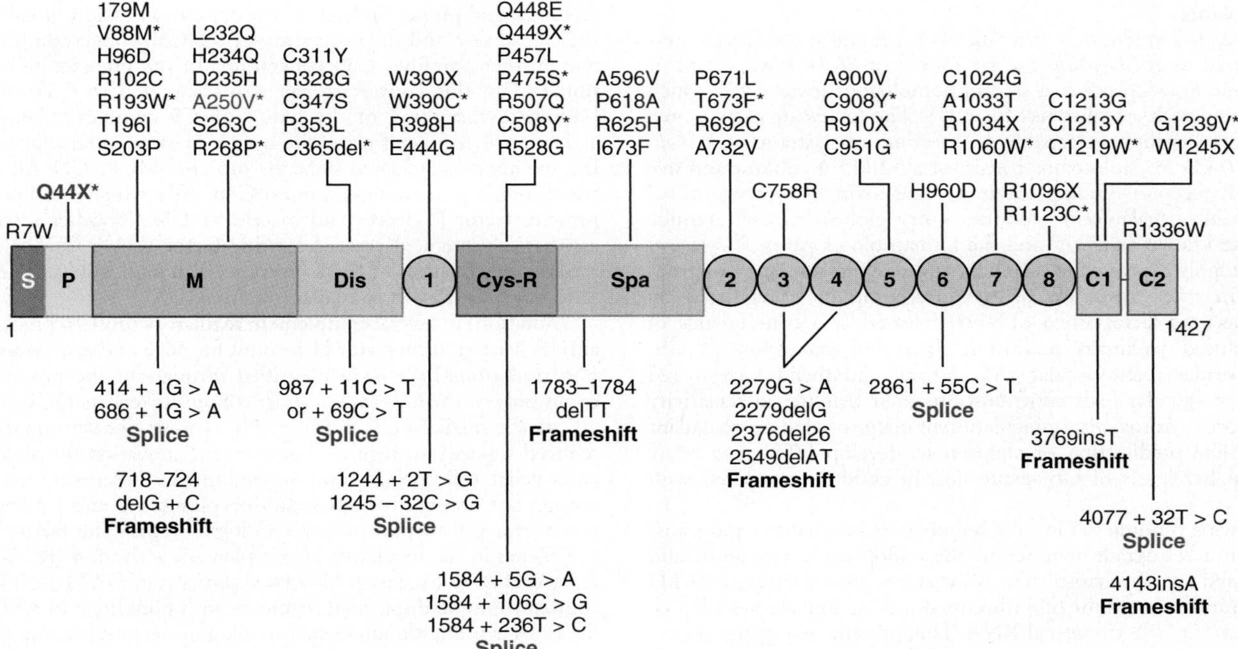

Figure 136-2 ADAMTS13 STRUCTURE AND LOCATION OF THE MUTATIONS FOUND IN PATIENTS WITH CONGENITAL THROMBOTIC THROMBOCYTOPENIC PURPURA. The point mutations that cause single amino acid substitutions and premature stop codons *(X)* are shown above the domain structure of ADAMTS13. The mutations that result in alternative splicing of *ADAMTS13* mRNA or frameshifts are listed under the domain structure of ADAMTS13. Those mutants expressed as recombinant proteins in cell culture *(*)* cause defects in ADAMTS13 secretion *(black)* or catalytic activity *(red)*. S, Signal peptide; P, propeptide; M, metalloprotease; Dis, disintegrin domain; 1, the first thrombospondin type 1 (TSP1) repeat; Cys-R, cysteine-rich domain; Spa, spacer domain; 2 through 8, the second to eighth TSP1 repeats; C1 and C2, the CUB domains 1 and 2. *(Reproduced from Zheng XL, Sadler JE: Pathogenesis of thrombotic microangiopathies.* Annu Rev Pathol *3:249, 2008.)*

plasma procoagulant activity; (6) increased endothelin and decreased nitric oxide, leading to vasoconstriction; and (7) diminished plasma fibrinolytic activity due to elevated levels of PAI-1.

Stx-HUS

HUS is caused by endothelial cell damage initiated by Shiga toxins and the inflammatory cytokines they induce. The type of Stx, as well as other virulence factors, contributes to risk.

The most common serotype of *E. coli* associated with HUS is O157:H7, although other serotypes including O26:H11, O103:H2, O111:NM, O21:H19, O145:NM, and O104:H4 have been reported. Enteropathic *E. coli* bacteria are noninvasive. After ingestion, organisms colonize the terminal ilium and follicle-associated epithelium of Peyer patches, after which they colonize the colon. Cross-talk between STEC and other commensal intestinal flora enhance STEC proliferation; these bacteria also respond to the host hormonal milieu, including elevated levels of epinephrine and norepinephrine that stimulate production of virulence factors by activating bacterial membrane histidine sensor kinases QseC and QseE. Once colonization is established, STEC bacteria express numerous virulence factors by horizontally transmitted gene cassettes termed *pathogenicity islands.* One pathogenicity island contains the locus of enterocyte effacement (LEE), which contains genes for the adhesin intimin, as well as a type III (three) secretion system (TTSS) that mediates transfer of bacterial proteins directly into enterocytes. These and other factors enable enteropathic bacteria to create a zone of tight attachment to the intestinal wall and enhance their proliferation. Their capacity to cause HUS is mediated by two 70-kD bacterial exotoxins named *verotoxins* for their cytotoxicity against African green monkey kidney (Vero) cells. The toxins are transported across the intestinal epithelium through specific para- and intercellular mechanisms and then circulate, most likely by binding with low affinity to the surface of neutrophils and platelets, before being transferred to receptors expressed on glomerular endothelial cells that are upregulated by proinflammatory cytokines.

Verotoxin-1 is identical to a Shigella toxin and is therefore generally referred to as *Shiga-like toxin 1 (SLT-1* or *Stx1).* Most strains of pathogenic *E. coli* produce a second homologous toxin, Stx2, which is associated with a higher risk for HUS. The toxins are carried on a lysogenic bacteriophage capable of infecting other strains of *E. coli.* Intact, 70-kD Stx holotoxins consist of a 32-kD A subunit and five 7.7-kD B receptor-binding subunits. The toxin binds to terminal Gala1-4Galb (galabiose) residues on globosyltriaosylceramide (Gb_3; also known as *CD77* and the human blood group *P^k antigen*) that are highly expressed on capillary endothelium in the glomerulus and brain; the expression of these receptors is upregulated by tumor necrosis factor-alpha (TNFα) released as a consequence of toxin-induced leukocyte activation. Increased expression of Gb_3 on glomerular microvascular and cerebral endothelium compared with other vascular beds contributes to their heightened sensitivity to apoptosis, cytotoxicity, upregulation of integrins, and procoagulant activity. The predilection of children to develop HUS may relate to the higher levels of Gb_3 expression in children compared with adults.

Following binding to Gb_3, the holotoxin is internalized and transported in a retrograde manner to the endoplasmic reticulum and translocated into the cytosol. The A subunit is proteolyzed to a 27-kD A1 subunit that binds the 60S ribosomal subunit and cleaves adenine 4323 from the 28S ribosomal RNA. This prevents elongation factor 1-dependent binding of aminoacyl tRNA, which inhibits protein synthesis and leads to endothelial cell apoptosis.

E. coli lipopolysaccharide and Stx also stimulate leukocyte and intrarenal expression of proinflammatory cytokines (including IL-1, -6, and -8; MCP-1; interleukin-1β; and interferon-γ) that exacerbate toxin- and leukocyte-induced endothelial dysfunction. Interactions between endothelial cell fractalkine and mononuclear leukocytes expressing the fractalkine receptor, CX(3)CR1, may play an important role in renal damage. Stx also acts in concert with lipopolysaccharide to trigger a procoagulant state early in the course of the disease that involves platelet activation, expression of tissue factor, release of unusually large vWF multimers, and elaboration of plasminogen activator-1.

Signal transduction through cross-linked B-unit/CD77 complexes may also contribute to cytotoxicity of the holotoxin. Recent studies demonstrated that both the Stx 1B and 2B subunits directly induce release of vWF from endothelial cells. Though Stx 1B binds Gb_3 with greater affinity than Stx 2B, the latter is a more potent inducer of endothelial cell vWF release, consistent with its ability to activate a different signaling pathway and its ability to induce acute TMA in ADAMTS13−/− mice.

Additional virulence factors, such as a cytolethal distending toxin that may interfere with the endothelial cell cycle, have been described, although their role in pathogenesis is undefined.

Atypical Hemolytic Uremic Syndrome

The pathogenesis of aHUS reflects aberrant activation of the alternative complement pathway leading to endothelial damage, resulting from mutations that lead to loss or functional impairment of complement regulatory proteins, or less commonly, activating mutations in alternative complement proteins. Such mutations have been detected in 70% of patients with aHUS and are transmitted in an autosomal manner, accounting for the commonly observed familial inheritance pattern, although disease penetrance is only 50%.

Complement may be activated via the classical (CP), alternative (AP) or lectin (LP) pathways. The AP plays an important role in protecting the intravascular space against bacterial infection and depends on potent amplification loops (Fig. 136-3). The AP is in a constant low-level activation state due to spontaneous hydrolysis of the thioester bond in C3, and regulation by complement inhibitory proteins is required to prevent pathologic activation and complement-mediated injury to host tissues. C3b is deposited on cell membranes, where an amplification loop consisting of complement factor B, factor D, and properdin leads to the deposition of additional C3b on the cell surface and the generation of the C3b convertase (C3bBbP) that further amplifies C3b generation. In the presence of an additional C3b, this convertase can also cleave C5 to C5a and C5b, leading to formation of the lytic C5b-C9 complex. Complement activation is regulated primarily by the plasma protein factor H, or the membrane-associated cofactor protein (MCP; CD46), each of which binds to membrane bound C3b, after which another plasma protein, factor I, cleaves and inactivates C3b. Another membrane-associated protein, decay-accelerating factor (DAF; CD55) accelerates the inactivation of C3 convertase, although mutations of DAF have not been shown to play a role in aHUS.

Mutations in several complement regulatory proteins predispose to aHUS. Mutations in factor H account for 30% of cases. Loss of function mutations have been identified throughout the protein, most commonly in the C-terminal short consensus repeats (SCRs) 19 and 20, which mediate cell binding (Fig. 136-4). These mutants have reduced capacity to regulate complement activation on platelet and endothelial cell surfaces and subendothelial basement membrane, though not necessarily in plasma; thus plasma C3 and C4 levels may not mirror cell surface pathophysiologic events. The factor H gene *(CFH)* lies in the regulators of complement activation (RCA) cluster at 1q32 close to five factor H–related proteins (*CFHR* 1-5). The latter contain multiple duplicated segments with homology to *CFH.* Thus the RCA is prone to nonallelic homologous recombination; this may lead to formation, for example, of a hybrid gene consisting of the first 21 exons of factor H (encoding the first 18 SCRs) and the last 2 exons of CFHR1 (encoding SCR 19 and 20), which has been associated with aHUS. In addition to genetic abnormalities of factor H, acquired deficiencies account for 5% to 10% of aHUS; these are most commonly due to inhibitory antibodies that recognize SCR 19 and 20 of factor H and occur in patients with deletions of *CFHR1* and *CFHR3.* The autoantibodies may cross react with factor H SCR 19 and 20 and CFHR1 SCR 4 and 5, which share extensive homology.

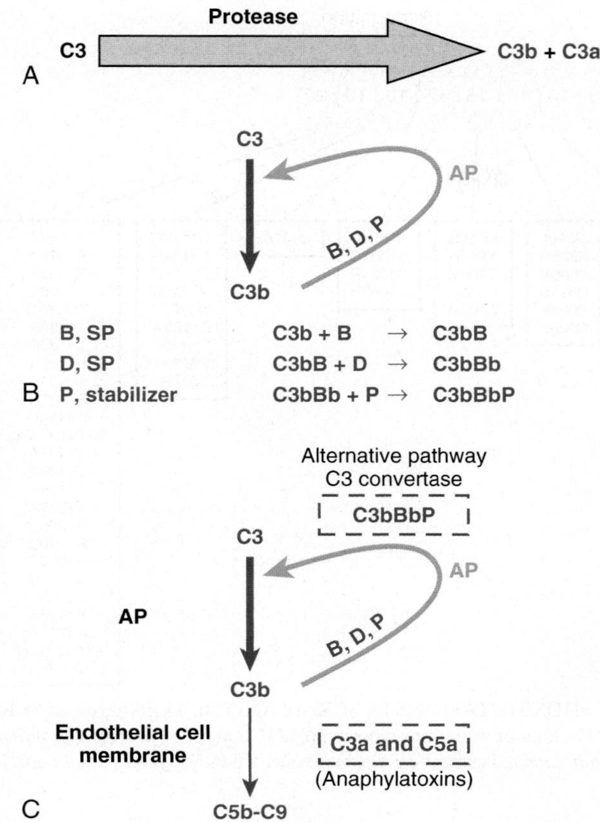

Figure 136-3 THE ALTERNATIVE PATHWAY OF COMPLEMENT ACTIVATION. **A,** The AP of the complement system originally consisted of a serine protease that cleaved C3 to the opsonin C3b and the proinflammatory anaphylatoxin C3a. **B,** An amplification loop was next evolved to more efficiently deposit C3b on a target and liberate C3a into the surrounding milieu. *B* indicates factor B; *D* indicates factor D, a serine protease; *P* indicates properdin, a stabilizer of the enzyme. **C,** Development of a C5 convertase. The same enzyme that cleaves C3 (AP C3 convertase) can cleave C5 to C5a and C5b with the addition of a second C3b to the enzyme complex (AP C5 convertase). *(From Liszewski MK, Atkinson JP: Too much of a good thing at the site of tissue injury: The instructive example of the complement system predisposing to thrombotic microangiopathy.* Hematology Am Soc Hematol Educ Program *2011:9, 2011, with permission.)*

Mutations in MCP are observed in approximately 15% of patients with aHUS. MCP is present on the surface of all nucleated cells except erythrocytes. Mutations are found throughout the protein (Fig. 136-5) and most commonly lead to diminished cell surface expression, although some impair protein activity.

MCP and factor H bind C3b and facilitate its cleavage on the cell membrane by factor I. Factor I mutations are observed in approximately 12% of aHUS patients, most commonly resulting in decreased protein expression, although some mutations cause decreased catalytic activity, which is mediated through the factor I light chain.

Activating mutations in factor B and C3 are observed in approximately 3% and 10% of aHUS patients, respectively. Mutations in factor B lead to enhanced formation or greater stability of the C3 convertase on cell surfaces. Mutations in C3 may result in enhanced resistance to regulation. Mutations in thrombomodulin, which block the ability to accelerate factor I–mediated inactivation of C3b, have also been observed in several patients.

The basis for incomplete penetrance of aHUS is not understood. Identified precipitating factors include infection, pregnancy, and additional single nucleotide genetic polymorphisms and haplotypes in complement regulatory genes. Approximately 20% of patients harbor more than one mutation in complement regulatory genes. The cause of aHUS in the 30% of patients with no identified complement protein mutations remains uncertain.

Clinical Manifestations of Thrombotic Microangiopathies

By definition, microangiopathic hemolytic anemia and thrombocytopenia are cardinal signs/features of all TMA syndromes. However, some syndromes display relatively specific features that may help in their identification.

TTP

The classic pentad of signs and symptoms that compose the TTP syndrome include microangiopathic hemolytic anemia (MAHA), thrombocytopenia, neurologic impairment, fever, and renal dysfunction. In early studies, approximately 75% of patients presented with a triad of MAHA, neurologic impairment, and thrombocytopenic purpura. However, earlier recognition and the established efficacy of plasma exchange have led to the appreciation that MAHA and thrombocytopenia, in the absence of an obvious precipitating condition, are sufficient to make a presumptive diagnosis of TTP. Indeed, the evolution of this diagnostic approach has led to a significant increase in the use of plasma exchange, and it is likely that TTP is now as frequently overdiagnosed as underdiagnosed.

Approximately 10% to 40% of patients with TTP recall an upper respiratory tract infection or flu-like syndrome in the weeks preceding diagnosis. Patients may present with malaise, fatigue, fever, or other nonspecific symptoms of days to weeks duration unresponsive to antibiotics or symptomatic management. The diagnosis of TTP may be overlooked until these prodromal symptoms become unrelenting or neurologic dysfunction develops. Neurologic symptoms ranging from headache and confusion to somnolence, seizures, aphasia, or coma often dominate the clinical picture in TTP and may fluctuate in severity, a characteristic attributed to the repetitive formation and dissolution of thrombi in the cerebral microvasculature. Other less common symptoms are abdominal pain and respiratory distress. Thrombocytopenia may be severe, with platelet counts below 20,000/μL, and mucocutaneous bleeding is common.

Stx-HUS

Stx-HUS occurs most commonly after *E. coli* O157:H7–induced gastroenteritis, with rare cases reported after infection of the urinary tract or skin, or infection with non-*E. coli* organisms. The disease begins with the sudden onset of abdominal pain and watery diarrhea, on average 3.7 days (range, 2-12 days) after toxin exposure. Abdominal pain may be severe and precede the onset of diarrhea. This presentation, particularly in the absence of fever, may be difficult to differentiate from inflammatory bowel disease, appendicitis, ischemic colitis, or intussusception. Bloody diarrhea generally ensues on the second day, accompanied in some cases by nausea and vomiting, though up to one-third of patients do not report blood in the stool. Fever is typically absent or mild. Colonoscopy reveals edematous colonic mucosa, with occasional ulceration and pseudomembrane formation. Thumbprinting in the distal ascending and proximal transverse colon, suggesting ischemic colitis, may be seen on barium enema and is attributed to exotoxin-induced thrombi in the microvasculature of the bowel wall.

E. coli–associated hemorrhagic gastroenteritis is complicated by HUS in 8% to 18% of sporadic cases, and over 20% in certain epidemic outbreaks. Thus the disease should be suspected in a patient who presents with characteristic clinical manifestations after an episode of bloody diarrhea, although the prototypic history of a preceding hemorrhagic gastroenteritis may be absent in up to 30%

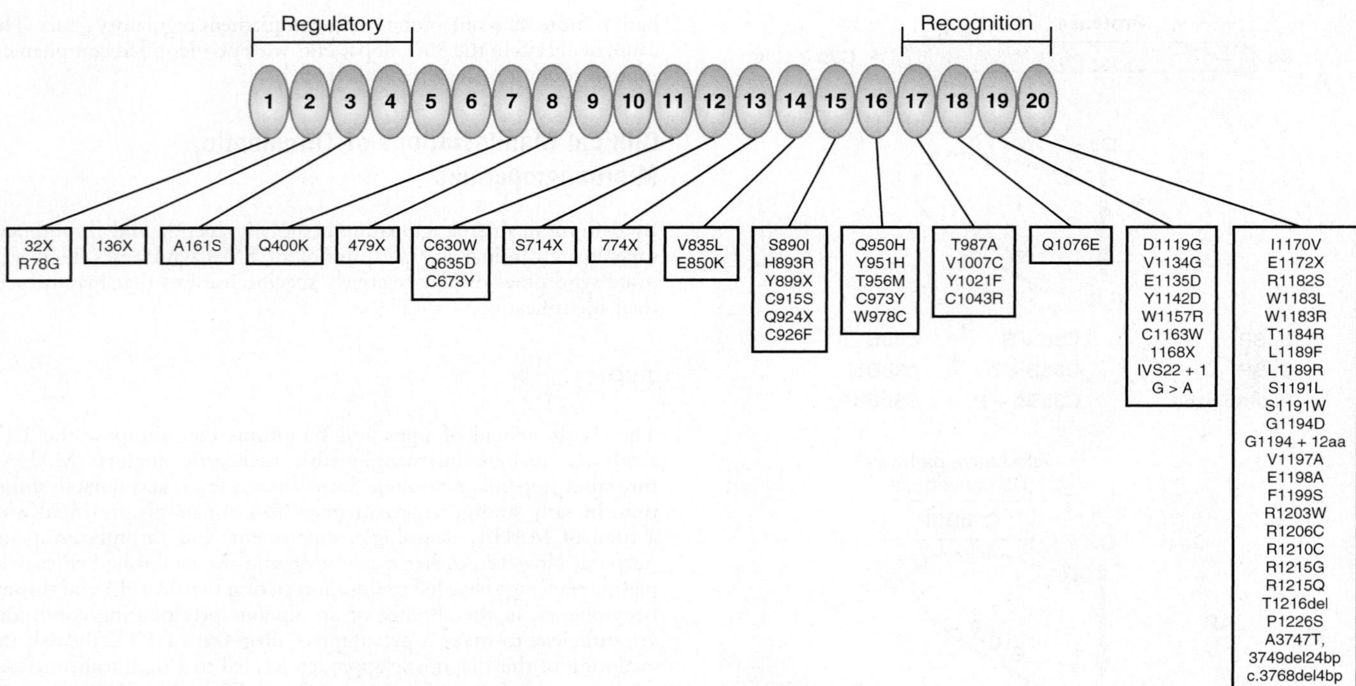

Figure 136-4 FACTOR H CONSISTS OF 20 SCRs, WITH THE MAJORITY OF aHUS MUTATIONS IN SCRs 19 AND 20. The N-terminal SCRs form the regulatory domain, and the C-terminal SCRs form the recognition domain. The sites of mutations reported in aHUS are shown. *(Reproduced from Kavanagh D, Goodship THJ: Atypical hemolytic uremic syndrome, genetic basis, and clinical manifestations.* Hematology Am Soc Hematol Educ Program *2011:15, 2011, with permission.)*

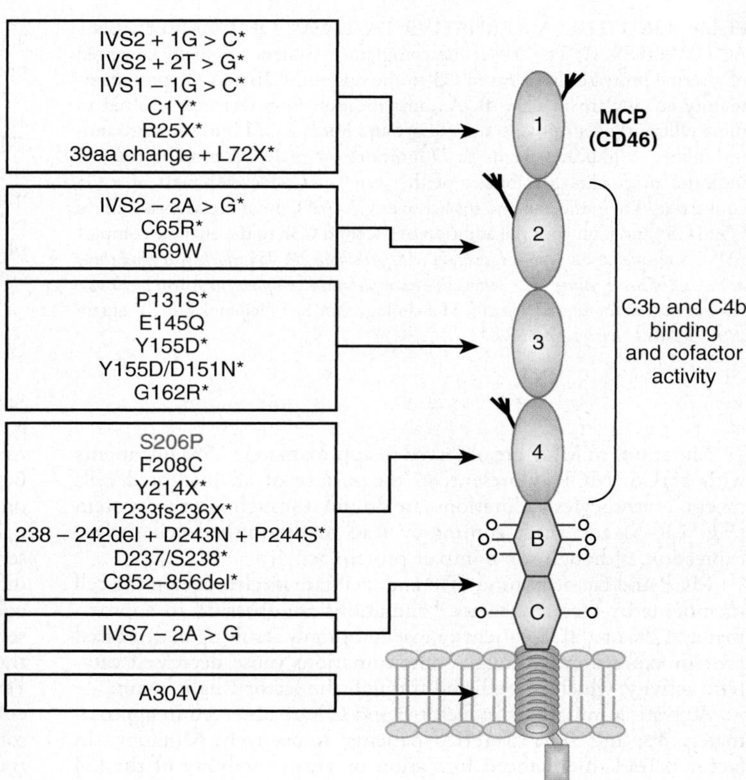

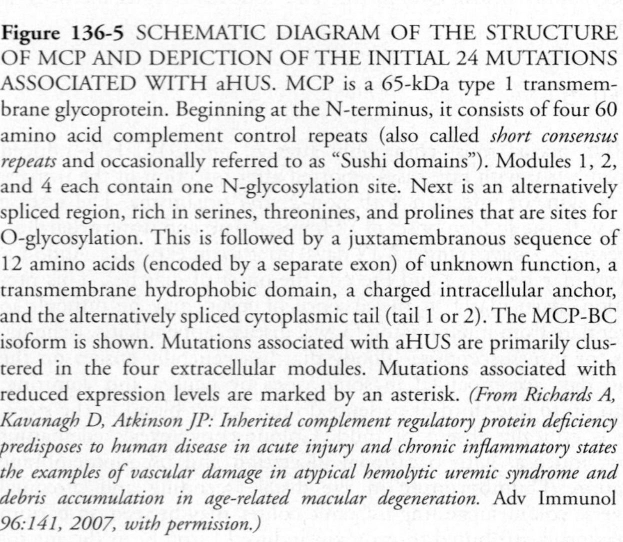

Figure 136-5 SCHEMATIC DIAGRAM OF THE STRUCTURE OF MCP AND DEPICTION OF THE INITIAL 24 MUTATIONS ASSOCIATED WITH aHUS. MCP is a 65-kDa type 1 transmembrane glycoprotein. Beginning at the N-terminus, it consists of four 60 amino acid complement control repeats (also called *short consensus repeats* and occasionally referred to as "Sushi domains"). Modules 1, 2, and 4 each contain one N-glycosylation site. Next is an alternatively spliced region, rich in serines, threonines, and prolines that are sites for O-glycosylation. This is followed by a juxtamembranous sequence of 12 amino acids (encoded by a separate exon) of unknown function, a transmembrane hydrophobic domain, a charged intracellular anchor, and the alternatively spliced cytoplasmic tail (tail 1 or 2). The MCP-BC isoform is shown. Mutations associated with aHUS are primarily clustered in the four extracellular modules. Mutations associated with reduced expression levels are marked by an asterisk. *(From Richards A, Kavanagh D, Atkinson JP: Inherited complement regulatory protein deficiency predisposes to human disease in acute injury and chronic inflammatory states the examples of vascular damage in atypical hemolytic uremic syndrome and debris accumulation in age-related macular degeneration.* Adv Immunol *96:141, 2007, with permission.)*

of cases. Young children and older adults are at greatest risk, perhaps in part because of slower clearance of the organism from the gastrointestinal tract. HUS typically develops 7 days (range, 5-13 days) after the onset of diarrhea. Patients often present with oliguria or other evidence of renal impairment; 50% of patients require dialysis, at least temporarily. The severity of MAHA varies considerably, but many affected individuals require red cell transfusions. Thrombocytopenia is common, with a median platelet count of 30,000/μL in one study, but may be mild or absent in up to 30% of cases at presentation. Up to 25% of patients develop neurologic manifestations, which may include irritability and somnolence and less commonly, confusion, paresis, and seizures.

Isolation of patient with Stx-HUS should be considered, because shedding of the pathogenic bacterium may continue for prolonged periods after cessation of diarrhea.

Atypical HUS

Like TTP, aHUS may present with a prodrome suggestive of an upper respiratory tract infection or nonspecific symptoms of malaise and fatigue, but severe abdominal pain and bloody diarrhea are absent. Neurologic manifestations are typically less common and severe than in TTP and are less likely to dominate the course. MAHA is universal, and the reticulocyte count and LDH concentration are elevated, but severe thrombocytopenia is less common than in TTP. aHUS does not display the seasonal variability characteristic of Stx-HUS. Renal involvement is more severe than in TTP, with up to 60% of patients requiring dialysis.

aHUS typically runs a chronic relapsing course, often complicated by hypertension and renal insufficiency. This disorder may resemble TMAs associated with pregnancy, cancer, and chemotherapy, which have similar clinical presentations, but different natural histories. Moreover, exacerbations are often preceded by infection, pregnancy, or other seemingly incidental events. Penetrance is approximately 50% in families with heterozygous mutations in complement regulatory proteins; thus aHUS may occur in siblings with identical genetic abnormalities at different times, or not at all. The prognosis of patients with factor H or factor I deficiency is poor, with a rate of recurrence and progression to end-stage renal disease or death of 70% in the former, whereas MCP deficiency carries a better prognosis. Aggressive treatment with plasma exchange or plasma infusions of 15 to 20 mL/kg weekly or biweekly may slow the progression of renal failure in some patients. However, there is limited evidence that plasma therapy or immunosuppression affects the clinical course.

Affected patients have a high risk for recurrence after renal allografting, and HUS occasionally presents in related donors after surgery. Since factor H is a soluble blood protein, factor H deficiency or dysfunction is not corrected by renal allografting, and HUS often recurs in the transplanted kidney, especially those from related donors.

Laboratory Manifestations of Thrombotic Microangiopathies

With improved understanding of the pathogenesis of TMA, laboratory evaluation is becoming increasingly important. Though the initial diagnosis of these disorders remains based on clinical features, the CBC, and peripheral blood film, faster turnaround times for laboratory studies, such as determination of ADAMTS13 levels, may improve diagnosis and management.

TTP

The presence of schistocytes on the peripheral blood smear is a characteristic laboratory finding of TTP (Fig. 136-6), although these may not be apparent in rare patients at disease onset. The markedly elevated levels of plasma lactate dehydrogenase (LDH) typically seen in patients with TTP reflect both hemolysis and tissue ischemia. Nucleated red blood cells are present in many patients, and their number may be disproportionately increased in comparison to the degree of reticulocytosis. With rare exceptions, the direct antiglobulin test is negative. The prothrombin time, partial thromboplastin time, and fibrinogen levels are usually normal or only mildly perturbed; mild elevations in fibrinogen degradation products occur in 50% of patients though more sensitive assays, such as those for prothrombin fragment 1+2. Thrombin-antithrombin and plasmin-antiplasmin complexes often demonstrate low-grade activation of coagulation and fibrinolytic pathways. Evidence of renal involvement may include hematuria, proteinuria, granular or red cell casts, and mild azotemia, though anuria and renal failure are uncommon presenting features. A severe deficiency (<5%) of ADAMTS13 in the appropriate clinical setting is considered diagnostic of TTP, though TTP is not excluded by a normal or only moderately decreased level (see box on ADAMTS13 in the Management of TTP).

The prototypic vascular lesions of TTP are characterized by platelet-rich thrombi within or beneath damaged endothelium. Involved microvascular endothelial cells are swollen and in some cases detached. The subendothelium contains hyaline material that is relatively poor

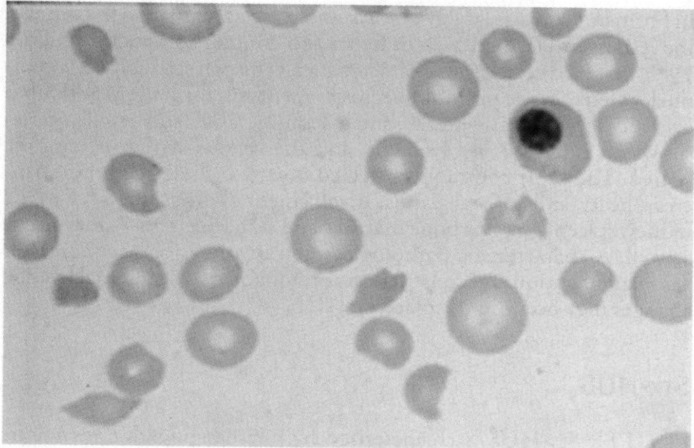

Figure 136-6 THIS PERIPHERAL BLOOD FILM WAS OBTAINED FROM A 28-YEAR-OLD WOMAN WHO PRESENTED WITH FEVER, EPISTAXIS, AND ALTERED MENTAL STATUS. Note the absence of platelets and the presence of a nucleated erythrocyte and schistocytes *(arrows)*, consistent with a microangiopathic process.

ADAMTS13 in the Management of TTP

A role for vWF in the pathogenesis of TTP was suspected in the early 1980s, when reports describing the presence of ultralarge vWF multimers in the plasma of affected patients first appeared. This finding led to the hypothesis that TTP might result from deficiency of a protease responsible for vWF cleavage, and almost 20 years later, the vWF cleaving protease was isolated and found to be deficient in most patients with TTP. This protease was subsequently cloned, found to be a member of the ADAMTS metalloprotease family, and denoted ADAMTS13. This advance raised expectations that a simple and accurate diagnostic test would soon be available for the diagnosis of TTP. However, the utility of ADAMTS13 testing remains undefined, due in part to issues such as a lack of assay standardization and the use of different inclusion criteria in studies that have assessed the relevance of ADAMTS13 measurements. Despite these obstacles, areas where this assay may be useful have begun to emerge. First, for patients with thrombotic microangiopathy, severe ADAMTS13 deficiency is specific for idiopathic TTP but may also occur, albeit uncommonly, in other disorders such as sepsis-induced DIC or severe liver failure. Thus although severe ADAMTS13 deficiency is consistent with TTP, it is not diagnostic in the absence of other clinical information. Moreover, normal or moderately reduced ADAMTS13 levels (20% to 40%) do not exclude the diagnosis of TTP. Second, severe ADAMTS13 deficiency at presentation correlates with an increased risk for relapsing TTP, approximately 30% during 2 years of follow-up. Conversely, patients without severe ADAMTS13 deficiency at presentation rarely relapse. Third, persistence or recurrence of severe ADAMTS13 deficiency further increases the risk for relapse, suggesting that monitoring ADAMTS13 activity may prove useful to select patients for additional intensive therapy. However, because these relationships are based on relatively small case series, they require validation in larger, prospective studies.

in fibrin but consists largely of vWF and platelet remnants. In contrast, the lesions of HUS are rich in fibrin and contain comparatively little vWF. Involved vessel walls characteristically display a paucity of mononuclear leukocytes; fibrinoid necrosis, aneurysm formation, and other evidence of vasculitis are absent. Medium- and large-sized arteries show less extensive involvement, and the venous system is typically spared. The most commonly affected organs include the brain, pancreas, heart, and adrenal glands. Involvement of other sites such as the kidney, spleen, gingiva, bone marrow, and skin (Fig. 136-7) may occur as well. A characteristic pathologic lesion involving adjacent areas of vascular dilatation and constriction accompanied by segmental hyaline changes may occur in the placenta.

Stx-HUS

Like TTP, Stx-HUS is characterized by microangiopathic hemolytic anemia and thrombocytopenia. A preceding history of gastroenteritis is common. Thrombocytopenia tends to be less severe than in TTP, and renal disease is the major clinical manifestation.

Renal biopsy, although rarely required for diagnosis in endemic areas, highlights the importance of endothelial damage. Involved glomeruli show widening of the subendothelial space, which is filled with cellular debris and fibrin. Glomerular capillary endothelial cells are swollen and occasionally detached, leading to obliteration of the capillary lumens.

Though clinical features are often sufficient for the diagnosis of Stx-HUS, bacteriologic confirmation should be sought through stool cultures, testing for Stx toxin, and acute and convalescent serologies. Stool should be tested as soon as possible after the onset of diarrhea. The recovery rate for STEC appears to be at least 90% during the first 6 days but less than 33% thereafter. *E. coli* O157:H7 ferments sorbitol slowly, appearing as colorless overnight colonies on sorbitol-MacConkey agar; sorbitol-negative cultures may be characterized further using commercially available O157:H7-specific antisera. Methods to detect Stx toxins or their structural genes improve diagnostic sensitivity and also can detect the rare sorbitol-fermenting O157:H7, as well as non-O157:H7 STEC. However, the risk for developing HUS associated with non-O157:H7 STEC varies and is often relatively low.

Antibody titers against *E. coli* O157:H7 antigens and Stx rise after infection, persist for 8 to 12 weeks, and may be useful to confirm STEC infection in selected cases; however, they are not widely available.

Atypical HUS

aHUS is characterized by microangiopathic hemolytic anemia and thrombocytopenia. Compared with TTP, thrombocytopenia and anemia may be less severe and renal insufficiency more prominent. Before the realization that complement activation plays a prominent role in most cases of aHUS, this disorder was primarily diagnosed clinically. However, recent guidelines have emphasized the importance of laboratory studies to diagnose aHUS and distinguish it from other thrombotic microangiopathies.

Diagnosis of aHUS requires several criteria, including: (1) the absence of other diseases associated with TMA, (2) no criteria for

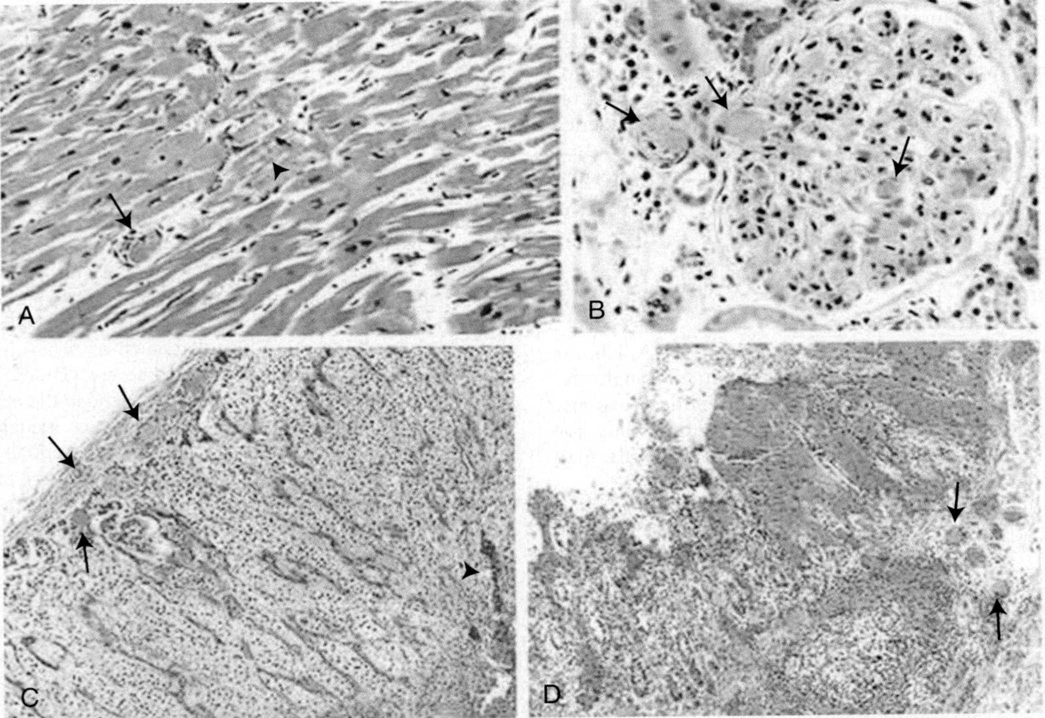

Figure 136-7 TISSUE SPECIMENS OBTAINED AT AUTOPSY FROM A PATIENT WITH ABNORMALITIES CHARACTERISTIC OF THROMBOTIC THROMBOCYTOPENIC PURPURA. A specimen from the heart **(A)** shows multiple intramyocardial microthrombi (*arrow*), hemorrhage, and early ischemic changes, with scattered foci of contraction-band necrosis (*arrowhead*). A specimen from the kidney **(B)** shows characteristic microthrombi in an afferent arteriole, the glomerular hilum, and glomerular capillaries (*arrows*), with vascular congestion and parenchymal hemorrhage in the surrounding interstitium. A tissue specimen from the adrenal gland **(C)** shows characteristic subcapsular microthrombi (*arrows*), with congestion of cortical arterioles and medullary parenchymal hemorrhage *(arrowhead)*. A specimen from the cecum **(D)** shows submucosal microthrombi *(arrows)* and hemorrhagic mucosal ulceration and necrosis. Microthrombi were also present in the pancreas, thyroid gland, and other organs. *(Reproduced from George, JN: Thrombotic thrombocytopenic purpura.* N Engl J Med *354:1927, 2006, with permission. Photographs and interpretation by Patrick Stangeby.)*

Stx-HUS (negative stool culture and Stx assays), and (3) no criteria for TTP (ADAMTS13 >10%). In addition, the complement system should be studied, since abnormalities of complement regulation are involved in at least 70% of cases. Real-time measurement of complement and complement inhibitory proteins are available in a few clinical laboratories. Investigations should include measurement of C3 and C4, as well as factors H, I, and B. MCP (CD46) can and should be measured on circulating mononuclear cells, and plasma should be screened for anti–factor H antibodies. Finally, mutation analyses of the nine genes that have been implicated in the pathogenesis of aHUS (CFH, CFI, C3, MCP, CFB, THBD, deletions of CFH1 and CFH3, or CFH1 and CFH4) should be pursued. The frequency of low C3 levels varies depending on the type of gene mutation present; C3 is reduced in essentially all patients with CFB mutations but in only 30% to 50% of patients with CFH mutations. Plasma concentrations of complement and complement inhibitory proteins in various subgroups of aHUS classified by mutation are shown in Table 136-2.

Differential Diagnosis

The differential diagnosis of MAHA and thrombocytopenia is extensive. Vascular damage secondary to systemic lupus erythematosus, scleroderma, septic or tumor emboli, immune complex-mediated vasculitis (e.g., infective endocarditis), malignant hypertension, cryoglobulinemia, or infection with rickettsial or, more rarely, hemorrhage-inducing viral organisms, may all mimic thrombotic microangiopathy. TMA may also be superimposed on preexisting immune vascular disorders such as systemic lupus erythematosus or the antiphospholipid syndrome (see Chapter 143). Occasional patients with disseminated intravascular coagulation secondary to malignancy or sepsis present with microangiopathy of sufficient severity to be confused with primary TMA (see Chapter 141). In the setting of renal transplantation, a biopsy may be required to distinguish TMA from allograft rejection or recurrence of a preexisting renal vascular disorder. Occasional patients present with acute pancreatitis, acute respiratory distress syndrome, memory and personality changes, or other poorly defined neurologic symptoms that themselves have a broad differential diagnosis.

TMA may also occur in other well-defined clinical settings. Some of these are considered part the category of "nonidiopathic TTP" because of their clinical associations, though the pathogenesis of these disorders is generally not well understood and their responses to various therapeutic interventions are not well defined.

Posttransplantation and Cyclosporine

Thrombotic microangiopathies occur most commonly in three transplant-related settings: (1) in association with the use of cyclosporine A (CyA), (2) as recurrent disease after transplantation for a TMA-related disorder, and (3) after hematopoietic stem cell transplantation.

Cyclosporine A

Cyclosporine A is a common cause of drug-induced thrombotic microangiopathy. CyA is cytotoxic to cultured endothelial cells at concentrations similar to the peak plasma levels and tissue concentrations achieved in vivo. Plasma levels of vWF and endothelin-1 are elevated during episodes of nephrotoxicity, consistent with endothelial cell injury. CyA also enhances platelet aggregation and thromboxane release.

TMA occurs in 1% to 5% of renal transplant recipients, as well as in occasional solid organ recipients treated with CyA or tacrolimus. CyA-induced TMA typically develops insidiously with progressive, otherwise unexplained renal insufficiency. MAHA or thrombocytopenia develops in only half these patients and is usually mild. The appearance of the glomerular capillary and arteriolar thrombotic lesions is similar to that in primary cases of TMA. The distinction of CyA-induced TMA from acute tubular necrosis or rejection can often be made only by biopsy, and an unequivocal distinction cannot be established in every case. Broad alloantibody reactivity and coinfection with cytomegalovirus may predispose to CyA-associated TMA.

CyA-induced TMA often responds to a reduction of the dose or temporary discontinuation of CyA. The prognosis is generally good, although some patients develop permanent renal failure. In many patients, CyA can be reintroduced at a lower dose; in others, tacrolimus has been substituted successfully, although the latter may also precipitate thrombotic microangiopathy. The utility of plasma exchange is uncertain.

Renal Transplantation

Approximately 50% of patients with aHUS develop end-stage renal insufficiency and become candidates for renal transplantation. Thrombotic microangiopathy may recur in up to 50% of transplanted kidneys, and 80% to 90% of these grafts will be lost. Recent studies from an Italian registry demonstrated that the risk for aHUS recurrence varies as a function of the complement abnormalities that originally contributed to aHUS. For example, the risk for

Table 136-2 **Plasma Concentration of C3, C4, CFH, CFI, and CFB and Expression of Membrane Cofactor Protein in the Various Subgroups of Atypical Hemolytic Uremic Syndrome**

	Protein Level or Expression					
	C4	**C3**	**CFH**	**CFI**	**CFB**	**MCP**
CFH mutation	N	Normal (decreased)	Normal (decreased)	Normal	Normal (decreased)	Normal
CFI mutation	N	Normal (decreased)	Normal	Normal (decreased)	Normal (decreased)	Normal
MCP mutation	N	Normal (decreased)	Normal	Normal	Normal	Decreased (normal)
CFB mutation	N	Decreased	Normal	Normal	Normal (decreased)	Normal
C3 mutation	N	Decreased	Normal	Normal	Normal (decreased)	Normal
THBD mutation	N	Normal or decreased	ND	ND	ND	Normal
Anti-CFH Ab	N	Decreased (normal)	Normal (decreased)	Normal	Normal (decreased)	Normal

Data from Loirat C, Frémeaux-Bacchi V: Atypical hemolytic uremic syndrome. *Orphanet J Rare Diseases* 6:60, 2011.
Note: Very low C3 levels are observed in patients with homozygous CFH mutation (complete CFH deficiency) or compound heterozygous CFH mutation, and in patients with CFB or C3 gain-of-function mutations. In most of the other patients, C3 concentration is mildly decreased or normal. Undetectable CFH concentrations are observed only in patients with homozygous CFH mutation. Decreased CFH concentration can be observed in patients with heterozygous type 1 *CFH* mutation, and during flares of anti-CFH antibodies-HUS. Decreased C4 plasma levels have been reported in zero to a few patients of the various subgroups.
"Normal" and "Decreased" without parentheses mean most frequently, normal or decreased. "Normal" and "Decreased" within parentheses mean possible, but not frequent. "Normal or decreased" without parentheses means that normal or decreased is equally frequent.
Ab, antibodies; *CFB*, factor B; *CFH*, Factor H; *CFI*, factor I; *ND*, not documented; *THBD*, thrombomodulin.

posttransplant HUS is 75% to 90% in patients with CFH, 45% to 80% in patients with CFI, and 40% to 70% in patients with C3 mutations, respectively. In contrast, the risk for recurrence in individuals with MCP mutations is 0% to 20%, since the transplanted organ provides wild-type MCP. The type of complement mutation is also associated with the timing of recurrence following transplantation. Thus for the hematologist evaluating posttransplant TMA, a careful, multigenerational history must be taken to exclude the possibility of familial TMA, and the possibility of an inherited mutation in complement regulatory genes must be considered.

Hematopoietic Stem Cell Transplantation

TMA occurs in approximately 6% of patients who undergo allogeneic marrow transplantation; the incidence is estimated to be 0.1% to 1% after autologous marrow or stem cell transplantation. Though guidelines have been developed, diagnosis is difficult since schistocytes and thrombocytopenia are common after bone marrow transplantation, and the differential diagnosis of fever, renal failure, and neurologic complications is extensive. The clinical manifestations typically begin months after transplantation. The pathophysiology is assumed to reflect systemic endothelial cell injury from a variety of causes. vWF protease activity may fall after transplantation, but severe deficiency as occurs in TTP is uncommon. Risk factors include use of an unrelated or mismatched donor, total body irradiation as part of the pretransplant conditioning regime, CyA or tacrolimus posttransplant, systemic cytomegalovirus or other infection, older age, female gender, and graft-versus-host disease (GVHD). Systemic microangiopathy is rare, but an intestinal biopsy may be needed to distinguish thrombotic microangiopathy from graft-versus-host disease in patients with refractory diarrhea.

Withdrawal or substitution of another immunosuppressive for CyA, if possible, should be considered, although at the risk for worsening of the underlying GVHD. Alternative causes should be sought, and aggressive treatment of infection and GVHD should be employed in all but the most overt cases. It is difficult to determine the prognosis because of variable inclusion criteria. Although patients may appear to show an initial response to plasma therapy, the effectiveness of plasma exchange has not been established and mortality exceeds 50%, often due to complications of GVHD or opportunistic infection. Defibrotide has been used with reported success in a few cases, and there have been anecdotal successes using rituximab or anti-CD25 antibodies.

Cancer and Chemotherapy-Associated Thrombotic Microangiopathy

TMA may terminate the course of some patients with disseminated malignant neoplasms and large tumor burdens, most commonly adenocarcinoma of the gastrointestinal tract, breast, or lung. Patients generally present with an abrupt onset of moderate to severe MAHA and thrombocytopenia. Renal insufficiency and neurologic dysfunction occur less commonly than in idiopathic or chemotherapy-induced thrombotic microangiopathy and may result from concurrent metabolic disturbances, central nervous system metastases, stroke, or hemorrhage.

The pathogenesis of cancer-associated thrombotic microangiopathy remains poorly understood. Laboratory evidence of DIC is found in 25% to 80% of patients based on findings of elevated fibrin-split products or more sensitive measures of fibrinogen turnover. However, the observation that TMA occurs in only 5% of patients with disseminated malignancy and DIC suggests the involvement of additional factors, such as microvascular occlusion, intimal proliferation induced by tumor emboli within the pulmonary vasculature, or formation of an incompletely endothelialized tumor vasculature that predisposes to platelet adhesion. Severe deficiency of ADAMTS13 is not typical. Survival is generally measured in weeks. The only effective therapy is reduction of the tumor burden, a goal often not attainable. A role for plasma exchange has not been established.

Specific cancer chemotherapeutic agents have also been implicated in the development of TMA. Patients are often receiving therapy for adenocarcinoma at the time TMA develops, making attribution to the neoplasm versus its therapy difficult to determine. However, unlike cancer-associated TMA, most patients with chemotherapy-associated TMA do not have a large tumor burden, and some may be in remission. Mitomycin-C, gemcitabine, cis-platinum, bleomycin, docetaxel, 5-fluourouracil, deoxycoformycin, carboplatin, and interferon-α, either alone or in combination, have been implicated.

Patients with chemotherapy-associated TMA generally present with moderate to severe MAHA, thrombocytopenia, and renal insufficiency (median creatinine value of 4.2 mg/dL). Approximately 15% to 20% of patients develop neurologic dysfunction. A unique feature in some series is noncardiogenic pulmonary edema in over 50% of patients. Pulmonary function may deteriorate rapidly after red blood cell or platelet transfusion, which should be used with caution.

Chemotherapy-associated TMA is presumed to result from direct toxicity to the endothelium. Mitomycin inhibits the production of prostacyclin by umbilical vein endothelium, and infusion of mitomycin-C into the rat kidney induces histologic changes similar to those of chemotherapy-induced TMA. ADAMST13 levels are not severely reduced. Fewer than 20% of affected patients appear to respond to plasma exchange and/or corticosteroids, and more than 50% die within 2 months.

Streptococcus Pneumonia and Disorders of Cobalamin Metabolism

Infection with *S. pneumonia* may lead to desialylation of the glycocalyx of cells that express the Thomsen-Freidenreich (T-F) antigen. A naturally occurring, cold reactive IgM may recognize the exposed antigen, leading to red cell agglutination in vitro. This disorder generally occurs in children less than 2 years of age and is associated with significant mortality. The pathogenesis is not well defined but may involve interactions among the IgM, red cells, platelets, and endothelium. Affected individuals have a positive antiglobulin test.

An autosomal recessive thrombotic microangiopathy associated with disordered cobalamin-C metabolism can occur in individuals during the first weeks to months of life. Deficiency of cobalamin-C may result in markedly elevated levels of homocysteine and methylmalonic acid, which may be responsible for vascular injury. Though many individuals develop a fulminant course leading to death, occasional patients display a more chronic form of the disease later in childhood.

Miscellaneous Drug-Associated Thrombotic Microangiopathy

TMA has been associated uncommonly with more than 50 other drugs, including penicillins, ciprofloxacin, clarithromycin, histamine H_2-receptor antagonists, the Norplant contraceptive, thienopyridines, and others. The mechanisms by which these agents induce TMA may differ, as may the natural history and response to therapy. Whereas mitomycin C, gemcitabine, and CyA appear to induce TMA in a cumulative dose-dependent manner, quinidine and thienopyridines (ticlopidine and clopidogrel) induce thrombotic microangiopathy through either idiosyncratic, immune-mediated mechanisms or acute endothelial toxicity (see Chapter 133).

An association of quinine with thrombotic microangiopathy was first reported by Gottschall and colleagues, who described the course of three patients with a syndrome resembling idiopathic HUS. Patients generally present with severe MAHA, platelet counts below 50,000/μL and renal insufficiency, usually requiring dialysis. Neurologic dysfunction occurs in a minority of patients, it but can be severe; granulocytopenia and lymphopenia have been reported. In earlier reports, the prognosis was favorable once quinine was withdrawn and plasma exchange instituted. However, in another series, 17 of 225 patients with HUS had quinine-associated thrombotic microangiopathy, 4 of whom died, and 7 survivors were left with chronic renal failure. Although this disorder occurs most commonly after the ingestion of quinine tablets, cases have been reported after exposure to quinine in beverages such as tonic water, and the syndrome may recur rapidly upon reexposure. The pathogenesis may involve idiosyncratic, quinine-dependent antibodies reactive with platelet glycoproteins IIb/IIIa and Ib/IX and related antigens on endothelial cells and neutrophils that promote neutrophil aggregation and binding to endothelial cells in a drug-dependent manner.

The thienopyridines are another common cause of drug-induced TTP. TTP occurs in a higher percentage of patients exposed to ticlopidine, with an incidence ranging from 1 : 600 to 1 : 4814 patient exposures in contrast to an estimated incidence of 4 per 1,000,000 to 1 per 8500 to 26,000 exposures in patients taking clopidogrel. No cases of clopidogrel-associated TTP were encountered in the CAPRIE and CURE studies, each of which enrolled more than 6200 patients. Despite the low incidence, the frequency with which clopidogrel is prescribed renders it the most commonly reported drug associated with TTP in the FDA's MedWatch database, accounting for more than 30% of all cases. The pathogenesis and natural history of TTP associated with ticlopidine and clopidogrel differ. Reductions in ADAMTS13 activity below 15% occur in 85% of patients with ticlopidine-associated TTP but in only 15% of patients with clopidogrel-associated TTP. Reduced ADAMTS13 reflects the development of anti-ADAMTS13 antibodies. TTP generally develops within 2 to 12 weeks of starting ticlopidine and responds relatively quickly to plasma exchange. Spontaneous relapses may occur. In contrast, 90% of patients exposed to clopidogrel but only 10% of patients exposed to ticlopidine develop a syndrome characterized primarily by MAHA and renal insufficiency, without severe thrombocytopenia; these individuals have normal levels of ADAMTS13, usually develop disease within the first 2 weeks of exposure, and may require several weeks of plasma exchange to achieve remission. Whether plasma exchange actually improves the clinical outcome is uncertain. Spontaneous relapses are uncommon.

Finally, the increasing use of anti-VEGF antibodies and other VEGF inhibitors has revealed a critical dependence of podocytes and glomerular endothelial cells on VEGF. Toxicity of these agents may include a thrombotic microangiopathy localized primarily to the kidney and manifested mainly by hypertension and proteinuria.

HIV-Associated Thrombotic Microangiopathy

An association between HIV infection and TMA has been recognized since 1984. Before the introduction of highly active antiretroviral therapy in the mid-1990s, TMA occurred in up to 7% of patients hospitalized with HIV infection. Conversely, the incidence of HIV infection in patients with TMA varied from 15% to 50% in endemic areas. Diagnosis was often difficult because fever, anemia, thrombocytopenia, nephropathy, neurologic dysfunction, and elevated LDH levels secondary to lymphoma, drug reactions, or pulmonary infection with *Pneumocystis carinii* occurred commonly in this population. In contrast, TMA is rare in HIV patients who are treated effectively with antiretroviral therapy. TMA that does occur in advanced or untreated HIV patients often responds quickly to the initiation of antiretroviral therapy and can relapse if therapy is discontinued.

In some patients with HIV infection, the associated immune dysfunction may predispose to the formation of autoantibodies against ADAMTS13, with severe ADAMTS13 deficiency and the development of TTP, despite adequate treatment for HIV. These patients may respond to plasma exchange.

PREGNANCY-ASSOCIATED THROMBOTIC MICROANGIOPATHY

The differential diagnosis of MAHA associated with gestation is complex. TMA may be difficult if not impossible to distinguish from other causes of MAHA unique to pregnancy, such as preeclampsia, acute fatty liver associated with DIC, and HELLP syndrome (which stands for hemolysis, elevated liver function tests, and low platelet counts). The severity of the renal and neurologic abnormalities and the time during gestation at which the signs and symptoms of TMA first appear may provide clues needed to prevent critical delays in therapy.

Approximately 10% of cases of idiopathic TTP occur in association with pregnancy. In one series, 40 of 45 cases of TTP in pregnancy were diagnosed antepartum, at a mean gestational age of 23.5 weeks. Additional studies have confirmed that TTP develops frequently in the second trimester, although some studies report more common occurrence in the third, or immediately postpartum. In the absence of appropriate therapy, maternal and fetal mortality approach 90%. There is no evidence that uterine evacuation leads to resolution. ADAMST13 levels fall progressively during pregnancy, but severe deficiency (<5%) is seen only in women with TTP. The prognosis of pregnancy-associated TTP has improved dramatically since the advent of plasma exchange, and continuing pregnancy does not impair response. Many patients carry to term successfully, although the overall risk for fetal loss remains significant.

Up to 20% of patients with chronic, relapsing TTP have recurrences during subsequent pregnancies, whereas recurrence occurs in almost all women with inherited ADAMTS13 deficiency. TTP during pregnancy carries an extremely high risk for fetal loss. Pregnancies in women with congenital ADAMTS13 deficiency have been carried to term successfully by treatment with prophylactic plasma infusions, sometimes combined with aspirin and low-molecular-weight heparin.

aHUS also occurs with increased frequency during pregnancy, and it is likely the underlying disorder previously referred to in various publications as *malignant nephrosclerosis, irreversible postpartum renal failure*, or *postpartum intravascular coagulation*. The disorder primarily affects primiparas who present with MAHA, thrombocytopenia, renal insufficiency and hypertension beginning with a mean time to onset of approximately 26 days after delivery in one series; this later onset may help to distinguish HUS from other causes of pregnancy-associated MAHA and thrombocytopenia, such as preeclampsia and HELLP, which occur late in gestation or soon after parturition. Recent studies have predictably noted a high incidence of complement regulatory protein mutations, particularly factor H, in patients with pregnancy-associated aHUS.

Prognosis

The prognosis for patients with thrombotic microangiopathies varies depending on the etiology and type of underlying genetic lesion, if any. Assuming timely diagnosis and effective therapy at initial presentation, the prognosis of primary TMAs is relatively favorable. For example, although older historic data suggest a response rate in TTP to plasma exchange of approximately 80%, a recent retrospective review of 134 episodes of TTP treated at Johns Hopkins Hospital found an all-cause mortality of only 4%. This apparent improvement in outcome may be generalized and reflects advances in supportive care as well as active therapies. Patients with acquired TTP continue to experience a significant relapse rate of 30% to 50%, though a recent report suggests that this may be reduced by therapy with rituximab during their initial treatment.

Though patients with congenital deficiency of ADAMTS13 may follow a chronic, relapsing course, relapses may be prevented by periodic plasma infusions. Insufficient numbers of patients have been followed to determine whether overall survival is reduced, although a natural history study identified individuals who survived into the seventh to eighth decades.

The outcomes of patients with Stx-HUS are generally favorable, although Stx-HUS remains the most common cause of acute renal failure in children and up to 60% of children require dialysis during the acute phase. However, Stx-HUS is usually self-limited and as a result of advances in supportive care, mortality has been reduced to

3% to 5%, with death usually due to severe involvement of the central nervous system, intestine, or myocardium. Renal insufficiency generally resolves within 2 to 3 weeks, although some patients have prolonged anuria, requiring several months before recovery. Despite a favorable short-term outcome, many children with Stx-HUS develop chronic renal insufficiency over time. In one report of 29 patients with "typical" childhood HUS followed for 15 to 28 years, 7 developed chronic renal failure and 12 developed hypertension, proteinuria, or reduced glomerular filtration rate, whereas only 10 showed no residual abnormalities. Thus 50% to 60% of patients have complete recovery with long-term preservation of renal function. Long-term outcome is worse in those presenting with prolonged anuria, an elevated leukocyte count, elevated levels of prothrombin fragment 1+2, tissue type plasminogen activator and PAI-1, and older age. Proteinuria persisting for more than 1 year after the initial episode of TMA is likewise associated with progressive renal disease. Given recent reports suggesting involvement of complement in the pathogenesis of Stx-HUS as well as aHUS, it is possible that the use of complement inhibitory drugs, such as eculizumab, might further reduce morbidity, though insufficient data are available to validate this hypothesis.

Atypical HUS has been historically associated with a poor prognosis, especially in older adults and those with severe renal dysfunction. The mortality rate approaches 25%, and 50% of surviving patients develop chronic renal insufficiency. However, as appreciation of the central role of complement in aHUS has expanded, prognostication based on genotype is becoming possible. For example, the observation that patients with CFH mutations may display a significant response rate to plasma exchange may explain the long-held but poorly understood clinical observation that a subfraction of aHUS patients do indeed respond to this intervention. Moreover, the recent approval of eculizumab for treatment of aHUS offers a new option (see the Therapy section, later in this chapter).

Pregnancy remains a significant risk factor for both TTP and aHUS, though gestation per se does not affect the response rates to therapy. The outcome of aHUS associated with pregnancy, in particular, has remained poor with mortality rates of as high as 50% and an additional 15% left with chronic renal insufficiency. Recent studies suggest that as in the nonpregnant setting, pregnancy-associated aHUS is closely tied to alternative complement pathway activation, and thus may respond to complement inhibitors.

Of the miscellaneous TMAs discussed in the Differential Diagnosis section earlier, prognosis depends on the underlying predisposition or etiology. Patients with quinine-induced TMA have a significant early mortality, though with appropriate supportive care and treatment of the acute episode, the disorder does not recur without reexposure to quinine. Likewise, TMA associated with CyA may respond to dose reduction or a change to another immunosuppressive agent and thus may be self-limited. Outcomes of patients who develop TMA in the setting of chemotherapy administration or advanced cancer are poor, because the TMA tends to be unrelenting and the comorbidity of the malignancy is significant. TMA associated with HSCT has a particularly poor prognosis, with mortality of 60% to 90%; this reflects an incomplete understanding of pathogenesis, limited response to plasma exchange, and only anecdotal responses to rituximab or anti-CD25 antibodies.

Therapy

Choosing the appropriate therapy depends on accurate diagnosis. However, the severity of thrombocytopenia, renal and neurologic involvement, and ADAMTS13 levels, if available, help to distinguish between TTP and aHUS, whereas the diagnosis of Stx-HUS is based on a compatible history and microbiologic testing. An ADAMTS13 level below 5% in the appropriate clinical context provides strong evidence for a diagnosis of TTP, although TTP should not be excluded in patients with characteristic/prototypic presentation whose levels of ADAMTS13 are not severely reduced.

TTP

The mortality rate of TTP exceeds 90% without therapy. Through the mid-1970s, splenectomy remained the only modality with more than an anecdotal response rate. Prognosis has been dramatically improved since the advent of plasma-based therapy, such that long-term survival now may exceed 90%.

Plasma Therapy

The beneficial effect of plasma therapy in TTP was first noted more than 3 decades ago. The results of a prospective trial reported in 1991 resolved the long-debated issue of the relative efficacy of plasma exchange versus infusion in favor of the former. At 6 months, complete remissions were seen in 78% of patients treated with exchange versus 31% of those treated with plasma infusion. This study did not resolve the question as to whether removal of a disease-inciting agent or replacement of a missing factor accounted for the superior response, particularly because patients in the exchange arm received a threefold greater volume of plasma. Indeed, a retrospective study demonstrated no significant difference in outcome in patients with acquired TTP who received equal volumes of plasma by exchange or infusion. However, the current model for the pathogenesis of acquired idiopathic TTP suggests that plasma exchange is superior because it both removes an IgG inhibitor of ADAMTS13 and replaces the deficient protein. In contrast, plasma infusion suffices for patients with genetic ADAMTS13 deficiency. Large volumes of plasma are more easily administered by exchange, and unless a genetic deficiency of ADAMTS13 has been documented, plasma infusion should be reserved for situations in which exchange is not immediately available. The recovery of ADAMTS13 levels may lag behind other indicators of clinical response, and the utility of monitoring ADAMTS13 levels during treatment has not been established (see box on ADAMTS13 in the Management of TTP).

Treatment is generally initiated with the goal of exchanging 1 to 1.5 plasma volumes (40 to 60 mL/kg) daily, although the optimal regimen has not been determined. The volume of exchange can be increased to 1.5 to 2 plasma volumes daily if the initial response is poor. Neurologic improvement occurs most rapidly, often within hours to days. The serum LDH level typically falls by 50% within 3 days in responders, and the platelet count begins to rise in a mean of 5 days, though normalization may take several weeks. Impaired renal function and disappearance of schistocytes are generally the last to improve.

Fresh frozen plasma (FFP) remains the most commonly used replacement product. There is no clear advantage to the use of cryo-poor plasma (CPP), which is depleted of vWF. These findings are consistent with a recent study showing similar concentrations and stability of ADAMTS13 during storage at 1° C to 5° C in CPP and FFP. Pilot studies indicate that solvent-detergent treated plasma (which contains ADAMTS13 at concentrations approximately 20% below FFP) appears to be as efficacious as FFP with fewer allergic/urticarial reactions.

Daily plasma exchange should be continued until neurologic symptoms have resolved and both a normal serum LDH and platelet count have been achieved; many experts recommend an additional 2 to 3 days of plasma exchange thereafter. Approximately 85% to 90% of patients show a clinical and laboratory response to plasma exchange within 3 weeks, most often within 10 days (mean 15.8; range 3 to 36 days). However, 20% to 40% of patients will experience an exacerbation of disease within 30 days of plasma exchange discontinuation, whereas approximately 30% will relapse at later dates, usually within the first year. The decision to switch to CPP or to introduce another form of therapy is empiric but in general is not considered until the patient has received a minimum of 10 to 14 days of daily exchange with FFP. One study suggests that administration of rituximab early in the course of disease in conjunction with plasma exchange induces more rapid responses and reduces relapses. Little or no data support either abrupt discontinuation or "tapering" of plasma exchange after remission.

Complication rates associated with plasma therapy may approach 30%, mostly related to central venous catheter insertion or infection. Thrombosis has also been reported, and some, but not all reports suggest a higher incidence with the use of solvent-detergent—treated plasma, which contains less protein S, as a replacement fluid.

Plasma exchange is effective for patients with or without inhibitors, and clinical responses frequently occur despite persistence of both the inhibitor and severe ADAMTS13 deficiency, although patients with high titer inhibitors may respond more slowly and relapse more often. Both congenital and acquired ADAMTS13 deficiency are characterized by unpredictable periods of stability between relapses, which probably reflects a role of stress in exacerbating the disease by activating or damaging endothelium, increasing the release of unusually large vWF multimers, and triggering microvascular thrombosis.

Rituximab

Several reports support the efficacy the anti-CD20 antibody, rituximab, for decreasing the level of autoantibodies and restoring normal ADAMTS13 activity in TTP. Rituximab is being used with increasing frequency, primarily as salvage therapy for patients refractory to plasma exchange. Rituximab also has been used in individuals in remission who exhibit falling ADAMTS13 activity and recurring inhibitors, although the natural history of such patients is not well defined. In a prospective, nonrandomized study, patients with acute TTP who received rituximab within 3 days of admission, in addition to standard plasma exchange, experienced a more than fivefold lower relapse rate at a median of 18 months compared with historic controls. However, because of the lack of randomized trials of rituximab in primary or relapsed TTP, optimal application remains uncertain and the drug has not received FDA approval for this indication.

Corticosteroids

Corticosteroids are often used as part of initial therapy or for patients who fail to show a brisk response to plasma-based therapy. These drugs are of little benefit on their own, and retrospective studies do not provide compelling evidence that they improve the response to plasma exchange. However, the antiinflammatory and immunosuppressive effects of corticosteroids make them logical adjunctive therapy for autoimmune TTP, and most experts continue to use them in patients receiving plasma exchange.

Splenectomy

Before the introduction of plasma therapy, splenectomy was the first-line treatment for TTP and induced remission in up to 50% of patients. Currently, open or laparoscopic splenectomy is generally reserved for patients refractory to plasma exchange and rituximab. Splenectomy may reduce the frequency of relapses in patients with chronic relapsing TTP. Plasma exchange should be continued after splenectomy until the thrombotic microangiopathy remits.

Other Modalities

The response rate to aspirin, dipyridamole, sulfinpyrazone, or ticlopidine as single antiplatelet agents approximates 10%, essentially indistinguishable from the natural history. Antiplatelet agents have not been convincingly shown to increase the response to plasma exchange and may promote bleeding in the setting of severe thrombocytopenia and invasive procedures. The efficacy of intravenous immunoglobulin remains unproven. Anecdotal reports exist of favorable responses to vincristine, as well as other immunosuppressive therapies such as azathioprine, cyclophosphamide, cyclosporine, mycophenylate mofitil, and staphylococcal protein A immunoadsorption. There is evidence that CyA reduces the incidence of TTP relapse and decreases ADAMTS13 antibody levels with parallel increases ADAMTS13 activity.

Starting low-dose aspirin (81 mg daily) once the platelet count exceeds 50,000/μL has been recommended in the 2003 guidelines of the British Committee for Standards in Haematology. Folate supplementation and administration of the hepatitis B vaccine should be considered routine components of supportive care. The role of platelet transfusion in patients with TTP is uncertain (see box on Transfusion Therapy in Thrombotic Microangiopathy).

Stx-HUS

Early volume expansion, within the first 4 days of the onset of diarrhea, significantly reduces the incidence of progression to oliganuric HUS. However, no therapy has been shown to prevent HUS or reduce the severity of kidney injury once established. In randomized trials, neither plasma infusion nor exchange was of benefit in children or adults with Stx-associated HUS. Corticosteroids, heparin, urokinase, aspirin, and dipyridamole are ineffective. A silicon dioxide particle covalently linked to a trisaccharide, designed to bind toxin in the intestine and block systemic effects, did not show benefit. Antimotility agents and narcotics delay clearance of *E. coli* and toxin from the GI tract and may increase the risk for progression to thrombotic microangiopathy; these agents should be avoided. Nonsteroidal antiinflammatory agents may reduce renal blood flow and should also be avoided. Most experts believe that antibiotics increase the risk for progression to HUS, probably by lysing bacteria, releasing Stx and inducing bacteriophages on which Stx genes are expressed.

Transfusion Therapy in Thrombotic Microangiopathy

Patients with TTP often develop symptomatic anemia because of bleeding and partially compensated hemolytic anemia. Packed red blood cells can be transfused safely in this setting. In older adult patients and in those with an impaired cardiovascular system, it may be prudent to provide an additional margin of safety when choosing a threshold for transfusion. In contrast, platelet transfusions have historically been considered to be contraindicated in TTP based on several reports of patients under treatment for TTP whose clinical situation deteriorated within 1 to 24 hours of receiving allogeneic platelets. Clinical deterioration after platelet transfusion can also occur in patients with HUS, as well as Stx-associated and drug-induced thrombotic microangiopathies, and postmortem examination of such patients has revealed widespread microthrombi involving the brain, heart, lung, kidney, and multiple other organs. Sudden death has also been reported on rare occasions in patients who responded to plasma therapy with a rapid rise in the platelet count. However, a recent study assessing the effects of platelet transfusions administered to patients in the Oklahoma TTP-HUS registry suggests that platelet transfusion in patients with TTP is not linked with poor overall outcomes. In this study of 54 consecutive patients (47 with ADAMTS13 activity <10%), 33 (61%) received platelet transfusions. Platelet transfusion had no effect on the frequency of death or severe neurologic events, and no consistent temporal relationship was identified between platelet transfusion and clinical deterioration, regardless of whether transfusion was administered before or after initiation of plasma exchange. Two patients died from hemorrhage during central venous catheter insertion, one of whom had received platelet transfusion. Thus although it remains possible that platelet transfusion may exacerbate the course of TTP in occasional patients, more recent data make it difficult to implicate platelet transfusion as a common cause of clinical demise in TTP. Although most experts and the authors continue to believe that platelet transfusion should be avoided or minimized in these patients, the paradigm that platelet transfusion should be reserved only for life-threatening bleeding may require reexamination. In light of this, it seems reasonable to administer platelets to patients with TTP who are bleeding or those who are facing surgery or other invasive procedures in the setting of severe thrombocytopenia.

Activation of complement may contribute to the pathogenesis of Stx-HUS. Stx2 directly activates the alternative pathway of complement and binds to SCR 6-8 and 19-20 of factor H, which mediate surface recognition, blocking its ability to inhibit complement activation on cell surfaces. In support of this concept, eculizumab was reported to reverse neurologic abnormalities, low platelet counts, and elevated LDH levels in three patients with Stx-HUS. However, the value of complement inhibition in Stx-HUS remains to be established.

Atypical HUS

With the recent understanding of the role of the alternative complement pathway in the pathogenesis of aHUS, along with the development of aHUS registries containing patients who have undergone genetic analyses for mutations in alternative pathway proteins and inhibitors, it has become apparent that long-appreciated differences in response rates to plasma exchange in patients with aHUS correlate with genotype. The highest response rates to plasma exchange, 63% in an Italian registry, were seen in patients with CFH mutations, although complete responses occurred in only 5%. In contrast, only 25% of patients with CFI mutations responded to plasma therapy, with 75% progressing to death or end-stage renal disease. Response to plasma therapy in patients with mutations in cell-associated MCP was low, as expected; however, flares of disease in these patients often resolve spontaneously.

These results suggest that plasma therapy has a role in the management of aHUS, even if responses are not durable or complete. Moreover, when first evaluating a patient with TMA, information on ADAMTS13 levels or complement mutational analyses are generally not available, and thus initiation of plasma exchange therapy is reasonable.

Therapy for aHUS, however, is rapidly evolving with the recent approval of eculizumab, a neutralizing antibody to C5. Approval was based on as-yet unpublished data from two single-arm studies involving 37 adults and adolescents and a retrospective review of 19 pediatric patients and 11 adults (for important drug information, refer to http://www.accessdata.fda.gov/drugsatfda_docs/label/2011/125166s172lbl.pdf). These studies demonstrated activity of eculizumab in the majority of treated patients, whether or not they were refractory to plasma therapy. Several patients with severe renal insufficiency were able to discontinue dialysis.

These results suggest that eculizumab is the treatment of choice for patients with established aHUS or with a high clinical likelihood in an appropriate setting (e.g., postpartum status, positive family history, younger than 2 years of age). Additional studies are needed to define the role of this agent in adults presenting with new onset of TMA or in patients with normal ADAMTS13 levels who are refractory to plasma exchange.

Generally, patients with aHUS who progress to end-stage renal disease are considered candidates for transplantation. Before proceeding, complement genotypes should be determined to predict the risk for recurrence, which ranges from 75% to 90% in patients with CFH mutations to as low as 0% to 15% in patients with MCP mutations. In patients at high risk for recurrence, plasma or complement inhibitor therapy is recommended during and after transplantation.

Living related donor transplants are not recommended for patients with CFH, CFI, CFB, C3, or THBD mutations, and these transplants are questionable for patients with MCP or no observed mutations. The risk for development of aHUS in the remaining donor kidney also must be considered, as aHUS within several months of donation has been reported.

FUTURE DIRECTIONS

Thrombotic microangiopathic syndromes are uncommon, but their associated morbidity and mortality are significant. Over the last 5 years, dramatic progress has been made in our understanding of the pathogenesis of these syndromes, and these discoveries are being translated into effective therapeutic interventions. Eculizumab and other complement inhibitors may well change the natural history of aHUS from that of a progressive disorder culminating in chronic renal failure or death to a manageable chronic disease. Recombinant ADAMTS13 and targeted disruption of the vWF-GP1b interaction may prevent microvascular occlusion in TTP, while expanded use of anti-CD20 and other immunomodulatory approaches may reduce relapses and induce durable remissions. Finally, complement factor H concentrates have received orphan drug designation in Europe. Phase II trials of Stx antibodies are currently in progress.

A critical gray area in the understanding of TMAs is the factors that trigger onset and relapse. Why do some patients with acquired TTP have multiple relapses whereas others have none? Clearly, Stx triggers acute episodes of Stx-HUS, but other factors must account for the fact that some individuals with congenital deficiency of ADAMTS13 present in early childhood, while others may not develop disease until the fifth or sixth decades of life, if at all. Why is the penetrance of aHUS only 50% in the presence of a complement inhibitor gene mutation known to predispose to disease? Clearly, a better understanding of genetic susceptibility factors is essential, but equally important is identification of the environmental agents that incite disease, about which we now have little information.

SUGGESTED READINGS

Allford SL, Hunt BJ, Rose P, et al: Guidelines on the diagnosis and management of the thrombotic microangiopathic haemolytic anaemias. *Brit J Haematol* 120:556; 2003.

Bennett CL, Kim B, Zakarija A, et al: Two mechanistic pathways for thienopyridine-associated thrombotic thrombocytopenic purpura: A report from the SERF-TTP Research Group and the RADAR Project. *J Am Coll Cardiol* 50:1138; 2007.

Bitzan M, Schaefer F, Reymond D: Treatment of typical (enteropathic) hemolytic uremic syndrome. *Semin Thromb Hemost* 36:594; 2010.

Buchholz U, Bernard H, Werber D, et al: German outbreak of Escherichia coli O104:H4 associated with sprouts. *N Engl J Med* 365:1763; 2011.

Fakhouri F, Roumenina L, Provot F, et al: Pregnancy-associated hemolytic uremic syndrome revisited in the era of complement gene mutations. *J Am Soc Nephrol* 21:859; 2010.

Fakhouri F, Vernant JP, Veyradier JP, et al: Efficiency of curative and prophylactic treatment with rituximab in ADAMTS13 deficient-thrombotic thrombocytopenic purpura: A study of 11 cases. *Blood* 106:1932; 2005.

Froissart A, Buffet M, Veyradier A, et al: Efficacy and safety of first-line rituximab in severe, acquired thrombotic thrombocytopenic purpura with a suboptimal response to plasma exchange. Experience of the French Thrombotic Microangiopathies Reference Center. *Crit Care Med* 40:104; 2012.

Furlan M, Robles R, Solenthaler M, et al: Deficient activity of von Willebrand factor-cleaving protease in chronic relapsing thrombotic thrombocytopenic purpura. *Blood* 89:3097; 1997.

Hosler GA, Cusanamo AM, Hutchins GM: Thrombotic thrombocytopenic purpura and hemolytic uremic syndrome are distinct pathologic entities. *Arch Path Lab Med* 127:834; 2003.

Hovinga JA, Vesely SK, Terrell DR, et al: Survival and relapse in patients with thrombotic thrombocytopenic purpura. *Blood* 115:1500; 2010.

Hunt JM: Shiga toxin-producing *Escherichia coli* (STEC). *Clin Lab Med* 30:21; 2010.

Karpman D, Sartz L, Johnson S: Pathophysiology of typical hemolytic uremic syndrome. *Semin Thromb Hemost* 36:575; 2010.

Kavanagh D, Goodship TH: Atypical hemolytic uremic syndrome, genetic basis, and clinical manifestations. *Hematology Am Soc Hematol Educ Program* 2011:15; 2011.

Kerr H, Richards A: Complement-mediated injury and protection of endothelium: Lessons from atypical haemolytic uraemic syndrome. *Immunobiology* 217:195; 2012.

Kose O, Zimmerhackl LB, Jungraithmayr T, et al: New treatment options for atypical hemolytic uremic syndrome with the complement inhibitor eculizumab. *Semin Thromb Hemost* 36:669; 2010.

Loirat C, Fremeaux-Bacchi V: Atypical hemolytic uremic syndrome. *Orphanet J Rare Dis* 6:60; 2011.

Loirat C, Garnier A, Sellier-Leclerc AL, et al: Plasmatherapy in atypical hemolytic uremic syndrome. *Semin Thromb Hemost* 36:673; 2010.

McCrae KR: Thrombocytopenia in pregnancy. *Hematology Am Soc Hematol Educ Program* 2010:397; 2010.

Obrig TG, Karpman D: Shiga toxin pathogenesis: Kidney complications and renal failure. *Curr Top Microbiol Immunol* 357:105; 2012.

Orth D, Wurzner R: Complement in typical hemolytic uremic syndrome. *Semin Thromb Hemost* 36:620; 2010.

Rock GA, Shumak KH, Buskard NA, et al: Comparison of plasma exchange with plasma infusion in the treatment of thrombotic thrombocytopenic purpura. *N Engl J Med* 325:393; 1991.

Sadler JE: von Willebrand factor, ADAMTS13, and thrombotic thrombocytopenic purpura. *Blood* 112:11; 2008.

Scully M, McDonald V, Cavenagh J, et al: A phase 2 study of the safety and efficacy of rituximab with plasma exchange in acute acquired thrombotic thrombocytopenic purpura. *Blood* 118:1746; 2011.

Tarr PI: Shiga toxin-associated hemolytic uremic syndrome and thrombotic thrombocytopenic purpura: Distinct mechanisms of pathogenesis. *Kidney Int Suppl* 112:S29; 2009.

Taylor CM, Machin S, Wigmore SJ, et al: Clinical practice guidelines for the management of atypical haemolytic uraemic syndrome in the United Kingdom. *Br J Haematol* 148:37; 2010.

Tsai H-M, Lian ECY: Antibodies to von Willebrand factor-cleaving protease in acute thrombotic thrombocytopenic purpura. *N Engl J Med* 339:1585; 1998.

Tschumi S, Gugger M, Bucher BS, et al: Eculizumab in atypical hemolytic uremic syndrome: Long-term clinical course and histological findings. *Pediatr Nephrol* 26:2085; 2011.

Wong CS, Jelacic S, Habeeb RL, et al: The risk of the hemolytic uremic syndrome after antibiotic treatment of Escherichia coli 0157:H7 infections. *N Engl J Med* 342:1930; 2000.

Zheng XL, Kaufman RM, Goodnough LT, et al: Effect of plasma exchange on plasma ADAMTS13 metalloprotease activity, inhibitor level, and clinical outcome in patients with idiopathic and nonidiopathic thrombocytopenic purpura. *Blood* 103:4043; 2004.

Zheng XL, Sadler JE: Pathogenesis of thrombotic microangiopathies. *Annu Rev Pathol* 3:249; 2008.

CHAPTER 137

HEMOPHILIA A AND B

Manuel Carcao, Paul Moorehead, and David Lillicrap

EPIDEMIOLOGY

Hemophilia is the most common, severe inherited bleeding disorder recognized in humans. The hereditary and sex-linked nature of the disease has been appreciated since prebiblical times, and the previous occurrence of the disease in the European Royal family has added further interest in this condition.

The prevalence of hemophilia is worldwide, with no major geographical variances aside from rare clusters of disease in areas where founder mutations have been propagated. In many parts of the developing world, the true prevalence of the condition is unknown because of inadequate diagnostic facilities, but from experiences in the developed world, we can probably assume that the prevalence of hemophilia A is approximately one in 10,000 males and for hemophilia B, one in 50,000 males (Table 137-1). These prevalence figures do show some variances among countries but except where local founder effects are important, these differences likely represent variable disease ascertainment and diagnosis. Although because of the X-linked recessive inheritance of the disease, the significant majority of affected subjects are male, there are also significant numbers of carrier women who manifest clinical symptoms of bleeding because of low clotting factor levels.

International studies in the past decade indicate that the numbers of persons with hemophilia in the population is increasing by approximately 2% each year. There are likely several reasons for this trend, including the overall increase in population numbers and the increasing longevity of persons with hemophilia.

The clinical signs and symptoms and inheritance patterns for hemophilia A and B are identical, and it was not until the early 1950s that the two forms of hemophilia were differentiated. Subsequently, in the early 1980s, the two genes encoding factor VIII (FVIII) and factor IX (FIX) were cloned, and the specific mutations responsible for hemophilia began to be determined.

FACTOR VIII (FVIII) BIOLOGY: GENETICS, STRUCTURE, FUNCTION, AND PATHOPHYSIOLOGY

The Factor VIII Gene

The FVIII gene *(F8)* encoding the FVIII protein is located at Xq28, the most distal band of the long arm of the X chromosome (Fig. 137-1). It is a large and complex structure, 186 kb in length, consisting of 9 kb of exonic DNA arranged into 26 exons and 177 kb of intronic DNA in 25 introns. Most of the exons are small, ranging in size from 69 base pairs (exon 5) to 313 base pairs (exon 1), but exons 26 and 14 (encoding the central B domain) are 1958 and 3106 base pairs, respectively. The correspondence of these exons to the domains of the FVIII protein is described later. The size of *F8* introns varies from 207 base pairs (intron 17) to 32.4 kb (intron 22).

In addition to the 9-kb FVIII transcript, this locus also encodes two additional mRNAs that, unlike FVIII, are expressed ubiquitously. Within intron 22 of the *F8* gene there are two further coding elements, *F8A* and *F8B*. The *F8A* transcript is made up entirely of intronic sequence from intron 22, and the *F8A* mRNA is transcribed in the opposite direction to *F8*. Although the function of the F8A transcript/protein is unknown, there is the potential that this mRNA could act as an antisense regulator of FVIII expression. In addition, two (or more) other copies of the *F8A* sequence are located further telomeric to *F8* and are involved in a frequent intrachromosomal recombination event in approximately 45% of patients with severe hemophilia A. The *F8B* transcript is expressed in the same orientation as the native *F8* mRNA, and this transcript comprises an initial intron 22 sequence that is spliced onto exons 23 to 26 of *F8*. As with F8A, the F8B transcript is also ubiquitously expressed, and the function of the protein is unknown, but because it contains the phospholipid binding region of FVIII, it may play a role in membrane binding.

Factor VIII Expression

Transcription of the *F8* gene is regulated by a promoter that contains binding sites for both tissue-specific and ubiquitous transcription factors. The mRNA transcribed from *F8* is 9 kb in length and contains 7053 nucleotides of coding sequence and short 5′ and long 3′ untranslated sequences. The cellular site of FVIII expression has long been a matter of controversy. The situation is complicated by the very low abundance and instability of the FVIII transcript and protein. Nevertheless, F8 mRNA has been found to be expressed in a variety of human tissues, including hepatocytes, splenocytes, kidney cells, and muscle. However most recently, evidence suggests that there are two principal sites of FVIII synthesis, the liver and the vascular endothelium. It has long been known that hemophilia can be cured by liver transplantation, but the cell types within the liver responsible for FVIII synthesis have been unclear. There is now good evidence that both liver sinusoidal endothelial cells and, probably to a lesser extent, hepatocytes, express and secrete FVIII.[1] During episodes of severe liver failure, FVIII levels are maintained, providing strong support for sites of extrahepatic FVIII expression. The most likely extrahepatic source of FVIII expression is the endothelium. There are reports of the pulmonary vasculature producing FVIII, and it may well be that other vascular beds may also be involved in this process under certain circumstances.[2]

Factor VIII is an acute phase reactant, and studies have shown that FVIII expression can be induced through a nuclear factor kappa-B (NFκB)–mediated mechanism. FVIII levels also increase with hormone induction (estrogen use), but the mechanistic basis for this increase is not known.

The Biosynthesis of Factor VIII

Factor VIII biosynthesis has been extensively investigated in vitro using cell types that do not normally express this protein. Therefore, conclusions about the details of this process in a physiological context should be made with some caution. After production of the primary polypeptide chain and cleavage of the 19 amino acid signal peptide, the protein undergoes a series of posttranslational modifications,

Table 137-1 2010 Canadian Hemophilia Registry*

Hemophilia A		
Severe	800	Total hemophilia A patients: 2722 (80 inhibitors)
Moderate	260	
Mild	1648	
Hemophilia B		
Severe	166	Total hemophilia B patients: 658 (four inhibitors)
Moderate	216	
Mild	273	

*Canadian population, 34 million.

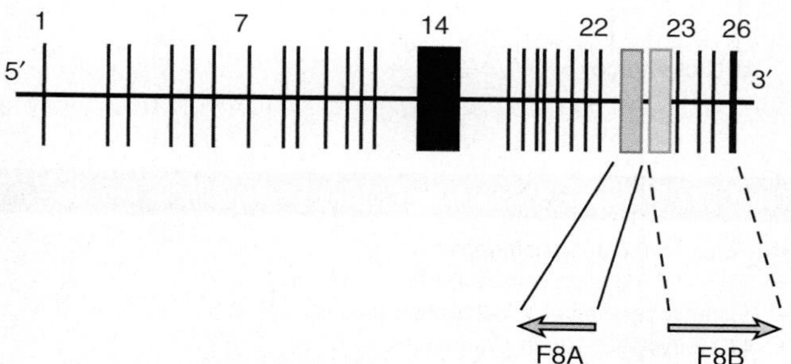

Figure 137-1 FACTOR VIII (FVIII) GENE. The FVIII gene *(F8)* is located on the X chromosome at cytogenic band Xq28-qter. The 26 exons span 184 kb of genomic DNA, and there are three open reading frames expressed from the locus: the 9 kb FVIII mRNA transcript incorporating all 26 exons of the gene; the F8A transcript that is transcribed in the opposite direction to FVIII and comprises sequences from intron 22; and finally, F8B comprising an initial 5′ exon derived from intron 22 sequence that is spliced to exons 23 to 26 of the *F8* gene.

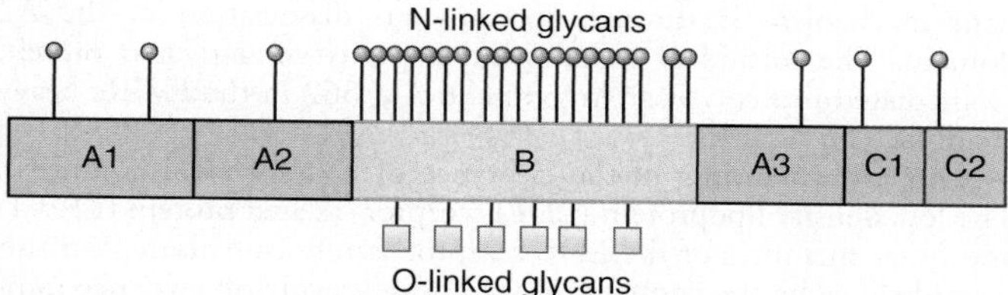

Figure 137-2 FACTOR VIII (FVIII) GLYCAN MODIFICATION (molecular weight, 260 kDa: plasma concentration, 100-200 ng/mL; 1 nM). The FVIII protein is modified by the addition of multiple N- and O-linked glycan chains. The majority of these glycan additions are located in the B domain and appear to play a role in facilitating intracellular trafficking and secretion of the protein.

including N- and O-linked glycosylation (mainly in the B domain) (Fig. 137-2) and sulfation of tyrosine residues. Furthermore, when the nascent protein transits the endoplasmic reticulum (ER), it interacts with ER chaperones, including calreticulin and immunoglobulin binding protein (BiP). Although these interactions limit the transport of malfolded or aggregated forms of the protein in heterologous cells with high levels of FVIII expression, their relevance in native FVIII-producing cells (i.e., a liver sinusoidal endothelial cell) is unknown. Indeed, under conditions of high-level FVIII expression, cells can activate a classical unfolded protein response and can succumb to apoptotic cell death.

The other detail of FVIII trafficking that has attracted attention is its transit between the ER and Golgi en route to secretion. Efficient transit through the ER–Golgi boundary appears to require an interaction with glycans within the B domain of the protein. Absence of these glycans or lack of specific transport proteins responsible for this trafficking event can significantly reduce the levels of secreted FVIII.

The Factor VIII Protein Structure

The DNA sequence of the *F8* gene predicts that the translated single chain polypeptide with a molecular weight of 260 kDa consisting of 2351 amino acid residues, including a 19-residue signal peptide. Upon translocation to the ER, the signal peptide is cleaved. The remaining polypeptide is 2332 residues long.

The FVIII protein consists of three types of domains: the three A domains, which have a 35% to 40% amino acid sequence homology to ceruloplasmin and factor V; a central B domain with no known homologues; and two C-terminal discoidin-like C domains that are also 35% to 40% homologous to factor V and ceruloplasmin (discoidin being a cell adhesion protein found in slime molds) (Fig. 137-3). There are also three small "a" domains (each between 20 and 40 amino acids) consisting of predominantly acidic residues. The sequence of these domains within the protein is NH2-A1-a1-A2-a2-B-a3-A3-C1-C2-COOH. Tyrosine residues in the a2 and a3 domains, when sulfated, contribute to the cofactor function of FVIII and enable its interaction with von Willebrand factor (vWF). As indicated, FVIII has structural similarities to coagulation factor V, which also has A and C domains 35% to 40% homologous to those in FVIII. However, FV does not contain a domain homologous to the B domain. Given these structural similarities, it is not surprising that both FVIII and FV function as cofactors for serine protease enzymes in the coagulation cascade, FVIII in the so-called intrinsic tenase complex and factor V in the prothrombinase complex.

Subsequent proteolysis of the FVIII polypeptide chain in the Golgi generates a light chain consisting of the A3-C1-C2 domains with a mass of 80 kDa (see Fig. 137-3).

Circulating FVIII exists as a heterodimer of the NH_2-terminus heavy chain and the COOH-terminus light chain. The two FVIII chains are bound to one another at the A1 and A3 domains by noncovalent bonds that are divalent metal ion dependent. The involved ion is likely copper, which has been found in association with FVIII.

Recently, two low-resolution crystal structures of B domain–deleted FVIII have been reported. These structures confirm prior proposals generated via molecular modeling in terms of the overall organization of the A and C domains, but higher resolution structures are required to resolve details of the location and orientation of individual residues.

Storage, Secretion, and Circulation of Factor VIII

After synthesis, FVIII is secreted into the circulation, where it forms a tight noncovalent complex with its multimeric partner vWF (Kd ≈0.2-0.5 nM). Whereas the plasma concentration of FVIII is 100 to 200 ng/mL (≈1 nM), the concentration of vWF is approximately 10 μg/mL (50 nM); thus the molar ratio of FVIII in the FVIII-vWF complex is about 1 to 50. The majority of vWF in plasma is synthesized and secreted by vascular endothelial cells. vWF binds to the a3 and C2 regions of FVIII through sequences in the D′/D3 region of the mature vWF monomer. Just as the cellular source of FVIII has long been argued, so, necessarily, has the site at which FVIII and vWF first interact. However, the recent finding that FVIII is expressed by at least some forms of endothelial cells suggests that some of the circulating FVIII may interact with vWF before secretion and may be co-stored with vWF in Weibel-Palade bodies. In the plasma, vWF protects FVIII from proteolysis by activated protein C. Without this interaction—for example, in cases of type 3 von Willebrand disease (in which vWF is absent) or type 2N von Willebrand disease (in which mutations occur in the FVIII binding region of vWF)—the plasma half-life of FVIII is reduced and, consequently, the plasma levels of FVIII are low.

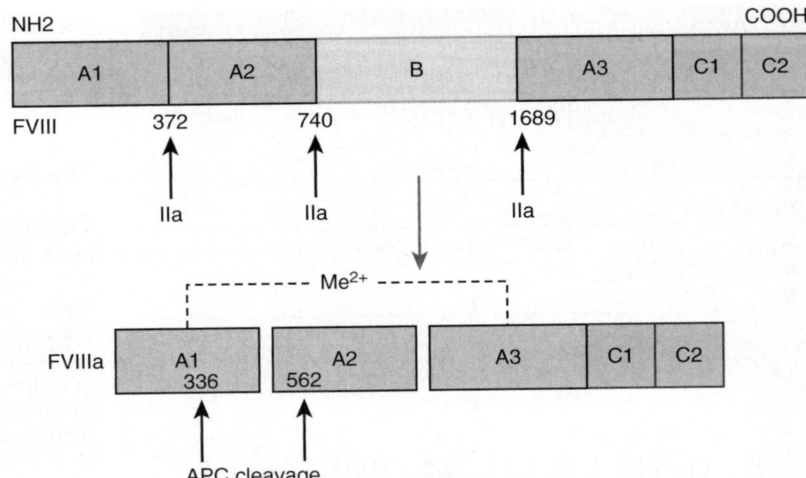

Figure 137-3 FACTOR VIII (FVIII) PROTEIN ACTIVATION AND INACTIVATION. The FVIII protein comprises a series of A and C domains that are homologous to FV and ceruloplasmin and a central B domain that does not show sequence homology. The inactive precursor protein is activated by thrombin through proteolytic cleavages at three locations. Inactivation of FVIIIa occurs through two mechanisms: spontaneous dissociation of the noncovalently bound A2 domain and proteolysis mediated by activated protein C (APC).

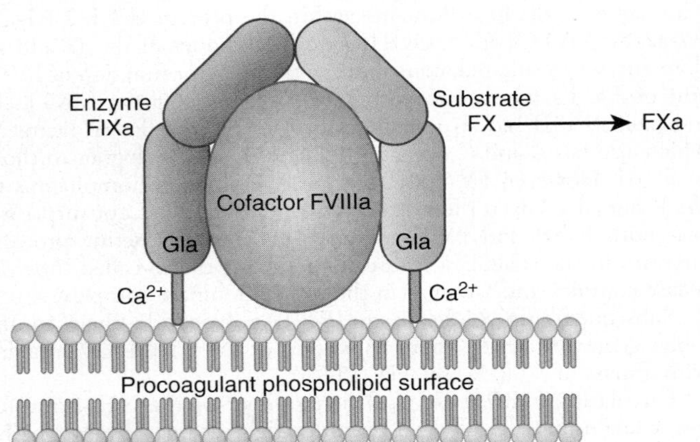

Figure 137-4 THE INTRINSIC TENASE COMPLEX. This membrane-bound complex plays an essential role in the amplification phase of hemostasis. Participation of all components of the complex enhances the catalytic efficiency of the factor Xa (FXa)–generating process by more than 200,000-fold. Deficiency or dysfunction of either the enzyme or cofactor involved in the complex results in a marked reduction in catalytic efficiency and the clinical manifestations of hemophilia. *FIXa,* Factor IXa; *FVIIIa,* factor VIIIa.

Table 137-2 Genetic Mechanisms Causing Hemophilia in Females

- *F8* or *F9* mutation homozygosity
- *F8* or *F9* mutation compound heterozygosity
- Extreme skewing of X inactivation process
- X/O karyotype: Turner syndrome
- X/autosome translocation

Activation and Coagulant Function of Factor VIII

Factor VIII plays a critical role in the propagation (amplification) phase of coagulation. The physiological activator of FVIII is thrombin, which proteolytically cleaves FVIII at three sites: Arg372 at the NH_2-terminus of the A2 domain, Arg740 at the NH_2-terminus of the B domain, and Arg1689 at the NH_2-terminus of the A3 domain (see Fig. 137-3). These cleavages release FVIII from vWF and result in the formation of a noncovalently associated A1-A2-A3/C1/C2 heterotrimeric activated FVIII (FVIIIa) molecule. FVIII can also be activated by FXa and FIXa, although the physiological contribution of activation by these proteases is less clear.

In its activated form, FVIII provides essential cofactor activity in the intrinsic tenase complex where FIXa is the serine protease and FX is the substrate (Fig. 137-4). This reaction takes place on a procoagulant phospholipid surface, which in normal hemostasis is likely the activated platelet. Participation of FVIIIa in the complex enhances the catalytic efficiency of this reaction about 200,000-fold, and thus severe FVIII deficiency profoundly reduces the rate of FXa generation and renders this reaction biologically futile. The exact details of the cofactor role of FVIIIa remain to be elucidated, but it is assumed that it acts as a "scaffold" protein that optimally aligns the enzymatic and substrate components of the complex on the phospholipid surface. Indeed, the FIXa and FX interactive regions of FVIII have been defined, and the cofactor binds to the phospholipid surface through hydrophobic residues in the C2 domain. Of note, the FVIII B domain is not required for cofactor function, and to date, it appears that the principal role of this region of the protein is to facilitate trafficking and secretion of the nascent polypeptide.

Factor VIIIa is inactivated through two processes. The predominant mechanism is through spontaneous dissociation of the A2 domain. The secondary inactivation event is via activated protein C–mediated proteolysis at Arg336 and Arg 562 in the FVIIIa heavy chain (see Fig. 137-3).

Our understanding of the clearance of FVIII/FVIIIa is limited. The low-density lipoprotein (LDL) receptor–related protein (LRP-1) and other members of the LDL receptor family contribute, but this is unlikely to be the complete story. Indeed, evolving evidence indicates that FVIII clearance may be mainly influenced by its multimeric partner, vWF, and that a group of receptors on macrophages, and possibly other cell types in the liver and spleen, may remove FVIII in complex with vWF.

PATHOPHYSIOLOGY OF HEMOPHILIA A

Hemophilia A is a disorder characterized by congenital deficiency of FVIII. Almost all patients with hemophilia A have *F8* gene mutations. Because *F8* is located on the X chromosome, hemophilia A typically follows an X-linked inheritance pattern. As a result, males are affected most often. Severe and moderately severe cases of hemophilia A are unusual in females but can result from genetic mechanisms, including the following (Table 137-2): inheritance of either homozygous or compound heterozygous *F8* mutations; inheritance of a single *F8* mutation together with a 46 XO karyotype (Turner syndrome); inheritance of a single *F8* mutation and an X/autosome translocation; and, rarely, a markedly skewed inactivation of the X chromosomes that may, in some instances, involve a second genetic defect that prevents inactivation of the hemophilic X chromosome. Approximately 30% of hemophilia A cases are caused by a sporadic mutation and occur without a family history of the disorder.

The molecular genetic basis of hemophilia A has been extensively characterized over the past 25 years. A comprehensive Internet database of hemophilia A mutations is maintained and updated at http://hadb.org.uk.

In contrast to hemophilia B, a significant proportion of hemophilia A cases are the result of a recurrent mutation, an inversion mutation involving sequences in intron 22 of the gene (Fig. 137-5). The mechanism involved in generating this mutation involves an intrachromosomal recombination event in which there is an exchange between the F8A gene in intron 22 and one of two extragenic copies of this sequence that are located 5′ and telomeric to *F8*. The origin of this recurrent mutation is almost exclusively in the male germline, where the single X chromosome has no partner to pair with, thereby potentially facilitating the F8A-mediated intrachromosomal recombination. The result of this event is the inversion of the *F8* gene between exons 1 and 22 and thus, although two distinct *F8* transcripts are expressed from separate promoters (exons 1-22 and exons 23-26), a contiguous FVIII protein sequence is not synthesized. The intron 22 inversion mutation is always associated with a severe phenotype and is responsible for approximately 45% of the cases of severe hemophilia A.

A second recurrent inversion mutation involving intron 1 of the *F8* gene is responsible for approximately 2% of the cases of severe hemophilia A.

The remainder of the mutations responsible for hemophilia A involve more than 1000 different alterations with a wide array of missense, nonsense, frameshift, insertion or deletion, and splicing mutations. In addition, two transcriptional mutations have been identified in the F8 promoter region. All regions of the gene are potential mutation targets, but, as elsewhere in the genome, certain sequences, such as the CpG dinucleotide in arginine codons, are more prone to mutation because of spontaneous methylation of the 5′ cytosine and spontaneous deamination to thymine. To date, approximately 98% of cases of hemophilia A have been associated with mutations of the *F8* locus. The location of the missing mutations is not yet resolved, but the likelihood of locus heterogeneity for hemophilia A seems small. Indeed, the recent identification of mutations deep within introns of the gene suggests that all hemophilia A mutations are quite likely to be found within or adjacent to *F8*.

There have been extensive genotype and phenotype studies of hemophilia A with, in general, a good correlation between null mutations and severe disease and with many missense mutations and a moderate or mild phenotype. The phenotype remains consistent with a specific mutation both within and among families.

In addition to its utility for family counseling issues, the *F8* genotype has also been found to be a predictive factor for the development of anti-FVIII antibody development (Table 137-3). Thus multidomain deletions are associated with an approximately 75% risk of inhibitor development, a group of mutations including the intron 22 and intron 1 inversions, nonsense and insertion or deletion mutations are associated with a 20% to 30% inhibitor risk. Finally, a group of mutations including most missense and splicing mutants have an inhibitor risk of less than 10%.

Table 137-3 Factor VIII Mutant Genotype and Inhibitor Risk in Previously Untreated Hemophilia A Patients

Multidomain deletions	≈75%
Light chain nonsense mutns	30%-40%
Intron 22 inversion	20%-25%
Single domain deletions	15%-25%
Small non-A run insertions/deltns	15%-20%
Heavy chain nonsense mutns	10%-20%
Factor VIII missense mutns	<10%
Small A run insertions/deltns	<5%
Splicing mutns	<5%

FACTOR IX BIOLOGY: GENETICS, STRUCTURE, FUNCTION, AND PATHOPHYSIOLOGY

Factor IX Gene and Factor IX Expression

The gene that encodes FIX was cloned and characterized by two groups in the early 1980s. The gene is located on the X chromosome at cytogenetic band Xq27 and spans 34 kb of genomic sequence (Fig. 137-6). The eight exons of the *F9* gene encode an mRNA transcript of 1.4 kb that is expressed exclusively in hepatocytes. The transcriptional regulatory elements of the *F9* gene have been well characterized, and indeed, there is a variant form of hemophilia B, hemophilia B Leyden, in which a postpubertal rescue of inherited FIX deficiency is the result of an activated androgen response element in the *F9* proximal promoter.[3] Aside from this hormone responsive element, the *F9* promoter contains a typical combination of predominantly liver-specific transcription factor binding sites.

Factor IX Protein

Factor IX is synthesized exclusively in hepatocytes and circulates in plasma at a concentration of approximately 5 μg/mL (90 nM). The mature circulating protein consists of 416 amino acids and has a molecular weight of 57 kDa (Fig. 137-7). The protein is initially synthesized as a pre-propolypeptide with a short signal sequence, which facilitates entry into the ER, and a propolypeptide sequence, which interacts with the γ-glutamylcarboxylase in the ER. The interaction with this microsomal enzyme catalyzes the posttranslational

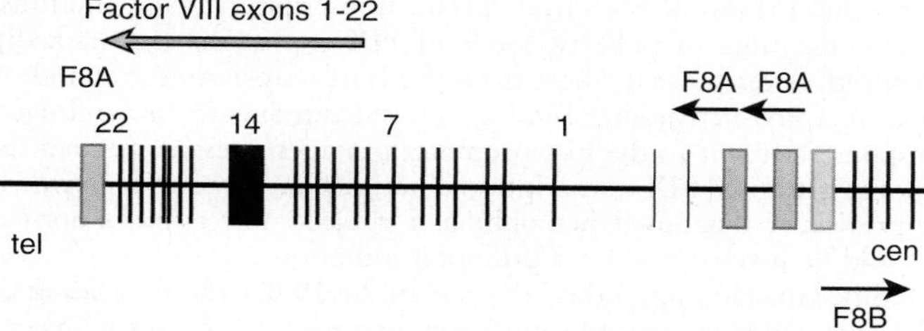

Figure 137-5 THE *F8* INTRON 22 INVERSION MUTATION. In about 45% of severe hemophilia A patients, there is a recurrent *F8* inversion mutation involving intrachromosomal recombination of F8A sequences within intron 22 of the gene and at a 5′ telomeric location. This mutation always results in a severe phenotype and almost always originates in the male germline.

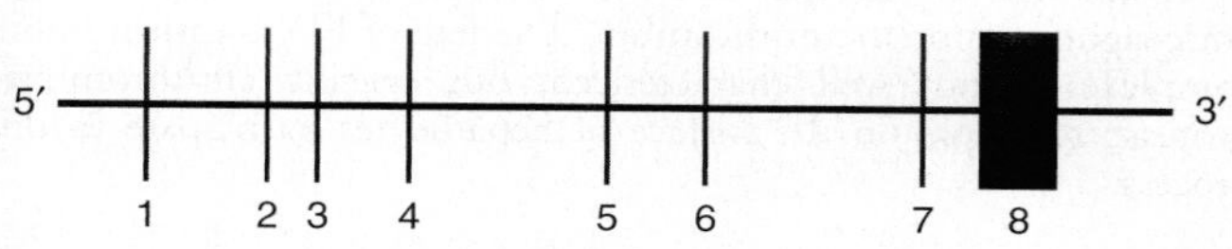

Figure 137-6 THE FACTOR IX GENE *(F9)*. The *F9* gene is located on the long arm of the X chromosome at cytogenetic band Xq27 centromeric to the *F8* gene and the common X chromosome fragile site. The gene comprises 34 kb of genomic DNA arranged in eight exons.

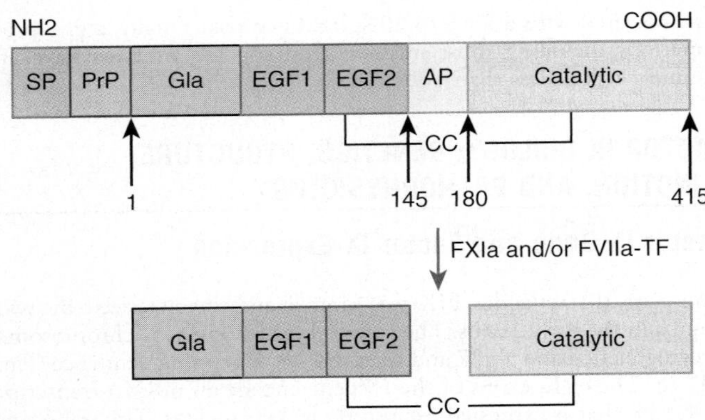

Figure 137-7 THE FACTOR IX (FIX) PROTEIN (415 amino acids; 57 kDa; plasma concentration, 5 μg/mL; 90 nM). FIX is synthesized exclusively in hepatocytes. The protein is produced initially as a pre-propolypeptide. The signal peptide (SP) is cleaved upon entry into the endoplasmic reticulum (ER), and the propeptide (PrP) is also removed in the ER after γ-carboxylation of 12 glutamic acid residues in the *N*-terminal Gla domain. Factor IX is activated by proteolytic removal of the activation peptide (AP), and FIXa is inactivated through complex formation with antithrombin *CC,* Disulfide linkage; *EGF,* epidermal growth factor-like domain..

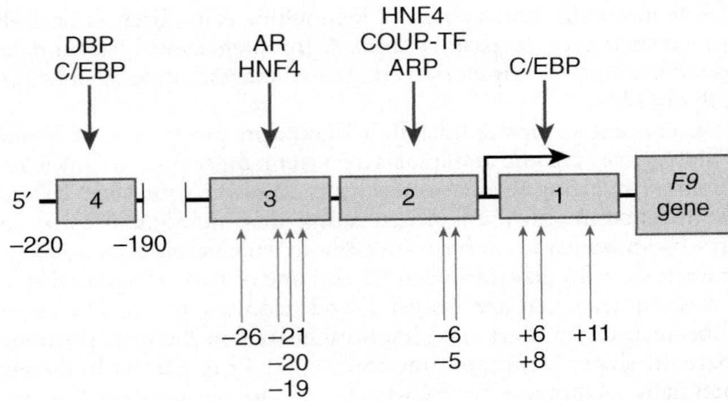

Figure 137-8 MUTATIONAL BASIS OF HEMOPHILIA B LEYDEN. In this variant form of hemophilia B, patients experience a spontaneous recovery of factor IX (FIX) levels after puberty. The disease results from mutations in the *F9* promoter that disrupt transcription factor binding. Postpubertal recovery is at least partly attributable to the expression of testosterone, with the subsequent activation and binding of the androgen receptor to its cognate sequence in the *F9* promoter. Sites 1 to 4 are transcription factor binding regions. *AR,* androgen receptor; *C/EBP,* CCAAT enhancer binding protein; *COUP-TF,* chicken ovalbumin upstream transcription factor; *DBP,* D site binding protein; *HNF-4,* hepatocyte nuclear factor 4.

conversion of the amino-terminal 12 glutamic acid residues of mature FIX into γ-carboxyglutamyl residues (the GLA domain). This posttranslational modification enables FIX to form calcium-dependent interactions with procoagulant phospholipid membranes. A second posttranslational modification at residue 64 in the first epidermal growth factor (EGF)–like domain of the mature polypeptide involves β-hydroxylation of asparagine. This modification also plays a role in facilitating interactions with calcium and phospholipid membranes.

The structure of FIX is homologous to that of other vitamin K–dependent coagulation proteins. The domain structure includes an amino-terminal GLA sequence followed by two EGF-like domains, an activation peptide and the carboxyl-terminus catalytic domain, which is similar to the organization of the procoagulant factors VII and X and to the anticoagulant protein C.

The FIX zymogen is activated by two processes, proteolytic cleavage mediated by FXIa and by a similar process involving the FVIIa–tissue factor complex. The activation of FIX involves sequential proteolysis of two peptide bonds at arginine residues 145/146 and 180/181 (see Fig. 137-7). These cleavages release the FIX activation peptide and result in the formation of the disulfide-linked FIXa enzyme with an NH_2-terminus light chain and COOH-terminus heavy chain. Whereas the light chain binds to procoagulant phospholipid surfaces through a calcium-mediated process involving the GLA domain, the C-terminus catalytic domain cleaves and activates the substrate factor X. This reaction involves the so-called intrinsic tenase complex in which activated FVIII participates as an essential cofactor. Absence of FVIIIa in the tenase complex reduces the catalytic efficiency of the reaction by approximately 200,000-fold.

Factor IXa is inhibited through an interaction with the natural anticoagulant protein antithrombin. The fate of FIXa–antithrombin complexes is not well characterized, but specific antithrombin–protease receptors on the surface of hepatocytes participate in this process.

Hemophilia B Molecular Pathology

To date, all of the mutations responsible for hemophilia B have involved the FIX gene. Although there is a combined vitamin K–dependent protein deficiency state that involves mutations of the γ-glutamylcarboxylase gene, this condition is characterized by low levels of FVII, FX, and prothrombin as well as FIX. Mutational analyses of large numbers of patients with hemophilia B have detected mutations in the FIX gene in more than 98% of cases, and it may well be that the remaining mutations are located within intronic sequences that have not yet been analyzed.

In marked contrast to hemophilia A, in which approximately 50% of mutations resulting in severe disease are caused by two recurrent gene inversion events, approximately 75% of mutations in hemophilia B are missense substitutions. There are no common recurrent FIX mutations, although mild forms of hemophilia B may show a founder effect of missense variants in some populations.

Aside from the predominance of missense mutations, multiple other mutations can produce hemophilia B ranging from large gene deletions to a mix of nonsense, insertion or deletion, and splicing changes. The full array of FIX mutations responsible for hemophilia B can be reviewed in an Internet-accessible database at http://www.kcl.ac.uk/ip/petergreen/haemBdatabase.html. The following text highlights several distinct and clinically important hemophilia B mutations.

The most biologically remarkable hemophilia B mutations are those that produce hemophilia B Leyden, a disorder wherein FIX levels gradually increase from less than 5% at birth to greater than 30% by early adulthood. Because of the low FIX levels early in life, boys with this disorder often have bleeding episodes and experience clinical symptoms and signs consistent with these. After puberty, these problems resolve or improve, and a frequent story told by individuals in these families is that a misdiagnosis of hemophilia was made during childhood. All of the hemophilia B Leyden point mutations are located in a 40-bp region of the FIX promoter around the transcriptional start site (Fig. 137-8). Each of these mutations interferes with the binding of a liver-specific transcription factor, and thus, up to the time of puberty, levels of FIX expression are markedly reduced. After puberty, there is synthesis of testosterone and androgen receptor activation. Binding of testosterone to an androgen response element in the FIX promoter provides a rescue mechanism for the disrupted FIX transcriptional status. Thus any family in which a previously diagnosed hemophilia B subject now appears normal should be investigated for a promoter mutation.

Since the cloning of the FIX gene in the 1980s, the association of *F9* gene deletions with FIX antibody formation has been well recognized. Thus, with partial and complete *F9* deletion mutations, the risk of development of a FIX antibody response is between 30% and 50%. In addition to neutralizing FIX enzymatic function, these antibodies can also be associated with anaphylactic or anaphylactoid reactions to FIX infusions.[4] The antibodies usually develop in young children (1-2 years old) after 10 to 20 exposures to FIX concentrate.

FIX concentrate use is no longer of benefit in most of these patients, and attempts at inducing immunologic tolerance to FIX may be complicated by the development of nephritic syndrome. The mechanism underlying this complication is currently unresolved.

Hemophilia is the bleeding disorder commonly associated with past members of the Royal families of Europe. Although the clinical picture in these individuals was consistent with severe hemophilia, the precise diagnosis was not reported until 2009. In fact, a diagnosis of hemophilia was confirmed, but not hemophilia A as had been thought and would have been expected on the basis of disease incidence, but hemophilia B (Fig. 137-9).[5] The "royal" *F9* mutation is a splicing variant occurring at the 3′ end of intron 3 that creates a new splice acceptor sequence that results in a novel out-of-frame transcript with 11 new amino acids followed by a premature stop codon. This mutation likely leads to either nonsense-mediated accelerated decay of the mutant FIX mRNA or to the translation of a significantly truncated nonfunctional FIX protein. In both instances, the clinical phenotype would likely have been severe.

Missense mutations elsewhere in the FIX gene have been informative with regards to our detailed understanding of protein structure and function. Mutations at both activation peptide cleavage sites have been described, and as with many genes, recurrent "hotspot" mutations have been documented at arginine codons with CpG dinucleotide sequences. Finally, some mild and frequently encountered FIX variants appear to be caused by founder mutations, as evidenced by a common adjacent polymorphic haplotype.

Hemophilia Diagnosis

The initial diagnosis of hemophilia depends to some extent on the family context. In families in which hemophilia has previously been identified, family counseling determines the risk of hemophilia transmission and usually results in a diagnosis being made in utero or early in neonatal life. In contrast, when there is no family history of the disease, the diagnosis will often not be made until there are signs of a bleeding diathesis, and the timing of this depends on the extent of factor deficiency. In severe deficiency states, the diagnosis is often made in the first 1 to 2 years of life, but with moderate and mild disease, the diagnosis may be made much later; with mild hemophilia, the diagnosis may be delayed until late adult life when bleeding occurs after a surgical intervention.

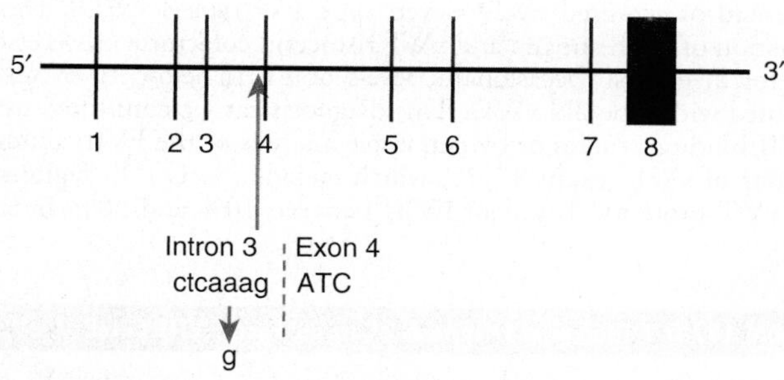

Figure 137-9 THE "ROYAL" HEMOPHILIA MUTATION. There is now definitive evidence that the hemophilia previously present in the European royal families was hemophilia B. The point mutation found in an affected male from the Russian royal family introduces a new acceptor splice site at the 3′ end of intron 3 of the *F9* gene. The consequence of this change is the translation of 11 novel amino acids from the exon 3/4 boundary followed by a premature stop codon. A severe phenotype would be expected either because of accelerated mRNA decay or the synthesis of a nonfunctional truncated factor IX protein. *(Data from Rogaev EI, Grigorenko AP, Faskhutdinova G, et al: Genotype analysis identifies the cause of the "royal disease."* Science *326:817, 2009.)*

Phenotypic Diagnosis of Hemophilia

Two diagnostic strategies can be used for hemophilia. In the vast majority of cases, this involves measurement of FVIII or FIX coagulant levels in platelet poor plasma using a functional clotting assay (usually a one-stage PTT-based assay). Although most clinical hemostasis laboratories use a one-stage PTT-based test to quantify FVIII, some laboratories use either a two-stage assay or a chromogenic substrate assay that measures the generation of FXa in a purified system (Table 137-4). In these latter assays, the incubation time is often longer, which may influence test results. For example, a group of mild hemophilia A missense mutations results in the synthesis of an unstable FVIII with enhanced dissociation of the A2 domain from the remainder of the protein. These unstable mutants can sometimes be missed when a one-stage FVIII assay is used but are readily apparent with two-stage or chromogenic assay protocols that use a prolonged incubation time.

The severity of hemophilia is based on the extent of clotting factor deficiency (severe, <1% [<0.01 U/mL]; moderate, 1%-5% [0.01-0.05 U/mL]; and mild, 5%-40% [0.05-0.40 U/mL]). When making a diagnosis of hemophilia B, caution must be taken in neonates because levels of FIX can be low in normal newborns as a result of an immature carboxylase system. It is advisable to wait for 1 month to confirm the baseline level of FIX in cases of apparent mild hemophilia B.

Genetic Diagnosis of Hemophilia

The other diagnostic strategy that can be used in hemophilia involves the use of DNA analysis. Since the cloning of the FVIII and FIX genes in the early 1980s, molecular genetic approaches to hemophilia diagnosis have advanced dramatically.

Currently, mutations responsible for hemophilia A and B can be identified in the F8 and F9 genes in approximately 98% of cases. In cases in which mutations have not been found, it is likely that sequence changes are deep within introns or within distant regulatory elements, regions of the genes that are not routinely examined in diagnostic laboratories.

The strategy for genetic analysis depends on the type of hemophilia and the severity of the phenotype. For example, all patients with severe hemophilia A should be screened initially for the recurrent F8 intron 22 and intron 1 inversion mutations. In contrast, most patients with hemophilia B require full-sequence analysis of the entire FIX promoter, coding region, and splice sites.

When a familial mutation has already been identified in the FVIII or FIX gene, a prenatal diagnosis can be made by either chorionic villus sampling or amniocentesis. Outside of the prenatal context, mutation testing in hemophilia can be used for carrier detection for family planning purposes and as one component of the risk analysis for inhibitor development. In hemophilia A and B, large gene deletions are associated with a higher risk of inhibitor formation soon after exposure to clotting factor therapy, and in hemophilia B, there is also the risk of anaphylactic reactions in these patients.

Table 137-4 Methods of Factor VIII Measurement

1. FVIII antigen ELISA (rarely used clinically)
2. FVIII functional assay
   a. One-stage clotting assay: >98% of clinical laboratories; assay CV <10%
   b. Chromogenic assay } May detect FVIII instability mutants
   c. Two-stage clotting assay } May detect FVIII instability mutants
3. Indirect measurement

Global assays (e.g., thrombin generation assay)

CV, Coefficient of variation; *ELISA,* enzyme-linked immunosorbent assay; *FVIII,* factor VIII.

Determination of the hemophilic genotype is now regarded as the standard of care in comprehensive hemophilia treatment centers (see box on Hemophilia Carrier Detection and Prenatal Diagnosis).

Diagnosis of the Carrier State in Hemophilia

The X-linked recessive nature of hemophilia naturally results in the majority of affected subjects being males. Females, however, carry and transmit the hemophilic trait and can sometimes also express clinical manifestations of the disease. Although there are rare genetic circumstances that can result in moderately severe or severe hemophilia in women (see Table 137-2), the majority of females with low FVIII or FIX levels do so because of variable skewing of the random X inactivation process that takes place early during embryonic development.

There are four ways in which hemophilia carriers can be identified. First, in light of the X-linked transmission of the disease, pedigree analysis will determine the carrier status of some women. Thus all daughters of hemophilic fathers are obligate carriers, and 50% of the daughters of a hemophilia carrier mother will also carry the mutant allele. The second mode of identification can be through the manifestation of abnormal bleeding caused by a low FVIII or FIX level. Estimates of the percentage of hemophilia carriers who experience excessive bleeding (most often demonstrated through menorrhagia) vary but likely approximate 20% to 30%. The third mode of carrier detection involves use of the laboratory phenotype, in which tests of the intrinsic pathway (PTT) may be abnormal and the plasma levels of FVIII or FIX may be reduced below the normal range. Finally, and most definitively, molecular genetic analysis provides precise determination of the hemophilic carrier state. This advance has significantly enhanced family counseling for hemophilic kindred and has also enabled women and their caregivers to prepare optimally for the delivery of newborns.

Hemophilia Carrier Detection and Prenatal Diagnosis

As an X-linked recessive trait, hemophilia most often manifests in males. However, females may be affected by the condition in two ways: through bleeding caused by low clotting factor levels and through transmission of the trait to later generations as a hemophilia carrier.

Women who are heterozygous carriers of a hemophilic mutation may have low levels of the implicated clotting factor. This depends on the ratio of inactivation of the hemophilic and normal X chromosomes, a random process that occurs early during embryonic development. If there is markedly skewed inactivation of the normal X chromosome, the plasma level of FVIII or FIX may be correspondingly reduced, and the carrier female may have evidence of a bleeding disorder. Thus FVIII or FIX levels should be determined in all potential carrier females before adolescence when they might first manifest with menorrhagia. A low plasma level of FVIII or FIX is predictive of the carrier state, and the lower the level, the more probable the carrier diagnosis.

Aside from using clotting factor levels to determine carrier status and bleeding risk, the most definitive approach to carrier diagnosis is to use molecular genetics to identify the causative FVIII or FIX mutation. Although carrier detection studies originally used analysis of linked polymorphisms to track mutant alleles, advances in sequencing technology now enable relatively easy access to direct mutation detection.

Ideally, carrier detection should be performed after puberty but before the woman is contemplating starting a family. In many countries, testing for the carrier status of genetic disease is prohibited before adolescence so that the girl can participate in discussions of testing options.

With current molecular genetic testing strategies, the results of mutation analyses are available within a few days in urgent circumstances. However, most often, results are returned within a few weeks.

Causative mutations in the FVIII or FIX genes are found in more than 95% of carriers. If a mutation is not found, it is possible that the mutation is deep within an intron or involves a distant transcriptional element.

Prenatal diagnosis of hemophilia should begin with an evaluation of the fetal sex, which can usually be determined through an ultrasound examination. If the fetus is female, no additional studies should be performed. If the fetus is male, molecular genetic analysis can be used to identify the hemophilic mutation. Fetal DNA can be isolated from chorionic villus samples obtained after 11 weeks of gestation or from amniocytes obtained by amniocentesis from 12 to 34 weeks. The risk of miscarriage with both of these procedures is approximately 1%. If the studies are being used for decision making concerning therapeutic abortion, the tests should be performed as soon as possible. Determination of the hemophilic status of the fetus will also help plan for delivery, although consensus about the optimal obstetric management of an affected baby is lacking. Finally, recent studies suggest that free fetal DNA can be isolated from the mother's blood, with levels increasing towards term. Examination of this material for the presence of Y chromosome sequences would allow definitive sex determination.

Differential Diagnosis of Hemophilia

The initial clinical suspicion of hemophilia will usually come from signs and symptoms of excessive bleeding, a family history of a bleeding problem, or abnormal coagulation test results.

There are many causes of mild bleeding manifestations, such as increased bruising and prolonged bleeding after dental and surgical procedures. These include either isolated or combined deficiencies of other clotting factors (i.e., FXI, FVII, FX, FII, FV deficiency; see Chapter 139), von Willebrand disease (vWD; see Chapter 140), or various quantitative or qualitative platelet pathologies (see Chapters 132 to 134). Acquired bleeding symptoms can be caused by antithrombotic drugs (e.g., antiplatelet agents and anticoagulants) or can result from autoantibodies against clotting factors (e.g., acquired hemophilia A or vWD).

The differential diagnosis of a low plasma FVIII level is relatively straightforward (Table 137-5). Levels of FVIII below 10% are likely the result of inherited or acquired hemophilia A or a severe form of inherited or acquired vWD (severe type 1 or type 3 vWD). Determination of vWF antigen and vWF ristocetin cofactor levels is essential for diagnosis. Occasionally, levels of FVIII below 10% can be attained with type 2N vWD. This diagnosis can be confirmed using FVIII binding studies or by genotypic analysis of the FVIII binding codons of vWF (exons 17-25, which encode the D′/D3 regions of the vWF protein).[6] Levels of FVIII between 10% and 50% are also

Table 137-5 Differential Diagnosis of a Low Factor VIII Level

1. FVIII <10%
   - Severe or moderately severe hemophilia A
   - Severe type 1 vWD
   - Type 3 vWD
   - Type 2N vWD
   - Acquired hemophilia A
   - Acquired vWD
2. FVIII: 10% to 50%
   - Mild hemophilia A
   - Type 1 vWD
   - Type 2N vWD
   - Combined FVIII and FV deficiency

FV, Factor V; *FVIII*, factor VIII; *vWD*, von Willebrand disease.

likely the result of either hemophilia A or vWD (types 1 or one of the type 2 variants, 2A, 2B, 2M, or 2N). Assessment of vWF levels must be undertaken in these cases; if the vWF:RCo/vWF:Ag ratio is below 0.6, further evaluation of a possible type 2 variant must be pursued. Rarely, mild or moderate FVIII deficiency can be co-inherited with FV deficiency (see Chapter 139). Combined inherited deficiency of FVIII and FV (levels are usually between 5% and 20%) has a prevalence of approximately 1 per million. This rare inherited trait is caused by recessive mutations in one of two genes involved in the facilitation of protein transport across the ER-Golgi interface: lectin mannose binding protein type 1 (LMAN1) or multiple coagulation factor deficiency 2 (MCFD2).

Isolated low plasma levels of FIX are almost always caused by congenital hemophilia B. Interestingly, in contrast to acquired hemophilia A, autoantibody development against FIX is rarely encountered. Other situations in which FIX deficiency is found usually involve concomitant reductions in the other vitamin K–dependent clotting factors, such as occurs with vitamin K antagonists, vitamin K deficiency, or significant liver disease. A much less common cause of a mild deficiency state of all of the vitamin K–dependent proteins is an inherited defect in the γ carboxylase enzyme required for the posttranslational modification of these proteins.

CLINICAL FEATURES OF HEMOPHILIA

The clinical symptoms and signs of hemophilia A and B are identical and relate to the propensity for prolonged and excessive bleeding. The bleeding tendency in hemophilia is determined in large part by the baseline level of the deficient or defective clotting factor. Thus, in severe hemophilia (A and B), in which the baseline level of clotting factor is below 1% (0.01 U/mL), spontaneous bleeding usually occurs multiple times each year. With a mild factor deficiency state of 1% to 5% (0.01-0.05 U/mL), spontaneous bleeding is infrequent, but excessive and prolonged bleeding can occur with trauma and invasive surgical or dental procedures. Finally, in mild disease, with factor levels of 5% to 40% (0.05-0.40 U/mL), excessive bleeding is usually only documented with trauma or invasive procedures.

Pathological bleeding can occur in the neonatal period, when intracranial bleeding can develop after traumatic delivery, especially in infants with severe hemophilia. However, most frequently, severe disease manifests with easy bruising or soft tissue or joint bleeding between 6 and 18 months of age when the young child becomes more mobile. In mild hemophilia, the disease may remain silent for many years, and occasionally a new diagnosis of hemophilia may be made in those older than 60 years of age when challenged with a surgical procedure.

The bleeding pattern in severe hemophilia is distinct and is not often seen in other bleeding disorders. In severe hemophilia, the development of hemarthroses is a classical clinical sign. Bleeding into the ankles, knees, and elbows is seen most frequently, although a hemarthrosis can occur in any joint (e.g., into the temporomandibular joint). The development of a hemarthrosis is accompanied by pain, swelling, and reduced mobility, but after repeated episodes of joint bleeding, most patients with hemophilia are able to discern intraarticular bleeding at a very early stage before any of the classical clinical signs are apparent. Repeated bleeding into a single joint results in the development of a "target joint," one in which further bleeding episodes are facilitated by previous events, leading to a vicious cycle of joint damage. With repeated episodes of bleeding, the joints become painful and less mobile. Eventually, this can result in immobility and muscle wasting of the affected limb (Fig. 137-10).

In addition to joint bleeding, patients with hemophilia are prone to excessive and prolonged soft tissue and mucocutaneous bleeding. Bleeding into unusual sites, such as the iliopsoas muscle, can result in prolonged disability, and rarely, intracranial bleeding can develop, most often after trauma.

Although bleeding is the hallmark of hemophilia, the types of bleeds and issues vary somewhat according to the age of the patient. This is particularly the case in newborns with hemophilia who have specific issues related to the birthing process not encountered later on in life. Also, the issues encountered in infancy (the highest risk period for developing inhibitors and the time for establishing home care and prophylaxis protocols) are different from those encountered in later childhood, adolescence, and the early and late adult years.

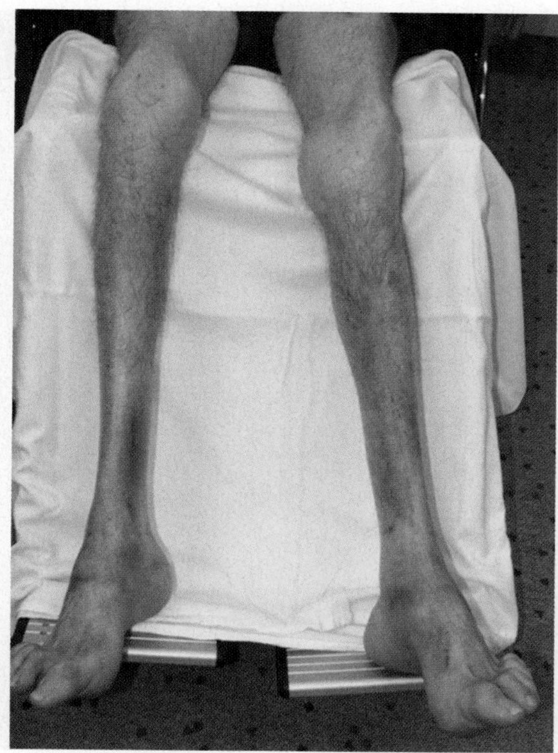

Figure 137-10 CLINICAL OUTCOME OF CHRONIC SEVERE HEMOPHILIC ARTHROPATHY. This picture shows the legs of a 55-year-old patient with severe hemophilia A who is a wheelchair user. After a lifelong experience of multiple hemarthroses, the patient has very limited mobility. His ankles and knees show deformities, and his leg muscles are markedly atrophic because of a lack of use.

Hemophilia in Newborns

The neonatal period is a particularly hazardous period for newborn children with severe hemophilia. Newborn babies with hemophilia can be born to mothers who are known or suspected of being carriers or can be born to mothers who are not known to be carriers. The latter occurs in about 30% of newborns with hemophilia. It is principally in the group of children born to families with no history of hemophilia that the risk of severe bleeding is greater because no precautions are taken to avoid bleeding. How best to deliver children known to have severe hemophilia is still a matter of debate. For the most part, physicians still recommend an atraumatic vaginal delivery because this can usually be performed safely and avoids the increased maternal morbidity associated with cesarean section. Furthermore, delivery of a child by cesarean section does not completely eliminate the risk of intracranial hemorrhage (ICH) (Fig. 137-11). The use of vacuum extraction or forceps should be avoided because these procedures increase the risk of both extracranial (e.g., subgaleal hemorrhage and cephalohematoma) and ICH. Fetal blood sampling has not been shown to be a significant risk factor for ICH.

Intracranial Hemorrhage in Newborns

The incidence of ICH in newborn children with severe hemophilia varies from 3.5% to 4%.[7] It is surprising that it is this low given the

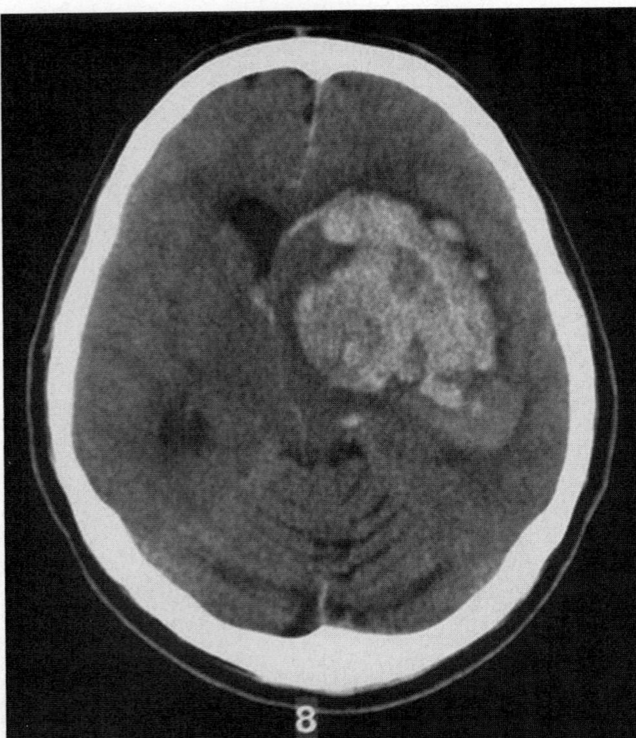

Figure 137-11 INTRACRANIAL BLEEDING IN HEMOPHILIA. A computed tomography scan shows an intracranial bleed in a person with hemophilia. This complication most often occurs after trauma with an incidence of five per 1000 per year in patients younger than age 5 years and 1% to 2% per year in persons with hemophilia older than age 55 years.

trauma of childbirth. Nevertheless, this is still 40- to 80-fold higher than that in the normal nonhemophilic population. If a child with known hemophilia shows any sign of ICH, prompt infusion of the appropriate factor concentrate should be undertaken. If the type of hemophilia is not known, fresh plasma can be given at a dose of 10 mL/kg. Because FVIII deficiency is more common than FIX deficiency, an alternative is to administer FVIII concentrate and determine the PTT 10 to 15 minutes later. If the patient has hemophilia A, the PTT should correct. If the PTT does not correct, then it can be assumed that the child has FIX deficiency, and an appropriate FIX concentrate can be given. If a FVIII concentrate is used, fresh plasma can be given while waiting for the PTT results to cover the possibility that the child has hemophilia B.

In newborn boys without a family history of hemophilia, signs of ICH (e.g., unequal pupils, seizures, vomiting, and lethargy) should prompt an urgent PTT determination along with central nervous system imaging. If the PTT is prolonged and imaging studies reveal an intracranial bleed, levels of FVIII, FIX, and vWF should be determined urgently. While waiting for the results of these levels, it is best to treat the patient with a FVIII concentrate, or plasma can be given.

Circumcision in Newborns

Surprisingly, bleeding after circumcision only occurs in about half of patients with severe hemophilia. Consequently, the lack of bleeding after circumcision does not exclude hemophilia. In children who are suspected of having hemophilia, the hemophilic status should be confirmed before circumcision. If hemophilia is proven and the family still wishes to undertake circumcision, the appropriate factor concentrate should be administered to the child before the procedure. Generally, a single dose is sufficient.

Other Bleeding Manifestations in Hemophilia

Although virtually all types of bleeds can occur in hemophilia, musculoskeletal bleeds (hemarthrosis, muscle bleeds, and hematomas) are most common and cause the most long-term complications. Other reasonably common bleeds include oral, dental, gastrointestinal (GI), genitourinary, and neurologic bleeding. Additionally, insufficiently treated muscle and soft tissue bleeds may develop into pseudotumors (see box on Hemophiliac Pseudotumors) or lead to compartment syndrome (see box on Compartment Syndrome). Finally, bleeds can occur in the context of surgery and dental procedures.

Bleeding in hemophilia is broadly correlated with the endogenous level of clotting factor. Patients with severe forms of hemophilia defined as having an endogenous FVIII or FIX level of less than 1% (<0.01 U/mL) will develop spontaneous bleeds throughout their lives beginning at about 6 to 12 months of age when beginning to crawl. Without prophylaxis, patients with severe hemophilia develop more bleeds as they age, and studies have shown that on average such patients experience 20 to 30 bleeds per year. Patients with moderate hemophilia (FVIII or FIX level of between 1% and 5% [0.01 and 0.05 U/mL]) and those with mild hemophilia (factor levels of >5% [>0.05 U/mL]) generally experience bleeding only in the context of trauma or surgery.

Both hemophilia A and hemophilia B are characterized by similar types of bleeds. However, the severity and frequency of bleeding may vary considerably among individuals with the same factor activity level, and the bleeding phenotype in hemophilia B seems to be less severe than that in hemophilia A with comparable factor levels. This is reflected in increased joint arthroplasty, increased use of prophylaxis, and a lower median age at start of prophylaxis in patients with severe hemophilia A compared with those with severe hemophilia B. Similarly, although a considerable proportion of children with moderate hemophilia A in Canada are on prophylaxis, few children with moderate hemophilia B are treated with prophylactic regimens, again suggesting a differential severity of hemophilia A and B. The reason for this difference in clinical bleeding severity between hemophilia A and B has not been well studied. For patients with severe hemophilia, one possible explanation is related to the genetics of hemophilia. Patients with severe hemophilia B generally have non-null mutations (e.g., missense mutations) and as such are likely to have some, albeit minimal, endogenous FIX activity. In contrast, most patients with severe hemophilia A have null mutations and produce no functional FVIII. Another theoretical reason to explain the difference in the severity of bleeding is that when patients with hemophilia B experience a bleed, their FVIII levels may rise because FVIII is an acute phase reactant. Because it serves as a cofactor for FIX, this increase in FVIII may augment the activity of the very low level of FIX that exists in patients with mild, moderate, or non-null mutation severe FIX deficiency, thereby improving the patients' hemostatic potential and limiting bleeding.

Even within patients with the same mutation and thus with the same endogenous level of clotting factor, there may be differences in bleeding predisposition. Reasons to account for this include the co-inheritance of other bleeding diatheses (e.g., vWD or mild functional platelet disorders) or prothrombotic disorders (e.g., factor V Leiden; prothrombin G20210A mutation; low levels of protein C, protein S, or antithrombin). Additional reasons to account for between-patient heterogeneity include varying levels of physical activity; differences in the pharmacokinetic handling of factor that might be associated with patients' ABO blood group and endogenous levels of vWF; and differences in the structural integrity of joints, making patients more or less susceptible to joint bleeds and joint damage. The latter may explain why some patients can experience one significant joint bleed and end up developing signs and symptoms of chronic hemophilic arthropathy but other patients may not develop joint damage despite repeated joint bleeding.

Soft Tissue Hemorrhages and Muscle Bleeds

Bleeding into soft tissues includes spontaneous and trauma-related bleeding into subcutaneous tissues and muscles. Superficial hematomas (bruises) may resolve spontaneously without the need for treatment, and as such, bruising is not an indication to treat the patient with clotting factor replacement. However, in moderate and severe hemophilia, soft tissue hematomas often undergo progressive enlargement and may need to be treated. Furthermore, some soft tissue bleeds (e.g., retroperitoneal bleeds or hematomas of the neck) may cause extensive blood loss and be life or organ threatening because of their propensity to expand, thus causing compression of adjacent organs, blood vessels, and nerves and, in the case of neck hematomas, compromise of the airway.

Muscle bleeds are quite common in hemophilia. The muscles most often involved are, in descending order of frequency, the calf, thigh, buttocks, and forearm. Bleeds into these locations can lead to compartment syndrome, which is an emergency situation (see box on Compartment Syndrome).

A particularly problematic muscle bleed is a bleed into the iliopsoas muscle, a large muscle in the hip region. Such bleeds can rapidly expand because there is no surrounding connective tissue to restrict their growth. Consequently, significant bleeding can occur into this muscle, potentially leading to the need for blood transfusion. Patients with iliopsoas muscle bleeds have pain and restriction of movement around the hip joint; they tend to maintain the leg in a flexed position. Because of increased pressure on the femoral nerve, they may complain of paresthesia, hyperesthesia, or weakness of the quadriceps muscle. An iliopsoas bleed can be confused with a hemarthrosis of the hip (see box on Hip Joint Bleeds). Urgent ultrasonography or magnetic resonance imaging (MRI) examination is required to differentiate between the two conditions. Iliopsoas muscle bleeds need prolonged treatment with factor concentrates, as well as immobilization and physical therapy. This may necessitate hospitalization (see box on Hemophilic Pseudotumors).[8]

Hemarthrosis

Bleeding into joints accounts for about 75% of all bleeding events in hemophilia and is the hallmark of hemophilia. Although any joints may be involved, the most commonly involved are the ankles, knees, and elbows. These three joints are therefore referred to as *index joints*. Less commonly involved joints are the shoulders, hips, and wrists. The least involved are the joints in the hands and feet.

There is significant variability in the time when children with severe hemophilia experience their first joint bleed. Although the median age to experience the first joint bleed is around 1.8 years, some children experience this within the first year of life (as they begin to ambulate) and others not until their fourth, fifth, or sixth years of life.[9] Hemarthroses become more common as children age if they are not placed on prophylactic therapy. Hemarthrosis can be either spontaneous or trauma related; the trauma may be imperceptible. Mild trauma may even occur while the child is asleep, causing the child to wake up with joint pain and swelling. The onset of a hemarthrosis is often signaled by a feeling of warmth and tingling in the joint. This may last for several hours before increasing pain and limitation of joint movement set in. In patients with severe hemophilia, bleeding into the joint will continue until the patient receives hemostatic therapy or the pressure within the joint increases to the point of causing occlusion of bleeding vessels and bleeding cessation. In the later scenario, the pain in the joint may be excruciating. In patients with moderate or mild hemophilia, the bleeding may stop without the administration of hemostatic replacement but only after substantial bleeding has occurred. Consequently, joint bleeds should be treated as soon as possible to minimize the extent of bleeding and reduce the risk of long-term disabling sequelae.

Blood in a joint leads to joint damage through at least three mechanisms: iron toxicity, inflammation, and mechanical distension of the joint. Repeated joint bleeds may result in inflammation and hyperplasia of the synovial tissue within the joint (a situation referred to as *synovitis*).[10] Synovitis is the first step toward the development of hemophilic arthropathy. Any joint that undergoes repeated bleeds is referred to as a *target joint*. The strict definition of a target joint is still under discussion, but in general, most clinicians tend to accept that a joint that bleeds three or four times in a 6-month period qualifies as a target joint. A target joint is a manifestation of synovitis, and if not managed with long-term prophylaxis, such a joint will continue to bleed and will ultimately become a chronically damaged, arthropathic joint. Early stage hemophilic arthropathy is characterized by synovial hyperplasia, extensive destruction of articular cartilage, progressive loss of joint space, cystic changes within the subchondral bone, osteoporosis, and atrophy of surrounding muscles. The final stage of hemophilic arthropathy is a deformed and dysfunctional joint. At this stage, joint bleeds become less frequent as synovial hypertrophy becomes less prominent.

Compartment Syndrome

A compartment syndrome arises when a bleed (usually trauma induced) occurs into a closed (encapsulated) space, such as the forearm or calf. The capsule restricts exit of blood, thereby raising the pressure within the compartment. This ultimately results in compression of blood vessels and obstruction of blood flow, leading to tissue ischemia and the potential for nerve and muscle damage. Compartment syndrome is characterized by severe pain and swelling, limb pallor, paresthesias, and reduced movement of the limb. Without treatment, a compartment syndrome may lead to permanent neuropathy, tissue necrosis, and even loss of the limb. This emergency condition requires urgent factor replacement and potentially surgical decompression (fasciotomy).

Hemophilic Pseudotumors

Pseudotumors are a rare but very problematic complication in hemophilia. The most common type of pseudotumor arises as a result of repeated hemorrhages into a muscle with insufficient resorption of blood between hemorrhages. Pseudotumors become walled-off cystic structures surrounded by a fibrous membrane. They may become multivacuolated over time, and parts may become calcified. These cystic lesions frequently expand into adjacent structures, leading to their destruction. Skeletal fractures and bony deformities may arise from such lesions. Another and rarer type of pseudotumor, generally only seen in adult patients, arises from within the bone itself and is often secondary to subperiosteal bleeding. This type of pseudotumor is typically observed in the long bones of the lower extremities and in the pelvis. Pseudotumors arising distally are more common in young children and most often occur in the hand. Pseudotumors may be associated with pain from rapid growth or nerve compression.

Pseudotumors are usually diagnosed by radiological means (ultrasonography or MRI). A pseudotumor may be misdiagnosed as a neoplasm (e.g., Ewing sarcoma or osteosarcoma) or as an infection (e.g., osteomyelitis or tuberculous abscess). Biopsy of such lesions is contraindicated because of the potential for significant bleeding or infection. Small pseudotumors, particularly distal ones or pseudotumors in patients with inhibitors, are often treated conservatively with aggressive clotting factor replacement along with immobilization of the affected limb.

Unfortunately, in some instances, factor replacement alone is insufficient, and complete surgical excision is needed. This carries potential morbidity and even mortality and should only be undertaken by skilled surgeons in conjunction with appropriate hemophilia specialists. Attempts have been made at embolization of such pseudotumors, and radiation therapy has been successfully used for treatment of small pseudotumors of the hand.

Determining the status of joints of patients with hemophilia at a given time or longitudinally over time necessitates both clinical and radiographic examinations. Over the past 10 to 20 years, clinical and radiographic scoring systems have been developed to objectively evaluate these findings (Table 137-6). Clinical scores are the most readily available, do not require expensive radiological equipment, and may be the most reflective of a patient's joint disability status. Plain radiographs are relatively inexpensive and widely available but are insensitive to the soft tissue changes seen in the early stages of joint disease and involve radiation exposure. MRI is the most sensitive to early joint (soft tissue) changes and does not expose patients to radiation but is limited by high cost, more limited availability, and the need for general anesthesia in very young children. Preliminary work is ongoing on the use of ultrasonography to evaluate acute and chronic changes in joints. Ultrasonography does not require sedation in young children; is much less expensive than MRI; and differentiates between synovium and hemosiderin, which is not always possible with MRI. However, ultrasonography also has limitations: (1) it is very operator dependent, and the interpretation of ultrasound findings can be subjective, and (2) some structures within a joint (e.g., cartilage) are not readily visualized.

Mucous Membrane Bleeding

Epistaxis is not a prominent feature of hemophilia, but it certainly can occur. Oral bleeding is, however, quite common in patients with hemophilia. Often, one of the first presentations of hemophilia is bleeding from the frenulum after trauma. Tongue bleeding, caused by a child biting the tongue, is also reasonably common. This can become an emergency, either because of significant blood loss or from tongue swelling to the point of airway obstruction. Excessive bleeding with loss of deciduous teeth and eruption of secondary dentition can occur but is not common in hemophilia. Fortunately, most bleeding from the mouth can be controlled with antifibrinolytic agents, such as tranexamic acid (Cyklokapron) or epsilon aminocaproic acid (Amicar). Factor replacement may be required for more serious cases. For dental surgery, particularly if it requires a nerve block, factor replacement or DDAVP (desmopressin) needs to be given to raise the factor level to at least 30% of normal.

Table 137-6 Hemophilia A and B

	Scores	Reference
Clinical	World Federation of Hemophilia Joint score (Gilbert score)	Gilbert, *Semin Hematol*, 1993
	The modified WFH joint score Colorado PE-1 and PE-0.5	Manco-Johnson et al, *Haemophilia*, 2000
	HJHS (Hemophilia Joint Health Score)	Feldman et al, *Arthritis Care Res*, 2011
Plain radiography	Arnold-Hilgartner	Arnold and Hilgartner 1977
	Pettersson	Petterson et al, *Acta Paediatrica*, 1981
MRI	Progressive Denver scoring system	Nuss et al, *Haemophilia*, 2000
	Additive European scoring system	Lundin et al, *Haemophilia*, 2004
	Single compatible IPSG MRI scoring system	Doria et al, *Haemophilia*, 2008

IPSG, International Prophylaxis Study Group; *MRI*, magnetic resonance imaging; *WFH*, World Federation of Hemophilia.

Hematuria

In the past, hematuria was a reasonably common occurrence in patients with hemophilia. Hematuria may be associated with trauma but most often is spontaneous, episodic, and usually painless. Hematuria can rarely be caused by renal calculi because these are thought to be more common in males with hemophilia compared with the normal nonhemophilic male population. There is no consensus on how best to manage hematuria in patients with hemophilia, but in general, increased oral fluids along with bed rest are recommended. If, despite these measures, bleeding continues or is particularly severe, factor replacement should be given; the use of steroids to manage hematuria in patients with hemophilia has been reported, but there is no conclusive evidence that steroids provide any additional benefit. Fortunately, hematuria in patients with hemophilia is not associated with progressive loss of renal function, and as such, its natural history is probably benign.

The use of antifibrinolytic agents (tranexamic acid or epsilon aminocaproic acid) is contraindicated with hematuria because of the risk of ureteral obstruction by clots.

Gastrointestinal Bleeding

Gastrointestinal bleeding can occur in patients with hemophilia, particularly in adults, in whom it is often associated with the chronic use of nonsteroidal antiinflammatory drugs (NSAIDs) for hemophilic arthropathy. Another potential explanation for GI tract bleeding is esophageal varices in patients with portal hypertension secondary to long-standing hepatitis C. Such patients may present with massive life-threatening melena or hematemesis.

Neurologic Bleeding

Intracranial hemorrhage is the most dangerous hemorrhagic event in hemophilic patients. It is at present, along with HIV and hepatitis C, one of the three leading causes of death in persons with hemophilia. In both neonates and children with hemophilia, ICH is the leading cause of death. ICH is also one of the leading causes of morbidity (mental retardation, seizure disorders, and motor dysfunction) in children with hemophilia.[11] The incidence of ICH is highest in neonates and is associated with the birthing process, particularly with a traumatic vaginal delivery. ICH is also seen in young children with severe hemophilia, particularly in those who are not on prophylaxis or have an inhibitor. In older adults, ICH again becomes more common, particularly in patients with coexisting HIV or hepatitis C. In such patients, mild to moderate thrombocytopenia is frequently seen either as a result of portal hypertension–induced splenomegaly or from HIV-associated immune thrombocytopenia. The combination of thrombocytopenia together with hemophilia increases the risk of CNS bleeding. ICH is rare in patients with mild or moderate hemophilia.

Most cases of ICH occur after trauma, but the trauma may be quite trivial, making the ICH appear to be spontaneous in nature. Patients with ICH usually present with neurologic symptoms soon after trauma, but bleeding may be delayed for several days or weeks. Typical neurologic symptoms suggestive of an ICH include drowsiness, loss of consciousness, seizures, headache, and vomiting. Any of these symptoms should alert the clinician to the potential for an ICH. In these circumstances, any person with hemophilia who has neurologic symptoms or signs should be presumed to have an ICH and should be immediately given a bolus of an appropriate factor concentrate to raise the patient's factor level to about 100%. This should always be done before any diagnostic procedure (e.g., computed tomography or MRI) to confirm the diagnosis of ICH. If an ICH is present, in addition to appropriate factor replacement, patients should be hospitalized for 10 to 14 days during which time they should be maintained on factor concentrate (by continuous infusion or frequent bolus infusions) to maintain a factor level over 100% at all times.

Lumbar punctures, which are almost never necessary in patients with hemophilia, and neurosurgical intervention, can safely be performed provided that 100% factor correction is achieved.

Intracranial bleeding may be subdural, epidural, subarachnoid, or intracerebral. Intraspinal (usually epidural) bleeding is rare, but when it occurs, can cause spinal cord compression.

Surgery and Bleeding

With the exception of circumcision in neonates, excessive bleeding is almost inevitable in patients with severe or moderate hemophilia who undergo surgery without adequate treatment with hemostatic agents. The bleeding can be acute or can be delayed for several hours or days. In addition to bleeding, surgery in such patients is characterized by poor wound healing as a result of poor clot formation along with prolonged bleeding and subsequent infection at the wound site. With appropriate management (factor replacement with or without other adjunctive hemostatic agents), intra- and postoperative hemorrhages can be prevented. With attention to the management of hemostasis, surgery can be performed safely in patients with hemophilia. Ideally, a multidisciplinary team is required to undertake surgery in a safe manner; physicians with expertise in the management of hemophilia patients should always be involved. Some surgeries might need to be adapted for patients with hemophilia (e.g., tissue cardiac valves are preferable to mechanical cardiac valves because of the relative contraindications of anticoagulant drugs in hemophilia).

CLINICAL MANAGEMENT OF HEMOPHILIA

As a lifelong, expensive, and disabling illness, the management of patients with hemophilia is complex and ideally best undertaken through comprehensive care in hemophilia treatment centers with multidisciplinary teams of health professionals. These teams should include a physician (usually a hematologist) with specialist training in hemophilia, a dedicated nurse, a physical therapist, and a social worker. Additional members that should be available for consultation include an orthopedic surgeon, a dentist, a genetic counselor, an obstetrician/gynecologist, a psychologist, a rheumatologist, a urologist, and (increasingly, for the management of elderly persons with hemophilia) a cardiologist. Fortunately, the role of the orthopedic surgeon in the management of hemophilia has been reduced in countries where prophylactic therapy can be provided.

Over the course of a lifetime, a patient and his family will experience numerous issues related to hemophilia. Significant psychological sequelae ensue for both affected children and their families. These children may be overprotected, and this may result in their experiencing difficulties in adjusting to the school environment and to society in general as they age. Hemophilia impacts children's school experience and what sports and recreational activities they are allowed to undertake. Some studies have shown lower academic performance and behavioral and emotional problems in school-aged children.[12] There may be multifactorial causes for this, including potentially silent ICH. These children may grow up with resentment toward their peers and nonhemophilic siblings and may harbor suppressed anger about having the condition. Hemophilia can also impact vocational choices and opportunities for adults with hemophilia with established arthropathy. In addition to all of the psychological sequelae of hemophilia, unfortunate men with hemophilia who acquired HIV and hepatitis C also have to deal with the myriad emotional and social ramifications of these devastating infectious illnesses.

For the family of people with hemophilia, the child's mother may experience considerable guilt knowing that as a carrier she passed the hemophilic mutation to her son. This can contribute to marriage breakdown, although it has not been ascertained whether separations occur more frequently in the marriages of parents of children with hemophilia than those of parents of children without the condition. Clearly, persons with hemophilia and their families require significant education, counseling, and support throughout the individual's lifetime.

For society in general, hemophilia with or without HIV or hepatitis C has a substantial impact, mainly because of the high cost of care.

The key aspects of hemophilia management are preventive therapy, treatment of bleeds, and care of the complications of hemophilic bleeding.

Preventive Therapy

Preventing trauma does much to reduce bleeding frequency in persons with hemophilia. One of the strategies involved in bleed prevention is restricting the child from high-risk sports (e.g., ice hockey, American-style football, rugby, and martial arts). A number of other sports (e.g., soccer, basketball, baseball, and tennis) also entail a certain amount of risk but for the child's psychological well-being are usually permitted. Other sports considered to be relatively safe include cycling (with a protective helmet), running, and swimming. Ideally, persons with hemophilia should be encouraged to keep active throughout their lives because osteoporosis and obesity are growing problems in this population as a result of inactivity. All patients with severe and moderately severe hemophilia should be told to wear helmets for bicycle riding, rollerblading, skateboarding, and downhill skiing. There is controversy regarding the use of helmets (outside of sports) in very young children as they are learning to walk and are unsteady on their feet and prone to falling. Some clinics advocate that patients between the ages of 1 and 2.5 years with severe forms of hemophilia wear a helmet at all times, with the exception of when they are sleeping. Whether this policy reduces the incidence of ICH is not known. Advising families on the importance of good dental hygiene is important because good oral hygiene may prevent or reduce the need for dental procedures (extractions, root canals), which entail a risk of bleeding. Unfortunately, dental care, including regular cleaning by a dentist, is often not subsidized by society and as such may be an expensive undertaking for families.

Vaccinations

Children with hemophilia have normal immune systems and should receive all routine vaccines. In addition, they should receive hepatitis B vaccinations at a young age because they are at a slightly higher risk of exposure to hepatitis B virus throughout their lives through the use of blood products. Recombinant factor concentrates and currently available plasma-derived factor concentrates do not transmit hepatitis B. However, patients with hemophilia are at a higher risk of requiring a routine blood transfusion because of trauma-associated blood loss, and there is still a small risk of acquiring hepatitis B from blood transfusions. It is not clear whether patients with hemophilia should receive the hepatitis A vaccination. However, the US National Hemophilia Foundation's Medical and Scientific Advisory Council has recommended that all persons with hemophilia who are seronegative for hepatitis A should be immunized against hepatitis A.

For persons with hemophilia, all vaccines should be given with care using the smallest gauge needle possible (#25 or #27) and applying pressure to the injection site for about 5 minutes. Vaccinations should be given subcutaneously rather than intramuscularly. This is a matter of some debate, however, because the majority of carefully administered intramuscular injections can be given safely. Nevertheless, there is an increased risk of hematoma formation after intramuscular injections subcutaneously administered. Vaccinations appear to produce the same immune response as those given intramuscularly.[13] Even if the immune response is slightly lower, the enhanced safety of subcutaneous injections renders this the preferred route.

Avoidance of Aspirin and Other Medications

Persons with hemophilia already have a severe bleeding disorder, and this can be exacerbated by aspirin. NSAIDS may also interfere with platelet function and should be avoided if possible. cyclooxygenase-2 inhibitors have less of an effect on platelet function than traditional NSAIDS. For older persons with hemophilia with coexistent cardiovascular disease, aspirin, other antiplatelet agents, or anticoagulants may be indicated, but such patients require coordinated care by an experienced cardiologist and a hemophilia specialist (see box on Home Care).

Treatment of Bleeds

When a bleed occurs in a patient with hemophilia, its immediate treatment is required to halt further bleeding. Rapid treatment prevents expansion of the bleed, accelerates healing, and reduces the risk of permanent disability. The longer the delay in providing treatment, the more bleeding will ensue and, consequently, the longer it will take to completely resorb the blood. If joint bleeds are treated rapidly, this will minimize the damage to the joint. Muscle bleeds if treated quickly tend not to become very big and have much less likelihood of transforming into pseudotumors or of causing a compartment syndrome. Rapid treatment of an ICH may save the life of the patient and minimize morbidity. Treatment of bleeds generally consists of more than just hemostatic support (factor concentrates or DDAVP). For example, whereas epistaxis and oral bleeding benefit greatly from the use of antifibrinolytic therapy, rest and physiotherapy are important components of the treatment of joint bleeds (see section on hemarthroses).

Coagulation Factor Concentrates

One of the main components of treating bleeds in hemophilia is replacement of the missing coagulation factor to achieve hemostasis. Until the 1970s, this entailed the use of plasma or cryoprecipitate. Plasma contains small amounts of FVIII and FIX. Consequently, when plasma is used as the source of clotting factor replacement, large volumes are needed. Cryoprecipitate contains a higher concentration of FVIII and, in the past, was commonly used for hemophilia A treatment. However, neither plasma nor cryoprecipitate is virally inactivated. Consequently, both of these blood products carry a risk of viral transmission. This limitation, together with issues of volume and convenience, has rendered these products obsolete management of bleeding in persons with hemophilia.

> **Home Care**
>
> Hemophilic treatment is best administered in the patient's home. Having a patient or other caregiver able to administer factor allows for prompt treatment of bleeds and facilitates prophylaxis. Teaching patients and families how to administer clotting factor concentrate is labor intensive and usually falls to the dedicated hemophilia clinic nurse. It often takes a long time before families become skilled at factor delivery. Most boys with hemophilia older than the age of 3 years can be treated at home after the parents are taught how to administer factor. In some children, poor venous access precludes routine factor delivery; these children often require implantation of a CVAD such as a port-a-cath or creation of an AVF. The teaching of home care is complex. Good sterile technique is critical to avoid CVAD or AVF infections. Later in life, children can be taught how to self-administer factor through peripheral veins. This is generally done in children between the ages of 8 and 12 years of age.

Plasma-derived clotting factor concentrates became available in the 1970s. In the early 1980s, it became evident that these concentrates were contaminated with HIV and hepatitis C. Consequently, thousands of hemophilia patients worldwide were exposed to these devastating viral illnesses, and many died of AIDS or of complications of hepatitis C. Out of this tragedy came the development of safer factor concentrates—plasma-derived concentrates that were subjected to effective viral inactivation methods, including solvent detergent, pasteurization, vapor treatment, nanofiltration, and dry heating—as well as recombinant clotting factors. Currently administered plasma-derived clotting factor concentrates are not associated with HIV, hepatitis B, or hepatitis C seroconversion. In theory, there still is a small possibility of transmission of viruses and prions from plasma-derived concentrates. Plasma-derived concentrates are generally classified as high purity (containing only the desired factor and very little else) or intermediate purity (containing the desired factor but with other factors present). In the case of FVIII, intermediate-purity products generally contain vWF (e.g., Alphanate [Grifols], Humate [CSL-Behring], and Wilate [Octapharma]), and intermediate-purity FIX products are prothrombin complex concentrates (e.g., Beriplex [CSL Behring], Octaplex [Octapharma], and Proplex [Baxter]), which, in addition to FIX, contain factors II, VII, and X, as well as protein C and S. In general, PCCs are no longer used for the management of bleeding in patients with hemophilia B because of the increased risk of thrombosis. In the late 1980s, recombinant factor concentrates were developed. First-generation recombinant products were stabilized by the inclusion of albumin in the final product. Second-generation products no longer contained albumin in the reconstituted preparation but were still exposed to human plasma-derived albumin during the manufacturing process. Third-generation products have no exposure to human or animal proteins and are stabilized with sucrose. Currently, all but one of the recombinant FVIII concentrates are derived from a full-length (as opposed to B domain–deleted) cDNA construct.

Recombinant factor concentrates are usually more expensive than their plasma-derived counterparts, but they have generally supplanted plasma-derived concentrates for hemophilia treatment because of increased safety and small volume of infusion. There is currently only one licensed recombinant FIX concentrate, but there are several different brands of recombinant FVIII. All brands of recombinant FVIII exhibit similar efficacy and are associated with similar rates of inhibitor development. With this in mind, the choice of FVIII concentrate is increasingly influenced by cost. There has been, however, some controversy over the incidence of inhibitors with the use of plasma-derived versus recombinant products. Currently, an international randomized study is evaluating this issue.

All currently available plasma-derived and recombinant concentrates have similar pharmacokinetic properties. The average half-life of FVIII concentrates (either plasma derived or recombinant) appears to be approximately 12 hours with no difference between currently licensed FVIII concentrates. The mean half-life of FIX is approximately 24 hours. The clotting factor half-life is affected by a number of factors. In the case of FVIII, it appears to be affected by the patient's endogenous vWF level, which in turn is related to the ABO blood group. The FVIII half-life appears to be shorter in children.

The recovery of factor concentrate refers to the increase in factor level achieved immediately after infusion of a given amount of factor. With FVIII concentrates, administration of 1 U/kg of FVIII increases the FVIII level by 2%. Therefore, achievement of a FVIII level of 100% in an individual with severe hemophilia requires a dose of 50 U/kg. For FIX, which has a volume of distribution twice that of FVIII, 1 U/kg increases the FIX level by 1%. Recovery of recombinant FIX is less, and in general, 1 U/kg increases the FIX level by 0.8%. Children exhibit lower recoveries of clotting factor, and dosing by body surface area may be more appropriate.

The dose and duration of substitution therapy depend on the severity of the bleed or the extent of the surgery. Table 137-7 shows the desired factor levels for various types of bleeding events and surgeries. After the initial bolus of factor, repeat doses are often necessary. For major bleeds, such as an ICH, or for major surgeries, such

Table 137-7 Recommendations for Clotting Factor Replacement

Site of Bleed	Level Desired (%)	Hemophilia A (rFVIII) (U/kg)	Hemophilia B (rFIX) (U/kg)
Oral mucosa	>30	20	40
Epistaxis	>30	20	40
Joint or muscle	>50	30	50
GI	>50	30	50
GU	>50	50	75
CNS	>100	75	125
Trauma or surgery	>100	75	125

CNS, Central nervous system; *GI,* gastrointestinal; *GU,* genitourinary; *rFIX,* recombinant factor IX; *rFVIII,* recombinant factor VIII.

as joint replacement, 10 to 14 days of full factor replacement may be required, but for less severe bleeds, such as an uncomplicated hemarthrosis, two or three treatments will usually be sufficient. For minor bleeds or minor surgeries (e.g., dental extraction) only 1 to 3 days of factor is required. For patients who require factor for a number of days, in addition to the initial dose of factor, bolus infusions are generally required every 6 to 24 hours depending on the severity of the bleed or the surgery. For major surgery it is generally desirable to maintain the factor level greater than 50% at all times in the postoperative period. This can be done with bolus infusions given approximately every 8 to 12 hours. In general, after the first infusion aiming for 100% replacement, subsequent infusions can be given at half the initial dose every 8 to 12 hours. Because of variable pharmacokinetics, factor levels should be monitored. This avoids high factor levels, which might be prothrombotic, and represent an unnecessary expense, as well as low factor levels, which increase the risk of bleeding. In addition, monitoring helps detect development of inhibitors. Determining the factor level at trough every several days ensures that the patient is achieving a hemostatic level of replacement.

An alternative method for maintaining hemostasis is by continuous clotting factor infusion. Substantially less factor is required with this form of treatment, and the peaks and troughs of repeated bolus administration are avoided. In general, a FVIII infusion rate of 2 to 3 U/kg/hr is sufficient after the FVIII level is increased to 100% with a bolus infusion of 50 U/kg. Although there has been concern about inhibitor development with the use of continuous infusion therapy, evidence that their treatment method increases the risk is lacking.

A number of long-acting FIX concentrates are currently undergoing prospective clinical studies. These studies are reported to have half-lives that are three to five times longer than those of the currently licensed FIX recombinant concentrate. In contrast, long-acting FVIII concentrates appear to have half-lives that are only 1.5- to 2.0-fold longer.

Adjunctive Treatments

Desmopressin

In the mid-1970s, Mannucci and colleagues showed that DDAVP (1-deamino-8 D-arginine vasopressin, desmopressin, Ferring Pharmaceuticals, Langley, UK), a synthetic analogue of the natural antidiuretic hormone, vasopressin, raises circulating levels of vWF and FVIII:C.[17] DDAVP causes the release of endogenous vWF from the Weibel-Palade bodies in endothelial cells into the blood. How DDAVP mobilizes FVIII is not well understood, but the recent discovery of endothelial sources of FVIII may help to explain this phenomenon. DDAVP also increases platelet adhesiveness and shortens the bleeding time independent of its effect on raising FVIII:C and vWF levels. Because DDAVP is not a blood-derived product or a factor concentrate, it is free of both infectious complications and potential inhibitor development. Furthermore, it is much less costly than factor concentrates and has few, generally mild and transient adverse events (flushing, headache, mild tachycardia, and hypotension). DDAVP, however, has antidiuretic activity and thus carries a risk of hyponatremia and seizures, particularly if given to very young children or to those with excessive fluid intake. Because of concern about hyponatremia, many clinicians do not give DDAVP to children younger than 3 years of age and administer DDAVP only once daily unless patients are hospitalized and serum sodium levels and fluid intake are monitored. The effectiveness of DDAVP decreases with repeated administration (tachyphylaxis) because of exhaustion of vWF/FVIII stores. Therefore, DDAVP should not be given for more than 3 consecutive days.

Most patients with mild hemophilia respond to DDAVP with a tripling of their FVIII:C levels to 30% or greater. In patients with moderate hemophilia, DDAVP rarely increases FVIII:C levels into a hemostatically effective range. All individuals with mild hemophilia A should be assessed for DDAVP responsiveness to determine whether they will benefit from this synthetic product. This involves determining FVIII and vWF levels before and 1 and 4 hours after DDAVP administration.

DDAVP can be administered intravenously, subcutaneously, or intranasally. The usual dose for intravenous administration is 0.3 μg/kg given in 50 mL of normal saline over 30 minutes. Intranasally, the usual dose is 150 μg (1 nasal puff) for patients weighing less than 50 kg and 300 μg (1 nasal puff into each nostril) for patients weighing 50 kg or more. The maximum effect of DDAVP is achieved within 30 minutes when given intravenously and within 60 minutes when given intranasally. In general, the safest approach to avoid hyponatremia is to restrict fluids in patients receiving DDAVP and to administer only isotonic solutions such as normal saline.

Because DDAVP stimulates vWF release from endothelial cells, it may increase platelet adhesiveness. In patients with hemophilia with risk factors for coronary or cerebral arterial thrombosis, this may result in angina, myocardial infarction, or stroke. Consequently, DDAVP should be used with caution in elderly men with hemophilia. Because DDAVP also stimulates the release of tissue plasminogen activator, it may exacerbate bleeding. Consequently, DDAVP is often administered in conjunction with antifibrinolytic agents.

Antifibrinolytic Agents

Antifibrinolytic agents are useful in the management of bleeding from mucosal sites where there is high fibrinolytic potential (e.g., the oropharynx, nose, GI tract, and uterine-vaginal lining). In hemophilia, antifibrinolytic agents (e.g., tranexamic acid or epsilon aminocaproic acid) are generally used in the context of oral bleeding or dental surgery. Oral tranexamic acid should be started 24 hours before the scheduled procedure or can be given intravenously immediately before the procedure. The dose of tranexamic acid is 10 mg/kg every 8 hours when given intravenously or 25 mg/kg every 6 to 8 hours when given orally. Tranexamic acid is available in 500-mg tablets, which can be crushed and dissolved in liquids for administration to young children. The usual dosage is 75 mg/kg every 6 hours. In general, antifibrinolytic agents should be administered for 3 to 10 days after a bleeding episode or an invasive procedure. Longer durations of therapy are required for tonsillectomy–adenoidectomy in which bleeding often occurs about 7 days after the procedure when the eschar detaches. The major contraindication to the use of antifibrinolytic agents is hematuria.

Fibrin Sealants

Experience with fibrin sealants in patients with hemophilia is increasing. Fibrin sealants function both as local hemostatic agents and as promoters of wound healing. They are particularly useful for dental procedures. Fibrin sealants have been used successfully to reduce bleeding with dental procedures, circumcision, and after excision of hemophilic pseudotumors.

Adjunctive and Alternative Management Strategies for Joint Bleeds

In the management of joint bleeds, appropriate hemostatic support is critical, but other important measures include appropriate joint rest, analgesia, and graduated physiotherapy. The application of rest, ice (for 20 minutes every 3-4 hours), compression, and elevation (RICE protocol) during the first 24 hours after a joint bleed can provide substantial benefits. The role of joint aspiration in the management of joint bleeds remains controversial, but the procedure is advocated by some groups for management of persistent pain in large-volume hemarthrosis or for exclusion of septic arthritis. Orthotics and physical therapy are of vital importance in the management of acute joint bleeds and in dealing with long-term joint damage in patients with hemophilia. Ankle guards and arch supports are useful for patients with ankle arthropathy to improve gait and weightbearing capacity. Shoe lifts can equalize the length of the lower extremities when there is a leg length discrepancy. Muscle strength training enhances the mechanics of joint movement and provides protection and stabilization of the joint.

Surgical Management of Joint Disease

Surgical approaches to manage the complications of joint bleeds include surgical or arthroscopic synovectomy, nonsurgical (chemical or radionucleotide) synovectomy, various arthrodesis procedures, and joint replacement.

An open surgical or arthroscopic synovectomy endeavors to remove the inflamed and thickened synovial tissue that is the source of bleeding within the joint. Although it may reduce the frequency of bleeding, it does not improve joint mobility and may even worsen it.

Radionucleotide synovectomy has largely replaced chemical synovectomy. This involves injection of a radioisotope (e.g., yttrium^{90}, chromic phosphate P^{32}) into the joint space to obliterate synovial tissue. Compared with surgical synovectomy, radionucleotide synovectomy is less invasive, necessitates a shorter period of hospitalization, and requires less clotting factor coverage. Consequently, the procedure is less costly than surgical synovectomy. Radionucleotide synovectomy is particularly useful for patients with inhibitors because there is a lower risk of bleeding. However, long-term safety data are lacking in hemophilia.

Arthrodesis (surgical joint fixation) is particularly useful for painful joints with greatly compromised mobility in which joint replacement is not easily undertaken (e.g., ankles).

Joint replacements (particularly of the knee and hip) are still commonly performed procedures in adult patients with hemophilia. The elbow, which is not amenable to arthrodesis or for the most part to joint replacement, is often the most difficult joint to manage in patients with hemophilia. It is likely that there will be less need for surgical procedures with the introduction of prophylaxis regimens beginning in early childhood (see box on Hip Joint Bleeds).

Hip Joint Bleeds

Hemorrhage into the hip joint is uncommon compared with other joints. However, the clinical features of hip bleeds are less distinctive than those of more exposed joints, and it is possible that the incidence of hip bleeding is underestimated. Patients with a hip bleed maintain the hip joint in a partially flexed position, the position of lowest pressure. This position is similar to that seen in patients with an iliopsoas muscle bleed, causing these entities to be confused.

The management of acute hemarthrosis of the hip joint is somewhat different from that of other joints because of the vascular anatomy of the hip joint, which renders the head of the femur vulnerable to ischemia in the context of a bleed, causing raised intraarticular pressure.

Pain in the hip joint region may be caused by a range of conditions (hip joint bleed, iliopsoas muscle bleed, bleeds of surrounding muscles, retroperitoneal bleed, and appendicitis). Consequently, without appropriate imaging, a hip joint bleed may be easily misdiagnosed. Ultrasonography remains the preferred modality for investigation of hip pain because plain radiographs lack sufficient sensitivity to detect a hip joint bleed. Persistent pain despite appropriate factor replacement may indicate impending avascular necrosis and urgent consideration for joint aspiration by an experienced interventionalist (using ultrasound guidance) or by a surgeon. Graded physiotherapy should be instituted when symptomatic improvement is observed. Follow-up imaging studies (MRI, bone scan, or both) should be considered for assessment of avascular necrosis.

Prophylactic Clotting Factor Replacement

Experience has shown that if treated solely on demand, patients with hemophilia will experience frequent bleeds and will, over time, develop disabling joint disease. Prophylaxis treatment regimens reduce bleeding and prevent or limit joint damage in patients with hemophilia. The longest experience with the use of prophylaxis comes from European centers in Sweden, The Netherlands, and Germany.[18] Based on numerous cohort studies, good evidence shows that patients with hemophilia who received prophylaxis experienced fewer bleeds and maintained better joint function than patients treated on demand. There are several different prophylaxis regimens distinguished by dose and frequency of factor administration. The full-dose prophylactic regimen, often referred to as the Malmo regimen, involves administration of 25 to 40 U/kg of FVIII every other day (minimum, 3 days/wk) for patients with hemophilia A and the same amount of FIX 2 days a week for those with hemophilia B. Less intense "intermediate-dose" prophylaxis regimens involve the administration of 15 to 25 U/kg two to three times a week, and low-dose prophylaxis regimens call for the administration of dosages of 10 to 15 U/kg given one or two times a week. Primary prophylaxis regimens are started at a very young age (usually 2 years of age or earlier) before joint disease has developed (generally, before or immediately after the first joint bleed) and are continued long term. Secondary prophylaxis includes continuous long-term prophylaxis started at a later age (after 2 years of age) or after more than one joint bleed has occurred. The term *prophylaxis* also encompasses short-term prophylaxis regimens given after surgery or an ICH.

Ample evidence shows that prophylaxis must be commenced early in life to prevent joint disease. In addition, comparisons of different starting prophylactic regimens have shown that patients can be started on less intensive prophylaxis regimens and gradually escalated to full-dose regimens. Although full-dose regimens prevent bleeds more effectively than intermediate- and low-dose schedules, they cost more and may not be feasible in less affluent countries. In these countries, intermediate- or low-dose prophylaxis regimens may be more affordable, and these still confer significant benefit.

Although prophylaxis has been used for years, a recent randomized study that compared primary full-dose prophylaxis with on-demand therapy in young children with severe hemophilia was the first to highlight the benefits of this approach. Patients given primary prophylaxis experienced 90% fewer bleeds and after only a few years already exhibited less joint damage than those treated on demand.[19] The benefits of prophylaxis include reduced hospitalization, less time lost from school or work, improved school performance, and a reduced need for orthopedic surgery. Because of these benefits, the World Health Organization, World Federation of Hemophilia, and many other national hemophilia organizations have endorsed primary prophylaxis as the standard of care for children with severe hemophilia.

The approach to prophylaxis varies by center and country. In some centers and countries, all patients are given full-dose prophylaxis, but in others, prophylaxis is individualized based on the severity and frequency of bleeding episodes.[20]

Burdens of prophylaxis include the need for venous access and cost. Patients receiving full-dose prophylaxis often require central venous access devices (CVADs) or arteriovenous fistulas (AVFs) for repeated factor administration, and full-dose regimens in young children are threefold more expensive than on-demand therapy. However, the cost of on-demand therapy increases over time because when joint bleeds occur, the subsequent joint damage triggers more bleeding. The social costs of joint damage are high in terms of lost time at school or work and limitations in vocational opportunities for adults with arthropathy. Whereas the costs of treating patients on demand rise over time, the cost of prophylaxis may stabilize or decrease when adults become less active. Although most children in Europe and North America are on prophylactic regimens, prophylaxis is less routinely used in adults.

Although there has been concern that starting prophylaxis early in life may increase the risk of development of inhibitors, mounting evidence shows that early initiation of prophylaxis reduces inhibitor development.

Considerations for Treatment of Hemophilic Bleeding in Adults

Although there is now little doubt that regular prophylactic infusions of clotting factor concentrate are the treatment approach of choice for children and adolescents, the role of prophylaxis in adults remains unclear. Although it may seem intuitive to maintain prophylaxis throughout life, this strategy is expensive, and its benefits have not been formally evaluated. Furthermore, some evidence indicates that not all children on prophylaxis required continued therapy as adults. Until more data are available, each case should be dealt with on its individual merits.

When prophylactic therapy in adult patients with hemophilia is undertaken, it should be administered in a manner best suited to the individual needs of the patient. Thus some patients prefer to treat themselves with a small amount of clotting factor every day (e.g., 500 U of FVIII/daily), but others prefer a once- or twice-weekly regimen with additional infusions before high-risk activities, such as sports. Prophylaxis should be used in patients with a target joint into which repeated bleeding is documented. In this instance, prophylactic concentrate infusions at regular intervals (three times a week for FVIII and twice a week for FIX) should be initiated and continued for several months or longer.

If an on-demand regimen is used, patients must be carefully counseled. Treatment should be started as soon as possible after the first signs of bleeding and, if appropriate, adjunctive measures such as rest, ice, compression, or limb elevation should be used to hasten symptom control.

Gene Therapy for Hemophilia

Since the cloning of the FVIII and FIX genes in the early 1980s, hemophilia has been a leading candidate for the application of somatic cell gene transfer.

The rationale for gene therapy in hemophilia includes the following: small increments in FVIII or FIX levels have a significant clinical benefit; regulation of FVIII or FIX levels is not critical as long as they do not reach supraphysiologic levels for extended periods of time; the site of coagulation transgene expression need not be restricted as long as sufficient amounts of the protein reach the circulation; and small (genetically modified hemophilic mice) and large (spontaneously generated hemophilic dogs) animal models of hemophilia are available for preclinical evaluation of gene transfer approaches.

Modes of Transgene Delivery

A key component to any gene transfer strategy is the development of a delivery system that enables efficient transfer of the therapeutic transgene to the recipient cell type of choice. After 30 years of investigation, viral vectors remain the most effective means of achieving high-level gene transfer. Although efforts have been made to enhance the efficiency of nonviral delivery methods such as liposome encapsulation, various physicochemical conjugates, and hydrodynamic injection, all of these approaches have limitations that preclude their advancement into the clinic at this time.

Hemophilia gene transfer studies have used three main types of viral vector: adenovirus, adeno-associated virus (AAV), and several forms of retrovirus. Trials of adenoviral gene transfer have been successful in animal models of hemophilia, but the single hemophilia A patient treated with an adenoviral vector experienced significant hematologic toxicity, and no further clinical studies have been undertaken with this vector type. Thus, although adenoviral gene transfer is highly efficient, these vectors elicit a major innate immune response upon cell entry, and the proinflammatory consequences of this response remain a significant safety concern. Therefore, until the innate immune reactivity of adenoviral gene delivery has been mitigated, this vector system will not be used for the treatment of hemophilia.

The second viral vector approach that has shown promise in hemophilia is the retroviral system. Initial studies were performed with replication-defective gammaretroviral vectors, and one human clinical study in hemophilia A also used this vector system. The major problem with these vectors is the requirement for recipient cell replication to facilitate nuclear entry of the vector. Consequently, gene transfer with these vectors is limited to tissues in which a significant proportion of cells are cycling. In contrast, lentiviral vectors are equally capable of transducing both postmitotic and replicating cells. For this reason, most of the more recent studies of retroviral hemophilia gene transfer have used lentiviral vector protocols in which the vector construct is usually derived from elements of the human immunodeficiency virus. The other major difference between lentiviral gene delivery and gene transfer with other viral vectors is that lentiviruses integrate their genome into the recipient cell genome as a natural part of their life cycle. Although viral vectors do not possess the structural components to enable further rounds of viral replication, there is a risk of insertional mutagenesis that can trigger activation of adjacent oncogenes or inactivation of tumor suppressor loci. Studies performed in the past 5 years indicate that lentiviral integrations are not random but tend to cluster in transcribed regions of the genome and more often occur within introns and coding regions of genes rather than in the upstream regulatory regions where γ-retroviruses insert.

In 2012, the lead candidate for hemophilia gene transfer is AAV (Table 137-8). This is a small nonpathogenic human parvovirus with a small, single-stranded DNA genome of approximately 4.8 kb. Infection in humans, which for some serotypes of the virus is frequent, is not associated with any clinical disease. The various serotypes of AAV have distinct tissue tropisms, and thus by using the

Table 137-8 Features of Adeno-Associated Virus–Mediated Gene Therapy

- AAV is a nonpathogenic virus.
- AAV rarely integrates into the host genome.
- There are no immediate adverse effects after AAV delivery.
- Innate immune reactivity to AAV is minimal.
- Vector readministration can be achieved with different vector serotypes (different capsids).
- Cytotoxic T-cell responses to capsid protein presentation can limit the duration of expression.
- Transgene size is limited to ~5 kb.

AAV, Adeno-associated virus.

capsid sequence for a particular serotype, gene therapists can target specific tissues for transgene expression. As one example, AAV-8 has excellent hepatotropic properties and has been successfully used for liver transgene delivery and expression. Upon entry into recipient cells, AAV is maintained within the nucleus in the form of stable extrachromosomal concatemers, and only a small proportion of the virus integrates into the recipient genome. Wild-type AAV preferentially integrates preferentially into a site on chromosome 19, but the replication-defective AAV vectors appear to insert into sites of natural chromosomal breakages. One significant limitation to AAV vectors is their small packaging capacity. Transgenes larger than 5 kb limit the capacity for viral particle assembly, and although this is not a problem for FIX (cDNA ≈1.4 kb), even the B domain deleted forms of FVIII (cDNA of ≈4.7 kb) are not easily accommodated by this vector type.

Clinical Trials of Hemophilia Gene Therapy

By the end of 2011, approximately 55 patients with hemophilia had undergone clinical evaluation of gene transfer strategies.[21] An initial trial of ex vivo gene transfer for FIX was performed on two subjects in China in the 1990s. A FIX gammaretroviral vector was used to transduce autologous skin-derived fibroblasts before reimplantation. No significant increases in FIX levels were observed. Since then, one patient has been treated with an intravenous FVIII adenoviral vector; a plasmid vector was used as a second ex vivo approach in which autologous fibroblasts were implanted into the omentum, and a small cohort of patients with hemophilia was treated with intravenous FVIII gammaretrovirus. Aside from the transient thrombocytopenia associated with adenoviral vector infusion, there were no adverse events, but none of those approaches increased FVIII or FIX levels beyond a few days, and even then, levels were in the 1% to 4% range.

In contrast, the AAV trials of gene transfer have shown evidence of therapeutic efficacy. There have now been three AAV FIX trials, the first into skeletal muscle and the latter two into liver. Both of the liver-directed trials, the first using hepatic artery delivery of AAV2 and the second systemic intravenous delivery of AAV8, have resulted in longer term expression of FIX at therapeutically relevant levels (between 2% and 10%) in some patients. Indeed, in the most recent AAV8 liver trial, the FIX levels have persisted beyond 5 months. Nevertheless, challenges persist. Most significant has been the recipient immune response against the vector capsid. This cytotoxic T cell–mediated response has resulted in transient hepatotoxicity in several patients and a subsequent loss of transgene expression in one patient. This immune response may be mitigated by transient immunosuppression, and recent evidence from the AAV8 trial suggests that a brief course of prednisone may be sufficient to minimize the hepatotoxicity. Of note, none of these patients has had an anti-FIX immune response.

The future for hemophilia gene therapy is promising. After 2 decades of excellent progress in preclinical studies, there is now realistic hope that clinical success will be achievable, at least for FIX gene therapy. Although AAV vector production will need to be scaled up and methods to limit the antivector immune response remain to be optimized, larger cohort studies are now possible. FVIII gene transfer may not be far behind, but the AAV packaging limitation and the inherent increased immunogenicity of FVIII are obstacles that need to be overcome (Table 137-9).

Table 137-9 Challenges to Successful Hemophilia Gene Therapy

1. Efficient transgene delivery
2. Persistent therapeutic transgene expression
3. Host immunologic responses
   a. To the transgene product: inhibitors
   b. To the vector
      - Antivector antibodies
      - Antivector cytotoxic T-cell response

Complications of Treatment

Until the mid-1970s, the biggest impediment to the management of patients with hemophilia was the lack of readily administered treatment, which virtually guaranteed that patients with severe hemophilia would develop hemophilic arthropathy, and many would die of bleeding, including ICH. By the 1980s, treatments were available, and prophylaxis programs were initiated in many countries. Unfortunately, the 1980s was the era of HIV and hepatitis C, and most patients with hemophilia treated before 1985 were infected with both, with smaller numbers also infected with hepatitis A and B. Many of these patients have died. This tragedy prompted widespread implementation of blood donor screening programs and viral inactivation processes and accelerated the development of recombinant clotting factor concentrates.

The management of HIV since the 1980s has undergone tremendous advances. Currently, patients infected with HIV who receive highly active antiretroviral therapy (HAART) live almost normal life spans. Infection with hepatitis C is more problematic, resulting in chronic disease in approximately 60% of infected subjects. A combination of interferon and ribavirin has been used with good results in patients with certain hepatitis C genotypes 2 and 3 and less satisfactory results in those with genotype 1.

However, there are still patients developing the long-term complications of chronic hepatic infection, including an incidence of hepatocellular carcinoma. Co-infection with HIV and alcohol use with hepatitis C make the development of these liver complications more common. There are now several new-generation anti-HCV therapies reaching the clinic, and this may facilitate the cure of increasing numbers of infected patients with hemophilia. In the meantime, all noninfected persons with hemophilia routinely receive hepatitis A and B vaccination.

Other Comorbidities in Patients With Hemophilia

With the progressive improvements to hemophilia care, persons with hemophilia are living longer, and the morbidities associated with aging are now complicating the clinical management of hemophilia. Although patients with hemophilia are somewhat protected from atherothrombotic events, there are increasing numbers of older patients with coronary artery disease. This problem is necessitating the development of new guidelines to safely introduce antiplatelet regimens for secondary prevention or for primary prevention in those undergoing percutaneous coronary interventions.

Table 137-10 Factors Associated With Successful Immune Tolerance Induction for Patients With Hemophilia A and Factor VIII Inhibitors

	Known or Probable Factors	Possible or Hypothesized Factors
Patient-related factors	Low Bethesda titer (<5 or 10 BU) at start of ITI Low historical peak Bethesda titer (<50 or 200 BU)	Low peak Bethesda titer during ITI Patient ethnicity Young age
Treatment-related factors	Short interval between inhibitor diagnosis and start of ITI	High FVIII dose (for patients with high Bethesda titers only) vWF-containing FVIII concentrate used for ITI

BU, Bethesda unit; *FVIII*, factor VIII; *ITI*, immune tolerance induction; *vWF*, von Willebrand factor.

Current Limitations to Treatment for Hemophilia

Currently, the biggest impediments in the management of patients with hemophilia are cost, inhibitor development, and the need for CVADs.

1. **Cost:** Worldwide, cost is the major issue. Currently available factor concentrates, particularly recombinant factor concentrates, are very expensive, and prophylaxis regimens can cost as much as $300,000 per patient per year.
2. **Inhibitor development:** Management of patients with inhibitors remains a challenge. Although inhibitor development is more common in patients with hemophilia A (particularly severe forms), patients with hemophilia B are difficult to manage because they often develop anaphylaxis and nephrotic syndrome. Although the genetic and environmental risk factors for inhibitor development are increasingly well understood, our capacity to prevent inhibitor development is limited.
3. **CVADs:** These are useful for the management of young children with severe hemophilia. They are of particular benefit in children who develop inhibitors and require immune tolerance therapy (ITT). Most ITT regimens call for daily administration of factor, which is not feasible through repeated peripheral venipunctures. CVAD complications include infections and thrombosis. Catheter infections caused by skin organisms can produce considerable morbidity, and the CVAD often needs to be removed. In a meta-analysis of studies evaluating CVAD complications, Valentino and colleagues reported a 40% CVAD infection rate with a mean of one CVAD infection for every four patients with hemophilia with a CVAD in place for 1 year.

Thrombi associated with CVADs vary in significance from small fibrin sheaths to thrombi that occlude large vessels and can lead to pulmonary embolism or death. Several studies have shown that radiographically proven CVAD associated thrombosis develops in up to 50% of patients with hemophilia with devices. Such thrombi may impair CVAD function, thereby necessitating their removal. Because of the complications associated with CVAD implantation, some institutions recommend arteriovenous fistulae (AVF) as an alternative. However, experience with AVF is still limited.

Immune Responses to Exogenous Factor VIII and Factor IX

Adverse immunologic responses to replacement products are a major complication for patients with hemophilia who have access to replacement factor concentrates. These responses occur because the infused factor contains foreign epitopes. However, not all patients develop an immune response to replacement; the reasons for this are unknown.

Immune responses include anaphylactic reactions and nonanaphylactic antibody-producing responses. The latter are classified according to their effects in vitro: whereas immunoglobulin G (IgG) antibodies that "inhibit" the coagulant function of the replacement factor are referred to as *inhibitors,* those that do not interfere with coagulant activity are called *nonneutralizing antibodies. Catalytic antibodies* directly hydrolyze the target protein.

Anaphylactic Reactions

Type I hypersensitivity reactions are rare in patients with hemophilia A but have been reported with infusion of either plasma-derived or recombinant FVIII concentrates. Rarely, there is evidence of IgE mediation, suggesting that in some cases, these reactions may reflect complement activation, immune complex formation, or other mechanisms.

Approximately 3% of patients with hemophilia B experience anaphylactic reactions to FIX products; these occur with equal frequency with plasma-derived and recombinant products. The median number of FIX exposure days at the time of anaphylactic reaction is 11.[22] These reactions often occur in patients who have FIX inhibitors and show evidence of IgE mediation. In some cases, transient IgG1 antibodies to FIX have been detected near the time of the allergic reaction. Because IgG1 antibodies can bind complement, this may point to an alternative mechanism for anaphylactic-type reactions without evidence of IgE mediation. Factors that may confer an increased risk for anaphylactic reactions to FIX include Hispanic race, personal or family history of other allergies, and severe hemophilia B (FIX:C <1%). Anaphylactic reactions appear to be predominantly associated with total deletions and nonsense mutations of *F9.*[23]

It is unclear why anaphylactic reactions are more common with FIX concentrates than with FVIII concentrates. It is possible that the extravascular distribution of FIX is more likely to provoke such a reaction. In addition, therapeutic doses of FIX contain much more protein than therapeutic doses of FVIII, which may trigger anaphylaxis. Total deletions of the *F9* gene may also include deletions of adjacent genes whose absence may predispose patients to anaphylaxis.

The acute management of anaphylaxis involves supportive care and the use of non–VIII or non–FIX-containing bypassing agents to treat bleeding. Desensitization by repeated administration of concentrate may be successful, particularly in patients with hemophilia B. Because of the timing of anaphylactic reactions in hemophilia B, it is recommended that the first 10 to 20 FIX treatments be given in a controlled setting.

Inhibitory Antibody Development

This important treatment-related complication is dealt with in detail in Chapter 138. The current chapter deals with selected issues concerning pathophysiologic mechanisms and inhibitor detection only.

Factor VIII Inhibitors: Pathophysiology

Factor VIII inhibitors in patients with hemophilia A are antibodies of the IgG isotype and are typically of the IgG4 subclass, although inhibitory antibodies of other subclasses are observed as well. Some evidence indicates that IgG4 antibodies are predominant in patients with high-titer inhibitors, but IgG1 antibodies are more abundant in patients with low-titer inhibitors. The predominance of IgG4 antibodies may be a consequence of prolonged exposure to exogenous FVIII because this phenomenon has been observed with repeated administration of other antigens.

Factor VIII epitopes for inhibitory antibodies have been identified in several locations in the FVIII molecule, such as in a site in the A2 domain that is involved in the function of the tenase complex, in the FIXa-binding site in the A3 domain, and in phospholipid-binding and vWF-binding sites in the C2 domain. The presence of these epitopes in areas of the FVIII molecule that have functional importance explains why antibodies to these epitopes have inhibitory activity (i.e., result in decreased coagulant activity of FVIII). In contrast, antibodies directed against the nonfunctional B domain do not appear to have inhibitory activity.

Inhibitors may be classified by the kinetics of their binding to FVIII. *Type I* inhibitors are characterized by a linear relationship between the antibody concentration and the logarithm of the residual FVIII activity; at high antibody concentrations, the inhibition of FVIII is near total. FVIII inhibitors in patients with congenital hemophilia A usually have type I kinetics. Inhibitors with *type II* kinetics do not display a linear relationship, and even high antibody concentrations do not result in complete inhibition of FVIII activity. Type II inhibitors are commonly autoantibodies seen in acquired hemophilia A, which is discussed later.

Inhibitors are produced when a FVIII-specific memory B cell is stimulated to differentiate into an anti-FVIII antibody secreting cell (plasma cell). This differentiation is dependent on binding of FVIII to the B-cell receptor, a membrane receptor in the immunoglobulin superfamily of receptors, to the antigen for which it has specificity, and subsequent interaction with a CD4 positive helper T cell. The important role of helper T cells in the genesis of inhibitors is supported by diverse data: T-cell proliferation in response to FVIII is increased in hemophilia A patients who have inhibitors compared with those without. Blockade of CD3, a component of the T-cell receptor complex, has been shown to decrease inhibitor formation in vitro, as has stimulation of cytotoxic T-lymphocyte antigen 4 (CTLA-4), an inhibitory receptor involved in the downregulation of T-cell stimulation. Decrease of inhibitor titers, and even loss of inhibitors altogether, has been observed in hemophilia A patients with inhibitors who have human HIV infection, particularly those with very low counts of CD4-positive T cells. T-cell activation that effectively produces inhibitors requires costimulation from antigen-presenting cells (e.g., via the CD40/CD40 ligand pathway or the CD28/B7 pathway).

Some observations suggest that the stimulation of memory B cells can be accomplished without FVIII-specific helper T cells. B cells have been stimulated in vitro by T cells that are specific for antigens other than FVIII ("bystander antigens"). Furthermore, B cells can be stimulated by Toll-like receptor (TLR) agonists without T-cell help. The significance of these findings for human patients with hemophilia is not known.

In humans, FVIII epitopes for CD4 positive T cells have been identified in the A2, A3, and C2 domains.

Regulatory T cells (Tregs), which can suppress the activity of helper T cells, may have a role in determining whether an individual patient will be immunologically reactive or tolerant to FVIII. T-cell proliferation in response to FVIII stimulation has been observed in Treg-depleted peripheral blood from normal (nonhemophiliac) human subjects. Hemophilia A mice treated with rapamycin (a small molecule inhibitor of the serine kinase mammalian target of rapamycin [mTOR]) failed to develop inhibitors on exposure to FVIII and had increased number of Tregs compared with control mice that did develop inhibitors. Hemophilia A mice had lower inhibitor titers in response to FVIII with infusion of Tregs taken from wild-type mice than without. These observations are consistent with Tregs perhaps having an important role in determining the immunologic response of hemophilia A patients to exogenous FVIII and intolerance to FVIII in normal individuals.

Immunologic tolerance to FVIII in people without hemophilia A is not complete. Rarely, usually as a result of autoimmune disease, immunologic tolerance to FVIII fails, and autoantibodies to FVIII develop; this is known as *acquired hemophilia A.* Furthermore, antibodies to FVIII, detectable by enzyme-linked immunosorbent assay (ELISA) and Bethesda assay as well as other methods, can be found in the plasma of some individuals who do not have hemophilia A. T cells that are reactive to FVIII can also be found in normal individuals, although this reactivity is transient and less intense than for hemophilia A patients. The relevance of these observations for hemophilia A patients who have inhibitors is not known. Further understanding of the mechanisms that might prevent normal individuals from developing clinically important autoantibodies to FVIII, such as T-cell suppression by Tregs or neutralization of inhibitory antibodies by anti-idiotypic antibodies (antibodies to the antigen-binding region of the inhibitory antibody), might provide insight into inhibitors in hemophilia A patients.

Not all patients with hemophilia A who are exposed to replacement FVIII products develop inhibitors. The reasons for tolerance to FVIII in some patients are not clear, although some of the known risk factors for inhibitor development suggest possible explanations. For example, patients with large *F8* gene deletions and other mutations that cause an absence of any synthesized FVIII protein have an increased inhibitor risk, suggesting that patients who do have some synthesized protein may be tolerant to the epitopes that they do produce. However, the mechanism and site of this tolerance are not known. It has been hypothesized that some patients are exposed in utero, via maternal–fetal hemorrhage, to small quantities of maternal FVIII that induce immunologic tolerance in the fetus. However, there has been no observed association between inhibitor risk and intrauterine procedures such as amniocentesis, or with breastfeeding.

Another theory to explain the development of FVIII inhibitors in some patients is that of immunologic "danger signals": if a patient has exposure to FVIII at the same time as exposure to pathogen-associated antigens, such as infectious agents or vaccines, or to tissue injury, such as surgical injury or acute bleeds, this may induce an immunogenic, rather than a tolerogenic, immune response to the FVIII antigen. Although specific danger signals, for example molecular patterns that are agonists for TLRs or other receptors in the innate immune system have not yet been definitively identified in association with FVIII inhibitor development, some clinical data are consistent with the danger signal hypothesis.

Transient Inhibitors

Some FVIII inhibitors may disappear spontaneously without specific management. Inhibitors may ultimately prove to be transient despite continued on-demand FVIII exposure. This typically occurs with low titer inhibitors (<5 Bethesda units [BU]) but can occur with higher titer inhibitors as well (≤10 BU). Transient inhibitors are also possible in patients with hemophilia B, but this phenomenon is not well characterized.

Catalytic Antibodies

Catalytic FVIII antibodies have been described that are capable of direct proteolysis of the FVIII protein.[24] These antibodies occur in approximately 50% of patients with FVIII inhibitors but have not been observed to occur in patients without inhibitors. The proteolysis caused by catalytic antibodies is specific to FVIII, and proteolytic cleavage sites have been identified at basic amino acids in the A1, A2, B, A3, and C1 domains. The rate of proteolysis by these antibodies is positively correlated with Bethesda titer and appears to be much slower than rates of other activating or inactivating enzymatic reactions involving FVIII, such as activation by thrombin or inactivation by protein C. It is possible to measure the effect of catalytic antibodies on the coagulant activity of FVIII with the Nijmegen assay, although the incubation time must be prolonged for proteolysis to occur.

The clinical importance of catalytic antibodies is unclear. It has been speculated that proteolysis of FVIII may create or expose neo-epitopes, resulting in the formation of new antibodies, but it is not known if this actually occurs. In an inhibitor-positive patient, it is unknown what fraction of total FVIII inhibition is caused by catalytic antibodies. Perhaps most importantly, the effect of catalytic antibodies on infused FVIII is unknown. It is possible that the proteolysis catalyzed by these antibodies occurs too slowly to inactivate FVIII given for acute bleeds; on the other hand, even a slow reaction, if it ultimately inactivates enough FVIII, might impair the effectiveness of FVIII given for prophylaxis. However, it may be that catalytic antibodies work too slowly to have any clinically important effect.

Factor IX Inhibitors: Pathophysiology

Hemophilia B is less common than hemophilia A, a smaller number of patients with hemophilia B have severe disease, and inhibitors are much less common in hemophilia B. As a result, much less is known about the basic science of FIX inhibitors than about FVIII inhibitors. There is, as previously described, a relationship between FIX inhibitors and anaphylaxis to FIX that generally does not occur with FVIII inhibitors.

Factor IX inhibitors are primarily antibodies of the IgG4 isotype, although some are of the IgG2 isotype.

Epitopes for FIX inhibitors have been identified in the γ-carboxyglutamic acid domain, which is involved in binding to phospholipid surfaces, the serine protease domain, and possibly in the activation peptide region, at which FIX is activated by activated factor XI. As is the case with inhibitory FVIII antibodies, the specificity of these antibodies for epitopes in functionally important regions of the FIX molecule explains their ability to inhibit FIX's coagulant activity.

Because FIX inhibitors are antibodies of the IgG subclass, they are products of interaction between FIX-specific B cells and helper T cells, but this process is less well described than is the case for FVIII inhibitors. The roles of costimulatory molecules, immunoregulatory genes, and Tregs in FIX inhibitors have not been demonstrated.

Detection of Inhibitors and Inhibitor Titers

Inhibitors are detected using the Bethesda assay (Fig. 137-12). In this assay, the ability of patient plasma, which may contain an inhibitor, to inhibit the coagulant activity of FVIII or FIX is measured using the activated partial thromboplastin time (aPTT). Plasma containing normal amounts of FVIII or FIX is used to create a standard curve that relates aPTT to FVIII or FIX activity. Patient plasma is incubated with the normal plasma for 2 hours at 37° C, the aPTT is measured, and the residual coagulant factor activity is then calculated. As a control, normal plasma is diluted with buffer, FVIII or FIX deficient plasma, or a 4% albumin solution, and the aPTT and coagulant factor activity are determined and compared with the result from the sample containing patient plasma. One Bethesda unit is defined as the amount of antibody required to reduce, in 1 mL of plasma, the coagulant factor activity to 50% of the activity present without antibody (or by a factor of 2^{-1}). By extension, 2 BU of inhibitory activity will decrease coagulant activity to 25% (by a factor of 2^{-2}), 3 BU to 12.5% (by a factor of 2^{-3}), and so on. In general: Bethesda titer (in BU) = $-\log_2$ (fraction of residual coagulant factor activity) = $-\log_{10}$ (fraction of residual coagulant factor activity)/$\log_{10}2$.

The Nijmegen modification of the Bethesda titer differs from the "classical" Bethesda assay in two respects: the normal plasma used is buffered to a pH of 7.4 with imidazole, and the control mixture is made by diluting normal plasma with FVIII deficient plasma rather than buffer. The Nijmegen modification is known to be more specific in detecting low-titer inhibitors than the classical Bethesda assay (i.e., it results in fewer false-positive results) and so is now the preferred assay for inhibitor quantification.

The Bethesda assay is poorly reproducible, although this can be minimized by rigorous standardization of laboratory reagents and procedures. The Bethesda assay will not, by definition, detect non-neutralizing antibodies (i.e., those antibodies to FVIII or FIX that do not inhibit the coagulant function of these proteins).

Both neutralizing and non-neutralizing antibodies to FVIII or FIX may also be detected by ELISA. This assay can only detect and quantify the antibodies present and cannot determine their inhibitory activity. It is possible that novel immunoassays with increased sensitivity will enter clinical practice in the future, but the importance and rational use of such assays will need to be determined.

An inhibitor may be categorized according to its titer: a low titer inhibitor has a Bethesda assay of less than or equal to 5 BU, but a high titer inhibitor has a Bethesda assay of greater than 5 BU. Whereas a low-responding inhibitor is one that remains at a low titer despite repeated FVIII exposure, a high-responding inhibitor is one that has a high titer (>5 BU) at any time after FVIII exposure even if the inhibitor titer decreases or becomes undetectable afterward.

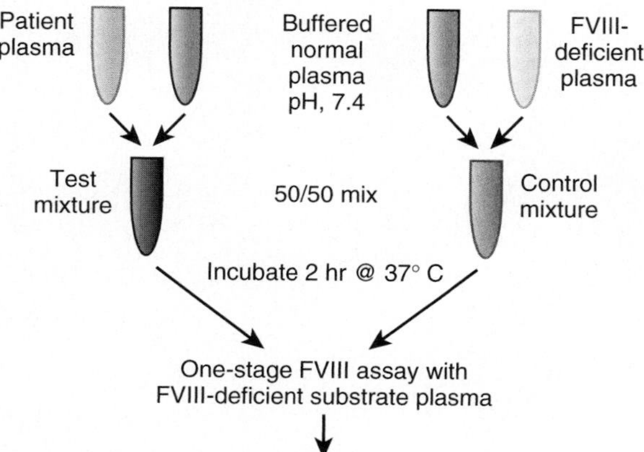

Figure 137-12 THE NIJMEGEN-MODIFIED BETHESDA ASSAY. This is the currently recommended methodology for quantifying anti–factor VIII (FVIII) inhibitory antibodies.

FUTURE DIRECTIONS

Already, in 2011, hemophilia represents a superb example of the application of molecular science to clinical benefit. Mutation-specific diagnosis is now being incorporated into the initial workup of many patients, and family counseling for kindreds with hemophilia has been dramatically enhanced by advances in the application of molecular genetic technology. In addition, use of the hemophilic mutation as a significant risk factor for inhibitor development is prompting clinicians to evaluate novel strategies to mitigate the likelihood of this treatment complication. As our ability to analyze the genome in far greater detail at greater speed and with reduced costs increases, we can look forward to an even greater potential for inhibitor risk definition.

The increasing use of recombinant factor concentrates worldwide is a strong indicator of our growing reliance on novel technologies to provide safe and effective therapies for hemophilia. In the next 5 to 10 years, we can look forward to a large number of additional innovations in the area of hemophilia treatment (Fig. 137-13). The first wave of novel products is aimed at extending the circulating half-life of the concentrates with the objective of reducing the frequency of replacement therapy. The two main approaches being used for this purpose are the conjugation of the clotting factor protein to hydrophilic polymers such as polyethylene glycol or the generation of recombinant fusion proteins using immunoglobulin or albumin as the fusion partner.

A second, more challenging approach to improving hemophilia therapy is to develop components of an improved intrinsic tenase complex. Currently, early phase investigations are exploring the

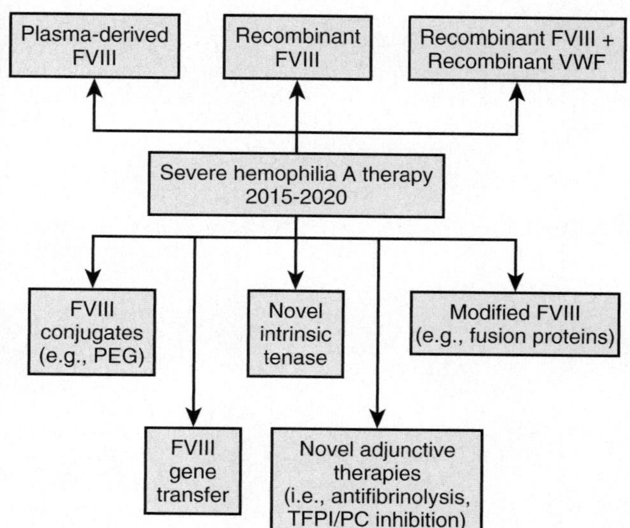

Figure 137-13 THE FUTURE OF HEMOPHILIA A TREATMENT. This figure speculates on the therapeutic options that may well face clinicians treating patients with hemophilia A within the next 5 to 10 years. *FVIII,* Factor VIII; *PC,* Protein C; *PEG,* polyethylene glycol; *TFPI,* tissue factor pathway inhibitor; *vWF,* von Willebrand factor.

potential of enhanced activity FIX variants and the development of FVIII mimetics that incorporate the various roles that FVIII plays as a "scaffold" protein in this membrane-bound complex.

Finally, various adjunctive strategies for hemophilia treatment are being pursued. These include inhibition of coagulation inhibitory proteins (tissue factor pathway inhibitor and protein C) with antibodies and nucleic acid strategies (siRNA) and the development of novel approaches to inhibit fibrinolysis.

Overall, the future for a more diverse array of hemophilia therapeutics seems highly promising. How each of these products will be used in individual patients will provide future hemophilia treaters with some interesting and ultimately gratifying challenges.

REFERENCES

1. Do H, Healey JF, Waller EK, et al: Expression of factor VIII by murine liver sinusoidal endothelial cells. *J Biol Chem* 274:19587, 1999.
2. Jacquemin M, Neyrinck A, Hermanns MI, et al: FVIII production by human lung microvascular endothelial cells. *Blood* 108:515, 2006.
3. Picketts DJ, Mueller CR, Lillicrap D: Transcriptional control of the factor IX gene: Analysis of five cis-acting elements and the deleterious effects of naturally occurring hemophilia B Leyden mutations. *Blood* 84:2992, 1994.
4. DiMichele D: Inhibitor development in haemophilia B: An orphan disease in need of attention. *Br J Haematol* 138:305, 2007.
5. Rogaev EI, Grigorenko AP, Faskhutdinova G, et al: Genotype analysis identifies the cause of the "royal disease." *Science* 326:817, 2009.
6. Mazurier C: Von Willebrand disease masquerading as haemophilia A. *Thromb Haemost* 67:391, 1992.
7. Ljung R, Chambost H, Stain A-M, et al: Haemophilia in the first years of life. *Haemophilia* 14:188, 2008.
8. Dauty M, Sigaud M, Trossaërt M, et al: Iliopsoas hematoma in patients with hemophilia: A single-center study. *Joint Bone Spine* 74:179, 2007.
9. van Dijk K, Fischer K, van der Bom JG, et al: Variability in clinical phenotype of severe haemophilia: The role of the first joint bleed. *Haemophilia* 11:438, 2005.
10. Valentino LA: Blood-induced joint disease: The pathophysiology of hemophilic arthropathy. *Journal of thrombosis and haemostasis: J Thromb Haemost* 8:1895, 2010.
11. Kulkarni R, Lusher JM: Intracranial and extracranial hemorrhages in newborns with hemophilia: A review of the literature. *J Pediatr Hematol Oncol* 21:289, 1999.
12. Shapiro AD, Donfield SM, Lynn HS, et al: Defining the impact of hemophilia: The academic achievement in children with hemophilia study. *Pediatrics* 108:E105, 2001.
13. Ragni MV, Lusher JM, Koerper MA, et al: Safety and immunogenicity of subcutaneous hepatitis A vaccine in children with haemophilia. *Haemophilia* 6:98, 2000.
14. Johnson RE, Lawrence DN, Evatt BL, et al: Acquired immunodeficiency syndrome among patients attending hemophilia treatment centers and mortality experience of hemophiliacs in the United States. *American Journal of Epidemiology* 121:797, 1985.
15. Brettler DB, Alter HJ, Dienstag JL, et al: Prevalence of hepatitis C virus antibody in a cohort of hemophilia patients. *Blood* 76:254, 1990.
16. Plug I, van der Bom JG, Peters M, et al: Mortality and causes of death in patients with hemophilia, 1992-2001: A prospective cohort study. *J Thromb Haemost* 4:510, 2006.
17. Mannucci PM, Aberg M, Nilsson IM, et al: Mechanism of plasminogen activator and factor FVIII increase after vasoactive drugs. *Br J Haematol* 30:81, 1975.
18. Van Creveld S: Prophylaxis of joint hemorrhages in hemophilia. *Acta Haematologica* 45:120, 1971.
19. Manco-Johnson MJ, Abshire TC, Shapiro AD, et al: Prophylaxis versus episodic treatment to prevent joint disease in boys with severe hemophilia. *N Engl J Med* 357:535, 2007.
20. Feldman BM, Pai M, Rivard GE, et al: Tailored prophylaxis in severe hemophilia A: Interim results from the first 5 years of the Canadian hemophilia primary prophylaxis study. *J Thromb Haemost* 4:1228, 2006.
21. Hough C, Lillicrap D: Gene therapy for hemophilia: An imperative to succeed. *J Thromb Haemost* 3:1195, 2005.
22. Warrier I, Ewenstein BM, Koerper MA, et al: Factor IX inhibitors and anaphylaxis in hemophilia B. *J Pediatr Hematol Oncol* 19:23, 1997.
23. Recht M, Pollmann H, Tagliaferri A, et al: A retrospective study to describe the incidence of moderate to severe allergic reactions to factor IX in subjects with haemophilia B. *Haemophilia* 17:494, 2011.
24. Lacroix-Desmazes S, Bayry J, Misra N, et al: The prevalence of proteolytic antibodies against factor FVIII in hemophilia A. *N Engl J Med* 346:662, 2002.

CHAPTER 138

INHIBITORS IN HEMOPHILIA A AND B

Guglielmo Mariani, Barbara A. Konkle, and Craig M. Kessler

With the availability of plasma-derived and recombinant replacement products safe from transmission of known infectious agents, the development of antibodies neutralizing factor VIII (FVIII) or FIX has become the major complication of hemophilia treatment.

The immune response to FVIII occurs and antibodies to FVIII can be detected in (1) healthy individuals, (2) patients suffering from an autoimmune disease, and (3) patients with factor VIII deficiency (hemophilia A). Clinically speaking, only those antibodies that affect the clotting activity, which are therefore termed *inhibitors,* are considered relevant because they render patients refractory to treatment. In hemophilias, inhibitors occur after factor replacement therapy with FVIII or factor IX concentrates. Patients with a severe deficiency (FVIII or FIX < 1% of normal) are particularly at risk.

Inhibitor formation in hemophilia was first reported in 1941.[1] A 44-year-old man with classic hemophilia had been treated numerous times with blood products, and his coagulation time subsequently became refractory to transfusions. The authors realized that transfusion may have caused this heretofore unknown complication and suggested that coagulation times should be checked after administration of blood products to monitor for the phenomenon. This report soon was followed by numerous cases[2-5] reporting the development of a substance that counteracted infused blood product components. The nature of the inhibitor was shown to be an IgG antibody of the IgG4 subclass.[6]

Alloantibody inhibitors arise much more frequently in patients with severe hemophilia A (15% to 20% with a range of 8% to 52%)[7] than in those with severe hemophilia B (≈1% to 3%). Their occurrence is associated with higher morbidity and mortality, increased cost of care, and more complicated treatment regimens.

HEMOPHILIA A

Epidemiology

It is curious that hemophilia A and B, which share an almost identical clinical phenotype, would have such a disparate incidence of alloantibody inhibitor development. The explanation may reside in the type of genetic mutation responsible for each disease. In hemophilia A, the severe phenotype most often is due to a null mutation, which is less common in hemophilia B. Null mutations result in complete absence of a translated protein product and are more likely to predispose to inhibitor formation. Also, FIX shares significant homology with the other vitamin K–dependent clotting factors, possibly protecting against inhibitor development.[8] Finally, it is hypothesized that because FIX is smaller and more abundant than FVIII, some FIX may cross the placenta, thereby inducing tolerance in the developing fetus.[8]

Among patients with severe hemophilia A, approximately 30% will develop an alloantibody inhibitor (compared with 3% of those with moderate hemophilia and 0.3% with mild hemophilia).[9] Inhibitor formation occurs early after initiation of replacement therapy. Data from prospective clinical trials of recombinant FVIII reveal that inhibitor development typically arises within a median of 8 to 10 "exposure days" (treatment days), but a wide range is not uncommon.[10] The risk for inhibitor development decreases inversely with increasing number of exposure days and is uncommon (≈2/1000 patient-years) after 150 exposure days.

There appears to be a bimodal distribution of inhibitor occurrence in severe hemophilia. The incidence peaks in early childhood in those younger than 5 years of age (64.3/1000 treatment-years), falls substantially between the ages of 10 and 49 years of age (5.3/1000 treatment-years), and rises again in older age (10.5/1000 treatment-years).[11] This finding raises the possibility that there is a breakdown of tolerance with aging.[11] Furthermore, inhibitor formation has a negative impact on overall mortality in severe hemophilia A patients, essentially canceling out the improved life expectancy realized in patients with severe hemophilia A population over the last 30 years.[12]

Genetic Factors

One of the most significant risk factors associated with the development of inhibitory alloantibodies in hemophilia A is the presence of a positive family history. The increased concordance rate of inhibitor occurrence in brother and twin pairs[13,14] provided the initial indication that genetic factors play a role in inhibitor development. Having a first-degree relative with an inhibitor raises the risk for inhibitor development threefold, resulting in an approximately 50% chance of inhibitor development compared with a control cohort in which there is a 15% risk.[13,14]

Patient ethnicity first emerged as a possible risk factor for inhibitor development in retrospective analyses of the prevalence of inhibitors in various racial cohorts included within large pooled populations of hemophiliacs.[14-17] African Americans and Latinos were observed to have a twofold higher rate of inhibitor formation compared with whites. For instance, in the Malmö International Brother Study (MIBS), inhibitors were noted in 27.4% of white patients and in 55.6% of African Americans.[14] This same racial trend was subsequently appreciated in prospective analyses of inhibitor development in the initial recombinant FVIII concentrate safety and efficacy trials.[18]

One potential and provocative explanation for the increased propensity of African Americans with hemophilia to produce FVIII relative to immunoreactivity is a mismatch between the host endogenous wild-type FVIII haplotype polymorphisms found only in blacks (H3, H4, and H5) and their exposure to the exogenous FVIII polymorphisms found in the commercially available brands of recombinant FVIII concentrates (either H1 or H2) used for replacement therapy. The risk for alloantibody inhibitor development is significantly higher among African Americans with haplotypes H3 or H4 than it is in those with the H1 or H2 haplotype (odds ratio [OR] of 3.4). These observations await confirmation in larger studies.[19]

Emerging data consistently indicate that certain FVIII mutations producing phenotypically severe hemophilia A[7,8] are strong predictors of inhibitor development.[20-22] Three general categories of mutations in FVIII place a patient at "high risk" for inhibitor formation: (a) inversions of intron 22 (intrachromosomal recombinations), (b) large deletions affecting more than one domain, and (c) nonsense mutations involving the light chain (the risk for inhibitor formation is twofold higher with light chain mutations than with heavy chain mutations).[7,20] All of these mutations either eliminate FVIII protein altogether or alter the molecular conformation of the FVIII protein in such a way that innate immune tolerance cannot be achieved during fetal development. Consequently, the immune system recognizes exogenously administered native FVIII protein as "foreign."[21] The "low-risk" FVIII mutations consist of small gene deletions/insertions, missense mutations, and splice site mutations. It is postulated that some "nonfunctional" FVIII protein is produced with these FVIII gene mutations, which may be sufficient to induce partial central immune tolerance.[20]

Even with genetic information, it is not possible to predict which patients are at highest risk for development of alloantibody inhibitors. Inhibitors in the high-risk category occur 7- to 10-fold more frequently for large deletions and nonsense mutations (pooled OR = 3.6; 95% confidence interval [CI] 2.3-5.7 and 1.4 CI 1.1-1.8, respectively)[20] (≈35%)[21] compared with those with intron 22 inversions. Furthermore, inhibitors occur less frequency with small FVIII gene deletions/insertions (≈7%)[21] or missense mutations (≈4%) (pooled OR 0.5 [95% CI 0.4-0.6] and 0.3, 95% CI 0.2-0.4, respectively).[20,21] Intron 22 inversions are associated with a lower inhibitor frequency than would be anticipated for a genotype, which produces no circulating FVIII protein. However, recent data suggest that some of these hemophiliacs may possess intrahepatocyte-endogenous FVIII protein fragments, which can induce partial immune tolerance.[20] There does not appear to be any relationship between the type of FVIII gene mutation and the relative risks for developing high titer versus low titer alloantibody FVIII inhibitors.[20]

Environmental Factors

Despite the strong FVIII genetic influences that underlie inhibitor formation, clinical observations indicate that various environmental or epigenetic pressures contribute to the development of alloantibody inhibitors. For example, within the MIBS cohort, there are discordant monozygotic twins (i.e., identical twin brothers with the same mutations) in which only one brother developed an inhibitor.[13] In addition, among families with high-risk gene mutations, only about 30% of siblings with severe hemophilia A due to the intron 22 inversion form inhibitors. Even with multidomain deletions, the highest estimated inhibitor risk only approaches 75%,[14] implying that other patients with the same mutation are somehow protected against inhibitor formation.

A concerted effort has been made to explore the importance of other genetic determinants in hemophilia A patients that may contribute to alloantibody inhibitor development. Of the immune response genes, the presence of a microsatellite polymorphism in the promoter region (134 base pair variant) of the interleukin (IL)-10 gene, which may lead to upregulated B-lymphocyte activity, has been associated with a 73% incidence of inhibitor formation (OR of 4.4). A G308A polymorphism in the promoter region of the tumor necrosis factor (TNF)-α gene (A/A genotype) has been associated with 72.7% inhibitors and an OR of 4.0. On the other hand, there is little consistent or robust evidence that polymorphisms of major histocompatibility complex (MHC) class II alleles or of other inflammatory cytokine genes contribute to alloantibody inhibitor development.[21-23]

Among possible environmental risk factors, the age at first treatment has been implicated as a major independent contributor for inhibitor development. Initial observations suggested that the earlier the first exposure to FVIII-containing products occurred, the greater the risk for alloantibody inhibitor formation.[23-26] Children treated before 6 months of age have a cumulative inhibitor incidence of 41% compared with a 12% incidence if initial exogenous FVIII exposure is delayed until after the first year of life. Results of a subsequent case-control study suggested that early age of first exposure to FVIII treatment reflected the severity of the hemophilia conveyed by the particular FVIII gene mutation. Thus more intense FVIII replacement and high-risk FVIII gene polymorphisms were more strongly associated with inhibitor formation than was age. In fact, there appeared to be a protective effect against the formation of inhibitors when children were started on primary FVIII prophylaxis regimens early in life.[27] The United Kingdom Haemophilia Centre Doctors' Organisation (UKHCDO) study reported that peak inhibitor formation occurs in children younger than 5 years of age.[11]

The method of FVIII infusion (continuous infusion versus bolus administration) and the clinical scenarios for FVIII replacement have also been examined for their contribution to inhibitor formation. Although administration of FVIII by continuous infusion has the advantage of requiring less factor replacement over time and avoids the peaks and troughs seen with bolus administration,[28] intense replacement of FVIII by continuous infusion was more likely to induce inhibitor development than bolus injections (57% versus 14%) in patients who were otherwise considered to be at low risk (i.e., mild hemophiliacs).[29,30] These results were gleaned from the retrospective examination of the medical records of 54 mild hemophiliacs, of whom only 7 had received FVIII by CI; a prospective study in a larger population remains to be conducted to confirm this finding. On the other hand, intensive FVIII replacement in the context of injury, surgery, or inflammation appears conducive to inhibitor formation. In the retrospective CANAL study (concerted action on neutralizing antibodies in severe hemophilia A) of previously untreated patients (PUPs), 65% of those whose first exposure to FVIII therapy was associated with surgery developed an allogeneic FVIII antibody inhibitor (relative risk, 3.7), compared with a 23% inhibitor incidence when first exposure was not related to a "danger signal" indication.[30]

Perhaps the most controversial "environmental" risk factor for alloantibody inhibitor development involves the type of FVIII concentrate replacement used by the patient (low- to intermediate-purity plasma-derived FVIII versus high-purity plasma-derived FVIII versus recombinant FVIII concentrates). After more than 20 years, the question of whether use of recombinant FVIII concentrates (highest purity) leads to a higher inhibitor incidence than the lower purity concentrates remains largely unresolved.[31,32] This debate originated with the prospective trials of first-generation recombinant FVIII concentrates in PUPs, which mandated frequent monitoring for inhibitor formation (at least every 3 months).[33,34] In the Kogenate trial, the total incidence of any inhibitor formation in patients with severe hemophilia A was 29.2% within a median of 9 exposure days.[35] A similar inhibitor incidence rate of 31.5% was found in a prospective trial of Recombinate.[36] Thus, when compared with the inhibitor incidence rate of approximately 10% reported in older retrospective studies, which employed low-purity plasma-derived FVIII concentrates and screened less frequently for inhibitors,[37] recombinant FVIII seemed to be significantly more immunogenic. Prospective monitoring of patients receiving high-purity plasma-derived FVIII concentrates revealed a similar inhibitor rate as seen in those given recombinant concentrates.[38]

A number of variables could potentially have contributed to these observations and thus attenuate their importance from the clinical perspective. The recombinant FVIII trials in PUPs were the first large prospective clinical trials of hemophilia treatment, so their comparison with results of anecdotal or retrospective case reports and case series is inappropriate.[30-35] These trials were also the first to employ routine and frequent prospective monitoring for inhibitor development. In prior studies, testing for inhibitors was done only when deemed clinically important. Continued analysis of the results of the recombinant FVIII trials showed that almost half (11/23) of the inhibitors in the Kogenate trial were transient in nature, decreasing the prevalence of inhibitors upon extended observation.[35] A similar pattern was observed in the Recombinate trial; alloantibodies disappeared in 14 of 22 study subjects who developed an inhibitor despite continued treatment, eventually reducing the prevalence rate to 11.1%.[36] The older studies likely missed these ephemeral inhibitors. A Dutch study suggested that although transient inhibitors may develop earlier during treatment with ultrapure plasma-derived and recombinant FVIII concentrates compared with lower-purity plasma products, the overall risk for inhibitor development is similar.[39] The debate continues with conflicting data in both

PUPs and previously treated patients.[40-42] The recent UKHCDO case-control study examined inhibitor occurrence over 25 years of observation and identified "high-intensity treatments" rather than the type of FVIII product as the main risk factor for inhibitor development.[43] Similarly, an analysis of pooled data from over 2900 hemophiliacs indicated that the duration of study observation and follow-up and testing frequency for inhibitor presence, but not the source or purity of concentrate, explained most of the differences in inhibitor development seen in earlier studies.[38]

Proposed causes of variable immunogenicity among FVIII products have included neoantigen formation during their manufacture and their content of von Willebrand factor (vWF) protein, which is present in low- and intermediate-purity plasma-derived products but absent in recombinant FVIII concentrates.[25] It has been suggested that vWF may interfere with FVIII-dendritic cell interactions, alter FVIII molecular conformation, or mask T- or B-lymphocyte epitopes. The former scenario has been illustrated by the fact that previously low immunogenic plasma-derived FVIII concentrates were rendered highly immunogenic after extra viral-attenuation steps were added to their manufacturing processes.[44-46] However, when recombinant FVIII products were administered to patients previously and extensively treated with lower-purity FVIII products, the rate of inhibitor formation was low, consistent with low immunogenicity in this setting (relative overall risk for inhibitors, 0.8; for high-titer inhibitors, 0.9; for plasma-derived products versus recombinant FVIII products, 1.0; for switching FVIII products, 1.1).[41,47] A large prospective, randomized study comparing the immunogenicity of vWF-containing concentrates with recombinant FVIII concentrates in PUPs and minimally treated patients is ongoing. Nonetheless, most experts believe that the risk for inhibitor formation with the various FVIII concentrates is similar.

Mild Hemophilia

For patients with mild or moderately severe hemophilia A, inhibitors appear to develop at a cumulative incidence of 3% to 13%, commonly after periods of intense FVIII replacement associated with surgery or inflammatory states.[48] Advanced age (>60 years) and the presence of a particular FVIII gene mutation (R539C) are other risk factors,[48-51] suggesting that the capacity for immune tolerance in these infrequently, if ever, treated individuals may be compromised with aging and that immune challenge with FVIII replacement should be avoided whenever possible by administration of desmopressin (DDAVP) to enhance endogenous FVIII activity levels.

Venous Access

A disturbingly high incidence of infections occurs in FVIII alloantibody inhibitor patients with central venous access catheter devices (CVAD), particularly those with external devices who are undergoing immune tolerance induction (ITI) (124 episodes in 41 patients).[52] This may be related to frequent catheter accessing for administration of replacement therapy. CVAD-associated infection did not seem to affect the ability to achieve tolerance.[52] The presence of CVADs per se does not appear to be associated with increased inhibitor formation.[43]

Other Factors

Other miscellaneous proposed environmental influences on inhibitor development, such as breastfeeding and receiving replacement therapy in the context of vaccination, remain to be confirmed as significant risk factors.

Pathobiology of FVIII Alloantibody Inhibitor Formation

Circulating antigens, provided by the exogenous FVIII contained in the replacement therapies administered to severe hemophiliacs, undergo initial endocytosis and subsequent proteolysis by antigen-presenting cells and digested peptides that bind to MHC II molecules for presentation to T-cell receptor on $CD4^+$ T lymphocytes.[53] Costimulation signals subsequently mediate differentiation of T-lymphocytes into either T_H1 or T_H2 subsets. T_H2 cells secrete IL-4, IL-5, and IL-10 cytokines, which promote the synthesis of non–complement-binding immunoglobulins, predominantly IgG4, by B lymphocytes.[53] This polyclonal antibody response can result in the inhibition of FVIII function via multiple mechanisms.[54]

The weak association between MHC II phenotypes and FVIII inhibitor formation is dependent on the availability of "risk" MHC class I/II alleles.[55,56] T-lymphocyte involvement in inhibitor formation is manifested by evidence of isotype switching and somatic hypermutation of the B cells.[57] There are several FVIII epitopes against which $CD4^+$ T cells react strongly.[57] In addition, non–FVIII-associated gene polymorphisms can exert a protective influence on inhibitor development—for example, the C→T single-nucleotide polymorphism (SNP) at position -318 in the promoter region of the gene encoding for cytotoxic T-lymphocyte–associated protein-4 (CTLA4).[58] This polymorphism "downregulates" the effects of the costimulatory signal of the B7-CD28 complex, which mediates T-cell immune responsiveness to infused FVIII. The MIBS study group reported an odds ratio of 0.3 for inhibitor formation among a cohort of severe hemophiliacs with the T allele SNP despite their high risk for inhibitors by virtue of FVIII intron 22 gene inversions.[58] MIBS also identified polymorphisms in the IL-10 cytokine gene that are associated with inhibitor formation in severe hemophiliacs.[59] In support of the polygenic nature of inhibitor formation, there is emerging evidence that the regulatory T cell (Treg) lymphocyte system downmodulates the immune reaction to FVIII and plays a role in ITI induction.[60]

FVIII exists as a heterodimer, with a heavy chain containing the A1, A2, and B domains connected to a light chain containing the A3, C1, and C2 domains (Fig. 138-1). Short intervening acidic regions (a1, a2, and a3) aid in FVIII binding to factor X and serve as important sites for FVIII proteolysis by thrombin and FXa.[61] By serving as a cofactor for FIX in the intrinsic tenase complex, FVIIIa aids in the conversion of FX to FXa, which together with factor Va forms the prothrombinase complex on the activated platelet surface. This complex then converts prothrombin to thrombin, which in turn amplifies the coagulation system (see Chapter 123).[62,63]

Normally, when FVIII is secreted, it is noncovalently bound to vWF via the light chain, particularly through interactions with the A3 and C2 domain.[63] Upon thrombin activation, FVIIIa dissociates from vWF and via the C2 domain, which is no longer bound by vWF, binds to phosphatidylserine on the platelet membrane.[64] Neutralizing alloantibody inhibitors can interrupt this process (see Fig. 138-1) by (a) preventing FVIII interaction with vWF, thereby significantly decreasing its circulating half-life, (b) impeding the release of FVIIIa from vWF after thrombin activation, (c) increasing the time for inactivation before association with the intrinsic tenase complex, and/or (d) preventing C2 domains from binding the phospholipid.[65-69]

Other FVIII alloantibody inhibitors interact with the A2 domain, predominantly at the Arg4844-Ile5085 epitope, and interrupt FVIIIa-FIXa interactions, thereby impairing intrinsic tenase activity.[70] Regions outside the A2 and C2 domains are minor epitopes for FVIII inhibitors; however, inhibitor binding to the A3 domain blocks the FVIIIa-FIXa interaction.[70] The inhibitors in most hemophilia A patients recognize multiple epitopes in both the A2 and C2 domains, in contrast to autoantibodies directed against FVIII, which target either the C2 or A2 domain but not both.[70] Although antibodies that target B domain epitopes have been reported, these do not neutralize FVIII coagulant activity.

Another mechanism of FVIII inhibition involves alloantibodies that catalyze the proteolysis of FVIII.[71,72] FVIII-hydrolyzing IgGs are detected in more than 50% of alloantibody inhibitor patients and functionally resemble serine proteases. In contrast to the A2, A3, and C2 epitope specificity of the classical alloantibody inhibitors in severe hemophilia A, IgG-mediated hydrolysis occurs evenly throughout the FVIII molecule with resultant loss of FVIII activity.[73]

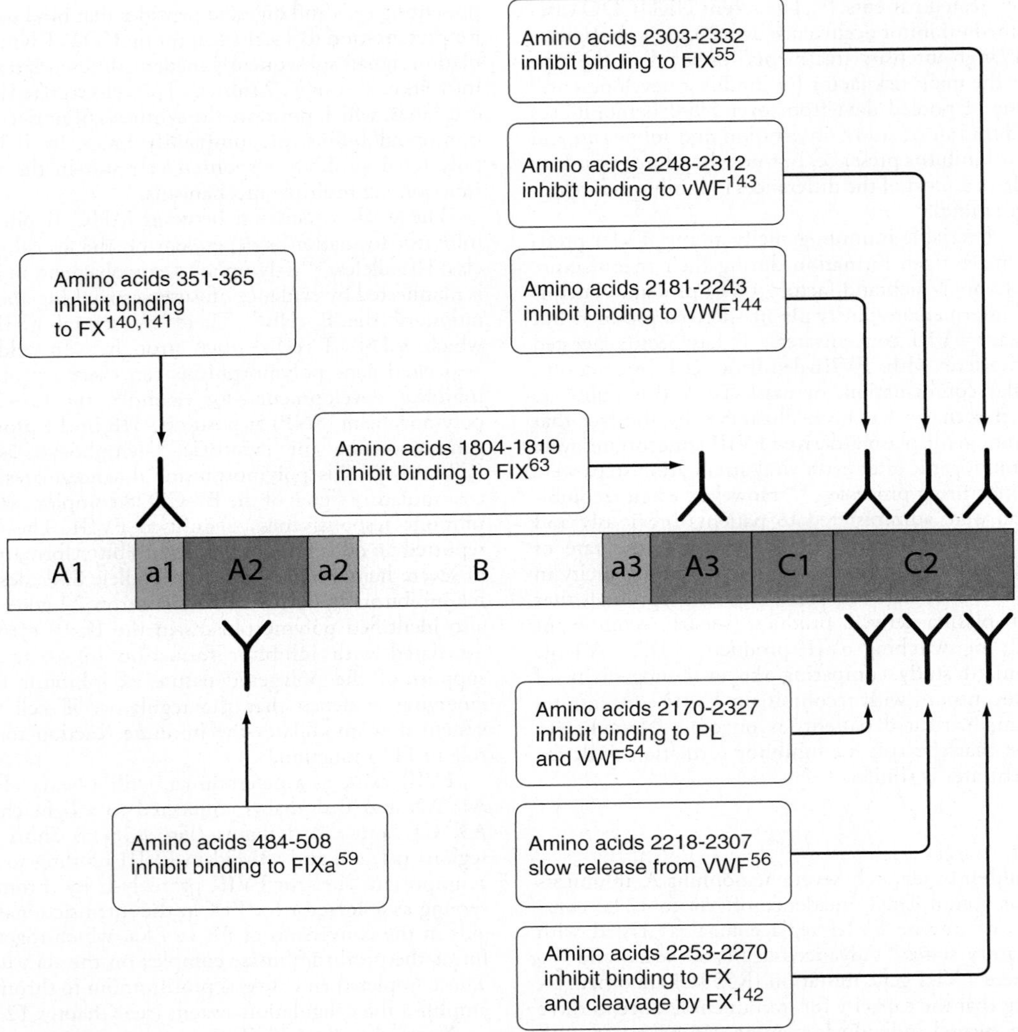

Figure 138-1 FACTOR VIII DOMAINS AND BINDING SITE BY AMINO ACID LOCATION AND EFFECT ON FACTOR VIII. Intensity of color reflects the frequency of inhibitors to the epitope.[140-144] *FIX,* Factor IX; *FIXa,* activated factor IX; *FX,* factor X; *PL,* phospholipid; *vWF,* von Willebrand factor.

Clinical Manifestations

The frequency and severity of bleeding complications do not necessarily increase when an alloantibody FVIII inhibitor develops in a severe hemophilia A patient. Similarly, no predictive relationship exists between the Bethesda unit (BU) titer and the severity of bleeding. Any person with hemophilia, regardless of severity, who is undergoing treatment and fails to respond to the FVIII dose that had previously been effective should be promptly evaluated for the development of an inhibitor.[74] Routine laboratory testing for the presence of an inhibitor is recommended before any major surgical procedure. A truncated pharmacokinetic study is also useful for inhibitor screening because even low-titer (<5 BU) asymptomatic inhibitors may be detected when less than 66% of the calculated incremental rise in FVIII activity is achieved within 30 minutes of administration of exogenous FVIII (i.e., decreased recovery). In general, patients with hemophilia A who have alloantibody FVIII inhibitors will experience more frequent hemarthroses, more severe and progressive arthropathy, and an overall reduced quality of life compared with noninhibitor patients.[75,76] Those with inhibitors have more hospital visits and absences from school or work, and they are more likely to require assistive devices, such as wheelchairs or crutches.[76] In the past, development of an inhibitor increased the mortality risk, but with current therapy the mortality rate is falling. However, the mortality rate for those with inhibitors still exceeds that for patients without an inhibitor.[77]

If patients with mild to moderately severe hemophilia A develop an alloantibody FVIII inhibitor, it usually occurs after a period of intense factor replacement. Genetic factors likely play a role as well. The clinical manifestations are the same as in severe hemophilia patients with inhibitors, including reduced recovery of FVIII activity after FVIII infusion. Thus a patient with mild disease may convert to a severe phenotype upon an inhibitor development and may present with spontaneous bleeding.

Laboratory Diagnosis

In 1975, the Bethesda assay was devised as a simple and reproducible method for determining antibody titer and quantifying the extent of its inhibitory/neutralizing capacity. The assay is based on the ability of patient plasma to inactivate FVIII in normal plasma. The result is expressed in BUs.[78] Patient plasma is serially diluted with normal plasma, incubated for 2 hours at 37° C, and residual FVIII activity is then measured using a one-stage assay. One BU correlates with patient FVIII activity of 50%. A standard curve is generated, and the patient's plasma is diluted until FVIII activity is between 25% and 75%, the linear portion of the standard curve. The inhibitor units are read from the graph and multiplied by the reciprocal of the dilution factor to determine the BU in undiluted plasma (Fig. 138-2).

To improve the specificity and reliability of the Bethesda assay, two groups developed the Nijmegen modification of the Bethesda assay.[79] The Bethesda assay can yield false-positive results, usually evidenced as low-titer inhibitors, because of decreased FVIII activity as pH increases and protein concentration decreases. The Nijmegen modification made two important changes to the Bethesda assay. First, the normal plasma and control mixtures were buffered with imidazole to a pH of 7.4, which prevents the FVIII:C inactivation that can occur at higher pH. Second, the imidazole buffer used in the control mixture was replaced with plasma depleted of FVIII in order to yield similar protein concentrations (Fig. 138-3). These modifications are now recommended for diagnosis of inhibitors.[80]

Care is needed to ensure that isolated prolongations of the activated partial thromboplastin time (aPTT) are not misdiagnosed as lupus anticoagulants or vice versa. The key maneuver to distinguish one from the other is based on the results obtained when patient and control plasma are mixed, and the aPTT is determined immediately or after 2 hours incubation at 37° C. Whereas the aPTT results determined immediately and after 2 hours incubation are similar to lupus anticoagulants, inhibitors exert an exaggerated effect upon incubation. This is a critical issue because patients with lupus anticoagulants do not usually bleed, whereas the bleeding with FVIII alloantibody inhibitors may be profound. In some instances, lupus anticoagulants and FVIII inhibitor may coexist.

Based on the results of the inhibitor assay, a value less than 5 BU is considered a low-titer inhibitor. If the inhibitor titer fails to rise despite repeated challenges with clotting factor protein, the patient is termed a *low responder*. In contrast, a patient with an inhibitor titer greater than 5 BU is considered a *high responder*.[80]

External quality control assessments examining the reliability of clotting-based inhibitor testing (Bethesda and Nijmegen) have noted considerable interlaboratory variability that could influence patient management and may contribute to differences in the incidence of FVIII inhibitors reported in various clinical settings.[81]

ELISA[82] or fluorescence immunoassay-based[83] assays may complement the clotting assays because these techniques also detect non-neutralizing antibodies against FVIII. The clinical implications of antibody-epitope interactions are unclear. There may be discordance between the results of ELISA-based inhibitor assays, which reveal the presence of an alloantibody, and functional clot-based assays, which determine the neutralizing capacity of the alloantibody. Pharmacokinetic studies may be useful in patients with antibodies that are not overtly neutralizing in the Bethesda assay because these antibodies may influence the circulating half-life of infused FVIII.[84]

Monitoring for inhibitor development in previously untreated patients is of paramount importance, especially when starting treatment or prophylaxis regimens because inhibitor development occurs early in the course of treatment. Guidelines recommend screening PUPs every 5th exposure day up to the 20th exposure day, and then every 3 months until the 150th exposure day.[85] Repeat testing should be performed before any invasive procedure or elective operation.[85]

Treatment

Patients with hemophilia should receive comprehensive and routine therapy at a hemophilia treatment center (HTC) of excellence, where expertise in the treatment of individuals with severe bleeding disorders and inhibitors is available. If emergency treatment or surgery is needed, patients should be transferred to the hemophilia treatment center as soon as possible and in a stabilized condition (see box on Treatment of Bleeding in a Patient With FVIII Deficiency and an Inhibitor). Typically, the HTC and its physicians serve as a community resource to help guide the care of complex inhibitor patients at other institutions when timely transport is not feasible due to active bleeding and hemodynamic instability.

Minor Bleeding Episodes

In established low-titer alloantibody FVIII inhibitor patients (consistently *less than* 5 BU after repeated challenges) or in patients with

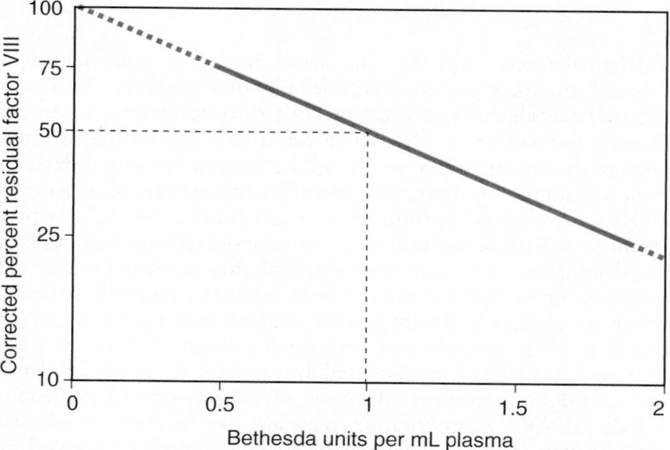

Figure 138-2 BETHESDA ASSAY FOR FACTOR VIII INHIBITOR QUANTITATION. Relationship between corrected residual factor VIII activity and Bethesda titer is shown. If the result is less than 25%, serial dilutions of the patient's plasma are tested until the result is between 25% and 75%. The result is multiplied by the dilution to assign the Bethesda titer. One Bethesda unit (BU) is defined by a corrected residual factor VIII of 50% in the assay *(dotted line). (From Konkle BA: Clinical approach to the bleeding patient. In Colman RW, Marder VJ, Clowes AW, et al, editors:* Hemostasis and thrombosis, *Philadelphia, 2006, Lippincott, Williams & Wilkins, p 1147.)*

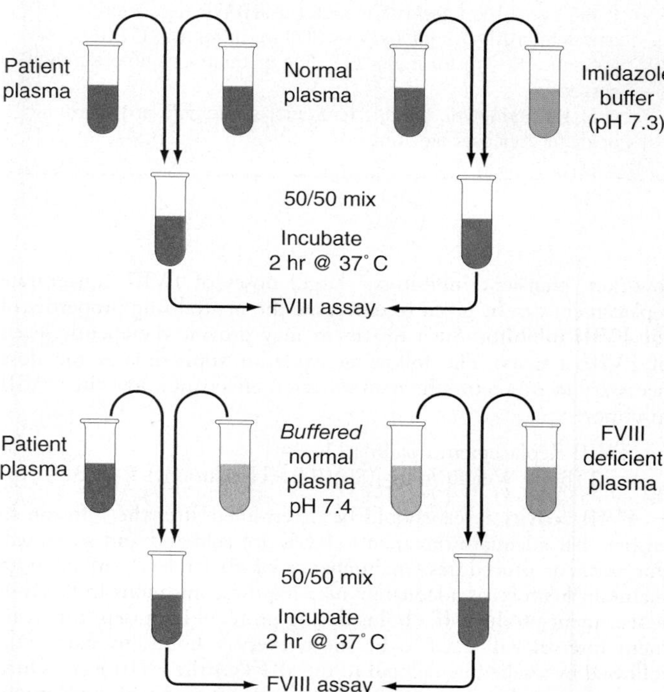

Figure 138-3 METHODOLOGIC DIFFERENCES BETWEEN THE CLASSIC BETHESDA ASSAY[80] AND THE MODIFIED NIJMEGEN ASSAY.[81] *(From Giles AR, Verbruggen B, Rivard GE, et al: A detailed comparison of the performance of the standard versus the Nijmegen modification of the Bethesda assay in detecting factor VIII:C inhibitors in the haemophilia A population of Canada. Association of Hemophilia Centre Directors of Canada. Factor VIII/IX Subcommittee of Scientific and Standardization Committee of International Society on Thrombosis and Haemostasis,* Thromb Haemost *9:872, 1998.)*

Treatment of Bleeding in a Patient With FVIII Deficiency and an Inhibitor

Low Titer, Low Responder
Mild Bleeding

- Local and conservative measures, such as rest, ice, compression, and elevation
- If the patient is known to respond to DDAVP (i.e., mild hemophilia A), 0.3 μg/kg IV or 300 μg intranasal (150 μg per nostril; 150 μg for patients <50 kg) for minor bleeding or treatment before minor surgery
- Oral antifibrinolytic therapy (ε-aminocaproic acid or tranexamic acid) for mucosal bleeding
- FVIII dosing to raise the level to 50%
- Recombinant FVIIa (90 to 120 μg/kg, followed by 90 μg/kg every 2 to 3 hours)
- Activated prothrombin complex concentrates (50 to 100 units/kg, with maximum daily dose of 200 units/kg)
- Concurrent treatment with antifibrinolytics should be administered with caution

Life- or Limb-Threatening Bleeding

- FVIII dosing to maintain FVIII activity levels at 100%
- Recombinant FVIIa (270 μg/kg for one dose may be considered with caution versus 90 μg/kg every 2 to 3 hours)
- Activated prothrombin complex concentrates (100 units/kg, with maximum daily dose of 200 units/kg)
- Concurrent treatment with antifibrinolytics should be administered with caution

Low Titer, High Responder
Mild Bleeding

- Local and conservative measures, such as rest, ice, compression, and elevation
- If the patient is known to respond to DDAVP (i.e., mild hemophilia A), 0.3 μg/kg IV or 300 μg intranasal (150 μg for patients <50 kg) for minor bleeding or treatment before minor surgery
- Oral antifibrinolytic therapy (ε-aminocaproic acid or tranexamic acid) for mucosal bleeding
- Recombinant factor VIIa (270 μg/kg, bolus may be considered with caution versus 90 μg/kg every 2 to 3 hours)
- Activated prothrombin complex concentrates (100 units/kg, with a maximum daily dose of 200 units/kg, may induce anamnesis)

Life- or Limb-Threatening Bleeding

- FVIII in high doses to maintain levels of 100%
- Frequent monitoring for an anamnestic response, usually within 5 to 7 days
- After the anamnestic response develops:
  - Recombinant FVIIa (270 μg/kg, may be considered with caution versus 90 μg/kg every 2 to 3 hours)
  - Activated prothrombin complex concentrates (50 to 100 units/kg, with a maximum daily dose of 200 units/kg)

High Titer, High Responder
Mild Bleeding

- Local and conservative measures, such as rest, ice, compression, and elevation
- Oral antifibrinolytic therapy (ε-aminocaproic acid or tranexamic acid) for mucosal bleeding
- Recombinant FVIIa (270 μg/kg, should be considered with caution versus 90 μg/kg every 2 to 3 hours)
- Activated prothrombin complex concentrates (100 units/kg, with a maximum daily dose of 200 units/kg)
- Concurrent treatment with antifibrinolytics should be administered with caution

Life- or Limb-Threatening Bleeding

- Recombinant FVIIa (270 μg/kg, should be considered with caution versus 90 μg/kg IV every 2 to 3 hours)
- Activated prothrombin complex concentrates (100 units/kg, with a maximum daily dose of 200 units/kg)
- If available, immunoadsorption can be attempted to rapidly lower the inhibitor titer so as to allow use of FVIII

low-titer "transient inhibitors," larger doses of FVIII concentrate replacement can be given to overcome the neutralizing properties of the FVIII inhibitor. Such treatment may provide therapeutic levels of FVIII activity. The following equation approximates the dose necessary to overcome the neutralization effects of a low titer FVIII inhibitor:

$$\text{FVIII Replacement Loading Dose} = 2\,(\text{Body Weight in kg}\,[(80)(100-\text{Hematocrit})/100]/\text{BU})$$

FVIII activity levels should be determined after the infusion to ensure that adequate therapeutic levels are achieved and sustained. For invasive procedures, maintenance of FVIII level sufficient to maintain hemostasis adequately may require continuous infusion of replacement product. If a bolus dosing protocol is chosen, the treatment interval will need to be short, every 4 hours, to start with, followed by a schedule tailored to the aPTT or the FVIII level. Once the optimal bolus dose of FVIII replacement is established, home therapy may be possible.

High-titer FVIII alloantibody inhibitors are characterized by titers above 5 BU and by anamnestic responsiveness after repeated exposures to exogenous FVIII. Often, high-titer inhibitors may spontaneously fall below 5 BU, especially after prolonged lapses in FVIII reexposure. In this scenario, FVIII replacement should be avoided, if possible, so that anamnesis can be abated and the chances for successful immune tolerance induction and eradication of the inhibitor can be enhanced.[86] On the other hand, in urgent situations when "bypass" products are not available, low-titer inhibitor expression (<5 BU) may allow for effective use of FVIII concentrate replacement therapy, particularly in bleeds that are threatening to life or limb, because the anamnestic response will be delayed for several days. In these situations, administration of sufficient amounts of exogenous FVIII to overcome the immediate neutralization by the low-titer inhibitor will allow hemostasis to be achieved. Anamnestic rises in FVIII inhibitor titers have been observed after infusion of activated prothrombin complex concentrates to high-titer antibody patients, which are administered to bypass the inhibitor and to treat or prevent bleeding. These products contain a small amount of FVIII.[86-89]

Low-titer FVIII alloantibody inhibitors never rise above 5 BU and do not exhibit anamnestic increases after reexposure to exogenous FVIII. DDAVP administration may also be effective in selected patients with mild to moderately severe hemophilia complicated by an inhibitor (high or low titer). A DDAVP "challenge" should be undertaken before any intervention in order to assess the adequacy of incremental rises in FVIII activity in such patients.

Severe Bleeding Episodes

For patients who have an inhibitor titer less than 5 BU, administration of exogenous FVIII should be considered if FVIII levels can be monitored closely. This approach provides the most specific and effective therapy; however, anamnesis can occur within a week in patients with a history of a high-titer inhibitor, and switching to a bypassing agent is indicated. Anamnesis may render subsequent use of exogenous FVIII therapy ineffective, so that even when exogenous FVIII replacement is anticipated to be effective in the short term, treatment should start with FVIIa or an activated prothrombin complex concentrate if prolonged periods of replacement therapy are necessary.

In the case of a severe bleed or a life-threatening emergency, the inhibitor titer should be determined as rapidly as possible, but treatment should not be delayed until the results are available. For patients with a known persistent high-titer antibody, prompt replacement treatment should consist of a bypass agent, either an activated prothrombin complex concentrate or recombinant FVIIa.

Surgery

Surgery in patients with hemophilia, especially those who have an inhibitor, requires the involvement of an entire facility experienced in the preoperative and postoperative care of such patients. Replacement therapy recommendations for surgical procedures are similar to those for hemorrhage. For known low responders, adequate hemostasis can be achieved with higher doses of FVIII. For the high-responding patient, activated prothrombin complex concentrate or FVIIa is most effective in the postoperative setting.[8-10]

Prothrombin Complex Concentrates

Prothrombin complex concentrates (PCCs) were designed for treatment of bleeding events associated with hemophilia B, congenital deficiencies of the other vitamin K–dependent clotting disorders, or with severe liver disease. PCCs were hypothesized to be useful to treat FVIII inhibitor-related bleeding because of their thrombogenic properties. Prepared from large pools of normal donor plasma, the PCCs contain the vitamin K–dependent clotting factors prothrombin, factor VII, factor IX, and factor X, as well as anticoagulant proteins C and S (action of the latter is unknown). Heparin or antithrombin is added to some preparations to limit activation of the coagulation factors during the manufacturing process and with administration. All PCCs undergo a viral inactivation process. In comparison with placebo, PCCs were shown to be partially effective in controlling approximately 50% of bleeding episodes in patients with FVIII alloantibody inhibitors, compared with 25% for product containing albumin alone.[90] A major caveat is that administration of PCCs to treat hemorrhage in hemophiliacs with inhibitors is *not* the treatment of choice and is justified *only* in the absence of more effective therapies.[90]

Activated Prothrombin Complex Concentrates and FVIIa

Activated prothrombin complex concentrates (APCCs) are PCCs that are "supercharged" by virtue of their partial "activation" during the manufacturing process with activated FVII credited for the maximum clotting potential. In a randomized, double-blind trial, an APCC showed significantly better control of bleeding events in severe hemophiliacs with FVIII alloantibody inhibitors than did PCCs ($P = 0.0085$); however, APCC was judged effective in only 64% of the episodes versus 52% effectiveness for PCC.[91] Uncontrolled clinical studies have shown that APCCs are effective in treating 81% to 93% of joint bleeds.[92,93] One should bear in mind, however, that APCCs are never as effective in inhibitor patients as is FVIII replacement in noninhibitor patients. Use of APCCs facilitates surgery in inhibitor patients and has been reported to be effective[93,94] and safe in large populations.[94]

APCC administration in a secondary prophylaxis regimen has also been deemed feasible, successful, and safe in reducing the frequency of bleeding events in severe hemophilia A patients with high-titer FVIII inhibitors. In the randomized, prospective, crossover Pro-FEIBA study, a statistically significant 62% reduction in all bleeding events was observed during the prophylaxis phase of the study (85 units/kg on 3 nonconsecutive days/week) compared with the on-demand period (85 units/kg every 6 to 12 hours).[95]

Use of PCCs and APCCs is hampered by the lack of laboratory tests to measure efficacy or to predict the potential for anamnesis (due to the presence of small amounts of FVIII) and the risk for precipitating thrombotic complications. The incidence of thrombosis is increased with regimens that exceed the recommended dosage and in patients at risk for thrombotic events, such as older individuals with coronary artery disease.

For acute bleeds, APCCs are administered at doses of 50 to 100 units/kg every 6 to 12 hours based on the clinical severity, with the maximum daily dose capped at 200 units/kg. This broader time frame allows for use at home for treatment of acute bleeds and for prophylaxis.

Recombinant FVIIa was purified from plasma and first used to treat a hemophilia A patient with an inhibitor in 1983.[96] Later, FVIIa produced by recombinant technology was found to be effective for preventing and treating acute bleeding. A randomized dose-finding trial determined that FVIIa effectively reversed 71% of joint and muscle bleeds within two to three doses, given every 2 to 3 hours.[97] Another prospective study established that 90 μg/kg FVIIa promoted adequate hemostasis during major surgical procedures, with an efficacy rate of 83% to 100%.[98]

Randomized prospective studies have directly compared the efficacy and safety of one dose of an APCC (factor eight inhibitor bypassing activity [FEIBA, Baxter], 85 to 90 international units/kg) with one to two doses of FVIIa (NovoSeven [Novo Nordisk Health Care AG] 90 to 105 μg/kg/dose) to treat acute joint bleeds. Although both products showed around 80% efficacy after 12 hours, equivalency was not shown at the 6-hour primary outcome point, but this was probably due to study design and underpowered cohorts.[99] When the primary outcome was the percentage of patients who required additional hemostatic replacement therapy 9 hours after initiation of treatment, significantly lower percentages of the 270 μg/kg (8.3%) and 3 × 90 μg/kg (9.1%) FVIIa treatment dose cohorts required rescue therapies compared with the aPCC treatment group (36.4%).[100]

Use of FVIIa is associated with some drawbacks, such as the lack of effective laboratory monitoring, very short half-life (≈2 to 3 hours, which necessitates frequent administration), potential for thrombotic events (more frequently observed in noninhibitor patients), and expense.

For acute bleeding events in inhibitor patients, debate exists as to whether the more convenient dosing regimen of a single large bolus dose of FVIIa (270 μg/kg) is as safe or efficacious as the multiple-dose regimen (90 μg/kg every 2 to 3 hours as recommended in the package insert). The initial concern was related to the thrombogenic potential of larger single doses, particularly in older individuals, since the large single-dose regimen was studied predominantly in children. In reality, a recent analysis of the FVIIa dosages used in FVIII inhibitor patients in the U.S.[101] ($n = 20{,}469$ doses, ranging from the 90 to 120 μg/kg FDA-recommended dose up to >270 μg/kg) revealed a very low incidence of thromboembolic complications (0.2%).[101] For serious life- and limb-threatening hemorrhages, a single 270 μg/kg bolus dose is recommended. Treatment of acute bleeds with FVIIa concentrate should be initiated as soon as possible because efficacy is inversely related to time to treatment. For surgery, some experts advise an initial dose of 120 μg/kg, followed by repeated 90 μg/kg doses every 2 to 3 hours.[102]

Parallel-Sequential Use of APCC and FVIIa Concentrates

For active inhibitor-associated bleeding episodes that are not totally responsive to treatment with either an APCC or rFVIIa concentrate alone, the administration of both products simultaneously or in an alternating regimen (within 12 hours) has been anecdotally successful.[103-105] This combination is not recommended by the product manufacturers, and its clinical utility has not been studied in a scientifically valid manner. In vitro sequential "spiking" experiments[106] or ex vivo systematic infusion studies employing plasma specimens from inhibitor patients who have received these two types of bypassing agents alone, simultaneously, or in tandem[107] have demonstrated enhanced hemostasis for the combined approach. One study suggests that individualized bypass replacement therapy regimens can be designed for inhibitor patients based on the ex vivo responses observed in thromboelastogram tracings.[107] Although the efficacy of parallel treatment with bypassing agents may be excellent in most inhibitor related refractory bleeds, such regimens may increase the risk for thrombotic complications. A recent critical review of 49 inhibitor patients (9 acquired and 40 congenital), who received both bypassing agents in combined or alternating dosing regimens, reported 10 thromboembolic events, of which 1 was fatal.[108]

Prophylaxis With APCC and FVIIa

Prophylaxis regimens employing either APCC or rFVIIa to prevent acute and chronic arthropathy in inhibitor patients can be classified as primary (children awaiting ITI) or secondary (patients in whom ITI failed). Though not formally compared, prophylaxis with bypassing agents in inhibitor patients is not as efficacious as FVIII replacement in patients without an inhibitor. However, an accumulation of case reports and small clinical studies has suggested that prophylaxis with bypassing agents is safe and feasible in the subset of inhibitor patients with frequent bleeds, such as in target joints. The first prospective controlled study of prophylaxis in FVIII inhibitor patients[109] showed that a daily bolus dose 270 μg/kg of FVIIa is superior to a 90 μg/kg FVIIa dose in reducing the bleeding frequency (59% versus 45%) observed in the preprophylaxis period. An uncontrolled study[110] described equivalent efficacy and safety for FVIIa and APCC for prophylaxis in hemophilia A patients with inhibitors. Patients were placed on prophylaxis while awaiting initiation of immune tolerance induction. In this context the investigators favored the use of FVIIa to avoid potential anamnestic responses with APCC.[110] A recent prospective controlled trial demonstrated that a prophylaxis APCC regimen of 85 international units/kg three times/week reduced bleeding events by 62% in FVIII inhibitor patients, compared with an on-demand treatment regimen.[87]

Fibrinolytic Inhibitors

ε-Aminocaproic and tranexamic acid have long safety records and are commonly used in hemophilia patients, including those with inhibitors, as a sole treatment modality or as adjuncts to factor replacement for mucosal bleeding, dental procedures, and some orthopedic surgeries.[111]

For children, ε-aminocaproic acid can be administered orally at doses of 50 to 100 mg/kg every 6 hours. If used prior to a surgical intervention, the first dose should be given 4 hours before the start of the procedure. In adults, a loading dose of 4 to 5 g can be given initially, followed by similar or lower doses every 6 to 12 hours until bleeding is controlled (total suggested dose is 100 mg/kg/day). Fibrinolytic inhibitors are useful adjuncts for the treatment or prevention of bleeds treated with DDAVP in patients with low-titer inhibitors but should be administered cautiously when APCCs are used for high-titer inhibitors. Antifibrinolytic inhibitors are considered to be safe for use in conjunction with FVIIa.[88]

Immune Tolerance Therapy

The ultimate therapy for a patient with hemophilia complicated by a neutralizing inhibitory alloantibody is ITI. The goal of ITI is to eradicate the alloantibody. Successful ITI enables reinitiation of FVIII replacement for treatment of bleeding episodes and for prophylaxis. ITI is considered the best treatment option for hemophilia A patients with high-titer inhibitors.

The first successful implementation of ITI was accomplished in 1974 when a child with a high-titer inhibitor (>500 BU) required emergency reversal of a life-threatening bleed.[112,113] Very large doses of FVIII concentrate and a PCC were administered, and the hemorrhage was eventually controlled. A serendipitous finding was that the inhibitor titer decreased to almost 40 BU. This was the first documentation that high-dose FVIII administration could decrease inhibitor titers and provide proof of principle for the "Bonn protocol," which originally used high doses of FVIII (100 international units/kg) twice daily.[112,113] Bypass agents are administered as needed to treat acute bleeds that occur during ITI. This regimen is continued until the inhibitor disappears, which can take up to a maximum of 3 years.[113,114]

The Malmö ITI protocol was developed to induce rapid elimination of an alloantibody inhibitor in a patient with severe hemophilia B who required urgent orthopedic surgery.[115] Unique among the ITI regimens, the Malmö protocol uses concurrent immunomodulatory therapies in conjunction with large doses of clotting factor concentrate to lower the inhibitor level.[116,117]

As experience with ITI regimens increased, it became evident that low-dose FVIII replacement protocols also induce tolerance. Such regimens start with a dose of 25 international units/kg every other day, a 16- to 24-fold lower dose than those used in high-dose ITI protocols.[118,119]

Because of different ITI treatment protocols, a retrospective International Immune Tolerance Registry (IITR) was established in 1989. The registry eventually collected 314 alloantibody inhibitor patients (>94% high-titer) who underwent either low- or high-dose ITI treatment regimens.[120] The success rate ranged from 50% to 60% over time. Predictors of successful ITI included a low maximum inhibitor titer (85% success with ≤20 BU titer); low immediate pre-ITI BU (59% failure rate for >20 BU); higher FVIII dosage (86% success with ≥200 international units/kg/day); age of patient at initiation of ITI (60% failure for age >20 years); and shorter time interval between inhibitor detection and ITI initiation (>70% success for <5-year interval).[121,122] Although other registries yielded similar findings,[123-125] uncertainty remains as to the optimal total daily dose of FVIII, the use of concomitant immunosuppressive/immune-modulating agents, and the type of clotting factor replacement therapy (plasma-derived versus recombinant concentrates). Another important difference among protocols reported in the registries was the definition of success: stringent criteria (disappearance of the inhibitor, normal FVIII recovery and half-life) were not always accepted and therefore had an impact on the registry outcome evaluation. Although never formally proven, some believe that low- and/or intermediate-purity factor concentrates containing vWF may be more efficacious than recombinant FVIII for successful ITI.[126,127]

Other treatment-related elements that may influence ITI outcomes cannot be addressed in registries. These include the number of acute bleeds during ITI, use of CVADs, onset of infections during ITI, and use of plasma-derived PCCs or FVIIa to treat bleeds. Most of these questions were addressed in a randomized prospective multinational ITI trial that compared high- and low-dose ITI regimens, with the decision to use recombinant or a vWF-containing FVIII replacement product left to the discretion of the treating physician.[128,129] The results published to date have confirmed that ITI can eradicate alloantibody inhibitors in almost 70% of cases, even when very stringent outcome definitions are applied. Recombinant FVIII preparations were used in 90% of enrolled individuals, making it very unlikely that plasma-derived vWF-containing concentrates are superior to recombinant FVIII. The success rates with high-dose (200 international units/kg) and low-dose (50 international units/kg thrice/week) ITI regimens were similar; however, successful ITI was achieved 50% earlier with the high-dose regimen. The low-dose regimen was associated with an increased frequency of breakthrough bleeding events during ITI. This safety signal led to premature discontinuation of the study.

A high proportion of patients (41/99, 41%) with a CVAD developed access device infection, but this complication did not affect the likelihood of ITI success[129] and therefore should not reduce ITI use; however, it pinpoints the need for training and professional device nursing when long-term treatments are needed. Further prospective studies are needed to determine the optimal and most cost-effective dosing regimens for ITI.

A number of high-risk and/or ITI-relapsed patients have been treated with ritruximab, an anti-CD20 monoclonal antibody, with or without FVIII concentrate. Success rates have ranged from 33% to 57%,[130] suggesting that rituximab may be useful for salvage of patients with little or no response to conventional ITI regimens.

HEMOPHILIA B

The development of alloantibody inhibitors to FIX in severe hemophilia B follows the same general principles as in hemophilia A. Inhibitory alloantibodies may arise after administration of FIX-containing replacement products, and this phenomenon was appreciated very soon after hemophilia B was documented to be a separate entity from hemophilia A.[131] However, several distinct features in the epidemiology and treatment of FIX alloantibody inhibitors in severe hemophilia B deserve mention. These include (1) the lower incidence and prevalence of FIX alloantibody inhibitors; (2) the increased risk for developing anaphylaxis after administration of FIX-containing concentrates to FIX alloantibody inhibitor patients; (3) the risk for developing nephrotic syndrome after exposure to FIX-containing replacement products; and (4) the lower success rate of ITI therapy for eradication of FIX alloantibodies.[132,133]

Epidemiology

Patients with severe hemophilia B have a 10-fold lower risk for developing alloantibody inhibitors compared with severe hemophilia A patients (3% and 30%, respectively).[134] FIX gene mutations associated with a very low risk for inhibitor formation are single amino acid substitutions, whereas the risk for inhibitor development approaches 20% with more significant mutations, such as frameshift mutations, premature stop codons, large deletions, and splice site mutations.[134] Patients with hemophilia B who are at highest risk for development of inhibitors have a severe phenotype as a result of large gene deletions or other aberrations of the gene product, such as nonsense mutations. Although the latter mutations are found only in a small fraction of the hemophilia B population, they account for approximately 50% of the inhibitor population.[134]

Diagnosis

As in hemophilia A, an inhibitor should be suspected in hemophilia B when a patient ceases to respond to conventional replacement treatment. Given the possibility of anaphylaxis that may occur with initial treatment of bleeding episodes, patients with high-risk FIX gene mutations should be regularly screened for alloantibody inhibitors. The laboratory diagnosis for inhibitors in hemophilia B involves a modification of the same Bethesda assay used for quantification of FVIII inhibitors. In this case, FIX-deficient plasma is used instead of FVIII-deficient plasma.[135] In contrast to the FVIII inhibitor scenario, FIX inhibitors act rapidly to neutralize FIX in the normal plasma/patient plasma mixing studies; there is no time-dependent increase in the inhibitory expression of FIX alloantibodies over a 2-hour incubation at 37° C with either high- or low-titer FIX inhibitors.

Treatment

Treatment of hemophilia B in patients with FIX inhibitors mirrors that of hemophilia A complicated by FVIII alloantibody inhibitors. Both APCC and FVIIa are the key therapeutic modalities to reverse, control, and prevent bleeding regardless of whether it is spontaneous in nature or induced by trauma or surgery.[135] However, because APCC contains significant amounts of FIX, which may induce anamnesis, some experts prefer FVIIa.

Few treatment options exist for patients with FIX alloantibody inhibitors who have experienced allergic reactions to the FIX antigenic material found in plasma, PCC, APCC, high-purity plasma-derived FIX concentrate, or even in recombinant FIX concentrates. Anaphylaxis is, in fact, a major complication that can occur soon after the infusion of FIX-containing replacement therapies, manifesting as either a type II (dyspnea and hypoxia, and generalized hypersensitivity) or a type III (anaphylaxis and hypotension) allergic reaction. The rarity of anaphylactic complications in hemophilia B patients with FIX alloantibody inhibitors (only an estimated 35 cases have been reported) does not negate the seriousness of this complication.[132,136,137] In addition, this is likely an underreported and perhaps underrecognized event. The major risk factor for developing an anaphylactic reaction is the presence of a FIX gene null mutation, leading to an absence of circulating factor IX antigenic material.[138]

Because these severe reactions occur only after initiation of treatment, they have been observed only in children (median age 12 months), occurring at a median of 11 exposure days. The development of anaphylaxis occurs at the same time as the appearance of an inhibitor. A recent survey on the topic has shown that allergic reactions can be elicited with either recombinant or plasma-derived FIX concentrates at similar rates (3.9%).[139]

Because experience with anaphylaxis is limited by its low incidence, some general practice guidelines have been developed:

1. For newly diagnosed hemophilia B patients, especially those with high-risk FIX gene mutations, the initial FIX replacement treatments should be conducted in a medical facility where hemophilia expertise and resuscitation equipment are immediately available.[132]
2. Once an FIX alloantibody inhibitor has been documented, FVIIa is the treatment of choice for active bleeding and for prophylaxis against bleeding.
3. ITI is generally ineffective in these FIX alloantibody patients, although tolerance to FIX has been reported with progressively increasing doses of FIX (desensitization procedure) administered with hydrocortisone.[132,137]
4. FIX alloantibody formation may be complicated by nephrotic syndrome, especially in patients who previously experienced an allergic reaction to FIX replacement. The limited data available suggest that this syndrome is not the result of immune complex deposition, and it does not respond to corticosteroid treatment.[140,141] If nephrosis occurs, FIX doses should be reduced or treatment should be discontinued and FVIIa therapy should be used instead.[141]
5. In a few refractory cases with or without nephrosis, immune modulation (anti-CD20,[142,143] cyclosporine A[144] or mycophenolate mofetil[145]) has resulted in temporary immune tolerance to FIX.
6. Prophylaxis regimens with FVIIa (or APCC, if anaphylaxis and/or anamnesis is not an issue) may be useful in the context of high-titer FIX alloantibody inhibitors; however, additional large, long-term controlled trials are necessary before this approach becomes the standard of care.

SUGGESTED READINGS

Alexander S, Hopewell S, Hunter S, et al: Rituximab and desensitization for a patient with severe factor IX deficiency, inhibitors and history of anaphylaxis. *J Pediatr Hematol Oncol* 30:93, 2008.

Darby SC, Kan SW, Spooner RJ, et al: Mortality rates, life expectancy and causes of death in people with haemophilia A or B in the United Kingdom who were not infected with HIV. *Blood* 110:815, 2007.

Fay PJ, Scandella D: Human inhibitor antibodies specific for the factor VIII A2 domain disrupt the interaction between the subunit and factor IXa. *J Biol Chem* 274:29826, 1999.

Hay CR, Brown S, Collins PW, et al: The diagnosis and management of factor VIII and IX inhibitors: A guideline from the United Kingdom Haemophilia Centre Doctors Organisation. *Br J Haematol* 133:591, 2006.

Hay CR, Dimichele DM: The principal results of the International Immune Tolerance Study: A randomized dose comparison. *Blood* 2011 (Epub ahead of print).

Hay CRM, Palmer B, Chalmers E, et al: On behalf of the United Kingdom Hemophilia Centre Doctor's Organisation (UKHCDO): Incidence of FVIII inhibitors throughout life in severe haemophilia A in the United Kingdom. *Blood* 117:6367, 2011.

Ingerslev J: Hemophilia. Strategies for the treatment of inhibitor patients. *Haematologica* 85:15, 2000.

Konkle B, Ebbesen LS, Erhardtsen E, et al: Randomized, prospective clinical trial of recombinant factor VIIa for secondary prophylaxis in haemophilia patients with inhibitors. *J Thromb Haemost* 5:1904, 2008.

Lacroix-Desmazes S, Bayry J, Misra N, et al: The prevalence of proteolytic antibodies against factor VIII in hemophilia A. *N Engl J Med* 346:662, 2002.

Mariani G, Ghirardini A, Bellocco R: Immunetolerance in hemophilia-principal results from the International Registry. Report of the factor VIII and IX Subcommittee. *Thromb Haemost* 72:155, 1994.

Mariani G, Siragusa S, Kroner B: Immunetolerance induction in hemophilia A: A review. *Seminars in Hemostasis and Thrombosis* 29:69, 2003.

Mauser-Bunschoten EP, Nieuwenhuis HK, Roosendaal G, et al: Low-dose immune tolerance induction in hemophilia A patients with inhibitors. *Blood* 86:983, 1995.

Miao CH: Immunemodulation for inhibitors in haemophilia A: The important role of Treg cells. *Expert Rev Hematol* 3:469, 2010.

Oldenburg J, Schroeder J, Brackmann HH, et al: Environmental and genetic factors influencing inhibitor development. *Semin Hematol* 41:82, 2004.

Oldenburg J, Schwaab R, Brackmann HH: Induction of immune tolerance in haemophilia A inhibitor patients by the "Bonn Protocol": Predictive parameter for therapy duration and outcome. *Vox Sang* 77:49, 1999.

Roberts HR, Monroe DM, White GC: The use of recombinant factor VIIa in the treatment of bleeding disorders. *Blood* 104:3858, 2004.

Thompson AR, Murphy ME, Liu M, et al: Loss of tolerance to exogenous and endogenous factor VIII in a mild hemophilia A patient with an Arg593 to Cys mutation. *Blood* 90:1902, 1997.

Warrier I, Ewenstein BM, Koerper MA, et al: Factor IX inhibitors and anaphylaxis in hemophilia B. *J Pediatr Hematol Oncol* 19:23, 1997.

For complete list of references log on to www.expertconsult.com.

CHAPTER 139

RARE COAGULATION FACTOR DEFICIENCIES

David Gailani and Anne T. Neff

Hemophilia A (factor VIII deficiency) and hemophilia B (factor IX deficiency) are the most common inherited deficiencies involving components of the plasma coagulation system (Fig. 139-1), with frequencies of 1 : 10,000 and 1 : 30,000 male births, respectively (Chapter 137). In comparison, frequencies of one in 500,000 to 2 million individuals are estimated for severe deficiency of other plasma coagulation factors, including fibrinogen; the protease zymogens prothrombin factors VII, X, XI, XII, and prekallikrein; the cofactors factor V and high-molecular-weight kininogen; and the transaminase factor XIII. These disorders are primarily autosomal recessive conditions, implying a carrier frequency of ≈1 : 1000, a value ≈10-fold higher than the mutant allele frequency for X-linked hemophilia A. Their rarity, therefore, is based on the fact that they are recessive conditions and not because of low allele frequencies. This is important to keep in mind, because partial (heterozygous) deficiencies of these proteins are relatively common and may be associated with mild bleeding symptoms in some cases. As with any recessive trait, incidences are up to 10-fold higher in areas where consanguinity is common. The conditions discussed in this chapter represent 3% to 5% of all coagulation factor deficiencies. A database (www.rbdd.org) has been established for the purpose of collecting clinical, genetic, and therapeutic information on these disorders to facilitate development of evidenced-based diagnostic and treatment recommendations.

Fig. 139-1, *A,* presents a scheme that reflects our current understanding of the reactions involved in thrombin generation and fibrin formation. Coagulation is triggered by binding of plasma factor VIIa to tissue factor in the wall of a damaged blood vessel. The factor VIIa/tissue factor complex converts factor X to Xa, which in turn converts prothrombin to thrombin in the presence of factor Va. Mice completely lacking prothrombin, factor VII, factor X, or factor V die in utero or soon after birth, demonstrating the importance of these proteins. Thrombin has many functions, including conversion of fibrinogen to fibrin. Factor IX is also activated by factor VIIa/tissue factor and, with factor VIIIa, sustains thrombin generation by activating factor X. In some situations, factor IX activation by factor XIa is required. The older model shown in Fig. 139-1, *B,* serves as the basis for the prothrombin time (PT) and partial thromboplastin time (PTT) assays. Here factor XI activation requires factor XII, prekallikrein and high-molecular-weight kininogen, the contact factors. Deficiency of a contact factor does not result in abnormal bleeding, however, indicating that other mechanisms exist for factor XI activation. For example, thrombin can activate factor XI (see Fig. 139-1, *A*). Finally, factor XIII is activated by thrombin and cross-links fibrin monomers to complete the process of fibrin formation. This chapter contains sections describing deficiency states for each coagulation factor. The number from the Online Mendelian Inheritance in Man (OMIM) database for the deficiency is given in the section title, and each section includes references to websites that compile updated lists of mutations associated with the factor deficiencies. Table 139-1 lists properties of each coagulation factor and features of the congenital deficiency states; Table 139-2 presents recommendations for treatment.

FIBRINOGEN DEFICIENCY (OMIM 202400)

Fibrinogen, the plasma precursor of the fibrin component of a clot, was first purified in the late 19th century. Fibrinogen and fibrin are designated *factor I* and *factor Ia,* respectively, by the International Committee for the Nomenclature of Blood Clotting. Congenital absence of fibrinogen (afibrinogenemia) was first described in 1920 and has an estimated incidence of one in 1 million to 2 million people (see Table 139-1).[1] Partial fibrinogen deficiency is called *hypofibrinogenemia.* Afibrinogenemia and hypofibrinogenemia represent the homozygous and heterozygous states, respectively, for mutations affecting plasma fibrinogen concentration.

Fibrinogen is a 340,000-Dalton protein composed of two heterotrimers, each containing an Aα, Bβ, and γ chain (Fig. 139-2). The three chains are encoded by separate genes (FGA, FGB, FGG) in a 50-kilobase region of chromosome 4. Thrombin converts fibrinogen to fibrin by cleaving fibrinopeptides A and B from the Aα and Bβ chains, respectively. Fibrinogen also binds glycoprotein IIb/IIIa, facilitating platelet aggregation. Fibrinogen is synthesized in hepatocytes. Fibrinogen in platelet α-granules is taken up from plasma via a glycoprotein IIb/IIIa-dependent mechanism. Between 8% and 15% of plasma fibrinogen contains at least one γ chain that is a product of an alternatively spliced mRNA and is referred to as γ′-fibrinogen. The γ′ chain modulates thrombin and factor XIII activity and influences clot architecture.

The normal plasma fibrinogen concentration is 150 to 400 mg/dL (1.5 to 4.0 gm/L). Afibrinogenemic patients have undetectable or very low levels of fibrinogen (<10 mg/dL) as determined by clotting and immunoreactive assays, due to homozygosity or compound heterozygosity for fibrinogen gene mutations. Hypofibrinogenemia is associated with partial deficiency due to heterozygosity for a mutation. Since the first report of a causative mutation in 1999, more than 70 fibrinogen gene abnormalities have been described in afibrinogenemic and hypofibrinogenemic patients (www.geht.org/databaseang/fibrinogen). Most affect the FGA gene and are deletion, frameshift, nonsense, or splicing mutations. Missense mutations are more prevalent in the FGB and FGG genes and cluster in the polypeptide C-termini, affecting formation of the fibrinogen D-domain (see Fig. 139-2) and interfering with secretion. In afibrinogenemia, fibrinogen is not secreted from hepatocytes; this is either a consequence of one of the fibrinogen chains not being synthesized or the result of a mutant chain altering the fibrinogen structure. In either case intracellular nonsecretable fibrinogen polypeptides are usually degraded. A few missense mutations in the FGG gene causing hypofibrinogenemia—for example, Gly284Arg (fibrinogen Brescia), Arg375Trp (fibrinogen Aguadilla), or Thr314Pro (fibrinogen Al DuPont)—are associated with accumulation of mutant γ-polypeptide in hepatocytes, leading to hepatic dysfunction and cirrhosis similar to the process associated with α_1-antitrypsin deficiency (endoplasmic reticulum storage disease).

Acquired hypofibrinogenemia is common in disseminated intravascular coagulation (DIC) and in primary fibrinolysis. Fibrinogen levels are usually normal or increased in liver disease, but levels may

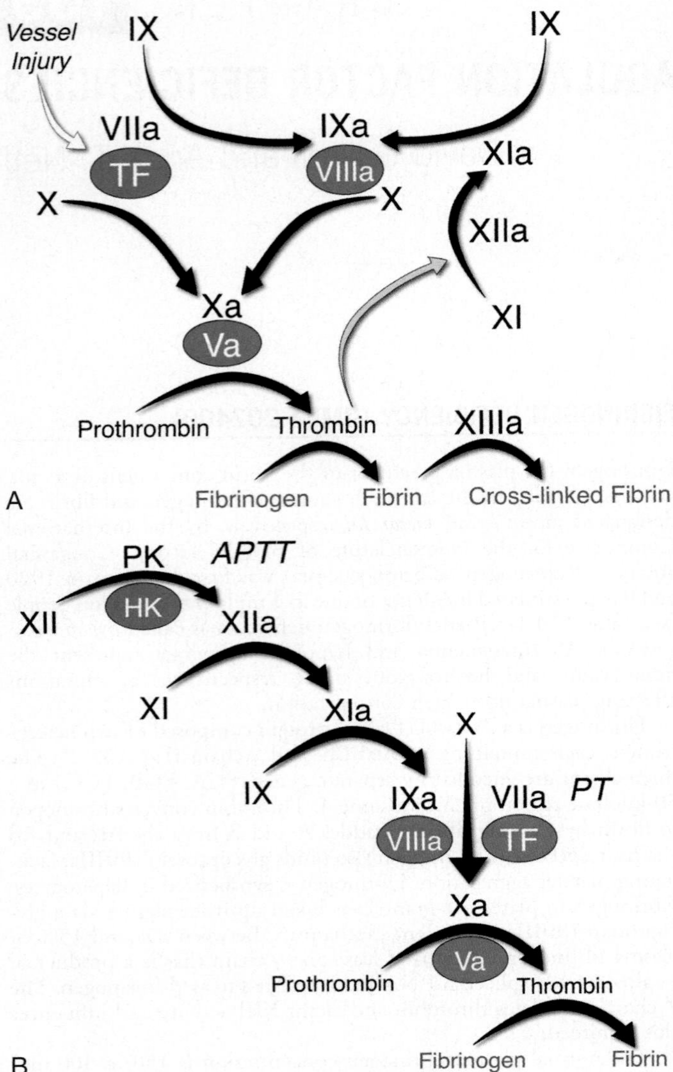

Figure 139-1 MODELS OF PLASMA COAGULATION. Unactivated plasma factors are indicated by Roman numerals and activated factors by Roman numerals followed by a lowercase *a*. Enzymes are indicated by black lettering and cofactors by white lettering in red ovals. Black arrows indicate reactions involving enzyme activation; gray arrow indicates feedback activation of factor XI by thrombin. **A,** A model of tissue factor initiated hemostasis. Please read the introduction to this chapter for a description of the events leading to formation and stabilization of a fibrin clot that are depicted in this figure. **B,** The cascade/waterfall model of hemostasis. This model serves as the basis for the prothrombin time (PT) and activated partial thromboplastin time (PTT) assays. In the PT assay a reagent containing TF is added to plasma, and the factor VIIa/TF complex induces clot formation through activation of factor X. In the PTT assay a reagent containing a negatively charged substance initiates clot formation through activation of factor XII (contact activation; see Fig. 139-3 for details). *TF,* Tissue factor; *HK,* high-molecular-weight kininogen; *PK,* prekallikrein.

be low (<100 mg/dL) in cirrhosis with hepatic failure or with fulminant hepatic necrosis. A low fibrinogen level in patients with hepatic insufficiency indicates a poor prognosis. Patients receiving L-asparaginase for hematologic malignancies may develop severe hypofibrinogenemia (<20 mg/dL), with other coagulation factors being normal or only slightly reduced.

Hemorrhagic symptoms in fibrinogen deficiency are most significant when the plasma level is below 50 mg/dL. Most afibrinogenemic patients (85%) have bleeding from the umbilical cord and from mucosal surfaces.[2] Menorrhagia and bleeding from the skin and the gastrointestinal and genitourinary tracts are common.[3] Hemarthroses and muscle hematomas were frequent in one series (54% and 72%, respectively), but hemarthroses were less frequent (25%) in another study, and hemarthrosis-related arthropathy appears to be less pronounced than in hemophilia. Intracranial bleeding is a major cause of death. Afibrinogenemic patients are also prone to spontaneous rupture of the spleen. Hypofibrinogenemic patients are often asymptomatic, but may have excessive bleeding with trauma or surgery, particularly if the fibrinogen level is <50 mg/dL.

The incidence Pregnancy loss is common in afibrinogenemic and hypofibrinogenemic women, usually in the first trimester.[4] Fibrinogen deficient mice also have difficulty sustaining pregnancies, confirming the importance of the maternal protein to fetal viability. Pre- and postpartum bleeding is common, and intraabdominal bleeding from ruptured corpus luteal cysts has been reported. Of note, arterial and venous thrombotic events have been described in afibrinogenemic patients. Although some cases are associated with other risk factors for thromboembolism (or with administration of replacement therapy), no identifiable risk factor is evident in most instances. Fibrinogen and fibrin have been shown to downregulate thrombin activity, providing a possible explanation for these events.

Assays that measure the time to clot formation, such as the PT, PTT, and thrombin time, will be infinitely prolonged in afibrinogenemia. The template bleeding time and tests of in vitro platelet aggregation are usually abnormal. Fibrinogen is absent, whereas other coagulation factor levels are normal. The von Clauss method is the most commonly used technique for measuring fibrinogen and is based on determining the time to clot formation after addition of thrombin to plasma. This assay is not reliable at low fibrinogen levels (<10 mg/dL) and may give falsely low readings with fibrinogen variants that polymerize slowly (dysfibrinogenemia) or if high levels of substances that interfere with fibrin polymerization (paraproteins, fibrin degradation products) are present. Therefore it is important to demonstrate absence of immunoreactive fibrinogen to confirm a diagnosis of afibrinogenemia. In hypofibrinogenemia functional and antigenic fibrinogen levels are proportionately decreased. A disproportionately low functional level suggests dysfibrinogenemia. The PT and PTT are relatively insensitive to fibrinogen and may not be prolonged with mild to moderate hypofibrinogenemia. The thrombin time is more sensitive in these situations. Afibrinogenemic patients have low erythrocyte sedimentation rates and develop little induration with skin tests for delayed hypersensitivity because of the absence of fibrin deposition.

In 1947, fibrinogen was identified as a major component of cryoprecipitate, which is the preparation used most often in the United States for treating fibrinogen deficiency (Table 139-2). Fresh frozen plasma (FFP) can also be used, although a large volume is required to correct significant fibrinogen deficiency. In 2009, the U.S. Food and Drug Administration (FDA) granted approval for a human fibrinogen concentrate (RiaSTAP) for treating congenital fibrinogen deficiency. In a study of 15 patients given 70 mg/kg of the concentrate, the median plasma fibrinogen concentration 1 hour postinfusion was 130 mg/dL and the half-life of infused fibrinogen was 77.1 hours. Measurement of clot firmness, a surrogate for efficacy, indicated effective treatment in 14 of 15 patients. The results supported those of an earlier study showing that the concentrate was effective in congenital fibrinogen deficiency in 26 of 26 bleeding episodes, 10 of 11 surgeries, and all of 90 prophylactic administrations. The required dose of the fibrinogen concentrate can be determined using the following formula:

$$\text{Dose (mg/kg body weight)} = \frac{\begin{array}{c}(\text{Target level [mg/dL]}\\ - \text{Measured level [mg/dL]})\end{array}}{1.7\ (\text{kg body weight/dL})}$$

In patients with a normal hematocrit, the plasma volume is ≈40 mL (0.04 liters) per kg body mass. A unit of cryoprecipitate

Table 139-1 Properties of Plasma Coagulation Factors and Characteristics of Deficiency States

Protein	Factor Plasma Half-Life (hr)	Vitamin K Dependent Modification	Factor Level in Pregnancy	Incidence of Severe Congenital Deficiency	Autosomal Inheritance Pattern of Deficiency	Other Names for Deficiency State	Bleeding Diathesis in Severe Deficiency	Screening Tests in Deficiency: PT	Screening Tests in Deficiency: PTT
Fibrinogen	72-120	No	↑	≈1:1-2 × 10^6	Recessive or dominant	Afibrino-genemia	Severe	↑	↑
Prothrombin	60-100	Yes	↔	≈1:2 × 10^6	Recessive	Hypopro-thrombinemia	Severe	↑	↑
Factor V	12-14	No	↔	≈1:1 × 10^6	Recessive	Parahemophilia	Moderate to severe	↑	↑
Factor VII	3-4	Yes	↑	≈1:5 × 10^5	Recessive	Serum prothrombin conversion accelerator deficiency	Moderate to severe	↑	↔
Factor X	20-40	Yes	↑	≈1:1 × 10^6	Recessive	Stuart-Prower factor deficiency	Severe	↑ ↔	↑ ↔
Factor XI	45-52	No	Inconsistent	≈1:1 × 10^6	Recessive or dominant	Hemophilia C, plasma thromboplastin antecedent deficiency	Asymptomatic to moderate	↔	↑
Factor XII	60	No	↑	Unknown	Recessive	Hageman trait	Asymptomatic	↔	↑
Prekallikrein	Not known	No	↔	Unknown	Recessive	Fletcher trait	Asymptomatic	↔	↑
High-molecular-weight kininogen	170	No	↔	Unknown	Recessive	Flaujeac trait Williams trait Fitzgerald trait	Asymptomatic	↔	↑
Factor XIII	150	No	↓	1:2 × 10^6	Recessive	Fibrin stabilizing factor deficiency	Severe	↔	↔

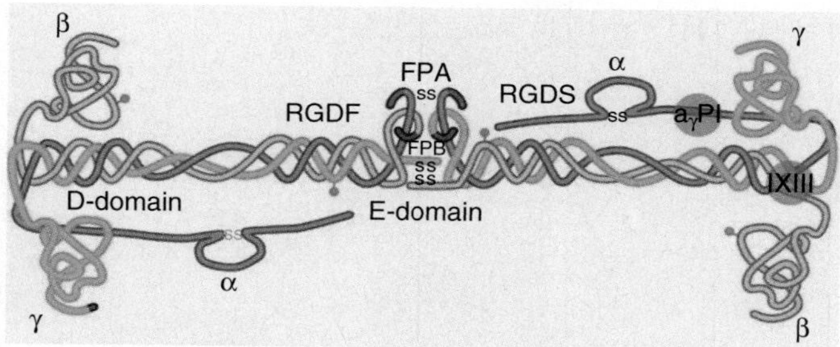

Figure 139-2 MODEL OF HUMAN FIBRINOGEN. A fibrinogen molecule consists of two trimers, each containing an Aα-chain *(blue),* a Bβ-chain *(pink),* and a γ-chain *(yellow).* The amino-termini of the six chains that compose the whole molecule are linked by disulfide bonds in the central E domain, and the C-termini of the polypeptides form two nodular D domains at opposite ends of the molecule. Fibrinopeptides A and B reside in the E domain and are removed by the proteolytic activity of thrombin during conversion of fibrinogen to fibrin monomer. *(Adapted from Mosesson MW: The roles of fibrinogen and fibrin in hemostasis and thrombosis.* Sem Hematol *29:177, 1992, with permission.)*

contains 300 mg of fibrinogen, and administering cryoprecipitate at 1 unit per 5 kg body mass will raise the fibrinogen level of an afibrinogenemic patient to ≈100 mg/dL.

For treatment of significant bleeding, the guidelines of the United Kingdom Haemophilia Centre Doctors Organization recommend that the plasma fibrinogen level be maintained at 100 mg/dL until hemostasis is achieved and above 50 mg/dL until wound healing is complete.[4] A similar strategy makes sense for managing surgical patients. A recent review of replacement therapy and outcomes for 50 patients with congenital fibrinogen deficiency generally agrees with these recommendations.[2] A fibrinogen concentration of 50 to 100 mg/dL was sufficient for prevention or treatment of bleeding in nonsurgical or obstetrical settings, whereas 100 to 200 mg/dL was effective for preventing bleeding during surgery. This review reported that thrombotic episodes (related or unrelated to replacement) occurred in 30% of patients.[2] The half-life of transfused fibrinogen is ≈3 days, and dosing every 2 to 4 days should be adequate to maintain levels in the absence of consumption. Increased dosing frequency may be necessary in cases of massive hemorrhage, major surgery or advanced pregnancy, and close monitoring of the fibrinogen level is recommended to facilitate dosing.

Prophylactic administration of fibrinogen at regular intervals is recommended to maintain pregnancies in afibrinogenemic women and to reduce postpartum hemorrhage.[2] Therapy should be initiated as early as possible, because fetal loss in the first trimester is common. One study suggested that initiating therapy before conception is beneficial.[2] Although some authors recommend keeping fibrinogen levels above 50 mg/dL during pregnancy and peripartum, others suggest a higher level (100 mg/dL) based on reports of fetal loss in patients with levels around 50 mg/dL. Long-term prophylaxis may also be useful in preventing initial bleeding in young patients or to prevent recurrence, particularly after central nervous system hemorrhage. Administration of fibrinogen every 7 to 14 days to maintain plasma levels around 50 mg/dL is recommended.[1]

Antifibrinolytic therapy with ε-amino caproic acid may be an effective replacement for blood products in the case of some mucosal bleeds and for dental extractions (see box on Adjuncts to Factor Replacement Therapy in Congenital Factor Deficiencies). However, this therapy is associated with an increased risk for thrombosis and must be used cautiously in patients with a history of thrombosis, as well as with pregnancy, surgery, or immobilization. Fibrin glue may be useful for tooth extraction, and estrogen/progesterone therapy may be helpful for controlling menorrhagia.

Table 139-2 Treatment Considerations for Rare Coagulation Factor Deficiencies

Protein	Blood Product Sources	Concentrate (Manufacturer)	Minimum Plasma Level Required for Hemostasis	Minimum Plasma Level Required for Surgery	Dose of Preferred Treatment For Surgery or Bleeding	Dosing Frequency for Surgery or Bleeding	Prophylaxis for Severe Deficiency	Pregnancy: Suggested Plasma Levels for Invasive Procedures and Delivery
Fibrinogen	CRYO FFP	RiaSTAP (CSL Behring)*	50 mg/dL	100 mg/dL	70 mg/kg[†]	Q 24-72 hr depending on consumption	Keep level 50 mg/dL for recurrent bleeders	Maintain at 100 mg/dL throughout pregnancy
Prothrombin	FFP	PCC*	≈5%	30%	20-30 factor IX units/kg	Q 48-72 hr	40 factor IX units/kg Q 5-6 days	20%-30%
Factor V	FFP* platelets	None	≈10%	25%	15-20 mL FFP/kg then 5-10 mL/kg q12 hr	Q 12-24 hr	Not usually required	15%-25%
Factor VII	FFP	NovoSeven* (recombinant factor VIIa, Novo Nordisk) PCC	5%-10%	15%-25%	15-30 mcg factor VIIa/kg	Q 2-6 hr	20-30 mcg/kg 2-3 times per wk	10%-20%
Factor X	FFP	PCC* Factor X concentrate (BioProducts Laboratory—Investigational)	≈10%	25%-40%	15-20 factor IX units/kg	Q 24 hr	15-20 factor X units/kg Q weekly	10%-20%
Factor XI	FFP	Hemoleven* (LFB Biomedicaments); Factor XI concentrate (BioProducts Laboratory)	15%	30%-40%	15-20 factor XI units/kg	Q 1-2 days	Not required	May withhold treatment unless bleeding. 20%-40% if bleeding occurs
Factor XIII	CRYO FFP	Corifact* (Formerly Fibrogammin P, CSL Behring) Recombinant Factor XIII (Novo Nordisk—Investigational)	1%-2%	20%-50%	20-30 factor XIII units/kg	Single dose may be sufficient	40 factor XIII units/kg Q 28 days	250 units/wk through wk 22, then 500 units/wk with a 1000 unit bolus during labor

FFP, Fresh frozen plasma; *CRYO*, cryoprecipitate; *PCC*, prothrombin complex concentrate.
*Preferred treatment for congenital deficiency.
[†]Assuming baseline fibrinogen is not known.

Adjuncts to Factor Replacement Therapy in Congenital Factor Deficiencies

The antifibrinolytic agents ε-amino caproic acid and tranexamic acid can be effective adjuncts to factor replacement when treating congenital or acquired bleeding disorders and may be useful alternatives to replacement therapy for mild bleeding or minor procedures. These drugs inhibit clot dissolution by blocking plasminogen activation and plasmin activity and are particularly valuable when bleeding involves tissues with high fibrinolytic activity such as the oral cavity. They are also useful for treating menorrhagia, limiting blood loss with surgery, controlling epistaxis, and reducing some types of gastrointestinal bleeding. A typical loading dose of ε-amino caproic acid is 50 to 100 mg/kg followed by 2 to 4 grams every 6 hours. If bleeding subsequently occurs, the dose can be increased to a maximum of 24 grams in 24 hours. ε-Amino caproic acid is available in oral and intravenous formulations. Identical dosing may be used for either preparation because of excellent bioavailability. For dental extraction in factor VIII or IX deficiency, many centers use a single 50% to 100% loading dose of clotting factor concentrate followed by seven days of ε-amino caproic acid as the sole prophylaxis, and it is reasonable to extrapolate this approach to patients with some of the rare bleeding disorders. Patients with factor XI deficiency do well with antifibrinolytic agents alone for tooth extractions. Dental procedures such as scaling or root canal can be performed safely using ε-amino caproic acid or tranexamic acid mouthwash prepared from the intravenous formulation three to four times daily with or without systemic antifibrinolytic therapy.

Prolonged therapy with antifibrinolytic agents must be undertaken with caution in patients who are not mobile, who have a history of thromboembolic events, or who have significant urogenital bleeding. These drugs interfere with urokinase-mediated fibrinolytic activity in the genitourinary tract and can cause renal outflow obstruction by thrombotic occlusion of the ureters. Concomitant use of antifibrinolytic agents with activated prothrombin complex concentrates or recombinant factor VIIa may result in a particularly high risk for thrombus formation. Patients may develop nausea or vertigo with high doses of ε-amino caproic doses, and rarely, rhabdomyolysis.

Hemorrhage may be controlled or prevented in rare bleeding disorders with recombinant factor VIIa. The mechanism by which this agent works is not completely understood in all situations, particularly for deficiencies of factors in the common pathway (prothrombin and factors V and X). For patients with rare bleeding disorders and an immunoglobulin inhibitor directed against the missing factor, factor VIIa may be the treatment of choice. Doses range from 15 to 120 mcg/kg every 2 to 6 hours depending upon the severity of bleeding. In factor XI–deficient patients without inhibitors, doses of 15 to 30 mcg/kg every 2 to 4 hours are often sufficient. A dose of 90 mcg/kg every 2 to 3 hours has been used in patients with congenital factor V deficiency or combined deficiencies of factors V and VIII, patients with acquired factor X deficiency associated with amyloidosis, and patients with antibody-mediated acquired prothrombin deficiency associated with lupus anticoagulants. An attractive aspect of using factor VIIa in place of FFP is the smaller volume of material infused. Factor VIIa is also associated with a lower risk for reactions associated with plasma infusions such as fever, urticaria, transfusion-related acute lung injury (TRALI), and anaphylaxis. Caution must be exercised when using factor VIIa in older patients with cardiovascular disease, because arterial thrombosis can result, particularly when therapy is combined with fibrinolytic inhibitors or prothrombin complex concentrate.

DYSFIBRINOGENEMIA (OMIM 134820 Aα-CHAIN, 134830 Bβ-CHAIN, AND 134850 γ-CHAIN)

In dysfibrinogenemia, structural variants of fibrinogen circulate in plasma. Cases in which the dysfunctional protein is present at low levels may be referred to as *hypodysfibrinogenemia*. The first family with dysfibrinogenemia (15 amino acid insertion after Gln350 in the γ-chain [fibrinogen Paris I]) was described in 1964. The actual incidence of congenital dysfibrinognemia is not known, because the majority of patients are probably asymptomatic and do not come to medical attention.

Congenital dysfibrinogenemias are almost all autosomal dominant conditions caused by a missense mutation in one of the fibrinogen genes, although some insertions and deletions have been identified (www.geht.or/databaseand/fibrinogen). Amino acid substitutions that alter fibrinopeptide release, fibrin cross-linking, fibrin polymerization, or fibrin degradation have been reported. The diagnosis of dysfibrinogenemia is established by identification of a low fibrinogen activity in a rate-based clotting assay relative to immunoreactive fibrinogen. The types of functional defects most often reported, therefore, are undoubtedly influenced by the assays available in clinical laboratories and are unlikely to represent the full spectrum of mutations that can cause fibrinogen dysfunction. Variants readily detected by the assays used in clinical laboratories typically have defects in fibrinopeptide release (e.g., FGA-Arg16His and FGA-Arg16Cys [fibrinogens Bicêtre and Metz]), or polymerize slowly (e.g., FGG-Ser434Asn [fibrinogen Caracas II], FGG-Arg275Cys and FGG-Arg275His). Indeed, ≈45% of the mutations associated with dysfibrinogenemia in the database involve substitutions at FGA-Arg16 or FGG-Arg275, at least partly reflecting the ease with which these variants can be detected with commonly used functional assays.

Most patients with dysfibrinogenemia (55% to 60%) are asymptomatic, and the condition is identified by an abnormal result on a coagulation screening assay. Excessive bleeding occurs in ≈25%, whereas 20% have thrombotic episodes. The correlation between functional abnormalities and symptoms is often weak. For example, the common FGA-Arg16His and FGA-Arg16Cys variants have been reported in asymptomatic individuals as well as patients with bleeding or thrombosis. Epistaxis, easy bruising, and menorrhagia are relatively common in those with symptoms. Although bleeding is often mild, soft tissue hematomas, hemarthroses, postoperative hemorrhage, and bleeding during pregnancy and peripartum may occur. Abnormal wound healing and spontaneous abortions have been reported. Thrombotic events primarily involve the venous circulation, although some arterial events have been reported. About one quarter of patients with thrombotic symptoms also experience excessive bleeding.

In 1995, a subcommittee of the International Society on Thrombosis and Haemostasis determined that a significant relationship exists between certain fibrinogen variants and venous thrombosis. However, in a review of 2376 patients with venous thrombosis, dysfibrinogenemia was found in less than 1%, so testing for dysfibrinogenemia is not widely recommended in this setting. Mutations associated with thrombosis tend to cluster at the C-terminus of the Aα-chain and near the thrombin cleavage site on the Bβ chain. Abnormalities in fibrin polymerization, cross-linking, clot structure, and susceptibility to fibrinolysis have been described. The "Dusart syndrome" caused by FGA-Arg554Cys (fibrinogen Paris V) has been associated with venous thrombosis and sudden death in teenagers and young adults in several families. Recently, dysfibrinogenemia was reported in 5 of 33 patients with chronic thromboembolic pulmonary hypertension.[5] The FGB-Pro235Leu mutation was found in three unrelated patients in this study. Dysfibrinogenemias were associated with altered fibrin polymer structure and/or susceptibility to lysis, suggesting that the involved fibrinogen variants predispose to incomplete clot dissolution.

A group of mutations in the C-terminus of the fibrinogen Aα-chain is associated with autosomal dominant hereditary amyloidosis. The amyloid deposits contain fragments of the variant fibrinogen.

The kidneys are initially affected, but wider visceral and nerve involvement may occur. Renal grafts subsequently become involved with amyloid, and liver transplantation may be a better treatment option. The allele for one responsible mutation, FGA-Glu526Val, is relatively common and may account for 5% of patients with apparent sporadic amyloid.

Acquired dysfibrinogenemia is most frequently diagnosed in severe liver disease, with 80% to 90% of patients with cirrhosis or liver failure showing some degree of fibrinogen dysfunction. Increased sialic acid content is likely responsible for impaired fibrin polymerization. Despite abnormalities in coagulation assays, the process probably does not contribute substantially to abnormal hemostasis. Homocysteine-induced modifications of fibrinogen have been proposed to contribute to the hypercoagulable state associated with elevated plasma levels of homocysteine. The monoclonal antibody in patients with multiple myeloma can interfere nonspecifically with fibrin polymerization but usually does not cause abnormal hemostasis. Acquired dysfibrinogenemia has been associated with other malignancies and bone marrow transplantation.

Most cases of dysfibrinogenemia present as abnormalities on routine coagulation tests such as the PT and PTT. The thrombin time is often used as a primary screening test for dysfibrinogenemia, although its sensitivity is not established. The test involves measuring the time to clot formation in citrated plasma after addition of a standard amount of thrombin. The specificity of the test is relatively poor; heparin, elevated fibrin degradation products, paraproteins, and low levels of fibrinogen all may affect results. The reptilase time has been used as an alternative screen for dysfibrinogenemia and is useful in combination with the thrombin time. The assay involves inducing clot formation with an enzyme from the venom of *Bothrops jararaca* or *Bothrops atrox* that cleaves fibrinopeptide A (but not fibrinopeptide B) from fibrinogen and is not sensitive to heparin. The apparent plasma concentration of clottable fibrinogen as determined by the von Clauss method (see section on Fibrinogen Deficiency) may be low in some types of dysfibrinogenemia. Levels of immunoreactive fibrinogen are usually normal, but they are decreased in cases of hypodysfibrinogenemia. With some variants, serum fibrin degradation products may appear to be elevated using certain assays because the variant fibrinogen is incompletely incorporated into the clot. This can lead to the false impression that DIC is present.

Most dysfibrinogenemic patients are asymptomatic, and symptoms correlate poorly with coagulation assay abnormalities, making it difficult to generalize regarding therapeutic recommendations. The patient's personal and family histories are useful for guiding therapy. Active bleeding can be treated with replacement therapy, as in afibrinogenemia, and such treatment may be indicated in some patients before invasive procedures. In general, patients with thrombosis and dysfibrinogenemia should be treated similarly to other patients with hypercoagulable conditions. There are no data on which to formulate recommendations as to duration of therapy; thus past history, family history, coexisting conditions, and the nature (idiopathic, pregnancy-related or postsurgery-related) and seriousness of the thrombosis must all be taken into consideration. As with any thrombotic event, the risk for bleeding associated with prolonged therapy must be considered. Recurrent spontaneous abortions have been associated with dysfibrinogenemia in several families, and some pregnancies have been carried to term using replacement therapy with cryoprecipitate.

PROTHROMBIN DEFICIENCY (OMIM 176930)

More than a century ago, Morawitz proposed that an insoluble fibrin clot is formed from fibrinogen through the activity of fibrin ferment or thrombin. Thrombin was generated from a precursor, prothrombin, by thrombokinase (probably factor Xa). Prothrombin and thrombin are designated *factors II* and *IIa*. Total prothrombin deficiency is probably not compatible with life, because complete absence of the protein has not been observed in humans and prothrombin-deficient mice succumb to bleeding in utero or shortly after birth. Severe congenital deficiency associated with reduced plasma prothrombin antigen (hypoprothrombinemia) or circulating dysfunctional prothrombin (dysprothrombinemia) affects an estimated 1 in 2 million people (see Table 139-1). Prothrombin deficiency is the third most common coagulation factor disorder in Puerto Rico (carrier frequency ≈1 in 700), accounting for 6% of non–von Willebrand disease congenital bleeding disorders at the University of Puerto Rico Hemophilia Center. In the North American Rare Bleeding Disorder Registry, 62% of patients with prothrombin deficiency were Latino, possibly reflecting the prevalence of the Arg457Gln variant prothrombin Puerto Rico I.

Prothrombin is a 72,000-Dalton protein that is converted to thrombin by factor Xa in complex with factor Va on phospholipid surfaces (see Fig. 139-1, *A*). Thrombin is a pivotal protease in hemostasis, with multiple procoagulant activities including cleavage of fibrinopeptides A and B from fibrinogen to form fibrin (see Fig. 139-2), activation of factors V, VIII, XI, and XIII, and cleavage of protease activated receptors on a variety of cells including platelets.[6] Thrombin forms a complex with thrombomodulin on endothelial cells to downregulate fibrinolysis by activating thrombin-activatable fibrinolysis inhibitor (TAFI) and to downregulate coagulation by activating protein C. Thrombin also has cytokine and growth factor–like properties.

Prothrombin deficiency is an autosomal recessive disorder manifested as hypoprothrombinemia (reduced activity and antigen; cross-reactive material–negative [CRM−] deficiency), dysprothrombinemia (activity reduced relative to antigen; cross-reactive material–positive [CRM+] deficiency) or a combination of both. Plasma prothrombin activity is typically 1% to 10% of normal in hypoprothrombinemia and 1% to 20% in dysprothrombinemia. Heterozygotes for either condition have 40% to 60% normal activity. More than 50 prothrombin gene mutations have been described (www.isth.org/default/index.cfm; www.hgmd.org) in patients with prothrombin deficiency, with ≈80% being missense mutations.[6] In dysprothrombinemia, missense mutations typically cause defects in prothrombin conversion to thrombin (e.g., prothrombin Arg457Gln [Puerto Rico I] and Arg271Cys [Madrid]), or result in functionally defective thrombin (e.g., prothrombin Arg418Trp [Tokushima]).

Prothrombin deficiency can be inherited in combination with deficiencies of other vitamin K–dependent proteins (see Combined Deficiency of Vitamin K–Dependent Proteins). Acquired prothrombin deficiency occurs with warfarin therapy, as well as in cases of poisoning with rodenticides such as brodifacoum, vitamin K deficiency, liver disease, and DIC. Cephalosporins, particularly those with N-methyl-thiotetrazole side chains, can decrease prothrombin levels. Antiprothrombin antibodies are common phospholipid-dependent antibodies found in patients with the lupus anticoagulant or the antiphospholipid antibody syndrome. More rarely, patients with a lupus anticoagulant or systemic lupus erythematosus have antibodies that enhance prothrombin clearance, causing true deficiency. No reports exist of neutralizing antibodies forming after replacement therapy in congenital prothrombin deficiency, consistent with severely affected patients having at least a trace of circulating prothrombin.

Severe hypoprothrombinemia is inevitably associated with bleeding that may be life threatening, although the correlation between plasma prothrombin activity and clinical severity is not particularly strong. Central nervous system hemorrhage was reported in 8% to 12% of patients, and in 20% of those with prothrombin levels below 1% of normal activity.[6] Soft tissue hematomas, bruising (60%), and hemarthroses (42%) are common. The bleeding diathesis can present at circumcision in neonates or as easy bruising, epistaxis, menorrhagia, or gastrointestinal hemorrhage, as well as with trauma or surgery. Heterozygotes occasionally have excessive bleeding with surgery or tooth extraction, but most are asymptomatic. Bleeding tends to be less severe in dysprothrombinemia, and some variants are particularly mild. For example, homozygosity for Arg67His causes severe reduction in plasma prothrombin activity (<20% of normal) but results in relatively few symptoms.

In the PT and PTT assays, prothrombin is converted to thrombin by factor Xa in complex with factor Va on phospholipids surfaces (see

Fig. 139-1, *B*), and severe prothrombin deficiency will prolong both test results. Some PT and PTT reagents are relatively insensitive to reductions in prothrombin, and mild deficiencies may be missed. The diagnosis is confirmed, and the degree of deficiency established, by a modified PT assay using prothrombin-deficient plasma. Prothrombin deficiency must be distinguished from deficiencies of fibrinogen, factor V, or factor X, which are also associated with a prolonged PT and PTT.

Prothrombin complex concentrate (PCC), approved for use in factor IX deficiency, contains varying amounts of prothrombin and factors VII and X (see Table 139-2) and is the preferred product for treating prothrombin deficiency. PCC is derived from human plasma and undergoes viral inactivation. The prothrombin activity in a typical PCC is usually comparable to, or higher than, factor IX activity. Hemostatic levels of prothrombin are estimated to be 20% to 40% of normal for major surgery or trauma, but 10% to 15% may be adequate for milder hemostatic challenges. A dose of 20 to 30 factor IX units/kg of PCC usually produces plasma prothrombin levels of 20% to 30% of normal. The half-life of prothrombin is about 3 days, and dosing every 2 to 3 days can maintain adequate levels until healing is complete. Alternatively, one-fourth of the loading dose each day should keep the level therapeutic. Prophylactic infusion of PCC every 5 to 6 days prevented spontaneous bleeding in one severely deficient patient. PCC administration has been associated with thrombosis, although a recent meta-analysis of studies using PCC preparations to reverse the anticoagulant effect of warfarin suggests the risk is relatively low (<2%).[7] It seems reasonable to maintain the factor VII, IX, and X levels at <150% of normal to reduce risk. Dental procedures or minor hemorrhage may respond to antifibrinolytic therapy with ε-amino caproic acid. Prothrombin deficiency may also be treated with FFP for bleeding episodes or surgical intervention (15 to 20 mL/kg loading dose followed by 3 mL/kg/day). Because of the long half-life, additional doses may not be required in all situations. Cryoprecipitate is not a source of prothrombin, and plasma prothrombin levels do not increase after infusion or inhalation of desmopressin (1-desamino-8-D-arginine vasopressin [DDAVP]).

Treatment of acquired prothrombin deficiency associated with lupus anticoagulants requires immunosuppression, most commonly with steroids. This is effective in most patients, although many relapse during weaning or after stopping treatment. Subsequent treatment with azathioprine or cyclophosphamide has successfully eradicated the antibody. Rituximab has also been reported to be effective, and we have observed this in our own practice. In a rare case of quinidine-induced lupus anticoagulant with concomitant antiprothrombin antibody, cessation of the drug led to spontaneous resolution of acquired prothrombin deficiency, but not the lupus anticoagulant. The low prothrombin activity in these patients may protect them from thrombosis, as reports of thrombosis after successful eradication of the antiprothrombin antibody suggest.

FACTOR V DEFICIENCY (OMIM 227400)

In 1943, Quick reported that aged plasma clotted more slowly than fresh plasma in a prothrombin time assay and proposed that a labile factor distinct from prothrombin was required for normal coagulation. At the same time, Owren noted that a patient with a lifelong bleeding problem lacked a factor normally found in plasma that, in contrast to prothrombin, did not adsorb onto aluminum hydroxide. Owren's patient was deficient in the labile factor described by Quick, which is now called factor V. Severe congenital factor V deficiency has been estimated to occur in 1 in 1 million persons (see Table 139-1).

Factor V is the 330,000-Dalton precursor of the cofactor factor Va, which facilitates prothrombin activation by factor Xa on phospholipid surfaces (Fig. 139-1, *A*). Severe factor V deficiency is an autosomal recessive trait with plasma factor V activity of 1% to 10% of normal.[8-10] More than 100 factor V gene mutations associated with factor V deficiency have been described (www.isth.org/default/index.cfm; www.hgmd.org). Nonsense and frameshift mutations are distributed throughout the gene, whereas missense mutations cluster in the A2 and C2 domains. Missense mutations usually result in abnormal polypeptides that are degraded within the cell, resulting in low plasma factor V antigen (CRM deficiency). The only well characterized CRM+ mutation is factor V New Brunswick [Ala221Val], which interferes with factor Va stability. Most (80%) of the factor V in blood is in plasma, with the remainder stored in a partially activated form in platelet α-granules. In humans, platelet factor V is primarily of plasma origin. After being taken up from the plasma, factor V is modified by platelets so that it is more procoagulant than plasma factor V. Some patients with very low plasma factor V levels and mild bleeding symptoms have sufficient platelet factor V to maintain thrombin generation. This implies that factor V is unstable in plasma but can still be taken up and stored by platelets. Patients with more severe bleeding symptoms may lack both plasma and platelet factor V activity.

Factor V deficiency can be inherited by mechanisms unrelated to mutations in the factor V gene. Combined factor V and factor VIII deficiency is caused by mutations in proteins required for secretion of both factors (discussed in Combined Factor V and Factor VIII Deficiency).[9,10] A few patients have been identified with abnormalities specific to platelet factor V. The Quebec platelet disorder is an autosomal dominant bleeding condition with low platelet factor V levels and normal plasma factor V. Proteolytic degradation of multiple α-granule proteins in this syndrome is due to overexpression of urokinase-type plasminogen activator. Platelet factor V activity is also reduced in Factor V New York, but the underlying mechanism is not known.

Acquired antibodies to factor V may present in a variety of ways ranging from asymptomatic laboratory abnormalities to life-threatening hemorrhage. Alloantibodies to factor V were often associated with exposure to topical bovine thrombin during surgery. These preparations contained bovine factor V, and the resulting antibodies cross-reacted with human factor V. This problem rarely occurs now because recombinant thrombin preparations are used instead of the bovine material. Alloantibodies to factor V also occur in some factor V–deficient patients exposed to human plasma. Factor V autoantibodies may develop after surgery or blood transfusions or with cancer, autoimmune disorders, or therapy with β-lactam or aminoglycoside antibiotics. Acquired factor V deficiency may occur with liver disease, DIC, and systemic amyloidosis.

There is considerable variation in bleeding among patients with severe factor V deficiency (1% to 10% of normal levels).[8-10] Although significant bleeding does occur, the frequency tends to be less than in cases of severe factor VIII or factor IX deficiency. Variability may be related partly to the amount of factor V associated with platelets. Mucosal bleeding is the primary abnormality, with 60% of patients experiencing epistaxis, menorrhagia, or oral bleeding. Hematomas and hemarthroses occur in 25% of patients, but debilitating arthropathy is uncommon. Severe bleeding in the central nervous system or gastrointestinal tract has been reported, but this is relatively rare. Postpartum hemorrhage is common. Trauma, surgery, and dental extraction are associated with a high risk for bleeding in untreated patients. Bleeding with surgery involving the urogenital tract, the nose, or the mouth may be particularly problematic because of high local fibrinolytic activity. Mild (heterozygous) factor V deficiency (25% to 60% of normal factor level) is usually not associated with excessive bleeding, although ≈10% of patients report some bleeding.

Thrombosis has been reported in factor V–deficient patients. In some cases, the deficiency may simply have not been sufficient to prevent thrombosis. Indeed, with the exception of deficiency of prothrombin or factor X, thrombotic events have been reported in all severe coagulation factor deficiency states. However, the situation with factor V is more complex. Deficiency can occur in patients with the common procoagulant factor V polymorphism Arg506Gln (factor V Leiden). If Arg506Gln and a mutation causing deficiency occur on opposite alleles (in-trans), most of the factor V in the blood will have the Gln506 substitution, which will significantly increase the risk for thrombosis (pseudohomozygous activated protein C resistance). Alternatively, Arg506Gln may occur on the same allele as a null mutation (in-cis), which will mask the prothrombotic effect of Arg506Gln. Such patients may have a bleeding tendency.

Factor V is required for normal prothrombin activation by factor Xa in the prothrombinase complex (see Fig. 139-1, *B*), and factor V deficiency causes prolongation of both the PT and PTT. The diagnosis and severity are established using a modified PT assay with factor V–deficient plasma. In some cases of severe deficiency, the template bleeding time is prolonged. Patients with factor V deficiency should be tested for factor VIII deficiency so that combined deficiency is not missed. Factor V inhibitors cause prolongations of the PT and PTT that do not correct on mixing with normal plasma. Like the situation with factor VIII inhibitors, factor V inhibitor titers are established using the Bethesda method. However, unlike the more common inhibitors to factor VIII, which typically take 1 to 2 hours of incubation to fully inactivate their target, factor V inhibitors inhibit factor V almost immediately. The thrombin time should be normal, except in cases of inhibition induced by bovine topical thrombin, where antithrombin antibodies against thrombin are also present.

No factor V concentrate is commercially available with which to treat deficient patients (see Table 139-2). Administration of FFP is recommended for serious bleeding or in preparation for surgery. The minimum factor V level for hemostasis is estimated to be ≈15%.[8] In a patient with less than 1% plasma factor V, this can be achieved by administering 15 to 20 mL/kg FFP, followed by 5 mL/kg every 12 hours. A plasma level of at least 25% is recommended for major surgery. Estimates of the factor V plasma half-life vary widely, but 12 to 14 hours can be assumed for replacement purposes. Infusion of 20 mL/kg FFP (over 3 to 4 hours) before surgery, followed by 5 to 10 mL/kg every 12 hours thereafter is usually adequate. Infusions should be continued for 7 to 10 days to establish wound healing. Care must be taken to avoid fluid overload from large volumes of FFP, particularly in older patients. Plasma exchange has been successful in a few factor V–deficient patients requiring surgery. Mucosal bleeding from the nose and mouth may respond to ε-amino caproic acid, and superficial lacerations often respond to local pressure. Although the defect caused by factor V deficiency would hypothetically render therapy with recombinant factor VIIa ineffective, this agent has been used successfully in a patient with severe factor V deficiency requiring surgery.

Menorrrhagia is common in a factor V–deficient women. Symptoms may be managed by antifibrinolytic therapy (ε-amino caproic acid 50 to 60 mg/kg every 4 to 6 hours or tranexamic acid 15 mg/kg every 6 to 8 hours), oral contraceptives, levonorgesterol intrauterine devices, replacement therapy, or surgical intervention (endometrial ablation or hysterectomy). Replacement should be adjusted to maintain a factor V level of ≈15% of normal. Factor V–deficient women may have significant bleeding with childbirth and should be treated in a similar manner.

Platelets are a source of factor V and may be particularly useful in patients with severe bleeding or factor V inhibitors. Platelet factor V may either be protected from inhibition or may be sufficiently different in structure from its plasma counterpart to not cross-react with antibodies directed at factor V. However, platelet transfusions are not recommended as routine first-line treatment for factor V deficiency because of the possibility of developing antiplatelet alloantibodies. Cryoprecipitate is not a source of factor V, and plasma levels do not respond to administration of DDAVP.

FACTOR VII DEFICIENCY (OMIM 227500)

Factor VII deficiency was first reported by Alexander and colleagues in 1951. Severe factor VII deficiency is the most common of the nonhemophilic coagulation factor deficiencies (see Table 139-1), with an estimated prevalence of 1 in 500,000 persons.[11-13]

Factor VII is the 50,000-Dalton precursor of the protease factor VIIa. Factor VII/VIIa binds to tissue factor to initiate coagulation through activation of factors X and IX (see Fig. 139-1, *A*). A cut-off value for severe factor VII deficiency has not been firmly established, but a value of less than 2% of normal has been proposed. A severity classification system based on clinical presentation has also been suggested.[11] Mice lacking factor VII develop normally in utero but succumb to bleeding at birth. An infant born with complete absence of factor VII died from intracranial hemorrhage 12 days after birth, whereas another survived with replacement therapy. Thus low levels of factor VII activity appear to be necessary to sustain life. Although factor VII deficiency is usually considered an autosomal recessive trait, the fact that bleeding symptoms occur in up to 36% of patients with heterozygous deficiency raises questions about this concept.[13]

More than 250 factor VII gene mutations associated with factor VII deficiency have been described (www.isth.org/default/index.cfm), two-thirds of which are missense mutations. Although most have been identified in single families, some are more widespread. In surveys of patients from Europe and Latin America, Ala244Val accounted for 84% of abnormal factor VII alleles in 88 unrelated Jewish patients and in 14% and 7% of abnormal factor VII alleles in Germany and France, respectively.[13] CRM+ variants are common. Some factor VII variants demonstrate variable activity in the PT assay, depending on the species of origin of the tissue factor in the thromboplastin reagent employed. The name "factor VII Padua" has been applied to these variants, and a number of cases are associated with a missense mutation (Arg304Gln) that causes a major defect in the interaction with rabbit tissue factor but not with human or ox tissue factor.

Factor VII deficiency may occur in combination with deficiencies of other vitamin K–dependent proteins (discussed in Combined Deficiency of Vitamin K–Dependent Proteins) and in combination with factor X deficiency as a result of loss of both genes due to a chromosome 13 q34 deletion. Factor VII deficiency has also been reported in cases of trisomy 8 and in conjunction with abnormalities of bilirubin metabolism, mental retardation, microcephaly, epicanthus, cleft palate, and patent ductus arteriosus.

Reduced levels of factor VII occur with warfarin therapy, liver disease, DIC, biliary tract disease, vitamin K deficiency, and cephalosporin therapy. In these situations other vitamin K–dependent factors are usually decreased, although the effect on factor VII is often the greatest because of its shorter half-life. Alloantibody inhibitors to factor VII have been reported in deficient patients after replacement therapy.[14] Acquired factor VII deficiency has been reported as a paraneoplastic syndrome with atrial myxoma and Wilms tumor. Other scenarios rarely associated with low factor VII include hematopoietic stem cell transplantation, aplastic anemia, and sepsis.

The clinical spectrum of bleeding in factor VII deficiency is broad. Not surprisingly, significant bleeding tends to be greatest with severe deficiency, and patients with levels less than 1% of normal may have a syndrome similar to severe hemophilia, with spontaneous joint and soft tissue bleeding and hemarthrosis-related arthropathy.[11-13] Of interest, a comparison of bleeding in factor VII and factor IX deficiency indicated that lower levels of factor VII sustain hemostasis better than comparable levels of factor IX. Central nervous system hemorrhage is relatively common (4% to 17%).[12,15] Patients with factor VII activity of ≥5% of normal tend to have milder symptoms such as epistaxis, menorrhagia, and bruising. Although little bleeding occurs in most patients with factor VII levels 10% to 15% of normal, some describe significant bleeding, either spontaneously or in response to hemostatic challenges. In one study, 36% of heterozygotes (factor VII activity 21% to 69%) reported bleeding problems, mostly involving skin and mucous membranes, whereas another study reported a greater risk for subcutaneous bleeding in heterozygotes. Excessive bleeding often complicates dental extraction and surgery on the oropharynx or urogenital tract in untreated patients. Abdominal surgery and hysterectomy are associated with fewer problems, likely reflecting varying levels of fibrinolytic activity in different tissues. Postpartum bleeding is not common in factor VII–deficient women because factor VII levels rise in late pregnancy in all but the most severely deficient patients. The need for prophylaxis to prevent bleeding correlates best with baseline factor VII levels less than 10% to 15% of normal.

Thrombosis associated with factor VII deficiency has been well documented. A study of 33 reported cases (6 arterial, 27 venous) revealed 15 with molecular studies. Nearly all patients had other thrombotic risk factors, usually acquired, and four had congenital thrombophilia. Of the 15 patients, 11 had either Arg304Gln (Factor VII Padua) or Ala294Val. Those with factor VII Padua had no bleeding history, whereas mild bleeding was reported with Ala294Val. Treatment of thrombosis with vitamin K antagonists is problematic in these cases because the baseline PT is abnormal as a result of the mutation. Therapy with low-molecular-weight heparin or one of the newer direct thrombin or factor Xa inhibitors may be a better option.

In the PT, factor VII/VIIa binds tissue factor supplied by the thromboplastin reagent. The factor VIIa/tissue factor complex then activates factor X (see Fig. 139-1, *B*). In factor VII deficiency, the PT is prolonged and the PTT is normal. The diagnosis is confirmed, and the severity determined, by a modified PT assay using factor VII–deficient plasma. With very sensitive thromboplastin reagents, the PT may be prolonged with factor VII levels at the lower end of the normal range. When assessing patients for factor VII deficiency, the source of the tissue factor must be considered, because some factor VII variants bind poorly to tissue factor from certain species. Factor VII Padua–type variants interact poorly with the rabbit tissue factor–based reagents widely used in North America; they function better with human tissue factor and best with ox tissue factor. We routinely retest patients with apparent factor VII deficiency in rabbit tissue factor-based assays with a human tissue factor thromboplastin reagent to detect Padua-type variants.

Major considerations when treating factor VII–deficient patients include the short plasma half-life of the protein (3 to 4 hours), relatively low recovery of infused material (possibly due to a large volume of distribution), and rapid clearance in children. A plasma factor VII level of 10% to 15% of normal is probably the minimum required for surgery, with 15% to 25% being adequate in most cases. Of 157 surgeries performed on 83 factor VII–deficient patients with a mean baseline activity of 5% who did not receive prophylaxis, 15.3% had bleeding complications.[16] The data suggest that supplementing patients with baseline levels below 10% should reliably exclude hemorrhage. Factor replacement can be accomplished with several products (see Table 139-2). FFP is widely used, but its effectiveness is limited because of the large volumes that must be administered. PCC contains variable amounts of factor VII. However, these products are not favored, because they contain other vitamin K–dependent factors in higher concentrations than factor VII, which could increase the risk for thrombosis. Recombinant factor VIIa is considered the optimal therapy for treating or preventing bleeding in factor VII deficiency. A dose of 15 to 30 mcg/kg body weight every 2 to 6 hours will usually achieve hemostasis, with the frequency adjusted to the clinical situation.[11,12] Hemarthroses often respond to single infusions. Prophylaxis for invasive procedures may require treatment every 2 to 3 hours. In a study of 41 surgeries in 34 factor VII–deficient subjects receiving factor VIIa, bleeding occurred in only three instances, and in those, the factor VIIa dose was considered low. Adequate replacement to prevent bleeding was determined to be at least 13 mcg/kg body weight per dose and no less than three doses administered on the day of surgery. Administration of factor VIIa by continuous infusion has been used successfully to cover surgical procedure and may reduce the total amount of drug administered by 70% to 90% compared with bolus infusions.

Patients with severe factor VII deficiency may benefit from secondary prophylaxis to prevent further life-threatening bleeding, particularly bleeding in the central nervous system, which is associated with a mortality rate of 50% to 70%. Although, several replacement products have been used in this situation, recombinant factor VIIa is the preferred agent. Despite its short half-life, factor VIIa can be effective at doses of 20 to 30 mcg/kg given 2 to 3 times per week.[17] Three cases of inhibitor formation have been reported. Not all bleeding episodes in factor VII–deficient patients require replacement therapy. Minor injuries may be controlled with local measures. Fibrinolytic inhibitors, such as ε-amino caproic acid, may be effective for minor bleeding, dental surgery, or other procedures involving mucous membranes. Fibrin glue may also be effective in some situations. Cryoprecipitate is not a source of factor VII, and plasma levels do not respond to administration of DDAVP.

FACTOR X DEFICIENCY (OMIM 227600)

Factor X deficiency was first described in two patients more than 50 years ago. The missing plasma factor was initially called *Stuart-Prower factor* after the two index cases and was subsequently designated *factor X*. Patient Stuart was originally thought to have factor VII deficiency, but mixing his plasma with factor VII–deficient plasma corrected the abnormal clotting assay results. Patient Prower had multiple coagulation assay abnormalities, including a prolonged thromboplastin generation test and PT. The prevalence of symptomatic factor X deficiency is thought to be about 1 in 1 million persons (Table 139-1).

Factor X is a 58,000-Dalton protein that is the precursor of the protease factor Xa. Factor X may be activated by the factor VIIa/tissue factor complex or by the factor IXa/factor VIIIa complex (see Fig. 139-1, *A*). Factor Xa converts prothrombin to thrombin in the presence of factor Va and phospholipid and calcium ions; it also catalyzes the conversion of factor V to factor Va.

Congenital factor X deficiency is an autosomal recessive trait. Factor X–deficient mice die in utero or shortly after birth from hemorrhage, indicating the protein is necessary for viability. Humans with severe factor X deficiency (<1% of normal) probably have at least a trace of factor X in plasma. Most of the more than 100 known factor X gene mutations (representing more than 60 families) identified in factor X–deficient patients are missense mutations (www.isth.org/default/index.cfm; www.hgmd.org). Many are CRM+ variants. A classification system based on clotting, chromogenic, and immunologic assays has been proposed. Type I deficiency includes CRM– mutations, including patient Stuart (homozygous for Val298Met). Type II deficiency includes CRM+ variants lacking activity and includes patient Prower (compound heterozygote for Arg287Trp and Asp282Asn). Type III deficiency is composed of mutations that affect specific aspects of factor X/Xa function. Within type III deficiency are variants that are activated by Russell Viper venom but are defective in activation by factor VIIa/tissue factor or factor IXa/VIIIa (e.g., Factor X Friuli [Pro343Ser]), variants defective only in activation by factor VIIa/tissue factor (e.g., Factor X Padua [Arg251Trp] or Vorarlberg [Gla14Lys and Glu102Lys in the same factor X gene]), variants defective only in activation by factor IXa/VIIIa (factor X Melbourne and factor X Roma [Thr358Met]), and variants with higher activity in chromogenic assays than clotting assays. Factor X deficiency can be inherited with deficiencies of other vitamin K–dependent proteins (see Combined Deficiency of Vitamin K–dependent Proteins) and in combination with factor VII deficiency as a result of loss of both genes due to a chromosome 13 q34 deletion.

Acquired factor X deficiency occurs with warfarin therapy, vitamin K deficiency, liver disease, and DIC, all of which also reduce the levels of other coagulation factors. Factor X deficiency has been reported with malignancy, infections, and medication. There are rare reports of acquired factor X inhibitors. Acquired factor X deficiency may accompany systemic amyloidosis, occurring in 8.7% of patients with AL amyloidosis in one study, but rarely in secondary (AA) amyloidosis. Factor X binds to amyloid fibrils, which reduces the plasma half-life of the protein. Distinguishing this type of factor X deficiency from the inherited disorder is based on the clinical setting and evidence of poor clinical response to infusion of factor X–containing products in amyloidosis patients.

A classification system for factor X deficiency has been proposed based on factor X activity (severe, <1%; moderate, 1% to 5%; mild, 6% to 10%). Bleeding in factor X deficiency is severe and occurs earlier in life in patients with the lowest plasma levels. There is an impression that factor X–deficient patients bleed more severely than patients with other rare congenital coagulopathies. In a series of 102 factor X–deficient patients, the most frequent symptom was easy bruising (55%) followed by hematomas (43%).[18] Epistaxis and hemarthrosis were common. Intracranial hemorrhage occurred in 21%

and was particularly prevalent in patients with the Gly380Arg, IVS7-1G>A, and Tyr163delAT mutations. Among homozygotes, hemarthrosis was the most common symptom, and all homozygous women suffered from menorrhagia. Umbilical stump bleeding occurred in 28% of newborns. Mildly affected persons (activity >15%) may have increased bruising or bleeding with trauma. Although most heterozygotes are asymptomatic, as many as one-third have excessive bleeding from mucous membranes with invasive procedures or with childbirth.[19]

Because factor X is the first coagulation protease in the common pathway (see Fig. 139-1, *B*), its deficiency typically prolongs the PT and PTT and must be distinguished from deficiencies of fibrinogen, prothrombin, and factor V, which are associated with similar test results. Definitive diagnosis and determination of severity are established using a modified PT or PTT assay with factor X–deficient plasma. As discussed earlier, some factor X variants preferentially prolong either the PT or the PTT. Congenital factor X deficiency cannot be distinguished from acquired deficiency associated with amyloidosis in the coagulation laboratory, because factor X-dependent assays correct after mixing with normal plasma in both conditions. The absence of a lifelong bleeding disorder, findings of a serum M-protein, signs of amyloidosis, and histologic confirmation of amyloid in tissues point toward AL amyloidosis. A poor response to factor X infusion in the absence of an inhibitor distinguishes the two conditions.

Factor X–deficient patients are treated with FFP or PCC for most bleeding episodes (see Table 139-2). A trough level of 10% to 20% is usually sufficient for hemarthroses and soft tissue bleeding. The half-life of factor X is ≈20 to 40 hours. FFP administered as a loading dose of 10 to 20 mL/kg followed by 3 to 6 mL/kg every 12 to 24 hours will usually keep trough levels above 10% to 20%. Higher factor X levels may be required for severe bleeding or surgery, and accumulation of factor X in plasma can be achieved by increasing the transfusion frequency to every 12 hours. PCC with a factor X/IX ratio of ≈1 : 1 will increase plasma factor X levels by 1.5% for each factor IX unit/kg body weight. A dose of 15 to 20 factor IX units/kg daily or every other day has been suggested for major surgery. Risk for thromboembolism and DIC is a concern when using PCC, and it is recommended that plasma factor X levels not exceed 50% of normal, unless absolutely necessary. Plasma exchange has been used successfully to increase plasma factor X levels in pregnant women before delivery. For patients with severe factor X deficiency and recurrent hemorrhage, prophylactic PCC infusion is effective in preventing bleeding. Minor bleeding episodes can be treated with local measures and/or ε-amino caproic acid. Cryoprecipitate lacks factor X, and DDAVP infusion does not affect factor X levels and should not be used. A factor X concentrate is under investigation in the United States and Europe and may become the treatment of choice. As with prothrombin deficiency, there are no reports of acquired alloantibody inhibitors to factor X after replacement therapy is given to congenitally deficient patients, consistent with the concept that these patients have trace amount of plasma factor X at baseline.

Patients with acquired factor X deficiency and amyloidosis usually respond poorly to infusion of products containing factor X. Treatment may involve chemotherapy, splenectomy, plasma exchange, PCC, and/or activated factor VIIa. The optimal hemostatic management for invasive procedures has not been determined, but in one series complications occurred in only 13% of procedures, and there was a poor correlation between the risk for bleeding and factor X levels.

FACTOR XI DEFICIENCY (OMIM 264900)

In 1953, Rosenthal and colleagues described three members of a family with abnormal hemostasis, prolonged time to clot formation in a glass tube, and a normal PT. In mixing studies, patient plasma shortened the clotting times of hemophilia A and B plasmas, indicating that the missing factor was distinct from factors VIII and IX. Unlike the X-linked hemophilias, the new disorder (sometimes referred to as hemophilia C) was transmitted as an autosomal trait. The missing factor was called *plasma thromboplastin antecedent* and subsequently designated *factor XI*. Estimates place the incidence of factor XI deficiency at 1 per million (see Table 139-1), although some suggest this would be higher if symptomatic cases with mild deficiency were included. Severe factor XI deficiency (<20% of normal plasma level) is common in persons of Ashkenazi Jewish ancestry (incidence of 1 in 450).[20-22]

Factor XI is the precursor of the 160,000-Dalton protease factor XIa. The protein is a dimer of identical polypeptides. This unusual feature has implications for inheritance patterns in factor XI deficiency. Factor XI is activated by factor XIIa in the PTT assay (see Fig. 139-1, *B*). However, factor XI must be activated by factor XII-independent processes in vivo because factor XII deficiency does not cause abnormal bleeding. Factor XI can also be activated by thrombin or factor XIa. Factor XIa contributes to clotting by activating factor IX (see Fig. 139-1, *A*).

Factor XI deficiency in the Jewish population and in many non-Jewish patients is an autosomal recessive condition.[20-22] Two point mutations account for more than 90% of abnormal factor XI alleles in Ashkenazi Jews. The nonsense mutation Glu117Stop encodes a truncated protein, and homozygotes lack factor XI protein in their plasma. The missense mutation Phe283Leu causes a defect in dimer formation, resulting in poor secretion. Phe283Leu homozygotes have ≈10% of normal plasma factor XI activity, and the plasma protein is dimeric. Compound heterozygotes for Glu117Stop and Phe283Leu have activity of ≈3%, whereas heterozygotes for either mutation have activities of 50% to 60%. The allele frequencies of Glu117Stop and Phe283Leu in Ashkenazi Jews (0.0217 and 0.0254, respectively) indicate a carrier frequency for an abnormal factor XI allele of ≈5% in this population. Although Phe283Leu occurs primarily in Jews of European ancestry and may be of relatively recent origin, Glu117Stop is at least 2500 years old and is found in Jews from different ethnic backgrounds, as well as in non-Jewish patients.

Since the discovery of Glu117Stop and Phe283Leu, more than 200 human factor XI gene mutations have been identified. Although most are unique to specific patients or families, several mutations are more widespread with evidence of founder effects. Cys38Arg has an allele frequency of ≈0.5% in French Basques, Cys128Stop accounts for ≈10% of abnormal factor XI alleles in Great Britain, and Gln88Stop is present in several families from Nantes, France. In most deficient patients, factor XI activity and antigen are comparably reduced (CRM−deficiency). A three-category scheme has been proposed for classifying CRM−factor XI deficiency. The first category contains mutations that prevent protein synthesis (e.g., Glu117Stop), whereas mutations in the second category interfere with dimer formation (e.g., Phe283Leu). Inheritance in both categories follows a recessive pattern, because mutant polypeptides do not interfere with the product of the normal allele in a heterozygote. The third category includes mutations that impair secretion but do not prevent dimer formation (e.g., Gly400Val). In heterozygotes, mutant and wild type polypeptides can form nonsecretable dimers, trapping normal protein in the cell (dominant negative effect). This may account for families in which severe to moderate factor XI deficiency appears to be a dominant trait. CRM+ factor XI mutations are rare, and they usually involve catalytic defects (e.g., Gly555Glu and Thr575Met). Factor XI Ser248Asn has normal activity in a PTT assay but binds poorly to platelets, possibly explaining the bleeding disorder associated with the mutation.

Factor XI levels decrease in liver disease and DIC but are not affected by vitamin K deficiency or warfarin therapy. Mild to moderate factor XI deficiency occurs in ≈25% of patients with Noonan syndrome and is also common in carbohydrate-deficient glycoprotein syndrome, a group of inherited disorders involving defects in glycosylation of secretory glycoproteins. Antibody inhibitors to factor XI are relatively common after replacement in deficient patients, with one-third of Glu117Stop homozygotes developing inhibitors, often after a single exposure to plasma.

Significant bleeding in severe factor XI deficiency is usually injury-related and is most frequent in tissues with robust fibrinolytic activity, such as the oral cavity, tonsils, and urinary tract.[20-22] Injury to these areas causes excessive bleeding in two-thirds of patients, regardless of genotype. Bleeding with injury at other locations is less frequent and tends to occur in those with the lowest factor XI levels.[20-23] Thus Glu117Stop homozygotes have more bleeding than Phe283Leu homozygotes. Excessive bleeding with skin laceration, circumcision, appendectomy, and orthopedic surgery is infrequent; and spontaneous bleeding (except for menorrhagia) is uncommon. Bleeding may start at the time of injury or be delayed by hours, and oozing from tooth extraction sites may persist for days. Bleeding correlates relatively poorly with plasma factor XI activity. Patients with severe deficiency may not bleed excessively, even during surgery without treatment, and a patient may exhibit different bleeding tendencies over time. Opinions differ regarding the propensity of patients with mild deficiency (20% to 50% of normal level) to bleed. Some studies describe minimal bleeding with tooth extraction, tonsillectomy, nasal surgery, and urologic surgery, whereas others report difficulty distinguishing severe from mild deficiency on clinical grounds. In a study of 45 families with factor XI deficiency, the odds ratios for excessive bleeding were 13.0 and 2.6 for homozygotes and heterozygotes, respectively. Thus mild factor XI deficiency may confer a slightly increased risk for bleeding but significantly less than the risk with severe deficiency.

In the PTT assay, factor XI is bound to the contact surface through high-molecular-weight kininogen and is activated by factor XIIa (see Fig. 139-1, *B,* and Fig. 139-3). Factor XIa, in turn, activates factor IX. Therefore factor XI deficiency prolongs the PTT, but not the PT. Diagnosis and severity are established by a modified PTT assay using factor XI–deficient plasma. The PTT is often normal in heterozygotes.

Perioperative therapy should be individualized for factor XI–deficient patients (see box on Treating Factor XI–Deficient Patients). Those requiring replacement may be treated with FFP or factor XI concentrate (Hemoleven or FXI concentrate) (see Table 139-2). The concentrates are effective in preventing bleeding with invasive procedures. Hemoleven received orphan drug-designation from the United States Food and Drug Administration in 2007. In the 1990s, use of factor XI concentrates was associated with thrombosis and evidence of DIC, primarily in older patients with cardiovascular disease receiving doses higher than 30 units/kg. To reduce procoagulant potential, current concentrates contain antithrombin and heparin, with or without C1-inhibitor. It is recommended that the factor XI level be raised no higher than 60% of the normal level with concentrates. Cryoprecipitate does not contain factor XI. The half-life of factor XI is 45 to 52 hours, facilitating daily or every-other-day administration. For major surgery or procedures involving the oropharynx or urinary tract, patients with severe deficiency should be treated to keep factor XI levels at ≈40% of normal for 7 days postoperation.[20-22] Minor surgery can be treated for 5 days to keep levels at ≈30% of normal. Circumcision, orthopedic surgery, and appendectomy carry a low bleeding risk, and replacement can be withheld unless bleeding occurs.[23] A similar "wait and see" approach has been proposed for factor XI–deficient women during labor and delivery, which are associated with a relatively low (≈20%) rate of excessive bleeding. However, others advocate replacement for childbirth. Dental procedures such as tooth extraction do not require FFP and should be covered with antifibrinolytic therapy. Patients with factor XI levels higher than 40% of normal do not require replacement for surgery. The effectiveness of DDAVP in mild factor XI deficiency is not established, but there are reports that factor XI levels increase in response to this drug. Factor XI–deficient patients with inhibitors do not usually have increased spontaneous bleeding. Recombinant factor VIIa has been used successfully for major surgery in factor XI–deficient patients with and without inhibitors and to cover epidural block in deficient women during labor and delivery.

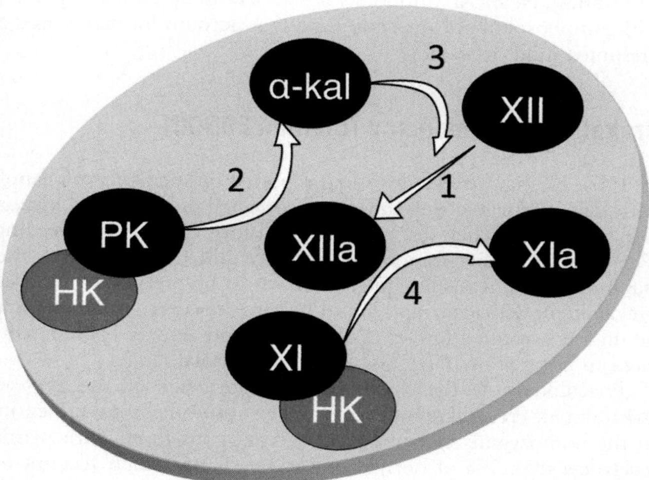

Figure 139-3 CONTACT ACTIVATION REACTIONS. In the PTT assay, contact activation is initiated by activation of factor XII (XII) to α-factor XIIa (XIIa) (reaction 1) when plasma is exposed to a negatively charged surface *(gray disk).* Factor XIIa converts prekallikrein (PK) to the active protease α-kallikrein (reaction 2), and α-kallikrein reciprocally activates additional factor XII (reaction 3). Factor XIIa initiates coagulation through conversion of factor XI (XI) to factor XIa (XIa) (reaction 4). Note that PK and factor XI require high-molecular-weight kininogen (HK) to bind properly to the negatively charged surface. Factor XIa ultimately promotes thrombin generation and fibrin clot formation through activation of factor IX (see Fig. 139-1).

DEFICIENCIES OF THE CONTACT FACTORS: FACTOR XII, PREKALLIKREIN, AND HIGH-MOLECULAR-WEIGHT KININOGEN

Factor XII, prekallikrein, and high-molecular-weight kininogen are required for normal activation of factor XI in the "contact phase" that initiates coagulation in the PTT assay (see Fig. 139-1, *B,* and Fig. 139-3). Patients with a deficiency in any one of these proteins have a prolonged PTT, but do not have abnormal hemostasis, even with major surgery or injury. Therefore these proteins either do not participate in hemostasis, or redundant mechanisms compensate for their absence. No specific therapy is required to prepare deficient patients for invasive procedures. However, it is important to distinguish factor XII, prekallikrein, or high-molecular-weight kininogen deficiency from deficiencies of factors VIII, IX, or XI, which also prolong the PTT, but cause abnormal hemostasis.

Factor XII Deficiency (OMIM 234000)

In 1955, Ratnoff and Colopy described three asymptomatic individuals with a novel abnormality of surface-induced coagulation. The missing plasma component was called *Hageman factor* (after the index case) and later designated *factor XII.* The incidence of severe factor XII deficiency is not known, because some deficient persons almost certainly go undiagnosed. Moderate to severe factor XII deficiency was reported in 1.5% to 3.0% of healthy blood donors. This unexpectedly high prevalence may be partly explained by anti–factor XII or antiphospholipid antibodies that interfere with factor XII activity assays.

Factor XIIa, the activated form of factor XII, is an 80,000-Dalton protease that activates factor XI and prekallikrein in the contact phase of the PTT assay (see Fig. 139-3). A C/T polymorphism in the 5′-untranslated region of the factor XII gene (referred to as 46C/T [or -4C/T]) strongly influences plasma factor XII levels, with the 46T allele associated with lower levels compared with 46C. The frequency of 46T is high (73%) in East Asians (compared with 20%

Treating Factor XI–Deficient Patients

When preparing patients with severe factor XI deficiency (plasma factor XI level <20% of normal) for an invasive procedure, it is important to keep in mind that (1) a negative bleeding history does not indicate a low risk with subsequent procedures, (2) certain procedures are associated with lower bleeding risks than others, and (3) patients with very low factor XI levels (<1%) often develop neutralizing inhibitors with replacement therapy. These observations have led to refinements in treatment recommendations that limit exposure to factor XI by targeting replacement therapy to certain clinical situations. Replacement therapy to reach appropriate target levels may be required for patients with mild factor XI deficiency (levels of 20% to 40% of normal) undergoing certain types of procedures.

Antiplatelet drugs should be stopped 1 week before surgery. The prothrombin time and platelet count should be normal, and the possibility of coexisting hemostatic abnormalities thoroughly investigated. Patients with factor XI levels greater than 40% to 45% generally do not experience bleeding, and a history of excessive bleeding in such an individual suggests other hemostatic abnormalities are present. If the patient has been exposed to factor XI in the recent past, the possibility that a neutralizing inhibitor is present should also be considered.

Factor replacement is required for most major surgery in factor XI–deficient patients and should be initiated before the procedure. Surgery on the oropharynx, nasopharynx, or urinary tract should be treated with FFP or factor XI concentrate to keep the plasma level at ≈40% of normal for at least 7 days. A similar strategy is appropriate for neurosurgery, head and neck surgery, cardiothoracic procedures, and major abdominal or pelvic surgery. For nasal surgery and oral procedures such as tonsillectomy, supplementing replacement therapy with antifibrinolytic therapy should be strongly considered. For prostatectomy and other surgery on the lower urinary tract, flushing the bladder with saline containing an antifibrinolytic agent may be beneficial. Minor surgery can be treated with replacement to maintain levels of 30% for 5 days.

A "wait and see" strategy, in which replacement is withheld unless bleeding occurs, appears to be appropriate for procedures such as circumcision, appendectomy, and some orthopedic surgery, as well as with normal vaginal deliveries. There are insufficient data to determine whether epidural anesthesia is safe in the absence of factor coverage, and replacement therapy should be used.

Factor XI concentrates are likely to become more popular in the near future for treating factor XI–deficient patients, and it is important to recognize that use of earlier versions of these preparations were associated with a high (10%) incidence of thromboembolism. The majority of thrombotic events occurred in older adult patients with preexisting cardiovascular disease, and these patients should probably not be treated with factor XI concentrate unless absolutely necessary. For other patients, the concentrates offer an effective form of treatment that requires a much smaller volume of infusion than does therapy with FFP.

Alternatives to factor replacement are recommended in several situations. Tooth extraction or skin biopsies can be managed with antifibrinolytic drugs alone (ε-amino caproic acid 5 to 6 g every 6 hours or tranexamic acid 1 g every 6 hours), starting 12 hours before the procedure and continuing for 7 days. Fibrin glues can be used in place of fibrinolytic therapy for skin biopsy or resection of skin lesions. Recombinant factor VIIa has been used successfully in factor XI–deficient patients with and without factor XI inhibitors and may be appropriate in situations in which exposure to plasma products needs to be limited.

Patients with factor XI deficiency can experience thromboembolic episodes. Aspirin or clopidogrel can be used in factor XI–deficient patients with myocardial infarction or other manifestations of atherosclerosis, whereas atrial fibrillation or venous thromboembolism should be treated with warfarin, with the goal of not allowing the INR to exceed 2.5.

in Caucasians), who have lower factor XII levels than other ethnic groups. Factor XII activity and antigen are usually reduced in parallel in deficient individuals, and circulating dysfunctional variants are rare.

Several factor XII gene mutations have been identified (www.hgmd.org). Factor XII deficiency is not associated with spontaneous or excessive posttraumatic bleeding, and most cases are identified by the incidental finding of a prolonged PTT. There is conflicting literature regarding an association between factor XII deficiency and thrombosis. Two recent studies reported an inverse relationship between plasma factor XII levels within the broad normal range and the risk for cardiovascular events. However, other work indicates that the increased risk does not apply to persons with severe factor XII deficiency or that low factor XII levels are more of a risk marker rather than a contributor to thrombosis. A metaanalysis of studies examining the 46C/T factor XII gene polymorphism, the major genetic determinant of plasma factor XII level, suggests that the correlation between the polymorphism and venous thrombosis or myocardial infarction, if present, is weak. Reports have linked low factor XII levels to pregnancy loss or failure of in vitro fertilization. Of interest, factor XII–deficient mice do not display an abnormality in reproduction. It is possible that antibodies that interfere with factor XII function, rather than true deficiency, are responsible for pregnancy-related complications in humans.

Factor XII undergoes autoactivation when exposed to the contact surface added to plasma to initiate clotting in the PTT assay. Factor XIIa activates prekallikrein to α-kallikrein, which reciprocally activates additional factor XII (see Fig. 139-3). Factor XIIa also activates factor XI to XIa. In severe factor XII deficiency, the PTT is very long. Definitive diagnosis is established using a modified PTT assay with factor XII–deficient plasma. Antiphospholipid antibodies may disproportionately affect factor XII measurements in PTT-based assays. In addition, factor XII antibodies are present in up to half of plasmas with antiphospholipid antibodies and may account for many cases of presumed mild deficiency.

Prekallikrein Deficiency (OMIM 229000)

In 1965, Hathaway and coworkers reported on members of a family with long plasma clotting times that corrected on prolonged incubation with glass. They did not have a history of excessive bleeding. The missing plasma component, initially called *Fletcher factor* after the index cases, was subsequently shown to be prekallikrein. Severe prekallikrein deficiency appears to be rare; however, mild cases may be missed because a low level of prekallikrein activity is often sufficient to bring many PTT assays into the normal range.

Prekallikrein is the 95,000-Dalton precursor of the protease α-kallikrein. Prekallikrein deficiency is an autosomal trait, presenting in the homozygous or compound heterozygous forms with plasma levels less than 1% of normal. CRM– variants, which account for about half of cases, are common in Caucasian and Japanese patients, whereas most black patients are CRM–. Few prekallikrein gene mutations have been identified (www.hgmd.org). Partial deficiency (10% to 50%) may be seen in patients with severe high-molecular-weight kininogen deficiency, likely due to increased catabolism or clearance because prekallikrein circulates in complex with high-molecular-weight kininogen. Severe prekallikrein deficiency presents as a prolongation of the PTT in a person without a history of excessive bleeding. Although thrombotic events have been described in deficient patients, it is not clear that the deficiency contributed to thrombosis. Indeed, recent studies in mice indicate that reducing prekallikrein levels can attenuate thrombus formation.

In the PTT, prekallikrein is converted to α-kallikrein by factor XIIa, which in turn reciprocally activates factor XII (see Fig. 139-3). Severe prekallikrein deficiency causes a prolonged PTT, and the diagnosis is confirmed using a modified PTT with prekallikrein–deficient plasma. The prolonged PTT in prekallikrein deficiency may be shortened by prolonged incubation with the contact reagent, which allows factor XII sufficient time to activate independently of prekallikrein. This distinguishes prekallikrein deficiency from deficiencies of factors VIII, IX, XI, XII, and high-molecular-weight kininogen, in which the prolonged PTT does not correct with prolonged incubation. PTT reagents using the contact activator ellagic acid are relatively insensitive to prekallikrein and may fail to detect some deficient patients.

High-Molecular-Weight Kininogen Deficiency (OMIM 228960)

In 1974, Schiffman and Lee reported that a plasma factor distinct from prekallikrein was required for factor XI activation by factor XIIa. In 1975, three asymptomatic patients from three separate families who appeared to lack the unknown factor were described with in vitro abnormalities of coagulation, fibrinolysis, and kinin generation. The condition, originally named for the affected families (Fitzgerald trait, Williams trait, and Flaujeac trait), was subsequently determined to be due to high-molecular-weight kininogen deficiency. The disorder appears to be very rare.

High-molecular-weight kininogen is a 110,000-Dalton protein that contains the vasoactive peptide bradykinin. Prekallikrein and factor XI circulate in complex with high-molecular-weight kininogen. Low-molecular-weight kininogen and high-molecular-weight kininogen are products of a single kininogen gene; however, low-molecular-weight kininogen does not play a role in coagulation in vitro. High-molecular-weight kininogen deficiency is an autosomal recessive trait. Depending on the genetic abnormality (www.hgmd.org), patients may have isolated high-molecular-weight kininogen deficiency or combined high-molecular-weight and low-molecular-weight kininogen deficiency. High-molecular-weight kininogen–deficient patients are usually identified by the incidental finding of a prolonged PTT, and they do not bleed excessively.

In the PTT assay, high-molecular-weight kininogen facilitates binding of prekallikrein and factor XI to the contact surface, thereby enhancing their activation by factor XIIa (see Fig. 139-3). Severe deficiency is characterized by a very prolonged PTT, and definitive diagnosis is established using a modified PTT with high-molecular-weight kininogen–deficient plasma. Partial prekallikrein deficiency is common in severe high-molecular-weight kininogen deficiency, likely due to increased catabolism of prekallikrein when it is not in complex with high-molecular-weight kininogen.

FACTOR XIII DEFICIENCY (OMIM 134570 [A SUBUNIT] AND 134580 [B SUBUNIT])

In 1944, Robbins demonstrated that fibrin formed from purified components was soluble in weak acid, whereas fibrin formed in the presence of serum or plasma was not. He proposed that a fibrin-stabilizing factor was present in plasma. In 1960, Duckert and colleagues described the first patient with deficiency of fibrin-stabilizing factor, which was subsequently designated *factor XIII*. The incidence of severe factor XIII deficiency is estimated at 1 in 2 million (see Table 139-1).[24-26]

Factor XIII in blood is distributed between plasma and platelets, with a small amount in monocytes. The plasma protein is a 330,000-Dalton tetramer composed of two catalytic A subunits and two carrier B subunits. Factor XIII in platelets, monocytes, and placenta has only A subunits. The A subunit in plasma appears to be synthesized primarily in hematopoietic cells, whereas the B subunit comes from the liver. Factor XIII is converted to the transglutaminase factor XIIIa by thrombin, and it catalyzes formation of γ-glutamyl-ε-lysyl bonds between fibrin monomers (see Fig. 139-1, *A*), resulting in a fibrin mesh that is resistant to dissolution in mild acids and urea. Factor XIIIa also cross-links fibrin to plasma, extracellular matrix, and cytoskeletal proteins, facilitating clot adherence to an injury site. Congenital factor XIII deficiency is an autosomal recessive condition. The currently recommended classification scheme recognizes factor XIII-A and factor XIII-B deficiencies. Factor XIII-A deficiency is divided into type I (quantitative) and type II (qualitative) deficiencies. Although earlier systems included a combined A and B deficiency category, low levels of the A subunit in these cases was the result of rapid clearance because of the absence of the B subunit.

Most cases of congenital factor XIII deficiency are due to mutations in the gene for the A subunit, with less than 5% in the B subunit gene.[25] More than 100 different mutations have been reported in the factor XIII-A gene, with less than 20 in the factor XIII-B gene. (www.isth.org/default/index.cfm; www.hgmd.org; www.f13-database.de). The incidence of factor XIII mutations affecting plasma activity is probably higher than suspected, considering that screening test abnormalities occur mostly in those with severely decreased plasma activity (<5% of normal). A few mutations show evidence of a founder effect, with the IVS5–1 G>A splice-site defect and Arg661Stop nonsense mutations each identified in 10 apparently unrelated individuals.

Plasma factor XIII levels decrease in DIC and liver disease. However, significant deficiency is rare in liver disease and may indicate a poor prognosis. Acquired deficiency has been reported in leukemia, Crohn disease, ulcerative colitis, and Henoch-Schönlein purpura, but levels are usually above 30% of normal and replacement is not required. Alloantibodies to factor XIII induced by replacement therapy are relatively rare in factor XIII–deficient patients. Neutralizing autoantibodies that block the activation, activity, or fibrin binding capacity of the factor XIII-A subunit, or that enhance factor XIII clearance from plasma, have been reported in older adults, in patients with systemic lupus erythematosus and lymphoproliferative disorders, and with medications such as isoniazid, penicillin, procainamide, phenytoin and practolol. An autoantibody to the B subunit that developed in a patient with lupus markedly enhanced clearance of the protein from plasma and was associated with life-threatening bleeding.

Delayed bleeding from the umbilical stump occurs in 80% to 90% of newborns with severe factor XIII deficiency and is considered a diagnostic feature of the disorder.[24-26] Ecchymoses, soft tissue hematomas, and prolonged bleeding with trauma are common, and recurrent soft tissue bleeding may lead to formation of hemorrhagic cysts (pseudotumors). Hemarthroses is less frequent than in factor VIII or IX deficiency. Bleeding that is delayed 12 to 36 hours postinjury is characteristic of factor XIII deficiency, although hemorrhage can be immediate in some cases. Bleeding at the time of invasive procedures may be minimal, but delayed hemorrhage often occurs. Intracranial bleeding is more frequent in factor XIII deficiency than in other inherited coagulation disorder, with an incidence as high as 30%, which justifies prophylactic replacement. Delayed wound healing has been observed in deficient patients, possibly related to a defect in angiogenesis. Recurrent spontaneous abortions occur with most pregnancies in untreated factor XIII–deficient women,[27] possibly due to abnormal formation of the cytotrophoblastic shell and poor attachment of the placenta to the uterus. The problems just described are recognized complications in patients with factor XIII levels less than 5% of normal. The issue of excessive bleeding in patients with milder factor XIII deficiency is more controversial. In at least two studies, patients heterozygous for factor XIII deficiency reported excessive bleeding. These studies lacked control groups, so it is difficult to determine whether the mild deficiency was responsible for symptoms. However, experience with pregnant women with severe factor XIII deficiency shows that the factor XIII level needs to be higher than 10% to reliably prevent pregnancy loss, indicating that clinically significant problems can occur in patients with levels higher than 5% of normal.

The PT and PTT measure time to fibrin clot formation; they do not assess clot stability. Results of these assays are therefore normal in factor XIII–deficient patients. Clots formed in plasma lacking factor XIII are soluble in 5 M urea or 1% monochloroacetic acid, whereas normal clots are stable for at least 24 hours. Solubility in 5 M urea (urea clot stability assay) is frequently used to screen for factor XIII deficiency or inhibitors. The assay is relatively insensitive to factor XIII deficiency and identifies only patients with factor XIII levels less than 5% of normal. Clots from plasma lacking α_2-antiplasmin can also show increased solubility in this assay, and can be identified with specific assays. Chromogenic assays for measuring factor XIIIa activity are commercially available and should strongly be considered as replacements for the urea clot lysis assay. These assays can also be used to detect and quantify neutralizing factor XIII inhibitors, using a mixing method with normal plasma.

The plasma half-life of factor XIII is 10 to 14 days,[20-22] facilitating prophylactic replacement therapy to prevent intracranial bleeding. Although some consider a plasma level of ≈5% adequate for hemostasis,[28] others suggest that levels in excess of 10% are required to significantly reduce bleeding risk. Both FFP and cryoprecipitate contain factor XIII; however, the factor XIII concentrate Fibrogammin P (marketed as Corifact in the United States; see Table 139-2) is the preferred replacement preparation.[24-29] Recombinant factor XIII has also undergone evaluation, and is awaiting approval. Fibrogammin P contains factor XIII purified from human plasma and is pasteurized. A regimen of 40 units/kg every 4 weeks is recommended for prophylaxis. A dose of 20 to 30 units/kg/day should be used with major surgery to keep the plasma activity higher than 20% to 50% of normal. For minor surgery, 10 to 20 units/kg/day for 2 to 3 days is sufficient, whereas bleeding episodes can be treated with 10 to 30 units/kg/day depending on the severity of the hemostatic abnormality. In pregnancy, factor XIII replacement should be started early, preferably before gestational week 5, because decidual bleeding from implantation will occur without replacement. The optimal plasma factor XIII concentration in pregnancy is not established, but at least 10% of normal is recommended. This can be achieved by infusing 250 units of concentrate every 7 days through week 22 of gestation, and 500 units per week for the remainder of pregnancy, with a bolus of 1000 units during labor. Although factor XIII concentrate is preferred for prophylaxis or treatment of acute bleeding, if it is not available, FFP (10-20 mL/Kg every 4 to 6 weeks) or cryoprecipitate (1 unit for every 10 to 20 kg body weight every 3 to 4 weeks) can be used.

CONGENITAL DEFICIENCIES INVOLVING MULTIPLE COAGULATION FACTORS

Numerous cases of congenital deficiencies of more than one coagulation factor have been described. Although most of these likely represent chance coinheritance of distinct deficiency states, several represent familial syndromes (see Table 139-3). Such syndromes are likely caused by abnormalities in intracellular processing of factors (e.g., type 1 deficiency) or alterations in the structure/activity of multiple factors due to abnormalities in posttranslational modification (e.g., type 3 deficiency). It must be remembered that common nonspecific inhibitors such as lupus anticoagulants interfere with coagulation assays and can lead to erroneous interpretations when they suggest multiple factor deficiencies (see box on Laboratory Testing in Rare Coagulation Factor Deficiencies). Similarly, potent inhibitors directed at a single coagulation factor (e.g., factor VIII) may occasionally interfere with assays for other factors. Two familial multiple factor deficiency states, combined factor V and VIII deficiency (type 1) and deficiency of vitamin K dependent factors (type 3), have been well characterized.

Combined Factor V and Factor VIII Deficiency (OMIM 227300)

Combined factor V and factor VIII deficiency was first reported in 1954. The familial form is an autosomal recessive trait caused by mutations in either the LMAN1 (mannose-binding lectin, formerly ERGIC-53) or MCFD2 (multiple combined factor deficiency protein) gene (www.isth.org/default/index.cfm). These proteins form a cargo receptor that is required for transport of factors V and VIII from the endoplasmic reticulum (ER) to the ER-Golgi intermediate compartment. Although the incidence of this disorder is thought to be 1 in 1 million persons, the allele frequency is particularly high (≈1%) in Tunisian Jews originating from a community on the island of Djerba.

Deficiency of either LMAN1 or MCFD2 activity causes a partial defect in factor V and factor VIII secretion, lowering plasma levels to ≈5% to 30% of normal. The mutation in Tunisian Jews is a T-to-C transition at a donor splice site in intron 9 of the LMAN1 gene. A history of consanguinity, co-segregation of the factor deficiencies, and similar reductions in factor V and VIII favor the familial disorder. Homozygotes or compound heterozygotes bleed primarily after trauma, although epistaxis, gingival bleeding, easy bruising, and menorrhagia are common. Non–trauma-related hemarthrosis may occur in 20% of patients, but bleeding from the GI tract or intracranial hemorrhage is less common. Postpartum hemorrhage occurs in most affected women, and invasive procedures, including dental extraction, are usually accompanied by excessive bleeding without replacement therapy. The disorder is associated with a prolonged PT and PTT (see Fig. 139-1, *B*). Isolated factor V deficiency also follows this pattern so it is recommended that patients with factor V deficiency have factor VIII levels measured to ensure that combined deficiency is not overlooked. Patients with mucosal bleeding and menorrhagia may respond to antifibrinolytic therapy. For more significant bleeding, or in preparation for surgical procedures or tooth extraction, a combination of FFP and factor VIII concentrate should be used. DDAVP can raise factor VIII, but not factor V levels. Trough levels of ≈50% for factor VIII and 25% for factor V have been recommended for surgery. Plasma exchange may be used to raise factor V levels in situations in which volume overload from large volumes of FFP is a concern.

Table 139-3 Combined Familial Deficiency States

Type	Deficient Factors	OMIM Designation	Underlying Cause
1	V and VIII	227300	Mutations in LMAN1 or MCFD2 genes
2	VIII and IX	134510	Unknown
3	II,VII, IX, X, protein C, and protein S	277450 (γ-glutamyl carboxylase) 607473 (vitamin K oxidoreductase)	Mutations in γ-glutamyl carboxylase (GGCX) or vitamin K epoxide reductase complex subunit 1 genes
4	VII and VIII	134430	Unknown
5	VIII, IX, and XI	134520	Unknown
6	IX and XI VII and X	134540	Unknown Gene deletion 13q34

OMIM, Online Mendelian Inheritance in Man.

Combined Deficiency of Vitamin K–Dependent Proteins (OMIM 277450 and 607473)

In 1966, McMillan and Roberts described a newborn girl with a prolonged PT and PTT; low levels of prothrombin and factors VII, IX, and X; and no evidence of liver disease or malabsorption. She had a partial response to large doses of vitamin K. In subsequent cases, low protein C and protein S levels were also noted in association with mutations in the γ-glutamyl carboxylase (GGCX) gene. Although the condition is considered to be a rare autosomal recessive trait, severe bleeding has been reported in a neonate who was heterozygous for a GGCX mutation.

Laboratory Testing in Rare Coagulation Factor Deficiencies

When deficiency of a coagulation factor is being considered, it is important to remember that (1) acquired conditions causing multiple factor deficiencies are more common than congenital deficiency of a single factor and (2) common nonspecific inhibitors of coagulation, such as lupus anticoagulants and heparin, will interfere with coagulation factor assays. Unexplained prolongation of the PT or PTT should be evaluated in a qualified laboratory. If at all possible, the plasma should be from blood collected by venipuncture. In our experience, the common practice of collecting blood from central venous catheters/ports or peripheral intravenous catheters frequently introduces fluids or drugs that adversely affect clotting assays and may contribute to misdiagnosis. Some laboratories use the thrombin time assay to screen samples for possible contamination with heparin or direct thrombin inhibitors to avoid this pitfall.

The initial evaluation of a plasma sample with a prolonged PT or PTT should start by repeating the abnormal test on a mixture of patient and normal plasma to determine whether the prolonged clotting time is related to a clotting factor deficiency (clotting time becomes normal with mixing) or an inhibitor that neutralizes clotting factor activity (clotting time remains prolonged with mixing). The mixing study should be performed with and without prolonged incubation (2 hours), because some antibody inhibitors show a time-dependent pattern of inhibition. Slight (a few seconds) prolongation of the PT or PTT can be difficult to evaluate with a mixing study. We evaluate such samples with assays for lupus anticoagulants before measuring specific levels of coagulation factors.

The antibodies to clotting factors that most physicians are familiar with neutralize factor activity and generate abnormal results on a mixing study (i.e., mixing with normal plasma fails to correct the abnormal clotting time). However, it is important to recognize that nonneutralizing antibodies can also be associated with severe factor deficiency. These antibodies typically enhance clearance of the clotting factor from the plasma in vivo and will not be detected by a mixing study. A failure to respond to replacement therapy in the absence of a clearly measurable inhibitor suggests this diagnosis. In our practice, we have observed severe acquired deficiencies of prothrombin, factor X, factor XI, and factor XIII caused by nonneutralizing antibodies.

If the level of a vitamin K–dependent protein (prothrombin or factors VII, IX, or X) is low, levels of factor V and at least one other vitamin K–dependent factor should be determined. If multiple vitamin K–dependent factors are low and factor V is normal, a process affecting vitamin K is likely. If factor V is also low, liver disease or DIC should be considered. Tests for hepatic function (albumin) or injury (transaminases) can facilitate interpretation of the coagulation factor studies. Distinguishing DIC from liver disease can be difficult, because results of standard tests such as the PT, PTT, platelet count, and fibrinogen and D-dimer levels may be abnormal in both conditions. Measuring factor V and factor VIII may be useful in this situation, because both factors are often low in DIC, whereas factor VIII is normal or elevated in liver disease.

Patients with factor XI, factor XII, prekallikrein, or high-molecular-weight kininogen deficiency may require anticoagulation for thromboembolism or other indications. Assays based on contact activation such as the PTT or the activated clotting time cannot be used for monitoring therapy with heparin or direct thrombin inhibitors such as argatroban or lepirudin in these patients, because the baseline test result will be abnormal. Many hospital laboratories now measure heparin with chromogenic assays based on factor Xa inhibition. Specific assays for argatroban and lepirudin are less readily available. Alternatively, low-molecular-weight heparin, fondaparinux or one of the new oral thrombin or factor Xa inhibitors that do not require monitoring may be used in these situations.

Prothrombin; factors VII, IX, and X; proteins C and S; and the bone proteins osteocalcin and matrix Gla protein require γ-carboxylation of glutamic acid residues in their N-terminal Gla-domains. γ-Carboxylation is mediated by GGCX (which uses reduced vitamin K as a cofactor) and results in formation of vitamin K 2,3-epoxide, which must be reduced vitamin K epoxide reductase complex subunit 1 to replenish the vitamin K pool. Mutations in the GGCX (e.g., Arg394Leu; see www.hgmd.org) or VKORC1 (e.g., Arg98Trp) genes can impair this process and result in reduced levels (10% to 50% of normal) of all vitamin K–dependent proteins, resulting in a variable bleeding tendency that may be severe. Some patients have skeletal abnormalities resembling warfarin embryopathy, possibly due to reduced activity of vitamin K–dependent bone proteins. Vitamin K–dependent proteins are reduced in patients taking warfarin, in poisoning with rodenticides such as brodifacoum, and with vitamin K deficiency. The levels of these proteins are also low in liver failure, in conjunction with other proteins synthesized in the liver, and in malabsorption syndromes. An acquired antibody that resulted in fatal bleeding in a patient with a lymphoproliferative disorder bound to an epitope on the Gla domain of prothrombin and factors IX and X.

The low levels of prothrombin and factors VII, IX, and X cause prolongation of the PT and PTT. Protein C and protein S are also reduced. The abnormalities correct on mixing with normal plasma. Failure to do so suggests that a nonspecific inhibitor such as a lupus anticoagulant is interfering with the assay. Patients with deficiencies of vitamin K–dependent proteins should be evaluated for liver disease, malabsorption, and exposure to warfarin or rodenticides containing vitamin-K antagonists such as brodifacoum. Toxicology screens can identify these agents in blood long after ingestion because of their long half-lives. Some patients have adequate clinical response to vitamin K_1 (10 mg weekly), but others require unusually high doses. Nonresponders, or responders with significant bleeding episodes, can be treated with FFP or PCC.

REFERENCES

1. de Moerloose P, Neerman-Arbez M: Congenital fibrinogen disorders. *Semin Thromb Hemost* 35:356, 2009.
   A review covering the biology, pathology, clinical presentation, diagnosis, and treatment of quantitative and qualitative congenital disorders of fibrinogen.
2. Bornikova L, Peyvandi F, Allen G, et al: Fibrinogen replacement therapy for congenital fibrinogen deficiency. *J Thromb Haemost* 9:1687, 2011.
   A literature review of replacement therapy and outcomes in patients with congenital fibrinogen deficiency over the past 50 years.
3. Peyvandi F, Haertel S, Knaub S, et al: Incidence of bleeding symptoms in 100 patients with inherited afibrinogenemia or hypofibrinogenemia. *J Thromb Haemost* 4:1634, 2006.
   Retrospective analysis of data from 100 patients with congenital fibrinogen deficiency, clearly demonstrating that bleeding becomes a major problem when the fibrinogen level is <50 mg/dL.
4. Lee CA, Chi C, Pavord SR, et al: The obstetric and gynaecological management of women with inherited bleeding disorders—review with guidelines produced by a taskforce of UK Haemophilia Centre Doctors' Organization. *Haemophilia* 12:301, 2006.
   Recommendations from a consensus panel for treatment and prophylaxis for obstetric and gynecological bleeding in women with rare coagulation factor deficiencies.
5. Morris TA, Marsh JJ, Chiles PG, et al: High prevalence of dysfibrinogenemia among patients with chronic thromboembolic pulmonary hypertension. *Blood* 114:1929, 2009.
   This study indicates that dysfibrinogenemia may be relatively common in patients with thromboembolic pulmonary hypertension, possibly because clots consisting of the abnormal fibrinogen lyse poorly.
6. Lancellotti S, De Cristofaro R: Congenital prothrombin deficiency. *Semin Thromb Hemost* 35:367, 2009.
   Review of the genetics, clinical manifestations, diagnosis, and treatment of prothrombin deficiency, including a section on the biology of prothrombin and thrombin.

7. Dentali F, Marchesi C, Pierfranceschi MG, et al: Safety of prothrombin complex concentrates for rapid anticoagulation reversal of vitamin K antagonists. A meta-analysis. *Thromb Haemost* 106:429, 2011.
Metaanalysis demonstrating that thrombotic complications associated with use of prothrombin complex concentrates, while possible, are relatively rare.
8. Asselta R, Peyvandi F: Factor V deficiency. *Sem Thromb Hemost* 35:382, 2009.
A review of the genetics, pathogenesis, laboratory, diagnosis, and treatment of factor V deficiency.
9. Lippi G, Favaloro EJ, Montagnana M, et al: Inherited and acquired factor V deficiency. *Blood Coagul Fibrinolysis* 22:160, 2011.
Review of clinical presentation, diagnosis, and treatment of patients with both inherited and acquired forms of factor V deficiency.
10. Camire RM: A new look at blood coagulation factor V. *Curr Opin Hematol* 18:338, 2011.
Concise review of the role of factor V in hemostasis and the biology of factor V deficiency.
11. Lapecorella M, Mariani G: International Registry on Congenital Factor VII Deficiency. Factor VII deficiency: Defining the clinical picture and optimizing therapeutic options. *Haemophilia* 14:1170, 2008.
Review of data from the International Registry of Congenital Factor VII Deficiency, including data on the clinical features and treatment outcomes for over 500 patients.
12. Mariani G, Bernardi F: Factor VII deficiency. *Semin Thromb Hemost* 35:400, 2009.
Review of the clinical presentation, diagnosis, and treatment of patients with congenital factor VII deficiency.
13. Herrmann FH, Wulff K, Auerswald G, et al: Factor VII deficiency: Clinical manifestation of 717 subjects from Europe and Latin America with mutations in the factor 7 gene. *Haemophilia* 15:267, 2009.
The largest reported study on clinical manifestations in patients with factor VII deficiency, including genetic studies to assess phenotype-genotype relationships.
14. Mariani G, Dolce A, Batorova A, et al: Recombinant, activated factor VII for surgery in factor VII deficiency: A prospective evaluation—the surgical STER. *Brit J Haematol* 152:340, 2010.
Prospective trial of recombinant factor VIIa is patients with factor VII deficiency.
15. Siboni SM, Zanon E, Sottilotta G, et al: Central nervous system bleeding in patients with rare bleeding disorders. *Haemophilia* 2011 (in press).
A retrospective analysis of patients with rare coagulation disorders and intracranial bleeding, indicating that the incidence of intracranial bleeds is relatively high in patients with severe factor V, VII, X, and XIII deficiencies.
16. Benlakhal F, Mura T, Schved JF, et al: A retrospective analysis of 157 surgical procedures performed without replacement therapy in 83 unrelated factor VII–deficient patients. *J Thromb Haemost* 9:1149, 2011.
Retrospective analysis of a large cohort of factor VII deficient patients undergoing invasive procedures without replacement therapy. Demonstrates the variability in hemostatic abnormalities associated with this disorder.
17. Todd T, Perry DJ: A review of long-term prophylaxis in the rare inherited coagulation factor deficiencies. *Haemophilia* 16:569, 2010.
A review of prophylaxis therapy in coagulation factor deficiencies other than hemophilia.
18. Herrmann FH, Auerswald G, Ruiz-Saez A, et al: Factor X deficiency: Clinical manifestation of 102 subjects from Europe and Latin America with mutations in the factor 10 gene. *Haemophilia* 12:479, 2006.
A large multinational study comparing the genotypes and phenotypes of patients with factor X deficiency.
19. Bachlechner C, Pechlaner C, Putz G, et al: Subclinical factor X deficiency may increase hemorrhage in women undergoing cesarean section. *Int J Obst Anest* 19:346, 2010.
A study showing that milder factor X deficiency can be associated with abnormal hemostasis.
20. Seligsohn U: Factor XI deficiency in humans. *J Thromb Haemost* 7:84, 2009.
A review of the natural history of factor XI deficiency, its diagnosis, and treatment.
21. Duga S, Salomon O: Factor XI deficiency. *Sem Thromb Haemost* 35:416, 2009.
Concise review of the genetics, clinical presentation, diagnosis, and treatment of congenital factor XI deficiency.
22. Bolton-Maggs PH: Factor XI deficiency—resolving the enigma? *Am Soc Hematol Educ Program* 97, 2009.
A review of our current understanding of the role of factor XI in hemostasis, along with recommendations for diagnosis and therapy of factor XI deficiency.
23. Salomon O, Steinberg DM, Seligsohn U: Variable bleeding manifestations characterize different types of surgery in patients with severe factor XI deficiency enabling parsimonious use of replacement therapy. *Haemophilia* 12:490, 2006.
A retrospective analysis of Ashkenazi Jewish patients with severe factor XI deficiency indicating that certain types of invasive procedures generally do not require factor replacement prior to the procedure.
24. Hsieh L, Nugent D: Factor XIII deficiency. *Haemophilia* 14:1190, 2008.
Review of the biochemistry of factor XIII, and the history, clinical presentation, diagnostic strategies and treatment for congenital factor XIII deficiency.
25. Karimi M, Bereczky Z, Cohan N, et al: Factor XIII deficiency. *Semin Thromb Hemost* 35:426, 2009.
Review of the presentation, genetics, diagnosis, and treatment of factor XIII deficiency.
26. Muszbek L, Bagoly Z, Cairo A, et al: Novel aspects of factor XIII deficiency. *Curr Opin Hematol* 18:366, 2011.
Review of the diagnosis and treatment of congenital factor XIII deficiency with a section discussing the current recommendations for classification.
27. Asahina T, Kobayashi T, Takeuchi K, et al: Congenital blood coagulation factor XIII deficiency and successful deliveries: A review of the literature. *Obstet Gynecol Surv* 62:255, 2007.
A review discussing the current understanding of how factor XIII deficiency compromises pregnancy, including current recommended treatment during pregnancy.
28. Castaman G: Prophylaxis of bleeding episodes and surgical interventions in patients with rare inherited coagulation disorders. *Blood Transfus* 6:s39, 2008.
Review of prophylactic and perioperative therapy for patients with rare coagulation factor deficiencies.
29. Dreyfus M, Barrois D, Borg JY, et al: Successful long-term replacement therapy with FXIII concentrate (Fibrogammin P) for severe congenital factor XIII deficiency: A prospective multicentre study. *J Thromb Haemost* 9:1264, 2011.
Results of a prospective study involving 19 patients with severe factor XIII deficiency demonstrating the efficacy of prophylactic treatment with the factor XIII concentrate Fibrogammin P (now Corifact).

CHAPTER 140

STRUCTURE, BIOLOGY, AND GENETICS OF VON WILLEBRAND FACTOR

Paula James and Natalia Rydz

von Willebrand factor (vWF) is an adhesive multimeric plasma glycoprotein that performs two major functions in hemostasis: it mediates platelet adhesion to injured subendothelium via glycoprotein 1bα (GP1bα), and it binds and stabilizes factor VIII (FVIII) in the circulation, protecting it from proteolytic degradation by enzymes. This important multifunctional protein was named after the Finnish physician, Dr. Erik von Willebrand, who first described von Willebrand disease (vWD) in 1926. In the original publication[1] he described a severe mucocutaneous bleeding problem in a family living on the Åland archipelago in the Baltic Sea. The index case, a young woman named Hjördis, bled to death during her fourth menstrual period at the age of 13. At least four other family members died from severe bleeding, and although the condition was originally referred to as *pseudohemophilia*, Dr. von Willebrand noted that in contrast to hemophilia, this condition affected both genders, with females typically being more severely affected. He also noted that affected individuals exhibited prolonged bleeding times despite normal platelet counts.

In the mid-1950s it was recognized that vWD was usually accompanied by a reduced level of FVIII activity and that the bleeding phenotype could be corrected by the infusion of normal plasma.[2] In the early 1970s the critical immunologic distinction between FVIII and vWF was made, and since that time significant progress has been made in our understanding of the molecular pathophysiology of this disorder. vWD is caused by qualitative or quantitative defects of vWF. Cloning and characterization of the vWF gene in the 1980s[3-6] has facilitated further investigation into the function of vWF and the genetic basis of vWD.

FUNCTIONS OF vWF

vWF is a multifunctional adhesive protein that plays an important role in both primary hemostasis and blood coagulation. In primary hemostasis, vWF initiates platelet adhesion at the site of endothelial injury, whereas in coagulation, vWF stabilizes FVIII in the circulation (Fig. 140-1).

Platelet Adhesion

At the site of endothelial injury, vWF secreted from local endothelial cells or recruited from the circulation adheres to exposed collagen. The most hemostatically important forms of collagen include types I, III, and VI, but vWF preferentially binds to type III collagen.[7] The interactions of vWF with collagen are predominately mediated by the A3 domain (See Figure 140-2). Once immobilized, vWF is subjected to the high shear rates of the arterial circulation and undergoes a conformational change that exposes the platelet GPIbα binding site within the A1 domain.[8] The high-affinity, rapid, and reversible interaction between vWF and GPIbα tethers platelets to the endothelium, where they roll until they are immobilized by integrin-mediated binding, which has slower binding kinetics. The Arg-Gly-Asp (RGD) sequence within the C1 domain also contributes to platelet adhesion by interacting with GPIIb-IIIa of activated platelets.[9]

FVIII Stabilization

vWF binds FVIII through the D'D3 domains and protects it from proteolytic degradation, thereby prolonging its half-life. In the absence of vWF, FVIII has a half-life of approximately 2 hours in contrast to a normal half-life of 12 to 20 hours when bound to vWF.[10]

BASAL vWF LEVELS

The normal level for vWF is highly variable and ranges from 50 to 200 IU/dL.[11] Factors that contribute to the variable vWF levels include ABO genotype (see section on ABO blood groups later), Secretor genotype, race, and age. Although plasma vWF concentrations have been reported to be approximately 20% higher in subjects homozygous for the Secretor (Se) allele as compared with those who are heterozygous,[12] studies exploring this relationship have yielded inconsistent results.[13] vWF levels in African Americans are 15% higher than those in whites.[14] Increased age has also been associated with higher vWF levels,[15,16] with studies suggesting that the levels may increase by as much as 15 to 17 units/mL per decade.[17] In addition, older age is associated with lower ADAMTS13 activity,[18] which together with the higher vWF levels, may contribute to the hypercoagulability that can be seen in older adults.

Within subjects, vWF levels often vary over time as a result of β-adrenergic stimuli, drugs, or more sustained physiologic factors, such as pregnancy, hypothyroidism, chronic illness, or long-term use of certain medications. The vasopressin analog, 1-deamino-(8-D-arginine)-vasopressin (DDAVP, desmopressin) transiently and reliably increases vWF and FVIII levels—a fact that, in addition to an acceptable side effect profile, has led to the use of desmopressin as first-line treatment in certain types of vWD and mild hemophilia A. Several physiologic stressors involving β-adrenergic stimulation, such as exercise[19,20] and psychologic distress, can produce an acute increase in vWF levels. Similarly, surgery and trauma are also associated with an immediate increase in vWF levels. vWF levels remain elevated for up to 6 days after surgery,[21] suggesting that after the acute secretory response, there is upregulation of vWF production. A sustained elevation of vWF levels can occur with chronic diseases, such as hyperthyroidism, renal failure, diabetes, liver disease, atherosclerosis, chronic inflammatory states, and cancer.[10] Conversely, acquired vWD, characterized by qualitative or quantitative vWF defects, can occur with certain medications, such as valproic acid, and with some chronic medical conditions (see section later on acquired vWD).

vWF levels are increased by estrogen. In premenopausal women, vWF levels vary in a cyclical fashion, with the lowest levels occurring in the early follicular phase of the menstrual cycle (days 1 to 7) and peak values occurring during the luteal phase.[17] Oral contraceptives increase vWF levels and dampen the cyclical variation. This dose-dependent effect is mediated by the estrogen component and evident with ethynylestradiol doses of 0.5 mcg or higher. Lower estrogen doses have little or no effect on vWF levels. vWF levels increase in pregnancy starting in the second trimester and achieve levels threefold higher than baseline values by the end of the third trimester.[11,22] vWF levels return to baseline 2 to 3 weeks after delivery.

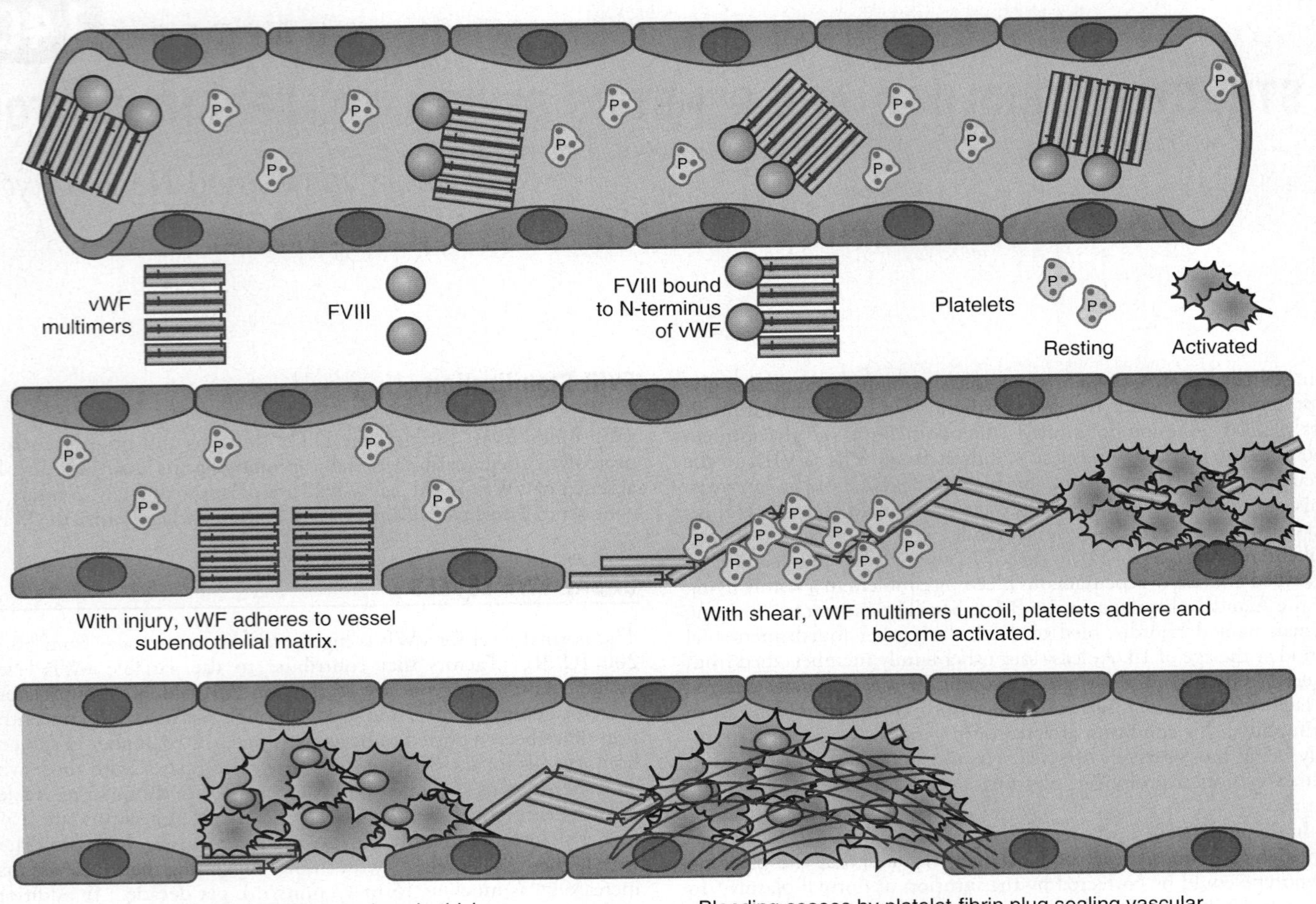

vWF multimers
FVIII
FVIII bound to N-terminus of vWF
Platelets
Resting
Activated
With injury, vWF adheres to vessel subendothelial matrix.
With shear, vWF multimers uncoil, platelets adhere and become activated.
Activated platelets expose phosphatidyl serine and bind FVIII to facilitate clotting.
Bleeding ceases by platelet-fibrin plug sealing vascular injury and is followed by thrombolysis and tissue repair.

Figure 140-1 FUNCTION OF vWF. Role of vWF in mediating the initial events in the hemostatic process. vWF is the carrier protein for FVIII *(top)*. After endothelial injury, vWF adheres to the exposed subendothelium, where it is uncoiled by the shear forces, thereby exposing GP1bα binding sites that interact with platelets *(middle)*. The bound platelets are activated, and the GpIIb-IIIa complex is exposed on the platelet surface. Interaction of fibrinogen and vWF with GpIIb-IIIa then consolidates the platelet adhesive event and initiates platelet aggregation *(bottom)*. *(Used with permission of Robert Montgomery.)*

vWF GENE

The vWF gene was cloned and characterized by four groups simultaneously in 1985.[3-6] Located on the short arm of chromosome 12 at p13.3, the vWF gene spans 178 kb and is composed of 52 exons that range in size from 1.3 kb (exon 28) to 40 bp (exon 50)[23] (Fig. 140-2). In humans, there is a partial, unprocessed pseudogene, vWFP, located on the long arm chromosome 22 at q 11.2, measuring 21 to 29 kb, which duplicates the vWF gene sequence for exons 23-34 with 97% sequence homology. The pseudogene contributes to the mutation spectrum of vWD through gene conversion,[24] although the frequency of this is unknown. The vWF gene is highly polymorphic. To date, more than 160 polymorphisms have been identified in the exons and closely flanking intronic sequences; these normal variants include promoter polymorphisms, a highly variable tetranucleotide repeat in intron 40, two insertion/deletion polymorphisms and 132 distinct single-nucleotide polymorphisms (SNPs) involving exon and intron sequences. An ISTH-SSC (International Society on Thrombosis and Haemostasis Scientific and Standardization Committee) database of both polymorphisms and mutations is maintained at the University of Sheffield (http://www.shef.ac.uk/vwf/). The high degree of polymorphism in the vWF gene, the large size of the gene, and the presence of the pseudogene render full gene sequencing and data interpretation challenging.

The vWF amino acid sequence contains four homologous repeated segments, named A through D, which make up approximately 90% of the precursor. These homologues also occur in a number of unrelated proteins. For example, vWF A domains appear in up to 22 human genes, such as leukocyte adhesion receptors, collagen receptors, and cartilage matrix protein. Likewise, homologues of vWF domains B, C, D, and CK exist throughout the genome, where they are found in proteins with various functions. This suggests that the vWF gene is the product of a complex series of partial gene duplications.[23]

The expression of the vWF gene is tightly restricted to endothelial cells, platelets, and megakaryocytes. Cell-specific transcriptional regulation is complex and poorly understood. A 734–base pair region, spanning approximately 500 bases of the 5′-flanking region and 247 bases into the first exon, functions as a promoter and includes a minimal core promoter, as well as negative and positive regulatory regions.[25] The positive regulatory region confers cell-specificity by relieving inhibition in specific cells, thereby allowing transcription of the vWF gene.

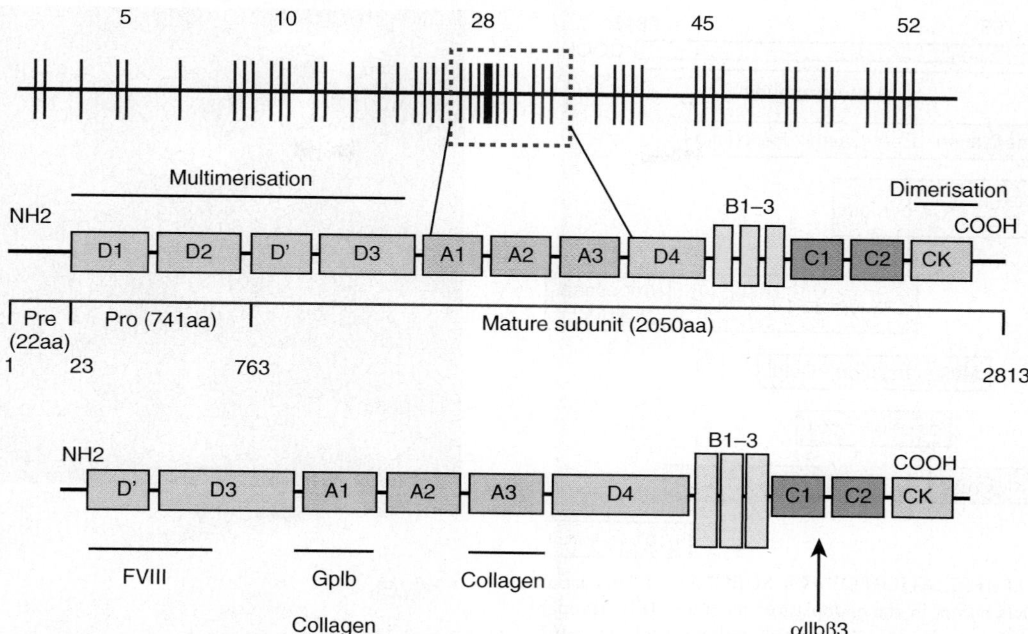

Figure 140-2 vWF GENE, mRNA AND PROTEIN. The vWF *gene* is located on chromosome 12 at p13.3 and spans 178 kb and includes 52 exons. The mRNA is 8.8 kb in length. Prepro-vWF contains 2813 amino acids (AA) with a 22-AA signal peptide, a 741-AA propeptide, and a 2050-AA mature subunit. The mature subunit consists of repeated domains *(A-D),* several of which have distinct functions and binding sites.

DOMAIN STRUCTURE

Encoded vWF mRNA is 8.8 kb in length and the translated prepro-vWF molecule contains 2813 amino acids (AA), comprising a 22 AA signal peptide, a 741 AA propeptide, and a 2050 AA secreted mature subunit that possesses all of the adhesive sites required for the hemostatic function of vWF.[26,27] The AA sequence is rich in cysteine residues, which make up 8.3% of the prepro-vWF and are abundant in all of the domains except the A domains, where only six cysteine residues are found. Cysteine residues are involved not only in interchain disulfide bonds, but also in intrachain disulfide bonds.

The domain structure of vWF, which consists of repeated domains, is arranged in the following sequence: S-D1-D2-D′-D3-A1-A2-A3-D4-B1-B2-B3-C1-C2-CK. Functional domains important for multimerization, cleavage, and binding have been identified. The signal peptide (S) targets prepro-vWF to the endoplasmic reticulum (ER), where it is promptly cleaved. The cysteine knot (CK) domains of adjacent vWF monomers form disulfide bonds, resulting in tail-to-tail dimers. The vWF pro-peptide (domains D1-D2), previously known as vWF antigen II, plays an important role in vWF multimer assembly by promoting the formation of head-to-head oligomers through disulfide bonds involving D3.[28] The A2 domain contains the Tyr1605-Met1606 cleavage site for ADAMTS13 (a disintegrin and metalloproteinase with a thrombospondin type 1 motif, member 13), which reduces both the size and the thrombogenicity of vWF multimers within the circulation.

Integral to vWF function, the vWF subunit possesses several binding sites, almost entirely encoded by exon 28 and including domains D′-D3-A1-A2-A3. In addition, the C1 domain, encoded by exons 42-44, contains a binding site. The D′ and D3 domains contain the FVIII-binding sites,[29] which interact with the N-terminus portion of the FVIII light chain.[30] vWF interacts with platelets via two platelet receptors; glycoprotein Ibα (GPIbα) and GPIIb/IIIa, which mediate platelet adhesion to injured subendothelium and the aggregation of activated platelets, respectively. The binding site for GPIbα is localized within the large disulfide loop of A1,[31] whereas the binding site for GPIIb/IIIa is found within the RGD sequence of C1.[9] The major binding site for collagen is found within the A3 domain, but the A1 domain has also been shown to bind collagen.[32,33]

BIOSYNTHESIS

von Willebrand factor is synthesized in endothelial cells[34] and megakaryocytes[35] as a protein subunit that undergoes a complex series of posttranslational modifications, including dimerization, glycosylation, sulfation, and ultimately, multimerization. The fully processed protein is then either released into the circulation or is stored in specialized organelles: the Weibel-Palade bodies (WPBs) of endothelial cells or the α-granules of platelets.

Dimerization of pro-vWF monomers occurs in the endoplasmic reticulum through the formation of disulfide bonds between CK domains monomers in a "tail-to-tail" fashion. The location of these intersubunit disulfide bonds has been localized to a subset of cysteine residues (Cys2771, Cys2773, and/or Cys2811).[36] In addition, the signal peptide is cleaved and most of the intrachain disulphide bonds are formed in the ER. Only pro-vWF dimers are then transported to the Golgi apparatus, where they make up the basic building blocks for further multimerization. Here, the propeptide (D1-D2) is cleaved by a propeptide processing protease, likely furin, between amino acids 763-764. The propeptide continues to be essential for vWF multimerization because under acidic conditions, it serves as an endogenous chaperone that promotes additional disulfide bond formation between D3 domains of adjacent dimers in a "head-to-head" orientation.[37] The intersubunit disulfide bonds are likely mediated by the alignment of the cysteine pairs C1099 and C1142.[38] The vWF subunit is approximately 250 kDa, whereas resulting disulfide-linked multimers can be more than 20,000 kDa (Fig. 140-3).

The mature vWF subunit is heavily glycosylated with carbohydrate making up approximately 20% of the mass of the mature subunit.[26] Although the function of these oligosaccharide chains is largely unknown, they appear to protect vWF from proteolytic degradation,[39] maintain the multimeric structure of vWF,[40] affect vWF

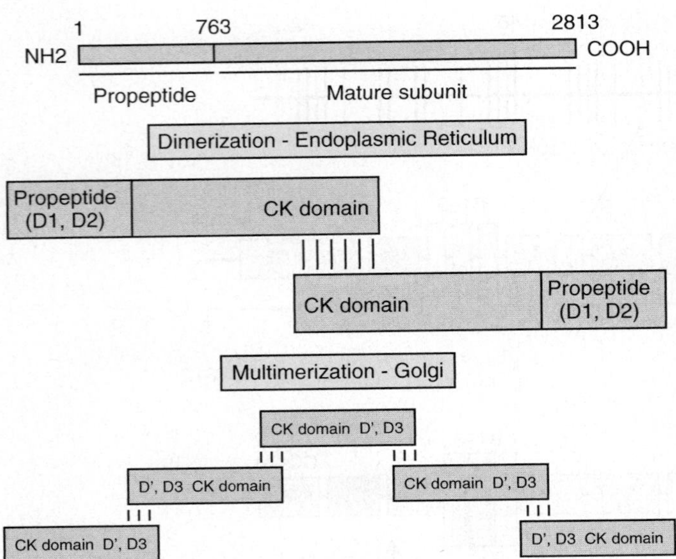

Figure 140-3 MULTIMERIZATION OF vWF SUBUNITS. Dimerization of pro-vWF monomers occurs in the endoplasmic reticulum (ER) through disulfide linkage of CK domains in a "tail-to-tail" fashion. Only pro-vWF dimers are transported to the Golgi, where they constitute the building blocks for further multimerization. Although the propeptide (D1-D2) is cleaved by a propeptide processing protease, it is essential for vWF multimerization because it serves as a chaperone that promotes further disulfide bond formation between adjacent D3 domains in a "head-to-head" orientation.

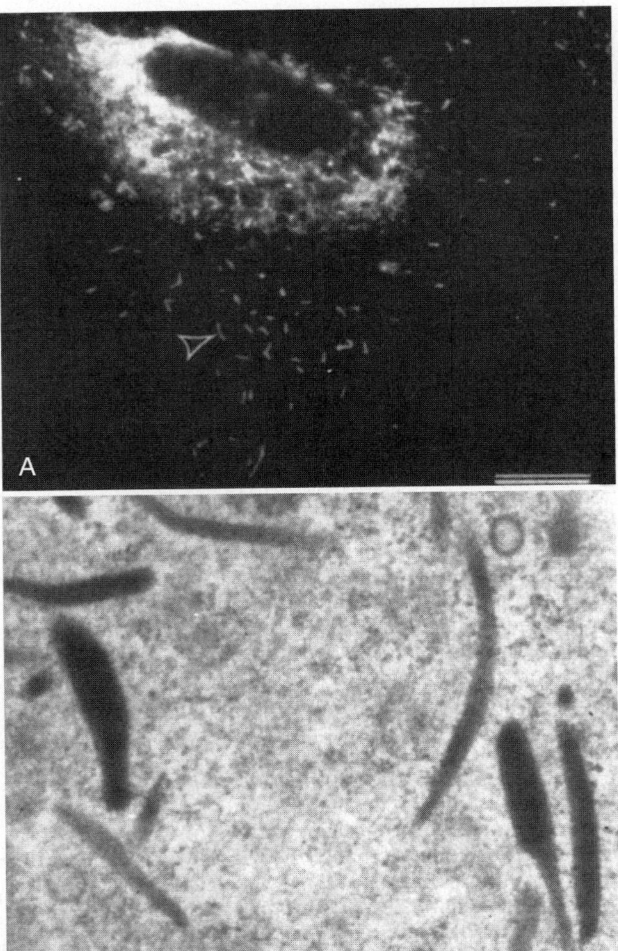

Figure 140-4 WEIBEL-PALADE BODIES OF ENDOTHELIAL CELLS. **A,** Immunofluorescence staining of a human umbilical vein endothelial cell with anti-vWF antiserum. vWF is present in the perinuclear region, where it is synthesized, and in the Weibel-Palade bodies *(arrowhead)* throughout the cytoplasm. Bar = 10 μm. **B,** Electron micrograph of Weibel-Palade bodies of the same origin. Bar = 0.5 μm. *vWF,* von Willebrand factor.

interaction with platelets and collagen, and influence plasma clearance of vWF.[41] In the ER, 12 N-linked high-mannose-containing oligosaccharide chains are added to each vWF subunit, and these appear to be necessary for vWF subunit dimerization. In addition, the propeptide has three additional potential N-glycosylation sites. Posttranslational modification continues in the Golgi with the addition of 10 O-linked oligosaccharides to the peptide chain, and the sulfation of certain N-linked oligosaccharides, such as Asn384 and Asn468.[27] The previously added N-linked glycans undergo further processing with the addition of ABO groups, as determined by the ABO genotype, in the post-Golgi compartment.[42] ABO blood groups affect the proteolysis of vWF by ADAMTS13[43] as well as the clearance of vWF from the circulation[41] (see the later section on ABO blood groups). The cleaved propeptide remains noncovalently associated with vWF multimers and is stored and secreted with the mature vWF in a 1 : 1 molar ratio.

STORAGE AND SECRETION

Most of the vWF in endothelial cells consists of small multimers that are constitutively secreted. The more biologically active high-molecular-weight (HMW) vWF multimers are preferentially targeted for storage in endothelium-specific cytoplasmic granules called *Weibel-Palade bodies.*[44] In addition to vWF and the vWF propeptide, WBPs also store P-selectin, CD63, IL-8,[45] tissue plasminogen activator (tPA),[46] and angiopoietin-2.[47] Thus WPBs store proteins that are involved not only in hemostasis, but also in inflammation, hemodynamics, and angiogenesis. WPBs have a characteristic cigar-like shape, measuring 0.2 μm wide and 5 μm long (Fig. 140-4), and are composed of tightly packed tubules, measuring 150 Å to 200 Å in cross-section. Platelet vWF is stored within similar tubules that are found in the periphery of α-granules[48] and constitutes approximately 15% of total blood vWF. Tubular packing condenses the length of vWF multimer by 50-fold[49] and is dependent on the acidic pH within the trans Golgi, as well as the propeptide (D1D2) and the NH_2-terminal region (D′D3A1).[50] Long vWF multimers, which can be up to 100 μm, are reversibly packaged into coils. With WPB exocytosis, the filamentous strings of vWF are secreted into the circulation, where they rapidly unfurl and are capable of binding to platelets. If the tubular structure is perturbed, WPBs release short, tangled vWF that does not support platelet binding to the endothelium.

A variety of agonists can induce the secretion of vWF from endothelial cells. These agonists include histamine, thrombin, fibrin, the terminal complement proteins C5b-9, and β-adrenergic agonists. With endothelial cell stimulation, WPBs fuse with the plasma membrane to form a secretion pore. This leads to a rapid rise in pH and release of intracellular calcium stores.[51] The freshly secreted unusually large (or ultra-large) vWF multimers (ULvWF) are highly active and can spontaneously bind platelets. Some of the released protein remains associated with the endothelial membrane,[52] and some self-associate.[53] The activity of these ULvWF multimers is regulated by ADAMTS13-mediated proteolysis.

ADAMTS13

ADAMTS13 is a plasma protease that cleaves circulating vWF between Tyr 1605 and Met 1606 in the A2 domain. ADAMTS13 regulates the function of vWF. Its main target is the ULvWF multimers, which spontaneously bind GPIbα platelet receptor; it cleaves these multimers when they under sufficient shear to unfold the A2 domain the cleavage site is exposed.[54] ULvWF multimers that appear in plasma after WPB secretion are cleaved within 2 hours by ADAMTS13 to form shorter, less hemostatically active multimers.[55] Proteolysis of vWF multimers is responsible for the characteristic "triplet" pattern of satellite bands flanking each main multimer band that is observed on multimer analysis gels.

vWF proteolysis is influenced by glycosylation and specific polymorphisms. For example, nonglycosylated recombinant vWF is degraded more rapidly than its plasma-derived glycosylated counterparts.[39] Likewise, addition of A or B blood group antigens to N-linked oligosaccharide chains of vWF reduces ADAMTS13 proteolysis compared with vWF bearing the O blood group antigen.[43] Single-nucleotide polymorphisms, such as the A/G polymorphism at position 24/1282 resulting in Tyr/Cys at 1584, have also been shown to affect the susceptibility of vWF to proteolysis.[56]

Alterations in the balance between ADAMTS13 activity and vWF proteolysis can lead to a number of disease states. Congenital or acquired deficiency of ADAMTS13 can result in thrombotic thrombocytopenic purpura (see Chapter 136). On the other hand, enhanced proteolysis can give rise to a bleeding phenotype. For example, mutant vWF in a subtype of type 2A vWD exhibits enhanced susceptibility to ADAMTS13 cleavage, which results in loss of large vWF multimers[57] (see the later section on vWD type 2A).

CLEARANCE

Although the mechanism and location of vWF clearance is largely unknown, data suggest that macrophages in the liver and spleen internalize and clear vWF in a process that is independent of multimer size.[58] In a recent metaanalysis of genome-wide association studies, loci outside of the vWF gene that contribute to the highly variable vWF levels in normal populations were identified.[59] CLEC4M (C-type lectin domain family 4, member M) and STAB2 (stabilin 2) are two transmembrane sinusoidal endothelial cell receptors that may be involved in vWF clearance. Further studies are needed to explore this possibility.

The cleaved propeptide remains associated with vWF multimers stored in WPB and is secreted in a 1:1 molar ratio with the mature vWF subunit. After secretion, the propeptide (vWFpp) dissociates from vWF and circulates at a concentration of approximately 1 mcg/mL. The propeptide has a half-life of 2 to 3 hours and no known function.[60] In contrast, vWF circulates at a plasma concentration of approximately 10 mcg/mL and has a half-life of approximately 8 to 12 hours. The ratio between vWFpp and mature vWF (vWFpp/vWF:Ag) can be used to estimate the relative half-life of mature vWF; elevated ratios indicate enhanced clearance.[61]

Changes in vWF glycosylation or point mutations can be associated with increased clearance. Blood group O subjects (see the following section on ABO Blood Groups) exhibit increased vWF clearance compared with the other blood types and have consistently elevated vWFpp/vWF:Ag ratios and shorter vWF survival after desmopresssin.[41]

Several point mutations may lead to increased vWF clearance and are associated with either a type 1 or type 2A vWD phenotype.[62] The vast majority of these are localized to the D3 domain (e.g., R1205H and C1130F), but point mutations in the A1 (I1416N), CK (C2617), and D4 domains (S2179F) have also been implicated.

vWF mutations associated with increased clearance are not necessarily associated with increased susceptibility to proteolysis by ADAMTS13 and vice versa.[63,64] For example, the vWD Vicenza mutation, R1205, is the prototypical clearance mutation. Patients with this mutation have severely reduced plasma FVIII and vWF levels, an increased vWFpp/vWF:Ag, and a marked increase in FVIII and vWF after desmopressin with a significantly shortened half-life of 1 to 2 hours. However, there is no association between increased clearance of this mutant vWF and altered susceptibility to ADAMTS13 proteolysis.[65]

ABO BLOOD GROUPS

Blood group O subjects have vWF levels that are on average 25% lower than those with non-O blood type: the mean vWF level in blood group O subjects is 74.8 IU/dL as compared with 105.9 IU/dL, 116.9 IU/dL and 123.3 IU/dL in blood group A, B and AB subjects, respectively.[15] ABO antigens are added to N-linked oligosaccharide chains on the vWF subunit. Thus patients with the type O blood group genotype lack a functional glycosyltransferase that adds *N*-acetylgalactosamine and *D*-galactose to the H antigen on vWF in blood group A and B subjects, respectively. Altered glycosylation of vWF in subjects with blood type O leads to lower plasma vWF levels as a result of increased proteolysis and/or increased clearance. Blood group O vWF is more susceptible to ADAMTS13 proteolysis,[43] and blood group O subjects have elevated vWFpp:vWFAg ratios and shorter vWF survival after desmopressin.[41] The mean half-life of vWF in type O subjects is approximately 10 hours compared with a half-life of approximately 25.5 hours in those with other ABO blood types. Clinically, the difference in vWF levels results in an overrepresentation of blood group O patients with type 1 vWD, which is defined by a reduction in vWF levels.

AREAS OF ONGOING INVESTIGATION

There is emerging evidence that vWF may have a role in the regulation of VEGF-dependent angiogenesis directly through its interaction with integrins on endothelial cells and indirectly via regulation of WPB formation and secretion of constituents such as angiopoietin-2.[66] In addition, vWF may protect against tumor metastasis.[67,68] Patients with increased vWF levels are at risk for cardiovascular events; it is unclear whether vWF contributes to atherosclerosis or whether it is a marker of endothelial dysfunction.[69] Nonetheless, vWF plays an important role in atherothrombosis, and drugs targeting vWF attenuate arterial thrombosis in animal models. Their utility in humans is unknown.

VON WILLEBRAND DISEASE

vWD, which is caused by deficient or defective plasma vWF, is the most common inherited bleeding disorder, affecting as much as 0.1 to 1% of the population.[70-72] The most common bleeding symptoms reflect the defect in primary hemostasis: mucocutaneous bleeding, especially epistaxis and menorrhagia. In some cases, FVIII levels may be sufficiently low that the bleeding phenotype overlaps with that of mild to moderate hemophilia; these patients may experience joint or muscle bleeds. The current vWD classification recognizes three subtypes.[73] Type 1 vWD is characterized by quantitative deficiency of essentially normal vWF, type 2 vWD is characterized by qualitative defects in vWF, and type 3 vWD is characterized by an almost complete quantitative deficiency of vWF. The classification incorporates important aspects of clinical phenotype, pathophysiologic mechanisms, and treatment considerations. The two main treatments are desmopressin (1-deamino-8-D-arginine vasopressin [DDAVP]) and clotting factor concentrates containing both vWF and FVIII (vWF/FVIII concentrate). Other treatment options include antifibrinolytic agents (tranexamic acid) and hormone therapy (oral contraceptive pill). Areas of ongoing research include defining the role of prophylaxis in vWD, optimizing the use of current therapies, such as tranexamic acid, and development of recombinant vWF replacement products.

Epidemiology

vWD is the most common inherited bleeding disorder. However, because vWF levels are highly variable in the populations and disease severity ranges from infrequent, mild bleeding symptoms to frequent, severe, or life-threatening bleeds, the prevalence of vWD depends on the diagnostic criteria and the study population. In two large epidemiologic studies, the prevalence of vWD was approximately 1% in healthy school-age children based on low vWF activity, measured as ristocetin cofactor, and a personal and family history of bleeding symptoms.[70,71] More recent studies suggest that the prevalence of vWD in individuals who present to a primary care physician with bleeding symptoms is approximately 0.1%,[74] whereas in patients whose bleeding symptoms are sufficiently severe to warrant referral to specialized centers, the prevalence of vWD ranges from 20 to 113 per million.[10]

Classification and Pathophysiology

The ISTH classification of vWD was updated in 2006.[73] This classification is clinically useful and relies on the vWF protein phenotype, which in turn often reflects the underlying pathophysiology and has implications on treatment approach. There are three primary categories: type 1, which is a partial quantitative deficiency; type 2 (with four subtypes—2A, 2B, 2M, and 2B), which is a qualitative defect; and type 3, which is a virtual deficiency of vWF (Table 140-1). In most cases, the diagnosis and categorization of vWD into a type can be achieved with widely available laboratory testing. However, further subcategorization, such as the differentiation among certain vWD type 2 subtypes, may require referral to a specialized laboratory. Because gene sequencing is not widely available, the current classification does not incorporate genotypic data. Also, the diagnosis of vWD is not limited to individuals with mutations within the vWF gene; vWF mutations may not be identified in vWD patients because of the complexity of the vWF gene, and mutations in other genes, such as those affecting secretion or clearance, also lead to a vWD phenotype. A third level of classification denoted by Roman numerals (e.g., vWD type 2A IIA) indicates specific phenotypes and is a remnant of an older classification system that is mainly used in the research setting (Table 140-2).

vWD Type 1

Type 1 vWD, a partial quantitative deficiency of vWF, represents approximately 70% of vWD cases. The vWF is functionally normal without a specific abnormality in ligand binding sites or a significant decrease in HMW multimers. Functional assays of vWF, such as vWF:RCo, are decreased in proportion to the decrease in vWF:Ag concentration, and the ratio of functional activity as compared with vWF:Ag is normal (i.e., vWF:RCo/vWF:Ag ratio is >0.6). Thus bleeding in this disorder is the result of decreases in the concentration of normal vWF.

Table 140-1 Classification of von Willebrand Disease

Type	Description
1	Partial quantitative deficiency of vWF. Mild abnormalities in multimer structure or distribution may occur.
2	Qualitative vWF defects.
2A	Decreased vWF-dependent platelet adhesion and deficiency of HMW vWF multimers.
2B	Increased affinity for platelet GPIbα.
2M	Decreased vWF-dependent platelet adhesion with a normal multimer distribution.
2N	Decreased affinity for FVIII.
3	Almost complete deficiency of vWF.

FVIII, Factor FVIII; *HMW*, high-molecular-weight; *vWF*, von Willebrand factor.

Point mutations, most frequently missense mutations, have been identified in approximately 65% of individuals with type 1 vWD and occur throughout the vWF gene.[75-77] Fully penetrant, dominantly inherited missense mutations are more often identified when vWF:Ag and vWF:RCo levels are less than 25 IU/dL. In contrast, incompletely penetrant, dominantly inherited missense mutations, such as p.Tyr1584Cys and p.Arg924Gln are identified in approximately 50% of individuals whose vWF:Ag and vWF:RCo levels are above 25 IU/dL.[77,78] The extent to which incompletely penetrant vWF mutations contribute to bleeding phenotype in individuals with vWF levels of about 50 IU/dL is not clear, and genetic analyses in such cases are difficult to interpret.

Missense mutations may affect vWF levels by reducing secretion and/or increasing clearance. The most frequently reported genetic mutation is a missense mutation that results in the substitution of tyrosine with cysteine at codon 1584 (Y1584C), which is found in 10% to 20% of type 1 vWD patients.[75-77] Intracellular retention is a common mechanism for type 1 vWD pathogenicity and can result from missense mutations in various vWF domains.[79] Haploinsufficiency from a heterozygous null allele results in reduced vWF expression in a small proportion of cases. A common heterozygous in-frame large deletion of exons 4-5 was reported in a cohort of type 1 vWD patients[80] in the United Kingdom, and this and similar partial gene deletions may contribute to the spectrum of mutation in a minority of cases. A well-described pathophysiologic mechanism for vWD type 1 is increased vWF clearance.[62] Patients with increased clearance typically have very low vWF levels, an increased vWFpp/vWF:Ag ratio, and a marked but short-lived response to desmopressin. Of note, the half-life of vWF/FVIII concentrates is normal in these individuals.[81] Missense mutations mainly occur in the D3 domain and reduce the half-life of vWF up to 15-fold. R1205H, which is known as the "Vicenza" variant, is the most common, most severe, and best characterized of these mutations.[82,83] Such mutations have been referred to as *type 1C* (C for increased clearance), although this designation is not included in the ISTH classification. Because of the transient response to desmopressin, the utility of this medication for treatment of major bleeds is questioned in this subgroup of patients. However, desmopressin may still be useful for management of most minor bleeds or minor surgical procedures.[84]

vWD Type 2

Type 2 vWD is characterized by a qualitative deficiency of vWF activity and is further classified into the qualitative variants that affect

Table 140-2 Subclassification of Type 2 vWD

Subtype	Location of Missense Mutations (Domains)	Inheritance	Mechanism
IIA	A1, A2	Dominant	Enhance susceptibility to ADAMTS13 proteolysis
IIC	D1, D2	Recessive	Affects the propeptide and results in impaired multimer assembly
IID	CK	Dominant	Impaired dimer assembly
IIE	D2, D3	Dominant	Usually involves a cysteine residue important for intersubunit disulfide bonds and multimerization

vWF-platelet interactions (2A, 2B, and 2M) and the rare type 2N characterized by defective vWF binding to FVIII. Type 2 vWD is often suspected when investigations demonstrate a function discordance: the vWF:RCo, a function of platelet GP1B binding, is decreased out of proportion to the decrease in vWF:Ag, and a vWF:RCo/vWF:Ag ratio of less than 0.6 occurs (Fig. 140-5).

Type 2A

vWD type 2A is the most common type 2 variant, accounting for approximately 10% of all vWD cases. vWD type 2A usually is inherited as a dominant trait (although some variants are recessive) and is characterized by disproportionately low functional activity compared with antigen level (i.e., vWF:RCo to vWF:Ag ratio of <0.6). The FVIII level may be low or normal. Ristocetin-induced platelet agglutination (RIPA) is reduced, and the multimer profile shows a loss of HMW and sometimes intermediate-molecular-weight (IMW) multimers. This subtype may encompass missense mutations that impair dimer (CK domain)[85] or multimer assembly (recessive mutations in the D1 and D2 domains),[86,87] disrupt intersubunit disulphide bonds (D3 and D2 domains), enhance susceptibility to ADAMTS13-mediated proteolysis (A2 and A1 domains),[88] and/or result in intracellular retention of vWF, particularly the HMW multimers (D3, A1, and A2 domains).[89] High-resolution multimer gel electrophoresis patterns can provide clues as to the specific disease mechanism and recognize the following categories: IIA, IIC, IID, and IIE (see Table 140-2). All patterns result in the synthesis of vWF that possesses fewer GpIbα binding sites and is less effective in platelet clot formation. Regardless of the mechanism, clinically affected individuals are treated similarly.

Type 2B

Type 2B vWD is the result of gain-of-function mutations within the GpIbα binding site on vWF. Missense mutations are located in exon 28, in or close to the A1 domain.[90] This results in spontaneous binding of vWF to platelets without the need for a vWF collagen interaction. The vWF-platelet interactions selectively depletes the HMW multimers by increasing ADAMTS13 proteolysis.[90,91] The increased binding of mutant vWF to platelets also triggers the formation of platelet aggregates, which are removed from the circulation resulting in thrombocytopenia. Altered megakaryocytopoiesis characterized by giant platelets with abnormal ultrastructure contributes to the thrombocytopenia.[92]

The laboratory profile reveals a decreased vWF:RCo to vWF:Ag ratio and absence of HMW multimers, but in contrast to 2A, RIPA reveals increased sensitivity to low doses of ristocetin. Although these features may be present to varying degrees in the majority of patients, not all cases demonstrate these classic features. For example, mutations affecting p.Pro1266Leu may enhance GpIbα binding (RIPA) without inducing thrombocytopenia or HMW multimer loss.[93]

Type 2M

Type 2M vWD (the *M* refers to *multimer*) is characterized by decreased vWF-platelet interactions. The laboratory workup shows a reduced ratio of vWF:RCo to vWF:Ag but a normal multimer pattern. RIPA is also reduced. A number of missense mutations are reported in exon 28, with case reports in exons 27, 30-31, and 52. vWF exhibits reduced affinity for GpIbα, because of mutations in the A1 domain that alter protein conformation, but HMW multimers are normal.[94] Mutations in the A3 domain that impair the vWF/collagen interaction[95,96] are also classified as 2M vWD. In these cases, vWF:RCo may be normal, and the diagnosis requires vWF/collagen binding assays (vWF:CB).

Type 2N

Type 2N vWD (with the *N* referring to *Normandy,* where the first cases were reported) has been described as an autosomal form of hemophilia A and is important in the differential diagnosis of individuals of either sex who present with low FVIII levels. The characteristic laboratory feature is a disproportionate reduction in the FVIII level relative to the vWF level (which may be low or normal) with a resultant FVIII/vWF:Ag ratio that is reduced.[97] Affinity of vWF for FVIII is reduced because of mutations of the FVIII binding site or conformational changes that impair the vWF-FVIII interaction. The majority of patients with vWD type 2N have a normal multimeric profile, but occasional cases will demonstrate loss of HMW multimers. The majority (≈ 80%) of missense mutations are located in exons 18-20 (D′ and D3) with a much lower proportion of mutations in exons 17 and 24-27.[98] Type 2N exhibits autosomal recessive inheritance, and affected individuals are either homozygous or compound heterozygous for missense mutations, or compound heterozygous for a missense mutation and a mutation resulting in a null allele. The latter mutations are found throughout the vWF gene; p.Arg854Gln occurs in 2% of white populations and frequently contributes to the phenotype.[99,100] Definitive diagnosis requires evidence of reduced FVIII binding to vWF (vWF:FVIIIB) or the identification of causative mutations in the FVIII binding region of the *vWF* gene.[101]

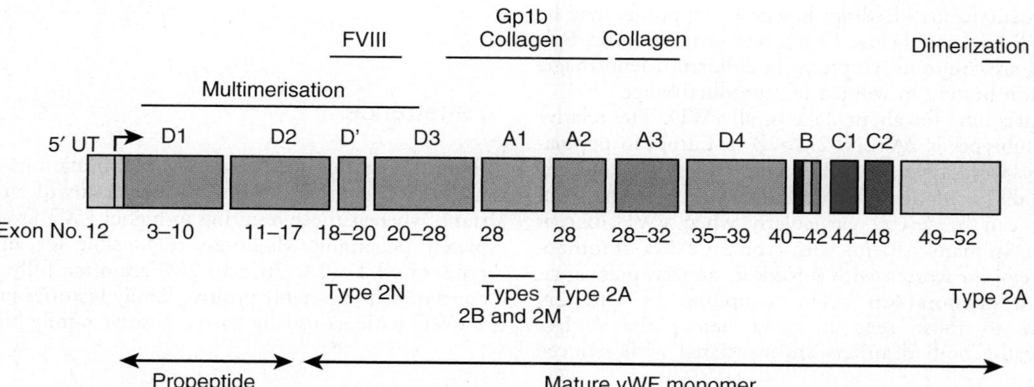

Figure 140-5 FUNCTIONAL DOMAINS OF vWF AND LOCATION OF TYPE 2 vWD MUTATIONS. vWF protein comprises a large N-terminal propeptide and mature subunit. Repeated protein domains are designated *A* through *D*. Highlighted are binding sites for factor VIII, platelet Gp1b, and collagen and the areas critical for dimerization and multimerization. Sites of the common mutations that result in type 2 vWD are shown. *Arrow* indicates translational start site.

Type 3 vWD

This subtype of vWD is defined by a virtual absence of vWF. The inheritance of type 3 vWD is autosomal recessive, and although parents of affected individuals are often asymptomatic, there is growing evidence that obligate carriers of type 3 vWD mutations have more mucocutaneous bleeding symptoms than normal individuals.[102] This condition is characterized by prolongation of the aPTT, undetectable levels of vWF : Ag, and vWF : RCo and FVIII levels less than 10 international units/dL (10%). Mutations associated with type 3 vWD are found throughout the coding region of vWF (i.e., exons 2-52). Up to 80% of type 3 vWD patients have two null alleles and produce little or no vWF. Null alleles can result from a variety of mutations, with nonsense mutations accounting for about one-third of these.[103] Approximately 20% of alleles carry missense mutations predominantly located in the D1-D2 (exons 3-11) and D4-CK (exons 37-52) domains. These mutations may impair dimer or multimer formation, resulting in intracellular vWF retention and decreased secretion into plasma.[104] Large deletions, predominantly resulting in frameshift mutations affecting one or more exons, contribute to approximately 12% of the type 3 vWD mutation spectrum. Because there is little or no circulating vWF, patients with these mutations may develop alloantibodies to infused vWF, which can complicate treatment.[105]

Clinical Manifestations

Although vWD is a congenital bleeding disorder, symptoms may manifest only when there is a hemostatic challenge. Consequently, bleeding symptoms become more obvious with increasing age. The bleeding history also depends on disease severity; type 3 vWD is often diagnosed early in life, whereas mild type 1 vWD may not be diagnosed until adulthood, despite a history of bleeding episodes. Individuals with vWD primarily complain of excessive mucocutaneous bleeding, such as bruising without recognized trauma, prolonged, recurrent nose bleeds, and oral cavity bleeding, including bleeding from the gums after brushing or flossing the teeth or prolonged bleeding after dental cleaning or extractions. In addition, prolonged or excessive bleeding after surgery or trauma is often reported. Affected females frequently experience menorrhagia, usually since menarche, and have prolonged or excessive bleeding after childbirth.[106,107] Musculoskeletal bleeding is unusual, except in type 2N or type 3 vWD when the FVIII : C level may be below 10 international units/dL. Clinical assessment scoring tools are helpful for vWD diagnosis (see Chapter 130) (see box on Case Example of the Presentation and Impact of Type 1 vWD).

Type 1 vWD accounts for up to 70% of vWD. It typically manifests as mild mucocutaneous bleeding; however, symptoms may be more severe if vWF levels are below 15 international units/dL. Epistaxis and bruising are common symptoms in children. Menorrhagia is the most common finding in women of reproductive age.

Type 2 vWD accounts for about 25% of all vWD. The relative frequency of the subtypes is 2A>2N>2M>2B in European populations. Individuals with type 2A, 2B, and 2M vWD usually present with mild to moderate mucocutaneous bleeding, but bleeding episodes can be severe, particularly when vWF : RCo is very low or absent. In many patients with type 2B vWD, thrombocytopenia can develop or worsen with infection, surgery, pregnancy, or treatment with desmopressin.[93] The symptoms of type 2N vWD are similar to those seen in mild hemophilia A (see Chapter 137) because both disorders are associated with reduced levels of FVIII : C.

Type 3 vWD is the most rare of the subtypes and accounts for less than 5% of vWD. Prevalence estimates range from 0.55 to 6 per million, with higher rates seen with consanguineous marriage.[10] Type 3 vWD manifests with severe bleeding, including excessive mucocutaneous bleeding and musculoskeletal bleeding.

Example of the Presentation and Impact of Type 1 vWD

J.C. is a 26-year-old female who presented with delayed postpartum hemorrhage (PPH) after the delivery of her first child. The pregnancy and delivery had been unremarkable. One week postpartum, the patient began to experience heavy bleeding, necessitating intervention on behalf of the obstetrician in the form of dilation and curettage. At the same time, J.C. was initiated on tranexamic acid, which was continued for 2 weeks. Complete cessation of bleeding occurred at approximately 3 weeks postpartum. This complication led to a referral to a hematologist. A bleeding history was significant for the following: excessive postsurgical bleeding as a child following tonsillectomy and adenoidectomy, which required nasal packing and RBC transfusion; excessive bleeding postdental extractions, requiring consultation with the dentist and repacking; mennorhagia from the time of menarche, which had been well controlled with the combined oral contraceptive pill. There is no family history of vWD. Investigations revealed vWF : Ag 0.45 international units/dL, vWF : RCo 0:39 IU/dL, and FVIII : C 0.60 IU/dL. Multimer gel was unremarkable. A DDAVP challenge demonstrated that the patient was a responder. Finally, ferritin was significantly decreased at 8 mcg/dL, with an associated microcytic anemia (hemoglobin 9.2 g/dL and MCV 72 fL). J.C. was initiated on iron supplementation with resolution of her iron deficiency. She became pregnant again 4 years later. At the time of delivery, she was treated with tranexamic acid and a dose of DDAVP after the cord was clamped. Her postpartum course was uncomplicated.

This case illustrates several important points. First, type 1 vWD is a mild to moderate bleeding disorder. Patients often do not have significant symptoms on a regular basis, or symptoms may be masked/ameliorated by concomitant combined oral contraceptive use, which is common in this patient demographic. A careful bleeding history, focusing on past hemostatic challenges and subsequent complications, is vital in making the diagnosis. A high index of suspicion in required for unusual bleeding complications, such as delayed PPH. The importance of making the diagnosis is highlighted here. With little burden of prophylactic treatment, bleeding complications can be avoided. Finally, women with vWD are at significantly increased risk for iron deficiency with subsequent anemia. This may have a significant impact on energy level and day-to-day physical and cognitive functioning.[160,161] In addition, iron deficiency is a risk factor for postpartum anemia, which itself is associated with impaired quality of life, reduced cognitive abilities, emotional instability, and depression.[162]

Penetrance

In autosomal dominant type 1 vWD, mutations resulting in plasma vWF level less than 25 international units/dL are often fully penetrant, whereas those resulting in higher vWF levels are often incompletely penetrant. Mutations responsible for autosomal dominant types of vWD (2A, 2B, and 2M) are often fully penetrant. Thus in contrast to the variably positive family histories in type 1 vWD, type 2 vWD patients usually have a positive family history.

Laboratory Investigations

The laboratory evaluation for vWD involves a battery of qualitative and quantitative measurements of vWF and FVIII that should be interpreted by a physician with experience in this area given the

Table 140-3 Table of Investigations

vWD Type	vWF : RCo IU/dL*	vWF : Ag IU/dL*	RCo/Ag IU/dL*	FVIII : C IU/dL*	Multimer Pattern†	Other
1	Low	Low	Equivalent	~1.5x vWF : Ag	Normal	
2A	Low	Low	vWF : RCo < vWF : Ag	Low or normal	Abnormal ↓ HMW	
2B	Low	Low	vWF : RCo < vWF : Ag	Low or normal	Abnormal ↓ HMW	↑RIPA‡ (↓ platelet count)
2M	Low	Low	vWF : RCo < vWF : Ag	Low or normal	Normal	
2N	Normal/low	Normal/low	Equivalent	<30	Normal	↓ vWF : FVIIIB§
3	Absent	Absent	NA	<10	Absent	

*Relative to the reference range (approximate values); vWF:RCo (50-200 IU/dL); vWF:Ag (50-200 IU/dL); FVIII:C (50-150 IU/dL).
†*HMW,* High-molecular-weight multimers.
‡Increased agglutination at low concentrations of ristocetin.
§The ability of vWF to bind and protect FVIII is reduced. vWF and FVIII levels can look exactly like those in males with mild haemophilia A or in symptomatic hemophilia A carrier females.

heterogeneity of possible results. Investigations should start with a complete blood count (CBC), along with determination of the activated partial thromboplastin time (aPTT) and prothrombin time (PT). The diagnosis is confirmed with assays of vWF : Ag, vWF : RCo, and FVIII, which are widely available. The last step is a battery of tests to distinguish among the subtypes of vWD (multimer gel electrophoresis, vWF : CB, RIPA, vWF : FVIIIB); these test are only available in specialized laboratories (Table 140-3).

Screening Tests

The CBC may show microcytic anemia as a result of iron deficiency or thrombocytopenia, particularly in type 2B vWD.[93] The aPTT is often normal, but may be prolonged if the FVIII level is reduced below 30 to 40 IU/dL, as can be seen in severe type 1, type 2N, or type 3 vWD. The PT is normal in vWD. Although some laboratories may also include a skin bleeding time and platelet function analysis (PFA closure time) in their evaluation of an individual with suspected vWD, these tests lack sensitivity in persons with mild bleeding or specificity for vWD.[108-110]

Confirming a Diagnosis of vWD

The following specific factor assays should be performed even if the screening tests are normal.[111]

vWF : Ag

This assay determines the quantity of vWF protein (antigen) in the plasma, measured using an enzyme-linked immunosorbant assay (ELISA) or latex immunoassay (LIA). The normal range (which should be determined independently by each laboratory) is approximately 50 to 200 IU/dL.

vWF : RCo

The ristocetin cofactor activity assay determines the capacity of vWF to agglutinate platelets in response to ristocetin. The normal range is approximately 50 to 200 IU/dL.

Factor VIII : C level

Functional FVIII assay determines the activity of FVIII in clot-bound assays. The normal range is approximately 50 to 150 IU/dL.

Normal plasma levels of vWF are approximately 100 IU/dL (100%, corresponds to approximately 10 mcg/mL) with a population range of 50 to 200 IU/dL (50% to 200%). These variations are influenced by a genetic and environmental factors, including ABO blood group (with vWF levels approximately 25% lower in type O individuals), physiologic stressors, and hormones. Several analytic variables also can complicate the diagnosis of vWD.[112] Based on established reference ranges, approximately 2.5% of the normal population will have low vWF levels. In addition, assay variability, particularly for vWF : RCo, renders differentiation of type 1 vWD from type 2 vWD difficult. vWF : RCo and vWF : Ag determined by latex immunoassay have limited sensitivity, which may result in the misdiagnosis of type 3 vWD as type 1 or type 2 vWD. Finally, preanalytic issues with sample handling can lead to decreases in vWF : Ag and vWF : RCo, which can complicate the diagnosis. All of these factors must be considered when interpreting vWF laboratory results and at least two sets of tests using fresh samples are needed to confirm the diagnosis of vWD. In addition, diagnostic testing should be avoided in stressed, ill, or pregnant patients (see box on Factors to Consider When Interpreting vWD Results).

Discriminating Tests to Identify vWD Subtype

vWF Multimer Analysis

SDS-agarose electrophoresis is used to assess vWF oligomers in plasma[113] (Fig. 140-6). Normal plasma contains multimers composed of over 40 vWF dimers. Multimers are classified as high, intermediate, or low molecular weight (HMW, IMW, LMW, respectively) by counting bands 1 to 5 as LMW, 6 to 10 as IMW and those above 10 as HMW (see www.isth.org/default/index.cfm/publication/ssc-minutes). HMW multimers are decreased or missing in types 2A and 2B vWD, and IMW multimers may also be absent in type 2A vWD. Abnormalities in satellite ("triplet") band patterns provide clues about pathogenesis and help to subclassify type 2A vWD, including IIA, IIC, IID, and IIE—for example, type 2A(IIE).[111,114]

Factors to Consider When Interpreting vWD Results

	Considerations	Results
Preanalytical	When was the sample collected and processed? Is there a significant length of time for travel/batching results before samples are run? Are they frozen in a timely fashion?	vWF:RCo may be decreased and result in a false-positive for type 2
Analytical	Convention of established references	False-positive diagnosis of vWD in 2.5% of population
	High degree of assay variability, particularly for vWF:RCo	False-positive diagnosis of type 2 in a type 1 patient may result in the misdiagnosis of type 3 for type 1 or type 2 vWD
	A high lower limit of detection (LOD) for certain vWF:Ag and vWF:RCo assays, in particular LIA-based assays	
Patient Factors	Drugs (OCP, HRT, or valproic acid)	False negative or positive
	ABO type	False negative
	Pregnancy	Reversible acquired von Willebrand syndrome (AvWS)
	Hypothyroidism	
	Comorbid illness (e.g., valvular heart disease, lymphoma)	

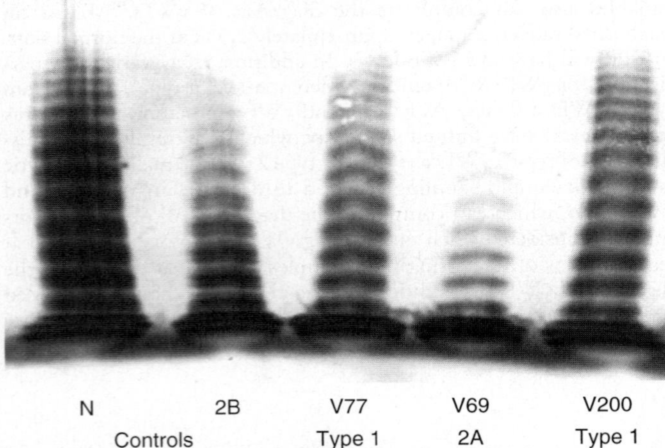

Figure 140-6 EXAMPLE OF A MULTIMER ANALYSIS. Lane 1 represents normal plasma multimer patterns. Lanes 2 and 4 show the plasma vWF multimer analysis for patients with type 2A and type 2B vWD, respectively. Both show variable loss of HMW multimers. On the other hand, lanes 3 and 5 represent type 1 patients and demonstrate the presence of HMW multimers and an overall decrease in vWF.

Ristocetin-Induced Platelet Aggregation

The RIPA assay tests the capacity of vWF to agglutinate platelets at varying concentrations of ristocetin. Agglutination with low concentrations of ristocetin (approximately 0.5 mg/mL) may indicate type 2B vWD or its phenocopy, platelet-type pseudo vWD (PT-vWD), resulting from mutations in GPIBA, in which enhanced vWF-platelet binding is present.[11,115] In contrast to the vWF:RCo (which evaluates the interaction between the patient's vWF and formalin-fixed platelets), the RIPA assay evaluates the sensitivity of the patient's platelets to low-dose ristocetin. In cases of type 2B or platelet-type vWD, the platelet membrane is "overloaded" with high-affinity mutant vWF, resulting in platelet agglutination at low ristocetin concentrations.[91] In some cases of type 2B vWD, all variables except RIPA may be normal.[116,117] RIPA should be normal in type 1 vWD unless vWF levels are below 10 to 20 units/dL.

Binding of FVIII by vWF (vWF:FVIIIB)

This test determines the ability of vWF to bind FVIII[118,119] and is useful for the diagnosis of type 2N vWD.[98] There are no standard units for the output of this test.

Collagen Binding Assay (vWF:CB)

This test determines the ability of vWF to bind to collagen and is dependent on HMW vWF multimers. Consequently, the test helps to identify functional vWF discordance (i.e., to distinguish between types 1 and 2 vWD). Reduced collagen binding reflects the loss of HMW multimer forms[120] (type 2A vWD) or can reflect a specific collagen-binding deficiency (type 2M vWD). The normal range is approximately 50 to 200 IU/dL.

vWF Propeptide/Antigen Ratio (vWFpp/vWF:Ag)

An increased ratio of steady-state plasma vWFpp to vWF:Ag identifies patients with mutations that increase vWF clearance.[61] The mean ratio in normal individuals is 1.3, with a normal range of 0.54 to 1.98.

Desmopressin (DDAVP) Responsiveness

DDAVP administration releases vWF stores from endothelial cells. The pattern of DDAVP response in vWD subtypes (Table 140-4) may help to assign vWD subtype.[112] In addition, a decrease in the duration of DDAVP response may indicate an increased clearance mutation.

Genotyping

The identification of a mutation is not necessary for the diagnosis of vWD. However, genotyping should be considered when specialized testing with the vWF:FVIIIB assay is unavailable and type 2N vWD is suspected. Genotyping is also useful to discriminate between type 2B vWD and platelet-type vWD for prenatal assessment and alloantibody risk assessment in type 3 vWD. In mild-type 1 vWD, the likelihood of finding a mutation is low because mutations are not localized to a particular domain or exon and the results are of little clinical utility. A recent guideline on vWD genetic testing has been published by the UK Haemophilia Centre Doctors Organisation.[121]

Differential Diagnosis

Hemophilia A

Both type 2N vWD and mild hemophilia A (caused by mutations in F8) result in reduced levels of FVIII:C (approximately 5-40 IU/dL) with normal or borderline low levels of vWF. Although the vWF:FVIIIB test distinguishes between the two disorders,[122] the test is not widely available and the results may be equivocal.

Table 140-4 DDAVP Responsiveness in the Various Subtypes of vWD

vWD Type	vWF:RCo	vWF:Ag	RCo/Ag	FVIII:C International Units/dL	vWF:CB	vWF:CB/vWF:Ag
1	Increase	Increase	Remains >0.7	Increase	Increase	Remains >0.7
2A	No/little change	Increase	Remains <0.7	Increase	No/little change	Remains <0.7
2M (GP1B binding dysfunction)	No/little change	Increase	Remains <0.7	Increase	Increase	Remains >0.7
3	No/little change	No/little change		No/little change	No/little change	

Modified from Favaloro EJ: Rethinking the diagnosis of von Willebrand disease. *Thromb Res* 2:17, 2011.

In families with reduced FVIII:C, an X-linked pattern of inheritance helps identify those with mild hemophilia A. When family history is uninformative and vWF levels and function are normal, it may be preferable to perform sequence analysis of F8 before vWF, even in symptomatic females who are simplex cases (i.e., a single occurrence in a family), because F8 mutation and skewed X-chromosome inactivation (lyonization) are often responsible for symptoms. In these cases, F8 intrachromosomal inversions may be sought and DNA sequence analysis or mutation scanning of F8 exons 1-26 undertaken.[123,124] In females, dosage analysis using MLPA can also be used to identify heterozygous partial or complete gene deletions or duplications. F8 mutations may be detected in more than 50% of cases referred for "possible 2N vWD or hemophilia A." When F8 mutations are absent, or if vWF level and function are also abnormal, vWF can be analyzed.

Platelet-Type vWD

Platelet-type pseudo vWD (PT-vWD, also called *pseudo vWD*) mimics type 2B vWD but is caused by mutations in *GPIBA*. The disorders can be distinguished by mixing patient platelets or plasma with control plasma or platelets and using aggregometry or flow cytometry to identify the defective compound. However, these assays are technically challenging.[113,125-127] In the absence of mutations in exon 28 of vWF, mutations in exon 2 of *GPIBA* may be identified in approximately 10% of persons misdiagnosed with type 2B vWD. To date, missense mutations reported to affect GpIbα include p.Gly249 and p.Met255 plus a 27bp in-frame deletion p.Pro449_Ser457del (c.1345_1371del27).[128] The PT-vWD registry is available at www.pt-vwd.org/. PT-vWD is probably underdiagnosed. Misdiagnosis of PT-vWD may result in ineffective treatment of patients. vWF concentrate is needed to correct the reduced vWF level, but platelet transfusion may also be required if there is significant thrombocytopenia.[115] The half-life of replaced vWF is reduced in PT-vWD because of binding to abnormal GpIbα. Consequently, vWF concentrate must be administered more frequently.

Acquired von Willebrand syndrome (AvWS)

This mild to moderate bleeding disorder is a result of an acquired deficiency or dysfunction of vWF.[129-131] Exclusion of a lifelong personal and family history of bleeding is an important aspect of the diagnosis. The prevalence of AvWS has not been established. Although AvWS was thought to be uncommon, cohort studies suggest that the prevalence may be significantly underestimated. For example, when selected patient populations were screened, approximately 10% of patients with hematologic disorders,[132] approximately 79% with aortic stenosis,[133] and up to 100% with left ventricular assist devices were diagnosed with AvWS.[134-136] The median age of diagnosis is 62 years, but the disorder may occur in any age group (range 2 to 96 years).[137] AvWS has diverse pathology and may result from autoantibodies that impair vWF function or increase its clearance, adsorption of HWM vWF multimers to malignant cells or platelets, proteolytic cleavage of vWF after shear stress-induced unfolding, or decreased synthesis. Diseases that have been implicated include (1) lymphoproliferative disorders and plasma cell dyscrasias, including monoclonal gammopathy of unknown significance, multiple myeloma, and Waldenstrom macroglobulinemia; (2) autoimmune disorders, including systemic lupus erythematosus, scleroderma, and antiphospholipid antibody syndrome; (3) aortic stenosis and ventricular septal defects, which can trigger shear-induced conformational changes that increase vWF proteolysis; (4) thrombocytosis, including essential thrombocythemia or other myeloproliferative disorders that lead to a type 2 phenotype; (5) Wilms tumor or lymphoproliferative disorders that can be associated with increased vWF clearance by aberrant binding to tumor cells; (6) decreased vWF synthesis, for instance, with hypothyroidism; and (7) drugs including valproic acid, ciprofloxacin, griseofulvin, and hydroxyethyl starch.[138] The treatment goals can be divided into two categories: treatment or prevention of bleeding or induction of long-term remission. The agents used for prevention and treatment of bleeding in AvWS overlap with those used in vWD and include DDAVP or vWF-containing concentrates, which can transiently increase vWF levels. Other options include recombinant factor VIIa, antifibrinolytic agents, IVIG, or plasmaphoresis for AvWS associated with monoclonal gammopathies. Often a combination of agents is required to effect hemostasis. Whenever possible, treatment of the underlying disorder should be considered and may result in remission of the AvWS.

Management of vWD

The approach to the management of vWD is summarized in Fig. 140-7.

Evaluations Following Initial Diagnosis

To establish the extent of disease in an individual diagnosed with vWD, the following evaluations are recommended: (1) a personal and family history of bleeding to help predict severity and tailor treatment (use of a standardized bleeding assessment tool can be helpful)[139-141]; (2) a joint and muscle evaluation for those with type 3 vWD (musculoskeletal bleeding is rare in types 1 and 2 vWD); (3) screening for hepatitis B and C, as well as HIV if the diagnosis is type 3 vWD or if the individual received blood products or plasma-derived clotting factor concentrates before 1985 (this screening should be followed by vaccinations for hepatitis A and B)[130]; (4) determination of serum iron and ferritin (to assess iron stores), because many individuals with vWD are iron deficient, particularly women with menorrhagia; and (5) gynecologic evaluation for women with menorrhagia.[142] Individuals with vWD benefit from referral to a comprehensive bleeding disorders program for education, treatment, and genetic counseling. In addition, individuals with type 3 vWD should have periodic evaluations by a physiotherapist to monitor joint mobility.

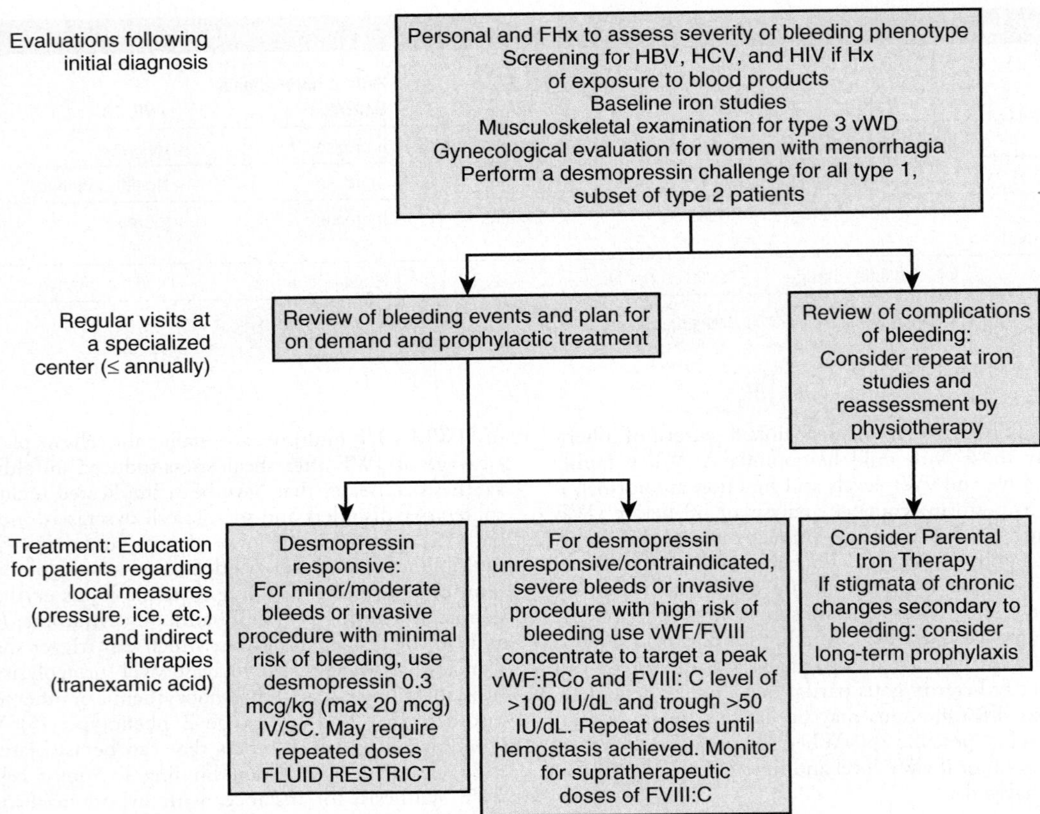

Figure 140-7 APPROACH TO THE MANAGEMENT OF vWD.

Treatment of vWD

In general, the management of vWD can be divided into three main categories: (1) localized measures to stop or minimize bleeding; (2) pharmacologic agents that provide indirect hemostatic benefit; and (3) treatments that directly increase plasma vWF and FVIII levels. Individuals with vWD should receive prompt treatment for severe bleeding episodes.

Localized Measures

The importance of localized measures to control bleeding in vWD, such as the application of direct pressure to a site of bleeding or injury, should not be understated. Biting down on a piece of gauze may halt bleeding from a tooth socket, and application of a compression bandage and cold pack to an injured limb may reduce subsequent hematoma formation. Management of nosebleeds can be particularly problematic for some affected children, and patients may benefit from a step-wise action plan that escalates from pressure to packing after a certain time period, including guidelines regarding how long to wait before seeking medical attention. In selected cases, nasal cautery may be required for prolonged or excessive epistaxis.

A number of topical hemostatic agents that are predominately used to achieve surgical hemostasis may have a limited role in the treatment of vWD and bleeding; these include gelatin foam/matrix, topical thrombin and fibrin sealants.

Indirect Therapies

A number of adjunctive therapies are of benefit in vWD, particularly at the time of minor surgical and dental procedures and to treat menorrhagia. Fibrinolytic inhibitors (e.g., tranexamic acid), which inhibit the conversion of plasminogen to plasmin, can be helpful for treatment or prevention of bleeding episodes.[11] These agents can be used either as sole therapy or as adjuncts to DDAVP or vWF/FVIII concentrates and may be particularly useful to control mucosal bleeding in the oral cavity or gastrointestinal or genitourinary tracts. The most common adverse events to tranexamic acid are gastrointestinal side effects and headache. Tranexamic acid is contraindicated in disseminated intravascular coagulation and bleeding from the upper urinary tract, where it can lead to urinary tract obstruction by clots. Hormonal treatments (i.e., the combined oral contraceptive pill) are effective for the treatment of menorrhagia. Nonmedical treatments, such as levonorgestrel-releasing intrauterine systems or endometrial ablation, may be useful in selected patients with vWD. A consensus document on the management of women with vWD was recently published.[142]

Desmopressin

Most individuals with type 1 vWD and some with type 2 vWD respond to intranasal, intravenous or subcutaneous treatment with desmopressin,[143,144] which promotes release of stored vWF and raises levels 3- to 10-fold. Peak effects are achieved 30 and 90 minutes after intravenous and intranasal delivery, respectively. The usual parenteral dose is 0.3 mcg/kg (maximum dose 20 mcg) infused in approximately 50 mL of normal saline over approximately 30 minutes. The dose of the highly concentrated intranasal preparation is 150 mcg for children under 50 kg and 300 mcg for larger children. It is important to note that highly concentrated products, (e.g., Stimate), deliver 150 mcg per spray, a much higher concentration than that used to treat enuresis.

After vWD diagnosis, a desmopressin challenge is advisable to assess vWF response. vWF and FVIII levels should be determined before and at several points after desmopressin administration (e.g., at baseline and at 1, 2, and 4 hours). A threefold increase in vWF and FVIII levels to at least 0.30 IU/mL (30%) is usually considered adequate for situations such as dental procedures, minor surgery, or the treatment of epistaxis or menorrhagia. Significantly decreased vWF:Ag or vWF:RCo at the 4-hour point may indicate a vWD phenotype with increased clearance. In such cases, the desmopressin response may be too transient to be of benefit.

Desmopressin is safe and generally well tolerated. Common side effects include facial flushing and headache. Tachycardia, lightheadedness and mild hypotension can occur. The most serious side effects are severe hyponatremia and seizures.[145] Reduction of fluid intake for 24 hours after DDAVP administration is an important precaution to prevent water intoxication. In patients receiving repeated desmopressin administrations, serum sodium levels should be monitored. Desmopressin should be used with caution in those younger than 2 years of age because of a higher risk for hyponatremia. Desmopressin is contraindicated in individuals with atherosclerotic disease and in those over 70 years of age; vWF/FVIII concentrate should be used in these patients. In persons who are intolerant to desmopressin or have a poor vWF response, clotting factor concentrate is required.

An important limitation in the use of desmopressin is the development of tachyphylaxis with repeated administration. When given repeatedly at intervals of less than 24 hours, the magnitude of the vWF and FVIII increments can fall to approximately 70% of that obtained with the initial dose.[146] For practical purposes, a single dose of desmopressin before dental extractions or minor procedures is usually sufficient. Although repeated doses can be given at 12 or 24 hours, the potential for tachyphylaxis must be considered. Additionally, in situations where repeat dosing is considered, more prolonged fluid restriction is required.

Most type 1 vWD patients respond adequately to desmopressin, type 3 vWD patients typically do not respond to this drug, and the response in type 2 vWD patients respond is variable. Type 2A patients often exhibit an adequate response and may benefit from a desmopressin trial. Type 2M patients typically do not respond well to desmopressin. Although desmopressin is generally contraindicated in type 2B vWD because of the transient thrombocytopenia that accompanies the release of mutant vWF, it is effective and can be considered on an individualized basis.[147,148] Desmopressin produces a two- to ninefold increase in vWF and FVIII in patients with type 2N vWD, but the increase in FVIII only persists for approximately 3 hours.[149] Therefore desmopressin should be reserved for situations in which a transient rise in FVIII is sufficient.

vWF/FVIII Concentrates

vWF/FVIII concentrates are required for patients who do not have an adequate response to desmopressin, those who experience side effects, or those have contraindications to desmopressin. Because of tachyphylaxis with desmopressin, patients with severe bleeding or those requiring major or repeated surgery often need vWF replacement therapy. Purified, viral-inactivated, plasma-derived vWF/FVIII are the products most frequently used (e.g., Humate-P, Wilate). The quantity of ristocetin cofactor activity (vWF:RCo) relative to factor VIII:C varies by product; Humate-P contains 2.4 vWF:RCo units for each 1 FVIII:C unit,[150] whereas Wilate contains a 1:1 ratio.[151] Both products contain a full spectrum of vWF multimers, including HMW multimers, and closely resemble normal plasma.[152] Highly purified FVIII concentrates (monoclonal antibody purified and recombinant) should not be used to treat vWD because they lack vWF.

Dosing recommendations are provided either in vWF:RCo (North America) or FVIII:C (Europe) units and are weight-based; repeat infusions can be given every 12 to 24 hours, depending on the clinical situation. The goal is to maintain vWF:RCo and FVIII:C at more than 100 IU/dL at peak and at more than 50 IU/dL at trough until hemostasis is achieved. With vWF/FVIII concentrates, the FVIII:C response is higher and more sustained than predicted from the dose because of the stabilizing effect of exogenous vWF on endogenous FVIII.[153] Details regarding dosing can be found in the product inserts. vWF:RCo and FVIII:C levels should be measured in patients receiving repeat infusions, not only to ensure adequate hemostasis but also to monitor for supraphysiologic levels of FVIII because thromboembolic events have been associated with high FVIII levels. The overall incidence is very low, and most cases occurred in surgical patients with other risk factors.[154] Therefore, mechanical and medical thromboprophylaxis should be considered on an case-by-case basis. Adverse reactions to vWF/FVIII concentrates are rare but include allergic and anaphylactic symptoms, such as urticaria, chest tightness, rash, pruritus and edema.[155]

vWF:FVIII concentrates are effective in over 97% of events.[150] In the rare event that infusion of a vWF/FVIII concentrate is ineffective at stopping bleeding, transfusion of platelet concentrates may be beneficial, presumably because they facilitate the delivery of small amounts of platelet vWF to the site of vascular injury.[11]

Prophylaxis

Short-term prophylaxis with a combination of an antifibrinolytic, desmopressin, and vWF/FVIII concentrates, in anticipation of a defined bleeding challenge, such as surgery, is the standard of care in the treatment of vWD. The role of long-term continuous prophylaxis, defined as primary if initiated before long-term sequelae have developed (e.g., joint damage) or secondary if initiated after the development of chronic changes, is less established in vWD than it is in severe hemophilia. Individuals with severe cases of vWD, in particular type 3 vWD and certain patients with severe type 1 or type 2 vWD, may experience significant joint bleeds with resultant hemophilic-like arthropathy, as well as severe and frequently recurrent nasal/oral, gastrointestinal, or menstrual bleeding. The resultant anemia, hospitalizations, and absences from school or work may have a significant impact on quality of life. Although there is limited evidence, several cohort and case studies[156-158] suggest that both primary and secondary long-term prophylaxis improve quality of life (by reducing the frequency of bleeding episodes or the need for transfusions), alleviate anemia, reduce hospitalizations, and prevent chronic joint disease. Complications are unusual aside from rare cases of vWF inhibitor formation (approximately 3%). Controversy exists about the specific indications, schedules, and dosing of prophylactic regimens. This is the subject of an ongoing international trial, known as the vWD International Prophylaxis (VIP) trial, which began recruitment of patients in 2007.

Pediatric Issues

Prenatal diagnosis for pregnancies at increased risk (generally only for type 3 vWD) is possible by analysis of DNA extracted from fetal cells obtained by chorionic villus sampling (CVS) at 11 to 13 weeks of gestation or amniocentesis, which is usually performed at 15 to 18 weeks of gestation. The disease-causing allele(s) of an affected family member must be identified before prenatal testing. Preimplantation genetic diagnosis (PGD) may be available for families in which the disease-causing mutation(s) have been identified.[159]

The diagnosis and care of infants and children with vWD requires special consideration. An accurate assessment of hemorrhagic symptoms is a key component in the diagnosis of vWD, but it often presents a significant challenge in the pediatric population. Bruising and epistaxis are common among children with vWD, but these symptoms are also reported by children without vWD. In addition, the classical symptoms of vWD in adults (e.g., menorrhagia, postsurgical bleeding) are clearly not prevalent in the pediatric population. Because a child may not have encountered many hemostatic challenges and may be prepubertal, the bleeding history may be unimpressive. The effect this negative history may have on perceived risk for bleeding is highlighted in two of the previously published bleeding scores,[139,140] which assign a negative value to lack of bleeding symptoms and are based on the accumulation of bleeding symptoms or complications. With a goal of addressing these issues, increasing interest exists in the development of new clinical tools for quantifying bleeding in the pediatric population.[141] Finally, the initial diagnostic

Assessment of a Neonate

A baby boy was born to a mother with known type 2B vWD. On the day of birth, investigations were performed and demonstrated the following: vWF:Ag 78 IU/dL, vWF:RCo 61 IU/dL, and FVIII:C 0.69 IU/dL. The mother was informed that the results were all within normal range and that her newborn infant was not affected by type 2B vWD. At approximately 18 months of age, the mother presented with her toddler boy with the complaint of excessive mucocutaneous bleeding. Blood work at that time demonstrated: vWF:Ag 50 international units/dL, vWF:RCo 20 international units/dL, and FVIII:C 51 international units/dL. Multimer analysis revealed an abnormal profile with a doublet patter. Finally, genotyping revealed that the boy was heterozygous for the same mutation, R1306W, that his mother carried.

This case illustrates several important points. Neonatal levels of vWF are increased over baseline; if investigations are performed, they should be interpreted using appropriate reference ranges. Alternatively, if a phenotypic diagnosis is being sought, it is preferable to postpone investigations, decreasing the likelihood of pretest analytical variables, such as difficulty in collecting an appropriate blood sample from a neonate, and the difficulties with interpretation of the results. Finally, in cases in which the mutation is known, genotyping is diagnostic and also the most straightforward.

assessment of an infant is complicated by the fact that vWF levels are higher in the neonatal period. Consequently, phenotypic testing of vWD should be delayed until later in childhood (see Fig. 140-7).

Desmopressin should be avoided in children younger than the age of 2 because of the potential difficulty in restricting fluids. Infant males should be circumcised only after consultation with a pediatric hemostasis specialist. Children with vWD may also experience bruising after routine immunizations and gum bleeding following the loss of primary teeth. Typically, only patients with type 3 vWD experience spontaneous musculoskeletal bleeding, such as that seen in patients with severe hemophilia, and should be considered for long-term prophylaxis with vWF/FVIII concentrates, as discussed in the preceding section (see box on Assessment of a Neonate).

SUGGESTED READINGS

Abshire T: The role of prophylaxis in the management of von Willebrand disease: Today and tomorrow. *Thromb Res* 124:S15, 2009.

Berntorp E: Haemate p / humate-p: A systematic review. *Thromb Res* 124:S11, 2009.

Bowen D: An influence of ABO blood group on the rate of proteolysis of von Willebrand factor ADAMTS13. *J Thromb Haemost* 33, 2003.

Bowman M, Mundell G, Grabell J, et al: Generation and validation of the condensed MCMDM-1VWD bleeding questionnaire for von Willebrand disease. *J Thromb Haemost* 6:2062, 2008.

Budde U, Pieconka A, Will K, et al: Laboratory testing for von Willebrand disease: Contribution of multimer analysis to diagnosis and classification. *Sem Thromb Hemost* 32:514, 2006.

Castaman G, Lethagen S, Federici AB, et al: Response to desmopressin is influenced by the genotype and phenotype in type 1 von Willebrand disease (vWD): Results from the European study MCMDM-1VWD. *Blood* 111:3531, 2008.

Castaman G, Tosetto A, Rodeghiero F: Pregnancy and delivery in women with von Willebrand's disease and different von Willebrand factor mutations. *Haematologica* 95:963, 2010.

Cumming A, Grundy P, Keeney S, et al: An investigation of the von Willebrand factor genotype in UK patients diagnosed to have type I von Willebrand disease. *Thromb Haemost* 96:630, 2006.

Eikenboom J, Van Marion V, Putter H, et al: Linkage analysis in families diagnosed with type 1 von Willebrand disease in the European study, molecular and clinical markers for the diagnosis and management of type 1 vWD. *J Thromb Haemost* 4:774, 2006.

Federici AB: The use of desmopressin in von Willebrand disease: The experience of the first 30 years (1977-2007). *Haemophilia* 14:5, 2008.

Federici AB, Mannucci PM, Castaman G, et al: Clinical and molecular predictors of thrombocytopenia and risk of bleeding in patients with von Willebrand disease type 2b: A cohort study of 67 patients. *Blood* 113:526, 2009.

Federici AB, Rand JH, Bucciarelli P, et al: Acquired von Willebrand syndrome: Data from an international registry. *Thromb Haemost* 84:345, 2000.

Giannini S, Cecchetti L, Mezzasoma AM, et al: Diagnosis of platelet-type von Willebrand disease by flow cytometry. *Haematologica* 95:1021, 2010.

Gill JC, Endres-Brooks J, Bauer PJ, et al: The effect of abo blood group on the diagnosis of von Willebrand disease. *Blood* 69:1691, 1987.

Ginsburg D, Sadler JE: von Willebrand disease: A database of point mutations, insertions, and deletions. For the consortium on von Willebrand factor mutations and polymorphisms, and the subcommittee on von Willebrand factor of the scientific and standardization committee of the International Society on Thrombosis and Haemostasis. *Thromb Haemost* 69:177, 1993.

Goodeve AC: The genetic basis of von Willebrand disease. *Blood Rev* 24:123, 2010.

Goodeve A, Eikenboom J, Castaman G, et al: Phenotype and genotype of a cohort of families historically diagnosed with type 1 von Willebrand disease in the European study, molecular and clinical markers for the diagnosis and management of type 1 von Willebrand disease (MCMDM-1VWD). *Blood* 109:112, 2007.

Haberichter SL, Castaman G, Budde U, et al: Identification of type 1 von Willebrand disease patients with reduced von Willebrand factor survival by assay of the vWF propeptide in the European study: Molecular and clinical markers for the diagnosis and management of type 1 vWD (MCMDM-1VWD). *Blood* 111:4979, 2008.

Halimeh S, Krümpel A, Rott H, et al: Long-term secondary prophylaxis in children, adolescents and young adults with von Willebrand disease. Results of a cohort study. *Thromb Haemost* 105:597, 2011.

James AH, Jamison MG: Bleeding events and other complications during pregnancy and childbirth in women with von Willebrand disease. *J Thromb Haemost* 5:1165, 2007.

James AH, Kouides PA, Abdul-Kadir R, et al: von Willebrand disease and other bleeding disorders in women: Consensus on diagnosis and management from an international expert panel. *Am J Obstet Gynec* 201:12, e1–8, 2009.

James PD, Notley C, Hegadorn C, et al: The mutational spectrum of type 1 von Willebrand disease: Results from a Canadian cohort study. *Blood* 109:145, 2007.

Keeney S, Bowen D, Cumming A, et al: The molecular analysis of von Willebrand disease: A guideline from the UK haemophilia centre doctors' organisation haemophilia genetics laboratory network. *Haemophilia* 14:1099, 2008.

Mazurier C, Goudemand J, Hilbert L, et al: Type 2N von Willebrand disease: Clinical manifestations, pathophysiology, laboratory diagnosis and molecular biology. Best practice & research. *Clin Haematol* 14:337, 2001.

Millar CM, Brown SA: Oligosaccharide structures of von Willebrand factor and their potential role in von Willebrand disease. *Blood Rev* 20:83, 2006.

Nichols WL, Hultin MB, James AH, et al: von Willebrand disease (vWD): Evidence-based diagnosis and management guidelines, the national heart, lung, and blood institute (NHLBI) expert panel report (USA). *Haemophilia* 14:171, 2008.

Ruggeri Z, Zimmerman T: The complex multimeric composition of factor VIII/von Willebrand factor. *Blood* 57:1140, 1981.

Sadler JE, Budde U, Eikenboom JCJ, et al: Update on the pathophysiology and classification of von Willebrand disease: A report of the subcommittee on von Willebrand factor. *J Thromb Haemost* 4:2103, 2006.

Springer TA: Biology and physics of von Willebrand factor concatamers. *Journal of Thromb Haemost* 9:130, 2011.

Tiede A, Rand JH, Budde U, et al: How I treat the acquired von Willebrand syndrome. *Blood* 117:6777, 2011.

For complete list of references log on to www.expertconsult.com.

CHAPTER 141

DISSEMINATED INTRAVASCULAR COAGULATION

Marcel Levi

A variety of disorders, including infectious or inflammatory conditions and malignant disease, lead to activation of coagulation. In many cases, this activation of coagulation will not lead to clinical complications and is not even detected by routine laboratory tests but can only be measured with sensitive molecular markers for activation of coagulation factors and pathways.[1,2] However, if activation of coagulation is sufficiently strong, the platelet count may decrease, and global clotting times may become prolonged. In its most extreme form, systemic activation of coagulation is known as disseminated intravascular coagulation (DIC). DIC is characterized by the simultaneous occurrence of widespread (micro)vascular thrombosis, thereby compromising blood supply to various organs, which may contribute to organ failure.[3,4] Because of ongoing activation of the coagulation system and other factors, such as impaired synthesis and increased degradation of coagulation proteins and protease inhibitors, consumption of clotting factors and platelets may occur, resulting in bleeding from various sites.

In view of the multiple, often contrasting mechanisms that occur in patients with DIC, a consensual definition of DIC had been a matter of debate. In 2001, the subcommittee on DIC of the International Society on Thrombosis and Hemostasis (ISTH) proposed a definition that reflects the central role of the microvascular milieu (i.e., endothelial cells, blood cells, and the plasma protease system) in the pathogenesis of DIC. This definition of DIC reads as follows: "DIC is an acquired syndrome characterized by the intravascular activation of coagulation without a specific localization and arising from different causes. It can originate from and cause damage to the microvasculature, which if sufficiently severe, can produce organ dysfunction."[5]

The diagnosis of DIC may be hampered by the nonspecific nature of many indicators of coagulation activation, although newly developed scoring algorithms based on readily available routine laboratory parameters show promising diagnostic accuracy.[5] Owing to the complexity of the clinical presentation, the variable and unpredictable course, and the multitude of therapies given to patients with DIC, properly conducted clinical trials are difficult to perform and even to devise. Management relies on limited evidence from clinical trials in combination with small studies using surrogate outcome endpoints and experience from case series, as well as from an understanding of the underlying pathophysiologic mechanisms.[6]

EPIDEMIOLOGY

Activation of coagulation in concert with inflammatory activation can result in microvascular thrombosis, which contributes to multiple organ failure in patients with severe sepsis.[7] In support of this concept, postmortem findings in patients with coagulation abnormalities and DIC on the background of severe sepsis include diffuse bleeding, hemorrhagic necrosis of tissues, microthrombi in small blood vessels, and thrombi in midsize and larger arteries and veins. Ischemia and necrosis were invariably the result of fibrin deposition in small- and midsize vessels. Importantly, intravascular thrombi appear to be the driver of the organ dysfunction. Fibrin deposition in various organs also is a characteristic finding in animal models of DIC. Thus experimental bacteremia or endotoxemia causes intra- and extravascular fibrin deposition in the kidneys, lungs, liver, brain, and other organs. Amelioration of the hemostatic defect by various interventions in these models reduces fibrin deposition; improves organ fraction; and, in some cases, reduces mortality. Finally, results of clinical studies also support the concept that activation of coagulation is as important a determinant of clinical outcome. DIC has shown to be an independent predictor of organ failure and mortality.[8] In a consecutive series of patients with severe sepsis, 43% of patients with DIC were compared with 27% in those without DIC. In this study, the severity of the coagulopathy was also directly related to mortality.[9]

In addition to microvascular thrombosis and organ dysfunction, coagulation abnormalities may have other harmful consequences. Thrombocytopenia in patients with sepsis places them at an increased risk of bleeding. For example, critically ill patients with a platelet count of below 50×10^9/L have a four- to fivefold higher risk for bleeding than those with higher platelet counts.[10] Although the overall risk of intracerebral bleeding in patients in the intensive care unit (ICU) is less than 0.5%, up to 88% of patients with this complication have platelet counts less than 100×10^9/L. The use of anticoagulants in patients with thrombocytopenia further increases the risk of bleeding. Regardless of the cause, multivariate analyses indicate that thrombocytopenia is an independent predictor of ICU mortality and increases the risk of death by 1.9- to 4.2-fold. In particular, thrombocytopenia that persists more than 4 days after ICU admission or 50% of greater decrease in platelet count during the ICU stay is associated with a four- to sixfold increase in mortality. In fact, the platelet count appears to be a stronger predictor for ICU mortality than composite scoring systems, such as the Acute Physiology and Chronic Evaluation (APACHE) II or Multiple Organ Dysfunction Score (MODS). Decreased levels of coagulation factors, as reflected by prolonged global coagulation times, also increase the risk of bleeding. Prolongation of the prothrombin time (PT) or activated partial thromboplastin time (aPTT) to over 1.5 times the control is associated with an increased risk of bleeding and mortality in critically ill patients.

PATHOBIOLOGY

Traditionally, DIC was thought to be the result of activation of both the extrinsic and intrinsic pathways of coagulation. The classical concept was that the extrinsic pathway was initiated by a tissue-derived component, which activated factor VII, leading to the direct conversion of prothrombin to thrombin. This process would proceed as long as there was tissue damage from systemic infection, trauma, solutio placentae, or malignancy. In contrast, the intrinsic or contact pathway of coagulation was initiated by contact activation of factor XII, which, together with its cofactors, kallikrein and kininogen, then activated factor XI with subsequent activation of factor IX. The initiators of contact activation were poorly understood until recently but were thought to include collagen and artificial surfaces. In recent years, the molecular mechanisms of coagulation pathways have been defined (Fig. 141-1). This has provided new insight into the

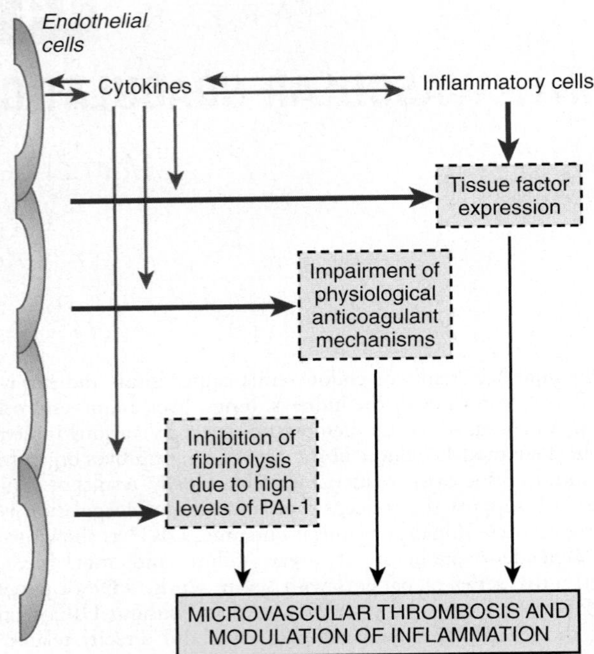

Figure 141-1 PATHOGENESIS OF DISSEMINATED INTRAVASCULAR COAGULATION (DIC). Pathways involved in the activation of coagulation in DIC. Both perturbed endothelial cells and activated mononuclear cells may produce proinflammatory cytokines that induce tissue factor expression, thereby initiating coagulation. In addition, downregulation of physiological anticoagulant mechanisms and inhibition of fibrinolysis promotes intravascular fibrin deposition. *PAI-1,* Plasminogen activator inhibitor, type 1.

pathogenesis of DIC. In general, current thinking is that thrombin and fibrin generation in patients with DIC is largely driven via the extrinsic pathway; the role of the contact system is uncertain.

Tissue Factor–Factor VII(a) Pathway

The extrinsic pathway is initiated by the tissue factor (TF)–factor VIIa complex. TF is a membrane-bound 4.5-kD protein that is constitutively expressed on cells that are mostly in tissues not in direct contact with blood, such as the adventitial layer of larger blood vessels.[11] Subcutaneous tissue also contains substantial amounts of TF. When expressed on the cell surface, TF interacts with factor VII, either in its zymogen or activated form. The TF–factor VIIa complex catalyzes the activation of both factor IX and factor X. Factors IXa and Xa enhance the activation of factors X and prothrombin, respectively. In cells in contact with the blood circulation, TF is induced by the action of mediators such as cytokines, C-reactive protein, and advanced glycosylation end products. Inducible TF is predominantly expressed by monocytes and macrophages. Monocyte TF expression is enhanced in the presence of platelets and granulocytes in a P-selectin dependent fashion. This may reflect nuclear factor kappa-B (NFκB) activation that occurs when activated platelets bind to neutrophils or mononuclear cells. These cell–cell interactions also stimulate the production of interleukin-1b (IL-1b), IL-8, MCP-1, and tumor necrosis factor-α (TNF-α). Under cell culture conditions, cytokines such as TNF-α, and IL-1, can induce TF expression by vascular endothelial cells, but the in vivo relevance of this finding is uncertain. Studies in vivo suggest that IL-6 is the dominant mediator of TF expression by mononuclear cells.

Increased monocyte TF expression and procoagulant activity have been demonstrated in DIC associated with sepsis, cancer, or coronary disease. Tissue expression of TF appears to be localized to certain organs and vascular beds, but it is uncertain whether its expression is under genetic control in an organ-specific fashion. With trauma, such as extensive surgery, brain injury, or burns, it is likely that constitutively expressed TF at the site of injury is the primary source of procoagulant material, but direct support for this concept is lacking.

The Intrinsic Pathway

The role of the intrinsic pathway in the pathogenesis of DIC is uncertain. Negatively charged substances, such as phospholipids, polyphosphates, and glycosaminoglycans, are potential activators of the contact pathway. Studies in patients with suspected DIC have identified elevated levels of markers of activation of the contact system. In patients with meningococcal septicemia, there was a negative correlation between plasma factor XII levels and factor XIIa–C1 inhibitor complexes. Although this finding implies consumption of factor XII and subsequent downstream activation of factor XI, an alternative explanation is that there is a negative acute phase effect with reduced synthesis of factor XII in conjunction with thrombin-mediated activation of factor XI.

However, blockade of the contact system with a factor XIIa-directed antibody failed to prevent DIC in a balloon model of *Escherichia coli* sepsis but diminished development of lethal hypotension. These findings provide reasonable support for the current view that the contact pathway does not contribute to DIC but may play important roles in proinflammatory mechanisms related to vascular permeability, vascular proliferation (kininogen induces smooth muscle cell proliferation), and enhancement of fibrinolysis.[12]

Cytokines and Other Amplification Pathways

Activation of blood coagulation requires several cofactors. For development of DIC, the surfaces of cell remnants or intact cells, inflammatory mediators, and coagulation proteins are required. The stimulus for activation depends on the underlying disease and may range from bacterial cell compounds, such as endotoxin, TF on host or cancer cells, other cancer cell procoagulants, or fat or amniotic fluid emboli by unknown pathways. Each of these triggers interacts with other mediators: TF assembles on anionic phospholipid surfaces, which can be provided by activated platelets, leukocytes, or cancer cells, and cytokines interact with receptors and induce signaling pathways that induce TF expression and other proinflammatory components via the NFκB complex.

Endotoxin is a lipopolysaccharide compound of gram-negative bacteria that induces the sepsis syndrome and DIC. Gram-negative bacteria liberate endotoxins from their membrane, which interact with cell surfaces via various pathways. In blood, endotoxin directly binds to CD 14 on monocytes and binds to endothelial cells after complexing with lipopolysaccharide binding protein (LBP) and the Toll-like receptor 4 (TLR 4) complex. Through these interactions, endotoxin induces signaling pathways that culminate in NFκB activation and initiates the expression of proinflammatory cytokines and TF. Likewise, exotoxins, such as lipoteichoic acid (LTA) from gram-positive bacteria, can induce proinflammatory cytokine expression in a similar fashion.

The molecular mechanisms underlying endotoxin-induced activation of coagulation have been studied in primates and baboons. In endotoxin or *E. coli* models of sepsis, inhibition of the TF pathway abolishes the activation of coagulation, highlighting the importance of TF. IL-6 is an important mediator of procoagulant effects, and TNF-α is involved in the fibrinolytic response to endotoxin. Inhibition of TF with TFPI reduces IL-6 levels in the baboon model, suggesting that there is extensive crosstalk between coagulation and inflammatory mediators (see later discussion). Monocytes that express TF bind factor VII(a), shed TF, or bind to the damaged vessel wall. After interacting with platelets, circulating monocytes may trigger DIC. Microvesicles may accelerate this process, and the complex interaction among cells, membrane fragments, soluble mediators, and proteins may trigger the DIC syndrome. The severity and duration of the consumptive process are mainly determined by the potency of the triggers and the capacity of inhibitory mechanisms.

Cross-Talk Among Coagulation Proteases Results in Proinflammatory Effects

In addition to activating coagulation protein zymogens, coagulation proteases also interact with specific cell receptors and trigger signaling pathways that elicit proinflammatory mediators.[7] Factor Xa, thrombin and the factor VIIa–TF complex have such effects. Factor Xa injection into rats induces localized inflammation, probably as a result of its interaction with effector cell protease receptor-1 (EPR-1) and not because of thrombin generation. Exposure of cultured endothelial cells to factor Xa stimulates the production of monocyte chemotactic protein 1 (MCP-1), IL-6, and IL-8 and upregulates the expression of adhesion proteins that tether neutrophils to the cell surface. Further evidence for the crosstalk between inflammation and coagulation comes from the observations that IL-6 and IL-8 elicit TF-dependent procoagulant activity in monocytes, and IL-6 has been identified as the critical mediator of procoagulant activity either on its own or after endotoxin challenge in vivo. Therefore, cytokine production induced by factor Xa may be an important driver of coagulation in DIC.

In addition to its procoagulant functions, thrombin has a variety of noncoagulant effects. Thrombin induces the release of MCP-1 and IL-6 from fibroblasts, epithelial cells, and mononuclear cells in vitro. Thrombin also induces IL-6 and IL-8 production in endothelial cells. When generated in whole blood, IL-8 production has a procoagulant effect that is TF dependent. Cell activation by thrombin is likely mediated by protease-activated receptor (PAR). The factor VIIa–TF complex also activates cells by binding PAR 2.

Direct evidence of the in vivo relevance of these phenomena comes from a study showing that recombinant factor VIIa infusion in volunteers induces an increase in plasma levels of IL-6 and IL-8. Although the concentrations of factor VIIa infused far exceed those found in patients with sepsis, it is possible that factor VIIa–induced cytokine production is of physiological importance. Thus this information adds to the concept that several coagulation proteases induce proinflammatory mediators that augment procoagulant activity and amplify the consumptive process. Endogenous anticoagulant pathways are essential to regulate these proteases and prevent uncontrolled DIC.

Endogenous Anticoagulant Pathways in Disseminated Intravascular Coagulation

The development of DIC is counteracted by several mechanisms. First, coagulation inhibitors regulate the coagulation mechanism. These inhibitors include antithrombin (AT), the proteins C system, and TF pathway inhibitor (TFPI) (Fig. 141-2).[7] AT, which complexes and inhibits thrombin and factor Xa, is one of the most important inhibitors, and reduced AT levels are a characteristic of DIC. Reduction in AT levels reflects a combination of reduced protein synthesis as well as increased clearance through the formation of protease–AT

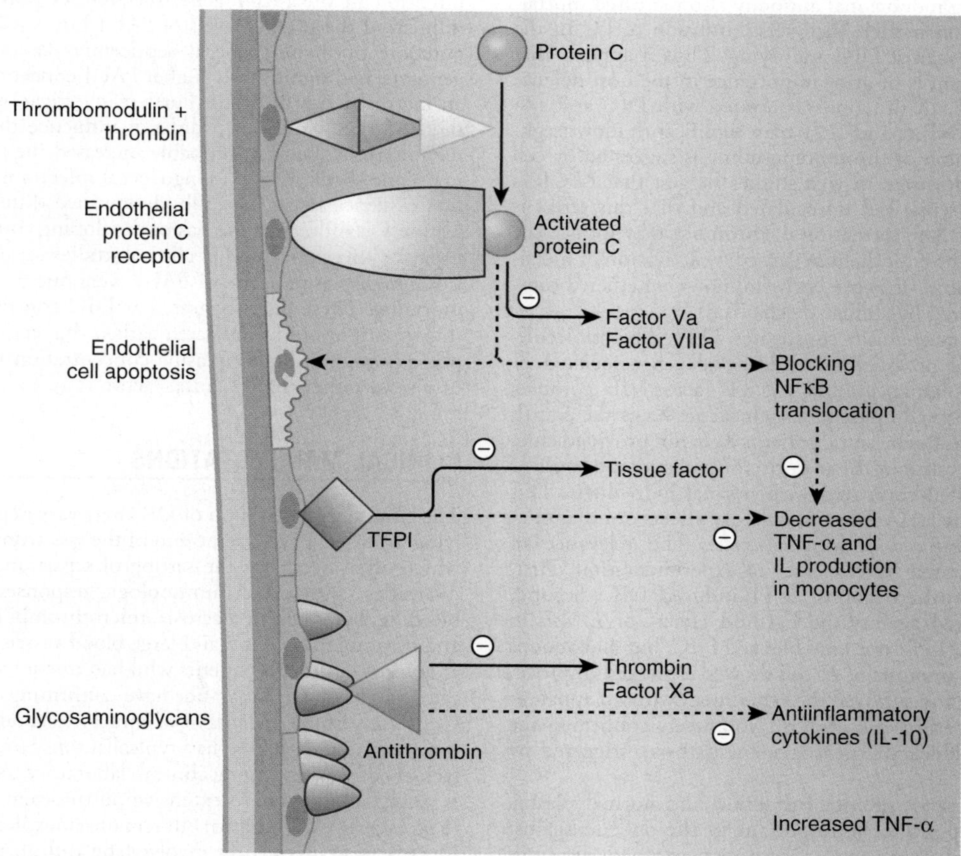

Figure 141-2 PHYSIOLOGICAL ANTICOAGULANT MECHANISMS IN DISSEMINATED INTRAVASCULAR COAGULATION. Physiological anticoagulant mechanisms (activated protein C system, tissue factor pathway inhibitor [TFPI], and antithrombin) are not only involved in blocking thrombin generation and thrombin activity but also affect inflammatory pathways. *IL,* Interleukin; *NFκB,* nuclear factor kappa-B; *TNF,* tumor necrosis factor.

complexes and by degradation by neutrophil elastase. In addition, cytokines may impair proteoglycan synthesis in the vessel wall, thereby reducing the availability of heparin sulphate for potentiation of AT activity.

In animal models of experimental bacteremia, AT concentrate infusion increases survival, reduces the severity of DIC, and lowers the levels of IL-6 and IL-8. Therefore, in addition to its anticoagulant function, AT may also have an antiinflammatory effect.

Activated protein C (APC) and its cofactor protein S form a second line of defense. Thrombin binds to the endothelial cell membrane–associated molecule thrombomodulin, and this complex converts protein C to its active form, APC.[13] In addition, the thrombin–thrombomodulin complex accelerates the conversion of TAFI. APC activates factors Va and VIIIa by proteolytic cleavage, thus slowing down the coagulation cascade. Endothelial cells, primarily of large blood vessels, express an endothelial protein C receptor (EPCR), which augments the activation of protein C at the cell surface. APC has antiinflammatory effects on mononuclear cells and granulocytes, which may be distinct from its anticoagulant activity. Administration of APC prevented thrombin-induced thromboembolism in mice, mainly through its antithrombotic effect. In addition, several studies have demonstrated antiinflammatory effects of APC.

In contrast, defects in the protein C mechanism enhance the vulnerability to inflammatory reactions and DIC. In patient studies, lowered levels of protein C and protein S are associated with increased mortality. Mice with a one allel targeted disruption of the protein C gene, causing heterozygous protein C deficiency, displayed a more severe DIC and associated inflammatory response. Blockade of the activity of protein C by infusion of C4 binding protein turns a sublethal model of *E. coli* in baboons into a lethal model. Blockade of EPCR by a neutralizing monoclonal antibody also increased mortality in the *E. coli* baboon model. Vice versa, infusion of PC in the same model protected against DIC and dying. Thus it appears that the protein C mechanism is of great importance in the host defense against sepsis and DIC. In situations associated with DIC and systemic inflammation, TNF-α and IL-1 may significantly downregulate the cellular expression of thrombomodulin, as suggested by cell culture experiments. However, in vivo studies suggest that EPCR is not downregulated in sepsis but upregulated and that this effect is mediated by thrombin. The formation of thrombin may induce the shedding of EPCR by the endothelium caused by activation of metalloproteinases by thrombin. It is presently unknown whether thrombomodulin is also cleaved by similar mechanisms.

A third inhibitory mechanism constitutes TFPI. This molecule, which exists in several pools either endothelial cell associated or lipoprotein bound in plasma, inhibits the TF–factor VIIa complex by forming a quaternary complex in which factor Xa is the fourth component. Clinical studies in septic patients have not provided clues as to its importance because in the majority of patients, the levels of TFPI are not diminished compared with normal individuals. This may be explained by the lack of downregulatory effects of inflammatory mediators on cultured endothelial cells. The relevance of TFPI in DIC is illustrated by two lines of experimentation. First, depletion of TFPI sensitized rabbits to TF-induced DIC. Second, TFPI infusion protected against the harmful effects of *E. coli* in primates. In this study, TFPI not only blocked DIC, but all baboons challenged with lethal amounts of *E. coli* showed a marked improvement in vital functions and survived the experiment without apparent complications. An experimental study in volunteers confirmed the potential of TFPI to block the procoagulant pathway triggered by endotoxin.

In general, the presence of intact function and normal plasma levels of inhibitors appears to be important in the defense against DIC. It should be noted, however, that there are no strong indications that humans with congenital deficiencies of inhibitors would have a greater chance of developing DIC, but this issue remains to be explored. In addition, the influence of inhibitors in modifying the interaction between coagulation and inflammation deserves further attention.

Fibrinolysis

In experimental models of DIC, fibrinolysis is activated, demonstrated by an initial activation of plasminogen activation, followed by a marked impairment caused by the release in blood of plasminogen activator inhibitor, type 1 (PAI-1). The latter inhibitor strongly inhibits fibrinolysis causing a net procoagulant situation. The molecular basis is cytokine-mediated activation of vascular endothelial cells; TNF-α and Il-1 decreased tissue plasminogen activator (t-PA) and increased PAI-1 production. TNF-α increased urokinase plasminogen activator (u-PA) production in endothelial cells. Endotoxin and TNF-α stimulated PAI-1 production in the livers, kidneys, lungs, and adrenal glands of mice. The net procoagulant state is illustrated by a late rise in fibrin breakdown fragments after *E. coli* challenge of baboons. Experimental data also indicate that the fibrinolytic mechanism is active in clearing fibrin from organs and circulation. Endotoxin-induced fibrin formation in the kidneys and adrenal glands was most dependent on a decrease in u-PA. PAI-1 knock-out mice challenged with endotoxin did not develop thrombi in the kidney in contrast to wild-type (WT) animals. Endotoxin administration to mice with a functionally inactive thrombomodulin gene (TMProArg mutation) and defective protein C activator cofactor function caused fibrin plugs in the pulmonary circulation, but WT animals did not develop macroscopic fibrin. This phenomenon proved to be temporary, with detectable thrombi at 4 hours after endotoxin and disappearance of clots at 24 hours in animals sacrificed at that time point. These experiments demonstrate that fibrinolytic action is required to reduce the extent of intravascular fibrin formation.

Fibrinolytic activity is markedly regulated by PAI-1, the principal inhibitor of this system. Recent studies have shown that a functional mutation in the PAI-1 gene, the 4G/5G polymorphism, not only influenced the plasma levels of PAI-1 but was also linked to clinical outcome of meningococcal septicemia. Patients with the 4G/4G genotype had significantly higher PAI-1 concentrations in plasma and an increased risk of death. Further investigations demonstrated that the PAI-1 polymorphism did not influence the risk of contracting meningitis as such but probably increased the likelihood of developing septic shock from meningococcal infection. These studies are the first evidence that genetically determined differences in the level of fibrinolysis influences the risk of developing complications of a gram-negative infection. In other clinical studies in cohorts of patients with DIC, high plasma levels of PAI-1 were one of the best predictors of mortality. These data suggest that DIC contributes to mortality in this situation, but as indicated earlier, the fact that PAI-1 is an acute phase protein, a higher plasma concentration may also be a marker of disease rather than a causal factor.

CLINICAL MANIFESTATIONS

The clinical manifestation of DIC may vary dependent on the underlying disorder. The extreme end of the spectrum is acute, severe DIC, which often occurs in the setting of sepsis, major trauma, obstetric calamities, and severe immunologic responses. Diffuse multiorgan bleeding, hemorrhagic necrosis, microthrombi in small blood vessels, and thrombi in medium and large blood vessels are common findings at autopsy, although patients who had unequivocal clinical and laboratory signs of DIC may not have confirming postmortem findings. Conversely, some patients in whom clinical and laboratory signs were not consistent with DIC had typical autopsy findings. This occasional lack of correlation among clinical, laboratory, and pathologic findings is partly attributable to extensive postmortem changes in the blood (e.g., excessive fibrinolysis) but remains unexplained in most instances. Organs most frequently involved by diffuse microthrombi are the lungs and kidneys, followed by the brain, heart, liver, spleen, adrenal glands, pancreas, and gut. Specific immunohistologic techniques and ultrastructural analysis have revealed that most thrombi consist of fibrin monomers or polymers in combination with platelets. In addition, involvement of activated mononuclear cells and other signs of inflammatory activation are frequently present. In cases of long-lasting DIC, organization and endothelialization of the microthrombi are often observed. Acute tubular necrosis is more frequent than renal cortical necrosis. Clinically, thrombotic occlusive events occur first as the result of microthrombi of fibrin or platelets that obstruct the microcirculation of organs. These thrombi result from clots that form either in the circulation or in situ in arterioles, capillaries, or venules. Circulatory obstruction produces organ hypoperfusion and even ischemia, infarction, and necrosis. The process is disseminated throughout the microcirculation; therefore, all organs are potentially vulnerable.

In contrast to acutely ill patients with complicated, severe DIC, other patients may have mild or protracted clinical manifestations of consumption or even subclinical disease manifest by only laboratory abnormalities.[1] The clinical picture of subacute to chronic DIC generally occurs in patients with malignancy, particularly with mucin-producing adenocarcinomas and acute promyelocytic leukemia (APL). The latter usually is dominated by a hemorrhagic presentation, but venous thrombotic manifestations are more common in the former. In addition, patients with solid tumors may develop nonbacterial thrombotic endocarditis with systemic arterial embolization and infarction. Another cause of subacute to chronic DIC is the retained dead fetus syndrome. These patients have an extremely variable presentation from asymptomatic to mild or moderate skin and mucous membrane bleeding.

It is important to stress that DIC is not a disease in itself but is always secondary to an underlying disorder that causes the activation of coagulation. The underlying disorders most commonly known to be associated with DIC are listed in the box on Clinical Conditions That Are Most Frequently Complicated by Disseminated Intravascular Coagulation and are described in detail below.

Clinical Conditions That Are Most Frequently Complicated by Disseminated Intravascular Coagulation

- Sepsis or severe infection
- Trauma, burn, or heatstroke
- Malignancy
  - Solid tumors
  - Acute leukemia
- Obstetric conditions
  - Amniotic fluid embolism
  - Abruptio placentae
  - HELLP syndrome
- Vascular abnormalities
  - Kasabach-Merritt syndrome
  - Other vascular malformations
  - Aortic aneurysms
- Severe allergic or toxic reactions
- Severe immunologic reactions (e.g., transfusion reaction)

Disseminated Intravascular Coagulation in Infectious Disease

Systemic infections are among the most common causes of DIC. Immunocompromised patients, asplenic patients whose ability to clear bacteria (particularly pneumococci) is impaired, and newborns whose anticoagulant systems are immature are particularly prone to infection-induced DIC. Infections may be superimposed on trauma or malignancies, which themselves are potential triggers of DIC. In addition, infections can aggravate bleeding and thrombosis by directly inducing thrombocytopenia, hepatic dysfunction, and shock, which can lead to diminished blood flow in the microcirculation.

Clinically overt DIC occurs in 30% to 50% of patients with gram-negative or -positive sepsis. Extreme examples of sepsis-related DIC are streptococcus A toxic shock syndrome, which is characterized by deep tissue infection, vascular collapse, vascular leakage, and multiple organ dysfunction. M protein released from streptococci forms complexes with fibrinogen that bind to β_2 integrins on neutrophils, leading to their activation and meningococcemia, a fulminant gram-negative infection characterized by extensive hemorrhagic necrosis, DIC, and shock. More frequent gram-negative infections associated with DIC are caused by *Pseudomonas aeruginosa, E. coli,* and *Proteus vulgaris.* Patients with these infections may only have laboratory evidence of activated coagulation or they may present with severe DIC.

Activation of the coagulation system has also been documented with nonbacterial pathogens, such as viruses, protozoa (malaria), and fungi.[14] Common viral infections, such as influenza, varicella, rubella, and rubeola, are rarely associated with DIC. Some viral infections can cause "hemorrhagic fevers" characterized by fever, hypotension, bleeding, and renal failure. Laboratory evidence of DIC can accompany Korean, rift valley, and dengue-related hemorrhagic fevers. Protozoan infections, such as cerebral malaria, may be associated with overt DIC. In these cases, secondary deficiency of a disintegrin and metalloproteinase with a thrombospondin type 1 motif, member 13 (ADAMTS13), the von Willebrand cleaving protease, may occur. Such deficiency may also complicate other types of sepsis-induced DIC and may enhance platelet–vessel wall interactions, thereby contributing to thrombosis in the microcirculation.[15]

An extreme form of DIC is represented by purpura fulminans, a severe, often lethal form of DIC in which extensive areas of the skin over the extremities and buttocks undergo hemorrhagic necrosis. The disease predominantly affects infants and children and is rare in adults. Diffuse microthrombi in small blood vessels leads to necrosis and vasculitis may also be found in biopsies of skin lesions. The disorder can occur 2 to 4 weeks after mild infection, such as scarlet fever, varicella, or rubella, or can occur during an acute viral or bacterial infection in patients with acquired or hereditary deficiencies of protein C or protein S. The syndrome mimics neonatal homozygous protein C or protein S deficiency, in which purpura fulminans, with or without extensive thrombosis, develops soon after birth.

Disseminated Intravascular Coagulation in Trauma, Brain Injury, Burns, and Heatstroke

The time interval between trauma and medical intervention correlates with the development and magnitude of DIC. Experience during wars proved that fast evacuation and prompt medical care reduce the risk of DIC. Extensive exposure of TF to the blood circulation and hemorrhagic shock probably are the most immediate triggers of DIC in such instances, although direct proof of this mechanism is lacking. An alternative hypothesis is that cytokines play a pivotal role in the occurrence of DIC in trauma patients. In fact, the changes in cytokine levels are virtually identical in trauma patients and septic patients.[16] The levels of TNF-α, IL-1β, PAI-1, circulating TF, plasma elastase derived from neutrophils, and soluble thrombomodulin all can be elevated in patients with signs of DIC, predicting multiple organ dysfunction (MOD) (ARDS included) and death. Careful monitoring of laboratory signs of DIC, reduced fibrinolytic activity, and perhaps low AT levels also are useful for predicting the outcome of such patients.

In adults and children with head injuries, a high rate of mortality occurred when DIC was present. A laboratory DIC score has predictive value for prognosis in patients with head injuries, thereby supplementing the Glasgow Coma Scale score. Brain injury can be associated with DIC, most likely because the injury exposes the abundant TF of the brain to blood. Specimens of contused brain, obtained during surgery in patients with head injury and of liver, lungs, kidneys, and pancreas obtained during autopsy, revealed microthrombi in arterioles and venules.

Bleeding, laboratory tests indicative of DIC, and vascular microthrombi in biopsies of undamaged skin have been described in patients with extensive burns. Kinetic studies with labeled fibrinogen and labeled platelets disclosed that in addition to systemic consumption of hemostatic factors, significant local consumption occurs in burned areas. TF exposed to blood at sites of burned tissue, the systemic inflammatory response syndrome induced by the burn, and the common presence of superimposed infections all can trigger DIC. Local activation of coagulation in the bronchoalveolar compartment may contribute to acute lung injury in these patients.

Severe hemorrhagic diathesis and multiple organ failure, indicative of DIC, may accompany heatstroke.[17] Diffuse fibrin deposition and hemorrhagic infarctions are found in fatal human cases. DIC associated with profound fibrin(ogen)olysis is evident in patients with heatstroke. The possible triggers of DIC in patients with heatstroke include endothelial cell damage and TF released from heat-damaged tissues. In a series of 18 critically ill patients from Paris with heatstroke during the 2003 heat wave in Western Europe that caused numerous deaths in France,[17] patients had very high levels of IL-6 and IL-8. In addition, there was a striking activation of white blood cells, as demonstrated by β2-integrin upregulation and increased production of reactive oxygen species. All patients also had evidence of a significant systemic activation of coagulation, and DIC was present in about 35% of patients. There was a marked correlation between the extent of inflammation and coagulation activation and the clinical severity of the heatstroke.

Disseminated Intravascular Coagulation in Obstetric Complications

Placental abruption is a leading cause of perinatal death.[18] Older multiparous women or patients with one of the hypertensive disorders of pregnancy are thought to be at highest risk. The severe hemostatic failure accompanying abruptio placentae is the result of acute DIC emanating from the introduction of large amounts of TF into the blood circulation from the damaged placenta and uterus. Amniotic fluid has been shown to be able to activate coagulation in vitro, and the degree of placental separation correlates with the extent of DIC, suggesting that leakage of thromboplastin-like material from the placental system is responsible for the occurrence of DIC. Abruptio placentae occurs in 0.2% to 0.4% of pregnancies, but only 10% of these cases are associated with DIC. Different grades of severity are found among those who develop DIC, with only the more severe forms resulting in shock and fetal death.

Amniotic fluid embolism is a rare but serious complication of pregnancy and delivery. A maternal mortality rate of 86% was reported in a 1979 review of 272 cases, but in a more recent population-based study, the maternal mortality rate (26.4%) was significantly lower. Patients predisposed to amniotic fluid embolism are multiparous women whose pregnancies are postmature with large fetuses and women undergoing a tumultuous labor after pharmacologic or surgical induction. Apparently, amniotic fluid is introduced into the maternal circulation through tears in the chorioamniotic membranes, rupture of the uterus, and injury of uterine veins. The trigger of DIC probably is TF present in amniotic fluid. The mechanical obstruction of pulmonary blood vessels by fetal debris, meconium, and other particulate matter in the amniotic fluid enhances local fibrin–platelet thrombus formation and fibrinolysis. The extensive occlusion of the pulmonary arteries and an acute anaphylactoid response reminiscent of severe systemic inflammatory response syndrome provoke sudden dyspnea, cyanosis, acute cor pulmonale, left ventricular dysfunction, shock, and convulsions. These symptoms are followed within minutes to several hours by severe bleeding in 37% of patients. Hemorrhage is particularly severe from the atonic uterus, puncture sites, gastrointestinal tract, and other organs.

Some studies provided evidence for significant activation of coagulation, in its most extreme form DIC, in preeclampsia and eclampsia. In a large series of patients, a good correlation was noted between the clinical severity and abnormalities in platelet counts and fibrin(ogen) degradation products. Also consistent with DIC were results of assays of sensitive parameters of thrombin generation and activation of fibrinolysis, such as thrombin-antithrombin (TAT) complexes, D-dimer, and fibrinopeptide Bβ1-42. Despite these observations, administration of heparin to patients with preeclampsia and eclampsia has not resulted in convincing benefits. The syndrome of hemolysis (H), elevated liver enzymes (EL), low platelet count (LP), and severe epigastric pain is another complication of pregnancy-induced hypertension. Liver biopsy findings of fibrin deposition in hepatic blood vessels and laboratory tests consistent with DIC in a significant proportion of patients imply that DIC plays a role in the pathogenesis of the syndrome. However, according to current insights, thrombotic microangiopathy rather than DIC causes the coagulation abnormalities seen in patients with hypertensive disorders of pregnancy.

Disseminated Intravascular Coagulation in Malignancy

Patients with solid tumors are vulnerable to risk factors and additional triggers of DIC that can aggravate thromboembolism and bleeding.[19] Risk factors include advanced age, stage of the disease, and use of chemotherapy or antiestrogen therapy. Triggers include septicemia, immobilization, and involvement of the liver by metastases that impede the function of the liver in controlling DIC. Microangiopathic hemolytic anemia frequently is induced by DIC in patients with malignancies and is particularly severe in patients with widespread intravascular metastases of mucin-secreting adenocarcinomas. Solid tumor cells can express different procoagulant molecules, including TF, which forms a complex with factor VII(a) to activate factors IX and X, and a cancer procoagulant (CP), a cysteine protease with factor X activating properties. In breast cancer, TF is expressed by vascular endothelial cells as well as the tumor cells. TF also appears to be involved in tumor metastasis and angiogenesis. Cancer procoagulant is an endopeptidase that can be found in extracts of neoplastic cells but also in the plasma of patients with solid tumors. The exact role of CP in the pathogenesis of cancer-related DIC is unclear. Interactions of P- and L-selectins with mucin from mucinous adenocarcinoma can induce formation of platelet microthrombi and probably constitute one-third mechanism of cancer-related thrombosis. Depending on the rate and quantity of exposure or influx of shed vesicles from tumors containing TF, a nonovert or overt DIC develops.

Numerous reports on DIC and fibrinolysis complicating the course of acute leukemias have been published. In 161 consecutive patients presenting with acute myeloid leukemia, DIC was diagnosed in 52 (32%). In acute lymphoblastic leukemia, DIC was diagnosed in 15% to 20%.[20] Some reports indicate that the incidence of DIC in acute leukemia patients might further increase during remission induction with chemotherapy. In patients with acute APL, DIC is present in more than 90% of patients at the time of diagnosis or after initiation of remission induction. The pathogenesis of hemostatic disturbance in APL is related to properties of the malignant cells and their interaction with the host's endothelial cells. APL cells express TF and the cancer procoagulant that can initiate coagulation, and they release IL-Iβ and TNF-α, which downregulate endothelial thrombomodulin, thereby compromising the protein C anticoagulant pathway. APL cells also express increased amounts of annexin II, which mediates augmented conversion of plasminogen to plasmin. The overall results of these processes are DIC and hyperfibrinolysis, ensued by major bleeding that can lead to death. All-*trans*-retinoic acid, used for induction and maintenance therapy of APL, inhibits in vitro and in vivo the deleterious effect of APL cells and has led to a reduced frequency of early hemorrhagic death.

Disseminated Intravascular Coagulation With Vascular Disorders

Rarely, vascular anomalies can trigger DIC. With some large aortic aneurysms, localized consumption of platelets and fibrinogen can produce coagulation abnormalities and bleeding.[21] In a series of patients with aortic aneurysms, 40% had elevated levels of fibrin(ogen) degradation products, but only 4% had laboratory evidence of DIC or bleeding.[21] Factors that predispose such patients to the development of DIC include a large aneurysm, dissection, and expansion.

Coagulation in these cases likely is triggered by the abundant TF in atherosclerotic plaques. Localized pain may occur, likely from thrombosis of vascular channels within the hemangiomas, and there may be bleeding after trauma or surgery because of the consumptive process. Increased fibrinogen consumption reflects hypofibrinolysis, which may be driven by t-PA release from the abnormal endothelium lining the tumor walls. Patients with this syndrome exhibit accelerated platelet turnover and accumulation of labeled platelets and fibrinogen in the hemangiomas.

Kasabach and Merritt were the first to describe bleeding in association with giant cavernous hemangiomas, benign tumors found in newborns or children that can evolve into convoluted masses of abnormal vascular channels that sequester and consume platelets and fibrinogen. Hemangiomas may regress spontaneously, and some respond to radiation or laser therapy.

Disseminated Intravascular Coagulation With Liver Disease

The levels of most coagulation factors, endogenous anticoagulants, and major components of the fibrinolytic system are reduced in patients with severe liver disease, reflecting reduced synthesis. In addition, the capacity of the liver to clear factors IXa, Xa, and XIa and t-PA is decreased. Thrombocytopenia is common because of hypersplenism and decreased hepatic production of thrombopoietin. The similarities between the hemostatic defects with liver disease and those with DIC have evoked controversy as to the contribution of DIC to the coagulopathy of liver disease. Several laboratory and clinical observations support the concept that DIC accompanies hepatic disorders. They include a reduced half-life of radiolabeled fibrinogen that is reversed by heparin administration, failure of replacement therapy to significantly increase the levels of hemostatic factors (suggesting ongoing consumption), and increased levels of markers of activation of coagulation. All of these findings are consistent with increased thrombin generation. Against the DIC hypothesis are the observation that microthrombi are found in only 2% of the tissues from patients who die of liver disease and the fact that the increased fibrinogen turnover can be explained by extravascular accumulation. Current thinking is that DIC is rare in patients with liver disease, but such patients are sensitive to the triggers of DIC because of the decreased synthetic capacity of the diseased liver and its inability to clear activated clotting factors. In patients who undergo peritoneovenous shunting for severe ascites, those with underlying liver disease are more likely to develop DIC than those who have normal livers.

Disseminated Intravascular Coagulation With Toxic Reactions or Snake Bites

The venom of certain snakes, particularly vipers and rattlesnakes, can produce a coagulopathy similar to that of DIC.[22] Prominent among these species are the *Vipera, Echis (Echis carinatus* or *Echis coloratus), Aspis, Crotalus, Bothrops,* and *Agkistrodon* spp. Venoms of these snakes contain enzymes or peptides that (1) release fibrinopeptide A *(Agkistrodon rhodostoma);* (2) activate prothrombin even in the absence of calcium *(E. carinatus);* (3) activate factors X and V (Russell viper venom); (4) degrade fibrinogen *(Agkistrodon acutus);* (5) induce platelet aggregation; (6) inhibit platelet aggregation because of the presence of arginine-glycine-aspartic acid–containing peptides; (7) activate protein C; and (8) damage endothelial cells, which leads to bleeding, tissue ischemia, and edema. Interestingly, victims of snake bites rarely have excessive bleeding or thromboembolism despite the abnormal coagulation tests and DIC-like picture.

LABORATORY MANIFESTATIONS

Thrombocytopenia or a rapidly declining platelet count is an important diagnostic hallmark of DIC. However, only 35% to 44% of critically ill patients develop thrombocytopenia (platelet count <150 × 10^9/L). Consequently, the specificity of thrombocytopenia for the diagnosis of DIC is limited.[10] A platelet count of less than 100 × 10^9/L is seen in 50% to 60% of DIC patients, and 10% to 15% of patients have a platelet count below 50 × 10^9/L. In surgical or trauma patients with DIC, more than 80% of patients have platelet counts less than 100 × 10^9/L.

Consumption of coagulation factors leads to low levels of coagulation factors in patients with DIC. In addition, impaired synthesis—for example, caused by impaired liver function or a vitamin K deficiency—and loss of coagulation proteins because of massive bleeding may play a role in DIC as well. Although the accuracy of the measurement of one-stage clotting assays in DIC has been contested (because of the presence of activated coagulation factors in plasma), the level of coagulation factors appears to correlate well with the severity of the DIC. The low level of coagulation factors is reflected by prolonged coagulation screening tests, such as the PT or the aPTT. A prolonged PT or aPTT occurs in 14% to 28% of intensive care patients but is present in more than 95% of patients with DIC.

Plasma levels of factor VIII are paradoxically increased in most patients with DIC, probably because of massive release of von Willebrand factor from the endothelium in combination with acute phase behavior of factor VIII. Recent studies have pointed to a relative insufficiency of the von Willebrand cleaving protease ADAMTS13, thereby causing high concentrations of ultra-large von Willebrand multimers in plasma, which may facilitate platelet–vessel wall interaction and the subsequent development of thrombotic microangiopathy, which may contribute to organ dysfunction.[15]

Measurement of fibrinogen has been widely advocated as a useful tool for the diagnosis of DIC but in fact is not very helpful to diagnose DIC in most cases.[23] Fibrinogen acts as an acute-phase reactant and despite ongoing consumption plasma levels can remain well within the normal range for a long period of time. In a consecutive series of patients, the sensitivity of a low fibrinogen level for the diagnosis of DIC was only 28%, and hypofibrinogenemia was detected in very severe cases of DIC only.

Markers of Fibrin Generation and Degradation

Plasma levels of fibrin split products are frequently used for the diagnosis of DIC.[24] Fibrin split products are detectable in 42% of a consecutive series of intensive care patients, in 80% of trauma patients, and in 99% of patients with sepsis and DIC. Fibrin degradation products (FDPs) may be detected by specific enzyme-linked immunosorbent assays (ELISAs) or by latex agglutination assays, allowing rapid and bedside determination in emergency cases. None of the available assays for FDPs discriminates between degradation products of cross-linked fibrin and fibrinogen degradation, which may cause spuriously high results. The specificity of high levels of fibrin degradation products is therefore limited, and many other conditions, such as trauma, recent surgery, inflammation, or venous thromboembolism, are associated with elevated FDPs. Because FDPs are metabolized by the liver and secreted by the kidneys, FDP levels are influenced by liver and kidney function. Other tests are specifically aimed at the detection of neoantigens on degraded cross-linked fibrin. One of such tests detects an epitope related to plasmin-degraded cross-linked chain, resulting in fragment D-dimer. These tests better differentiate degradation of cross-linked fibrin from fibrinogen or FDPs. D-dimer levels are high in patients with DIC but also poorly distinguish patients with DIC from patients with venous thromboembolism, recent surgery, or inflammatory conditions. Theoretically, measurement of soluble fibrin or fibrin monomers in plasma could be helpful to diagnose intravascular fibrin formation in DIC. Indeed, initial clinical studies indicate that if the concentration of soluble fibrin has increased above a defined threshold, a diagnosis of DIC can be made. The only problem so far is that a reliable test is not available for quantitating soluble fibrin in plasma. Because soluble fibrin in plasma can only be generated intravascularly, this test will not be influenced by extravascular fibrin formation, which, for example, may occur during local inflammation or trauma.

Endogenous Coagulation Inhibitors

Plasma levels of physiological coagulation inhibitors, such as protein C and AT, may be useful indicators of ongoing coagulation activation.[24] Low levels of these coagulation inhibitors are found in 40% to 60% of critically ill patients and in 90% of DIC patients.

Levels of protein C may indicate the severity of the DIC. In patients with meningococcal septicemia, very low plasma levels of protein C are observed, and this may play a pivotal role in the occurrence of purpura fulminans in these patients. In fact, the plasma level of protein C may also be regarded as a strong predictor for the outcome in DIC patients. Observations in patients with severe gram-negative septicemia indeed confirmed the downregulation of thrombomodulin in vivo and impaired activation of protein C. Low levels of free protein S (the cofactor of APC) may further compromise an adequate function of the protein C system.

Antithrombin is the principal inhibitor of thrombin and may be readily exhausted during continuous thrombin generation. Plasma levels of AT have been shown to be potent predictors for survival in patients with sepsis and DIC. During severe inflammatory responses, AT levels are markedly decreased not only because of consumption but also because of impaired synthesis (as a result of a negative acute phase response) and degradation by elastase from activated neutrophils.

Fibrinolytic Markers

Fibrinolytic activation in DIC may be monitored by measurement of plasma levels of plasminogen and α2-antiplasmin. Low levels may indicate consumption of these proteins. Because of the relatively low plasma concentration of α_2-antiplasmin, the determination of this protease inhibitor is a helpful test for judging the dynamics of fibrinolysis. Plasmin generation may be best judged by measurement of plasmin-α2-antiplasmin (PAP) complexes, which are indeed moderately elevated in patients with DIC. However, because the concentration of α2-antiplasmin is relatively low and therefore sensitive to relatively rapid exhaustion, this test may underestimate total fibrinolytic activity. At low concentrations of α2-antiplasmin, other protease inhibitors, such as AT, α2-macroglobulin, α1-antitrypsin, and C1-inhibitor, may act as plasmin inhibitors as well. The apparent insufficient fibrinolytic activity in patients with DIC is attributed to high levels of the inhibitor of plasminogen activation, PAI-1. Indeed, plasma levels of PAI-1 are elevated in patients with DIC and various underlying conditions and are strongly correlated with an unfavorable outcome. Of interest, studies have shown that a functional mutation in the PAI-1 gene, the 4G/5G polymorphism, not only influenced the plasma levels of PAI-1 but was also linked to clinical outcome of meningococcal septicemia and associated DIC. Patients with the 4G/4G genotype had significantly higher PAI-1 concentrations in plasma and an increased risk of death.

Point-of-Care Tests

Thrombelastography (TEG), a method that was developed decades ago, provides an overall picture of ex vivo coagulation. Modern techniques, such as rotational thrombelastography (ROTEM), enable bedside performance of this test and have again become popular in acute care settings.[25] The theoretical advantage of TEG over conventional coagulation assays is that it provides an index of platelet function as well as fibrinolytic activity. Hyper- and hypocoagulability as demonstrated with TEG was shown to correlate with clinically relevant morbidity and mortality in several studies, although its superiority over conventional tests has not unequivocally been established. Also, TEG seems to be overly sensitive to some interventions in the coagulation system, such as administration of fibrinogen, of which the therapeutic benefit remains to be established. There are no systematic studies on the diagnostic accuracy of TEG for the diagnosis of DIC, but the test may be useful for assessing the global status of the coagulation system in critically ill patients.

A new method that has proved sensitive and specific for hypercoagulability in critically ill patients is the activated partial thromboplastin time (aPTT) biphasic waveform analysis. This test, which requires specific instrumentation, detects the presence of precipitates of a complex of very-low-density lipoprotein and C-reactive protein that appears very early in DIC. When such complexes first appear in the plasma of individuals with diseases known to predispose to hypercoagulability, they confer a greater than 90% sensitivity and specificity for subsequent development of DIC and fatal outcome.

Diagnostic Algorithm for Disseminated Intravascular Coagulation

For the diagnosis of overt DIC, a simple scoring system has been developed by the subcommittee on DIC of the ISTH (see box on Diagnostic Algorithm for the Diagnosis of Overt Disseminated Intravascular Coagulation).[5] The score can be calculated based on routinely available laboratory tests, that is, platelet count, PT, a fibrin-related marker (usually D-dimer), and fibrinogen. Tentatively, a score of 5 or more is compatible with DIC, and a score of less than 5 may be indicative but is *not* affirmative for non-overt DIC. For non-overt DIC, more refined scoring systems have been developed, which are currently being evaluated. A recent study showed that the international normalized ratio (INR) can be used (instead of PT prolongation), further facilitating international exchange and standardization. By using receiver-operating characteristics curves, an optimal cutoff for a quantitative D-dimer assay was determined, thereby optimizing sensitivity and the negative predictive value of the system. Prospective studies show that the sensitivity of the DIC score is 93% and the specificity is 98%. Studies in series of patients with specific underlying disorders causing DIC (e.g., cancer, obstetric complications) show similar results. The severity of DIC according to this scoring system is related to the mortality in patients with

Diagnostic Algorithm for the Diagnosis of Overt Disseminated Intravascular Coagulation*

1. Presence of an underlying disorder known to be associated with DIC (see box on Clinical Conditions That Are Most Frequently Complicated by Disseminated Intravascular Coagulation)
   (no = 0; yes = 2)
2. Score global coagulation test results:
   - Platelet count (>100 = 0; <100 = 1; <50 = 2)
   - Level of fibrin markers (e.g., D-dimer, fibrin degradation products)
     (no increase: 0; moderate increase: 2; strong increase: 3)†
   - Prolonged prothrombin time
     (<3 sec = 0; >3 sec but <6 sec = 1; >6 sec = 2)
   - Fibrinogen level
     (>1.0 g/L = 0; <1.0 g/L = 1)
3. Calculate score
4. If >5: compatible with overt DIC; repeat scoring daily
   If <5: suggestive (not affirmative) for non-overt DIC; repeat in the next 1 or 2 days

*According to the Scientific Standardization Committee of the International Society of Thrombosis and Haemostasis.[5]

†Strong increase greater than five times the upper limit of normal; moderate increase is greater than upper limit of normal but less than five times the upper limit of normal

sepsis.[9] Linking prognostic determinants from critical care measurement scores such as APACHE-II to DIC scores is an important means to assess prognosis in critically ill patients. Similar scoring systems have been developed and extensively evaluated in Japan. The major difference between the international and Japanese scoring systems seems to be a slightly higher sensitivity of the Japanese algorithm, although this may be attributable to different patient populations because Japanese series typically include relatively large numbers of patients with hematologic malignancies.

DIFFERENTIAL DIAGNOSIS

There are several other causes of coagulation abnormalities in patients with underlying disorders known to be associated with DIC. A complicating factor is that more than one diagnosis for the coagulopathy may be present in one patient; for example, a septic patient with DIC may have liver failure and a vitamin K deficiency as well.

The differential diagnosis of thrombocytopenia in patients with suspected DIC is shown in Table 141-1. Sepsis itself is a clear risk factor for thrombocytopenia in critically ill patients, and the severity of sepsis correlates with the decrease in platelet count. The principal factors that contribute to thrombocytopenia in patients with sepsis are impaired platelet production, increased consumption or destruction, or sequestration platelets in the spleen or along the endothelial surface. Impaired production of platelets from within the bone marrow may seem contradictory to the high levels of platelet production-stimulating proinflammatory cytokines, such as TNF-α and IL-6, and high concentration of circulating thrombopoietin in patients with sepsis. These cytokines and growth factors should theoretically stimulate megakaryopoiesis in the bone marrow.

Table 141-1 Differential Diagnosis of Thrombocytopenia in Suspected Disseminated Intravascular Coagulation

Differential Diagnosis	Additional Diagnostic Clues
DIC	Prolonged aPTT and PT, increased FDP, low levels of AT or protein C
Sepsis without DIC	Positive (blood) cultures, positive sepsis criteria, hematophagocytosis in BM aspirate
Massive blood loss	Major bleeding, low hemoglobin, prolonged aPTT and PT
Thrombotic microangiopathy	Schistocytes in blood smear, Coombs-negative hemolysis, fever, neurologic symptoms, renal insufficiency, coagulation test results usually normal, ADAMTS13 levels decreased
Heparin-induced thrombocytopenia	Use of heparin, venous or arterial thrombosis, positive HIT test (usually immunoassay for heparin-platelet factor 4 antibodies), increase in platelet count after cessation of heparin; coagulation tests usually normal
Immune thrombocytopenia	Antiplatelet antibodies, normal or increased number of megakaryocytes in BM aspirate, TPO decreased; coagulation tests usually normal
Drug-induced thrombocytopenia	Decreased number of megakaryocytes in BM aspirate or detection of drug-induced antiplatelet antibodies, increase in platelet count after cessation of drug; coagulation test results usually normal

ADAMTS13, A disintegrin and metalloproteinase with a thrombospondin type 1 motif, member 13; *aPTT,* activated partial thromboplastin time; *AT,* antithrombin; *BM,* bone marrow; *DIC,* disseminated intravascular coagulation; *FDP,* fibrin degradation product; *HIT,* heparin-induced thrombocytopenia; *PT,* prothrombin time; TPO, thrombopoietin.

However, in a substantial number of patients with sepsis, marked hemophagocytosis may occur. This pathologic process consists of active phagocytosis of megakaryocytes and other hematopoietic cells by monocytes and macrophages, hypothetically because of stimulation with high levels of macrophage colony-stimulating factor (M-CSF) in sepsis.

Heparin-induced thrombocytopenia (HIT) is caused by a heparin-induced antibody that binds to the heparin–platelet factor IV complex on the platelet surface. This may result in massive platelet activation and as a consequence a consumptive thrombocytopenia and arterial and venous thrombosis occur. A consecutive series of critically ill patients who received heparin revealed an incidence of 1% in this setting. Unfractionated heparin (UFH) carries a higher risk of HIT than low-molecular-weight (LMW) heparin. Thrombosis may occur in 25% to 50% of patients with HIT (with fatal thrombosis in 4%-5%). The diagnosis of HIT is based on the detection of HIT antibodies in combination with the occurrence of thrombocytopenia in a patient receiving heparin with or without concomitant arterial or venous thrombosis. It should be mentioned that the commonly used ELISA for HIT antibodies has a high negative predictive value (100%) but a very low positive predictive value (10%).The gold standard for the diagnosis of HIT is a sensitive platelet activation assay; however, this test is usually not routinely available. Normalization in the number of platelets in 1 to 3 days after discontinuation of heparin may further support the diagnosis of HIT.

The group of thrombotic microangiopathies encompasses syndromes such as thrombotic thrombocytopenic purpura, hemolytic uremic syndrome, severe malignant hypertension, chemotherapy-induced microangiopathic hemolytic anemia, and the HELLP (hemolysis, elevated liver enzymes, low platelet count) syndrome. A common pathogenetic feature of these clinical entities appears to be endothelial damage, causing platelet adhesion and aggregation, thrombin formation, and an impaired fibrinolysis. The multiple clinical consequences of this extensive endothelial dysfunction include thrombocytopenia; mechanical fragmentation of red blood cells with hemolytic anemia; and obstruction of the microvasculature of various organs, such as the kidneys and brain (leading to renal failure and neurologic dysfunction, respectively). Despite this common final pathway, the various thrombotic microangiopathies have different underlying etiologies.

Drug-induced thrombocytopenia is another frequent cause of thrombocytopenia in critically ill patients. Thrombocytopenia may be caused by drug-induced myelosuppression, by cytostatic agents, or by immune-mediated mechanisms. Drug-induced thrombocytopenia is a difficult diagnosis in patients suspected of DIC because these patients are often exposed to multiple agents and have numerous other potential reasons for platelet depletion. Drug-induced thrombocytopenia is often diagnosed based on the timing of initiation of a new agent in relationship to the development of thrombocytopenia after exclusion of other causes of thrombocytopenia. The observation of rapid restoration of the platelet count after discontinuation of the suspected agent is highly suggestive of drug-induced thrombocytopenia.

A prolongation of global coagulation tests may be caused by a deficiency of one or more coagulation factors (Table 141-2). In addition, but more rarely, the presence of an inhibiting antibody, which can have major in vivo relevance (e.g., in acquired hemophilia) but can also be a clinically insignificant laboratory phenomenon, should be considered. The presence of lupus anticoagulants may cause a prolongation of the aPTT and can be associated with thrombocytopenia as well. Paradoxically, lupus anticoagulants may dramatically increase the risk of thrombosis. The presence of an inhibiting antibody can be confirmed by a simple mixing experiment. As a general rule, if a prolongation of a global coagulation test cannot be corrected by mixing 50% of patient plasma with 50% of normal plasma, then an inhibiting antibody is likely to be present.

In general, acquired deficiencies in coagulation factors may be caused by impaired synthesis, massive loss, or increased turnover (consumption). Impaired synthesis is often caused by liver insufficiency or vitamin K deficiency. Vitamin K deficiency may be caused by poor nutrition in combination with the use of antibiotics that affect intestinal flora and thereby bacterial vitamin K production. The PT is most sensitive to both conditions because this test is highly dependent on the plasma levels of factor VII (a vitamin K–dependent coagulation factor with a shortest half-life of the clotting factors). Liver failure may be differentiated from vitamin K deficiency by measuring factor V, which is not vitamin K dependent. In fact, factor V plays an important role in various scoring systems for severe acute liver failure. Uncompensated loss of coagulation factors may occur after massive bleeding, such as in trauma patients and patients undergoing major surgical procedures. This is particularly common in patients with major blood loss in whom intravascular volume is rapidly replaced with crystalloids, colloids, and red blood cells without simultaneous administration of coagulation factors. This resulting depletional form of coagulopathy may persist and exacerbate the bleeding. In addition, transfusion in these patients may lead to systemic activation of inflammatory processes and may contribute to further coagulation derangements. In hypothermic patients (e.g., trauma patients), measurement of the global coagulation tests may underestimate coagulation in vivo because in the laboratory test tube assays are standardized and performed at 37°C to mimic normal body temperature.

Table 141-2 Differential Diagnosis of Prolonged Activated Partial Thromboplastin Time or Prothrombin Time in Suspected Disseminated Intravascular Coagulation

Test Result	Cause
PT prolonged; aPTT normal	Factor VII deficiency Mild vitamin K deficiency Mild liver insufficiency Low doses of vitamin K antagonists
PT normal; aPTT prolonged	Factor VIII, IX, or XI deficiency UFH Inhibitory antibody or antiphospholipid antibody Factor XII or prekallikrein deficiency
both PT and aPTT prolonged	Factor X, V, or II or fibrinogen deficiency Severe vitamin K deficiency Vitamin K antagonists Global clotting factor deficiency Decreased synthesis: liver failure Increased loss: massive bleeding, DIC

aPTT, Activated partial thromboplastin time; *DIC,* disseminated intravascular coagulation; *PT,* prothrombin time; *UFH,* unfractionated heparin.

THERAPY

Adequate management of patients with DIC depends on vigorous treatment of the underlying disorder to alleviate or remove the inciting injurious cause. For sepsis-induced DIC, treatment includes aggressive use of intravenous organism-directed antibiotics and source control (e.g., by surgery or drainage). Other examples of vigorous treatment of underlying conditions are cancer surgery or chemotherapy, uterus evacuation in patients with abruptio placentae, resection of aortic aneurysm, and debridement of crushed tissue in case of trauma. In addition, intensive support of vital function supportive treatment aimed at the coagulopathy may be helpful (see box on Mainstays of Supportive Treatment of Disseminated Intravascular Coagulation),[6] as outlined in the following.

Platelet and Plasma Transfusion

Low levels of platelets and coagulation factors may increase the risk of bleeding. However, plasma or platelet substitution therapy should not be instituted on the basis of laboratory results alone; it is indicated only in patients with active bleeding and in those requiring an invasive procedure or in those at risk for bleeding complications.[6] The presumed efficacy of treatment with plasma, fibrinogen concentrate, cryoprecipitate, or platelets is not based on randomized controlled trials but appears to be rational therapy in bleeding patients or in patients at risk of bleeding who have a significant depletion of these hemostatic factors. The suggestion that administration of blood components might "add fuel to the fire" has never been proven in clinical or experimental studies.

Replacement therapy for thrombocytopenia should consist of 5 to 10 U of platelet concentrate to raise the platelet count to 20 to 30 $\times 10^9$/L and, in cases in patients who need an invasive procedure, to 50 $\times 10^9$/L.

One of the major challenges of infusion of fresh-frozen plasma (FFP) in DIC and bleeding is the propensity of the added volume, which is necessary to correct the coagulation defect, to exacerbate capillary leak. This situation can increase the risk of inducing or worsening pulmonary edema and, by extension, predisposes to acute respiratory distress syndrome and induces ascites. Coagulation factor

Mainstays of Supportive Treatment of Disseminated Intravascular Coagulation

Modality	*Details*	*Expectations/Rationale*
Treating the underlying disorder	Dependent on the primary diagnosis	Inhibit or block the complicating pathologic mechanism of DIC in parallel with the response (if any) of the disorder
Antithrombotic agents	Prophylactic heparin to prevent venous thromboembolic complications (Low-dose) therapeutic heparin in case of confirmed thromboembolism or if clinical picture is dominated by (micro)vascular thrombosis and associated organ failure	Risk of thromboembolism is increased in critically ill patients, trauma patients, and patients with cancer Prevent fibrin formation; tip the balance within the microcirculation toward anticoagulant mechanisms and physiologic fibrinolysis; allow reperfusion of the skin, kidneys, and brain
Transfusion	Infuse platelets, plasma and fibrinogen (cryoprecipitate) if there is overt bleeding or a high risk of bleeding	Bleeding should diminish and stop over the course of hours Platelet count, coagulation test results, and fibrinogen should return toward normal
Anticoagulant factor concentrates	Recombinant human activated protein C may be effective in sepsis and DIC (24 μg/kg/hr for 4 days)	Restore anticoagulation in microvascular environment and may have antiinflammatory activity
Fibrinolytic inhibitors	Tranexamic acid (e.g., 500-1000 mg every 8-12 hr or ε-aminocaproic acid 1000-2000 mg every 8-12 hr)	May be useful if there is (hyper)fibrinolysis Bleeding ceases, but there is a risk of microvascular thrombosis and renal failure

concentrates, such as prothrombin complex concentrate, may partially overcome this obstacle but do not contain essential factors, such as factor V. Moreover, caution is advocated with the use of prothrombin complex concentrates in DIC because it may worsen the coagulopathy because of traces of activated factors that are present in these concentrates. Specific deficiencies of coagulation factors, such as fibrinogen, may be corrected by administration of purified coagulation factor concentrates.

Cryoprecipitate (if available) can be used to rapidly raise the fibrinogen and von Willebrand or factor VIII levels, particularly when bleeding is part of the DIC and fibrinogen level is less than 1 g/L. Cryoprecipitate has at least four to five times the mass of fibrinogen per milliliter of infusate compared with FFP. FFP contains fibrinogen in sufficient amounts for treatment of patients with mild to moderate hypofibrinogenemia.

Anticoagulant Treatment

Heparin therapy in patients with DIC remains controversial. Experimental studies have shown that heparin can at least partly inhibit the activation of coagulation in DIC. However, a beneficial effect of heparin on clinically important outcome events in patients with DIC has not been demonstrated in controlled clinical trials. Also, the safety of heparin treatment is debatable in DIC patients who are prone to bleeding. A large trial in patients with severe sepsis showed a slight but nonsignificant benefit of low-dose heparin on 28-day mortality in patients with severe sepsis and no major safety concerns.[26]

There is general consensus that administration of heparin is beneficial in some categories of DIC, such as metastatic carcinomas, purpura fulminans, and aortic aneurysm (before resection). Heparin also is indicated for treating thromboembolic complications in large vessels and before surgery in patients with chronic DIC. Heparin administration may be helpful in patients with acute DIC when intensive blood component replacement fails to improve excessive bleeding or when thrombosis threatens to cause irreversible tissue injury (e.g., acute cortical necrosis of the kidney or digital gangrene).

Heparin should be used cautiously in all these conditions. In patients with chronic DIC because of metastatic carcinoma or aortic aneurysm, continuous infusion of UFH 500 to 750 U/hr without a bolus injection has been advocated. If no response is obtained within 24 hours, escalating dosages can be used. In hyperacute DIC cases, such as amniotic fluid embolism, septic abortion, and purpura fulminans, intravenous bolus injection of 5000 to 10,000 U heparin may be given simultaneously with replacement therapy with blood products. Some experts, however, would not administer a bolus dose of heparin even under these circumstances. Continuous infusion of 500 to 1000 U/hr of heparin may be necessary to maintain the benefit until the underlying disease responds to treatment. Apart from all of these considerations, current guidelines dictate the universal use of prophylactic doses of heparin or low-molecular-weight heparin to prevent venous thromboembolic events in critically ill patients.[6]

Theoretically, the most logical anticoagulant agent to use in DIC is directed against TF activity. Potential agents include recombinant TFPI; inactivated factor VIIa; and recombinant NAPc2, a potent and specific inhibitor of the ternary complex of TF/factor VIIa and factor Xa. Phase II trials of recombinant TFPI in patients with sepsis showed promising results, but phase III trials in patients with severe sepsis or severe pneumonia and organ failure did not show an overall survival benefit in patients who were treated with TFPI.[27]

Recombinant human soluble thrombomodulin binds to thrombin to form a complex that inactivates thrombin's coagulant activity and activates protein C and thus is a potential drug for the treatment of patients with DIC. In a phase III, randomized, double-blind clinical trial in patients with DIC, administration of the soluble thrombomodulin had a significantly better effect on bleeding manifestations and coagulation parameters than heparin. Currently ongoing trials with soluble thrombomodulin focus on DIC, organ failure, and mortality rate.

Physiological Anticoagulant Factor Concentrates

Restoration of the levels of physiological anticoagulants in DIC may be a rational approach.[28,29] Based on successful preclinical studies, the use of AT concentrates and heparin in patients with DIC has been examined mainly in randomized controlled trials that included patients with sepsis, septic shock, or both. All trials have shown some beneficial effect in terms of improvement of laboratory parameters, shortening of the duration of DIC, or even improvement in organ function. In several small clinical trials, use of very high doses of AT concentrate showed even a modest reduction in mortality, however, without being statistically significant. A large-scale, multicenter, randomized, controlled trial also showed no significant reduction in mortality of patients with sepsis.[30] Interestingly, post-hoc subgroup analyses of the latter study indicated some benefit in patients who did not receive concomitant heparin, but this observation needs validation. In a small randomized trial in patients with burns and DIC, AT administration decreased mortality, reduced multiple organ failure, and improved coagulation parameters compared with placebo-control patients.

Because a decreased function of the protein C system contributes to the pathogenesis of DIC, therapy by APC was predicted to be beneficial.[31] Indeed, a dose-ranging controlled trial using continuous infusion of recombinant human APC disclosed that a dose of 24 μg/kg/hr was optimal, judged by a decrease of D-dimer level in plasma. A subsequent phase III trial of APC concentrate in patients with sepsis was prematurely stopped because of efficacy in reducing mortality in these patients.[32] All-cause mortality at 28 days after inclusion was 24.7% in the APC group versus 30.8% in the control group (a 19.4% relative risk reduction). Amelioration of coagulation abnormalities and less organ failure were noted in patients who received the concentrate. Part of the success of therapy could be ascribed to the anti-inflammatory effect of APC. Interestingly, patients who manifested "overt DIC" (see Diagnosis) benefited more from the therapy with APC than patients who did not have overt DIC.[9] The relative risk reduction in mortality of patients with both sepsis and DIC was 38%, but patients with sepsis and no DIC had a risk reduction of 18%. This seems to underscore the importance of the coagulation derangement in the pathogenesis of sepsis and implies that the restoration of the protein C pathway in the microvasculature is essential for cure in patients with sepsis. However, meta-analyses of published literature conclude that the basis for treatment with APC even in patients with a high disease severity, is not very strong or even insufficient. The series of negative trials in specific populations of patients with severe sepsis has added to the skepticism regarding the use of APC. In addition, there is uncertainty regarding the bleeding risk of APC in patients with severe sepsis. In a phase 3 study conducted in patients with severe sepsis, the incidence of major bleeding (i.e., bleeding reported as a serious adverse event) during the infusion period was 2.4% in the APC group compared with 1.0% in the control group ($P = .02$). During the 28-day study period, the incidence of major bleeding was 3.5% in the APC group and 2.0% in the placebo group ($P = .06$). Gastrointestinal bleeding was the most frequent bleeding complication in both groups. Most bleeding episodes were procedure related or occurred in patients with a severely deranged coagulation system (partial thromboplastin time >120 sec or INR >3.0), but spontaneous bleeding was rare. The bleeding rate in the clinical trials seems to be acceptable, but it may be that in the "real world," the risk of bleeding, including intracranial bleeding, is higher. A recently completed placebo-controlled trial in patients with severe sepsis and septic shock was prematurely stopped because of the lack of any significant benefit of APC. Subsequently, the manufacturer of APC has decided to withdraw the product from the market, which has resulted in a revision of current guidelines for treatment of DIC.

Fibrinolytic Inhibitors

Most guidelines recommend against the use of antifibrinolytic agents, such as ε-aminocaproic acid or tranexamic acid, in patients with

DIC. This is because these drugs block already suppressed endogenous fibrinolysis, and may further compromise tissue perfusion. In support of this concept, there are reports of severe thrombosis in DIC patients treated with these agents. However, in patients with DIC accompanied by primary fibrino(geno)lysis, as in some cases of APL, giant cavernous hemangioma, heatstroke, and metastatic carcinoma of the prostate, the use of fibrinolytic inhibitors can be considered if the patient has profuse bleeding that does not respond to replacement therapy and there is evidence of excessive fibrino(geno)lysis.[33] In these situations, it is important to replace depleted blood components before initiating treatment with fibrinolytic inhibitors.

REFERENCES

1. Seligsohn U: Disseminated intravascular coagulation. In Handin RI, Lux SE, Stossel TP, editors: *Blood: Principles and practice of hematology,* Philadelphia, 2000, J.B. Lippincott.
2. Levi M, Seligsohn U: Disseminated intravascular coagulation. In Kaushansky K, Lichtman M, Beutler E, et al, editors: *Williams hematology,* New York, 2010, McGraw Hill, chapter 130.
3. Levi M, ten Cate H: Disseminated intravascular coagulation. *N Engl J Med* 341:586, 1999.
4. Levi M: Disseminated intravascular coagulation. *Crit Care Med* 35:2191, 2007.
5. Taylor FBJ, Toh CH, Hoots WK, et al: Towards definition, clinical and laboratory criteria, and a scoring system for disseminated intravascular coagulation. *Thromb Haemost* 86:1327, 2001.
6. Levi M, Toh CH, Thachil J, et al: Guidelines for the diagnosis and management of disseminated intravascular coagulation. *Br J Haematol* 145:24, 2009.
7. Levi M, van der Poll T: Inflammation and coagulation. *Crit Care Med* 38:S26, 2010.
8. Fourrier F, Chopin C, Goudemand J, et al: Septic shock, multiple organ failure, and disseminated intravascular coagulation. Compared patterns of antithrombin III, protein C, and protein S deficiencies. *Chest* 101:816, 1992.
9. Dhainaut JF, Yan SB, Joyce DE, et al: Treatment effects of drotrecogin alfa (activated) in patients with severe sepsis with or without overt disseminated intravascular coagulation. *J Thromb Haemost* 2:1924, 2004.
10. Levi M, Opal SM: Coagulation abnormalities in critically ill patients. *Crit Care* 10:222, 2006.
11. Osterud B, Bjorklid E: The tissue factor pathway in disseminated intravascular coagulation. *Semin Thromb Hemost* 27:605, 2001.
12. Colman RW, Schmaier AH: Contact system: A vascular biology modulator with anticoagulant, profibrinolytic, antiadhesive, and proinflammatory attributes. *Blood* 90:3819, 1997.
13. Esmon CT: The regulation of natural anticoagulant pathways. *Science* 235:1348, 1987.
14. Keller TT, Mairuhu AT, de Kruif MD, et al: Infections and endothelial cells. *Cardiovasc Res* 60:40, 2003.
15. Lowenberg EC, Meijers JC, Levi M: Platelet-vessel wall interaction in health and disease. *Neth J Med* 68:242, 2010.
16. Gando S, Nakanishi Y, Tedo I: Cytokines and plasminogen activator inhibitor-1 in posttrauma disseminated intravascular coagulation: Relationship to multiple organ dysfunction syndrome. *Crit Care Med* 23:1835, 1995.
17. Huisse MG, Pease S, Hurtado-Nedelec M, et al: Leucocyte activation: The link between inflammation and coagulation during heatstroke. A study of patients during the 2003 heat wave in Paris. *Crit Care Med* 36:2288, 2008.
18. Levi M: Disseminated intravascular coagulation (DIC) in pregnancy and the peri-partum period. *Thromb Res* 123:S63, 2009.
19. Colman RW, Rubin RN: Disseminated intravascular coagulation due to malignancy. *Seminars in Oncology* 17:172, 1990.
20. Barbui T, Falanga A: Disseminated intravascular coagulation in acute leukemia. *Semin Thromb Hemost* 27:593, 2001.
21. Fisher DF, Jr, Yawn DH, Crawford ES: Preoperative disseminated intravascular coagulation associated with aortic aneurysms. A prospective study of 76 cases. *Arch Surg* 118:1252, 1983.
22. Isbister GK: Snake bite doesn't cause disseminated intravascular coagulation: Coagulopathy and thrombotic microangiopathy in snake envenoming. *Semin Thromb Hemost* 444, 2010.
23. Levi M, de Jonge E, Meijers J: The diagnosis of disseminated intravascular coagulation. *Blood Rev* 16:217, 2002.
24. Levi M, Meijers JC: DIC: Which laboratory tests are most useful? *Blood Rev* 2010.
25. Dempfle CE, Borggrefe M: Point of care coagulation tests in critically ill patients. *Semin Thromb Hemost* 34:445, 2008.
26. Levi M, Levy M, Williams MD, et al: Prophylactic heparin in patients with severe sepsis treated with drotrecogin alfa (activated). *Am J Respir Crit Care Med* 176:483, 2007.
27. Abraham E, Reinhart K, Opal S, et al: Efficacy and safety of tifacogin (recombinant tissue factor pathway inhibitor) in severe sepsis: A randomized controlled trial. *JAMA* 290:238, 2003.
28. Levi M, de Jonge E, van der Poll T: Rationale for restoration of physiological anticoagulant pathways in patients with sepsis and disseminated intravascular coagulation. *Crit Care Med* 29:S90, S90-S94, 2001.
29. de Jonge E, van der Poll T, Kesecioglu J, et al: Anticoagulant factor concentrates in disseminated intravascular coagulation: Rationale for use and clinical experience. *Semin Thromb Hemost* 27:667, 2001.
30. Warren BL, Eid A, Singer P, et al: Caring for the critically ill patient. High-dose antithrombin III in severe sepsis: A randomized controlled trial. *JAMA* 286:1869, 2001.
31. Levi M: Activated protein C in sepsis: A critical review. *Curr Opin Hematol* 15:481, 2008.
32. Bernard GR, Vincent JL, Laterre PF, et al: Efficacy and safety of recombinant human activated protein C for severe sepsis. *N Engl J Med* 344:699, 2001.
33. Mannucci PM, Levi M: Prevention and treatment of major blood loss. *N Engl J Med* 356:2301, 2007.

CHAPTER 142

HYPERCOAGULABLE STATES

Julia A. Anderson and Jeffrey I. Weitz

Arterial and venous thromboses are common problems for all clinicians. Some patients with thrombosis have an underlying hypercoagulable state. These hypercoagulable states can be divided into three categories: inherited disorders, acquired disorders and those that are mixed in origin.[1,2]

Inherited hypercoagulable states, which are also known as thrombophilic disorders, can be due to loss of function of natural anticoagulant pathways or gain of function in procoagulant pathways (Table 142-1). Acquired hypercoagulable states represent a heterogeneous group of disorders in which the risk for thrombosis appears to be higher than that in the general population. These include such diverse risk factors as a prior history of thrombosis, obesity, pregnancy, cancer and its treatment, antiphospholipid antibody syndrome, drug-induced thrombosis such as heparin-induced thrombocytopenia or thrombosis associated with chemotherapeutic agents and myeloproliferative disorders. The pathogenesis of thrombosis in these situations is largely unknown and, in many cases, is likely multifactorial in origin. Mixed disorders are those with both an inherited and an acquired component; one example is hyperhomocysteinemia. Although severe hyperhomocysteinemia and associated homocysteinuria are rare genetic disorders, most cases of mild to moderate hyperhomocysteinemia result from acquired folate and/or vitamin B_{12} deficiency superimposed on common genetic mutations in biochemical pathways involved in methionine metabolism.[2]

Genetic hypercoagulable states and acquired risk factors combine to establish an intrinsic risk for thrombosis for each individual.[3,4] This risk can be modified by extrinsic or environmental factors, such as surgery, immobilization, or hormonal therapy, which also increase the risk for thrombosis. When the intrinsic and extrinsic forces exceed a critical threshold, thrombosis occurs (Fig. 142-1). Appropriate thromboprophylaxis can prevent the thrombotic risk from exceeding this critical threshold, but breakthrough thrombosis can occur if procoagulant stimuli overwhelm protective mechanisms.

This chapter describes the inherited, acquired, and mixed hypercoagulable states, details their laboratory evaluation, and provides practical advice for the management of these conditions.

INHERITED HYPERCOAGULABLE STATES

Inherited disorders are found in up to half of patients who present with venous thromboembolism before the age of 40, particularly those whose event occurred either in the absence of well-recognized risk factors, such as surgery or immobilization, or with minimal provocation, such as after minor trauma, after a long distance flight, or after taking estrogens.[5] Patients with inherited thrombophilic disorders often have a family history of thrombosis. Of greatest significance is a family history of sudden death due to pulmonary embolism or a history of multiple family members requiring long-term anticoagulation therapy because of recurrent thrombosis. Patients who present with venous thrombosis in unusual sites, such as the cerebral venous sinuses or mesenteric veins, those with recurrent thrombosis, and patients who develop skin necrosis upon initiation of warfarin therapy should also be suspected of having an inherited hypercoagulable state.[6,7]

From a pathophysiologic perspective, inherited hypercoagulable states fall into two categories. First are those associated with loss of function of endogenous anticoagulant proteins. These include deficiencies of antithrombin, protein C, and protein S. The second category involves gain of function in procoagulant pathways. These disorders include factor V_{Leiden} and the FIIG20210A mutation, as well as increased levels of procoagulant proteins, such as factors VIII, IX, and XI. Each of these conditions will be briefly described.

Loss of Function of Endogenous Anticoagulants

Antithrombin Deficiency

Antithrombin, a single-chain glycoprotein with a molecular weight of 52,000 Da, is a member of the serine proteinase inhibitor (serpin) superfamily that was first described by Brinkhous in 1939.[8] Antithrombin is synthesized in the liver[9] and endothelial cells, and its gene (SERPINC1, previously known as *AT3*)[10] is localized on the long arm of chromosome 1 (1q23-1q25). SERPINC1 is composed of 7 exons and 7 introns and spans 16 kb.

Antithrombin plays a critical role in regulating coagulation by forming a 1 : 1 covalent complex with thrombin, factor Xa, and other activated clotting factors. Once covalent complexes are generated, they are cleared from the circulation via the liver. The rate of antithrombin interaction with its target proteases is accelerated by heparin by 1000-fold.[11] Heparan sulfate proteoglycan, which coats the vasculature, is the physiologic counterpart of medicinal heparin.[12]

Newborn infants have approximately 50% of normal adult antithrombin levels, and much lower levels are found in preterm infants because of liver immaturity; adult levels are attained at 6 months.[13-16]

Antithrombin deficiency can be inherited or acquired[17,18] and congenital deficiency of antithrombin was the first reported inherited risk factor for venous thromboembolism.[19] Congenital antithrombin deficiency is relatively rare, occurring in about 1 in 2000,[20,21] and can be one of two types (Table 142-2),[10] both of which are inherited in an autosomal dominant fashion[17] and affect both sexes equally.[22,23] Type I deficiency, which represents the classic deficiency state, is the result of reduced synthesis of biologically normal antithrombin.[24] Heterozygotes with this condition have parallel reductions in antithrombin antigen and activity with levels reduced to about 50% those of normal. A heterogeneous group of nonsense mutations, small deletions, insertions, or single-base substitutions are the molecular cause of most cases, although gene deletions can also be responsible. In total, more than 113 mutations have been identified as causes of type I antithrombin deficiency.[25] An antithrombin mutation database compiled by members of the Plasma Coagulation Inhibitors Subcommittee of the Scientific and Standardization Committee of the International Society on Thrombosis and Hemostasis summarizes the mutations and can be accessed on the Imperial College London website (www1.imperial.ac.uk/medicine/about/divisions/department ofmedicine/experimentalmedicine/haematology/coag/antithrombin/) or in the human gene mutation database (www.hgmd.cf.ac.uk).

Table 142-1 Classification of Hypercoagulable States

Hereditary	Mixed	Acquired
LOSS OF FUNCTION		
Antithrombin deficiency Protein C deficiency Protein S deficiency	Hyperhomocysteinemia Obesity Cancer	Previous venous thromboembolism Pregnancy, puerperium Drug-induced: Heparin-induced thrombocytopenia Prothrombin complex concentrates L-asparaginase Hormonal therapy
GAIN OF FUNCTION		
Factor V Leiden Prothrombin FII20210A Elevated factor VIII, IX, or XI	Postoperative Myeloproliferative disorders	

Table 142-2 Types of Inherited Antithrombin Deficiency

Type	Antigen	Activity (no heparin)	Activity (with heparin)
I	Low	Low	Low
II (active site defect)	Normal	Low	Low
II (heparin-binding site defect)	Normal	Normal	Low

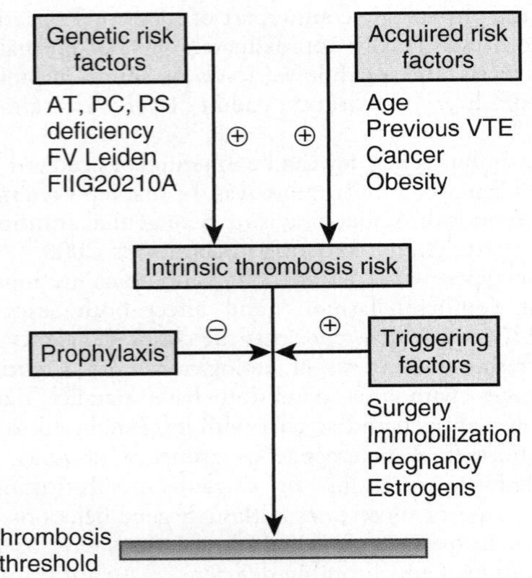

Figure 142-1 THROMBOSIS THRESHOLD. Genetic and acquired risk factors continue to determine an intrinsic risk for thrombosis for each individual. This risk is increased by extrinsic or environmental factors and decreased by thromboprophylaxis. If the intrinsic and extrinsic forces exceed a critical threshold at which thrombin generation overwhelms the protective mechanisms, thrombosis will result. *(From Anderson JA, Weitz JI: Hypercoagulability and uncommon vascular diseases. In Jaff MR, White CJ, editors:* Vascular disease: Diagnostic and therapeutic approaches, *Minneapolis, Minn, 2011, Cardiotext Publishing.)*

Table 142-3 Causes of Acquired Antithrombin Deficiency

Decreased Synthesis	Increased Consumption	Enhanced Clearance
Hepatic cirrhosis	Major surgery	Heparin
Severe liver disease	Acute thrombosis	Nephrotic syndrome
L-asparaginase	Disseminated intravascular coagulation Severe sepsis Multiple trauma Malignancy Prolonged extracorporeal circulation	

Type II antithrombin deficiencies are characterized by normal levels of antithrombin with impaired functional activity due to the presence of a variant protein. This condition is mainly caused by missense mutations that result in single amino acid substitutions.[17] The clinical consequences of type II antithrombin deficiency depend on the location of the mutation,[26,27] which may involve the reactive center loop or the heparin-binding domain. For example, some mutations in the reactive center loop of antithrombin slow its interaction with target proteases and are characterized by reduced antithrombin activity in the absence or presence of heparin. In contrast, mutations in the heparin-binding domain are associated with reduced antithrombin activity in the presence of heparin but normal activity in its absence.[28] Unlike other inherited forms of antithrombin deficiency, which are embryonic lethal in the homozygous state, mutations in the heparin-binding domain have clinical consequences only in individuals homozygous for these mutations[29] and do not increase the risk for thrombosis in the heterozygous state.

Because of the wide variety of heritable forms of antithrombin deficiency, functional antithrombin assays are the preferred method for screening. Most functional assays use synthetic substrates to monitor the rates at which added thrombin or factor Xa are inhibited in patient plasma.[16,30] However, the assays differ in terms of whether bovine or human thrombin is used and whether or not heparin is added. Defects in the heparin-binding domain of antithrombin will be detected only in the presence of heparin. When antithrombin deficiency is identified with functional assays, immunologic assays are performed to distinguish between type I and type II deficiency.

Congenital antithrombin deficiency can cause spontaneous venous thromboembolism, but thrombosis often occurs in the setting of pregnancy and the puerperium; the use of the combined oral contraceptive pill; or after major trauma or surgery. Thrombotic events are rare in children with events typically occurring from mid- to late teenage years and into the early twenties. The European Prospective Cohort on Thrombophilia (EPCOT) study compared the risks of a first episode of venous thromboembolism in asymptomatic individuals with antithrombin, protein C, or protein S deficiency with that in subjects with factor V_{Leiden} over a 6-year period. The annual incidence of venous thromboembolism was highest in those with antithrombin deficiency.[31]

The most common sites for venous thrombosis are the deep veins of the leg, but thrombosis can occur in mesenteric veins, as well as the renal and retinal veins. The risk for recurrent thrombosis is high. The risk for recurrence is not well correlated with the antithrombin level but appears to vary depending on the subtype of antithrombin deficiency.

Acquired antithrombin deficiency can reflect decreased antithrombin synthesis, increased consumption, or enhanced clearance (Table 142-3). Decreased synthesis can occur in patients with severe hepatic disease, particularly cirrhosis, or in those given L-asparaginase,[32] the latter as a result of drug-induced retention of antithrombin within the endoplasmic reticulum.[33] Increased thrombin generation can result in antithrombin consumption. Disorders associated with excessive thrombin generation include acute thrombosis, disseminated intravascular coagulation, severe sepsis, multiple trauma, disseminated malignancy, extensive burns, or prolonged extracorporeal circulation.[34,35] Heparin treatment can reduce antithrombin levels up to 20% by enhancing its clearance.[36] Severe antithrombin deficiency can also occur in some patients with nephrotic syndrome because of the loss of protein in the urine.[37]

Users of oral contraceptive pills or hormone replacement therapy may have moderate reductions in antithrombin levels; during pregnancy, the antithrombin levels do not fall significantly but decreases are found in preeclampsia and pregnancy-induced hypertensive illnesses.

Protein C Deficiency

The protein C pathway is an important natural anticoagulant pathway.[38] This on-demand pathway is activated when thrombin is generated (Fig. 142-2). Thrombin binds to thrombomodulin, a transmembrane thrombin receptor found on the surface of endothelial cells. Once bound to thrombomodulin, the substrate specificity of thrombin is altered so that it no longer serves as a procoagulant enzyme, but becomes a potent activator of protein C, a vitamin K–dependent glycoprotein. Thus thrombin bound to thrombomodulin activates protein C 1000-fold more efficiently than free thrombin.[39] The endothelial cell protein C receptor (EPCR), another transmembrane receptor on the endothelial cell surface, binds protein C and presents it to the thrombin-thrombomodulin complex for activation, thereby producing an additional 20-fold increase in the rate of protein C activation.[40,41] The physiologic importance of thrombomodulin and EPCR is highlighted by the fact that deficiency of either receptor results in embryonic lethality in mice, as does deficiency of protein C.

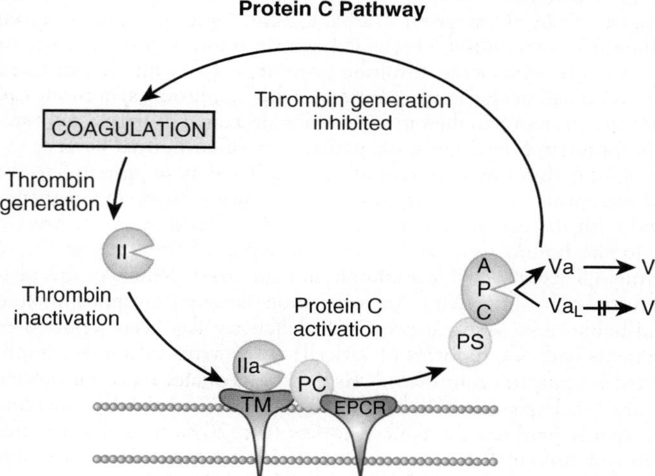

Figure 142-2 PROTEIN C PATHWAY. Activation of coagulation triggers thrombin (IIa) generation. Excess thrombin binds to thrombomodulin (TM) on the endothelial cell surface. Once bound, the substrate specificity of thrombin is altered so that it no longer acts as a procoagulant but becomes a potent activator of protein C (PC). Endothelial protein C receptor (EPCR) binds protein C and presents it to thrombomodulin-bound thrombin, where it is activated. Activated protein C (APC), together with its cofactor, protein S (PS), binds to the activated platelet-surface and proteolytically degrades factor Va (Va) into inactive fragments (Vi). Because factor Va is a critical component of the prothrombinase complex, factor Va inactivation by activated protein C attenuates thrombin generation. Because factor Va_{Leiden} (FVa_L) is resistant to inactivation by activated protein C, patients with the factor V_{Leiden} mutation have reduced capacity to regulate thrombin generation. *(From Anderson JA, Weitz JI: Hypercoagulability and uncommon vascular diseases. In Jaff MR, White CJ, editors:* Vascular disease: Diagnostic and therapeutic approaches, *Minneapolis, Minn, 2011, Cardiotext Publishing.)*

Activated protein C (APC) dissociates from this activation complex and acts as an anticoagulant by proteolytically degrading and inactivating factors Va and VIIIa, thereby attenuating thrombin generation. For efficient inactivation of factors Va and VIIIa, APC must bind to protein S, its cofactor. This interaction facilitates APC binding to activated cell surfaces, particularly the platelet surface, where factors Va and VIIIa are localized.[39]

APC has a half-life in the circulation of about 15 minutes, whereas thrombin has a half-life of about 10 seconds. APC is inhibited by protein C inhibitor and α_1-proteinase inhibitor (α_1-antitrypsin), both of which are relatively slow inhibitors. Only the activity of protein C inhibitor is enhanced by heparin, but both inhibitors appear to contribute to APC inhibition in vivo.

Protein C deficiency can be inherited or acquired. Like antithrombin deficiency, protein C deficiency is inherited in an autosomal-dominant fashion[42] and has a proven association with recurrent venous thrombosis.[43] Based on studies in healthy blood donors, heterozygous protein C deficiency can be found in 1 in 200 to 500 of the adult population,[44,45] but many of these individuals do not have a history of thrombosis. Thus the phenotypic expression of hereditary protein C deficiency is highly variable and may depend on other, as yet unrecognized, modifying factors.[5] In contrast to antithrombin deficiency in which the homozygous state is embryonic lethal, homozygous or doubly heterozygous protein C deficiency can occur. The prevalence of homozygous protein C deficiency is estimated to be 1:160,000 to 1:360,000 births.[46] Newborns with these disorders may present with purpura fulminans characterized by widespread thrombosis.[47]

Individuals with heterozygous protein C deficiency can develop skin necrosis upon initiation of warfarin therapy.[48-50] Typically, skin lesions are found on the extremities, breasts, or trunk. Starting as erythematous macules, the central regions of the cutaneous lesions become purpuric and then necrotic over a period of hours unless protein C is administered. Biopsies reveal fibrin thrombi within the vessels of the skin associated with interstitial hemorrhage. The skin lesions are clinically and histologically similar to those seen in infants with purpura fulminans and are attributable to the transient hypercoagulable state that is induced by warfarin, thereby explaining why they occur early during the course of warfarin therapy. The half-life of protein C is short and similar to that of factor VII. Starting warfarin in patients with protein C deficiency causes a further reduction in protein C levels, particularly if loading doses of warfarin are given. Thus the activity of the natural anticoagulant protein C pathway is compromised before warfarin lowers the levels of the vitamin K procoagulant proteins into the range required for its antithrombotic effects. Warfarin-induced skin necrosis has also been reported in association with acquired deficiency of protein C.[51]

Hereditary protein C deficiency can be further delineated into two subtypes using immunologic and functional assays (Table 142-4). Most functional assays use Protac, a snake venom protease, to activate protein C in plasma.[52] The enzymatic activity of APC can then be assayed directly using an APC-directed synthetic substrate, or it can be indirectly quantified by measuring the extent of prolongation of the activated partial thromboplastin time (aPTT).[53] The most common form of hereditary protein C deficiency is the classic or type I deficiency state. This disorder reflects reduced synthesis of a normal protein and is characterized by a parallel reduction in protein C antigen and activity, a quantitative deficiency due to reduced synthesis or stability of protein C.[54] A variety of genetic defects can produce type I protein C deficiency, including promoter mutations, splice-site

Table 142-4 Types of Inherited Protein C Deficiency

Type	Antigen	Activity
I	Low	Low
II	Normal	Low

abnormalities, in-frame deletions, frameshift deletions, in-frame insertions, and frameshift insertions in the protein C gene (PROC), but missense or nonsense mutations are the most common.

Type II protein C deficiency reflects synthesis of a dysfunctional protein and is characterized by normal protein C antigen with reduced functional activity, a qualitative deficiency. Most type II protein C deficiency states are caused by point mutations. Mutations in the active site of APC reduce its activity against synthetic substrates and decrease its capacity to prolong the aPTT. In contrast, mutations that affect other protein C domains essential for its activity may reduce its anticoagulant activity but may not affect its amidolytic activity. Therefore coagulation-based functional assays are preferred when screening patients for protein C deficiency.

Diagnosis of protein C deficiency is complicated. Protein C circulates in human plasma at an average concentration of 4 μg/mL. Protein C antigen levels are distributed in healthy adults so that 95% of the values range from 70% to 140%.[46] Furthermore, protein C levels increase with age by about 4% per decade with no influence of gender. The wide range of values makes it difficult to establish a normal range. Levels less than 55%, however, are likely to reflect deficiency, whereas those between 55% and 70% are considered borderline[7,38,55] and may be consistent with a deficiency state or the lower end of the normal distribution.[46] Acquired causes of protein C deficiency must be excluded, and to document the presence of protein C deficiency, it is necessary to repeat the testing. Family studies may also be helpful to highlight the autosomal dominant pattern of inheritance.

Acquired protein C deficiency can be due to decreased synthesis or increased consumption. Decreased synthesis can occur in patients with liver disease or in those given warfarin.[56] Warfarin decreases functional activity more than immunologic activity; newborns have protein C levels 20% to 40% lower than those of adults, and premature infants have even lower levels.[57,58] Protein C consumption can occur with severe sepsis, with disseminated intravascular coagulation, and after surgery.[58] Reduced protein C levels have also been reported in cancer patients receiving cyclophosphamide, methotrexate, 5-fluorouracil, or L-asparaginase.[59] A particularly severe form of acquired protein C deficiency has been described in association with meningococcal septicemia.[60] In contrast to antithrombin, which is excreted in the urine of patients with nephrotic syndrome, the levels of protein C are normal or elevated in patients with nephrotic syndrome.[61]

Protein S Deficiency

Protein S serves as a cofactor for APC and enhances its capacity to inactivate factors Va and VIIIa.[40,62] In addition, protein S may have direct anticoagulant activity by inhibiting prothrombin activation through its capacity to bind anionic phospholipid, factor Va or factor Xa, components of the prothrombinase complex.[39,63] The importance of the direct anticoagulant activity of protein S is uncertain.

In the circulation, about 60% of total protein S is bound to C4b-binding protein, an acute phase complement component. Only the 40% of the protein S that is free is functionally active.[7] The diagnosis of protein S deficiency, therefore, requires measurement of both free and bound forms of protein S. Total protein S levels can be measured immunologically under conditions that dissociate protein S from C4b-binding protein.[64] A monoclonal antibody that only recognizes noncomplexed protein S can then be used to measure free protein S.[65] The functional activity of protein S can be measured using an APC cofactor assay. This assay depends on prolongation of the aPTT when diluted patient plasma is added to protein S-depleted plasma containing APC and factor Va.[53,66]

Protein S deficiency can be inherited or acquired. Heterozygous protein S deficiency is inherited in an autosomal dominant manner; the prevalence varies between 1% and 7% among patients with thrombotic events,[67] and there is a proven association with recurrent thrombosis.[68] Based on measurements of total and free protein S antigen and protein S activity, three subtypes of inherited protein S deficiency have been identified (Table 142-5). Type I or classical deficiency results from decreased synthesis of a normal protein and is characterized by reduced levels of total and free protein S antigen together with reduced protein S functional activity. Molecular analysis of protein S deficiency is complicated because there are two homologous protein S genes, one of which is likely a pseudogene. Nonetheless, most cases of type I protein S deficiency are caused by partial gene deletions, missense mutations, base pair insertions or deletions, premature stop codons, or mutations affecting a splice site in the gene encoding protein S (PROS1).[69] Type II protein S deficiency is characterized by normal levels of total and free protein S, associated with reduced protein S activity. This type of deficiency is uncommon, and most of the causative mutations encode protein S domains involved in its interaction with APC.[70]

Table 142-5 Types of Inherited Protein S Deficiency

Type	Total Protein S	Free Protein S	Protein S Activity
I	Low	Low	Low
II	Normal	Normal	Low
III	Normal	Low	Low

Type III protein S deficiency is characterized by normal levels of total protein S, but low levels of free protein S associated with reduced protein S activity. The molecular basis of this type of deficiency appears to be similar to that of the type I deficiency states.[71] In fact, type I and type III protein S deficiency are likely to be manifestations of the same disease because they often coexist in families. Thus younger family members present with type I deficiency, whereas older family members have type III deficiency because protein S levels increase with age.

Acquired protein S deficiency can be due to decreased synthesis, increased consumption, loss, or shift of free protein S to the bound form. Decreased synthesis can occur in patients with severe liver disease,[72,73] in those given L-asparaginase,[74] and in patients given vitamin K antagonists.[72] Increased consumption of protein S occurs in patients with acute thrombosis or in those with disseminated intravascular coagulation.[73] Patients with nephrotic syndrome can lose free protein S in their urine, causing decreased protein S activity.[75] Total protein S levels in these patients are often normal because the levels of C4b-binding protein increase, shifting more protein S to the bound form. C4b-binding protein levels also increase in pregnancy and with the use of oral contraceptives.[76,77] This shifts more protein S to the bound form and lowers the levels of free protein S and protein S activity.[78,79] The pathophysiologic consequences of this phenomenon are uncertain. An association between antiphospholipid antibodies and acquired protein S deficiency has been reported in patients with severe forms of varicella zoster virus infection complicated by purpura fulminans.[80] In healthy neonates the total protein S antigen levels are 15% to 30% of normal, and the C4b-binding protein is significantly reduced to less than 20%, such that the free form of protein S predominates and the functional levels are only slightly reduced compared with normal adult levels.[81]

Gain of Function Mutations

Gain of function mutations include factor V_{Leiden}, FIIG20210A, elevated levels of procoagulant proteins, and other less well-characterized genetic disorders. The gain of function mutations are more prevalent in the general population than those associated with loss of function.

Factor V_{Leiden}

In 1993, Dahlback and colleagues described three families with a history of venous thromboembolism.[82,83] Affected family members exhibited limited prolongation of the aPTT when APC was added to their plasma. Accordingly, this phenotype was designated APC resistance (APCR). Bertina and colleagues demonstrated that APCR co-segregated with the factor V gene and was due to a single base substitution, guanine to adenine at position 1691, that produced an Arg 506 Gln mutation at one of the APC cleavage sites on factor Va.[84-86] This mutation, which is designated factor V_{Leiden}, endows activated factor V_{Leiden} with a 10-fold longer half-life in the presence of APC than its wild-type counterpart.

The factor V_{Leiden} mutation is responsible for most cases of APCR.[87,88] Other causes are mutations at Arg 306, another APC cleavage site. Arg 306 is replaced by a Gly residue in factor $V_{Hong\ Kong}$[89] and by a Thr residue in factor $V_{Cambridge}$.[90] Neither of these mutations is strongly associated with thrombosis.

The factor V_{Leiden} mutation is inherited in an autosomal-dominant fashion. The prevalence of the mutation ranges from 2% to 5% in whites,[91] but it is rare in Asians and Africans.[92,93] This racial difference likely reflects a founder effect with the mutation arising 20,000 to 30,000 years ago, after the divergence of non-Africans from Africans and Caucasoids from Mongoloid subpopulations.[94] The prevalence of factor V_{Leiden} homozygosity is about 1 in 2500.[7] The risk for thrombotic complications is lower with factor V_{Leiden} than it is with deficiencies of antithrombin, protein C, or protein S.[95-97] Heterozygotes with the factor V_{Leiden} mutation have a yearly risk of 0.1% to 0.3%, whereas the risk with deficiencies of antithrombin, protein C, or protein S ranges from 0.5% to 1.5% per year. The risk for thrombosis is higher in homozygotes than in heterozygotes. Acquired APC resistance may be caused by hormonal changes during pregnancy[98] or by the administration of estrogens, such as oral contraceptive pills[99] or hormone replacement therapy.[54,98]

A diagnosis of APCR is established using a functional assay based on the ratio of the aPTT after APC addition divided by that determined before APC addition.[100] Second-generation tests, which add dilute patient plasma to factor V-deficient plasma, are more specific for factor V_{Leiden}.[101] A normal functional test excludes factor V_{Leiden}; a positive functional test for APCR should be confirmed with a genetic test for the factor V_{Leiden} mutation.[102]

FIIG20210A Mutation

After extensive screening of 28 families with unexplained venous thromboembolism, Poort and colleagues identified a heterozygous G to A nucleotide transition at position 20210 in the 3′-untranslated region of the prothrombin gene in 5 of the probands.[103] This mutation, FIIG20210A, results in elevated levels of prothrombin. Elevated levels of prothrombin, in turn, may increase the risk for thrombosis by enhancing thrombin generation[104,105] or by inhibiting factor Va inactivation by APC.[106]

The mechanism by which the FIIG20210A mutation causes increased prothrombin levels appears to vary. Enhanced protein synthesis may result from more efficient 3′-end formation, increased messenger RNA stability, increased translation efficiency, or some combination of these mechanisms.[107] An intronic FII gene polymorphism, A19911G, which influences splicing efficiency, may modulate the effect of the FIIG20210A mutation such that heterozygous carriers of both mutations have a greater risk for thrombosis than those with only the FIIG20210A mutation.[108]

Like the factor V_{Leiden} mutation, the prevalence of the FIIG20210A mutation is higher in whites and low in Asians, American Indians, and African Americans.[109] A founder effect likely explains the higher prevalence in whites. The mutation may have provided a survival advantage based on a protective effect with childbirth or severe sepsis.[110,111]

FIIG20210A is found in 1% to 6% of whites.[103,112] The mutation is more common in southern Europe than in northern Europe, a gradient opposite to that of factor V_{Leiden}.[113] Rare individuals homozygous for the FIIG20210A mutation have been identified.[114,115] In the Leiden Thrombophilia Study, 6.2% of venous thrombosis patients and 2.3% of healthy matched controls had the FIIG20210A mutation.[116] The mutation independently confers a 2.8-fold increased risk for venous thrombosis, with no gender bias. Similar to the factor V_{Leiden} mutation, the risk for venous thrombosis is increased by the use of oral contraceptives.[117]

Laboratory diagnosis of FIIG20210A depends on genetic screening after PCR amplification of the 3′-untranslated region of the FII gene.[53] Although FIIG20210A heterozygotes have 30% higher levels of prothrombin than noncarriers, the wide range of prothrombin levels in healthy individuals precludes the use of this phenotype to identify carriers.[116,118]

Elevated Levels of Procoagulant Proteins

Elevated levels of factor VIII and other coagulation factors, including factors XI, IX and VII, have been implicated as independent risk factors for thrombosis.[119-122] Although the molecular bases for the high levels of these coagulation factors have yet to be identified, genetic mechanisms are likely responsible because the hereditability of these quantitative abnormalities is high.

Other Hereditary Disorders

The dysfibrinogenemias represent a heterogeneous group of disorders characterized by abnormal fibrinogen structure and are diagnosed by low functional and/or immunologic levels of fibrinogen, in association with prolonged thrombin and reptilase times. Acquired causes of dysfibrinogenemia, such as liver disease, must be excluded in the diagnostic work-up. Most congenital dysfibrinogenemias are asymptomatic, and they are often identified as an incidental finding when coagulation testing is performed for other reasons. Up to 40% of the known dysfibrinogenemias are associated with a bleeding diathesis. Approximately 15 variant fibrinogens, which represent less than 10% of known dysfibrinogenemias, have been reported to be associated with thrombotic complications, including fibrinogen Marburg, Caracas V, Chapel Hill III, Hannover II, Nijmegen, New York I, Christchurch II and III, and Milano III.[123] The exact mechanism by which these dysfibrinogenemias increase the risk for thrombosis depends on the nature of the fibrinogen defect. Most affect the C-terminal domain of the Aα chains or the thrombin cleavage site on the Bβ chains.[124] Some biochemical defects have been further characterized, such as defects in the release of fibrinopeptides A or B by thrombin, impaired binding of thrombin or tissue plasminogen activator to fibrin,[125,126] or resistance to lysis by plasmin.[124,127] It is likely that acquired and/or other hereditary factors contribute to thrombosis that occurs in patients with dysfibrinogenemia. For example, a woman heterozygous for fibrinogen Cedar Rapids and the factor V_{Leiden} mutation was reported to have thrombosis during pregnancy, but family members with only one hereditary defect were asymptomatic.[128]

Polymorphisms in the gene encoding EPCR have been associated with thrombosis. An EPCR polymorphism associated with high levels of soluble EPCR has been identified. By binding circulating protein C and APC, soluble EPCR competes with cell surface EPCR for protein C and prevents circulating APC from functioning as an anticoagulant.[129,130]

ACQUIRED HYPERCOAGULABLE STATES

Acquired hypercoagulable states include antiphospholipid antibody syndrome and cancer, as well as pregnancy and estrogen therapy (oral contraception or hormone replacement therapy). These disorders can occur in isolation or can be superimposed on hereditary hypercoagulable states. Heparin-induced thrombocytopenia is an immune-mediated adverse drug reaction, and is a strong, independent risk factor for arterial and venous thrombosis.

Lupus Anticoagulants and the Antiphospholipid Syndrome

First described in a study by Wasserman and colleagues in 1906 among patients with positive serologic tests for syphilis,[131] antiphospholipid antibodies are a heterogeneous group of autoantibodies directed against proteins that bind phospholipid.[132] Antibodies can be categorized into those that prolong phospholipid-dependent coagulation assays, known as lupus anticoagulants (LAs), or anticardiolipin antibodies (ACLs), which target cardiolipin. A subset of ACL recognizes other phospholipid-bound proteins, particularly β_2-glycoprotein I.

Patients who have thrombosis in association with an LA and/or ACL (antibodies of the IgG or IgM subclass directed against cardiolipin, or β_2-glycoprotein I–directed antibodies of the IgG or IgM subclass) are diagnosed with antiphospholipid syndrome (APS). The criteria for diagnosis of APS were developed in 1999[133] through international consensus and were updated in 2004.[134] APS is considered primary when it occurs in isolation and secondary when it is associated with autoimmune disorders, such as systemic lupus erythematosus or other connective tissue diseases. Clinical manifestations of APS include one or more episode of thrombosis, one or more unexplained fetal deaths at 10 or more weeks of gestation, or three or more first-trimester miscarriages (less than 10 weeks of gestation).[135] Placental thrombosis is hypothesized to be the root cause of the pregnancy-related complications that characterize APS. Intrauterine growth retardation, preeclampsia, and eclampsia have also been associated with APS. APS can also occur with cancer, with some infections, and with drugs, such as phenothiazines, phenytoin, hydralazine, or amoxicillin. Thrombosis in APS patients can be arterial, venous, or placental.[136]

To make the diagnosis of APS, at least one clinical criterion and one laboratory criterion must be met. Laboratory diagnosis of APS requires the presence of LA or ACL on tests taken at least 6 to 12 weeks apart.[137] LAs are detected using phospholipid-dependent clotting tests. Most screening assays are based on the aPTT. aPTT reagents differ in their sensitivity for detection of LA, and many laboratories have adopted less-sensitive aPTT reagents for routine aPTT testing. LA is suspected when the aPTT is prolonged. To explore the cause of the prolonged aPTT, patient plasma is mixed with normal plasma and the aPTT is again determined. If the aPTT remains prolonged, an LA is suspected. The diagnosis is confirmed by demonstrating that addition of excess hexagonal-phase phospholipid normalizes the aPTT, thereby documenting the phospholipid dependence of the abnormal test result. In addition to the aPTT, a battery of phospholipid-dependent clotting tests is often used for diagnosis of LA. These include the dilute Russell viper venom time and kaolin clotting time.[138]

ACL antibodies are detected using immunoassays.[139] Only ACL of medium to high titer and of the IgG or IgM subclass, or anti–β_2 glycoprotein-1 antibodies of the IgG or IgM subclass, are associated with thrombosis. For ACL, the amount of IgG or IgM antibody binding to cardiolipin-coated platelets is expressed in standardized GPL or MPL units, with 1 unit representing the cardiolipin-binding capacity of 1 μg/mL affinity-purified antiphospholipid antibody from reference sera. The extent of antibody binding is influenced by both the titer of the antibody and its affinity for cardiolipin. Lack of standardization of ACL assays makes it difficult to compare results between laboratories.[140,141]

ACL antibodies are found in 3% to 10% of healthy individuals. They also are common with certain infections (such as mycobacterial pneumonia, malaria, or parasitic disorders) and after exposure to some medications. Often, these antibodies are of low titer and are transient. ACL antibodies are detected in about 30% to 50% of patients with systemic lupus erythematosis.[142] Of these, 10% to 20% also have an LA.[143]

The mechanism by which antiphospholipid antibodies trigger thrombin is unclear. In cell culture systems, these antibodies can directly activate endothelial cells and induce the expression of adhesion molecules that can tether tissue factor-bearing leukocytes or microparticles onto their surface. Tissue factor can then induce clotting in vitro. Antiphospholipid antibodies also have been shown to (a) interfere with the protein C pathway, (b) inhibit antithrombin catalysis by vessel wall heparan sulfate, and (c) impair fibrinolysis.[141,144-146] Whether these mechanisms are operative in vivo has yet to be established.

In contrast to most hypercoagulable states, APS can be associated with spontaneous arterial thrombosis, as well as with venous thromboembolism.[6] Arterial thrombosis can manifest as a stroke or transient ischemic attack.[147,148] Thrombosis of the sagittal sinus, a form of venous thrombosis, also can cause stroke in these patients.[149]

Heparin-Induced Thrombocytopenia

A clinico-pathologic syndrome, heparin-induced thrombocytopenia (HIT) is diagnosed on the basis of clinical features (Table 142-6) and laboratory detection of HIT antibodies. The risk for HIT is higher with unfractionated heparin than with low-molecular-weight heparin (LMWH) and almost never occurs with fondaparinux. HIT is more common in surgical patients than in medical patients and occurs more frequently in women.

Typical clinical features of HIT include thrombocytopenia and thrombosis (arterial or venous). Less common features include necrotic skin lesions at the site of subcutaneous heparin injection, acute systemic reactions to heparin, and rarely, disseminated intravascular coagulation.[150,151] Thrombocytopenia is the most common finding, occurring in 90% of patients. Typically, the platelet count falls 5 to 10 days after heparin is started. However, thrombocytopenia can occur earlier if the patient has been exposed to heparin in the past 3 months. Rarely, the onset of HIT can be delayed and occurs several days after stopping heparin.[152]

HIT is an autoimmune-like disorder and is caused by heparin-dependent, platelet-activating antibodies of the IgG subclass. These antibodies are directed against neoantigens that are exposed on platelet factor 4 (PF4) when it forms a complex with heparin.[151] By binding to FcγII receptors on platelets, these antibodies trigger platelet activation. Activated platelets and platelet-derived microparticles provide an anionic phospholipid surface on which coagulation factors assemble and promote thrombin generation. This produces a hypercoagulable state and explains why 30% to 70% of HIT patients develop thrombosis.[153,154]

The diagnosis of HIT is supported by assays that capitalize on the platelet-activating properties of HIT antibodies. The platelet serotonin release assay is the gold standard for the diagnosis of HIT.[155] Enzyme immunoassays for detection of antibodies against PF4 are more sensitive, but are less specific than the serotonin release assay.[156]

When the diagnosis of HIT is established, heparin must be stopped and an alternative anticoagulant should be given. Options include direct thrombin inhibitors (such as lepirudin, argatroban, or bivalirudin) or factor Xa inhibitors (such as fondaparinux or danaparoid). Treatment with these agents should be continued until the platelet count returns to baseline levels at which point, low-dose warfarin can be initiated.

Cancer and Its Treatment

About 25% of patients who present with venous thromboembolism have cancer.[157] Cancer patients who develop venous

Table 142-6 Features of Heparin-Induced Thrombocytopenia

Feature	Details
Thrombocytopenia	Platelet count of 100,000/μl or less or a decrease in platelet count of 50% or more
Timing	Platelet count falls 5 to 10 days after starting heparin
Type of heparin	More common with unfractionated heparin than LMWH
Type of patient	More common in surgical patients than medical patients; more common in women than in men
Thrombosis	Venous thrombosis more common than arterial thrombosis

thromboembolism have reduced survival compared with those without this complication.[158] Patients with brain tumors, pancreatic cancer, and advanced ovarian, lung, gastrointestinal tract, or prostate cancer have particularly high rates of venous thromboembolism.[159] Treatment with chemotherapy, hormonal therapy, and biologic agents, such as erythropoietin and antiangiogenic drugs, further increases the risk for venous thromboembolism.

The pathogenesis of thrombosis in cancer patients is multifactorial in origin and represents a complex interplay among the tumor, patient characteristics, and the host hemostatic system. Tumor cells often express tissue factor or other procoagulants that can initiate coagulation.[160,161] In addition to its role in coagulation, tissue factor also acts as a cell-signaling molecule that promotes tumor proliferation and spread.

Patient factors that contribute to venous thromboembolism include immobility and venous stasis secondary to extrinsic compression of major veins by tumor. Surgical procedures, indwelling central venous catheters, and chemotherapy can produce vessel wall injury.[162] In addition, tamoxifen, selective estrogen receptor modulators (SERM), L-asparaginase, and other drugs may induce an acquired hypercoagulable state by reducing the levels of natural anticoagulant proteins.[163]

L-asparaginase and combination chemotherapeutic regimens, such as breast cancer regimens of cyclophosphamide, methotrexate, and 5-fluorouracil[164] increase the risk for thrombosis. The incidence of thromboembolic events in children receiving L-asparaginase for treatment of acute lymphocytic leukemia ranges from 1.1% to 36.7%, depending on whether or not catheter-related events are included; the overall mean is 3.2%.[165] The mechanism likely involves decreased synthesis of antithrombin, protein C, and protein S, in addition to the retention of antithrombin within the endoplasmic reticulum.[33] Concomitant administration of steroids increases the risk for thrombosis,[165] and age seems to be an important risk factor; older children demonstrate a more marked decrease in anticoagulant and fibrinolytic proteins than younger children, as well as a slower recovery to normal.[166]

Patients with multiple myeloma and other plasma cell dyscrasias are at increased risk for arterial and venous thrombosis. The reason for this is unclear, but may include acquired activated protein C resistance, elevated levels of factor VIII and/or von Willebrand factor, and the influence of the paraprotein on blood viscosity and fibrinolysis.[167,168] Patients treated with thalidomide or lenalidomide are at high risk for venous thromboembolism,[169] particularly when these drugs are given in combination with dexamethasone.[170] Several thromboprophylaxis regimens have been investigated in an attempt to mitigate this risk, including aspirin, LMWH, fixed low-dose warfarin, and therapeutic doses of warfarin, but the optimal regimen remains elusive. A recent randomized clinical trial compared aspirin, low-dose warfarin and LMWH in myeloma patients who were receiving combination therapy with lenalidomide, steroids, and melphalan. Although the results suggested that aspirin and fixed low-dose warfarin were as effective as LMWH for reducing serious venous or arterial thromboembolic events and sudden death,[171] additional studies are needed to confirm these findings.

A proportion of patients who present with unprovoked venous thromboembolism have occult cancer. This observation has prompted some experts to recommend extensive screening for cancer in such patients. Any benefits of this approach, however, are offset by potential harms. These include procedure-related morbidity, the psychologic impact of false-positive tests and the cost of screening. Furthermore, early detection of cancer is only of benefit if there is potentially curative therapy. To date, only screening for breast, cervical, and possibly colon cancer have been shown to reduce mortality.[172]

Small studies comparing extensive cancer screening with no screening in patients with unprovoked venous thromboembolism have yet to demonstrate that extensive screening reduces cancer-related mortality. Therefore it is difficult to recommend extensive screening at this time.[5] Instead, a careful history should be taken to identify any symptoms suggestive of underlying cancer. If such symptoms are present, further investigation is warranted. If there are no symptoms suggestive of underlying cancer, patients should be encouraged to undergo age-appropriate screening tests for breast, cervical, colon, or prostate cancer.

Myeloproliferative Disorders

The most common Philadelphia chromosome-negative (Ph-neg) myeloproliferative disorders, essential thrombocythemia (ET) and polycythemia vera (PV), are associated with an increased risk for thrombosis, especially arterial thrombosis, and venous thrombosis affecting the splanchnic vessels, including the hepatic and portal veins, which can lead to the Budd-Chiari syndrome, or the mesenteric veins. Thrombosis involving the microcirculation is common in patients with ET, and patients may complain of erythromelalgia, characterized by burning pain, redness and swelling of the fingers and toes, transient visual defects, or recurrent headache. Although ET and PV may evolve to myelofibrosis or transform into acute myeloid leukemia, fatal cardiovascular events are a leading cause of mortality.[173] The reported cumulative risk for thrombosis ranges from 2.5% to 5.0% per patient-year in PV and from 1.9% to 3% per patient-year in ET, depending on the patient risk category.[173-175] Age over 60 years and a previous history of thrombosis are risk factors for serious thrombosis, whereas usual cardiovascular risk factors, such as hypertension, diabetes, dyslipidemia and smoking, may place patients at intermediate risk.

The pathogenesis of thrombosis in patients with myeloproliferative disorders is multifactorial in origin and includes leukocytosis,[176] leukocyte activation, rheologic abnormalities due to raised red cell mass in PV, abnormal platelet function, and a prothrombotic endothelial phenotype.[177]

An acquired point mutation in the Janus kinase 2 gene (JAK2 G1849T) is found in up to 95% of patients with Ph-neg PV and in 50% to 60% of those with ET.[178-182] The JAK2 gene encodes a cytoplasmic tyrosine kinase that is critical for signaling between type 1 cytokine receptors and intracellular proliferation mechanisms. Currently, it is uncertain whether patients with the JAK2 mutation are at higher risk for thrombosis.[183,184] Clinical observations, supported by laboratory studies, suggest an association between the JAK2 mutation and increased leukocyte and platelet activation, as well as a correlation between the burden of the mutant allele and thrombin generation or activated protein C resistance secondary to a reduction in free protein S levels has been demonstrated in patients with ET and PV.[185] Overall, there is little to support routine JAK2 screening unless splenomegaly or an elevated hemoglobin, white blood cell, and/or platelet count raises the possibility of an underlying myeloproliferative disorder. However, it may be justifiable to check for the JAK2 mutation in patients with unexplained splanchnic or mesenteric vein thrombosis, even in the absence of evidence of these findings.[186]

Current management of PV and ET is aimed at prevention of major cardiovascular events and is based on the patient's risk category. Low-risk patients with PV are managed with phlebotomy, whereas high-risk patients are given cytoreductive therapy. Low-dose aspirin (70-100 mg daily) is recommended for all PV patients regardless of risk category, and such therapy is highly effective for treatment of the microcirculatory disturbances in patients with ET.

Paroxysmal Nocturnal Hemoglobinuria

A rare, but serious disorder, paroxysmal nocturnal hemoglobinuria (PNH) is associated with intravascular hemolysis and cytopenia.[187,188] PNH is caused by the clonal expansion of a hematopoietic stem cell that has a somatic mutation in the X-linked PIGA gene, which encodes cell surface proteins that serve as phosphatidylinositol anchors.[189] Patients with PNH may have life-threatening thrombosis that can be difficult to recognize when it affects the splanchnic or cerebral veins. Severe persistent abdominal pain or headache in patients with PNH should prompt appropriate radiologic investigations to exclude thrombosis.[188] Although patients with PNH who have documented thrombosis should be treated with anticoagulants, phlebotomy, cytoreductive therapy, and eculizumab are important adjunctive measures to reduce the risk for recurrence.[188]

Pregnancy

Pregnancy is an independent risk factor for venous thromboembolism, and the risk for venous thromboembolism in pregnant women is five- to sixfold higher than that in age-matched nonpregnant women.[7] About 1 in 1000 pregnancies are complicated by venous thromboembolism, and about 1 in 1000 women develop venous thromboembolism in the postpartum period.[190,191] Thus venous thromboembolic disease is the leading cause of maternal morbidity and mortality and is estimated to account for 12% of fatalities in pregnancy.[192-194]

The individual risk for venous thromboembolism in pregnancy and the puerperium, defined as the 6-week period after delivery, is influenced by patient-related factors. These factors include age over 35 years, body mass index over 29, Cesarean delivery, prolonged immobilization, obesity, and thrombophilia or family history of venous thromboembolism.[190,195,196] Multiparity, ovarian hyperstimulation, and a past history of venous thromboembolism[197] are other risk factors.

Over 90% of deep vein thrombosis in pregnancy occurs in the left leg because the enlarged uterus further compresses the left iliac vein by placing pressure on the overlying right iliac and ovarian arteries.[198,199] A similar mechanism likely explains the isolated left iliofemoral thrombosis that can occur in pregnancy.

Hypercoagulability of the blood occurs in pregnancy and reflects a combination of venous stasis and changes in the hemostatic system. The enlarging uterus reduces venous blood flow from the lower extremities. This is not the only mechanism responsible for venous stasis because blood flow from the lower extremities begins to decrease by the end of the first trimester, likely reflecting hormonally induced venous dilatation. Systemic factors also contribute to hypercoagulability. Thus the levels of circulating procoagulant proteins increase in the third trimester of pregnancy. These include factor VIII, fibrinogen, and von Willebrand protein, among others.[200,201] Coincidentally, suppression of natural anticoagulant pathways and decreased fibrinolytic activity occur. Thus there is an acquired resistance to activated protein C that is related, at least in part, to reduced levels of free protein S.[76,202,203] The net effect of these changes is enhanced thrombin generation, in addition to release of tissue factor from the uteroplacental circulation, as evidenced by elevated levels of prothrombin fragments and thrombin/antithrombin complexes.[204,205] Platelet activation and increased platelet turnover occur, and mild thrombocytopenia, likely secondary to consumption, occurs in 8.3% of women at term.[206] The altered levels of hemostatic proteins normalize 4 to 6 weeks after delivery.

About half of the episodes of venous thromboembolism in pregnancy occur in women with thrombophilia.[207,208] The risk for venous thromboembolism in women with thrombophilic defects depends on the type of abnormality and the presence of other risk factors.[209] The risk appears to be highest in women with antithrombin, protein C, or protein S deficiency and lower in those with heterozygosity for the factor V_{Leiden} or FIIG20210A mutations.[210-212] In general, the daily risk for venous thromboembolism in these women is higher in the postpartum period than it is during pregnancy.[213,214] The risk during pregnancy is similar in all three trimesters.[209] Therefore, if thromboprophylaxis is given during pregnancy, it must be administered throughout the pregnancy and continued for at least 6 weeks postpartum.[215]

Assisted Conception and Ovarian Hyperstimulation Syndrome

The overall risk for venous thrombosis in women undergoing ovarian hyperstimulation is small (estimated as 0.1% per treatment cycle).[216] Often, thrombosis affects veins of the upper extremities or the jugular veins; the explanation for this phenomenon remains unclear. Thrombophilia testing is not routinely recommended in women undergoing ovarian stimulation as its predictive value is low.

Hormonal Therapy

Oral contraceptives, estrogen replacement therapy,[217] and SERM are all associated with an increased risk for thrombosis.[217,218] The relatively high risk for venous thromboembolism associated with early oral contraceptives prompted development of low-dose formulations containing reduced doses of estrogen and progestin. Currently available low-estrogen combination oral contraceptives contain 20 to 50 μg of ethinylestradiol and one of several different progestins. Even these low-dose combination contraceptives are associated with a three- to fourfold increased risk for venous thromboembolism compared with the risk in nonusers. In absolute terms, this translates to an incidence of 3 to 4 per 10,000 compared with 5 to 10 per 100,000 in nonusers of reproductive age.[219]

Although smoking increases the risk for myocardial infarction and stroke in women taking oral contraceptives, it is unclear whether smoking affects the risk for venous thromboembolism.[220] In contrast, obesity increases the risk for both arterial and venous thrombosis.[221] The risk for venous thromboembolism is highest during the first year of oral contraceptive use and persists only for the duration of use.[222,223]

Case-control studies suggest that the risk for venous thromboembolism is 20- to 30-fold higher in women with inherited thrombophilia who use oral contraceptives than the risk for nonusers with thrombophilia or users without these defects.[219,224-226] Despite the increased risk, however, routine screening for thrombophilia is not indicated in women considering the use of oral contraceptives. Based on the estimated incidence and case fatality rate of thrombotic events, it is estimated that 400,000 women would need to be screened to detect 20,000 carriers of factor V_{Leiden}. Oral contraceptives would need to be withheld in all of these women to prevent a single death.[227] For less prevalent thrombophilic defects, even large numbers of women would need to be screened. Based on these considerations, routine screening cannot be recommended.

Oral contraceptive pills may cause prothrombotic side effects by inducing modest increases in levels of procoagulant factors (such as factors VII, VIII, X, prothrombin, and fibrinogen) and decreases in the levels of anticoagulant proteins (such as antithrombin and protein S). Acquired APC resistance is an almost universal finding in women taking oral contraceptives; the clinical significance of this phenomenon is uncertain.

In recent years, mounting evidence suggests that hormonal replacement therapy with conjugated equine estrogen (with or without a progestin) increases the risk for myocardial infarction, ischemic stroke, and venous thrombosis. Carriers of the factor V Leiden mutation receiving hormone replacement therapy have a significantly increased risk for venous thromboembolism.[162,228] Data from the Heart and Estrogen Replacement Study (HERS) and the Estrogen Replacement and Atherosclerosis Trial indicate that heterozygous carriers of the factor V_{Leiden} mutation who were taking hormone replacement therapy had a 14-fold higher risk for venous thromboembolism compared with noncarriers receiving placebo.[229,230] Based on this information, the use of hormone replacement therapy has markedly decreased.

SERMs are estrogen-like compounds. The prototypical SERM is tamoxifen, which serves as an estrogen antagonist in the breast, but has an estrogen agonist in other tissues, such as bone and uterus.[231] Like estrogens, tamoxifen increases the risk for venous thromboembolism three- to fourfold.[232] The risk is higher in postmenopausal women, particularly those also receiving systemic combination chemotherapy.[163]

Aromatase inhibitors are replacing tamoxifen for treatment of estrogen receptor–positive breast cancer. These newer agents are associated with a lower risk for venous thromboembolism than is tamoxifen.[233] Raloxifene, a SERM used to prevent osteoporosis, increases the risk for venous thromboembolism threefold compared with placebo.[234] Therefore this agent is contraindicated for prevention of osteoporosis in women with a prior history of venous thromboembolism.[214]

Prior History of Venous Thromboembolism

A history of previous venous thromboembolism places patients at risk for recurrence.[235,236] Those with unprovoked venous thromboembolism have a particularly high risk for recurrence when anticoagulant treatment is stopped.[237] Their risk for recurrence is about 10% at 1 year and 30% at 5 years. This risk occurs regardless of whether or not there is an underlying thrombophilic defect, such as factor V_{Leiden} or the FIIG20210A mutation.

The risk for recurrent venous thromboembolism is lower in patients whose incident event occurred in association with a well-recognized and transient risk factor, such as major surgery or prolonged immobilization. These patients have a risk for recurrence of about 4% at 1 year and 10% at 5 years. Patients whose initial venous thromboembolic event was associated with minor risk factors, such as oral contraceptive use or following a long distance flight, likely have an intermediate risk for recurrence.[238,239] Patients at highest risk for recurrence are those homozygous for factor V_{Leiden} or the FIIG20210A mutation and those with antiphospholipid antibody syndrome, advanced malignancy, or inherited deficiencies of antithrombin, protein C, or protein S. These patients' risk for recurrence is likely to be 15% at 1 year and up to 50% at 5 years.[95-97]

COMBINED INHERITED AND ACQUIRED HYPERCOAGULABLE STATES

Hyperhomocysteinemia is the prototypical hypercoagulable state that occurs due to a combination of inherited and acquired factors.[240,241] Homocysteine is an intermediate sulfur-containing amino acid that acts as a methyl group donor during the metabolism of methionine, an essential amino acid derived from the diet. The interconversion of methionine and homocysteine depends on the availability of 5-methyltetrahydrofolate, a methyl group donor, vitamin B_{12} and folate, cofactors in the interconversion, and the enzyme methionine synthase.[242] Increased levels of homocysteine can be the result of increased production or reduced metabolism. Severe hyperhomocysteinemia and cysteinuria are rare and are usually caused by deficiency in the enzyme, cystathione β-synthetase.[243] More common is mild to moderate hyperhomocysteinemia. This can be caused by genetic mutations in methyltetrahydrofolate reductase (MTHFR) when they are accompanied by nutritional deficiency of folate, vitamin B_{12}, or vitamin B_6.[244] Common polymorphisms in MTHFR, C677T and A1298C, are associated with reduced enzymatic activity and increased thermolability. The cofactor requirements are therefore increased with these mutations.[2] Hyperhomocysteinemia also can be associated with certain drugs, such as methotrexate, theophylline, cyclosporine, and most anticonvulsants, as well as some chronic diseases, such as end-stage renal disease, severe hepatic dysfunction, and hypothyroidism.[245]

A fasting serum homocysteine level over 15 mmol/L is considered elevated. Although elevated levels were a common finding, routine fortification of flour with folic acid has resulted in lower homocysteine levels in the general population.[246,247] Elevated serum levels of homocysteine have been associated with an increased risk for arterial thrombosis (myocardial infarction, stroke, and peripheral arterial disease) and venous thromboembolism.[245,248]

Elevated levels of homocysteine can be reduced by administration of folate with vitamin B_{12} and vitamin B_6.[249] Recent randomized trials, however, have shown that reduction of homocysteine levels with vitamin therapy does not reduce the risk for recurrent cardiovascular events in patients with coronary artery disease or stroke,[250] nor does it lower the risk for recurrent venous thromboembolism. Based on these negative trials and the declining incidence of hyperhomocysteinemia, the enthusiasm for screening for hyperhomocysteinemia has rapidly declined.

CLINICAL EVALUATION OF PATIENTS WITH HYPERCOAGULABLE STATES

A carefully taken history is essential to evaluate a patient with a history of thrombosis. The patient's age at the time of thrombosis, the location of the thrombosis and results of objective diagnostic tests should be recorded. A historical record of previous thromboses and sites, and potential risk factors, such as recent surgery, trauma, prolonged immobility, pregnancy, or estrogen use should be noted. A family history of thrombosis, especially in first-degree relatives may point to a heritable thrombophilic defect; systemic symptoms, such as anorexia, weight loss, change in bowel habits, or gastrointestinal bleeding may suggest an underlying malignant condition.

A full physical examination should be conducted with attention to abdominal or pelvic masses, lymphadenopathy, and skin changes such as skin necrosis and livedo reticularis. Basic investigations are necessary to exclude acquired causes of thrombosis and to assess the patient's general health and tolerance to anticoagulation (see box on Routine Investigations to Evaluate a Patient With [Venous] Thrombosis).

THROMBOPHILIA SCREENING

In the past, the indications for thrombophilia screening were somewhat controversial,[251,252] and the implications of such tests were often misinterpreted.[253] It is now apparent that testing for heritable thrombophilia does not predict the likelihood of recurrence in unselected

Routine Investigations to Evaluate a Patient With (Venous) Thrombosis

Test	*Abnormality*	*Diagnostic Information*
Complete blood count	Elevated hematocrit Increased white count Increased platelet count Leukopenia Thrombocytopenia	Myeloproliferative disorder (e.g., essential thrombocythemia, polycythemia vera); may be found in paroxysmal nocturnal hemoglobinuria; if associated with heparin administration, consider heparin-induced thrombocytopenia
Blood film	Leukoerythroblastic film	Underlying neoplasm invading bone marrow
Liver function tests	Abnormal tests	May point to malignancy
Renal function	Impaired renal function	Assess prior to anticoagulation with heparin or LMWH
Urinalysis	Proteinuria	Nephrotic syndrome; may be associated with venous thromboembolism or renal vein thrombosis
PT and aPTT	Prolonged PT and aPTT	To enable safe anticoagulation to proceed if required Need to exclude lupus anticoagulant

patients with symptomatic venous thrombosis.[254,255] For patients with a first episode of venous thromboembolism, thrombophilia screening is indicated only if the results influence the duration of treatment or have an impact on family counseling regarding use of estrogen-containing compounds.[53] It is reasonable to screen patients whose first episode of thrombosis occurred before the age of 40 years, patients with thrombosis in an unusual site,[256] such as cerebral or mesenteric veins, and those with two or more first-degree relatives with unprovoked thrombosis. Women with a previous unprovoked episode of thrombosis and those who develop thrombosis during pregnancy or in association with estrogen treatment qualify for thromboprophylaxis on the basis of clinical history alone, but it is not unreasonable to perform a thrombophilia screen in such situations. It also is reasonable to screen women with a history of more than one second-trimester pregnancy loss or intrauterine death.[7] Neonates and children with purpura fulminans should be urgently tested for protein C or S deficiency, as should adults who develop skin necrosis in association with vitamin K antagonists[257] (see box on When to Perform a Thrombophilia Screen).

LABORATORY EVALUATION OF THROMBOPHILIA

Screening should include functional assays for antithrombin and protein C, an immunoassay for free protein S, testing for activated protein C resistance using the modified APC sensitivity ratio with DNA testing for the factor V_{Leiden} mutation if the screening test is positive, DNA testing for the FIIG20210A gene mutation, phospholipid-based clotting tests to detect a lupus anticoagulant and enzyme immunoassay for ACL[5] (see box on Essential Tests for Thrombophilia Screening). The benefits and potential harms of thrombophilia testing should always be discussed in advance with the patient because the psychologic impact of knowing that they are a carrier of a genetic defect is one of the disadvantages of testing,[54,258] and test results may also impact on the cost of life insurance.

When to Perform a Thrombophilia Screen

Clinical Scenario

- First episode of unprovoked venous thromboembolism in individuals younger than 40 years of age
- Thrombosis in an unusual site (e.g., cerebral or mesenteric thrombosis)
- Two or more first-degree relatives with unprovoked thrombosis
- Females with a history of more than one second-trimester pregnancy loss or intrauterine death

Essential Tests for Thrombophilia Screening

Basic coagulation screen
- International Normalized Ratio (INR): to exclude warfarin effect—warfarin will lower protein C and S levels
- Activated partial thromboplastin time (aPTT): to exclude heparin effect—heparin will lower antithrombin levels

Functional assay for antithrombin: (with heparin to detect type II defects)
Functional assay for protein C
Functional assay for protein S: (immune assays for total and free protein S)
APC resistance assay: with genetic test for factor V_{Leiden} for confirmation of abnormal results
Genetic test for FIIG20210A gene mutation

The timing of thrombophilia screening is critical. Levels of natural anticoagulants may be lower at the time of an acute thrombotic event; additionally, heparin can reduce the level of antithrombin, while vitamin K antagonists, such as warfarin, reduce the levels of protein C and protein S. Therefore testing is best performed after the acute event and when anticoagulant treatment has stopped. During pregnancy, protein S levels fall, which complicates the diagnosis of protein S deficiency. The investigation of other family members may be helpful to exclude an acquired cause.

MANAGEMENT OF THROMBOSIS IN PATIENTS WITH HYPERCOAGULABLE STATES

Thrombosis treatment is usually divided into two overlapping stages, initial treatment and extended therapy. The impact of hypercoagulable states on these two stages is discussed separately as is their impact on duration of anticoagulant therapy and recommendations for prevention of recurrence.

Initial Treatment

With few exceptions, management of initial thrombotic events in patients with hypercoagulable states is no different from the management of these events in patients without underlying hypercoagulable disorders.[101] The exceptions are purpura fulminans in newborns with homozygous protein C or protein S deficiency, warfarin-induced skin necrosis, and thrombosis in patients with severe antithrombin deficiency. Newborns with purpura fulminans require protein C or protein S concentrates or sufficient amounts of plasma to increase the levels of protein C or protein S.[259,260]

Patients with severe antithrombin deficiency can usually be managed with low-molecular-weight-heparin (LMWH) or unfractionated heparin, although some patients may require considerably higher doses to achieve therapeutic anticoagulation. Some individuals may require antithrombin concentrates to increase plasma levels of antithrombin to a point where heparin or LMWH can be used for treatment.[113,261] Antithrombin concentrates are commercially available in plasma-derived and recombinant forms. The aim of treatment with antithrombin concentrate is to initially increase antithrombin activity to greater than 120% of the normal level (based on an expected 1.4% increase above baseline activity level per IU/kg of antithrombin administered) and to then maintain antithrombin activity at over 80% of the normal level.[262] Plasma antithrombin levels need to be monitored to ensure that levels over 80% are maintained; antithrombin has a half-life of 2 to 4 days. A recombinant human antithrombin concentrate produced in the milk of transgenic goats has recently become available; due to differences in glycosylation, transgenic antithrombin has a shorter half-life of 11 hours and a fourfold higher affinity for heparin.[263]

The management of acute venous thromboembolism in patients with APS is similar to that in other patients. However, monitoring treatment with heparin or vitamin K antagonists can be problematic because the aPTT or INR may be prolonged at baseline. Under these circumstances, heparin can be monitored using an anti-Xa assay. Alternatively, LMWH or fondaparinux can be used in place of heparin because these agents do not require coagulation monitoring. In asymptomatic subjects with laboratory evidence of ACL or LA, but no history of venous or arterial thrombosis, appropriate thromboprophylaxis should be given at time of thrombotic challenge, such as major surgical procedures, prolonged immobilization, or pregnancy and the puerperium. There is no indication for primary preventive treatment with anticoagulants or antiplatelet agents in such individuals.

Extended Therapy

Extended treatment of thrombosis in patients with hypercoagulable states is similar to that of patients without these underlying disorders. Caution is needed when starting patients with protein C or protein

S deficiency on warfarin or other vitamin K antagonists to prevent skin necrosis.[264] Warfarin should not be started in these patients until therapeutic anticoagulation has been fully achieved with heparin or LMWH. Once started, low doses of warfarin should be given to prevent precipitous decreases in the levels of protein C or protein S; the heparin or LMWH should only be stopped when the INR has been therapeutic for at least 2 consecutive days.

Recent randomized trials have shown that usual-intensity warfarin (target INR of 2.0 to 3.0) is as effective as higher-intensity warfarin in patients with antiphospholipid antibody syndrome. The risk for major bleeding is lower with usual-intensity warfarin than it is with higher-intensity regimens.[265,266] A target INR of 2.5 with an INR range from 2.0 to 3.0 is appropriate for patients with other hypercoagulable states as well.[267]

Patients with thrombosis who have a history of metastatic cancer may do better with extended treatment with LMWH. Randomized clinical trials have shown that, compared with warfarin, LMWH reduces the risk for recurrent venous thromboembolism without increasing bleeding.[268] Furthermore, LMWH simplifies treatment because it can be given subcutaneously once-daily without coagulation monitoring. The drug can be held before invasive procedures, and the dose may be reduced if thrombocytopenia is present. The major drawbacks of LMWH are cost and its requirement for parenteral administration, although the drug has been shown to be cost-effective in patients at high risk for recurrent venous thromboembolism (see box on Clinical Scenarios That Merit Long-Term Anticoagulation).

In patients with APS, warfarin is effective for prevention of recurrent thrombosis, and randomized clinical trials have demonstrated that a target INR of 2 to 3 is as effective as an INR of 3 to 4 in prevention of recurrent venous thromboembolism.[269,270] If the baseline INR is prolonged because of LA, vitamin K antagonists can be monitored by following the levels of factor X and titrating the dose of warfarin to maintain factor X levels less than 25% of normal; extended treatment with LMWH is another option.

Duration of Treatment

The presence of a hypercoagulable state has no influence on the duration of anticoagulant treatment in patients whose venous thromboembolic event occurred in the setting of a well-recognized and transient risk factor, such as major surgery or prolonged immobilization due to medical illness. These patients are treated with anticoagulants for at least 3 months.[271] For those with unprovoked venous thromboembolism, a minimum of 3 months of anticoagulation treatment is recommended, but most patients are given long-term treatment provided that they are not at high risk for bleeding.[237,272] Heterozygosity for factor V_{Leiden} or the FIIG20210A mutation does not influence the risk for recurrence. In contrast, patients with deficiency of antithrombin, protein C, or protein S or those homozygous for factor V_{Leiden} or the FIIG20210A mutation appear to be at higher risk for recurrence and likely should receive longer-term anticoagulation treatment.[273-275] Likewise, patients with APS with a persistent ACL or LA are also at high risk for recurrence and require long-term treatment.[132]

The decision to continue anticoagulation indefinitely requires consideration of the site and severity of the first episode of venous thromboembolism, information on whether or not the event was provoked, consideration of other risk factors, and an assessment of the risk for anticoagulant-related bleeding.[257] The decision should also take into account patient adherence and patient preferences. Commonly cited criteria for indefinite anticoagulation include the following: two or more unprovoked venous thrombotic events within a relatively short space of time (i.e., less than 2 years); one unprovoked event in an individual with antithrombin, protein C or S deficiency, persistently positive LA and/or ACL, or active cancer; a single unprovoked event in an individual with combined heterozygosity or homozygosity for factor V_{Leiden} or the prothrombin gene mutation; and a single unprovoked severe pulmonary embolism.

Clinical Scenarios That Merit Long-Term Anticoagulation*

- Two or more unprovoked venous thrombotic events in less than 2 years, or within a relatively short space of time
- A single unprovoked thrombosis in an individual with antithrombin deficiency, APS, dual heterozygosity for the factor V_{Leiden} and FIIG20210A gene mutations, or homozygosity for these mutations
- A single unprovoked massive or submassive pulmonary embolism
- An episode of venous thrombosis in a patient with active malignancy

*Note: Each clinical scenario requires an individual assessment of the balance between the risks for recurrent thrombosis and major hemorrhage and should consider patient preference.

Treatment and Prevention of Thrombosis During Pregnancy

Thrombophilic disorders have no influence on the treatment of venous thrombosis during pregnancy. These women require therapeutic doses of subcutaneous heparin, LMWH, or fondaparinux throughout pregnancy.[215,276] Heparin is given once daily with the dose titrated to achieve a therapeutic midinterval aPTT. LMWH can be given once or twice daily in a weight-adjusted fashion.[209] Monitoring with anti–factor Xa levels is recommended, particularly in the third trimester. Fondaparinux is given once daily. It is uncertain whether monitoring is required. After delivery, LMWH or warfarin should be given for at least 4 to 6 weeks. In total, treatment should be given for 6 months from the time of diagnosis. Warfarin and LMWH can be safely administered in nursing mothers, with no detectable anticoagulant effect in breast milk.[135]

Women with a past history of unprovoked or recurrent venous thromboembolism, those homozygous for factor V_{Leiden} or the FIIG20210A mutation, and those with deficiencies of antithrombin, protein C, or protein S should receive antepartum prophylaxis with heparin or LMWH.[215] Postpartum, LMWH or warfarin should be given for 4 to 6 weeks.[277] Postpartum treatment with LMWH or warfarin for 4 to 6 weeks is likely adequate for women with a history of venous thrombosis secondary to a well-defined risk factor.[278] Prophylaxis during pregnancy, as well as postpartum, should be considered for women who developed venous thromboembolism after taking oral contraceptives particularly if they have underlying thrombophilia. Women with thrombophilic defects and no prior history of venous thromboembolism likely do not require antepartum prophylaxis or postpartum treatment, but definitive data are lacking.[215] A summary of these recommendations is provided in Table 142-7.

Thrombophilia and Fetal Loss

About 30% of women have at least one fetal loss, and approximately 5% of women of reproductive age experience recurrent fetal loss.[279] Women with hereditary thrombophilia have a two- to fivefold increased risk for fetal loss.[280] Acquired hypercoagulable states, particularly antiphospholipid antibody syndrome, also increase the risk for fetal loss.[281-283] The use of once-daily heparin or LMWH in prophylactic doses, with or without aspirin, is often prescribed for women with recurrent fetal loss on the background of an underlying thrombophilic defect, although no adequate clinical trial assessing the efficacy of such an approach is available.[277]

CONCLUSIONS AND FUTURE DIRECTIONS

Inherited or acquired hypercoagulable states can now be identified in up to 50% of patients with venous thromboembolism thanks to an

Table 142-7 Management of Women With a History of Venous Thrombosis During Pregnancy and the Puerperium

Clinical History	Thrombophilia	Antepartum	Postpartum*
Prior VTE due to a transient risk factor	No	Surveillance	Yes
Prior VTE due to pregnancy or estrogens	Yes or no	Prophylactic heparin or LMWH	Yes
Prior idiopathic VTE	Yes or no	Prophylactic heparin or LMWH	Yes
Recurrent VTE	Yes or no	Treatment-dose heparin or LMWH	Resume long-term anticoagulation
No prior VTE	Antithrombin deficiency; homozygous FIIG20210A; or Factor V leiden; or dual heterozygosity for both mutations	Treatment-dose heparin or LMWH	Yes Consider antithrombin concentrate in antithrombin deficiency

*Postpartum prophylaxis involves a 4- to 6-week course of warfarin with the dose adjusted to achieve an INR of 2.0 to 3.0. Prophylactic doses of LMWH can be used as an alternative.

increased understanding of the regulation of coagulation. The role of these disorders in the pathogenesis of arterial thrombosis is less clear, and further research is necessary to identify those individuals vulnerable to arterial thrombosis after plaque rupture. Despite an improved ability to diagnose hypercoagulable states, the impact of this information on clinical decisions remains limited. Common congenital hypercoagulable states increase the risk for a first thrombotic episode but appear to have little impact on the risk for recurrence. Identification of biomarkers for patients at risk for recurrent thrombosis and elucidating new hypercoagulable states are goals for the future.

SUGGESTED READINGS

Austin SK, Lambert JR: The JAK2 V617F mutation and thrombosis. *Br J Haematol* 143:307, 2008.

Baglin T, Gray E, Greaves M, et al: Clinical guidelines for testing for heritable thrombophilia. *Br J Haematol* 149:209, 2009.

Baglin T, Luddington R, Brown K, et al: Incidence of recurrent venous thromboembolism in relation to clinical and thrombophilic risk factors: Prospective cohort study. *Lancet* 362:523, 2003.

Brill Edwards P, Ginsberg JA, Gent M, et al: Safety of withholding heparin in pregnant women with a history of venous thromboembolism: Recurrence of clot in this pregnancy study group. *N Engl J Med* 343:1439, 2000.

Comp PC, Nixon RR, Cooper MR, et al: Familial protein S deficiency is associated with recurrent thrombosis. *J Clin Invest* 74:2082, 1984.

Crowther MA, Ginsberg JS, Julian J, et al: A comparison of two intensities of warfarin for the prevention of recurrent thrombosis in patients with the antiphospholipid antibody syndrome. *N Engl J Med* 349:1133, 2003.

Crowther MA, Kelton JG: Congenital thrombophilic states associated with venous thrombosis: A qualitative overview and proposed classification system. *Ann Intern Med* 138:128, 2003.

Dahlback B: The discovery of activated protein C resistance. *J Thromb Haemost* 1:3, 2003.

Esmon CT: The protein C pathway. *Chest* 124:26S, 2003.

Lowering blood homocysteine with folic acid based supplements: Meta-analysis of randomised trials. Homocysteine Lowering Trialists' Collaboration. *BMJ* 316:894, 1998.

Griffin JH, Evatt B, Zimmerman TS, et al: Deficiency of protein C in congenital thrombotic disease. *J Clin Invest* 68:1370, 1981.

Jennings I, Kitchen S, Woods TA, et al: Multi-laboratory testing in thrombophilia through the United Kingdom National External Quality Assessment Scheme (Blood Coagulation) Quality Assurance Program. *Semin Thromb Hemost* 31:66, 2005.

Kearon C, Gent M, Hirsh J, et al: A comparison of three months of anticoagulation with extended anticoagulation for a first episode of idiopathic venous thromboembolism. *N Engl J Med* 340:901, 1999.

Lane DA, Bayston T, Olds RJ, et al: Antithrombin mutation database: 2nd (1997) update. For the Plasma Coagulation Inhibitor Subcommittee of the Scientific and Standardization Committee of the International Society on Thrombosis and Haemostasis. *Thromb Haem* 77:197, 1997.

Lee AYY, Levine MN, Baker R, et al: Low-molecular weight heparin versus a coumarin for the prevention of recurrent venous thromboembolism in patients with cancer. *N Engl J Med* 349:146, 2003.

Lim W, Crowther MA, Eikelboom JW: Management of Antiphospholipid antibody syndrome. *JAMA* 295:1050, 2006.

Lonn E, Yusuf S, Arnold MJ, et al: Homocysteine lowering with folic acid and B vitamins in vascular disease. *N Engl J Med* 354:1567, 2006.

Luzzatto L, Gianfaldoni G, Notaro R: Management of Paroxysmal Nocturnal Haemoglobinuria: A personal view. *Br J Haematol* 153:709, 2011.

Manco-Johnson MJ, Marlar RA, Jacobson LY: Severe protein C deficiency in newborn infants. *J Pediatr* 113:359, 1988.

Middeldorp S, van Hylckama Vlieg A: Does thrombophilia testing help in the clinical management of patients? *Br J Haematol* 143:321, 2008.

Miyakis S, Lockshin MD, Atsumi T, et al: International consensus statement on an update of the classification criteria for definite antiphospholipid syndrome (APS). *J Thromb Haemost* 4:295, 2006.

Muszbek L, Bereczky Z, Kovacs B, et al: Antithrombin deficiency and its laboratory diagnosis. *Clin Chem Lab Med* 48:S67, 2010.

Prandoni P, Lensing AW, Cogo A, et al: The long-term clinical course of acute deep venous thrombosis. *Ann Intern Med* 125:1, 1996.

Poort SR, Rosendaal FR, Reisma PH, et al: A common genetic variation in the 3'-untranslated region of the prothrombin gene is associated with elevated prothrombin levels and an increase in venous thrombosis. *Blood* 88:3698, 1996.

Tripodi A: A review of the clinical and diagnostic utility of laboratory tests for the detection of congenital thrombophilia. *Semin Thromb Hemost* 31:25, 2005.

Vandenbroucke JP, Rosing J, Bloemenkamp KWM: Oral contraceptives and the risk of venous thrombosis. *N Engl J Med* 344:1527, 2001.

Vossen CY, Conard J, Fontcuberta J, et al: Risk of a first venous thrombotic event in carriers of a familial thrombophilic defect: The European Prospective Cohort on Thrombophilia (EPCOT). *J Thromb Haemost* 3:459, 2005.

Warkentin TE: Drug-induced immune-mediated thrombocytopenia—from purpura to thrombosis. *N Engl J Med* 356:891, 2007.

Warkentin TE: Heparin-induced thrombocytopenia: Pathogenesis and management. *Br J Haematol* 121:535, 2003.

Wolberg AS, Monroe DM, Roberts HR, et al: Elevated prothrombin results in clots with an altered fiber structure: A possible mechanism of the increased thrombotic risk. *Blood* 101:3008, 2003.

For complete list of references log on to www.expertconsult.com.

CHAPTER 143

ANTIPHOSPHOLIPID SYNDROME

Jacob H. Rand and Lucia R. Wolgast

The antiphospholipid (aPL) syndrome (APS) is an autoimmune thrombophilic condition that is defined by a combination of clinical and laboratory criteria. This chapter reviews the current understanding of aPL-mediated pathogenic mechanisms, diagnostic tests for the condition, its clinical manifestations, and current treatment approaches.

DEFINITION AND DIAGNOSTIC CATEGORIES

In general terms, APS can be described as an autoimmune thrombophilic condition in which patients have circulating antibodies against plasma proteins that bind to phospholipids. The formal investigational criteria for APS (often referred to as the Sydney Criteria), detailed in Table 143-1, require that patients have documented evidence of vascular thrombosis or obstetric complications attributable to placental vascular insufficiency. The latter include otherwise unexplained recurrent miscarriages, intrauterine growth restriction, intrauterine fetal demise, preeclampsia or toxemia, placental abruption, and preterm labor. The laboratory criteria require persistent abnormality of one or more of the aPL assays (i.e., at least two abnormal measurements at least 12 weeks apart), which include elevated anticardiolipin (aCL) immunoglobulin G (IgG) or IgM antibodies, anti–β_2-glycoprotein I (anti-β_2GPI) IgG or IgM antibodies, or a lupus anticoagulant (LA). As described in this chapter, the diagnosis of APS in a patient with thrombosis may have an impact on the duration and intensity of anticoagulant treatment.

It is important for readers to understand that these criteria were not designed as requirements for the clinical diagnosis of APS. Rather, the intent was to provide a uniformly rigorous definition of APS for standardization of research on the disorder. In clinical practice, some patients may be appropriately diagnosed with presumptive APS without meeting the strict investigational criteria. Occasional patients may even have negative test results on aPL assays but have typical clinical manifestations of the disorder, a situation referred to as *seronegative APS* (SNAPS).

Patients with APS may also have clinical manifestations that have been associated with aPL antibodies but were not included in the clinical criteria. These "noncriteria manifestations" include thrombocytopenia, livedo reticularis, skin ulcers, nephropathy, migraine, cognitive defects, diffuse alveolar hemorrhage and valvular heart disease (Libman-Sachs endocarditis). Some patients with APS may also test positive for "noncriteria" clinical laboratory tests (described later) that have not been included by consensus panels as diagnostic criteria for the disorder.

At the present time, APS may be divided into the following subcategories: (1) primary APS is "stand-alone" APS in the absence of systemic lupus erythematosus (SLE); (2) secondary APS occurs in the presence of SLE; (3) SNAPS includes patients who test entirely negative for the disorder but are nevertheless suspected of having it on clinical grounds; and (4) catastrophic APS (CAPS), which manifests as disseminated thrombosis in large and small vessels with resulting multiorgan failure (Table 143-2).

ANTIGENIC SPECIFICITIES OF ANTIPHOSPHOLIPID ANTIBODIES

β_2Glycoprotein I

β_2-Glycoprotein I, a 50-kd glycoprotein member of the complement control protein (CCP) superfamily, is believed to be a major antigenic target for aPL antibodies. The protein consists of five homologous CCP domains, each consisting of about 60 amino acids, with a fifth domain that includes a phospholipid binding site near the NH_2-terminal of the protein (Fig. 143-1). Recently, it has been reported that the protein undergoes a conformational change when it binds to membranes. Transmission electron microscopy analysis of negatively stained β_2GPI molecules indicates that the free unbound protein has a circular confirmation that is caused by the affinity of its COOH-terminal domain (domain V) for the NH_2-terminal domain (domain I); when membrane bound, the protein assumes an open "fishhook" conformation in which the portion of domain I that is inaccessible in the coiled fishhook conformation becomes exposed for recognition by autoantibodies (see Fig. 143-1). This domain I epitope appears to be a major target for thrombogenic aPL antibodies. Binding of β_2GPI to membranes that express anionic phospholipids occurs via the affinity of cationic residues near the NH_2-terminus for anionic polar heads of phospholipids and by a hydrophobic loop that inserts into the lipid bilayer.

Several properties have been ascribed to β_2GPI, although its biologic function has not been resolved. Among these, β_2GPI binds to apoptotic cells and may aid in their phagocytosis and clearance. Recent evidence suggests that, consistent with its structure, the protein may have a complement control function. β_2GPI can also bind to oxidized low-density lipoprotein (oxLDL) and may play a role in their clearance. Recently, a new role for β_2GPI has been identified in innate immunity; the protein binds to and clears lipopolysaccharide (LPS), thereby reducing LPS binding to the Toll-like receptor 4 (TLR4), and the triggering of downstream endotoxin effects.

Although the protein has several effects on coagulation and hemostatic reactions, genetic deficiency of β_2GPI is not associated with bleeding or thrombosis in humans. Likewise, homozygous β_2GPI null mice also do not display any obvious disease phenotype. Although not yet tested, it is possible that these mice may be more susceptible to LPS challenge. The heterozygous pregnant female mice were reported to produce fewer than expected numbers of homozygous β_2GPI-null offspring, which suggested that the protein might contribute to—but not be absolutely required for—successful pregnancy. A recent study in humans suggested an atheroprotective role for the protein since elevated levels of β_2GPI-protected older (but not younger) men from myocardial infarction (MI).

All five domains of β_2GPI have been reported to be recognized by anti-β_2GPI antibodies isolated from patients. Of these, IgG antibodies directed against an epitope on domain I comprising Gly40-Arg43 has correlated with LA activity and had a strong association with thrombosis; that study also found that antibodies with heterogeneous reactivities for the other domains were not correlated with an increased risk for thrombotic complications.

Table 143-1 Sydney Investigational Criteria for the Diagnosis of the Antiphospholipid Syndrome*

CLINICAL

- Vascular thrombosis (one or more episodes of arterial, venous, or small vessel thrombosis). For histopathologic diagnosis, there should be no evidence of inflammation in the vessel wall.
- Pregnancy morbidities attributable to placental insufficiency, including: (1) three or more otherwise unexplained recurrent spontaneous miscarriages before 10 weeks of gestation; (2) one or more fetal losses after the 10th week of gestation; (3) stillbirth; and (4) episode of preeclampsia, preterm labor, placental abruption, intrauterine growth restriction, or oligohydramnios that are otherwise unexplained.

LABORATORY

- Medium- or high-titer aCL or anti-β_2GPI IgG or IgM antibody present on two or more occasions, at least 12 weeks apart, measured by standard ELISAs.
- Lupus anticoagulant in plasma on two or more occasions at least 12 weeks apart detected according to the guidelines of the ISTH SSC Subcommittee on Lupus Anticoagulants and Phospholipid-Dependent Antibodies.

Modified from Miyakis S, Lockshin MD, Atsumi T, et al: International consensus statement on an update of the classification criteria for definite antiphospholipid syndrome (APS). *Thromb Haemost* 4:295, 2006.
aCL, Anticardiolipin; *aPL,* antiphospholipid; *β_2GPI,* β_2-glycoprotein I; *ELISA,* enzyme-linked immunosorbent assay; *Ig,* immunoglobulin, *ISTH SSC,* International Society on Thrombosis and Haemostasis, Scientific and Standardization Subcommittee.
*"Definite APS" is considered to be present if at least one of the clinical criteria and one of the laboratory criteria are met.

Table 143-2 Proposed Criteria for the Classification of Catastrophic Antiphospholipid Syndrome

1. Evidence of involvement of three or more organs, systems, or tissues*
2. Development of manifestations simultaneously or in less than 1 week
3. Confirmation by histopathology of small vessel occlusion in at least one organ or tissue†
4. Laboratory confirmation of the presence of aPL antibodies (lupus anticoagulant or anticardiolipin antibodies)‡

Definite catastrophic APS
- All four criteria

Probable catastrophic APS
- All four criteria except for only two organs, systems, or tissues involvement
- All four criteria except for the absence of laboratory confirmation at least 6 weeks apart caused by the early death of a patient never previously tested for aPL before the catastrophic APS event
- Criteria 1, 2, and 4
- Criteria 1, 3, and 4 and the development of a third event in more than 1 week but less than 1 month despite anticoagulation

Modified from Asherson RA, Cevera R, de Groot PG, et al: Catastrophic antiphospholipid syndrome: International consensus statement on classification criteria and treatment guidelines. *Lupus* 12:530, 2003.
aPL, Antiphospholipid; *APS,* antiphospholipid syndrome.
*Usually, clinical evidence of vessel occlusions, confirmed by imaging techniques when appropriate. Renal involvement is defined by a 50% rise in serum creatinine, severe systemic hypertension (N180/100 mm Hg), or proteinuria (N500 mg/24 h).
†For histopathologic confirmation, significant evidence of thrombosis must be present, although in contrast to Sydney criteria, vasculitis may coexist occasionally.
‡If the patient had not been previously diagnosed as having an APS, the laboratory confirmation requires that the presence of antiphospholipid antibodies must be detected on two or more occasions at least 6 weeks apart (not necessarily at the time of the event), according to the proposed preliminary criteria for the classification of definite APS.

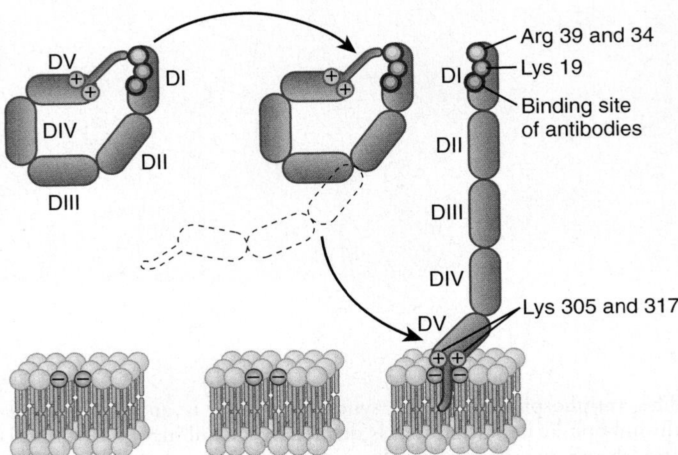

Figure 143-1 SCHEMATIC REPRESENTATIONS OF THE CONFORMATIONAL STATES OF β_2GPI. The protein circulates as a "coiled fish-hook" in which the epitope on domain I (DI) is shielded by a portion of domain V (DV). Binding to phospholipid membranes via a "barb" near the carboxyterminus of DV opens the protein and exposes an immunogenic epitope near the aminoterminal portion of the molecule. *(From Rand JH: A snappy new concept for APS.* Blood *116:1193, 2010. Inside* Blood *commentary on Agar C, van Os GM, Morgelin M, et al: Beta2-glycoprotein I can exist in 2 conformations: Implications for our understanding of the antiphospholipid syndrome.* Blood *116:1336, 2010. Professional illustration by Paulette Dennis. Reprinted with permission from Agar C, van Os GM, Morgelin M, et al: β2-Glycoprotein I can exist in 2 conformations: Implications for our understanding of the antiphospholipid syndrome.* Blood *116:1336, 2010.)*

Additional Antigenic Targets

Targets other than β_2GPI that have been identified for aPL antibodies include prothrombin, factor V, protein C, protein S, annexin A2, annexin A5, high- and low-molecular-weight (LMWH) kininogen, heparin, factor VII/VIIa, and plasmin. Recently, the cytoskeletal intermediate filament, vimentin, was also shown to be a target for aPL antibodies; in that study, about half of patients with clinical manifestations but lacking positivity for the standard aPL antibodies (i.e., patients with SNAPS) had serologic evidence for antivimentin/cardiolipin antibodies. Antibodies to lyso(bis)phosphatidic acid (LBPA), a hydrophobic isomer of phosphatidylglycerol, have also been shown to exert LA activity. Autoantibodies have also been found to bind sulfatides, acidic glycosphingolipids, which can interact with sulfatide-binding proteins such as von Willebrand factor (vWF), thrombospondin, and P-selectin.

β_2GPI appears to have both beneficial and harmful effects on the toxicity of oxLDL, which promote endothelial dysfunction and cytokine release and contribute to atherosclerosis. On the one hand, β_2GPI can bind to oxLDL to form oxLDL–β_2GPI complexes that may promote oxLDL clearance. On the other hand, recent data have indicated that binding of β_2GPI to oxLDL promotes aPL autoimmunity by facilitating dendritic cell presentation of β_2GPI epitopes to autoreactive T cells.

PATHOGENIC MECHANISMS

Several different mechanisms have been proposed to explain the thrombotic manifestations of APS (Table 143-3).

Pathogenic Effects of Anti-β_2GPI Antibodies on Endothelial Cells

Antiphospholipid antibodies can bind to, injure, or activate cultured vascular endothelial cells. Antibody binding to β_2GPI on the

Table 143-3 Proposed Pathogenic Mechanisms of Antiphospholipid Syndrome

I. Pathogenic effects of anti-β_2GPI antibodies on endothelial cells
  A. Direct injury and subsequent anti-β_2GPI binding on endothelial cells
  B. Signaling via annexin A2/TLR4/ApoER2′ inducing proadhesive prothrombotic phenotype
  C. Induction of adhesion molecules and TF on endothelial cells and cytokine release
II. Activation of platelets by aPL antibodies
  A. Activation of platelets via ApoER2′, GPIbα, or β_2GPI–platelet factor 4 interaction
  B. Interference of vWF-mediated platelet adhesion
III. Inhibition of endogenous anticoagulant and fibrinolytic mechanisms
  A. Disruption of the annexin A5 anticoagulant shield
  B. Interference with fibrinolysis via annexin A2, β_2GPI cofactor activity, autoactivation of XIIa, direct inhibition of plasmin, and increase of PAI-1
  C. Inhibition of the protein C pathway: decreased activation of protein C, barrier of APC proteolysis of factor Va and VIIIa, prevention of protein C, and EPCR binding
  D. Interference with TFPI
IV. aPL-mediated activation of complement

aPC, Activated protein C; *aPL,* antiphospholipid; *β_2GPI,* β_2-glycoprotein I; *EPCR,* endothelial cell protein C receptor; *GP,* glycoprotein; *PAI-1,* plasminogen activator inhibitor 1; *TF,* tissue factor; *TFPI,* tissue factor pathway inhibitor; *TLR4,* Toll-like receptor 4; *vWF,* von Willebrand factor.

endothelial surface can also trigger signaling cascades that promote increased expression of tissue factor (TF) and adhesion molecules (Fig. 143-2). Evidence indicates that annexin A2, which forms tetramers with S100 and is an endothelial surface receptor for tissue plasminogen activator (t-PA) and plasminogen, serves as a receptor for β_2GPI on vascular endothelium. Annexin A2 is not a transmembrane protein, and the signaling coreceptors, TLR4/TLR2 and CD14 have been implicated as triggering of the signaling cascade. In support of this aPL-mediated mechanism, a mutation in murine TLR4 that disrupts LPS binding attenuated the prothrombotic state in wild-type mice induced by aPL antibody administration.

Antiphospholipid-mediated promotion of TF expression induces trophoblast injury and fetal death in mice. In addition, TF contributes to the C5a-induced oxidative burst in neutrophils, which leads to trophoblast and fetal injury in APS. A mAb against factor B that disrupts the alternative pathway of complement activation, protects against aPL antibody–induced fetal loss in mice by preventing complexation of C3b and factor B.

Apolipoprotein E receptor 2′ (ApoER2′), a member of the LDL receptor family and a multiligand receptor with a wide tissue distribution, may also be a target for anti-β_2GPI–β_2GPI complexes that trigger TF and cell adhesion molecule expression on the endothelial surfaces (see Fig. 143-2). ApoER2′ is expressed on endothelial cells, platelets and monocytes, where it may mediate the pathogenic effects of the antibodies. Evidence from ApoER2′$^{-/-}$ knockout mice supports such a role raising the possibility that treatments that interfere with antibody binding to this receptor may be of value in APS.

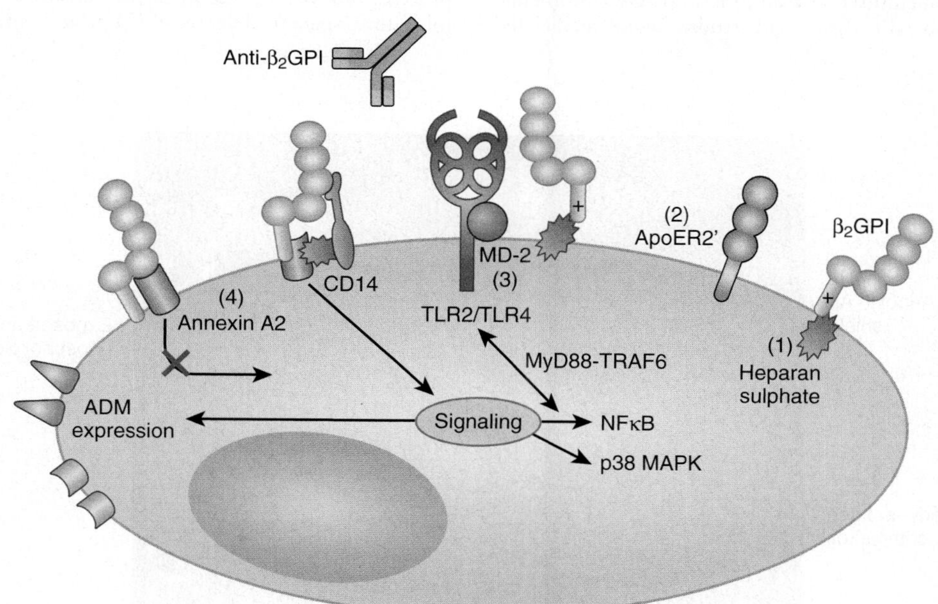

Figure 143-2 ENDOTHELIAL CELL SURFACE AND RECEPTOR ACTIVATION BY ANTI-β_2GPI–β_2GPI COMPLEXES. In this model, anti-β_2GPI–β_2GPI complexes bind to the endothelial membrane through the cationic DV of β_2GPI to a number of receptors, including (1) anionic structures, such as heparan sulfate; (2) apolipoprotein E receptor 2′ (ApoER2′); (3) Toll-like receptor 2 or 4 (TLR2/TLR4); and (4) annexin A2, to promote downstream signaling pathways involving p38 mitogen-activated protein kinase (p38 MAPK) and nuclear factor kappa-B (NFκB), leading to the upregulation of tissue factor and adhesion molecules (ADM) and a proinflammatory and prothrombotic phenotype. Annexin A2 does not have a transmembrane domain; therefore, other membrane proteins such as CD14, TLR2/TLR4, and ApoER2′, may act as accessory molecules. *β_2GPI,* β_2 glycoprotein I; *MyD88,* myeloid differentiation primary response protein MyD88; *TRAF6,* tumor necrosis factor receptor–associated factor 6. *(Adapted from Meroni PL, Borghi MO, et al: Pathogenesis of antiphospholipid syndrome: Understanding the antibodies.* Nat Rev Rheumatol *7:330, 2011.)*

Activation of Platelets by aPL Antibodies

Antiphospholipid antibodies can induce platelet activation and aggregation. The binding of β_2GPI dimers to ApoER2′ on platelets increases the sensitivity of platelets to low concentrations of agonists. Recombinant dimers of β_2GPI, which were designed to model anti-β_2GPI antibody-mediated dimerization of β_2GPI, increase platelet adhesion to collagen and thrombus formation in flow systems, effects that are abrogated by inhibiting thromboxane A2 synthesis. aPL antibodies may also interfere with the inhibitory effect of β_2GPI on the platelet–vWF interaction; this "inhibition of an inhibitor" effect may result in increased platelet adhesion.

Inhibition of Endogenous Anticoagulant and Fibrinolytic Mechanism

Antiphospholipid antibodies accelerate coagulation reactions on endothelial cells and trophoblasts by disrupting an antithrombotic shield composed of annexin A5. Annexin A5 is a potent anticoagulant protein with high affinity for phospholipid membranes that contain anionic phospholipids, specifically phosphatidylserine. The protein forms two-dimensional crystalline arrays over the phospholipid bilayers (Fig. 143-3) that render anionic phospholipids available for coagulation factor complex assembly. Annexin A5 is highly expressed by endothelial cells and on the apical membranes of placental syncytiotrophoblasts, the location where maternal blood interfaces with fetal cells. Annexin A5 binds to these cells and inhibits thrombin formation. This may explain why pregnant mice given anti–annexin A5 antibodies develop placental necrosis, fibrosis, and pregnancy loss.

Numerous studies indicate a reduction in cell surface annexin A5 in APS, including immunohistochemical analysis of placental villi in APS patients, exposure of cultured human umbilical vein endothelial cells or trophoblasts to aPL IgG, and studies with artificially reconstituted phospholipid bilayers. The reduction of cell surface annexin A5 is the result of competitive displacement by aPL IgG–β_2GPI immune complexes (see Fig. 143-3). Loss of all surface annexin A5 induces a prothrombotic phenotype.

Antiphospholipid antibodies can affect fibrinolytic mechanisms in several ways. Patients with APS have high annexin A2–directed antibodies that can interfere with t-PA or plasminogen binding to the endothelial cell surface, thereby attenuating plasmin generation. In addition, mAbs isolated from APS patients can directly inhibit plasmin activity. Finally, β_2GPI serves as a cofactor for t-PA–mediated activation of plasminogen. Consequently, aPL antibodies directed against β_2GPI can downregulate plasmin generation.

Antiphospholipid antibodies can interfere with several steps in the protein C anticoagulant pathway. These include (1) reducing the activation of protein C by the thrombomodulin–thrombin complex; (2) inhibiting the assembly of the protein C complex; (3) inhibiting the activity of protein C, or cofactor protein S; and (4) binding to factors Va and VIIIa and protecting them from proteolysis by activated protein C (APC). Some aPL antibodies can recognize protein C or protein S (or both) and may reduce their levels by accelerating their clearance. One study found an association between anti–protein C IgM and venous thrombosis. In addition, antibodies against β_2GPI may crossreact with APC and vice versa. APC resistance has been described in APS plasma and correlates with anti-β_2GPI domain I antibodies.

Autoantibodies against TF pathway inhibitor (TFPI) have also been reported in patients with APS; dysregulation of TF–factor VIIa activity may also contribute to the increased risk of thrombosis.

Antiphospholipid-Mediated Activation of Complement

Complement activation may also play a role in the APS disease process. Blockade of complement activation with a C3 convertase inhibitor or genetic deletion of C3 protects mice from the pregnancy

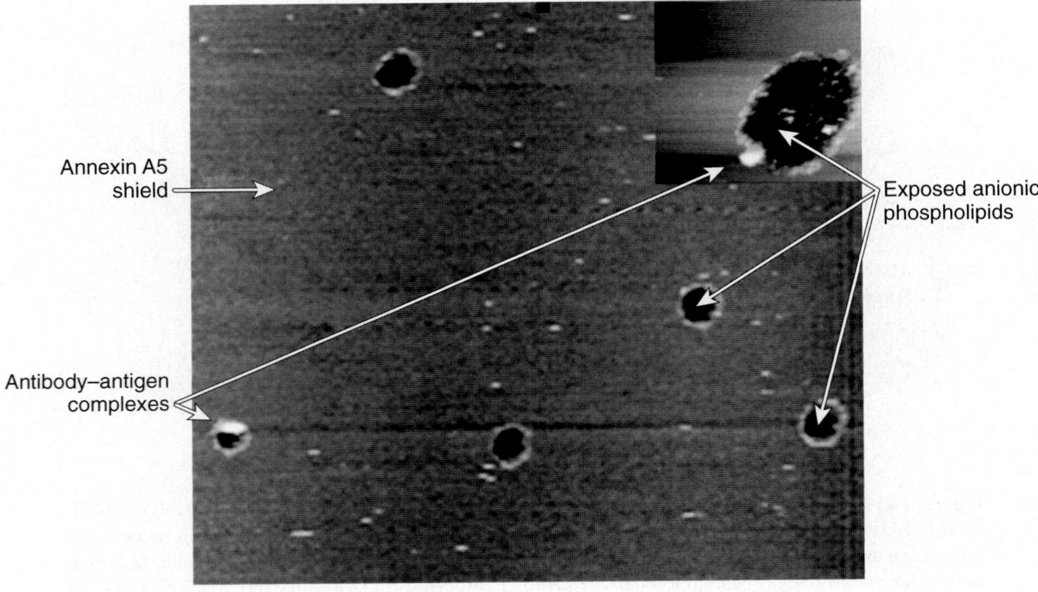

Figure 143-3 DISRUPTION OF ANNEXIN A5 SHIELD BY MONOCLONAL ANTIPHOSPHOLIPID (aPL) ANTIBODIES AND β_2 GLYCOPROTEIN I (β_2GPI). Atomic force microscopy picture showing the effect of aPL mAB IS3 on a preformed annexin A5 crystal. The figure demonstrates the smooth lipid bilayer covered by the annexin A5 crystals, disrupted by antibody–β_2GPI complexes *(white rims)* and exposing anionic phospholipids *(black holes)* to coagulation factors and accelerated coagulation. *(Adapted from Rand JH, Wu XX, Quinn AS, et al: Human monoclonal antiphospholipid antibodies disrupt the annexin A5 anticoagulant crystal shield on phospholipid bilayers: Evidence from atomic force microscopy and functional assay.* Am J Pathol *163:1193, 2003.)*

complications induced by aPL antibodies. Complement activation in APS appears to involve (1) direct aPL antibody–induced injury to endothelial cells and monocytes, which promotes cell lysis and inflammation, and (2) protease activated receptor 2 (PAR-2) signaling with upregulation of TF expression by monocytes.

Genetic, Genomic, and Proteomic Studies in Antiphospholipid Syndrome

Although familial APS is rare, genetic factors appear to influence development of aPL antibodies. In a study of seven families that included 30 individuals who met the consensus criteria for APS, the inheritance pattern of aPL antibodies appeared to be autosomal dominant. However, no specific linkages could be identified. A recent study using peripheral blood mononuclear cells isolated from aPL antibody–positive patients found a gene expression pattern that correlated with the predisposition for thrombosis. Some of these genes encoded proteins involved in thrombogenesis, including apolipoprotein E, factor X, and thromboxane. Other genes, such as hypoxia inducible factor-1 α (HIF-1α), zinc finger proteins, matrix metalloproteinase 19 (MMP19), interleukin-22 (IL-22) receptor, and hematopoietic progenitor cell antigen (CD34) precursor, had no clear connection with the disease process.

Proteomic studies also provide some insights into the pathogenesis of thrombosis in APS patients. Proteins to be differentially expressed by monocytes of APS patients with a history thrombosis, include annexin A1, annexin A2, ubiquitin Nedd8, Rho A protein, protein disulfide isomerase, and Hsp60. How these proteins might conspire to increase the thrombosis risk remains to be determined.

LABORATORY ASSAYS

Development Paths

The current assays for APS began with descriptive reports of two laboratory artifacts, the biologic false-positive (BFP) serologic test for syphilis (STS) and an unusual inhibitor to the activated partial thromboplastin time (aPTT) that was not directed against a specific coagulation factor. The immunoassays were developed in the early 1980s in an effort to quantify the BFP-STS, a laboratory phenomenon known to be associated with autoimmunity. Because cardiolipin (diphosphatidyl glycerol) is the key antigen in the STS assay, quantitative immunoassays identify and quantify antibodies in the test serum that bind to cardiolipin. Subsequent clinical studies revealed that elevated levels of aCL antibodies were associated with an increased risk of thrombosis, spontaneous abortion, and neurologic deficits. This constellation of clinical and laboratory abnormalities was recognized as a new disorder, named APS. It was subsequently discovered that the antibodies from patients with this syndrome did not directly bind to cardiolipin. Instead, the antibodies bind β_2GPI, and β_2GPI mediates the interaction with cardiolipin. It was later determined that although β_2GPI is the primary target antigen, aPL antibodies also may recognize several other phospholipid-binding proteins.

The LA assays were derived from a report by Conley and Hartmann in the early 1950s that two patients with SLE had prolonged partial thromboplastin time tests. It was these anticoagulants that were later associated with the biologic false-positive STS recurrent pregnancy loss and thrombosis. Ultimately, there was recognition that the anticoagulant reflected antibody-induced inhibition of phospholipid-dependent coagulation reactions and was part of APS. The term *lupus anticoagulant* was mistakenly coined to describe these antibodies because initial studies were done in SLE patients.

Antiphospholipid tests are inherently limited because they were not designed to measure known disease mechanisms. Nevertheless, these assays serve as surrogate reporters of thrombotic risk. Strong positivity for more than one of the aPL antibody–detection assays is indicative of an increased risk of clinical events.

Lupus Anticoagulant Tests

Overview

The various LA tests use different coagulation systems to report the inhibition of phospholipid-dependent blood coagulation reactions, These include modifications of the aPTT with LA-sensitive and LA-insensitive reagents, the kaolin clotting time (KCT), the dilute Russell viper venom time (dRVVT), the tissue thromboplastin inhibition time (TTIT), the hexagonal phase array test, and the platelet neutralization procedure. The results of LA tests may vary among laboratories; although most laboratories are able to identify plasmas containing strongly positive LA activity, they frequently disagree about samples with weak LA activity (which are missed in approximately half of the cases), and laboratories may often misdiagnose factor-deficient LA-negative plasmas as being LA positive.

Despite these limitations, the presence of LA activity is a more sensitive and specific marker for thrombosis or pregnancy loss than aCL immunoassays, both in patients with or without SLE. For example, based on a meta-analysis of studies examining the association of aPL antibodies in patients without autoimmune disease with subsequent thrombosis over a 15-year period reported mean odds ratio (OR) of 11 for LA, 3.2 for high-titer aCL antibodies and 1.6 for elevated aCL antibodies generally. In a systematic literature review, 12 of 12 studies showed significant associations between LA and thrombosis, with ORs ranging from 5.7 to 9.4. LA increased the risk of arterial and venous events to a similar extent. In contrast, only 15 of 28 studies showed significant associations between aCL antibodies and thrombosis. In the Antiphospholipid Antibodies Stroke Study (APASS), positivity for both LA and aCL antibodies, but not for aCL antibodies alone, predicted a higher risk of recurrent thrombo-occlusive events in patients with a first ischemic stroke. In the Risk of Arterial Thrombosis In relation to Oral contraceptives (RATIO) study, the presence of LA was found to be a major risk factor for arterial thrombotic events in young women, including ORs of 5.3 for MI and 43.1 for ischemic stroke. In LA-positive women taking oral contraceptives, the ORs for MI and ischemic stroke were 21.6 and 201.0, respectively. For LA-positive women who were also cigarette smokers, the ORs for MI and ischemic stroke increased to 33.7 and 87.0, respectively.

Indications for Testing

Lupus anticoagulants should not be included in routine testing panels of patients without a history of SLE, thrombosis, or pregnancy complications typical of APS. The Antiphospholipid Antibodies Subcommittee of the ISTH has prioritized the appropriateness of testing for LA into low, moderate, and high groups. The *low appropriateness group* includes elderly patients with venous or arterial thromboembolism; the *moderate group* includes asymptomatic patients with a prolonged aPTT on routine testing or young women with recurrent spontaneous early pregnancy loss and provoked venous thromboembolism (VTE); and the *high appropriateness group* includes patients with unprovoked or unexplained VTE, arterial thrombosis in young patients (<50 years of age), thrombosis in unusual sites, late pregnancy loss, and any thrombosis or pregnancy morbidity in patients with autoimmune diseases (SLE, rheumatoid arthritis, autoimmune thrombocytopenia, autoimmune hemolytic anemia). In the authors' opinion, these same guidelines may also be applied to the PL immunoassays.

The same subcommittee recommends performing two LA tests that are based on different assay principles, specifically, the dRVVT and an aPTT that uses silica as an activator and has a low phospholipid content.

Dilute Russell Viper Venom Time

The dRVVT is considered one of the most sensitive of the LA tests. The assay uses Russell viper venom (RVV) in a system containing limiting quantities of diluted rabbit brain phospholipid. RVV directly activates coagulation factor X, leading to the formation of fibrin. aPL antibodies can prolong the dRVVT by interfering with assembly of the prothrombinase complex; this prolongation is reversed by adding excess phospholipid (sometimes referred to as a "confirmatory test"). To ensure that prolongation of the clotting time is not the result of a factor deficiency, the procedure includes a mixture of patient and control plasma. Treatment with heparin, warfarin, or direct thrombin inhibitors can produce false-positive test results.

Activated Partial Thromboplastin Time

Prolonged aPTTs in otherwise healthy individuals without bleeding tendencies are most frequently caused by LAs. Different commercial aPTT reagents vary widely with respect to their sensitivities to LA, so it is important to know the characteristics of the reagent that is used. LA needs to be differentiated from inhibitors of specific coagulation factors and from anticoagulants such as heparin. Aside from specific assays to exclude the latter two possibilities, the clinician should determine whether the aPTT normalizes when an LA-insensitive aPTT reagent is used or when the assay is performed using frozen washed platelets as a source of phospholipid, a procedure referred to as the *platelet neutralization procedure*. The effects of incubation with normal plasma may be helpful to distinguish between LAs and coagulation factor inhibitors. aPTTs performed on a mixture of normal plasma with plasma containing a factor VIII inhibitor usually require incubation for 1 to 2 hours at 37° C to show prolongation, but LA-containing plasmas usually prolong the aPTT immediately after mixing with normal plasma and show no further prolongation with incubation. The clinician should be aware that, in rare patients, both types of anticoagulants (i.e., LA and specific coagulation factor inhibitors) may coexist and yield a confusing laboratory picture. LAs may cause artifactual decreases in the levels of contact activation pathway coagulation factors because those assays are based on the aPTT; these patients are sometimes misdiagnosed as having multiple coagulation factor deficiencies. This problem can be handled by repeating the coagulation factor assays after dilution of the plasma samples or by using an aPTT reagent that is insensitive to LA for coagulation factor assays.

Antiphospholipid Immunoassays

Anticardiolipin Antibody Assays

The quantities of bound aCL IgG and aCL IgM are expressed in GPL or MPL units, respectively, one unit representing the cardiolipin-binding activity of 1 μg/mL of affinity-purified aPL antibody from reference sera. Binding reflects both the titer and affinity or avidity of the antibody. aCL antibody levels in reference sera may vary among laboratories, particularly when measured with different commercial enzyme-linked immunosorbent assay (ELISA) kits.

It is important to recognize that most patients with elevated aCL antibodies encountered during the course of general screening studies do not have APS. The prevalence of positive immunoassays in the asymptomatic "normal" population has ranged from approximately 3% to nearly 20%. In a prospective study of 2132 consecutive Spanish patients with VTE, 4.1% had elevated levels of aCL antibodies (i.e., about the same prevalence as in the asymptomatic healthy population). In a group of healthy young women, 18.2% had elevated levels of aCL antibodies, and 12.8% tested LA positive. Many individuals have transient elevations in antibody levels in response to infections; these are not associated with thrombotic complications. Patients with syphilis, Lyme disease, and other infections may be misdiagnosed with APS based on elevated aCL antibody levels, particularly if they present with a stroke or arterial thrombosis.

High levels of aCL antibodies are associated with an increased risk of thrombosis. During a 10-year follow-up of patients with elevated levels of aCL antibodies, approximately 50% of those who had no clinical manifestations of APS at the outset went on to develop APS. The presence of elevated titers of aCL antibodies 6 months after an episode of VTE is a predictor of increased risk of recurrence and of death. In a systematic literature review, 15 of 28 studies showed significant associations between aCL antibodies and thrombosis. In all cases, a correlation existed between higher antibody titers and high ORs for thrombosis. Elevated levels of aCL antibodies, whether high or low titer, were significantly associated with both MI and stroke. Only high-titer aCL antibodies significantly increased the risk of deep venous thrombosis (DVT). With respect to pregnancy losses, a meta-analysis of 25 studies that examined aPL antibodies in women with recurrent fetal losses showed significant correlation; however, the highest OR was seen in those who were LA positive.

Elevated aCL antibodies of IgG or IgM isotype were reported to be significant risk factors for stroke. aPL antibodies were also reported to be an independent risk factor for stroke in young women. In the APASS, 41% of patients who were within 30 days of having an ischemic stroke tested aCL antibody positive.

Anti-β_2GPI Antibody Assay

β_2GPI is the major protein cofactor recognized by aPL antibodies. ELISAs for anti-β_2GPI antibodies are considered to be more specific but less sensitive for APS than aCL antibody assays. Although anti-β_2GPI antibodies are usually found in conjunction with abnormal aCL and antiphosphatidylserine antibodies, patients with APS may only have antibodies against β_2GPI. Despite their higher specificity for APS (98%), β_2GPI antibodies alone cannot be relied upon for the diagnosis because of their low sensitivity (40%-50%), and concurrent testing for both antibodies along with LA is advised.

In a systematic literature review, 34 of 60 studies, of which none were prospective, showed significant associations between anti-β_2GPI antibodies and thrombosis. Of 10 studies that included multivariate analysis, only two confirmed that IgG anti-β_2GPI antibodies were independent risk factors for venous thrombosis. Anti-β_2GPI antibodies were more often associated with venous than arterial events.

Multipositivity for Antiphospholipid Tests and Clinical Risk

Strong positivity for more than one of the aPL antibody assays has been correlated with an increased risk for developing clinical events in several retrospective studies and in one recent prospective study. One study showed that multipositivity for aPL antibodies, but not single positivity, was associated with antenatal and postnatal DVT. Another study of pregnant women with APS reported that patients with triple aPL antibody positivity, or previous thromboembolism appeared to have a higher probability of poor neonatal outcomes than patients with double or single aPL antibody positivity and no thrombosis history. A retrospective analysis of 162 APS patients who were positive for LA, aCL, and anti-β_2GPI antibodies reported a higher risk of recurrent thromboembolic events with a cumulative incidence of events of 44.2% after 10 years. This finding was confirmed in a recent prospective analysis of 104 triple-positive patients without a history of thrombosis or pregnancy complications who were followed for a mean of 4.5 years. The cumulative incidence for a first thrombotic event after 10 years was 37.1% (95% confidence interval [CI], 19.9%-54.3%. The annual rate of a first cardiovascular event (including VTE) was 0.4% in the patients without abnormal aPL assays, 1.36% in single aPL antibody positive carriers, and 5.3% in triple antibody positive carriers (Fig. 143-4). Male sex and the presence of other risk factors for venous thrombosis were associated with an increased risk of developing a first thrombotic event in this cohort.

A risk scale has been proposed in order to aid in the diagnosis and management of patients with APS (Table 143-4). Overall, both

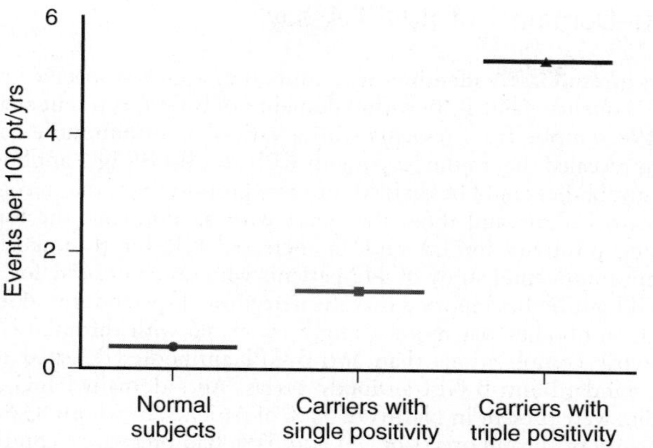

Figure 143-4 AVERAGE ANNUAL RATES OF FIRST CARDIOVASCULAR EVENTS (INCLUDING VENOUS THROMBOEMBOLISM) IN A WHITE NORMAL POPULATION IN SINGLE-POSITIVE ANTIPHOSPHOLIPID CARRIERS AND IN TRIPLE-POSITIVE CARRIERS. *(Modified from Pengo V, Ruffatti A, Legnani C, et al: Incidence of a first thromboembolic event in asymptomatic carriers of high-risk antiphospholipid antibody profile: A multicenter prospective study.* Blood *118:4714, 2011.)*

symptomatic and asymptomatic patients with triple-positive laboratory results (LA positive, aCL [IgG or IgM >40 GPL or MPL units], and anti-β_2GPI [IgG or IgM >99th percentile]) should be considered at high risk for future manifestations of APS. Those who are double positive for LA, aCL (IgG or IgM >40 GPL or MPL units) or anti-β_2GPI (IgG or IgM >99th percentile) or single positive for LA should be considered at medium risk for APS, and those with single positivity for aCL (IgG or IgM >40 GPL or MPL units) or anti-β_2GPI (IgG or IgM >99th percentile) should be considered at low risk for APS. Even in those at medium or low risk, treatment may be warranted in the presence of thrombosis or pregnancy complications or other high-risk factors.

"Noncriteria" Antiphospholipid Assays

IgA Antibodies to Cardiolipin and β_2-Glycoprotein I

The clinical utility of testing aPL antibodies of IgA isotype remains controversial. The prevalence of true positivity to aCL IgA antibodies has been reported to be very low; for example, one study of 795 patients reported positive aCL IgA in only two patients, both of

Table 143-4 Laboratory Interpretation in Antiphospholipid Syndrome Diagnosis and Treatment

Risk	Laboratory Result*	Clinical Manifestation	Treatment
High risk (OR >9)	Triple positive for LA, aCL (IgG or IgM >40 GPL or MPL), and anti-β_2GPI (IgG or IgM >99th percentile)	VTE Arterial thromboembolism	Long-term VKA: INR, 2.0-3.0 Stroke: Long–term VKA: INR, 2.0-3.0 plus aspirin 100 mg/day MI: Long-term VKA: INR, 2.0-3.0 plus aspirin 100 mg/day *or* Long-term VKA: INR, 3.0-4.0 MI with PCI and stent placement: Long-term VKA: INR, 2.0-3.0; aspirin 100 mg/day; and clopidogrel 75 mg/day
		Pregnant women with history of pregnancy complications or thrombotic events	UFH plus low-dose aspirin
		Asymptomatic	Consider anticoagulant prophylaxis for high-risk situations (e.g., immobilization, surgery, air travel) Consider long-term VKA; recommended to prevent thromboembolic events Consider low-dose aspirin and possible UFH for pregnant patients
Medium risk (OR, 5-9)	Double positive for LA, aCL (IgG or IgM >40 GPL or MPL), or anti-β_2GPI (IgG or IgM >99th percentile) *or* Single positive for LA	Venous thromboembolism Arterial thromboembolism Pregnant women with history of pregnancy complications Asymptomatic	Long-term VKA: INR, 2.0-3.0 Long-term VKA: INR, 2.0-3.0 plus aspirin 100 mg/day UFH plus low-dose aspirin No treatment; consider prophylaxis treatment in situations with increased risk (e.g., surgery, prolonged immobilization)
Low risk (OR, 1-5)	Single positive for aCL (IgG or IgM >40 GPL or MPL) or anti-β_2GPI (IgG or IgM >99th percentile)†	VTE	Long-term VKA: INR, 2.0-3.0
		Arterial thromboembolism	Long-term VKA: INR, 2.0-3.0
		Pregnant women with history of pregnancy complications	Early miscarriage (does not meet clinical criteria for obstetric APS); consider low-dose aspirin Late miscarriage: UFH plus low-dose aspirin
		Asymptomatic	No treatment but consider prophylaxis treatment in situations with increased risk (e.g., surgery, prolonged immobilization)

Adapted from Sciascia S, Cosseddu D, Montaruli B, et al: Risk scale for the diagnosis of antiphospholipid syndrome. *Ann Rheum Dis* 70:1517, 2011; Pengo V, Banzato A, Bison E, et al: Antiphospholipid syndrome: Critical analysis of the diagnostic path. *Lupus* 19:428, 2010; Pengo V, Ruffatti A, Legnani C, et al: Incidence of a first thromboembolic event in asymptomatic carriers of high risk antiphospholipid antibody profile: A multicenter prospective study. *Blood* 118:4714, 2011; Tripodi A, de Groot PG, Pengo V: Antiphospholipid syndrome: Laboratory detection, mechanisms of action and treatment. *J Intern Med* 270:110, 2011.

β_2GPI, β_2-Glycoprotein I; *Ig,* immunoglobulin; *INR,* international normalized ratio; *LA,* lupus anticoagulant; *MI,* myocardial infarction; *OR,* odds ratio; *PCI,* percutaneous coronary intervention; *UFH,* unfractionated heparin; *VKA,* vitamin K antagonist; *VTE,* venous thromboembolism.

*Laboratory tests should be deferred until at least 12 weeks after the clinical event to avoid interferences of the acute phase of the disease. Earlier testing may yield false-positive results.

†More information from clinical studies on homogeneous cohort of patients with single positivity is needed.

whom were also positive for IgG aCL. However, anti-β2GPI IgA antibodies were reported to be significantly associated with thrombosis. A recent retrospective case-control study of 56 patients with isolated anti-β_2GPI IgA found that patients with this marker had significantly more thromboembolic events and higher polyclonal IgA levels than control participants. Anti-β_2GPI IgA was also found to be associated with an increased risk of thromboembolic events in patients with SLE.

Antiphospholipid antibodies of IgA isotype (either aCL or anti-β_2GPI) were not included in the international consensus statement on the criteria for APS classification. However, testing for the IgA isotype (particularly IgA anti-β_2GPI) was recommended in cases in which APS is suspected but the IgG and IgM test results are negative.

Annexin A5 Resistance Assay

The "annexin A5 resistance" (A5R) assay was designed to test for a specific pathogenic mechanism—the aPL antibody–mediated disruption of annexin A5 crystallization on phospholipid surfaces. As discussed earlier (see Pathophysiologic Mechanisms), annexin A5 forms a crystal shield on endothelial surfaces that is disrupted by anti-β_2GPI–β_2GPI complexes, thereby exposing more anionic phospholipids and accelerating coagulation reactions. The failure of annexin A5 to sufficiently prolong coagulation times because of interference by aPL antibodies is referred to as A5R. A study of 96 patients demonstrated significantly lower A5R values in APS patients with a history of thrombosis than in aPL antibody-positive patients with no thrombosis history, aPL antibody–negative patients with a thrombosis history, and healthy control participants. A recent study of 166 patients demonstrated a significantly lower A5R ratio in obstetric primary APS patients and thrombotic primary APS patients than in healthy control participants (Fig. 143-5).

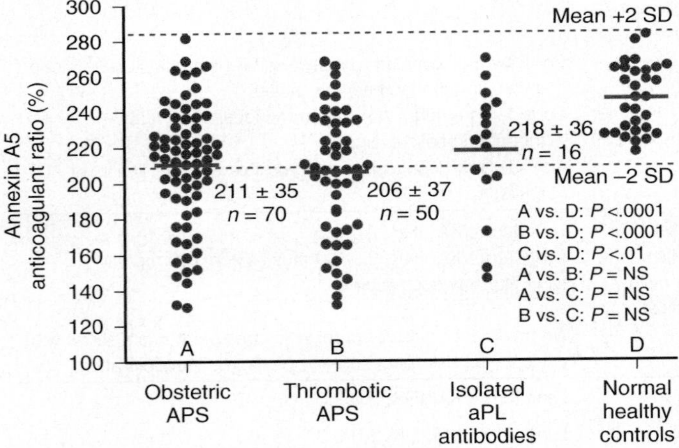

Figure 143-5 REDUCTION OF ANNEXIN A5 (AnxA5) ANTICOAGULANT RATIO ("ANNEXIN A5 RESISTANCE") IN PLASMAS FROM PATIENTS WITH ANTIPHOSPHOLIPID (aPL) SYNDROME (APS). The mean AnxA5 anticoagulant ratio for obstetric primary APS patients (group A) and thrombotic primary APS patients (group B) was significantly decreased compared with normal healthy control participants (both P <.0001). The patients with isolated aPL antibodies (group C) also showed significant reduction of AnxA5 anticoagulant ratios compared with the normal control participants (P = .007). There were no significant differences in AnxA5 anticoagulant ratio between groups A and B, between groups A and C, and between groups B and C. The *horizontal lines* show the mean of each group; the *dashed lines* show the mean ±2 standard deviation (SD) of the 30 normal healthy control participants. *(From Hunt BJ, Wu XX, de LB, et al: Resistance to annexin A5 anticoagulant activity in women with histories for obstetric antiphospholipid syndrome.* Am J Obstet Gynecol *205:485, 2011.)*

Anti–Domain I of β_2GPI Assay

This immunoassay identifies IgG antibodies against a specific amino acid sequence, G40-R30, within domain I of β_2GPI. A recent analysis of 198 samples from patients with a variety of autoimmune conditions revealed that in the 52 patients with anti-β_2GPI IgG antibodies, the antibodies could be divided into two groups: those that recognize domain I alone and those that react with all domains, the former having positivity for LA and an increased OR for thrombosis. A recent multicenter study of 442 patients who tested positive for anti-β2GPI antibodies reported that the detection of specific anti–domain I IgG antibodies was more strongly associated with thrombosis and obstetric complications than anti-β_2GPI antibodies detected using the standard anti-β_2GPI antibody assays. Anti–domain I IgG antibodies were present in plasma of 55% of patients, of whom 83% had a history of thrombosis (OR, .5) and 57% had pregnancy complications (OR, 2.4).

Antiprothrombin Antibody Assay

Prothrombin is considered the second major cofactor for aPL antibodies after β_2GPI. However, the evidence regarding the potential association of antiprothrombin antibodies and thrombosis is mixed. In a systematic literature review, a minority of studies (17 of 46) showed statistically significant associations. Overall, antiprothrombin antibody assays have not been considered to have sufficient clinical utility to be included in standard screening panels for aPL antibodies.

In a possible improvement over the standard antiprothrombin assay, it was recently reported that antibodies against the phosphatidylserine–prothrombin complex (aPS/PT) were closely associated with APS and LA. The presence of aPS/PT antibodies strongly correlated with the presence of LA, had a higher sensitivity and specificity than antiprothrombin antibodies alone for the diagnosis of APS and had comparable sensitivity and specificity to aCL for the diagnosis of APS. In addition, IgG aPS/PT antibodies were highly prevalent in APS patients compared with patients with other diseases with an OR of 12.8. Additional studies are needed to confirm these findings.

Antiphosphatidylserine Antibody Assay

Cardiolipin is normally present in mitochondrial membranes and is unlikely to be exposed to plasma coagulation proteins in vivo. Consequently, it was hypothesized that antibodies against phosphatidylserine may be more relevant pathophysiologically because this phospholipid is expressed on apoptotic cells, activated platelets, and syncytial cells. The utility of antiphosphatidylserine antibody determination is unclear. Although these studies have shown a relationship between antiphosphatidylserine antibodies and pregnancy complications, mainly recurrent miscarriages and reproductive failure, others have not. However, in patients with arterial thrombosis, antiphosphatidylserine antibodies have shown better correlation with APS than aCL antibodies.

Assays for Antibodies Against Other Phospholipids

Antibodies against the zwitterionic phospholipid phosphatidylethanolamine have been associated with thrombosis and with APC resistance. Some studies have suggested that antiphosphatidyethanolamine antibodies can occur in APS in the absence of antibodies against aCL or other anionic phospholipids. Antibodies against phosphatidylinositol antibodies were reported in young patients with cerebral ischemia. In a recent study of nearly 3000 women, IgG antibodies against phosphatidylinositol, phosphatidic acid, phosphatidylserine, and IgM antibodies against phosphatidylcholine were reported to be significantly elevated in patients with recurrent pregnancy loss, implantation failure, and unexplained fertility compared with fertile control participants. Although some investigators have advocated testing for such antibodies, the most recent consensus statement concluded that testing patients for antibodies other than those directed against cardiolipin and β_2GPI was not worthwhile.

CLINICAL MANIFESTATIONS OF ANTIPHOSPHOLIPID SYNDROME

The clinical manifestations of APS can be categorized into "criteria manifestations" and "noncriteria manifestations." The "criteria manifestations" include vascular thrombotic events, obstetric APS, and CAPS. The "noncriteria manifestations" include other pathologic conditions that have been associated with aPL antibodies or with APS.

Criteria Manifestations of Antiphospholipid Syndrome

Systemic Vascular Thrombosis

Thrombosis in APS may occur spontaneously or in the presence of provoking factors such as estrogen replacement therapy, oral contraceptives, pregnancy, the postpartum state, vascular stasis, surgery, or trauma. Some patients with venous thrombosis—but generally not with arterial thrombosis—have concurrent genetic thrombophilic conditions such as heterozygosity for the factor V Leiden mutation. Patients may present with venous or arterial thromboembolism, but about 50% present with DVT of the lower extremities; other sites of venous thrombosis include the superior vena cava, axillary or subclavian veins, jugular vein, or abdominal or pelvic veins. In one study of patients with aPL antibodies and radiologic evidence of thrombosis, 59% had thrombosis limited to the venous circulation, 28% only had arterial thrombosis, and 13% had both.

The most significant risk factor for thromboembolic events in APS is a history of thromboembolism. The risk of recurrence in such patients is about 30% at 4 years and is particularly high in those who have both aCL and LA. The presence of anti-β_2GPI domain I antibodies also increases the risk of recurrence.

Reproductive Manifestations

Routine aPL antibody screening of asymptomatic obstetric patients is not warranted because of the high frequency of false-positive test results with the current tests and the absence of any specified treatment for asymptomatic patients who test positive. Most studies have estimated the prevalence of aPL antibodies among general obstetric populations to be less than 5%, and most of these aPL antibody-positive patients are not clinically affected. Reports from cohorts of obstetric patients with recurrent fetal losses indicate that approximately 16% to 38% had elevated aPL antibodies. Compared with aPL antibody–negative pregnant women, those with elevated aPL antibodies had significantly more obstetric complications, including preeclampsia, placental abruption, miscarriage, prematurity, intrauterine fetal death, intrauterine growth restriction, and oligohydramnios.

Women with obstetric APS generally present with a history of recurrent (i.e., three or more) miscarriages. In approximately half of patients, the pregnancy losses occur in the first trimester; other patients present with later losses, most in the second trimester, but some even later, including stillbirth. The specific pregnancy complications that define obstetric APS include the absence of an alternative explanation for the complications; three or more recurrent spontaneous first trimester miscarriages; or one midtrimester loss or stillbirth, episode of preeclampsia, preterm labor, placental abruption, intrauterine growth restriction, or oligohydramnios. Pregnant women with APS are also more likely to develop DVT during pregnancy or the puerperium. Rarely, pregnant patients develop CAPS.

A prior history of adverse clinical events—specifically, a history of previous pregnancy loss, complications, or thrombosis—is a better predictor for future pregnancy loss than the degree of laboratory abnormality. As mentioned previously, recent studies have shown that positivity for more than one assay—so called "multipositivity"—correlates with increased pregnancy-related morbidities. For example, one study showed that multipositivity but not single positivity for aPL antibodies was associated with antenatal and postnatal DVT. Another retrospective study of 128 pregnant women with APS found that patients with triple aPL positivity or previous thromboembolism appeared to have a higher likelihood of poor neonatal outcome than those with double or single positivity and no thrombosis history.

The current consensus is that aPL antibodies *do not* contribute to early reproductive failure (i.e., infertility). The Practice Committee of the American Society for Reproductive Medicine stated that "the assessment of aPL antibodies is not indicated among couples undergoing IVF [in vitro fertilization], and therapy is not justified on the basis of existing data." However, although an older study showed no relationship between the presence of aPL antibodies and implantation or ongoing pregnancy rates, a recent study reported that 8% to 9% of women with a history of unexplained infertility and recurrent implantation failure had more than one positive aPL antibody compared with only 1.5% of fertile negative control women and 11% of positive control women experiencing recurrent pregnancy loss. Studies suggest a possible nonthrombogenic mechanism of impaired trophoblastic differentiation, proliferation, and migration that may lead to the recurrent implantation failure seen in infertile women.

Neurologic Manifestations

Strokes are common in APS. In a large European cohort, stroke or transient ischemic attack (TIA) was the initial presentation in 29.9% of adults with APS, and recurrent stroke contributed to a significant proportion of deaths. In a study of Latin American adults with APS, 18% presented with stroke or TIA. A multinational lupus cohort showed that aPL antibody–associated stroke accounted for 11.8% of deaths. In the European CAPS registry, cerebral manifestations occurred in 62% of patients and were responsible for 13% of deaths.

Prospective analysis for the presence of aPL antibodies in stroke patients in the APASS demonstrated that elevated levels of aCL are associated with an increased risk of stroke but not other thromboembolic events. Patients who tested positive for *both* aCL and LA appeared to have more subsequent thrombo-occlusive events (with a trend that approached, but did not reach, statistical significance) than patients who tested negative for both (31.7% vs. 24.0%; $P = .07$). A subsequent study from the same group reported that elevated antibodies against β_2GPI and LA—and not aCL or antiphosphatidylserine—were the most significant risk factors for stroke. It is important to recognize that the presence of conventional risk factors for vascular disease adds to the baseline risk associated with the antibodies. In the RATIO study, women with LA positivity and other modifiable risk factors such as smoking or use of oral contraceptives had a higher risk of ischemic stroke. Patients with lupus and those with APS should undergo echocardiography because a high proportion have cardiac valve abnormalities (see later discussion).

The diagnosis of APS should be suspected in young patients with stroke or TIA, particularly those without other risk factors. Rates of stroke were higher in younger patients with APS, with a rate of up to 32% in a multinational childhood registry versus 16% to 21% in adult APS patients. Case-control and prospective studies have shown strong associations between aPL antibody positivity or LA positivity and ischemic strokes in young adults with an OR of 43.1 for positive LA test results. Younger patients presenting with stroke tended to have venous, rather than arterial, thrombosis with 7% of children presenting with cerebral vein thrombosis in the multinational childhood registry. In addition to their immediate impact, recurrent strokes may lead to multi-infarct dementia.

Cardiovascular Manifestations

Antiphospholipid syndrome should be considered in patients who present with coronary artery thrombosis in the absence of evidence of atherosclerosis and without typical risk factors. In the RATIO study, the presence of an LA was a significant risk factor for arterial thrombosis; the OR for MI was 5.3 and increased to 21.6 in women who used oral contraceptives and to 33.7 in those who smoked. Elevated anti-β_2GPI correlated with a small increase in the risk of stroke, but not MI. Antiprothrombin antibodies were reported to be a predictor of MI in middle-aged men, and one study found that these antibodies together with conventional cardiovascular risk factors increased the risk of MI in a multiplicative fashion.

Hepatic and Gastrointestinal Manifestations

The liver is the most commonly affected abdominal organ in APS, mainly via occlusion of hepatic vessels, including those supplying the biliary tree. The latter may present as acute acalculous cholecystitis with gallbladder necrosis. Gastrointestinal manifestations of APS also include esophageal necrosis with perforation, intestinal ischemia and infarction, pancreatitis, colonic ulceration, and giant gastric ulceration. APS has been reported in patients with mesenteric inflammatory venoocclusive disease and with mesenteric and portal vein thrombosis.

Renal Abnormalities

Patients with APS may present with vasoocclusive manifestations in the kidneys, including renal artery stenosis or thrombosis, renal infarction, renal vein thrombosis, and nonthrombotic manifestations (described in the section below). An entity known as *APS nephropathy* consists of vasoocclusive disease involving small intrarenal vessels; the features include fibrous intimal hyperplasia, focal cortical atrophy, and thrombotic microangiopathy. The acute form of this vascular nephropathy resembles other thrombotic microangiopathies, such as hemolytic uremic syndrome or thrombotic thrombocytopenic purpura (see Chapter 136). A chronic form is often clinically silent and consists of a vasoocclusive process that involves the entire renal vasculature, including the main renal artery and its branches, arterioles, glomerular capillaries, and renal veins.

Retinal Abnormalities

The diagnosis of APS retinopathy should be suspected in patients with diffuse retinal vasoocclusion, particularly when they have involvement of arteries and veins, neovascularization, and symptoms suggestive of a systemic rheumatologic disease. Elevated aPL antibody levels were present in 5% to 33% of patients with retinal vein occlusion. Cilioretinal artery occlusion, optic neuropathy, and severe vasoocclusive retinopathy have also been described with APS.

Other Organ Manifestations

Skin manifestations may be the first sign of APS in up to 3.5% of cases. Patients present with skin ulceration associated with skin necrosis.

Antiphospholipid antibodies have been described in patients with pulmonary hypertension. A multi-institutional study of 687 patients with chronic thromboembolic pulmonary hypertension reported that aPL antibodies were a significant risk factor. In one prospective trial of 38 consecutive patients with precapillary pulmonary hypertension, 30% had aPL antibodies with various phospholipid specificities.

Acute adrenal failure secondary to bilateral adrenal infarction or hemorrhage has been reported as the first manifestation of primary APS. aPL antibodies have also been associated with osteonecrosis.

Catastrophic Antiphospholipid Syndrome

Rare patients present with a *catastrophic* form of APS, which is characterized by severe widespread vascular occlusions and high mortality. The formal diagnostic criteria include involvement of at least three organs, systems, or tissues; development of manifestations simultaneously or within 1 week, histopathologic confirmation of small vessel occlusion; and laboratory confirmation of the presence of aPL antibodies (see Table 143-2). In contrast to the diagnostic criteria for APS, which exclude the diagnosis when histopathology reveals evidence of vasculitis, the diagnostic criteria for CAPS permit histologic evidence of vasculitis in association with thrombosis.

Of the 280 patients with CAPS reported in "The Registry of the European Forum on Antiphospholipid Antibodies for Patients With CAPS" (http://www.med.ub.es/mimmun/forum/caps.htm), 72% were female, with a mean age of 37 years (range, 11-60), 46% had primary APS, and 40% had SLE. In 46%, CAPS was their first manifestation of APS. The most common presentations were pulmonary (24%), neurologic (18%), and renal (18%) complications. Thrombosis affecting the renal, adrenal, splenic, intestinal, or pancreatic vessels was most commonly encountered. CAPS patients present with extensive VTE, respiratory failure, stroke, abnormal liver enzymes, renal impairment, adrenal insufficiency, and areas of cutaneous infarction. The respiratory failure is usually the result of acute respiratory distress syndrome and diffuse alveolar hemorrhage. Laboratory evidence of disseminated intravascular coagulation is frequently present (see Chapter 141). Table 143-5 describes the reported clinical manifestations from the CAPS registry. In marked contrast

Table 143-5 Clinical Manifestations Reported From the Catastrophic Antiphospholipid Syndrome Registry

Systemic vascular thrombosis	Extensive thrombosis affecting the renal, adrenal, splenic, intestinal, or pancreatic vessels was most commonly encountered with resultant multiorgan ischemia or infarction
Pulmonary manifestations	ARDS, diffuse alveolar damage, pulmonary embolism, dyspnea, hemoptysis
Neurologic manifestation	Stroke, TIA, seizures, encephalopathy, coma, psychosis, headache, vertigo, mononeuritis, peripheral neuropathy
Renal manifestations	Renal failure caused by thrombosis of renal arteries or veins, glomerulonephritis, interstitial nephritis, proteinuria, hematuria, hypertension
Dermatologic manifestations	Ulcerations attributable to microvascular infarction, livedo reticularis, skin ulcerations, skin necrosis, purpura rash, petechiae
Cardiovascular manifestations	Thrombotic occlusion of nonatherosclerotic coronary artery, thrombotic MI, valvular abnormalities, congestive heart failure, dilated cardiomyopathy, arrhythmia, pericardial effusion, atrial thrombosis
Hepatic and GI manifestations	Thrombotic occlusion of hepatic and mesenteric arteries and veins, Budd-Chiari syndrome, elevated liver enzymes, ascites, jaundice, cholestasis, cholecystitis, GI bleeding, diarrhea, vomiting, abdominal pain
Other manifestations	Acute adrenal failure caused by bilateral adrenal hemorrhagic infarction, avascular osteonecrosis, pancreatitis, blurred vision, decreased vision, diplopia

ARDS, Acute respiratory distress syndrome; *GI,* gastrointestinal; *MI,* myocardial infarction; *TIA,* transient ischemic attack.

to thrombotic thrombocytopenic purpura, another autoimmune thrombotic microangiopathy (see Chapter 136), in which recurrences are common, patients with CAPS who respond to treatment rarely experience a subsequent event.

Pediatric Antiphospholipid Syndrome

Antiphospholipid syndrome is increasingly recognized as a significant cause of thrombosis in the pediatric population. A European registry that included 121 cases described thrombotic manifestations similar to those seen in adults with APS. However, patients with primary APS tended to be younger and had a higher frequency of arterial thrombotic events. In contrast, those with secondary APS were older and had a higher frequency of venous thrombotic events associated with hematologic and skin manifestations. Children with rheumatic diseases who have persistently positive aPL are more likely to have resistance to annexin A5 anticoagulant activity than those with transiently positive antibodies. Although the catastrophic form of the syndrome has been reported in children, it is rare.

"Noncriteria" Clinical Manifestations Associated With Antiphospholipid Antibodies and Antiphospholipid Syndrome

"Noncriteria" Cardiovascular Manifestations

Cardiac Valve Abnormalities

About 35% of patients with primary APS have cardiac valve abnormalities that can be detected by echocardiography. When patients with cardiac valve disorders were evaluated for aPL antibodies, about 20% had aPL antibodies compared with 10% of matched control participants. Valvular abnormalities were reported in about 50% of patients with the combination of SLE and aPL antibodies; these abnormalities include leaflet thickening, vegetations, regurgitation, and stenosis. The mitral valve is most often affected followed by the aortic valve. In a prospective follow-up of 89 patients with severe, nonspecific valvular heart disease, thromboembolic events were significantly more frequent in the aPL antibody–positive group than in the aPL antibody–negative group; however, the presence of aPL antibodies was not an independent risk factor for thromboembolic events.

Coronary Artery Disease in the Absence of Thrombotic Occlusion

Antiphospholipid antibodies have been associated with increased susceptibility to coronary artery disease, particularly premature atherosclerosis. aPL antibodies appear to be a risk factor for adverse outcomes after percutaneous or surgical coronary revascularization procedures and for restenosis after coronary angioplasty. A carotid ultrasound study showed a correlation between aPL antibodies in young primary APS patients (age 37 years ± 11 years) and increased intimal thickness.

Peripheral Arterial Disease

Approximately one-third of patients with peripheral arterial disease undergoing bypass grafting procedures have elevated aPL antibody levels (mostly aCL antibodies). In one study, however, such patients did not have an increased risk for reocclusion compared with those who were aPL antibody negative, possibly because both groups received anticoagulant therapy.

"Noncriteria" Neurologic Manifestations

Other aPL antibody–associated neurologic abnormalities include migraines, seizures, chorea, Guillain-Barré syndrome, transient global amnesia, dementia, diabetic peripheral neuropathy, and orthostatic hypotension. In the pediatric APS registry, migraines (7%), chorea (4%), and epilepsy (3%) were the most common nonthrombotic neurologic manifestations.

In SLE patients, recurrent seizures are more common in those who have persistently elevated aCL antibodies. aPL antibody positivity has also been associated with cognitive impairment in lupus patients, especially in the areas of attention, psychomotor speed, and executive abilities. It has been proposed that aPL antibody–mediated damage to white matter tracts and basal ganglia structures may account for the multiple sclerosis–like features and movement disorders in APS patients.

Elevated aCL antibodies also occur in patients with multiple sclerosis, and these do not appear to be associated with an increased risk for thrombosis or stroke. In one series of patients with multiple sclerosis, 9% had IgG antibodies, and 44% had IgM antibodies, but there was no clinical distinction between aPL antibody–positive and –negative patients. Patients with psychotic disorders have also been reported to have an increased prevalence of LA and aCL antibodies that is not associated with antipsychotic medications. In this study, 32% (11 of 34) of the unmedicated psychotic patients had elevated aPL antibodies. These were not associated with an increased risk of thrombosis. Optic neuritis with elevated aPL antibodies has been described in the absence of retinal vasoocclusion. Sudden acute sensorineural hearing loss in patients with SLE or lupuslike syndromes has been described as a manifestation of APS.

"Noncriteria" Pulmonary Manifestations

Patients with APS may bleed into the acinar portions of the lung, which can lead to diffuse alveolar hemorrhage. Biopsy specimens reveal microvascular thrombosis, septal thickening caused by edema, neutrophilic septal infiltrates, and extravasation of red blood cells into the alveolar spaces. Because acute diffuse alveolar hemorrhage can occur in anticoagulated APS patients, it is thought that the lesions may be caused by vasculitis rather than thrombosis.

"Noncriteria" Gastrointestinal Manifestations

Antiphospholipid antibody levels are frequently elevated in patients with a variety of chronic liver diseases. In one prospective study of patients with liver disease, approximately half of the patients with alcoholic liver disease and one-third of those with chronic hepatitis C virus had elevated aPL antibody levels. The frequency was even higher in patients with severe cirrhosis. One review reported that about 20% of patients with chronic hepatitis B and hepatitis C had elevated aPL antibodies, most of which were cofactor independent (i.e., similar to the antibodies found in infections, which directly recognize phospholipid). Hepatitis C may be an exception because some patients present with "true" autoimmune aPL antibodies; the most common features reported were intraabdominal thrombosis and MI. Primary biliary cirrhosis has also been associated with aPL antibodies.

"Noncriteria" Renal Manifestations

Several nonthrombotic types of renal lesions have also been identified in APS patients. Patients with aPL antibodies may present with glomerulonephritis without vasoocclusive disease. A review of 29 consecutive renal biopsies from patients with primary APS performed at two institutions over 22 years described 20 cases of APS nephropathy and identified nine cases with distinct pathologic features, including membranous nephropathy, minimal change disease or focal segmental glomerulonephritis, mesangial C3 nephropathy, and pauci-immune crescentic glomerulonephritis.

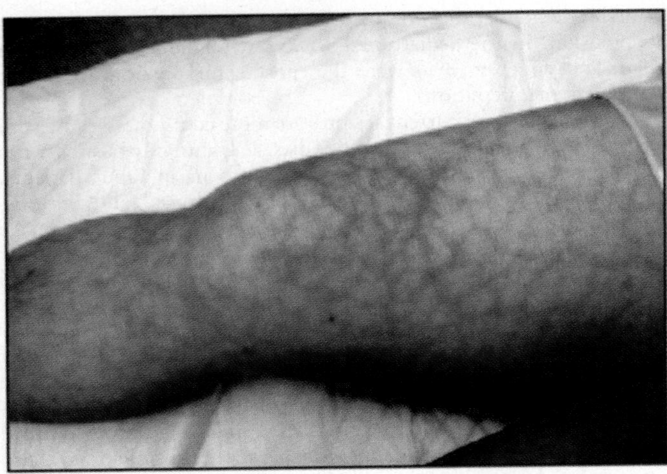

Figure 143-6 LIVEDO RETICULARIS IN A WOMAN WITH ANTIPHOSPHOLIPID SYNDROME. *(From Ruiz-Irastorza G, Crowther M, Branch W, et al: Antiphospholipid syndrome.* Lancet *376:1498, 2010.)*

"Noncriteria" Dermatologic Manifestations

Livedo reticularis (Fig. 143-6) is relatively common, occurring in 24% of patients in a series that included 1000 patients with aPL. On rare occasions, patients present with a necrosing form. Livedo reticularis is usually widespread and can localize on nonadjacent areas on the limbs, trunk, and buttocks. Its prevalence is higher in APS associated with SLE compared with primary APS, in women compared with men, and in patients with high levels of aCL antibodies. Livedo reticularis may be associated with other manifestations of APS, such as cerebral or ocular ischemic arterial events (OR, 10.8; 95% CI, 5.2-22.5), seizures (OR, 6.5; 95% CI, 2.6-16), arterial events (OR, 6; 95% CI, 2.9-12.6), heart valve abnormalities (OR, 7.3; 95% CI, 3.6-14.7), and arterial systemic hypertension (>160-90 mm Hg; OR, 2.9; 95% CI, 1.5-5.7). Necrotizing vasculitis, livedoid vasculitis, superficial vein thrombosis, cutaneous ulceration and necrosis, erythematous macules, purpura, ecchymoses, painful skin nodules, and subungual splinter hemorrhages, anetoderma (macular atrophy), discoid lupus erythematosus, and cutaneous T-cell lymphoma have all been reported.

Other "Noncriteria" Hematologic Abnormalities

Thrombocytopenia

Thrombocytopenia occurs in a large proportion of APS patients, but the count is rarely low enough to cause bleeding complications or to preclude anticoagulant therapy. Most cases appear to be immune mediated (see Chapter 133). According to one study, the majority of patients with APS and thrombocytopenia were found to have antibodies against the platelet membrane glycoproteins, GPIIb/IIIa or GPIb/IX complexes (or both). However, in another study, no correlation was found between the presence of antibodies against platelet GPIIb/IIIa or GPIb/IX and thrombocytopenia, and the eluted platelet antibodies did not have any LA activity. Conversely, aPL antibodies and antibodies against platelet membrane GPs were present simultaneously in about 70% of patients with immune-mediated thrombocytopenia (ITP). In a prospective cohort study, the 5-year, thrombosis-free survivals of aPL antibody-positive and -negative ITP patients were 39% and 98%, respectively, indicating that thrombocytopenia itself is not protective against thrombosis in these patients.

Bleeding

The presence of a concurrent coagulopathy must be considered when patients with APS exhibit a bleeding tendency. Acquired hypoprothrombinemia can result in severe bleeding. This diagnosis may be missed if abnormal coagulation screening tests are attributed solely to the LA. To address this possibility, the level of prothrombin should be determined in patients with prolonged prothrombin times who are not receiving anticoagulant medications. Other causes of bleeding in the setting of APS include acquired thrombocytopathies (see Chapter 132), thrombocytopenia, acquired inhibitors against specific coagulation factors such as factor VIII (see Chapter 138), and acquired von Willebrand syndrome (see Chapter 140). It is important to note that the mechanism for AVWS in autoimmunity has not been established and that this deficiency of vWF is rarely associated with a demonstrable inhibitor.

TREATMENT OF PATIENTS WITH ANTIPHOSPHOLIPID SYNDROME

There is general agreement that patients with recurrent or spontaneous thrombosis require long-term anticoagulant therapy and that patients with recurrent spontaneous pregnancy losses require antithrombotic therapy for most of the gestational period and for the puerperium. There are differences of opinion regarding the approach to treatment of patients with single thrombotic events, a remote history of thrombosis, or a past history of provoked VTE. The recent categorization of patients into high-, medium-, and low-risk groups based on multipositivity of laboratory test results may help to guide management (see Table 143-4).

Thrombosis

The accumulated evidence from randomized controlled trials indicates that, in general, patients with APS and thrombosis should be treated with warfarin for the long term with doses adjusted to achieve a target international normalized ratio (INR) of 2.0 to 3.0.

Although there is a general consensus on this therapeutic range for venous thrombosis, there is controversy as to whether patients with arterial thrombosis warrant a higher intensity of anticoagulation because a retrospective study of a variety of patients with APS showed that an INR above 3.0 was necessary to prevent recurrences in this group of patients. Although two prospective, randomized, controlled trials reported no benefit and an increased risk of bleeding with higher intensity warfarin, neither study included a large number of APS patients with arterial thrombosis. Recent recommendations suggest that patients with MI and triple positivity should be treated with higher intensity warfarin (INR, 3.0-4.0) or usual intensity warfarin (INR, 2.0-3.0) plus low-dose aspirin. In addition, the triple-positive MI patients who undergo coronary stenting should receive triple therapy with warfarin (INR, 2.0-3.0), low-dose aspirin, and clopidogrel.

The LA may complicate monitoring of warfarin and heparin. The INR and aPTT can be artifactually elevated in some patients with APS and LA. A multicenter study reported that all but one of the commercial thromboplastins in use at nine centers provided acceptable INR values for APS patients with LA. If APS patients are given intravenous heparin, the baseline aPTT needs to be determined. If it is prolonged because of the LA, the heparin level can be monitored either by using an LA-insensitive aPTT reagent or with an anti–factor Xa assay. The need for monitoring can, in most patients, be obviated by the use of an LMWH.

Fibrinolytic therapy has been used in patients with primary APS with extensive DVT, acute ischemic stroke, or acute MI. The antimalarial drug hydroxychloroquine (HCQ) has been associated with a reduced risk of thrombosis in patients with APS and SLE. The potential effectiveness of this treatment is supported by findings in an animal model of aPL antibody thrombosis and by recent reports that HCQ directly disrupts aPL IgG–β_2GPI complexes and reverses the aPL antibody-mediated disruption of annexin A5 binding. At the time of writing, a prospective controlled, randomized trial is being planned by the APS ACTION! Network (http://www.apsaction.org)

to test whether this drug may be useful for treating asymptomatic individuals with positive aPL antibody assays who are considered to be at high risk for an initial thrombotic event.

The new oral thrombin and factor Xa inhibitors have not been evaluated in APS patients.

Stroke

There is controversy about the appropriate antithrombotic treatment of aPL antibody–associated stroke. Currently, most hematologists and rheumatologists view an APS-related stroke as no different than other arterial manifestations of APS, and they treat such patients with warfarin, although there is debate about the optimal intensity. Most stroke neurologists view APS-related strokes the same way they do strokes of other causes, and they accept the APASS study conclusion that treatment with aspirin is equivalent to warfarin but is associated with a lower risk of bleeding. Guidelines issued in 2006 from the American Heart Association and American Stroke Association stated that for patients with cryptogenic ischemic stroke or TIA associated with aPL antibodies, antiplatelet therapy is reasonable, and for patients who meet the criteria for APS with venous and arterial occlusive disease in multiple organs, miscarriages, and livedo reticularis, warfarin (target INR, 2.0-3.0) is reasonable.

Pregnancy Complications

A systematic review of treatments for women with a history of prior miscarriages and aPL antibodies concluded that combined unfractionated heparin (UFH) and aspirin reduces pregnancy loss by 54% compared with aspirin alone. Three trials of treatment with aspirin alone showed no significant reduction in pregnancy loss; intravenous immunoglobulin (IVIG), with or without UFH and aspirin, was associated with an increased risk of pregnancy loss or premature birth compared with UFH or LMWH combined with aspirin. Recently, a meta-analysis of five studies that included a total of 398 women concluded that adding UFH to low-dose aspirin significantly reduces first trimester losses but does not reduce late-pregnancy losses.

Despite the absence of "head-to-head" trials comparing LMWH with UFH, LMWH is often prescribed because it can be given once daily and the risk of heparin-induced thrombocytopenia and osteoporosis is lower than with heparin.

Women with a history of three or more spontaneous pregnancy losses and evidence of aPL antibodies should be treated with a combination of low-dose aspirin (75-81 mg/day) and prophylactic doses of UFH or LMWH. Treatment should be started as soon as pregnancy is documented and, when UFH is used, continued until delivery to reduce the rate of late complications. For patients treated with LMWH, clinicians frequently discontinue the drug in the last month of pregnancy and switch to treatment with UFH because of its advantages compared with LMWH (i.e., the shorter half-life and because the presence of significant concentrations in the bloodstream can be monitored with the simple aPTT assay) in case the patient goes into earlier labor. Low-dose UFH (i.e., 5000 U twice daily) or prophylactic dose LMWH should be started approximately 4 to 6 hours after delivery, provided that bleeding is not excessive, and continued until the patient is fully ambulatory. For patients with a history of VTE, anticoagulant therapy is warranted for at least 6 weeks after delivery. The optimal duration of postpartum treatment for patients without a history of thrombosis is unknown, but many physicians recommend prophylaxis for 6 weeks after delivery (see Chapter 142).

With the possible exception of women with SLE and high-titer triple-positive tests, the presence of elevated aPL antibodies in pregnant women without any history of spontaneous pregnancy losses, other attributable pregnancy complications, thrombosis, or embolism is not a sufficient indication for treatment. A prospective study of an untreated general obstetric population found that 2% to 3% of nonpregnant patients had low-titer increases of aCL antibodies, with a live birth rate of approximately 60% among these patients. It is therefore recommended that physicians should not include screening for aPL antibodies or LA in their routine prenatal screening panels.

Although prednisone was reported to improve the outcomes of pregnant patients with APS, any benefits were associated with significant toxicity. Corticosteroids or IVIG should be reserved for patients who are refractory to anticoagulant therapy, who have a severe immune thrombocytopenia or other significant bleeding problem, or who have a significant contraindication to heparin therapy. Treatment with prednisone and heparin increases risks of osteoporosis and vertebral fractures.

Catastrophic Antiphospholipid Syndrome

Patients with CAPS require aggressive treatment because of the high mortality. Conventional anticoagulant therapy is usually insufficient, and treatment modalities may include anticoagulation and immunosuppressive therapy with high-dose glucocorticoids, IVIG, cyclophosphamide, azathioprine, or rituximab. Plasmapheresis may be a helpful adjunct in some patients. According to the CAPS Registry, anticoagulation together with corticosteroids was most often used followed by the combination of anticoagulation, corticosteroids, and plasma exchange and/or IVIG. The highest recovery rate was obtained with the combination of anticoagulation, corticosteroids, and plasma exchange (77.8%) followed by anticoagulation, corticosteroids, plasma exchange, and/or IVIG (69%). The higher rate of the use of the last combination of treatment seems to be the main explanation for the reduction in mortality rate to 30% in CAPS.

Asymptomatic Antiphospholipid Antibody–Positive Patients

A recent, multicenter prospective study of 104 asymptomatic patients with triple positivity for aPL antibodies showed them to be at increased risk for a first thromboembolic event. Because aspirin alone did not effectively reduce this risk, it is recommended that anticoagulation be considered for some of these high-risk patients. After a careful risk-to-benefit analysis, anticoagulant therapy may be considered for some asymptomatic patients who are considered to be at very high risk, such as those with convincing family histories for thromboembolic complications of APS who themselves manifest significant laboratory abnormalities, patients with SLE who have significant multipositive aPL laboratory abnormalities, and patients who have other reasons for being at increased risk for thrombosis (e.g., severe valvular heart disease).

ASH evidence-based guidelines do not recommend prophylactic treatment with aspirin in asymptomatic aPL antibody–positive patients because the benefit is uncertain and there is a small risk of bleeding. However, some experts recommend low-dose aspirin prophylaxis in persistently aPL antibody–positive patients, in aPL antibody–positive patients with SLE, and in patients with obstetric APS. Heparin prophylaxis, which should be considered for all patients during periods of increased thrombotic risk (surgery or prolonged immobilization) are likely to be even more important for high-risk patients who also have aPL antibodies. The guidelines stress the importance of individual assessment of thrombotic risk in aPL antibody–positive patients. As with all patients, reversible thrombotic risk factors should also be addressed because these add to the risks of vascular occlusion in patients with positive aPL antibodies.

SUGGESTED READINGS

Agar C, van Os GM, Morgelin M, et al: Beta-2-glycoprotein I can exist in two conformations: Implications for our understanding of the antiphospholipid syndrome. *Blood* 116:1336, 2010.

Avcin T, Cimaz R, Silverman ED, et al: Pediatric antiphospholipid syndrome: Clinical and immunologic features of 121 patients in an international registry. *Pediatrics* 122:e1100, 2008.

Branch DW, Silver RM, Porter TF: Obstetric antiphospholipid syndrome: Current uncertainties should guide our way. *Lupus* 19:446, 2010.

Bucciarelli S, Espinosa G, Cervera R: The CAPS Registry: Morbidity and mortality of the catastrophic antiphospholipid syndrome. *Lupus* 18:905, 2009.

Cervera R: Catastrophic antiphospholipid syndrome (CAPS): Update from the "CAPS Registry." *Lupus* 19:412, 2010.

Conley CL, Hartmann RC: A hemorrhagic disorder caused by circulating anticoagulant in patients with disseminated lupus erythematosus. *J Clin Invest* 31:621, 1952.

Crowther MA, Ginsberg JS, Julian J, et al: A comparison of two intensities of warfarin for the prevention of recurrent thrombosis in patients with the antiphospholipid antibody syndrome. *N Engl J Med* 349:1133, 2003.

de Laat B, Wu XX, van Lummel M, et al: Correlation between antiphospholipid antibodies that recognize domain I of ß2-glycoprotein I and a reduction in the anticoagulant activity of annexin A5. *Blood* 109:1490, 2007.

de Laat HB, Pengo V, Pabinger I, et al: The association between circulating antibodies against domain I of beta2-glycoprotein I and thrombosis: An international multicenter study. *J Thromb Haemost* 7:1767, 2009.

Derksen R, de Groot PG: Towards evidence-based treatment of thrombotic antiphospholipid syndrome. *Lupus* 19:470, 2010.

Erkan D, Lockshin MD: Non-criteria manifestations of antiphospholipid syndrome. *Lupus* 19:424, 2010.

Finazzi G, Marchioli R, Brancaccio V, et al: A randomized clinical trial of high-intensity warfarin vs. conventional antithrombotic therapy for the prevention of recurrent thrombosis in patients with the antiphospholipid syndrome (WAPS). *J Thromb Haemost* 3:848, 2005.

Galli M, Luciani D, Bertolini G, et al: Lupus anticoagulants are stronger risk factors for thrombosis than anticardiolipin antibodies in the antiphospholipid syndrome: A systematic review of the literature. *Blood* 101:1827, 2003.

Hunt BJ, Wu XX, de LB, et al: Resistance to annexin A5 anticoagulant activity in women with histories for obstetric antiphospholipid syndrome. *Am J Obstet Gynecol* 205:485, e17, 2011.

Levine SR, Brey RL, Tilley BC, et al: Antiphospholipid antibodies and subsequent thrombo-occlusive events in patients with ischemic stroke. *JAMA* 291:576, 2004.

Meroni PL, Borghi MO, Raschi E, et al: Pathogenesis of antiphospholipid syndrome: Understanding the antibodies. *Nat Rev Rheumatol* 7:330, 2011.

Miyakis S, Lockshin MD, Atsumi T, et al: International consensus statement on an update of the classification criteria for definite antiphospholipid syndrome (APS). *J Thromb Haemost* 4:295, 2006.

Pengo V, Banzato A, Bison E, et al: Antiphospholipid syndrome: Critical analysis of the diagnostic path. *Lupus* 19:428, 2010.

Pengo V, Ruffatti A, Legnani C, et al: Clinical course of high-risk patients diagnosed with antiphospholipid syndrome. *J Thromb Haemost* 8:237, 2010.

Pengo V, Ruffatti A, Legnani C, et al: Incidence of a first thromboembolic event in asymptomatic carriers of high-risk antiphospholipid antibody profile: A multicenter prospective study. *Blood* 118:4714, 2011.

Pengo V, Tripodi A, Reber G, et al: Update of the guidelines for lupus anticoagulant detection. Subcommittee on Lupus Anticoagulant/Antiphospholipid Antibody of the Scientific and Standardisation Committee of the International Society on Thrombosis and Haemostasis. *J Thromb Haemost* 7:1737, 2009.

Petri M: Update of anti-phospholipid antibodies on SLE: The Hopkins' Lupus Cohort. *Lupus* 19:419, 2010.

Rand JH, Wu XX, Lapinski R, et al: Detection of antibody-mediated reduction of annexin A5 anticoagulant activity in plasmas of patients with the antiphospholipid syndrome. *Blood* 104:2783, 2004.

Rand JH, Wu XX, Quinn AS, et al: Human monoclonal antiphospholipid antibodies disrupt the annexin A5 anticoagulant crystal shield on phospholipid bilayers: Evidence from atomic force microscopy and functional assay. *Am J Pathol* 163:1193, 2003.

Rand JH, Wu XX, Quinn AS, et al: Hydroxychloroquine protects the annexin A5 anticoagulant shield from disruption by antiphospholipid antibodies: Evidence for a novel effect for an old antimalarial drug. *Blood* 115:2292, 2010.

Ruffatti A, Calligaro A, Hoxha A, et al: Laboratory and clinical features of pregnant women with antiphospholipid syndrome and neonatal outcome. *Arthritis Care Res (Hoboken)* 62:302, 2010.

Sacco RL, Adams R, Albers G, et al: Guidelines for prevention of stroke in patients with ischemic stroke or transient ischemic attack: A statement for healthcare professionals from the American Heart Association/American Stroke Association Council on Stroke: Co-sponsored by the Council on Cardiovascular Radiology and Intervention: The American Academy of Neurology affirms the value of this guideline. *Circulation* 113:e409, 2006.

Saha SP, Bhattacharjee N, Ganguli RP, et al: Prevalence and significance of antiphospholipid antibodies in selected at-risk obstetrics cases: A comparative prospective study. *J Obstet Gynaecol* 29:614, 2009.

Sciascia S, Cosseddu D, Montaruli B, et al: Risk scale for the diagnosis of antiphospholipid syndrome. *Ann Rheum Dis* 70:1517, 2011.

Urbanus RT, Siegerink B, Roest M, et al: Antiphospholipid antibodies and risk of myocardial infarction and ischaemic stroke in young women in the RATIO study: A case-control study. *Lancet Neurol* 8:998, 2009.

Ziakas PD, Pavlou M, Voulgarelis M: Heparin treatment in antiphospholipid syndrome with recurrent pregnancy loss: A systematic review and meta-analysis. *Obstet Gynecol* 115:1256, 2010.

CHAPTER 144

VENOUS THROMBOEMBOLISM

Wendy Lim

Venous thromboembolism (VTE), encompassing both deep venous thrombosis (DVT) of the lower extremities and pulmonary embolism (PE), remains a common medical condition that is associated with significant morbidity and mortality.

Although VTE can occur in any vein, it most commonly occurs in the leg veins. Superficial venous thrombosis occurs most frequently in varicosities and usually is self-limiting and benign. In contrast, DVT is a more serious condition. Thrombi localized to the deep calf veins often are small and therefore less commonly associated with clinically important PE or postthrombotic syndrome, but proximal DVT involving the popliteal, femoral, or iliac venous system is complicated by PE in approximately 50% of cases.

The diagnosis of acute VTE is now being made more frequently because of increased diagnostic suspicion and the availability of reliable, noninvasive diagnostic tests. In hospitalized patients, this condition is largely preventable through the use of anticoagulant prophylaxis. In patients with established VTE, treatment is increasingly outpatient-based because of advances in anticoagulant therapy.

PATHOGENESIS OF VENOUS THROMBOEMBOLISM AND CLINICAL RISK FACTORS

Venous thrombi are composed predominantly of fibrin and red cells[1] and usually arise in the large venous sinuses in the calf, in valve cusp pockets in the deep veins of the calf or at sites of vessel damage. Pathologic or physiologic venous thrombosis occurs when activation of blood coagulation exceeds the ability of the natural anticoagulant mechanisms and the fibrinolytic system to prevent clot formation.[1] The current understanding of the pathogenesis of VTE was first described by Virchow more than 150 years ago.[2] He proposed that thrombotic disorders were associated with the triad of stasis, vascular injury, and hypercoagulability and that abnormalities in this triad result in thromboembolism. Stasis and vascular injury are the most frequent precipitants of VTE. In addition to activating coagulation, tissue damage can also impair fibrinolysis by reducing synthesis of tissue plasminogen activator (t-PA) and by increasing endothelial cell production of plasminogen activator inhibitor type 1 (PAI-1), the major inhibitor of the fibrinolytic pathway.[3]

Under normal circumstances, activated coagulation factors are diluted in the flowing blood and are neutralized by inhibitors on the surface of endothelial cells or by circulating antiproteinases.[4] Activated coagulation factors that escape regulation as a result of either reduced levels of inhibitors or because of generation of overwhelming amounts of these coagulation factors, trigger the coagulation system and fibrin formation. Homeostatic mechanisms, including activation of the fibrinolytic system with release of t-PA[5] and urokinase, are immediately invoked to reduce the likelihood of pathologic thrombus formation.

THROMBOGENIC FACTORS

Activation of Blood Coagulation

With the exception of small amounts of factor VII, the coagulation factors circulate as inactive protein precursors, or zymogens. Each zymogen is converted into an active enzyme that then activates the next zymogen in the coagulation pathway (see Chapter 124).[6] Traditionally, the coagulation system has been divided into the intrinsic, extrinsic, and common pathways. Although these pathways reflect the way coagulation is measured in the laboratory, they do not reflect how coagulation occurs in vivo. In vivo, coagulation is primarily initiated via the tissue factor pathway. In this pathway, a proportion of the circulating activated factor VII—factor VIIa—binds to tissue factor at sites of vascular injury. The tissue factor–factor VIIa complex then activates both factor IX and factor X.[7] Levels of factor VIIa can be increased by factor Xa; however, this reaction is rapidly downregulated by tissue factor pathway inhibitor (TFPI). TFPI renders factor Xa inactive by complexing with it; the TFPI–factor Xa complex then binds the factor VIIa–tissue factor complex and prevents further activation of factor X.[8]

In the presence of activated factor V, phospholipid, and calcium, factor Xa completes the coagulation system by converting prothrombin to thrombin. Thrombin then converts fibrinogen to fibrin, activates platelets, and activates factor XIII, which, in the presence of calcium, cross-links fibrin and stabilizes the fibrin clot. To ensure continuous generation of thrombin, thrombin and, to a lesser extent, factor Xa activate factor VIII and factor V, markedly accelerating the coagulation reactions involving these two cofactors. Thrombin also activates factor XI, which in turn activates additional factor IX, establishing a positive feedback loop.[6]

Coagulation may be activated by contact of factor XII with collagen on exposed subendothelium of damaged vessels, by contact with prosthetic surfaces, or by polyphosphates released from activated platelets. The importance of this pathway in thrombosis is uncertain, but studies in mice deficient in factor XII or factor XI exhibit attenuated thrombus formation at sites of injury, suggesting that the contact pathway plays a part in thrombus stabilization. Under most situations, coagulation is initiated by the exposure of blood to tissue factor made available locally as a result of vascular wall damage,[7] by activation of endothelial cells, or by activated monocytes that migrate to areas of vascular injury.[9] Factor X can be activated directly by extracts of malignant cells that contain a cysteine protease,[10] which may be one of the mechanisms by which thrombosis is induced in patients with cancer. A factor elaborated by hypoxic endothelial cells also can directly activate factor X,[11] potentially leading to thrombosis in patients with severe venous stasis in whom stagnant hypoxia occurs in the valve cusps.

Venous Stasis

Venous stasis is produced by immobility, venous obstruction, increased venous pressure, venous dilation, and increased blood viscosity. Venous return from the lower extremities is enhanced by venous valves, which prevent blood from pooling in the lower legs, and by contraction of the calf muscles, which propels blood upward from the extremities. Venous stasis may contribute to thrombogenesis by allowing stagnation of the blood with associated local hypoxia, which stimulates endothelial cell release of an activator of blood coagulation.[11]

Immobility

Venous thrombosis can occur in immobilized persons because blood pools in the intramuscular sinuses of the calf, which are dilated during recumbency. Many clinical examples highlight the role of stasis in the pathogenesis of VTE. For example, the prevalence of VTE found at autopsy is markedly increased in persons who were confined to bed for more than 1 week before death. Preoperative immobility is associated with a higher frequency of perioperative VTE, and postoperative immobility contributes to the high incidence of postoperative VTE in patients who have undergone hysterectomy, transabdominal prostatectomy, hip surgery, knee surgery, or surgery for fractures of the lower limb. The effect of immobility on thrombus formation is well illustrated by comparing the location of thrombosis in patients with paraplegia with that in patients who have had a stroke. Whereas thrombosis occurs with equal frequency in both legs in patients with paraplegia, it occurs more frequently in the paralyzed limb in patients who have had a stroke.

Venous Obstruction and Increased Venous Pressure

Venous obstruction contributes to the risk of VTE in patients with pelvic tumors and to recurrent venous thrombosis in patients with persistent obstruction because of proximal vein thrombosis. Raised central venous pressure produces venous stasis in the extremities, which may explain the high prevalence of venous thrombosis in patients with congestive heart failure. A similar mechanism may underlie the propensity for thrombosis in the left leg during pregnancy, presumably from obstruction of the left common iliac vein by the right common iliac artery, which is accentuated by the presence of the gravid uterus.[12]

Increased Blood Viscosity and Venous Dilation

Venous stasis can be caused by increased blood viscosity or venous dilation. The blood viscosity can be increased by polycythemia, hypergammaglobulinemia, dysproteinemias, or increased fibrinogen levels. Stasis because of venous dilation may contribute to the increased risk of thromboembolism in patients with varicose veins and in elderly patients, particularly if they are bedridden. The capacity of estrogens to cause venous dilation may contribute to the increased prevalence of thrombosis during pregnancy,[13] in patients taking estrogen-containing oral contraceptive pills,[13] and in women taking postmenopausal estrogen replacement therapy.[14-16]

Vessel Wall Damage

Damage or injury to the vascular endothelium exposes tissue factor, which triggers coagulation. Furthermore, the exposure of blood to the subendothelium leads to platelet adhesion, activation, and aggregation.

The vascular endothelium can be damaged by direct trauma, or it can be perturbed by exposure to endotoxin, inflammatory cytokines such as interleukin-1 and tumor necrosis factor, thrombin, or low oxygen tension. Perturbed endothelial cells synthesize tissue factor and PAI-1 and internalize thrombomodulin, promoting thrombogenesis.[17] Furthermore, damaged endothelial cells may produce less t-PA, the principal activator of intravascular fibrinolysis.

Direct venous damage may lead to venous thrombosis in patients undergoing hip surgery, knee surgery, or varicose vein stripping and in patients with severe burns or lower limb trauma.

PROTECTIVE MECHANISMS

Endothelial Protective Mechanisms

Normal vascular endothelium is nonthrombogenic to flowing blood. Endothelial cell surface glycosaminoglycans, thrombomodulin, and endothelial protein C receptor (EPCR) are potent inhibitors of coagulation, and vessel wall generation of prostacyclin, nitric oxide and synthesis of plasminogen activators limit platelet aggregation and fibrin deposition.

Heparan sulphate, thrombomodulin, and EPCR present on the luminal surface of endothelial cells are important modulators of thrombin activity. Heparan sulfate, a glycosaminoglycan similar to heparin, catalyzes the inhibition of thrombin and factor Xa by antithrombin.[4] Thrombomodulin serves as a surface-bound receptor for thrombin.[17] After being complexed with thrombomodulin, thrombin undergoes a conformational change that markedly alters its substrate specificity such that thrombin is no longer capable of activating platelets, of converting fibrinogen to fibrin, or of activating factors V, VIII, and XIII.[4] Rather, complexed thrombin acquires enhanced ability to activate protein C, which in turn proteolytically inactivates factors Va and VIIIa. This reaction requires protein S as a cofactor. Thus, when bound to thrombomodulin, thrombin not only loses its procoagulant activity but, by activating protein C, triggers a potent anticoagulant pathway. EPCR enhances protein C activation by binding protein C and presenting it to the thrombin–thrombomodulin complex for activation.

Generation of plasminogen activators[18] by vascular endothelium limits fibrin deposition, and platelet aggregation is inhibited by the release of prostacyclin (prostaglandin I2) and endothelium-derived nitric oxide.[19] Endothelial cell affinity for t-PA, plasminogen, and activated protein C and protein S also may contribute to the resistance of the vessel wall to thrombosis.[4] Plasminogen binds to the cell surface, where it can be activated to plasmin by t-PA, thereby promoting local fibrinolytic activity.

Inhibitors of Blood Coagulation

Activated coagulation factors are serine proteases, and their activity is modulated by several naturally occurring plasma inhibitors. The most important inhibitors of the blood coagulation system are antithrombin, protein C, and protein S.[4] An inherited deficiency of one of these three proteins was found in 11% of patients enrolled in a prospective study of 2132 consecutive patients presenting with VTE.[20] Abnormalities in the fibrinolytic system, including congenital dysfibrinogenemias and deficiency of plasminogen, can also predispose the affected person to thromboembolism.

HYPERCOAGULABLE STATES

Other potential causes of VTE are hypercoagulable states, including those associated with deficiencies of antithrombin and proteins C and S, the factor V Leiden and prothrombin G20210A mutations, hyperhomocysteinemia, and the presence of antiphospholipid antibodies. Hypercoagulable states are the subject of Chapter 142.

NATURAL HISTORY OF VENOUS THROMBOEMBOLISM

Most thrombi are asymptomatic and confined to the intramuscular veins of the calf. These calf vein thrombi often undergo spontaneous lysis and rarely produce long-term sequelae.[21] In contrast, complete lysis of proximal vein thrombosis is uncommon even when heparin treatment is given.[22]

The symptoms and signs of VTE are caused by obstruction to venous outflow, inflammation of the vessel wall or perivascular tissues, or embolization of thrombus into the pulmonary circulation. Asymptomatic PE is detected by perfusion lung scanning in approximately 50% of patients with documented proximal vein thrombosis.[23] Most clinically significant and fatal pulmonary emboli probably arise from DVT in the proximal veins of the legs. Although PE also may complicate calf vein thrombosis, these emboli tend to be smaller in size, and PE occurs less commonly than in patients with proximal DVT.[23] Asymptomatic DVT is found in 70% of patients who present with confirmed PE.[24] These thrombi usually are large and involve the proximal veins.

Extensive DVT causes venous valvular damage, which leads to the postthrombotic syndrome.[25] Patients with a previous history of DVT are at increased risk of recurrence, particularly when patients are exposed to high-risk situations.[26]

PROGNOSIS OF VENOUS THROMBOEMBOLISM

Untreated or inadequately treated VTE is associated with a high complication rate, which can be decreased markedly by adequate anticoagulant therapy. Approximately 20% of untreated asymptomatic calf vein thrombi and 20% to 30% of untreated symptomatic calf vein thrombi extend into the popliteal vein. When extension occurs and is untreated, it is associated with a 40% to 50% risk of clinically detectable PE.[21] Patients with proximal vein thrombosis who receive inadequate treatment[27] have a 47% frequency of recurrent VTE over 3 months, and patients with symptomatic calf vein thrombosis who receive a 5-day course of intermittent intravenous unfractionated heparin (UFH) without continuing oral anticoagulants have a recurrence rate greater than 20% over the next 3 months.[28]

By contrast, clinically detectable recurrence occurs in fewer than 2% of patients with proximal vein thrombosis during the initial period of UFH therapy[23] if an adequate anticoagulant response is achieved, and the recurrence rate during the subsequent 3 months of treatment with oral anticoagulants or moderate doses of subcutaneous UFH is 2% to 4%.[27,29,30] After 3 months of anticoagulant therapy, the recurrence rate is 5% to 10% in the subsequent year.[27,29,30] Patients whose first episode of VTE was idiopathic and those who have ongoing risk factors, such as prolonged immobilization or cancer, have a higher risk of recurrence.

The significance of asymptomatic calf DVT discovered incidentally by screening venography after orthopedic surgery is unclear, but the risk of clinical sequelae from these thrombi is low.[31] As a result, if adequate perioperative thromboprophylaxis is given, it is probably unnecessary to perform screening tests for DVT in asymptomatic patients at the time of hospital discharge.

POSTTHROMBOTIC SYNDROME

The postthrombotic syndrome is caused by venous hypertension, usually resulting from valve damage. Valve damage results in malfunction of the muscular pump mechanism, which leads to increased pressure in the deep calf veins during ambulation. The high pressure ultimately renders the perforating veins of the calf incompetent, so that blood flow is directed from the deep veins into the superficial venous system during muscular contraction. This leads to edema and impaired viability of subcutaneous tissues and, in its most severe form, to venous ulceration. Outflow obstruction initially may be bypassed by the development of collateral veins, but with time, the veins distal to the obstruction become dilated, and their valves become incompetent.

In patients whose thrombosis extends into the iliofemoral veins, the leg swelling at initial presentation may not resolve entirely. This is in contrast to patients with less extensive proximal vein thrombosis, in whom the swelling may subside after initial treatment but recur months or years later. Other symptoms and signs of the postthrombotic syndrome may be delayed for 5 to 10 years after the initial thrombotic event. These symptoms include pain in the calf that is relieved with rest and leg elevation, skin pigmentation and induration around the ankle and lower third of the calf, and ulceration in the region of the medial malleolus.

Patients with extensive thrombosis involving the iliofemoral vein frequently have greater disability and may have venous claudication, characterized by incapacitating, bursting pain with exercise.[32] This complication rarely occurs in patients with thrombosis involving the more distal veins.

The frequency with which postthrombotic syndrome occurs after VTE is controversial. Prandoni and colleagues[33] demonstrated that 29% of patients with acute DVT will develop the syndrome after 8 years of follow-up; however, other investigators have found a much lower rate.[34] The development of ipsilateral recurrent thrombosis was associated with a large increase in risk for the development of postthrombotic syndrome.

Treatment for acute DVT may reduce the long-term risk of postthrombotic syndrome. In addition, the use of below-knee graduated compression stockings has been shown to reduce the risk of postthrombotic syndrome in patients with DVT.[35]

DIAGNOSIS OF VENOUS THROMBOEMBOLISM

The diagnosis of VTE is based on objective testing, as opposed to clinical assessment, which may be subjective.

DEEP VENOUS THROMBOSIS

Clinical Manifestations

Deep venous thrombosis classically causes swelling, pain and erythema of the affected extremity. Proximal DVT is more likely to be symptomatic than calf vein thrombosis. Patients with massive thrombosis involving the iliac and femoral veins may present with phlegmasia cerulea dolens, which is severe leg pain with swelling, cyanosis, venous gangrene, compartment syndrome, and arterial compromise. Patients with phlegmasia cerulea dolens may experience circulatory collapse and shock, which may result in death or loss of the affected limb.

Differential Diagnosis

The differential diagnosis of patients with suspected DVT includes musculoskeletal disorders (muscle or tendon strains or tears), lymphatic obstruction, venous insufficiency, a ruptured popliteal (Baker) cyst, cellulitis, sciatica, muscle hematoma, and the postthrombotic syndrome.

OBJECTIVE DIAGNOSTIC TESTS FOR DEEP VENOUS THROMBOSIS

Both invasive and noninvasive tests are useful for the diagnosis of DVT. Venography is the only invasive test of proven value, and venous compression ultrasonography is the most widely studied and used noninvasive test. Although other imaging modalities have been studied (e.g., magnetic resonance direct thrombus imaging), these are not commonly performed.

Venography

Venography remains the reference standard for the diagnosis of DVT, although it is performed increasingly less frequently.[36] It is technically difficult, and its proper execution and interpretation require considerable experience. Venography may produce superficial phlebitis and can cause DVT,[36] but with good technique, ascending venography outlines the entire deep venous system of the lower extremities, including the calf and iliac veins. It is currently used only when noninvasive testing is not feasible or the results of such testing are inconclusive.

Venous Compression Ultrasonography

Venous ultrasonography is performed using a high-resolution real-time scanner equipped with a 5-MHz electronically focused linear array transducer. The common femoral vein and femoral artery are first located in the groin, with the patient in a supine position. The superficial femoral vein is then examined along its course. Next, the popliteal vein is located and examined down to the level of its trifurcation into the peroneal and tibial veins. At each of these locations, the vein being examined is compressed gently but firmly with the transducer probe, and the results are observed on the monitor. Hard copies from freeze-frame images of both stages of the procedure are obtained and serve as a permanent record.

In symptomatic patients, venous compression ultrasonography has a sensitivity and specificity for detection of proximal DVT (femoral or popliteal vein) of more than 95%.[37] However, ultrasonography is less sensitive for detection of calf vein thrombosis.[38] Ultrasound examination can be repeated 7 days after the initial study to increase its sensitivity for detection of clinically important calf vein thrombosis and to improve the safety of diagnostic strategies that do not include venography in patients with suspected calf vein thrombosis. This strategy will detect the 10% to 30% of calf vein thrombi that extend proximally. If the ultrasound examination result remains negative after 7 days, the risk of clinically important proximal extension is negligible, and it is safe to withhold antithrombotic treatment.[39-42]

If the field of examination is extended to the distal popliteal vein and the proximal deep calf veins, venous ultrasonography detects approximately 50% of calf vein thrombi in symptomatic patients.[44,45] Although there are reports that ultrasound examination of the calf can reliably detect thrombi, most such reports have not used venography as their reference standard. Furthermore, whether the value of this test is maintained when it moves from highly specialized vascular laboratories into community ultrasonography laboratories is unknown. A potential limitation of venous ultrasonography is its inability to visualize the iliac veins and the segment of the superficial femoral vein within the femoral canal. This is not a serious limitation because isolated thrombi within the femoral canal or the iliac vein are rare.[46] Furthermore, the obstruction produced by iliac vein thrombi often limits the compressibility of the common femoral vein segment and hence will be detected indirectly. Doppler color flow can also be used to assess for blood flow and occlusion within a vein. The combination of compression ultrasonography and Doppler is often referred to as duplex ultrasonography.

D-Dimer Assays

D-dimer assays use mono- or polyspecific antibodies against D-dimer to provide quantitative or qualitative data on the concentration of D-dimer in whole blood or plasma. D-dimer is the product of lysis of cross-linked fibrin and the levels of D-dimer are increased in patients with acute VTE. However, the test is nonspecific because the level of D-dimer is increased in a variety of other conditions, including malignancy, inflammatory conditions, and infections. Therefore, the D-dimer assay is most useful as a tool to rule out suspected DVT.[47,48]

D-dimer assays have two principal limitations: (1) A positive test result is nonspecific and should not be used as the sole criterion for diagnosis of VTE, and (2) numerous test kits are available that have different sensitivities for VTE. Thus D-dimer results are not interchangeable between kits. (Assays also use different standards; some use fibrinogen, others use D-dimer. This leads to confusion in reporting because the cut-offs are different depending on which standard is used.) This has led to confusion among clinicians regarding the use of D-dimer assays, and this confusion is exacerbated by the fact that the use of an insensitive D-dimer assay to rule out VTE could result in omission of required diagnostic testing, placing patients at risk for PE and death.

The optimal setting for use of a D-dimer assay is in the assessment of patients with a low clinical pretest probability of VTE. The combination of a low pretest probability (determined using a validated scoring system) and a negative result with a validated D-dimer assay rules out the diagnosis of acute DVT, obviating the need for additional testing. Some D-dimer kits have been studied in patients with low and moderate pretest probabilities of DVT and have been shown to reliably exclude DVT in both patient groups.[49,50] Evaluation of the levels of D-dimer may be of particular value in patients with suspected recurrent VTE, and it may assist in decision making about optimal duration of anticoagulation.[51]

DIAGNOSTIC STRATEGIES FOR DEEP VENOUS THROMBOSIS

Diagnostic algorithms for the noninvasive diagnosis of clinically suspected VTE are presented in Fig. 144-1. If compression ultrasonography is not immediately available, patients can be empirically

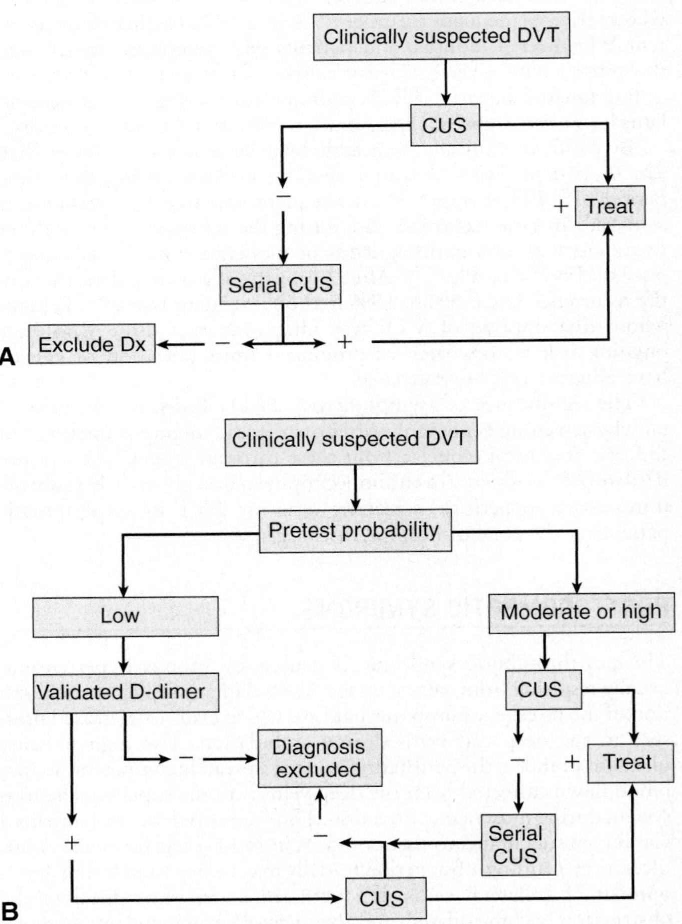

Figure 144-1 DIAGNOSTIC ALGORITHMS FOR THE MANAGEMENT OF PATIENTS WITH SUSPECTED DEEP VENOUS THROMBOSIS (DVT). **A**, Ultrasound examination–based strategy. **B**, Clinical probability–based strategy. *CUS,* Compression ultrasound.

anticoagulated with a therapeutic dose of low-molecular-weight heparin (LMWH) and can then return for diagnostic testing on the subsequent day. In assessing patients with suspected DVT, patients can be classified into high-, intermediate-, or low-probability groups based on their clinical manifestations and the presence or absence of risk factors such as recent immobilization, hospitalization within the past 6 months, or malignancy.[43] In one series, patients with the classic symptoms and signs of DVT and who had at least one risk factor had an 85% probability of DVT, but those with atypical symptoms and no risk factors had only a 5% probability of DVT. These low- and high-pretest probabilities can be combined with the results of objective noninvasive tests to make clinical decisions. A low clinical pretest probability and a negative result on noninvasive testing can be used to exclude a diagnosis of DVT and obviate further testing, but a high clinical pretest probability and a negative noninvasive test result should prompt further investigation with either venography or serial ultrasonography.

In approximately 70% of patients referred for clinically suspected DVT, the diagnosis will be excluded by objective tests.[39,40] Of the 30% who have DVT, approximately 85% will have proximal vein thrombosis, and the remainder will have thrombosis confined to the calf.[39,40]

PULMONARY EMBOLISM

Clinical Manifestations

The most frequently reported symptom of PE is dyspnea.[52,53] Chest pain is common and typically pleuritic in nature but may be substernal and compressing. Hemoptysis is a less frequent feature.[24,52,53]

The physical signs of PE are nonspecific. Syncope usually is associated with massive PE and is caused by a reduction in cardiac output. This in turn results in hypotension and transient impairment of cerebral blood flow.

Although 70% of patients with PE have venographic evidence of thrombosis at presentation, fewer than 20% of these patients have leg symptoms.[24] Massive PE causes tachypnea, tachycardia, cyanosis, and hypotension. In these patients, cardiac examination may reveal a right ventricular heave, a loud pulmonary second sound, and a gallop rhythm. Physical examination of the chest may be normal, or nonspecific abnormalities may be detected. Patients with pulmonary infarction or atelectasis may have reduced movement of the affected portion of the chest.

Differential Diagnosis

The differential diagnosis of dyspnea and pleuritic chest pain, in addition to PE, includes pneumonia, pleurisy, chest wall pain, pericarditis, atelectasis, pneumothorax, acute bronchitis, acute bronchiolitis, and acute bronchial obstruction as a result of mucous plugging or bronchoconstriction.

Diagnosis

The clinical diagnosis of PE requires objective testing. The chest radiograph is not specific for PE and usually does not show any diagnostic abnormality. Nevertheless, it is useful in excluding other causes for the presenting symptoms (e.g., pneumothorax) and is essential for interpreting ventilation/perfusion (V/Q) lung scan findings. The electrocardiogram (ECG) findings are frequently normal or show nonspecific abnormalities. However, in the appropriate clinical setting, ECG evidence of right ventricular strain is strongly suggestive of PE. Elevated levels of cardiac troponin can result from right ventricular strain and associated myocardial ischemia.[54]

OBJECTIVE DIAGNOSTIC TESTS FOR PULMONARY EMBOLISM

Pulmonary Angiography

Pulmonary angiography is the reference standard for establishing the presence or absence of PE. However, similar to venography of the lower extremities, it requires technical expertise and is done only when noninvasive testing is not feasible or the results of such testing are nondiagnostic. Selective angiography and magnification views improve resolution and reduce the risk of the procedure. When pulmonary angiography is adequately performed, a negative result excludes the diagnosis of PE. Unless the tertiary pulmonary arteries are visualized in a patient with a small perfusion defect, however, the diagnosis of PE cannot be excluded.[55]

Arrhythmias, cardiac perforation, cardiac arrest, and hypersensitivity reactions to contrast material occur in 3% to 4% of patients undergoing pulmonary angiography.[56] Patients with a history of allergy to radiopaque dye should not undergo pulmonary angiography.

Helical Computed Tomography Scanning

Helical or spiral computed tomography (CT) scanning of the chest has emerged as the preferred test for the diagnosis of PE. When performed in experienced clinical centers with use of validated scanning protocols, helical CT scanning is a useful tool to rule out PE in patients with compatible clinical symptoms. For example, in one study in which patients with suspected PE were evaluated with single-detector helical CT scanning and those with negative or inconclusive findings on CT scanning underwent ultrasonography of the lower extremities on the day of presentation and on days 4 and 7 after scanning, 124 of 510 enrolled patients had PE.[58] In 130 patients, an alternate diagnosis for their chest symptoms was found with the CT scan, 10 patients either could not have a CT performed or had a uninterpretable scan, and 248 patients had normal scans. Two of these 248 patients had proximal DVT on their initial ultrasound study, and all other patients had normal findings on serial ultrasound examinations. This and other similar studies suggest that if used correctly, helical CT scanning is a useful test in patients with suspected PE. In fact, systematic reviews suggest that a correctly done spiral CT effectively rules out PE in patients suspected to be at low or moderate risk of this complication.[59]

Ventilation/Perfusion Lung Scan

The lung scan consists of a perfusion and a ventilation component. For the perfusion component, particles of isotopically labeled microaggregates of human albumin are injected intravenously and become trapped in the pulmonary capillary bed. Their distribution reflects lung blood flow and is recorded with an external photoscanner. A normal perfusion scan excludes PE, but an abnormal perfusion scan is nonspecific.[24,53,57]

Ventilation lung scanning is performed using either radioactive gases or aerosols that are inhaled and exhaled by the patient while a gamma camera records the distribution of radioactivity within the alveolar gas exchange units. The purpose of ventilation imaging is to improve the specificity of perfusion scanning for the diagnosis of PE. A high-probability V/Q scan (in which a segmental or greater area is ventilated but not perfused) has a positive predictive value for PE of more than 90%, obviating the need for angiography.

The relative ease and accessibility of CT scanning has reduced the use of V/Q scanning for the diagnosis of PE. However, V/Q scanning is frequently preferred in two patient populations: patients with impaired renal function and young women. In patients with impaired renal function, contrast dye administration for the CT scan can induce contrast nephropathy, increasing mortality up to 30% after such a procedure. Furthermore, CT scanning results in radiation exposure, which is associated with a small increase in the risk of subsequent cancer. Although this risk varies depending on a number of factors, concern about increasing the risk of breast cancer in young women has prompted use of V/Q scanning preferentially in this population. V/Q lung scanning should ideally be reserved for patients with normal chest radiographs because preexisting lung disease may result in indeterminate scans.

Diagnostic Strategy for Pulmonary Embolism

Patients with large perfusion defects (involving one or more segments or more extensive defects) and a V/Q mismatch have a 90% probability of PE. Patients with a normal perfusion scan have less than a 2% probability of having PE, excluding the diagnosis. However, most patients who have V/Q scanning performed will have neither of these findings; rather, they will have either matched defects or small perfusion defects (indeterminate scan).[24,53,57] Patients with these findings require further investigation with either pulmonary angiography or objective tests for DVT of the lower extremities. A patient with suspected PE, an indeterminate V/Q scan result, and positive findings on compression ultrasound examination of the lower extremities can be assumed to have PE. A patient with suspected PE, an indeterminate scan, and a negative result on leg ultrasound examination requires additional testing because the thrombus may have completely embolized to the lungs.[24,53]

A diagnostic algorithm for the management of clinically suspected PE is shown in Fig. 144-2. After a history and physical examination, ECG, and chest radiography, all patients with suspected PE should undergo helical CT scanning or V/Q lung scanning. A negative helical CT or a normal perfusion lung scan result rules out clinically significant PE, and anticoagulant therapy can be withheld. If an intraluminal filling defect is seen on helical CT or the perfusion scan demonstrates one or more segmental (or larger) defects and ventilation to these regions is normal, a diagnosis of PE is made. Although a V/Q mismatch supports a diagnosis of PE, a V/Q "match" does not exclude PE, and further objective testing is required in these patients. Similarly, the diagnosis of PE cannot be excluded in patients with small perfusion defects (one or more subsegmental defects) or those with indeterminate lung scan findings (in which the perfusion defects correspond with abnormalities on the chest radiograph). In these patients, venous ultrasonography should be performed. If DVT is documented, a diagnosis of PE can be assumed, and anticoagulant therapy should be started. However, if results on these tests are negative, additional objective investigations (e.g., pulmonary angiography) are required in patients with a high clinical pretest probability. For those with a lower pretest probability of PE, an alternative strategy is to withhold anticoagulants and to perform serial noninvasive tests to detect venous thrombosis. In patients with a low or low to moderate pretest probability of PE, a D-dimer test may prove useful. If the D-dimer assay result is negative, further testing can be avoided, but if it is positive (increasing the likelihood of acute thrombosis), further testing (e.g., venous compression ultrasonography) is warranted.[60,61]

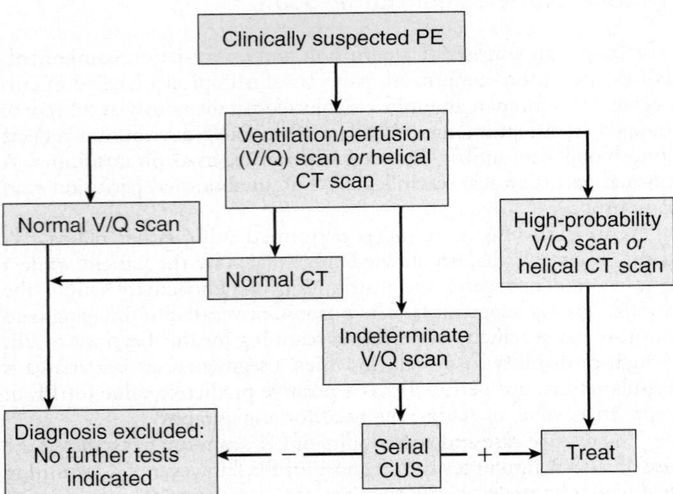

Figure 144-2 DIAGNOSTIC ALGORITHM FOR THE MANAGEMENT OF PATIENTS WITH SUSPECTED PULMONARY EMBOLISM (PE). *CT,* Computed tomography; *CUS,* compression ultrasound; *V/Q,* ventilation/perfusion.

DIAGNOSIS OF ACUTE RECURRENT VENOUS THROMBOEMBOLISM

The diagnosis of acute recurrent VTE is difficult to make because the clinical manifestations of recurrence are nonspecific. In addition, all of the validated diagnostic tests for acute VTE have limitations in this setting because the venous occlusion produced by the initial episode of venous thrombosis makes it difficult to identify new abnormalities.

The most appropriate diagnostic strategy for suspected recurrent DVT has yet to be determined. The patient's history may be helpful in determining the likelihood of recurrent thrombosis. Leg pain with ambulation and leg swelling that is relieved with overnight rest is typical of the postthrombotic syndrome. New clinically significant and persistent leg swelling, particularly if the symptoms do not abate overnight, is consistent with recurrent thrombosis and should prompt diagnostic evaluation. In patients taking vitamin K antagonists such as warfarin, it may also be useful to determine the international normalized ratio (INR) at the time of presentation and to assess the INR measurements in recent weeks. Warfarin is a very effective antithrombotic agent, and the risk of recurrent thrombosis in therapeutically anticoagulated patients irrespective of their symptoms is very low. Nevertheless, recurrent thrombosis despite therapeutic anticoagulation occasionally is seen in patients with cancer or those with antiphospholipid antibodies.

Many patients with a history of VTE will have a heightened level of concern about the risk of recurrent thrombosis. This heightened concern will lead these patients to seek testing for recurrent thrombosis even with incompatible symptoms. Such patients require careful clinical and radiologic evaluation. If there is no evidence of acute recurrence, they may require counseling and education about their condition.

To establish a diagnosis of recurrent DVT, one must demonstrate a new thrombus in a previously unaffected venous segment, either through lack of compressibility on ultrasonography or an intraluminal filling defect on venography. A normal venogram result rules out recurrence, and normal findings on ultrasound examination rule out proximal thrombus. A normal result on ultrasound study does not rule out recurrent calf vein thrombosis and requires that additional testing with serial ultrasonography be performed if this is suspected. If the lack of compressibility of the veins or an intraluminal filling defect with flow seen on Doppler ultrasound studies is visualized in the venous segment previously affected, these tests are not sufficiently reliable to either confirm or rule out acute thrombosis. In these cases, serial testing to detect extension may be useful. Alternately, if the patient had a follow-up ultrasound examination, comparison with previous imaging may be useful.

D-dimer–based testing strategies are very attractive in patients with suspected recurrence, because they may obviate the need for additional diagnostic testing. A quantitative D-dimer assay was evaluated in a prospective cohort of 300 patients with suspected recurrent DVT in which patients with a negative D-dimer had heparin withheld and patients with a positive D-dimer underwent compression ultrasonography.[62] This appears to be a safe strategy among symptomatic patients with suspected recurrence but must be validated with different D-dimer assays.

DIAGNOSIS OF THE POSTTHROMBOTIC SYNDROME

The clinical spectrum of the postthrombotic syndrome varies from a course that may mimic acute DVT to one of persistent leg pain that is worse at the end of the day and is associated with dependent edema; stasis pigmentation; and, in its most severe form, skin ulceration.[63] Rarely, patients may complain of venous claudication on walking.[64] When symptoms are acute or subacute in onset, a diagnosis of postthrombotic syndrome should be considered only after recurrent DVT has been excluded by objective testing. There is no single definitive diagnostic test for the postthrombotic syndrome, but a history of objectively documented DVT, appropriate clinical findings, and evidence of venous reflux or outflow obstruction on venous ultrasonography constitute sufficient evidence to make this diagnosis.

PROPHYLAXIS OF VENOUS THROMBOEMBOLISM

PE is a common preventable cause of death in hospitalized patients.[65] Hospitalized patients can be classified as having a low, moderate, or high risk for developing VTE. Effective prophylaxis is cost effective and is available for most high-risk groups.[66]

Low-Molecular-Weight Heparins and Fondaparinux

Low-molecular-weight heparins exert their anticoagulant effect by preferentially catalyzing the inactivation of factor Xa by antithrombin. When used in prophylactic doses once or twice daily, LMWH is an effective and safe agent for prophylaxis in medical and surgical patients. Anticoagulant monitoring is not required when used in prophylactic doses. It is as or more effective than standard low-dose UFH and warfarin in most patient populations.[67]

The anticoagulant effect of LMWH is mediated by a unique pentasaccharide sequence in the heparin molecule that binds antithrombin. The pentasaccharide moiety has been synthesized chemically as fondaparinux. Fondaparinux has been shown to be superior to LMWH for the prevention of VTE in patients undergoing hip fracture surgery. Extended use of fondaparinux in this patient population significantly reduces the risk of clinical VTE over an extended follow-up period.[68] Fondaparinux has also been shown in clinical trials to be as effective and safe as unfractionated intravenous heparin for the treatment of acute symptomatic PE,[69] as effective and safe as twice-daily LMWH for the treatment of DVT[70] and as effective as therapeutic dose enoxaparin in patients with unstable coronary syndromes. In this latter study, fondaparinux was also safer than enoxaparin.

Low-Dose Unfractionated Heparin

Low doses of UFH prevent thrombosis by antithrombin-mediated inhibition of thrombin, factor Xa, and other serine proteases. UFH is usually given subcutaneously at 5000 units 2 hours before surgery and continued postoperatively at 5000 units every 8 to 12 hours. Low-dose UFH prophylaxis does not require laboratory monitoring and is simple and convenient to administer. It is an acceptable option for moderate risk general surgical and medical patients, and it reduces the risk of VTE by 50% to 70%.[65,71-73] When used in these doses, UFH is both highly effective and associated with only a small increase in the risk of bleeding. Although low-dose UFH is effective in patients undergoing elective hip surgery and reduces the incidence of venous thrombosis by approximately 40%, it is less effective than other current prophylactic strategies and thus should not be used as the sole form of prophylaxis in such patients. Low-dose UFH has not been shown to be effective in patients with hip fractures or those undergoing major knee surgery. In addition, use of subcutaneous heparin may be associated with heparin induced thrombocytopenia, particularly in the postoperative period.

Vitamin K Antagonists

When administered in doses that prolong the prothrombin time to an INR of 2.0 to 3.0, vitamin K antagonists effectively prevent postoperative VTE in patients in all risk categories.[65,73] Vitamin K antagonists can be given preoperatively, at the time of surgery, or in the early postoperative period. The antithrombolytic effect of vitamin K antagonists is not achieved until the fourth or fifth day of administration. Nevertheless, when used in this fashion, vitamin K antagonists are effective in very high-risk patient groups.[74] Prophylaxis with vitamin K antagonists is relatively inconvenient, however, because careful laboratory monitoring using the INR is necessary.

Oral Direct Factor Xa or Thrombin Inhibitors for Orthopedic Thromboprophylaxis

Rivaroxaban is an oral direct factor Xa inhibitor with excellent bioavailability that has been studied in patients undergoing total knee or hip replacement surgery.[75-78] In a pooled analysis of these randomized trials, 10 mg/day of rivaroxaban was superior to enoxaparin for prevention of symptomatic VTE and all-cause mortality with similar major bleeding rates.[79] Although rivaroxaban has also been evaluated for prophylaxis in medically ill patients, its benefit-to-risk profile is less certain in this setting.

Dabigatran etexilate is an oral direct thrombin inhibitor that also has been used in patients undergoing total knee or hip replacement surgery. Dabigatran etexilate is a prodrug that is converted to the active agent dabigatran, which binds both free and clot-bound thrombin. In large clinical trials, once-daily dabigatran was noninferior to enoxaparin 40 mg once daily but was inferior when enoxaparin was dosed at 30 mg twice daily.[80-82]

Rivaroxaban is licensed in the United States, Europe, and Canada for orthopedic thromboprophylaxis. Although licensed in Europe and Canada, dabigatran etexilate is not approved in the United States for orthopedic thromboprophylaxis.

Intermittent Pneumatic Compression

Intermittent pneumatic compression of the legs enhances blood flow in the deep veins and increases systemic fibrinolytic activity.[65] Although few methodologically rigorous studies support the effectiveness of intermittent pneumatic compression for VTE prophylaxis, this modality has few clinically important side effects and is particularly useful in patients who have a high risk of bleeding. It also is frequently used, albeit with little supporting evidence, during the operative procedure in patients undergoing extended-duration surgery and in patients after trauma. Intermittent compression is the prophylactic measure of choice in selected patients undergoing neurosurgical procedures[83]; however, most of these patients should eventually receive pharmacologic thromboprophylaxis as well.[84]

Graduated Compression Stockings

Graduated compression stockings also reduce venous stasis in the legs and are effective for preventing postoperative VTE in low- and moderate-risk general surgical patients[72] and in medical or surgical patients with neurologic disorders, including paralysis of the lower limbs.[83] In surgical patients, the combination of graduated compression stockings and low-dose UFH is significantly more effective than low-dose UFH alone.[85,86] Use of graduated compression stockings alone, however, constitutes inadequate prophylaxis in patients undergoing surgery associated with a very high risk of thromboembolism.[87] Graduated compression stockings are inexpensive and should be considered for use in all high-risk surgical patients even if other forms of prophylaxis are used.

TREATMENT OF VENOUS THROMBOEMBOLISM

The goals of treatment for VTE are to prevent death from PE, reduce morbidity from the acute event, minimize development of postthrombotic symptoms, and prevent chronic thromboembolic pulmonary hypertension. All of these goals can be achieved with adequate anticoagulant therapy. Use of thrombolytic therapy or surgical approaches are reserved for patients with severe disease or severe complications.

ANTICOAGULANT THERAPY FOR TREATMENT OF ACUTE VENOUS THROMBOEMBOLISM

The treatment of acute VTE currently involves administration of effective doses of a parenteral anticoagulant as soon as the diagnosis is confirmed (or if testing is delayed and the clinical likelihood of disease is moderate or high, before confirmation of the diagnosis).

Traditionally, patients with acute VTE were admitted to hospital and given intravenous UFH, administered to achieve a therapeutic activated partial thromboplastin time (aPTT). A vitamin K antagonist, typically warfarin, was then started and the heparin continued until the INR was more than 2.0 on two consecutive measurements. This treatment strategy remains a practice standard. However, the vast majority of patients with proximal DVT, calf vein thrombosis, and minimally symptomatic PE are now eligible to receive outpatient LMWH or fondaparinux treatment. These agents are preferred given the ease in administration and ability to be administered on an outpatient basis without the need for anticoagulant monitoring. Treatment with LMWH or fondaparinux involves administration of weight-adjusted, once- or twice-daily subcutaneous injections. If anticoagulant-related complications develop or if the patient is at the extremes of weight (<40 kg or >100 kg) or has severe renal insufficiency (creatinine clearance <30 ml/min), then the anticoagulant effect of the LMWH can be assessed using an anti(factor)-Xa assay. Typically, one would target a peak anti-Xa level of 0.5 to 1.0 unit/mL measured 4 hours after a subcutaneous injection of LMWH using a twice-daily dosing schedule. LMWH and fondaparinux do not have predictable effects on the aPTT and therefore cannot be monitored using this test.

Although increasingly less common, selected patients may be admitted to the hospital for intravenous UFH therapy. There is no evidence that UFH therapy is superior to LMWH in any clinical setting. Hence, intravenous UFH is typically reserved for patients with comorbid conditions that preclude outpatient treatment, including those with significantly symptomatic PE and patients at high risk of bleeding in whom rapid anticoagulant reversal may be necessary.[88] Patients with significant renal impairment are also typically treated with UFH because LMWH is predominantly renally eliminated and there is a risk of anticoagulant accumulation in these patients.

Unfractionated heparin therapy can be monitored using the activated clotting time, the aPTT, or by heparin assays that measure the ability of heparin to accelerate the inactivation of factor Xa or thrombin. It is important to give adequate doses of UFH at initial presentation because the risk of recurrent VTE is increased if insufficient doses are given. Accordingly, the aPTT should be maintained above a level equivalent to a heparin level of 0.3 unit/mL as determined by measuring the antifactor Xa activity. For most currently used aPTT reagents, this is equivalent to an aPTT ratio of 1.8 to 2.5 times the control value.[89] To monitor UFH given by continuous intravenous infusion, the aPTT should be measured 6 hours after the bolus dose so that it reflects the anticoagulant effects of the infusion. If twice-daily subcutaneous UFH is given, a mid-interval aPTT is typically measured 6 hours after the injection. However, UFH can also be used without laboratory monitoring; in a study of more than 700 patients, UFH was administered using a fixed, weight-adjusted dose without aPTT monitoring. The risk of bleeding and recurrent thrombosis was found to be similar to that seen in patients treated with twice-daily LMWH.[90]

After an initial course of parenteral therapy (heparin or fondaparinux), patients with VTE require ongoing anticoagulant therapy to prevent recurrence.[27,28] Patients with cancer-associated thrombosis may be treated with ongoing LMWH to decrease recurrence,[91] but most other patients should be transitioned to oral anticoagulant therapy. The most commonly used oral anticoagulants are the vitamin K antagonists, such as warfarin. In most cases, warfarin therapy can be initiated on the same day as the institution of the parenteral agent. The parenteral agent should be continued for at least 5 days and until the INR has been between 2.0 and 3.0 on 2 consecutive days.

Optimal warfarin dosing must consider the patient age and gender. An initial dose of 5 to 10 mg can be given to most individuals, and initial doses less than 5 mg should be used for elderly patients. Women generally require lower warfarin doses than men. The warfarin dose variability is also affected by variation in the genotypes of the cytochrome P450 CYP2C9 and the vitamin K epoxide reductase complex, VKORC1. These enzymes influence the rate of warfarin metabolism and sensitivity, respectively. Studies using warfarin genotyping to optimize warfarin dosing have yielded conflicting results, and further study along with economic evaluation is ongoing.

At the present time, novel oral anticoagulants are in development that do not require anticoagulant monitoring and have fewer interactions with food and drugs compared with warfarin. Dabigatran was noninferior to warfarin for the treatment of acute VTE. Rivaroxaban was also noninferior to combination treatment with enoxaparin and warfarin for treatment of DVT. However, neither of these agents is currently approved in the United States for treatment of VTE.

The optimal duration of oral anticoagulant therapy for treatment of VTE is unknown. Patients with a secondary thrombosis (provoked by a clear transient risk factor) are generally treated for 3 months. Patients with unprovoked (idiopathic) VTE should be treated for a minimum of 3 months, although consideration may be given for a longer duration of therapy. Patients with a persistent, major risk factor for recurrence and patients who prefer to decrease their thrombotic risk should receive warfarin for longer periods or indefinitely. At this time, there are no absolute predictors of recurrence, but recurrence appears to be more common in patients with an elevated D-dimer assay at or around the time of anticoagulant discontinuation, in the male sex, and possibly in patients with residual DVT seen on ultrasonography at the time of anticoagulant discontinuation.

INFERIOR VENA CAVA FILTER

Anticoagulants are effective in reducing mortality from PE.[92] However, some patients have relative or absolute contraindications to anticoagulant therapy. In these cases, there may be a role for inferior vena cava filters (see Chapter 145). These filters do not treat VTE but are used to prevent PE. In patients with a transient risk factor for bleeding, such as surgery for resection of a bowel tumor or active ulcer disease, insertion of a temporary inferior vena cava filter followed by its removal and subsequent therapeutic anticoagulation when the bleeding risk is diminished should be considered. Although not formally evaluated in randomized trials, this strategy likely reduces the initial risk of bleeding while eliminating the long-term increase in the risk of DVT associated with permanent caval interruption. In contrast, patients who have a persistent major risk factor for bleeding, such as angiodysplasia of the gastrointestinal tract, should be considered for insertion of a permanent inferior vena cava filter because the mortality rate associated with major bleeding occurring during therapeutic anticoagulation is approximately 20%. This procedure is associated with a significant risk of immediate worsening of leg symptoms because of blockage of the inferior vena cava by thrombus and a long-term increase in the risk of recurrent DVT.

THROMBOLYTIC THERAPY FOR MASSIVE PULMONARY EMBOLISM

Thrombolytic therapy with streptokinase, urokinase, or t-PA is more effective than UFH alone in correcting the angiographic defects produced by PE[92] and may be better than UFH in preventing death in patients with massive PE associated with shock.[93,94] Based on these findings, thrombolytic therapy is the treatment of choice for patients with massive PE associated with cardiovascular collapse and in those with underlying cardiac or pulmonary disease, in whom even a small or moderate-sized embolus may be life threatening.

Bleeding occurs more frequently with thrombolytic therapy than with UFH.[92,95] The risk of hemorrhage increases with the duration of thrombolytic infusion and usually occurs at a site of previous surgery or trauma. Intracranial hemorrhage occurs in approximately 1% of patients at risk, approximately twice as frequently as with UFH treatment.

THROMBOENDARTERECTOMY FOR PULMONARY EMBOLISM

Thromboendarterectomy is effective in selected cases of chronic thromboembolic pulmonary hypertension with proximal pulmonary arterial obstruction.[96] Urgent pulmonary embolectomy is usually reserved for patients with a saddle embolism lodged in the main pulmonary artery or for those with massive embolism whose blood pressure cannot be maintained despite thrombolytic therapy and vasopressor agents.[92] Although this procedure can be successfully performed by experienced surgical teams, in inexperienced hands, it is associated with high complication and mortality rates. Patients with repeated episodes of PE and significant chronic pulmonary hypertension with right ventricular compromise should be anticoagulated and monitored. If pulmonary pressures do not decrease, patients should be evaluated for surgical fitness. If deemed necessary, thromboendarterectomy should be carried out in centers with expertise with optimal perioperative management, within which the likelihood of success of the procedure is high.[96]

SUGGESTED READINGS

Kearon C, Ginsberg JS, Anderson DR, et al: SOFAST Investigators: Comparison of 1 month with 3 months of anticoagulation for a first episode of venous thromboembolism associated with a transient risk factor. *J Thromb Haemost* 2:743, 2004.

Prandoni P, Lensing AW, Prins MH, et al: Below-knee elastic compression stockings to prevent the post-thrombotic syndrome: A randomized, controlled trial. *Ann Intern Med* 141:249, 2004.

Ridker PM, Goldhaber SZ, Danielson E, et al: Long-term, low-intensity warfarin therapy for the prevention of recurrent venous thromboembolism. *N Engl J Med* 348:1425, 2003.

Van Strijen MJ, De Monye W, Schiereck J, et al: Single-detector helical computed tomography as the primary diagnostic test in suspected pulmonary embolism: A multicenter clinical management study of 510 patients. *Ann Intern Med* 138:307, 2003.

For complete list of references log on to www.expertconsult.com.

CHAPTER 145

MECHANICAL INTERVENTIONS IN ARTERIAL AND VENOUS THROMBOSIS

Steven Sauk and Suresh Vedantham

Arterial and venous thromboses are common medical conditions that are associated with significant morbidity. Patients who suffer from acute occlusions of the peripheral arteries may present with ischemic extremities, culminating in limb loss or death if left untreated. Those who suffer from venous thrombosis are at significant risk not only for pulmonary embolism (PE), but also for a chronic condition known as the postthrombotic syndrome (PTS), which can cause significant impairment of patients' quality of life (QOL).

For many patients with symptomatic arterial or venous occlusions, surgical therapies are required in addition to standard medical treatments to provide optimal patient outcomes. Spurred by advances in vascular imaging and catheter/device technology and driven by the clinical needs of the large number of vascular patients with concomitant comorbidities, many patients are now referred for nonsurgical, imaging-guided endovascular interventions to eliminate thrombi and to treat associated vascular lesions. In this chapter, we discuss the use of catheter-based interventions in the management of arterial and venous thromboses.

OVERVIEW OF CATHETER-BASED THROMBOLYTIC INTERVENTIONS

Systemic thrombolysis, which refers to the dissolution of thrombus via the administration of a fibrinolytic drug into an intravenous line distant from the affected site, can be a valuable treatment option for acute myocardial infarction (MI), massive PE, and acute ischemic stroke. A primary advantage of the systemic administration route is the ability to rapidly initiate therapy in almost any clinical setting, without the need for specialized technical expertise or hospital resources. However, only a fraction of systemically administered drug reaches the target vessel. This problem is compounded when there is complete occlusion of blood flow in the target vessel such that access of the fibrinolytic drug to the interior of the thrombus is precluded. For acute MI and stroke, this limitation is overcome by the use of relatively high concentrations of fibrinolytic drugs (e.g., 50-100 mg of recombinant tissue plasminogen activator [rt-PA]) and the ability of arterial pulsations to force sufficient amounts of the drug into the fresh thrombus that occludes a small (2-4 mm) coronary or cerebral artery to effect fibrinolysis. However, with these high doses of fibrinolytic drugs, there is a small, but significantly increased risk for major bleeding, a price that physicians are willing to pay given the potentially fatal consequences of ongoing vascular occlusion in these critical sites.

For occlusions in the peripheral arteries and veins, however, systemic fibrinolysis is not sufficiently effective to justify the attendant risks, presumably because of the larger vessel size, greater thrombus burden, and the presence of mature thrombus that is less susceptible to dissolution. For these reasons, catheter-directed fibrinolysis and mechanical methods for thrombus extraction and dissolution have been developed.

Catheter-Directed Intrathrombus Thrombolysis

Catheter-directed intrathrombus thrombolysis (CDT) refers to the infusion of a fibrinolytic drug directly into the thrombosed vessel via a catheter that has been inserted into that vessel using imaging guidance.[1] The rationale for CDT is to improve the efficacy of thrombus dissolution by achieving a higher intrathrombus concentration of fibrinolytic drug, and to reduce the risk for hemorrhage by enabling the use of lower total fibrinolytic drug doses than those required for systemic fibrinolysis. Although several catheters and devices have been approved by the Food and Drug Administration (FDA) for this purpose, none of the currently available fibrinolytic drugs is FDA-approved for the specific indication of peripheral arterial or venous thrombosis.

Although the procedural details are beyond the scope of this chapter, the principles of CDT are reviewed here[2,3] (Fig. 145-1). First, a vascular access site is selected based on the thrombus location and extent, and needle access into the vessel is obtained. With ultrasound-guided venipuncture, access site bleeding is rare. Under fluoroscopic guidance, the needle is exchanged over a guidewire for an angiographic catheter, and iodinated contrast is injected to delineate the location, extent, and morphology of the thrombus and the status of other relevant vessels in the limb. The angiographic catheter is then exchanged for a specially designed infusion catheter with multiple side holes (akin to a soaking garden hose) that is positioned so that the side holes are embedded within the thrombus-containing vascular segment. Fibrinolytic drug is then infused. The drugs and doses commonly used for this purpose include rt-PA (0.5-1.0 mg/hr), reteplase (0.25-0.75 units/hr), and tenecteplase (0.25-0.50 mg/hr).[4,5] The procedure is done under conscious sedation and with local anesthesia, and the heart rate, blood pressure, and oxygen saturation are continuously monitored.

Patients are then transferred to an observation unit, usually an intensive care or step-down unit, for monitoring during the fibrinolytic drug infusion. Typically, a concomitant infusion of unfractionated heparin at subtherapeutic doses is administered, and the hemoglobin, partial thromboplastin time (PTT), and in some centers, the fibrinogen level are determined every 6 to 8 hours while the fibrinolytic drug is given. Patients are monitored closely for evidence of bleeding and for changes in limb status, and the drug infusion rate is adjusted (or stopped entirely) as necessary. After 6 to 18 hours, patients return to the procedure room for a follow-up venogram or angiogram to assess the extent of thrombus dissolution. The infusion catheter may be repositioned and the infusion continued if there is residual thrombus. Once thrombolysis is nearly complete, the fibrinolytic drug infusion is stopped, and based on the results of the venogram or angiogram, a decision is made as to whether adjunctive treatment with balloon angioplasty or stent placement is needed—if so, this is performed, usually through the same vascular access site during the same procedure session. The catheter and sheath are then removed, and systemic anticoagulation at fully therapeutic levels is reinstituted. The treated limb is closely monitored for improvement in pain, perfusion abnormalities (arterial), and/or swelling (venous).

Although few changes have been made to the CDT technique over the past 25 years, there has been a switch from biologically derived fibrinolytic drugs (streptokinase and urokinase) to recombinant drugs that are less allergenic and have greater affinity for fibrin. Recently, a multi–side-hole catheter (the Ekosonic Mach 4e catheter) that not only enables drug infusion, but also emits low-power

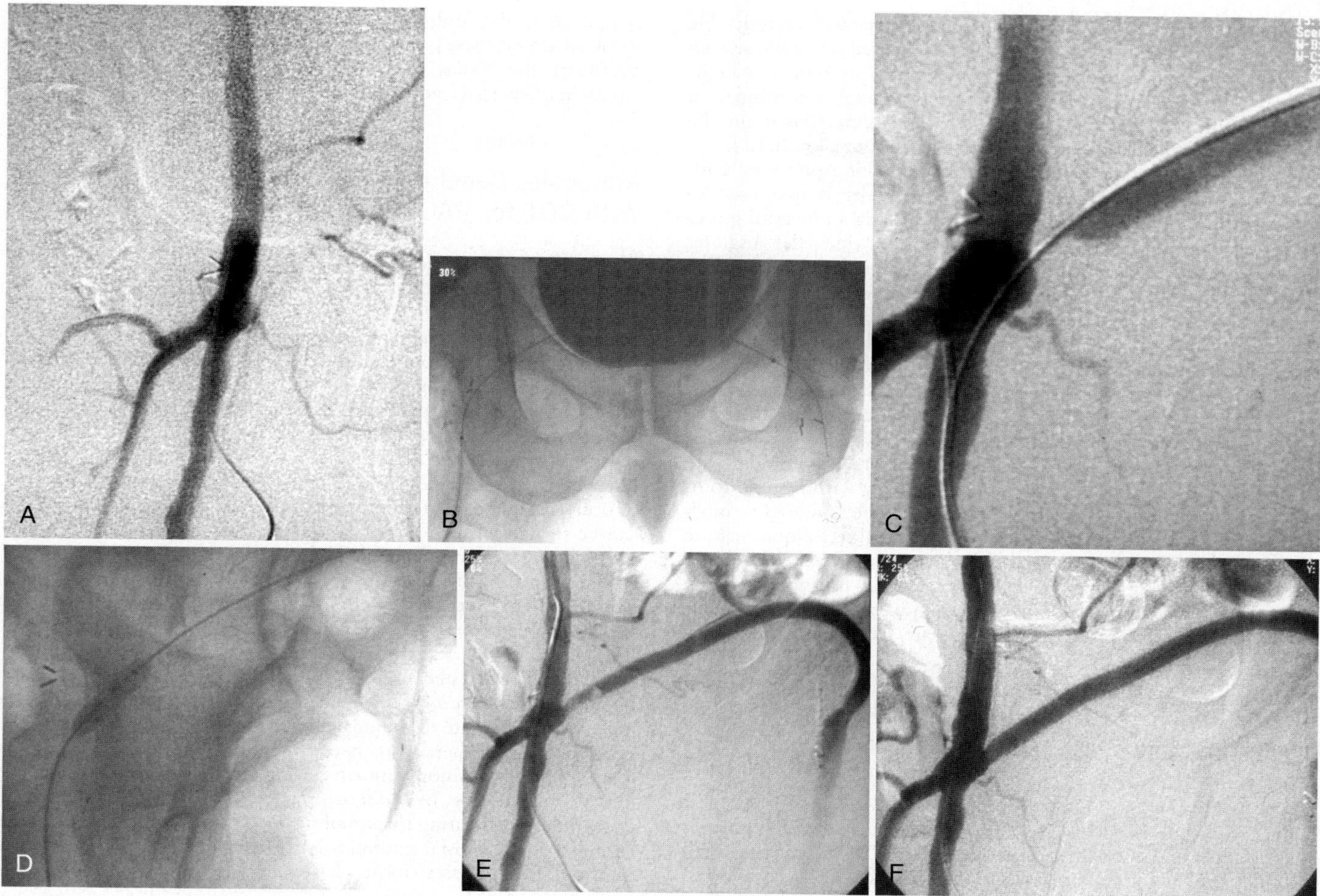

Figure 145-1 A 67-YEAR-OLD MAN WITH A CHRONIC LEFT ILIAC ARTERY OCCLUSION AND A RIGHT-TO-LEFT FEMORAL–FEMORAL ARTERIAL BYPASS GRAFT PRESENTS WITH LEFT FOOT PAIN AND PULSELESSNESS. **A,** Digital subtraction arteriography reveals patency of the right iliac artery, but only a "stump" of the bypass graft is seen, consistent with graft thrombosis. **B,** The lowermost aspect of the right common femoral artery was accessed, and a multi–side-hole infusion catheter was positioned across the occluded graft. The radiopaque markers show the infusion zone. An infusion of rt-PA was given at 0.5 mg/hr through this catheter. The patient received heparin (500 units/hr) through a peripheral intravenous catheter. **C,** After 16 hours of thrombolysis, a repeat arteriogram reveals successful thrombus removal with residual tight focal stenosis at the proximal graft anastomosis. **D,** The stenosis was subjected to angioplasty using a 6-mm balloon. **E,** Repeat arteriogram shows improvement in the stenosis, but small thrombi are evident within the graft. **F,** After use of the AngioJet Rheolytic Thrombectomy System to aspirate residual thrombus, the graft is widely patent. Subsequent physical examination revealed good pedal pulses and capillary refill, consistent with successful reperfusion of the limb.

ultrasound energy to ostensibly loosen fibrin strands and permit more rapid intrathrombus drug dispersion has been introduced.[6] Although limited evidence suggests that this catheter permits successful thrombolysis with reasonably good treatment times (16-21 hours), conclusive evidence of improved patient outcomes is lacking.

Variation on a Theme—Percutaneous Mechanical Thrombectomy

Hemorrhagic complications are the Achilles' heel of currently available thrombolytic agents. To reduce exposure to these drugs, specialized catheters, known as percutaneous mechanical thrombectomy (PMT) devices, have been developed. PMT is the use of a percutaneous catheter-based device that contributes to thrombus removal via thrombus fragmentation, maceration, and/or aspiration.[1] Although the devices were originally developed to supplant thrombolytic drugs, none of the available PMT devices enables safe, successful clot removal when used as a stand-alone treatment.[5] Consequently, fibrinolytic drugs are used in conjunction with PMT, except in situations in which absolute contraindications to the use of fibrinolytic drugs exist and no other treatment options are available.

Variations on a Theme—Pharmacomechanical Catheter-Directed Thrombolysis

Pharmacomechanical catheter-directed thrombolysis (PCDT) refers to thrombus dissolution via the combined use of CDT and PMT devices.[1] The rationale for utilizing both modalities is twofold. First, fibrinolytic drugs given via CDT soften the thrombus, rendering it more susceptible to mechanical fragmentation and removal with PMT, while also dissolving thrombus fragments that may otherwise embolize. Second, PMT devices macerate the thrombus, enhance dispersion of the fibrinolytic drug, and can accelerate pharmacologic thrombolysis. Although a broad range of PCDT techniques have been used, these techniques largely fall into two general categories: (1) "first-generation" PCDT techniques incorporate PMT devices to assist traditional CDT—either a PMT device is first used to de-bulk thrombus before starting the CDT infusion, or a PMT device is used after initial CDT to aspirate and/or macerate residual thrombus; (2) "single-session" PCDT techniques use PMT devices that can rapidly disperse the thrombolytic drug within the thrombus to enable the entire clot removal treatment to be completed in a single on-table procedure session, thereby obviating the need for an overnight thrombolytic infusion with the required ICU monitoring.

Single-session PCDT techniques have attracted considerable interest. Two currently available devices can be used for single-session PCDT. The AngioJet Rheolytic Thrombectomy System uses high-velocity saline jets to fracture the thrombus through a combination of rapid fluid streaming and hydrodynamic forces. Based on the Bernoulli principle of low pressure, these jets create a localized negative pressure zone at the catheter tip, enabling clot aspiration. With the "Powerpulse" PCDT technique, the Angiojet is first used to deliver a thrombolytic drug into the thrombus via a powerful pulse-spray injection.[7] After a 20- to 30-minute dwell time, the AngioJet is then used to aspirate and remove the softened thrombus. The "Isolated Thrombolysis" technique refers to the use of the Trellis Peripheral Infusion System to provide single-session PCDT[8] (Fig. 145-2). The Trellis device is composed of a multilumen catheter with two balloons, which when inflated, effectively isolate a thrombus-containing treatment zone from the remainder of the venous circulation. After the device is advanced across the venous thrombus, the occluding balloons are inflated and a thrombolytic drug is injected into the thrombus via side holes in the catheter. A sinusoidal wire within the catheter oscillates to disperse the drug within the thrombus, after which liquefied thrombotic debris can be aspirated through a port in the catheter. Both single-session PCDT techniques feature rapid intrathrombus drug dispersion that promotes faster thrombolysis, thereby reducing patient exposure to the fibrinolytic drug. Because the mechanical manipulation can induce thrombus fragmentation and embolization, these methods are best suited for venous applications.

Mechanical Interventions in Peripheral Arterial Occlusion

Acute peripheral arterial occlusion (PAO) is associated with high rates of morbidity and mortality. Up to 15% to 20% of patients with chronic peripheral arterial disease will develop acute exacerbation of symptoms (acute limb ischemia), usually due to thrombosis of the involved artery; these patients are at high risk for limb loss. Even with treatment, the 30-day mortality rate of acute arterial thrombosis is approximately 15%, and the amputation rate ranges from 10% to 30%.[9]

Rationale, Benefits, and Risks Associated With CDT for PAO

The traditional treatment for acute limb ischemia is open surgery. However, the emergent nature of these procedures and the characteristics of affected patients, who tend to have high rates of concomitant coronary and cerebrovascular disease, have contributed to significant rates of perioperative complications and death. By dissolving platelet-fibrin aggregates in the microcirculation and thrombi in collateral vessels, CDT allows rapid but gradual reperfusion of the distal limb, thereby minimizing the risk for reperfusion complications and compartment syndrome.[4] CDT enables both rapid restoration of arterial blood flow to the ischemic limb and unmasking of arterial stenotic or occlusive lesions that require treatment. Because many such lesions can be treated with endovascular techniques, such as balloon angioplasty or stent placement, CDT allows many patients to avoid the risks and inconveniences of open surgery. When surgery is required, a more limited procedure can often be performed on an elective basis in a well-prepared patient, with reduced rates of complications and death.

The major complication of CDT is bleeding.[10] In the setting of PAO, the incidence of CDT-related hemorrhagic stroke is approximately 1%. The rate of major hemorrhage, defined by hypotension, need for surgical therapy, or need for blood transfusion, is approximately 5%, with minor hemorrhage (e.g., local hematoma) occurring in 15% of patients. In modern practice, the use of subtherapeutic doses of heparin during thrombolysis may help to minimize bleeding complications.[11] Distal embolization of thrombus fragments occurs in about 5% of cases; most of these resolve with continued lytic

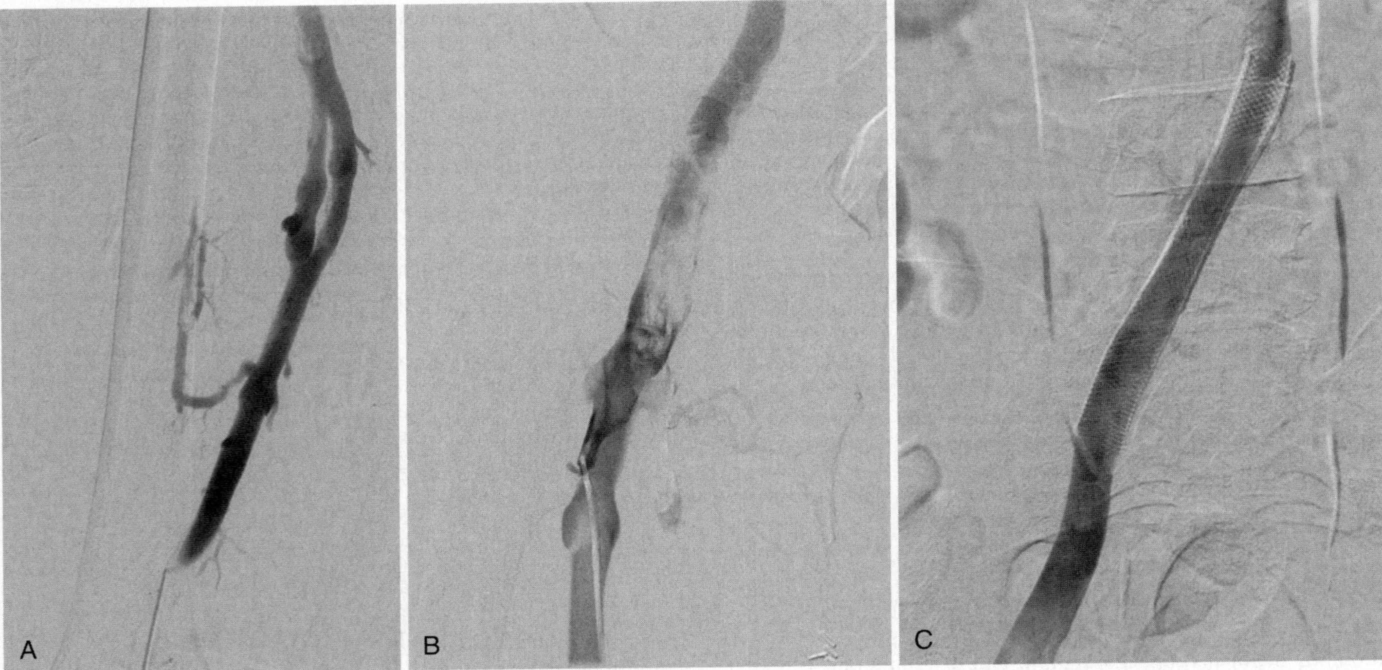

Figure 145-2 A 35-YEAR-OLD MAN PRESENTS WITH A 3-DAY HISTORY OF SEVERE LEFT LOWER EXTREMITY PAIN AND SWELLING. **A,** Digital subtraction venogram from a left popliteal vein approach shows patency of the lower part of the femoral vein with a short segment of duplication, a normal variant. **B,** The left common femoral and iliac veins have large globular filling defects, consistent with acute iliofemoral DVT. **C,** The Trellis device was used to deliver and disperse 10 mg of rt-PA into the thrombus. After balloon maceration of the thrombus and subsequent placement of two 12-mm stents to treat stenosis of the left common iliac vein, the left common femoral vein and iliac vein are seen to be widely patent. The pain and swelling resolved within a few days.

therapy. However, worsening ischemia can occur and generally requires percutaneous thrombus aspiration or operative intervention if the condition does not improve with thrombolysis within a few hours. Compartment syndrome, a complication that results from rapid reperfusion of the ischemic limb, occurs in 2% of patients. Death occurs in less than 1% of patients, usually in the setting of intracranial or abdominal hemorrhage, or reperfusion syndrome. Complications of CDT, which usually are minor, can also be related to intraarterial catheter insertion. Catheter-related trauma, resulting in mural dissection, puncture-site pseudoaneurysm, and/or major hematoma occurs in 1% to 2% of patients.

Randomized Trials—CDT Versus Surgery for Arterial Thrombosis

Three randomized controlled trials compared clinical outcomes in patients with acute PAO who were randomized to receive either CDT or surgical intervention. The Rochester Trial randomized 114 patients presenting with acute limb ischemia to catheter-directed urokinase infusion or surgery.[12] Although there was no difference in limb salvage rates at 1 year, mortality at 1 year was significantly lower with urokinase than with surgery. However, there was more bleeding with CDT than with surgery.

The STILE (surgery versus thrombolysis for ischemia of the lower extremity) trial included 393 patients who either underwent CDT with urokinase or rt-PA or surgery.[13] In patients with acute ischemia, CDT was associated with significantly fewer amputations, increased amputation-free survival at 1 year, and a shorter hospital stay. However, in those with chronic ischemia, surgery was associated with fewer amputations and improved amputation-free survival (Table 145-1). In a subgroup analysis, the patients with acute bypass graft occlusions had a significantly lower rate of amputations compared with those patients who underwent surgery. These data suggest that patients with acute bypass occlusion may derive the greatest benefit from CDT.

The TOPAS (thrombolysis or peripheral arterial surgery) trial randomized 544 patients with acute limb ischemia to CDT with recombinant urokinase or to surgery.[11] No difference in amputation-free survival was evident at 1 year. However, CDT was associated with more bleeding complications, including a 1.6% rate of intracranial hemorrhage.

In summary, the results of these three trials suggest that CDT reduces the need for amputation and surgical intervention in patients with acute limb ischemia, particularly those with acute bypass graft occlusion. However, the risk for bleeding is higher with CDT than with surgery. Although outcomes in patients with acute limb ischemia are better with CDT, surgery is recommended for those with chronic ischemia.

PMT, PCDT, and Ultrasound-Assisted CDT for Arterial Thrombosis

A paucity of data exists concerning the relative effectiveness and safety of newer thrombolytic techniques for PAO. The AngioJet device is FDA-approved for peripheral arterial thrombus removal and is routinely utilized as an adjunct to CDT.[14] Limited data are available related to the safety and efficacy of the AngioJet, Trellis, and Ekosonic devices for the treatment of PAO. Aside from bleeding, the major complications associated with PMT and PCDT are distal embolization and local vascular injury (i.e., dissection or rupture).

Summary: Indications and Contraindications for Thrombolytic Therapy in PAO

The use of arterial CDT should be individualized. Reasonable candidates include those with (1) acute (<14 days) thrombosis of a previously patent bypass graft or native artery; (2) acute embolus in a vessel not readily accessible to surgical embolectomy; (3) acute thrombosis of a popliteal artery aneurysm resulting in severe ischemia when all distal run-off vessels are also thrombosed; and (4) acute arterial thromboembolic occlusions in patients who are poor surgical candidates.[11,15,16] The clinical status of PAO patients should be categorized using the Rutherford classification scheme (Table 145-2). Patients

Table 145-1 Clinical Outcomes in Patients With Acute or Chronic Limb Ischemia Treated by Catheter-Directed Thrombolysis or Surgery in the STILE Trial

	Acute Ischemia (≤14 days), n = 112			*Chronic Ischemia (>14 days), n = 266*		
	Surgery (%)	**Lysis (%)**	**P-value**	**Surgery (%)**	**Lysis (%)**	**P-value**
Death	10.0	5.6	0.45	7.9	6.9	0.81
Amputation	30.0	11.1	0.02	3.0	12.1	0.01
Death and Amputation	37.5	15.3	0.01	9.9	17.8	0.08

Table 145-2 Rutherford Classification of Acute Limb Ischemia

		Clinical Examination		*Doppler Signal*	
Category	**Description / Prognosis**	**Sensory Loss**	**Muscle Weakness**	**Arterial**	**Venous**
I. Viable	Not immediately threatened	None	None	Audible	Audible
IIa. Marginally threatened	Salvageable if promptly treated	Minimal (toes) or none	None	(Often) Audible	Audible
IIb. Immediately threatened	Salvageable with immediate revascularization	More than toes, associated with rest pain	Mild, Moderate	(Usually) Audible	Audible
III. Irreversible	Major tissue loss or permanent nerve damage inevitable	Profound, anesthetic	Profound, paralysis (rigor)	Inaudible	Inaudible

From [no authors listed]: Results of a prospective randomized trial evaluating surgery versus thrombolysis for ischemia of the lower extremity. The STILE trial. *Ann Surg* 220:251, 1994, discussion 266–268.

with Rutherford category I, category IIa, and in specific cases, category IIb disease are potential candidates for CDT. In patients with irreversible limb ischemia, mild to moderate ischemia with claudication, early postoperative bypass graft thrombosis, or large vessel thrombi that are easily accessible by surgery, open surgery is preferred over CDT. Absolute and relative contraindications to CDT are outlined in Table 145-3.

Mechanical Interventions in Deep Vein Thrombosis

Venous thromboembolism (VTE) occurs in 350,000 to 600,000 persons per year in the United States alone, of which more than 250,000 cases represent a first-episode of deep vein thrombosis (DVT). The management of DVT has traditionally been anchored in a longstanding view of the disease as an "acute" condition involving an initial period of high risk for PE (which is estimated to kill over 100,000 persons in the United States each year), followed by a steadily diminishing risk over time that ultimately permits discontinuation of anticoagulant therapy in most patients. In recent years, there is better appreciation of the long-term impact of DVT in terms of the risk for recurrence, particularly in those with unprovoked VTE, and the high incidence of PTS in patients with extensive DVT.

For most patients, initial DVT therapy consists of administration of a parenteral anticoagulant drug (unfractionated heparin, low-molecular-weight heparin [LMWH], or fondaparinux) with subsequent transition to long-term oral vitamin K antagonist therapy for at least 3 months, with the duration of therapy dependent on the presence or absence of ongoing risk factors for recurrence.[17] The preferred initial approach for most patients with cancer-related DVT is LMWH monotherapy for at least 3 to 6 months. The therapeutic goals of anticoagulant therapy are to prevent symptomatic and fatal PE, thrombus progression, and late recurrent DVT. Currently available anticoagulants are effective in achieving these goals in most patients. In general, during the first year after discontinuation of anticoagulant therapy, recurrent VTE events occur in 3% to 5% of patients whose DVT episode was provoked by a major reversible risk factor and in 10% to 15% of patients with unprovoked/idiopathic DVT or cancer-related DVT.

Table 145-3 Contraindications to Thrombolytic Therapy

ABSOLUTE CONTRAINDICATIONS
Active bleeding
History of stroke within the previous 3 months
Neurosurgery (intracranial, spinal) within the previous 3 months
Intracranial trauma within the previous 3 months
RELATIVE CONTRAINDICATIONS
Recent (<7-10 days) major surgery, trauma, CPR, obstetrical delivery, or cataract surgery
Recent (<7-10 days) major invasive procedure or puncture of uncompressible vessel
Recent (<3 months) internal eye surgery or hemorrhagic retinopathy
Acute gastroduodenal ulcer or recent (<7-10 days) gastrointestinal bleeding
Intracranial neoplasm, arteriovenous malformation, aneurysm, or other lesion
Uncontrolled hypertension (systolic >180 mm Hg or diastolic >110 mm Hg)
Hepatic failure, particularly in cases with coagulopathy
Bacterial endocarditis or septic thrombophlebitis
Pregnancy
Severe anemia or thrombocytopenia

Rationale, Benefits, and Risks Associated With CDT for DVT

PTS develops in 20% to 50% of patients after a first episode of lower extremity DVT.[18] The symptoms and signs of PTS include chronic aching, swelling, fatigue, heaviness, edema, hyperpigmentation, and/or subcutaneous fibrosis in the affected limb. In severe cases, patients may experience short-distance venous claudication and venous leg ulcers—both of which limit ambulation and the ability to work and perform the activities of daily living. Consequently, PTS reduces health-related QOL. In fact, in a recent large prospective cohort study, the presence and severity of PTS were the leading determinants of QOL 2 years after an initial lower extremity DVT.[19] PTS also occurs with moderate frequency in patients with upper extremity DVT, particularly those who present with axillosubclavian involvement in the dominant arm. The management of PTS results in major economic costs to patients and society because of the direct medical costs of caring for its clinical sequelae (e.g., venous ulcers) and the indirect costs of work disability.

The pathogenesis of PTS is complex and incompletely understood. Inflammatory mediators, growth factors, extracellular matrix components, blood-borne elements, and endothelial cell factors contribute to the inflammatory response to DVT, which influences thrombus resolution, organization, and subsequent venous wall injury.[20] Even with anticoagulant therapy, incomplete clearance of thrombus is common, and residual thrombus often blocks venous blood flow. In addition, venous valves may be damaged, resulting in valvular reflux. The combination of valvular reflux and obstruction causes ambulatory venous hypertension, which leads to edema, tissue hypoxia and injury, progressive calf pump dysfunction, subcutaneous fibrosis, and skin ulceration. Therefore it is logical to postulate that rapid thrombus elimination and restoration of deep venous flow may prevent these untoward physiologic effects and preserve long-term venous function.

In support of this "open vein" hypothesis are studies that have observed a strong correlation between the amount of residual thrombus after a course of anticoagulant therapy and the subsequent incidence of recurrent venous thromboembolism. Moreover, data from a number of small randomized trials suggest that systemic thrombolysis and contemporary surgical venous thrombectomy are associated with improved long-term venous patency, preservation of venous valvular function, and reduced PTS compared with anticoagulation alone. However, these studies are small and have methodologic limitations. For patients with DVT, CDT is performed using the same procedures as those used for arterial thrombosis. Ultrasound-guided access to an extremity vein, usually the popliteal vein for the lower extremity, is obtained.[3] A venogram is performed, and the CDT or PCDT methods described earlier are used to remove the thrombus. After clot lysis, venography is performed to evaluate the underlying vein. Any residual stenosis is then treated with angioplasty or stenting. In general, the use of stents after DVT thrombolysis is optimally limited to the iliac vein, although it is sometimes necessary to extend contiguous stents into the common femoral vein. Patients with femoral vein stenosis, or isolated common femoral vein lesions that do not extend into the iliac vein, are best treated with angioplasty. Axillosubclavian venous thrombosis of known cause (e.g., previous central venous catheter) is amenable to balloon angioplasty if there is underlying stenosis. In patients with primary axillosubclavian venous thrombosis ("effort thrombosis"), stenosis of the subclavian vein is typically identified and is best treated with surgical thoracic outlet decompression rather than aggressive balloon angioplasty or stenting. With rare exceptions, stent placement in the subclavian vein is contraindicated because of the high frequency of stent fractures.

In a 473-patient multicenter registry, the use of CDT resulted in successful clot lysis in more than 80% of patients with acute proximal DVT.[21] However, major bleeding was observed in 11.4% of patients, mostly access site bleeding. Intracranial bleeding was observed in 0.4% of patients, and fatal PE occurred in 0.2% of patients. Adjunctive CDT or PCDT plus anticoagulant therapy has been compared with anticoagulant therapy alone. In a case-control study that included 68 patients with acute iliofemoral DVT who underwent technically successful CDT, Comerota and colleagues reported fewer PTS symptoms and improved QOL at 16-month follow-up compared with a similar group of 30 patients who received anticoagulant therapy alone.[22] In a nonrandomized study, AbuRahma and colleagues[23] reported higher rates of symptom resolution at 5 years in iliofemoral DVT patients treated with CDT than in controls (78% versus 30%, $p = 0.0015$). A small randomized trial reported a higher rate of normal venous function with CDT at 6 months than with anticoagulation alone (72% versus 12%, $p < 0.001$) and less valvular reflux (11% versus 41%, $p = 0.04$).[24] Finally, a preliminary report from an ongoing Norwegian multicenter randomized trial[25] reported a lower rate of late venous obstruction with CDT compared with anticoagulation alone (64% versus 36%, $p < 0.001$). These studies highlight the potential for CDT to restore venous patency in patients with extensive DVT, as well as the risks and inconveniences of such treatment. However, these studies have limitations, including surrogate outcome measures, inclusion of only a single-center, small sample size, and/or nonrandomized design. Advances in CDT techniques, such as routine ultrasound-guided venipuncture and the use of PCDT to accelerate treatment and limit fibrinolytic drug exposure, have the potential to reduce bleeding. As a result, more recent studies with low-dose rt-PA report major bleeding rates of 3% to 4%.[25] Therefore contemporary methods of PCDT have been integrated into pivotal multicenter randomized trials, including the ongoing NIH-sponsored ATTRACT (acute venous thrombosis: thrombus removal with adjunctive catheter-directed thrombolysis) trial.

Acute Iliofemoral DVT as a High-Risk Condition

It is important for physicians to recognize the range of clinical presentations of proximal DVT. The extent of thrombosis is an important predictor of clinical course and long-term outcome with anticoagulant therapy. In particular, with femoral vein thrombosis, the primary collateral route by which blood leaves the limb (and by which the venous obstruction is decompressed) is the deep (profunda) femoral vein, which empties into the common femoral vein in the groin. Consequently, thrombosis above the entry point of the deep femoral vein (i.e., in or above the common femoral vein) causes more severe outflow obstruction, which often results in more leg swelling and pain and a higher incidence of late clinical sequelae.

Iliofemoral DVT is defined as DVT involving the iliac vein and/or common femoral vein, with or without involvement of other lower extremity veins.[1] Although physicians typically classify DVT as either distal or proximal because the risk for PE is higher with proximal DVT, patients with iliofemoral DVT have poorer clinical outcomes than patients with less extensive proximal DVT. In a prospective study of 1149 DVT patients, involvement of the common femoral vein and/or iliac vein portended a 2.4-fold increased risk for recurrent VTE during 3 months follow-up.[26] Likewise, in a large prospective cohort study, patients with iliofemoral DVT had 2 to 3 times more severe PTS than those with less extensive DVT.[18] Hence it is important to view iliofemoral DVT as a high-risk condition and to ensure the utilization of evidence-based PTS prevention measures, including therapeutic anticoagulation of appropriate intensity and duration and the use of elastic compression stockings. These patients are readily identified because they usually present with swelling of the entire limb and most have compression ultrasound evidence of thrombus in the common femoral vein.

Patients with acute (symptom duration ≤4 days) iliofemoral DVT who are not at increased risk for bleeding are the best candidates for CDT and PCDT.[17] In a large registry of DVT patients receiving CDT, patients with acute iliofemoral DVT were the most likely group to experience successful removal of thrombus, and many of the small studies supporting use of thrombus removal for DVT were performed in patients with iliofemoral DVT.[21-23] There are no well-designed prospective studies of CDT for treatment of upper extremity DVT; generally, such treatment is restricted to symptomatic patients with axillosubclavian thrombosis of recent onset.

Summary: Indications and Contraindications for CDT in DVT

The lack of data to establish the utility and proper indications for CDT in DVT patients does not absolve physicians of their responsibility to ensure that the long-term risks of PTS are carefully considered when crafting an individualized treatment strategy for DVT patients. The strategy should incorporate a high degree of confidence in anticoagulation drugs and compression therapy, a familiarity with the available (albeit imperfect) data that suggest that CDT is reasonable for selected DVT patients, and an individualized assessment of the clinical DVT severity, extent of thrombosis, comorbidities, and personal preferences of the patient.

Patients who do not meet a clinical threshold justifying the use of CDT include those with asymptomatic DVT or DVT isolated to the calf (because the risk for PTS is relatively low in these groups) and patients with chronic femoropopliteal DVT (because studies have shown that organized thrombus is not susceptible to thrombolytic drugs).[21]

The most important safety factor to consider in a patient being evaluated for DVT thrombolysis is the risk for major bleeding. Factors associated with an increased risk for bleeding include ongoing or recent bleeding; recent major surgery, trauma, pregnancy, obstetrical delivery, or cardiopulmonary resuscitation; or the presence of lesions in critical areas such as the central nervous system that may bleed. Because CDT involves the administration of iodinated contrast material for venography, renal function is also an important consideration, as are life expectancy, baseline ambulatory capacity, and comorbidities.[5,27] Patients with limited long-term mobility or those with a life expectancy of less than 6 months are unlikely to benefit from aggressive therapy to prevent PTS. Comorbidities that increase procedure risks, such as respiratory compromise that limits the use of sedation, may also render CDT less attractive.

Urgent endovascular thrombolysis is indicated to prevent life-, limb-, or organ-threatening complications of acute DVT in situations such as phlegmasia cerulea dolens or extensive inferior vena cava (IVC) thrombosis (especially with suprarenal extension, which may lead to fatal PE or acute renal failure). The use of endovascular thrombolysis in these situations is justifiable when other treatment options are lacking. In contrast, significant uncertainty exists regarding the appropriate indications for nonurgent CDT for the treatment of DVT. In 2008, guidelines from the American College of Chest Physicians and the Society of Interventional Radiology suggested that CDT/PCDT may be appropriate as an adjunct to anticoagulant therapy for selected patients with major symptomatic axillosubclavian DVT or extensive proximal lower extremity DVT, such as those with acute iliofemoral DVT, who have a low risk for bleeding and a long life expectancy.[5,17] The 2011 guidelines from the American Heart Association concurred and suggest that CDT also may be reasonable for patients with progression of DVT symptoms or rapid thrombus extension despite initial anticoagulation.[27]

Treatment of Established Postthrombotic Syndrome

Patients with established PTS suffer major symptoms that significantly impair their ability to conduct their daily activities and to enjoy a normal QOL. Unfortunately, once PTS has developed, no treatments have consistently been shown to be effective. Despite limited evidence of benefit, elastic compression stockings are often used because of their low risk and ready availability. Low-dose diuretics may be useful to reduce edema. Patients with venous ulcers can be treated with pentoxifylline, multilayer compression bandaging,

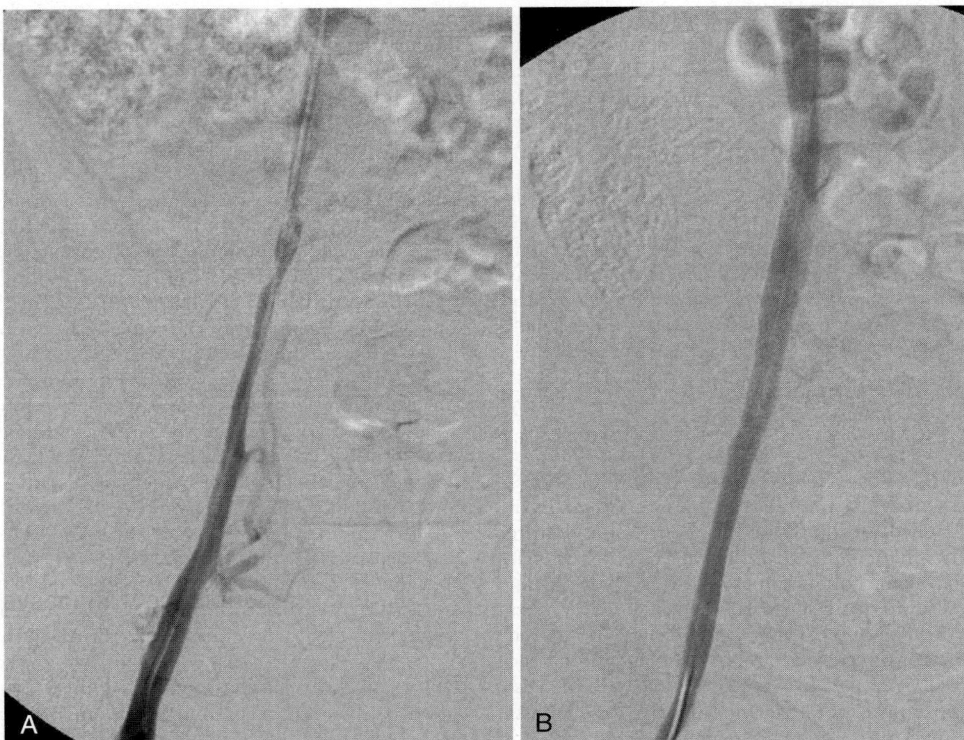

Figure 145-3 A 46-YEAR-OLD WOMAN WITH A PAST HISTORY OF RIGHT ILIOFEMORAL DVT 2 YEARS AGO NOW PRESENTS TO THE CLINIC COMPLAINING OF DAILY ACHING AND SWELLING IN THE RIGHT LOWER EXTREMITY THAT PRECLUDE AMBULATION FOR EVEN ONE BLOCK AND RENDER HER UNABLE TO WORK. These symptoms have been present since her previous DVT. **A,** A transjugular pelvic venogram demonstrates chronic narrowing of the right iliac vein with collateral formation. **B,** After placement of four 12-mm stents, the right iliac vein is widely patent. The pain and swelling improved, and the patient was subsequently able to return to work.

and dedicated wound care with topical antibiotics, exfoliants, and growth factors.[17] Despite these measures, PTS symptoms and venous ulcers often resist improvement and cause long-term hardships.

Because the severity of PTS symptoms often parallels the degree of ambulatory venous hypertension, endovascular interventions that eliminate venous obstruction and valvular reflux have been used for treatment of patients with severe PTS. Studies suggest that stent recanalization of chronically occluded iliac veins in patients with advanced PTS can be achieved in over 80% of patients and can reduce PTS symptoms, improve QOL, and enhance healing of venous ulcers[28] (Fig. 145-3). Accordingly, physicians who see patients with severe PTS, with or without ulcers, should consider consulting a venous endovascular specialist.

Inferior Vena Cava Filters

IVC filters are indicated for patients with proximal DVT or PE who have contraindications to or complications of anticoagulation, who develop symptomatic PE despite therapeutic-level anticoagulation, and/or who have severe cardiorespiratory compromise. In other circumstances, caution should be used when placing IVC filters because of ongoing uncertainty about their long-term risk-benefit ratio.[17] In the only available recent clinical trial, which was done in patients concomitantly receiving anticoagulant therapy and which was underpowered to detect an effect on fatal PE, filters appeared to provide additional protection against symptomatic PE but did not alter mortality.[29] Symptomatic recurrent DVT was increased in the filter group, but the overall rates of PTS and symptomatic recurrent VTE did not differ significantly. Because fatal PE rarely occurs in DVT patients who are properly anticoagulated, IVC filters should not be routinely placed in DVT patients. Patients who experience clinical failure of a first-line anticoagulant (e.g., warfarin therapy) can usually be switched to an effective alternative regimen, such as LMWH or a direct thrombin inhibitor.[30]

Retrievable IVC filters have the intended advantages of allowing PE prophylaxis during the period of highest risk, with subsequent removal thereafter. However, it should be noted that the stability and mechanical integrity of retrievable devices do not yet match those of older filters designed for permanent implantation and that many cases of retrievable filter migration have been reported.[27] Therefore if there is a strong likelihood that permanent IVC filtration will be needed, it is best to select a permanent nonretrievable IVC filter device. In DVT patients with a time-limited indication for an IVC filter, placement of a retrievable IVC filter is reasonable. However, it is important that the need for the IVC filter be reassessed every few weeks after placement so that the filter can be removed when it is no longer needed. Although many filters are placed with the intent to be retrieved, less than 50% are removed. Consequently, physicians must monitor patients with these devices to ensure that they are removed when appropriate.

At the health care system level, better studies of the use of IVC filters in different clinical scenarios should be considered an urgent priority because these devices are being used more frequently. The balance between PE prophylaxis and the long-term risks of IVC filter placement is complex and deserves more rigorous evaluation (Fig. 145-4).

FUTURE DIRECTIONS

Imaging-guided endovascular interventions have evolved significantly over the last 25 years and now offer the potential for improved patient outcomes in several disease states. For PAO, randomized trials have

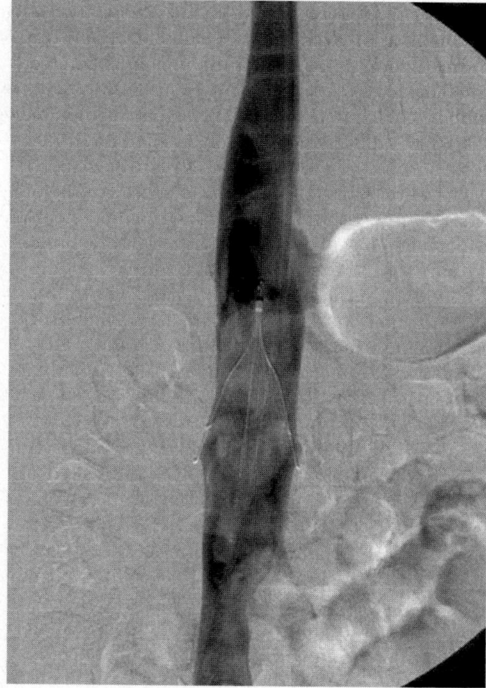

Figure 145-4 ILLUSTRATING THE COMPLEXITIES OF DETERMINING WHETHER IVC FILTERS ARE OF BENEFIT, A DIGITAL SUBTRACTION VENOGRAM SHOWS A LARGE GLOBULAR FILLING DEFECT WITHIN AN IVC FILTER THAT WAS PLACED 3 DAYS AGO. Filter proponents might argue that this represents a large, potentially fatal PE trapped within the filter, whereas filter opponents might propose that this is a case of filter-induced IVC thrombosis, a major complication. Who would be right?

defined the role for CDT for the treatment of acute limb ischemia. For DVT, a robust body of preliminary research supports the potential for catheter-based thromboreductive therapies to improve long-term patient outcomes, but randomized trials have not yet been completed to establish this benefit. Therefore an individualized approach is recommended to ensure that harms are minimized and appropriate patients are selected for intervention. Multidisciplinary collaboration between internists and endovascular physicians is needed to ensure optimal patient care.

REFERENCES

1. Vedantham S, Grassi CJ, Ferral H, et al: Reporting standards for endovascular treatment of lower extremity deep vein thrombosis. *J Vasc Interv Radiol* 17:437, 2006.
2. McNamara TO, Fischer JR: Thrombolysis of peripheral arterial and graft occlusions: Improved results using high-dose urokinase. *AJR Am J Roentgenol* 144:769, 1985.
3. Semba CP, Dake MD: Iliofemoral deep venous thrombosis: Aggressive therapy with catheter-directed thrombolysis. *Radiology* 191:487, 1994.
4. Rajan DK, Patel NH, Valji K, et al: Quality improvement guidelines for percutaneous management of acute limb ischemia. *J Vasc Interv Radiol* 20:S208, 2009.
5. Vedantham S, Thorpe PE, Cardella JF, et al: Quality improvement guidelines for the treatment of lower extremity deep vein thrombosis with use of endovascular thrombus removal. *J Vasc Interv Radiol* 17:435, 2006.
6. Wissgott C, Richter A, Kamusella P, et al: Treatment of critical limb ischemia using ultrasound-enhanced thrombolysis (PARES Trial): Final results. *J Endovasc Ther* 14:438, 2007.
7. Cynamon J, Stein EG, Dym J, et al: A new method for aggressive management of deep vein thrombosis: Retrospective study of the power pulse technique. *J Vasc Interv Radiol* 17:1043, 2006.
8. O'Sullivan GJ, Lohan DG, Gough N, et al: Pharmacomechanical thrombectomy of acute deep vein thrombosis with the Trellis-8 isolated thrombolysis catheter. *J Vasc Interv Radiol* 18:715, 2007.
9. Dormandy J, Heeck L, Vig S: Acute limb ischemia. *Semin Vasc Surg* 12:148, 1999.
10. Working Party on Thrombolysis in the Management of Limb Ischemia. Thrombolysis in the management of lower limb peripheral arterial occlusion—a consensus document. *J Vasc Interv Radiol* 14:S337, 2003.
11. Ouriel K, Veith FJ, Sasahara AA: A comparison of recombinant urokinase with vascular surgery as initial treatment for acute arterial occlusion of the legs. Thrombolysis or Peripheral Arterial Surgery (TOPAS) Investigators. *N Engl J Med* 338:1105, 1998.
12. Ouriel K, Shortell CK, DeWeese JA, et al: A comparison of thrombolytic therapy with operative revascularization in the initial treatment of acute peripheral arterial ischemia. *J Vasc Surg* 19:1021, 1994.
13. Results of a prospective randomized trial evaluating surgery versus thrombolysis for ischemia of the lower extremity. The STILE trial. *Ann Surg* 220:251, discussion 266–268, 1994.
14. Silva JA, Ramee SR, Collins TJ, et al: Rheolytic thrombectomy in the treatment of acute limb-threatening ischemia: Immediate results and six-month follow-up of the multicenter AngioJet registry. Possis Peripheral AngioJet Study AngioJet Investigators. *Cathet Cardiovasc Diagn* 45:386, 1998.
15. Hirsch AT, Haskal ZJ, Hertzer NR, et al: ACC/AHA guidelines for the management of patients with peripheral arterial disease (lower extremity, renal, mesenteric, and abdominal aortic): A collaborative report from the American Associations for Vascular Surgery/Society for Vascular Surgery, Society for Cardiovascular Angiography and Interventions, Society for Vascular Medicine and Biology, Society of Interventional Radiology, and the ACC/AHA Task Force on Practice Guidelines—summary of recommendations. *J Vasc Interv Radiol* 17:1383; quiz 98, 2006.
16. Costantini V, Lenti M: Treatment of acute occlusion of peripheral arteries. *Thromb Res* 106:V285, 2002.
17. Kearon C, Kahn SR, Agnelli G, et al: Antithrombotic therapy for venous thromboembolic disease: American College of Chest Physicians evidence-based clinical practice guidelines (8th edition). *Chest* 133:454S, 2008.
18. Kahn SR, Shrier I, Julian JA, et al: Determinants and time course of the postthrombotic syndrome after acute deep venous thrombosis. *Ann Intern Med* 149:698, 2008.
19. Kahn SR, Shbaklo H, Lamping DL, et al: Determinants of health-related quality of life during the 2 years following deep vein thrombosis. *J Thromb Haemost* 6:1105, 2008.
20. Roumen-Klappe EM, Janssen MC, Van Rossum J, et al: Inflammation in deep vein thrombosis and the development of post-thrombotic syndrome: A prospective study. *J Thromb Haemost* 7:582, 2009.
21. Mewissen MW, Seabrook GR, Meissner MH, et al: Catheter-directed thrombolysis for lower extremity deep venous thrombosis: Report of a national multicenter registry. *Radiology* 211:39, 1999.
22. Comerota AJ, Throm RC, Mathias SD, et al: Catheter-directed thrombolysis for iliofemoral deep venous thrombosis improves health-related quality of life. *J Vasc Surg* 32:130, 2000.
23. AbuRahma AF, Perkins SE, Wulu JT, et al: Iliofemoral deep vein thrombosis: Conventional therapy versus lysis and percutaneous transluminal angioplasty and stenting. *Ann Surg* 233:752, 2001.
24. Elsharawy M, Elzayat E: Early results of thrombolysis vs anticoagulation in iliofemoral venous thrombosis. A randomised clinical trial. *Eur J Vasc Endovasc Surg* 24:209, 2002.
25. Enden T, Sandvik L, Kløw NE, et al: Catheter-directed venous thrombolysis in acute iliofemoral vein thrombosis—the CaVenT study: Rationale and design of a multicenter, randomized, controlled, clinical trial (NCT00251771). *Am Heart J* 154:808, 2007.
26. Douketis JD, Crowther MA, Foster GA, et al: Does the location of thrombosis determine the risk of disease recurrence in patients with proximal deep vein thrombosis? *Am J Med* 110:515, 2001.

27. Jaff MR, McMurtry MS, Archer SL, et al: Management of massive and submassive pulmonary embolism, iliofemoral deep vein thrombosis, and chronic thromboembolic pulmonary hypertension: A scientific statement from the American Heart Association. *Circulation* 123:1788, 2011.
28. Raju S, Neglen P: Percutaneous recanalization of total occlusions of the iliac vein. *J Vasc Surg* 50:360, 2009.
29. The PREPIC Study Group: Eight-year follow-up of patients with permanent vena cava filters in the prevention of pulmonary embolism. *Circulation* 112:416, 2005.
30. Schulman S, Kearon C, Kakkar AK, et al: Dabigatran versus warfarin in the treatment of acute venous thromboembolism. *N Engl J Med* 361:2342, 2009.

CHAPTER 146

ATHEROTHROMBOSIS

Roy L. Silverstein

Morbidity and mortality from atherosclerosis, the pathologic process underlying acute myocardial infarction, sudden death, stroke, and limb loss, represent an enormous burden on society and health care systems. Even though death rates from heart attack and stroke have dropped precipitously over the past 60 years (69% and 76%, respectively, from 1950 to 2006), cardiovascular diseases are still the number one cause of death in the United States, accounting for more than 25% of all deaths—approximately 2300 per day.[1] Unfortunately, as the developing world adopts a more "Western" lifestyle (i.e., one marked by a high-fat, calorie-rich diet and limited physical activity), these statistics are becoming the norm worldwide. The annual financial burden of cardiovascular disease in the United States in 2010 was estimated by the American Heart Association (AHA) to be $445 billion, including $172 billion due to lost productivity.[2] These costs are predicted to triple over the ensuing 20 years; analyses of population survey data predict an increase in cardiovascular disease prevalence from 36.9% to 40.5%. It is interesting to note that as treatment of the acute complications of atherosclerosis improves, the burden of chronic complications, particularly heart failure, is expected to increase by as much as 25% over the next 20 years.[3]

Much of our knowledge of the epidemiology of cardiovascular disease comes from large-scale, long-term population studies, the most important being the Framingham Heart Study sponsored by the National Heart, Lung, and Blood Institute (NHLBI).[4] This ongoing prospective study began in 1948 with a cohort of ≈5200 men and women between the ages of 30 and 62 in Framingham, Massachusetts, and has since added two subsequent generations and several other cohorts. Through this study and others it elsewhere in the United States and in Europe, major risk factors for cardiovascular disease have been identified, including cigarette smoking, low-density lipoprotein (LDL) cholesterol, systolic blood pressure, male sex, menopause, physical inactivity, body mass index, and high-sensitivity C-reactive protein (hsCRP). Additionally, high-density lipoprotein (HDL) was identified as a protective factor. Based on these data, risk scores have been developed to guide physicians and patients, and public health campaigns developed targeting hypertension, elevated cholesterol, and lifestyle modifications. These have clearly contributed to the reductions in cardiovascular mortality just noted.

PATHOBIOLOGY

Atherosclerosis is caused by the progressive formation of arterial plaques, which are characterized by accumulation of lipids, in particular cholesterol and its derivatives, and inflammatory cells in the tunica intima of large- and medium-sized arteries (Fig. 146-1). Although occlusion of blood flow by plaque encroachment into the lumen can occur and cause ischemia of downstream tissues, most of the severe clinical events associated with atherosclerosis derive from acute or subacute thrombosis at a site of an unstable, inflamed, or ruptured plaque or at a site of recent mechanical or pharmacologic intervention. The past 40 years have seen a remarkable increase in our understanding of the basic pathophysiologic mechanisms that govern plaque formation, plaque progression and acute arterial thrombosis.[5,6] Translation of this knowledge into diagnostic, preventive, and therapeutic strategies has been impressive, but there is still much unmet need for improvement. This chapter will summarize the current prevailing models of atherogenesis and atherothrombosis, highlighting some key knowledge gaps and potential new therapeutic targets.

LIPOPROTEIN HOMEOSTASIS AND THE "CHOLESTEROL HYPOTHESIS"

Human epidemiologic and clinical trial data and animal model studies show unequivocally that elevated levels of plasma lipids, especially LDL cholesterol, are essential for plaque development. Atherosclerotic lesions can be induced in "atheroresistant" animals, including mice and rabbits, by manipulating their diets and/or genomes to cause hypercholesterolemia.[7] In humans, raising LDL cholesterol levels increases the risk for atherosclerosis proportionally and lowering levels either by lifestyle change or pharmacologic intervention reduces risk proportionally. In general, lowering LDL cholesterol levels by 10% reduces risk for cardiovascular events by 25% and cardiovascular death by 10%.

Normally, cholesterol levels are tightly controlled in response to diet and cellular needs by a complex transcriptional pathway mediated by sterol response element–binding protein 2 (SREBP2).[8] At low levels of cellular cholesterol, SREBP2 is activated and binds to specific DNA sequences in target genes known as *sterol response elements* to activate their transcription. Two key target genes are HMGCR and LDLR, which encode 3-hydroxy-3-methylglutaryl coenzyme A (HMGCoA) reductase (the rate-limiting enzyme in cholesterol biosynthesis) and the LDL receptor, respectively, thereby increasing both cholesterol production and cellular LDL uptake. At high levels of cellular cholesterol, SREBP2 is inactive, cholesterol biosynthesis is turned off, and LDL receptor expression is downregulated. As shown in Fig. 146-2, statin drugs decrease cellular cholesterol biosynthesis by inhibiting HMGCoA reductase and thereby induce an increase in LDL receptor expression, driving down plasma LDL cholesterol levels.

Multiple randomized clinical trials have demonstrated efficacy of statin class drugs in reducing risk for cardiovascular events in high-risk individuals. Initial studies focused on secondary prevention in patients with a history of a previous atherosclerotic event, but more recent trials have demonstrated efficacy as part of a primary prevention strategy in subjects with elevated LDL cholesterol or in subjects with normal LDL cholesterol in the setting of other risk factors, such as diabetes, hypertension, or elevated plasma levels of hsCRP.[9] The latter studies, along with those showing benefit of lowering LDL cholesterol to levels well below "normal" (e.g. to 70 mg/dL in high-risk individuals),[10] are consistent with the concept that "normal" levels of LDL cholesterol, as defined by population means in the Western world, are not reflective of a true normal biology.

Recent genetic studies of rare individuals with extremely low LDL cholesterol levels identified a null mutation in a gene known as *PCSK9* that encodes an enzyme involved in downregulating LDL receptor expression.[11] These individuals seem to be otherwise normal, despite nearly absent LDL, suggesting that targeting this enzyme could represent a new strategy for cholesterol-lowering therapeutics. Phase I and II trials of PCSK9 inhibitors are, in fact, already underway.

Cells in the periphery have the capacity to eliminate excess cholesterol through a process known as *reverse cholesterol transport (RCT)*.[12] In this pathway, summarized in Fig. 146-3, postlysosomal trafficking of intracellular cholesterol to the plasma membrane, mediated in part by actions of acyl-CoA cholesterol acyltransferase (ACAT) and Neimann-Pick type C (NPC) protein, allows the cell surface adenosine triphosphate (ATP)–binding cassette (ABC) proteins ABCA1 and ABCG1 to transport excess cholesterol to apolipoprotein A (apoA) containing lipoproteins, either nascent HDL (in the case of ABCA1) or mature HDL (in the case of ABCG1). HDL then "delivers" the cholesterol back to the liver, where it is selectively taken up by hepatocytes through a protein known as *scavenger receptor B1 (SRB1)* and ultimately secreted into bile and excreted in feces. The role of HDL in RCT probably accounts for its association with lowered risk for cardiovascular disease, but HDL particles also contain antiinflammatory and antioxidant proteins that may also contribute to lowering atherosclerosis risk.

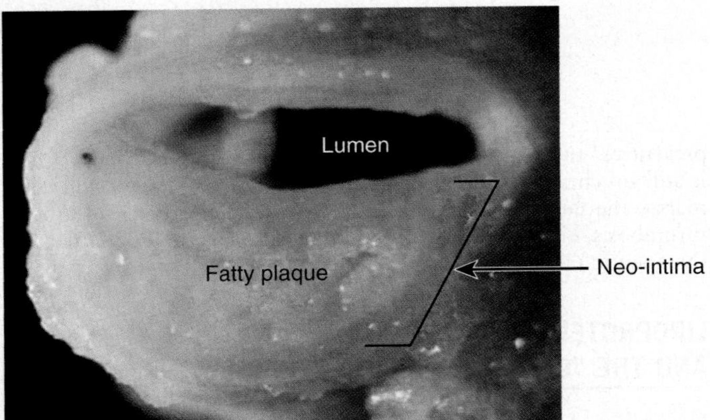

Figure 146-1 ATHEROMATOUS PLAQUE. Cross-sectional view of a human artery taken from an autopsy, showing accumulation of yellow-colored fatty materials in neointima.

Pharmacologic and lifestyle approaches to enhance RCT have received significant attention as potential antiatherosclerosis strategies. HDL levels can be raised by physical exercise, as well as by moderate alcohol ingestion. The only FDA-approved pharmacologic agent capable of raising HDL is niacin, but high doses are required and these are not easily tolerated because of side effects, especially facial flushing. A combination of high-dose niacin with a prostaglandin D_2 receptor antagonist to block facial flushing is currently under study.

The circulating plasma enzyme, cholesterol ester transfer protein (CETP), functions to transfer cholesterol esters from HDL to VLDL (very low-density lipoprotein) and LDL (Fig. 146-3). Inhibiting this enzyme raises HDL levels (and lowers LDL) significantly in humans, but a large phase III randomized clinical trial with the initially developed pharmacologic CETP inhibitor torcetrapib was halted in 2006

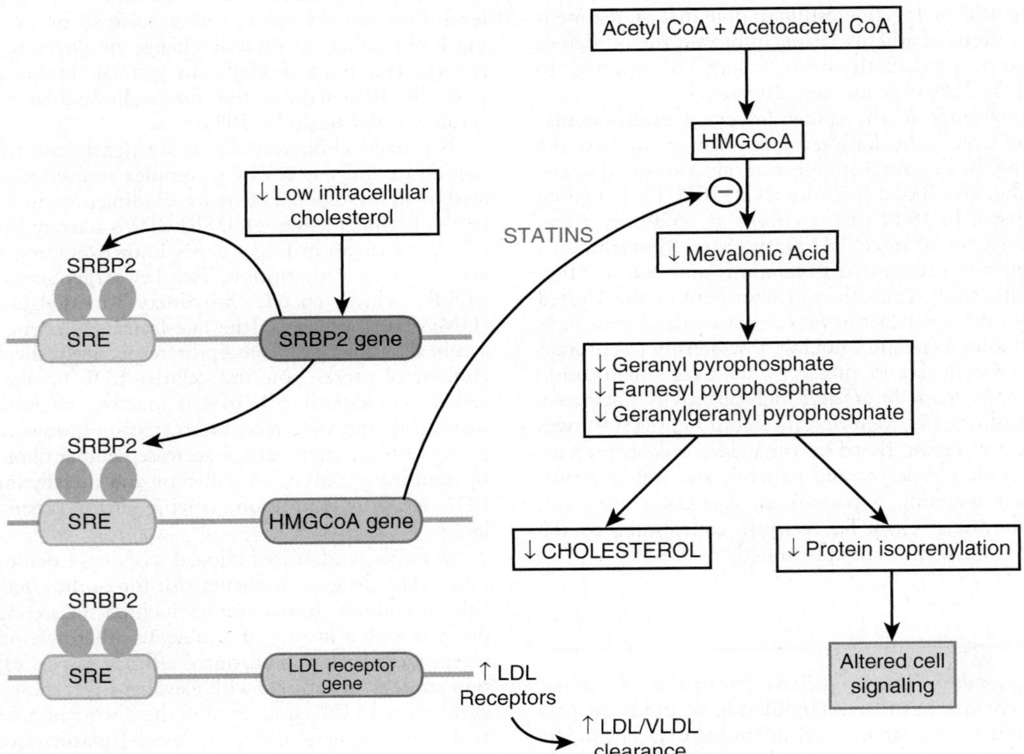

Figure 146-2 STATINS TARGET CHOLESTEROL AND ISOPRENYLATION PATHWAYS. The statin class of drugs inhibits the intracellular enzyme 3-hydroxy-3-methylglutaryl coenzyme A (HMGCoA) reductase. This enzyme converts HMGCoA to mevalonic acid, which is a precursor in the biosynthesis of the isoprenoids geranyl and farnesyl pyrophosphates, which in turn are precursors of cholesterol, as well as intermediates in isoprenyl modification of proteins, including small-molecular-weight G proteins. Since HMGCoA reductase is the rate-limiting step in these pathways, its inhibition leads to decreases in cholesterol biosynthesis, hepatic VLDL production, and protein isoprenylation *(arrows)*. Low levels of intracellular cholesterol activate the SRBP2 gene *(green)*, which encodes a transcription factor that binds to sterol response elements (SRE) in multiple genes, including HMGCoAR and LDL receptor. The ensuing increased expression of LDL receptor results in increased clearance of apoB-containing lipoproteins (LDL and VLDL) from plasma, further lowering plasma cholesterol levels.

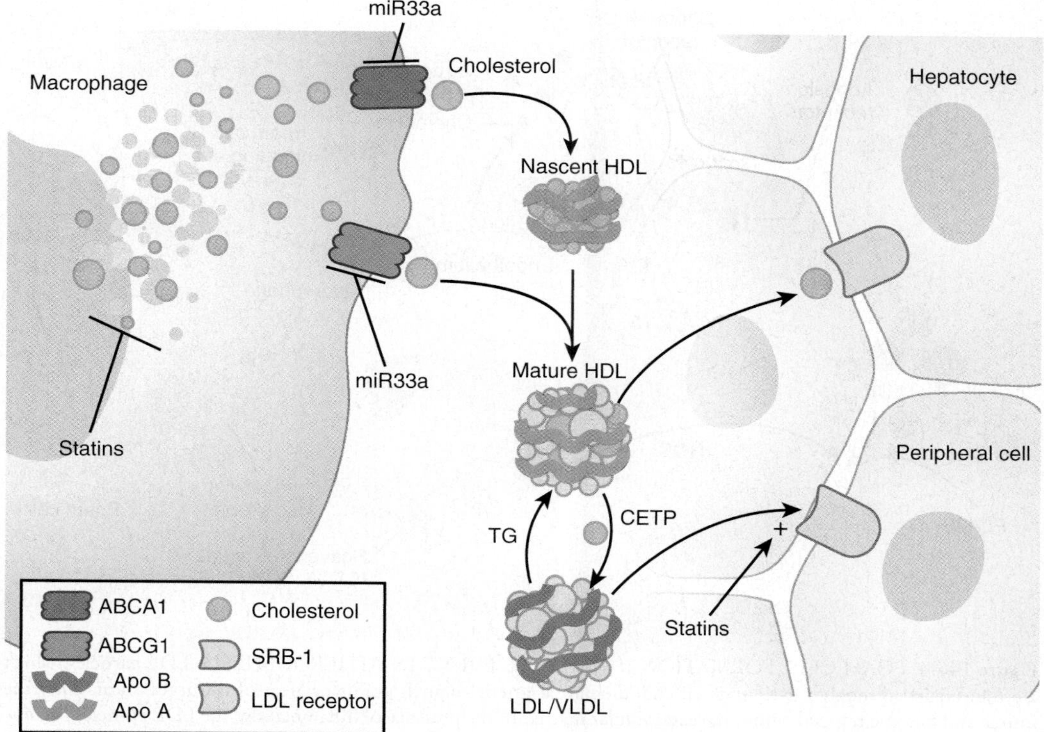

Figure 146-3 REVERSE CHOLESTEROL TRANSPORT. Cells in the periphery, including macrophage foam cells, have the capacity to unload intracellular cholesterol via two members of the ATP-binding cassette (ABC) transporter family: ABCA1 and G1. The former transfers cholesterol to apoA and/or nascent HDL particles, whereas the latter transfers cholesterol to mature HDL. HDL interacts with scavenger receptor B1 (SRB1) on liver cells, and through a process known as *selective cholesterol uptake,* the cholesterol within the HDL is internalized, where it can ultimately be reused or excreted via bile. The cholesterol in HDL can exchange with triglycerides (TG) in LDL and VLDL particles through the action of an enzyme, cholesterol ester transfer protein (CETP). Inhibitors of CETP thus raise plasma HDL levels and lower LDL levels. LDL and VLDL are normally cleared by cells in the periphery via internalization by LDL receptor. Statin drugs, by inhibiting HMGCoA reductase, lower intracellular cholesterol levels and raise LDL levels, thus lowering plasma LDL. A microRNA miR33a encoded within the SREBP gene blocks expression of ABCA1 and ABCG1.

because of excessive all-cause mortality in the treatment group receiving a combination of atorvastatin and the study drug.[13] This result may have been due to an off-target effect of the drug, but nevertheless, development of this strategy has been significantly slowed. Several other CETP inhibitors are, however, under development and in phase II studies showed efficacy in raising HDL and lowering LDL. Of interest, a microRNA, miR-33a, encoded by a DNA sequence embedded in the SREBP2 gene was found to repress several key genes involved in cholesterol homeostasis (see Fig. 146-3), including ABCA1 and ABCG1, as well as genes involved in fatty acid oxidation and glucose metabolism.[14] Blocking miR-33a in mice increased HDL levels and inhibited atherosclerosis, suggesting that this could be a good target for therapeutic development. Other strategies under development to enhance RCT include direct infusion of cholesterol acceptors from ABCA1 or G1, including recombinant apoA, or a "hyperfunctioning" apoA mutant known as *apoA Milano,* or a small apoA mimetic amphipathic peptide.

FOAM CELL FORMATION AND THE FATTY STREAK

Atherosclerotic plaque develops in a geographically discontinuous manner very slowly and is continuously evolving over many decades.[5,6] Autopsy studies of motor vehicle accident victims showed early "preatherosclerotic" lesions present in the aorta of otherwise healthy young children. These small superficial lesions consist predominantly of lipid-laden macrophages and are termed *fatty streaks.*

The initial event in atherogenesis is most likely transudation of apolipoprotein B–containing lipoproteins across the endothelial cell monolayer into the arterial wall (Fig. 146-4). These lipoproteins are predominantly LDL, which is derived by remodeling of VLDL particles secreted into the plasma by hepatocytes. So-called remnant lipoproteins derived from chylomicrons produced by the intestinal epithelium may also play a role. The primary sites of lipoprotein entry are at arterial branch points or curvatures, explaining the discontinuous nature of atherosclerotic lesions. These locations are where normal laminar blood flow is disturbed. Normal laminar flow activates a specific genetic "protection" program in endothelial cells that enhances barrier function and promotes an antiinflammatory, antioxidant, antiatherogenic phenotype.[15] Loss of these shear-dependent signals disrupts the normal endothelial architecture and increases permeability, allowing unregulated entry of lipoproteins into the tunica intima. Within the intima the lipoproteins become "trapped" by specific interactions with normal components of the vessel wall, such as glycosoaminoglycans, and undergo structural modifications, including aggregation, oxidation, and in settings of hyperglycemia, glycation.[16]

Just as data show an unequivocal role for LDL cholesterol in atherogenesis, equally compelling studies in humans and animal models show that mononuclear phagocytes are necessary for plaque formation and progression and that atherosclerosis is associated with a chronic inflammatory state in the vessel wall and in the systemic circulation.[17,18] Targeted genetic mutations that block monocyte development from hematopoietic precursors or that prevent

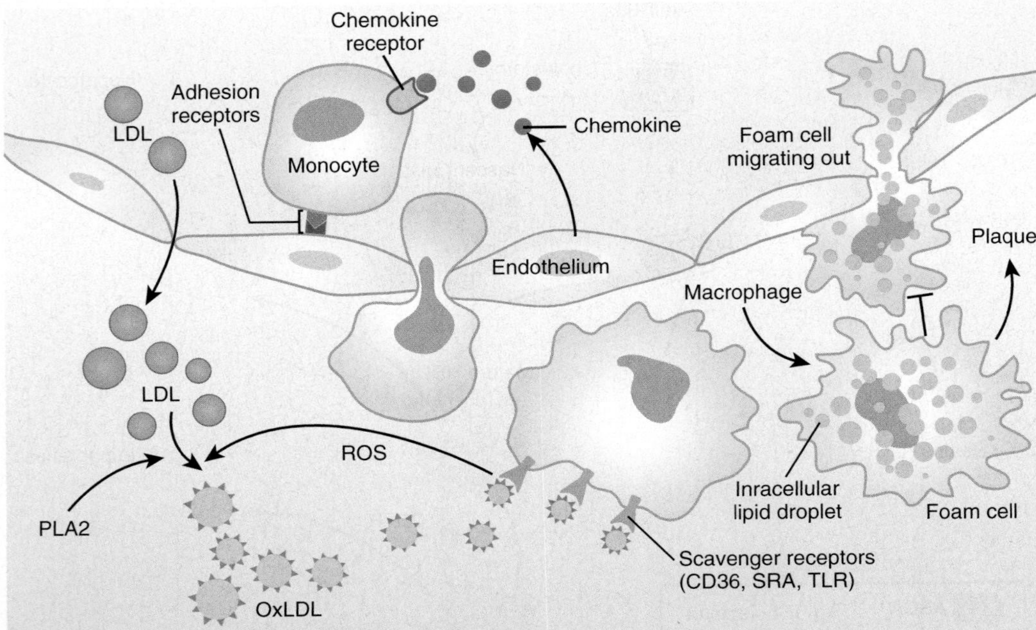

Figure 146-4 FOAM CELL FORMATION IS AN EARLY EVENT IN ATHEROGENESIS. LDL particles, which are transudated through a dysfunctional endothelium at arterial branch points or areas of disrupted shear, enter the intima and become trapped within the extracellular matrix. In the presence of inflammation, the LDL particles become oxidized or otherwise modified and contribute to endothelial dysfunction by interacting with receptors on endothelial cells, such as LOX1. Monocytes, in response to chemokines secreted by activated endothelial cells and/or inflammatory leukocytes and platelets, adhere to the endothelium via selectin family adhesion receptors, as well as β2 integrins and their counter receptors (ICAM and VCAM). The monocytes then diapedese into the intima, where they differentiate into inflammatory macrophages that generate oxidant stress within the vessel wall and release proinflammatory mediators. Scavenger receptors, in particular CD36, expressed on macrophages recognize and internalize oxidized LDL, leading to a feed-forward loop of increased LDL oxidation and increased scavenger receptor expression, resulting ultimately in the formation of cholesterol-laden foam cells. These accumulate in the intima, in part because of signals induced by oxLDL that inhibit migration, forming plaque.

monocyte trafficking into tissues dramatically protect mice from experimental atherosclerosis. The earliest and most prominent cell type in human and mouse atherosclerotic lesions are monocytes and macrophages. Initial monocyte entry into the arterial intima is in response to poorly understood cues related to endothelial cell dysfunction. Environmental and genetic influences, such as hypertension, angiotensin II production, cigarette smoke, diabetes, metabolic syndrome, and chronic periodontal infection may contribute to generalized endothelial dysfunction, but it is likely that the modified lipoproteins, particularly oxidized LDL (oxLDL), trapped in the vessel wall play a major initiating role. The oxLDL can activate an endothelial cell receptor known as *LOX1* to induce expression of monocyte adhesion molecules and this response is dramatically amplified in the presence of angiotensin II.[19] Other components of the "dysfunctional" endothelial cell phenotype include von Willebrand factor release from Weibel-Palade bodies and altered homeostasis of nitric oxide and eicosanoid pathways.

Monocyte recruitment to the vessel wall (see Fig. 146-4) begins with their capture and rolling along the activated endothelium mediated by specific interaction of selectin family adhesion molecules (L-selectin on circulating monocytes and P-selectin on activated endothelial cells) with their counter receptors, including PSGL1. Subsequent signals induced by endothelial-derived chemokines, including CCL5/RANTES, CCL2/MCP1, IL-8, and CXCL1, lead to further recruitment of monocytes and facilitate firm adhesion of the rolling monocytes to the vessel wall.[18,20] The latter is mediated by interaction of ICAM1 and VCAM on the activated endothelial surface with specific integrin family counter receptors on monocytes, β2 integrins for ICAM1 and α4β1 for VCAM. The adherent monocytes then diapedese through disrupted endothelial junctions and enter the intima. Recent studies have suggested that a particular subset of circulating "inflammatory" monocytes, defined by high expression of the Ly6C antigen (in mice) or CD14 (in humans), are the predominant source of entering cells.[18] The normal vasculature also contains a small number of resident macrophages, as well as "patrolling" monocytes. The latter are distinct from the $Ly6C^+$/$CD14^{hi}$ cells and exhibit a less inflammatory phenotype.

The ultimate fate of monocytes within the intima is probably determined in part by lineage commitment programs carried by the entering monocytes and in part by local environmental cues. Most, however, seem to polarize toward the so-called M1 inflammatory macrophage phenotype. Investigators have, however, detected dendritic cell-like phenotypes (expressing CD11c), as well as M2-like (expressing arginase and eNOS) and proangiogenic (expressing VEGF) macrophage phenotypes within plaque. In addition to monocytes, small numbers of lymphocytes, particularly T cells, also enter the intima, where they contribute to plaque formation by secreting cytokines and other mediators.

Reactive oxygen species (ROS) generated by the inflammatory milieu within the atherogenic vessel wall modify the trapped LDL by oxidizing both protein and lipid moieties (see Fig. 146-4), creating what are called collectively *oxLDL*.[16] Modified LDL lose their affinity for the LDL receptor but gain affinity for a genetically unrelated family of receptors known as *scavenger receptors (SR)*, including SRA1 and CD36, which are present at high levels on the macrophage surface. These receptors are part of the innate immune system, and their recognition of specific structures within oxLDL presumably relates to their mimicry of similar structures found on pathogenic organisms. CD36, for example,[21] also recognizes mycobacterial and *Staphylococcus* cell wall components, certain fungal structures, and falciparum malaria–infected erythrocytes. TLR family members, including TLR2, TLR4, and TLR6, can also recognize modified LDL and can partner with CD36 in these functions. Unlike the LDL receptor, which is downregulated in the setting of excess ligand, SR expression is increased in the presence of oxLDL, in part via internalization of oxidized fatty acids that serve as ligands for PPAR family transcription factors, particularly PPARγ, which is a major positive regulator of CD36 expression.[22] Thus over many months and years, the continued entry and oxidation of LDL in the intima coupled with upregulated expression of SRs leads to massive intracellular accumulation of cholesterol and formation of lipid-laden cells known as *foam cells*.

OxLDL-SR interactions initiate a cascade of events in macrophages, including internalization of the bound oxLDL, activation of proinflammatory pathways, and activation of transcriptional pathways. The CD36-oxLDL interaction, in addition to promoting ROS formation, also decreases expression of endogenous antioxidant pathways and inhibits macrophage migration.[21] These events result in a feed forward loop that increases leukocyte recruitment into the vessel wall, inhibits macrophage migration out of the vessel wall, and increases oxLDL formation. The net effect is formation and accumulation of lipid-laden foam cells and proinflammatory immune cells, which together form plaque (see Fig. 146-4). In mouse models, genetic deletion of scavenger receptors, especially CD36, provides substantial protection from plaque formation.

Although abundant data from animal models and correlative human studies support the oxidative stress hypothesis, considerable controversy remains because large- and medium-sized interventional trials of antioxidant therapy in humans have generally failed to prevent the complications of atherosclerosis.[19] These trials, however, are difficult to interpret because of lack of convincing evidence that the tested "antioxidant" therapies actually targeted the relevant vascular or circulating oxidant pathways. These oxidant systems include NADPH oxidase, xanthine oxidase, myeloperoxidase (MPO), and uncoupled nitric oxide synthase. MPO is of particular interest because it generates a highly specific oxidized phospholipid ligand for CD36 from LDL and because circulating MPO levels associate with risk for atherosclerosis and with risk for acute cardiovascular events.

Another potential problem with the antioxidant clinical trials is that the choice of antioxidants may have been flawed. Most used vitamin E formulations containing mainly α-tocopherol. Recent studies showed that tocopherols, in addition to having activity as antioxidants, have important cell-signaling functions mediated by specific cellular receptors. Therapy with formulations containing primarily α-tocopherol may downregulate endogenous γ-tocopherol levels, leading to imbalance in natural tocopherol signaling pathways. Furthermore, tocopherols are lipid-based structures that are themselves subject to oxidation, producing lipid peroxides that can actually promote further oxidative stress. Nevertheless, it is possible that pathways of cholesterol uptake unrelated to LDL oxidation and SR expression, such as by micro- and macro-pinocytosis of "native" LDL or aggregated LDL, may play a significant role in foam cell formation.

Important unresolved issues in the pathogenesis of early atherosclerotic lesions include understanding why macrophages do not exit the vessel wall and travel to regional nodes after ingesting modified LDL, as they would after ingesting exogenous pathogens, and why cholesterol efflux cannot keep up with LDL uptake to maintain a homeostatic state.[23] OxLDL inhibition of macrophage migration (see Fig. 146-4) may explain the former, suggesting that blocking oxLDL-mediated signaling pathways might have therapeutic potential by facilitating macrophage exit from developing plaque. In experimental animals, transplantation of atherosclerotic aortae from hypercholesterolemic animals into normal recipients induces migration of lipid-laden macrophages out of the vessel wall and plaque regression.[24] The second issue might relate to differential gene regulation of SRs compared with cholesterol efflux transporters, and/or to intracellular cholesterol trafficking that might make it inaccessible to efflux transporters. In addition, HDL particles, similar to LDL, are sensitive to oxidative modification and such oxidation may produce what is termed "dysfunctional" HDL—that is, HDL particles that do not function optimally in RCT and that may lose some of their other atheroprotective activity.[25]

LESION EVOLUTION: REMODELING AND THE VULNERABLE PLAQUE

In humans, plaque develops and evolves very slowly over many decades, explaining in part why animal models in which advanced lesions develop rapidly over weeks and months may not accurately reflect the human condition. Accumulation of foam cells is only one component of the atherogenic process. Early on, signals from macrophages (Fig. 146-5) and the injured endothelium, primarily platelet-derived growth factor (PDGF), stimulate adventitial smooth muscle cells to migrate into the intima and proliferate.[6] These cells contribute to the mass of the lesions and also secrete collagen and other factors that change the nature of the intimal extracellular matrix. Lymphocytes infiltrating from the circulation and mast cells from the adventitia also contribute to the inflammatory milieu and matrix remodeling. Platelet antigens are also readily detectable in plaque,[26] suggesting that platelets enter the intima, where they may contribute to matrix remodeling and the inflammatory state by secreting PDGF, transforming growth factor-β, and other growth factors, along with platelet factor 4, which is a potent chemokine, also known as *CXCL4,* for monocytes. Animal studies suggest that platelets may facilitate monocyte recruitment, acting as a bridge between the endothelium and circulating monocytes (see Fig. 146-5). Sophisticated single-cell imaging studies in mice showed that monocytes continue to traffic through the "shoulders" of even advanced stage lesions.

Plaque generally grows in an eccentric pattern within the intima and in certain instances can create significant obstruction to blood flow (Fig. 146-6, *left*). In such cases, as oxygen demand increases, tissue ischemia results, leading to angina and/or lower extremity claudication. Recent in vivo studies using sophisticated imaging techniques, such as intravascular ultrasound, however, demonstrate that in most cases, the vessel wall remodels as plaque grows (Fig. 146-6, *right*) so that the arterial lumen is mostly preserved and the bulk of the atheromatous mass is ablumenal.[10,27] These studies show that traditional two-dimensional angiographic techniques vastly underestimate plaque burden. Of note, such studies along with careful histopathologic examinations, have led to the concept that the "quality" of the plaque may be more important than its quantity in predicting cardiovascular outcomes. Some plaques, particularly those with thick fibrous caps and cellular cores seem to be "stable" (Fig. 146-7), whereas others, particularly those with thin fibrous caps, abundant leukocytes, and necrotic, lipid-rich cores seem to be "unstable" and vulnerable to erosion and rupture (see Fig. 146-7). Rupture refers to the sudden loss of integrity of the fibrous cap with release of plaque material into the lumen, often followed by acute occlusive thrombosis. Erosion is a more subtle concept referring to loss of endothelial cells at the shoulder of the lesion or minimal leakage of plaque through a partially disrupted cap. Plaque erosion may lead to subocclusive thrombus formation and/or intraplaque hemorrhage and thrombosis. Repeated cycles of erosion and intraplaque hemorrhage/thrombosis may account for the apparent stepwise growth of some lesions.

Understanding factors that contribute to plaque vulnerability is an extremely important topic of research, but one that is difficult to model in animals. Some key features that have emerged are the degree of angiogenesis within the plaque, the balance of matrix-degrading enzymes and enzyme inhibitors, the level of apoptosis of cells within the plaque, and the deposition of calcium within the plaque.

Plaque angiogenesis is a recently appreciated process that can be visualized by certain imaging modalities, such as ultrafast CT and MRI, in real time.[27] Based on analogy to tumor growth, it is not surprising that growing plaque requires a blood supply and also that the neovessels within plaque may, similar to their counterparts in cancer, be leaky and unstable. This neovascular instability may

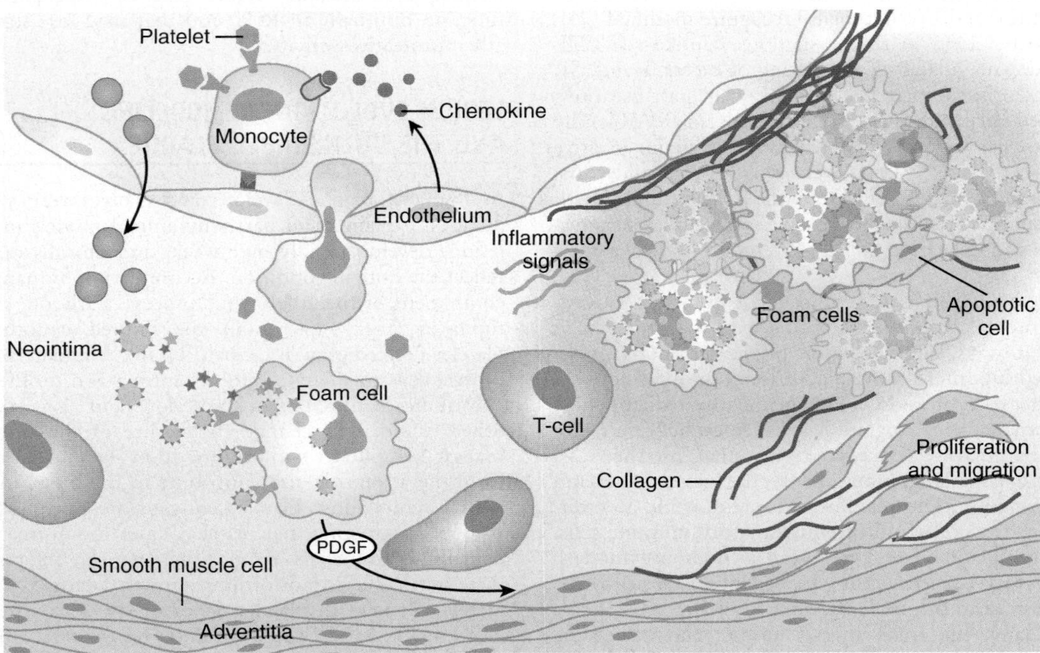

Figure 146-5 LATER EVENTS IN ATHEROGENESIS. Fatty streaks formed in the vessel wall via accumulation of foam cells (see Fig. 146-4) evolve over many years into complex plaque. In response to chemokines, monocytes continue to enter plaque, perhaps accompanied by platelets. T cells, B cells, and other inflammatory cells also accumulate. Cholesterol loading of macrophages induces apoptosis and apoptotic cells accumulate because of dysfunction of normal efferocytotic clearance pathways. Smooth muscle cells respond to PDGF, TGFβ, and other signals and proliferate and migrate into the neointima. These cells produce collagen and other matrix components, contributing to plaque growth and formation of a fibrous cap. To support plaque growth, an angiogenic response is elicited from vasa vasora within the adventitia.

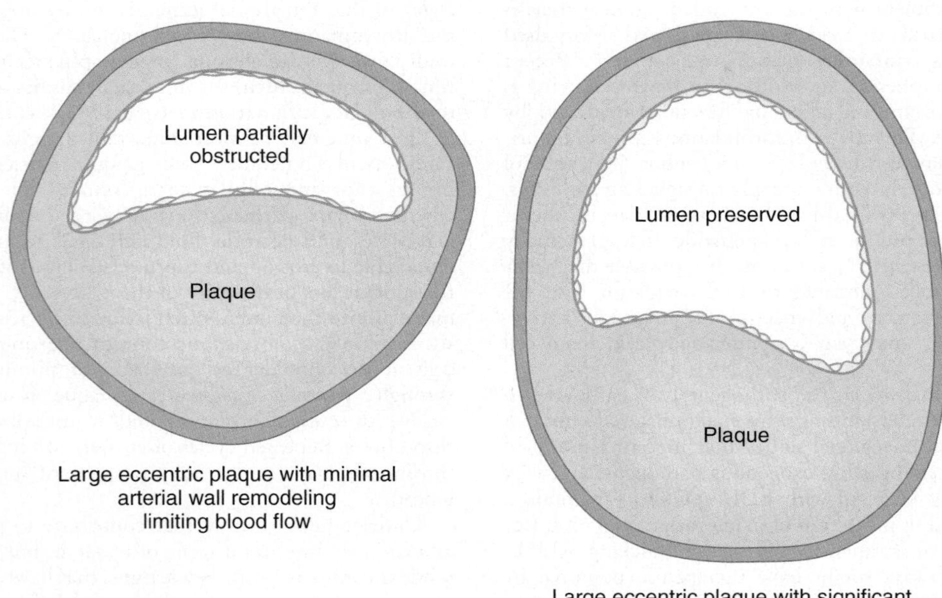

Figure 146-6 VESSEL WALL REMODELING CAN PRESERVE ARTERIAL LUMEN. On the left is a cross-section cartoon image of an artery containing a large eccentric plaque *(orange)*. The vessel has undergone minimal remodeling. The atheromatous lesion is extending into the arterial lumen and would be visible on an angiogram as an obstructing lesion. On the right is a lesion of similar mass, but its formation was accompanied by significant vessel wall remodeling so that the lesion extends mainly into the vessel wall, preserving the lumen. On an angiogram this would be nearly invisible.

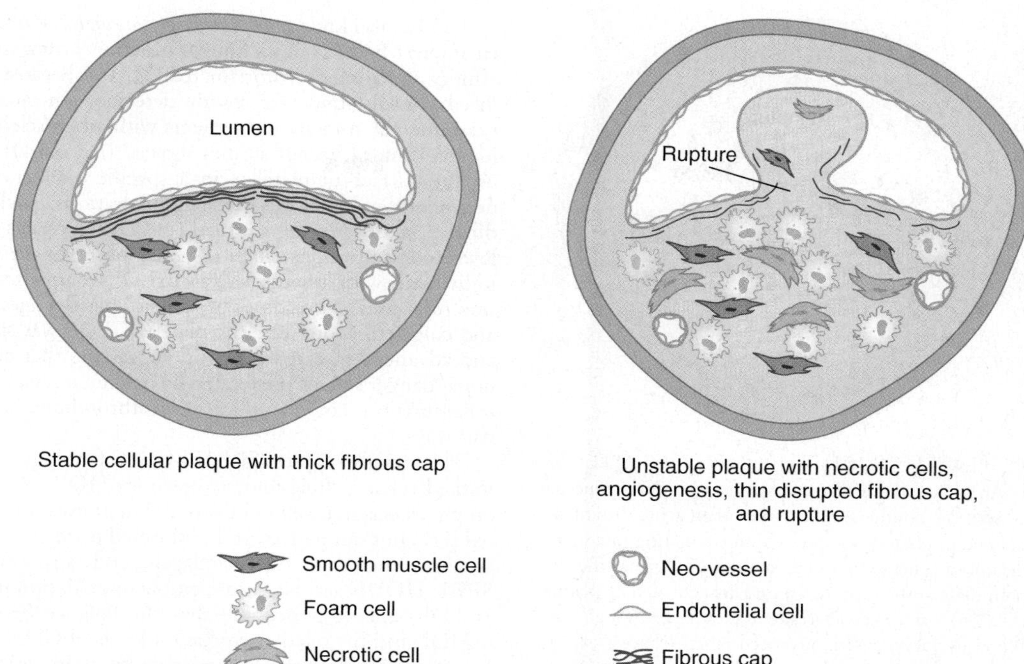

Figure 146-7 UNSTABLE PLAQUE IS PRONE TO RUPTURE. On the left is a cross-section cartoon image of an artery with a plaque containing abundant smooth muscle cells and foam cells and a thick fibrous cap. On the right is a similar-size plaque, but with a thin fibrous cap that has ruptured allowing plaque contents to extrude into the lumen. This plaque contains smooth muscle cells and foam cells, as in the stable plaque on the left, but there is abundant angiogenesis, along with apoptotic and necrotic cells.

contribute to plaque instability by facilitating entry of inflammatory cells, platelets, and plasma components, such as fibrinogen and cell-derived microparticles (MP). In animal models, treatment with anti-angiogenic agents significantly slows plaque growth. In some diseases states, such as diabetes, accelerated atherosclerosis may reflect a "microvascular" disease of the vasa vasorum.

Integrity of the fibrous cap is maintained by a balance between collagen synthesis by smooth muscle cells and fibroblasts and collagenolysis by matrix-degrading enzymes. The latter is maintained by a balance between enzymes and their endogenous inhibitors. The predominant enzymes are members of the large family of zinc-dependent matrix metalloproteinases (MMPs) that are capable of degrading most matrix components, including collagen. These enzymes are tightly regulated by a network of activators and inhibitors and in settings in which activation exceeds inhibition, excessive matrix degradation may occur. Metalloproteases of the ADAM (a disintegrin and metalloprotease domain) family and ADAMTS (a disintegrin and metalloprotease domain with thrombospondin structural homology domains) family may also contribute to plaque instability. Although several clinical trials have studied MMP inhibitors in atherosclerosis, none has shown clear benefit to date.

A prominent feature of advanced atherosclerotic lesions is the presence of apoptotic cells, mostly of macrophage and smooth muscle cell origin. The nature of the proapoptotic signals within plaque is incompletely understood, but excess intracellular cholesterol can initiate the endoplasmic reticulum stress response leading to apoptosis.[28] OxLDL signaling through SRs and/or TLRs can also induce apoptosis.[17] A recent study showed that lipoprotein(a), a known risk factor for cardiovascular disease can function as a "carrier" for oxLDL and thereby activate the CD36/TLR2 signaling complex to trigger apoptosis in the setting of ER stress. In most inflammatory sites, apoptotic leukocytes are quickly removed by phagocytes in a process known as *efferocytosis*. The efferocytotic macrophages are generally thought to be of the M2, antiinflammatory type; thus their engagement by apoptotic cells not only removes the apoptotic cell from the microenvironment, but also directly contributes to downregulation of the inflammatory state by inducing secretion of antiinflammatory cytokines and effectors. In atherosclerotic plaque, this process seems to be inefficient so that apoptotic cells accumulate, contributing to the lipid load and releasing potentially toxic contents.

Although therapeutic interventions to stabilize vulnerable plaque or prevent plaques from becoming vulnerable have not yet materialized, several imaging approaches have been studied in attempt to develop useful biomarkers to identify vulnerable plaque and therefore to identify patients who might benefit from aggressive antithrombotic and lipid-lowering therapeutic interventions. Neovascular imaging by CT or MRI are promising technologies, as are plaque characterization by optical coherence tomography, near infrared imaging, and thermography.[27]

PLAQUE RUPTURE AND ACUTE ARTERIAL THROMBOSIS

The devastating complications of atherosclerosis, including acute coronary syndromes (ACS), stroke, gangrene, and sudden death result primarily from acute and subacute thrombosis occurring at the site of plaque rupture (Fig. 146-8). As described in later chapters in this section, treatment and prevention strategies using aggressive antiplatelet, anticoagulant, fibrinolytic, and/or mechanical approaches have been remarkably effective at reducing major cardiovascular events, but tremendous unmet need still exists, particularly in the areas of primary and secondary prevention of thrombosis.

The pathophysiologic mechanisms underlying acute arterial thrombosis center on two key concepts: (1) exposure of prothrombotic materials to the local circulation as a consequence of plaque rupture acts as a thrombotic trigger, and (2) advanced atherosclerosis is associated with a systemic prothrombotic state that accelerates or enhances pathologic thrombosis.[29,30] The former mechanism undoubtedly plays a major role. Immunohistochemical studies have convincingly shown that plaque contains abundant tissue factor (TF), and acute anticoagulation therapy directed toward blocking thrombin generation or inhibiting thrombin has proven to be effective in ACS.

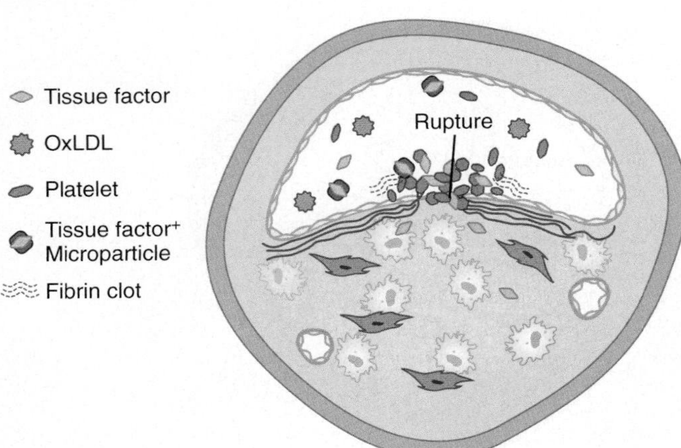

Figure 146-8 ACUTE PLATELET-RICH THROMBUS AT SITE OF PLAQUE RUPTURE. An atherosclerotic artery with a ruptured plaque (as described in Fig. 146-7) serves as a nidus for formation of an acute thrombus. Tissue factor (TF) contained in plaque or expressed on circulating microparticles (MPs) leads to thrombin generation and formation of fibrin at the site of rupture. Platelets accumulate at the rupture site and are activated by plaque components, such as collagen, forming an aggregate that, if large enough, can obstruct blood flow. Blood in patients with advanced atherosclerosis is prothrombotic, in part because of oxidized LDL–induced release of TF-positive MPs from monocytes. Oxidized LDL also interacts with platelets to make them more sensitive to activation and aggregation by plaque contents.

Plaque TF is derived mainly from smooth muscle cells, fibroblasts, and activated macrophages. Recent studies have also suggested that platelets can synthesize TF after stimulation by inflammatory mediators and thus may also contribute to the plaque procoagulant load. A significant proportion of plaque TF may be in the form of membrane-bound microparticles (MP) derived from apoptotic and/or activated cells (see next section for more detailed explanation). Exposure of flowing blood to TF exposed in or released from ruptured plaque leads to rapid activation of factor Xa, thrombin generation, and activation of platelets. In addition to TF, other components of plaque that become exposed to blood at sites of rupture include collagen and oxidized phospholipids, both of which can activate platelets directly. Thus aggressive antiplatelet therapy with aspirin, ADP receptor P2Y12 inhibitors, and glycoprotein $\alpha IIb\beta 3$ inhibitors are mainstays of the pharmacologic approach to treatment of ACS, and aspirin and P2Y12 inhibitors are of proven efficacy for secondary prevention.

HYPERLIPIDEMIA, ATHEROSCLEROSIS, AND A SYSTEMIC PROTHROMBOTIC STATE

Platelet hyperreactivity has long been thought to play a role in acute atherothrombosis. Clinical studies support an association between in vitro platelet reactivity and prognosis in patients with coronary disease, and it was shown in the 1970s that platelets from patients with familial hypercholesterolemia were more sensitive to activation by epinephrine or ADP. Similar findings were seen in platelets from mouse models of hyperlipidemia, such as the apoE-null strain, which was fed a high-fat diet. Of note, the time to form occlusive thrombi after arterial injury in vivo was accelerated in hyperlipidemic mice compared with controls. In that context, much attention has been paid to identifying and characterizing receptors on the platelet surface that recognize specific classes of lipids and lipoproteins.[31] The receptors fall into two main groups: pattern recognition innate immune receptors, including CD36, SRA, TLR4, and LDL receptor–like protein (LRP)-8 (also known as *apoER2*), and G-protein coupled receptors, including receptors for lysophosphatidic acid (LPA), platelet-activating factor, and thromboxane.

CD36 (also known as *platelet glycoprotein IV* or *IIIb*) is of particular interest because of its known function on macrophages as a high affinity signaling receptor for oxLDL and because oxLDL and oxidized phospholipids are readily detectable in circulating plasma of experimental animals and patients with atherosclerosis and hyperlipidemia. Indeed, recent studies showed that oxLDL bound to CD36 on the surface of platelets in a specific, concentration, and time-dependent manner. At high concentrations, such as might occur during acute plaque rupture, oxLDL activates platelets and at lower concentrations, such as those observed in the circulation of individuals with atherosclerosis, oxLDL-augmented platelet aggregation responses to low doses of "classic" platelet agonists, such as ADP and collagen. More recently, platelet CD36 was shown to bind MP and advanced glycated proteins, suggesting that circulating endogenous "danger signals" generated by oxidant stress, hyperglycemia, and inflammation could induce a prothrombotic state through this pathway.

Platelets also express SRB1, a CD36 family protein that functions in the liver as a cholesterol acceptor for HDL. The function of SRB1 on platelets is not well understood, but at least one study showed that oxHDL, but not native HDL, inhibited platelet reactivity to multiple agonists, including ADP, collagen, and thrombin via binding to SRB1. HDL is at least as susceptible to oxidation in vitro and in vivo as LDL, and it is possible that the balance between oxLDL and oxHDL and the relative expression levels of CD36, SRB1, and other receptors may determine platelet reactivity in patients with hyperlipidemia and oxidant stress.

Atherosclerotic plaque and so-called "minimally" oxidized LDL contain LPA, a biologically active lipid generated by the action of phospholipases on LDL and cell membrane lipids. Platelets express at least three different G-protein-coupled LPA receptors but the in vivo relevance of this system has not been demonstrated. Ex vivo studies, however, demonstrated that minimally oxidized LDL at high concentrations could induce platelet shape change and sensitize platelets to aggregate in response to other agonists. Epidemiologic studies have also associated levels of soluble phospholipase A2 with cardiovascular risk.[32] In addition to participating in LPA biosynthesis, this family of enzymes generates free fatty acids from phospholipids that serve as substrates for cyclooxygenase and lipoxygenases, producing both pro- and antiatherogenic eicosanoids.

LRP-8 (particularly a splice variant known as apoER2) binds lipidated apoE3 (e.g., chylomicrons and remnant particles) resulting in enhanced nitric oxide production and inhibition of platelet activation by ADP and other agonists. On the other hand, LRP-8 has also been shown to bind apoB-containing lipoproteins, leading to enhanced thromboxane generation and sensitization of platelets to other agonists. Consistent with this, in mice genetic deletion of LRP-8 has an antithrombotic effect in models of arterial injury.

In addition to platelet hyperreactivity, it is also quite likely that systemic activation of the coagulation cascade contributes to the prothrombotic state associated with advanced atherosclerosis. This is consistent with studies showing that atherosclerosis is associated with increased risk for venous thromboembolic disorders, as well as arterial thrombosis.[9] Elevated levels of circulating D-dimer and thrombin-antithrombin complexes have been reported in patients with ACS and D-dimer levels tend to track with hsCRP. Large-scale population studies have identified elevated fibrinogen and factor VIII levels as risk factors for atherosclerosis. Recent studies suggest that a key initiator of thrombin generation in these settings is circulating TF (see Fig. 146-8) in the form of TF-expressing MPs. MPs are vesicular fragments that bud off from cells during either activation or apoptosis. They are 200 to 1000 nm in size and possess different antigenic properties depending on the cell from which they are derived. MPs can be generated from platelets, monocytes, erythrocytes, leukocytes, or endothelial cells during vascular injury and have been shown to become incorporated into developing thrombi in vivo. MPs, mostly of platelet origin, can be detected in the circulation of normal human subjects, but markedly increased numbers of circulating MPs have been reported in patients with a variety of inflammatory and prothrombotic disorders including ACS.[29]

MPs contribute to thrombus formation through several mechanisms. A general feature of MP generation is loss of membrane asymmetry so that anionic phospholipids normally oriented in the inner membrane leaflet become exposed on the outer leaflet. Surface-exposed phosphatidylserine (PS) is a site for catalytic assembly of the prothrombinase complex and thrombin generation. Furthermore, PS on the surface of MP also has the capacity to bind to platelet CD36 and enhance platelet reactivity via the same mechanism as does oxLDL.

It is important to note that MPs derived from some cells (e.g., monocytes, macrophages, smooth muscle cells, and tumor cells) are a source of circulating TF. An important mechanistic link between atherogenesis and thrombosis may be oxLDL, which in vitro can induce TF-positive MP generation from blood-derived monocytes.[33] Of interest, a recent large clinical trial testing the efficacy of statins in subjects with normal LDL, but elevated levels of hsCRP, showed that rates of venous thrombosis, as well as coronary events, were significantly decreased.[9] In animal models, statins decrease circulating levels of oxLDL and also decrease circulating MP levels and levels of other prothrombotic and proinflammatory biomarkers, even in the absence of lowering cholesterol, suggesting that oxLDL-mediated prothrombotic activities may be important targets for thromboprevention in patients with atherosclerosis.[33] These studies also support those showing that statins may have antiinflammatory and antithrombotic activities independent of lipid lowering. Since HMGCoA reductase is also the limiting step in biosynthesis of isoprenoids, it has been postulated that statins may dampen signaling pathways mediated by small molecular weight G proteins (e.g., Ras) in which membrane targeting by protein isoprenylation is required (see Fig. 146-2).

In mice, the contact activating system and intrinsic coagulation cascade have been shown to participate in arterial thrombosis after injury and to have proatherogenic properties.[30] Targeting these systems is attractive in that patients with known deficiencies in factor XII or contact system proteins have no obvious phenotype and do not have a bleeding diathesis, thus presumably an antithrombotic effect could be achieved without altering normal hemostasis.

CROSS TALK BETWEEN COAGULATION AND INFLAMMATION SYSTEMS IMPACT ATHEROGENESIS

As noted previously, atherosclerosis can be thought of as a chronic, low-grade inflammatory disease of the artery wall. Clinical studies based on biomarkers, such as hsCRP, MPO, and IL6, also suggest that advanced atherosclerosis is associated with a systemic state of chronic inflammation and that the degree of inflammation reflects the level of risk for major complications, possibly because the more inflamed the plaque, the more vulnerable the lesion. It is also now clear that mediators of inflammation, such as IL1, LPA, oxLDL, and circulating MPs may interact with platelets and the coagulation cascade to promote a hypercoagulable, prothrombotic state.[20] Furthermore, mediators of coagulation, such as thrombin, TF-factor VIIa complexes, and factor Xa, may contribute to the proinflammatory state by interacting with protease-activated receptors on endothelial cells and leukocytes. Activated platelets can contribute to inflammation by facilitating monocyte adhesion to endothelium and by secreting small molecules (ATP, pyrophosphates, and serotonin), cytokines and growth factors that have proinflammatory activity. Thus bidirectional cross-talk between the inflammation and coagulation systems serves to enhance each other and to promote atherosclerosis.

Not surprisingly, patients with systemic autoimmune inflammatory disorders, including rheumatoid arthritis, Wegener's granulomatosis, and lupus erythematosus have been shown to have accelerated atherosclerosis, as assessed by biomarkers, such as ultrasound evidence of carotid artery intima-medial thickening, as well as major cardiovascular events. Obesity, a risk factor for atherosclerosis, is now also known to be a systemic inflammatory disorder, with evidence of inflammation readily detectable within obese central adipose tissue. Obese patients also have elevated, circulating levels of coagulation and inflammation biomarkers, including plasminogen activator inhibitor-1 (PAI-1).

Given these observations, there has been renewed interest in exploring the use of antiinflammatory agents and antithrombotic agents to slow the progress of atherosclerosis. The approach has been tempered by clinical studies showing small increases in atherosclerotic complications in patients taking COX inhibitors (especially those with preferential activity against COX2), but this may relate to the specific target and the complication of altered eicosanoid production, perhaps changing the balance away from antiatherothrombotic end products, such as prostacyclin and resolvins, towards proatherothrombotic products, such as thromboxane, HETE, and lipoxins. Also, although aspirin and ADP receptor antagonists definitively reduce risk for major cardiovascular events, no studies have shown an impact on burden of atheroma. Nevertheless, novel agents targeted to more specific atherothrombotic pathways, such as chemokines, LDL oxidation, scavenger receptors, lipoxygenases, phospholipase 2, leukotrienes, selectins, and IL1 are being considered.

Although B cells are not prominent cellular constituents of plaque, humans and experimental animals often develop humoral immune responses to plaque constituents, particularly modified LDL. Antibodies against oxLDL may be protective, perhaps by facilitating clearance via pathways that do not lead to foam cell formation, and/or by interfering with oxLDL-mediated activation of circulating monocytes and platelets.[16] Based on these observations, passive immunization strategies against oxLDL are also being considered.

PLAQUE REGRESSION AND FUTURE DIRECTIONS

Finding pharmacologic approaches to decrease the amount of arterial plaque has proved to be an elusive goal. Intravenous ultrasound has shown that very aggressive lowering of LDL cholesterol with high-dose statins and extremely rigorous dietary alterations can halt plaque progression and, in some cases, cause some regression.[10] As noted previously, strategies to enhance RCT or to induce macrophage emigration from plaque are being developed and strategies to stabilize plaque by targeting the neovasculature, cellular apoptosis and efferocytosis are being considered. Specific antioxidant approaches based on fundamental understanding of the oxidation processes relevant to atherosclerosis remain viable as well. Finally, it is hoped that the large investment of research funds in large-scale genome-wide association studies (GWAS) may lead to identification of novel genes and pathways (such as miR-33a and PCSK9) that can be targeted with therapeutic or preventive effect. At present the most consistent data to come from GWAS identified a fairly large genomic region on chromosome 9p21 as a risk site, but specific gene identification has not yet been accomplished.

REFERENCES

1. National Institutes of Health, National Heart, Lung, and Blood Institute: *Morbidity and mortality: 2009 Chart book on cardiovascular, lung, and blood diseases,* 2009, NIH. http://www.nhlbi.nih.gov/resources/docs/2009_ChartBook_508.pdf.
2. Lloyd-Jones D, Adams RJ, Brown TM, et al: Executive summary: Heart disease and stroke statistics—2010 update: A report from the American Heart Association. *Circulation* 121:e46, 2010.
3. Heidenreich PA, Trogdon JG, Khavjou OA, et al: Forecasting the future of cardiovascular disease in the United States: A policy statement from the American Heart Association. *Circulation* 123:933, 2011.
4. Pencina MJ, D'Agostino RB, Sr, Larson MG, et al: Predicting the 30-year risk of cardiovascular disease: The Framingham Heart Study. *Circulation* 119:3078, 2009.
5. Ross R, Glomset JA: The pathogenesis of atherosclerosis (first of two parts). *N Engl J Med* 295:369, 1976.
6. Libby P, Ridker PM, Hansson GK: Progress and challenges in translating the biology of atherosclerosis. *Nature* 473:317, 2011.

7. Plump AS, Smith JD, Hayek T, et al: Severe hypercholesterolemia and atherosclerosis in apolipoprotein E-deficient mice created by homologous recombination in ES cells. *Cell* 71:343, 1992.
8. Sato R: Sterol metabolism and SREBP activation. *Arch Biochem Biophys* 501:177, 2010.
9. Ridker PM, Danielson E, Fonseca FA, et al; JUPITER Study Group: Rosuvastatin to prevent vascular events in men and women with elevated C-reactive protein. *N Engl J Med* 359:2195, 2008.
10. Nicholls SJ, Ballantyne CM, Barter PJ, et al: Effect of two intensive statin regimens on progression of coronary disease. *N Engl J Med* 365:2078, 2011.
11. Cohen JC, Boerwinkle E, Mosley TH, Jr, et al: Sequence variations in PCSK9, low LDL, and protection against coronary heart disease. *N Engl J Med* 354:1264, 2006.
12. Tall AR, Yvan-Charvet L, Terasaka N, et al: HDL, ABC transporters, and cholesterol efflux: Implications for the treatment of atherosclerosis. *Cell Metab* 7:365, 2008.
13. Nissen SE, Tardif JC, Nicholls SJ, et al; ILLUSTRATE Investigators: Effect of torcetrapib on the progression of coronary atherosclerosis. *N Engl J Med* 356:1304, 2007.
14. Fernández-Hernando C, Moore KJ: MicroRNA modulation of cholesterol homeostasis. *Arterioscler Thromb Vasc Biol* 31:2378, 2011.
15. Dai G, Kaazempur-Mofrad MR, Natarajan S, et al: Distinct endothelial phenotypes evoked by arterial waveforms derived from atherosclerosis-susceptible and -resistant regions of human vasculature. *Proc Natl Acad Sci U S A* 101:14871, 2004.
16. Steinberg D, Witztum JL: Oxidized low-density lipoprotein and atherosclerosis. *Arterioscler Thromb Vasc Biol* 30:2311, 2010.
17. Moore KJ, Tabas I: Macrophages in the pathogenesis of atherosclerosis. *Cell* 145:341, 2011.
18. Ley K, Miller YI, Hedrick CC: Monocyte and macrophage dynamics during atherogenesis. *Arterioscler Thromb Vasc Biol* 31:1506, 2011.
19. Mitra S, Deshmukh A, Sachdeva R, et al: Oxidized low-density lipoprotein and atherosclerosis implications in antioxidant therapy. *Am J Med Sci* 342:135, 2011.
20. Charo IF, Taub R: Anti-inflammatory therapeutics for the treatment of atherosclerosis. *Nat Rev Drug Discov* 10:365, 2011.
21. Silverstein RL, Febbraio M: CD36, a scavenger receptor involved in immunity, metabolism, angiogenesis, and behavior. *Science Signaling* 2, re3, 2009.
22. Nagy L, Tontonoz P, Alvarez JG, et al: Oxidized LDL regulates macrophage gene expression through ligand activation of PPARgamma. *Cell* 93:229, 1998.
23. Curtiss LK: Reversing atherosclerosis? *N Engl J Med* 360:1144, 2009.
24. Llodrá J, Angeli V, Liu J, et al: Emigration of monocyte-derived cells from atherosclerotic lesions characterizes regressive, but not progressive, plaques. *Proc Natl Acad Sci U S A* 101:11779, 2004.
25. Undurti A, Huang Y, Lupica JA, et al: Modification of high density lipoprotein by myeloperoxidase generates a pro-inflammatory particle. *J Biol Chem* 284:30825, 2009.
26. Massberg S, Brand K, Grüner S, et al: A critical role of platelet adhesion in the initiation of atherosclerotic lesion formation. *J Exp Med* 196:887, 2002.
27. Fayad ZA: Cardiovascular molecular imaging. *Arterioscler Thromb Vasc Biol* 29:981, 2009.
28. Scull CM, Tabas I: Mechanisms of ER stress-induced apoptosis in atherosclerosis. *Arterioscler Thromb Vasc Biol* 31:2792, 2011.
29. Rautou PE, Vion AC, Amabile N, et al: Microparticles, vascular function, and atherothrombosis. *Circ Res* 109:593, 2011.
30. Borissoff JI, Spronk HM, ten Cate H: The hemostatic system as a modulator of atherosclerosis. *N Engl J Med* 364:1746, 2011.
31. Silverstein RL: Type 2 scavenger receptor CD36 in platelet activation: The role of hyperlipidemia and oxidative stress. *Clinical Lipidology* 4:767, 2009.
32. Thompson A, Gao P, Orfei L, et al: Lipoprotein-associated phospholipase A(2) and risk of coronary disease, stroke, and mortality: Collaborative analysis of 32 prospective studies. *Lancet* 375:1536, 2010.
33. Owens AP 3rd, Passam FH, Antoniak S, et al: Monocyte tissue factor-dependent activation of coagulation in hypercholesterolemic mice and monkeys is inhibited by simvastatin. *J Clin Invest* 2012; Jan 3 Epub ahead of print.

CHAPTER 147

STROKE

Michelle Canavan, Emer McGrath, and Martin O'Donnell

Stroke is the leading cause of acquired adult disability worldwide and the second most common cause of death after coronary heart disease. Primary stroke subtypes include ischemic stroke, intracerebral hemorrhage, and subarachnoid hemorrhage. Each stroke subtype has differing etiologies, outcomes, and management strategies. The past 20 years has seen considerable advances in diagnosis (emergence of widely available neuroimaging) and treatment of acute stroke. In addition, there is an increased awareness of the importance of covert stroke (stroke on neuroimaging in the absence of a history of acute clinical stroke). In this chapter, we provide an overview of stroke, with a primary focus on ischemic stroke, which is the most common cause of stroke worldwide.

DEFINITION

Stroke is defined by the World Health Organization (WHO) as "rapidly developing clinical signs of focal (at times global) disturbance of cerebral function, lasting more than 24 hours or leading to death with no apparent cause other than that of vascular origin." This definition is conventionally considered to include ischemic stroke, intracerebral hemorrhage, and subarachnoid hemorrhage. Clinical presentations lasting less than 24 hours are classified as transient ischemic attacks (TIA). Recently, it has been proposed that the definitions of stroke and TIA be revised to more tissue-based definitions—that is, based on the presence or absence of acute ischemia or hemorrhage on neuroimaging.

EPIDEMIOLOGY

Frequency

The WHO estimates that 15 million people suffer a stroke each year, and of these, 5 million people are left with permanent disability. In 2005, an estimated 5.7 million stroke-related deaths occurred, accounting for approximately 10% of total deaths worldwide. A small decrease in the age-specific stroke mortality rates has been projected from 2005 to 2030, which is largely due to a decline in mortality rates in high-income countries. However, considering the increasingly ageing population worldwide, the crude stroke mortality rates are projected to increase across all ages, from 89 per 100,000 in 2005 to an estimated 98 per 100,000 in 2030. In the absence of further effective population-based interventions, a projected 6.5 million stroke deaths will occur in 2015 and 7.8 million deaths in 2030. The increase in stroke mortality will be most marked in developing countries, where increases in stroke incidence are most prominent. Worldwide, stroke shows significant geographic variation, in terms of incidence (and temporal trends), case fatality, and case mix (i.e., stroke subtypes). A recent systematic review of population-based studies reported that from 1970 to 2008 a 42% decrease occurred in the incidence of stroke in high-income countries, compared with a more than 100% increase in the incidence of stroke in middle- and low-income countries. Therefore the projected increase in stroke incidence will occur largely in low- and middle-income countries.

Traditional Risk Factors for Stroke

Both ischemic stroke and intracerebral hemorrhage are associated with a number of potentially modifiable risk factors—namely, hypertension, smoking, diet, sedentary lifestyle, obesity, diabetes mellitus, and exercise. The INTERSTROKE study, which included 6000 participants from 22 countries, reported that 10 key risk factors were associated with 90% of the population-attributable risk (PAR) of ischemic stroke: hypertension, smoking, waist-to-hip ratio, diet, physical activity level, diabetes mellitus, alcohol intake, psychosocial stress and depression, cardiac causes such as atrial fibrillation, and ratio of apolipoprotein B to A1 (Table 147-1). Of these risk factors, five (hypertension, smoking, abdominal obesity, physical inactivity, and diet) were associated with 80% of the PAR for all strokes, and each of these five risk factors was important for both ischemic stroke and hemorrhagic stroke. Therefore a large proportion of stroke is potentially preventable, emphasizing the importance of developing effective population-based interventions to modify these key risk factors. Hypertension is the strongest risk factor for both ischemic stroke and intracranial hemorrhage, and it is arguably the most modifiable factor by lifestyle intervention (e.g., reduced salt intake) and medications.

PATHOBIOLOGY

Stroke can be primarily classified into ischemic stroke (Fig. 147-1) and hemorrhagic stroke. Hemorrhagic stroke is further subtyped into intracerebral hemorrhage (Fig. 147-2) and subarachnoid hemorrhage. In North America and Europe, approximately 87% of strokes are due to ischemia, with the remaining 13% occurring as a result of hemorrhage. In developing countries, a larger proportion of strokes are due to intracerebral hemorrhage.

Etiologic Classification of Ischemic Stroke

Unlike acute coronary syndrome, which is primarily due to large vessel atherosclerosis, the underlying mechanisms for ischemic stroke are more heterogeneous. The most commonly used etiologic classification is the Trial of Org 10172 in Acute Stroke Treatment (TOAST) classification system, which focuses on the pathophysiologic mechanism of ischemic stroke based on clinical features and the results of diagnostic investigations (brain imaging, cardiac investigations, and neurovascular imaging). The five etiologic subcategories in the TOAST classification system are large-artery stroke, cardioembolism, small-artery occlusion (or lacunar ischemic stroke), ischemic stroke of other determined etiology, and stroke of undetermined etiology.

Large-Artery Stroke

Large-artery stroke is usually a consequence of atherosclerosis in the extracranial (carotid or vertebral) and/or intracranial arteries (e.g., middle cerebral or basilar artery), with plaque rupture and

Table 147-1 Traditional Risk Factors for Ischemic Stroke

Risk Factor	OR (99% CI)
Hypertension (self-reported history)	2.37 (2.00-2.79)
Current smoking*	2.32 (1.91-2.81)
Diabetes mellitus	1.60 (1.29-1.99)
Ratio of apoB to apoA1	2.40 (1.86-3.11)
Obesity (waist-to-hip ratio)	1.69 (1.38-2.07)
Regular physical activity	0.68 (0.51-0.91)
Diet risk score	1.34 (1.09-1.65)
Alcohol consumption*	
1-30 Drinks per month	0.79 (0.63-1.00)
>30 Drinks per month	1.41 (1.09-1.82)
Psychosocial factors	
Psychosocial stress	1.30 (1.04-1.62)
Depression	1.47 (1.19-1.83)

From O'Donnell MJ, Xavier D, Lisheng L, et al: Risk factors for ischaemic and intracerebral haemorrhagic stroke in 22 countries (the INTERSTROKE study): A case-control study, *Lancet* 376:112, 2010.
apo, Apolipoprotein; *CI*, confidence interval; *OR*, odds ratio.
*Comparator for current smoker and alcohol intake is never or former.

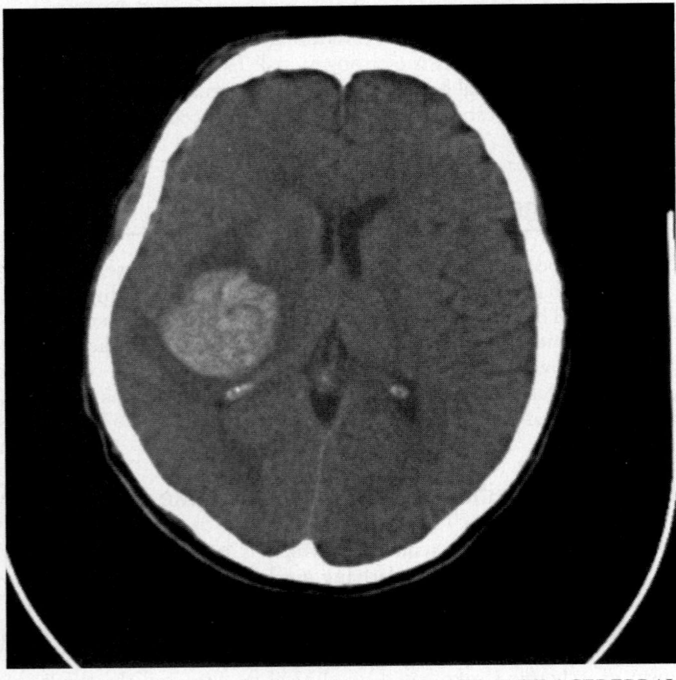

Figure 147-1 CT OF BRAIN WITH RIGHT INTRACEREBRAL HEMORRHAGE.

superimposed thrombus formation. Ischemic stroke may result from artery-to-artery thromboembolism with distal occlusion or, less commonly, by acute occlusion with resultant hypoperfusion (e.g., watershed infarction). Large-vessel atherosclerosis accounts for about 20% of all ischemic stroke in high-income countries and is predominantly extracranial in origin. Intracranial atherosclerosis has been reported to account for as high as 33% to 50% of ischemic strokes in parts of Asia (e.g., China and Thailand), but it is a less common cause of ischemic stroke in North America and Europe. Arterial dissection, the third leading cause of ischemic stroke in young people, can lead

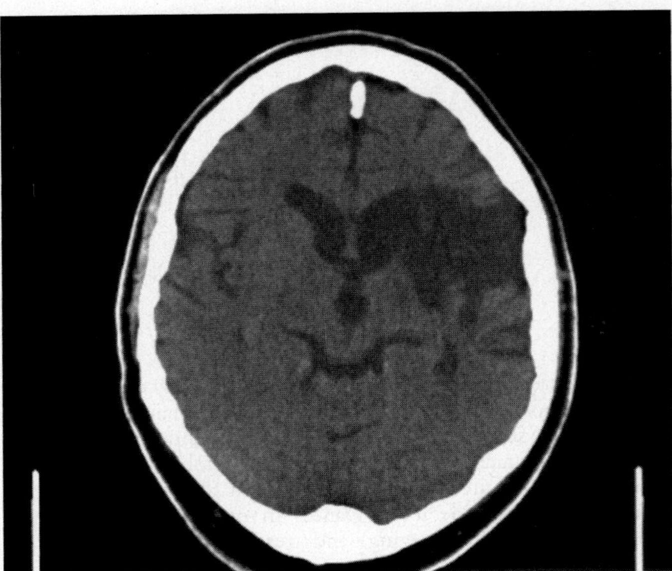

Figure 147-2 CT OF BRAIN WITH LEFT HEMISPHERIC ISCHEMIC STROKE.

to ischemic stroke by either local occlusion or distal thromboembolism. Predisposing factors for dissection are trauma and underlying arteriopathies, such as fibromuscular dysplasia. Less common large-vessel mechanisms of ischemic stroke include Moyamoya disease, Fabry disease, and large vessel arteritis (e.g., Takayasu arteritis and giant-cell arteritis).

Cardioembolism

This mechanism is responsible for approximately 14% to 30% of all ischemic strokes, with marked regional variations. There are a number of conditions that predispose to cardioembolism; emboli may originate from precardiac sources in the venous system (e.g., paradoxical embolism), intracardiac sources (e.g., atrial fibrillation) or postcardiac sources (e.g., aortic arch disease).

Precardiac. Paradoxical emboli are proposed to occur when emboli that arise in the venous circulation (e.g., from a deep vein thrombus) cross into the arterial circulation through a patent foramen ovale (PFO) or atrial septal defect (ASD), or through a pulmonary arteriovenous malformation (AVM). PFO is a common finding in the general population; occurring in about 20% of people have this finding. A number of observational studies have reported an association between first ischemic stroke and PFO, particularly in younger patients, but a PFO has not been shown to be a risk factor for recurrent ischemic stroke. An atrial septal aneurysm, which is a protrusion of part of the atrial septum through the fossa ovalis into the right and/or left atrium, is associated with an increased risk for ischemic stroke, especially in association with a PFO.

Intracardiac. Left-sided cardiac sources of emboli include left atrial thrombus secondary to atrial fibrillation or flutter; left ventricle thrombus subsequent to a transmural myocardial infarction, or akinetic segments of myocardium with a low ejection fraction; cardiac tumors such as left atrial myxoma; and abnormalities of the mitral valve (both native and artificial). Atrial fibrillation or flutter is a significant risk factor for stroke, and it is associated with a fivefold increase in risk. In North America and Europe, about 25% of all ischemic strokes are attributed to atrial fibrillation, a proportion that increases with advancing age. After acute myocardial infarction, mural thrombi can arise as a result of the presence of left ventricular aneurysms, akinetic segments of the left ventricular myocardium, or new-onset atrial fibrillation or flutter. Congestive heart failure is also an independent risk factor for stroke and is associated with a two- to threefold increase in the relative risk for ischemic stroke.

Valvular heart disease may involve native (e.g., rheumatic) or prosthetic heart valves. Of native valvular disease, mitral stenosis has the strongest association with ischemic stroke; mitral annular calcification and mitral valve prolapse have weaker associations. Mitral stenosis is commonly associated with atrial fibrillation, which further increases the risk of ischemic stroke. Emboli can also arise from valvular vegetations in nonbacterial thrombotic endocarditis or infective endocarditis. Mechanical mitral and aortic valves are associated with a sufficiently high risk for ischemic stroke that indefinite oral anticoagulant therapy is indicated; the risk for stroke is highest with mechanical mitral valves. Rheumatic heart disease still accounts for half of all cases of endocarditis in some regions of the world (e.g., India and Africa). Several epidemiologic studies have shown a link between ischemic stroke and *Trypanosoma cruzi* infection (Chagas disease) in South America.

Postcardiac. Postcardiac sources of embolism include atherosclerotic plaques in the aortic arch, proximal to the left subclavian artery; atheromatous debris or platelet emboli arising from these plaques may enter the cerebral circulation, leading to an ischemic stroke. The prevalence of severe atheromata of the aortic arch (>4 mm) in patients with ischemic stroke is approximately 30%, and their presence is associated with a fourfold increase in the risk for ischemic stroke and peripheral embolism. Although anatomically a large vessel source, aortic arch disease is usually included in cardiac causes of ischemic stroke, as it is most often identified by transesophageal echocardiography.

Small-Artery Occlusion

Approximately 20% of all ischemic strokes are due to lacunar or small-vessel infarcts. Lacunar infarcts are the result of occlusion of small, deep-penetrating arteries, such as the lenticulostriate branches of the anterior cerebral and middle cerebral arteries. The terminal pathophysiologic mechanism underlying small artery occlusion is believed to be local thrombosis secondary to microatheroma (lipid-laden macrophages, cholesterol deposits, and subintimal fibroblast proliferation) and lipohyalinosis (the intermediate stage between fibrinoid necrosis and microatheroma, which has characteristics of both arterial atheromatous lipid deposits and arteriolar [hyalinization] disease). Growing evidence supports a concept that damage to the glycocalyx by factors such as hyperglycemia, hypertension, and smoking contributes to vascular endothelial damage. Other causes of small-artery occlusion include microemboli from atherosclerotic plaques, polycythemia rubra vera, antiphospholipid antibodies, amyloid angiopathy, cerebral autosomal dominant arteriopathy with subcortical infarcts and leukoencephalopathy (CADASIL), cerebral autosomal recessive arteriopathy with subcortical infarcts and leukoencephalopathy (CARASIL), Sneddon syndrome, and various types of small-vessel arteritis. The combination of mitochondrial myopathy, encephalopathy, lactic acidosis, and stroke-like episodes (MELAS) is an inherited progressive disorder characterized by mitochondrial dysfunction and onset of stroke, typically before the age of 40. The mitochondrial angiopathy hypothesis suggests that the lesions are secondary to ischemia, which is caused by mitochondrial and vascular dysfunction in small cerebral arteries.

Ischemic Stroke of Other Determined Etiology

Cerebral Venous Sinus Thrombosis. Cerebral venous sinus thrombosis accounts for less than 1% of ischemic strokes and typically affects younger people. The superior sagittal, transverse and cavernous sinuses are those most commonly affected by thrombosis. Venous thrombosis in these sites results in localized edema and venous infarction, which often becomes hemorrhagic and may raise intracranial pressure. Reported risk factors for cerebral venous sinus thrombosis include inherited thrombophilias; acquired prothrombotic states such as antiphospholipid antibodies, pregnancy, and the puerperium; infections such as otitis, sinusitis, and mastoiditis; chronic inflammatory conditions such as Wegener granulomatosis and sarcoidosis; trauma such as head injury, dehydration, or injury to the jugular veins or sinuses during neurosurgical procedures.

Intracerebral Hemorrhage. Intracerebral hemorrhage accounts for approximately 10% to 15% of all strokes (a larger proportion is reported in middle- and low-income countries) and can be classified as either primary or secondary, depending on the underlying cause. Primary intracerebral hemorrhage accounts for about 80% to 90% of cases and is the result of spontaneous rupture of small intracerebral blood vessels, usually those damaged by chronic hypertension (and other vascular risk factors) or amyloid angiopathy. Antithrombotic therapy, particularly anticoagulant therapy, is an important risk factor for intracerebral hemorrhage. Secondary intracerebral hemorrhage occurs as a result of vascular abnormalities (e.g., ruptured saccular aneurysm, arteriovenous malformation), tumors (e.g., cavernous angioma, intracerebral neoplasm), impaired coagulation (e.g., due to oral anticoagulant drug use or bleeding disorders such as hemophilia or von Willebrand disease), hemorrhagic transformation of ischemic stroke, septic emboli, vasculitis, Moyamoya disease, or alcohol and/or illicit drug use (e.g., cocaine, amphetamines).

Subarachnoid Hemorrhage. Subarachnoid hemorrhage refers to bleeding within the subarachnoid space, which is the space between the arachnoid and pia mater. It accounts for about 5% of all strokes and is most commonly caused by rupture of an intracranial aneurysm (approximately 80% to 85% of cases). Idiopathic nonaneurysmal perimesencephalic hemorrhage accounts for about 10% of cases, whereas the remaining 5% are due to rare disorders, such as inflammatory lesions of cerebral arteries (e.g., mycotic aneurysm, polyarteritis nodosa, primary angiitis), noninflammatory lesions of intracerebral vessels (e.g., arterial dissection, cerebral arteriovenous malformations, cerebral amyloid angiopathy, cerebral venous thrombosis, Moyamoya disease), vascular lesions of the spinal cord (e.g., saccular aneurysm of the spinal artery, spinal arteriovenous malformation), coagulopathy (e.g., hemophilia, von Willebrand disease), sickle cell disease, tumors (e.g., malignant glioma), trauma, and drug use (cocaine, anticoagulants).

Stroke of Undetermined Etiology

In some cases, the cause of stroke cannot be definitively determined and the stroke is classified as "stroke of undetermined etiology". A stroke may be classified in this category when one of the following two conditions are met: (1) an extensive evaluation is negative, that includes large vessel imaging and complete cardiovascular assessment or; (2) the diagnostic evaluation is incomplete. Clearly, the most important determinant of the proportion of patients labeled as cryptogenic is the extent of the diagnostic testing, which makes between-study comparisons difficult.

Covert Stroke

Clinically overt stroke is considered to represent only a fraction of all episodes of stroke. The advent of contemporary magnetic resonance imaging (MRI) sequences has identified a large burden of subclinical cerebrovascular disease, which includes covert infarction, white matter hyperintensities, cerebral atrophy, and microbleeds. Covert stroke is common; for example, a systematic review of eight population-based studies reported a prevalence of "silent" brain infarcts in the general older adult population of 8% to 28%. Moreover, covert stroke has been associated with an increased risk of cognitive decline, dementia, depression, and gait impairment. Accordingly, the term *covert* has been adopted to replace the term *silent.*

Hematologic Disorders and Ischemic Stroke

Inherited Thrombophilias

In general, studies have reported either no association or a modest association between inherited thrombophilias and ischemic stroke. Metaanalyses of observational studies have failed to demonstrate a significant association between the factor V Leidin mutation and ischemic stroke in adults, although some small case-control studies have reported an increased risk for ischemic stroke in women with the Factor V Leiden mutation using oral contraceptives. Two large prospective population-based studies failed to demonstrate a significant association between the prothrombin mutation G20210A and ischemic stroke risk, although a large metaanalysis of 19 case control studies reported a modest association. There is no evidence to support an association between protein C, protein S, or antithrombin deficiency and ischemic stroke in adults.

Antiphospholipid Syndrome

Antiphospholipid syndrome is reviewed in Chapter 143. Stroke is the main acute arterial thrombotic complication of antiphospholipid syndrome and is reported to be the initial clinical manifestation in 13% of patients subsequently diagnosed with antiphospholipid antibody syndrome. However, the overall association between antiphospholipid antibodies (in the absence of other feature of the syndrome) and ischemic stroke is less certain. Anticardiolipin antibodies have been associated with ischemic stroke in some studies, especially in young women, but not in others. The lupus anticoagulant is a more potent risk factor for ischemic stroke than are antiphospholipid antibodies. For example, in the RATIO (Risk of Arterial Thrombosis in Relation to Oral Contraceptives) study, the odds ratio for lupus anticoagulant was 43.1 (95% CI, 12.2-152.2) compared with an odds ratio of 2.3 (95% CI, 1.4-3.7) for anti–β_2-glycoprotein I antibodies, with no significant association reported for anticardiolipin antibodies. Current American Heart Association (AHA) guidelines recommend oral anticoagulant therapy for the secondary prevention of ischemic stroke in patients with antiphospholipid syndrome; antiplatelet therapy is recommended for patients with ischemic stroke and anticardiolipin antibodies without other clinical features of antiphospholipid syndrome.

Sickle Cell Disease

This disorder is associated with an increased risk for stroke, particularly in those homozygous for the sickle cell gene. The risk for stroke is 11% at 20 years of age, increasing to 15% by 30 years and 24% by 45 years of age. Stroke may also be a clinical manifestation of heparin-induced thrombocytopenia. In one cohort study ($n = 906$), stroke was reported in 3.1% of patients with heparin-induced thrombocytopenia after 1 month of follow-up, with a reported 94% occurring due to ischemia.

Myeloproliferative Disorders

These disorders are associated with an increased risk for stroke. A large stroke registry reported that stroke was the presenting manifestation of a hematologic disorder in 1.3% (14/1099) of patients with acute stroke; myeloproliferative disorders were the most common hematologic disorder. Polycythemia vera is a risk factor for ischemic stroke. A randomized controlled trial of aspirin (100 mg daily) versus placebo in 518 patients with polycythemia rubra vera reported a rate of stroke (ischemic and hemorrhagic) of 1.2% in the aspirin group compared with 3.8% in the control group (RR 0.32; 95% CI, 0.09-1.16) over approximately 3 years of follow-up. Defective platelet function in patients with myeloproliferative conditions increases the risk for bleeding, and so intracerebral hemorrhage can also occur.

Thrombotic Thrombocytopenic Purpura

The risk for ischemic stroke is increased in this disorder, which is characterized by thrombocytopenia, microangiopathic hemolytic anemia, fever, renal failure, and neurologic abnormalities, including ischemic stroke.

Paraproteinemias

Waldenström macroglobulinemia, multiple myeloma, and POEMS syndrome (plasma-cell proliferative disorders, typically myeloma, polyneuropathy, and effects on many other organ systems) can be associated with an increased risk for stroke.

Genetic Risk Factors

A substantial body of evidence from twin, family, and animal studies supports a genetic contribution to stroke risk. However, very few genetic variants have shown convincingly positive associations with ischemic stroke in epidemiologic studies. According to a recent metaanalysis, the concordance rate for stroke is 65% higher in monozygotic twins than in dizygotic twins, ranging from 12.8% to 19.0% in monozygotic twins and 3.6% to 13.0% in dizygotic twins. Family history of stroke increases the risk for ischemic stroke by about 75%, and the presence of a first-degree relative with a history of hemorrhagic stroke is associated with a sixfold increase in the risk for hemorrhagic stroke. Rare Mendelian forms of stroke, such as CADASIL and CARASIL, have been described. These disorders manifest as small-vessel ischemic stroke. However, most single-gene disorders are uncommon and thus have limited impact on the wider population, despite their marked effect on individual risk in young populations. Beyond Mendelian forms of inheritance, very few common genetic variants have reliably been associated with sporadic, multifactorial cases of stroke.

CLINICAL MANIFESTATIONS

Clinical Presentation

Stroke is a clinical diagnosis, supported by the results of neuroimaging (CT or MRI of brain), but CT of the brain may be normal in patients with acute ischemic stroke. Stroke is characterized by a rapid onset, usually presenting with a focal neurologic deficit, lasting more than 24 hours or leading to death of a presumed vascular cause. Clinical episodes lasting less than 24 hours are classified as TIA. In about one-quarter of cases of TIA, there is evidence of ischemia on MRI imaging. Common presenting features include lateralizing weakness of the arms and/or legs, facial weakness, speech abnormalities (aphasia, dysarthria), visual loss (monocular visual loss or homonymous hemanopia), reduced level of consciousness, ataxia, diplopia, vertigo, and headache. A number of clinical conditions may mimic stroke. Among patients admitted to the hospital with a suspected stroke, only about two-thirds are subsequently diagnosed with stroke. Common mimics of stroke include migraine, seizures, syncope, hypoglycemia, primary or secondary brain tumors, transient global amnesia, or toxic-metabolic disturbances with delirium.

Ischemic Stroke Versus Intracerebral Hemorrhage

Patients with ischemic stroke and intracerebral hemorrhage have similar presentations. Although some clinical features are more typically associated with intracerebral hemorrhage (e.g., coma, neck stiffness, seizures, vomiting, and headache) than with ischemic stroke, neuroimaging is required to discriminate between ischemia and hemorrhage. Therefore CT or MRI imaging of the brain is mandatory in all patients with acute stroke.

Measuring Severity of Stroke

Many scales are available to determine stroke severity. Examples include the Scandinavian Stroke Scale, the Canadian Stroke Scale, and the National Institutes of Health Stroke Scale (NIHSS). Of these, the one most widely studied and most often used in clinical practices is the NIHSS. Other scales (e.g., Hunt and Hess; Fisher) are used to measure stroke severity in patients with subarachnoid hemorrhage.

Risk for Stroke After Transient Ischemic Attack

The ABCD2 score is a validated clinical prediction for stroke in patients with TIA. Points are scored for each of the following factors: age 60 years or older (1); blood pressure 140/90 mm Hg or higher on first evaluation (1); clinical symptoms of focal weakness with the spell (2) or speech impairment without weakness (1); duration of 10 to 59 minutes (1) or duration of 60 minutes or longer (2); and diabetes (1). In combined validation cohorts, the 2-day risks for stroke were 0% for scores of 0 or 1; 1.3% for scores of 2 or 3; 4.1% for scores of 4 or 5; and 8.1% for scores of 6 or 7. The presence of a new infarct on brain imaging in patients with a classic time definition of TIA is associated with a 2- to 15-fold increase in the subsequent short-term risk for stroke.

INVESTIGATIONS

CT of the Brain

Neuroimaging is required for valid distinction between ischemic and hemorrhagic stroke. CT of the brain is widely available in most acute hospital settings and reliably excludes intracerebral hemorrhage. On CT of the brain, early features of ischemia include loss of distinction between grey and white matter, sulcal effacement, loss of definition of the insula, and evolving areas of hypodensity. Scoring systems (e.g., ASPECT score) may be used to quantify the burden of ischemia, which predicts the risk for intracerebral hemorrhage in patients receiving thrombolysis. However, subarachnoid hemorrhage is not reliably excluded by CT alone; therefore a lumbar puncture and CSF analysis are also needed to reliably exclude this diagnosis in those with suspected subarachnoid hemorrhage who have a normal CT of the brain.

Magnetic Resonance Imaging

MRI is superior to CT for detecting acute ischemia, but in practice it is limited by patient contraindications and availability, especially in the acute setting. Diffusion-weighted imaging (DWI) may identify acute ischemia within 3 to 6 hours of symptom onset. For the diagnosis of intracerebral hemorrhage, MRI with GRE sequence has been reported to be similar to CT of brain (96% concordance).

Neurovascular Imaging

Extracranial and intracranial stenosis may be detected using ultrasound, CT angiography, MR angiography, or formal angiography. Ultrasound is a noninvasive, relatively inexpensive, and widely available imaging modality, but it is dependent on ultrasonographer experience and skill. Transcranial Doppler may be used to detect intracranial large vessel stenosis and has also been shown to risk-stratify patients with carotid stenosis by identifying those with microembolic signals. CT and MR angiography provide more precise measurements of large vessel stenosis than does ultrasound imaging.

Cardiac Workup

An electrocardiogram to identify atrial fibrillation/flutter or evidence of previous myocardial infarction should be performed in all patients. In addition, Holter/cardiac monitoring will reveal atrial fibrillation in a further 5% of patients with acute ischemic stroke. Transthoracic echocardiography has a low yield in patients without a previous cardiac history and with a normal cardiac examination. The routine use of transesophageal echocardiography is controversial, but this investigation is essential in patients with suspected endocarditis. A patent foramen ovale can be identified with a bubble study while performing transthoracic or transesophageal echocardiography. Although transesophageal echocardiography will detect potential etiologies of ischemic stroke in a relatively large proportion of patients, such as patent foramen ovale, atrial septal aneurysm, or aortic arch disease, the treatment implications of these findings are less certain (see later section on secondary prevention).

All patients should be screened for vascular risk factors, including hypertension, fasting lipid profile, serum glucose, and HbA1c. Coagulation profiles are required in all patients with acute ischemic stroke. Other investigations may include a complete blood count and erythrocyte sedimentation rate (ESR), as well as tests for C-receptive protein, antiphospholipid antibodies, lupus anticoagulant, troponin, blood cultures, antineutrophil cytoplasmic antibodies (ANCA), and antinuclear antibodies (ANA).

THERAPY

A complete review of the management of stroke is beyond the scope of this chapter. Instead, we will provide an overview of acute and chronic management of patients with acute stroke.

Reperfusion Therapy for Acute Ischemic Stroke

Thrombolysis for Acute Ischemic Stroke

Intravenous tPA is the most rigorously evaluated thrombolytic intervention in acute ischemic stroke. Current guidelines recommend administration of tPA to patients with acute ischemic stroke within 3 hours of symptom onset or within 3 hours since patient was last seen normal (e.g., patient presents with symptoms on waking). The recently published European Cooperative Acute Stroke Study (ECASS III) trial reported a reduction in stroke severity even when tPA was administered between 3 and 4.5 hours. A recent metaanalysis of trials (n = 3670) that evaluated tPA in acute ischemic stroke reported adjusted odds ratio for favorable 3-month outcomes of 2.55 (95% CI, 1.44-4.52) for tPA administration within 0 to 90 minutes, 1.64 (1.12-2.40) for 91 to 180 minutes, 1.34 (1.06-1.68) for 181 to 270 minutes, and 1.22 (0.92-1.61) for 271 to 360 minutes. The main complication of tPA is intracerebral hemorrhage. In the above metaanalysis, large parenchymal hemorrhage was seen in 96 (5.2%) of 1850 patients assigned to tPA compared with 18 (1.0%) of 1820 controls (Table 147-2). An ongoing randomized controlled trial (International Stroke Trial [IST]-3) is evaluating tPA administered within 6 hours of symptoms onset in 3100 patients with acute ischemic stroke; this trial should provide key information on the effectiveness of tPA administration between 3 and 6 hours and in older adults.

Intraarterial Thrombolysis

Intraarterial thrombolysis within 6 hours of acute ischemic stroke has been evaluated in three small clinical trials (n = 334). This treatment is associated with an increased odds of a good functional outcome. However, no trials have compared intraarterial thrombolysis with intravenous thrombolysis. Current guidelines suggest intraarterial thrombolysis within 6 hours of symptom onset for patients with a contraindication to intravenous thrombolysis and who have proximal

Table 147-2 Eligibility Criteria and Contraindications for Acute Thrombolysis in Acute Ischemic Stroke

ELIGIBILITY CRITERIA
Diagnosis of ischemic stroke causing measurable neurologic deficit
Neurologic signs not minor or isolated (caution to be exercised in treating patients with major deficits)
Onset of symptoms <3 hours before beginning treatment (some guidelines suggest up to 4.5 hours)
Neurologic signs not clearing spontaneously
Symptoms of stroke not suggestive of subarachnoid hemorrhage
Patient and/or family members aware of potential risks and benefits of treatment
CONTRAINDICATIONS FOR THROMBOLYSIS
Evidence of intracranial hemorrhage on CT
Head trauma or prior stroke in previous 3 months
Myocardial infarction in previous 3 months
Gastrointestinal or urinary tract hemorrhage in previous 21 days
Arterial puncture at a noncompressible site in previous 7 days
Major surgery in previous 14 days
History of previous intracranial hemorrhage
Blood pressure elevated (systolic >185 mm Hg and diastolic >110 mm Hg)
Evidence of active bleeding or acute trauma (fracture) on examination
Taking an oral anticoagulant or, if anticoagulant being taken, INR ≥ 1.7
If received heparin in previous 48 hours, aPTT outside the normal range.
Platelet count ≤ 100 000 mm^3
Blood glucose concentration ≤ 50 mg/dL (2.7 mmol/L)
Seizure with postictal residual neurologic impairments
CT showing a multilobar infarction (hypodensity >1/3 cerebral hemisphere)

cerebral artery occlusions. However, limited access to interventional neuroradiology services has been a major limitation to the use of this intervention and to its evaluation in large-scale trials.

Mechanical Clot Retrieval

Mechanical thrombectomy has been evaluated in cohort studies but there are no randomized controlled trials to date.

Acute Stroke Unit

Organized stroke unit care in a dedicated, geographically identified ward with multidisciplinary teams that exclusively manage patients with stroke is associated with improved outcomes in patients with acute stroke. A metaanalysis of 26 trials ($n = 5592$) reported a reduction in death at 1 year (OR 0.86; 95% CI, 0.76-0.98) and death or dependency at 1 year (OR 0.82; 95% CI, 0.73-0.92). Unlike acute thrombolysis, stroke unit care is generalizable to the majority of patients with acute stroke. Beneficial results were independent of age, sex, or stroke severity and appeared to be more likely when the stroke unit was located in a separate geographic area within the hospital. Organized stroke care is associated with improved outcomes for several reasons, including early mobilization, reduced risk of medical complications such as aspiration pneumonia, fever prevention, and reduced frequency of urinary tract infections, falls, and delirium. Prompt evaluation of swallow function and compliance with speech pathology guidelines in relation to safe swallow practices have been shown to reduce the risk for aspiration pneumonia in stroke patients.

Blood Pressure in Acute Stroke

Although hypertension is the most important risk factor for both ischemic and hemorrhagic stroke, the optimal approach to managing elevated blood pressure in the acute setting remains uncertain. The recently published Scandinavian Candesartan Acute Stroke Trial (SCAST) randomized 2029 patients with acute stroke (ischemic or hemorrhagic) and systolic blood pressures of 140 mm Hg or higher to escalating doses of candesartan (4-16 mg on day 1 to days 3-7) or to placebo. No difference was observed in the rate of recurrent cardiovascular events, and there was a suggestion that lower blood pressures were associated with poorer functional outcome at 6 months. The Intensive Blood Pressure Reduction in Acute Cerebral Haemorrhage Trial (INTERACT), a phase II trial of patients with intracerebral hemorrhage and high blood pressure (150-220 mm Hg systolic), suggested that early intensive blood pressure reduction was safe and associated with reduced hematoma growth. A phase III trial (INTERACT II) is now underway to examine the effect of this blood pressure strategy on clinical outcomes.

Antithrombotic Therapy in Acute Ischemic Stroke

Based on the results of two large randomized controlled trials (IST and the Chinese Acute Stroke Trial [CAST]), aspirin reduces the risk for recurrent stroke and mortality in patients with acute ischemic stroke. The risk of the composite outcome of recurrent stroke of any type (including hemorrhagic stroke and hemorrhagic transformation of ischemic stroke), and death from any cause was reduced by 11% during the treatment period. In general, treatment doses of parenteral anticoagulants are not indicated in acute ischemic stroke, other than in patients with cerebral venous sinus thrombosis. Although treatment doses of heparins are commonly used in patients with extracranial dissection, clinical trials comparing antiplatelet therapy with anticoagulant therapy in these patients have not been performed.

Carotid Endarterectomy and Stenting

The European Carotid Surgery Trial (ECST) and the North American Symptomatic Carotid Endarterectomy Trial (NASCET) are the largest trials to evaluate carotid endarterectomy (CEA) in patients with recent ischemic stroke and TIA. Based on the results of these trials, current guidelines recommend CEA in patients with 70% to 99% stenosis of the ipsilateral carotid artery, provided that the perioperative morbidity and mortality are estimated to be less than 6%. Although patients with stenosis of 50% to 69% also benefit from CEA, the benefit is more modest and CEA is only recommended for selected patients based on age, comorbidities, time from stroke/TIA onset, and operative risk. Time from symptom onset to CEA is the primary determinant of the absolute risk reduction obtained with the procedure, with most of the benefit realized when CEA is performed within 2 weeks of presentation. Carotid stenting, which has been compared with CEA in patients with recent stroke and TIA, is not superior to CEA. However, although CEA remains the gold standard for patients with symptomatic significant carotid stenosis, carotid stenting is an alternative for patients with over 70% stenosis who are considered unsuitable for CEA (e.g., estimated to be at high operative risk).

Intracranial Stenting

For patients with large-vessel intracranial disease, a recent clinical trial (SAMMPRIS) did not report a benefit of endovascular stenting (plus aggressive medical management) over aggressive medical management alone. This trial was stopped early because of a higher rate of stroke and death at 30 days in the endovascular group.

Prevention of Venous Thromboembolism

See Chapter 144 for this discussion.

Acute Management of Intracerebral Hemorrhage

Management of intracerebral hemorrhage includes both medical and surgical components. Initial strategies include monitoring in an intensive care setting in appropriate patients, intubation in those with reduced consciousness, discontinuation of antithrombotic therapy and immediate reversal of anticoagulant therapy (see Chapter 151), administration of antipyretic medications to febrile patients, insulin for hyperglycemia, and venous thromboembolism prophylaxis (e.g., compression stockings). Raised intracranial pressure (ICP) can occur as a result of the hemorrhage itself or because of secondary edema. Management of increased ICP includes elevating the head of the bed to 30 degrees, analgesia, and sedation. More aggressive therapies include osmotic diuresis with mannitol, drainage of cerebrospinal fluid using a ventricular catheter (ventriculostomy), hyperventilation, and neuromuscular blockade. Antiepileptic therapy should be administered to control seizures in patients with intracerebral hemorrhage. Seizure prophylaxis is not recommended in current guidelines. The Surgical Trial in IntraCerebral Haemorrhage (STICH trial; n = 1033), which compared early surgery with medical management in patients with intracerebral hemorrhage within 72 to 96 hours of onset, failed to demonstrate a significant benefit of early surgery. However, uncertainty remains in some patient groups, and current guidelines suggest craniotomy for those with a lobar bleed of more than 30 mL located within 1 cm of the brain surface. Surgical evacuation of intracerebral hemorrhages is recommended for patients with cerebellar hemorrhages over 3 cm in diameter who have evidence of deterioration, brainstem compression, or hydrocephalus. Ventriculostomy with external drainage may be required for patients with intraventricular extension of an intracranial hemorrhage and a deteriorating level of consciousness. Although initial studies with recombinant factor VIIa (rFVIIa) yielded promising results, such treatment failed to reduce in death or severe disability at 90 days compared with placebo in a large phase III study, and higher-dose FVIIa administration (80 mcg/kg) was associated with a higher rate of serious adverse arterial thromboembolic events (myocardial infarction or cerebral infarction) in the 80 mcg/kg group compared with placebo. Current guidelines suggest that rFVIIa is investigational and should not be used outside of a clinical trial.

Stroke Rehabilitation

Stroke rehabilitation should commence as soon as possible. Animal models of neuroplasticity suggest that training results in upregulation of growth-promoting factors primarily in the first 4 weeks after the stroke, but recovery can continue for months or years after stroke. Good outcomes from stroke rehabilitation are associated with high patient (and family) motivation and engagement. Substantial evidence supports well-coordinated multidisciplinary team care (nursing, physiotherapy, occupational therapy, speech therapy, dietetics, and social work) as the basis for delivery of stroke rehabilitation. This care can be provided in the stroke unit setting or by early supported discharge teams in the patient's own home. Both strategies have been shown to improve independence in stroke patients. For older patients with stroke, physical rehabilitation in long-term care facilities is effective and has been shown to improve independence.

Chronic Secondary Prevention of Ischemic Stroke

Case Study

A 72-year-old man presented with right-sided weakness and expressive aphasia 4 weeks ago. CT scan of the brain revealed an ischemic stroke in the left hemisphere. He was admitted to a stroke unit, and after completing a rehabilitation program, he was discharged home. Etiologic investigations included ultrasound of carotids (<20% stenosis), Holter monitor (no arrhythmia), and transthoracic echocardiogram with bubble study, which revealed a small patent foramen ovale. He is known to have hypertension; his serum glucose level and HbA1c were normal. He was initiated on aspirin at the time of diagnosis. His blood pressure in the clinic today is 152/92 mm Hg, and he is currently taking perindopril (8 mg daily). His fasting LDL level was 140 mg/dL.

Antithrombotic Therapy

Acceptable regimens include aspirin, clopidogrel, or aspirin-dipyridamole; any one of these is recommended by current guidelines for secondary prevention of noncardioembolic ischemic stroke. The combination of aspirin plus clopidogrel should not be used because this regimen was not superior to clopidogrel alone in the MATCH trial and was associated with a higher risk of bleeding. If the patient had atrial fibrillation or a mechanical heart valve, oral anticoagulation therapy should be given for secondary prevention of ischemic stroke (see box on When Should Warfarin Be Started After Acute Ischemic Stroke in Patients With Atrial Fibrillation?). Although the new oral thrombin or factor Xa inhibitors (see Chapter 151) have not been specifically evaluated for secondary prevention in patients with atrial fibrillation, they are likely to provide the same risk reduction compared with warfarin as they do in primary prevention. Oral anticoagulants are not superior to aspirin for secondary prevention of stroke in patients with noncardioembolic ischemic stroke (WARSS and ESPRIT trials) or in patients with intracranial stenosis (WASID trial).

Lipid Modification

Current guidelines recommend statin therapy in patients with LDL levels of 100 mg/dL or higher. The SPARCL trial, which randomized 4731 patients with stroke/TIA and LDL levels between 100 and 190 mg/dL to atorvastatin 80 mg daily or placebo, reported a 16% reduction in recurrent stroke over approximately 5 years of follow-up with statin therapy (HR 0.84; 95% CI, 0.71-0.99).

Blood Pressure

The largest secondary prevention blood pressure study was the PROGRESS trial, which evaluated the use of perindopril plus indapamide. The combination reduced blood pressure by 12/5 mm Hg

When Should Warfarin Be Started After Acute Ischemic Stroke in Patients With Atrial Fibrillation?

The optimal timing of introduction of oral anticoagulation in patients with acute ischemic stroke and atrial fibrillation is uncertain, and there are variations in clinical practice. We initiate all patients on aspirin in the acute setting, and we base the timing of warfarin on the severity of stroke, the size of infarction, and comorbidities that may increase the risk for intracerebral hemorrhage. In patients with acute transient ischemic attack or in those with a minor ischemic stroke who do not have a large area of acute infarction, we usually initiate warfarin within 1 to 2 days, provided there are no other contraindications. For those with moderate or severe stroke with a moderate to large area of infarction, aspirin without anticoagulant therapy is recommended in the acute phase. Warfarin may be initiated 5 to 7 days after stroke onset—after excluding hemorrhagic transformation on neuroimaging. In patients with large infarcts or in those with evidence of hemorrhagic transformation, progressing stroke, or uncontrolled hypertension, initiation of warfarin should be delayed beyond 14 days. We stop aspirin once a therapeutic anticoagulant effect with warfarin is achieved, unless there is an indication for the combination of aspirin plus warfarin (e.g., coronary stent).

and stroke risk by 43% (CI 30%-54%). The combination of perindopril plus a diuretic produced greater reductions in blood pressure and larger risk reductions than therapy with perindopril alone. Current guidelines recommend a target blood pressure of 140/90 mm Hg or less.

Patent Foramen Ovale Closure

The recent CLOSURE trial failed to demonstrate a benefit of patent foramen ovale closure after acute ischemic stroke, and the risk for new atrial fibrillation was higher in the closure group than in those managed medically. Studies evaluating other closure devices after ischemic stroke are ongoing.

Lifestyle Modification

Lifestyle modification remains a cornerstone of stroke prevention. These measures include smoking cessation, moderate physical activity, weight reduction in those who are overweight or obese, a heart-healthy diet with increased fruit and vegetable intake, reduced salt intake in those who consume high-salt diets, and moderate alcohol consumption.

PROGNOSIS

Prognosis after stroke depends on the age of the patients, the etiology of the stroke, the severity of the neurologic deficits (and consequent level of dependence), and the burden of comorbid conditions. In a large cohort study that included 10,399 patients hospitalized with stroke in the United States, the 1- and 4-year mortality rates were 24.5% and 41.3%, respectively, and the 1- and 4-year risks of recurrent stroke were 8.0% and 18.1%, respectively. In that study, and in others, mortality was higher in patients with intracerebral or subarachnoid hemorrhage. Early causes of death are usually neurologic in origin (cerebral edema, raised intracranial pressure) or medical complications of dependence (e.g., aspiration pneumonia). On longer-term follow-up, most deaths are cardiovascular in origin. Of patients who survive stroke, two-thirds are left with chronic disability. In addition, patients with stroke are at increased risk for myocardial infarction, hip fracture, pneumonia, and repeated hospital admission. Other common chronic complications of stroke include seizure disorders, cognitive impairment and dementia, depression, and chronic pain syndromes (e.g., central post-stroke pain).

FUTURE DIRECTIONS

Most of our knowledge about the epidemiology of stroke comes from studies in North America and Europe, with considerably less data derived from middle and low-income countries. Ongoing large epidemiologic studies (e.g., INTERSTROKE) will provide data on regional variations in the importance of risk factors for stroke. In addition, a number of large ongoing epidemiologic collaborative studies (International Stroke Genetics Consortium) will clarify the role of genetics in the pathogenesis of stroke. Population-based interventions to reduce the burden of stroke will be an important focus of future research and will include interventions to reduce excess salt intake and the use of combination cardioprotective therapies (e.g., Polycap) in high-risk populations. In patients with TIA and minor ischemic stroke, a phase II trial (FASTER) suggests that the combination aspirin plus clopidogrel may be superior to aspirin alone; a phase III trial will clarify the role of dual antiplatelet therapy in this setting. The Efficacy of Nitric Oxide in Stroke (ENOS) trial is evaluating the effectiveness of transdermal glyceryl trinitrate in acute stroke. Other ongoing trials will determine the role of acute interventions designed to reduce the severity of stroke (e.g., albumin, hypothermic interventions, magnesium, or erythropoietin). For secondary prevention, ongoing trials will help to clarify the optimal antithrombotic therapy and target blood pressure for patients with small-vessel disease (Secondary Prevention of Small Subcortical Strokes [SPS-3]), the utility of closure devices in patients with a patent foramen ovale, and the usefulness of anticoagulant therapy for aortic arch disease (Aortic Arch-Related Cerebral Hazard [ARCH] trial).

SUGGESTED READINGS

Albers GW, Amarenco P, Easton JD, et al: Antithrombotic and thrombolytic therapy for ischemic stroke: American College of Chest Physicians Evidence-Based Clinical Practice Guidelines (8th Edition). *Chest* 133:630S, 2008.

Amarenco P, Bogousslavsky J, Callahan A, III, et al: High-dose atorvastatin after stroke or transient ischemic attack. *N Engl J Med* 355:549, 2006.

Berge E, Sandercock P: Anticoagulants for acute ischemic stroke. *Adv Neurol* 92:257, 2003.

Broderick JP, Meyers PM: Acute stroke therapy at the crossroads. *JAMA* 306:2026, 2011.

Chimowitz MI, Lynn MJ, Derdeyn CP, et al: Stenting versus aggressive medical therapy for intracranial arterial stenosis. *N Engl J Med* 365:993, 2011.

Diener HC, Sacco RL, Yusuf S, et al: Effects of aspirin plus extended-release dipyridamole versus clopidogrel and telmisartan on disability and cognitive function after recurrent stroke in patients with ischaemic stroke in the Prevention Regimen for Effectively Avoiding Second Strokes (PRoFESS) trial: A double-blind, active and placebo-controlled study. *Lancet Neurol* 7:875, 2008.

Ederle J, Dobson J, Featherstone RL, et al: Carotid artery stenting compared with endarterectomy in patients with symptomatic carotid stenosis (International Carotid Stenting Study): An interim analysis of a randomised controlled trial. *Lancet* 375:985, 2010.

Furie KL, Kasner SE, Adams RJ, et al: Guidelines for the prevention of stroke in patients with stroke or transient ischemic attack: A guideline for healthcare professionals from the American Heart Association/American Stroke Association. *Stroke* 42:227, 2011.

Goldstein LB, Bushnell CD, Adams RJ, et al: Guidelines for the primary prevention of stroke: A guideline for healthcare professionals from the American Heart Association/American Stroke Association. *Stroke* 42:517, 2011.

Halkes PH, van GJ, Kappelle LJ, et al: Aspirin plus dipyridamole versus aspirin alone after cerebral ischaemia of arterial origin (ESPRIT): Randomised controlled trial. *Lancet* 367:1665, 2006.

Koton S, Rothwell PM: Performance of the ABCD and ABCD2 scores in TIA patients with carotid stenosis and atrial fibrillation. *Cerebrovasc Dis* 24:231, 2007.

Langhorne P, Bernhardt J, Kwakkel G: Stroke rehabilitation. *Lancet* 377:1693, 2011.

Lees KR, Bluhmki E, von KR, et al: Time to treatment with intravenous alteplase and outcome in stroke: An updated pooled analysis of ECASS, ATLANTIS, NINDS, and EPITHET trials. *Lancet* 375:1695, 2010.

Lip GY, Tse HF, Lane DA: Atrial fibrillation. *Lancet* 379:648, 2011.

Morgenstern LB, Hemphill JC, III, Anderson C, et al: Guidelines for the management of spontaneous intracerebral hemorrhage: A guideline for healthcare professionals from the American Heart Association/American Stroke Association. *Stroke* 41:2108, 2010.

O'Donnell MJ, Xavier D, Liu L, et al: Risk factors for ischaemic and intracerebral haemorrhagic stroke in 22 countries (the INTERSTROKE study): A case-control study. *Lancet* 376:112, 2010.

Rothwell PM, Algra A, Amarenco P: Medical treatment in acute and long-term secondary prevention after transient ischaemic attack and ischaemic stroke. *Lancet* 377:1681, 2011.

Rothwell PM, Eliasziw M, Gutnikov SA, et al: Endarterectomy for symptomatic carotid stenosis in relation to clinical subgroups and timing of surgery. *Lancet* 363:915, 2004.

Sandercock P, Lindley R, Wardlaw J, et al: Update on the third international stroke trial (IST-3) of thrombolysis for acute ischaemic stroke and baseline features of the 3035 patients recruited. *Trials* 12:252, 2011.

Sandercock PA, Counsell C, Gubitz GJ, et al: Antiplatelet therapy for acute ischaemic stroke. *Cochrane Database Syst Rev* CD000029, 2008.

Sandercock PA, Counsell C, Tseng MC: Low-molecular-weight heparins or heparinoids versus standard unfractionated heparin for acute ischaemic stroke. *Cochrane Database Syst Rev* CD000119, 2008.

Sandset EC, Bath PM, Boysen G et al: The angiotensin-receptor blocker candesartan for treatment of acute stroke (SCAST): A randomised, placebo-controlled, double-blind trial. *Lancet* 377:741, 2011.

Tomaselli GF: Prevention of cardiovascular disease and stroke: Meeting the challenge. *JAMA* 306:2147, 2011.

Yuan ZH, Jiang JK, Huang WD, et al: A meta-analysis of the efficacy and safety of recombinant activated factor VII for patients with acute intracerebral hemorrhage without hemophilia. *J Clin Neurosci* 17:685, 2010.

CHAPTER 148

ACUTE CORONARY SYNDROMES

John W. Eikelboom and Jeffrey I. Weitz

Acute coronary syndromes (ACS) lead to millions of hospital admissions worldwide each year and are a leading cause of death. Antithrombotic therapies are a cornerstone in the immediate and long-term management of ACS, reducing the risk of myocardial infarction (MI) and death in both medically and invasively managed patients. This chapter reviews fibrinolytic, antiplatelet, and anticoagulant therapies in the treatment of patients with ACS and provides a practical guide to several common hemostatic and thrombotic problems encountered in this patient population.

CLASSIFICATION

The clinical classification of ACS is based on the electrocardiogram (ECG) at the time of presentation and on blood levels of cardiac biomarkers (creatine kinase, troponin). Patients with ST-segment elevation on the ECG and elevated cardiac biomarkers are diagnosed with ST-segment elevation MI (STEMI). Patients with non–ST-segment elevation (NSTE) ACS are subdivided according to whether or not they have elevated blood levels of cardiac biomarkers; those with elevated cardiac biomarkers are diagnosed with non–ST-segment elevation MI (NSTEMI), and those without elevated cardiac biomarkers are diagnosed with unstable angina (UA).[1-3]

PATHOPHYSIOLOGY

Atherothrombosis plays a central role in the pathogenesis of ACS.[4] Hypertension, abnormal blood glucose levels, dyslipidemia, and toxins contained in tobacco cause endothelial injury. Lipid accumulation and the recruitment of macrophages, smooth muscle cells, and fibroblasts to the site of injury results in the formation of increasingly complex and unstable plaques with a necrotic core and fibrous cap. Disruption of the fibrous cap by shear forces and its degradation by enzymatic and cellular processes expose the plaque contents to the blood. Platelets adhere to exposed subendothelial proteins and become activated and aggregate. Exposed tissue factor promotes thrombin generation on cellular surfaces, further promoting the formation of a platelet-fibrin thrombus that can occlude coronary blood flow. These processes are described in more detail in Chapter 146.

The clinical manifestations of coronary atherothrombosis are influenced by the extent and duration of obstruction to blood flow and the presence or absence of a collateral circulation. Patients with minor plaques that do not significantly impair blood flow generally remain asymptomatic. Patients with significant flow-limiting plaques may develop ischemic symptoms (e.g., chest pain, breathlessness) during exertion when myocardial oxygen demand exceeds supply. Patients with acute plaque rupture with superimposed thrombus formation that completely obstructs coronary blood flow typically present with STEMI unless there is an adequate collateral circulation. If obstruction to blood flow is transient or partial, patients typically present with NSTE ACS. If myocardial ischemia results in ventricular fibrillation, sudden cardiac death supervenes.

ANTITHROMBOTIC MANAGEMENT

The goal of antithrombotic therapies in patients with ACS is to facilitate lysis of intracoronary thrombus and prevent new thrombus formation at the site of plaque disruption. Antithrombotic drugs are also used to prevent thrombus formation on catheters and stents and to prevent and treat left ventricular thrombus formation.

Although the pathophysiology is similar irrespective of whether patients present with STEMI or NSTE ACS, only STEMI patients benefit from immediate reperfusion therapy. Most patients with NSTEMI do not have an occluded infarct-related coronary artery. Instead, they develop infarction as a consequence of distal embolization of thrombus.

REPERFUSION THERAPY FOR ST-SEGMENT ELEVATION MYOCARDIAL INFARCTION

Effective approaches to coronary reperfusion include mechanical (primary percutaneous coronary intervention) and pharmacologic (fibrinolytic therapy) methods.

Primary Percutaneous Coronary Intervention

Primary percutaneous coronary intervention (PCI) is preferred over fibrinolytic therapy in patients with STEMI because it produces higher patency rates and does not cause intracranial bleeding. Unlike fibrinolysis, which only treats the thrombus, primary PCI also allows treatment of the underlying atherosclerotic plaque. However, many centers lack the facilities and expertise to perform urgent coronary interventions, and only a minority of STEMI patients worldwide is treated with primary PCI.[5,6] Patients undergoing primary PCI are routinely treated with anticoagulant and antiplatelet therapy (discussed in sections on antiplatelet therapy and anticoagulant therapy).

Fibrinolytic Therapy

Fibrinolytic drugs are plasminogen activators that initiate fibrinolysis by converting plasminogen to plasmin. Plasmin degrades fibrin resulting in clot lysis and recanalization of thrombotic occlusion. Restoration of coronary blood flow limits infarct size and improves myocardial function and survival.

The pharmacologic characteristics of the fibrinolytic drugs most commonly used in the management of ACS are summarized in Table 148-1. Streptokinase was the first agent to be evaluated in large-scale randomized controlled trials. A non–fibrin-specific agent, streptokinase, indirectly activates plasminogen, but the more fibrin-specific agents alteplase, reteplase, and tenecteplase directly convert plasminogen to plasmin. Reteplase and tenecteplase have longer half-lives than alteplase, enabling them to be given by double- or single-bolus injection, respectively, which simplifies administration. The direct-acting fibrinolytic agents are more fibrin specific than streptokinase because

Table 148-1 Pharmacologic Characteristics of Fibrinolytic Drugs Used in the Management of Patients With ST-Segment Elevation Myocardial Infarction

Characteristic	Streptokinase	Alteplase	Reteplase	Tenecteplase
Fibrin specificity*	–	++	+	+++
Dose	1.5 million units	100 mg	20 U	30-50 mg
Administration	Infusion over 30-60 minutes	Bolus 15 mg; then infusion 0.75 mg/kg (maximum, 50 mg) over 30 minutes, 0.5 mg/kg (maximum, 35 mg) over the next 60 minutes	Double bolus, 10 U over 2 minutes; then repeat 10 U bolus at 30 minutes	Single weight-adjusted bolus, <60 kg = 30 mg, 60 to 69 kg = 35 mg, 70 to 79 kg = 40 mg, 80 to 89 kg = 45 mg, ≥90 kg = 50 mg
Half-life (min)	18-23	3-4	18	20
Adjunctive antiplatelet therapy[†]	Aspirin	Aspirin	Aspirin	Aspirin
Adjunctive anticoagulant therapy	Heparin in patients at high risk of thromboembolism[‡]	Heparin 60 U/kg bolus (maximum, 4000 U); 12 U/kg/hr (maximum, 1000 U/hr)	Heparin 60 U/kg bolus (maximum, 4000 U); 12 U/kg/hr (maximum, 1000 U/hr)	Heparin 60 U/kg bolus (maximum, 4000 U); 12 U/kg/hr (maximum, 1000 U/hr)

*Less fibrin specificity is associated with more systemic fibrinogen depletion.
[†]Fibrinolytic drugs were evaluated on a background of aspirin, but the addition of clopidogrel to aspirin was subsequently shown to provide incremental benefit.
[‡]High-risk patients include those with large or anterior myocardial infarction, atrial fibrillation, known left ventricular thrombus, or previous thromboembolism.

they bind to fibrin where they convert fibrin-bound plasminogen to plasmin. Consequently, these agents produce a less marked systemic lytic state than streptokinase, which has no fibrin affinity. Avoidance of a systemic lytic state is an important potential advantage of fibrin-specific drugs because this can be expected to be associated with a lower risk of bleeding complications.

Initial trials with streptokinase established the efficacy of fibrinolytic therapy for reduction in the risk of MI and death; subsequent trials compared the efficacy and safety of newer fibrinolytic drugs with those of streptokinase or alteplase.

Streptokinase

Streptokinase is a single-chain polypeptide derived from β-hemolytic streptococcus cultures. After intravenous (IV) administration, streptokinase binds to plasminogen, and the resulting streptokinase–plasminogen enzymatic complex cleaves plasminogen to form plasmin. Because plasmin nonspecifically degrades circulating fibrinogen as well as fibrin, streptokinase induces a systemic lytic state. Streptokinase induces the formation of antistreptokinase antibodies and can cause allergic reactions, particularly with repeated administration. Severe reactions are rare, but rash, shivering, pyrexia, and mild hypotension occur in up to 10% of patients. It is uncertain whether neutralizing antibodies reduce the efficacy of streptokinase.

The GISSI-1 (Gruppo Italiano per lo Studio della Sopravvivenza nell'Infarto Miocardico 1) trial, which was conducted in 11,806 patients with STEMI, demonstrated that streptokinase (1.5 million units over 1 hour) compared with no lytic therapy significantly reduced 21-day in-hospital mortality (10.7% vs. 13.0%; $P = .0002$). A similar reduction in mortality was seen when the same dose of streptokinase was compared with no lytic therapy in 17,187 patient with suspected MI in the ISIS-2 (International Studies of Infarct Survival 2) trial (9.2% vs. 12.0%; $P < .00001$).

Alteplase

Alteplase is a recombinant tissue-type plasminogen activator that directly converts plasminogen to plasmin. Although more fibrin-specific than streptokinase, alteplase still induces a systemic lytic state. It has a circulating half-life of 3 to 4 minutes.

The ISIS-3 (n = 41,299) and GISSI-2 (20,891) trials found no benefit of alteplase over streptokinase, findings possibly explained by the suboptimal use of heparin in conjunction with a short-acting fibrinolytic agent (heparin was given subcutaneously after a delay of 4 to 12 hours) and lack of front-loading of alteplase. The GUSTO-1 (Global Utilization of Streptokinase and Tissue Plasminogen Activator to Treat Occluded Arteries 1) trial (n = 41,021) demonstrated that front-loaded alteplase (15 mg bolus, 0.75 mg/kg infusion [maximum, 50 mg] over 30 minutes and then 0.50 mg/kg [maximum 35 mg] over 60 minutes [maximum, 100 mg over 90 minutes]) plus IV heparin (5000 U bolus, 1000 U/hr, with the dose titrated to achieve an activated partial thromboplastin time [aPTT] of 60 to 85 seconds) compared with streptokinase (1.5 million units over 1 hour) with or without IV heparin, reduced 30-day mortality (6.3% vs. 7.3%; $P = .001$). The mortality benefits of alteplase were greatest in patients younger than the age of 75 years and in those with anterior MI. Despite its enhanced fibrin specificity, alteplase was not associated with less bleeding than streptokinase.

The greatest benefits of fibrinolytic therapy are seen in patients treated within 1 hour of symptom onset; there is a much smaller benefit or no benefit if treatment is commenced more than 6 hours after symptom onset.[7]

Reteplase

Reteplase is a second-generation nonglycosylated deletion mutant of alteplase. Reteplase is less fibrin specific than alteplase but has a longer half-life (18 minutes) that enables administration by bolus injection.

The INJECT trial (n = 6,010) demonstrated that reteplase and streptokinase were associated with similar 35-day rates of mortality (9.0% vs. 9.5%), in-hospital stroke (1.2% vs. 1.0%), and major bleeding (0.7% vs. 1.0%), although reteplase was associated with a twofold higher rate of intracranial bleeding (0.8% vs. 0.4%). The GUSTO-III trial (n = 15,059) demonstrated that reteplase (two 10 mg IV injections 30 minutes apart) and front-loaded alteplase were associated with similar 30-day rates of mortality (7.5% vs. 7.2%) and stroke (1.6% vs. 1.7%).

Tenecteplase

Tenecteplase is a third-generation multiple point mutant of alteplase. Tenecteplase has a half-life of 20 minutes and is given by single bolus injection. Tenecteplase is the most fibrin-specific fibrinolytic drug approved for clinical use.

The ASSENT-2 (Assessment of the Safety and Efficacy of a New Thrombolytic) study, which enrolled 16,949 STEMI patients, showed that tenecteplase and alteplase were associated with similar 30-day rates of mortality (6.2% vs. 6.2%) and stroke (1.8% vs. 1.7%). Tenecteplase did not increase the risk of intracerebral bleeding (1% vs. 1%) and reduced major noncerebral bleeding (4.7% vs. 5.9%; $P < .0002$), possibly reflecting its enhanced fibrin-specificity.

Adjunctive Antithrombotic Therapy in Patients Receiving Fibrinolytic Drugs

A compelling rationale exists to administer adjunctive antithrombotic therapy to STEMI patients treated with fibrinolytic therapy. Platelet-rich thrombi that form after plaque rupture are relatively resistant to lysis, and the use of concomitant antiplatelet therapy may help to promote clot lysis. Fibrinolytic drugs have a proaggregatory effect on platelets, and the plaque rupture site remains prothrombotic after successful reperfusion therapy. Evidence in support of the efficacy of adjuvant antiplatelet and anticoagulant therapy in patients with STEMI is summarized in the sections on antiplatelet and anticoagulant therapy.

Intracranial Bleeding

The most important side effect of fibrinolytic therapy is intracranial bleeding, which affects up to 1% of patients and, in the majority of cases, is either fatal or permanently disabling.[8] Risk factors for intracranial bleeding include increasing age (particularly patients older than the age of 75 years), history of prior stroke, uncontrolled blood pressure, female sex, and low body weight. Bolus dose fibrinolytic therapy may be associated with a higher risk of intracranial bleeding than fibrinolytic therapy administered by continuous IV infusion (see Table 148-2 and box on Case 1: Bleeding After Fibrinolytic Therapy).[9]

ANTIPLATELET THERAPY

Aspirin and the second-generation thienopyridine, clopidogrel, are the foundation antiplatelet therapies for the management of ACS. IV glycoprotein IIb/IIIa (GP IIb/IIIa) inhibitors were introduced during the 1980s. Although their use has fallen since the introduction of clopidogrel, they retain a role in high-risk ACS, particularly in STEMI patients undergoing primary PCI.[5,6,10] Many countries have recently approved the new $P2Y_{12}$ receptor antagonists prasugrel and ticagrelor as alternatives to clopidogrel. The pharmacologic characteristics of antiplatelet drugs commonly used in the management of ACS are summarized in Tables 148-3 (oral drugs) and 148-4 (IV GP IIb/IIIa inhibitors).

Oral Antiplatelet Drugs

Aspirin

Aspirin inhibits platelets by irreversibly blocking the platelet enzyme cyclooxygenase-1 (COX-1), thereby preventing the formation of thromboxane A_2, a potent platelet agonist and vasoconstrictor. Despite having a half-life of only 20 minutes, the antiplatelet effect of aspirin lasts for the lifetime of the platelet (5–10 days) because platelets are anucleate and lack the machinery to synthesize new enzyme.[11]

Multiple randomized trials have demonstrated the efficacy of aspirin for the prevention of recurrent MI, stroke, or death in patients with ACS.[12] The ISIS-2 investigators evaluated the efficacy and safety of aspirin in 17,187 STEMI patients who were also randomized to receive or not to receive fibrinolytic therapy. Aspirin (162 mg/day), compared with no aspirin, significantly reduced 35-day mortality

Case 1: Bleeding After Fibrinolytic Therapy

A 63-year-old man with a history of hypertension presents to a rural hospital with sudden onset of severe retrosternal chest pain. An ECG performed in the emergency department demonstrates 4-mm anterior ST segment elevation. The nearest hospital with a cardiac catheterization laboratory is more than 6 hours away. He is treated with aspirin (300 mg loading dose), clopidogrel (300 mg loading dose), and an IV infusion of front-loaded alteplase, with rapid resolution of pain and normalization of ST-segment elevation. Toward the end of the alteplase infusion, he complains of abdominal pain, becomes hypotensive, and develops melena. Hemoglobin is 10.2 g/dL, the aPTT is 89 seconds, the international normalized ratio (INR) is 1.7, and the fibrinogen level is below 100 mg/dL.

Aspirin and clopidogrel are held; the patient receives 10 units of cryoprecipitate and is started on an IV infusion of a proton pump inhibitor. He undergoes urgent upper gastrointestinal tract endoscopy with injection of a bleeding ulcer. He does not receive platelets because of concerns about the risk of recurrent MI. No further bleeding occurs, and after 48 hours, he resumes aspirin. Clopidogrel is restarted 1 week later after repeat endoscopy demonstrates a healing ulcer.

Comment

Fibrinolytic trials report a 1% to 6% incidence of major bleeding and a 10% incidence of moderate bleeding during the first 30 days. The most common sources of major bleeding are the gastrointestinal tract and procedure-related bleeding. The principles of management of major bleeding in STEMI patients treated with fibrinolytic therapy are summarized in Table 148-2. Steps include (1) stop antithrombotic therapies; (2) use local measures when possible to control bleeding; (3) draw blood to measure fibrinogen, prothrombin time (PT), aPTT, and possibly anti-Xa levels (to measure the anticoagulant effect of low-molecular-weight heparin) and to crossmatch blood; and (4) administer therapies to mitigate or reverse the effects of fibrinolytic, antiplatelet, and anticoagulant drugs.

The extent and duration of the lytic effects of fibrinolytic drugs is determined by their fibrin specificity. Whereas streptokinase produces profound and sustained depletion of fibrinogen (<100 mg/dL) that lasts for up to 24 to 48 hours, alteplase and other more fibrin-specific agents exert a less pronounced and more short-lived effect on fibrinogen levels. The aPTT and PT can be markedly prolonged in patients with hypofibrinogenemia. Normal coagulation can be restored by elevating fibrinogen level to at least 100 mg/dL. This can be readily achieved by infusing cryoprecipitate (recommended dose, 10 units). Fresh-frozen plasma also contains fibrinogen but requires administration of much larger volumes.

Platelet dysfunction caused by aspirin, clopidogrel, and fibrinolytic therapy cannot be specifically reversed, but infusion of donor platelets can help to restore platelet function. Platelet transfusion is generally reserved for patients with life-threatening bleeding because of concerns about the risk of recurrent MI. A single unit of single donor platelets can be expected to increase the platelet count by 50 to 60 × 10^9/L. Even a small number (e.g., 10%-20%) of functional (nonaspirinated) platelets are sufficient to generate sufficient thromboxane to sustain normal platelet aggregation, but a much larger number of transfused platelets are need to overcome the antiplatelet effects of clopidogrel. In this case, bleeding was controlled with cryoprecipitate, and local measures and platelet infusions were not required.

Table 148-2 Management of Major Bleeding in Patients With ST-Segment Elevation Myocardial Infarction Treated With Fibrinolytic Therapy

Steps	Approach	Considerations
Stop treatment	Stop fibrinolytic drug Stop antiplatelet drugs Stop anticoagulant	Recovery of fibrinogen levels can take 24 to 48 hours after stopping streptokinase Antiplatelet effects of aspirin and clopidogrel last for life of platelet (5-10 days) Heparin has a half-life of about 40 minutes; LMWH has a half-life of 3 to 6 hours
Local measures	Local pressure Endoscopy and local injection* Embolization*	Sustained local pressure (e.g., for 30 minutes) may be required Can be used for upper or distal lower GI bleeding Used in rare situations such as life-threatening pulmonary or intra-abdominal bleeding
Laboratory evaluation	Fibrinogen PT and aPTT Anti-Xa level Crossmatch blood	Levels may be undetectable (<0.1 g/L) Results are uninterpretable if fibrinogen levels are low PT (INR) is elevated by warfarin; aPTT is prolonged by heparin but not with LMWH or fondaparinux Chromogenic assay for LMWH and fondaparinux Unaffected by low fibrinogen To restore blood volume and maintain hemoglobin
Reversal of fibrinolytic effect	Cryoprecipitate FFP	Recommended initial dose is 10 U; monitor by repeat fibrinogen level The half-life of fibrinogen is about 4 days Requires large volumes (e.g., 2 L) to restore fibrinogen levels
Reversal of antiplatelet effect	Platelet transfusion	Increases the number of functional platelets but does not reverse the antiplatelet effects of aspirin and clopidogrel Also see text under heading "Antiplatelet Therapy"
Reversal of anticoagulant effect	Protamine	Protamine reverses heparin and partially reverses LMWH; also see Table 148-6

aPTT, Activated partial thromboplastin time; *FFP,* fresh-frozen plasma; *GI,* gastrointestinal; *INR,* international normalized ratio; *LMWH,* low-molecular-weight heparin; *PT,* prothrombin time
*Also requires restoration of adequate hemostasis.

Table 148-3 Pharmacologic Characteristics of Oral Antiplatelet Drugs Commonly Used in the Management of Acute Coronary Syndromes

		ADP Receptor Antagonists		
Characteristic	**Aspirin**	**Clopidogrel**	**Prasugrel**	**Ticagrelor**
Class	COX inhibitor	Thienopyridine (second generation)	Thienopyridine (third generation)	Cyclopentyltriazolopyrimidine
Target	COX-1	P2Y12	P2Y12	P2Y12
Dose	162-325 mg loading dose; 75-325 mg/day maintenance dose	300-600 mg loading dose; 75 mg/day maintenance dose	60 mg loading dose; 10 mg/d maintenance dose	180 mg loading dose; 90 mg bid maintenance dose
Prodrug	No	Yes	Yes	No
Time to effect*	<1 hr	4-6 hr†	<1 hr	<1 hr
Drug half-life	20 min	Minutes	Minutes	12 hr
Reversible	No	No	No	Yes

ADP, Adenosine diphosphate; *bid,* twice daily; *COX,* cyclooxygenase.
*After loading dose.
†Increased antithrombotic benefit was seen after the first hour in patients enrolled in the COMMIT trial who did not receive a loading dose, but maximum effect is not seen until after 4 to 6 hours.

Table 148-4 Pharmacologic Characteristics of Intravenous Glycoprotein IIb/IIIa Inhibitors Used in the Management of Acute Coronary Syndrome

Characteristic	Abciximab	Eptifibatide	Tirofiban
Class	Fab fragment	Nonpeptide	Cyclic heptapeptide
Onset	Rapid	Rapid	Rapid
Drug half-life	10-30 min	2 hr	2.5 hr
Reversibility of platelet inhibition	Slow	Rapid	Rapid
Excretion	Unknown	40%-70% renal	50% renal

(9.4% vs. 11.8%; *P* <.00001) as well as nonfatal reinfarction (1.0% vs. 2.0%) and stroke (0.3% vs. 0.6%) without increasing bleeding. The Antithrombotic Trialists' Collaboration (ATTC) pooled the data from 15 randomized trials of antiplatelet therapy (predominantly aspirin) involving 19,302 patients with acute MI who were also treated with fibrinolytic therapy. Antiplatelet therapy given for a mean duration of 1 month compared with placebo or no antiplatelet therapy significantly reduced the composite outcome of MI, stroke, or death (10.4% vs. 14.2%; *P* <.0001).

At least four randomized controlled trials have demonstrated the efficacy of aspirin in patients with NSTE ACS. Pooled data from the four trials involving a combined total of 3096 patients indicate that aspirin compared with placebo or no aspirin significantly reduced the composite endpoint of MI, stroke, or vascular death (6.4% vs. 12.5%; *P* = .0005).

The efficacy and safety of aspirin have been evaluated in combination with dipyridamole in PCI patients in one randomized controlled trial involving 376 patients. Aspirin (300 mg) plus dipyridamole (75 mg), given orally three times daily (except during a 24-hour period around the time of the procedure when dipyridamole was given intravenously), compared with placebo, reduced the risk of MI by more than half (1.6% vs. 6.9%; *P* = .01). These results led to the adoption of aspirin as standard therapy for patients undergoing PCI.

The CURRENT OASIS-7 (Clopidogrel Optimal Loading Dose Usage to Reduce Recurrent EveNTs/Optimal Antiplatelet Strategy for InterventionS) trial explored the optimal dose of aspirin in 25,086 ACS patients with or without ST-segment elevation on the presenting ECG and included 17,263 patients undergoing early PCI.[13] After an initial aspirin loading dose, aspirin 300 to 325 mg/day and 75 to 100 mg/day were associated with similar rates of MI, stroke, or death at 30 days (4.2% vs. 4.4%), but the higher aspirin dose increased gastrointestinal bleeding (0.4% vs. 0.2%; *P* = .04). Based on these results, the optimal dose of aspirin for the management of patients with ACS (after an initial loading dose of 160-325 mg) appears to be 75 to 100 mg/day.

Clopidogrel

Clopidogrel is metabolized via the liver to form the active moiety that irreversibly blocks the platelet P2Y12 receptor to prevent adenosine diphosphate–induced platelet activation and aggregation. Similar to aspirin, the antiplatelet effect of clopidogrel lasts for the lifetime of the platelet. Clopidogrel is an effective antiplatelet drug for the prevention of MI and death when used in combination with aspirin but has a slow onset of action and a variable antiplatelet effect that may limit its effectiveness.

The COMMIT trial, which involved 45,582 patients with STEMI, all of whom were treated with aspirin (162 mg/day) demonstrated that 30 days of treatment with clopidogrel (75 mg/day) compared with placebo reduced the risk of MI, stroke, or death (9.2% vs. 10.1%; *P* = .002) with no increase in major bleeding (0.58% vs. 0.55%).[14] There was no age restriction in the COMMIT trial, and clopidogrel was given without a loading dose. In the CLARITY (Clopidogrel as Adjunctive Reperfusion Therapy) trial (*n* = 3,491), which was conducted in parallel with COMMIT, clopidogrel was given as a loading dose of 300 mg followed by 75 mg/day for 2 to 8 days and was compared with placebo in patients receiving fibrinolysis. Clopidogrel reduced the risk of MI or death (15% vs. 21.7%; *P* <.001). Consistent benefits of clopidogrel were demonstrated in the 1863 patients who underwent PCI after mandated angiography.

The CURE (Clopidogrel in Unstable Angina to Prevent Recurrent Events) trial, which involved 12,562 patients with NSTE ACS, all of whom were treated with aspirin (recommended dose 75-325 mg/day), demonstrated that a median of 9 months treatment with clopidogrel (300 mg loading dose followed by 75 mg/day) compared with placebo reduced the risk of MI, stroke, or death (9.3% vs. 11.4%; *P* <.001) at the cost of an increase in major bleeding (3.7% vs. 2.7%; *P* = .001).[15] Consistent benefits of clopidogrel were seen in the 2658 patients who underwent PCI irrespective of whether or not they underwent stenting.

Prompted by concerns that some patients achieve suboptimal inhibition of platelet function with conventional doses of clopidogrel, the CURRENT-OASIS 7 trial evaluated the efficacy and safety of a higher loading and maintenance dose of clopidogrel compared with standard dose clopidogrel in 25,086 patients with ACS referred for an invasive management strategy.[13] Clopidogrel, 600-mg loading dose followed by 150 mg/day for 6 days ("double-dose clopidogrel") and 75 mg/day for 23 days compared with a 300-mg loading dose and 75 mg daily thereafter ("standard dose clopidogrel") for 30 days were associated with similar rates of the primary outcome, MI, stroke, or vascular death (4.2% vs. 4.4%) and an increase in major bleeding (2.5% vs. 2.0%; *P* = .01). However, in the 17,263 patients who underwent PCI, double-dose compared with standard-dose clopidogrel reduced MI, stroke, or vascular death (3.9% vs. 4.5%; *P* = .039) and stent thrombosis (0.7% vs. 1.3%; *P* = .0001).

Prasugrel

Prasugrel is a third-generation thienopyridine that is more potent and has a more rapid onset of action than clopidogrel. Prasugrel is a prodrug, but unlike clopidogrel, it requires only single-step bioconversion to form the active metabolite that irreversibly blocks the platelet P2Y12 receptor.

The TRITON-TIMI 38 (Trial to Assess Improvement in Therapeutic Outcomes by Optimizing Platelet Inhibition With Prasugrel–Thrombolysis In Myocardial Infarction 38) trial evaluated the efficacy and safety of prasugrel in 13,608 patients with ACS with or without ST-segment elevation who were undergoing PCI, all of whom were treated with aspirin (recommended dose, 75-162 mg/day).[16] Prasugrel (60 mg followed by 10 mg once daily) compared with clopidogrel (300 mg followed by 75 mg once daily) continued for a median of 14.5 months reduced the risk of MI, stroke, or cardiovascular death (9.9% vs. 12.1%; *P* <.001) and stent thrombosis (1.1% vs. 2.4%; *P* <.001) but did not reduce mortality and increased non–coronary artery bypass graft (CABG) major bleeding (2.4% vs. 1.8%; *P* = .03) as well as intracranial and fatal bleeding.

Ticagrelor

Ticagrelor is nonthienopyridine platelet P2Y12 receptor antagonist. Similar to prasugrel, ticagrelor is more potent and has a more rapid onset of action than clopidogrel, but unlike both clopidogrel and prasugrel, ticagrelor binds reversibly to the platelet P2Y12 receptor.

The PLATO trial evaluated the efficacy and safety of ticagrelor in 18,624 patients with ACS with or without ST-segment elevation.[17] Ticagrelor (180 mg loading dose followed by 90 mg twice daily) compared with clopidogrel (300 or 600 mg loading dose followed by 75 mg once daily) reduced the risk of MI, stroke, or vascular death by 16% (9.8% vs. 11.7%; *P* <.001) and produced a significant reduction in vascular death (4.0% vs. 5.1%; *P* = .001) and stent thrombosis (1.3% vs. 1.9%; *P* = .009). There was no increase in major bleeding (11.6% vs. 11.2%) or in intracranial or fatal bleeding, but ticagrelor increased non-CABG major bleeding (4.5% vs. 3.8%; *P* = .03).

Intravenous Antiplatelet Drugs

Glycoprotein IIb/IIIa Inhibitors

Three IV GP IIb/IIIa inhibitors are available for clinical use (see Table 148-4). Abciximab is a humanized version of a Fab fragment of a murine antibody directed against GP IIb/IIIa. Tirofiban is a nonpeptide tyrosine derivative that selectively binds to GP IIb/IIIa. Eptifibatide is a synthetic disulfide-linked cyclic heptapeptide with high specificity for GP IIb/IIIa.

The efficacy and safety of GP IIb/IIIa inhibitors has been extensively evaluated in patients with ACS. Meta-analysis restricted to trials (*n* = 6) involving at least 1000 patients suggests a modest effect of these agents for the prevention of MI, urgent revascularization, or vascular death in patients with NSTE ACS (10.8% vs. 11.8%; *P* = .015).[18] Pooled data from a meta-analysis of 16 randomized trials involving 10,085 STEMI patients undergoing primary PCI demonstrated that adjunctive GP IIb/IIIa blockade did not reduce 30-day mortality (2.8 vs. 2.9%; *P* = 0.75) or reinfarction (1.5 vs. 1.9%; *P* = .22) and increased major bleeding (4.1 vs. 2.7%; *P* = .0004). However, meta-regression analysis confirmed the impression from individual trials of a mortality benefit of IV GP IIb/IIIa inhibitors in those at highest risk (see boxes on Case 2: Stent Thrombosis and Case 3: Thrombocytopenia After Stenting).[19]

Case 2: Stent Thrombosis

A 49-year-old man with a history of type 2 diabetes presents with NSTEMI and undergoes PCI with placement of a drug-eluting stent in the left anterior descending coronary artery. He receives a 300-mg loading dose of aspirin and a 600-mg loading dose of clopidogrel and is discharged on aspirin 100 mg/day and clopidogrel 75 mg/day. He presents to the emergency department 3 weeks later with recurrent chest pain and anterior ST-segment elevation on the ECG. He denies missing any doses of clopidogrel. He is taken urgently to the cardiac catheterization laboratory, where a diagnosis of stent thrombosis is confirmed, and he undergoes repeat PCI with thrombus aspiration.

Prompted by concern about the possibility of "clopidogrel resistance," genotyping studies are performed and demonstrate heterozygosity for the CYP2C19 *2 loss-of-function allele. Clopidogrel is stopped, and he is started on prasugrel (10 mg once daily) instead. He is discharged on indefinite dual antiplatelet therapy with aspirin and prasugrel.

Comment

Stent thrombosis is a potentially life-threatening complication of PCI, affecting 1% to 2% of patients during the first year and presenting in almost all cases as death or MI.[20] Risk factors for stent thrombosis can be categorized as patient related, technical (procedure, stent, or lesion), or drug related. The single most important predictor of stent thrombosis is premature discontinuation of clopidogrel. High on-treatment platelet reactivity during clopidogrel therapy has also emerged as a predictor of stent thrombosis and is affected by clinical (e.g., age, diabetes, renal insufficiency) and genetic factors. Carriers of reduced function CYP2C19 alleles have low levels of the active metabolite of clopidogrel, diminished platelet inhibition, and an increased risk of stent thrombosis. Unlike clopidogrel, which undergoes two-step, cytochrome P450-dependen, metabolic conversion in the liver, prasugrel and ticagrelor are not affected by CYP polymorphisms and consistently produce a greater and more consistent level of platelet inhibition than standard clopidogrel doses. Higher doses of clopidogrel (e.g., 225 or 300 mg/day) in patients heterozygous for CYP2C19*2 alleles achieve levels of platelet inhibition similar to those seen with standard (75 mg) doses but have not been evaluated in clinical outcome studies.

The role of genetic testing to detect poor clopidogrel responders remains controversial. Although observational studies have demonstrated an independent association between CYP2C19 loss-of-function alleles and risk of stent thrombosis, analyses from multiple randomized controlled trials provide no evidence of an interaction between genotype and treatment for major cardiovascular events, including stent thrombosis.[21] It is reasonable to switch (without laboratory testing) patients who have experienced stent thrombosis despite clopidogrel therapy to one of the newer P2Y12 receptor antagonists (i.e., prasugrel or ticagrelor) that have been demonstrated to reduce the risk of stent thrombosis compared with clopidogrel.

ANTICOAGULANT THERAPY

Anticoagulant therapy is effective for the initial and long-term management of patients with ACS with or without ST-segment elevation.[5,6,10] The pharmacologic characteristics of parenteral anticoagulants commonly used in the management of ACS are summarized in Table 148-5. Early trials suggested that heparin and aspirin were similarly effective for the prevention of MI, but aspirin was adopted as the foundation antithrombotic therapy because it caused less bleeding than heparin. Subsequent randomized controlled trials demonstrated that the combination of heparin plus aspirin provided additive benefit. More recent trials have established the efficacy and safety of

Case 3: Thrombocytopenia After Stenting

A 65-year-old woman presenting with STEMI undergoes primary PCI with placement of a bare metal stent in her circumflex coronary artery. During the procedure, she receives an IV bolus of abciximab in addition to aspirin, clopidogrel, and heparin. A blood count performed after returning to the coronary care unit (within 6 hours of the procedure) reveals a platelet count of 6×10^9/L, which is confirmed on repeat testing using a sample collected in sodium citrate (to eliminate platelet clumping as a cause of spurious thrombocytopenia). She is diagnosed with abciximab-induced thrombocytopenia.

Heparin is stopped, and the patient receives 1 unit of single donor platelets with a prompt increase in her platelet count. She is continued on aspirin and clopidogrel and is started in a proton pump inhibitor. The platelet count begins to rise spontaneously on day 4 and returns to baseline levels within 1 week.

Comment

Severe thrombocytopenia (platelet count $<50 \times 10^9$/L) occurs in about 0.5% and less severe thrombocytopenia in 2% to 4% of patients treated with GP IIb/IIIa inhibitors.[22] Thrombocytopenia caused by GP IIb/IIIa inhibitors is readily distinguished from other causes by its rapid onset, typically within 24 hours of exposure and sometimes within with first hour, and severity (count often $<10 \times 10^9$/L). By contrast, heparin-induced thrombocytopenia is usually delayed until at least 4 days after starting heparin therapy (with the exception of patients with prior exposure to heparin in the past 3 months) and platelet counts rarely fall below 30×10^9/L. The very rapid onset of thrombocytopenia is believed to be caused by preformed antibodies that react with GP IIb/IIIa inhibitor–coated platelets. Spontaneous recovery of the platelet count usually occurs within days but can take several weeks. Patients with GP IIb/IIIa inhibitor–induced thrombocytopenia respond normally to platelet transfusions, which should be considered when the count is below 10×10^9/L to reduce the risk of spontaneous bleeding. There is no evidence that steroids or IV gamma globulin alter the natural history of GP IIb/IIIa inhibitor–induced thrombocytopenia. Repeated exposure to GP IIb/IIIa inhibitors should be avoided because there is a risk of recurrent thrombocytopenia, which may be more severe than the initial episode.

newer parenteral anticoagulants, low-molecular-weight heparin (LMWH), fondaparinux, or bivalirudin, on a background of single- or dual-agent antiplatelet therapy in the initial management of patients with ACS.

The pharmacologic characteristics of warfarin and new oral anticoagulants evaluated in the management of ACS are summarized in Table 148-6.[23] Warfarin is effective for the prevention of major cardiovascular events for the long-term management of patients with ACS who are also treated with aspirin, but no adequately powered randomized controlled trials have evaluated the efficacy and safety of warfarin in the context of dual antiplatelet therapy. Two new oral anticoagulants (rivaroxaban and apixaban) have been evaluated in phase III trials for the long-term management of ACS, but neither agent is currently approved for this indication.[24,25]

Heparin

Heparin is derived from porcine intestinal mucosa and is administered by IV or subcutaneous injection. It inhibits coagulation by binding to antithrombin to produce a conformational change that converts antithrombin from a slow to a rapid inhibitor of thrombin and factor Xa.

Table 148-5 Pharmacologic Characteristics of Parenteral Anticoagulants Commonly Used in the Management of Patients With Acute Coronary Syndromes

	Unfractionated heparin	Enoxaparin	Bivalirudin	Fondaparinux
Route of administration	IV	SC (first dose IV*)	IV	SC (first dose IV*)
Frequency of dosing	Continuous IV infusion	Twice daily; once daily if CrCl <30 mL/min	Continuous IV infusion	Once-daily injection
Clearance	Primarily nonrenal	Renal	Renal, proteolytic cleavage	Renal
Use in ACS patients with moderate renal impairment	Yes	Yes (dose reduction)	Yes (dose reduction)	Yes[†]
Use in ACS patients undergoing dialysis	Yes	No experience	Yes (dose reduction)	No experience[‡]
Routine laboratory monitoring	Yes	No	No[§]	No
Dose	Adjust dose according to the results of the aPTT	Fixed weight adjusted	Fixed weight adjusted	Fixed
Accumulation in renal failure	No	Yes	Yes	Yes
Non-anticoagulant side effects	Allergy, HIT	HIT (rare)	—	—
Nonbleeding contraindications	Allergy, immune HIT	Allergy, immune HIT	Allergy	Allergy
Antidote	Protamine sulfate	No	No	No

ACS, acute coronary syndromes; *aPTT,* activated partial thromboplastin time; *CrCl,* creatinine clearance; *HIT,* heparin-induced thrombocytopenia; *IV,* intravenous; *SC,* subcutaneous.

*The first dose of enoxaparin was given by the intravenous route in the TIMI-11B (Thrombolysis In Myocardial Infarction 11B) and EXTRACT-TIMI 25 (Enoxaparin and Thrombolysis Reperfusion for Acute Myocardial Infarction Treatment, Thrombolysis in Myocardial Infarction 25) studies. The first dose of fondaparinux was given by the intravenous route in the OASIS-6 (Optimal Antiplatelet Strategy for InterventionS 6) trial.

[†]Acute coronary syndrome patients with creatinine up to 265 μmol/L were eligible for inclusion in the OASIS-5 and -6 trials (equivalent to an estimated creatinine clearance of 15 to 20 mL/min in a 70-kg patient who is 70 years of age).

[‡]Fondaparinux is contraindicated in patients with venous thromboembolism who have severe renal impairment.

[§]Monitoring and dose adjustment required in patients with creatinine clearance below 30 mL/min.

Table 148-6 Pharmacological Characteristics of Warfarin and New Oral Anticoagulants Evaluated in Phase 3 Trials for the Long-Term Management of Acute Coronary Syndromes

Characteristic	Warfarin	Rivaroxaban	Apixaban
Target	VKOR	fXa	fXa
Prodrug	No	No	No
Bioavailability, %	100	80	60
Dosing	Variable, once daily	Fixed, 2.5 or 5 mg twice daily*	Fixed, 5 mg twice daily (2.5 mg twice daily in selected patients)
Half-life	Mean, 40 hours (range, 20-60 hr)	7-11 hr	12 hr
Renal clearance, %	Nil	66[†]	25
Routine coagulation monitoring	Yes (INR)	No	No
Drug interactions	Multiple	Potent inhibitors of CYP3A4 and P-gp[‡]	Potent inhibitors of CYP3A4[‡]
Antidote	Yes (vitamin K, PCC, FFP)	No	No

CYP-3A4, Cytochrome p-450 3A4; *FFP,* fresh-frozen plasma; *fXa,* activated factor X; *INR,* international normalized ratio; *PCC,* prothrombin complex concentrates; *P-gp,* P-glycoprotein; *VKOR,* vitamin K epoxide reductase.

*A once-daily regimen was tested in atrial fibrillation.

[†]Half of renally cleared rivaroxaban is cleared as unchanged drug and half as inactive metabolites.

[‡]Potent inhibitors of both CYP3A4 and P-glycoprotein include azole antifungals (e.g., ketoconazole, itraconazole, voriconazole, posaconazole) and protease inhibitors, such as ritonavir. Potent inhibitors of CYP3A4 include azole antifungals, macrolide antibiotics (e.g., clarithromycin), and protease inhibitors (e.g., atanazavir).

Heparin has several limitations, including immune-mediated platelet activation, which leads to heparin-induced thrombocytopenia, and nonspecific protein binding, resulting in a variable anticoagulant response and the need for routine coagulation monitoring. Despite these limitations, heparin remains widely used because it has important advantages over more recently introduced anticoagulants. First, the anticoagulant effect of heparin can be rapidly and completely reversed with protamine sulfate. Second, heparin is suitable for use in patients with renal failure because it is predominantly nonrenally cleared. Third, unlike LMWH and fondaparinux, heparin is also highly effective for prevention of contact activation of coagulation induced by catheters and stents.[26]

Meta-analysis of four randomized controlled trials involving 1239 STEMI patients treated with aspirin and fibrinolytic therapy demonstrated that short-term IV heparin (given for about 1 week) compared with placebo or no heparin did not significantly reduce death or reinfarction but increased bleeding.[27] However, these trials were underpowered to demonstrate a benefit of heparin. Definitive data concerning the efficacy of heparin in STEMI patients treated with fibrinolysis come from a meta-analysis of 26 trials involving 73,000 patients, in which heparin, given either intravenously or subcutaneously, compared with placebo or no heparin reduced mortality and reinfarction.[28] Consistent benefits were evident in a subset of five trials in which patients also received aspirin; heparin compared with placebo or no heparin reduced both mortality (8.6% vs. 9.1%; $P = .03$) and reinfarction (3.0% vs. 3.3%; $P = .04$).

Short-term heparin therapy is also beneficial when added to aspirin in patients with NSTE ACS. A meta-analysis of six trials involving 1353 patients demonstrated that up to 7 days of IV heparin compared with placebo or no heparin reduced death or MI (4.5% vs. 7.4%; $P = .045$) with a nonsignificant excess of major bleeding.[29] Heparin has not been rigorously evaluated in ACS patients undergoing PCI but is routinely used in this setting.

Low-Molecular-Weight Heparin

Low-molecular-weight heparin is derived from heparin by enzymatic or chemical methods, yielding shorter polysaccharide chains that produce a more predictable anticoagulant effect than heparin and a lower propensity for thrombocytopenia. LMWH is given in fixed weight-adjusted doses without routine coagulation monitoring. The anticoagulant effects of LMWH can be partially reversed with protamine sulfate.

The CREATE trial ($n = 15{,}570$) was the largest of four trials that evaluated the efficacy and safety of various LMWH preparations in patients with STEMI also treated with aspirin and fibrinolysis.[30] Approximately half of patients in the CREATE trial were treated with dual antiplatelet therapy. The pooled data ($n = 16{,}943$) demonstrated that initial LMWH continued for up to 7 days compared with placebo reduced the risk of reinfarction (1.6% vs. 2.2%; $P < .05$) and death (7.8% vs. 8.7%; $P < .05$) at the cost of an increase in major bleeding (1.1% vs. 0.4%; $P < .05$).

Most of the trials comparing LMWH with heparin for the treatment of STEMI tested enoxaparin. Pooled data from eight trials involving 27,758 patients demonstrated that initial LMWH compared with heparin reduced the risk of MI (2.1% vs. 3.9%; $P < .05$) with similar rates of death (5.3% vs. 5.8%) at the cost of an increase in major bleeding (2.2% vs. 1.6%).[31] Consistent results were evident at 30 days.

The FRISC-1 (Fragmin during Instability in Coronary Artery Disease 1) trial evaluated the efficacy and safety of dalteparin in patients with NSTE ACS. Pooled data from FRISC-1 ($n = 1539$) and a second much smaller phase 2 study demonstrated that LMWH compared with placebo or no LMWH reduced the risk of MI or death (1.6% vs. 5.2%; $P < .0001$) with no significant increase in major bleeding.

Multiple trials have compared LMWH with heparin in patients with NSTE ACS. A pooled analysis of five trials involving 12,171 patients demonstrated that LMWH and heparin were associated with similar rates of MI or death (2.2% vs. 2.3%) and major bleeding.[29] A subsequent meta-analysis involving 21,946 patients with NSTE ACS demonstrated that enoxaparin compared with heparin reduced the risk of death or MI (10.1% vs. 11.0%; $P < .05$) with no increase in major bleeding.[32] The latter meta-analysis included some trials that did not involve the use of GP IIb/IIIa inhibitors and other trials in which they were widely used. The proportion of patients who underwent an invasive management strategy also varied among the trials.

Fondaparinux

Fondaparinux is a synthetic pentasaccharide that contains the essential five-sugar chain that interacts with antithrombin to inhibit factor Xa. Fondaparinux has a half-life of 17 hours, which enables once-daily administration and produces an even more predictable anticoagulant effect than LMWH and does not appear to cause thrombocytopenia. Fondaparinux does not have an antidote.

Fondaparinux has been evaluated in patients with ACS in three large phase 3 randomized controlled trials. The OASIS-6 trial evaluated fondaparinux in 12,092 STEMI patients treated with single or dual antiplatelet therapy and fibrinolytic therapy.[33] Fondaparinux (2.5 mg/day) compared with placebo or heparin reduced the risk of reinfarction or death (9.7% vs. 11.2%; $P = .008$) with consistent effects in patients with or without an indication for heparin therapy and in patients who received aspirin alone or the combination of aspirin and clopidogrel. Fondaparinux did not increase major bleeding. However, fondaparinux was associated with no benefit and a trend for harm in patients undergoing primary PCI.

The OASIS-5 trial evaluated fondaparinux in 20,078 patients with NSTE ACS treated with aspirin with or without clopidogrel. Fondaparinux (2.5 mg once daily) and enoxaparin (1 mg/kg twice a day) given for a mean of 6 days were associated with similar rates of the primary outcome of refractory ischemic, MI, or death at 9 days (5.8% vs. 5.7%), but there was a lower rate of major bleeding with fondaparinux (2.2% vs. 4.1%; $P < .001$).[34] At 30 days, fondaparinux compared with enoxaparin was associated with a reduced rate of death (2.9% vs. 3.5%; $P = .02$), which appeared to be explained primarily by the lower rate of bleeding. In 6238 invasively managed patients, fondaparinux and enoxaparin were associated with similar rates of the primary outcome but fondaparinux was associated with a small excess of catheter-related thrombosis (0.9% vs. 0.4%) and a reduction in major bleeding (2.4% vs. 5.1%; $P < .00001$). The risk of catheter thrombosis was largely prevented by the administration of heparin at the time of intervention.

The FUTURA OASIS-8 (Fondaparinux Trial With Unfractionated Heparin During Revascularization in Acute Coronary Syndromes) study evaluated the effect of standard dose heparin (85 units/kg bolus with additional boluses based on an activated clotting time dosing algorithm) compared with reduced dose heparin (50 units/kg without activated clotting time adjustment) on the primary composite outcome, bleeding or major vascular site access complications, in 2026 patients with NSTE ACS who were treated with fondaparinux and scheduled to undergo PCI within 72 hours.[35] The incidences of the primary outcome and of catheter-related thrombosis were similar in the two heparin dose groups, but death, MI, or target vessel revascularization occurred more often in the low-dose group. These data support the use of standard dose heparin in patients with NSTE ACS who are treated with fondaparinux and scheduled to undergo PCI.

Bivalirudin

Bivalirudin is an IV direct thrombin inhibitor that blocks the interaction between thrombin and its substrates. Bivalirudin has a short half-life of only 25 minutes after IV injection, making the lack of an antidote less problematic than for longer acting anticoagulants. It is about 20% renally cleared, and the half-life is prolonged in patients with renal impairment. Bivalirudin does not cause heparin-induced thrombocytopenia.

The efficacy and safety of direct thrombin inhibitors in ACS patients and those undergoing PCI was examined in the Direct Thrombin Inhibitor Trialists' Collaboration meta-analysis involving data from 11 trials and 35,970 patients.[36] The pooled data indicated a significant benefit of direct thrombin inhibitors (including bivalirudin) compared with heparin for the prevention of MI or death. Clopidogrel and GP IIb/IIIa inhibitors were not used in the trials included in this meta-analysis.

The HORIZONS AMI (Harmonizing Outcomes with Revascularization and Stents in Acute Myocardial Infarction) trial evaluated the use of bivalirudin in 3600 STEMI patients treated with the combination of aspirin and clopidogrel and undergoing PCI.[37] Bivalirudin plus provisional GP IIb/IIIa inhibitor compared with heparin plus GP IIb/IIIa were associated with similar rates of the primary outcome, MI, target vessel revascularization, stroke, or death (5.4% vs. 5.5%) at 30 days, but bivalirudin significantly reduced major bleeding (4.9 vs. 8.3%; $P < .0001$).

The ACUITY (Acute Catheterization and Urgent Intervention Triage Strategy) trial evaluated the use of bivalirudin in 13,819 patients with NSTE ACS undergoing PCI who were treated with the combination of aspirin plus clopidogrel as well as a GP IIb/IIIa inhibitor.[38] Bivalirudin was non-inferior to heparin or enoxaparin plus a GP IIb/IIIa inhibitor for the prevention of MI, unplanned revascularization, or death at 30 days (7.8% vs. 7.3%) but was associated with a lower rate of major bleeding (3.0% vs. 5.7%; $P < .001$).

Oral Anticoagulation

Warfarin is an oral vitamin K antagonist that has been evaluated in the long-term management of patients with ACS who are treated with aspirin but has not been rigorously tested on a background of dual antiplatelet therapy. Furthermore, the efficacy and safety of the combination of aspirin plus warfarin have not been compared with those of dual antiplatelet therapy.

The results from a meta-analysis of 14 trials involving 25,307 patients demonstrated that long-term warfarin (target INR, 2.0-3.0) compared with placebo or no warfarin reduced the risk of MI, ischemic stroke or death (9.4% vs. 12.3%; $P < 0.0001$) at the cost of a 2-fold increase in major bleeding (2.6% vs. 1.1%; $P < .00001$).[39]

Rivaroxaban and apixaban are orally active factor Xa inhibitors that have undergone evaluation in phase 3 trials for the long-term management of patients with ACS. The ATLAS TIMI-51 trial compared rivaroxaban (2.5 or 5 mg twice a day) with placebo in 15,526 ACS patients, the majority of whom were also treated with the combination of aspirin and clopidogrel.[24] Treatment was started a median of 4.7 days after onset of symptoms and was continued for a mean of 13 months. Rivaroxaban significantly reduced the risk of MI, stroke, or cardiovascular death (8.9% vs. 10.7%; $P = .008$) at the cost of an increase in non-CABG major bleeding (2.1% vs. 0.6%; $P < .001$) and intracranial bleeding (0.6% vs. 0.2%; $P = .009$). The APPRAISE trial compared apixaban (5 mg twice a day; 2.5 mg twice a day in selected patients) with placebo in patients with ACS. The trial was stopped early because of an excess of bleeding with no significant reduction in ischemic events.[25] The oral direct thrombin inhibitor dabigatran etexilate has been tested in a phase 2 trial but has not undergone evaluation in a phase 3 trial in ACS patients (see Table 148-7 and box on Case 4: Triple Therapy).

Table 148-7 Strategies Aimed at Minimizing the Risk of Bleeding in Patients Treated With Triple Therapy (Dual Antiplatelet Therapy and an Oral Anticoagulant)

Proposed Approach	Rationale
Aspirin maintenance dose ≤100 mg/day	Higher aspirin maintenance doses increase bleeding, and there is no evidence that they improve efficacy.
PPI with a preference for agents that interfere less with CYP 2C19 (e.g., pantoprazole)	Much of the excess bleeding is from the GI tract. The use of acid-suppressive agents that interfere less with CYP 2C19 minimizes the potential for a negative interaction with clopidogrel.
For warfarin, use a target INR of 2 to 2.5	Some evidence that a restricted target INR range reduces the risk of bleeding.
Manage warfarin in a specialized anticoagulation clinic	Compared with usual care, specialist clinics achieve a higher time-in-therapeutic-range of the INR.
Minimize duration of triple therapy	The risk of bleeding is highest during the first 30 days but remains elevated with long-term treatment.
Avoid NSAIDs	NSAIDs are a common cause of upper GI bleeding.
Avoid prasugrel and ticagrelor	Prasugrel and ticagrelor cannot be recommended because they are more potent and cause more bleeding than clopidogrel.

CYP, Cytochrome P450; *GI,* gastrointestinal; *INR,* international normalized ratio; *NSAID,* nonsteroidal antiinflammatory drug; *PPI,* proton pump inhibitor.

Case 4: Triple Therapy

A 55-year-old woman with a recent anterior MI treated who underwent primary PCI with implantation of a drug-eluting stent in the left anterior descending coronary artery is found to have a left ventricular thrombus on transthoracic echocardiogram. She is taking aspirin and clopidogrel. She is started on IV heparin, which is overlapped with warfarin until an INR of 2 is achieved. She is discharged home on triple antithrombotic therapy with aspirin, clopidogrel, and warfarin.

Comment

Anticoagulation is indicated for the management of left ventricular thrombosis, and the combination of aspirin and clopidogrel is indicated for the management of patients with drug-eluting stents. The combination of anticoagulation and dual antiplatelet therapy is associated with a 2% to 3% incidence of major bleeding during the first 30 days and a 4% to 12% incidence during the first year.[40] Strategies that may help to minimize the risk of bleeding in patients receiving triple antithrombotic are summarized in Table 148-7. The new oral anticoagulants dabigatran etexilate (110 mg twice a day) and apixaban (5 mg twice a day) may offer an advantage if they are used instead of warfarin in patients who require triple antithrombotic therapy because they cause less bleeding than warfarin in direct head-to-head comparisons.[41,42] However, all anticoagulants, including the new oral agents, increase the risk of bleeding when added to dual antiplatelet therapy.

CONCLUSIONS AND FUTURE DIRECTIONS

Antiplatelet and anticoagulant drugs are effective for the prevention of MI and death across the spectrum of patients presenting with ACS, including STEMI patients treated with fibrinolytic therapy and those undergoing mechanical reperfusion. Aggressive antithrombotic treatment regimens involving multiple antiplatelet drugs given in combination with an anticoagulant during the acute phase have substantially reduced the risk of early and late recurrent ischemic events and stent thrombosis in ACS patients but at the cost of an increased risk of bleeding. Clinicians require detailed knowledge of the pharmacology and side effects profile of antithrombotic therapies used in the management of patients with ACS to optimize clinical outcomes. Comparative effectiveness studies are urgently required to further define those combinations of antithrombotic drugs that will maximize the net clinical benefit for patients with ACS by minimizing the risk of both thrombotic and bleeding events.

REFERENCES

1. White HD, Chew DP: Acute myocardial infarction. *Lancet* 372:570, 2008.
2. Sami S, Willerson JT: Contemporary treatment of unstable angina and non-ST-segment-elevation myocardial infarction (part 1). *Tex Heart Inst J* 37:141, 2010.
3. Sami S, Willerson JT: Contemporary treatment of unstable angina and non-ST-segment-elevation myocardial infarction (part 2). *Tex Heart Inst J* 37:262, 2010.
4. Davi G, Patrono C: Platelet activation and atherothrombosis. *N Engl J Med* 357:2482, 2007.
5. Antman EM, Anbe DT, Armstrong PW, et al: ACC/AHA guidelines for the management of patients with ST-elevation myocardial infarction: A report of the American College of Cardiology/American Heart Association Task Force on Practice Guidelines (Committee to Revise the 1999 Guidelines for the Management of Patients with Acute Myocardial Infarction). *Circulation* 110:e82, 2004.
6. Kushner FG, Hand M, Smith SC Jr, et al: 2009 focused updates: ACC/AHA guidelines for the management of patients with ST-elevation myocardial infarction (updating the 2004 Guideline and 2007 Focused update) and ACC/AHA/SCAI guidelines on percutaneous coronary intervention (updating the 2005 guideline and 2007 focused update): A report of the American College of Cardiology Foundation/American Heart Association Task Force on Practice Guidelines. *Circulation* 120:2271, 2009.
7. Indications for fibrinolytic therapy in suspected acute myocardial infarction: Collaborative overview of early mortality and major morbidity results from all randomised trials of more than 1000 patients. Fibrinolytic Therapy Trialists' (FTT) Collaborative Group. *Lancet* 343:311, 1994.
8. Patel SC, Mody A: Cerebral hemorrhagic complications of thrombolytic therapy. *Prog Cardiovasc Dis* 42:217, 1999.
9. Mehta SR, Eikelboom JW, Yusuf S: Risk of intracranial haemorrhage with bolus versus infusion thrombolytic therapy: A meta-analysis. *Lancet* 356:449, 2000.
10. Anderson JL, Adams CD, Antman EM, et al: 2011 ACCF/AHA focused update incorporated into the ACC/AHA 2007 guidelines for the management of patients with unstable angina/non-ST-elevation myocardial infarction: A report of the American College of Cardiology Foundation/American Heart Association Task Force on Practice Guidelines. *Circulation* 123:e426, 2011.
11. Patrono C, Garcia Rodriguez LA, Landolfi R, et al: Low-dose aspirin for the prevention of atherothrombosis. *N Engl J Med* 353:2373, 2005.
12. Antithrombotic Trialists' Collaboration: Collaborative meta-analysis of randomised trials of antiplatelet therapy for prevention of death, myocardial infarction, and stroke in high risk patients. *BMJ* 324:71, 2002.
13. Mehta SR, Bassand JP, Chrolavicius S, et al: Dose comparisons of clopidogrel and aspirin in acute coronary syndromes. *N Engl J Med* 363:930, 2010.
14. Chen ZM, Jiang LX, Chen YP, et al: Addition of clopidogrel to aspirin in 45,852 patients with acute myocardial infarction: Randomised placebo-controlled trial. *Lancet* 366:1607, 2005.
15. Yusuf S, Zhao F, Mehta SR, et al: Effects of clopidogrel in addition to aspirin in patients with acute coronary syndromes without ST-segment elevation. *N Engl J Med* 345:494, 2001.
16. Wiviott SD, Braunwald E, McCabe CH, et al: Prasugrel versus clopidogrel in patients with acute coronary syndromes. *N Engl J Med* 357:2001, 2007.
17. Wallentin L, Becker RC, Budaj A, et al: Ticagrelor versus clopidogrel in patients with acute coronary syndromes. *N Engl J Med* 361:1045, 2009.
18. Boersma E, Harrington RA, Moliterno DJ, et al: Platelet glycoprotein IIb/IIIa inhibitors in acute coronary syndromes: A meta-analysis of all major randomised clinical trials. *Lancet* 359:189, 2002 .
19. De LG, Navarese E, Marino P: Risk profile and benefits from Gp IIb-IIIa inhibitors among patients with ST-segment elevation myocardial infarction treated with primary angioplasty: A meta-regression analysis of randomized trials. *Eur Heart J* 30:2705, 2009.
20. Marchini JF, Manica A, Croce K: Stent thrombosis: Understanding and managing a critical problem. *Curr Treat Options Cardiovasc Med* 14:91, 2012.
21. Holmes MV, Perel P, Shah T, et al: CYP2C19 genotype, clopidogrel metabolism, platelet function, and cardiovascular events: A systematic review and meta-analysis. *JAMA* 306:2704, 2011.
22. Aster RH, Curtis BR, Bougie DW, et al: Thrombocytopenia associated with the use of GPIIb/IIIa inhibitors: Position paper of the ISTH working group on thrombocytopenia and GPIIb/IIIa inhibitors. *J Thromb Haemost* 4:678, 2006.
23. Eikelboom JW, Weitz JI: New anticoagulants. *Circulation* 121:1523, 2010.
24. Mega JL, Braunwald E, Wiviott SD, et al: Rivaroxaban in patients with a recent acute coronary syndrome. *N Engl J Med* 366:9, 2011.
25. Alexander JH, Lopes RD, James S, et al: Apixaban with antiplatelet therapy after acute coronary syndrome. *N Engl J Med* 365:699, 2011 .
26. Hirsh J, O'Donnell M, Eikelboom JW: Beyond unfractionated heparin and warfarin: Current and future advances. *Circulation* 116:552, 2007.
27. Eikelboom JW, Quinlan DJ, Mehta SR, et al: Unfractionated and low-molecular-weight heparin as adjuncts to thrombolysis in aspirin-treated patients with ST-elevation acute myocardial infarction: A meta-analysis of the randomized trials. *Circulation* 112:3855, 2005.
28. Collins R, MacMahon S, Flather M, et al: Clinical effects of anticoagulant therapy in suspected acute myocardial infarction: Systematic overview of randomised trials. *BMJ* 313:652, 1996.
29. Eikelboom JW, Anand SS, Malmberg K, et al: Unfractionated heparin and low-molecular-weight heparin in acute coronary syndrome without ST elevation: A meta-analysis. *Lancet* 355:1936, 2000.
30. Yusuf S, Mehta SR, Xie C, et al: Effects of reviparin, a low-molecular-weight heparin, on mortality, reinfarction, and strokes in patients with acute myocardial infarction presenting with ST-segment elevation. *JAMA* 293:427, 2005.

For complete list of references log on to www.expertconsult.com.

CHAPTER 149

ATRIAL FIBRILLATION

Stavros Apostolakis and Gregory Y.H. Lip

Atrial fibrillation (AF) is a supraventricular arrhythmia characterized by uncoordinated atrial activation and loss of synchronous atrial mechanical activity. Typically, AF occurs in patients with underlying heart disease, such as hypertension or coronary or valvular heart disease; pulmonary pathology and thyroid disease; or other noncardiac causes. Nevertheless, a substantial proportion of patients with AF have no overt cardiovascular disease.

EPIDEMIOLOGY

AF is the most common sustained arrhythmia, affecting 5% of people older than 65 years. An analysis of the Framingham study indicates that the lifetime risk of developing AF from age 40 years onward is approximately 25% for the general population.[1] The estimated overall prevalence of AF is 0.9% in the United States and increases steadily to 3% to 5% in people older than 65 years and to 10% or higher in people older than 80 years of age. A similar prevalence has been reported in most regions of Western Europe.

The incidence of AF follows a similar pattern and also has a propensity to increase with age. The Framingham study, over a 38-year follow-up period, found an overall incidence of three in 1000 person-years in men and two in 1000 person-years in women ages 55 to 64 years.[1,2] The Manitoba follow-up study in Canada reported a similar overall incidence rate of two in 1000 person-years. The incidence of AF increases exponentially with advancing age to 20 to 30 per 1000 patient-years in individuals 85 years of age and older.[3]

AF is 1.5 times more common in men than in women. Moreover, the onset of AF in women occurs at a later age than in men (mean age, 65 years versus 60 years). Interestingly, the incidence pattern of AF shows racial and geographical variations.[2] The Cardiovascular Health Study reported that incidence of AF among white subjects was twice that among African Americans. The incidence and prevalence of AF appear to be similar in the United States and Western Europe but possibly lower in Asia.

Projected data from population-based studies, such as the ATRIA (Anticoagulation and Risk Factors in Atrial Fibrillation) study in California and analysis from the Mayo Clinic in Olmsted County, Minnesota, suggest that the number of adults with AF may reach 5.6 to 12.1 million by 2050. In fact, this number could be as high as 15.9 million if a continuous rise in the incidence of AF is present.

PATHOPHYSIOLOGY: A BRIEF OVERVIEW

Genesis and Preservation of Atrial Fibrillation

The pathophysiology of AF includes triggers that provoke the arrhythmia and a variety of electromechanical phenomena that sustain it. The triggers are diverse, and it is unclear whether they can induce AF in the absence of other contributors.[4] Triggers include sympathetic or parasympathetic stimulation, bradycardia or tachycardia, and atrial premature beats and acute atrial stretch. Ectopic foci occurring in areas of atrial tissue within the pulmonary veins or vena caval junctions have also been considered triggers of the arrhythmia.[5] When triggered, AF may be brief; however, a variety of factors may act as perpetuators to promote the persistence of AF. One is persistence of trigger factors and initiators that induce AF; nevertheless, AF often persists in their absence. This is probably the result of electrical and structural remodeling, characterized by atrial dilatation and shortening of the atrial effective refractory period. The longer AF persists, the more difficult it is to restore and maintain sinus rhythm. Early cardioversion progressively reduces the total time that patients are in AF and progressively increases the time between recurrences. The latter observation is attributed to the prevention of long-lasting AF paroxysms and subsequently to the prevention of electrophysiological remodeling.

Advanced age is also a perpetuating factor for AF with an obscure pathophysiological background. Age and atrial disease are associated with increases in connective tissue degeneration and atrial scarring. Fibrotic myocardium exhibits slow conduction; thus, reentrant circuits—only a few millimeters in diameter—can develop in discontinuously conducting tissue. Atrial regions with advanced fibrosis can be local "sources" for AF.

Thrombosis and Embolism

Thromboembolic events related to AF result in significant morbidity and mortality. Thrombi have a predilection to form within the left atrial appendage (LAA) in patients with AF (Fig. 149-1). Approximately 90% of atrial thrombi in nonvalvular AF and 60% of thrombi in patients with mitral valve disease are formed within the LAA. The LAA is a long, tubular, hooked structure that is usually crenulated and has a narrow junction with the main atrial cavity. The LAA is the remnant of the original embryonic left atrium that develops during the third week of gestation. The main smooth-walled cavity of the left atrium develops later and is formed from the outgrowth of the pulmonary veins.[6]

In sinus rhythm, the LAA contracts to a greater extent than the rest of the left atrium and has a distinct pattern of contraction. Blood flow within the LAA has been studied with transesophageal echocardiography (TEE), which provides better views of the appendage and its orifice than transthoracic echocardiography (TTE). Doppler-measured LAA flow in patients with sinus rhythm was initially described as biphasic, but additional emptying and filling waves resulting in quadriphasic appendage flow have been described in 40% to 70% of patients.[6]

Thrombus formation in AF is consistent with the fulfillment of the Virchow triad of thrombogenesis, with intraatrial stasis, endothelial dysfunction, and a prothrombotic or hypercoagulable state. Reduced or absent LAA inflow and outflow velocities and low LAA ejection fractions are commonly observed in patients in AF (Fig. 149-2). Mechanical dysfunction leads to blood stasis and thrombus formation. The cause of LAA dysfunction, however, has not been fully elucidated. It is likely to be related in part to a myopathic process that results in AF or that occurs as a result of the AF itself. Endothelial dysfunction has also been recognized as a contributor to thrombus formation in AF, and along with stasis, contributes to a

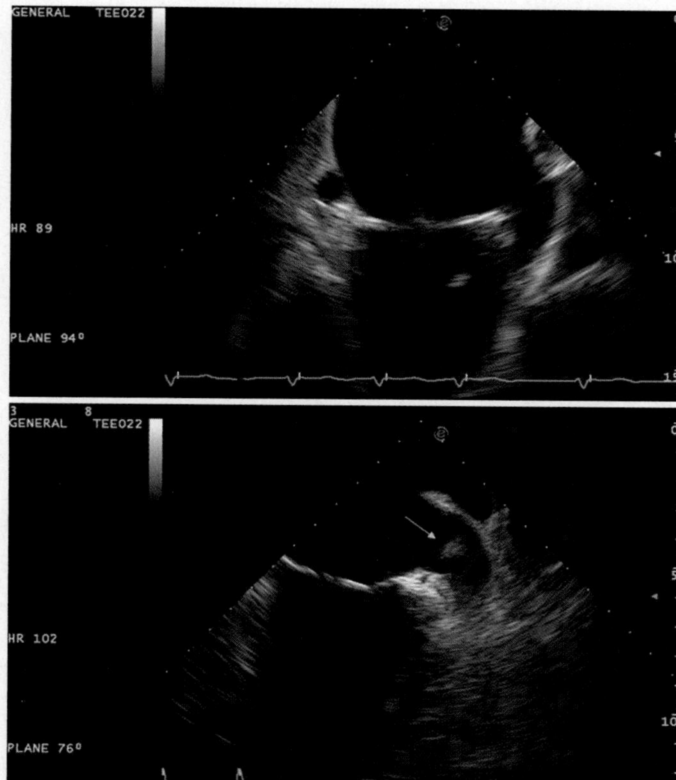

Figure 149-1 TRANSESOPHAGEAL VIEWS OF LEFT ATRIAL APPENDAGE (LAA). The LAA is a long, tubular, hooked structure that is usually crenulated and has a narrow junction with the venous component of the atrium. Thrombi have a predilection to form within the LAA *(yellow arrow)*.

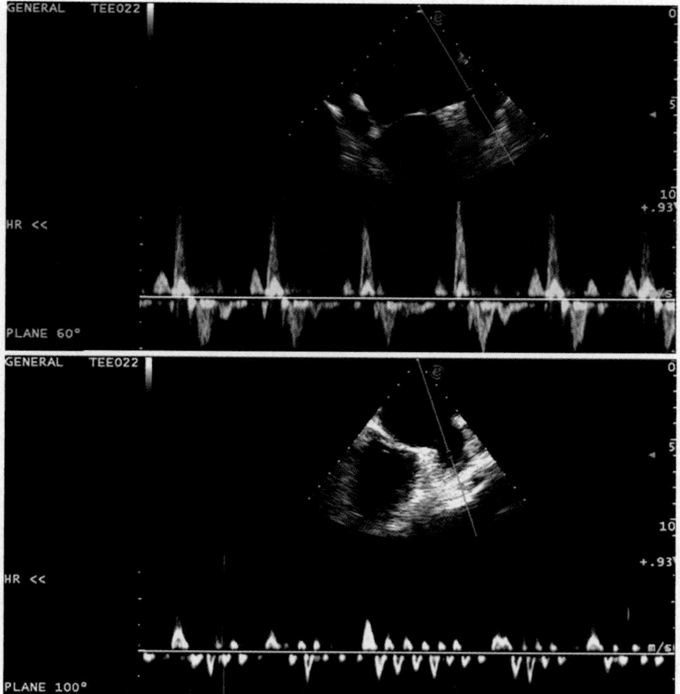

Figure 149-2 DOPPLER MEASURED LEFT ATRIAL APPENDAGE (LAA) FLOW IN A PATIENT WITH SINUS RHYTHM *(UPPER)*. Reduced LAA inflow and outflow velocities are observed in patients in atrial fibrillation.

hypercoagulable state. Elevated plasma and atrial tissue levels of prothrombotic markers, such as D-dimer, P-selectin, and von Willebrand factor, have been reported in patients with AF independent of associated comorbidities or structural heart disease, leading to the concept that AF induces a systemic hypercoagulable state.

The size and mobility of the LAA thrombus are other determinants of thromboembolic risk. Mobile thrombi with a diameter greater than 15 mm have been associated with an increased risk of thromboembolism.[6]

Functional indices of LAA stasis are restored after conversion to sinus rhythm. However, patients with AF who are successfully cardioverted with drugs or DC shock show depressed AF mechanical function for a variable period after restoration of sinus rhythm. These findings support the concept that such patients require antithrombotic therapy for at least 4 weeks after successful cardioversion.

CLINICAL MANIFESTATION AND DIAGNOSIS

History and Physical Examination

AF is often asymptomatic, and it is not unusual for a patient to first become aware of AF during a routine physical examination. When symptoms occur, they are commonly associated with rapid ventricular rate. Rapid and irregular heart rates may be experienced as palpitations, exercise intolerance, or vague chest discomfort. In some patients with persistently elevated ventricular rates, cardiomyopathy may occur, leading to heart failure as the prominent manifestation of AF. Syncope is a rare complication of AF that can occur in patients with sinus node dysfunction, with rapid ventricular rates in patients with left ventricular outflow obstruction, or when an accessory pathway exists. It is not uncommon for patients with AF to present with an acute ischemic stroke, transient ischemic attack (TIA), or systemic embolism (see Chapter 147).[7]

Common findings suggestive of AF during physical examination are an irregular pulse, variation in the intensity of the first heart sound, or absence of a previously heard fourth heart sound. Examination may also reveal associated valvular heart disease, myocardial abnormalities, or heart failure. A pulse deficit may be present if the left ventricular stroke volume is insufficient to produce a palpable peripheral pressure wave with rapid ventricular rates.

Because most cases of AF are secondary to other medical conditions, a detailed medical history is important to assess the presence of angina, hyperthyroidism, or lung disease. A previous history of stroke or TIA, as well as hypertension, diabetes, heart failure, and rheumatic fever, may indicate whether a patient is at a higher risk of thromboembolism.[7]

Additional Testing and Cardiac Imaging

The diagnosis of AF is based on a detailed history and clinical examination, and electrocardiographic (ECG) recordings confirm the arrhythmia. The initial evaluation of a patient with suspected or documented AF involves defining the pattern of the arrhythmia, identifying its cause, and revealing associated cardiac and noncardiac factors relevant to the etiology.

Electrocardiography is the gold standard for the diagnosis of AF. A single-lead recording during the arrhythmia is sufficient to establish the diagnosis. Diagnostic ECG criteria include absence of P waves, irregular timing, fibrillatory (F) waves between QRS complexes, and irregularly irregular R-R intervals (Fig. 149-3).

Echocardiography and thyroid function tests are important in the initial evaluation. A chest radiograph may detect enlargement of the cardiac chambers and heart failure; however, it is less important than echocardiography for routine evaluation of patients with AF. As part of the initial evaluation, all patients with AF should undergo two-dimensional and Doppler echocardiography to assess left atrial and left ventricular dimensions and function and to reveal underlying

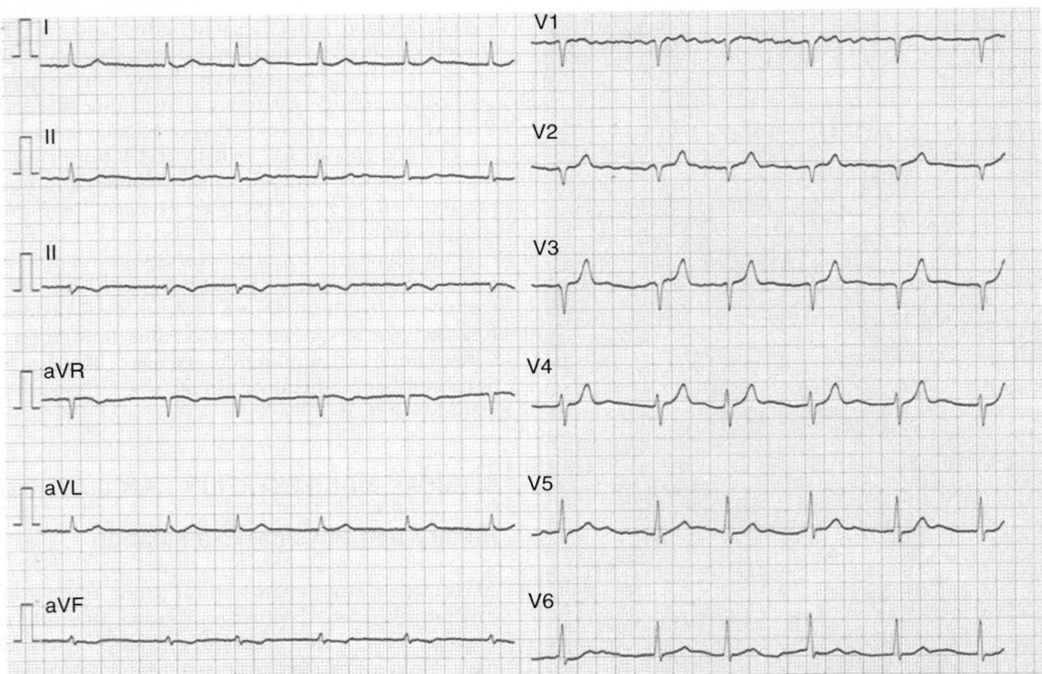

Figure 149-3 TYPICAL 12-LEAD ELECTROCARDIOGRAM OF ATRIAL FIBRILLATION. Absence of P waves, irregular timing, and morphology fibrillatory (F) waves and irregularly irregular R-R intervals are evident.

structural heart disease. Quantification of left ventricular systolic function further assists decision making regarding antiarrhythmic and antithrombotic therapy.[7]

Blood tests are important in initial assessment but can be limited to tests of thyroid, renal, and hepatic function, serum electrolytes, and a hemogram. These tests should be performed at least once in the course of the patient's evaluation. Novel markers of cardiovascular disease have been assessed in AF, but their prognostic and diagnostic impact remains obscure. Natriuretic peptides have been found to be elevated in patients with paroxysmal and persistent AF and decline rapidly after sinus rhythm is restored. Although high levels of B-type natriuretic peptide have been associated with thromboembolism and recurrences of AF, further studies are needed to evaluate their prognostic significance.

Prolonged ECG monitoring may be necessary to reveal episodes of asymptomatic AF. Ambulatory ECG monitoring may also document the adequacy of rate control and further guide therapy. Exercise testing is recommended when myocardial ischemia is suspected before the initiation of type Ic antiarrhythmic agents and when the adequacy of rate control on activity needs to be assessed.

Transesophageal echocardiography is the most sensitive and specific technique to detect sources of cardiogenic embolism and has been most effectively used to stratify stroke risk in patients with AF scheduled for cardioversion. However, TEE is not recommended as part of the routine initial evaluation of patients with AF. Contrast-enhanced magnetic resonance imaging is a promising technique for the detection of intracardiac thrombi with a reported sensitivity higher than TTE and comparable to TEE. Finally, an electrophysiological study can be useful in cases in which AF is a consequence of reentrant tachycardia such as atrial flutter, intraatrial reentry, or atrioventricular (AV) reentry involving an accessory pathway.

Differential Diagnosis

Other irregular rhythms may resemble AF on ECG, but these can easily be distinguished by the presence of discrete P waves. Atrial flutter, in the typical form, is characterized by a saw-tooth pattern of regular atrial activation, called flutter (F) waves on the ECG, which is particularly visible in leads II, III, aVF, and V1, especially with vagal maneuvers. With atrial flutter, the atrial rate typically ranges from 240 to 320 stimuli per minute. Atrial flutter commonly occurs with 2:1 AV block, resulting in a regular or irregular ventricular rate of approximately 150 beats/min.

In most other atrial tachycardias, P waves can readily be identified in one or more ECG leads. The morphology and the arrangement of the P waves relative to the preceding and the forthcoming QRS complexes may help identify the origin of the tachycardia.[7]

Prognosis

AF is clinically relevant. It may indicate underlying heart disease or cause symptoms related to hemodynamic impairment or palpitations. However, the most important reason to make the diagnosis of AF is because of the increased risk of stroke and systemic thromboembolism. On average, the overall risk of stroke among individuals with AF is about 5% per year and is about five or six times greater than the risk among age-matched subjects in sinus rhythm.

AF is also an accurate marker of future morbidity. Large-scale studies have demonstrated increased risk of all-cause mortality and death from cardiovascular causes in AF patients, ranging from a 1.3- to 1.8-fold increase for men and 1.9- to 2.8-fold increase for women. AF imposes a substantial cost burden on the health care system because of the increased arrhythmia-related morbidity and mortality and the significant cost associated with management strategies.[7]

AF can occur after acute myocardial infarction or cardiac surgery, and it can be found in association with pericarditis, myocarditis, hyperthyroidism or acute pulmonary disease. In these settings, AF is not the culprit condition, and treatment of the underlying disorder usually terminates the arrhythmia and diminishes the chance of recurrences. The term *lone AF* has been generally applied to young individuals without evidence of cardiovascular disease. These patients have a favorable prognosis regarding both thromboembolism and mortality.

THERAPY

General Considerations

There are two ways to approach arrhythmia-related symptoms in patients with AF: rate control and rhythm control. Whereas rhythm control strategies aim to restore and maintain sinus rhythm, rate control uses interventions to maintain the heart rate within normal range with no commitment to restoring sinus rhythm. The wide heterogeneity in both the clinical presentation and the clinical background of AF necessitates a personalized approach to its management. Such an approach requires selection of the appropriate rhythm control or rate control strategy, taking into account the impact of each strategy on prognosis, quality of life, and financial resource utilization. In general, antiarrhythmic drugs and invasive procedures have proven to be effective for rate and rhythm control, and for selected patients, intervention may be the preferred option. Regardless of the initial approach, the need for anticoagulation is based on individualized stroke risk and not on whether sinus rhythm is restored and maintained. For rhythm control, drugs are typically the first choice. However, in young symptomatic patients, radiofrequency ablation may be preferable to long-term drug therapy. Few patients are candidates for a stand-alone surgical procedure to cure AF using the Cox-maze procedure or left atrial ablation techniques; however, these approaches can be valuable additions to coronary bypass or valve repair surgery to prevent recurrences of AF.

Rhythm or Rate Control

Prophylactic antiarrhythmic drug therapy should ideally maintain sinus rhythm, minimize symptoms, improve exercise capacity, and prevent tachycardia-induced cardiomyopathy. Nevertheless, maintenance of sinus rhythm does not seem to prevent thromboembolism or heart failure or reduce mortality. Trials comparing rate versus rhythm control approaches in patients with persistent or paroxysmal AF concluded that rhythm control offered no benefits in terms of reduction in death, disabling stroke, hospitalizations, new arrhythmias, or thromboembolic complications. The AFFIRM (Atrial Fibrillation Follow-up Investigation of Rhythm Management) trial, which randomized 4060 patients to either strategy, demonstrated no difference in mortality or stroke rate with rhythm versus rate control.[8] Similarly, the RACE (Rate Control versus Electrical cardioversion for persistent atrial fibrillation) trial recruited 522 patients and concluded that rate control is noninferior to rhythm control for prevention of death and morbidity.[9] Therefore, pharmacologic therapy to maintain sinus rhythm should only be considered in symptomatic patients who can tolerate antiarrhythmic drugs and have a high probability of retaining sinus rhythm for an extended period. Physicians should not insist on antiarrhythmic medication when it does not improve symptoms or is poorly tolerated.

Direct current cardioversion is the most effective method for restoring sinus rhythm. However, whether cardioversion by electrical shock has advantages over medical cardioversion has never been subjected to a randomized clinical trial.

General Approaches to Pharmacologic Antiarrhythmic Therapy

As an initial approach, every reversible precipitant of AF should be corrected before the administration of any antiarrhythmic agent. Indefinite antiarrhythmic treatment is usually not recommended after a first episode of AF. Selection of an appropriate agent is based on safety, tolerability, the underlying cardiovascular pathology, and the individual characteristics of AF. A drug that is initially safe may become proarrhythmic if coronary disease or heart failure develops or if the patient begins other potentially proarrhythmic medication. Consequently, patients should be regularly reassessed and informed about the potential significance of symptoms suggestive of rhythm disorders.

There is general agreement between the European and the North American cardiovascular societies on the antiarrhythmic management of AF. According to the latest consensus documents, β-adrenergic antagonists may be effective in patients who only develop AF during exercise. Likewise, in patients with lone AF, a β-blocker may be initially recommended, although flecainide, propafenone, and sotalol are particularly effective for rhythm maintenance. Amiodarone may also be instituted for chronic treatment when conventional measures are ineffective, but it may cause severe extracardiac adverse events, including thyroid dysfunction and bradycardia. Dronedarone has a better long-term safety profile than amiodarone and according to the latest guidelines should be considered before amiodarone for rhythm maintenance in patients with acute coronary syndromes, chronic stable angina, hypertensive heart disease, and stable New York Heart Association class I to II heart failure. Quinidine, procainamide, and disopyramide are not favored unless amiodarone is ineffective or contraindicated. In patients in whom treatment with a single antiarrhythmic agent fails, combination therapy may be considered. Effective combinations include a β-blocker, such as sotalol, or amiodarone with a class Ic agent. The addition of a calcium channel blocker, such as diltiazem, to a class Ic agent, such as flecainide or propafenone, is also beneficial for some patients, especially to avoid 1:1 atrial flutter with the class I agent.[10]

The safety of dronedarone has been questioned lately based on data derived both from postmarketing surveillance and clinical trials. In the PALLAS (Permanent Atrial fibriLLAtion Study) trial, dronedarone increased rates of heart failure, stroke, and death from cardiovascular causes in patients with permanent AF who were at risk for major vascular events.[10] The PALLAS investigators concluded that this drug should not be used in such patients. Moreover, the Food and Drug Administration (FDA) has received several case reports of hepatocellular liver injury and hepatic failure in patients treated with dronedarone, including two postmarketing reports of acute hepatic failure requiring transplantation.

Pharmacologic management to achieve rate control in AF patients should be tailored to the potential concomitant cardiac disease states, particularly coronary artery disease or heart failure. β-Blockers may be especially useful when high adrenergic tone or symptomatic myocardial ischemia occurs in association with AF. Nondihydropyridine calcium channel antagonists (i.e., verapamil or diltiazem) are particularly effective for acute and chronic rate control in AF; however, these drugs are contraindicated in patients with systolic dysfunction because of their negative inotropic effect. Digoxin is effective for control of heart rate at rest but not during exercise, but it may be effective in combination with a β-blocker in patients with heart failure. Digoxin may cause adverse effects in patients with heart failure and can interact with other drugs. Amiodarone is an effective rate control drug even though it is often started for rhythm control. Class I antiarrhythmic drugs are not effective for rate control.[10]

The optimum way for monitoring antiarrhythmic therapy varies depending on the agent and the patient's cardiovascular comorbidities. In patients given class Ic agents, prolongation of the QRS interval should not exceed 50%. Exercise testing may help to detect QRS widening that occurs only with rapid heart rates. In patients treated with class IA or class III drugs, with the possible exception of amiodarone, the corrected QT interval in sinus rhythm should be kept below 520 msec. During follow-up, plasma potassium and magnesium levels and renal function should be checked periodically.[10]

Nonpharmacologic Approaches

The limited efficacy and potential toxicity of antiarrhythmic drugs have lead to the exploration of alternative, nonpharmacologic strategies for the management of AF.

The Cox-maze procedure was developed by James Cox and associates and was first performed at St. Louis' Barnes Hospital in 1987.[11]

This surgical approach creates conduction barriers within the atria and reduces the mass of the left and right atrium to prevent or block the microreentry circuits that maintain the arrhythmia. From the technical standpoint, the procedure involves encircling the pulmonary veins with multiple linear incisions over both atria using either the cut-and-sew technique or different energy probes. The success rate of the procedure ranges from 85% to 95%. Moreover, removal or closure of the LAA together with maintenance of sinus rhythm reduces the long-term stroke rate to less than 1%. However, the procedure is invasive. Recent modifications use minimally invasive thoracoscopic techniques and different energy ablation probes to shorten the procedure time and improve safety.

Device Therapies—Atrial Pacing and Defibrillation

There is no evidence to support the use of permanent atrial pacing to treat paroxysmal AF in patients without a conventional indication for pacing. However, in patients with sinus node disease, symptomatic bradycardia, or chronotropic incompetence in need of permanent pacing, the use of dual-chamber or atrial pacemakers reduces the occurrence of AF. Although many modern pacemakers and implantable ventricular defibrillators have features such as overdrive pacing, antitachycardia atrial pacing, and atrial defibrillation that are designed to prevent or terminate AF, data from large randomized trials do not support their routine use.[10,12]

Catheter Ablation

Ablation of the AV node and permanent pacing is an effective method for rate control and symptomatic relief in patients with antiarrhythmic drug-resistant AF and for those who cannot tolerate drug therapy. A meta-analysis, involving 1181 patients, reported significant improvement in quality-of-life and clinical outcome measures after ablation and pacing therapy with acceptable 1-year total and sudden death mortality rates. However, this approach leads to pacemaker dependency, a requirement for indefinite anticoagulation, and is associated with proarrhythmia.

Catheter ablation strategies to treat AF aim to eliminate the triggers that initiate or promote the arrhythmia and to modify the electrophysiological background that sustains it. In patients with paroxysmal AF, arrhythmogenic foci in the pulmonary veins, or less commonly from other atrial sites, may be important triggers of the disease and subsequently therapeutic targets. Isolation of these arrhythmogenic sites can eliminate recurrences in 80% to 90% of the treated patients.[13,14] Different catheter ablation techniques are used to electrically isolate the pulmonary veins from the left atrium or to modify the left atrial tissue around the pulmonary veins (circumferential ablation). The safety and efficacy of pulmonary vein isolation has been compared with antiarrhythmic drug therapy in a few randomized trials with promising results. However, catheter ablation procedures are technically challenging and operator dependent. This is reflected in the inconsistent rates of success and adverse events in clinical trials and in clinical practice. In addition, the long-term effectiveness of catheter ablation procedures remains obscure. Development of new catheter ablation techniques and the use of different imaging and navigation systems may improve the success and safety of the procedure.

PREVENTION OF THROMBOEMBOLISM

Cardioversion and Thromboembolism Prevention

Patients who have been in AF for more than 48 hours—or those in whom the onset of the arrhythmia cannot be accurately defined—may be considered for anticoagulation therapy and strategies to restore and maintain sinus rhythm. Adjusted-dose warfarin within the therapeutic range should be administered for 3 weeks before cardioversion is attempted. If cardioversion cannot be postponed, a TEE should be performed. Cardioversion can be undertaken with an acceptable risk of stroke if TEE excludes LAA thrombus.[15] However, if TEE identifies LAA thrombus, cardioversion should be delayed until the patient has been anticoagulated for at least 3 to 4 weeks and a repeat TEE reveals thrombus dissolution. If the thrombus persists, cardioversion should not be performed.

After successful cardioversion, warfarin therapy should be continued for at least 4 weeks to prevent thrombus formation in the "stunned" left atrium. If the patient has a low risk of recurrent AF and remains in sinus rhythm for 1 month after cardioversion, anticoagulation therapy with warfarin can be stopped. In patients at higher risk of thromboembolism, it may be more appropriate to continue warfarin therapy indefinitely.[10,12]

Long-Term Primary and Secondary Prevention of Thromboembolism

Risk Stratification

Patients with AF have a substantial risk of stroke and systemic thromboembolism compared with age-matched people in sinus rhythm. This risk depends on comorbidities and demographic factors and ranges from less than 1% to more than 20% per year.[16] The important independent prognostic factors for an increased risk of AF-related stroke are increasing age, a history of previous TIA or stroke, hypertension, diabetes mellitus, and evidence of moderate to severe left ventricular systolic dysfunction. Echocardiographic evidence of left atrial enlargement and left atrial spontaneous echo contrast have also been associated with increased risk for AF-related stroke.[17] Moreover, these risk factors are cumulative: for people younger than 65 years old with no risk factors, the annual risk of stroke is about 1%. For the same age group, the untreated risk exceeds 12% if multiple risk factors are present. The complexity of the factors that influence thromboembolic risk in patients with AF necessitated the development of risk stratification schemas to identify the subgroup of patients who will benefit from anticoagulation.

The most widely used stroke risk classification scheme, known as $CHADS_2$ (Table 149-1 defines $CHADS_2$), was developed in 2001 and adapted by the American College of Cardiology/American Heart Association/European Society of Cardiology (ACC/AHA/ESC) guideline committee in 2006.[7] The $CHADS_2$ score classifies patients with 0 points as low risk, 1 point as moderate risk, and 2 points or more as high risk. Such a practice translates to better outcomes in AF patients because there is a clear relationship between $CHADS_2$ score and stroke rate.

In 2008, the Stroke in AF Working Group compared the predictive value of 12 published risk-stratification schemes, including the $CHADS_2$ score. The investigators concluded that most of these clinical tools had very modest predictive value for stroke, especially if patients were artificially categorized into low-, moderate-, and high-risk strata. The $CHADS_2$ score categorized most subjects as "moderate risk" and had a low c-statistic to predict stroke. Moreover, the $CHADS_2$ score did not include several stroke risk factors that have been substantiated in randomized studies and registries.[12]

The CHA_2DS_2-VASc scoring system was developed to overcome these problems (see Table 149-1). In this system, the "major" risk factors are defined as prior stroke, TIA, or systemic thromboembolism and older age (75 years or older). The presence of mitral stenosis or prosthetic heart valves also identifies AF patients as high risk. Clinically relevant nonmajor risk factors include heart failure—particularly moderate to severe systolic LV dysfunction—hypertension, or diabetes. Other clinically relevant nonmajor risk factors include female sex, age 65 to 74 years; vascular disease defined as myocardial infarction; and complex aortic plaque or peripheral arterial disease. That risk factors are still cumulative, and the simultaneous presence of two or more clinically relevant nonmajor risk factors justifies anticoagulation.

The ESC guidelines recommend the use of both $CHADS_2$ and CHA_2DS_2-VASc score. The $CHADS_2$ stroke risk stratification scheme

Table 149-1 CHA_2DS_2-VASc and $CHADS_2$ Scores*

CHA_2DS_2-VASc Score		$CHADS_2$ Score	
Major Risk Factors	**Points**	**Risk Factors**	**Points**
Previous stroke, TIA, or systemic embolism	2	Congestive heart failure or LV dysfunction	1
Age >75 years	2	Hypertension	1
Clinically Relevant Nonmajor Risk Factors		Age >75 years	1
Congestive heart failure or left ventricular dysfunction*	1	Diabetes mellitus	1
Hypertension	1	Previous stroke, TIA, or systemic embolism	2
Diabetes mellitus	1		
Vascular disease†	1		
Age 65-74 years	1		
Sex category (i.e., female sex)	1		
Maximum points	9		6

LV, Left ventricular; *TIA*, transient ischemic attack;
*Especially moderate to severe systolic LV dysfunction, defined arbitrarily as LV ejection fraction of 40% or less.
†Defined as myocardial infarction, complex aortic plaque, or peripheral arterial disease (PAD), including prior revascularization, amputation because of PAD, or angiographic evidence of PAD.

Table 149-2 The HAS-BLED score

	Clinical Characteristic	**Point**
H	Hypertension*	1
A	Abnormal renal† and liver function‡ (1 point each)	1 or 2
S	Stroke	1
B	Bleeding§	1
L	Labile INRs¶	1
E	Elderly (e.g., age >65 years)	1
D	Drugs¶ or alcohol (1 point each)	1 or 2
	Maximum points	9

*Systolic blood pressure >160 mm Hg.
†The presence of chronic dialysis or renal transplantation or serum creatinine ≥200 mmol/L.
‡Chronic hepatic disease (e.g., cirrhosis) or biochemical evidence of significant hepatic derangement.
§Previous bleeding history or predisposition to bleeding.
¶Unstable or high international normalized ratio (INR) or poor time in the therapeutic range.
¶Concomitant use of drugs, such as antiplatelet agents or nonsteroidal antiinflammatory drugs.

should be used as a simple initial means of assessing stroke risk, particularly suited to primary care physicians and nonspecialists. In patients with a $CHADS_2$ score of 2 or greater, chronic oral anticoagulation therapy should be prescribed unless contraindicated. In patients with a $CHADS_2$ score of 0 to 1 or when a more detailed stroke risk assessment is indicated, the CHA_2DS_2-VASc score can be used. A pragmatic view is also recommended in the guideline for certain patient groups. For example, in women ages 65 years with no other risk factors and normal echocardiography, aspirin (or no antithrombotic therapy) rather than oral anticoagulation therapy may be considered.

Risk factors predisposing to anticoagulant-associated hemorrhage have also been identified. These include previous symptomatic cerebrovascular disease; computed tomography scan evidence of small vessel disease; poorly controlled hypertension; and excessive anticoagulation, including factors predisposing to it, such as confusion, dementia, inadequate monitoring, and alcoholic liver disease. Increasing age predisposes to all of these risk factors; thus, it is considered a potent risk factor for anticoagulant-associated hemorrhage.[7]

In the latest edition of the ESC guidelines, a simple and user-friendly clinical tool was developed to assess 1-year risk of major bleeding in patients with AF based on analysis of data from 3978 participants of the EuroHeart Survey. The clinical tool was given the acronym HAS-BLED and includes most of the clinical predictors that have been associated with hemorrhagic complications related to antithrombotic therapy (Table 149-2). A score of 3 or greater indicates high risk. Regular patient review and HAS-BLED score calculation are needed to balance the risk of bleeding with the benefits of anticoagulant therapy.[12]

Warfarin for Stroke Prevention in Atrial Fibrillation

Strategies for reducing the risk of stroke and systemic thromboembolism in patients with chronic AF have been studied in many randomized controlled trials over the previous decades. Five large randomized primary prevention trials have shown that in people with chronic nonvalvular AF, warfarin reduces the overall risk of stroke from 4.5% to 1.4% per year with an acceptable increase in major bleeding rates. This translates to 30 strokes prevented per 1000 patient-years of treatment at a cost of at least two serious bleeds per 1000 patients per year.[18-22]

For secondary prevention, the European Atrial Fibrillation Trial investigators randomized 1007 patients with a recent TIA or minor ischemic stroke to open anticoagulation or double-blind treatment with either aspirin or placebo.[23] The authors concluded that in patients with chronic nonvalvular AF and a history of stroke or TIA, the annual risk of stroke is reduced from 12% to 4% with warfarin. The annual incidence of major bleedings was 2.8% in the anticoagulant group and 0.7% in the placebo group. Thus, in the secondary prevention setting, warfarin prevents 80 strokes per 1000 patient-years, at a cost of at least 20 major bleeds per 1000 patients treated for one year.

The optimal time to initiate anticoagulation therapy after a recent cerebrovascular accident depends on the risk of recurrent thromboembolism and the risk of hemorrhagic transformation of the infarct. Two randomized trials have demonstrated no benefit from early anticoagulation because any net gain obtained from reduction in recurrent ischemic stroke was offset by the excess hazard of hemorrhagic stroke. Thus, in the absence of evidence, common practice is to begin warfarin 3 to 14 days after patients present with an acute stroke (see Chapter 147).[7]

New Oral Anticoagulants for Stroke Prevention in Atrial Fibrillation

Dabigatran etexilate is an oral prodrug that is rapidly converted by a serum esterase to dabigatran, a potent, direct inhibitor of thrombin (see Chapter 151). In the RE-LY (Randomized Evaluation of Long Term Anticoagulant Therapy) study, 18,113 patients with AF and a risk of stroke were randomly assigned to fixed doses of 110 mg or 150 mg dabigatran twice daily or adjusted-dose warfarin. The primary outcome was stroke or systemic embolism. The results based on the criterion of noninferiority indicated that the dose of 150 mg twice a day was significantly more effective than warfarin in the prevention of ischemic stroke with similar rates of major hemorrhage. The dose of 110 mg twice a day was similar to warfarin in the prevention of thromboembolism and was associated with significantly lower rates of hemorrhagic events.[24]

Rivaroxaban is the first available orally active direct factor Xa inhibitor (see Chapter 151). It possesses impressive pharmacologic properties, including once-daily oral administration, rapid onset of action, and predictable pharmacokinetics. The ROCKET-AF (Rivaroxaban Once-daily oral direct factor Xa inhibition Compared with vitamin K antagonism for prevention of stroke and Embolism Trial in Atrial Fibrillation) recruited 14,264 patients with nonvalvular AF at increased risk for stroke. Patients were randomly assigned to receive either rivaroxaban at a daily dose of 20 mg or dose-adjusted warfarin. The investigators concluded that in patients with AF, rivaroxaban was noninferior to warfarin for the prevention of stroke or systemic embolism. Moreover, there was no significant between-group difference in the risk of major bleeding. Nevertheless, intracranial and fatal bleeding occurred less frequently in the rivaroxaban group.[25]

Apixaban is the second direct inhibitor of activated factor X that completed successfully phase III trials (see Chapter 151). The AVERROES (Apixaban versus Acetylsalicylic Acid to Prevent Strokes) trial was a double-blind study that recruited 5599 patients with AF who were at increased risk for stroke and for whom vitamin K antagonist (VKA) therapy was considered unsuitable. The study participants were randomly assigned to receive either 5 mg of apixaban twice daily or aspirin. The primary outcome was stroke or systemic embolism. Treatment with apixaban was associated with a 55% reduction in the risk of stroke or systemic embolism compared with aspirin. The risk of major bleeding was not significantly different between apixaban and aspirin.[26] In the ARISTOTLE (Apixaban for Reduction In Stroke and other ThromboemboLic Events in atrial fibrillation) study, apixaban 5 mg twice daily was compared with adjusted dose warfarin in a randomized, double-blind trial involving 18,201 patients with AF and at least one additional risk factor for stroke. The primary outcome was ischemic or hemorrhagic stroke or systemic embolism. In ARISTOTLE, apixaban reduced the primary outcome by 21% compared with warfarin. The reduction was significant and supports the superiority of apixaban over warfarin. Apixaban also significantly reduced all-cause mortality and major bleeding rates.[27]

Antiplatelet Drugs for Stroke Prevention in Atrial Fibrillation

Three primary prevention and three secondary prevention trials have shown that in patients with AF, aspirin reduces the annual incidence of stroke from 5.2% to 3.7% for primary prevention and from 12.9% to 10.4% for secondary prevention. Aspirin was not associated with any significant increase in the rate of intracranial hemorrhage or the rate of major extracranial bleeding. This means that aspirin might prevent about 10 to 20 strokes per 1000 patient-years of treatment, depending on baseline patient characteristics and baseline risk of stroke. The relative benefits and risks of aspirin versus warfarin have been studied in three trials, all of which showed that dose-adjusted warfarin (target INR, 2.0-3.0) was associated with half the risk of stroke compared with aspirin monotherapy. Similarly, for patients with AF who are at high risk of stroke, adding aspirin to low-intensity, fixed-dose warfarin was not as effective in preventing stroke or systemic thromboembolism as adjusted-dose warfarin monotherapy targeting to an INR of 2.0 to 3.0. There was no difference in major bleeding rates.

Dual antiplatelet therapy has been compared with warfarin for the prevention of thromboembolism in patients with AF in the ACTIVE W (Atrial Fibrillation Clopidogrel Trial with Irbesartan for Prevention of Vascular Events) trial. The trial was stopped prematurely because of a clear benefit of warfarin arm over the combination of clopidogrel plus aspirin. Of note, the incidence of major bleeding was similar in the two groups.[28] The ACTIVE-A study compared the clopidogrel–aspirin combination with aspirin alone in moderate- to high-risk patients with AF for whom VKA therapy was unsuitable. The trial showed that the addition of clopidogrel to aspirin reduced the risk of major vascular events and concluded that combination antiplatelet therapy was better than aspirin alone for the prevention of thromboembolism in patients with AF. Nonetheless, major bleeding rates with aspirin plus clopidogrel were more than 50% greater than with aspirin alone and were similar to rates seen with anticoagulation.[29]

Practical Considerations

The decision to treat an individual patient should be based on the balance between the risk of thromboembolism if left untreated and the risks of thromboembolism and hemorrhage if treated. The patient's willingness to accept the potential risks, costs, and inconvenience related to treatment and the limitations of the available health care system should also be considered. Finally, one should also keep in mind that the current profile of individual risk of thromboembolism and bleeding complications (see above) is imperfect and continues to be refined as new data emerge.

The choices of thromboprophylaxis for AF patients include warfarin, which is the most effective but also the most risky treatment, and aspirin, which is less effective but safer than warfarin. The ideal treatment strategy is the one in which patients at high risk of stroke and low risk of hemorrhage are treated with warfarin and patients at low risk of stroke or high risk of hemorrhage are treated with aspirin or no antithrombotic treatment.

Based on current guidelines, aspirin or no antithrombotic therapy (the latter preferred) should be considered for individuals in AF who are at "truly low risk" of stroke, such as those without any of the independent risk factors listed earlier (i.e., CHA_2DS_2-VASc score of 0). Oral anticoagulation therapy (whether with warfarin or one of the new oral anticoagulants) is the treatment of choice for individuals with chronic AF who have an annual risk of stroke greater than 4% (i.e., CHA_2DS_2-VASc score >1) and an acceptable risk of hemorrhage. For patients at intermediate risk (i.e., CHA_2DS_2-VASc score of 1), either treatment is reasonable, but oral anticoagulation therapy is preferred. For patients whose risks of thromboembolism and hemorrhage are both high, identifying a treatment strategy can be difficult and may ultimately be guided by the patient's preferences.[10]

Patients on aspirin or no antithrombotic therapy should be reviewed regularly, and their treatment may change because individualized risk changes over time; such change occurs in 10% to 15% of people being treated with aspirin per year.

The range of VKA therapy intensity (INR) that provides the best balance between the prevention of thromboembolism and the occurrence of bleeding appears to be between 2.0 and 3.0 but may be higher in patients at greater risk of thromboembolism, particularly those with prosthetic valves. Although some advocate a lower INR intensity for those at risk of bleeding (e.g., INR 1.8-2.5), the bleeding rate is lowest with an INR below 3.0 with no further decline with an INR below 2.0. Hence, there is little reason to aim for a lower target INR, especially because the risk of thromboembolism increases with an INR below 2.0.

When cessation of warfarin is required because of scheduled invasive procedures, it is necessary to stratify the bleeding risk associated with the procedure and the short-term risk of thromboembolism. Warfarin can be ceased 5 days before a high bleeding risk procedure and continued at a decreased dose for a minor bleeding risk procedure. In either case, therapy should be reinstituted as soon as possible. For patients at high risk of thromboembolism, heparin or low-molecular-weight bridging during warfarin cessation is the preferred strategy.[10,12]

Nonpharmacologic Approaches to Prevention of Thromboembolism

A promising option for patients with AF who cannot safely be subjected to oral anticoagulation is obliteration of the LAA to remove the main anatomic source of thrombus formation. In addition to direct surgical amputation or truncation of the LAA, several methods are under development to achieve this with intravascular catheters or via a transpericardial approach. The most recent study, PROTECT-AF

(Protection in Patients With Atrial Fibrillation), reported that the WATCHMAN LAA occlusion device was noninferior to warfarin for stroke prevention, suggesting that this option could be considered or patients could not tolerate anticoagulants. However, the long-term safety and efficacy of these procedures remain to be determined.[30]

FUTURE DIRECTIONS

Future studies are planned to evaluate the safety and effectiveness of new antiarrhythmic drugs and procedures as well as new thromboprophylaxis strategies in AF patients. New oral anticoagulants—such as oral direct thrombin inhibitors and oral factor Xa inhibitors—are promising alternatives to warfarin. In general, these new drugs have fewer drug or food interactions and, most importantly, do not require anticoagulation monitoring. In fact, dabigatran and rivaroxaban have already been approved for stroke prevention in AF, and based on evidence from recent clinical trials, apixaban will get approval, too.

In conclusion, antithrombotic management of AF patients will change dramatically the following years. Available evidence indicates that dabigatran and apixaban are better than warfarin for stroke prevention in patients with AF. Rivaroxaban was proved as effective as warfarin in an exceedingly high-risk population, and patients can also benefit from its optimal pharmacokinetic profile. Warfarin remains a safe and effective option, limited by its narrow therapeutic range, the need for close monitoring, and the multiple food and drug interactions. The low cost of VKAs remains their strongest and most appreciated quality. Finally, for patients not suitable for anticoagulant treatments, closure of the LAA with a percutaneous LAA occluder seems a promising alternative, with encouraging initial results.

REFERENCES

1. Lloyd-Jones DM, Wang TJ, Leip EP, et al: Lifetime risk for development of AF: The Framingham Heart Study. *Circulation* 110:1042, 2004.
2. Feinberg WM, Blackshear JL, Laupacis A, et al: Prevalence, age distribution and gender of patients with atrial fibrillation. *Arch Intern Med* 155:469, 1995.
3. Krahn AD, Manfreda J, Tate RB, et al: The natural history of atrial fibrillation: Incidence, risk factors and prognosis in the Manitoba follow-up study. *Am J Med* 98:476, 1995.
4. Allessie MA, Boyden PA, Camm AJ, et al: Pathophysiology and prevention of atrial fibrillation. *Circulation* 103:769, 2001.
5. Mandapati R, Skanes A, Chen J, et al: Stable microreentrant sources as a mechanism of atrial fibrillation in the isolated sheep heart. *Circulation* 101:194, 2000.
6. Qamruddin S, Shinbane J, Shriki J, et al: Left atrial appendage: Structure, function, imaging modalities and therapeutic options. *Expert Rev Cardiovasc Ther* 8:65, 2010 Jan.
7. Fuster V, Rydén LE, Cannom DS, et al; American College of Cardiology; American Heart Association Task Force; European Society of Cardiology Committee for Practice Guidelines; European Heart Rhythm Association; Heart Rhythm Society: ACC/AHA/ESC 2006 guidelines for the management of patients with atrial fibrillation: Full text: A report of the American College of Cardiology/American Heart Association Task Force on practice guidelines and the European Society of Cardiology Committee for Practice Guidelines (Writing Committee to Revise the 2001 guidelines for the management of patients with atrial fibrillation) developed in collaboration with the European Heart Rhythm Association and the Heart Rhythm Society. *Europace* 8:651, 2006.
8. Wyse DG, Waldo AL, DiMarco JP, et al; Atrial Fibrillation Follow-up Investigation of Rhythm Management (AFFIRM) Investigators: A comparison of rate control and rhythm control in patients with atrial fibrillation. *N Engl J Med* 347:1825, 2002.
9. Van Gelder IC, Hagens VE, Bosker HA, et al; Rate Control Versus Electrical Cardioversion for Persistent Atrial Fibrillation Study Group: A comparison of rate control and rhythm control in patients with recurrent persistent atrial fibrillation. *N Engl J Med* 347:1834, 2002.
10. European Heart Rhythm Association; European Association for Cardio-Thoracic Surgery; Camm AJ, Kirchhof P, Lip GY, et al: Guidelines for the management of atrial fibrillation: The Task Force for the Management of Atrial Fibrillation of the European Society of Cardiology (ESC). *Europace* 12:1360, 2010.
11. Cox JL, Schuessler RB, D'Agostino HJ, Jr, et al: The surgical treatment of atrial fibrillation. III. Development of a definitive surgical procedure. *J Thorac Cardiovasc Surg* 101:569, 1991.
12. Lip GY, Tse HF: Management of atrial fibrillation. *Lancet* 370:604, 2007.
13. Wazni OM, Marrouche NF, Martin DO, et al: Radiofrequency ablation vs antiarrhythmic drugs as first-line treatment of symptomatic atrial fi-brillation: A randomized trial. *JAMA* 293:2634, 2005.
14. Oral H, Pappone C, Chugh A, et al: Circumferential pulmonary-vein ablation for chronic atrial fibrillation. *N Engl J Med* 354:934, 2006.
15. Klein AL, Grimm RA, Murray RD, et al: Assessment of Cardioversion Using Transesophageal Echocardiography Investigators. Use of transesophageal echocardiography to guide cardioversion in patients with atrial fibrillation. *N Engl J Med* 344:1411, 2001.
16. Wolf PA, Abbott RD, Kannel WB: Atrial fibrillation as an independent risk factor for stroke: The Framingham Study. *Stroke* 22:983, 1991.
17. Atrial Fibrillation Investigators: Echocardiographic predictors of stroke in patients with atrial fibrillation. A prospective study of 1066 patients from 3 clinical trials. *Arch Intern Med* 158:1316, 1998.
18. Risk factors for stroke and efficacy of antithrombotic therapy in atrial fibrillation. Analysis of pooled data from five randomised controlled trials. *Arch Intern Med* 154:1449, 1994.
19. The Stroke Prevention in Atrial Fibrillation Investigators: Bleeding during antithrombotic therapy in patients with atrial fibrillation. *Arch Intern Med* 156:409, 1996.
20. Petersen P, Boysen G, Godtfredsen J, et al: Placebo-controlled randomised trial of warfarin and aspirin for prevention of thromboembolic complications in chronic atrial fibrillation. *Lancet* i:175, 1988.
21. Connolly SJ, Laupacis A, Gent M, et al; Joyner C for the CAFA Study Coinvestigators: Canadian atrial fibrillation anticoagulation (CAFA) study. *J Am Coll Cardiol* 18:349, 1991.
22. Ezekowitz MD, Bridgers SL, James KE, et al; Radford MJ for the Veterans Affairs Stroke Prevention in Nonrheumatic Atrial Fibrillation (SPINAF) Investigators: Warfarin in the prevention of stroke associated with atrial fibrillation. *N Engl J Med* 327:1406, 1992.
23. Secondary prevention in nonrheumatic atrial fibrillation and transient ischaemic attack or minor stroke. EAFT (European Atrial Fibrillation Trial) Study Group. *Lancet* 342:1255, 1993.
24. Connolly SJ, Ezekowitz MD, Yusuf S, et al; RE-LY Steering Committee and Investigators: Dabigatran versus warfarin in patients with atrial fibrillation. *N Engl J Med* 361:1139, 2009.
25. Patel MR, Mahaffey KW, Garg J, et al; the ROCKET AF Investigators: Rivaroxaban versus Warfarin in Nonvalvular Atrial Fibrillation. *N Engl J Med* 365:883, 2011.
26. Connolly SJ, Eikelboom J, Joyner C, et al; AVERROES Steering Committee and Investigators: Apixaban in patients with atrial fibrillation. *N Engl J Med* 364:806, 2011.
27. Granger CB, Alexander JH, McMurray JJ, et al; ARISTOTLE Committees and Investigators: Apixaban versus warfarin in patients with atrial fibrillation. *N Engl J Med* 365:981, 2011.
28. The ACTIVE Writing Group on behalf of the ACTIVE Investigators: Clopidogrel plus aspirin versus oral anticoagulation for atrial fibrillation in the Atrial fibrillation Clopidogrel Trial with Irbesartan for prevention of Vascular Events (ACTIVE W): A randomized controlled trial. *Lancet* 367:1903, 2006.
29. Connolly SJ, Pogue J, Hart RG, et al: The ACTIVE Investigators: Effect of clopidogrel added to aspirin in patients with atrial fibrillation. *N Engl J Med* 360:2066, 2009.
30. Holmes DR, Reddy VY, Turi ZG, et al; PROTECT AF Investigators: Percutaneous closure of the left atrial appendage versus warfarin therapy for prevention of stroke in patients with atrial fibrillation: A randomised non-inferiority trial. *Lancet* 374:534 2009.

CHAPTER 150

PERIPHERAL ARTERY DISEASE

Reena L. Pande and Mark A. Creager

Peripheral artery disease (PAD) is an important manifestation of systemic atherosclerosis with significant morbidity and mortality.[1,2] PAD affects the lower extremities and is defined as a stenosis or occlusion in the aorta or in the arteries supplying blood to the legs, including the iliac, femoral, popliteal, or infrapopliteal vessels (peroneal, posterior tibial, and anterior tibial arteries). Stenosis is typically caused by atherosclerosis. Nonatherosclerotic causes of vascular disease also can obstruct the peripheral arteries (see later discussion). There are two major clinical consequences of PAD. First, PAD can cause leg symptoms that include intermittent claudication, which impairs walking ability and diminishes quality of life, and rest pain, which occurs when there is critical limb ischemia. Second, as an atherosclerotic disorder, PAD is associated with as much as a four- to sixfold increased risk of cardiovascular death, myocardial infarction (MI), and stroke. This chapter reviews the epidemiology, pathophysiology, and management of PAD.

EPIDEMIOLOGY

Prevalence and Incidence

The prevalence of PAD has been determined from several epidemiologic studies. Early studies determined the prevalence of PAD from the presence of symptoms, such as intermittent claudication, or history of peripheral revascularization. Many patients with PAD are asymptomatic, and the use of noninvasive diagnostic testing, specifically measurement of the ankle-brachial index (ABI), has provided further clarification of the overall prevalence of disease. In most of these studies, an ABI of 0.90 or less was used to define PAD. Based on data from the National Health and Nutrition Examination Survey (NHANES), the prevalence of PAD in adults 40 years of age or older is estimated to be 5.9%, accounting for approximately 7.1 million adults in the United States alone.[3] There is a sharp increase in the prevalence of PAD with increasing age.[4,5] In the Rotterdam study, which enrolled 7715 subjects ages 55 years and older, the prevalence of PAD ranged from 6.6% in men 55 to 59 years of age to 52.0% in men ages 85 years or older and from 9.5% to 59.6% in the corresponding age categories in women.[4] A San Diego population study determined the prevalence of PAD to be 11.7% among an older adult population with a mean age of 66 years.[5] The German Epidemiological Trial on ABI (get ABI study), which evaluated an unselected group of 6880 individuals older than 65 years of age, found a prevalence of PAD of 19.8% in men and 16.8% in women.[6] The PARTNERS (PAD Awareness, Risk, and Treatment: New Resources for Survival) study was a United States–based observational study that examined a more selected population, including older adults (older than 70 years) and adults ages 50 to 69 years with a history of diabetes or smoking. The prevalence of PAD, determined by an office-based ABI measurement, was as high as 29% in this targeted primary care population.[7]

The incidence of PAD, which is largely based on the development of symptomatic disease, is less well established. Data from the Framingham Heart Study show an incidence rate of intermittent claudication of less than 0.4 per 100 per year in younger men (35-45 years) and a rate as high as 6 per 100 per year in older men (older than 65 years).[8] The incidence of symptomatic PAD is lower in women at most age groups, although the estimates are more comparable in the oldest age group. Estimates of the incidence of PAD based on ABI are less commonly reported. One such study reports an incidence of 1.7 per 1000 person-years for ages 40 to 54 years, 1.5 per 1000 person-years for ages 55 to 64 years, and 17.8 per 1000 person-years for ages 65 years and older.[9] When the diagnosis of PAD is based on ABI alone, the differences in incidence between men and women are less evident. In the Cardiovascular Health Study, for example, there are no gender differences in the incidence of PAD based on ABI after adjusting for cardiovascular risk factors.[10] At the other end of the spectrum, critical limb ischemia (CLI) represents only 1% to 2% of the patients with PAD. The incidence of CLI is estimated to be approximately 400 to 1000 per million individuals per year.[2]

Risk Factors

Atherosclerotic risk factors, including smoking, diabetes, hypertension, hyperlipidemia, and inflammation, contribute to the development of PAD.

In virtually all population-based studies, smoking has been one of the strongest risk factors for PAD. The risk is highest for current smokers compared with nonsmokers, with a two to four times increased odds of PAD,[11] and the risk of PAD increases in a dose-dependent manner relative to the number of cigarettes smoked and the duration of tobacco use.[12-14] In the Women's Health Study, smoking more than 15 cigarettes per day increased the risk of incidence of PAD approximately 17-fold, and the risk was lower in former smokers than in active smokers.[15] In the Edinburgh Artery Study, smoking was two to three times more likely to cause lower extremity PAD compared with coronary artery disease (CAD).[12,16]

Diabetes is also a potent risk factor for PAD and increases the risk of PAD by two- to fourfold. Data from the Rotterdam study and the San Luis Valley Diabetes study reveal that upwards of 12% to 20% of individuals with PAD have coexisting diabetes.[4,17] Moreover, the risk of PAD increases depending on the duration and severity of diabetes. In the Strong Heart Study, individuals with PAD had a more than twofold higher prevalence of diabetes compared with those without PAD, and the diabetes tended to be of longer duration (11.7 vs. 8.4 years, $P < .001$) and associated with higher glycosylated hemoglobin levels.[18] Patients with PAD who have concomitant diabetes are also more likely to develop intermittent claudication and ischemic ulceration and to require major amputation compared with those without diabetes.[19,20]

Hypertension is a more modest risk factor for the development of PAD compared with its importance as a risk factor for coronary and cerebrovascular disease.[1] Although evidence suggests that hypertension increases the prevalence of PAD by 1.5- to 2.2-fold, the association of hypertension with incident or symptomatic PAD is less clear. Among American Indians in the Strong Heart Study, those with PAD had a higher mean systolic blood pressure, and the prevalence of PAD was significantly higher in those with established hypertension.[18] In the Framingham Heart Study, hypertension increased the risk of developing intermittent claudication.[8] However, in the Whitehall study of more than 18,000 men ages 40 to 64 years, there was no significant association between elevated blood pressure and claudication symptoms.[21] Similarly, in the ARIC (Atherosclerosis Risk in Communities) study, there was no association of hypertension with incident PAD in subjects with diabetes.[22] In the Women's Health Study, however, the risk of incident PAD increased by 43% with every 10-mm Hg increase in systolic blood pressure.[23]

Dyslipidemia, specifically elevated total cholesterol, low-density lipoprotein (LDL) cholesterol and triglycerides, and reduced high-density lipoprotein (HDL) cholesterol, is associated with PAD. Epidemiologic studies, such as the Cardiovascular Health Study and the Framingham Heart Study, have shown that a 10-mg/dL increase in total cholesterol increases the risk of PAD by 5% to 10%.[10,24] In the Strong Heart study, individuals with PAD had significantly higher levels of total cholesterol, triglycerides, and LDL cholesterol.[18] The Whitehall study also demonstrated that an elevated total cholesterol level is associated with symptoms of intermittent claudication.[21]

Chronic renal insufficiency has been recognized to be significantly associated with PAD in several studies. In the NHANES, renal insufficiency (defined as a glomerular filtration rate <60 mL/min) was associated with a 2.5-fold higher odds of PAD even after adjustment for other cardiovascular risk factors.[25] In the Heart and Estrogen/Progesterone Replacement (HERS) study, renal insufficiency was also associated with an increased risk of incident peripheral vascular events, including revascularization and amputation.[26] Moreover, renal insufficiency increases the mortality risk in patients with PAD irrespective of other risk factors, including diabetes.[27,28]

Several other nontraditional factors have been associated with PAD. Markers of systemic inflammation, such as C-reactive protein (CRP), are elevated in patients with PAD. In the Physicians' Health Study, the risk of developing symptomatic PAD was approximately twofold higher in those in the highest CRP quartile compared with those in the lowest quartile.[29] Other markers of inflammation, such as soluble intercellular adhesion molecule 1 (sICAM-1), a leukocyte adhesion molecule, are also associated with PAD in this population and in the Women's Health Study.[30,31] Insulin resistance is also associated with PAD. In NHANES, individuals in the highest quartile of HOMA-IR (homeostasis model of insulin resistance) had a twofold increased odds of PAD compared with those in the lowest quartile.[32] The protective effect of bilirubin, an endogenous antioxidant, was explored in NHANES; there was evidence of an inverse association between total serum bilirubin levels and PAD.[33] The impact of genetics on the development of PAD has not been well explored, but a family history of PAD has been associated with development of PAD.[34]

PATHOBIOLOGY

Atherosclerosis is a progressive vascular disease characterized by lipid accumulation and formation of plaque in the arterial walls (see Chapter 146). The pathophysiology of atherosclerosis includes endothelial dysfunction, vascular inflammation, and cellular proliferation.[35] Early in the atherogenic process, recruitment of inflammatory cells and accumulation of lipids promote development of a lipid-rich atheroma. Inflammation promotes the elaboration of proteases that weaken the vessel wall and allow positive remodeling with outward expansion of the arterial wall to accommodate the intimal expansion that occurs as a result of plaque formation. Although positive remodeling initially preserves the arterial lumen, continued plaque growth results in progressive narrowing of the lumen, which then limits blood flow and oxygen supply to target organs. This process may be enhanced by biomechanical factors, such as turbulent blood flow, particularly in areas of altered shear stress. This phenomenon is of particular significance at branch points along the arterial tree, which are predisposed to atherosclerotic plaque formation.

Increasingly, it has been recognized that atherosclerotic plaque formation is a dynamic biologic process that exhibits marked heterogeneity; some plaques remain "stable", but others have a more "unstable" pathophysiology. Stable atherosclerotic plaques may be asymptomatic or symptoms can occur with exertion if demand exceeds supply. On the other hand, "vulnerable" or unstable plaques are prone to acute rupture, and superimposed thrombi may cause sudden arterial insufficiency. Studies have shown that acute thrombosis is not restricted to plaques that produce stenosis; many lesions without flow-limiting disease are prone to rupture. Evidence suggests that disruption of the fibrous cap overlying the atheroma is promoted by proinflammatory cytokines. Plaque disruption exposes the highly prothrombotic lipid-rich core of the atheroma to the blood, a process that triggers platelet aggregation and fibrin formation.

Although PAD is mostly caused by atherosclerosis, other causes include thromboembolism, atheroembolism, vasculitides (e.g., thromboangiitis obliterans, giant cell arteritis, Takayasu arteritis), trauma, popliteal artery entrapment, cystic adventitial disease, fibromuscular dysplasia, and endofibrosis of the iliac artery (Table 150-1). Nonvascular causes of leg pain should also be considered in the differential diagnosis, including lumbosacral spine disease (causing pseudoclaudication), acute and chronic venous diseases, hip or knee osteoarthritis, myositis, and others (Table 150-2).

Table 150-1 Nonatherosclerotic Causes of Peripheral Artery Disease

- Thromboembolism
- Atheroembolism
- Vasculitides
  - Large vessel vasculitides, such as giant cell arteritis and Takayasu arteritis
  - Small vessel vasculitides, such as thromboangiitis obliterans (Buerger disease)
- Trauma
- Popliteal artery entrapment
- Cystic adventitial disease
- Fibromuscular dysplasia
- Iliac artery endofibrosis

Table 150-2 Nonarterial Causes of Leg Pain (Differential Diagnosis for Intermittent Claudication Symptoms)

- Lumbar radiculopathy
- Spinal stenosis
- Hip or knee osteoarthritis
- Myositis
- Venous claudication

CLINICAL MANIFESTATIONS

The majority of patients with PAD are asymptomatic at presentation. Typical claudication symptoms are present in only 10% to 35% of patients and CLI in 1% to 2%.[1] The classic symptoms of PAD include intermittent claudication and rest pain, the latter occurring in patients with CLI. Intermittent claudication is defined as exertional discomfort in the muscles of the lower extremities that is variably described as pain, aching, burning, fatigue, or heaviness. Symptoms arise with leg exercise, typically walking, and are relieved after a predictable duration of rest (usually <10 minutes). Intermittent claudication occurs with effort and not at rest, and symptoms do not abate until activity ceases; a change in position is unnecessary. Although many patients with PAD report atypical symptoms, most have impaired walking ability exemplified by reduced walking speed or distance.[36] CLI arises when there is inadequate perfusion to meet the resting metabolic demands of the tissues. Patients with CLI have pain at rest, typically affecting the toes, feet, or both; they may have accompanying tissue loss with nonhealing ulcers, tissue necrosis, or gangrene.

DIAGNOSIS

The diagnosis of PAD is often evident from the history and physical examination. An important diagnostic feature is diminished or absent pulses in the legs. The examiner should palpate the femoral, popliteal, dorsalis pedis, and posterior tibial pulses. Absence of selected pulses provides insight into the location of critical stenoses. The groin should be auscultated for femoral artery bruits, which may be indicative of turbulent flow from atherosclerotic plaque. Other findings suggestive of PAD include pallor of the soles of the feet upon leg elevation and the development of rubor when the feet are then placed in the dependent position. Signs of chronic limb ischemia include muscle atrophy; hair loss; thickened nails; and in severe stages, cyanosis, pallor, and coolness of the skin of the feet.

Ankle-Brachial Index

The ABI is a simple, noninvasive test for the diagnosis of PAD. Normally when measured in the supine position, the systolic blood pressure in the legs is the same as that in the arms. However, pulse wave amplification may yield a higher systolic pressure at the ankle. Therefore, the ratio of the ankle to the brachial systolic pressure, designated as the ABI, should be 1.0 or slightly higher. A diminution of the ankle systolic blood pressure relative to the brachial artery pressure indicates a stenosis or occlusion in the aorta or in arteries of the lower extremities.

The ABI is determined by measuring the systolic blood pressure in both arms (brachial arteries) and in both ankle vessels (dorsalis pedis and posterior tibial arteries) after the patient has been in the supine position for at least 5 to 10 minutes.[1] To measure these pressures, sphygmomanometric cuffs are sequentially inflated at each location to suprasystolic pressures. The onset of systole with subsequent cuff deflation is determined with a Doppler device that is placed over the artery. The ABI for each leg is calculated by dividing the higher of the two ankle pressures by the higher of the two arm pressures. Taking into account the intrinsic variability in blood pressure over time, an ABI of 0.90 or less is indicative of PAD. At this threshold, the ABI has excellent sensitivity (90%) and specificity (>95%) compared with angiography.[37] An ABI of 0.91 to 1.0 is considered borderline.[38] Vascular calcification, as often occurs in patients with diabetes or renal insufficiency, may preclude accurate determination of systolic blood pressure at the ankle. For this reason, an ABI that is markedly elevated (e.g., >1.4) is considered inaccurate and indicative of vascular calcification. In this circumstance, other simple noninvasive diagnostic tests, such as assessment of the toe-brachial index or pulse volume recordings, may be useful to detect PAD. In some cases of PAD, the ABI is normal at rest. This is particularly common in patients who have proximal disease, such as iliac artery stenosis, and an extensive collateral circulation. In such cases, measurement of the ABI after walking will detect a decrease in the ankle systolic pressure relative to brachial artery systolic pressure, thereby revealing the presence of PAD.

Noninvasive Imaging for Diagnosis

Several other noninvasive tests may help in the diagnosis of PAD and in the identification of sites of stenosis. These tests include segmental pressures with pulse volume recordings, duplex ultrasonography, computed tomography angiography (CTA), magnetic resonance angiography (MRA), and conventional contrast angiography. When measuring segmental leg pressures, systolic blood pressure measurements are obtained at multiple levels in the leg, typically in the upper thigh, lower thigh, upper calf, ankle, and across the metatarsal region of the foot. Systolic blood pressures in these sites are then compared with the higher of the arm systolic blood pressures. A significant drop in blood pressure (>20 mm Hg) from one level to the next can localize arterial stenosis with a high degree of precision. An upper thigh pressure that is lower than the arm pressure indicates stenosis in the distal aorta or in the iliac or femoral arteries (or both). In patients with vascular calcification, measurement and interpretation of segmental pressures are unreliable. Pulse volume recordings can also be obtained at each level using a plethysmographic instrument that records the change in volume of that limb segment with each arterial pulsation. A normal waveform resembles an arterial waveform with a brisk upstroke and a prominent dicrotic notch in the downstroke (Fig. 150-1). Abnormal waveforms, which appear distal to a hemodynamically significant stenosis, have a parvus et tardus appearance with a blunted upstroke and decreased pulse amplitude.

Duplex ultrasonography is used both for diagnosis of PAD and for the surveillance of bypass grafts or stents after revascularization procedures. Color Doppler can identify abnormal flow with turbulence and Doppler aliasing suggesting an area of stenosis (Fig. 150-2). Pulse Doppler sampling can then confirm flow acceleration in a diseased segment. A peak systolic velocity (PSV) in a diseased segment that is more than twice the PSV in the proximal segment indicates a hemodynamically significant stenosis of at least 50%. Duplex ultrasonography has been shown to be accurate and reproducible with a sensitivity and specificity of 82% and 92%, respectively, compared with angiography.[39] However, duplex ultrasonography is a time-consuming procedure and is operator dependent.

The most commonly used imaging modalities for diagnosis of PAD are MRA and CTA. The two tests have comparable diagnostic accuracy for identification of arterial stenosis. MRA takes advantage of the inherent magnetic properties of human tissue. Pulsed magnetic sequences cause protons within cells to spin and align, generating a frequency of energy that can be detected by the scanner. Various tissues have different frequencies that allow delineation of the structures and tissues within the body. The addition of the paramagnetic contrast agent gadolinium allows selective imaging of moving blood (Fig. 150-3). This flow-related enhancement of the vasculature produces angiographic images. Although MRA has the advantage of using nonionizing radiation, it has several limitations. The test cannot be performed in patients with implanted cardiac devices or other metal objects. Although MRA can be used in patients with vascular stents, ferromagnetic metals in the stents may produce artifacts that limit assessment of the stented vessel. MRA is contraindicated with renal insufficiency because gadolinium administration in such patients can be associated with nephrogenic systemic fibrosis (NSF).[40] Claustrophobia may also preclude MRA.

Similar to MRA, CTA also has excellent specificity and sensitivity for detection of arterial stenosis. The advent of large-volume imaging with multidetector scanners enables rapid image acquisition and high resolution. Advantages of CTA include the capacity to rapidly visualize the entire arterial tree and to delineate vascular calcification and intraluminal thrombus. Limitations of the test include the exposure to ionizing radiation and the need for iodinated contrast agents, which is problematic in patients with renal impairment. In addition, extensive arterial calcification may prevent accurate determination of the degree of stenosis.

Magnetic resonance angiography and CTA have largely supplanted conventional angiography for PAD diagnosis. Nonetheless, invasive contrast angiography remains the gold standard for the diagnosis of PAD. Conventional angiography is most useful in situations in which concurrent endovascular interventions are planned or in preparation for surgical revascularization. Limitations to conventional angiography include the invasive nature of the procedure, the need to administer iodinated contrast, and the radiation exposure. Potential complications include arteriovenous fistula or pseudoaneurysm formation at the access site, atheroembolism, dissection, and contrast-induced renal insufficiency. Alternatives to iodine-based contrast agents, such as carbon dioxide and gadolinium, can be used when administration of iodinated contrast is contraindicated.

PROGNOSIS

Prognostic considerations are broadly divided into limb outcomes and overall cardiovascular outcomes. Limb prognosis is dependent on

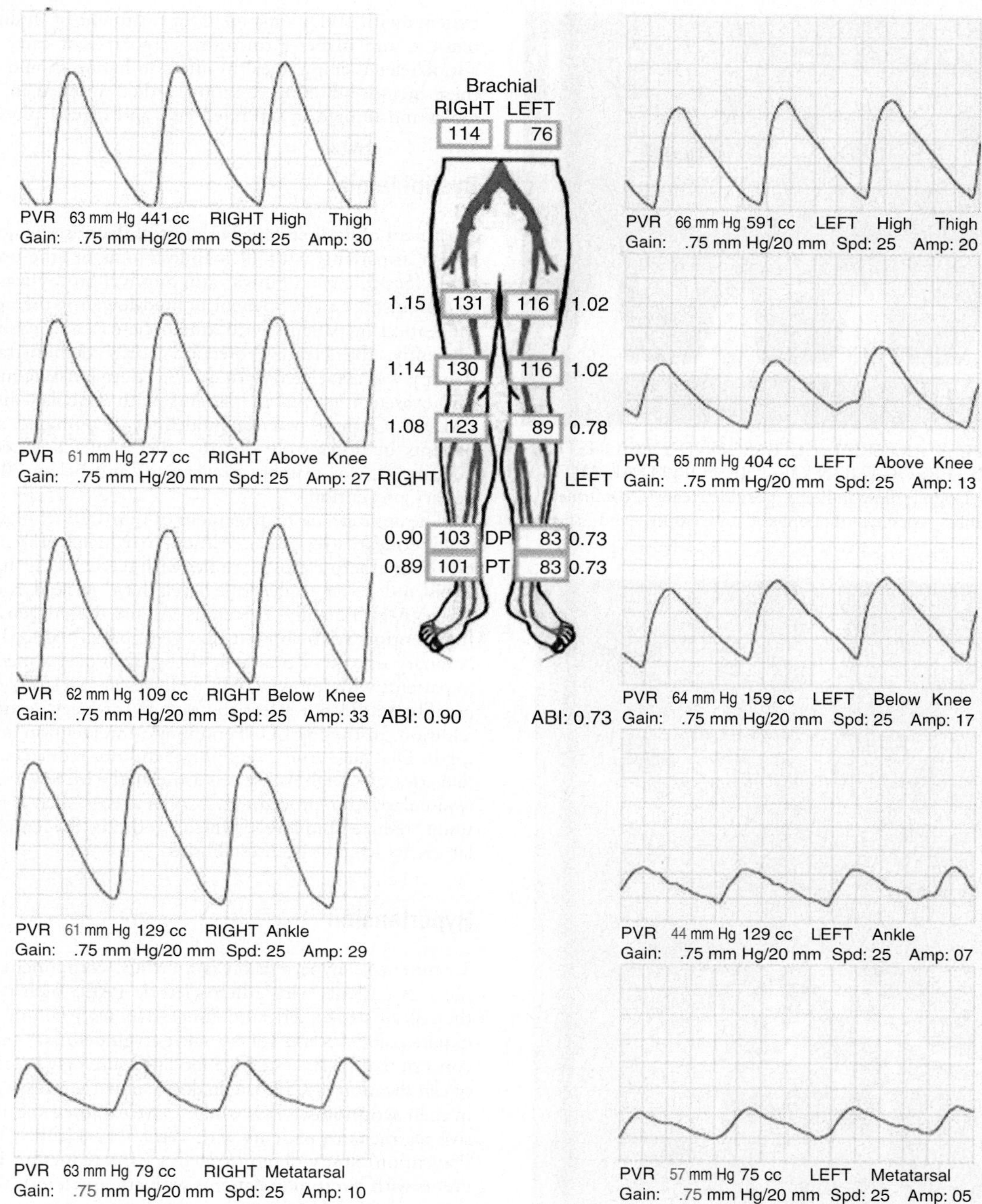

Figure 150-1 SEGMENTAL LEG PRESSURE MEASUREMENTS AND PULSE VOLUME RECORDINGS (PVRs). The ankle-brachial index (ABI) is normal in the right leg. The greater than 20-mm Hg drop in systolic blood pressure between the lower thigh and the calf in the left leg suggests stenosis involving the distal left femoral artery, popliteal artery, or both. There is also evidence of blunting of the pulse volume recording with a parvus et tardus waveform. The significant difference in brachial artery systolic blood pressure is suggestive of left subclavian artery stenosis. *Amp,* amplitude; *Spd,* speed.

the severity of symptoms at initial presentation; concurrent risk factors, such as cigarette smoking and diabetes; and the likelihood of successful revascularization in those with threatened limb viability. Among patients with claudication symptoms, leg discomfort remains stable in the majority (≈70%-80%), worsens in about 10% to 20%, and progresses to CLI in a small percentage.[1] Prognosis is worst for those with CLI, which is associated with a mean amputation-free survival at 1 year of only 50%. Outcomes are worse for PAD patients who continue to smoke or have coexisting diabetes; such patients have even higher rates of ischemic ulceration and amputation.

Given the high risk of concomitant coronary and cerebrovascular disease, individuals with PAD are also at increased risk of MI, stroke, and cardiovascular death. The mortality rate is increased two- to fourfold in patients with PAD compared with those without this complication. A meta-analysis of 16 cohort studies from the ABI collaboration confirmed the association between PAD and mortality and firmly established a graded association of lower ABI with increased mortality.[41] In PAD patients, the risk of MI is increased by 20% to 60%, and the risk of stroke is increased by 40%.[42-45] The REACH registry found that the 1-year event rate for the composite of cardiovascular death, MI, and stroke was 6.2% in individuals with

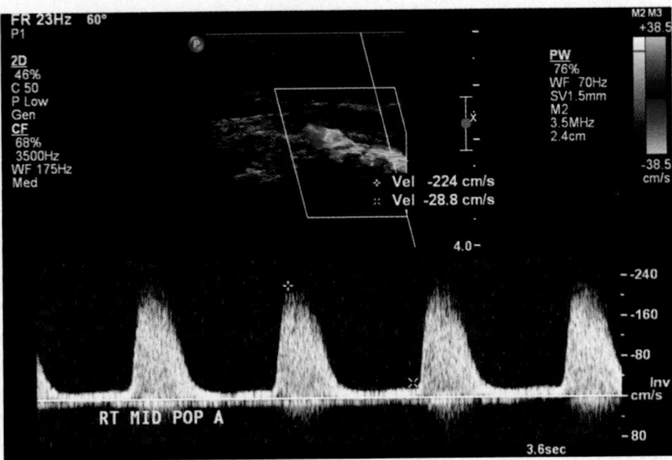

Figure 150-2 DUPLEX ARTERIAL ULTRASOUND DEMONSTRATING DOPPLER INTERROGATION OF THE POPLITEAL ARTERY. Turbulence of color Doppler flow indicates possible stenosis, confirmed by elevated peak systolic velocity, monophasic waveform, and spectral broadening.

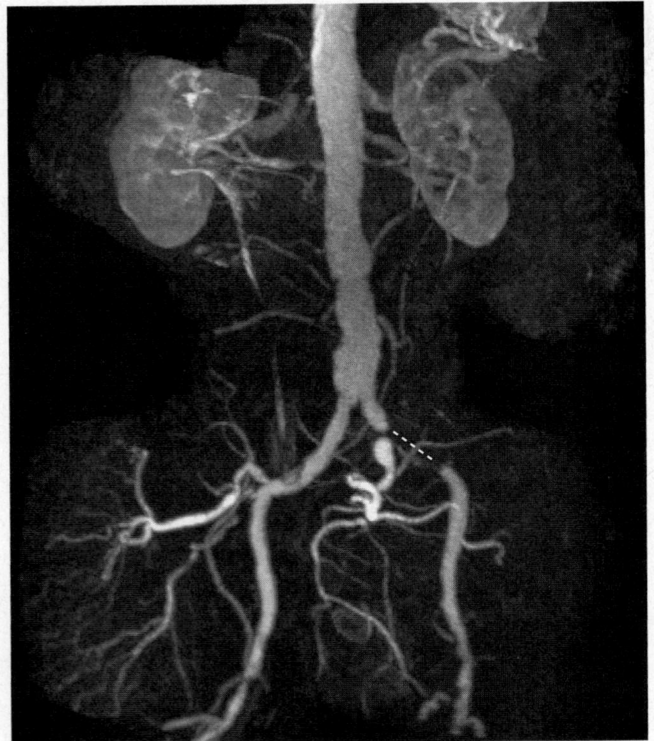

Figure 150-3 Representative projection imaging from a gadolinium-enhanced magnetic resonance angiogram demonstrating segmental occlusion of the left common iliac artery (indicated by *dashed white line*), as well as nonobstructive atherosclerotic disease in the distal aorta and more distally in the external iliac arteries.

PAD. The highest event rates were in those with polyvascular disease compared with rates in patients with atherosclerosis involving only one vascular bed.[46,47]

THERAPY

The major goals in the management of patients with PAD are to (1) reduce the risk of cardiovascular morbidity and mortality and (2) improve lower extremity symptoms and preserve limb viability. Aggressive cardiovascular risk factor modification is indicated for all patients with PAD. This includes treatment of dyslipidemia, hypertension, and diabetes (including regular foot care) and the use of antiplatelet therapy. Healthy lifestyle habits should be encouraged; these include smoking cessation, a diet enriched in fruits and vegetables and limited in saturated fats, and regular physical activity.[1]

Dyslipidemia

Treatment of dyslipidemia with statins decreases major cardiovascular events in patients with all manifestations of atherosclerosis. The 4S study (Scandinavian Simvastatin Survival Study) was one of the first to demonstrate a clear benefit of lipid-lowering therapy for secondary prevention in patients with atherosclerosis and dyslipidemia.[48] Subsequently, the Heart Protection Study demonstrated that statin therapy was associated with a 22% relative risk reduction in adverse cardiovascular events in patients with vascular disease, including PAD.[49,50] Current practice guidelines recommend statins for PAD patients in doses sufficient to lower LDL cholesterol levels below 100 mg/dL (for primary prevention) and below 70 mg/dL for secondary prevention.[1,51]

The appropriate management of non-LDL cholesterol (HDL and triglycerides) is less clear. Although reduced HDL levels are a risk factor for atherosclerosis, studies with medications that increase HDL levels and lower triglyceride levels have yielded conflicting results. The VA-HIT study (Veterans Affairs High-Density Lipoprotein Intervention Trial) showed that gemfibrozil reduced the risk of fatal coronary disease or nonfatal MI by 22% over a median of 5.1 years in patients with known CAD.[52] However, in a study of PAD patients, bezafibrate did not affect the rate of coronary events or stroke.[53] In addition, in the FIELD (Fenofibrate Intervention and Event Lowering in Diabetes) study, fenofibrate did not reduce coronary events in diabetics, although its use was associated with fewer nonfatal MIs and revascularization procedures.[54] Other agents, such as niacin or binding resins, reduce lipid levels, but their efficacy for reducing cardiovascular events has not been established.[55]

Hypertension

Treatment of hypertension is a critical component of the management of patients with atherosclerotic PAD. Such treatment reduces the risk of stroke, MI, and congestive heart failure. Management of hypertension should follow current guidelines.[56] Although there is concern that lower systemic blood pressure may exacerbate symptoms of claudication or CLI, the majority of patients experience no change in their symptoms.[57] Few studies have explored specific antihypertensive regimens in patients with PAD. The HOPE (Heart Outcomes Prevention) study demonstrated a 22% reduction in cardiovascular events with ramipril in patients with atherosclerotic disease, including patients with PAD defined as claudication symptoms, revascularization, or ABI below 0.90.[58,59] ONTARGET (Ongoing Telmisartan Alone and in Combination with Ramipril Global Endpoint Trial) demonstrated that telmisartan and ramipril produced similar reductions in the composite cardiovascular endpoint that included cardiovascular death, MI, stroke, or hospitalization for heart failure (16.7% and 16.5%, respectively; relative risk [RR], 1.01; 95% confidence interval, 0.94-1.09). However, the combination of telmisartan and ramipril was associated with more adverse events, including hypotension, syncope, and renal insufficiency.[60] In a substudy of the ABCD (Appropriate Blood Pressure Control in Diabetes) trial, intensive blood pressure lowering in PAD patients was associated with a 65% relative reduction in the risk of MI, stroke, or cardiovascular death compared with modest blood pressure–lowering therapy.[61]

Diabetes

In PAD patients with concomitant diabetes, the goals of diabetes care include control of hyperglycemia and special attention to diabetic foot care. Not only is diabetes associated with adverse limb outcomes (increased risk of ischemic ulceration and amputation in PAD patients), but it also is associated with increased mortality. Aggressive glycemic control reduces both macrovascular events (MI, stroke, and death) and microvascular events (nephropathy, neuropathy, and retinopathy) in patients with type I diabetes.[62] Although aggressive glycemic control reduces microvascular events in individuals with type II diabetes, reductions in macrovascular events have not been shown.[63] Several recent studies, such as the ADVANCE (Action in Diabetes and Vascular Disease: Preterax and Diamicron Modified Release Controlled Evaluation), ACCORD (Action to Control Cardiovascular Risk in Diabetes) and Veterans Affairs Diabetes trials, have failed to show a reduction in cardiovascular events with aggressive treatments aimed at lowering the hemoglobin A1C to 6%.[64,65] Likewise, the PROactive study (Prospective Pioglitazone Clinical Trial In Macrovascular Events) failed to show a reduction in cardiovascular or limb outcomes (lower rates of extremity revascularization or amputation with pioglitazone) in patients with type II diabetes who were at risk for cardiovascular events. However, the study did show a significant 16% reduction in the secondary endpoint, a composite of total mortality, nonfatal MI, or stroke, with pioglitazone.[66] Consequently, although the optimal glycemic control required to reduce macrovascular complications in patients with type II diabetes remains unclear, guidelines recommend treatments that maintain the level of hemoglobin A1c below 7%.

Foot care is a critical component of diabetes management, particularly in those with PAD. Diabetes increases the risk of foot injury because of the associated peripheral neuropathy and decreased sensation, thereby increasing the risk of ulcer formation. Resting limb ischemia and amputation are more frequent in PAD patients with diabetes than in those without diabetes. Therefore, careful attention to foot care is imperative to prevent skin breakdown, infections, ulceration, and amputation.

Antiplatelet Therapy

Antiplatelet therapy is recommended for patients with atherosclerosis, including patients with symptomatic PAD.[38] The Anti-platelet Trialists' Collaboration meta-analysis showed a 22% to 32% reduction in the relative risk of stroke, MI, or vascular death in patients with high-risk vascular disease, including prior stroke or transient ischemic attack or MI.[67] In a subset of patients with evidence of PAD based on symptoms of claudication or prior lower extremity bypass or angioplasty, antiplatelet therapy also produced a 22% relative risk reduction. The meta-analysis included studies that evaluated a variety of antiplatelet agents, such as aspirin, dipyridamole, picotamide, and ticlopidine. The benefits of aspirin have been called into question with a recent meta-analysis showing no significant effect of aspirin on cardiovascular events in patients with PAD.[68] The largest of the studies included in this meta-analysis was the POPADAD (The Prevention Of Progression of Asymptomatic Diabetic Arterial Disease) study, which randomized patients with ABI below 0.99 and no known cardiovascular disease to 100 mg of aspirin or placebo and showed no significant difference between the groups (hazards ratio [HR], 0.98; 95% CI, 0.76-1.26). The AAA (Aspirin for Asymptomatic Atherosclerosis Trial) explored whether aspirin (100 mg/day) was of benefit in asymptomatic individuals with PAD diagnosed solely on the basis of an abnormal ABI.[69] Compared with placebo, aspirin had no effect on the composite endpoint of fatal or nonfatal MI, stroke, or revascularization. When clopidogrel was compared with aspirin in the CAPRIE trial, clopidogrel was associated with an 8% reduction in endovascular events.[70] The CHARISMA study showed no benefit of dual antiplatelet therapy with aspirin plus clopidogrel in patients with established CAD, cerebrovascular disease, or PAD or in patients with risk factors for these disorders.[71] In a post-hoc analysis that focused on patients with symptomatic or asymptomatic PAD, there also was no benefit of dual antiplatelet therapy for the primary endpoint. However, the risk of MI and repeat hospitalization for ischemic events were lower for dual antiplatelet therapy (HR, 0.63; 95% CI, 0.42-0.96 and HR, 0.81; 95% CI, 0.68-0.95, respectively).

Treatment of Lower Extremity Symptoms

Treatments that target the symptoms and signs of PAD are implemented to improve function and mobility and preserve limb viability. Established treatments can be broadly categorized into supervised exercise therapy, pharmacotherapy, and revascularization. Therapeutic angiogenesis has also been explored as a potential therapeutic option.

Exercise Therapy

Supervised exercise therapy improves walking distance by as much as 100% to 150% in patients with PAD.[72,73] Patients are recommended to walk on a treadmill or track three to five times per week for a duration of at least 45 minutes per session for 3 to 6 months. Exercise should continue until patients develop moderate to severe claudication; after a rest period, they should resume walking with the cycle repeated until the session is over. As patients improve, walking speed and treadmill grade can be increased. Supervised exercise programs are of greater benefit in PAD patients than home-based unsupervised training. However, a recent study showed that home-based therapy quantified by monitoring home activities can be of benefit.[74] The CLEVER (The Claudication: Exercise Versus Endoluminal Revascularization) trial showed that a 6-month supervised exercise training program in patients with aortoiliac disease and claudication produced a greater improvement in walking time than optimal medical therapy alone or stenting.[75] The mechanisms responsible for the benefits of exercise remain unclear. Potential mechanisms include collateral blood vessel development as a consequence of upregulation of angiogenic growth factors, endothelium-dependent vasodilation because of enhanced nitric oxide bioavailability, more efficient walking biomechanics, and improved skeletal muscle metabolism.

Pharmacologic Therapies

Although many medications have been evaluated, few have improved the symptoms of claudication in PAD patients. Only two medications are approved by the Food and Drug Administration; cilostazol and pentoxifylline. Cilostazol is a phosphodiesterase 3 (PDE3) inhibitor that has both vasodilator and antiplatelet properties. The precise mechanism by which cilostazol confers benefit in patients with PAD is unknown. Several randomized trials have shown that compared with placebo, cilostazol produces an approximately 50% increase in walking time and improves perceived quality of life.[76] Because other PDE3 inhibitors (e.g., milrinone) have been linked to increased mortality in patients with congestive heart failure, cilostazol should not be used in this subpopulation of PAD patients. However, cilostazol has not been associated with an increase in mortality.[77] Evidence for the efficacy of pentoxifylline, a hemorrheologic agent, is less robust than that for cilostazol, and pentoxifylline is less likely to be of clinical benefit.[76]

Statins have also been explored for the treatment of claudication to exploit their pleiotropic effects, such as attenuation of inflammation. One study showed an improvement in pain-free walking time with atorvastatin but no significant increase in maximal walking time.[78] Other studies revealed an increase in walking time with simvastatin.[79,80] A recent study, however, showed no benefit of niacin plus lovastatin on walking times compared with placebo.[81]

Revascularization

Lower extremity revascularization is reserved for patients with CLI or lifestyle-limiting claudication symptoms despite maximal medical therapy. For those with CLI, prompt revascularization is necessary. Revascularization in such patients may alleviate resting limb pain, accelerate the healing of ulcers, and reduce infection. In patients with claudication, revascularization can lessen leg discomfort and improve quality of life. Options for revascularization include endovascular (percutaneous) intervention or open surgical revascularization.

Endovascular intervention, which includes percutaneous transluminal balloon angioplasty (PTA) and endovascular stenting, is increasingly being used as a less invasive option for revascularization in patients with PAD. The advances in technology of balloon-expandable and self-expanding stents have widened the population of patients with suitable anatomic lesions that stands to benefit from these procedures. Eligible patients include those with severe or disabling symptoms of claudication and those with limb-threatening ischemia. Clinical outcomes for endovascular revascularization depend on the type and length of the lesions. Treatment of stenoses is more likely to be successful than treatment of total occlusions, and success is influenced by a variety of morphologic characteristics, as delineated in the TASC (TransAtlantic Inter-Society Consensus) Working Group classification for iliac and for femoropopliteal lesions.[2] Durability and patency are greatest for iliac artery lesions; the likelihood of long-term patency with endovascular interventions is lower with disease in more distal arteries. Patency rates decrease with increasing lesion length, the presence of diffuse disease or multiple lesions, and poor run-off, as well as other adverse patient characteristics, such as diabetes, active smoking, and renal failure.[1]

For aortoiliac interventions, endovascular treatment affords excellent long-term patency, especially when combined with stenting. Five-year patency rates are approximately 94% and are comparable to rates achieved with surgical intervention. Results are less durable for femoropopliteal PTA, with patency rates of 50% to 70% at 3 to 5 years. It is less clear that stenting improves outcomes in the femoropopliteal arteries. One study comparing nitinol stents with PTA alone in patients with femoropopliteal artery stenosis with lesions averaging approximately 130 mm in length revealed lower rates of restenosis and improved walking time in patients treated with stenting.[82] However, for shorter lesions, data from the FAST study (Femoral Artery Stenting Trial) found no difference in restenosis rates with nitinol stents versus PTA.[83] Compared with bare-metal stents, drug-eluting stents (DES) have shown promise for femoral artery revascularization; a recent study showed improved survival free of major vascular events (death, amputation, or revascularization) with DES.[84] The role for drug-eluting balloons is unclear. Preliminary data suggest that local application of paclitaxel with a drug-eluting balloon during femoropopliteal artery revascularization reduces the rates of restenosis and target vessel revascularization at 6 months compared with uncoated balloon angioplasty.[85] Endovascular treatment of infrapopliteal artery stenosis is typically reserved for patients with limb ischemia. Recent studies have shown that DES use is safe for below-knee limb ischemia and may improve outcomes. For example, in the PARADISE (Preventing Amputations Using Drug Eluting Stents) study, a prospective, nonrandomized study of 106 patients, the 3-year amputation-free survival rate after DES implantation for treatment of limb ischemia involving the infrapopliteal vessels was 68%.[86] Several randomized clinical trials are currently underway to further address the utility of DES in the peripheral vasculature.

Surgical revascularization remains the gold standard for peripheral revascularization with the choice of operation depending on the location of the stenosis. Options include (1) aortoiliac or aortofemoral reconstruction for proximal disease involving the aorta or iliofemoral vessels, (2) femoral-popliteal bypass (either above- or below-knee popliteal) for superficial femoral artery or popliteal artery disease, and (3) femoral-distal (tibial or peroneal) for distal arterial stenosis. Aortobiiliac or aortobifemoral bypass graft surgery for aortoiliac occlusive disease ("inflow") produces excellent long-term results with 5-year patency rates ranging from 85% to 90%.[87] Surgical treatment of infrainguinal disease ("outflow") also produces durable results, although outcomes depend on the type of bypass conduit used. Vein grafts are the most durable; femoral-popliteal vein bypass grafts have an expected 5-year patency rate of approximately 66%. The 5-year patency rate for prosthetic grafts, such as polytetrafluoroethylene (PTFE), is lower, about 47%.[1] Limitations of surgical interventions include the need for general anesthesia and the attendant risk of cardiovascular events and death associated with major noncardiac surgery in patients with atherosclerosis. Given the potential for coexistent cardiovascular disease, preoperative assessment is important to identify and limit the risk of cardiovascular events in vascular surgery patients.[88]

Therapeutic Angiogenesis

Several clinical trials have explored the utility of angiogenic growth factors for improvement of walking time in patients with claudication or for promotion of healing and preservation of limb viability in patients with CLI. Angiogenic factors investigated have included vascular endothelial growth factor, fibroblast growth factor, hepatocyte growth factor, and hypoxia inducible factor-1 α.[89,90] Despite encouraging results with these agents in animal models of hindlimb ischemia, none of the human studies has demonstrated a benefit of gene therapy. It is not known whether the lack of success is due to the choice of gene, mode of delivery, or other factors.

Early data on infusion of endothelial progenitor cells (EPCs) has been more promising. In experimental models, EPC infusion in hindlimb ischemia models promotes angiogenesis, as indicated by capillary density, and reduces the need for amputation.[91] Preliminary studies in humans suggest that infusion of autologous CD34 cells may reduce amputation rates in patients with CLI.[92]

FUTURE DIRECTIONS

A better understanding of the factors that contribute to intermittent claudication and CLI is needed to craft innovative and durable therapeutic interventions for management of the limb complications of PAD. More studies are needed to explore the role of therapeutic angiogenesis and to identify the optimal growth factors, stem cells, and modes of delivery. A critical component of PAD management is treatment to reduce the risk of cardiovascular events. Greater knowledge dissemination regarding PAD diagnosis is key to early diagnosis and implementation of risk factor modification therapies.

SUGGESTED READINGS

Comprehensive Guidelines for the Management of Patients With Atherosclerotic Vascular Disease, Including Epidemiology, Pathophysiology, and Management of Peripheral Artery Disease

Hirsch AT, Haskal ZJ, Hertzer NR, et al: ACC/AHA 2005 Practice Guidelines for the Management of Patients with Peripheral Arterial Disease (Lower Extremity, Renal, Mesenteric, and Abdominal Aortic): A Collaborative Report from the American Association for Vascular Surgery/Society for Vascular Surgery, Society for Cardiovascular Angiography and Interventions, Society for Vascular Medicine and Biology, Society of Interventional Radiology, and the ACC/AHA Task Force on Practice Guidelines (Writing Committee to Develop Guidelines for the Management of Patients with Peripheral Arterial Disease): Endorsed by the American Association of Cardiovascular and Pulmonary Rehabilitation; National Heart, Lung, and Blood Institute; Society for Vascular Nursing; Transatlantic Inter-Society Consensus; and Vascular Disease Foundation. *Circulation* 113:e463, 2006.

Norgren L, Hiatt WR, Dormandy JA, et al: Inter-Society Consensus for the Management of Peripheral Arterial Disease (TASC II). *J Vasc Surg* 45:S5, 2007.

Rooke TW, Hirsch AT, Misra S, et al: 2011 ACCF/AHA Focused Update of the Guideline for the Management of Patients with Peripheral Artery Disease (Updating the 2005 Guideline): A Report of the American College of Cardiology Foundation/American Heart Association Task Force on Practice Guidelines. *Circulation* 124:2020, 2011.

Prevalence, Incidence, and Risk Factors for Peripheral Artery Disease

Hirsch AT, Criqui MH, Treat-Jacobson D, et al: Peripheral arterial disease detection, awareness, and treatment in primary care. *JAMA* 286:1317, 2001.

Murabito JM, D'Agostino RB, Silbershatz H, et al: Intermittent Claudication. A Risk Profile from the Framingham Heart Study. *Circulation* 96:44, 1997.

Pande RL, Perlstein TS, Beckman JA, et al: Secondary Prevention and Mortality in Peripheral Artery Disease: National Health and Nutrition Examination Study, 1999 to 2004. *Circulation* 124:17, 2011.

Prognosis and Outcomes in Peripheral Artery Disease

Cacoub PP, Abola MT, Baumgartner I, et al: Cardiovascular Risk Factor Control and Outcomes in Peripheral Artery Disease Patients in the Reduction of Atherothrombosis for Continued Health (REACH) Registry. *Atherosclerosis* 204:e86, 2009.

Criqui MH, Coughlin SS, Fronek A: Noninvasively Diagnosed Peripheral Arterial Disease as a Predictor of Mortality: Results from a Prospective Study. *Circulation* 72:768, 1985.

Fowkes FG, Murray GD, Butcher I, et al: Ankle Brachial Index Combined with Framingham Risk Score to Predict cardiovascular Events and Mortality: A Meta-Analysis. *JAMA* 300:197, 2008.

Newman AB, Shemanski L, Manolio TA, et al: Ankle-Arm Index as a Predictor of Cardiovascular Disease and Mortality in the Cardiovascular Health Study. The Cardiovascular Health Study Group. *Arterioscler Thromb Vasc Biol* 19:538, 1999.

Zheng ZJ, Sharrett AR, Chambless LE, et al: Associations of Ankle-Brachial Index with Clinical Coronary Heart Disease, Stroke and Preclinical Carotid and Popliteal Atherosclerosis: The Atherosclerosis Risk in Communities (ARIC) Study. *Atherosclerosis* 131:115, 1997.

Therapy for Patients With Peripheral Artery Disease

Belch J, Hiatt WR, Baumgartner I, et al: Effect of Fibroblast Growth Factor Nv1FGF on Amputation and Death: A Randomised Placebo-Controlled Trial of Gene Therapy in Critical Limb Ischaemia. *Lancet* 377:1929, 2011.

Berger JS, Krantz MJ, Kittelson JM, et al: Aspirin for the Prevention of Cardiovascular Events in Patients with Peripheral Artery Disease: A Meta-Analysis of Randomized Trials. *JAMA* 301:1909, 2009.

Bhatt DL, Flather MD, Hacke W, et al: Patients with Prior Myocardial Infarction, Stroke, or Symptomatic Peripheral Arterial Disease in the Charisma Trial. *J Am Coll Cardiol* 49:1982, 2007.

Collaborative Overview of Randomised Trials of Antiplatelet Therapy–I: Prevention of Death, Myocardial Infarction, and Stroke by Prolonged Antiplatelet Therapy in Various Categories of Patients. Antiplatelet Trialists' Collaboration. *BMJ* 308:81, 1994.

de Vries SO, Hunink MG: Results of aortic bifurcation grafts for aortoiliac occlusive disease: A meta-analysis. *J Vasc Surg* 26:558, 1997.

Fowkes FG, Price JF, Stewart MC, et al: Aspirin for Prevention of Cardiovascular Events in a General Population Screened for a Low Ankle Brachial Index: A Randomized Controlled Trial. *JAMA* 303:841, 2010.

Krankenberg H, Schluter M, Steinkamp HJ, et al: Nitinol stent implantation versus percutaneous transluminal angioplasty in superficial femoral artery lesions up to 10 cm in length: The femoral artery stenting trial (fast). *Circulation* 116:285, 2007.

Mohler ER 3rd, Hiatt WR, Creager MA: Cholesterol reduction with atorvastatin improves walking distance in patients with peripheral arterial disease. *Circulation* 108:1481, 2003.

MRC/BHF Heart Protection Study of Cholesterol Lowering with Simvastatin in 20,536 High-Risk Individuals: A Randomised Placebo-Controlled Trial. *Lancet* 360:7, 2002.

Murphy TP, Cutlip DE, Regensteiner JG, et al: Supervised Exercise Versus Primary Stenting for Claudication Resulting from Aortoiliac Peripheral Artery Disease: Six-Month Outcomes from the Claudication: Exercise Versus Endoluminal Revascularization (CLEVER) Study. *Circulation* 125:130, 2011.

Pande RL, Hiatt WR, Zhang P, et al: A pooled analysis of the durability and predictors of treatment response of cilostazol in patients with intermittent claudication. *Vasc Med* 15:181, 2010.

A Randomised, Blinded, Trial of Clopidogrel Versus Aspirin in Patients at Risk of Ischaemic Events (CAPRIE): Caprie Steering Committee. *Lancet* 348:1329, 1996.

Randomized Trial of the Effects of Cholesterol-Lowering with Simvastatin on Peripheral Vascular and Other Major Vascular Outcomes in 20,536 People with Peripheral Arterial Disease and Other High-Risk Conditions. *J Vasc Surg* 45:645, 2007.

Schillinger M, Sabeti S, Loewe C, et al: Balloon angioplasty versus implantation of nitinol stents in the superficial femoral artery. *N Engl J Med* 354:1879, 2006.

Stewart KJ, Hiatt WR, Regensteiner JG, et al: Exercise training for claudication. *N Engl J Med* 347:1941, 2002.

Tepe G, Zeller T, Albrecht T, et al: Local delivery of paclitaxel to inhibit restenosis during angioplasty of the leg. *N Engl J Med* 358:689, 2008.

Yusuf S, Sleight P, Pogue J, et al: Effects of an Angiotensin-Converting-Enzyme Inhibitor, Ramipril, on Cardiovascular Events in High-Risk Patients. The Heart Outcomes Prevention Evaluation Study Investigators. *N Engl J Med* 342:145, 2000.

For complete list of references log on to www.expertconsult.com.

CHAPTER 151

ANTITHROMBOTIC DRUGS

Jeffrey I. Weitz

Arterial or venous thromboembolism is a major cause of morbidity and mortality. Arterial thrombosis is the most common cause of acute myocardial infarction, ischemic stroke, and limb gangrene, whereas deep venous thrombosis leads to pulmonary embolism, which can be fatal, and to the postthrombotic syndrome. Most arterial thrombi are superimposed on disrupted atherosclerotic plaque because plaque rupture exposes thrombogenic material in the plaque core to the blood.[1] This material then triggers platelet aggregation and fibrin formation, which results in the generation of a platelet-rich thrombus that can temporarily or permanently occlude blood flow. In contrast to arterial thrombi, venous thrombi rarely form at sites of obvious vascular disruption.[1] Although they can develop after surgical trauma to veins, or secondary to indwelling central venous catheters, venous thrombi usually originate in the valve cusps of the deep veins of the calf or in the muscular sinuses where they are triggered by stasis. Sluggish blood flow in these veins reduces the oxygen supply to the avascular valve cusps. Endothelial cells lining the valve cusps become activated and express adhesion molecules on their surface. These adhesion molecules tether tissue factor–bearing leukocytes and microparticles to the surface of activated endothelial cells, where the tissue factor triggers coagulation. Local thrombus formation is exacerbated by reduced clearance of activated clotting factors as a result of impaired blood flow. If the calf vein thrombi extend into more proximal veins of the leg, thrombus fragments can dislodge, travel to the lungs, and produce a pulmonary embolism.

Arterial and venous thrombi are composed of platelets and fibrin, but the proportions differ. Arterial thrombi are rich in platelets because of the high shear in the injured arteries. In contrast, venous thrombi, which form under low-shear conditions, contain relatively few platelets and are predominantly composed of fibrin and trapped red cells. Because of the predominance of platelets, arterial thrombi appear white, whereas venous thrombi are red, reflecting the trapped red cells.

Antithrombotic drugs are used for prevention and treatment of thrombosis. Targeting the components of thrombi, these agents include (1) antiplatelet drugs, which inhibit platelets; (2) anticoagulants, which attenuate coagulation; and (3) fibrinolytic agents, which induce fibrin degradation (Fig. 151-1). With the predominance of platelets in arterial thrombi, strategies to inhibit or treat arterial thrombosis focus mainly on antiplatelet agents, although in the acute setting they often include anticoagulants and fibrinolytic agents. Anticoagulants are the mainstay of prevention and treatment of venous thromboembolism because fibrin is the predominant component of venous thrombi. Antiplatelet drugs are less effective than anticoagulants in this setting because of the limited platelet content of venous thrombi. Fibrinolytic therapy is used in selected patients with venous thromboembolism. For example, patients with massive or submassive pulmonary embolism can benefit from systemic or catheter-directed fibrinolytic therapy. Catheter-directed fibrinolytic therapy also can be used as an adjunct to anticoagulants for treatment of certain patients with extensive iliofemoral vein thrombosis.

This chapter focuses on antithrombotic agents. In addition to describing antiplatelet, anticoagulant, and fibrinolytic drugs that are in current use, new agents in advanced stages of development also are discussed.

ANTIPLATELET DRUGS

Role of Platelets in Arterial Thrombosis

In healthy vasculature, circulating platelets are maintained in an inactive state by nitric oxide and prostacyclin released by endothelial cells lining the blood vessels. In addition, endothelial cells also express ADPase on their surface, which degrades adenosine diphosphate (ADP) released from activated platelets (see Chapter 125). When the vessel wall is damaged, release of these substances is impaired and subendothelial matrix is exposed. Platelets adhere to exposed collagen and von Willebrand factor via $\alpha_2\beta_1$ and glycoprotein (GP) Ib-IX, respectively, receptors constitutively expressed on the platelet surface (see Chapter 127). Adherent platelets undergo a change in shape, secrete ADP from their dense granules, and synthesize and release thromboxane A_2. Released ADP and thromboxane A_2, which are platelet agonists, activate ambient platelets and recruit them to the site of vascular injury.

Disruption of the vessel wall also exposes tissue factor–expressing cells to the blood. Tissue factor initiates coagulation. Activated platelets potentiate coagulation by binding clotting factors and supporting the assembly of activation complexes that enhance thrombin generation. In addition to converting fibrinogen to fibrin, thrombin amplifies its own generation and serves as a potent platelet agonist, thereby recruiting additional platelets to the site of injury.

When platelets are activated, GPIIb/IIIa, the most abundant receptor on the platelet surface, undergoes a conformational change that enables it to ligate fibrinogen. Divalent fibrinogen molecules bridge adjacent platelets together to form platelet aggregates. Fibrin strands, generated through the action of thrombin, then weave these aggregates together to form a platelet/fibrin mesh.

Antiplatelet drugs target various steps in this process (Fig. 151-2). The commonly used drugs include aspirin, thienopyridines (ticlopidine, clopidogrel, and prasugrel), ticagrelor, dipyridamole, and GPIIb/IIIa antagonists. Each is briefly described.

Aspirin

The most widely used antiplatelet agent worldwide is aspirin. As a cheap and effective antiplatelet drug, aspirin serves as the foundation of most antiplatelet strategies.

Mechanism of Action

Aspirin produces its antithrombotic effect by irreversibly acetylating and inhibiting platelet cyclooxygenase (COX)-1, a critical enzyme in the biosynthesis of thromboxane A_2 (see Fig. 151-2). At high doses (about 1 g/day), aspirin also inhibits COX-2, an inducible COX isoform found in endothelial cells and inflammatory cells. In endothelial cells, COX-2 initiates the synthesis of prostacyclin, a potent vasodilator and inhibitor of platelet aggregation.

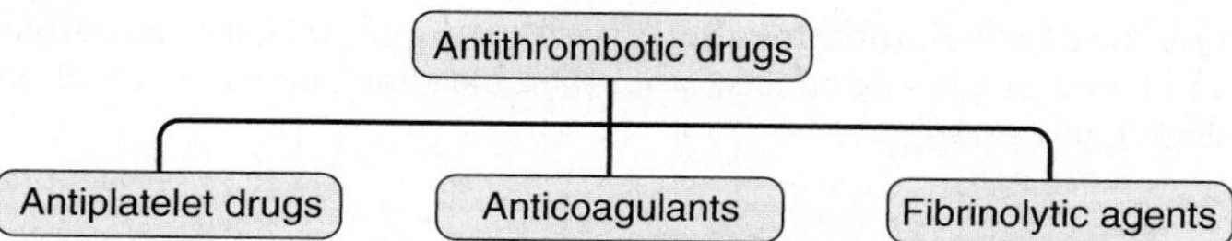

Figure 151-1 CLASSIFICATION OF ANTITHROMBOTIC DRUGS.

Indications

Aspirin is widely used for secondary prevention of cardiovascular events in patients with coronary artery disease, cerebrovascular disease, or peripheral vascular disease. Compared with placebo, aspirin produces about a 25% reduction in the risk for cardiovascular death, myocardial infarction, or stroke in these patients. There is controversy about the use of aspirin for primary prevention in subjects without clinical evidence of cardiovascular disease.[2] Although metaanalyses demonstrate a reduction in nonfatal myocardial infarction with daily aspirin use, this benefit is partially offset by an increase in gastrointestinal bleeding. Nonetheless, there also is evidence that aspirin reduces cancer mortality. If used for primary prevention, aspirin should be restricted to those at moderate to high risk for cardiovascular events.

Dosages

Aspirin is usually administered at doses of 75 to 325 mg once daily. There is no evidence that higher-dose aspirin is more effective than lower aspirin doses, and some analyses suggest reduced efficacy with higher doses. Because the side effects of aspirin are dose related, daily aspirin doses of 75 to 150 mg are recommended for most indications. When rapid platelet inhibition is required, an initial aspirin dose of at least 160 mg should be given.

Side Effects

Most common side effects are gastrointestinal and range from dyspepsia to erosive gastritis or peptic ulcers with associated bleeding. These side effects are, at least to some extent, dose related. Use of enteric-coated or buffered aspirin in place of plain aspirin does not eliminate the gastrointestinal side effects. The risk for major bleeding with aspirin ranges from 1% to 3% per year and is higher when aspirin is used in conjunction with anticoagulants, such as warfarin. When dual therapy is used, low-dose aspirin should be given (75 to 100 mg daily). Eradication of *Helicobacter pylori* infection and concomitant administration of proton pump inhibitors may reduce the risk for upper gastrointestinal bleeding, particularly in patients with a history of peptic ulcer disease.

Aspirin should not be administered to patients with aspirin allergy characterized by bronchospasm. This problem occurs in about 0.3% of the general population but is more common in those with chronic urticaria or asthma, particularly in subjects with coexisting nasal polyps or chronic rhinitis. Hepatic and renal toxicity are observed with aspirin overdose.

Aspirin Resistance

The term *aspirin resistance* has been used to describe both clinical and laboratory phenomena.[3] Clinical aspirin resistance is defined as the failure of aspirin to protect patients from ischemic vascular events. This is not a helpful definition because it is made after the event occurs. Furthermore, it is not realistic to expect aspirin, which only blocks thromboxane A_2–induced platelet activation, to prevent all vascular events.

Aspirin resistance also has been described biochemically as failure of the drug to produce its expected inhibitory effects on tests of platelet function, such as thromboxane A_2 synthesis or arachidonic acid–induced platelet aggregation. However, the tests used for the diagnosis of aspirin resistance are not well standardized. Furthermore, there is no definitive evidence that these tests identify patients at risk for recurrent vascular events, or that resistance can be reversed either by giving higher doses of aspirin or by adding other antiplatelet drugs. Until such information is available, testing for aspirin resistance remains a research tool.

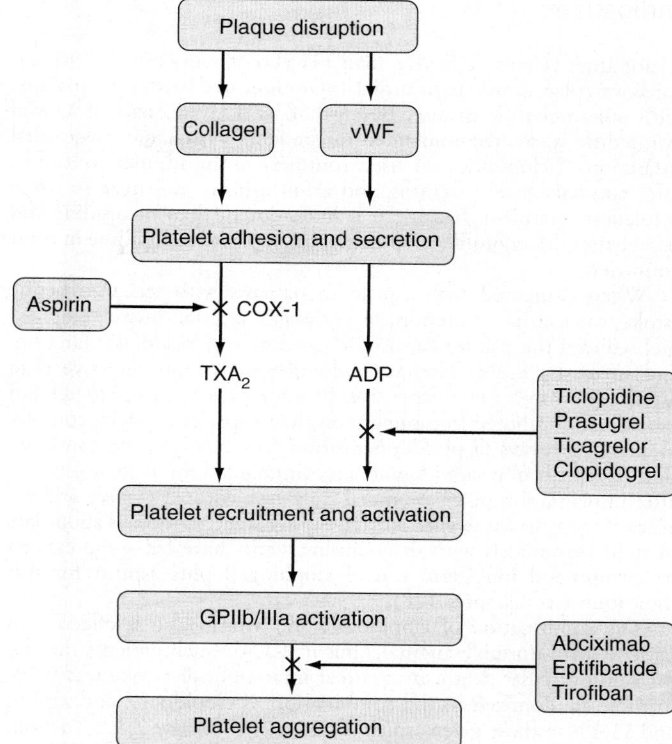

Figure 151-2 SITE OF ACTION OF ANTIPLATELET DRUGS. Aspirin inhibits thromboxane A_2 (TXA_2) synthesis by irreversibly acetylating cyclooxygenase-1 (COX-1). Reduced TXA_2 release attenuates platelet activation and recruitment to the site of vascular injury. Ticlopidine, clopidogrel, and prasugrel irreversibly block $P2Y_{12}$, a key adenosine diphosphate (ADP) receptor on the platelet surface whereas ticagrelor reversibly inhibits this receptor. Therefore these agents also attenuate platelet recruitment. Abciximab, eptifibatide, and tirofiban inhibit the final common pathway of platelet aggregation by blocking fibrinogen binding to activated glycoprotein (GP) IIb/IIIa. *vWF,* von Willebrand factor.

Thienopyridines

The thienopyridines include ticlopidine, clopidogrel, and prasugrel, drugs that target $P2Y_{12}$, the major ADP receptor on platelets.

Mechanism of Action

The thienopyridines are structurally related drugs that selectively inhibit ADP-induced platelet aggregation by irreversibly blocking $P2Y_{12}$ (see Fig. 151-2). Ticlopidine, clopidogrel, and prasugrel are prodrugs that must be metabolized by the hepatic cytochrome P450 (CYP) enzyme system to acquire activity. Consequently their onset of action is delayed unless loading doses are given. The metabolic activation of prasugrel is more efficient than that of ticlopidine or clopidogrel. Consequently prasugrel produces more rapid, higher, and more uniform $P2Y_{12}$ blockade than the other thienopyridines.

Indications

Ticlopidine is more effective than placebo at reducing the risk for cardiovascular death, myocardial infarction, and stroke in patients with atherosclerotic disease. Because of its delayed onset of action, ticlopidine is not recommended for patients with acute myocardial infarction. Ticlopidine was used routinely as an adjunct to aspirin after coronary artery stenting and as an aspirin substitute in those intolerant to aspirin. Because it is more potent than ticlopidine and has a better safety profile, clopidogrel has replaced ticlopidine in most countries.

When compared with aspirin in patients with recent ischemic stroke, myocardial infarction, or peripheral arterial disease, clopidogrel reduced the risk for cardiovascular death, myocardial infarction, and stroke by 8.7%. Therefore, clopidogrel is more effective than aspirin but also is more expensive. In some patients, clopidogrel and aspirin are combined to capitalize on their capacity to block complementary pathways of platelet activation. For example, the combination of aspirin plus clopidogrel is recommended for at least 4 weeks after implantation of a bare metal stent in a coronary artery and for at least 1 year in those with a drug-eluting stent. Concerns about late in-stent thrombosis with drug-eluting stents have led some experts to recommend long-term use of clopidogrel plus aspirin for this indication (see Chapter 148).

The combination of clopidogrel and aspirin also is effective in patients with unstable angina. Thus in 12,562 such patients the risk for cardiovascular death, myocardial infarction, or stroke was 9.3% in those randomized to the combination of clopidogrel and aspirin and 11.4% in those given aspirin alone, a 20% relative risk reduction. However, combining clopidogrel with aspirin increases the risk for major bleeding to about 2% per year. This bleeding risk persists even if the daily dose of aspirin is 100 mg or less. Therefore the combination of clopidogrel and aspirin should be used only when there is a clear benefit. For example, this combination has not proven to be superior to clopidogrel alone in patients with acute ischemic stroke or to aspirin alone for primary prevention in those at risk for cardiovascular events.

When compared with clopidogrel in 13,608 patients with acute coronary syndromes undergoing percutaneous coronary interventions, prasugrel reduced the combined rate of cardiovascular death, myocardial infarction, or stroke from 12.1% to 9.9%, a decrease mainly driven by a reduction in nonfatal myocardial infarction. However, prasugrel increased the rate of major bleeding and fatal bleeding, particularly in patients over the age of 65 years, those weighing less than 60 kg, and in those with a history of stroke. Prasugrel should not be used in patients with these characteristics.

Dosing

Ticlopidine is given twice-daily at a dose of 250 mg, whereas clopidogrel is given once-daily at a dose of 75 mg. Because its onset of action is delayed for several days, loading doses of clopidogrel are given when rapid ADP receptor blockade is desired. For example, patients undergoing coronary artery stenting are often given a loading dose of 600 mg, which produces inhibition of ADP-induced platelet aggregation within 6 hours. Prasugrel is given as a loading dose of 60 mg followed by 10 mg once daily. Partial inhibition of ADP-induced platelet aggregation is evident within 1 hour of prasugrel administration.

Side Effects

The most common side effects of ticlopidine are gastrointestinal. More serious are the hematologic side effects, which include neutropenia, thrombocytopenia, and thrombotic thrombocytopenic purpura. These side effects usually occur within the first few months of starting treatment. Therefore blood counts must be carefully monitored when initiating therapy with ticlopidine. Gastrointestinal and hematologic side effects, other than bleeding, are rare with clopidogrel and prasugrel.

Clopidogrel Resistance

There is between-subject variability in the capacity of clopidogrel to inhibit ADP-induced platelet aggregation.[4] This variability reflects, at least in part, genetic polymorphisms in CYP2C19, which is involved in the metabolic activation of clopidogrel. For example, subjects with the loss-of-function CYP2C19*2 and CYP2C19*3 alleles exhibit decreased responsiveness to clopidogrel. These alleles are found in 2% of white, 4% of black and 14% of Asian racial groups. Based on these findings, it is possible that pharmacogenetic profiling and point-of-care devices that assess the extent of platelet inhibition may help to identify clopidogrel-resistant patients. Such patients may benefit from a switch to prasugrel, which produces more uniform inhibition of ADP-induced platelet aggregation, or to ticagrelor.

Ticagrelor

An orally active agent belonging to the cyclopentyl-triazolopyrimidine class, ticagrelor acts as a direct inhibitor of $P2Y_{12}$.

Mechanism of Action

Ticagrelor binds to $P2Y_{12}$, at a location distinct from the ADP binding site and blocks ADP-mediated receptor activation in a noncompetitive fashion, likely through an allosteric mechanism. Because it does not require metabolic activation, ticagrelor has a more rapid onset of action than clopidogrel or prasugrel.

Dosing

Ticagrelor is given as a 180-mg oral loading dose followed by 80 mg twice daily. Although the trial with ticagrelor was not designed to stratify outcomes by geographic regions, patients enrolled from North America did not have the same benefit as those from other countries. Based on post-hoc analysis, the only baseline covariate associated with this difference was the higher dose of aspirin used in the United States. Consequently it is recommended that when combined with aspirin, the daily aspirin dose should be less than 100 mg.

When compared with clopidogrel in 18,624 patients with acute coronary syndromes, ticagrelor reduced the rate of cardiovascular death, myocardial infarction, or stroke from 11.7% to 9.8%.[5] All-cause mortality was also reduced with ticagrelor compared with clopidogrel (4.5% and 5.9%, respectively; $P < .001$), but ticagrelor produced more major bleeding not related to bypass surgery (2.8% and 2.2%, respectively).[5]

An invasive strategy was planned for 72% of the 18,624 patients entered in the trial. In this subset, the primary composite end point occurred in 9.0% of patients randomized to ticagrelor and in 10.7% of those given clopidogrel, a 16% reduction.[6] Rates of major bleeding were similar with ticagrelor and clopidogrel (11.6% and 16.5%, respectively; $P = .88$). Therefore ticagrelor is superior to clopidogrel.

Indications

If cost is not an issue and patients are compliant with twice-daily dosing, ticagrelor is a reasonable alternative to clopidogrel in patients with acute coronary syndrome regardless of whether they have been managed medically or have undergone a percutaneous coronary intervention with stent insertion. For these indications, ticagrelor should be given for at least a year. It also is reasonable to use ticagrelor in place of clopidogrel in patients with increased platelet reactivity on clopidogrel or in those who developed in-stent thrombosis despite clopidogrel therapy.

Side Effects

Ticagrelor produces dyspnea, which is usually mild and dose related, asymptomatic bradycardia with ventricular pauses, and a modest increase in the levels of uric acid. The mechanisms responsible for these side effects are unclear. One possible explanation relates to the capacity of ticagrelor to inhibit adenosine reuptake by erythrocytes, thereby increasing circulating levels of adenosine. In addition to explaining the dyspnea and the bradycardia, the resultant adenosine-induced vasodilation and increased myocardial perfusion could also endow ticagrelor with beneficial effects that are independent of $P2Y_{12}$ blockade.

Dipyridamole

A relatively weak antiplatelet agent on its own, an extended-release formulation of dipyridamole combined with low-dose aspirin, a preparation known as Aggrenox, is used for prevention of stroke in patients with transient ischemic attacks.

Mechanism of Action

By inhibiting phosphodiesterase, dipyridamole blocks the breakdown of cyclic adenosine monophosphate (cAMP). Increased levels of cAMP reduce intracellular calcium and inhibit platelet activation. Dipyridamole also blocks the uptake of adenosine by platelets and other cells. This produces a further increase in local cAMP levels because the platelet adenosine A_2 receptor is coupled to adenylate cyclase (Fig. 151-3).

Dosing

Aggrenox is given twice daily. Each capsule contains 200 mg of extended-release dipyridamole and 25 mg of aspirin.

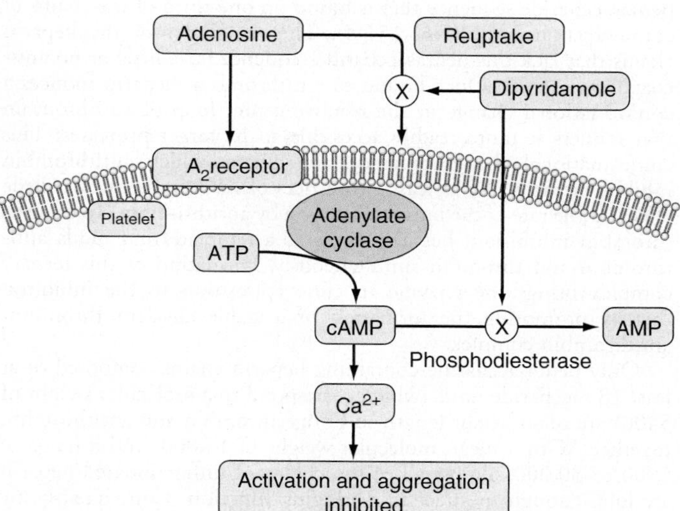

Figure 151-3 MECHANISM OF ACTION OF DIPYRIDAMOLE. Dipyridamole increases levels of cyclic adenosine monophosphate (cAMP) in platelets by (1) blocking the reuptake of adenosine and (2) inhibiting phosphodiesterase-mediated cAMP degradation. By promoting calcium uptake, cAMP reduces intracellular levels of calcium. This, in turn, inhibits platelet activation and aggregation. *AMP,* Adenosine monophosphate; *ATP,* adenosine triphosphate.

Side Effects

Because dipyridamole has vasodilatory effects, it must be used with caution in patients with coronary artery disease. Gastrointestinal complaints, headache, facial flushing, dizziness, and hypotension also can occur. These symptoms often subside with continued use of the drug.

Indications

Dipyridamole plus aspirin was compared with aspirin or dipyridamole alone, or with placebo, in patients with an ischemic stroke or transient ischemic attack. The combination reduced the risk for stroke by 22.1% compared with aspirin alone and by 24.4% compared with dipyridamole alone. A second trial compared dipyridamole plus aspirin with aspirin alone for secondary prevention in patients with ischemic stroke. Vascular death, stroke, or myocardial infarction occurred in 13% of patients given combination therapy and in 16% of those treated with aspirin alone. When Aggrenox was compared with clopidogrel, however, there was no difference in efficacy and there was more intracranial bleeding with Aggrenox.[7] Although Aggrenox is used for stroke prevention, because of its vasodilatory effects and the paucity of data supporting the use of dipyridamole in patients with symptomatic coronary artery disease, Aggrenox should not be used for stroke prevention in such patients (see Chapter 147).

GPIIb/IIIa Antagonists

As a class, parenteral GPIIb/IIIa antagonists have an established niche in patients with acute coronary syndromes. The three agents in this class are abciximab, eptifibatide, and tirofiban.

Mechanism of Action

A member of the integrin family of adhesion receptors, GPIIb/IIIa is found on the surface of platelets and megakaryocytes. With about 40,000 to 80,000 copies per platelet, GPIIb/IIIa is the most abundant receptor (see Chapter 127). Consisting of a noncovalently linked heterodimer, GPIIb/IIIa is inactive on resting platelets. When platelets are activated, inside-outside signal transduction pathways trigger a conformational activation of the receptor. Once activated, GPIIb/IIIa binds adhesive molecules, such as fibrinogen and, under high-shear conditions, von Willebrand factor. Binding is mediated by Arg-Gly-Asp (RGD) sequences found on the fibrinogen and von Willebrand factor and by the Lys-Gly-Asp (KGD) sequence located within a unique dodecapeptide domain on the γ-chains of fibrinogen. Once bound, fibrinogen and/or von Willebrand factor bridge adjacent platelets together to induce platelet aggregation.

Although abciximab, eptifibatide, and tirofiban all target the GPIIb/IIIa receptor, they are structurally and pharmacologically distinct (Table 151-1). Abciximab is a Fab fragment of a humanized murine monoclonal antibody directed against the activated form of GPIIb/IIIa. Abciximab binds to the activated receptor with high affinity and blocks the binding of adhesive molecules. In contrast to abciximab, eptifibatide and tirofiban are synthetic small molecules. Eptifibatide is a cyclic heptapeptide that binds GPIIb/IIIa because it incorporates the KGD motif, whereas tirofiban is a nonpeptidic tyrosine derivative that acts as an RGD mimetic. Abciximab has a long half-life and can be detected on the surface of platelets for up to 2 weeks. Eptifibatide and tirofiban have shorter half-lives.

In addition to targeting the GPIIb/IIIa receptor, abciximab also inhibits the closely related $\alpha v\beta 3$ receptor, which binds vitronectin, and $\alpha M\beta 2$, a leukocyte integrin. In contrast, eptifibatide and tirofiban are specific for GPIIb/IIIa. Inhibition of $\alpha v\beta 3$ and $\alpha M\beta 2$ may endow abciximab with antiinflammatory and/or antiproliferative properties that extend beyond platelet inhibition.

Table 151-1 Features of GPIIb/IIIa Antagonists

Feature	Abciximab	Eptifibatide	Tirofiban
Description	Fab fragment of humanized mouse monoclonal antibody	Cyclical KGD-containing heptapeptide	Nonpeptidic RGD mimetic
Specific for GPIIb/IIIa	No	Yes	Yes
Plasma half-life	Short (min)	Long (2.5 hr)	Long (2.0 hr)
Platelet-bound half-life	Long (days)	Short (sec)	Short (sec)
Renal clearance	No	Yes	Yes
Dosing	0.25-mg/kg bolus followed by a 12-hr infusion of 10 mcg/min	Two 180-mcg/kg boluses given 10 min apart	25-mcg/kg bolus followed by an18-hr infusion of 0.15 mcg/kg/min
Adjustment for renal impairment	No	Yes	Yes

KGD, Lys-Gly-Asp; *RGD*, Arg-Gly-Asp.

Dosing

All of the GPIIb/IIIa antagonists are given as an intravenous bolus followed by an infusion. Because they are cleared by the kidneys, the doses of eptifibatide and tirofiban must be reduced in patients with renal impairment.

Side Effects

In addition to bleeding, thrombocytopenia is the most serious complication (see Chapter 134). Thrombocytopenia is immune mediated and is caused by antibodies directed against neoantigens on GPIIb/IIIa that are exposed upon antagonist binding. With abciximab, thrombocytopenia occurs in up to 5% of patients. Thrombocytopenia is severe in about 1% of these individuals. Thrombocytopenia is less common with the other two agents, occurring in about 1% of treated patients.

Indications

These agents are used in patients undergoing percutaneous coronary interventions, particularly those with ST-segment elevation acute myocardial infarction. Tirofiban and eptifibatide are also used in high-risk patients with unstable angina.

New Antiplatelet Agents

Vorapaxar and atopaxar are orally active inhibitors of protease-activated receptor 1 (PAR1), the major thrombin receptor on platelets. Vorapaxar has been compared with placebo as an adjunct to standard of care in patients undergoing percutaneous coronary interventions[8] or for prevention of cardiovascular events in those with a history of stroke, myocardial infarction, or peripheral arterial disease.[9] Although vorapaxar shows promise for these indications, it causes excessive bleeding, including intracranial bleeding, in patients with a prior history of stroke, and its role has not yet been defined.

ANTICOAGULANTS

There are both parenteral and oral anticoagulants. Currently available parenteral anticoagulants include heparin, low-molecular-weight heparin (LMWH), and fondaparinux, a synthetic pentasaccharide. The oral anticoagulants include the vitamin K antagonists, of which warfarin is the agent most often used in North America, and new agents that target thrombin (dabigatran etexilate) or factor Xa (rivaroxaban and apixaban).[10]

Parenteral Anticoagulants

Heparin

A sulfated polysaccharide, heparin is isolated from mammalian tissues rich in mast cells. Most commercial heparin is derived from porcine intestinal mucosa and is a polymer of alternating D-glucuronic acid and N-acetyl-D-glucosamine residues.

Mechanism of Action

Heparin acts as an anticoagulant by activating antithrombin (previously known as antithrombin III) and accelerating the rate at which antithrombin inhibits clotting enzymes, particularly thrombin and factor Xa (see Chapter 128). Antithrombin, the obligatory plasma cofactor for heparin, is a 58,000-Da single-chain polypeptide that is a member of the serine protease inhibitor (serpin) superfamily. Synthesized in the liver and circulating in plasma at a concentration of 2.6 ± 0.4 μM, antithrombin acts as a suicide substrate for its target enzymes.

To activate antithrombin, heparin binds to the serpin via a unique pentasaccharide sequence that is found on one-third of the chains of commercial heparin (Fig. 151-4). The remainder of the heparin chains that lack this pentasaccharide sequence have little or no anticoagulant activity. Once bound to antithrombin, heparin induces a conformational change in the reactive center loop of antithrombin that renders it more readily accessible to its target proteases. This conformational change enhances the rate at which antithrombin inhibits factor Xa by at least two orders of magnitude but has little effect on the rate of thrombin inhibition by antithrombin. To catalyze thrombin inhibition, heparin serves as a template that binds antithrombin and thrombin simultaneously. Formation of this ternary complex brings the enzyme in close apposition to the inhibitor, thereby promoting the formation of a stable covalent thrombin-antithrombin complex.

Only pentasaccharide-containing heparin chains composed of at least 18 saccharide units (which correspond to a molecular weight of 5400) are of sufficient length to bridge thrombin and antithrombin together. With a mean molecular weight of 15,000, and a range of 5000 to 30,000, almost all of the chains of unfractionated heparin are long enough to affect this bridging function. Consequently, by definition, heparin has equal capacity to promote the inhibition of thrombin and factor Xa by antithrombin and is assigned an anti–factor Xa to anti–factor IIa (thrombin) ratio of 1 : 1 (Fig. 151-5).

In addition to activating antithrombin, heparin also can catalyze heparin cofactor II. This 66,000-Da serpin, which is found in plasma at a concentration of 1.2 ± 0.4 μM, is a specific inhibitor of thrombin. Two features account for the specificity of heparin cofactor II. First, the reactive site of heparin cofactor II contains the sequence

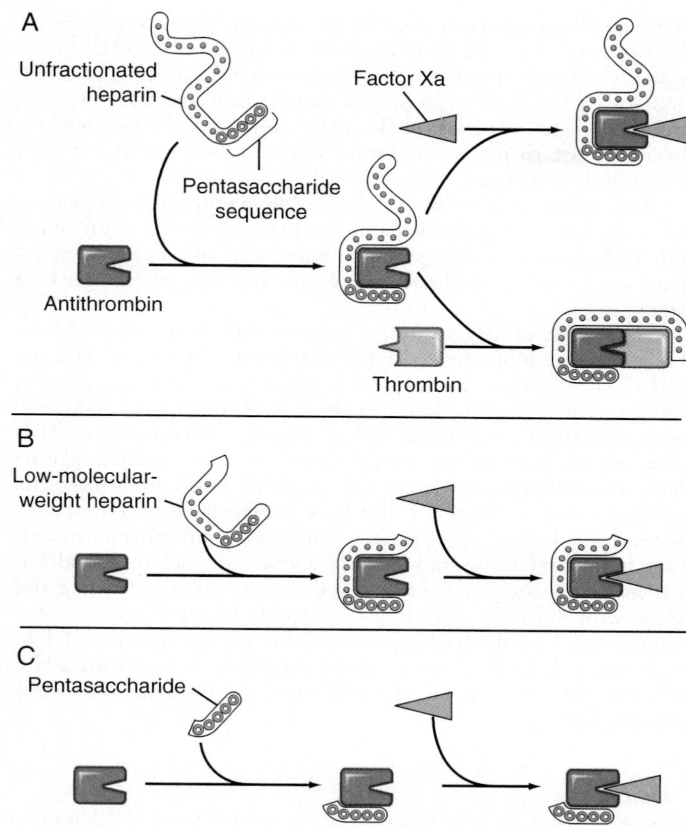

Figure 151-4 MECHANISM OF ACTION OF HEPARIN, LOW-MOLECULAR-WEIGHT HEPARIN (LMWH), AND FONDAPARINUX, A SYNTHETIC PENTASACCHARIDE. **A,** Heparin binds to antithrombin via its pentasaccharide sequence. This induces a conformational change in the reactive center loop of antithrombin that accelerates its interaction with factor Xa. To potentiate thrombin inhibition, heparin must simultaneously bind to antithrombin and thrombin. Only heparin chains composed of at least 18 saccharide units, which corresponds to a molecular weight of 5400, are of sufficient length to perform this bridging function. With a mean molecular weight of 15,000, all of the heparin chains are long enough to do this. **B,** LMWH has greater capacity to potentiate factor Xa inhibition by antithrombin than thrombin because, with a mean molecular weight of 4500 to 5000, at least half of the LMWH chains are too short to bridge antithrombin to thrombin. **C,** The pentasaccharide only accelerates factor Xa inhibition by antithrombin because the pentasaccharide is too short to bridge antithrombin to thrombin.

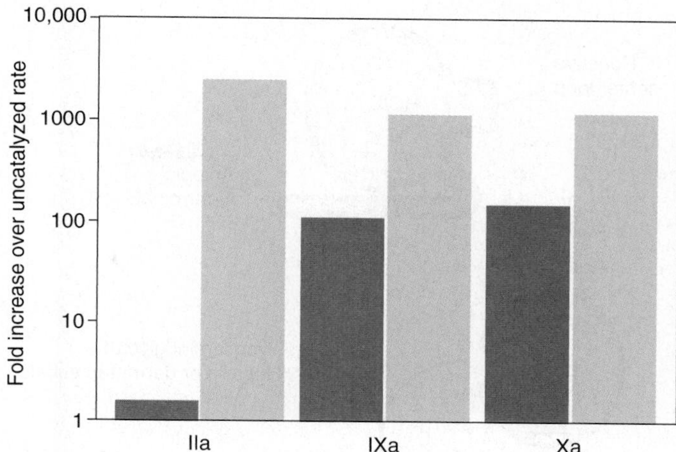

Figure 151-5 COMPARISON OF THE STIMULATORY EFFECTS OF PENTASACCHARIDE AND UNFRACTIONATED HEPARIN ON CATALYSIS OF ANTITHROMBIN-MEDIATED INHIBITION OF THROMBIN (IIa), FACTOR IXA (IXa), AND FACTOR XA (Xa). Second-order rate constants of inhibition of IIa, IXa, or Xa by antithrombin, measured in the presence of heparin *(green bars)* or fondaparinux *(pink bars),* were divided by those determined in the absence of glycosaminoglycan and are plotted as fold increase over the uncatalyzed rate of inhibition. *(Reprinted with permission from Wiebe EM, Stafford AR, Fredenburgh JC, et al: Mechanism of catalysis of inhibition of factor IXa by antithrombin in the presence of heparin or pentasaccharide,* J Biol Chem *278:35767, 2003.)*

Leu444-Ser445, a peptide bond that is not readily susceptible to cleavage by coagulation proteases other than thrombin. Second, heparin cofactor II possesses a unique anionic sequence at its N-terminal. In its unactivated state, this sequence forms an intramolecular bond with the positively charged glycosaminoglycan binding site located on the body of heparin cofactor II. When heparin or dermatan sulfate, a glycosaminoglycan that interacts only with heparin cofactor II, binds to heparin cofactor II, this N-terminal sequence is displaced, which enables its tethering to a positively charged domain on thrombin known as exosite 1. This tethering interaction occurs only with thrombin and facilitates thrombin inhibition by heparin cofactor II (Fig. 151-6).

Maximum catalysis of heparin cofactor II by heparin requires heparin chains composed of at least 26 saccharide units, which corresponds to a molecular weight of 7800. Longer heparin chains activate heparin cofactor II to a greater extent than shorter chains because the longer chains are of sufficient length to not only bind to heparin cofactor II, but to also bind to thrombin to form a ternary complex. Formation of this complex brings thrombin and heparin cofactor II into close apposition.

The interaction of heparin with heparin cofactor II is not mediated by the antithrombin-binding pentasaccharide sequence. Because heparin lacks a specific heparin cofactor II binding domain, heparin's affinity for heparin cofactor II is lower than that for antithrombin. Consequently 10-fold higher heparin concentrations are needed to accelerate thrombin inhibition by heparin cofactor II in plasma than are necessary to enhance thrombin's inactivation by antithrombin. Therefore it is likely that heparin cofactor II only contributes to the anticoagulant activity of heparin when the drug is given in high doses.

Heparin causes the release of tissue factor pathway inhibitor (TFPI) from the endothelium (see Chapters 128 and 129). A factor Xa–dependent inhibitor of tissue factor–bound factor VIIa, TFPI may contribute to the antithrombotic activity of heparin. Longer heparin chains induce the release of more TFPI than shorter chains.

Pharmacology

Heparin must be given parenterally. It is usually administered subcutaneously or by continuous intravenous infusion. When used for therapeutic purposes, the intravenous route is most often employed. If heparin is given subcutaneously for treatment of thrombosis, the dose of heparin must be high enough to overcome the limited bioavailability associated with this method of delivery.

After entering the circulation, heparin binds to a variety of plasma proteins other than antithrombin, which decreases the anticoagulant activity of heparin. The levels of heparin-binding proteins vary between patients because some of these proteins are acute-phase reactants whose levels are elevated in ill patients, whereas others, such as high-molecular-weight multimers of von Willebrand factor, are released when platelets or endothelial cells are activated by thrombin. Activated platelets also release platelet factor 4 (PF4), a highly cationic protein that binds heparin with high affinity. The large amount of PF4 found in the vicinity of platelet-rich arterial thrombi has the potential to locally neutralize the anticoagulant activity of heparin.

Because the levels of heparin-binding proteins are so variable between patients, the anticoagulant response to fixed or weight-adjusted doses of heparin is unpredictable. Consequently coagulation monitoring is essential to ensure that a therapeutic response is obtained when heparin is administered for treatment purposes.

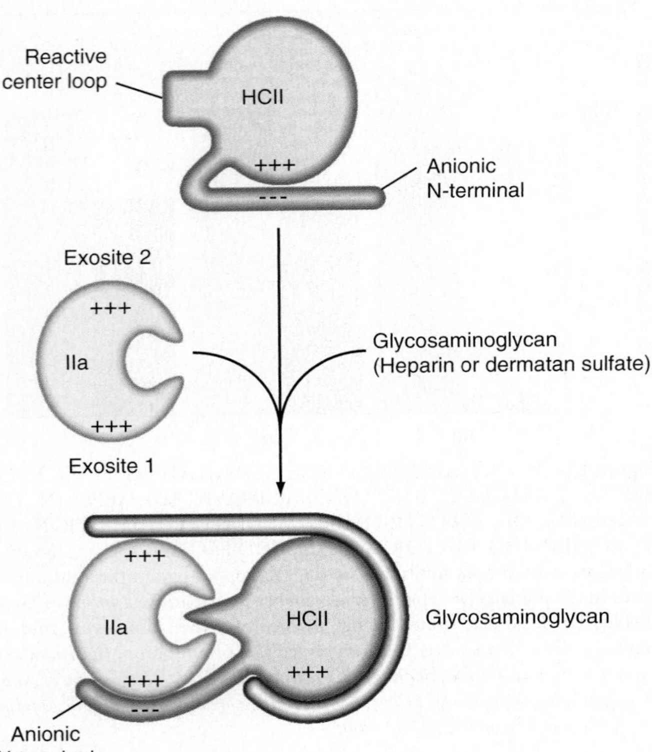

Figure 151-6 CATALYSIS OF HEPARIN COFACTOR II (HCII) BY GLYCOSAMINOGLYCANS. In its unactivated form, the acidic N-terminal tail of HCII is tethered to the positively charged glycosaminoglycan-binding site on the body of the serine protease inhibitor (serpin). The binding of heparin or dermatan sulfate to this binding site displaces the N-terminal tail, thereby facilitating the interaction of this anionic domain with exosite 1 on thrombin. Glycosaminoglycan binding also evokes a conformational change in the reactive center loop of HCII that contributes to the formation of the HCII-thrombin complex. Longer heparin chains not only bind to HCII, but also bind to the heparin-binding domain on thrombin, so-called exosite 2. Heparin-mediated bridging of HCII to thrombin enhances the rate of inhibition. Consequently, longer heparin chains that contain at least 26 saccharide units promote thrombin inhibition by HCII to a greater extent than shorter chains. Unlike heparin, dermatan sulfate does not need to bind to thrombin for maximal enhancement in the rate of thrombin inhibition because shorter dermatan sulfate fragments are just as active as longer ones.

Heparin is cleared through a combination of a rapid saturable and a much slower first-order mechanism. The saturable phase of heparin clearance is thought to be due to binding to endothelial cell receptors and macrophages. Bound heparin is internalized and depolymerized. The slower nonsaturable mechanism of clearance is largely renal. At therapeutic doses, a large proportion of heparin is cleared through the rapid saturable, dose-dependent mechanism. The complex kinetics of clearance make the anticoagulant response to heparin nonlinear at therapeutic doses, with both the intensity and duration of effect rising disproportionately with increasing dose. Thus the apparent biologic half-life of heparin increases from approximately 30 minutes after an intravenous bolus of 25 units/kg, to 60 minutes with an intravenous bolus of 100 units/kg, to 150 minutes with a bolus of 400 units/kg.

Monitoring

Heparin therapy can be monitored using the activated partial thromboplastin time (aPTT) or anti–factor Xa level. Although the aPTT is the test most often employed for this purpose, there are problems with this assay. aPTT reagents vary in their sensitivity to heparin, and the type of coagulometer used for testing can influence the results. Consequently laboratories must establish a therapeutic aPTT range with each reagent-coagulometer combination by measuring the aPTT and anti–factor Xa level in plasma samples collected from heparin-treated patients. For most of the aPTT reagents and coagulometers in current use, therapeutic heparin levels are achieved with a twofold to threefold prolongation of the aPTT.

Anti–factor Xa levels also can be used to monitor heparin therapy. With this test, therapeutic heparin levels range from 0.3 to 0.7 units/mL. Although this test is gaining in popularity, anti–factor Xa assays have yet to be standardized, and results can vary widely between laboratories.

Up to 25% of heparin-treated patients with venous thromboembolism require more than 35,000 units/day to achieve a therapeutic aPTT. These patients are considered heparin resistant. It is useful to measure anti–factor Xa levels in these patients because many will have a therapeutic anti–factor Xa level despite a subtherapeutic aPTT. This dissociation in test results occurs because elevated plasma levels of fibrinogen and factor VIII, both of which are acute-phase proteins, shorten the aPTT but have no effect on anti–factor Xa levels. Heparin therapy in patients who exhibit this phenomenon is best monitored using anti–factor Xa levels instead of the aPTT. Patients with congenital or acquired antithrombin deficiency and those with unusually high levels of heparin-binding proteins often require very high doses of heparin to achieve a therapeutic aPTT or anti–factor Xa level. If there is good correlation between the aPTT and the anti–factor Xa levels, either test can be used to monitor heparin therapy.

Dosing

For prophylaxis, heparin is usually given in fixed doses of 5000 units subcutaneously two or three times daily. With these low doses, coagulation monitoring is unnecessary. In contrast, monitoring is essential when heparin is given in therapeutic doses because a subtherapeutic anticoagulant response has been associated with a higher risk for recurrent thrombosis. Fixed-dose or weight-based heparin nomograms are used to standardize heparin dosing and to shorten the time required to achieve a therapeutic anticoagulant response. At least two heparin nomograms have been validated in patients with venous thromboembolism and reduce the time required to achieve a therapeutic aPTT. Weight-adjusted heparin nomograms also have been evaluated in patients with acute coronary syndromes.

Unmonitored twice-daily subcutaneous heparin proved as effective and safe as once-daily LMWH for initial treatment of venous thromboembolism in one study. High doses of heparin were used; treatment was started with a dose of 333 units/kg followed by 250 units/kg twice daily thereafter. This regimen may be an option for patients with renal insufficiency where LMWH or fondaparinux is problematic.

Limitations

Heparin has pharmacokinetic and biophysical limitations (Table 151-2). The pharmacokinetic limitations reflect heparin's propensity to bind in a pentasaccharide-independent fashion to cells and plasma proteins. Heparin binding to cells explains its dose-dependent clearance, whereas binding to plasma proteins results in a variable anticoagulant response and can lead to heparin resistance.

The biophysical limitations of heparin reflect the inability of the heparin-antithrombin complex to (1) inhibit factor Xa when it is incorporated into the prothrombinase complex, the complex that converts prothrombin to thrombin, and (2) to inhibit thrombin bound to fibrin. Consequently factor Xa bound to activated platelets within platelet-rich thrombi has the potential to generate thrombin, even in the face of heparin. Once this thrombin binds to fibrin, it too is protected from inhibition by the heparin-antithrombin complex. Clot-associated thrombin can then trigger thrombus growth by locally activating platelets and amplifying its own generation through feedback activation of factors V, VIII, and XI. Further

Table 151-2 Pharmacokinetic and Biophysical Limitations of Heparin

Limitations	Mechanism
Poor bioavailability at low doses	Limited absorption of long heparin chains
Dose-dependent clearance	Binds to endothelial cells
Variable anticoagulant response	Binds to plasma proteins whose levels vary from patient to patient
Reduced activity in the vicinity of platelet-rich thrombi	Neutralized by platelet factor 4 released from activated platelets within platelet-rich thrombi
Limited activity against factor Xa incorporated in the prothrombinase complex and thrombin bound to fibrin	Reduced capacity of heparin-antithrombin complex to inhibit factor Xa bound to activated platelets and thrombin bound to fibrin

compounding the problem is the potential for heparin neutralization by the high concentrations of PF4 released from activated platelets within the platelet-rich thrombus.

Side Effects

The most common side effect of heparin is bleeding. Other complications include thrombocytopenia, osteoporosis, and elevated levels of transaminases.

Bleeding

The risk for heparin-induced bleeding increases with higher heparin doses. Concomitant administration of drugs that affect hemostasis, such as antiplatelet or fibrinolytic agents, increases the risk for bleeding, as does recent surgery or trauma. Heparin-treated patients with serious bleeding can be given protamine sulfate to neutralize the heparin. Protamine sulfate, a mixture of basic polypeptides isolated from salmon sperm, binds heparin with high affinity, and the resultant protamine-heparin complexes are then cleared. Typically 1 mg of protamine sulfate neutralizes 100 units of heparin. Protamine sulfate is given intravenously. Anaphylactoid reactions to protamine sulfate can occur, and drug administration by slow intravenous infusion is recommended to reduce the risk for these problems.

Thrombocytopenia

Heparin can cause thrombocytopenia. Heparin-induced thrombocytopenia (HIT) is an antibody-mediated process that is triggered by antibodies directed against neoantigens on PF4 that are exposed when heparin binds to this protein (see Chapter 135). These antibodies, which usually are of the immunoglobulin G (IgG) subtype, bind simultaneously to the heparin-PF4 complex and to platelet Fc receptors. Such binding activates the platelets and generates platelet microparticles. Circulating microparticles are prothrombotic because they express anionic phospholipids on their surface and can bind clotting factors, thereby promoting thrombin generation.

HIT can be associated with thrombosis, either arterial or venous (Table 151-3). Venous thrombosis, which manifests as deep venous thrombosis and/or pulmonary embolism, is more common than arterial thrombosis. Arterial thrombosis can manifest as ischemic stroke or acute myocardial infarction. Rarely, platelet-rich thrombi in the distal aorta or iliac arteries can cause critical limb ischemia.

The diagnosis of HIT is established using enzyme-linked assays to detect antibodies against heparin-PF4 complexes or with platelet activation assays. Enzyme-linked assays are sensitive but can be positive in the absence of any clinical evidence of HIT. The most specific diagnostic test is the serotonin-release assay. This test is performed by quantifying serotonin release when washed platelets loaded with labeled serotonin are exposed to patient serum in the absence or presence of varying concentrations of heparin. If the patient serum contains the HIT antibody, heparin addition induces platelet activation and subsequent serotonin release.

Table 151-3 Features of Heparin-Induced Thrombocytopenia

Features	Details
Thrombocytopenia	Platelet count of 100,000/μL or less or a decrease in platelet count of 50% or more
Timing	Platelet count falls 5-10 days after starting heparin
Type of heparin	More common with unfractionated heparin than low-molecular-weight heparin
Type of patient	More common in surgical patients than medical patients. More common in women than in men
Thrombosis	Venous thrombosis more common than arterial thrombosis

Table 151-4 Management of Heparin-Induced Thrombocytopenia

Stop all heparin.
Give an alternative anticoagulant, such as lepirudin, argatroban, bivalirudin, danaparoid, or fondaparinux.
Do not give platelet transfusions.
Do not give warfarin until the platelet count returns to its baseline level. If warfarin is administered, give vitamin K to restore the INR to normal.
Evaluate for thrombosis, particularly deep venous thrombosis.

INR, International normalized ratio.

Management of HIT is outlined in Table 151-4. Heparin should be stopped in patients with suspected or documented HIT, and an alternative anticoagulant should be administered to prevent or treat thrombosis.[11] The agents most often used for this indication are parenteral direct thrombin inhibitors, such as lepirudin, argatroban, or bivalirudin, or factor Xa inhibitors, such as fondaparinux or danaparoid (see Chapter 135).

Patients with HIT, particularly those with associated thrombosis, often have evidence of increased thrombin generation that can lead to consumption of protein C. If these patients are given warfarin without a concomitant parenteral anticoagulant to suppress thrombin generation, the further decrease in protein C levels induced by warfarin can trigger skin necrosis. To avoid this problem, patients with HIT should be treated with a direct thrombin inhibitor or fondaparinux until the platelet count returns to normal levels. At this point, low-dose warfarin therapy can be introduced, and the thrombin inhibitor or fondaparinux can be discontinued when the anticoagulant response to warfarin has been therapeutic for at least 2 days.

Osteoporosis

Treatment with therapeutic doses of heparin for over a month can cause a reduction in bone density. This complication has been reported in up to 30% of patients given long-term heparin therapy, and symptomatic vertebral fractures occur in 2% to 3% of these individuals.

Studies in vitro and in laboratory animals have provided insights into the pathogenesis of heparin-induced osteoporosis. These investigations suggest that heparin causes bone resorption both by decreasing bone formation and by enhancing bone resorption. Thus heparin affects the activity of both osteoblasts and osteoclasts.

Elevated Levels of Transaminases

Therapeutic doses of heparin frequently cause modest elevation in the serum levels of hepatic transaminases, without a concomitant increase in the level of bilirubin. The levels of transaminases rapidly return to normal when the drug is stopped. The mechanism responsible for this phenomenon is unknown.

Low-Molecular-Weight Heparin

Consisting of smaller fragments of heparin, LMWH is prepared from unfractionated heparin by controlled enzymatic or chemical depolymerization. The mean molecular weight of LMWH is between 4500 and 5000, about one-third the mean molecular weight of unfractionated heparin. LMWH has advantages over heparin (Table 151-5) and has replaced heparin for most indications.

Mechanism of Action

Like heparin, LMWH exerts its anticoagulant activity by activating antithrombin. With a mean molecular weight of 4500 to 5000, which corresponds to about 17 saccharide units, at least half of the pentasaccharide-containing chains of LMWH are too short to bridge thrombin to antithrombin (see Fig. 151-4). However, these chains retain the capacity to accelerate factor Xa inhibition by antithrombin because this activity is largely the result of the conformational changes in antithrombin evoked by pentasaccharide binding. Consequently LMWH catalyzes factor Xa inhibition by antithrombin more than thrombin inhibition. Depending on their unique molecular weight distributions, LMWH preparations have anti–factor Xa to anti–factor IIa ratios ranging from 2:1 to 4:1.

Pharmacology

Although usually given subcutaneously, LMWH also can be administered intravenously if a rapid anticoagulant response is needed. LMWH has pharmacokinetic advantages over heparin. These advantages reflect the fact that shorter heparin chains bind less avidly to endothelial cells, macrophages, and heparin-binding plasma proteins. Reduced binding to endothelial cells and macrophages eliminates the rapid, dose-dependent, and saturable mechanism of clearance that is a characteristic of unfractionated heparin. Instead, the clearance of LMWH is dose independent, and its plasma half-life is longer. Based on measurement of anti–factor Xa levels, LMWH has a plasma half-life of about 4 hours. LMWH is cleared almost exclusively by the kidneys, and the drug can accumulate in patients with renal insufficiency.

LMWH exhibits about 90% bioavailability after subcutaneous injection. Because LMWH binds less avidly to heparin-binding proteins in plasma than heparin, LMWH produces a more predictable dose response and resistance to LMWH is rare. With a longer half-life and more predictable anticoagulant response, LMWH can be given subcutaneously once or twice daily without coagulation monitoring, even when the drug is given in treatment doses. These properties render LMWH more convenient than unfractionated heparin. Capitalizing on this feature, studies in patients with venous thromboembolism have shown that home treatment with LMWH is as effective and safe as in-hospital treatment with continuous intravenous infusions of heparin. Outpatient treatment with LMWH streamlines care, reduces health care costs, and increases patient satisfaction.

Table 151-5 Advantages of Low-Molecular-Weight Heparin Over Heparin

Advantage	Consequence
Better bioavailability and longer half-life after subcutaneous injection	Can be given subcutaneously once or twice daily for both prophylaxis and treatment
Dose-independent clearance	Simplified dosing
Predictable anticoagulant response	Coagulation monitoring is unnecessary in most patients
Lower risk for heparin-induced thrombocytopenia	Safer than heparin for short- or long-term administration
Lower risk for osteoporosis	Safer than heparin for extended administration

Monitoring

In the majority of patients, LMWH does not require coagulation monitoring. If monitoring is necessary, anti–factor Xa levels must be measured because most LMWH preparations have little effect on the aPTT. Therapeutic anti–factor Xa levels with LMWH range from 0.5 to 1.2 units/mL when measured 3 to 4 hours after drug administration. When LMWH is given in prophylactic doses, peak anti–factor Xa levels of 0.2 to 0.5 units/mL are desirable.

Indications for LMWH monitoring include renal insufficiency and morbid obesity. LMWH monitoring in patients with a creatinine clearance of 50 mL/min or less is advisable to ensure that there is no drug accumulation. Although weight-adjusted LMWH dosing appears to produce therapeutic anti–factor Xa levels in patients who are overweight, this approach has not been extensively evaluated in those with morbid obesity. It may also be advisable to monitor the anticoagulant activity of LMWH during pregnancy because dose requirements can change, particularly in the third trimester. Monitoring also is important in high-risk settings, such as in patients with mechanical mitral valves who are given LMWH for prevention of valve thrombosis.

Dosing

The doses of LMWH recommended for prophylaxis or treatment vary depending on the LMWH preparation. For prophylaxis, once-daily subcutaneous doses of 4000 to 5000 units are often used, whereas doses of 2500 to 3000 units are given when the drug is administered twice daily. For treatment of venous thromboembolism, a dose of 150 to 200 units/kg is given if the drug is administered once daily. If a twice-daily regimen is employed, a dose of 100 units/kg is given. In patients with unstable angina, LMWH is given subcutaneously on a twice-daily basis at a dose of 100 to 120 units/kg.

Side Effects

The major complication of LMWH is bleeding. Recent metaanalyses suggest that the risk for major bleeding may be lower with LMWH than with unfractionated heparin. HIT and osteoporosis are less common with LMWH than with unfractionated heparin.

Bleeding

Like the situation with heparin, bleeding with LMWH is more common in patients receiving concomitant therapy with antiplatelet or fibrinolytic drugs. Recent surgery, trauma, or underlying hemostatic defects also increase the risk for bleeding with LMWH.

Although protamine sulfate can be used as an antidote for LMWH, protamine sulfate incompletely neutralizes the anticoagulant activity of LMWH because it binds only the longer chains of LMWH. Because longer chains are responsible for catalysis of thrombin inhibition by antithrombin, protamine sulfate completely reverses the anti–factor IIa activity of LMWH. In contrast, protamine sulfate only partially reverses the anti–factor Xa activity of LMWH because the shorter pentasaccharide-containing chains of LMWH do not bind to protamine sulfate. Consequently patients at high risk for bleeding may be more safely treated with continuous intravenous unfractionated heparin than with subcutaneous LMWH. In addition to the potential for complete reversal with protamine sulfate, the short half-life of intravenous heparin also is an advantage if major bleeding occurs.

Thrombocytopenia

The risk for HIT is about fivefold lower with LMWH than with heparin. LMWH binds less avidly to platelets and causes less PF4 release. Furthermore, with lower affinity for PF4 than heparin, LMWH is less likely to induce the conformational changes in PF4 that trigger the formation of HIT antibodies.

LMWH should not be used to treat patients with HIT because most HIT antibodies exhibit cross-reactivity with LMWH and there are case reports of thrombosis when HIT patients were treated with LMWH (see Chapter 135).

Osteoporosis

The risk for osteoporosis is lower with long-term LMWH than with heparin. For extended treatment therefore LMWH is a better choice than heparin because of the lower risk for both osteoporosis and HIT.

Fondaparinux

A synthetic analogue of the antithrombin-binding pentasaccharide sequence, fondaparinux differs from LMWH in several ways (Table 151-6). Fondaparinux is licensed for (1) thromboprophylaxis in medical, general surgical, and high-risk orthopedic patients and (2) as an alternative to heparin or LMWH for initial treatment of patients with established venous thromboembolism. In some countries, fondaparinux also is approved as an alternative to heparin or LMWH for treatment of patients with acute coronary syndromes.

Mechanism of Action

As a synthetic analogue of the antithrombin-binding pentasaccharide sequence found in heparin and LMWH, fondaparinux has a molecular weight of 1728. Fondaparinux binds only to antithrombin (see Fig. 151-4) and is too short to bridge thrombin to antithrombin. Consequently fondaparinux catalyzes factor Xa inhibition by antithrombin and does not enhance the rate of thrombin inhibition.

Pharmacology

Fondaparinux exhibits complete bioavailability after subcutaneous injection. With no binding to endothelial cells or plasma proteins, the clearance of fondaparinux is dose independent and its plasma half-life is about 17 hours. The drug is given subcutaneously once daily. Because fondaparinux is cleared unchanged via the kidneys, it is contraindicated in patients with a creatinine clearance of less than 30 mL/min and it should be used with caution in those with a creatinine clearance of less than 50 mL/min.

Table 151-6 Comparison of Low-Molecular-Weight Heparin and Fondaparinux

Features	LMWH	Fondaparinux
Molecular weight	4500 to 5000	1728
Catalysis of factor Xa inhibition	Yes	Yes
Catalysis of thrombin inhibition	Yes	No
Bioavailability after subcutaneous administration (%)	90	100
Plasma half-life (hr)	4	17
Renal excretion	Yes	Yes
Induces release of tissue factor pathway inhibitor	Yes	No
Neutralized by protamine sulfate	Partially	No

LMWH, Low-molecular-weight heparin.

Fondaparinux produces a predictable anticoagulant response after administration in fixed doses because it does not bind to plasma proteins. The drug is given at a dose of 2.5 mg once daily for prevention of venous thromboembolism. For initial treatment of established venous thromboembolism, fondaparinux is given at a dose of 7.5 mg once daily. The dose can be reduced to 5 mg once daily for those weighing less than 50 kg and increased to 10 mg for those over 100 kg. When given in these doses, fondaparinux is as effective as heparin or LMWH for initial treatment of patients with deep venous thrombosis or pulmonary embolism and produces similar rates of bleeding.

Fondaparinux is used at a dose of 2.5 mg once daily in patients with acute coronary syndromes. When this prophylactic dose of fondaparinux was compared with treatment doses of enoxaparin in patients with non–ST segment elevation acute coronary syndromes, there was no difference in the rate of cardiovascular death, myocardial infarction, or stroke at 9 days.[12] However, the rate of major bleeding was 50% lower with fondaparinux than with enoxaparin, a difference that likely reflects the fact that the dose of fondaparinux was lower than that of enoxaparin. In acute coronary syndrome patients who require percutaneous coronary interventions, there is a risk for catheter thrombosis with fondaparinux unless adjunctive heparin is given.

Side Effects

Fondaparinux does not cause HIT, and, in contrast to LMWH, there is no cross-reactivity of fondaparinux with HIT antibodies. Interestingly, fondaparinux induces the formation of HIT antibodies to the same extent as LMWH. In contrast to heparin or LMWH, however, fondaparinux is too short to cluster PF4 tetramers together, which is a prerequisite for HIT antibody binding. This phenomenon not only explains why HIT antibodies do not cross-react with fondaparinux, but also explains why fondaparinux does not cause HIT despite the fact that it induces the formation of HIT antibodies. Although fondaparinux has been successfully used for HIT treatment, large clinical trials are lacking and the drug is not licensed for this indication.

The major side effect of fondaparinux is bleeding. There is no antidote for fondaparinux. Protamine sulfate has no effect on the anticoagulant activity of fondaparinux because it fails to bind to the drug. Recombinant activated factor VII reverses the anticoagulant effects of fondaparinux in volunteers, but it is unknown whether this agent will control fondaparinux-induced bleeding.

Parenteral Direct Thrombin Inhibitors

Heparin and LMWH are indirect inhibitors of thrombin because their activity is mediated by antithrombin. In contrast, direct thrombin inhibitors do not require a plasma cofactor; instead, these agents bind directly to thrombin and block its interaction with its substrates. Approved parenteral direct thrombin inhibitors include hirudin derivatives (lepirudin and desirudin), argatroban and bivalirudin (Table 151-7). Lepirudin and argatroban are licensed for treatment

Table 151-7 Comparison of the Properties of Hirudin, Bivalirudin, and Argatroban

	Hirudin	Bivalirudin	Argatroban
Molecular mass	7000	1980	527
Site(s) of interaction with thrombin	Active site and exosite 1	Active site and exosite 1	Active site
Renal clearance	Yes	No	No
Hepatic metabolism	No	No	Yes
Plasma half-life (min)	60	25	45

of patients with HIT, whereas bivalirudin is approved as an alternative to heparin in patients undergoing percutaneous coronary interventions, including those with HIT (see Chapter 135). Desirudin is licensed for thromboprophylaxis after elective hip replacement surgery.

Lepirudin and Desirudin

Recombinant forms of hirudin, lepirudin, and desirudin are bivalent direct thrombin inhibitors that interact with both the active site and exosite 1, the substrate binding site, on thrombin. Lepirudin is given by continuous intravenous infusion, whereas desirudin is administered subcutaneously twice daily. Lepirudin has a plasma half-life of 60 minutes after intravenous infusion, whereas the half-life of desirudin is about 2 hours. Both drugs are cleared by the kidneys and can accumulate in patients with renal insufficiency. A high proportion of lepirudin-treated patients develop antibodies against the drug. Although these antibodies rarely cause problems, in a small subset of patients they can delay lepirudin clearance and prolong its anticoagulant activity. Serious bleeding has been reported in some of these patients.

Desirudin is given subcutaneously in low doses and does not require monitoring. In contrast, lepirudin is usually monitored using the aPTT, and the dose is adjusted to maintain an aPTT that is 1.5 to 2.5 times the control. The aPTT is not an ideal test for monitoring lepirudin therapy because the clotting time plateaus with higher drug concentrations. Although the ecarin clotting time provides a better index of lepirudin dose than does the aPTT, the ecarin clotting time has yet to be standardized.

Argatroban

A univalent inhibitor that targets the active site of thrombin, argatroban is metabolized in the liver. Consequently this drug must be used with caution in patients with hepatic insufficiency. Argatroban is not cleared via the kidneys, so this drug is safer than lepirudin for HIT patients with renal insufficiency.

Argatroban is administered by continuous intravenous infusion and has a plasma half-life of about 45 minutes. The aPTT is used to monitor its anticoagulant effect, and the dose is adjusted to achieve an aPTT 1.5 to 3 times the baseline value, but not to exceed 100 seconds. Argatroban also prolongs the international normalized ratio (INR), a feature that can complicate the transitioning of patients from argatroban to warfarin. This problem can be circumvented by using the levels of factor X to monitor warfarin in place of the INR. Alternatively, the argatroban infusion can be stopped for 2 to 3 hours before INR determination.

Bivalirudin

A synthetic 20–amino acid analogue of hirudin, bivalirudin is a divalent thrombin inhibitor. Thus the N-terminal portion of bivalirudin interacts with the active site of thrombin, whereas its C-terminal tail binds to exosite 1. Bivalirudin has a plasma half-life of 25 minutes, the shortest half-life of all the parenteral direct thrombin inhibitors. Bivalirudin is degraded by peptidases and is partially excreted via the kidneys. When given in high doses in the cardiac catheterization laboratory, the anticoagulant activity of bivalirudin is monitored using the activated clotting time. With lower doses, its activity can be assessed using the aPTT.

Studies comparing bivalirudin with heparin plus GPIIb/IIIa antagonists suggest that bivalirudin produces less bleeding. This feature plus its short half-life make bivalirudin an attractive alternative to heparin in patients undergoing percutaneous coronary interventions, and it is licensed for this indication. Bivalirudin also is approved for management of HIT patients who require percutaneous coronary interventions (see Chapter 135).

ORAL ANTICOAGULANTS

Current oral anticoagulant practice dates back almost 60 years to when the vitamin K antagonists were discovered as a result of investigations into the cause of hemorrhagic disease in cattle. Characterized by a decrease in prothrombin levels, this disorder is caused by ingestion of hay containing spoiled sweet clover. Hydroxycoumarin, which was isolated from bacterial contaminants in the hay, interferes with vitamin K metabolism, thereby causing a syndrome similar to vitamin K deficiency. A variety of coumarin derivatives are available. The agent most widely used in North America is warfarin.

The repertoire of oral anticoagulants has expanded with the introduction of new oral anticoagulants that target thrombin or factor Xa.[10] These agents are now licensed for thromboprophylaxis after hip or knee replacement, stroke prevention in patients with atrial fibrillation, and, in some countries, for treatment of venous thrombosis. The drugs in this class include dabigatran, rivaroxaban, and apixaban.

Warfarin

A water-soluble vitamin K antagonist, warfarin was initially developed as a rodenticide. Like other vitamin K antagonists, warfarin interferes with the synthesis of the vitamin K–dependent clotting proteins, which include prothrombin (factor II) and factors VII, IX, and X. The synthesis of the vitamin K–dependent anticoagulant proteins, proteins C, S, and Z, also is reduced by vitamin K antagonists (see Chapter 128).

Mechanism of Action

All of the vitamin K–dependent clotting factors possess glutamic acid residues at their N-terminals. A posttranslational modification adds a carboxyl group to the γ-carbon of these residues to generate γ-carboxyglutamic acid (see Chapter 128). This modification is essential for expression of the activity of these clotting factors because it permits their calcium-dependent binding to negatively charged phospholipid surfaces. The γ-carboxylation process is catalyzed by a vitamin K–dependent carboxylase. Thus vitamin K from the diet is reduced to vitamin K hydroquinone by vitamin K reductase (Fig. 151-7). Vitamin K hydroquinone serves as a cofactor for the carboxylase enzyme, which in the presence of carbon dioxide replaces the hydrogen on the γ-carbon of glutamic acid residues with a carboxyl group. During this process, vitamin K hydroquinone is oxidized to vitamin K epoxide, which is then reduced to vitamin K by vitamin K epoxide reductase.

Warfarin inhibits vitamin K–epoxide reductase (VKOR), thereby blocking the γ-carboxylation process. This results in the synthesis of vitamin K–dependent clotting proteins that are only partially γ-carboxylated. Warfarin acts as an anticoagulant because these partially γ-carboxylated proteins have reduced or absent biologic activity. The onset of action of warfarin is delayed until the newly synthesized clotting factors with reduced activity gradually replace their fully active counterparts.

The antithrombotic effect of warfarin depends on a reduction in the functional levels of factor X and prothrombin, clotting factors that have half-lives of 24 and 72 hours, respectively. Because of the delay in achieving an antithrombotic effect, initial treatment with warfarin is supported by concomitant administration of a rapidly acting parenteral anticoagulant, such as heparin, LMWH, or fondaparinux, in patients with established thrombosis or at high risk for thrombosis.

Pharmacology

Warfarin is a racemic mixture of R and S isomers; of these, the S isomer is more active. Warfarin is rapidly and almost completely

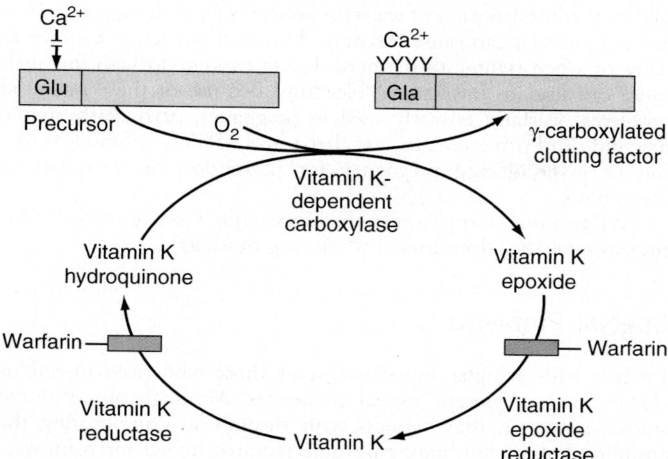

Figure 151-7 THE VITAMIN K CYCLE AND ITS INHIBITION BY WARFARIN. Dietary vitamin K is reduced by vitamin K reductase to generate vitamin K hydroquinone. Vitamin K hydroquinone serves as a cofactor for the vitamin K–dependent carboxylase that converts glutamic acid (Glu) residues at the N-terminals of the vitamin K–dependent precursors to γ-carboxyglutamic acid (Gla) residues, thereby creating the so-called Gla domain. By binding calcium, the Gla domain is critical for the interaction of the vitamin K–dependent clotting factors with negatively charged phospholipid membranes. During vitamin K–dependent carboxylation, vitamin K hydroquinone is oxidized to vitamin K epoxide. Vitamin K epoxide is then converted to vitamin K by vitamin K epoxide reductase. Vitamin K antagonists, such as warfarin, interfere with this cycle by inhibiting vitamin K epoxide reductase and vitamin K reductase. Of these two enzymes, vitamin K epoxide reductase is more readily blocked by vitamin K antagonists than vitamin K reductase. Consequently, supplemental vitamin K can overcome the inhibitory effects of vitamin K antagonists.

absorbed from the gastrointestinal tract. Levels of warfarin in the blood peak about 90 minutes after drug administration. Racemic warfarin has a plasma half-life of 36 to 42 hours, and over 97% of circulating warfarin is bound to albumin. It is only the small fraction of unbound warfarin that is biologically active.

Warfarin accumulates in the liver, where the two isomers are metabolized via distinct pathways. Oxidative metabolism of the more active S isomer is effected by CYP2C9.[13] Two relatively common variants, CYP2C9*2 and CYP2C9*3, have reduced activity. Patients with these variants require lower maintenance dose of warfarin. The target of warfarin is VKOR. Polymorphisms in the C1 subunit of this enzyme (VKORC1) also can render patients less or more responsive to the anticoagulant effects of warfarin.[13] These findings have prompted a recommendation that patients starting on warfarin should be tested for these polymorphisms and that this information should be incorporated into their warfarin-dosing algorithms. Whether this approach will increase the efficacy and/or safety of warfarin therapy is uncertain.

In addition to genetic factors, the anticoagulant effect of warfarin is influenced by diet, drugs, and various disease states. Fluctuations in dietary vitamin K intake affect the activity of warfarin. A wide variety of drugs can alter absorption, clearance, or metabolism of warfarin. Because of the variability in the anticoagulant response to warfarin, coagulation monitoring is essential to ensure that a therapeutic response is obtained.

Monitoring

Warfarin therapy is most often monitored using the prothrombin time, a test that is sensitive to reductions in the levels of prothrombin, factor VII, and factor X.[14] The test is performed by adding thromboplastin, a reagent that contains tissue factor, and phospholipid, and calcium to citrated plasma and determining the time to clot formation. Thromboplastins vary in their sensitivity to reductions in the levels of the vitamin K–dependent clotting factors. Consequently, less sensitive thromboplastins will prompt the administration of higher doses of warfarin to achieve a target prothrombin time. This is problematic because higher doses of warfarin increase the risk for bleeding.

The INR was developed to circumvent many of the problems associated with the prothrombin time assay (see Chapter 128). To calculate the INR, the patient's prothrombin time is divided by the mean normal prothrombin time and this ratio is then multiplied by the international sensitivity index (ISI), an index of the sensitivity of the thromboplastin used for prothrombin time determination to reductions in the levels of the vitamin K–dependent clotting factors. Highly sensitive thromboplastins have an ISI of 1.0. Most current thromboplastins have ISI values that range from 1.0 to 1.4.

Although the INR has helped to standardize anticoagulant practice, problems persist. The precision of INR determination varies depending on reagent-coagulometer combinations. This leads to variability in the INR results. Also complicating INR determination is unreliable reporting of the ISI by thromboplastin manufacturers. Furthermore, every laboratory must establish the mean normal prothrombin time with each new batch of thromboplastin reagent. To accomplish this, the prothrombin time must be measured in fresh plasma samples from at least 20 healthy volunteers using the same coagulometer that is used for patient samples.

For most indications, warfarin is administered in doses that produce a target INR of 2.0 to 3.0.[14] An exception is patients with mechanical heart valves, for whom a target INR of 2.5 to 3.5 is recommended.[14] Vitamin K antagonists have a narrow therapeutic window. Thus studies in atrial fibrillation demonstrate an increased risk for cardioembolic stroke when the INR falls below 1.7 and an increase in bleeding with INR values over 4.5. Likewise, a study in patients receiving long-term warfarin therapy for unprovoked venous thromboembolism demonstrated a higher rate of recurrent venous thromboembolism when the warfarin dose was adjusted to achieve a target INR of 1.5 to 1.9 than with a target INR of 2.0 to 3.0. Rates of major bleeding were similar.

Dosing

Warfarin is usually started at a dose of 5 to 10 mg. The dose is then titrated to achieve the desired target INR. Because of warfarin's delayed onset of action, patients with established thrombosis or those at high risk for thrombosis are given concomitant treatment with a rapidly acting parenteral anticoagulant, such as heparin, LMWH, or fondaparinux. Initial prolongation of the INR reflects reduction in the functional levels of factor VII. Consequently concomitant treatment with the parenteral anticoagulant should be continued until the INR has been therapeutic for at least 2 consecutive days. A minimum 5-day course of parenteral anticoagulation is recommended to ensure that the levels of prothrombin have been reduced into the therapeutic range with warfarin.

Because warfarin has a narrow therapeutic window, frequent coagulation monitoring is essential to ensure that a therapeutic anticoagulant response is obtained. Even patients with stable warfarin dose requirements should have their INR determined every 2 to 4 weeks.[14] More frequent monitoring is necessary when new medications are introduced because many drugs enhance or reduce the anticoagulant effects of warfarin.

Side Effects

The major side effect of warfarin, like all anticoagulants, is bleeding. A rare complication is skin necrosis. Warfarin crosses the placenta and can cause fetal abnormalities. Consequently warfarin should be avoided during pregnancy.

Bleeding

At least half of the bleeding complications with warfarin occur when the INR exceeds the therapeutic range. Bleeding complications may be mild, such as epistaxis or hematuria, or more severe, such as retroperitoneal or gastrointestinal bleeding. Life-threatening intracranial bleeding also can occur.

To minimize the risk for bleeding, the INR should be maintained in the therapeutic range. In asymptomatic patients whose INR is between 3.5 and 4.5, warfarin should be withheld until the INR returns to the therapeutic range. If the INR is over 4.5, a therapeutic INR can be achieved more rapidly by administration of low doses of sublingual vitamin K.

Patients with serious bleeding need more aggressive treatment. These patients should be given 5 to 10 mg of vitamin K by slow intravenous infusion. Additional vitamin K should be given until the INR is in the normal range. Treatment with vitamin K should be supplemented with fresh frozen plasma as a source of the vitamin K–dependent clotting proteins. For life-threatening bleeds, or if patients cannot tolerate the volume load, prothrombin complex concentrates can be used.[14]

Warfarin-treated patients who experience bleeding when their INR is in the therapeutic range require investigation into the cause of the bleeding. Those with gastrointestinal bleeding often have underlying peptic ulcer disease or a tumor. Similarly, investigation of hematuria or uterine bleeding in patients with a therapeutic INR may unmask a tumor of the genitourinary tract.

Skin Necrosis

A rare complication of warfarin, skin necrosis usually is seen 2 to 5 days after initiation of therapy. Well-demarcated erythematous lesions form on the thighs, buttocks, breasts, or toes. Typically the center of the lesion becomes progressively necrotic. Examination of skin biopsy specimens taken from the border of these lesions reveals thrombi in the microvasculature.

Warfarin-induced skin necrosis is seen in patients with congenital or acquired deficiencies of protein C or protein S (see Chapters 128, 129, and 142). Initiation of warfarin therapy in these patients produces a precipitous fall in plasma levels of proteins C or S, thereby eliminating this important anticoagulant pathway before warfarin exerts an antithrombotic effect through lowering of the functional levels of factor X and prothrombin. The resultant procoagulant state triggers thrombosis. Why the thrombosis is localized to the microvasculature of fatty tissues is unclear.

Treatment involves discontinuation of warfarin and reversal with vitamin K, if needed. An alternative anticoagulant, such as heparin or LMWH, should be given in patients with thrombosis. Protein C concentrates or recombinant activated protein C can be given to protein C–deficient patients to accelerate healing of the skin lesions; fresh frozen plasma may be of value for those with protein S deficiency. Occasionally skin grafting is necessary when there is extensive skin loss.

Because of the potential for skin necrosis, patients with known protein C or protein S deficiency require overlapping treatment with a parenteral anticoagulant when initiating warfarin therapy. Warfarin should be started in low doses in these patients, and the parenteral anticoagulant should be continued until the INR is therapeutic for at least 2 to 3 consecutive days.

Pregnancy

Warfarin crosses the placenta and can cause fetal abnormalities or bleeding. The fetal abnormalities include a characteristic embryopathy, which consists of nasal hypoplasia and stippled epiphyses. The risk for embryopathy is highest if warfarin is given in the first trimester of pregnancy. Central nervous system abnormalities also can occur with exposure to coumarins at any time during pregnancy. Finally, maternal administration of warfarin produces an anticoagulant effect in the fetus that can cause bleeding. This is of particular concern at delivery, when trauma to the head during passage through the birth canal can lead to intracranial bleeding. Because of these potential problems, warfarin is rarely used in pregnancy, particularly in the first and third trimesters. Instead, heparin, LMWH, or fondaparinux can be given during pregnancy for prevention or treatment of thrombosis.

Warfarin does not pass into the breast milk. Consequently warfarin can safely be administered to nursing mothers.

Special Problems

Patients with a lupus anticoagulant or those who need urgent or elective surgery present special challenges. Although observational studies suggested that patients with thrombosis complicating the antiphospholipid antibody syndrome required higher-intensity warfarin regimens to prevent recurrent thromboembolic events, two randomized trials demonstrated that targeting an INR of 2.0 to 3.0 is as effective as higher-intensity treatment and produces less bleeding. Monitoring warfarin therapy can be problematic in patients with antiphospholipid antibody syndrome if the lupus anticoagulant prolongs the baseline INR (see Chapter 143).

If patients receiving long-term warfarin treatment require an elective invasive procedure, warfarin can be stopped 5 days before the procedure to allow the INR to return to normal levels. Those at high risk for recurrent thrombosis can be bridged with once- or twice-daily subcutaneous injections of LMWH when the INR falls below 2.0. The last dose of LMWH should be given 12 to 24 hours before the procedure, depending on whether LMWH is administered twice or once daily, respectively. After the procedure, warfarin can be restarted.

Dabigatran

The active moiety of dabigatran etexilate, dabigatran targets the active site of thrombin and blocks its procoagulant activities. Dabigatran inhibits both free and fibrin-bound thrombin.

Mechanism of Action

Dabigatran etexilate is a prodrug with an oral bioavailability of 6% to 7%. Once absorbed, the drug is rapidly biotransformed by esterases to dabigatran, the levels of which peak 1 to 2 hours after oral administration. Dabigatran has a half-life of 14 to 17 hours. About 80% of the drug is excreted unchanged by the kidneys. Potent P-glycoprotein inhibitors, such as ketoconazole, are contraindicated.

Dosing

For thromboprophylaxis after hip or knee replacement surgery, dabigatran is given once daily at a dose of 220 or 150 mg; a half-dose is given on the day of surgery. In patients with atrial fibrillation, dabigatran is given at a dose of 150 mg or 110 mg twice daily. A dose of 75 mg twice daily is used in the United States for patients with a creatinine clearance of 15 to 30 mL/min, whereas the 150 mg twice-daily dose is recommended for those with a creatinine clearance over 30 mL/min; the 110-mg twice-daily dose is not licensed in the United States (see Chapters 147 and 149). For treatment of venous thromboembolism, dabigatran is given at a dose of 150 mg twice daily (see Chapter 144).

Side Effects

Dabigatran can be associated with dyspepsia. Taking the drug with food often helps to alleviate this problem. Compared with warfarin, there may be a small increase in the risk for myocardial infarction with dabigatran. This increase translates into 2 additional myocardial infarcts for every 1000 patients treated. However, mortality appears to be lower with dabigatran.

There is no antidote for dabigatran. Unactivated prothrombin complex concentrates do not reverse the anticoagulant effects of dabigatran (i.e., prolongation of the aPTT or thrombin time) but attenuate dabigatran-induced bleeding in animal models. Unactivated or activated prothrombin complex concentrates or factor VIIa are reasonable choices in patients on dabigatran who have life-threatening bleeding.

Indications

In many countries, dabigatran is licensed for prophylaxis after hip or knee replacement surgery. Although not inferior to once-daily low-molecular-weight heparin for this indication, once-daily dabigatran was inferior to twice-daily low-molecular-weight heparin for thromboprophylaxis after elective knee replacement surgery.

At the 150-mg twice-daily dose, dabigatran was superior to warfarin for reduction in both hemorrhagic and ischemic stroke.[15] Rates of major and life-threatening bleeding were similar and lower, respectively, with dabigatran than with warfarin. In those over the age of 75 years, there is more gastrointestinal bleeding with this dose of dabigatran than with warfarin.[16]

When used at the 110-mg twice-daily dose, dabigatran is not inferior to warfarin for stroke prevention but is associated with significantly less intracranial and major bleeding.[15] In those over the age of 75 years, the rates of gastrointestinal bleeding with this dose of dabigatran and warfarin are similar.[16] The 75-mg twice-daily dose, which is only licensed in the United States, has not been tested in humans. However, the dose was selected because pharmacokinetic data revealed similar drug exposure in those with reduced renal function as produced by the 150-mg twice-daily dose in those with a creatinine clearance over 30 mL/min. Although drug exposure is similar, the half-life of dabigatran is prolonged to several days in those with impaired renal function.

For treatment of venous thromboembolism, dabigatran is not inferior to warfarin and is associated with reduced major plus clinically relevant nonmajor bleeding. Dabigatran is started after a 5- to 7-day course of heparin or low-molecular-weight heparin.[17]

Rivaroxaban

An oral factor Xa inhibitor, rivaroxaban is an active drug that targets the active site of factor Xa even when the enzyme is incorporated in the prothrombinase complex.

Mechanism of Action

Rivaroxaban has an oral bioavailability of 80%, and plasma levels peak 2 to 3 hours after drug administration. The terminal half-life is 7 to 11 hours, and one-third of the drug is cleared unchanged by the kidneys. The remainder is metabolized in the liver; half is cleared by the kidneys as inactive metabolites, and the rest is excreted in the feces. The pharmacokinetic and pharmacodynamic profile is dose dependent and is not influenced by age, gender, or body weight. Potent inhibitors of both P-glycoprotein and CYP3A4, such as ketoconazole or ritonavir, are contraindicated because they increase drug exposure.

Dosing

For thromboprophylaxis after hip or knee replacement surgery, rivaroxaban is given once daily at a dose of 10 mg.[18] When used for stroke prevention in atrial fibrillation, the dose is 20 mg once daily. The dose is reduced to 15 mg once daily for those with a creatinine clearance of 15 to 49 mL/min. For treatment of venous thromboembolism, rivaroxaban is started at a dose of 15 mg twice daily for 3 weeks and the dose is then reduced to 20 mg once daily thereafter. When used as an adjunct to antiplatelet therapy in stabilized patients with acute coronary syndrome, rivaroxaban is given at a dose of 2.5 mg twice daily.

Side Effects

Rivaroxaban is well tolerated and is not associated with dyspepsia or hepatic toxicity. The major side effect is bleeding. There is no specific antidote for rivaroxaban. Although prothrombin complex concentrate reverses the anticoagulant effects of rivaroxaban, its utility for treatment of bleeding is uncertain. Nonetheless, unactivated or activated prothrombin complex concentrate or factor VIIa should be considered in patients with life-threatening bleeding.

Indications

When used for thromboprophylaxis after hip or knee replacement surgery, the risk for major bleeding is similar to that with low-molecular-weight heparin.[18] Compared with warfarin for stroke prevention in atrial fibrillation, rivaroxaban is associated with less intracranial bleeding and hemorrhagic stroke, but similar rates of major bleeding (see Chapters 147 and 149).[19] In patients with acute venous thromboembolism, rivaroxaban is as effective as conventional anticoagulant therapy but is associated with less major bleeding (see Chapter 144).[20,21] When compared with placebo as an adjunct to antiplatelet therapy in stabilized patients with acute coronary syndromes, rivaroxaban (at a dose of 2.5 mg twice daily) reduced the primary efficacy end point—the composite of cardiovascular death, myocardial infarction, and stroke—from 10.7% to 9.1%.[22] There was more bleeding with rivaroxaban, including intracranial bleeding, but there was no increase in fatal bleeding.

Current licensed indications for rivaroxaban include (1) thromboprophylaxis after hip or knee replacement surgery, situations in which the drug is usually given for 2 and 4 weeks, respectively, and (2) as an alternative to warfarin for stroke prevention in atrial fibrillation. The drug also is licensed in some countries for treatment of deep venous thrombosis and is under consideration for treatment of pulmonary embolism and for secondary prevention in stabilized patients with acute coronary syndromes.

Apixaban

Another oral factor Xa inhibitor, apixaban is licensed in many countries, but not the United States, for thromboprophylaxis after hip or knee replacement surgery. It is under consideration for licensing as an alternative to aspirin or warfarin for stroke prevention in atrial fibrillation.

Mechanism of Action

Like rivaroxaban, apixaban targets the active site of free factor Xa or factor Xa incorporated in the prothrombinase complex. The drug has about 50% oral bioavailability, and plasma levels peak 3 to 4 hours after drug administration. The half-life of apixaban is 8 to 14 hours. Apixaban is metabolized in the liver via CYP3A4/5-dependent and independent pathways. About 25% of the drug is cleared unchanged by the kidneys, and the remainder is excreted in the feces. Potent inhibitors of CYP3A4/5 and P-glycoprotein increase drug exposure and should be avoided.

Dosing

Apixaban is given twice daily at a dose of 2.5 mg for thromboprophylaxis after hip or knee replacement surgery and at 5 mg for stroke prevention in patients with atrial fibrillation. For the latter indication, the dose is reduced to 2.5 mg twice daily in patients with impaired renal function.

Side Effects

Apixaban has excellent tolerability, and the rate of discontinuation due to adverse events is similar to or lower than that with aspirin. The drug does not cause dyspepsia and is not associated with hepatic toxicity. The major side effect is bleeding. Like the situation with dabigatran and rivaroxaban, there is no specific antidote for apixaban. Unactivated or activated prothrombin complex concentrates or factor VIIa may be of benefit in patients with life-threatening bleeding.

Indications

Although not licensed in the United States, apixaban is licensed in many countries for thromboprophylaxis after hip or knee replacement surgery. The drug is under consideration for licensing as an alternative to aspirin or warfarin for stroke prevention in patients with atrial fibrillation.

For thromboprophylaxis after hip or knee replacement surgery, apixaban has efficacy and safety similar to those of low-molecular-weight heparin.[23-25] Apixaban was superior to aspirin for stroke prevention in atrial fibrillation patients unwilling or unable to take warfarin and did not significantly increase the risk for bleeding.[26] When compared with warfarin for stroke prevention in patients with atrial fibrillation, apixaban produced a greater reduction in hemorrhagic stroke, but not ischemic stroke, and was associated with less major bleeding and lower all-cause mortality.[27]

Other New Oral Anticoagulants

Edoxaban and betrixaban are other oral factor Xa inhibitors under development. Edoxaban is being evaluated as an alternative to warfarin for stroke prevention in atrial fibrillation and for treatment of venous thromboembolism. Betrixaban has entered phase III evaluation for thromboprophylaxis in medically ill patients where it is being compared with low-molecular-weight heparin.

FIBRINOLYTIC DRUGS

Role of Fibrinolytic Therapy

Used to degrade thrombi, fibrinolytic drugs can be administered systemically, or they can be delivered via catheters directly into the substance of the thrombus (see Chapter 145). Systemic delivery is used for treatment of acute myocardial infarction (see Chapter 148), acute ischemic stroke (see Chapter 147), and most cases of massive pulmonary embolism (see Chapter 144). The goal of therapy is to produce rapid thrombus dissolution, thereby restoring antegrade blood flow. In the coronary circulation, restoration of blood flow reduces morbidity and mortality by limiting myocardial damage, whereas in the cerebral circulation, rapid thrombus dissolution decreases the neuronal death and brain infarction that produce irreversible brain injury. For patients with massive pulmonary embolism, the goal of fibrinolytic therapy is to restore pulmonary artery perfusion.

Peripheral arterial thrombi and thrombi in the proximal deep veins of the leg are most often treated using a catheter-directed approach. Catheters with multiple side holes can be used to deliver fibrinolytic drugs. In some cases, intravascular devices that fragment and extract the thrombus are used to hasten treatment (see Chapter 145).

Mechanism of Action

Commonly used fibrinolytic agents include streptokinase, recombinant tissue plasminogen activator (rt-PA), which is also known as *alteplase* (Activase), and two recombinant derivatives of rt-PA, tenecteplase and reteplase. All of these agents act by converting the proenzyme, plasminogen, to plasmin, the active enzyme (Fig. 151-8). Plasmin then degrades the fibrin matrix of thrombi, thereby producing soluble fibrin degradation products.

Endogenous fibrinolysis is regulated at two levels. Plasminogen activator inhibitors, particularly the type 1 form, known as PAI-1, prevent excessive plasminogen activation by regulating the activity of t-PA and urokinase plasminogen activator (uPA). Once plasmin is generated, it is regulated by plasmin inhibitors, the most important of which is α_2-antiplasmin. The plasma concentration of plasminogen is twofold higher than that of α_2-antiplasmin. Consequently with pharmacologic doses of plasminogen activators, the concentration of plasmin that is generated can exceed that of α_2-antiplasmin. In addition to degrading fibrin, unregulated plasmin also can degrade fibrinogen and other clotting factors. This process, which is known as the systemic lytic state, reduces the hemostatic potential of the blood and increases the risk for bleeding.

The endogenous fibrinolytic system is geared to localize plasmin generation to the fibrin surface. Both plasminogen and t-PA bind to fibrin to form a ternary complex that promotes efficient plasminogen activation. In contrast to free plasmin, plasmin generated on the fibrin surface is relatively protected from inactivation by α_2-antiplasmin, a feature that promotes fibrin dissolution. Furthermore, C-terminal lysine residues exposed as plasmin degrades fibrin serve as binding sites for additional plasminogen and t-PA molecules. This creates a positive feedback that enhances plasmin generation. When used pharmacologically, the various plasminogen activators capitalize on these mechanisms to a lesser or greater extent.

There are two pools of plasminogen: circulating plasminogen and fibrin-bound plasminogen (Fig. 151-9). Plasminogen activators that preferentially activate fibrin-bound plasminogen are considered fibrin specific. In contrast, nonspecific plasminogen activators do not discriminate between fibrin-bound and circulating plasminogen. Activation of circulating plasminogen results in the generation of unopposed plasmin that can trigger the systemic lytic state. Alteplase and its derivatives are fibrin-specific plasminogen activators, whereas streptokinase is a nonspecific agent.

Streptokinase

Unlike other plasminogen activators, streptokinase is not an enzyme and does not directly convert plasminogen to plasmin. Instead, streptokinase forms a 1 : 1 stoichiometric complex with plasminogen. Formation of this complex induces a conformational change in

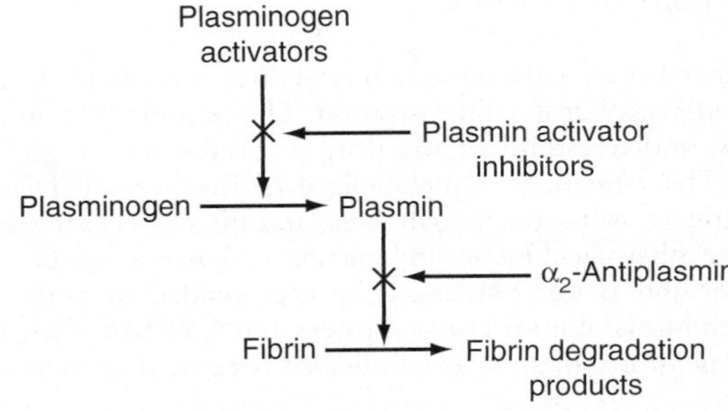

Figure 151-8 FIBRINOLYTIC SYSTEM AND ITS REGULATION. Plasminogen activators convert plasminogen to plasmin. Plasmin then degrades fibrin into soluble fibrin degradation products. The system is regulated at two levels. Type 1 plasminogen activator inhibitor (PAI-1) regulates the plasminogen activators, whereas α_2-antiplasmin serves as the major inhibitor of plasmin.

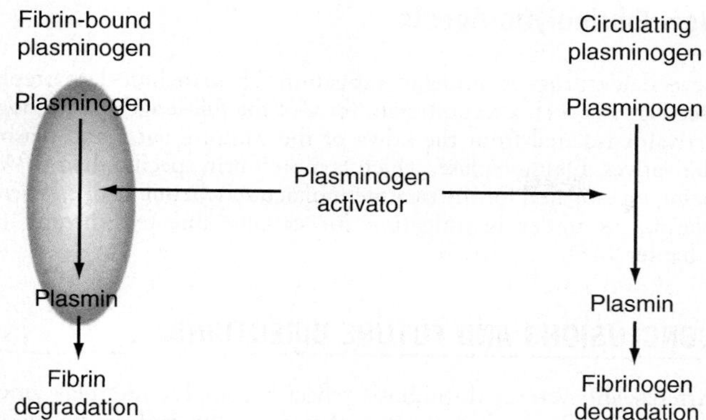

Figure 151-9 CONSEQUENCES OF ACTIVATION OF FIBRIN-BOUND OR CIRCULATING PLASMINOGEN. The fibrin specificity of plasminogen activators reflects their capacity to distinguish between fibrin-bound and circulating plasminogen. This, in turn, reflects their affinity for fibrin. Plasminogen activators with high affinity for fibrin preferentially activate fibrin-bound plasminogen. This results in the generation of plasmin on the fibrin surface. Fibrin-bound plasmin, which is protected from inactivation by α_2-antiplasmin, degrades fibrin to yield soluble fibrin degradation products. In contrast, plasminogen activators with little or no affinity for fibrin do not distinguish between fibrin-bound and circulating plasminogen. Activation of circulating plasminogen results in systemic plasminemia and subsequent degradation of fibrinogen and other clotting factors.

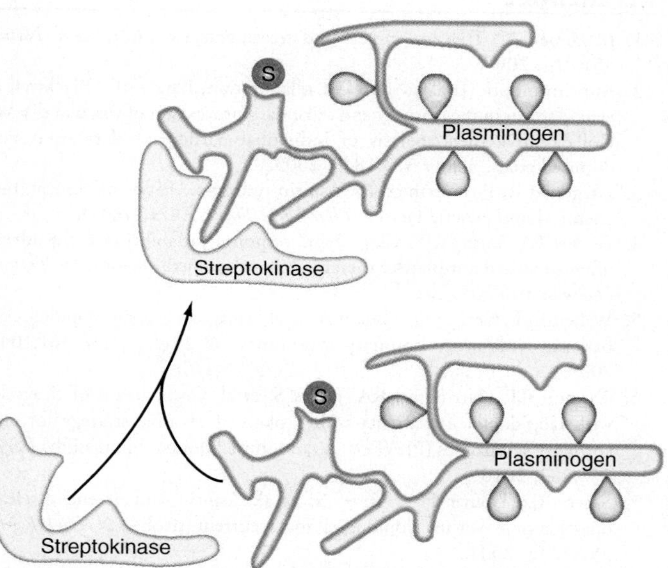

Figure 151-10 MECHANISM OF ACTION OF STREPTOKINASE. Streptokinase binds to plasminogen and induces a conformational change in plasminogen that exposes its active site serine (S). The streptokinase/plasmin(ogen) complex then serves as the activator of additional plasminogen molecules.

plasminogen that exposes its active site (Fig. 151-10). This conformationally altered plasminogen then converts additional plasminogen molecules to plasmin.

Streptokinase has no affinity for fibrin, and the streptokinase-plasminogen complex activates both free and fibrin-bound plasminogen. Activation of circulating plasminogen generates sufficient amounts of plasmin to overwhelm α_2-antiplasmin. Unopposed plasmin not only degrades fibrin in the occlusive thrombus but also induces a systemic lytic state.

When given systemically to patients with acute myocardial infarction, streptokinase reduces mortality. For this indication the drug is usually given as an intravenous infusion of 1.5 million units over 30

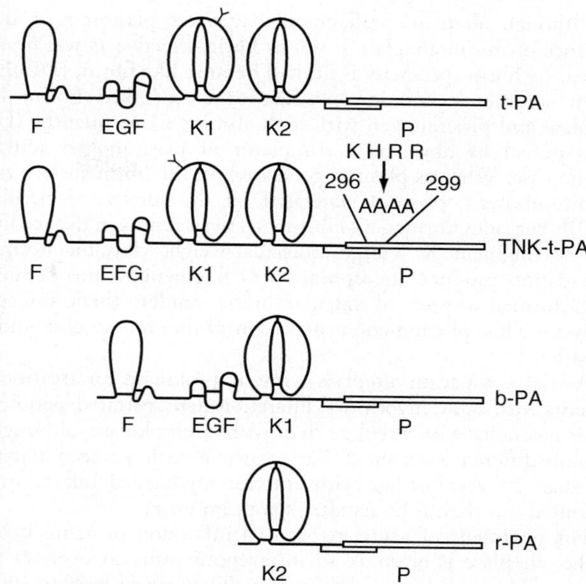

Figure 151-11 DOMAIN STRUCTURES OF ALTEPLASE (t-PA), TENECTEPLASE (TNK-t-PA), DESMOTEPLASE (b-PA), AND RETEPLASE (r-PA). The finger (F), epidermal growth factor (EGF), first and second kringles (K1 and K2, respectively), and protease (P) domains are illustrated. The glycosylation site (Y) on K1 has been repositioned in tenecteplase to endow it with a longer half-life. In addition, a tetraalanine substitution in the protease domain renders tenecteplase resistant to PAI-1 inhibition. Desmoteplase differs from alteplase and tenecteplase in that it lacks a K2 domain. Reteplase is a truncated variant that lacks the F, EGF, and K1 domains.

to 60 minutes. Patients who receive streptokinase can develop antibodies against the drug as can patients with prior streptococcal injection. These antibodies can reduce the effectiveness of streptokinase.

Allergic reactions occur in about 5% of patients treated with streptokinase. These may manifest as a rash, fever, chills, and rigors. Although anaphylactic reactions can occur, these are rare. Transient hypotension is common with streptokinase and has been attributed to plasmin-mediated release of bradykinin from kallikrein. The hypotension usually responds to leg elevation and administration of intravenous fluids and low-doses of vasopressors, such as dopamine or norepinephrine.

Alteplase

A recombinant form of single-chain t-PA, alteplase has a molecular weight of 68,000. Alteplase is rapidly converted into its two-chain form by plasmin. Although single- and two-chain forms of t-PA have equivalent activity in the presence of fibrin, in its absence, single-chain t-PA has 10-fold lower activity.

Alteplase consists of five discrete domains (Fig. 151-11). The N-terminal A-chain of two-chain alteplase contains four of these domains. Residues 4 to 50 make up the finger domain, a region that resembles the finger domain of fibronectin; residues 50 to 87 are homologous with epidermal growth factor; whereas residues 92 to 173 and 180 to 261, which have homology to the kringle domains of plasminogen, are designated as the first and second kringle, respectively. The fifth alteplase domain is the protease domain; it is located on the C-terminal B-chain of two-chain alteplase.

The interaction of alteplase with fibrin is mediated by the finger domain, and to a lesser extent by the second kringle domain. The affinity of alteplase for fibrin is considerably higher than that for fibrinogen. Consequently the catalytic efficiency of plasminogen activation by alteplase is two to three orders of magnitude higher in the presence of fibrin than in the presence of fibrinogen. This phenomenon helps to localize plasmin generation to the fibrin surface.

Although alteplase preferentially activates plasminogen in the presence of fibrin, alteplase is not as fibrin-selective as was first predicted. Its fibrin specificity is limited because like fibrin, (DD)E, the major soluble degradation product of cross-linked fibrin, binds alteplase and plasminogen with high affinity. Consequently, (DD)E is as potent as fibrin as a stimulator of plasminogen activation by alteplase. Whereas plasmin generated on the fibrin surface results in thrombolysis, plasmin generated on the surface of circulating (DD)E degrades fibrinogen. Fibrinogenolysis results in the accumulation of fragment X, a high-molecular-weight clottable fibrinogen degradation product. Incorporation of fragment X into hemostatic plugs formed at sites of vascular injury renders them susceptible to lysis. This phenomenon may contribute to alteplase-induced bleeding.

A trial comparing alteplase with streptokinase for treatment of patients with acute myocardial infarction demonstrated significantly lower mortality with alteplase than with streptokinase, although the absolute difference was small. The greatest benefit was seen in patients less than 75 years of age with anterior myocardial infarction who presented less than 6 hours after symptom onset.

For treatment of acute myocardial infarction or acute ischemic stroke, alteplase is given as an intravenous infusion over 60 to 90 minutes. The total dose of alteplase usually ranges from 90 to 100 mg. Allergic reactions and hypotension are rare, and alteplase is not immunogenic.

Tenecteplase

A genetically engineered variant of t-PA, tenecteplase was designed to have a longer half-life than t-PA and to be resistant to inactivation by PAI-1. To prolong its half-life, a new glycosylation site was added to the first kringle domain (see Fig. 151-11). Because addition of this extra carbohydrate side chain reduced fibrin affinity, the existing glycosylation site on the first kringle domain was removed. To render the molecule resistant to inhibition by PAI-1, a tetraalanine substitution was introduced at residues 296 to 299 in the protease domain, the region responsible for the interaction of t-PA with PAI-1.

Tenecteplase is more fibrin specific than t-PA. Although both agents bind to fibrin with similar affinity, the affinity of tenecteplase for (DD)E is significantly lower than that of t-PA. Consequently (DD)E does not stimulate systemic plasminogen activation by tenecteplase to the same extent as t-PA. As a result, tenecteplase produces less fibrinogenolysis than t-PA.

For coronary fibrinolysis, tenecteplase is given as a single intravenous bolus. In a large phase III trial that enrolled almost 17,000 patients, the 30-day mortality rate with single-bolus tenecteplase was similar to that with accelerated dose t-PA.[28] Although rates of intracranial hemorrhage also were similar with both treatments, patients given tenecteplase had fewer noncerebral bleeds and a reduced need for blood transfusions than those treated with t-PA. The improved safety profile of tenecteplase likely reflects its enhanced fibrin specificity. These properties have prompted its recent compression with alteplase in patients with acute ischemic stroke.[29]

Reteplase

A recombinant t-PA derivative, reteplase is a single-chain variant that lacks the finger, epidermal growth factor, and first kringle domains (see Fig. 151-11). This truncated derivative has a molecular weight of 39,000. Reteplase binds fibrin more weakly than t-PA because it lacks the finger domain. Because it is produced in *Escherichia coli,* reteplase is not glycosylated. This endows it with a plasma half-life longer than that of t-PA. Consequently reteplase is given as two intravenous boluses, which are separated by 30 minutes. Clinical trials have demonstrated that reteplase is at least as effective as streptokinase for treatment of acute myocardial infarction, but the agent is not superior to t-PA.[29]

New Fibrinolytic Agents

Several new drugs are under investigation. These include desmoteplase (see Fig. 151-11), a recombinant form of the full-length plasminogen activator isolated from the saliva of the vampire bat,[30] and plasmin derivatives. Desmoteplase, which is more fibrin specific than t-PA, is being investigated for the treatment of acute ischemic stroke, whereas plasmin is under investigation for catheter-directed therapy (see Chapter 145).

CONCLUSIONS AND FUTURE DIRECTIONS

Arterial and venous thrombosis reflect a complex interplay among the vessel wall, platelets, the coagulation system, and the fibrinolytic pathways. Activation of coagulation also triggers inflammatory pathways that may contribute to thrombogenesis. A better understanding of the biochemistry of blood coagulation and advances in structure-based drug design have identified new targets and resulted in the development of novel antithrombotic drugs. Well-designed clinical trials have provided detailed information on which drugs to use and when to use them. Despite these advances, however, arterial and venous thromboembolic disorders remain a major cause of morbidity and mortality. Therefore the search for better targets and more potent or more convenient antiplatelet, anticoagulant, and fibrinolytic drugs continues.

REFERENCES

1. Mackman N: Triggers, targets and treatments for thrombosis. *Nature* 451:914, 2008.
2. Antithrombotic Trialists' (ATT) Collaboration, Baigent C, Blackwell L, et al: Aspirin in the primary and secondary prevention of vascular disease: Collaborative meta-analysis of individual participant data from randomised trials. *Lancet* 373:1849, 2009.
3. Fitzgerald R, Pirmohamed M: Aspirin resistance: Effect of clinical, biochemical and genetic factors. *Pharmacol Ther* 130:213, 2011.
4. Gurbel PA, Tantry US: Clopidogrel response variability and the advent of personalized antiplatelet therapy. A bench to bedside journey. *Thromb Haemost* 106:265, 2011.
5. Wallentin L, Becker RC, Budaj A, et al: Ticagrelor versus clopidogrel in patients with acute coronary syndromes. *N Engl J Med* 361:1045, 2009.
6. Cannon CP, Harrington RA, James S, et al: Comparison of ticagrelor with clopidogrel in patients with a planned invasive strategy for cute coronary syndromes (PLATO): A randomised double-blind study. *Lancet* 375:283, 2010.
7. Sacco RL, Diener HC, Yusuf S, et al: Aspirin and extended-release dipyridamole versus clopidogrel for recurrent stroke. *N Engl J Med* 359:1238, 2008.
8. Tricoci P, Huang Z, Held C, et al: Thrombin-receptor antagonist vorapaxar in acute coronary syndromes. *N Engl J Med* 366:20, 2012.
9. Morrow DA, Braunwald E, Bonaca MP, et al: Vorapaxar in the secondary prevention of atherothrombotic events. *N Engl J Med* 366:1404, 2012.
10. Eikelboom JW, Weitz JI: New anticoagulants. *Circulation* 121:1523, 2010.
11. Cuker A, Cines DB: How I treat heparin-induced thrombocytopenia *Blood* 119:2209, 2012.
12. Fifth Organization to Assess Strategies in Acute Ischemic Syndromes Investigators, Yusuf S, Mehta SR, et al: Comparison of fondaparinux and enoxaparin in acute coronary syndromes. *N Engl J Med* 354:1464, 2006.
13. Manolopoulos VG, Ragia G, Tavridou A: Pharmacogenetics of coumarinic oral anticoagulants. *Pharmacogenomics* 11:493, 2010.
14. Ageno W, Gallus AS, Wittkowsky A, et al: Oral anticoagulant therapy: Antithrombotic Therapy and Prevention of Thrombosis, 9th ed: American College of Chest Physicians Evidence-based Clinical Practice Guidelines. *Chest* 141:44S, 2012.
15. Connolly SJ, Ezekowitz MD, Yusuf S, et al: Dabigatran versus warfarin in patients with atrial fibrillation. *N Engl J Med* 361:1139, 2009.

16. Eikelboom JW, Wallentin L, Connolly SJ, et al: Risk of bleeding with 2 doses of dabigatran compared with warfarin in older and younger patients with atrial fibrillation: An analysis of the randomized evaluation of long-term anticoagulant therapy (RE-LY) trial. *Circulation* 123:2363, 2011.
17. Schulman S, Kearon C, Kakkar AK, et al: Dabigatran versus warfarin in the treatment of acute venous thromboembolism. *N Engl J Med* 361:2342, 2009.
18. Duggan ST, Scott LJ, Plosker GL: Rivaroxaban: A review of its use for the prevention of venous thromboembolism after total hip or knee replacement surgery. *Drugs* 69:1829, 2009.
19. Patel MR, Mahaffey KW, Garg J, et al: Rivaroxaban versus warfarin in nonvalvular atrial fibrillation. *N Engl J Med* 365:883, 2011.
20. EINSTEIN Investigators, Bauersachs R, Berkowitz SD, et al: Oral rivaroxaban for symptomatic venous thromboembolism. *N Engl J Med* 363:2499, 2010.
21. EINSTEIN-PE Investigators, Buller HR, Prins MH, et al: Oral rivaroxaban for the treatment of symptomatic pulmonary embolism. *N Engl J Med* 366:1287, 2012.
22. Mega JL, Braunwald E, Wiviott SD, et al: Rivaroxaban in patients with a recent acute coronary syndrome. *N Engl J Med* 366:9, 2012.
23. Lassen MR, Raskob GE, Gallus A, et al: Apixaban or enoxaparin for thromboprophylaxis after knee replacement. *N Engl J Med* 361:594, 2009.
24. Lassen MR, Raskob GE, Gallus A, et al: Apixaban versus enoxaparin for thromboprophylaxis after knee replacement (ADVANCE-2): A randomised double-blind trial. *Lancet* 375:807, 2010.
25. Lassen MR, Gallus A, Raskob GE, et al: Apixaban versus enoxaparin for thromboprophylaxis after hip replacement. *N Engl J Med* 363:2487, 2010.
26. Connolly SJ, Eikelboom J, Joyner C, et al: Apixaban in patients with atrial fibrillation. *N Engl J Med* 364:906, 2011.
27. Granger CB, Alenander JH, McMurray JJ, et al: Apixaban versus warfarin in patients with atrial fibrillation. *N Engl J Med* 365:981, 2011.
28. Assessment of the Safety and Efficacy of a New Thrombolytic (ASSENT-2) Investigators, Van De Werf F, Adgey J, et al: Single-bolus tenecteplase compared with front-loaded alteplase in acute myocardial infarction: The ASSENT-2 double-blind randomised trial. *Lancet* 354:716, 1999.
29. Parsons M, Spratt N, Bivard A, et al: A randomized trial of tenecteplase versus alteplase for acute ischemic stroke. *N Engl J Med* 366:1099, 2012.
30. Medcalf RL: Desmoteplase: Discovery, insights and opportunities for ischaemic stroke. *Br J Pharmacol* 165:75, 2012.

CHAPTER 152

DISORDERS OF COAGULATION IN THE NEONATE

Christine A. Macartney, Nethnapha Paredes, and Anthony K.C. Chan

The neonatal stage is a period of rapid physiologic changes, some of which affect the hemostatic system. The hemostatic system is a dynamic system that evolves gradually from birth into the mature adult form. Evaluation of disorders of coagulation in the neonate requires an understanding of the evolution of physiologic normal values for age, the congenital disorders that present in early life, and the clinical settings common in neonatology that affect hemostasis and thrombosis risks. The rapid evolution of the blood coagulation system after birth leads to a dynamic group of age-dependent reference ranges for the levels of the various components that should be considered physiologically normal. *Developmental hemostasis* is the term applied to the evolution of the hemostatic and fibrinolytic systems through infancy and childhood.

DEVELOPMENTAL HEMOSTASIS

The coagulation system in children provides innate protection from thrombosis without an increased risk for bleeding. The hemostatic system evolves throughout childhood and most rapidly during the neonatal period. Changes in the plasma concentrations of proteins involved in blood coagulation lead to a dynamic group of reference ranges for preterm and term infants. Although different from adult values, these reference ranges are neither abnormal nor pathologic. The relative rarity of hemorrhagic or thrombotic complications in this population argues that the neonatal coagulation system is physiologically replete.

Laboratory Evaluation

The pioneering work of the late Dr. Maureen Andrew paved the way for research into pediatric hemostasis. The concept of developmental hemostasis is now widely accepted, and her seminal papers describing the reference ranges for healthy premature and full-term neonates are still widely quoted.[1,2] Laboratory evaluation of thrombosis or bleeding in neonates must take into account the age-related reference ranges for healthy newborns, which differ significantly from adult levels. Thus prior publications of defined reference ranges for neonates may not be relevant because coagulation assay results vary depending on the type of analyzer and reagents used.[3] Each laboratory that performs coagulation tests on neonatal samples must therefore develop their own age-related reference ranges specific to their analyzer and reagent combination in order to effectively diagnose and manage neonates with suspected hemostatic abnormalities. Neonatal samples should be drawn by experienced staff. Samples are processed in 1-mL tubes containing 0.1 mL of 3.2% buffered sodium citrate, aiming for a final ratio of one part citrate to nine parts blood.

Functional assays are predominantly used in pediatric studies. Although the absolute values are reagent- and analyzer-specific, the changes in functional protein levels lead to corresponding changes in global tests of coagulation. The prothrombin time (PT), expressed in seconds, in full-term neonates is similar to that in adults, despite the fact that neonates have relative deficiencies of the vitamin K–dependent coagulation factors. However, samples from premature infants and cord blood exhibit a prolonged PT compared with adults.[1] The activated partial thromboplastin time (aPTT) is prolonged in newborns, which is attributed to relative deficiencies in the contact factors. Other tests, such as the thrombin time (TT) and thromboelastography, are less sensitive to age-related changes. The TT in neonates is similar to that in adults when measured in the presence of calcium, which compensates for the unique fetal form of fibrinogen that has increased sialic acid content. Thromboelastography values vary very little with age. The template bleeding time is reported to be normal in neonates, but this is an unreliable test in neonatology and is not recommended for bleeding evaluations. Investigations into neonatal hemostatic pathology are limited by the lack of normal reference values for the neonatal population and the difficulties associated with obtaining clean blood samples for testing.

Blood Coagulation Proteins

The synthesis of fetal and neonatal coagulation proteins begins at approximately 10 weeks of gestation, and plasma concentrations of these proteins increase with gestational age. Maternal coagulation proteins cannot cross the placenta. However, maternal drug intake can affect the synthesis of fetal vitamin K–dependent coagulation proteins, with warfarin, phenytoin, barbiturates, and antibiotics serving as examples.

In the healthy newborn, plasma levels of procoagulant factors such as thrombin, factor (F)VII, FIX, FX, and prothrombin (the vitamin K–dependent coagulation factors) and FXI, FXII, prekallikrein, and high-molecular-weight kininogen (the contact factors) are about 50% lower than adult values (Table 152-1).[1,2] The levels rise as the infant ages, and they reach about 80% of normal adult values by 6 months of age but remain decreased throughout childhood.[4] The levels of fibrinogen, FV, FVIII, and FXIII in neonates are similar to those in adults and remain so throughout childhood.[2,4] The levels of von Willebrand factor (vWF) in newborns are about twofold higher than adult values and gradually decrease over the first 6 months of life,[2] whereas the levels of antithrombin (AT) are lower than adult levels in the first 3 months of life and are comparable to the levels seen in patients with heterozygous AT deficiency. The physiologic ranges for coagulation factors in healthy newborns who have received intramuscular vitamin K after delivery are shown in Table 152-2.

Regulation of Thrombin

Despite decreased and delayed thrombin generation, neonates have excellent hemostasis. Thrombin regulation in neonatal plasma is similar to that in plasma from adults who are receiving therapeutic doses of anticoagulants. The concentration of thrombin generated in neonatal plasma is proportional to the available prothrombin concentration, whereas the rate of thrombin generation depends on the level of other procoagulant proteins. Neonatal fibrin clots bind less thrombin than clots formed in adult plasma, in part because of lower levels of thrombin generation. Reduced thrombin generation and less fibrin-bound thrombin may protect neonates from thrombosis.

Table 152-1 Neonatal Versus Adult Hemostasis

Component	Neonatal Versus Adult Level	
Primary hemostasis	↔	Platelet count
	↑	vWF
Coagulation factors	↓	FII, FVII, FIX, FX
	↓	FXI, FXII
	↓ to ↔	FV, FXIII
	↔	Fibrinogen
	↑	FVIII
Anticoagulant factors	↓	TFPI, AT, PC, PS
	↑	α_2M
Fibrinolysis	↓	Plasminogen
	↔ to ↑	PAI

Modified from Guzzetta NA, Miller BE: Principles of hemostasis in children: Models and maturation. *Paediatr Anaesth* 21:3, 2011.
α_2M, α_2-Macroglobulin; *AT,* antithrombin; *F,* factor; *PAI,* plasminogen activator inhibitor; *PC,* protein C; *PS,* protein S; *TFPI,* tissue factor pathway inhibitor; *vWF,* von Willebrand factor.

Thrombin is inhibited by α_2-macroglobulin, AT, and heparin cofactor II. In neonates the α_2-macroglobulin concentration is twofold higher than that in adults. The overall capacity of newborn plasma to inhibit thrombin is similar to that of adult plasma due in part to the increased binding of thrombin by α_2-macroglobulin. Thrombin inhibition by heparin cofactor II is catalyzed by a dermatan sulfate–like proteoglycan, which is produced by the placenta and is found in both the maternal and the fetal plasma.

Regulation of thrombin generation is accomplished by upstream inhibition of the clotting proteins in the prothrombinase and tenase complexes (see Chapters 128 and 129). Plasma concentrations of protein C are low at birth and gradually increase to adult levels by 6 months of age. Although the total concentration of protein S is low at birth, the functional activity of protein S is comparable to that in adults because low levels of C4b-binding protein result in more free protein S. The interaction of protein S with activated protein C in neonatal plasma may be limited by the elevated levels of α_2-macroglobulin. Free tissue factor pathway inhibitor levels are lower than in adults, despite total tissue factor pathway inhibitor levels being similar in neonatal and adult plasma.

The Fibrinolytic System

Although the levels of some of the components of the fibrinolytic system in neonates are different from those in adults, the clinical relevance of this finding is probably minimal. The fibrinolytic system regulates fibrin deposition by generating plasmin, which solubilizes fibrin. At birth the fibrinolytic system has all the key components, but there are important age-related differences in the quantity and quality of the fibrinolytic proteins and enzymes. Plasma concentrations of plasminogen, tissue plasminogen activator (tPA), and α_2-antiplasmin (α_2AP) are decreased, whereas plasma concentrations of plasminogen activator inhibitor 1 (PAI-1) are increased. As well, plasmin generation and overall fibrinolytic activity are decreased.[5] The capacity to generate plasmin in newborn plasma is generally reduced compared with adult plasma, which likely reflects the decreased plasminogen concentration. Despite lower levels of fibrinolytic components, the newborn fibrinolytic system is still effective.

The whole-blood clotting time and euglobulin clot lysis time are global assays of fibrinolytic activity but reflect only part of the physiologic fibrinolytic potential. Maneuvers that induce the release of endogenous fibrinolytic components, such as venous occlusion, desmopressin infusion, or exercise, provide more sensitive measures in vivo fibrinolytic activity.[5]

Plasminogen levels are lower in neonates than in adults, and fetal plasminogen binds to cellular receptors with lower affinity because of its increased sialic acid and mannose content. Whereas healthy neonates have lower plasmin-generating potential than adults, baseline levels of tPA can increase up to eightfold with illness. Neonates with severe plasminogen deficiency have only a minimal increased risk for thrombosis, and most of their clinical findings are the result of impaired extravascular fibrinolysis. The major plasmin inhibitors circulate at near adult levels in the neonate.

Imbalance in the fibrinolytic system, whether hereditary or acquired, can lead to thrombotic or bleeding complications. Hereditary disorders, although rare, include plasminogen deficiency, PAI-1 deficiency, and α_2AP deficiency. The efficacy and safety of fibrinolytic therapy may be influenced by age-dependent differences in the fibrinolytic system. Data are lacking on the optimal doses of fibrinolytic agents for the pediatric population, especially for neonates. The contribution of differences between the neonatal and adult fibrinolytic systems to the protection from thromboembolic complications in childhood remains to be elucidated.

Platelets

The platelet count and mean platelet volume in neonates are similar to those in adults as is platelet ultrastructure. Neonatal platelets exhibit reduced phospholipid metabolism, calcium mobilization, granule secretion, and aggregation in response to agonists compared with adult platelets.[6] Although thrombocytopenia is common in neonates, thrombocytosis is rare and is associated with prematurity.

Platelet function is reduced at birth, which may reflect the platelet activation and degranulation that occurs during labor and delivery. Flow cytometric studies using monoclonal antibodies directed against platelet activation markers indicate that platelets from cord blood or from neonates on the first postnatal day are hyporeactive compared with adult platelets.[6] This hyporesponsiveness is transient, and the platelets regain normal reactivity 10 to 14 days after delivery.

Despite the reduced platelet reactivity at birth, platelet adhesion may be enhanced because of the presence of higher-molecular-weight vWF multimers in the plasma. Consistent with this concept, the bleeding time and the platelet function analyzer (PFA-100) closure time are shorter in neonates than adults.[6] In healthy neonates, enhanced platelet adhesion immediately after delivery may compensate for the reduced platelet activation in response to agonists. Nonetheless, sick neonates may be at an increased risk for bleeding.[6]

If available, the PFA-100 closure time is preferred over the bleeding time as a means of assessing platelet-related hemostasis. Bleeding times are variable in neonates as they are in adults. Consequently the bleeding time is rarely determined. Although the PFA-100 will not detect mild defects in platelet function, such defects rarely cause serious bleeding in neonates.

The Vessel Wall

Studies in vitro and in neonatal animals suggest that the endothelium from neonates has greater antithrombotic potential than endothelium from adult vessels. In both rabbit venous and aortic models, neonatal endothelium expresses more heparan sulfate proteoglycan than adult endothelium, which results in greater AT-mediated anticoagulant activity in rabbit pups compared with adults. Circulating levels of endothelial cell adhesion markers vary with age, implying dynamic expression and/or secretion of these proteins as a function of age.

NEONATAL HEMORRHAGIC DISORDERS

Significant bleeding in neonates should prompt clinical evaluation. In sick infants, acquired factor deficiencies or thrombocytopenia are frequently to blame, but rare congenital factor deficiencies can also manifest with neonatal bleeding. Attention to maternal factors (e.g.,

Table 152-2 Reference Values (Ranges) for Common Coagulation Tests and Blood Coagulation Protein Levels by Age, Comparing Two Comprehensive Prospective Studies With Different Methodologies

	Day 1		Day 3 (Ref 3) Versus Day 5 (Ref 2)		1 Month to 1 Year		Adult (Measured)	
	Ref 3	***Ref 2***	***Ref 3***	***Ref 2***	***Ref 3***	***Ref 2***	***Ref 3***	***Ref 2***
Prothrombin time (sec)	15.6 (14.4-16.4)	13 (11.6-14.4)	14.9 (13.5-16.4)	12.4 (10.5-13.9)	13.1 (11.5-15.3)	12.3 (10.7-13.9)	13 (11.5-14.5)	12 (11-14)
PTT (sec)	38.7 (34.3-44.8)	42.9 (31.3-54.5)	36.3 (29.5-42.2)	42.6 (25.4-59.8)	39.3 (35.1-46.3)	35.5 (28.1-42.9)	33.2 (28.6-38.2)	33 (27-40)
Thrombin time (sec)	N/A	23.5 (19-28.3)	N/A	23.1 (18-29.2)	17.1 (16.3-17.6)	24.3 (19.4-29.2)	16.6 (16.2-17.2)	N/A
Fibrinogen (mg/dL)	280 (192-374)	283 (225-341)	330 (283-401)	312 (237-387)	242 (82-383)	251 (150-387)	310 (190-430)	278 (156-400)
Prothrombin (%)	54 (41-69)	48 (37-59)	62 (50-73)	63 (48-78)	90 (62-103)	88 (60-116)	110 (78-138)	108 (70-146)
Factor V (%)	81 (64-103)	72 (54-90)	122 (92-154)	95 (70-120)	113 (94-141)	91 (55-127)	118 (78-152)	106 (62-150)
Factor VII (%)	70 (52-88)	66 (47-85)	86 (67-107)	89 (62-116)	128 (83-160)	87 (47-127)	129 (61-199)	105 (67-143)
Factor VIII (%)	182 (105-329)	100 (61-139)	159 (83-274)	88 (55-121)	94 (54-145)	73 (53-109)	160 (52-290)	99 (50-149)
Factor IX (%)	48 (35-56)	53 (34-72)	72 (44-97)	53 (34-72)	71 (43-121)	86 (36-139)	130 (59-254)	109 (55-163)
Factor X (%)	55 (46-67)	40 (26-54)	60 (46-75)	49 (34-64)	95 (77-122)	78 (38-118)	124 (96-171)	106 (70-152)
Factor XI (%)	30 (7-41)	38 (24-52)	57 (24-79)	55 (39-71)	89 (62-125)	86 (49-134)	112 (67-196)	97 (67-127)
Factor XII (%)	58 (43-80)	53 (33-73)	53 (14-80)	47 (29-65)	79 (20-135)	77 (39-115)	115 (35-207)	108 (52-164)
Antithrombin III (%)	76 (58-90)	63 (51-75)	74 (60-89)	67 (54-80)	109 (72-134)	104 (84-124)	96 (66-124)	100 (74-126)
Protein C activity (%)	36 (24-44)	35 (26-44)	44 (28-54)	42 (31-53)	71 (31-112)	59 (37-81)	104 (74-164)	96 (64-128)
Protein S activity (%)	36 (28-47)	36 (24-48)	49 (33-67)	50 (36-64)	102 (29-162)	87 (55-119)	75 (54-103)	81 (60-113)
D-dimer (mcg/mL)	1.47 (0.41-2.47)	N/A	1.34 (0.58-2.74)	N/A	0.22 (0.11-0.42)	N/A	0.18 (0.05-0.42)	N/A

Modified from Monagle P, Barnes C, Ignjatovic V, et al: Developmental haemostasis: Impact for clinical haemostasis laboratories. *Thromb Haemost* 95:362, 2006; and Andrew M, Paes B, Milner R, et al: Development of the human coagulation system in the full-term infant. *Blood* 70:165, 1987 (range inferred from published statistical documentation).
N/A, Not available; *PTT,* partial thromboplastin time.

infection, thrombocytopenia, drugs) is critical when evaluating neonates. Initial empirical therapy consists of platelet and/or factor supplementation, which is often administered while diagnostic studies are under way.

Evaluation of the Bleeding Neonate

Neonatal, peripartum, maternal, and family history are each important in the evaluation of a newborn with hemorrhagic complications. Maternal history of prior pregnancies, medications, and illnesses can provide clues to the hemostatic disorder in the neonate. The family history, such as parental ethnicity and consanguineous marriage, may help to identify congenital bleeding disorders. Maternal infection, drug use, or immune thrombocytopenia can lead to neonatal thrombocytopenia. Maternal deficiency of vitamin K or consumption of drugs that impair vitamin K metabolism can reduce the levels of the vitamin K–dependent coagulation proteins at birth. Vitamin K administration in the delivery room should be confirmed.

On physical examination, the location and characteristics of bleeding (e.g., procedural, mucosal, cutaneous, intraventricular), whether diffuse or localized, and the general appearance of the baby as sick or well will help to identify the underlying etiology of the hemorrhage. In ill-appearing newborns, disseminated intravascular coagulation (DIC) or liver disease may result in acquired factor deficiencies. These disorders tend to present with diffuse bleeding. Well-appearing newborns are more likely to have localized bleeding or ecchymoses because of thrombocytopenia from a transplacental antibody, vitamin K deficiency, or a rare inherited factor deficiency.

Laboratory evaluation of the hemorrhage in newborns should include sepsis evaluation and determination of the platelet count, PT, aPTT, TT, and fibrinogen concentration. If the test results are normal,

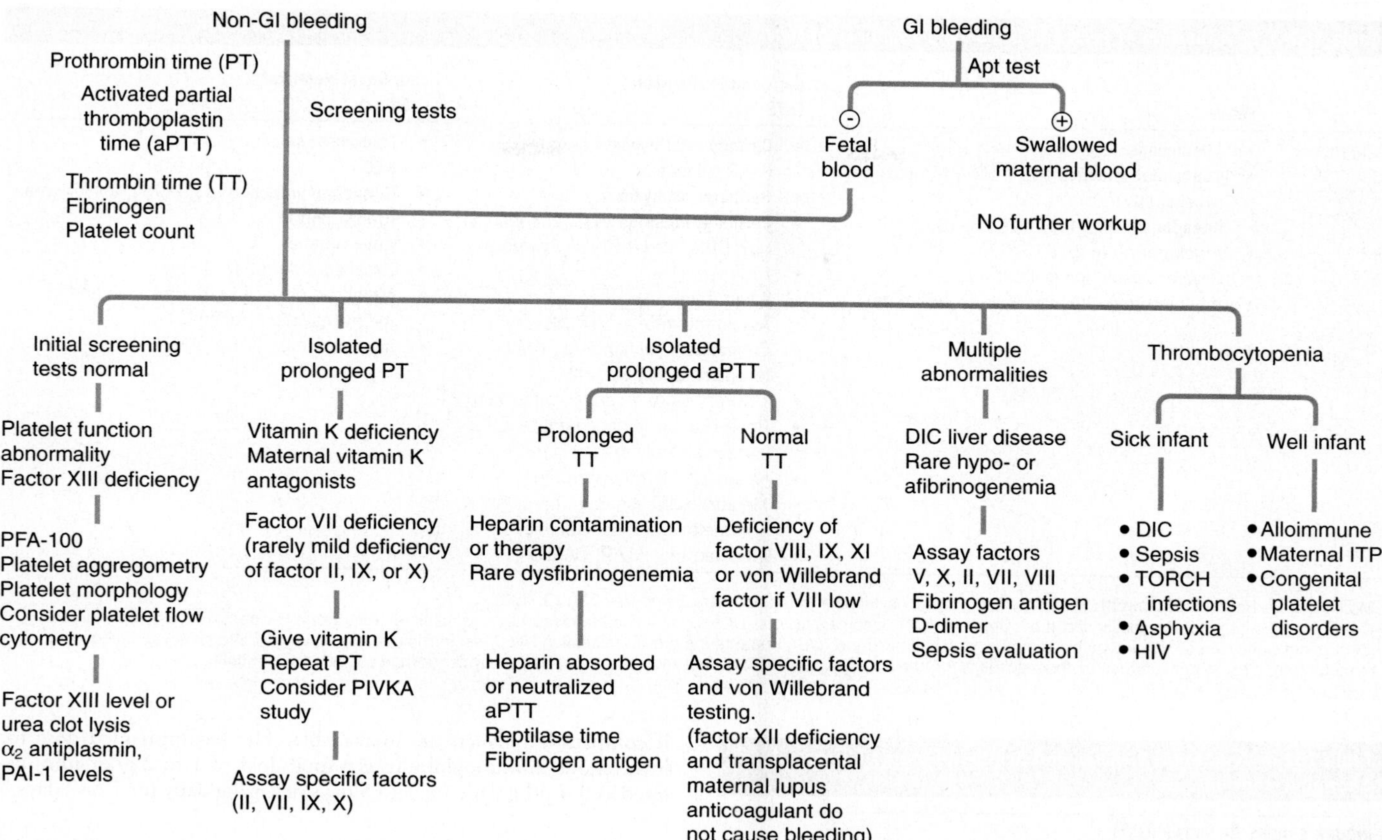

Figure 152-1 DIAGNOSTIC APPROACH TO THE BLEEDING NEONATE. *DIC,* Disseminated intravascular coagulation; *GI,* gastrointestinal; *HIV,* human immunodeficiency virus; *ITP,* immune thrombocytopenia purpura; *PAI-1,* plasminogen activator inhibitor 1; *TORCH,* toxoplasmosis, other agents, rubella, cytomegalovirus, herpes simplex. *(Modified from Blanchette VS , Rand ML: Platelet disorders in newborn infants: diagnosis and management.* Semin Perinatol *21:53, 1997.)*

bleeding neonates or infants should be assessed for FXIII and α_2AP activity. Deficiencies of FXIII, α_2AP, or PAI-1 are not detected with routine screening, and specific testing is needed if deficiencies are suspected. The approach to laboratory screening is summarized in Fig. 152-1, which has been modified from Blanchette and Rand.[7] Platelet function should be evaluated when primary hemostatic defects are suspected.[8] In male infants with a family history of hemophilia or when hemophilia is suspected, the levels of FVIII and FIX should be determined regardless of the degree of aPTT prolongation.

Neonatal Thrombocytopenia

The following factors are important to consider when evaluating neonates with thrombocytopenia: congenital or acquired, sick or well, maternal antibody or drug, and platelet size. A classification of neonatal thrombocytopenia is provided in Table 152-3. Thrombocytopenia is defined as a platelet count of less than 150×10^9/L.[9] Platelet counts in the range of 100 to 150×10^9/L are common in healthy neonates; these mostly reflect transient thrombocytopenias and require no further investigation unless there is a further decrease in the count. More severe thrombocytopenia (platelet count of $<50 \times 10^9$/L) in neonates rarely manifests with bleeding, particularly in the absence of maternal antiplatelet antibodies. The estimated prevalence of thrombocytopenia is in the range of 1% to 5% of all newborns. The prevalence of thrombocytopenia increases to 22% to 35% in neonates admitted to the neonatal intensive care unit (NICU), with the rates increasing with decreasing gestational age. With severe thrombocytopenia, platelet transfusion may be necessary to treat or decrease the risk for bleeding.

Causes of neonatal thrombocytopenia include decreased platelet production, increased platelet consumption, and/or hypersplenism. Other contributing factors include infection, placental insufficiency, genetic disorders, medications, DIC, or immune deficiency. In well-appearing newborns, thrombocytopenia is usually immune mediated and related to maternal transplacental immunoglobulin G antibodies or drugs (e.g., quinine, hydralazine, thiazides, tolbutamide). In sick newborns, platelet destruction is often related to infection, DIC, extracorporeal membrane oxygenation (ECMO), thrombosis, or mechanical ventilation for hyaline membrane disease. Large vessel thrombosis can also lead to thrombocytopenia, as can specific syndromes, such as renal vein thrombosis (RVT), necrotizing enterocolitis, or vascular anomalies (Kasabach-Merritt syndrome). Platelet production can be impaired with hypoxic-ischemic injury, perhaps because fetal megakaryocytes are particularly sensitive to hypoxia. Newborns from pregnancies complicated by intrauterine growth restriction or pregnancy-induced hypertension frequently exhibit transient mild to moderate thrombocytopenia. Other rare causes of decreased platelet production in neonates include primary congenital platelet or marrow disorders and infiltrative disorders. These are summarized in Table 152-4.

Neonatal Alloimmune Thrombocytopenia

Neonatal alloimmune thrombocytopenia is the platelet equivalent of hemolytic disease of the newborn. The transplacental passage of maternal antibodies directed against fetal platelets that express paternal antigens (HPA) that the mother lacks can result in severe neonatal thrombocytopenia (platelet count $<30 \times 10^9$/L). This may result in major bleeding, particularly intracranial hemorrhage (ICH), which

Table 152-3 Classification of Fetal and Neonatal Thrombocytopenia

	Fetal	Early-Onset Neonatal (<72 hr)	Late-Onset Neonatal (>72 hr)
Conditions	• **Alloimmune** • **Congenital infection** (e.g., CMV, toxoplasma, rubella, HIV) • **Aneuploidy** (e.g., trisomies 18, 13, 21) • Autoimmune (e.g., ITP, SLE) • Severe rhesus hemolytic disease • Inherited (e.g., Wiskott-Aldrich syndrome)	• **Chronic fetal hypoxia** (e.g., PIH, IUGR, diabetes) • **Perinatal asphyxia** • **Perinatal infection** (e.g., *Escherichia coli*, GBS, *Haemophilus influenzae*) • DIC • Alloimmune • Autoimmune (e.g., ITP, SLE) • Congenital infection (e.g., CMV, toxoplasma, rubella, HIV) • Thrombosis (e.g., aortic, renal vein) • Bone marrow replacement (e.g., congenital leukemia) • Kasabach-Merritt syndrome • Metabolic disease (e.g., propionic and methylmalonic acidemia) • Inherited (e.g., TAR, CAMT)	• **Late-onset sepsis** • **NEC** • Congenital infection (e.g., CMV, toxoplasma, rubella, HIV) • Autoimmune • Kasabach-Merritt syndrome • Metabolic disease (e.g., propionic and methylmalonic acidemia) • Inherited (e.g., TAR, CAMT)

Modified from Roberts I, Stanworth S, Murray NA: Thrombocytopenia in the neonate. *Blood Rev* 22:173, 2008.
CAMT, Congenital amegakaryocytic thrombocytopenia; *CMV*, cytomegalovirus; *DIC*, disseminated intravascular coagulation; *GBS*, group B *Streptococcus; HIV*, human immunodeficiency virus; *ITP*, idiopathic thrombocytopenic purpura; *IUGR*, intrauterine growth restriction; *NEC*, necrotizing enterocolitis; *PIH*, pregnancy-induced hypertension; *SLE*, systemic lupus erythematosus, *TAR*, thrombocytopenia with absent radii. The most frequently occurring conditions are in **bold.**

Table 152-4 Syndromic, Genetic, and Acquired Causes of Neonatal Thrombocytopenia

INBORN ERRORS OF METABOLISM
Isovaleric acidemia
Methylmalonic acidemia (with acute acidosis) and cobalamin metabolic defects
Holocarboxylase deficiency
Mitochondrial disorders
Pearson syndrome
Kearns-Sayre syndrome
GENETIC MARROW FAILURE SYNDROMES
Amegakaryocytic thrombocytopenia
Fanconi anemia
OTHER SYNDROMIC THROMBOCYTOPENIAS
Thrombocytopenia with absent radii syndrome
Paris-Trousseau syndrome
X-linked thrombocytopenias
Wiskott-Aldrich syndrome
GATA1 mutations
ANEUPLOIDY
Trisomy 21, 13, or 18
GENETIC MACROTHROMBOCYTOPENIAS
May-Hegglin, Sebastian, Fechtner syndromes
Bernard-Soulier syndrome
ACQUIRED MARROW DISORDERS
Oncologic
Neonatal leukemia
Neuroblastoma
Histiocytic lymphohistiocytosis

can occur in 10% to 20% of untreated pregnancies.[9] About half of the cases of neonatal alloimmune thrombocytopenia occur in the first pregnancy. Treatment options include transfusion of antigen-negative platelets if available (HPA-1a ± 5b), administration of high-dose intravenous immunoglobulin and/or a trial of random donor platelets if compatible platelets are unavailable. The recommended dose for intravenous immunoglobulin is a total dose of 1 to 2 g/kg administered as 0.4 g/kg daily for 3 to 5 days or 1 g/kg daily for 1 or 2 days.[10]

Inherited Thrombocytopenia

Most cases of inherited thrombocytopenia are the result of decreased platelet production because of abnormal hematopoietic stem or progenitor cell development. Such disorders are often associated with congenital anomalies, which can direct the course of investigation and aid in the diagnosis.[9] Disorders that present with neonatal thrombocytopenia include Bernard-Soulier syndrome, type 2B von Willebrand disease (vWD), Wiskott-Aldrich syndrome, Fanconi anemia, thrombocytopenia with absent radii syndrome, amegakaryocytic thrombocytopenia with radioulnar synostosis, congenital amegakaryocytic thrombocytopenia, X-linked macrothrombocytopenia due to GATA1 mutation, giant platelet syndromes, Kasabach-Merritt syndrome, thrombotic disorders, and metabolic disorders.

Platelet Abnormalities

Qualitative platelet disorders are rarely associated with overt neonatal bleeding. Patients who present with bleeding and have normal coagulation test results and platelet counts require further investigation. Bleeding may be from mucocutaneous sites, sites of capillary blood sampling, cephalohematoma, umbilical stump, or at sites of procedures. Only the most severe genetic disorders of platelet function present in the neonatal period. These include Glanzmann thrombasthenia and Bernard-Soulier syndrome (see Chapters 127 and 132). Maternal medications may affect platelet function, most notably aspirin, although low-dose aspirin does not appear to alter neonatal platelet function. Neonatal medications may also affect platelet function. Common offenders include nitric oxide, prostaglandin E_2, indomethacin, and aspirin.

Suspected platelet function disorders should be evaluated by platelet morphology and platelet aggregation studies after initial screening by PFA-100. Although PFA-100 testing is a sensitive test for detecting hemostatic disorders in the pediatric population, it is relatively nonspecific. Flow cytometry to evaluate specific surface glycoproteins or electron microscopy studies for granule morphology may be necessary. Platelet transfusions are often given if bleeding is present. The potential risk for allosensitization from normal platelets in congenital deficiencies of platelet surface antigens must be weighed against the severity of bleeding when functional defects are suspected. Recombinant activated factor VIIa (rFVIIa) has been used to avoid allosensitization.

Vitamin K Deficiency Bleeding

Vitamin K is a necessary cofactor for γ-glutamyl carboxylase, the enzyme required for posttranslational carboxylation of prothrombin, FVII, FIX, and FX, and proteins C, S, and Z. Many newborns are deficient in vitamin K, whether measured in cord blood or indirectly by measuring the levels of vitamin K–dependent coagulation proteins. Vitamin K deficiency bleeding can be acquired or congenital. Risk factors for bleeding include maternal malabsorption, maternal intake of drugs that impair vitamin K metabolism, exclusive breastfeeding, and neonatal malabsorption. Classification is based on the time of presentation. Bleeding in the first 24 to 48 hours of life is usually associated with maternal intake of drugs (e.g., phenytoin, barbiturates, antibiotics), which cross the placenta and impair vitamin K synthesis. Typically bleeding from vitamin K deficiency manifests from days 2 to 7 of life. Gastrointestinal bleeding is the most common presentation, but procedural bleeding, bruising, or ICH can occur. Late-onset vitamin K–related bleeding can occur at up to 12 weeks of age, usually in association with exclusive breastfeeding or with neonatal fat malabsorption, and often manifests as catastrophic bleeding, including ICH. Congenital vitamin K deficiency is an autosomal recessive disorder that occurs because of mutations in the genes encoding γ-glutamyl carboxylase or vitamin K2,3–epoxide reductase complex. Neonates with this disorder often have severe bleeding, including ICH. Genotype analysis is necessary to confirm the defect.[11]

The diagnostic criteria for vitamin K deficiency bleeding include an elevated international normalized ratio (INR) and normal levels of fibrinogen and a normal platelet count. The diagnosis is confirmed if the INR normalizes after administration of vitamin K and the bleeding is stopped. The aPTT is prolonged in severe vitamin K deficiency. Prophylaxis with a single dose of vitamin K (0.5 to 1 mg) in the delivery room prevents early- and classic-onset bleeding. Although oral dosing may be effective because of the potential for impaired absorption, regurgitation, or noncompliance, parenteral administration by the intramuscular, subcutaneous, or intravenous route is preferred. Additional doses of oral vitamin K should be given at days 7 and 28 in breastfed infants.

Vitamin K–induced coagulopathy should be treated with vitamin K, which can be given by intravenous infusion (to minimize anaphylactoid reactions) or by subcutaneous injection. Intramuscular injection should be avoided with severe deficiency because of the potential for hematoma formation. If there is bleeding, fresh frozen plasma (FFP) at a dose of 10 to 15 mL/kg body weight can be given. Because of the potential for thrombotic complications, prothrombin complex concentrates (PCCs) should be reserved for life-threatening bleeding or situations where FFP may produce volume overload. PCC has the added benefit of decreased volumetric load. In the absence of published guidelines, extrapolation from adult data suggests that a PCC dose of 50 units/kg is sufficient. The overall prognosis of vitamin K deficiency bleeding is good.

Inherited Coagulation Disorders

Prolonged aPTT

In neonates the aPTT is physiologically prolonged compared with adult values. Hemophilia is the most common inherited coagulation disorder, as discussed in detail in Chapter 137. Evaluation for FVIII, FIX, and FXI deficiencies should be undertaken immediately in any neonate bleeding with an isolated prolongation of the aPTT or a positive family history. Cord blood samples can be used in those with a family history, thereby avoiding the need for peripheral venipuncture, but careful sampling is important to avoid maternal contamination of the sample. In term and preterm infants, FVIII levels are within the normal adult range despite physiologic differences in the hemostatic system. Thus confirmation of hemophilia A is possible in the neonatal period regardless of gestational age of the child or severity of the condition. However, because the levels of the vitamin K–dependent clotting factors, including FIX, are reduced at birth (and even lower in preterm infants), diagnosis of hemophilia B, particularly mild hemophilia B, is difficult in the neonatal period.

Male newborns with a family history of hemophilia should be evaluated before intramuscular injections, including vitamin K. Typically newborns with hemophilia and bleeding are well appearing. Male infants far outnumber females, given the location of both FVIII and FIX genes on the X chromosome. However, severe FVIII or FIX deficiency can, albeit rarely, present in females, such as in Turner syndrome or extreme lyonization. Approximately one-third of cases of hemophilia are the result of spontaneous mutations; consequently a family history may be lacking. FXI deficiency is an autosomal recessive disorder, so female newborns with bleeding and isolated prolongation of the aPTT should also be tested. Evaluation of hemophilia carrier status in mothers of unknown status (e.g., single prior affected child or positive history in maternal grandmother) can be performed genetically because factor levels in carriers are variable and can overlap with normal levels. Most bleeding episodes in newborn males occur after circumcision or umbilical stump separation, although ICH is reported in approximately 3.5% of hemophiliac newborns,[12] and cephalhematomas are common. Joint bleeding is unusual in the neonatal period. Patients with known or suspected hemophilia and those with severe deficiencies of FVII, FX, or FXIII should be screened for ICH. Although cranial ultrasonography is often used for screening purposes, computed tomography (CT) or magnetic resonance (MR) scanning is more sensitive for detection of small parafalcine bleeds, which can also occur in a small percentage of normal neonates.[8] Neonates with hemophilia A or B are treated with recombinant FVIII or FIX concentrates, respectively. Routine prophylaxis is controversial after uncomplicated term delivery but is recommended for high-risk situations, such as prolonged labor, forceps delivery, or preterm infants.

Isolated Prolonged PT

In term neonates, the PT is normal. Inherited FVII deficiency is a rare, autosomal recessive condition with a strong gene dosage effect. Neonatal bleeding can occur in severe cases (i.e., homozygosity or compound heterozygosity for two mutations in the FVII gene). FVII deficiency can be associated with microcephaly or midline defects because disruption of chromosome 13q can lead to loss of adjacent genes. As a vitamin K–dependent protein, FVII deficiency can occur in association with deficiencies of the other vitamin K–dependent clotting proteins with abnormalities of the vitamin K pathways. Low doses of rFVIIa can be used for treatment of isolated FVII deficiency; FFP and/or vitamin K can be used for management of combined deficiencies.

Prolonged PT and aPTT

The association of bleeding with prolongation of both the PT and aPTT in a healthy newborn may indicate vitamin K deficiency or congenital deficiencies of prothrombin, FV or FX, as well as rare combined deficiencies. Routine prophylactic administration of vitamin K_1 to newborns can complicate the diagnosis of vitamin K deficiency bleeding in neonates.[13] More commonly, combined PT and aPTT prolongation occurs in sick newborns with DIC or severe hepatic decrease. Combined factor deficiencies are rare but must be considered when the laboratory findings or clinical course is confusing. Autosomal recessive mutations in LMAN1 (ERGIC-53) or MCFD2 result in combined FV and FVIII deficiency because of defective intracellular processing of the factors. Mutations in γ-glutamyl carboxylase are associated with inherited combined deficiencies of all vitamin K–dependent proteins. FVII deficiency has rarely been reported in combination with FV, FVIII, FIX, FX, FXI, and protein C defects, as reviewed by Girolami.[14]

FXIII Deficiency

FXIII is a transpeptidase that cross-links fibrin, thereby rendering it resistant to lysis. FXIII deficiency is inherited in an autosomal recessive fashion, and the prevalence of FXIII deficiency is estimated to be 1 in 3 to 5 million. Homozygotes usually have FXIII levels of less than 1% and have a severe bleeding diathesis. Patients with heterozygous FXIII deficiency are usually asymptomatic but have reduced levels of FXIII.[15] Neonates with FXIII deficiency may present with umbilical bleeding a few days after birth, a frequent finding that occurs in 80% of cases. More severe bleeding, including ICH, occurs in 25% to 30% of patients, a frequency higher than that in patients with hemophilia. ICH is the major cause of death and disability in neonates with FXIII deficiency, and ICH in a child with no other risk factors should prompt a search for FXIII deficiency.

FXIII deficiency is not detected with screening PT, aPTT, or TT assays. Specific assays for FXIII or urea clot solubility testing are used for diagnosis. The clot solubility test is sensitive to very low levels of FXIII (<1%) but is normal if FXIII levels are in the 1% to 3% range. Consequently FXIII immunoassays are perferable.[15]

Treatment of FXIII deficiency includes FFP, cryoprecipitate, or plasma-derived FXIII concentrate. Prognosis is excellent, but affected patients face a lifelong risk for bleeding and those with severe deficiency require prophylaxis.

Other Inherited Deficiencies Associated With Neonatal Bleeding

vWD, which is the most common inherited bleeding diathesis, is in detail in Chapter 140. vWD is rarely associated with neonatal bleeding and may be associated with the most severe subtypes. In a case series that included 55 newborns with vWD, there were no bleeding complications, although cases of scalp hematomas and bleeding after vitamin K injection or umbilical stump detachment were reported. Acquired forms of vWD also are rare but may complicate obstetric management of affected mothers and can affect their newborn babies. A family history of vWD, especially type 2, should prompt vWD evaluation in the neonate before circumcision and possibly before intramuscular injections. There is possible association of vWD with acute idiopathic pulmonary hemorrhage. The diagnosis of vWD may be difficult because vWF concentrations are high at birth and there is a large proportion of high-molecular-weight vWF multimers. Children with a diagnosis of type 3 vWD should be tested for mutations that predispose them to inhibitory alloantibody formation before aggressive replacement with exogenous vWF.[16] Treatment of neonates with vWF involves administration of plasma-derived concentrates that contain vWF (e.g., Humate-P or Alphanate), dosed initially at 40 to 60 ristocetin cofactor units/kg.

Although most of the bleeding problems in neonates are acquired, patients with severe deficiencies of coagulation factors can present in the neonatal period. Autosomal recessive deficiencies, in either homozygous or compound heterozygous state, are grouped as rare coagulation disorders that can manifest as severe bleeding diatheses. In the neonatal period, severe deficiencies of fibrinogen, FVII, FX, and FXIII are the most likely disorders to present with bleeding conditions. One common feature of these disorders is the association with intracranial bleeding.[17] Deficiency of fibrinogen can manifest with bleeding in the soft tissues, after circumcision, or after umbilical stump detachment. The diagnosis can be established with fibrinogen assays, and treatment involves replacement with cryoprecipitate or, if available, fibrinogen concentrate (see box on Recommended Dosing for Transfusion in Neonatal Hemorrhage). Severe FXI deficiency is more prevalent in Ashkenazi Jews and can present with bleeding in newborns after hemostatic challenges, such as circumcision. FV and prothrombin deficiencies are the other rare autosomal recessive homozygous deficiencies that can cause hemorrhagic symptoms.[8]

Not all deficiencies result in a bleeding diathesis. Even complete deficiencies of the contact factors, high-molecular-weight kininogen, prekallikrein, and FXII, are not associated with a bleeding phenotype. Autosomal recessive deficiencies of α_2AP and PAI-1 have been associated with bleeding, but not in the neonatal period.

Liver Disease

Acute liver disease or hepatic failure is uncommon in neonates. Liver disease in neonates may be caused by viral hepatitis, parenteral nutrition, cholestasis, hypoxic injury, or metabolic disease. Rare disorders that cause liver failure in neonates include hereditary tyrosinemia, neonatal hemochromatosis, and hemophagocytic lymphohistiocytosis. Liver dysfunction can affect the hemostatic balance resulting in activation of the coagulation and fibrinolytic systems, reduced synthesis of coagulation factors, poor clearance of activated hemostatic components, thrombocytopenia, platelet dysfunction, loss of coagulation proteins into ascitic fluid, and failure to utilize vitamin K.[18]

Because of reduced synthesis of multiple coagulation proteins, laboratory workup typically reveals a prolonged PT and aPTT. Acute liver disease also results in elevated liver enzyme levels, direct hyperbilirubinemia, and elevated ammonia concentrations. The platelet count may be reduced, especially if hypersplenism is present, and platelet dysfunction is common. Hypofibrinogenemia is a late manifestation of liver disease, and elevated fibrin degradation products and D-dimer occur because of delayed hepatic clearance. Assays of FV, FVII, and FVIII can help distinguish between liver disease, vitamin K deficiency, and consumptive coagulopathy (e.g., DIC). FV and FVIII are not vitamin K dependent. FV is synthesized in the liver, whereas FVIII is synthesized in multiple cell types, and have neonatal concentrations similar to adult levels. Deficiency of all three implies consumption, whereas decreased levels of FV and FVII with a normal FVIII level is consistent with liver disease.

Treatment should include replacement with FFP and/or cryoprecipitate, as well as platelet transfusion. Fibrinogen concentrate has been used as an alternative to cryoprecipitate. Patients with biliary atresia or other cholestatic liver failure syndromes may also benefit from parenteral vitamin K. The outcome is dependent on treatment of the underlying cause of liver disease.

Intraventricular Hemorrhage

Intraventricular hemorrhage (IVH) is associated with significant morbidity and mortality in the newborn period, particularly in premature infants. In the United States, it is estimated that approximately 12,000 premature infants and 20% to 25% of very low-birth-weight infants develop IVH each year. With improvements in neonatal care, the incidence of IVH is decreasing.

The etiology of IVH is multifactorial and includes prematurity of the cerebral vasculature and ischemia-reperfusion injury related to ventilatory support, blood pressure lability, and ECMO. Other risk factors for IVH include vaginal delivery, severe respiratory distress syndrome (RDS), low Apgar scores, pneumothorax, hypoxia, hypercapnia, seizures, patent ductus arteriosus, and infection. Many of these risk factors induce IVH by altering cerebral blood flow. Coagulopathy and thrombocytopenia can contribute to IVH, but their role in the pathogenesis of IVH is uncertain. One study reported hypofibrinogenemia, thrombocytopenia, or prolonged clotting time in 11 of 15 neonates with IVH and in only 5 of 35 unaffected newborns. Hemorrhage complicating cerebral thrombosis may explain some cases of IVH (especially in full-term infants), and heterozygosity for the FV Leiden mutation was reported in 18% of neonates with grade 2 to 4 IVH compared with 3% of controls.

Vitamin K, indomethacin, AT, FFP, FXIII, tranexamic acid, or ethamsylate have all been evaluated for prevention of IVH with mixed results. Cerebellar hemorrhage should raise suspicion of organic acidemia, such as methylmalonic, propionic, or isovaleric acidemia. rFVIIa may be useful for treatment of IVH, but additional studies are needed to determine its efficacy and safety.

Extracorporeal Membrane Oxygenation

ECMO is occasionally used for treatment of neonates with severe pulmonary hypertension or cardiomyopathy. The ECMO pump, oxygenation membrane, and large-bore catheters can induce thrombosis, which necessitates administration of high-dose systemic anticoagulation, thereby imposing the risk for bleeding. Thrombosis and hemorrhage are common complications in pediatric ECMO patients, particularly if ECMO is initiated after open heart surgery. Approximately 15% of neonates on ECMO sustain an ICH.[19]

With the doses of heparin used during ECMO, the PT and aPTT may not correlate with the activated clotting time (ACT). Furthermore, there is evidence that the heparin dose provides prognostic information in ECMO patients independent of the ACT, suggesting that an ACT of 180 to 220 seconds may not provide adequate anticoagulation. Prolonged ECMO is associated with depletion of clotting factors and high levels of fibrin degradation products. Consequently the aPTT and ACT are prolonged and the levels of D-dimer are increased even when low doses of heparin are administered.

A retrospective study of 29 nonsurvivors of ECMO revealed that most patients have a coagulopathy characterized by a prolonged PT and aPTT, as well as being thrombocytopenic, and most had generally low levels of fibrinogen despite ACT values that were within the acceptable range of 180 to 220 seconds in the final 24 hours of ECMO. Thus routine laboratory testing is inadequate for predicting or preventing thrombotic or hemorrhagic complications in pediatric ECMO patients. Thrombin generation assays, anti-FXa heparin levels, and thromboelastography have been suggested as alternatives to the ACT. Data supporting the use of these tests are lacking.

In neonates with established thrombosis or at risk for thrombosis, daily FFP infusion is sometimes used as a source of plasminogen and anticoagulant proteins. Data supporting this approach are lacking.

Respiratory Distress Syndrome

RDS, also known as hyaline membrane disease, is an acute pulmonary process that is common in premature neonates. The disorder is characterized by hyaline membrane formation and fibrin deposition in diffuse areas of atelectasis. Although increased thrombin generation and decreased levels of AT are found in severe RDS, therapeutic interventions aimed at addressing abnormalities in the coagulation system have yielded inconclusive results. Plasmin or plasminogen may enhance survival; heparin is of uncertain benefit, and AT supplementation may increase mortality. Additional studies are needed to explore the utility of anticoagulant or thrombolytic therapies in RDS. A laboratory profile consistent with mild DIC is common in RDS; fibrinogen levels are decreased, and levels of D-dimer are elevated. An unexpected increase in ventilatory support should raise the suspicion of pulmonary embolism in this population.

NEONATAL THROMBOEMBOLIC DISORDERS

The incidence of thromboembolism in newborns is higher than that in older infants or children. Medical advances have improved neonatal survival at the expense of an increase in the incidence of thrombosis. Venous or arterial access devices are the major acquired risk factor for thromboembolism. The risk is higher in neonates with congenital heart defects or RDS and in those undergoing interventions or ECMO. Dehydration, sepsis, heart failure, congenital nephritic syndrome, necrotizing enterocolitis, and asphyxia are other risk factors for thromboembolism.

Laboratory workup often reveals a hypercoagulable state with a short aPTT; decreased levels of AT, protein C, and protein S; defective fibrinolysis; hyperactive platelets; elevated levels of clotting factors (i.e., fibrinogen, FVII, FVIII); and the presence of antiphospholipid antibodies or thrombophilic defects, such as FV Leiden or the prothrombin gene mutation. A family history of thrombosis or miscarriages may indicate a hereditary thrombophilia.

Consensus guidelines for therapy of neonates with thrombosis have been developed.[20] Heparin, either unfractionated heparin (UFH) or low-molecular-weight heparin (LMWH), remains the mainstay of treatment in newborns. If the thrombus is limb- or life-threatening, thrombolytic therapy may be considered. Because much of the information in this patient population is derived from case reports, case series, registries, and extrapolation from studies in adults, recommendations are mostly of low grade. Large, multicenter, prospective controlled clinical trials are needed to generate evidence-based guidelines; such studies are problematic in neonates.

Incidence

Current estimates of the incidence of neonatal thrombosis are derived from three international registries, each with different inclusion criteria. Based on the data from the German,[21] Dutch,[22] and Canadian[23] registries, it is estimated that clinically relevant neonatal thromboembolism occurs in approximately 24 of 10,000 patients in the NICU and in 0.29 to 0.51 of 10,000 newborn infants. Two-thirds of thromboembolic events are venous, and 80% are either catheter associated or develop after a severe illness.[24] Arterial thromboembolic events in neonates usually present as strokes or emboli to the limbs from catheter-associated thrombi. Neonatal thrombosis is associated with significant mortality and morbidity.

Acquired Thrombophilia

Indwelling Catheters

Central venous and arterial access is essential for the advanced care provided in modern neonatology. The most common acquired thrombotic risk factor in neonates is the presence of an indwelling vascular catheter. The risk for thrombosis depends on catheter location, size, material, duration of placement, and type of fluid delivered. A Canadian registry reported that 80% of episodes of deep venous thrombosis (DVT) in newborns were related to indwelling central venous catheters.[25] Inferior and superior vena cava thrombosis are common complications of central venous catheters, including Broviac and umbilical venous catheters.[23] The incidence of catheter-associated DVT is influenced by the method of detection. When catheters are used for total parenteral nutrition, it is estimated that DVT is diagnosed in 1% on clinical grounds, in 35% by echocardiography, and in 75% by venography. In cases involving central venous catheters, contrast venography is regarded as the reference standard for the diagnosis of thrombosis but ultrasonography is most often used because it is noninvasive, easily performed by the bedside, and there is no ionizing radiation exposure.

DVT often causes pain, swelling, and discoloration of the affected limb. Loss of catheter patency, evidence of collateral circulation, and/or unexplained thrombocytopenia should raise the suspicion of DVT. Prospective imaging studies performed before central access catheter removal demonstrate thrombi in up to 86% of patients.[22] Treatment often begins with removal of the catheter, although consideration of anticoagulation before catheter removal is warranted, especially in infants with right-to-left intracardiac or intrapulmonary shunting. Small catheter-associated thrombi may resolve without specific therapy. Larger thrombi or those in locations associated with greater morbidity (e.g., sinovenous, renal, portal) may warrant short courses of heparin or thrombolytic agents. Platelets should never be administered through arterial catheters because of the potential risk for thromboembolism.

Disseminated Intravascular Coagulation

Neonates are susceptible to DIC because of their immature anticoagulant and fibrinolytic systems. Most cases of neonatal DIC are associated with tissue ischemia and acidosis secondary to sepsis, low-output cardiac failure, perinatal asphyxia, severe RDS, or necrotizing enterocolitis. Other causes of consumptive coagulopathy include large vascular anomalies, severe liver disease, massive hemolysis, or hereditary thrombophilia. DIC may present with hemorrhage and/or thrombosis. Bleeding in a well-appearing neonate is usually the result of an inherited deficiency of a coagulation protein or immune-mediated thrombocytopenia rather than DIC. In contrast, bleeding in a sick preterm neonate is more likely the result of DIC. Patients with DIC often exhibit a prolonged PT, aPTT, and thrombin clotting time, a decreased fibrinogen and FVIII level, thrombocytopenia, and increased levels of D-dimer.

Definitive therapy requires identification and reversal of the trigger for DIC. FFP, platelets (if bleeding is severe), and cryoprecipitate (if the fibrinogen concentration is low) are given to replace the consumed factors. Reasonable treatment targets include maintaining the fibrinogen level over 100 mg/dL, the platelet count over 50×10^9/L, and the PT close to normal. Heparin should be given if there is thrombosis along with AT concentrate if indicated. Successful treatment of DIC depends on reversal of the trigger and provision of aggressive supportive care. Therapy aimed at reversing the coagulopathy has little effect on DIC outcome.

Hereditary Thrombophilia

Spontaneous thrombosis is rare in healthy newborns, and this presentation should prompt evaluation for hereditary thrombophilia. Among the known causes of hereditary thrombophilia, only homozygous or compound heterozygous protein C and/or protein S deficiency is sufficient to induce neonatal thrombosis. Other inherited thrombophilic conditions include FV Leiden, the prothrombin mutation, AT deficiency, elevated lipoprotein(a), maternal anticardiolipin antibodies, and nonspecific inhibitors.

Hereditary thrombophilia should be suspected in patients with spontaneous and extensive thrombosis, ischemic skin lesions, or purpura fulminans. The Subcommittee for Perinatal and Pediatric Thrombosis of the Scientific and Standardization Committee of the International Society on Thrombosis and Haemostasis recommended that pediatric patients with thrombosis be tested for a full panel of genetic and acquired thrombophilic defects.[26] However, because of the difficulty in obtaining a large volume of blood, one can consider performing these tests in stages unless the result of the testing has immediate impact on patient management. On initial presentation of thrombosis, DNA-based assays can be performed. Testing for levels of natural coagulation inhibitors should be delayed until 6 months of age when the levels approach those in adults and until anticoagulant treatment is discontinued.

Specific Neonatal Thrombotic Syndromes

Renal Vein Thrombosis

The renal vein is one of the most common sites of neonatal thrombosis. The incidence of renal vein thrombosis (RVT) is estimated to be 0.5 per 1000 admissions to NICUs and 2.2 per 100,000 live births.[21] RVT is more common in males and in the left renal vein, although 28% to 44% occur bilaterally. In term neonates, RVT usually presents 3 days postnatally; 7% of neonates present with RVT in utero.[27] Clinical manifestations of RVT include hematuria, proteinuria, a palpable abdominal mass, edema, hypertension, renal failure, anuria, adrenal hemorrhage, thrombocytopenia, and anemia. RVT is associated with prematurity, umbilical venous catheters, diabetic mothers, asphyxia, and infections. FV Leiden, prothrombin gene mutation, and elevated lipoprotein(a) have also been found in association with RVT. However, these are common traits, and it would be inaccurate to say they are proven to be causal, despite the associations. Most infants with RVT will experience complete, cortical, or segmental infarction of the affected kidney(s) and/or hypertension.[18]

Diagnosis is reliably confirmed by Doppler ultrasound examination. There are no evidence-based treatment guidelines, and most cases of RVT result in loss of renal tissue regardless of the treatment. Neonates with RVT should be followed for persistent hypertension and progressive renal insufficiency. Unilateral RVT without uremia or clot extension into the inferior vena cava can be managed with heparin or LMWH. Treatment should be given for at least 3 months if there is extension into the inferior vena cava. Bilateral RVT with renal failure should be treated with thrombolytic therapy followed by heparin or LMWH.[20]

Portal Vein Thrombosis

The true incidence of portal vein thrombosis (PVT) is unknown, but it is estimated to range from 1% to 43% of neonates with umbilical venous catheters. The wide variation in incidence reflects differences in imaging protocols. In another study, the incidence of PVT was estimated to be at least 36 cases per 10,000 NICU admissions.[28] When ultrasonography is performed prospectively, 43% of neonates with umbilical venous catheters have asymptomatic PVT.

Major risk factors for PVT include umbilical venous catheters and sepsis/omphalitis. The role of inherited thrombophilia in PVT is controversial. Long-term complications of PVT include lobar atrophy and portal hypertension with associated gastrointestinal bleeding. Complications are more frequent with ectopic umbilical venous catheter placement (below or in the liver) or when thrombi are occlusive. Ultrasonography may reveal evidence of prior PVT with cavernous transformation of the portal vein and subsequent splenomegaly and reversal of portal flow.[29] Spontaneous resolution of PVT is common, but detection of PVT is important, even in asymptomatic patients, because PVT can lead to portal hypertension, which may manifest up to 10 years later.[29] Neonates with umbilical venous catheters should be monitored by ultrasonography, and catheter removal and/or anticoagulation should be considered for PVT.

Purpura Fulminans

Purpura fulminans is characterized by disseminated purpuric lesions, often associated with bullae and necrosis. The histopathology of these lesions reveals diffuse cutaneous microthrombi with surrounding hemorrhage. Diffuse thrombosis, including stroke, retinal infarcts, limb gangrene, and DIC, can occur in purpura fulminans. Causes include severe protein C, protein S, or AT deficiency, either acquired as a complication of sepsis or inherited as homozygous or compound heterozygous conditions. Some infants with severe protein C deficiency do not develop thrombosis until adulthood, suggesting that additional factors influence the neonatal presentation. Treatment with heparin and replacement with protein C concentrate or FFP are indicated. Long-term anticoagulation is often needed.[30]

Arterial Ischemic Stroke

Perinatal arterial ischemic stroke (AIS) is an important cause of cerebral palsy, epilepsy, and cognitive impairment. Perinatal AIS mostly occurs in full-term neonates with a prevalence of 28.6 to 93 cases per 100,000 live births. Presenting features include seizures and lethargy. In the neonatal period, AIS often presents with focal or generalized seizures, although pathologic hand preference before 1 year of age is most common if the stroke was asymptomatic in the newborn period. Ischemic injury is usually detected by MR angiography, and unilateral lesions favor the left hemisphere. Diffusion-weighted MR imaging is superior to cranial ultrasonography or CT scanning.[20]

Risk factors for perinatal AIS are different from thrombosis risk factors in older infants and children because maternal and placental factors play a more important role, and some events even occur in utero.[31] The most common acquired risk factors for perinatal AIS are perinatal asphyxia, fetal distress, chorioamnionitis or other infections, preeclampsia, congenital heart disease, and dehydration. The contribution of congenital thrombophilia to perinatal AIS risk is unclear, although maternal anticardiolipin antibodies may be present for a brief period. In most cases of perinatal AIS, a hypercoagulable state is not detected. One potential mechanism of stroke is embolism of placental thrombi via the umbilical vein and through the patent foramen ovale of the fetus or neonate. Evaluation of placental pathologic conditions is important because demonstration of placental thrombi or abruption may be indicative of maternal prothrombotic state. Furthermore, if placental thrombi are seen histologically, the risk for recurrent events is especially low. Long-term developmental outcomes depend on the extent of the stroke and location of the lesion; strokes involving Broca and Wernicke areas, the internal capsule, or the basal ganglia have a poor outcome.

Treatment depends on whether the stroke is embolic or nonembolic in origin. For nonembolic AIS, current guidelines recommend against anticoagulation or aspirin for neonates with a first AIS, especially if the infarct is large or there is evidence of hemorrhage. Anticoagulant or aspirin therapy is recommended for neonates with recurrent AIS.[20] In a patient with a documented cardioembolic stroke, anticoagulant therapy is suggested.

Sinovenous Thrombosis

Based on data from the Canadian Pediatric Ischemic Stroke Registry, the prevalence of sinovenous thrombosis is 0.67 per 100,000 children, with 43% occurring in the neonatal period.[32] The clinical presentation may be relatively silent, or patients may manifest with diffuse neurologic changes, seizures, and IVH. The most frequently involved vessels are the superior and lateral sinuses, and up to one-third of cases have associated venous infarction and subsequent hemorrhage.[18] Up to 31% of full-term neonates with IVH have associated sinovenous thrombosis, suggesting that the pathophysiology of IVH in full-term neonates is different from that in premature infants.

Risk factors for neonatal sinovenous thrombosis include perinatal asphyxia, diffuse hypoxic injury, dehydration, infection, congenital heart disease, and severe illness, with ECMO now recognized as a specific risk factor. The frequency of hereditary thrombophilias in neonates with sinovenous thrombosis ranges from 20% to 40%, with FV Leiden and MTHFR C677T occurring most often. In contrast to purpura fulminans, no cases of congenital deficiencies of protein C, protein S, or AT have been reported in association with sinovenous thrombosis. Multiple risk factors (maternal, neonatal, perinatal, or prothrombotic) are found in over half of neonates with sinovenous thrombosis.[20] Although the diagnosis of sinovenous thrombosis in neonates is often made by transcranial ultrasonography, MR venography is the most sensitive diagnostic test. Based on data from the Canadian Pediatric Ischemic Stroke Registry, neonatal sinovenous thrombosis is associated with cerebral parenchymal infarcts in 42% of cases, and 83% of these are hemorrhagic infarcts.[32]

Aside from treatment of the underlying conditions, when relevant, there are no standard treatment guidelines. Nonetheless, good results have been obtained with anticoagulant therapy, and UFH or LMWH is given provided that there is no significant ICH. Extended treatment with LMWH or a vitamin K antagonist is recommended for a minimum of 6 weeks and no longer than 3 months.[20] For those with significant hemorrhage, radiologic monitoring at 5 to 7 days is recommended, and anticoagulation should be initiated if there is evidence of thrombus propagation.[20] Anticoagulation is associated with a high rate of hemorrhage, so treatment plans should be individualized. In older patients, punctate hemorrhage behind a cerebral venous infarct is not an absolute contraindication to anticoagulation, but studies in neonates are lacking. Nevertheless, in the Canadian registry, 36% of neonates were treated with UFH or LMWH, mostly for 3 months, and no cases of death or neurologic compromise from hemorrhage were reported.[32] Overall, neurologic impairment was reported in up to two-thirds of cases, and approximately 2% died.

Principles of Therapy

Supportive Therapy

As with other age-groups, therapeutic modalities available to neonates include supportive care, anticoagulation, thrombolytic agents, and surgical thrombectomy. The British Haemostasis and Thrombosis Task Force and the American College of Chest Physicians have proposed guidelines for the management of neonatal thrombosis.[33] Supportive therapy is recommended for clinically silent thrombi, including catheter-associated events. As soon as practical, clotted catheters should be removed, and all documented thrombi should be followed by serial imaging. If venous access is required, one can either monitor the clot closely or provide anticoagulation therapy.

Vitamin K Antagonist Therapy

Vitamin K antagonists, such as warfarin, are not recommended for neonates because liquid preparations are not available, monitoring is complicated, and doses are variable because of alterations in the dietary intake of vitamin K.

Heparin (UFH or LMWH)

UFH or LMWH is the mainstay of anticoagulant therapy in neonates. UFH can be used for the initial treatment of DVT. The rate of heparin clearance is different in newborns compared with adults or older children. Newborns generally have lower levels of AT, which renders them relatively resistant to the anticoagulant effects of heparin. Consequently supplementation with AT concentrate or FFP may be necessary, particularly if there is evidence of heparin resistance. The UFH and LMWH dosing regimens are outlined in the box on Treatment of Neonatal Thrombosis. Anticoagulation is monitored using anti-FXa assays with added AT to compensate for the low levels of AT in neonatal plasma. Therapeutic anti-FXa levels are 0.3 to 0.7 units/mL for UFH and 0.5 to 1 unit/mL for LMWH. The aPTT can also be used to monitor UFH; aPTT values that correlate with anti-FXa levels of 0.3 to 0.7 units/mL are considered therapeutic.

LMWH has emerged as the anticoagulant of choice in the pediatric setting both for prophylaxis and for treatment. The advantages of LMWH include subcutaneous delivery, minimal monitoring, and a lower risk for heparin-induced thrombocytopenia (HIT) and osteoporosis compared with UFH. In the pediatric population, the anticoagulant response to weight-adjusted doses of LMWH appears to be less predictable than that in adults. Prophylactic UFH is recommended to maintain patency of umbilical arterial lines (0.25-1 unit/mL, 25-200 units/kg/day, use lowest dose possible) and for cardiac catheterization (bolus 100 to 150 units/kg with catheter insertion, repeat for prolonged procedures). More studies are needed to define the optimal doses of LMWH. Based on a review of data from 240 neonates treated with enoxaparin, starting doses of 1.75 mg/kg twice daily are recommended for term neonates and 2.0 mg/kg twice daily for preterm neonates, provided that the bleeding risk is low.[34]

HIT antibodies are found in up to 1.5% of neonates, particularly in those who have undergone cardiac surgery. Overt HIT with thrombosis, however, is rare, but it can occur. Mothers with HIT can passively immunize their fetuses. Diagnostic criteria for HIT are described in detail in Chapter 135. Treatment includes cessation of heparin and anticoagulation with argatroban, danaparoid, or lepirudin.[35] Fondaparinux may be a reasonable option in selected cases, but experience in neonates is limited.

Treatment of Neonatal Thrombosis

Unfractionated Heparin
Bolus: 75 units/kg over 10 minutes
Maintenance: 28 units/kg/hr; therapeutic goal, anti-FXa of 0.3 to 0.7 units/mL
Prophylaxis: 10 units/kg/hr
Follow platelet count to detect possible HIT (risk is low)

Enoxaparin
1.5 mg/kg subcutaneously every 12 hours (with normal renal function; round dose to nearest milligram; consider higher dose [see text][34])
Check anti-FXa level by peripheral venipuncture 4 to 6 hours after second or third dose; therapeutic goal, anti-FXa of 0.5 to 1 unit/mL (0.4 to 0.6 unit/mL if concurrent thrombocytopenia or other bleeding risk factor)
Follow platelet count to detect possible HIT (risk is low)
Hold for 24 hours before procedures

Prophylaxis With Enoxaparin
0.75 mg/kg subcutaneously every 12 hours
If checked, anti-FXa level 4 to 6 hours after second or third dose should be less than 0.4 units/mL
Hold for 12 hours before procedures

Purpura Fulminans
Concurrent heparin: UFH dose of 28 units/kg/hr with target anti-FXa of 0.3 to 0.7 units/mL; LMWH dose of 1.0 to 1.5 mg/kg every 12 hours with therapeutic target anti-FXa range of 0.5 to 1 units/mL and replacement with FFP or protein C concentrate
FFP: 10 to 20 mL/kg every 6 to 12 hours for purpura fulminans
Protein C concentrate for severe protein C deficiency: load with 100 to 120 units/kg, then 60 to 80 units/kg every 6 hours × three doses (goal protein C activity 100%). Once therapeutic anticoagulation is achieved, maintenance therapy with 45 to 60 units/kg every 6 to 12 hours (goal protein C activity >25%)

Antithrombin Repletion
Antithrombin (functional) should be maintained at greater than 50% of normal levels for effective heparin-based anticoagulation
Dose in international units = (desired − current AT*) × weight (kg)

AT, Antithrombin; *FFP*, fresh frozen plasma; *HIT*, heparin-induced thrombocytopenia; *LMWH*, low-molecular-weight heparin; *UFH*, unfractionated heparin.
*Expressed as percentage of normal level based on functional ATIII level.

Thrombolytic Therapy

Guidelines for thrombolytic management of neonatal thrombosis are provided by the British Haemostasis and Thrombosis Task Force[33] and the Scientific Subcommittee on Perinatal and Pediatric Thrombosis of the International Society of Thrombosis and Haemostasis.[36] Both groups agree that thrombolysis should be considered for extensive thrombosis associated with organ dysfunction or limb-threatening ischemia. Low-dose thrombolysis is recommended to open occluded catheters. tPA is the drug that has been most widely studied in pediatric patients. Transfusion support for hypofibrinogenemia and thrombocytopenia should be provided to minimize the bleeding risk. Contraindications for thrombolytic therapy include active bleeding and major surgery or bleeding within the past 10 days, whereas relative contraindications include severe asphyxia within 7 days, generalized seizures within the last 48 hours, sepsis or prematurity of less than 32 weeks of gestation. If UFH or LMWH is given concomitantly with tPA, it should be administered at prophylactic doses (0.75 mg/kg every 12 hours for LMWH or 10 units/kg/hr for UFH; see box on Tissue Plasminogen Activator Thrombolysis for Neonatal Thrombosis). Surgical thrombectomy is reserved for organ-, limb-, or life-threatening thrombosis when tPA administration is impractical or predicted to be ineffective. Thrombolytic therapy may be of benefit in a select group of pediatric patients with massive pulmonary embolism or extensive DVT.

Tissue Plasminogen Activator Thrombolysis for Neonatal Thrombosis

Concurrent Heparin (UFH or Enoxaparin) Should Be Considered at Prophylactic Dosing; UFH Preferred
Life- or limb-threatening thrombi: starting dose of 0.1 to 0.5 mg/kg/hr for up to 6 hours
If no response, consider increase by 0.1 mg/kg/hr increments to maximum 0.5 mg/kg/hr
Consider using fresh frozen plasma 10 mL/kg before thrombolytic therapy
Maintain fibrinogen greater than 100 mg/dL
Maintain platelet count above 100
Reversal of severe bleeding with aminocaproic acid at 100 mg/kg intravenously every 6 hours

UFH, Unfractionated heparin.

Recommended Dosing for Transfusion in Neonatal Hemorrhage

PRBC: 10 to 15 mL/kg single-donor PRBC infused over 4 hours
Platelets*: 10 mL/kg raises platelet count by 75,000 (goal >50,000 if bleeding, >20,000 if not bleeding)
FFP: 10 to 20 mL/kg every 6 to 12 hours for purpura fulminans
Cryoprecipitate: 0.15 units/kg raises fibrinogen about 100 mg/dL (goal >150 mg/dL if bleeding, >50 mg/dL if not bleeding)
von Willebrand factor: 40 to 60 ristocetin cofactor units/kg of plasma-derived FVIII/vWF preparations
Factor VIII: for hemophilia A—50 units/kg load, then 25 units/kg every 12 hours; recombinant factor preferred (monitor FVIII)
Factor IX: for hemophilia B—80 to 100 units/kg daily; recombinant factor preferred (monitor FIX)
Factor VIIa: for severe factor VII deficiency—20 to 30 mcg/kg every 6 to 12 hours

FFP, Fresh frozen plasma; *PRBC*, packed red blood cells; *vWF*, von Willebrand factor.
*Volume limits transfusion of platelets by the "unit" in small neonates. Practices vary—follow institutional guidelines for volume dosing or volume reduction.

SUGGESTED READINGS

Kenet G, Chan AK, Soucie JM, et al: Bleeding disorders in neonates. *Haemophilia* 16:168, 2010.
Male C, Johnston M, Sparling C, et al: The influence of developmental haemostasis on the laboratory diagnosis and management of haemostatic disorders during infancy and childhood. *Clin Lab Med* 19:39, 1999.
Monagle P, Chan AK, Goldenberg NA, et al: Antithrombotic therapy in neonates and children: Antithrombotic therapy and prevention of thrombosis, ed 9: American College of Chest Physicians evidence-based clinical practice guidelines. *Chest* 141:e737S, 2012.

For complete list of references log on to www. expertconsult.com.

PART XIII

CONSULTATIVE HEMATOLOGY

CHAPTER 153

HEMATOLOGIC CHANGES IN PREGNANCY

Caroline Cromwell

Hematologic conditions are often seen during pregnancy. These range from the simple to the complex. The primary physiological hematologic changes during pregnancy relate to the expansion of plasma volume.[1] In addition to physiologic changes of pregnancy, a prothrombotic state develops as the pregnancy advances that is thought to prepare the mother and fetus for eventual placental separation.[2] All require proper planning, anticipation, and discussion with the treating physicians as well as the patient. The effect of the condition on the pregnancy and conversely the effect of the pregnancy on the condition should be considered. The evolving clinical picture as the pregnancy progresses must also be taken into account. Multidisciplinary planning and communication are essential.

More common hematologic problems and dilemmas in management are discussed in this chapter.

ANEMIA IN PREGNANCY

Anemia in pregnancy is quite common and affects approximately half of all pregnancies worldwide. It is more prevalent in underdeveloped countries.

The World Health Organization classifies anemia in pregnancy as hemoglobin below 11 g/dL, although in developing countries, it is clinically defined as hemoglobin below 10 g/dL.[1] Physiologic anemia occurs during pregnancy as blood volume increases a greater proportion than red blood cell (RBC) mass, resulting in a dilutional anemia. Total circulatory volume increases to approximately 50% greater than prepregnancy volume. Plasma volume and RBC mass return to baseline during the first and second postpartum months. Common maternal signs of anemia include pallor, tachypnea, fatigue, and headache. Hemoglobin levels less than 6 g/dL in pregnant women can be associated with significant maternal and fetal complications. At these levels, tissue oxygenation decreases and may lead to a state of high-output congestive heart failure in the mother.[2-4] Multiple studies have shown a correlation between maternal anemia and increased rates of both preterm (<37 weeks' gestation) and low-birth-weight deliveries.[5-13]

There are varied etiologies behind anemia in pregnancy.

Iron-Deficiency Anemia

Iron-deficiency anemia is the most common cause of anemia in pregnancy. It has been identified as a risk factor for preterm delivery and low birth weight. Iron requirements increase during pregnancy because of maternal and fetal erythropoiesis. Generally, hemoglobin levels decrease throughout pregnancy and then may increase in the last month of pregnancy. Ferritin levels also increase in the last month of pregnancy because it is an acute phase reactant. Erythropoietin levels increase throughout pregnancy. The clinical symptoms of iron deficiency are similar to those in nonpregnant patients and include fatigue, pallor, tachycardia, and poor exercise tolerance. The diagnosis and treatment are generally similar to those in nonpregnant patients. Anemia and a low ferritin level are considered diagnostic. Ferritin levels may be increased in the third trimester.

Because the typical diet in the United States provides only 50% of daily iron requirements for pregnant women and because of the relatively high prevalence of iron deficiency among women of childbearing age, routine iron supplementation in pregnancy is recommended.[16] Currently, the Centers for Disease Control and Prevention, American Dietetic Association, and American College of Obstetrics and Gynecology recommend 15 to 30 mg/day of elemental iron to prevent adverse outcomes from iron-deficiency anemia.[15-19] Treatment should be from the beginning of gestation to 3 months postpartum. Based on the results of a study by Casanueva et al,[20] weekly therapy with 120 mg of iron appears to be a safe and effective alternative to daily therapy. The side effects associated with iron therapy—constipation, diarrhea, nausea—are well known.

Intravenous iron is appropriate in certain circumstances; evidence from a recently published randomized trial by Al et al supports the use of intravenous iron therapy to replenish iron stores in appropriately selected patients, including those who have not tolerated a trial of oral iron therapy and those with severe iron deficiency.[21]

Multiple studies have shown that routine iron supplementation in pregnancy decreases the incidence of iron-deficiency anemia. Furthermore, in a recent randomized, double-blind study in which 275 iron-replete pregnant women received either a daily iron supplement or placebo from the time of enrollment (all women were enrolled before week 20) to 28 weeks' gestation, the incidence of both low-birth-weight and preterm low-birth-weight infants was lower among women who received daily iron.[22] Nonetheless, there are limits to the effectiveness of routine iron supplementation. After all, the recommendation by prominent public health organizations for universal iron supplementation has not led to a commensurate decrease in the incidence of iron-deficiency anemia in pregnancy[23,24] or an increase in maternal hemoglobin levels.[25,26] Compliance is an important factor in this discussion. A large, multicenter, randomized, controlled trial on the benefits of iron supplementation during pregnancy in the United States is needed to draw more definitive conclusions.

Other Nutritional Deficiencies

Folate deficiency and vitamin B_{12} deficiency are the next most common causes of anemia in pregnancy. Cobalamin and folate are critical for fetal growth because they are necessary for the production of tetrahydrofolate. Tetrahydrofolate is key in the DNA synthesis pathway.

Folate deficiency accounts for 95% of megaloblastic anemias in pregnancy.[27] Folate deficiency complicates between 1% and 4% of pregnancies in the United States and affects approximately one-third of pregnancies worldwide.[28] Similar to iron-deficiency anemia, the incidence of megaloblastic anemia in pregnancy is increased in adolescents, women of low socioeconomic status, and women with multiple closely-spaced births.[29] The folic acid requirement for nonpregnant women is 50 to 100 μg/day, but this increases to 150 μg during pregnancy as RBC mass in the mother increases and as fetal demands for folate grow with cell proliferation.[30]

Diagnosis of folate deficiency is best based on RBC folate levels. An elevated homocysteine level also helps confirm the diagnosis. Pregnant women should at least receive 400 μg of folic acid a day. Vitamin B_{12} deficiency is much less common during pregnancy. Diagnosis of vitamin B_{12} deficiency can be aided by the assessment of homocysteine and methylmalonic acid. If a woman is found to be deficient in vitamin B_{12} during pregnancy, vitamin B_{12} injections are indicated. These are usually injected weekly for 4 to 8 weeks and then monthly.

HEMOGLOBINOPATHIES AND PREGNANCY

Sickle Cell Disease

Every year more than 300,000 children are born with either sickle cell disease or thalassemia. Prenatal counseling now exists in many countries. In the United States, all newborns are screened for sickle cell disease. Management of pregnant patients with sickle cell disease requires coordination of care between the hematologist and obstetrician. Many women with sickle cell disease experience more frequent vasoocclusive crises and other sickle cell–related complications during pregnancy.[31] The increased frequency of vasoocclusive crises, particularly during the latter half of pregnancy, likely results from heightened metabolic requirements in pregnancy, increased venous stasis, and the physiologic prothrombotic state of pregnancy. In addition, pathophysiologic changes in the renal and immune function of patients with sickle cell disease increase their susceptibility to urinary tract infections and pyelonephritis. In a recently published retrospective cohort study, Thurman and colleagues[32] compared rates of asymptomatic bacteriuria and pyelonephritis among women with sickle cell trait with those among a cohort of pregnant control patients. The implications of such a study are noteworthy because in the general population, bacteriuria in pregnant women is associated with increased morbidity and mortality for both the mother and fetus. The authors found equivalent rates of asymptomatic bacteriuria in the two groups. On the other hand, they detected a higher prevalence of pyelonephritis among the cohort with sickle cell trait.

Other significant complications occur in pregnant women with sickle cell disease as well. For example, the incidences of preeclampsia, thromboembolic events, placental abruption, intrauterine growth retardation, low birth weight, and postpartum infections are higher among women with hemoglobin SS, SC, and Sb-thalassemia compared with women without sickle cell disease. One study noted a higher incidence of stillbirths and perinatal mortality among patients with sickle cell disease,[33] but another study revealed an increased risk of preterm labor and premature rupture of membranes in women with hemoglobin SS disease.[34] By causing tissue hypoxia, sickling of RBCs within the placental vasculature causes deleterious effects on the fetus.[35]

Because of the increased risk for such complications, women with sickle cell disease should receive close medical attention throughout the prenatal period. This includes counseling about intrauterine diagnosis of sickle cell disease when appropriate. Pregnant women can undergo chorionic villi sampling as early as the ninth week of gestation or amniocentesis in the 15th to 16th weeks. A reticulocyte count along with hemoglobin, iron, and folate levels should be obtained to assess for deficiency states and bone marrow suppression. Urinalysis with urine culture is performed as often as every trimester to monitor for asymptomatic bacteriuria. Finally, beginning around 28 weeks' gestation, patients should make weekly clinic visits and begin serial ultrasonography.

Treatment of sickle cell disease during pregnancy warrants careful consideration. With regard to maintenance therapy, hydroxyurea has been used safely throughout pregnancy in patients with sickle cell anemia, although formal studies of its use in this setting have not been performed to date.[36] Generally, the medication is discontinued. Women should receive 5 mg/day of supplemental folic acid. Studies examining the benefit of prophylactic blood transfusions or exchange transfusions have not led to definitive conclusions.[36] Although they may lead to alloimmunization, prophylactic transfusions appear to decrease the incidence of vasoocclusive crises and decrease maternal and fetal morbidity and mortality.[37] A conservative approach reserves transfusions for patients whose hemoglobin levels fall below 6 g/dL, patients who develop progressive complications related to sickle cell disease, and patients with obstetric complications.[38] Following this approach, 60% to 75% of women with sickle cell disease will require transfusion therapy during pregnancy. Patients with sickle cell crisis during pregnancy should receive aggressive analgesic therapy, hydration, and oxygen while undergoing evaluation of infection or other precipitating influence.

At the time of delivery, pregnant women with sickle cell disease are managed in a manner similar to those with high cardiac output anemia. Supplemental oxygen, hydration, and adequate anesthesia should be given to prevent sickling of RBCs and the associated complications. During the postpartum period, hemoglobin levels are followed closely and prophylaxis for venous thromboembolism (VTE) is administered unless contraindications preclude it.

Thalassemias

Pregnant women with an underlying thalassemia typically have β-thalassemia minor or α-thalassemia trait—conditions with a relatively benign clinical phenotype—rather than β-thalassemia major or hemoglobin H disease. Because of delayed pubertal growth or hypogonadism with associated anovulation, women with β-thalassemia major and hemoglobin H disease rarely become pregnant. Case reports indicate that when it does occur, pregnancy in women with hemoglobin H disease can be complicated by severe hemolytic anemia and hepatosplenomegaly. Pregnancy outcomes among women with β-thalassemia intermedia were examined in a recently published study by Nassar et al. After nine pregnancies in five patients with β-thalassemia intermedia, the authors noted a high incidence of intrauterine growth restriction (IUGR) and frequent requirement for RBC transfusion, even among women who had not been transfusion dependent before pregnancy.[39] One pregnancy resulted in intrauterine fetal demise at 36 weeks. These findings are consistent with previous observations made in reference to a population of pregnant women with thalassemia; an earlier review of the literature found that 50% of pregnancies in this patient population were complicated by preterm delivery, third trimester stillbirth, or IUGR.[40]

Pregnancy is a common setting for the diagnosis of β-thalassemia minor or α-thalassemia trait in previously asymptomatic women who are found to be anemic on routine laboratory evaluation during pregnancy. Several studies indicate that the physiologic anemia of pregnancy may be exacerbated in women with thalassemia minor, although findings from at least one study suggest otherwise.[41] β-Thalassemia minor and α-thalassemia traits do not have an adverse effect on fetal development, fetal morbidity and mortality, or maternal morbidity and mortality.[42]

Similar to those with sickle cell disease, women with thalassemia require vigilant follow-up throughout their pregnancies. This includes interval monitoring of maternal vital signs and fetal heart rate, maternal hemoglobin levels, and fetal growth as assessed by ultrasonography beginning around the 24th week of gestation. Patients are screened for folate and iron deficiency. They should also be assessed for iron overload, which can develop in individuals with thalassemia as a result of increased intestinal iron absorption, frequent blood transfusions, and rapid turnover of plasma iron.[43] Prenatal genetic testing can be performed if desired, with results used to counsel parents of the child and guide optimal care of the fetus. In terms of therapy, there are no specific treatment recommendations for women with thalassemia during pregnancy aside from folate supplementation and supportive care. In pregnant women with evidence of iron overload, chelation therapy using deferoxamine has been safely used, although the potential for teratogenicity associated with the agent must be considered in this setting.[44]

OTHER HEMOLYTIC ANEMIAS

Hereditary Spherocytosis

Hereditary spherocytosis is the most common inherited hemolytic anemia among people of northern European descent.[45] Few cases of pregnancy in individuals with hereditary spherocytosis have been reported. Published reports indicate there may be an increased incidence of first trimester fetal loss in patients with hereditary spherocytosis.[46] Because some patients have only low levels of hemolysis under normal conditions, the disease may not become clinically apparent until pregnancy. Pregnant women with hereditary spherocytosis can exhibit a variety of clinical manifestations. These include folate deficiency related to the increased requirements of pregnancy superimposed on chronic hemolysis, hemolytic crisis, and aplastic crisis.[47,48] The results of two small series suggest that pregnancy outcomes for women with hereditary spherocytosis are generally good, with improvements in outcomes for splenectomized patients.[49] Care is primarily supportive.

Glucose 6-Phosphate Dehydrogenase Deficiency

Favorable pregnancy outcomes observed in women with hereditary spherocytosis and pyruvate kinase deficiency stand in contrast to those in women with glucose 6-phosphate dehydrogenase (G6PD) deficiency. The deficiency of G6PD in this disorder leads to hemolytic anemia in the face of oxidative stress. The condition increases the risk of spontaneous abortion, low birth weight, and neonatal jaundice.[50] Women with G6PD deficiency should be instructed to strictly avoid medications with oxidative potential. Complications after the ingestion of oxidative drugs can even occur in a carrier of the G6PD deficiency gene if her male fetus has inherited the disease.[51]

Paroxysmal Nocturnal Hemoglobinuria

Paroxysmal nocturnal hemoglobinuria (PNH) is a rare clonal disorder caused by somatic mutation in the membrane-anchoring protein *PIGA*. *PIGA* mutation leads, in turn, to deficient function of critical membrane proteins that in wild-type individuals are anchored by the gene product of *PIGA*. Features of the clinical phenotype include hemolysis, thrombosis, and bone marrow failure. Hemolysis results from deficiency in the membrane proteins CD55 and CD59, which renders affected individuals susceptible to complement-mediated intravascular hemolysis.

The clinical manifestations of PNH can have a devastating impact on pregnancy. Reported cases highlight the significant pregnancy-associated morbidity and mortality in women with this condition. Complications include severe anemia, thrombocytopenia, thrombotic events, preterm delivery, low-birth-weight infants, neonatal death, and maternal death.[52,53] A study by Ray and colleagues[53] reviewed pregnancy outcomes in 24 women with PNH and found a 20% maternal mortality rate.

Owing to the high-risk nature of their pregnancies, women with PNH require close medical attention in the antenatal, perinatal, and postnatal periods. Prophylactic anticoagulation is recommended because of the high incidence of thrombotic events during pregnancy. Warfarin is contraindicated because of its teratogenicity. Low-molecular-weight heparin (LMWH) is favored over unfractionated heparin because it less frequently causes heparin-induced thrombocytopenia. Anticoagulation should be interrupted during the perinatal period but, in the absence of contraindications, reinitiated thereafter and continued for 6 weeks postpartum.[54]

Results of a phase III trial by Hillmen and colleagues[55] demonstrated that eculizumab, a humanized monoclonal antibody against the terminal complement protein C5, can reduce levels of hemolysis, stabilize hemoglobin, minimize transfusion requirement, and improve quality of life in patients with PNH. There are case reports describing success in patients chronically receiving eculizamb throughout pregnancy with uncomplicated deliveries. However, a large randomized trial has not been performed. Supportive care is used as needed throughout pregnancy. RBC transfusions are used in the treatment of anemia. In the setting of thrombocytopenia and bleeding, platelet transfusions may also be necessary.

Autoimmune Hemolytic Anemia

Autoimmune hemolytic anemia can occur during pregnancy and lead to anemia. The relatively small size of immunoglobulin G (IgG) immunoglobulin molecules allows them to cross the placenta; thus the IgG subtype of autoimmune hemolytic anemia can adversely affect fetuses. In contrast, the larger IgM antibodies do not cross the placenta. Patients with autoimmune hemolytic anemia are treated with glucocorticoids and, if necessary, intravenous immunoglobulin (IVIG). Supportive transfusions are administered when needed.[56] In rare instances, pregnancy appears to precipitate the development of autoimmune hemolytic anemia in a previously unaffected woman. The etiology of this phenomenon is not known.[57] Women in this circumstance have been treated in the standard fashion with favorable results.

THROMBOCYTOPENIA

Thrombocytopenia during pregnancy is quite common. It occurs in approximately 10% of pregnancies.[58] Although there is not one clear value to define thrombocytopenia in pregnancy, generally a platelet count less than 100,000 is considered cause for concern. There is some physiologic thrombocytopenia that occurs during pregnancy. Gestational thrombocytopenia (GT) is the most common cause of thrombocytopenia in pregnancy followed by preeclampsia and immune thrombocytopenia. Much rarer causes include disseminated intravascular coagulation (DIC), thrombotic thrombocytopenic purpura (TTP) and hemolytic uremic syndrome (HUS), and medication induced.

The evaluation of thrombocytopenia is essential to rule out any systemic disorders that may affect pregnancy management

Gestational Thrombocytopenia

Gestational thrombocytopenia is quite common during pregnancy. The platelet count is generally never lower than 70,000/μL. This occurs mainly in the third trimester. Patients are asymptomatic and have no history of thrombocytopenia. The platelet count normalizes within 3 months of delivery but often normalizes within 1 week. The etiology of GT remains unclear, but it is thought in part to be autoimmune in nature and demonstrates a clear overlap with mild idiopathic thrombocytopenic purpura (ITP).

The management of patients with GT is uncomplicated. Typically, they can receive epidural anesthesia. However, practice varies at each institution in terms of platelet threshold for epidural anesthesia. Platelet counts greater than 100,000/μL are considered safe for epidural anesthesia. There are studies demonstrating safe administration of epidural anesthesia in pregnant patients with platelet counts as low as 70,000/μL.[60]

Immune Thrombocytopenia

Responsible for pregnancy-associated thrombocytopenia in approximately 3% of cases, ITP represents an important diagnostic consideration in this patient population. It is the most common cause of thrombocytopenia during the first two trimesters of pregnancy.[61] ITP can recur in women with previously documented disease or can develop de novo during pregnancy.

Idiopathic thrombocytopenic purpura is usually not diagnosed during pregnancy. Pregnant patients with ITP usually have a longstanding history of thrombocytopenia. ITP may be difficult to distinguish from GT because patients with these conditions can present with similar clinical and laboratory findings. Elevated levels of platelet-associated IgG and antibody titers can be found in both conditions.[62] Furthermore, assays that detect antibodies against the glycoprotein receptors IIb/IIIa and Ib/IX are not specific for ITP.[63] Whereas thrombocytopenia in the first trimester or early portion of the second trimester should raise suspicion for ITP, thrombocytopenia that develops later in pregnancy should raise suspicion for GT. A preconception platelet count can also be helpful in distinguishing between the two. It is important to attempt to distinguish between ITP and GT because there is a small but significant risk of neonatal thrombocytopenia in the setting of ITP.[64]

In terms of diagnostic evaluation, HIV, hepatitis, and lupus should be tested for if clinically indicated. Platelet antibody testing is not considered helpful. The peripheral smear may demonstrate an increased platelet size but should otherwise be normal. Bone marrow biopsy and aspirate are not indicated unless there are other hematologic abnormalities present.

Treatment options are generally similar to those for nonpregnant ITP patients (Table 153-1). Platelet transfusions are reserved for life-threatening bleeding because the lives of transfused platelets are usually short in ITP. Glucocorticoids are considered first-line treatment; prednisone is usually initiated at 1 mg/kg based on the patient's baseline weight. Side effects of prednisone should be discussed with the patient and include weight gain, bone loss, hypertension, and gestational diabetes. IVIG can also be used. It is a means of rapid increase in platelet count. It is particularly used to help increase platelet counts a few days before delivery.[65] It is usually administered at a dose of 2 g/kg over 2 days. However, the improvement in platelet count is fairly transient. Splenectomy is also an option indicated for refractory thrombocytopenia; it is best performed during the second trimester.

Other agents such as danazol, cyclophosphamide, and vinca alkaloids—although used in the management of ITP in nonpregnant individuals—are teratogenic and should be avoided during pregnancy.[66] Use of cyclophosphamide has been associated with birth defects. Danazol may cause clitoral enlargement and labial fusion in female fetuses when given in the first trimester.[67,68] The use of rituximab has never been systematically studied in this setting and is considered pregnancy class C. Although case reports exist of its use, it is not generally recommended in this case. Animal data indicates thrombopoietin mimetics may cause fetal harm, and little is known about their use in pregnant patients. A registry has been developed for pregnant patients treated with thrombopoietin mimetics.

As discussed previously, maternal antiplatelet IgG can cross the placenta and cause thrombocytopenia in fetuses. Percutaneous umbilical blood sampling is the most accurate means to obtain the fetal platelet count. However, the procedure is associated with a high complication rate and 1% fetal mortality.[69] Intrapartum fetal scalp sampling represents an alternative, but the accuracy of this technique is only 50% to 70%.[70] The maternal platelet count and antiplatelet antibody level do not accurately predict the fetal platelet count.[71] Overall, 10% of babies born to mothers with ITP have a platelet count less than 50,000/μL, but fewer than 5% have a platelet count less than 20,000/μL.[72] Treatment of pregnant women with IVIG or steroids does not appear to affect the platelet count of fetuses.[72,73] Thrombocytopenia places neonates at risk for bleeding events, including intracranial hemorrhage, although this complication is rare.[74]

Table 153-1 Initiation of Treatment in Pregnant Patients With Idiopathic Thrombocytopenic Purpura

Platelet Count	Treatment
<10,000/μL	Platelet transfusion for life-threatening bleeding
10,000-30,000/μL	Consider monitoring in first trimester; treat in second or third trimester
>30,000/μL	Clinically monitor

In terms of delivery, at present, available guidelines on the subject suggest that obstetric factors, rather than hematologic ones, should guide the manner of delivery.[75] After the delivery of a child, cord blood platelet is checked and the newborn platelet count followed because thrombocytopenia most often peaks 4 to 6 days after delivery and resolves as maternal antiplatelet IgG is cleared.

Preeclampsia and HELLP Syndrome

Thrombocytopenia in pregnant woman also occurs in association with preeclampsia and HELLP syndrome (hemolysis, elevated liver enzymes, low platelet count), potentially severe multisystem disorders associated with pregnancy. In previously healthy nulliparous women, the incidence of preeclampsia is between 2% and 7%.[76] Thrombocytopenia is observed in 15% to 50% of patients with this condition.[59,77] Clinical manifestations include a maternal syndrome characterized by hypertension, proteinuria, and systemic abnormalities as well as a fetal syndrome characterized by fetal growth restriction, preterm delivery, and hypoxia-induced neurologic damage.[76,77]

In most instances, preeclampsia occurs during a woman's first pregnancy, but it can recur in a subsequent pregnancy or occur for the first time in a woman with one or more previously unaffected pregnancies. Risk factors for the disorder include, but are not limited to, preeclampsia in a previous pregnancy, a family history of preeclampsia, chronic hypertension, obesity, multifetal gestation, rheumatic disease, and preexisting thrombophilia.[76] With respect to thrombophilia, a case control study by Mello and colleagues[78] suggests that the prevalence of an underlying thrombophilia is significantly higher among women who develop preeclampsia during pregnancy than among those who have uneventful pregnancies.

HELLP syndrome represents a severe variant of preeclampsia. In the majority of cases, patients who develop the syndrome are white and multiparious.[79] The median age of affected patients is 25 years. The time of presentation during pregnancy ranges from the midtrimester (15%) to term (18%). Thirty percent of patients develop HELLP within 2 days after delivery.[80] Patients typically exhibit vague symptoms such as malaise, fatigue, epigastric or right upper quadrant pain, nausea, vomiting, and flulike symptoms. Because of the nonspecific nature of these symptoms, diagnosis is often delayed; one study found an average time to diagnosis of 8 days in women with HELLP syndrome.[81] Clinical findings at the time of diagnosis—weight gain or edema, hypertension, and proteinuria—are similar to those observed in preeclampsia.[80]

Although various criteria have been used in diagnosing HELLP syndrome, they generally share the following features: signs of microangiopathic hemolytic anemia, serum lactate dehydrogenase greater than 600 U/L or serum total bilirubin greater than 1.2 mg/dL, aspartate aminotransferase greater than 70 IU/L, and a platelet count lower than 100,000/μL.[82] Martin and colleagues[80] have further defined HELLP syndrome on the basis of platelet count. According to this classification, patients with class 1 HELLP syndrome have a platelet count lower than 50,000/μL, those with class 2 disease have a platelet count between 50,000 and 100,000/μL, and individuals with class 3 HELLP syndrome have a platelet count higher than 100,000/μL. As might be expected, women with class 1 HELLP syndrome required a recovery period in the aftermath of their illness.

Although the precise mechanism through which preeclampsia develops is uncertain, research in the field continues to advance understanding of the underlying pathophysiology. Endothelial cell dysfunction after placentation appears to play a central role in the pathogenesis of the disease. During development of the placenta, placental trophoblast cells interface with the epithelial layer of the uterus, forming the decidua. Penetration and remodeling of maternal spiral arteries beginning at week 9 during pregnancy increase placental perfusion and improve oxygenation for the developing fetus under normal conditions.[83]

Cellular abnormalities such as those described impair placental implantation and vasculogenesis, leading to fetal hypoxia and the release of vasoactive compounds such as endothelin, nitric oxide, and prostaglandins. High levels of endothelin, a potent vasoconstrictor, are seen in preeclamptic patients, and injection of endothelin into rabbits produces a syndrome similar to HELLP syndrome.[84,85] The activity of endothelin, nitric oxide, and prostaglandins leads to hypertension and platelet activation. Angiogenic factors such as vascular endothelial growth factor 1 (VEGF 1) are elevated in preeclampsia compared with normal pregnancy. Injury to the vascular endothelium results in fibrin deposition, further platelet activation, and the release of additional vasoactive agents such as serotonin and thromboxane A_2. The etiology of thrombocytopenia in preeclampsia is likely related to increased antiplatelet IgG levels[86] or to activation of the coagulation cascade with subsequent consumption of platelets.[87,88]

These events lead to the multisystem dysfunction seen in patients with HELLP syndrome. Fibrin deposition in the hepatic sinusoids causes hepatocellular injury. Patients can develop right upper quadrant pain if intraparenchymal or subcapsular hemorrhage occurs. DIC was observed in 21% of patients with HELLP in one series, and placental abruption was seen in 16% of patients.[89] Other manifestations of HELLP syndrome include acute renal failure, pulmonary edema, shock, cerebrovascular accident (CVA), eclampsia, retinal detachment, diabetes insipidus, and increased incidence of cesarean section.

HELLP syndrome is associated with high maternal and neonatal mortality rates. Maternal mortality rates range from 1.1% to 24.2%.[90] The immediate cause of death is most often rupture of the liver, DIC, acute renal failure, pulmonary edema or acute respiratory distress syndrome (ARDS), shock, or CVA. Perinatal deaths resulting from placental abruption, asphyxia, or extreme prematurity occur in 10% to 15% of patients. After delivery, infants born to women with preeclampsia or HELLP can develop a self-limited neonatal thrombocytopenia. Uncertainty exists as to whether infant thrombocytopenia in these instances results from preeclampsia or HELLP itself or from a related complication such as neonatal sepsis.[91-93] HELLP recurs in subsequent pregnancies of affected women in 3% to 27% of cases. There is also an increased risk of preeclampsia, placental abruption, and preterm delivery in these pregnancies.[94-103]

In caring for a patient with preeclampsia or HELLP syndrome, the clinician's primary concerns are the mother's health and safety. The clinician must also consider the stage of pregnancy at time of diagnosis, the condition of the fetus, and desires of the patient in making management decisions. Definitive treatment for preeclampsia and HELLP involves delivery of the fetus; it is indicated for women who present after 34 weeks' gestation and those with evidence of multisystem dysfunction. However, conservative, supportive care without immediate delivery can be pursued for women who are relatively asymptomatic, hemodynamically stable, less than 32 to 34 weeks' gestation, and without evidence of abnormal coagulation.[103,104] Magnesium sulfate, which reduces cerebral vasoconstriction and ischemia, should be administered for seizure prophylaxis.[105] Parenteral labetalol or hydralazine is given for blood pressure control. Systemic corticosteroids appear to lessen the risk of maternal ARDS and reduce neonatal complications when administered to women who present at less than 34 weeks' gestation.[106] In addition to these measures, volume status is closely monitored to prevent overexpansion of plasma volume and ensure adequate urine output.

Persistent right upper quadrant pain—which may herald a liver hematoma or rupture, hemodynamic instability, coagulation profile abnormalities, or a decline in clinical status—should prompt delivery by cesarean section. As mentioned previously, delivery is also indicated if the fetus is at least 32 to 34 weeks' gestation at the time signs and symptoms of preeclampsia or HELLP develop. In a clinically stable woman, vaginal delivery can be attempted.[107] When cesarean section is required, transfusion of RBCs, platelets, and fresh-frozen plasma (FFP) is performed as necessary before and during surgery. Severe hypofibrinogenemia should be treated with cryoprecipitate.

Patients are monitored closely in the postpartum period. Magnesium should be continued for 12 to 48 hours after delivery and blood pressure controlled appropriately. Although hypertension typically resolves within 6 weeks after delivery, some women require long-term antihypertensive therapy.[105] Coagulation and platelet abnormalities tend to resolve within the 24 to 48 hours after delivery. Some patients, however, experience an ongoing decline in the platelet count and should be followed until counts normalize. Postpartum eclampsia can occur for up to 48 hours after delivery; thus patients and health care providers should remain vigilant in monitoring for suggestive signs and symptoms.[108] Treatment options in the setting of severe postpartum preeclampsia and HELLP include corticosteroids and plasmapheresis.[109,110]

In light of the morbidity and mortality associated with preeclampsia and HELLP, considerable research has focused on prevention of these conditions. The efficacy of various preventive strategies, including magnesium supplementation, low-dose aspirin, zinc supplementation, antihypertensive drugs, and heparin therapy among others, has been the focus of observational studies, systematic reviews, and randomized trials. Initial small studies suggested that low-dose aspirin reduces the risk of preeclampsia, although patients who received aspirin had a higher incidence of placental abruption and bleeding.[111-118] Larger, randomized trials failed to confirm the benefit of low-dose aspirin.[112,113]

Thrombotic Thrombocytopenic Purpura–Hemolytic Uremic Syndrome

Thrombotic thrombocytopenic purpura and HUS are also important considerations in the evaluation of pregnant women with thrombocytopenia. Similar to preeclampsia and HELLP syndrome, they are multisystem disorders associated with high morbidity and mortality rates in the absence of appropriate therapy. Microvascular injury and platelet agglutination with resulting thrombocytopenia and microangiopathic hemolytic anemia are pathologic hallmarks of TTP and HUS (Fig. 153-1). They are rare conditions overall, but the incidence of both increases in pregnancy.[119] In the case of TTP, in fact, estimates suggest that approximately 10% of cases occur in pregnant or postpartum women.[120]

Because they share many common clinical features, TTP and HUS are often categorized as a single entity, TTP-HUS. However, the pathophysiology underlying the two conditions appears to be distinctive. TTP is associated with unusually large multimers of circulating von Willebrand factor (vWF), which foster platelet aggregation and thrombus formation. Under normal circumstances, a vWF-cleaving protease referred to as ADAMTS13 (a disintegrin and metalloproteinase with a thrombospondin type 1 motif, member 13) cleaves these multimers into smaller multimers of normal size. In TTP, function of the cleaving protease is impaired. ADAMTS13 deficiency characterizes familial TTP. Inhibition of ADAMTS13 protease activity by an autoantibody characterizes the acquired form of TTP. An inhibitory autoantibody can be found in 70% to 85% of patients with TTP.[121] On the other hand, impaired vWF-cleaving protease activity does not appear to play a role in the pathogenesis of HUS.[122]

There can be some similarity found between the features of TTP-HUS and HELLP syndrome. It can be difficult to distinguish TTP and HUS from HELLP syndrome because they both have signs of microangiopathy. TTP tends to occur earlier in pregnancy, with a mean onset at 23.5 weeks, although it can occur at any point from the first trimester through the postpartum period.[123] HUS primarily occurs after delivery; 90% of cases occur in the postpartum period, with a mean onset at 26 days after delivery.[124] TTP and HUS do not cause hypertension or liver necrosis. Furthermore, TTP and HUS frequently persist after delivery, but HELLP syndrome typically resolves in the postpartum period.

Treatment of TTP-HUS involves emergent plasmapheresis within 24 to 48 hours of diagnosis. The response rate among pregnant women treated with plasmapheresis for TTP is approximately 75%. By comparison, the overall response rate in patients with TTP is approximately 80% to 90%.[125–128] Long-term sequelae in surviving patients include chronic renal failure, hypertension, and recurrence of TTP-HUS. TTP-HUS recurs in approximately 50% of subsequent pregnancies.[129] Infusion of FFP represents an alternative to plasmapheresis, although plasmapheresis is the preferred treatment modality.

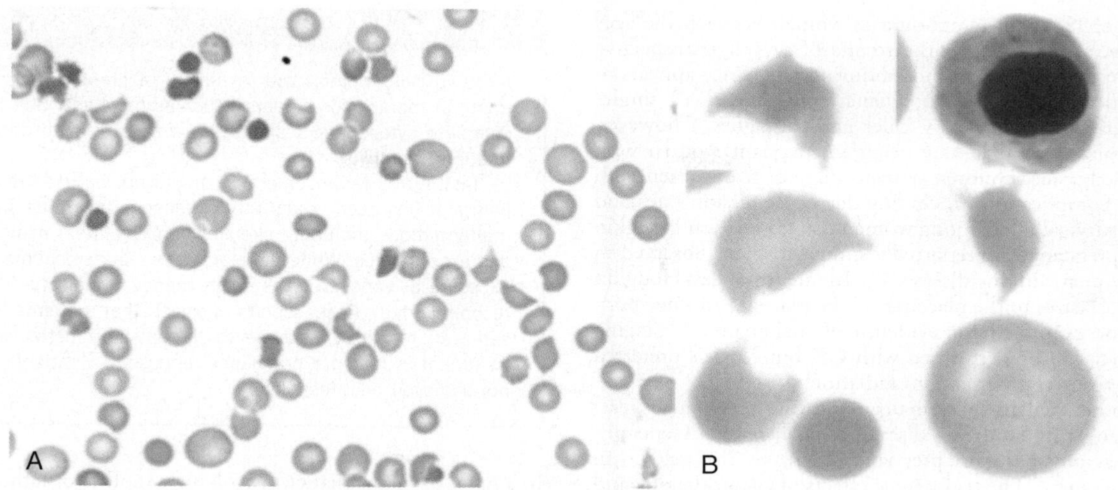

Figure 153-1 MICROANGIOPATHIC HEMOLYTIC ANEMIA. Microangiopathic hemolytic anemia in pregnancy, peripheral blood smear (**A** and **B**). Evidence of microangiopathy with the formation of schistocytes, fragmented forms and spherocytes, associated with polychromasia and nucleated red blood cells (**A** and **B,** detail).

The response rate after FFP infusion is 64%.[130] Corticosteroids (prednisolone 200 mg/day intravenously or prednisone 200 mg/day orally) have also been successfully used in the treatment of pregnancy-associated TTP-HUS, with a response rate of 26%.[128] Conversely, antiplatelet agents such as aspirin do not play a role in the treatment of pregnancy-associated TTP-HUS.[131]

Disseminated Intravascular Coagulation

Disseminated intravascular coagulation in pregnant women can occur in various clinical settings, including HELLP syndrome, TTP-HUS, placental abruption, amniotic fluid embolism, uterine rupture, intrauterine fetal demise, sepsis, elective abortion, and acute fatty liver of pregnancy (AFLP).

Severe placental abruption sufficient to cause fetal death occurs in 0.12% of all pregnancies.[132] This condition leads to a consumptive hypofibrinogenemia, and—when fibrinogen levels fall below 100 to 150 mg/dL—bleeding may ensue. Maintenance of adequate urine output and a hematocrit level greater than 30% are important components of care for women who have had a placental abruption. Either vaginal delivery or cesarean section is appropriate in the context of severe placental abruption. In a woman undergoing cesarean section after abruption, the platelet count should be maintained at 50,000/μL or above through platelet transfusion and fibrinogen replaced with FFP or cryoprecipitate.

Amniotic fluid embolism is a rare but often lethal condition with a mortality rate of approximately 80%.[133] About 10% to 15% of these patients develop a coagulopathy. DIC in this setting most likely follows the release of thromboplastin-rich material into the maternal circulation. DIC seen in association with uterine rupture and intrauterine fetal demise presumably occurs through a similar mechanism.[134] On the contrary, bacterial endotoxin or exotoxin mediates sepsis-associated DIC in pregnant women with pyelonephritis, chorioamnionitis, endometritis, or septic abortion.[135] On rare occasions, elective abortions that use hypertonic solution and those complicated by hemorrhage can be associated with DIC.[136]

Acute fatty liver of pregnancy, or acute yellow atrophy, occurs in one of every 5000 to 10,000 pregnancies, most often in the third trimester of primiparous women.[137] Maternal and fetal mortality are 5% and 15%, respectively. Although the pathogenesis of AFLP is not clear, microvesicular fatty infiltration of the liver's central zone is observed and presumably plays a central role in the development of this disease.[138] In some cases, fatty infiltration can be detected by ultrasonography or computed tomography (CT).[139] Patients present with a variety of symptoms, including malaise, fatigue, right upper quadrant pain, dyspnea, and mental status changes. Laboratory findings include abnormal liver function test results consistent with cholestatic disease, elevated ammonia, low fibrinogen and antithrombin levels, and elevated prothrombin time, with evidence of DIC. Hepatic dysfunction can impair gluconeogenesis. Diabetes insipidus may be present. The clinical course of AFLP resembles those of HELLP syndrome, TTP, and HUS, although the microangiopathy and thrombocytopenia are not as severe.[140] With supportive care, the condition typically resolves within 10 days after delivery.

LEUKEMIA AND LYMPHOMA

The diagnosis of hematologic malignancy during pregnancy can be incredibly traumatic for a pregnant patient and her family, and it is a treatment challenge for the physician. Although great strides have been made in the treatment of this heterogeneous group of diseases, the treatment of pregnant patients is limited because of the lack of research in this area and limited pregnancy safety data. The need to treat the patient and risk to the fetus must both be taken into account. Diagnosis can be difficult because many of the nonspecific signs that accompany these disorders, including fatigue, anemia, loss of appetite, and weight loss, can occur at various times during a normal pregnancy. Diagnostic imaging is mainly limited to ultrasonography and magnetic resonance imaging (MRI). Although the radiation dose from a CT scan is considered low, it is usually avoided. Diagnostic procedures such as bone marrow or lymph node biopsy can usually be safely performed during pregnancy.

In terms of treatment, the risk of teratogenicity from treatment appears highest during fetal organogenesis, which occurs mainly during the first trimester of pregnancy.[141] Ideal dosing is unknown, but dosing is usually based on the woman's prepregnancy weight.

In the largest study of its kind, Aviles and Neri[142] followed 84 children born to mothers with hematologic malignancies, including 29 women with acute leukemia and 38 who received treatment during the first trimester. Assessing growth and development, hematologic parameters, psychological characteristics, and cognitive function over 19 years, the authors found no significant, long-term, deleterious consequences related to treatment. The risk of childhood malignancies was not increased

Hodgkin Lymphoma

That hematologic malignancies are among the most commonly diagnosed cancers during pregnancy reflects to a large extent the relatively high incidence of Hodgkin lymphoma in women between the ages of 15 and 24 years.[143] Based on the results of several retrospective studies, Hodgkin lymphoma diagnosed during pregnancy appears to have no significant effect on pregnancy outcome.[144] A single-institution experience published by Dilek and colleagues,[145] however, highlights complications that may occur in pregnant women with Hodgkin disease because children born to three of five women with the disease had complications, including death. Remission rates and 20-year overall survival rates among women diagnosed with Hodgkin disease during pregnancy are reportedly similar to those observed in nonpregnant women with the disease.[146,147] In rare instances, Hodgkin lymphoma metastasizes to the placenta, so the placenta and newborn infant should be examined for evidence of malignancy.[148] Staging during pregnancy can be performed with CT, but MRI is preferred to reduce to exposure of the fetus to radiation.

Similar to other malignancies managed during pregnancy, treatment of women with Hodgkin disease is challenging. Generally, chemotherapy at any point in pregnancy increases the risk of an unfavorable outcome.[145] The teratogenic effects of chemotherapy and radiation during pregnancy are a primary concern. However, the standard regimen of Adriamycin, bleomycin, vinblastine, and dacarbazine does not appear to increase teratogenic risk when given in the second or third trimesters.

Non-Hodgkin lymphoma (NHL) rarely occurs during pregnancy. There are case reports and case series of women with NHL who have been successfully treated with chemotherapy during the second and third trimesters of pregnancy.[148] Alkylating agents given in the first trimester can result in fetal malformations or death,[149,150] although there are reports of children who received chemotherapy in the first trimester with no subsequent deficits.[151] Based on the available data, response and recurrence rates among women treated for NHL during pregnancy are similar to those seen in the treatment of pregnant women with Hodgkin disease

Acute and Chronic Leukemias

Treatment of acute myeloid leukemia cannot be delayed. Minimal data are available on the treatment of patients with acute leukemia, but in patients treated with chemotherapy during the first trimester, outcomes were poor. For patients in the first trimester, planned abortion should be discussed, followed by treatment with standard induction chemotherapy.[152]

Patients in the second and third trimesters should be treated immediately. There is an association of preterm delivery, IUGR, and spontaneous abortion with treatment in the second and third trimesters.[153] In terms of treatment options, daunorubicin is preferred because idarubicin has increased placental transfer. Amphotericin B is considered the antifungal of choice in pregnancy because there have been no reports of teratogenicity.[154,155] If treatment is not delayed, pregnant women can have similar outcomes as nonpregnant patients.

Among acute leukemias arising within the myeloid lineage, acute promyelocytic leukemia is unique in terms of clinical features—particularly DIC and associated bleeding complications—and therapy, which involves all-trans retinoic acid (ATRA) in conjunction with traditional chemotherapy. Concern regarding the teratogenic effects of ATRA is warranted. In the 1980s, Lammer and colleagues[156] noted an increased risk of fetal malformation after in utero exposure to the retinoid isotretinoin. And a recent case report by Carradice et al[157] describes a bleeding complication that occurred even after ATRA initiation in a pregnant woman with acute promyelocytic anemia. However, a review of 13 women treated during pregnancy with ATRA for acute promyelocytic anemia found no evidence that the agent leads to fetal malformation when used in the treatment of pregnant women.[158]

Similar concerns regarding toxicity of therapy arise in managing pregnancies conceived before and during treatment of chronic myeloid leukemia (CML). Imatinib, a small molecule inhibitor against the BCR-ABL tyrosine kinase, is the standard of care for treatment of CML. In animal studies, imatinib exhibited teratogenicity in rats and impaired spermatogenesis in dogs, monkeys, and rats.[159]

Imatinib Therapy

A 38-year-old woman with a history of chronic phase CML on imatinib therapy for 5 years becomes pregnant. She has had a complete cytogenetic response. She asks what to do about her imatinib therapy.

Imatinib is teratogenic and should not be used during pregnancy. It has been linked to spontaneous abortions and to fetal malformations including skeletal abnormalities, hydrocephalus, and exopthalmos. While there are case reports documenting fetal exposure at various stages of pregnancy without harm, it is not recommended. Case reports suggest that patients who have achieved maximal response to therapy fare better when their treatment is held for pregnancy, opposed to patients who have not achieved best response.

In a series of 19 pregnancies involving a mother or father undergoing imatinib-based therapy for CML, three pregnancies resulted in a spontaneous abortion, and two others produced children with minor malformations.[160] The remaining 13 pregnancies resulted in the delivery of a healthy child. Among mothers in this study who had previously achieved a complete hematologic remission with imatinib and interrupted therapy during pregnancy, a majority (five of nine) lost the hematologic remission. These findings highlight the important therapy-related implications for mother and fetus, which must be weighed carefully in determining an appropriate course of management (see box on Imatinib Therapy). Currently, it is recommended by specialists in the field that patients undergoing treatment with imatinib for CML use proper contraception.[160]

The Myeloproliferative Neoplasms: Essential Thrombocythemia, Polycythemia Vera, and Myelofibrosis

Essential thrombocythemia (ET) has a bimodal peak of distribution, so it is the most common myeloproliferative neoplasm (MPN) in women of childbearing age. Although evidenced-based guidelines do not exist for the management of pregnancy in this setting, more and more information regarding this topic is being reported.[161] Although some variation is seen in the rates of complications among various studies, overall, all of the studies noted a consistent increase in the rate of complications compared with pregnant women without MPN.[161] Pregnancy alone is a risk factor for thrombosis, and pregnancy confers a sixfold increase in the rate of thrombosis in pregnant patients *without* MPN. Thrombosis is a major source of morbidity and mortality in patients with MPN. It is thought that the prothrombotic state that exists in MPN is behind a majority of the morbidity that can develop during pregnancy. Thrombotic occlusion of placental circulation has been found.

In a study documenting 103 pregnancies occurring in 62 patients with MPN, the rate of live birth was 60%, and the first trimester abortion rate was 32%. Fetal complications occurred in 40% of cases and maternal complications in 9%. The risk of fetal loss for patients with ET was 3.4-fold higher than for those in the aged-matched control population.[162]

A pooled outcome analysis of 461 pregnant patients with ET demonstrated that first trimester loss occurred in 25% to 40% of patients with a live birth rate of 50% to 70%. Late pregnancy loss occurred in 10% of cases.[163] Postpartum thrombotic complications occurred in 5.2% of patients. In a recent analysis of all publications of pregnant patients with ET that had more than 30 patients per study, a mean rate of live birth obtained from the literature was 60.6% (50%-75.4%).[164]

Studies of pregnancy in the setting of polycythemia vera (PV) are much fewer and consist mainly of case reports. One of the largest studies to date consisted of 18 pregnancies. There were 11 live births and seven miscarriages.[165] First trimester loss is the most frequent complication in patients with PV.[164] Information regarding pregnancy in PMF is even more sparse, with overall fewer than 20 cases reported in the literature. However, based on these, fetal loss is common.[166] In women of childbearing age with an MPN, a discussion when the patient is not pregnant should occur, outlining pregnancy management and risks. Women should be informed if they are taking a drug with teratogenic potential, and the risk of unplanned pregnancy should be recognized.

Continuing aspirin is considered standard if there is no clear contraindication, extrapolating from the results of the ECLAP study, which confirmed the importance of aspirin in the management of MPN.[167] Certain features may confer a patient at more risk of maternal or fetal complications during pregnancy. These include cardiovascular risk factors, prior thrombosis, and prior pregnancy-related complications that may have been caused by MPN or for which no other cause can be identified. In these settings, cytoreductive therapy or LMWH can be considered. There are no clear evidence-based management guidelines in these settings, but local practice is to use LMWH. It is clear that management of these patients requires close collaboration with a hematologist and high-risk obstetrician.

BLEEDING DISORDERS

von Willebrand Disease

Affecting approximately 1% of the population, von Willebrand disease (vWD) is the most common inherited disorder of coagulation. By mediating platelet adhesion and functioning as a carrier for circulating factor VIII, vWF plays a vital role in hemostasis. According to the most widely used classification by Sadler,[168] there are three types of vWD: type 1 (partial deficiency of vWF); type 3 (severe deficiency of vWF); and type 2, which includes four subtypes that involve qualitative defects in vWF. Factor VIIIc, vWF antigen (vWF : Ag), and the ristocetin cofactor activity (vWF : Rock) are important components of the laboratory diagnosis. vWD does not impair fertility or increase the likelihood of miscarriage.[169] Thus the management of pregnancy in patients with the condition is an important feature of the overall care for these individuals.

For pregnant women with vWD, bleeding at parturition and in the postpartum period is of primary concern. Related concerns include the administration of anesthesia, perineal hematoma, episiotomy blood loss and healing, and bleeding at surgical sites. Approximately 75% of women with moderate to severe vWD experience significant peripartum bleeding.[170] And overall, there is a 20% risk of postpartum hemorrhage in women with vWD. In a normal pregnancy, FVIIIc and vWF levels increase, beginning in the second trimester.[171] They peak as the pregnancy nears term. Among many pregnant women with vWD, particularly those with type 1 disease, a similar increase in FVIII and vWF levels is observed. Factor VIIIc levels in pregnant women with vWD peak at 29 to 32 weeks' gestation, but vWF : Ag levels peak at approximately 35 weeks' gestation.[172] The risk of peripartum bleeding is related to the level of these factors.[173] In most instances, vWF : Ag, factor VIIIc, and vWF : RCo levels should be assessed during the first and third trimesters to determine the bleeding risk for individuals with vWD. However, this may be less relevant for patients with type 3 vWD, wherein levels tend to remain low throughout pregnancy. Patients without a documented bleeding disorder who have bleeding complications during pregnancy should be evaluated for vWD because many with the disorder have a mild clinical course and remain undiagnosed for a long period.[174]

As a general rule, therapy can be rendered either in the setting of a spontaneous bleeding event or in a prophylactic context for the high-risk individual. Mainstays of therapy for pregnant women with vWD include DDAVP (1-deamino-8-D-arginine-vasopressin; desmopressin), a synthetic analogue of vasopressin, and vWF-FVIII concentrates (Humate-P, Alphanate). Cryoprecipitate can be used on an emergent basis if vWF–FVIII concentrates are unavailable but is avoided if possible during pregnancy because it poses a small risk of bloodborne infection.[175] Although antifibrinolytic therapy plays a role in the management of individuals with vWD, it is also generally avoided during pregnancy and lactation because of its potential teratogenicity and effects on newborns. Data concerning the toxicity of antifibrinolytic therapy in pregnancy are limited.

Exerting its effect through the type 2 vasopressin receptors, DDAVP rapidly and transiently increases levels of factor VIII and vWF.[176] It is administered by continuous intravenous infusion over 30 minutes in the setting of an acute bleeding event. On a prophylactic basis, it can be given subcutaneously or inhaled nasally.[177] Although highly effective when used in an appropriate clinical context, DDAVP does have limitations. Patients who have never received DDAVP therapy should be tested for responsiveness to the agent during the second trimester. Because of its potential oxytocic effect, DDAVP is pregnancy risk category B.[178] Owing to its antidiuretic effect, DDAVP can cause fluid retention and hyponatremia. Finally, DDAVP has uncertain utility in the management of women with type 2 and type 3 vWD because of an underlying genetic defect in these individuals. VWF–factor VIII concentrate is indicated for these patients.

Multidisciplinary care by an experienced obstetrician and hematologist should be provided for pregnant women with vWD. This becomes particularly important as parturition nears. In providing care for this population of patients, clinicians aim to control disease effects in the pregnant and postpartum mother. Factor VIIIc and vWF : RCo levels, PTT, type and crossmatch, and a complete blood count are obtained at the time of hospital admission. Women with vWD should be monitored for bleeding at the time of delivery, with transfusional products and DDAVP available for use as needed. vWF : RCo and factor VIIIc levels of 50 IU/dL generally serve as a target at parturition and in the postpartum period; expert opinion suggests that women with levels below this should receive replacement products.[178]

In the management of pregnant women with vWD, the provision of regional anesthesia during delivery is an important topic. Some anesthesiologists use epidural anesthesia in patients with mild disease with or without the use of DDAVP.[179,180] For patients with moderate to severe disease, an alternative form of analgesia may be considered. If epidural analgesia is used in a patient with moderate to severe disease, prophylactic therapy is indicated. The epidural catheter should be removed soon after delivery because falling factor levels in the postpartum period increase the bleeding risk.[176]

The route of delivery is also an important matter in patients with vWD. To minimize the risk of neonatal hemorrhage, some obstetricians recommend cesarean delivery for patients with type 2, type 3, and clinically moderate type 1 disease. However, neonatal bleeding occurs in the setting of cesarean delivery as well, and delivery methods have not been rigorously compared.[170,179]

Prenatal testing is a challenge in women with vWD. The specific mutations involved in the pathogenesis of type 1 and type 3 vWD are not known. And multiple mutations are involved in the pathogenesis of type 2 vWD. Fetal blood vWF levels can be obtained if necessary, but inherent risks are associated with the procedure.[181] Expectant mothers should be informed of these risks in making decisions about prenatal genetic testing.

HEMOPHILIAS

The hemophilias (A and B) are X-linked recessive diseases characterized by hemarthrosis and subcutaneous and intramuscular bleeding.[182] Hemophilia A results from deficient production of factor VIII, and hemophilia B, from deficient production of factor IX. As X-linked disorders, hemophilia A and B occur most often in men, but they can occur in women under several circumstances, including X-chromosome inactivation (lyonization), X hemizygosity, and double heterozygosity as can occur in the female offspring of an affected father and carrier mother.[182] In the United States, women account for 1.7% of patients with hemophilia A and 3.2% of patients with hemophilia B.[183] Fifty percent of male offspring from a female carrier inherit the disorder, whereas 100% of male offspring from an affected mother inherit the disease. Female carriers in both disorders can be detected through laboratory screening and pedigree analysis.[184] Women with hemophilia and pregnant women with an affected fetus must be monitored closely during pregnancy for bleeding events that compromise the well-being of either the mother or fetus. Fetal umbilical blood sampling can be used to check factor VIII and factor IX levels. Chorionic villus sampling may also be used.[185]

At parturition, women with hemophilia A whose factor VIIIc level lies below 50% of the normal range should receive purified factor VIII. Levels should be greater than 80% for surgery and maintained at 30% to 40% for 3 to 4 days postoperatively. Rarely, thrombosis can occur in the aftermath of factor VIII replacement therapy.[186] Six to 10% of neonates with hemophilia have hemorrhagic complications in the perinatal period, including intracranial hemorrhage. Vacuum extractors, forceps delivery, and scalp electrodes should be avoided. To date, no studies have rigorously compared vaginal and cesarean delivery in this patient population. Neonatal blood should be assayed for factor VIIIc levels and PTT immediately after birth. Neonates with low factor VIIIc levels may require serial cranial ultrasounds to rule out bleeding.[187]

Hemophilia B is treated in a similar fashion. However, it should be noted that cryoprecipitate contains low levels of factor IX and should not be used as replacement therapy in the management of this condition. Purified factor IX is the agent of choice for patients with hemophilia B. Meanwhile, individuals with other clotting factor deficiencies should receive fresh frozen plasma or specific clotting factor products to maintain factor levels at greater than 25%.[188] One exception to this pertains to the management of patients with factor XIII deficiency; the occurrence of spontaneous recurrent abortions and uterine bleeding in these individuals necessitates regular infusions of fresh frozen plasma or factor XIII concentrate to maintain pregnancy.[189]

Table 153-2 Hemostatic Changes in Pregnancy

Factor XIII	↑/↓
Protein C, antithrombin	=
Protein S	↓
Factor XI	↓/ =
Factors V, VII, VIII, IX, X, XII	↑
von Willebrand factor, fibrinogen	↑
Tissue plasminogen activator	↓
Prothrombin, D-dimer	↑

Bleeding Associated With Factor XI Deficiency

A 25-year-old female is referred for prolonged PTT discovered during pregnancy. Evaluation reveals severe factor XI deficiency. She has no history of easy bruising or bleeding. She is at 30 weeks' gestation and is here for evaluation prior to delivery.

Bleeding associated with factor XI deficiency can be quite variable, ranging from no bleeding symptoms to bleeding associated with trauma or surgery. For a patient without a history of bleeding, prophylaxis is not necessary but fresh frozen plasma should be available if needed. Epidural is usually contraindicated in patients with severe factor XI deficiency, and women should be advised to speak with the treating anesthesiologist prior to delivery in order to plan alternative strategies. If consideration for regional block anesthesia is made, it is usually administered with FFP prior and with documentation of normalization of the PTT.

In patients with a bleeding history, FFP should be administered prior to delivery, as well as 2 to 3 days later to reduce the risk of delayed hemorrhage.

VENOUS THROMBOEMBOLIC DISEASE AND PREGNANCY

Venous thromboembolic (VTE) disease is a leading cause of maternal morbidity and mortality.[189] The risk of VTE increases two- to fourfold during pregnancy and the early postpartum period.[190] In women who have had a previous VTE event, pregnancy appears to increase the risk of a recurrent thromboembolic event.[191] Various factors account for the prothrombotic state associated with pregnancy. Increased estrogen levels early in pregnancy increase venous distention and contribute to venous stasis.[192] Increased plasma volume and compression of the inferior vena cava by the gravid uterus contribute to venous stasis as well.[193] In addition, studies have demonstrated decreased blood flow velocity in pregnant women, particularly in the left leg when pregnant women lie in a supine position. This phenomenon likely explains the increased risk of left leg thrombosis among pregnant women.[194] Furthermore, whereas the concentration of coagulation factors changes during pregnancy, the concentration of vWF, fibrinogen, and prothrombin, along with factors V, VII, VIII, IX, X, and XII increases, and the concentration of factor XI and protein S decreases (Table 153-2).[195–197] Finally, fibrinolytic activity decreases during pregnancy as the levels of plasminogen activator inhibitors 1 and 2 increase.[198] Other factors—including high body mass index, smoking, immobilization, and age older than 35 years—should also be considered when assessing the thrombotic risk of a pregnant woman (see box on Bleeding Associated With Factor XI Deficiency).

Because of the prothrombotic physiology associated with pregnancy, a clinician's concern for VTE in a pregnant woman should prompt immediate evaluation. To assess for lower extremity thrombosis, venous compression ultrasonography remains the initial test of choice. Ultrasonography poses no threat to the fetus and can detect thrombosis of the proximal common femoral and popliteal veins with a sensitivity of 95% and specificity of 96%. Despite the efficacy of ultrasonography, limitations to its use do exist. The test is less effective for the diagnosis of calf vein thrombosis, with a sensitivity and specificity in the 60% to 70% range.[199] For this reason, a woman with suspected lower extremity deep venous thrombosis should undergo serial ultrasonography if the initial evaluation is nondiagnostic.[200] Similarly, thrombus in the common iliac vein can evade diagnosis by venous compression ultrasonography.

In such cases, other modalities such as contrast venography and magnetic resonance venography (MRV) can be considered. Although contrast venography exposes the fetus to radiation and should thus be used with caution during pregnancy, its use may be warranted when clinical suspicion for an underlying thrombotic event is high.[199] Serum D-dimer tests are often used in conjunction with imaging studies to assess for thrombosis in nonpregnant patients. The sensitivity of D-dimer tests for the presence of thrombus ranges from 85% to 95%.[201] However, several pregnancy-associated conditions elevate D-dimer levels, including preterm labor, placental abruption, and hypertension of pregnancy, thus undermining the utility of the test somewhat in pregnant women by decreasing its specificity.[198] Nonetheless, when normal, the D-dimer assay provides the clinician with useful information.

When lower extremity imaging reveals no evidence of thrombus in a pregnant woman with suspected pulmonary embolism (PE), the clinician has several options. Helical CT has become the standard modality for the diagnosis of PE in nonpregnant individuals at many centers. However, even with abdominal shielding, the procedure results in fetal radiation exposure (≈16 mrad) because of internal scatter.[202] Although this low level of radiation exposure probably does not cause harm to the fetus, repeated imaging during the course of pregnancy is to be avoided.[200] Ventilation/perfusion (V/Q) scanning is frequently used in the evaluation of pregnant women with suspected PE but has limitations as well. Results of a prospective study indicate that when used in this patient population, V/Q scanning infrequently yields a conclusively positive result (1.8% of cases) and is often nondiagnostic (24.8% of cases).[203] Finally, pulmonary angiography can be used in the evaluation of PE in rare instances when the previously described diagnostic tests yield nondiagnostic results in the face of a high clinical suspicion.

Venous thromboembolism in pregnancy is treated with heparin. Until LMWH was introduced in the late 1980s, unfractionated heparin (UFH) was the anticoagulant of choice for treatment of pregnant women with VTE. Because it does not cross the placenta, UFH is nonteratogenic. However, drawbacks to UFH therapy, including heparin-associated osteoporosis, heparin-induced thrombocytopenia (HIT), and the drug's unpredictable pharmacokinetics, are well documented.[189] Heparin-associated osteoporosis can develop in women who receive at least 1 month of therapy; it is likely related to a toxic effect of heparin on osteoblasts.[204] Because of its more favorable side effect profile, reliable pharmacokinetics, and equal efficacy in treating VTE, LMWH now represents the most commonly used anticoagulant for treatment of VTE in pregnancy.[205] The risk of osteoporosis and HIT appears to be less with LMWH-based anticoagulation than with UFH-based anticoagulation.[206,207] Although practice patterns vary, it is reasonable to base the initial dose of LMWH on early pregnancy—rather than current—weight.[207] Because clearance of LMWH increases during pregnancy, twice-daily dosing regimens are preferred to once-daily regimens.[208] In terms of duration of therapeutic anticoagulation, many clinicians continue therapy at full dose through the entire pregnancy and puerperium based on the rationale that pregnancy itself represents a risk factor for recurrent VTE.[205] In contrast, other clinicians advocate initial anticoagulation with full-dose LMWH for a designated period followed by conversion to an intermediate dose. This approach may be beneficial for individuals susceptible to side effects of anticoagulation such as bleeding or osteoporosis.[189] The risk of significant bleeding with LMWH during pregnancy is estimated to be around 2%.

Warfarin is contraindicated in pregnant women. It crosses the placenta and can cause both fetal hemorrhage and nervous system abnormalities and other teratogenic effects.[209] Warfarin can be used in the postpartum period after initiating therapy with concurrent heparin and in this setting does not appear to increase the risk of bleeding in children of lactating mothers.[199]

Anticoagulation should be discontinued at the time of parturition. UFH and LMWH should, in most circumstances, be stopped 12 to 24 hours before delivery. If the risk of recurrent VTE is particularly high in a woman receiving LMWH, the clinician can convert to intravenous UFH and treat until 4 to 6 hours before delivery, minimizing the time off anticoagulation.

The risks of regional anesthesia must be weighed carefully in women receiving anticoagulation because therapy increases the likelihood of bleeding, hematoma formation, and potential neurologic compromise. In a woman undergoing elective delivery with discontinuation of anticoagulation 12 to 24 hours prior, epidural anesthesia may be used. UFH or LMWH may be reinitiated 6 to 12 hours after delivery or after removal of the epidural catheter. Then, after therapeutic levels of UFH or LMWH have been achieved, warfarin may be initiated.

PROPHYLACTIC ANTICOAGULATION DURING PREGNANCY

Given the prothrombotic state associated with pregnancy itself, prophylactic anticoagulation should be considered in pregnant women with a history of VTE. Recurrence rates for VTE during pregnancy may be as high as 12% based on the results of retrospective studies.[210] Conversely, Brill-Edwards and colleagues[211] prospectively studied 125 pregnant women with prior VTE in a study that excluded women with known thrombophilia. Study subjects did not receive prophylactic anticoagulation during the antenatal period, but did receive anticoagulation therapy for 4 to 6 weeks postpartum. The authors documented a VTE recurrence rate of 2.4%. Women who had a temporary risk factor at the time of their initial VTE event and lacked laboratory evidence of an underlying hypercoagulable disorder at the time of study enrollment experienced no recurrences during pregnancy. Based on the results of this study, routine prophylactic anticoagulation for women with a single previous VTE event is not recommended. However, patients with a known hypercoagulable state, those with multiple previous VTE events, and those considered high risk for recurrent VTE should receive prophylactic anticoagulation during pregnancy and for 4 to 6 weeks postpartum. As previously discussed, prophylactic anticoagulation can be discontinued at parturition and reinitiated 6 to 12 hours postpartum.

The management of pregnant women with prosthetic heart valves is controversial and deserves special attention, although a full review of the topic is beyond the scope of this review. Coupled with the prothrombotic physiology of pregnancy, the presence of a prosthetic valve places such women in an ultra-high risk category. Before the introduction of LMWH, options for anticoagulation in this patient population included (1) warfarin throughout pregnancy, (2) warfarin with UFH during weeks 6 to 12, the period of major organogenesis, and (3) UFH throughout pregnancy.[189] More recently, LMWH has been used in this setting, although its safety and efficacy have been questioned on the basis of several studies. Overall, a lack of rigorous, comparative studies hinders evidence-based management of women with prosthetic heart valves. Current recommendations allow for one of three therapeutic strategies, initiated after a thorough discussion of risks and benefits with the patient: (1) warfarin, with LMWH or UFH substituted during weeks 6 to 12, (2) dose-adjusted UFH throughout pregnancy, or (3) dose-adjusted LMWH throughout pregnancy.[189]

THROMBOPHILIA AND PREGNANCY

Thrombophilias, inherited and acquired, increase the risk of VTE in pregnant women and adversely affect pregnancy outcomes. Included within this category of diseases are factor V Leiden, prothrombin gene polymorphisms, antiphospholipid antibody syndrome, antithrombin deficiency, and protein S and C deficiency. In addition, hyperhomocysteinemia and methylenetetrahydrofolate reductase C677T mutation have been studied. There are varied results when assessing the literature in regards to the risk of pregnancy-associated VTE in the setting of an inherited thrombophilia. A meta-analysis in 2005 reviewed the risk of VTE during pregnancy by the specific thrombophilia present. The inherited thrombophilias (with the exception of *MTHFR* mutation) were associated with a statistically significant increase in the risk of VTE during pregnancy.[212] But because the overall incidence of VTE in pregnancy is low, in women without a history of thrombosis, the absolute risk conferred by thrombophilias is generally low. The positive predictive value of factor V Leiden heterozygosity was one in 500. Prothrombin heterozygosity was one in 200. Women with homozygosity for these mutations, double heterozygosity and antithrombin III deficiency were at highest risk. Given the increased risk of VTE in those particular settings, aggressive management with prophylactic anticoagulation is warranted.

Screening for inherited thrombophilia in patients with recurrent miscarriage or pregnancy complications such as preeclampsia or placental abruption is not indicated. Thrombophilia screening is only indicated in patients with a prior thromboembolic event or a high likelihood of thrombophilia. Selective screening based on personal and family history is recommended (see box on Thrombophilia During Pregnancy).

Prophylactic treatment of carriers of low-risk mutations with any personal or family history of VTE is not indicated. In patients with recurrent miscarriage, anticoagulation has been used in efforts to improve rates of live birth. There have been varied results in clinical trials using anticoagulation in the setting of recurrent miscarriage. However, in the large, multicenter, randomized, placebo-controlled study examining the use of aspirin or aspirin plus heparin in women with unexplained miscarriage, there was no improvement in the live birth rate compared with placebo.[213]

Thrombophilia During Pregnancy

A 25-year-old female wishes to become pregnant. Her mother suffered from a PE at the age of 60, underwent thrombophilia evaluation, and was found to be heterozygous for the factor V Leiden mutation. She herself has never suffered thrombotic episode, just recently discontinued her birth control, and was told to see a hematologist before she became pregnant. Her primary care physician tested her for Factor V Leiden and she is heterozygous for the mutation. She is asking if she should be on anticoagulation during her pregnancy.

Every case of thrombophilia during pregnancy needs to be assessed on a case by case basis. Asymptomatic women who harbor thrombophilic conditions, but have never manifested clinical manifestations, do not require anticoagulation. In women with a personal history of thrombosis an inherited thrombophilia, anticoagulation during and in the postpartum setting should be used.

Table 153-3 Antiphospholipid Antibody Syndrome

Vascular Thrombosis
One or more episodes of arterial or venous thrombosis confirmed by imaging
Pregnancy Morbidity
Death of a fetus beyond 10 weeks' gestation with normal fetal morphology
Premature birth before 34 weeks' gestation
Three or more consecutive spontaneous abortions before 10 weeks' gestation
Laboratory Criteria (All Measured on Two or More Occasions at Least 12 Weeks Apart)
Lupus anticoagulant on two or more occasions at least 12 weeks apart
Anticardiolipin antibody
Anti-B2 glycoprotein IgM or IgG

Ig, Immunoglobulin.

Antiphospholipid Antibody Syndrome

The antiphospholipid antibody syndrome (Table 153-3) is the most common form of acquired thrombophilia.[214] Antiphospholipid antibodies include lupus anticoagulant antibodies and anticardiolipin antibodies. They can occur as a manifestation of various conditions, such as systemic lupus erythematosus (SLE) and other rheumatic diseases, infection, and drug reactions. Antiphospholipid antibodies exert their prothrombotic effect through several mechanisms. For example, they inhibit the activity of anticoagulants thrombomodulin, protein S, protein C, β2-glycoprotein I, and prostacyclin.[215-217] They interact with phospholipids on the surface of platelets, increasing platelet adhesiveness and production of von Willebrand mulitmers.[218,219] And in pregnant patients, antiphospholipid antibodies decrease levels of annexin V, a potent vascular endothelial anticoagulant produced by placental trophoblasts.[220] Nonpregnant individuals with antiphospholipid antibody syndrome can develop arterial and venous thromboses. In pregnant women, antiphospholipid antibody syndrome can manifest as thrombotic events, spontaneous abortion, preeclampsia, and HELLP syndrome, as well as IUGR.[221-224]

Antiphospholipid antibodies can be detected in 5% of healthy pregnant women and 37% of pregnant women with SLE.[225] Thrombotic events occur in approximately 5% of pregnant women with antiphospholipid antibodies.[224] All pregnant women with SLE should undergo testing for antiphospholipid antibodies. Women who sustain recurrent spontaneous abortions or a thromboembolic event during pregnancy should also undergo evaluation for the disorder. A history of either vascular thrombosis or fetal loss coupled with the presence of either lupus anticoagulant antibodies or anticardiolipin antibodies establishes the diagnosis of antiphospholipid antibody syndrome.[226]

False-negative laboratory results do occur and do so more frequently in pregnant than in nonpregnant women. This may be because of the increased concentration of clotting factors observed in pregnancy.[227] Women with antiphospholipid antibody syndrome who have sustained prior thrombotic events receive therapeutic anticoagulation during pregnancy. Those with antiphospholipid antibodies but no manifestations of the clinical syndrome should receive prophylactic anticoagulation.

FUTURE DIRECTIONS

Managing of the hematologic complications of pregnancy continue to be a challenge. The physicians and patient involved all benefit from a multidisciplinary approach. In certain disorders, the management is clear and will likely remain unchanged in the future. In other disorders, treatment paradigms may shift as new treatments are discovered for the nonpregnant patient. In all instances, further well-designed studies will continue to advance evidence-based management of the pregnant patient.

SUGGESTED READINGS

Al RA, Unlubilgin E, Kandamir O, et al: Intravenous verses oral iron for treatment of anemia in pregnancy: A randomized trial. *Obstet Gynecol* 106:1335, 2005.

Allen LH: Nutritional supplementation for the pregnant woman. *Clin Obstet Gynecol* 37:587, 1994.

Bothwell TH: Overview and mechanisms of iron regulation. *Nutr Rev* 53:237, 1995.

Casanueva E, Viteri FE, Mares-Galindo M, et al: Weekly iron as a safe alternative to daily supplementation for nonanemic pregnant women. *Arch Med Res* 12:674, 2006.

Centers for Disease Control: Recommendations to prevent and control iron deficiency in the United States. *MMWR* 47(No. RR-3), 1998.

Chanarin I: Folate and cobalamin. *Clin Haematol* 14:729, 1985.

Chanarin I, MacGibbon BM, O'Sullivan WJ, et al: Folic acid deficiency in pregnancy—The pathogenesis of megaloblastic anemia of pregnancy. *Lancet* 2:634, 1959.

Chanarin I, Rothman D: Further observations on the relation between iron and folate status in pregnancy. *Br Med J* 2:81, 1971.

Cogswell ME, Parvanta I, Ickes L, et al: Iron supplementation during pregnancy, anemia, and birth rate: A randomized trial. *Am J Clin Nutr* 78:773, 2003.

Council on Foods and Nutrition Committee on Iron Deficiency: Iron deficiency in the United States. *JAMA* 203:119, 1968.

Crowley J: Coagulopathy bleeding in the parturient patient. *R I Med* 72:135, 1989.

Garn SM, Ridella SA, Petzold AS, et al: Maternal hematologic levels and pregnancy outcomes. *Semin Perinatol* 5:155, 1981.

Galloway R, McGuire J: Determinants of compliance with iron supplementation: Supplies, side effects, or psychology? *Soc Sci Med* 39:381, 1994.

Hiss RG: Evaluation of the anemic patient. In Laros RK, editor: *Blood disorders in pregnancy,* Philadelphia, 1986, Lea & Febiger, p 1.

Hytten F: Blood volume changes in normal pregnancy. *Clin Haematol* 14:601, 1985.

Institute of Medicine: *Nutrition services in perinatal care,* Washington, DC, 1992, National Academy Press.

Klebanoff MA, Shiono PH, Selby JV, et al: Anemia and spontaneous preterm birth. *Am J Obstet Gynecol* 164:59, 1991.

Lieberman E, Ryan KJ, Monson RR, et al: Association of maternal hematocrit with premature labor. *Am J Obstet Gynecol* 159:107, 1988.

Lu ZM, Goldenberg RL, Oliver SP, et al: The relationship between maternal hematocrit and pregnancy outcome. *Obstet Gynecol* 77:190, 1991.

Milman N, Agger AI, Nielson OJ: Iron status markers and serum erythropoietin in 120 mothers and newborn infants: Effect of iron supplementation and normal pregnancy. *Acta Obstet Gynecol Scand* 73:200, 1994.

Milman N: Iron and pregnancy—a delicate balance. *Ann Hematol* 85:559, 2006.

Morbidity and Mortality Weekly Report: CDC criteria for anemia in children and childbearing-aged women. *MMWR Morb Mortal Wkly Rep* 38:400, 1989.

Murphy JF, O'Riordan J, Newcombe RG, et al: Relation of haemoglobin levels in first and second trimesters to outcome of pregnancy. *Lancet* 1:992, 1986.

Perry GS, Yip R, Zyrkowski C: Nutritional risk factors among low-income pregnant US women: The Centers for Disease Control and Prevention (CDC) Pregnancy Nutrition Surveillance System, 1979 through 1993. *Semin Perinatol* 19:211, 1995.

Romslo I, Haram K, Sagen N, et al: Iron requirement in normal pregnancy as assessed by serum ferritin, serum transferring saturation, and erythrocyte protoporphyrin determinations. *Br J Obstet Gynaecol* 90:101, 1983.

Rothman D: Folic acid in pregnancy. *Am J Obstet Gynecol* 108:149, 1970.

Singh K, Fong YF, Arulkumaran S: Anaemia in pregnancy—a cross-sectional study in Singapore. *Eur J Clin Nutr* 52:65, 1998.

Scholl TO, Hediger ML: Anemia and iron deficiency anemia: Complication of data on pregnancy outcome. *Am J Clin Nutr* 59:492S, 1994.

Scholl TO, Hediger ML, Fischer RL, et al: Anemia vs iron deficiency: Increased risk of preterm delivery in a prospective study. *Am J Clin Nutr* 55:985, 1992.

World Health Organization: *The prevalence of anaemia in women: A tabulation of available information,* ed 2, Geneva, 1992, World Health Organization.

Zhou LM, Yang WW, Hua JZ, et al: Relation of hemoglobin measured at different times in pregnancy to preterm birth and low birth weight in Shanghai, China. *Am J Epidemiol* 148:998, 1998.

For complete list of references log on to www.expertconsult.com.

CHAPTER 154

HEMATOLOGIC MANIFESTATIONS OF CHILDHOOD ILLNESS

Arthur Kim Ritchey, Frank G. Keller, and Sarah H. O'Brien

The hematologic response to systemic illness in children is similar to that in adults. A number of disorders occur more frequently in children, however, and some are unique to the pediatric population. In addition, interpretation of the hematologic response is predicated on knowledge of the normal developmental changes that occur within the hematopoietic system throughout childhood (Table 154-1). This chapter focuses on the hematologic manifestations of common or unique systemic diseases that occur in neonates, children, and adolescents. Illnesses that often require hematologic consultation are emphasized. Systemic diseases that produce hematologic abnormalities that are similar in adults and children are discussed in other chapters (see Chapters 155 to 160). For a comprehensive review of the subject, readers are referred to a published textbook.[1]

INFECTIOUS DISEASE

Infection, especially viral infection, is the most common problem encountered by pediatricians. Although most infections do not produce significant hematologic sequelae, all classes of microorganisms have been implicated in the pathogenesis of hematologic abnormalities that range from mild and clinically irrelevant to severe and life threatening. This section describes the changes seen in red blood cells (RBCs), white blood cells (WBCs), platelets, and the coagulation system that are routinely encountered, are associated with a specific infection, or have a potentially serious clinical impact.

Changes in Red Blood Cells

The anemia of chronic inflammation or infection in children is similar to that seen in adults in terms of both clinical and hematologic findings and pathogenesis.[2] However, anemia with acute infections occurs more commonly in children than in adults.

Anemia of Acute Infections

A mild to moderate anemia of uncertain etiology may occur in the setting of both acute viral infections and more serious bacterial infections. In a study of children with mild viral or bacterial infections in the outpatient setting, anemia was documented in 5% of children 4 to 12 years of age, 17% of children 6 months to 4 years of age, and 33% of infants 6 to 11 months of age.[3] In 14 of 15 young children, the anemia resolved within 3 to 4 weeks. However, multiple mild infections may predispose infants to the development of a more chronic, mild anemia or low-normal hemoglobin that may be caused by iron deficiency, thus warranting a trial of iron supplementation.

Among children hospitalized with moderately severe inflammatory processes, the incidence of mild anemia (hemoglobin, 10.1-11.0 g/dL) is as high as 78%.[4] In a study of hospitalized children with either pyelonephritis bacteremia, average age 5 to 6 years, 60% had anemia.[5] No evidence of hemolysis was seen in this group of children. Follow-up hemoglobin in a subset of patients returned to normal without specific intervention. These data suggest that there is no indication to investigate the mild anemia of acute infection. Specific acute bacterial infections associated with a high incidence of anemia (44%-74%) include bone and joint infections, typhoid fever, brucellosis, and invasive *Haemophilus influenzae* infections.

The anemia associated with *H. influenzae* meningitis has been the most thoroughly studied of the anemias of acute infection. A majority of children with *H. influenzae* meningitis have mild anemia on admission, with hemoglobin in the 9 to 11 g/dL range, and up to 90% become anemic during the course of the illness.[6] This is in contrast with meningitis secondary to *Streptococcus pneumoniae* or *Neisseria meningitidis,* in which anemia is uncommon. The pathophysiology of the anemia of *H. influenzae* disease appears to be multifactorial. Shurin and associates[7] have shown that *H. influenzae* capsular polysaccharide, polyribosyl ribitol phosphate, binds to erythrocytes, which, in the presence of antibody and complement, can result in intravascular and extravascular hemolysis. They further hypothesize that polyribosyl ribitol phosphate alone may induce more rapid clearance of RBCs, perhaps on the basis of decreased RBC deformability. In addition, hypoferremia may limit bone marrow response to hemolysis.

Acute Hemolytic Anemia

Acute hemolysis has been observed with infections from all classes of microorganisms but is relatively uncommon. The anemia may be mild to severe, and the condition is manifested in children in either of two ways: (1) clinical presentation with symptoms and signs of infection predominating in a child subsequently found to have anemia or (2) clinical presentation with the manifestations of acute hemolytic anemia.

The mechanism of hemolysis in patients presenting with an infectious disorder depends on the infecting organism, but in most cases, hemolysis is extravascular.[8] Reported mechanisms include the following:

- Release of hemolysins (*Clostridium perfringens* sepsis)
- Invasion of the RBC (malaria)
- Alteration of the RBC surface:
  - Direct adherence by the organism (*Bartonella* spp.)
  - Alterations of antigenic phenotype by neuraminidase (influenza virus)
  - Cold agglutinins (*Mycoplasma* spp., *Listeria* spp., Epstein-Barr virus [EBV], *Leptospira* spp., *Rubella* spp.[8])
  - Absorption of capsular polysaccharide *(H. influenzae)*
- Mechanical mechanisms (microangiopathy associated with disseminated intravascular coagulation [DIC] or hemolytic uremic syndrome [HUS])
- Oxidative damage in persons with congenital enzyme deficiencies (e.g., hepatitis or brucellosis[9] with glucose-6-phosphate dehydrogenase [G6PD] deficiency, *Campylobacter jejuni* infection in neonates)

Acute, infection-associated hemolytic anemia in one study lagged behind the clinical infection by 3 to 7 days.[10] Most children were shown to have adsorption of microbial antigens to the RBC surface,

Table 154-1 Normal Hematologic Values in Childhood

									White Cells		Coagulation			
	Hb (g/dL)		RBCs Hct (%)		MCV (fl)		Total (×10³/μL)		Neutrophils (%)	Lymphocytes (%)	PT (sec)*		aPTT (sec)*	
Age	**Mean**	**(Range)**	**Mean**	**(Range)**	**Mean**	**(Range)**	**Mean**	**(Range)**	**Mean**	**Mean**	**Mean**	**(Range)**	**Mean**	**(Range)**
Birth (term)	18.5	(14.5-22.5)	56	(45-69)	108	(95-121)	18.1	(9.3-30.0)	61	31	16	(13-20)	55	(45-65)
2 mo	11.2	(9.4-14.0)	35	(28-42)	96	(77-115)								
6 mo-2 years	12.5	(11.0-14.0)	37	(33-41)	77	(70-84)	11.3	(6.0-17.5)	32	61				
2-6 yr	12.5	(11.5-13.5)	37	(34-40)	81	(75-87)	8.5	(5.0-15.5)	42	50				
6-12 yr	13.5	(11.5-15.5)	40	(35-45)	86	(77-95)	8.1	(4.5-13.5)	53	39				
12-18 yr							7.8	(4.5-13.5)	57	35				
Male	14.5	(13.0-16.0)	43	(37-49)	88	(78-98)								
Female	14.0	(12.0-16.0)	41	(36-46)	90	(78-102)								

Data from Rudolph AM, Hoffman JIE, eds: *Pediatrics,* ed 17, East Norwalk, Conn, Appleton-Century-Crofts, 1982, p 1036, and from Nathan DG, Oski FA, eds: *Hematology of infancy and childhood,* ed 3, Philadelphia, WB Saunders, 1987, p 1679.
aPTT, Activated partial thromboplastin time; *Hb,* hemoglobin; *Hct,* hematocrit; *MCV,* mean corpuscular volume; *PT,* prothrombin time; *RBC,* red blood cell.
*The normal range for the PT and APTT varies between laboratories. The time at which normal adult values are attained is 1 week for the PT and 2 to 9 months for the APTT. The platelet count is within the adult range from birth.

suggesting an "innocent bystander" mechanism of erythrocyte sensitization, ultimately leading to hemolysis. A minority of patients in this series had classic autoantibody-mediated hemolytic anemia.

Autoimmune hemolytic anemia (AIHA) in children usually is transient, is not associated with underlying systemic disease, and carries a low mortality rate. Children frequently have a history of concurrent or recently resolved infection, especially viral upper respiratory tract infection. Anti-cytomegalovirus (CMV) immunoglobulin G (IgG) has been implicated as the cause of acute AIHA in infants with CMV disease. Although mycoplasma pneumonia is usually associated with cold agglutinin syndrome, there is a report of multiple episodes of warm antibody-mediated hemolytic anemia in a child with Down syndrome.[11] Parvovirus has been rarely associated with AIHA. In some, but not all, cases, the Donath-Landsteiner antibody was identified.[12] In the typical acute, transient cases, 59% to 68% of children have a history of recent infection, but only 0% to 20% of those with the less common chronic course have such a history of infection.

Aplastic Crisis

Temporary arrest of RBC production has been observed in children with infections, but anemia is uncommon because of the long RBC lifespan. In two situations, however, severe anemia has been linked with infection and cessation of erythropoiesis: (1) B19 parvovirus infection in patients with an underlying hemolytic anemia and (2) transient erythroblastopenia of childhood.

The B19 parvovirus has been a known pathogen in animals for years but has only recently been linked with human disease.[13] It is the etiologic agent of fifth disease (erythema infectiosum), a mild illness with a characteristic "slapped cheek" facial erythema and a generalized reticular rash. In normal volunteers infected with B19 parvovirus, a mild, transient, and clinically irrelevant drop in the hemoglobin and reticulocyte count was observed.[14] In normal children, this infection usually is not associated with hematologic abnormalities, although reports of both hematologic and nonhematologic effects are increasing.[15] In children with sickle cell disease, spherocytosis, and other hemolytic anemias, B19 parvovirus infection can produce a severe anemia associated with peripheral reticulocytopenia and marrow erythroblastopenia—the "aplastic crisis." There may be other transient cytopenias noted during the RBC aplastic crisis.[16] Recovery within 1 to 2 weeks is the rule, but transfusion may be necessary.

B19 parvovirus infection also has been associated with prolonged anemia and reticulocytopenia in children with acute lymphoblastic leukemia (ALL) in remission, those with solid tumors receiving chemotherapy, those with immunodeficiency, those who have undergone renal transplantation, those with AIHA, and as the initial manifestation of human immunodeficiency virus (HIV) infection. Human parvovirus also has been identified as a cause of nonimmune hydrops fetalis.[17]

Transient erythroblastopenia of childhood (TEC) is a syndrome characterized by temporary arrest of RBC production with moderate to severe anemia in previously normal infants and toddlers. Although no specific infectious agent has been proved to cause TEC, the frequency of a history of infection within 1 to 3 months, the seasonal clustering, and the similarity to childhood idiopathic thrombocytopenic purpura (ITP) all suggest a possible viral etiology. B19 parvovirus has not been definitively associated with TEC.[18]

Changes in White Blood Cells

Children, as a rule, have the expected leukocyte response to infection. Infants and young children normally have a lymphocyte predominance (see Table 154-1), however, and any leukocyte response to infection must be judged on the basis of age-related normal values.

The predictive value of the peripheral WBC and differential counts in suspected bacterial infections has been extensively evaluated in infants and children. Todd has shown that in hospitalized children, a neutrophil count greater than 10,000/μL or band count greater than 500/μL is associated with an 80% chance of having a bacterial infection.[19] In children undergoing evaluation for possible meningitis, Lembo and colleagues[20] found that a ratio of immature to total neutrophils greater than 0.12 was more strongly associated with and more sensitive for bacterial meningitis than was the total WBC count or the total band count. Febrile children between the ages of 3 and 48 months are at increased risk for bacteremia, especially with *S. pneumoniae.* McCarthy and associates[21] demonstrated a threefold increase in risk of bacteremia in febrile (temperatures >40°C) children younger than 2 years of age who had a WBC count of 15,000/μL or greater. In this setting, the WBC count was a more sensitive indicator of the presence of pneumonia or bacteremia than was the absolute neutrophil or band count. The degree of leukocytosis (i.e., >25,000/mm^2 vs. <15,000/mm^2) probably has no further discriminating ability.[22] Other studies have found both the WBC count and absolute neutrophil count (ANC) to be of value in differentiating bacterial from nonbacterial infection; the band count was not helpful.

There are recognized exceptions to the anticipated leukocyte response to infection that may serve as a clue to the diagnosis. In typhoid fever and brucellosis, leukopenia and neutropenia are prominent early in the illness. Shigellosis is associated with a variable leukocyte count, but the count often is normal, with a greater percentage of bands than neutrophils. Illnesses associated with lymphocytosis include pertussis (whooping cough), infectious lymphocytosis, infectious mononucleosis, and other viral infections. Neutropenia can be seen in bacterial sepsis from meningococci, pneumococci, staphylococci, and other bacteria and is associated with a poor prognosis. Black children (and adults) normally have lower WBC and neutrophil counts than those seen in whites; leukocyte and neutrophil response to serious infection may be decreased.[23]

Neutropenia

The most common cause of neutropenia (neutrophil count <1500/μL) in children is viral infection. A number of specific viruses are associated with neutropenia, including hepatitis virus, roseola virus, rubella virus, mumps virus, adenovirus, coxsackievirus A21, EBV, human herpesvirus-6 (HHV-6), and influenza virus.[24] The most common clinical setting, however, is the incidental discovery of neutropenia in a child with a nonspecific viral syndrome. Usually the neutropenia in this situation continues for less than 30 days and is rarely associated with infectious complications. In one large study of 1888 otherwise healthy children with fever and ANCs below 1000 cells/μL, there was only a 1.3% incidence of serious bacterial infection in children older than 3 months of age (one bacteremia, 13 urinary tract infections). The risk was higher in infants younger than 3 months of age (3.3%), similar to the risk of febrile infants of the same age without neutropenia.[25] Neutropenia also has been associated with a number of bacterial, rickettsial, and fungal infections.[26]

Eosinophilia

The most common cause of eosinophilia worldwide is parasitic infection. In the United States, visceral larva migrans *(Toxocara infestation)* is the most common cause of exaggerated eosinophilia (WBC count, 30,000-100,000/μL with 50%-90% mature eosinophils) in children.[27] Mild to moderate eosinophilia (≥600/μL) is most often seen in children with allergic rhinitis or asthma but also is characteristic of Chlamydia pneumonitis in infants.

Changes in Platelets or Coagulation

Thrombocytosis

Thrombocytosis (platelet count >500,000/μL) is known as an acute-phase reaction to infection, but it has been infrequently identified in children in the past. There is a particularly high incidence of reactive thrombocytosis in patients with bacterial infections, especially pneumonia with emphysema, and *H. influenzae* meningitis. Inflammatory cytokines, such as interleukin (IL)-1, IL-6, and thrombopoietin, may play an etiologic role in the reactive thrombocytosis of infection.[28] The vast majority of children with thrombocytosis have platelet counts between 500 and 700,000/μL, but 6% to 8% have counts between 700 and 900,000/μL and only 0.5% to 3% have platelet counts above 1,000,000/μL.[29] Thrombocytosis may be more common in simple acute infections than was previously recognized. Heath and Pearson[30] documented a 13% incidence of thrombocytosis in ambulatory patients; children with an increased platelet count were more likely to have a diagnosis of infection. In a Japanese study of more than 7500 hospitalized patients with platelet counts greater than 15,000, 6% of patients had thrombocytosis with an age-dependent incidence: 12.5% in neonates, 35.8% in 1-month-old babies, 12.9% in 6- to 12-month-old infants, then decreasing to 0.6% in 11- to 15-year-old children. Infection was the cause of the thrombocytosis in 67.5% of the cases.[31] Complications of reactive thrombocytosis are rare, but hemorrhagic or thrombotic complications may occur if there are additional acquired risk factors. Antiplatelet therapy is not indicated in patients with reactive thrombocytosis secondary to infection. Although the most common cause of thrombocytosis in children is infection, the list of considerations in the differential diagnosis of an elevated platelet count is extensive[32] and rarely includes underlying childhood malignancy.

Thrombocytopenia

Thrombocytopenia can be seen in patients who have infections with all types of organisms. Common viral agents include varicella virus, EBV, influenza virus, rubella virus, mumps virus, measles virus (wild or vaccine strains), HHV-6, hepatitis A virus, and CMV. The primary mechanism of the thrombocytopenia is immune destruction, although a direct viral effect on the platelet, megakaryocyte, or hematopoietic stem cell has been demonstrated. Because childhood ITP is thought to be secondary to infection in most instances, the definitions of "thrombocytopenia with infection" and "childhood ITP" tend to merge. Thrombocytopenia from infection usually is transient, although instances of chronic thrombocytopenia from specific viral infections (e.g., varicella or CMV) have been documented.[33,34]

Thrombocytopenia also is associated with bacterial sepsis. The low platelet count may be an isolated finding or associated with DIC. Corrigan[35] documented a 61% incidence of thrombocytopenia in 45 children with sepsis. The degree of thrombocytopenia was mild to moderate (64% had platelet counts >50,000/μL), but platelet counts ranged as low as 8000/μL. There was no evidence of DIC in 39% of those with low platelet counts. Thrombocytopenia in the setting of bacterial sepsis probably is also mediated by an immune mechanism with elevated platelet-associated IgG.

Petechial bleeding without thrombocytopenia can be seen in both bacterial and viral disease, especially that caused by meningococci, streptococci, and echoviruses. The explanation for the petechial rash in these infections is either vasculitis or platelet dysfunction.

Disseminated Intravascular Coagulation and Purpura Fulminans

Disseminated intravascular coagulation is uncommon after childhood infections and, if present, usually is accompanied by shock, with at least a 50% mortality rate. The most common organisms producing DIC are bacterial, especially the gram-negative bacteria (meningococci, *H. influenzae, Aerobacter* spp., and others) but also gram-positive organisms (*Staphylococcus aureus;* group B streptococci; *S. pneumoniae,* particularly in asplenic hosts; and *Bacillus anthracis*). DIC also is associated with disseminated viral (varicella, measles, rubella), rickettsial (Rocky Mountain spotted fever), fungal, mycoplasmal, and parasitic infections.

Purpura fulminans is a rare syndrome, seen in extremely ill children with DIC. Purpura fulminans is characterized by the rapid progression of ecchymotic skin lesions, especially of the extremities, that may progress to gangrene, ultimately resulting in amputation.[36] This syndrome has been described as a postinfectious purpura, with scarlet fever, upper respiratory tract infection, and varicella as the most common preceding illnesses and a latent period of 0 to 90 days after infection. A similar clinical picture can be seen in children with DIC and acute bacterial sepsis, especially meningococcemia.

Increasing evidence indicates that DIC with purpura fulminans is associated with deficiency of the naturally occurring anticoagulants. Children with postviral purpura fulminans have been shown to have acquired protein S deficiency, anti–protein S antibody, or the presence of a lupus anticoagulant.[37,38] In children with infectious purpura, protein C activation is impaired as reflected in low levels of protein C, protein S, and antithrombin. These findings are consistent with downregulation of the endothelial thrombomodulin–protein C receptor pathway.[39] The severity of protein C deficiency has been associated with increased morbidity and mortality.[40] There are minimal data on the frequency of inherited thrombophilia in children who develop purpura fulminans. In one report, the frequency of factor V Leiden was not different from that in healthy children; the presence of factor V Leiden was not associated with an increased mortality rate, although complications were increased.[41] In another study of 16 children with purpura fulminans, six of 16 (37%) patients studied had the actor V Leiden mutation. All of the children in this study survived, but 10 (63%) required amputation.[42]

Treatment of purpura fulminans consists of antibiotics for suspected bacterial infection, volume replacement for shock, and heparin. Although there is controversy regarding the routine use of heparin in DIC, its use in purpura fulminans has been associated with an improved outcome when it is started early in the course of the disease and continued for 2 to 3 weeks.[43] Theoretically, to improve the efficacy of heparin, it is reasonable to infuse fresh-frozen plasma or antithrombin III (AT III) concentrates[44] if the AT III level is low. There is anecdotal evidence that infusion of AT III concentrates or protein C concentrates partially correct or normalize the hemostatic abnormalities.[45,46] However, the KyberSept trial, a double-blind placebo-controlled trial of the use of ATIII concentrates in 2300 adults with sepsis, found no difference in mortality at day 28 after diagnosis.[47] In a phase II trial of protein C concentrate in the treatment of sepsis and purpura fulminans in children, there was dose-dependent activation of protein C and normalization of coagulation imbalances. Although there was no improvement in the mortality rate, the study was not powered to detect these changes.[48]

In initial trials recombinant human activated protein C (drotrecogin alfa activated) reduced the mortality rate in adults with severe sepsis,[49] but in pediatric trials, there was no noticeable improvement in mortality (children have a lower mortality rate than adults), and there were significant bleeding risks.[50,51] Although activated protein C has been used in patients with purpura fulminans, the data do not suggest a beneficial effect on mortality.[52,53] In October 2011, this agent was withdrawn from the market after a major study showed no efficacy for the treatment of sepsis. Recombinant tissue plasminogen activator (tPA) has been used in an attempt to restore organ perfusion by dissolution of diffuse microvascular thrombosis[54]; however, in a retrospective multicenter study of 62 patients with meningococcal purpura fulminans treated with systemic tPA, there was a high incidence of intracerebral hemorrhage without proven efficacy in reduction of mortality or incidence of amputation.[55] Other treatments, such as regional sympathetic blockade, topical nitroglycerin, and local infusion of tPA, have been used to improve regional blood flow to the affected part. The mortality rate for postinfectious purpura fulminans has declined from 90% in the past to 18%,[56] but the amputation rate has remained high.[42] The outcome for patients with acute bacterial sepsis and purpura fulminans has also improved, but a mortality rate as high as 50% continues to be reported.

Coagulation Inhibitors

Acquired inhibitors of coagulation in children with infection are usually transient and mild but may be associated with severe bleeding.[56] They are often detected after a viral illness, during antibiotic therapy, or incidentally (frequently before tonsillectomy or adenoidectomy). Both specific inhibitors of coagulation factors (especially factors VIII and IX) and lupus anticoagulants have been demonstrated. Although previously thought to be uncommon, studies have found 50% to 90% of children with infection have at least one positive test result for an antiphospholipid antibody (aPL).[57,58] Significant bleeding is usually seen only in children with specific factor inhibitors, although hemorrhage also has been described with lupus anticoagulants.[59] In symptomatic patients, treatment with prednisone has been associated with remission of bleeding manifestations. Complete resolution without recurrence is the most common event. Thrombosis in the setting of transient postinfectious coagulation inhibitors is rare, although splenic infarction from aPLs has been reported during infection with EBV and mycoplasma pneumonia.[60,61]

Pancytopenia

Pancytopenia in a child should alert the clinician to the possibility of disorders such as leukemia, aplastic anemia, or disseminated neuroblastoma. Infectious causes of pancytopenia are uncommon, and disseminated disease is most often present. Organisms implicated in patients with pancytopenia include *Mycobacterium tuberculosis,* atypical mycobacteria, *Histoplasma capsulatum, Leishmania* spp., *Salmonella typhi, Mucor* spp., Brucella spp., *Fusobacterium necrophorum, Mycoplasma pneumoniae,* and *Ehrlichia canis.*[26] Virus-associated or reactive hemophagocytic syndrome is an additional, although rare, cause of pancytopenia. Children with HIV infection and concomitant infection with *Mycobacterium avium-intracellulare* or parvovirus B19 have been reported to have pancytopenia.

Human Immunodeficiency Virus Infection in Children and Adolescents

Infection with HIV is more common in adults but is now recognized as a leading cause of immunodeficiency in infants and children.[62] Acquisition of HIV in a majority of infected children (most of whom are younger than 2 years of age) is by vertical transmission from an infected mother to her infant. Of children younger than 13 years with acquired immunodeficiency syndrome (AIDS), 80% have a parent with AIDS or AIDS-related complex (ARC), 13% have a history of blood transfusion, and 5% have hemophilia or another coagulation disorder.[63] With improvement in screening blood and blood donors for HIV, it is expected that vertical transmission from mother to infant will remain the primary method of transmission. Other "adult" routes of infection (homosexuality, intravenous needle use) are possible, especially in adolescents and sexually abused children.

Significant advances in the treatment of HIV infection in children have been made since the availability of antiretroviral therapy (ART). The transmission rate of HIV from an infected mother to her child has dropped to less than 2%. Rates of death, AIDS, opportunistic infection, and organ-specific disease (including thrombocytopenia) have all decreased since the advent of ART.[64] A review of HIV infection in children is available.[65]

The hematologic manifestations of AIDS in children are similar to those in adults (see Chapter 159) and depend on the stage of the HIV infection and the presence of coexistent disease.[66,67] Anemia is by far the most common finding (seen in 70%-90% of cases), although the incidence has decreased with effective antiviral therapy.[68] Moderate anemia (hemoglobin <8-9 g/dL) has been identified as an independent risk factor for disease progression in children.[69] Although there have been few studies of severe anemia (hematocrit <25%), in one study it correlated with development of an opportunistic infection and death within 7 months.[70] As in adults, inadequate RBC production is the most important pathogenetic mechanism for the anemia. The etiology for reduced erythropoiesis is multifocal, including direct effect of HIV, associated infections, medications, and deficiency of micronutrients.[69] Although Coombs-positive hemocytic anemia has been described,[71] studies suggest that the finding of a positive direct antiglobulin test result is more likely a reflection of hypergammaglobulinemia. Although evidence indicates that erythropoietin may improve the hemoglobin and quality of life patients with HIV and anemia,[72] the evidence is not strong.[73]

Leukopenia and neutropenia are commonly seen in HIV-infected children (occurring in 47% and 41%, respectively), with severe neutropenia associated with opportunistic infections. Immune neutropenia and also circulating anticoagulants have been described. Lymphopenia is progressive but less prominent in children than in adults until late in the course.

Thrombocytopenia is present in 13% to 30% of pediatric AIDS patients and can be associated with clinically significant and even fatal hemorrhage. The mechanism of the thrombocytopenia in most cases is immune destruction, with a high percentage of patients having antiplatelet antibodies or immune complexes,[74] although amegakaryocytic thrombocytopenia has been reported.[60] Variable therapeutic responses to both corticosteroids and intravenous IgG have been demonstrated; some children have spontaneous remissions.[74,75] Thrombosis has also been described and is associated with severe disease.[76]

Isolated thrombocytopenia as a presenting manifestation of HIV infection has been reported in a number of children, usually infants and even in a neonate.[63,77] There have been no associated clinical stigmata of AIDS or ARC, and patients have been responsive to standard treatment (intravenous IgG or prednisone), often with sustained remissions. In a few patients with prolonged follow-up, no further manifestations of HIV infection were seen. Although it has been suggested that HIV testing may be indicated in all children with ITP, it seems most reasonable to check the HIV status of those with risk factors for AIDS and those outside the typical age group for ITP, especially infants.

COLLAGEN VASCULAR DISEASE AND ACUTE VASCULITIS

Juvenile Idiopathic Arthritis

Juvenile idiopathic arthritis (JIA) (formerly juvenile rheumatoid arthritis) includes a group of disorders with varied clinical presentation, course, and outcome. Systemic JIA, which occurs in 10% of patients, is a multisystem disease characterized by fever, rash, polyarticular (often destructive) arthritis, hepatosplenomegaly, and lymphadenopathy. New understanding of the pathogenesis of systemic JIA points to abnormalities in innate immunity (cytokines IL-1, IL-6, IL-18, neutrophils, and macrophages), distinguishing it from other forms of JIA, suggesting systemic JIA is an autoinflammatory syndrome rather than an autoimmune disease.[78] Another distinguishing feature of JIA is the association with macrophage activation syndrome (MAS) (see later discussion). Patients with JIA commonly demonstrate hematologic abnormalities that are proportional to disease activity. In the polyarticular presentation, more than four joints are involved, but the systemic findings are absent. This group, which accounts for 25% of patients, also may exhibit hematologic abnormalities. Pauciarticular JIA is characterized by involvement of fewer than four joints and is rarely associated with hematologic abnormalities.

Children with acute lymphoblastic leukemia may have a similar presentation as children with systemic JIA, which includes fever, joint pain, hepatosplenomegaly, and isolated cytopenias. Because about 5% of children with ALL are misdiagnosed as having JIA, it is important to perform bone marrow aspiration to rule out leukemia in any patient thought to have systemic JIA before initiation of corticosteroid therapy. Distinguishing features of children ultimately diagnosed with ALL after referral to a rheumatologist include atypical pattern of pain (nonarticular bone pain and night pain with no morning stiffness) and cytopenias, especially thrombocytopenia.[63]

The incidence of anemia is 50% to 60% in patients with systemic or polyarticular JIA and 10% in those with pauciarticular arthritis. The anemia usually correlates with disease activity, worsening during acute flare-ups; however, there is no relationship to the duration of illness. RBCs may be normochromic/normocytic or microcytic/hypochromic. The reticulocyte count usually is low. Iron studies often show low serum iron, increased free erythrocyte protoporphyrin, low-normal or elevated total iron-binding capacity, and normal or low serum ferritin. Serum erythropoietin levels usually are mildly elevated (but not as high as in iron deficiency). The bone marrow does not show erythroid hyperplasia in response to the anemia and has diminished (but not absent) iron stores. The etiology of the anemia may be chronic disease, iron deficiency, or both.

Although it is difficult to differentiate anemia of chronic disease from iron-deficiency anemia, studies in patients with systemic-onset chronic JIA suggest defective iron supply as the primary cause.[79] Transferrin receptor levels are inversely related to hemoglobin levels in this population. The finding of elevated serum transferrin receptor levels may be a reliable indicator for diagnosis of iron deficiency in JIA.[80] Oral iron has been effective in raising the hemoglobin in iron-deficient anemic patients with JIA, and intravenous iron has been effective in raising the hemoglobin level in children unresponsive to oral iron.[79] Excessive production of IL-6, tumor necrosis factor-α (TNF-α), and other inflammatory cytokines has been documented in patients with JIA and may provide an explanation for the abnormalities in iron metabolism. IL-6 may enhance ferritin synthesis and increase hepatic uptake of serum iron. Increased ferritin results in reticuloendothelial iron blockage and diminished iron absorption.[79] In one study, treatment with anti–TNF-α therapy, the hemoglobin as well as markers of abnormal iron metabolism, improved significantly.[81] Less common causes of anemia in patients with JIA include erythroid aplasia, suppression of erythropoiesis by circulating inhibitors, hemolysis, and a macrocytic anemia probably related to increased folate clearance and low plasma and RBC folate levels.

In systemic JIA, leukocytosis with mean WBC counts up to 30,000/μL and neutrophilia with a left shift occur in 90% of patients, especially those with active disease. Leukocytosis is less common in polyarticular arthritis and usually absent in pauciarticular disease. Leukocytosis is so prevalent in systemic JIA that the presence of neutropenia should alert the clinician to question the diagnosis and ensure that other possibilities such as systemic lupus erythematosus (SLE) and ALL are not overlooked. Nonetheless, neutropenia has been reported in several patients with JIA.[82] Other causes of neutropenia are bone marrow suppression due to therapy with gold or nonsteroidal antiinflammatory drugs (NSAIDs)[83] and, in adults, Felty syndrome, the triad of rheumatoid arthritis, splenomegaly, and neutropenia.

The platelet count is elevated in about half of the patients with systemic JIA. IL-6, a cytokine that stimulates thrombopoiesis, is elevated in patients with active systemic JIA, and increased levels of IL-6 are correlated with elevated platelet counts.[84] Persistent thrombocytosis may serve as an adverse prognostic marker for long-term outcome in JIA.

Thrombocytopenia may result from bone marrow suppression by gold therapy, the rare consumptive coagulopathy, or platelet trapping in Felty syndrome. Thrombocytopenia is also seen in the potentially life-threatening complication of MAS (see MAS below). Because thrombocytopenia is uncommon in JIA, however, an unexplained low platelet count should lead the clinician to consider alternative diagnoses, such as SLE or ALL. On the other hand, isolated thrombocytopenia may be the only presenting sign in a child who later develops JIA or another collagen vascular disease. Therefore, JIA and SLE should be considered in the differential diagnosis of ITP in children who are older than 9 years of age and female. Appropriate screening tests for autoantibodies (e.g., antinuclear antibody assay, direct Coombs test) should be performed at diagnosis and periodically if new symptoms develop.

Disseminated intravascular coagulation may occur in children with systemic JIA after hepatic damage, as part of the MAS, from aspirin or gold therapy, or during disease flare-ups treated with NSAIDs when serum albumin is low.[85] These patients often are very ill and may require early and aggressive medical therapy as well as platelet and coagulation factor replacement to control the coagulopathy. The incidence of coagulation abnormalities in nonbleeding patients with systemic JIA is controversial. One study demonstrated prolonged prothrombin time (PT) and activated partial thromboplastin time (aPTT) and elevated fibrinogen, factor VIII, and fibrinopeptide A levels in up to 50% of these patients,[86] but other reports have not confirmed such findings. Another study found elevation of D-dimer levels in 96% of systemic-onset JIA patients; serial measurements of D-dimer levels appeared to parallel response to treatment.[87] In apparent distinction, decreased fibrinolytic activity and increased plasminogen activator inhibitor have been found in patients with active JIA, especially those with the systemic form. Antibodies against factor VIII and the lupus anticoagulant are occasionally seen in children with JIA.

Macrophage Activation Syndrome

Macrophage activation syndrome is a life-threatening multisystem disorder most closely resembling hemophagocytic lymphohistiocytosis (HLH) that occurs primarily in patients with systemiconset juvenile idiopathic arthritis (sJIA). This syndrome usually occurs early in the course of active sJIA and can even be a presenting feature,[88] although it has been reported to occur later and during a quiescent phase.[89] It is estimated that approximately 7% of patients with sJIA develop MAS, and the mortality rate is between 10% and 20%.[90] MAS has also been reported in other systemic inflammatory disorders, including SLE and Kawasaki disease.[88]

The main clinical features of MAS include a high unremitting fever, hepatosplenomegaly, lymphadenopathy, bleeding, rash, and central nervous system manifestations. Neurologic symptoms include lethargy, irritability, disorientation, headache, seizures, and coma. Children with MAS are acutely ill, and almost 50% require intensive care unit care.[91] The diagnosis may be delayed because the presentation mimics an acute exacerbation of sJIA or severe infection. Of interest, some patients have shown a paradoxical improvement in the underlying inflammatory disease at the onset of MAS. Precipitating factors that have been implicated include a flare-up of the underlying disease, aspirin or other NSAID toxicity, viral infections, a second injection of gold salts, methotrexate, and sulfasalazine therapy.[91]

Typical laboratory features include pancytopenia, hypofibrinogenemia (<250 mg/dL), elevated liver enzymes (>40 IU/mL), hypertriglyceridemia (>160 mg/dL), and marked elevation of ferritin (>10,000 ng/mL). Other laboratory findings with less sensitivity and specificity include coagulopathy, hyponatremia, and hypoalbuminemia. The hallmark of this disorder is the presence of hemophagocytic histiocytes usually seen in the bone marrow, although they can also be found in the liver and other organs. These characteristic macrophages are regarded as confirmatory evidence rather than a requirement for a diagnosis because they have not been documented in as many as 20% of patients with the classical clinical and laboratory findings of MAS.[91,92]

There are no accepted diagnostic criteria for MAS in sJIA. Preliminary diagnostic guidelines have been proposed (Table 154-2), although they have not been validated in prospective studies.[92] An international consensus survey of diagnostic criteria for MAS was completed by 232 physicians.[93] The top nine diagnostic criteria identified by more 50% of respondents in order of frequency were:

1. Falling platelet count
2. Hyperferritinemia
3. Bone marrow hemophagocytosis
4. Increased live enzymes
5. Falling leukocyte count
6. Persistent continuous fever >38°C
7. Falling erythrocyte sedimentation rate
8. Hypofibrinogenemia
9. Hypertriglyceridemia

Table 154-2 Preliminary Diagnostic Guidelines for Macrophage Activation Syndrome in Systemic Juvenile Idiopathic Arthritis*

Laboratory Criteria
1. Decreased platelet count (≤262 × 10^9/L)
2. Elevated levels of aspartate aminotransferase (>59 IU/L)
3. Decreased white blood cell count (≤4.0 × 10^9/L)
4. Hypofibrinogenemia (≤250 mg/dL)
Clinical Criteria
1. Central nervous system dysfunction (irritability, disorientation, lethargy, headache, seizures, coma)
2. Hemorrhages (purpura, easy bruising, mucosal bleeding)
3. Hepatomegaly (≥3 cm below the costal margin)
Histopathologic Criterion
Evidence of macrophage hemophagocytosis in the bone marrow aspirate
Diagnostic Rule
The diagnosis of MAS requires the presence of any two or more laboratory criteria or of ≥2 clinical or laboratory criteria. A bone marrow aspirate for the demonstration of hemophagocytosis may be required only in doubtful cases.

From Ravelli A, Magni-Manzoni S, Pistorio A, et al: Preliminary diagnostic guidelines for macrophage activation syndrome complicating systemic juvenile idiopathic arthritis. *J Pediatr* 146:598, 2005.
MAS, Macrophage activation syndrome.
*The suggested criteria are useful only in patients with active systemic-onset juvenile idiopathic arthritis. The laboratory thresholds are examples only and are not specific for the diagnosis (see text).

These features may give us the best candidates for future refinement of diagnostic criteria. The diagnostic guidelines are similar to criteria for the diagnosis of HLH,[94] although a number of differences should be emphasized. In MAS, clinical features are weaker discriminators than laboratory features. Although the presence of fever was universal in patients with MAS, it had a low specificity rate because of the high incidence of fever in patients with sJIA without MAS. The pattern of fever may be of more importance because patients with MAS tend to have nonremitting fever as opposed to the high spiking fevers seen in sJIA. The other clinical criteria may occur late in the course of MAS, resulting in abnormal laboratory findings being more helpful in making a diagnosis early in the course of the illness. Because blood counts are usually elevated in patients with sJIA, the decrease in counts seen with MAS may actually result in a "normal" blood count, although in patients with HLH, cytopenias are usually well below the normal levels. Laboratory markers of T-cell activation (soluble IL-2 receptor [SCD25]) and of macrophage activation (soluble CD163 [SCD163]) have been shown to be elevated in patients with MAS and may serve as useful diagnostic markers in the future.[95]

The pathogenesis of MAS is similar to that proposed for HLH.[94,96] Indeed, it has been proposed that MAS be considered one of the subtypes of acquired HLH.[90] The presentation of MAS is a result of an ineffective immune response to an endogenous or exogenous stimulus leading to an exaggerated inflammatory state produced by a release of high levels of cytokines. These proinflammatory cytokines include TNF-α, IL-1, IL-6, IL-8, IL-12, IL-18, macrophage inflammatory protein (MIP 1-a), and interferon-γ (INF-γ) released by stimulated lymphocytes and histiocytes. Defective natural killer (NK) cell function and cytotoxic T-cell activity has been documented in patients with MAS as well as HLH and may be the common pathway leading to the clinical presentation.[97] NK function in patients with active sJIA but without MAS has also been found to be abnormal.[98] This may explain why MAS is almost exclusively seen in the systemic form of JIA and not the other subtypes of the disease. Mutations in the perforin gene and the *MUNC 13-4* gene have been described in some patients with HLH. The cytotoxic function of NK cells is mediated by the release of perforin and other cytolytic granules into the target cell, leading to cell death. Abnormalities of both perforin gene and *MUNC 13-4* polymorphisms have been found in patients with MAS.[97,99,100]

Treatment of MAS should be started promptly and not delayed for lack of hemophagocytosis if the clinical and laboratory features are consistent with the diagnosis. The initial treatment should be high-dose corticosteroid therapy followed by cyclosporine A if there is not a rapid response. Intravenous methylprednisolone with doses from 2 to 30 mg/kg/day has been the most common corticosteroid reported in the literature and is usually effective in controlling hyperinflammation.[91] The corticosteroid of choice used in the treatment of HLH is dexamethasone, but its use has not been reported in MAS. Cyclosporine A has been very effective in inducing remissions either when used as initial treatment or in cases of corticosteroid failure.[89,91] In addition to immunosuppression, there should be withdrawal of any suspected triggering medications and treatment of infection. Intravenous immunoglobulin (IVIG) therapy has usually been ineffective, although it has been reported to induce a full recovery in one case of a child who failed high-dose corticosteroids.[101] For unresponsive patients treatment with etoposide or other HLH salvage therapy may be necessary. Etanercept and infliximab have also been reported to induce clinical responses in patients with MAS.[102-104] These drugs are recombinant soluble TNF-α receptor fusion proteins that bind to TNF-α, blocking its effect. Although use of these agents to reduce the elevated levels of TNF-α found in this disorder is attractive, they should be used with caution because there are case reports of MAS developing after the initiation of etanercept.[105] Anakinra, a recombinant IL-1 receptor antagonist, has shown promising results in treatment of systemic JIA as well as MAS.[105,106]

Kawasaki Syndrome

Kawasaki syndrome is an acute multisystem disorder characterized by an abrupt onset of fever unresponsive to antibiotics; bilateral conjunctival injection; reddening of the lips, tongue, or oral mucosa; reddening, induration, or peeling of the skin on the hands or feet; polymorphous truncal rash; and cervical lymphadenopathy. This disorder occurs most commonly in children younger than 2 years and has many features of a severe vasculitis. The most serious complication is development of coronary artery aneurysms, which occurs in 20% of children and is responsible for the 3% mortality rate; death often is caused by coronary artery thrombosis or rupture. The etiology of Kawasaki disease is unknown. The immunologic and clinical characteristics of this disorder are similar to those of diseases associated with superantigen production, of which toxic shock syndrome is a classic example.[107]

Children with Kawasaki syndrome may have a mild normochromic, normocytic anemia with reticulocytopenia. Rare patients with AIHA have been reported. Leukocytosis is almost universal, with mean neutrophil counts of 21,000/μL. Ninety-five percent of patients have neutrophilia, with a left shift persisting up to 3 weeks. The finding of vacuoles and toxic granulation in neutrophils is a helpful adjunct in the diagnosis of Kawasaki disease. Activated neutrophils and monocytes may play a role in aneurysm development through the production of elastase. Granulocyte colony-stimulating factor levels have been correlated with coronary artery dilatation during the acute phase of Kawasaki syndrome.[108]

Studies of cellular immunity show normal total T-cell numbers but decreased suppressor T cells, causing relatively elevated T helper–cell levels during the first 4 weeks of disease.[109] The change of T-cell subsets plus B-lymphocyte stimulation may contribute to the exaggerated production of all major immunoglobulin classes during the first 8 weeks of the disease.[110] An unusual infiltration of IgA-producing plasma cells within vascular tissue in Kawasaki syndrome, with an oligoclonal IgA response, suggests that the immune stimulation is antigen driven.[111] Circulating immune complexes and high C3 (but not C4) levels are found during weeks 1 and 3. During the acute phase, increased levels of the cytokines IL-1, IL-6, IL-8, INF-γ, and TNF are noted in the circulation, and IL-1, IL-2, INF-γ, and TNF in blood vessels and skin biopsies.[107] Declining serum IL-6 levels appear to correlate with clinical response after treatment with IVIG.[112]

Impressive thrombocytosis occurs in 85% of patients by the second week, peaking during the third. Platelet counts of up to 2 million/μL are not uncommon, and the mean platelet count is 700,000/μL. Thrombocytosis may serve as a marker of possible atypical Kawasaki disease in infants younger than 1 year of age. In a study of more than 25,000 infants with unexplained fever, 8.8% with a platelet count greater than 800,000/μL were found to have Kawasaki disease as opposed to 0.4% of those with a platelet count less than 800,000/μL.[113] Thrombocytosis is preceded by elevated thrombopoietin levels.[114] However, 2% of patients may have thrombocytopenia caused by a consumptive coagulopathy. Platelets demonstrate hyperaggregation on exposure to adenosine diphosphate, epinephrine, and collagen in vitro. These abnormalities may persist for as long as 9 months after diagnosis.[115] During the first month, levels of factor VIII, fibrinogen, thromboxane B_2, and thromboglobulin are increased. AT III and fibrinolysis activity are decreased. The PT, aPTT, and thrombin time usually are normal.[116]

Prevention and treatment of existing coronary aneurysms constitute the primary therapeutic goal. Aspirin suppresses platelet aggregation but does not affect aneurysm formation. Combining aspirin with high-dose IVIG infusions reduces aneurysm formation, decreases fever, and normalizes laboratory signs of inflammation.[117] The use of corticosteroids is controversial, with conflicting data regarding increased aneurysm formation after steroid usage.[118-120] However, in a randomized, double-blind, placebo-controlled trial, a single pulsed dose of intravenous methylprednisolone, in addition to conventional therapy, did not improve coronary artery outcomes.[121,122] In subgroup analysis of children with persistent fever, coronary outcomes were better in the corticosteroid group. If children at highest risk of primary treatment failure could be identified initially, corticosteroid use may be of benefit in this group. Infliximab has been used in the treatment of IVIG-resistant patients with limited success.[123] Guidelines for the diagnosis, treatment, and long-term management of patients with Kawasaki syndrome have been published.[121,124]

Henoch-Schönlein Purpura

Henoch-Schönlein purpura (HSP) (anaphylactoid purpura) is a systemic vasculitis characterized by unique purpuric skin lesions, transient arthralgias or arthritis (especially affecting the knees and ankles), colicky abdominal pain, and nephritis. Recognition of HSP is important, not so much for its hematologic abnormalities (which are rare) as for the unusual nonthrombocytopenic purpuric lesions, which are frequently confused with the hemorrhagic rash of ITP. This vasculitis occurs most commonly in children 3 to 7 years old, often 1 to 3 weeks after an upper respiratory tract illness. The presenting sign in 50% of children is a characteristic rash, which may begin as urticaria. As these eruptions fade, they are replaced by brownish-red maculopapular lesions and petechiae. The petechiae coalesce, forming areas of raised or "palpable" purpura on the buttocks, legs, and extensor surfaces of the arms, with a symmetrical distribution. The rash may fade but can recur for months, especially with increased activity. Children younger than 3 years of age often have painful soft tissue swellings of the scalp and face (especially periorbital areas) and on the dorsa of the hands and feet. Infantile acute hemorrhagic edema is an acute vasculitis affecting infants younger than 2 years, which may be a benign form of HSP.

Sixty-seven percent of patients experience colicky abdominal pain, often associated with vomiting, hematemesis, or melena from submucosal hemorrhage and edema of the small bowel wall. With severe edema, the bowel wall may become a leading point for intussusceptions.[125]

Renal involvement occurs in 50% of patients, especially boys and older children, and may present after initial systemic symptoms. Hematuria, either microscopic or gross, may occur with proteinuria during the first 3 weeks of the illness but rarely after 6 months. With progressive involvement, hypertension, impaired renal function, and renal failure can occur in up to 15% of children, with an associated mortality rate of 3%. In occasional patients, an acute scrotum that mimics testicular torsion may develop; however, surgical exploration may not be necessary if appropriate clinical and radiographic features are present. Other rare manifestations of HSP include neurologic, cardiac, and pulmonary events.

Anemia occasionally develops as a result of gastrointestinal (GI) tract blood loss or decreased RBC production caused by renal failure. The leukocyte count is normal. Despite the impressive purpura, the platelet count is normal or increased with normal platelet function. Coagulation factor levels usually are normal, although transient decreases in factor XIII activity and vitamin K deficiency from severe vasculitis-induced intestinal malabsorption have been reported. Signs of increased fibrinolysis, as evidenced by elevation of D-dimer and other markers, have been described.[126] Bleeding in the GI tract; the lungs; or, rarely, the central nervous system is caused by a necrotizing vasculitis and not a hemostatic defect.[125] Hypercoagulability does not play a role with normal frequency of MTHFR, prothrombin, and factor V Leiden gene mutations.[127]

Henoch-Schönlein purpura is considered an IgA-mediated inflammation of small vessels. Biopsy of skin or other involved tissue reveals a leukocytoclastic vasculitis. Immune complexes of IgA with complement, IgG, or IgM have been found circulating in the serum[128] and deposited in blood vessel walls of the kidneys and in intestinal and skin lesions.[129] The mechanism of production, accumulation, and deposition of IgA immune complexes in the blood vessel is unclear. It has been suggested that HSP may be a systemic form of IgA nephropathy.[130] Both disorders have identical features on renal biopsy and are characterized by mesangial proliferation, occasional focal sclerosis, and crescent formation.[131]

Treatment is mainly supportive, although corticosteroids have been found to provide symptomatic relief with severe joint, scrotal, or abdominal pain.[132,133] They do not alter skin involvement or prevent renal involvement. Recent studies have suggested that corticosteroids plus azathioprine, cyclosporin A, or cyclophosphamide may have a role in the management of severe renal involvement.[134-138] Rituximab has been reported to be effective in decreasing the symptoms of three patients with severe, refractory chronic HSP.[139] The prognosis is good for full recovery except in children with renal failure.

CARDIOPULMONARY DISEASE

Congenital Heart Disease

Congenital heart disease (CHD) occurs in about 1% of live births. Structural heart malformation usually follows predictable patterns such that six defects account for 70% of all cardiac disorders: ventricular septal defect, atrial septal defect, tetralogy of Fallot, patent ductus arteriosus, pulmonary stenosis, and aortic stenosis. Children with cardiac abnormalities may be acyanotic or cyanotic, depending on the underlying lesion. Hematologic abnormalities occur most often in children with cyanotic CCHD. Polycythemia is the bone marrow response to chronic hypoxemia in patients with CCHD. The decreased arterial oxygen content stimulates erythropoietin production, which in turn increases erythropoiesis. The resultant increased RBC mass increases the oxygen-carrying capacity of the blood, resulting in improved tissue oxygenation. With adequate compensation, erythropoietin levels fall to normal, and higher RBC production is maintained. A second compensatory mechanism is an increase in 2,3-diphosphoglycerate (2,3-DPG) levels in the RBC when the arterial oxygen tension is less than 70 mm Hg. The higher 2,3-DPG level causes a right shift of the oxyhemoglobin curve, resulting in greater oxygen release to the tissues.

Polycythemia in cyanotic children is beneficial up to a point. Because the relationship between the hematocrit and blood viscosity is hyperbolic, minor increases in the hematocrit above 70% cause marked increases in blood viscosity. This higher viscosity results in impaired perfusion within the microvasculature with ultimately less tissue oxygen delivery. The impairment is magnified in severe polycythemia (hematocrit level >75%) such that headache; irritability; dyspnea; and even formation of pulmonary, renal, or central nervous system thrombi may result.[140] To prevent these complications, the hematocrit level should be maintained around 60% through the use of exchange transfusions. Small aliquots of the patient's blood are slowly removed and replaced by equal volumes of plasma or 5% albumin. Care should be taken to remove blood slowly because vascular collapse, cyanosis, stroke, and seizures have been reported with too rapid an exchange. Apheresis (erythrocytapheresis) also has been shown to be an effective means of decreasing viscosity in polycythemic patients.

Infants with CCHD are at risk of developing iron-deficiency anemia. The deficiency may result from the combination of poor iron stores at birth (especially in premature infants), increased iron needed for enhanced erythropoiesis, poor iron intake because of poor feeding, and ongoing iron losses as a consequence of phlebotomy or exchange transfusion. These children may exhibit symptoms of iron deficiency (irritability, anorexia, poor weight gain) or worsening cyanosis. The hemoglobin may be normal for age but inappropriately low for the degree of hypoxemia. Low RBC indices and hypochromic, microcytic RBCs are the best indices of iron deficiency in this setting.[141] Polycythemic children with iron-deficiency anemia are at increased risk for cerebral vein thrombosis because of the poor deformability of the iron-deficient RBC, which further increases blood viscosity.[142] To prevent this complication and to allow for maximal tissue oxygenation, all infants should be fed iron-rich infant formula and receive iron replacement therapy as needed to normalize RBC indices.

Hemolytic anemia, characterized by mechanical destruction of RBCs and manifested by the presence of schistocytes in the peripheral blood smear, is occasionally seen after the placement of prosthetic heart valves.

Routine screening of patients with CHD has demonstrated coagulation abnormalities in 20% to 59% of children with acyanotic defects and in 40% to 50% of those with cyanotic heart disease (Table 154-3).[143] Only 11% of children with CCHD have any clinical evidence of bleeding preoperatively. However, children with underlying hemostatic defects have a greater frequency and severity of postoperative bleeding.[143,144] Presurgical screening tests should include at least a platelet count, platelet function assay (e.g., closure time), PT, and aPTT. Further investigations may be indicated if there is a history of bleeding or abnormal results on screening tests. Acquired von Willebrand syndrome has been reported in patients with CHD and is possibly associated with an increased bleeding risk, especially in those receiving aspirin. The multimer pattern reveals decreased large-molecular-weight multimers.[145] Children with polycythemia have contracted plasma volumes; therefore, when blood samples are collected, extra care should be taken to ensure the proper 1:9 ratio of 3.8% sodium citrate to blood to prevent artificial abnormalities in coagulation test results.

The etiology of the coagulation abnormalities in CCHD is unclear. Earlier reports suggesting a role for consumptive coagulopathy have not been confirmed. Protein C levels in eight of 29 term infants with CCHD were significantly lower than in control participants with no evidence of familial deficiency. Of these infants, two had thrombotic complications, and four had consumptive coagulopathy.[146] Platelets have shortened survival times (even with normal counts), and normal to increased numbers of megakaryocytes in the bone marrow are reported.[147] This increased platelet destruction does not appear to be attributable to DIC. Both the platelet and coagulation abnormalities are directly proportional to the degree of hypoxemia and polycythemia. For example, whereas children with oxygen saturations greater than 60% have a mean platelet count of 315,000/μL, those with saturations less than 60% have a mean count of 185,000/μL.[147] The mild platelet and coagulation abnormalities usually are decreased or corrected after surgical repair of the heart defect.[143,148] With bleeding or if surgery is not possible, the coagulopathy may be treated by correction of polycythemia to a hematocrit level of 60% by using slow plasma-exchange transfusion.[149]

Table 154-3 Coagulation Abnormalities in Congenital Heart Disease

	Incidence (%)	
Abnormality	Acyanotic CHD	Cyanotic CHD
Prolonged bleeding time	11	28
Prolonged PT		20
Prolonged aPTT		19
Thrombocytopenia	12-40	0-36
Abnormal platelet aggregation	14	38-70
Increased fibrinolysis	12	0-10
Abnormal clot retraction	10	
Low fibrinogen	16	12
Increased fibrin split products		Occasionally
Decreased factors II, V, VII, VIII, IX, X, XI, XII		Occasionally
Decreased protein C		25*

Adapted from Lascari AD: *Hematologic manifestations of childhood diseases,* New York, Thieme-Stratton, 1984, with permission.
aPTT, Activated partial thromboplastin time; *CHD,* congenital heart disease; PT, prothrombin time.
*Data from MacDonald PD, Gibson BE, Braunlie J, et al: Protein C activity in severely ill newborns with congenital heart disease. *J Perinatal Med* 20:421, 1992.

Cystic Fibrosis

Cystic fibrosis (CF) is a multisystem disorder of exocrine gland dysfunction characterized by chronic pulmonary disease, pancreatic exocrine insufficiency, hepatic dysfunction, abnormal reproductive organ function, and intestinal obstruction associated with abnormally high sweat electrolyte levels. It is an autosomal recessive disease with an incidence of one in 2000 live births.

Severe hemolytic anemia caused by vitamin E deficiency may be the presenting manifestation of CF. Dolan[150] initially linked deficiency of vitamin E with severe hemolytic anemia in infants who presented with pallor, edema, hypoproteinemia, and thrombocytosis. This complication can be seen as early as 6 weeks of age.

Many children with CF are chronically hypoxic, yet they do not have the expected augmented erythroid response. In a study by Vichinsky and colleagues,[151] none of 42 children with CF had polycythemia, and 30% (especially the boys and the older children) had a normochromic, normocytic or hypochromic microcytic anemia with reticulocytopenia. In contrast with children with CCHD, there was no appropriate increase in RBC 2,3-DPG levels, no right shift of the oxyhemoglobin curve, and either a low or a normal erythropoietin level. In vitro assays showed normal erythroid progenitor cell numbers and no serum inhibitor of erythropoiesis. Up to 66% of the children studied had abnormalities consistent with iron deficiency, and all responded to oral or parenteral iron therapy.

It appears that the etiology of anemia in CF is multifactorial. A blunted erythropoietic response to hypoxia plus iron deficiency secondary to iron malabsorption or poor dietary iron intake may each be partially responsible for the development of anemia. If iron deficiency persists despite adequate oral supplementation, the possibility of ongoing blood loss or of iron malabsorption that may necessitate parenteral iron replacement should be considered. Soluble transferrin receptor levels may be helpful in distinguishing iron deficiency from anemia of chronic inflammation in CF because, unlike serum ferritin and transferrin, soluble transferrin receptor does not appear to be an acute phase reactant.[152,153]

Use of multiple antibiotics in patients with CF is routine. There have been a number of case reports of adult patients with severe, life-threatening hemolytic anemia attributed to piperacillin.[154,155] This complication has not been reported in children at this time.

Findings of studies of neutrophil function in children with CF are conflicting. Some reports indicate impaired chemotaxis, chemiluminescence, granule release, and superoxide production,[156-158] but others have demonstrated factors in patient sputum that actually enhance neutrophil and monocyte responses to stimulants.[159,160] Although these sputum factors may improve neutrophil killing ability, they also may worsen neutrophil-mediated lung damage through increased release of neutrophil elastase.[161] Evaluation of immune function has revealed impaired lymphoproliferative responses to *Pseudomonas* spp. and other gram-negative bacterial antigens, defective opsonization, increased levels of circulating immune complexes, and decreased numbers of T-helper cells in 30% of patients.[138,162] The contribution of these findings to frequent pulmonary infection is still under investigation.

Children with CF usually do not experience clinically significant bleeding owing to impaired hemostasis despite the risk of liver disease and vitamin K deficiency from malabsorption. An exception may be infants younger than 1 year of age, in whom rare case reports of vitamin K–deficient hemorrhage have been reported in association with CF.[163-165] Routine coagulation tests usually yield normal results, with an occasional prolonged PT reported. A study by Corrigan and colleagues[142,166] revealed that 60% of 24 patients had a more subtle deficiency of prothrombin activity, thought to be caused by vitamin K deficiency. Other investigators, using direct measurement of vitamin K and PIVKA-II (protein induced by vitamin K absence-II), have reported conflicting percentages of patients to be vitamin K deficient,[167,168] with another uncontrolled study demonstrating normalization of PIVKA-II values in many patients by routine administration of daily oral vitamin K.[169] Routine vitamin K supplementation is recommended for all patients with CF,[170] although there are inadequate data to define the ideal dose.[171]

Children with CF appear to have a particularly high predisposition to recurrent venous thrombosis. In one study of 19 patients with recurrent venous thrombosis, six had CF, but none of 101 thrombosis patients without recurrence had CF. A striking association with respiratory tract colonization with *Burkholderia cepacia* was noted, as was the frequent presence of a central venous catheter. Several of the recurrences occurred while on therapeutic anticoagulation.[172] Studies of small populations of both children and adults had documented an increased incidence of protein C and protein S deficiency, as well as lupus anticoagulants.[173-175] These abnormalities are likely acquired defects in most CF patients because of the potential for having subclinical vitamin K deficiency, liver function abnormalities, and recurrent infections. Follow-up studies have not shown persistent abnormalities in many patients. The incidence of activated protein C resistance and factor V Leiden was similar to the general population. Although it would be anticipated there would be an increased frequency of venous thrombosis because of the increased use of central venous catheters, at least one large study in older adolescents and adults with CF who had totally implanted venous access devices revealed a very low incidence of complications.[176] Whether patients with CF have a greater risk of venous thrombosis than the control population awaits a larger prospective controlled trial.

HEMATOLOGIC MANIFESTATIONS OF CHILDHOOD GASTROINTESTINAL DISEASE

Milk Protein–Induced Enteropathy and Heiner Syndrome

The association of iron deficiency with dietary intake of cow's milk in young infants is established. A major contributing factor is the relatively poor bioavailability of iron in cow's milk compared with breast milk. In addition, the rapid growth of infants and corresponding rapid increase in RBC mass necessitate an increased requirement for dietary iron. The role of cow's milk in inducing occult GI blood loss in infants was carefully documented more than 3 decades ago in a sentinel paper that also demonstrated a correlation between the amount of milk ingested and the amount of fecal blood lost.[177] GI blood loss in response to cow's milk ingestion appears to be most prevalent in infants younger than 6 months of age and occurs with diminishing frequency in older infants.[178] The majority of affected infants outgrow their milk protein sensitivity by 3 years of age. The GI blood loss may be ameliorated by heat denaturing of the milk proteins. Occasionally, toddlers and older children have been documented to have milk-induced GI bleeding with associated iron-deficiency anemia.[179,180] Substantially limiting cow's milk consumption and prescribing iron supplementation is sufficient to correct the iron deficiency and associated hypoproteinemia with edema in most children.[181]

A variety of GI syndromes associated with cow's milk sensitivity, with varying manifestations and severity, has been described. Associated findings may include vomiting, diarrhea, poor growth, and hypoproteinemia; however, some patients may have occult blood loss and iron-deficiency anemia without associated complaints. At the severe end of the spectrum, cow's milk protein–induced enterocolitis may occur.[182] Such patients may present with acute, severe bloody diarrhea; vomiting; abdominal distention; methemoglobinemia; and shock even in the absence of anemia.[182] Even minute amounts of cow's milk protein in human breast milk may be sufficient to precipitate a severe event.[183] In patients with chronic occult GI blood loss, esophagogastroduodenoscopy may reveal gastritis or gastroduodenitis, and colonoscopy may demonstrate modest histologic abnormalities in the proximal colon.[177,180] The immunopathobiology of cow's milk protein allergy syndromes has not been fully elucidated. Most of these syndromes affecting the intestinal tract only are non–IgE mediated.[177] Wilson et al[177] reported the frequent presence of precipitating antibodies to milk proteins in the study population as a whole. However, the presence of such antibodies did not appear to predict milk-induced GI bleeding. The roles that genetic predisposition, intestinal and immunologic immaturity in young infants, exposure to cow's milk protein in breast milk, GI infections, or other factors may play in the development of milk protein enteropathy are not fully understood.

In 1962, Heiner et al described a syndrome in infants and young children that included chronic cough, recurrent lung infiltrates, poor growth, GI symptoms and blood loss, iron-deficiency anemia, and pulmonary hemosiderosis associated with multiple serum precipitins to cow's milk proteins. Others have confirmed and further detailed this rare syndrome. Additional manifestations may include intermittent wheezing; hilar lymphadenopathy; eosinophilia; elevated levels of serum IgE, IgM, or IgA; chronic rhinitis; adenoidal hypertrophy; hypercapnia; and cor pulmonale. A feature of this syndrome is rapid improvement of the pulmonary manifestations after eliminating cow's milk from the diet.

Celiac Disease

Celiac disease, or gluten sensitive enteropathy, is an inflammatory and malabsorptive process resulting from an aberrant intestinal T-cell immune response to ingested dietary gluten, leading to injury of the mucosa of the small intestine.[177] Classical celiac disease has been characterized as frequently affecting infants and young children, leading to steatorrhea, failure to thrive, weight loss, and nutritional deficiency. With the advent of improved screening techniques, the prevalence is recognized to be greater than previous estimates. Celiac disease broadly affects both children and adults, many of whom may have minimal classical symptoms of the disorder. Treatment is usually institution of a gluten-free diet, with resolution of the process in the majority of cases.

Iron deficiency is frequently present in celiac disease in children and adults and may be the sole recognized manifestation of the disorder.[165] Dietary iron absorption primarily occurs within the proximal small intestine, the same region most affected by celiac disease. As a result, iron deficiency in celiac disease appears to be primarily caused by impaired absorption of dietary iron, although a component of chronic GI blood loss may also apply in a minority of patients. Iron deficiency in celiac disease may be refractory to iron supplementation, and a significant percentage of children and adults with iron-deficiency anemia that does not respond to therapeutic oral iron replacement have celiac disease.

Folic acid and, to a lesser frequency, vitamin B_{12} deficiency may also result from the malabsorptive process in celiac disease. Manifestations may include macrocytic anemia, leukocytopenia, and pancytopenia. Neurologic findings may be present with vitamin B_{12} deficiency. Other vitamin and micronutrient deficiencies, including copper and vitamin K deficiency, have been observed in celiac disease. Splenic hypofunction may occur with some frequency in adults with celiac disease but appears to be less common in children. A number of case reports have suggested an association of pulmonary hemosiderosis with celiac disease. The pathophysiology of this association is not known, but the pulmonary process may improve with initiation of a gluten-free diet.

A high index of suspicion is important for diagnosing celiac disease in children, particularly those who are minimally symptomatic or who may be at increased risk for development of celiac disease. The latter group includes children with trisomy,[21] Turner syndrome, IgA deficiency, autoimmune thyroiditis, and type 1 diabetes, and those with a family history of celiac disease. In addition to correcting the nutritional deficiencies and growth failure in children with celiac disease, recognition of the disease and institution of a gluten-free diet may minimize the risk of some of the associated conditions of celiac disease, including the development of non-Hodgkin lymphoma involving the intestinal tract.

Inflammatory Bowel Disease

Anemia is a very common extraintestinal manifestation of inflammatory bowel disease (IBD), particularly in children with Crohn disease, in whom the historical prevalence of anemia approaches 70% to 80%. A more recent series of studies suggests that the prevalence of anemia may be declining in Crohn disease, perhaps because of more effective therapy.[178] The etiology of anemia in IBD appears to be multifactorial, but the most common contributing factors are iron deficiency related to chronic GI blood loss or iron malabsorption caused by intestinal mucosal injury and decreased absorption and sequestration of iron stores as is seen in the anemia of chronic inflammation. These broad mechanisms for anemia may coexist, and it is sometimes difficult to determine the predominant mechanism. Measurement of serum soluble transferrin receptor and the hemoglobin content of reticulocytes can be helpful in this setting.[178] Other contributing factors to anemia in IBD may also be present in individual patients, including immune-mediated hemolytic anemia, hemophagocytosis, malnutrition, folate and vitamin B_{12} deficiency, and the suppressive effects of medications on hematopoiesis.[178]

Specific treatment of anemia in IBD may be difficult. Oral iron supplementation is not always effective. Comparative studies of oral versus intravenous iron supplementation suggest the intravenous route may result in better short-term improvement in anemia; however, long-term outcome data are lacking.[178] Some patients may respond to supplemental erythropoietin administration as well.[178] Patients with IBD may have impaired enterocyte-mediated intestinal absorption of iron, the degree of which appears to correlate with disease activity.[184] The role that induction of hepcidin expression by mediators of inflammation, particularly IL-6, plays in the anemia of IBD is an intriguing area of ongoing investigation.

Other hematologic manifestations of IBD include leukocytosis and thrombocytosis, hyposplenism, an increased propensity toward thrombosis, and therapy-related leucopenia and thrombocytopenia. There may be an increased incidence of immune-mediated thrombocytopenia associated with IBD. The recently described potential association between infliximab, an anti-TNF antibody, and hepatosplenic T-cell lymphoma bears close observation and suggests that biologic agents such as infliximab should be used only after careful consideration of the potential benefits and risks of the agent in the individual patient.

Other Gastrointestinal Disorders

In addition to the disorders already discussed, other GI disorders that occur in children and adolescents may be associated with the development of anemia. Examples include antral gastritis, duodenal and colonic polyps, parasitic infestations, and GI malignancies. GI stromal tumors, although rare, usually present in teenage girls with anemia related to GI blood loss.[185] In a recent small experience of endoscopic evaluation of the upper GI system in children and teenagers between the ages of 9 and 17 years presenting with iron-deficiency anemia who did not have hematologic or chronic diseases, heavy menstrual flow or obvious blood loss demonstrated abnormal finding in 57% of patients.[186] This small study suggests that careful evaluation of the GI system should be considered in children and adolescents with unexplained iron-deficiency anemia and in those in whom the iron deficiency does not correct appropriately with oral iron supplementation.

ENDOCRINE DISEASE

Hematologic Manifestations of Thyroid Disorders

The associations between thyroid disorders and hematologic abnormalities are diverse.[177] The most commonly reported findings include anemia of several etiologies and abnormalities of hemostasis. Specific associations in childhood and adolescence appear to be less common than in adults. However, some rare disorders with both hematologic and thyroid manifestations appear to be particularly pertinent to the pediatric population.

Congenital hypothyroidism has multiple etiologies, including thyroid agenesis, thyroid-stimulating hormone resistance, disorders in thyroid hormone production, and central hypothyroidism. Screening programs for congenital hypothyroidism have been widely adopted as part of neonatal screening programs for several decades, resulting in marked improvement in the clinical manifestations of congenital hypothyroidism. A series of 50 infants with congenital hypothyroidism identified by neonatal screening found that modest normocytic, normochromic anemia, correlating with the severity of the hypothyroidism, is present during the first year of life despite thyroid hormone replacement.[178] By comparison, a separate publication of infants also identified by neonatal screening demonstrated no anemia, and six of 23 infants were found to be polycythemic.[179] The differences in these reports is not understood but may reflect, in part, the differences in the pathophysiology of congenital hypothyroidism.

The association between autoimmune thyroid disease and anemia is well recognized. The anemia may be exacerbated by several mechanisms, including iron deficiency, pernicious anemia, and AIHA. In adults, the anemia of uncomplicated hypothyroidism is typically normocytic or macrocytic, with modest anisocytosis present on the peripheral smear.[177] In children and adolescents, the same findings appear to be present. Additionally, children may have a decrease in linear growth velocity as a manifestation of hypothyroidism, suggesting that investigation of thyroid function is appropriate for children with macrocytic anemia and declining growth rate.[180] Pernicious anemia and iron deficiency may be less common in children with autoimmune thyroid disease than in adults. However, parietal cell antibodies are found in a significant percentage of children and adolescents with autoimmune thyroid disease, a finding that may predispose them to the development of both iron-deficiency and pernicious anemia during young adulthood.[181]

Disturbances of hemostasis are also well recognized as a manifestation of thyroid dysfunction. Overt hypothyroidism and hyperthyroidism modify the hemostatic balance in opposite directions, with hypothyroid patients having an increased risk of bleeding and hyperthyroid patients having an increased risk of thrombosis.[182] There are few reports of bleeding or thrombosis in children and adolescents attributed to uncomplicated overt thyroid dysfunction. Of interest is the association between acquired von Willebrand disease and hypothyroidism reported in several adolescent girls, which may be a cause of menorrhagia.[183,187,188] This hemostatic imbalance may improve with thyroid hormone replacement.

More global immune dysregulation syndrome may result in both endocrine dysfunction, including thyroid abnormalities, and cytopenias. The association of the autoimmune polyglandular syndrome, a heterogenous group of disorders, and pernicious anemia has been reported in children.[189] Additionally the immunodysregulation, polyendocrinopathy, and enteropathy, X-linked (IPEX) syndrome, which is caused by loss-of-function mutations of the *FOXP3* gene, has been associated with immune cytopenias, including hemolytic anemia, neutropenia, and thrombocytopenia.[190]

ANOREXIA NERVOSA

Anorexia nervosa is a psychiatric disorder occurring in about one in 800 adolescent girls; it is characterized by an inability to maintain a minimal normal body weight, intense fear of being fat, body image distortion, and amenorrhea. The profound weight loss is accompanied by hypothermia, hypotension, edema, lanugo, and metabolic changes and is associated with a mortality rate of 5% to 18%. A mild, normochromic, normocytic anemia with reticulocytopenia occurs in 30% of patients.[191] Acanthocytes or spur cells have been reported and may be caused by low serum α-lipoprotein levels. The causes of the anemia probably are decreased RBC production and a relative increase in plasma volume. A few patients have had slightly decreased RBC survival. Serum vitamin B_{12} and folate levels usually are normal. Despite low serum iron and decreased bone marrow iron stores in 80% of patients, iron-deficiency anemia is uncommon except during recovery, when iron supplementation is necessary. The severe hypophosphatemia seen during refeeding of severely malnourished patients has been associated with hemolytic anemia.

Fifty percent of patients have leukopenia, with an absolute decrease in numbers of neutrophils, lymphocytes, and monocytes.[192,193] The neutropenia may be quite severe. An increased incidence of infection is not usual, although with increasing use of central venous catheters, more serious bacterial infections are being reported.[193] Bone marrow reserves are normal despite marrow hypoplasia and a normal to slightly decreased size of the marginal pool. Impaired neutrophil chemotaxis, intracellular killing of staphylococci, and decreased complement levels have been demonstrated in patients with anorexia. These findings are associated with occasional skin abscess formation.

Patients with anorexia nervosa have no apparent bleeding diathesis. The platelet count is normal to slightly decreased,[191,194] and the in vitro platelet aggregation response to epinephrine, adenosine diphosphate, and collagen is exaggerated. Coagulation defects are uncommon except for that related to vitamin K deficiency reported in bulimia.

The hematologic changes in anorexia nervosa are directly correlated with total body fat mass depletion.[195] A bone marrow pattern on magnetic resonance imaging suggestive of gelatinous transformation of bone marrow (serous atrophy) is seen in patients with the lowest hematologic parameters. Direct examination of the bone marrow reveals hypoplasia with loss of fat stores and replacement by a gelatinous acid mucopolysaccharide ground substance. Focal or extensive necrosis may be present.[196] Bone marrow histiocytes are relatively increased in number and have prominent blue-green granules. With nutritional supplementation, bone marrow hypoplasia reverses, the gelatinous material disappears, and the hematologic abnormalities, including neutrophil defects and low complement levels, resolve by 8 weeks.

THROMBOEMBOLIC COMPLICATIONS IN CHILDHOOD ILLNESS

Improvements in medical and surgical care, particularly advances in critical and supportive care, have led to increased survival among children with malignancy and chronic illnesses. However, the extended survival of these children has led to comorbidities such as thromboembolic complications. The increased risk of thromboembolism in children with chronic illnesses is multifactorial and can include the illness itself, medical and surgical interventions, or the central venous line used to administer therapy.

In a recent analysis of 13,449 admissions at United States children's hospitals, the majority (63%) of patients with venous thromboembolism had one or more complex chronic conditions, most commonly cardiovascular disease (28%), followed by malignancy (14%), neuromuscular (11%), and respiratory (7%).[172] This review focuses on four childhood illnesses commonly associated with thromboembolism: malignancy, CHD, nephrotic syndrome, and SLE. In addition to the diseases discussed in this review, other chronic illnesses of childhood have been associated with thromboembolism, including sickle cell anemia, IBD, diabetes, and CF. Children receiving home total parental nutrition also have an increased risk of thrombosis due to the combination of a central venous catheter and infusion of hyperosmolar solutions that can injure the vascular endothelium.[197,198] As the incidence of pediatric venous thromboembolism increases, the concept of thromboprophylaxis in hospitalized children is receiving increased attention. The end of this section will review the small but growing body of literature on this topic.

Thromboembolism in Pediatric Cancer

Although thrombosis is a well-known complication of pediatric malignancy, the overall incidence is low compared with adults with cancer. Most epidemiologic studies in this area have been limited to single-center experience or specific cancer types. The reported incidence of thromboembolism in pediatric cancer ranges from 2% to 14% when based on clinical symptoms and up to 44-50% when children undergo routine radiographic screening.[199-206] In a report of 17 years' experience at McMaster's Children's Hospital, 7.9% (95% confidence interval, 6.0%-10.0%) of oncology patients experienced thromboembolism. Increasing age, certain cancer types (hematologic malignancies and sarcomas), intrathoracic disease, and catheter dysfunction were associated with a higher risk of thromboembolism.[206] Because many thrombotic events in pediatric cancer are catheter related, the majority of thrombosis described in the literature is located in the upper venous system. Factors associated with an increased risk of catheter-related thrombosis include insertion of peripherally inserted central catheters or Hickman catheters and a history of catheter occlusion and infection.[207] Right atrial thrombi are also frequently seen, with a reported incidence of 9% to 14% in children with indwelling catheters.[203,208] Typically asymptomatic, these thrombi are often found incidentally on routine surveillance echocardiograms for children receiving anthracycline chemotherapy. Patients with asymptomatic catheter-related thrombosis are at risk for post-thrombotic syndrome (persistent pain, swelling, or skin changes) after catheter removal, and screening cancer survivors for these symptoms should be part of the long-term follow-up care for these patients.[207]

There are several mechanisms by which malignancy increases the risk of thromboembolism.[209] These include direct activation of the coagulation system; inhibition of fibrinolysis through secretion of plasminogen activator inhibitor-1; and the release of cytokines, which themselves induce procoagulant and antifibrinolytic activity. Malignant cells can also adhere to platelets, leukocytes, and the endothelium through adhesion molecules present on their surfaces. Finally, as tumors increase in size, they may compress or occlude blood vessels, leading to reduced blood flow and stasis.

Published studies indicate that patients with hematologic malignancies and sarcomas appear to have the highest risk of thromboembolism. In a meta-analysis including 1752 children with ALL, the incidence rate for thrombosis was 5.2%.[210] As opposed to other types of cancer, cerebral venous thrombosis and stroke are frequently seen in ALL, particularly in the setting of asparaginase therapy. Asparaginase, an essential component of induction chemotherapy, reduces the synthesis of both coagulation factors and inhibitors as a consequence of asparagine depletion.[211] Higher incidences of thrombosis appear to be associated with lower doses of asparaginase given over longer treatment durations, as well as prednisone (when given instead of dexamathasone).[210]

The incidence of thromboembolism in sarcoma ranges from 14% to 16%.[212,213] Thrombotic events in sarcoma are frequently detected at the time of presentation and may be asymptomatic. Patients with greater disease burden or metastatic disease appear to be at highest risk. Brain tumors, the most common solid tumor in children, have a relatively lower risk of thrombosis in children compared with adults. Pediatric and adolescent studies have reported incidences of 0.5%, 0.6%, and 2.8% as opposed to the 18% to 28% incidence of thrombosis in adults with brain tumors.[206,214-216] Because the incidence of thromboembolism increases with age, this complication is of particular concern in adolescents and young adults with cancer, an increasing number of whom are cared for at children's hospitals. In a study of 2001 to 2008 national discharge data from U.S children's hospitals, 5.3% of adolescents and young adults (15-24 years of age) with cancer had a discharge diagnosis of venous thromboembolism.[217] Large prospective cohort studies including pediatric patients with all types of malignancies are needed to better understand the true incidence of thromboembolism in pediatric cancer.

Thromboembolism in Congenital Heart Disease

Although CHD affects only 1% of live births, almost 50% of infants younger than 6 months of age and 30% of older children who develop venous thromboembolism have underlying cardiac disorders.[218] Also, the majority of children receiving prophylactic anticoagulation are those with complex CHD or severe acquired cardiac diseases such as cardiomyopathy. Children with CHD are at risk of venous, arterial, and intracardiac thrombosis, as well as embolism to the central nervous system. CHD is the most common associated diagnosis among children hospitalized with arterial ischemic stroke in the United States.[219]

Cardiac catheterization is the most common procedure performed in children with CHD, and it is used for both diagnostic and therapeutic purposes. Access is typically obtained through the femoral artery. Historically, thromboembolism of the femoral artery was a common complication of this procedure, particularly in younger patients. In the 1970s, a randomized clinical trial demonstrated that the use of unfractionated heparin prophylaxis reduced the incidence of femoral artery thrombosis from 40% to 8% in children younger than 10 years of age.[220] The current recommendation from the American College of Chest Physicians (ACCP) is that all children should receive prophylaxis with unfractionated heparin before cardiac catheterization, using a bolus of 100 to 150 U/kg, with additional doses recommended for prolonged catheterizations.[221,222]

The Fontan procedure, which diverts systemic venous return directly to the pulmonary arteries, is the definitive palliative surgical treatment for most congenital univentricular heart lesions.[223] Unfortunately, thromboembolic events continue to be a major cause of morbidity and mortality in this procedure. The reported incidence of these complications in cohort studies ranges from 1% to 19% and includes venous thrombosis of the Fontan circuit, right atrial thrombosis, and stroke.[223] Thromboembolic events may occur anytime after the procedure but often present months to years later.[224] There is no consensus as to the optimal type or duration of anticoagulation that Fontan patients should receive, nor are there data that any one prophylactic regimen is effective in reducing thromboembolic complications. Institutional protocols, if they exist, range from no anticoagulation to aspirin to warfarin. The ACCP guidelines suggest either therapy with aspirin (1-5 mg/kg/day) or therapeutic heparin followed by warfarin to achieve a target international normalized ratio (INR) of 2.5 but state that the optimal duration of therapy is unknown.[221,222] In a recently published international randomized trial of aspirin (5 mg/kg/day) versus warfarin as primary thromboprophylaxis in the first 2 years after Fontan surgery, there was no difference in thrombosis rates between groups.[225] However, the overall thrombosis rate was suboptimal, suggesting that alternative approaches need to be considered.

There are even less data on the role of anticoagulation or antiplatelet therapy in other cardiac procedures with the potential risk of thromboembolism. These include the placement of endovascular stents and Blalock-Taussig shunts as well as Norwood and Glenn procedures, which are typically performed before the definitive Fontan procedure. The ACCP recommends perioperative heparin therapy for these procedures.[221,222] However, the need for antiplatelet therapy after these procedures remains unknown.

Recombinant activated factor VII (rVIIa) is increasingly used as a hemostatic adjunct in pediatric cardiac surgery. In two of three single-center studies, thrombotic complications were not increased in patients receiving rFVIIa compared with those who did not receive rFVIIa during surgery.[226-228] However, prospective adequately powered studies are required to properly assess the safety of this prothrombotic agent in patients with CHD.

Long-term anticoagulation therapy is clearly indicated for children with prosthetic heart valves. This population is currently treated according to adult recommendations.[229] Children with mitral bioprosthetic valves should receive three months of warfarin followed by long-term aspirin therapy, but those with aortic bioprosthetic valves can be managed with aspirin alone. Those with mechanical valves must remain on long-term warfarin, with target INRs of 2.5 or 3.0 depending on the specific type of valve. Patients with mechanical valves and a history of thromboembolism or additional thrombotic risk factors should also receive low-dose aspirin.

Thromboembolism in Nephrotic Syndrome

The increased risk of thromboembolism in pediatric nephrotic syndrome is multifactorial.[230] The same urinary losses that lead to profound hypoalbuminemia in these patients also cause acquired deficiencies of anticoagulant proteins such as antithrombin and free protein S. In addition to deficiencies of anticoagulants, increased levels of procoagulants (fibrinogen, factor V, and factor VIII), hypercholesterolemia, and increased platelet aggregation have all been described in nephrotic syndrome. Finally, the therapeutic interventions for nephrotic syndrome can increase the risk of thromboembolism. Diuretics cause reduced intravascular volume, leading to hemoconcentration, and steroids and cyclosporine increase procoagulant activities.

The incidence of thromboembolism in pediatric nephrotic syndrome ranges from 1.8% to 9.2% in published series.[230-233] This contrasts with adult nephrotic syndrome, in which incidence rates as high as 44% have been reported.[231] The most common locations in children are the deep veins of the lower extremities and renal veins, and events are frequently associated with the use of central venous catheters. Although pulmonary embolism is clinically diagnosed in fewer than 1% of patients, a frequency of 27% (seven of 26) was found in a series of nephrotic children who underwent screening with ventilation–perfusion scans.[234] These data suggest that pulmonary symptoms may not always be caused by fluid overload in this population and that pulmonary embolism should at least be considered in any nephrotic patient with a significant change in respiratory status.

Prophylactic anticoagulation is recommended for adult nephrotic syndrome as long as the patient has proteinuria or severe hypoalbuminemia. However, no studies have been performed to evaluate the efficacy or safety of this practice in pediatric patients, and prophylaxis is generally not used in children without a history of thrombosis.[235] One reason for the controversy is that predictors of thrombosis have not been clearly established in this population. Even decreased plasma concentrations of antithrombin, a well-recognized risk factor, is not a consistent finding in nephrotic children who develop thromboembolism.[236] The most consistent biologic risk factor to date is the presence of severe hypoalbuminemia.[230] Age 12 years or older at diagnosis of nephrotic syndrome, severe proteinuria, and history of thromboembolism preceding the diagnosis of nephrotic syndrome have also been identified as significant predictors of thromboembolism.[233]

Although the traditional duration of anticoagulation for a deep venous thrombosis (DVT) is 3 months, some form of anticoagulation should be continued or resumed in the setting of active disease.[222] To avoid hemoconcentration, diuretics must be avoided or used judiciously in patients who have experienced a thromboembolic event. Finally, it is important to remember that the efficacy of heparin can be impaired in the setting of decreased antithrombin levels.

Thromboembolism in Systemic Lupus Erythematosus and Antiphospholipid Syndrome

The reported incidence of thromboembolism in pediatric SLE ranges from 9% to 17%, similar to rates reported in adult SLE patients.[237,238] Although DVT of the lower extremities is still the most common manifestation, patients with SLE are more likely to experience arterial and central nervous system thrombosis compared with those with malignancy, CHD, or nephrotic syndrome. In approximately half of cases, thrombosis occurs before or at the time of SLE diagnosis.[239] The significant association between the presence of aPLs and thromboembolism is well described in patients with SLE.[240] aPLs are a heterogenous group of antibodies directed against plasma proteins and phospholipid complexes. They most frequently occur in the setting of SLE but are also associated with JIA, epilepsy, and other diseases.[241] There are multiple aPLs subtypes, including lupus anticoagulants, anticardiolipin antibodies, anti-β_2-glycoprotein I antibodies, and antiprothrombin antibodies. The exact mechanism of aPL-associated thromboembolism has not been elucidated, but recent data suggest that lupus anticoagulant antibodies interfere with the function of the protein C pathway, leading to an acquired activated protein C resistance.[242]

Antiphospholipid antibodies are quite common in the pediatric SLE population. An analysis of 12 published series of children with SLE reported a global prevalence of 48% for anticardiolipin antibodies and 23% for lupus anticoagulants.[241] Recent work has focused on the predictive value of aPL subtypes for the risk of thromboembolic events. In a cohort of 58 children with SLE, the presence of lupus anticoagulants had the highest predictive power for thromboembolism.[243] The presence of anticardiolipin antibodies was also predictive but only if they were persistent (positive on at least two occasions 3 months apart). Other studies have confirmed the strong predictive power of aPLs, particularly lupus anticoagulants, for the risk of thromboembolism.[237,244,245] However, pediatric SLE patients who are negative for aPLs rarely develop thrombotic events.

Based on these data, it is recommended that children with SLE be routinely screened for lupus anticoagulants, and if antibodies are present on more than one occasion, families should be counseled on the presenting symptoms of stroke and other thrombotic events.[245] Prophylaxis with low-dose aspirin may be reasonable, especially in the setting of other thrombotic risk factors. However, there are not yet data to support routine prophylactic anticoagulation in SLE patients with lupus anticoagulants in the absence of a history of thromboembolism.[237] Patients who develop DVT can be treated with the standard 3 months of anticoagulation. However, all children with systemic inflammatory disorders such as SLE, rheumatoid arthritis, and IBD are at risk for recurrent thrombus when their inflammatory process is exacerbated. Therefore, children with systemic inflammation and a history of thrombosis should receive prophylactic anticoagulation until the inflammation is well controlled.[221,246]

It is important to note that transient lupus anticoagulants, likely the result of infections or immunizations, have been well described in healthy children. These incidentally found antibodies are not associated with an increased risk of thrombosis or bleeding. There are also patients with antiphospholipid syndrome (APS), defined as a thrombotic event and persistence of aPL positivity for at least 12 weeks after diagnosis, who do not have underlying SLE, although they may develop the disease later.

The management of thromboembolism in primary and secondary APS is different from most other pediatric thromboembolisms. Patients with APS have a high risk of thrombus recurrence off therapy, and most affected children are treated indefinitely.[239,246] However, the appropriate duration or intensity of prolonged therapy is not known. The international Ped-APS registry was established in 2004, and a published report of the first 121 patients has provided insight into the clinical and immunologic manifestations of pediatric APS.[239] As opposed to adults, pediatric APS is only slightly more frequent in girls (female:male ratio, 1.2 : 1), likely because women with recurrent fetal losses are not included in this population. Similar to adults, approximately half of patients present with primary APS. Thrombotic events are diverse and include DVT of the lower extremities (40%), arterial ischemic stroke (26%), and cerebral sinus vein thrombosis (7%). Multiple aPL positivity is frequent (81% with anticardiolipin antibodies, 72% with lupus anticoagulants, and 67% with anti–β_2-glycoprotein I antibodies), but two-thirds of patients tested negative for one or more of the aPL tests, emphasizing the importance of testing for all subtypes in clinical practice. Nineteen percent of pediatric patients with APS experienced a recurrent thrombotic event, even higher than the numbers reported in adult patients.[247,248]

Thromboprophylaxis During Childhood Illness

The use of thromboprophylaxis to prevent hospital-acquired venous thromboembolism has become the standard of care in adult institutions. Even though the risk of thrombosis in hospitalized children is much lower than in adults, there are patients in pediatric hospitals (particularly adolescents and young adults) who deserve systematic screening for thrombosis risk and application of prophylactic measures.[249] Multicenter prospective studies are required to determine the safety and efficacy of prophylaxis, as well as the age cutoff at which prophylaxis should begin to be considered, yet these studies will be very difficult to complete because of the relative rarity of thrombosis in the pediatric setting. In a single-center prospective safety evaluation of anticoagulation prophylaxis in high-risk patients 14 years of age and older, there have been no major bleeding complications.[249]

The 2008 ACCP guidelines discuss the use of thromboprophylaxis in only a few specified settings.[222] The guidelines recommend prophylaxis for children receiving long-term home parenteral nutrition and for patients with complex cardiac conditions and associated procedures. Routine prophylaxis is not recommended in children with central venous lines (including those with cancer).

Most studies of thromboprophylaxis in children with chronic disease have been in the setting of ALL. Because central venous catheters are the most important risk factor in the development of cancer-related thrombosis, investigators have sought to determine if thromboprophylaxis is effective in preventing this complication. Studies have shown that thromboprophylaxis is well tolerated in children with cancer.[205,250,251] However, a randomized trial demonstrated no difference in the incidence of line-related thrombosis between pediatric cancer patients receiving low-dose warfarin (goal INR, 1.3-1.9) and those in the control group.[252] A predictive model incorporating high-dose prednisone, asparaginase in combination with steroids, the presence of a central venous catheter, and the presence of inherited thrombophilias has demonstrated validity in the ability to identify children at high risk of thrombosis in a large population of children with ALL.[253] As a secondary outcome of this study, high-risk patients without low-molecular-weight (LMWH) prophylaxis showed significantly reduced thrombosis-free survival during induction therapy compared with those who did receive prophylaxis (LMWH was administered according to preference of the treating physician) (see box How to Manage Thromboembolism in the Setting of Pediatric Cancer).

How to Manage Thromboembolism in the Setting of Pediatric Cancer

When treating thromboembolism in a patient with cancer, LMWH is the preferred choice. Warfarin, although it is less expensive and can be given orally, is difficult to regulate in the setting of multiple chemotherapy agents, frequent invasive procedures, and changing vitamin K stores because of antibiotics and illness.[205,254,255] A randomized clinical trial in adult cancer patients demonstrated that LMWH was more efficacious and as safe as warfarin in preventing recurrent thromboembolism.[256] The 2008 ACCP guidelines recommend the use of LMWH in the treatment of cancer-related venous thromboembolism for a minimum of 3 months and until the precipitating factor (e.g., use of asparaginase) has resolved.[222] Other practical suggestions have been reported, but none are supported by any systematic observations.[213,222,254]

- A minimum of two doses of LMWH should be held before lumbar punctures and other invasive procedures.
- For intramuscular asparaginase injections, applying firm pressure and administering the medication at the trough of the anti-Xa level are probably adequate to avoid bleeding.
- Clinicians should maintain platelet counts above 50,000/μL in the first 2 weeks of anticoagulation. After that time period, the LMWH dose should be adjusted according to platelet count (50% dosing for platelet counts 20-50,000/μL; hold doses for platelet counts <20,000/μL).

Asparaginase-Related Thrombosis

Management of asparaginase-related thrombosis in ALL can be particularly challenging, and the Dana-Farber Cancer Institute has recently published its experience rechallenging pediatric and adult patients with asparaginase after a first thrombosis.[257] In this retrospective review, survival was similar in patients with and without thrombosis, and the following guidelines were suggested:

- Asparaginase can be resumed when symptoms of thrombosis have resolved and there is evidence of clot stabilization or improvement on repeat imaging, typically after about 4 weeks of anticoagulation.
- Because of the protein depletion experienced by patients receiving asparaginase, anti-Xa levels should be monitored frequently.
- If LMWH at previously adequate doses no longer adequately anticoagulates the patient, antithrombin levels should be checked and antithrombin repleted as necessary.

HEMATOLOGIC COMPLICATIONS OF SOLID ORGAN TRANSPLANTATION IN CHILDREN

The frequency and the success of solid organ transplantation in children have been increasing over the past decade. In 2004, there were 1816 transplants in children representing 7% of all recipients.[258,259] This is an increase of 13% over the previous decade. Of the transplants in 2004, the majority were renal transplants (765) followed by liver (529) and then heart (250-290). The success rate has been also improving impressively, with 5-year survival after kidney transplant at 95% to 96%, liver transplant 79% to 83%, and cardiac transplant 70% to 75%.

Hematologic complications after solid organ transplantation are a common problem. Although most of the evidence regarding the type, frequency, and etiology of these complications has been studied in adults,[260] there are increasing reports in children. After renal transplantation, 60% of children are reported to be anemic. After liver transplant, 36% of children will have a hematologic problem, and of these, 54% are anemic events, 19% anemia and neutropenia, 12% thrombocytopenia, 8% neutropenia, and 2% pancytopenia.[261] After heart, heart–lung, or double lung transplant, 51% of patients have been reported to have hematologic problems, including 49% anemia, 14% neutropenia, 14% thrombocytopenia, and 23% anemia plus neutropenia with or without thrombocytopenia.[262] The etiology of these hematologic problems is most commonly a result of infection followed by medication effect. Miscellaneous causes include blood loss, microangiopathic hemolytic anemia, autoimmune cytopenias, posttransplant lymphoproliferative disease (PTLD), and multifactorial.

In the next section, discussion of the hematologic complications of solid organ transplantation is divided into cell type and by organ type when feasible. The incidence, etiology, and natural history of the problem are addressed. Much of the data are derived from adult studies, but information from pediatric studies is emphasized.

Red Blood Cells

Anemia is a common problem after transplantation, occurring in 66% of kidney transplant recipients at the time of transplant[263] and 60% to 84% after transplant.[264] In liver transplant recipients, the incidence is 20% to 35%,[261,265,266] and in recipients of heart or heart–lung or double lung, it is 30% to 70%.[262,267] There are distinct patterns of presentation of the problems associated with RBCs, including early posttransplant anemia, HUS/microangiopathic hemolytic anemia (MAHA), late anemia from immunosuppressant drugs (ISDs), late anemia from other causes, and pure RBC aplasia (PRBCA).

Early Posttransplant Anemia

Early posttransplant anemia is defined as anemia that occurs within 6 months from the time of transplant. The etiologies include:

1. Postoperative hemorrhage
2. Hemolytic anemia secondary to passenger lymphocyte syndrome or HUS/MAHA
3. Infection including bacterial sepsis or viral infections such as CMV, EBV, or parvovirus
4. Medication, including immunosuppressive drugs and other drugs
5. After renal transplantation, additional causes are iron deficiency or prior uremia or bone disease

Passenger Lymphocyte Syndrome

Passenger lymphocyte syndrome is a graft-versus-host reaction.[268,269] Antibodies made by donor B cells ("passengers") transplanted with the organ are made against host RBCs. This direct antiglobulin-positive immune hemolytic anemia occurs within 3 to 24 days after transplant. Rh antibodies, especially anti-D, are the most common type of antibody. The anemia can be mild to severe but is self-limited, lasting about 1 month. The incidence of this complication increases as the size of the transplanted organ increases:

	Antibody + (%)	Hemolysis (%)
Kidney	17	9
Liver	40	29
Heart–lung	70	70

The incidence also varies depending on the blood type of the donor and recipient:

- 61% with O donor and A recipient
- 22% with O donor and B recipient
- 17% with AB donor and non-AB recipient

Pediatric cases have been reported after all types of solid organ transplant, and the incidence appears to be the same in children and adults, at least after liver transplantation.

Treatment consists of observation alone if mild and transfusion if severe.[268] When transfusing RBCs, the ABO type of the transfused product should be identical to or compatible with the recipient serum, regardless of donor type. When transfusing platelets or fresh-frozen plasma, the product should be compatible with both the recipient and donor. Empiric therapy used in the management of severe cases includes corticosteroids, plasma exchange, and RBC exchange.

Hemolytic Uremic Syndrome/Microangiopathic Hemolytic Anemia

HUS/MAHA after solid organ transplant has been described most often in adults who have the typical clinical presentation for this disorder.[270-272] The majority of cases have been described in renal transplant recipients (90% of cases reported), but it has been seen with all transplant types. The median time of onset is 30 days after transplant, ranging from 8 days to 9 months,[270] and 80% of cases are within 90 days and 96% within 1 year.[272] After renal transplant for HUS, 23% of patients have a recurrence, but the incidence varies depending on the original type of HUS. When transplant is for diarrhea-associated HUS, the recurrence rate is less than 10%. The incidence increases when the original diagnosis is atypical adult HUS and increases even more with familial HUS (60% recurrence rate). In children transplanted for HUS, there was an 8.8% recurrence rate,[271] although it was 80% for those transplanted for atypical HUS and factor H or I deficiency. However, other genetic abnormalities of the complement system are not associated with this high rate of recurrence. Genetic screening is recommended before transplantation not only to determine risk but to develop posttransplant management plans[273] (see later).

The calcineurin inhibitors cyclosporine A (CsA) and tacrolimus (TAC) have triggered the HUS in all of the nonrenal transplant cases and half of the renal transplant cases. Sirolimus alone and especially in combination with cyclosporin has been associated with development of thrombotic microangiopathy.[274] The possibility of an infectious trigger has been suggested for the development of MAHA.

Treatment consists of discontinuing or decreasing the dose or switching the calcineurin inhibitor. Plasma exchange is an unproven therapy. The outcome for graft survival is 60% for de novo HUS but only about 33% for recurrent HUS. In children transplanted for atypical HUS, especially those with a known high risk genetic mutation, perioperative plasma exchange and the use of the terminal complement inhibitor eculizumab have shown promising efficacy in preventing HUS recurrence.[273] Eculizumab has been approved by the U.S. Food and Drug Administration for the treatment of pediatric and adult patients with atypical HUS.

Late Posttransplant Anemia

Anemia occurring greater than 6 months after transplant is termed late *posttransplant anemia*. Causes of late anemia that are common to all solid organ transplants include:[261-263,265,267]

1. Infection with viruses, particularly EBV and parvovirus, and more rarely, CMV
2. Drug effect caused by myelosuppression, hemolytic anemia, or other drug effects (e.g., trimethoprim–sulfamethoxazole, dapsone)

3. Rejection or PTLD
4. Anemia of chronic disease
5. Iron deficiency
6. Acute renal failure
7. Uncommon or multifactorial

Etiologies of late anemia in the renal transplant setting include: end-stage renal disease or low erythropoietin levels (68% of patients will have levels <2 standard deviation [SD] below the norm).[263] After renal transplant, young children have less anemia than older children and young adults. This may be because of the large donor kidney with higher erythropoietin levels and creatinine clearance relative to the size of the patient.

Immunosuppressant Drugs

There is a wide variation—1% to 53%—in the reported incidence of anemia secondary to ISDs. This variation may be a result of the lack of a specific test for drug-associated anemia and the lack of prospective studies. Indirect evidence for the association, however, is quite strong—that is, the ISD is stopped or changed and the anemia improves. There is a clear association of HUS/MAHA with the ISDs CsA and TAC in the early posttransplant period, but a number of studies have documented the association of late anemia with these agents as well. In a study of children after liver transplant, half of the cases of anemia were attributed to ISD.[261] The diagnosis was usually made by excluding other causes of anemia plus evidence of resolution of the anemia after a change in the ISD dose or switch to an alternative drug (median time for resolution, 4 months).

In a study of children and young adults after cardiothoracic transplantation, approximately 25% of the cases of anemia were attributed to tacrolimus, primarily because no other cause was found.[262] The nadir hemoglobin in these patients was 7.3 to 8.8 g/dL, with reticulocytes from 1.5% to 6.7%. Only one patient had a direct antiglobulin study performed, and the results were negative. Four of five patients with simultaneous anemia and neutropenia recovered counts within 5 weeks of switching to CsA. In another study of 50 pediatric renal transplant patients, the prevalence of anemia was 60%, with 30% having hemoglobin levels below 10 g/dL. The TAC dose was found to be significantly associated with the presence of anemia.[275]

The association of PRCA and TAC was first reported in adults. Two children were reported to develop PRCA while taking TAC 8 and 47 months after liver transplantation.[276] Neither had evidence of parvovirus B19 infection. When there was no evidence of spontaneous recovery after 2 to 3 months of observation, they were switched from TAC to CsA, and both recovered within 3 weeks. Of interest, in a study of adults after liver transplantation, erythropoietin production was found to be reduced in patients receiving cyclosporin but not tacrolimus.[277]

There are a number of case reports of AIHA associated with the use of TAC and other ISDs in both children and adults. AIHA has been seen after liver, small bowel, multivisceral, kidney, and heart transplants. Onset of severe anemia has been from 2 months to many years after transplant. The direct antiglobulin test has revealed warm, mixed, or cold antibodies. The common finding in all cases was use of tacrolimus immunosuppression, although in a few cases, other ISDs were also used. Treatment was variable, including corticosteroids, IVIG, plasmapheresis, rituximab, and splenomegaly. TAC was discontinued in many cases with alternative ISD, including cyclosporine or sirolimus initiated. Resolution of the AIHA was the usual outcome with some rapid and apparently sustained responses to rituximab and switching to an alternative ISD.[278-282]

Nonimmune hemolysis has also been documented in adults. In a retrospective study of 81 patients (median age, 39 years; range, 12-66 years) after lung transplantation, 20% developed hemolytic anemia in the first year after transplant.[283] All were taking CsA, and none received TAC. The anemia was mild to moderate, there was no evidence of autoantibody formation or MAHA, and other causes of anemia were excluded. The authors postulate an auto- or alloimmune mechanism to explain this phenomenon.

Anemia has been reported to be associated with all of the currently used ISDs, including mycophenolate mofetil (MMF) and sirolimus. Although direct comparison of all of the drugs has not been performed, it appears that TAC and CsA have a similar incidence,[284] with anemia occurring less commonly with the others. One possible mechanism of the development of autoimmune antibodies posttransplant is the chronic T-cell suppression resulting from the use of these agents followed by release of B-cell control. As noted earlier, treatment has been empiric and has included the standard treatments for AIHA, including rituximab. Reduction in dose or switching the type of the ISD appears to be an effective therapy.

Pure Red Blood Cell Aplasia Associated With Parvovirus B19

Pure RBC aplasia was initially reported in adults in 1986 with multiple reports since that time. Review of the literature in 2006 revealed 91 cases of parvovirus B19 infection posttransplant reported in adults.[283] Seventy-four were in solid organ recipients, with the majority after kidney transplant (71%) followed by heart–lung transplant (16%) and then liver transplant (12%). A total of 99% were anemic, with one-third also having leukopenia and 18% thrombocytopenia. The average time to onset was 1.75 months posttransplant with a range of 1 week to 96 months. The most reliable test to diagnose infection was the parvovirus B19 PCR, with results being positive in 85% of cases; IgM results were positive in 78% and IgG in 39%. Treatment with IVIG was used in 84% of patients, and there was a recurrence in 28%. The three deaths were only seen in patients after liver transplant who developed myocarditis and cardiogenic shock. Of interest, in a prospective study of 47 solid organ transplant recipients, none were found to have molecular evidence of parvovirus B19 in the first year posttransplant.[285]

In a review of parvovirus B19 infection in children after transplantation, there were 16 case reports: five after liver, heart, and renal transplant each and one after bone marrow transplantation.[286] The onset was at a median of 8 months with a range of 1 to 24 months. Although only three of 14 tested were IgM positive, all were PCR positive. There were no associated symptoms in seven of 14, but other reported symptoms include cytopenias, rash, myocarditis, and pneumonia. All 10 patients who received IVIG treatment were cured, although recurrences have been reported.

Platelets

Problems with platelets including thrombocytopenia and thrombocytopathy have been reported after transplant primarily in adults. After liver transplantation, almost all patients develop a transient thrombocytopenia. Delayed thrombocytopenia is much less frequent. It has been reported in 12% of children after liver transplant,[261] 8% after cardiothoracic transplant,[259] and outside of the setting of HUS/MAHA very infrequently after kidney transplantation. Causes of platelet problems posttransplant include medication effect, immune etiology, HUS/MAHA, infection, and other miscellaneous causes.

Immediate Thrombocytopenia After Liver Transplantation

More than 90% of adults have been reported to have thrombocytopenia within the first week after liver transplantation.[287-291] Nadir counts usually occur between days 4 and 6 posttransplant, with an average count of 58,000/μL (range, 19,000-330,000/μL). An increase in thrombopoietin is seen on days 4 to 6, and increased reticulated platelets are noted on days 7 and 8. There are few reported clinical sequelae from the mild thrombocytopenia, although the lowest platelet counts have been associated with the most severe and complicated posttransplant course. Resolution is usually seen in 2 weeks. Lack of resolution is associated with a poor prognosis for graft and overall survival.

There is controversy regarding the etiology of this transient thrombocytopenia. One theory is that it is a nonimmune consumptive process reflected by increased markers of thrombin generation.[291] The liver may be the site of platelet sequestration. A second theory is that it is unlikely to be a consumptive process because of the lack of platelet activation after day 1. The thrombocytopenia is more likely a result of low levels of thrombopoietin seen pretransplant. With new production and rising levels of thrombopoietin from the new liver, there is a subsequent increase in platelet production, resulting in normalization of the platelet count soon after transplantation. Although the specific etiology has not been clarified, there is general consensus that it is not immune mediated.

Lymphocyte-depleting antibodies such as rabbit antithymocyte globulin (rATG) are being used with increasing frequency as induction type therapy in pediatric liver and intestine transplantation. rATG does exacerbate the transient thrombocytopenia seen immediately after solid organ transplant but resolves in a similar 1- to 2-week period. Treatment of this transient thrombocytopenia is supportive. Platelet transfusions are of uncertain benefit. Although originally azathioprine was believed to be a cause of this thrombocytopenia, there is no evidence that alteration of azathioprine dose is necessary.

Delayed Posttransplantation Thrombocytopenia

Delayed thrombocytopenia is not a major problem after solid organ transplantation, and most of the data are published in adult series. In one retrospective study of 36 adult liver transplant recipients, mild thrombocytopenia (<140,000/μL) was seen in 54% of patients at 1 year and 25% at 3 years after transplant.[292] However, severe thrombocytopenia (<50,000/μL) was only seen in 9% of patients at 1 year and in no patients at 3 years after transplant. The thrombocytopenia was associated with splenomegaly in some patients. No clinical bleeding problems were noted after 1 year from transplant. In one report, three of 25 (12%) pediatric liver transplant recipients were found to have isolated thrombocytopenia.[261] The etiology of the thrombocytopenia in these children was cavernous transformation of the portal vein, autoimmune, and unknown. In two other children in this series, thrombocytopenia was associated with additional cytopenias, and the cause was possibly related to TAC. In an additional study of 126 children who underwent cardiothoracic transplantation, nine (8%) were noted to have isolated thrombocytopenia. Infection was the most common etiology (262). In patients with combined cytopenias, including thrombocytopenia, two-thirds were related to either infection or PTLD and 20% possibly secondary to TAC.

Sirolimus has been associated with mild thrombocytopenia in adults, although the reported frequency has varied. In a study of renal transplant recipients, 23% were reported to have mild thrombocytopenia,[293] but no liver transplant patients taking the drug were found to be thrombocytopenic.[294] In 66 pediatric kidney transplant recipients taking sirolimus, there were no reported cases of thrombocytopenia.[295] Low platelet counts are usually seen within the first 4 weeks of treatment and are associated with higher sirolimus blood levels.[296,297] Similar to TAC and CsA, sirolimus has been shown to potentiate agonist-induced platelet aggregation, although this is not the proven explanation for the thrombocytopenia.[298] A 25% to 50% dose reduction is often effective in resolving sirolimus-mediated thrombocytopenia.

Immune-Mediated Thrombocytopenia Posttransplantation

There are many case reports of immune-mediated thrombocytopenia after all types of solid organ transplantation in children and adults and either alone or in combination with other cytopenias. Eight adults after liver transplant were reported to have immune thrombocytopenia (incidence, 0.7%).[299] The low platelets were seen on average 53 months after transplantation with a range of 1.9 to 173 months. Three patients had demonstrable antiplatelet antibodies. Steroids provided effective therapy in four and rituximab in four, although splenectomy was ultimately necessary in three. Seven of the eight survived with normal platelet counts. Five children were reported to have severe thrombocytopenia (<10,000/μL) within 2 to 4 months after starting TAC.[280,300] All were documented to have antiplatelet antibodies. Responses were seen to steroids, rituximab, or anti-D.

After heart or lung transplantation, two cases in adults have been reported.[301] These cases occurred 60 to 460 days after transplant and responded to prednisone and IVIG. Acquired Glanzmann thromboasthenia has been reported in two children after cardiac transplantation.[281,302] Both were receiving TAC and had demonstrable antibodies against glycoprotein IIb/IIIa. One patient had multiple autoantibodies, and the other subsequently developed additional antiplatelet antibodies. One child responded to prednisone therapy and switching from TAC to CsA. The other responded to rituximab after failing prednisone and IVIG.

Alloimmune thrombocytopenia was reported in three recipients of organs from the same donor (two kidneys and a liver).[303] Development of HPA-1a (PL^{A1}) antibodies from donor B cells were documented in an example of passenger lymphocyte syndrome. The thrombocytopenia in these cases was particularly refractory to standard treatment except transfusion of HPA-1a–negative platelets. One patient died, another required splenectomy, and one patient's thrombocytopenia resolved after an episode of severe graft rejection (see box on Treatment of Immune-Mediated Thrombocytopenia After Solid Organ Transplantation in Children).

Treatment of Immune-Mediated Thrombocytopenia After Solid Organ Transplantation in Children

There is no standard approach to the treatment of immune-mediated thrombocytopenia that occurs after solid organ transplantation. First, all other causes of thrombocytopenia should be ruled out before beginning therapy for what is often a presumptive diagnosis of immune-mediated thrombocytopenia. If the thrombocytopenia is mild to moderate (>20,000-30,000/μL) with no associated bleeding symptoms, we usually observe without intervention and monitor the platelet count on at least a weekly basis. If the platelet count is lower than 10,000 to 15,000/μL or if there is bleeding, immediate treatment is initiated with high-dose corticosteroids: 4 mg/kg/day of prednisone (or intravenous equivalent) divided in three or four doses and continued for 4 days. If there is a response (i.e., platelet count >20,000/μL), the corticosteroid is dropped to 2 mg/kg/day divided in two or three doses and then slowly tapered to zero over the subsequent 2 to 3 weeks. IVIG or anti-D in standard doses used for childhood ITP can be used if there is no response to high-dose corticosteroids.

For patients who have recurrent or chronic thrombocytopenia requiring multiple courses of treatment to maintain platelet counts greater than 10,000 to 15,000/μL, we have used vincristine (1.5 mg/M^2 [maximum dose, 2 mg] intravenously weekly for 6 weeks) with success. Rituximab (375 mg/M^2 IV weekly for 4 weeks) has infrequently been used in this situation. For patients taking tacrolimus with refractory thrombocytopenia, serious consideration should be given to switching to an alternative ISD because this may be necessary for resolution of the thrombocytopenia. Involvement of both the transplant team and the hematology team is necessary for ideal management of these complex patients.

Infection-Associated Thrombocytopenia Posttransplantation

Although there are few published reports, one would expect the same hematologic problems, including thrombocytopenia, associated with bacterial sepsis or other serious infections as seen in nontransplant patients. Infection with HHV-6 and the herpesvirus group has been studied closely. HHV-6 is commonly seen after transplant, mostly in stem cell transplant recipients. In adults after liver transplant, there are case reports of a syndrome of HHV-6 infection with thrombocytopenia, fever, and encephalopathy.[304] This syndrome has not been reported in children with HHV-6 infection.[305,306]

Herpesvirus infection after kidney transplantation in children is seen in about one-third of patients, with CMV being the most common infection.[307] The hematologic abnormalities associated with herpesvirus infection include thrombocytopenia and leukopenia, with an incidence of 31% and 24%, respectively. These and other symptoms of herpesvirus infection occur at the same frequency as nontransplant patients.

There is a case report of a child after liver transplant who developed measles complicated by autoimmune thrombocytopenia and neutropenia.[308]

White Blood Cells

Leukopenia and neutropenia are uncommonly reported in the literature after solid organ transplantation, although this may not reflect the true incidence seen in practice.[309] In two reviews of hematologic complications in children after transplantation, isolated neutropenia was seen in two of 70 (3%) patients after liver transplant and nine of 106 (8%) patients after cardiothoracic transplant.[261,262] Neutropenia was also seen in combination with other cytopenias. Although there are predominantly case reports in the pediatric literature, in one review of neutropenia after 400 renal transplants in adults, 35 cases (9%) were reported.[310] The etiology of leukopenia or neutropenia is similar in children and adults and includes immunosuppressive agents; other myelosuppressive drugs (e.g., ganciclovir); infection (e.g., CMV, sepsis); and less frequently, INF, PTLD, hypersplenism, INF, and idiopathic. Use of TAC is often implicated as a possible contributing factor.

Both filgrastim (granulocyte colony-stimulating factor) and sargramostim (granulocyte macrophage colony-stimulating factor) have been used to treat neutropenia in adults and children. In adults, it has resulted in improvement of the WBC count in more than 90% of patients after three to four doses.[310,311] There was no evidence of precipitation of rejection. In the case reports in children, both agents have been found to be effective in most patients, but there is a suggestion that efficacy may be affected by continuation of TAC.[309,312,313] Although cytokine therapy has been shown to increase the neutrophil count, there are insufficient data to prove effectiveness of preventing or treating infection or decreasing mortality.[314]

There has been one report on the use of granulocyte transfusions in solid organ transplant recipient, including one child. Of the 14 patients studied, 11 showed an increase in ANC greater than 1000/μL by the end of the course. Of 12 patients with infections, four (33%) showed a clinical response. Additional studies will be needed to evaluate the efficacy of granulocyte transfusions in transplant patients.[314]

Azathioprine is well known to cause myelosuppression and has been associated with moderate to severe neutropenia. Azathioprine is catabolized in vivo by xanthine oxidase and thiopurine methyltransferase (TPMT). TPMT activity can vary considerably depending on a genetic polymorphism. Approximately 0.3% of whites are homozygous and 11% heterozygous for deficiency of TPMT. Severe myelosuppression, including fatal neutropenia, has been documented in transplant patients who are homozygous for TMPT deficiency and receiving azathioprine.[315] Some data suggest that monitoring 6-thioguanine nucleotides (the metabolites of azathioprine) may allow for individualized management of azathioprine dosing with fewer side effects, although this has not become common practice.[316,317]

Neutropenia has also been associated with the use of MMF and sirolimus. Neutropenia and thrombocytopenia have been noted as side effects of MMF since 1998.[318] Leukopenia may affect 5% to 11% of patients taking the drug, and pseudo Pelger-Huet anomaly has also been noted.[319,320] The leukopenia is often seen within 2 to 8 months after starting the drug. Filgrastim has been effective in reversing the neutropenia, although some patients required decreasing the dose or stopping the drug. Ganciclovir and valacyclovir are commonly used simultaneously with MMF to treat or prevent CMV disease. These drugs are also known to be associated with neutropenia.[321] There may be an interaction between these drugs that increases the risk for neutropenia.[322,323] It may be necessary to stop ganciclovir as well as MMF for the neutropenia to improve.[319] Of note, serious infections are infrequently encountered.

In two reports of the use of sirolimus in children, neutropenia was the most common toxicity along with hepatitis, hyperlipidemia, and mouth ulcers.[324,325] It is not clear whether the neutropenia is directly related to serum level of the drug. Most counts improve with a decrease in the drug dose, although a few patients need to have the drug discontinued.

Pancytopenia

Pancytopenia is seen in two settings after solid organ transplantation. The first is early after liver transplant for acute liver failure from acute infectious hepatitis.[326,327] This represents the known aplastic anemia that can be seen in as many as one-third of patients after non-A-E hepatitis. Treatment and outcome are similar to those in patients with posthepatitic aplastic anemia who do not require liver transplantation. The second setting is delayed pancytopenia, which may be secondary to infection with or without PTLD.[328] A number of cases have been associated with the use of TAC.[261,329] Hemophagocytic syndrome has also been reported in the posttransplant setting, usually caused by an acquired viral infection.[330]

HEMATOLOGIC ASPECTS OF POISONING

It has been estimated that about 6 million children, most younger than 5 years of age, ingest some toxin each year. The effects of toxins on the blood are diverse, usually nonspecific, and in most situations overshadowed by the nonhematologic manifestations of the exposure.[331] With certain toxins, however, bleeding, anemia, or change in the appearance (color) of the blood may be an important component of the clinical sequelae of an acute exposure.

The abnormalities of hemostasis after poisoning are numerous, and the mechanisms vary. Bleeding may be the only manifestation of warfarin toxicity secondary to an overdose of the drug or ingestion of a rodenticide containing warfarin. Any hepatotoxic substance (e.g., iron, acetaminophen) may lead to decreased synthesis of clotting factors and resultant coagulopathy. Bleeding in these circumstances is delayed for at least 24 hours, although there appears to be an early coagulopathy in iron poisoning that may be caused by a direct effect on clotting protein function and not hepatotoxicity.[332] DIC has been seen after ingestion of mushrooms of the *Amanita* genus or after a bite from the brown recluse spider *(Loxosceles reclusa)*. Poisonous snake bites can result in coagulation abnormalities characterized by hypofibrinogenemia with or without thrombocytopenia or a DIC-like syndrome.[331] Severe thrombocytopenia has been described with elemental mercury poisoning.

Acute hemolytic anemia may be the presenting manifestation after exposure to drugs and toxins in children with G6PD deficiency or hemoglobin Zürich or (rarely) in normal children. Severe hemolytic anemia has been seen after the bite of the brown recluse spider and of a rattlesnake and after a wasp sting.

Exposure to certain toxins may result in characteristic color changes of the blood, which in turn may be reflected clinically in abnormal skin color. The child with methemoglobinemia (see next paragraph) presents with a slate-gray cyanosis unresponsive to 100%

oxygen administration. On exposure to air, the blood retains a distinct brown color. Patients with toxic exposure to carbon monoxide or cyanide have increased levels of carboxyhemoglobin or cyanhemoglobin, respectively, resulting in a cherry-red color of the blood and skin, but only with high concentrations of the offending hemoglobin.

Infants (up to 4 months of age) are at particular risk for developing methemoglobinemia because of a reduced amount (≈60% of normal) of cytochrome b5 reductase present in neonatal RBCs. Methemoglobinemia has been described in infants with diarrheal illness and in infants exposed to exogenous agents.[333]

Yano and colleagues[334] described 11 patients with transient methemoglobinemia, all infants younger than 1 month of age, who presented with vomiting, diarrhea, and acidosis. In prospective studies of infants younger than 6 months of age with diarrheal disease, 64% had elevated levels of methemoglobin (with a mean ± SD of 10.5% ± 12.3%), 31% were cyanotic, most infants were small or failing to thrive, there was no association of methemoglobinemia and acidosis, and all children recovered from their illness.[335,336] Although most infants with endogenous methemoglobinemia can be managed with support and hydration, treatment with methylene blue (1 mg/kg) is indicated in symptomatic or more severely affected children (i.e., with methemoglobin >20%-30%).

Nursery epidemics of methemoglobinemia have been reported in normal newborns exposed to disinfectants or aniline dyes used to mark diapers. Infants fed formulas made with well water containing a high concentration of nitrates have developed methemoglobinemia. EMLA cream, a eutectic mixture of the local anesthetics lidocaine and prilocaine, has been effective in decreasing pain in infants undergoing circumcision. Methemoglobinemia has been reported with EMLA use in this situation but only in overdose.[337] Other ingestions associated with methemoglobinemia include phenazopyridine (Pyridium), dapsone, metoclopramide, and nitroethane (an artificial fingernail remover). Although the list of oxidants reported to cause methemoglobinemia is long, methemoglobinemia caused by exogenous agents is uncommonly seen in infants and children.[338]

Lead Poisoning

Lead poisoning in children has been a serious public health problem for decades. However, the most serious toxic effects of lead (e.g., encephalopathy) commonly seen in the past are rarely encountered today, primarily because of measures instituted to decrease lead exposure (no-lead paint, no-lead gasoline) and screening programs in high-risk areas. Mean blood lead levels in the United States have declined, from 15 μg/dL between 1976 and 1982 to 3.6 μg/dL between 1988 and 1991.[328] Nonetheless, lead toxicity remains a problem, especially in high-risk children. Additionally, children arriving from other countries with less stringent public health requirements regarding lead exposure remain at risk for significant lead toxicity.[339] Increasing evidence shows that even low levels of lead exposure are associated with a significant decline in neurodevelopmental outcome, and in 1991, the Centers for Disease Control and Prevention (CDC) lowered the intervention level of lead in the blood from 25 to 10 μg/dL.[339,340] Reviews of the public health issues relating to lead poisoning in children have been published.[341]

The occurrence of lead poisoning in children with sickle cell disease may be underrecognized. Pica may be a manifestation of sickle cell anemia, even in the absence of iron deficiency, predisposing children to lead ingestion.[342] Additionally, some children with sickle cell disease may be at risk for environmental lead exposure, including substandard housing with lead paint. The signs and symptoms of lead toxicity may resemble those of sickle cell disease, including abdominal pain, peripheral neuropathy with extremity pain, constipation, and hyponatremia.[343] Lead toxicity should be considered in the differential diagnosis of children with unusual manifestations of sickle cell disease.

The primary hematologic effect of lead is interference at multiple points along the heme synthetic pathway. The two most important effects are inhibition of δ-aminolevulinic acid (ALA) dehydratase and ferrochelatase, resulting in the accumulation of heme intermediates such as protoporphyrin. A shortened RBC survival time accompanies lead poisoning and probably is caused by decreased activity of pyrimidine 5-nucleotidase (also resulting in basophilic stippling of the RBC) and possibly inhibition of G6PD and the pentose shunt.[344]

The anemia of lead poisoning has classically been described as a hypochromic, microcytic anemia, as might be expected from the effects of lead on heme synthesis. Although anemia has been said to be a common finding in lead intoxication, in reality, anemia is uncommon unless the lead poisoning is severe or there is associated iron deficiency.

A strong association exists between lead poisoning and iron deficiency in children. Both tend to occur in the same population of predominantly lower socioeconomic status. Experimentally, iron deficiency has been shown to increase lead absorption, retention in tissues, and toxicity. Iron deficiency also decreases lead excretion during chelation.[345] Lead may impede iron absorption and metabolism, leading to a vicious circle of increasing lead toxicity and worsening iron deficiency. In a study of children with lead poisoning (blood lead ≥30 μg/dL), 86% were found to have iron deficiency, and 100% of those with more severe lead poisoning (CDC risk classification III) were iron deficient.[346]

A number of reports in children with lead toxicity have documented the infrequent occurrence of anemia without concomitant iron deficiency. Cohen and colleagues[346] found anemia in 12% and microcytosis in 21% of iron-sufficient children with severe lead poisoning (CDC classes III and IV). The combination of anemia plus microcytosis, however, was found in only one of the 58 children in their series. In less severely affected children (CDC classes I to III), Yip and associates[347] found a 30% incidence of anemia, but of those with either mild or no iron deficiency, only 6% were anemic. Clark and coworkers,[348] using multiple linear regression analysis, found transferrin saturation to be the most important predictor of mean corpuscular volume, hemoglobin, and zinc protoporphyrin levels in children with lead poisoning.

Two important points emerge from the foregoing information: (1) children with significant lead poisoning may have neither anemia nor microcytosis, and (2) children with documented lead poisoning should be screened for underlying iron deficiency. The immediate treatment and long-term management of patients with lead poisoning can be found in a recent review.[349]

HEMATOLOGIC ASPECTS OF METABOLIC DISEASES

A number of congenital disorders of metabolism may manifest hematologic abnormalities as part of the clinical presentation. Such global metabolic defects have diverse manifestations; especially prominent are neurologic abnormalities, failure to thrive, and unexplained metabolic acidosis. Although the hematologic findings may be overshadowed by the systemic illness, the recognition of a characteristic pattern of signs and symptoms may lead expeditiously to the correct diagnosis. Table 154-4 is a compilation of inborn disorders of metabolism that may manifest in infancy or childhood with hematologic cytopenias.[350] Additional information regarding metabolic disorders is available through the Online Mendelian Inheritance in Man (http://www.ncib.nlm.nih.gov/omim).

SPLENOMEGALY IN CHILDREN

Splenomegaly is a problem frequently encountered by both pediatricians and pediatric hematologists. Although the spleen is rarely a site of primary disease, it may reflect systemic involvement in a variety of disorders. The spleen is the largest collection of lymphoid tissue in the body, with a unique association between the bloodstream and the reticuloendothelial compartment of the spleen. Splenomegaly may result when there is antigenic stimulation of the lymphoid

Table 154-4 Hematologic Manifestations of Metabolic Disease With Onset in Infancy and Childhood

Category	Disease	Defect	Hematologic Finding(s)	Associated Findings
Lysosomal enzyme defects	Gaucher disease, type 1	Glucocerebrosidase deficiency	Anemia, thrombocytopenia	Splenomegaly, bone abnormalities, delayed puberty, lipid engorged macrophages (Gaucher cell) in BM
	Niemann-Pick disease, type A	Acid sphingomyelinase deficiency	Anemia	Feeding difficulties, hepatosplenomegaly, developmental delay, neurodegenerative course, cherry-red macula, lipid-laden macrophages (foam cells) in BM
	Wolman disease	Acid lipase deficiency	Anemia, thrombocytopenia	Emesis, diarrhea, hepatosplenomegaly, vacuolization of lymphocytes, lipid-laden macrophages in BM, adrenal calcification
	Aspartylglycosaminuria	Aspartylglycosaminidase deficiency	Neutropenia	Recurrent infections, diarrhea, hernias, lens opacities, neurologic abnormalities, vacuolated lymphocytes
Defects of heme synthesis	Congenital erythropoietic porphyria	Uroporphyrinogen III cosynthase deficiency	Anemia, thrombocytopenia	Hemolysis, staining of diapers, photosensitivity, developmental delay, splenomegaly, erythrodontia
	Erythropoietic protoporphyria	Ferrochelatase deficiency	Anemia, thrombocytopenia	Hemolysis, photosensitivity, neurologic abnormalities, hepatobiliary dysfunction
Defect of amino acid metabolism	Tyrosinemia, type 1	Fumarylacetoacetate hydrolase deficiency	Anemia, thrombocytopenia	Failure to thrive, emesis, hepatopathy, neurologic abnormalities, bleeding, "cabbage-like" odor, renal tubular dysfunction
Defects of organic acid metabolism	Isovaleric academia	Isovaleryl-CoA dehydrogenase deficiency	Anemia, thrombocytopenia, neutropenia, pancytopenia	Acidosis, emesis, neurologic abnormalities, odor of "sweaty feet"
	Methylmalonic academia	Methylmalonyl-CoA mutase deficiency	Anemia, thrombocytopenia, leukopenia, pancytopenia	Acidosis, neurologic abnormalities, failure to thrive, emesis
	Mevalonic aciduria	Mevalonate kinase deficiency	Anemia, thrombocytopenia	Acidosis, cataracts, neurologic abnormalities, hepatosplenomegaly
Defects of organic acid metabolism	Propionic academia	Propionyl CoA carboxylase deficiency	Anemia, thrombocytopenia neutropenia, pancytopenia	Ketotic hyperglycinemia, acidosis, neurologic abnormalities
	Pyroglutamic aciduria	Glutathione synthetase deficiency	Anemia, neutropenia	Hemolysis, neurologic abnormalities, metabolic acidosis
Membrane transport defect	Lysinuric protein intolerance	*SLC7A7* gene mutations	Anemia, thrombocytopenia, leukopenia, pancytopenia	Malabsorption, protein intolerance, hyperammonemia, neurologic abnormalities, glomerulonephritis, pulmonary hemorrhage, hemophagocytosis
Glycolytic pathway defects	Triosephosphate isomerase deficiency	Triosephosphate isomerase deficiency	Anemia	Hemolysis, neurologic abnormalities, myopathy
	Phosphoglycerate kinase deficiency	Phosphoglycerate kinase deficiency	Anemia	Hemolysis, neurologic abnormalities
Defects of vitamin metabolism	Cobalamin metabolic defects	Cobalamin transport and utilization defects	Anemia, thrombocytopenia, neutropenia, pancytopenia	Megaloblastosis, failure to thrive, neurologic abnormalities
	Folate metabolic defects	Folate transport and utilization defects	Anemia, thrombocytopenia	Megaloblastosis, ringed sideroblasts, diarrhea, failure to thrive, neurologic abnormalities
	Holocarboxylase synthetase deficiency	Holocarboxylase synthetase deficiency	Thrombocytopenia	Acidosis, hyperammonemia, respiratory distress, neurologic abnormalities, skin rash
Defect in metal metabolism	Wilson disease	*ATP7B* gene mutation	Anemia	Hemolysis, liver dysfunction, neurologic abnormalities, Kayser-Fleischer rings, arthropathy
Defects of purine and pyrimidine metabolism	Hereditary orotic aciduria synthase deficiency	Uridine-5′-monophosphate	Anemia, leukopenia	Megaloblastosis, orotic acid crystalluria, immunodeficiency
	Lesch-Nyhan syndrome	Hypoxanthine-guanine phosphoribosyltransferase deficiency	Anemia	Megaloblastosis, hyperuricemia, nephrolithiasis, neurologic abnormalities, self-mutilation

Continued

Table 154-4 Hematologic Manifestations of Metabolic Disease With Onset in Infancy and Childhood—cont'd

Category	Disease	Defect	Hematologic Finding(s)	Associated Findings
Defects of carbohydrate metabolism	Galactosemia	Galactose-1 phosphate uridyltransferase deficiency	Anemia	Hemolysis, failure to thrive, neurologic findings, jaundice, emesis, diarrhea, hepatic dysfunction, cataracts, gram-negative sepsis
	Glycogen storage disease type 1b	Deficient hepatic transport of glucose-phosphate	Anemia, neutropenia	Hypoglycemia, acidosis, hepatomegaly, xanthomas, inflammatory bowel disease
	Hereditary fructose intolerance	Aldolase B deficiency	Anemia, thrombocytopenia	Poor feeding, emesis, failure to thrive, neurologic findings, hypoglycemia, liver dysfunction, ringed sideroblasts, coagulopathy, hemophagocytosis, shock
Mitochondrial disorders	DIDMOAD syndrome (Wolfram syndrome)	Mitochondrial DNA deletion	Anemia, thrombocytopenia, neutropenia, pancytopenia	Megaloblastosis, ringed sideroblasts, diabetes insipidus, diabetes mellitus, optic atrophy, deafness
	Pearson syndrome	Mitochondrial DNA deletions	Anemia thrombocytopenia, neutropenia, pancytopenia	Ringed sideroblasts, vacuolization of BM precursors, exocrine pancreatic dysfunction, metabolic acidosis
Lipoprotein disorder	Abetalipoproteinemia	Microsomal triglyceride transfer protein defects	Anemia	Hemolysis, acanthocytosis, bleeding, emesis, diarrhea, failure to thrive, neurologic findings
Miscellaneous disorders	Barth syndrome (endocardial fibroelastosis-2)	Tafazzin gene mutations	Neutropenia	Cardiomyopathy, endocardial fibroelastosis, skeletal myopathy, short stature, 3-myethylglutaconicaciduria, abnormal mitochondria
	Cyclic hematopoiesis	Neutrophil elastase gene mutation	Neutropenia	Recurrent oral ulcers, poor dentition, recurrent fever, malaise
	Severe congenital neutropenia (Kostmann syndrome)	Neutrophil elastase gene mutation	Neutropenia	Severe invasive infections, acute leukemia
	Wiscott-Aldrich syndrome	*WAS* gene mutations	Thrombocytopenia	Eczema, infections, small platelets

BM, Bone marrow; *CoA,* coenzyme A; *DIDMOAD,* diabetes insipidus, diabetes mellitus, optic atrophy, deafness.

Evaluation and Management of Children With Splenomegaly

When evaluating a child with chronic splenomegaly, the clinician must consider all of the possibilities noted in Table 154-5. Clues from the history and physical examination may suggest a specific etiology and direct a tailored approach to the diagnostic laboratory evaluation. If, on the other hand, there is no apparent cause of the enlarged spleen, a number of screening laboratory tests should be performed, including a complete blood count with differential, platelet count, and reticulocyte count; evaluation of the peripheral smear; determination of sedimentation rate; liver function tests; determination of antibody titers to EBV, CMV, and *Toxoplasma* spp.; antinuclear antibody assay; and ultrasound evaluation of the liver, spleen, and portal system (the last with Doppler flow technique). Further evaluation, including bone marrow examination, may be necessary if the screening tests do not reveal the cause of the splenic enlargement.

Management of splenomegaly usually is that of the underlying disease, when such treatment exists. Splenectomy may be indicated in selected conditions, but the potential benefits from splenectomy must be weighed against the risk of postsplenectomy sepsis, a rapidly progressive bacteremia, most commonly from *S. pneumoniae,* with a mortality rate of approximately 50%. The risk of postsplenectomy sepsis depends on the age of the patient and the nature of the underlying disorder. Patients younger than 3 years of age and those with a compromised immune or reticuloendothelial system are most susceptible. When elective splenectomy is indicated, it is advisable to (1) postpone surgery until the patient is at least 5 to 6 years of age; (2) administer pneumococcal, meningococcal, and *H. influenzae* vaccines (if the patient was not previously immunized) at least 1 to 2 weeks before splenectomy; (3) consider use of prophylactic penicillin for at least 4 years; and (4) manage significant febrile illnesses as possible postsplenectomy sepsis at all times. In addition to the risk of postsplenectomy sepsis, the rare complication of postsplenectomy portal or splenic vein thrombosis must also be considered.

For children younger than 5 years of age with severe symptoms from hemolytic anemia, hemoglobinopathy, or hypersplenism, partial splenectomy should be considered. In a number of studies, up to 90% of the spleen has been removed safely, with a high rate of success and preservation of splenic function.[351,352] Regrowth of the spleen to variable degrees has been noted, with occasional need for reoperation.

Table 154-5 Causes of Splenomegaly in Children

DISORDERS OF THE BLOOD
Hemolytic anemia: congenital or acquired
Thalassemia
Sickle cell disease
Leukemia
Osteopetrosis
Myelofibrosis, myeloid metaplasia, thrombocythemia
INFECTIONS: ACUTE AND CHRONIC
Viral
Congenital (e.g., TORCH association)
Mononucleosis (e.g., EBV, CMV infection)
Virus-associated hemophagocytic syndrome
Human immunodeficiency virus
Bacterial
Sepsis or abscess
Brucellosis
Salmonellosis
Tularemia
Tuberculosis
Subacute bacterial endocarditis
Syphilis
Lyme disease
Fungal
Histoplasmosis (disseminated)
Rickettsial
Rocky Mountain spotted fever
Cat scratch disease
Parasitic
Toxoplasmosis
Malaria
Leishmaniasis (kala-azar)
Schistosomiasis
Echinococcosis
HEPATIC AND PORTAL SYSTEM DISORDERS
Acute or chronic active hepatitis
Cirrhosis, hepatic fibrosis, biliary atresia
Portal or splenic venous obstruction (Banti syndrome)
AUTOIMMUNE DISEASE
Juvenile rheumatoid arthritis
Systemic lupus erythematosus
Autoimmune lymphoproliferative syndrome (Canale-Smith syndrome)
NEOPLASMS AND CYSTS
Lymphomas (Hodgkin and non-Hodgkin)
Hemangiomas and lymphangiomas
Hamartomas
Congenital or acquired (posttraumatic) cysts
STORAGE DISEASES AND INBORN ERRORS OF METABOLISM
Lipidoses: Gaucher disease, Niemann-Pick disease, others
Mucopolysaccharidoses
Defects in carbohydrate metabolism: galactosemia, fructose intolerance
Sea-blue histiocyte syndrome
MISCELLANEOUS DISORDERS
Histiocytoses
Reactive
Langerhans cell
Malignant
Sarcoidosis
Congestive heart failure
Familial Mediterranean fever

CMV, Cytomegalovirus; *EBV,* Epstein-Barr virus; *TORCH,* toxoplasmosis, other infections, rubella, cytomegalovirus infection, herpes simplex.

system (e.g., infection), obstruction of blood flow within or distal to the spleen (e.g., portal vein obstruction), exaggeration of one of the normal functions of the spleen because of an underlying abnormality (e.g., hemolytic anemia, splenic sequestration), or infiltration of the spleen by a foreign cell (e.g., leukemia, storage diseases).

The spleen tip normally is palpable in preterm infants; up to 30% of full-term neonates have a palpable spleen. A spleen can be felt in up to 5% to 10% of normal children, but most of these are in the infant or toddler age group. As a general rule, a spleen easily palpable below the costal margin in any child older than the age of 3 to 4 years must be considered abnormal until proven otherwise. That some palpable spleens may indeed be normal is attested to by the study of McIntyre and Ebaugh,[353] who found that 3% of healthy college freshmen have palpable spleens, of which about one-third persist. "Pretenders" of splenomegaly include the left lobe of the liver, a left upper quadrant tumor such as Wilms tumor or neuroblastoma, the "wandering spleen," and the proptotic spleen (seen in children with a depressed diaphragm from obstructive pulmonary disease, such as asthma or bronchiolitis).

The most common cause of acute splenomegaly in children, especially young children, is a viral infection. Splenic enlargement in this setting is mild to moderate and usually transient. When the history and physical findings suggest a viral etiology, a complete blood count with differential, platelet count, and reticulocyte count should be performed to rule out unsuspected leukemia or hemolytic anemia and to determine whether there is an atypical lymphocytosis. The child should be reevaluated in approximately 4 weeks (or sooner if symptoms persist). If splenomegaly persists beyond 4 to 6 weeks, the splenic enlargement may be considered chronic.

A list of causes of splenomegaly in children is presented in Table 154-5.[354] Symptoms from splenic enlargement are uncommon, although massive splenomegaly may cause abdominal discomfort and early satiety. If the spleen is sufficiently large, there may be increased destruction or sequestration of one or more of the formed elements of the blood (hypersplenism). Cytopenias tend to be mild to moderate, with the platelet count affected the most.

An approach to the pediatric patient with splenic enlargement is outlined in the box on Evaluation and Management of Children With Splenomegaly.

SUGGESTED READINGS

General

Lascari AD: *Hematologic manifestations of childhood diseases,* New York, 1984, Thieme-Stratton.

Infectious Disease

Ballin A, Lotan A, Serour F, et al: Anemia of acute infection in hospitalized children–no evidence of hemolysis. *J Pediatr Hematol Oncol* 31:750, 2009.

Calis JC, van Hensbroek MB, de Hann RJ, et al: HIV-associated anemia in children: A systematic review from a global perspective. *AIDS* 22:1099, 2008.

Melendez E, Harper MB: Risk of serious bacterial infection in isolated and unsuspected neutropenia. *Acad Emerg Med* 2:163, 2010.

Buranski B, Young N: Hematologic consequences of viral infections. *Hematol Oncol Clin North Am* 1:167, 1987.

Strausbaugh LJ: Hematologic manifestations of bacterial and fungal infections. *Hematol Oncol Clin North Am* 1:185, 1987.

Collagen Vascular Disease and Acute Vasculitis

Cazzola M, Panchio L, deBenedetti F, et al: Defective iron supply for erythropoiesis and adequate endogenous erythropoietin production in the anemia associated with systemic-onset juvenile chronic arthritis. *Blood* 87:4824, 1996.

Newburger JW, Fulton DR: Kawasaki disease. *Curr Treat Options Cardio Vasc Med* 9:148, 2007.

Ravelli R: Macrophage activation syndrome. *Curr Opin Rheumatol* 14:548, 2002.

Jordan MB, Allen CE, Weitzman S, et al: How we treat hemophagocytic lymphohistiocytosis. *Blood* 118:4041, 2011.

Cardiopulmonary Disease

Khalid S, McGrowder D, Kemp M, et al: The use of soluble transferin receptor to assess iron deficiency in adults with cystic fibrosis. *Clinica Chimica Acta* 378:194, 2007.

West D, Scheel J, Stove R, et al: Iron deficiency in children with cyanotic congenital heart disease. *J Pediatr* 17:266, 1990.

Gastrointestinal Disease

Halfdanarson T, Litzow MR, Murray JA: Hematologic Manifestations of Celiac Disease. *Blood* 109:412, 2007.

Semrin G, Fishman D, Gousvaros A, et al: Impaired intestinal iron absorption in Crohn's disease correlates with disease activity and markers of inflammation. *Inflamm Bowel Dis* 12:1101, 2006.

Tunnessen WW, Oski FA: Consequences of starting whole cow milk at 6 months of age. *J Pediatr* 111:813, 1987.

Thromboembolic Complications in Childhood Illness

Monagle P, Chan AK, Goldenberg NA, et al: Antithrombotic therapy in neonates and children: Antithrombotic therapy and prevention of thrombosis, ed 9: American College of Chest Physicians Evidence-Based Clinical Practice guidelines. *Chest* 141:e7375, 2012.

Bajzar L, Chan AK, Massicotte MP, et al: Thrombosis in children with malignancy. *Curr Opin Pediatr* 18:1, 2006.

Monagle P: Thrombosis in pediatric cardiac patients. *Semin Thromb Hemost* 29:547, 2003.

Kerlin BA, Blatt NB, Fuh B, et al: Epidemiology and risk factors for thromboembolic complications of childhood nephrotic syndrome: A Midwest Pediatric Nephrology Consortium (MWPNC) study. *J Pediatr* 155:105, 2009.

Avcin T, Cimaz R, Silverman ED, et al: Pediatric antiphospholipid syndrome: Clinical and immunologic features of 121 patients in an international registry. *Pediatrics* 122:e1100, 2008.

Hematologic Complications of Solid Organ Transplantation in Children

Dobrolet NC, Webber SA, Blatt J, et al: Hematologic abnormalities in children and young adults receiving tacrolimus-based immunosuppression following cardiothoracic transplantation. *Pediatr Transplant* 5:125, 2001.

Iglesias-Berengue J, Lopez-Espinosa JA, Ortega-Lopez J, et al: Hematologic abnormalities in liver-transplanted children during medium- to long-term follow-up. *Transplant Proc* 35:1904, 2003.

Taylor RM, Bockenstedt P, Su GL, et al: Immune thrombocytopenic purpura following liver transplantation: A case series and review of the literature. *Liver Transplant* 12:781, 2006.

Marinella MA: Hematologic abnormalities following renal transplantation. *Int Urol Nephrol* 42:151, 2010.

Hematologic Aspects of Poisoning

Sauter D, Goldfrank L: Hematologic aspects of toxicology. *Hematol Oncol Clin North Am* 1:335, 1987.

For complete list of references log on to www.expertconsult.com.

CHAPTER 155

HEMATOLOGIC MANIFESTATIONS OF LIVER DISEASE

Andrea Lee and Wendy Lim

From a hematologic perspective, the liver is essential for heme metabolism and extramedullary hematopoiesis, affects the structure of the red blood cell (RBC) membrane through lipid metabolism, and is involved in the production of hematopoietic growth factors such as thrombopoietin. The liver plays a major role in hemostasis through synthesis of coagulation factors, coagulation inhibitors, and fibrinolytic proteins and is involved in the clearance of activated coagulation factors, proteolytic enzyme–inhibitor complexes, fibrin, and fibrinogen degradation products. As a consequence, chronic liver disease is frequently associated with multiple hematologic abnormalities.

Progressive liver disease can lead to cirrhosis, which is often associated with portal hypertension and splenomegaly. Portal hypertension can lead to the formation of portal gastropathy or gastric, esophageal, or rectal varices, resulting in gastrointestinal bleeding. Sequestration of hematopoietic cells caused by splenomegaly may manifest as any combination of leukopenia, thrombocytopenia, and anemia.

This chapter discusses several common hematologic abnormalities encountered in liver disease, including RBC, leukocyte, and platelet abnormalities; coagulopathy; and thrombosis.

RED BLOOD CELL ABNORMALITIES

Morphologic Abnormalities

The size and shape of the RBC membrane can be affected by abnormal lipid metabolism caused by liver disease. Excess cholesterol content of the outer leaflet of the RBC membrane bilayer is thought to be responsible for the common morphologic findings observed, including macrocytosis, target cells, and acanthocytes (spur cells) (Fig. 155-1), and is associated with a loss of RBC membrane fluidity and deformability. When these less deformable RBCs traverse through the splenic microcirculation, cytoskeletal damage and permanent deformation can occur, resulting in the formation of spur cells.[1]

Spur cell anemia is a type of hemolytic anemia, with the most common cause being chronic or severe liver disease.[1] Life-threatening hemolysis can ensue, as well as disseminated intravascular coagulation (DIC), gastrointestinal bleeding, or liver failure depending on the primary cause.[1] Spur cell anemia associated with hereditary diseases such as neuroacanthocytosis syndromes or lipoprotein disorders, however, tends to be milder (see Chapter 45). Treatment options for spur cell anemia associated with liver disease are limited and suboptimal. The most effective therapy is liver transplantation.[2] Clinical improvement using flunarizine, pentoxifylline, and cholestyramine has been documented in case reports.[3]

Anemia

Cytopenias are detected in approximately 75% of patients with liver disease. The etiology of anemia is multifactorial, although gastrointestinal hemorrhage is a primary contributor.[4] Hemodilution can occur due to fluid retention related to cirrhosis. Hypersplenism or splenomegaly results in sequestration of erythrocytes. Reduced erythropoiesis may exist secondary to nutritional deficiencies in folate or vitamin B_{12} resulting from poor intake or malabsorption, bone marrow suppression from alcohol or viral hepatitis, hepatitis-associated aplastic anemia, treatment-related toxicities for viral hepatitis (e.g., interferon), and anemia of chronic disease. Patients with chronic liver disease or cirrhosis can also experience nonimmune hemolysis because of acquired alterations in the RBC membrane (e.g., spur cell anemia), Zieve syndrome, or treatment-related toxicities (e.g., ribavirin).[4]

The therapeutic approach to anemia in liver disease includes transfusional support for symptomatic disease; identification and treatment of any gastrointestinal bleeding; supplementation for documented iron, vitamin B_{12}, or folate deficiencies; discontinuation of bone marrow suppressive medications or alcohol; and appropriate treatment for the primary cause of liver disease.

Small studies have suggested that inadequate production or response to erythropoietin (EPO) also contributes to chronic anemia in hepatic disease, although the association is controversial.[5] Nonetheless, EPO supplementation has demonstrated clinical efficacy, cost-effectiveness, and increased quality of life in patients with hemoglobin less than 12 g/dL undergoing hepatitis C antiviral therapy.[6] The use of EPO to maintain a hemoglobin greater than 10 g/dL may obviate the need for dose reduction or discontinuation of ribavirin, either of which reduce rates of sustained viral response. It may take up to 6 weeks to observe a significant rise in hemoglobin in response to EPO.

WHITE BLOOD CELL ABNORMALITIES

Leukopenia

Leukopenia, particularly neutropenia, has been observed in up to 55% of patients with cirrhosis.[7] Splenic sequestration is considered to be the main culprit; however, reduced production of leukocytes may also be a consequence of altered granulocyte colony-stimulating factor (G-CSF) and granulocyte macrophage colony-stimulating factor (GM-CSF) levels, bone marrow suppression mediated by primary infections or toxins (e.g., hepatitis B or C, alcohol), or an iatrogenic effect from treatment with interferon. Immune-mediated neutropenia can occur in the context of hepatitis C or autoimmune hepatitis, and increased apoptosis may also be responsible for a shortened neutrophil lifespan.[8] Furthermore, impairment in neutrophil recruitment and phagocytic function may contribute to an increased susceptibility for severe and recurrent infections in patients with cirrhosis.[9] G-CSF and GM-CSF have been safely used in patients with cirrhosis and neutropenia in the setting of hypersplenism or treatment of viral hepatitis, resulting in improvements in white blood cell counts. The impact on risk of infection or response to antiviral therapy, however, is unclear.[10,11]

PLATELET ABNORMALITIES

Thrombocytopenia

Thrombocytopenia alone or in combination with other cytopenias is the most common cytopenia associated with liver disease, occurring in up to 77% of patients with cirrhosis.[7] Platelet counts are usually mildly to moderately reduced; severe thrombocytopenia ($<30\text{-}40 \times 10^9/L$) and spontaneous bleeding are uncommon.

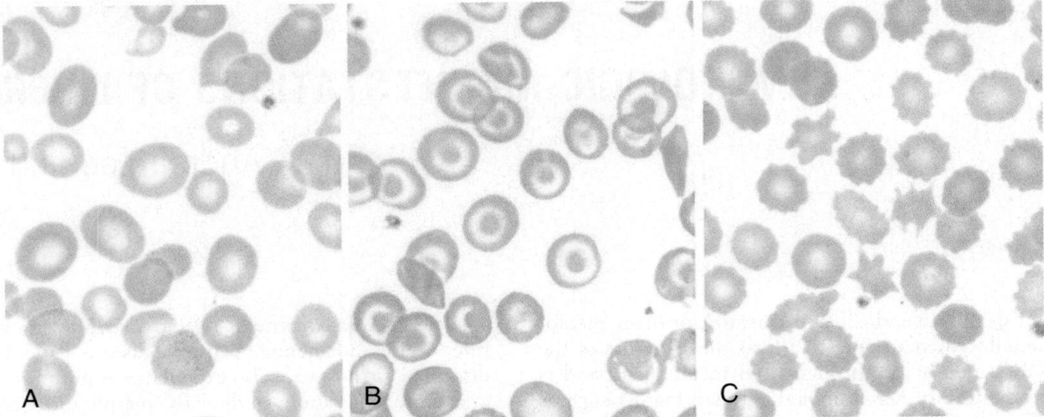

Figure 155-1 RED BLOOD CELL (RBC) MORPHOLOGY IN LIVER DISEASE. **A,** Macrocytes have a mean corpuscular volume greater than 100 fL and can be oval shaped. Commonly associated disorders include liver disease and vitamin B_{12} and folate deficiency. **B,** Target cells are characterized by the bull's-eye appearance of the RBC. They are a result of an increased surface-to-volume ratio related to excess RBC membrane (e.g., liver disease) or disproportionate reduction of cytoplasmic content (e.g., hemoglobinopathies, iron deficiency). **C,** Acanthocytes, or spur cells, typically appear as contracted RBCs lacking central pallor with multiple irregular membrane projections. The morphologic appearance reflects the irreversible cytoskeletal damage that has occurred because of passage of nondeformable RBCs through the reticuloendothelial system. They are most commonly seen in severe liver disease but can also be features of rare neuroacanthocytosis syndromes or lipoprotein disorders.

Many factors contribute to thrombocytopenia in liver disease. Decreased platelet counts may result from splenomegaly and hypersplenism. There may be impaired platelet production in the bone marrow related to nutritional deficiencies in folate or vitamin B_{12}; direct toxicity of alcohol, viral hepatitis, or interferon treatment; or reduced hepatic synthesis of thrombopoietin. Accelerated destruction of platelets can occur via immune-mediated mechanisms because autoantibodies to platelet antigens have been demonstrated in patients with cirrhosis. Although controversial, the presence of low-grade DIC may contribute to platelet consumption.[12] Thrombocytopenia in patients with cirrhosis, especially in combination with leukopenia, has been associated with increased morbidity and mortality.[7]

Platelet Dysfunction

Laboratory evaluation of platelet function has demonstrated abnormal bleeding times (BTs), PFA-100 results, and platelet aggregation in response to multiple agonists in some individuals with liver disease, implying that there may be a component of platelet dysfunction.[12] Intrinsic platelet defects leading to abnormal platelet aggregation or adhesion include impaired transmembrane signaling and thromboxane A2 synthesis, storage pool deficiency, or defects in platelet glycoprotein Ib or $\alpha_{IIb}\beta_3$ receptors.[12] Extrinsic defects resulting in platelet dysfunction include circulating fibrin(ogen) degradation products, bile salts, abnormal high-density lipoproteins, reduced hematocrit, and excess production of nitric oxide and prostacyclin.[12]

The clinical significance of platelet dysfunction demonstrated in vitro is unclear. Although prolonged BTs are present in up to 40% of patients with cirrhosis and appear to be correlated with disease severity, they have not been predictive of bleeding.[13] Improvement in BT in randomized trials of DDAVP (desmopressin) did not translate into reductions in surgical blood loss, transfusion requirements, or improved control of variceal hemorrhage.[14,15] This discordance between laboratory findings and clinical bleeding may be explained by two observations. First, platelets studied under physiologic flow conditions show normal adhesion to fibrinogen and collagen even in cirrhosis.[16] Second, elevated levels of von Willebrand Factor (vWF) are commonly found in patients with cirrhosis and may compensate for thrombocytopenia or platelet dysfunction.

Platelet transfusions can be used to treat thrombocytopenia caused by liver disease but are generally not indicated unless the patient has severe thrombocytopenia less than 10 to 20 × 10^9/L or platelets less than 50 × 10^9/L with bleeding symptoms.[17] Platelet counts greater than 50 to 70 × 10^9/L are usually considered adequate for invasive procedures.[17] Less commonly attempted interventions for thrombocytopenia secondary to liver disease include splenectomy, partial splenic arterial embolization, and transjugular intrahepatic portosystemic shunt (TIPS), which are associated with unpredictable results and procedural risks. Thrombopoietin mimetic agents (e.g., eltrombopag, romiplostim) may offer potential treatment for these patients. In a phase II trial of 74 patients with hepatitis C–related cirrhosis and platelet counts of 20 to 70 × 10^9/L randomized to eltrombopag (30, 50, or 75 mg/day) or placebo, the primary endpoint of achieving a platelet count greater than 100 × 10^9/L at week 4 was seen in 75% to 95% of patients taking eltrombopag compared with 0% in the placebo group. Furthermore, 36% to 65% of patients taking eltrombopag were able to complete a 12-week course of antiviral treatment compared with 6% of the placebo group.[18] However, another trial evaluating eltrombopag in chronic liver disease was stopped because of an increase in portal vein thrombosis, highlighting some of the toxicities that can be associated with these new agents. Further study is required before recommendations can be made about their use.

COAGULATION AND LIVER DISEASE

The manifestations of aberrant coagulation in liver disease reflect a complex interplay between procoagulant and anticoagulant mechanisms. Patients with cirrhosis are recognized not only to be at increased risk of bleeding but also thrombosis.

Deficiencies in coagulation factors, vitamin K deficiency, dysfibrinogenemia, and systemic fibrinolysis can all contribute to impaired hemostasis.[19] Clinical manifestations can range from asymptomatic laboratory abnormalities to life-threatening hemorrhage.

Cirrhosis is marked by reduced synthesis of most coagulation factors. The number and degree of clotting factor deficiencies reflect the severity of liver damage. With the shortest half-life of approximately 6 hours, factor VII levels often decline early and are reflected by prolongation of the prothrombin time (PT). Factor VIII levels may be normal or elevated because of extrahepatic synthesis, increased vWF levels, or impaired hepatic clearance. Being an acute phase reactant, fibrinogen synthesis is generally preserved unless liver disease is severe.

Reductions in factors II, VII, IX, and X may also result from vitamin K deficiency. For these coagulation factors, vitamin K is required as a cofactor in γ-carboxylation, a process that converts inactive precursors to biologically active factors. Vitamin K deficiency associated with liver disease can occur as a consequence of malnutrition, malabsorption, use of antibiotics, or biliary tract obstruction.

Defects in coagulation factors are suggested by prolonged PT and partial thromboplastin time (PTT) measurements and confirmed by individual factor levels. PT can also be expressed as the international normalized ratio (INR), a measure developed and validated to standardize PT measurements across laboratories for monitoring of vitamin K antagonist (VKA) therapy. Both the PT and INR have been incorporated into prognostic indices (Child-Pugh and model of end-stage liver disease [MELD]) to estimate the severity of liver disease and stratify patients for transplant, respectively. Furthermore, these parameters have been applied to estimate bleeding risk and guide therapy. Several significant limitations exist in applying these laboratory parameters in the context of liver disease. First, PT, PTT, and INR have been shown to correlate poorly with gastrointestinal or procedural bleeding.[20,21] Second, the INR has not been validated for patients with cirrhosis. Wide variations in INR have been observed in cirrhosis and may therefore undermine the utility and objectivity of the MELD index. Third, because these parameters suboptimally predict bleeding, the value of correcting these abnormal values with plasma or procoagulant agents becomes uncertain. Several reasons may account for the lack of correlation between PT or PTT with bleeding. Liver disease results in deficiencies of procoagulant proteins but also deficiencies in the natural anticoagulant proteins, including antithrombin and proteins C and S. PT and PTT assays are designed to be sensitive to procoagulant protein levels and do not reflect these alterations in anticoagulant proteins. Small studies have demonstrated normal thrombin generation and potential resistance to thrombomodulin in cirrhotic patients. Furthermore, factor VIII levels are increased in cirrhosis.[22]

Acquired dysfibrinogenemia has been described in approximately 75% of patients with chronic liver disease, acute liver failure, and cirrhosis. Aberrant polymerization of fibrin monomers may be related to excess sialic acid residues on fibrinogen, interfering with the activity of thrombin.[23] Laboratory findings in dysfibrinogenemia include elevated PT, PTT, or thrombin time; low or normal fibrinogen by immunologic assay; and reduced fibrinogen by functional assay. Despite these objective abnormalities, dysfibrinogenemia is not thought to contribute significantly to bleeding in most patients with liver disease.

The presence of hyperfibrinolysis in liver disease and its contribution to bleeding risk is controversial. Triggers of increased fibrinolysis may involve release of tissue plasminogen activator (tPA) in the setting of infection or surgery, reabsorption of ascitic fluid with fibrinolytic activity, and altered synthetic or metabolic functions of the liver.[24] With the exception of tPA and plasminogen activator inhibitor-1 (PAI-1), all fibrinolytic and antifibrinolytic proteins are synthesized in the liver. Paradoxically, low levels of plasminogen, plasmin inhibitor, factor XIII, and thrombin activatable fibrinolysis inhibitor (TAFI) and high levels of tPA and PAI-1 have been reported in cirrhosis. Decreased hepatic clearance of tPA and reduced synthesis of α2 anti-plasmin and TAFI favor an increase in circulating plasmin and a hyperfibrinolytic state in cirrhosis. Available laboratory tests measure individual components but cannot adequately assess the overall activity of profibrinolytic and antifibrinolytic components. Shortened whole blood euglobulin clot lysis time and elevated levels of D-dimer, fibrin, and fibrinogen degradation products are suggestive of increased fibrinolysis. These abnormal laboratory indices have been observed in nonbleeding patients but are seen more frequently in bleeding patients and have been reported to correlate with gastrointestinal bleeding, severity of liver failure, and variceal size. Hyperfibrinolysis may theoretically aggravate bleeding through secondary effects on other aspects of hemostasis, such as consumption of coagulation factors, inhibition of fibrin polymerization, and reduced platelet aggregation via degradation of vWF and glycoprotein Ib and $\alpha_{IIb}\beta_3$. Hyperfibrinolysis likely plays a more important role in hemostasis in the context of liver transplantation.[24]

TREATMENT OF LIVER DISEASE–RELATED BLEEDING

Because there is minimal correlation between laboratory abnormalities and bleeding, treatment and correction of asymptomatic hemostatic abnormalities is generally not indicated. Intervention is indicated when there is active bleeding or a planned invasive procedure or surgery.

Red blood cell transfusions should be provided to maintain an adequate hemoglobin or hematocrit and for symptomatic anemia. Generally, platelet transfusions are not indicated for isolated thrombocytopenia in the absence of bleeding. An effort should be made to maintain platelet counts greater than 50 to 70 × 10^9/L with active bleeding or before invasive procedures.[17] Platelet transfusion may be effective if there is suspected platelet dysfunction. Patients with cirrhosis often have smaller platelet increments in response to transfusions caused by splenic sequestration.

A trial of oral vitamin K can be considered in patients with prolonged PT or INR. Vitamin K can be given intravenously for earlier onset of action but carries the small risk of anaphylaxis. Subcutaneous and intramuscular administrations are not preferred because of inconsistent absorption and risk of hematoma formation, respectively. If no improvement is seen after 10 to 20 mg of vitamin K, additional

Hemostatic Indices in Liver Disease

Laboratory Changes	*PT*	*PTT*	*TCT*	*Fib*	*Clauss*	*Plt*	*Platelet Aggregation*	*FVII*	*DD*	*ELT*
Thrombocytopenia	N	N	N	N	N	↓	N	N	N	N
Platelet dysfunction	N	N	N	N	N	N	abnormal	N	N	N
Vitamin K deficiency*	↑	↑	N	N	N	N	N	↓	N	N
Factor deficiency	↑	↑	N	N	N	N	N	↓	N	N
Hypofibrinogenemia	N/↑	N/↑	↑	↓	↓	N	N	N	N	N
Dysfibrinogenemia	N/↑	N/↑	↑	N	↓	N	N	N	N	N
Hyperfibrinolysis	N/↑	N/↑	N/↑	N/↓	N/↓	N	N	↓	↑	↓
DIC	N/↑	N/↑	N/↑	↓	↓	↓	N	N/↓	↑	↓

Clauss, Clauss fibrinogen; *DD,* D-dimer; *DIC,* disseminated intravascular coagulation; *ELT,* euglobulin lysis time (measure of fibrinolysis); *Fib,* fibrinogen; *FVII,* factor VII functional assay; *N,* normal; *Plt,* platelet; *PT,* prothrombin time; *PTT,* partial thromboplastin time; *TCT,* thrombin clotting time.

*Differentiating between vitamin K deficiency and liver disease can be challenging with conventional laboratory tests. If available, performing a factor II assay with and without Echis venom (factor II biological and factor II Echis) may be useful. Ecarin is derived from Echis carinatus snake venom and can activate prothrombin irrespective of γ-carboxylation. Factor II activity (biological) is reduced in both vitamin K deficiency and liver disease. In contrast, the factor II Echis is reduced in liver disease but is normal in vitamin K deficiency.

vitamin K is unlikely to be beneficial. Although it may be reasonable to use vitamin K replacement alone in asymptomatic patients, it should be considered as an adjunct to other therapy in actively bleeding patients.

Fresh-frozen plasma (FFP) has traditionally been used to correct liver-related coagulopathy because it replaces all the coagulation and fibrinolytic factors. Despite its widespread use, its clinical effectiveness in reducing bleeding has not been supported by data from randomized controlled trials.[25] Guidelines variably support the use of 10 to 20 mL/kg of FFP for major hemorrhage, prevention of bleeding before major invasive procedures, or prevention of bleeding in acute liver failure.[17,26,27] Laboratory parameters, including a complete blood count (CBC), PT, PTT, fibrinogen, and D-dimer, should be followed to assess therapeutic effect. Generally, moderate correction of the PT and PTT is achieved after FFP transfusion but is transient, and repeat doses may have to be administered every 6 to 12 hours to maintain the effect. Patients should be monitored for complications of FFP, including transfusion reactions, risk of blood-borne infections, transfusion-related lung injury, and volume overload.[26] It may not be well tolerated in patients with liver disease who already have expanded intravascular plasma volume. Plasma exchange in addition to FFP has been described primarily in the setting of acute liver failure and in preparation for liver transplantation. However, the efficacy of this approach has not been thoroughly studied in controlled trials.

The presence of hyperfibrinolysis, DIC, and dysfibrinogenemia may exacerbate bleeding and are inadequately treated with FFP alone. These disorders should be suspected if coagulation parameters fail to correct with FFP or there is persistent bleeding. Administration of cryoprecipitate, rich in fibrinogen, vWF, factor VIII, and factor XIII, may help control bleeding. One unit of cryoprecipitate for every 10 kg of body weight increases plasma fibrinogen by approximately 50 mg/dL. Cryoprecipitate carries similar risks to FFP. Although antifibrinolytic agents could be considered in the setting of hyperfibrinolysis, no randomized trials have demonstrated efficacy or safety outside the setting of liver transplantation. Aprotinin and tranexamic acid have been shown to reduce blood loss and the need for transfusion in liver resection and transplantation.[28] Because of concerns regarding an increased risk of renal failure, stroke, heart failure, and death, aprotinin has been withdrawn from the market. Furthermore, thrombotic risks must be weighed and DIC must be excluded before usage.

Three- and four-factor prothrombin complex concentrates (PCCs) contain the vitamin K–dependent factors II, IX, and X and may or may not contain variable amounts of factor VII. They have proven to be effective in reversing anticoagulation with VKAs, but they have not been widely studied in liver disease. Data are limited to case reports and small, uncontrolled studies describing improvement in coagulation parameters, subjective clinical improvement, and safe administration in patients with liver disease.[29,30] Still, the use of PCCs in liver disease should be undertaken cautiously because of the risk of DIC, thrombotic complications, and anaphylaxis; its use should be restricted to emergency situations such as refractory bleeding or if FFP administration is limited by risk of circulatory overload.[31]

Recombinant FVIIa (rFVIIa) is formally approved for the treatment and prevention of bleeding episodes in patients with hemophilia and inhibitors, acquired hemophilia, and congenital factor VII deficiency. Because of proven efficacy in these other disorders, rFVIIa has been investigated for gastrointestinal or variceal bleeding in liver disease, liver resection or biopsy, and liver transplantation.[32-34] Studies have demonstrated transient normalization of the PT after rFVIIa, yet correlation with improved clinical outcomes has been inconsistent.[34,35] The only two randomized trials examining rFVIIa in active gastrointestinal and variceal bleeding did not show any benefit over placebo.[32] rFVIIa appears to reduce blood loss and blood product requirements when used prophylactically in invasive procedures or surgery; however, there is no clear mortality benefit.[36] These potential benefits may be offset by an observed increase in arterial thromboembolic events, particularly in elderly adults.[37] Compared with FFP, rFVIIa can be given in small volumes and has no infectious risk. Additional research is required to establish the overall benefit and risk of rFVIIa, and clinicians should proceed with the use of rFVIIa judiciously in the interim.

Management of Coagulopathy in Liver Disease

- Actively bleeding patients should be adequately resuscitated and stabilized with crystalloid or colloid solutions (or both). Admission to the intensive care setting may be appropriate.
- Basic coagulation tests should be ordered to identify the cause of bleeding; these include CBC, PT (INR), PTT, thrombin clotting time, fibrinogen, D-Dimer, FDP, and mixing studies. The need for more specialized tests will be dictated by the clinical situation and response to therapy.
- It is important to identify any localized source of bleeding (e.g., varices) amenable to procedural intervention because this will assist in achieving hemostasis.
- A trial of 5 to 10 mg of vitamin K is reasonable in asymptomatic patients with prolonged PT and PTT but should be used with other therapies in actively bleeding patients.
- Platelet transfusions can be used, targeting counts greater than 50×10^9/L.
- In patients who can tolerate volume, FFP 4 to 6 units (1000-1500 mL) given over 1 to 2 hours can be used to replace coagulation factors. Coagulation parameters should be monitored to document effect and determine the timing and need for additional units.
- Dysfibrinogenemia or hypofibrinogenemia should be suspected if coagulation assays do not correct with FFP or fibrinogen levels are low, respectively. Replacement can be attempted with 10 to 20 units of cryoprecipitate while following laboratory results.
- Patients who are intravascularly overloaded or who do not respond to FFP should be considered for rFVIIa. Low doses of rFVIIa (25-50 μg/kg) are generally used, and repeated doses may be required because of the short half-life of 2 to 3 hours. rFVIIa may thus be most suitable as a temporizing measure to enable invasive procedures or hemostasis to be achieved by other means. Avoid use in the setting of DIC.

HYPERCOAGULABILITY AND THROMBOSIS IN PATIENTS WITH LIVER DISEASE

Although retrospective studies have reported variable rates of venous thromboembolism (VTE) in patients with cirrhosis, it is clear that these patients are not immune to thrombotic events as once believed. Reported incidences of deep venous thrombosis (DVT) or pulmonary embolism (PE) have ranged from 0.5% to 6.3%.[38] Thrombotic complications can also involve portal, mesenteric, and hepatic veins. Portal vein thrombosis (PVT) occurs in approximately 8 to 15% of patients with cirrhosis and is associated with both severity of disease and inferior prognosis in liver transplantation.

The frequency of thrombotic events in patients with liver disease indicates that some patients may benefit from prophylactic or therapeutic anticoagulation. Hepatic or portal vein thrombosis may result in worsening liver function, ascites, varices, and hemorrhage. Furthermore, microvascular thrombosis has been proposed to promote hepatic fibrosis and progression of cirrhosis.[39] Clinical decisions are limited by a paucity of studies establishing the optimal dose, duration, monitoring, or choice of anticoagulant and, more importantly, clear clinical benefit and safety.

With respect to prophylactic anticoagulation, there are currently no standard means of identifying high-risk patients and reconciling the perceived increased risk of bleeding in these patients. Guidelines

Hemostatic Balance in Liver Disease

	Promotes Thrombosis	*Promotes Bleeding*
Primary hemostasis	• Increased vWF • Decreased ADAMTS13	• Thrombocytopenia • Platelet dysfunction
Secondary hemostasis	• Increased factor VIII • Decreased protein C, protein S, antithrombin	• Factor deficiencies: II, V, VII, IX, XI • Vitamin K deficiency • Hypofibrinogenemia • Dysfibrinogenemia
Fibrinolysis	• Reduced plasminogen • Increased PAI-1	• Reduced α2-antiplasmin, TAFI, factor XIII • Increased tPA

PAI-1, Plasminogen activator inhibitor-1; *TAFI*, thrombin activatable fibrinolysis inhibitor; *tPA*, tissue plasminogen activator; *vWF*, von Willebrand factor

on antithrombotic prophylaxis do not specifically address cirrhosis, so decisions to proceed with prophylactic anticoagulation remain individualized. Patients who may particularly benefit from primary prophylaxis are those awaiting liver transplantation because portal vein thrombosis worsens the long-term posttransplant prognosis. Small trials have recently suggested that low-molecular-weight heparins may be safe for thromboprophylaxis in cirrhosis.[38] Use of VKAs for thromboprophylaxis in patients with liver disease may be complicated by unreliable INR measurements. Trials involving newer anticoagulants such as direct thrombin and factor Xa inhibitors have usually excluded patients with liver disease.

A similar risk–benefit analysis must be completed before therapeutic anticoagulation for confirmed thrombosis. Expert opinion recommends screening for varices and appropriate treatment with β-blockers or endoscopic therapy before anticoagulant initiation to mitigate bleeding potential.[40] There are several indications for therapeutic anticoagulation in the setting of cirrhosis, including DVT or PE, acute PVT, and Budd-Chiari syndrome. The comprehensive management of these disorders is beyond the scope of this chapter. Treatment options for portal vein or hepatic vein thromboses may include one or more of anticoagulation, systemic or local thrombolysis, or TIPS. The American Association for the Study of Liver Diseases' 2009 guidelines recommended a minimum of 3 months of anticoagulation for acute PVT in the absence of cirrhosis, with consideration for long-term anticoagulation in patients with persistent thrombotic risk factors or concerns for extension into mesenteric veins.[40] Individualized assessment has been recommended for patients with PVT with cirrhosis.[40] Overall recanalization after 6 months has been observed in up to 75% of PVT patients with cirrhosis and minimal major bleeding.[41] The value of anticoagulation for chronic PVT is uncertain, particularly in patients with cirrhosis with varices. Hepatic vein thrombosis is more uncommon than PVT, and even less evidence exists to guide therapy. Anticoagulation is usually instituted acutely and maintained long term to prevent recurrence in the absence of contraindications. Symptomatic patients may go on to have additional interventional therapies as mentioned above, as well as possible liver transplantation.[40]

FUTURE DIRECTIONS

Liver disease can cause a variety of hematologic manifestations. Patients may have concurrent coagulopathic, hypercoagulable, and hyperfibrinolytic features. Bleeding or thrombosis may be the end result of a reduced capacity of the hemostatic system to maintain homeostasis in the face of physiologic stress. Advancements in patient care will evolve with improved understanding of pathophysiology and refinement of laboratory assays.

REFERENCES

1. Vassiliadis T, Mpoumponaris A, Vakalopoulou S, et al: Spur cells and spur cell anemia in hospitalized patients with advanced liver disease: Incidence and correlation with disease severity and survival. *Hepatol Res* 40:161, 2010.
2. Chitale AA, Sterling RK, Post AB, et al: Resolution of spur cell anemia with liver transplantation: A case report and review of the literature. *Transplantation* 65:993, 1998.
3. Aihara K, Azuma H, Ikeda Y, et al: Successful combination therapy–flunarizine, pentoxifylline, and cholestyramine–for spur cell anemia. *Int J Hematol* 73:351, 2001.
4. Gonzalez-Casas R, Jones EA, Moreno-Otero R: Spectrum of anemia associated with chronic liver disease. *World J Gastroenterol* 15:4653, 2009.
5. Bruno CM, Neri S, Sciacca C, et al: Plasma erythropoietin levels in anaemic and non-anaemic patients with chronic liver diseases. *World J Gastroenterol* 10:1353, 2004.
6. Afdhal NH, Dieterich DT, Pockros PJ, et al: Epoetin alfa maintains ribavirin dose in HCV-infected patients: A prospective, double-blind, randomized controlled study. *Gastroenterology* 126:1302, 2004.
7. Qamar AA, Grace ND, Groszmann RJ, et al: Incidence, prevalence, and clinical significance of abnormal hematologic indices in compensated cirrhosis. *Clin Gastroenterol Hepatol* 7:689, 2009.
8. Ramirez MJ, Titos E, Claria J, et al: Increased apoptosis dependent on caspase-3 activity in polymorphonuclear leukocytes from patients with cirrhosis and ascites. *J Hepatol* 41:44, 2004.
9. Fiuza C, Salcedo M, Clemente G, et al: In vivo neutrophil dysfunction in cirrhotic patients with advanced liver disease. *J Infect Dis* 182:526, 2000.
10. Gurakar A, Fagiuoli S, Gavaler JS, et al: The use of granulocyte-macrophage colony-stimulating factor to enhance hematologic parameters of patients with cirrhosis and hypersplenism. *J Hepatol* 21:582, 1994.
11. Gronbaek K, Krarup HB, Ring-Larsen H, et al: Interferon alfa-2b alone or combined with recombinant granulocyte-macrophage colony-stimulating factor as treatment of chronic hepatitis C. *Scand J Gastroenterol* 37:840, 2002.
12. Witters P, Freson K, Verslype C, et al: Review article: Blood platelet number and function in chronic liver disease and cirrhosis. *Aliment Pharmacol Ther* 27:1017, 2008.
13. Basili S, Ferro D, Leo R, et al: Bleeding time does not predict gastrointestinal bleeding in patients with cirrhosis. The CALC Group. Coagulation Abnormalities in Liver Cirrhosis. *J Hepatol* 24:574, 1996.
14. de Franchis R, Arcidiacono PG, Carpinelli L, et al: Randomized controlled trial of desmopressin plus terlipressin vs. terlipressin alone for the treatment of acute variceal hemorrhage in cirrhotic patients: A multicenter, double-blind study. New Italian Endoscopic Club. *Hepatology* 18:1102, 1993.
15. Wong AY, Irwin MG, Hui TW, et al: Desmopressin does not decrease blood loss and transfusion requirements in patients undergoing hepatectomy. *Can J Anaesth* 50:14, 2003.
16. Lisman T, Adelmeijer J, de Groot PG, et al: No evidence for an intrinsic platelet defect in patients with liver cirrhosis—studies under flow conditions. *J Thromb Haemost* 4:2070, 2006.
17. Polson J, Lee WM: AASLD position paper: The management of acute liver failure. *Hepatology* 41:1179, 2005.
18. McHutchison JG, Dusheiko G, Shiffman ML, et al: Eltrombopag for thrombocytopenia in patients with cirrhosis associated with hepatitis C. *N Engl J Med* 357:2227, 2007.
19. Roberts LN, Patel RK, Arya R: Haemostasis and thrombosis in liver disease. *Br J Haematol* 148:507, 2010.
20. Segal JB, Dzik WH: Paucity of studies to support that abnormal coagulation test results predict bleeding in the setting of invasive procedures: An evidence-based review. *Transfusion* 45:1413, 2005.

21. Tripodi A, Chantarangkul V, Mannucci PM: Acquired coagulation disorders: Revisited using global coagulation/anticoagulation testing. *Br J Haematol* 147:77, 2009.
22. Lisman T, Porte RJ: Rebalanced hemostasis in patients with liver disease: Evidence and clinical consequences. *Blood* 116:878, 2010.
23. Martinez J, MacDonald KA, Palascak JE: The role of sialic acid in the dysfibrinogenemia associated with liver disease: Distribution of sialic acid on the constituent chains. *Blood* 61:1196, 1983.
24. Ferro D, Celestini A, Violi F: Hyperfibrinolysis in liver disease. *Clin Liver Dis* 13:21, 2009.
25. Stanworth SJ, Brunskill SJ, Hyde CJ, et al: Is fresh frozen plasma clinically effective? A systematic review of randomized controlled trials. *Br J Haematol* 126:139, 2004.
26. Hellstern P, Muntean W, Schramm W, et al: Practical guidelines for the clinical use of plasma. *Thromb Res* 107:S53, 2002.
27. O'Shaughnessy DF, Atterbury C, Bolton Maggs P, et al: Guidelines for the use of fresh-frozen plasma, cryoprecipitate and cryosupernatant. *Br J Haematol* 126:11, 2004.
28. Molenaar IQ, Warnaar N, Groen H, et al: Efficacy and safety of antifibrinolytic drugs in liver transplantation: A systematic review and meta-analysis. *Am J Transplant* 7:185, 2007.
29. Lorenz R, Kienast J, Otto U, et al: Efficacy and safety of a prothrombin complex concentrate with two virus-inactivation steps in patients with severe liver damage. *Eur J Gastroenterol Hepatol* 15:15, 2003.
30. Bick RL, Schmalhorst WR, Shanbrom E: Prothrombin complex concentrate: Use in controlling the hemorrhagic diathesis of chronic liver disease. *Am J Dig Dis* 20:741, 1975.
31. Liumbruno G, Bennardello F, Lattanzio A, et al: Recommendations for the use of antithrombin concentrates and prothrombin complex concentrates. *Blood Transfus* 7:325, 2009.
32. Bosch J, Thabut D, Albillos A, et al: Recombinant factor VIIa for variceal bleeding in patients with advanced cirrhosis: A randomized, controlled trial. *Hepatology* 47:1604, 2008.
33. Jeffers L, Chalasani N, Balart L, et al: Safety and efficacy of recombinant factor VIIa in patients with liver disease undergoing laparoscopic liver biopsy. *Gastroenterology* 123:118, 2002.
34. Lodge JP, Jonas S, Jones RM, et al: Efficacy and safety of repeated perioperative doses of recombinant factor VIIa in liver transplantation. *Liver Transpl* 11:973, 2005.
35. Planinsic RM, van der Meer J, Testa G, et al: Safety and efficacy of a single bolus administration of recombinant factor VIIa in liver transplantation due to chronic liver disease. *Liver Transpl* 11:895, 2005.
36. Lin Y, Stanworth S, Birchall J, et al: Recombinant factor VIIa for the prevention and treatment of bleeding in patients without haemophilia. *Cochrane Database Syst Rev* CD005011, 2011.
37. Levi M, Levy JH, Andersen HF, et al: Safety of recombinant activated factor VII in randomized clinical trials. *N Engl J Med* 363:1791, 2010.
38. Tripodi A, Anstee QM, Sogaard KK, et al: Hypercoagulability in Cirrhosis: Causes and Consequences(1). *J Thromb Haemost* 2011.
39. Northup PG: Hypercoagulation in liver disease. *Clin Liver Dis* 13:109, 2009.
40. DeLeve LD, Valla DC, Garcia-Tsao G: Vascular disorders of the liver. *Hepatology* 49:1729, 2009.
41. Amitrano L, Guardascione MA, Menchise A, et al: Safety and efficacy of anticoagulation therapy with low molecular weight heparin for portal vein thrombosis in patients with liver cirrhosis. *J Clin Gastroenterol* 44:448, 2010.

CHAPTER 156

HEMATOLOGIC MANIFESTATIONS OF SYSTEMIC DISEASE: RENAL DISEASE

Peter W. Marks, Rachel Rosovsky, and Edward J. Benz, Jr.

Disorders of the kidney can be associated with very significant hematologic effects. Significant compromises of renal function have major adverse effects on red blood cell production and platelet function but can also affect red cell morphology and survival, leukocyte function, and coagulation factors. Understanding the pathogenesis of these changes facilitates accurate diagnosis and management of hematologic abnormalities encountered in patients with renal disease.

Because the kidney is the locus for the production of erythropoietin, the primary driver of red blood cell production, it is hardly surprising that renal injury is almost always accompanied by anemia. Indeed anemia is usually the most prominent hematologic manifestation encountered in patients with renal dysfunction. It is widely appreciated that end-stage renal disease is associated with severe anemia (see later). However, even modest renal damage, such as that seen in diabetic patients with very modestly elevated serum creatinine levels, can be associated with impaired erythropoietin production.

Renal disease can also lead to defects in red blood cells, platelets, leukocytes, and coagulation factors. In addition, acquired disorders arising outside of the kidney, such as hemolytic uremic syndrome (HUS), can manifest simultaneously as hematologic and renal disturbances.

Abnormal red blood cell morphology due to uremia is usually manifested by the presence of echinocytes (burr cells) on the peripheral blood smear (Fig. 156-1). The pathogenesis underlying this morphologic change remains unknown despite many efforts to provoke the abnormal erythrocyte topology with substances accumulating in renal failure plasma. Uremic toxins are likely the culprit responsible for significant impairments in platelet function that are often encountered in these patients. The abnormality closely resembles an acquired aspirin-like platelet release defect. This finding, in combination with a decreased quantity and/or function of certain clotting proteins, including von Willebrand factor, can lead to significant bleeding complications. Cellular and humoral immunity mediated via lymphocytes are also adversely affected in renal disease,[1] and a wide variety of leukocyte defects have been reported in this setting.[2] In clinical practice, however, hypoproliferative anemia, bleeding complications, and HUS are the most frequent clinically relevant entities encountered, so they are covered in greater detail here.

MANAGEMENT OF HYPOPROLIFERATIVE ANEMIA

End-stage renal disease is a major health problem in the United States, with incidence increasing every year. The associated anemia is thus a cause of significant morbidity and mortality on a public health scale. Although the cause of the anemia is multifactorial, reduced erythropoietin production is primarily responsible. Erythropoietin is a glycoprotein hormone synthesized primarily in the kidney.[3,4] This crucial component in the regulation of hematopoiesis is essential for the proliferation, maturation, and differentiation of erythroid precursors (see Chapter 24).[5]

Previously the great majority of patients on dialysis required chronic blood transfusions. This situation has changed dramatically with the introduction of recombinant human erythropoietin (rHuEPO) into clinical practice (see box on Management of the Anemia of Renal Disease). In addition to accelerating erythropoiesis and reducing allogeneic blood transfusions, rHuEPO has been shown to increase exercise capacity and improve quality of life, sleep, cognitive function, and sexual function in anemic patients with chronic renal failure.[6-10] A small number of prospective and retrospective clinical studies has also shown that treatment with rHuEPO decreases the rise in creatinine, slows the decline of glomerular filtration rate, and delays initiation of dialysis in patients with chronic renal failure. The results from these few exploratory clinical trials support the hypothesis that using rHuEPO and correcting anemia may slow the rate of progression of renal failure.[11-13]

Treatment of anemia may also have significant cardiovascular benefits in this population. A few recent studies have shown that left ventricular hypertrophy is directly related to the level of anemia in chronic renal failure patients.[8-10] In addition, left ventricular mass has been shown to be an independent determinant in the survival of patients on dialysis.[14] Thus treatment with rHuEPO may have benefits in terms of cardiac function and subsequently survival for these patients.[15] However, data also suggest that excessive correction of the hemoglobin level to values greater than approximately 12 g/dL is associated with an increased incidence of cardiovascular and thromboembolic events. There are also theoretical concerns, supported by animal and cell culture data, that erythropoietin might stimulate the proliferation of some neoplastic cells. Therefore the use of erythropoiesis-stimulating agents to increase hemoglobin values to greater than 12 g/dL is not routinely recommended.

Although rHuEPO can be administered intravenously or subcutaneously, the subcutaneous route appears to be advantageous. It is easier to administer and can be given less frequently. Hypertension and, to a much lesser degree, thrombosis have been reported in patients on dialysis.[13,16] In addition, a short-lived influenza-like syndrome has been described.[17] Rare side effects include allergic reactions, seizures, hyperkalemia, and thrombocytosis. Pure red blood cell aplasia, thought to be due to the development of antierythropoietin antibodies, is also a rare but serious complication that has primarily been reported with certain preparations of rHuEPO.[14,15,18]

An increase in the hemoglobin level to greater than 10 g/dL after a 4-week course of therapy is frequently the target goal when administering rHuEPO. Some patients may fail to respond or may be resistant to the effects of rHuEPO. The most common cause for a failure in response is iron deficiency anemia.[19] Other contributing factors that may affect the response are cobalamin or folate deficiency, infection, chronic inflammation, secondary hyperparathyroidism, malnutrition, hemoglobinopathies, aluminum toxicity, or bone marrow fibrosis.[17,20-22]

Iron deficiency is almost universal in the dialyzed patient. Gastrointestinal bleeding, blood draws, and hemodialysis all contribute to this iron-deficient state.[23] In addition, by accelerating erythropoiesis, rHuEPO actually can cause functional iron deficiency.[19,20] As a result, iron supplementation in chronic renal failure patients is usually essential. Even with the most rigorous protocols, oral iron preparations have not been as effective as intravenous ones, largely because of poor absorption resulting in failure to maintain adequate hematologic parameters (hemoglobin level >11 to 12 g/dL, transferrin saturation >20%, plasma ferritin concentration >100 ng/mL). Thus intravenous iron is often administered.[24,25] There are now multiple formulations of intravenous iron available for administration, including iron

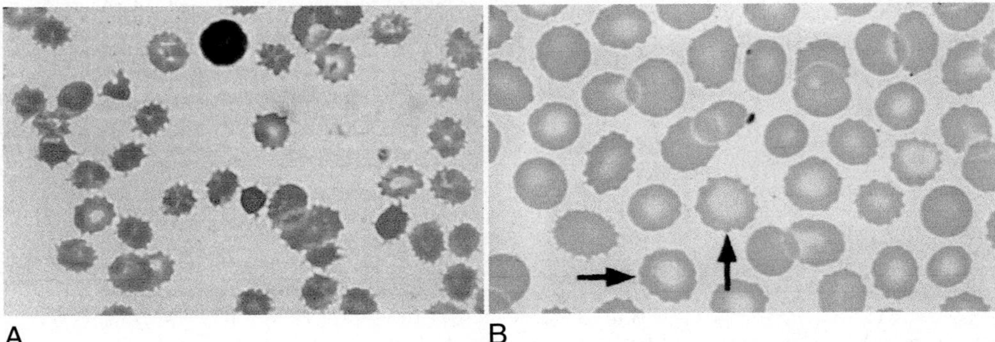

Figure 156-1 MORPHOLOGY OF ACANTHOCYTES AND ECHINOCYTES. **A,** Acanthocytes, or spur cells, are most commonly observed in significant numbers on the peripheral blood smear in cases of liver disease, although they may also be prominent in certain rare disorders (e.g., alpha, beta-lipoproteinemia). Their characteristic features are spines that seemingly project from the surface of the cell. Such morphologic change represents the result of irreversible cytoskeletal damage due to passage of abnormally stiff cells through the reticuloendothelial system. **B,** Echinocytes, or burr cells, are the hallmark of uremia, although they may be observed as an artifact on less than optimally prepared smears. An undulating or bumpy red blood cell surface *(arrows)* characterizes this morphologic change, the cause of which is unknown.

Management of the Anemia of Renal Disease

Recombinant human erythropoietin (rHuEPO) and the longer-acting modified erythropoietin, darbepoetin, have revolutionized treatment of the anemia of renal disease. However, owing to their potential for adverse events, the potential inconvenience of their administration by the parenteral route, and their expense, they should be used thoughtfully and judiciously.

Regardless of the extent of renal insufficiency, patients who are candidates for erythropoietin replacement should have an assessment of their iron stores. Analysis of serum parameters, such as ferritin, iron, and transferrin, generally suffice for this purpose. If there is any hint that iron deficiency may be present, it should be addressed before, or at least concomitantly with, the administration of rHuEPO. Although oral replacement may be reasonable in a patient with borderline iron stores and renal insufficiency, intravenous replacement with iron dextran, iron gluconate, or iron sucrose should be considered in patients with more severe iron deficiency or renal failure.

In the setting of mild to moderate renal insufficiency, such as that often seen in diabetic patients, it is not unreasonable to initiate therapy on a weekly basis if using rHuEPO or every other week when using darbepoetin when the hemoglobin level is less than 9 g/dL. After the hemoglobin concentration increases to greater than 10 g/dL, the frequency of administration or dose can be tapered to maintain a level between 10 and 11 g/dL. In some exceptional circumstances, such as in patients with significant congestive heart failure or pulmonary disease, maintenance of hemoglobin at a higher level (between 11-11.5 g/dL, but not above) may be determined to be beneficial. However, this should only be done with extreme caution, since the use of rHuEPO to raise levels above 11 g/dl has been associated with increase risk of cardiovascular events and death.

If there is no response to erythropoietin after 4 to 8 weeks of weekly therapy with rHuEPO or biweekly therapy with darbepoetin, iron stores should be reevaluated. If adequate, dose escalation of rHuEPO or darbepoetin by 50% and an additional trial for 4 to 8 weeks is reasonable. After that time, however, the drug should be discontinued and consideration be given to the cause for the lack of response, which is otherwise rare in the setting of anemia purely due to renal insufficiency. New formulations of rHuEPo are appearing; doing will vary by preparation. Dosing should be adjusted to maintain hemoglobin levels in the aforementioned target ranges.

dextran (InFeD), sodium ferric gluconate complex (Ferrlecit), and iron sucrose (Venofer). The latter two preparations are often used because they would appear to have more favorable safety profiles.[22,26-28] In particular, anaphylactic reactions appear to be somewhat less common.[29]

A hyperglycosylated rHuEPO, darbepoetin (Aranesp), is available.[30] It has the same mechanism of action as rHuEPO with the advantage of having a twofold to threefold longer half-life.[31,32] Consequently it can be dosed less frequently, allowing for fewer injections.[33,34] Darbepoetin appears to be equivalent to rHuEPO in terms of its clinical outcomes in patients with chronic renal failure, specifically in reaching a target hemoglobin level, the time it takes to reach that target, and the percentage of patients who reach that goal.[35,36] It is also a well-tolerated medication and has a safety profile that is similar to that of rHuEPO.[37,38] There have been no antibodies to native or recombinant erythropoietin detected to date in patients treated with darbepoetin.

HEMOSTATIC AGENTS FOR USE IN UREMIA

Bleeding from uremia is one of the major causes of morbidity in patients with end-stage renal disease.[32,33] There are multiple factors contributing to the pathogenesis of this bleeding risk, but recent focus has centered on platelet dysfunction,[35,36,39] abnormal platelet–vessel wall interactions,[37] retention of uremic toxins,[38] presence of anemia, and increased levels of nitrous oxide.[40-42]

The hemorrhagic manifestations commonly seen with uremia include epistaxis, gastrointestinal and genitourinary bleeding, subdural hematomas, hemorrhagic pericarditis, ecchymoses, and prolonged bleeding from skin puncture sites. A number of therapeutic options exist for the treatment of the hemorrhagic diathesis caused by uremia, and these should be considered in any patient who is actively bleeding or about to undergo a surgical procedure.

Correction of anemia with either red blood cell transfusions or recombinant human erythropoietin contributes significantly to reducing the bleeding tendency. Raising the hematocrit to 27% or greater has been shown to decrease the bleeding time and improve platelet function.[43-45] Similarly, hemodialysis has been shown to partially correct the bleeding time and potentially decrease the risk for bleeding.[46]

Perhaps the most convenient and safest treatment for bleeding in the setting of uremia, regardless of whether a patient is being dialyzed, is the use of desmopressin (DDAVP). Possibly through release of von Willebrand factor from endothelial stores and through improved platelet signal transduction, it frequently improves hemostasis. In a randomized placebo-controlled trial, administration of 0.3 mcg/kg of DDAVP resulted in a decrease in the bleeding time 1 hour after the infusion. However, the duration of action was relatively short and the improvement lasted only 6 to 12 hours.[47] If a longer duration of action is needed, administration of conjugated estrogens can be considered.[42,48] An intravenous dose of 0.6 mg/kg is given daily for 5 days. Although estrogens are slower in their onset of action, and perhaps somewhat less reproducible in terms of response, their effect can last 7 to 10 days. The mechanism of action of estrogens is not well understood but may be related to their effects on nitrous oxide. Finally, cryoprecipitate, rich in von Willebrand factor and fibrinogen, can also sometimes temporarily correct the bleeding time. It appears to act as quickly and last as long as DDAVP. A commonly used dose is 10 units every 12 to 24 hours.[49]

MANAGEMENT OF HEMOLYTIC UREMIC SYNDROME AND THROMBOTIC THROMBOCYTOPENIC PURPURA

Hematologic and renal abnormalities can manifest nearly simultaneously and suddenly in two disorders: HUS and thrombotic thrombocytopenic purpura (TTP)(see Chapter 136). Distinguishing between these two entities can be difficult.[50,51] They are both characterized by thrombocytopenia, microangiopathic hemolytic anemia, and platelet aggregation ultimately leading to end-organ dysfunction.[52] In HUS, the microvascular thrombi tend to occur within the renal microcirculation, causing acute renal failure. In TTP, the microvascular ischemia occurs in many organs and may affect the cerebral circulation, causing neurologic abnormalities.

Although not infrequently idiopathic, both HUS and TTP have been associated with the administration of various medications such as cyclosporine (HUS) and clopidogrel (TTP). In addition, the occurrence of HUS has been associated with Shiga toxin–producing bacteria (*Escherichia coli* 0157:H7).[47] Interestingly, the clinical course of HUS appears to depend on cause. Children who suffer from postdiarrheal HUS generally improve on their own with supportive care, and they only occasionally require short-term dialysis.[53] Patients with medication-related HUS tend to have poorer prognoses.

Deficiencies in factors of the alternative complement pathway have been associated with HUS, and ADAMTS13 deficiency has been found in some patients with TTP.[49,54,55] However, rapid determination of the level of these proteins is not yet routinely available, so the distinction between HUS and TTP, when made, generally relies on associated clinical findings.

In adults, HUS and TTP are often managed similarly by clinicians. Plasma-based therapies have been demonstrated to significantly decrease the mortality rates associated with HUS-TTP, and studies have documented the value of plasma exchange over simple plasma infusion.[56,57] The efficacy of plasma exchange possibly comes from its ability to remove the toxic factors implicated in the initiation of these disorders as well as to replace a depleted, missing, or inhibited factor such as the ADAMTS13 protease.[58,59] Some clinicians advocate that plasma exchange should begin promptly in any individual suspected of having HUS or TTP, regardless of whether the former or the latter is more strongly suspected.[60] Daily therapy with total plasma exchange is recommended until remission is evident, as determined by resolution of any renal and/or neurologic failure, normalization of platelet count and lactate dehydrogenase level, and a stable hematocrit level reflecting absence of ongoing hemolysis, or until it is clear that no further clinical benefit is being derived. Further research will hopefully better elucidate the pathogenesis of HUS and TTP and thereby facilitate the development of tailored therapies for each of these entities.

FUTURE DIRECTIONS

There are numerous hematologic manifestations of renal disease ranging from morphologic changes of red blood cells to coagulation abnormalities affecting hemostasis. Optimal patient care is facilitated by an understanding of these associated complications and their appropriate management.

SUGGESTED READINGS

Bailie GR, Clark JA, Lane CE, et al: Hypersensitivity reactions and deaths associated with intravenous iron preparations. *Nephrol Dial Transplant* 20:1443, 2005.

Lodge JPA, Jonas S, Jones RM, et al: Efficacy and safety of repeated perioperative doses of recombinant factor VIIa in liver transplantation. *Liver Transpl* 11:973, 2005.

Niemann CU, Behrends M, Quan D, et al: Recombinant factor VIIa reduces transfusion requirements in liver transplant patients with high MELD scores. *Transfus Med* 16:93, 2006.

Planinsic RM, van der Meer J, Testa G, et al: Safety and efficacy of a single bolus administration of recombinant factor VIIa in liver transplantation due to chronic liver disease. *Liver Transpl* 11:895, 2005.

Xia VW, Steadman RH: Antifibrinolytics in orthotopic liver transplantation: Current status and controversies. *Liver Transpl* 11:10, 2005.

Zipfel PF, Misselwitz J, Licht C, et al: The role of defective complement control in hemolytic uremic syndrome. *Semin Thromb Hemost* 32:146, 2006.

For complete list of references log on to www.expertconsult.com.

CHAPTER 157

HEMATOLOGIC MANIFESTATIONS OF CANCER

Gerald A. Soff, David L. Green, and Lawrence B. Gardner

Hematologic abnormalities are often seen in a variety of nonhematologic cancers. These manifestations range from trivial to life-threatening and may complicate management and require additional therapy. Some of these abnormalities can be the initial manifestation of cancer, providing a crucial diagnostic clue (e.g., Trousseau syndrome or erythrocytosis). Finally, the hematologic aspects of cancer can provide insight into the biology of tumorigenesis. This chapter focuses on the role of nonhematologic malignancies on red cells, platelets, and coagulation. Abnormalities seen with hematologic malignancies (e.g., the hemolytic anemia noted with chronic lymphocytic leukemia, or microangiopathic hemolytic anemias during bone marrow transplant) are addressed within those specific chapters.

CYTOPENIAS AND CANCER

Anemia

The most common hematologic manifestation of cancer is anemia, with studies demonstrating 30% to 90% of patients with cancer having anemia before treatment, including 40% of patients with early-stage colon cancer and 80% of patients with advanced colon cancer.[1] The causes of this anemia are varied. In gastrointestinal cancers, or cancers metastatic to the gastrointestinal tract, as well as in bladder cancer, iron deficiency from bleeding is common. More rarely, tumors involving the small bowel can interfere with iron absorption and/or vitamin B_{12} absorption. Most cancers are associated with systemic inflammation, manifested by elevated levels of cytokines, which can directly inhibit erythropoiesis and suppress iron available for erythropoiesis, both features of the anemia of chronic inflammation (see Chapter 35). Specifically, serum erythropoietin concentrations are not as elevated in patients with cancer as they are in patients with the same degree of anemia due to iron deficiency, and cancer patients often demonstrate increased hepcidin levels. Hepcidin decreases the iron transporter ferroportin, which results in increased iron stores (in the form of ferritin) and a decrease of free iron available for erythropoiesis, classic serologic findings in patients with cancer and anemia.

Another common cause of anemia in patients with cancer is bone marrow suppression due to chemotherapy. The European Cancer Anaemia Survey prospectively studied over 15,000 patients with a variety of solid tumors and treatments for 6 months.[2] Before therapy 10% of patients had hemoglobin levels below 10 g/dL, and during therapy this increased to almost 40% and correlated with poor performance status. In this study, radiation therapy alone did not dramatically increase the prevalence of anemia, but the combination of chemotherapy and radiation led to a greater degree of anemia than chemotherapy alone. Anemia due to chemotherapy is related to cumulative dose (e.g., there is a significant correlation of anemia with total cisplatinum dose), drug combinations (there is more anemia when cisplatinum is added to paclitaxel), and drug schedule (e.g., there is more anemia when paclitaxel is given over 24 hours compared to shorter time courses).[3] In contrast to iron deficiency and the anemia of chronic disease, anemia due to chemotherapy is generally associated with a similar or even greater decrease in platelets and neutrophils (due to their shorter half-lives), and it is important to note that specific chemotherapeutic agents are associated with particular cytopenias (e.g., gemcitabine and thrombocytopenia).[3] Although anemia in cancer patients plays an important clinical role because the degree of anemia correlates with quality of life, anemia can be treated with red cell transfusions and erythropoietin (see Treatment of Cytopenias Due to Cancer), whereas myelosuppression resulting in neutropenia and/or thrombocytopenia can be more difficult to treat and may result in significant morbidity and/or delay in treatment.

Thrombocytopenia

Although chemotherapeutic and immunosuppressive agents typically cause thrombocytopenia by suppressing hematopoiesis, they can also cause immune thrombocytopenia, and this diagnosis should be considered particularly when there is a sudden drop in platelets alone. For example, trastuzumab and oxaliplatin have both been shown to cause immune thrombocytopenia. Thrombocytopenia *independent* of treatment effect may be seen as a result of bone marrow infiltration by tumor cells, thrombotic microangiopathy, consumption coagulopathy, or rarely as an associated autoimmune manifestation. Bone marrow involvement, often occult, is common in prostate, lung, and breast cancer, although thrombocytopenia is not usually the sole presenting cytopenia. The laboratory features of disseminated intravascular coagulation (DIC) (elevated D-dimer and fibrinogen degradation products) are commonly seen in cancer patients (up to 90% of advanced cancers[4]), and DIC is the most common cause of non–treatment-related thrombocytopenia, although it is a relatively uncommon cause of bleeding in the cancer patient (see later).

Although thrombocytopenia often has a clinical impact because of bleeding or delays in the administration of chemotherapy, reactive thrombocytosis is actually more common than thrombocytopenia in cancer patients. Although in general thrombocytosis has not been associated with either bleeding or thrombotic events, prechemotherapy platelet count greater than 350,000 was a risk factor for venous thromboembolism (VTE) in a large prospective observational study of cancer patients undergoing chemotherapy.[5] Cancer-related thrombocytosis is likely to be a cytokine-mediated effect, and elevated levels of cytokines known to stimulate protein production, including interleukin-6 (IL-6), IL-11, and thrombopoietin (TPO), are often documented in cancer. In most tumor types, such as breast, renal cell, and gastric, elevated platelet counts confer an adverse prognosis.[6]

Multiple Cytopenias Due to Bone Marrow Metastases

When cancer is associated with the decrease of multiple lineages, the metastases of cancer to the bone marrow must be considered (Fig. 157-1). There are some data showing that platelet size can help differentiate thrombocytopenias due to bone marrow metastases from thrombocytopenia due to other causes, including immune thrombocytopenia, and decreased survival due to platelet activation and/or DIC seen in cancer.[7] Although all malignancies, even glioblastomas,

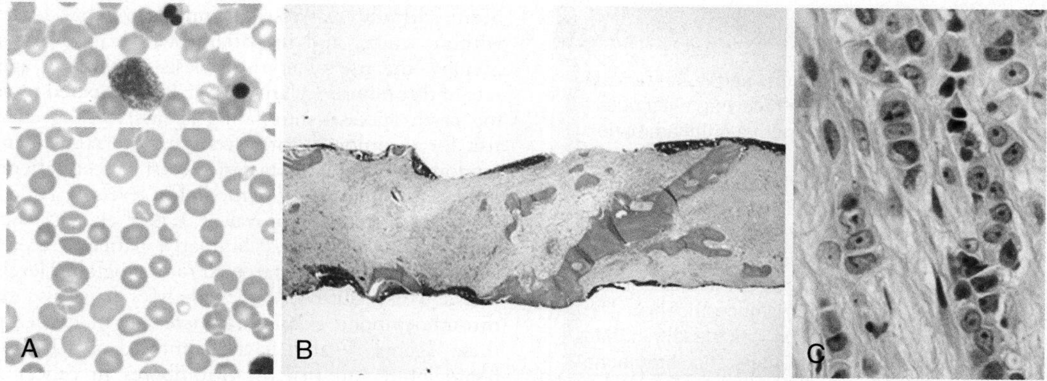

Figure 157-1 PERIPHERAL BLOOD AND BONE MARROW FROM A PATIENT WITH METASTATIC BREAST CANCER. THE PATIENT WAS A 77-YEAR-OLD WOMAN WHO PRESENTED WITH ANEMIA AND THROMBOCYTOPENIA. On physical examination she was found to have a breast mass. **A,** The peripheral smear showed a leukoerythroblastosis *(top)* with nucleated red blood cells and immature granulocytic precursors. Platelets were reduced, and red blood cells exhibited anisopoikilocytosis *(bottom)* with occasional teardrop forms and rare schistocytes. **B,** The bone marrow biopsy was fibrotic and had thickened bone with new bone formation. **C,** The bone marrow cavity was replaced by tumor cells infiltrating through bands of fibrosis.

have been reported to metastasize to the marrow, the most common malignancies include breast, gastric, lung, and prostate cancer. In one study, 8% of the time no primary tumor was identified at the time of bone marrow metastases, and only 13% of patients had normal blood counts at the time bone marrow involvement was noted.[8]

As expected, patients with bone marrow involvement of their solid tumor are more likely to experience cytopenias from chemotherapy, and bone marrow metastases carry a poor prognosis in virtually all solid malignancies.[8] For example, one study in patients with extensive small cell lung cancer found that those with bone marrow metastases had significantly shorter time to progression and significantly shorter survival time than other patients with extensive disease.[9] Although the poor prognosis in patients with bone marrow metastases is in large part due to tumor burden, the ability of a tumor to metastasize and grow in the bone marrow niche may indicate that the tumor has biologic features that render it particularly aggressive and/or resistant to therapy. Such tumor cell characteristics could include homing, adhesion, immune escape, and angiogenic potential. Laboratory data suggest that tumors that secrete more proangiogenic and proinflammatory cytokines may be more likely to metastasize to the bone marrow. Clinical data support the concept that the marked heterogeneity that exists within tumors includes characteristics that are required for growth with the bone marrow. One such example is the bone marrow micrometastases seen in women with early-stage breast cancer; 30.6% of women who have stage I to III breast cancer were found to have bone marrow micrometastases, and this was an independent poor prognosis in multivariable analysis.[10] Although bone marrow metastases also conferred a poor prognosis on women with small tumors and uninvolved lymph nodes, there was survival of patients even in the absence of chemotherapy, suggesting more factors may be necessary for cancer cells to grow in the bone marrow, and this may be an indicator of more aggressive disease rather than burden of disease. Indeed, a recent study of over 5000 women with T1N0M0 to T2N0M0 invasive breast carcinoma found that the presence of bone marrow metastases (found in 3% of patients) was an indicator of poor prognosis on univariate analysis, but not in multivariate analysis.[11]

The pathophysiology by which marrow involvement by cancer causes cytopenias is not fully understood. Total marrow replacement by tumor is rare, and only a small percentage of marrow can support normal peripheral blood counts, as indicated by the normal counts found in older adults with hypocellular marrows. Cancer may disrupt bone marrow niches required for normal hematopoiesis. Indeed, tumor growth in bone marrow may depend on specific niches that include osteoclasts as well as specific bone marrow stromal cell populations.

Other Cytopenias in Cancer

As noted, immune cytopenias, including immune thrombocytopenia, can occur as a complication of cancer treatment. Cancers can also cause autoimmune disorders resulting in cytopenias. Although this is commonly seen with thymomas and pure red cell aplasia, a variety of nonhematologic cancers can rarely lead to this phenomenon, including breast and lung cancer. Cytopenias can also be due to microangiopathic hemolytic anemias, leading to thrombocytopenia and anemia. Typically the white blood cell count is normal. Although a true incidence is difficult to determine, there are reports that 5% to 10% of mucin-producing disseminated adenocarcinomas result in a microangiopathic hemolytic anemia.[12] Although these microangiopathic syndromes are commonly referred to as thrombotic thrombocytopenic purpura (TTP), the pathophysiology appears distinct from idiopathic TTP, as suggested by the absence of very low levels of a disintegrin and metalloproteinase with thrombospondin motifs-13 (ADAMTS-13) and associated antibody inhibitors, and by the poor response to therapeutic plasma exchange. Some data suggest that cancer associated microangiopathy may result from endothelial damage. A microangiopathic hemolytic anemia may also be seen with the use of some drugs used in the treatment of cancer, including cyclosporine, mitomycin, and gemcitabine and anti–vascular endothelial growth factor (VEGF) agents.

EVALUATION OF CANCER-ASSOCIATED CYTOPENIAS

As in all cases of cytopenias, the initial step in the evaluation of cytopenias in a patient with cancer is a careful history and physical. Special emphasis should be placed on whether the patient suffers from an isolated cytopenia (e.g., anemia) or whether multiple lineages are affected, suggesting marrow suppression or involvement. Similarly, the temporal nature of the cytopenia, whether it correlates to therapy or is progressive, may suggest that it is therapy related or due to marrow involvement of cancer, respectively (see box on Evaluation of Cytopenias).

An examination of the peripheral blood smear is crucial. Appearance of a microangiopathy (fragmented red cells, thrombocytopenia, reticulocytosis) can suggest a TTP-like condition, DIC, or marrow replacement by tumor. In this case coagulation tests may be helpful, and a bone marrow aspirate and biopsy may be necessary. Finally, readily treatable causes of cytopenias that are common in the general population (e.g., iron deficiency) should be ruled out in all patients with cancer.

Evaluation of Cytopenias

The evaluation of cytopenias can be difficult, particularly in the complex patient who has cytopenia before receiving chemotherapy that is worsened with treatment. The anemia of inflammation and the anemia of iron deficiency, both of which are microcytic, can be difficult to differentiate, particularly because the serum ferritin level is an unreliable assessment of iron stores in inflammatory conditions such as cancer (as reviewed in Chapter 35). Marrow-occupying tumors are often associated with microangiopathic features, including schistocytes, teardrops, and bizarre red cell forms, leukoerythroblastosis, and thrombocytopenia. The peripheral smear and laboratory evaluation can be difficult to distinguish from primary bone marrow disorders and thrombotic thrombocytopenic purpura (TTP), and in some cases a bone marrow examination may be necessary, particularly if the involvement of marrow has prognostic or treatment implications.

TREATMENT OF CYTOPENIAS DUE TO CANCER

Cytopenias resulting from cancer and/or chemotherapy can be asymptomatic. However, anemia (particularly hemoglobin level below 8 to 10 g/dL) is thought to be a major contributor to fatigue and thus quality of life, leukopenia can lead to infections, and thrombocytopenia can either lead to spontaneous bleeding or make procedures, including intrathecal treatments, more dangerous. Cytopenias can also commonly cause delays in treatment or alterations in treatment.

The treatment of cytopenias is dependent on the underlying cause. For example, cytopenias due to marrow infiltration of a chemosensitive cancer are best treated with chemotherapy, although less-myelosuppressive regimens are most appropriate. In contrast, if the cytopenias are *due* to treatment, holding or delivering an alternative therapy is best. For cytopenias due to immune-mediated effects, steroids and other standard therapies are appropriate.

Because of the limitations and potential morbidities of transfusions, for almost two decades hematopoietic growth factors have been frequently used for therapy. Although erythropoietin and granulocyte colony-stimulating factor (G-CSF) have been most studied and used clinically, other growth factors (including platelet factors) have been developed. These therapies have primarily been studied in those receiving chemotherapy, although several studies using erythropoietin have included cancer patients not receiving chemotherapy, many of whom had an inflammatory anemia. Initial trials of erythropoietin treatment of thrice-weekly injections of erythropoietin, and later trials using weekly erythropoietin or longer-acting agents such as darbepoietin, have unequivocally demonstrated that the use of erythropoiesis-stimulating agents during myelosuppressive treatment increases hemoglobin level and decreases transfusion requirements by approximately 50%. Although many of these studies with these agents demonstrate an improvement of quality of life, most of these studies were not blinded, prospective, or definined a minimal quality-of-life metric that would be considered clinically relevant.

Despite the biologic effectiveness of erythropoietin in a variety of noncancer patients, several trials using erythropoietic growth factors led to no clinical improvement, or decreased improvement, in intensively ill patients, patients with heart failure, patients requiring hemodialysis, patients with severe renal dysfunction, and patients with a variety of other noncancer conditions (see Chapter 35). Similarly, a randomized trial showed that patients with cancer not receiving chemotherapy had increased cardiovascular and thromboembolic events and decreased survival over 4 months of treatment with darbopoietin, though the increased risks were not significant in multivariate analyses.[13] These studies and others had led to a consensus recommendation that erythropoiesis-stimulating agents not be used in those patients with cancer *not* receiving chemotherapy.[14]

Recently the prevalent use of erythroid, and even myeloid, growth factors in patients with cancer receiving chemotherapy has also been critically reassessed. Similar to what was seen in patients without cancer and in patients with cancer not receiving chemotherapy, the use of erythropoiesis-stimulating agents increases the rate of thrombosis (relative risk 1.67, compared to patients not receiving erythropoiesis-stimulating agents) during chemotherapy.[15] This risk for thrombosis correlates with the target hemoglobin. A large randomized trial in metastatic breast cancer patients of patients with mild anemia, targeting hemoglobin levels of 12 to 14 g/dL, demonstrated a decreased survival at 1 year, in part because of increased cardiovascular toxicity.[16] Similarly, patients receiving radiation for head and neck cancer, targeted to hemoglobin levels of over 14 g/dL, had a worse survival.[17] Metaanalyses have also demonstrated that thromboembolic events are increased in cancer patients receiving these agents[18-20] and have confirmed a relationship with target hemoglobin and risk for thromboses in cancer patients receiving erythropoietin.[21]

Of great concern is that both the breast cancer and head and neck studies cited earlier also demonstrated decreased tumor control with these, albeit high, doses of erythropoietin. Several randomized trials and metaanalyses, including one assessing almost 14,000 patients, have also found that the use of erythropoiesis-stimulating agents worsened overall survival, particularly in patients undergoing chemotherapy.[22] In other studies, although overall survival was not affected by concomitant erythropoietin use, local tumor control was decreased. However, it is important to note that this correlation has not been found in all analyses,[20,21] and in recent randomized trials of patients receiving radiation and chemotherapy erythropoietin did not alter survival (though hemoglobin was minimally increased).[23,24] A recent consensus stresses that reversible causes of anemia be ruled out before erythropoietin usage, that the minimal amount of erythropoietin be used to aim for a target hemoglobin level of 10 g/dL, and that erythropoietin only be used for patients receiving chemotherapy when palliation is the ultimate goal.[14]

The pathobiology of the increased rate of thromboses and the poorer rate of tumor control with erythropoiesis-stimulating agents is unknown. Although hemoglobin concentration correlates with thrombosis risk, suggesting that an increase in viscosity could be a causative factor, hemoglobin concentration could also serve as a surrogate for either effective erythropoietin dose or target cell (nonerythroid) responsiveness. In terms of the poor tumor control noted in some trials of erythropoietin, it has been noted that many tumor cells express erythropoietin receptors, and in fact increased erythropoietin receptor expression may be a poor prognostic indicator in many tumors. Erythropoietin signaling can serve as a survival signal, suggesting that targeting the erythropoietin receptor may be a therapeutic strategy in cancer therapy. Although it is reasonable to think that exogenous erythropoietin can promote tumor growth in this way, it is also possible that increased red cell mass and/or increased tumor oxygenation could play a role.

Myeloid growth factors (most commonly G-CSF) have also been used intensively in patients receiving chemotherapy over the past decade, with the goal of improving survival by intensifying the chemotherapy regimen, decreasing delays in chemotherapy administration, and decreasing infections and hospitalizations with neutropenic fever. G-CSF administration has also been suggested for regimens when the risk for neutropenia is greater than 20%. It is clear that many dose-intensive regimens, some of which may be more effective than less intensive regimens, are possible only with the support of myeloid growth factors. G-CSF receptors have been found on tumors, and there is a theoretic concern that exogenous G-CSF may increase proliferation and/or improve survival of these tumors. Use of myeloid growth factors during chemotherapy for solid tumors has been theorized to promote leukemia risk, by acting as a survival signal to hematopoietic progenitor cells damaged by chemotherapy. A recent metaanalysis of 25 randomized clinical trials found that there was an almost twofold increase in acute myeloid leukemia in those patients assigned to receive chemotherapy with growth factor support, compared to those who did not receive growth factor support, although all-cause mortality was actually decreased in those who received growth factor support.[25]

THROMBOSIS AND CANCER

Relationship of Cancer and Thrombosis

The association of thrombosis and cancer is widely recognized, dating to the middle of the 19th century, and can be considered the first recognized paraneoplastic syndrome. Armand Trousseau was the first to associate thrombosis and malignancy, the first to suggest screening for malignancy in recurrent or idiopathic thromboembolic disease, the first to suggest that the pathophysiology was not mechanical obstruction, but a change in the character in the coagulation system itself, and the first to suggest that the association may be integral to the cancer growth itself. What has made this association particularly poignant was the fact that Trousseau predicted his own occult malignancy when he developed "phlebitis," dying 6 months later of gastric cancer. More recently, some of the biologic mechanisms underlying the increased risk for thrombosis in patients with cancer have been better delineated (see later).

Patients with active malignancy have a higher risk for thrombosis than other medical patients, and surgical oncology patients have a higher thrombosis rate than other surgical patients undergoing major procedures. Although reports of thrombosis rates vary, it is generally accepted that about 15% to 20% of cancer patients will develop VTE at some point during their illness and about 20% of VTEs occur in cancer patients.[26] Cancer is a potent situational risk factor for venous thrombosis, increasing the risk about 6- to 10-fold. In comparison, the common hereditary thrombophilia, heterozygous factor V Leiden, increases the risk for venous thrombosis by approximately 5-fold (see Chapter 142). Arterial and venous thrombosis are second only to progression of disease as a cause of death among cancer patients, accounting for 9.2% of deaths among patients receiving outpatient chemotherapy.[27] There have been a number of reports characterizing the strength of the association of thrombosis with different cancer types, and these have yielded variable findings. The reported adjusted odds ratios for thrombosis for a given tumor type varies greatly, based on the methodology to capture the thrombosis diagnosis. But several important conclusions may be drawn. Virtually all solid tumor types, as well as hematologic malignancies, result in a significantly increased risk for thrombosis, and secondly, certain tumor types consistently appear to have particularly high risk for thrombosis, including lung, pancreas and other gastrointestinal cancers, and brain tumor.[28]

Not only does the diagnosis of thrombosis in the cancer patient require specific therapy that can complicate overall treatment strategies, it also serves as an important prognostic indicator. In patients with advanced cancer, those who present with venous thromboembolic disease have a 1-year survival of 12%, compared with 1-year survival of 36% in patients with advanced cancer presenting without thrombosis.[29] Similar studies have noted that the diagnosis of thrombosis during the first year after cancer diagnosis was a significant predictor of death for most cancer types and stages analyzed. One key question is whether the thrombotic tendency in some patients is mostly a marker of a more aggressive disease or the development of thrombosis is a major cause of increased mortality. Thrombosis is the second leading cause of death in outpatient chemotherapy patients, but of the 9.2% of total deaths attributable to thromboembolism, 3.5% were venous and 5.6% were arterial.[27] The preponderance of VTE events occur within the first 3 months of diagnosis, and not in the later stages of disease.[28] This can be interpreted as the thrombotic tendency is a property of the underlying cancer biology more than a reflection of tumor burden or a specific treatment strategy. And interestingly, in a recent study of gastroesophageal malignancy patients undergoing chemotherapy, multivariate analysis showed that development of a VTE during the course of chemotherapy was not associated with reduced survival.[30] These findings suggest that much of the mortality burden of venous thrombosis in cancer reflects the more severe underlying cancer biology rather than simply death from complications of the thrombosis itself.

Diagnosis of Coagulopathies in Cancer Patients

Thrombotic episodes in patients with cancer are typically diagnosed similarly to thrombotic events in patients without cancer. However, several subtleties exist. For example, thromboses may be confused with either intravascular disease progression and/or intravascular fungal infections. In many cases, the diagnosis of thromboses or an abnormality in coagulation may be made in an asymptomatic patient, leading to a difficult decision regarding the risks and benefits of correction. The constitutive activation of the coagulation system by cancer has been well documented. Elevated levels of markers of in vivo coagulation activation, including thrombin-antithrombin complexes, prothrombin F1+2 activation peptide, and fibrin degradation products, including fibrinopeptide A and D-dimer have been described.[31] A process of fibrin formation and degradation is continuous in the setting of many patients with malignancy. Thus cancer is often felt to be a process of "chronic DIC." It should be noted, however, that the levels of the coagulation factors and platelets are often actually elevated, not diminished as is typically noted in DIC. In two prospective studies of routine coagulation parameters in cancer patients, *elevated* fibrinogen and platelet counts were the most frequent alterations.[31] Furthermore, the increase in the levels of these two markers, observed prospectively every month, directly correlated with disease progression. The clinical spectrum of DIC in cancer varies from asymptomatic to a life-threatening thrombohemorrhagic disorder. Thrombotic manifestations of DIC include arterial and venous thromboembolism, migratory thrombophlebitis, and marantic endocarditis and microvascular thrombosis with organ failure or skin necrosis. The consumptive phase of DIC may manifest with bleeding and may respond favorably to low-dose heparin, plasma therapy, or successful treatment of the underlying malignancy. In one study of patients with prostate cancer, a clinical picture of DIC with excessive fibrinolysis and decreased levels of fibrinogen was noted.[32] In contrast to the thrombotic tendency observed in most solid tumor patients who exhibit evidence of activation of the coagulation system, the prostate cancer patients with DIC with excessive fibrinolysis did not exhibit thrombosis, and 30% died of hemorrhage.[32] When DIC is not associated with bleeding in the patient with a solid tumor, the best strategy is treatment of the underlying tumor.

With increased use of high-resolution computed tomographic imaging studies, pulmonary emboli (PEs) are increasingly being identified incidentally, in the absence of clinical suspicion. This has led to the question of how to treat these incidental PEs. Two recent studies have provided valuable guidance. A retrospective cohort study of the period from 2004 to 2010, comparing the rate of recurrent VTE and overall survival between those patients whose PEs were detected on incidental imaging studies with those whose PEs were suspected by classic clinical criteria did not identify a significant difference in these two end points.[33] A separate prospective observational study enrolling consecutive cancer patients newly diagnosed with combined deep venous thrombosis and PE from 2006 to 2009 found that 60% of the incidental thrombosis events were PEs, but only 26% of the symptomatic events were PEs.[34] This study also noted that a lower risk for recurrent thrombosis was observed in patients with incidental thrombosis compared with symptomatic thrombosis, with no differences in major bleeding and overall survival compared with symptomatic venous thrombosis patients.[34] Taken together, these two studies would support the routine anticoagulation treatment of an incidentally found thrombosis, but as always, one must balance the risks and benefits of anticoagulation.

Management of Thrombosis in Patients With Cancer

In the general population, management of venous thromboembolic disease has consisted of an acute course of heparin, or more recently a low-molecular-weight heparin (LMWH), followed by an oral vitamin K antagonist. This regimen has been the mainstay of thrombosis management since 1960, and countless patients have benefited from this treatment regimen. However, it is now well recognized that cancer

Use of Low-Molecular-Weight Heparin in Cancer Patients With Thromboses

Because of several factors, including the pharmacokinetics and varied absorption of warfarin in patients receiving chemotherapy, the use of low-molecular-weight-heparin (LMWH) in cancer patients with thromboses is suggested. In general, anticoagulation should continue as long as the patient has a hypercoagulable state. In some patients with solid tumors, this means lifelong therapy. However, the clinician should regularly reassess the risks and benefits of anticoagulation for each patient.

patients have a much higher rate of recurrent thrombosis while managed with warfarin than the population without cancer. Prandoni et al[35] compared recurrent thrombosis and major bleeding rates in thrombosis with and without cancer, managed with dose-adjusted intravenous unfractionated heparin or weight-adjusted LMWH, followed by warfarin. The 12-month cumulative incidence of recurrent thromboembolism in cancer patients was 20.7% versus 6.8% in patients without cancer, with a hazard ratio of 3.2. The 12-month cumulative incidence of major bleeding was 12.4% in patients with cancer and 4.9% in patients without cancer, with a hazard ratio of 2.2.[35]

Warfarin by its very nature is difficult to use safely and effectively in cancer patients for several reasons. There are numerous and unpredictable drug interactions. Cancer patients have variable nutritional intake, with variable vitamin K in their diets, and frequent use of antibiotics leads to highly variable bioavailability of the dietary vitamin K. Further, there is a frequent need to interrupt anticoagulation for procedures and coexisting thrombocytopenia, and the long half-life of warfarin makes these interruptions problematic. Improved treatment strategies for thrombosis in cancer have been reported with chronic use of LMWH. The seminal study was the "CLOT" study by Lee et al, published in 2003.[36] Patients with cancer and VTE received dalteparin 200 International Units/kg, subcutaneously once daily for 5 to 7 days, then randomized to either continued dalteparin 150 International Units/kg subcutaneously once daily or dose-adjusted warfarin with target international normalized ratio (INR) of 2 to 3. The hazard ratio for recurrent thromboembolism in the dalteparin group compared with the oral-anticoagulant group was 0.48, and major bleeding (6% versus 4%) and all bleeding (14% versus 19%) rates were similar. Of note, despite the marked reduction in the rate of recurrent thrombosis by the dalteparin, the overall survival rate was not affected. Based on the significant reduction in rate of recurrent thrombosis and comparable safety of LMWH compared with warfarin, this study has now established the acute and chronic use of LMWH as the standard of care for thrombosis in cancer. A similar study that compared enoxaparin with warfarin for treatment of venous thrombosis in cancer was published in 2002.[37] This study also showed an approximately 50% reduction of combined outcome of major bleeding or recurrent VTE within 3 months with enoxaparin compared with warfarin (10.5% versus 21.1%).[37] However, the study was underpowered, and the effect was not statistically significant. But the similar trend of benefit does reinforce the now-standard use of LMWH for both acute and chronic management of thrombosis in the cancer patient (see box on Use of Low-Molecular-Weight Heparin in Cancer Patients With Thromboses).

BIOLOGIC MECHANISMS UNDERLYING THROMBOSIS IN CANCER

The etiology of thrombosis is best understood in the context of the classic Virchow triad. Virchow described three classes of risk factors for thrombosis: stasis or altered blood flow, changes in the vessel wall, or changes in the blood. Cancer contributes to thrombosis by mechanisms within all three of these categories. Physical compression and/or disruption of blood vessels by a tumor may cause disrupted flow or stasis. Upon interaction with cancer cells, monocytes or macrophages release cytokines, including tumor necrosis factor, IL-1, and IL-6, which damage vascular endothelial cells.[38] The damaged vessel surface has reduced expression of naturally occurring anticoagulants, such as thrombomodulin, heparin sulfate, CD39/ecto-ADPase, nitric oxide, and prostacyclin, and increased expression of procoagulant proteins, particularly tissue factor (TF), and the blood is exposed to the procoagulant subendothelial matrix, all of which contribute to the thrombotic tendency.[38]

Tumor-Derived Tissue Factor

Despite the contributions of stasis and vessel changes in cancer-associated thrombosis, the best-documented contributing factor to thrombosis in the cancer patient is elevated procoagulant plasma factors, many of which are generated by the tumor itself. TF is the primary protein that initiates the coagulation cascade, by binding to and activating factor VII (see Chapter 128). TF is increased in a number of cancer types, including pancreatic cancer, breast cancer, and non–small cell lung cancer, compared with the nontransformed epithelium. Low oxygen levels often found in the tumor microenvironment, activation of oncogenes, such as RAS or MET, and inactivation of suppressor genes such as TP53 or PTEN directly induce TF, as well as other genes controlling hemostasis.[39] Targeting the human MET oncogene to mouse liver using lentiviral vector[40] driven by a tissue-specific promoter results in a cancer-associated coagulopathy and striking thrombotic events, which may serve as a model of Trousseau syndrome. Elevated TF expression and activation of the coagulation system correlate with both thrombotic tendency and disease progression (see later).

In addition to TF expression in tumors, activated endothelium, and tumor-associated macrophages, TF is increased in platelets and microparticles from cancer patients compared to healthy controls.[41] The generation of TF-expressing microparticles may be an important mechanism of cancer hypercoagulability. Microparticles are vesicular structures released from cell membranes under a range of situations, including activation, malignant transformation, stress, or death and are detected in plasma in a wide range of disease states, including sepsis and cancer.[42] There is no precise definition of the size and nature of microparticles, but they are generally considered to be between 100 nm and 1000 nm in diameter. Microparticles have been reported to arise from platelets, monocytes, endothelial cells, and tumor cells and carry on their surfaces a range of proteins that derived from the cell of origin, including TF. Cancer cells, directly and indirectly, lead to the generation and circulation of TF-bearing microparticles, and the levels of circulating TF-bearing microparticles in pancreatic cancer patients strongly correlates with the subsequent risk for venous thromboembolic disease. In one recent report, 34.8% of patients with detectable TF-bearing microparticles developed venous thrombosis, compared with no thrombosis in those without detectable TF-bearing microparticles.[42]

Coagulation's Role in Tumor Progression

Although the interplay between the coagulation pathway and cancer is best appreciated to result in an increase in thrombosis in cancer patients, the activation of coagulation in cancer may also play a role in tumor progression. For example, TF expression levels often correlate with a more aggressive tumor phenotype, and both clotting-dependent and clotting-independent signaling mechanisms of TF may be important in regulating tumor metastasis.[43] TF promotes angiogenesis and coexpresses with VEGF on malignant cells. Each is also able to upregulate the other. Interestingly, TF and VEGF knockout mice are embryologic lethal at the same stage with a similar phenotype, disorganized yolk sac vasculature,[44,45] implying functions that are overlapping.

Thrombin not only is the key terminal enzyme of coagulation resulting in fibrin deposition and platelet activation but also is a growth factor for a number of cell types such as fibroblasts, endothelial cells, smooth muscle cells, and tumor cells. The cellular effects of thrombin are mediated through seven transmembrane-spanning G protein–coupled protease-activated receptors (PARs), principally PAR1. PAR1 is activated by thrombin through cleavage of its N-terminal, which exposes a tethered ligand that then binds to the second transmembrane domain of the receptor. PARs are expressed on platelets and other cells, as well as on tumor cells and human tumor specimens.[43] Thrombin-activated tumor cells have PAR1-dependent enhanced expression of multiple integrins. Thrombin may enhance tumor progression by several mechanisms, including enhancing tumor cell proliferation; activating tumor-platelet adhesion; tumor adhesion to the matrix or endothelium; tumor implantation, growth, and metastasis; and tumor angiogenesis.[43] Thrombin alters tumor cell gene expression with upregulation of angiogenesis-related genes such as VEGF, VEGFRs, matrix metalloproteinase 2 (MMP-2), angiopoietin 2 (ANG2), and other genes and micro-ribonucleic acids (miRNAs) affecting tumor cell proliferation and invasion such as SKP2, Twist, cathepsin D, and growth-regulated oncogene-α (GRO-α).

Platelets and Cancer

In addition to the abnormalities in platelet number seen in cancer, described earlier, platelet function has been noted to be altered in cancer, and these alterations may contribute to tumor progression. Platelets derived from cancer patients are activated as measured by increased surface P-selectin expression and elevated serum levels of platelet factor 4 and β-thromboglobulin. Not only may the activation of platelets contribute to coagulation abnormalities seen in cancer patients (see later), but activated platelets can interact with leukocytes, endothelial cell as well as tumor cells, and contribute to the early stages of tumor cell dissemination. Visualization of tumor cells arrested in the pulmonary vasculature reveals interaction with platelets and fibrinogen, and in fact the ability of tumor cells to aggregate platelets in vitro correlates with metastatic potential.[46] In blood-borne models of hematogenous metastasis, platelets are necessary for efficient metastasis.[47] In these classic studies platelet reduction by antiplatelet antibody markedly reduces experimental hematogenous metastasis. The importance of platelet number and function in metastasis was confirmed by more recent studies in NF-E2$^{-/-}$ mice that have few circulating platelets, in mice whose platelets are rendered nonfunctional by knockout of Gαq$^{-/-}$, and in PAR4$^{-/-}$ mice that are unable to respond to thrombin.[48]

A number of platelet receptors may contribute to the platelet support of metastasis, including GPIIb/IIIa, adenosine diphosphate (ADP) receptors, P-selectin and thrombin receptors, and others, and there are likely multiple mechanisms underlying the platelet effects on malignancy[48]. (1) Platelets stabilize otherwise short-lived tumor cells in the circulation; (2) Platelet–tumor cell interaction enhances tumor cell adhesion to the vessel wall and results in distal embolization and downstream ischemic endothelial damage; (3) Platelets in the vicinity of tumor cells alter vessel wall permeability and tumor cell invasion; (4) Platelets protect tumor cells from immune surveillance and destruction, in part by shielding tumor cells from natural killer cells, although other mechanisms are likely; (5) Platelets provide nutrient support (growth factors) and release proangiogenic factors. Platelets contain numerous growth factors, coagulation factors and adhesive molecules, chemokines, and bioactive lipids that may enhance metastatic efficiency. Platelets are enriched in angiogenic growth factors such as basic fibroblast growth factor and VEGF, as well as several inhibitors, and may regulate angiogenesis, which is a hallmark of malignancy. Selective P-selectin and thrombin receptor activation on platelets may release α-granules enriched in either VEGF or endostatin; (6) Platelet-derived transforming growth factor-β and direct platelet–tumor cell contacts promote epithelial mesenchymal transformation and tumor metastases; (7) Platelet activation by tumor cells provides a surface for local thrombin generation.

FUTURE DIRECTIONS

Future research on the interplay of cancer, hematopoiesis, and coagulation not only will provide effective therapies for the hematologic manifestations of cancer, but also will provide insight into the biology of tumorigenesis and may lead to new strategies to treat cancer. For example, understanding how the use of exogenous erythropoietin may promote tumor survival and/or growth may lead not only to a better appreciation of which tumors may be more sensitive to this untoward effect (e.g., localized versus metastatic, tumors expressing the erythropoietin receptor versus tumors not expressing this receptor), but to novel agents that bypass this effect and even to agents that can disrupt this signaling and have antitumor effect. Better understanding of the role that platelets and/or thrombin play in tumor promotion may one day lead to an effective antitumor strategy that incorporates antiplatelet or antithrombotic agents.

SUGGESTED READINGS

Aapro M, Osterwalder B, Scherhag A, et al: Epoetin-beta treatment in patients with cancer chemotherapy-induced anaemia: The impact of initial haemoglobin and target haemoglobin levels on survival, tumour progression and thromboembolic events. *Br J Cancer* 101:1961, 2009.

Bennett CL, Silver SM, Djulbegovic B, et al: Venous thromboembolism and mortality associated with recombinant erythropoietin and darbepoetin administration for the treatment of cancer-associated anemia. *JAMA* 299:914, 2008.

Bohlius J, Wilson J, Seidenfeld J, et al: Recombinant human erythropoietins and cancer patients: Updated meta-analysis of 57 studies including 9353 patients. *J Natl Cancer Inst* 98:708, 2006.

Bohlius J, Schmidlin K, Brillant C, et al: Recombinant human erythropoiesis-stimulating agents and mortality in patients with cancer: A meta-analysis of randomised trials. *Lancet* 373:1532, 2009.

Blom JW, Doggen CJ, Osanto S, et al: Malignancies, prothrombotic mutations, and the risk of venous thrombosis. *JAMA* 293:715, 2005.

Braun S, Vogl FD, Naume B, et al: A pooled analysis of bone marrow micrometastasis in breast cancer. *N Engl J Med* 353:793, 2005.

Chandra S, Chandra H, Saini S: Bone marrow metastasis by solid tumors—probable hematological indicators and comparison of bone marrow aspirate, touch imprint and trephine biopsy. *Hematology* 15:368, 2010.

Chang JC, Naqvi T: Thrombotic thrombocytopenic purpura associated with bone marrow metastasis and secondary myelofibrosis in cancer. *Oncologist* 8:375, 2003.

Giuliano AE, Hawes D, Ballman KV, et al: Association of occult metastases in sentinel lymph nodes and bone marrow with survival among women with early-stage invasive breast cancer. *JAMA* 306:385, 2011.

Glaspy J, Crawford J, Vansteenkiste J, et al: Erythropoiesis-stimulating agents in oncology: A study-level meta-analysis of survival and other safety outcomes. *Br J Cancer* 102:301, 2010.

Groopman JE, Itri LM: Chemotherapy-induced anemia in adults: Incidence and treatment. *J Natl Cancer Inst* 91:1616, 1999.

Henke M, Laszig R, Rube C, et al: Erythropoietin to treat head and neck cancer patients with anaemia undergoing radiotherapy: Randomised, double-blind, placebo-controlled trial. *Lancet* 362:1255, 2003.

Hillen HF: Thrombosis in cancer patients. *Ann Oncol* 11:273, 2000.

Hoskin PJ, Robinson M, Slevin N, et al: Effect of epoetin alfa on survival and cancer treatment–related anemia and fatigue in patients receiving radical radiotherapy with curative intent for head and neck cancer. *J Clin Oncol* 27:5751, 2009.

Khorana AA, Francis CW, Culakova E, et al: Frequency, risk factors, and trends for venous thromboembolism among hospitalized cancer patients. *Cancer* 110:2339, 2007.

Khorana AA, Kuderer NM, Culakova E, et al: Development and validation of a predictive model for chemotherapy-associated thrombosis. *Blood* 111:4902, 2008.

Kilickap S, Erman M, Dincer M, et al: Bone marrow metastasis of solid tumors: Clinicopathological evaluation of 73 cases. *Turk J Cancer* 37:85, 2007.

Knight K, Wade S, Balducci L: Prevalence and outcomes of anemia in cancer: A systematic review of the literature. *Am J Med* 116:11S, 2004.

Leyland-Jones B: Semiglazov V, Pawlicki M, et al: Maintaining normal hemoglobin levels with epoetin alfa in mainly nonanemic patients with metastatic breast cancer receiving first-line chemotherapy: A survival study. *J Clin Oncol* 23:5960, 2005.

Ludwig H, Van Belle S, Barrett-Lee P, et al: The European Cancer Anaemia Survey (ECAS): A large, multinational, prospective survey defining the prevalence, incidence, and treatment of anaemia in cancer patients. *Eur J Cancer* 40:2293, 2004.

Lyman GH, Dale DC, Wolff DA, et al: Acute myeloid leukemia or myelodysplastic syndrome in randomized controlled clinical trials of cancer chemotherapy with granulocyte colony–stimulating factor: A systematic review. *J Clin Oncol* 28:2914, 2010.

Nash GF, Turner LF, Scully MF, et al: Platelets and cancer. *Lancet Oncol* 3:425, 2002.

Rizzo JD, Brouwers M, Hurley P, et al: American Society of Hematology/American Society of Clinical Oncology clinical practice guideline update on the use of epoetin and darbepoetin in adult patients with cancer. *Blood* 116:4045, 2010.

Sallah S, Wan JY, Nguyen NP, et al: Disseminated intravascular coagulation in solid tumors: Clinical and pathologic study. *Thromb Haemost* 86:828, 2001.

Shah MA, Capanu M, Soff G, et al: Risk factors for developing a new venous thromboembolism in ambulatory patients with non-hematologic malignancies and impact on survival for gastroesophageal malignancies. *J Thromb Haemost* 8:1702, 2010.

Smith RE, Jr, Aapro MS, Ludwig H, et al: Darbepoetin alpha for the treatment of anemia in patients with active cancer not receiving chemotherapy or radiotherapy: Results of a phase III, multicenter, randomized, double-blind, placebo-controlled study. *J Clin Oncol* 26:1040, 2008.

Sorensen HT, Mellemkjaer L, Olsen JH, et al: Prognosis of cancers associated with venous thromboembolism. *N Engl J Med* 343:1846, 2000.

Tonelli M, Hemmelgarn B, Reiman T, et al: Benefits and harms of erythropoiesis-stimulating agents for anemia related to cancer: A meta-analysis. *CMAJ* 180:E62, 2009.

Tsuboi M, Ezaki K, Tobinai K, et al: Weekly administration of epoetin beta for chemotherapy-induced anemia in cancer patients: Results of a multicenter, phase III, randomized, double-blind, placebo-controlled study. *Jpn J Clin Oncol* 39:163, 2009.

Zych J, Polowiec Z, Wiatr E, et al: The prognostic significance of bone marrow metastases in small cell lung cancer patients. *Lung Cancer* 10:239, 1993.

For complete list of references log on to www.expertconsult.com.

CHAPTER 158

INTEGRATIVE THERAPIES IN PATIENTS WITH HEMATOLOGIC DISEASES

David S. Rosenthal, Kara M. Kelly, and Donald I. Abrams

Complementary and alternative medicine, more popularly known as CAM, is tremendously popular in the United States and many parts of the world in helping people deal with wellness and health concerns.[1] In the United States alone, an estimated $36 to $47 billion is spent annually by the public on CAM methods of therapy,[2] and in a National Health Interview Survey in 2007, 37% of adults used at least one form of CAM. Over the past decade, CAM practices have become even more popular, especially in individuals with a chronic disease such as hematologic malignancies and cancer.[3] The National Center for Complementary and Alternative Medicine (NCCAM) at the National Institutes of Health studies the efficacy and safety of CAM practices.

Unfortunately, the term *CAM* causes consternation in many of our professional colleagues who perceive that their patients are forgoing conventional therapy. That is generally not the case. The term *CAM* is controversial because the words *complementary* and *alternative* have completely different meanings and should not be connected by an "and" but by an "or." Whereas complementary therapies as defined by NCCAM are therapies used to complement or to be used *alongside* conventional methods of therapy, alternative methods refer to those therapies that are used *instead* of known conventional therapies and have not been shown to be effective. The term *integrative medicine* (IM) is used to more accurately describe the complementary therapies being used in U.S. medical settings today. These therapies are used alongside conventional therapies in a therapeutic environment.

Integrative therapies is the term used in this chapter. The components of IM include (1) combining the best of both conventional and evidence-based complementary therapies, (2) emphasizing patient participation, (3) promoting the primacy of the patient–provider relationship and the importance of shared decision making, (4) emphasizing the contribution of the therapeutic encounter itself, and (5) optimizing the individual's innate healing capacity.[4a] In contrast, alternative medicine includes therapies such as the use of laetrile or amygdalin, which are proven to be toxic and ineffective.

Although many integrative therapies such as acupuncture, massage, and meditation are quite beneficial for cancer patients by helping them to cope with the disease, reducing their stress and symptoms related to conventional therapy or to the disease process itself, many interventions are unproven and could be harmful for patients who may believe that these interventions can cure them of their malignancy. An American Cancer Society study concluded that as many as 61% of cancer survivors used some form of complementary or alternative therapies.[3] Unfortunately, the majority of people do not share this information with their primary care providers. According to a survey by Eisenberg et al,[4b] patients do not think that their physician needs to know about their usage of these interventions or the physician never asked about such use. Because there are many potential drug–drug, drug–herb, drug–radiation, and antioxidant–drug interactions, it is extremely important for patients to share their use of integrative therapies and alternative treatments with their providers and similarly for physicians to ask about their patients' usage.[5]

Through the NCCAM and IM centers, more information and education has been going out not only to the public but also to physicians, alerting both groups to the importance of physicians' "asking" about the use of integrative therapies and alternative therapies and patients "telling" about the use of these therapies (http://www.nccam.nih.gov). Many hematology/oncology centers have established IM programs where complementary therapies such as acupuncture, massage, nutrition, physical activity, and stress management are offered alongside conventional therapies such as chemotherapy and radiation. These programs provide guidance to patients in choosing the safest and most effective integrative therapies to incorporate into their plans of care.

Despite the level of evidence supporting standard treatment, some patients still do not want chemotherapy, radiation, or surgery. Instead, they choose to pursue an alternative therapy. Sometimes this choice is because of cultural belief, because they believe that natural products are potentially less toxic, or because they believe that the alternative treatment will offer a "cure" for their disease. Alternative medicine practitioners and clinics exist in our country and around the world that, usually for a significant amount of out-of-pocket fees, suggest that they can offer a "cure" for individuals' hematologic malignancies. Unfortunately, these clinics rarely ever provide any evidence that they are curing disease and typically do not conduct research or report their results except in advertisements.

There is small but increasing body of research on the benefits of many integrative practices. Clinical studies provide evidence that some integrative therapies are beneficial to patients by improving their quality of life and reducing their symptoms from the disease and side effects from treatment. Research on botanicals and herbs is often aimed at efficacy and safety.

Clinical studies demonstrate concerns regarding the safe use of some botanicals in conjunction with chemotherapy and radiation therapy. Some may reduce the effectiveness of certain chemotherapies, and others may reduce metabolism of an active drug, enhancing its potential toxicity.

INTEGRATIVE THERAPY DOMAINS AND THEIR USE

The four major categories of integrative therapies include mind–body approaches, energy-based therapies, body-based manipulative therapies, and natural products (Table 158-1). There is also an abundance of whole-systems practices that include ayurvedic medicine, naturopathy, homeopathy, and traditional Chinese medicine. The whole-systems approaches incorporate many of the above integrative therapies. Mind–body approaches include meditation, mindfulness meditation, guided imagery, music therapy, creative arts therapy, self-hypnosis, yoga, tai chi, and qigong, among many other types of spiritual practices. Energy-based therapies include reiki and healing touch. Body-based manipulative therapies include chiropractic and massage therapy. Examples of natural products include dietary supplements, antioxidants, herbs, and botanicals.

In the literature, there is a paucity of information on the use of integrative therapies in the treatment of hematologic malignancies.[6] In India, there is a significant use of ayurvedic medicine. In a German study of a large group of chronic lymphocytic leukemia (CLL) patients, approximately 44% used integrative therapies with 26%

Table 158-1 Integrative Therapies Domain

• Mind–body programs	• Whole Systems
• Energy therapies	• Traditional Chinese medicine
• Body based or manipulative	• Ayurvedic
• Natural products	

using vitamin supplementation, 18% mineral supplementation, 14% homeopathy, 7% acupuncture, and 9% mistletoe therapy. In the United States, 30% to 80% of pediatric hematology/oncology patients used one or more complementary therapies in conjunction with their conventional care. In the U.S. pediatric group, there is an especially high use of vitamin and nutritional supplements,[6,7] with mind–body therapies a close second. Because many patients do not report their use of complementary therapies to their primary care hematologist/oncologist, there is markedly disparate data from one study to another. In a review by Wesa and Cassileth,[8] the major reason why leukemia patients use integrative therapies or remedies not prescribed by their hematologist/oncologist is in an effort to improve their treatment outcome and to manage their symptoms. For those with leukemia, the integrative therapies that were most beneficial included mind–body interventions such as self-hypnosis, meditation, guided imagery, and breath awareness. Massage and reflexology are also frequently used to decrease symptoms (see discussion of massage below). Acupuncture is very beneficial for symptom management with minimal side effects (see discussion of acupuncture below).

RESEARCH TECHNIQUES OF INTEGRATIVE THERAPIES

Over the past several years, there has been a gradual increase in research in the United States on integrative therapies. Supported by the National Institutes of Health (NIH) thru NCCAM and Office of Cancer Complementary and Alternative Medicine at the National Cancer Institute, investigators have often tried to apply the same research principles used to evaluate new chemotherapy programs for leukemias and lymphomas (i.e., the traditional randomized clinical trial).[9] This approach has been problematic because it is often difficult to identify the proper controls for integrative therapies such as mind–body techniques, acupuncture, and massage. As a result, meta-analyses on integrative therapies reveal an abundance of pilot studies and nonrandomized clinical studies that are criticized on the basis that any positive result may be attributable to the placebo effect.[10] In the case of acupuncture, practitioners have used sham or "fake" acupuncture as a control in which nontraditional needles are not placed in the meridian spots and not stimulated.

In randomized clinical trials of acupuncture effectiveness, comparing active acupuncture with "sham" or acupuncture, only those who are naïve to acupuncture can participate. With massage therapy, randomized clinical trials have used an educational program of equivalent attention time to attempt to control for the placebo effect. This has been similarly true for research on reiki and many of the mind–body programs.

Whole-systems research is another approach taken by integrative therapists.[10] This involves combining nutrition, physical activity, and stress and symptom management therapies together as an intervention in determining quality of life measures over a period of time. This type of research creates many variables and is totally contrary to the current widely accepted reductionist method of research.

The study of herbs and other over-the-counter (OTC) unregulated products has been fraught with confounding variables, including the standardization of the product studied.[11] For example, PC-SPES, an eight-herbal compound manufactured by a single company, was demonstrated in a pilot study in men undergoing active surveillance for prostate cancer to be associated with a decrease in their prostate-specific antigen levels. The promising trends of this phase I and later a phase II study led to a randomized clinical trial of PC-SPES. During the phases of this randomized clinical trial, there were complications that led to the reevaluation of the constituents of PC-SPES. Previous evaluations showed no evidence of any phytoestrogens in any of the eight herbal compounds, but during the randomized clinical trial, phytoestrogens were found, and patients began to demonstrate breast engorgement. Other lots did not contain phytoestrogens but were demonstrated to have contaminants such as dicoumarol, and individuals taking them were noted because of their increased bruisability. Investigators have attempted to overcome the standardization issue of herbs by studying individual proteins in in vitro models, and others have attempted to closely monitor the constituents of the herbs by protein fractionation, ensuring that the product remains constant during the research study. Most herbs and botanicals are not regulated by the U.S. Food and Drug Administration, potentiating issues of quality control, possible contamination, and stability issues. The United States Pharmacopeia (USP) does verify the identity, strength, purity, and quality of some supplements and applies its USP verification label (http://www.usp.org/uspverified).

REVIEW OF RESULTS OF INTEGRATIVE THERAPIES IN HEMATOLOGY/ONCOLOGY PATIENTS

Most studies on the use of integrative therapies in hematology/oncology disorders have been used to investigate the effect on patients' general quality of life and symptomatic relief of stress, pain, fatigue, and anxiety. The results discussed here will be reviewed in terms of improvement in symptoms and quality of life, and when appropriate, the effect on immune function and survival if investigated. In most studies, the major symptoms for which integrative therapies are used include anxiety, fatigue, pain, chemotherapy-induced nausea and vomiting (CINV), worsening immune system, stress, and depression.

Literature on Outcomes: Science, Safety, and Efficacy

In making decisions about what integrative therapies physicians should recommend, Weiger et. al[12] suggest that decisions be based on safety and efficacy. If an intervention is safe and effective such as acupuncture for CINV, it can be appropriately recommended. If a therapy is unsafe or toxic and has been demonstrated to be ineffective, it should not be recommended, and patients should be cautioned about its use. For example, laetrile (Amygdalin), which contains varying amounts of cyanide, is toxic and in studies has been shown to be ineffective in treating disease.

In addition, many interventions, products, and substances are safe, but their effectiveness is unknown. With these, the physician should be cautious and recommend their use with the following proviso. If this is a substance taken orally, it should be evaluated as to whether it has any unfavorable interactions with chemotherapy or medications that the patient is already taking or whether it interacts with a disease process such as causing hypoglycemia in a diabetic patient. Taking one new OTC substance at a time is common sense, and patients should be told to observe any change in symptoms, whether they are favorable or unfavorable, before adding another substance to their oral regimens. With respect to drug–drug and drug–herb interactions, websites are available for professionals as well as for individual patients. A list of these websites is given in Table 158-2. Most of these websites list the various terms by which a given agent is known and provide information on each agent's constituents, reasons for use, evidence for safety or toxicity, and evidence of effectiveness. Most importantly, these websites list the adverse effects of these substances and the drug–drug, drug–herb, and drug–disease interactions when known. When asked about the use of an OTC substance that is not FDA regulated, physicians should consult one of the databases to ensure safety and lack of adverse interactions (see Table 158-2).

Table 158-2 Herbs and Botanicals: Educational Websites

- Memorial Sloan-Kettering Cancer Center: http://www.mskcc.org/mskcc/html/5707.cfm?Criteria=about+herbs&x=13&y=
- The University of Texas MD Anderson Cancer Center: http://www.mdanderson.org/departments/CIMER/
- American Cancer Society: http://www.cancer.org/docroot/ETO/ETO_5.asp
- National Center for Complementary and Alternative Medicine: http://nccam.nih.gov/
- National Cancer Institute's Office of Cancer Complementary and Alternative Medicine: http://www.cancer.gov/cam/
- Natural Medicines Comprehensive Database: http://www.naturaldatabase.com
- Natural Standard: http://www.naturalstandard.com

Table 158-3 Mind–Body Therapies

- Relaxation response and biofeedback
- Mindfulness meditation
- Guided imagery
- Self-hypnosis
- Self-expression in words
- Music therapy
- Expressive arts therapy
- Dance
- Yoga
- Tai chi
- Qi gong
- Support groups

INDIVIDUAL INTEGRATIVE THERAPY MODALITIES

Mind–Body Therapies

Mind–body therapies are frequently studied interventions in patients with chronic diseases such as hematology/oncology malignancies.[13,14] Stress is part of normal physiologic body function and can be subdivided into good stress and bad stress. Chronic stress can be caused by an unexpected situation one is faced with such as experiencing a new diagnosis (e.g., leukemia), an uncomfortable interaction with a colleague, or the loss of a job. Chronic stress has been shown to decrease immune function, perhaps through the mechanism of decreasing natural killer (NK) cells and impairing the effectiveness of DNA repair. In the 1970s, Dr. Herbert Benson popularized the "relaxation response," the performance of "a time out" in normal daily functions. Benson coined this term after observing that when monks meditated, they experienced decreases in their pulse, blood pressure, and respirations. Although there are now known genetic, environmental, and dietary factors that play a significant role in causation of chronic disease, stress may be a lesser but significant factor. Frequently studied, mind–body techniques (Table 158-3) include meditation or the relaxation response, mindfulness meditation, guided imagery, and hypnosis. In addition, music therapy, physical activities such as yoga, tai chi, and chi gong also are related mind–body programs.

There are three common forms of meditation: (1) concentrative meditation, which focuses on a phrase or a visual image such as the relaxation response; (2) mindfulness meditation or awareness, in which the client becomes aware of his or her thoughts and feelings and focuses on those issues; and (3) expressive meditation used in tribal societies consisting of fast deep breathing, shaking, whirling, and dancing.[13]

Mind–body interventions are often self-taught or presented by a professional. Double-blinded trials are difficult to conduct partly because the presence of an empathetic professional giving the therapeutic modality may be considered a placebo effect. Mind–body interventions are often accompanied by other integrative therapy interventions, making pure studies unevaluable; however, randomized clinical trials have demonstrated that relaxation training and guided imagery significantly reduce nausea and anxiety.[14a]

Compared with medication, relaxation therapy showed similar decreases in anxiety and depression, although medication might have been slightly faster in its effect. Other randomized trials have shown decreases in tension, depression, anger, and fatigue during relaxation training or imagery. In children, hypnosis has been found to be especially effective. In a randomized clinical trial comparing hypnosis or nonhypnotic distraction such as the relaxation techniques versus joining a placebo attention control group, the children in the hypnosis group reported significant reduction in anticipatory and CINV.

Mind–body therapies have also been used to alleviate pain. In a study of children undergoing bone marrow or lumbar puncture procedures, hypnosis significantly reduced the pain as well as anxiety. In a randomized clinical trial examining the effects of the relaxation response therapy (RRT) versus reiki therapy in men being treated with external-beam radiotherapy for prostate cancer, RRT improved emotional well-being and eased anxiety, and reiki therapy had a positive effect on anxiety. Expressive arts therapy and music therapy as well as repetitive exercise, yoga, tai chi, qigong, and Pilates also can reduce stress and anxiety.

Music therapy is considered a mind–body therapy that reduces stress and anxiety because it uses a variety of active and passive music experiences, live or recorded. This technique can be used either independently or with a music therapist. Randomized trials have shown statistically significant improvements in mood and physical discomfort. In patients with hematologic malignancies admitted for autologous stem cell transplantations, patients receiving an individualized program of live music therapy had a significant improvement in mood. Music therapy has also been shown to be an effective adjunct to antiemetic therapy. Studies of immune function have yet to show any statistically significant improvement in immune function.

Yoga and physical activity have been studied to determine whether there is a related reduction in symptoms of depression and anxiety. In a 12-week yoga intervention in healthy subjects, it was demonstrated that there was greater improvement in mood and anxiety than a metabolically matched walking exercise. The authors demonstrated an acute increase in thalamic GABA (γ-aminobutyric acid) levels alongside the improvement in mood and anxiety scales. White et al[14b] demonstrated the potential benefits of physical activity for children with acute lymphocytic leukemia.

Mind–body therapies can reduce anxiety, temper the adverse effects of chemotherapy and radiation treatments, relieve pain, and possibly stimulate immune responses. By reducing stress and anxiety, these therapies can help patients deal with a wide range of relationship issues and decision making as they move through the diagnostic and therapeutic phases of their malignancy. Mind–body approaches have very minimal risk and potentially significant benefits. Most importantly, they are often self-taught and therefore low cost. Anderson and Taylor[14c] reviewed three clinical trials addressing the use of mind–body therapies for management of the metabolic syndrome as defined by an increased risk of type II diabetes, cardiovascular disease, and other chronic conditions. Findings in these studies support the potential clinical effectiveness of mind–body practices in improving indices of the metabolic system. Mind–body practices should be considered as an adjunct to usual care regardless of whether patients are beginning or recovering from chemotherapy.

Acupuncture

Overview and Definitions

One of the major components of traditional Chinese medicine has been the use of acupuncture. For more than 2.5 millennia, this traditional practice has been used in the Far East to "correct an imbalance in yin-yang and qi [energy].” It is believed that with acupuncture, “blocked” channels can be unblocked, reducing symptoms. Acupuncture is the stimulation of certain points on the body by a needle or alternatively by pressure called acupressure. Both techniques take advantage of the meridians described by traditional Chinese medicine. Acupuncture points are situated along meridians, which are channels for “qi.” Sham or “fake” acupuncture implies the use of needles that are not inserted to the same depth, not put in the meridian points, and not given stimulation. Electroacupuncture implies the use of added electrical pulses to create additional or accentuated stimulation. Several studies have shown that electroacupuncture provides greater symptom relief than regular acupuncture.

Research on Usage and Effectiveness

Most acupuncture in the Western world is used to manage symptoms, not treat disease.[15] Research studies have demonstrated release of neurotransmitters and change of brain functional magnetic resonance imaging signals during acupuncture. Acupuncture was confirmed as an effective intervention for CINV at an NIH consensus conference in 1997. Whether this beneficial effect is attributable to an induced relaxation response or a direct antiemetic effect is not known.

Randomized clinical trials on acupuncture have been used in a variety of settings. As mentioned earlier, only individuals who are naïve to acupuncture can take part in acupuncture studies because they will note the difference between active acupuncture and its sham component. Acupuncture has been shown to be effective in randomized clinical trials in cancer-related fatigue, cancer-related pain, and postoperative pain as well as reduced CINV.

Several randomized clinical trials conducted in China have suggested that acupuncture could be effective in reducing the marrow suppression in patients on aggressive chemotherapy. Analysis of these trials performed by Lu et al[16] suggest that acupuncture is associated with an increase in neutrophils and total white blood cell count in patients during chemotherapy or chemoradiation therapy. The weighted mean difference of over 1000/μL white blood cells on average is a statistically significant difference. Lu et al[17] carried out a small, randomized, sham-controlled clinical trial in the United States exploring this issue in ovarian and breast cancer patients receiving aggressive chemotherapy. In a pilot randomized, sham-controlled trial using manual and electrostimulation two to three times per week for a total of 10 sessions beginning 1 week before the second cycle of chemotherapy, the media leukocyte count in the active acupuncture arm at the first day of the next cycle was significantly higher than in the sham arm. The median leukocyte nadir, neutrophil nadir, and recovering absolute neutrophil counts were all higher but not statistically different. The result showed improved neutrophil count both at the nadir and rebound points during chemotherapy, but the study was not statistically significant and was underpowered.

Uncontrolled pilot studies of acupuncture have shown effectiveness in reducing anxiety and improving mood and other quality of life measures in patients with both oncologic and hematologic disorders. These studies have also shown improvement in sleeplessness, depression, and xerostomia. Acupuncture enhanced xerostomia inventory scores in 18 patients who received radiation therapy and had pilocarpine-resistant xerostomia. However, a randomized clinical trial failed to show any significant difference between active acupuncture and sham acupuncture in xerostomia. In patients with hot flashes and vasomotor symptoms caused by chemotherapy, acupuncture attenuated some of the hot flashes. In a controlled study comparing venlafaxine and acupuncture, no statistical difference was found between the favorable response to acupuncture and the medication.

Safety

With the increasing use of acupuncture in the United States because of evidence of its effectiveness, there are concerns about its safety when used in the community, especially with hematology patients and those getting chemotherapy and radiotherapy. However, reports of major side effects of acupuncture are rare and usually are evident when performed by untrained practitioners. In closely monitored clinical trials, there is a low incidence of adverse events. In one study, the rate of minor adverse events was 14 per 10,000 sessions; serious events were 0.05 per 10,000 treatments and 0.55 per 10,000 individual patients. Common adverse events include bloodborne infections and internal organ and tissue injury. Generally, acupuncture should be avoided in patients with severe neutropenia and thrombocytopenia (absolute neutrophil count <500/μL and platelets <25,000/μL). However, in one study of acupuncture given during stem cell transplantation, there were no bleeding side effects in individuals with severe thrombocytopenia (platelet counts <20,000/μL). Currently in the United States, there are several schools of traditional Chinese medicine emphasizing the practice of acupuncture. These are 3- to 4-year certificate programs well versed not only in understanding effectiveness but also safety.

Massage and Touch Therapies

Overview and Definitions

Massage has been defined by some as “rhythmic and methodical stretching and compressing of the muscles and connective tissue through the touch of the therapist's hands.” There are many types of massage and hands-on soft tissue therapies (Table 158-4). Therapies include Swedish massage, aromatherapy massage, reflexology, acupressure, and manual lymphatic drainage massage. Swedish massage provides broad, flowing, soothing strokes (effleurage) generally applied with a lotion or massage oil from distal to proximal areas on extremities. In addition, there is usually gentle kneading of soft tissues (petrissage). Aromatherapy has often been combined with massage in which selected scented oils are blended with the usual massage oil to enhance the beneficial effects of both physical and emotional well-being. Reflexology focuses on manual pressure to specific areas of the feet that, in traditional Chinese medicine, are linked with remote areas of the body. Acupressure massage uses the meridian theory of traditional Chinese medicine in which focal pressure is applied to acupuncture needle sites with the goal of adjusting the flow of energy similar to the theory in acupuncture. Manual lymphatic drainage is the application of light, flowing strokes of massage in specific patterns with the goal of alleviating lymph edema after lymph node resection or radiation therapy.

Research on Usage and Effectiveness

Corbin[18a] has reviewed the value of massage as well as the difficulties in performing scientific research. Many randomized clinical trials use a cross-over arm and attempt interventions that try to control for the placebo effect. The various measurement tools used to assess outcomes involve numerical rating scales, visual analog scales, profile of mood status, the S state trait anxiety inventory, the European Organization for Research and Treatment of Cancer quality of life

Table 158-4 Massage or Body Manipulation

- Swedish massage
- Aromatherapy massage
- Reflexology
- Acupressure
- Shiatsu
- Manual lymphatic drainage
- Reiki
- Deep tissue massage
- Rolfing

questionnaire, and so on. In a critical review of potential benefits of massage, Joske et al[18b] identified eight randomized controlled clinical studies in hematology/oncology patients totaling more than 357 patients. Specifically, there was evidence of anxiety reduction with less benefit for analgesia. In autologous bone marrow transplantation patients, the massage group had significantly decreased distress and nausea scores early on in the trial, but these were not long standing. Massage therapy has been found to reduce state anxiety in many meta-analyses, probably its most beneficial attribute. Pain may be alleviated, but this has not been demonstrated to be statistically significant. Numerous studies have shown trends not only in decreased anxiety but also in nausea, pain, fatigue, and depression.

To date, there is little evidence suggesting that massage therapies have any effect on immune function or survival outcomes in hematology/oncology patients. A small randomized study did find higher NK cells and lymphocyte cells in a massage. Similarly, in a study in HIV patients, there was a significant increase in NK cell fighter toxicity during the massage period. In some trials, there is a short-term effect on NK cell activity; however, long-term clinical effect has not been demonstrated. A significant effect of effleurage massage on cellular immunity, cortisol, oxytocin, anxiety, depression, or quality of life also has not been demonstrated in more rigorous randomized clinical trials. In another randomized clinical study, dopamine levels, NK cells, and lymphocytes increased from the first to last day of the massage therapy. In a study of children with HIV, a control arm had a greater relative risk of CD4 count decline than the massage therapy children. Lymphocyte loss was also more extensive in the control participants, and more of the control group than the massage group lost greater than 50/mm^3 CD8 lymphocytes. The immediate effects of massage therapy are decreased anxiety, depressed mood, and anger. The long-term effects of massage include reduced depression and hostility as well as increased urine meridopamine, serotonin values and NK cell number, and lymphocytes. However, it is not clear that these results were statistically significant.

Weaknesses exist in many of the massage therapy studies reported to date such as small sample sizes and lack of controls. Most of the practitioners have not been blinded to the hypothesis of the studies. Furthermore, no systematic approach has been identified to determine the optimal number of massage treatments in a trial and within-group comparisons. Strong evidence shows that massage therapy can be very helpful in alleviating anxiety and stress in patients. However, more rigorous study designs, adequate statistical power, better identification of predictors for response to massage, and study of the psychologic and biologic mechanisms are needed. There is also a need for larger sample sizes and rigorous design reporting on massage therapy.

Safety

The concern that massage therapy can spread a tumor is unfounded. However, direct pressure over known tumor sites is usually discouraged. In general, massage therapy of all types is quite safe.

Nutrition and Supplements

Nutrition

Nutritional guidelines for patients with hematologic malignancies should be based on the recommendations of the American Cancer Society and the American Institute for Cancer Research (AICR)/World Cancer Research Fund.[19] The AICR clearly states that cancer survivors should follow its nine nutrition and physical activity guidelines for risk reduction. The first recommendation is to be as lean as possible without being underweight. Although hematologic malignancies are not among those listed as being most associated with obesity (breast, esophagus, pancreas, gallbladder, colorectal, endometrial, and kidney), a review suggests that being overweight or obese probably does increase the risk of non-Hodgkin lymphoma (NHL), diffuse large B-cell lymphoma, follicular lymphoma, and CLL, although results are inconsistent among studies. In general, because obesity is related to increased inflammation and decreased immune function, it is best for patients with hematologic malignancies to aim to maintain a body mass index of less than 25.

The second AICR recommendation is to be physically active for 30 minutes every day. Although few studies have evaluated physical activity and hematologic malignancies, data suggest that low physical activity may increase the risk of NHL and increasing activity may reduce the risk, especially for follicular and small lymphocytic lymphoma.

The third recommendation is to avoid sugary drinks and limit consumption of energy-dense foods. This is obviously linked with the body weight guideline because sugary drinks contribute many empty calories to the standard American diet. In addition, the contribution of insulin and insulin-like growth factor type 1 to the development of malignant disease is being increasingly appreciated in a number of cancers, leading to the investigation of blockade of the insulin-like growth factor 1 receptor as a novel treatment for some malignant diagnoses.

Fourth, the AICR suggests that people eat a greater variety of fruits, vegetables, whole grains, and legumes such as beans. Data from the U.S. Centers for Disease Control and Prevention demonstrate that the American public falls far short on the conservative recommendation to consume at least five servings of fruits and vegetables daily with only 14% of adults meeting the guideline. Plants are rich sources of fiber, antioxidants, and phytonutrients, many of which are believed to be useful in cancer risk reduction. In one study, dietary fiber intake was associated with a lower risk of all NHL subtypes. Another analysis found that high consumption of fruits and vegetables was associated with a lower risk of all NHL subtypes, particularly follicular lymphoma, in women but not men.[20]

Fifth, the AICR recommends limiting consumption of red meats (beef, pork, and lamb) and avoiding processed meats. Epidemiologic studies suggest that consumption of fried red meats as well as dairy products leads to an increased risk of NHL.[20] Conversely, consumption of higher levels of omega-3 or marine fatty acids has been shown to be inversely correlated with lymphoma risk. Additional studies suggest that a diet high in fish may also be protective against the development of other hematopoietic malignancies—leukemias and multiple myeloma as well as NHL—in an Australian cohort.[21]

Sixth, the AICR guidelines state that if consumed at all, alcoholic drinks should be limited to two for men and one for women per day.

Although moderate alcohol consumption may be associated with cardiovascular benefits, alcohol use has been associated with an increased risk of a number of malignancies. A pooled analysis of nine case-control studies of NHL revealed that ever drinkers, compared with never drinkers, had a 17% lower risk of NHL, a finding the investigators attributed to a possible beneficial effect of moderate alcohol consumption on immune function. A cohort study in 126,293 multiethnic adults used lifelong abstainers and infrequent drinkers as the referent and reported a relative risk of 0.5 for the development of both lymphocytic and myeloid leukemias in those consuming three or more drinks daily without any contribution of choice of beverage (wine, beer, or liquor). With regards to patients already diagnosed, a cohort of 575 female NHL cases in Connecticut was followed for a median of 7.75 years. Compared with never drinkers, wine drinkers experienced better overall survival (75% vs. 69% five-year survival; $P = .030$) and disease-free survival (70% vs. 67%; $P = .049$). The favorable effect for wine drinkers was seen mainly in patients with diffuse large B-cell lymphoma. Resveratrol, a red wine polyphenol known for its potential cardioprotective effects, is also believed to have potential in cancer risk reduction and perhaps even as an adjunct to conventional therapy. An in vitro study involving acute lymphoblastic leukemia (ALL) cell lines demonstrated that red wine polyphenols caused growth inhibition and apoptosis. Although these cell line experiments often produce elegant results regarding mechanism of observed in vitro action, whether the phytonutrients have the same benefits in humans consuming the whole foodstuffs or concentrated supplements remains uncertain.

Supplements

Most conventional medical and radiation oncologists recommend that their cancer patients avoid all supplements, especially during active radiation and chemotherapy. This recommendation is primarily based on the absence of convincing data supporting therapeutic benefit. Three other valid concerns about supplement use are (1) the potential for supplement–drug interactions via a pharmacokinetic or pharmacodynamics pathway; (2) the oxidant–anti-oxidant issue; and (3) the impact of supplements on clotting, a particular problem for patients with hematologic malignancies on or off anticoagulants.

Concurrent use of a supplement, particularly a botanical, with chemotherapy could lead to a clinically important interaction that could yield an increase or decrease in the effects of either component. Considering that 35% of currently prescribed oncology drugs are metabolized by the CYP3A4 isoform of the hepatic cytochrome p450 enzyme system, use of supplements that either induce or inhibit the pathway can be problematic.[22] In treatment of hematologic toxicities, cyclophosphamide, the epipodophyllotixins, and the vinca alkaloids are all dependent of CYP3A4 for their metabolism. For example, the botanical supplement St. John's wort used for the treatment of mild depression is a strong inducer of many CYP isoforms. In a classic pharmacokinetic interaction study, 10 healthy volunteers were administered a single 400-mg oral dose of imatinib before and after 2 weeks of treatment with 300 mg of St. John's wort three times daily. The investigators found that the pharmacokinetics of imatinib were significantly altered by St. John's wort, with reductions of 32% in the median area under the concentration-time curve ($P = .0001$), 29% in maximum observed concentration ($P = .005$), and 21% in half-life ($P = .0001$). The conclusion was that coadministration of St. John's wort might compromise the clinical efficacy of imatinib. It is generally recommended that cancer patients receiving any intervention avoid taking St. John's wort.

Patients with hematologic malignancies are often at increased risk for bleeding problems. There has been a long-standing tendency to attribute thrombocytopenias of unclear etiology in cancer patients to botanical supplements that they are taking, particularly traditional Chinese medicine herbs. Warfarin is a frequently prescribed anticoagulant, itself derived from a botanical, which can be impacted in a number of ways by diet and dietary supplements. Inappropriate control of anticoagulation because of fluctuation in warfarin effect exposes the patient to risks of increased bleeding or thromboembolic complications. Warfarin is metabolized by the cytochrome p450 system isoforms, including CYP3A4. In addition, it is also highly protein bound and hence can interact with medications or supplements that are also highly protein bound, resulting in displacement and causing increases in international normalized (INR) ratio and necessitating warfarin dose reduction. Finally, the anticoagulant effect of warfarin can be antagonized by vitamin K intake. Patients prescribed warfarin are often advised not to eat green leafy and cruciferous vegetables or to consume green tea because they are rich in vitamin K and might interfere with the anticoagulant effect. An alternative is to allow the patient to consume a healthful diet and adjust the warfarin dose accordingly to maintain the desired INR.

Omega-3 Fatty Acids

Omega-3 fatty acids have been reported in isolated cases to potentiate the anticoagulant effects of warfarin. Omega-3 fatty acids may lower thromboxane A(2) levels within the platelet as well as decrease factor VII levels. These factors, which make the omega-3s attractive as anti-inflammatory and cardiovascular agents, need to be borne in mind in patients on warfarin therapy. Taken in the absence of warfarin, omega-3s are not believed to be a significant cause of bleeding at doses of less than 4000 mg/day. Epidemiologic data suggest an inverse relationship between the intake of marine omega-3 fatty acids and the development of a number of hematologic malignancies and the good risk-to-benefit profile.

Vitamin D3

Vitamin D is one of the few remaining vitamins that has not been shown to be ineffective in protecting against malignant disease. An ongoing randomized clinical trial is currently looking at a two-by-two factorial design of omega-3 fatty acids and vitamin D3 supplementation in older adults to assess cancer risk reduction, among other endpoints. At the same time, increasing evidence suggests that vitamin D deficiency may be related to the risk of a number of solid tumors, particularly breast, colon, prostate, and pancreas. An inverse relationship has been described between the development of NHL and sun exposure, particularly recreational, non-occupational sun exposure. One proposed explanation for this unexpected finding is that sun exposure is actually a surrogate marker of vitamin D status, and it is actually vitamin D sufficiency that is protective against lymphoma.[23] In a meta-analysis of eight studies to date, the investigators found no conclusive evidence that vitamin D was providing the observed benefit, although serum levels were not available in any of the studies. Hence, it may be appropriate in view of the widespread incidence of vitamin D insufficiency, especially in older adults, for integrative oncologists to measure 25-hydroxy-vitamin D levels in patients with hematologic malignancies and supplement with a fat-soluble vitamin D3 preparation to bring the levels into sufficient or optimal range.

Green Tea

Green tea *(Camellia sinensis)* is an increasingly consumed beverage being sought after for multiple potential beneficial health effects. An inhibitor of CYP3A4 metabolism as well as a potent source of vitamin K, green tea may interact with prescribed anticancer drugs or anticoagulant therapies. However, green tea polyphenols have been shown to have antiproliferative activity against a wide variety of cell lines, including CLL,[24] multiple myeloma, and human promyelocytic leukemia HL-60. Epigallocathechin-3-gallate (EGCG) is the specific green tea polyphenol that is an antioxidant with chemopreventive and chemotherapeutic actions. Present in situ in the beverage, EGCG has also been prepared as green tea extract (GTE) supplements and even more concentrated EGCG capsules that patients can purchase in health food and supplement emporiums. The publication of the CLL data has led to increased use of EGCG in patients with low-grade lymphomas. A phase I study in patients with asymptomatic stage 0 to II CLL demonstrated that the Polyphenon E preparation use was well tolerated in 33 participants and that the majority of participants had decreased total lymphocyte counts, lymphadenopathy, or both. Of note, when taken on an empty stomach, GTE preparations have been associated with a risk of hepatotoxicity. The question of whether health benefits against hematologic malignancies can be achieved by simply drinking an as yet undetermined quantity of the beverage or higher dose preparations such as GTE or EGCG is not known.

Patients with multiple myeloma are now frequently advised by their oncologists not to consume green tea at all because of its potential to negate the treatment effects of bortezomib, found in mouse studies.

Other commonly used OTC products include turmeric, melatonin, medicinal mushrooms, and Chinese herbs. Studies are being conducted regarding their efficacy and safety.

Antioxidants

Antioxidants (e.g., beta-carotene; lycopene; vitamins C, E, and A) are substances that counteract free radicals and prevent them from causing tissue and organ damage. They are among the most common classes of supplements used by patients with hematologic malignancies. Their use is directed for cytotoxic effects, for synergy with conventional therapy, or to lessen the toxicity of conventional therapy. Estimates of antioxidant use by patients with cancer have varied considerably, with rates ranging from 13% to 87% depending on the survey, the type of disease studied, and a variety of other individual and demographic factors.[25] Specific prevalence data on the use of antioxidants among patients with only hematologic malignancies has generally not been reported in the surveys.

Evidence supporting the potential role of antioxidants in preventing and treating disease include preclinical studies. These studies have correlated oxidative stress and an antioxidant-depleted diet with the development of diseases, including cancer. Increased consumption of green tea (which contains the anticarcinogenic agent, EGCG) has been associated with a reduced incidence of leukemia. In addition, decreases in antioxidant enzymes or the micronutrients, thiol, vitamin E, vitamin C, beta-carotene, or zinc and increases in the production of reactive oxygen species have been reported in leukemia patients. In one study in children with ALL, higher levels of oxidative stress at diagnosis were associated with a poor prognosis.

In another prospective observational study conducted among children with ALL, low plasma[26] and dietary antioxidant[27] levels directly correlated with treatment-related toxicity. These types of data have led many patients with hematologic malignancies to take antioxidant supplements primarily in conjunction with conventional cancer treatment.

Much of the controversy surrounding antioxidants and cancer therapy has arisen because radiation therapy and certain classes of chemotherapy agents exert some of their anticancer effects through the generation of reactive oxygen species or free radicals. Some of these agents include the anthracyclines (e.g., doxorubicin), platinum-containing complexes (e.g., cisplatin and carboplatin), and alkylating agents (e.g., cyclophosphamide and ifosfamide). The theoretical concern is that antioxidants might somehow interfere with or counteract the activities of these anticancer agents. However, to date, preclinical experiments and clinical studies have not definitively shown impact on treatment outcome.[28] Of particular note, an observational cohort study from the Fred Hutchinson Cancer Research Center in Seattle evaluating the prevalence of supplement use in persons before receiving hematopoietic stem cell transplant and the association of select supplements with outcomes found that pretransplant intake of vitamin C (≥500 mg/day) or vitamin E (≥400 IU/day) was associated with increased risk of relapse or mortality.[29]

Recent studies have shown interactions of antioxidant supplements with the proteasome inhibitor bortezomib. Vitamin C, at orally achievable concentrations (equivalent to 1 g/day, a dose frequently used by patients), inhibited the in vitro multiple myeloma cell cytotoxicity of bortezomib and blocked its inhibitory effect on 20S proteasome activity. In addition, green tee polyphenols and dietary supplements carrying hydroxyl groups, including flavonoid compounds such as quercetin, bind and inhibit the activity of bortezomib on malignant B cells and multiple myeloma cells in vitro, although by mechanisms independent of their antioxidant activity. Taken together, these studies suggest that antioxidant supplements should be avoided in patients taking bortezomib and other boronic acid proteasome inhibitor therapy.

The precise role of antioxidant supplementation in the patients with hematologic malignancies remains to be determined. Studies adequately evaluating the impact of supplementation on toxicity and disease free survival have not yet adequately demonstrated that the benefits of supplementation clearly outweigh the risks; therefore, the possibility of harm must be strongly considered. Recommendations for clinical practice at the present time include the following:

- Patients should be advised to avoid dietary antioxidant supplements above the basic nutritional requirements during radiation therapy and stem cell transplantation.
- Patients should avoid dietary antioxidant supplements while receiving bortezomib and other boronic acid proteasome inhibitor therapy. Counseling patients to avoid supplementation while receiving chemotherapy associated with high oxidative stress (anthracyclines, alkylating agents, platinum-containing agents, topoisomerase I and II inhibitors) is encouraged.
- Use of antioxidant supplements while receiving chemotherapy associated with low oxidative stress (purine or pyrimidine analogues, antimetabolites, monoclonal antibodies, vinca alkaloids, taxanes, and corticosteroids) is less likely to be associated with interactions. Caution should be taken with other agents (e.g., anti-angiogenic agents, tyrosine kinase inhibitors) for which there is insufficient information.

Recommendations for Patients

"All patients with hematological problems should be asked specifically about their use of complementary and alternative therapies."

"All patients with hematological problems should receive guidance about the advantages and limitations of complementary therapies in an open, evidence based, and patient-centered manner by a qualified professional."

Adapted from Deng GE, Cassileth BR, Cohen L, et al: Integrative Oncology Practice Guidelines. *J Soc Integr Oncol* 5:65, 2007.

REFERENCES

1. Schultz AM, Chao SM, McGinnis JM: *Integrative Medicine and the Health of the Public: A Summary of the February 2009 Summit,* Washington, DC, National Academies Press 2009, Institute of Medicine.
2. McGuire S: *Complementary and Alternative Medicine in the United States,* Washington, DC, 2005, National Academies Press: Institute of Medicine.
3. Gansler T, Kaw C, Crammer C, et al: A population-based study of prevalence of complementary methods use by cancer survivors: A report from the American Cancer Society's studies of cancer survivors. *Cancer* 113:1048, 2008.

4a. Snyderman R, Weil AT: Integrative medicine: Bringing medicine back to its roots. *Arch Intern Med* 162:395, 2002.

4b. Eisenberg DM, Kessler RC, Van Rompay M, et al: Perceptions about complementary therapies relative to conventional therapies among adults who use both; results from a national survey. *Ann Intern Med* 135:344, 2001.

5. Sparreboom A: Herbal remedies in the United States: Potential interactions with anticancer agents. *J Clin Oncol* 22:2489, 2004.
6. Kelly KM: Bringing evidence to complementary and alternative medicine in children with cancer: Focus on nutrition-related therapies. *Pediatr Blood Cancer* 50:490; discussion 8, 2008.
7. Sencer SF, Kelly KM: Bringing evidence to complementary and alternative medicine for children with cancer. *J Pediatr Hematol Oncol* 28:186, 2006.
8. Wesa KM, Cassileth BR: Is there a role for complementary therapy in the management of leukemia? *Expert Rev Anticancer Ther* 9:1241, 2009.
9. Barton DL, Loprinzi C, Jatoi A, et al: Can complementary and alternative medicine clinical cancer research be successfully accomplished? The Mayo Clinic-North Central Cancer Treatment Group experience. *J Soc Integr Oncol* 4:143, 2006.
10. Verhoef MJ, Leis A: From studying patient treatment to studying patient care: Arriving at methodologic crossroads. *Hematol Oncol Clin North Am* 22:671, viii–ix, 2008.
11. Yeung KS, Gubili J, Cassileth B: Evidence-based botanical research: Applications and challenges. *Hematol Oncol Clin North Am* 22:661, viii, 2008.
12. Weiger W, Smith M, Boon H, et al: Advising patients who seek complementary and alternative medical therapies for cancer. *Ann Int Med* 137:889, 2002.
13. Gordon JS: Mind-body medicine and cancer. *Hematol Oncol Clin North Am* 22:683, ix, 2008.

14a. Rossman M, Shrock D: Mind-body medicine in integrative cancer care. In Abrams D, Weil A, editors: *Integrative Oncology,* New York, 2009, Oxford University Press, p 244.

14b. White J, Flohr JA, Winter SS, et al: Potential benefits of physical activity for children with acute lymphoblastic leukemia. *Pediatric Rehabilitation* 8:53, 2005.

14c. Anderson JG, Taylor AG: The metabolic syndrome andnmind-body therapies: Unsystematic review. *J Nutr Metab* 2011:276419, 2011.

15. Lu W, Dean-Clower E, Doherty-Gilman A, et al: The value of acupuncture in cancer care. *Hematol Oncol Clin North Am* 22:631, viii, 2008.

16. Lu W, Hu D, Dean-Clower E, et al: Acupuncture for chemotherapy-induced leukopenia: Exploratory meta-analysis of randomized controlled trials. *J Soc Integr Oncol* 5:1, 2007.

17. Lu W, Matulonis UA, Doherty-Gilman A, et al: Acupuncture for chemotherapy-induced neutropenia in patients with gynecologic malignancies: A pilot randomized, sham-controlled clinical trial. *J Altern Complement Med* 15:745, 2009.

18a. Corbin L: Massage Therapy. In DI A, Weil A, editors: *Integrative Oncology*, New York, 2009, Oxford University Press.

18b. Joske DJL, Rao A, Kristjanson L: Critical review of complementary therapies in haemato-oncology. *Int Med J* 36:579, 2006.

19. Kushi LH, Byers T, Doyle C, et al: American Cancer Society Guidelines on Nutrition and Physical Activity for cancer prevention: Reducing the risk of cancer with healthy food choices and physical activity. *CA Cancer J Clin* 56:254; quiz 313-314, 2006.

20. Chang ET, Smedby KE, Zhang SM, et al: Dietary factors and risk of non-Hodgkin lymphoma in men and women. *Cancer Epidemiol Biomarkers Prev* 14:512, 2005.

21. Fritschi L, Ambrosini GL, Kliewer EV, et al: Dietary fish intake and risk of leukaemia, multiple myeloma, and non-Hodgkin lymphoma. *Cancer Epidemiol Biomarkers Prev* 13:532, 2004.

22. Sparreboom A, Baker S, editors: *CAM: Chemo Interactions: What Is Known*, New York, 2009, Integrative Oncology, Oxford University Press.

23. Kelly JL, Friedberg JW, Calvi LM, et al: Vitamin D and non-Hodgkin lymphoma risk in adults: A review. *Cancer Invest* 27:942, 2009.

24. Lee YK, Bone ND, Strege AK, et al: VEGF receptor phosphorylation status and apoptosis is modulated by a green tea component, epigallocatechin-3-gallate (EGCG), in B-cell chronic lymphocytic leukemia. *Blood* 104:788, 2004.

25. Ladas E, Kelly KM: The antioxidant debate. *Explore (NY)* 6:75, 2010.

26. Kennedy DD, Ladas EJ, Rheingold SR, et al: Antioxidant status decreases in children with acute lymphoblastic leukemia during the first six months of chemotherapy treatment. *Pediatr Blood Cancer* 44:378, 2005.

27. Kennedy D, Tucker KL, Ladas E, et al: Low antioxidant vitamin intakes are associated with increases in adverse effects of chemotherapy in children with acute lymphoblastic leukemia. *Am J Clin Nutr* 79:1029, 2004.

28. Lawenda BD, Kelly KM, Ladas EJ, et al: Should supplemental antioxidant administration be avoided during chemotherapy and radiation therapy? *J Natl Cancer Inst* 100:773, 2008.

29. Bruemmer B, Patterson RE, Cheney C, et al: The association between vitamin C and vitamin E supplement use before hematopoietic stem cell transplant and outcomes to two years. *J Am Diet Assoc* 103:982, 2003.

CHAPTER 159

HEMATOLOGIC MANIFESTATIONS OF HIV/AIDS

Howard A. Liebman and Anil Tulpule

Human immunodeficiency virus type 1 (HIV-1) is the pathogenic infectious agent responsible for the development of acquired immunodeficiency syndrome (AIDS). Chronic HIV infection leads to progressive immunodeficiency and immune dysregulation, resulting in an increased risk for opportunistic infections, increased incidence of certain malignancies, autoimmune disorders, and varied organ system dysfunction. Although nearly every organ system can be affected by HIV infection, hematologic manifestations involving the bone marrow and peripheral blood occur in all patients in the course of the disease. This chapter will provide a general overview of the epidemiology of AIDS, HIV virology and immunopathogenesis, and a more comprehensive review of the hematologic manifestations of HIV infection.

DEFINITION AND EPIDEMIOLOGY OF HIV INFECTION

Although the original definition of AIDS was based upon clinical symptoms and signs alone, knowledge of the viral pathogenesis has lead to a series of revised case definitions by the U.S. Public Health Service and Centers for Disease Control and Prevention (CDC). The present case definition for HIV-1 infection divides the disease into three stages as defined by $CD4^+$ lymphocyte counts and the presence of AIDS-defining conditions (Tables 159-1 and 159-2). A diagnosis of AIDS can be made by recognition of well-characterized clinical symptoms and signs (see Table 159-2) with evidence of HIV infection (clinical AIDS). HIV infection in an individual with a blood CD4 lymphocyte count of less than 0.2×10^9/L classifies the patient as having "immunologic AIDS." With the advent of routine testing for HIV infection in developed countries, a significant proportion of individuals with HIV infection who are receiving highly active antiretroviral therapy (HAART) have little or no clinical manifestations of viral infections and can maintain near-normal immunologic function. However, many of the same individuals suffer from HAART-related toxicities. The World Health Organization (WHO) originally used an alternate case definition because of the limited availability for serologic, virologic, and immunologic testing of patients in resource-poor countries but after 2007 required serologic confirmation of HIV-1 infection. Therefore the early estimates of HIV-related disease worldwide were limited by this more clinically based definition.

The CDC estimates the 2008 prevalence of HIV infection in the United States at 1,178,350 Americans with a 2009 incidence of 48,000 new infections. WHO has estimated that there were 2.7 million new HIV infections in 2009 with an estimated prevalence worldwide of 38 to 45 million people infected by HIV. However, WHO estimates a 16% decline in new infections worldwide since the year 2000; with a stable rate of new infections in Africa and Asia, but an increased incidence of new infections in Eastern Europe and central Asia. Vertical transmission from mother to infant continues in Africa and areas in Asia because of a lack of antiviral medications.

A second, but molecularly distinct HIV, human immunodeficiency virus type 2 (HIV-2), is endemic to regions of West Africa. HIV-2 and the simian immunodeficiency virus of sooty mangabeys are essentially identical, confirming its simian origin that subsequently crossed over into man. Less is known about the epidemiology of HIV-2, but infection appears to result in a less virulent clinical course than HIV-1 infection. Despite being structurally closely related to HIV-1, infection with HIV-2 does not provide protection against HIV-1 infection, and coinfection is frequent in sex workers in West Africa.

TRANSMISSION OF HIV-1

HIV may be transmitted by sexual contact with an infected individual, use of a contaminated needle in parenteral drug use, exposure to infected blood products, or prenatal transmission from infected mother to her infant.

HIV-1 has been recovered both from semen of HIV-infected men and from cervical and vaginal secretions of HIV-infected women. Virus can be detected in seminal fluid during the first 4 weeks of infection. Several factors are associated with increased viral content of seminal fluid, including advanced symptomatic HIV infection, higher plasma viral loads, CD4 lymphocyte counts less than 0.2×10^9/L, and the presence of leukocytes in the seminal fluid. Factors that influence the levels of HIV-1 in female vaginal secretions include advanced HIV stage of HIV infection, menstruation, concomitant vaginal infection, ulcerative and nonulcerative sexually transmitted diseases and a high HIV-1 viral plasma load. Prevention and treatment of sexually transmitted disease has been associated with a decrease in HIV-1 transmission.

The risk for HIV infection with transfusion of a single unit of infected blood is estimated at greater than 90%. The use of coagulation factor concentrate prepared before routine screening of blood products for HIV-1 in the United States resulted in an unfortunately high incidence of HIV infection in patients with congenital bleeding disorders. With active blood product screening and inactivation protocols used in the preparation of coagulation factor concentrate, HIV transmission has been essentially eliminated. With screening of all blood units in the United States, receipt of a unit of screened blood is associated with an estimated risk for transmission of approximately 1 in 500,000.

HIV may be transmitted to a fetus or infants from the mother in utero, at the time of delivery, or postpartum through breastfeeding. The risk is greatest when the mother has advanced HIV disease, higher HIV viral load in the plasma, and active injection drug use. At the time of delivery, active chorioamnionitis, premature rupture of amniotic membranes (>4 hours), and vaginal delivery, as opposed to elective cesarean section, have been associated with an increased risk for maternal-infant transmission. Prematurity, low gestational age, and breastfeeding have been reported as risk factors for HIV transmission. The use of antiretroviral agents in pregnancy, during delivery, and during the first 6 weeks of life has resulted in a significant reduction in transmission from an estimated 25% to 8% with zidovudine alone and even greater benefit with the use of HAART. To date, except for the use of efavirenz, there is no evidence to suggest an increased risk for congenital birth defects with the use of antiretroviral agents for this indication. The use of antiretroviral therapy during pregnancy has resulted in a nearly 50% reduction in the number of children with perinatal-acquired HIV infection.

Table 159-1 Surveillance Case Definition for HIV Infection in Adults and Adolescents (Age Over 13 Years)

Stage	Laboratory Evidence	Clinical Evidence
Stage1	Laboratory confirmation of HIV infection and $CD4^+$ T-lymphocyte count of ≥500 cells/μL or $CD4^+$ T-lymphocyte percentage of ≥29*	No AIDS-defining condition (see Table 159-2)
Stage 2	Laboratory confirmation of HIV infection and $CD4^+$ T-lymphocyte count of 200-499 cells/μL or $CD4^+$ T-lymphocyte percentage of 14-28*	No AIDS-defining condition (see Table 159-2)
Stage 3	Laboratory confirmation of HIV infection and $CD4^+$ T-lymphocyte count of <200 cells/μL or $CD4^+$ T-lymphocyte percentage of <14*	Documentation of an AIDS-defining condition with laboratory confirmation of HIV infection (see Table 159-2)
Stage unknown	Laboratory confirmation of HIV infection and no information on $CD4^+$ T-lymphocyte count or percentage	No information on presence of an AIDS-defining condition

AIDS, Acquired immunodeficiency syndrome; *HIV,* human immunodeficiency virus.
*The $CD4^+$ T-lymphocyte percentage is the percentage of the total lymphocyte count.

Table 159-2 Surveillance Definitions of AIDS-Defining Conditions

Opportunistic infections
Pneumocystis jiroveci (carinii)
Mycobacterium avium complex
Mycobacterium tuberculosis
Toxoplasmosis
Candidiasis: esophageal and systemic
Histoplasmosis
Cryptococcosis
Cryptosporidiosis and isosporiasis
Leishmaniasis
Cytomegalovirus disease
Recurrent bacterial infections (≥2 episodes/yr)
Lymphomas
Kaposi sarcoma
Cervical cancer
AIDS dementia syndrome
Wasting syndrome

AIDS, Acquired immunodeficiency syndrome.

Transmission can also occur by the sharing of needles and syringes between injection drug users. The use of cocaine and other noninjection drugs can be associated with an increased risk for HIV infection in that their use is frequently associated with high-risk sexual behaviors. Needlestick exposures can also result in transmission of HIV from infected patients to health care workers. The risk for transmission is increased if the patient who is the source of the contaminated needle has more advanced disease with a high plasma viral load, if the needle injury is deep, if there is visible blood on the needle, or if the injury directly enters a vein or artery. The estimated risk for acquiring HIV is approximately 0.3% per needle injury exposure if the source of the blood is a patient with advanced HIV infection (stage 3 AIDS). The use of a 4-week course of antiretroviral therapy as postexposure prophylaxis has been shown to significantly reduce the risk for transmission. Prophylaxis using drug regimens recommended by the CDC should be initiated within 72 hours of exposure and continued for a duration that is based upon the stage of the patient who was the source of the exposure and the type of exposure.

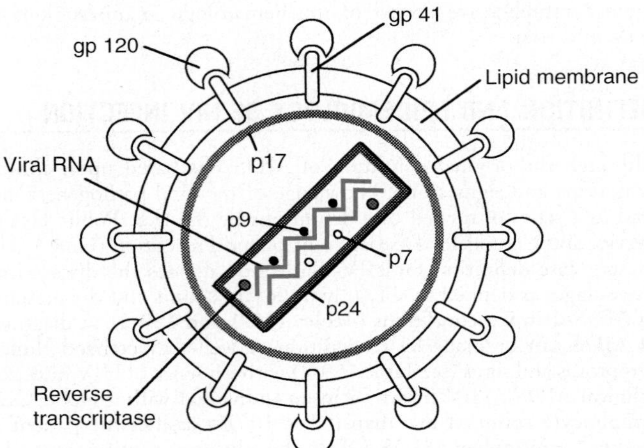

Figure 159-1 STRUCTURE OF THE HIV VIRION. Two coding strands of genomic ribonucleic acid (RNA) are packaged in the nucleoid core with p7, p9, and p24 proteins and reverse transcriptase. The core is surrounded by the p17 matrix protein lining the inner surface of the envelope. The envelope consists of a lipid bilayer derived from the infected cell and glycoprotein spikes that consist of the outer gp120 molecule, which contains the binding site for CD4, and gp41, which anchors the glycoprotein complex to the envelope and mediates fusion of the viral membrane with the cell membrane during viral penetration. *HIV,* Human immunodeficiency virus.

ETIOLOGY AND PATHOGENSIS

Human Immunodeficiency Virus Type 1

HIV-1 is a member of the primate Lentivirinae subfamily of retroviruses. Retroviruses are ribonucleic acid (RNA) viruses that induce a chronic cellular infection by converting their RNA genome into a deoxyribonucleic acid (DNA) provirus that is integrated into the genome of the host cell. The genome of the virus contains three major genes necessary for viral replication and cellular invasion. The env gene codes for a 160-kD precursor protein that is processed into a 120-kD surface glycoprotein (gp) noncovalently linked to a 41-kD transmembrane protein. The gp120-gp41 complex is necessary for virus binding to CD4 and CCR5 on the cell membrane and fusion of the viral envelope with the cell membrane, allowing for the release of the viral genome into the host cell. The gag gene codes for the four viral structural core proteins. These proteins form the nucleocapsid for the viral genome and assist in assembly of the replicating virus before viral release from the cell membrane. The pol gene codes for three functional enzymes; a reverse transcriptase necessary for formation of the proviral double-strand DNA, an integrase necessary for stable integration of the proviral DNA into the host cellular DNA, and viral protease necessary for processing viral membrane and core proteins (Figs. 159-1 and 159-2).

In addition to these three essential genes, the 9-kD genome of HIV-1 contains six additional genes (vif, vpu, vpr, tat, ref, nef) necessary for the regulation of viral gene expression, cellular latency, and each gene product playing an important role in the life cycle of HIV.

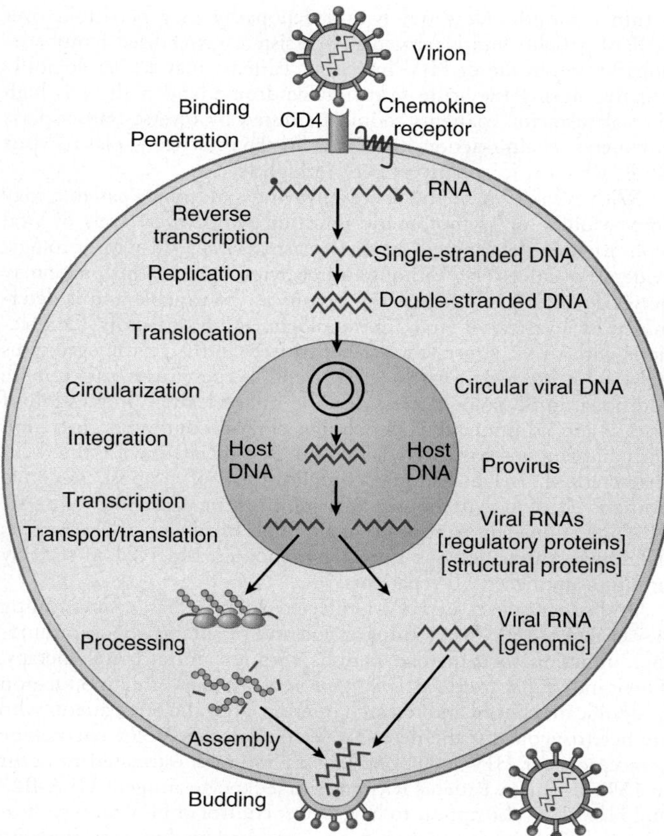

Figure 159-2 HIV LIFE CYCLE. Binding of the virion to the cell surface is mediated by a specific interaction of the gp120 envelope glycoprotein with cellular CD4 and members of the chemokine receptor family of proteins (CCR5 or CXCR4). Penetration occurs as the viral membrane fuses with the cellular membrane in a process that requires the gp41 transmembrane protein. The viral capsid is uncoated, and viral genomic ribonucleic acid (RNA) is reverse transcribed and duplicated by the viral reverse transcriptase to produce a double-stranded copy of viral deoxyribonucleic acid (DNA). The viral DNA is transported to the nucleus, where it integrates into the host chromosomes. After appropriate activating signals, the provirus is transcribed by cellular RNA polymerase and transported to the cytoplasm. Proteins are translated and processed through biochemical steps that, depending on the protein, involve glycosylation (gp120 and gp41), cleavage (envelope proteins, gag, pol), myristoylation (p17), and phosphorylation (rev, nef). Packaging of genomic RNA with viral proteins occurs as envelope glycoproteins are inserted into the cell membrane and new virion subsequently buds outward from the plasma membrane. Viral protease continues protein processing to completion during viral budding. *HIV,* Human immunodeficiency virus.

Life Cycle of HIV-1

Cellular infection begins with engagement of HIV-1 gp120 binding to CD4 surface membrane protein, resulting in a conformational change in gp120 allowing for further high-affinity binding to chemokine CCR5 receptor (see Fig. 159-2). Thymic helper-inducer (CD4) lymphocytes, macrophage-monocytes, Langerhans cells, follicular dendritic cells, megakaryocytes, and thymic cells express both CD4 and CCR5 receptors molecules and are susceptible to HIV-1 infection. Rare individuals who are homozygotes for the delta32 deletion in CCR5 are highly resistant to HIV-1 infection. The structural diversity of gp120 viral receptor has resulted in HIV-1 strains with selective or restricted patterns of infection with strains that readily infect monocytes, whereas others are tropic for CD4 lymphocytes. Some CD4$^+$-tropic strains may also use the CXCR4 chemokine receptor in addition to the CCR5 receptor.

Upon binding to the CD4 and CCR5 receptors, the viral transmembrane gp41 mediates fusion with the host cell membrane. The internalized viral nucleocapsid dissociates after binding to cellular cyclophilin, releasing the diploid viral RNA genome that is associated with the viral reverse transcriptase. Reverse transcription proceeds to synthesis of a single-strain complementary DNA (cDNA), followed by degradation of the viral RNA by ribonuclease H activity of p66. The reverse transcriptase then acts as a DNA polymerase, forming a double-stranded DNA provirus. The reverse transcriptase of HIV has a significant rate of base substitution errors estimated as high as 1 in 1700 to 1 in 2000 nucleoside bases, resulting in an average of 5 to 10 nucleoside mutations for each replication cycle. This explains the high degree of genomic diversity observed between HIV-1 viral isolates.

A linear form of the provirus is integrated into the host DNA by the viral integrase. In kinetic studies of HIV-1 infection, viral DNA is present in the cytoplasm within 2 to 3 hours of infection, whereas viral nuclear DNA has been detected by 24 hours. The gene product of vpr assists in transport of the proviral DNA into the nucleus for subsequent integration. After integration of the viral genome, the HIV-1 infected cell may develop either a latent or persistent form of infection.

HIV-1 does not replicate readily in resting lymphocytes and macrophages. Cellular transactivation, by NF-κB, for example, can enhance proviral transcription. HIV-1 proviral transcription leads to the expression of regulatory proteins tat, rev, and nef. Tat is a protein essential for HIV replication, and in conjunction the cellular proteins TAK (Tat-associated kinase) and Cyc T (cyclin T) promote viral RNA elongation resulting in a 1000-fold increase in HIV-1 expression. Rev is a viral protein that is also essential to replication by regulating nuclear export of unspliced viral RNA. Nef and vpu proteins modulate the downregulation of cellular CD4.

The structural proteins of the gag, pol, and env genes are expressed as precursor proteins and subsequently cleaved by viral protease, yielding mature viral proteins. This final step in protein processing is essential for the assembly of mature infectious virus. For this reason, inhibition of the viral protease has proven a fruitful target for ART. The products of the env gene, gp120, and gp 41, are transported to the cell membrane and the assembled ribonucleoprotein core moved from the cytoplasm to the membrane surface for subsequent budding. The efficient packaging of the viral RNA is dependent upon packaging signals in the gag region of the viral RNA. Final budding is dependent upon the product of the vpu gene, which also assists in transport of env products to the cell membrane and association with the ribonucleoprotein core.

Pathogenesis of HIV Infection

HIV infection results in progressive immunodeficiency and immune dysregulation. By progressive depletion of helper CD4 thymic lymphocytes there is decreased response to soluble antigens, decreased helper response to immunoglobulin synthesis, and impaired delayed hypersensitivity. Decreased interferon-γ production leads to decreased cytoplasmic killing of intracellular organisms. There is also defective natural killer (NK) function and decreased T lymphocyte–mediated cytotoxicity of viral infected cells. An imbalance of CD4, CD25, Foxp2$^+$ regulatory cells, and CD4/interleukin (IL)-17 lymphocytes may result in the expression of autoreactive T and B lymphocytes, accounting for the increased incidence of autoimmune disorders associated with HIV infection and defective CD8 responses against HIV-infected lymphocytes. Viral expression in activated CD4 lymphocytes results in rapid cell death, whereas infection of macrophages, dendritic cells, and nonreplicating CD4 lymphocytes accounts for a persistent and long-lived reservoir of HIV-1 infected cells. High-level viral replication and budding associated with potent immunostimulation from acute and chronic infections may contribute to accelerated lymphocyte cytotoxicity.

In addition to the direct cytopathic effect of viral replication in CD4 lymphocytes, formation of syncytial multinucleated giant cells by fusion of infected CD4 lymphocytes expressing gp120 on their membrane with uninfected CD4⁺ lymphocytes is another mechanism for CD4 depletion. Viral strains capable of forming such syncytia in vitro appear to be associated with a more aggressive clinical course. The host immunologic response against HIV-infected lymphocytes by cytotoxic T lymphocytes and antibody-mediated cellular cytotoxicity may also contribute to CD4 lymphocyte loss in HIV disease. Some CD4 lymphocytes may also be destroyed by an "innocent-bystander" mechanism secondary to the binding of free gp120 to their surface CD4 protein. In vitro studies have found that binding of the gp120 with anti-gp120 antibodies to the CD4 receptor can induce in the lymphocyte programmed cell death or apoptosis. Defective production of immune-stimulatory cytokines (IL-2) and expression of inhibitors of T-lymphocyte proliferation such as transforming growth factor-β (TGFβ) may also contribute to the progressive loss of CD4 lymphocytes.

The development of progressive CD4 lymphocyte depletion and its resulting immunodeficiency is closely linked to the degree of viral production. The level of plasma HIV-1 viral RNA, in addition to the CD4 lymphocyte count, is a major prognostic indicator of disease progression. The advent of HAART capable of marked suppression of viral replication has radically changed the natural history of HIV infection. Efficient viral suppression with reduction in blood and tissue viral reservoirs has resulted in prolonged immunologic reconstitution characterized by increased CD4 lymphocyte numbers, reduced opportunistic infections, and prolonged survival. However, significant immune defects do persist, and complete immunologic reconstitution with normal immune regulation does not occur.

There appears to be a more selective effect of HIV cytotoxicity on memory CD4 lymphocytes and Th1 lymphocyte subsets. This contributes to a profound imbalance in host immune responses with resulting B-lymphocyte dysregulation leading to polyclonal hypergammaglobulinemia and defective cellular immune responses against malignant or viral infected cells (including HIV-infected lymphocytes). Infection of monocytes, macrophages, and dendritic cells not only provide a long-lived reservoir for HIV, but further contribute to the immunologic dysfunction because of their role in antigen presentation and cytokine production.

CLINICAL COURSE OF HIV-1 INFECTION

Serial assessment of HIV-1 RNA in plasma and CD4⁺ lymphocytes has proven to be a reliable means for following HIV-1 infection and predicting the course of disease in individual patients. The use of HAART has significantly changed the natural history of HIV disease. With active surveillance programs that can find HIV-1 infected individuals before the development of symptomatic disease, the early use of HAART based upon U.S. Public Health Service guidelines has resulted in significant decreases in the incidence of HIV-defining opportunistic infections. Based upon laboratory markers of disease progression, guidelines from the U.S. Public Health Service recommend the initiation of HAART in all symptomatic HIV-1-infected patients and asymptomatic patients with CD4⁺ lymphocyte counts less than 0.35×10^9/L or when plasma HIV viral load reaches 55×10^6 copies/L or greater.

Three general stages of HIV infection have been characterized: an acute retroviral syndrome, an asymptomatic stage, and a period of symptomatic conditions that may or may not fulfill criteria for classification as symptomatic AIDS. The acute retroviral syndrome occurs in approximately 50% to 80% percent of infected individuals. The onset of symptoms occurs 1 to 3 weeks (range, 5 days to 3 months) after primary infection. Symptoms last from 1 to 2 weeks and can include significant fatigue, headache, malaise, fever as high as 40° C, sore throat, and myalgias. A morbilliform rash can be observed in 40% to 50% of patients with generalized lymphadenopathy occurring toward the end of the acute illness. Symptoms are similar to those observed in other viral syndromes such as mononucleosis. Laboratory findings may include lymphocytosis, occasional neutropenia, and mild thrombocytopenia. Most symptoms subside within a month. However, lymphadenopathy may persist in over 50% of patients and is termed the persistent generalized lymphadenopathy syndrome of HIV infection. Patients may be serologically negative during the acute retroviral syndrome, and if there is high clinical suspicion, patients should be tested by reverse-transcriptase polymerase chain reaction (RT-PCR) for the presence of plasma virus RNA, which is frequently present in high levels.

With resolution of the acute retroviral syndrome, patients may enter a phase of asymptomatic infection with lower levels of viral replication as determined by their plasma viral load with serologic evidence of infection. Without antiretroviral therapy, this phase may persist for nearly a decade. Progression can be variable and is determined by a variety of viral, immunologic, and host factors. Coinfections with other viruses such a hepatitis B and C, cytomegalovirus (CMV), Epstein-Barr virus (EBV), and herpesviruses can impose additional immunologic stress, leading to accelerated progression of disease and additional AIDS-defining clinical conditions. Infection with human herpesvirus 8 (HHV-8) is associated with the well-characterized AIDS-defining complications of Kaposi sarcoma, primary effusion lymphoma, and multicentric Castleman disease. EBV infection may contribute to the high incidence of lymphoma, including central nervous system lymphomas, observed in severely immunosuppressed HIV patients.

A distinct subset of HIV-1-infected patients has a significantly slower rate of HIV disease progression and maintains good immunologic function for extended periods without antiretroviral therapy. These individuals, termed *long-term nonprogressors,* are a population of significant clinical and research interest. They include patients who are heterozygous for the delta 32 deletion in the CCR5 chemokine coreceptors for HIV infection. This mutation is estimated to occur in 15% of whites. Patients with human leukocyte antigens HLA-B27 and HLA-B57 also appear to have better control of HIV viral replication and slower disease progression. This may be due to an inability of these patients' T regulatory lymphocytes to suppress CD8 cytotoxic–lymphocyte HIV-specific responses.

In the absence of antiretroviral therapy, HIV-infected patients develop progressive immunodeficiency with the development of opportunistic infections, central and peripheral neurologic symptoms, HIV-associated malignancies, fatigue, weight loss, and a general wasting syndrome (see Table 159-2).

HEMATOLOGIC AND BONE MARROW ABNORMALITIES IN HIV-1 INFECTION

The hallmark of HIV infection is the CD4⁺ lymphopenia. However, during the course of the disease about 70% to 80% of patients with HIV/AIDS will develop anemia, 50% will develop neutropenia, and 40% will develop thrombocytopenia. The presence of cytopenias in addition to the CD4⁺ T lymphopenia of HIV disease has long suggested that the suppressive effects of HIV on the hematopoietic compartment are far more broadly based than just a select subset of T cells. A number of studies have assessed the bone marrow microenvironment, the cytokine milieu, and the number and the function of primitive hematopoietic elements in HIV disease. A low fraction of progenitor cells can be infected ex vivo by HIV under some conditions. The growth of these few cells infected by HIV may not be impaired as a result of infection. However, in vivo infection of progenitor cells rarely if ever occurs. Progenitor populations such as those yielding megakaryocytes or monocytes can be infected.

HIV infection leads to hematopoietic inhibition in vivo by depleting myeloid and erythroid colony-forming precursor activity. This activity may be due to an indirect mechanism rather than direct infection of CD34⁺ cells. The presence of messenger RNA for and cell surface expression of HIV receptor CD4 and the chemokine receptors CXCR4 and CCR5 have been demonstrated in fractionated cells representing multiple stages of hematopoietic development. Productive infection by HIV via these receptors is observed with the notable exception of stem cells, in which case the presence of CD4, CXCR4, and CCR5 is insufficient for infection.[1] Although direct infection of stem cells does not occur, alterations in stem cell number and function have been documented. HIV replication in the bone marrow microenvironment is believed to be the essential component causing decreased hematopoietic cell production in HIV infection.[2] The exact mechanism by which the microenvironment induces these alterations is unknown. Mononuclear macrophage cells can develop productive HIV infection, and the resultant aberrant release of cytokines, such as TGFβ, tumor necrosis factor-α (TNF-α), and IL-1, can contribute to the suppression of hematopoiesis. TNF-α is a potent mediator of inflammation and host response to infectious diseases, with pleiotropic effects such as tissue damage, caloric wasting, and impairment of hematopoiesis. It has been observed that HIV suppresses hematopoiesis through induction of TNF-α. TNF-binding protein has been shown to reverse in vitro hematopoietic defects.[3] The relationship of virus replication to inducing the hematopoietic defects is most readily apparent in the clinical changes seen when patients initiate potent antiretroviral therapy. When patients begin HAART therapy, an increase in white blood cells, polymorphonuclear neutrophils, and platelets in addition to an increase in $CD4^+$ T cells occurs as plasma HIV RNA levels decline.[4] T cell–kinetics studies have demonstrated a markedly shortened half-life of peripheral blood T cells from approximately 82 days to 23 days. Initiation of antiretroviral therapy does not improve lymphocyte half-life. The increase in T cell numbers in the peripheral blood of patients treated with HAART appears to be a result of improved production, which in turn may be due to one of several mechanisms: expansion or redistribution of existing subsets of cells or de novo production of T cells from the thymus. The increase in T cells following initiation of HAART is biphasic. In the interval immediately following the start of therapy, there is a prompt increase in both $CD4^+$ and $CD8^+$ cells that is composed predominantly of cells of a memory phenotype ($CD45RO^+$ or $CD45RA^+$ $CD62L^-$). This increase is slightly different for $CD4^+$ cells, which increase more briskly (0.027/day) and plateau at approximately 3 weeks compared with $CD8^+$ cells (increase of 0.008/day), which plateau at 8 weeks.[5] This increase is thought to be due largely to redistribution from peripheral tissues, perhaps related to a changing level of activation of the cells with declining viral antigen stimulation. This initial increase in circulating cell numbers does not achieve normal blood levels of lymphocytes. The secondary, much slower phase of T-cell increase tends to be sustained for months to years with a greater contribution of cells with a naive phenotype ($CD45RA^+$ $CD62L^+$). The naive population rises along with cells bearing the T cell–receptor excision circle, an indicator of recent T cell–receptor rearrangement that accompanies early T-cell differentiation. It is this population that is generally regarded as thymus dependent and that is capable of truly expanding the immune repertoire. In addition, in vivo models have further defined that T-cell generation from precursor populations both endogenous and exogenous to the thymus accompanies control of viremia.

Evaluation of Cytopenias in HIV-Infected Individuals

The evaluation of cytopenias in patients infected with HIV requires a review of the complete blood cell count and thorough examination of the peripheral blood smear (see box on Peripheral Blood Smear and Bone Marrow Morphology in HIV/AIDS). Although there is a gradual fall in CD4-positive lymphocytes during the asymptomatic phase of HIV infection, a mild lymphocytosis may at times be seen because of an increase in CD8-positive lymphocytes. Atypical or activated lymphocytes may frequently be seen. Lymphopenia is present in the advanced stage of disease. Anemia, when present, is usually normocytic and normochromic. It can be at times macrocytic, either due to the effect of certain antiretroviral drugs such as zidovudine or stavudine or seen in patients with advanced HIV disease (Fig. 159-3). Occasionally red blood cell (RBC) anisocytosis, poikilocytosis, and rouleaux can be seen in patients with untreated advanced HIV disease. Also, hypogranular neutrophils and Pelger-Huët forms may rarely be present in patients with advanced HIV disease. However, in comparison to patients with myelodysplastic syndrome (MDS), agranular neutrophils and neutrophils with the acquired Pelger-Huët anomaly are not a predominant feature in patients with HIV infection. Thrombocytopenia is associated with normal-sized platelets, except occasional large platelets may be seen when there is immune-mediated destruction of platelets with preserved marrow function.

The bone marrow in patients with HIV can be hypercellular, normocellular, or hypocellular (see Fig. 159-3). In a majority of cases the normal bone marrow architecture is often disturbed with dysplastic changes similar to what is seen in MDS.[6] Associated stromal changes include edema, gelatinous transformation and lymphoid infiltrates, and granuloma with increased reticulin fibers. Dense collagen fibrosis, however, is not a feature of the HIV bone marrow.

There are some important features distinguishing the morphology of the bone marrow of an HIV-infected individual from that of patients with MDS. Dyserythropoiesis is usually less severe in HIV disease than observed in MDS and occurs predominantly in patients treated with HAART. Megaloblastic changes are usually associated with zidovudine and stavudine therapy. In contrast to MDS, in which erythropoiesis maybe hyperplastic, the myeloid/erythroid ratio in HIV is usually normal, and there may even be neutrophilic and megakaryocytic hyperplasia. An increase in blasts can be seen in MDS, but never in bone marrow in HIV-infected patients, unless they have an associated leukemia. In contrast to MDS, the bone marrow in HIV patients often shows eosinophilia, lymphohistiocytic infiltrates, and reactive plasmacytosis.

Although a bone marrow examination is not routinely required to evaluate isolated anemia, thrombocytopenia, or neutropenia in patients with HIV infection, a bone marrow examination can be useful in the evaluation of unexplained fever and in patients with pancytopenia suspected of having marrow infiltration with an infectious agent or malignancy. Granulomas are observed in approximately 15% of bone marrow trephines and may be due to the HIV infection

Peripheral Blood Smear and Bone Marrow Morphology in HIV/AIDS

The peripheral blood smear of a patient with HIV/AIDS might show anisocytosis, poikilocytosis, and rouleaux formation. Anemia when present is usually normocytic and normochromic. Sometimes macrocytic anemia can be seen even in the absence of zidovudine therapy. Lymphopenia is seen in advanced disease. Hypogranular neutrophils and Pelger-Huët forms are rarely present. Platelets can be normal or hypogranular. In cases of thrombocytopenia the platelets can be normal-sized or large when thrombocytopenia is due to immune destruction with preserved marrow function.

The bone marrow is usually hypercellular but can be normocellular or hypocellular. Interstitial and perivascular polyclonal plasmacytosis is usually present. HIV-associated stromal changes include edema, gelatinous transformation, and increased reticulin fibers (dense collagen fibers are not a feature of HIV). Normal bone marrow architecture is often disturbed, and dysplastic changes can be seen, including dyserythropoiesis, dysgranulopoiesis, and abnormal megakaryocytes (including clusters and bare megakaryocytic nuclei). However, the following features distinguish the bone marrow morphology in HIV from that of myelodysplastic syndrome (MDS): Dysplasia is less severe in HIV. Dyserythropoiesis occurs mainly in patients on highly active antiretroviral therapy (HAART). Megaloblastic changes are associated with zidovudine therapy. Whereas erythropoiesis is usually hyperplastic in MDS, myeloid/erythroid ratio is usually normal in HIV. Increased blasts can be seen in MDS but never in HIV. Lastly, in contrast to MDS, the basement membrane in HIV often shows eosinophilia, lymphohistiocytic infiltrates, and plasmacytosis.

AIDS, Acquired immunodeficiency syndrome; *HIV,* human immunodeficiency virus.

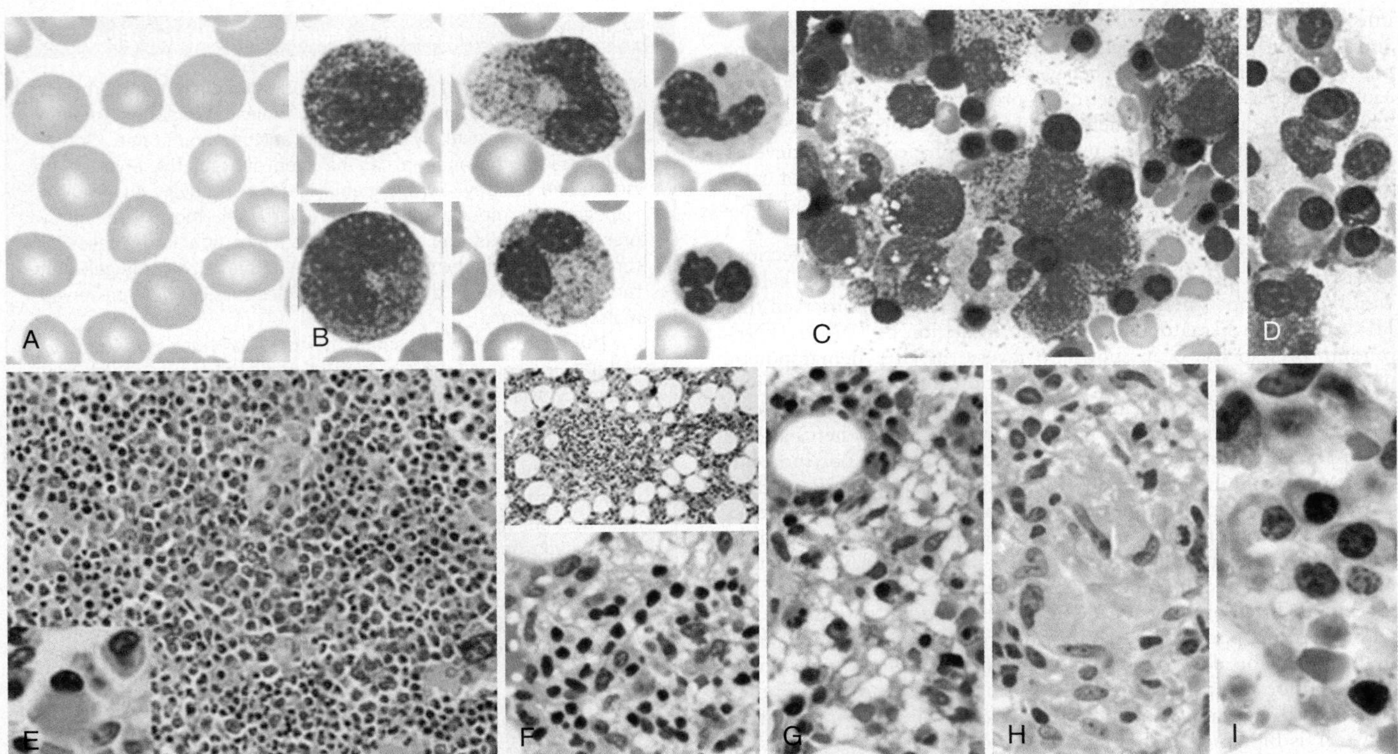

Figure 159-3 TYPICAL PERIPHERAL BLOOD AND BONE MARROW FINDINGS IN HIV. The peripheral smear not uncommonly shows anemia, which is sometimes macrocytic (**A**), but can be normochromic and normocytic. There frequently is a neutrophilia with left shift, toxic granulation, and some mild dysplastic change in the granulocytes (**B**). In some patients, particularly those with severe disease, some of the segmented neutrophils show cytoplasmic inclusions similar to Howell-Jolly bodies seen in red cells (**B**, *top, right cell*). These are nuclear in origin and are not microorganisms. The bone marrow can show granulocytic hyperplasia with left shift and megaloblastoid change in the myeloid and erythroid cell lines (**C**). Typically, there is also a reactive plasmacytosis (**D**). The biopsy specimen can be hypocellular, normocellular, or hypercellular (**E**) and commonly shows cellular atypia/dysplasia *(insert)* and atypical reactive lymphoid infiltrates (**F**), poorly formed (**G**) or well-formed granuloma (**H**), and increased plasma cells (**I**).

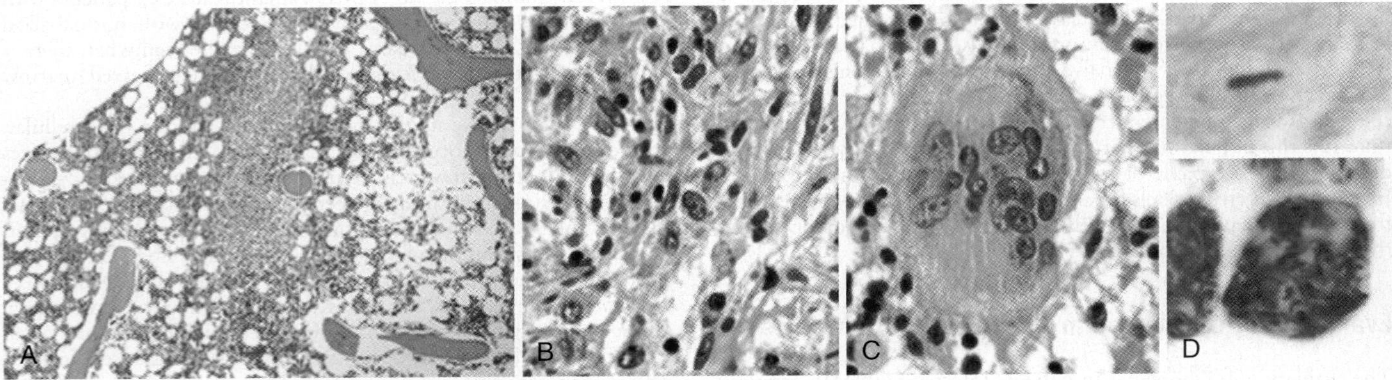

Figure 159-4 ACID-FAST ORGANISMS IN GRANULOMA. Large poorly formed granuloma in the bone marrow (**A**), is composed of loosely aggregated histiocytes, lymphocytes, and plasma cells (**B**), with occasional giant cells (**C**). The acid-fast stain shows rare elongated, slightly beaded organisms, typical of *Mycobacterium tuberculosis* (**D**, *top*). In *Mycobacterium avium* complex, the organisms frequently stuff histiocytes (**D**, *bottom*).

alone, but a thorough search for mycobacterium and other infections is required. A particular effort should be made to identify bone marrow involvement with opportunistic infections, which could include mycobacterial (Fig. 159-4), fungal, protozoal, and/or viral infections.[6] Cytopenias in HIV-infected individuals may also be due to bone marrow involvement by non-Hodgkin lymphoma (Fig. 159-5), Hodgkin lymphomas (Fig. 159-6), Kaposi sarcoma, and Castleman disease.

The etiology of cytopenias in HIV/AIDS is frequently multifactorial. In addition to HIV infection, the medications often prescribed to HIV-infected patients can account for a significant proportion of cytopenias. A thorough review of the medications and supplements taken by an HIV/AIDS patient with a cytopenia is essential. Tables 159-3 and 159-4 list antiretroviral and antiinfective medications prescribed for prophylaxis/treatment of opportunistic infections and their association with hematologic toxicities.

The clinical presentation and management of individual cytopenias can be unique, and therefore the diagnosis and management of anemia, thrombocytopenia, and neutropenia in HIV/AIDS are addressed separately later. In addition, the emerging issue of thrombosis in HIV and principles of antiretroviral therapy management will also be discussed in this chapter.

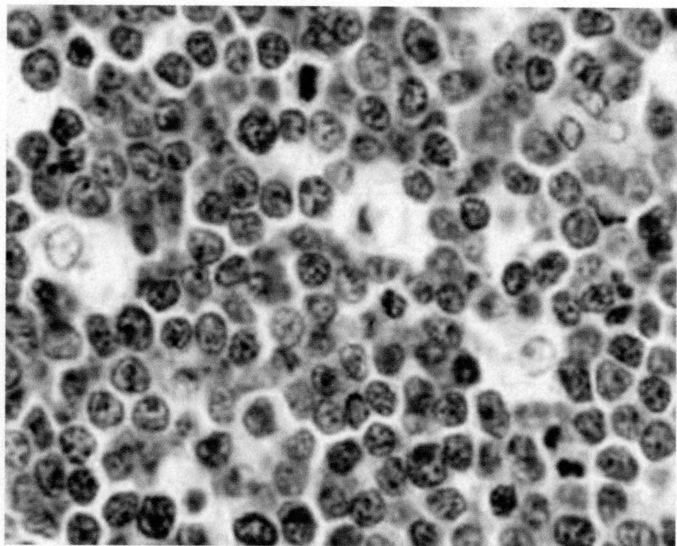

Figure 159-5 BURKITT LYMPHOMA INVOLVING THE BONE MARROW OF A PATIENT WITH ACQUIRED IMMUNODEFICIENCY SYNDROME (AIDS). *(Zhao X, Sun NC, Witt MD, et al: Changing pattern of AIDS: A bone marrow study. Am J Clin Pathol 121:393, 2004.)*

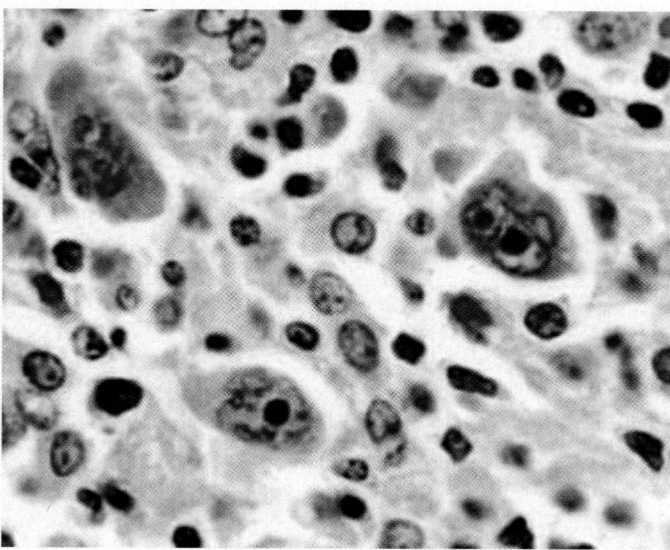

Figure 159-6 CLASSIC HODGKIN LYMPHOMA INVOLVING THE BONE MARROW OF A PATIENT WITH ACQUIRED IMMUNODEFICIENCY SYNDROME (AIDS). *(Zhao X, Sun NC, Witt MD, et al: Changing pattern of AIDS: A bone marrow study. Am J Clin Pathol 121:393, 2004.)*

Anemia in HIV/AIDS

Anemia can occur at any stage of HIV disease but is more frequent and severe in advanced disease. Anemia in HIV disease is independently associated with an increased risk for disease progression and mortality. In general, the etiology of anemia seen in HIV infection is often multifactorial, with several mechanisms playing a role in an individual patient. Anemia could be due to decreased red blood cell (RBC) production, ineffective RBC production, or increased RBC destruction. A methodical workup of anemia in a patient with HIV should be similar to that for anemia in the HIV-negative individual.

The most common cause of anemia in HIV disease is decreased RBC production. Frequently encountered mechanisms responsible for decreased RBC production in patients with HIV include anemia of acute and chronic inflammation (chronic disease anemia), infection or infiltration of bone marrow by infectious agents such as atypical mycobacterium, tuberculosis, cytomegalovirus, and/or fungal organisms or malignancies such as lymphoma. Parvovirus B19 can cause isolated red cell aplasia in the more severely immunocompromised individuals. Medications used for treatment of HIV or other illnesses and for prophylaxis of opportunistic infections can cause anemia mostly due to decreased RBC production. The list of medications as in Tables 159-3 and 159-4 is extensive. Hence it is very important that a thorough review of all the medications is done. Nutritional deficiencies, including vitamin B_{12} and folic acid deficiency, are causes of anemia due to ineffective production.

Other causes of anemia include anemia secondary to blood loss or hemolysis. Causes of hemolysis include medications such as sulfonamides and dapsone in individuals with glucose-6-phosphate dehydrogenase (G6PD) deficiency, thrombotic thrombocytopenic purpura or hemophagocytic syndrome. Patients with advanced HIV infection (AIDS) appear to acquire gastrointestinal defects resulting in B_{12} malabsorption.

Diagnosing the cause or causes of anemia is essential to proper therapy. Treatment of anemia should be directed toward correcting the underlying cause whenever possible. The use of blood transfusion should be minimized and reserved for patients who have rapid decreases in hemoglobin levels, extremely low hemoglobin levels, or pronounced anemia-related symptoms. Antiretroviral medication combinations (highly active antiretroviral therapy [HAART]) have shown that suppression of HIV replication is associated with improvement in anemia. Erythropoietin supplementation has been shown to be beneficial in HIV-infected patients with well-established anemia and when the hemoglobin level is decreasing or has decreased slowly. The primary goal of treating anemia should be to maintain quality of life and functional status.

AIDS, Acquired immunodeficiency syndrome; *HIV,* human immunodeficiency virus.

Red Blood Cell Abnormalities and Anemia

Anemia can occur at any stage of HIV disease but is more frequent and severe in advanced disease[7] (see box on Anemia in HIV/AIDS). There is increasing evidence suggesting that anemia in HIV disease is independently associated with an increased risk for disease progression and mortality.[7,8] Anemia is associated with an increased risk for death in HIV-infected patients regardless of CD4 count, and survival is not significantly different between patients with drug-related anemia and anemia attributed to other causes.[7] Correction of anemia in HIV-infected patients has been associated with measurable improvements in quality of life[7] and increased survival.[7]

Detection and treatment of the underlying cause of the anemia should be an immediate goal, which may involve the treatment of opportunistic infections or gastrointestinal blood loss. In general, the etiology of anemia seen in HIV infection is often multifactorial, with several mechanisms playing a role in an individual patient. Diagnosing the cause or causes of anemia is essential to proper therapy.

Anemia Due to Decreased Production

The most common cause of anemia in HIV disease is decreased RBC production. Frequently encountered mechanisms responsible for decreased RBC production in patients with HIV disease are listed in Table 159-5. Examples include anemia of acute and chronic inflammation (chronic disease anemia) with a blunted production of and response to erythropoietin and cytokine suppression of bone marrow

Table 159-3 Hematologic Toxicities of Antiretroviral Agents

MULTICLASS COMBINATIONS

Combination	Brand Name	Hematologic Toxicities
EFV + TDF + FTC	Atripla	

NUCLEOSIDE/NUCLEOTIDE REVERSE TRANSCRIPTASE INHIBITORS

Abbreviation	Generic Name	Brand Name	Hematologic Toxicities
3TC	Lamivudine	Epivir	Neutropenia Thrombocytopenia
ABC	Abacavir	Ziagen	Thrombocytopenia
AZT or ZDV	Zidovudine	Retrovir	Pancytopenia Anemia Thrombocytopenia Neutropenia Pure red cell aplasia
d4T	Stavudine	Zerit	
ddI	Didanosine	Videx EC	
FTC	Emtricitabine	Emtriva	Neutropenia Anemia
TDF	Tenofovir	Viread	Neutropenia

COMBINED NUCLEOTIDE REVERSE TRANSCRIPTASE INHIBITORS

Combination	Brand Name	Hematologic Toxicities
ABC + 3TC	Epzicom (United States) Kivexa (Europe)	Neutropenia Anemia Thrombocytopenia
ABC + AZT + 3TC	Trizivir	Neutropenia Anemia Thrombocytopenia
AZT + 3TC	Combivir	Neutropenia Anemia Thrombocytopenia
TDF + FTC	Truvada	Neutropenia Anemia

NONNUCLEOSIDE REVERSE TRANSCRIPTASE INHIBITORS

Abbreviation	Generic Name	Brand Name	Hematologic Toxicities
DLV	Delavirdine	Rescriptor	Anemia
EFV	Efavirenz	Sustiva (United States) Stocrin (Europe)	Neutropenia
ETR	Etravirine	Intelence	
NVP	Nevirapine	Viramune	Neutropenia

PROTEASE INHIBITORS

Abbreviation	Generic Name	Brand Name	Hematologic Toxicities
APV	Amprenavir	Agenerase	
FOS-APV	Fosamprenavir	Lexiva (United States) Telzir (Europe)	Neutropenia
ATV	Atazanavir	Reyataz	Neutropenia Anemia Thrombocytopenia
DRV	Darunavir	Prezista	Anemia
IDV	Indinavir	Crixivan	Neutropenia Anemia Thrombocytopenia
LPV/RTV	Lopinavir + ritonavir	Kaletra Aluvia (developing world)	Neutropenia Anemia Thrombocytopenia
NFV	Nelfinavir	Viracept	Neutropenia Anemia Lymphopenia
RTV	Ritonavir	Norvir	Anemia
SQV	Saquinavir	Invirase	
TPV	Tipranavir	Aptivus	Neutropenia Anemia

FUSION OR ENTRY INHIBITORS

Abbreviation	Generic Name	Brand Name	Hematologic Toxicities
T20	Enfuvirtide	Fuzeon	Neutropenia Anemia Eosinophilia
MVC	Maraviroc	Celsentri (Europe) Selzentry (United States)	Neutropenia

INTEGRASE INHIBITORS

Abbreviation	Generic Name	Brand Name	Hematologic Toxicities
RAL	Raltegravir	Isentress	Anemia Thrombocytopenia

colony-forming unit–granulocyte, erythrocyte, macrophage, megakaryocyte (CFU-GEMM). Infection or infiltration of bone marrow by infectious agents such as atypical mycobacterium, tuberculosis, cytomegalovirus, and/or fungal organisms can result in profound anemia, although most often associated with pancytopenia. Parvovirus B19 can cause isolated red cell aplasia in the more severely immunocompromised individuals. Bone marrow infiltration by HIV-associated lymphomas, in addition to anemia, can cause neutropenia and thrombocytopenia. Nutritional deficiencies, including vitamin B_{12} and folic acid deficiency, are not uncommon. Other causes of anemia, including anemia secondary to blood loss or hemolysis as seen in the non–HIV patient population, can also occur in patients infected with HIV. Most significant is that most patients with advanced HIV disease are often treated with one or more medications that can affect RBC production and survival.

Before the HAART era, treatment of HIV disease with high doses of zidovudine was a major cause of myelosuppression and anemia in patients with AIDS. More recent studies, even in the era of HAART, continue to report a high prevalence of anemia among HIV-infected patients.[9] Acute and chronic inflammation is the most frequent cause of anemia in HIV infection. This is characterized by the classic findings of decreased serum iron concentration, reduced total iron-binding capacity, a normal or high ferritin level, an inappropriately low reticulocyte count for the degree of anemia, and reduced blood levels of erythropoietin. HIV infection itself may account for anemia. Therefore initiation of HAART may result in improvement or normalization of hemoglobin levels in patients who are anemic at baseline. Frequently this occurs in parallel with improvement in $CD4^+$ lymphocyte count but can occur with only marginal increase in $CD4^+$ lymphocyte numbers. The use of HIV protease inhibitors in HAART

Table 159-4 Agents for Treatment and Prevention of Opportunistic Infections With Hematologic Toxicities

Drug Class	Drug Toxicities	Hematologic
Antifungal agents	Amphotericin B deoxycholate and lipid formulations	Anemia
	Anidulafungin	Deep venous thrombosis (rare)
	Flucytosine	Bone marrow suppression
	Micafungin	Hemolysis, leukopenia
Anti-*Pneumocystis* pneumonia (PCP) agents	Dapsone	Methemoglobinemia, hemolytic anemia (especially in patients with G6PD deficiency), neutropenia
	Primaquine	Methemoglobinemia, hemolytic anemia (especially in patients with G6PD deficiency)
	Trimethoprim-sulfamethoxazole (TMP-SMX)	Bone marrow suppression
Antitoxoplasmosis agents	Pyrimethamine	Neutropenia, thrombocytopenia, megaloblastic anemia
	Sulfadiazine	Bone marrow suppression
Antimycobacterial agents	Rifampin	Thrombocytopenia, hemolytic anemia.
	Rifabutin	Neutropenia anemia, thrombocytopenia
Antiviral agents	Ganciclovir	Neutropenia, thrombocytopenia, anemia
	Interferon-α and peginterferon-α	Neutropenia, thrombocytopenia
	Ribavirin	Hemolytic anemia
	Valacyclovir	At a high dose of 8 g/day: thrombotic thrombocytopenic purpura/hemolytic uremic syndrome reported in advanced human immunodeficiency virus patients and in transplant recipients
	Valganciclovir	Neutropenia, thrombocytopenia, anemia
Antiparasitic agents	Albendazole	Neutropenia
	Benznidazole	Bone marrow suppression
	Fumagillin (investigational)	Oral therapy: neutropenia, thrombocytopenia Ocular therapy: minimal systemic effect or local effect
	Miltefosine	Leukocytosis, thrombocytosis
Treatment for syphilis	Pentavalent antimony (sodium stibogluconate)	Leukopenia, anemia, thrombocytopenia
	Penicillin G	Bone marrow suppression (rare), drug fever

PCP, Pneumocystis carinii pneumonia.

therapy also appears to improve hematopoiesis.[10] A report by the Women's Interagency HIV Study has shown that the use of HAART is associated with decreased prevalence of anemia among women.[11] HAART may also decrease the risk for anemia developing in patients who are not anemic at the initiation of therapy. Although the use of HAART is associated with decreased prevalence among people with AIDS generally, the prevalence of anemia remains high among persons with low CD4 counts.

Parvovirus B19 is a member of the Parvoviridae family and is responsible for several diseases in humans, including erythema infectiosum (fifth disease) in children, hydrops fetalis, acute arthropathy in adults, aplastic crisis in patients with chronic hemolytic disorders, and pure red cell aplasia in immunocompromised individuals. Parvovirus-induced pure red cell aplasia in association with HIV infection was described over a decade ago.[12] Parvovirus B19 infection is generally limited to human erythroid progenitor cells and leads to erythroid cell death. In hosts with normal immune responses and normal erythrocyte production, acute infection causes a self-limited (4 to 8 days) interruption in the production of erythrocytes that does not result in significant anemia. However, if host immune responses are impaired, this can result in persistent infection of erythroid precursors, leading to a prolonged and severe anemia.

The seroprevalence of parvovirus B19 infection is similar among HIV-infected and noninfected individuals. Furthermore, HIV-infected individuals who have serologic evidence of parvovirus B19 infection usually do not have evidence of active infection (i.e., Parvovirus B19 viremia). Parvovirus B19–induced red cell aplasia seen in HIV patients often occurs in individuals with low or absent levels of B19-specific antibodies.[13]

Clinically the disease presents in patients with findings consistent with profound anemia characterized by weakness, pallor, dyspnea, and tachycardia. Hemoglobin values as low as 4 to 5 g/dL and absolute reticulocyte counts of less than 5×10^9/L (<0.1%) are commonly reported. Detection of parvovirus immunoglobulin G (IgG) and IgM is not reliable because levels of antibodies may be low or undetectable among patients and are not diagnostic of acute parvovirus B19 red cell aplasia. The most reliable diagnostic study of parvovirus B19 infection is the detection of parvovirus DNA by either PCR or dot blot hybridization. Because the high sensitivity of PCR may lead to positive test results for months after the original infection, dot blot hybridization may be a better test for making a diagnosis of acute infection resulting in red cell aplasia. Histologic examination of bone marrow aspirates reveals hypocellularity, markedly decreased maturing erythrocytes, and occasional giant pronormoblasts. The presence of giant pronormoblasts in a bone marrow aspirate or biopsy specimen as shown in Fig. 159-7 is diagnostic of parvovirus B19 infection.[6]

Initial therapy for parvovirus-induced red cell aplasia should be aimed at correcting the anemia through red blood cell transfusions. Treatment with intravenous immunoglobulin (IgG) 0.4 g/kg daily for 5 days can lead to a rapid decrease in the level of parvovirus viremia, improvement in the reticulocyte count, and resolution of the anemia. Recurrence is commonly seen if there is no improvement in the patient's immunologic function. If the anemia recurs within 6 months of the initial therapy, monthly maintenance therapy with 0.4 g/kg intravenous IgG may be required. Immune reconstitution resulting from the successful use of HAART may lead to complete remission of this condition.

Anemia Due to Ineffective Red Blood Cell Production

Ineffective production of red cells can occur with deficiencies of folate or vitamin B_{12}. Ineffective production of red blood cells is frequently characterized by concomitant decreases in platelets and neutrophils accompanied by megaloblastic red cell morphology with large oval macrocytes and hypersegmented neutrophils. In addition to a low reticulocyte count, there may be elevations in indirect bilirubin and serum lactate dehydrogenase. Because of the relatively small tissue stores of folate, patients with advanced HIV disease who have poor dietary intake, excessive alcohol ingestion, and/or jejunal disease may become deficient in folate. More commonly reported in patients with advanced HIV infection is decreased serum B_{12} levels. Low serum B_{12} level has been documented in approximately one-third of patients with AIDS. Patients with advanced HIV infection (AIDS) appear to acquire gastrointestinal defects resulting in B_{12} malabsorption. The mechanisms responsible for decreased B_{12} absorption observed in these patients include both infections of and other acquired disorders of the small intestine and ileum, food B_{12} malabsorption secondary to inadequate gastric acid production, and true pernicious anemia with antibodies to the H^+/K^+ parietal cell pump and intrinsic factor. However, not all cases of low serum levels of B_{12} are associated with true metabolic B_{12} deficiency as characterized by elevated methylmalonic acid. This may be due to the finding that some patients with neutropenia secondary to a hypocellular bone marrow may have low serum levels of transcobalamin I (TCI), the major serum B_{12} carrier protein that is found in the specific granules of neutrophils. However, transport of B_{12} into cells is mediated by transcobalamin II (TCII), which carries only 25% to 30% of serum B_{12}, and for that reason the newer assays that measure B_{12} bound to TCII (holotranscobalamin II assays) may be more reflective of serum B_{12} status in neutropenic HIV-infected patients.

A diagnosis of B_{12} deficiency should include not only a low serum B_{12} level, but normal or elevated blood levels of folic acid, and elevated blood homocysteine and methylmalonic acid levels in a patient with normal renal function. With a diagnosis of B_{12} deficiency an effort should be made to determine the causes of B_{12} malabsorption and treatment begun with monthly administration of parenteral B_{12} to correct the deficiency. If anemia and cytopenias are due to the B_{12} deficiency alone, treatment should result in correction within 4 to 6 weeks. Because B_{12} deficiency is also associated with a variety of neurologic defects, including motor and sensory neuropathy; cognitive defects, including dementia; and the most severe neurologic manifestation of subacute combined degeneration of the spinal cord, the possibility of B_{12} deficiency should be considered in any HIV-infected patient with neurologic symptoms.

Table 159-5 Etiology of Anemia in HIV

HIV RELATED	
HIV Infection	
Anemia of chronic disease	
Blunted production/response to erythropoietin	
Suppression of CFU-GEMM (HIV/inflammatory cytokines)	
Neoplasms Infiltrating the BM	
Non-Hodgkin lymphoma, Kaposi sarcoma, Hodgkin lymphoma	
Infections of the BM	
Parvovirus B19	
Atypical mycobacterium (MAI/MAC)	
Mycobacterium tuberculosis	
Histoplasma	
Cytomegalovirus	
Medications Causing Decreased Production	**Medications Causing Hemolysis**
RT inhibitors	Indinavir
Ganciclovir	Bactrim and dapsone in G6PD deficiency
Bactrim	
Amphotericin B	
HIV UNRELATED	
B_{12} and/or folic acid deficiencies	
Iron deficiency due to chronic blood loss	

BM, Basement membrane; *CFU-GEMM,* colony-forming unit–granulocyte, erythrocyte, macrophage, megakaryocyte; *HIV,* human immunodeficiency virus, *MAI/MAC, Mycobacterium avium-intracellulare/Mycobacterium avium* complex; *RT,* reverse transcriptase.

Anemia Due to Increased Red Blood Cell Destruction

Anemia resulting from hemolysis of RBCs can result from processes either intrinsic or extrinsic to the RBC. Examples of intrinsic defects include hemoglobinopathies, RBC membrane defects, or RBC enzyme functional deficiencies such as glucose-6-phosphate dehydrogenase (G6PD) deficiency. Exclusive of G6PD deficiency, the majority of patients with these RBC defects have a lifelong history of anemia. Diagnosis in most circumstances can be made by careful

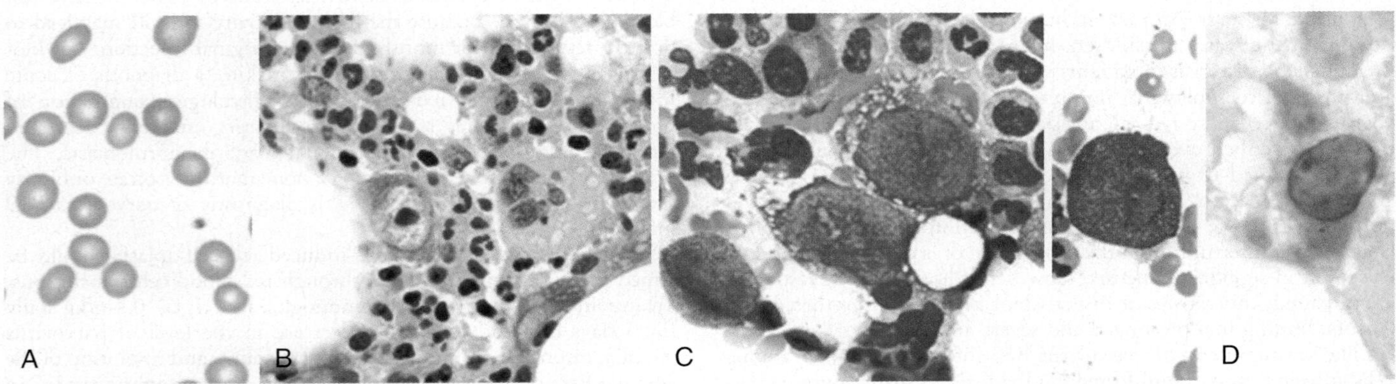

Figure 159-7 HUMAN PARVOVIRUS INFECTION IN HIV. The peripheral blood smear shows anemia with no polychromasia **(A)**. The marrow biopsy shows mostly granulocytic and megakaryocytic elements with a lack of erythroid forms **(B)**, except for rare large pronormoblasts with nuclear inclusions **(B,** *center***)**. On the aspirate, the large degenerating pronormoblasts have nuclear inclusions that resemble large nucleoli **(C)**. These are viral inclusions. Sometimes the pronormoblasts are totally degenerated and present as only bare nuclei with the viral inclusion still obvious **(C,** *right***)**. An immunostain for parvovirus in a degenerated pronormoblast is illustrated **(D)**.

review of the peripheral blood smear. G6PD deficiency is an X-linked disorder and found predominately in men. Hemolysis occurs when erythrocytes are exposed to oxidative stress. Depending upon the degree of enzyme deficiency, patients may not have had a previous documented episode of hemolysis. G6PD deficiency–associated hemolysis can occur in HIV-infected patients who are taking dapsone or trimethoprim and sulfamethoxazole combinations for pneumocystis prophylaxis or treatment. In some patients the degree of hemolysis does not result in significant anemia because RBC destruction is well compensated by effective RBC production, and patients can continue on treatment. However, patients with the Mediterranean form of G6PD may develop severe hemolysis, and treatment with such medications is contraindicated.

Extrinsic causes of RBC hemolysis observed in patients with HIV infection include microangiopathic hemolytic disorders such as thrombotic thrombocytopenic purpura (TTP; see Thrombocytopenia in HIV Infection), vasculitis, or disseminated intravascular coagulation. Patients will have associated thrombocytopenia and demonstrate RBC fragmentation on the peripheral blood smear. Autoimmune hemolytic anemia rarely occurs in HIV-infected individuals, although a positive antiglobulin (Coombs) test result is not uncommon. Patients with documented autoimmune hemolysis may respond to treatment with corticosteroids, rituximab, or splenectomy. The risk for HIV progression with the use of corticosteroids and rituximab does not appear to be an issue in patients receiving HAART.

Impact of Anemia on HIV Disease Progression and Survival

Anemia has been shown to be an independent risk factor for clinical progression of HIV disease. In patients in whom antiretroviral therapy (HAART) is to be initiated, anemia, a CD4 cell count that is less than 0.2×10^9/L, HIV viral load, and a pretreatment diagnosis of clinical AIDS are well-established risk factors for rapid disease progression. A moderate anemia with a hemoglobin level of 8 to 14 g/dL in men or 8 to 12 g/dL in women is associated with a relative hazard of disease progression or death of 2.2 (95% CI, 1.6 to 2.9; $P<0.0001$), whereas a more severe anemia with a hemoglobin level of less than 8 g/dL has a relative hazard of 7.1 (95% CI, 2.5 to 20.1; $P<0.0002$).

Anemia has a significant impact on overall survival in HIV-infected patients. A Baltimore study of 2348 HIV-infected patients found that a hemoglobin level of 6.5 to 8 g/dL was predictive of a threefold increased risk for death, and a hemoglobin of less than 6.5 g/dL was predictive of a fourfold increased risk for death. A European study of 6725 HIV-infected patients found the hemoglobin level at baseline was an independent prognostic factor for survival along with the $CD4^+$ lymphocyte count and HIV plasma viral load. For each 1 g/dL decrease in hemoglobin level, the relative hazard of death was 1.39 (95% CI, 1.34 to 1.43; $P<0.0001$). Additional cohort studies from the United States, including the Multistate Adult and Adolescent Spectrum of HIV Disease Surveillance Project and the Women's Interagency HIV Study, have also confirmed that anemia is an independent risk factor for mortality in HIV-infected individuals.

Management of Anemia and the Use of Erythropoietin in HIV-Infected Patients

Treatment of anemia should be directed toward correcting the underlying cause whenever possible. The use of blood transfusion should be minimized and reserved for patients who have rapid decreases in hemoglobin levels, extremely low hemoglobin levels, or pronounced anemia-related symptoms. A number of clinical trials of antiretroviral medication combinations (HAART) have shown that suppression of HIV replication is associated with improvement in anemia. In addition, improvement of anemia on HAART has been found to occur independent of the patients' sex, race, mode of HIV infection, change in $CD4^+$ lymphocyte count, and additional therapies for anemia. Improvement in anemia, with an increase in the reticulocyte count, can be seen as early as 8 to 12 weeks, with maximum improvement usually obtained by 12 months.

Erythropoietin supplementation has been shown to be beneficial in HIV-infected patients with well-established anemia and when the hemoglobin level is decreasing or has decreased slowly. A blunted response to erythropoietin, as observed in anemia of acute and chronic inflammation, is common in HIV-infected patients with anemia. However, erythropoietin (Epogen, Procrit) therapy should be considered for refractory anemia in symptomatic patients with a hemoglobin level of less than 11 g/dL in men and less than 10 g/dL in women. The primary goal should be to maintain quality of life and functional status. Many patients may be asymptomatic with lower hemoglobin levels (9 to 10 g/dL), and physicians should use erythropoietic agents only for symptomatic patients with these lower hemoglobin levels. The initial adult dose is 40,000 units subcutaneously per week which has been shown to be equivalent to treatment three times a week at 100 to 200 units/kg.[14] Also, darbepoietin alfa given at a dose of 3.0 mcg/kg every 2 weeks has been shown to be equally effective. Onset of action as characterized by an increase in the reticulocyte count is within 1 to 2 weeks, with increased hemoglobin noted in 2 to 6 weeks. The baseline level of endogenous serum erythropoietin has been shown to be predictive of response to the therapeutic use of erythropoietin. A baseline erythropoietin level of greater than 500 International Units/L is associated with a significantly lower response to treatment. Response to erythropoietin therapy also depends on the severity of anemia, presence of active infection, and available iron stores. If the hemoglobin level fails to increase more than 1 g/dL after 4 weeks of therapy, the dose may be increased to 60,000 units weekly. After an additional 4 weeks, if the hemoglobin level does not increase by at least 1 g/dL from baseline, therapy should be discontinued. When combined with the use of HAART, erythropoietin treatment may result in a more rapid improvement in hemoglobin level but has not been shown to improve survival or statistically reduce the total number of transfusions. This may be due to the marginal contribution that erythropoietin supplementation may have in the background of the significant improvement in immune status and bone marrow function provided by effective antiretroviral therapy.[10]

LEUKOPENIA AND NEUTROPENIA: INCIDENCE AND PATHOGENESIS

Leukopenia is common in patients with advanced HIV infection, occurring in up to 85% of patients with clinical AIDS. In such patients low white blood cell counts are frequently a result of both decreased lymphocytes and neutrophils. Neutropenia ($<1.5 \times 10^9$/L) is reported in 5% to 10% of HIV-infected patients with the highest prevalence in patients with advanced HIV infection (AIDS) (see box on Neutropenia in HIV/AIDS). In a 7.5-year longitudinal study of 1729 women with HIV infection an absolute neutrophil count (ANC) of less than 1×10^9/L was documented in 31%. HIV-related risk factors for the development of neutropenia include a high level of plasma HIV viral RNA and a low $CD4^+$ lymphocyte count. In turn, the use of HAART is associated with a lower risk for developing neutropenia. Decreases in the neutrophil count are often transient, self-limiting, and rarely of clinical significance, but a neutrophil count of less than 0.5×10^9/L of prolonged duration does pose a significant risk for infection. In a study of 87 consecutive HIV-infected patients who developed neutrophil counts of less than 1×10^9/L, the median duration of neutropenia was 13 days and the nadir neutrophil count was 0.66×10^9/L. Infection occurred in only 6 (8%) of 71 evaluable patients, of which 4 patients had neutrophil counts less than 0.5×10^9/L. Ten (14%) patients had neutrophil counts less than 0.5×10^9/L and received granulocyte colony-stimulating factor (G-CSF) treatment, which artificially altered the natural history of neutropenia in this patient population.

Decrease in vitro colony growth of the colony-forming unit—granulocyte-macrophage progenitor cell has been reported, which

Neutropenia in HIV/AIDS

Leukopenia is common in patients with advanced HIV infection. Low white blood cell counts are frequently a result of both decreased lymphocytes and neutrophils. HIV-related risk factors for the development of neutropenia include a high level of plasma HIV viral RNA and a low $CD4^+$ lymphocyte count. The use of highly active antiretroviral therapy (HAART) is associated with a lower risk for developing neutropenia. Decreases in the neutrophil count are often transient, self-limiting, and rarely of clinical significance, but a neutrophil count of less than 0.5×10^9/L of prolonged duration does pose a significant risk for infection. The most common cause of neutropenia in HIV-infected patients is medication-related myelosuppression. Neutropenia is a common complication reported with many of the drugs used to treat opportunistic infections such as *Pneumocystis carinii*, toxoplasmosis, or cytomegalovirus (CMV) infection. Although neutropenia resulting from HIV-related myelosuppression often improves with HAART, antiretroviral-associated neutropenia can be observed with higher doses of zidovudine. Rare cases of agranulocytosis have been reported with the use of the antiretroviral drugs abacavir and indinavir. Other causes of neutropenia include bone marrow involvement by opportunistic infections such as *Mycobacterium avium* or CMV or bone marrow involvement with HIV-associated malignancies and their subsequent treatment. A number of acquired functional defects have been described in both neutrophils and monocytes from patients with HIV infection. Many of these defects are observed in patients with advanced disease with high levels of plasma viral RNA and $CD4^+$ lymphopenia.

Treatment of neutropenia should be guided by the underlying cause. This may require treatment of active infection or removal of medications associated with the development of neutropenia. The use of HAART has clearly been shown to reduce the risk for developing leukopenia and neutropenia and to significantly increase the neutrophil counts in treated patients. Sargramostim, or granulocyte-macrophage colony-stimulating factor (GM-CSF; Leukine), and filgrastim, or granulocyte colony-stimulating factor (G-CSF; Neupogen), are the primary pharmacologic agents used in the treatment of severe neutropenia in HIV-infected patients and have been shown in clinical studies to be safe and effective. G-CSF is indicated for drug-induced, cancer-related, and HIV-related neutropenia with an absolute neutrophil count (ANC) of less than 0.5×10^9/L. Common side effects of treatment with GM-CSF include fever, fatigue, myalgias, bone pain, and headache.

AIDS, Acquired immunodeficiency syndrome; *HIV,* human immunodeficiency virus.

may explain the neutropenia observed with HIV infection alone. Inhibitory substances produced by HIV-infected cells have been reported to suppress neutrophil growth and differentiation in vitro. A number of inflammatory cytokines, including TGF-β and TNF-α, may directly suppress myelopoiesis or inhibit the production of important myeloid growth factors, G-CSF and granulocyte-macrophage colony-stimulating factor (GM-CSF). Decreased serum levels of G-CSF have been observed in afebrile neutropenic HIV-infected patients. The HIV proteins tat and p24 have also been reported capable of suppressing myelopoiesis.

The most common causes of neutropenia in HIV-infected patients are medication-related myelosuppression. In a study of 87 consecutive HIV-infected patients with neutrophil counts of less than 2×10^9/L, only 3 patients were not receiving medications associated with a risk for neutropenia and 66% were receiving three or more myelosuppressive medications. Neutropenia is a common complication reported with many of the drugs used to treat opportunistic infections such as *Pneumocystis carinii,* toxoplasmosis, or CMV infection. These medications are listed in Table 159-4. Although neutropenia resulting from HIV-related myelosuppression often improves with HAART, antiretroviral-associated neutropenia can be observed with higher doses of zidovudine. Zidovudine-associated neutropenia resolves with dose reduction or discontinuation of the medication. In a study of 62 HIV-infected patients with neutrophil counts of 1×10^9/L or less, cancer chemotherapy, zidovudine, trimethoprim-sulfamethoxazole, and ganciclovir were the medications most commonly responsible for neutropenia. In the same report, medication-related neutropenia associated with infection was most often seen in the patients receiving cancer chemotherapy. Rare cases of agranulocytosis have been reported with the use of the antiretroviral drugs abacavir and indinavir.

Neutropenia is often observed in patients with bone marrow involvement by opportunistic infections such as *Mycobacterium avium* or CMV. Bone marrow involvement with HIV-associated malignancies and their subsequent treatment can also result in significant and prolonged neutropenia. However, malignancy treatment–related neutropenia in clinical trials appears to be less severe in patients receiving simultaneous HAART.

Abnormalities of Neutrophil and Monocyte Function

A number of acquired functional defects have been described in both neutrophils and monocytes from patients with HIV infection. Many of these defects are observed in patients with advanced disease with high levels of plasma viral RNA and $CD4^+$ lymphopenia. Impaired chemotaxis and reduced expression of leukocyte adhesion molecules necessary for migration of neutrophils to sites of infection have been reported. Decreased opsonization of antibody-coated bacteria due to Fc-receptor dysfunction and decreased superoxide production necessary for optimal intracellular killing of bacterial and fungal organisms have been observed in both neutrophils and macrophages from HIV-infected patients. Defective intracellular killing of mycobacterial and fungal organisms may also be due in part to defective production of interferon-γ.

Management of Neutropenia in HIV-Infected Patients

Impact of HAART and Use of GM-CSF and G-CSF

Treatment of neutropenia should be guided by the underlying cause. This may require treatment of active infection or removal of medications associated with the development of neutropenia. The use of HAART has clearly been shown to reduce the risk for developing leukopenia and neutropenia and significantly increasing the neutrophil counts in treated patients. The Women's Interagency HIV Study of 1729 HIV-infected women found that the use of HAART, without zidovudine, was associated with protection against developing neutropenia. In addition, HAART therapy, even incorporating zidovudine, was associated with resolution of neutropenia in women with advanced HIV disease. Another study of 66 HIV-infected patients treated with HAART reported statistically significant increases in total leukocyte and neutrophil counts after 6 months of treatment. These studies support the use of effective HAART therapy as the initial approach to the management of mild to moderate leukopenia and neutropenia in HIV-infected patients.

Sargramostim, or GM-CSF (Leukine), and filgrastim, or G-CSF (Neupogen), are the primary pharmacologic agents used in the treatment of severe neutropenia in HIV-infected patients and have been shown in clinical studies to be safe and effective. A long-term study of 105 HIV-infected patients randomized to receive weekly injections of GM-CSF (125 mcg/m^2) or placebo while receiving zidovudine antiretroviral therapy reported after 6 months of treatment that GM-CSF–treated patients were more likely to have an HIV plasma RNA level below level of detection and less zidovudine resistance mutations. A study that compared 123 HIV-infected leukopenic patients treated for 12 weeks with GM-CSF to 121 untreated leukopenic patients showed that the total leukocyte count, including neutrophils and monocytes, increased by 65% at week 12 when compared to baseline values ($P<0.001$). In the untreated leukopenic HIV-infected patients, the total leukocyte count decreased by 24% below baseline values at week 12 ($P<0.001$). Common side effects of treatment with GM-CSF include fever, fatigue, myalgias, bone pain, and headache.

A randomized study of 258 HIV-infected patients with $CD4^+$ lymphocyte counts below $0.2 \times 10^9/L$ and neutrophil counts of less than $1 \times 10^9/L$ were randomized to one of two dose regimens of G-CSF (1 mcg/kg/day or 300 mcg three times a week) versus no treatment. Patients in the control group who developed severe neutropenia ($<0.5 \times 10^9/L$) were then randomized to one of the treatment regimens. The intention-to-treat analysis found the incidence of severe neutropenia ($<0.5 \times 10^9/L$) was 1.7% in the treated group versus 22% in the untreated controls. The incidence of bacterial infections was 31% lower in the treated group, with fewer severe bacterial infections and significantly fewer hospital days (45% reduction) for bacterial infections.

The use of G-CSF has been associated with a reduction in severe neutropenia in patients treated for CMV infection with ganciclovir (Cytovene), but the evidence is unclear as to whether it offers a clear clinical benefit. However, in general it has been shown to be safe and effective in raising leukocyte counts when administered to patients with HIV infection receiving antiretroviral therapy. G-CSF is indicated for drug-induced, cancer-related, and HIV-related neutropenia with an ANC of less than $0.5 \times 10^9/L$. The initial dose is 1 to 10 mcg/kg/day and should be titrated by 1 mcg/kg/day to obtain a neutrophil count of $1.0 \times 10^9/L$. Most patients will respond to a dose of 1 mcg/kg/day. G-CSF use should be carefully monitored and the dose reduced or stopped when the neutrophil count exceeds $1.0 \times 10^9/L$.

THROMBOCYTOPENIA IN HIV INFECTION

Thrombocytopenia, alone or in association with anemia and/or leukopenia, is frequently seen in approximately 40% of HIV-infected patients in the course of their disease. Thrombocytopenia has been reported to be the first sign of HIV infection in up to 10% of infected individuals. The most common cause of thrombocytopenia in HIV infection is HIV-related autoimmune thrombocytopenia, which is clinically indistinguishable from classic immune thrombocytopenia purpura (ITP) (see box on Thrombocytopenia in HIV Infection).

An association between AIDS and ITP was described before HIV had been isolated and characterized. HIV infects $CD4^+$ lymphocytes, monocytes, and macrophages, and some experimental evidence also documents infection of megakaryocytes. Although a number of different mechanisms have been reported by which HIV infection can produce thrombocytopenia, the ability of effective antiretroviral therapy to improve platelet counts demonstrates a clear relationship between viral replication, the expression of viral-related proteins, and the host response to platelets.

Thrombocytopenia in HIV Infection

The most common cause of thrombocytopenia in HIV infection is HIV-related autoimmune thrombocytopenia, which is clinically indistinguishable from classic immune thrombocytopenia purpura (ITP). HIV infects $CD4^+$ lymphocytes, monocytes, and macrophages, and some experimental evidence also documents infection of megakaryocytes. Thrombocytopenia is more prevalent in patients with advanced HIV infection and among intravenous drug abusers. The clinical picture of HIV-associated ITP (HIV-ITP) is often mild, with only a minority of patients having platelet counts of less than $50 \times 10^9/L$. Major bleeding is rare, and only a few cases of fatal hemorrhage have been reported. HIV-ITP is generally responsive to therapeutic interventions used in classic ITP. Despite the initial anxiety regarding the use of corticosteroids in HIV-infected, immune-suppressed patients, no deleterious effects of short-term treatment with prednisone have become evident. However, long-term treatment with corticosteroids should still be avoided, and other coinfections such as tuberculosis, cytomegalovirus, or hepatitis C should be excluded before initiating treatment with corticosteroids. Intravenous immunoglobulin (IVIg) and anti-Rh(D) are equally effective in increasing platelet counts acutely in severely affected patients. Splenectomy has proven to be safe and effective in refractory patients. Highly active antiretroviral therapy (HAART) induces sustained platelet responses in association with effective viral suppression and is the front line of treatment for HIV-associated thrombocytopenia. At present there are no data evaluating the efficacy of the newly approved thrombopoietin receptor agonists, romiplostim and eltrombopag, in the management of HIV-related thrombocytopenia, but long-term efficacy and safety data regarding the use of these agents in primary ITP would suggest that they would be effective in the management of HIV-ITP.

AIDS, Acquired immunodeficiency syndrome; *HIV,* human immunodeficiency virus.

Epidemiology

Thrombocytopenia was first associated with AIDS before the discovery of HIV. Before the use of HAART, HIV-associated thrombocytopenia (HIV-ITP; platelet count $<150 \times 10^9/L$) was identified in approximately 5% to 30% of HIV-1 infected patients. Thrombocytopenia is more prevalent in patients with advanced HIV infection defined as a CD4 lymphocyte count of less than $0.2 \times 10^9/L$, clinical AIDS, and among intravenous drug abusers. The Multicenter AIDS Cohort Study of 1611 HIV-positive homosexual and bisexual men reported a platelet count of less than $150 \times 10^9/L$ in 6.7%. The incidence of thrombocytopenia was only 2.8% in men with CD4 lymphocyte counts greater than $0.7 \times 10^9/L$, but rose to 10.8% in those with $CD4^+$ lymphocyte counts of less than $0.2 \times 10^9/L$. A review of 1004 HIV-infected patients seen in two HIV/AIDS clinics identified platelet counts of less than $150 \times 10^9/L$ on at least one determination in 110 (11%) patients; 42 (4.2%) patients had platelet counts of less than $100 \times 10^9/L$, and 15 (1.5%) had a platelet count of less than $50 \times 10^9/L$. Thrombocytopenia was more prevalent in patients with clinical AIDS (21.2%) and a $CD4^+$ lymphocyte count of less than $0.2 \times 10^9/L$ (20%).

A review of the medical records of 36,515 HIV-infected participants in the Multistate Adult and Adolescent Spectrum of HIV Disease Surveillance Project reported a 1-year incidence of thrombocytopenia of 3.7%, defined as a platelet count of less than $50 \times 10^9/L$. The incidence and severity of thrombocytopenia was associated with the stage of disease with an incidence of 1.7% among patients with HIV infection, but not clinical or immunologic AIDS, 3.1% among persons with immunologic AIDS ($CD4^+$ lymphocytes less than $0.2 \times 10^9/L$), and 8.7% in patients with clinical AIDS. By logistic regression analysis, clinical AIDS, CD4 lymphocyte count of less than $0.2 \times 10^9/L$, age above 45 years, intravenous drug use, lymphoma, and/or anemia, were associated with a platelet count of less than $50 \times 10^9/L$.

An increased incidence and severity of thrombocytopenia in HIV-infected intravenous drug users compared to HIV-infected homosexuals has been reported. Mientjes et al[14] reported a platelet count of less than $150 \times 10^9/L$ in 29/182 (16.4%) homosexual HIV-infected men compared with 38/103 (36.9%) HIV-infected intravenous drug users. None of the homosexual men had a platelet count of less than $50 \times 10^9/L$, whereas 6 (5.8%) intravenous drug users had a count of less than $50 \times 10^9/L$. These differences may be explained in part by the higher incidence of coinfection with hepatitis C and underlying liver disease in HIV-infected intravenous drug users.

In a prospective multicenter cohort study of 738 HIV-infected hemophilia patients, the incidence over time of HIV-related conditions was determined in 130 children and 193 adults. The 10-year cumulative incidence of thrombocytopenia (platelets <100 × 10^9/L) after seroconversion was 43% ± 7% in adults and 27% ± 6% in children. The mean CD4 counts were significantly higher in children (514 ± 61 cells/μL) than adults (260 ± 24 cells/μL) with thrombocytopenia (P = .0004).

Most clinical data were obtained before the widespread use of HAART therapy in patients with early HIV infection. There is little data on the current prevalence of thrombocytopenia in patients under active antiviral treatment. However, recent prospective data from the Women's Interagency HIV Study have documented a reduction in the incidence of anemia and neutropenia in HIV-infected women on HAART therapy. These findings are in accord with the impression that there has been a similar reduction in the incidence of thrombocytopenia, especially platelet counts of less than 50 × 10^9/L in compliant patients.

Pathophysiology

Multiple mechanisms may contribute to the development of chronic ITP (CITP) in the HIV-infected patient, and these have recently been reviewed. Proposed mechanisms include accelerated platelet clearance due to immune complex disease, and antiplatelet glycoprotein antibodies and/or anti-HIV antibodies that cross-react with platelet membrane glycoproteins (antigenic mimicry). The ability of HIV-1 to rapidly mutate may facilitate both its ability to escape immune surveillance and to mimic host antigens. Direct infection of megakaryocytes results in defective platelet production and megakaryocytic apoptosis.

Epidemiologic studies suggest that the pathogenesis of thrombocytopenia is partially dependent on disease burden. HIV-ITP developing early after infection more often resembles classic ITP in which thrombocytopenia is mediated primarily by peripheral destruction, whereas thrombocytopenia in patients with immunologic AIDS (CD4 lymphocytes <2 × 10^9/L) is attributable predominately to decreased platelet production and ineffective hematopoiesis. Although platelet counts may improve with antiretroviral therapy in both patient populations, patients with advanced disease are less likely to respond to classic primary ITP therapy such as splenectomy, corticosteroids, intravenous immunoglobulin, or anti-Rh(D). Initial studies of HIV-associated ITP suggested that an immune complex mechanism was responsible for the thrombocytopenia, wherein platelets were cleared from the circulation as "innocent bystanders." More recent studies have shown that these immune complexes contain antibodies that cross-react with both HIV and platelet glycoproteins. These antibodies also cross-reacted with sequences on HIV nef, gag, env, and pol proteins. Similar cross-reactivity between HIV viral proteins and platelet glycoproteins has been reported in the studies of Bettlaieb et al,[15] who eluted immunoglobulin from platelets from patients with HIV-ITP and found these antibodies bound to antigenic epitopes common to both platelet GPIIIa and HIV GP160.

Studies of platelet kinetics have demonstrated that HIV-ITP is frequently associated with decreased platelet production. Megakaryocytes express the CD4 receptor and coreceptors necessary for HIV infection. Cytopathic infection of HIV of the megakaryocyte has been demonstrated and is the postulated primary mechanism for impaired megakaryopoiesis. However, the potential of cross-reactive antibodies between HIV-related proteins and platelet glycoproteins capable of inducing apoptosis of megakaryocytes as has been described with primary ITP has not been studied.

Clinical Manifestations

HIV-seropositive patients can develop thrombocytopenia several years before the development of overt AIDS, and the early disease is clinically indistinguishable from classic ITP. However, the clinical picture of HIV-ITP is often mild, with only a minority of patients having platelet counts of less than 50 × 10^9/L. Major bleeding is rare, and only a few cases of fatal hemorrhage have been reported. There has been greater variability in patients with hemophilia A. For example, in one report of thrombocytopenia (platelets <100 × 10^9/L) in 14 of 124 (11%) hemophiliacs, only 1 patient had a major hemorrhage. In contrast, in another report of patients with a platelet count of less than 100 × 10^9/L in 30 of 87 (34%) hemophiliac patients, with 11 (13%) having a platelet count of less than 50 × 10^9/L, 9 of the 11 patients (82%) had major bleeding complications and 3 suffered fatal hemorrhage.

Severe thrombocytopenia in patients with advanced HIV infection is frequently associated with additional cytopenias. In a study of 52 HIV-infected intravenous drug users with thrombocytopenia, 4 patients (8%) with advanced HIV infection had a hypocellular bone marrow examination and pancytopenia. HIV-infected drug users were also more likely to have antibodies to both hepatitis B and C and to have abnormal liver function studies. The role of immune-mediated platelet destruction versus bone marrow failure in patients with advanced HIV disease is still uncertain.

Treatment of HIV-ITP

HIV-ITP is generally responsive to therapeutic interventions used in classic ITP. Therapy with prednisone produces a major hematologic response (platelet count >100 × 10^9/L) in over half of all patients, although only a minority will maintain a platelet count of greater than 50 × 10^9/L after cessation of steroids. Despite the initial anxiety regarding the use of corticosteroids in HIV-infected, immune-suppressed patients, no deleterious effect of short-term treatment with prednisone has become evident. However, long-term treatment with corticosteroids should still be avoided, and other coinfections such as tuberculosis, CMV, or hepatitis C should be excluded before initiating treatment with corticosteroids. Intravenous immunoglobulin (IVIg) and anti-Rh(D) are equally effective in increasing platelet counts acutely in severely affected patients, but a crossover study clearly demonstrated a longer duration of response with the latter agent.

Splenectomy has proven to be safe and effective in refractory patients with HIV-TP. After splenectomy, there is a transient increase in the peripheral blood CD4 lymphocyte count, which reflects redistribution from the splenic pool into the circulation rather than an improvement in the patient's immunologic status.

HIV-related hematologic cytopenias have been shown to correlate with plasma viral load. Effective antiretroviral therapies have resulted in improvement in several HIV-related cytopenias, including HIV-CITP. Zidovudine monotherapy increased platelet counts in 60% to 70% of HIV-CITP patients. Although other antiretroviral drugs have been shown to improve hematologic parameters in patients with advanced HIV infection, their efficacy as monotherapy for the management of HIV-CITP is less well documented. Use of HAART in both de novo and zidovudine-refractory HIV-CITP has induced sustained platelet responses in association with effective viral suppression.

Responses to zidovudine and HAART may be more limited in HIV-infected intravenous drug users, possibly reflecting the impact of associated liver disease and infection with hepatitis C virus. In a prospective placebo-controlled, double-blind, randomized trial, 12 of 14 (86%) zidovudine-refractory HIV-infected intravenous drug users with elevated serum alanine aminotransferase levels suggestive of underlying liver disease who were treated with interferon-α had a statistically significant increase in their platelet counts by week 4 of therapy. Similar responses to interferon-α therapy alone have been reported in HIV-seronegative, hepatitis C virus–infected patients. An open label trial of interferon-α in a cohort of predominately homosexual men documented responses in 9 of 16 (56%) patients, with responses occurring as early as 2 weeks after the initiation of treatment. Such rapid responses preclude the possibility that improvement in the platelet count is due solely to suppression of concomitant hepatitis C virus infection. At present there are no data evaluating the efficacy of the new approved thrombopoietin receptor agonists, romiplostim and eltrombopag, in the management of HIV-related thrombocytopenia, but long-term efficacy and safety data regarding the use of these agents in primary ITP would suggest that they would be effective in the management of HIV-ITP.

THROMBOTIC MICROANGIOPATHY AND THROMBOTIC THROMBOCYTOPENIC PURPURA

Thrombotic microangiopathy, including both TTP and the hemolytic uremic syndrome (HUS), is a well-described complication of HIV infection seen in approximately 1% of patients. The incidence of this complication appears to have decreased with the advent of HAART therapy. The incidence of TTP appears to be similar to that observed in the general population, whereas HUS appears more frequently in patients with advanced HIV infection.

TTP can occur anytime in the course of HIV infection and has been reported in some patients to be the initial manifestation of HIV infection. This life-threatening disorder is characterized by thrombocytopenia and microangiopathic (fragmentation) hemolytic anemia. The original description of this disorder emphasized a classic pentad of fever, thrombocytopenia, microangiopathic hemolytic anemia, renal failure, and neurologic abnormalities. However, most patients present with only one or two manifestations of the original pentad, and isolated thrombocytopenia may be the initial finding. Therefore it is essential that the evaluation of thrombocytopenia include a careful review of the peripheral blood smear.

TTP is the result of a failure to process endothelial-derived high-molecular-weight von Willebrand factor due to an absence of or inhibitor to the von Willebrand factor cleaving protease (a disintegrin and metalloproteinase with thrombospondin motifs [ADAMTS13]). Measurement of ADAMTS13 activity before the initiation of plasma exchange will report levels nearly always less than 10%, and additional assays will often detect an inhibitor to the protease. First-line therapy is daily plasma exchange until remission and maintenance of platelet count at 150×10^9/L, though there are a number of reported differences in how to use plasma exchange in the management of this disorder. Initial plasma exchanges should be at least a 1.5 plasma volume exchange. Corticosteroids such as prednisone (1 mg/kg/day) also can be given with the exchanges. If plasma exchange is not immediately available, infusion of fresh frozen plasma alone has been shown to be effective in patients with HIV-associated TTP. In classic TTP, relapses can occur in up to 30% of patients; however, relapse in HIV-associated TTP appears to be less frequent. Patients who relapse can be treated with repeat exchange combined with immunosuppressive therapy including agents such as vincristine or rituximab.

HUS most likely results from endothelial perturbation secondary to either HIV or other viral infections such as CMV or is drug or toxin induced, such as observed with *Escherichia coli* 0157:H7 infection. Recent data suggest that the primary event leads to unregulated complement activation due to either inhibitors of complement regulatory protein such as complement H or congenital abnormalities in complement regulation. In these patients measurement of ADAMTS13 activity will uniformly report levels near normal and above 30%. Many patients will respond to aggressive plasma exchange, but complete remissions are rare. Recently the inhibitor of complement C5a, eculizumab, has been approved for the treatment of atypical HUS, but there are no reports of its use in HIV-associated HUS.

THROMBOEMBOLIC DISEASE

Since the beginning of the AIDS epidemic, an unexpectedly high incidence of venous thromboembolism (VTE) has been observed among people with HIV disease (see box on Thromboembolic Disease in HIV/AIDS). The most compelling data in support of an increased risk for VTE in HIV disease estimated the incidence of thrombosis in their HIV-infected population to be about 2.6 per 1000 person-years. Given the fact that cohorts of patients with HIV infection tend to include a disproportionate number of younger individuals compared with the general population, this figure represents an increased incidence of VTE. The increased incidence in venous thrombosis was disproportionately greater among patients with clinical AIDS, those older than 45 years, those with AIDS-defining illnesses (particularly CMV infection), and those taking indinavir (Crixivan) or megestrol acetate (Megace). However, 53% of the thrombotic events occurred in individuals without history of recent hospitalization.

In a study comparing the risk for VTE in HIV-infected patients to an age-matched uninfected control population, there was no statistical difference in the overall risk for VTE (2.8% HIV-infected patients versus 1.8% controls) except in the HIV-infected patients less than 50 years of age (3.31% HIV-infected patients versus 0.53% controls; P <0.0001). A study of 37,535 HIV-infected veterans compared to 37,535 age-, race-, and site-matched uninfected controls found a 39% increased incidence in VTE in the pre-HAART era (before 1996) and a 33% increased incidence in the era of HAART therapy. The increased risk for thrombosis was independent of a diagnosis of malignancy, HIV-related opportunistic infections, or the use of central catheters. The development of a thromboembolic event was associated with statistically increased mortality in all groups.

Thromboembolic Disease in HIV/AIDS

The estimated incidence of thrombosis in the HIV-infected population is about 2.6 per 1000 person-years. Given the fact that cohorts of patients with HIV infection tend to include a disproportionate number of younger individuals compared with the general population, this figure represents an increased incidence of venous thromboembolism (VTE). The increased incidence in venous thrombosis is disproportionately greater among patients with clinical AIDS, those older than 45 years, those with AIDS-defining illnesses, and those taking indinavir (Crixivan) or megestrol acetate (Megace). With advancing HIV disease, there are progressive prothrombotic hemostatic changes, specifically a decrease in protein S and an increase in factor VIII. It is well established that antiphospholipid antibodies (anticardiolipin antibodies [ACA] and lupus anticoagulant) are associated with a hypercoagulable state. The incidence of elevated ACA in asymptomatic HIV disease is reported to be as high as 50% and even higher in patients with clinical AIDS. Certain protease inhibitors (indinavir) have been found to be associated with VTE. The overall management principles and goals of therapy for VTE are the same for people with and without HIV infection, although extra caution is needed to anticipate possible drug interactions with highly active antiretroviral therapy (HAART), particularly with the use of warfarin.

AIDS, Acquired immunodeficiency syndrome; *HIV,* human immunodeficiency virus.

Role of Inflammation and Its Effect on the Protein C and S Anticoagulant System

With advancing HIV disease, there are progressive prothrombotic hemostatic changes, specifically a decrease in protein S and an increase in factor VIII. There is a well-documented association between acute and chronic inflammation and activation of the hemostatic system. Inflammatory cytokines such as TNF-α, IL-1, and IL-6 have been shown to activate coagulation and downregulate activation of protein C. Activated protein C (APC) is a major inhibitor of coagulation, degrading activated coagulation factors VIIIa and Va. Inflammation can also result in a decrease in functional protein S, the cofactor of APC, which most likely explains the acquired protein S deficiency observed in some HIV-infected patients, without and with thrombosis.

An important additional component of the inflammatory state, which further contributes to an increased risk for thrombosis, is the inflammation-induced increase in factor VIII coagulant protein. Factor VIII levels greater than 1500 units/L (150%) are an independent risk factor for idiopathic VTE. A study of 94 HIV-infected women and 50 HIV-negative controls who were participants in the Women's Interagency HIV Study documented a progressive prothrombotic state with advancing HIV disease characterized by progressive decreases in protein S activity associated with a progressive increase in factor VIII activity. The decreases in protein S activity and reciprocal increases in factor VIII activity closely correlated with decreasing $CD4^+$ lymphocyte count and were most significant in the women with clinical AIDS. This study provides evidence for a link between advancing HIV disease characterized by decreasing $CD4^+$ lymphocyte count and the development of clinical AIDS with opportunistic infections and hemostatic changes associated with an increased risk for venous thrombosis. This acute and chronic inflammatory state is the most likely pathogenic mechanism for development of VTE in HIV-infected individuals.

Anticardiolipin Antibodies

It is well established that antiphospholipid antibodies (anticardiolipin antibodies [ACAs] and lupus anticoagulant) are associated with a hypercoagulable state. The incidence of elevated levels of ACA in asymptomatic HIV disease is reported to be as high as 50% and even higher in patients with clinical AIDS. Recent reports have documented the presence of ACAs in HIV-infected individuals with VTE. However, two small studies reported no correlation between high levels of ACA and thrombosis in HIV infection. Because the increased thrombotic risk associated with the antiphospholipid antibody syndrome is predominantly associated with the lupus anticoagulant and β_2-glycoprotein 1, it is not surprising that increased level of ACA alone was not associated with a significantly increased risk for thrombosis. Thus the contribution of antiphospholipid antibodies to the development of VTE in HIV disease remains unknown and will require larger prospective studies that include assays for the lupus anticoagulant and anti–β_2-glycoprotein antibodies.

Role of Protease Inhibitors

Several investigators have found protease inhibitors to be associated with VTE. Sullivan et al[16] reported that the use of indinavir was associated with an increased risk for VTE. In a case series, George et al[17] reported unexplained thrombosis in HIV patients receiving protease inhibitors. Abnormalities of glucose metabolism and serum lipids are commonly observed with protease inhibitor therapy. These include acquired insulin resistance, increased levels of low-density–lipoprotein cholesterol, and decreased levels of high-density–lipoprotein cholesterol. Insulin resistance is associated with acquired defects in the fibrinolytic system, including increased levels of plasminogen activator inhibitor and tissue plasminogen activator. Similar fibrinolytic abnormalities have been observed in patients with documented insulin resistance who are treated with protease inhibitors.

High-density–lipoprotein cholesterol has been shown to significantly enhance the activity of the APC complexed with protein S. This APC complex plays an essential role in downregulating thrombin generation. The lipoprotein abnormalities associated with the use of protease inhibitors, when combined with other acquired defects in the protein C anticoagulant pathway, may further depress the anticoagulant activity of the APC complex and subsequently promote increased thrombin generation. Thus there are a number of pathogenic mechanisms that could predispose HIV-infected patients to VTE. The majority of reported hemostatic abnormalities appear primarily to affect the protein C and S inhibitory mechanisms. However, the available studies reporting an increased risk for VTE in HIV disease are only suggestive at present because most supporting data come from case reports and one uncontrolled retrospective study. Larger prospective studies are needed to assess the true relative risk for VTE in HIV-infected individuals and to determine the primary pathogenic mechanisms responsible for thrombosis in this population.

Management of VTE With HIV Infection

The overall management principles and goals of therapy for VTE are the same for people with and without HIV infection, although extra caution is needed to anticipate possible drug interactions with HAART, particularly with the use of warfarin. Initial therapy for the patient presenting with deep vein thrombosis and/or pulmonary emboli involves the use of either intravenous unfractionated heparin (UFH) or preferentially subcutaneous low-molecular-weight heparin (LMWH). Oral anticoagulants can be started immediately upon achieving therapeutic heparin levels, and under optimal circumstances heparin treatment can be completed and the patient discharged from the hospital within 5 to 7 days. LMWH preparations given subcutaneously without monitoring have been shown to be safe and effective treatment for VTE and may be preferable because they also allow for safe outpatient management. In a metaanalysis of clinical trials comparing LMWH with UFH, LMWH preparations were associated with a lower risk for major bleeding compared with adjusted-dose intravenous UFH.

The greatest difficulties in the management of VTE in HIV-infected patients occur with the use of oral anticoagulants. The optimal therapeutic range for oral anticoagulation with warfarin in patients with VTE is a prothrombin time (PT) international normalized ratio (INR) of 2 to 3. No data suggest that HIV-infected patients require a different degree of anticoagulation. However, most studies have found that general medical patients managed as outpatients have a therapeutic INR in only 60% of assays. Although there are no published data regarding the use of oral anticoagulants in HIV-infected patients, individuals receiving HAART appear to have greater difficulty in maintaining therapeutic anticoagulation, most likely due to complex drug interactions. With a reported annual risk for major bleeding with oral anticoagulants of 2% to 3% and bleeding-related fatality of 20%, careful PT monitoring of HIV-infected patients is mandatory. They should be monitored at least weekly for the first 6 to 8 weeks and should then have their PT checked every 2 weeks. In patients in whom maintaining therapeutic levels is difficult, home monitoring using devices approved by the U.S. Food and Drug Administration may be indicated. Patients who have significant difficulty maintaining a therapeutic INR or have had bleeding complications because of poor control of their anticoagulation can be treated with long-term LMWH as has been recommended for the long-term management of cancer-related VTE. In both HIV-infected and HIV-negative patients with malignancies who develop VTE, long-term management with LMWH appears to be associated with a significantly lower risk for recurrent VTE.

Oral anticoagulation in the patient with VTE should be maintained for at least 6 months. Patients with unprovoked VTE who have had major pulmonary emboli, recurrent thromboemboli, or underlying inherited or acquired prothrombotic defects may benefit from longer courses of oral anticoagulation. However, the decision to extend anticoagulation to prevent recurrence of thrombosis must be weighed against the significant risk for bleeding in this population.

REFERENCES

1. Shen H, Cheng T, Preffer FI, et al: Intrinsic human immunodeficiency virus type 1 resistance of hematopoietic stem cells despite coreceptor expression. *J Virol* 73:728, 1999.
2. Bahner I, Kearns K, Coutinho S, et al: Infection of human marrow immunodeficiency virus-1 (HIV-1) is both required and sufficient for HIV-1 inducted hematopoietic suppression in vitro: Demonstration by gene modification of primary human stroma. *Blood* 90:1787, 1997.

3. Gradstein S, Hahn T, Barak Y, et al: In vitro effects of recombinant TNF-alfa binding protein (rTBP-1) on hematopoiesis of HIV-infected patients. *J Acquir Immune Defic Syndr* 26:111, 2001.
4. Huang SS, Barbour JD, Deeks SG, et al: Reversal of immunodeficiency virus type 1-associated hematosuppression by effective antiretroviral therapy. *Clin Infect Dis* 30:504, 2000.
5. Parker NG, Notermans DW, de Boer RG, et al: Biphasic kinetics of peripheral blood T cells after triple combination therapy in HIV-1 infection: A composite of redistribution and proliferation. *Nat Med* 4:208, 1998.
6. Zhao X, Sun NC, Witt MD, et al: Changing pattern of AIDS: A bone marrow study. *Am J Clin Pathol* 121:393, 2004.
7. Sullivan PS, Hanson DL, Chu SY, et al: Epidemiology of anemia in human immunodeficiency virus (HIV)-infected persons: Results from the Multistate Adult and Adolescent Spectrum of HIV Disease Surveillance Project. *Blood* 91:301, 1998.
8. Abrams DI, Steinhart C, Frascino R: Epoetin alfa therapy for anaemia in HIV-infected patients: Impact on quality of life. *Int J STD AIDS* 11:659, 2000.
9. Coyle TE: Hematological complications of human immunodeficiency virus infection and the acquired immunodeficiency syndrome. *Med Clin North Am* 81:449, 1997.
10. Isgrò I, Auiti A, Mezzaroma I, et al: HIV type I protease inhibitors enhance bone marrow progenitor cell activity in normal subjects and HIV type 1-infected patients. *AIDS Res Hum Retroviruses* 21:51, 2005.
11. Berhane K, Karim R, Cohen MH, et al: Impact of highly active antiretroviral therapy on anemia and relationship between anemia and survival in a large cohort of HIV-infected women. *J Acquir Immune Defic Syndr* 37:1245, 2004.
12. de Mayolo JA, Temple JD: Pure red cell aplasia due to parvovirus B19 infection in a man with HIV infection. *South Med J* 83:1480, 1990.
13. Chen M, Chien-Ching H, Fang C, et al: Reconstituted immunity against persistent parvovirus B19 infection in a patient with acquired immunodeficiency syndrome after highly active antiretroviral therapy. *Clin Infect Dis* 32:1361, 2001.
14. Mientjes GH, van Ameijden EJ, Malder JW, et al: Prevalence of thrombocytopenia in HIV-infected and non-HIV infected drug users and homosexual men. *Br J Haematol* 82:615, 1992.
15. Battaieb A, Fromont P, Louache F, et al: Presence of cross-reactive antibody between HIV and platelet glycoproteins in HIV-realted immune thrombocytopenic purpura. *Blood* 80:162, 1992.
16. Sullivan PS, Dworkin MS, Jones JL, et al: Epidemiology of thrombosis in HIV-infected individuals. *AIDS* 14:321, 2000.
17. George S, Swindells S, Knudson R, et al: Unexplained thrombosis in HIV-infected patients receiving protease inhibitors: Report of seven cases. *Am J Med* 107:624, 1999.

CHAPTER 160

HEMATOLOGIC ASPECTS OF PARASITIC DISEASES

David J. Roberts

Parasitic diseases are not common in medical, let alone hematologic, practice in North America or Europe. However, much of the world's population are infected and become symptomatic from a plethora of parasites, and many of these infections represent global public health problems.

Although some significant parasitic diseases are transmitted in temperate climates, the majority of parasites of significance to human health are endemic in the tropical world. This reflects not only socioeconomic circumstances but also the origin of our species in tropical Africa, where the human host, parasites, and also vectors have established complex relationships over evolutionary timescales.[1] Notwithstanding such geographic variation in the incidence of parasitic disease, both travelers and recent immigrants now present to hematology clinics and laboratories all over the world with increasing frequency. Even here, there are marked variations in practice in North America and Europe, where the United Kingdom reports more cases of imported malaria than the United States and indeed has a 10-fold greater incidence of malaria per capita, reflecting the increased frequency of travel to and from endemic areas compared to North American populations.

Malaria, leishmaniasis, trypanosomiasis, and babesiosis may present directly or indirectly to hematologists. This account will concentrate on the biologic, clinical, and hematologic features of these infections and the hematologic aspects or complications of their treatment. Comprehensive accounts of the general medical aspects of these diseases are provided in many recent textbooks.[2-4]

MALARIA

Malaria is a major public health problem in tropical areas, and it is estimated that it is responsible for 600,000 to 900,000 deaths annually and 150 to 300 million infections.[5] The vast majority of morbidity and mortality from malaria is caused by infection with *Plasmodium falciparum,* although *Plasmodium vivax, Plasmodium ovale,* and *Plasmodium malariae* also are responsible for human infections. Recently a fifth species, *Plasmodium knowlesi,* has been shown to cause human infection in some parts of Southeast Asia (for review see reference 5). In endemic areas, a significant proportion of the mortality and morbidity is due to anemia. In Europe and North America, malaria is not infrequently a clinical problem in travelers or recent arrivals from malaria-endemic areas, and hematologists may be involved in the diagnosis and management of the disease. Moreover, in nonendemic areas, malaria may cause a fatal transfusion-transmitted infection, and detection of blood donors who may be carrying the disease represents a major challenge for blood services.

Epidemiology

Approximately 1000 million people live in areas of endemic or epidemic malaria. The global mortality and morbidity have been revised to 350 million cases and 1 million deaths per year following an evaluation of the prevalence of infection in Southeast Asia (Fig. 160-1). There is substantial evidence that the incidence of severe disease is now falling, sometimes spectacularly, in many parts of Africa following the widespread introduction of artemisinin combination treatment, impregnated bed nets, and residual spraying because the resources available for malaria control have increased substantially through the Global Fund and the World Health Organization's "Roll Back Malaria" campaign (www.rbm.who.int/).[6]

The distribution of malaria is determined by features of host, vector, and parasite. In summary, the global distribution of autochthonous or endogenous malaria is limited by the lower temperature limits for development of the parasite in the mosquito (sporogony) of 20° C for *P. falciparum* and 15° C for other human malarias. Within these limits transmission does not occur above 1500 m in arid regions or in the Central and South Pacific (due to the absence of suitable vectors). In addition, *P. vivax* malaria is rare in Africa where the population frequency of the blood group Duffy negative (Fya^-Fyb^-) is high. *P. ovale* requires a lengthy period of sporogony and is confined to areas of Africa and Southeast Asia with a high density of susceptible *Anopheles* spp. *P. knowlesi* is transmitted from macaque monkeys in forest areas of Borneo, Malaysia, Thailand, and Vietnam.[5]

In some malarious areas the seasonal pattern of clinical malaria is determined by the increase in vector density after rainfall, leading to an increase in new infections as transmission increases. In naive individuals, parasites can cause chronic infection lasting many months.

The intensity of transmission determines the distribution of clinical symptoms in different age-groups.[7] In general, in areas of high transmission younger children suffer from severe disease. Where transmission is less intense, older children suffer from severe disease. Finally, if the rate of transmission is very low, few cases of malaria are seen in any age-group and such populations would have little natural immunity. In such areas, a sudden increase in vectorial capacity (through the accidental introduction of efficient vectors or higher density, biting, or survival of the resident vectors), more rapid parasite sporogony, or migration of infected or nonimmune populations can result in epidemics where large numbers fall ill in all age-groups. The transition from high to low transmission has been classified by holoendemicity, hyperendemicity, mesoendemicity, and hypoendemicity. These categories can be related epidemiologically to age-specific rates of parasite prevalence or splenomegaly and theoretically to the reproductive ratio of malarial infection.[8]

Malaria exerts a substantial selection for human traits that protect from infection. Sickle cell trait and thalassemia traits protect from infection and are truly polymorphic characteristics in many parts of the world. Understanding the genetic epidemiology has provided the foundation of population genetics and has provided classic examples of principles of genetic selection in vivo—for example, balancing selection for sickle cell trait and negative epistasis for sickle cell trait and α-thalassemia. The homozygous forms of these characteristics cause significant clinical disease, for example, sickle cell disease, β-thalassemia, and glucose-6-phosphate dehydrogenase reduced (G6PDH) deficiency. In endemic areas, these genetic diseases represent major public health problems (for review see references 9 and 10).

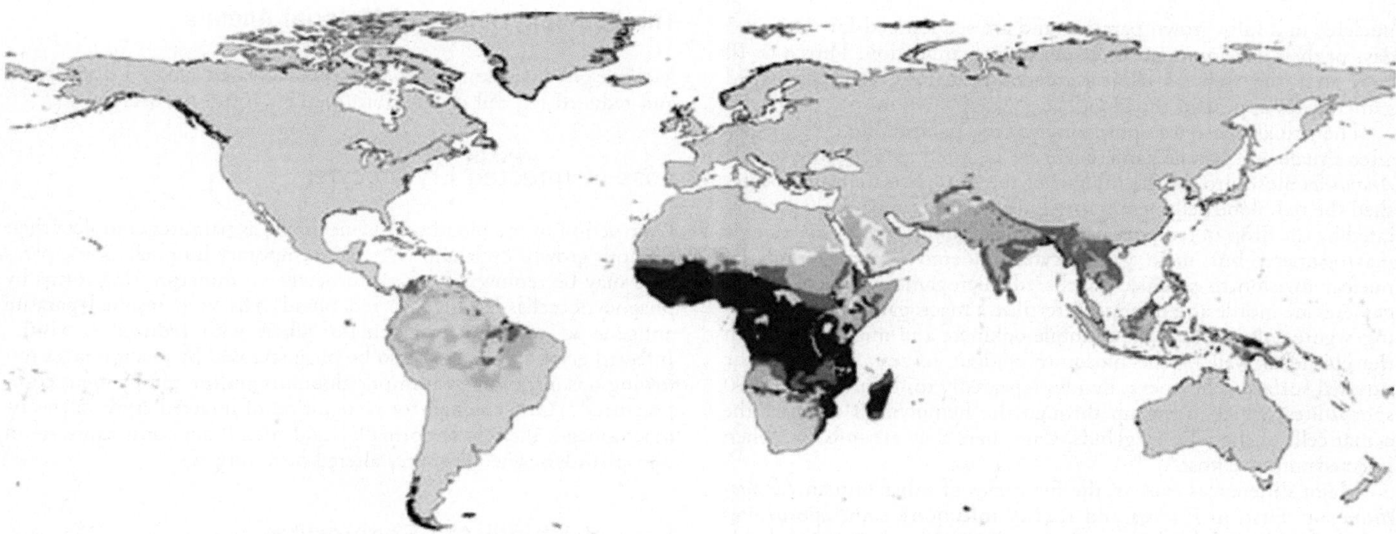

Figure 160-1 GLOBAL MALARIA ENDEMICITY. Areas are colored according to malaria endemicity (prevalence): *light green,* hypoendemic (areas in which childhood infection prevalence is less than 10%); *medium green,* mesoendemic (areas with infection prevalence between 11% and 50%); *dark green,* hyperendemic and holoendemic (areas with an infection prevalence of 50% or more); unclassified areas *(yellow)* represent only 6% of the global population at risk and are due to discrepancies in recent data. Grey areas are a combined mask of areas outside of the transmission limits and areas of population density less than 1 person/km^2. *(Data from Snow RW, Guerra CA, Noor AM, et al: The global distribution of clinical episodes of* Plasmodium falciparum *malaria,* Nature *434:214, 2005.)*

Parasitology

In *P. falciparum* (see later for a discussion of the other human parasites) the infective sporozoite forms are inoculated into the bloodstream from the salivary glands of a female *Anopheles* mosquito (Fig. 160-2). These thin, needle-shaped cells, 10 to 12 μm in length, circulate briefly with a half-life of approximately 30 minutes, before traversing macrophages and several hepatocytes before residing in a single hepatocyte.[11,12] Here rapid multiplication takes place over 5 to 8 days to produce a liver schizont, 80 μm in diameter and containing 30,000 ± 10,000 merozoites that are released into the bloodstream, where they infect erythrocytes.[13] When ready to leave hepatocytes, the parasite induces cell death in the hepatocytes and causes the release of merozoites in membrane-enclosed structures or merosomes that are extruded from the infected cell, so avoiding host cell defense mechanisms.[14]

The merozoites bind and then invade red blood cells (for review of red cell and merozoite interactions see reference 15). The host plasma membrane is invaginated to form the parasitophorous vacuole. For the first 10 hours, the developing parasites appear as fine "ring forms." Between 10 and 15 hours, the cytoplasm thickens, and 16 hours after invasion granules of the black pigment hematin, the end product of hemoglobin digestion, begin to appear. Ligands are expressed at the surface of the infected red blood cell that mediate adhesion to host receptors on venular endothelium. These trophozoites no longer circulate throughout the body but are sequestered in the peripheral circulation. Nuclear division begins, at approximately 30 hours, to form schizonts, containing up to 32 merozoites. At 48 hours, the red blood cell is ruptured to release the merozoites into the circulation to continue further cycles of asexual multiplication.

The erythrocytic cycle of schizogony may achieve a 10-fold increase in parasitemia in vivo and a patent or microscopically detectable infection 6 days after the liver stage is completed. After two or more cycles, the infection becomes clinically apparent by the paroxysms of fever that accompany the release of merozoites. Cycles of schizogony continue until the rate of parasite multiplication is reduced by chemotherapy, specific or nonspecific defense mechanisms, or occasionally, the demise of the host.

Some merozoites do not multiply but become committed during the previous erythrocytic cycle to form male or female gametocytes.[16] Gametocytes are distinguished by dispersed pigment in a single

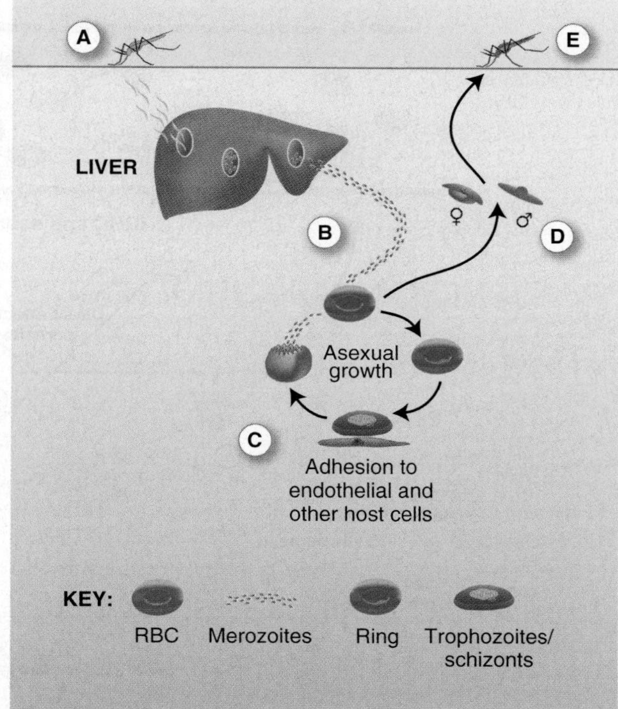

Figure 160-2 PLASMODIUM LIFE CYCLE. **A,** The asexual life cycle begins when sporozoites from a female mosquito taking a blood meal enter the circulation and invade hepatocytes. **B,** Up to 10,000 merozoites are formed. Following rupture of the hepatocyte, infective merozoites are released and invade erythrocytes (RBC). **C,** Within RBC, the parasite develops through the stages of rings, trophozoites, and schizonts. Mature schizonts burst to release erythrocytic merozoites that invade new RBC. **D,** A small proportion of merozoites in RBC transform into male and female gametocytes that are ingested by the mosquito. **E,** The male and female gametes fuse and transform into an oocyst, which divides asexually into many sporozoites that migrate to the salivary gland from where they are released during the next blood meal.

nucleus, in a fully grown parasite, and are sequestered for the first 5 days of their development in the peripheral circulation. Thus 8 to 10 days after the start of clinical infection, mature, crescent-shaped gametocytes appear in the blood.

The sexual phase (or sporogony) of the parasite life cycle begins after a male and female gametocyte are ingested by a feeding female *Anopheles* mosquito. In the midgut of the mosquito the gametocytes shed the red blood cell membrane. This change is apparently precipitated by the drop in temperature. A female gametocyte forms a single macrogamete, but male gametocytes undergo several rounds of nuclear division to produce flagellated microgametes. These microgametes are motile and migrate to fertilize a macrogamete. The resulting zygote enlarges to form a mobile ookinete and migrates through the epithelial wall of the mosquito midgut to rest finally on the external surface. The oocyst divides repeatedly to form up to 10,000 sporozoites, which travel up through the hemolymph to enter the acinar cells of the salivary glands. Once here they are infective when injected into the host.

Major differences exist in the life cycles of other human *Plasmodium* spp. First, in *P. vivax* and *P. ovale* infections, some sporozoites entering the liver form dormant hypnozoites that only begin to divide after a variable period of some months to cause further blood-stage infections or relapses. Second, the cycle of erythrocytic development in *P. malariae* takes 72 hours and thus causes quartan fever (i.e., on days 1 and 4).

The Pathophysiology of Malarial Anemia

Malaria gives ample reasons for both increased red cell destruction and reduced red cell production (see Fig. 160-3 for overview).

Loss of Infected Erythrocytes

Destruction of red blood cells is inevitable as parasites complete their 48-hour growth cycle and lyse their temporary host cell. Some parasites may be removed from erythrocytes as immature ring forms by phagocytic cells, leaving the red blood cells with residual parasite antigens to continue to circulate, albeit with reduced survival.[17] Infected erythrocytes may also be phagocytosed by macrophages following opsonization by immunoglobulins and/or complement components.[18,19] Other signals for recognition of infected erythrocytes by macrophages include abnormally rigid membranes and exposure of phosphatidylserine and other altered host antigens.[20-22]

Loss of Uninfected Erythrocytes

The activity and the number of macrophages are increased in malarial infection, and increased removal of uninfected cells may occur. Moreover, the signals for recognition of uninfected erythrocytes for removal

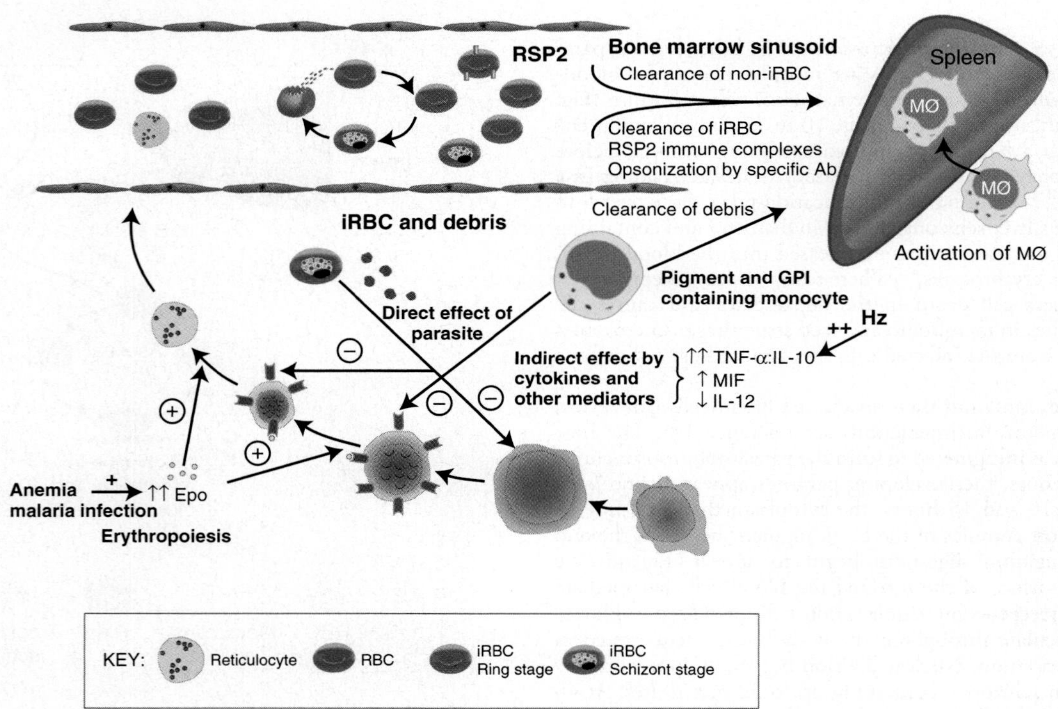

Figure 160-3 PATHOGENESIS OF MALARIAL ANEMIA. Severe malarial anemia is characterized by destruction of infected red blood cell (iRBC) following schizogony and clearance of both iRBC and uninfected RBC. During malarial infection, changes in membrane protein composition occur, and the resultant immune complexes of RBC, Ag, and immunoglobulin (Ig) (e.g., RBC-RSP2-Ig) are cleared by macrophages to the spleen, where they become activated. Pigment-containing macrophages may release inflammatory cytokines and other biologically active mediators such as 4-hydroxynonenal (HNE). Macrophage inhibitory factor (MIF) may be released by macrophages or a plasmodial homologue may suppress erythropoiesis. Malarial pigment or other parasite products may have a direct inhibitory effect on erythropoiesis. Inhibition of erythropoiesis may be at one or more sites in the growth and differentiation of hematopoietic progenitors. Both indirect and direct effects may cause suppression of the bone marrow and spleen resulting in inadequate reticulocyte counts for the degree of anemia. *Ab,* Antibody; *Ag,* antigen; *Epo,* erythropoietin; *GPI,* glycosylphosphatidylinositol anchors of merozoite proteins; *Hz,* hemozoin; *IL,* interleukin; *Mϕ,* macrophage; *RSP2,* ring surface protein-2; *TNF-α,* tumor necrosis factor-α.

by macrophages are enhanced. Uninfected erythrocytes bind increased amounts of immunoglobulin and/or complement as detected in the direct antiglobulin test (DAT or Coombs test).[23] These antibodies do not have a particular specificity but are more likely to represent immune complexes absorbed onto the surface of red blood cells.[23] Furthermore, hemozoin may activate complement directly and cause deposition of C3b on uninfected red blood cells.[24] However, an association between positive DAT results and severe anemia has not been established.[25] More recent studies have shown that red cells from malaria patients were not only more susceptible to phagocytosis but also red cells from children with acute malaria showed increased surface IgG and low levels of red cell CR1 and CD55 compared with controls.[26]

Role of the Spleen

Some degree of splenomegaly is a normal feature of malarial infection, and the prevalence of splenomegaly in regions of malarial transmission is used as a major indicator of the level of malarial endemicity. The importance of the spleen in host defense against malaria has been demonstrated in experimental systems, and individuals whose spleens have been surgically removed are thought to be more susceptible to severe infection. Indeed, the phenomenon of parasitic sequestration is thought to have evolved primarily as an immune evasion strategy so the mature parasite can avoid passing through the spleen.[27]

Active erythrophagocytosis is a conspicuous feature within the bone marrow during *P. vivax* and *P. falciparum* malaria,[28,29] and it is highly probable that this also occurs within the spleen. Cytokines may be responsible for activating macrophages during malarial infection. Children with acute *P. falciparum* malaria have high circulating levels of interferon-γ (IFN-γ) and tumor necrosis factor-αTNF-α,[30] a synergistic combination of cytokines that activate macrophages.

Several studies have attempted to define the pathophysiologic changes in the spleen during acute malaria. In animal models, malaria is accompanied by increased intravascular clearance of infected or rigid, heat-treated cells by the spleen,[31] and alterations in the splenic microcirculation.[32] In studies of human malaria it has been found that increased splenic clearance of heated red cells occurs during acute attacks.[33] More recent, histologic studies and ex vivo models of splenic function suggest that the spleen removes not only mature infected red blood cells but also uninfected cells marked for clearance by low deformability, aggregated band 3, complement deposition, or phosphatidylserine exposure. Moreover, "pitting" of ring-stage infected cells may remove the parasite and leave the red cell marked with parasite antigen to return to the circulation (reviewed in Reference 34).

Changes to the uninfected red blood cells during infection also contribute to their own enhanced clearance by phagocytes. Uninfected red cells in children and adults with severe disease are less deformable, and this is a significant predictor of the severity of anemia and indeed outcome, consistent with the notion that these cells are being removed by the spleen.[20] It has also been found that immunoglobulin (Ig) G–sensitized red cells are rapidly removed from the circulation by the spleen and that unusually rapid clearance persists well into the convalescent phase.[35]

Thus all the available evidence points to increased reticuloendothelial clearance in *P. falciparum* malaria, persisting long after recovery. These changes are presumably a host defense mechanism, maximizing the clearance of parasitized erythrocytes.

The Role of Ineffective Erythropoiesis in Severe Malarial Anemia

Reticulocytopenia has been confirmed in numerous clinical studies of malarial anemia.[36-38] The histopathologic study of the bone marrow of children with malarial anemia shows erythroid hyperplasia with increased numbers of erythroid precursors (Fig. 160-4). However, the maturation is abnormal by light and electron microscopy. Abdalla et al[39,40] described the hallmark characteristics of such abnormal maturation, namely cytoplasmic and nuclear bridging and irregular nuclear outline. They later confirmed that the distribution of the erythroid progenitors through the cell cycle is abnormal in malarial anemia, with an increased proportion of cells in the G2 phase compared with normal controls.[41] Dormer et al[38] confirmed these findings using the same criteria as Abdalla et al; they studied six patients with falciparum malaria before and after treatment.

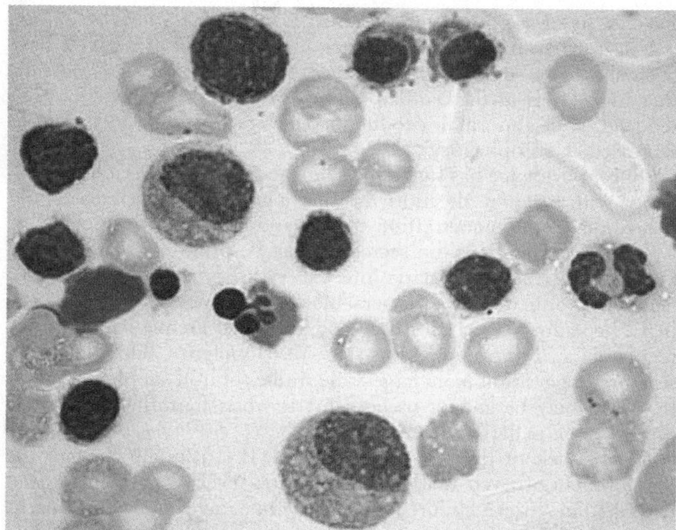

Figure 160-4 BONE MARROW ASPIRATE IN MALARIA. Although erythropoiesis is usually normoblastic in individuals with acute or chronic malaria, the examination of bone marrow frequently shows changes reflecting dyserythropoiesis, such as the irregular nuclei and cytoplasmic bridges in erythroblasts seen in this figure. Two young rings of *Plasmodium falciparum* can be seen in an erythrocyte. *(Courtesy Dr. Saad H. Abdalla.)*

Ineffective erythropoiesis also contributes to anemia in animal models of malaria. A recent study has shown that vaccinated *Aotus* monkeys, after a challenge infection, may develop moderate to severe anemia following rapid clearance of uninfected erythrocytes but with low reticulocyte counts, indicating bone marrow dysfunction.[42] Erythropoiesis is disrupted in mice during malarial infection. Mice infected with *Plasmodium berghei* show reduced bone marrow cellularity, erythroblasts, burst-forming units–erythroid (BFU-E), and colony-forming units–erythroid (CFU-E) as early as 24 hours postinfection.[43] The cellularity and colony-forming unit–spleen (CFU-S) content of the femoral marrow of BALB/c mice infected with *Plasmodium chabaudi adami* decreases as the parasitemia increases.[44]

Modulation of Erythropoiesis by Cytokines

Given the importance of erythropoietin (Epo) to erythropoiesis, attention has been focused on the levels of this crucial cytokine in malarial infection. Serum Epo was appropriately raised in a single study of African children suffering from malarial anemia.[45,46] However, other studies in adults from Thailand and Sudan have suggested that the Epo concentration, although raised, was inappropriate for the degree of anemia.[47,48] The most recent studies of the level of Epo in African children have shown a supraphysiologic rise in Epo levels compared to age-matched community controls with nonmalarial anemia.[49] There is now evidence that these high levels of Epo in children with malarial anemia may exert a cytoprotective effect and reduce the risk for neurologic sequelae or death in children with cerebral malaria.[50]

The prime candidates for the host factors mediating dyserythropoiesis are imbalances of TNF-α, IFN-γ, and interleukin-10 (IL-10). The concentrations of TNF-α and IFN-γ have been correlated with the severity of the disease.[51-53] Whereas low concentrations of TNF-α (<1 ng/mL) stimulate erythropoiesis, higher levels of TNF-α have been shown to suppress erythropoiesis.[53] Furthermore, it is possible that high levels of these inflammatory cytokines may contribute to reduced and abnormal production of erythrocytes and also to increased erythrophagocytosis.

Recent evidence has suggested that the release of hepcidin is associated with malarial infection and that high levels of hepcidin could contribute to the sequestration of iron and impair erythropoiesis.[54,55] The stimulus for hepcidin secretion may be proinflammatory cytokines such as IL-6, but malaria-infected erythrocytes may also enhance hepcidin production by peripheral blood mononuclear cells.[56] Intriguingly, hepcidin released during blood-stage parasitemia may be a key regulator of *P. falciparum* liver-stage development.[57] This data now supports suggestions from large-scale studies of iron supplementation that iron may be at best useless and at worst harmful when given during acute malarial infection.

High levels of the Th2-type cytokine, IL-10, might prevent the development of severe malarial anemia. Low levels of IL-10 have been described in African children with severe malarial anemia.[51] Similarly, defective IL-12 production has been shown experimentally to be associated with increased severity of malaria in a rodent model, and low IL-12 levels have been associated with severe malaria in African children.[58,59]

Modulation of Erythropoiesis by Infected Erythrocytes

There is also substantial evidence that lysate of infected erythrocytes may directly modulate the function of host cells. During its blood stage, the malaria parasite proteolyses host hemoglobin in an acidic vacuole to obtain amino acids, releasing heme as a by-product, which is auto-oxidized to potentially toxic hematin (aquaferriprotoporphyrin IX, H_2O–Fe(III)PPIX). β-Hematin forms as a crystalline cyclic dimer of Fe(III)PPIX and is complexed with protein and lipid products as malarial pigment or hemozoin. Schwarzer et al[60-62] showed that the function of monocytes and of monocyte-derived macrophages is severely inhibited after ingestion of malaria pigment or hemozoin. These cells were unable to repeat phagocytosis and to generate oxidative burst when appropriately stimulated. Furthermore, after phagocytosis of hemozoin, human and murine myeloid cells were unable to kill ingested fungi, bacteria, and tumor cells[63] and to respond to IFN-γ stimulation, but instead responded by increased release of IL-1β and TNF-α,[64] macrophage inflammatory protein-1α (MIP-1α) and MIP-1β.[65]

The hemozoin polymer of heme moieties may be complexed with biologically active compounds. The oxidation of membrane lipids catalyzed by the ferric heme produces the lipoperoxides.[62,66] There is accumulating evidence that 4-hydroxynonenal (HNE) and other lipoperoxides, including 15-hydroxy-arachidonic acid (15-(*R,S*)-HETE), may play a role in the pathophysiology of malaria. It has been shown that HNE and HETE are generated in parasitized erythrocytes and that HNE and endoperoxides produced in pigment-containing monocytes or macrophages may cause cell cycle arrest and impair erythroid growth.[66,67] Hemozoin may also directly inhibit erythroid development in vitro and cause apoptosis of erythroid precursors. Furthermore, increased levels of plasma hemozoin and pigment in monocytes have been associated with anemia.[50,68]

Modulation of Erythropoiesis by Infection

In children presenting with acute malaria, bacteremia is associated not only with anemia but also with excess mortality.[69] Parvovirus B19 may cause a transient reticulocytopenia and thus severe and sudden anemia in those suffering from a hemolytic anemia or fetal anemia and intrauterine death. Most children in Africa have serologic evidence of infection early in life. However, acute infection with this virus is uncommon in those presenting with severe malarial anemia.[47,70]

Prevalence and Etiology of Anemia in the Developing World

In endemic areas the etiology of anemia is complex. Acute or chronic malarial infection is a major precipitating factor in children with severe anemia causing admission to hospital.[47]

Longitudinal studies from The Gambia have shown that whereas the mean hemoglobin levels in children vary significantly through the year, anemia is much more common in the rainy season, when malaria transmission is at its highest.[71] However, the rains are also associated with an increase in water-borne diarrheal disease and poor food supplies. So the seasonal increase in anemia in malaria-endemic areas arises on a background of low or frankly deficient stores of hematinics and/or other micronutrients. Iron deficiency, which affects at least 20% of the world's population, is a major factor in the seasonal surge of anemia in the tropical rainy season. Low iron stores at birth and dietary iron deficiency may be exacerbated by hookworm or schistosomal infection. It is now also clear that malarial infection is associated with reduced uptake of available iron and reduced incorporation of iron into developing erythroid cells.[54,55] Folate deficiencies and/or increased requirements may occur in many populations, although frank folate deficiency is uncommon.

A low baseline hemoglobin level at the start of the season for malaria transmission is a major risk factor for developing severe malarial anemia and has encouraged studies aimed at preventing the development of anemia by hematinic supplementation with or without antimalarial prophylaxis or surveillance.[72]

Quantifying the contribution of these individual factors to anemia reliably requires intervention studies. In Tanzania, Menendez et al[73] and Schellenberg et al[74] have shown that iron supplementation and antimalarial prophylaxis prevented 30% and 60%, respectively, of all cases of moderate anemia presenting during the malaria transmission season in children and in infants.

Translating the results of these studies from well-defined and carefully controlled study areas has not been easy. Considerable concerns about iron supplementation programs for children have been raised in sub-Saharan Africa and in areas of high malaria endemicity. One large trial of iron supplementation was stopped because of increased hospital admission and death in the group receiving iron. However, metaanalysis of iron supplementation in malaria-endemic areas has shown that iron alone or with antimalarial treatment does not increase the risk for clinical malaria or death when regular malaria surveillance and treatment services are provided.[75] It is increasingly clear that iron supplementation in these areas must be based on either defining iron-deficient children or combining iron administration with effective infection control and treatment strategies.[76]

Features of Malarial Anemia

The Spectrum of Disease Caused by Malarial Infection

The signs and symptoms of malarial infection in humans are caused by the asexual blood stage of the parasite. Infection with blood-stage parasites may result in a wide range of outcomes and pathologic conditions. Indeed, the spectrum of severity ranges from asymptomatic infection to rapidly progressive, fatal illness. The clinical presentation of malarial infection is also wide and influenced by age, immune status, and pregnancy and by the species, genotype, and perhaps the geographic origin of the parasite. In endemic areas, many infections present as an uncomplicated febrile illness. In more severe forms of the disease, children may present with prostration or inability to take oral fluids or in younger children an inability to suckle. Alternatively, they may exhibit a number of syndromes of severe disease, including anemia, coma, respiratory distress, and hypoglycemia and may also have a high rate of bacteremia.[69,77]

In most age-groups, anemia is frequently accompanied by more than one syndrome of severe disease, and the already substantial case fatality rate of 15% to 20% for severe malaria in African children rises significantly when multiple syndromes of severe disease are present.[77]

The age distribution of anemia and other syndromes of severe disease is a consistent but puzzling feature of the epidemiology of clinical malaria. Children born in endemic areas are protected from severe malaria in the first 6 months of life by the passive transfer of maternal immunoglobulins and by fetal hemoglobin. Beyond infancy, the most common form of presentation of severe disease changes from anemia in children ages 1 to 3 years old, in areas of high transmission, to cerebral malaria in older children, in areas of lower transmission.[78] As transmission intensity declines further, severe malaria is most frequently found in older age-groups.

The Clinical Features of Malarial Anemia

The blood stage of falciparum malaria may cause life-threatening anemia; a hemoglobin level of less than 5 g/dL is considered to represent severe disease. Children with anemia may present with malaise, fatigue, and dyspnea or respiratory distress, which usually represents metabolic acidosis, but in an ill child acute respiratory infection must be carefully excluded.[77,79]

Acidosis is largely due to excessive lactic acid and other anions. Salicylate toxicity and dehydration may also play a role. However, the majority of children presenting with respiratory distress are severely anemic, have a metabolic acidosis secondary to reduced oxygen-carrying capacity, and respond to rapid transfusion of fresh blood (for review see reference 80). A minority of those with respiratory distress do not respond to appropriate resuscitation. They probably represent a heterogeneous clinical group and may have renal failure, systemic bacterial infection, or a more profound syndrome of systemic disturbance due to malarial parasites.

However, a large randomized trial of a bolus of fluids in the treatment of African children with shock and life-threatening infections showed somewhat surprisingly that fluid boluses significantly increased 48-hour mortality in these critically ill children with impaired perfusion.[81] Fluid resuscitation must be carefully supervised.

Hemolytic Syndromes, Including Blackwater Fever

The sudden appearance of hemoglobin in the urine, indicating severe intravascular hemolysis leading to hemoglobinemia and hemoglobinuria or blackwater fever, received particular attention in early studies of anemia in expatriates living in endemic areas.[82] There was an association between blackwater fever and the irregular use of quinine for chemoprophylaxis. This drug can act as a hapten and stimulate production of a drug-dependent complement-fixing antibody. Recent studies of sudden intravascular hemolysis have shown that it is rare in Africa but more common in Southeast Asia and Papua New Guinea, where some cases are associated with G6PD deficiency and treatment with variety of drugs, including quinine, mefloquine, and artesunate.[83] However, in the majority of cases, the cause of sudden hemolysis cannot be accounted for, and it seems likely that unidentified hemolytic mechanism(s) may operate.

The Hematologic Features of Malarial Infection

The anemia of falciparum malaria is typically normocytic and normochromic, with a notable absence of reticulocytes, although microcytosis and hypochromia may be present because of the very high frequency of α- and β-thalassemia traits and/or iron deficiency in many endemic areas.[47,71]

The anemia of malaria may be accompanied by changes in the white cell and platelet counts and in clotting parameters, but these changes are not in themselves diagnostic nor do they guide management. Malaria is accompanied by a modest leukocytosis, although leukopenia may also occur. Occasionally leukemoid reactions have been observed. Leukocytosis has been associated with severe disease.[84,85] A high neutrophil count may also suggest intercurrent bacterial infection. Monocytosis and increased numbers of circulating lymphocytes are also seen in acute infection, although the significance of these changes is not established.[86] However, malarial pigment is often seen in neutrophils and in monocytes and has been associated with severe disease and unfavorable outcome.[87,88]

Thrombocytopenia is almost invariable in malaria and so may be helpful as a sensitive, but nonspecific, marker of active infection. However, severe thrombocytopenia (platelet count $<50 \times 10^9/L$) is rare. Increased removal of platelets may follow absorption of immune complexes or platelet activation, but there is no evidence for platelet-specific alloantibodies.[89] By analogy with erythropoiesis, there may be a defect in thrombopoiesis but this has not been established. Thrombocytopenia is not associated with disease severity, although somewhat paradoxically platelets have been shown to contribute to disease pathology in animal and in human malaria.[90,91] Moreover, in human infections, platelets may form clumps with infected erythrocytes.[92] One explanation of this paradox could be that low levels of platelets might not only be a marker of parasite burden but also be protective from severe disease and/or be associated with antiinflammatory cytokine responses.[93]

Disordered coagulation and clinical evidence of bleeding are not infrequent in nonimmune adults contracting malaria and presenting with severe disease. Patients may present with bleeding at injection sites, gums, or epistaxis. Abnormal test results for laboratory tests of hemostasis, suggesting activation of the coagulation cascade, occur in acute infection. However, histologic evidence of intravascular fibrin deposition is notably absent in adults dying from severe malaria.[94] Factor XIII, normally responsible for cross-linking fibrin, is inactivated during malarial infection, and these data may explain low levels of fibrin deposition in the face of increased procoagulant activity.[95]

During acute disease the levels of a disintegrin and metalloproteinase with thrombospondin motifs 13 (ADAMST13) protease are moderately reduced, and the concentration of high-molecular-weight von Willebrand multimers is increased. Such multimers may play a role in the adherence of infected red blood cells and platelets to endothelium, but the role of this adhesive pathway in the etiology of severe and cerebral malaria has not been established.[96]

The bone marrow is typically hypercellular. The most striking findings are of grossly abnormal development of erythroid precursors or dyserythropoiesis. The developing erythroid cells typically demonstrate cytoplasmic and nuclear bridging and irregular nuclear outline.[39,40] These changes are probably central to the pathophysiology of malarial anemia and are discussed in detail later. The proportion of abnormal erythroid precursors and the degree of dyserythropoiesis are markedly greater in chronic compared to acute infection, suggesting that the inhibition and abnormal maturation of erythroid precursors may have somewhat differing etiologies in acute and chronic infection.[39]

The role of hematinic deficiency in children presenting with malaria and anemia may be difficult to assess. The relative importance of absolute and functional iron deficiency have not been defined. Iron will not be absorbed during acute infection because hepcidin levels are raised.[54,55] Nevertheless, many hospitals give a course of iron supplementation after an episode of acute malaria, although no general guidelines have been established. Chronic hemolysis may increase folate requirements, but frank deficiency is uncommon in children presenting with acute malaria, at least in East Africa.[47] Folate deficiency may be more common in West Africa, and protocols for folate supplementation after malaria must reflect local experience.

Malarial Anemia in Pregnancy

Pregnancy is accompanied by a series of physiologic changes that predispose not only to anemia but also to malaria. Hemodilution causes a physiologic decrease in hemoglobin. Moreover, the demand for both iron and folate increases as the fetus grows and often precipitates frank folate or iron deficiency, particularly in multigravid women.

Occult malarial infection, often without fever, may cause anemia and placental dysfunction. This effect is greatest in primigravidas and has been attributed to the adhesion of parasitized erythrocytes to chondroitin sulfate A and hyaluronic acid in the placenta[97,98] (for review see reference 99). Fetal growth is impaired, and babies born to women with placental malaria are on average 100 g lighter than controls born to women without malaria. The subsequent contribution of malaria to infant mortality is substantial.[100] Furthermore, the increase in hematopoiesis demanded by hemolysis during malarial infection may precipitate frank folate deficiency. Finally, women who are not immune to malaria are more likely to develop hypoglycemia and pulmonary edema during pregnancy.

The increase in maternal and fetal morbidity and mortality secondary to malaria may be prevented by routine hematinic supplementation and by intermittent treatment with antimalarials during the second and third trimesters with sulphadoxine-pyrimethamine (Fansidar).[101]

Hyperreactive Malarial Splenomegaly

Although splenomegaly secondary to malarial infection usually regresses as immunity is acquired, some people living in endemic areas develop progressive, massive splenomegaly.[102] The pathophysiology of such hyperreactive malarial splenomegaly (HMS) is poorly understood but certainly results in B-cell hyperplasia with high levels of polyclonal IgM, reaching a level greater than 2 standard deviations (SDs) above the local reference mean. The specific antimalarial antibody titer is high, although only a small proportion of the polyclonal IgM response is directed at malarial antigens. B-cell hyperplasia may provoke proliferation of both T cells and macrophages, and IgM levels may cause cryoglobulinemia and stimulate erythrophagocytosis.

Patients may present typically between 20 and 40 years old, with massive splenomegaly without lymphadenopathy, anemia that may be severe, neutropenia, and thrombocytopenia. The anemia may cause life-threatening hemolytic crises and/or neutropenia associated with severe bacterial infection. Thrombocytopenia is rarely symptomatic. The bone marrow shows hypercellularity, with a lymphocytosis in marrow and peripheral blood. The high IgM levels distinguish HMS from chronic lymphocytic leukemia or other lymphoproliferative disorders. However, the polyclonal proliferation of B cells may transform to a true clonal lymphoproliferative disorder. This appears to be derived from a naive B cell, although the exact classification of such lymphoproliferative disorders is poorly defined[103]; however, there is a single report of a high incidence of B prolymphocytic leukemia in one population.

Treatment for HMS is lifelong antimalarial prophylaxis. Signs and symptoms usually subside over 1 to 2 years, but relapse may occur if antimalarial therapy ceases. Splenectomy is contraindicated because it is technically difficult, with considerable interoperative mortality and may predispose to severe infection.

Anemia and *P. vivax*, *P. ovale*, and *P. malariae* Infection

In *P. vivax* and *P. ovale* malaria, high parasitemias are rare because invasion of erythrocytes is limited to reticulocytes. However, there is an emerging consensus that *P. vivax* monoinfection may cause severe disease with cerebral malaria and/or anemia (for review see reference 104). The vivax-infected red blood cell can adhere to host cells, but sequestration in the peripheral circulation and organ-specific syndromes of disease are much less common than in falciparum malaria.

P. vivax malaria has been associated with anemia during pregnancy and with low birth weight of children of affected mothers. Here cytokines or other inflammatory mediators appear to cause placental dysfunction.[105] *P. malariae* infection is also rarely fatal but is distinguished by the persistence of blood-stage parasites for up to 40 years. It can, however, cause a progressive and fatal nephrotic syndrome.[106]

Malaria Diagnosis

The diagnosis of malaria is based on the identification of circulating blood-stage parasites. The standard methods of preparing thick and thin films are straightforward and allow a simple method to diagnose infection (Table 160-1).[107-109] However, malaria diagnosis poses particular problems for inexperienced staff. The main biologic problem is that the level of circulating parasites is only weakly associated with the overall parasite burden because falciparum-infected erythrocytes are sequestered in capillary venules; thus the parasitemia is not a reliable guide to the severity of disease. Second, missing or delaying the diagnosis of falciparum malaria may result in serious morbidity and mortality. Finally, the most sensitive methods for diagnosis of infection, namely microscopy, require both skill and time.

In endemic areas, laboratory staff are skilled at the examination of thick films and routinely are able to detect 1 parasite in 100 high-power fields of a thick film, which corresponds to a sensitivity of approximately 5 to 50 parasites/μL.[107,110] Thin films are used for determining the species of the parasites, and the circulating asexual forms of the four main malaria species can be readily identified, whereas the sexual forms (gametocytes) of the species require some skill and regular practice (Figs. 160-5 and 160-6).

Nevertheless, diagnosis of malaria by microscopy in nonendemic countries has proven problematic. Routine laboratories may only achieve sensitivities of the order of 500 parasites/μL using thick films.[110,111] Quality assurance schemes show that performance of routine hematology laboratories in the recognition of and species determination of malaria parasites is poor.[109,111]

There has therefore been a strong drive to use nonmicroscopy methods for malaria diagnosis. It is now apparent that these methods are not sufficiently sensitive for clinical diagnosis, although they may have a role in detecting parasites of more than 500 parasites/μL when experienced staff are not available and/or as part of an out-of-hours service. However, it must be emphasized that these tests are no substitute for careful microscopy. Operationally this means that hematology laboratories need to make the diagnosis of malaria and must maintain the skills needed for reliable examination of thick films.

Table 160-1 Malaria Diagnosis

Thick and thin films should be prepared for cases of suspected malaria.

Immunochromographic tests lack sensitivity to detect low levels of parasites that may be highly clinically significant.

Routine Giemsa or May-Grünwald-Giemsa stains are unlikely to give satisfactory results because the pH is too low.

Films can be stained with Giemsa or Leishman stain (thin films) or Field stain (thick films). (For details see *Guideline: The Laboratory Diagnosis of Malaria*, www.bcshguidelines.org.)

Two hundred high-power fields (×100 objectives) should be examined in a thick film.

Asexual parasitemia should be reported after counting 1000 RBCs in a thin film. A graticule or grid may help counting.

If parasitemia is less than 1 : 1000 RBCs, parasitemia may be counted in a thick film in relation to the number of WBCs.

During active infection, daily parasite count should be obtained.

Counting and species determination of malaria parasites should be verified by a second observer.

Reports on negative films despite a strong clinical suspicion of malaria should be qualified that negative films do not exclude a diagnosis of malaria. Repeat films should be requested if clinically appropriate.

Thrombocytopenia may heighten suspicion of malaria.

RBC, Red blood cell; *WBC*, white blood cell.

A number of methods based on the fluorescent staining of parasite deoxyribonucleic acid (DNA) and/or ribonucleic acid (RNA) and the concentration of parasites have been devised.[112-114] However attractive these methods may appear, their sensitivity is limited by background staining of cellular debris, and the limit of their sensitivity is approximately 100 parasites/μL. The time taken in preparing samples and the specialized equipment and skills needed to use these methods limit their effectiveness in routine practice.

Detection of circulating malarial antigens is another potentially attractive, but ultimately limited, alternative to the laborious method of screening blood films. The widely available tests detect *Plasmodium* histidine-rich protein 2 (BinaxNow malaria test) and *Plasmodium*-specific lactate dehydrogenase (OptiMal-IT test) by immunochromatography.[115] The formulation of the tests using dipstick antigens allows rapid testing to be performed by laboratory staff. However, the sensitivity is 100 to 1000 parasites/μL, and this is comparable to the sensitivity achieved by inexperienced but not experienced microscopists. The current recommendations for malaria diagnosis in the United Kingdom emphasize clearly that these tests only have a place when experienced staff are not available or to provide a rapid diagnosis that will be later confirmed by microscopy to exclude low-level infection and/or determine the species and quantify the infection.[116]

Amplification of circulating parasite DNA using the repeated ribosomal RNA (rRNA) genes is an extremely sensitive method of malaria diagnosis.[117] The sensitivity may be as low as 0.005 parasites/μL or 5 parasites/mL.[118,119] Undoubtedly, this is a useful tool for reference laboratories but is not yet in routine diagnostic use.

Treatment

Malaria requires urgent effective chemotherapy to prevent progression of disease and may be the most crucial public health intervention to reduce global mortality from malaria. The drug treatment of malaria must take account of the expected pattern of drug resistance in the area where infection was contracted, the severity of clinical disease, and the species of parasite. The spread of drug-resistant parasites and the optimal use of affordable, effective drugs are of continual concern, and these have recently been reviewed (Table 160-2).[116,120,121] Artemisinin-based combination treatments have been the mainstay of treatment for falciparum malaria in Southeast Asia for more than 10 years and are now recommended as first-line treatment throughout the rest of the world.[122] The hematologic side effects of antimalarial drugs in use today are few. Amodiaquine is associated with neutropenia and agranulocytosis. Artemisinin-based treatments may cause reticulocytopenia, but this is not clinically significant.

In severely ill patients, good nursing care is vital. Monitoring and treatment of fits and hypoglycemia is essential, and antipyretics should be given.[123]

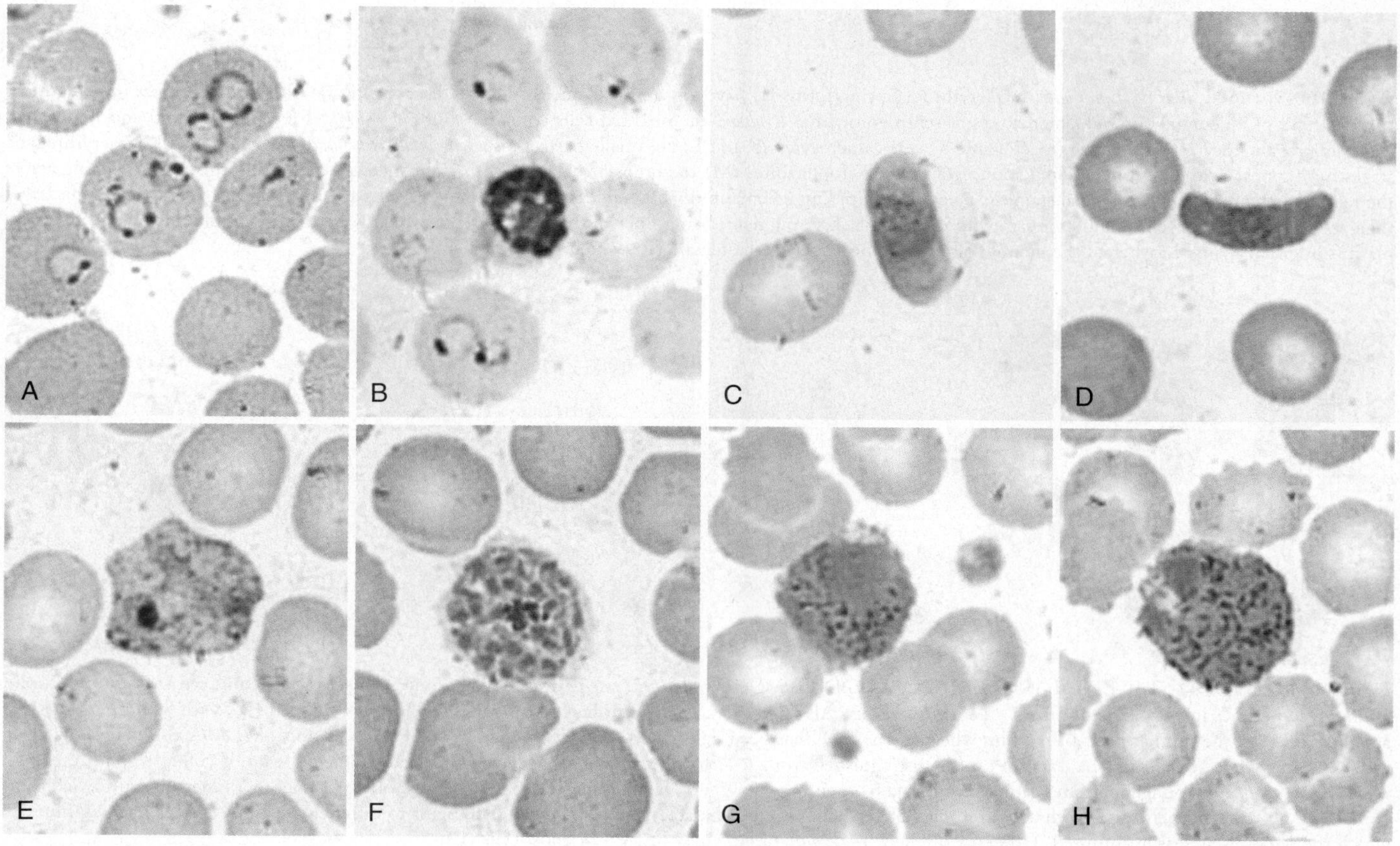

Figure 160-5 BLOOD STAGE MALARIA (THIN BLOOD FILMS). *Plasmodium falciparum:* Fine rings **(A)** predominate, with mature trophozoites and schizonts **(B)** appearing uncommonly in the peripheral circulation because infected cells adhere to postcapillary venules. Host cells are not enlarged. Basophilic clefts and spots of irregular shape and size (Maurer clefts and dots) may be seen in erythrocytes containing more mature parasites. They are thought to be aggregates of parasite proteins that are being exported from the parasite to the surface of the red cell. Crescent-shaped male **(C)** and female gametocytes **(D)** are diagnostic. *Plasmodium vivax:* All stages of asexual parasites—from young trophozoites **(E)** to schizonts—appear in the peripheral circulation in vivax malaria together with gametocytes. The parasites are large and ameboid and produce schizonts with approximately 16 daughter cells (merozoites) **(F)**. Pigment is well developed. Host red cells are enlarged and uniformly covered with fine eosinophilic stippling (Schüffner dots). Gametocytes are round, with the male (microgametocytes; **G**) being approximately 7 μm and the female (macrogametocytes; **H**) being 10 μm or more in diameter.

Continued

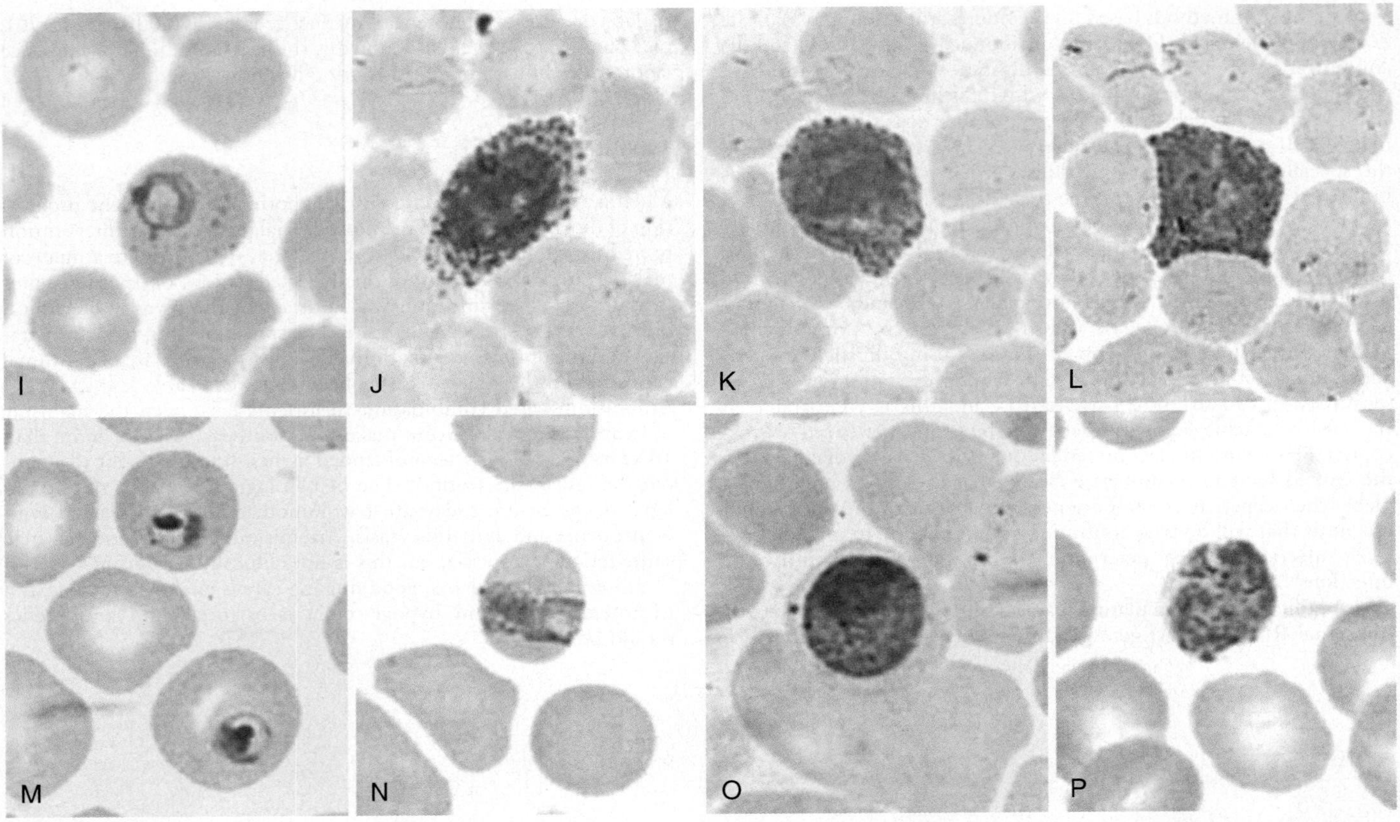

Figure 160-5, cont'd *Plasmodium ovale:* Intraerythrocytic ring forms **(I)** have a prominent nucleus. The older parasites **(J)** differ from *P. vivax* in being more compact and producing about eight merozoites at schizogony. Like *P. vivax*, the host red cells contain Schüffner dots and tend to be ovoid and fimbriated. Male (microgametocytes) and female (macrogametocytes) gametocytes (**K** and **L**) are smaller than those of *P. vivax. Plasmodium malariae:* All intraerythrocytic stages may appear in the peripheral circulation, from young trophozoites **(M)** to compact schizonts with eight merozoites. Band forms **(N)** stretching across the red cell are common. With special staining, a very fine stippling (Ziemann dots) is sometimes seen. Host red cells are not enlarged. Gametocytes, no larger than their host cells, are round and compact with distinct blackish pigment, being finer in the males **(O)**, in which the nucleus is more diffuse and the cytoplasm somewhat mauvish, whereas the granules are fewer and larger in the female **(P)**, which stains a bluer color.

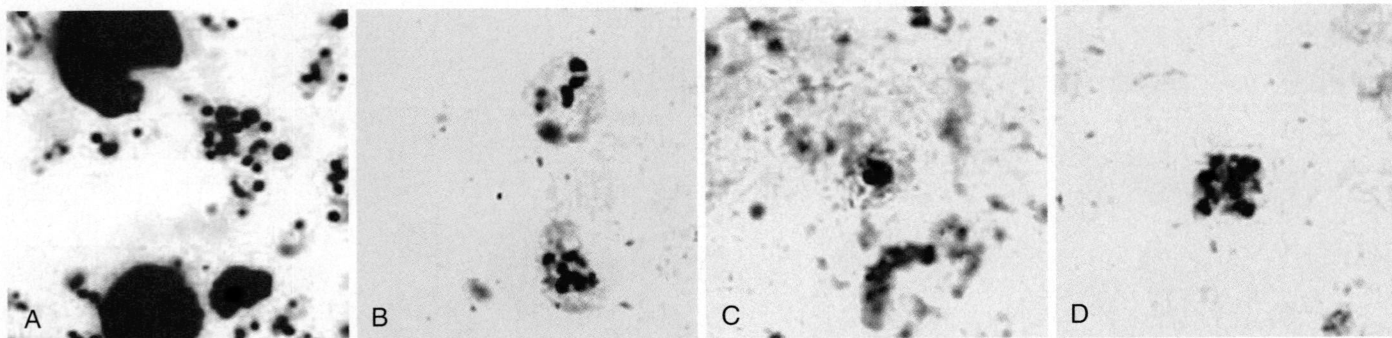

Figure 160-6 BLOOD-STAGE MALARIA (THICK BLOOD FILMS). *Plasmodium falciparum:* Usually only young rings **(A)** are seen in acute infections, although sometimes in very large numbers. *Plasmodium vivax:* All stages may be present; here two young trophozoites are seen **(B)**, with Schüffner dots seen as "ghost cells" in the thinner parts of the film where the host cell has been hemolyzed. *Plasmodium ovale:* The Schüffner dots of *P. ovale* also may show up in a thick film as a ghost cell, but the parasite can be distinguished from *P. vivax* by the solid appearance and heavy pigment even of young trophozoites **(C)**. *Plasmodium malariae:* Younger parasites can be recognized by their heavy pigment, but this may be so heavy that it obscures the other inner structures. Schizonts containing up to eight merozoites with a central mass of pigment **(D)** are characteristic. *P. malariae* is difficult to differentiate from *P. ovale* in thick films, in which the parasites are easily confused. However, unlike *P. malariae, P. ovale* may be seen in ghost cells **(C)**.

Certainly, blood transfusion is in principle a straightforward solution to the treatment of severe malarial anemia, although controversy exists over the trigger for transfusion and the rate of administration of blood. The standard regimens of cautious and slow delivery of blood have been challenged by the demonstration that rapid initial flow rates may correct lactic acidosis and hypovolemia. However, in nonimmune patients and in pregnant women, blood transfusion must be accompanied by careful hemodynamic monitoring to avoid precipitating or exacerbating pulmonary edema.

No formal controlled trials for the transfusion of patients with malaria have been performed. Whatever clinical guidelines emerge, in reality blood transfusion in the heartland of malaria-endemic areas

Table 160-2 Commonly Used Antimalarial Drugs and Their Side Effects

	Oral Dose	Parenteral Dose	Side Effects
Sulphadoxine-pyrimethamine	Sulphadoxine 25 mg/kg Pyrimethamine 1.25 mg/kg as a single dose (max 1500 mg sulphadoxine and 75 mg pyrimethamine)	For IM injection, doses as for oral	Use with caution in first trimester Causes kernicterus in neonates Skin rashes, fatal Stevens-Johnson syndrome
Artemether	3.2 mg/kg day 1 1.6 mg/kg days 2-7	3.2 mg/kg IM day 1, then 1.6 mg/kg for 3 days, then oral	Reticuolcytopenia
Artesunate	4 mg/kg OD for 7 days	2.4 mg/kg IM day 1, then 1.2 mg/kg for 3 days, then oral	Reticulocytopenia
Artemether/ lumofantrine	Fixed-dose combination: artemether (20 mg) with lumofantrine (120 mg), adults give 4 tablets initially, followed by 5 further doses of 4 tablets each given at 8, 24, 36, 48, and 60 hours (total 24 tablets over 60 hours) If 5-15 kg, then 1 tablet initially followed by 5 further doses of 1 tablet each, given at 8, 24, 36, 48, and 60 hours (total 6 tablets over 60 hours); 15-25 kg, then 2 tablets initially, followed by 5 further doses of 2 tablets each given at 8, 24, 36, 48, and 60 hours (total 12 tablets over 60 hours); bodyweight 25-35 kg, 3 tablets initially, followed by 5 further doses of 3 tablets each given at 8, 24, 36, 48, and 60 hours (total 18 tablets over 60 hours)		
Quinine	10 mg/kg of salt (max 600 mg) 8 hourly for 7 days, together with or followed by either doxycycline 200 mg once daily for 7 days or clindamycin 450 mg every 8 hours for 7 days [unlicensed indication]	20 mg/kg in 10 mL/kg isotonic fluid over 4 hours, then 10 mg/kg over 2 hours given 12 hourly in children and 8 hourly in adults, together with or followed by either doxycycline 200 mg once daily for 7 days or clindamycin 450 mg every 8 hours for 7 days [unlicensed indication]	Thrombocytopenia, intravascular hemolysis (blackwater fever) when used prophylactically, nausea, tinnitus, deafness

IM, Intramuscular; *max,* maximum; *OD,* once a day.

is beset by many practical and theoretic problems. First, the absence of well-characterized donor panels (and thus systematic blood collection) frequently jeopardizes the supply of blood. Second, even when standard screening for HIV is in place, the residual risk for human immunodeficiency virus (HIV) transmission in the serologic window of infectivity remains at 1 in 2000.[124] At a practical level, positive indirect antiglobulin tests in acute infection may make the exclusion of alloantibodies difficult. Depending on the clinical urgency and transfusion history, the least serologically incompatible blood may have to be given.

One therapeutic option available in North America and in Europe for the urgent treatment of nonimmune patients with severe disease would be an exchange blood transfusion. This procedure removes nonsequestered, infected erythrocytes and possibly circulating toxins. In the absence of evidence from trials for the use of exchange transfusion in malaria, some have suggested that this treatment could be given for hyperparasitemia (>20%) in severely ill nonimmune patients.[125,126]

The salient features that make this clinical problem a major public health concern are the very large numbers of children affected and the difficulty of satisfactory treatment by blood transfusion outside specialist centers.

Malaria as a Transfusion-Transmitted Infection

Malaria is undoubtedly the most common transfusion-transmitted infection in the world. In endemic areas a large proportion of adult donors will be parasitemic, perhaps 20% to 80%, depending on the rate of transmission. Here donor deferral is impractical, and treatment of recipients with a course of effective antimalarials is the most practical alternative.

In nonendemic areas, transmission of malaria is an occasional but potentially devastating complication of blood transfusion, and considerable thought and resources are required to combat the problem effectively.

The first case of transfusion-transmitted malaria (TTM) was in 1911.[127] Between 1911 and the mid-1970s the incidence of TTM rose to more than 140 cases per year, with *P. vivax* the most common species causing infection, although the proportion of cases due to *P. falciparum* has steadily increased, perhaps reflecting the speed and destination of international travel. It is striking that the background problem, namely, malaria in returned travelers, is much more common in the United Kingdom than the United States, with the per capita incidence differing by nearly a factor of 10 and a higher proportion of cases due to *P. falciparum* in Europe and the United Kingdom compared with the United States.[128]

Recent experience in the United Kingdom and the United States has emphasized the seriousness of TTM. Two of the last five cases of malaria due to blood transfusion in the United Kingdom were fatal.[129-131] In the United States, 14 cases of TTM were reported between 1990 and 1999, but only 5 cases between 2000 and 2009.[132,133]

Detecting these cases after transfusion is frequently delayed because malarial infection acquired in nonendemic countries rarely figures in immediate differential diagnosis and requires careful examination of the blood film.

The mainstay of preventing TTM in the United Kingdom is donor deferral backed up by detection of circulating antibodies to

Table 160-3 UK Donor Selection Guidelines for Donors "At-Risk" of Transmitting Malaria

Donor "Risk" Category	Guidelines
Resident	Defined as having lived in sub-Saharan Africa (except South Africa) or Papua New Guinea for a continuous period of 6 months at any time of life Permanent deferral unless malaria antibody test results are negative at least 6 months after returning from a malarious area Any subsequent visits to any malarious area each require a 6-month deferral period and negative antibody test results before reinstatement
History of malaria	Permanent deferral unless malarial antibody test results are negative at least 3 years after cessation of treatment or last negative test results
Undiagnosed febrile illness	While abroad or within 4 weeks of return Deferral for 12 months or 6 months if malarial antibody test results are negative
All other risks	Deferral for 12 months or 6 months if malarial antibody test results are negative

malaria antigens. The guidelines for donor deferral were carefully revised after analysis of circumstances of recent TTM (Table 160-3).[134] These criteria recognize that malaria in the nonimmune patient is likely to present within 6 months of return from an endemic area and that significant immunity to falciparum malaria may be acquired by residence after 6 months in a malarious area.

The criteria also required that residents, those having had malaria or an undiagnosed febrile illness, may be reinstated if antimalarial antibodies cannot be detected. The importance of antimalarial antibody testing rests on the fact that it is a very sensitive method to detect chronic infection, whereas the identification of circulating malarial antigens or nucleic acids or microscopy would fail to detect a level of 1 parasite/mL, which would still give a highly infectious dose in a unit of blood.

The assays for antimalarial antibodies previously used indirect immunofluorescence antibody tests (IFATs) to detect reactivity to a crude parasite lysate as a target antigen. However, an enzyme-linked immunosorbent assay (ELISA) using recombinant malarial antigens has proved to be a more practical if slightly less sensitive alternative to IFAT.[131,134,135] These tests detect antimalarial antibodies in less than 2% of donors who have visited endemic areas. It has been calculated that the return of 90% of malarial antibody–positive visitors to the donor pool releases an extra 50,000 units a year in the United Kingdom, and this is a highly cost-effective process to reduce the attrition of eligible blood donors. In the United States, over 200,000 donors a year are deferred after travel to malaria-endemic areas.

Donor deferral is based on the potential of a donor to carry malaria and is therefore based on the area of travel, length of stay or residence, elapsed time since leaving the endemic area, and history of malaria. It has been repeatedly shown that application of even the most thorough donor questionnaires allows some of those carrying malaria to give blood because guidelines are frequently incorrectly applied or questions answered inaccurately in routine practice.[133,136]

In Canada donors reporting diagnosis or treatment of malaria defer permanently, and in the United States donors are deferred for 3 years after treatment.[133] The criteria will inevitably cause unnecessary deferral of those who never actually had malaria but also permits some individuals with low-level chronic infection to donate because malaria not infrequently presents more than 3 years after returning from endemic areas.[133,132] The last case of malaria transmitted in the United Kingdom was by someone who left a malarious area 8 years previously, and the longest recorded case of recrudescence of malarial infection is 44 years for *P. malariae*.

In conclusion, permanent deferral of all those visiting malaria-endemic areas is unlikely to be a viable strategy to prevent TTM because donor bases are declining. Preventing malaria transmission through blood transfusion requires comprehensive, regularly reviewed, and effectively implemented guidelines for donor deferral and laboratory testing. Even the best strategy is a compromise, and medical laboratory staff should be aware of the rarely, but potentially serious, possibility of fever after transfusion that could be caused by malaria.

VISCERAL LEISHMANIASIS

Leishmaniasis is a generic term of infection by 30 or so species of the obligate intracellular parasites from the genus *Leishmania*. Visceral leishmaniasis (VL), or kala-azar, presents with a wide spectrum of systemic and hematologic features.

Epidemiology

VL occurs in all countries bordering the Mediterranean and across the Middle East, including Saudi Arabia and Yemen. Indian VL occurs in the eastern regions (particularly Assam, Bengal, Bihar, Uttar Pradesh, Madras, and Sikkim) and in Nepal and Bangladesh. African kala-azar is endemic in Kenya, Ethiopia, and the Sudan and sporadically elsewhere in tropical Africa. In the Americas, VL occurs in foci across Mexico, Central America, Colombia, Venezuela, Guyana, Brazil, Bolivia, and northern Argentina (Fig. 160-7).

The total burden of disease is difficult to estimate but significant. Leishmaniasis burden is endemic in 88 countries, with 500,000 new cases of VL per year, with the vast majority occurring in India, Bangladesh, Nepal, Northern Sudan, and northeastern Brazil.[137] VL is associated with poverty and undernutrition in endemic areas, particularly in the hyperendemic foci of southern Sudan and the Ganges river basin. In the Mediterranean area, it is increasingly seen in association with HIV infection, where infection rates in HIV-infected people may be as high as 10%.

VL is caused by a number of species of the *Leishmania donovani* complex.[138,139] In the Mediterranean and areas in the Middle East and Central Asia through to China, *Leishmania infantum* predominates, whereas *L. donovani* is more prevalent in India. *Leishmania tropica* is a less common cause of VL in these areas. Throughout their range in the Old World, parasites are transmitted by the female sandfly of the *Phlebotomus* genus.

Leishmaniasis is caused by different parasites and vectors in the New World, where *Leishmania chagasi* and *Leishmania amazonensis* are transmitted by the *Lutzomyia* genus of sandfly.

Leishmania organisms are present in blood, and so the disease can be transmitted by blood transfusion, as a sexually transmitted disease, as a congenital infection, by needle sharing for intravenous drug abuse, or within a laboratory by intradermal inoculation of *L. donovani* promastigotes.[140,141] Very few cases of leishmaniasis have occurred as transfusion-transmitted infections in Europe or North America, with under 10 cases in infants or immunocompromised patients over the last 50 years. In endemic areas, this problem represents a much greater but unquantified risk.

Parasitology

Leishmania amastigotes live and multiply within macrophages by binary fission. They are round or ovoid bodies, approximately 2 to 3 μm in diameter. Occasional rupture of cells allows invasion of uninfected monocytes and macrophages by free forms. Sandflies ingest amastigotes within macrophages from blood or skin. In the insect's stomach, free amastigotes multiply and divide asexually, becoming elongated and developing flagella as metacyclic promastigotes. Within 2 weeks, such infective forms migrate through the lining of the stomach and enter the proboscis of the sandfly, allowing

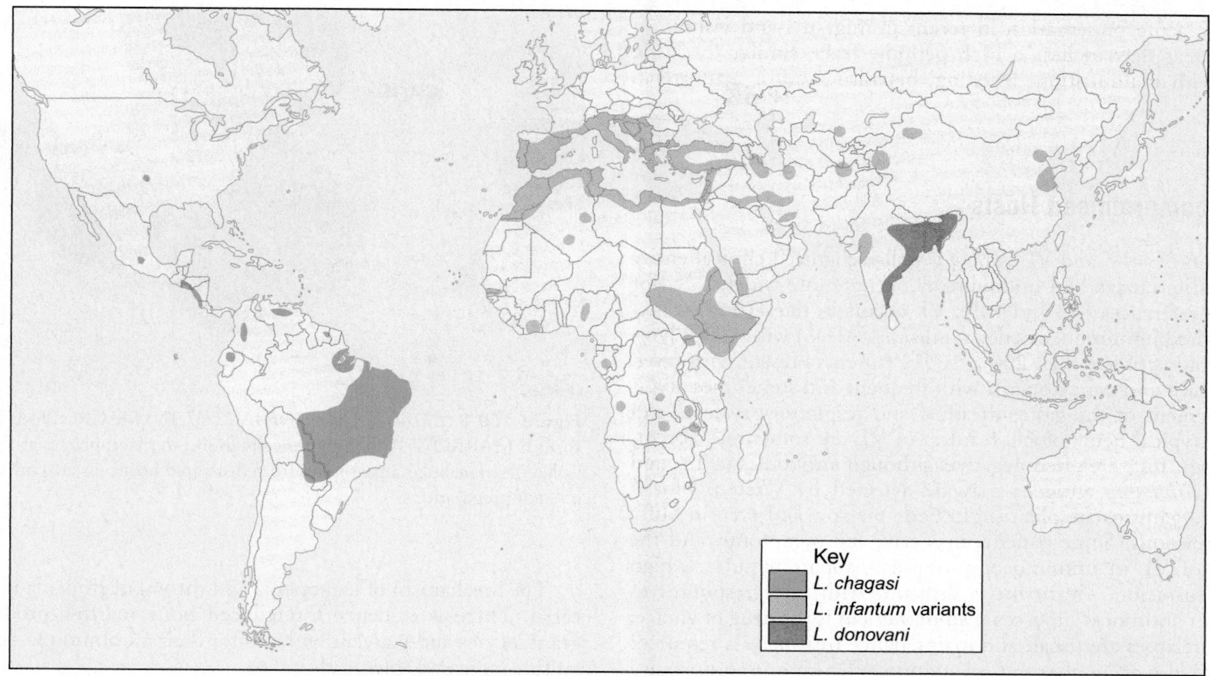

Figure 160-7 EPIDEMIOLOGY OF VISCERAL LEISHMANIASIS (VL). VL caused by parasites of the *Leishmania donovani–Leishmania infantum* complex occurs in the Mediterranean littorals, the Middle East, and adjacent parts of the former Soviet Union, the Sudan, East Africa, the Indian subcontinent and China, and South America *(Leishmania chagasi)*. An arid, warm environment provides ideal ecologic conditions for the breeding of many species of sandfly. Zoonotic kala-azar due to *L. infantum* and *L. chagasi* is commonly associated with dry, rocky, hill country, where cases are typically scattered. In India, *L. donovani* is essentially an anthroponosis. This type of kala-azar may occur in severe epidemic fashion, as can kala-azar in the Sudan.

them to be inoculated in the human host while the sandfly takes a blood meal. Promastigotes are taken up by macrophages, where they become amastigotes by simple fission.

The large elongated fusiform promastigote measures 15 to 20 μm in length and 0.5 to 3.5 μm in width. Cultured promastigotes may also demonstrate rounded forms 4 to 5 μm in diameter. In Giemsa or other Romanovsky stains, a large nucleus and smaller distinct rod-like kinetoplast are obvious. The organisms must be distinguished from *Histoplasma capsulatum*.

Pathology

Parasites spread within macrophages to local lymph nodes and then to the liver, spleen, and bone marrow. They are also present more widely, in particular in the gastrointestinal tract and epidermis. In the subclinical cases, a cellular-mediated immune response causes a granulomatous lesion and resolution of the infection. However, in clinical VL little if any inflammatory response to the rapidly extensive and expanding parasite-laden macrophages is seen. Where it shows, a granuloma develops at the site of the initial inoculation but may not be apparent at the time of presentation.

Clinical Features of Visceral Leishmaniasis

The spectrum of clinical disease is wide, from asymptomatic infection to acute or chronic illness. Perhaps only 1% to 3% of all infections are symptomatic, with an incubation period of 10 days to 10 years, but it is typically between 3 and 6 months.

The high number of seropositive individuals in relation to clinical cases suggests that spontaneous cure without symptoms or with mild systemic symptoms and hepatosplenomegaly occurs in the majority of individuals. In a large series of children with VL in Brazil, the overall case fatality rate was 10%, and mucosal bleeding, jaundice, dyspnea, bacterial infections, and low neutrophil count of less than $500/mm^3$ or low platelet count of less than $50,000/mm^3$ were associated with a poor outcome.[142]

In endemic areas, a significant number of seropositive children, who do not develop classic VL, suffer a subclinical form of disease with malaise, fever, poor weight gain, intermittent cough, diarrhea, hepatomegaly, and variable splenomegaly. In these cases, leishmania were neither cultured nor seen in bone marrow aspirates.[143] There are also reports of VL presenting as mild nonspecific illness with fever, fatigue, cough, and abdominal pain in returning army personnel from the Middle East. In these cases, *Leishmania tropica* was isolated from bone marrow or lymph nodes.[144]

Patients with typical chronic VL often present with malaise and considerable fatigue and the slow onset of low-grade fever, anorexia, and weight loss. They usually have anemia, progressive and occasionally massive splenomegaly, hepatomegaly, lymphadenopathy, and hypergammaglobulinemia, with increasing skin pigmentation (hence the name *kala-azar* from the Hindi for "black sickness"). Patients may have jaundice, petechia, or purpura, heart murmurs, and edema. The size of the spleen is related to the length of infection and severity of the pancytopenia. In Africa, patients may have diffuse polymorphic papular lesions at presentation. Oral, nasal, nasopharyngeal, and laryngeal ulcers may occur during active disease or after treatment. The large spleen, often extending to the right iliac fossa, may be painful. Other features of acute disease include cough, epistaxis, and in some severe cases concurrent infection of the respiratory or gastrointestinal tracts and/or tuberculosis.

The typical features of VL may be preceded by bacteremia, bacterial infection, acute hepatitis, or Guillain-Barré syndrome. VL may be associated with hepatic necrosis, cholecystitis, or neuropathy. Occasionally lymphadenopathy may occur without systemic features of the disease. Here histology shows noncaseating granulomas and amastigotes within macrophages.

A more acute presentation in recent immigrants and visitors to endemic areas may include a high periodic fever, similar to classic malaria, with malnutrition, bleeding, hepatitis, and/or acute renal failure.

Immunocompromised Hosts

Coinfection of HIV and VL is now a well-recognized clinical entity in the Mediterranean and undoubtedly occurs more widely[145-147] (for review see references 148 and 149). VL occurs in the setting of late-stage acquired immunodeficiency syndrome (AIDS) with $CD4^+$ lymphocyte counts of less than 200×10^6/L. Patients present with fever, splenomegaly, and pancytopenia with frequent and sometimes atypical involvement of the gastrointestinal and respiratory systems and skin. The typical hematologic features of VL are sometimes absent, and serologic tests are often negative, although antibodies to 14- and 16-kDa *Leishmania* antigens may be detected by Western blot.[150] However, organisms are plentiful in bone marrow and even in buffy coat preparations. Some patients may have few symptoms, and the diagnosis of VL in immunocompromised patients requires a high index of suspicion. Treatment is difficult, with poor responses to pentavalent antimony. Liposomal amphotericin is the drug of choice. However, relapses are usual, and maintenance treatment is required.

VL may also occur after transplantation, after immunosuppressive treatments, including chemotherapy, rituximab, or other immunodeficiency states.[151,152] Although patients present with a typical combination of fever, pancytopenia, and splenomegaly, the diagnosis may be missed if not considered.

Hematologic Features

VL causes a moderate normocytic, normochromic anemia.[153] The pathogenesis of anemia is multifactorial and includes hemodilution, shortened red cell survival, and reduced erythropoiesis.[154] The plasma is low, with plentiful stored iron typical of the anemia of chronic disease.[155] One report has suggested that Epo levels are reduced compared to what would be expected for the degree of anemia.[156] Occasionally folate deficiency secondary to malabsorption and/or increased cell turnover or coexistent iron deficiency are associated with macrocytic or microcytic anemia, respectively.[157]

The direct Coombs test results are usually positive for C3 components, and IgG and anti-I agglutinins may be present, but the presence and strength of the test is not correlated with the severity of the anemia. The positive direct Coombs test results appear to be due to absorbed immune complexes onto erythrocytes.[158] The neutrophil survival is reduced, and the differential white blood cell count shows neutropenia, relative lymphocytosis, and low eosinophil levels, with a white blood cell count typically in the range 2 to 4×10^9 L.

Neutrophil function may be impaired.[159] Pancytopenia is more severe in those with concurrent HIV infection. A leukemoid reaction to infection has been reported.

Typically the platelet count is reduced to 50 to 200 10^9/L as platelet survival is reduced. Mucosal bleeding may occur, but extensive purpura is uncommon.

The prothrombin time is usually mildly prolonged to 2 to 4 seconds longer than control, secondary to impaired liver function. Fibrinolytic activity is increased, and in advanced cases fibrinogen levels may be reduced. Disseminated intravascular coagulation or vasculitis may occur.[153,159] Full coagulation screening is advisable if a splenic aspirate or bone marrow biopsy is planned.

The bone marrow is usually hypercellular, with increased erythroid, myeloid, and platelet precursors. Lymphocytes may be increased, and macrophages contain Leishman-Donovan bodies (Fig. 160-8).[160] If weight loss and malabsorption are extensive, the marrow may undergo gelatinous transformation.

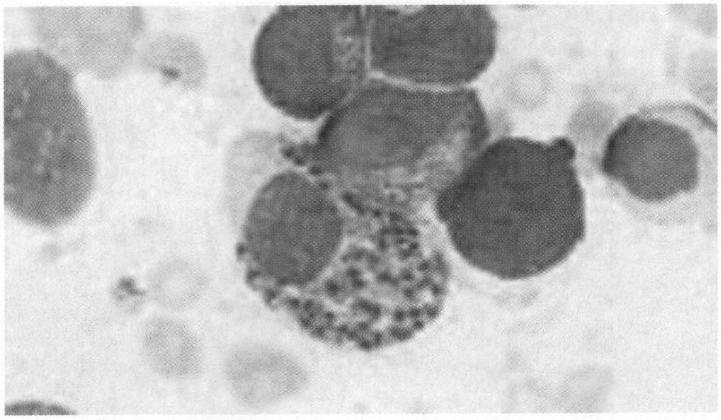

Figure 160-8 *LEISHMANIA INFANTUM* IN MACROPHAGE FROM BONE MARROW. Although typically found in macrophages as shown here, isolated extracellular amastigotes from disrupted host cells are commonly seen in such preparations.

The mechanism of leukopenia and thrombocytopenia is multifactorial. There is evidence for reduced bone marrow production of granulocytes and platelets and also for their autoimmune destruction and/or increased splenic clearance.

After treatment, hematologic recovery is slow and full recovery may take many months.[155]

Laboratory Features

The epidemiologic context and clinical features can suggest a diagnosis of leishmaniasis. Hematologic and biochemical tests are nonspecific; biochemical tests may show mild elevation of bilirubin and transaminase levels and more commonly raised level of alkaline phosphatase. Previously the nonspecific formol gel test was used to indicate hypergammaglobulinemia. Diagnosis is confirmed by direct examination of parasites by microscopy, culture, or polymerase chain reaction (PCR) (for a detailed review see references 161 to 163).

Morphology

The pathognomic amastigotes of *Leishmania* spp. can be found in a variety of sources. The diagnosis is often made by splenic puncture or by bone marrow aspiration where large numbers of amastigotes may be seen within macrophages. Amastigotes are stained using Giemsa or other Romanovsky stains and demonstrate a purple nucleus and the large anterior kinetoplast (see Fig. 160-8).

In nonimmunocompromised patients, splenic aspirates are positive in more than 95%, bone marrow aspirates positive in more than 85%, buffy coat macrophages positive in more than 70%, and lymph nodes positive in more than 60% of patients with VL. In practice, samples are taken from the least invasive sites first, although lymphadenopathy is not invariable.

Where coinfection of HIV and leishmania occurs, amastigotes are more reliably found in bone marrow than in peripheral blood and may also be demonstrated in biopsy specimens from a wide variety of sites. Biopsy material can be stained with polyclonal anti-*Leishmania* serum and indirect immunofluorescence. However, direct demonstration of parasites is less sensitive than culture or PCR.

Splenic Aspiration

Splenic aspiration is rarely performed in North America and Europe but is a common diagnostic procedure in endemic areas. Aspiration is contraindicated in the presence of a bleeding tendency, portal hypertension, or a splenic hydatid cyst. Splenic aspirates are obtained from the middle of the long axis of the spleen. After cleaning the skin, a 21-gauge needle attached to a 5-mL syringe is inserted subcutaneously in line with the long axis of the spleen. The needle should be swiftly inserted to a depth of approximately 2 or 3 cm at an angle of roughly 45 degrees to the skin, applying negative pressure. The needle should be withdrawn immediately while maintaining negative pressure and only taking a few seconds for the entire procedure. The splenic tissue may be expelled from the needle using a small amount of air and by fixing the stain using standard procedures.

Culture

Amastigotes may be grown as motile promastigotes from aspirates on the classic Novy-MacNeal-Nicolle medium or other suitable media at 22° to 24° C, and populations double only every 2 to 3 days.[164,165] Inoculation of material into the susceptible golden hamster is no longer used to grow parasites.

Molecular Methods

The PCR may detect low levels of infection and has been used for diagnosis and monitoring of treatment and to determine the genotype of the parasites.[166,167] Blood from filter paper can be used to prepare DNA, but as for direct morphology, PCR from bone marrow samples is a more sensitive method to demonstrate parasites.[168] It may be particularly useful for monitoring treatment and relapse in HIV- and *Leishmania*-infected patients.[168] Isothermal DNA amplification methods are being applied to develop tests to be used where sophisticated equipment is not available.[169]

Serologic Tests

Serologic tests have to be interpreted in light of the clinical findings. The tests are useful to screen suspected cases or populations for VL. However, they are unreliable in immunocompromised patients, who frequently are seronegative in spite of patent infection. Conversely, those harboring a subclinical infection may be seropositive, but samples may fail to yield evidence of parasites. Finally, serologic findings are positive many years after treatment or self-cure.

An indirect IFAT or ELISA using freeze-dried *Leishmania* antigen has sensitivity and specificity greater than 95%. A DAT is also available with purified freeze-dried antigen and is a highly sensitive and specific test.[170] The freeze-dried antigen is very stable even when stored in extreme conditions.

The ELISA and immunochromatographic tests using *Leishmania* recombinant K39 antigen are 100% sensitive and more than 98% specific in Asia.[171,172] The sensitivity and specificity of the DAT and K39 immunochromatographic test are broadly similar, although the K39 test was less sensitive in the Sudan than in Asia.[173] An alternative target antigen for serologic tests such a recombinant K28 and rapid point-of-care test are now being developed.[21]

Treatment in patients without HIV coinfection may be monitored using urine antigen tests using detection of the K39 and K26 *Leishmania* antigens. These test results become negative 3 weeks after commencing treatment.

Management

General supportive care is important and includes correction of nutritional and hematinic deficiencies, blood transfusion in severe anemia, and antibiotics for secondary infections (for review of diagnosis, therapy, and management, see reference 162).

Specific chemotherapy for VL uses a number of potentially toxic drugs. Intercurrent infections must be identified and treated, and general measures include improvement of nutritional status (for review of treatment see references 174 and 175). Use of pentavalent antimonials, including sodium stibogluconate (Pentostam) and meglumine antimonate (Glucantime) are now limited, especially in South Asia, by increasing drug resistance. There is concern that drug resistance will develop to the alternative therapies, and combination treatment aiming at short courses that also delay the development of drug resistance are in progress.[53]

Amphotericin B is effective against *Leishmania* and is used in endemic areas where high levels of resistance to pentavalent antimonials are present. It may be given as a slow intravenous infusion in 5% dextrose over 4 to 6 hours, beginning at 250 micrograms/kg a day, increasing to 1 mg/kg until a total dose of 20 mg/kg has been given. Side effects include anaphylaxis, anemia, fever, bone chills, bone pain, and thrombophlebitis. Hypokalemia and hypomagnesemia are significant problems, and potassium loss and supplementation may be reduced by the concurrent use of amiloride to prevent renal tubular potassium leakage.[176]

Reduced toxicity from amphotericin is achieved using a liposomal amphotericin preparation (AmBisome), which has been made more widely available through preferential pricing in endemic areas. It is an effective and safe treatment and is used when affordable. A test dose of 1 mg should be given and then the recommended dose is 3 mg/kg/day on days 1 to 5, 14, and 21. Studies have shown a short course of treatment of the single infusion at 5 mg/kg or 5 daily infusions of 1 mg/kg have cure rates of over 90%. In patients with HIV, a dose of liposomal amphotericin at 4 mg/kg/day on days 1 to 5 followed by 4 mg/kg/day on days 10, 17, 24, 31, and 38 is recommended. The relapse rate is high, and close monitoring of patients is required.

Miltefosine is a new drug and effective orally against VL in India and Africa.[177,178] The current regime is 2.5 mg/kg/day for adults and children older than 2 years for 4 weeks. Higher than 95% cure rates have been achieved. Gastrointestinal upset occurs frequently. Miltefosine is teratogenic and may reduce fertility. It has a long half-life and has a low therapeutic index, which may contribute to the development of resistance, and so combination chemotherapy is being investigated to combat development of resistance.

Intramuscular paromomycin has been used at a dose of 20 mg/kg/day for 21 days. It has been shown to be equivalent to amphotericin B for the treatment of VL in India.[179] Moreover, patients treated for VL in Africa with sodium stibogluconate and paromomycin have an improved outcome compared with therapy with sodium stibogluconate alone.[180]

Post–kala-azar dermal leishmaniasis may occur in up to 10% of patients after treatment for VL. It is seen mainly in India and is common in Africa. It occurs after treatment of VL and may appear up to 10 years after treatment. It presents as a maculopapular rash spreading around the mouth, trunk, and limbs. These nodules and papules contain amastigotes. Prolonged treatment may be required to eliminate infection.

Leishmaniasis as a Transfusion-Transmitted Infection

Leishmaniasis poses problems as a potential transfusion-transmitted infection in endemic areas. The disease can be transmitted by blood and platelet concentrates, although leukodepletion by filtration reduces organisms by many orders of magnitude and so probably also the risk for transmission. In Europe, given the low absolute risk for transmission, donor deferral is used to reduce the risk for donation by anyone who is parasitemic.[181] However, surveys of blood donors in areas where the parasite is transmitted suggest parasite DNA can be detected in 0.3% to 1.75% of blood donors. It has been noted that service personnel returning from the Middle East represent a group of potential donors who may have been exposed to infection.[182]

AFRICAN TRYPANOSOMIASIS

African trypanosomiasis is caused by the flagellate protozoa *Trypanosoma brucei* ssp, named after David Bruce, a Scottish parasitologist who first demonstrated the parasite in the blood of cattle affected by nagana. In man, Aldo Castellani demonstrated trypanosomes in the cerebrospinal fluid of patients with sleeping sickness. Bruce was able to show the protozoa in blood and showed that they were transmitted from antelopes to cattle by the tsetse fly and blood of patients suffering from sleeping sickness.

Epidemiology

Trypanosomes are transmitted by some species of the large and distinctive tsetse flies (*Glossina* spp.) in a sporadic distribution south of the Sahara and north of the Zambezi River. Of the three subspecies, *Trypanosoma brucei brucei* infects animals, whereas *Trypanosoma brucei gambiense* causes infection and sleeping sickness in Central and West Africa, and *Trypanosoma brucei rhodesiense* causes disease in East and Central Africa. *T. b. gambiense* is transmitted mainly between humans by the *Glossina palpalis* group in foci along watercourses in West and Central Africa. *T. b. rhodesiense* is transmitted by the *Glossina morsitans* groups widely distributed in the East African savannah. Here the disease is clearly a zoonosis, with antelopes and domestic cattle as reservoir hosts; it afflicts mainly hunters, guides, and game wardens and may occasionally occur in tourists on safari in the game parks of East Africa (Fig. 160-9).

Historically the disease has caused major epidemics, causing hundreds of thousands of deaths, and has prevented human settlement in large areas of Africa. Over 50 million people are now at risk for trypanosomiasis, and it has been estimated that the disease causes over 50,000 deaths each year. Most cases are reported in Zaire and northwestern Uganda, with a few hundred or fewer each year in neighboring East African countries.

Case finding and control measures have substantially reduced the risk for epidemics. Epidemics of disease have been associated with a breakdown in health services, for example, in villages in the areas of Lake Victoria in Uganda and more recently in Zaire, Angola, and southern Sudan (for review of current epidemiologic and clinical aspects of this disease see references 183 to 185).

Parasitology

The small, mobile trypomastigotes circulate and may be seen in peripheral blood. These flattened, fusiform organisms are pleomorphic, but are typically of a size similar to a red blood cell, approximately 20 μm long, and have an undulating membrane, attached to the protruding flagellum, extending from the anterior pole of the elongated body (Fig. 160-10).

Parasites multiply by binary fission and may cause chronic parasitemia and evade humoral immune responses by clonal antigenic variations of the major surface glycoprotein.[186]

When trypomastigotes are taken up in a blood meal by the tsetse fly, they multiply in the midgut by simple fission. Later they penetrate the wall of the gut and migrate to the salivary glands. There, as morphologically distinct epimastigotes, they become infective (or metacyclic) trypomastigotes 15 to 30 days after first infecting the fly. In endemic areas, up to 1% to 5% of flies may be infected. Flies remain infective until they die, several months later.

Pathology

The lymphatic, cardiac, and central nervous systems are involved by the disease. Initially proliferation of trypanosomes within lymph nodes and the spleen is accompanied by expansion of the lymphocytes, macrophages, and erythrophagocytosis. Polyclonal activation of lymphocytes results in high production of IgM and rheumatoid factor, and anti-DNA antibodies may appear. Later fibrosis and endarteritis supervenes with proliferation of endothelial cells and perivascular infiltration of plasma cells and lymphocytes. The liver shows infiltration of the portal tracts and fatty degeneration.

In *T. b. rhodesiense,* cardiac involvement may be extensive, with endocarditis, myocarditis, and pericarditis leading to extensive damage and death.

In the second stage of the disease, trypanosomes multiply within the central nervous system (CNS) and cause a chronic meningoencephalitis. Edema, hemorrhages, granulomatous lesions, and

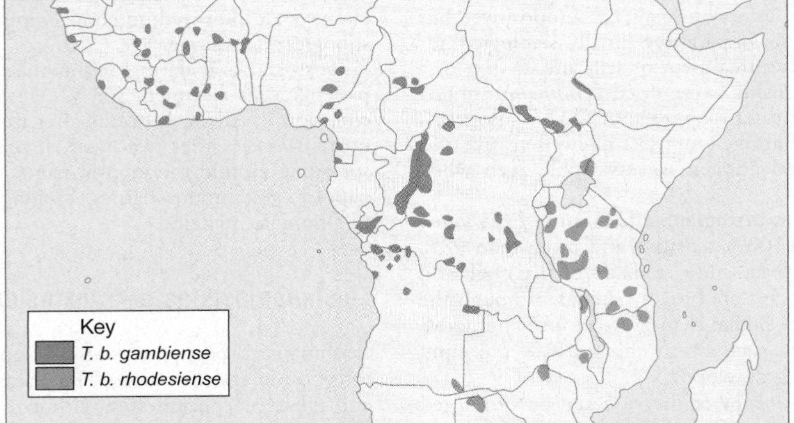

Figure 160-9 DISTRIBUTION OF *TRYPANOSOMA BRUCEI* INFECTION IN HUMANS. African trypanosomiasis is confined to equatorial Africa, with a patchy distribution depending on detailed topographic conditions. It is caused by two subspecies of *T. brucei*: *T. b. gambiense* infection is widespread in West and Central Africa, mainly by riverine species of tsetse fly *(Glossina),* but *T. b. rhodesiense,* transmitted mostly by savannah species, is restricted to the east and east-central areas, with some overlaps between the two. Although domestic pigs form an important reservoir for *T. b. gambiense* infection, various wild ruminants are the major sources for *T. b. rhodesiense*. The epidemic reemergence of African trypanosomiasis in recent years is exemplified by the death of at least 96 people in Angola in 2003, when 3115 cases were confirmed among a suspected 270,000 new cases in that country. In the same year it was estimated that some 500,000 people across Africa were suffering from trypanosomiasis, which was likely to have a mortality rate of approximately 80%. Recent reports indicate a spread of transmission from the northern toward the southern parts of Angola. *(Modified from WHO Map No. 98005.)*

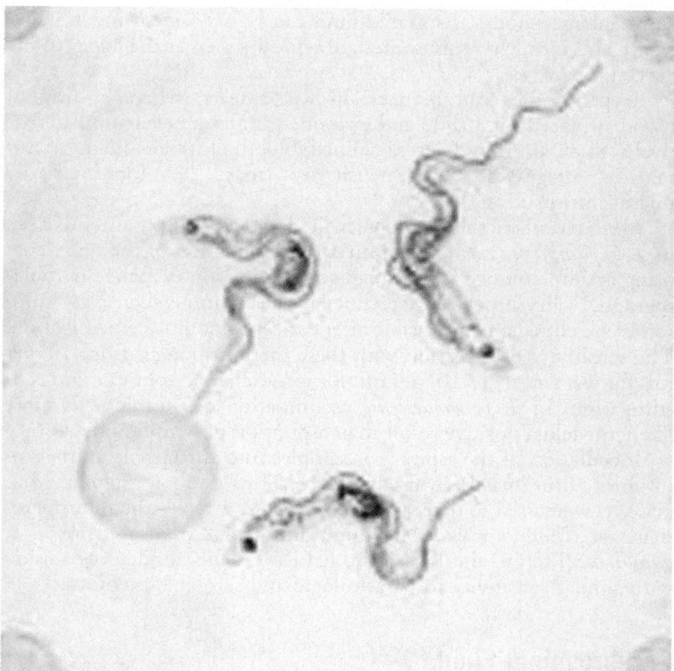

Figure 160-10 ORIGINAL ILLUSTRATION OF *TRYPANOSOMA (TRYPANOZOON) BRUCEI GAMBIENSE* IN HUMAN BLOOD BY J. EVERETT DUTTON. Polymorphic trypanosomes were first discovered more than a century ago, in 1895, by David Bruce in the blood of domestic cattle suffering from the wasting disease nagana in South Africa. The first observation of these protozoa in humans was by R. M. Forde, who noted, in 1902, "small worm-like, extremely active bodies" in the blood of a sick European seaman in The Gambia. The parasites seen here in a Romanovsky-stained, thin blood film, which were described and named by Dutton in the same year, are responsible for sleeping sickness in West Africa. *(Reproduced by kind permission of the Director, Liverpool School of Tropical Medicine.)*

thrombosis contribute to cerebral degeneration. Lymphocytosis and plasma cells with large eosinophilic inclusions (Mott cells) may be found in the CNS.

Intriguingly, nonpathogenic species of African trypanosomes may be killed by the human high-density-lipoprotein particles astonishingly subverting a parasite pathway for heme uptake. The complex of haptoglobin-related protein and apolipoprotein L-1 (apoL1) are taken up into the parasite by a parasite glycoprotein receptor, which binds the haptoglobin-hemoglobin complex.[187-190] *T. b. rhodesiense* is resistant to killing by human sera because the apoL1, which induces parasite apoptosis, is neutralized in the lysosome by serum resistance–associated protein, which binds to a specific apoL1 domain. The selection of trypanolytic apoL1 variants have a cost. In African Americans, focal segmental glomerulosclerosis and hypertension-attributed end-stage kidney disease are associated with two independent sequence variants in the APOL1 gene.[191]

Clinical Features

T. brucei gambiense

Local inflammation at the site of inoculation causes a distinctive chancre or painful, indurated ulcer appearing 2 to 3 days after an infective bite and lasting for up to a month.

Trypanosomes multiply in the lymphatic system for 6 to 14 days before causing patent infection in the blood, characterized by waves of parasitemia and fever. Later, invasion of the CNS may occur by transit of organisms through the choroid plexus and/or endothelial cells.

In the blood stage of infection, fever, headache, and arthralgia are prominent. Lymphadenopathy is common, particularly in the posterior triangle of the neck (Winterbottom sign). There may be intermittent rashes (often circinate erythema), pruritus, or edema. Moderate splenomegaly occurs in 10% to 20% of patients. A few infected patients are asymptomatic.

This early stage of infection may last for up to 2 years or more before CNS involvement, although rapidly progressive disease may occur. The CNS phase of disease is marked by the progressive onset of headache, disinhibited behavioral changes, and mood, thought, and sleep disturbance. Wasting is prominent. Signs of diffuse CNS damage in the last phases of the disease include dementia, extrapyramidal and cerebellar dysfunction, and hyperesthesia. Tendon reflexes are increased and signs of upper motor neuron lesions widespread. Death usually occurs by intercurrent infection.

T. brucei rhodesiense

T. b. rhodesiense is more virulent, causing a more serious acute disease, with systemic features including serous effusions, hepatocellular jaundice, and a mild normocytic, normochromic anemia. Hepatosplenomegaly and lymphadenopathy are common, but involvement of cervical lymph nodes is less typical. Myocarditis is rare but may cause death before CNS involvement. Here CNS disease occurs sooner and is more rapidly progressive than *T. b. gambiense* infection and is fatal within 1 to 3 months.

Infection with *T. b. gambiense* may resolve in the vast majority of cases. Where infection persists, there is typically a long asymptomatic phase. Numerous lymph nodes are enlarged to 1 to 2 cm in diameter and are soft, mobile, and painless.

The differential diagnosis of trypanosomiasis includes malaria, typhoid, fever, and viral hepatitis in the acute phase, whereas lymphadenopathy may suggest infectious mononucleosis or tuberculosis. In the cerebral phase of the disease, syphilis, tuberculosis, HIV-associated cryptococcal meningitis, or chronic viral encephalitis must be considered.

Children

Those affected in utero may be born with CNS abnormalities. In children the disease is more rapidly progressive, and epileptic seizures and psychomotor retardation are the principal features of the disease.

HIV

The frequency of HIV seropositivity has been reported to show no significant differences between those presenting with trypanosomiasis and age-matched controls.[192,193] These results do not exclude that coinfections may modulate the course of the disease or the effectiveness of treatment.

Hematologic and Laboratory Features

The main hematologic features are a normocytic, normochromic anemia and moderate thrombocytopenia.[194] The anemia of trypanosomiasis is multifactorial. Hemodilution, hemolysis, and dyserythropoiesis or ineffective erythropoiesis all contribute to the pathogenesis. Hemolysis may be caused directly by lytic factors released by trypanosomes or indirectly by deposition of immune complexes and subsequent clearance of coated erythrocytes. In vitro studies have suggested that the variant surface glycoprotein from trypanosomes may be shed and taken up onto the erythrocyte membrane, where antibody and complement deposition could contribute to hemolysis. Bone marrow response is inadequate, and although the nature of the defect is unclear, there is failure in incorporation of iron into erythroid precursors as is seen in many forms of the anemia of chronic disease. In mice infected with human trypanosomiasis, TNF-α contributes to bone marrow suppression, but detailed studies of the pathogenesis of anemia in human infections have not been reported. Serum IgM levels may be elevated to four times normal and with raised IgG levels cause an increased erythrocyte sedimentation rate.

The white blood cell count may be elevated with monocytosis, lymphocytosis, and circulating plasma cells, but eosinophilia is absent. Plasma cells with eosinophilic inclusion or Mott morular cells may occasionally be seen.

Petechia and purpura may be secondary to vascular injury, thrombocytopenia, and a complex but poorly defined coagulopathy. Abnormal liver function may cause prolonged clotting times. Functionally both thrombosis and fibrinolysis are increased, and fibrin degradation products (D dimers) are raised in acute disease, and in *T. b. rhodesiense* a frank disseminated intravascular coagulation may become evident.[195]

Examination of the bone marrow shows hypercellularity. Gelatinous degeneration may be seen in wasted patients.

Mononuclear cells are present late in the disease, and the cell count corresponds to the degree of neurologic involvement and may reach more than 300/μL in severely ill patients. The cerebral spinal fluid (CSF) protein levels are elevated (0.4 to 1.0 g/L).

As disease progresses, the circulating parasites become scarce. However, anemia and endocrine dysfunction, including amenorrhea, reduced libido, and impotence become apparent.

Parasitologic Assays

Direct detection of the parasite is particularly important in the light of the toxicity of the treatment.

Trypanosomes may be detected in lymph node aspirates and in wet and thick blood smears (Fig. 160-11). An aspirate may be taken from enlarged nodes. Aspirated fluid can be examined under a coverslip, and motile trypanosomes are typically seen at the edges of the coverslip.

Trypanosomes can be seen in wet smears, where a drop of blood is placed on a slide and examined under a coverslip. Alternatively, thick or thin Giemsa-stained blood films are made as for malaria diagnosis. The sensitivity may be increased by microcentrifugation.[196]

More recent methods to detect the low levels of parasitemia seen in *T. b. gambiense* include quantitative examination of the buffy coat using acridine orange[197] and small-scale ion-anion exchange chromatography.[198] Erythrocytes are retained in the column, whereas trypanosomes are eluted and are visible after concentration by centrifugation. The sensitivity of detection with these methods ranges from 10^4 per mL for wet smears to 10^2 per mL for ion-exchange columns and centrifugation. In *T. b. rhodesiense,* examination of the blood is more likely to yield a positive result than aspiration of lymph nodes.

Inoculation of the aspirate or samples into susceptible animals or in vitro culture has been used to detect low-level parasitemia. Mice and rats were used to detect *T. b. rhodesiense*, whereas the multimammate rat *(Mastomys natalensis)* and guinea pigs were used for *T. b. gambiense.* PCR of the 18S ribosomal RNA gene can detect parasites with similar sensitivity to parasitologic and serologic methods.[199]

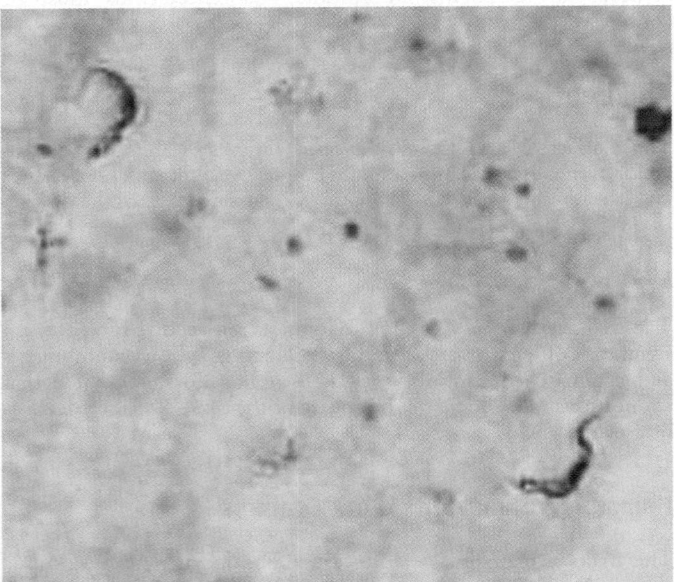

Figure 160-11 *TRYPANOSOMA BRUCEI RHODESIENSE* IN HUMAN BLOOD. *T. brucei brucei* parasitizes wild and domestic animals but does not infect humans. The different subspecies can be distinguished with certainty only by biochemical techniques, such as electrophoretic typing of their isoenzymes or by the use of deoxyribonucleic acid (DNA) probes. *T. brucei gambiense* and *T. b. rhodesiense* (and *T. b. brucei* of animals) are virtually indistinguishable in blood films. Note the small kinetoplast and free flagellum. Both subspecies from humans will infect guinea pigs, but only *T. b. rhodesiense* is infective to rats, in which the parasites are polymorphic, that is, long, thin, intermediate and short, stumpy forms of trypomastigotes may coincide.

Cerebrospinal Fluid

Trypanosomes may be found in the CSF as disease progresses, although a double centrifugation technique may be required to demonstrate organisms. In this technique 5 to 10 mL of CSF is centrifuged and the sediment taken up into a capillary tube and recentrifuged before examining the capillary tube under a coverslip (Fig. 160-12).[200] Specific molecular markers for this stage of CNS disease are being sought by proteomic analysis of the CSF.

Serology

Serologic tests are used for passive population screening in control programs (for review see reference 201). A Card Agglutination Test for Trypanosomiasis (CATT) is robust and can be used without extensive laboratory facilities.[202,203] The test contains freeze-dried trypanosomes with the LiTat 1.3 variant antigens and can be obtained from the Institute of Tropical Medicine, Antwerp (www.itg.be/itg/). It is quite sensitive (>95%) but lacks specificity due to cross-reactivities with animal *Trypanosoma* spp. Although useful as a patient screening

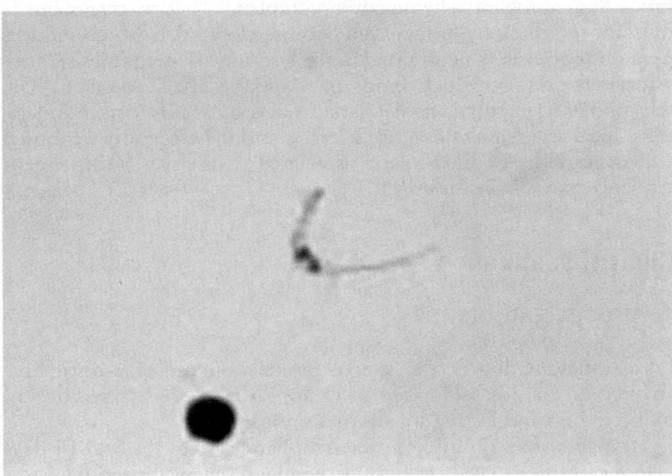

Figure 160-12 TRYPOMASTIGOTE OF *TRYPANOSOMA BRUCEI BRUCEI* IN CEREBROSPINAL FLUID. A single organism is seen in this sample taken from cerebrospinal fluid filtered in a "minicolumn."

test in a hospital for suspected cases of trypanosomiasis, the predictive value for positive test results falls when screening populations for active cases. It has nevertheless been reported to double the number of active cases found. Some patients may have false-negative results using this test if they are infected by parasites that do not express this variant antigen. Further versions of this assay have been developed to use dried blood on filter paper, namely the micro-CATT and macro-CATT, but these are less sensitive than the whole blood assay.

In *T. b. gambiense* serologic tests are not widely available, and direct examination of blood and CSF for parasites is the first line of investigation.

The card indirect agglutination trypanosomiasis test (TrypTect CIATT) can detect circulating antigens in *T. b. gambiense* and *T. b. rhodesiense* infection by latex agglutination. The sensitivity of the test is 95.8% for *T. b. gambiense* and 97.7% for *T. b. rhodesiense* and so significantly higher than that of lymph node puncture, microhematocrit centrifugation, and CSF examination after single and double centrifugation.[204]

A rapid latex agglutination test (LATEX/*T. b. gambiense*) contains a mixture of three variable surface antigens of the bloodstream form of trypanosomes and has been used to detect antibodies in patients infected with *T. b. gambiense*. At 1 : 16 serum dilution, test specificity was 99%, whereas sensitivity ranged from 83.8% to 100% depending on the geographic origin of the samples. The test sensitivity falls to 66% for CSF samples from second-stage patients.[205] A rapid latex agglutination test, LATEX/IgM, for the semiquantitative detection of IgM in CSF is available.[206] Finally, immunofluorescence assays and ELISA tests for antibodies using whole parasites are highly sensitive and specific, although less practical for mass screening.[207]

Treatment

Treatment of trypanosomiasis depends on the subspecies of trypanosome present. The drugs may be difficult to source and are toxic, so treatment requires expert help.

Early-stage *T. b. gambiense* may be treated with pentamidine for 14 days (intravenously [IV] or more usually intramuscularly [IM], 4 mg/kg/day). Hematologic side effects include neutropenia, and more general side effects include hypotension, hypercalcemia, hyperkalemia, renal failure, and hyperglycemia. Pentamidine will not cure CNS disease, and so examination of the CSF is required after initial treatment of the blood-stage disease.

Eflornithine (α-difluoromethylornithine) for 14 days (IV; 100 mg/kg, 6 hourly) is effective for CNS treatment for *T. b. gambiense*.[208] It is a toxic drug suppressing DNA replication by inhibition of ornithine decarboxylase and thus polyamine synthesis and DNA replication. It causes dose-dependent bone marrow suppression with anemia, neutropenia, and thrombocytopenia in the majority of patients. The effects are reversible and are rarely dose limiting. It is effective neither in children nor in coinfection with HIV, where melarsoprol is required.

Melarsoprol is a trivalent organic arsenical compound and is more toxic but cheaper than eflornithine. It is used in Africa for the treatment of late-stage CNS trypanosomiasis. It is given as three daily IV injections, at a dose of 3.6 mg/kg up to 180 mg, on two occasions a week apart. If the CNS leukocyte count is greater than 20/mm^3, a further three injections are given a week later.

Melarsoprol causes a secondary encephalopathy in 5% to 10% of treated cases and is fatal in half of these.[209] The incidence and severity of encephalopathy may be reduced by concurrent administration of prednisolone (1 mg/kg/day up to 40 mg) started 1 to 2 days before melarsoprol treatment.[210] When steroids are used, it is necessary to give patients antimalarial and antihelminthic therapy, especially if *Strongyloides stercoralis* is present.

Prior treatment of blood-stage disease with pentamidine may reduce antigen levels and possibly adverse events. Promethazine, anticonvulsants, and antiemetics are important adjunctive treatments before commencing CNS therapy.

Polyneuropathy occurs in 10% of cases treated with melarsoprol and may be severe, causing quadriplegia. If neuropathy is suspected, melarsoprol should be stopped immediately and thiamine (100 mg, three times a day) given until symptoms subside.

Patients require prolonged specialist follow-up over 2 years, including blood and CSF examination for parasites. A rising CSF leukocyte count is a good guide to CSF relapse even in the absence of a demonstration of parasites.[211]

In treatment for early-stage *T. b. rhodesiense*, suramin is given as five IV injections (20 mg/kg, up to 1.5 g) on days 1, 3, 6, 14, and 21. Adverse effects include fever, proteinuria, paresthesia, pruritus, and urticaria. Hemolytic anemia, agranulocytosis, and thrombocytopenia have been reported as side effects.

Combination therapies of the antitrypanosomal drugs nifurtimox and eflornithine and also the combination of melarsoprol and nifurtimox are under trial for the treatment of second-stage disease to increase the efficacy of treatment and to overcome increasing drug resistance.[212]

Trypanosomiasis as a Transfusion-Transmitted Infection

Trypanosomiasis is a transfusion-transmitted infection. Asymptomatic or early-stage patients with trypanosomiasis are clearly a threat to the blood supply. Patients are excluded in the United Kingdom, Europe, and North America by the general donor queries relating to fever and constitutional symptoms.

In endemic areas, exclusion of infected donors with early-stage *T. b. gambiense* is clearly a more complex problem because patients may be asymptomatic for long periods of time if the degree of risk is unknown and no specific screening procedures are in place.

In summary, hematologic involvement in trypanosomiasis is peripheral to the main two features of the disease, but examination of lymph node aspirates, blood, and CSF is essential for diagnosis and management of the disease. Occasional patients may become severely ill and have complex hematologic abnormalities. In endemic areas, trypanosomiasis may pose a risk to the blood supply.

AMERICAN TRYPANOSOMIASIS

American trypanosomiasis (or Chagas disease, named after the Brazilian parasitologist Carlos Chagas) is caused by infection with *Trypanosoma cruzi*. This flagellated protozoon is transmitted by the triatomine insects, the reduviid bugs. The acute phase of infection is characterized by fever and high parasitemia, followed by a chronic phase with positive serologic results and low parasitemia but with end-organ damage to the heart, peripheral nervous system, and gastrointestinal tract, causing a chronic cardiomyopathy, neuropathy, and megaesophagus and megacolon.

Epidemiology

Chagas disease may occur in the Americas from the southern United States to Chile, but the highest prevalence is in Bolivia and Brazil (Fig. 160-13). There are approximately 10 million seropositive people in Latin America, and the number of people infected and the incidence of new infection is falling rapidly.[213] Infections are found not only in rural areas but also in recent immigrants to urban areas in North and South America and to Europe.[214] It is estimated that approximately 100,000 seropositive individuals are living in the United States. True, endogenous (autochthonous) infection in the United States is vanishingly rare, but seven such human infections have been reported in Texas, California, Tennessee, and Louisiana. Visitors to endemic areas are only rarely infected, with only a handful of cases being recorded in intrepid travelers spending time in traditional housing in rural areas. The range of reservoir hosts and species of triatomine bugs transmitting infection is wide.

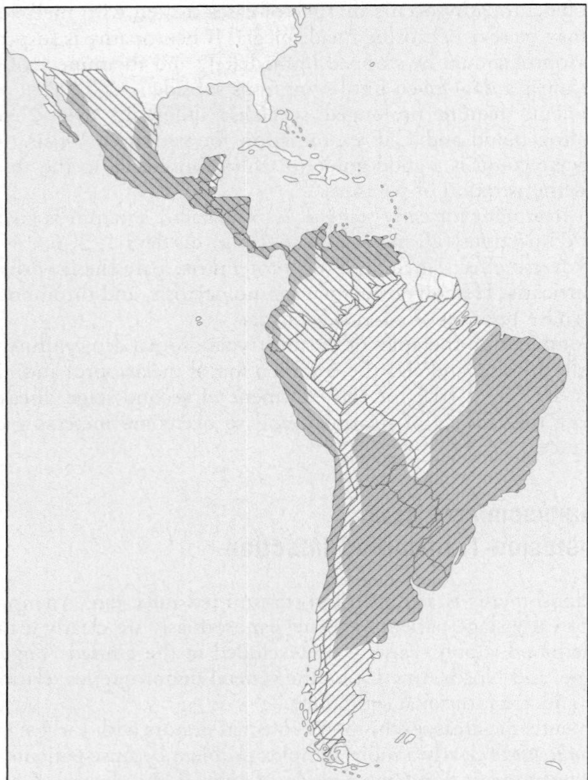

Figure 160-13 DISTRIBUTION OF CHAGAS DISEASE. Human infection is endemic in parts of Central and South America from the Andes to the Atlantic coast and as far south as the latitude of the River Plate (Río de la Plata) shown here in green. Two major intergovernmental programs were started in 1991 to eliminate domestic vectors by a combination of spraying residual insecticides in houses, the use of insecticidal paints, and the deployment of fumigant canisters. The countries covered in the two initiatives, the second of which started in 1997, are shown in the figure. The latter program instituted universal blood screening to avoid transmission from infected blood donors. In less than a decade, remarkable progress has been made. Transmission (by the major vector, *Triatoma infestans*) was eliminated in Uruguay by 1997 and in Chile by 1999. Major reductions in transmission have also been reported from other endemic countries but, to date, not complete control. *(Southern Cone Initiative; Andean and American Initiative areas.)*

Parasites may also be transmitted by blood transfusion (see later), vertically from mother to child by breastfeeding, organ transplantation, and rarely by sexual transmission. Several outbreaks in Brazil have been reported after contamination of food by triatomine bugs and their feces. Laboratory infection by accidental ingestion or inoculation of parasites is well recorded.

Parasitology

T cruzi parasites are from the order Kinetoplastida and family Trypanosomatidae, existing as infective trypomastigotes in the bloodstream of vertebrate hosts. These organisms are fusiform cells, 10 to 20 μm in length, with a distinctive large posterior kinetoplast, containing mitochondrial DNA. They can enter phagocytes, muscle and nerve cells, and a wide variety of other cell types and here transform to oval amastigotes 2 to 5 μm in diameter. They multiply by fission, and amastigotes develop into mature trypomastigotes released on rupture of the cell to begin a new cycle of invasion and multiplication.

Slender, highly motile and broader, less motile trypomastigotes have been distinguished, which may be relatively more infective for host cells and insects, respectively.

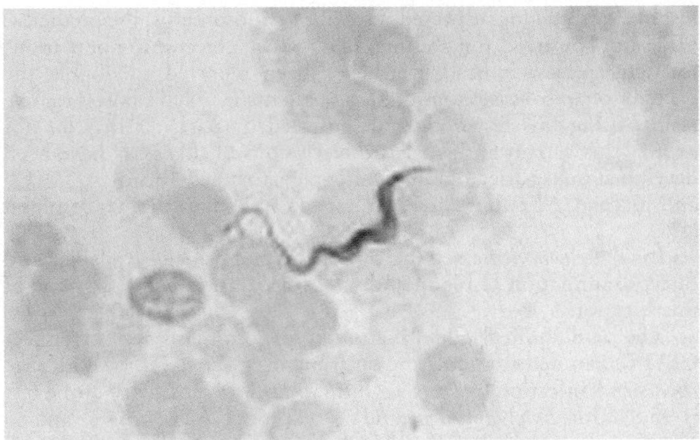

Figure 160-14 *TRYPANOSOMA RANGELI. T. rangeli* is a long, slender trypanosome also transmitted by reduviid bugs from wild animals to humans. It is readily distinguished by its shape from *Trypanosoma cruzi* in blood films and appears to be nonpathogenic to humans.

The species of triatomine bugs that commonly transmits disease is able to cause extensive infestation of simple mud-and-wattle thatched houses in rural Latin America,[215] where Chagas disease is a disease of poverty associated with poor housing. These bugs are infected by circulating trypomastigotes after taking a blood meal on sleeping victims. In the mid gut, trypomastigotes transform into epimastigotes and multiply by fission, before migrating to the hind gut where they develop into metacyclic trypomastigotes, adherent to the epithelium of the rectum. These infective forms are excreted into the feces and people are infected by rubbing this infected material from the bug into the skin or conjunctival membranes. In the human host, multiplication into macrophages is followed by rapid dissemination of trypomastigotes into the blood and hence to tissues.

The genome sequence of *T. cruzi* has stimulated a plethora of comparative and genomic approaches to the study of the parasite.[216,217]

Trypanosoma rangeli Infections

The nonpathogenic trypanosomes can be transmitted directly to people by the bite of the triatomine bugs, and they exist only as circulating trypomastigotes. No tissue amastigotes exist. Circulating organisms are sparse, but sometimes diagnosis can be made by careful microscopic examination of the distinctive morphology of these organisms in blood smears. The anterior position of the nucleus and small kinetoplast distinguish it from *T. cruzi* (Fig. 160-14). The antibodies produced to *T. rangeli* cross-react with those from *T cruzi* and hence cause false-positive serologic test results for *T. cruzi*. However, the species may be differentiated by xenodiagnosis or molecular genetics in specialized laboratories.[218] The importance of recognizing this nonpathogenic infection is to avoid unnecessary treatment for *T. cruzi*.

Pathology

There is a wide variation in the pathogenicity of isolates and some regional variation in the clinical spectrum of acute and chronic illness. Molecular typing has demonstrated considerable heterogeneity of *T. cruzi* isolates, although the association between strains of parasite and the outcome of infection are unclear. Clearly the organism must have many mechanisms of the immune evasion to cause chronic infections in a high proportion of individuals. Some of these have been elegantly defined, including resistance to activation of the alternate pathway of complement, specific mechanisms of entering the host cells, and evasion of intracellular killing by the oxidative burst and lysozymes.

Both CD4+ and CD8+ T cells are important for killing *T. cruzi*–infected cells, and interferon-γ has shown to be important to controlling disease, whereas transforming growth factor-β (TGF-β) and IL-10 enhance parasite replication (for review see reference 219).

End-organ damage occurs after tissues have been infected by *T. cruzi* amastigotes, but the mechanisms leading to extensive cell damage are not clear. After multiplication, tissue amastigotes form pseudocysts in the heart with little or no inflammatory reaction, although occasionally acute myocarditis with focal hemorrhage and inflammation may lead to heart failure. As the disease progresses, the inflammatory response is increased and is associated with increased tissue damage. There may be an autoimmune component to this inflammatory response, but the precise pathogenesis is poorly understood.[220] In the heart, chronic myocarditis leads to a decline in cardiac function. In late-stage disease, amastigotes can be found in almost all organs. Acute myocarditis with focal hemorrhage and inflammation may also lead to heart failure. Involvement of the brain, meninges, liver, lymph nodes, and spleen is common. Damage to the muscle walls and intramural nerve plexus in the esophagus and colon leads to dilation of these structures in the later phases of the disease.

Clinical Features

In about half the patients, a granuloma (or chagoma) occurs where parasites have been inoculated. The tender erythematous papule becomes keratotic and later heals, forming a hyperpigmented scar. When the conjunctiva are inoculated, the extensive unilateral periorbital edema may be prolonged (Romaña sign).

The severity of the acute illness is variable and ranges from asymptomatic infection or a mild febrile illness to a severe, potentially fatal illness with cardiac failure and meningoencephalitis in a minority of cases. Myalgia, generalized lymphadenopathy, hepatosplenomegaly, headaches, facial or generalized edema, vomiting, diarrhea, and anorexia are common features of the acute disease. The disease may be worse in children. The acute illness typically resolves in 4 to 8 weeks.

Chagas disease must be distinguished from typhoid fever, VL, brucellosis, toxoplasmosis, and malaria in cases of chronic, febrile illness in endemic areas.

Chronic Disease

The acute phase of *T. cruzi* infection is followed by a variable latent or indeterminate phase with no clinical symptoms. Indeed, patients may never present with signs of end-organ damage. However, up to a third of clinically infected patients may develop cardiac involvement and show right bundle branch block, AV conduction abnormalities, and/or abnormal T and Q waves. The patient may experience palpitations, chest pain, edema, and dizziness or syncope or dyspnea. The heart is enlarged, and intramural thrombus may cause sudden death.

In a further minority of chronically infected patients, the gastrointestinal tract is infected with abnormal motility of the esophagus and colon, leading to dysphagia and/or severe constipation. Occasionally other hollow organ systems may be affected.

Pregnancy and Congenital Infection

In pregnant women, Chagas disease can cause spontaneous abortion, premature birth, intrauterine growth retardation, and stillbirth. Congenital infection occurs in 1% to 2% of women with chronic infection. Prompt diagnosis of circulating parasites in neonates at risk for congenital Chagas disease is essential to beginning early treatment. It is recognized that infection can also be transmitted by breastfeeding. Most children are asymptomatic, but 10% to 20% of children have a mild systemic illness with hepatosplenomegaly. More severely affected newborn children have pneumonitis, meningoencephalitis, and diffuse dermal granulomas. Petechiae, purpura, and a generalized bleeding tendency may occur.[221]

Immunocompromised Patients

The disease may recrudesce after chemotherapy for malignant disease, immunosuppressive therapy, or after organ transplantation. The clinical disease may be fulminating with obvious parasitemia. Irregular erythematous indurated lesions have been described during *T. cruzi* recrudescence after solid organ transplantation. Here tissue amastigotes can be demonstrated by fine-needle aspiration.

HIV

Coinfection with *T. cruzi* and HIV has been reported from urban centers in Brazil. *T. cruzi* develops in end-stage disease with CD4+ T-cell counts of less than 400/μL. Patients may be severely ill, the majority with meningoencephalitis and often with a space-occupying lesion. Typically the CSF shows a mild lymphocytosis (<100 cells/μL). Parasites may be seen in the blood and occasionally the CSF. Cardiac involvement and heart failure is common.

Hematologic and Laboratory Features

A mild normocytic, normochromic anemia is typical of acute illness. The pathogenesis of the anemia and contributions of hemolysis and bone marrow depression have not been studied in humans, but in experimental infections in mice, uncontrolled infection and TNF-α can be shown to contribute to depressed hematopoiesis. A modest lymphocytosis and increases in liver and muscle enzymes may be present. Nonspecific electrocardiographic changes, first-degree heart block, and cardiomegaly suggest early myocardial involvement.

Hematologic abnormalities are not usually found in the late stage of disease, in which cardiomyopathy with cardiac failure, rhythm disturbance, and angina and systemic emboli from intramural thrombus may occur. Trials of systemic anticoagulation have not been conducted.

Diagnosis

Microscopy

During the acute phase of the disease, motile trypanosomes can be identified in wet preparations or buffy coat preparations using concentration methods and detailed morphologic examination, including Giemsa-stained gently prepared thick and thin films to avoid damage to parasites (Fig. 160-15). Trypanosomes can be aspirated from the chagoma in the acute phase of disease and visualized in a wet preparation of needle aspirates. Parasites may occasionally be found in lachrymal fluid.

Sensitivity is increased by the concentration methods described for *T. brucei* earlier. Organisms may also be sought in centrifuged serum after blood has clotted or by centrifugation after lysis of red blood cells with 0.8% ammonium chloride. Trypomastigotes can also be detected in other specimens, including CSF, bone marrow, pericardiac fluid, and tissue biopsy specimens. Organisms must be distinguished from the morphologically similar nonpathogenic *T. rangeli* (see Fig. 160-14 and earlier).

After the acute phase, circulating parasites are not visible, although inoculation of blood into susceptible animals (xenodiagnosis), in vitro culture, or molecular methods may demonstrate patent infection. Parasitemia may be obvious in immunocompromised patients in the chronic phase of disease.

Xenodiagnosis

Infection of laboratory triatomine bugs by a seropositive patient is more sensitive than morphologic examination in chronically infected

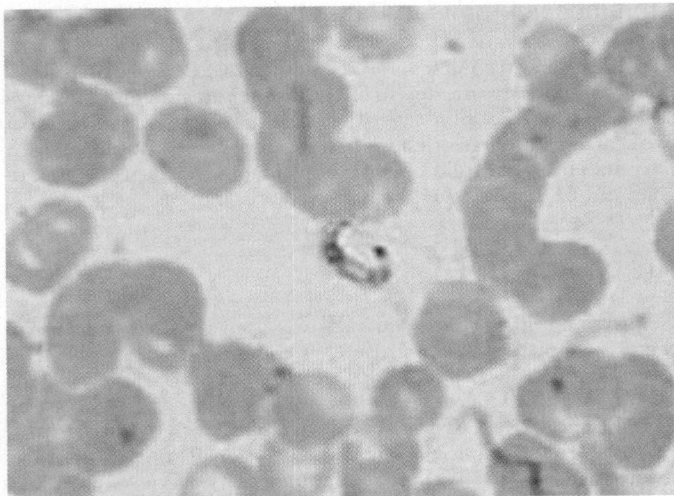

Figure 160-15 *TRYPANOSOMA CRUZI* IN HUMAN BLOOD FILM. The causative agent occurs in blood films characteristically as short C-shaped or S-shaped trypomastigotes with a prominent kinetoplast. It is otherwise monomorphic.

patients. It is also possible to infect susceptible laboratory animals. However, these techniques are only available in specialized centers in Latin America.

In Vitro Culture

Epimastigotes can be cultured using blood agar (Novy Nichol MacNeal [NNN]) medium or other media such as Schneider insect medium. After 4 weeks or more culture at 26° C, epimastigotes may be detected.[222,223]

Serology

Serologic testing is a sensitive method of detecting infection after the acute phase. In Latin America, a number of commercial assays are available using crude epimastigote lysates in a variety of different formats. Serologic tests have used IFAT and ELISA using crude antigen prepared from in vitro cultures of epimastigotes. These tests must be carefully controlled with appropriate positive or negative sera. Chronically infected patients usually give a positive test result if titers are greater than 1 : 80.[224] These have a sensitivity and specificity of more than 95%. These antibodies may cross-react with antibodies to malaria, leishmaniasis, syphilis, and some autoimmune conditions. ELISA should be used in conjunction with a confirmatory test such as a Western blot.

In South and North America, a number of companies market ELISA-based assays using recombinant antigens, synthetic peptides, or a concentrated extract of excretory-secretory antigens from either Brazil or Tulahuen strain *T. cruzi* trypomastigotes (total trypomastigote excretory-secretory antigens [TESAs]). These assays may provide more rapidly available and cheaper tests without loss of sensitivity and specificity (see Trypanosomiasis as a Transfusion-Transmitted Infection for further discussion).

Serologic testing may be useful in the evaluation of people who may have been exposed to Chagas disease, pregnant women, and patients about to undergo immunosuppressive treatment or to receive chemotherapy or who have been diagnosed with HIV or other immunosuppressive illness. Children born to seropositive women will have maternally derived IgG anti–*T. cruzi* antibodies but demonstrate IgM anti–*T. cruzi* antibodies if congenitally infected.[225]

Molecular Diagnosis

Amplification of *T. cruzi*–specific sequences by PCR is potentially the most widely applicable, sensitive, and specific method for detecting parasites. A number of assays have been developed, based on the application of repetitive sequences in kinetoplast DNA. A metaanalysis has suggested that PCR is not more sensitive than ELISA for detection of *T. cruzi* in chagasic patients.[226]

Treatment

The detailed treatment of Chagas disease is beyond the scope of this chapter. Treatment of the acute, intermediate, and chronic phases requires expert supervision because parasitologic cure is achieved in only half the cases and monitoring progress requires specialist testing and evaluation and where necessary treatment of end-organ damage. The current and potential future chemotherapy[227-229] have recently been reviewed.

Nifurtimox is a synthetic nitrofuran that inhibits pyruvic acid synthesis by inhibition of lactic dehydrogenase. It is given for 30 to 120 days at 3 to 5 mg/kg three times a day. The most serious side effects are peripheral neuropathy, mental disturbance (including psychosis), and hemolytic anemia associated with G6PD.

Benznidazole is widely available in Latin America and is given at 2.5 to 5 mg/kg twice a day for 30 to 60 days. Severe hematologic complications are common, and bone marrow depression is a serious side effect. Thrombocytopenia may be severe, and neutropenia may progress to agranulocytosis. Other serious complications include photosensitivity, neuropathy, and weight loss.[230]

Supportive therapy is required for heart failure and acute meningoencephalitis. Surgery may be required for alleviation of esophageal and chronic dysfunction. In the absence of effective or simple therapy, control of triatomine bugs and an improvement in the housing stock are essential to prevent and control disease.

Trypanosomiasis as a Transfusion-Transmitted Infection

Chagas disease may occur as a transfusion-transmitted infection and represents a real threat to the safety of the blood supply in endemic areas. It is estimated that 1.5% to 50% of contaminated units cause infection in recipients, a wide range that may reflect the stage of infection in the donor, the type and processing of the component, and the immune status of the recipient.[231]

In endemic areas, seropositivity is high, reaching 50% in some areas of Bolivia and 1% to 2% in major areas in Brazil. Control of blood transfusion–transmitted infection is part of the World Health Organization strategy for control of Chagas disease.[232-234] Serologic screening, tests using synthetic peptide antigens, or a mixture of recombinant antigens to detect anti–*T cruzi* antibodies in chronically infected blood donors, are more than 95% sensitive.[235,236] These serologic tests, replacing those based on crude antigens, have allowed improved coverage of screening of blood donors throughout Latin America.[237,238]

It is possible to treat blood with gentian violet (0.25 g/L for 24 hours at 4° C) or with methylene blue to kill circulating organisms. It has also been shown that amotosalen or riboflavin plus ultraviolet A photochemical inactivation technology is effective in inactivating *T. cruzi* in platelet concentrates and plasma.[238,239] In addition, prophylactic benznidazole can be given to immunosuppressed patients receiving blood products in endemic areas.

Outside Latin America, Chagas disease is an occasional cause of transfusion-transmitted infection, mainly in immunosuppressed patients. It is possible that minor infections are not recognized in healthy individuals. Clearly the high rates of seropositivity in individuals from endemic areas suggest that recent immigrants may easily transmit the disease.

In the United Sates, the overall seropositive rate among blood donors is 1 : 250,000, with local incidence rates reaching 1 : 7500 or greater in Los Angeles and Miami.[231] These rates are probably underestimates because immigration from endemic areas has recently increased. Surveys of blood donors in France have shown seropositivity of *T. cruzi* can be detected by PCR in about half the seropositive donors and remain viable for at least 20 days, surviving cryopreservation and thawing. *T. cruzi* has been reported to be transmitted after organ transplantation[240,241] and after blood transfusion in seven patients who were immunosuppressed.[242-246]

Donors can be excluded by a medical questionnaire eliciting obvious symptoms of acute or chronic disease. Prospective studies have shown these questionnaires would miss many infected donors,[247,248] including those infected congenitally.[249] Nevertheless, in Europe screening for anti–*T. cruzi* antibodies is targeted at at-risk blood donors who originated from an endemic area, donors with mothers originating from such an area, and individuals who have lived in or traveled to endemic areas. In France the seropositivity in these selected donors was 1 : 32,000.[250]

In the United States, new tests have been requested by the Food and Drug Administration to combat this threat. A radioimmunoprecipitation assay (RIPA) is the most sensitive method to detect anti–*T cruzi* antibodies,[251] although RIPA cross-reactivity has been reported in patients with VL.[252] It is, however, unsuitable for mass screening. An ELISA based in a concentrated extract of excretory-secretory antigens from either Brazil or Tulahuen strain *T. cruzi* trypomastigotes (TESAs)[253,254] had an overall sensitivity of 100% and specificity of more than 94%, and a prototype *T. cruzi* lysate–based ELISA has been developed and appears to be 97.7% sensitive and 100% specific.[251]

It is only to be hoped that sensitive screening tests are consistently applied to reduce transmission of Chagas disease by blood products in endemic and nonendemic countries. On a more general note, it is encouraging that the initiatives to control *T. cruzi* infection across Latin America are showing real evidence of success.[213,255]

BABESIOSIS

Babesiosis is an intraerythrocytic infection caused by parasites from the order Piroplasmida and the family Babesiidae. It was first observed as causing parasitic inclusions in erythrocytes of cattle in Romania by Victor Babes at the end of the 19th century.[256] The infection is zoonosis transmitted by hard-bodied ticks and causes fever and hemolytic anemia.[257] Several distinct *Babesia* spp. cause disease in different geographic areas.[257,258]

There are two well-defined *Babesia* species that cause human infection. *Babesia microti* is a parasite of small rodents in the northeastern United States and is spread by nymphs, larvae, and adult forms of the hard-bodied ixodid ticks *(Ixodes dammini)*. Infection of the white-tailed deer by ticks allows multiplication and spread of the infected ticks. Infections can be transferred to humans by all forms of the tick after prolonged feeding. The infection is therefore most common in people holidaying or working in forested areas of the northeastern United States. The offshore islands of Nantucket, Martha's Vineyard, Block Island, and Shelter Island are foci of disease, but it also occurs in northeastern and upper midwestern states, particularly Connecticut, Rhode Island, Delaware, and New York State. Hundreds of cases have been recorded since the first identified case in 1969. Visitors and workers in endemic areas should avoid tick bites using appropriate clothing and repellents.

In Europe, *Babesia divergens* and the morphologically indistinguishable parasite *Babesia bovis* are transmitted to humans by ticks *(Ixodes ricinus)* from cattle. Less than 50 cases have been recorded. European cases of *B. microti* and *Babesia canis* infection have also been reported.[257]

A handful of cases of infections with poorly defined *Babesia* spp. have been reported from the western United States. These organisms are morphologically indistinguishable from *B. microti* but are distinguished by molecular methods. The MO1-type piroplasm has caused illness in an index case in Missouri in 1992, and the WA1-type and CA1-4 piroplasms caused disease in five cases reported from Washington State and California, respectively, in 1994.[259,260] A further *B. microti*–like organism has been isolated from an asymptomatic woman in Taiwan.[261]

B. microti and the WA1-type piroplasms have been transmitted by blood and platelet transfusions. Transplacental infection by *B. microti* has been reported.

Parasitology

Parasites appear to be introduced into the bloodstream, where they invade erythrocytes. There they multiply by asexual fission to produce two to four merozoites. These infective forms are released after lysis of the erythrocyte and begin another cycle of invasion multiplication. Parasites are cleared by macrophages. The contribution of antibodies and cell-mediated immune response has not been defined, although *B. bovis* expresses clonally variant antigens on the surface of infected erythrocytes.[27]

Clinical Features

The North American *B. microti* infections have an incubation period of several weeks, and after infection by blood transfusion clinical symptoms have taken from 17 days to many months to become manifest.[262-265]

The spectrum of clinical disease is wide. *B. microti* may cause asymptomatic infection or present with a mild flu-like illness in most cases in people with normal immune and splenic function.[266] The cardinal manifestations are fever and hemolytic anemia. Splenectomy, old age, and immunosuppression, including HIV, may increase the risk for more severe clinical disease.[267-269] The disease may progress to adult respiratory distress syndrome (ARDS), disseminated intravascular coagulation, or renal failure.[262] Patients who have had a splenectomy should avoid exposure to ticks in forested areas where the disease is transmitted.

B. divergens in Europe predominantly causes symptomatic infection in people who have had a splenectomy.[270,271] Here, the case fatality rate is on the order of 50%. However, symptomatic disease does also occur in immunocompetent individuals.[272]

Patients present with high fever, often with chills and sweats, jaundice, fatigue, malaise, headache, arthralgia, and myalgia. Gastrointestinal disturbances are common, and people may complain of dark urine secondary to hemoglobinuria. In some cases, the disease progresses with respiratory failure secondary to ARDS, disseminated intravascular coagulation, and renal failure requiring the appropriate supportive care.[273] Such severe cases resemble severe malaria in nonimmune persons, and it has been suggested that the pathophysiology, like malaria, includes adhesion and sequestration of infected erythrocytes and the release of proinflammatory cytokines. These diseases may be confused with falciparum malaria, leptospirosis, or viral hepatitis.

Hematologic and Laboratory Features

The hematologic features of the disease are dominated by substantial intravascular hemolysis.[273] Physical examination shows pallor, jaundice, and mild hepatosplenomegaly.

The laboratory findings are those of a compensated intravascular hemolytic anemia and thus feature low hemoglobin and haptoglobin levels and increased reticulocyte count, serum lactate dehydrogenase, and hemoglobinuria and proteinuria. Moderate thrombocytopenia is common.[265,274] Electron microscopy suggests uninfected erythrocytes are damaged during infection and so likely to be cleared more rapidly than normally.[275] The white blood cell count is usually decreased with atypical lymphocytosis and occasional evidence of hemophagocytosis. However, leukocytosis may occur, particularly in *B. divergens* infections.

The direct Coombs test is frequently positive for both C3 components and IgG. Polyclonal hypergammaglobulinemia is seen, and levels of C3 and C4 are reduced in acute infection.[276] Liver function tests show raised indirect bilirubin and mildly raised transaminase levels.

Diagnosis

The blood films stained with Giemsa or Romanovsky stain show ring-like intraerythrocytic parasites. Morphology is variable, and ring, rod, and ameboid forms of *Babesia* parasites may be seen (Fig. 160-16).[277] Occasionally, multiple intraerythrocytic forms can be seen, linked to form a tetrad or colloquially "Maltese Cross." However, at low parasitemia, *Babesia* parasites may easily be mistaken for ring-stage forms of *P. falciparum*. Moreover, false-positive sightings of *Babesia* spp. may be due to platelets, nonspecific stain deposit overlying erythrocytes, or indeed other intraerythrocytic inclusions.

Parasitemias are variable, and in *B. microti* infections may be low or transient.[266] In symptomatic infection, parasitemias typically range from less than 1% to 10% and rarely much higher, more than 70%, in severe infections.

Low-level parasitemias may be detected by inoculation of the blood into susceptible animals, including the golden hamster (*Mesocricetus auratus*), but this is not routinely available.

An indirect fluorescent antibody test using crude antigen is available in the United States through the Division of Parasitic Diseases at the Centers for Disease Control and Prevention (CDC).[278] Titers greater than 1:64 are regarded as positive and have been reported to be 88% to 96% sensitive and 90% to 100% specific.

PCR analysis is the most useful method of detecting or confirming low levels of parasitemia when serologic tests are positive, and it can also be used to monitor treatment.[279] Species-specific PCR primers are available to provide precise identification of infected parasites. Nevertheless, some rare forms of piroplasm parasites cannot be classified.

Treatment

Many *B. microti* infections are self-limiting, and therapy is used for moderate or severe disease.[280-282] The combination of atovaquone and azithromycin is the treatment of choice for mild-to-moderate illness, whereas clindamycin and quinine and exchange transfusion are indicated for severe disease.

B. divergens infections are often fatal in splenectomized patients, and therapy is based on somewhat limited experience. Pentamidine with cotrimoxazole has been used successfully, whereas individual patients treated with pentamidine and cotrimoxazole or quinine, chloroquine, and pyrimethamine have been unsuccessful. Three cases have been treated successfully with large-volume exchange transfusions (two to three blood volumes) and IV clindamycin and oral quinine.[283] This regimen of clindamycin and IV and oral quinine gives the best chance of success in the absence of randomized controlled trial evidence.

Exchange transfusion has been suggested as a useful adjunctive treatment if the parasitemia rises to greater than 10% and/or in severely ill patients. *B. divergens* infections can run a rapidly progressive course, and early exchange transfusion should be considered. A prolonged course of treatment may be required in immunocompromised patients.[284]

The parasite and hemoglobin levels should be regularly monitored during treatment.

Serologic testing and PCR testing of seropositive cases may be helpful in making a diagnosis. An indirect IFAT is available for *B. divergens* and *B. microti*. The IFAT titer is usually greater than 1:64 in acute infection. The reported sensitivity of the *B. microti* IFAT is 88% to 96% and specificity 90% to 100%.[278] Antimalarial antibodies may cross-react in this test.

Babesia and Transfusion-Transmitted Infection

Babesia infection poses a substantial and increasing threat to the blood supply. Between 150 and 170 cases of transfusion-transmitted babesiosis have been reported from 1979 to 2009 with 12 recorded fatalities.[285-287] There are no approved serologic screening tests for donors, and prevention of transfusion-transmitted babesiosis in the United States requires screening donors about a previous history of babesiosis and excluding patients with fever and a low hematocrit level. The scale of infection can be gauged from surveys of blood donors in the northeastern United States, where 1% to 2% of donors in some panels are seropositive for babesia.[288] In the United Kingdom, a conservative approach has been taken, and all donors who have

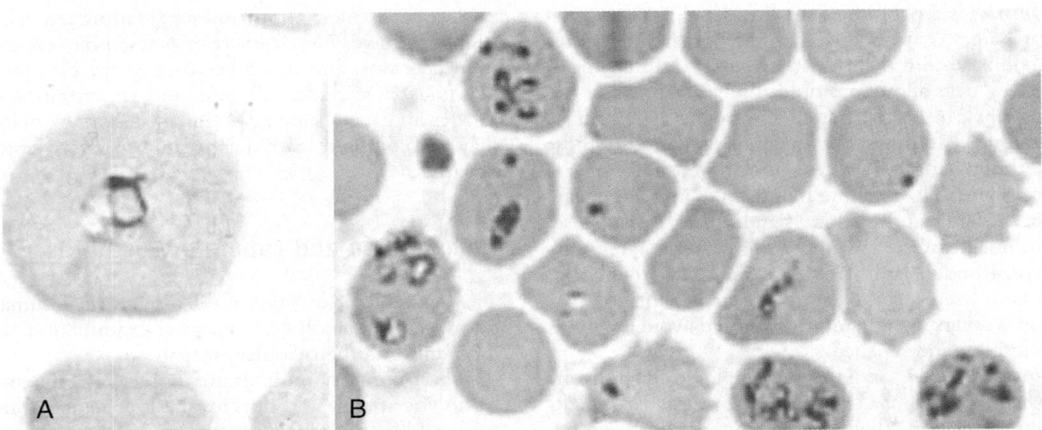

Figure 160-16 *BABESIA* PARASITES. Human infection with species of piroplasm transmitted by the bite of the tick *Ixodes ricinus* infected from cattle is a rare occurrence. Infection in normal people with this piroplasm may give rise to a self-limiting fever and parasitemia, as in the case of infection with the rodent parasite *Babesia microti* on the northeastern seaboard of the United States via the tick *Ixodes scapularis* **(A)**. Heavy red-cell infection may develop, however, in splenectomized patients, leading to fatal hemolytic anemia. This patient died of an infection acquired from the cattle parasite *Babesia divergens* in Scotland **(B)**. Other species of *Babesia* that occasionally infect humans, for example, the WA1, CA1, and MO1 isolates from the United States, are distinguished by molecular means.

visited the northeastern United States between May and October are excluded, in addition to the standard criteria of screening out febrile and/or anemic donors.

EOSINOPHILIA

Eosinophilia may be caused by a wide variety of systemic diseases and parasitic infections. The association with parasitic disease is through part of the Th2 T-cell response stimulated by helminths (worms), filaria, and cestodes. In general, protozoan infections, such as malaria, amebiasis, and giardiasis, are not associated with eosinophilia. However, case reports do exist suggesting isosporosis, toxoplasmosis, and infection with *Dientamoeba fragilis* can cause eosinophilia.

The rise in absolute eosinophil count depends on the degree of tissue invasion and is therefore modest with tapeworms and adult roundworms resident in the bowel but much higher where invasion occurs, for example, *Toxocara canis* or filaria. Some parasites have migratory larval stages, for example, ascariasis (roundworms) and clonorchiasis.

The differential diagnosis of eosinophilia in those who have lived in tropical areas is therefore wide. Evaluating the patients must begin by establishing the degree of eosinophilia (minimal, $<1 \times 10^9$/L; moderate, 1 to 3×10^9/L; high, $>3 \times 10^9$/L), the relation to travel (where necessary), and the presence of symptoms. A wide range of systemic diseases are associated with eosinophilia, and the eosinophil count may be high in drug allergy, pulmonary infiltrate with eosinophilia, and vasculitides.

Eosinophilia in Travelers

Evaluating the cause of eosinophilia in travelers to tropical areas where many parasitic diseases are endemic requires a systematic approach to narrow down likely possibilities by considering existing systemic diseases that may cause eosinophilia (particularly allergy, drug ingestion and autoimmune disease, vasculitis, or arthritis), the areas visited, duration of stay and history of exposure to soil-transmitted nematodes, freshwater potentially infected with schistosomiasis, and rural areas where loiasis, onchocerciasis, and hydatid disease may be contracted.

Physical examination may show subcutaneous swellings associated with filaria or hepatosplenomegaly consistent with schistosomiasis, hydatid disease, or toxocara.

Laboratory examination requires a stepwise approach given the breadth of the differential diagnosis (Table 160-4). The details of specific parasitologic tests are beyond the scope of this chapter, and detailed investigation would certainly require consultation with colleagues in infectious diseases.

Some parasitic causes of eosinophilia may not be diagnosed during the incubation period because larval stages of nematode worms may cause eosinophilic drug migration, but eggs will not be excreted in stools for many months. Moreover, filarial infections do not produce detectable parasites in blood or skin for many months after exposure.

In immunocompromised patients or those about to receive diagnosis, eosinophilia may be crucial, given the risks of giving immunosuppressive therapy such as chemotherapy or hematopoietic stem cell or solid organ transplantation to a patient with a chronic parasitologic infection. Patients with undiagnosed eosinophilia and possible exposure to *Strongyloides* should be given empirical course of treatment.

OTHER PARASITIC DISEASES

Many parasitic diseases cause some minor hematologic disturbance. A few may present with distinct hematologic features or indeed syndromes.

Table 160-4 Approach to Investigation of Eosinophilia in a Returning Traveler

History	Allergy Drugs and vitamins (L-tryptophan) Regions, localities, and duration of exposure
Physical examination	Skin, subcutaneous tissues Liver/spleen Signs of other systemic disease
Initial investigations	Full blood count and differential white blood cell count Stool examination for ova and parasites (×3) Urine analysis Examination of midday urine for ova and parasites (×3) (in those who have traveled to Africa or the Middle East)
Further investigations as suggested by travel and exposure from history	As suggested by travel and exposure from history *Strongyloides* culture and serologic testing Duodenal aspirate (strongyloidiasis, hookworm) Serologic testing (schistosomiasis, filariasis) Day/night blood films (filariasis)
Further studies if suggested by history and physical examination	Skin snips (onchocerciasis) Chest x-ray examination (hydatid cyst, tropical pulmonary eosinophilia, paragonimiasis) Soft tissue x-ray examination (cysticercosis) Sputum examination for ova and parasites (paragonimiasis) Abdominal ultrasound examination (hydatid cyst) Cystoscopy with or without biopsy (schistosomiasis) Rectal snips (schistosomiasis)

Filariasis

Lymphatic filariasis is caused by *Wuchereria bancrofti* and *Brugia malayi*. Infection with *W. bancrofti* occurs throughout the tropics, but by far the majority of cases are in Asia. The distribution of *B. malayi* is more restricted to China, Southeast Asia, and Southern India. The male and female adult worms live in the lymphatics, and the female worm releases a vast number of microfilariae, each 250 to 300 μm in length. Microfilariae develop but do not appear to multiply in the mosquito.

Infection may present with lymphangitis; often recurrent and unlike bacterial infections, the inflammatory features may spread distally. Over time, lymphatic obstruction may cause hydrocele, lymphedema (if severe elephantiasis), chyluria, and tropical pulmonary eosinophilia. *B. malayi* causes neither hydrocele nor chyluria.

Filariasis is most easily diagnosed by finding microfilariae in peripheral blood in a wet preparation. Motile microfilariae can be seen under low power and may be concentrated by centrifugation or filtration using a 3-μm filter. They are speciated in thin or thick films by their nuclear distribution and sheath characteristics (Fig. 160-17), and the two pathogenic species must be distinguished from the nonpathogenic species *Mansonella perstans* and *Mansonella ozzardi,* which do not have sheaths. Circulating *W. bancrofti* antigens can also be detected in the circulation by ELISA or immunochromatographic methods. Adult worms can sometimes be imaged by ultrasound. Filarial DNA from all species can be detected by PCR. Serologic testing is unhelpful because many people become exposed without developing clinical symptoms.

The worms cause marked or severe eosinophilia (see later) with counts greater than 1×10^9/L. Migration of worms through the lungs may exacerbate the eosinophil count and cause minor respiratory

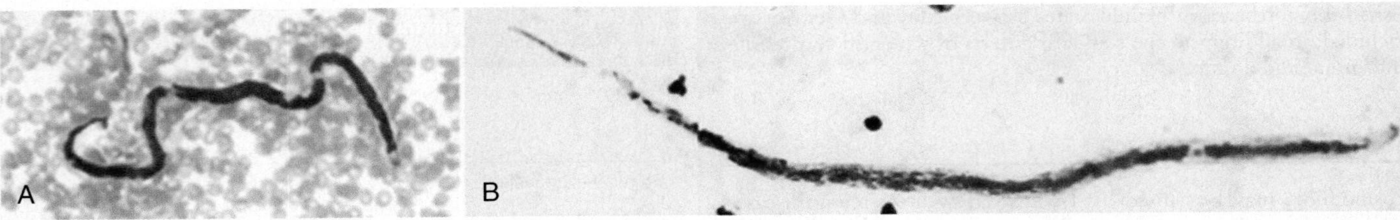

Figure 160-17 MICROFILARIA *(BRUGIA MALAYI)* ON THICK **(A)** AND THIN PREP **(B)**. The species is determined by the nuclear distribution and sheath characteristics.

symptoms and fluctuating radiologic signs. Other causes of tropical pulmonary eosinophilia are the worms (helminths) *Ascaris, Strongyloides, Schistosoma,* and *Toxocara.* Of these organisms causing pulmonary symptoms and signs, filariasis alone is responsive to diethylcarbamazine. Albendazole and ivermectin may also be used against filarial infection.

Toxoplasmosis

Toxoplasmosis may cause a mild illness or a more prolonged course with constitutional symptoms, atypical lymphocytes, and thrombocytopenia. Congenital toxoplasmosis as a result of infection acquired during pregnancy is a cause of neonatal thrombocytopenia, where it may be accompanied by cerebral calcification, hepatitis, and pneumonitis. In immunocompromised patients, new or reactivated toxoplasmosis may cause severe disease, including encephalitis, pneumonitis, and hepatitis. Thrombocytopenia is frequently accompanied by anemia and leukopenia.

Amebiasis

Amebiasis causes hypochromic, microcytic anemia both as a result of chronic blood loss and as an anemia of chronic disease in which disease progresses to formation of a liver abscess. Neutrophilia accompanies severe tissue damage caused by perforation of the bowel or a liver abscess or may be present in a secondary bacterial infection. Sometimes a leukemoid reaction with high white blood cell count and extreme left-shifted myeloid cells can be seen. Prolonged and/or extensive liver damage may cause prolongation of the prothrombin time.

Giardiasis

Acute giardiasis causes folate deficiency through malabsorption of folate in the small intestine. Chronic infection can cause vitamin B_{12} deficiency because ileal absorption of the vitamin is impaired.

Hookworm Infection

Adult hookworms attach themselves to the lining of the small bowel and take blood meals. The accumulated blood loss may be extensive because worms consume 2.0 mL *(Necator americanus)* or 0.5 mL of blood *(Ancylostoma duodenale)* each day. These infections are a common contributing factor to iron deficiency anemia in children, in whom infection is acquired by eating or walking barefoot on larva-infected soil. The disease is usually diagnosed by finding excreted eggs in stool samples, and treatment is with albendazole.

Tapeworm Infection

The fish tapeworm *(Diphyllobothrium latum)* is a rare cause of vitamin B_{12} deficiency. This tapeworm is transmitted in the Far East by eating raw or partially cooked fish. Infection has to be extensive and causes vitamin B_{12} deficiency; however, such cases are rare, even in endemic areas.

Schistosomiasis

Schistosoma haematobium causes blood loss in urine. Infection is acquired by swimming in freshwater, where cercariae from the infected snail host enter the skin and migrate to the blood vessels of the bladder. Chronic blood loss is a cause of iron deficiency anemia in children in endemic areas, but infection is likely to be diagnosed at an early stage in travelers because of the striking symptoms of painless hematuria. Treatment is with praziquantel.

FUTURE DIRECTIONS

Parasitic diseases present many problems for global heath. They cause a wide spectrum of hematologic abnormalities, and in endemic areas, a broad knowledge of the parasitic disease is vital for everyday practice. In nonendemic areas, there are a few situations where the diagnosis or management of these diseases may fall within the remit of hematologists and hematology laboratories, particularly malaria and the diagnosis of anemia, cytopenias, eosinophilia, and hepatosplenomegaly. Here, a high index of suspicion is often needed for the diagnosis to be made. A good travel history is crucial in order to establish exposure to parasitic disease and to prompt the search for the appropriate organisms. Several parasitic diseases pose a threat for the safe supply of blood, and the problems of screening of these infections are far from solved. Beyond everyday practice the pathophysiology and prevention of these diseases pose major challenges for biomedical research and public health.

SUGGESTED READINGS

Alvar J, Aparicio P, Aseffa A, et al: The relationship between leishmaniasis and AIDS: The second 10 years. *Clin Microbiol Rev* 21:334, 2008.

Bailey JW, Williams JE, Bain BJ, et al: Guideline: The laboratory diagnosis of malaria. 2007. wwwbcshguidelinescom. Accessed 1st June 2008.

Bern C: Antitrypanosomal therapy for chronic Chagas' disease. *N Engl J Med* 364:2527, 2011.

Brun R, Blum J, Chappuis F, et al: Human African trypanosomiasis. *Lancet* 375:148, 2011.

Collins WE: *Plasmodium knowlesi*: A malaria parasite of monkeys and humans. *Annu Rev Entomol* 57:107, 2011.

Coura JR, Borges-Pereira J: Chagas disease: 100 years after its discovery. A systemic review. *Acta Trop* 115:5, 2010.

Cowman AF, Crabb BS: Invasion of red blood cells by malaria parasites. *Cell* 124:755, 2006.

Cox FE: History of human parasitology. *Clin Microbiol Rev* 15:595, 2002.

Croft SL, Olliaro P: Leishmaniasis chemotherapy—challenges and opportunities. *Clin Microbiol Infect* 17:1478, 2010.

Genovese G, Friedman DJ, Ross MD, et al: Association of trypanolytic apoL1 variants with kidney disease in African Americans. *Science* 329:841, 2010.

Gubernot DM, Lucey CT, Lee KC, et al: Babesia infection through blood transfusions: Reports received by the US Food and Drug Administration, 1997-2007. *Clin Infect Dis* 48:25, 2009.

Lalloo DG, Shingadia D, Pasvol G, et al: UK malaria treatment guidelines. *J Infect* 54:111, 2007.

Leiby DA: Transfusion-transmitted *Babesia* spp.: Bull's-eye on *Babesia microti*. *Clin Microbiol Rev* 24:14, 2011

Maitland K, Kiguli S, Opoka RO, et al: Mortality after fluid bolus in African children with severe infection. *N Engl J Med* 364:2483, 2011.

Mandell GL, Bennett JE, Dolin R: *Principles and practice of infectious diseases,* London, 2009, Churchill Livingstone.

Marsh K, Forster D, Waruiru C, et al: Indicators of life-threatening malaria in African children. *N Engl J Med* 332:1399, 1995.

Mungai M, Tegtmeier G, Chamberland M, et al: Transfusion-transmitted malaria in the United States from 1963 through 1999. *N Engl J Med* 344:1973, 2001.

Pays E, Vanhollebeke B: Human innate immunity against African trypanosomes. *Curr Opin Immunol* 21:493, 2009.

Portugal S, Carret C, Recker M, et al: Host-mediated regulation of superinfection in malaria. *Nat Med* 17:732, 2011.

Prentice AM: Iron metabolism, malaria, and other infections: What is all the fuss about? *J Nutr* 138:2537, 2008.

Simarro PP, Cecchi G, Paone M, et al: The atlas of human African trypanosomiasis: A contribution to global mapping of neglected tropical diseases. *Int J Health Geogr* 9:57, 2010.

Vannier E, Gewurz BE, Krause PJ: Human babesiosis. *Infect Dis Clin North Am* 22:469, 2008.

Wendel S: Transfusion transmitted Chagas disease: Is it really under control? *Acta Trop* 115:28, 2010.

World Health Organization: Control of the leishmaniases. *World Health Organ Tech Rep Ser* 949:1, 2010.

For complete list of references log on to www.expertconsult.com.

CHAPTER 161

HEMATOLOGIC PROBLEMS IN THE SURGICAL PATIENT: BLEEDING AND THROMBOSIS

Mark T. Reding and Nigel S. Key

Surgical patients often present unique challenges to the consulting hematologist. They may develop hemostatic disorders ranging from unexpected bleeding to pathologic thrombosis, both of which can be potentially life-threatening. Consultation may be sought to assess preoperative bleeding risk and/or to recommend strategies to prevent postoperative thrombosis. The hematologist may be called upon to assist in the management of patients with a previous history of bleeding or thrombosis and in those with unexplained bleeding or thrombosis in the postoperative period. This chapter will review the preoperative evaluation of bleeding risk, the management of patients with hemostatic abnormalities, perioperative management of patients on long-term oral anticoagulation, and strategies to prevent surgery-induced venous thromboembolism (VTE).

PREOPERATIVE EVALUATION OF HEMOSTATIC RISK

Preoperative evaluation of hemostatic risk begins with a carefully taken history. Particular attention should be directed at specific bleeding symptoms and any history of bleeding associated with surgical procedures, including circumcision, tonsillectomy, and dental extractions. For women, it is important to inquire about a history of menorrhagia or excessive bleeding associated with childbirth. A detailed family history and record of medication use, including nonprescription medications, should be obtained. In adults, an interview to assess for the presence or absence of bleeding symptoms has a high discriminating power when used in a screening situation, where no bleeding disorder is suspected, but may be less discriminatory for those referred for specialty evaluation.[1] In the pediatric population, the medical history may be less reliable as a screening method because of fewer previous hemostatic challenges.[2]

Obtaining an adequate bleeding history may be complicated by the fact that many hemostatically normal people consider their bleeding to be excessive. Surveys of healthy individuals frequently report excessive nosebleeds (5% to 39%), gingival bleeding (7% to 51%), easy bruising (12% to 24%), menorrhagia (23% to 44%), postpartum bleeding (6% to 23%), and bleeding following dental extraction (up to 13%) and tonsillectomy (up to 11%).[1,3-5] Thus a thorough search for objective confirmation of reported symptoms is essential. Also, a constellation of bleeding symptoms, rather than any single symptom, is most helpful in suggesting the presence and etiology of an underlying bleeding disorder.

The need for routine coagulation testing before surgical or invasive procedures has been controversial for many years. Those in favor of testing point to the asymptomatic nature of some hemostatic abnormalities that may cause surgical bleeding and the occasional failure to obtain a detailed history.[6-8] A prospective study of preoperative screening in children before tonsillectomy found both history and laboratory screening to have high specificity but a low positive predictive value for perioperative bleeding.[7] Another study found that perioperative blood loss in adult cardiothoracic surgery patients could be predicted with a model, which included the bleeding time, prothrombin time (PT), and platelet count.[9] Given the variety of potential hemostatic defects, however, no simple screening system will identify all patients at increased risk for bleeding. Those against routine laboratory testing[10] point to retrospective studies indicating that they rarely detect unexpected bleeding disorders[11,12] and also emphasize the problems in evaluating false-positive abnormalities. A literature review found insufficient evidence to conclude that an abnormal prothrombin time/international normalized ratio (PT/INR) predicts bleeding during invasive procedures.[13] A retrospective review[14] of the value of preoperative platelet count, PT, and activated partial thromboplastin time (aPTT) in 828 patients undergoing major noncardiac surgery found that only 2% had abnormal results, and most were expected on the basis of history and physical examination. Furthermore, no relation between abnormal laboratory test results and intraoperative blood loss or postoperative bleeding complications was found.[14] This is not surprising, given the lack of studies using an evidence-based approach to determine the degree of abnormality in the PT/INR or aPTT at which an invasive procedure may be unsafe.[15] A number of prospective studies have also concluded that routine laboratory screening tests in asymptomatic patients are not predictive of perioperative or postoperative bleeding.[16-20] Thus for an unselected population, in the absence of historical risk factors or physical examination findings suggestive of an underlying bleeding tendency, the likelihood of an unsuspected, clinically significant congenital or acquired coagulopathy is low enough that routine laboratory screening is not warranted,[21] particularly for those undergoing low-risk procedures. The British Committee for Standards in Haematology recently issued guidelines reiterating this position: indiscriminate coagulation testing before surgical or invasive procedures is a poor predictor of bleeding risk and is not recommended in the absence of a positive personal or family bleeding history.[22] However, it has been suggested that Ashkenazi Jews should receive special consideration, because of the relatively high prevalence of factor XI deficiency. In this population, a screening aPTT might be reasonable.[21]

There are a variety of reasons why routine coagulation tests such as the PT/INR and aPTT may be poorly predictive of underlying coagulopathy and bleeding risk.[22] First, these tests are designed to measure time to clot formation in an artificial in vitro assay and may not reliably depict the global hemostatic situation in vivo (see Liver Disease). More importantly, the PT/INR and aPTT may be insensitive to mild but clinically relevant bleeding disorders such as von Willebrand disease or mild hemophilia. Conversely, they may detect conditions such as factor XII deficiency or a lupus inhibitor that do not increase the risk for bleeding.

The bleeding time had long been used to assess primary hemostasis and to predict the risk for hemorrhage associated with invasive procedures. However, there is now general consensus that in the absence of a history of a bleeding disorder, the bleeding time is not useful,[23] and many laboratories no longer perform this test. The platelet function analyzer (PFA-100) has been developed for rapid, quantitative, in vitro global testing of platelet function.[24-28] The clinical sensitivity (94% to 95%) and specificity (88% to 89%) of this instrument are virtually identical to platelet aggregometery,[28] and it is clearly superior to the bleeding time.[25,29] Although some have suggested that the PFA-100 could be used for screening for primary hemostatic defects,[30] such testing has limitations. The PFA-100 has high sensitivity for moderate to severe von Willebrand disease and severe platelet defects, such as Glanzmann thrombasthenia and Bernard-Soulier syndrome, but it has poor sensitivity for milder intrinsic platelet disorders like storage pool disease, Hermansky-Pudlak syndrome, and primary secretion defects.[29] Although the PFA-100 is most useful when a hemostatic defect is clinically likely, in such cases additional testing is usually necessary to establish a specific diagnosis.[29-31] If clinical suspicion is high, further testing is indicated even with normal PFA-100 results.[29] Thus the PFA-100 should not be used for general unselected screening.[31] It had been hoped that platelet function testing of this sort might provide a convenient and inexpensive means to reliably predict surgical bleeding, but clinical studies have yielded disappointing results. Although some studies have demonstrated the ability of the PFA-100 to predict recurrent ischemic events following percutaneous coronary interventions[32] and coronary artery bypass graft surgery,[33] such testing has been inadequate to predict bleeding events following coronary stent placement.[34] Similarly, PFA-100 testing has not proven useful in predicting perioperative bleeding in patients undergoing heart surgery[35,36] or hip fracture surgery.[37]

Notwithstanding the ongoing controversy regarding the value of preoperative laboratory screening, it seems reasonable to adopt an approach that is a compromise, in which the level of hemostatic risk for the proposed surgery or invasive procedure (Table 161-1) forms the basis for an approach to preoperative evaluation (Table 161-2). A hemostatic history should be obtained in all patients, and in those about to undergo a low-risk procedure no laboratory tests are required. For moderate- to high-risk procedures, additional screening could include a PT/INR, aPTT, and assessment of the platelet count.

In practice, a hematologist is rarely consulted for routine screening because surgeons have adopted approaches based on their own training and local practice patterns. Rather, consultation is sought because of a history suggesting a bleeding disorder or an abnormal test result that is found on screening. The approach of the consultant cannot be one of "routine screening" because the judgment of the referring physician that a bleeding disorder may be present indicates an increased probability of finding an abnormality. If a referral is obtained as a result of an abnormal screening test result, this finding must be pursued and the abnormality fully explained. However, for all referrals the history is still of central importance and must include a thorough review of any bleeding episodes, including hospital records and results of prior hemostatic testing, as well as careful attention to the family history. The physical examination should focus on evidence of bleeding and on identifying systemic disorders such as hepatic or renal disease. If the history of bleeding is negative or minimal, appropriate laboratory testing would include a PT/INR, aPTT, and a biochemical profile to evaluate hepatic and renal function. A complete blood count and examination of the peripheral blood smear are useful to identify myeloproliferative disorders, gray platelet syndrome, or thrombocytopenia. If the history is suggestive of a hemostatic abnormality, a full evaluation is indicated and additional specific testing is usually required because von Willebrand disease; mild deficiencies of factors VIII, IX, and XI; severe factor XIII deficiency; platelet function defects; and fibrinolytic abnormalities may not be identified by global screening tests (see Table 161-2).

Table 161-1 Risk for Bleeding With Surgical or Invasive Procedures

Risk	Type of Procedure	Examples
Low	Nonvital organs involved, exposed surgical site, limited dissection	Lymph node biopsy, dental extraction, cataract extraction, most cutaneous surgery, laparoscopic procedures, coronary angiography
Moderate	Vital organs involved, deep or extensive dissection	Laparotomy, thoracotomy, mastectomy, major orthopedic surgery, pacemaker insertion
High	Bleeding likely to compromise surgical result, bleeding complications frequent	Neurosurgery, ophthalmic surgery, cardiopulmonary bypass, prostatectomy or bladder surgery, major vascular surgery, renal biopsy, bowel polypectomy

Table 161-2 Preoperative Hemostatic Evaluation

	Routine Screening
Surgical Risk	***Approach***
Low	History only
Moderate or high	History, PT, aPTT, platelet count
Consultation History	
Negative or minimal for bleeding	PT, aPTT, platelet count, biochemical profile, complete blood count with differential, review of peripheral smear
Suggestive of bleeding disorder	Add to above as indicated: platelet function tests, von Willebrand antigen, ristocetin cofactor, factor VIII, factor IX, factor XI, factor XIII assays

aPTT, Activated partial thromboplastin time; *PT,* prothrombin time.

HEMOSTATIC AGENTS

A variety of hemostatic agents are available and may be useful for the prevention or treatment of bleeding in the surgical patient. These agents work through a variety of mechanisms to facilitate hemostasis, including enhancement of primary hemostasis, stimulation of thrombin generation and fibrin formation, and inhibition of fibrinolysis.[38] However, it is important to note that there is a paucity of safety data involving hemostatic agents, because most trials have been designed to assess therapeutic efficacy rather than potential complications, including thrombosis.[38,39] The use of desmopressin, topical hemostatic agents, antifibrinolytics, and recombinant factor VIIa (rFVIIa) will be discussed here. Blood products (platelets, fresh frozen plasma, cryoprecipitate) and clotting factor VIII and IX concentrates are discussed elsewhere (see Chapters 118 and 137).

Desmopressin

Desmopressin (1-deamino-8-D-arginine vasopressin, or DDAVP) is a synthetic analogue of the antidiuretic hormone arginine vasopressin. Intravenous, subcutaneous, or intranasal administration of DDAVP results in transient increases in plasma concentrations of factor VIII and von Willebrand factor as a result of their release from vascular endothelium.[40] Peak levels (typically two to four times basal) are achieved 30 to 60 minutes after intravenous and 60 to 90 minutes after subcutaneous or intranasal administration.[41] Doses may be repeated at intervals of 12 to 24 hours, but tachyphylaxis may occur after three or four doses,[42] limiting further usefulness of DDAVP. Expression of glycoprotein Ib (GPIb) and GPIIb/IIIa on platelet membranes is also enhanced following administration of DDAVP.[43]

DDAVP is the treatment of choice for patients with mild hemophilia A or type 1 von Willebrand disease who require low-risk surgical procedures. Moderate- or high-risk procedures usually require administration of clotting factor concentrates.[42] DDAVP may also be useful for patients with congenital or acquired platelet function disorders.[41,43,44] A recent prospective, randomized, controlled trial comparing intranasal DDAVP with transfusion of fresh frozen plasma and/or platelets in cirrhotic patients with platelet counts of 30,000 to 50,000/μL and/or INRs of 2.0 to 3.0 undergoing dental extraction found that DDAVP was equally effective, less expensive, and well tolerated.[45]

Although initially felt to be promising,[46] the efficacy of DDAVP in reducing blood loss and transfusion requirements associated with cardiopulmonary bypass has not been supported by subsequent clinical trials[47-50] or metaanalyses.[51,52] Worrisome also is the fact that metaanalysis has shown a 2.4-fold increase in perioperative myocardial infarction in cardiac surgery patients treated with DDAVP.[52] Thus the routine use of DDAVP in cardiac, orthopedic, or other elective surgical procedures generally has not been recommended.[39,53] A more recent metaanalysis of 38 randomized placebo-controlled trials including nearly 2500 surgical patients found that DDAVP slightly reduced blood loss (approximately 80 mL per patient) and transfusion requirements (approximately 0.3 units per patient) without a reduction in the proportion of patients receiving transfusions.[54] The authors acknowledge that the clinical impact of this finding may be questioned yet still should be considered in view of the low cost of DDAVP. They found a similar incidence of thromboembolic events (5.4% versus 4.6%) in the DDAVP and placebo groups, respectively, but point out that identification of harm from DDAVP is limited by study design and that safety concerns remain unresolved.[54] However, certain subgroups of patients, such as those with platelet dysfunction, may benefit.[43,53-57] Because of the small but important risk for myocardial infarction,[58] DDAVP should be used with caution in any surgical patient with a history of, or risk factors for, coronary artery disease.

Topical Hemostatic Agents

Although some forms of topical hemostatic agents have been in routine clinical use for many years, a sharp increase in the number of available products has occurred over the last decade. These agents have found broad application across a wide range of surgical specialties, including cardiovascular, orthopedic, urologic, hepatic, reconstructive, laparoscopic, bariatric, and dental surgery.[59-62]

Choice of one topical hemostatic agent over another depends largely on individual experience and product availability.[63] There are few randomized controlled trials in the literature to guide clinical practice, and the methodologic quality of the available studies has been criticized.[39,64] The fact that many of the published studies in this field are industry funded further contributes to the lack of a solid evidence base from which clinical practice guidelines can emerge.[63]

Topical hemostatic agents can be grouped into several categories: physical agents (bone wax, Ostene), absorbable agents (gelatin foams, oxidized cellulose, microfibrillar collagen), biologic agents (thrombin, fibrin sealants, platelet gel), synthetic agents (polyethylene glycol hydrogels, cyanoacrylates, glutaraldehyde cross-linked albumin), and hemostatic dressings.[65] A brief overview of the different types of topical hemostatic agents follows. A thorough discussion of the currently available products, including mechanisms of action, specific advantages and disadvantages, and recommendations for use is provided in a recent comprehensive review.[65]

Physical Agents

Bone wax (first used in the 1880s) and alkylene oxide copolymers (Ostene, introduced in 2001) control hemorrhage by occluding bleeding channels on bone surfaces. The latter is preferred because it does not impede bone growth and is eventually absorbed. Both can increase the risk for local infection.[65]

Absorbable Agents

Gelatin foams, which have been in use since 1945, are derived from animal products and provide a physical matrix upon which coagulation can initiate. These products expand to double their volume, an attractive feature for use in penetrating wounds, but potentially problematic if used near nerves or in confined spaces.[65]

Oxidized cellulose was also introduced in the 1940s, and is derived from wood pulp. It provides a physical matrix for clotting initiation and has excellent handling characteristics. By lowering surrounding pH, oxidized cellulose exerts antimicrobial effect, but this property limits its ability to be used with biologic agents such as thrombin that are pH sensitive, and it can also contribute to local inflammation.[65]

Microfibrillar collagen was developed in 1970 and is derived from bovine components. It contributes to hemostasis through platelet adherence and activation and is effective in controlling wide-area parenchymal bleeding. Therefore it can be useful even in the face of heparin therapy, although it is less effective in the setting of thrombocytopenia.[65]

Biologic Agents

Thrombin derived from bovine plasma has been used for more than 40 years as a topical hemostatic agent in surgical patients. However, bovine thrombin can trigger the formation of antibodies that cross-react with human blood proteins, leading to hemorrhagic complications.[66-68] Because of these issues, human plasma–derived and subsequently recombinant forms of thrombin were developed. A phase III randomized double-blind comparative trial found that recombinant human thrombin had comparable efficacy and safety, but with fewer immunologic complications compared with bovine thrombin.[69] In 2008, recombinant human thrombin was licensed in the United States and is now the preferred form of topical thrombin.

Fibrin sealants are topical hemostatic agents composed of purified virally inactivated human fibrinogen, human thrombin, and sometimes added components such as human factor XIII and antifibrinolytic agents.[60] They have been available in Europe and Japan since the 1960s, but concern about viral transmission halted development and use of fibrin sealants in the United States until 1998, when licensing was approved by the Food and Drug Administration (FDA). The components of fibrin sealants are supplied in separate chambers of a dual-syringe delivery device that combines them at the time of administration. The final steps of the coagulation cascade are reproduced, resulting in formation of a stable fibrin clot. These products are particularly effective for controlling oozing from raw surfaces.[65]

Approved by the FDA in 2000, platelet gel combines microfibrillar collagen and thrombin with patient-derived plasma that contains fibrinogen and platelets. It is also applied with a dual-chamber syringe device, similar to fibrin sealants. The presence of platelets improves clot strength and provides growth factors, but the need for centrifugation of patient blood and processing before use are disadvantages.[65]

Synthetic Agents

Cyanoacrylates are liquid monomers that rapidly polymerize in the presence of water and attach adjacent surfaces together. Approved in the United States in 1998, octyl-2-cyanoacrylate is useful for closing small wounds or incisions and provides good cosmetic results.[65]

Polyethylene glycol hydrogel was approved for use in the United States in 2001 and can be sprayed onto tissue, where it rapidly forms a cross-linked polymer matrix and serves as a sealant and inhibits cell ingrowth and adhesion formation. It is useful for preventing pericardial adhesions and as a mechanical sealant for vascular reconstructions in which swelling and expansion are not a concern.[65]

Glutaraldehyde cross-linked albumin (bovine) received FDA approval in 1999. It has a rapid onset of action and is primarily used to seal sutures or staple lines in complex cardiovascular procedures. However, it can restrict tissue growth and should therefore not be used circumferentially around developing structures, particularly in children.[65]

Hemostatic Dressings

Progress in the field of topical hemostatic agents over the last decade has expanded into the development of hemostatic dressings. Several products containing combinations of gauze and lyophilized fibrinogen and thrombin, chitin and chitosan (polysaccharides found in arthropod skeletons and produced by fermenting algae), and mineral zeolite are available. In general, the use of hemostatic dressings is still under investigation, primarily by the military and emergency first responders.[65]

Antifibrinolytics

Antifibrinolytic agents include the synthetic lysine analogues 6-aminohexanoic acid (aminocaproic acid) and 4-(aminomethyl) cyclohexanecarboxylic acid (tranexamic acid), and the serine protease inhibitor aprotinin. Although both types of antifibrinolytic agents have been used in managing surgical bleeding, the lysine analogues are available in oral forms that facilitate their use in other clinical situations as well.

Aminocaproic Acid and Tranexamic Acid

Both aminocaproic acid and tranexamic acid bind reversibly to the lysine binding site on plasminogen, thereby interfering with fibrin binding, which is required for activation by plasminogen activators.[41] Although tranexamic acid is approximately 10 times more potent than aminocaproic acid and has a longer half-life, both drugs have similar hemostatic effects even in the absence of laboratory signs of excessive fibrinolysis.[70] Extravascular accumulation with inhibition of tissue fibrinolysis and subsequent clot stabilization is thought to explain the efficacy of these drugs.[41]

Because the oral form of tranexamic acid was not commercially available in the United States for a number of years, aminocaproic acid became the lysine derivative of choice. It is commonly used to treat mucosal hemorrhage (menorrhagia, epistaxis, dental bleeding) in patients with congenital coagulopathies and is also effective for prevention of oral bleeding in those who require dental work while receiving long-term oral anticoagulant therapy. Although aminocaproic acid is sometimes used to treat bleeding in patients with thrombocytopenia, randomized controlled trials are lacking.[45] The use of antifibrinolytic drugs in patients with gastrointestinal bleeding would seem rational given the high concentration of fibrinolytic enzymes in the digestive tract, and a metaanalysis found reductions in recurrent bleeding, need for surgery, and mortality.[71] However, improvements in the efficacy of other medical and endoscopic treatments have limited the use of these drugs in this setting, although they are still useful for some patients with underlying bleeding disorders.[41] The urinary tract is also rich in plasminogen activators, and some clinical trials comparing tranexamic acid or aminocaproic acid with placebo in patients undergoing prostatectomy have shown reduced blood loss, but not a reduced need for transfusion or decreased mortality.[41] Additional data from appropriately designed clinical trials are needed before the routine use of antifibrinolytic agents in urologic surgery can be recommended.[56] As noted earlier, oral antifibrinolytics are effective in the treatment of menorrhagia, and oral tranexamic acid received FDA approval for this indication in late 2009.

The largest experience with aminocaproic acid in surgical patients is in those undergoing cardiac surgery. Older metaanalyses have consistently shown that prophylactic treatment of cardiac surgery patients with aminocaproic acid results in a 30% to 40% reduction in postoperative bleeding, without an increase in thromboembolic complications.[52,72-74] Similar results have been shown with tranexamic acid.[43] Other metaanalyses have shown that aminocaproic acid and tranexamic acid are effective in reducing surgical blood loss but have yielded inconsistent results in reducing transfusion requirements.[53,75] A wide variety of dosing schedules may partly explain these heterogeneous results.[53] A recent metaanalysis showed that both agents were effective in reducing blood loss and transfusion requirements in those undergoing cardiac surgery.[76]

A number of studies have demonstrated that antifibrinolytic agents reduce blood loss in orthopedic surgery. A metaanalysis of 43 randomized controlled trials in total hip and knee arthroplasty, spine fusion, musculoskeletal infection, or tumor surgery found that aprotinin and tranexamic acid significantly reduced the number of patients requiring transfusion, with a dose–effect relationship suggested for tranexamic acid.[77] Aminocaproic acid was not found to be effective, although the data were sparse. Similarly, data were too limited to make any definitive conclusions about the safety of these agents in orthopedic surgery patients. A recent metaanalysis of 11 clinical trials involving total hip replacement found that the use of tranexamic acid significantly reduced intraoperative blood loss and transfusion requirements, without any increase in venous thromboembolism or other complications.[78] A recent double-blind, randomized, placebo-controlled trial demonstrated that intraoperative treatment with tranexamic acid was also effective in reducing the need for transfusion in patients undergoing retropubic prostatectomy.[79]

Antifibrinolytics, particularly tranexamic acid, have also been studied in the treatment of trauma patients, in whom 30% of deaths are attributed to hemorrhage.[80] A recent landmark trial, Clinical Randomisation of an Antifibrinolytic in Significant Haemorrhage 2 (CRASH-2), evaluated the safety and efficacy of tranexamic acid in the setting of trauma.[81] This randomized, placebo-controlled, multinational trial that included more than 20,000 trauma patients demonstrated a significant reduction in all-cause mortality and death due to bleeding in the treatment group. More severely injured patients and those treated within 3 hours of injury derived the greatest benefit, and there was no difference in the rate of vascular occlusive events between the two groups.[81] A subsequent review has argued for the immediate incorporation of tranexamic acid into trauma clinical practice guidelines and treatment protocols given that it is the only drug with prospective clinical trial evidence to support this application.[82]

Two randomized controlled trials have shown that high-dose tranexamic acid significantly reduces surgical blood loss and transfusion requirements in liver transplant recipients.[83,84] A recent metaanalysis identified 23 studies with a total of 1407 liver transplant patients who received aminocaproic acid, tranexamic acid, or aprotinin compared with each other or with controls/placebo. This review found that tranexamic acid and aprotinin reduced transfusion requirements without any increased risk for hepatic artery thrombosis, VTE, or perioperative mortality.[85] Additional studies comparing the efficacy of tranexamic acid with aminocaproic acid and/or aprotinin are needed in this population.[44]

There are case reports of thrombosis associated with both aminocaproic acid and tranexamic acid. However, no significant increase in thrombotic complications has been observed when these drugs have been used in patients undergoing cardiac, liver transplant, or orthopedic surgery, although those studies were not specifically powered to evaluate for thrombotic complications.[42,44,77,79,86]

Aprotinin

Aprotinin is a polypeptide extracted from bovine lung that inhibits the action of serine proteases, including plasmin and kallikrein.[42] In addition to its antifibrinolytic activity, aprotinin is also thought to preserve platelet function and have antiinflammatory effects, both of which may be mediated by inhibition of protease-activated receptors expressed on platelets, vascular endothelium, and neutrophils.[86] The pharmacokinetics of aprotinin are complex, and there is wide between-patient variability.[54] Renal failure results in reduced clearance and prolonged half-life of this drug. Because neither the optimal dose nor the appropriate therapeutic concentration required for effective hemostasis has been established, many different dosing regimens have been used.[54] Because of its bovine origin, aprotinin may cause hypersensitivity reactions. The incidence is less than 1%, increasing to approximately 3% upon reexposure. Thus retreatment within 6 months is not recommended.[58,87]

The bulk of clinical experience with aprotinin is in cardiac surgery. A large number of clinical trials have consistently shown that prophylactic administration of aprotinin improves hemostasis and reduces requirements for transfusion of red blood cells, platelets, and fresh frozen plasma in the majority of patients undergoing cardiopulmonary bypass.[40,44,54] A large metaanalysis of randomized controlled trials using aprotinin in cardiac surgery also demonstrated decreased mortality and a reduced incidence of repeat thoracotomy, without any increased risk for perioperative myocardial infarction.[53] Furthermore, another metaanalysis of randomized controlled trials showed a lower incidence of stroke in cardiac surgery patients treated with high-dose aprotinin.[88]

Although there is abundant evidence that aprotinin reduces blood loss and transfusion requirements in cardiac surgery patients, recent literature highlights the risk for serious adverse events associated with this drug. A nonrandomized observational study involving 4374 patients who underwent elective coronary revascularization compared aprotinin, aminocaproic acid, and tranexamic acid with no treatment.[89] Aprotinin was associated with a doubling of the risk for renal failure requiring dialysis, a 55% increase in the risk for myocardial infarction or heart failure, and a nearly doubled increase in the risk for stroke or encephalopathy. Aminocaproic acid and tranexamic acid reduced blood loss to a similar degree, but without any increased risk for adverse renal, cardiac, or cerebrovascular events. The same investigators subsequently reported that aprotinin use is associated with an increased risk for long-term (5 years) mortality following coronary artery bypass graft surgery.[90] In another cohort study of 3348 patients who underwent cardiothoracic surgery in a single center that reserves aprotinin use for complex surgeries and for those patients whose religious beliefs forbid blood transfusion confirmed an increased risk for postoperative renal dysfunction but found no increased risk for myocardial or cerebrovascular events.[91] Although aminocaproic acid and tranexamic acid appear to be relatively safe, it is important to note that the numbers of trials and study participants are much smaller for these drugs than for aprotinin. Moreover, trials directly comparing aprotinin with aminocaproic acid and tranexamic acid have been few in number and small in size.

To address these issues, the Blood Conservation Using Antifibrinolytics in a Randomized Trial (BART) study was launched in 2002.[92] Over the subsequent 5 years, this blinded multicenter trial randomly assigned 2331 cardiac surgical patients to receive aprotinin, tranexamic acid, or aminocaproic acid during surgical procedures for which cardiopulmonary bypass was required. The study was terminated prematurely in October 2007 due to a higher death rate in the aprotinin group, and the drug was subsequently withdrawn from the market in both Europe and the United States. In the years following BART, debate has continued about the optimal use of antifibrinolytics in cardiac surgery. A 2009 metaanalysis of 49 trials involving over 7400 subjects found that, compared with placebo or no treatment, aprotinin, tranexamic acid, and aminocaproic acid were all effective in reducing the need for transfusion but that the risk for death was consistently higher with the use of aprotinin than with either of the lysine analogues.[93] In contrast, a 2010 multicenter database analysis of over 30,000 children undergoing congenital heart operations at 35 children's hospitals found no difference in postoperative mortality, need for dialysis, or length of stay in the 44% of total subjects who received aprotinin versus those who did not.[94] This study serves as a reminder that extrapolation from clinical trial data in adults may not be appropriate for the pediatric population.

A potentially important issue that may not have been adequately addressed in earlier trials of antifibrinolytic agents in cardiac surgery is the risk category of the patients being studied. Most studies in the literature are limited to coronary artery bypass graft patients, a generally low- to moderate-risk population. Although the BART study specifically aimed to include high-risk cases, complex or emergency surgeries were not included, leaving a population of predominantly low- or moderate-risk patients.[95] A recent single-center cohort study compared outcomes of 772 cardiac surgery patients who received aprotinin with the same number of propensity score–matched patients who received tranexamic acid and found that aprotinin was associated with lower massive blood loss and fewer adverse events in high-risk, but not in low- to moderate-risk patients.[96] This suggests that aprotinin, with its greater hemostatic potency and antiinflammatory properties, may be the antifibrinolytic agent of choice in high-risk patients, who tend to develop more severe coagulopathy and systemic inflammatory response syndrome.[96] Randomized controlled trials in high-risk cardiac surgery patients are needed to test this hypothesis.

In spite of the large number of studies and amount of effort put forth, debate remains about the optimal use of antifibrinolytic agents in cardiac surgery. There appears to be no appreciable difference in efficacy between tranexamic acid and aminocaproic acid, and most studies were not designed to properly evaluate safety. Aprotinin remains unavailable in 2012 but may have a role in high-risk patients. For now, clinical decisions about use of antifibrinolytic agents in this setting should be individualized based on anticipated blood loss and the risk characteristics of each patient.[96]

Although the use of aprotinin in orthotopic liver transplantation was first reported more than 20 years ago, its routine use in this setting has also been long debated. Two randomized controlled trials have shown a 30% to 40% reduction in transfusion requirements in liver transplant recipients.[97,98] Aprotinin may also have favorable hemodynamic effects following graft reperfusion,[99] possibly because of inhibition of the release of bradykinin and other vasodilating substances. More recently, a retrospective analysis of 150 patients from a single center who underwent liver transplant between 2004 and 2008 found that those who received prophylactic aprotinin (n = 111) required significantly fewer units of red blood cell transfusion than the group not treated with aprotinin (n = 39).[100] Comparative studies of antifibrinolytic agents in this setting are limited, but a similar study comparing 300 patients who received aprotinin and 100 patients who received tranexamic acid found no differences in intraoperative blood loss, transfusion requirements, renal function, and 1-year survival.[101] A 2011 Cochrane database review found that aprotinin may potentially reduce blood loss and transfusion requirements in liver transplantation, but methodologic shortcomings and high risk for bias in the available studies severely limit the strength of these conclusions.[102] Clearly, properly designed trials are needed to address these issues. Prophylactic administration of aprotinin has also been shown to significantly reduce perioperative bleeding in patients undergoing noncardiac thoracic surgery and orthopedic surgery, although the data are limited.[44,103]

Recombinant Factor VIIa

rFVIIa is a hemostatic agent currently licensed in the United States only for the prevention and treatment of bleeding in hemophilia patients with factor VIII or factor IX inhibitors, acquired hemophilia, and in those with congenital factor VII deficiency. This drug is believed to induce hemostasis at local sites of tissue injury through enhancement of thrombin generation on the surface of thrombin-activated platelets.[104] rFVIIa also activates thrombin activatable fibrinolysis inhibitor (TAFI), which in turn stabilizes the clot by inhibiting fibrinolysis.[105] The use of rFVIIa in the management of hemophilia and factor VII deficiency is reviewed in Chapters 138 and 139.

Following its approval by the FDA in 1999, encouraging anecdotal experience and case series generated much interest in the use of rFVIIa for a variety of off-license indications, such as to control refractory bleeding after surgery or major trauma and to prevent bleeding in surgeries where blood loss is expected to be excessive. A recently published retrospective database analysis found that from 2000 to 2008, the off-label use of rFVIIa in hospitals increased more than 140-fold. The most common off-label uses include trauma, adult and pediatric cardiovascular surgery, and intracranial hemorrhage.[106]

Difficult-to-control "coagulopathic" hemorrhage commonly occurs without preexisting coagulation deficits in those who suffer major trauma, and roughly half of all early trauma deaths are due to hemorrhage. Such bleeding is typically multifactorial, with contributions from the dilution of platelets and clotting factors secondary to large-volume transfusions, excessive transfusion of citrate anticoagulant, hyperfibrinolysis, hypothermia with subsequent slowing of the enzymatic coagulation reactions, and acidosis. In 1999 a report of the successful treatment of a bleeding soldier with rFVIIa[107] generated widespread interest in the use of rFVIIa in areas other than hemophilia. A number of case reports and series followed, describing favorable results with the use of rFVIIa in trauma patients. A prospective, multicenter, randomized, controlled trial published in 2005[108] that included 143 blunt and 134 penetrating trauma patients found that in the group with blunt trauma, three successive doses of rFVIIa significantly decreased red blood cell transfusion (mean reduction of 2.6 units) and decreased by approximately half the number of patients requiring massive transfusion (more than 20 units of red blood cells). Although similar trends were observed in the patients with penetrating trauma, the differences were not statistically significant. In spite of the reduction in the need for blood products, there was no survival benefit. After these initial encouraging reports of the use of rFVIIa in trauma patients, questions regarding optimal dosing and timing of administration remained. In an attempt to address these issues, the Western Trauma Association Multi-Center Trials Group (with support from the drug manufacturer) conducted a case registry of 380 adult trauma patients who received rFVIIa as an adjunct for hemorrhage control in 21 level I and II U.S. trauma centers between 2003 and 2008.[109] This registry was unable to define the precise role of rFVIIa in traumatic bleeding. However, a pH of less than 7.2, platelet count of less than 100,000/μL, and blood pressure less than or equal to 90 mm Hg were each found to be predictors of poor response to rFVIIa, suggesting that correction of shock, acidosis, and thrombocytopenia should precede the use of rFVIIa in bleeding trauma patients.[109] The CONTROL trial is the largest placebo-controlled study of rFVIIa in trauma patients to date. This multicenter trial randomized 560 actively bleeding trauma patients and found no differences in overall mortality, organ system failure, or adverse events in either group.[110] Thus, although initial reports were encouraging, there is currently insufficient evidence to support a role for the routine use of rFVIIa in the setting of trauma.

The use of rFVIIa in cardiac surgery remains a topic of much debate, with a number of conflicting reports and opinions in the literature. Significant hemostatic alterations may result from cardiopulmonary bypass, leading to excessive postoperative bleeding. Hypothermia, hemodilution, and activation of the coagulation, fibrinolytic, and inflammatory pathways all contribute to the complex hemostatic defect associated with cardiopulmonary bypass. In addition, use of newer anticoagulant drugs, including direct thrombin inhibitors, low-molecular-weight heparins (LMWHs), pentasaccharides, and platelet inhibitors, may also contribute to hemorrhagic risk in cardiac surgery patients.[111] Conversely, by virtue of the disease process itself and the nature of the surgical procedures undertaken, cardiac surgery patients are also at risk for both arterial and venous thrombosis.[112] Because perioperative bleeding is a major cause of morbidity and mortality, there is increasing off-label use of rFVIIa in this patient population.[113] A number of case reports and uncontrolled case series in both adult and pediatric populations have suggested that rFVIIa is effective in decreasing blood loss and transfusion requirements in many patients with intractable bleeding following cardiopulmonary bypass. However, well-designed randomized placebo-controlled trials are lacking. Although a randomized placebo-controlled study in adult complex noncoronary cardiac surgical patients[114] found that rFVIIa significantly reduced the need for transfusion, the study has major methodologic limitations.[113] Another randomized placebo-controlled study using two different doses of rFVIIa found that it may be beneficial for treating bleeding after cardiac surgery but also noted an increase in the number of serious adverse events, including stroke.[115] Although use of rFVIIa in cardiac surgery patients has been increasingly common, there now appears to be general consensus that prophylactic or routine use is not warranted.[113,116,117]

Outside of trauma and cardiac surgery, rFVIIa has been used in a variety of other surgical settings, with conflicting results. A randomized, double-blind, placebo-controlled trial of 36 patients undergoing retropubic prostatectomy demonstrated a greater than 50% reduction in surgical blood loss in patients treated with a single intraoperative dose of rFVIIa.[118] Conversely, however, in a similarly designed trial in 204 noncirrhotic patients undergoing partial hepatectomy, treatment with rFVIIa resulted in only a modest reduction in blood loss.[119] In another study involving 221 noncirrhotic patients undergoing partial hepatectomy, the use of rFVIIa before and every 2 hours during surgery failed to decrease transfusion requirements or the number of patients needing transfusion.[120] Overall, the published experience with the use of rFVIIa in urologic, orthopedic, vascular, and obstetric/gynaecologic surgery is still too limited and subject to bias to draw meaningful conclusions.[114] High-quality clinical trials are needed but are unlikely to be performed.

Neurosurgical patients are distinct from other groups in that rather than treating massive hemorrhage, the goal is to treat relatively small bleeds within a closed space where even mild or modest benefit may result in significantly better outcomes.[114] A randomized placebo-controlled study of 399 patients with intracerebral hemorrhage showed that treatment with rFVIIa within 4 hours after the onset of symptoms limits growth of the hematoma, reduces mortality, and improves functional outcomes at 90 days, albeit with a small increase in the frequency of thromboembolic events.[121] However, the same investigators subsequently reported the results of a larger phase III trial (Factor Seven for Acute Hemorrhagic Stroke [FAST]) involving 821 patients. In this study, rFVIIa failed to improve the primary outcomes of mortality and disability at 90 days.[122] Following this, the manufacturer of rFVIIa abandoned plans to seek FDA approval for use in the treatment of acute intracranial hemorrhage.[123]

The primary safety concern with the use of rFVIIa is thrombosis. Most of the initially reported thrombotic events were associated with other risk factors such as preexisting atherosclerotic vascular disease or advanced age.[124] In hemophilia, the risk for thrombosis is estimated to be less than 1%.[125,126] However, with the increasing off-label use of rFVIIa, concerns about the thrombogenic potential of this drug have remained. Much of the published literature describing off-label use of rFVIIa reports a very low incidence of thrombotic complications, but it is important to recognize that most of these studies involved patients with already impaired coagulation and were not specifically designed to assess thrombotic risk. A 2006 review based on the FDA MedWatch database[127] heightened awareness about the thrombogenic potential of rFVIIa. Both arterial and venous thromboembolic events have been reported, and the vast majority have occurred with off-label use of rFVIIa. Thromboembolic events were the probable cause of death in 72% of the reported fatalities. Half of the thromboembolic events occurred within 24 hours of the last dose of rFVIIa, and many occurred within 2 hours.[128] Similar concerns were raised by a report describing a 9.4% incidence of thromboembolic complications after administration of rFVIIa to trauma patients, with 10 of 14 deaths attributed at least in part to the thromboembolic event.[128] A recently published systematic review and metaanalysis also concluded that off-label use of rFVIIa for intracranial hemorrhage and cardiac surgery is associated with an increased risk for thromboembolism.[118]

In summary, rFVIIa represents a major advance in the management of hemophilia A and B patients with inhibitors, acquired hemophilia, and congenital factor VII deficiency. The off-label use of this drug has been the subject of much debate, driven in part by its very high cost. Although rFVIIa was once touted as a "universal hemostatic agent,"[129] numerous clinical trials over the last decade have illustrated that it is more appropriately considered to be a potent but specific prohemostatic agent that requires the presence of adequate amounts of hemostatic substrates in order to be effective.[130] A 2011 Cochrane database review of 25 randomized controlled trials found that the use of rFVIIa, either therapeutically or prophylactically, in patients without hemophilia was of unproven effectiveness and recommended that the use of the drug outside its current licensed indications be restricted to clinical trials.[131]

MANAGEMENT OF PATIENTS WITH HEMOSTATIC ABNORMALITIES

Patients with known hemostatic abnormalities are often referred before surgery for assessment of bleeding risk and recommendations regarding perioperative management. The approach to these patients should be according to the following considerations: (1) evaluation of the risk for bleeding associated with the specific surgery or procedure (see Table 161-1); (2) careful consideration of the need for surgery and its urgency; greater risks are more warranted for correction of life-threatening conditions than for purely elective procedures; (3) recognition of the nature and severity of the patient's hemostatic abnormality and the ability to correct it; and (4) consideration of the duration of replacement that will be required, with appreciation of potential bleeding that may be associated with events in the postoperative period such as removal of sutures and deep drains and the need for physical therapy, especially after orthopedic surgery. The following sections discuss perioperative management of some common coagulation abnormalities; the management of congenital factor deficiencies and von Willebrand disease are discussed elsewhere in this text (see Chapters 137, 139, and 140).

Thrombocytopenia

Thrombocytopenia is one of the most common acquired hemostatic abnormalities, and the availability of platelet transfusion makes consideration of both emergency and elective surgery reasonable even in severely thrombocytopenic patients. The best index of bleeding risk in thrombocytopenic patients is the platelet count. In nonsurgical patients a threshold platelet count of 10,000/μL is widely used for prophylactic transfusions, yet there is inadequate scientific evidence to determine the platelet count below which the risk for surgical bleeding is increased.[132,133] The American Society of Anesthesiologists Task Force on Blood Component Therapy concluded that prophylactic platelet transfusion in surgical patients is usually indicated when the count is below 50,000/μL and is rarely indicated when the count is above 100,000/μL.[133] Clinical trials addressing this issue are still lacking.[134,135] For low-risk surgery, a single transfusion to increase the platelet count to more than 50,000/μL followed by close observation may suffice, whereas transfusion to maintain the platelet count at greater than 50,000/μL for moderate-risk surgery and greater than 100,000/μL for high-risk surgery is usually appropriate. The optimal duration of postoperative platelet support has not been carefully studied, but even for moderate- or high-risk surgery, platelets may be needed for less than 1 week because they are principally required for primary hemostasis. The platelet count should be monitored closely during the postoperative period, with the expectation that platelet survival will be shortened by infection, fever, or bleeding. In addition, platelet transfusion may be indicated for surgical patients despite an apparently adequate count in the presence of known or suspected platelet dysfunction and microvascular bleeding.

When thrombocytopenia is due to increased platelet destruction (e.g., immune thrombocytopenic purpura), prophylactic platelet transfusion is largely ineffective and is indicated only for active, serious bleeding. In preparation for surgery, therapy with steroids and/or intravenous γ-globulin often will increase the platelet count to a satisfactory level so that transfusion is not needed. $Rh_o(D)$ immune globulin (WinRho) may also be useful in this setting.

Platelet Dysfunction

Patients with platelet dysfunction represent a large group for whom preoperative consultation is sought, typically because of an abnormal bleeding history or the discovery of a prolonged bleeding time or other laboratory assessment of platelet function with a normal platelet count. Drugs are the most common cause of acquired platelet dysfunction. Many commonly used types of medications, including aspirin and other nonsteroidal antiinflammatory drugs (NSAIDs), antibiotics, antidepressants (selective serotonin reuptake inhibitors), cardiovascular drugs, and newer antiplatelet agents, including adenosine diphosphate (ADP) receptor or GPIIb/IIIa antagonists, can cause platelet dysfunction. Ethanol as well as certain foods and herbal supplements can also inhibit platelets; a careful history is therefore essential. Any drugs that interfere with platelet function should be discontinued before surgery and avoided in the perioperative period if possible.

A number of medical conditions can cause acquired platelet dysfunction. The etiology may be fairly obvious in cases of renal or liver disease, myeloproliferative disorders, leukemias, myelodysplastic syndromes, or dysproteinemias, but consideration of undiagnosed intrinsic platelet defects (storage pool disease or platelet release defects) or von Willebrand disease may be necessary. Treatment of the underlying disease is the most effective approach, if possible. If not, platelet transfusion may be indicated, but the dose required to achieve hemostasis is difficult to predict and depends in part on the severity of the underlying platelet abnormality. As discussed earlier, treatment with DDAVP may be appropriate in selected patients. The exact mechanism of action of DDAVP in acquired platelet dysfunction is not well understood, but one study suggests that DDAVP interacts directly with platelets and exerts a priming effect on platelet aggregation stimulated by ADP or collagen.[136] Expression of GPIb and GPIIb/IIIa on platelet membranes is also enhanced following administration of DDAVP.[44]

Renal Disease

Impaired hemostasis has long been recognized in patients with chronic renal failure and is discussed in greater detail in Chapter 156. The pathogenesis is multifactorial but is due in large part to alterations in platelet function.[137] Anemia also contributes to platelet dysfunction in chronic renal failure. Red blood cells release ADP, which in turn inactivates vascular prostacyclin, an inhibitor of platelet function.[138] Correction of anemia, now routinely accomplished through the use of recombinant erythropoietin, also improves the rheologic factors that facilitate platelet interaction with the vessel wall. Increase in hematocrit, whether by the use of erythropoietin or transfusions, is accompanied by significant shortening of the bleeding time and improvement of platelet adhesion.[139] In addition to platelet dysfunction and altered balance between mediators of normal endothelial function, the pathophysiology of uremic bleeding is complicated by the comorbidities in this patient population, such as vascular disease and hypertension, and the medical treatment of those conditions.[140]

Owing to the success of erythropoietin, other hemostatic agents now play a smaller, yet still important, role in the management of bleeding in patients with renal insufficiency, particularly those with acute or subacute renal failure. DDAVP was shown in a randomized placebo-controlled trail to normalize bleeding times within 1 hour in uremic patients.[141] DDAVP may be useful for treating acute bleeding and for prophylaxis before biopsy or urgent surgery. Conjugated estrogens also improve bleeding times and reduce or stop bleeding in uremic patients through unknown mechanisms.[142,143] Unlike DDAVP, the clinical effect of conjugated estrogens is delayed for several hours, but they have a much longer duration of action (10 to 15 days).[42] Thus conjugated estrogens are more useful for management of chronic recurrent bleeding and perhaps before elective surgery. DDAVP and conjugated estrogens may be given concurrently, thereby taking advantage of the different timing of their hemostatic effects.[42] Conjugated estrogens may be given orally or intravenously, usually as five to seven daily doses, and are usually well tolerated, with negligible side effects. Cryoprecipitate can also shorten the bleeding time in patients with renal failure, but concerns about viral transmission and the effectiveness of other hemostatic agents have limited its routine use in this setting.

Liver Disease

Hemostatic alterations in patients with acute or chronic liver disease (see Chapter 155) are complex and involve both procoagulant and anticoagulant pathways.[144,145] Although patients with liver disease are typically felt to have deficient hemostasis, this concept has been challenged in the recent literature.[146] These patients are not "autoanticoagulated" as often assumed. In fact, they are not protected from and may even be at increased risk for thrombosis, particularly in the portal venous system.[147-151] The presence of genetic thrombophilic mutations may further increase this risk.[152] The procoagulant tendency associated with chronic liver disease[153-155] suggests that prophylaxis against venous thromboembolism may be warranted in high-risk situations.[147] However, the perceived bleeding risk often limits the use of prophylaxis,[156] and appropriately designed pharmacologic clinical studies are clearly needed here.[147]

The coagulopathy of liver disease is usually the result of a combination of several defects,[157,158] including the following: (1) There is reduced synthesis of procoagulant and anticoagulant clotting factors, which is proportional to the extent of hepatocyte damage.[158] Minimal prolongation of the PT/INR occurs in mild to moderate liver disease, primarily reflecting decreased factor VII synthesis, whereas more advanced liver disease can lead to reductions in factors II, IX, and X, followed by fibrinogen and factor V. Conversely, factor VIII levels are typically preserved (and are often elevated) even in severe liver disease. This is likely the result of decreased clearance of factor VIII, mediated by increased levels of von Willebrand factor and decreased expression of low-density lipoprotein receptor–related protein, both of which occur in advanced liver disease.[147] (2) Vitamin K deficiency due to impaired enterohepatic recirculation of bile salts and subsequent malabsorption may compound the reduction in clotting factor synthesis. (3) Dysfibrinogenemia due to synthesis of abnormally glycosylated fibrinogen occurs in 60% to 70% of patients with liver disease.[159] This results in a disproportionate prolongation of the thrombin time relative to a mildly prolonged PT/INR and aPTT. (4) Thrombocytopenia is common in advanced chronic liver disease and occurs in up to 65% of those with cirrhosis.[160,161] Platelet counts rarely fall below 30,000 to 40,000/μL, and spontaneous bleeding on this basis alone is uncommon. Thrombocytopenia results from both hypersplenism and reduced hepatic synthesis of thrombopoietin.[162] Ethanol toxicity and folate deficiency may also impair platelet production. (5) Platelet dysfunction through a variety of mechanisms is also seen in liver disease,[159] although this may be offset by elevated von Willebrand factor levels.[163] (6) Hyperfibrinolysis due to impaired hepatic clearance of plasminogen activators and/or reduced synthesis of endogenous inhibitors of fibrinolysis (α_2-antiplasmin, TAFI) is also common with advanced liver disease.[158,159]

In spite of all the potential defects in hemostasis that may occur in association with liver disease, results of routine coagulation tests such as the PT/INR and aPTT correlate poorly with clinical bleeding, and these patients may indeed have thrombotic events. An emerging concept to explain this is that the coagulation system is "rebalanced," due to the coexisting alterations of both procoagulant and anticoagulant factors.[147] In support of this notion, plasma from cirrhotic patients has been shown to have comparable thrombin-generating ability as plasma from healthy subjects when measured with assays that reflect the action of both procoagulant and anticoagulant factors.[164,165] Although it may be rebalanced, the coagulation system in patients with chronic liver disease is clearly in a more tenuous state than that of healthy individuals.[147]

Patients with severe decompensated liver disease and markedly abnormal coagulation test results are at increased risk for bleeding, and surgery should be avoided except as a lifesaving measure. In evaluating hemostasis in patients with less severe disease, the PT/INR and aPTT may be good indicators of decreased synthesis of clotting factors and vitamin K deficiency, but they are poor predictors of bleeding risk. Several studies have shown the failure of the PT/INR and aPTT to predict bleeding following liver biopsy.[13,166-170] Similarly, preoperative hemostatic testing has generally not been shown to be clinically useful in predicting bleeding during liver transplantation.[171] A study in patients with liver disease found that INR values in the range of 1.3 to 2.0 generally correspond to levels of factors II, V, and VII that are adequate for hemostasis.[172] A preoperative platelet count is needed to identify thrombocytopenia, and some assessment of platelet function may be useful to determine whether platelet function is abnormal in the setting of a normal or near-normal platelet count. A thrombin time or fibrinogen level should also be performed to evaluate for dysfibrinogenemia. Tests for fibrinogen/fibrin degradation products, D-dimer, euglobulin clot lysis time, or thromboelastography may be useful in evaluating for disseminated intravascular coagulation (DIC) or accelerated fibrinolysis.

In patients with mild liver disease and mild-moderate PT/INR prolongation (<2.0), serious surgical bleeding is unlikely in the absence of other hemostatic abnormalities, and prophylactic intervention is generally not necessary for low- or moderate-risk surgery. For high-risk surgery or greater degrees of hemostatic abnormality, transfusion of fresh frozen plasma is the most commonly used approach for correcting the coagulation abnormality, although there are no good prospective studies to guide the use of fresh frozen plasma in this situation, and there are guidelines that caution against the indiscriminate use of plasma before invasive procedures.[173] It should be noted that the PT of fresh frozen plasma is approximately 15 seconds, so complete correction of the patient's PT/INR cannot usually be achieved.[174] Administration of platelets should be considered for more severe degrees of thrombocytopenia, although recovery will be decreased in the presence of splenomegaly. Administration of DDAVP may be useful in correcting abnormal platelet function in some cases.[175] Administration of 5 to 10 mg vitamin K will usually shorten the PT/INR if vitamin K deficiency is a contributory factor. As discussed earlier, antifibrinolytic agents may also be useful in the reduction of perioperative hemorrhage in patients with liver disease.

INTRAOPERATIVE AND POSTOPERATIVE BLEEDING

Excessive bleeding during or after surgery is a serious and potentially life-threatening complication that requires immediate evaluation and a rapid approach to diagnosis and institution of treatment. The first consideration should be to differentiate between "surgical" and "coagulopathic" causes of bleeding. Failure to surgically control bleeding vessels at the operative site is the most frequent cause of postoperative bleeding and is suggested by evidence of hemorrhage only at the operative site and seen as expanding hematoma, excessive blood in surgical drains, or saturated wound dressings. Conversely, coagulopathic bleeding is suggested by slower "oozing" at the operative site in addition to evidence of bleeding outside the operative field that may be seen as petechiae, purpura, or bleeding at sites of venipuncture, urinary or vascular catheters, or nasogastric and endotracheal tubes.[176] In addition to careful physical examination, laboratory tests, including PT/INR, aPTT, and platelet count, are an essential part of the evaluation. Other useful tests may include a fibrinogen level, a test for fibrin degradation products or D-dimer, euglobulin clot lysis time, or thromboelastography to search for evidence of DIC or fibrinolysis. The peripheral blood smear should also be reviewed to examine platelet morphology and number and to identify possible red blood cell fragmentation that may occur in DIC. The possibility of a preexisting hemostatic abnormality that may have been undetected before surgery should also be considered. Revisiting the patient's family and past medical history, along with a thorough review of preoperative medication use, may yield important diagnostic clues.

When evaluating hemostatic test results in surgical patients, changes that normally occur in response to surgery must be considered. These vary depending on the extent of tissue dissection and duration of the procedure. Consumption as well as hemodilution from crystalloid and blood product infusion both lead to acute reductions of coagulation factors and platelets during surgery and in the initial postoperative period. This is typically followed by changes resulting from the acute phase response, including increases in fibrinogen, platelet count, factor VIII, and plasminogen activator inhibitor I during the first postoperative week.[177]

Alterations in coagulation factor levels that occur during surgery and in the initial postoperative period can limit the reliability of the PT/INR and aPTT in evaluating the bleeding surgical patient. Clinical practice guidelines have consistently recommended transfusion of fresh frozen plasma when PT/INR and aPTT results exceed the mean reference range by 1.5 times.[133,178-183] However, a prospective study of 16 patients with bleeding caused by dilutional coagulopathy following spinal surgery found significant variability in the PT/INR and aPTT and suggested that depending on which test system was used, clinical decisions regarding coagulation factor replacement therapy might differ.[184] Conversely, another and larger retrospective study in a similar patient population found that the PT/INR and aPTT had sufficient sensitivity and specificity to be helpful in guiding transfusion therapy,[185] and some consensus panel guidelines do recommend that transfusion of fresh frozen plasma and cryoprecipitate in the bleeding surgical patient be guided by coagulation studies.[186] Additional prospective studies of patients undergoing other types of surgery are needed to more clearly define the role of coagulation testing in the management of surgical bleeding. In addition, assays that measure thrombin generation or global hemostasis such as thromboelastography may be useful in this setting but await further study and clinical validation.

Coagulopathy Associated With Massive Blood Loss/Transfusion

Massive bleeding (loss of one or more blood volumes in a 24-hour period) may occur in the setting of severe trauma or major surgery and requires aggressive fluid resuscitation and transfusion of blood products. The mechanisms involved in the coagulopathy that accompanies massive transfusion have not yet been fully elucidated but are multifactorial in nature.[187] Similar to chronic liver disease, procoagulant, anticoagulant, profibrinolytic, and antifibrinolytic factors are all affected, resulting in a complex coagulopathy. Impaired thrombin generation is compensated in part by reduction in the activity of antithrombin and other protease inhibitors. Fibrinogen levels can fall rapidly and are proportional to the degree of hemodilution. Antifibrinolytic protein levels are decreased, rendering clots more susceptible to fibrinolysis.[188] In addition to a dilutional coagulopathy, other complications, including consumptive coagulopathy, hypothermia, electrolyte abnormalities (due to citrate intoxication), and acid-base disturbances, may also develop.[188]

In patients without a preexisting coagulopathy, replacement of approximately 1.5 blood volumes is the threshold for the development of dilutional coagulopathy.[189] At that point, PT/INR, aPTT, fibrinogen level, and platelet count should be determined. If the PT/INR or aPTT is prolonged greater than 1.5 times control, the fibrinogen level is below 100 mg/dL, or the platelet count is reduced to 50,000 to 70,000/μL, clinical coagulopathy is suspected and appropriate blood product administration is indicated, particularly if additional blood loss is expected. The same coagulation parameters should be measured again with the replacement of each additional half blood volume (i.e., 5 to 6 units of red blood cells).[190]

Over the last several years, there has been an increased emphasis on more aggressive blood component therapy, driven by data from both military and civilian trauma populations.[191-196] These studies have demonstrated that higher ratios (approaching 1 : 1) of plasma and platelets to red blood cells are associated with improved outcomes in massively transfused patients. Patients receiving less than massive transfusion may also benefit from higher plasma to red blood cell ratios.[197] Furthermore, maintaining an adequate fibrinogen level is essential for successful management of dilutional coagulopathy.[188]

With prolonged hypotension, acidosis, or extensive tissue trauma and ischemia, tissue factor and tissue plasminogen activator may be released into the bloodstream, initiating DIC. Obstetric catastrophes also commonly result in DIC. Consumptive coagulopathy results in hemostatic failure at lower volumes of blood loss or replacement, and simple administration of blood components may not correct the coagulopathy. In these circumstances, restoration of systemic and hepatic perfusion (the liver is an important site of clearance of fibrin degradation products and activated coagulation factors) is essential for regaining control of hemostasis.

Cardiopulmonary Bypass

Cardiopulmonary bypass is associated with unique hemostatic changes. Perfusion through the extracorporeal membrane oxygenator has profound effects on platelets and clotting factors: platelet count, hematocrit, and levels of coagulation and fibrinolytic factors are reduced to approximately 50% of baseline after starting bypass and remain reduced throughout the procedure, with the exception of factor V, which may be further reduced to less than 20%.[198-201] These changes may be caused in part by exposure to artificial surfaces and also by a tissue factor–dependent pathway related to surgical trauma.[202] Cardiopulmonary bypass results in significant platelet dysfunction[203] reflected by release of α-granule contents, the generation of platelet microparticles, abnormal in vitro platelet aggregation test results, and a prolonged bleeding time that usually corrects within 1 hour postoperatively.[199-204] In addition to quantitative and qualitative defects, cardiopulmonary bypass also results in platelet activation, which may contribute to thrombotic and inflammatory complications.[204] Patients with acute ischemic coronary syndromes (who may be candidates for urgent cardiac surgery) are often given GPIIb/IIIa inhibitors, which may further impair platelet function. If surgery cannot be delayed, consideration of prophylactic platelet transfusions may be required.[205] Inadequate neutralization of heparin with protamine sulfate may result in a prolonged aPTT and thrombin time with a normal reptilase time and is an indication for administration of additional protamine sulfate. The use of DDAVP, antifibrinolytic drugs, and rFVIIa to reduce the hemorrhagic complications of cardiac surgery was discussed earlier. Fibrinogen concentrate has also been shown to reduce blood loss and transfusion requirements during cardiac surgery.[206]

Orthotopic Liver Transplantation

In addition to the complex coagulopathy of end-stage liver disease, orthotopic liver transplantation is accompanied by major alterations in hemostasis. The surgical procedure itself can be divided into three stages, each with its own profile of coagulation abnormalities.[207] Bleeding during the preanhepatic stage, while the host liver is surgically isolated, is due primarily to the patient's preexisting coagulopathy and is determined by the severity of the underlying liver disease. Excessive fibrinolysis may be encountered during this stage in 10% to 20% of those with cirrhosis. The anhepatic stage begins with surgical removal of the liver. Bleeding during this stage is primarily hemostatic because of DIC and excessive fibrinolysis.[208] As the donor liver is reperfused, the postanhepatic stage begins, and serious bleeding is often encountered as a result of a combination of hyperfibrinolysis, metabolic acidosis, hypothermia, electrolyte abnormalities, and sometimes impaired cardiac function.[208,209]

The multifactorial nature of the coagulopathy associated with orthotopic liver transplantation requires a combination of therapeutic interventions. In addition to transfusion of blood products, other hemostatic agents such as DDAVP and antifibrinolytics may be useful and were discussed earlier. There has also been much interest in the use of rFVIIa, and some randomized placebo-controlled trials have been completed. In one study, a single dose of rFVIIa before surgery failed to reduce the number of red blood cell transfusions required.[210] Another study used repeated doses of rFVIIa during surgery, which also failed to reduce the number of red blood cell units transfused or intraoperative blood loss. However, a small but significant increase in the number of patients who avoided red blood cell transfusion entirely was observed in the treatment group.[211] A recent systematic review of these, plus three additional studies, evaluating a total of 215 patients who received prophylactic rFVIIa at the time of liver transplantation, found no effect on mortality or thromboembolism.[118]

Although there may be a trend toward reduced red blood cell transfusion requirements, neither operating room time nor length of stay in the intensive care unit is reduced by the prophylactic use of rFVIIa in this setting.[118] As for other types of surgery, questions about optimal dosing, cost-effectiveness, and safety remain to be fully answered, and it is still questionable whether rFVIIa should be used as prophylaxis in liver transplant patients outside of a prospective clinical trial.[212]

Perioperative Anticoagulation Management

Hematologists are frequently consulted for advice on the perioperative management of patients who are taking oral anticoagulants. Important considerations to be taken into account include (1) the bleeding risk associated with the surgery; (2) the underlying indication for anticoagulant therapy; (3) in the case of secondary antithrombotic prophylaxis, the remoteness of the most recent thrombotic event; (4) other comorbid conditions that may increase the risk for thrombosis and/or the potential consequences of thrombosis while oral anticoagulation is temporarily interrupted; and (5) the half-life of the anticoagulant agent. Regarding the first point, experience has accumulated in recent years suggesting that many relatively minor procedures can be carried out without any interruption of warfarin therapy.[213] These include minor dental procedures (single or multiple extraction, endodontic procedure), cataract removal, minor dermatologic procedures, and low-risk endoscopy procedures. Audits have suggested that discontinuation of anticoagulation is excessively frequent in these situations and discordant with guidelines.[214] Apart from the risk for thromboembolism, the inappropriate use of bridging therapy may also conversely place the patient at risk for bleeding complications, which can set in motion a potentially morbid chain of clinical events. Suggested management strategies are summarized in Table 161-3.

Traditionally, patients on chronic oral anticoagulation with vitamin K antagonists were admitted to hospital several days before surgery for "bridging" anticoagulation, at which time warfarin was discontinued and dose-adjusted unfractionated heparin (UFH) was administered by continuous infusion. The short half-life of UFH allows it to be safely discontinued approximately 4 to 6 hours ahead of the procedure. More recently, there has been a trend toward the use of LMWHs in place of UFH.[215-218] LMWHs have the advantage that in most patients with normal renal function, no monitoring is required, so that therapy can be administered in the outpatient setting. In addition, the risk for heparin-induced thrombocytopenia (HIT) is less with LMWHs.[219] However, the longer half-life (generally in the range of 4 to 6 hours) necessitates withdrawal of these agents at least 12 hours (for prophylactic doses) or 24 hours (for full therapeutic doses) preoperatively, although even then significant circulating anticoagulant activity may remain in the plasma.[220] Bridging with UFH may still be appropriate for some patients, for example, those with an estimated creatinine clearance less than 30 mL/min in whom the half-life of LMWHs may be prolonged, some patients with mechanical prosthetic heart valves (see later), or those at increased risk for bleeding if treated on an outpatient basis. To date there are no published randomized controlled trials data on which to base decisions regarding the relative efficacy and bleeding risks of perioperative anticoagulation management. One concern with the lack of randomized studies is the fact that it has been assumed that heparins are equally efficacious as warfarin in reducing the risk for arterial thromboembolism in patients with atrial fibrillation (AF) or mechanical heart valves, whereas in fact there are few data to support this assumption.[221]

In recent years, oral anticoagulants that directly inhibit thrombin or factor Xa have been licensed for the prevention of stroke and systemic embolism in patients with nonvalvular AF (see Chapter 149). At the time of writing, both dabigatran etexilate (Pradaxa, a direct thrombin inhibitor) at a dose of 150 mg twice daily (75 mg twice daily for patients with a creatinine clearance <30 mL/min),[222-224] and rivaroxaban (Xarelto, a factor Xa inhibitor) at a dose of 20 mg once daily (15 mg for patients with creatinine clearance of 15 to 49 mL/min)[225,226] have been licensed in the United States for these indications. Based on the results of the recently published Apixaban for Reduction in Stroke and Other Thromboembolic Events in Atrial Fibrillation (ARISTOTLE) trial,[227] the licensure of apixaban (Eliquis), another oral factor Xa inhibitor, can also be anticipated. All of these agents have a more rapid onset (within 1 to 3 hours) of action than warfarin,[228] whose peak action occurs after 4 to 5 days. In addition, they share a low potential for drug-food and drug-drug interaction and a predictable response that eliminates the need for routine coagulation monitoring. A consistent finding with these agents is a lower rate of intracranial hemorrhage compared with warfarin.[228-230] Based on the completed or soon-to-be-completed phase III trials in the treatment of venous thromboembolism,[231-233] it can be anticipated that one or more of these agents will also soon receive approval for this indication.

Table 161-3 Perioperative Management Strategies for Patients on Chronic Oral Anticoagulant Therapy

Clinical Situation	Suggested Anticoagulation Management
Low-bleeding-risk surgery (dental, cataract, skin)	Reduce dose of OAT to achieve INR ≤2.0
Low thrombotic risk Aortic valve prosthesis without other thrombotic risk factors* or AF with low stroke risk or VTE > 3 months previously	Stop OAT 4 nights before surgery Safe to operate when INR ≤1.5 Restart OAT on evening of surgery Use prophylactic perioperative UFH/LMWH if indicated (depends on type of surgery)
Moderate thrombotic risk Mitral or multiple prostheses or Aortic prosthesis with risk factors for thrombosis or AF at high stroke risk or VTE within past 3 months	Stop OAT 4 days before surgery Begin IV UFH† when INR < 2.0 (target aPTT = 2-3 × control) Stop heparin 5 hours before surgery Begin UFH prophylaxis and OAT as soon as possible postoperatively; continue heparin until INR has been therapeutic for >48 hours

Modified from Dorman BH, Spinale FG, Bailey MK, et al: Identification of patients at risk for excessive blood loss during coronary artery bypass surgery: Thromboelastography versus coagulation screen. *Anesth Analg* 76:694, 1993.
AF, Atrial fibrillation; *INR,* international normalized ratio; *LMWH,* low-molecular-weight heparin; *OAT,* oral anticoagulant therapy; *UFH,* unfractionated heparin; *VTE,* venous thromboembolism.
*Risk factors include caged-ball or single tilting-disk valve, AF, history of stroke/transient ischemic attack/other embolic event, left ventricular failure, underlying hypercoagulable state, including cancer.
†LMWH at full-treatment doses may also be used for bridging, although a Food and Drug Administration warning about their use in patients with mechanical valve prostheses was issued in 2002 (discussed in text).

Temporary interruption of oral anticoagulants is often required for more major surgery. Even with a normal diet, 4 to 5 days should be allowed for full or near-full reversal of warfarin when it is being targeted to an INR of 2.0 to 3.0. A more rapid reversal over 24 to 36 hours can be achieved if necessary by administration of a small oral dose of vitamin K_1 (1.0 to 2.5 mg).[234,235] Large doses of vitamin K_1 (>10 mg) are generally unnecessary for this purpose and will lead to prolonged refractoriness to warfarin after it is reinitiated. Although frequently used, subcutaneous administration of vitamin K_1 is associated with highly variable absorption and should be avoided. Intravenous vitamin K_1 has the advantage of more rapid INR reversal compared to the oral route,[236] but it should be administered slowly to avoid anaphylactoid reactions. Urgent reversal of oral anticoagulation before surgery may call for the administration of fresh frozen plasma, although large volumes (15 to 20 mL/kg) are usually required to reverse the INR, and indeed complete normalization cannot usually be achieved. Furthermore, the effect is relatively short-lived because of the short half-life (approximately 6 hours) of transfused factor VII. Therefore concomitant vitamin K_1 administration is required to ensure maintenance of adequate hemostasis. Prothrombin complex concentrates (PCCs; 25 to 50 units/kg) may be used to control hemorrhage in warfarin-treated patients with active bleeding,[235,237-239] and they have been used to expeditiously reverse warfarin therapy before emergency surgery.[169] These concentrates are manufactured by fractionation of pooled plasma and contain the vitamin K–dependent factors II, VII, IX, and X. However, it is important to be aware that there is significant heterogeneity among these agents, with some (three-factor PCCs[238]) having a low concentration of factor VII, which may leave the INR prolonged following administration.[240] At the time of writing, practice in the United States is at variance with most other developed nations in the lack of an available four-factor PCC, although licensure of at least one product for warfarin reversal is anticipated in the near future. PCCs also vary in their content of heparin and antithrombin, and the vitamin K–dependent anticoagulant proteins C and/or S.[238,241] They are all subjected to one or more virucidal processes. Concern has been raised that PCCs may be associated with an increased risk for thrombosis. However, the reports of thrombosis with these agents generally preceded the availability of modern-day nonactivated concentrates and occurred in patients with hemophilia who had received greater than 200 units/kg/day for several days. Nonetheless, because the thrombotic risk might be accentuated in the perioperative period, the risks and benefits of these agents to reverse anticoagulation before surgery need to be carefully weighed. The use of rFVIIa to reverse anticoagulation before emergency surgery has also been reported,[242] but further experience has shown that although rFVIIa will correct the INR, this may not equate to hemostatic efficacy in vivo.[243]

Thus far, there has been scarce published experience on outcomes following reversal of oral direct thrombin and Xa inhibitors before elective or emergency surgery.[244] A working knowledge of the respective elimination half-lives of these agents is important in deciding when to discontinue before elective procedures. In addition, an appreciation of the dominant mechanism(s) of clearance that may affect the elimination half-life is essential (Table 161-4). In general, when the procedure is considered to be more than minor, and the aim is to have negligible amounts of drug (<10%) in the circulation at the time of surgery, the drug should be discontinued at a time before surgery equivalent to four to five half-lives. This would imply 2 to 3 days (48 to 60 hours) for dabigatran.[222,223,228,245-247] Patients undergoing minor surgery could omit the drug for 1 day, expecting that there will still be some residual anticoagulant effect at the time of surgery. These recommendations may need to be amended for patients with reduced renal function or in those over the age of 75. Given the shorter half-life of rivaroxaban, omission of the drug on the day before surgery should be sufficient to ensure normal hemostasis.[225,244,246] Notably, in the event of emergency surgery or life-threatening bleeding, none of the new oral anticoagulants has a specific antidote and there remains significant uncertainty about the optimal urgent reversal strategy. Both PCCs and rFVIIa have been suggested, but as yet there is very limited clinical experience with either.[244,246]

Table 161-4 Suggested Timing of Interruption of Oral Xa or Thrombin Inhibitor Before Surgery

Calculated Creatinine Clearance (mL/Min)	Half-Life (Hr)	Standard Risk for Bleeding (e.g., Colonoscopy, Cholecystectomy)	High Risk for Bleeding (e.g., Neurosurgery, Cardiac Surgery)
DABIGATRAN			
>80	13 (11-22)	24 hr	2 days
>50-<80	15 (12-34)	24 hr	2 days
>30-<50	18 (13-23)	2 days	4 days
<30	27 (22-35)	4 days	6 days
RIVAROXABAN			
>30	12 (11-23)	24 hr	2 days
<30	Unknown	2 days	4 days

Modified from Schulman S, Crowther MA: How I treat with anticoagulants in 2012: New and old anticoagulants, and when and how to switch. *Blood* 119:3016, 2012.

Depending on the estimated risk for thrombosis when long-term oral anticoagulation is temporarily discontinued, bridging with LMWH (or UFH) may be required while the INR is in the subtherapeutic range.[213,218,248,249] In this regard, a number of specific issues, which are considered in the next several paragraphs, surround each of the three most common indications for long-term oral anticoagulation therapy, namely VTE, AF, and mechanical cardiac valve prostheses.[250] Although no LMWH yet has FDA approval for this purpose, large case series support the safety of this approach.[249,251-253] Regardless of whether bridging anticoagulation with UFH or LMWH is employed, the INR should be checked preoperatively to ensure that the pharmacologic effect of warfarin has been adequately reversed. As a rule, most surgeries can be safely carried out when the INR is less than 1.5.

Venous Thromboembolism

Patients are generally anticoagulated with warfarin to a target INR of 2.0 to 3.0 for several months to years after an acute episode of VTE (here defined as deep venous thrombosis [DVT] with or without pulmonary embolism [PE]) (see Chapter 151). Before deciding on a perioperative anticoagulation management strategy in these patients, it is helpful to assess separately the risks for bleeding and recurrent VTE in the preoperative and postoperative periods.[215] Although somewhat dependent on the type and magnitude of the intervention and method and duration of anesthesia, the risk for thrombosis may be magnified up to 100-fold during the postoperative period.[254] In some individuals, for example, those with a critically reduced cardiopulmonary reserve, even a minimal risk for PE may be unacceptable. Conversely, the potential consequences of even a modest amount of bleeding may be unacceptable in certain situations, for example, bleeding into an enclosed space such as the central nervous system in a patient undergoing neurosurgery.

It has been estimated that the risk for a recurrent event after an acute VTE without anticoagulant therapy is approximately 40% at 1 month.[215] Even in patients appropriately treated with anticoagulants, the cumulative risk for recurrent VTE at 3 months is on the order of 6% to 8%, with approximately three-quarters of events occurring within the first 3 to 4 weeks.[254-256] The risk gradually recedes thereafter, such that it is essentially back to baseline by approximately 3 months. However, the baseline risk may itself vary considerably. For example, in the case of an individual with a history of idiopathic VTE (i.e., not associated with surgery, pregnancy/oral contraceptive therapy, or trauma), it may be as high as 10% to 15% per year, at least during the first 2 to 3 years.[257,258] Especially high rates of recurrence may also be seen with underlying cancer, chronic cardiorespiratory disease, or antiphospholipid syndrome.[258] Therefore wherever possible it is usually preferable to delay elective surgery for at least 2 to 3 months after an acute episode of VTE. In the extreme situation where surgery is unavoidable within the first month after an acute VTE, the risk-benefit ratio usually favors bridging with full-dose UFH or LMWH before surgery and resuming again as soon as possible after surgery.[213,215,218] When the bleeding risk precludes the use of anticoagulation, the use of an inferior vena cava (IVC) filter may need to be considered. Generally speaking, a delay of 12 hours is sufficient to ensure adequate hemostasis after surgery before prophylactic doses of heparin are reinitiated, although of course this will also depend on the type of surgery and its customary bleeding risks. However, when therapeutic-dose anticoagulation is indicated, the ninth edition of the American College of Chest Physicians (ACCP) guidelines recommend that resumption be delayed until 48 to 72 hours following surgery.[239] When UFH is used, no bolus dose should be administered to avoid overanticoagulation and the attendant increased risk for bleeding. In the second or third month after an acute VTE, the heightened risk for VTE after surgery still favors full-intensity heparin therapy initiated as soon as possible in the postoperative period. However, the preoperative risk for recurrence has receded to the point where prophylactic doses of subcutaneous heparin or LMWH are probably sufficient.[215] One of these agents should be initiated when the INR is less than 2.0 and continued until approximately 12 hours preoperatively. In most patients who are 3 or more months remote from their most recent episode of VTE, preoperative bridging anticoagulation is usually unnecessary. Standard postoperative prophylaxis with LMWH/UFH is then administered with simultaneous reinitiation of warfarin.

Atrial Fibrillation

Several large prospective studies have established the major risk factors for and rates of embolic stroke and bleeding for patients with nonvalvular AF.[259-261] The $CHADS_2$ score[261] (Congestive heart failure, Hypertension, Age >75 years, and Diabetes mellitus, and 2 points for prior Stroke/transient ischemic attack) is the most widely used risk stratification model to define the risk for embolization in nonvalvular AF. Thus low-thrombotic-risk patients include those who are younger (<75 years) with "lone" AF and no additional risk factors for stroke, such as a previous history of stroke or transient ischemic attack, hypertension, diabetes, or left ventricular dysfunction. Their risk for stroke without anticoagulant therapy (and while not in the postoperative period) is estimated to be less than 1% per year, although there are limited clinical trials data on this topic.[262] At the opposite end of the spectrum, the estimated risk for stroke may approach 15% per year in older adult patients (>75 years) with a previous history of stroke and one or more of the risk factors listed.

Depending on the procedure, a reasonable approach to perioperative anticoagulation management in patients with AF is to discontinue oral anticoagulation 4 to 5 days ahead of a planned major surgery, with no bridging therapy except for those at high risk (stroke or transient ischemic attack within previous month, rheumatic mitral valvular disease, nonvalvular AF with two or more risk factors). A large single-center series, using a standardized algorithm of full-treatment-dose LMWH bridging in patients at risk for arterial thromboembolism (mechanical heart valve, AF, or thromboembolic stroke), reported a thromboembolism rate of 0.4%, and a 0.7% incidence of major bleeding.[263] Other studies and registries have reported rates of major bleeding as high as 8%.[249] In the case of the oral thrombin and Xa inhibitors, a time frame for discontinuation dependent on the respective elimination half-life has already been discussed. However, of some concern in the clinical trials was the increased risk for stroke in AF patients discontinuing rivaroxaban,[264] which led to a black box warning from the FDA that another agent be considered for bridging if the drug is discontinued for a reason other than bleeding.

Mechanical Prosthetic Heart Valves

The major thrombotic risks associated with mechanical prosthetic heart valves are systemic embolization and valve thrombosis, which usually presents as acute congestive heart failure. These risks are dependent on the location of the valve (higher in the mitral position than the aortic position), number of valves, and type of valve.[265] The earlier model ball-and-cage valves (e.g., Starr-Edwards) are considered to be more thrombogenic than the single-leaflet tilting-disk models (e.g., Björk-Shiley, Medtronic-Hall), which in turn are more thrombogenic than the bileaflet tilting-disk models (e.g., St. Jude Medical). The annual risk for thrombosis in patients with mechanical valves not receiving oral anticoagulation will therefore vary with (1) the type and location of the valve(s) and (2) certain comorbidities that increase the thrombotic risk, such as AF, congestive heart failure, enlarged left atrium, left ventricular aneurysm, and intracardiac thrombus. Estimates of the risk for thrombosis without anticoagulation are generally in the range of 8% to 15% per year, but these figures may be exaggerated owing to the overrepresentation of older-model valves in these series.[265]

It is generally agreed that bridging with UFH or LMWH is unnecessary for the patient with an isolated prosthetic valve in the aortic position without any other major risk factors who is to undergo elective surgery. Warfarin therapy is discontinued 4 to 5 days ahead of the procedure and is reinitiated as soon as possible after surgery along with prophylactic doses of UFH or LMWH.[252,266-268] On the other hand, bridging may be indicated for patients with an aortic valve prosthesis and other risk factors for thrombosis, for mitral valve prosthesis, and for multiple valvular prostheses. A growing experience with outpatient LMWH bridging (given at full therapeutic doses) suggests that it may be as effective and safe as UFH, at a lower overall cost.[249] However, in 2002, the manufacturers of enoxaparin issued a drug label warning indicating that the use of enoxaparin was not recommended for thromboprophylaxis for patients with prosthetic heart valves.[269] This action was prompted by the deaths of two pregnant patients with prosthetic valves from thrombotic complications while taking enoxaparin. The warning was subsequently reworded to acknowledge that the standard approach—infusional dose-adjusted UFH—has also been associated with adverse thrombotic outcomes in pregnant women with prosthetic heart valves, and that this topic has not been studied adequately.[267,270,271] It is therefore likely that pregnancy represents a very different situation with respect to the failure rate of all heparins in bridging. The accompanying hypercoagulable state and increased plasma volume and glomerular filtration rate (which can affect the volume of distribution of the drug) contribute to the uniqueness of the pregnant patient with a prosthetic valve.[272,273] In the absence of data from randomized controlled trials, consensus is moving toward recommending the use of LMWH without routine monitoring for bridging anticoagulation in nonpregnant patients, based on an absence of evidence of any lesser efficacy or safety.[213,218,266] LMWH is probably also a reasonable option for longer-term prophylaxis in the pregnant patient who cannot take warfarin, although in this situation routine periodic monitoring of anti-Xa activity is recommended with appropriate dose adjustments to target a peak anti-Xa activity (4 to 6 hours after dosing) of 0.7 to 1.2 units/mL.[267,271] The relatively low enrollment of subjects with mechanical heart valves receiving LMWH in registries of bridging anticoagulation suggests that there remains some reluctance to use this approach.[249,274] Indeed, recommendations from the American College of Cardiology and American Heart Association continue to recommend UFH given by continuous infusion rather than LMWHs for bridging in patients at high risk for thrombosis.[267] This category would include all patients with mitral or tricuspid valve replacements and those with an aortic valve replacement and additional risk factors (AF, previous thromboembolism, a "hypercoagulable condition," older-generation mechanical valves, more than one mechanical valve, or a left ventricular ejection fraction <0.3). It is clear that there is clinical equipoise in the optimal choice of bridging for higher-risk patients, and data from prospective randomized clinical trials are urgently required to resolve the issue.

Management of Anticoagulation in Patients Undergoing Dental Surgery

A common reason for hematologic consultation is to provide recommendations for the patient on long-term oral anticoagulation therapy for whom dental surgery, including dental extraction(s), is scheduled. In a randomized clinical trial, a nonsignificant increase in bleeding complications occurred in patients continued on oral anticoagulation without adjustment (other than ensuring that the INR was <4.0), compared to an intervention group in which anticoagulation was discontinued for 2 days to achieve an INR less than 2.0.[275] Similar results were reported from a large prospective case-control study in Italy, where no difference in bleeding complications after dental extraction was observed in patients taking oral anticoagulant therapy (with INRs in the range of 1.8 to 4.0) compared to controls.[276] In this study, local hemostatic measures (fibrin sponges, silk sutures, and tranexamic-soaked gauzes) were used in anticoagulated patients. It is likely also that the concurrent use of an antifibrinolytic agent mouthwash—which has independently been shown to reduce blood loss in this situation[277,278]—would further diminish the bleeding risk.

Management of Anticoagulation in Patients Undergoing Gastrointestinal Endoscopic Procedures

When a clinician is deciding on the most appropriate periprocedural management of oral anticoagulant therapy in patients undergoing gastrointestinal endoscopy, a working knowledge of the bleeding risk associated with the various interventional procedures is required (Table 161-5). Although simple diagnostic colonoscopy is associated with a very low bleeding risk (approximately 0.1%), colonic polyps will be identified in approximately one-third of patients undergoing routine screening. Endoscopic polypectomy may be associated with a significant (1% to 5%) bleeding risk.[279] Risk factors for hemorrhage include hypertension, polyp size, sessile morphology, and location in the ascending colon. Bleeding in patients on anticoagulation is frequently delayed, with a median onset at approximately 5 days, although it may be encountered up to 14 days after the procedure.[280] Current guidelines are based on smaller trials and expert opinion. The guidelines of the American Society for Gastrointestinal Endoscopy[281] and the European Society of Gastrointestinal Endoscopy[282] recommend continuing warfarin in the therapeutic range in patients who have a low risk for bleeding (e.g., upper- or lower-gastrointestinal endoscopy with or without biopsy). On the other hand, interruption of anticoagulation (either temporary cessation or halving the dose for several days preoperatively in all but the highest-thrombotic-risk patients[283]) is recommended in those undergoing high-risk procedures (see Table 161-5). In those patients with the highest risk for thromboembolism (e.g., AF with valvular disease and/or prior history of stroke), bridging anticoagulation with heparin is recommended before and after high-risk procedures.[284]

Similarly, the decision whether to temporarily interrupt antiplatelet agents should be made after weighing the risks for thrombosis if withheld and bleeding if continued (which will depend to some extent on the type of procedure). Current guidelines[281,282] recommend continuation of aspirin irrespective of polyp size, but discontinuation of thienopyridines (5 days for clopidogrel, 7 days for prasugrel) for polyps greater than 1 cm in patients in whom the risk for thrombosis is not judged to be excessive. For patients who cannot discontinue these agents, the judicious use of topical hemostatic devices should be considered.

Table 161-5 Risk for Bleeding Associated With Various Endoscopic Procedures

Low-Risk Procedures	High-Risk Procedures (Approximate Bleeding Risk [%])
Diagnostic esophagogastroduodenoscopy	Colonoscopic polypectomy (1%-2.5%)
Flexible sigmoidoscopy and colonoscopy ± biopsy	Gastric polypectomy (4%)
Diagnostic endoscopic retrograde cholangiopancreatography	Laser ablation and coagulation (<6%)
Biliary stent insertion without endoscopic sphincterotomy	Endoscopic sphincterotomy (2.5%-5%)
Endosonography	Dilation of benign or malignant strictures
Push enteroscopy	Percutaneous endoscopic gastrostomy

Management of Anticoagulation in Patients Receiving Neuraxial Anesthesia

A special situation concerns the management of perioperative anticoagulation, particularly LMWHs, in patients receiving neuraxial (spinal and epidural) anesthesia or analgesia for surgery or delivery. The advantages of these forms of regional anesthesia compared to systemic anesthesia (superior analgesia, decreased transfusion requirements, and lower incidence of thrombotic complications) must be weighed against the risk for spinal hematoma. This rare but potentially disastrous complication is a result of needle- or catheter-induced vascular trauma during placement into the subarachnoid or epidural space. Bleeding usually occurs into the epidural space, probably because of the prominent epidural venous plexus.[285] It presents more frequently as a delayed but progressive sensory or motor deficit, or bladder or bowel dysfunction, rather than radicular back pain. Attention was drawn to this problem in the mid-1990s when multiple cases of spinal hematoma associated with the use of the LMWH enoxaparin were reported to the FDA. Significant risk factors that have been identified include the timing of both needle or catheter placement and removal in relation to the last dose of LMWH, the concurrent use of antiplatelet agents, and trauma during the regional anesthetic procedure.[286] Spinal hematomas have been reported with both single-dose and continuous neuraxial anesthesia, although the risk is considered to be much lower with the former procedure. Recommendations designed to minimize the risk for spinal hematoma include the following: (1) placement of the needle should occur at least 10 to 12 hours after the last prophylactic dose, or longer (e.g., 20 to 24 hours) after the last full therapeutic dose of LMWH, and (2) similarly, removal of an indwelling catheter should be delayed for at least 10 to 12 hours after a dose of LMWH, most of which have a half-life in the range of 4 to 6 hours.[286,287] Once-daily prophylactic LMWH regimens are associated with lower trough anticoagulant levels than twice-daily regimens, and they may be a safer choice in patients in whom indwelling catheters are employed,[288] with removal of the catheter scheduled for 20 or more hours after the last dose of drug. It is generally considered safe to administer the next dose of LMWH 2 hours after catheter removal. The synthetic pentasaccharide fondaparinux (Arixtra) also carries a black box warning from the FDA, although in fact very little is known about the associated risk for spinal hematoma formation. The long plasma half-life of the agent (17 hours) should be borne in mind when making treatment decisions about its use when regional anesthesia is being concurrently employed.[286] As a rule, fondaparinux should be discontinued 36 hours before catheter insertion and not restarted before 6 to 8 hours following the procedure. Avoidance of the simultaneous use of antiplatelet agents, including aspirin and NSAIDs, is advisable in the case of all of these anticoagulants, even though the use of aspirin or NSAIDs in isolation likely does not lead to any increased risk for procedure-related bleeding. It is, however, recommended that thienopyridines be discontinued at an appropriate interval before catheter insertion (e.g., 5 to 7 days in the case of clopidogrel). For further information about this topic, the reader is referred to one of the North American or European guidelines.[286-289]

In the case of the new anticoagulants, there are minimal data on which to base recommendations. However, expert recommendations on the timing of administration of dabigatran and rivaroxaban, based on their pharmacologic profiles, have been published.[290,291]

Prophylaxis for Venous Thromboembolism After Surgery and Trauma

Epidemiology and Natural History

The overall incidence rate of VTE in the community is approximately 1 in 1000 per year. It has been estimated that hospitalization for surgery accounts for about one-quarter of cases of VTE and is associated with an almost 22-fold increased risk. Trauma accounts for about half as many additional cases, with a 13-fold increased risk.[254] Additional identified risk factors (which may coexist in these individuals) include malignancy, central vein catheterization, and neurologic disease with extremity paresis. Older age is also a strong independent risk factor, whereas hormonal therapies (oral contraceptives, hormone replacement therapy, tamoxifen, and raloxifene) compound the risk in women.[255] In hospitalized patients, DVT is often clinically silent, and PE may be rapidly fatal. It has been estimated that more than 12 million hospitalized patients per year are at risk for VTE.[292] Because screening for asymptomatic DVT by ultrasonography is expensive yet relatively insensitive,[293] widespread use of prophylaxis is widely acknowledged to be the most effective strategy to minimize the burden of venous thromboembolic disease. This strategy has also been shown to be a cost-effective approach.

Although patients on the surgical and trauma services represent a significant proportion of VTE disease burden, they also provide an important opportunity for prevention through the appropriate design and use of validated VTE prophylaxis regimens. A comprehensive treatise with updated recommendations was recently published in the ninth edition of the ACCP guidelines.[294] The reader is referred to these guidelines for details of recommended regimens, frequency, and duration of therapy graded according to level of evidence. Some general principles from this document will be discussed here, with a focus on more recent developments and recent controversies in the field.

Using sensitive techniques such as ascending venography, much has been learned about the frequency and natural history of DVT formation after surgical procedures. In many studies, venography was performed at 7 to 14 days postoperatively, to coincide with the termination of pharmacologic prophylaxis. Recently, however, it has become clear that DVT formation may continue for several weeks after surgery, and the trend in the last several years in certain situations, such as after hip replacement or abdominal/pelvic cancer surgery, has been toward longer duration of therapy, up to 28 to 35 days (discussed further later). These studies have defined the absolute risks for VTE according to these end points and allowed a given individual's risk for VTE to be assessed preoperatively (Table 161-6). Low-risk individuals are defined as those less than 40 years of age undergoing minor surgery lasting less than 30 minutes, with no additional risk factors. At the other end of the spectrum, very high-risk individuals are those more than 40 years of age undergoing major orthopedic lower extremity or spinal surgery, or who have suffered major trauma. A history of prior VTE, use of estrogen-containing therapies, and presence of certain thrombophilic disorders or cancer may further heighten the risk in this group.[295]

Nonpharmacologic Methods of Venous Thrombosis Prophylaxis

Early ambulation should be a routine component of postoperative care whenever possible. It has been shown to be associated with a lower risk for postoperative VTE, for example, after hip replacement surgery.[296] Properly fitted elastic stockings (i.e., those not leading to venous compression above the knee) are a useful adjunct in VTE prophylaxis but are generally insufficient as the sole prophylactic modality. On the other hand, intermittent pneumatic compression devices, both those that provide intermittent calf and/or thigh compression or foot pumping action, may be used as the primary modality in all but the highest-risk group of patients undergoing high-risk general surgery, or hip or knee surgery, and some forms of neurosurgery. These devices presumably reduce the risk for VTE by preventing venostasis in the immobilized limb(s). Although it has been postulated that they also enhance fibrinolysis by stimulating endothelial release of plasminogen activators, it has been difficult to support this hypothesis with experimental data.[297,298] Compliance is a constant concern with these devices, as is the possibility of reduced efficacy in significantly overweight individuals. Intermittent pneumatic compression is often used as an adjunct to pharmacologic prophylaxis in high-risk individuals.[299]

IVC filters are occasionally used to prevent pulmonary embolization in patients with extensive trauma in whom the bleeding risks are (sometimes incorrectly) perceived to be too high for the use of pharmacologic prophylaxis.[300-302] There are very few prospective randomized trials to support the use of IVC filters in this or any other surgical situations, and in one of the few such trials, filter placement was associated with a significantly greater risk for late-onset DVT.[303] Filter deployment may still be a reasonable approach in a patient with a very recent VTE who requires urgent surgery in whom aggressive anticoagulant prophylaxis is not considered feasible. Temporary (retrievable) IVC filters, which generally require removal within 2 to 3 months, are being increasingly used in this type of situation, despite an absence of data from randomized clinical trials.[300] An all-too-frequent issue with these filters is that they are not removed once the indication for their placement has resolved.[304] Furthermore, as the experience with retrievable IVC filters has matured, it has become

Table 161-6 Recommendations for Prophylaxis of Deep Vein Thrombosis

Approximate Risk Category*	Patients	Calf DVT	DVT	PE	Recommendation
Low	Surgical patients under 40, surgery lasting <30 minutes, no additional risk factors	1%-2%	0.5%-1%	0%-0.1%	Ambulation, leg exercises
Moderate	Surgical patients older than 40, having abdominal or thoracic surgery lasting >30 minutes	20%-30%	2%-10%	1%-3%	Low-dose heparin
	Neurosurgery or other patients with high bleeding risk				Pneumatic compression
High	Hip fracture	40%-80%	20%-40%	5%-10%	Warfarin,† LMWH
	Hip replacement				Warfarin,† adjusted-dose heparin, LMWH
	Knee replacement				LMWH, external pneumatic compression
	Open prostatectomy				Pneumatic compression
	Gynecologic malignancy				Pneumatic compression

DVT, Deep venous thrombosis; *LMWH,* low-molecular-weight heparin; *PE,* pulmonary embolism.
*Without prophylaxis.
†Given in low-dose regimen.

clear that long-term complications (including filter limb fracture and/or migration, distal DVT, and IVC thrombosis and/or stenosis) with nonretrieved filters are a serious concern.[305]

Pharmacologic Methods of Prophylaxis

The surgical situations in which there exist the largest body of accumulated clinical trials data are in major orthopedic surgery (total hip and knee arthroplasty, hip fracture, and spinal surgery). As mentioned, the primary end point for VTE in these antithrombotic agent trials has been DVT detected by venography, which occurs in 40% to 70% of patients not receiving prophylaxis.[306] Until the recent publication of the ninth edition of the ACCP guidelines, this surrogate end point for clinically apparent symptomatic DVT was the basis of recommendations for antithrombotic prophylaxis because of its sensitivity and reproducibility. However, the most recent iteration of the guidelines saw a marked shift toward patient-relevant outcomes, even if these outcomes needed to be estimated/extrapolated from the existing evidence. In addition, an emphasis on patient values and preferences was introduced to the panels' deliberations.[307]

Prophylactic UFH is administered subcutaneously, either 5000 units two to three times daily without monitoring or every 8 hours with dose adjustment to maintain a high-normal midinterval aPTT, LMWH (enoxaparin, tinzaparin, or dalteparin) is given subcutaneously once or twice daily (depending on the agent), and warfarin is given postoperatively and adjusted to a target INR of 2.0 to 3.0. Fondaparinux, a synthetic pentasaccharide that selectively inhibits factor Xa in an antithrombin-dependent manner, is also licensed for VTE prophylaxis in total hip and knee arthroplasty surgery and hip fracture surgery.[308] An advantage of LMWHs and other structurally unrelated molecules over UFH is a reduced or absent risk for HIT. For example, clinically apparent HIT was present in 2.7% of patients receiving prophylactic doses of UFH after hip surgery, compared with 0% in the cohort who received LMWH ($P = .0018$).[309] However, HIT may occur as a rare complication of LMWHs such as enoxaparin, tinzaparin, or dalteparin.[219] On the other hand, although HIT has been very rarely described as a result of fondaparinux therapy,[310] accumulating data from case series suggest that fondaparinux can paradoxically be used for the treatment of HIT.[311,312]

In general, all these forms of thromboprophylaxis are associated with roughly a 70% risk reduction in perioperative VTE, but there are some important differences in efficacy that have been demonstrated in specific types of surgery,[295] which are briefly outlined later. Conversely, the bleeding risks are principally related to dose and host risk factors, and to a lesser extent the choice of agent and timing of administration in relation to surgery. For example, in orthopedic surgery in the United States, LMWH is traditionally initiated 12 hours postoperatively, compared to European regimens in which these agents are initiated in close proximity to surgery (between 2 hours preoperatively and 6 to 8 hours postoperatively).[313] Details of suggested dosing schedules are shown in Table 161-7.

Table 161-7 Suggested Dosing Regimens for Prophylactic Low-Molecular-Weight Heparins and Pentasaccharide for Orthopedic or General Surgery

Drug	Orthopedic Surgery	General Surgery
Enoxaparin	30 mg (3000 International Units) every 12 hr Begin 12-24 hr after surgery Continue for 7-10 days Consider extended prophylaxis After THA (40 mg once daily until 28-35 days after surgery)	40 mg (4000 International Units) once daily Begin 1-2 hr before surgery
Dalteparin	5000 International Units once daily	2500 International Units once daily Begin 1-2 hr before surgery
Tinzaparin	75 International Units/kg once daily Begin 1-2 hr preoperatively	
Fondaparinux	2.5 mg once daily Begin 6 hr after surgery	

THA, Total hip arthroplasty.

Orthopedic Surgery

Among the various types of surgery, the efficacy and safety of pharmacologic VTE prophylaxis has been most extensively studied in major orthopedic surgery. However, as discussed later, it has also recently become a highly controversial topic. As mentioned, the primary (surrogate) end point of venographically detected DVT is in the range of 40% to 70% in patients not receiving prophylaxis. The corresponding rates of death due to PE are 0.1% to 0.4% of patients undergoing total hip replacement, 0.2% to 0.7% undergoing total knee replacement, and 3.6% to 12.9% following hip fracture surgery.

In 2007 the American Academy of Orthopaedic Surgeons (AAOS) published their own guidelines for the prevention of perioperative symptomatic PE (www.aaos.org/guidelines). These guidelines differ from those of the eighth edition of the ACCP document by recommending that (1) mechanical prophylaxis be used in all patients; (2) warfarin is a suitable alternative in most patients; and (3) in patients with an increased risk for bleeding, warfarin, aspirin, or mechanical prophylaxis alone is a suitable alternative. A major impetus for the AAOS guidelines was the concern among orthopedic surgeons about bleeding risks associated with antithrombotic agents. Indeed, it has been noted that the lack of standardization of the definition of "major bleeding" in pharmacoprophylaxis clinical trials may result in seriously flawed conclusions about bleeding rates when comparing treatment groups.[314] Although vigorously refuted at first,[315] the principles of the AAOS recommendations—in particular, that only the clinically relevant end points of symptomatic VTE and serious bleeding should be considered when recommending thromboprophylaxis strategies—have been incorporated into the ninth edition of the ACCP guidelines.[307] One acknowledged practical difficulty is determining the relative importance ascribed to these opposing events. As a result of the revised grading criteria, the quality of evidence for many recommendations was downgraded in the ninth edition. One novel recommendation was the inclusion of aspirin as an acceptable method of pharmacoprophylaxis for total hip or knee arthroplasty. In fact, it was assigned a grade 1B recommendation on the basis of the very large Pulmonary Embolization Prevention trial.[316] In this study, 160 mg a day of aspirin initiated preoperatively as an adjunctive therapy to conventional prophylaxis was associated with a reduction in symptomatic PE from 1.2% with placebo to 0.7% ($P < .001$), although there was an increased rate of bleeding requiring transfusion.[317] In contrast, intermittent pneumatic compression (applied for at least 18 hours daily) as the sole method of prophylaxis received a grade 1C recommendation.[316]

Metaanalysis has demonstrated that the protection against proximal DVT afforded by low-dose UFH may be inferior to LMWH, and LMWH is recommended over UFH.[316] An acceptable alternative to LMWH is warfarin, which is preferred by many orthopedic surgeons. Most commonly, warfarin is initiated the evening of surgery, although in some protocols it is begun on the evening before surgery, without any apparent difference in efficacy. Dose adjustment is performed to achieve a target INR of 2.5 ± 0.5. The efficacy of LMWH is either equivalent or slightly superior to warfarin in total hip arthroplasty and more definitively superior in total knee arthroplasty, albeit at the expense of a mildly increased risk for bleeding.[295]

Fondaparinux (2.5 mg once daily) was compared with enoxaparin (40 mg once daily or 30 mg twice daily) in hip and knee arthroplasty and in hip fracture repair.[318-320] In a metaanalysis of the major trials, which included 7344 patients, there was a statistically significant 55% relative risk reduction (6.8% versus 13.7%) in the incidence of venographically detected DVT (and proximal DVT).[308] However, there was no difference in the incidence of symptomatic VTE or fatal PE, and major bleeding was more frequently encountered in the fondaparinux group compared to the enoxaparin group (2.7% versus 1.7%). It is likely that the higher efficacy at the expense of greater bleeding with fondaparinux is explained by the fact that the first dose was usually administered earlier than enoxaparin (6 hours versus 12 hours postoperatively). Prolonged prophylaxis beyond the usual 7 to 10 days is a pertinent consideration for total hip arthroplasty patients, where the median time to diagnosis of symptomatic VTE (occurring in 2.8% of patients within 3 months) is 17 days postoperatively. In contrast, VTE after total knee arthroplasty (occurring in 2.1% of patients within 3 months) tends to occur much earlier, after a median of 7 days.[306] By metaanalysis, trials in which LMWH prophylaxis was extended for 30 to 42 days were associated with a significant reduction in the frequency of symptomatic VTE, without any increase in major bleeding.[313,321] This was especially true in total hip arthroplasty, where the absolute risk reduction in symptomatic VTE was approximately 2%.[321] Prolonged therapy with warfarin may be similarly effective, although some studies,[322] but not others,[323] have raised concerns about the bleeding risks. As yet, despite early indications of favorable cost-effectiveness, long-term prophylaxis with LMWH or warfarin is not widely used.

The new oral anticoagulants (dabigatran, rivaroxaban, and apixaban) have all been tested against the common comparator, enoxaparin, in phase III clinical trials of VTE prophylaxis in hip or knee replacement surgery.[324-330] A pooled analysis of these studies, which included more than 32,000 randomized patients undergoing total hip or knee arthroplasty, concluded that the new anticoagulants demonstrated significantly better efficacy (considering the end points of total VTE and all-cause mortality, major VTE, and proximal DVT) with an equivalent safety profile (i.e., bleeding).[331] Rivaroxaban (10 mg once daily) has received approval in the United States and elsewhere for the prevention of VTE in patients undergoing elective total hip or knee replacement surgery. Apixaban (2.5 mg twice daily) has also been approved for these indications, as has dabigatran (220 mg once daily) in the European Union and in Canada.[228] In the ninth edition of the ACCP guidelines, LMWH, fondaparinux, apixaban, dabigatran, rivaroxaban, low-dose UFH, or adjusted-dose vitamin K antagonists all received a grade 1B recommendation when used for VTE prophylaxis in these situations.

Recently it has been demonstrated that patients with comparatively minor forms of lower-extremity orthopedic surgery, such as therapeutic arthroscopic knee procedures, are also at increased risk for VTE.[332,333] A recent metaanalysis concluded that the total incidence of asymptomatic DVT after knee arthroscopy was 9.9% (95% confidence interval [CI], 8.1% to 11.7%), with a proximal DVT incidence of 2.1% (95% CI, 1.2% to 3.0%).[334] Routine use of pharmacologic prophylaxis is probably not warranted, although it would be appropriately considered in a patient with a previous history of VTE or other risk factors, such as prolonged tourniquet time (>60 minutes), a known thrombophilic disorder, or on estrogen therapy.[316]

Trauma

Trauma is the leading cause of death in people less than 40 years of age, and PE is the third most common cause of death in subjects who survive the first 24 hours.[335] A recent analysis of almost 900,000 patients in the National Trauma Data Bank suggests that although the incidence of posttrauma PE is increasing (possibly due to a more liberal use of chest computed tomography scanning), mortality from PE is decreasing, and PE now accounts for the death of about 1 in every 500 patients with trauma.[336]

Up to 60% of trauma patients suffer venographically demonstrated DVT within 14 days of admission,[337] although the range of reported VTE complication rate in trauma varies enormously in the literature, possibly reflecting not only variable study methodologies but also study subject heterogeneity.[338-340] Factors that appear to be independently associated with a greater risk for thrombosis following trauma include (1) age over 40 years, (2) lower-extremity fracture, (3) major head injury, (4) more than 3 ventilator days, (5) venous injury, and (6) major surgical procedure.[336] Although there is general agreement that some form of prophylaxis is routinely warranted, there is confusion (even from prospective randomized clinical trials) whether pharmacologic prophylaxis is superior to nonpharmacologic prophylaxis[341-343] and whether LMWH has a specific advantage over UFH.[335,344] There is general agreement that warfarin should not be used in the acute situation, although it may have a role during the rehabilitation phase in selected patients. Nonpharmacologic methods of prophylaxis may be difficult to apply in some cases with external fixation devices in the lower extremities, and it is therefore recommended that intermittent pneumatic compression alone be used only when both lower extremities are available. Routine surveillance using duplex ultrasound scans are not recommended unless VTE prophylaxis cannot be employed.[295] An extensive review of the scientific evidence and development of evidence-based practice consensus guidelines in trauma surgery published in 2002 recommended that, where feasible, prophylaxis using LMWH rather than UFH be preferred for patients with pelvic, complex lower-extremity, or spinal fractures,[345] especially with partial or complete motor paralysis. However, these Eastern Association for the Surgery of Trauma (EAST) guidelines acknowledge a paucity of Level I evidence to support the prophylaxis algorithms. A subsequent registry of 743 high-risk trauma patients prescribed once-daily prophylactic dose LMWH, regardless of the need for invasive procedures and including those with stable intracranial injuries, did not document any exacerbations of head injury due to bleeding.[346] Notably in this study, the LMWH was initiated an average of 3.3 days after admission. However, for patients at very high risk for both VTE and bleeding with anticoagulation, IVC filter placement—generally using retrievable devices—may occasionally be justified.[347] However, given the lack of randomized controlled trials in this area, it is not surprising that the rate of filter deployment varies widely among major trauma centers.[348]

Even without the associated risks of surgery, bony fracture and immobilization may be sufficient stimuli to increase the incidence of VTE. For example, a 19% rate of venographically demonstrated DVT was noted in patients requiring plaster immobilization or bracing after a leg fracture or ruptured Achilles tendon. This was reduced to 9% in a matched group treated with prophylactic LMWH throughout the period of immobilization.[349] Here again, however, the evidence overall does not clearly support the need for routine pharmacologic VTE prophylaxis in all patients treated for lower-extremity fracture.

Neurosurgery

Patients undergoing neurosurgery involving craniotomy, particularly when performed for high-grade glioma,[350] are also at high risk for VTE. Symptomatic events occur in as many as 6% of patients within the first 3 months postoperatively.[351] In patients with high-grade glioma, the incidence of symptomatic VTE is in the range of 20% to 30%; although the incidence is highest in the first few weeks postoperatively, it does continue throughout the course of the disease.[352] The need for pharmacologic prophylaxis is tempered by the potentially disastrous consequences of intracranial bleeding as a complication of therapy. This concern has led some to recommend a conservative strategy of nonpharmacologic prophylaxis only. However, a landmark randomized placebo-controlled trial demonstrated that enoxaparin 40 mg daily (initiated within 24 hours postoperatively) was associated with a 49% relative risk reduction in venographically demonstrated DVT compared to placebo in patients undergoing elective cranial or spinal surgery (97% for tumors). The rate of symptomatic VTE was reduced from 6% to 1%, with no increase in bleeding. A more recent metaanalysis concluded that a combination of LMWH and intermittent pneumatic compression significantly reduced perioperative VTE risk by 40% without any increase in intracranial hemorrhage.[353] Yet concerns remain that preoperative or early postoperative administration of LMWH is associated with an increased risk for bleeding.[354,355] In this more than in other areas of surgery, the timing of initiation of heparin/LMWH, dosing, and duration of therapy are critical factors in determining the risk-benefit ratio.[356]

General and Gynecologic Surgery

Rates of asymptomatic VTE in all patients undergoing general surgery without VTE prophylaxis (approximately 20% to 25%) are lower than in major orthopedic surgery, although it should be noted that the rates are substantially lower in certain minor forms of surgery, such as appendectomy or abdominal wall surgery. The increasing use of laparoscopic techniques has tended to lower the risks that were previously encountered with the corresponding open procedures. Patient-related risk factors include cancer, advancing age, a history of previous VTE, obesity, varicose veins, and estrogen use.[294]

In several metaanalyses, thrombosis prophylaxis using LMWH is uniformly superior to placebo and equivalent to subcutaneous UFH.[295,357,358] UFH is also equivalent to LMWH in high-risk urologic or gynecologic surgery. In moderate-risk gynecologic surgery, nonpharmacologic prophylaxis with intermittent pneumatic compression is as efficacious as LMWH,[359] although patients with a history of cancer or DVT or age more than 60 years may be more prone to fail intermittent pneumatic compression alone.[360] Although bleeding rates are purportedly higher with LMWH than UFH in general surgery, this may be a function of administered dose. A lower dose of LMWH (<3500 anti-Xa units/day) may be as efficacious as UFH, with a bleeding rate that is actually somewhat lower.[361]

Cancer increases the risk for postoperative VTE by a factor of approximately 2,[255] and patients undergoing major abdominal or pelvic surgery for neoplastic disorders should be considered to be at high risk. This risk may be related to enhanced activation of coagulation, more prolonged immobilization, and/or greater extent of surgery and duration of anesthesia. Low-dose UFH or LMWH combined with intermittent pneumatic compression appears to be ideal VTE prophylaxis.[361,362] Therapy is typically initiated 2 hours preoperatively. Approximately 40% of VTE occurs following discharge, suggesting a need for prolonged therapy. Indeed, prolonged administration of enoxaparin (40 mg once daily) results in a reduction of venographically demonstrated DVT (from 12.0% in the 1-week treatment group to 4.8% in the 4-week treatment group), without any increased risk for bleeding.[363]

IVC filters are not recommended for VTE prophylaxis in patients undergoing general and abdominal or pelvic surgery.[294] Instead, in the high-risk patient who cannot receive LMWH or UFH, fondaparinux, low-dose aspirin, or mechanical forms of prophylaxis should be considered.[294]

Renal Transplantation

In the United States, approximately 14,000 renal transplants are performed annually. Published estimates of the incidence of postoperative VTE have varied from 0.6% to 25%.[364] A retrospective analysis of more than 2000 renal allograft recipients found a 6.2% incidence of symptomatic DVT in patients undergoing kidney or simultaneous kidney-pancreas transplant without prophylaxis in the period between 1985 and 1995.[365] In this study, the incidence of symptomatic DVT following kidney transplantation (4.5%) did not appear to be significantly higher than the rate in general surgical procedures of a comparable magnitude; however, the rate in patients receiving kidney-pancreas allografts (18.1%) was considered to be excessively high. In another series of 518 transplant recipients, a similar rate of first VTE (9%) was recorded, at a median time of 17 months postoperatively.[366]

A number of special considerations apply to the use of prophylactic anticoagulation in renal transplant recipients. Because renal function may remain impaired for several days or more following the procedure, impaired clearance of LMWHs may increase the risk for bleeding. Therefore UFH may be a better choice for prophylaxis. Furthermore, prophylactic anticoagulation may be of theoretical benefit in the prevention of other vascular complications of renal transplantation. Specifically, it has been demonstrated that common inherited and acquired thrombophilias (factor V Leiden [FV G1691A], prothrombin G20210A mutation, and antiphospholipid antibodies) are associated with an increased risk for primary renal graft thrombosis and acute vascular rejection. Primary renal graft thrombosis, defined as thrombosis of the renal graft vasculature in the absence of histopathologic evidence of rejection, usually occurs within 10 days of renal transplant and virtually always results in loss of the graft. Thrombosis is as likely to be arterial as venous and occurs in approximately 2% (range 1% to 6%) of recipients. The usual presentation is with sudden-onset oliguria or anuria associated with a falloff in graft function. In the case of renal vein thrombosis, there may be pain at the graft site, hematuria, and even graft rupture. A number of retrospective case-control studies[367-369] and a prospective study[370] have demonstrated that one or more of these thrombophilias are associated with an estimated 3- to 10-fold increased risk for renal graft thrombosis.

It has not been established by appropriate prospective randomized study whether antithrombotic prophylaxis can prevent early renal graft thrombosis. However, small series have suggested that UFH, LMWH, or aspirin (>75 mg daily) may diminish the rate of early allograft thrombosis, compared with historical controls.[371,372] Prophylaxis may be particularly vital in high-risk patients, for example, those with identified thrombophilia and/or a previous history of early graft loss or VTE.[373] However, the optimal intensity, duration, and composition of prophylactic regimens has not been determined, and opinions differ considerably, from long-term full-intensity anticoagulation begun in the early postoperative period to short-term lower-intensity heparin followed by longer-term aspirin therapy.[374,375]

COMPLIANCE WITH VENOUS THROMBOEMBOLISM PROPHYLAXIS

Most studies examining the rates of compliance with nationally developed guidelines for VTE prophylaxis have concluded that thromboprophylaxis is underutilized, both in terms of the absolute number of eligible but undertreated patients and the appropriateness (ranging from total omission to suboptimal choice, dose, or duration) of therapy. In the past, orthopedic services tended to be more (>85%) compliant with published guidelines, probably reflecting the longer history of use.[376-378] This pattern may, however, be changing, as orthopedic surgeons are faced with selecting potentially conflicting guidelines.[315] In general surgery in the United States, compliance with grade A recommendations may be much lower, sometimes in the 30% to 50% range.[379,380] This reluctance to use prophylaxis may be explained by a tendency to underestimate the thrombotic risk in high-risk patients.[292,376] Conversely, despite uncertainties regarding the optimal approach to prophylaxis in neurosurgical patients, 85% of practitioners in the United Kingdom regularly used some form of prophylaxis.[381] Improvement in compliance is probably best achieved by the application of guidelines developed by every hospital, including consideration of orders that all patients receive VTE prophylaxis unless they have contraindications.[382] Like all guidelines, the recommendations should be flexible enough to allow informed physicians to exercise their clinical judgment when assessing risks and benefits of a specific regimen in the case of an individual patient.

Treatment of Postsurgical Venous Thromboembolism

The principles of treatment of acute VTE occurring in the postoperative period do not differ materially from treatment under other circumstances (see Chapter 144), with the exception that the bleeding risks associated with anticoagulation are increased. Not surprisingly, patients who develop postoperative VTE after major orthopedic surgery have a higher risk for mortality, bleeding, and rehospitalization.[383] Although virtually all series agree that recent surgery is a risk factor for bleeding,[384] it is difficult to find relevant literature that quantifies the risk (with respect to the rate of decline in the risk after surgery). It is generally recommended that if surgery has involved a vital organ (e.g., brain, eye), it is inappropriate to risk full-intensity anticoagulation for 5 to 7 days[350] (or longer—e.g., at least 7 to 10 days—when thrombolytic therapy is to be used). This recommendation is supported by animal data demonstrating that the risk for intracranial hemorrhage with full-intensity heparin anticoagulation in the postoperative period following craniotomy dropped off sharply between the 7th and 10th postoperative day.[385] If anticoagulation is strongly contraindicated, placement of an IVC filter may be the only available option. At the other end of the spectrum, anticoagulation after minor procedures in patients judged to be at low risk for bleeding can probably be initiated after 12 to 24 hours. UFH may have certain advantages over LMWH in these circumstances, most notably its short half-life and susceptibility to more complete reversal with protamine, which dictate that it will be more reversible in the event of bleeding.

SUGGESTED READINGS

Achneck HE, Sileshi B, Jamiolkowski RM, et al: A comprehensive review of topical hemostatic agents: Efficacy and recommendations for use. *Ann Surg* 251:217, 2010.

Angel LF, Tapson V, Galgon RE, et al: Systematic review of the use of retrievable inferior vena cava filters. *J Vasc Interv Radiol* 22:1522, 2011, e1523.

Bonow RO, Carabello BA, Kanu C, et al: ACC/AHA 2006 guidelines for the management of patients with valvular heart disease: A report of the American College of Cardiology/American Heart Association Task Force on Practice Guidelines (writing committee to revise the 1998 Guidelines for the Management of Patients With Valvular Heart Disease): Developed in collaboration with the Society of Cardiovascular Anesthesiologists: Endorsed by the Society for Cardiovascular Angiography and Interventions and the Society of Thoracic Surgeons. *Circulation* 114:e84, 2006.

Borgman MA, Spinella PC, Perkins JG, et al: The ratio of blood products transfused affects mortality in patients receiving massive transfusions at a combat support hospital. *J Trauma* 63:805, 2007.

Chee YL, Crawford JC, Watson HG, et al: Guidelines on the assessment of bleeding risk prior to surgery or invasive procedures. British Committee for Standards in Haematology. *Br J Haematol* 140:496, 2008.

Crescenzi G, Landoni G, Biondi-Zoccai G, et al: Desmopressin reduces transfusion needs after surgery: A meta-analysis of randomized clinical trials. *Anesthesiology* 109:1063, 2008.

Douketis JD: Pharmacologic properties of the new oral anticoagulants: A clinician-oriented review with a focus on perioperative management. *Curr Pharm Des* 16:3436, 2010.

Douketis JD, Spyropoulos AC, Spencer FA, et al: Perioperative management of antithrombotic therapy: Antithrombotic Therapy and Prevention of Thrombosis, 9th ed: American College of Chest Physicians Evidence-Based Clinical Practice Guidelines. *Chest* 141:e326S, 2012.

Eubanks JD: Antifibrinolytics in major orthopaedic surgery. *J Am Acad Orthop Surg* 18:132, 2010.

Falck-Ytter Y, Francis CW, Johanson NA, et al: Prevention of VTE in orthopedic surgery patients: Antithrombotic Therapy and Prevention of Thrombosis, 9th ed: American College of Chest Physicians Evidence-Based Clinical Practice Guidelines. *Chest* 141:e278S, 2012.

Gould MK, Garcia DA, Wren SM, et al: Prevention of VTE in nonorthopedic surgical patients: Antithrombotic Therapy and Prevention of Thrombosis, 9th ed: American College of Chest Physicians Evidence-Based Clinical Practice Guidelines. *Chest* 141:e227S, 2012.

Guyatt GH, Eikelboom JW, Gould MK, et al: Approach to outcome measurement in the prevention of thrombosis in surgical and medical patients: Antithrombotic Therapy and Prevention of Thrombosis, 9th ed: American College of Chest Physicians Evidence-Based Clinical Practice Guidelines. *Chest* 141:e185S, 2012.

Horlocker TT, Wedel DJ, Rowlingson JC, et al: Regional anesthesia in the patient receiving antithrombotic or thrombolytic therapy: American Society of Regional Anesthesia and Pain Medicine Evidence-Based Guidelines (Third Edition). *Reg Anesth Pain Med* 35:64, 2010.

Kearon C, Hirsh J: Management of anticoagulation before and after elective surgery. *N Engl J Med* 336:1506, 1997.

Kwok A, Faigel DO: Management of anticoagulation before and after gastrointestinal endoscopy. *Am J Gastroenterol* 104:3085, quiz 3098, 2009.

Leissinger CA, Blatt PM, Hoots WK, et al: Role of prothrombin complex concentrates in reversing warfarin anticoagulation: A review of the literature. *Am J Hematol* 83:137, 2008.

Logan AC, Yank V, Stafford RS: Off-label use of recombinant factor VIIa in U.S. hospitals: Analysis of hospital records. *Ann Intern Med* 154:516, 2011.

Paikin JS, Eikelboom JW, Cairns JA, et al: New antithrombotic agents–insights from clinical trials. Nature reviews. *Cardiology* 7:498, 2010.

Schulman S, Crowther MA: How I treat with anticoagulants in 2012: New and old anticoagulants, and when and how to switch. *Blood* 119:3016, 2012.

Tripodi A, Mannucci PM: The coagulopathy of chronic liver disease. *N Engl J Med* 365:147, 2011.

Yank V, Tuohy CV, Logan AC, et al: Systematic review: Benefits and harms of in-hospital use of recombinant factor VIIa for off-label indications. *Ann Intern Med* 154:529, 2011.

For complete list of references log on to www.expertconsult.com.

CHAPTER 162

THE SPLEEN AND ITS DISORDERS

Nathan T. Connell, Susan B. Shurin, and Fred J. Schiffman

Galen described the spleen as the "organ of mystery," with functions related to mood and good or ill humors. It was not until the 18th century that the spleen's relationship to the immune and hematologic systems was appreciated. The complexities of splenic function continue to be the focus of research and observation. Although the spleen is not necessary to life because many of its functions overlap with or can be assumed by other organs, it is an important part of immune and hematologic systems and part of many disease processes. The spleen efficiently phagocytoses erythrocytes, recycles iron, recognizes and destroys pathogens, and induces adaptive immune responses. An appreciation for the subtleties of its anatomy and function is important for the physician evaluating patients with many hematologic, immunologic, hepatic, and infectious diseases.

NORMAL SPLENIC ANATOMY AND FUNCTION

Embryology

The spleen arises from the mesoderm. By the ninth week of gestation, layers of the left dorsal mesogastrium condense and blood vessels appear. Sheaths are formed around arterioles by reticular cells and fibers.[1] Macrophages are present and are phagocytic by the end of the first trimester. Lymphocytes appear during the fourth month, and red and white pulp can be identified by the sixth month. Germinal centers do not develop during fetal life, but primitive inactive follicles are evident at birth. In mice, a homeobox gene, Tlx1 (formerly known as Hox11), which controls the genesis of the splanchnic mesodermal plate, is essential for development of the spleen.[2] Both the basic helix-loop-helix transcription factor capsulin and the Wilms tumor suppressor 1 gene (WT1) are necessary for formation of the spleen. The genetic basis for development of the human spleen is less well understood. The spleen is capable of supporting hematopoiesis during fetal life and, in a variety of pathologic states, postnatally. The circulation of primitive hematopoietic stem cells in peripheral blood during prenatal life through birth makes it difficult to distinguish hematopoiesis arising from stem cells in the spleen as opposed to the incidental presence of hematopoietic cells within the circulation.

Anatomy

The spleen is the body's largest filter of the blood.[3,4] Located directly below the diaphragm and adjacent to the stomach, it is covered by a fibrous capsule with blood vessels, lymphatics, and nerves coated by peritoneal mesothelium. The splenic artery arises from the celiac axis, enters the capsule at the hilum, and branches into trabecular arteries. The trabecular arteries then branch into central arteries and enter the white pulp. The periarterial lymphatic sheath consists of a cuff of T lymphocytes, plasma cells, and macrophages around the central arteries. As the arteries branch, the sheath narrows. B-lymphocyte clusters appear in follicles along the periarterial lymphatic sheath at arterial branch points (Fig. 162-1).

The components of the white pulp are connected by a reticular network and supporting stromal cells. On the cut surface of the normal spleen, white pulp is visible as white nodules 1 to 2 mm in diameter. Their size varies with age and antigenic stimulation. The nodules are fully developed at birth, increase in size in childhood (especially with immunizations and infections), peak at puberty, and involute in adulthood. Immunologically normal, uninfected adults normally have no evident germinal centers. A mantle zone of B lymphocytes surrounds the follicle, or secondary germinal center. Antigen trapping and processing take place in the marginal zone of the white pulp.

The red pulp of the spleen consists of vascular sinuses, the cords of Billroth, and the terminal branches of the penicilliary arteries (Fig. 162-2). Vascular sinuses are lined with $CD8^+$ endothelial cells with long processes and a basement membrane with ring fibers that attach to macrophage-derived dendritic processes. No tight junctions or interdigitations connect the cytoplasmic processes. Intact leukocytes, erythrocytes, and platelets are able to squeeze through the potential spaces between these cells and between the ring fibers (Fig. 162-3). Processes of the reticular cells of the cords of Billroth are outside the sinus walls. Endothelial cells line pulp veins but not the cords.

The reticular structure of the spleen facilitates its immune response. Venous sinus endothelial cells contain a plasma membrane-associated network of stress fibers composed of actin and myosin-like filaments. These filaments may cross the plasma membrane and insert into the mesh-like basement membrane. As the fibers tense, they create fenestrations through which erythrocytes must pass if they hope to continue their journey. Cells infected by parasites or simply worn from age become trapped by the fibers and will not continue in the circulation. This mechanism combined with mannose receptors and Toll-like receptors helps the infrastructure of the spleen play a part in the host's overall immune response.

Circulation of blood through red pulp lined with endothelial cells represents a closed circulation, which is rapid. Circulation into the cords, or open circulation, is slower and permits the macrophages lining the cord to remove damaged or aged cells.

Accessory spleens are present in up to a third of the population and result from failure of precursor cells to fuse during embryologic development. They often receive blood flow from the splenic artery and are located near the spleen but can be distant and confused with a tumor when noted on imaging studies or even physical examination. They can develop similar conditions as the spleen proper and may result in continued abnormalities even after splenectomy.

Functions

The functions of the spleen and their anatomic locations are summarized in Table 162-1.

The Red Pulp

Splenic macrophages dominate the function of the red pulp and are responsible for filtering blood, removing bacteria, and recycling iron.

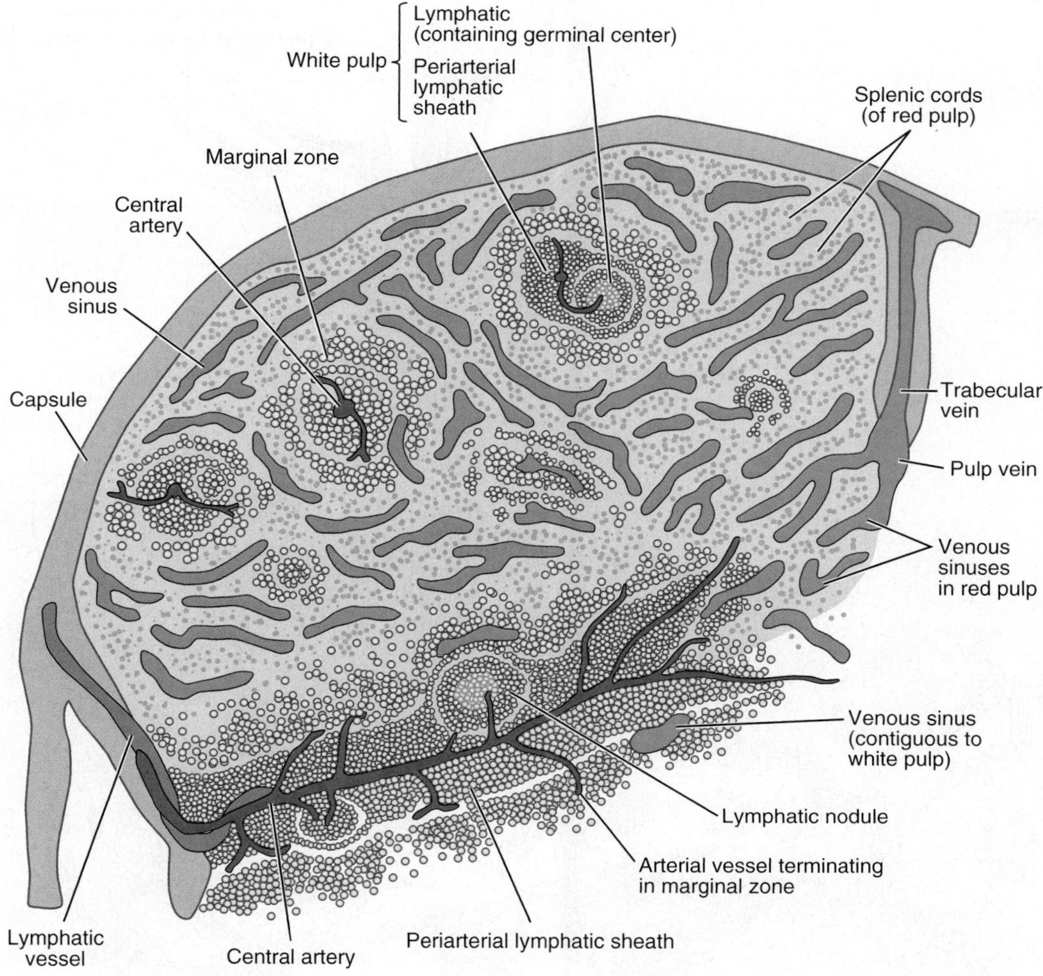

Figure 162-1 ORGANIZATION OF THE HUMAN SPLEEN PRESENTED SCHEMATICALLY. See text for description of blood flow and cell distribution. *(From Emerson SG: Hematopoiesis: The development of blood cells. In Schiffman FJ, editor:* Hematologic pathophysiology, *Philadelphia, 1998, Lippincott-Raven, p 10. Used with permission.)*

Table 162-1 Functions of the Spleen

Category	Function	Effector Cells/Areas
Clearance/Filtration	Antibody-mediated clearance Culling and pitting	Macrophages Reticular meshwork
Immune Response		
Marginal zone	Interaction of antigens with effector cells Antigen processing Immune recognition	Monocytes, lymphocytes Macrophages T cells (periarteriolar sheath)
White pulp	Immunoregulation, antibody production Antigen processing, preservation	B cells (lymphoid follicles) Macrophages
Red pulp	Phagocytosis	Macrophages, monocytes, neutrophils
Hematologic	Hematopoiesis Storage of erythrocytes, platelets, leukocytes Finishing/polishing of erythrocytes	Cords and sinuses Reticular meshwork, red pulp Reticular meshwork, macrophages
Hemostasis	Production of factor VIII, von Willebrand factor	Endothelial cells

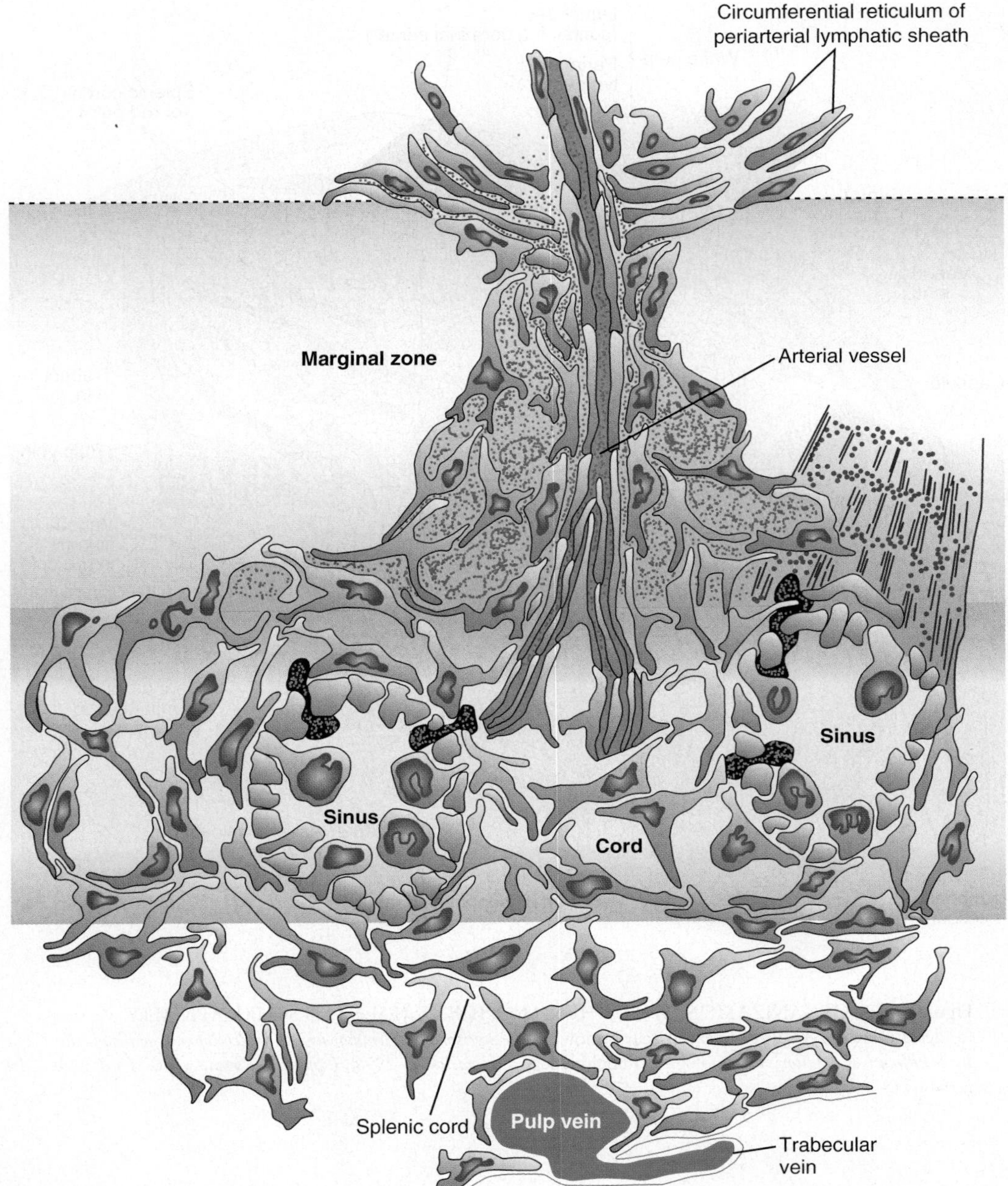

Figure 162-2 DIAGRAM OF THE SPLENIC ARTERY. Arterial blood pools in the splenic cords before entering the splenic sinuses and returning to systemic circulation. *(From Emerson SG: Hematopoiesis: The development of blood cells. In Schiffman FJ, editor:* Hematologic pathophysiology, *Philadelphia, 1998, Lippincott-Raven, p 12. Used with permission.)*

Removal of Damaged and Aged Formed Elements

The venous system of the red pulp enables it to filter whole blood, removing senescent erythrocytes and other blood cells. Arterial blood is delivered to the cords of the red pulp through an open system of reticular fibers, fibroblasts, and macrophages without an endothelial lining. Blood then passes from the cords into the efferent venous sinuses, which are lined with endothelium with a discontinuous structure. Stress fibers extend beneath the basal plasma membrane and run parallel to the axis of the endothelial cells. These cords direct the blood into sinuses through slits modulated in size by the stress fibers. In many animals, these stress fibers and the splenic capsule are contractile and enable the spleen to serve as a reservoir of red cells and reduce blood viscosity when the animal is at rest. In humans, however, there is no evidence that the spleen serves such a function or is capable of significant changes in volume with rest and exercise. To return to the circulation, cells must pass through the slits between venous sinus endothelial cells (see Fig. 162-3), the size of which may be controlled by actin and myosin filaments within the stress fibers in the basal portion of endothelial cells. This surface is probably an important site for the culling and pitting of aged or damaged cells.

As erythrocytes and platelets age, they are less able to tolerate the hostile splenic environment than when they are younger and have a healthy metabolic reserve. The spleen is acidotic (pH 6.8 to 7.2), hypoxic (partial pressure of oxygen [P_{O_2}] 54 mm Hg), and hypoglycemic (glucose concentration approximately 60% of that in venous blood). With age, damaged enucleated cells develop changes in complex membrane carbohydrates; these changes facilitate recognition by splenic macrophages and removal from the circulation. *Culling* describes the destruction of erythrocytes: the normal removal of aging cells or the removal of damaged cells in pathologic states. Most platelets and leukocytes are not removed by the spleen as they

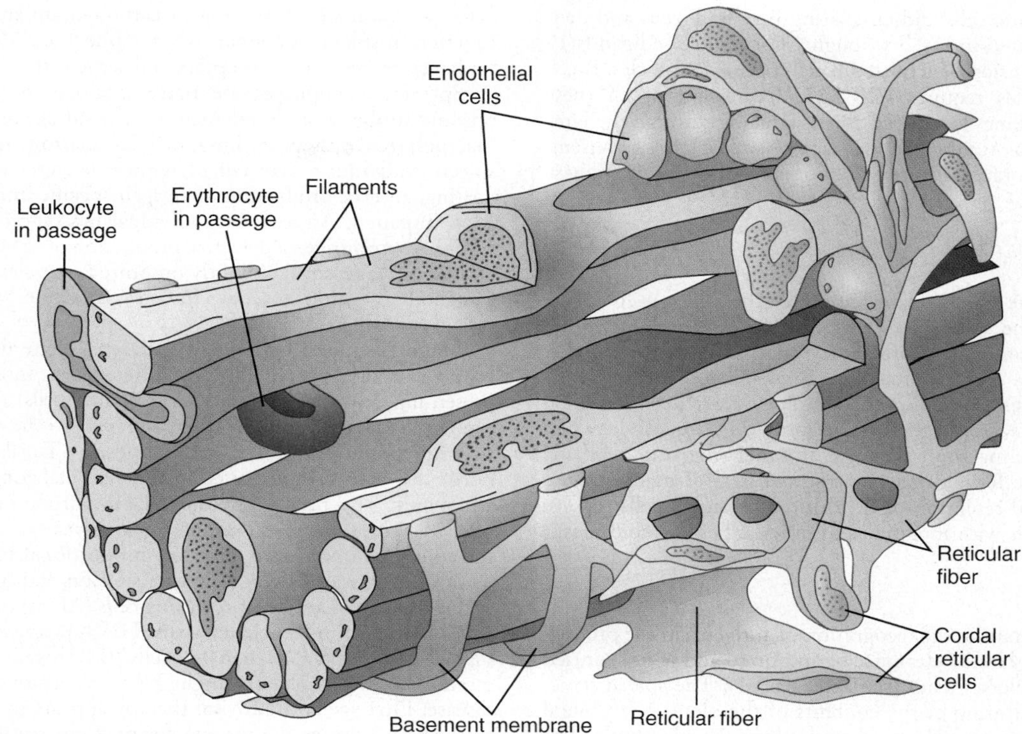

Figure 162-3 ORGANIZATION OF THE SPLENIC SINUSES. Erythrocytes and leukocytes are scrutinized as they squeeze through the reticular fibers of endothelial cells to enter the splenic sinuses. The fenestrae contract and relax according to sympathetic stimuli to regulate cell passage. *(From Emerson SG: Hematopoiesis: The development of blood cells. In Schiffman FJ, editor:* Hematologic pathophysiology, *Philadelphia, 1998, Lippincott-Raven, p 13. Used with permission.)*

age but adhere to vessel walls and migrate into tissues, where they die. *Pitting* refers to the removal of inclusions from within erythrocytes, which are then released back into the circulation. The erythrocyte membrane is in close apposition to the macrophage membrane, so that aged or damaged glycoproteins, antibody, or complement on the surface of the cell are easily recognized and activate phagocytosis. Particulate matter—Howell-Jolly bodies, Heinz bodies, Pappenheimer bodies, and malarial and other parasites—can be removed and the cell returned to the bloodstream. Membrane-containing adsorbed antibody can be removed and the remainder of the cell released with changes in shape and volume. Internal vesicles near the erythrocyte membrane appear as if they were on the surface of the cell and are termed *pits* or *pocks*. The spleen also normally removes these, with the polished erythrocyte returned to the circulation. The lack of this polishing function can be used to assess splenic dysfunction as the number of pits or pocks per erythrocyte is increased when the spleen fails to remove them. The number of cells with pits and pocks is also increased.

Recycling of Iron

Macrophages in the liver and spleen are important for recycling iron as erythrocytes are phagocytized and hydrolyzed in the phagolysosome. Degradation of hemoglobin releases heme, which is catabolized into biliverdin, carbon monoxide, and ferrous iron (Fe^{2+}). Iron is then either released as a low-molecular-weight species for rapid reuse or stored as ferritin. As ferritin accumulates, it aggregates into hemosiderin. Iron-laden macrophages are a feature of iron overload states in both the liver and spleen. Erythrocytes that are destroyed intravascularly release hemoglobin that binds to haptoglobin. CD163 on the surface of splenic macrophages mediates endocytosis of circulating hemoglobin and haptoglobin-bound hemoglobin.

Iron is released from stores in splenic macrophages in response to the erythropoietic drive expressed by the bone marrow. The precise mechanisms are not well understood. Uptake of iron is mediated in most cells by a divalent cation transporter, the natural resistance–associated macrophage protein 2 (NRAMP2), in recycling endosomes that express the transferrin receptor. NRAMP2 transports ferritin into the cytoplasm across the endosomal membrane. In addition to the more widely expressed NRAMP2, macrophages and monocytes express NRAMP1, which was initially described as an iron-transporting protein affecting resistance to intracellular pathogens. A third molecule involved in iron metabolism in the spleen is lipocalin-2, which is secreted by macrophages and other myeloid cells when activated by exposure to bacterial metabolites. Lipocalin-2 binds to bacterial siderophores and sequesters iron from microorganisms. These and other related molecules tightly link the iron-recycling and host resistance functions of the red pulp of the spleen.

Antibody Production

After stimulation and differentiating in the follicles of the white pulp, antigen-specific plasmablasts and plasma cells lodge in the red pulp, where they are closer to macrophages. A similar translocation occurs in lymph nodes, where plasmablasts migrate to the medullary cords. This translocation occurs after upregulation of expression of CXC-chemokine receptor 4 (CXCR4), which binds CXC-chemokine ligand 12 (CXCL12) expressed in red pulp.

The White Pulp

The lymphoid region of the spleen incorporates multiple components of the immune system that are organized to enhance recognition and/or response to pathogens.[5] The white pulp contains lymphoid sheaths around branching arterial vessels, similar to the structure of lymph nodes. Specific chemokines attract B and T cells to their appropriate domains. The periarteriolar lymphatic sheath contains T cells that interact with dendritic cells and circulating B cells. T cells and dendritic cells are attracted to PALS through CC-chemokine ligands 19 and 21. Clonal expansion of activated B cells occurs in follicles. B-cell migration to follicles requires CXCL13. Expression of all these homeostatic chemokines is reduced when signaling through the lymphotoxin receptor or tumor necrosis factor-α receptor 1 is absent, which results in disorganization of the domains of the white pulp.

Marginal Zone

Leukocytes leave the bloodstream and enter the white pulp in the marginal zone of the spleen via G protein–coupled receptor functions, similar to the migration of leukocytes across endothelial barriers in inflammation. The marginal zone is an area for cells in transit as well as home to resident cells with complex interactions. Marginal zone metallophilic macrophages form an inner ring close to the white pulp, marginal zone macrophages form an outer ring, and dendritic cells and B cells are located between the two sets of macrophages. Both trafficking and retention of dendritic cells and B cells involve complex interactions with integrins and other adhesion molecules.

Innate Immunity

The spleen is important in the recognition of antigens, in the production of antibody, and in the clearance of opsonized and nonopsonized particles from the bloodstream (see Table 162-1). The spleen structure facilitates monitoring of the contents of the blood, with blood flowing through the marginal zone directly along the white pulp. The white pulp is involved in adaptive immunity, whereas the marginal zone is involved in both innate and adaptive immunity (Table 162-2).

Trapping and processing antigens is a major function of the marginal zone. Macrophages are abundant here and the spleen may capture more than 5% of the cardiac output (greater than 250 ml/minute), allowing a large volume of blood to be immunologically scrutinized. Antigens penetrate the germinal center where T lymphocytes predominate. Processing of carbohydrate antigens is a special function of splenic marginal zone lymphocytes. Marginal zone macrophages express lectin receptors and scavenger.

Splenic macrophages are more sensitive to small amounts of opsonic antibody or complement on the surface of particles than are macrophages in the liver, lung, or bone marrow. In the absence of a spleen, individuals may fail to remove bacteria with little opsonic coating, and the production of antigen-specific immunoglobulin (Ig) M is impaired. An asplenic individual has defective recognition of carbohydrate antigens, defective production of IgM early in infection, and defective removal of lightly opsonized particles—all crucial components of response to an invasive infection with encapsulated organisms.

Marginal zone B lymphocytes are sensitive to detection of blood-borne pathogens and rapidly differentiate into either antigen-presenting cells or IgM-producing plasma cells. After activation in the marginal zone, some B cells migrate into the white pulp, where they function to activate naive CD4-positive T cells. Similarly, blood-borne dendritic cells activated in the marginal zone migrate into the white pulp. This process appears to be important in control of certain parasitic infections. For example, in *Leishmania donovani* infection, the spread of infection is inversely proportional to the upregulation or downregulation of CCR7 expression on activated dendritic cells and migration of antigen-presenting cells (APCs) into the white pulp. In human immunodeficiency virus (HIV)–positive patients with low CD4 T-cell counts (less than 300 cells/μL), there is evidence that IgM memory B cell–depletion might be a risk factor for pneumococcal disease. Effective antiretroviral therapy appears to reverse this depletion, in turn decreasing the risk for pneumococcal infection.

Adaptive Immunity

Although the white pulp is both anatomically and functionally similar to lymph nodes, all cells enter the white pulp via the marginal zone rather than through high endothelial venules and afferent lymphatic vessels, exposing them to an environment highly sensitive to detection of blood-borne pathogens. Circulating dendritic cells capture bacteria

Table 162-2 Innate Immune Pattern Recognition Receptors That Are Highly Expressed on Splenic Phagocytic Cells*

Name	Abbreviation	Function	Splenic Cells Expressing	Recognizes or Affects	Pathogens Recognized
Toll-like receptor networks	TLR	Pattern recognition of pathogen-associated molecular patterns	Marginal zone macrophages Dendritic cells	Lipopolysaccharide Flagellin Double-stranded RNA	Multiple bacteria, especially gram negative
Natural resistance–associated macrophage protein-1	NRAMP1	Solute carrier family 11 (proton-coupled divalent metal ion transporters); phagolysosomal function	Macrophages	Lysosomal targeting	*Mycobacterium tuberculosis* *Mycobacterium avium* *Mycobacterium leprae*
Natural resistance–associated macrophage protein-2	NRAMP2	Proton-dependent cation transporter; iron absorption	Macrophages (apical duodenal cells, erythroid cells)	Impairs bacterial gene expression, protein synthesis	*Brucella* spp
Sialic acid–binding Ig-like lectin-1; sialoadhesin	SIGLEC1, CD169	Immunoglobulin superfamily	Splenic and peritoneal macrophages Many hematopoietic cells	Mannose	*Streptococcus pneumoniae*
Specific intercellular adhesion molecule 3–grabbing nonintegrin related 1	SIGNR1, CD209b	ICAM3-binding nonintegrin homologue, mannose receptor	Dendritic cells	Polysaccharide antigens, mannosylated lipoarabinomannan (ManLAM)	Fungi, other pathogens
Macrophage receptor with collagenous structure	MARCO	Type 1 scavenger	Marginal zone macrophages	Lipopolysaccharide	*Staphylococcus aureus* *Escherichia coli*

ICAM, Intercellular adhesion molecule; *RNA,* ribonucleic acid.
*These receptors contribute to resistance to infection with pathogens in the absence of prior exposure, specific immune responses, or surface opsonic immunoglobulin or complement.

from the blood and transport them to the spleen, where they mediate the initial differentiation of B cells to plasmablasts or antigen presenting cells (APCs). Activated APCs entering the white pulp activate T cells, resulting in changes in receptor expression that enable them to migrate to the edge of B-cell follicles. Contact with activated T cells induces an isotype switch in follicular B cells, which then migrate to the red pulp and marginal zones or remain in splenic germinal centers. The white pulp of the spleen is the largest mass of lymphoid tissue in the body. The B lymphocytes, which ultimately produce antibodies, predominate in the nearby germinal centers and mantle zones. These areas all increase in size and activity with immunization or infection. The complex interaction between the cells in close apposition, autocrine and paracrine signaling, and migration of cells into, within and ultimately out of the spleen contributes to the extraordinary repertoire of innate and adaptive immunity within the organ. Changes in splenic architecture are quite dramatic with septicemia; the most marked being depletion of splenic B areas that occurs during overwhelming enterococcemia. Bacterial virulence factors appear to contribute to depletion of B- and T-cell areas.

Hematopoiesis

Active hematopoiesis can be seen in the fetal spleen throughout the second trimester, decreasing during the third trimester. Erythropoiesis and megakaryocytopoiesis predominate, with myelopoiesis present to a lesser extent. As hematopoiesis transitions from the hepatic phase into the bone marrow, it becomes less evident within the fetal spleen. The spleen is not normally a site of hematopoiesis in postnatal life in humans, but it is a rich source of hematopoietic stem cells and can support hematopoiesis in a number of pathologic states. Extramedullary hematopoiesis is a significant cause of splenomegaly primarily in bone marrow disorders (e.g., myelofibrosis or osteopetrosis) and chronic hemolytic anemias (e.g., thalassemia). The stromal cells of the spleen appear to be capable of supporting hematopoiesis and may produce the C-KIT ligand, as do marrow stromal cells. When splenic hematopoiesis occurs, the erythrocytes and platelets that circulate tend to be less mature than when hematopoiesis occurs in the bone marrow, which suggests that egress from the spleen is easier than from the marrow.

In higher mammals, including primates, the resident stem cells are capable of restoring hematopoietic and immunologic function after lethal irradiation.[6]

Stem Cells

Recently the spleen has been shown to be a source of multipotent stem cells in humans as well as other animals. These stem cells have been shown to contribute to the regeneration of multiple types of tissue, including pancreatic islet cells, bone, cranial nerves, and salivary glands. In addition, undifferentiated splenic monocytes assembled in clusters in the cords of the subcapsular red pulp and were shown to accumulate in injured myocardial tissue.[7] These stem cells are considered to have limited potential to undergo malignant transformation.

Storage of Cells

The normal adult human spleen contains 20 to 40 mL of blood and does not serve as a reservoir for blood or erythrocytes. However, in many conditions associated with splenomegaly, especially portal hypertension, the pulp cords widen to create an organ with more storage volume. Vascular pooling of blood and formed elements occurs, regardless of the underlying cause of the splenomegaly. Platelets and granulocytes, however, are normally stored in the red pulp of the spleen. As much as one-third of the total platelet mass may be stored in the spleen and released when cytokines affecting platelet adhesiveness are released. The lack of musculature in the human splenic capsule prevents the distention and contraction that occur in many animals, such as dogs, although the spleen appears to contract in divers during periods of breath-hold apnea. Platelet counts and granulocyte counts rise significantly after splenectomy, then fall. The circulating masses of these cell pools are chronically increased post-splenectomy, which may contribute to an increased incidence of atherosclerosis years after splenectomy.

EXAMINATION OF THE SPLEEN

Maneuvers for examination of the spleen involve inspection, percussion, and palpation, but their sensitivity and specificity vary based on patient factors (such as body habitus) and operator skill.[8] The pretest probability of splenomegaly, based on associated historical and clinical data, influences the positive predictive value of finding splenomegaly on physical examination. If the pretest probability of splenomegaly is less than 10%, then physical examination maneuvers are inadequate for determining the presence or absence of splenomegaly. For those patients with a greater than 10% pretest probability of splenomegaly (for instance, patients with suspected infectious mononucleosis), the examination begins with inspection and then percussion of Traube's space. For adequate examination of the spleen, the patient must be fully supine, relaxed, with arms adjacent to the trunk. Dullness to percussion in Traube's space—defined by the sixth rib superiorly, the anterior axillary line, and the costal margin—should be followed by palpation. Beginning in the right iliac fossa, the examiner's hand gently advances toward the left upper quadrant. This minimizes the likelihood that a grossly enlarged spleen will be missed, and the lower pole and medial border should be easily appreciated. If the spleen cannot be felt with this approach, the left hand of the examiner is placed on the left flank, lifting the lower part of the rib cage to displace the spleen medially toward the examiner's right hand. The splenic notch should be felt in the inferior medial border. Rotating the patient into the right lateral decubitus position while still recumbent may make it easier to palpate the spleen. The spleen should move with deep inspiration. The degree of enlargement is usually measured in centimeters below the costal margin. Depending on the position of the spleen within the abdomen, it may be difficult to appreciate even significant enlargement. Normal splenic size in an adult is up to 250 g and up to 13 cm in its long axis. Up to half of spleens weighing 600 to 750 g are not palpable. Greater degrees of splenomegaly are easier to appreciate on physical examination. In terms of sensitivity and specificity, there appears to not be a difference between examination in the supine position and examination in the right lateral decubitus position.

Up to 15% of normal children and 3% of young adults have palpable spleens, up to 2 cm below the left costal margin, without evidence of illness. The spleen involutes with age, and a spleen that is palpable in an older person is less likely to be a normal variant and more likely to be associated with clinical disease.

IMAGING OF THE SPLEEN

Radionuclide scintigraphy assesses anatomic and functional aspects of the spleen. The most common procedure is a liver-spleen scan in which technetium-99m sulfur colloid is injected intravenously and taken up by hepatic and splenic macrophages. It is the phagocytic activity of macrophages—rather than the presence of the spleen itself or any aspects of lymphoid function—that is assessed. A dynamic ^{99m}Tc scan can also assess the distribution of blood within the portal system and suggest the presence of portal hypertension. Infusion of ^{99m}Tc-labeled or Indium-111–labeled platelets with scintigraphy to determine their relative distribution in the liver and spleen has been used with considerable, but not absolute, success to predict the clinical efficacy of splenectomy in patients with immune thrombocytopenia purpura (ITP).

Ultrasonography readily shows the size, shape, and several aspects of splenic anatomy, including the presence of cysts and abscesses. The procedure is noninvasive, painless, of low cost, avoids radiation exposure for patients, and is a good screening study when the spleen is thought to be enlarged. In 95% of the normal population, the long axis of the spleen measures less than 12 cm on ultrasound examination. Accessory spleens tend not to be well visualized on routine ultrasonography. In the hands of a skilled operator, endoscopic ultrasound-guided biopsy permits accurate diagnosis of lesions as small as a centimeter or less, which compares well with results obtained using computed tomography (CT). High-frequency sonography has significantly better resolution and can visualize both nodularity within the spleen, which occurs in childhood as immunity is acquired, and accessory spleens and splenosis after splenic rupture or trauma.

CT imaging has the advantage of showing the anatomy and some aspects of splenic function. Contrast material in the stomach, small bowel, and colon, given enterally, helps delineate splenic tissue when it impinges on these organs. Intravenous contrast material is required to delineate splenic lesions whose density is the same as normal splenic tissue. Abscesses have a rim of contrast agent enhancement.

CT can be used to estimate the volume of the spleen. Accessory spleens have the same attenuation as a normal spleen, which is somewhat less than that of liver. Accessory spleens are usually located in the gastrosplenic ligament near the hilum. Subcapsular and intrasplenic hematomas and splenic lacerations are clearly seen on CT. Leukemias and many inflammatory diseases produce diffuse splenomegaly. Granulomas and infarcted areas eventually calcify. Cysts, abscesses, and some malignancies have inhomogeneous patterns on CT scan. Although not replacing other methods of staging, splenic enlargement on CT may direct follow-up studies and indicate prognosis.

In addition to imaging the spleen, CT can be used to direct therapeutic interventions. Abscesses, hematomas, and cysts can be drained (see box on Management of Splenic Cysts). As long as portal hypertension is not present and vascular lesions have been excluded, thin-needle aspiration under CT guidance is generally a safe intervention.

CT scanning of the abdomen, performed as part of the initial emergency department evaluation of patients with abdominal trauma, may avert hospital admission and prevent exploratory laparotomy.[10]

Magnetic resonance imaging (MRI) is useful for identifying vascular lesions, which would otherwise require angiography, and splenic infections. It is more difficult to image the contents of the upper abdomen with MRI than with CT because of respiratory motion. With more rapid imaging technology, MRI has gained considerable utility for imaging infectious and vascular lesions of the spleen. Hepatosplenic candidiasis and other infections to which immunocompromised patients are susceptible can be identified noninvasively with modern MRI technology.

Perhaps the most valuable use of MRI imaging of the spleen is to obtain a quantitative measurement of iron burden in organs that accumulate iron.[11]

Positron emission tomography (PET) scanning using ^{18}F-2-deoxyglucose (FDG) has an increasing role in the diagnosis, staging, and monitoring of lymphoma, both non-Hodgkin and Hodgkin disease. It is more sensitive than CT scanning at identifying nodal disease and superior to both lymphangiography and CT scanning at imaging the spleen. The availability of more sensitive, specific, and less toxic approaches to imaging permits more precise staging of Hodgkin lymphoma without the complications of splenectomy (Fig. 162-4).[12,13]

The role of PET scanning is expanding in other disorders as whole-body PET scanners and appropriate small-molecule markers

Management of Splenic Cysts

A 37-year-old woman with no past medical history comes in for evaluation of early satiety and left shoulder pain. She reports that she feels full after only a few bites of any meal and sometimes becomes nauseated and vomits. Physical examination is remarkable for an enlarged nontender spleen. Imaging shows a large splenic cyst.

- Many conditions can lead to cyst formation in the spleen, including parasitic infections, trauma, hemangiomas, and polycystic kidney disease.
- Asymptomatic nonparasitic cysts may be observed with careful attention and development of a plan for intervention should they become symptomatic, rupture, or become infected.
- Symptomatic cysts may require percutaneous drainage with radiologic guidance or sometimes surgical procedures, including partial or total splenectomy.[9]
- Parasitic cysts should be treated in consultation with infectious disease specialists because the particular parasitic infection, radiologic appearance, and patient comorbidities will guide choice of therapies.

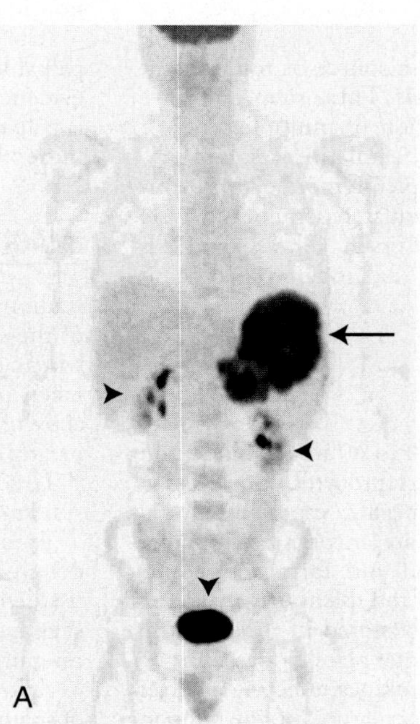

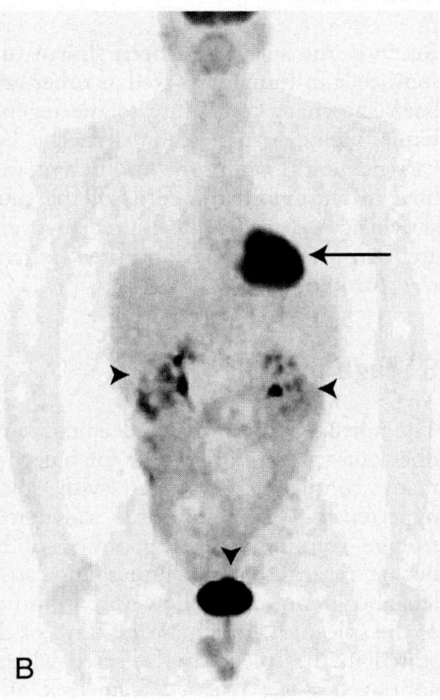

Figure 162-4 PET SCANNING TO IMAGE AREAS OF INVOLVEMENT IN HODGKIN DISEASE. **A,** Pretreatment imaging showing the spleen *(large mass in left upper quadrant with arrow)* and activity in the kidney and bladder *(arrowheads)*. **B,** The same patient after three cycles of chemotherapy. The *arrow* now points to normal activity in the myocardium not seen previously while arrowheads point to persistent urinary tract activity. The spleen is particularly well imaged on PET scan. *PET,* Positron emission tomography. *(From Friedberg JW, Chengazi V: PET scans in the staging of lymphoma: Current status,* Oncologist *8:438, 2003. Used with permission.)*

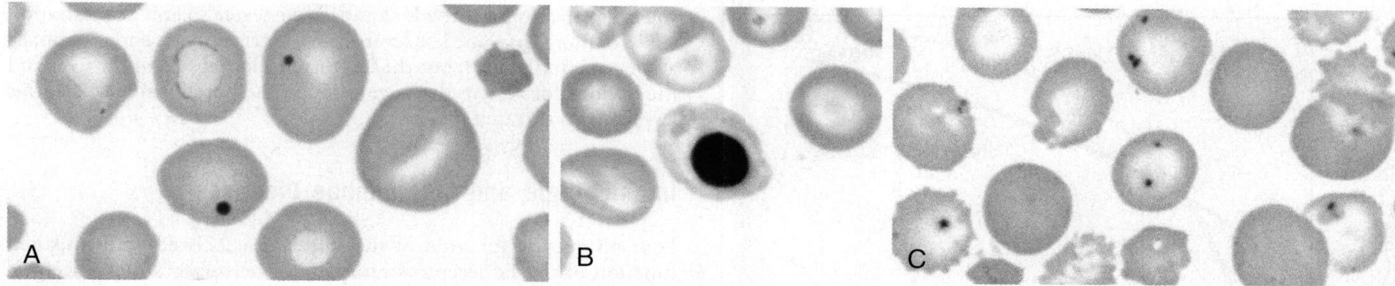

Figure 162-5 RED BLOOD CELL FINDINGS IN HYPOSPLENISM. **A,** Red blood cells with Howell-Jolly bodies. **B,** Nucleated red blood cell. **C,** Cells with Pappenheimer bodies. Red blood cells with Howell-Jolly bodies are seen in patients with hyposplenism. The cytoplasmic inclusions **(A)** are nuclear remnants that are usually round and stain similar to the nucleus of a nucleated red blood cell **(B)**. They occur normally during red cell maturation but are typically removed by a normal spleen. Their presence in the blood indicates less-than-normal splenic function. Pappenheimer bodies **(C)**, which can also be seen in hyposplenism, are siderotic granules that are irregular in shape and frequently multiple.

for individual diseases are more widely available. Imaging studies in small-animal models are very promising; splenic involvement can be identified with high sensitivity in mice.[14]

TESTS OF SPLENIC FUNCTION

The peripheral blood smear may be the most sensitive tool for identification of functional or anatomic hyposplenia. The presence of Howell-Jolly bodies, which are nuclear remnants normally removed by the spleen, is an excellent indicator of hyposplenism (Fig. 162-5). These are rarely seen until the spleen is largely nonfunctional or overwhelmed by other phagocytic functions, such as extravascular hemolysis. Newborn infants commonly have visible Howell-Jolly bodies, and splenic function appears to be at least somewhat impaired in the first week of life. Pappenheimer bodies (siderotic granules normally removed by the spleen) are often seen in hyposplenic states, particularly when a component of hemolysis exists. Erythrocyte morphologic features reflect the lack of membrane polishing by the spleen, with the presence of acanthocytes and target cells. Granulocyte and platelet numbers are increased during asplenic states, including splenic infarction and surgical splenectomy.

To confirm suspected hyposplenism, the simplest test is a count of pitted or pocked erythrocytes. Fixation in 0.5% to 1.0% glutaraldehyde and examination under interference optics should reveal endocytic vesicles containing hemoglobin, ferritin, and remnants of mitochondria. These form in mature erythrocytes and are normally removed by the functioning spleen. The number of pitted cells (not the number of pits per cell) is inversely proportional to splenic function, with normal persons having less than 2% pitted cells.[15] It should be noted that the *absence* of Howell-Jolly bodies on a peripheral blood smear cannot be used as evidence of adequate splenic immune function.[16]

ASPLENIA AND HYPOSPLENIA

Congenital asplenia may be an isolated lesion or associated with severe cyanotic congenital heart disease and bilateral right-sidedness. Life-threatening cardiac lesions, including transposition of the great vessels, pulmonary artery atresia or stenosis, septal defects, anomalous venous drainage, and a single atrioventricular valve, are components of bilateral right-sidedness. The liver is central, and both lungs have three lobes. The peripheral blood smear shows Howell-Jolly bodies and other signs of hyposplenism. There is considerable variation in the anatomic and functional findings, and it is difficult to predict with accuracy the degree of splenic dysfunction on the basis of the anatomy alone. Children who survive the cardiac difficulties in the neonatal period have a significant incidence of sepsis secondary to a variety of organisms.

Polysplenia is associated with bilateral left-sidedness. Dextrocardia, bilateral superior venae cavae, septal defects, and anomalous pulmonary venous return are associated cardiac lesions. Both lungs have two lobes, the liver is midline, and bowel malrotation is common. The splenic tissue is divided into two to nine masses. The peripheral blood smear usually does not suggest hyposplenism, and no clear association with an increased risk for infection has been documented.

Asplenia occurring without heart disease is less likely to be detected before an infection develops than when associated cardiac lesions bring the patient to medical attention. Some of these patients also have situs inversus. Isolated cases of asplenia discovered after death of an otherwise healthy adult or child from overwhelming sepsis with encapsulated organisms have been reported. Familial instances of congenital asplenia are likely to be instances of genetic abnormalities (e.g., Hox11/Tlx1), but these have not yet been documented. Examination of a blood smear for Howell-Jolly bodies is a simple procedure and may be lifesaving in the rare patients affected with these disorders.

If Howell-Jolly bodies are observed on the blood smear of an otherwise healthy person, imaging should be performed to assess for the presence of a spleen. Immunization with polysaccharide vaccines and early intervention with antibiotics for apparent infection may prove lifesaving for these individuals. Because approximately 20% of invasive pneumococcal infections in these patients are nonvaccine strains, a high degree of vigilance remains essential, even with more widespread immunization of healthy children.

ACQUIRED HYPOSPLENISM

Infarction in Sickle Cell Disease

The course of sickle cell disease is marked by progressive dysfunction of multiple organs over many years, and one of the earliest organs to be affected is the spleen. Serial measurements of the numbers of pitted erythrocytes in patients with sickle cell disease demonstrate that splenic dysfunction develops progressively over the first few years of life in the major sickle syndromes (Figs. 162-6 and 162-7). The hypoxic, acidotic, hypoglycemic environment of the spleen creates optimal conditions for tactoid formation and for sickling of the poorly deformable erythrocytes, which then block splenic blood vessels and infarct the tissues. Splenic environmental conditions that enhance acidosis or hypoxia, or additional erythrocyte membrane or enzyme abnormalities that promote irreversible sickling, increase splenic infarction. The hyposplenism is reversible with transfusion for at least the first few years of life but becomes irreversible with progressive damage to blood vessels by 6 years of age in patients with sickle cell disease.

Splenic sequestration is a manifestation of the infarctive process of sickling in the spleen that extends to involve larger veins. Distensible splenic tissues results in pooling of a large amount of blood, whereas the venous drainage is occluded by sickled hypoxic erythrocytes. Patients with sickle cell disease who have not yet had multiple episodes

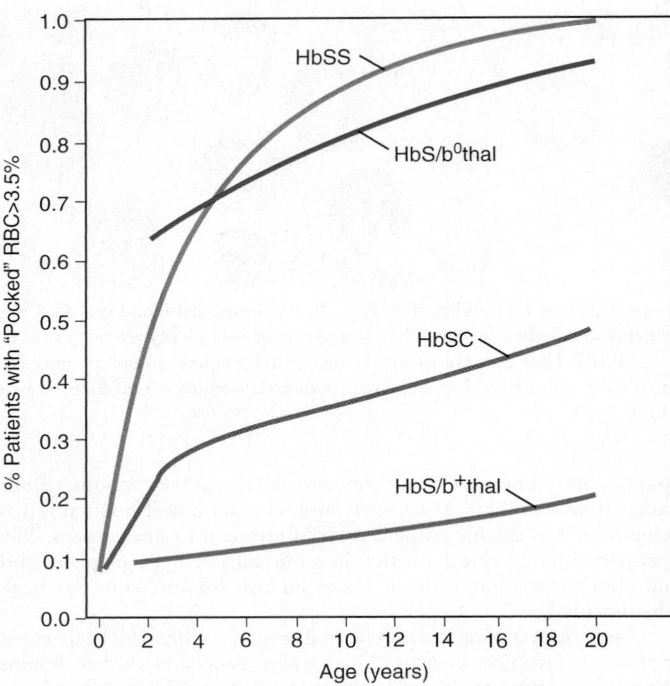

Figure 162-6 DEVELOPMENT OF FUNCTIONAL ASPLENIA IN SICKLE CELL DISORDERS. *(From Pearson HA, Gallagher D, Chilcote R, et al: Developmental pattern of splenic dysfunction in sickle cell disorders,* Pediatrics *76:392, 1985. Used with permission.)*

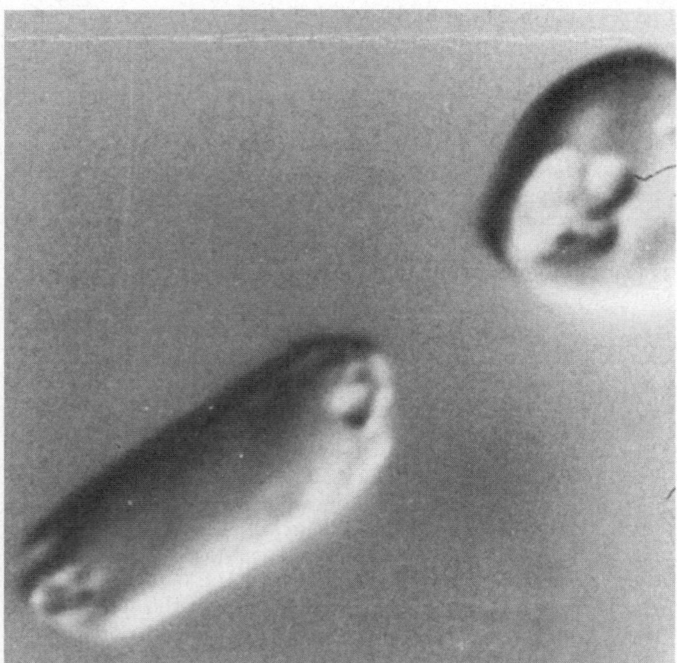

Figure 162-7 POCKED ERYTHROCYTES IN THE SICKLE HEMOGLOBINOPATHIES. *(From Sills R, Oski FA: RBC surface pits in the sickle hemoglobinopathies,* Am J Dis Child *133:526, 1979. Used with permission.)*

of infarction and whose spleens have not undergone fibrosis are susceptible to this syndrome. Unlike the chronic process of smaller-vessel infarction, the acute splenic sequestration crisis can be life threatening because a large amount of blood can collect in the highly distended spleen. The tendency to recurrence and the potential for fatal outcome lead to the Propensity for recurrence and the high-associated morbidity and mortality has resulted in the common recommendation for splenectomy in a patient who has had one severe splenic sequestration crisis, or more than one less severe crisis. Occlusion of venous drainage also occurs in the liver, but the less distensible capsule of the liver and the options for venous drainage through the portal system make this less likely to threaten life.

Immunologic and Autoimmune Diseases

Poor phagocytic function of the spleen is associated with impaired function of the Fc receptors on splenic macrophages in a variety of immunologic, rheumatic, and inflammatory disorders. Among those disorders in which hyposplenism has been clearly defined and associated with a risk for infection are systemic lupus erythematosus, rheumatoid arthritis, sarcoidosis, systemic vasculitis, ulcerative colitis, celiac disease, amyloidosis, chronic graft-versus-host disease, mastocytosis, and congenital and acquired immunodeficiency. The diseases themselves and the immunosuppressive therapies that are used in their management may contribute to the risk for infection in these conditions. Immunization with polysaccharide antigens and recognition of the risk of bacterial infection are important steps in reducing the risks of splenic hypofunction.

Splenomegaly and the production of autoantibodies (such as to platelets) are features of the acquired immunodeficiency syndrome (AIDS). In the late stages of AIDS, atrophy of lymphoid follicles and depletion of T cell–dependent areas are common. It is not clear that impairment of phagocytic function is a component of splenic atrophy in AIDS.

Therapy-Induced Splenic Hypofunction

Radiation therapy affects splenic function depending on the dose administered. In general, phagocytic cells are not affected by irradiation, but lymphoid cells are extremely sensitive. B-cell function is nearly ablated with as little as 500 cGy. T-cell lymphoblastogenesis is eliminated by administration of 3000 cGy. With doses of 2000 cGy, splenic hypofunction is usually transient because the macrophages and splenic stroma are not affected, and circulating B and T lymphocytes can repopulate the splenic follicles. Permanent splenic hypofunction may develop with doses of 4000 cGy or higher. The risk for infection is significant after such therapy.

Corticosteroid therapy impairs the affinity of the Fc receptors of splenic macrophages for opsonized IgG and decreases the adhesiveness of granulocytes and monocytes. This can result in an acute pharmacologic splenectomy, even at commonly administered therapeutic dosages. The function of the Fc receptors on hepatic, pulmonary, and bone marrow macrophages is far less affected than that of splenic macrophages. The acute rise in platelet count or hemoglobin values seen with corticosteroid therapy in ITP or autoimmune hemolytic anemia is due to decreased clearance of sensitized cells. With prolonged therapy, the production of antibodies by splenic lymphocytes is also affected, and splenic function continues to be impaired.

Intravenous IgG appears to decrease the phagocytic function of the spleen by binding to Fc receptors and impeding their recognition of opsonized particles. This is a transient effect because the Fc receptors are internalized and recycled, and opsonic function returns to normal within 2 to 3 weeks. Occupancy and impairment of function of Fc receptors is also seen with administration of anti-D immunoglobulin to Rh-positive patients, which induces a transient hemolytic anemia. Reticuloendothelial blockade, or occupancy of these receptors, refers to the impaired ability of the spleen to recognize and remove other IgG-coated particles, including bacteria, in the presence of these agents.

SPLENOMEGALY AND HYPERSPLENISM

An enlarged spleen is not a disease state in itself but usually indicates some underlying pathologic state.[17] The processes run the gamut from

Timing of Return to Contact Sports in Athletes Who Have Had Infectious Mononucleosis

A 17-year-old male high school student is diagnosed by his primary care physician with infectious mononucleosis. The patient is concerned about the upcoming soccer season and wants to be able to start training with the team in 4 weeks.

- More than half of patients with infectious mononucleosis develop splenomegaly within the first 14 days of illness.
- Most reports of splenic rupture in the setting of infectious mononucleosis occur in the first 21 days of illness.
- There is a paucity of data to support imaging the spleen to document resolution of splenomegaly before returning to contact sports.
- Noncontact sports may be safely resumed after at least 21 days from the onset of initial symptoms, and contact sports should be safe in most cases after at least 28 days. Infectious mononucleosis–associated splenic rupture has been reported as far as 7 weeks after symptom onset.
- The timing of return to sports and the risks should be discussed with the patient, especially if the patient may not have returned to baseline after prolonged fatigue.

minor to life threatening, from congenital disorders to those at the end of life. It is useful to approach the differential diagnosis of splenomegaly by considering the processes that may cause splenic enlargement and then to focus on the specific diagnoses within those categories. The spleen may be enlarged as a result of infiltration, hypertrophy of normal elements (macrophages and lymphoid components), extramedullary hematopoiesis, inflammatory or immunologic processes, and systemic or portal congestion (see box on Timing of Return to Contact Sports in Athletes Who Have Had Infectious Mononucleosis). The degree of splenomegaly correlates well with involvement of the spleen in many malignant disorders, such as Hodgkin disease. Rarely, anatomic abnormalities will cause splenomegaly. Splenomegaly is important to investigate because it is frequently the presenting finding of a serious disorder whose earlier recognition and treatment may prevent significant long-term morbidity and mortality. The diseases associated with splenomegaly are detailed in Table 162-3. Patients with splenomegaly do not necessarily have hypersplenism, and patients with hypersplenism may indeed have normal-sized spleens, such as those seen in ITP.

Hypersplenism refers to nonimmune, indiscriminate destruction of the formed elements of the blood by a spleen that is usually enlarged, affected by portal hypertension, or both. The bone marrow is hyperplastic, and the peripheral blood cell counts are decreased as a consequence of destruction of mature formed elements. Splenectomy corrects the cytopenia. Any of the formed elements of the blood—erythrocytes, neutrophils, or platelets—can be affected, alone or in combination. Splenic hypertrophy in cirrhosis is due to an increase in splenic macrophages and their activity. Because a normal function of splenic macrophages is to remove senescent cells, this is an exaggeration of a physiologic process.

Hypersplenism develops in patients who receive chronic transfusions. There are several components that contribute to the development of hypersplenism. The antigenic load of allogeneic transfused cells stimulates the immune system. Transfused cells have shorter survival than normal red cells (mean of 60 instead of 120 days, unless specially prepared neocytes are used), which increases the work of splenic macrophages. Finally, iron overload causes hemosiderosis of both the spleen and the liver, so that portal hypertension may develop and further increase splenic pathology. Hypersplenism increases the transfusion requirement in patients who are already transfusion dependent.

Table 162-3 Causes of Splenomegaly

Primary Process	Pathogenesis	Examples
Anatomic	Developmental abnormalities	Cysts, pseudocysts, hamartomas, peliosis, hemangiomas
Hematologic	Hemolysis	Intrinsic (membrane, enzyme, hemoglobin disorders), extrinsic (immune)
	Extramedullary hematopoiesis	Myeloproliferative diseases/myelodysplasias, myelofibrosis, osteopetrosis
Infectious	Bacteria	Acute and chronic systemic infection, abscesses, subacute bacterial endocarditis
	Mycobacteria	Miliary tuberculosis
	Spirochetes	Syphilis, Lyme disease, leptospirosis
	Viruses	Epstein-Barr virus; cytomegalovirus; human immunodeficiency virus; hepatitis A, B, C
	Rickettsia	Rocky Mountain spotted fever, Q fever, typhus
	Fungi	Disseminated candidiasis, histoplasmosis, South American blastomycosis
	Parasites	Malaria, babesiosis, toxoplasmosis, *Toxocara canis, Toxocara cati,* leishmaniasis, schistosomiasis, trypanosomiasis
Immunologic	Collagen vascular diseases	Felty syndrome, systemic lupus erythematosus, mixed connective tissue disorder, systemic vasculitis, Sjögren syndrome, systemic mastocytosis
	Immunodeficiency	Common variable immunodeficiency
	Immune/inflammatory	Graft-versus-host disease, serum sickness, large granular lymphocyte lymphocytosis, Weber-Christian panniculitis
Neoplastic	Primary malignancies	Lymphomas, leukemias
	Metastatic malignancies	Breast, lung, skin, colon
Infiltrative	Storage diseases	Gaucher disease, Niemann-Pick disease, GM_1 gangliosidosis, glycogen storage disease type IV, Tangier disease, Wolman disease, mucopolysaccharidoses, hyperchylomicronemia types I and IV
Congestive	Portal hypertension	Intrahepatic cirrhosis, extrahepatic cirrhosis (Budd-Chiari syndrome)
	Systemic	Congestive heart failure
	Local	Splenic vein thrombosis

SPLENECTOMY

Indications and Timing

Splenectomy should be performed for clinical indications rather than for specific diagnoses. In many instances, removal of the spleen will improve the condition of patients with hemolytic anemia due to intrinsic disorders of erythrocyte membranes and enzyme disorders, and of those with chronic conditions, such as storage diseases and portal hypertension. Specific clinical indices that require intervention should be identified, and parameters that can be used to identify clinical improvement (usually an increase in peripheral blood cell counts, growth, or energy level) should be determined before the procedure is performed. For patients with inherited erythrocyte membrane or enzyme disorders, such as hereditary spherocytosis or pyruvate kinase deficiency, marked reticulocytosis indicating significant metabolic energy required for erythropoiesis, somatic growth failure, or lack of exercise tolerance would be potential indications for splenectomy. Avoidance of formation of gallstones, formerly often considered an indication for splenectomy when a diagnosis of hereditary spherocytosis was made, is less important today because minimally invasive surgical procedures have improved the management of cholelithiasis. Patients with storage disorders such as Gaucher disease with splenomegaly and hypersplenism develop cytopenias requiring intervention. The clinical benefit to be obtained from splenectomy should at least balance, and preferably outweigh, the potential long-term risks of postsplenectomy septicemia, an increased risk for thrombosis, and the shift of storage cells from the spleen to other organs, such as the bone marrow, where they may do more harm in the absence of the spleen. Not all patients with hemolytic anemias, require splenectomy. If such patients develop an aplastic crisis due to parvovirus B19 infection while their spleens are intact, they may require a transfusion. Many patients with mild chronic hemolysis and well-compensated anemia may be better off with their spleens remaining intact. Patients with ITP should undergo surgical splenectomy when the risks of bleeding or of medical therapies (such as long-term corticosteroids) are such that the benefits of splenectomy exceed the risks. The indications for splenectomy are different in adults than in children and are affected by the presence of underlying disorders, such as systemic lupus erythematosus and HIV. In an attempt to avoid immunologic consequences of a total splenectomy, several centers are performing partial splenectomies for hereditary spherocytosis, although in some cases a second procedure is later required.[18]

Splenectomy for sickle cell disease is usually performed for splenic sequestration that is severe, persistent, or recurrent. In some sickle syndromes, the spleen does not autoinfarct in childhood, and persistent splenomegaly may increase the degree of anemia. The risk for subsequent development of gallstones should be considered in patients with hemoglobinopathies and other hemolytic anemias so that cholecystectomy can be performed simultaneously, if deemed indicated.[19]

The timing of splenectomy—when it is to be performed—should again be chosen to minimize risks and maximize benefits. Immunity to carbohydrate antigens, such as those in the cell walls of encapsulated organisms such as *Streptococcus pneumoniae, Neisseria meningitidis,* and *Haemophilus influenzae* type b, develops over the first 2 to 3 years of life. When splenectomy can be delayed until the patient is at least 2 and preferably more than 5 years of age, specific immunity and response to administered polysaccharide vaccines will improve host defenses and lessen the risk for postsplenectomy sepsis. When patients have a disease, such as Gaucher disease, or hemolytic anemia predisposing to iron overload, such as thalassemia, the presence of the spleen as a preferential site for the storage of harmful cellular breakdown products may protect other organs from damage. Delaying splenectomy until a clear clinical indication is present will balance risks and benefits to an optimal degree.

Surgical Options

When splenectomy is clearly indicated, acute complications are rarely a consideration in the decision to perform surgery. Nevertheless, advances in surgical procedures have minimized the short-term risks of the procedure itself and of postoperative complications, such as intestinal obstruction from adhesions. Subtotal splenectomy can be performed when total splenectomy is not desirable, such as for the removal of a cyst, a pseudocyst, or tumors, after trauma, or for Gaucher disease. Wedge resection with mattress sutures and cyanoacrylate adhesions and microfibrillar collagen omental packs have greatly improved partial splenectomy procedures in the past decade. Laparotomy is required when extensive peritoneal adhesions are present and for removal of massively enlarged spleens. A sufficiently large incision to permit full visualization and mobilization is essential when the spleen is very large or when inspection is a major part of the surgical procedure. A retroperitoneal approach is useful when the spleen is not massively enlarged but needs to be fully removed, such as when cytopenias are the indication for the procedure. This approach shortens the postoperative recovery time and avoids induction of peritoneal adhesions.

Minimally invasive procedures have become standard for most splenectomies. Laparoscopy is now the procedure of choice for splenectomy. Although the operative time is significantly greater than for laparotomy, the postoperative recovery time, the risk for damage to the pancreas, the likelihood of developing a subphrenic abscess and peritoneal adhesions postoperatively, and the nutritional and metabolic challenges to the patient are considerably reduced. Laparoscopic splenectomy can be performed even in thrombocytopenic patients. The outcome of laparoscopic splenectomy in ITP is affected by the experience and skill of the surgeon and by the patient's obesity. Prolonged presurgical use of corticosteroids may induce obesity and impair tissue healing, resulting in a higher risk for complications from laparoscopic splenectomy than when splenectomy is performed before the adverse drug effects develop.

Appreciation of the risk for postsplenectomy septicemia and refinements in noninvasive, accurate radiologic monitoring techniques have led to more conservative approaches to splenic injury. Nonoperative management has increased over time and has an acceptable mortality and complication rate in selected patients, although early discharge may put patients at risk for the later complications.[20] Noninvasive imaging and minimally invasive surgical procedures have greatly affected these trends. After traumatic rupture, splenic tissue may regenerate minisplenules in the peritoneal cavity, a process termed *splenosis*. Although splenosis appears to be partially protective against overwhelming postsplenectomy infection in animals, its protective value in humans is not known and may depend on the adequacy of splenic tissue perfusion. If poorly vascularized, the ectopic splenic tissue may not provide adequate contact between macrophages and the antigens of the infecting organism. It is generally valuable to attempt preservation of splenic function when possible after traumatic rupture. Some surgeons attempt to induce splenosis when traumatic splenectomy is unavoidable, in the hope of minimizing late complications.

As the late complications of splenectomy are better appreciated, surgeons have become increasingly creative at performing procedures that preserve or restore splenic function. Even large cysts that were indications for splenectomy until recently have been managed with spleen-conserving procedures, such as partial or total cyst removal, which can often be performed laparoscopically.[21] Pancreatic surgery often requires sacrifice of the spleen; however, increasing numbers of procedures are being performed with salvage of the spleen.[22,23]

Splenic transplantation is being used as a means of developing immune tolerance, as well as a means of reducing the risk for infection following organ transplantation.[24] Allograft spleen has been transplanted within multivisceral grafts with only minimal graft-versus-host disease. To date there are more animal than human data, and it is unclear how large an impact this approach will have on visceral, especially small bowel and pancreatic, allotransplantation.[25] If protection against infection is the main consideration, an intact spleen is superior to a repaired or autotransplanted spleen, whereas accessory spleens and splenosis may be only marginally better than asplenia.[16]

Complications After Splenectomy

Acute complications in the perioperative period include rupture of the spleen, the development of a subphrenic abscess, and injury to the pancreas during the operative procedure. In a healthy patient, the immediate risk of splenectomy is limited. The degree of splenomegaly greatly affects the risk for rupture and pancreatic injury. The technical difficulty of performing a splenectomy is much greater when the spleen is massively enlarged than when the spleen is small. Rupture of the spleen once the arterial supply has been ligated is rarely a problem. The splenic hilum is retroperitoneal, so if the spleen is very large, mobilization to gain access to the splenic artery and vein can be difficult. After recovery from surgery, intestinal obstruction due to formation of peritoneal adhesions is a complication that, if it is to occur at all, usually occurs within the first few months.

Two late complications of splenectomy give the greatest concern: overwhelming postsplenectomy septicemia and atherosclerotic heart disease. Both of these complications may develop many years after the splenectomy (Fig. 162-8). The precise risk is not known, and preventive interventions are probably underused because patients may not be aware of the risks of splenectomy performed early in life.

Postsplenectomy septicemia is rare but may be rapidly lethal. In the absence of protective levels of opsonic IgG antibodies produced in the spleen, hepatic and pulmonary macrophages are unable to effectively clear organisms from the bloodstream. Organisms that enter the bloodstream and would ordinarily be removed by splenic macrophages are able to evade recognition by macrophages whose Fc and C3b receptors appear to be less avid than those of splenic macrophages. Circulation of the blood through the liver and lung is more rapid than through the spleen, and there is little opportunity for macrophages to recognize organisms with surfaces containing little IgG and only small amounts of C3bi. The important filtration function of the venous sinus endothelial cells is absent following splenectomy. The generation of cytokines, including tumor necrosis factor-α, and bacterial endotoxins leads to cardiovascular collapse and shock. It is rare to revive an asplenic patient once the patient is in shock, even with effective antibiotic therapy. The risk that this will happen varies with the indication for splenectomy (Table 162-4) and the patient's medical condition. Factors that impair host defenses significantly increase the risk for infection. These include deficient opsonins (hypogammaglobulinemia and specific antibody production deficiency), reticuloendothelial blockade related to increased phagocytic activity of macrophages in other organs, impaired antigen processing or recognition (AIDS, lymphoma, other malignancies, and some collagen vascular diseases), neutropenia, and high iron load (thalassemia). The tetrapeptide tuftsin, primarily produced in the spleen, enhances the phagocytic activity of monocytes and neutrophils; its absence in asplenic patients appears to contribute to depressed neutrophil function and the subsequent increased risk for infection.

Patients at the lowest risk for overwhelming postsplenectomy sepsis are those in whom splenectomy cures the underlying problem, such as isolated ITP, hereditary spherocytosis, and trauma. Patients undergoing splenectomy for trauma have a 50-fold greater risk for subsequent septic death than trauma patients with spleens intact, whereas the risk in patients with sickle cell disease is increased 350-fold over that of the general population, and other authors report the risk to be 600 times greater.

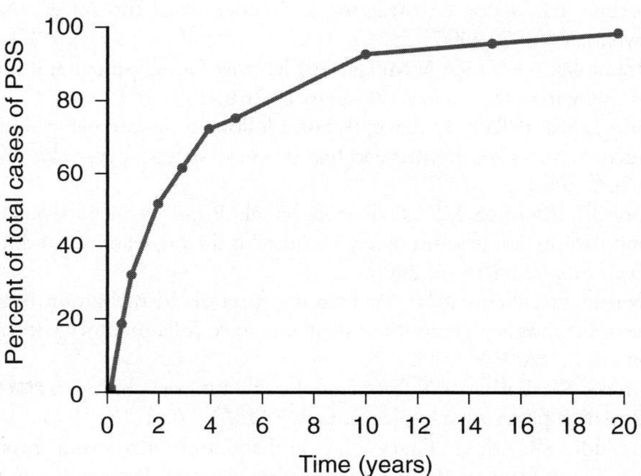

Figure 162-8 THE INTERVAL FROM SPLENECTOMY TO POSTSPLENECTOMY SEPSIS (PSS). Of the total (N = 288), 3.1% occurred more than 20 years after splenectomy. *(From Lutwick LI: Infections in asplenic patients. In Mandell GL, Bennett JE, Dolin R, editors:* Principles and practice of infectious diseases, *ed 7, Philadelphia, 2009, Churchill Livingstone. Used with permission.)*

An increased risk for vascular complications may result from splenectomy. Acute portal vein thrombosis occurs within 2 months of splenectomy in 5% to 37% of patients, which is probably the result of local surgical factors. Patients with thalassemia and prior splenectomy appear to also have an increased incidence of venous thromboembolism beyond the portal venous system. In addition, splenectomy appears to be a risk factor for the development of pulmonary hypertension. Vascular events after splenectomy are likely multifactorial in origin, being attributed to a combination of hypercoagulability, platelet activation, activation of endothelium due to the persistence of particulate matter, and damaged cells in the bloodstream.

Atherosclerosis that develops many years after splenectomy in patients with hereditary spherocytosis or hereditary stomatocytosis may be related to subsequent thrombocytosis that leads to enhancement of plaque formation. Statistically the increased risk for atherosclerosis is not great, but for individuals with other risk factors, such as hypertension, diabetes, high levels of cholesterol or homocysteine, heterozygous protein C or S deficiency, or factor V Leiden, splenectomy may pose a more significant risk. Although no human data are currently available in this area, some studies have suggested that the spleen might be involved in lipid metabolism in both rats and rabbits.

Prevention of Complications

Postsplenectomy Septicemia

The major risk for postsplenectomy sepsis is infection with encapsulated organisms such as *Staphylococcus pneumoniae, Haemophilus influenzae* type b, and *Neisseria meningitidis,* which require opsonization for effective phagocytosis. Polysaccharide vaccines are available for all three bacteria.[26,27] The highest risk period for children is in the first 2 years of life, when their ability to mount an antibody response to purified polysaccharides has not developed completely, so protein-conjugated vaccines are now in widespread use. This has significant potential benefit for patients when asplenia is not recognized, because they might then be immunized as part of their routine care. The antibody responses to vaccines, especially the conjugated vaccines, differ in IgG subclasses from those produced following natural infection. Overwhelming postsplenectomy sepsis and death from sepsis in functionally hyposplenic patients should be preventable.[28] It is recommended that immunization be done 2 to 3 weeks before the anticipated splenectomy to optimize antigen recognition and processing and induce more effective immunity. If emergency

Table 162-4 Incidence of Postsplenectomy Sepsis

Indication for Splenectomy	Cumulative Incidence of Bacterial Sepsis (%)
Trauma	1.5
Hematologic disorders	3.4
Portal hypertension	8.2
Hodgkin disease	10
Sickle cell disease	15
Thalassemia	25

Data from Gorse GJ: The relationship of the spleen to infection. In Bowlder AJ, editor: *The spleen: Structure, function, and clinical significance,* New York, 1990, Van Nostrand Reinhold, p 269, with permission.

Vaccination of a Patient Scheduled for Elective Versus Emergency Splenectomy

A 50-year-old man with refractory immune thrombocytopenia purpura is scheduled for splenectomy. Having heard that there is a risk for different types of infection after splenectomy, he asks what he can do to reduce his risk.

Patients scheduled for elective splenectomy should receive the following at least 14 days before the procedure:

- *Streptococcus pneumoniae* vaccine
- *Haemophilus influenzae* vaccine
- *Neisseria meningitis* vaccine

Consider administration of the influenza vaccine because influenza is a risk factor for secondary bacterial infection.

If the procedure is done emergently, wait until at least the 14th postoperative day.

splenectomy is performed, it is recommended that vaccination be postponed until at least 2 weeks postsplenectomy to avoid the transient immune suppression often seen with general anesthesia and surgery (see box on Vaccination of a Patient Scheduled for Elective Versus Emergency Splenectomy). Adults are generally presumed to be immune to *Haemophilus influenzae* type b and may receive the 23-valent pneumococcal polysaccharide vaccine (PPSV23) and meningococcal vaccines alone. Reimmunization for children is recommended 2 to 5 years after initial immunization. Splenectomized adults should be revaccinated with the PPSV23 once after 5 years, whereas meningococcal revaccination should occur every 5 years. Conjugating polysaccharides to pneumococcal surface peptides may offer a novel approach. Because these recommendations change with experience and vaccine use, it is wise to consult current guidelines for individual patients. Additional organisms to consider in postsplenectomy sepsis include *Escherichia coli, Pseudomonas aeruginosa,* and *Capnocytophaga canimorsus.*[29]

There are fewer data on the efficacy of prophylactic antibiotics for asplenic patients, except for young children with sickle cell disease, in whom antibiotics should be initiated as soon as the diagnosis is established. Present recommendations are that twice-daily oral penicillin V potassium or amoxicillin be continued in sickle cell patients until 5 years of age or 3 years postsplenectomy. High-risk patients with surgical or functional asplenia, including those with diagnoses of thalassemia, Hodgkin disease, other malignancies, immunodeficiency disease, or chronic graft-versus-host disease, should receive prophylactic antibiotics unless specific contraindications exist. Patients who have a history of pneumococcal postsplenectomy sepsis may be considered candidates for lifelong daily prophylaxis as well. Whether or not such patients receive prophylactic antibiotics, and regardless of their immunization status, they may develop overwhelming infections with other organisms, including gram-negative organisms and *Staphylococcus aureus.* Updated recommendations should be consulted for specific circumstances.

The single most important measure to prevent postsplenectomy septicemia is education of the patient, family, and physician. Recognition of the risk, the institution of appropriate preventive measures, and the rapid administration of antibiotics to a patient who is showing signs of infection (fever and chills) can be lifesaving. Some experts recommend that at the time of febrile illness, asplenic patients take immediate antibiotics at home before quickly traveling to an emergency room for evaluation.

Atherosclerosis

The magnitude of the risk for development of atherosclerosis is not clear.[9,30,31] Appropriate preventive measures include identifying and minimizing concurrent risk factors, such as obesity, dietary patterns, a sedentary lifestyle, and the presence of other hereditary factors that would predispose to thrombosis. Low-dose aspirin could be considered, but no data exist regarding its efficacy in this situation.

CONCLUSIONS AND FUTURE DIRECTIONS

Although very little novel information has emerged about clinical aspects of splenic function in recent years, appreciation of many subtleties of splenic function and advances in supportive care in several fields have had significant impacts on the management of disorders of the spleen. Better education and more effective immunizations have helped prevent serious complications related to splenic disorders. Advances in imaging and surgery have transformed the diagnosis and management of congenital and traumatic splenic disorders.

Enhanced understanding of the complexity of communication interaction between the cells of the immune and hematopoietic system has improved our appreciation of the molecular, cellular, system, and network basis for clinical observations about splenic function. The ability of splenic macrophages, in concert with dendritic cells and B cells, to recognize and ingest a variety of microorganisms—even in patients without previous exposure to the pathogens—provides great insight into the reasons that the spleen provides protection against a variety of very specific infections. More detailed understanding of the impact of the splenic microenvironment on cellular functions, the role of stromal infrastructure on the ability of cells to interact with and respond to invading pathogens, and the integration of components of the immune system has contributed to an appreciation of clinical observations about the role the spleen plays in normal biology. The intersection of hematopoiesis, recycling of aging cells, and iron metabolism is most clearly demonstrated in the spleen.

Although not necessary to life under baseline circumstances, the contribution of the spleen to homeostasis under stress is considerable. Ongoing efforts to preserve and manage splenic function will continue to benefit from enhanced appreciation of the underlying biology.

REFERENCES

1. Weiss L: The spleen. In Weiss L, editor: *Cell, and tissue biology: A textbook of histology,* ed 6, Baltimore, 1988, Urban & Schwarzenberg, p 515.
2. Kanzler B, Dear TN: Hox11 acts cell autonomously in spleen development and its absence results in altered cell fate of mesenchymal spleen precursors. *Dev Biol* 234:231, 2001.
3. Mebius RE, Kraal G: Structure and function of the spleen. *Nat Rev Immunol* 5:606, 2005.
4. Brendolan A, Rosado MM, Carsetti R, et al: Development and function of the mammalian spleen. *Bioessays* 29:166, 2007.
5. Junt T, Scandella E, Ludewig B: Form follows function: Lymphoid tissue microarchitecture in antimicrobial immune defence. *Nat Rev Immunol* 8:764, 2008.
6. Dor FJ, Ramirez ML, Parmar K, et al: Primitive hematopoietic cell populations reside in the spleen: Studies in the pig, baboon, and human. *Exp Hematol* 34:1573, 2006.
7. Swirski FK, Nahrendorf M, Etzrodt M, et al: Identification of splenic reservoir monocytes and their deployment to inflammatory sites. *Science* 325:612, 2009.
8. Grover SA, Barkun AN, Sackett DL: The rational clinical examination. Does this patient have splenomegaly? *JAMA* 270:2218, 1993.
9. Troendle SB, Adix L, Crary SE, et al: Laboratory markers of thrombosis risk in children with hereditary spherocytosis. *Pediatr Blood Cancer* 49:781, 2007.
10. Haan JM, Boswell S, Stein D, et al: Follow-up abdominal CT is not necessary in low-grade splenic injury. *Am Surg* 73:13, 2007.
11. Hackett S, Chua-anusorn W, Pootrakul P, et al: The magnetic susceptibilities of iron deposits in thalassaemic spleen tissue. *Biochim Biophys Acta* 1772:330, 2007.

12. Juweid ME, Stroobants S, Hoekstra OS, et al: Use of positron emission tomography for response assessment of lymphoma: Consensus of the Imaging Subcommittee of International Harmonization Project in Lymphoma. *J Clin Oncol* 25:571, 2007.
13. Valette F, Querellou S, Oudoux A, et al: Comparison of positron emission tomography and lymphangiography in the diagnosis of infradiaphragmatic Hodgkin's disease. *Acta Radiol* 48:59, 2007.
14. Cai W, Olafsen T, Zhang X, et al: PET imaging of colorectal cancer in xenograft-bearing mice by use of an 18F-labeled T84.66 anti-carcinoembryonic antigen diabody. *J Nucl Med* 48:304, 2007.
15. Corazza GR, Ginaldi L, Zoli G, et al: Howell-Jolly body counting as a measure of splenic function. A reassessment. *Clin Lab Haematol* 12:269, 1990.
16. Connell NT, Brunner AM, Kerr CA, et al: Splenosis and sepsis: The born-again spleen provides poor protection. *Virulence* 2:4, 2011.
17. Yongxiang W, Zongfang L, Guowei L, et al: Effects of splenomegaly and splenic macrophage activity in hypersplenism due to cirrhosis. *Am J Med* 113:428, 2002.
18. Buesing KL, Tracy ET, Kiernan C, et al: Partial splenectomy for hereditary spherocytosis: A multi-institutional review. *J Pediatr Surg* 46:178, 2011.
19. Al-Salem AH: Indications and complications of splenectomy for children with sickle cell disease. *J Pediatr Surg* 41:1909, 2006.
20. Crawford RS, Tabbara M, Sheridan R, et al: Early discharge after nonoperative management for splenic injuries: Increased patient risk caused by late failure? *Surgery* 142:337, 2007.
21. Mattioli G, Pini Prato A, Cheli M, et al: Italian multicentric survey on laparoscopic spleen surgery in the pediatric population. *Surg Endosc* 21:527, 2007.
22. Matsumoto CS, Fishbein TM: Modified multivisceral transplantation with splenopancreatic preservation. *Transplantation* 83:234, 2007.
23. Salvia R, Bassi C, Festa L, et al: Clinical and biological behavior of pancreatic solid pseudopapillary tumors: Report on 31 consecutive patients. *J Surg Oncol* 95:304, 2007.
24. Wluka A, Olszewski WL: Innate and adaptive processes in the spleen. *Ann Transplant* 11:22, 2006.
25. Kato T, Tzakis AG, Selvaggi G, et al: Transplantation of the spleen: Effect of splenic allograft in human multivisceral transplantation. *Ann Surg* 246:436; discussion 445–436, 2007.
26. Grijalva CG, Nuorti JP, Arbogast PG, et al: Decline in pneumonia admissions after routine childhood immunisation with pneumococcal conjugate vaccine in the USA: A time-series analysis. *Lancet* 369:1179, 2007.
27. Stephens DS: Conquering the meningococcus. *FEMS Microbiol Rev* 31:3, 2007.
28. Price VE, Blanchette VS, Ford-Jones EL: The prevention and management of infections in children with asplenia or hyposplenia. *Infect Dis Clin North Am* 21:697, viii–ix, 2007.
29. Di Sabatino A, Carsetti R, Corazza GR: Post-splenectomy and hyposplenic states. *Lancet* 378:86, 2011.
30. Crary SE, Buchanan GR: Vascular complications after splenectomy for hematologic disorders. *Blood* 114:2861, 2009.
31. Ahmed S, Horton KM, Fishman EK: Splenic incidentalomas. *Radiol Clin North Am* 49:323, 2011.

CHAPTER 163

HEMATOLOGY IN AGING

Andrew S. Artz and William B. Ershler

Although most classifications consider patients "older" once the age exceeds 65 or 70 years, age-related changes are not discrete and certainly do not occur at any specific age. A central tenet of gerontology (the study of normal aging) is that biologic measures show increased variation with advancing age, but that these variations are of insufficient magnitude to result in disease per se. Hematologic conditions in older adults have unique features and frequently require a modified approach relative to younger adults. We will focus on anemia in older adults, because this is the most frequent clinically defined hematologic problem among older adults.

EPIDEMIOLOGY

Aging

The median life expectancy continues to rise throughout the world. In the United States, the Centers for Disease Control and Prevention estimates life expectancy at 77.9 years for children born in 2007. For those who survive to age 75 years in this cohort, they may expect to live until 86 years of age (www.cdc.gov/nchs/data/hus/hus10.pdf#022). Therefore the proportion and absolute number of older adults is increasing, and the life expectancy of adults who have reached an advanced age may be considerable. Accordingly we advocate estimating life expectancy for older adults found to have hematologic conditions, and several calculators are available online for this purpose (e.g., http://gosset.wharton.upenn.edu/mortality/perl/CalcForm.html).

Anemia Definition

Historically criteria for diagnosing anemia in older and younger adults applied the World Health Organization (WHO) hemoglobin (Hb) threshold below 13 g/dL for men and less than 12 g/dL for women.[1] Because it was widely recognized that the criteria required modification, Beutler and Waalen[2] evaluated two large databases (the third U.S. National Health and Nutrition Examination Survey [NHANES] and the Scripps-Kaiser database) to develop population-based thresholds, defining the fifth percentile as the lower limit of normal as shown in Table 163-1. Importantly, they excluded patients with low iron stores, vitamin deficiencies, elevated creatinine level of 1.4 mg/dL, and increased markers of inflammation. Therefore the remaining adults were mostly devoid of anemia-related conditions, and actual population prevalence would be higher.

Anemia Prevalence

Most reports of anemia prevalence use the historical WHO thresholds of less than 13 g/dL of Hb for men and less than 12 g/dL for women. For adults 65 years and older residing in the community, the prevalence of anemia is around 10% to 11% and rises with advancing age to around 20% to 25% for those 85 years and older.[3,4] As expected, older adults admitted to the hospital or chronically residing in a nursing-home have lower Hb values and a higher prevalence of anemia.[5]

Race/ethnicity also influences anemia prevalence. Studies from Europe and Japan[3,6] indicate a fairly similar anemia prevalence in older adults. Blacks have lower median Hb values and almost three times higher prevalence of anemia by WHO cutoff points.[4] In a substantial portion of blacks with lower Hb levels α-thalassemia trait with one or two deletions is likely a contributory factor.

Neutropenia and Thrombocytopenia

The incidence of thrombocytopenia, defined as a platelet count below 150×10^9/L, does not appreciably change with age with an average reduction of 19×10^9/L in those 70 to 90 years of age.[7,8] A study of Sardinian villages revealed an increasing incidence of thrombocytopenia with aging, approaching 6% in the seventh decade and 8% for octogenarians.[9] Interestingly, neutropenia (less than 1.5×10^9/L) appears less common with advancing age, such that the prevalence in community-dwelling older adults 75 years and older has been approximated at 0.5%.[10] This does not account for the higher incidence of cytopenias among patients undergoing myelosuppressive challenges such as drugs or infection.

PATHOBIOLOGY

Hematopoietic Changes With Aging

The study of older adults illustrates an overriding paradox that although aging alone does not cause clinically significant cytopenias, aging predisposes to reduced hematopoietic reserve and to diseases, both of which increase the tendency to encounter significantly lower counts in older adults. Major hematopoietic changes occurring with aging are listed in Table 163-2.

The attention to the hematopoietic system must be understood in the context that organ systems are integrated to maintain homeostasis. For example, decreased bone mass and heightened systemic inflammation may adversely influence hematopoiesis.[11,12] Functional decline and the development of frailty with aging relates to a global loss of reserve. Whether hematopoietic perturbations are linked to global decline or the factors promoting functional decline attenuate marrow function cannot be easily deciphered. Reduced neutrophil responses to granulocyte colony-stimulating factors have long been appreciated as predisposing to infection with advancing age, but this occurs in the setting of decline in immune function with aging.[13,14] Further, the prevalence of anemia exceeds 50% in frail older adult patients, and poor functional status or functional limitations predict hematologic toxicities after chemotherapy.

Anemia as a Model of Aging

Anemia may be an ideal model for the interaction of the influence of hematopoietic aging and organ disease. Although anemia is not a normal finding in older adults, the prevalence increases markedly from the seventh decade to the ninth decade of life.[4] For the majority, anemia is related to an underlying cause such as iron deficiency/

Table 163-1 Anemia Definitions*

Group	Hemoglobin (g/dL)
MEN, 60 YEARS OR OLDER	
White	13.2
Black	12.7
WOMEN, 50 YEARS OR OLDER	
White	12.2
Black	11.5

Adapted from Beutler E, Waalen J: The definition of anemia: what is the lower limit of normal of the blood hemoglobin concentration? *Blood* 107:1747, 2006.

Table 163-2 Hematopoietic Changes Associated With Advancing Age

Diminished bone marrow cellularity
Reduced CD34+ cell mobilization to G-CSF administration in healthy donors
Decreased stem cell telomeres
Reduced hematopoietic cell proliferative capacity
Increased numbers of hematopoietic stem cells
Reduction in lymphocyte function
Reduced response to vaccination
Development of unexplained anemia[4]

G-CSF, Granulocyte colony-stimulating factor.

bleeding, chronic disease/inflammation, or renal insufficiency.[4] An intensive hematologic evaluation of anemia in older adults reveals a wider range of causes than previously appreciated, including 5% to 10% with hematologic neoplasms.[15,16] Nevertheless 30% to 40% of anemic adults lack a discernible cause despite a thorough investigation, and this has become commonly termed *unexplained anemia in the elderly* (Fig. 163-1). Renal insufficiency, hypogonadism, or undiagnosed myelodysplastic syndromes do not seem to account for most cases.[15,17,18] Our recommended approach for anemia in older adults differs from that for younger adults (see box on Evaluating Anemia in Older Adults).

Leukopenia and Thrombocytopenia

The causes of thrombocytopenia and neutropenia, as with anemia, are vast. Although the causes of cytopenias are not unique to older adults, the possibility of more than one cause should not be overlooked. For example, a patient with an emerging bone marrow failure syndrome may be prone to develop severe pancytopenia at the time of a serious infection or other insult.

CLINICAL MANIFESTATIONS

In the industrialized countries, the detection of cytopenias is often encountered after routine laboratory testing or accompanies minor or nonspecific symptoms. Especially for anemia, one may not be able to disentangle anemia symptoms from other conditions that coexist or underlie the anemia (e.g., rheumatoid arthritis). Although fatigue may be the most obvious symptom of anemia, the potential signs and symptoms are protean. Patients frequently attribute fatigue to "growing old." Observational studies demonstrate a clear association between mild hemoglobin reduction (e.g., less than 14 g/dL for women and less than 15 g/dL for men) and reduced quality of life, strength, and mobility.[19-21] Signs and symptoms may also direct one toward a cause, such as a pica suggesting iron deficiency or weight loss directing the clinician toward a systemic illness.

Specific hemoglobin thresholds do not permit one to validate symptoms because patients have different levels of reserve and organ function, pace of hemoglobin fall, and underlying cause for the

Evaluating Anemia in Older Adults

Anemia in older adults is a common finding and frequently results in a request for hematology consultation.

To define anemia, we follow the hemoglobin criteria defined by Beutler and Waalen in Table 163-1. However, hemoglobin trajectory over time is as important. Based on the fact that the average hemoglobin level declines in older adults about 1 g/dL over 15 years or more, we consider decline of 1 g/dL in less than 5 years or 2 g/dL over 10 years significant and supports a complete evaluation. We work diligently to retrieve remote blood counts. Older adults frequently have had blood counts obtained either routinely in the past, before a procedure, or at the time of hospital admission. Counts at the time of hospital admission may be the least reliable because they occur in the context of an illness.

To elicit symptoms, both the patient and family members or caregivers who know the patient are asked about functional changes (walking, naps, activity level) over the short-term (weeks) and longer term (months to years). Many older adults will often attribute functional changes to "old age."

Our basic evaluation begins with a complete blood count, red cell indices, and review of the peripheral smear. The red cell size by mean corpuscular volume is helpful but imperfect. We also perform a reticulocyte count, but 95% or more of anemias in older adults are hypoproliferative. Because anemia can be mixed or multifactorial, we routinely perform the same panel on most patients: serum ferritin, serum iron, total iron-binding capacity, serum creatinine (and estimated renal function), vitamin B_{12}, and thyrotropin levels. We also have found c-reactive protein and serum erythropoietin to be very useful. High c-reactive protein level, such as above 10 mg/L, is frequently associated with inflammatory illnesses and raises caution in interpreting the serum ferritin level. Serum erythropoietin levels are typically in the reference range (i.e., inappropriately low) for most older anemic adults except for iron deficiency, hematologic malignancy, or hyperproductive anemias. Folate levels are rarely low, at least in the United States, where dietary folate supplementation is universal. The remainder of the laboratory tests will be performed as indicated. We do not routinely evaluate for a serum monoclonal gammopathy unless unexplained renal dysfunction, elevated total protein level, elevated calcium level, or bone pain is present.

A ferritin level of less than 50 ng/mL will prompt a complete evaluation for iron deficiency. At a minimum, we embark on an oral iron trial and fecal tests for blood. The lower the iron stores and more evidence for iron deficiency anemia, the more we recommend endoscopic gastrointestinal evaluation, assuming no other cause is clearly established. Other measures exist for diagnosing iron deficiency, such as reticulocyte counts, serum transferrin receptor, or intravenous iron trials. We also empirically treat if vitamin B_{12} levels are less than 200 pg/mL with oral vitamin B_{12} at 1000 mcg for 8 to 12 weeks. If there is no response, we discontinue therapy.

A bone marrow examination is recommended if any of the following are present: unexplained requirement for red blood cell transfusion therapy, unexplained mean corpuscular volume of 97 fL or greater, thrombocytopenia below $120 \times 10^9/L$, neutropenia below $1000 \times 10^9/L$, or suspicious peripheral smear. If the bone marrow is nondiagnostic, we only repeat the marrow examination at the time of clinical progression (e.g., red blood cell transfusion required, the development of more significant cytopenias).

When the anemia has no established cause, the hemoglobin level is above 10 g/dL, the patient lacks major symptoms, and the hemoglobin kinetics are stable (i.e., fall of less than 1 g/dL over 5 years), we follow up with blood cell counts every 6 months and then annually. Any significant fall in hemoglobin will prompt repeat evaluation. We do not routinely administer erythropoiesis-stimulating agents for unexplained anemia.

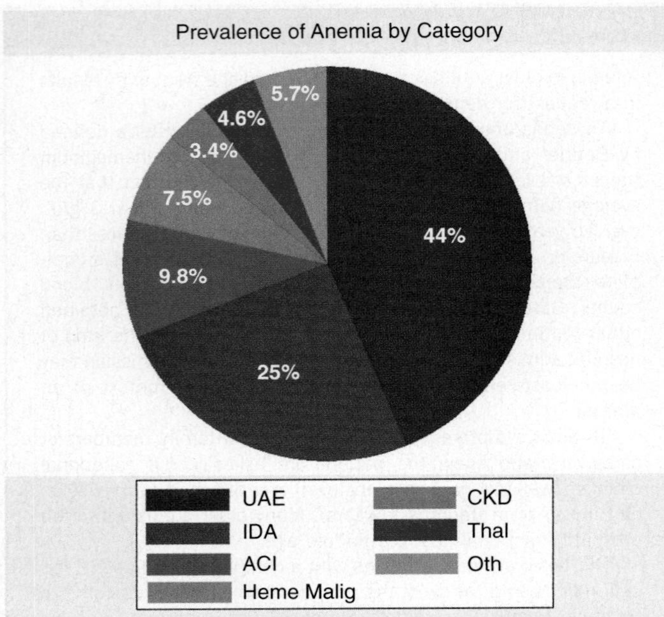

Figure 163-1 CATEGORIZATION OF PRIMARY ANEMIA ETIOLOGY OR UNEXPLAINED ANEMIA IN THE ELDERLY (UAE) IS SHOWN. *IDA,* Iron deficiency anemia; *ACI,* anemia of chronic inflammation; *Heme malig,* hematologic malignancy; *CKD,* chronic kidney disease; *Thal,* thalassemia trait; *Oth,* other. (Other includes hemolysis, 4; alcohol, 3; hypothyroidism, 1; vitamin B_{12} deficiency, 1; medication, 1.) *(From Artz AS, Thirman MF: Unexplained anemia predominates despite an intensive evaluation in a racially diverse cohort of older adults from a referral anemia clinic.* J Gerontol A Biol Sci Med Sci *66:925, 2011.)*

anemia. A more rapid pace of hemoglobin decline is at least as important in provoking symptoms relative to anemia severity. Overall functional reserve and organ function also determines compensation for the stress of anemia. In contrast, a chronic stable anemia, even if severe, may be well compensated. Moreover, patients may adjust their activity level and be unaware of limitations.

Neutropenia and Thrombocytopenia

Because of immune alterations with aging, one expects older adults at a given degree of neutropenia to suffer more infections and/or more serious infections. For example, not only do older adults have a greater probability of developing neutropenia, they also have a heightened risk for life-threatening complications.[22] Thrombocytopenia in older adults increases bleeding risks compared with younger adults, best illustrated in chronic autoimmune thrombocytopenic purpura.[23,24]

LABORATORY MANIFESTATIONS

Diagnosis

The use of age-adjusted norms remains quite controversial because normal aging itself has only a small impact on normal values. For cytopenias, blood counts are mandatory for diagnosis, to establish severity, and to guide the etiologic evaluation. For anemia, we advocate applying the hemoglobin thresholds published by Beutler and Waalen as seen in Table 163-1. Thresholds to define neutropenia and thrombocytopenia should not differ from younger adults.

Laboratory Evaluation for Anemia

To the extent significant cytopenias are uncommon among community-dwelling adults and the decline with normal aging is modest, a cause should always be sought and will often be found. Remote blood counts are of enormous value, not only to ensure the acquired nature, but to assess the tempo of change over time. Most older adults in industrialized countries will have prior blood counts. An evaluation of worsening neutropenia or thrombocytopenia, similar to anemia, will typically yield a cause. Review of the blood smear can be enormously useful, if not simply to exclude a high-risk hematologic disorder (e.g., lack of peripheral blood blasts and significant dysplasia or cytosis).

Table 163-3 Differential Diagnosis for Common Causes of Cytopenias in Older Adults

Cytopenia of one or more lineages
Hematologic neoplasm
Vitamin B_{12} deficiency
Autoimmune disorder
Consumptive coagulopathy
Systemic inflammation
Alcohol
Splenomegaly
Thyroid dysfunction
Human immunodeficiency virus

Bone Marrow Evaluation

Although a bone marrow examination may be invaluable in excluding serious marrow-related conditions, all cytopenias in older adults do not warrant a bone marrow examination. We favor delaying bone marrow examination until recovery from acute events unless a high-grade hematologic malignancy that would warrant immediate treatment is suspected. Mild fluctuations of counts, particularly within the range found over years, without other evidence of a hematologic malignancy may allow one to safely defer a bone marrow examination.

DIFFERENTIAL DIAGNOSIS

It is important to distinguish true and clinically important findings from false or transiently low values by having serial blood counts and/or a review of the peripheral smear.

In addition to causes delineated in Table 163-3, other causes specific for anemia in older adults include unexplained iron deficiency/blood loss, folate deficiency, hemolysis, and androgen deprivation.

PROGNOSIS

The underlying condition driving the hematologic abnormality usually dictates prognosis. There is now a wealth of data that suggests that even a mildly low hemoglobin concentration is an independent adverse prognostic factor in older adult patients. It is likely anemia, rather than an obscure or unrecognized condition, imparts an adverse prognosis because a serious underlying condition is typically not found in patients with isolated mild anemia. A lower hemoglobin concentration independently increases the risks for hospitalization and mortality, even in those 85 years and older.[20,21,25-29]

THERAPY

To the extent possible, the underlying illness should be treated. Particularly for anemia, the cause often remains obscure or the underlying illness may not be amenable to therapy. We favor diagnostic and therapeutic trials of iron or vitamins but for a defined period of 3 months and discontinuing if ineffective. One must be attuned to

Assessment of Older Adults With Hematologic Malignancies

Optimal treatment for a hematologic condition in an older patient must be measured in terms of both efficacy and anticipated toxicity. Assessing patients' reserve before treatment not only promotes tailoring treatment, but also provides an objective baseline assessment and an opportunity to direct interventions for these limitations.

For all adults over 50 years, we screen for age-associated vulnerabilities. Cataloging comorbid conditions and assessing performance status (PS) play a central role. Estimating PS alone provides only a crude estimate of tolerance to treatment. An Eastern Cooperative Oncology Group (ECOG) PS of 2 or more suggests important health limitations, but one must recognize that a PS of 0 to 1 covers a broad range of health, from robust to substantial limitations. In older patients, it is important to estimate PS before the current illness, because this is more likely to provide insight into vulnerability. We find insufficient data to recommend a specific comorbidity tool or index. However, certain tools such as the Charlson comorbidity index or hematopoietic cell transplantation–comorbidity index have been validated in the context of certain diseases and their treatments and thus may be invaluable in specific situations.

The PS and comorbidity index should be complemented by screening for other vulnerabilities, particularly in those older patients with a PS of 0 to 2 for whom intensive therapy is under consideration. Limitations in the following domains also suggest vulnerability:

- Instrumental activities of daily living, which are the skills required to live independently in the community (e.g., transportation, paying bills, shopping)
- Poor caregiver support
- Cognition
- Age 70 years and older

One should not overlook inquiring specifically about whether patients perceive problems for the recommended treatment. Patients will often relay difficulties not recognized by a standard medical examination (e.g., caring for an ill-spouse, limited prescription coverage, and poor perceived health). More formal screening instruments are available and useful if familiarity can be achieved (e.g., Vulnerable Elders Survey-13).

Knowledge of disease-based response rates will allow further individualizing treatment decisions. Responses to imatinib for chronic-phase chronic myeloid leukemia do not differ substantially by age, whereas acute myeloid leukemia induction results in lower responses, shorter disease-free survival, and greater toxicity relative to younger adults, even among relatively "young" healthy adults in their seventh decade of life.

Although disease-based therapy exists on a spectrum, we generally divide therapy into low-intensity, intermediate-intensity, or high-intensity therapy. High-intensity treatment entails strategies such as AML induction and autologous or allogeneic hematopoietic cell transplantation, and these have high rates of early death for patients with health limitations. Prior treatment and disease status influence the expected complication rate. Refractory or relapsed disease or multiple prior regimens may escalate the expected complications and may warrant providing traditionally less-intensive therapy instead of high-intensity treatment strategies. We typically reserve high-intensity therapy for patients with a preserved PS. We recommend that a patient with any vulnerability on screening undergo a more comprehensive geriatric assessment, if available, before curative-intent intensive therapy. Clinics focusing on issues and research in geriatric oncology are becoming available, and identifying experts (physician and nonphysician) in aging with an interest in oncology is invaluable. They often can connect patients with resources for specific problems (e.g., home care, transportation, financial help, assisted living).

Intermediate-intensity therapy such as CHOP (cyclophosphamide, hydroxydaunomycin, vincristine [Oncovin], and prednisone)-like regimens and fludarabine plus cyclophosphamide may be somewhat more likely to produce manageable toxicity-related morbidity in older patients, but they remain efficacious and can be administered safely to those with a PS of 2 or better. Demethylating agents span the gap between low- and intermediate-intensity therapy. Low-intensity therapies, such as imatinib or supportive care alone, generally require only a reasonable nondisease life expectancy of more than a couple of months and can be given with an ECOG PS of 3 or less.

Patient support often extends past the traditional nuclear family and may include friends, business associates, or extended relatives. We strongly encourage a family meeting before initiating treatment at which goals and expectations are clearly discussed. Not only will insights be gained into the available support system, but communicating to the entire team harmonizes goals for providers and patients alike. Supportive care should be addressed prospectively before treatment plans and with the entire "treatment family." Standard guidelines for infectious disease prophylaxis and growth factor support should be supplemented with plans to address limitations found in the initial assessment.

fluctuations, normal variation, or confounding factors in assessing response. For example, anemia detected immediately after a hospitalization may reflect phlebotomy, dilution, and an acute inflammatory response. The anemia may improve slowly after hospitalization even without therapy.

For unexplained or idiopathic cytopenias, caution should be exercised in employing erythropoiesis-stimulating agents because of concerns for toxicity. Although not clearly established, it is unlikely that toxicity to these agents would be less in older patients. The data are sparse for erythropoiesis-stimulating agents and unexplained anemia in older adults.[30,31] More importantly, erythropoiesis-stimulating agent treatment for anemia associated with renal insufficiency not requiring dialysis has been associated with neutral to negative results.[32,33]

Polypharmacy remains a frequent problem in older adults and may either cause hematologic abnormalities or adversely interact with the detected blood abnormality. The primary physician, once prompted, may determine many medications are unnecessary and can simply be discontinued.

For older adults with an established hematologic malignancy for which aggressive therapy may be entertained, a detailed assessment may guide decision making (see box on Assessment of Older Adults With Hematologic Malignancies).

FUTURE DIRECTIONS

The availability of large databases that contain representative populations or sometimes primarily older populations (e.g., U.S. Medicare program) represents a tremendous opportunity for intensive study in older adults. Studies of normal healthy aging individuals are of tremendous value. Although interventional trials among older persons remain challenging, the growing number of older and often relatively healthy adults mandates efforts to study older adults to inform clinical practice.

REFERENCES

1. World Health Organization: Nutritional anemias. Report of a WHO scientific group. *World Health Organ Tech Rep Ser* 405:5, 1968.
2. Beutler E, Waalen J: The definition of anemia: What is the lower limit of normal of the blood hemoglobin concentration? *Blood* 107:1747, 2006.
3. Ferrucci L, Guralnik JM, Bandinelli S, et al: Unexplained anaemia in older persons is characterised by low erythropoietin and low levels of pro-inflammatory markers. *Br J Haematol* 136:849, 2007.

4. Guralnik JM, Eisenstaedt RS, Ferrucci L, et al: Prevalence of anemia in persons 65 years and older in the United States: Evidence for a high rate of unexplained anemia. *Blood* 104:2263, 2004.
5. Artz AS, Fergusson D, Drinka PJ, et al: Prevalence of anemia in skilled-nursing home residents. *Arch Gerontol Geriatr* 39:201, 2004.
6. Ishine M, Wada T, Akamatsu K, et al: No positive correlation between anemia and disability in older people in Japan. *J Am Geriatr Soc* 53:733, 2005.
7. Segal JB, Molterno AR: Platelet Counts Vary by Ethnicity, Sex, and Age: Analysis of NHANES III Data. *Blood:Abstract* 3937, 2004.
8. Nilsson-Ehle H, Jagenburg R, Landahl S, et al: Haematological abnormalities and reference intervals in the elderly. A cross-sectional comparative study of three urban Swedish population samples aged 70, 75 and 81 years. *Acta Med Scand* 224:595, 1988.
9. Biino G, Balduini CL, Casula L, et al: Analysis of 12,517 inhabitants of a Sardinian geographic isolate reveals that predispositions to thrombocytopenia and thrombocytosis are inherited traits. *Haematologica* 96:96, 2011.
10. Hsieh MM, Everhart JE, Byrd-Holt DD, et al: Prevalence of neutropenia in the U.S. population: Age, sex, smoking status, and ethnic differences. *Ann Intern Med* 146:486, 2007.
11. Ershler WB, Keller ET: Age-associated increased interleukin-6 gene expression, late-life diseases, and frailty. *Annu Rev Med* 51:245, 2000.
12. Brockstedt H, Kassem M, Eriksen EF, et al: Age- and sex-related changes in iliac cortical bone mass and remodeling. *Bone* 14:681, 1993.
13. Chatta GS, Price TH, Allen RC, et al: Effects of in vivo recombinant methionyl human granulocyte colony-stimulating factor on the neutrophil response and peripheral blood colony-forming cells in healthy young and elderly adult volunteers. *Blood* 84:2923, 1994.
14. Pawelec G, Larbi A: Immunity and ageing in man: Annual Review 2006/2007. *Exp Gerontol* 43:34, 2008.
15. Artz AS, Thirman MJ: Unexplained anemia predominates despite an intensive evaluation in a racially diverse cohort of older adults from a referral anemia clinic. *J Gerontol A Biol Sci Med Sci*, 66:925, 2011.
16. Price EA, Mehra R, Holmes TH, et al: Anemia in older persons: Etiology and evaluation. *Blood Cells Mol Dis* 46:159, 2011.
17. Ble A, Fink JC, Woodman RC, et al: Renal function, erythropoietin, and anemia of older persons: The InCHIANTI study. *Arch Intern Med* 165:2222, 2005.
18. Ferrucci L, Maggio M, Bandinelli S, et al: Low testosterone levels and the risk of anemia in older men and women. *Arch Intern Med* 166:1380, 2006.
19. Chaves PH, Ashar B, Guralnik JM, et al: Looking at the relationship between hemoglobin concentration and prevalent mobility difficulty in older women. Should the criteria currently used to define anemia in older people be reevaluated? *J Am Geriatr Soc* 50:1257, 2002.
20. Denny SD, Kuchibhatla MN, Cohen HJ: Impact of anemia on mortality, cognition, and function in community-dwelling elderly. *Am J Med* 119:327, 2006.
21. Patel KV, Harris TB, Faulhaber M, et al: Racial variation in the relationship of anemia with mortality and mobility disability among older adults. *Blood* 109:4663, 2007.
22. Klastersky J, Paesmans M, Rubenstein EB, et al: The Multinational Association for Supportive Care in Cancer risk index: A multinational scoring system for identifying low-risk febrile neutropenic cancer patients. *J Clin Oncol* 18:3038, 2000.
23. Cortelazzo S, Finazzi G, Buelli M, et al: High risk of severe bleeding in aged patients with chronic idiopathic thrombocytopenic purpura. *Blood* 77:31, 1991.
24. Cohen YC, Djulbegovic B, Shamai-Lubovitz O, et al: The bleeding risk and natural history of idiopathic thrombocytopenic purpura in patients with persistent low platelet counts. *Arch Intern Med* 160:1630, 2000.
25. Izaks GJ, Westendorp RG, Knook DL: The definition of anemia in older persons. *JAMA* 281:1714, 1999.
26. Penninx BW, Pahor M, Woodman RC, et al: Anemia in old age is associated with increased mortality and hospitalization. *J Gerontol A Biol Sci Med Sci* 61:474, 2006.
27. Culleton BF, Manns BJ, Zhang J, et al: Impact of anemia on hospitalization and mortality in older adults. *Blood* 107:3841, 2006.
28. Chaves PH, Xue QL, Guralnik JM, et al: What constitutes normal hemoglobin concentration in community-dwelling disabled older women? *J Am Geriatr Soc* 52:1811, 2004.
29. Zakai NA, Katz R, Hirsch C, et al: A prospective study of anemia status, hemoglobin concentration, and mortality in an elderly cohort: The Cardiovascular Health Study. *Arch Intern Med* 165:2214, 2005.
30. Agnihotri P, Telfer M, Butt Z, et al: Chronic anemia and fatigue in elderly patients: Results of a randomized, double-blind, placebo-controlled, crossover exploratory study with epoetin alfa. *J Am Geriatr Soc* 55:1557, 2007.
31. Ershler WB, Artz AS, Kandahari MM: Recombinant erythropoietin treatment of anemia in older adults. *J Am Geriatr Soc* 49:1396, 2001.
32. Singh AK, Szczech L, Tang KL, et al: Correction of anemia with epoetin alfa in chronic kidney disease. *N Engl J Med* 355:2085, 2006.
33. Pfeffer MA, Burdmann EA, Chen CY, et al: A trial of darbepoetin alfa in type 2 diabetes and chronic kidney disease. *N Engl J Med* 361:2019, 2009.

INDEX

Page numbers followed by "f" indicate figures, "t" indicate tables, and "b" indicate boxes.

A

B

D

E

F

H

I

J

M

O

P

Q

R

S

T

U

W

X

Y

Z